D0952808

THE MERCK MANUAL

18TH EDITION

1st Edition – 1899
2nd Edition – 1901
3rd Edition – 1905
4th Edition – 1911
5th Edition – 1923
6th Edition – 1934
7th Edition – 1940
8th Edition – 1950
9th Edition – 1956
10th Edition – 1961
11th Edition – 1966
12th Edition – 1972
13th Edition – 1977
14th Edition – 1982
15th Edition – 1987
16th Edition – 1992
17th Edition – 1999
18th Edition – 2006

FOREIGN LANGUAGE EDITIONS
of *The Merck Manual*

Arabic—Larike Publications Services, Cyprus
Chinese—People's Medical Publishing House, Beijing
Croatian—Placebo, Split
Czech—Egem, Prague
French—Editions d'Après, Paris
German—Elsevier, Ltd., Munich
Greek—Medical & Scientific Publishing, Athens
Hungarian—Melania, Budapest
Italian—Springer-Verlag Italia Srl (Medicom), Milan
Japanese—Nikkei Business Publications, Tokyo
Korean—Hanwoori Publishing Co., Seoul
Polish—Elsevier, Ltd, Wroclaw
Portuguese—Editora Roca Ltda., São Paulo
Romanian—All Publishers, Bucharest
Russian—MIR Publishers, Moscow
Spanish—Elsevier España, S.A., Madrid
Turkish—Yüce, Istanbul

OTHER MERCK BOOKS

THE MERCK INDEX
First Edition, 1889

THE MERCK VETERINARY MANUAL
First Edition, 1955

THE MERCK MANUAL OF GERIATRICS
First Edition, 1990

THE MERCK MANUAL OF MEDICAL INFORMATION—HOME EDITION
First Edition, 1997

THE MERCK MANUAL OF HEALTH & AGING
First Edition, 2004

Merck books are published as a service to the scientific community and the public.

EIGHTEENTH EDITION

THE MERCK MANUAL OF DIAGNOSIS AND THERAPY

MARK H. BEERS, MD, Editor-in-Chief
ROBERT S. PORTER, MD, Editor
THOMAS V. JONES, MD, MPH, Associate Editor
JUSTIN L. KAPLAN, MD, Senior Assistant Editor
MICHAEL BERKWITS, MD, MSCE, Assistant Editor

Published by MERCK RESEARCH LABORATORIES
Division of MERCK & CO., INC.
Whitehouse Station, NJ
2006

Editorial and Production Staff

Executive Editor: Keryn A.G. Lane
Senior Staff Writer: Susan T. Schindler
Senior Staff Editor: Susan C. Short
Staff Editor: Michelle A. Hoffman
Production Editor: Melody Sadighi
Textbook Operations Manager: Diane C. Zenker
Manager, Electronic Publications: Barbara Amelia Nace
Project Manager: Diane Cosner-Bobrin
Executive Assistant: Jean Perry
Administrative Assistant: Marcia Yarbrough

Designer: Lorraine B. Kilmer
Illustrators: Michael Reingold
Christopher C. Butts
Indexer: Susan Thomas, PhD

Publisher: Gary Zelko
Advertising and Promotions Supervisor: Pamela J. Barnes-Paul
Subsidiary Rights Coordinator: Jeanne Nilsen
Sales and Service Specialist: Leta S. Bracy

Library of Congress Catalog Card Number 1-31760
ISBN 0911910-18-2
ISSN 0076-6526

Printed in the USA.

FOREWORD

The previous edition of *The Merck Manual* celebrated our 100th anniversary and an illustrious history of providing information to health care practitioners around the world. With this new edition, we are implementing the changes necessary to ensure that *The Merck Manual* meets your information needs through the next century. Your needs have changed, and so *The Merck Manual* must change.

Today, readers want to find what they are looking for quickly and hone in on specific topics. Yet, readers want a complete resource containing all the information needed, now or later. Because the generation of new medical information occurs rapidly, a book too quickly becomes out of date. *The Merck Manual* can no longer wait five years to appear with updates. The revolution has arrived, and with it, *The Merck Manual* starts a new chapter in its history.

In 1899, Merck published a 192-page reference called *Merck's Manual of the Materia Medica*, which later became known as *The Merck Manual of Diagnosis and Therapy.* That book was printed and bound, distributed to users, and ultimately rewritten and published as a 2nd edition a few years later. More editions followed at intervals of two to 12 years, making the advances in medical care all the more apparent for the time lag between editions. If that lag were proportional to the speed at which medical care advanced, one edition would have followed the next more and more quickly, with intermittent bursts of editions as antibiotics were discovered, open heart surgery perfected, and computer-assisted imaging studies developed. Today, important progress in medical care is made continually; old information is potentially dangerous information; lag time in distributing information is unacceptable. The book must change or die.

This edition of *The Merck Manual* has been organized and structured to help you find what you want more easily. The index is complete and detailed. Information has been separated even more clearly into separate entities describing pathophysiology, etiology, symptoms and signs, diagnosis, prognosis, treatment, and prevention. A summary of key points introduces every major discussion. While you can use this new edition to browse and read through topics at your leisure, it will now be even more useful to look up what you want and get the information you need quickly.

The edition of *The Merck Manual* printed and bound here is as up-to-date as a printed book can be. While it is the 18th edition, more importantly it is the 2006 edition. It was reviewed and finalized just before printing. However, over the months after its release, it will become out-of-date. Of course, the vast majority of information in it will be correct and relevant to health care practitioners for many years. Yet, in some areas of practice, new information will become available. As quickly as possible, we will update that information on our web site at www.merckmanuals.com, available to all free of charge.

That electronic source of *The Merck Manual* will be more up-to-date than this printed one. Electronic publishing makes such a process possible, even if it robs the book of some of its allure. The web site is an electronic resource, however, providing none of the charm and comfort of a printed volume. Almost certainly, such complaints were targeted at Guttenberg by the scribes who asserted that books were works of art rather than mass-produced, utilitarian objects. The book changed, and we are grateful that it did.

At some time in the near future, we will print a new edition of the content of *The Merck Manual* and bind and distribute it as a book. It will be the printed edition of the up-to-date content of our web site. We will do so for all those who cherish holding a book in their hands, leafing through its pages, folding back its corners, and scribbling in its margins. We hope that those who enjoy such pleasures will remain a sizeable number for a long time to come.

We hope this edition of *The Merck Manual* will serve as an aid to you, our readers, compatible with your needs and worthy of frequent use. We thank the many hundreds of contributors who have poured their knowledge into this volume. Suggestions for improvements will be warmly welcomed and carefully considered.

MARK H. BEERS, MD, and ROBERT S. PORTER, MD

Committed to Providing Medical Information: Merck and The Merck Manuals

In 1899, the American drug manufacturer Merck & Co. first published a small book titled *Merck's Manual of the Materia Medica*. It was meant as an aid to physicians and pharmacists, reminding doctors that "Memory is treacherous." Compact in size, easy to use, and comprehensive, *The Merck Manual* (as it was later known) became a favorite of those involved in medical care and others in need of a medical reference. Even Albert Schweitzer carried a copy to Africa in 1913, and Admiral Byrd carried a copy to the South Pole in 1929.

By the 1980s, the book had become the world's largest selling medical text and was translated into more than a dozen languages. While the name of the parent company has changed somewhat over the years, the book's name has remained constant, known officially as *The Merck Manual of Diagnosis and Therapy* but usually referred to as *The Merck Manual* and sometimes "The Merck."

In 1990, the editors of *The Merck Manual* introduced *The Merck Manual of Geriatrics*. This new book quickly became the best-selling textbook of geriatric medicine, providing specific and comprehensive information on the care of older people. The 3rd edition was published in five languages. The creation of this book reflects Merck's commitment to the world's aging population and the company's desire to improve geriatric care globally.

In 1997, *The Merck Manual of Medical Information–Home Edition* was published. In this revolutionary book, the editors translated the complex medical information in *The Merck Manual* into plain language, producing a book meant for all those people interested in medical care who did not have a medical degree. The book received critical acclaim and sold over 2 million copies. *The Second Home Edition* was released in 2003 and continued Merck's commitment to providing comprehensive, understandable medical information to all people.

The Merck Manual of Health & Aging, published in 2004, continued Merck's commitment to education and geriatric care, providing information on aging and the care of older people in words understandable by the lay public.

As part of its commitment to ensuring that all who need and want medical information can get it, Merck provides the content of these Merck Manuals on the web for free (visit www.merckmanuals.com). Registration is not required, and use is unlimited. The web publications are continuously updated to ensure that the information is as up-to-date as possible.

Merck also supports the community of chemists and others with the need to know about chemical compounds with *The Merck Index*. First published in

1889, this publication actually predates *The Merck Manual* and is the most widely used text of its kind. *The Merck Veterinary Manual* was first published in 1955. It provides information on the health care of animals and is the preeminent text in its field.

Merck & Co., Inc. is one of the world's largest pharmaceutical companies. Merck is committed to providing excellent medical information and, as part of that effort, continues to proudly provide all of The Merck Manuals as a service to the community.

CONTENTS

GUIDE FOR READERS

The **Contents** (p. ix) shows the pages on which readers will find listed the Editors and Editorial Board members, consultants, additional reviewers, and contributors, as well as abbreviations, titles of sections, appendixes, and the index. **Thumb tabs** with appropriate abbreviations and section numbers mark each section and the index.

Each **Section** begins with its own table of contents, listing chapters and subchapters in that section. **Chapters** are numbered serially from the beginning to the end of the book.

The **Index** contains many cross-entries; page numbers in boldface signify major discussions of the topics. In addition, readers will find many cross-references throughout the text to specific pages where additional or related information can be found.

Running heads carry the section number and title on left-hand pages and the chapter number and title on right-hand pages.

Abbreviations and symbols, used throughout the text as essential space savers, are listed on pages xi and xii. Other abbreviations in the text are expanded at first mention in the chapter or subchapter.

Tables and figures are referenced appropriately in the index but are not listed in a table of contents.

Section 22, **Special Subjects,** has discussions on complementary and alternative medicine, dietary supplements, genetics, smoking cessation, rehabilitation, geriatric medicine, care of the surgical patient, care of the dying patient, and clinical decision making, among others.

Laboratory values in the book are given in conventional units. In most cases, however, SI units follow in parentheses.

Drugs are designated in the text by generic (nonproprietary) names. In Appendix II, many of the drugs mentioned in the book are listed alphabetically, with each generic term followed by one or more trade names.

Important: The authors, reviewers, and editors of this book have made extensive efforts to ensure that treatments, drugs, and dosage regimens are accurate and conform to the standards accepted at the time of publication. However, constant changes in information resulting from continuing research and clinical experience, reasonable differences in opinions among authorities, unique aspects of individual clinical situations, and the possibility of human error in preparing such an extensive text require that the reader exercise individual judgment when making a clinical decision and, if necessary, consult and compare information from other sources. In particular, the reader is advised to check the product information provided by the manufacturer of a drug product before prescribing or administering it, especially if the drug is unfamiliar or is used infrequently.

Note: Readers can find up-to-date information, additional tables and figures, as well as multimedia enhancements at www.merckmanuals.com. Visit the web site frequently for new enhancements and the latest information on clinical developments.

ABBREVIATIONS

The following abbreviations are used throughout the text; other abbreviations are expanded at first mention in the chapter or subchapter.

ABG arterial blood gas
ACE angiotensin converting enzyme
ACTH adrenocorticotropic hormone
ADH antidiuretic hormone
AIDS acquired immunodeficiency syndrome
ALT alanine aminotransferase (formerly SGPT)
AST aspartate aminotransferase (formerly SGOT)
ATP adenosine triphosphate
BCG bacille Calmette-Guérin
bid 2 times a day
BMR basal metabolic rate
BP blood pressure
BSA body surface area
BUN blood urea nitrogen
C Celsius; centigrade; complement
Ca calcium
cAMP cyclic adenosine monophosphate
CBC complete blood count
cGy centigray
Ci curie
CK creatine kinase
Cl chloride; chlorine
cm centimeter
CNS central nervous system
CO_2 carbon dioxide
COPD chronic obstructive pulmonary disease
CPK creatine phosphokinase
CPK-MB creatine phosphokinase muscle band isoenzyme
CPR cardiopulmonary resuscitation
CSF cerebrospinal fluid
CT computed tomography
cu cubic
D & C dilation and curettage
dL deciliter (= 100 mL)
DNA deoxyribonucleic acid
DTP diphtheria-tetanus-pertussis (toxoids/vaccine)
D/W or D dextrose in water
ECF extracellular fluid
ECG electrocardiogram
EEG electroencephalogram
ENT ear, nose, and throat
ERCP endoscopic retrograde cholangiopancreatography
ESR erythrocyte sedimentation rate
F Fahrenheit
FDA U.S. Food and Drug Administration
ft foot; feet (measure)
FUO fever of unknown origin
g gram
GFR glomerular filtration rate
GI gastrointestinal
G6PD glucose-6-phosphate dehydrogenase
GU genitourinary
Gy gray
h hour
Hb hemoglobin
HCl hydrochloric acid; hydrochloride
HCO_3 bicarbonate
Hct hematocrit
Hg mercury
HIV human immunodeficiency virus
HLA human leukocyte antigen
HMG-CoA hydroxymethyl glutaryl coenzyme A
Hz hertz (cycles/second)
ICF intracellular fluid
ICU intensive care unit
IgA, etc immunoglobin A, etc
IL interleukin
IM intramuscular(ly)
INR international normalized ratio
IPPB intermittent positive pressure breathing
IU international unit
IV intravenous(ly)
IVU intravenous urography
K potassium
kcal kilocalorie (food calorie)

kg kilogram
L liter
lb pound
LDH lactic dehydrogenase
M molar
m meter
MCH mean corpuscular hemoglobin
MCHC mean corpuscular hemoglobin concentration
mCi millicurie
MCV mean corpuscular volume
mEq milliequivalent
Mg magnesium
mg milligram
MI myocardial infarction
MIC minimum inhibitory concentration
mIU milli-international unit
mL milliliter
mm millimeter
mmol millimole
mo month
mol wt molecular weight
mOsm milliosmole
MRI magnetic resonance imaging
N nitrogen; normal (strength of solution)
Na sodium
NaCl sodium chloride
ng nanogram (= millimicrogram)
nm nanometer (= millimicron)
nmol nanomole
npo nothing by mouth
NSAID nonsteroidal anti-inflammatory drug
O_2 oxygen
OTC over-the-counter (pharmaceuticals)
oz ounce
P phosphorus; pressure
$PACO_2$ alveolar carbon dioxide partial pressure
$PaCO_2$ arterial carbon dioxide partial pressure
PAO_2 alveolar oxygen partial pressure
PaO_2 arterial oxygen partial pressure
PAS periodic acid-Schiff
PCO_2 carbon dioxide partial pressure (or tension)
PCR polymerase chain reaction
PET positron emission tomography
pg picogram (= micromicrogram)
pH hydrogen ion concentration
PMN polymorphonuclear leukocyte
po orally
PO_2 oxygen partial pressure (or tension)
PPD purified protein derivative (tuberculin)
ppm parts per million
prn as needed
PT prothrombin time
PTT partial thromboplastin time
q every
qid 4 times a day
RA rheumatoid arthritis
RBC red blood cell
RNA ribonucleic acid
SaO_2 arterial oxygen saturation
SBE subacute bacterial endocarditis
sc subcutaneous(ly)
SI International System of Units
SIDS sudden infant death syndrome
SLE systemic lupus erythematosus
soln solution
sp species (singular)
spp species (plural)
sp gr specific gravity
sq square
SSRI selective serotonin reuptake inhibitor
STS serologic test(s) for syphilis
TB tuberculosis
tid 3 times a day
TPN total parenteral nutrition
URI upper respiratory infection
UTI urinary tract infection
WBC white blood cell
WHO World Health Organization
wt weight
μ micro-; micron
μCi microcurie
μg microgram
μL microliter
μm micrometer (= micron)
μmol micromole
μOsm micro-osmole
mμ millimicron (= nanometer)

EDITORS

Editor-in-Chief

MARK H. BEERS, MD
Executive Director of Geriatrics and Clinical Literature, Merck & Co., Inc. and Clinical Professor of Medicine, Drexel University College of Medicine

Editor

ROBERT S. PORTER, MD
Merck & Co., Inc. and Clinical Assistant Professor, Department of Emergency Medicine, Jefferson Medical College

Associate Editor

THOMAS V. JONES, MD, MPH
Merck & Co., Inc. and Adjunct Clinical Associate Professor of Medicine, Temple University School of Medicine

Senior Assistant Editor

JUSTIN L. KAPLAN, MD
Merck & Co., Inc. and Clinical Associate Professor, Department of Emergency Medicine, Jefferson Medical College

Assistant Editor

MICHAEL BERKWITS, MD, MSCE
Merck & Co., Inc. and Adjunct Assistant Professor of Medicine, University of Pennsylvania School of Medicine

EDITORIAL BOARD

Editorial Board continues on the next page.

CONSULTANTS

INA CALLIGARO, PharmD
Assistant Dean for Education and Associate Professor of Clinical Pharmacy, Temple University School of Pharmacy
Pediatric Pharmaceutical Preparations and Dosages

ROBERT B. COHEN, DMD
Associate Professor of Dentistry and Practice Coordinator, Tufts University School of Dental Medicine
Dental Disorders

RALPH E. CUTLER, MD
Professor of Medicine (Emeritus), Loma Linda University School of Medicine; Consultant in Nephrology, Loma Linda VAMC
Genitourinary Disorders

DAVID P. HUSTON, MD
Cullen Professor of Immunology, Departments of Medicine and Immunology, Baylor College of Medicine
Immunologic Disorders

SIDNEY N. KLAUS, MD
Professor of Medicine, Section of Dermatology, Dartmouth Medical School
Dermatologic Disorders

JOANNE LYNN, MD, MA, MS
Senior Researcher, RAND Health, Arlington
Death and Dying Issues

NAYAHMKA MCGRIFF-LEE, PharmD
Senior Regional Medical Scientist, GlaxoSmithKline
Adult Pharmaceutical Preparations and Dosages

MELVIN I. ROAT, MD
Assistant Surgeon, Wills Eye Hospital, Philadelphia
Eye Disorders

JAMES R. ROBERTS, MD, FACEP, FAAEM, FACMT
Professor and Vice Chair, Department of Emergency Medicine and Director, Division of Medical Toxicology, The Drexel University College of Medicine; Chair, Department of Emergency Medicine and Director, Division of Medical Toxicology, Mercy Catholic Medical Center
Injuries and Poisoning

ROBERT J. RUBEN, MD, FACS, FAAP
Distinguished University Professor, Albert Einstein College of Medicine, Department of Otolaryngology, Montefiore Medical Center
Ear, Nose, and Throat Disorders

Reviewers for Selected Chapters

Steven Berney, MD
William C. Black, MD
Jerrold T. Bushberg, PhD, DABMP
John J. Caronna, MD
Patricia Coyle, MD
Dwight L. Evans, MD
Margery Gass, MD
Laura C. Hanson, MD, MPH
Mary L. Hardy, MD
Jerome M. Hershman, MD
Helen Hoenig, MD
Randall Hughes, MD
Gail P. Jarvik, MD, PhD
Peter Laibson, MD
Allen S. Levine, PhD
Colonel David F. Murchison, DDS, MMS
John S. Oghalai, MD
Ann Ouyang, MB, BS
Stewart Shankel, MD
David R. Thomas, MD
Elise W. van der Jagt, MD, MPH
James Wayne Warnica, MD, FRCP(C)
Eric C. Westman, MD, MHS

Acknowledgments

We thank the following for their editorial assistance: Rosalyn Carson-Dewitt, MD, J. Ricker Polsdorfer, MD, Susan Spitz, MD, MSJ, and Oren Traub, MD, PhD. We also thank Andrew J. Fletcher, MB, BChir, Sandra J. Masse, Debra G. Share, and Jonathan S. Simmons, who assisted with initial editing of this book, and Maureen Howard, Mary Evangelisto Miller, J. Donna LeBlanc, Beth A. Mescolotto, Nicole L. Paul, and Regina A. Stamatis, who assisted with copyediting and proofreading.

CONTRIBUTORS

MOIRA L. AITKEN, MD
Professor of Medicine, University of Washington
Bronchiectasis

ROY D. ALTMAN, MD
Professor of Medicine, Division of Rheumatology and Immunology, David Geffen School of Medicine at University of California, Los Angeles
Joint Disorders; Paget's Disease of Bone

BRADLEY D. ANAWALT, MD
Associate Professor of Medicine, University of Washington; Assistant Chief of Medicine, VA Puget Sound
Male Reproductive Endocrinology

KENNETH C. ANDERSON, MD
Kraft Family Professor of Medicine, Harvard Medical School; Chief, Division of Hematologic Neoplasia, Dana-Farber Cancer Institute
Plasma Cell Disorders

GERALD L. ANDRIOLE, MD
Professor and Chief of Urologic Surgery, Washington University School of Medicine; Urologist-in-Chief, Barnes-Jewish Hospital, St. Louis
Prostate Disease

BRIAN R. APATOFF, MD, PhD
Director, Multiple Sclerosis Clinical Care and Research Center, Department of Neurology and Neuroscience, New York Presbyterian Hospital; Weill Medical College of Cornell University
Demyelinating Disorders

NOEL A. ARMENAKAS, MD
Clinical Associate Professor of Urology, Cornell Weill Medical School; Attending Surgeon, Lenox Hill Hospital and New York Presbyterian Hospital
Genitourinary Tract Trauma

J. MALCOLM O. ARNOLD, BSc, MD, FRCP, FACC
Professor of Medicine, Physiology and Pharmacology, University of Western Ontario; Program Leader, Circulation Group, Lawson Health Research Institute; Research Director, Division of Cardiology, London Health Sciences Center
Heart Failure and Cardiomyopathies

JOHN A. ASTIN, PhD
California Pacific Medical Center, San Francisco
Complementary and Alternative Medicine

GEORGE L. BAKRIS, MD
Professor of Preventive Medicine and Internal Medicine and Director, Hypertension/Clinical Research Center, Rush Medical Center
Arterial Hypertension

DAVID H. BARAD, MD, MS
Associate Clinical Professor, Albert Einstein College of Medicine, Bronx
Approach to the Gynecologic Patient

JOHN G. BARTLETT, MD
Professor of Medicine and Chief, Division of Infectious Diseases, Johns Hopkins University School of Medicine
Acute Bronchitis; Pneumonia; Lung Abscess

ROSEMARY BASSON, MD, FRCP (UK)
Clinical Professor, Department of Psychiatry, University of British Columbia
Sexual Dysfunction in Women

BYRON E. BATTEIGER, MD
Professor of Medicine and Microbiology and Immunology, Division of Infectious Diseases, Indiana University School of Medicine
Chlamydia and Mycoplasmas

J. BRAD BELLOTTE, MD
Department of Neurosurgery, Allegheny General Hospital, Pittsburgh
Spinal Trauma

CHESTON M. BERLIN, JR., MD
University Professor of Pediatrics, Penn State Children's Hospital, M. S. Hershey Medical Center, Hershey
Principles of Drug Treatment in Children

BRIAN M. BERMAN, MD
Professor of Family Medicine; Director, Center for Integrative Medicine, University of Maryland School of Medicine
Complementary and Alternative Medicine

RICHARD W. BESDINE, MD
Professor of Medicine, Greer Professor of Geriatric Medicine, and Director, Division of Geratrics (Medicine) and Director of Center for Gerontology and Healthcare Research, Brown Medical School
Geriatric Medicine

ALBERT BIGLAN, MD
Adjunct Associate Professor of Ophthalmology, University of Pittsburgh School of Medicine; Staff Physician, Children's Hospital of Pittsburgh
Eye Defects and Conditions

JOSEPH J. BIUNDO, MD
Medical Director of Rehabilitation, Kenner Regional Medical Center
Bursitis, Tendinitis, and Fibromyalgia

SEAN BLACKWELL, MD
Assistant Professor, Department of Obstetrics and Gynecology, Wayne State University School of Medicine, Hutzel Women's Hospital
Pregnancy Complicated by Disease

ANN S. BOTASH, MD
Professor of Pediatrics, State University of New York, Upstate Medical University
Child Maltreatment

ALFRED A. BOVE, MD, PhD
Chief of Cardiology, Cardiology Section, Temple University School of Medicine
Injury During Diving or Work in Compressed Air

KAREN BOWEN, MD
Assistant Clinical Professor of Medicine, The George Washington University; Associate Medical Director, Community Hospices of The Washington Home
The Dying Patient

THOMAS G. BOYCE, MD, MPH
Assistant Professor of Pediatrics, Mayo Clinic College of Medicine; Consultant in Pediatric Infectious Diseases, Mayo Clinic
Gastroenteritis

PETER C. BRAZY, MD
Professor of Medicine, University of Wisconsin-Madison
Abnormal Renal Transport Syndromes; Anomalies in Kidney Transport

CHRISTIAN M. BRIERY, MD
Fellow, Maternal-Fetal Medicine, University of Mississippi Medical Center
High-Risk Pregnancy

GEORGE R. BROWN, MD
Professor and Associate Chairman, Department of Psychiatry, East Tennessee State University; Chief of Psychiatry, Mountain Home VAMC
Sexuality and Sexual Disorders

HAYWOOD L. BROWN, MD
Professor and Chair, Department of Obstetrics and Gynecology, Duke University Medical Center
Normal Pregnancy, Labor, and Delivery

ROBERT G. BRZYSKI, MD, PhD
Associate Professor of Obstetrics and Gynecology, The University of Texas Health Science Center at San Antonio
Female Reproductive Endocrinology

REBECCA H. BUCKLEY, MD
J. Buren Sidbury Professor of Pediatrics and Professor of Immunology, Duke University Medical Center
Immunodeficiency Disorders

ANGELA CAFIERO, PharmD, CGP
Assistant Professor of Clinical Pharmacy, University of the Sciences in Philadelphia, Philadelphia College of Pharmacy; Clinical Pharmacy Specialist-Geriatrics, Philadelphia VA Medical Center
Pharmacodynamics

CHARLES LEE CAPERTON II, MD
Assistant Professor of Obstetrics and Gynecology, The University of Texas Health Science Center at San Antonio
Female Reproductive Endocrinology

JOHN J. CARONNA, MD
Professor of Clinical Neurology and Vice Chairman, Department of Neurology and Neuroscience, Weill Medical College of Cornell University
Stupor and Coma

MARY T. CASERTA, MD
Associate Professor of Pediatrics, University of Rochester School of Medicine and Dentistry; Attending Physician, Golisano Children's Hospital at Strong
Enteroviruses; Other Viruses; Neonatal Infections

BRUCE A. CHABNER, MD
Professor of Medicine and Clinical Director, Massachusetts General Hospital Cancer Center and Harvard Medical School
Principles of Cancer Therapy

IAN M. CHAPMAN, MBBS, PhD
Associate Professor of Endocrinology, University of Adelaide; Department of Medicine, Royal Adelaide Hospital
Pituitary Disorders

RACHEL L. CHAPMAN, MD
Assistant Professor, Department of Pediatrics, Yale University School of Medicine
Perinatal Physiology; Approach to the Care of Infants and Children; Caring for Sick Children and Their Families

LAN X. CHEN, MD, PhD
Clinical Assistant Professor and Attending Rheumatologist, University of Pennsylvania Medical Center-Presbyterian and VAMC
Infections of Joints and Bones

WILLIAM D. CHEY, MD, FACG, FACP
Associate Professor, Director of Gastrointestinal Physiology Laboratory, University of Michigan
Bezoars and Foreign Bodies

JILL M. CHOLETTE, MD
Critical Care Pediatrics Fellow, University of Rochester School of Medicine and Dentistry
Perinatal Hematologic Disorders

WILLIAM J. COCHRAN, MD
Vice Chairman, Department of Pediatrics, Geisinger Clinic, Danville, PA
Congenital Gastrointestinal Anomalies; Gastrointestinal Disorders in Neonates and Infants

ALAN S. COHEN, MD
Distinguished Professor of Medicine (Emeritus), Boston University School of Medicine; Editor-in-Chief, *Amyloid: The Journal of Protein Folding Disorders*
Amyloidosis

ROBERT B. COHEN, DMD
Associate Professor of Dentistry and Practice Coordinator, Tufts University School of Dental Medicine
Approach to the Dental Patient; Dental Emergencies; Common Dental Disorders; Approach to the Patient With Nasal, Oral, and Pharyngeal Symptoms; Facial Trauma

SIDNEY COHEN, MD
Professor of Medicine and Director, Research Programs, Thomas Jefferson University
Gastritis and Peptic Ulcer Disease; Esophageal and Swallowing Disorders

NANANDA F. COL, MD, MPP, MPH, FACP
Associate Professor of Medicine, Brown University Medical School
Clinical Decision Making

KATHRYN COLBY, MD, PhD
Assistant Professor of Ophthalmology, Harvard Medical School; Attending Surgeon, Cornea Service and Director of the Joint Clinical Research Center, Massachusetts Eye and Ear Infirmary
Approach to the Ophthalmologic Patient

DANIEL W. COLLISON, MD
Associate Professor of Medicine and Surgery, Section of Dermatology, Dartmouth Medical School
Psoriasis and Scaling Diseases; Pigmentation Disorders; Sweating Disorders; Benign Tumors; Pressure Ulcers

EVE R. COLSON, MD
Associate Professor of Pediatrics, Yale University School of Medicine; Director, Well Newborn Nursery, Yale-New Haven Hospital
Perinatal Physiology; Approach to the Care of Infants and Children; Caring for Sick Children and Their Families

MARY ANN COOPER, MD
Professor, Department of Emergency Medicine, University of Illinois at Chicago
Electrical and Lightning Injuries

BRYAN D. COWAN, MD
Professor and Chairman, Department of Obstetrics and Gynecology; University of Mississippi Medical Center
Uterine Fibroids

JILL P. CRANDALL, MD
Assistant Professor, Division of Endocrinology, Diabetes Research and Training Center, Albert Einstein College of Medicine
Diabetes Mellitus and Disorders of Carbohydrate Metabolism

RICARDO CRUCIANI, MD, PhD
Clinical Assistant and Professor, Department of Neurology and Anesthesiology, Albert Einstein College of Medicine; Director, Research Division, Department of Pain Medicine and Palliative Care, Beth Israel Medical Center
Neurotransmission

BURKE A. CUNHA, MD
Professor of Medicine, State University of New York School of Medicine; Chief, Infectious Disease Division, Winthrop-University Hospital, Mineola
Spirochetes; Gram-Negative Bacilli

EMMETT T. CUNNINGHAM, JR., MD, PhD, MPH
Professor of Ophthalmology and Director, The Uveitis Service, New York University School of Medicine; Senior Vice President, Medical Strategy, Eyetech Pharmaceuticals
Uveitis

DREW C. CUTLER, MD
Associate Professor of Pediatrics, Loma Linda University School of Medicine
Cystic Kidney Disease

RALPH E. CUTLER, MD
Professor of Medicine (Emeritus), Loma Linda University School of Medicine; Consultant in Nephrology, Loma Linda VAMC
Approach to the Genitourinary Patient; Renal Replacement Therapy; Tubulointerstitial Diseases; Urinary Tract Infections

PATRICIA A. DALY, MD
Assistant Professor of Clinical Medicine, University of Virginia; Clinical Endocrinologist, Front Royal, VA
Multiple Endocrine Neoplasia Syndromes

JOHANNA P. DAILY, MD
Associate Physician, Brigham and Women's Hospital; Instructor, Harvard Medical School
Viruses

DANIEL F. DANZL, MD
Professor and Chair of Emergency Medicine, University of Louisville School of Medicine
Cold Injury

NORMAN L. DEAN, MD, FCCP
Pulmonologist, Internal Medicine, Geriatrics, North Carolina Department of Corrections; Director of Airway Clinics, North Carolina Correctional Institution for Women
Near Drowning

ALAN H. DeCHERNEY, MD
Professor of Obstetrics and Gynecology, Division of Reproductive Endocrinology, David Geffen School of Medicine at University of California, Los Angeles
Endometriosis

RONALD DEE, MD
Associate Clinical Professor of Surgery, Albert Einstein College of Medicine, Bronx
Peripheral Venous and Lymphatic Disorders

PETER J. DELVES, PhD
Reader in Immunology, Department of Immunology and Molecular Pathology, Division of Infection and Immunity, University College London
Biology of the Immune System

CRAIG S. DERKAY, MD
Professor, Otolaryngology and Pediatrics, Eastern Virginia Medical School; Director, Pediatric Otolaryngology, Children's Hospital of the King's Daughters, Norfolk
Oropharyngeal Disorders

ARA DerMARDEROSIAN, PhD
Professor of Pharmacognosy and Medicinal Chemistry, Roth Chair of Natural Products, Scientific Director, Complementary and Alternative Medicine Institute, University of the Sciences in Philadelphia, Philadelphia College of Pharmacy
Dietary Supplements

DEEPINDER KAUR K. DHALIWAL, MD
Associate Professor, University of Pittsburgh School of Medicine; Director of Cornea/External Disease and Director of Refractive Surgery, University of Pittsburgh Medical Center Eye Center; Medical Director, University of Pittsburgh Medical Center Laser Center
Refractive Error

DAMIAN DHAR, MD
Private Practice
Bacterial Skin Infections; Fungal Skin Infections

JAMES G. H. DINULOS, MD
Assistant Professor of Medicine and Pediatrics (Dermatology), Dartmouth Medical School and Children's Hospital at Dartmouth
Parasitic Skin Infections; Viral Skin Diseases; Cornification Disorders

CAROLINE CARNEY DOEBBELING, MD, MSc
Associate Professor of Psychiatry and Internal Medicine, Indiana University School of Medicine; Research Scientist, Regenstrief Institute
Approach to the Patient With Mental Complaints

KARL DOGHRAMJI, MD
Professor of Psychiatry and Human Behavior, Jefferson Medical College; Director, Sleep Disorders Center, Thomas Jefferson University
Sleep and Wakefulness Disorders

SOUMITRA R. EACHEMPATI, MD
Associate Professor of Surgery, Weill Medical College of Cornell University
Approach to the Critically Ill Patient

JOHN E. EDWARDS, JR., MD
Professor of Medicine, David Geffen School of Medicine at University of California, Los Angeles; Los Angeles Biomedical Research Institute at Harbor-UCLA
Fungi

DAVID EIDELBERG, MD
Professor, Departments of Neurology and Neurosurgery, New York University School of Medicine; Director, Center for Neuroscience, North Shore–Long Island Jewish Research Institute
Movement and Cerebellar Disorders

SHERMAN ELIAS, MD
John J. Sciarra Professor and Chair, Department of Obstetrics and Gynecology, Northwestern University, Feinberg School of Medicine; Chairman, Obstetrics and Gynecology, Prentice Women's Hospital of Northwestern Memorial Hospital
Prenatal Genetic Counseling and Evaluation

JAN FAWCETT, MD
Professor of Psychiatry, University of New Mexico School of Medicine
Mood Disorders

NORAH C. FEENY, PhD
Assistant Professor, Department of Psychiatry and Psychology, University Hospitals of Cleveland and Case Western Reserve University
Medical Examination of the Rape Victim

WAYNE S. FENTON, MD
Associate Director for Clinical Affairs, National Institute of Mental Health, Bethesda
Schizophrenia and Related Disorders

THOMAS M. FILE, JR., MD, MS
Professor of Internal Medicine and Master Teacher, Northeastern Ohio Universities College of Medicine; Chief, Infectious Disease Service, Summa Health System
Gram-Positive Cocci; Gram-Positive Bacilli

MICHAEL C. FIORE, MD
Professor of Medicine and Director, Center for Tobacco Research and Intervention, University of Wisconsin Medical School
Smoking Cessation

CHIN-TO FONG, MD
Associate Professor of Pediatrics, Biochemistry & Biophysics, and Dentistry, and Chief, Division of Pediatric Genetics, University of Rochester School of Medicine and Dentistry
Inherited Disorders of Metabolism

STEVEN D. FREEDMAN, MD, PhD
Associate Professor of Medicine, Harvard Medical School; Director, The Pancreas Center, Beth Israel Deaconess Medical Center
Pancreatitis

EUGENE P. FRENKEL, MD
Professor of Internal Medicine and Radiology, Patsy R. and Raymond D. Nasher Distinguished Chair in Cancer Research; Elaine Dewey Sammons Distinguished Chair in Cancer Research in honor of Eugene P. Frenkel, MD; and A. Kenneth Pye Professorship in Cancer Research, Harold C. Simmons Comprehensive Cancer Center, The University of Texas Southwestern Medical Center at Dallas
Overview of Cancer; Spleen Disorders; Anemias Caused by Hemolysis; Anemias Caused by Deficient Erythropoiesis; Approach to the Patient With Anemia; Iron Overload

MARVIN P. FRIED, MD
Professor and University Chairman, Department of Otolaryngology, Albert Einstein College of Medicine, Montefiore Medical Center
Facial Trauma; Nose and Paranasal Sinus Disorders

STEVEN M. FRUCHTMAN, MD
Medical Director of Hematology, Tibotec Therapeutics, Bridgewater, NJ
Myeloproliferative Disorders

DMITRY GABRILOVICH, MD, PhD
Professor of Interdisciplinary Oncology, Immunology, Molecular Biology, and Biochemistry, H. Lee Moffitt Cancer Center, University of South Florida
Tumor Immunology

MARC GALANTER, MD
Professor of Psychiatry and Director, Division of Alcoholism and Drug Abuse, New York University
Drug Use and Dependence

JAMES GARRITY, MD
Professor of Ophthalmology and Consultant, Department of Ophthalmology, Mayo Clinic
Optic Nerve Disorders; Orbital Disorders

BRIAN K. GEHLBACH, MD
Assistant Professor of Medicine, University of Chicago
Respiratory Failure and Mechanical Ventilation

JAMES N. GEORGE, MD
Presidential Professor, Presbyterian Health Foundation; Professor of Medicine, Hematology-Oncology Section, The University of Oklahoma Health Sciences Center
Thrombocytopenia and Platelet Dysfunction; Bleeding Due to Abnormal Blood Vessels

DAVID M. GERSHENSON, MD
Professor and Chairman, Department of Gynecologic Oncology and J. Taylor Wharton, MD, Distinguished Chair in Gynecologic Oncology, The University of Texas M. D. Anderson Cancer Center
Gynecologic Tumors

ELIAS A. GIRALDO, MD
Assistant Professor of Neurology and Neurosurgery, University of Tennessee College of Medicine; Director, Comprehensive Stroke Center and Neurological Critical Care, University of Tennessee Health Science Center
Stroke

BARRY STEVEN GOLD, MD
Associate Professor of Medicine, Johns Hopkins University School of Medicine; Assistant Professor, Division of Emergency Medicine, Department of Surgery, University of Maryland School of Medicine
Bites and Stings

ANNE CAROL GOLDBERG, MD, FACP
Associate Professor of Medicine, Washington University School of Medicine
Lipid Disorders

STEPHEN E. GOLDFINGER, MD
Professor of Medicine, Harvard Medical School; Physician, Massachusetts General Hospital
Hereditary Periodic Fever Syndrome

STEVEN R. GOLDSTEIN, MD
Professor of Obstetrics and Gynecology, New York University School of Medicine; Director of Gynecologic Ultrasound, Co-Director, Bone Densitometry, New York University Medical Center
Menstrual Abnormalities

M. JAY GOODKIND, MD
Associate Professor (Emeritus) of Clinical Medicine, University of Pennsylvania School of Medicine; Chairman (Emeritus) of Clinical Cardiology, Capital Health System, Mercer Hospital Campus, Trenton
Cardiac Tumors

NORTON J. GREENBERGER, MD
Clinical Professor of Medicine, Harvard Medical School; Senior Physician, Brigham and Women's Hospital
Approach to the Patient With Upper GI Complaints; Diagnostic and Therapeutic GI Procedures

JOHN H. GREIST, MD
Clinical Professor of Psychiatry, University of Wisconsin; Distinguished Senior Scientist, Madison Institute of Medicine
Anxiety Disorders

ASHLEY B. GROSSMAN, BA, BSc, MD, FRCP, FMedSci
Professor of Neuroendocrinology and Honorary Consultant Physician, St. Bartholomew's Hospital, London
Adrenal Disorders

JOHN G. GUNDERSON, MD
Professor of Psychiatry, Harvard Medical School; Director of Center for Treatment and Research on Borderline Personality Disorder, McLean Hospital
Personality Disorders

JERRY H. GURWITZ, MD
Chief, Division of Geriatric Medicine, University of Massachusetts Medical School; Executive Director, Meyers Primary Care Institute, Worcester
Drug Therapy in the Elderly

JESSE HALL, MD
Professor of Medicine, Department of Anesthesia and Critical Care and Section Chief, Pulmonary and Critical Care Medicine, University of Chicago
Respiratory Failure and Mechanical Ventilation

JUDITH G. HALL, OC, MD, FRCP(C), FAAP, FCCMG, FABMG
Professor of Pediatrics and Medical Genetics (Emeritus), The University of British Columbia and Children's and Women's Health Centre of British Columbia; Department of Pediatrics, British Columbia's Children's Hospital
Chromosomal Abnormalities; General Principles of Medical Genetics

JOHN W. HALLETT, JR., MD, FACS
Clinical Professor of Surgery, Medical University of South Carolina; Medical Director, Roper St. Francis Heart and Vascular Center, Charleston
Diseases of the Aorta and Its Branches; Peripheral Arterial Disorders

KEVIN C. HAZEN, PhD, D(ABMM)
Professor of Pathology and Microbiology and Director of Clinical Microbiology, University of Virginia Health System
Laboratory Diagnosis of Infectious Disease

DAVID M. HEIMBACH, MD
Professor of Surgery, University of Washington Burn Center, Harborview Medical Center
Burns

R. PHILLIPS HEINE, MD
Associate Professor and Director, Division of Maternal-Fetal Medicine, Duke University Medical Center, Department of Obstetrics and Gynecology
Approach to the Pregnant Woman and Prenatal Care

SUSAN L. HENDRIX, DO
Professor, Department of Obstetrics and Gynecology, Wayne State University School of Medicine, Hutzel Women's Hospital
Menopause

JEROME M. HERSHMAN, MD
Distinguished Professor of Medicine, University of California, Los Angeles School of Medicine; Associate Chief, Endocrinology and Diabetes Division, West Los Angeles VA Medical Center
Thyroid Disorders

MARTIN HERTL, MD
Assistant Professor of Surgery, Transplantation Unit, Massachusetts General Hospital
Transplantation

ROBERT M. A. HIRSCHFELD, MD
Titus H. Harris Chair, Professor and Chair, Department of Psychiatry and Behavioral Sciences, University of Texas Medical Branch, Galveston
Suicidal Behavior

BRIAN D. HOIT, MD
Professor of Medicine, Case Western Reserve University; Director of Echocardiography, University Hospitals of Cleveland
Pericarditis

WAUN KI HONG, MD
American Cancer Society Professor and Samsung Distinguished University Chair in Cancer Medicine; Professor of Medicine, Department of Thoracic/Head and Neck Medical Oncology, and Head, Division of Cancer Medicine, The University of Texas M. D. Anderson Cancer Center
Tumors of the Lungs

CYNTHIA R. HOWARD, MD, MPH
Associate Professor of Pediatrics, University of Rochester School of Medicine and Dentistry
Approach to the Care of Infants and Children

DANIEL A. HUSSAR, PhD
Remington Professor of Pharmacy, University of the Sciences in Philadelphia, Philadelphia College of Pharmacy
Concepts in Pharmacotherapy

MICHAEL G. ISON, MD, MS
Assistant Professor, Northwestern University, Feinberg School of Medicine
Arboviridae, Arenaviridae, Bunyaviridae, and Filoviridae

MASAYOSHI ITOH, MD
Clinical Professor of Rehabilitation Medicine, New York University School of Medicine; Senior Management Consultant, Coler-Goldwater Specialty Hospital and Nursing Facility
Rehabilitation

MICHAEL JACEWICZ, MD
Professor of Neurology, University of Tennessee Health Science Center and Veterans Administration Medical Center, Memphis
Neuro-ophthalmologic and Cranial Nerve Disorders; Approach to the Neurologic Patient; Meningitis; Brain Infections

JON A. JACOBSON, MD
Associate Professor of Radiology and Director, Division of Musculoskeletal Radiology, University of Michigan
Principles of Radiologic Imaging

JAMES W. JEFFERSON, MD
Clinical Professor of Psychiatry, University of Wisconsin; Distinguished Senior Scientist, Madison Institute of Medicine
Anxiety Disorders

LARRY E. JOHNSON, MD, PhD
Associate Professor of Geriatrics and Family and Preventive Medicine, University of Arkansas for Medical Sciences; Attending Physician, Central Arkansas Veterans Healthcare System
Vitamin Deficiency, Dependency, and Toxicity

ROBERT G. JOHNSON, MD
C. Rollins Hanlon Professor and Chairman, Department of Surgery, Saint Louis University School of Medicine
Care of the Surgical Patient

BRIAN D. JOHNSTON
Director of Education and President, International Association of Resistance Trainers Fitness Certification Institute, Ontario
Exercise and Sports Injury

HUGH F. JOHNSTON, MD
Clinical Associate Professor, Department of Psychiatry and Office of Continuing Medical Education, University of Wisconsin Medical School
Mental Disorders in Children and Adolescents

NICHOLAS JOSPE, MD
Associate Professor of Pediatrics, Department of Pediatrics, University of Rochester School of Medicine and Denistry
Metabolic, Electrolyte, and Toxic Disorders in Neonates; Endocrine and Metabolic Disorders in Children

ANAND D. KANTAK, MD
Clinical Associate Professor of Pediatrics, Northeast Ohio College of Medicine, Rootstown; Director, Division of Neonatology, Children's Hospital Medical Center of Akron
Respiratory Disorders in Neonates, Infants, and Young Children

KENNETH M. KAYE, MD
Assistant Professor, Division of Infectious Diseases, Department of Medicine, Brigham and Women's Hospital, Harvard Medical School
Herpesviruses

MICHAEL J. KEATING, MBBS
Professor of Medicine, The University of Texas M. D. Anderson Cancer Center
Leukemias

JAMES W. KENDIG, MD
Professor of Pediatrics, Penn State University College of Medicine, Hershey
Perinatal Problems

TALMADGE E. KING, JR., MD
Chief, Medical Services, San Francisco General Hospital; The Constance B. Wofsy Distinguished Professor and Vice-Chairman, Department of Medicine, University of California, San Francisco
Interstitial Lung Diseases

JOEL KLINE, MD, MSC
Professor, Division of Pulmonary, Critical Care & Occupational Medicine, University of Iowa College of Medicine; Professor, Department of Occupational Environmental Health, College of Public Health, University of Iowa
Interstitial Lung Diseases

JAMES P. KNOCHEL, MD
Clinical Professor of Internal Medicine, University of Texas, Southwestern Medical Center, Dallas; Past Chairman, Department of Internal Medicine, Presbyterian Hospital of Dallas
Heat Illness

MARCI KOCH, MD
Resident, Department of Neurosurgery, University of Cincinnati College of Medicine
Traumatic Brain Injury

DAVID N. KORONES, MD
Associate Professor of Pediatrics, Oncology, and Neurology, University of Rochester School of Medicine and Dentistry
Pediatric Cancers

JULES Y. T. LAM, MD, FRCP(C)
Associate Professor of Medicine, University of Montreal; Cardiologist, Montreal Heart Institute
Arteriosclerosis

LEWIS LANDSBERG, MD
Vice President for Medical Affairs and Dean, Northwestern University, Feinberg School of Medicine
Multiple Endocrine Neoplasia Syndromes

NANCY E. LANPHEAR, MD
Director of the Developmental Assessment Team for Infants and Toddlers and Pediatric Developmental Specialist, Cincinnati Children's Hospital Medical Center
Behavioral Concerns and Problems

NOAH LECHTZIN, MD, MHS
Assistant Professor, Department of Medicine, Division of Pulmonary and Critical Care Medicine, Johns Hopkins University School of Medicine
Approach to the Patient With Pulmonary Symptoms

MATHEW H. M. LEE, MD
Howard A. Rusk Professor of Rehabilitation Medicine and Chairman, Department of Rehabilitation Medicine, New York University School of Medicine
Rehabilitation

HARVEY LEMONT, DPM
Professor, Department of Medicine, Pennsylvania College of Podiatric Medicine
Foot and Ankle Disorders

JOSEPH R. LENTINO, MD, PhD
Professor of Medicine, Loyola University Stritch School of Medicine; Chief, Infectious Diseases, Hines VA Hospital
Anaerobic Bacteria

NORMA B. LERNER, MD
Associate Professor of Pediatrics, Division of Pediatric Hematology/Oncology, Golisano Children's Hospital at Strong
Perinatal Hematologic Disorders

MATTHEW E. LEVISON, MD
Professor of Medicine and Public Health, Division of Infectious Diseases, Drexel University College of Medicine
Bacteria and Antibacterial Drugs

JAMES L. LEWIS III, MD
Nephrology Associates, P.C. of Birmingham; Baptist Health System, Princeton and Montclair, Birmingham
Fluid and Electrolyte Metabolism

PAUL LAWRENCE LIEBERT, MD
Private Practice
Exercise and Sports Injury

RICHARD W. LIGHT, MD
Professor of Medicine, Vanderbilt University; Director, Pulmonary Disease Program, Saint Thomas Hospital
Mediastinal and Pleural Disorders

GREGORY S. LIPTAK, MD, MPH
Professor of Pediatrics, University of Rochester Medical Center; Medical Director, Kirch Developmental Services Center
Congenital Neurologic Anomalies; Congenital Craniofacial and Musculoskeletal Abnormalities

JEFFREY M. LIPTON, MD, PhD
Chief, Division of Pediatric Hematology/Oncology and Stem Cell Transplantation, Schneider Children's Hospital; Professor of Pediatrics, Albert Einstein College of Medicine
Histiocytic Syndromes

ELLIOT M. LIVSTONE, MD, FACP, FACG
Attending Physician, Sarasota Memorial Hospital, Sarasota, FL
Tumors of the GI Tract

CHARLES J. LOCKWOOD, MD
The Anita O'Keefe Young Professor and Chair, Department of Obstetrics, Gynecology and Reproductive Sciences, Yale University School of Medicine; Chief, Department of Obstetrics and Gynecology, Yale-New Haven Hospital
Abnormalities of Pregnancy

MICHAEL LONDNER, MD, MPH, MBA
Assistant Professor, Department of Emergency Medicine, Johns Hopkins University
Acid-Base Regulation and Disorders

PHILIP LOW, MD
Professor of Neurology, Mayo Clinic College of Medicine
Autonomic Nervous System

PAUL D. LUI, MD
Associate Professor of Surgery, Division of Urology, Loma Linda University School of Medicine
Voiding Disorders; Penile and Scrotal Disorders

JOANNE LYNN, MD, MA, MS
Senior Researcher, RAND Health, Arlington
The Dying Patient

EDWARD R. MARCANTONIO, MD
Associate Professor of Medicine, Harvard Medical School; Director of Research, Division of General Medicine, Beth Israel Deaconess Medical Center
Delirium and Dementia

RICHARD J. MARTIN, MD
Professor of Medicine, National Jewish Medical and Research Center and University of Colorado Health Sciences Center
Asthma

MICHAEL A. MATTHAY, MD
Professor of Medicine and Anesthesia, University of California at San Francisco and The Cardiovascular Research Institute
Acute Lung Injury and Acute Respiratory Distress Syndrome

JOHN T. McBRIDE, MD
Professor and Vice-Chair of Pediatrics, Northeast Ohio College of Medicine, Rootstown; Vice-Chair, Department of Pediatrics, Akron Children's Hospital
Respiratory Disorders in Neonates, Infants, and Young Children

MARGARET C. McBRIDE, MD
Professor of Pediatrics, Northeast Ohio College of Medicine; Director, Neurodevelopmental Center and Chief, Division of Neurology, Akron Children's Hospital
Neurologic Disorders in Children

DANIEL J. McCARTY, MD
Will and Cava Ross Professor of Medicine (Emeritus), Medical College of Wisconsin
Crystal-Induced Arthritides

J. ALLEN McCUTCHAN, MD, MSc
Professor of Medicine, Division of Infectious Diseases, University of California at San Diego School of Medicine
Sexually Transmitted Diseases; Human Immunodeficiency Virus

ROBERT S. McKELVIE, MD, PhD, FRCP(C)
Professor of Medicine, Division of Cardiology, McMaster University and Hamilton Health Sciences
Sports and the Heart

KAREN McKOY, MD
Clinical Instructor, Department of Dermatology, Harvard Medical School; Senior Staff, Department of Dermatology, Lahey Clinic
Dermatitis; Acne and Related Disorders; Principles of Topical Dermatologic Therapy

JAMES I. McMILLAN, MD
Associate Professor of Medicine, Loma Linda University; Chief, Nephrology Section, VA Loma Linda Healthcare System
Glomerular Diseases

S. GENE McNEELEY, MD
Professor of Obstetrics, Gynecology and Urology, Wayne State University School of Medicine, Hutzel Women's Hospital
Benign Gynecologic Lesions; Pelvic Relaxation Syndromes

NOSHIR R. MEHTA, DMD, MDS, MS
Professor and Chairman of General Dentistry and Director, Craniofacial Pain Center, Tufts University School of Dental Medicine
Temporomandibular Disorders

DANIEL MENKES, MD
Associate Professor of Neurology, University of Tennessee, Health Sciences Center at Memphis; Director, Clinical Neurophysiology Service and Winston Wolfe Peripheral Neuropathy Research Laboratory
Seizure Disorders; Peripheral Nervous System Disorders

DANIEL R. MISHELL, JR., MD
The Lyle G. McNeile Professor and Chairman, Department of Obstetrics and Gynecology, Keck School of Medicine, University of Southern California
Family Planning

L. BRENT MITCHELL, MD
Professor and Head, Department of Cardiac Sciences, University of Calgary; Professor and Head, Department of Cardiac Sciences, Calgary Health Region; Director, Libin Cardiovascular Institute of Alberta
Arrhythmias and Conduction Disorders

RICHARD T. MIYAMOTO, MD
Arilla Spence DeVault Professor and Chairman, Department of Otolaryngology–Head and Neck Surgery, Indiana University School of Medicine
Middle Ear and Tympanic Membrane Disorders

JOEL L. MOAKE, MD
Professor of Medicine, Baylor College of Medicine; Associate Director, Biomedical Engineering Laboratory, Rice University
Hemostasis; Coagulation Disorders; Thrombotic Disorders

JULIE S. MOLDENHAUER, MD
Assistant Professor, Department of Obstetrics and Gynecology, University of Chicago
Postpartum Care

JOHN E. MORLEY, MB, BCh
Dammert Professor of Gerontology, Saint Louis University Health Sciences Center; Director, Geriatric Research, Education and Clinical Center, St. Louis VA Medical Center
Undernutrition; Principles of Endocrinology; Mineral Deficiency and Toxicity

JOHN MORRISON, MD
Professor of Obstetrics/Gynecology and Pediatrics, University of Mississippi Medical Center
High-Risk Pregnancy

CARLENE A. MUTO, MD, MS
Assistant Professor of Medicine and Epidemiology, University of Pittsburgh; Medical

Director, Division of Hospital Epidemiology and Infection Control, University of Pittsburgh Medical Center
Neisseriaceae

RAJ K. NARAYAN, MD
Frank H. Mayfield Professor and Chairman, Department of Neurosurgery, University of Cincinnati College of Medicine, The Neuroscience Institute, and Mayfield Clinic, Cincinnati
Traumatic Brain Injury

EDWARD A. NARDELL, MD
Associate Professor, Harvard Medical School, Harvard School of Public Health; Department of Social Medicine and Health Inequalities, Brigham and Women's Hospital
Mycobacteria

LAWRENCE F. NAZARIAN, MD
Clinical Professor of Pediatrics, University of Rochester School of Medicine and Dentistry
Approach to the Care of Infants and Children; Approach to the Care of Adolescents; Physical Growth and Development

JOHN H. NEWMAN, MD
Professor of Medicine, Vanderbilt University School of Medicine
Pulmonary Embolism; Pulmonary Hypertension

LEE S. NEWMAN, MD, MA
Professor of Medicine and Head, Division of Environmental and Occupational Health Sciences, National Jewish Medical and Research Center; Professor of Medicine and Professor of Preventive Medicine and Biometrics, Division of Pulmonary Sciences and Critical Medicine, University of Colorado at Denver Health Sciences Center
Environmental Pulmonary Diseases; Sarcoidosis

JENNIFER R. NIEBYL, MD
Professor and Head, Department of Obstetrics and Gynecology, University of Iowa College of Medicine
Conception and Prenatal Development

MARY LYNN R. NIERODZIK, MD
Associate Professor, New York University School of Medicine
Eosinophilic Disorders

DEBORAH L. NUCATOLA, MD
Fellow, Family Planning, Department of Obstetrics and Gynecology, Keck School of Medicine, University of Southern California
Family Planning

JAMES M. O'BRIEN, MD
Instructor/Fellow, Division of Pulmonary Sciences and Critical Care Medicine, University of Colorado Health Sciences Center
Tests of Pulmonary Function

GERALD F. O'MALLEY, DO
Clinical Associate Professor, Department of Emergency Medicine, Thomas Jefferson University Hospital; Director of Toxicology, Department of Emergency Medicine, Albert Einstein Medical Center; Faculty Consultant, Division of Emergency Medicine, Children's Hospital of Philadelphia
Poisoning

JOHN S. OGHALAI, MD
Assistant Professor, Department of Otolaryngology and Communicative Sciences, Baylor College of Medicine
Inner Ear Disorders; Facial Trauma

ELIZABETH J. PALUMBO, MD
Private Practice, The Pediatric Group, Fairfax, VA
Miscellaneous Disorders in Infants and Children

MYUNG K. PARK, MD
Professor (Emeritus), Division of Pediatric Cardiology, University of Texas Health Science Center, San Antonio; Staff Cardiologist, Driscoll Children's Hospital, Corpus Christi
Congenital Cardiovascular Anomalies

STEPHEN G. PAUKER, MD, MACP
Sara Murray Jordan Professor of Medicine, Tufts University School of Medicine; Associate Physician-in-Chief, Tufts–New England Medical Center
Clinical Decision Making

RICHARD D. PEARSON, MD
Professor of Medicine and Pathology, University of Virginia School of Medicine
Nematodes (Roundworms); Intestinal Protozoa; Extraintestinal Protozoa; Approach to Parasitic Infections; Cestodes (Tapeworms); Trematodes (Flukes)

LAWRENCE L. PELLETIER, JR., MD
Professor, Internal Medicine, University of Kansas School of Medicine; Staff Physician, Robert J. Dole VA Medical and Regional Office Center, Wichita
Endocarditis

FRANK PESSLER, MD, PhD
Fellow, Rheumatology and Immunology, The Children's Hospital of Philadelphia
Rheumatic Fever; Bone and Connective Tissue Disorders in Children

WILLIAM A. PETRI, JR., MD, PhD
Wade Hampton Frost Professor of Epidemiology and Chief, Division of Infectious Diseases and International Health, University of Virginia School of Medicine
Rickettsiae and Related Organisms

KATHARINE A. PHILLIPS, MD
Professor of Psychiatry and Human Behavior, Brown Medical School; Director, Body Dysmorphic Disorder Program, Butler Hospital
Somatoform and Factitious Disorders

SIDNEY F. PHILLIPS, MD
Professor of Medicine, Karl F. and Marjory Hasselmann Professor of Research, Mayo Clinic
Approach to the Patient With Lower GI Complaints

RUSSELL K. PORTENOY, MD
Professor of Neurology and Anesthesiology, Albert Einstein College of Medicine; Chairman, Department for Pain Medicine and Palliative Care, Beth Israel Medical Center
Pain

CAROL S. PORTLOCK, MD
Attending Physician, Lymphoma Service, Memorial Sloan-Kettering Cancer Center
Lymphomas

GLENN M. PREMINGER, MD
Professor of Urologic Surgery and Director, Duke Comprehensive Kidney Stone Center, Duke Medical Center
Urinary Calculi

DOUGLAS J. PRITCHARD, MD
Consultant of Orthopedic Surgery and Oncology, Mayo Foundation, Rochester
Tumors of Bones and Joints

SALLY PULLMAN-MOOAR, MD
Clinical Associate Professor, Department of Medicine, Division of Rheumatology, University of Pennsylvania; Philadelphia Veterans Administration Medical Center
Neck and Back Pain

RONALD RABINOWITZ, MD
Professor of Urology and Pediatrics and Chief of Pediatric Urology, University of Rochester School of Medicine and Dentistry
Congenital Renal and Genitourinary Anomalies

LAWRENCE G. RAISZ, MD
Professor of Medicine and Director, UConn Center for Osteoporosis
Osteoporosis

PEDRO T. RAMIREZ, MD
Assistant Professor, Gynecologic Oncology Department, The University of Texas M. D. Anderson Cancer Center
Gynecologic Tumors

ROBERT W. REBAR, MD
Executive Director, American Society for Reproductive Medicine; Volunteer Clinical Professor, Department of Obstetrics and Gynecology, University of Alabama
Infertility

ALICIA M. REESE, PharmD, MS
Assistant Professor of Clinical Pharmacy, Philadelphia College of Pharmacy, University of the Sciences in Philadelphia
Trade Names of Some Commonly Used Drugs

WINGFIELD E. REHMUS, MD, MPH
Co-Director of Clinical Trials and Clinical Instructor, Stanford University Department of Dermatology
Bullous Diseases; Hypersensitivity and Inflammatory Disorders; Nail Disorders; Hair Disorders

NORMAN RELKIN, MD, PhD
Associate Professor of Neurology and Neuroscience, Weill Medical College of Cornell University; Director, Cornell Memory Disorders Program, Weill Medical College of Cornell University
Function and Dysfunction of the Cerebral Lobes

DOUGLAS J. RHEE, MD
Assistant Professor of Opthalmology, Wills Eye Hospital; Assistant Professor of Pathology,

Anatomy, and Cell Biology, Jefferson Medical College
Glaucoma

MELVIN I. ROAT, MD
Assistant Surgeon, Wills Eye Hospital, Philadelphia
Eyelid Disorders; Corneal Disorders; Conjunctival and Scleral Disorders; Cataract; Eye Injuries

KENNETH B. ROBERTS, MD
Professor of Pediatrics, University of North Carolina School of Medicine; Director, Pediatric Teaching Program, Moses Cone Health System, Greensboro
Dehydration and Fluid Therapy

BERYL J. ROSENSTEIN, MD
Professor of Pediatrics, Johns Hopkins University School of Medicine; Johns Hopkins Hospital, Cystic Fibrosis Center
Cystic Fibrosis

LANNY J. ROSENWASSER, MD
Marjorie and Stephen Raphael Chair in Asthma Research; Professor, Division of Allergy and Immunology, National Jewish Medical and Research Center; Professor of Medicine and Immunology, University of Colorado Health Science Center
Allergic and Other Hypersensitivity Disorders

ROBERT J. RUBEN, MD, FACS, FAAP
Distinguished University Professor, Albert Einstein College of Medicine, Department of Otolaryngology, Montefiore Medical Center
Hearing Loss

FRED H. RUBIN, MD
Professor of Medicine, University of Pittsburgh, School of Medicine; Chair, Department of Medicine, University of Pittsburgh Medical Center Presbyterian Shadyside Hospital, Shadyside Campus
Immunization

MICHAEL RUBIN, MD, FRCP(C)
Professor of Clinical Neurology, Weill Cornell Medical College; Director, Neuromuscular Service, New York Presbyterian Hospital-Cornell Medical Center
Craniocervical Junction Abnormalities; Inherited Muscular Disorders; Spinal Cord Disorders

ATENODORO R. RUIZ, JR., MD
Associate Physician, Department of Medicine, The Permanente Medical Group, Inc., Santa Clara
Malabsorption Syndromes

PAUL S. RUSSELL, MD
John Homans Distinguished Professor of Surgery, Harvard Medical School and Massachusetts General Hospital
Transplantation

CHARLES SABATINO, JD
Adjunct Professor, Georgetown University Law Center; Director, Commission on Law and Aging, American Bar Association
Medicolegal Issues

DAVID B. SACHAR, MD, FACP, MACG
Clinical Professor of Medicine, Mount Sinai School of Medicine; Director (Emeritus), Division of Gastroenterology, The Mount Sinai Hospital
Inflammatory Bowel Disease

SEYED-ALI SADJADI, MD
Associate Professor of Medicine, Loma Linda University School of Medicine
Renal Replacement Therapy; Renovascular Disorders

CHRISTOPHER SANFORD, MD, MPH, DTM&H
Clinical Assistant Professor, Department of Family Medicine, University of Washington; Co-Director, Travel Clinic, Hall Health Center, University of Washington
Medical Aspects of Travel

RAVINDRA SARODE, MD
Associate Professor of Pathology and Director, Transfusion Medicine and Coagulation Laboratory, The University of Texas Southwestern Medical Center at Dallas
Transfusion Medicine

CLARENCE T. SASAKI, MD
The Charles W. Ohse Professor, Yale School of Medicine; Chief, Section of Otolaryngology, Yale-New Haven Hospital
Laryngeal Disorders

H. RALPH SCHUMACHER, JR., MD
Professor of Medicine, University of Pennsylvania School of Medicine; Chief of Rheumatology,

Department of Veterans Affairs Medical Center, Philadelphia
Approach to the Patient With Joint Disease; Autoimmune Rheumatic Disorders; Vasculitis; Infections of Joints and Bones

MARVIN I. SCHWARZ, MD
The James C. Campbell Professor of Pulmonary Medicine, Division of Pulmonary Sciences and Critical Care Medicine, University of Colorado Health Sciences Center
Diffuser Alveolar Hemorrhage and Pulmonary-Renal Syndromes

KATHY SCHWARZENBERGER, MD
Associate Professor of Medicine (Dermatology), Dartmouth Medical School
Reactions to Sunlight; Approach to the Dermatologic Patient

ELDON A. SHAFFER, MD, FRCP(C), FACP, FACG, DIPABIM
Professor of Medicine, Faculty of Medicine, University of Calgary
Vascular Disorders; Fibrosis and Cirrhosis; Testing for Hepatic and Biliary Disorders; Alcoholic Liver Disease; Gallbladder and Bile Duct Disorders

WILLIAM R. SHAPIRO, MD
Professor of Clinical Neurology, University of Arizona College of Medicine, Tucson; Chief, Neuro-oncology, Division of Neurology, Barrow Neurological Institute
Intracranial and Spinal Tumors

MICHAEL J. SHEA, MD
Professor of Internal Medicine, University of Michigan
Cardiovascular Tests and Procedures

DAVID D. SHERRY, MD
Professor of Pediatrics, University of Pennsylvania; Director, Pediatric Rheumatology, The Children's Hospital of Philadelphia
Rheumatic Fever; Bone and Connective Tissue Disorders in Children

DAPHNE SIMEON, MD
Associate Professor, Mount Sinai School of Medicine
Dissociative Disorders

JEROME B. SIMON, MD, FRCP(C), FACP
Professor of Medicine (Emeritus), Division of Gastroenterology, Queen's University, Kingston, Ontario
Liver Masses and Granulomas; Drugs and the Liver; Hepatitis; Approach to the Patient with Liver Disease

ROBERT SIMON, MD
Professor and Executive FAAEM Chairman, Department of Emergency Medicine, Cook County Hospital, Rush Medical College, Rush University Medical Center
Fractures, Dislocations, and Sprains

TAMMY L. HARRIS SIMS, MD, MS
Assistant Professor of Pediatrics, Center for Tobacco Research and Intervention; University of Wisconsin Medical School
Smoking Cessation

CARL V. SMITH, MD
Professor and Chair, Department of Obstetrics and Gynecology, University of Nebraska College of Medicine
Abnormalities and Complications of Labor and Delivery

NORMAN SOHN, MD
Clinical Assistant Professor of Surgery, New York University School of Medicine
Anorectal Disorders

DAVID E. SOPER, MD
Professor and Vice Chairman, Department of Obstetrics and Gynecology, Medical University of South Carolina
Vaginitis and Pelvic Inflammatory Disease

STEVEN SPENCER, MD
Professor of Medicine and Surgery, Department of Dermatology, Dartmouth Medical School
Cancers of the Skin

SCOTT M. STEIDL, MD
Associate Professor and Director of Vitreoretinal Services, Department of Ophthalmology, University of Maryland School of Medicine
Retinal Disorders

DAVID R. STEINBERG, MD
Associate Professor, Department of Orthopaedic Surgery and Director, Hand & Upper Extremity Fellowship, University of Pennsylvania
Hand Disorders

KINGMAN P. STROHL, MD
Professor of Medicine and Director, Center for Sleep Disorders Research, Case Western Reserve University
Sleep Apnea

ALBERT STUNKARD, MD
Professor of Psychiatry, University of Pennsylvania
Eating Disorders

STEPHEN BRIAN SULKES, MD
Professor of Pediatrics, Strong Center for Developmental Disabilities, Golisano Children's Hospital at Strong, University of Rochester School of Medicine and Dentistry
Learning and Developmental Disorders

GEETA K. SWAMY, MD
Associate Professor, Division of Maternal-Fetal Medicine, Department of Obstetrics and Gynecology, Duke University Medical Center
Approach to the Pregnant Woman and Prenatal Care

DAVID A. SWANSON, MD
N.G. and Helen Hawkins Distinguished Professor for Cancer Research; Department of Urology, The University of Texas M. D. Anderson Cancer Center
Genitourinary Cancer

PAUL H. TANSER, MD, FRCP(C), FRCP (GLASGOW)
Professor of Medicine (Emeritus), McMaster University; Medical Head of Cardiology, Palmerston North Hospital, New Zealand
Valvular Disorders; Approach to the Cardiac Patient

SYED H. TARIQ, MD
Assistant Professor of Medicine, Division of Geriatric Medicine, Saint Louis University School of Medicine
Polyglandular Deficiency Syndromes

JOAN B. TARLOFF, PhD
Professor, Department of Pharmaceutical Sciences, University of the Sciences in Philadelphia, Philadelphia College of Pharmacy
Drug Toxicity

MARY TERRITO, MD
Professor of Medicine, Director of Hematopoietic Stem Cell Transplantation, University of California, Los Angeles
Neutropenia and Lymphocytopenia

WENDY THEOBALD, PhD
Assistant Researcher, Center for Tobacco Research and Intervention, University of Wisconsin
Smoking Cessation

DAVID R. THOMAS, MD
Professor of Internal Medicine and Geriatrics, Saint Louis University Health Sciences Center
Nutritional Support

ELIZABETH CHABNER THOMPSON, MD, MPH
21st Century Oncology, Yonkers, NY
Principles of Cancer Therapy

STIG THUNELL, MD, PhD
Professor, Karolinska Institute; Senior Consultant, Porphyria Center Sweden, Karolinska University Hospital Huddinge, Stockholm
Porphyrias

SHELLY D. TIMMONS, MD, PhD
Assistant Professor and Chief of Neurotrauma Division, University of Tennessee College of Medicine; Private Practice, Semmes-Murphey Neurological & Spine Institute
Traumatic Brain Injury

RONALD GARY TOMPKINS, MD, ScD
John F. Burke Professor of Surgery, Harvard Medical School, Visiting Surgeon, Massachusetts General Hospital
Diverticular Disease; Acute Abdomen and Surgical Gastroenterology; GI Bleeding

COURTNEY M. TOWNSEND, JR., MD
Professor and John Woods Harris Distinguished Chairman, Department of Surgery, The University of Texas Medical Branch
Carcinoid Tumors

ANNE S. TSAO, MD
Assistant Professor, The University of Texas M. D. Anderson Cancer Center
Tumors of the Lungs

DEBARA L. TUCCI, MD
Associate Professor, Division of Otolaryngology-Head and Neck Surgery, Duke University Medical Center
Approach to the Patient With Ear Problems

ALLAN R. TUNKEL, MD, PhD
Professor of Medicine and Senior Associate Dean for Academic Campuses, Drexel University College of Medicine
Biology of Infectious Disease

RONALD B. TURNER, MD
Professor of Pediatrics, University of Virginia School of Medicine
Respiratory Viruses

PAUL J. VANKEVICH, DMD
Assistant Professor of Oral Diagnosis and Oral Medicine, Tufts University School of Dental Medicine
Tumors of the Head and Neck

EVA M. VIVIAN, PharmD
Associate Professor of Pharmacy Practice, Western University of Health Sciences, College of Pharmacy, Pomona
Pharmacokinetics

VICTOR G. VOGEL, MD, MHS
Professor of Medicine and Epidemiology, University of Pittsburgh School of Medicine; Director, Breast Cancer Prevention Program, University of Pittsburgh Cancer Institute/ Magee-Womens Hospital
Breast Disorders

AARON D. WALFISH, MD
Division of Digestive Diseases, Department of Medicine, Beth Israel Medical Center, Manhattan Campus of Albert Einstein College of Medicine
Inflammatory Bowel Disease

JAMES WAYNE WARNICA, MD, FRCP(C)
Professor of Medicine, University of Calgary; Director, Cardiac Intensive Care Unit, Foothills Medical Center
Coronary Artery Disease

YASMINE WASFI, MD
Instructor, Department of Medicine, Parker B. Francis Fellow, National Jewish Medical and Research Center; Instructor, Division of Pulmonary Sciences and Critical Care Medicine, University of Colorado at Denver Health Sciences Center
Sarcoidosis

MAX HARRY WEIL, MD, PhD
Distinguished University Professor and President of the Institute of Critical Care Medicine, Rancho Mirage and Palm Springs
Sepsis and Septic Shock; Respiratory and Cardiac Arrest; Shock and Fluid Resuscitation

GEOFFREY A. WEINBERG, MD
Associate Professor of Pediatrics, University of Rochester School of Medicine and Dentistry; Director, Pediatric HIV Program, Golisano Children's Hospital at Strong
Infections in Infants and Children

HOWARD D. WEISS, MD
Associate Professor of Neurology, Johns Hopkins-Sinai Hospital of Baltimore
Headache

JOHN B. WEST, MD, PhD, DSc
Professor of Medicine and Physiology, University of California, San Diego
Altitude Sickness

JACK WILBERGER, MD
Professor and Chairman, Department of Neurosurgery, Allegheny General Hospital, Pittsburgh; Vice Dean, Drexel University College of Medicine
Spinal Trauma

MARGARET-MARY G. WILSON, MD
Associate Professor of Internal and Geriatric Medicine, Saint Louis University Health Sciences Center
Nutrition: General Considerations; Syndromes of Uncertain Origin

ROBERT A. WISE, MD
Professor of Medicine, Johns Hopkins University School of Medicine
Chronic Obstructive Pulmonary Disease

GARY WITTERT, MBBCh, MD, FRCP
Associate Professor and Head, Department of Medicine, University of Adelaide; Senior Consultant Endocrinologist, Royal Adelaide Hospital
Obesity and The Metabolic Syndrome

EIJI YANAGISAWA, MD
Clinical Professor of Otolaryngology, Yale University School of Medicine
External Ear Disorders; Facial Trauma

THOMAS MICHAEL ZIZIC, MD
Associate Professor of Medicine, The Johns Hopkins University School of Medicine; Co-Director, Chesapeake Medical Research
Avascular Necrosis

DOROTHEA ZUCKER-FRANKLIN, MD
Professor of Medicine, New York University School of Medicine
Eosinophilic Disorders

SECTION 1
NUTRITIONAL DISORDERS

1 NUTRITION: GENERAL CONSIDERATIONS

Nutrition is the science of food and its relationship to health. Nutrients are chemicals in foods that are used by the body for growth, maintenance, and energy. Nutrients that cannot be synthesized by the body and thus must be derived from the diet are considered essential. They include vitamins, minerals, some amino acids, and fatty acids. Nutrients that the body can synthesize from other compounds, although they may also be derived from the diet, are considered nonessential. Macronutrients are required by the body in relatively large amounts; micronutrients are needed in minute amounts.

Lack of nutrients can result in deficiency syndromes (eg, kwashiorkor, pellagra) or other disorders (see Ch. 2 on p. 10). Excess intake of macronutrients can lead to obesity (see p. 56); excess intake of micronutrients can be toxic.

Macronutrients

Macronutrients constitute the bulk of the diet and supply energy and many essential nutrients. Carbohydrates, proteins (including essential amino acids), fats (including essential fatty acids), macrominerals, and water are macronutrients. Carbohydrates, fats, and proteins are interchangeable as sources of energy; fats yield 9 kcal/g (37.8 kJ/g); proteins and carbohydrates yield 4 kcal/g (16.8 kJ/g).

Carbohydrates: Dietary carbohydrates are broken down into glucose and other monosaccharides. Carbohydrates increase blood glucose levels, supplying energy. Simple carbohydrates are composed of small molecules, generally monosaccharides or disaccharides, which are rapidly absorbed. Complex carbohydrates are composed of larger molecules, which are broken down into monosaccharides. Complex carbohydrates increase blood glucose levels more slowly but for a longer time. Glucose and sucrose are simple carbohydrates; starches and fiber are complex carbohydrates.

The glycemic index measures how rapidly a carbohydrate increases blood glucose levels. Values range from 1 (the slowest increase) to 100 (the fastest increase, equivalent to pure glucose—see TABLE 1–1). However, the actual rate of increase also depends on what foods are combined with the carbohydrate.

Carbohydrates with a high glycemic index may increase blood glucose to high levels rapidly. As a result, insulin levels increase, inducing hypoglycemia and hunger, which tends to lead to consumption of excess calories and weight gain. Carbohydrates with a low glycemic index increase blood glucose levels slowly, resulting in lower postprandial insulin levels and less hunger, which makes consumption of excess calories less likely. These effects result in a more favorable lipid profile and a decreased risk of obesity, diabetes mellitus, and complications of diabetes if present.

Proteins: Dietary proteins are broken down into peptides and amino acids. Proteins are required for tissue maintenance, replacement, function, and growth. However, if the body is not getting enough calories from tissue stores (particularly of fat) or dietary sources, protein may be used for energy.

As the body uses dietary protein for tissue production, there is a net gain of protein (positive nitrogen balance). During catabolic states (eg, starvation, infections, burns), more protein may be used (because body tissues are broken down) than is absorbed, resulting in a net loss of protein (negative nitrogen balance). Nitrogen balance is best determined by subtracting the amount of nitrogen excreted in urine and feces from the amount of nitrogen consumed.

Of the 20 amino acids, 9 are essential amino acids (EAAs); they cannot be synthesized and must be obtained from the diet. All people require 8 EAAs; infants also require histidine.

The weight-adjusted requirement for dietary protein correlates with growth rate, which decreases from infancy until adulthood. The protein requirement decreases from 2.2 g/kg in 3-mo-old infants to 1.2 g/kg in 5-yr-old children and to 0.8 g/kg in adults. Protein requirements correspond to EAA requirements (see TABLE 1–2). Adults trying to increase muscle mass need very little extra protein.

The amino acid composition of protein varies widely. Biological value (BV) reflects the similarity in amino acid composition of protein to that of animal tissues. A perfect match is egg protein, with a value of 100. Animal proteins in milk and meat have a high BV (~90); proteins in cereal and vegetables have a lower BV (~40), and some derived proteins (eg, gelatin) have a BV of 0. The extent to which dietary proteins supply each other's missing amino acids (complementarity) determines the overall BV of the diet. The recommended daily allowances (RDA) for protein assumes that the average mixed diet has a BV of 70.

Fats: Fats are broken down into fatty acids and glycerol. Fats are required for tissue growth and hormone production. Saturated fatty acids, common in animal fats, tend to be solid at room temperature. Except for palm and coconut oil, fats derived from plants tend to be liquid at room temperature; they contain high levels of monounsaturated fatty acids or polyunsaturated fatty acids (PUFAs). Partial hydrogenation of unsaturated fatty acids produces trans fatty acids.

Essential fatty acids (EFAs) are linoleic acid, an ω-6 (n-6) fatty acid, and linolenic acid, an ω-3 (n-3) fatty acid. Other ω-6 acids (eg, arachidonic acid) and other ω-3 fatty acids (eg, eicosapentaenoic acid, docosahexaenoic acid) are required by the body but can be synthesized from EFAs.

EFAs are needed for the formation of various eicosanoids, including prostaglandins, thromboxanes, prostacyclins, and leukotrienes (see also p. 20). ω-3 Fatty acids appear to decrease the risk of coronary artery disease.

Requirements for EFAs vary by age. Adults require amounts of linoleic acid equal to at least 2% of total caloric needs and linolenic acid equal to at least 0.5%. Vegetable oils provide linoleic acid and linolenic acid. Oils made from safflower, sunflower, corn, soya, primrose, pumpkin,

TABLE 1–1. GLYCEMIC INDEX OF SOME FOODS

CATEGORY	FOOD	INDEX
Beans	Kidney	33
	Red lentils	27
	Soy	14
Bread	Pumpernickel	49
	White	69
	Whole wheat	72
Cereals	All bran	54
	Corn flakes	83
	Oatmeal	53
	Puffed rice	90
	Shredded wheat	70
Dairy	Milk, ice cream, yogurt	34–38
Fruit	Apple	38
	Banana	61
	Orange	43
	Orange juice	49
	Strawberries	32
Grains	Barley	22
	Brown rice	66
	White rice	72
Pasta	—	38
Potatoes	Instant mashed (white)	86
	Mashed (white)	72
	Sweet	50
Snacks	Corn chips	72
	Oatmeal cookies	57
	Potato chips	56
Sugar	Fructose	22
	Glucose	100
	Honey	91
	Refined sugar	64

TABLE 1–2. ESSENTIAL AMINO ACID REQUIREMENTS IN MG/KG BODY WEIGHT

REQUIREMENT	INFANT (4–6 mo)	CHILD (10–12 yr)	ADULT
Histidine	29	—	—
Isoleucine	88	28	10
Leucine	150	44	14
Lysine	99	49	12
Methionine and cystine	72	24	13
Phenylalanine and tyrosine	120	24	14
Threonine	74	30	7
Tryptophan	19	4	3
Valine	93	28	13
Total essential amino acids (excluding histidine)	715	231	86

and wheat germ provide large amounts of linoleic acid. Marine fish oils and oils made from flaxseeds, pumpkin, soy, and canola provide large amounts of linolenic acid. Marine fish oils also provide some other ω-3 fatty acids in large amounts.

In the US, the main dietary source of trans fatty acids is partially hydrogenated vegetable oils. Trans fatty acids may elevate LDL cholesterol and lower HDL; they also independently increase the incidence of coronary artery disease.

Macrominerals: Na, Cl, K, Ca, P, and Mg are required in relatively large amounts per day (see TABLES 1–3, 1–4, and 5–2).

Water: Water is considered a macronutrient because it is required in amounts of 1 mL/kcal (0.24 mL/kJ) of energy expended, or about 2500 mL/day. Needs change with fever, warm or cold climates, and high or low humidity.

Micronutrients

Vitamins and minerals required in minute amounts (trace minerals) are micronutrients (see Chs. 4 and 5).

Water-soluble vitamins are vitamin C (ascorbic acid) and eight members of the vitamin B complex: thiamin (vitamin B_1), riboflavin (vitamin B_2), niacin, pyridoxine (vitamin B_6), folic acid, cobalamin (vitamin B_{12}), biotin, and pantothenic acid.

Fat-soluble vitamins are retinol (vitamin A), cholecalciferol and ergocalciferol (vitamin D), α-tocopherol (vitamin E), and phylloquinone and menaquinone (vitamin K). Only vitamins A, E, and B_{12} are stored to any significant extent in the body.

Essential trace minerals include iron, iodine, zinc, chromium, selenium, manganese, molybdenum, and copper. Except for chromium, each of these is incorporated into enzymes or hormones required in metabolism. Except for deficiencies of iron and zinc, micromineral deficiencies are uncommon in industrialized countries (see Ch. 4 on p. 26 and Ch. 5 on p. 47).

Other minerals (eg, aluminum, arsenic, boron, cobalt, fluoride, nickel, silicon, vanadium) have not been proved essential for people. Fluoride, although not essential, helps prevent tooth decay by forming a compound with Ca (CaF_2), which stabilizes the mineral matrix in teeth.

All trace minerals are toxic at high levels, and some (arsenic, nickel, and chromium) may cause cancer.

Other Dietary Substances

The daily human diet typically contains as many as 100,000 chemicals (eg, coffee contains 1000). Of these, only 300 are nutrients, only some of which are essential. However, many nonnutrients in foods are useful. For example, food additives (eg, preservatives, emulsifiers, antioxidants, stabilizers) improve the production and stability of foods. Trace components (eg, spices, flavors, odors, colors, phytochemicals, many other natural products) improve appearance and taste.

Fiber, which occurs in various forms (eg, cellulose, hemicellulose, pectin, gums), increases GI motility, prevents constipation, and helps control diverticular disease. Fiber is thought to accelerate the elimination of cancer-causing substances produced by bacteria in the large intestine. Epidemiologic evidence strongly supports an association between colon cancer and low fiber intake and a beneficial effect of fiber in functional bowel disorders, Crohn's disease, obesity, and hemorrhoids. Soluble fiber (present in fruits, vegetables, oats, barley, and legumes) reduces the postprandial increase in blood glucose and insulin and can reduce cholesterol levels.

The typical Western diet is low in fiber (about 12 g/day) because of a high intake of highly refined wheat flour and a low intake of fruits and vegetables. Increasing fiber intake to about 30 g/day by consuming more vegetables, fruits, and high-fiber cereals is generally recommended.

NUTRITIONAL REQUIREMENTS

Proper nutrition aims to achieve and maintain a desirable body composition and high potential for physical and mental work. Balancing energy intake with energy expenditure is necessary for a desirable body weight. Energy expenditure depends on age, sex, weight (see TABLE 1–4), and metabolic and physical activity. If energy intake exceeds expenditure, weight is gained. If energy intake is less than expenditure, weight is lost.

Daily dietary requirements for essential nutrients also depend on age, sex, weight, and metabolic and physical activity. Every 5 yr, the Food and Nutrition Board of the National Academy of Sciences/National Research Council and the US Department of Agriculture (USDA) issues the recommended dietary allowances for protein, energy, and some vitamins and minerals (RDAs–see TABLES 1–4, 4–2, and 5–2). For vitamins and minerals about which less is known, safe and adequate daily dietary intakes are estimated (see Ch. 4 and TABLE 5–2).

TABLE 1–3. MACROMINERALS

NUTRIENT	PRINCIPAL SOURCES	FUNCTIONS
Ca	Milk and milk products, meat, fish, eggs, cereals, beans, fruits, vegetables	Bone and tooth formation, blood coagulation, neuromuscular irritability, muscle contractility, myocardial conduction
Cl	Many foods, mainly animal products but some vegetables; similar to Na	Acid-base balance, osmotic pressure, blood pH, kidney function
K	Many foods, including whole and skim milk, bananas, prunes, raisins, meats	Muscle activity, nerve transmission, intracellular acid-base balance, water retention
Mg	Green leaves, nuts, cereals, grains, seafood	Bone and tooth formation, nerve conduction, muscle contraction, enzyme activation
Na	Many foods, including beef, pork, sardines, cheese, green olives, corn bread, potato chips, sauerkraut	Acid-base balance, osmotic pressure, blood pH, muscle contractility, nerve transmission, maintenance of cell membrane gradients
P	Milk, cheese, meat, poultry, fish, cereals, nuts, legumes	Bone and tooth formation, acid-base balance, energy production

TABLE 1–4. RECOMMENDED DIETARY ALLOWANCES* FOR SOME MACRONUTRIENTS, Food and Nutrition Board, National Academy

CATEGORY	AGE (YR) OR TIME FRAME	PROTEIN (g/kg)	ENERGY (kcal/kg)	CALCIUM (mg/kg)	PHOSPHORUS (mg/kg)	MAGNESIUM (mg/kg)
Infants	0.0–0.5	2.2	108.3	66.7	50.0	6.7
	0.5–1.0	1.6	94.4	66.7	55.6	6.7
Children	1–3	1.2	100.0	61.5	61.5	6.2
	4–6	1.2	90.0	40.0	40.0	6.0
	7–10	1.0	71.4	28.6	28.6	6.1
Males	11–14	1.0	55.6	26.7	26.7	6.0
	15–18	0.9	45.5	18.2	18.2	6.1
	19–24	0.8	40.3	16.7	16.7	4.9
	25–50	0.8	36.7	10.1	10.1	4.4
	51+	0.8	29.9	10.4	10.4	4.5
Females	11–14	1.0	47.8	26.1	26.1	6.1
	15–18	0.8	40.0	21.8	21.8	5.5
	19–24	0.8	37.9	20.7	20.7	4.8
	25–50	0.8	34.9	12.7	12.7	4.4
	51+	0.8	29.2	12.3	12.3	4.3
Pregnant		0.9	4.6	18.5	18.5	4.9
Breastfeeding	1st yr	1.0	7.9	19.0	19.0	5.4

*The allowances, expressed as average daily intakes over time, are intended to provide for individual variations among most healthy people living in the US under usual environmental stresses.

Pregnant women (see p. 2152) and infants (see p. 2224) have special nutritional needs.

The USDA publishes the Food Guide Pyramid, which specifies the number of recommended daily servings of various food groups (see TABLES 1–5 and 1–6). Some nutritionists recommend eating a higher proportion of fruits and vegetables. A separate food guide pyramid has been developed for the elderly, who have different nutritional requirements (see FIG. 1–1). Adequate fluid intake is emphasized as the base of that pyramid.

Fats should constitute ≤ 30% of total calories, and saturated and trans fatty acids should constitute < 10%. Excess intake of saturated fats contributes to atherosclerosis. Substituting PUFAs for saturated fats can decrease the risk of atherosclerosis. Routine use of nutritional supplements is not necessary or beneficial; some supplements can be harmful.

NUTRITION IN CLINICAL MEDICINE

Nutritional deficiencies can often worsen health outcomes (whether a disorder is present or not), and some disorders (eg, malabsorption) can cause nutritional deficiencies. Also, many patients (eg, elderly patients during acute hospitalization) have unsuspected nutritional deficiencies that require treatment. Many medical centers have multidisciplinary nutrition support teams of physicians, nurses, dietitians, and pharmacists to help the clinician prevent, diagnose, and treat occult nutritional deficiencies.

Overnutrition may contribute to chronic disorders, such as cancer, hypertension, obesity, diabetes mellitus, and coronary artery disease. Dietary restrictions are necessary in many hereditary metabolic disorders (eg, galactosemia, phenylketonuria).

Evaluation of Nutritional Status

Indications for nutritional evaluation include undesirable body weight or body composition, suspicion of specific deficiencies or toxicities of essential nutrients and, in infants and children, insufficient growth or development. However, nutritional status should be evaluated routinely as part of the clinical examination for infants and children, the elderly, people taking several drugs, people with psychiatric disorders,

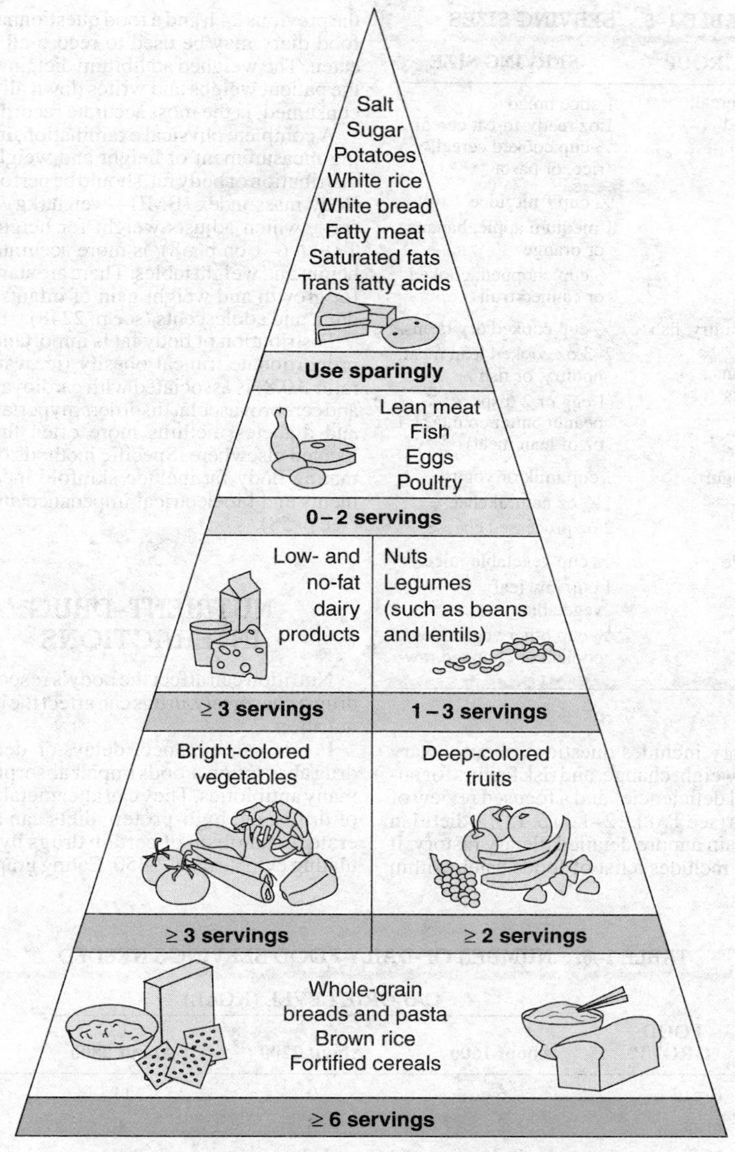

Fig. 1–1. Daily food guide pyramid for older adults.

and people with systemic diseases that last longer than several days.

Evaluating general nutritional status includes history, physical examination, and sometimes tests. If undernutrition is suspected, laboratory tests and skin anergy tests may be done (see p. 12). Body composition analysis is used to evaluate obesity.

TABLE 1–5. SERVING SIZES

FOOD GROUP	SERVING SIZE
Bread, cereal, rice, and pasta	1 slice bread 1 oz ready-to-eat cereal ½ cup cooked cereal, rice, or pasta
Fruit	¾ cup fruit juice 1 medium apple, banana, or orange ½ cup chopped, cooked, or canned fruit
Meat, poultry, fish, eggs, dry beans, and nuts	½ cup cooked dry beans 2–3 oz cooked lean meat, poultry, or fish (1 egg or 2 tbsp peanut butter counts as 1 oz of lean meat)
Milk, yogurt, and cheese	1 cup milk or yogurt 1½ oz natural cheese 2 oz processed cheese
Vegetable	¾ cup vegetable juice 1 cup raw leafy vegetables ½ cup other vegetables, cooked or chopped raw

History includes questions about dietary intake, weight change, and risk factors for nutritional deficiencies and a focused review of systems (see TABLE 2–1 on p. 13). A dietitian can obtain a more detailed dietary history. It usually includes a list of foods eaten within the previous 24 h and a food questionnaire. A food diary may be used to record all foods eaten. The weighed ad libitum diet, in which the patient weighs and writes down all foods consumed, is the most accurate record.

A complete physical examination, including measurement of height and weight and distribution of body fat, should be performed. Body mass index (BMI)—weight(kg)/height $(m)^2$, which adjusts weight for height (see TABLE 6–1 on p. 58), is more accurate than height and weight tables. There are standards for growth and weight gain of infants, children, and adolescents (see p. 2248).

Distribution of body fat is important. Disproportionate truncal obesity (ie, waist/hip ratio > 0.8) is associated with cardiovascular and cerebrovascular disorders, hypertension, and diabetes mellitus more often than fat located elsewhere. Specific methods of estimating body fat include skinfold measurements and bioelectrical impedance analysis (see p. 58).

NUTRIENT–DRUG INTERACTIONS

Nutrition can affect the body's response to drugs; conversely, drugs can affect the body's nutrition.

Foods can enhance, delay, or decrease drug absorption. Foods impair absorption of many antibiotics. They can alter metabolism of drugs; eg, high-protein diets can accelerate metabolism of certain drugs by stimulating cytochrome P-450. Eating grapefruit

TABLE 1–6. NUMBER OF DAILY FOOD SERVINGS NEEDED

FOOD GROUP	CALORIE LEVEL (KCAL) About 1600	About 2200	About 2800
Bread	6	9	11
Fruit	2	3	4
Milk	2–3*	2–3*	2–3*
Meat	2 (total, 5 oz)	2 (total, 6 oz)	3 (total, 7 oz)
Vegetable	3	4	5

*Women who are pregnant or breastfeeding, adolescents, and young adults (up to age 24 yr) need 3 servings.

can inhibit cytochrome P-450, slowing metabolism of the same drugs. Diets that alter the bacterial flora may markedly affect the overall metabolism of certain drugs. Some foods affect the body's response to drugs. For example, tyramine, a component of cheese and a potent vasoconstrictor, can cause hypertensive crisis in some patients who take monoamine oxidase inhibitors and eat cheese.

Nutritional deficiencies can affect drug absorption and metabolism. Severe energy and protein deficiencies reduce enzyme tissue concentrations and may impair the response to drugs by reducing absorption or protein binding and causing liver dysfunction. Changes in the GI tract can impair absorption and affect the response to a drug. Deficiency of Ca, Mg, or zinc may impair drug metabolism. Vitamin C deficiency decreases activity of drug-metabolizing enzymes, especially in the elderly.

Many drugs affect appetite, food absorption, and tissue metabolism (see TABLE 1–7). Some drugs (eg, metoclopramide) increase GI motility, decreasing food absorption. Other drugs (eg, opioids, anticholinergics) decrease GI motility.

Certain drugs affect mineral metabolism. For example, diuretics, especially thiazides, and corticosteroids can deplete body K, increasing susceptibility to digoxin-induced cardiac arrhythmias. Repeated use of laxatives may deplete K. Cortisol, desoxycorticosterone, and aldosterone cause marked Na and water retention, at least temporarily; retention is much less with prednisone, prednisolone, and some other corticosteroid analogs. Estrogen-progesterone oral contraceptives also cause Na and water retention. Sulfonylureas and lithium can impair the uptake or release of iodine by the thyroid. Oral contraceptives can lower plasma zinc levels and increase copper levels.

Certain drugs affect vitamin absorption or metabolism. Ethanol impairs thiamin utilization, and isoniazid interferes with niacin and pyridoxine metabolism. Ethanol and oral contraceptives inhibit folate absorption. Most patients receiving phenytoin, phenobarbital, primidone, or phenothiazines develop folate deficiency, probably because hepatic microsomal drug-metabolizing enzymes are affected. Folate

TABLE 1–7. EFFECTS OF DRUGS ON NUTRITION

EFFECT	DRUGS
Increases appetite	Alcohol, antihistamines, corticosteroids, dronabinol, insulin, megestrol acetate, mirtazapine, psychoactive drugs, sulfonylureas, thyroid hormone
Decreases appetite	Antibiotics, bulk agents (methylcellulose, guar gum), cyclophosphamide, digoxin, glucagon, indomethacin, morphine, fluoxetine
Decreases absorption of fats	Orlistat
Increases blood glucose levels	Octreotide, opioids, phenothiazines, phenytoin, probenecid, thiazide diuretics, corticosteroids, warfarin
Decreases blood glucose levels	Aspirin, barbiturates, β-blockers, monoamine oxidase inhibitors (MAOIs), oral antihyperglycemic drugs, phenacetin, phenylbutazone, sulfonamides
Decreases plasma lipid levels	Aspirin and *p*-aminosalicylic acid, L-asparaginase, chlortetracycline, colchicine, dextrans, glucagon, niacin, phenindione, statins, sulfinpyrazone, trifluperidol
Increases plasma lipid levels	Adrenal corticosteroids, chlorpromazine, ethanol, growth hormone, oral contraceptives (estrogen-progestogen type), thiouracil, vitamin D
Decreases protein metabolism	Chloramphenicol, tetracycline

supplements may make anticonvulsants less effective, but yeast tablet supplements seem to increase folate levels without this effect. Anticonvulsants can cause vitamin D deficiency. Malabsorption of vitamin B_{12} can occur with use of aminosalicylic acid, slow-release K iodide, colchicine, trifluoperazine, ethanol, and oral contraceptives. Oral contraceptives with high progestogen content can cause depression, probably because of metabolically induced tryptophan deficiency.

Nutrient metabolism may be affected by other dietary substances. For example, nonheme iron absorption is impaired or facilitated by a number of dietary substances (see p. 1037).

FOOD ADDITIVES AND CONTAMINANTS

Additives are chemicals combined with foods to facilitate their processing and preservation or to enhance their desirability. Only amounts of additives shown to be safe by laboratory tests are permitted in commercially prepared foods.

Weighing the benefits of additives (eg, reduced waste, increased variety of available foods, protection against foodborne illness) against the risks is often complex. For example, nitrite, which is used in cured meats, inhibits the growth of *Clostridium botulinum* and improves flavor. However, nitrite converts to nitrosamines, which are carcinogens in animals. On the other hand, the amount of nitrite added to cured meat is small compared with the amount from naturally occurring food nitrates converted to nitrite by the salivary glands. Dietary vitamin C can reduce nitrite formation in the GI tract. Rarely, some additives (eg, sulfites) cause food hypersensitivity (allergy) reactions. Most reactions are caused by ordinary foods (see p. 1358).

Contaminants sometimes cannot be completely eliminated without damaging foods; so limited quantities are allowed. Common contaminants are pesticides, heavy metals (lead, cadmium, mercury), nitrates (in green leafy vegetables), aflatoxins (in nuts and milk), growth-promoting hormones (in dairy products and meat), animal hairs and feces, and insect parts. FDA-estimated safe levels are those that have not caused illness or adverse effects in people. However, demonstrating a causal relationship between extremely low level exposures and adverse effects is difficult; long-term adverse effects, although unlikely, are still possible. Safe levels are often determined by consensus rather than by hard evidence.

2 UNDERNUTRITION

Undernutrition is a form of malnutrition (which also includes overnutrition—see Ch. 6 on p. 56). Undernutrition can result from inadequate ingestion of nutrients, malabsorption, impaired metabolism, loss of nutrients due to diarrhea, or increased nutritional requirements (as occurs in cancer or infection). Undernutrition progresses in stages; each stage usually takes considerable time to develop. First, nutrient levels in blood and tissues change, followed by intracellular changes in biochemical functions and structure. Ultimately, symptoms and signs appear.

Risk Factors

Undernutrition is associated with many disorders and circumstances, including poverty and social deprivation. Risk is also greater at certain times (ie, during infancy, early childhood, adolescence, pregnancy, breastfeeding, and old age).

Infancy and childhood: Infants and children are particularly susceptible to undernutrition because of their high demand for energy and essential nutrients. If vitamin K is inadequate, newborns may develop hemorrhagic disease of the newborn, a life-threatening disorder (see p. 46). An infant fed only breast milk can develop vitamin B_{12} deficiency if the mother is a vegan. Inadequately fed infants and children are at risk of protein-energy malnutrition and deficiencies of iron, folic acid, vitamins A and C, copper, and zinc. During adolescence, nutritional requirements increase because the growth rate accelerates. Anorexia nervosa (see p. 1701) may affect adolescent girls.

Pregnancy and breastfeeding: Requirements for nutrients increase during pregnancy and breastfeeding. Aberrations of diet, including pica (the consumption of nonnutritive substances, such as clay and charcoal), may occur during pregnancy. Anemia due to iron deficiency is common as is anemia due to folic acid deficiency, especially among women who have taken oral contraceptives.

Old age: Aging—even when disease or dietary deficiency is absent—leads to sarcopenia (progressive loss of lean body mass), starting after age 40 and eventually amounting to a muscle loss of about 10 kg (22 lb) in men and 5 kg (11 lb) in women. Causes include decreased physical activity and food intake and increased cytokine levels (particularly interleukin-6). In men, decreasing androgen levels are a cause. Aging decreases basal metabolic rate (due mainly to decreased fat-free mass), total body weight, height, and skeletal mass and increases mean body fat (as a percentage of body weight) from about 20 to 30% in men and 27 to 40% in women.

From age 20 to 80, food intake decreases, especially in men. Anorexia due to aging itself has many causes, including reduced adaptive relaxation of the stomach's fundus, increased release and activity of cholecystokinin (which produces satiation), and increased leptin (an anorectic hormone produced by fat cells). Diminished taste and smell can decrease eating pleasure but usually decrease food intake only slightly. Anorexia may have other causes (eg, loneliness, inability to shop or prepare meals, dementia, some chronic disorders, use of certain drugs). Depression is a common cause. Occasionally, anorexia nervosa, paranoia, or mania interferes with eating. Dental problems limit the ability to chew and subsequently to digest foods. Swallowing difficulties are common (eg, due to strokes, other neurologic disorders, esophageal candidiasis, or xerostomia). Poverty or functional impairment limits access to nutrients.

The institutionalized elderly are at particular risk of protein-energy malnutrition (PEM). They are often confused and may be unable to express hunger or preferences for foods. They may be physically unable to feed themselves. Chewing or swallowing may be very slow, making it tedious for another person to feed them enough food. Inadequate intake and decreased absorption of vitamin D and inadequate exposure to sunshine contribute to osteomalacia (see p. 41).

Disorders and medical procedures: Diabetes, some chronic disorders that affect the GI tract, bowel resections, and certain other GI surgical procedures tend to impair absorption of fat-soluble vitamins, vitamin B_{12}, Ca, and iron. Gluten enteropathy, pancreatic insufficiency, or other disorders can result in malabsorption. Decreased absorption possibly contributes to iron deficiency and osteoporosis. Liver disorders impair storage of vitamins A and B_{12} and interfere with metabolism of protein and energy sources. Renal insufficiency predisposes to protein, iron, and vitamin D deficiencies. Anorexia causes some patients with cancer or depression and many with AIDS to consume inadequate amounts of food. Infections, trauma, hyperthyroidism, extensive burns, and prolonged fever increase metabolic demands.

Vegetarian diets: Iron deficiency can occur in ovo-lacto vegetarians (although such a diet can be compatible with good health). Vegans may develop vitamin B_{12} deficiency unless they consume yeast extracts or Asian-style fermented foods. Their intake of Ca, iron, and zinc also tends to be low. A fruit-only diet is not recommended because it is deficient in protein, Na, and many micronutrients.

Fad diets: Some fad diets result in vitamin, mineral, and protein deficiencies; cardiac, renal, and metabolic disorders; and sometimes death. Very low calorie diets (< 400 kcal/day) cannot sustain health for long.

Drugs and nutritional supplements: Many drugs (eg, appetite suppressants, digoxin) decrease appetite; others impair nutrient absorption or metabolism. Some drugs (eg, stimulants) have catabolic effects. Certain drugs can impair absorption of many nutrients; eg, anticonvulsants can impair absorption of vitamins.

Alcohol or drug dependency: Patients with alcohol or drug dependency may neglect their nutritional needs. Absorption and metabolism of nutrients may also be impaired. IV drug addicts typically become undernourished as do alcoholics who consume ≥ 1 quart of hard liquor/day. Alcoholism can cause deficiencies of Mg, zinc, and certain vitamins, including thiamin.

Symptoms and Diagnosis

Symptoms vary depending on the cause and type of undernutrition (see p. 15 and Ch. 4 on p. 26).

Diagnosis is based on results of medical and diet histories, physical examination, body composition analysis (see p. 58), and selected laboratory tests.

History: History should include questions about dietary intake (see FIG. 2–1), recent changes in weight, and risk factors for undernutrition, including drug and alcohol use. Unintentional loss of ≥ 10% of usual body weight during a 3-mo period indicates a high probability of undernutrition. Social history should include questions about whether money is available for food and whether the patient can shop and cook.

Review of systems should focus on symptoms of nutritional deficiencies (see TABLE 2–1). For example, headache, nausea, and diplopia may indicate vitamin A toxicity.

Physical examination: Physical examination should include measurement of height and weight, inspection of body fat distribution, and anthropometric measurements of lean body mass. Body mass index (BMI = weight(kg)/height(m)^2) adjusts weight for height (see TABLE 6–1 on p. 58). If weight is < 80% of what is predicted for the patient's height or if BMI is ≤ 18, undernutrition should be suspected. Although these findings are useful in diagnosing undernutrition, they lack specificity.

The mid upper arm muscle area estimates lean body mass. This area is derived from the triceps skinfold thickness (TSF) and mid upper arm circumference. Both are measured at the same site, with the patient's right arm in a relaxed position. The average mid upper arm circumference is about 32 ± 5 cm for men and 28 ± 6 cm for women. The formula for calculating the mid upper arm muscle area in cm^2 is shown below.

This formula corrects the upper arm area for fat and bone. Average values for the mid upper arm muscle area are 54 ± 11 cm^2 for men and 30 ± 7 cm^2 for women. A value < 75% of this standard (depending on age) indicates depletion of lean body mass (see TABLE 2–2). This measurement may be affected by physical activity, genetic factors, and age-related muscle loss.

Physical examination should focus on signs of specific nutritional deficiencies. Signs of PEM (eg, edema, muscle wasting, rash) should be sought. Examination should also focus on signs of conditions that could predispose to nutritional deficiencies, such as dental problems. Mental status should be assessed, because depression and cognitive impairment can lead to weight loss.

The widely used Subjective Global Assessment (SGA) uses information from the patient history (eg, weight loss, change in intake, GI symptoms), physical examination findings (eg, loss of muscle and subcutaneous fat, edema, ascites), and the clinician's judgment of the patient's nutritional status. The Mini Nutritional Assessment (MNA) has been validated and is widely used, especially for elderly patients (see FIG. 2–1).

Testing: The extent of laboratory testing needed is unclear and may depend on the patient's circumstances. If the cause is obvious and correctable (eg, a wilderness survival situation), testing is probably of little benefit. Other patients may require more detailed evaluation.

Serum albumin measurement is the laboratory test most often used. Decreases in albumin and other proteins (eg, prealbumin [transthyretin], transferrin, retinol-binding protein) may indicate protein deficiency or PEM. As undernutrition progresses, albumin decreases slowly; prealbumin, transferrin, and retinol-binding protein decrease rapidly. Albumin measurement is inexpensive and predicts morbidity and mortality better than measurement of the other proteins. However, the correlation of albumin with morbidity and mortality may be related to nonnutritional as well as nutritional factors. Inflammation produces cytokines that cause albumin and other nutritional protein markers to extravasate, decreasing serum levels. Because prealbumin, transferrin, and retinol-binding protein decrease more rapidly during starvation than

$$\frac{[\text{midarm circumference (cm)} - (3.14 \times \text{TSF cm})]^2}{4\pi} - 10 \text{ (males) or } - 6.5 \text{ (females)}$$

TABLE 2–1. SIGNS AND SYMPTOMS OF NUTRITIONAL DEFICIENCY

AREA/SYSTEM	SYMPTOM OR SIGN	DEFICIENCY
General appearance	Wasting	Energy
Skin	Rash	Many vitamins, zinc, essential fatty acids
	Rash in sun-exposed areas	Niacin (pellagra)
	Easy bruising	Vitamin C or K
Hair and nails	Thinning or loss of hair	Protein
	Premature whitening of hair	Selenium
	Spooning of nails	Iron
Eyes	Impaired night vision	Vitamin A
	Corneal keratomalacia	Vitamin A
Mouth	Cheilosis and glossitis	Riboflavin, niacin, pyridoxine, iron
	Bleeding gums	Vitamin C, riboflavin
Extremities	Edema	Protein
Neurologic	Paresthesias or numbness in a stocking-glove distribution	Thiamin
	Tetany	Ca, Mg
	Cognitive and sensory deficits	Thiamin (beriberi), niacin (pellagra), pyridoxine, vitamin B_{12}
	Dementia	Thiamin, niacin, vitamin B_{12}
Musculoskeletal	Wasting of muscle	Protein
	Bone deformities (eg, bowlegs, knocked knees, curved spine)	Vitamin D, Ca
	Bone tenderness	Vitamin D
	Joint pain or swelling	Vitamin C
GI	Diarrhea	Protein, niacin, folic acid, vitamin B_{12}
	Diarrhea and dysgeusia	Zinc
	Dysphagia or odynophagia (due to Plummer-Vinson syndrome)	Iron
Endocrine	Thyromegaly	Iodine

does albumin, their measurements are sometimes used to diagnose or assess the severity of acute starvation. However, whether they are more sensitive or specific than albumin is unclear.

Total lymphocyte count, which often decreases as undernutrition progresses, may be determined. Undernutrition produces a marked decline in $CD4^+$ T lymphocytes, so this count is more useful in patients who do not have AIDS.

Skin tests using antigens can detect impaired cell-mediated immunity in PEM and in some other disorders of undernutrition (see p. 1337).

Other laboratory tests, such as measuring vitamin and mineral levels, are used selectively to diagnose specific deficiencies.

NESTLÉ NUTRITION SERVICES

Last name: ______ First name: ______ Sex: ______ Date: ______

Age: ______ Weight, kg: ______ Height, cm: ______ I.D. Number: ______

Complete the screen by filling in the boxes with the appropriate numbers.
Add the numbers for the screen. If score is 11 or less, continue with the assessment to gain a Malnutrition Indicator Score.

SCREENING

A Has food intake declined over the past 3 months due to loss of appetite, digestive problems, chewing or swallowing difficulties?
0 = severe loss of appetite
1 = moderate loss of appetite
2 = no loss of appetite ☐

B Weight loss during last months
0 = weight loss greater than 3 kg (6.6 lbs)
1 = does not know
2 = weight loss between 1 and 3 kg (2.2 and 6.6 lbs)
3 = no weight loss ☐

C Mobility
0 = bed or chair bound
1 = able to get out of bed/chair but does not go out
2 = goes out ☐

D Has suffered psychological stress or acute disease in the past 3 months
0 = yes 2 = no ☐

E Neuropsychological problems
0 = severe dementia or depression
1 = mild dementia
2 = no psychological problems ☐

F Body Mass Index (BMI) (weight in kg) / (height in m)^2
0 = BMI less than 19
1 = BMI19 to less than 21
2 = BMI 21 to less than 23
3 = BMI 23 or greater ☐

Screening Score (subtotal max. 14 points) ☐☐

12 points or greater	Normal—not at risk—no need to complete assessment
11 points or below	Possible malnutrition—continue assessment

ASSESSMENT

G Lives independently (not in a nursing home or hospital)
0 = no 1 = yes ☐

H Takes more than 3 prescription drugs per day
0 = yes 1 = no ☐

I Pressure sores or skin ulcers
0 = yes 1 = no ☐

J How many full meals does the patient eat daily?
0 = 1 meal
1 = 2 meals
2 = 3 meals ☐

K Selected consumption markers for protein intake
- At least one serving of dairy products (milk, cheese, yogurt) per day? yes ☐ no ☐
- Two or more servings of legumes or eggs per week? yes ☐ no ☐
- Meat, fish or poultry every day yes ☐ no ☐

0.0 = if 0 or 1 yes
0.5 = if 2 yes
1.0 = if 3 yes ☐.☐

L Consumes two or more servings of fruits or vegetables per day?
0 = no 1 = yes ☐

M How much fluid (water, juice, coffee, tea, milk. . .) is consumed per day?
0.0 = less than 3 cups
0.5 = 3 to 5 cups
1.0 = more than 5 cups ☐.☐

N Mode of feeding
0 = unable to eat without assistance
1 = self-fed with some difficulty
2 = self-fed without any problem ☐

O Self view of nutritional status
0 = views self as being malnourished
1 = is uncertain of nutritional state
2 = views self as having no nutritional problem ☐

P In comparison with other people of the same age, how do they consider their health status?
0.0 = not as good
0.5 = does not know
1.0 = as good
2.0 = better ☐.☐

Q Mid-arm circumference (MAC) in cm
0.0 = MAC less than 21
0.5 = MAC 21 to 22
1.0 = MAC 22 or greater ☐.☐

R Calf circumference (CC) in cm
0 = CC less than 31 1 = CC 31 or greater ☐

Assessment (max. 16 points) ☐☐.☐

Screening score ☐☐

Total Assessment (max. 30 points) ☐☐.☐

Malnutrition Indicator Score

17 to 23.5 points	at risk of malnutrition	☐
Less than 17 points	malnourished	☐

FIG. 2–1. SEE LEGEND ON THE OPPOSITE PAGE.

TABLE 2–2. MID UPPER ARM MUSCLE AREA IN ADULTS

STANDARD (%)	MEN (cm^2)	WOMEN (cm^2)	MUSCLE MASS
100 ± 20*	54 ± 11	30 ± 7	Adequate
75	40	22	Marginal
60	32	18	Depleted
50	27	15	Wasted

*Mean mid upper arm muscle mass ± 1 standard deviation. From National Health and Nutrition Examination Surveys I and II.

PROTEIN-ENERGY MALNUTRITION

Protein-energy malnutrition (PEM), or protein-calorie malnutrition, is an energy deficit due to chronic deficiency of all macronutrients. It commonly includes deficiencies of many micronutrients. PEM can be sudden and total (starvation) or gradual. Severity ranges from subclinical deficiencies to obvious wasting (with edema, hair loss, and skin atrophy) to starvation. Multiple organ systems are often impaired. Diagnosis usually involves laboratory testing, including serum albumin. Treatment consists of correcting fluid and electrolyte deficits with IV solutions, then gradually replenishing nutrients, orally if possible.

In developed countries, PEM is common among the institutionalized elderly (although often not suspected) and among patients with disorders that decrease appetite or impair nutrient digestion, absorption, or metabolism. In developing countries, PEM affects children who do not consume enough calories or protein.

Classification and Etiology

PEM is graded as mild, moderate, or severe. Grade is determined by calculating weight as a percentage of expected weight for length or height using international standards (normal, 90 to 110%; mild PEM, 85 to 90%; moderate, 75 to 85%; severe, <75%).

PEM may be primary or secondary. Primary PEM is caused by inadequate nutrient intake. Secondary PEM results from disorders or drugs that interfere with nutrient use.

Primary PEM: Worldwide, primary PEM occurs mostly in children and the elderly who lack access to nutrients, although a common cause in the elderly is depression. It can also result from fasting or anorexia nervosa. Child or elder abuse may be a cause.

In children, chronic primary PEM has three common forms: marasmus, kwashiorkor, and a form with characteristics of both (marasmic kwashiorkor). The form depends on the balance of nonprotein and protein sources of energy. Starvation is an acute severe form of primary PEM.

Fig. 2–1. Mini nutritional assessment. Guigoz Y and Garry PJ 1994. Mini nutritional assessment. A practical assessment tool for grading the nutritional status of elderly patients. Facts and Research in Gerontology. Supplement 2:15–59. Rubenstein LZ, Jarker J, Guigoz Y, and Vellas B. Comprehensive geriatric assessment (CGA) and the MNA: An overview of the CGA, nutritional assessment and development of a shortened version of the MNA. In "Mini nutritional assessment (MNA): Research and practice in the elderly." Vellas B, Garry PJ, and Guigoz Y, editors. Nestlé Nutrition Workshop Series. Clinical & Performance Programme, vol. 1, Karger, Bale, 1997. ® Société des Produits Nestlé S.A., Vevey, Switzerland, trademark owners. Reprinted with permission.

Marasmus (also called the dry form of PEM) causes weight loss and depletion of fat and muscle. In developing countries, marasmus is the most common form of PEM in children.

Kwashiorkor (also called the wet, swollen, or edematous form) is associated with premature abandonment of breastfeeding, which typically occurs when a younger sibling is born, displacing the older child from the breast. So children with kwashiorkor tend to be older than those with marasmus. Kwashiorkor may also result from an acute illness, often gastroenteritis or another infection (probably secondary to cytokine release), in a child who already has PEM. A diet that is more deficient in protein than energy may be more likely to cause kwashiorkor than marasmus. Less common than marasmus, kwashiorkor tends to be confined to specific parts of the world, such as rural Africa, the Caribbean, and the Pacific islands. In these areas, staple foods (eg, yams, cassavas, sweet potatoes, green bananas) are low in protein and high in carbohydrates. In kwashiorkor, cell membranes leak, causing extravasation of intravascular fluid and protein, resulting in peripheral edema.

Marasmic kwashiorkor is characterized by features of marasmus and kwashiorkor. Affected children have some edema and more body fat than those with marasmus.

Starvation is a complete lack of nutrients. It is occasionally voluntary (as in fasting or anorexia nervosa) but usually due to external factors (eg, famine, wilderness exposure).

Secondary PEM: This type most commonly results from disorders that affect GI function, wasting disorders, and conditions that increase metabolic demands (eg, infections, hyperthyroidism, Addison's disease, pheochromocytoma, other endocrine disorders, burns, trauma, surgery, other critical illnesses). In wasting disorders (eg, AIDS, cancer) and renal failure, catabolism causes cytokine excess, resulting in undernutrition. End-stage heart failure can cause cardiac cachexia, a severe form of undernutrition; mortality rate is particularly high. Wasting disorders can decrease appetite or impair metabolism of nutrients. Disorders that affect GI function can interfere with digestion (eg, pancreatic insufficiency), absorption (eg, enteritis, enteropathy), or lymphatic transport of nutrients (eg, retroperitoneal fibrosis, Milroy's disease).

Pathophysiology

The initial metabolic response is decreased metabolic rate. To supply energy, the body first breaks down adipose tissue. However, later, visceral organs and muscle also are broken down and decrease in weight. Loss of organ weight is greatest in the liver and intestine, intermediate in the heart and kidneys, and least in the nervous system.

Symptoms and Signs

Symptoms of moderate PEM can be constitutional or involve specific organ systems. Apathy and irritability are common. The patient is weak, and work capacity decreases. Cognition and sometimes consciousness are impaired. Temporary lactose deficiency and achlorhydria develop. Diarrhea is common and can be aggravated by deficiency of intestinal disaccharidases, especially lactase (see p. 143). Gonadal tissues atrophy. PEM can cause amenorrhea in women and loss of libido in men and women.

Wasting of fat and muscle is common in all forms of PEM. In adult volunteers who fasted for 30 to 40 days, weight loss was marked (25% of initial weight). If starvation is more prolonged, weight loss may reach 50% in adults and possibly more in children.

Wasting (called cachexia in adults) is most obvious in areas where prominent fat depots normally exist. Muscles shrink and bones protrude. The skin becomes thin, dry, inelastic, pale, and cold. The hair is dry and falls out easily, becoming sparse. Wound healing is impaired. In elderly patients, risk of hip fractures and decubitus ulcers increases.

With acute or chronic severe PEM, heart size and cardiac output decrease; pulse slows and blood pressure falls. Respiratory rate and vital capacity decrease. Body temperature falls, sometimes contributing to death. Edema, anemia, jaundice, and petechiae can develop. Liver, kidney, or heart failure may occur.

Cell-mediated immunity is impaired, increasing susceptibility to infections. Bacterial infections (eg, pneumonia, gastroenteritis, otitis media, UTIs, sepsis) are common in all forms of PEM. Infections result in release of cytokines, which produce anorexia, worsen muscle wasting, and cause a marked decrease in serum albumin levels.

Marasmus in infants causes hunger, weight loss, growth retardation, and wasting of subcutaneous fat and muscle. Ribs and facial bones appear prominent. Loose, thin skin hangs in folds.

Kwashiorkor is characterized by peripheral edema. The abdomen protrudes, but there is no ascites. The skin is dry, thin, and wrinkled; it can become hyperpigmented and fissured and later hypopigmented, friable, and atrophic. Skin in different areas of the body may be affected at different times. The hair can become thin, reddish brown, or gray. Scalp hair falls out easily, eventually becoming sparse, but eyelash hair may grow excessively. Alternating episodes of undernutrition and adequate nutrition may cause the hair to have a dramatic "striped flag" appearance. Affected children may be apathetic but become irritable when held.

Total starvation is fatal in 8 to 12 wk. Thus, certain symptoms of PEM do not have time to develop.

Diagnosis

Diagnosis can be based on history when dietary intake is markedly inadequate. The cause of inadequate intake, particularly in children, needs to be identified. In children and adolescents, child abuse and anorexia nervosa should be considered.

Physical examination findings can usually confirm the diagnosis. Laboratory tests are required to identify causes of secondary PEM. Measurement of plasma albumin, total lymphocyte count, $CD4^{+}$ T lymphocytes, and response to skin antigens may help determine the severity of PEM (see TABLE 2–3) or confirm the diagnosis in borderline cases. Measurement of C-reactive protein or soluble interleukin-2 receptor should be measured when the cause of undernutrition is unclear; these measurements can help determine whether there is cytokine excess. Many other test results may be abnormal: eg, decreased levels of hormones, vitamins, lipids, cholesterol, prealbumin, insulin growth factor-1, fibronectin, and retinol-binding protein. Urinary creatine and methylhistidine levels can be used to gauge the degree of muscle wasting. Because protein catabolism slows, urinary urea level also decreases. These findings rarely affect treatment.

Other laboratory tests can detect associated abnormalities that may require treatment. Serum electrolytes, BUN, glucose, and possibly levels of Ca, Mg, phosphate, and Na should be measured. Levels of blood glucose and electrolytes (especially K, phosphate, Ca, and Mg and occasionally Na) are usually low. BUN is often low unless renal failure is present. Metabolic acidosis may be present. CBC is usually obtained; normocytic anemia (usually due to protein deficiency) or microcytic anemia (due to simultaneous iron deficiency) is usually present.

Stool cultures should be obtained and checked for ova and parasites if diarrhea is severe or does not resolve with treatment. Sometimes urinalysis, urine culture, blood cultures, tuberculin testing, and a chest x-ray are used to diagnose occult infections because people with PEM may have a muted response to infections.

Prevention and Treatment

Worldwide, the most important preventive strategy is to reduce poverty and improve nutritional education and public health measures.

Mild or moderate PEM, including brief starvation, can be treated by providing a balanced diet, preferably orally. Liquid oral food supplements (usually lactose-free) can be used when solid food cannot be adequately ingested. Diarrhea often complicates oral feeding because starvation makes the GI tract more likely to move bacteria into Peyer's patches, facilitating infectious diarrhea. If diarrhea persists (suggesting lactose intolerance), yogurt-based rather than milk-based formulas are given because people with lactose intolerance can tolerate yogurt. Patients should also be given a multivitamin supplement.

Severe PEM or prolonged starvation requires treatment in a hospital with a controlled diet. The first priority is to correct fluid and electrolyte abnormalities (see Ch. 156 on p. 1233) and treat infections. Next is to supply macronutrients orally or, if necessary, through a feeding tube, a nasogastric tube (usually), or a gastronomy (G) tube. Parenteral nutrition is indicated if malabsorption is severe (see p. 23).

Other treatments may be needed to correct specific deficiencies, which may become evident as weight increases. To avoid deficiencies, patients should continue to take micronutrients at about twice the recommended daily allowance (RDA) until recovery is complete.

In children: Underlying disorders should be treated. For children with diarrhea, feeding may be delayed for 24 to 48 h to avoid making the diarrhea worse. Feedings are

TABLE 2–3. VALUES COMMONLY USED TO GRADE THE SEVERITY OF PROTEIN-ENERGY MALNUTRITION

MEASUREMENT	NORMAL	MILD MALNUTRITION	MODERATE MALNUTRITION	SEVERE MALNUTRITION
Normal weight (%)	90–110	85–90	75–85	< 75
Body mass index	19–24*	18–18.9	16–17.9	< 16
Serum albumin (g/dL)	3.5–5.0	3.1–3.4	2.4–3.0	< 2.4
Serum transferrin (mg/dL)	220–400	201–219	150–200	< 150
Total lymphocyte count (per mm^3)	2000–3500	1501–1999	800–1500	< 800
Delayed hypersensitivity index†	2	2	1	0

*In the elderly, BMI < 21 may increase mortality risk.

†Delayed hypersensitivity index quantitates the amount of induration elicited by skin testing using a common antigen, such as those derived from *Candida* sp or *Trichophyton* sp. Induration grade 0 = < 0.5 cm, 1 = 0.5–0.9 cm, 2 = ≥ 1.0 cm.

given often (6 to 12 times/day) but, to avoid overwhelming the limited intestinal absorptive capacity, are limited to small amounts (< 100 mL). During the first week, milk-based formulas with supplements added are usually given in progressively increasing amounts; after a week, the full amounts of 175 kcal/kg and 4 g of protein/kg can be given. Twice the RDA of micronutrients should be given, using commercial multivitamin supplements. After 4 wk, the formula can be replaced with whole milk plus cod liver oil and solid foods, including eggs, fruit, meats, and yeast.

Energy distribution among macronutrients should be about 16% protein, 50% fat, and 34% carbohydrate. An example is a combination of powdered cow's skimmed milk (110 g), sucrose (100 g), vegetable oil (70 g), and water (900 mL). Many other formulas (eg, whole [full-fat] fresh milk plus corn oil and maltodextrin) can be used. Milk powders used in formulas are diluted with water.

Usually, supplements should be added to formulas: Mg 0.4 mEq/kg/day IM is given for 7 days; B-complex vitamins at twice the RDA are given parenterally for the first 3 days, usually with vitamin A, phosphorus, zinc, manganese, copper, iodine, fluoride, molybdenum, and selenium. Because absorption of oral iron is poor in children with PEM, oral or IM iron supplementation may be necessary. Parents are taught about nutritional requirements.

In adults: Disorders associated with PEM should be treated. For example, if AIDS or cancer results in excess cytokine production, megestrol acetate or medroxyprogesterone may improve food intake. However, because these drugs dramatically decrease testosterone in men (possibly causing muscle loss), testosterone should be replaced. Because these drugs can cause adrenal insufficiency, they should be used only short-term (< 3 mo). In patients with functional limitations, home delivery of meals and feeding assistance are key.

An orexigenic drug, such as the cannabis extract dronabinol, should be given to patients with anorexia when no cause is obvious or to patients at the end of life when anorexia impairs quality of life. Anabolic steroids have positive effects (eg, increase lean body mass, possibly improve function) in patients with cachexia due to renal failure and possibly in elderly patients.

Correction of PEM in adults generally resembles that in children. For most adults, feeding does not need to be delayed; small volumes are given often. A commercial formula for oral feeding can be used. Nutrient supply should be given at a rate of 60 kcal/kg and 1.2 to 2 g of protein/kg. If liquid oral supplements are used with solid food, they should be given at least 1 h before meals so that the amount of food eaten at the meal is not reduced.

Treatment of institutionalized elderly patients with PEM requires multiple interventions, including environmental measures (eg, making the dining area more attractive); feeding assistance; changes in diet (eg, use of food enhancers and caloric supplements between meals); treatment of depression and other underlying disorders; and the use of orexigenics, anabolic steroids, or both. The long-term use of gastrostomy tube feeding is essential for patients with severe dysphagia; its use in patients with dementia is controversial. Increasing evidence supports the avoidance of unpalatable therapeutic diets (eg, low salt, diabetic, low cholesterol) in institutionalized patients because these diets decrease food intake and may cause severe PEM.

Complications of treatment: Treatment of PEM can cause complications (refeeding syndrome), including fluid overload, electrolyte deficits, hyperglycemia, cardiac arrhythmias, and diarrhea. Diarrhea is usually mild and resolves; however, diarrhea in patients with severe PEM occasionally causes severe dehydration or death. Causes of diarrhea (eg, sorbitol used in elixir tube feedings, *Clostridium difficile* if the patient has received an antibiotic) may be correctable. Osmotic diarrhea due to excess calories is rare in adults and should be considered only when other causes have been excluded.

Because PEM can impair cardiac and renal function, hydration can cause intravascular volume overload. Treatment decreases extracellular K and Mg. Depletion of K or Mg may cause arrhythmias. Carbohydrate metabolism that occurs during treatment stimulates insulin release, which drives phosphate into cells. Hypophosphatemia can cause muscle weakness, paresthesias, seizures, coma, and arrhythmias. With parenteral feeding, phosphate levels should be measured regularly.

During treatment, endogenous insulin may become ineffective, leading to hyperglycemia. Dehydration and hyperosmolarity can result. Fatal ventricular arrhythmias can develop, possibly caused by a prolonged QT interval.

Prognosis

In children, mortality varies from 5 to 40%. Mortality rates are lower in children with milder PEM and those given intensive care. Death in the first days of treatment is usually due to electrolyte deficits, sepsis, hypothermia, or heart failure. Impaired consciousness, jaundice, petechiae, hyponatremia, and persistent diarrhea are ominous signs. Resolution of apathy, edema, and anorexia are favorable signs. Recovery is more rapid in kwashiorkor than in marasmus.

Long-term effects of PEM in children are not fully documented. Some children develop chronic malabsorption and pancreatic insufficiency. Very young children may develop mild mental retardation, which may persist until at least school age. Permanent cognitive impairment may occur, depending on the duration, severity, and age at onset of PEM.

In adults, PEM can result in morbidity and mortality (eg, progressive weight loss increases mortality rate by 10% for elderly people in nursing homes). Except when organ failure occurs, treatment is uniformly successful. In elderly patients, PEM increases the risk of morbidity and mortality due to surgery, infections, or another disorder.

CARNITINE DEFICIENCY

Carnitine deficiency results from inadequate intake of or inability to metabolize the amino acid carnitine. It can cause a heterogeneous group of disorders. Muscle metabolism is impaired, causing myopathy, hypoglycemia, or cardiomyopathy. Most often, treatment consists of dietary L-carnitine.

The amino acid carnitine is required for the transport of long-chain fatty acyl coenzyme A (CoA) esters into myocyte mitochondria, where they are oxidized for energy. Carnitine is obtained from foods, particularly animal-based foods, and via endogenous synthesis.

Causes of carnitine deficiency include inadequate intake (eg, due to fad diets, lack of access, or long-term TPN); inability to metabolize carnitine due to enzyme deficiencies (eg, carnitine palmitoyltransferase deficiency, methylmalonicaciduria, propionicacidemia, isovalericacidemia); decreased endogenous synthesis of carnitine due to a severe liver disorder; excess loss of carnitine due to diarrhea, diuresis, or hemodialysis; a hereditary disorder in which carnitine leaks from renal tubules; increased requirements for carnitine in states of ketosis and high demand for fat oxidation; and use of valproate. Deficiency may be generalized (systemic) or may affect mainly muscle (myopathic).

Symptoms and the age at which symptoms appear depend on the cause. Carnitine deficiency may cause muscle necrosis, myoglobinuria, lipid-storage myopathy, hypoglycemia, fatty liver, and hyperammonemia with muscle ache, fatigue, confusion, and cardiomyopathy.

In neonates, carnitine palmitoyltransferase deficiency is diagnosed using mass spectrometry to screen blood. Prenatal diagnosis may be possible using amniotic villous cells. In adults, the definitive diagnosis is based on acylcarnitine levels in serum, urine, and tissues (muscle and liver for systemic deficiency; muscle only for myopathic deficiency).

Carnitine deficiency due to inadequate dietary intake, increased requirements, excess losses, decreased synthesis, and (sometimes) enzyme deficiencies can be treated by giving L-carnitine 25 mg/kg po q 6 h.

ESSENTIAL FATTY ACID DEFICIENCY

Essential fatty acid (EFA) deficiency is rare, occurring most often in infants fed diets deficient in EFAs. Signs include scaly dermatitis, alopecia, thrombocytopenia, and, in children, growth retardation. Diagnosis is clinical. Dietary replenishment of EFAs reverses the deficiency.

The EFAs linoleic and linolenic acid are substrates for the endogenous synthesis of other fatty acids that are needed for many physiologic processes, including maintaining the integrity of skin and cell membranes and synthesizing prostaglandins and leukotrienes. For example, eicosapentaenoic acid and docosahexaenoic acid, synthesized from EFAs, are important components of the brain and retina.

For EFA deficiency to develop, dietary intake must be very low. Even small amounts of EFAs can prevent EFA deficiency. Cow's milk has only about 25% of the linoleic acid in human milk, but when ingested in normal amounts, it has enough linoleic acid to prevent EFA deficiency. Total fat intake of people in many developing countries may be very low, but the fat is often vegetable based, with large amounts of linoleic acid and enough linolenic acid to prevent EFA deficiency.

Babies fed a formula low in linoleic acid, such as a skim-milk formula, can develop EFA deficiency. EFA deficiency used to result from long-term TPN if fat was not included. But now, most TPN solutions include fat emulsions to prevent EFA deficiency. In patients with fat malabsorption or increased metabolic needs (eg, because of surgery, multiple trauma, or burns), laboratory evidence of EFA deficiency may be present without clinical signs.

Dermatitis due to EFA deficiency is generalized and scaly; in infants, it can resemble congenital ichthyosis. The dermatitis increases water loss from the skin.

Diagnosis is usually clinical; however, laboratory assays are now available in large research centers. Treatment consists of dietary EFAs, reversing the deficiency.

3 NUTRITIONAL SUPPORT

Many undernourished patients need nutritional support, which aims to increase lean body mass. Oral feeding can be difficult for some patients with anorexia or with eating or absorption problems. Behavioral measures, including encouraging eating, heating or seasoning foods, providing favorite or strongly flavored foods, encouraging small portions, scheduling around meals, and assisting patients with feeding, are sometimes effective.

If behavioral measures are ineffective, nutritional support—oral, enteral tube, or parenteral nutrition—is indicated. Nutritional support may not be indicated for dying or severely demented patients.

Predicting Nutritional Requirements

Nutritional requirements can be predicted by formulas or measured by indirect calorimetry. Total energy expenditure (TEE) and protein requirements are usually predicted. TEE is commonly predicted based on the patient's weight, activity level, and degree of metabolic stress (metabolic demands); TEE ranges from 25 kcal/kg/day for people who are sedentary and not under stress to about 40 kcal/kg/day for people who are critically ill. TEE equals resting energy expenditure (REE, normally about 70% of TEE), energy dissipated by metabolism of food (10% of TEE), plus energy expended during physical activity (20% of TEE). Undernutrition can decrease REE up to 20%. Conditions that increase metabolic stress, such as critical illness, infection, inflammation, trauma, or surgery, can increase REE but rarely by > 50%.

The Harris-Benedict equation shown at the bottom of this page estimates REE.

TEE can also be estimated by adding about 10% (for sedentary people) to about 40% (for people who are critically ill) to REE.

For healthy people, protein requirements are estimated at 0.8 g/kg/day. However, for patients with metabolic stress or kidney failure and for elderly patients, requirements may be higher (see TABLE 3–1).

Total caloric expenditure can be measured by indirect calorimetry using a metabolic cart (a closed rebreathing system that determines energy expenditure based on total CO_2 production). A metabolic cart requires special expertise and is not always available. Calorimetry can also be used to monitor caloric expenditure.

TABLE 3–1. ESTIMATED ADULT DAILY PROTEIN REQUIREMENT

CONDITION	REQUIREMENT (g/kg of ideal body weight/day)
Normal	0.8
Age > 70 yr	1.0
Kidney failure without dialysis	0.8–1.0
Kidney failure with dialysis	1.2–1.5
Metabolic stress (eg, critical illness, trauma, burns, surgery)	1.0–1.8

Assessing Response to Nutritional Support

There is no gold standard to assess response. Indicators of lean body mass, such as body mass index (BMI), body composition analysis, and body fat distribution, can help (see pp.12 and 58). Nitrogen balance, response to skin antigens, muscle strength measurement, and indirect calorimetry can also be used.

Nitrogen balance, which reflects the balance between protein needs and supplies, is the difference between amount of nitrogen ingested and amount lost. A positive balance (ie, more ingested than lost) implies adequate intake. Precise measurement is impractical, but estimates help assess response to nutritional support. Estimated nitrogen losses consist of urinary nitrogen losses (estimated by measuring urea nitrogen content of an accurately obtained 24-h urine collection) plus stool losses (estimated at 1 g/day if stool is produced; negligible if stool is not produced) plus insensible and other unmeasured losses (estimated at 3 g).

Response to skin antigens, a measure of delayed hypersensitivity, often increases to normal as an undernourished patient responds to nutritional support. However, other factors can affect response to skin antigens.

Muscle strength indirectly reflects increases in lean body mass. It can be measured quantitatively, by hand-grip dynamometry, or electrophysiologically (typically by stimulating the ulnar nerve with an electrode).

Measurement of serum proteins, particularly short-lived proteins such as prealbu-

Men: kcal/day = 66 + (13.7 × wt [kg]) + (5 × height [cm]) – (6.8 × age)

Women: kcal/day = 665 + (9.6 × wt [kg]) + (1.8 × height [cm]) – (4.7 × age)

min, retinol-binding protein, and transferrin, helps assess response (see p. 12).

ENTERAL TUBE NUTRITION

Enteral tube nutrition is indicated for patients who have a functioning GI tract and cannot ingest enough nutrients orally because they require intensive protein and caloric support or they are unable or unwilling to take oral feedings. Enteral nutrition, unlike parenteral nutrition, helps preserve the structure and function of the GI tract; it is also cheaper and probably causes fewer complications.

Specific indications include prolonged anorexia, severe protein-energy malnutrition, coma or depressed sensorium, liver failure, inability to take oral feedings due to head or neck trauma or neurologic disorders, and critical illnesses (eg, burns) causing metabolic stress. Other indications may include preparation of the bowel for surgery in seriously ill or undernourished patients, closure of enterocutaneous fistulas, and small-bowel adaptation after massive intestinal resection or in disorders that may cause malabsorption (eg, Crohn's disease).

Procedure: If tube feeding is needed for ≤ 6 wk, a small-caliber, soft nasogastric or nasoenteric (eg, nasoduodenal) tube made of silicone or polyurethane is usually used. If a nasal injury or deformity makes nasal placement difficult, an orogastric or other oroenteric tube can be placed.

Tube feeding for > 6 wk usually requires a gastrostomy or jejunostomy tube. This tube is usually placed endoscopically, surgically, or radiologically. Choice depends on physician capabilities and patient preference. Jejunostomy tubes are useful for patients with contraindications to gastrostomy (eg, gastrectomy, bowel obstruction proximal to the jejunum). However, they do not pose less risk of tracheobronchial aspiration than gastrostomy tubes, as is often thought. Jejunostomy tubes are easily dislodged and are usually used only for inpatients.

Surgical placement of feeding tubes is particularly helpful if endoscopic and radiologic placement is unavailable, technically impossible, or unsafe (eg, because of overlying bowel). Open or laparoscopic techniques can be used.

Formulas: Liquid formulas commonly used include feeding modules and polymeric or other specialized formulas.

Feeding modules are commercially available products that contain a single nutrient, such as proteins, fats, or carbohydrates. Feeding modules may be used individually to treat a specific deficiency or combined with other formulas to completely satisfy nutritional requirements.

Polymeric formulas (including blenderized food and milk-based or lactose-free commercial formulas) are commercially available and generally provide a complete, balanced diet. They can be used for oral or tube feedings. In hospitalized patients, lactose-free formulas are the most commonly used polymeric formulas. However, milk-based formulas tend to taste better than lactose-free formulas. Patients with lactose intolerance may be able to tolerate milk-based formulas given slowly by continuous infusion.

Hydrolyzed protein or sometimes amino acid formulas are used for patients who have difficulty digesting complex proteins. However, these formulas are expensive and usually unnecessary. Most patients with pancreatic insufficiency, if given enzymes, and most patients with malabsorption can digest complex proteins.

Other specialized formulas (eg, calorie and protein-dense formulas for patients whose fluids are restricted; fiber-enriched formulas for constipated patients) may be helpful.

Administration: Patients should be sitting upright at 30 to 45° during tube feeding and for 2 h afterward. Tube feedings are given in boluses several times a day or by continuous infusion. Bolus feeding is indicated for patients who cannot sit upright continuously. Continuous infusion is necessary if boluses produce nausea; this method may reduce the incidence of diarrhea and aspiration.

For bolus feeding, total daily volume is divided into 4 to 6 separate feedings, which are injected through the tube with a syringe or infused by gravity from an elevated bag. After feedings, the tube is flushed with water to prevent clogging.

Because nasogastric or nasoduodenal tube feeding often causes diarrhea initially, feedings are usually started with small amounts of dilute preparations and increased as tolerated. Most formulas contain

0.5, 1, or 2 kcal/mL. Feeding often begins by giving a 0.5-kcal/mL solution (often obtained by a 50% dilution of a 1-kcal/mL commercially prepared solution) at 50 mL/h. An alternative is a 1-kcal/mL solution at 25 mL/h. Usually, these solutions do not supply enough water, particularly if vomiting, diarrhea, sweating, or fever has increased water loss. Extra water is supplied as boluses via the feeding tube or IV. After a few days, the rate or concentration can be increased to supply 1 kcal/mL at 50 mL/h or more as needed to meet caloric and water needs. Jejunostomy tube feeding requires even greater dilution and smaller volumes. Feeding usually begins at a concentration ≤ 0.5 kcal/mL and a rate of 25 mL/h. After a few days, concentrations and volumes can be increased to eventually meet caloric and water needs. Usually, the maximum that can be tolerated is 0.8 kcal/mL at 125 mL/h for 2400 kcal/day.

Complications: Complications are common and can be serious. Tubes, particularly large tubes, can erode tissues, damaging the nose, pharynx, or esophagus. Sinusitis occasionally develops. Thick feedings or pills can block the lumen, particularly of small tubes. Sometimes blockages can be dissolved by instilling a solution of pancreatic enzymes or other commercial products.

Tubes can become dislodged, particularly jejunostomy tubes. Feeding tube replacement is more difficult and more likely to cause complications if the tube was placed invasively rather than noninvasively.

Nasogastric tubes can be misplaced intracranially if the cribriform plate is disrupted by severe facial trauma. Nasogastric or orogastric tubes can be misplaced into the tracheobronchial tree, causing coughing and gagging in responsive patients. Tracheobronchial misplacement may produce few symptoms in obtunded patients. If tracheobronchial misplacement is not recognized, feedings enter the lung, causing pneumonia. A dislodged gastrostomy or jejunostomy tube may be replaced into the peritoneal cavity; intraperitoneal feedings cause peritonitis.

In up to 20% of patients and 50% of critically ill patients, diarrhea and GI discomfort develop because the intestine cannot tolerate one of the formula's main nutrient components, particularly with bolus feeding. Sorbitol, often contained in liquid drug preparations given through feeding tubes, can exacerbate diarrhea. Nausea, vomiting, abdominal pain, and occasionally mesenteric ischemia may also develop.

Aspiration may occur, even though tubes are placed correctly, because of refluxed tube feedings or oropharyngeal secretions unrelated to feedings. Aspiration can usually be avoided by keeping the upper body elevated.

Electrolyte disturbances, hyperglycemia, volume overload, and hyperosmolarity can develop. Frequently monitoring weight and blood electrolytes, glucose, Mg, and phosphate (daily during the first week) is recommended.

TOTAL PARENTERAL NUTRITION

Parenteral nutrition is by definition given IV. Partial parenteral nutrition supplies only part of daily nutritional requirements, supplementing oral intake. Many hospitalized patients receive dextrose or amino acid solutions by this method. Total parenteral nutrition (TPN) supplies all daily nutritional requirements. TPN can be used in the hospital or at home. Because TPN solutions are concentrated and can cause thrombosis of peripheral veins, a central venous catheter is usually required.

Indications: TPN is indicated for patients whose GI tract is not functional. A general but untested indication is anticipation of undernutrition (< 50% of metabolic needs met) for > 7 days. TPN is given before and after treatment to severely undernourished patients who cannot ingest large volumes of oral feedings and are being prepared for surgery, radiation therapy, or chemotherapy. TPN may reduce morbidity and mortality after major surgery, severe burns, and head trauma, especially in patients with sepsis. Patients with disorders requiring complete bowel rest (eg, some stages of Crohn's disease, ulcerative colitis, severe pancreatitis) or with pediatric GI disorders (eg, congenital anomalies; prolonged diarrhea, regardless of its cause) often respond well to TPN.

Nutritional content: TPN requires water (30 to 40 mL/kg/day), energy (30 to 60 kcal/kg/day, depending on energy expenditure), amino acids (1 to 2.0 g/kg/day, depending on the degree of catabolism), essential fatty acids, vitamins, and minerals (see TABLE 3–2). Children who need TPN may have different fluid requirements and need

TABLE 3–2. BASIC ADULT DAILY REQUIREMENTS FOR TOTAL PARENTERAL NUTRITION

NUTRIENT	AMOUNT
Water (/kg body wt/day)	30–40 mL
Energy*	
Medical patient	30 kcal
Postoperative patient	30–45 kcal
Hypercatabolic patient	45–60 kcal
Amino acids (/kg body wt/day)	
Medical patient	1.0 g
Postoperative patient	2.0 g
Hypercatabolic patient	3.0 g
Minerals	
Acetate/gluconate	90 mEq
Calcium	15 mEq
Chloride	130 mEq
Chromium	15 µg
Copper	1.5 mg
Iodine	120 µg
Magnesium	20 mEq
Manganese	2 mg
Phosphorus	300 mg
Potassium	100 mEq
Selenium	100 µg
Sodium	100 mEq
Zinc	5 mg
Vitamins	
Ascorbic acid	100 mg
Biotin	60 µg
Cobalamin	5 µg
Folic acid	400 µg
Niacin	40 mg
Pantothenic acid	15 mg
Pyridoxine	4 mg
Riboflavin	3.6 mg
Thiamin	3 mg
Vitamin A	4000 IU
Vitamin D	400 IU
Vitamin E	15 mg
Vitamin K	200 µg

*Requirements for energy increase by 12% per 1° C of fever.

more energy (120 kcal/kg/day) and amino acids (2.5 to 3.5 g/kg/day).

Basic TPN solutions are prepared using sterile techniques, usually in liter batches according to standard formulas. Normally, 2 L/day of the standard solution is needed. Solutions may be modified based on laboratory results, underlying disorders, hypermetabolism, or other factors. Commercially available lipid emulsions are often added to supply essential fatty acids and triglycerides; 20 to 30% of total calories is usually supplied as lipids. However, withholding lipids and their calories may help obese patients mobilize endogenous fat stores, increasing their insulin sensitivity.

Solutions: Many solutions are commonly used. Electrolytes can be added to meet the patient's needs.

Patients who have renal insufficiency and are not receiving dialysis or who have liver failure require solutions with reduced protein content and a high percentage of essential amino acids. For patients with heart or kidney failure, volume (liquid) intake must be limited. For patients with respiratory failure, a lipid emulsion must provide most of nonprotein calories to minimize CO_2 production by carbohydrate metabolism. Neonates require lower dextrose concentrations (17 to 18%).

Beginning TPN administration: Because the central venous catheter needs to remain in place for a long time, strict sterile techniques must be used during insertion and maintenance. The TPN line should not be used for any other purpose. External tubing should be changed q 24 h with the first bag of the day. In-line filters are controversial and may not help. Dressings should be kept sterile and are usually changed q 48 h using strict sterile techniques. For TPN given outside the hospital, patients must be taught to recognize symptoms of infection, and qualified home nursing must be arranged.

The solution is started slowly at 50% of the calculated requirements, using 5% dextrose to make up the balance of fluid. Energy and nitrogen should be given simultaneously. The amount of regular insulin given (added directly to the TPN solution) depends on the blood glucose level; if the level is normal and the final solution contains the usual 25% dextrose concentration, the usual starting dose is 5 to 10 units of regular insulin/L of TPN fluid.

Monitoring: Progress should be followed on a flowchart. An interdisciplinary nutrition team, if available, should monitor the patient. Weight, CBC, electrolytes, and BUN should be monitored often (eg, daily for inpatients). Blood glucose should be monitored q 6 h until stable. Fluid intake and output should be monitored continuously. When the patient becomes stable, blood tests can be done much less often.

Liver function tests should be done. Plasma proteins (eg, serum albumin, possibly transthyretin or retinol-binding protein);

prothrombin time; plasma and urine osmolality; and Ca, Mg, and phosphate (not during glucose infusion) should be measured twice/wk. Full nutritional assessment (including BMI calculation and anthropometric measurements—see pp. 12 and 58) should be repeated at 2-wk intervals.

Complications: With close monitoring by a nutrition team, the complication rate may be < 5%. Complications may be related to the central venous catheter (see TABLE 63–5 on p. 519) or to the provision of nutrition.

Glucose abnormalities are common. Hyperglycemia can be avoided by monitoring blood glucose often, adjusting the insulin dose in the TPN solution, and giving subcutaneous insulin as needed. Hypoglycemia can be precipitated by suddenly discontinuing constant concentrated dextrose infusions. Treatment, depending on the degree of hypoglycemia, may consist of 50% dextrose IV or infusion of 5 or 10% dextrose for 24 h before resuming TPN via the central venous catheter.

Abnormalities of serum electrolytes and minerals should be corrected by modifying subsequent infusions or, if correction is urgently required, by beginning appropriate peripheral vein infusions. Vitamin and mineral deficiencies are rare if solutions are given correctly. Elevated BUN may reflect dehydration, which can be corrected by giving free water as 5% dextrose via a peripheral vein.

Volume overload (suggested by > 1 kg/day weight gain) may occur when high daily energy requirements require large fluid volumes.

Metabolic bone disease, or bone demineralization (osteoporosis or osteomalacia), develops in some patients receiving TPN for > 3 mo. The mechanism is unknown. Advanced disease can cause severe periarticular, lower extremity, and back pain. Temporarily or permanently discontinuing TPN is the only known treatment.

Adverse reactions to lipid emulsions (eg, dyspnea, cutaneous allergic reactions, nausea, headache, back pain, sweating, dizziness) are uncommon but may occur early, particularly if lipids are given at > 1.0 kcal/kg/h. Temporary hyperlipidemia may occur, particularly in patients with kidney or liver failure; treatment is usually not required. Delayed adverse reactions to lipid emulsions include hepatomegaly, mild elevation of liver enzymes, splenomegaly, thrombocytopenia, leukopenia, and, especially in premature infants with respiratory distress syndrome, pulmonary function abnormalities. Temporarily or permanently slowing or stopping lipid emulsion infusion may prevent or minimize these adverse reactions.

Hepatic complications include liver dysfunction, painful hepatomegaly, and hyperammonemia. They can develop at any age but are most common among infants, particularly premature ones (whose livers are immature). Transient liver dysfunction, evidenced by increased transaminases, bilirubin, and alkaline phosphatase, is common with the initiation of TPN. Delayed or persistent elevations may result from excess quantities of amino acids. Pathogenesis is unknown. Contributing factors probably include cholestasis and inflammation. Progressive fibrosis occasionally develops. Reducing protein delivery may help. Painful hepatomegaly suggests fat accumulation; carbohydrate delivery should be reduced. Hyperammonemia can develop in infants. Signs include lethargy, twitching, and generalized seizures. Correction consists of arginine supplementation at 0.5 to 1.0 mmol/kg/day. For infants who develop any hepatic complication, limiting amino acids to 1.0 g/kg/day may be necessary.

Gallbladder complications include cholelithiasis, gallbladder sludge, and cholecystitis. These complications can be caused or worsened by prolonged gallbladder stasis. Stimulating contraction by providing about 20 to 30% of calories as fat and stopping glucose infusion several hours a day is helpful. Oral or enteral intake also helps. Treatment with metronidazole, ursodeoxycholic acid, phenobarbital, or cholecystokinin helps some patients with cholestasis.

NUTRITIONAL SUPPORT FOR DYING OR SEVERELY DEMENTED PATIENTS

Anorexia or loss of appetite is common among dying patients. Behavioral measures (eg, using flexible feeding schedules, feeding slowly, giving small portions or favorite or strongly flavored foods) can often increase oral intake. A small amount of a favorite alcoholic drink, given 30 min before meals, may also help. Certain antidepressants, megestrol acetate, and dronabinol may stimulate appetite. Metoclopramide enhances gastric emptying, which can increase appetite, but it may take 1 to 2 wk to reach peak effectiveness.

Advanced dementia eventually leads to inability to eat; sometimes affected patients are given tube feedings. However, there is no convincing evidence that tube feedings prolong life, provide comfort, improve function, or prevent complications (eg, aspiration, pressure sores).

Tube feedings and parenteral nutrition cause discomfort and are usually not indicated for patients who are dying or too demented to eat. Forgoing nutritional support may be difficult for family members to accept, but they should understand that patients are usually more comfortable eating and drinking as they choose. Sips of water and easy-to-swallow foods may be useful. Supportive care, including good oral hygiene (eg, brushing the teeth, moistening the oral cavity with swabs and ice chips as needed, applying lip salve), can physically and psychologically comfort the patient and the family members who provide the care. Counseling may help family members who are dealing with anxieties over the decision about whether to use invasive nutritional support.

4 VITAMIN DEFICIENCY, DEPENDENCY, AND TOXICITY

In developed countries, vitamin deficiencies result mainly from poverty, food faddism, drugs (see p. 8 and TABLE 4–1), alcoholism, or prolonged and inadequately supplemented parenteral feeding. Vitamin dependency results from a genetic defect involving metabolism of a vitamin. In some cases, vitamin doses as high as 1000 times the daily recommended intake (DRI) improve function of the altered metabolic pathway. Vitamin toxicity (hypervitaminosis) usually results from taking megadoses of vitamin A, D, C, B_6, or niacin.

Foods alone may provide suboptimal amounts of some vitamins. In these cases, the risk of certain cancers or other disorders may be increased. Because of this risk, routine daily multivitamin supplements are sometimes recommended.

Dietary requirements, sources, functions, effects of deficiencies and toxicities, blood levels, and usual therapeutic dosages for vitamins are listed in TABLES 4–2 and 4–3. Vitamins may be fat soluble (vitamins A, D, E, and K) or water soluble (B vitamins and vitamin C). The B vitamins include biotin, folate, niacin, pantothenic acid, riboflavin, thiamin, pyridoxine, and B_{12}.

BIOTIN

Biotin acts as a coenzyme for carboxylation reactions essential to fat and carbohy-

TABLE 4–1. POTENTIAL VITAMIN-DRUG INTERACTIONS

NUTRIENT	DRUG
Folate	Alcohol, 5-fluorouracil, metformin, methotrexate, phenobarbital, phenytoin, primidone, sulfasalazine, triamterene, trimethoprim
Niacin	Aspirin
Riboflavin	Phenothiazines
Thiamin	Thiamin antagonists in coffee, tea, raw fish, and red cabbage; alcohol
Vitamin A	Cholestyramine, mineral oil
Vitamin B_6	Cycloserine, hydralazine, isoniazid, levodopa, penicillamine
Vitamin B_{12}	Antacids, metformin, nitrous oxide
Vitamin D	Cholestyramine, corticosteroids, mineral oil, phenytoin, primidone
Vitamin E	Warfarin
Vitamin K	Antibiotics

TABLE 4–2. RECOMMENDED DAILY INTAKES FOR VITAMINS*

CATEGORY	AGE (yr)	FOLATE (µg)	RIBOFLAVIN (mg)	THIAMIN (mg)	VITAMIN A (µg)	VITAMIN B_6 (mg)	VITAMIN B_{12} (µg)	VITAMIN C (mg)	VITAMIN D (IU)†	VITAMIN E (mg)	VITAMIN K (µg)
Infants	0–6 mo	**65**	**0.3**	**0.2**	**400**	**0.1**	**0.4**	**40**	**200**	**4**	**2.0**
	7–12 mo	**80**	**0.4**	**0.3**	**500**	**0.3**	**0.5**	**50**	**200**	**5**	**2.5**
Children	1–3 yr	150	0.5	0.5	300	0.5	0.9	15	**200**	6	**30**
	4–8	200	0.6	0.6	400	0.6	1.2	25	**200**	7	**55**
Males	9–13	300	0.9	0.9	600	1.0	1.8	45	**200**	11	**60**
	14–18	400	1.3	1.2	900	1.3	2.4	75	**200**	15	**75**
	19–50	400	1.3	1.2	900	1.3	2.4	90	**200**	15	**120**
	>51	400	1.3	1.2	900	1.7	2.4	90	**400‡**	15	**120**
Females	9–13	300	0.9	0.9	600	1.0	1.8	45	**200**	11	**60**
	14–18	400	1.0	1.0	700	1.2	2.4	65	**200**	15	**75**
	19–50	400	1.1	1.1	700	1.3	2.4	75	**200**	15	**90**
	>51	400	1.1	1.1	700	1.5	2.4	75	**400‡**	15	**90**
Pregnant (19–50 yr)		600	1.4	1.4	770	1.9	2.6	85	**200**	15	**90**
Lactating (19–50 yr)		500	1.6	1.4	1200	2.0	2.8	120	**200**	19	**90**
Upper limit (UL)		1000	ND	ND	3000	100	ND	2000	2000	1000	ND

*This table lists recommended dietary allowances (RDAs) in regular type and adequate intakes (AIs) in bold type. RDAs are set to meet the needs of 97 to 98% of healthy people. When data to calculate the RDA for a nutrient are insufficient, AI is estimated as accurately as possible. UL is the largest amount of a nutrient that most adults can ingest daily without risk of adverse effects. The more the UL is exceeded, the greater risk of adverse effects.

†200 IU of vitamin D = 5 µg.

‡600 IU of vitamin D is recommended for people > 70 yr.

ND = Not determinable because of lack of data; sources of intake should be limited to foods.

Adapted from Dietary Reference Intakes, Standing Committee on the Scientific Evaluation of Dietary Reference Intakes, Food and Nutrition Board, Institute of Medicine. Washington, DC: National Academy Press.

drate metabolism. Adequate intake for adults is 30 µg/day.

Deficiency and dependency: Anticonvulsants can increase the metabolic demand for biotin but probably do not cause deficiency. Rarely, isolated biotin deficiency occurs when total parenteral nutrition (TPN) solutions are not supplemented with biotin. Very rarely, prolonged consumption of large amounts of raw egg whites (which contain avidin, a biotin antagonist) causes deficiency, resulting in seborrheic dermatitis and glossitis; these symptoms respond rapidly to 150 to 300 µg biotin po daily. People taking anticonvulsants may benefit from daily supplementation with the DRI (30 µg).

Impaired metabolism (dependency) results from mutations in holocarboxylase synthetase (the enzyme required to link biotin to four carboxylases necessary for metabolism) or in biotinidase (the enzyme required to remove biotin from the same four carboxylases for catabolism). Retarded physical and mental development, a facial rash similar to cutaneous candidiasis and zinc deficiency (with seborrheic and eczematous components), seizures, alopecia, keratoconjunctivitis, and defects in immunity have

TABLE 4–3. SOURCES, FUNCTIONS, AND EFFECTS OF VITAMINS

NUTRIENT	PRINCIPAL SOURCES	FUNCTIONS	EFFECTS OF DEFICIENCY AND TOXICITY
Biotin	Liver, kidney, egg yolks, yeast, cauliflower, nuts, legumes	Carboxylation reactions	**Deficiency:** Dermatitis, glossitis, metabolic acidosis
Folate (folic acid)	Fresh green, leafy vegetables; fruits; organ meats (eg, liver); enriched cereals and breads	Maturation of RBCs; synthesis of purines, pyrimidines, and methionine; development of fetal nervous system	**Deficiency:** Megaloblastic anemia, neural tube birth defects
Niacin (nicotinic acid, niacinamide)	Liver, red meat, fish, poultry, milk, legumes, whole-grain or enriched cereals and breads	Oxidation-reduction reactions, carbohydrate and cell metabolism	**Deficiency:** Pellagra (dermatitis, glossitis, GI and CNS dysfunction) **Toxicity:** Flushing
Riboflavin (vitamin B_2)	Milk, cheese, liver, meat, eggs, enriched cereal products	Many aspects of carbohydrate and protein metabolism, integrity of mucous membranes	**Deficiency:** Cheilosis, angular stomatitis, corneal vascularization
Thiamin (vitamin B_1)	Whole grains, meat (especially pork and liver), enriched cereal products, nuts, legumes, potatoes	Carbohydrate, fat, amino acid, glucose, and alcohol metabolism; central and peripheral nerve cell function; myocardial function	**Deficiency:** Beriberi (peripheral neuropathy, heart failure), Wernicke-Korsakoff syndrome
Vitamin A (retinol)	As preformed vitamin: fish liver oils, liver, egg yolks, butter, vitamin A–fortified dairy products As provitamin carotenoids: dark green leafy and yellow vegetables, carrots, yellow fruits	Formation of rhodopsin (a photoreceptor pigment in the retina), integrity of epithelia, lysosome stability, glycoprotein synthesis	**Deficiency:** Night blindness, perifollicular hyperkeratosis, xerophthalmia, keratomalacia, increased morbidity and mortality in young children **Toxicity:** Headache, peeling of skin, hepatosplenomegaly, bone thickening
Vitamin B_6 group (pyridoxine, pyridoxal, pyridoxamine)	Organ meats (eg, liver) whole-grain cereals, fish, legumes	Many aspects of nitrogen metabolism (eg, transaminations, porphyrin and heme synthesis, tryptophan conversion to niacin); nucleic acid biosynthesis; linoleic acid, lipid, carbohydrate, and amino acid metabolism	**Deficiency:** Seizures, anemias, neuropathies, seborrheic dermatitis **Toxicity:** Peripheral neuropathy

TABLE 4–3. SOURCES, FUNCTIONS, AND EFFECTS OF VITAMINS—Continued

NUTRIENT	PRINCIPAL SOURCES	FUNCTIONS	EFFECTS OF DEFICIENCY AND TOXICITY
Vitamin B_{12} (cobalamins)	Meats (especially beef, pork, and organ meats [eg, liver]), fish, poultry, eggs, fortified cereals, milk and milk products	Maturation of RBCs, neural function, DNA synthesis, methionine synthesis, methyl transfer, myelin synthesis and repair	**Deficiency:** Megaloblastic anemia, neurologic deficits (confusion, paresthesias, ataxia)
Vitamin C (ascorbic acid)	Citrus fruits, tomatoes, potatoes, broccoli, strawberries, sweet peppers	Collagen formation; bone and blood vessel health; carnitine, hormone, and amino acid formation; wound healing	**Deficiency:** Scurvy (hemorrhages, loose teeth, gingivitis, bone defects)
Vitamin D (cholecalciferol, ergocalciferol)	Ultraviolet irradiation of the skin (main source); fortified milk (main dietary source), fish liver oils, butter, egg yolks, liver	Ca and P absorption; resorption, mineralization, and maturation of bone; tubular reabsorption of Ca; chemical messengers in many organs	**Deficiency:** Rickets (sometimes with tetany), osteomalacia **Toxicity:** Anorexia, renal failure, metastatic calcifications
Vitamin E group (α-tocopherol, other tocopherols)	Vegetable and wheat germ oils, nuts	Intracellular antioxidant, scavenger of free radicals in biologic membranes	**Deficiency:** RBC hemolysis, neurologic deficits, creatinuria **Toxicity:** Tendency to bleed; increased risk of premature death
Vitamin K group (phyloquinone, menaquinones)	Green, leafy vegetables (especially collards, spinach, and salad greens); pork; liver; soy beans; vegetable oils; bacteria in the GI tract after neonatal period	Formation of prothrombin, other coagulation factors, and bone proteins	**Deficiency:** Bleeding due to deficiency of prothrombin and other factors, osteopenia

been reported in children with dependency. No assays of biotin status are readily available. Children with biotinidase deficiency respond well to biotin 50 to 150 μg po once/day. Other biotin-responsive inborn errors of metabolism may require up to 200 mg po or 20 mg IV once/day.

FOLATE

Folate (folic acid) is now added to enriched grain foods in the US. Folate is also plentiful in various plant foods and meats, but its bioavailability is greater when it is in supplements or enriched foods than when it occurs naturally in food.

Folates are involved in RBC maturation and synthesis of purines and pyrimidines. They are required for development of the fetal nervous system. Absorption occurs in the duodenum and upper jejunum. Enterohepatic circulation of folate occurs. Whether folate supplementation protects against coronary artery disease (by lowering homocysteine levels) or various cancers is unclear. The upper limit for folate is 1000 μg. Folate is essentially nontoxic.

FOLATE DEFICIENCY

Deficiency is common; it may result from inadequate intake, malabsorption, and use of various drugs. Deficiency produces megaloblastic anemia (indistinguishable from that

TABLE 4–4. CAUSES OF FOLATE DEFICIENCY

CAUSE	SOURCE
Inadequate intake	Diet lacking fresh, green vegetables or enriched grains; chronic alcoholism; TPN
Impaired absorption	Celiac disease, sprue, other malabsorption syndromes, drugs (phenytoin, primidone, barbiturates), congenital or acquired folate malabsorption
Inadequate utilization	Folate antagonists (methotrexate, triamterene, trimethoprim), anticonvulsants, congenital or acquired enzyme deficiency, alcoholism
Increased demand	Pregnancy, lactation, infancy, increased metabolism
Increased excretion	Renal dialysis (peritoneal or hemodialysis)

due to vitamin B_{12} deficiency). Maternal deficiency increases the risk of neural tube birth defects. Diagnosis usually requires laboratory testing to confirm. Measurement of neutrophil hypersegmentation is sensitive and readily available. If available, other tests can provide greater accuracy. Treatment with oral folate is usually successful.

Etiology and Pathophysiology

The most common causes are inadequate intake (usually associated with undernutrition or alcoholism), increased demand (eg, due to pregnancy or lactation), and impaired absorption (eg, in tropical sprue or due to certain drugs). Deficiency can also result from inadequate bioavailability and increased excretion (see TABLE 4–4).

Prolonged cooking destroys folate, predisposing to inadequate intake. Liver stores provide only a 3- to 6-mo supply. Intake of folate is often barely adequate (eg, in alcoholism).

Alcohol interferes with folate absorption, metabolism, renal excretion, and enterohepatic reabsorption. 5-Flurouracil, metformin, methotrexate, phenytoin, phenobarbital, sulfasalazine, and trimethoprim impair folate metabolism.

Symptoms and Signs

Folate deficiency may cause glossitis, diarrhea, depression, and weight loss. Anemia may develop insidiously and, because of compensatory mechanisms, be more severe than symptoms suggest.

Folate deficiency during pregnancy increases the risk of fetal neural tube defects and perhaps other brain defects (see p. 2441).

Diagnosis

Tests include CBC and measurement of plasma vitamin B_{12} and folate levels. CBC may indicate megaloblastic anemia indistinguishable from that of vitamin B_{12} deficiency. If serum folate is < 3 μg/L (< 7 nmol/L), deficiency is likely. Serum folate reflects folate status unless intake has recently increased or decreased. If intake has changed, erythrocyte (RBC) folate level better reflects tissue stores. A level of < 140 μg/L (< 305 nmol/L) indicates inadequate status. Also, an increase in the homocysteine level suggests tissue folate deficiency (but the level is also affected by vitamin B_{12} and vitamin B_6 levels, renal insufficiency, and genetic factors). A normal methylmalonic acid level may differentiate folate deficiency from vitamin B_{12} deficiency.

Treatment

Folate 400 to 1000 μg po once/day replenishes tissues and is usually successful even if deficiency has resulted from malabsorption. The normal requirement is 400 μg/day. (CAUTION: *In megaloblastic anemia, vitamin B_{12} deficiency must be ruled out before treating with folate, which, if vitamin B_{12} deficiency is present, can alleviate the anemia but does not arrest or reverse neurologic deficits.*) For pregnant women, the recommended daily allowance (RDA) is 600 μg/day. For women who have had a fetus or infant with a neural tube defect, the recommended dose is 1000 to 5000 μg/day.

NIACIN

Niacin (nicotinic acid) derivatives include nicotinamide adenine dinucleotide (NAD, coenzyme I) and nicotinamide adenine dinucleotide phosphate (NADP, coenzyme II), which are coenzymes in oxidation-reduction reactions. They are vital in cell metabolism. Because dietary tryptophan can be metabolized to niacin, foods rich in tryptophan (eg, dairy products) can compensate for inadequate dietary niacin.

Niacin Deficiency

Dietary niacin deficiency (causing pellagra) is uncommon in developed countries. Clinical manifestations include the "three Ds": diffuse, pigmented rash (dermatitis); gastroenteritis (diarrhea); and widespread neurologic deficits, including cognitive decline (dementia). However, constipation is more common than diarrhea. Diagnosis is usually clinical, and dietary supplementation is usually successful.

Etiology

Primary deficiency results from extremely inadequate intake of both niacin and tryptophan, which usually occurs in areas where maize (Indian corn) constitutes a substantial part of the diet. Bound niacin, found in maize, is not assimilated in the GI tract unless it has been previously treated with alkali, as when tortillas are prepared. Corn protein is also deficient in tryptophan. The high incidence of pellagra in India among people who eat millet with a high leucine content has led to the hypothesis that amino acid imbalance may contribute to deficiency. Deficiencies of protein and several B vitamins commonly accompany primary niacin deficiency.

Secondary deficiency may be due to diarrhea, cirrhosis, or alcoholism. Pellagra also may occur during prolonged isoniazid therapy, in carcinoid syndrome (tryptophan is diverted to form 5-hydroxytryptophan), and in Hartnup disease.

Symptoms and Signs

Pellagra is characterized by skin, mucous membrane, CNS, and GI symptoms. Advanced pellagra can cause a symmetric photosensitive rash, stomatitis, glossitis, diarrhea, and mental aberrations. Symptoms may appear alone or in combination.

Skin symptoms include several types of lesions, which are usually bilaterally symmetric. The distribution of lesions—at pressure points or sun-exposed skin—is more pathognomonic than the form of the lesions. Lesions can develop in a glovelike distribution on the hands (pellagrous glove) or in a boot-shaped distribution on the feet and legs (pellagrous boot). Sunlight causes Casal's necklace and butterfly-shaped lesions on the face.

Mucous membrane symptoms affect primarily the mouth but may also affect the vagina and urethra. Glossitis and stomatitis characterize acute deficiency. As the deficiency progresses, the tongue and oral mucous membranes become bright scarlet (called scarlet glossitis), followed by pain in the mouth, increased salivation, and edema of the tongue. Ulcerations may appear, especially under the tongue, on the mucosa of the lower lip, and opposite the molar teeth.

GI symptoms early in the deficiency include burning in the pharynx and esophagus and abdominal discomfort and distention. Constipation is common. Later, nausea, vomiting, and diarrhea may occur. Diarrhea is often bloody because of bowel hyperemia and ulceration.

CNS symptoms include psychosis (characterized by memory impairment, disorientation, confusion, and confabulation; the predominant symptom may be excitement, depression, mania, delirium, or paranoia), encephalopathy (characterized by impaired consciousness), and cognitive decline (dementia).

Diagnosis and Treatment

Diagnosis is clinical and may be straightforward when skin and mouth lesions, diarrhea, delirium, and dementia occur simultaneously. More often, the presentation is not so specific. Differentiating the CNS changes from those in thiamin deficiency is difficult. A history of a diet lacking niacin and tryptophan may help establish the diagnosis. A favorable response to treatment with niacin can usually confirm it. If available, laboratory testing can help confirm the diagnosis, particularly when the diagnosis is otherwise unclear. Urinary excretion of N′-methylnicotinamide (NMN) is decreased; < 0.8 mg/day (< 5.8 μmol/day) suggests a niacin deficiency.

Because multiple deficiencies are common, a balanced diet, including other B vitamins (particularly riboflavin and pyridoxine), is needed. Nicotinamide is usually used to treat deficiency, because nicotinamide, unlike nicotinic acid (the most common form of niacin), does not cause flushing, itching, burning, or tingling sensations. Nicotinamide 40 to 250 mg/day po should be given in divided doses (tid to qid). If diarrhea or lack of patient cooperation precludes oral therapy, 100 to 250 mg IM bid or tid should be given.

NIACIN TOXICITY

Niacin (nicotinic acid) in large amounts is sometimes used to lower LDL cholesterol and triglyceride levels and to increase HDL cholesterol levels. Symptoms may include flushing and, rarely, hepatotoxicity.

Immediate- and sustained-release preparations of niacin (but not nicotinamide) may improve lipid levels. Flushing, which is prostaglandin-mediated, is more common with immediate-release preparations. It may be more intense after alcohol ingestion, aerobic activity, sun exposure, and consumption of spicy foods. Flushing is minimized if niacin is taken after meals or if aspirin (325 mg) is taken 30 to 45 min before niacin. The chance of severe flushing can be reduced by starting immediate-release niacin at a low dose (eg, 50 mg tid) and increasing it very slowly. At intermediate doses (1000 mg/day), triglyceride levels decrease 15 to 20%, and HDL cholesterol levels increase 15 to 30%. Reductions in LDL cholesterol are modest (< 10%). Higher doses of niacin (3000 mg/day) reduce LDL cholesterol 15 to 20%. Higher doses may be associated with jaundice, abdominal discomfort, blurred vision, worsening of hyperglycemia, and precipitation of preexisting gout. People with a liver disorder probably should not take high-dose niacin.

Hepatotoxicity, which appears to be more common with sustained-release preparations, appears to be dose-related (eg, > 3 g/day). Some authorities recommend checking levels of uric acid, blood glucose, and plasma transaminases q 6 to 8 wk until the dose of niacin has been stabilized.

PANTOTHENIC ACID

Pantothenic acid is widely distributed in foods; it is an essential component of coenzyme A. Adults probably require about 5 mg/day. A beneficial role for pantothenic acid supplementation in lipid metabolism, RA, or athletic performance remains unproved.

Deficiency: Isolated pantothenic acid deficiency is rare. A diet deficient in pantothenic acid produces malaise, abdominal discomfort, and burning hands and feet with paresthesias; these symptoms respond to pantothenic acid. However, in clinical practice, these nonspecific symptoms rarely respond to the vitamin because they rarely result from pantothenic deficiency.

RIBOFLAVIN

Riboflavin (vitamin B_2) is involved in carbohydrate metabolism as an essential coenzyme in many oxidation-reduction reactions. Riboflavin is essentially nontoxic.

RIBOFLAVIN DEFICIENCY

Riboflavin deficiency usually occurs with other B-vitamin deficiencies. Symptoms and signs include sore throat, lesions of the lips and mucosa of the mouth, glossitis, conjunctivitis, seborrheic dermatitis, and normochromic-normocytic anemia. Diagnosis is usually clinical. Treatment consists of oral or, if needed, IM riboflavin.

Primary riboflavin deficiency results from inadequate intake of fortified cereals, milk, and other animal products. The most common causes of secondary deficiency are chronic diarrhea, liver disorders, hemodialysis, peritoneal dialysis, and chronic alcoholism.

Symptoms and Signs

The most common signs are pallor and maceration of the mucosa at the angles of the mouth (angular stomatitis) and vermilion surfaces of the lips (cheilosis), eventually replaced by superficial linear fissures. The fissures can become infected with *Candida albicans*, causing grayish white lesions (perlèche). The tongue may appear magenta. Seborrheic dermatitis develops, usually affecting the nasolabial folds, ears, eyelids, and scrotum or labia majora. These areas become red, scaly, and greasy.

Rarely, neovascularization and keratitis of the cornea occur, causing lacrimation and photophobia.

Diagnosis and Treatment

The lesions characteristic of riboflavin deficiency are nonspecific. Riboflavin deficiency should be suspected if characteristic signs develop in a patient with other B vitamin deficiencies. Diagnosis can be confirmed by a therapeutic trial or laboratory testing, usually by measuring urinary excretion of riboflavin.

Riboflavin 2 to 10 mg po tid is given until a response is evident; then 2 to 4 mg once/day is given until recovery. If oral supplementation is ineffective, riboflavin 5 to 20 mg/day IM in single or divided doses can be given. In most cases, other water-soluble vitamins should also be given.

THIAMIN

Thiamin (vitamin B_1) is widely available in the diet. Thiamin is involved in carbohydrate, fat, amino acid, glucose, and alcohol metabolism. Thiamin is essentially nontoxic.

THIAMIN DEFICIENCY

Thiamin deficiency (causing beriberi) is most common among people subsisting on highly refined rice or other carbohydrates in developing countries and among alcoholics. Symptoms include diffuse polyneuropathy, high-output heart failure, and Wernicke-Korsakoff syndrome. Thiamin is given to help diagnose and treat deficiency.

Etiology

Primary thiamin deficiency is caused by inadequate intake of thiamin. It is commonly due to a diet of highly refined carbohydrates (eg, polished rice, white flour, white sugar). It also develops when intake of other nutrients is inadequate; it often occurs with other B vitamin deficiencies.

Secondary thiamin deficiency is caused by increased demand (eg, due to hyperthyroidism, pregnancy, lactation, strenuous exercise, or fever), impaired absorption (eg, in prolonged diarrhea), or impaired metabolism (eg, due to hepatic insufficiency). Many mechanisms contribute to thiamin deficiency in alcoholics, including decreased intake, impaired absorption and use, increased demand, and possibly an apoenzyme defect.

Pathophysiology

Deficiency causes degeneration of peripheral nerves. Neurons in the spinal cord, especially the posterior columns and the anterior and posterior nerve roots, may also degenerate. Severe deficiency results in brain lesions. Cerebral blood flow is markedly reduced, and vascular resistance is increased.

The heart may become dilated; muscle fibers become swollen, fragmented, and vacuolized, with interstitial spaces dilated by fluid. Vasodilation occurs and can result in edema in the feet and legs. Arteriovenous shunting of blood increases. Eventually, high-output heart failure may occur.

Symptoms and Signs

Early symptoms are nonspecific: fatigue, irritability, poor memory, sleep disturbances, precordial pain, anorexia, and abdominal discomfort.

Dry beriberi refers to peripheral neurologic deficits due to thiamin deficiency. These deficits are bilateral and roughly symmetric, occurring in a stocking-glove distribution. They affect predominantly the lower extremities, beginning with paresthesias in the toes, burning in the feet (particularly severe at night), muscle cramps in the calves, pains in the legs, and plantar dysesthesias. Calf muscle tenderness, difficulty rising from a squatting position, and decreased vibratory sensation in the toes are early signs. Muscle wasting occurs. Continued deficiency worsens polyneuropathy, which can eventually affect the arms.

Cerebral beriberi (Wernicke-Korsakoff syndrome), which combines Wernicke's encephalopathy (see p. 1688) and Korsakoff's psychosis (see p. 1689), occurs in alcoholics who do not consume foods fortified with thiamin. Wernicke's encephalopathy consists of nystagmus, ataxia, ophthalmoplegia, impaired consciousness, and, if untreated, coma and death. It probably results from severe acute deficiency superimposed on chronic deficiency. Korsakoff's psychosis consists of mental confusion, listlessness, dysphonia, and confabulation with impaired memory of recent events. It probably results from chronic deficiency and may develop after repeated episodes of Wernicke's encephalopathy.

Cardiovascular (wet) beriberi is myocardial disease due to thiamin deficiency. The first effects are vasodilation, tachycardia, a wide pulse pressure, sweating, warm skin, and lactic acidosis. Later, heart failure develops, causing orthopnea and pulmonary and peripheral edema. Vasodilation can continue, sometimes resulting in shock.

Infantile beriberi occurs in infants (usually by age 3 to 4 wk) who are breastfed by thiamin-deficient mothers. Heart failure (which may occur suddenly), aphonia, and absent deep tendon reflexes are characteristic.

Because thiamin is necessary for glucose metabolism, glucose infusions may precipitate or worsen symptoms of deficiency in thiamin-deficient people.

Diagnosis

Diagnosis is usually based on a favorable response to treatment with thiamin in a patient with symptoms or signs of deficiency. Similar bilateral lower extremity polyneuropathies due to other disorders (eg, diabetes, alcoholism, vitamin B_{12} deficiency, heavy metal poisoning) do not respond to thiamin. Single-nerve neuritides (mononeuropathies—eg, sciatica) and multiple mononeuropathies (mononeuritis multiplex) are unlikely to result from thiamin deficiency.

Electrolytes, including Mg, should be measured to exclude other causes. For confirmation in equivocal cases, erythrocyte transketolase activity and 24-h urinary thiamin excretion may be measured.

Diagnosis of cardiovascular beriberi can be difficult if other disorders that cause heart failure are present. A therapeutic trial of thiamin can help.

Treatment and Prognosis

Ensuring dietary supplies of thiamin are adequate is important regardless of symptoms. Because IV glucose can worsen thiamin deficiency, alcoholics and others at risk of thiamin deficiency should receive IV thiamin 100 mg before receiving IV glucose solutions.

For mild polyneuropathy, thiamin 10 to 20 mg po once/day is given for 2 wk. For moderate or advanced neuropathy, the dose is 20 to 30 mg/day; it should be continued for several weeks after symptoms disappear. For edema and congestion due to cardiovascular beriberi, thiamin 100 mg IV once/day is given for several days. Heart failure is also treated.

For Wernicke-Korsakoff syndrome, thiamin 50 to 100 mg bid IM or IV must usually be given for several days, followed by 10 to 20 mg once/day until a therapeutic response is obtained. Anaphylactic reactions to IV thiamin are rare. Symptoms of ophthalmoplegia may resolve in a day; improvement in patients with Korsakoff psychosis may take 1 to 3 mo. Recovery from neurologic deficits is often incomplete in Wernicke-Korsakoff syndrome and in other forms of thiamin deficiency.

Because thiamin deficiency often occurs with other B vitamin deficiencies, multiple water-soluble vitamins are usually given for several weeks. Patients should continue to consume a nutritious diet, supplying 1 to 2 times the daily recommended intake (DRI) of vitamins; all alcohol intake should stop.

VITAMIN A

Vitamin A (retinol) is required for the formation of rhodopsin, a photoreceptor pigment in the retina. Vitamin A helps maintain epithelial tissues. Normally, the liver stores 90% of the body's vitamin A. To use vitamin A, the body releases it into the circulation bound to prealbumin (transthyretin) and retinol-binding protein. β-carotene and other provitamin carotenoids, contained in green leafy and yellow vegetables and deep- or bright-colored fruits, are converted to vitamin A. Carotenoids are absorbed better from vegetables when they are cooked or homogenized and served with some fats or oils.

Retinol 1 μg equals vitamin A 3.3 IU and is equivalent to 10 IU β-carotene. Other provitamin carotenoids are half as active as β-carotene.

Synthetic vitamin analogs (retinoids) are used increasingly in dermatology. The possible protective role of β-carotene, retinol, and retinoids against some epithelial cancers is under study. However, risk of certain cancers may be increased after β-carotene supplementation.

VITAMIN A DEFICIENCY

Deficiency can result from inadequate intake, fat malabsorption, or liver disorders. Deficiency impairs immunity and causes skin rashes and typical ocular effects (eg, xerophthalmia, night blindness). Diagnosis is based on typical ocular findings and low vitamin A levels. Treatment consists of vitamin A given orally or, if symptoms are severe or malabsorption is the cause, parenterally.

Etiology

Primary vitamin A deficiency is usually caused by prolonged dietary deprivation. It is endemic in areas such as southern and eastern Asia, where rice, devoid of β-carotene, is the staple food. Xerophthalmia due to primary deficiency is a common cause of blindness among young children in developing countries.

Secondary vitamin A deficiency may be due to inadequate conversion of β-carotene to vitamin A or to interference with absorption, storage, or transport of vitamin A. Interference with absorption or storage is likely in sprue, cystic fibrosis, pancreatic insufficiency, duodenal bypass, chronic diarrhea, bile duct obstruction, giardiasis, and cirrhosis. Vitamin A deficiency is common in prolonged protein-energy malnutrition not only because the diet is deficient but also because vitamin A storage and transport is defective.

Symptoms and Signs

Impaired dark adaptation of the eyes, which can lead to night blindness, is an early symptom. Xerophthalmia (which is nearly pathognomonic) results from keratinization of the eyes. It involves drying (xerosis) and thickening of the conjunctivae and corneas. The cornea becomes hazy and can develop erosions, which can lead to its destruction (keratomalacia). In advanced deficiency, superficial foamy patches composed of epithelial debris and secretions on the exposed bulbar conjunctiva (Bitot's spots) develop.

Keratinization of the skin and of the mucous membranes in the respiratory, GI, and urinary tracts can occur. Drying, scaling, and follicular thickening of the skin and respiratory infections can result. Immunity is generally impaired.

The younger the patient, the more severe the effects of vitamin A deficiency. Growth retardation is common among children. Mortality can exceed 50% in children with severe vitamin A deficiency.

Diagnosis

Ocular findings suggest the diagnosis. Dark adaptation can be impaired in other disorders (eg, zinc deficiency, retinitis pigmentosa, severe refractive errors, cataracts, diabetic retinopathy). Rod scotometry and electroretinography can be used to test for vitamin A deficiency.

Plasma levels of vitamin A and retinol-binding protein decrease in vitamin A deficiency; they may also decrease in acute infections. Because the liver contains large stores, vitamin A levels do not decrease until deficiency is advanced, unless an infection is also present. The normal range is 20 to 80 μg/dL (0.7 to 2.8 μmol/L). A therapeutic trial of vitamin A may help confirm the diagnosis.

Prevention

The diet should include dark green leafy vegetables, deep- or bright-colored fruits (eg, papayas, oranges), carrots, and yellow vegetables (eg, squash, pumpkin). Vitamin A–fortified milk and cereals, liver, egg yolks, and fish liver oils are helpful. Carotenoids are absorbed better when consumed with some dietary fat. If milk allergy is suspected, infants should be given adequate vitamin A in formula feedings. In developing countries, prophylactic doses of vitamin A palmitate in oil 66,000 μg (200,000 IU) po once q 4 to 6 mo are advised for all children > 1 yr; infants < 6 mo can be given a one-time dose of 17,000 μg (50,000 IU), and those aged 6 to 12 mo can be given a one-time dose of 33,000 μg (100,000 IU).

Treatment

Dietary deficiency is traditionally treated with vitamin A palmitate in oil 20,000 μg (60,000 IU) po once/day for 2 days, followed by 1500 μg (4500 IU) po once/day. If vomiting, malabsorption, or possibly xerophthalmia is present, a dose of 17,000 μg (50,000 IU) for infants < 6 mo, 33,000 μg (100,000 IU) for infants 6 to 12 mo, or 66,000 μg (200,000 IU) for children > 12 mo and adults should be given for 2 days, with a third dose at least 2 wk later. Prolonged daily administration of large doses, especially to infants, must be avoided because toxicity may result.

For pregnant or lactating women, prophylactic or therapeutic doses should not exceed 4500 μg (13,500 IU)/day to avoid possible damage to the fetus or infant.

VITAMIN A TOXICITY

Vitamin A toxicity can be acute (usually due to accidental ingestion by children) or chronic. Both types usually cause headache and increased intracranial pressure. Acute toxicity also causes nausea and vomiting. Chronic toxicity also causes changes in skin, hair, and nails; abnormal liver test results; and, in a fetus, birth defects. Diagnosis is usually clinical. Unless birth defects are present, adjusting the dose almost always leads to complete recovery.

Acute vitamin A toxicity in children may result from taking large doses (> 100,000 μg [> 300,000 IU]), usually accidentally. In adults, acute toxicity has occurred when arctic explorers have ingested polar bear or seal livers, which contained several million units of vitamin A.

Chronic toxicity in older children and adults usually develops after doses of > 33,000 μg (> 100,000 IU)/day have been taken for months. Megavitamin therapy is a possible cause, as are massive daily doses (50,000 to 120,000 μg [150,000 to 350,000 IU]) of vitamin A or its metabolites, which are sometimes given for nodular acne or other skin disorders. Adults who consume > 1500 μg (>4500 IU)/day of vitamin A may develop osteoporosis. Infants who are given excessive doses (6,000 to 20,000 μg [18,000 to 60,000 IU]/day) of water-miscible vitamin A may develop toxicity within a few weeks. Birth defects occur in children of women receiving isotretinoin (which is related to vitamin A) for acne treatment during pregnancy.

Although carotene is converted to vitamin A in the body, excessive ingestion of carotene causes carotenemia, not vitamin A toxicity. Carotenemia is usually asymptomatic but may lead to carotenodermia, in which the skin becomes yellow.

Symptoms, Signs, and Diagnosis

Although symptoms may vary, headache and rash usually develop during acute or chronic toxicity. Acute toxicity causes increased intracranial pressure. Drowsiness, irritability, abdominal pain, nausea, and vomiting are common. Sometimes the skin subsequently peels.

Early symptoms of chronic toxicity are sparsely distributed, coarse hair; alopecia of the eyebrows; dry, rough skin; dry eyes; and cracked lips. Later, severe headache, pseudotumor cerebri, and generalized weakness develop. Cortical hyperostosis of bone and arthralgia may occur, especially in children. Fractures may occur easily, especially in the elderly. In children, toxicity can cause pruritus, anorexia, and failure to thrive. Hepatomegaly and splenomegaly may occur.

In carotenodermia, the skin (but not the sclera) becomes deep yellow, especially on the palms and soles.

Diagnosis is clinical. Blood vitamin levels correlate poorly with toxicity. However, if clinical diagnosis is equivocal, laboratory testing may help. In vitamin A toxicity, fasting plasma retinol levels may increase from normal (20 to 80 μg/dL [0.7 to 2.8 μmol/L]) to > 100 μg/dL (> 3.49 μmol/L), sometimes to > 2000 μg/dL (> 69.8 μmol/L). Hypercalcemia is common.

Differentiating vitamin A toxicity from other disorders may be difficult. Carotenodermia may also occur in severe hypothyroidism and anorexia nervosa, possibly because carotene is converted to vitamin A more slowly.

Prognosis and Treatment

Complete recovery usually occurs if vitamin A ingestion stops. Symptoms and signs of chronic toxicity usually disappear within 1 to 4 wk. However, birth defects in the fetus of a mother who has taken megadoses of vitamin A are not reversible.

VITAMIN B_6

Vitamin B_6 includes a group of closely related compounds: pyridoxine, pyridoxal, and pyridoxamine. They are metabolized in the body to pyridoxal phosphate, which acts as a coenzyme in many important reactions in blood, CNS, and skin metabolism. Vitamin B_6 is important in heme and nucleic acid biosynthesis and in lipid, carbohydrate, and amino acid metabolism.

VITAMIN B_6 DEFICIENCY AND DEPENDENCY

Because vitamin B_6 is present in most foods, dietary deficiency is rare. Secondary deficiency may result from various conditions. Symptoms can include peripheral neuropathy, a pellagra-like syndrome, anemia, and seizures, which, particularly in infants, may not resolve with anticonvulsants. Impaired metabolism (dependency) is rare; it produces various symptoms, including seizures, mental retardation, and anemia. Diagnosis is usually clinical; no laboratory test readily assesses vitamin B_6 status. Treatment consists of giving oral vitamin B_6 and, when possible, treating the cause.

Dietary deficiency, though rare, can develop because extensive processing can deplete foods of vitamin B_6. Secondary deficiency most often results from protein-energy malnutrition, malabsorption, alcoholism, use of pyridoxine-inactivating drugs (eg, anticonvulsants, isoniazid, cycloserine, hydralazine, corticosteroids, penicillamine), or excessive loss. Rarely, it results from increased metabolic demand (eg, in hyperthyroidism).

Rare inborn errors of metabolism can affect pyridoxine metabolism.

Vitamin B_6 deficiency can alter platelet function. The role of vitamin B_6 deficiency in increasing plasma homocysteine levels or in contributing to vascular disorders is under study.

Symptoms and Signs

Deficiency causes a pellagra-like syndrome, seborrheic dermatitis, glossitis, cheilosis, and lymphopenia and can cause depression, confusion, EEG abnormalities, and seizures in adults. Rarely, deficiency or dependency cause seizures in infants. Seizures, particularly in infants, may be refractory to treatment with anticonvulsants. Normocytic, microcytic, or sideroblastic anemia can also develop.

Diagnosis

Vitamin B_6 deficiency should be considered in any infant who has seizures, any patient who has seizures refractory to treatment with anticonvulsants, and any patient with deficiencies of other B vitamins, particularly if associated with alcoholism or protein-energy malnutrition. Diagnosis is usually clinical. There is no generally accepted laboratory test of vitamin B_6 status.

Tryptophan is sometimes given to help with diagnosis. Tryptophan 2 g po results in urinary excretion of large amounts of xanthurenic acid over 24 h in patients with vitamin B_6 deficiency but < 65 μmol in patients without deficiency.

Prevention and Treatment

For secondary deficiency, causes (eg, use of pyridoxine-inactivating drugs, malabsorption) should be corrected if possible. Usually, pyridoxine 50 to 100 mg po once/day corrects the deficiency in adults. Most people taking isoniazid should also receive pyridoxine 30 to 50 mg/day. For deficiency due to increased metabolic demand, amounts larger than the DRI may be required. For most cases of inborn errors of metabolism, high doses of pyridoxine may be effective.

Vitamin B_6 Toxicity

The ingestion of megadoses (1 to 6 g/day) of pyridoxine (eg, taken to treat carpal tunnel syndrome or premenstrual syndrome although efficacy is unproved) may cause peripheral neuropathy with deficits in a stocking-glove distribution, including progressive sensory ataxia and severe impairment of position and vibration senses. Senses of touch, temperature, and pain are less affected. Motor and central nervous systems are usually intact. Diagnosis is clinical; treatment is to stop taking vitamin B_6. Recovery is slow and, for some patients, incomplete.

VITAMIN B_{12}

Cobalamin is a general term for compounds with biologic vitamin B_{12} activity. These compounds are involved in nucleic acid metabolism, methyl transfer, and myelin synthesis and repair. They are necessary for the formation of normal RBCs.

Food-bound vitamin B_{12} is released in the stomach's acid environment and is bound to R protein. Pancreatic enzymes cleave this B_{12} complex (B_{12}-R protein) in the small intestine. After cleavage, intrinsic factor, secreted by parietal cells in the gastric mucosa, binds with vitamin B_{12}. Intrinsic factor is required for absorption of vitamin B_{12}, which takes place in the terminal ileum.

Vitamin B_{12} in plasma is bound to transcobalamins I and II. Transcobalamin II is responsible primarily for delivering vitamin B_{12} to tissues. The liver stores large amounts of vitamin B_{12}. Enterohepatic reabsorption helps retain vitamin B_{12}. Liver vitamin B_{12} stores can normally sustain physiologic needs for 3 to 6 yr if intrinsic factor is absent and for months to 1 yr if enterohepatic reabsorption capacity is absent.

Large amounts of vitamin B_{12} should not be used as a general tonic but otherwise appear to be nontoxic.

Vitamin B_{12} Deficiency

Dietary vitamin B_{12} deficiency usually results from inadequate absorption, but deficiency can develop in vegans who do not take vitamin supplements. Deficiency causes megaloblastic anemia, damage to the white matter of the spinal cord and brain, and peripheral neuropathy. Diagnosis is usually made by measuring plasma

TABLE 4–5. CAUSES OF VITAMIN B_{12} DEFICIENCY

CAUSE	SOURCE
Inadequate diet	Vegan diet, breastfeeding of infants by vegan mothers, fad diets
Impaired absorption	Lack of intrinsic factor (due to pernicious anemia, destruction of gastric mucosa, gastric surgery, or endocrinopathy), intrinsic factor inhibition, decreased acid secretion, small-bowel disorders (eg, inflammatory bowel disease, sprue, malignancy, biliary or pancreatic disorders), competition for vitamin B_{12} (in fish tapeworm infestation or blind loop syndrome), AIDS
Inadequate utilization	Enzyme deficiencies, liver disorders, transport protein abnormality

vitamin B_{12} levels. The Schilling test helps determine etiology. Treatment consists of oral or parenteral vitamin B_{12}. Folate should not be used instead of vitamin B_{12} because folate may alleviate the anemia but allow neurologic deficits to progress.

If liver stores (which are normally extensive) are limited and demand is high because of rapid growth rate (eg, in breastfed babies of vegan mothers), deficiency may develop by age 4 to 6 mo.

Etiology and Pathophysiology

Inadequate vitamin B_{12} intake is possible in vegans but is otherwise unlikely. Vitamin B_{12} deficiency usually results from inadequate absorption (see TABLE 4–5 and p. 140), which, in the elderly, most commonly results from decreased acid secretion. In such cases, crystalline vitamin B_{12} (such as that available in vitamin supplements) can be absorbed, but food-bound vitamin B_{12} is not liberated and absorbed normally. Inadequate absorption may occur in the blind loop syndrome (with overgrowth of bacteria) or fish tapeworm infestation; in these cases, bacteria or parasites use ingested vitamin B_{12} so that less is available for absorption. Vitamin B_{12} absorption may be inadequate if ileal absorptive sites are destroyed by inflammatory bowel disease or surgically removed. Less common causes of inadequate vitamin B_{12} absorption include chronic pancreatitis, gastric surgery, malabsorption syndromes, AIDS, use of certain drugs (eg, antacids, metformin), repeated exposure to nitrous oxide, and a genetic disorder causing malabsorption in the ileum (Imerslund-Gräsbeck syndrome).

Pernicious anemia is often used synonymously with vitamin B_{12} deficiency. However, pernicious anemia specifically refers to vitamin B_{12} deficiency caused by an autoimmune gastritis with loss of intrinsic factor (see p. 120). Classic pernicious anemia, most common in younger adults, is associated with an increased risk of stomach and other GI cancers.

Subacute combined degeneration refers to degenerative changes in the nervous system due to vitamin B_{12} deficiency; they affect mostly brain and spinal cord white matter. Demyelinating or axonal peripheral neuropathies can occur.

Symptoms and Signs

Anemia usually develops insidiously. It is often more severe than its symptoms indicate because its slow evolution allows physiologic adaptation. Occasionally, splenomegaly and hepatomegaly occur. Various GI symptoms, including anorexia, constipation, and poorly localized abdominal pain, may occur. Glossitis, usually described as burning of the tongue, is uncommon.

Neurologic symptoms develop independently from and often without hematologic abnormalities. In early stages, decreased position and vibratory sensation in the extremities is accompanied by mild to moderate weakness and hyporeflexia. In later stages, spasticity, extensor plantar responses, greater loss of position and vibratory sensation in the lower extremities, and ataxia emerge. These deficits may develop in a stocking-glove distribution. Tactile, pain, and temperature sensations are usually spared but may be difficult to assess in the elderly.

Some patients are also irritable and mildly depressed. Paranoia (megaloblastic madness), delirium, confusion, spastic ataxia, and, at times, postural hypotension may occur in advanced cases. The confusion may be difficult to differentiate from age-related dementias, such as Alzheimer's disease.

Diagnosis

Diagnosis is based on CBC and vitamin B_{12} and folate levels. If symptoms suggest spinal cord compression or multiple sclerosis, a neurologic imaging study, such as MRI, may be needed.

CBC detects megaloblastic anemia. Tissue deficiency and macrocytic indexes may precede the development of anemia. A vitamin B_{12} level < 200 pg/mL (< 145 pmol/L) indicates vitamin B_{12} deficiency. The folate level is measured because vitamin B_{12} deficiency must be differentiated from folate deficiency as a cause of megaloblastic anemia; folate supplementation can mask vitamin B_{12} deficiency and can alleviate megaloblastic anemia but allow the neurologic deficits to progress.

When clinical judgment suggests vitamin B_{12} deficiency but the vitamin B_{12} level is low-normal (200 to 350 pg/mL [145 to 260 pmol/L]) or hematologic indexes are normal, other tests can be done. Measuring serum methylmalonic acid (MMA) levels may be useful. An elevated MMA level supports vitamin B_{12} deficiency but may be due to renal failure. MMA levels can also be used to monitor the response to treatment. Homocysteine levels may be elevated. Less commonly, holotranscobalamin II (transcobalamin II–B_{12} complex) content is measured; when holotranscobalamin II is < 40 pg/mL (< 30 pmol/L), vitamin B_{12} is deficient.

After deficiency is diagnosed, additional tests may be indicated for younger adults but usually not for the elderly. Unless dietary vitamin B_{12} is obviously inadequate, upper GI endoscopy and measurement of serum autoantibodies to gastric parietal cells may be done to rule out autoimmune metaplastic atrophic gastritis (see p. 120).

Schilling test: The Schilling test is useful only if diagnosing intrinsic factor deficiency is important, as in classic pernicious anemia. This test is not necessary for most elderly patients. The Schilling test measures absorption of free oral radiolabeled vitamin B_{12}. Radiolabeled vitamin B_{12} is given orally, followed in 1 to 6 h by 1000 μg (1 mg) of parenteral vitamin B_{12}, which reduces uptake of radiolabeled vitamin B_{12} by the liver. Absorbed radiolabeled vitamin B_{12} is then excreted by the urine, which is collected for 24 h. The percentage of total radiolabeled vitamin B_{12} is measured. If absorption is normal, ≥ 9% of the dose given appears in the urine. Reduced urinary excretion (< 5% if kidney function is normal) indicates inadequate vitamin B_{12} absorption. The test is often difficult to perform or interpret because of incomplete urine collection or renal insufficiency. In addition, because the Schilling test does not measure absorption of protein-bound vitamin B_{12}, the test does not detect defective liberation of vitamin B_{12} from foods, which is common among the elderly. The Schilling test repletes vitamin B_{12} and can mask deficiency, so it should be performed only after all other diagnostic tests and therapeutic trials.

The Schilling test can be repeated after a 2-wk trial of an oral antibiotic. If antibiotic therapy corrects malabsorption, the likely cause is intestinal overgrowth of bacteria (eg, blind-loop syndrome).

Treatment

Vitamin B_{12} 1000 to 2000 μg po can be given once/day to patients who do not have severe deficiency or neurologic symptoms or signs. These large oral doses can be absorbed by mass action, even when intrinsic factor is absent. If the MMA level (sometimes used to monitor treatment) does not decrease, the patient may not be taking vitamin B_{12}. For more severe deficiency, vitamin B_{12} 1 mg IM is usually given 1 to 4 times/wk for several weeks until hematologic abnormalities are corrected; then it is given once/mo. Although hematologic abnormalities are usually corrected within 6 wk (reticulocyte count may improve within 1 wk), resolution of neurologic symptoms may take much longer. Neurologic symptoms that persist for months or years become irreversible. In most elderly people with vitamin B_{12} deficiency and dementia, cognition does not improve after treatment. Vitamin B_{12} treatment must be continued for life unless the pathophysiologic mechanism for the deficiency is corrected.

Infants of vegan mothers should receive supplemental vitamin B_{12} from birth.

VITAMIN C

Vitamin C (ascorbic acid) plays a role in collagen, carnitine, hormone, and amino acid formation. It is essential for wound healing and facilitates recovery from burns. Vitamin C is also an antioxidant, supports immune function, and facilitates the absorption of iron.

VITAMIN C DEFICIENCY

In developed countries, deficiency can occur with general undernutrition, but severe deficiency (causing scurvy) is uncommon. Symptoms include fatigue, depression, and connective tissue defects (eg, gingivitis, petechiae, rash, internal bleeding, impaired wound healing). In infants and children, bone growth may be impaired. Diagnosis is usually clinical. Treatment consists of oral vitamin C.

Severe deficiency results in scurvy, an acute or chronic disorder characterized by hemorrhagic manifestations and abnormal osteoid and dentin formation.

Etiology

In adults, primary deficiency is usually due to inadequate diet. The need for dietary vitamin C is increased by febrile illnesses, inflammatory disorders (particularly diarrheal disorders), achlorhydria, smoking, thyrotoxicosis, iron deficiency, cold or heat stress, surgery, burns, and protein deficiency. Heat (eg, sterilization of formulas, cooking) can destroy some of the vitamin C in food.

Pathophysiology

Formation of intercellular cement substances in connective tissues, bones, and dentin is defective, resulting in weakened capillaries with subsequent hemorrhage and defects in bone and related structures.

Bone tissue formation becomes impaired, which, in children, causes bone lesions and poor bone growth. Fibrous tissue forms between the diaphysis and the epiphysis, and costochondral junctions enlarge. Densely calcified fragments of cartilage are embedded in the fibrous tissue. Subperiosteal hemorrhages, sometimes due to small fractures, may occur in children or adults.

Symptoms and Signs

In adults, symptoms develop only after months of vitamin C depletion. But lassitude, weakness, irritability, weight loss, and vague myalgias and arthralgias may develop early.

Later, symptoms related to defects in connective tissues develop. Follicular hyperkeratosis, coiled hair, and perifollicular hemorrhages may develop. Gums may become swollen, purple, spongy, and friable; they bleed easily in severe deficiency. Eventually, teeth become loose and avulsed. Secondary infections may develop. Wounds heal poorly and tear easily, and spontaneous hemorrhages may occur, especially as ecchymoses in the skin of the lower limbs or bulbar conjunctival hemorrhage.

Other symptoms and signs include femoral neuropathy due to hemorrhage into femoral sheaths (which may mimic deep vein thrombosis), lower extremity edema, bleeding within joints, effusions, and arthralgias.

Diagnosis

Diagnosis is usually made clinically in a patient who has skin or gingival signs and is at risk of vitamin C deficiency. Laboratory confirmation may be available. Anemia is common. Bleeding, coagulation, and prothrombin times are normal.

Skeletal x-rays can help diagnose childhood (but not adult) scurvy. Changes are most evident at the ends of long bones, particularly at the knee. Early changes resemble atrophy. Loss of trabeculae results in a ground-glass appearance. The cortex thins. A line of calcified, irregular cartilage (white line of Fraenkel) may be visible at the metaphysis. A zone of rarefaction or a linear fracture proximal and parallel to the white line may be visible as only a triangular defect at the bone's lateral margin but is specific. The epiphysis may be compressed. Healing subperiosteal hemorrhages may elevate and calcify the periosteum.

Laboratory diagnosis, which requires measuring plasma ascorbic acid, is sometimes done at academic centers. A fall in plasma ascorbic acid from the normal range to < 0.6 mg/dL (< 34 μmol/L) is considered marginal, and a fall to < 0.2 mg/dL (< 11 μmol/L) indicates vitamin C deficiency. Measurement of ascorbic acid levels in the WBC-platelet layer of centrifuged blood is not widely available or standardized.

In adults, scurvy must be differentiated from arthritis, hemorrhagic disorders, gingivitis, and protein-energy malnutrition. Hyperkeratotic hair follicle with surrounding hyperemia or hemorrhage is almost pathognomonic. Bleeding gums, conjunctival hemorrhages, most petechiae, and ecchymoses are nonspecific.

Prevention and Treatment

Vitamin C 75 mg po once/day for women and 90 mg po once/day for men prevents deficiency. Smokers should consume an additional 35 mg/day. For scurvy in adults, ascorbic acid 500 mg po once/day to qid is given for 1 to 2 wk, until signs disappear, and followed by a nutritious diet supplying 1 to 2 times the DRI for several more weeks. In scurvy, therapeutic doses of ascorbic acid restore the functions of vitamin C in a few days. The symptoms and signs usually disappear over 1 to 2 wk. Chronic gingivitis with extensive subcutaneous hemorrhage persists longer.

Vitamin C Toxicity

The upper limit of vitamin C is 2000 mg/day. Up to 10 g/day of vitamin C are sometimes taken for unproven health benefits, such as preventing or shortening the duration of viral infections or slowing or reversing the progression of cancer or atherosclerosis. Such doses may acidify the urine, cause nausea and diarrhea, and, in patients with thalassemia or hemochromatosis, promote iron overload. Intake below the upper limit does not have toxic effects in healthy adults.

VITAMIN D

Vitamin D has two main forms: D_2 (ergocalciferol) and D_3 (cholecalciferol). Vitamin D_3 is synthesized in skin by exposure to sunlight (ultraviolet radiation) and obtained in the diet chiefly in fish liver oils and egg yolks. In some developed countries, milk and other foods are fortified with vitamin D. Human breast milk is low in vitamin D, containing an average of only 10% of the amount in fortified cow's milk. Requirements for vitamin D increase with aging.

Vitamin D is a prohormone with several active metabolites that act as hormones. Vitamin D_3 is metabolized by the liver to 25(OH)D, which is then converted by the kidneys to $1,25(OH)_2D$ (1,25-dihydroxycholecalciferol, calcitriol, or active vitamin D hormone). 25(OH)D, the major circulating form, has some metabolic activity, but $1,25(OH)_2D$ is the most metabolically active. The conversion to $1,25(OH)_2D$ is regulated by its own concentration, parathyroid hormone (PTH), and the serum concentrations of Ca and phosphate.

Vitamin D affects many organ systems (see TABLE 4–6), but mainly it increases Ca and P absorption from the intestine and promotes normal bone formation and mineralization. Vitamin D and related analogs may be used to treat psoriasis, hypoparathyroidism, renal osteodystrophy, and possibly leukemia, breast, prostate, or colon cancer; they may also be used for immunosuppression.

Vitamin D Deficiency and Dependency

Inadequate exposure to sunlight predisposes to vitamin D deficiency. Deficiency impairs bone mineralization, causing rickets in children and osteomalacia in adults and possibly contributing to osteoporosis. Treatment usually consists of oral vitamin D, Ca, and phosphate. Prevention is often possible. Rarely, hereditary disorders cause impaired metabolism of vitamin D (dependency).

Rickets and osteomalacia may also result from other conditions (eg, various renal tubular disorders, familial hypophosphatemic [vitamin D–resistant] rickets [see p. 2440], chronic metabolic acidosis, hypoparathyroidism [which reduces vitamin D absorption], inadequate dietary Ca, and disorders or drugs that impair the mineralization of bone matrix).

Etiology and Pathophysiology

Vitamin D deficiency may result from inadequate intake, reduced absorption, abnormal metabolism, or resistance to the effects of vitamin D.

Inadequate sunlight exposure and inadequate intake usually must occur simultaneously to result in clinical deficiency. Susceptible people include the elderly (who are often undernourished and are not exposed to enough sunlight), and certain communities (eg, women and children who are confined to the home or who wear clothing that covers the entire body and face). Inadequate vitamin D stores are common among the elderly, particularly those who are housebound, institutionalized, or hospitalized or who have had a hip fracture. Rarely, very low intake of Ca or P may cause vitamin D deficiency. Malabsorption can deprive the body of dietary vitamin D and 25(OH)D (the latter undergoes a small amount of enterohepatic recirculation).

Vitamin D deficiency may result from defects in the production of 25(OH)D. Conditions that interfere with production of active vitamin D metabolites (eg, liver or kidney disorders) do not respond to normal amounts of supplemental vitamin D (ie, are vitamin D–resistant).

TABLE 4–6. ACTIONS OF VITAMIN D AND ITS METABOLITES

ORGAN	ACTIONS
Bone	Promotes bone formation by stimulating osteoblasts to produce more alkaline phosphatase and osteocalcin (a vitamin K–dependent bone protein) and less collagen Stimulates mononuclear cells to differentiate into macrophages, which fuse with osteoclasts and increase Ca mobilization
Immune system	Stimulates immunogenic and antitumor activity
Intestine	Enhances Ca and phosphate transport (absorption)
Kidneys	Enhances Ca reabsorption by the tubule
Parathyroid glands	Inhibits parathyroid hormone secretion

Vitamin D deficiency also results from resistance to the effects of 1,25(OH)$_2$D. Type I hereditary vitamin D–dependent rickets is an autosomal recessive disorder characterized by absent or defective conversion of 25(OH)D to 1,25(OH)$_2$D in the kidneys. Type II hereditary vitamin D–dependent rickets has several forms and is due to mutations in the 1,25(OH)$_2$D receptor. This receptor affects the metabolism of gut, kidney, bone, and other cells. Although 1,25(OH)$_2$D is abundant, it is ineffective because the receptor is not functional. Anticonvulsants (eg, phenytoin, phenobarbital) can cause end-organ resistance to 1,25(OH)$_2$D, resulting in osteomalacia.

People with a renal disorder commonly develop rickets or osteomalacia because of decreased renal production of 1,25 (OH)$_2$D and elevated phosphate levels. Rickets refractory to vitamin D may also be caused by renal tubular acidosis, X-linked familial hypophosphatemia, or Fanconi's syndrome.

Vitamin D deficiency causes hypocalcemia, which stimulates production of PTH, causing hyperparathyroidism. Hyperparathyroidism increases absorption, bone mobilization, and renal conservation of Ca but increases excretion of phosphate. As a result, the serum level of Ca may be normal, but because of hypophosphatemia, bone mineralization is impaired.

Symptoms and Signs

Vitamin D deficiency can cause muscle aches, muscle weakness, and bone pain at any age.

Vitamin D deficiency in a pregnant woman causes deficiency in the fetus. Occasionally, deficiency severe enough to cause maternal osteomalacia results in rickets with metaphyseal lesions in a newborn. In young infants, rickets causes softening of the entire skull (craniotabes). When palpated, the occiput and posterior parietal bones feel like a ping pong ball. In older infants with rickets, sitting and crawling are delayed, as is fontanelle closure; there is bossing of the skull and costochondral thickening. Costochondral thickening can look like beadlike prominences along the lateral chest wall (rachitic rosary). In children 1 to 4 yr, epiphyseal cartilage at the lower ends of the radius, ulna, tibia, and fibula enlarge; kyphoscoliosis develops, and walking is delayed. In older children and adolescents, walking is painful; in extreme cases, deformities such as bowlegs and knock-knees develop.

Rachitic tetany is caused by hypocalcemia and may accompany infantile or adult vitamin D deficiency. Tetany may produce paresthesias of the lips, tongue, and fingers; carpopedal and facial spasm; and, if very severe, seizures. Maternal deficiency can cause tetany in newborns.

Osteomalacia predisposes to fractures. In the elderly, hip fractures may result from only minimal trauma.

Diagnosis

Diagnosis may be suspected based on a history of inadequate sunlight exposure or dietary intake; on symptoms and signs of rickets, osteomalacia, or neonatal tetany; or on characteristic bone changes seen on x-ray. X-rays of the radius and ulna plus serum levels of Ca, phosphate, alkaline phosphatase, PTH, and 25(OH)D are needed to differentiate vitamin D deficiency from other causes of bone demineralization.

Infants with craniotabes should have serologic tests for syphilis, even though congenital syphilis causes craniotabes most often in newborns, and rickets causes craniotabes most often in infants 2 to 4 mo. Rickets can be distinguished from chondrodystrophy because the latter is characterized by a large head, short extremities, thick bones, and normal serum Ca, phosphate, and alkaline phosphatase levels.

Tetany due to infantile rickets may be clinically indistinguishable from seizures due to other causes. Blood tests and clinical history may help distinguish them.

Bone changes, seen on x-rays, precede clinical signs. In rickets, changes are most evident at the lower ends of the radius and ulna. The diaphyseal ends lose their sharp, clear outline; are cup-shaped; and show a spotty or fringy rarefaction. Later, because the ends of the radius and ulna have become noncalcified and radiolucent, the distance between them and the metacarpal bones appears increased. The bone matrix elsewhere also becomes more radiolucent. Characteristic deformities result from the bones bending at the cartilage-shaft junction because the shaft is weak. As healing begins, a thin white line of calcification appears at the epiphysis, becoming denser and thicker as calcification proceeds. Later, the bone matrix becomes calcified and opacified at the subperiosteal level.

In adults, bone demineralization, particularly in the spine, pelvis, and lower extremities, can be seen on x-rays; the fibrous lamellae also can be seen, and incomplete ribbonlike areas of demineralization (pseudofractures, Looser's lines, Milkman's syndrome) appear in the cortex.

Because levels of serum 25(OH)D reflect body stores of vitamin D and correlate with symptoms and signs of vitamin D deficiency better than levels of other vitamin D metabolites, 25(OH)D measurement is generally considered the best way to diagnose deficiency. In healthy people, levels are 25 to 40 ng/mL (60 to 100 nmol/L).

If the diagnosis is unclear, serum levels of $1,25(OH)_2D$ and urinary Ca concentration can be measured. In severe deficiency, serum $1,25(OH)_2D$ is abnormally low, usually undetectable. Urinary Ca is low in all forms of the deficiency except those associated with acidosis.

In vitamin D deficiency, serum Ca may be low or, because of secondary hyperparathyroidism, may be normal. Serum phosphate usually decreases, and serum alkaline phosphatase usually increases. Serum PTH is elevated.

Type I hereditary vitamin D–dependent rickets results in normal serum 25(OH)D, low serum $1,25(OH)_2D$ and Ca, and normal or low serum phosphate.

Prevention

Dietary counseling is particularly important in communities whose members are at risk of vitamin D deficiency. Breastfed infants should be given supplemental vitamin D 5.0 μg (200 IU) once/day from birth to 6 mo; at 6 mo, a more diversified diet is available. Fortifying unleavened chapati flour with vitamin D (125 μg/kg) has been effective among Indian immigrants in Britain. Among adolescents at risk, a single IM dose of ergocalciferol 2.5 mg (100,000 IU) given in the fall can maintain adequate 25(OH)D levels throughout the winter.

Treatment

As long as Ca and P intake is adequate, adults with osteomalacia and children with uncomplicated rickets can be cured by giving vitamin D 40 μg (1600 IU) po once/day. Serum 25(OH)D and $1,25(OH)_2D$, which need not be routinely measured, begin to increase within 1 or 2 days. Serum Ca and phosphate increase and serum alkaline phosphatase decreases within about 10 days. During the 3rd wk, enough Ca and P are deposited in bones to be visible on x-rays. After about 1 mo, the dose can be reduced gradually to the usual maintenance level of 10 μg (400 IU) once/day. If tetany is present, vitamin D should be supplemented with IV Ca salts for up to 1 wk (see p. 1253).

Rickets and osteomalacia that result from defective production of vitamin D metabolites are vitamin D–resistant; they do not respond to the doses usually effective for rickets due to inadequate intake. Endocrinologic evaluation is required. Some cases respond to massive doses (600 to 1200 μg vitamin D_2 or D_3 once/day), but toxicity may result. When 25(OH)D production is defective, 50 μg of 25(OH)D once/day increases serum levels and results in clinical improvement. People with kidney disorders may need $1,25(OH)_2D$ supplementation.

Type I hereditary vitamin D–dependent rickets responds to $1,25(OH)_2D$ 1 to 2 μg po once/day. Some patients with type II hereditary vitamin D–dependent rickets respond to very high doses (eg, 10 to 24 μg/day) of $1,25(OH)_2D$; others require long-term infusions of Ca.

Vitamin D Toxicity

Usually, vitamin D toxicity results from taking excessive amounts. Marked hypercalcemia commonly causes symptoms. Diagnosis is typically based on elevated blood levels of 25(OH)D. Treatment consists of discontinuing vitamin D, restricting dietary Ca, restoring intravascular volume deficits, and, if toxicity is severe, giving corticosteroids or bisphosphonates.

Because synthesis of its potent metabolite $1,25(OH)_2D$ is tightly regulated, vitamin D toxicity usually occurs only if excessive doses (prescription or megavitamin) are taken. Vitamin D 1000 μg (40,000 IU)/day produces toxicity within 1 to 4 mo in infants; as little as 50 to 75 μg (2000 to 3000 IU)/day, if taken for years, can produce toxicity. In adults, taking 2500 μg (100,000 IU)/day for several months can produce toxicity. Vitamin D toxicity can occur iatrogenically when hypoparathyroidism is treated (see p. 1253).

Symptoms and Diagnosis

The main symptoms of vitamin D toxicity result from hypercalcemia. Anorexia, nausea, and vomiting can develop, often followed by polyuria, polydipsia, weakness, nervousness, pruritus, and eventually renal failure. Proteinuria, urinary casts, azotemia, and metastatic calcifications (particularly in the kidneys) can develop.

A history of excessive vitamin D intake may be the only clue differentiating vitamin D toxicity from other causes of hypercalcemia. Elevated serum Ca levels of 12 to 16 mg/dL (3 to 4 mmol/L) are a constant finding when toxic symptoms occur. Serum 25(OH)D levels are elevated as much as 15-fold in vitamin D toxicity. Levels of $1,25(OH)_2D$, which need not be measured to confirm the diagnosis, are usually normal.

Serum Ca should be measured often (weekly at first, then monthly) in all patients receiving large doses of vitamin D, particularly the potent $1,25(OH)_2D$.

Treatment

After stopping vitamin D intake, corticosteroids or bisphosphonates (which inhibit bone resorption) are used to reduce blood Ca levels.

Kidney damage or metastatic calcifications, if present, may be irreversible.

VITAMIN E

Vitamin E is a group of compounds (including tocopherols and tocotrienols) that have similar biologic activities. The most biologically active is a-tocopherol, but β-, γ-, and δ-tocopherols, four tocotrienols, and several stereoisomers may also have important biologic activity. These compounds act as antioxidants, which prevent lipid peroxidation of polyunsaturated fatty acids in cellular membranes. Plasma tocopherol levels vary with the total plasma lipid levels. Normally, the plasma α-tocopherol level is 5 to 20 μg/mL (11.6 to 46.4 μmol/L). Whether vitamin E protects against cardiovascular disorders, Alzheimer's disease, tardive dyskinesia, and prostate cancer among smokers is controversial. Although the amount of vitamin E in many fortified foods and supplements is given in IU, current recommendations are to use mg or μmol.

Vitamin E Deficiency

Dietary vitamin E deficiency is common in developing countries; deficiency among adults in developed countries is uncommon and usually due to fat malabsorption. The main symptoms are hemolytic anemia and neurologic deficits. Diagnosis is based on measuring the ratio of plasma α-tocopherol to total plasma lipids; a low ratio suggests vitamin E deficiency. Treatment consists of oral vitamin E, given in high doses if there are neurologic deficits or if deficiency results from malabsorption.

Vitamin E deficiency causes fragility of RBCs and degeneration of neurons, particularly peripheral axons and posterior column neurons.

Etiology

In developing countries, the most common cause is inadequate intake of vitamin E. In developed countries, the most common causes are disorders that cause fat malabsorption, including abetalipoproteinemia (Bassen-Kornzweig syndrome, due to genetic absence of apolipoprotein B), chronic cholestatic hepatobiliary disease, pancreatitis, short bowel syndrome, and cystic fibrosis. A rare genetic form of vitamin E deficiency without fat malabsorption results from defective liver metabolism.

Symptoms and Signs

The main symptoms are mild hemolytic anemia and nonspecific neurologic deficits. Abetalipoproteinemia results in progressive neuropathy and retinopathy in the first two decades of life (see p. 1309).

Vitamin E deficiency may contribute to retinopathy of prematurity (also called retrolental fibroplasia) in premature infants and to some cases of intraventricular and subependymal hemorrhage in newborns. Affected premature newborns have muscle weakness.

In children, chronic cholestatic hepatobiliary disease or cystic fibrosis causes neurologic deficits, including spinocerebellar ataxia with loss of deep tendon reflexes, truncal and limb ataxia, loss of vibration and position senses, ophthalmoplegia, muscle weakness, ptosis, and dysarthria.

In adults with malabsorption, vitamin E deficiency very rarely causes spinocerebellar ataxia because adults have large vitamin E stores in adipose tissue.

Diagnosis

Without a history of inadequate intake or a predisposing condition, vitamin E deficiency is unlikely. Confirmation usually requires measuring the vitamin level. Measuring RBC hemolysis in response to peroxide can suggest the diagnosis but is nonspecific. Hemolysis increases as vitamin E deficiency impairs RBC stability.

Measuring the plasma α-tocopherol level is the most direct method of diagnosis. In adults, vitamin E deficiency is suggested if the α-tocopherol level is < 5 μg/mL (< 11.6 μmol/L). Because abnormal plasma lipid levels can affect vitamin E status, a low ratio of plasma α-tocopherol to plasma lipids (< 0.8 mg/g total lipid) is the most accurate indicator in adults with hyperlipidemia.

In children and adults with abetalipoproteinemia, plasma α-tocopherol levels are usually undetectable.

Prevention and Treatment

Although premature newborns may require supplementation, human milk and commercial formulas have enough vitamin E for full-term newborns.

If malabsorption causes clinically evident deficiency, α-tocopherol 15 to 25 mg/kg po once/day should be given. However, larger doses given by injection are required to treat neuropathy during its early stages or to overcome the defect of absorption and transport in abetalipoproteinemia.

Vitamin E Toxicity

Many adults take relatively large amounts of vitamin E (α-tocopherol 400 to 800 mg/day) for months to years without any apparent harm. Occasionally, muscle weakness, fatigue, nausea, and diarrhea occur. The most significant risk is bleeding. However, bleeding is uncommon unless the dose is > 1000 mg/day or the patient takes oral coumarin or warfarin. Thus, the upper limit for adults aged ≥ 19 yr is 1000 mg (2326 μmol) for any form of α-tocopherol. Recent reviews of previous studies report that high vitamin E intakes may increase the risk of premature death.

VITAMIN K

Vitamin K_1 (phylloquinone) is dietary vitamin K. Dietary fat enhances its absorption. Infant formulas contain supplemental vitamin K. Vitamin K_2 refers to a group of compounds (menaquinones) synthesized by bacteria in the intestinal tract; the amount synthesized does not satisfy the vitamin K requirement.

Vitamin K controls the formation of coagulation factors II (prothrombin), VII, IX, and X in the liver. Other coagulation factors dependent on vitamin K are protein C, protein S, and protein Z; proteins C and S are anticoagulants. Metabolic pathways conserve vitamin K; once vitamin K has participated in formation of coagulation factors, the reaction product, vitamin K epoxide, is enzymatically converted to the active form, vitamin K hydroquinone.

The actions of vitamin K–dependent proteins require Ca. The vitamin K–dependent proteins, osteocalcin and matrix γ-carboxyglutamyl (Gla) protein, may have important roles in bone and other tissues.

Vitamin K Deficiency

Vitamin K deficiency results from extremely inadequate intake, fat malabsorption, or use of coumarin anticoagulants. Deficiency is particularly common among breastfed infants. It impairs clotting. Diagnosis is suspected based on routine coagulation study findings and confirmed by response to vitamin K. Treatment consists of vitamin K given orally or, when fat mal-

absorption is the cause or risk of bleeding is high, parenterally.

Vitamin K deficiency decreases levels of prothrombin and other vitamin K–dependent coagulation factors, causing defective coagulation and, potentially, bleeding.

Etiology

Worldwide, vitamin K deficiency can cause infant morbidity and mortality. Vitamin K deficiency causes hemorrhagic disease of the newborn, which usually occurs 1 to 7 days postpartum. In affected newborns, birth trauma can cause intracranial hemorrhage. Newborns are prone to vitamin K deficiency because (1) the placenta transmits lipids and vitamin K relatively poorly; (2) the neonatal liver is immature with respect to prothrombin synthesis; (3) breast milk is low in vitamin K, containing about 2.5 μg/L (cow's milk contains 5000 μg/L); and (4) the neonatal gut is sterile during the first few days of life. Late hemorrhagic disease (occurring 3 to 8 wk postpartum) is usually associated with breastfeeding, malabsorption, or a liver disorder. If the mother has ingested phenytoin anticonvulsants, coumarin anticoagulants, or cephalosporin antibiotics, the risk of both types of hemorrhagic disease is increased.

In healthy adults, dietary vitamin K deficiency is uncommon because vitamin K is widely distributed in green vegetables and the bacteria of the normal gut synthesize menaquinones. Biliary obstruction, malabsorption, cystic fibrosis, and resection of the small intestine can contribute to vitamin K deficiency.

Coumarin anticoagulants interfere with the synthesis of vitamin–K dependent coagulation proteins (factors II, VII, IX, and X) in the liver. Certain antibiotics (particularly some cephalosporins and other broad-spectrum antibiotics), salicylates, megadoses of vitamin E, and hepatic insufficiency increase risk of bleeding in patients with vitamin K deficiency.

Symptoms and Signs

Bleeding is the usual manifestation. Easy bruisability and mucosal bleeding (especially epistaxis, GI hemorrhage, menorrhagia, and hematuria) can occur. Oozing of blood from puncture sites or incisions may occur.

In infants, hemorrhagic disease of the newborn and late hemorrhagic disease may cause cutaneous, GI, intrathoracic, or, in the worst cases, intracranial bleeding. If obstructive jaundice develops, bleeding—if it occurs—usually begins after the 4th or 5th day. It may begin as a slow ooze from a surgical wound, the gums, the nose, or GI mucosa, or it may begin as massive bleeding into the GI tract.

Diagnosis

Vitamin K deficiency or antagonism (due to coumarin anticoagulants) is suspected when abnormal bleeding occurs in a patient at risk. Blood coagulation studies can preliminarily confirm the diagnosis. Prothrombin time (PT), usually reported as the INR, is prolonged, but partial thromboplastin time (PTT), thrombin time, platelet count, bleeding time, and levels of fibrinogen, fibrin-split products, and D-dimer are normal. If phytonadione (USP generic name for vitamin K_1) 1 mg IV significantly decreases PT within 2 to 6 h, a liver disorder is not the likely cause, and the diagnosis of vitamin K deficiency is confirmed. Some centers can detect vitamin K deficiency more directly by measuring the plasma vitamin level. The plasma level of vitamin K_1 ranges from 0.2 to 1.0 ng/mL in healthy people consuming adequate quantities of vitamin K_1 (50 to 150 μg/day). Knowing vitamin K intake can help interpret plasma levels; recent intake affects levels in plasma but not in tissues.

More sensitive indicators of vitamin K status, such as PIVKA (*P*rotein *I*nduced in *V*itamin *K* *A*bsence or *A*ntagonism) and undercarboxylated osteocalcin, are under study.

Prevention

Phytonadione 0.5 to 1 mg IM is recommended for all newborns within 1 h of birth to reduce the incidence of intracranial hemorrhage due to birth trauma. It is also used prophylactically before surgery. Some clinicians recommend that pregnant women taking anticonvulsants receive phytonadione 10 mg po once/day for the 1 mo or 20 mg po once/day for the 2 wk before delivery. The low vitamin K_1 content in breast milk can be improved by increasing maternal dietary intake of phylloquinone to 5 mg/day.

Treatment

Whenever possible, phytonadione should be given po or sc. The usual adult dose is 5 to 20 mg. (Rarely, even when phytonadione is correctly diluted and given slowly, IV replacement can result in anaphylaxis or anaphylactoid reactions.) INR usually decreases within 6 to 12 h. The dose may be repeated in 6 to 8 h if INR has not decreased satisfactorily. Phytonadione 2.5 to 10 mg po is indicated for nonemergency correction of a prolonged INR in patients taking anticoagulants. Correction usually occurs within 6 to 8 h. When only partial correction of INR is desirable (eg, when INR should remain slightly elevated because of a prosthetic heart valve), lower doses (eg, 1 to 2.5 mg) of phytonadione can be given.

In infants, bleeding due to deficiency can be corrected by giving phytonadione 1 mg sc or IM once. The dose is repeated if INR remains elevated. Higher doses may be necessary if the mother has been taking oral anticoagulants.

VITAMIN K TOXICITY

Vitamin K_1 (phylloquinone) is not toxic when consumed orally, even in large amounts. However, menadione (a synthetic, water-soluble vitamin K precursor) can cause toxicity and should not be used to treat vitamin K deficiency.

5 MINERAL DEFICIENCY AND TOXICITY

Six macrominerals are required by people in gram amounts. Four (Na, K, Ca, and Mg) are cations; two (P and Cl) are accompanying anions. Daily requirements range from 0.3 to 2.0 g.

Nine trace minerals (microminerals) are required by people in minute amounts: chromium, copper, iodine, iron, fluorine, manganese, molybdenum, selenium, and zinc. (For sources, functions, effects of deficiency and toxicity, therapeutic doses, and dietary requirements, see TABLES 5–1 and 5–2.) All trace minerals are toxic at high levels; some (arsenic, nickel, and chromium) may be carcinogens.

Mineral deficiencies (except of iron, zinc, and iodine) do not often develop spontaneously in adults on ordinary diets; infants are more vulnerable because their growth is rapid and intake varies. Trace mineral imbalances can result from hereditary disorders (eg, hemochromatosis, Wilson's disease), kidney dialysis, parenteral nutrition, or restrictive diets prescribed for people with inborn errors of metabolism. Excess intake of trace minerals (eg, selenium) can cause toxicity.

CHROMIUM

Only 1 to 3% of biologically active trivalent chromium (Cr) is absorbed. Normal plasma levels are 0.05 to 0.50 μg/L (1.0 to 9.6 nmol/L). Chromium combined with a dinicotinic-glutathione complex forms the biologically active glucose tolerance factor (present in Brewer's yeast, liver, and kidneys).

Four patients receiving long-term TPN developed possible chromium deficiency, with glucose intolerance, weight loss, ataxia, and peripheral neuropathy. Symptoms resolved in three who received trivalent chromium 150 to 250 mg.

High doses of trivalent chromium given parenterally causes skin irritation, but lower doses given orally are not toxic. Exposure to hexavalent chromium (CrO_3) in the workplace may irritate the skin, lungs, and GI tract and may cause perforation of the nasal septum and lung carcinoma.

COPPER

About half of ingested copper is absorbed. Copper absorbed in excess of metabolic requirements is excreted through bile. Copper is a component of many body proteins; almost all of the body's copper is bound within copper proteins. Unbound (free) copper ions are toxic. Genetic mechanisms control the incorporation of copper into apoproteins and the processes that prevent toxic accumulation of copper in the body.

TABLE 5–1. MINERALS

NUTRIENT	PRINCIPAL SOURCES	FUNCTIONS	EFFECTS OF DEFICIENCY AND TOXICITY	USUAL THERAPEUTIC DOSAGE
Chromium	Brewer's yeast, liver, processed meats, whole-grain cereals, spices	Promotion of glucose tolerance	**Deficiency:** Possible impaired glucose tolerance	**Deficiency:** Chromium chloride 150–250 μg/day po
Copper	Organ meats, shellfish, nuts, dried legumes, dried fruits, whole-grain cereals, peas, cocoa, mushrooms	Enzyme component, hematopoiesis, bone formation	**Deficiency:** Anemia in undernourished children, Menkes' (kinky-hair) syndrome **Toxicity:** Wilson's disease, copper poisoning	**Deficiency:** Copper sulfate 1.5–3 mg/day po
Fluorine	Seafood, vegetables, grains, tea, coffee, fluoridated water (sodium fluoride 1.0–2.0 ppm)	Bone and tooth formation	**Deficiency:** Predisposition to dental caries, possibly osteoporosis **Toxicity:** Fluorosis, mottling and pitting of permanent teeth, exostoses of spine	**Deficiency:** Sodium fluoride 1.1–2.2 mg/day po to prevent dental caries
Iodine	Seafood, iodized salt, eggs, dairy products, drinking water (content varies)	Thyroxine (T4) and triiodothyronine (T3) synthesis, development of fetus	**Deficiency:** Simple (colloid, endemic) goiter, cretinism, deaf-mutism, impaired fetal growth and brain development **Toxicity:** Hyperthyroidism or myxedema	**Primary deficiency:** Iodine 0.15 mg/day (RDA) as potassium iodide indefinitely
Iron	Many foods (except dairy products)—soybean flour, beef, kidney, liver, beans, clams, peaches	Hemoglobin and myoglobin formation, cytochrome enzymes, iron-sulfur proteins	**Deficiency:** Anemia, pica, glossitis, angular cheilosis	**Deficiency:** Ferrous sulfate or gluconate 300 mg po tid for 4–8 wk

			Toxicity: Hemochromatosis, cirrhosis, diabetes mellitus, skin pigmentation	
Manganese	Whole-grain cereals, green leafy vegetables, nuts, tea	Healthy bone structure; component of manganese-specific enzymes: glycosyltransferases, phosphoenolpyruvate carboxykinase, manganese-superoxide dismutase	**Primary deficiency:** Questionable **Toxicity:** Neurologic symptoms resembling those of parkinsonism or Wilson's disease	**Deficiency:** Manganese sulfate 10 mg/day po for several weeks or until symptoms abate
Molybdenum	Milk, legumes, whole-grain breads and cereals	Component of coenzyme for sulfite oxidase, xanthine dehydrogenase, and one aldehyde oxidase	**Deficiency:** Tachycardia, headache, nausea, obtundation (sulfite toxicity)	**Deficiency:** Ammonium molybdate 300 μg/day (IV or po) for 4 wk
Selenium	Many foods—meats, other animal products, plant-based foods (selenium content varying with soil concentration)	Component of glutathione peroxidase and thyroid hormone iodinase	**Deficiency:** Keshan disease (viral cardiomyopathy), muscle weakness **Toxicity:** Hair loss, abnormal nails, nausea, dermatitis, peripheral neuropathy	**Deficiency:** Sodium selenite 100 μg/day po
Zinc	Meat, liver, eggs, oysters, peanuts, whole grains (bioavailability variable in plant sources)	Component of enzymes, skin integrity, wound healing, growth	**Deficiency:** Impaired growth and delayed sexual maturation, hypogonadism, hypogeusia **Toxicity:** RBC microcytosis, neutropenia, impaired immunity	**Deficiency:** Elemental zinc 15–70 mg/day po for 6 mo

TABLE 5–2. RECOMMENDED DAILY INTAKES FOR MINERALS*

CATEGORY	AGE (yr) OR TIME FRAME	CHROMIUM (μg)	COPPER (μg)	FLOURIDE (mg)	IODINE (μg)	IRON (mg)	MANGANESE (mg)	MOLYBDENUM (μg)	SELENIUM (μg)	ZINC (mg)
Infants	0.0–0.6	**0.2**	**200**	NR	**110**	**0.27**	**0.3**	**2**	**15**	**2**
	0.7–1.0	**5.5**	**220**	**0.01–0.5**	**130**	11	**0.6**	**3**	**20**	**3**
Children	1–3	**11**	340	**0.7**	90	7	1.2	17	20	3
	4–8	**15**	440	**1**	90	10	1.5	22	30	5
Males	9–13	**25**	700	**2**	120	8	1.9	34	40	8
	14–18	**35**	890	**3**	150	11	2.2	43	55	11
	19–30	**35**	900	**4**	150	8	2.3	45	55	11
	31–50	**35**	900	**4**	150	8	2.3	45	55	11
	51+	**30**	900	**4**	150	8	2.3	45	55	11
Females	9–13	**21**	700	**2**	120	8	1.6	34	40	8
	14–18	**24**	890	**3**	150	15	1.6	43	55	9
	19–30	**25**	900	**3**	150	18	1.8	45	55	8
	31–50	**25**	900	**3**	150	18	1.8	45	55	8
	51+	**20**	900	**3**	150	8	1.8	45	55	8
	Pregnant	**30**	1000	**3**	220	27	2.0	50	60	11
	Breast-feeding	45	1300	**3**	290	9	2.6	50	70	12
Upper limit (UL)	Infants (< 1)	ND	ND	0.7–0.9	ND	40	ND	ND	45–60	4–5
	Children (1–8)	ND	1000–3000	1.3–2.2	200–300	40	2–3	300–600	90–150	7–12
	People (≥ 9)	ND	5,000–10,000	10	600–1100	40–45	6–11	1100–2000	280–400	23–40

*This table lists recommended dietary allowances (RDAs) in regular type and adequate intakes (AIs) in bold type. RDAs are set to meet the needs of 97 to 98% of people in a group. For healthy breastfed infants, the AI is the mean intake. The AI for other groups is believed to meet the needs of all people in the group, but because of lack of data, the percentage of people covered cannot be specified with confidence.

NR = Not recommended; ND = Not determinable because of lack of data; sources of intake should be limited to foods.

Adapted from *Dietary Reference Intakes for Vitamin A, Vitamin K, Arsenic, Boron, Chromium, Copper, Iodine, Iron, Manganese, Molybdenum, Nickel, Silicon, Vanadium, and Zinc,* Food and Nutrition Board, Institute of Medicine. Washington, DC, National Academies Press, 2002, p. 772–773.

Acquired Copper Deficiency

If the genetic mechanisms controlling copper metabolism are normal, dietary deficiency rarely causes clinically significant copper deficiency. The only reported causes are kwashiorkor, persistent infantile diarrhea (usually associated with a diet limited to milk), severe malabsorption (as in sprue), and excessive zinc intake. Deficiency may cause neutropenia, impaired bone calcification, and hypochromic anemia not responsive to iron supplements. Diagnosis is based on low serum levels of copper and ceruloplasmin. Treatment is directed at the deficiency's cause, and copper 1.5 to 3 mg/day po (usually as copper sulfate) is given.

Inherited Copper Deficiency

Inherited copper deficiency (Menkes' syndrome) occurs in male infants who inherit a mutant X-linked gene. Incidence is about 1 in 50,000 live births. Copper is deficient in the liver, serum, and essential copper proteins, including cytochrome-c oxidase, ceruloplasmin, and lysyl oxidase. Symptoms are severe mental retardation; vomiting; diarrhea; protein-losing enteropathy; hypopigmentation; bone changes; arterial rupture; and sparse, steely, or kinky hair. Diagnosis is based on low copper and ceruloplasmin levels, usually in infants < 2 wk old. Parenteral copper (given as cupric sulfate) 20 to 30 mg/kg IV once/day is the usual treatment. However, parenteral copper does not enter the copper-containing enzymes. Copper histidine 100 to 600 mg sc once/day may be more effective; monitoring is essential during treatment.

Acquired Copper Toxicity

Acquired copper toxicity can result from ingesting or absorbing excess copper (eg, from ingesting an acidic food or beverage that has had prolonged contact with a copper container). Self-limited gastroenteritis with nausea, vomiting, and diarrhea may occur. More severe toxicity results from ingestion (usually with suicidal intent) of gram quantities of a copper salt (eg, copper sulfate) or from absorption of large amounts through the skin (eg, if compresses saturated with a solution of a copper salt are applied to large areas of burned skin). Hemolytic anemia and anuria can result and may be fatal.

Indian childhood cirrhosis, non-Indian childhood cirrhosis, and idiopathic copper toxicity are probably identical disorders in which excess copper causes cirrhosis. All appear to be caused by ingesting milk that has been boiled or stored in corroded copper or brass vessels. Recent studies suggest that idiopathic copper toxicity may develop only in infants with an unknown genetic defect. Diagnosis usually requires liver biopsy, which shows Mallory hyalin bodies.

Treatment

For copper toxicity due to ingesting grams of copper, prompt gastric lavage followed by daily IM injections of at least 300 mg of dimercaprol may prevent death. The chelating drug penicillamine binds copper, facilitating its excretion. Doses of 1 to 4 g/day po may promote excretion of copper absorbed from burned skin (see also TABLE 326–4 and copper salts in TABLE 326–8). If used early, hemodialysis may be effective. Occasionally, copper toxicity is fatal despite treatment.

For Indian childhood cirrhosis, treatment with penicillamine may be curative.

Inherited Copper Toxicity

Inherited copper toxicity (Wilson's disease) results in accumulation of copper in the liver and other organs. Hepatic or neurologic symptoms develop. Diagnosis is based on a low serum ceruloplasmin level, high urinary excretion of copper, and sometimes liver biopsy results. Treatment consists of chelation, usually with penicillamine.

Wilson's disease is a progressive disorder of copper metabolism that affects 1 person in 30,000. Affected people are homozygous for the mutant recessive gene, located on chromosome 13. Heterozygous carriers, who constitute about 1.1% of the population, are asymptomatic.

Pathophysiology

Beginning at birth, copper accumulates in the liver. Serum levels of the copper protein ceruloplasmin decrease. Hepatic fibrosis develops, ultimately producing cirrhosis. Copper diffuses out of the liver into the blood, then into other tissues. It is most destructive to the brain but also damages the kidneys and reproductive organs and causes hemolytic anemia. Some copper is deposited in Descemet's membrane of the cornea.

Symptoms and Signs

Symptoms usually develop between ages 6 and 30. In almost half of patients, particularly adolescents, the first symptom is hepatitis—acute, chronic active, or fulminant. But hepatitis may develop at any time. In about 40% of patients, particularly young adults, the first symptoms reflect CNS involvement. Motor deficits are common, including any combination of tremors, dystonia, dysarthria, dysphagia, chorea, drooling, and incoordination. Sensory disturbances do not occur. Sometimes the first symptoms are behavioral or cognitive abnormalities. In 5 to 10% of patients, the first symptom is incidentally noted gold or greenish gold Kayser-Fleischer rings or crescents (due to copper deposits in the cornea), amenorrhea or repeated miscarriages, or hematuria.

Diagnosis

Wilson's disease should be suspected in a person < 40 with any of the following: an otherwise unexplained hepatic, neurologic, or psychiatric disorder; an otherwise unexplained persistent elevation in hepatic transaminase; a sibling, parent, or cousin with Wilson's disease; or fulminant hepatitis and Coombs'-negative hemolytic anemia (see p. 1047).

If Wilson's disease is suspected, slit lamp examination for Kayser-Fleischer rings is required, and serum ceruloplasmin and copper levels and 24-h urinary copper excretion are measured.

Serum ceruloplasmin (normally 20 to 35 mg/dL) is usually low in Wilson's disease but can be normal. It can also be falsely low, particularly in heterozygous carriers. If serum ceruloplasmin is low and urinary copper excretion is high, diagnosis is clear. If levels are equivocal, measuring urinary copper excretion after penicillamine is given (penicillamine provocation test) may confirm the diagnosis. If it does not, biopsy to measure hepatic copper concentration is necessary.

A low ceruloplasmin level usually means that total serum copper is low. However, the free (unbound) copper level is usually increased. Free copper can be calculated by subtracting the amount of copper in ceruloplasmin from total serum copper, or it can be measured directly.

Kayser-Fleischer rings rarely occur in other liver disorders (eg, biliary atresia, primary biliary cirrhosis). However, Kayser-Fleischer rings combined with typical motor neurologic abnormalities or a decrease in ceruloplasmin are nearly pathognomonic for Wilson's disease.

In Wilson's disease, urinary copper excretion (normally, ≤ 30 µg/day) is usually > 100 µg/day. Administration of penicillamine 500 mg po tid or qid increases excretion to > 1200 µg/day in patients with Wilson's disease but to < 500 µg/day in patients without Wilson's disease. In borderline cases, the diagnosis is made by detecting a decreased incorporation of radioactive copper into ceruloplasmin.

Hepatic copper concentration (normally, < 50 µg/g dry weight) is usually > 250 µg/g dry weight in patients with Wilson's disease. However, false-negative results may occur, because of a sampling error (due to large variations in copper concentrations in the liver) or fulminant hepatitis (causing necrosis that releases large amounts of copper).

The serum uric acid level may be low because its excretion in urine is increased.

Treatment

Continual, lifelong treatment is mandatory regardless of whether symptoms are present. Accumulated copper should be removed with chelating drugs. Copper accumulation should be prevented by a low copper diet (eg, avoiding beef liver, cashews, black-eyed peas, vegetable juice, shellfish, mushrooms, and cocoa) and by either low-dose chelation therapy or oral zinc.

Penicillamine is the chelating drug of choice. Patients aged > 5 yr receive 500 mg po tid or qid on an empty stomach (> 1 h before meals and at bedtime). Younger children receive 50 mg/kg po qid. Occasionally, use of penicillamine is associated with worsening neurologic symptoms. Pyridoxine 25 mg po once/day is given with penicillamine.

Trientine hydrochloride is less potent than penicillamine. It is started immediately at 500 mg po bid, given on an empty stomach, if penicillamine is discontinued because of an adverse effect.

Zinc acetate 50 mg po tid can prevent reaccumulation of copper in patients who cannot tolerate penicillamine or trientine or who have neurologic symptoms that do not respond to the other drugs. CAUTION: *Penicillamine or trientine must not be given with zinc because either drug can bind zinc, forming a compound with no therapeutic effect.*

Ammonium tetrathiomolybdate has an evolving role. It decreases copper absorption, binds with plasma copper, and is relatively nontoxic. It is particularly useful for neurologic symptoms because, unlike penicillamine, it does not appear to worsen neurologic symptoms during treatment.

Liver transplantation may be lifesaving for patients who have Wilson's disease with fulminant hepatic failure or severe hepatic insufficiency unresponsive to drugs.

Prognosis and Screening

Prognosis is usually good, unless disease is advanced before treatment begins. Untreated Wilson's disease is fatal, usually by age 30.

Because early treatment is most effective, screening is indicated for anyone who has a sibling, cousin, or parent with Wilson's disease. Screening consists of a slit lamp examination, liver function tests, and measurement of serum copper and ceruloplasmin and 24-h urine copper excretion. If any results are abnormal, liver biopsy is done to measure hepatic copper concentration. Infants should not be tested until after age 1 yr because ceruloplasmin levels are low during the first few months of life. Children < 6 yr with normal test results should be retested 5 to 10 yr later. Genetic testing is not feasible.

FLUORINE

Most of the body's fluorine (F) is contained in bones and teeth. Fluoride (the ionic form of fluorine) is widely distributed in nature. The main source of fluoride is drinking water.

Deficiency: Fluorine effectively prevents dental caries and possibly osteoporosis. Fluoridation of water that contains < 1 ppm (the ideal) reduces the incidence of dental caries. If a child's drinking water is not fluoridated, oral fluoride supplements can be prescribed.

Toxicity: Excess fluorine can accumulate in teeth and bones, causing fluorosis. Drinking water containing > 10 ppm is a common cause. Permanent teeth that develop during high fluorine intake are most likely to be affected. Exposure must be much greater to affect deciduous teeth. The earliest signs are chalky-white, irregularly distributed patches on the surface of the enamel; these patches become stained yellow or brown, producing a characteristic mottled appearance. Severe toxicity weakens the enamel, pitting its surface. Bony changes, including osteosclerosis, exostoses of the spine, and genu valgum, can develop but only in adults after prolonged high intake of fluorine. No tests to diagnose toxicity are available.

IODINE

In the body, iodine (I) is primarily involved in the synthesis of two thyroid hormones, thyroxine and triiodothyronine. In adults, about 80% of the iodide absorbed is trapped by the thyroid gland.

Most environmental iodine occurs in seawater; a small amount enters the atmosphere and, through rain, enters ground water and soil near the sea. Thus, people living far from the sea and at higher altitudes are at particular risk of deficiency. Fortifying table salt with iodide (typically 70 μg/g) helps ensure adequate intake (100 μg/day).

Deficiency: Deficiency is rare in areas where iodized salt is used but common worldwide. Iodine deficiency develops when iodide intake is < 20 μg/day. In mild or moderate deficiency, the thyroid gland, influenced by thyroid-stimulating hormone (TSH), hypertrophies to concentrate iodide in itself, resulting in colloid goiter. Usually, the patient remains euthyroid; however, severe iodine deficiency in adults may cause hypothyroidism (endemic myxedema). Mild or moderate deficiency decreases IQ by about 10 to 15 points. It can decrease fertility and increase risk of stillbirth, spontaneous abortion, and prenatal and infant mortality. Severe maternal iodine deficiency retards fetal growth and brain development, sometimes resulting in birth defects and, in infants, causes hypothyroidism (endemic cretinism) and deaf-mutism in a neurologic or myxedematous form.

Diagnosis is usually based on thyroid function test and imaging study findings identifying abnormalities in thyroid function and structure (see p. 1192). For large populations, urinary iodine excretion may be more specific for iodine deficiency than thyroid function abnormalities, but urinary iodine excretion may be inaccurate for individuals. These levels (normally, 100 to 200 μg/L) are 50 to 99 μg/L for mild deficiency, 20 to 49 μg/L for moderate deficiency, and < 20 μg/L for severe deficiency. WHO criteria for diagnosis in school-aged children are goiter detected by palpation, increased thyroid volume (> 97th percentile) detected by ultrasonography, and decreased urinary iodine excretion. All newborns should be screened by measuring the TSH level.

Infants with iodine deficiency are given L-thyroxine 3 μg/kg po once/day for a week plus iodide 50 μg po once/day for several weeks to quickly restore a euthyroid state. Plasma TSH levels are monitored until they are normal (ie, < 5 μIU/mL). Adults with deficiency are given iodide 150 μg once/day.

Toxicity: Chronic toxicity develops only when intake is > 2 mg/day. Use of amiodarone can also cause toxicity.

Most people who ingest excess amounts of iodine remain euthyroid. Some people who ingest excess amounts of iodine, particularly those who were previously deficient, develop hyperthyroidism (Jod-Basedow phenomenon). Paradoxically, excess uptake of iodine by the thyroid may inhibit thyroid hormone synthesis (called Wolff-Chaikoff effect). Thus, iodide toxicity can eventually cause iodide goiter, hypothyroidism, or myxedema. Very large amounts of iodide may cause a brassy taste, increased salivation, GI irritation, and acneiform skin lesions.

Diagnosis is usually based on thyroid function test and imaging study findings (see p. 1192). Iodine excretion may be more specific but is not usually measured. Treatment consists of correcting thyroid abnormalities and, if intake is excessive, dietary modification.

IRON

Iron (Fe) is a component of hemoglobin, myoglobin, and many enzymes in the body. Heme iron, contained mainly in animal products, is absorbed much better than nonheme iron, which accounts for > 85% of iron in the average diet. However, absorption of nonheme iron is increased when it is consumed with animal protein and vitamin C.

Deficiency: Iron deficiency, which can cause microcytic anemia (see p.1036), is the most common nutritional deficiency in the world. It may result from inadequate iron intake, common in infants, adolescent girls, and pregnant women. It may also result from malabsorption (eg, celiac disease). Chronic bleeding may also cause iron deficiency. Chronic bleeding due to colon cancer is a common cause in middle-aged people and the elderly. When deficiency is advanced, microcytic anemia develops. Iron toxicity can damage many organs, particularly the GI tract. All people with iron deficiency require iron supplementation.

Toxicity: Iron may accumulate in the body when a person receives iron therapy in excessive amounts or for too long, is given repeated blood transfusions, has chronic alcoholism, or takes an overdose of iron. Excess iron is toxic, causing vomiting, diarrhea, and damage to the intestine and other organs. Toxicity can also result from iron overload disease (hemochromatosis—see p. 1131), a potentially fatal but easily treatable genetic disorder in which too much iron is absorbed. Hemochromatosis affects > 1 million Americans.

MANGANESE

Manganese (Mn), necessary for healthy bone structure, is a component of several enzyme systems, including manganese-specific glycosyltransferases and phosphoenolpyruvate carboxykinase. Usual intake is 2 to 5 mg/day; absorption is 5 to 10%.

Deficiency has not been conclusively documented, although one experimental case in a volunteer resulted in transient dermatitis, hypocholesterolemia, and increased alkaline phosphatase levels. Toxicity is usually limited to people who mine and refine ore; prolonged exposure causes neurologic symptoms resembling those of parkinsonism or Wilson's disease.

MOLYBDENUM

Molybdenum (Mo) is a component of coenzymes necessary for the activity of xanthine oxidase, sulfite oxidase, and aldehyde oxidase.

Genetic and nutritional deficiencies of molybdenum have been reported but are rare. Genetic sulfite oxidase deficiency was described in 1967 in a child. It resulted from the inability to form the molybdenum coenzyme despite the presence of adequate molybdenum. The deficiency caused mental retardation, seizures, opisthotonus, and lens dislocation.

Molybdenum deficiency resulting in sulfite toxicity occurred in a patient on long-term TPN. Symptoms were tachycardia, tachypnea, headache, nausea, vomiting, and coma. Laboratory tests showed high levels of sulfite and xanthine and low levels of sulfate and uric acid in the blood and urine. Ammonium molybdate 300 μg/day IV produced dramatic recovery.

A case of molybdenum toxicity may have occurred in 1961; it caused goutlike symptoms and abnormalities of the GI tract, liver, and kidneys.

SELENIUM

Selenium (Se) is a part of the enzyme glutathione peroxidase, which metabolizes hydroperoxides formed from polyunsaturated fatty acids. Selenium is also a part of the enzymes that deiodinate thyroid hormones. Generally, selenium acts as an antioxidant that works with vitamin E. Some epidemiologic studies associate low selenium levels with cancer. In children with Down syndrome, selenium supplements help prevent bacterial infections. Plasma levels vary from 8 to 25 µg/dL, depending on selenium intake. Diagnosis is usually clinical; sometimes blood glutathione peroxidase is measured.

Deficiency: Deficiency is rare, even in New Zealand and Finland, where selenium intake is 30 to 50 µg/day, compared with 100 to 250 µg/day in the US and Canada. In certain areas of China, where intake averages 10 to 15 µg/day, selenium deficiency predisposes patients to Keshan disease, an endemic viral cardiomyopathy affecting primarily children and young women. This cardiomyopathy can be prevented but not cured by sodium selenite supplements of 50 µg/day po. Patients receiving long-term TPN have developed selenium deficiency with muscle pain and tenderness that responded to a selenomethionine supplement. In Siberian Russia and China, growing children with selenium deficiency may develop chronic osteoarthropathy (Kashin-Beck disease). Selenium deficiency may contribute synergistically with iodine deficiency to the development of goiter and hypothyroidism. Diagnosis is made by measuring selenium levels in RBCs or hair and glutathione peroxidase activity. Measuring serum selenium is less useful. Treatment consists of sodium selenite 100 µg/day po.

Toxicity: At high doses (> 900 µg/day), selenium produces toxicity. Manifestations include hair loss, abnormal nails, dermatitis, peripheral neuropathy, nausea, diarrhea, fatigue, irritability, and a garlic odor of the breath. The plasma levels may be > 100 µg/dL (> 1.27 µmol/L); however, no sensitive or specific biochemical tests for selenium are available.

ZINC

Zinc (Zn) is contained mainly in bones, teeth, hair, skin, liver, muscle, leukocytes, and testes. Zinc is a component of several hundred enzymes, including many nicotinamide adenine dinucleotide (NADH) dehydrogenases, RNA and DNA polymerases, and DNA transcription factors as well as alkaline phosphatase, superoxide dismutase, and carbonic anhydrase. A diet high in fiber and phytate (eg, containing whole-grain bread) reduces zinc absorption.

Deficiency: Dietary deficiency is uncommon in developed countries; secondary deficiency is more common. Secondary zinc deficiency develops in some patients with hepatic insufficiency (because the ability to retain zinc is lost), patients receiving diuretics, and those with diabetes mellitus, sickle cell disease, chronic renal failure, malabsorption, or stressful conditions (eg, septicemia, burns, head injury). Zinc deficiency is extremely common among elderly institutionalized and homebound patients and patients with lung cancer. Maternal zinc deficiency may cause fetal malformations and low birth weight.

Zinc deficiency in children causes impaired growth and impaired taste (hypogeusia). Other signs and symptoms in children include delayed sexual maturation and hypogonadism. In children or adults, symptoms include hypospermia, alopecia, impaired immunity, anorexia, dermatitis, night blindness, anemia, lethargy, and impaired wound healing. With secondary deficiency, testosterone deficiency, night blindness, apathy, and irritability may develop.

Zinc deficiency should be suspected in undernourished patients with typical symptoms or signs. However, because many of the symptoms and signs are nonspecific, clinical diagnosis of mild zinc deficiency is difficult. Laboratory diagnosis is also difficult. Serum levels are often inaccurate; diagnosis usually requires the combination of low levels of zinc in serum or tissues (eg, in RBCs, WBCs, platelets, saliva, hair, or nails) and increased urinary zinc excretion. If available, isotope studies can measure zinc status more accurately. Treatment consists of elemental zinc 15 to 70 mg/day po for 6 mo.

Acrodermatitis enteropathica (a rare, once fatal autosomal recessive disorder) causes malabsorption of zinc. The disorder causes psoriasiform dermatitis around the eyes, nose, and mouth; on the buttocks; and in an acral distribution. It causes hair loss, paronychia, impaired immunity, recurrent infection, impaired growth, and diarrhea. Symptoms and signs usually develop after an infant is weaned from breast milk. In such cases, doctors suspect the diagnosis, which is confirmed by measuring a low plasma, WBC, or hair zinc level. Zinc sulfate 30 to 150 mg/day po results in complete remission.

Toxicity: Toxicity is extremely rare. Ingesting doses of elemental zinc ranging from 100 to 150 mg/day interferes with copper metabolism and causes low blood copper levels, RBC microcytosis, neutropenia, and impaired immunity. Ingesting large amounts (200 to 800 mg/day), usually by consuming acidic food or drink from a galvanized (zinc-coated) container, can cause vomiting and diarrhea. Metal fume fever, also called brass-founders' ague or zinc shakes, is caused by inhaling industrial zinc oxide fumes; it results in neurologic damage. Symptoms resolve after 12 to 24 h in a zinc-free environment.

6 OBESITY AND THE METABOLIC SYNDROME

OBESITY

Obesity is severe excess body fat. Complications include cardiovascular disorders, diabetes mellitus, many cancers, cholelithiasis, fatty liver and cirrhosis, osteoarthritis, psychologic disorders, and premature death. Diagnosis is based on body mass index (BMI—calculated from height and weight) and waist circumference. Blood pressure, fasting blood glucose, and lipid levels should be measured. Treatment includes exercise, dietary and behavior modification, and sometimes drugs or surgery.

Prevalence of obesity in the US is high and is increasing. Age-adjusted prevalence was 22.9% in 1988 to 1994, increasing to 30.5% in 1999 to 2000. Prevalence of overweight (less severe excess body fat) increased from 55.9 to 64.5% during this period. Prevalence is more than twice as high at age 55 than at age 20. Obesity is twice as common among women with a lower socioeconomic status as among those with a higher status. Prevalence among black and white men does not differ significantly, but it is higher among black women than white women. More than half of black women aged ≥ 40 yr are obese; > 80% are overweight. Obesity and its complications cause as many as 300,000 premature deaths each year, making it second to cigarette smoking as a cause of death.

Etiology

Almost all cases of obesity result from chronic overeating plus inadequate exercise and a genetic predisposition. Genetic, metabolic, and other determinants usually play minor roles.

Genetic determinants: Heritability of BMI is about 33%. Genetic factors may affect the many signaling molecules and receptors used by parts of the hypothalamus and GI tract to regulate food intake (see sidebar 6–1). Rarely, obesity results from abnormal levels of peptides that regulate food intake (eg, leptin) or abnormalities in their receptors (eg, melanocortin-4 receptor). Genetic factors also regulate energy expenditure, including BMR, diet-induced thermogenesis, and nonvoluntary activity–associated thermogenesis. Genetic factors may play a larger role in determining body fat distribution, particularly abdominal fat (see Metabolic Syndrome on p. 61), than the amount of body fat.

Environmental determinants: Overweight results much more often from excess caloric intake than from slow metabolism.

Diets high in fat and refined carbohydrates promote weight gain; those high in fresh fruit and vegetables, fiber, and complex carbohydrates minimize weight gain. A sedentary lifestyle promotes weight gain.

Regulatory determinants: Maternal obesity, maternal smoking, intrauterine growth restriction, drugs, and, rarely, brain damage and endocrine disorders can disturb weight regulation. About 15% of women permanently gain ≥ 20 lb with each pregnancy. Infant or childhood obesity makes weight loss in later life more difficult.

Drugs, including corticosteroids, lithium, traditional antidepressants (tricyclics, tetracyclics, and monoamine oxidase inhibitors [MAOIs]), benzodiazepines, and antipsychotic drugs, often cause weight gain.

Rarely, brain damage caused by a tumor (especially a craniopharyngioma) or an infection (particularly affecting the hypothalamus) can stimulate consumption of excess calories. Hyperinsulinism due to pancreatic tumors may result in weight gain. Hypercortisolism due to Cushing's syndrome produces predominantly abdominal obesity. Hypothyroidism is rarely a cause of substantial weight gain.

Psychologic and behavioral determinants: Psychologic and behavioral factors are believed to be limited largely to two pathologic eating patterns: binge eating disorder and night-eating syndrome. Similar but less extreme patterns, classified as eating disorders not otherwise specified, probably contribute to excess weight gain in more people.

Binge eating disorder is consumption of large amounts of food quickly with a subjective sense of loss of control during the binge and distress after it (see p. 1703). This disorder does not include compensatory behaviors, such as vomiting. Prevalence is 1 to 3% among both sexes and 10 to 20% among people entering weight reduction programs. Obesity is usually severe, large amounts of weight are frequently gained or lost, and pronounced psychologic disturbances are present.

The **night-eating syndrome** consists of morning anorexia, evening hyperphagia, and insomnia. At least 25 to 50% of daily intake occurs after the evening meal. About 10% of people seeking treatment for severe obesity may have this disorder. However, nocturnal eating contributes to excess weight gain in many other people.

Sidebar 6–1. PATHWAYS REGULATING FOOD INTAKE

Preabsorptive and postabsorptive signals from the GI tract and changes in plasma nutrient levels provide short-term feedback to regulate food intake. GI hormones (eg, glucagon-like peptide 1 [GLP-1], cholecystokinin [CCK]) reduce food intake. Ghrelin increases food intake. Leptin, secreted from adipose tissue, informs the brain as to the state of fat stores; high leptin levels correlate with increased body fat.

The hypothalamus integrates various signals involved in the regulation of energy balance and consequently activates pathways that increase or decrease food intake. Neuropeptide Y (NPY), agouti-related peptide (ARP), α-melanocyte-stimulating hormone (α-MSH), cocaine- and amphetamine-related transcript, (CART), orexin, and melanin-concentrating hormone (MCH) increase food intake. Corticotropic hormone (CRH) and urocortin decrease it.

Complications

Insulin resistance, dyslipidemias, and hypertension develop, ultimately predisposing to diabetes mellitus and coronary artery disease. Complications are more likely if fat is concentrated abdominally. Obesity is also a risk factor for nonalcoholic fatty liver, which may lead to cirrhosis.

Obstructive sleep apnea can result if excess fat in the neck compresses the airway during sleep. Breathing stops for moments, as often as hundreds of times a night (see p. 499). This disorder, often undiagnosed, can cause loud snoring and excessive daytime sleepiness.

In the obesity-hypoventilation syndrome (Pickwickian syndrome), impaired breathing leads to hypercapnia, reduced sensitivity to CO_2 in stimulating respiration, hypoxia, cor pulmonale, and risk of premature death. This syndrome may occur alone or secondary to obstructive sleep apnea.

Degenerative arthritis, particularly affecting weight-bearing joints, may result from obesity. Skin disorders are common; increased sweat and skin secretions, trapped in thick folds of skin, are conducive to fungal and bacterial growth, making intertriginous infections especially common. Being overweight probably predisposes to cholelithiasis, polycystic ovary syndrome, gout, deep venous thrombosis and pulmonary embolism, and many cancers.

Obesity leads to social, economic, and psychologic problems as a result of prejudice, discrimination, poor body image, and low self-esteem.

Diagnosis

In adults, overweight or obesity is determined by BMI, defined as weight (kg) divided by height $(m)^2$. BMI of 25 kg/m^2 to 29.9 kg/m^2 indicates overweight; BMI $\geq$ 30 kg/m^2 indicates obesity (see TABLE 6–1). BMI is age- and race-specific; its use is limited in children and the elderly. In children and adolescents, overweight is BMI $\geq$ 95th percentile based on age- and sex-specific CDC growth charts. Asians, Japanese, and many aboriginal populations have a lower cut-off (23 kg/m^2) for overweight. Large muscle mass without excess body fat may result in a high BMI.

In whites, a waist circumference > 93 cm (> 36.3 in), particularly > 101 cm (> 39.4 in), in men or > 79 cm (> 30.8 in), particularly > 87 cm (> 33.9 in), in women is a risk factor for complications of obesity.

Body composition analysis: Body composition—the percentage of body fat and muscle—is also considered when obesity is diagnosed. The percentage of body fat can be estimated by measuring skinfold thickness or determining mid upper arm area (see p. 12). The appropriate percentage is based on the patient's demographic group. Ranges are higher for women and the elderly.

Skinfold thickness estimates body fat stores. On average, about 50% of adipose tissue is beneath the skin. This figure can vary in the elderly because of age-related atrophic changes. Skinfold thickness (consisting of a double layer of skin and subcutaneous fat) can be measured with a special caliper at subscapular, posterior triceps (triceps skinfold [TSF]), lower thoracic, iliac, and abdominal sites. A single measurement of the TSF is acceptable; this area is easily accessible and usually edema-free. Typical ranges for TSF are 0.5 to 2.5 cm (average, 1.2 cm) in healthy men and 1.2 to 3.4 cm (average, 2.0 cm) in healthy women. TSF varies with age. In the elderly, the subscapular region is more reliable.

Bioelectrical impedance analysis (BIA) can estimate percentage of body fat simply and non-

TABLE 6–1. BODY MASS INDEX (BMI)

BMI	NORMAL* 19–24	OVERWEIGHT 25–29	OBESE 30–34	35–39	EXTREMELY OBESE 40–47	48–54
Height (inches)	**Body Weight (pounds)**					
60–61	97–127	128–153	153–180	179–206	204–248	245–285
62–63	104–135	136–163	164–191	191–220	218–265	262–304
64–65	110–144	145–174	174–204	204–234	232–282	279–324
66–67	118–153	155–185	186–217	216–249	247–299	297–344
68–69	125–162	164–196	197–230	230–263	262–318	315–365
70–71	132–172	174–208	209–243	243–279	278–338	334–386
72–73	140–182	184–219	221–257	258–295	294–355	353–408
74–75	148–192	194–232	233–272	272–311	311–375	373–431
76	156–197	205–238	246–279	287–320	328–385	394–443

*BMIs less than those listed as normal are considered underweight.

invasively. BIA estimates percentage of total body water directly; percentage of body fat is derived indirectly. BIA is most reliable in healthy people and people with a limited number of chronic disorders that do not change the percentage of total body water (eg, moderate obesity, diabetes mellitus). Whether measuring BIA poses risks in people with implanted defibrillators is unclear.

Underwater (hydrostatic) weighing is the most accurate method for measuring percentage of body fat. Costly and time-consuming, it is used more often in research than in clinical care. To be weighed accurately while submerged, a person must fully exhale beforehand.

Imaging procedures, including CT, MRI, and dual-energy x-ray absorptiometry (DEXA), can also estimate the percentage and distribution of body fat but are usually used only for research.

Other testing: Obese patients should be screened for sleep apnea with an instrument such as the Epworth Sleepiness Scale. If the respiratory distress index is > 6, a polysomnographic sleep study should be done. Fasting blood glucose and plasma lipids should be measured routinely in obese patients.

Prevention

Exercise, healthful eating, and behavior changes, which improve general health, are recommended. They can control weight even in healthy people and help prevent obesity and diabetes mellitus. Also, exercise decreases the risk of cardiovascular disorders; dietary fiber decreases the risk of colon cancer and cardiovascular disorders.

Prognosis

Untreated, obesity tends to progress. After weight loss, most people return to their pretreatment weight within 5 yr. The probability and severity of complications are proportional to the severity of obesity and, independently of sex, to the waist circumference. In men, mortality and morbidity are worse, probably because abdominal adiposity is greater. However, most people treated for obesity are women, who are less likely to develop its complications.

Treatment

Weight loss of even 5 to 10% seems to improve health, increase longevity, and decrease risk of complications. In obstructive sleep apnea, a much greater weight loss is required.

Support from health care practitioners, peers, and family members and various structured programs can help with weight loss and weight maintenance.

Weight loss requires dietary modification and increased physical activity, usually with behavioral therapy. Sometimes drugs or surgery is required.

Diet: Low-fat and healthful diets, modest calorie restriction (to 1000 to 1400 kcal/day), and the substitution of some protein for carbohydrate appear to have the best long-term outcome. Fresh fruits and vegetables and fiber should be substituted for refined carbohydrates and processed food, and water for soft drinks or juices. Foods with a low glycemic index (see TABLE 1–1 on p. 3) and marine fish oils or monounsaturated fats derived from plants (eg, olive oil) reduce the risk of cardiovascular disorders and diabetes.

Diets that require atypical eating habits should be avoided. They are unlikely to be maintained, and weight increases when the patient resumes previous poor eating habits. Calorie restriction to < 1200 kcal/day cannot be sustained, but such diets are sometimes needed to achieve rapid short-term weight loss (eg, before surgery or for obstructive sleep apnea). Diets of < 800 kcal do not produce greater weight loss and are less well tolerated.

Physical activity: Exercise increases energy expenditure, BMR, and diet-induced thermogenesis. Exercise also seems to regulate appetite to more closely match caloric needs. Other benefits include increased insulin sensitivity, improved plasma lipid profile, reduced blood pressure, better aerobic fitness, and improved psychologic well-being. Strengthening (resistance) exercises increase muscle mass. Because muscle tissue burns more calories at rest than fat tissue, increasing muscle mass produces lasting increases in BMR. Exercise that is interesting and enjoyable is more likely to be sustained.

Behavioral therapy: Behavioral therapy aims to improve eating habits and physical activity level. Rigid dieting is discouraged in favor of healthy eating. Common-sense measures include avoiding high-calorie snacks, choosing healthful foods when dining out, eating slowly, and substituting a physically active hobby for a passive one. Social support, cognitive therapy, and stress management may help, particularly during the lapses usually experienced during any long-term weight loss program.

Drugs: Drugs are indicated if BMI is > 30 or if BMI is > 27 and there are complications (eg, hypertension, insulin resistance). Most weight loss due to drug treatment is modest (5 to 10%) and occurs during the first 6 mo; drugs are more useful for maintaining weight loss. Premenopausal women taking systemically acting drugs for weight control should use contraception.

Sibutramine is a centrally acting appetite suppressant that produces dose-related weight loss. The usual starting dose is 10 mg po once/day; the dose can be decreased to 5 mg or increased to 15 mg. Common adverse effects are headache, dry mouth, insomnia, and constipation; the most common serious one is hypertension. Cardiovascular disorders, particularly poorly controlled hypertension, are contraindications.

Orlistat inhibits intestinal lipase, decreasing fat absorption and improving blood glucose and lipids. Because orlistat is not absorbed, systemic effects are rare. Flatus, oily stools, and diarrhea are common but tend to resolve during the second year of treatment. A dose of 120 mg po tid should be taken with meals that include fat. A vitamin supplement should be taken at least 2 h before or after taking orlistat. Malabsorption and cholestasis are contraindications; irritable bowel syndrome and other GI disorders may make orlistat difficult to tolerate.

OTC weight-loss drugs are not recommended. Some (eg, caffeine, ephedrine, guarana, phenylpropanolamine) may be marginally effective, but their adverse effects outweigh their advantages. Others (eg, brindleberry, L-carnitine, chitosan, pectin, grapeseed extract, horse chestnut, chromium picolinate, fucus vesiculosus, ginkgo biloba) have not been shown to be effective and may have adverse effects.

Surgery: Surgery is indicated if exercise, diet, and behavioral therapy are ineffective in patients who are very obese (BMI > 40) or have serious complications. Weight loss (usually 40 to 60 kg) is proportional to the severity of obesity; losses appear to be maintained for the long term. The Roux-en-Y gastric bypass is most effective. Adjustable gastric bands placed via a laparoscope, a reversible procedure, are also effective.

Weight loss after surgery is rapid at first, slowing gradually over 2 yr. Many complications of obesity resolve; mood, self-esteem, body image, activity levels, and interpersonal and vocational effectiveness improve. If experienced surgeons perform surgery, preoperative and operative mortality is usually < 1% and operative complications are < 10%. Chronic complications depend on the procedure and may include vomiting, diarrhea, and dumping syndrome (see p. 123). Vitamin and iron deficiencies may occur but are rare if the diet is nutritionally balanced and supplements are taken.

Special Populations

Obesity is a particular concern in children and the elderly.

Children: Childhood obesity is even more worrisome than adult obesity. For obese children, complications are more likely because they are obese longer. About 20 to 25% of children and adolescents are overweight or obese. Risk factors for obesity in infants are low birth weight and maternal obesity, diabetes, and smoking. After puberty, food intake increases; in boys, the extra calories are used to increase protein deposition, but in girls, fat storage is increased.

For obese children, psychologic and musculoskeletal complications can develop early. Respiratory, metabolic, and hepatic complications may also develop. Some musculoskeletal complications, such as slipped capital femoral epiphyses, occur only in children. The risk of cardiovascular, respiratory, and other obesity-related complications increases during adulthood.

The risk of obesity persisting into adulthood is low if obesity first develops during infancy, 25% if between 6 mo and 5 yr, > 50% if after 6 yr, and > 80% if during adolescence and a parent is obese.

In children, preventing further weight gain, rather than losing weight, is a reasonable goal. Diet should be modified, and physical activity increased. Increasing general activities and play is more likely to be effective than a structured exercise program. Participating in physical activities during childhood may promote a lifelong physically active lifestyle. Drugs and surgery are avoided but, if complications of obesity are life threatening, may be warranted.

Measures that control weight and prevent obesity in children may benefit public health the most. Such measures should be implemented in the family, schools, and primary care programs.

The elderly: With aging, body fat increases and is redistributed to the abdomen, and muscle mass is lost, largely because of physical inactivity. The risk of complications depends on body fat distribution (increasing with a predominantly abdominal distribution), history of obesity, and associated sarcopenia. Increased waist circumference better predicts morbidity and mortality risk in the elderly than BMI. For the elderly, mortality risk is greater when BMI decreases; thus, increased physical activity is preferable to dietary restriction unless mobility is restricted. Physical activity also improves muscle strength, endurance, and overall well-being. Activity should include strengthening and endurance exercises. Use of weight-loss drugs has not been evaluated in the elderly; surgery is best avoided.

METABOLIC SYNDROME

Metabolic syndrome, also called syndrome X, is characterized by excess abdominal fat causing at least two of the following: insulin resistance, dyslipidemia, and hypertension. Causes, complications, diagnosis, and treatments are similar to those of obesity.

Metabolic syndrome is very common, possibly affecting almost half of people aged > 50 yr in the US. Distribution as well as amount of fat is important. The syndrome develops more often in people whose fat accumulates around the abdomen (called apple shape) and who have a high waist-to-hip ratio. The syndrome is less common among people whose fat accumulates around the hips (called pear shape) and who have a low waist-to-hip ratio.

Excess abdominal fat leads to excess free fatty acids in the portal vein, increasing fat accumulation in the liver and muscle cells. Hepatic and muscle insulin resistance, hyperinsulinemia, dyslipidemias, hypertension, and, ultimately, diabetes mellitus and coronary artery disease result. Typically, serum uric acid levels are elevated, and a prothrombotic state (with increased levels of fibrinogen and plasminogen activator inhibitor I) develops.

Patients with a higher-than-normal BMI or waist circumference should be screened for metabolic syndrome by measuring blood pressure, fasting plasma glucose, and blood lipid levels (see TABLE 6–2). Treatment is similar to that of obesity, although insulin "sensitizers" such as metformin and peroxisome peroxidase reductase receptor (PPAR) agonists may also have a role.

TABLE 6–2. CRITERIA OFTEN USED FOR DIAGNOSIS OF METABOLIC SYNDROME*

PARAMETER	VALUE
Waist circumference (cm [in])	> 102 (40) for men > 88 (34. 6) for women
Fasting glucose (mg/dL [mmol/L])	≥ 110 (6.1)
2-h postprandial glucose (mg/dL [mmol/L])	≥ 140 (7.7)
Blood pressure (mm Hg)	≥ 130/85
Triglycerides, fasting (mg/dL [mmol/L])	≥ 150 (1.7)
Low-density lipoprotein (LDL) cholesterol (mg/dL [mmol/L])	≥ 100 (2.59)
High-density lipoprotein (HDL) cholesterol (mg/dL [mmol/L])	≤ 40 (1.04) for men ≤ 50 (1.29) for women

*At least three of the parameters must be present for the diagnosis.

SECTION 2
GASTROINTESTINAL DISORDERS

7 APPROACH TO THE PATIENT WITH UPPER GI COMPLAINTS

Upper GI complaints include chest pain, chronic and recurrent abdominal pain, dyspepsia, globus sensation, halitosis (see p. 812), hiccups, nausea and vomiting, and rumination. Some upper GI complaints represent functional illness (ie, no physiologic cause found after extensive evaluation).

History: Using open-ended, interview-style questions, the physician identifies the location and quality of symptoms and any aggravating and alleviating factors. Psychologic stress factors must be specifically sought. Because a psychiatric disorder does not preclude physiologic disease, the significance of vague, dramatic, or bizarre complaints should not be minimized.

Patients report symptoms differently depending on their personality, the impact of the illness on their life, and sociocultural influences. For example, nausea and vomiting may be minimized or reported indirectly by a severely depressed patient but presented with dramatic urgency by a histrionic one.

Physical examination: Inspection of the abdomen with the patient supine may show a convex appearance when bowel obstruction, ascites, or rarely, a large mass is present. Auscultation to assess bowel sounds and determine presence of bruits should follow. Percussion elicits hyperresonance (tympany) in the presence of bowel obstruction and dullness with ascites and can determine the span of the liver. Palpation proceeds systematically, beginning gently to identify areas of tenderness and, if tolerated, palpating deeper to locate masses or organomegaly. Digital rectal examination with testing for occult blood and (in women) pelvic examination complete the evaluation of the abdomen.

Testing: Patients with acute, nonspecific symptoms (eg, dyspepsia, nausea) and an unremarkable physical examination rarely require testing. Findings suggesting significant disease (eg, hepatomegaly, blood in the stool, fever, anemia, metabolic disturbance) should prompt further evaluation. Chronic or recurrent symptoms, even with an unremarkable examination, also warrant evaluation. Specific GI tests are discussed in Ch. 9 on p. 85.

CHEST PAIN

Etiology and Pathophysiology

Midline chest pain has many causes, including GI and cardiovascular (see p. 580) disorders. Pain from esophageal disease can mimic angina pectoris.

About 50% of patients undergoing esophageal studies for chest pain have gastroesophageal reflux disease (GERD). Other esophageal disorders that cause pain include infections (bacterial, viral, or fungal), tumors, and motility disorders (eg, hyperkinetic esophageal motor disorder, achalasia, diffuse esophageal spasm).

Increased sensitivity of esophageal nerve receptors (visceral hypersensitivity) or amplification of normal afferent input (allodynia) by the spinal cord or CNS may contribute to esophageal chest pain.

Evaluation

Because symptoms overlap, many patients with esophageal disease undergo cardiac evaluation (including coronary arteriography) to exclude heart disease; some patients with coronary artery disease undergo GI studies to exclude esophageal disease.

History: Chest pain of esophageal and cardiac origin can be very similar. In both, pain can be severe and associated with exertion. Episodes last minutes to hours and can recur for days.

Heartburn is a substernal burning pain that rises in the chest and may radiate into the neck, throat, or face. It usually occurs after meals or when lying down. Heartburn may be accompanied by regurgitation into the mouth and subsequent water brash (hypersalivation occurring via vagal stimulation when acid irritates the lower esophagus). Typical heartburn suggests gastroesophageal reflux (see p. 112); however, some patients use "heartburn" for any discomfort in the mid chest and must be queried about specific symptoms.

Odynophagia is pain occurring promptly with swallowing (particularly very hot or cold food or beverages) and suggests an esophageal etiology. It occurs with or without dysphagia. The pain is described as a burning sensation or a substernal tightness.

Dysphagia is the sensation of difficulty swallowing and strongly suggests an esophageal etiology. Patients with esophageal motility disorders often have both dysphagia and odynophagia.

Physical examination: Few physical findings indicate an esophageal cause of chest pain. Cardiovascular findings are discussed on p. 580.

Testing: Chest discomfort should prompt ECG, chest x-ray, and—depending on patient age, symptoms, and risk factors—stress ECG or stress imaging studies. If cardiac disease is excluded, further studies are often deferred in favor of symptomatic treatment.

If treatment fails or dysphagia is present, the upper GI tract should be evaluated with endoscopy or contrast studies. Ambulatory pH monitoring (to exclude GERD) and esophageal manometry (with or without edrophonium) can help identify an esophageal motor disorder (see p. 110). In some centers, assessment of sensation thresholds with a balloon barostat can identify visceral hypersensitivity. Psychosocial assessment for treatable psychiatric disorders (eg, panic disorder, depression) may be helpful.

Treatment

If no etiology is discovered, symptomatic treatment includes Ca channel blockers for possible esophageal dysmotility or H_2 blockers or proton pump inhibitors for possible GERD. Psychologic treatments (eg, relaxation techniques, hypnosis, cognitive-behavioral therapy) may help if anxiety is a factor. Finally, if symptoms are frequent or disabling, low-dose antidepressants may be effective, although the mechanism is unclear.

CHRONIC AND RECURRENT ABDOMINAL PAIN

Chronic abdominal pain (CAP) persists for more than 3 mo either continuously or intermittently. Intermittent pain may be referred to as recurrent abdominal pain (RAP). Acute abdominal pain is discussed on p. 94. CAP occurs any time after 5 yr of age. Up to 10% of children require evaluation for RAP. About 2% of adults, predominantly women, have CAP.

Nearly all patients with CAP have had prior medical evaluation that did not yield a diagnosis after history, physical, and basic testing. Perhaps 10% of these patients have an occult physiologic illness, but many have a functional process. Determining whether a particular abnormality (eg, adhesions, ovarian cyst, endometriosis) is the cause of symptoms or an incidental finding can be difficult.

Etiology and Pathophysiology

CAP can have physiologic causes (see TABLE 7–1) or be a functional illness.

Functional abdominal pain syndrome (FAPS) is pain that persists > 6 mo without evidence of physiologic disease, shows no relationship to physiologic events (eg, meals, defecation, menses), and interferes with daily functioning. FAPS is poorly understood but appears to involve altered nociception. Sensory neurons in the dorsal horn of the spinal cord may become abnormally excitable and hyperalgesic from a combination of factors. Cognitive and psychologic factors (eg, depression, stress, culture, secondary gain, coping and support mechanisms) may cause efferent stimulation that amplifies pain signals, resulting in perception of pain with low level inputs and persistence of pain long after the stimulus has ceased. Additionally, the pain itself may function as a stressor, perpetuating a positive feedback loop.

Evaluation

Determining whether CAP is physiologic or functional can be difficult.

TABLE 7–1. PHYSIOLOGIC CAUSES OF CHRONIC ABDOMINAL PAIN

CAUSE	DIAGNOSTIC APPROACH
GU disorders	
Congenital abnormalities	IV urography, ultrasound
UTI	Urine culture
Pelvic inflammatory disease	Pelvic examination
Ovarian cyst, endometriosis	Gynecologic consultation
GI disorders	
Hiatus hernia	Barium swallow, fluoroscopy
Hepatitis	Liver function tests
Cholecystitis	Ultrasound
Pancreatitis	Serum amylase and lipase levels, CT
Peptic ulcer disease	Endoscopy, *Helicobacter pylori* breath test, stool examination for occult blood
Parasitic infestation (eg, giardiasis)	Stool examination for ova or parasites
Meckel's diverticulum	Technetium scan
Granulomatous enterocolitis	ESR, barium enema
Intestinal TB	Tuberculin test
Ulcerative colitis	Sigmoidoscopy, rectal biopsy
Crohn's disease	Endoscopy, x-rays, biopsy of colon or small bowel
Postoperative adhesive bands	Upper GI series, SBFT, or enteroclysis
Pancreatic pseudocyst	Ultrasound
Chronic appendicitis	Abdominal x-ray, ultrasound
Systemic disorders	
Lead intoxication	Blood lead, free RBC protoporphyrin levels
Henoch-Schönlein purpura	History, urinalysis
Sickle cell disease	Sickle preparation, Hb electrophoresis
Food allergy	Elimination diet
Abdominal epilepsy	EEG
Porphyria	Urine porphyrins
Familial Mediterranean anemia, familial angioneurotic edema, migraine equivalent	Family history

SBFT = Small-bowel follow through

Adapted from Barbero GJ: "Recurrent abdominal pain." *Pediatrics in Review* 4:30, 1982; reproduced by permission of *Pediatrics in Review*.

History and physical examination: Physiologic causes produce pain that is well localized, especially to areas other than the periumbilical region. It frequently wakes the patient and may radiate to the back. Associated findings that indicate a high risk of significant underlying disease include anorexia; recurrent or persistent fever; jaundice; anemia; hematuria; joint symptoms; edema; weight loss; blood in the stools; hematemesis; changes in bowel consistency, color, or elimination pattern; and abdominal distention, mass, or hepatomegaly. Intermittent pain from a structural cause tends to occur with particular activities or is related to diet, eating, or defecation.

Functional CAP may result in pain similar to that of physiologic origin. However, there are no associated findings indicating high risk, and psychosocial features are prominent. A history of physical or sexual abuse further suggests functional CAP. An unresolved loss, such as divorce, miscarriage, or death of a family member, may be a clue. Patients often have a psychologic or personality disorder and may have evidence of impaired functioning in work, school, family, and social settings. Pain is often a central feature of the patient's life, resulting in a "pain career." A family history of chronic somatic complaints or pain, peptic ulcer disease, headaches, "nerves," or depression is common.

Children with functional CAP may demonstrate immaturity, unusual dependence on parents, anxiety or depression, apprehension, tension, and perfectionism. Often, parents perceive the child as special because of the position in the family (eg, only child, youngest child, only male or female in a large sibship) or because of a medical problem (eg, colic, eating difficulty). Parents are often anxious, overprotective, authoritarian, and preoccupied with the child.

Testing: In general, simple tests (including urinalysis, CBC, liver function tests, ESR, amylase, and lipase) should be performed. Abnormalities in these tests, or the presence of high-risk symptoms and signs, mandate further testing, even if previous work-ups have been negative. Specific tests depend on the findings but typically include CT of the abdomen and pelvis with contrast, upper GI endoscopy or colonoscopy, and perhaps small-bowel x-rays.

The benefits of testing patients with no high-risk symptoms and signs are unclear. Those > 50 should probably have a colonoscopy; those ≤ 50 can be observed or have CT of the abdomen and pelvis with contrast if an imaging study is desired. ERCP and laparoscopy are rarely helpful in the absence of specific indications.

Between the initial evaluation and the follow-up visit, the patient (or family, if the patient is a child) should record any pain, including its nature, intensity, duration, and precipitating factors. Diet, defecation pattern, and any remedies tried (and the results obtained) should also be recorded. This record may reveal inappropriate behavior patterns and exaggerated responses to pain or otherwise suggest a diagnosis. A specific inquiry as to whether milk and milk products cause abdominal cramps, bloating, or distention is needed, as lactose intolerance is common, especially in blacks.

Prognosis and Treatment

Physiologic conditions are treated. If the diagnosis of functional CAP is made, frequent examinations and tests should be avoided because they may focus on or magnify the physical complaints or imply that the physician lacks confidence in the diagnosis.

There are no modalities to cure functional CAP; however, many palliative measures are available. These measures rest on a foundation of a trusting, empathic relationship between the physician, patient, and family. The patient should be reassured that he is not in danger; specific concerns should be sought and addressed. The physician should explain the laboratory findings and the nature of the problem and describe how the pain is generated and how the patient perceives it (ie, that there is a constitutional tendency to feel pain at times of stress). It is important to avoid perpetuating the negative psychosocial consequences of chronic pain (eg, prolonged absences from school or work, withdrawal from social activities) and to promote independence, social participation, and self-reliance. These strategies help the patient control or tolerate the symptoms while participating fully in everyday activities.

Except for occasional use of NSAIDs and perhaps tricyclic antidepressants, drugs are ineffective. Opioids should be avoided as they invariably lead to dependency.

Cognitive methods (eg, relaxation training, biofeedback, hypnosis) may help by contributing to the patient's sense of well-being and control. Regular follow-up visits should be scheduled weekly, monthly, or bimonthly, depending on the patient's needs, and should continue until well after the problem has resolved. Psychiatric referral may be required if symptoms persist, especially if the patient is depressed or there are significant psychologic difficulties in the family.

School personnel should become involved for children with CAP. The child can rest briefly in the nurse's office during the school day, with the expectation that he will return to class after 15 to 30 min. The school nurse can be authorized to dispense a mild analgesic (eg, acetaminophen). The nurse can sometimes allow the child to call a parent, who should encourage the child to stay in school. However, as parents stop treating their child as special or ill, the symptoms may worsen before they abate.

DYSPEPSIA

Dyspepsia is a sensation of pain or discomfort in the upper abdomen. It may be described as indigestion, gassiness, early satiety, postprandial fullness, gnawing, or burning.

Etiology

Common causes of dyspepsia include peptic ulcer disease, motility disorders, gastroesophageal reflux, drugs (eg, erythromycin, NSAIDs, alendronate), and esophageal or gastric malignancy. However, many patients have no physical abnormalities (functional or nonulcer dyspepsia). Others have findings (eg, duodenitis, pyloric dysfunction, motility disturbance, *Helicobacter pylori* gastritis, lactose deficiency, cholelithiasis) that correlate poorly with symptoms (ie, correction of the condition does not alleviate dyspepsia).

Evaluation

History: Symptoms are sometimes classified as ulcer-like, dysmotility-like, or reflux-like; these classifications suggest but do not confirm an etiology. Ulcer-like symptoms consist of pain that is localized in the epigastrium, frequently occurs before meals, and is relieved by food, antacids, or H_2 blockers. Dysmotility-like symptoms consist of discomfort rather than pain, along with early satiety, postprandial fullness, nausea, vomiting, bloating, and symptoms that are worsened by food. Reflux-like symptoms consist of heartburn or acid regurgitation. However, symptoms often overlap.

Alternating constipation and diarrhea with dyspepsia suggests irritable bowel syndrome or abuse of over-the-counter laxatives or antidiarrheals.

Alarm symptoms in dyspepsia include anorexia, nausea, emesis, weight loss, anemia, blood in the stools, dysphagia, odynophagia, and failure to respond to standard therapy such as H_2 blockers.

Physical examination: Examination rarely suggests a cause of dyspepsia, although occult blood in the stool should prompt further testing.

Testing: Routine tests include CBC and stool testing for occult blood (to exclude GI blood loss) and routine blood chemistries. If results are abnormal, additional tests (eg, imaging studies, endoscopy) should be considered. Because of the risk of malignancy, patients > 45 and those with new onset of alarm symptoms should undergo upper GI endoscopy. For patients < 45 without alarm symptoms, some authorities recommend empiric therapy with antisecretory or prokinetic agents followed by endoscopy in treatment failures. Others recommend screening for *H. pylori* infection with a C_{14}-urea breath test or stool assay (see p. 116). However, caution is required in using *H. pylori* or any other nonspecific findings to explain symptoms.

Esophageal manometry and pH studies are indicated if reflux symptoms persist after upper GI endoscopy and a 2- to 4-wk trial with a proton pump inhibitor.

Treatment

Specific conditions are treated. Patients without identifiable conditions are observed over time and reassured. Symptoms are treated with proton pump inhibitors, H_2 blockers, or a cytoprotective agent (eg, sucralfate). Prokinetic drugs (eg, metoclopramide, erythromycin) given as a liquid suspension also may be tried in patients with dysmotility-like dyspepsia. However, there is no clear evidence that matching the drug class to the specific symptoms (eg, reflux vs. dysmotility) makes a difference. Misoprostol and anticholinergics are not effective in functional dyspepsia. Drugs that alter sensory perception (eg, tricyclic antidepressants) may be helpful.

GLOBUS SENSATION

Globus sensation ("lump in the throat," globus hystericus) is the sensation of a lump or mass in the throat, unrelated to swallowing, when no mass is present.

Etiology

No specific etiology or physiologic mechanism has been established. Some studies suggest that elevated cricopharyngeal (upper esophageal sphincter) pressure or abnormal hypopharyngeal motility occur during the time of symptoms. The sensation may also result from gastroesophageal reflux disease (GERD) or from frequent swallowing and drying of the throat associated with anxiety or another emotional state. Although not associated with stress factors or a specific psychiatric disorder, globus sensation may be a symptom of certain mood states (eg, grief, pride); some patients may have a predisposition to this response.

Disorders that can be confused with globus sensation include cricopharyngeal (upper esophageal) webs, symptomatic diffuse esophageal spasm, GERD, skeletal muscle disorders (eg, myasthenia gravis, myotonia dystrophica, polymyositis), and mass lesions in the neck or mediastinum that cause esophageal compression.

Evaluation

True dysphagia, which suggests a structural or motor disorder of the pharynx or esophagus, can usually be identified clinically.

History: Symptoms of globus sensation do not worsen during swallowing. Food does not stick in the throat, and eating or drinking often provides relief. Pain or weight loss does not occur. Chronic symptoms may occur during unresolved or pathologic grief and may be relieved by crying.

Physical examination: Palpation of the neck and floor of the mouth and inspection of the oropharynx (including direct laryngoscopy) are unremarkable in patients with globus sensation. Observed swallowing and swallowing time (see p. 108) are normal.

Testing: If the diagnosis is unclear or the clinician cannot adequately visualize the pharynx, specialty referral is appropriate. Plain or video esophagography, chest x-ray, or esophageal manometry as indicated by the clinical data may exclude other disorders.

Treatment

Treatment involves reassurance and sympathetic concern. No drug is of proven benefit. Underlying depression, anxiety, or other behavioral disturbances should be managed supportively, with psychiatric referral if necessary. At times, communicating to the patient the association between symptoms and mood state can be beneficial.

HICCUPS

Hiccups (hiccough, singultus) are repeated involuntary spasms of the diaphragm followed by sudden closure of the glottis, which checks the inflow of air and produces the characteristic sound. Transient episodes are very common. Persistent (> 2 days) and intractable (> 1 mo) hiccups are uncommon but quite distressing.

Etiology

Hiccups follow irritation of afferent or efferent diaphragmatic nerves or of medullary centers that control the respiratory muscles, particularly the diaphragm. Hiccups are more common in men.

Cause is generally unknown, but transient hiccups are often caused by gastric distention, alcohol consumption, or swallowing hot or irritating substances. Persistent and intractable hiccups have myriad causes, including often gastroesophageal reflux disease (GERD) and other esophageal disorders. Additional abdominal causes are bowel diseases, pancreatitis, pregnancy, gallbladder disease, hepatic metastases, hepatitis, and abdominal surgery. Thoracic and mediastinal lesions, including diaphragmatic pleurisy, pneumonia, pericarditis, or surgery may be responsible. Metabolic disorders include uremia and alcoholism. Posterior fossa tumors or infarcts may cause hiccups by stimulating centers in the medullary reticular formation.

Evaluation and Treatment

No specific evaluation is required for acute hiccups if routine history and physical examination are unremarkable; abnormalities are pursued with appropriate testing. Hiccups of longer duration and no obvious cause should have testing, probably including serum electrolytes, BUN and creatinine, chest x-ray, and ECG. Upper GI endoscopy and perhaps esophageal pH monitoring should be considered. If these are unremarkable, MRI of the brain and CT of the chest may be performed. Identified problems are treated (eg, proton pump inhibitors for GERD, dilation for esophageal stricture).

Symptomatic relief: Many simple measures can be tried, although none are more than slightly effective: $Paco_2$ can be increased and diaphragmatic activity inhibited by a series of deep breath-holdings or by breathing deeply into and out of a paper bag. (CAUTION: *Plastic bags can cling to the nostrils and should not be used.*) Vagal stimulation by pharyngeal irritation (eg, swallowing dry bread, granulated sugar, or crushed ice, applying traction on the tongue, stimulating gagging) may work. Numerous other folk remedies exist.

Persistent hiccups are often recalcitrant to treatment. Many drugs have been used in anecdotal series. Baclofen, a γ-aminobutyric acid agonist, 5 mg po q 6 h increasing to 20 mg/dose, may be effective. Other drugs include chlorpromazine 25 to 50 mg IV q 6 h, metoclopramide 10 mg po bid to qid, and various anticonvulsants. Additionally, an empiric trial of proton pump inhibitors may be given. In intractable cases, the phrenic nerve may be blocked by small amounts of 0.5% procaine solution, with caution being taken to avoid respiratory depression and pneumothorax. Even bilateral phrenicotomy does not cure all cases.

NAUSEA AND VOMITING

Nausea, the unpleasant feeling of needing to vomit, represents awareness of afferent stimuli (including increased parasympathetic tone) to the medullary vomiting center. Vomiting is the forceful expulsion of gastric contents produced by involuntary contraction of the abdominal musculature when the gastric fundus and lower esophageal sphincter are relaxed. Vomiting should be distinguished from regurgitation, the spitting up of gastric contents without associated nausea or forceful abdominal muscular contractions.

Etiology and Pathophysiology

Nausea and vomiting occur in response to conditions that affect the vomiting center. Some conditions originate in the GI tract (eg, gastric or intestinal obstruction, acute gastroenteritis, peptic ulcer disease, gastroparesis, cholecystitis, choledocholithiasis, perforated viscus or other acute abdomen, ingestion of noxious substances); others originate in other parts of the body (eg, pregnancy, systemic infection, radiation exposure, drug toxicity, diabetic ketoacidosis, cancer) or the CNS (eg, increased intracranial pressure, stimulation of the vestibular center, pain, meningitis, head trauma, tumor).

Psychogenic vomiting can be self-induced or occur involuntarily in stressful or unpleasant situations. Psychologic factors leading to vomiting can be culturally determined (eg, eating food considered repulsive). Vomiting can express hostility, as when a child vomits during a temper tantrum, or be a symptom of a conversion disorder.

Cyclic vomiting syndrome is an uncommon disorder characterized by severe, discrete attacks of vomiting or sometimes only nausea that occur at varying intervals, with normal health between episodes. It is most common in childhood (mean age of onset 5 yr) and tends to remit with adulthood. The condition may be associated with migraine headaches, possibly representing a migraine variant.

Acute, severe vomiting can lead to symptomatic dehydration and electrolyte abnormalities. Chronic vomiting can result in malnutrition, weight loss, and metabolic abnormalities.

Evaluation

History and physical examination: Diarrhea and fever suggest infectious gastroenteritis. Vomiting undigested food suggests achalasia or a Zenker's diverticulum. Vomiting partially digested food more than a few hours after ingestion suggests gastric outlet obstruction or gastroparesis. Headache, mental status change, or papilledema suggests a CNS etiology. Tinnitus or vertigo suggests a labyrinthine disorder. Obstipation and abdominal distention suggest bowel obstruction.

Vomiting that occurs at the thought of food or is not temporally related to eating suggests a psychogenic cause, as does personal or family history of functional nausea and vomiting. Patients should be questioned about the relationship between vomiting and stressful events because they may not recognize the association or even admit to feeling distress at those times.

Testing: All females of childbearing age should have a urine pregnancy test. Patients with severe vomiting, vomiting lasting over 1 day, or signs of dehydration on examination should have other laboratory tests (eg, electrolytes, BUN, creatinine, glucose, urinalysis, and sometimes liver function tests). Patients with symptoms or signs of obstruction or perforation should have flat and upright abdominal x-rays. The work-up of chronic vomiting usually includes upper GI endoscopy, small-bowel x-rays, and tests to assess gastric emptying and antral-duodenal motility.

Treatment

Specific conditions, including dehydration, are treated. Even without significant dehydration, IV fluid therapy (0.9% saline 1 L, or 20 mL/kg in children) often leads to reduction of symptoms. In adults, antiemetics (eg, prochlorperazine 5 to 10 mg IV or 25 mg per rectum) are effective for most acute vomiting. Additional useful drugs include metoclopramide 5 to 20 mg po or IV tid to qid and a scopolamine patch (1 mg over 72 h). Drugs are usually avoided in children because of side effects. Antihistamines (eg, dimenhydrinate 50 mg po q 4 to 6 h and meclizine 25 mg po q 8 h) are useful in treating vomiting of labyrinthine origin. Vomiting secondary to chemotherapeutic drugs may require 5-HT_3 antagonists (eg, ondansetron, granisetron); for highly emetogenic chemotherapeutic drugs, a new substance-P neurokinin 1 inhibitor, prepitant, can be added.

For psychogenic vomiting, reassurance indicates awareness of the patient's discomfort and a desire to work toward relief of symptoms, regardless of cause. Comments such as "nothing is wrong" or "the problem is emotional" should be avoided. Brief symptomatic treatment with antiemetics can be tried. If long-term management is necessary, supportive, regular office visits may help resolve the underlying problem.

RUMINATION

Rumination is the (usually involuntary) regurgitation of small amounts of food from the stomach (most often 15 to 30 min after eating) that are re-chewed and, in most cases, again swallowed.

Rumination is commonly observed in infants. The incidence in adults is unknown, as it is rarely reported by patients themselves. The pathophysiology is poorly understood. The reverse peristalsis in ruminants has not been reported in humans. The disorder is probably a learned, maladaptive habit and may be part of an eating disorder. The person learns to open the lower esophageal sphincter and propel gastric contents into the esophagus and throat by increasing gastric pressure via rhythmic contraction and relaxation of the diaphragm.

Symptoms and Diagnosis

Nausea, pain, and dysphagia do not occur. During periods of stress, the patient may be less careful about concealing rumination. Seeing the act for the first time, others may refer the patient to a physician. Rarely, patients regurgitate and expel enough food to lose weight.

Rumination is usually diagnosed through observation. A psychosocial history may disclose underlying emotional stress. Endoscopy or an upper GI series is necessary to exclude disorders causing mechanical obstruction or Zenker's diverticulum. Esophageal manometry and tests to assess gastric emptying and antral-duodenal motility may be used to identify a motility disturbance.

Treatment

Treatment is supportive. Drug therapy generally does not help. Motivated patients may respond to behavioral techniques (eg, relaxation, biofeedback). Psychiatric consultation may be helpful.

FUNCTIONAL GI ILLNESS

Often, no physiologic cause for GI complaints is found, even after extensive evaluation. Such patients are said to have functional illness, which accounts for 30 to 50% of referrals to gastroenterologists. Functional illness may manifest with upper and/or lower GI symptoms.

The reasons for functional symptoms are not clear. Some evidence suggests that such patients have visceral hypersensitivity, a disturbance of nociception in which they experience discomfort from sensations (eg, luminal distention, peristalsis) that other people do not find distressing. In some patients, psychologic conditions such as anxiety (with or without aerophagia), conversion disorder, somatization in depression, or hypochondriasis are associated with GI symptoms. Psychologic theories hold that functional symptoms may satisfy certain psychologic needs. For example, some patients with chronic illness derive secondary benefits from being sick. For such patients, successful treatment of symptoms may lead to development of other symptoms.

Many referring physicians and GI specialists find functional GI complaints difficult to understand and treat, and uncertainty may lead to frustration and judgmental attitudes. Physicians should avoid ordering repeated studies or multiple drug trials for the insistent patient with inexplicable complaints. When symptoms are not suggestive of serious illness, the physician should wait rather than embark on another diagnostic or therapeutic plan. In time, new information may direct evaluation and management. Functional complaints are sometimes present in patients with physiologic disease (eg, peptic ulcer, esophagitis); such symptoms may not remit even when a physiologic illness is addressed.

8 APPROACH TO THE PATIENT WITH LOWER GI COMPLAINTS

Lower GI complaints include constipation, diarrhea, gas and bloating, abdominal pain (see also p. 94), and rectal pain or bleeding (see Ch. 20 on p. 162). As with upper GI complaints, complaints result from physiologic illness or represent a functional disorder (ie, no physiologic cause found even after extensive evaluation). The reasons for functional symptoms are not clear. Evidence suggests that patients with functional symptoms have a disturbance of nociception; ie, they perceive as uncomfortable sensations (eg, luminal distention, peristalsis) that other people do not find distressing.

No bodily function is more variable and subject to external influences than defecation. Bowel habits vary considerably from person to person and are affected by age, physiology, diet, and social and cultural influences. Some individuals have unwarranted preoccupation with bowel habits. In Western society, normal stool frequency ranges from 2 to 3/day to 2 to 3/wk. Changes in stool frequency, consistency, volume, or composition (ie, presence of blood, mucus, pus, or excess fatty material) may indicate disease.

CONSTIPATION

Constipation is difficult or infrequent passage of stool, hardness of stool, or a feeling of incomplete evacuation.

Many people incorrectly believe that daily defecation is necessary and complain of constipation if stools occur less frequently. Others are concerned with the appearance (size, shape, color) or consistency of stools. Sometimes the major complaint is dissatisfaction with the act of defecation. Constipation is blamed for many complaints (abdominal pain, nausea, fatigue, anorexia) that are actually symptoms of an underlying problem (eg, irritable bowel syndrome, depression). Patients should not expect all symptoms to be relieved by a daily bowel movement.

Because of these concerns, many people abuse the colon with laxatives, suppositories, and enemas. This can result in colonic inertia and physical changes in the colon, including cathartic colon (a "pipe stem" colon lacking haustra seen on barium enema examination, thus mimicking ulcerative colitis) and melanosis coli (deposits of brown pigment in the mucosa, seen on endoscopy and in colonic biopsy specimens).

Obsessive-compulsive patients often feel the need to rid the body daily of "unclean" wastes. Depression may result from the failure to defecate daily. A cycle may develop in which depression reduces stool frequency and failure to defecate augments depression. Such patients often spend excessive time on the toilet or become chronic users of cathartics.

Etiology

Acute constipation suggests a physiologic cause; chronic constipation can be physiologic or functional (see TABLE 8–1).

In colonic inertia, the colon does not respond to the usual stimuli—eating and physical activity—that promote evacuation, or those stimuli are lacking. The patient passes stool infrequently but does not feel a need to defecate. Inertia typically occurs when rectal sensitivity to fecal masses is dulled by habitual disregard of the urge to defecate or by prolonged use of laxatives or enemas. It is common in elderly people because of age-related decreases in intrinsic colonic reflexes, low-fiber diets, lack of exercise, and use of constipating drugs.

Fecal impaction, which may cause or develop from constipation, is particularly common in elderly patients. With aging, rectal capacity increases, and colonic motility decreases, particularly with prolonged bed rest or decreased physical activity. It is also common after barium has been given by mouth or enema. The patient has rectal pain and tenesmus and makes repeated but futile attempts to defecate. The patient may have cramps and may pass watery mucus or fecal material around the impacted mass, mimicking diarrhea (paradoxic diarrhea). Rectal examination discloses a firm, sometimes rocklike, but often puttylike mass.

TABLE 8–1. CAUSES OF CONSTIPATION

CAUSE	EXAMPLES
Acute constipation	
Acute bowel obstruction	Volvulus, hernia, adhesions, fecal impaction
Adynamic ileus	Peritonitis, head or spinal trauma, bed rest
Drugs	Anticholinergics (antipsychotics, antiparkinsonians, antispasmodics), cations (iron, aluminum, Ca, barium, bismuth), opioids, general anesthesia
Chronic constipation	
Colonic tumor	
Metabolic disorders	Diabetes mellitus, hypothyroidism, hypercalcemia, uremia, porphyria
Central nervous system disorders	Parkinson's disease, multiple sclerosis, stroke, spinal cord lesions
Peripheral nervous system disorders	Hirschsprung's disease, neurofibromatosis, autonomic neuropathy
Systemic disorders	Systemic sclerosis, amyloidosis, dermatomyositis, myotonic dystrophy
Functional	Colonic inertia, irritable bowel syndrome

Evaluation

History: A lifetime history of the patient's stool frequency, consistency, and color should be obtained, including use of laxatives or enemas. Some patients deny previous constipation but, when questioned specifically, admit to spending 15 to 20 min per bowel movement. Symptoms of metabolic or neurologic conditions should be sought. Prescription and nonprescription drug use should be queried.

Chronic constipation with frequent laxative use suggests colonic inertia. Chronic constipation without the sensation of a need to defecate suggests a neurologic disorder. Chronic constipation alternating with diarrhea and associated with intermittent abdominal pain suggests irritable bowel syndrome (see p. 82). New-onset constipation that persists for weeks or occurs intermittently with increasing frequency or severity suggests colonic tumor or other causes of partial obstruction. Reduced stool size suggests an obstructive lesion in the distal colon or irritable bowel syndrome.

Physical examination: A general examination is performed for signs of systemic disease, including fever and cachexia. A tense, distended, tympanitic abdomen indicates mechanical obstruction. Abdominal masses should be sought by palpation, and a rectal examination should be performed to evaluate tone; sensation; and presence of fissures, strictures, blood, or masses (including fecal impaction).

Testing: Constipation with a clear etiology (drugs, trauma, bed rest) may be treated symptomatically without further study. Patients with symptoms of bowel obstruction require flat and upright abdominal x-rays and possibly a CT scan (see also p. 104). Most patients without a clear etiology should have sigmoidoscopy or colonoscopy and a laboratory evaluation (CBC, thyroid-stimulating hormone, fasting glucose, electrolytes, and Ca).

Further tests are usually reserved for patients with abnormal findings on the above tests or who do not respond to symptomatic treatment. If the primary complaint is infrequent defecation, colonic transit times should be measured with radiopaque markers. If the primary complaint is straining with defecation, anorectal manometry is best.

Treatment

Any identified conditions should be treated. Whenever possible, drugs that cause constipation should be stopped.

Agents used to treat constipation are summarized in TABLE 8–2. Adequate water intake (generally at least 2 L/day) is essential.

TABLE 8–2. AGENTS USED TO TREAT CONSTIPATION

TYPE	AGENT	DOSAGE	SIDE EFFECTS
Fiber	Bran	Up to 1 cup/day	Bloating, flatulence, iron and Ca malabsorption
	Psyllium	Up to 30 g/day in divided doses of 2.5–7.5 g	Bloating, flatulence
	Methylcellulose	Up to 9 g/day in divided doses of 0.45–3 g	Less bloating than other fiber agents
	Ca polycarbophil	2–6 tablets/day	Bloating, flatulence
Emollients	Docusate Na	100 mg bid or tid	Ineffective for severe constipation
	Glycerin	2–3 g suppository, once/day	Rectal irritation
	Mineral oil	15–45 mL po once/day	Lipid pneumonia, malabsorption of fat-soluble vitamins, dehydration, fecal incontinence
Osmotic agents	Sorbitol	15–30 mL po of 70% solution once/day or bid; 120 mL rectally of 25–30% solution	Transient abdominal cramps, flatulence
	Lactulose	10–20 g (15–30 mL) once/day up to qid	Same as for sorbitol
	Polyethylene glycol	Up to 3.8 L during a 4-h period	Fecal incontinence (related to dosage)
Stimulants	Anthraquinones	Depends on brand used	Degeneration of Meissner's and Auerbach's plexus, malabsorption, abdominal cramps, dehydration, melanosis coli
	Bisacodyl	10-mg suppositories up to 3 times/wk; 5–15 mg/day po	Fecal incontinence, hypokalemia, abdominal cramps, rectal burning with daily use of suppository form
Saline laxative	Mg	Mg sulfate 15–30 g/day or bid; milk of Mg, 30–60 mL/day; Mg citrate, 150–300 mL/day (up to 360 mL)	Mg toxicity, dehydration, abdominal cramps, fecal incontinence
Enemas	Mineral oil/olive oil retention	100–250 mL/day rectally	Fecal incontinence, mechanical trauma
	Tap water	500 mL rectally	Mechanical trauma
	Phosphate	60 mL rectally	Accumulated damage to rectal mucosa, hyperphosphatemia, mechanical trauma
	Soapsuds	1500 mL rectally	Accumulated damage to rectal mucosa, mechanical trauma

Adapted from Romero Y, Evans JM, Fleming KC, Phillips SF: Constipation and fecal incontinence in the elderly population. *Mayo Clinic Proceedings* 71:81-92, 1996; by permission.

The diet should contain enough fiber (typically 20 to 30 g/day) to ensure adequate stool bulk. Vegetable fiber, which is largely indigestible and unabsorbable, increases stool bulk. Certain components of fiber also absorb fluid, making stools softer and facilitating their passage. Fruits and vegetables are recommended sources, as are cereals containing bran.

Laxatives should be used carefully. Some (eg, phosphate, bran, cellulose) bind drugs and interfere with absorption. Rapid fecal transit may rush some drugs and nutrients beyond their optimal absorptive locus. Contraindications to laxative and cathartic use include acute abdominal pain of unknown origin, inflammatory bowel disorders, intestinal obstruction, GI bleeding, and fecal impaction.

Behavioral changes may help. The patient should try to move the bowel at the same time daily, preferably 15 to 45 min after breakfast, because food ingestion stimulates colonic motility. Initial efforts at regular, unhurried bowel movements may be aided by glycerin suppositories.

Explanation is important, but it is difficult to convince obsessive-compulsive patients that their attitude toward defecation is abnormal. Physicians must explain that daily bowel movements are not essential, that the bowel must be given a chance to function, and that frequent use of laxatives or enemas (> once/3 days) denies the bowel that chance.

Types of laxatives: Bulking agents (eg, psyllium, Ca polycarbophil, methylcellulose) are the only laxatives acceptable for long-term use. Some patients prefer unrefined miller's bran 16 to 20 g (2 to 3 tsp) on fruit or cereal. Bulking agents act slowly and gently and are the safest agents for promoting elimination. Proper use involves gradually increasing the dose—ideally, taken tid or qid with sufficient liquid (eg, 500 mL/day of extra fluid) to prevent impaction—until a softer, bulkier stool results. Bulking agents produce natural effects and, unlike other laxatives, do not lead to colonic inertia.

Emollient agents (eg, docusate, mineral oil, glycerine suppositories) act slowly to soften stools, making them easier to pass. However, they are not potent stimulators of defecation. Docusate is a surfactant, which allows water to enter the fecal mass to soften and increase its bulk. Increased bulk may stimulate peristalsis, which moves the softened stool more easily. Mineral oil softens fecal matter but may decrease absorption of fat-soluble vitamins. Emollients may be useful after MI or anorectal surgery and when prolonged bed rest is required.

Osmotic agents are used to prepare patients for some diagnostic bowel procedures and occasionally to treat parasitic diseases. They are also effective in constipation. They contain poorly absorbed polyvalent ions (eg, Mg, phosphate, sulfate) or carbohydrates (eg, lactulose, sorbitol) that remain in the bowel, increasing intraluminal osmotic pressure and thereby drawing water into the intestine. The increased volume stimulates peristalsis. These agents usually work within 3 h.

The occasional use of osmotic laxatives is harmless. However, Mg and phosphate are partially absorbed and may be detrimental in some conditions (eg, renal insufficiency). Na (in some preparations) may exacerbate heart failure. In large or frequent doses, these drugs may upset fluid and electrolyte balance. Another approach to cleansing the bowel for diagnostic tests or surgery uses large volumes of a balanced osmotic agent (eg, polyethylene glycol–electrolyte solution) taken by mouth or nasogastric tube.

Secretory or stimulant cathartics (eg, senna and its derivatives, cascara, phenolphthalein, bisacodyl, castor oil, anthraquinones) act by irritating the intestinal mucosa or by directly stimulating the submucosal and myenteric plexus. Some are absorbed, metabolized by the liver, and returned to the bowel in bile. Peristalsis and intraluminal fluid both increase, with cramping and passage of semisolid stool in 6 to 8 h. In addition to treating constipation, these agents are often used to cleanse the bowel for diagnostic tests. With continued use, melanosis coli, neuronal degeneration in the colon, "lazy bowel" syndrome, and serious fluid and electrolyte disturbances may develop. Phenol-phthalein has been removed from the US market because of teratogenicity in animals.

Enemas can be used, including tap water and commercially prepared hypertonic solutions.

Fecal impaction: Fecal impaction is treated initially with enemas of tap water followed by small enemas (100 mL) of commercially prepared hypertonic solutions (eg, Na phosphate). If these fail, manual fragmentation and disimpaction of the mass will be necessary. This procedure is painful, so perirectal and intrarectal application of local anesthetics (eg, lidocaine 5% ointment or dibucaine 1% ointment) is recommended. Some patients require sedation.

DYSCHEZIA

(Disordered Evacuation; Dysfunction of Pelvic Floor or Anal Sphincters)

Dyschezia is difficulty defecating. Patients sense the presence of stool and the need to defecate but are unable. It results from a lack of coordination of pelvic floor muscles and anal sphincters. Diagnosis is by anorectal manometry. Treatment is difficult, but biofeedback may be of benefit.

Etiology

Normally, when a person tries to defecate, rectal pressure rises in coordination with relaxation of the external anal sphincter. This process may be altered by impairment of rectal contraction, paradoxic anal contraction, or failure of anal relaxation. Physiologic causes include rectal prolapse and Hirschsprung's disease. However, in most patients the disorder appears to be an acquired behavioral problem or a manifestation of irritable bowel syndrome; in 1/3 of these patients, the behavioral problem began in childhood.

Symptoms, Signs, and Diagnosis

The patient senses that stool is present and wants to defecate but cannot, even with prolonged straining and digital evacuation. Even soft stools are difficult to pass. Actual stool frequency may or may not be decreased.

Rectal and pelvic examinations may show hypertonia of the pelvic floor muscles and anal sphincters. With bearing down, patients may not demonstrate the expected anal relaxation and perineal descent. A rectocele or enterocele may be present but is usually not of prime pathogenic importance. Long-standing dyschezia with chronic straining may produce a solitary rectal ulcer or varying degrees of rectal prolapse. Special x-rays (defecatory proctography) and anorectal manometry and balloon expulsion help diagnose the condition.

Treatment

Treatment with laxatives is unsatisfactory. Relaxation exercises and biofeedback can help, although a group approach (physiotherapists, dietitians, behavior therapists, gastroenterologists) may be needed.

DIARRHEA

(See also Chs. 17 and 18 and, for diarrhea in children, p. 2238.)

Stool is 60 to 90% water. In Western society, stool amount is 100 to 300 g/day in healthy adults and 10 g/kg/day in infants, depending on amount of unabsorbable dietary material (mainly carbohydrates). Generally, stool amount > 300 g/day is considered diarrhea. However, the lay public uses the term variably.

Etiology and Pathophysiology

Diarrhea results mainly from excess fecal water, which can have infectious, drug-induced, food-related, surgical, inflammatory, transit-related, or malabsorptive causes. These causes produce diarrhea by 4 distinct mechanisms: increased osmotic load, increased secretion, inflammation, and decreased absorption time. Paradoxic diarrhea results from stool oozing around a fecal impaction. Acute diarrhea (< 4 days) is predominantly caused by self-limited conditions such as food poisoning or infections (see Ch. 16 on p. 133).

Complications may result from diarrhea of any etiology. Fluid loss with consequent dehydration, electrolyte loss (Na, K, Mg, Cl), and even vascular collapse sometimes occur. Collapse can develop rapidly in patients who have severe diarrhea (eg, patients with cholera) or are very young, very old, or debilitated. HCO_3 loss can cause metabolic acidosis. Hypokalemia can occur in severe or chronic diarrhea or if the stool contains excess mucus. Hypomagnesemia after prolonged diarrhea can cause tetany.

Osmotic diarrhea occurs when unabsorbable, water-soluble solutes remain in the bowel and retain water. Such solutes include polyethylene glycol, Mg salts (hydroxide and sulfate), and Na phosphate, which are used as laxatives. Osmotic diarrhea occurs with sugar intolerance (eg, lactose intolerance caused by lactase deficiency). Ingesting large amounts of hexitols (eg, sorbitol, mannitol, xylitol), which are used as sugar substitutes in candy and gum, causes osmotic diarrhea because hexitols are poorly absorbed. Lactulose, which is used as a laxative, causes diarrhea by a similar mechanism. Overingesting certain fruits (see TABLE 8–3) can produce osmotic diarrhea.

Secretory diarrhea occurs when the bowels secrete more electrolytes and water than

TABLE 8–3. DIETARY FACTORS THAT MAY WORSEN DIARRHEA

DIETARY FACTOR	SOURCE
Caffeine	Coffee, tea, cola, OTC headache remedies
Fructose (in quantities surpassing the gut's absorptive capacity)	Apple juice, pear juice, grapes, honey, dates, nuts, figs, soft drinks (especially fruit flavored)
Hexitols, sorbitol, and mannitol	Apple juice, pear juice, sugar-free gum, mints
Lactose	Milk, ice cream, frozen yogurt, yogurt, soft cheeses
Magnesium-containing antacids	Antacids
Sucrose	Table sugar

Adapted from Bayless T: Chronic diarrhea. *Hospital Practice* Jan. 15, 1989, p 131; used with permission.

they absorb. Secretagogues include bacterial toxins (eg, in cholera and *Clostridium difficile* colitis), enteropathogenic viruses, bile acids (eg, after ileal resection), unabsorbed dietary fat, and many drugs (eg, quinidine, quinine, colchicine, SSRIs, cholinesterase inhibitors, anthraquinone cathartics, castor oil, prostaglandins). Various endocrine tumors produce secretagogues, including vipomas (vasoactive intestinal peptide), gastrinomas (gastrin), mastocytosis (histamine), medullary carcinoma of the thyroid (calcitonin and prostaglandins), and carcinoid tumors (histamine, serotonin, and polypeptides). Rarely, microscopic colitis (collagenous or lymphocytic colitis) causes secretory diarrhea, particularly in women > 60.

Inflammatory diarrhea occurs with some infections and diseases that cause mucosal inflammation or ulceration (eg, Crohn's disease, ulcerative colitis, TB, lymphoma, cancer). The resultant outpouring of plasma, serum proteins, blood, and mucus increases fecal bulk and fluid content. Involvement of the rectal mucosa may cause urgency and increased stool frequency because the inflamed rectum is more sensitive to distention.

Diarrhea due to decreased absorption time occurs when chyme is not in long enough contact with an adequate absorptive surface of the GI tract, causing too much water to remain in the stool. Factors that decrease contact time include small- or large-bowel resection, gastric resection, pyloroplasty, vagotomy, surgical bypass of intestinal segments, and drugs (eg, Mg-containing antacids, laxatives) or humoral agents (eg, prostaglandins, serotonin) that speed transit by stimulating intestinal smooth muscle.

Malabsorption-related diarrhea may be the result of osmotic or secretory mechanisms. The mechanism may be osmotic if the unabsorbed material is abundant, water-soluble, and of low molecular weight. Lipids are not osmotic, but some (fatty acids, bile acids) act as secretagogues and produce secretory diarrhea. In generalized malabsorption (eg, nontropical sprue), fat malabsorption causes colonic secretion, and carbohydrate malabsorption causes osmotic diarrhea. Malabsorption-related diarrhea may also develop when transport of chyme is prolonged and fecal bacteria proliferate in the small bowel, as occurs in strictured segments, sclerodermatous intestinal disease, and stagnant loops created by surgery.

Evaluation

History: Duration and severity of diarrhea, circumstances of onset (including recent travel, food ingested, source of water, and drug use—including any antibiotics within the previous 3 mo), abdominal pain or vomiting, frequency and timing of bowel movements, changes in stool characteristics (eg, presence of blood, changes in color or consistency, evidence of steatorrhea), associated changes in weight or appetite, and rectal urgency or tenesmus should be noted.

The symptoms can help identify the affected part of the bowel. Generally, in small-bowel diseases, stools are voluminous and watery or fatty. In colonic diseases, stools are frequent, sometimes small in volume, and possibly accompanied by blood, mucus, pus, and abdominal discomfort. In rectal mucosal diseases, the rectum may be more sensitive to distention, and stools may be small and frequent.

Physical examination: Fluid and hydration status should be evaluated. A full examination with attention to the abdomen and a digital rectal examination for sphincter competence and occult blood testing are important. Extra-abdominal findings that suggest an etiology include skin lesions or flushing (mastocytosis), thyroid nodules (medullary carcinoma of the thyroid), right-sided heart murmur (carcinoid), lymphadenopathy (lymphoma, AIDS), and arthritis (inflammatory bowel disease, celiac disease).

Testing: Acute diarrhea (< 4 days) typically does not require testing. Exceptions are patients with signs of dehydration, bloody stool, fever, severe pain, hypotension, or toxic features—particularly those who are very young or very old. These patients should have a CBC and measurement of electrolytes, BUN, and creatinine. Stool samples should be collected for microscopy, culture, fecal leukocyte testing, and, if antibiotics were taken recently, *Clostridium difficile* toxin assay.

Chronic diarrhea (> 4 wk) requires evaluation, as does a shorter (1 to 3 wk) bout of diarrhea in immunocompromised patients or those who appear significantly ill. Initial stool testing should include culture, fecal leukocytes (detected by smear or measurement of fecal lactoferrin), microscopic examination for ova and parasites, pH (bacterial fermentation of unabsorbed carbohydrate lowers stool pH < 6.0), fat (by Sudan stain), and electrolytes (Na and K). If no standard pathogens are found, specific tests for *Giardia* antigen and *Aeromonas, Plesiomonas*, coccidia, and microsporidia should be requested. Sigmoidoscopy or colonoscopy with biopsies should follow to look for inflammatory causes.

If no diagnosis is apparent and Sudan stain is positive for fat, fecal fat excretion should be measured, followed by small-bowel enteroclysis or abdominal CT (structural disease) and endoscopic small-bowel biopsy (mucosal disease). If evaluation still yields negative findings, assessment of pancreatic structure and function (see p. 130) is needed.

The stool osmotic gap, which is calculated $290 - 2 \times$ (stool Na + stool K), indicates whether diarrhea is secretory or osmotic. An osmotic gap < 50 mEq/L indicates secretory diarrhea; a larger gap suggests osmotic diarrhea. Patients with osmotic diarrhea may have covert Mg laxative ingestion (detectable by stool Mg levels) or carbohydrate malabsorption (diagnosed by H_2 breath test, lactase assay, and dietary review).

Undiagnosed secretory diarrhea requires testing (eg, plasma gastrin, calcitonin, VIP levels, histamine, and urinary 5-hydroxyindole acetic acid [5-HIAA]) for endocrine-related causes. A review for signs and symptoms of thyroid disease and adrenal insufficiency should be done. Surreptitious laxative abuse must be considered; it can be ruled out by a fecal laxative assay.

Treatment

Severe diarrhea requires fluid and electrolyte replacement to correct dehydration, electrolyte imbalance, and acidosis. Parenteral fluids containing NaCl, KCl, and glucose are generally required. Salts to counteract acidosis (Na lactate, acetate, HCO_3^-) may be indicated if serum HCO_3^- is < 15 mEq/L. An oral glucose-electrolyte solution can be given if diarrhea is not severe and nausea and vomiting are minimal (see p. 2293). Oral and parenteral fluids are sometimes given simultaneously when water and electrolytes must be replaced in massive amounts (eg, in cholera).

Diarrhea is a symptom. When possible, the underlying disorder should be treated, but symptomatic treatment is often necessary. Diarrhea may be decreased by oral loperamide 2 to 4 mg tid or qid, diphenoxylate 2.5 to 5 mg (tablets or liquid) tid or qid, codeine phosphate 15 to 30 mg bid or tid, or paregoric (camphorated opium tincture) 5 to 10 mL once/day to qid.

Because antidiarrheals may exacerbate *C. difficile* colitis or increase the likelihood of hemolytic-uremic syndrome in Shiga toxin–producing *Escherichia coli* infection, they should not be used in bloody diarrhea of unknown cause. Their use should be restricted to patients with watery diarrhea and no signs of systemic toxicity. However, there is little evidence to justify previous concerns about prolonging excretion of possible bacterial pathogens with antidiarrheals.

Psyllium or methylcellulose compounds provide bulk. Although usually prescribed for constipation, bulking agents given in small doses decrease the fluidity of liquid stools. Kaolin, pectin, and activated attapulgite adsorb fluid. Osmotically active dietary substances (see TABLE 8–3) and stimulatory drugs should be avoided.

GAS-RELATED COMPLAINTS

Gas is normally present in the gut, either as a result of swallowed air (aerophagia), production in the lumen, or diffusion from the blood into the lumen. Gas diffuses between the lumen and the blood in a direction dependent on the difference in partial pressures. Thus, most nitrogen (N_2) in the lumen originates from the bloodstream, and most hydrogen (H_2) in the bloodstream originates from the lumen.

Etiology and Physiology

There are three main "gas"-related complaints: excessive belching, distention (bloating), and excessive flatus. Infants 2 to 4 mo of age with recurrent crying spells often appear to observers to be in pain, which in the past has been attributed to abdominal cramping or gas and termed "colic." However, studies show no increase in H_2 production or in mouth-to-cecum transit times in colicky infants. Hence, the cause of infantile colic remains unclear (see p. 2236).

Excessive belching: Belching (eructation) results from swallowed air or from gas generated by carbonated beverages. Aerophagia occurs normally in small amounts during eating and drinking, but some people unconsciously swallow air repeatedly while eating or smoking and at other times, especially when anxious. Excessive salivation increases aerophagia and may be associated with various GI disorders (gastroesophageal reflux disease), ill-fitting dentures, certain drugs, gum chewing, or nausea of any cause.

Most swallowed air is eructated. Only a small amount of swallowed air passes into the small bowel; the amount is apparently influenced by position. In an upright person, air is readily belched; in a supine person, air trapped above the stomach fluid tends to be propelled into the duodenum. Excessive eructation may also be voluntary; patients who belch after taking antacids may attribute the relief of symptoms to belching rather than to antacids and may intentionally belch to relieve distress.

Distention (bloating): The sensation of bloating can result from a number of GI (eg, aerophagia, nonulcer dyspepsia, gastroparesis, irritable bowel syndrome) and non-GI (eg, myocardial ischemia) conditions. However, excessive intestinal gas is not clearly linked to these complaints. In most healthy people, 1 L/h of gas can be infused into the gut with minimal symptoms. It is likely that many symptoms are incorrectly attributed to "too much gas."

On the other hand, some patients with recurrent GI symptoms often cannot tolerate small quantities of gas: Retrograde colonic distention by balloon inflation or air instillation during colonoscopy often elicits severe discomfort in some patients (eg, those with irritable bowel syndrome) but minimal symptoms in others. Similarly, patients with eating disorders (eg, anorexia nervosa, bulimia) often misperceive and are particularly stressed by symptoms such as bloating. Thus, the basic abnormality in patients with "gas"-related symptoms may be a hypersensitive intestine. Altered motility may contribute further to symptoms.

Excessive flatus: There is great variability in the quantity and frequency of rectal gas passage. As with stool frequency, people who complain of flatulence often have a misconception of what is normal. The average number of gas passages is about 13 to 21/day. Objectively recording flatus frequency (using a diary kept by the patient) is a first step in evaluation.

Flatus is a metabolic byproduct of intestinal bacteria; almost none originates from swallowed air or back-diffusion of gases (primarily N_2) from the bloodstream. Bacterial metabolism yields significant volumes of H_2, methane (CH_4), and CO_2.

H_2 is produced in large quantities after ingestion of certain fruits and vegetables containing indigestible carbohydrates (eg, baked beans) and in patients with malabsorption syndromes. In patients with disaccharidase deficiencies (most commonly lactase deficiency), large amounts of disaccharides pass into the colon and are fermented to H_2. Celiac disease, tropical sprue, pancreatic insufficiency, and other causes of carbohydrate malabsorption should also be considered in cases of excess colonic gas.

CH_4 is produced by bacterial metabolism of exogenous (dietary fiber) and endogenous (intestinal mucus) substances in the colon; the production rate is influenced by food ingestion. Some people consistently excrete large quantities of CH_4. The tendency to produce large quantities is familial, appearing during infancy and persisting for life.

CO_2 is also produced by bacterial metabolism and generated in the reaction of HCO_3^- and H^+. H^+ may come from gastric HCl or from fatty acids released during digestion of fats—the latter sometimes produces several hundred mEq of H^+. The acid products released by bacterial fermentation of unabsorbed carbohydrates in the colon may also react with HCO_3^- to produce CO_2. Although bloating may occasionally occur, the rapid diffusion of CO_2 into the blood generally prevents distention.

Diet accounts for much of the variation in flatus production between individuals, but poorly understood factors (eg, differences in colonic flora and motility) may also play a role.

Despite the flammable nature of the H_2 and CH_4 in flatulence, working near open flames is not hazardous. However, gas explosion, even with fatal outcome, has been reported during jejunal and colonic surgery and colonoscopy, when diathermy was used during procedures in patients with incomplete bowel cleaning.

Essay on Flatulence
(first printed in the 14th Edition of *The Merck Manual*)

Flatulence, which can cause great psychosocial distress, is unofficially described according to its salient characteristics: (1) the "slider" (crowded elevator type), which is released slowly and noiselessly, sometimes with devastating effect; (2) the open sphincter, or "pooh" type, which is said to be of higher temperature and more aromatic; (3) the staccato or drumbeat type, pleasantly passed in privacy; and (4) the "bark" type (described in a personal communication) is characterized by a sharp exclamatory eruption that effectively interrupts (and often concludes) conversation. Aromaticity is not a prominent feature. Rarely, this usually distressing symptom has been turned to advantage, as with a Frenchman referred to as "Le Petomane," who became affluent as an effluent performer who played tunes with the gas from his rectum on the Moulin Rouge stage.

Evaluation

History: Patients with belching should have the history directed at finding the cause of aerophagia, especially dietary causes. Patients complaining of gas or bloating must have a history aimed at discovering physiologic causes (particularly cardiac causes in at-risk patients). Long-standing symptoms in an otherwise well young person who has not lost weight are unlikely to be caused by serious physiologic disease, although an eating disorder should be considered, particularly in young women. Older patients, especially those with onset of new symptoms, merit thorough examination before excessive gas, real or imagined, is treated.

Physical examination: Examination is rarely rewarding in patients with belching or flatus. Individuals with bloating and gas require a more detailed examination for objective signs of GI or other pathology.

Testing: Unless there is suspicion of a particular physiologic etiology, testing is limited. Rarely, unsuspected bacterial overgrowth in the small bowel, diagnosed by H_2 breath testing, may present this way.

Treatment

Belching and bloating are difficult to relieve because they are usually caused by unconscious aerophagia or increased sensitivity to normal amounts of gas. To reduce aerophagia, the patient should avoid habits such as gum chewing or smoking. Upper GI diseases (eg, peptic ulcer) that may cause reflex hypersalivation should be treated. Carbonated beverages or antacids should be eliminated if associated with belching. Foods containing unabsorbable carbohydrates should be avoided. Dairy products should be excluded from the diet of lactose-intolerant patients.

The mechanism of repeated belching should be explained and demonstrated. When aerophagia is troublesome, biofeedback and relaxation therapy can retrain the patients to swallow and chew more effectively and break the cycle of aerophagia-discomfort-belch-relief.

Drugs provide little benefit. Simethicone, an agent that breaks up small gas bubbles, and various anticholinergic drugs demonstrate poor results. Some patients with dyspepsia and postprandial upper abdominal fullness benefit from antacids.

Complaints of excess flatus are treated with avoidance of triggering substances. Roughage (eg, bran, psyllium seed) may be added to the diet to try to increase colonic transit; however, in some patients, worsening of symptoms may result. Activated charcoal can sometimes help reduce gas and unpleasant odor; however, its tendency to stain clothing and the oral mucosa makes it undesirable. Chlorophyll tablets may reduce odor and are better accepted by patients.

In general, functional bloating, distention, and flatus run an intermittent, chronic course that is only partially relieved by therapy. Reassurance that these problems are not detrimental to health is important.

IRRITABLE BOWEL SYNDROME

(Spastic Colon)

Irritable bowel syndrome consists of recurring upper and lower GI symptoms, including variable degrees of abdominal pain, constipation or diarrhea, and abdominal bloating. The cause is unknown, and the pathophysiology is incompletely understood. Diagnosis is clinical. Treatment is symptomatic, consisting of dietary management and drugs, including anticholinergics and agents active at serotonin receptors.

Etiology

The cause of irritable bowel syndrome (IBS) is unknown. No anatomic cause can be found. Emotional factors, diet, drugs, or hormones may precipitate or aggravate GI symptoms. Some patients have anxiety disorders (particularly panic disorder, major depressive disorder, and somatization disorder). However, stress and emotional conflict do not always coincide with symptom onset and recurrence. Some patients with IBS appear to have a learned aberrant illness behavior (ie, they express emotional conflict as a GI complaint, usually abdominal pain). The physician evaluating patients with IBS, particularly those with refractory symptoms, should investigate for unresolved psychologic issues, including the possibility of sexual or physical abuse.

Pathophysiology

There are no consistent motility abnormalities. Some patients have an abnormal gastrocolonic reflex, with delayed, prolonged colonic activity. There may be reduced gastric emptying or disordered jejunal motility. Some patients have no demonstrable abnormalities, and in those that do, the abnormalities may not correlate with symptoms. Small-bowel transit varies: sometimes the proximal small bowel appears to be hyperreactive to food or parasympathomimetic drugs. Intraluminal pressure studies of the sigmoid show that functional constipation can occur with hyperreactive haustral segmentation (ie, increased frequency and amplitude of contractions). In contrast, diarrhea is associated with diminished motor function. Thus strong contractions can, at times, accelerate or delay transit.

Excess mucus production, which often occurs in IBS, is not related to mucosal injury. Its cause is unclear but may be related to cholinergic hyperactivity.

Hypersensitivity to normal amounts of intraluminal distention and heightened perception of pain in the presence of normal quantity of intestinal gas exist. Pain seems to be caused by abnormally strong contractions of the intestinal smooth muscle or by increased sensitivity of the intestine to distention. Hypersensitivity to the hormones gastrin and cholecystokinin may also be present. However, hormonal fluctuations do not correlate with symptoms. Meals of high caloric density may increase the magnitude and frequency of myoelectrical activity and gastric motility. Fat ingestion may cause a delayed peak of motor activity, which can be exaggerated in IBS. The first few days of menstruation can lead to transiently elevated prostaglandin E_2, resulting in increased pain and diarrhea, probably by the release of prostaglandins.

Symptoms and Signs

IBS tends to begin in the teens and 20s, causing bouts of symptoms that recur at irregular periods. Onset in late adult life is less common but not rare. Symptoms rarely rouse the sleeping patient. Symptoms can be triggered by stress or food.

Features of IBS include abdominal pain related to or relieved by defecation, change in stool frequency or consistency, abdominal distention, mucus in the stool, and the sensation of incomplete evacuation after defecation. In general, the character and location of pain, precipitating factors, and defecatory pattern are distinct for each patient. Variations or deviations from the usual symptoms may suggest intercurrent physiologic disease and should be thoroughly investigated. Patients with IBS may also have extra-intestinal symptoms (eg, fibromyalgia, headaches, dyspareunia, temporomandibular joint syndrome).

Two major clinical types of IBS have been described.

In **constipation-predominant IBS,** most patients have pain over at least one area of the colon and periods of constipation alternating with a more normal stool frequency. Stool often contains clear or white mucus. Pain is either colicky, coming in bouts, or a continuous dull ache; it may be relieved by a bowel movement. Eating commonly triggers symptoms. Bloating, flatulence, nausea, dyspepsia, and pyrosis can also occur.

Diarrhea-predominant IBS is characterized by precipitous diarrhea that occurs immediately on rising or during or immediately after eating, especially rapid eating. Nocturnal diarrhea is unusual. Pain, bloating, and rectal urgency are common, and incontinence may occur. Painless diarrhea is not typical and should lead the physician to consider other diagnostic possibilities (eg, malabsorption, osmotic diarrhea).

Diagnosis

Diagnosis is based on characteristic bowel patterns, time and character of pain, and exclusion of other disease processes through physical examination and routine diagnostic tests. Diagnostic testing should be more intensive when "red flags" are present: older age, weight loss, rectal bleeding, vomiting. Common illnesses that may be confused with IBS include lactose intolerance, diverticular disease, drug-induced diarrhea, biliary tract disease, laxative abuse, parasitic diseases, bacterial enteritis, eosinophilic gastritis or enteritis, microscopic colitis, and early inflammatory bowel disease.

Hyperthyroidism, carcinoid syndrome, medullary cancer of the thyroid, vipoma, and Zollinger-Ellison syndrome are additional possibilities in patients with diarrhea. The bimodal age distribution of patients with inflammatory bowel disease makes it imperative to evaluate both younger and older patients. In patients > 60, ischemic colitis should be considered. Patients with constipation and no anatomic lesion should be evaluated for hypothyroidism and hyperparathyroidism. If the patient's symptoms suggest malabsorption, tropical sprue, celiac disease, and Whipple's disease must be considered. Elimination disorders (eg, pelvic floor dyssynergia) should be considered as a cause of constipation in patients who report excessive straining on defecation.

History: Particular attention should be given to the character of the pain, bowel habits, familial interrelationships, and drug and dietary histories. Equally important are the patient's interpretation of personal problems and overall emotional state. The quality of the patient-physician interaction is key to diagnostic and therapeutic efficacy.

The Rome criteria are standardized symptom-based criteria for diagnosing IBS; the criteria are met by the presence for at least 3 mo of the following symptoms: (1) abdominal pain or discomfort that is relieved by defecation or is associated with a change in frequency or consistency of stool, and (2) disturbed defecation involving at least two of the following: altered stool frequency, altered stool form, altered stool passage, passage of mucus, and bloating or feeling of distention.

Physical examination: Patients generally appear to be healthy. Palpation of the abdomen may reveal tenderness, particularly in the left lower quadrant, at times associated with a palpable, tender sigmoid. A digital rectal examination, including a test for occult blood, should be performed on all patients. In women, a pelvic examination helps rule out ovarian tumors and cysts or endometriosis, which may mimic IBS.

Testing: Proctosigmoidoscopy with a flexible fiberoptic instrument should be performed. Introduction of the sigmoidoscope and air insufflation frequently trigger bowel spasm and pain. The mucosal and vascular patterns in IBS usually appear normal. Colonoscopy is preferred for patients > 40 with a change in bowel habits, particularly those with no previous IBS symptoms, to exclude colonic polyps and tumors. In patients with chronic diarrhea, particularly older women, mucosal biopsy can rule out possible microscopic colitis.

Many patients with IBS are overtested. Laboratory studies do not aid diagnosis in patients meeting Rome criteria who have no other signs or symptoms suggestive of another etiology. If symptoms are inconclusive, the following tests should be obtained: CBC, ESR, biochemical profile (including liver function tests and serum amylase), urinalysis, and thyroid-stimulating hormone.

Additional studies (such as ultrasound, CT, barium enema x-ray, upper GI esophagogastroduodenoscopy, and small-bowel x-rays) should be undertaken only when there are other objective abnormalities. If structural studies show an abnormality, H_2

breath tests may be indicated. Stool cultures or examinations for ova and parasites are rarely indicated without a supporting travel history or supporting symptoms (eg, fever, bloody diarrhea, acute onset of severe diarrhea).

Intercurrent disease: Patients may develop additional GI disorders, and the clinician must not summarily dismiss their complaints. Changes in symptoms (eg, in the location, type, or intensity of pain; in bowel habits; in constipation and diarrhea) and new symptoms or complaints (eg, nocturnal diarrhea) may signal another disease process. Other symptoms that require investigation include fresh blood in the stool, weight loss, very severe abdominal pain or unusual abdominal distention, steatorrhea or noticeably foul-smelling stools, fever or chills, persistent vomiting, hematemesis, symptoms that wake the patient from sleep (eg, pain, the urge to defecate), and a steady progressive worsening of symptoms. Patients > 40 are more likely than younger patients to develop an intercurrent physiologic illness.

Treatment

Therapy is supportive and palliative. Sympathetic understanding and guidance are of overriding importance. The physician must explain the underlying condition and convincingly demonstrate that no physiologic disease is present. This requires explaining normal bowel physiology and the bowel's hypersensitivity to stress, food, or drugs. These explanations form the foundation for attempting to reestablish regular bowel routine and individualizing therapy. The prevalence, chronicity, and need for continuing care should be emphasized.

Psychologic stress, anxiety, or mood disorders should be identified, evaluated, and treated. Regular physical activity helps relieve stress and assists in bowel function, particularly in patients with constipation.

Diet: In general, a normal diet should be followed. Meals should not be overly large, and eating should be slow and paced. Patients with abdominal distention and increased flatulence may benefit from reducing or eliminating beans, cabbage, and other foods containing fermentable carbohydrates. Reduced intake of apple and grape juice, bananas, nuts, and raisins may also lessen the incidence of flatulence. Patients with evidence of lactose intolerance should reduce their intake of milk and dairy products. Bowel function may also be disturbed by the ingestion of sorbitol, mannitol, or fructose. Sorbitol and mannitol are artificial sweeteners used in dietetic foods and as drug vehicles, whereas fructose is a common constituent of fruits, berries, and plants. Patients with postprandial abdominal pain may try a low-fat diet supplemented with increased protein.

Dietary fiber can help many patients by absorbing water and solidifying stool. It may benefit patients with either constipation or diarrhea. A bland bulk-producing agent may be used (eg, raw bran, starting with 15 mL [1 tbsp] with each meal, supplemented with increased fluid intake). Alternatively, psyllium hydrophilic mucilloid with two glasses of water may be used. However, excessive use of fiber can lead to bloating and diarrhea. Fiber doses must therefore be adjusted to individual needs.

Drug therapy: Drug therapy is rarely advisable except for short-term use during periods of increased activity. Anticholinergic drugs (eg, hyoscyamine 0.125 mg 30 to 60 min before meals) may be used for their antispasmodic effects. New selective M3 muscarinic receptor antagonists, including zamifenacin and darifenacin, have fewer cardiac and gastric effects.

Serotonin receptor modulation may be of benefit. The $5HT_4$ agonists tegaserod and prucalopride may help patients with constipation. $5HT_3$ antagonists (eg, alosetron) may benefit female patients with diarrhea.

In patients with diarrhea, oral diphenoxylate 2.5 to 5 mg or loperamide 2 to 4 mg may be given before meals. However, chronic use of antidiarrheals is discouraged because tolerance to the antidiarrheal effect may occur. For many patients, tricyclic antidepressants (eg, desipramine, imipramine, amitriptyline 50 to 150 mg po once/day) help relieve symptoms of constipation, diarrhea, abdominal pain, and bloating. These drugs are thought to reduce pain by down-regulating the activity of spinal cord and cortical afferent pathways arriving from the intestine. Finally, certain aromatic oils (carminatives) can relax smooth muscle and relieve pain caused by cramps in some patients. Peppermint oil is the most commonly used agent in this class.

9 DIAGNOSTIC AND THERAPEUTIC GI PROCEDURES

Diagnostic tests and therapeutic procedures available for patients with GI disorders include acid-related tests, endoscopy, laparoscopy, manometry, nuclear scans, x-ray contrast studies, nasogastric or intestinal intubation, anoscopy and sigmoidoscopy, abdominal paracentesis, electrogastrography, and electrical impedance testing. CT, MRI, and ultrasound are also commonly done for GI disorders, and sometimes angiography is used. The selection of procedures is discussed in subsequent chapters. ERCP, percutaneous transhepatic cholangiography, and liver biopsy are discussed in Ch. 23 on p. 201.

ACID-RELATED TESTS

Acid-related tests are used to ascertain the effectiveness of acid-blocking drugs. All require nasogastric or nasoesophageal intubation. Complications are very rare. Patients must have nothing by mouth (npo) after midnight.

AMBULATORY pH MONITORING

Ambulatory 24-h esophageal pH monitoring is currently the best available test for quantifying esophageal acid exposure. The principal indications are (1) to document excessive acid exposure in patients without endoscopic evidence of esophagitis, and (2) to evaluate the effectiveness of medical or surgical treatments. A thin tube containing a pH probe is positioned 5 cm above the lower esophageal sphincter. The patient records symptoms, meals, and sleep for 24 h. Esophageal acid exposure is defined by the percentage of the 24-h recording time that the pH is <4.0. Values $>3.5\%$ are considered abnormal. However, symptoms may not correlate with acid exposure or the presence of esophagitis. This may be because symptoms may result from nonacidic as well as acidic refluxate.

GASTRIC ANALYSIS

Samples of stomach contents obtained via nasogastric tube are used to measure gastric acid output in a basal and stimulated state. This may be useful in a patient who develops a recurrent ulcer following surgical vagotomy for peptic ulcer disease. In this case, a positive acid response to stimulation (sham feeding) indicates an incomplete vagotomy. The test is also used to evaluate a patient with elevated serum gastrin levels. Hyperchlorhydria in the presence of elevated gastrin indicates Zollinger-Ellison syndrome. Hypochlorhydria in the presence of elevated gastrin indicates impairment of acid output, such as occurs in pernicious anemia, atrophic gastritis, and Ménétrier's disease and after inhibition of gastric acid secretion by potent antisecretory drugs.

To perform gastric analysis, a nasogastric tube is inserted and the gastric contents are aspirated and discarded. Gastric juice is then collected for 1 h, divided into four 15-min samples. These samples represent basal acid output.

ENDOSCOPY

Flexible endoscopes equipped with video cameras can be used to view the upper GI tract from pharynx to upper duodenum and the lower GI tract from anus to cecum (and, sometimes, terminal ileum). Several other diagnostic and therapeutic interventions can also be performed endoscopically. The potential to combine diagnosis and therapy in one procedure gives endoscopy a significant advantage over procedures that provide only imaging (eg, x-ray contrast studies, CT, MRI) and often outweighs endoscopy's higher cost and need for sedation.

Diagnostic procedures include the use of ultrasound-equipped endoscopes to evaluate blood flow or provide imaging of lesions. Endoscopic ultrasound can provide information (eg, the depth and extent of lesions) that is not available via conventional endoscopy. Other diagnostic procedures include cell and tissue sample collection by brush or biopsy forceps.

Screening flexible sigmoidoscopy or colonoscopy is recommended for patients at high risk for colon cancer and for everyone ≥ 50. Sigmoidoscopy should be done every 5 yr, colonoscopy every 10 yr.

Therapeutic endoscopic procedures include removal of foreign bodies; hemostasis by thermal coagulation, laser photocoagulation, variceal banding, or sclerotherapy; debulking of tumors by laser or bipolar electrocoagulation; dilation of webs or strictures; stent placement; reduction of volvulus or intussusception; and decompression of acute or subacute colonic dilatation.

Absolute contraindications to endoscopy include shock, acute MI, peritonitis, acute perforation, and fulminant colitis. Relative contraindications include poor patient cooperation, coma (unless the patient is intubated), and cardiac arrhythmias or recent myocardial ischemia.

Patients on anticoagulants or chronic NSAID therapy can safely undergo diagnostic endoscopy. However, if there is a possibility that biopsy or photocoagulation will be performed, these drugs should be discontinued for an appropriate interval before the procedure. Oral iron-containing drugs should be stopped 4 to 5 days before colonoscopy, because certain green vegetables interact with iron to form a sticky residue that is difficult to remove with a bowel preparation and interferes with visualization. Because bacteremia may occur with endoscopy, antibiotic pretreatment is recommended for patients requiring endocarditis prophylaxis (see TABLE 77–2 on p. 728).

Routine preparations for endoscopy include no solids for 6 to 8 h and no liquids for 4 h before the procedure. Additionally, colonoscopy requires cleansing of the colon. A variety of regimens may be used, but all typically include a full or clear liquid diet for 24 to 48 h and some type of laxative, with or without an enema. A common laxative preparation involves having the patient drink a high-volume (4 L) balanced electrolyte solution over a period of 3 to 4 h before the procedure. Patients who cannot tolerate this solution may be given Mg citrate, Na phosphate, lactulose, or other laxatives. Enemas can be performed with either Na phosphate or tap water.

Endoscopy generally requires IV sedation and, for upper endoscopy, topical anesthesia of the throat. Exceptions are anoscopy and sigmoidoscopy (see p. 88), which generally require nothing. The overall complication rate of endoscopy is 0.1 to 0.2%; mortality is about 0.03%. Complications are usually drug related (eg, respiratory depression); procedural complications (eg, aspiration, perforation, significant bleeding) are less common.

LAPAROSCOPY

Diagnostic laparoscopy is a surgical procedure used to evaluate intra-abdominal or pelvic pathology (eg, tumor, endometriosis) in patients with acute or chronic abdominal pain and operability in patients with cancer. It is also used for lymphoma staging and liver biopsy. Absolute contraindications include a coagulation or bleeding disorder, poor patient cooperation, peritonitis, intestinal obstruction, and infection of the abdominal wall. Relative contraindications include severe cardiac or pulmonary disease, large abdominal hernias, multiple abdominal operations, and tense ascites.

CBC, coagulation studies, and type and Rh testing are obtained before laparoscopy. X-rays of the chest, kidneys, ureters, and bladder are also obtained. Laparoscopy is performed with sterile technique in an operating room or a well-equipped endoscopy suite. The patient is given local anesthesia plus IV sedation and analgesia with an opioid and short-acting sedative (eg, midazolam or propofol).

The procedure involves insertion of a pneumoperitoneum needle into the peritoneal cavity and infusion of nitrous oxide to distend the abdomen. After the opening is enlarged, a peritoneoscope is inserted into the abdomen and the abdominal contents are examined. Surgical instruments for biopsy and other procedures are inserted through separate openings. When the procedure is completed, the nitrous oxide is expelled by the patient with a Valsalva maneuver and the cannula is removed. Complications can include bleeding, bacterial peritonitis, and perforation of a viscus.

MANOMETRY

Manometry is measurement of pressure within various parts of the GI tract. It is performed by passing a catheter containing solid-state or liquid-filled pressure transducers through the mouth or anus into the lumen of the organ to be studied. Manometry is typically performed to evaluate motility disorders in patients in whom structural lesions have been ruled out by other studies. Manometry is used in the esophagus, stomach and duodenum, sphincter of Oddi, and rectum. Aside from minor discomfort, complications are very rare. Patients must have nothing by mouth (npo) after midnight.

Esophageal manometry is used to evaluate patients with dysphagia, heartburn, or chest pain. It measures the pressure in the upper and lower esophageal sphincters, determines the effectiveness and coordination of propulsive movements, and detects abnormal contractions. Manometry is used to diagnose achalasia, diffuse spasm, systemic sclerosis, and lower esophageal sphincter hypotension and hypertension. It is also used to evaluate esophageal function prior to certain therapeutic procedures (eg, antireflux surgery, pneumatic dilation for achalasia).

In **gastroduodenal manometry,** transducers are placed in the gastric antrum, duodenum, and proximal jejunum. Pressure is monitored for 5 to 24 h in both fasting and fed states. This test is used mainly in patients who have symptoms suggestive of dysmotility but normal gastric emptying studies.

A **barostat** is a pressure-sensing device that is placed in the stomach to measure gastric accommodation. The device consists of a plastic balloon and an electronic controller that varies the amount of air in the balloon to maintain constant pressure. This device is mainly used in research studies assessing sensory threshold and altered visceral perception, particularly in functional GI disorders.

Anorectal manometry evaluates the anorectal sphincter mechanism and rectal sensation in patients with incontinence (and sometimes constipation) by means of a pressure transducer in the anus. It can help diagnose Hirschsprung's disease and provide biofeedback training for fecal incontinence.

NUCLEAR SCANS

Gastric emptying can be measured by having the patient ingest a radiolabeled meal (solid or liquid) and observing its passage out of the stomach with a gamma camera. Because this test cannot differentiate physical obstruction from gastroparesis, further diagnostic studies are typically performed if emptying is delayed. The test is also useful in monitoring response to promotility drugs (eg, metoclopramide, erythromycin).

Bleeding scans use ^{99m}Tc-labeled RBCs, or occasionally ^{99m}Tc-labeled colloid, to determine the origin of lower GI hemorrhage before surgery or angiography. Active bleeding sites are identified by focal areas of tracer that conform to bowel anatomy, increase with time, and move with peristalsis. Bleeding scans are useful mainly for colonic bleeding in patients with significant hemorrhage and an unprepared bowel, in whom endoscopic visualization is difficult.

A **Meckel scan** identifies ectopic gastric mucosa using an injection of ^{99m}Tc pertechnetate, which is taken up by mucus-secreting cells of the gastric mucosa. Focal uptake outside of the stomach indicates a Meckel's diverticulum.

X-RAY CONTRAST STUDIES

X-ray contrast studies visualize the entire GI tract from pharynx to rectum and are most useful for detecting mass lesions and structural abnormalities (eg, tumors, strictures). Single-contrast studies fill the lumen with radiopaque material, outlining the structure. Better, more detailed images are obtained from double-contrast studies, in which a small amount of high-density barium coats the mucosal surface and gas distends the organ and enhances contrast. The gas is injected by the operator in double-contrast barium enema, whereas in other studies, intrinsic GI tract gas is adequate. In all cases, the patient turns himself to properly distribute the gas and barium. Fluoroscopy can monitor the progress of the contrast material. Either video or plain films can be taken for documentation, but video is particularly useful when assessing motor disorders (eg, cricopharyngeal spasm, achalasia).

The main contraindication to x-ray contrast studies is suspected perforation, because free barium is highly irritating to the mediastinum and peritoneum; water-soluble contrast is less irritating and may be used if perforation is possible. Older patients may have difficulty turning themselves to properly distribute the barium and intraluminal gas.

Patients having upper GI x-ray contrast studies must have nothing by mouth (npo) after midnight. Patients having barium enema follow a clear liquid diet the day before, take an oral Na phosphate laxative in the afternoon, and take a bisacodyl suppository in the evening. Other laxative regimens are effective.

Complications are rare. Perforation can occur if barium enema is performed in a patient with toxic megacolon. Barium impaction may be prevented by postprocedure oral fluids and sometimes laxatives.

An **upper GI examination** is best performed as a biphasic study beginning with a double-contrast examination of the esophagus, stomach, and duodenum, followed by a single-contrast study using low-density barium. Glucagon 0.5 mg IV can facilitate the examination by producing gastric hypotonia.

A **small-bowel meal** is performed using fluoroscopy and provides a more detailed evaluation of the small bowel. Shortly before the examination, the patient is given metoclopramide 20 mg po to hasten transit of the contrast material.

Enteroclysis (small-bowel enema) provides still better visualization of the small bowel but requires intubation of the duodenum with a flexible, balloon-tipped catheter. A barium suspension is injected, followed by a solution of methylcellulose, which functions as a double-contrast agent that enhances visualization of the small-bowel mucosa.

A **barium enema** can be performed as a single- or double-contrast study. Single-contrast barium enemas are used for potential obstruction, diverticulitis, fistulas, and megacolon. Double-contrast studies are preferred for detection of tumors.

GI PROCEDURES FOR THE GENERALIST

Nasogastric or Intestinal Intubation

Nasogastric or intestinal intubation is used to decompress the stomach. It is used to treat gastric atony, ileus, or obstruction; remove ingested toxins; obtain a sample of gastric contents for analysis (volume, acid content, blood); and supply nutrients. Contraindications include nasopharyngeal or esophageal obstruction, severe maxillofacial trauma, and uncorrected coagulation abnormalities. Esophageal varices have previously been considered a contraindication, but evidence of adverse effects is lacking.

Several types of tubes are available. A Levin or Salem sump tube is used for gastric decompression or analysis and rarely for short-term feeding. A variety of long, thin, intestinal tubes are used for long-term enteral feeding (see p. 20).

For intubation, the patient sits upright or, if unable, lies in the left lateral decubitus position. A topical anesthetic sprayed in the nose and pharynx helps reduce discomfort. With the patient's head partially flexed, the lubricated tube is inserted through the nares and aimed back and then down to conform to the nasopharynx. As the tip reaches the posterior pharyngeal wall, the patient should sip water through a straw. Violent coughing with flow of air through the tube during respiration indicates that the tube is misplaced in the trachea. Aspiration of gastric juice verifies entry into the stomach. The position of larger tubes can be confirmed by instilling 20 to 30 mL of air and listening with the stethoscope under the left subcostal region for a rush of air.

Some smaller, more flexible intestinal feeding tubes require the use of stiffening wires or stylets. These tubes usually require fluoroscopic or endoscopic assistance for passage through the pylorus.

Complications are rare and include nasopharyngeal trauma with or without hemorrhage, pulmonary aspiration, traumatic esophageal or gastric hemorrhage or perforation, and (very rarely) intracranial or mediastinal penetration.

Anoscopy and Sigmoidoscopy

Anoscopy and sigmoidoscopy are used to evaluate symptoms referable to the rectum or anus (eg, bright rectal bleeding, discharge, protrusions, pain). There are no absolute contraindications. Patients with cardiac arrhythmias or recent myocardial ischemia should have the procedure postponed until the comorbid conditions improve; otherwise, they will need cardiac monitoring. Antibiotics are given to patients requiring endocarditis prophylaxis.

The perianal area and distal rectum can be examined with a 7-cm anoscope, and the rectum and sigmoid with either a rigid 25-cm or a flexible 60-cm instrument. Flexible sigmoidoscopy is much more comfortable for the patient and readily permits photography and biopsy of tissue. Considerable skill is required to pass a rigid sigmoidoscope beyond the rectosigmoid junction (15 cm) without producing discomfort.

Sigmoidoscopy is performed after a phosphate enema to empty the rectum. IV medication is usually not needed. The patient is placed in the left lateral position. After external inspection and digital rectal examination, the lubricated instrument is gently inserted 3 to 4 cm past the anal sphincter. At this point, the obturator of the rigid sigmoidoscope is removed, and the instrument is inserted under direct vision.

Anoscopy may be performed without preparation. The anoscope is inserted its full length as described above for rigid sigmoidoscopy, usually with the patient in the left lateral position. Complications are exceedingly rare when properly performed.

Abdominal Paracentesis

Abdominal paracentesis is used to obtain ascitic fluid for testing. It can also be used to remove tense ascites causing respiratory difficulties or pain or as a treatment for chronic ascites. Absolute contraindications include severe, uncorrectable disorders of blood coagulation; intestinal obstruction; and an infected abdominal wall. Poor patient cooperation, surgical scarring over the puncture area, and severe portal hypertension with abdominal collateral circulation are relative contraindications.

CBC, platelet count, and coagulation studies are obtained before the procedure. After emptying the bladder, the patient sits in bed with the head elevated 45 to 90°. In patients with obvious and marked ascites, a point is located at the midline between the umbilicus and the pubic bone and is cleaned with an antiseptic solution and alcohol. In patients with moderate ascites, precise location of ascitic fluid by abdominal ultrasound is indicated. Under sterile technique, the area is anesthetized to the peritoneum with lidocaine 1%. For diagnostic paracentesis, an 18-gauge needle attached to a 50-mL syringe is inserted through the peritoneum (generally a popping sensation is noted). Fluid is gently aspirated and sent for cell count, protein or amylase content, cytology, or culture as needed. For therapeutic (large-volume) paracentesis, a 14-gauge cannula attached to a vacuum aspiration system is used to collect up to 8 L of ascitic fluid. Postprocedure hypotension caused by fluid redistribution is rare as long as interstitial (leg) edema is present.

Hemorrhage is the most common complication. Occasionally, with tense ascites, prolonged leakage of ascitic fluid occurs through the needle site.

OTHER TESTING PROCEDURES

Electrogastrography measures gastric electrical activity with adhesive cutaneous electrodes. This is useful in patients with gastroparesis.

In **electrical impedance testing,** an electrical sensor is placed in the distal esophagus to assess nonacid reflux, which is common in patients receiving gastric antisecretory drugs and in infants with reflux disease.

10 GI BLEEDING

GI bleeding can originate anywhere from the mouth to the anus and can be overt or occult. There are many possible causes (see TABLE 10–1), which are divided into upper GI (above the ligament of Treitz) and lower GI.

Bleeding of any cause is more likely, and potentially more severe, in patients with chronic liver disease or hereditary coagulation disorders or in those who are taking certain drugs. Drugs associated with GI bleeding include anticoagulants (heparin, warfarin), those affecting platelet function (eg, aspirin and certain other NSAIDs, clopidogrel, SSRIs), and those affecting mucosal defenses (eg, NSAIDs).

Symptoms and Signs

The manifestations of GI bleeding depend on the location and rate of bleeding.

Hematemesis is vomiting of red blood and indicates upper GI bleeding, usually from an arterial source or varix. Coffee-ground emesis results from bleeding that has slowed or stopped, with conversion of red Hb to brown hematin by gastric acid.

Hematochezia is the passage of gross blood from the rectum and usually indicates lower GI bleeding but may result from vigorous upper GI bleeding with rapid transit of blood through the intestines.

Melena is black, tarry stool and typically indicates upper GI bleeding, but bleeding from a source in the small bowel or right colon may also be the cause. About 100 to 200 mL of blood in the upper GI tract is required to produce melena, which may persist for several

TABLE 10–1. COMMON CAUSES OF GI BLEEDING

Upper GI tract
- Duodenal ulcer (20–30%)
- Gastric or duodenal erosions (20–30%)
- Varices (15–20%)
- Gastric ulcer (10–20%)
- Mallory-Weiss tear (5–10%)
- Erosive esophagitis (5–10%)
- Angioma (5–10%)
- Arteriovenous malformation (< 5%)

Lower GI tract (percentages vary with the age group sampled)
- Anal fissures
- Angiodysplasia (vascular ectasia)
- Colitis: radiation, ischemic
- Colonic carcinoma
- Colonic polyps
- Diverticular disease
- Inflammatory bowel disease: ulcerative proctitis/colitis, Crohn's disease, infectious colitis
- Internal hemorrhoids

Small-bowel lesions (rare)
- Angiomas
- Arteriovenous malformations
- Meckel's diverticulum
- Tumors

days after bleeding has ceased. Black stool that does not contain occult blood may result from ingestion of iron, bismuth, or various foods and should not be mistaken for melena.

Chronic occult bleeding can occur anywhere in the GI tract and is detectable by chemical testing of a stool specimen.

Patients with severe bleeding may present with signs of shock (eg, tachycardia, tachypnea, pallor, diaphoresis, oliguria, confusion). Patients with underlying ischemic heart disease may develop angina or MI because of hypoperfusion.

Patients with lesser degrees of bleeding may simply have mild tachycardia (heart rate > 100). Orthostatic changes in pulse (a change of > 10 beats/min) or BP (a drop of ≥ 10 mm Hg) often develop after acute loss of ≥ 2 units of blood. However, orthostatic measurements are unwise in patients with severe bleeding (possibly causing syncope) and unreliable as a measure of intravascular volume in patients with mild bleeding, especially elderly patients.

Patients with chronic blood loss may present with symptoms and signs of anemia (eg, weakness, easy fatigability, pallor, chest pain, dizziness). GI bleeding may precipitate hepatic encephalopathy (see p. 197) or hepatorenal syndrome (kidney failure secondary to liver failure).

Evaluation

Stabilization with IV fluid, transfusions, or other treatment is essential before and during diagnostic evaluation. In addition to history and physical examination, testing is typically required.

History: The history suggests a diagnosis in about 50% of patients, but confirmatory testing is required. Epigastric abdominal pain relieved by food or antacids suggests peptic ulcer disease. However, many patients with bleeding ulcers have no history of pain. Weight loss and anorexia suggest a GI malignancy. A history of cirrhosis or chronic hepatitis suggests esophageal varices. Dysphagia suggests esophageal cancer or stricture. Vomiting and retching before the onset of bleeding suggests a Mallory-Weiss tear of the esophagus, although about 50% of patients with Mallory-Weiss tears do not have this history.

A history of bleeding (eg, purpura, ecchymosis, hematuria) may indicate a bleeding diathesis (eg, hemophilia, hepatic failure). Bloody diarrhea, fever, and abdominal pain suggest inflammatory bowel disease (ulcerative colitis, Crohn's disease) or an infectious colitis (eg, *Shigella, Salmonella, Campylobacter,* amebiasis). Hematochezia suggests diverticulosis or angiodysplasia. Fresh blood only on toilet paper or the surface of formed stools suggests internal hemorrhoids, whereas blood mixed with the stool indicates a more proximal source.

A drug history may reveal use of drugs that break the gastric barrier and damage the gastric mucosa (eg, aspirin, NSAIDs, alcohol).

Physical examination: Blood in the nose or trickling down the pharynx suggests the nasopharynx as the source. Spider angiomas, hepatosplenomegaly, or ascites is consistent with chronic liver disease and hence possible esophageal varices. Arteriovenous malformations, especially of the mucous membranes, suggest hereditary hemorrhagic telangiectasia (Rendu-Osler-Weber syndrome). Cutaneous nail bed and GI telangiectasia may indicate systemic sclerosis or mixed connective tissue disease.

A digital rectal examination is necessary to search for stool color, masses, fissures, and hemorrhoids. Chemical testing of a stool specimen for occult blood completes the examination. Occult blood in the stool may be the first sign of colon cancer or a polyp, particularly in patients > 45.

Testing: CBC should be obtained in patients with occult blood loss. Those with more significant bleeding also require coagulation studies (platelet count, PT, PTT), and liver function tests (bilirubin, alkaline phosphatase, albumin, AST, ALT). Type and crossmatch are performed if bleeding is ongoing. Hb and Hct may be repeated up to q 6 h in patients with severe bleeding. Additionally, one or more diagnostic procedures are typically required.

Nasogastric aspiration and lavage should be performed in all patients with suspected upper GI bleeding (eg, hematemesis, coffee-ground emesis, melena, massive rectal bleeding). Bloody nasogastric aspirate indicates active upper GI bleeding, but about 10% of patients with upper GI bleeding have no blood in the nasogastric aspirate. Coffee-ground material indicates bleeding that is slow or stopped. If there is no sign of bleeding, and bile is returned, the nasogastric tube is removed; otherwise, it is left in place to monitor continuing or recurrent bleeding.

Upper endoscopy (examination of the esophagus, stomach, and duodenum) should be performed for upper GI bleeding. Because endoscopy may be therapeutic as well as diagnostic, it should be performed rapidly for significant bleeding but may be deferred for 24 h if bleeding stops or is minimal. Upper GI barium x-rays have no role in acute bleeding. Angiography has a limited role in the diagnosis of upper GI bleeding (mainly for bleeding from hepatobiliary fistulas), although it does permit certain therapeutic maneuvers (eg, embolization, vasoconstrictor infusion).

Flexible sigmoidoscopy and rigid anoscopy may be all that is required acutely for patients with symptoms typical of hemorrhoidal bleeding. All other patients with hematochezia should have colonoscopy, which can be done electively after routine preparation unless there is significant ongoing bleeding. In such patients, a rapid prep (5 to 10 L of polyethylene glycol solution delivered via nasogastric tube or by mouth over 3 to 4 h) often allows adequate visualization. If colonoscopy cannot visualize the source and ongoing bleeding is sufficiently rapid (> 0.5 to 1 mL/min), angiography may localize the source. Some angiographers first perform a radionuclide scan to focus the examination, although the benefit of this is unproven.

Diagnosis of occult bleeding can be difficult, because heme-positive stools may result from bleeding anywhere in the GI tract. Endoscopy is the preferred method, with symptoms determining whether the upper or lower GI tract is examined first. Double-contrast barium enema and sigmoidoscopy can be used for the lower tract when colonoscopy is unavailable or the patient refuses it. If the results of upper endoscopy and colonoscopy are negative and occult blood persists in the stool, an upper GI series with small-bowel follow-through, small-bowel endoscopy (enteroscopy), technetium-labeled colloid or RBC scan, and angiography should be considered.

Treatment

Hematemesis, hematochezia, or melena should be considered an emergency. Admission to an ICU, with consultation by both a gastroenterologist and a surgeon, is recommended for all patients with severe GI bleeding. General treatment is directed at maintenance of the airway and restoration of circulating volume. Hemostasis and other treatment depend on the cause of the bleeding.

Airway: A major cause of morbidity and mortality in patients with active upper GI bleeding is aspiration of blood with subsequent respiratory compromise. To prevent this, endotracheal intubation should be considered in patients who have inadequate gag reflexes or are obtunded or unconscious—particularly if they will be undergoing upper endoscopy or placement of a Sengstaken-Blakemore tube.

Fluid resuscitation: IV fluids are initiated as for any patient with hypovolemia or hemorrhagic shock (see p. 564): healthy adults are given normal saline IV in 500- to 1000-mL aliquots until signs of hypovolemia remit—up to a maximum of 2 L (for children 20 mL/kg, which may be repeated once). Patients requiring further resuscitation should receive transfusion with packed RBCs. Transfusions continue until intravascular volume is restored and then are given as needed to replace ongoing blood loss. Transfusions may be stopped when Hct is stable at 30 unless the patient is symptomatic. Patients with chronic bleeding are usually not transfused unless Hct is < 21 or they have symptoms such as dyspnea or coronary ischemia.

Platelet count should be monitored closely; platelet transfusion may be required with severe bleeding. Patients who are taking antiplatelet drugs (eg, clopidogrel, aspirin) have platelet dysfunction, often resulting in increased bleeding. Platelet transfusion should be considered when patients taking these drugs have severe ongoing bleeding, although residual circulating drug (particularly clopidogrel) may inactivate transfused platelets.

Hemostasis: GI bleeding stops spontaneously in about 80% of patients. The remaining patients require some type of intervention. Specific therapy depends on the bleeding site. Early intervention to control bleeding is important to minimize mortality, particularly in elderly patients.

For peptic ulcer, ongoing bleeding or rebleeding is treated with endoscopic coagulation (with bipolar electrocoagulation, injection sclerotherapy, heater probes, or laser). Nonbleeding vessels that are visible within an ulcer crater are also treated. If endoscopy fails to stop the bleeding, surgery is required to oversew the bleeding site. Some surgeons perform acid-reduction surgery (see p. 123) at the same time.

Active variceal bleeding can be treated with endoscopic banding, injection sclerotherapy, or a transjugular intrahepatic portosystemic shunting (TIPS) procedure.

Severe, ongoing lower GI bleeding from diverticula or angiomas can sometimes be controlled colonoscopically by electrocautery, coagulation with a heater probe, or injection with dilute epinephrine. Polyps can be removed by snare or cautery. If these methods are ineffective or unfeasible, angiography with embolization or vasopressin infusion may be successful. However, because collateral blood flow to the bowel is limited, angiographic techniques have a significant risk of bowel ischemia or infarction. Vasopressin infusion has about an 80% success rate for stopping bleeding, but bleeding recurs in about 50% of patients. Also, there is a risk of hypertension and coronary ischemia. Surgery may be used in patients with continued bleeding (requiring > 4 units transfusion/24 h), but localization of the bleeding site is very important. Blind hemicolectomy (with no preoperative identification of the bleeding site) carries a much higher mortality risk than does directed segmental resection. However, work-up must be expeditious so that surgery is not unnecessarily delayed.

Acute or chronic bleeding of internal hemorrhoids stops spontaneously in most cases. Patients with refractory bleeding are treated via anoscopy with rubber band ligation, injection, coagulation, or surgery.

VARICES

Varices are dilated veins in the distal esophagus or proximal stomach caused by elevated pressure in the portal venous system, typically from cirrhosis. They may bleed massively but cause no other symptoms. Diagnosis is by upper endoscopy, and treatment is primarily with endoscopic banding and intravenous octreotide. Sometimes a transjugular intrahepatic portosystemic shunting procedure is needed.

Portal hypertension (see p. 195) results from a number of conditions, predominantly liver cirrhosis. If portal pressure remains higher than inferior vena caval pressure for a significant period, venous collaterals develop. The most dangerous collaterals occur in the distal esophagus and gastric fundus, producing engorged, serpentine submucosal vessels known as varices. These varices partially decompress portal hypertension but can rupture, causing massive GI bleeding. The trigger for variceal rupture is unknown, but bleeding almost never occurs unless the portal/systemic pressure gradient is > 12 mm Hg. Coagulopathies from liver disease may facilitate bleeding. Nasogastric tube passage in a patient with varices has not been shown to trigger bleeding.

Symptoms and Signs

Patients typically present with sudden painless upper GI bleeding, often massive. Signs of shock may be present. Bleeding is usually from the distal esophagus, less often from the gastric fundus. Bleeding from gastric varices also may be acute but is more often subacute or chronic.

Bleeding into the GI tract may precipitate hepatic encephalopathy in patients with impaired hepatic function.

Diagnosis

Both esophageal and gastric varices are best diagnosed by endoscopy, which may also identify varices at high risk of bleeding (eg, those with red markings). Endoscopy is also critical to exclude other causes of acute bleeding (eg, peptic ulcer), even in patients known to have varices; perhaps ⅓ of patients with known varices who have upper GI bleeding have a nonvariceal source.

Because varices are typically associated with significant hepatic disease, evaluation for possible coagulopathy is important. Laboratory tests include CBC with platelets, PT, PTT, and liver function tests. Bleeding patients should have type and crossmatch for 6 units of packed RBCs.

Prognosis

In about 80% of patients, variceal bleeding stops spontaneously. Nevertheless, mortality is high, often > 50%. Mortality depends primarily on severity of the associated liver disease rather than on the bleeding itself; bleeding is often fatal in patients with severe hepatocellular impairment (eg, advanced cirrhosis), whereas patients with good hepatic reserve usually recover.

Surviving patients are at high risk of further variceal bleeding, typically 50 to 75% have recurrence within 1 to 2 yr. Ongoing endoscopic or drug therapy significantly lowers this risk, but the overall effect on long-term mortality appears to be marginal, probably because of the underlying hepatic disease.

Treatment

Management of hypovolemia and hemorrhagic shock is as described above and in Ch. 67 (see p. 559). Patients with coagulation abnormalities (eg, elevated INR) should be given 1 to 2 units of fresh frozen plasma IV and 2.5 to 10 mg vitamin K IM (or IV if severe).

Because varices are invariably diagnosed during endoscopy, primary treatment is endoscopic. Endoscopic banding of varices is preferred over injection sclerotherapy. At the same time, intravenous octreotide (a synthetic analog of somatostatin, which may also be used) should be given. Octreotide increases splanchnic vascular resistance by inhibiting the release of splanchnic vasodilator hormones (eg, glucagon and vasoactive intestinal peptide). The usual dose is a 50 μg IV bolus, followed by infusion of 50 μg/h. Octreotide is preferred over previously used agents such as vasopressin and terlipressin, because it has fewer adverse effects.

If bleeding continues or recurs despite these measures, emergency techniques to shunt blood from the portal system to the vena cava can lower portal pressure and diminish bleeding. A transjugular intrahepatic portosystemic shunting (TIPS) procedure is the emergency intervention of choice: it is an invasive radiologic procedure in which a guidewire is passed from the vena cava through the liver parenchyma into the portal circulation. The resultant passage is dilated by a balloon catheter, and a metallic stent is inserted, creating a bypass between the portal and hepatic venous circulations. Stent size is crucial: if it is too large, hepatic encephalopathy results because of diversion of too much portal blood flow from the liver. On the other hand, small stents are more likely to occlude. Surgical portacaval shunts, such as the distal spleno-renal shunt, work by a similar mechanism but are more invasive and have a higher immediate mortality.

Mechanical compression of bleeding varices with a Sengstaken-Blakemore tube or one of its variants is associated with considerable morbidity and should not be used as primary management. However, such a tube may provide life-saving tamponade pending decompression with a TIPS or surgical procedure. The tube is a flexible nasogastric tube with two balloons, gastric and esophageal. After insertion, the gastric balloon is inflated with a fixed volume of air, and traction is applied to the tube to pull the balloon snug against the gastroesophageal junction. This is often sufficient to control bleeding, but if not, the esophageal balloon is inflated to a pressure of 25 mm Hg. The procedure is quite uncomfortable and may result in esophageal perforation and aspiration; thus, endotracheal intubation and IV sedation are often recommended.

Liver transplantation can also decompress the portal system but is a practical option only for patients already on a transplant list.

Long-term medical therapy of portal hypertension (with β-blockers and nitrates) is described on p. 197. Treatment of hepatic encephalopathy may be needed (see p. 198).

VASCULAR GI LESIONS

Several distinct congenital or acquired syndromes involve abnormal mucosal or submucosal blood vessels in the GI tract. These vessels may cause recurrent bleeding, which is rarely massive. Diagnosis is by endoscopy and sometimes angiography. Treatment is endoscopic hemostasis; occasionally angiographic embolization or surgical resection may be needed.

Vascular ectasias (angiodysplasias) are dilated, tortuous vessels that typically develop in the cecum and ascending colon. They occur mainly in people > 60 and are the most common cause of lower GI bleeding in that age group. They are thought to be degenerative and do not occur in association with other vascular abnormalities. Most patients have two or three lesions, which are typically 0.5 to 1.0 cm, bright red, flat or slightly raised, and covered by very thin epithelium. Vascular ectasias also occur in association with a number of systemic diseases (eg, renal failure, cirrhosis, CREST syndrome—see p. 270) and after radiation to the bowel.

Gastric antral vascular ectasia (watermelon stomach) consists of large dilated veins running linearly along the stomach, creating a striped appearance suggestive of a watermelon. The condition occurs mainly in older women and is of unknown etiology.

Hereditary hemorrhagic telangiectasia (Rendu-Osler-Weber syndrome—see also p. 1089) is an autosomal dominant disorder that causes multiple vascular lesions in various parts of the body, including the entire GI tract. GI bleeding rarely occurs before age 40.

Dieulafoy's lesion is an abnormally large artery that penetrates the gut wall, occasionally eroding through the mucosa and causing massive bleeding. It occurs mainly in the proximal stomach.

Arteriovenous malformations (AVMs) and **hemangiomas,** both congenital disorders of blood vessels, can occur in the GI tract but are rare.

Symptoms, Signs, and Diagnosis

Vascular lesions are painless and often present with heme-positive stools or modest amounts of bright red blood from the rectum. Bleeding is often intermittent, sometimes with long periods between episodes. Upper GI lesions may present with melena. Major bleeding is unusual.

Vascular lesions are most commonly diagnosed endoscopically. If routine endoscopy is nondiagnostic, small-bowel endoscopy, capsule endoscopy, intraoperative endoscopy, or visceral angiography may be required. ^{99m}Tc-labeled RBC scans are less sensitive but may help localize the lesion enough to facilitate endoscopy.

Treatment

Endoscopic coagulation (with heater probe, laser, argon plasma, or bipolar electrocoagulation) is effective for many vascular lesions. Vascular ectasias often recur, although there is some evidence that oral estrogen-progesterone combinations may limit this.

Mild recurrent bleeding can be treated simply with chronic iron therapy. More significant bleeding that is unresponsive to endoscopic measures may require angiographic embolization or surgical resection. However, rebleeding occurs in about 15 to 25% of surgically treated patients.

11 ACUTE ABDOMEN AND SURGICAL GASTROENTEROLOGY

Acute abdomen refers to abdominal symptoms and signs of such severity or concern that disorders requiring surgery should be considered. The primary symptom is acute abdominal pain. Chronic abdominal pain is discussed on p. 66.

ACUTE ABDOMINAL PAIN

Abdominal pain is common and often inconsequential. Acute and severe abdominal pain, however, is almost always a symptom of intra-abdominal disease. It may be the sole indicator of the need for surgery and must be attended to swiftly: Gangrene and perforation of the gut can occur < 6 h from onset of symptoms in certain conditions (eg, interruption of the intestinal blood supply from a strangulating obstruction or an arterial embolus). Abdominal pain is of particular concern in patients who are very young or very old and those who have HIV infection or are taking immunosuppressants.

Textbook descriptions of abdominal pain have limitations because people react to pain differently. Some, particularly elderly people, are stoic, whereas others exaggerate their symptoms. Infants, young children, and some elderly people may have difficulty localizing the pain.

Pathophysiology

Visceral pain comes from the abdominal viscera, which are innervated by autonomic nerve fibers and respond mainly to the sensations of distention and muscular contraction—not to cutting, tearing, or local irritation. Visceral pain is typically vague, dull, and nauseating. It is poorly localized and tends to be perceived in areas corresponding to the embryonic origin of the affected structure. Foregut structures (stomach, duodenum, liver, and pancreas) cause upper abdominal pain. Midgut structures (small bowel, proximal colon, and appendix) cause periumbilical pain. Hindgut structures (distal colon and GU tract) cause lower abdominal pain.

Somatic pain comes from the parietal peritoneum, which is innervated by somatic nerves, which respond to irritation from infectious, chemical, or other inflammatory processes. Somatic pain is sharp and well localized.

Referred pain is pain perceived distant from its source and results from convergence of nerve fibers at the spinal cord. Common examples of referred pain are scapular pain due to biliary colic, groin pain due to renal colic, and shoulder pain due to blood or infection irritating the diaphragm.

Peritonitis is inflammation of the peritoneal cavity. Most serious cause is perforation of the GI tract (see p. 100), which produces immediate chemical inflammation followed shortly by infection from intestinal organisms. Peritonitis can also result from any abdominal condition that produces marked inflammation (eg, appendicitis, diverticulitis, strangulating intestinal obstruction, pancreatitis, pelvic inflammatory disease, and mesenteric ischemia). Intraperitoneal blood from any source (eg, ruptured aneurysm, trauma, surgery, ectopic pregnancy) is irritating and results in peritonitis. Barium causes severe peritonitis and should never be given to a patient with suspected GI tract perforation. Peritoneo-systemic shunts, drains, and dialysis catheters in the peritoneal cavity predispose a patient to infectious peritonitis, as does ascitic fluid. Rarely, spontaneous bacterial peritonitis occurs, in which the peritoneal cavity is infected by blood-borne bacteria. Peritonitis causes fluid shift into the peritoneal cavity and bowel leading to severe dehydration and electrolyte disturbances. Adult respiratory distress syndrome can develop rapidly. Kidney failure, liver failure, and disseminated intravascular coagulation follow. The patient's face becomes drawn into the masklike appearance typical of hippocratic facies. Death occurs within days.

TABLE 11–1. EXTRA-ABDOMINAL CAUSES OF ABDOMINAL PAIN

Abdominal wall
- Rectus muscle hematoma

Genitourinary
- Testicular torsion

Infectious
- Herpes zoster

Metabolic
- Alcoholic ketoacidosis
- Diabetic ketoacidosis
- Porphyria
- Sickle cell disease

Thoracic
- Myocardial infarction
- Pneumonia
- Pulmonary embolism
- Radiculitis

Toxic
- Black widow spider bite
- Heavy metal poisoning
- Methanol poisoning
- Scorpion sting

Etiology

Many intra-abdominal disorders produce abdominal pain (see Fig 11–1); some are trivial but some are immediately life threatening, requiring rapid diagnosis and surgery. These include ruptured abdominal aortic aneurysm (AAA), perforated viscus, mesenteric ischemia, and ruptured ectopic pregnancy. Others (eg, intestinal obstruction, appendicitis, severe acute pancreatitis) are also serious and nearly as urgent. Several extra-abdominal disorders also produce abdominal pain (see Table 11–1).

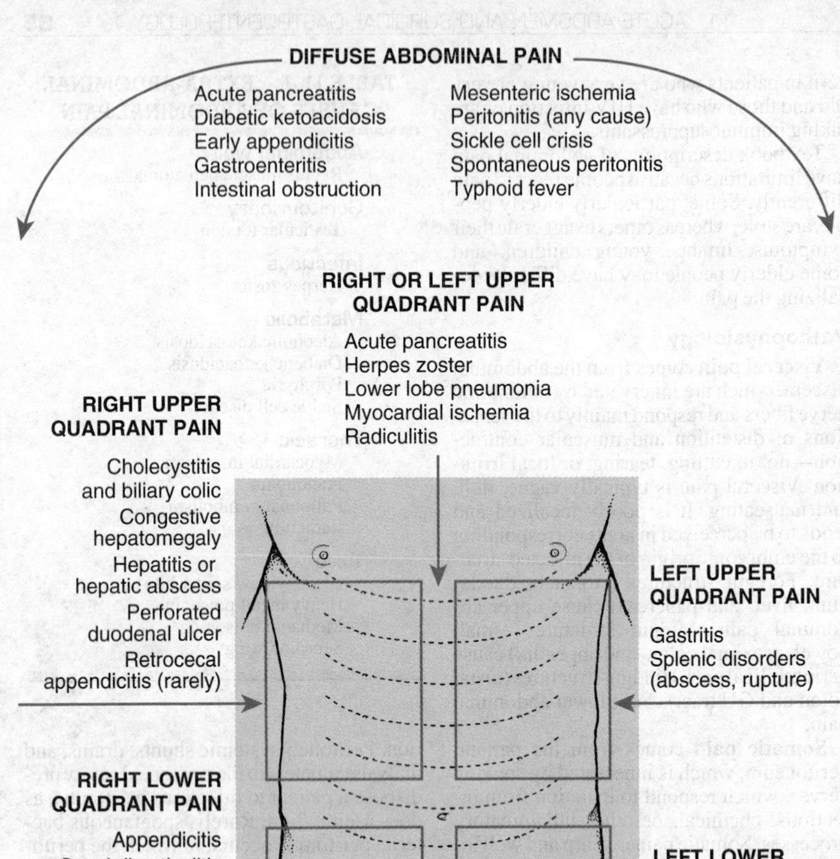

DIFFUSE ABDOMINAL PAIN
Acute pancreatitis
Diabetic ketoacidosis
Early appendicitis
Gastroenteritis
Intestinal obstruction
Mesenteric ischemia
Peritonitis (any cause)
Sickle cell crisis
Spontaneous peritonitis
Typhoid fever
RIGHT OR LEFT UPPER QUADRANT PAIN
Acute pancreatitis
Herpes zoster
Lower lobe pneumonia
Myocardial ischemia
Radiculitis
RIGHT UPPER QUADRANT PAIN
Cholecystitis and biliary colic
Congestive hepatomegaly
Hepatitis or hepatic abscess
Perforated duodenal ulcer
Retrocecal appendicitis (rarely)
LEFT UPPER QUADRANT PAIN
Gastritis
Splenic disorders (abscess, rupture)
RIGHT LOWER QUADRANT PAIN
Appendicitis
Cecal diverticulitis
Meckel's diverticulitis
Mesenteric adenitis
LEFT LOWER QUADRANT PAIN
Sigmoid diverticulitis
RIGHT OR LEFT LOWER QUADRANT PAIN
Abdominal or psoas abscess
Abdominal wall hematoma
Cystitis
Endometriosis
Incarcerated or strangulated hernia
Inflammatory bowel disease
Mittelschmerz
Pelvic inflammatory disease
Renal stone
Ruptured abdominal aortic aneurysm
Ruptured ectopic pregnancy
Torsion of ovarian cyst or teste

Fig. 11–1. Location of abdominal pain and possible causes.

Abdominal pain in neonates, infants, and young children has numerous causes not encountered in adults, including meconium peritonitis, pyloric stenosis, esophageal webs, volvulus of a gut with a common mesentery, imperforate anus, intussusception, and intestinal obstruction from atresia.

Evaluation

Evaluation of mild and severe pain follows the same process, although with severe abdominal pain, therapy sometimes proceeds simultaneously and involves early consultation with a surgeon. History and physical examination usually exclude all but a few possible causes, with final diagnosis confirmed by judicious use of laboratory and imaging tests. Life-threatening causes should always be ruled out before focusing on less serious diagnoses. In seriously ill patients with severe abdominal pain, the most important diagnostic measure may be expeditious exploratory laparotomy. In mildly ill patients, watchful waiting may be best.

History: A thorough history usually suggests the diagnosis (see TABLE 11–2). Of particular importance are pain location (see FIG 11–1) and characteristics, history of similar symptoms, and associated symptoms. Concomitant symptoms such as gastroesophageal reflux, diarrhea, constipation, jaundice, melena, hematuria, hema-temesis, weight loss, and mucus or blood in the stool help direct subsequent evaluation.

A drug history should include details concerning prescription and illicit drug use as well as alcohol. Many drugs cause GI upset. Prednisone or immunosuppressants may inhibit the inflammatory response to perforation or peritonitis and result in less pain and leukocytosis than might otherwise be expected. Anticoagulants can increase the chances of bleeding and hematoma formation. Alcohol predisposes to pancreatitis.

Known medical conditions are important. Previous abdominal surgery makes obstruction from adhesions more likely. Generalized atherosclerosis increases the possibility of MI, AAA, and mesenteric ischemia. HIV infection makes infectious causes and drug adverse effects likely.

Physical examination: The general appearance is important. A happy, comfortable-appearing patient rarely has a serious problem, unlike one who is anxious, pale, diaphoretic, or in obvious pain. BP, pulse, state of consciousness, and other signs of peripheral perfusion must be evaluated. However, the focus of the examination is the abdomen, beginning with inspection and auscultation. Distention, especially when surgical scars are present, suggests bowel obstruction. Ecchymoses of the costovertebral angles (Grey Turner's sign) or around the umbilicus (Cullen's sign) sometimes appear in hemorrhagic pancreatitis. Active peristalsis of normal pitch suggests a nonsurgical disease (eg, gastroenteritis). High-pitched peristalsis or borborygmi in rushes suggests intestinal obstruction. Severe pain with a silent abdomen suggests peritonitis. Back pain with shock suggests ruptured AAA.

Palpation begins gently, away from the area of greatest pain, detecting areas of particular tenderness, as well as the presence of guarding, rigidity, and rebound (all suggesting peritoneal irritation) and any masses. Guarding is an involuntary contraction of the abdominal muscles that is slightly slower and more sustained than the rapid, voluntary flinch exhibited by sensitive or anxious patients. The inguinal area and all surgical scars should be palpated for hernias. Rectal and pelvic examinations are essential.

Testing: Standard tests (eg, CBC, chemistries, urinalysis) are often performed but are of little value due to poor sensitivity: patients with significant disease may have normal results. Abnormal results do not provide a specific diagnosis (the urinalysis in particular may show pyuria or hematuria in a wide variety of conditions), and they can also occur in the absence of significant disease. An exception is serum lipase, which suggests strongly the diagnosis of acute pancreatitis. A bedside urine pregnancy test should be obtained in all women of childbearing age because a negative result effectively excludes ruptured ectopic pregnancy.

An abdominal series, consisting of flat and upright abdominal x-rays and upright chest x-rays (left lateral recumbent abdomen and anteroposterior chest x-ray for patients unable to stand), should be obtained when perforation or obstruction is suspected. However, these plain x-rays are seldom diagnostic for other conditions and need not be automatically obtained. Ultrasound should be performed for suspected biliary tract disease or ectopic pregnancy (transvaginal probe). Ultrasound can also detect AAA but cannot reliably identify rupture. Noncontrast helical

TABLE 11–2. HISTORY IN PATIENTS WITH ACUTE ABDOMINAL PAIN

QUESTION	POTENTIAL RESPONSES AND INDICATIONS
Where is the pain?	See FIG. 11–1
What is the pain like?	Acute waves of sharp constricting pain that "takes the breath away" (renal or biliary colic) Waves of dull pain with vomiting (intestinal obstruction) Colicky pain that becomes steady (appendicitis, strangulating intestinal obstruction, mesenteric ischemia) Sharp, constant pain, worsened by movement (peritonitis) Tearing pain (dissecting aneurysm) Dull ache (appendicitis, diverticulitis, pyelonephritis)
Have you had it before?	Yes suggests recurrent problems such as ulcer disease, gallstone colic, diverticulitis, or mittelschmerz
Was the onset sudden?	Sudden: "like a light switching on" (perforated ulcer, renal stone, ruptured ectopic pregnancy, torsion of ovary or testis, some ruptured aneurysms) Less sudden: most other causes
How severe is the pain?	Severe pain (perforated viscus, kidney stone, peritonitis, pancreatitis) Pain out of proportion to physical findings (mesenteric ischemia)
Does the pain travel to any other part of the body?	Right scapula (gallbladder pain) Left shoulder region (ruptured spleen, pancreatitis) Pubis or vagina (renal pain) Back (ruptured aortic aneurysm)
What relieves the pain?	Antacids (peptic ulcer disease) Lying as quietly as possible (peritonitis)
What other symptoms occur with the pain?	Vomiting precedes pain and is followed by diarrhea (gastroenteritis) Delayed vomiting, absent bowel movement and flatus (acute intestinal obstruction; the delay increases with a lower site of obstruction) Severe vomiting precedes intense epigastric, left chest, or shoulder pain (emetic perforation of the intra-abdominal esophagus)

CT is the modality of choice for suspected renal stones. CT with oral contrast is diagnostic in about 95% of patients with significant abdominal pain and has markedly lowered the negative laparotomy rate. However, advanced imaging must not be allowed to delay surgery in patients with definitive symptoms and signs.

Treatment

Some clinicians feel that providing pain relief before a diagnosis is made interferes with their ability to evaluate. However, moderate doses of IV analgesics (eg, fentanyl 50 to 100 μg, morphine 4 to 6 mg) do not mask peritoneal signs and, by diminishing anxiety and discomfort, often make examination easier.

ACUTE MESENTERIC ISCHEMIA

Acute mesenteric ischemia is interruption of intestinal blood flow by embolism, thrombosis, or a low-flow state. It leads to mediator release, inflammation, and ultimately infarction. Abdominal pain is out of proportion to physical findings. Early diagnosis is difficult, but angiography and exploratory

laparotomy have the most sensitivity; other imaging modalities often become positive only late in the disease. Treatment is by embolectomy, revascularization of viable segments, or resection; sometimes vasodilator therapy is successful. Mortality is high.

Etiology and Pathophysiology

The intestinal mucosa has a high metabolic rate and, accordingly, a high blood flow requirement (normally receiving 20 to 25% of cardiac output), making it very sensitive to the effects of decreased perfusion. Ischemia disrupts the mucosal barrier, allowing release of bacteria, toxins, and vasoactive mediators, which in turn leads to myocardial depression, systemic inflammatory response syndrome (see p. 566), multisystem organ failure, and death. Mediator release may occur even before complete infarction. Necrosis can occur as soon as 10 to 12 h after the onset of symptoms.

Three major vessels serve the abdominal contents: the celiac trunk, the superior mesenteric artery (SMA), and the inferior mesenteric artery (IMA). The celiac trunk supplies the esophagus, stomach, proximal duodenum, liver, gallbladder, pancreas, and spleen. The SMA supplies the distal duodenum, jejunum, ileum, and colon to the splenic flexure. The IMA supplies the descending and sigmoid colon and the rectum. Collateral vessels are abundant in the stomach, duodenum, and rectum; these areas rarely develop ischemia. The splenic flexure is a watershed between the SMA and IMA and is at particular risk for ischemia.

Mesenteric blood flow may be disrupted on either the venous or arterial sides. In general, patients > 50 are at greatest risk and have the following types of occlusions and risk factors. (1) Arterial embolus (50%), risk factors: coronary artery disease, heart failure, valvular heart disease, atrial fibrillation, and history of arterial emboli. (2) Arterial thrombosis (10%), risk factor: generalized atherosclerosis. (3) Venous thrombosis (10%), risk factors: hypercoagulable state, inflammatory conditions (eg, pancreatitis, diverticulitis), trauma, heart failure, renal failure, portal hypertension, and decompression sickness. (4) Nonocclusive ischemia (25%), risk factors: low flow states (heart failure, shock, cardiopulmonary bypass) and splanchnic vasoconstriction (vasopressors, cocaine). However, many patients have no identifiable risk factors.

Symptoms and Signs

The early hallmark of mesenteric ischemia is severe pain but minimal physical findings. The abdomen remains soft, with little or no tenderness. Mild tachycardia may be present. Later, as necrosis develops, signs of peritonitis appear, with marked abdominal tenderness, guarding, rigidity, and no bowel sounds. The stool may be heme-positive (increasingly likely as ischemia progresses). The usual signs of shock develop and are frequently followed by death.

Sudden onset of pain suggests but is not diagnostic of an arterial embolism, whereas a more gradual onset is typical of venous thrombosis. Patients with a history of postprandial abdominal discomfort (which suggests intestinal angina) may have arterial thrombosis.

Diagnosis

Early diagnosis is particularly important because mortality increases significantly once intestinal infarction has occurred. Mesenteric ischemia must be considered in any patient > 50 with known risk factors or predisposing conditions who develops sudden, severe abdominal pain.

Patients with clear peritoneal signs should proceed directly to laparotomy for both diagnosis and treatment. For others, selective mesenteric angiography is the diagnostic procedure of choice. Other imaging studies and serum markers can demonstrate abnormalities but lack sensitivity and specificity early in the course of the disease when diagnosis is most critical. Plain abdominal x-rays are useful mainly to rule out other causes of pain (eg, perforated viscus), although late in the disease portal venous gas or pneumatosis intestinalis may be seen. These findings also appear on CT, which may also directly visualize vascular occlusion—more accurately on the venous side. Doppler ultrasonography can sometimes identify arterial occlusion, but sensitivity is low. MRI is very accurate in proximal vascular occlusion, less so in distal vascular occlusion. Serum markers (eg, creatine phosphokinase and lactate) rise with necrosis but are nonspecific and later findings. Serum intestinal fatty acid binding protein may prove valuable in the future as an early marker.

Prognosis and Treatment

If diagnosis and treatment take place before infarction occurs, mortality is low;

after intestinal infarction, mortality approaches 70 to 90%.

If diagnosis is made during exploratory laparotomy, options are surgical embolectomy, revascularization, or resection. If diagnosis is made by angiography, infusion of the vasodilator papaverine through the angiography catheter may improve survival in both occlusive and nonocclusive ischemia. A 60-mg bolus is given over 2 min, followed by an infusion of 30 to 60 mg/h. Papaverine is useful even when surgical intervention is planned and is sometimes given during and after surgery as well. In addition, for arterial occlusion, thrombolysis or surgical embolectomy may be performed. The development of peritoneal signs at any time during the evaluation suggests the need for immediate surgery. Mesenteric venous thrombosis without signs of peritonitis can be treated with papaverine followed by anticoagulation with heparin and then warfarin.

Patients with arterial embolism or venous thrombosis require long-term anticoagulation with warfarin. Patients with nonocclusive ischemia may be treated with antiplatelet therapy.

ACUTE PERFORATION

Any part of the GI tract may become perforated from a variety of causes, releasing gastric or intestinal contents into the peritoneal space. Symptoms develop suddenly, with severe pain followed shortly by signs of shock. Diagnosis is usually made by the presence of free air in the abdomen on imaging studies. Treatment is with fluid resuscitation, antibiotics, and surgery. Mortality is high, varying with the underlying disorder and the patient's general health.

Etiology

Both blunt and penetrating trauma can result in perforation of any part of the GI tract. Swallowed foreign bodies, even sharp ones, rarely cause perforation unless they become impacted, causing ischemia and necrosis from local pressure.

Esophageal perforation usually occurs above the diaphragm (Boerhaave's syndrome) but may occur into the abdomen either from forceful vomiting or iatrogenic causes (eg, perforation with an esophagoscope, balloon dilator, or bougie). Ingestion of large amounts of corrosive material perforates the esophagus or stomach.

Gastric or duodenal perforation is usually the result of peptic ulcer disease, although about $\frac{1}{3}$ of patients have not had previous ulcer symptoms.

Perforated intestine may arise from strangulating obstruction. Acute appendicitis and Meckel's diverticulitis also may perforate.

Perforated colon is caused by obstruction, diverticulitis, ulcerative colitis, Crohn's disease, and toxic megacolon. Sometimes perforation occurs spontaneously. In the presence of colonic obstruction, perforation typically occurs at the cecum; this catastrophe is imminent if the cecum is ≥ 13 cm in diameter. Patients receiving prednisone or other immunosuppressants are apt to have such perforations, which may be essentially silent.

Perforated gallbladder rarely occurs with acute cholecystitis. The biliary tree may be perforated by iatrogenic damage during cholecystectomy. Perforation of the gallbladder usually leads to a local abscess contained by the omentum and rarely leads to generalized peritonitis.

Symptoms and Signs

Esophageal, gastric, and duodenal perforation tend to present suddenly and catastrophically, with abrupt onset of acute abdomen with severe generalized abdominal pain, tenderness, and peritoneal signs. Pain may radiate to the shoulder.

Perforation at other GI sites often occurs in the setting of other painful, inflammatory conditions. Because perforations are often small initially and frequently walled off by the omentum, pain often develops gradually and may be localized. Tenderness also is more focal.

In all types of perforation, nausea, vomiting, and anorexia are common. Bowel sounds are quiet to absent.

Diagnosis and Treatment

An abdominal series (flat and upright abdominal x-rays and chest x-rays) may be diagnostic, showing free air under the diaphragm in 50 to 75% of cases. As time passes, this sign becomes more common. A lateral chest x-ray is more sensitive for free air than a posteroanterior x-ray. If the abdominal series is nondiagnostic, CT with oral and perhaps IV contrast may be helpful.

If a perforation is noted, immediate surgery is necessary because mortality from peritonitis increases rapidly the longer treatment is delayed. If an abscess or an inflammatory mass has formed, the operation may be limited to drainage of the abscess.

A nasogastric tube is inserted before operation. Patients with signs of volume depletion should have urine output monitored with a catheter. Fluid status is maintained by adequate IV fluid and electrolyte replacement. IV antibiotics effective against intestinal flora should be given (eg, cefotetan 1 to 2 g bid, or amikacin 5 mg/kg tid plus clindamycin 600 to 900 mg qid).

APPENDICITIS

Appendicitis is acute inflammation of the vermiform appendix, typically resulting in abdominal pain, anorexia, and abdominal tenderness. Diagnosis is clinical, often supplemented by CT or ultrasound. Treatment is surgical removal.

Etiology and Pathophysiology

Appendicitis is thought to result from obstruction of the appendiceal lumen, typically by lymphoid hyperplasia, but occasionally by a fecalith, foreign body, or even worms. The obstruction leads to distention, bacterial overgrowth, ischemia, and inflammation. If untreated, necrosis, gangrene, and perforation occur. If the perforation is contained by the omentum, an appendiceal abscess results.

In the US, acute appendicitis is the most common cause of acute abdominal pain requiring surgery. Over 5% of the population develops appendicitis at some point. It is most common in the teens and 20s but may occur at any age.

Other conditions affecting the appendix include carcinoids, cancer, villous adenomas, and diverticula. The appendix may also be affected by Crohn's disease or ulcerative colitis with pancolitis.

Symptoms and Signs

The classic symptoms of acute appendicitis are epigastric or periumbilical pain followed by brief nausea, vomiting, and anorexia; after a few hours, the pain shifts to the right lower quadrant. Pain increases with cough and motion. Classic signs are right lower quadrant direct and rebound tenderness located at McBurney's point (junction of the middle and outer thirds of the line joining the umbilicus to the anterior superior spine). Additional signs are pain felt in the right lower quadrant with palpation of the left lower quadrant (Rovsing's sign), an increase in pain from passive extension of the right hip joint that stretches the iliopsoas muscle (psoas sign), or pain produced by passive internal rotation of the flexed thigh (obturator sign). Low-grade fever (rectal temperature 37.7 to 38.3° C [100 to 101° F]) is common.

Unfortunately, these classic findings appear in < 50% of patients. Many variations in symptoms and signs occur. Pain may not be localized, particularly in infants and children. Tenderness may be diffuse or, in rare instances, absent. Bowel movements are usually less frequent or absent; if diarrhea is a sign, a retrocecal appendix should be suspected. RBCs or WBCs may be present in the urine. Atypical symptoms are common in elderly patients and pregnant women; in particular, pain is less severe and local tenderness is less marked.

Diagnosis

When classic signs and symptoms are present, the diagnosis is clinical. In such patients, delaying laparotomy to perform imaging tests only increases the likelihood of perforation and subsequent complications. In patients with atypical or equivocal findings, imaging studies should be performed without delay. Contrast-enhanced CT has reasonable accuracy in diagnosing appendicitis and can also reveal other causes of an acute abdomen. Graded compression ultrasound can usually be obtained more quickly than CT but is occasionally limited by the presence of bowel gas and is less useful for recognizing nonappendiceal causes of pain. Use of these studies has lowered the rate of negative laparotomy.

Laparoscopy can be used for diagnosis; it may be especially helpful in women with lower abdominal pain of unclear etiology. Laboratory studies typically show leukocytosis (12,000 to 15,000/μL), but this finding is highly variable; a normal WBC count should not be used to exclude appendicitis.

Prognosis and Treatment

With early surgery, the mortality rate is < 1%, and convalescence is normally rapid and complete. With complications (rupture and development of an abscess or peritonitis), the prognosis is worse: Repeat operations and long convalescence may follow.

Treatment of acute appendicitis is appendectomy; because treatment delay increases mortality, a negative appendectomy rate of 10% is considered acceptable. The surgeon can usually remove the appendix even if perforated. Occasionally, the appendix is difficult to locate: In these cases, it usually lies behind the cecum or the ileum and mesentery of the right colon. A contraindication to appendectomy is inflammatory bowel disease involving the cecum. However, in cases of terminal ileitis and a normal cecum, the appendix should be removed.

Appendectomy should be preceded by IV antibiotics. Third-generation cephalosporins are preferred. For nonperforated appendicitis, no further antibiotics are required. If the appendix is perforated, antibiotics should be continued until the patient's temperature and WBC count have normalized (about 5 days). If surgery is impossible, antibiotics—although not curative—markedly improve the survival rate. Without surgery or antibiotics, mortality is > 50%.

When a large inflammatory mass is found involving the appendix, terminal ileum, and cecum, resection of the entire mass and ileocolostomy are preferable. In late cases in which a pericolic abscess has already formed, the abscess is drained either by an ultrasound-guided percutaneous catheter or by open operation (with appendectomy to follow at a later date). A Meckel's diverticulum should be removed concomitantly with the appendectomy unless extensive inflammation around the appendix prevents the procedure.

HERNIAS OF THE ABDOMINAL WALL

A hernia of the abdominal wall is a protrusion of the abdominal contents through an acquired or congenital area of weakness or defect in the wall. Many hernias are asymptomatic, but some become incarcerated or strangulated, causing pain and requiring immediate operation. Diagnosis is clinical. Treatment is elective surgical repair.

Abdominal hernias are extremely common, particularly in males, necessitating about 700,000 operations each year in the US.

Location and Type

Abdominal hernias are classified as either abdominal wall or groin hernias. Strangulated hernias are ischemic from physical constriction of their blood supply. Gangrene, perforation, and peritonitis may develop. Incarcerated and strangulated hernias cannot be reduced manually.

Abdominal wall hernias include umbilical hernias, epigastric hernias, Spigelian hernias, and incisional (ventral) hernias. Umbilical hernias (protrusions through the umbilical ring) are mostly congenital, but some are acquired in adulthood secondary to obesity, ascites, pregnancy, or chronic peritoneal dialysis. Epigastric hernias occur through the linea alba. Spigelian hernias occur through defects in the transversus abdominis muscle lateral to the rectus sheath, usually below the level of the umbilicus. Incisional hernias occur through an incision from previous abdominal surgery.

Groin hernias include inguinal hernias and femoral hernias. Inguinal hernias occur above the inguinal ligament. Indirect inguinal hernias traverse the internal inguinal ring into the inguinal canal, and direct inguinal hernias extend directly forward and do not pass through the inguinal canal. Femoral hernias occur below the inguinal ligament and go into the femoral canal.

About 50% of all abdominal hernias are indirect inguinal hernias and 25% are direct inguinal hernias. Incisional hernias comprise another 10 to 15%. Femoral and unusual hernias account for the remaining 10 to 15%.

Symptoms and Signs

Most patients complain only of a visible bulge, which may cause vague discomfort or be asymptomatic. Most hernias, even large ones, can be manually reduced with persistent gentle pressure; placing the patient in the Trendelenburg position may help. An incarcerated hernia cannot be reduced but has no additional symptoms. A strangulated hernia causes steady, gradually increasing pain, typically with nausea and vomiting. The hernia itself is tender, and peritonitis may develop depending on location, with diffuse tenderness, guarding, and rebound.

Diagnosis

The diagnosis is clinical. Because the hernia may be apparent only when abdominal pressure is increased, the patient should be examined in standing position. If no hernia is palpable, the patient should cough or perform a Valsalva maneuver as the examiner palpates the abdominal wall. Examination focuses on the umbilicus, the inguinal area (with a finger in the inguinal canal in males), the femoral triangle, and any incisions that are present.

Inguinal masses that resemble hernias may be the result of adenopathy (infectious or malignant), an ectopic testis, or lipoma. These masses are solid and are not reducible. A scrotal mass may be a varicocele, hydrocele, or testicular tumor. Ultrasound may be obtained if physical examination is equivocal.

Prognosis and Treatment

Congenital umbilical hernias rarely strangulate and are not treated; most resolve spontaneously within several years. Very large defects may be repaired electively after age 2 yr. Umbilical hernias in adults cause cosmetic concerns and can be electively repaired; strangulation and incarceration are unusual but, if happen, usually contain omentum rather than intestine.

Groin hernias should be repaired electively because of the risk of strangulation, which results in higher morbidity (and possible mortality in elderly patients). Repair may be through a standard incision or laparoscopically.

ILEUS

(Paralytic Ileus; Adynamic Ileus; Paresis)

Ileus is a temporary arrest of intestinal peristalsis. It occurs most commonly after abdominal surgery, particularly when the intestines have been manipulated. Symptoms are nausea, vomiting, and vague abdominal discomfort. Diagnosis is based on x-ray findings and clinical impression. Treatment is supportive, with nasogastric suction and IV fluids.

Etiology

In addition to postoperative causes, ileus also results from intraperitoneal or retroperitoneal inflammation (eg, appendicitis, diverticulitis, perforated duodenal ulcer), retroperitoneal or intra-abdominal hematomas (eg, ruptured abdominal aortic aneurysm, lumbar compression fracture), metabolic disturbances (eg, hypokalemia), or drugs (eg, opioids, anticholinergics, sometimes Ca channel blockers). Ileus sometimes occurs in association with renal or thoracic disease (eg, lower rib fractures, lower lobe pneumonias, MI).

Gastric and colonic motility disturbances after abdominal surgery are common. The small bowel is typically least affected, with motility and absorption returning to normal within hours after surgery. Stomach emptying is usually impaired for about 24 h or more; the colon is often most affected and may remain inactive for 48 to 72 h or more.

Symptoms and Signs

Symptoms and signs include abdominal distention, vomiting, and vague discomfort. Pain rarely has the classic colicky pattern present in mechanical obstruction. There may be obstipation or passage of slight amounts of watery stool. Auscultation reveals a silent abdomen or minimal peristalsis. The abdomen is not tender unless the underlying cause is inflammatory.

Diagnosis

The most essential task is to distinguish ileus from intestinal obstruction. In both conditions, x-rays show gaseous distention of isolated segments of intestine. In postoperative ileus, however, gas may accumulate more in the colon than in the small bowel. Postoperative accumulation of gas in the small bowel often implies development of a complication (eg, obstruction, peritonitis). In other types of ileus, x-ray findings are similar to obstruction; differentiation can be difficult unless clinical features clearly favor one or the other. Water-soluble contrast studies may help differentiate.

Treatment

Treatment involves continuous nasogastric suction, npo, IV fluids and electrolytes, a minimal amount of sedatives, and avoidance of opioids and anticholinergic drugs. Maintaining an adequate serum K level (> 4 mEq/L [> 4 mmol/L]) is especially important. Ileus persisting > 1 wk probably has a mechanical obstructive cause, and laparotomy should be considered. Sometimes colonic ileus can be relieved by colonoscopic decompression; rarely, cecostomy is required. Colonoscopic decompression is helpful in treating pseudo-obstruction (Ogilvie's syndrome), which consists of apparent obstruction at the splenic flexure, although no cause can be found by contrast enema or colonoscopy for the failure of gas and feces to pass this point.

INTESTINAL OBSTRUCTION

Intestinal obstruction is significant impairment or complete arrest of the passage of contents through the intestine. Symptoms include cramping pain, vomiting, obstipation, and lack of flatus. Diagnosis is clinical, confirmed by abdominal x-rays. Treatment is fluid resuscitation, nasogastric suction, and, in most cases of complete obstruction, surgery.

Mechanical obstruction is divided into obstruction of the small bowel (including the duodenum) and obstruction of the large bowel. Obstruction may be partial or complete. About 85% of partial small-bowel obstructions resolve with nonoperative treatment, while about 85% of complete small-bowel obstructions require operation.

Etiology

Overall, the most common causes of mechanical obstruction are adhesions, hernias, and tumors. Other general causes are diverticulitis, foreign bodies (including gallstones), volvulus (twisting of bowel on its mesentery), intussusception (telescoping of one segment of bowel into another—see p. 2285), and fecal impaction. Specific segments of the intestine are affected differently (see TABLE 11–3).

Pathophysiology

In simple mechanical obstruction, blockage occurs without vascular compromise. Ingested fluid and food, digestive secretions, and gas accumulate above the obstruction. The proximal bowel distends, and the distal segment collapses. The normal secretory and absorptive functions of the mucosa are depressed, and the bowel wall becomes edematous and congested. Severe intestinal distention is self-perpetuating and progressive, intensifying the peristaltic and secretory derangements and increasing the risks of dehydration and progression to strangulating obstruction.

Strangulating obstruction is obstruction with compromised blood flow; it occurs in nearly 25% of patients with small-bowel obstruction. It is usually associated with hernia, volvulus, and intussusception. Strangulating obstruction can progress to infarction and gangrene in as little as 6 h. Venous obstruction occurs first, followed by arterial occlusion, resulting in rapid ischemia of the bowel wall. The ischemic bowel becomes edematous and infarcts, leading to gangrene and perforation. In large-bowel obstruction, strangulation is rare (except with volvulus).

Perforation may occur in an ischemic segment (typically small bowel) or when marked dilation occurs. The risk is high if the cecum is dilated to a diameter ≥ 13 cm. Perforation of a tumor or a diverticulum may also occur at the obstruction site.

Symptoms and Signs

Obstruction of the small bowel produces symptoms shortly after onset: abdominal cramps centered around the umbilicus or in the epigastrium, vomiting, and—in patients with complete obstruction—obstipation. Patients with partial obstruction may develop diarrhea. Severe, steady pain suggests that strangulation has occurred. In the absence of strangulation, the abdomen is not tender. Hyperactive, high-pitched peristalsis with rushes coinciding with cramps is typical. Sometimes, dilated loops of bowel are palpable. With infarction, the abdomen becomes tender and auscultation reveals a silent abdomen or minimal peristalsis. Shock and oliguria are serious signs that indicate either late simple obstruction or strangulation.

Obstruction of the large bowel usually produces milder symptoms that develop more gradually than those produced by small-bowel obstruction. Increasing constipation leads to obstipation and abdominal distention. Vomiting may occur (usually several hours after onset of other symptoms) but is not common. Lower abdominal cramps unproductive of feces occur. Physical examination typically shows a distended abdomen with loud borborygmi. There is no tenderness, and the rectum is usually empty. A mass corresponding to the site of an obstructing tumor may be palpable. Systemic symptoms are relatively mild, and fluid and electrolyte deficits are uncommon.

Volvulus often has an abrupt onset. Pain is continuous, sometimes with superimposed waves of colicky pain.

Diagnosis

Supine and upright abdominal x-rays should be obtained and are usually adequate to diagnose obstruction. Although only laparotomy can definitively diagnose strangulation, careful serial clinical examination and tests (eg, CBC and serum chemistries, including lactate levels) may provide early warning.

On plain x-rays, a ladderlike series of distended small-bowel loops is typical of small-bowel obstruction but may also occur with obstruction of the right colon. Fluid levels in the bowel can be seen in upright views. Similar although perhaps less dramatic x-ray findings and symptoms occur in ileus (paralysis of the intestine without obstruction—see p. 103); differentiation can be difficult. Distended loops and fluid levels may be absent with an obstruction of the upper jejunum or with closed-loop strangulating obstructions (as may occur with volvulus). Infarcted bowel may produce a mass effect on x-ray. Gas in the bowel wall (pneumatosis intestinalis) indicates gangrene.

In large-bowel obstruction, abdominal x-ray shows distention of the colon proximal to the obstruction. In cecal volvulus there may be a large gas bubble in the mid-abdomen or the left upper quadrant. With both cecal and sigmoidal volvulus, a contrast enema shows the site of obstruction by a typical "bird-beak" deformity at the site of the twist; the procedure may actually reduce a sigmoid volvulus. If contrast enema is not performed, colonoscopy can be used to decompress a sigmoid volvulus but rarely works with a cecal volvulus.

Treatment

Patients with possible intestinal obstruction should be hospitalized. Treatment of acute intestinal obstruction must proceed simultaneously with diagnosis. A surgeon should always be involved.

Supportive care is similar for small- and large-bowel obstruction: nasogastric suction, IV fluids (0.9% saline or lactated Ringer's solution for intravascular volume repletion), and a urinary catheter to monitor fluid output. Electrolyte replacement should be guided by test results, although in cases of repeated vomiting serum Na and K are likely to be depleted. If bowel ischemia or infarction is suspected, antibiotics should be given (eg, a 3rd-generation cephalosporin, such as cefotetan 2 g IV).

Specific measures: Obstruction of the duodenum in adults is treated by resection or, if the lesion cannot be removed, palliative gastrojejunostomy (for treatment in children, see p. 2428).

TABLE 11–3. CAUSES OF INTESTINAL OBSTRUCTION

LOCATION	CAUSES
Colon	Tumors (usually at splenic or sigmoid flexure), diverticulitis (usually in sigmoid), volvulus of sigmoid or cecum, fecal impaction, Hirschsprung's disease
Duodenum	
Adults	Cancer of the duodenum or head of pancreas
Neonates	Atresia, volvulus, bands, annular pancreas
Jejunum and ileum	
Adults	Hernias, adhesions (common), tumors, foreign body, Meckel's diverticulum, Crohn's disease (uncommon), *Ascaris* infestation, midgut volvulus, intussusception by tumor (rare)
Neonates	Meconium ileus, volvulus of a malrotated gut, atresia, intussusception

Complete obstruction of the small bowel is preferentially treated with early laparotomy, although surgery can be delayed 2 or 3 h to improve fluid status and urine output in a very ill, dehydrated patient. The offending lesion is removed whenever possible. If a gallstone was the cause of obstruction, cholecystectomy can be performed either simultaneously or later. Procedures to prevent recurrence should be performed, including repair of hernias, removal of foreign bodies, and lysis of adhesions. In some patients with early postoperative obstruction or repeated obstruction caused by adhesions, simple intubation with a long intestinal tube (many consider a standard nasogastric tube to be equally effective), rather than surgery, may be attempted in the absence of peritoneal signs.

Disseminated intraperitoneal cancer obstructing the small bowel is a major cause of death in adult patients with GI tract malignancy. Bypassing the obstruction, either surgically or with endoscopically placed stents, may palliate symptoms briefly.

Obstructing colon cancers can often be treated by a single-stage resection and anastomosis. Other options include a diverting ileostomy and distal anastomosis. Occasionally, a diverting colostomy with delayed resection is required.

When diverticulitis causes obstruction, perforation is often present. Removal of the involved area may be very difficult but is indicated if perforation and general peritonitis are present. Resection and colostomy are performed, and anastomosis is postponed.

Fecal impaction usually occurs in the rectum and can be removed digitally and with enemas. However, a fecal concretion alone or in a mixture (ie, with barium or antacids) that produces complete obstruction (usually in the sigmoid) requires laparotomy.

Treatment of cecal volvulus consists of resection and anastomosis of the involved segment or fixation of the cecum in its normal position by cecostomy in the frail patient. In sigmoidal volvulus, an endoscope or a long rectal tube can often decompress the loop, and resection and anastomosis may be deferred for a few days. Without a resection, recurrence is almost inevitable.

INTRA-ABDOMINAL ABSCESSES

Abscesses can occur anywhere in the abdomen and retroperitoneum. They mainly follow operation, trauma, or conditions involving abdominal infection and inflammation, particularly when peritonitis or perforation occurs. Symptoms are malaise, fever, and abdominal pain. Diagnosis is by CT. Treatment is with drainage, either surgical or percutaneous. Antibiotics are ancillary.

Etiology and Pathophysiology

Intra-abdominal abscesses are classified as intraperitoneal, retroperitoneal, or visceral (see TABLE 11–4). Many intra-abdominal abscesses develop following perforation of a hollow viscus (see p. 100) or colonic malignancy. Others develop by extension of infection or inflammation resulting from conditions such as appendicitis, diverticulitis, Crohn's disease, pancreatitis, pelvic inflammatory disease, or indeed any condition causing generalized peritonitis. Abdominal surgery, particularly that involving the digestive or biliary tract, is another significant risk factor: The peritoneum may be contaminated during or after surgery from such events as anastomotic leaks. Traumatic abdominal injuries—particularly lacerations and hematomas of the liver, pancreas, spleen, and intestines—may develop abscesses, whether treated operatively or not.

The infecting organisms typically reflect normal bowel flora and are a complex mixture of anaerobic and aerobic bacteria. Most frequent isolates are aerobic gram-negative bacilli (eg, *Escherichia coli* and *Klebsiella*) and anaerobes (especially *Bacteroides fragilis*).

Undrained abscesses may extend to contiguous structures, erode into adjacent vessels (causing hemorrhage or thrombosis), rupture into the peritoneum or bowel, or form a cutaneous fistula. Subdiaphragmatic abscesses may extend into the thoracic cavity, causing an empyema, lung abscess, or pneumonia. Splenic abscess is a rare cause of sustained bacteremia in endocarditis that persists despite appropriate chemotherapy.

Symptoms and Signs

Abscesses may form within 1 wk of perforation or significant peritonitis, whereas postoperative abscesses may not occur until 2 to 3 wk after operation and rarely not for several months. Although manifestations vary, most abscesses cause fever and abdominal discomfort ranging from minimal to severe (usually near the abscess). Paralytic ileus, either generalized or localized, may develop. Nausea, anorexia, and weight loss are common.

Abscesses in the Douglas' cul-de-sac, adjacent to the colon, may cause diarrhea; contiguity to the bladder may result in urinary urgency and frequency.

Subphrenic abscesses may produce chest symptoms such as nonproductive cough, chest pain, dyspnea, and shoulder pain. Rales, rhonchi, or a friction rub may be audible. Dullness to percussion and decreased breath sounds are typical when basilar atelectasis, pneumonia, or pleural effusion occurs.

Generally, there is tenderness over the location of the abscess. Large abscesses may be palpable as a mass.

TABLE 11–4. INTRA-ABDOMINAL ABSCESSES

LOCATION	ETIOLOGY	ORGANISMS
Intraperitoneal		
Subphrenic Right or left lower quadrant Interloop Pelvic	Postoperative; perforation of hollow viscus, appendicitis, diverticulitis, or tumor; Crohn's disease; pelvic inflammatory disease; generalized peritonitis of any etiology	Bowel flora, often polymicrobial
Retroperitoneal		
Anterior	Perforation of appendicitis, diverticulitis, or tumor; Crohn's disease; pancreatitis	Bowel flora, often polymicrobial
Perinephric	Spread of renal parenchymal abscess (complication of pyelonephritis or rarely hematogenous from remote source)	Aerobic gram-negative bacilli
Visceral		
Hepatic	Trauma, ascending cholangitis, portal bacteremia	Aerobic gram-negative bacilli if biliary origin; polymicrobial bowel flora, if portal bacteremia; amebic infection may occur (see p. 1565)
Pancreatic	Trauma, acute pancreatitis	Bowel flora, often polymicrobial
Splenic	Trauma, hematogenous, infarction (as in sickle cell disease, malaria)	Staphylococci, streptococci, anaerobes, aerobic gram-negative bacilli including *Salmonella, Candida* in immunocompromised patients

Diagnosis

CT of the abdomen and pelvis with oral contrast is the preferred diagnostic modality for suspected abscess. Other imaging studies, if obtained, may show abnormalities; plain abdominal x-rays may reveal extraintestinal gas in the abscess, displacement of adjacent organs, a soft-tissue density representing the abscess, or loss of the psoas muscle shadow. Abscesses near the diaphragm may result in chest x-ray abnormalities such as ipsilateral pleural effusion, elevated or immobile hemidiaphragm, lower lobe infiltrates, and atelectasis.

CBC and blood cultures should be obtained. Leukocytosis occurs in most patients, and anemia is common.

Occasionally, radionuclide scanning with indium^{111}-labeled leukocytes may be helpful in identifying intra-abdominal abscesses.

Prognosis and Treatment

Intra-abdominal abscesses have a mortality rate of 10 to 40%. Outcome depends mainly on the patient's primary illness or injury and general medical condition rather than on the specific nature and location of the abscess.

All intra-abdominal abscesses require drainage, either by percutaneous catheters or surgery. Drainage through catheters (placed with CT or ultrasound guidance) may be appropriate given the following conditions: Few abscess cavities are present; the drainage route does not traverse bowel or uncontaminated organs, pleura, or peritoneum; the source of contamination is controlled; and the pus is thin enough to pass through the catheter.

Antibiotics are not curative but may limit hematogenous spread and should be given before and after intervention. Therapy requires drugs active against bowel flora, such as a combination of an aminoglycoside (eg, gentamicin 1.5 mg/kg q 8 h) and metronidazole 500 mg q 8 h. Single-agent therapy with cefotetan 2 g q 12 h is also reasonable. Patients previously given antibiotics or those who have hospital-acquired infections should receive drugs active against resistant aerobic gram-negative bacilli (eg, *Pseudomonas*) and anaerobes.

Nutritional support is important, with the enteral route preferred. Parenteral nutrition should begin early if the enteral route is not feasible.

ISCHEMIC COLITIS

Ischemic colitis is a transient reduction in blood flow to the colon.

Necrosis may occur but is usually limited to the mucosa and submucosa, only occasionally producing full-thickness necrosis necessitating surgery. It occurs mainly in older people (> 60) and is of unknown etiology, although there is some association with the same risk factors as for acute mesenteric ischemia.

Symptoms are milder and of slower onset than those of acute mesenteric ischemia and consist of left lower quadrant pain followed by rectal bleeding. Diagnosis is made by colonoscopy; angiography is not indicated. Treatment is supportive with IV fluids, bowel rest, and antibiotics. Surgery is rarely required. About 5% of patients have a reoccurrence. Occasionally, strictures develop at the site of the ischemia, necessitating surgical resection.

12 ESOPHAGEAL AND SWALLOWING DISORDERS

(See also Esophageal Cancer on p. 168 and Esophageal Atresia on p. 2427.)

The swallowing apparatus consists of the pharynx, upper esophageal (cricopharyngeal) sphincter, the body of the esophagus, and the lower esophageal sphincter (LES). The upper third of the esophagus and the structures proximal to it are composed of skeletal muscle; the distal esophagus and LES are composed of smooth muscle. These components work as an integrated system that transports material from the mouth to the stomach and prevents its reflux into the esophagus. Physical obstruction or disorders that interfere with motor function (motility disorders) can affect the system.

The patient's history suggests the diagnosis almost 80% of the time. The only physical findings in esophageal disorders are cervical and supraclavicular lymphadenopathy caused by metastasis, swellings in the neck from large pharyngeal diverticula, and prolonged swallowing time (the time from the act of swallowing to the sound of the bolus of fluid and air entering the stomach—normally ≤ 12 sec—heard by auscultation with the stethoscope over the epigastrium). Watching the patient swallow may help diagnose aspiration or nasal regurgitation. Most esophageal disorders require specific tests for diagnosis.

DYSPHAGIA

Dysphagia is difficulty swallowing. The usual complaint is that food "gets stuck" on the way down.

The condition results from impeded transport of liquids, solids, or both from the pharynx to the stomach. Dysphagia is classified as oropharyngeal or esophageal, depending on where it occurs. Dysphagia should not be confused with globus sensation (see p. 69), a feeling of having a lump in the throat, which is unrelated to swallowing and occurs without impaired transport.

OROPHARYNGEAL DYSPHAGIA

Oropharyngeal dysphagia is difficulty emptying material from the oropharynx into the esophagus; it results from abnormal function proximal to the esophagus.

Most often, this occurs in patients with neurologic conditions or muscular disorders that affect skeletal muscles. Neurologic conditions include Parkinson's disease, stroke, multiple sclerosis, amyotrophic lateral sclerosis, bulbar poliomyelitis, pseudobulbar palsy, and other CNS lesions. Muscular disorders include dermatomyositis, myasthenia gravis, and muscular dystrophy.

Symptoms include difficulty initiating swallowing, nasal regurgitation, and tracheal aspiration followed by coughing. Diagnosis is by direct observation and videotaped barium swallow. Treatment is directed at the underlying condition.

ESOPHAGEAL DYSPHAGIA

Esophageal dysphagia is difficulty passing food down the esophagus. It can result from either a mechanical obstruction or a motility disorder.

Causes of mechanical obstruction include intrinsic disorders such as peptic strictures, esophageal cancer, and lower esophageal rings. Mechanical obstruction can also result from extrinsic disorders that compress the esophagus, including an enlarged left atrium, aortic aneurysm, vascular abnormalities such as an aberrant subclavian artery (dysphagia lusoria), substernal thyroid, cervical bony exostosis, and a thoracic tumor—most commonly lung cancer. Rarely, the esophagus is involved by lymphoma, leiomyosarcoma, or metastatic cancer. Caustic ingestion often results in significant stricture.

Motility disorders cause dysphagia by disrupting function of esophageal smooth muscle (ie, impairing esophageal peristalsis and lower esophageal sphincter function). Motility disorders include achalasia and diffuse esophageal spasm. Systemic sclerosis may cause a motility disorder.

Symptoms and Signs

Motility disorders produce dysphagia for both solids and liquids; mechanical obstruction produces dysphagia for solids alone. Meat and bread cause the most difficulty; however, some patients cannot tolerate any solids. Patients who complain of dysphagia in the lower esophagus are usually correct about the condition's location, whereas patients who complain of dysphagia in the upper esophagus are often incorrect.

Dysphagia can be intermittent (eg, from lower esophageal ring or diffuse esophageal spasm), progress rapidly over weeks to months (eg, from esophageal cancer), or progress over years (eg, from peptic stricture). Patients whose dysphagia is caused by peptic stricture usually have a prominent history of gastroesophageal reflux disease.

Diagnosis and Treatment

Dysphagia for both liquids and solids helps distinguish motor from obstructive causes. A barium swallow (with a solid bolus, usually a marshmallow or tablet) should be performed. If this shows obstruction, endoscopy (and possibly biopsy) should be performed to rule out malignancy. If the barium swallow is negative or suggestive of a motility disorder, esophageal motility studies should be performed. Treatment is directed at the specific cause.

CRICOPHARYNGEAL INCOORDINATION

In cricopharyngeal incoordination, the cricopharyngeal muscle (the upper esophageal sphincter) is uncoordinated. It can cause a Zenker's diverticulum; repeated aspiration of material from the diverticulum can lead to chronic lung disease. The condition can be treated by surgical section of the cricopharyngeal muscle.

OBSTRUCTIVE DISORDERS

(See also Benign Esophageal Tumors and Esophageal Cancer on p.168.)

LOWER ESOPHAGEAL RING

(Schatzki's Ring, B Ring)

A lower esophageal ring is a 2- to 4-mm mucosal stricture, probably congenital, causing a ringlike narrowing of the distal esophagus at squamocolumnar junction.

These rings cause intermittent dysphagia for solids. Symptoms usually occur only when the esophageal lumen is < 12 mm in diameter and never when it is > 20 mm. If the distal esophagus is adequately distended, barium x-rays usually demonstrate the ring. Instructing the patient to chew food thoroughly is usually the only treatment required in wider rings, but narrow-lumen rings require dilation by endoscopy or bougienage. Surgical resection is rarely required.

ESOPHAGEAL WEB

(Plummer-Vinson or Paterson-Kelly Syndrome; Sideropenic Dysphagia)

An esophageal web is a thin mucosal membrane that grows across the lumen.

Rarely, webs develop in patients with untreated severe iron-deficiency anemia; they develop even more rarely in patients without anemia. Webs usually occur in the upper esophagus, producing dysphagia for solids. They are best diagnosed by barium swallow. Webs resolve with treatment of the anemia but can be easily ruptured during esophagoscopy.

DYSPHAGIA LUSORIA

Dysphagia lusoria is caused by compression of the esophagus from any of several congenital vascular abnormalities.

The vascular abnormality is usually an aberrant right subclavian artery arising from the left side of the aortic arch, a double aortic arch, or a right aortic arch with left ligamentum arteriosum. The dysphagia may develop in childhood or later in life as a result of arteriosclerotic changes in the aberrant vessel. Barium swallow shows the extrinsic compression, but arteriography is necessary for absolute diagnosis. Most require no treatment, but surgery is sometimes performed.

MOTILITY DISORDERS

ACHALASIA

(Cardiospasm; Esophageal Aperistalsis; Megaesophagus)

Achalasia is a neurogenic esophageal motility disorder characterized by impaired esophageal peristalsis and a lack of lower esophageal sphincter relaxation during swallowing. Symptoms are slowly progressive dysphagia, usually to both liquids and solids, and regurgitation of undigested food. Evaluation typically includes barium swallow, endoscopy, and sometimes manometry. Treatments include dilation, chemical denervation, and surgical myotomy.

Achalasia is thought to be caused by a loss of ganglion cells in the myenteric plexus of the esophagus, resulting in denervation of esophageal muscle. Etiology of the denervation is unknown, although a viral cause is suspected, and certain tumors may cause achalasia either by direct obstruction or as a paraneoplastic process. Chagas' disease, which causes destruction of autonomic ganglia, may result in achalasia.

Increased pressure at the lower esophageal sphincter (LES) produces obstruction with secondary dilation of the esophagus. Esophageal retention of undigested food is common.

Symptoms and Signs

Achalasia occurs at any age but usually begins between ages 20 and 40. Onset is insidious, and progression is gradual over months or years. Dysphagia for both solids and liquids is the major symptom. Nocturnal regurgitation of undigested food occurs in about 33% of patients and may cause cough and pulmonary aspiration. Chest pain is less common but may occur on swallowing or spontaneously. Mild to moderate weight loss occurs; when weight loss is pronounced, particularly in elderly patients whose symptoms of dysphagia developed rapidly, achalasia secondary to a tumor of the gastroesophageal junction should be considered.

Diagnosis

The preferred test is barium x-ray, which demonstrates absence of progressive peristaltic contractions during swallowing. The esophagus is dilated, often enormously, but is narrowed and beaklike at the LES. If esophagoscopy is performed, there is dilation but no obstructing lesion. The esophagoscope usually passes readily into the stomach; resistance raises the possibility of an inapparent malignancy or stricture. To exclude malignancy, a retroflexed view of the gastric cardia, biopsies, and brushings for cytology should be obtained. Esophageal manometry is not usually performed but typically shows aperistalsis, increased LES pressure, and incomplete sphincteric relaxation during swallowing.

Achalasia must be differentiated from a distal stenosing carcinoma and a peptic stricture, particularly in patients with systemic sclerosis (see p. 270), in whom esophageal manometry may also show aperistalsis. Systemic sclerosis is usually accompanied by a history of Raynaud's phenomenon and symptoms of gastroesophageal reflux disease (GERD).

Achalasia due to cancer at the gastroesophageal junction can be diagnosed by CT of the chest and abdomen or endoscopic ultrasound.

Prognosis

Pulmonary aspiration and the presence of cancer are the determining prognostic factors. Nocturnal regurgitation and coughing suggest aspiration. Pulmonary complications secondary to aspiration are difficult to manage. Incidence of esophageal cancer in patients with achalasia may be increased; this point is controversial.

Treatment

No therapy restores peristalsis; treatment aims at reducing the pressure (and thus the obstruction) at the LES. Pneumatic balloon dilation of the LES is indicated initially. Results are satisfactory in about 85% of patients, but repeated dilations may be needed. Esophageal rupture and secondary mediastinitis requiring surgery occur in < 2% of patients. Nitrates (eg, isosorbide dinitrate 5 to 10 mg sublingually before meals) or Ca channel blockers (eg, nifedipine 10 mg po tid) are of limited effectiveness but may reduce LES pressure enough to prolong the time between dilations.

Achalasia can also be treated by chemical denervation of cholinergic nerves in the distal esophagus by direct injection of botulinum toxin into the LES. Clinical improvement occurs in 70 to 80% of patients, but results may last only 6 mo to 1 yr.

A Heller myotomy, in which the muscular fibers in the LES are cut, is usually reserved for patients who do not respond to dilation; its success rate is about 85%. It can be performed via laparoscopy or thoracoscopy and may be a viable alternative to dilation as primary therapy. Symptomatic GERD follows surgery in about 15% of patients.

SYMPTOMATIC DIFFUSE ESOPHAGEAL SPASM

(Spastic Pseudodiverticulosis; Rosary Bead or Corkscrew Esophagus)

Symptomatic diffuse esophageal spasm is part of a spectrum of motility disorders characterized variously by nonpropulsive contractions, hyperdynamic contractions, or elevated lower esophageal sphincter pressure. Symptoms are chest pain and sometimes dysphagia. Diagnosis is by barium swallow or manometry. Treatment is difficult but includes nitrates, Ca channel blockers, botulinum toxin injection, and antireflux therapy.

Abnormalities in esophageal motility correlate poorly with patient symptoms; similar abnormalities may produce different or no symptoms in different people. Furthermore, neither symptoms nor abnormal contractions are definitively associated with histopathologic abnormalities of the esophagus.

Symptoms and Signs

Diffuse esophageal spasm typically causes substernal chest pain with dysphagia for both liquids and solids. The pain may waken the patient from sleep. Very hot or cold liquids may aggravate the pain. Over many years, this disorder may evolve into achalasia.

Esophageal spasms can produce severe pain in the absence of dysphagia. This pain is often described as a substernal squeezing pain and may occur in association with exercise. Such pain may be indistinguishable from angina pectoris.

Some patients have symptoms that combine those of achalasia and diffuse spasm. Some of these complexes have been called vigorous achalasia because they feature both the food retention and aspiration of achalasia and the severe pain and spasm of diffuse spasm.

Diagnosis

Alternative diagnoses include coronary ischemia. Definitive confirmation of an esophageal origin for symptoms is difficult. Barium swallow may show poor progression of a bolus and disordered, simultaneous contractions or tertiary contractions. Severe spasms may mimic the radiographic appearance of diverticula but vary in size and position. Esophageal manometry (see p. 86) provides the most specific description of the spasms. Contractions are usually simultaneous, prolonged or multiphasic, and possibly of very high amplitude ("nutcracker esophagus"). However, spasms may not occur during testing. Lower esophageal sphincter (LES) pressure elevation or impaired relaxation is present in 30% of patients. Esophageal scintigraphy and provocative tests with drugs (eg, edrophonium chloride 10 mg IV) have not proven helpful.

Treatment

Esophageal spasms are often difficult to treat, and controlled studies of treatment methods are lacking. Anticholinergics, nitroglycerin, and long-acting nitrates have had limited success. Ca channel blockers given orally (eg, verapamil 80 mg tid, nifedipine 10 mg tid) may be useful, as may injection of botulinum toxin into the LES.

Medical management is usually sufficient, but pneumatic dilation and bougienage, or even surgical myotomy along the full length of the esophagus, may be tried in intractable cases.

ESOPHAGEAL DIVERTICULA

An esophageal diverticulum is an outpouching of mucosa through the muscular layer of the esophagus. It can be asymptomatic or cause dysphagia and regurgitation. Diagnosis is made by barium swallow; surgery is rarely required.

There are several types of esophageal diverticula, each of different origin. Zenker's (pharyngeal) diverticula are posterior outpouchings of mucosa and submucosa through the cricopharyngeal muscle, probably resulting from an incoordination between pharyngeal propulsion and cricopharyngeal relaxation. Midesophageal (traction) diverticula are caused by traction from mediastinal inflammatory lesions or, secondarily, by motility disorders. Epiphrenic diverticula occur just above the diaphragm and usually accompany a motility disorder (achalasia, diffuse esophageal spasm).

Symptoms and Signs

A Zenker's diverticulum fills with food that might be regurgitated when the patient bends or lies down. Aspiration pneumonitis may result if regurgitation is nocturnal. Rarely, the pouch becomes large, causing dysphagia and sometimes a palpable neck mass. Traction and epiphrenic diverticula are rarely symptomatic, although their underlying cause may be.

Diagnosis and Treatment

All diverticula are diagnosed by videotaped barium swallow. Specific treatment is usually not required, although resection is occasionally necessary for large or symptomatic diverticula. Diverticula associated with motility disorders require treatment of the primary disorder. For example, case reports suggest the performance of cricopharyngeal myotomy at the time of resection of a Zenker's diverticulum.

GASTROESOPHAGEAL REFLUX DISEASE

Incompetence of the lower esophageal sphincter allows reflux of gastric contents into the esophagus, causing burning pain. Prolonged reflux may lead to esophagitis, stricture, and rarely metaplasia. Diagnosis is clinical, sometimes with endoscopy, with or without acid testing. Treatment involves lifestyle modification, acid suppression using proton pump inhibitors, and sometimes surgery.

Gastroesophageal reflux disease (GERD) is common, occurring in 30 to 40% of adults. It also occurs frequently in infants, typically beginning at birth.

Etiology and Pathophysiology

The presence of reflux implies lower esophageal sphincter (LES) incompetence, which may result from a generalized loss of intrinsic sphincter tone or from recurrent transient relaxations (unrelated to swallowing). Transient LES relaxations are triggered by gastric distention or subthreshold pharyngeal stimulation.

Factors that contribute to the competence of the gastroesophageal junction include the angle of the cardioesophageal junction, the action of the diaphragm, and gravity (ie, an upright position). Factors contributing to reflux include weight gain, fatty foods, caffeinated or carbonated beverages, alcohol, tobacco smoking, and drugs. Drugs that lower LES pressure include anticholinergics, antihistamines, tricyclic antidepressants, Ca channel blockers, progesterone, and nitrates.

GERD may lead to esophagitis, peptic esophageal ulcer, esophageal stricture, and Barrett's esophagus (a premalignant condition, see p. 168). Factors that contribute to the development of esophagitis include the caustic nature of the refluxate, the inability to clear the refluxate from the esophagus, the volume of gastric contents, and local mucosal protective functions. Some patients, particularly infants, aspirate the reflux material.

Symptoms and Signs

The most prominent symptom of GERD is heartburn, with or without regurgitation of gastric contents into the mouth. Infants present with vomiting, irritability, anorexia, and sometimes symptoms of chronic aspiration. Both adults and infants with chronic aspiration may have cough, hoarseness, or wheezing.

Esophagitis may cause odynophagia and even esophageal hemorrhage, which is usually occult, but can be massive. Peptic stricture causes a gradually progressive dysphagia for solid foods. Peptic esophageal ulcers cause the same type of pain as gastric or duodenal ulcers, but the pain is usually localized to the xiphoid or high substernal region. Peptic esophageal ulcers heal slowly, tend to recur, and usually leave a stricture on healing.

Diagnosis

A detailed history points to the diagnosis. Patients with typical symptoms of GERD may be given a trial of therapy. Patients who do not improve, or have long-standing symptoms or symptoms of complications, should be studied. Endoscopy, with cytologic washings and biopsy of abnormal areas, is the test of choice. Endoscopic biopsy is the only test that consistently detects the columnar mucosal changes of Barrett's esophagus. Patients with unremarkable endoscopy findings and symptoms despite treatment with proton pump inhibitors should undergo pH testing (see p. 85). Although barium swallow readily shows esophageal ulcers and peptic strictures, it is less useful for mild to moderate reflux; in addition, most patients with abnormalities require subsequent endoscopy. Esophageal manometry may be used to guide pH probe placement and to evaluate esophageal peristalsis before surgical treatment.

Treatment

Management of uncomplicated GERD consists of elevating the head of the bed 6 inches and avoiding the following: eating within 2 to 3 h of bedtime, strong stimulants of acid secretion (eg, coffee, alcohol), certain drugs (eg, anticholinergics), specific foods (eg, fats, chocolate), and smoking.

Drug therapy is with a proton pump inhibitor. Adults can be given omeprazole 20 mg, lansoprazole 30 mg, or esomeprazole 40 mg 30 min before breakfast. In some cases, proton pump inhibitors must be given bid. Infants and children may be given these drugs at an appropriate lower single daily dose (ie, omeprazole 20 mg in children > 3 yr, 10 mg in children < 3 yr; lansoprazole 15 mg in children ≤ 30 kg, 30 mg in children > 30 kg). These drugs may be continued long-term, but the dose should be adjusted to the minimum required to prevent symptoms. H_2 blockers (eg, ranitidine 150 mg at bedtime) or promotility agents (eg, metoclopramide 10 mg po 30 min before meals and at bedtime) are less effective.

Antireflux surgery (usually via laparoscopy) is performed on patients with serious esophagitis, hemorrhage, stricture, ulcer, or intractable symptoms. Esophageal strictures are managed by repeated balloon dilation.

Barrett's esophagus may or may not regress with medical or surgical therapy. Because Barrett's esophagus is a precursor to adenocarcinoma, endoscopic surveillance for malignant transformation is recommended every 1 to 2 yr. Surveillance has uncertain cost-effectiveness in patients with low-grade dysplasia but is important in high-grade dysplasia. Alternatively, Barrett's esophagus may be treated with surgical resection or laser ablation.

HIATUS HERNIA

Hiatus hernia is a protrusion of the stomach through the diaphragmatic hiatus. Most hernias are asymptomatic, but an increased incidence of acid reflux may lead to symptoms of gastroesophageal reflux disease (GERD). Diagnosis is by barium swallow. Treatment is directed at symptoms of GERD if present.

Etiology and Pathophysiology

Etiology is usually unknown, but a hiatus hernia is thought to be acquired through stretching of the fascial attachments between the esophagus and diaphragm at the hiatus (the opening through which the esophagus traverses the diaphragm). In a sliding hiatus hernia, the most common type, the gastroesophageal junction and a portion of the stomach are above the diaphragm. In a paraesophageal hiatus hernia, the gastroesophageal junction is in the normal location, but a portion of the stomach is adjacent to the esophagus. Hernias may also occur through other parts of the diaphragm (see p. 2427).

A sliding hiatus hernia is common and is an incidental finding on x-ray in >40% of the population. Ergo, the relationship of hernia to symptoms is unclear. Although most patients with GERD have some degree of hiatus hernia, <50% of patients with hiatus hernia have GERD.

Symptoms and Signs

Most patients with a sliding hiatus hernia are asymptomatic, but chest pain and other reflux symptoms can occur. A paraesophageal hiatus hernia is generally asymptomatic but, unlike a sliding hiatus hernia, may incarcerate and strangulate. Occult or massive GI hemorrhage may occur with either type.

Diagnosis and Treatment

A large hiatus hernia is often discovered incidentally on chest x-ray. Smaller hernias are diagnosed with a barium swallow. An asymptomatic sliding hiatus hernia requires no specific therapy. Patients with accompanying GERD should be treated. A paraesophageal hernia should be reduced surgically because of the risk of strangulation.

INFECTIOUS ESOPHAGEAL DISORDERS

Esophageal infection occurs mainly in patients with impaired host defenses. Primary agents include *Candida albicans*, herpes simplex virus, and cytomegalovirus. Symptoms are odynophagia and chest pain. Diagnosis is by endoscopic visualization and culture. Treatment is with antifungal or antiviral drugs.

Esophageal infection is rare in patients with normal host defenses. Primary esophageal defenses include saliva, esophageal motility, and cellular immunity. Thus, at-risk patients include those with AIDS, organ transplants, alcoholism, diabetes, malnutrition, malignancy, and motility disorders. *Candida* infection may occur in any of these patients. Herpes simplex virus (HSV) and cytomegalovirus (CMV) infections occur mainly in AIDS and transplant patients.

Patients with *Candida* esophagitis usually complain of odynophagia and, less commonly, dysphagia. About ⅔ have signs of oral thrush (thus its absence does not exclude esophageal involvement). Patients with odynophagia and typical thrush may be given empiric treatment, but if significant improvement does not occur in 5 to 7 days, endoscopic evaluation is required. Barium swallow is less accurate. Treatment is with fluconazole 200 mg po or IV for one dose, then 100 mg po or IV q 24 h for 14 to 21 days. Alternatives include ketoconazole and itraconazole. Topical therapy has no role.

HSV and CMV infections are equally likely in transplant patients, but HSV occurs early after transplantation (reactivation) and CMV occurs 2 to 6 mo out. In AIDS patients, CMV is much more common than HSV, and viral esophagitis occurs mainly when the $CD4^+$ count is < 200/μL. Severe odynophagia results from either infection.

Endoscopy, with cytology or biopsy, is usually necessary for diagnosis. HSV is treated with IV acyclovir 5 mg/kg q 8 h for 7 days or valacyclovir 1 g po tid. CMV is treated with ganciclovir 5 mg/kg IV q 12 h for 14 to 21 days with maintenance at 5 mg/kg IV 5 days/wk in immunocompromised patients. Alternatives include foscarnet and cidofovir.

MALLORY-WEISS SYNDROME

Mallory-Weiss syndrome is a nonpenetrating mucosal laceration of the distal esophagus and proximal stomach caused by vomiting, retching, or hiccuping.

Initially described in alcoholics, Mallory-Weiss syndrome can occur in any patient who vomits forcefully. It is the cause of about 5% of episodes of upper GI hemorrhage. Most episodes of bleeding stop spontaneously; severe bleeding occurs in about 10% of patients who require significant intervention, such as transfusion or endoscopic hemostasis (by injection of ethanol, polidocanol, or epinephrine or by electrocautery). Intra-arterial infusion of pitressin or therapeutic embolization into the left gastric artery during angiography may also be used to control bleeding. Surgery is rarely required.

ESOPHAGEAL RUPTURE

Esophageal rupture may be iatrogenic during endoscopic procedures or other instrumentation or may be spontaneous (Boerhaave's syndrome). Patients are seriously ill, with symptoms of mediastinitis. Diagnosis is by esophagography with a water-soluble contrast agent. Immediate surgical repair and drainage are required.

Endoscopic procedures are the primary cause of esophageal rupture, but spontaneous rupture may occur, typically related to vomiting, retching, or swallowing a large food bolus. The most common site of rupture is the distal esophagus on the left side. Acid and other stomach contents cause a fulminant mediastinitis and shock. Pneumomediastinum is common.

Symptoms and Signs

Symptoms include chest and abdominal pain, vomiting, hematemesis, and shock. Subcutaneous emphysema is palpable in about 30% of patients. Mediastinal crunch (Hamman's sign), a crackling sound synchronous with the heartbeat, may be present.

Diagnosis and Treatment

Chest and abdominal x-rays showing mediastinal air, pleural effusion, or mediastinal widening suggest the diagnosis. Diagnosis is confirmed by esophagography with a water-soluble contrast agent, which avoids potential mediastinal irritation from barium. CT of the thorax detects mediastinal air and fluid but does not localize the perforation well. Endoscopy may miss a small perforation.

Pending surgical repair, patients should receive broad-spectrum antibiotics (eg, gentamicin plus metronidazole or piperacillin/tazobactam) and fluid resuscitation as needed for shock. Even with treatment, mortality is high.

13 GASTRITIS AND PEPTIC ULCER DISEASE

Acid is secreted by parietal cells in the proximal two thirds (body) of the stomach. Gastric acid aids digestion by creating the optimal pH for pepsin and gastric lipase and by stimulating pancreatic bicarbonate secretion. Acid secretion is initiated by food: the thought, smell, or taste of food effect vagal stimulation of the gastrin-secreting G cells located in the distal one third (antrum) of the stomach. The arrival of protein to the stomach further stimulates gastrin output. Circulating gastrin triggers the release of histamine from enterochromaffin-like cells in the body of the stomach. Histamine stimulates the parietal cells via their H_2 receptors. The parietal cells secrete acid and the resulting drop in pH causes the antral D cells to release somatostatin, which inhibits gastrin release (negative feedback control).

Acid secretion is present at birth and reaches adult levels (on a weight basis) by age 2. There is a decline in acid output in elderly patients who develop chronic gastritis, but it is otherwise maintained throughout life.

Normally, the GI mucosa is protected by several distinct mechanisms: (1) Mucosal production of mucus and HCO_3 creates a pH gradient from the gastric lumen (low pH) to the mucosa (neutral pH). The mucus serves as a barrier to the diffusion of acid and pepsin. (2) Epithelial cells remove excess hydrogen ions (H^+) via membrane transport systems and have tight junctions, which prevent back diffusion of H^+ ions. (3) Mucosal blood flow removes excess acid that has diffused across the epithelial layer. Several growth factors (eg, epidermal growth factor, insulin-like growth factor I) and prostaglandins have been linked to mucosal repair and maintenance of mucosal integrity.

Factors that interfere with these mucosal defenses (particularly NSAIDs and *Helicobacter pylori* infection) predispose to gastritis and peptic ulcer disease.

NSAIDs promote mucosal inflammation and ulcer formation (sometimes with GI bleeding) both topically and systemically. By inhibiting prostaglandin production via blockage of the enzyme cyclooxygenase (COX), NSAIDs reduce gastric blood flow, reduce mucus and HCO_3 secretion, and decrease cell repair and replication. Also, because NSAIDs are weak acids and are nonionized at gastric pH, they diffuse freely across the mucus barrier into gastric epithelial cells, where H^+ ions are liberated, leading to cellular damage. Because gastric prostaglandin production involves the COX-1 isoform, NSAIDs that are selective COX-2 inhibitors have fewer adverse gastric effects than other NSAIDs.

HELICOBACTER PYLORI INFECTION

H. pylori **is a common gastric pathogen that causes gastritis, peptic ulcer disease, gastric adenocarcinoma, and low-grade gastric lymphoma. Infection may be asymptomatic or result in varying degrees of dyspepsia. Diagnosis is by urea breath test and testing of endoscopic biopsy samples. Treatment is with a proton pump inhibitor plus two antibiotics.**

H. pylori is a spiral-shaped, gram-negative organism that has adapted to thrive in acid. In developing countries, it commonly causes chronic infections and is usually acquired in childhood. In the US, infection is less common in children but increases with age: by age 60 about 50% of people are infected. Infection is most common in blacks and Hispanics.

The organism has been cultured from stool, saliva, and dental plaque, which suggests oral-oral or fecal-oral transmission. Infections tend to cluster in families and in residents of custodial institutions. Nurses and gastroenterologists appear to be at high risk: bacteria can be transmitted by improperly disinfected endoscopes.

Pathophysiology

Effects of *H. pylori* infection vary depending on the location within the stomach. Antral-predominant infection results in increased gastrin production, probably via local impairment of somatostatin. Resultant hypersecretion of acid predisposes to prepyloric and duodenal ulcer. Body-predominant infection leads to gastric atrophy and decreased acid production, possibly via increased local production of interleukin-1β. Patients with body-predominant infection are predisposed to gastric ulcer and adenocarcinoma. Some patients have mixed infection of both antrum and body with varying clinical effects. Many patients with *H. pylori* infection have no noticeable clinical effects.

Ammonia produced by *H. pylori* enables the organism to survive in the acidic environment of the stomach and may erode the mucus barrier. Cytotoxins and mucolytic enzymes (eg, bacterial protease, lipase) produced by *H. pylori* may play a role in mucosal damage and subsequent ulcerogenesis.

Infected people are 3 to 6 times more likely to develop stomach cancer. *H. pylori* infection is associated with intestinal-type adenocarcinoma of the gastric body and antrum but not cancer of the gastric cardia. Other associated malignancies include gastric lymphoma and mucosa-associated lymphoid tissue (MALT) lymphoma, a monoclonally restricted B-cell tumor.

Diagnosis

Screening of asymptomatic patients is not warranted. Tests are performed during evaluation for peptic ulcer and gastritis. Post-treatment testing is typically performed to confirm eradication of the organism. Different tests are preferred for initial diagnosis and post-treatment.

Noninvasive tests: Laboratory and office-based serologic assays for antibodies to *H. pylori* have sensitivity and specificity of > 85% and are considered the noninvasive tests of choice for initial documentation of *H. pylori* infection. However, because qualitative assays remain positive for up to 3 yr after successful treatment and because quantitative antibody levels do not decline significantly for 6 to 12 mo after treatment, serologic assays are not usually used to assess cure.

Urea breath tests use an oral dose of ^{13}C- or ^{14}C-labeled urea. In an infected patient, the organism metabolizes the urea and liberates labeled CO_2, which is exhaled and can be quantified in breath samples taken 20 to 30 min after ingestion of the urea. Sensitivity and specificity are > 90%. Urea breath tests are well suited for confirming eradication of the organism after therapy. False-negative results are possible with recent antibiotic use or concomitant proton pump inhibitor therapy; therefore, follow-up testing should be delayed ≥ 4 wk after antibiotic therapy and 1 wk after proton pump inhibitor therapy. H_2 blockers do not affect the test.

Invasive tests: Gastroscopy is used to obtain mucosal biopsy samples for a rapid urease test (RUT) or histologic staining. Bacterial culture is of limited use because of the fastidious nature of the organism.

The RUT, in which presence of bacterial urease in the biopsy sample causes a color change on a special medium, is the diagnostic method of choice on tissue samples. Histologic staining of biopsy samples should be done for patients with negative RUT results but suspicious clinical findings, recent antibiotic use, or treatment with proton pump inhibitors. RUT and histologic staining each have a sensitivity and specificity of > 90%.

Treatment

Patients with complications (eg, gastritis, ulcer, malignancy) should have the organism eradicated. Eradication of *H. pylori* can even cure some cases of MALT lymphoma (but not other infection-related malignancies). Treatment of asymptomatic infection has been controversial, but the recognition of the role of *H. pylori* in cancer has led to a recommendation for treatment.

H. pylori eradication requires multi-drug therapy, typically antibiotics plus acid suppressants. Proton pump inhibitors suppress *H. pylori*, and the increased gastric pH accompanying their use can enhance tissue concentration and efficacy of antimicrobials, creating a hostile environment for *H. pylori*.

Triple therapy is recommended. Oral omeprazole 20 mg bid or lansoprazole 30 mg bid, plus clarithromycin 500 mg bid, plus either metronidazole 500 mg bid or amoxicillin 1 g bid for 14 days, cures infection in > 95% of cases. This regimen has excellent tolerability. Ranitidine bismuth citrate 400 mg po bid may be substituted for the proton pump inhibitor.

Quadruple therapy with a proton pump inhibitor bid, tetracycline 500 mg and bismuth subsalicylate or subcitrate 525 mg qid, and metronidazole 500 mg tid is also effective but more cumbersome.

Infected patients with duodenal or gastric ulcer require continuation of the acid suppression for at least 4 wk.

Treatment is repeated if *H. pylori* is not eradicated. If two courses are unsuccessful, some authorities recommend endoscopy to obtain cultures for sensitivity testing.

GASTRITIS

Gastritis is inflammation of the gastric mucosa caused by any of several conditions, including infection (*Helicobacter pylori*), drugs (NSAIDs, alcohol), stress, and autoimmune phenomena (atrophic gastritis). Many cases are asymptomatic, but dyspepsia and GI bleeding sometimes occur. Diagnosis is by endoscopy. Treatment is directed at the underlying cause but often includes acid suppression and, for *H. pylori* infection, antibiotics.

Gastritis is classified as erosive or nonerosive based on the severity of mucosal injury. It is also classified according to the site of involvement (ie, cardia, body, antrum). Gastritis can be further classified histologically as acute or chronic based on the inflammatory cell type. No classification scheme matches perfectly with the pathophysiology; a large degree of overlap exists. Some forms of gastritis involve acid-peptic and *H. pylori* disease. Additionally, the term is often loosely applied to nonspecific (and often undiagnosed) abdominal discomfort and gastroenteritis.

Acute gastritis is characterized by PMN infiltration of the mucosa of the antrum and body.

Chronic gastritis implies some degree of atrophy (with loss of function of the mucosa) or metaplasia. It predominantly involves the antrum (with subsequent loss of G cells and decreased gastrin secretion) or the corpus (with loss of oxyntic glands, leading to reduced acid, pepsin, and intrinsic factor).

EROSIVE GASTRITIS

Erosive gastritis is gastric mucosal erosion caused by damage to mucosal defenses. It is typically acute, presenting with bleeding, but may be subacute or chronic with few or no symptoms. Diagnosis is by endoscopy. Treatment is supportive, with removal of the inciting cause. Certain ICU patients (eg, ventilator bound, head trauma, burn, multisystem trauma) benefit from prophylaxis with acid suppressants.

Causes of erosive gastritis include NSAIDs, alcohol, stress, and less commonly radiation, viral infection (eg, cytomegalovirus), vascular injury, and direct trauma (eg, nasogastric tubes).

Superficial erosions and punctate mucosal lesions occur. These may develop as soon as 12 h after the initial insult. Deep erosions, ulcers, and sometimes perforation may occur in severe or untreated cases. Lesions typically occur in the body, but the antrum may also be involved.

Acute stress gastritis, a form of erosive gastritis, occurs in about 5% of critically ill patients. The incidence increases with duration of ICU stay and length of time the patient is not receiving enteral feeding. Pathogenesis likely involves hypoperfusion of the GI mucosa, resulting in impaired mucosal defenses. Patients with head injury or burns may also have increased secretion of acid.

Symptoms, Signs, and Diagnosis

Patients with mild erosive gastritis are often asymptomatic, although some complain of dyspepsia, nausea, or vomiting. Often, the first sign is hematemesis, melena, or blood in the nasogastric aspirate, usually within 2 to 5 days of the inciting event. Bleeding is usually mild to moderate, although it can be massive if deep ulceration is present, particularly in acute stress gastritis. Acute and chronic erosive gastritis are diagnosed endoscopically.

Prevention

Prophylaxis can reduce the incidence of acute stress gastritis. However, it mainly benefits certain high-risk ICU patients, including those with severe burns, CNS trauma, coagulopathy, sepsis, shock, multiple trauma, mechanical ventilation for > 48 h, hepatic or renal failure, multiorgan dysfunction, and history of peptic ulcer or GI bleeding.

Prophylaxis consists of IV H_2 blockers, proton pump inhibitors, or oral antacids to raise intragastric pH > 4.0. Repeated pH measurement and titration of therapy are not required. Early enteral feeding also can decrease the incidence of bleeding.

Acid suppression is not recommended for patients simply taking NSAIDs unless they have previously had an ulcer.

Treatment

In severe gastritis, bleeding is managed with IV fluids and blood transfusion as needed. Endoscopic hemostasis should be attempted, with surgery (total gastrectomy) a fallback procedure. Angiography is unlikely to stop severe gastric bleeding because of the many collateral vessels supplying the stomach. Acid suppression should be started if the patient is not already receiving it.

For milder gastritis, removing the offending agent and using drugs to reduce gastric acidity (see p. 124) may be all that is required.

Nonerosive Gastritis

Nonerosive gastritis refers to a variety of histologic abnormalities that are mainly the result of *H. pylori* infection. Most patients are asymptomatic. The condition is discovered by endoscopy. Treatment is eradication of *H. pylori* and sometimes acid suppression.

Pathology

Superficial gastritis: Lymphocytes and plasma cells mixed with neutrophils are the predominant infiltrating inflammatory cells. Inflammation is superficial and may involve the antrum, body, or both. It is usually not accompanied by atrophy or metaplasia. Prevalence increases with age.

Deep gastritis: Deep gastritis is more likely to be symptomatic (eg, vague dyspepsia). Mononuclear cells and neutrophils infiltrate the entire mucosa to the level of the muscularis, but exudate or crypt abscesses seldom result, as might be expected by such infiltration. Distribution may be patchy. Superficial gastritis may be present, as may partial gland atrophy and metaplasia.

Gastric atrophy: Atrophy of gastric glands may follow in gastritis, most often long-standing antral (sometimes referred to as type B) gastritis. Some patients with gastric atrophy manifest autoantibodies to parietal cells, usually in association with corpus (type A) gastritis and pernicious anemia.

Atrophy may occur without specific symptoms. Endoscopically, the mucosa may appear normal until atrophy is advanced, when submucosal vascularity may be visible. As atrophy becomes complete, secretion of acid and pepsin diminishes and intrinsic factor may be lost, resulting in vitamin B_{12} malabsorption.

Metaplasia: Two types of metaplasia are common in chronic nonerosive gastritis: mucous gland and intestinal.

Mucous gland metaplasia (pseudopyloric metaplasia) occurs in the setting of severe atrophy of the gastric glands, which are progressively replaced by mucous glands (antral mucosa), especially along the lesser curve. Gastric ulcers may be present (typically at the junction of antral and corpus mucosa), but whether they are the cause or consequence of these metaplastic changes is not clear.

Intestinal metaplasia typically begins in the antrum in response to chronic mucosal injury and may extend to the body. Gastric mucosa cells change to resemble intestinal mucosa—with goblet cells, endocrine (enterochromaffin or enterochromaffin-like) cells, and rudimentary villi—and may even assume functional (absorptive) characteristics. It is classified histologically as complete (most common) or incomplete. With complete metaplasia, gastric mucosa is completely transformed into small-bowel mucosa, both histologically and functionally, with the ability to absorb nutrients and secrete peptides. In incomplete metaplasia, the epithelium assumes a histologic appearance closer to that of the large intestine and frequently exhibits dysplasia. Intestinal metaplasia may lead to stomach cancer.

Symptoms and Diagnosis

Most patients with *H. pylori*–associated gastritis are asymptomatic, although some have mild dyspepsia or other vague symptoms. Often the condition is discovered during endoscopy performed for other purposes. Testing of asymptomatic patients is not indicated. Once gastritis is identified, testing for *H. pylori* is appropriate.

Treatment

Treatment of chronic nonerosive gastritis is *H. pylori* eradication (see p. 117). Treatment of asymptomatic patients is somewhat controversial given the high prevalence of *H. pylori*–associated superficial gastritis and the relatively low incidence of clinical sequelae (ie, peptic ulcer disease). However, *H. pylori* is a class J carcinogen; eradication removes the cancer risk. In *H. pylori*–negative patients, treatment is directed at symptoms using acid-suppressive drugs (eg, H_2 blockers, proton pump inhibitors) or antacids.

Postgastrectomy Gastritis

Postgastrectomy gastritis is gastric atrophy developing after partial or subtotal gastrectomy (except in cases of gastrinoma).

Metaplasia of the remaining corpus mucosa is common. The degree of gastritis is usually greatest at the lines of anastomosis.

Several mechanisms are responsible: bile reflux, which is common after such surgery, damages the gastric mucosa; loss of antral gastrin decreases stimulation of parietal and peptic cells, causing atrophy; and vagotomy may result in a loss of vagal trophic action.

There are no specific symptoms of gastritis. Postgastrectomy gastritis often progresses to severe atrophy and achlorhydria. Production of intrinsic factor may cease with resultant vitamin B_{12} deficiency (which may be worsened by bacterial overgrowth in the afferent loop). The relative risk of gastric adenocarcinoma appears to increase 15 to 20 yr after partial gastrectomy; however, given the low absolute incidence of postgastrectomy cancer, routine endoscopic surveillance is probably not cost effective, but upper GI symptoms or anemia in such patients should prompt endoscopy.

Uncommon Gastritis Syndromes

Ménétrier's disease: This rare idiopathic disorder affects adults aged 30 to 60 and is more common among men. It manifests as a significant thickening of the gastric folds of the gastric body but not the antrum. Gland atrophy and marked foveolar pit hyperplasia occur, often accompanied by mucous gland metaplasia and increased mucosal thickness with little inflammation. Hypoalbuminemia (the most consistent laboratory abnormality) caused by GI protein loss may be present (protein-losing gastropathy). As the disease progresses, the secretion of acid and pepsin decreases, producing hypochlorhydria.

Symptoms are nonspecific and commonly include epigastric pain, nausea, weight loss, edema, and diarrhea. Differential diagnosis includes (1) lymphoma, in which multiple gastric ulcers may occur, (2) mucosa-associated lymphoid tissue (MALT) lymphoma, with extensive infiltration of monoclonal B lymphocytes, (3) Zollinger-Ellison syndrome with associated gastric fold hypertrophy, and (4) Cronkhite-Canada syndrome, a mucosal polypoid protein-losing syndrome associated with diarrhea. Diagnosis is made by endoscopy with deep mucosal biopsy or full-thickness laparoscopic gastric biopsy.

Various treatments have been used, including anticholinergics, antisecretory drugs, and corticosteroids, but none have proven fully effective. Partial or complete gastric resection may be necessary in cases of severe hypoalbuminemia.

Eosinophilic gastritis: Extensive infiltration of the mucosa, submucosa, and muscle layers with eosinophils often occurs in the antrum. It is usually idiopathic but may result from nematode infestation. Symptoms include nausea, vomiting, and early satiety. Diagnosis is by endoscopic biopsy of involved areas. Corticosteroids can be successful in idiopathic cases; however, if pyloric obstruction develops, surgery may be required.

Mucosa-associated lymphoid tissue (MALT) lymphoma (pseudolymphoma): This rare condition is characterized by massive lymphoid infiltration of the gastric mucosa, which can resemble Ménétrier's disease.

Gastritis caused by systemic disorders: Sarcoidosis, TB, amyloidosis, and other granulomatous diseases can cause gastritis, which is seldom of primary importance.

Gastritis caused by physical agents: Radiation and ingestion of corrosives (especially acidic compounds) can cause gastritis. Exposure to > 16 Gy of radiation produces marked deep gastritis, usually involving the antrum more than the corpus. Pyloric stenosis and perforation are possible complications of radiation-induced gastritis.

Infectious (septic) gastritis: Except for *H. pylori* infection, bacterial invasion of the stomach is rare and mainly occurs following ischemia, ingestion of corrosives, or exposure to radiation. On x-ray, gas outlines the mucosa. The condition can present as an acute surgical abdomen and has a very high mortality rate. Surgery is often necessary.

Debilitated or immunocompromised patients may develop viral or fungal gastritis with cytomegalovirus, *Candida*, histoplasmosis, or mucormycosis; these diagnoses should be considered in patients with exudative gastritis, esophagitis, or duodenitis.

AUTOIMMUNE METAPLASTIC ATROPHIC GASTRITIS

Autoimmune metaplastic atrophic gastritis is an inherited autoimmune disease that attacks parietal cells, resulting in hypochlorhydria and decreased production of intrinsic factor. Consequences include atrophic gastritis, B_{12} malabsorption, and frequently pernicious anemia. Risk of gastric carcinoma increases threefold. Diagnosis is by endoscopy. Treatment is with parenteral vitamin B_{12}.

Patients with autoimmune metaplastic atrophic gastritis (AMAG) have antibodies to parietal cells and their components (which include intrinsic factor and the proton pump H^+,K^+-ATPase). AMAG is inherited as an autosomal dominant trait. Some patients also develop Hashimoto's thyroiditis and 50% have thyroid antibodies; conversely, parietal cell antibodies are found in 30% of patients with thyroiditis.

The lack of intrinsic factor leads to vitamin B_{12} deficiency that can result in a megaloblastic anemia (pernicious anemia—see p. 1044) or neurologic symptoms (subacute combined degeneration—see p. 38).

Hypochlorhydria leads to G-cell hyperplasia and elevated serum gastrin levels (often >1000 pg/mL). Elevated gastrin levels lead to enterochromaffin-like cell hyperplasia, which occasionally undergoes transformation to a carcinoid tumor.

In some patients, AMAG may be associated with chronic *H. pylori* infection, although the relationship is not clear. Gastrectomy and chronic acid suppression with proton pump inhibitors cause similar deficiencies of intrinsic factor secretion.

The areas of atrophic gastritis in the body and fundus may manifest metaplasia. Patients with AMAG have a threefold increased relative risk of developing gastric adenocarcinoma.

Diagnosis is made by endoscopic biopsy. Serum B_{12} levels should be obtained. Parietal cell antibodies can be detected but are not measured routinely. The issue of surveillance endoscopy for cancer screening is unsettled; follow-up examinations are unnecessary unless histologic abnormalities (eg, dysplasia) are present on initial biopsy or symptoms develop. No treatment is needed other than parenteral replacement of vitamin B_{12}.

PEPTIC ULCER DISEASE

A peptic ulcer is an erosion in a segment of the GI mucosa, typically in the stomach (gastric ulcer) or the first few centimeters of the duodenum (duodenal ulcer), that penetrates through the muscularis mucosae. Nearly all ulcers are caused by *Helicobacter pylori* infection or NSAID use. Symptoms typically include burning epigastric pain that is often relieved by food. Diagnosis is by endoscopy and testing for

***H. pylori*. Treatment involves acid suppression, eradication of *H. pylori* (if present), and avoidance of NSAIDs.**

Ulcers may range in size from several millimeters to several centimeters. Ulcers are delineated from erosions by the depth of penetration; erosions are more superficial and do not involve the muscularis mucosae. Ulcers can occur at any age, including infancy and childhood, but are most common in middle-aged adults.

Etiology and Pathophysiology

H. pylori and NSAIDs disrupt normal mucosal defense and repair, making the mucosa more susceptible to acid. *H. pylori* infection is present in 80 to 90% of patients with duodenal ulcers and 70 to 90% of patients with gastric ulcers. If *H. pylori* is eradicated, only 10 to 20% of patients have recurrence of peptic ulcer disease, compared with 70% recurrence in patients treated with acid suppression alone.

Cigarette smoking is a risk factor for the development of ulcers and their complications. Also, smoking impairs ulcer healing and increases the incidence of recurrence. Risk correlates with the number of cigarettes smoked per day. Although alcohol is a strong promoter of acid secretion, no definitive data link moderate amounts of alcohol to the development or delayed healing of ulcers. Very few patients have hypersecretion of gastrin (Zollinger-Ellison syndrome—see p. 181).

A family history exists in 50 to 60% of children with duodenal ulcer.

Symptoms and Signs

Symptoms depend on ulcer location and patient age; many patients, particularly elderly patients, have few or no symptoms. Pain is most common, often localized to the epigastrium and relieved by food or antacids. The pain is described as burning or gnawing, or sometimes a sensation of hunger. The course is usually chronic and recurrent. Only about half of patients present with the characteristic pattern of symptoms.

Gastric ulcer symptoms often do not follow a consistent pattern (eg, eating sometimes exacerbates rather than relieves pain). This is especially true for pyloric channel ulcers, which are often associated with symptoms of obstruction (eg, bloating, nausea, vomiting) caused by edema and scarring.

Duodenal ulcers tend to produce more consistent pain. Pain is absent when the patient awakens but appears in mid-morning, is relieved by food, but recurs 2 to 3 h after a meal. Pain that awakens a patient at night is common and is highly suggestive of duodenal ulcer. In neonates, perforation and hemorrhage may be the first manifestation of duodenal ulcer. Hemorrhage may also be the first recognized sign in later infancy and early childhood, although repeated vomiting or evidence of abdominal pain may be a clue.

Diagnosis

Diagnosis of peptic ulcer is suggested by patient history and confirmed by endoscopy. Empiric therapy is often begun without definitive diagnosis. However, endoscopy allows for biopsy or cytologic brushing of gastric and esophageal lesions to distinguish between simple ulceration and ulcerating stomach cancer. Stomach cancer may present with similar manifestations and must be excluded, especially in patients who are > 45, have lost weight, or report severe or refractory symptoms. The incidence of malignant duodenal ulcer is extremely low, so biopsies of lesions in that area are generally not warranted. Endoscopy can also be used to definitively diagnose *H. pylori* infection, which should be sought when an ulcer is detected.

Gastrin-secreting malignancy and Zollinger-Ellison syndrome should be considered when there are multiple ulcers, when ulcers develop in atypical locations (eg, postbulbar) or are refractory to treatment, or when the patient has prominent diarrhea or weight loss. Serum gastrin levels should be measured in these patients.

Complications

Hemorrhage: Mild to severe hemorrhage is the most common complication of peptic ulcer disease. Symptoms include hematemesis (vomiting of fresh blood or "coffee ground" material); passage of bloody or black tarry stools (hematochezia and melena, respectively); and weakness, orthostasis, syncope, thirst, and sweating caused by blood loss.

Penetration (confined perforation): A peptic ulcer may penetrate the wall of the stomach. If adhesions prevent leakage into the peritoneal cavity, free penetration is avoided and confined perforation occurs. Still, the ulcer may penetrate into the duodenum and enter the adjacent confined space (lesser sac) or another organ (eg, pancreas, liver). Pain may be intense, persistent, referred to sites other than the abdomen (usually the back when caused by penetration of a posterior duodenal ulcer into the pancreas), and modified by body position. CT or MRI is usually needed to confirm the diagnosis. When therapy does not produce healing, surgery is required.

Free perforation: Ulcers that perforate into the peritoneal cavity unchecked by adhesions are usually located in the anterior wall of the duodenum or, less commonly, in the stomach. The patient presents with an acute abdomen. There is sudden, intense, continuous epigastric pain that spreads rapidly throughout the abdomen, often becoming prominent in the right lower quadrant and at times referred to one or both shoulders. The patient usually lies still because even deep breathing worsens the pain. Palpation of the abdomen is painful, rebound tenderness is prominent, abdominal muscles are rigid (boardlike), and bowel sounds are diminished or absent. Shock may ensue, heralded by increased pulse rate and decreased BP and urine output. Symptoms may be less striking in elderly or moribund patients and those receiving corticosteroids or immunosuppressants.

Diagnosis is confirmed if an x-ray shows free air under the diaphragm or in the peritoneal cavity. Upright views of the chest and abdomen are preferred. The most sensitive view is the lateral x-ray of the chest. Severely ill patients may be unable to sit upright and should have a lateral decubitus x-ray of the abdomen. Failure to detect free air does not exclude the diagnosis.

Immediate surgery is required. The longer the delay, the poorer is the prognosis. When surgery is contraindicated, the alternatives are continuous nasogastric suction and broad-spectrum antibiotics.

Gastric outlet obstruction: Obstruction may be caused by scarring, spasm, or inflammation from an ulcer. Symptoms include recurrent, large-volume vomiting, occurring more frequently at the end of the day and often as late as 6 h after the last meal. Loss of appetite with persistent bloating or fullness after eating also suggests gastric outlet obstruction. Prolonged vomiting may cause weight loss, dehydration, and alkalosis.

If the patient's history suggests obstruction, physical examination, gastric aspiration, or x-rays may provide evidence of retained gastric contents. A succussion splash heard > 6 h after a meal or aspiration of fluid or food residue > 200 mL after an overnight fast suggests gastric retention. If gastric aspiration shows marked retention, the stomach should be emptied and endoscopy or x-ray performed to determine site, cause, and degree of obstruction.

Edema or spasm from an active pyloric channel ulcer is treated with gastric decompression by nasogastric suction and acid suppression (eg, IV H_2 blockers). Dehydration and electrolyte imbalances resulting from protracted vomiting or continued nasogastric suctioning should be vigorously sought and corrected. Prokinetic agents are not indicated. Generally, obstruction resolves within 2 to 5 days of treatment. Prolonged obstruction may result from peptic scarring and may respond to endoscopic pyloric balloon dilation. Surgery is necessary to relieve obstruction in selected cases.

Recurrence: Factors that affect recurrence of ulcer include failure to eradicate *H. pylori*, NSAID use, and smoking. Less commonly, a gastrinoma (Zollinger-Ellison syndrome) may be the cause. The 1-yr recurrence rate for gastric and duodenal ulcers is < 10% when *H. pylori* is successfully eradicated but > 60% when it is not. Thus, a patient with recurrent disease should be tested for *H. pylori* and treated again if the tests are positive.

Although long-term treatment with H_2 blockers, proton pump inhibitors, or misoprostol reduces the risk of recurrence, their routine use for this purpose is not recommended. However, patients who require NSAIDs after having had a peptic ulcer are candidates for long-term therapy, as are those with a marginal ulcer or prior perforation or bleeding.

Stomach cancer: Patients with *H. pylori*–associated ulcers have a 3- to 6-fold increased risk of gastric malignancy later in life. There is no increased risk of malignancy with ulcers of other etiology.

Treatment

Treatment of gastric and duodenal ulcers requires eradication of *H. pylori* when present (see p. 117) and a reduction of gastric acidity. For duodenal ulcers, it is particularly important to suppress nocturnal acid secretion.

Methods of decreasing acidity include a number of drugs, all of which are effective but which vary in cost, duration of therapy, and convenience of dosing. In addition, mucosal protective drugs (eg, sucralfate) and acid-reducing surgical procedures may be used. Drug therapy is discussed on p. 124.

Adjuncts: Smoking should be discontinued, and alcohol consumption discontinued or limited to small amounts of dilute alcohol. There is no evidence that changing the diet speeds ulcer healing or prevents recurrence. Thus, many physicians recommend eliminating only foods that cause distress.

Surgery: With current drug therapy, the number of patients requiring surgery has declined dramatically. Indications include perforation, obstruction, uncontrolled or recurrent bleeding, and symptoms that do not respond to drug therapy.

Surgery consists of a procedure to reduce acid secretion, often combined with a procedure to ensure gastric drainage. The recommended operation for duodenal ulcer is highly selective, or parietal cell, vagotomy (which is limited to nerves at the gastric body and spares antral innervation, thereby obviating the need for a drainage procedure). This procedure has a very low mortality rate and avoids the morbidity associated with resection and traditional vagotomy. Other acid-reducing surgical procedures include antrectomy, hemigastrectomy, partial gastrectomy, and subtotal gastrectomy (ie, resection of 30 to 90% of the distal stomach). These are typically combined with truncal vagotomy. Patients who undergo a resective procedure or who have an obstruction require gastric drainage via a gastroduodenostomy (Billroth I) or gastrojejunostomy (Billroth II).

The incidence and type of postsurgical symptoms vary with the type of operation. After resective surgery, up to 30% of patients have significant symptoms, including weight loss, maldigestion, anemia, dumping syndrome, reactive hypoglycemia, bilious vomiting, mechanical problems, and ulcer recurrence.

Weight loss is common after subtotal gastrectomy; the patient may limit food intake because of early satiety (because the residual gastric pouch is small) or to prevent dumping syndrome and other postprandial syndromes. With a small gastric pouch, distention or discomfort may follow a meal of even moderate size; patients should be encouraged to eat smaller and more frequent meals.

Maldigestion and steatorrhea caused by pancreaticobiliary bypass, especially with Billroth II anastomosis, may contribute to weight loss.

Anemia is common (usually from iron deficiency, but occasionally from vitamin B_{12} deficiency caused by loss of intrinsic factor or bacterial overgrowth) in the afferent limb, and osteomalacia may occur. IM vitamin B_{12} supplementation is recommended for all patients with total gastrectomy but may also be given to patients with subtotal gastrectomy if deficiency is suspected.

Dumping syndrome may follow gastric surgical procedures, particularly resections. Weakness, dizziness, sweating, nausea, vomiting, and palpitation occur soon after eating, especially hyperosmolar foods. This phenomenon is referred to as early dumping, the cause of which remains unclear but likely involves autonomic reflexes, intravascular volume contraction, and release of vasoactive peptides from the small intestine. Dietary modifications, with smaller, more frequent meals and decreased carbohydrate intake, usually help.

Reactive hypoglycemia or **late dumping** (another form of the syndrome) results from rapid emptying of carbohydrates from the gastric pouch. Early high peaks in blood glucose stimulate excess release of insulin, which leads to symptomatic hypoglycemia several hours after the meal. A high-protein, low-carbohydrate diet and adequate caloric intake (in frequent small feedings) are recommended.

Mechanical problems (including gastroparesis and bezoar formation—see p. 126) may occur secondary to a decrease in phase III gastric motor contractions, which are altered after antrectomy and vagotomy. Diarrhea is especially common after vagotomy, even without a resection (pyloroplasty).

Ulcer recurrence occurs in 5 to 12% after highly selective vagotomy and 2 to 5% after resective surgery. Recurrent ulcers are diagnosed by endoscopy and generally respond to either proton pump inhibitors or H_2 blockers. For ulcers that continue to recur, the completeness of vagotomy should be tested by gastric analysis, *H. pylori* eliminated if present, and Zollinger-Ellison syndrome ruled out by serum gastrin studies.

DRUG TREATMENT OF GASTRIC ACIDITY

Drugs for decreasing acidity are used for peptic ulcer, gastroesophageal reflux disease (GERD–see p. 112), and many forms of gastritis. Some drugs are used in regimens for treating *H. pylori* infection. Drugs include proton pump inhibitors, H_2 blockers, antacids, and prostaglandins.

Proton pump inhibitors: These drugs are potent inhibitors of H^+,K^+-ATPase. This enzyme, located in the apical secretory membrane of the parietal cell, plays a key role in the secretion of H^+ (protons). These drugs can completely inhibit acid secretion and have a long duration of action. They promote ulcer healing and are also key components of *H. pylori* eradication regimens. Proton pump inhibitors have replaced H_2 blockers in most clinical situations because of greater rapidity of action and efficacy.

Proton pump inhibitors include omeprazole, lansoprazole, rabeprazole, esomeprazole, all available orally; and pantoprazole, available orally and IV (see TABLE 13–1). For uncomplicated duodenal ulcers, omeprazole 20 mg po once/day or lansoprazole 30 mg po once/day is given for 4 wk. Complicated duodenal ulcers (ie, multiple ulcers, bleeding ulcers, those > 1.5 cm, or those occurring in patients with serious underlying illness) respond better to higher doses (omeprazole 40 mg once/day, lansoprazole 60 mg once/day or 30 mg bid). Gastric ulcers require treatment for 6 to 8 wk. Gastritis and GERD require 8 to 12 wk of therapy; GERD additionally requires long-term maintenance.

Long-term proton pump inhibitor therapy produces elevated gastrin levels, which lead to enterochromaffin-like cell hyperplasia. However, there is no evidence of dysplasia or malignant transformation in patients receiving this treatment. Some may develop vitamin B_{12} malabsorption.

H_2 blockers: These drugs (cimetidine, ranitidine, famotidine, available IV and orally; and nizatidine available orally) are competitive inhibitors of histamine at the H_2 receptor, thus suppressing gastrin-stimulated acid secretion and proportionately reducing gastric juice volume. Histamine-mediated pepsin secretion is also decreased.

H_2 blockers are well absorbed from the GI tract, with onset of action 30 to 60 min after ingestion and peak effects at 1 to 2 h. IV administration produces a more rapid onset of action. Duration of action is proportional to dose and ranges from 6 to 20 h. Doses should often be reduced in elderly patients.

For duodenal ulcers, once daily oral administration of cimetidine 800 mg, ranitidine 300 mg, famotidine 40 mg, or nizatidine 300 mg given at bedtime or after dinner for 6 to 8 wk is effective. Gastric ulcers may respond to the same regimen continued for 8 to 12 wk, but because nocturnal acid secretion is less important, morning administration may be equally or more effective. Children ≥ 40 kg may receive adult doses. Below that weight, the oral dosage is ranitidine 2 mg/kg q 12 h and cimetidine 10 mg/kg q 12 h. For GERD, H_2 blockers are now mostly used for pain management. Gastritis heals with famotidine or ranitidine given bid for 8 to 12 wk.

Cimetidine has minor antiandrogen effects expressed as reversible gynecomastia and, less commonly, erectile dysfunction with prolonged use. Mental status changes, diarrhea, rash, drug fever, myalgias, thrombocytopenia, and sinus bradycardia and hypotension after rapid IV administration have been reported with all H_2 blockers, generally in < 1% of treated patients but more commonly in elderly patients.

Cimetidine and, to a lesser extent, other H_2 blockers interact with the P-450 microsomal enzyme system and may delay metabolism of other drugs eliminated through this system (eg, phenytoin, warfarin, theophylline, diazepam, lidocaine).

Antacids: These agents neutralize gastric acid and reduce pepsin activity (which diminishes as gastric pH rises to > 4.0). In addition, some antacids adsorb pepsin. Antacids may interfere with the absorption of other drugs (eg, tetracycline, digoxin, iron).

Antacids relieve symptoms, promote ulcer healing, and reduce recurrence. They are relatively inexpensive but must be taken 5 to 7 times/day. The optimal antacid regimen for ulcer healing appears to be 15 to 30 mL of liquid or 2 to 4 tablets 1 and 3 h after each meal and at bedtime. The total daily dosage of antacids should provide 200 to 400 mEq neutralizing capacity. However, antacids have been superseded by acid suppressive therapy in the treatment of peptic ulcer and are used only for short-term symptom relief.

In general, there are two types of antacids: absorbable and nonabsorbable. Absorbable

TABLE 13–1. PROTON PUMP INHIBITORS

DRUG	MOST CONDITIONS*	COMPLICATED DUODENAL ULCERS
Esomeprazole	40 mg once/day	40 mg bid
Lansoprazole	30 mg once/day (Pediatric doses: < 10 kg 7.5 mg once/day 10–20 kg 15 mg once/day ≥ 20 kg 30 mg once/day)†	30 mg bid
Omeprazole	20 mg once/day (Pediatric dose: 1 mg/kg/day in a single dose or divided bid)†	40 mg once/day
Pantoprazole	40 mg once/day	40 mg bid
Rabeprazole	20 mg once/day	20 mg bid

*Gastritis, gastroesophageal reflux disease, uncomplicated duodenal ulcers.
†Representative doses. Data are limited on the use of proton pump inhibitors in children.

antacids (eg, Na bicarbonate, Ca carbonate) provide rapid, complete neutralization but may cause alkalosis and should be used only briefly (1 or 2 days). Nonabsorbable antacids (eg, aluminum or Mg hydroxide) cause fewer systemic side effects and are preferred.

Aluminum hydroxide is a relatively safe, commonly used antacid. With chronic use, phosphate depletion occasionally develops as a result of binding of phosphate by aluminum in the GI tract. The risk of phosphate depletion increases in alcoholics, malnourished patients, and patients with renal disease (including those receiving hemodialysis). Aluminum hydroxide causes constipation.

Mg hydroxide is a more effective antacid than aluminum but may cause diarrhea. To limit diarrhea, many proprietary antacids combine Mg and aluminum antacids. Because small amounts of Mg are absorbed, Mg preparations should be used with caution in patients with renal disease.

Prostaglandins: Certain prostaglandins (especially misoprostol) inhibit acid secretion and enhance mucosal defense. Synthetic prostaglandin derivatives are used predominantly to decrease the risk of NSAID-induced mucosal injury. Patients at high risk for NSAID-induced ulcers (ie, elderly patients, those with a history of ulcer or ulcer complication, those also taking corticosteroids) are candidates to take misoprostol 200 μg po qid with food along with their NSAID. Common side effects of misoprostol are abdominal cramping and diarrhea, which occur in 30% of patients. Misoprostol is a powerful abortifacient and is absolutely contraindicated in women of childbearing age who are not using contraception.

Sucralfate: This drug is a sucrose-aluminum complex that dissociates in stomach acid and forms a physical barrier over an inflamed area, protecting it from acid, pepsin, and bile salts. It also inhibits pepsin-substrate interaction, stimulates mucosal prostaglandin production, and binds bile salts. It has no effect on acid output or gastrin secretion. Sucralfate appears to have trophic effects on the ulcerated mucosa, possibly by binding growth factors and concentrating them at an ulcer site. Systemic absorption of sucralfate is negligible. Constipation occurs in 3 to 5% of patients. Sucralfate may bind to other drugs and interfere with their absorption.

14 BEZOARS AND FOREIGN BODIES

Food and other ingested materials may collect and form solid masses within the GI tract.

BEZOARS

A bezoar is a tightly packed collection of partially digested or undigested material that is unable to exit the stomach. It often occurs in patients with abnormal gastric emptying, as may occur following gastric surgery. Many bezoars are asymptomatic, but some produce symptoms of gastric outlet obstruction. Some can be dissolved enzymatically, others removed endoscopically, and some require surgery.

Partially digested agglomerations of vegetable matter or hair are called phytobezoars or trichobezoars, respectively. Pharmacobezoars are concretions of medication (particularly sucralfate and aluminum hydroxide gel). Many other substances have been found in bezoars.

Etiology

Trichobezoars, which can weigh several kg, most commonly occur in patients with psychiatric disturbances who chew and swallow their own hair. Phytobezoars often occur in patients who have undergone a Billroth I or II partial gastrectomy, especially when accompanied by vagotomy. Hypochlorhydria, diminished antral motility, and incomplete mastication are the main predisposing factors. Others include diabetic gastroparesis and gastroplasty for morbid obesity. Finally, consumption of persimmons (a fruit containing the tannin shibuol, which polymerizes in the stomach) has been known to cause bezoars that require surgery in > 90% of cases. Persimmon bezoars often occur in epidemics in regions where the fruit is grown.

Symptoms, Signs, and Diagnosis

Most bezoars cause no symptoms, although postprandial fullness, nausea and vomiting, pain, and GI bleeding may occur. Bezoars are detectable as a mass lesion on most tests (eg, x-ray, ultrasound, CT) that may be performed to evaluate upper GI symptoms. They may be mistaken for tumors; upper endoscopy is usually performed. On endoscopy, bezoars have an unmistakable irregular surface and may range in color from yellow-green to gray-black. An endoscopic biopsy that yields hair or plant material is diagnostic.

Treatment

If initial diagnosis was made by endoscopy, removal can be attempted at that time. Fragmentation with forceps, wire snare, jet spray, or even laser may break up bezoars, allowing them to pass or be extracted. Metoclopramide 40 mg IV over 24 h or 10 mg IM q 4 h for several days may increase peristalsis and aid gastric emptying of fragmented material.

If endoscopy was not initially performed, treatment is based on the symptoms. Asymptomatic patients, with a bezoar discovered incidentally during testing for other reasons, do not necessarily require intervention. In some cases, a trial of enzymatic therapy can be attempted. Enzymes include papain (10,000 U with each meal), meat tenderizer (5 mL [1 tsp] in 8 oz of clear liquid before each meal), or cellulase (10 g dissolved in 1 L water, consumed over 24 h for 2 to 3 days). If enzymatic therapy is unsuccessful, or if patients are symptomatic, endoscopic removal may be tried. Rocklike concretions and trichobezoars usually require laparotomy.

FOREIGN BODIES

A variety of foreign bodies may enter the GI tract. Many pass spontaneously, but some become impacted, causing symptoms of obstruction. Perforation may occur. The esophagus is the most common (75%) site of impaction. Nearly all impacted objects can be removed endoscopically, but surgery is occasionally necessary.

Undigestible objects may be intentionally swallowed by children and demented adults. Denture wearers, the elderly, and inebriated people are prone to accidentally swallowing inadequately masticated food (particularly meat), which may become impacted in the esophagus. Smugglers who swallow drug-filled balloons, vials, or packages to escape detection (body packers or body stuffers) may develop intestinal obstruction. The packaging may rupture, leading to drug overdose.

Esophageal foreign bodies: Foreign bodies usually lodge in an area of esophageal narrowing such as at the cricopharyngeus or aortic arch or just above the gastroesophageal junction. If obstruction is complete, patients retch or vomit. Some patients drool because they are unable to swallow secretions.

Immediate endoscopic removal is required for sharp objects, coins in the proximal esophagus, and any obstruction causing significant symptoms. Also, button batteries lodged in the esophagus may cause direct corrosive damage, low-voltage burns, and pressure necrosis and thus require prompt removal.

Other esophageal foreign bodies may be observed for a maximum of 12 to 24 h. Glucagon 1 mg IV sometimes relaxes the esophagus enough to allow spontaneous passage. Other methods, such as use of effervescent agents, meat tenderizer, and bougienage, are not recommended. Removal is best achieved using a forceps, basket, or snare with an overtube placed in the esophagus to prevent aspiration. Endoscopic removal is the treatment of choice.

Sometimes, foreign bodies scratch the esophagus but do not become lodged. In such cases, patients may report a foreign body sensation even though no foreign body is present.

Gastric and intestinal foreign bodies: Foreign bodies that pass through the esophagus are asymptomatic unless obstruction or perforation occurs. Of the foreign bodies that reach the stomach, 80 to 90% pass spontaneously, 10 to 20% require nonoperative intervention, and ≤ 1% require surgery. Thus, most intragastric foreign bodies can be ignored. However, objects larger than 5 × 2 cm rarely pass the stomach. Sharp objects should be retrieved from the stomach because 15 to 35% will cause intestinal perforation, but small round objects (eg, coins and button batteries) can simply be observed. The patient's stools should be searched, and if the object does not appear, x-rays are taken at 48-h intervals. A coin that remains in the stomach for > 4 wk, or a battery showing signs of corrosion on x-ray that remains in the stomach for > 48 h, should be removed. A hand-held metal detector can localize metallic foreign bodies and provide information comparable to that yielded by plain x-rays.

Patients with symptoms of obstruction or perforation require laparotomy. Ingested drug packages are of great concern because of the risk of leakage and consequent drug overdose. Patients with symptoms of drug toxicity should have immediate laparotomy. Asymptomatic patients should be admitted to the hospital. Some clinicians advocate oral polyethylene glycol solution as a cathartic to enhance passage of the material; others suggest surgical removal. The best practice is unclear.

Most foreign objects that have passed into the small intestine usually traverse the GI tract without problem, even if they take weeks or months to do so. They tend to be held up just before the ileocecal valve or at any site of narrowing, as is present in Crohn's disease. Sometimes objects such as toothpicks remain within the GI tract for many years, only to turn up in a granuloma or abscess.

Rectal foreign bodies: Gallstones, fecaliths, and swallowed foreign bodies (including toothpicks and chicken and fish bones) may lodge at the anorectal junction. Urinary calculi, vaginal pessaries, or surgical sponges or instruments may erode into the rectum. Foreign bodies, sometimes bizarre and/or related to sexual play, may be introduced intentionally but become lodged unintentionally. Some objects are caught in the rectal wall, and others are trapped just above the anal sphincter.

Sudden, excruciating pain during defecation should arouse suspicion of a penetrating foreign body, usually lodged at or just above the anorectal junction. Other manifestations depend on the size and shape of the foreign body, its duration in situ, and the presence of infection or perforation.

Foreign bodies usually become lodged in the mid rectum, where they cannot negotiate the anterior angulation of the rectum. They can be felt on digital examination. Abdominal examination and chest x-rays may be necessary to exclude possible intraperitoneal rectal perforation.

If the object can be palpated, a local anesthetic is given by subcutaneous and submucosal injections of 0.5% lidocaine or bupivacaine. The anus can be dilated with a rectal retractor and the foreign body grasped and removed. If the object cannot be palpated, the patient should be hospitalized. Peristalsis generally moves the foreign body down to the mid rectum, and the above routine can be followed. Removal via a sigmoidoscope or proctoscope is rarely successful, and sigmoidoscopy usually forces the foreign body proximally, delaying its extraction. Regional or general anesthesia is infrequently necessary, and laparotomy with milking of the foreign body toward the anus or colotomy with extraction of the foreign body is rarely necessary. After extraction, sigmoidoscopy should be performed to rule out significant rectal trauma or perforation. Removal of a rectal foreign body may be of high risk and should be done by a surgeon or gastroenterologist skilled in foreign body removal.

15 PANCREATITIS

Pancreatitis is classified as either acute or chronic. Acute pancreatitis is inflammation that resolves both clinically and histologically. Chronic pancreatitis is characterized by histologic changes that are irreversible and progressive and that result in considerable loss of exocrine and endocrine pancreatic function. Patients with chronic pancreatitis may have a flare-up of acute disease.

Pancreatitis can affect both the exocrine and endocrine functions of the pancreas. Pancreatic acinar cells secrete bicarbonate and digestive enzymes into ducts that connect the pancreas to the duodenum at the ampulla of Vater (exocrine function). Pancreatic beta cells secrete insulin directly into the bloodstream (endocrine function).

ACUTE PANCREATITIS

Acute pancreatitis is inflammation of the pancreas (and, sometimes, adjacent tissues) caused by the release of activated pancreatic enzymes. The most common triggers are biliary tract disease and chronic heavy alcohol intake. The condition ranges from mild (abdominal pain and vomiting) to severe (pancreatic necrosis and a systemic inflammatory process with shock and multiorgan failure). Diagnosis is based on clinical presentation and serum amylase and lipase levels. Treatment is supportive, with IV fluids, analgesics, and fasting.

Etiology and Pathophysiology

Biliary tract disease and alcoholism account for ≥ 80% of acute pancreatitis cases. The remaining 20% result from myriad causes (see TABLE 15–1).

The precise mechanism by which obstruction of the sphincter of Oddi by a gallstone or microlithiasis (sludge) causes pancreatitis is unclear, although it probably involves increased ductal pressure. Prolonged alcohol intake (> 100 g/day for > 3 to 5 yr) may cause the protein of pancreatic enzymes to precipitate within small pancreatic ductules. Ductal obstruction by these protein plugs may cause premature activation of pancreatic enzymes. An alcohol binge in such patients can trigger pancreatitis by activating pancreatic enzymes.

A number of genetic mutations predisposing to pancreatitis have been identified. One, an autosomal dominant mutation of the cationic trypsinogen gene, causes pancreatitis in 80% of carriers; an obvious familial pattern is present. Other mutations have lesser penetrance and are not readily apparent clinically except through genetic testing. The genetic abnormality responsible for cystic fibrosis increases the risk of recurrent acute pancreatitis.

Regardless of the etiology, pancreatic enzymes (including trypsin, phospholipase A2, and elastase) become activated within the gland itself. The enzymes damage tissue and activate complement and the inflammatory cascade, producing cytokines. This causes inflammation, edema, and sometimes necrosis. In mild pancreatitis, inflammation is confined to the pancreas; the mortality rate is < 5%. In severe pancreatitis, there is significant inflammation, with necrosis and hemorrhage of the gland and a systemic inflammatory response; the mortality rate is 10 to 50%. After 5 to 7 days, necrotic pancreatic tissue may become infected by enteric bacteria.

Activated enzymes and cytokines that enter the peritoneal cavity cause a chemical burn and third spacing of fluid; those that enter the systemic circulation produce a systemic inflammatory response that can result in acute respiratory distress syndrome and renal failure. The systemic effects are mainly the result of increased capillary permeability and decreased vascular tone. Phospholipase A2 is thought to injure alveolar membranes of the lungs.

In about 40% of patients, collections of enzyme-rich pancreatic fluid and tissue debris form in and around the pancreas. In about half, the collections resolve spontaneously. In others, the collections become infected or form pseudocysts. Pseudocysts have a fibrous capsule without an epithelial lining. Pseudocysts may hemorrhage, rupture, or become infected.

Death during the first several days is usually caused by cardiovascular instability (with refractory shock and renal failure) or respiratory failure (with hypoxemia and at times adult respiratory distress syndrome). Occasionally, death results from heart failure secondary to an unidentified myocardial depressant factor. Death after the first week is usually caused by pancreatic infection or rupture of a pseudocyst.

Symptoms and Signs

An acute attack causes steady, boring upper abdominal pain, typically severe enough to require large doses of parenteral opioids. The pain radiates through to the back in about 50%; rarely, pain is first felt in the lower abdomen. Pain usually develops suddenly in gallstone pancreatitis; in alcoholic pancreatitis, pain develops over a few days. The pain usually persists for several days. Sitting up and leaning forward may reduce pain, but coughing, vigorous movement, and deep breathing may accentuate it. Nausea and vomiting are common.

The patient appears acutely ill and sweaty. Pulse rate is usually 100 to 140 beats/min. Respiration is shallow and rapid. BP may be transiently high or low, with significant postural hypotension. Temperature may be normal or even subnormal at first but may increase to 37.7 to 38.3° C (100 to 101° F) within a few hours. Sensorium may be blunted to the point of semicoma. Scleral icterus is occasionally present. The lungs may have limited diaphragmatic excursion and evidence of atelectasis.

About 20% of patients experience upper abdominal distention caused by gastric distention or displacement of the stomach by a pancreatic inflammatory mass. Pancreatic duct disruption may cause ascites (pancreatic ascites). Marked abdominal tenderness occurs, most often in the upper abdomen. There may be mild tenderness in the lower abdomen, but the rectum is not tender and the stool is usually negative for occult blood. Mild-to-moderate muscular rigidity may be present in the upper abdomen but is rare in the lower abdomen. Rarely, severe peritoneal irritation results in a rigid and boardlike abdomen. Bowel sounds may be hypoactive. Grey Turner's sign and Cullen's sign are ecchymoses to the flanks and umbilical region, respectively, and indicate extravasation of hemorrhagic exudate.

Infection in the pancreas or in an adjacent fluid collection should be suspected if the patient has a generally toxic appearance with elevated temperature and WBC count or if deterioration follows an initial period of stabilization.

TABLE 15–1. SOME CAUSES OF ACUTE PANCREATITIS

CAUSE	EXAMPLE
Drugs	ACE inhibitors, asparaginase, azathioprine, 2′, 3′–dideoxyinosine, furosemide, 6-mercaptopurine, pentamidine, sulfa drugs, valproate
Infectious	Coxsackie B virus, cytomegalovirus, mumps
Inherited	Multiple known gene mutations, including a small percentage of cystic fibrosis patients
Mechanical/ structural	Gallstones, ERCP, trauma, pancreatic or periampullary cancer, choledochal cyst, sphincter of Oddi stenosis, pancreas divisum
Metabolic	Hypertriglyceridemia, hypercalcemia (including hyperparathyroidism)
Toxins	Alcohol, methanol
Other	Pregnancy, postrenal transplant, ischemia from hypotension or atheroembolism, tropical pancreatitis

Diagnosis

Pancreatitis is suspected whenever severe abdominal pain occurs, especially in a person with significant alcohol use or known gallstones. Conditions producing similar symptoms include perforated gastric or duodenal ulcer, mesenteric infarction, strangulating intestinal obstruction, dissecting aneurysm, biliary colic, appendicitis, diverticulitis, inferior wall MI, and hematoma of the abdominal muscles or spleen.

Diagnosis is made by clinical suspicion, serum markers (amylase and lipase), and the absence of other causes for the patient's symptoms. Thus, a broad range of tests is obtained, typically including CBC, electrolytes, Ca, Mg, glucose, BUN, creatinine, amylase, and lipase. Other routine tests include ECG and an abdominal series (chest, flat, and upright abdomen). A urine dipstick for trypsinogen-2 has sensitivity and specificity of > 90% for acute pancreatitis. Ultrasound and CT are not generally obtained specifically to diagnose pancreatitis but are often used to evaluate acute abdominal pain (see p. 97) and are indicated once pancreatitis has been diagnosed.

Laboratory tests: Serum amylase and lipase concentrations increase on the first day of acute pancreatitis and return to normal in 3 to 7 days. Lipase is more specific for pancreatitis, but both enzymes may be increased in renal failure and various abdominal conditions (eg, perforated ulcer, mesenteric vascular occlusion, intestinal obstruction). Other causes of increased serum amylase include salivary gland dysfunction, macroamylasemia, and tumors that secrete amylase. Both amylase and lipase levels may remain normal if destruction of acinar tissue during previous episodes precludes release of sufficient amounts of enzymes. The serum of patients with hypertriglyceridemia may contain a circulating inhibitor that must be diluted before an elevation in serum amylase can be detected.

Amylase:creatinine clearance ratio does not have sufficient sensitivity or specificity to diagnose pancreatitis. It is generally used to diagnose macroamylasemia when no pancreatitis exists. In macroamylasemia, amylase bound to serum immunoglobulin falsely elevates the serum amylase level.

Fractionation of total serum amylase into pancreatic type (p-type) and salivary-type (s-type) isoamylase increases the accuracy of serum amylase. However, the level of p-type also increases in renal failure and in other severe abdominal conditions in which amylase clearance is altered.

The WBC count usually increases to 12,000 to 20,000/μL. Third space fluid losses may increase the Hct to as high as 50 to 55%, indicating severe inflammation. Hyperglycemia may occur. Serum Ca concentration falls as early as the first day because of the formation of Ca "soaps" secondary to excess generation of free fatty acids, especially by pancreatic lipase. Serum bilirubin increases in 15 to 25% of patients because pancreatic edema compresses the common bile duct.

Imaging: Plain x-rays of the abdomen may disclose calcifications within pancreatic ducts (evidence of prior inflammation and hence chronic pancreatitis), calcified gallstones, or localized ileus in the left upper quadrant or the center of the abdomen (a "sentinel loop" of small bowel, dilation of the transverse colon, or duodenal ileus). Chest x-ray may reveal atelectasis or a pleural effusion (usually left-sided or bilateral but rarely confined to the right pleural space).

If not obtained initially, ultrasound should be performed to detect gallstones or dilation of the common bile duct (which indicates biliary tract obstruction). Edema of the pancreas may be visualized, but overlying gas frequently obscures the pancreas.

CT with IV contrast is generally obtained to identify necrosis, fluid collections, or pseudocysts once pancreatitis has been diagnosed. It is particularly recommended for severe pancreatitis or if a complication ensues (eg, hypotension or progressive leukocytosis and elevation of temperature). IV contrast facilitates the recognition of pancreatic necrosis; however, it may cause pancreatic necrosis in areas of low perfusion (ie, ischemia). Thus, contrast-enhanced CT should be performed only after the patient has been adequately hydrated.

If pancreatic infection is suspected, fluid obtained by percutaneous CT-guided needle aspiration of cysts or areas of fluid collection or necrosis may reveal organisms on Gram stain or culture. The diagnosis is supported by positive blood cultures and, particularly, by the presence of air bubbles in the retroperitoneum on abdominal CT. The advent of MRI cholangiopancreatography (MRCP) may make the selection of pancreatic imaging simpler.

Prognosis

In edematous pancreatitis, mortality is < 5%. In pancreatitis with necrosis and hemorrhage, mortality is 10 to 50%. In pancreatic infection, the mortality rate is usually 100% without extensive surgical debridement or drainage of the infected area.

CT findings correlate with prognosis. If CT is normal or shows only mild pancreatic edema (Balthazar class A or B), the prognosis is excellent. Patients with peripancreatic inflammation or one area of fluid collection (class C and D) have a 10 to 15% incidence of abscess formation; the incidence is over 60% in patients with two or more areas of fluid collection (Class E).

Ranson's prognostic signs help predict the prognosis of acute pancreatitis. Five of Ranson's signs can be documented at admission: age > 55 yr, serum glucose > 200 mg/dL (> 11.1 mmol/L), serum LDH > 350 IU/L, AST > 250 U, and WBC count > 16,000/µL. The rest are determined within 48 h of admission: Hct decrease > 10%, BUN increase > 5 mg/dL (> 1.78 mmol/L), serum Ca < 8 mg/dL (< 2 mmol/L), Pa_{O_2} < 60 mm Hg (< 7.98 kPa), base deficit > 4 mEq/L (> 4 mmol/L), and estimated fluid sequestration > 6 L. Mortality increases with the number of positive signs: If fewer than three signs are positive, the mortality rate is < 5%; if three or four are positive, it is 15 to 20%.

The APACHE II index (see TABLE 63–4 on p. 517), calculated on the 2nd hospital day, also correlates with prognosis.

Treatment

Adequate fluid resuscitation is essential; up to 6 to 8 L/day of fluid containing appropriate electrolytes may be required. Inadequate fluid therapy increases the risk of pancreatic necrosis.

Fasting is indicated until acute inflammation subsides (ie, cessation of abdominal tenderness and pain, normalization of serum amylase, return of appetite, feeling better). Fasting can last from a few days in mild pancreatitis to several weeks. To prevent malnutrition, TPN should be initiated in severe cases within the first few days.

Pain relief requires parenteral opioids, which should be given in adequate doses. Although morphine may cause the sphincter of Oddi to contract, this is of doubtful clinical significance. Antiemetic agents (eg, prochlorperazine 5 to 10 mg IV q 6 h) should be given to alleviate vomiting. A nasogastric tube is required only if significant vomiting persists or ileus is present.

Parenteral H_2 blockers or proton pump inhibitors are given. Efforts to reduce pancreatic secretion with drugs (eg, anticholinergics, glucagon, somatostatin, octreotide) have no proven benefit.

Severe acute pancreatitis should be treated in an ICU, particularly in patients with hypotension, oliguria, Ranson's score ≥ 3, APACHE II ≥ 8, or pancreatic necrosis on CT scan > 30%. In the ICU, vital signs and urine output are monitored hourly; metabolic parameters (Hct, glucose, and electrolytes) are reassessed q 8 h; arterial blood gases are determined prn; central venous pressure line or Swan-Ganz catheter measurements are determined q 6 h if the patient is hemodynamically unstable or if fluid requirements are unclear. CBC, platelet count, coagulation parameters, total protein with albumin, BUN, creatinine, Ca, and Mg are measured daily.

Hypoxemia is treated with humidified oxygen via mask or nasal prongs. If hypoxemia persists or adult respiratory distress syndrome develops, assisted ventilation may be required. Glucose > 170 to 200 mg/dL (9.4 to 11.1 mmol/L) should be treated cautiously with subcutaneous or IV insulin and carefully monitored. Hypocalcemia generally is not treated unless neuromuscular irritability occurs; 10 to 20 mL of 10% Ca gluconate in 1 L of IV fluid is given over 4 to 6 h. Chronic alcoholics and patients with documented hypomagnesemia should receive Mg sulfate 1 g/L of replacement fluid for a total of 2 to 4 g, or until levels normalize. If renal failure occurs, serum Mg levels are monitored and IV Mg given cautiously. With restoration of normal Mg levels, serum Ca levels usually return to normal.

Heart failure should be treated (see p. 658). Prerenal azotemia should be treated by increased fluid replacement. Renal failure may require dialysis (usually peritoneal).

Antibiotic prophylaxis with imipenem can prevent infection of sterile pancreatic necrosis, although the effect on reducing mortality is unclear. Infected areas of pancreatic necrosis require surgical debridement, but infected fluid collections outside the pancreas may be drained percutaneously. A pseudocyst that is expanding rapidly, infected, bleeding, or likely to rupture requires drainage. Whether drainage is percutaneous, surgical, or endoscopic depends on location of the pseudocyst and institutional expertise. Peritoneal lavage to wash out activated pancreatic enzymes and inflammatory mediators has no proven benefit.

Surgical intervention during the first several days is justified for severe blunt or penetrating trauma or uncontrolled biliary sepsis. Although > 80% of patients with gallstone pancreatitis pass the stone spontaneously, ERCP with sphincterotomy and stone removal is indicated for patients who do not improve after 24 h of treatment. Patients who spontaneously improve generally undergo elective laparoscopic cholecystectomy. Elective cholangiography remains controversial.

CHRONIC PANCREATITIS

Chronic pancreatitis is persistent inflammation of the pancreas that results in permanent structural damage with fibrosis and ductal strictures, followed by a decline in exocrine and endocrine function. It can occur as the result of chronic alcohol abuse but may be idiopathic. Initial symptoms are recurrent attacks of pain. Later in the disease, some patients develop malabsorption and glucose intolerance. Diagnosis is usually made by imaging studies such as ERCP, endoscopic ultrasound, or secretin pancreatic function testing. Treatment is supportive, with dietary modification, analgesics, and enzyme supplements. In some cases, surgery is helpful.

Etiology and Pathophysiology

In the US, 70 to 80% of cases result from alcoholism and 15 to 25% are idiopathic. Rare causes include hereditary pancreatitis, hyperparathyroidism, and obstruction of the main pancreatic duct caused by stenosis, stones, or cancer. In India, Indonesia, and Nigeria, idiopathic calcific pancreatitis occurs among children and young adults ("tropical pancreatitis").

Similar to acute pancreatitis, the mechanism of disease may be ductal obstruction by protein plugs. The protein plugs may result from excess secretion of glycoprotein-2 or a deficiency of lithostatin, a protein in pancreatic fluid that inhibits Ca precipitation. If obstruction is chronic, persistent inflammation leads to fibrosis and alternating areas of ductal dilation and stricture, which may become calcified. Neuronal sheath hypertrophy and perineural inflammation occur and may contribute to chronic pain. After several years, progressive fibrosis leads to loss of exocrine and endocrine function. Diabetes develops in 20 to 30% of patients within 10 to 15 yr of onset.

Symptoms and Signs

Most patients present with episodic abdominal pain. About 10 to 15% have no pain and present with malabsorption. Pain is epigastric, severe, and may last many hours or several days. Episodes typically subside spontaneously after 6 to 10 yr as the acinar cells that secrete pancreatic digestive enzymes are progressively destroyed. When lipase and protease secretions are reduced to < 10% of normal, the patient develops steatorrhea, passing greasy stools or even oil droplets, and creatorrhea. Symptoms of glucose intolerance may appear at this time.

Diagnosis

Diagnosis can be difficult because amylase and lipase levels are frequently normal because of significant loss of pancreatic function. In a patient with a typical history of alcohol abuse and recurrent episodes of acute pancreatitis, detection of pancreatic calcification on plain x-ray of the abdomen may be sufficient. However, such calcifications typically occur late in the disease and then are visible in only about 30% of cases. In patients without a typical history, pancreatic malignancy must be excluded as the cause of pain: abdominal CT is recommended. CT can demonstrate calcifications and other pancreatic abnormalities (eg, pseudocyst or dilated ducts) but still may be normal early in the disease.

The primary options for patients with normal CT findings include ERCP, endoscopic ultrasound, and secretin pancreatic function testing. These tests are quite sensitive, but ERCP precipitates acute pancreatitis in about 5% of patients. MRI cholangiopancreatography (MRCP) may prove an acceptable alternative.

Late in the disease, tests of pancreatic exocrine function become abnormal. A 72-h test for stool fat is diagnostic for steatorrhea but cannot establish a cause. The secretin test collects pancreatic secretions via a duodenal tube for analysis but is performed in only a few centers. Levels of serum trypsinogen and fecal chymotrypsin and elastase may be decreased. In the bentiromide test and the pancreolauryl test, substances are administered orally and the urine is analyzed for cleavage products generated by pancreatic enzymes. All such exocrine tests are less sensitive than ERCP or endoscopic ultrasound early in the disease.

Treatment

A relapse requires treatment similar to acute pancreatitis with fasting, IV fluids, and analgesics. When feeding resumes, the patient must eschew alcohol and consume a low-fat (< 25 g/day) diet (to reduce secretion of pancreatic enzymes). An H_2 blocker or proton pump inhibitor may reduce acid-stimulated release of secretin, thereby decreasing the flow of pancreatic secretions. Too often, these measures do not relieve pain, requiring increased amounts of opioids, with the threat of addiction. Medical treatment of chronic pancreatic pain is often unsatisfactory.

Pancreatic enzyme supplementation may reduce chronic pain by inhibiting the release of cholecystokinin, thereby reducing the secretion of pancreatic enzymes. This is more likely to be successful in mild idiopathic pancreatitis than in alcoholic pancreatitis. Enzymes are also used to treat steatorrhea. Various preparations are available, and a dose providing at least 30,000 U of lipase should be used. Nonenteric coated tablets should be used, and they should be taken with meals. An H_2 blocker or proton pump inhibitor should be given to prevent acid breakdown of the enzymes.

Favorable clinical responses include weight gain, fewer bowel movements, elimination of oil droplet seepage, and improved well-being. Clinical response can be documented by showing a decrease in stool fat after enzyme therapy. If steatorrhea is particularly severe and refractory to these measures, medium-chain triglycerides can be provided as a source of fat (they are absorbed without pancreatic enzymes), reducing other dietary fats proportionally. Supplementation with fat-soluble vitamins (A, D, K) should be given, including vitamin E, which may minimize inflammation.

Surgery may be effective for pain relief. A pancreatic pseudocyst, which may cause chronic pain, can be decompressed into a nearby structure to which it firmly adheres (eg, the stomach) or into a defunctionalized loop of jejunum (via a Roux-en-Y cystojejunostomy). If the main pancreatic duct is dilated > 5 to 8 mm, a lateral pancreaticojejunostomy (Puestow procedure) relieves pain in about 70 to 80% of patients. If the duct is not dilated, a partial resection is similarly effective; either distal pancreatectomy (for extensive disease at the tail of the pancreas) or Whipple's operation (for extensive disease at the head of the pancreas) is used. Operative approaches should be reserved for patients who have discontinued using alcohol and who can manage diabetes that may be intensified by pancreatic resection.

Some pseudocysts can be drained endoscopically. Endoscopic ultrasound–guided denervation of the celiac plexus with alcohol and bupivacaine may provide pain relief. If there is significant stricture at the papilla or distal pancreatic duct, ERCP with sphincterotomy, stent placement, or dilatation may be effective.

Oral hypoglycemic drugs rarely help treat diabetes caused by chronic pancreatitis. Insulin should be given cautiously because the coexisting deficiency of glucagon secretion by α-cells means that the hypoglycemic effects of insulin are unopposed and prolonged hypoglycemia may occur.

Patients are at increased risk for pancreatic cancer. Worsening of symptoms, especially with development of a pancreatic duct stricture, should prompt an examination for malignancy. This may include brushing of strictures for cytologic analysis or measurement of serum markers (eg, CA 19-9, carcinoembryonic antigen).

16 GASTROENTERITIS

(See also Food Allergy on p. 1358.)

Gastroenteritis is inflammation of the lining of the stomach and small and large intestines. Most cases are infectious, although gastroenteritis may follow ingestion of drugs and chemical toxins (eg, metals, plant substances). Symptoms include anorexia, nausea, vomiting, diarrhea, and abdominal discomfort. Diagnosis is clinical or by stool culture, although immunoassays are increasingly used. Treatment is symptomatic, although parasitic and some bacterial infections require specific anti-infective therapy.

Gastroenteritis is usually uncomfortable but self-limited. Electrolyte and fluid loss is usually little more than an inconvenience to an otherwise healthy adult but can be grave for people who are very young (see p. 2289), elderly, or debilitated or who have serious concomitant illnesses. Worldwide, an estimated 3 to 6 million children die each year from infectious gastroenteritis.

Etiology and Pathophysiology

Infectious gastroenteritis may be caused by viruses, bacteria, or parasites. Many specific organisms are discussed further in § INF (see p. 1386).

Viruses: Viruses are the most common cause of gastroenteritis in the US. They infect enterocytes in the villous epithelium of the small bowel. The result is transudation of fluid and salts into the intestinal lumen; sometimes, malabsorption of carbohydrates worsens symptoms by causing osmotic diarrhea. Diarrhea is watery. Inflammatory diarrhea (dysentery), with fecal WBCs and RBCs or gross blood, is uncommon. Four categories of viruses cause most gastroenteritis: rotavirus, calicivirus (which includes norovirus [formerly Norwalk virus]), astrovirus, and enteric adenovirus.

Rotavirus is the most common cause of sporadic severe, dehydrating diarrhea in young children (peak incidence, 3 to 15 mo). Rotavirus is highly contagious; most infections occur by the fecal-oral route. Adults may be infected after close contact with an infected infant. The illness in adults is generally mild. Incubation is 1 to 3 days. In temperate climates, most infections occur in the winter. Each year in the US, a wave of rotavirus illness begins in the Southwest in November and ends in the Northeast in March.

Caliciviruses most commonly infect older children and adults. Infections occur year-round. Caliciviruses are the principal cause of sporadic viral gastroenteritis in adults and of epidemic viral gastroenteritis in all age groups; large waterborne and food-borne outbreaks occur. Person-to-person transmission also occurs because the virus is highly contagious. Incubation is 24 to 48 h.

Astrovirus can infect people of all ages but usually infects infants and young children. Infection is most common in winter. Transmission is by the fecal-oral route. Incubation is 3 to 4 days.

Adenoviruses are the 4th most common cause of childhood viral gastroenteritis. Infections occur year-round, with a slight increase in summer. Children < 2 yr are primarily affected. Transmission is by the fecal-oral route. Incubation is 3 to 10 days.

In immunocompromised hosts, additional viruses (eg, cytomegalovirus, enterovirus) can cause gastroenteritis.

Bacteria: Bacterial gastroenteritis is less common than viral. Bacteria cause gastroenteritis by several mechanisms. Certain species (eg, *Vibrio cholerae,* enterotoxigenic strains of *Escherichia coli*) adhere to intestinal mucosa without invading and produce enterotoxins. These toxins impair intestinal absorption and cause secretion of electrolytes and water by stimulating adenylate cyclase, resulting in watery diarrhea. *Clostridium difficile* produces a similar toxin when overgrowth follows antibiotic use (see p. 1500).

Some bacteria (eg, *Staphylococcus aureus, Bacillus cereus, Clostridium perfringens*) produce an exotoxin that is ingested in contaminated food. The exotoxin can cause gastroenteritis without bacterial infection. These toxins generally cause acute nausea, vomiting, and diarrhea within 12 h of ingestion of contaminated food. Symptoms abate within 36 h.

Other bacteria (eg, *Shigella, Salmonella, Campylobacter,* some *E. coli* strains) invade the mucosa of the small bowel or colon and produce microscopic ulceration, bleeding, exudation of protein-rich fluid, and secretion of electrolytes and water. The invasive process and its results can occur whether or not the organism produces an enterotoxin. The resulting diarrhea contains WBCs and RBCs and sometimes gross blood.

Salmonella and *Campylobacter* are the most common bacterial causes of diarrheal illness in the US. Both infections are most frequently acquired through undercooked poultry; unpasteurized milk, undercooked eggs, and contact with reptiles are also sources. *Campylobacter* is occasionally transmitted from dogs or cats with diarrhea. Species of *Shigella* are the 3rd most common bacterial cause of diarrhea in the US and are usually transmitted person to person, although food-borne epidemics occur. *Shigella dysenteriae* type 1 (not present in the US) produces Shiga toxin, which can cause hemolytic-uremic syndrome (see p. 1070).

Several different subtypes of *E. coli* cause diarrhea. The epidemiology and clinical manifestations vary greatly depending on the subtype: (1) Enterohemorrhagic *E. coli* is the most clinically significant subtype in the US. It produces Shiga toxin, which causes bloody diarrhea. *E. coli* O157:H7 is the most common strain of this subtype in the US. Undercooked ground beef, unpasteurized milk and juice, and contaminated water are possible sources. Person-to-person transmission is common in the day care setting. Hemolytic-uremic syndrome is a serious complication that develops in 2 to 7% of cases, most commonly in the young and old. (2) Enterotoxigenic *E. coli* produces two toxins (one similar to cholera toxin) that cause watery diarrhea. This subtype is the most common cause of traveler's diarrhea. (3) Enteropathogenic *E. coli* causes watery diarrhea. Once a common cause of diarrhea outbreaks in nurseries, this subtype is now rare. (4) Enteroinvasive *E. coli* causes bloody or nonbloody diarrhea, primarily in the developing world. It is rare in the US.

Several other bacteria cause gastroenteritis, but most are uncommon in the US. *Yersinia enterocolitica* can cause gastroenteritis or a syndrome that mimics appendicitis. It is transmitted by undercooked pork, unpasteurized milk, or contaminated water. Several *Vibrio* species (eg, *V. parahaemolyticus*) cause diarrhea after ingestion of undercooked seafood. *V. cholerae* sometimes causes severe dehydrating diarrhea in the developing world. *Listeria* causes food-borne gastroenteritis. *Aeromonas* is acquired from swimming in or drinking contaminated fresh or brackish water. *Plesiomonas shigelloides* can cause diarrhea in patients who have eaten raw shellfish or traveled to tropical regions of the developing world.

Parasites: Certain intestinal parasites, notably *Giardia lamblia* (see p. 1567), adhere to or invade the intestinal mucosa, causing nausea, vomiting, diarrhea, and general malaise. Giardiasis occurs in every region of the US and throughout the world. The infection can become chronic and cause a malabsorption syndrome. It is usually acquired via person-to-person transmission (often in day care centers) or from contaminated water.

Cryptosporidium parvum causes watery diarrhea sometimes accompanied by abdominal cramps, nausea, and vomiting. In healthy people, the illness is self-limited, lasting about 2 wk. In immunocompromised patients, illness may be severe, causing substantial electrolyte and fluid loss. *Cryptosporidium* is usually acquired through contaminated water.

Other parasites that can produce symptoms similar to those of cryptosporidiosis, especially in immunocompromised hosts, include *Cyclospora cayetanensis, Isospora belli,* and a collection of organisms referred to as microsporidia (eg, *Enterocytozoon bieneusi, Encephalitozoon intestinalis*). *Entamoeba histolytica* (amebiasis) is a common cause of subacute bloody diarrhea in the developing world and occasionally occurs in the US.

Symptoms and Signs

The character and severity of symptoms vary. Generally, onset is sudden, with anorexia, nausea, vomiting, borborygmi, abdominal cramps, and diarrhea (with or without blood and mucus). Malaise, myalgias, and prostration may occur. The abdomen may be distended and mildly tender; in severe cases, muscle guarding may be present. Gas-distended intestinal loops may be palpable. Borborygmi are present even without diarrhea (an important differential feature from paralytic ileus). Persistent vomiting and diarrhea can result in intravascular fluid depletion with hypotension and tachycardia. In severe cases, shock, with vascular collapse and oliguric renal failure, occurs.

If vomiting is the main cause of fluid loss, metabolic alkalosis with hypochloremia can occur. If diarrhea is more prominent, acidosis is more likely. Both vomiting and diarrhea can cause hypokalemia. Hyponatremia may develop, particularly if hypotonic fluids are used in replacement therapy.

In viral infections, watery diarrhea is the most common symptom; stools rarely contain mucus or blood. Rotavirus gastroenteritis in infants and young children may last 5 to 7 days. Vomiting occurs in 90% of patients, and fever > 39° C (> 102.2° F) occurs in about 30%. Calicivirus typically causes acute onset of vomiting, abdominal cramps, and diarrhea, with symptoms lasting only 1 to 2 days. In children, vomiting is more prominent than diarrhea, whereas in adults, diarrhea usually predominates. Patients may also experience fever, headache, and myalgias. The hallmark of adenovirus gastroenteritis is diarrhea lasting 1 to 2 wk. Affected infants and children may have mild vomiting that typically starts 1 to 2 days after the onset of diarrhea. Low-grade fever occurs in about 50% of patients. Astrovirus causes a syndrome similar to mild rotavirus infection.

Bacteria that cause invasive disease (eg, *Shigella, Salmonella*) are more likely to result in fever, prostration, and bloody diarrhea. Bacteria that produce an enterotoxin (eg, *S. aureus, B. cereus, C. perfringens*) usually cause watery diarrhea.

Parasitic infections typically cause subacute or chronic diarrhea. Most cause nonbloody diarrhea; an exception is *E. histolytica,* which causes amebic dysentery. Fatigue and weight loss are common when diarrhea is persistent.

Diagnosis

Other GI disorders that cause similar symptoms (eg, appendicitis, cholecystitis, ulcerative colitis) must be excluded. Findings suggestive of gastroenteritis include copious, watery diarrhea; ingestion of potentially contaminated food (particularly during a known outbreak), untreated surface water, or a known GI irritant; recent travel; or contact with similarly ill people. *E. coli* O157:H7–induced diarrhea is notorious for appearing to be a hemorrhagic rather than an infectious process, presenting as GI bleeding with little or no stool. Hemolytic-uremic syndrome may follow as evidenced by renal failure and hemolytic anemia (see p. 1070). Recent oral antibiotic use (within 3 mo) must raise suspicion for *C. difficile* infection (see p. 1500). Acute abdomen is unlikely without abdominal muscle spasm and localized tenderness.

Stool testing: If a rectal examination shows occult blood or if watery diarrhea persists > 48 h, stool examination (fecal WBCs, ova, parasites) and culture are indicated. However, for the diagnosis of giardiasis or cryptosporidiosis, stool antigen detection using an enzyme immunoassay has a higher sensitivity. Rotavirus and enteric adenovirus infections can be diagnosed using commercially available rapid assays that detect viral antigen in the stool, but these are usually performed only to document an outbreak.

All patients with grossly bloody diarrhea should be tested for *E. coli* O157:H7, as should patients with nonbloody diarrhea during a known outbreak. Specific cultures must be requested because this organism is not detected on standard stool culture media. Alternatively, a rapid enzyme assay for the detection of Shiga toxin in stool can be performed; a positive test indicates infection with *E. coli* O157:H7 or one of the other serotypes of enterohemorrhagic *E. coli.* (NOTE: *Shigella* species in the US do not produce Shiga toxin.)

Adults with grossly bloody diarrhea should usually have sigmoidoscopy with cultures and biopsy. Appearance of the colonic mucosa may help diagnose amebic dysentery, shigellosis, and *E. coli* O157:H7 infection, although ulcerative colitis may produce similar lesions. Patients with recent antibiotic use should have stool assay for *C. difficile* toxin.

General tests: Serum electrolytes, BUN, and creatinine should be obtained to evaluate hydration and acid-base status in patients who appear seriously ill. CBC is nonspecific, although eosinophilia may indicate parasitic infection.

Treatment

Supportive treatment is all that is needed for most patients. Bed rest with convenient access to a toilet or bedpan is desirable. Oral glucose-electrolyte solutions, broth, or bouillon may prevent dehydration or treat mild dehydration. Even if vomiting, the patient should take frequent small sips of such fluids: vomiting may abate with volume replacement. Children may become dehydrated more quickly and should be given an appropriate rehydration solution (several are available commercially—see also p. 2293). Carbonated beverages and sports drinks lack the correct ratio of glucose to Na and thus are not appropriate for children < 5 yr. If the child is breastfed, breastfeeding should continue. If vomiting is protracted or if severe dehydration is prominent, IV replacement of volume and electrolytes is necessary (see p. 564).

When the patient can tolerate fluids without vomiting and the appetite has begun to return, food may be gradually restarted. There is no demonstrated benefit from restriction to bland food (cereal, gelatin, bananas, toast). Some patients have temporary lactose intolerance.

Antidiarrheal agents are safe for patients > 5 yr with watery diarrhea (as demonstrated by heme-negative stool). However, antidiarrheals may cause deterioration of patients with *C. difficile* or *E. coli* O157:H7 infection and thus should not be given to any patient with recent antibiotic use or heme-positive stool, pending specific diagnosis. Effective antidiarrheals include loperamide 4 mg po initially, followed by 2 mg po for each subsequent episode of diarrhea (maximum of 6 doses/day or 16 mg/day); diphenoxylate 2.5 to 5 mg tid or qid in tablet or liquid form; or bismuth subsalicylate 524 mg (two tablets or 30 mL) po 6 to 8 times/day.

If vomiting is severe and a surgical condition has been excluded, an antiemetic may be beneficial. Agents useful in adults include prochlorperazine 5 to 10 mg IV tid or qid, or 25 mg per rectum bid; and promethazine 12.5

to 25 mg IM tid or qid, or 25 to 50 mg per rectum qid. These agents are usually avoided in children because of lack of demonstrated efficacy and the high incidence of dystonic reactions.

Antimicrobials: Empiric antibiotics are generally not recommended except for certain cases of traveler's diarrhea or when suspicion of *Shigella* or *Campylobacter* infection is high (eg, contact with a known case). Otherwise, antibiotics should await results of stool culture, particularly in children, who have a higher rate of *E. coli* O157:H7 infection (antibiotics increase the risk of hemolytic-uremic syndrome in patients infected with *E. coli* O157:H7).

In proven bacterial gastroenteritis, antibiotics are not always required. They do not help with *Salmonella* and prolong the duration of shedding in the stool. Exceptions include immunocompromised hosts, neonates, and patients with *Salmonella* bacteremia. Antibiotics are also ineffective against toxic gastroenteritis (eg, *S. aureus*, *B. cereus*, *C. perfringens*). Indiscriminate use of antibiotics fosters the emergence of drug-resistant organisms. However, certain infections do require antibiotics (see TABLE 16–1).

The use of probiotics, such as lactobacillus, is generally safe and may have some benefit in relieving symptoms. They can be given in the form of yogurt with active cultures.

For cryptosporidiosis, nitazoxanide may be helpful in immunocompetent children. The dose is 100 mg po bid for children 12 to 47 mo and 200 mg po bid for children 4 to 11 yr.

Prevention

Prevention of infection is complicated by the frequency of asymptomatic infection and the ease with which many agents, particularly viruses, are transmitted from person to person. In general, proper procedures for handling and preparing food must be followed. Travelers (see below) must avoid potentially contaminated food and drink.

Breastfeeding affords some protection to newborns and infants. Caregivers should wash their hands thoroughly with soap and water after changing diapers, and diaper-changing areas should be disinfected with a freshly prepared solution of 1:64 household bleach (¼ cup diluted in 1 gallon of water). Children with diarrhea should be excluded from child-care facilities for the duration of symptoms. Children infected with enterohemorrhagic *E. coli* or *Shigella* should also have two negative stool cultures before readmission to the facility.

TRAVELER'S DIARRHEA

(Turista)

Traveler's diarrhea is gastroenteritis that is usually caused by bacteria endemic to local water. Symptoms include vomiting and diarrhea. Diagnosis is mainly clinical. Treatment is with ciprofloxacin, loperamide, and replacement fluids.

Etiology

Traveler's diarrhea may be caused by any of several bacteria, viruses, or parasites. However, enterotoxigenic *E. coli* is most common. *E. coli* is common in the water supplies of areas that lack adequate purification. Infection is common in people traveling to developing countries. Travelers who avoid drinking local water may still become infected by brushing their teeth with an improperly rinsed toothbrush, drinking bottled drinks with ice made from local water, or eating food washed with local water.

Symptoms, Signs, and Diagnosis

Nausea, vomiting, borborygmi, abdominal cramps, and diarrhea begin 12 to 72 h after ingesting contaminated food or water. Severity is variable. Some people develop fever and myalgias. Most cases are mild and self-limited, although dehydration can occur, especially in warm climates. Specific diagnostic measures are usually not necessary. However, fever, severe abdominal pain, and bloody diarrhea suggest more serious disease and should prompt immediate evaluation.

Prevention and Treatment

Travelers should dine at restaurants with a reputation for safety and avoid foods and beverages from street vendors. They should consume only cooked foods that are still steaming hot, fruit that can be peeled, and carbonated beverages without ice served in sealed bottles (bottles of noncarbonated beverages can contain tap water added by unscrupulous vendors); uncooked vegetables should be avoided. Hot buffets and fast food restaurants pose an increased risk.

TABLE 16–1. SELECTED ORAL ANTIBIOTICS FOR INFECTIOUS GASTROENTERITIS*

ORGANISM	ANTIBIOTIC	ADULT DOSAGE	PEDIATRIC DOSAGE
Vibrio cholerae	Ciprofloxacin	1 g once	NA
	Doxycycline†	300 mg single dose	6 mg/kg x 1 dose
	TMP-SMX	1 DS tablet bid for 3 days	4–6 mg‡/kg bid for 5 days
Clostridium difficile	Metronidazole	250 mg qid or 500 mg tid for 10 days	7.5 mg/kg qid for 10 days
	Vancomycin (if fail metronidazole)	125–250 mg qid for 10 days	10 mg/kg qid for 10 days
Shigella	Ciprofloxacin	500 mg po bid for 5 days	NA
	TMP-SMX	1 DS tablet bid	4–6 mg‡/kg bid for 5 days
Giardia lamblia	Metronidazole	250 mg tid for 5 days	5 mg/kg tid for 5 days (maximum 750 mg/day)
Entamoeba histolytica	Metronidazole§	750 mg tid for 5–10 days	12–16 mg/kg tid for 10 days (maximum 750 mg/day)
Campylobacter jejuni	Ciprofloxacin	500 mg bid for 5 days	NA
	Azithromycin	500 mg once/day for 3 days	10 mg/kg once/day for 3 days

*Antibiotics are not indicated in most cases but may be used supportively with IV fluids to treat infections caused by specific organisms.

†Should not be given to children aged < 8 yr.

‡Based on trimethoprim component.

§Treatment should be followed by iodoquinol 10–13 mg/kg tid for 20 days or paromomycin 500 mg po tid for 7 days.

TMP-SMX = trimethoprim-sulfamethoxazole; DS = double-strength; NA = not applicable.

Prophylactic antibiotics are effective in preventing diarrhea, but, because of concerns about adverse effects and development of resistance, they should probably be reserved for immunocompromised patients.

The mainstay of treatment is fluid replacement and an antimotility agent such as diphenoxylate or loperamide (see p. 136), with or without bismuth subsalicylate. Antimotility agents are contraindicated in patients with fever or bloody stools and in children < 2 yr. Iodochlorhydroxyquin, which may be available in some developing countries, should not be used, as it may cause neurologic damage. Generally, antibiotics are not necessary for mild diarrhea. In patients with moderate to severe diarrhea (≥ 3 loose stools over 8 h), antibiotics are given, especially if vomiting, abdominal cramps, fever, or bloody stools are present. Ciprofloxacin 500 mg po bid for 3 days or levofloxacin 500 mg po once/day is recommended. Azithromycin 5 to 10 mg/kg po once/day may be used for children.

DRUG-RELATED GASTROENTERITIS

Many drugs produce nausea, vomiting, and diarrhea as adverse effects. A detailed drug history must be obtained. In mild cases, cessation followed by reuse of the drug may establish a causal relationship. Commonly responsible drugs include antacids containing Mg, antibiotics, antihelminthics, cytotoxics (used in cancer therapy), colchicine, digoxin, heavy metals, laxatives, and radiation therapy. Use of antibiotics may lead to *C. difficile* diarrhea (see p. 1500).

Iatrogenic, accidental, or intentional heavy-metal poisoning frequently produces nausea, vomiting, abdominal pain, and diarrhea.

Laxative abuse, sometimes denied by patients, may lead to weakness, vomiting, diarrhea, electrolyte depletion, and metabolic disturbances.

17 MALABSORPTION SYNDROMES

Malabsorption is inadequate assimilation of dietary substances due to defects in digestion, absorption, or transport. Malabsorption affects macronutrients (eg, proteins, carbohydrates, fats) or micronutrients (eg, vitamins, minerals), causing excessive fecal excretion and producing nutritional deficiencies and GI symptoms.

Pathophysiology

Digestion and absorption occur in three phases: (1) intraluminal hydrolysis of fats, proteins, and carbohydrates by enzymes—bile salts enhance the solubilization of fat in this phase; (2) digestion by brush border enzymes and uptake of end-products; (3) lymphatic transport of nutrients. Malabsorption occurs when any of these phases is impaired.

Fats: Pancreatic enzymes split long-chain triglycerides into fatty acids and monoglycerides, which combine with bile acids and phospholipids to form micelles that pass through jejunal enterocytes. Absorbed fatty acids are resynthesized and combined with protein, cholesterol, and phospholipid to form chylomicrons, which are transported by the lymphatic system. Medium-chain triglycerides can be absorbed directly.

Unabsorbed fats trap fat-soluble vitamins (A, D, E, K) and possibly some minerals, causing deficiency. Bacterial overgrowth results in deconjugation and dehydroxylation of bile salts, limiting their absorption. Unabsorbed bile salts stimulate the colon, causing diarrhea.

Carbohydrates: Enzymes on microvilli lyse carbohydrates and disaccharides into constituent monosaccharides. Colonic bacteria ferment unabsorbed carbohydrates into CO_2, methane, H_2, and short-chain fatty acids (butyrate, propionate, acetate, and lactate). These fatty acids cause diarrhea. The gases cause abdominal distention and bloating.

Proteins: Enterokinase, a brush border enzyme, activates trypsinogen into trypsin, which converts many pancreatic proteases into their active forms. Active pancreatic enzymes hydrolyze proteins into oligopeptides, which are absorbed directly or hydrolyzed into amino acids.

Etiology

Malabsorption has many causes (see TABLE 17–1). Some malabsorptive disorders (eg, celiac sprue) impair the absorption of most nutrients, vitamins, and trace minerals (global malabsorption); others (eg, pernicious anemia) are more selective.

Pancreatic insufficiency causes malabsorption if > 90% of function is lost. Increased luminal acidity (eg, Zollinger-Ellison syndrome) inhibits lipase and fat digestion. Cirrhosis and cholestasis reduce hepatic bile synthesis or delivery of bile salts to the duodenum, causing malabsorption. Other causes are discussed below.

Symptoms and Signs

The effects of unabsorbed substances include diarrhea, steatorrhea, abdominal bloating, and gas. Other symptoms result from nutritional deficiencies. Patients often lose weight despite adequate food intake.

Chronic diarrhea is the most common symptom. Steatorrhea—fatty stool, the hallmark of malabsorption—occurs when > 6 g/day of fat are excreted. Steatorrhea produces foul-smelling, pale, bulky, and greasy stools.

TABLE 17–1. CAUSES OF MALABSORPTION

MECHANISM	CAUSE
Inadequate gastric mixing and/or rapid emptying	Billroth II gastrectomy Gastrocolic fistula Gastroenterostomy
Insufficient digestive agents	Biliary obstruction Chronic liver failure Chronic pancreatitis Cholestyramine-induced bile acid loss Cystic fibrosis Lactase deficiency Pancreatic cancer Pancreatic resection Sucrase-isomaltase deficiency
Improper milieu	Abnormal motility secondary to diabetes, scleroderma, hyperthyroidism Bacterial overgrowth—blind loops (deconjugation of bile salts), diverticula Zollinger-Ellison syndrome (low duodenal pH)
Acutely abnormal epithelium	Acute intestinal infections Alcohol Neomycin
Chronically abnormal epithelium	Amyloidosis Celiac disease Crohn's disease Ischemia Radiation enteritis Tropical sprue Whipple's disease
Short bowel	Jejunoileal bypass for obesity Intestinal resection (eg, for Crohn's disease, volvulus, intussusception, or infarction)
Impaired transport	Abetalipoproteinemia Addison's disease Blocked lacteals—lymphoma, tuberculosis Lymphangiectasia

Severe vitamin and mineral deficiencies occur in advanced malabsorption; symptoms are related to the specific nutrient deficiency (see TABLE 17–2). Vitamin B_{12} deficiency may occur in blind loop syndrome or after extensive resection of the distal ileum or stomach.

Amenorrhea may result from malnutrition and is an important presentation of celiac sprue in young women.

Diagnosis

Malabsorption is suspected in a patient with chronic diarrhea, weight loss, and anemia. The etiology is sometimes obvious. Chronic pancreatitis may be preceded by bouts of acute pancreatitis. Patients with celiac sprue usually have lifelong diarrhea exacerbated by gluten products and may have dermatitis herpetiformis. Cirrhosis and pancreatic cancer usually present with jaundice. Abdominal distention, excessive flatus, and watery diarrhea 30 to 90 min after carbohydrate ingestion suggest deficiency of a disaccharidase enzyme, usually lactase. Previous abdominal operations suggest short bowel syndrome.

If the history suggests a specific cause, testing should be directed to that condition. If no cause is readily apparent, blood tests (eg, CBC, RBC indices, ferritin, Ca, Mg, albumin, cholesterol, PT) may suggest a diagnosis.

Macrocytic anemia should prompt measurement of serum folate and B_{12} levels. Folate deficiency is common in mucosal disorders involving the proximal small bowel (eg, celiac sprue, tropical sprue, Whipple's disease). Low B_{12} levels can occur in pernicious anemia, chronic pancreatitis, bacterial overgrowth, and terminal ileal disease. A combination of low B_{12} and high folate is suggestive of bacterial overgrowth, because intestinal bacteria use vitamin B_{12} and synthesize folate.

Microcytic anemia suggests iron deficiency, which may occur with celiac sprue. Albumin is a general indicator of nutritional state. Low albumin can result from poor intake, decreased synthesis, or protein wasting. Low serum carotene (a precursor of vitamin A) suggests malabsorption if intake is adequate.

Confirming malabsorption: Tests to confirm malabsorption are appropriate when symptoms are vague and etiology is not apparent. Most tests for malabsorption assess fat malabsorption because it is relatively easy to measure. Confirmation of carbohydrate malabsorption is not helpful once steatorrhea is documented. Tests for protein malabsorption are rarely used because fecal nitrogen is difficult to measure.

Direct measurement of fecal fat from a 72-h stool collection is standard for establishing steatorrhea but unnecessary with gross steatorrhea of obvious cause. Stool is collected for a 3-day period during which the patient consumes ≥ 100 g fat/day. Total fat in the stool is measured. Fecal fat > 6 g/day is abnormal. Although severe fat malabsorption (fecal fat ≥ 40 g/day) suggests pancreatic insufficiency or small-bowel mucosal disease, this test cannot determine the specific cause of malabsorption. Because the test is messy, unpleasant, and time consuming, it is unacceptable to most patients and difficult to perform.

Sudan III staining of a stool smear is a simple and direct, but nonquantitative, screening test for fecal fat. Acid steatocrit is a gravimetric assay performed on a single stool sample; it has a reported sensitivity of 100% and specificity of 95% (using 72-h collection as the standard). Near-infrared reflectance analysis simultaneously tests stool for fat, nitrogen, and carbohydrates and may become the preferred test.

The D-xylose absorption test should also be performed if the etiology is not obvious. It is the best noninvasive test to assess intestinal mucosal integrity and differentiate mucosal from pancreatic disease. This test has a reported specificity of 98% and sensitivity of 91% for small-bowel malabsorption.

D-Xylose is absorbed by passive diffusion and does not require pancreatic enzymes for digestion. A normal D-xylose test in the presence of moderate to severe steatorrhea indicates pancreatic exocrine insufficiency rather than small-bowel mucosal disease. Bacterial overgrowth syndrome can produce abnormal results because the enteric bacteria metabolize pentose, thus decreasing the D-xylose available for absorption.

After fasting, the patient is given 25 g of D-xylose in 200 to 300 mL of water po. Urine is collected over 5 h, and a venous sample is obtained after 1 h. Serum D-xylose < 20 mg/dL or < 4 g in the urine sample indicates abnormal absorption. Falsely low levels can also occur in renal diseases, portal hypertension, ascites, or delayed gastric emptying time.

TABLE 17–2. SYMPTOMS OF MALABSORPTION

SYMPTOM	MALABSORBED NUTRIENT
Anemia (hypochromic, microcytic)	Iron
Anemia (macrocytic)	Vitamin B_{12}, folate
Bleeding, bruising, petechiae	Vitamins K and C
Carpopedal spasm	Ca, Mg
Edema	Protein
Glossitis	Vitamins B_2 and B_{12}, folate, niacin, iron
Night blindness	Vitamin A
Pain in limbs, bones, pathologic fractures	K, Mg, Ca, vitamin D
Peripheral neuropathy	Vitamins B_1, B_6, B_{12}

Diagnosing the cause of malabsorption: Endoscopy with small-bowel biopsy is performed when mucosal disease of the small bowel is suspected or if the D-xylose test is abnormal in a patient with massive steatorrhea. Aspirate from the small bowel should be sent for bacterial culture and colony count to document bacterial overgrowth. Histologic features on small-bowel biopsy (see TABLE 17–3) can establish the specific mucosal disease.

Small-bowel x-rays can detect anatomic conditions that predispose to bacterial overgrowth. These include jejunal diverticula, fistulas, surgically created blind loops and anastomoses, ulcerations, and strictures. Abdominal flat plate x-ray may show pancreatic calcifications indicative of chronic pancreatitis. Barium contrast studies of the small bowel (small-bowel follow-through or enteroclysis) are neither sensitive nor specific but may have findings suggestive of mucosal disease (eg, dilated small-bowel loops, thinned or thickened mucosal folds, coarse fragmentation of the barium column).

TABLE 17–3. JEJUNAL HISTOLOGY IN CERTAIN MALABSORPTIVE DISORDERS

DISORDER	HISTOLOGIC CHARACTERISTICS
Normal	Fingerlike villi with a villous: crypt ratio of about 4:1; columnar epithelial cells with numerous regular microvilli (brush border); mild round cell infiltration in the lamina propria
Celiac sprue (untreated)	Virtual absence of villi and elongated crypts; increased intraepithelial lymphocytes and round cells (especially plasma cells) in the lamina propria; cuboidal epithelial cells with scanty, irregular microvilli
Intestinal lymphangiectasia	Dilation and ectasia of the intramucosal lymphatics
Tropical sprue	
Mild	Minimal changes in villous height; moderate epithelial cell damage
Severe	Similar to untreated celiac disease, except that lymphocytes predominate in the lamina propria
Whipple's disease	Lamina propria densely infiltrated with PAS-positive macrophages; villous structure may be obliterated in severe lesions

Tests for pancreatic insufficiency (eg, secretin stimulation test, bentiromide test, pancreolauryl test, serum trypsinogen, fecal elastase, fecal chymotrypsin—see p. 132) are performed if history suggests but is not sensitive for mild pancreatic disease.

The ^{14}C-xylose breath test helps diagnose bacterial overgrowth. ^{14}C-xylose is given orally, and the exhaled $^{14}CO_2$ concentration measured. Catabolism of ingested xylose by the overgrowth flora causes $^{14}CO_2$ to appear in exhaled breath. The hydrogen breath test measures the exhaled hydrogen produced by the bacterial degradation of carbohydrates. In patients with disaccharidase deficiencies, enteric bacteria degrade nonabsorbed carbohydrates in the colon, increasing exhaled hydrogen. The lactose-H_2 breath test is only useful to confirm lactase deficiency (see p. 144) and is not used as an initial diagnostic test in the work-up of malabsorption.

The Schilling test assesses malabsorption of vitamin B_{12}. Its four stages determine whether the deficiency results from pernicious anemia, pancreatic exocrine insufficiency, bacterial overgrowth, or ileal disease. The patient is given 1 µg of radiolabeled cyanocobalamin po concurrent with 1000 µg of nonlabeled cobalamin IM to saturate hepatic binding sites. A 24-h urine collection is analyzed for radioactivity; urinary excretion of < 8% of the oral dose indicates malabsorption of cobalamin (stage 1). If this stage is abnormal, the test is repeated with the addition of intrinsic factor (stage 2). Pernicious anemia is present if this normalizes absorption. Stage 3 is performed after adding pancreatic enzymes; normalization in this stage indicates cobalamin malasorption secondary to pancreatic insufficiency. Stage 4 is performed after antimicrobial therapy with anaerobic coverage; normalization after antibiotics suggests bacterial overgrowth. Cobalamin deficiency secondary to ileal disease or ileal resection results in abnormalities in all stages.

Tests for less common causes of malabsorption include serum gastrin (Zollinger-Ellison syndrome), intrinsic factor and parietal cell antibodies (pernicious anemia), sweat chloride (cystic fibrosis), lipoprotein electrophoresis (abetalipoproteinemia), and plasma cortisol (Addison's disease).

BACTERIAL OVERGROWTH SYNDROME

Small-bowel bacterial overgrowth can occur from alterations in intestinal anatomy or GI motility or lack of gastric acid secretion. This condition can lead to vitamin deficiencies, fat malabsorption, and

malnutrition. Diagnosis is by ^{14}C-xylose breath test. Treatment is with oral antibiotics.

Under normal conditions, the proximal small bowel contains < 10^5 bacteria/mL, mainly gram-positive aerobic bacteria. This low bacterial count is maintained by normal peristalsis, normal gastric acid secretion, mucus, secretory IgA, and an intact ileocecal valve.

Usually, bacterial overgrowth occurs when anatomic alterations promote stasis of intestinal contents. These conditions include small-bowel diverticulosis, surgical blind loops, postgastrectomy states (especially in the afferent loop of a Billroth II), strictures, or partial obstruction. Intestinal motility disorders associated with diabetic neuropathy, systemic sclerosis, amyloidosis, and idiopathic intestinal pseudo-obstruction can also impair bacterial clearance. Achlorhydria and idiopathic changes in intestinal motility may cause bacterial overgrowth in elderly people.

The excess bacteria consume nutrients, including vitamin B_{12} and carbohydrates, leading to caloric deprivation and vitamin B_{12} deficiency. However, because the bacteria produce folate, folate deficiency is rare. The bacteria deconjugate bile salts, causing failure of micelle formation and subsequent fat malabsorption. Severe bacterial overgrowth also damages the intestinal mucosa.

Symptoms, Signs, and Diagnosis

Many patients are asymptomatic and present with only weight loss or nutrient deficiencies. Some have significant diarrhea or steatorrhea.

Some clinicians advocate response to empiric antibiotic therapy as a diagnostic test. However, because bacterial overgrowth can mimic other malabsorptive disorders (eg, Crohn's disease) and side effects of the antibiotics can worsen symptoms, establishing a definitive etiology is preferred.

The standard for diagnosis is quantitative culture of intestinal fluid aspirate showing bacterial count > 10^5/mL. This method, however, requires endoscopy. Breath tests are noninvasive and easy to perform. The ^{14}C-xylose breath test is probably the most sensitive and specific. In addition, an upper GI series with small-bowel follow-through should be performed to identify predisposing anatomical lesions.

Treatment

Treatment is with 10 to 14 days of oral antibiotics. Empiric regimens include tetracycline 250 mg qid, amoxicillin/clavulanic acid 250 to 500 mg tid, cephalexin 250 mg qid, trimethoprim-sulfamethoxazole 160/800 mg bid, and metronidazole 250 to 500 mg tid or qid. Antibiotics should be changed based on culture and sensitivity results. Underlying conditions and nutritional deficiencies (eg, vitamin B_{12}) should be corrected.

CARBOHYDRATE INTOLERANCE

Carbohydrate intolerance is an inability to digest certain carbohydrates due to a lack of one or more intestinal enzymes. Symptoms include diarrhea, abdominal distention, and flatulence. Diagnosis is clinical and by H_2 breath test. Treatment is removal of the causative disaccharide from the diet.

Pathophysiology

Disaccharides are normally split into monosaccharides by disaccharidases (eg, lactase, maltase, isomaltase, sucrase [invertase]) located in the brush border of small-bowel enterocytes. Undigested disaccharides cause an osmotic load that attracts water and electrolytes into the bowel, producing watery diarrhea. Bacterial fermentation of carbohydrates in the colon produces gases (hydrogen, carbon dioxide, and methane), resulting in excessive flatus, bloating and distention, and abdominal pain.

Etiology

Enzyme deficiencies can be congenital, acquired (primary), or secondary. Congenital deficiencies are rare.

Acquired lactase deficiency (primary adult hypolactasia) is the most common form of carbohydrate intolerance. Lactase levels are high in neonates, permitting digestion of milk; in most ethnic groups (80% of blacks and Hispanics, almost 100% of Asians), the levels decrease in the post-weaning period rendering older children and adults unable to digest significant amounts of lactose. However, 80 to 85% of whites of Northwest European descent produce lactase throughout life and are thus able to digest milk and milk products. It is unclear why the normal state of

>75% of the world's population should be labeled a "deficiency."

Secondary lactase deficiency occurs in conditions that damage the small-bowel mucosa (eg, celiac sprue, tropical sprue, acute intestinal infections). In infants, temporary secondary disaccharidase deficiency may complicate enteric infections or abdominal surgery. Recovery from the underlying disease is followed by an increase in activity of the enzyme.

Symptoms and Signs

Symptoms and signs are similar in all disaccharidase deficiencies. A child who cannot tolerate lactose develops diarrhea after ingesting significant amounts of milk and may not gain weight. An affected adult may have watery diarrhea, bloating, excessive flatus, nausea, borborygmi, and abdominal cramps after ingesting lactose. The patient often recognizes this early in life and avoids eating dairy products. Symptoms typically require ingestion of the equivalent of 8 to 12 oz of milk. Diarrhea may be severe enough to purge other nutrients before they can be absorbed. Symptoms may be similar to and can be confused with irritable bowel syndrome (see p. 82).

Diagnosis

Lactose intolerance can usually be diagnosed with a careful history supported by dietary challenge. Patients usually have a history of intolerance to milk and dairy foods. The diagnosis is also suggested if the stool from chronic or intermittent diarrhea is acidic ($pH < 6$) and can be confirmed by a H_2 breath or a lactose tolerance test.

In the H_2 breath test, 50 g of lactose is given orally and the H_2 produced by bacterial metabolism of undigested lactose is measured with a breath meter at 2, 3, and 4 h postingestion. Most affected patients have an increase in expired H_2 of > 20 ppm over baseline. Sensitivity and specificity are > 95%.

The lactose tolerance test is less specific. Oral lactose (1.0 to 1.5 g/kg body weight) is given. Blood glucose is measured before ingestion and 60 and 120 min after. Lactose-intolerant patients develop diarrhea, abdominal bloating, and discomfort within 20 to 30 min, and their blood glucose levels do not rise > 20 mg/dL (< 1.1 mmol/L) above baseline. Low lactase activity in a jejunal biopsy specimen is diagnostic, but endoscopy is needed to obtain a specimen and is not routine.

Treatment

Carbohydrate malabsorption is readily controlled by avoiding dietary sugars that cannot be absorbed (eg, following a lactose-free diet in cases of lactase deficiency). However, because the degree of lactose malabsorption varies greatly, many patients can ingest up to 12 oz (18 g of lactose) of milk daily without symptoms. Yogurt is usually tolerated because it contains an appreciable amount of lactase produced by intrinsic *Lactobacilli*.

For symptomatic patients wishing to drink milk, lactose in milk can be predigested by the addition of a commercially prepared lactase, and pretreated milk is now available. Enzyme supplements should be an adjunct to, not a substitute for, dietary restriction. Lactose-intolerant patients must take Ca supplements (1200 to 1500 mg/day).

CELIAC SPRUE

(Nontropical Sprue; Gluten Enteropathy; Celiac Disease)

Celiac sprue is an immunologically mediated disease in genetically susceptible individuals caused by intolerance to gluten, resulting in mucosal inflammation, which causes malabsorption. Symptoms usually include diarrhea and abdominal discomfort. Diagnosis is by small-bowel biopsies demonstrating characteristic though not specific pathologic changes of villous atrophy that improve with a strict gluten-free diet.

Etiology and Epidemiology

Celiac sprue is a hereditary disorder caused by sensitivity to the gliadin fraction of gluten, a protein found in wheat; similar proteins occur in rye and barley. In a genetically susceptible individual, gluten-sensitive T cells are activated when gluten-derived peptide epitopes are presented. The inflammatory response produces characteristic mucosal villous atrophy in the small bowel.

Prevalence varies from about 1/150 in southwest Ireland to 1/5000 in North America. The disease affects about 10 to 20% of first-degree relatives. Female-to-male ratio is 2:1. Onset is generally in childhood but may occur later.

Symptoms and Signs

No typical presentation exists. Some patients are asymptomatic or only have signs of nutritional deficiency. Others have significant GI symptoms.

Celiac sprue can present in infancy and childhood after introduction of cereals into the diet. The child has failure to thrive, apathy, anorexia, pallor, generalized hypotonia, abdominal distention, and muscle wasting. Stools are soft, bulky, clay-colored, and offensive. Older children may present with anemia or failure to grow normally.

In adults, lassitude, weakness, and anorexia are most common. Mild and intermittent diarrhea is sometimes the presenting symptom. Steatorrhea ranges from mild to severe (7 to 50 g fat/day). Some patients have weight loss, rarely enough to become underweight. Anemia, glossitis, angular stomatitis, and aphthous ulcers are usually seen in these patients. Manifestations of vitamin D and Ca deficiencies (eg, osteomalacia, osteopenia, osteoporosis) are common. Both men and women may have reduced fertility.

About 10% have dermatitis herpetiformis, an intensely pruritic papulovesicular rash that is symmetrically distributed over the extensor areas of the elbows, knees, buttocks, shoulders, and scalp. This rash can be induced by a high-gluten diet. Celiac sprue is also associated with diabetes mellitus, autoimmune thyroid disease, and Down syndrome.

Diagnosis

The diagnosis is suspected clinically and by laboratory abnormalities suggestive of malabsorption. Family incidence is a valuable clue. Celiac sprue should be strongly considered in a patient with iron deficiency without obvious GI bleeding.

Confirmation requires a small-bowel biopsy from the second portion of the duodenum. Findings include lack or shortening of villi (villous atrophy), increased intraepithelial cells, and crypt hyperplasia. However, such findings can also occur in tropical sprue, severe intestinal bacterial overgrowth, eosinophilic enteritis, lactose intolerance, and lymphoma.

Because biopsy lacks specificity, serologic markers can aid diagnosis. Anti-gliadin antibody (AGA) and anti-endomysial antibody (EMA, an antibody against an intestinal connective tissue protein) in combination have a positive and negative predictive value of nearly 100%. These markers can also be used to screen populations with high prevalence of celiac sprue, including 1st-degree relatives of affected patients and patients with diseases that occur at a greater frequency in association with celiac sprue. If either test is positive, the patient should have a diagnostic small-bowel biopsy. If both are negative, celiac sprue is extremely unlikely. These antibodies decrease in titer in patients on a gluten-free diet and are thus useful in monitoring dietary compliance.

Other laboratory abnormalities often occur and should be sought. These include anemia (iron-deficiency anemia in children and folate-deficiency anemia in adults); low albumin, Ca, K, and Na; and elevated alkaline phosphatase and PT.

Malabsorption tests are not specific for celiac sprue. If performed, common findings include steatorrhea of 10 to 40 g/day and abnormal D-xylose and (in severe ileal disease) Schilling tests.

Treatment

Treatment is gluten-free diet (avoiding foods containing wheat, rye, or barley). Gluten is so widely used (eg, in commercial soups, sauces, ice creams, hot dogs) that a patient needs a detailed list of foods to avoid. Patients are encouraged to consult a dietitian and join a celiac support group. The response to a gluten-free diet is usually rapid, and symptoms resolve in 1 to 2 wk. Ingesting even small amounts of food containing gluten may prevent remission or induce relapse.

Small-bowel biopsy should be repeated after 3 to 4 mo of a gluten-free diet. If abnormalities persist, other causes of villous atrophy (eg, lymphoma) should be considered. Improvement of symptoms and small-bowel morphology is accompanied by a decrease in AGA and EMA titers.

Supplementary vitamins, minerals, and hematinics may be given, depending on the deficiencies. Mild cases may not require supplementation, whereas severe cases may require comprehensive replacement. For adults, this includes ferrous sulfate 300 mg po once/day to tid, folate 5 to 10 mg po once/day, Ca supplements, and any standard multivitamin. Sometimes children (but rarely adults) who are seriously ill on initial diagnosis require bowel rest and TPN.

If a patient responds poorly to gluten withdrawal, either the diagnosis is incorrect or the disease has become refractory. Corticosteroids can control symptoms in the latter case.

Prognosis

Mortality is 10 to 30% without a gluten-free diet. With proper diet, mortality is < 1%, mainly in adults who had severe disease at the outset. Complications include refractory sprue, collagenous sprue, and the development of intestinal lymphomas. Intestinal lymphomas affect 6 to 8% of patients with celiac sprue, usually presenting in the patient's 50s. The incidence of other GI malignancies (eg, carcinoma of the esophagus or oropharynx, small-bowel adenocarcinoma) increases. Adherence to a gluten-free diet can significantly reduce the risk of malignancy.

INFECTION AND INFESTATION

Acute bacterial, viral, and parasitic infections may cause transient malabsorption, probably as a result of temporary, superficial damage to the villi and microvilli. Chronic bacterial infections of the small bowel are uncommon, apart from blind loops, systemic sclerosis, and diverticula. Intestinal bacteria may use up dietary vitamin B_{12} and other nutrients, perhaps interfere with enzyme systems, and cause mucosal injury.

INTESTINAL LYMPHANGIECTASIA

(Idiopathic Hypoproteinemia)

Intestinal lymphangiectasia is obstruction or malformation of the intramucosal lymphatics of the small bowel. It primarily affects children and young adults. Symptoms include those of malabsorption, with edema and growth retardation. Diagnosis is by small-bowel biopsy. Treatment is usually supportive.

Malformation of the lymphatic system is congenital or acquired. Congenital cases usually present in children and young adults (mean age of onset: 11 yr). Males and females are equally affected. In acquired cases, the defect may be secondary to retroperitoneal fibrosis, constrictive pericarditis, pancreatitis, neoplastic tumors, and infiltrative disorders that block the lymphatics.

Impaired lymphatic drainage leads to increased pressure and leakage of lymph into the intestinal lumen. Impairment of chylomicron and lipoprotein absorption results in malabsorption of fats and protein. Because carbohydrates are not absorbed through the lymphatic system, their uptake is not impaired.

Symptoms, Signs, and Diagnosis

Early manifestations include massive, often asymmetric, peripheral edema, intermittent diarrhea, nausea, vomiting, and abdominal pain. Some patients have mild to moderate steatorrhea. Chylous pleural effusions (chylothorax) and chylous ascites may be present. Growth is retarded if onset is in the 1st decade of life.

Diagnosis usually requires endoscopic small-bowel biopsy, which demonstrates marked dilation and ectasia of the mucosal and submucosal lymphatic vessels. Alternatively, contrast lymphangiography (injection of contrast material via the pedal vein) can demonstrate the abnormal intestinal lymphatics.

Laboratory abnormalities include lymphocytopenia and low levels of serum albumin, cholesterol, IgA, IgM, IgG, transferrin, and ceruloplasmin. Barium studies may demonstrate thickened, nodular mucosal folds that resemble stacked coins. D-Xylose absorption is normal. Intestinal protein loss can be demonstrated using chromium 51-labeled albumin.

Treatment

Abnormal lymphatics cannot be corrected. Supportive treatment includes a low-fat (< 30 g/day), high-protein diet containing medium-chain triglyceride supplements. Supplemental Ca and fat-soluble vitamins are given. Intestinal resection or anastomosis of the abnormal lymphatics to the venous channels may be beneficial. Pleural effusions should be drained by thoracentesis.

SHORT BOWEL SYNDROME

Short bowel syndrome is malabsorption resulting from extensive resection of the small bowel. Symptoms depend on the length and function of the remaining small bowel, but diarrhea can be severe and nutritional deficiencies are common. Treatment is with small feedings, antidiarrheals, and sometimes TPN or intestinal transplantation.

Common reasons for extensive resection are Crohn's disease, mesenteric infarction, radiation enteritis, malignancy, volvulus, and congenital anomalies.

Because the jejunum is the primary digestive and absorptive site for most nutrients, jejunal resection significantly reduces nutrient absorption. In response, the ileum adapts by increasing the length and absorptive function of its villi, resulting in gradual improvement of nutrient absorption.

The ileum is the site of vitamin B_{12} and bile acid absorption. Severe diarrhea and malabsorption result when > 100 cm of the ileum is resected. Notably, there is no compensatory adaptation of the remaining jejunum. Consequently, malabsorption of fat, fat-soluble vitamins, and vitamin B_{12} occurs. In addition, unabsorbed bile acids in the colon result in secretory diarrhea. Preservation of the colon can significantly reduce water and electrolyte losses. Resection of the terminal ileum and ileocecal valve can predispose to bacterial overgrowth.

Treatment

In the immediate postoperative period, diarrhea is typically severe, with significant electrolyte losses. Patients typically require TPN and intensive monitoring of fluid and electrolytes (including Ca and Mg). An oral iso-osmotic solution of Na and glucose (similar to WHO oral rehydration formula—see p. 2293) is slowly introduced in the postoperative phase once the patient stabilizes and stool output is < 2 L/day.

Patients with extensive resection (< 100 cm of remaining jejunum) and those with excessive fluid and electrolyte losses require TPN for life.

Patients with > 100 cm of jejunum left can achieve adequate nutrition through oral feeding. Fat and protein in the diet are usually well tolerated, unlike carbohydrates, which contribute a significant osmotic load. Small feedings reduce the osmotic load. Ideally, 40% of calories should consist of fat.

Patients who have diarrhea after meals should take antidiarrheals (eg, loperamide) 1 h before eating. Cholestyramine 2 to 4 g taken with meals reduces diarrhea associated with bile acid malabsorption. Monthly IM injections of vitamin B_{12} should be given to patients with a documented deficiency. Most patients should take supplemental vitamins, Ca, and Mg.

Gastric acid hypersecretion can develop, which can deactivate pancreatic enzymes; thus, most patients are given H_2 blockers or proton pump inhibitors.

Small-bowel transplantation is advocated for patients who are not candidates for long-term TPN and in whom adaptation does not occur.

TROPICAL SPRUE

Tropical sprue is an acquired disease, probably of infectious etiology, characterized by malabsorption and megaloblastic anemia. Diagnosis is clinical and by small-bowel biopsy. Treatment is with tetracycline and folate for 6 mo.

Etiology

Tropical sprue occurs chiefly in the Caribbean, southern India, and Southeast Asia, affecting both natives and visitors. The illness is rare in visitors spending < 1 mo in areas where the disease is endemic. Although etiology is unclear, it is thought to result from chronic infection of the small bowel by toxigenic strains of coliform bacteria. Malabsorption of folate and vitamin B_{12} deficiency result in megaloblastic anemia. The incidence of tropical sprue is decreasing, perhaps because of increasing use of antibiotics for acute traveler's diarrhea.

Symptoms and Signs

Patients commonly have acute diarrhea with fever and malaise. A chronic phase of milder diarrhea, nausea, anorexia, abdominal cramps, and fatigue follows. Steatorrhea is common. Nutritional deficiencies, especially of folate and vitamin B_{12}, eventually develop after several months to years. The patient may also have weight loss, glossitis, stomatitis, and peripheral edema.

Diagnosis

Tropical sprue is suspected in people who live in or have visited areas where the disease is endemic and who have megaloblastic anemia and symptoms of malabsorption. The definitive test is upper GI endoscopy with small-bowel biopsy. Characteristic histologic changes (see TABLE 17–3) usually involve the entire small bowel and include blunting of the villi with infiltration of chronic inflammatory cells in the epithelium and lamina propria. Celiac disease and parasitic infection must be ruled out.

Additional laboratory studies (eg, CBC; albumin; Ca; PT; iron, folate, and B_{12} levels) help evaluate nutritional status. Barium small-bowel follow-through may show segmentation of the barium, dilation of the lumen, and thickening of the mucosal folds. D-Xylose absorption is abnormal in >90% of cases. However, these tests are not specific or essential for diagnosis.

Treatment

Treatment is tetracycline 250 mg po qid for 1 or 2 mo, then bid for up to 6 mo, depending on disease severity and response to treatment. Folate 5 to 10 mg po once/day should be given for the first month along with vitamin B_{12} 1 mg IM weekly for several weeks. Megaloblastic anemia promptly improves, and the clinical response is dramatic. Other nutritional replacements are given as needed. Relapse may occur in 20%. Failure to respond after 4 wk of therapy suggests another condition.

WHIPPLE'S DISEASE

(Intestinal Lipodystrophy)

Whipple's disease is a rare systemic illness caused by the bacterium *Tropheryma whippelii*. Main symptoms are arthritis, weight loss, and diarrhea. Diagnosis is by small-bowel biopsy. Treatment is with a minimum 1 yr of trimethoprim-sulfamethoxazole.

Whipple's disease predominately affects white men aged 30 to 60. Although it affects many parts of the body (eg, heart, lung, brain, serous cavities, joints, eye, GI tract), the mucosa of the small bowel is almost always involved. Affected patients may have subtle defects of cell-mediated immunity that predispose to infection with *T. whippelii*. About 30% of patients have HLA-B27.

Symptoms and Signs

Clinical presentation varies depending on the organ systems affected. Usually, the first symptoms are arthritis and fever. Intestinal symptoms (eg, watery diarrhea, steatorrhea, abdominal pain, anorexia, weight loss) usually manifest later, sometimes years after the initial complaint. Gross or occult intestinal bleeding may occur. Severe malabsorption may be present in patients diagnosed late in the clinical course. Other findings include increased skin pigmentation, anemia, lymphadenopathy, chronic cough, serositis, peripheral edema, and CNS symptoms.

Diagnosis

The diagnosis may be missed in patients without prominent GI symptoms. Whipple's disease should be suspected in middle-aged white men who have arthritis and abdominal pain, diarrhea, weight loss, or other symptoms of malabsorption. Such patients should have upper endoscopy with small-bowel biopsy; the intestinal lesions are specific and diagnostic. The most severe and consistent changes are in the proximal small bowel. Light microscopy shows PAS-positive macrophages that distort the villus architecture. Gram-positive, acid fast–negative bacilli (*T. whippelii*) are seen in the lamina propria and in the macrophages. Confirmation by electron microscopy is recommended.

Whipple's disease should be differentiated from intestinal infection with *Mycobacterium avium-intracellulare* (MAI), which has similar histologic findings. However, MAI stains positive with acid fast. Polymerase chain reaction testing may be useful for confirmation.

Treatment

Untreated disease is progressive and fatal. Many antibiotics are curative (eg, tetracycline, trimethoprim-sulfamethoxazole, chloramphenicol, ampicillin, penicillin, cephalosporins). One recommended regimen is ceftriaxone (2 g IV daily) or procaine (1.2 million units IM once/day) or penicillin G (1.5 to 6 million units IV q 6 h) plus streptomycin (1.0 g IM once/day for 10 to 14 days) followed by trimethoprim-sulfamethoxazole (160/800 mg po bid for 1 yr). Sulfa-allergic patients may substitute oral penicillin VK or ampicillin. Prompt clinical improvement occurs, with fever and joint pains resolving in a few days. Intestinal symptoms usually improve within 1 to 4 wk.

Some authorities do not recommend repeat small-bowel biopsies because macrophages may persist for years after treatment. However, others recommend repeat biopsy after 1 yr. In the latter approach, electron microscopy is needed to document bacilli (not just macrophages). Relapses are common and may occur years later. If relapse is suspected, small-bowel biopsies should be obtained (regardless of affected organ systems) to determine presence of free bacilli.

18 INFLAMMATORY BOWEL DISEASE

Inflammatory bowel disease (IBD), which includes Crohn's disease and ulcerative colitis (UC), is a relapsing and remitting condition characterized by chronic inflammation at various sites in the GI tract that results in diarrhea and abdominal pain.

Inflammation results from a cell-mediated immune response in the GI mucosa. The precise etiology is unknown; evidence suggests that the normal intestinal flora trigger an immune reaction in patients with a multifactorial genetic predisposition (perhaps involving abnormal epithelial barriers and mucosal immune defenses). No specific environmental, dietary, or infectious causes have been identified. The immune reaction involves the release of inflammatory mediators, including cytokines, interleukins, and tumor necrosis factor (TNF).

Although Crohn's disease and UC are similar, they can be distinguished in most cases (see TABLE 18–1). About 10% of colitis cases are considered indeterminate. The term colitis applies only to inflammatory disease of the colon (eg, ulcerative, granulomatous, ischemic, radiation, infectious). Spastic (mucous) colitis is a misnomer sometimes applied to a functional disorder, irritable bowel syndrome (see p. 82).

Epidemiology

IBD affects people of all ages but usually begins before age 30, with peak incidence from 14 to 24. UC may have a second smaller peak between ages 50 and 70; however, this later peak may include some cases of ischemic colitis.

IBD is most common in people of Northern European and Anglo-Saxon origin and is several times more common in Jews. The incidence is lower in central and southern Europe and lower still in South America, Asia, and Africa. However, the incidence is increasing in blacks and Latin Americans living in North America. Both sexes are equally affected. First-degree relatives of patients with IBD have a 4- to 20-fold increased risk; their absolute risk may be as high as 7%. Familial tendency is much higher in Crohn's disease than UC. A specific gene mutation conferring a high risk of Crohn's disease (but not UC) has been identified.

Cigarette smoking seems to contribute to development or exacerbation of Crohn's disease but decreases risk of UC. NSAIDs may exacerbate IBD.

Extraintestinal Manifestations

Crohn's disease and UC both affect organs other than the intestines. Most extraintestinal manifestations are more common in UC and Crohn's colitis than in Crohn's disease limited to the small bowel. Extraintestinal manifestations are categorized in three ways:

1. Disorders that usually parallel (ie, wax and wane with) IBD flare-ups. These include peripheral arthritis, episcleritis, aphthous stomatitis, erythema nodosum, and pyoderma gangrenosum. Arthritis tends to involve large joints and be migratory and transient. One or more of these parallel disorders develops in > 1/3 of patients hospitalized with IBD.

2. Disorders that probably result from IBD but appear independently of IBD flare-ups. These include ankylosing spondylitis, sacroiliitis, uveitis, and primary sclerosing cholangitis. Ankylosing spondylitis occurs more commonly in IBD patients with the HLA-B27 antigen. Most patients with spinal or sacroiliac involvement have evidence of uveitis and vice versa. Primary sclerosing cholangitis is a risk factor for cancer of the biliary tract, which may appear even 20 yr after colectomy. Liver disease (eg, fatty liver, autoimmune hepatitis, pericholangitis, cirrhosis) occurs in 3 to 5% of patients, although minor abnormalities in liver function tests are more common. Some of these conditions (eg, primary sclerosing cholangitis) may precede IBD by many years and, when diagnosed, should prompt an evaluation for IBD.

3. Disorders that are consequences of disrupted bowel physiology. These occur mainly in severe Crohn's disease of the small bowel. Malabsorption may result from extensive ileal resection and produce vitamin B_{12} and mineral deficiencies, leading to anemia, hypocalcemia, hypomagnesemia, clotting disorders, bone demineralization, and, in children, retarded growth and development. Other disorders include kidney stones from excessive dietary oxalate absorption, hydroureter and hydronephrosis from ureteral compression by the intestinal inflam-

TABLE 18–1. DIFFERENTIATING CROHN'S DISEASE AND ULCERATIVE COLITIS

CROHN'S DISEASE	ULCERATIVE COLITIS
Small bowel is involved in 80% of cases.	Disease is confined to the colon.
Rectosigmoid is often spared; colonic involvement is usually right-sided.	Rectosigmoid is invariably involved; colonic involvement is usually left-sided.
Gross rectal bleeding is rare, except in 75 to 85% of cases of Crohn's colitis.	Gross rectal bleeding is always present.
Fistula, mass, and abscess development are common.	Fistulas do not occur.
Perianal lesions are significant in 25 to 35% of cases.	Significant perianal lesions never occur.
On x-ray, bowel wall is affected asymmetrically and segmentally, with "skip areas" between diseased segments.	Bowel wall is affected symmetrically and uninterruptedly from rectum proximally.
Endoscopic appearance is patchy, with discrete ulcerations separated by segments of normal-appearing mucosa.	Inflammation is uniform and diffuse.
Microscopic inflammation and fissuring extend transmurally; lesions are often highly focal in distribution.	Inflammation is confined to mucosa except in severe cases.
Epithelioid (sarcoid-like) granulomas are detected in bowel wall or lymph nodes in 25 to 50% of cases (pathognomonic).	Typical epithelioid granulomas do not occur.

matory process, gallstones from impaired ileal reabsorption of bile salts, and amyloidosis secondary to long-standing inflammatory and suppurative disease.

Thromboembolic disease may occur as a result of multiple factors in all three categories.

Treatment

Several classes of drugs are helpful for IBD. Details of their selection and use are discussed under each disorder.

5-Aminosalicylic acid (5-ASA, mesalamine): 5-ASA blocks production of prostaglandins and leukotrienes and has other beneficial effects on the inflammatory cascade. Because 5-ASA is active only intraluminally and is rapidly absorbed by the proximal small bowel, it must be formulated for delayed absorption when given orally. Sulfasalazine, the original agent in this class, delays absorption by complexing 5-ASA with a sulfa moiety, sulfapyridine. The complex is cleaved by bacterial flora in the lower ileum and colon, releasing the 5-ASA. The sulfa moiety, however, causes numerous adverse effects (eg, nausea, dyspepsia, headache), interferes with folic acid absorption, and occasionally causes serious adverse reactions (eg, hemolytic anemia or agranulocytosis, and, rarely, hepatitis or pneumonitis). Reversible decreases in sperm count and motility occur in up to 80% of men. If used, sulfasalazine should be given with food, initially in a low dosage (eg, 0.5 g po bid) and gradually increased over several days to 1 to 2 g bid to tid. Patients should take daily folate supplements 1 mg po and have CBC and liver tests every 6 to 12 mo.

Newer drugs that complex 5-ASA with other vehicles appear almost equally effective but have fewer adverse effects. Olsalazine (a 5-ASA dimer) and balsalazide (5-ASA conjugated to an inactive compound) are cleaved by bacterial azoreductases (as is sulfasalazine). These drugs are activated mainly in the colon and are less effective for proximal small-bowel disease. Olsalazine dosage is 500 to 1500 mg bid, and balsalazide is 2.25 g tid. Olsalazine sometimes causes diarrhea, especially in patients with pancolitis. This problem is minimized by gradual escalation of dose and administration with meals.

Other forms of 5-ASA use delayed-release coatings. Asacol (typical dose 800 to 1200 mg tid) is 5-ASA coated with an acrylic polymer whose pH solubility delays release of the drug until entry into the distal ileum and colon. Pentasa (1 g qid) is 5-ASA encapsulated in ethylcellulose microgranules that release 35% of the drug in the small bowel. Acute interstitial nephritis secondary to mesalamine occurs rarely; periodic monitoring of renal function is advisable since most cases are reversible if recognized early.

5-ASA is also available as a suppository (500 mg bid or tid) or enema (4 g at bedtime or bid) for proctitis and left-sided colon disease. These rectal preparations are effective for acute treatment and long-term maintenance and may have incremental benefit in combination with oral 5-ASA.

Corticosteroids: Corticosteroids are useful for acute flares of most forms of IBD when 5-ASA compounds are inadequate but are not appropriate for maintenance. IV hydrocortisone 300 mg/day or methylprednisolone 60 to 80 mg/day by continuous drip or in divided doses is used for severe disease; oral prednisone or prednisolone 40 to 60 mg once/day may be used for moderate disease. Treatment is continued until symptoms remit (usually 7 to 28 days) and tapered by 5 to 10 mg weekly to 20 mg once/day, and then further tapered by 2.5 to 5 mg weekly while instituting maintenance therapy with 5-ASA or immunomodulators. Adverse effects of short-term corticosteroids in high doses include hyperglycemia, hypertension, insomnia, hyperactivity, and acute psychotic episodes.

Hydrocortisone enemas or foam may be used for proctitis and left-sided colon disease; as an enema, 100 mg in 60 mL of isotonic solution is given once/day or bid. It should be retained in the bowel as long as possible; instillation at night, with the patient lying on the left side with hips elevated, may prolong retention and extend distribution. Treatment, if effective, should be continued daily for about 2 to 4 wk, then every other day for 1 to 2 wk, then discontinued gradually over 1 to 2 wk.

Budesonide is a corticosteroid with a high (>90%) first-pass liver metabolism; thus oral administration may have significant effect on GI tract disease but minimal adrenal suppression. Oral budesonide has fewer adverse effects than prednisolone but is not as rapidly effective and is typically used for less severe disease. Dosage is 9 mg once/day. It is also available outside the US as an enema. Like other corticosteroids, budesonide is not effective for long-term maintenance.

Immunomodulating drugs: Azathioprine and its metabolite 6-mercaptopurine inhibit T-cell function. They are effective long-term and may diminish corticosteroid requirements and maintain remission for years. These drugs often require 1 to 3 mo to produce clinical benefits, so corticosteroids cannot be withdrawn until at least the 2nd month. Dosage of azathioprine is usually 2.5 to 3.0 mg/kg po once/day and 6-mercaptopurine 1.5 to 2.5 mg/kg po once/day, but dosage varies depending on individual metabolism. Signs of bone marrow suppression must be monitored with regular WBC count (biweekly for 1 mo, then q 1 to 2 mo). Pancreatitis or high fever occurs in about 3 to 5% of patients; either is an absolute contraindication to rechallenge. Hepatotoxicity is rarer and can be screened by blood tests every 6 to 12 mo.

Methotrexate 15 to 25 mg po, IM, or sc weekly benefits some patients with severe corticosteroid-refractory disease, even those who failed to respond to azathioprine or 6-mercaptopurine. Nausea, vomiting, and asymptomatic liver function test abnormalities are common. Folate 1 mg po once/day may diminish some of the adverse effects. Alcohol use, obesity, and diabetes are risk factors for hepatotoxicity. Patients with these conditions should have a liver biopsy after a total dose of 1.5 g.

Cyclosporine, which blocks lymphocyte activation, may benefit patients with severe UC unresponsive to corticosteroids who may otherwise require colectomy. Its only well-documented use in Crohn's disease is for patients with refractory fistulas or pyoderma. Initial dose is 4 mg/kg IV once/day; responders are converted to an oral dose of 6 to 8 mg/kg once/day and are soon shifted to azathioprine or 6-mercaptopurine. Long-term use (> 6 mo) is contraindicated by multiple adverse effects (eg, renal toxicity, seizures, opportunistic infections). Generally, patients are not offered cyclosporine unless there is a reason to avoid the safer curative option of colectomy. If the drug is used, trough blood levels should be kept between 200 to 400 ng/mL and *Pneumocystis jiroveci* (formerly called *P. carinii*) prophylaxis considered. Tacrolimus, an immunosuppressant used in transplant patients, appears as effective as cyclosporine.

Anticytokine drugs: Infliximab, CDP571, CDP870, and adalimumab are antibodies against TNF. Natalizumab is an antibody against a leukocyte adhesion molecule. These agents may be useful in Crohn's disease but are of unknown benefit in UC.

Infliximab is given as a single IV infusion of 5 mg/kg over 2 h. Some clinicians begin 6-mercaptopurine concomitantly, using infliximab as a bridge until the slower-acting drug begins working. Corticosteroid tapering may begin after 2 wk. If needed, infliximab may be repeated every 8 wk. Adverse effects include delayed hypersensitivity reactions, headache, and nausea. Several patients have died of sepsis following infliximab use, so it is contraindicated when uncontrolled bacterial infection is present. Furthermore, TB reactivation has been attributed to this drug; therefore, screening by PPD and chest x-ray is required before its use.

Thalidomide decreases production of TNF-α and interleukin-12 and has some anti-angiogenesis action. It may benefit some patients with Crohn's disease, but teratogenicity and other adverse effects (eg, rash, hypertension, neurotoxicity) limit its use to research studies. Other anticytokine, anti-integrin, and growth factors are under investigation.

Antibiotics and probiotics: Antibiotics are helpful in Crohn's disease but of limited use in UC. Metronidazole 500 to 750 mg po tid for 4 to 8 wk may control mild disease and help heal fistulas. However, adverse effects (particularly neurotoxicity) may preclude completion of treatment. Ciprofloxacin 500 to 750 mg po bid may prove less toxic. Some experts recommend metronidazole and ciprofloxacin in combination.

Various nonpathogenic microorganisms (eg, commensal *Escherichia coli, Lactobacillus species, Saccharomyces*) administered daily serve as probiotics and may be effective in preventing pouchitis (see p. 158), but other therapeutic roles have yet to be clearly defined.

Supportive care: Most patients and their families are interested in diet and stress management. Although there are anecdotal reports of clinical improvement on certain diets, including one with rigid carbohydrate restrictions, controlled trials have shown no benefit. Stress management may be helpful.

CROHN'S DISEASE

(Regional Enteritis; Granulomatous Ileitis or Ileocolitis)

Crohn's disease is a chronic transmural inflammatory disease that usually affects the distal ileum and colon but may occur in any part of the GI tract. Symptoms include diarrhea and abdominal pain. Abscesses, internal and external fistulas, and bowel obstruction may arise. Extraintestinal symptoms, particularly arthritis, may occur. Diagnosis is by colonoscopy and barium contrast studies. Treatment is with 5-ASA, corticosteroids, immunomodulators, anticytokines, antibiotics, and often surgery.

Pathophysiology

Disease begins with crypt inflammation and abscesses, which progress to tiny focal aphthoid ulcers. These mucosal lesions may develop into deep longitudinal and transverse ulcers with intervening mucosal edema, creating a characteristic cobblestoned appearance to the bowel.

Transmural spread of inflammation leads to lymphedema and thickening of the bowel wall and mesentery. Mesenteric fat typically extends onto the serosal surface of the bowel. Mesenteric lymph nodes often enlarge. Extensive inflammation may result in muscle hypertrophy, fibrosis, and stricture formation, which can cause bowel obstruction. Abscesses are common, and fistulas often penetrate into adjoining structures, including other loops of bowel, the bladder, or psoas muscle; fistulas may even extend to the skin of the anterior abdomen or flanks. Independently of intra-abdominal disease activity, perianal fistulas and abscesses occur in ¼ to ⅓ of cases; these complications are frequently the most troublesome aspects of Crohn's disease.

Noncaseating granulomas can occur in lymph nodes, peritoneum, the liver, and all layers of the bowel wall. Although pathognomonic when present, granulomas are not found in up to 50% of patients with Crohn's disease. Their presence does not appear to be related to the clinical course.

Segments of diseased bowel are sharply demarcated from adjacent normal bowel ("skip areas"); hence, the name regional enteritis. About 35% of Crohn's disease cases involve the ileum alone (ileitis); about 45% involve the ileum and colon (ileocolitis), with a predilection for the right side of the colon; and about 20% involve the colon alone (granulomatous colitis), most of which, unlike ulcerative colitis (UC), spare the rectum. Occasionally, the entire small bowel is involved (jejunoileitis). Rarely, the stomach, duodenum, or esophagus is involved. In the absence of surgical intervention, the disease does not usually extend into areas of small bowel that are not involved at first diagnosis.

There is an increased risk of cancer in affected small-bowel segments. Patients with colonic involvement have a long-term risk of colorectal cancer equal to that of UC, given the same extent and duration of disease.

Symptoms and Signs

The most common initial presentation is chronic diarrhea with abdominal pain, fever, anorexia, and weight loss. The abdomen is tender, and a mass or fullness may be palpable. Gross rectal bleeding is unusual except in isolated colonic disease, which may present similar to UC. Some patients present with an acute abdomen that simulates acute appendicitis or intestinal obstruction. About ⅓ of patients have perianal disease (especially fissures and fistulas), which is sometimes the most prominent or even initial complaint. In children, extraintestinal manifestations frequently predominate over GI symptoms; arthritis, FUO, anemia, or growth retardation may be a presenting symptom, and abdominal pain or diarrhea may be absent.

With recurrent disease, symptoms vary. Pain is most common and occurs with both simple recurrence and abscess formation. Patients with severe flare-up or abscess are likely to have marked tenderness, guarding, rebound, and a general toxic appearance. Stenotic segments may cause bowel obstruction, with colicky pain, distention, obstipation, and vomiting. Adhesions from previous surgery also may produce bowel obstruction, which begins rapidly, without the prodrome of fever, pain, and malaise typical of obstruction due to a Crohn's disease flare-up. An enterovesical fistula may produce air bubbles in the urine (pneumaturia). Draining cutaneous fistulas may be present. Free perforation into the peritoneal cavity is unusual.

Chronic disease produces a variety of systemic symptoms, including fever, weight loss, malnutrition, and extraintestinal manifestations (see p. 149).

The "Vienna Classification" classifies Crohn's disease into three principal patterns: (1) primarily inflammatory, which after several years commonly evolves into either (2) primarily stenotic or obstructing or (3) primarily penetrating or fistulizing. These different clinical patterns dictate different therapeutic approaches. Some genetic studies suggest a molecular basis for this classification.

Diagnosis

Crohn's disease should be suspected in a patient with inflammatory or obstructive symptoms or in a patient without prominent GI symptoms but with perianal fistulas or abscesses or with otherwise unexplained arthritis, erythema nodosum, fever, anemia, or (in a child) stunted growth. A family history of Crohn's disease also increases the index of suspicion. Similar signs and symptoms (eg, abdominal pain, diarrhea) may be produced by other GI disorders. Differentiation from UC (see TABLE 18–1 and discussion below) may be difficult in the 20% of cases in which Crohn's disease is confined to the colon. However, because treatment is similar, this distinction is critical only when surgery or experimental therapy is contemplated.

Patients presenting with an acute abdomen (either initially or on relapse) should have flat and upright abdominal x-rays and an abdominal CT scan. These studies demonstrate obstruction, abscesses or fistulas, and other possible causes of an acute abdomen (eg, appendicitis). Ultrasound may better delineate gynecologic pathology in women with lower abdominal and pelvic pain.

If initial presentation is less acute, an upper GI series with small-bowel follow-through and spot films of the terminal ileum is preferred over CT. A GI series is diagnostic if it demonstrates strictures (by producing the "string sign"), fistulas, or separation of bowel loops. If findings are questionable, enteroclysis or video capsule enteroscopy may show superficial aphthous and linear ulcers. Barium enema x-ray may be used if symptoms appear predominantly colonic (eg, diarrhea) and may show reflux of barium into the terminal ileum with irregularity, nodularity, stiffness, wall thickening, and a narrowed lumen. Similar x-ray findings occur in cancer of the cecum, ileal carcinoid, lymphosarcoma, systemic vasculitis, radiation enteritis, ileocecal TB, and ameboma.

In atypical cases (eg, predominantly diarrhea, with minimal pain), evaluation is similar to suspected UC, with colonoscopy (including biopsy, sampling for enteric pathogens, and, when possible, visualization of the terminal ileum). Upper GI endoscopy may identify gastroduodenal involvement even in the absence of upper GI symptoms.

Laboratory tests should be obtained to screen for anemia, hypoalbuminemia, and electrolyte abnormalities. Liver function tests should be obtained; elevated alkaline phosphatase and γ-glutamyl transpeptidase levels suggest possible primary sclerosing cholangitis. Leukocytosis or increased levels of acute-phase reactants (eg, ESR, C-reactive protein) are nonspecific but may be used serially to monitor disease activity.

Perinuclear antineutrophil cytoplasmic antibodies are present in 60 to 70% of UC patients and in only 5 to 20% of Crohn's disease patients. Anti-*Saccharomyces cerevisiae* antibodies are relatively specific for Crohn's disease. However, these tests do not reliably separate the two diseases. They have uncertain value in cases of "indeterminate colitis" and are not recommended for routine diagnosis.

Prognosis

Established Crohn's disease is rarely cured and is characterized by intermittent exacerbations and remissions. Some suffer severe disease with frequent, debilitating periods of pain. However, with judicious medical and, where appropriate, surgical therapy, most patients function well and adapt successfully. Disease-related mortality is very low. GI cancer, including cancer of the colon and small bowel, is the leading cause of Crohn's disease–related death.

Treatment

See above for details of specific drugs and dosages.

General management: Cramps and diarrhea may be relieved by oral administration up to qid (ideally before meals) of loperamide 2 to 4 mg. Such symptomatic treatment is safe, except in cases of severe, acute Crohn's colitis, which may progress to toxic megacolon as in UC. Hydrophilic mucilloids (eg, methylcellulose or psyllium preparations) sometimes help prevent anal irritation by increasing stool firmness. Dietary roughage is to be avoided in stricturing disease or active colonic inflammation.

Mild to moderate disease: This category includes ambulatory patients who tolerate oral intake and have no signs of toxicity, tenderness, mass, or obstruction. 5-Aminosalicylic acid (5-ASA, mesalamine) is commonly used as first-line treatment, although its benefits for small-bowel disease are modest at best. Pentasa is the most effective formulation for disease proximal to the terminal ileum; Asacol is effective in distal ileal disease; all formulations are roughly equivalent for Crohn's colitis, although none of the newer preparations rival sulfasalazine for efficacy on a dose-for-dose basis.

Antibiotics are considered a first-line agent by some clinicians, or they may be reserved for patients not responding to 4 wk of 5-ASA; their use is strictly empiric. With any of these drugs, 8 to 16 wk of treatment may be required.

Responders are converted to maintenance therapy.

Moderate to severe disease: Patients without fistulas or abscesses but with significant pain, tenderness, fever, or vomiting, or those who have not responded to treatment for mild disease, require corticosteroids, either oral or parenteral, depending on severity of symptoms and frequency of vomiting. Oral prednisone or prednisolone may act more rapidly and reliably than oral budesonide, but the latter has somewhat fewer adverse effects. Patients not responding to corticosteroids, or those who cannot be tapered, should receive azathioprine, 6-mercaptopurine, or possibly methotrexate. Infliximab is preferred by some as a second-line agent after corticosteroids but is contraindicated in active infection.

Obstruction, whether due to adhesions or to Crohn's disease, is managed initially with nasogastric suction, IV fluids, and sometimes parenteral nutrition. Obstruction due to uncomplicated Crohn's disease resolves within a few days; absence of prompt response indicates a complication or another etiology and demands immediate surgery.

Fulminant disease or abscess: Patients with toxic appearance, high fever, persistent vomiting, rebound, or a tender or palpable mass must be hospitalized for administration of IV fluids and antibiotics. Abscesses must be drained, either percutaneously or surgically. IV corticosteroids should be administered only when infection has been ruled out or controlled. If there is no response to corticosteroids in 5 to 7 days, surgery is usually indicated.

Fistulas: Fistulas are treated initially with metronidazole and ciprofloxacin. Patients who do not respond in 3 to 4 wk may receive an immunomodulator (eg, azathioprine, 6-mercaptopurine), with or without an induction regimen of infliximab for more rapid response. Cyclosporine is an alternative, but fistulas often relapse after treatment. Severe refractory perianal fistulas may require temporary diverting colostomy but almost invariably recur following reconnection; hence, diversion is more appropriately considered an adjunct to definitive surgery rather than a primary treatment.

Maintenance therapy: Patients who require only 5-ASA to achieve remission can be maintained on this drug. Patients requiring acute treatment with corticosteroids or infliximab generally require azathioprine, 6-mercaptopurine, or methotrexate for maintenance. Corticosteroids are neither safe nor effective for long-term maintenance. Patients who respond to infliximab for acute disease but who are not well maintained on antimetabolites may stay in remission with repeat doses of inflximab 5 to 10 mg/kg at 8-wk intervals. Monitoring during remission can be done by symptoms and blood tests and does not require x-rays or colonoscopy (other than routine yearly dysplasia surveillance) after 7 yr of disease.

Surgery: Even though about 70% of patients ultimately require surgery, surgery is always performed reluctantly. It is best reserved for recurrent intestinal obstruction or intractable fistulas or abscesses. Resection of the involved bowel may ameliorate symptoms but does not cure the disease, since Crohn's disease is likely to recur even after resection of all clinically apparent disease. The recurrence rate, defined by endoscopic lesions at the anastomotic site, is > 70% at 1 yr and > 85% at 3 yr; defined by clinical symptoms, it is about 25 to 30% at 3 yr and 40 to 50% at 5 yr. Ultimately, further surgery is required in nearly 50% of cases. However, recurrence rates appear to be reduced by early postoperative prophylaxis with 6-mercaptopurine, metronidazole, or possibly 5-ASA. When surgery is performed for appropriate indications, almost all patients experience an improved quality of life.

ULCERATIVE COLITIS

Ulcerative colitis is a chronic inflammatory and ulcerative disease arising in the colonic mucosa, characterized most often by bloody diarrhea. Extraintestinal symptoms, particularly arthritis, may occur. Long-term risk of colon cancer is high. Diagnosis is by colonoscopy. Treatment is with 5-ASA, corticosteroids, immunomodulators, anticytokines, antibiotics, and occasionally surgery.

Pathophysiology

Ulcerative colitis (UC) usually begins in the rectum. It may remain localized to the rectum (ulcerative proctitis) or extend proximally, sometimes involving the entire colon. Rarely, it involves most of the large bowel at once.

The inflammation of UC affects the mucosa and submucosa, and there is a sharp border between normal and affected tissue. Only in severe disease is the muscularis involved. In early cases, the mucous membrane is erythematous, finely granular, and friable, with loss of the normal vascular pattern and often with scattered hemorrhagic areas. Large mucosal ulcers with copious purulent exudate characterize severe disease. Islands of relatively normal or hyperplastic inflammatory mucosa (pseudopolyps) project above areas of ulcerated mucosa. Fistulas and abscesses do not occur.

Fulminant colitis occurs when transmural extension of ulceration results in localized ileus and peritonitis. Within hours to days, the colon loses muscular tone and begins to dilate.

Toxic megacolon (or toxic dilation) is a medical emergency in which severe transmural inflammation leads to colonic dilation and sometimes perforation. It is considered present when the diameter of the transverse colon exceeds 6 cm during an exacerbation. This condition usually occurs spontaneously in the course of very severe colitis but may be precipitated by opioid or anticholinergic antidiarrheal drugs. Colonic perforation increases mortality significantly.

Symptoms and Signs

Bloody diarrhea of varied intensity and duration is interspersed with asymptomatic intervals. Usually an attack begins insidiously, with increased urgency to defecate, mild lower abdominal cramps, and blood and mucus in the stools. Some cases develop after an infection (eg, amebiasis, bacillary dysentery).

When ulceration is confined to the rectosigmoid, the stool may be normal or hard and dry, but rectal discharges of mucus loaded with RBCs and WBCs accompany or occur between bowel movements. Systemic symptoms are absent or mild. If ulceration extends proximally, stools become looser and the patient may have > 10 bowel movements/day, often with severe cramps and distressing rectal tenesmus, without respite at night. The stools may be watery or contain mucus and frequently consist almost entirely of blood and pus. In severe cases, patients may hemorrhage enough over several hours to require emergency transfusion.

Fulminant colitis presents with sudden violent diarrhea, fever to 40° C (104° F), abdominal pain, signs of peritonitis (eg, rebound tenderness), and profound toxemia.

Systemic symptoms, more common with severe UC, include malaise, fever, anemia, anorexia, and weight loss. Extraintestinal manifestations (particularly joint and skin complications—see p. 149) are most common when systemic symptoms are present.

Diagnosis

Initial presentation: Diagnosis is suggested by typical signs and symptoms, particularly when accompanied by extraintestinal manifestations or a history of previous similar attacks. UC must be distinguished from Crohn's disease (see TABLE 18–1 and discussion above) and other causes of acute colitis (eg, infection; in elderly patients, ischemia).

In all patients, stool cultures for enteric pathogens should be obtained, and *Entamoeba histolytica* should be excluded by examination of fresh stool specimens. When amebiasis is suspected because of epidemiologic or travel history, serologic titers and biopsies should be obtained. History of prior antibiotic use or recent hospitalization should prompt stool assay for *Clostridium difficile* toxin. Patients at risk should be tested for HIV, gonorrhea, herpesvirus, chlamydia, and amebiasis. Opportunistic infections (eg, cytomegalovirus, *Mycobacterium avium-intracellulare*) or Kaposi's sarcoma must also be considered in immunosuppressed patients. In women using oral contraceptives, contraceptive-induced colitis is possible; it usually resolves spontaneously after hormone therapy is stopped.

Sigmoidoscopy should be performed; it allows visual confirmation of colitis and permits direct sampling for culture and microscopic evaluation, as well as biopsy of affected areas. However, both visual inspection and biopsies may be nondiagnostic, as there is much overlap in appearance between different types of colitis. Severe perianal disease, rectal sparing, absence of bleeding, and asymmetric or segmental involvement of the colon indicate Crohn's disease rather than UC (see TABLE 18–1). Colonoscopy is usually unnecessary initially but should be performed electively if inflammation has extended proximal to the reach of the sigmoidoscope.

Laboratory tests should be obtained to screen for anemia, hypoalbuminemia, and electrolyte abnormalities. Liver function tests should be obtained; elevated alkaline phosphatase and γ-glutamyl transpeptidase levels suggest possible primary sclerosing cholangitis. Perinuclear antineutrophil cytoplasmic antibodies are relatively specific (60 to 70%) for UC. Anti–*Saccharomyces cerevisiae* antibodies are relatively specific for Crohn's disease. However, these tests do not reliably separate the two diseases and are not recommended for routine diagnosis.

X-rays are not diagnostic but occasionally show abnormalities. Plain x-rays of the abdomen may show mucosal edema, loss of haustration, and absence of formed stool in the diseased bowel. Barium enema shows similar changes, albeit more clearly, and may also demonstrate ulcerations but should not be performed during an acute presentation. A shortened, rigid colon with an atrophic or pseudopolypoid mucosa is often seen after several years' illness. X-ray findings of thumbprinting and segmental distribution are more suggestive of intestinal ischemia or possibly Crohn's colitis rather than of UC.

Recurrent symptoms: Patients with known disease and a recurrence of typical symptoms should be examined, but extensive testing is not always required. Depending on duration and severity of symptoms, sigmoidoscopy or colonoscopy may be performed and a CBC obtained. Cultures, ova and parasite examination, and *C. difficile* toxin assay should be performed when there are atypical features to the relapse or when there is an exacerbation after prolonged remission, during a contagious outbreak, after antibiotic exposure, or whenever the clinician is suspicious.

Fulminant symptoms: Patients require further evaluation during severe flares. Flat and upright abdominal x-rays should be obtained; they may show megacolon or intraluminal gas accumulated over a long, continuous, paralyzed segment of colon—a result of lost muscle tone. Colonoscopy and barium enema should be avoided because of the risk of perforation. CBC, ESR, electrolytes, PT, PTT, and type and crossmatch should be obtained.

The patient must be watched closely for progressive peritonitis or perforation. Percussion over the liver is important because loss of hepatic dullness may be the first clinical sign of free perforation, especially in a patient whose peritoneal signs are suppressed by high-dose corticosteroids. Abdominal x-rays are obtained every 1 or 2 days to follow the course of colonic distention and to detect free or intramural air.

Prognosis

Usually, UC is chronic with repeated exacerbations and remissions. In about 10% of patients, an initial attack becomes fulminant with massive hemorrhage, perforation, or sepsis and toxemia. Complete recovery after a single attack occurs in another 10%.

Patients with localized ulcerative proctitis have the best prognosis. Severe systemic manifestations, toxic complications, and malignant degeneration are unlikely, and late extension of the disease occurs in only about 20 to 30%. Surgery is rarely required, and life expectancy is normal. The symptoms, however, may prove stubborn and refractory. Moreover, because extensive UC may begin in the rectum and spread proximally, proctitis should not be considered localized until it has been observed for ≥ 6 mo. Localized disease that later extends is often more severe and more refractory to therapy.

Colon cancer: The risk of colon cancer is proportional to the duration of disease and amount of colon affected, but not necessarily to disease activity. Cancer begins to appear by 7 yr from onset of illness in patients with extensive colitis. The cumulative likelihood of cancer is about 3% at 15 yr, 5% at 20 yr, and 9% at 25 yr, representing an annual risk of about 0.5 to 1% after the 10th yr. There is probably no higher absolute cancer risk among patients with childhood-onset colitis independent of the longer duration of disease.

Regular colonoscopic surveillance, preferably during remission, is advised for patients with disease duration > 8 to 10 yr (except for isolated proctitis). Endoscopic biopsies should be taken every 10 cm throughout the colon. Any grade of definite dysplasia within an area affected by colitis is liable to progress to more advanced neoplasia and even cancer and is a strong indication for total colectomy unless the dysplasia is strictly confined to a discrete, completely excisable polyp. It is important to distinguish definite neoplastic dysplasia from reactive or regenerative atypia secondary to inflammation. However, if the dysplasia is unequivocal, delaying colectomy in favor of repeated follow-up surveillance is a risky strategy. Pseudopolyps have no prognostic significance but may be difficult to distinguish from neoplastic polyps; thus, any suspect polyp should undergo excision biopsy.

The optimal frequency of colonoscopic surveillance has not been established, but some authorities recommend every 2 yr during the 2nd decade of disease and annually thereafter.

Long-term survival after diagnosis of colitis-related cancer is about 50%, a figure comparable to that for colorectal cancer in the general population.

Treatment

See above for details of specific drugs and regimens.

General management: Avoiding raw fruits and vegetables limits trauma to the inflamed colonic mucosa and may lessen symptoms. A milk-free diet may help but need not be continued if no benefit is noted. Loperamide 2.0 mg po bid to qid is indicated for relatively mild diarrhea; higher oral doses (4 mg in the morning and 2 mg after each bowel movement) may be required for more intense diarrhea. Antidiarrheal drugs must be used with extreme caution in severe cases because they may precipitate toxic dilation.

Mild left-sided disease: Patients with proctitis, or colitis that does not extend proximally beyond the splenic flexure, are treated with 5-aminosalicylic acid (5-ASA, mesalamine) enemas once/day or bid depending on severity. Suppositories are effective for more distal disease and are usually preferred by patients. Corticosteroid and budesonide enemas are slightly less effective but should be used if 5-ASA is unsuccessful or not tolerated. Once remission is achieved, dosage is slowly tapered to maintenance levels. Oral 5-ASA drugs theoretically have some incremental benefit in lessening the probability of proximal spread of disease.

Moderate or extensive disease: Patients with inflammation proximal to the splenic flexure or left-sided disease unresponsive to topical agents should receive an oral 5-ASA formulation in addition to 5-ASA enemas. High-dose corticosteroids are added for more severe symptoms; after 1 to 2 wk, the daily dose is reduced by about 5 to 10 mg each wk.

Severe disease: Patients with > 10 bloody bowel movements per day, tachycardia, high fever, or severe abdominal pain require hospitalization for high-dose IV corticosteroids. 5-ASA may be continued. IV fluids and blood transfusion are given as needed for dehydration and anemia. The patient must be observed closely for the development of toxic megacolon. Parenteral hyperalimentation is sometimes used for nutritional support but is of no value as primary therapy; patients who can tolerate food should eat.

Patients who do not respond within 3 to 7 days should be considered for IV cyclosporine or surgery. Patients who do respond are switched within a week or so to prednisone 60 mg po once/day, which may be gradually reduced at home based on clinical response.

Fulminant colitis: If fulminant colitis or toxic megacolon is suspected: (1) discontinue all antidiarrheal drugs; (2) give nothing by mouth and pass a long intestinal tube attached to intermittent suction; (3) give aggressive IV fluid and electrolyte therapy, with 0.9% NaCl, and potassium chloride and blood as needed; (4) give high-dose IV corticosteroids; and (5) give antibiotics (eg, metronidazole 500 mg IV q 8 h and ciprofloxacin 500 mg IV q 12 h).

Having the patient roll over in bed from the supine to prone position every 2 to 3 h may help redistribute colonic gas and prevent progressive distention. Passage of a soft rectal tube may also be helpful but must be done with extreme caution to avoid bowel perforation.

If intensive medical measures do not produce definite improvement within 24 to 48 h, immediate surgery is required or the patient may die of sepsis caused by perforation.

Maintenance therapy: Following effective treatment of a flare-up, corticosteroids are tapered based on clinical response and discontinued; they are ineffective as maintenance. Patients should remain on 5-ASA drugs indefinitely—oral or rectal, depending on location of disease—because stopping maintenance therapy often allows disease relapse. Dosage intervals for rectal preparations may be gradually lengthened to every second or third day.

Patients who cannot be withdrawn from corticosteroids should be given azathioprine or 6-mercaptopurine.

Surgery: Nearly $\frac{1}{3}$ of patients with extensive UC ultimately require surgery. Total proctocolectomy is curative: Life expectancy and quality of life are restored to normal, the disease does not recur (unlike Crohn's disease), and the risk of colon cancer is eliminated.

Emergency colectomy is indicated for massive hemorrhage, fulminating toxic colitis, or perforation. Subtotal colectomy with ileostomy and rectosigmoid closure or mucous fistula is usually the procedure of choice because most critically ill patients cannot tolerate more extensive surgery. The rectosigmoid stump may be electively removed later or may be used for ileoanal anastomosis with a pouch. The intact rectal stump should not be allowed to remain indefinitely because of the risk of disease activation and malignant transformation.

Elective surgery is indicated for high-grade mucosal dysplasia confirmed by two pathologists, definite cancer, all symptomatic strictures, growth retardation in children, or most commonly, intractable chronic disease resulting in invalidism or corticosteroid dependence. Rarely, severe colitis-related extraintestinal manifestations (eg, pyoderma gangrenosum) are also indications for surgery. The elective procedure of choice in patients with normal sphincter function is restorative proctocolectomy with ileoanal anastomosis. This procedure creates a pelvic reservoir or pouch from distal ileum, which is connected to the anus. The intact sphincter allows continence, typically with 8 to 10 bowel movements/day. Pouchitis is an inflammatory reaction occurring after this procedure in about 50% of patients. It is thought to be related to bacterial overgrowth and is treated with antibiotics (eg, quinolones). Probiotics may be protective. Most cases of pouchitis are readily controlled, but 5 to 10% may prove refractory to all medical therapy. Alternative surgical procedures include a continent ileostomy

(Kock pouch) or, more often, traditional (Brooke) ileostomy.

The physical and emotional burdens imposed by any form of colon resection must be recognized, and care should be taken to see that the patient receives all the instructions and psychologic support that are necessary before and after surgery.

19 DIVERTICULAR DISEASE

Diverticula are saclike mucosal outpouchings that protrude from a tubular structure. True diverticula contain all layers of the parent structure. False or pseudodiverticula are mucosal projections through the muscular layer. Esophageal (see p. 112) and Meckel's diverticula are true diverticula. Colonic diverticula are pseudodiverticula; they cause symptoms by trapping feces and becoming inflamed or infected, bleeding, or rupturing.

DIVERTICULOSIS

Diverticulosis is the presence of multiple diverticula in the colon, probably resulting from a lifelong low-fiber diet. Most diverticula are asymptomatic, but some become inflamed or bleed. Diagnosis is by colonoscopy or barium enema. Treatment varies depending on presentation.

Diverticula occur anywhere in the large bowel—usually in the sigmoid but rarely below the peritoneal reflection of the rectum. They vary in diameter from 3 mm to > 3 cm. Patients with diverticula usually have several of them. Diverticulosis is uncommon in people < 40 but becomes common rapidly thereafter; essentially every 90-yr-old person has many diverticula. Giant diverticula, which are rare, range in diameter from 3 to 15 cm and may be single.

Etiology and Pathophysiology

Diverticula are probably caused by increased intraluminal pressure leading to mucosal extrusion through the weakest points of the muscular layer of the bowel—areas adjacent to intramural blood vessels. Diverticula are more common in people who eat a low-fiber diet; however, the mechanism is not clear. One theory is that increased intraluminal pressure is required to move low-bulk stool through the colon; another is that low-stool bulk produces a smaller diameter colon, which by Laplace's law would have increased pressure.

The etiology of giant diverticula is unclear: one theory is that a valvelike abnormality exists at the base of the diverticulum, so bowel gas can enter but escapes less freely.

Symptoms, Signs, and Diagnosis

Most (70%) diverticula are asymptomatic, 15 to 25% become painfully inflamed (diverticulitis), and 10 to 15% bleed painlessly. The bleeding is probably caused by erosion of the adjacent vessel by local trauma from impacted feces in the diverticulum. Although most diverticula are distal, 75% of bleeding occurs from diverticula proximal to the splenic flexure. In $\frac{1}{3}$ of patients (5% overall), bleeding is serious enough to require transfusion.

Asymptomatic diverticula are usually found incidentally during barium enema or colonoscopy. Diverticulosis is suspected when painless rectal bleeding develops, particularly in an elderly patient. Evaluation of rectal bleeding typically includes colonoscopy, which can be done electively after routine preparation unless there is significant ongoing bleeding. In such patients, a rapid preparation (5 to 10 L of polyethylene glycol solution delivered via nasogastric tube over 3 to 4 h) often allows adequate visualization. If colonoscopy cannot visualize the source and ongoing bleeding is sufficiently rapid (> 0.5 to 1 mL/min), angiography may localize the source. Some angiographers first perform a radionuclide scan to focus the examination.

Treatment

Treatment of diverticulosis aims at reducing segmental spasm. A high-fiber diet helps and may be supplemented by psyllium seed preparations or bran. Low-fiber diets are contraindicated. The intuitive injunction to avoid seeds or other dietary material that might become impacted in a diverticulum has no established medical basis. Antispasmodics (eg, belladonna) are not of benefit and may cause adverse effects. Surgery is unwarranted for uncomplicated disease. Giant diverticula, however, require surgery.

Diverticular bleeding stops spontaneously in 75% of patients. Treatment is often administered during diagnostic procedures. If angiography was performed for diagnosis, ongoing bleeding can be controlled in 70 to 90% of patients by intra-arterial injection of vasopressin. In some cases, bleeding recurs within a few days and requires surgery. Angiographic embolization effectively stops bleeding but leads to bowel infarction in up to 20% of patients and is not recommended. Colonoscopy allows heat or laser coagulation of vessels or injection of epinephrine. If these measures fail to stop bleeding, segmental resection or subtotal colectomy is indicated.

DIVERTICULITIS

Diverticulitis is inflammation of a diverticulum, which can result in phlegmon of the bowel wall, peritonitis, perforation, fistula, or abscess. The primary symptom is abdominal pain. Diagnosis is by CT scan. Treatment is with antibiotics (ciprofloxacin, or a 3rd-generation cephalosporin plus metronidazole) and occasionally surgery.

Diverticulitis occurs when a micro or macro perforation develops in a diverticulum, releasing intestinal bacteria. The resultant inflammation remains localized in about 75% of patients. The remaining 25% may develop abscess, free intraperitoneal perforation, bowel obstruction, or fistulas. The most common fistulas involve the bladder but may also involve the small bowel, uterus, vagina, abdominal wall, or even the thigh.

Diverticulitis is most serious in elderly patients, especially those taking prednisone or other drugs that increase the hazards of infection. Nearly all serious diverticulitis occurs in the sigmoid.

Symptoms and Signs

Diverticulitis usually presents with pain, tenderness in the left lower quadrant of the abdomen, and fever. Peritoneal signs may be present, particularly with abscess or free perforation. Fistulas may manifest as pneumaturia, feculent vaginal discharge, or a cutaneous or myofascial infection of the abdominal wall, perineum, or upper leg. Patients with bowel obstruction have nausea, vomiting, and abdominal distention. Bleeding is uncommon.

Diagnosis

Clinical suspicion is high in patients with known diverticulosis. However, because other disorders (eg, appendicitis, colon or ovarian cancer) may produce similar symptoms, testing is required. Abdominal CT scan with oral and IV contrast is preferred, although findings in about 10% of patients cannot be distinguished from colon cancer. Exploratory laparotomy may be necessary for definitive diagnosis.

Treatment

A patient who is not very ill is treated at home with rest, a liquid diet, and oral antibiotics (eg, ciprofloxacin 500 mg bid, or amoxicillin/clavulanate 500 mg tid plus metronidazole 500 mg qid). Symptoms usually subside rapidly. The patient gradually advances to a soft low-fiber diet and a daily psyllium seed preparation. The colon should be evaluated after 2 to 4 wk with a barium enema. After 1 mo, a high-fiber diet is resumed.

Patients with more severe symptoms (pain, fever, marked leukocytosis) should be hospitalized, as should patients taking prednisone (who are at higher risk for perforation and general peritonitis). Treatment is bed rest, nothing by mouth, IV fluids, and IV antibiotics (eg, ceftazidime 1 g IV q 8 h plus metronidazole 500 mg IV q 6 to 8 h).

About 80% of patients can be treated successfully without surgery. An abscess may respond to percutaneous drainage (CT guided). If response is satisfactory, the patient remains hospitalized until symptoms are relieved and a soft diet is resumed. A barium enema is performed ≥ 2 wk after symptoms have resolved.

Surgery: Surgery is required immediately for patients with free perforation or general peritonitis and for patients with severe symptoms that do not respond to nonsurgical treatment within 48 h. Increasing pain, tenderness, and fever are other signs that surgery is needed. Surgery should also be considered in patients with any of the following: two or more previous attacks of mild diverticulitis (or one attack in a patient < 50); a persistent tender mass; clinical, endoscopic, or x-ray signs suggestive of cancer; and dysuria associated with diverticulitis in men (or in women who have had a hysterectomy), because this symptom may presage perforation into the bladder.

The involved section of the colon is resected. The ends can be reanastomosed immediately in healthy patients without perforation, abscess, or significant inflammation. Other patients have a temporary colostomy with anastomosis carried out in a subsequent operation after inflammation resolves and the patient's general condition improves.

MECKEL'S DIVERTICULUM

Meckel's diverticulum is a congenital sacculation of the distal ileum occurring in 2 to 3% of people. It is usually located within 100 cm of the ileocecal valve and often contains heterotopic gastric and/or pancreatic tissue. Symptoms are uncommon but include bleeding, bowel obstruction, and inflammation (diverticulitis). Diagnosis is difficult and often involves radionuclide scanning and barium studies. Treatment is surgical resection.

Etiology and Pathophysiology

In early fetal life, the vitelline duct running from the terminal ileum to the umbilicus and yolk sac is normally obliterated by the 7th wk. If the portion connecting to the ileum fails to atrophy, a Meckel's diverticulum results. This congenital diverticulum arises from the antimesenteric margin of the intestine and contains all layers of the normal bowel. About 50% of diverticula also contain heterotopic tissue of the stomach (and thus contain parietal cells that secrete HCl), pancreas, or both.

Only about 2% of people with Meckel's diverticulum develop complications. Although diverticula are equally common in males and females, males are 2 to 3 times more likely to have complications. Complications include bleeding, obstruction, diverticulitis, and tumors. Bleeding is more common in young children (< 5 yr) and occurs when acid secreted from ectopic gastric mucosa in the diverticulum ulcerates the adjacent ileum. Obstruction can occur at any age but is more common in older children and adults. In children, intussusception of the diverticulum is the most likely cause. Obstruction may also result from adhesions, volvulus, retained foreign bodies, tumors, or incarceration in a hernia (Littre's hernia). Acute Meckel's diverticulitis can occur at any age, but its incidence peaks in older children. Tumors, including carcinoids, are rare and occur mainly in adults.

Symptoms, Signs, and Diagnosis

In all ages, intestinal obstruction is manifested by cramping abdominal pain, nausea, and vomiting. Acute Meckel's diverticulitis is characterized by abdominal pain and tenderness typically localized below or to the left of the umbilicus; it is often accompanied by vomiting and is similar to appendicitis except for location of pain.

Children may present with repeated episodes of painless, bright red rectal bleeding, which is usually not severe enough to produce shock. Adults may also bleed, typically resulting in melena rather than frank blood.

Diagnosis is difficult, and tests are chosen based on presenting symptoms. If rectal bleeding is suspected to originate from a Meckel's diverticulum, a ^{99m}Tc pertechnetate scan will identify ectopic gastric mucosa and hence the diverticulum. Patients presenting with abdominal pain and focal tenderness should have a CT scan with oral contrast. If vomiting and signs of obstruction are predominant, flat and upright x-rays of the abdomen are performed. Sometimes diagnosis is made only during surgical exploration for presumed appendicitis; whenever a normal appendix is found, Meckel's diverticulum should be suspected.

Treatment

Patients with intestinal obstruction from Meckel's diverticulum require early surgery. For detailed treatment of intestinal obstruction, see p. 105.

A bleeding diverticulum with an indurated area in the adjacent ileum requires resection of this section of the bowel and the diverticulum. A bleeding diverticulum without ileal induration requires only resection of the diverticulum.

Meckel's diverticulitis also requires resection. Small, asymptomatic diverticula encountered incidentally at laparotomy need not be removed.

DIVERTICULAR DISEASE OF THE STOMACH AND SMALL BOWEL

Diverticula rarely involve the stomach but occur in the duodenum in up to 25% of people. Most duodenal diverticula are solitary and occur in the second portion of the duodenum near the ampulla of Vater (periampullary). Jejunal diverticula occur in about 0.26% of patients and are more common in patients with disorders of intestinal motility. Meckel's diverticulum occurs in the distal ileum.

Duodenal and jejunal diverticula are asymptomatic in >90% of cases and are usually detected incidentally during radiologic or endoscopic investigation of the upper GI tract for an unrelated disease. Rarely, small-bowel diverticula bleed or become inflamed, causing pain and nausea. Some even perforate. For poorly understood reasons, patients with periampullary diverticula are at increased risk for gallstones and pancreatitis. Treatment is surgical resection; however, the clinician should be cautious of recommending surgery for patients with a diverticulum and vague GI symptoms (eg, dyspepsia).

20 ANORECTAL DISORDERS

(See also Foreign Bodies on p. 126 and Anorectal Cancer on p. 177.)

The anal canal begins at the anal sphincter and ends at the anorectal junction (pectinate line, mucocutaneous junction, dentate line), where there are 8 to 12 anal crypts and 5 to 8 papillae. The canal is lined with anoderm, a continuation of the external skin. The anal canal and adjacent skin are innervated by somatic sensory nerves and are highly susceptible to painful stimuli. Venous drainage from the anal canal occurs through the caval system, but the anorectal junction can drain into both the portal and caval systems. Lymphatics from the anal canal pass to the internal iliac nodes, the posterior vaginal wall, and the inguinal nodes. The venous and lymphatic distributions determine how malignant disease and infection spread.

The rectum is a continuation of the sigmoid colon beginning at the level of the 3rd sacral vertebra and continuing to the anorectal junction. The rectal lining consists of red, glistening glandular mucosa, which has an autonomic nerve supply and is relatively insensitive to pain. Venous drainage occurs through the portal system. Lymphatic return from the rectum occurs along the superior hemorrhoidal vascular pedicle to the inferior mesenteric and aortic nodes.

The sphincteric ring encircling the anal canal is composed of the internal sphincter, the central portion of the levators, and components of the external sphincter. Anteriorly, it is more vulnerable to trauma, which can result in incontinence. The puborectalis forms a muscular sling around the rectum for support and assistance in defecation.

History should include the details of bleeding, pain, protrusion, discharge, swelling, abnormal sensations, bowel movements, stool characteristics, use of cathartics and enemas, and abdominal and urinary symptoms. All patients should be asked about anal intercourse and other possible causes of trauma and infection.

Physical examination should be performed gently and with good lighting. It consists of external inspection, perianal and intrarectal digital palpation, abdominal examination, and rectovaginal bidigital palpation. Anoscopy and rigid or flexible sigmoidoscopy to 15 to 60 cm above the anal verge are often included. Inspection, palpation, and anoscopy and sigmoidoscopy are best performed with the patient in the left lateral (Sims') or knee-chest position or inverted on a tilt table (see p. 88). In cases of painful anal lesions, topical (lidocaine 5% ointment), regional, or even general anesthesia may be required. If it can be tolerated, a cleansing phosphate enema may facilitate sigmoidoscopy. Biopsies, smears, and cultures may be taken, and x-ray examination ordered if indicated.

ANAL FISSURE

(Fissure in Ano; Anal Ulcer)

An anal fissure is an acute longitudinal tear or a chronic ovoid ulcer in the squamous epithelium of the anal canal. It produces severe pain, sometimes with bleeding, particularly with defecation. Diagnosis is by inspection. Treatment is local hygiene, stool softeners, and sometimes botulinum toxin injection.

Anal fissures are believed to result from laceration by a hard or large stool, with secondary infection. Trauma (eg, anal intercourse) is a rare cause. The fissure may cause internal sphincter spasm, decreasing blood supply and perpetuating the fissure.

Symptoms, Signs, and Diagnosis

Anal fissures usually lie in the posterior midline but may occur in the anterior midline. Those off the midline may have specific etiologies, particularly Crohn's disease. An external skin tag (the sentinel pile) may be present at the lower end of the fissure, and an enlarged (hypertrophic) papilla may be present at the upper end.

Infants may develop acute fissures, but chronic fissures are rare. Chronic fissures must be differentiated from cancer, primary lesions of syphilis, TB, and ulceration from Crohn's disease.

Fissures cause pain and bleeding. The pain typically occurs with or shortly after defecation, lasts for several hours, and subsides until the next bowel movement. Examination must be gentle but with adequate spreading of the buttocks to allow visualization.

Treatment

Fissures often respond to conservative measures that minimize trauma during defecation (eg, stool softeners, psyllium, fiber). Healing is aided by use of protective zinc oxide ointments or bland suppositories (eg, glycerin) that lubricate the lower rectum and soften stool. Topical anesthetics (eg, benzocaine, lidocaine) and warm (not hot) sitz baths for 10 or 15 min after each bowel movement and prn give temporary relief.

Topical nitroglycerin 0.2% ointment, nifedipine cream 0.2% or 0.3%, arginine gel, and injections of botulinum toxin into the internal sphincter relax the anal sphincter and decrease maximum anal resting pressure, allowing healing. When conservative measures fail, surgery (internal anal sphincterotomy or controlled anal dilation) is needed to interfere with the cycle of internal anal sphincter spasm.

ANORECTAL ABSCESS

An anorectal abscess is a localized collection of pus in the perirectal spaces. Abscesses usually originate in an anal crypt. Symptoms are pain and swelling. Diagnosis is by examination and CT scan or pelvic MRI for deeper abscesses. Treatment is surgical drainage.

An abscess may be located in various spaces surrounding the rectum and may be superficial or deep. A perianal abscess is superficial and points to the skin. An ischiorectal abscess is deeper, extending across the sphincter into the ischiorectal space below the levator ani; it may penetrate to the contralateral side, forming a "horseshoe" abscess. An abscess above the levator ani (ie, supralevator abscess) is quite deep and may extend to the peritoneum or abdominal organs; this abscess often results from diverticulitis or pelvic inflammatory disease. Crohn's disease (especially of the colon) sometimes causes anorectal abscess. A mixed infection usually occurs, with *Escherichia coli*, *Proteus vulgaris*, *Bacteroides*, streptococci, and staphylococci predominating.

Symptoms, Signs, and Diagnosis

Superficial abscesses can be very painful; perianal swelling, redness, and tenderness are characteristic. Deeper abscesses may be less painful but cause toxic symptoms (eg, fever, chills, malaise). There may be no perianal findings, but digital rectal examination may reveal a tender, fluctuant swelling of the rectal wall. High pelvirectal abscesses may cause lower abdominal pain and fever without rectal symptoms. Sometimes fever is the only symptom.

Treatment

Prompt incision and adequate drainage are required and should not wait until the abscess points. Many abscesses can be drained as an outpatient procedure; deeper abscesses may require drainage in the operating room. Febrile or diabetic patients should also receive antibiotics (eg, ciprofloxacin 500 mg IV q 12 h and metronidazole 500 mg IV q 8 h, ampicillin/sulbactam 1.5 g IV q 8 h), which are not indicated for healthy patients with superficial abscesses. Anorectal fistulas may develop after drainage.

ANORECTAL FISTULA

(Fistula in Ano)

An anorectal fistula is a tubelike tract with one opening in the anal canal and the other usually in the perianal skin. Symptoms are discharge and sometimes pain. Diagnosis is by examination and sigmoidoscopy. Treatment often requires surgery

Fistulas arise spontaneously or occur secondary to drainage of a perirectal abscess.

Predisposing causes include Crohn's disease and TB. Most fistulas originate in the anorectal crypts; others may result from diverticulitis, tumors, or trauma. Fistulas in infants are congenital and are more common in boys. Rectovaginal fistulas may be secondary to Crohn's disease, obstetric injuries, radiotherapy, or malignancy.

Symptoms, Signs, and Diagnosis

A history of recurrent abscess followed by intermittent or constant discharge is usual. Discharge material is purulent, serosanguineous, or both. Pain may be present if there is infection. On inspection, one or more secondary openings can be seen. A cordlike tract can often be palpated. A probe inserted into the tract can determine the depth and direction and often the primary opening. Sigmoidoscopy should follow. Hidradenitis suppurativa, pilonidal sinus, dermal suppurative sinuses, and urethroperineal fistulas must be differentiated from cryptogenic fistulas.

Treatment

In the past, the only effective treatment was surgery. The primary opening and the entire tract are unroofed and converted into a "ditch." Partial division of the sphincters may be necessary. Some degree of incontinence may occur if a considerable portion of the sphincteric ring is divided. In the presence of diarrhea or Crohn's disease, fistulotomy is inadvisable because of delayed wound healing. For patients with Crohn's disease, metronidazole, other appropriate antibiotics, and suppressive therapies can be given (see p. 154). Infliximab is very effective in closing Crohn's fistulas. Advancement flaps or fibrin glue instillations into the fistulous tract are alternatives to conventional surgery.

FECAL INCONTINENCE

Fecal incontinence is a loss of voluntary control of defecation.

Fecal incontinence can result from injuries or diseases of the spinal cord, congenital abnormalities, accidental injuries to the rectum and anus, procidentia, diabetes, severe dementia, fecal impaction, extensive inflammatory processes, tumors, obstetric injuries, and operations involving division or dilation of the anal sphincters.

Physical examination should evaluate gross sphincter function and perianal sensation and rule out fecal impaction. Anal sphincter ultrasound, pelvic and perineal MRIs, pelvic floor electromyography, and anorectal manometry are also useful.

Treatment

Treatment includes a bowel management program to develop a predictable pattern of defecation. The program includes intake of adequate fluid and sufficient dietary bulk. Sitting on a toilet or using another customary defecatory stimulant (eg, coffee) encourages defecation. A suppository (eg, glycerin, bisacodyl) or a phosphate enema may also be used. If a regular defecatory pattern does not develop, a low-residue diet and oral loperamide may reduce the frequency of defecation.

Simple perineal exercises, in which the patient repeatedly contracts the sphincters, perineal muscles, and buttocks, may strengthen these structures and contribute to continence, particularly in mild cases. Biofeedback (to train the patient to use the sphincters maximally and to better appreciate physiologic stimuli) should be considered before recommending surgery in well-motivated patients who can understand and follow instructions and who have an anal sphincter capable of recognizing the cue of rectal distention. About 70% of such patients respond to biofeedback.

A defect in the sphincter can be sutured directly. When there is insufficient residual sphincter for repair, particularly in patients < 50, a gracilis muscle can be transposed. Some centers apply a pacemaker to the gracilis muscle, as well as an artificial sphincter; these or other experimental procedures are available only in a few centers in the US, as experimental protocols. Alternatively, a Thiersch wire or other material can be used to encircle the anus. When all else fails, a colostomy can be considered.

HEMORRHOIDS
(Piles)

Hemorrhoids are dilated veins of the hemorrhoidal plexus in the lower rectum. Symptoms include irritation and bleeding. Thrombosed hemorrhoids are painful. Diagnosis is by inspection or anoscopy. Treatment is symptomatic or with endo-

scopic banding, injection sclerotherapy, or sometimes surgery.

External hemorrhoids are located below the dentate line and are covered by squamous epithelium. Internal hemorrhoids are located above the dentate line and are lined by rectal mucosa. Hemorrhoids typically occur in the right anterior, right posterior, and left lateral zones. They occur in adults and children.

Symptoms, Signs, and Diagnosis

Hemorrhoids are often asymptomatic, or they may simply protrude. Pruritus ani is uncommonly caused by hemorrhoids.

External hemorrhoids may become thrombosed, resulting in a painful, purplish swelling. Rarely, they ulcerate and produce minor bleeding. Cleansing the anal region may be difficult.

Internal hemorrhoids typically present with bleeding following defecation; blood is noted on toilet tissue and sometimes in the toilet bowl. Rectal bleeding should be attributed to hemorrhoids only after more serious conditions are excluded. Internal hemorrhoids may be uncomfortable but are not as painful as thrombosed external hemorrhoids. Internal hemorrhoids sometimes cause mucus discharge and a sensation of incomplete evacuation.

Strangulated hemorrhoids occur when protrusion and constriction occlude the blood supply. They cause pain that is occasionally followed by necrosis and ulceration.

Most painful hemorrhoids, thrombosed, ulcerated or not, are seen on inspection of the anus and rectum. Anoscopy is essential in evaluating painless or bleeding hemorrhoids.

Treatment

Symptomatic treatment is usually all that is needed. It is accomplished with stool softeners (eg, docusate, psyllium), warm sitz baths (ie, sitting in a tub of tolerably hot water for 10 min) after each bowel movement and prn, anesthetic ointments containing lidocaine, or witch hazel (hamamelis) compresses (which soothe by an unknown mechanism). Pain caused by a thrombosed hemorrhoid can be treated with NSAIDs. Infrequently, simple incision and evacuation of the clot may relieve pain rapidly; after infiltration with 1% lidocaine, the hemorrhoid is opened and the clot expressed or extracted with forceps. Bleeding hemorrhoids can be treated by injection sclerotherapy with 5% phenol in vegetable oil. Bleeding should cease at least temporarily.

Rubber band ligation is used for larger internal hemorrhoids or those that fail to respond to injection sclerotherapy. With mixed internal and external hemorrhoids, only the internal component should be rubber band ligated. The internal hemorrhoid is grasped and withdrawn through a stretched ¼-inch diameter band, which is released to ligate the hemorrhoid, resulting in its necrosis and sloughing. One hemorrhoid is ligated every 2 wk; 3 to 6 treatments may be required. Sometimes, multiple hemorrhoids can be ligated at a single sitting.

Infrared photocoagulation is useful for ablating small internal hemorrhoids, hemorrhoids that cannot be rubber band ligated because of pain sensitivity, or hemorrhoids that are not cured with rubber band ligation. Laser destruction, cryotherapy, and various types of electrodestruction are of unproven efficacy. Surgical hemorrhoidectomy is required for those that do not respond to other forms of therapy.

LEVATOR SYNDROME

Episodic rectal pain caused by spasm of the levator ani muscle.

Proctalgia fugax (fleeting pain in the rectum) and **coccydynia** (pain in the coccygeal region) are variants of levator syndrome. Rectal spasm causes pain, typically unrelated to defecation, usually lasting < 20 min. The pain may be brief and intense or a vague ache high in the rectum. It may occur spontaneously or with sitting and can waken the patient from sleep. The pain may feel as if it would be relieved by the passage of gas or a bowel movement. In severe cases, the pain can persist for many hours and recur frequently. The patient may have undergone various rectal operations for these symptoms, with no benefit.

Diagnosis and Treatment

Physical examination can exclude other painful rectal conditions (eg, hemorrhoids, fissures, abscesses). Physical examination is often normal, although tenderness or tightness of the levator muscle, usually on the left, may be present. Occasional cases are caused by low back or prostate disorders.

Treatment consists of explanations to the patient of the benign nature of the condition.

An acute episode may be relieved by the passage of gas or a bowel movement, by a sitz bath, or by a mild analgesic. When the symptoms are more intense, physical therapy with electrogalvanic stimulation applied to the lower rectum is usually effective. Skeletal muscle relaxants or anal sphincter massage under local or regional anesthesia can be tried, but the benefit is unclear.

PILONIDAL DISEASE

Pilonidal disease refers to an acute abscess or chronic draining sinus in the sacrococcygeal area.

Pilonidal disease usually occurs in young, hirsute, white males. One or several midline or adjacent-to-the-midline pits or sinuses occur in the skin of the sacral region and may form a cavity, often containing hair. The lesion is usually asymptomatic; infected lesions are painful.

Treatment of an acute abscess is by incision and drainage. Usually, one or more chronic draining sinuses persist and must be extirpated by excision and primary closure or, preferably, by an open technique (eg, cystotomy, marsupialization). Antibiotics are generally not needed.

PROCTITIS

Proctitis is inflammation of the rectal mucosa, which may result from infection, inflammatory bowel disease, or radiation. Symptoms are rectal discomfort and bleeding. Diagnosis is by sigmoidoscopy, usually with cultures and biopsy. Treatment depends on etiology.

Proctitis may be a manifestation of sexually transmitted disease, certain enteric infections (eg, *Campylobacter*, *Shigella*, *Salmonella*), inflammatory bowel disease, or radiation treatments; it may be associated with prior antibiotic use. Sexually transmitted pathogens produce proctitis more commonly in homosexual males. Immunocompromised patients are at particular risk for infections with herpes simplex and cytomegalovirus.

Symptoms, Signs, and Diagnosis

Typically, patients report rectal bleeding or passage of mucus. Proctitis resulting from gonorrhea, herpes simplex, or cytomegalovirus may cause intense anorectal pain.

Diagnosis requires proctoscopy or sigmoidoscopy, which may reveal an inflamed rectal mucosa. Small discrete ulcers and vesicles suggest herpes infection. Smears should be sent for culture of *Neisseria gonorrhoeae, Chlamydia* sp, enteric pathogens, and viral pathogens. Serologic tests for syphilis and stool tests for *Clostridium difficile* toxin are performed. Sometimes mucosal biopsy is needed. Colonoscopy may be valuable in some patients.

Treatment

Infective proctitis can be treated with antibiotics. Homosexual males with nonspecific proctitis may be treated empirically with ceftriaxone 125 mg IM once (or ciprofloxacin 500 mg po bid for 7 days) plus doxycycline 100 mg po bid for 7 days. Antibiotic-associated proctitis is treated with metronidazole (250 mg po qid) or vancomycin (125 mg po qid) for 7 to 10 days.

Radiation proctitis is usually effectively treated with topical formalin carefully applied to the affected mucosa. Alternative treatments include topical corticosteroids as foam (hydrocortisone 90 mg) or enemas (hydrocortisone 100 mg or methylprednisolone 40 mg) bid for 3 wk, or mesalamine (4 g) enema at bedtime for 3 to 6 wk. Mesalamine suppositories 500 mg once/day or bid, mesalamine 800 mg po tid, or sulfasalazine 500 to 1000 mg po qid for ≥ 3 wk alone or in combination with topical therapy may also be effective. Patients unresponsive to these forms of therapy may benefit from a course of systemic corticosteroids.

PRURITUS ANI

Pruritus ani is anal and perianal itching.

The perianal skin tends to itch, which can result from numerous causes (see TABLE 20–1).

Diagnosis is made from the appearance of the anal skin and relevant information from the history. The skin typically shows dullness and thickening, although the underlying pathology is often obscured by excoriation caused by scratching and secondary infection. A scraping of local skin may help disclose fungal infection, and a stool sample may help find parasites. Visible lesions may be biopsied.

TABLE 20–1. CAUSES OF PRURITUS ANI

CATEGORY	EXAMPLES
Dermatologic disorders	Psoriasis, atopic dermatitis
Topical irritants	Local anesthetics, soaps, ointments
Ingested irritants	Spices, citrus, caffeinated beverages
Fungal infection	*Candida*
Bacterial infection	Secondary infection caused by scratching
Parasites	Pinworms, scabies
Local disease	Bowen's disease, extramammary Paget's disease, cryptitis, draining fistulas
Systemic disease	Diabetes mellitus, liver disease
Hygiene-related	Poor cleansing, tight undergarments
Psychogenic	—

Foods suspected of causing pruritus ani should be eliminated from the diet. Clothing should be loose, and bed clothing light. After bowel movements, the patient should cleanse the anal area with absorbent cotton or plain soft tissue moistened with water. Liberal, frequent dusting with nonmedicated talcum powder helps combat moisture. Hydrocortisone acetate 1% ointment, applied sparingly qid, may relieve symptoms. Systemic causes and parasitic or fungal infections must be treated specifically.

RECTAL PROLAPSE AND PROCIDENTIA

Rectal prolapse is painless protrusion of the rectum through the anus. Procidentia is complete prolapse of the entire thickness of the rectum. Diagnosis is by inspection. Surgery is required to correct rectal prolapse or procidentia.

Transient, minor prolapse of just the rectal mucosa often occurs in otherwise normal infants. Mucosal prolapse in adults persists and may progressively worsen.

Procidentia is complete prolapse of the entire thickness of the rectum. The primary cause is unclear. Most patients are women > 60.

Symptoms, Signs, and Diagnosis

The most prominent symptom is protrusion. It may only occur while straining or while walking or standing. Rectal bleeding can occur, and incontinence is frequent. Pain is uncommon.

To determine the full extent of the prolapse, the doctor should examine the patient while the patient is standing or squatting and straining. Rectal procidentia can be distinguished from hemorrhoids by the presence of mucosal folds. Anal sphincter tone is usually diminished. Colonoscopy or barium enema x-rays of the colon must be performed to search for other disease. Primary neurologic disorders (eg, spinal cord tumors) must be ruled out.

Treatment

In infants and children, conservative treatment is most satisfactory. Causes of straining should be eliminated. Firmly strapping the buttocks together with tape between bowel movements usually facilitates spontaneous resolution of the prolapse. For simple mucosal prolapse in adults, the excess mucosa can be excised. For procidentia, an abdominal operation may be required. In patients who are very old or in poor health, a wire or synthetic plastic loop can encircle the sphincteric ring (Thiersch's procedure). Other perineal operations (eg, Delorme or Altemeier procedure) can be considered.

21
TUMORS OF THE GI TRACT

Various benign and malignant tumors can develop anywhere in the GI tract. Tumors of the mouth are covered on p. 842.

BENIGN ESOPHAGEAL TUMORS

Although there are many types of benign esophageal tumors, most are of little consequence except for producing annoying swallowing symptoms (see p. 108) and rarely ulceration or bleeding. Leiomyoma, the most common, may be multiple but usually has an excellent prognosis.

ESOPHAGEAL CANCER

The most common malignant esophageal tumor is squamous cell carcinoma, followed by adenocarcinoma. Symptoms are progressive dysphagia and weight loss. Diagnosis is by endoscopy, followed by CT and endoscopic ultrasound for staging. Treatment varies with stage and generally includes surgery with or without chemotherapy and radiation. Long-term survival is poor except for those with local disease.

Esophageal cancer accounts for about 13,500 cases and 12,500 deaths in the US annually.

Squamous cell carcinoma: About 8000 cases occur annually in the US. It is more common in parts of Asia and in South Africa. In the US, it is 4 to 5 times more common among blacks than whites, and 2 to 3 times more common among men than women.

The primary risk factors are alcohol ingestion and tobacco use (in any form). Other factors include achalasia, human papillomavirus, lye ingestion (resulting in stricture), sclerotherapy, Plummer-Vinson syndrome, irradiation of the esophagus, and esophageal webs. Genetic causes are unclear, but 50% of patients with tylosis (hyperkeratosis palmaris et plantaris), an autosomal dominant disorder, have esophageal cancer by age 45, 95% by age 55.

Adenocarcinoma: Adenocarcinoma occurs in the distal esophagus. Its incidence is increasing; it accounts for 50% of esophageal carcinoma in whites. It is 4 times more common among whites than blacks. Alcohol is not an important risk factor, but smoking is contributory. Adenocarcinoma of the distal esophagus is difficult to distinguish from adenocarcinoma of the gastric cardia invading the distal esophagus.

Most adenocarcinomas arise in Barrett's esophagus, which results from chronic gastroesophageal reflux disease and reflux esophagitis. In Barrett's esophagus, a metaplastic, columnar, glandular, intestine-like mucosa replaces the stratified squamous epithelium of the distal esophagus during the healing phase of acute esophagitis.

Other malignant tumors: Less common malignant tumors include spindle cell carcinoma (a poorly differentiated variant of squamous cell carcinoma), verrucous carcinoma (a well-differentiated variant of squamous cell carcinoma), pseudosarcoma, mucoepidermoid carcinoma, adenosquamous carcinoma, cylindroma (adenoid cystic carcinoma), primary oat cell carcinoma, choriocarcinoma, carcinoid tumor, sarcoma, and primary malignant melanoma.

Metastatic cancer constitutes 3% of esophageal cancer. Melanoma and breast cancer are most likely to metastasize to the esophagus; others include cancers of the head and neck, lung, stomach, liver, kidney, prostate, testis, and bone. These tumors usually seed the loose connective tissue stroma around the esophagus, whereas primary esophageal cancers begin in the mucosa or submucosa.

Symptoms and Signs

Early-stage esophageal cancer tends to be asymptomatic. When the lumen of the esophagus becomes constricted to < 14 mm, dysphagia commonly occurs. The patient first has difficulty swallowing solid food, then semisolid food, and finally liquid food and saliva; this steady progression suggests a growing malignant process rather than a spasm, benign ring, or peptic stricture. Chest pain may be present, usually radiating to the back.

Weight loss, even when the patient maintains a good appetite, is almost universal. Compression of the recurrent laryngeal nerve may lead to vocal cord paralysis and hoarseness. Compression of sympathetic nerves may lead to Horner's syndrome, and nerve compression elsewhere may produce spinal pain, hiccups, or paralysis of the diaphragm. Malignant pleural effusions or pulmonary metastasis may cause dyspnea. Intraluminal tumor involvement may produce odynophagia, vomiting, hematemesis, melena, iron deficiency anemia, aspiration, and cough. Fistulas between the esophagus and tracheobronchial tree may produce lung abscess and pneumonia. Other findings may include superior vena cava syndrome, malignant ascites, and bone pain.

Lymphatic spread to internal jugular, cervical, supraclavicular, mediastinal, and celiac nodes is common. The tumor usually metastasizes to lung and liver and occasionally to distant sites (eg, bone, heart, brain, adrenal glands, kidneys, peritoneum).

Diagnosis

There are no screening tests. Patients suspected of having esophageal cancer should have endoscopy with cytology and biopsy. Although barium x-ray may demonstrate an obstructive lesion, endoscopy is required for biopsy and tissue diagnosis.

Patients in whom cancer is identified require CT of the chest and abdomen to determine extent of tumor spread. If results are negative for metastasis, endoscopic ultrasound should be performed to determine the depth of the tumor in the esophageal wall and regional lymph node involvement. Findings guide therapy and help determine prognosis.

Basic blood tests, including CBC, electrolytes, and liver function, should be performed.

Prognosis and Treatment

Prognosis depends greatly on stage, but overall is poor (5-yr survival: < 5%) because many patients present with advanced disease. Patients with cancer restricted to the mucosa have about an 80% survival rate, which drops to < 50% with submucosal involvement, 20% with extension to the muscularis propria, 7% with extension to adjacent structures, and < 3% with distant metastases.

Treatment decisions depend on tumor staging, size, location, and the patient's wishes (many choose to forgo aggressive treatment).

General principles: Patients with stage 0, I, or IIa disease (see TABLE 21–1) respond well to surgical resection; chemotherapy and radiation provide no additional benefit. Those with stage IIb and III have poor survival with surgery alone; response and survival are enhanced by preoperative (neoadjuvant) use of radiation and chemotherapy to reduce tumor volume prior to surgery. Patients unable or unwilling to undergo surgery may receive some benefit from combined radiation and chemotherapy. Radiation or chemotherapy alone is of little benefit. Patients with stage IV disease require palliation and should not undergo surgery.

After treatment, patients are screened for recurrence by endoscopy and CT of the neck, chest, and abdomen at 6-mo intervals for 3 yr and annually thereafter.

Patients with Barrett's esophagus require intense long-term treatment for gastroesophageal reflux disease (see p. 112) and endoscopic surveillance for malignant transformation at 3- to 12-mo intervals depending on the degree of metaplasia.

Surgery: En bloc resection for cure requires removal of the entire tumor, proximal and distal margins of normal tissue, all potentially malignant lymph nodes, and a portion of the proximal stomach sufficient to contain the distal draining lymphatics. The procedure requires gastric pull-up with esophagogastric anastomosis, small-bowel interposition, or colonic interposition. Pyloroplasty is required to ensure proper gastric drainage because esophagectomy necessarily results in bilateral vagotomy. This extensive surgery may be poorly tolerated by patients > 75 yr, particularly those with underlying cardiac or pulmonary disease (ejection fraction < 40%, or FEV_1 < 1.5 L/min). Overall, operative mortality is about 5%.

Complications of surgery include anastomotic leaks, fistulas, and strictures, bilious gastroesophageal reflux, and dumping syndrome. The burning chest pain of bile reflux after distal esophagectomy can be more annoying than the original symptom of dysphagia and may require subsequent Roux-en-Y jejunostomy for bile diversion. An interposed segment of small bowel or colon in the chest has a tenuous blood supply, and torsion, ischemia, or gangrene of the interposed bowel may result.

External beam radiation therapy: Radiation is usually used in combination with chemotherapy for patients who are poor candidates for curative surgery, including those with advanced disease. Radiation is contraindicated in patients with tracheoesophageal

TABLE 21–1. STAGING ESOPHAGEAL CANCER

STAGE	TUMOR (Maximum Penetration)	REGIONAL LYMPH NODE METASTASIS	DISTANT METASTASIS
0	Tis	N0	M0
I	T1	N0	M0
II	T2 or T3	N0	M0
III	T3 or T4	N1	M0
IV	Any T	Any N	M1

TNM classification: Tis = carcinoma in situ; T1 = lamina propria or submucosa; T2 = muscularis propria; T3 = adventitia; T4 = adjacent structures.
N0 = none; N1 = present.
M0 = none; M1 = present.

fistula because tumor shrinkage enlarges the fistula. Similarly, patients with vascular encasement by tumor may experience massive hemorrhage with tumor shrinkage. During the early stages of radiation therapy, edema may worsen esophageal obstruction, dysphagia, and odynophagia. This problem may require esophageal dilation or preradiation placement of a percutaneous gastrostomy feeding tube. Other side effects of radiation therapy include nausea, vomiting, anorexia, fatigue, esophagitis, excess esophageal mucus production, xerostomia, stricture, radiation pneumonitis, radiation pericarditis, myocarditis, and myelitis (spinal cord inflammation).

Chemotherapy: Tumors are poorly responsive to chemotherapy alone. Response rates (defined as ≥ 50% reduction in all measurable areas of tumor) vary from 10 to 40%, but responses generally are incomplete (minor shrinkage of tumor) and temporary. No drug is notably more effective than another.

Most commonly, cisplatin and 5-fluorouracil are used in combination. However, several other drugs, including mitomycin, doxorubicin, vindesine, bleomycin, and methotrexate, also are active against squamous cell carcinoma.

Palliation: Palliation is directed at reducing esophageal obstruction sufficiently to allow oral intake. Suffering from esophageal obstruction can be significant, with salivation and recurrent aspiration. Options include manual dilation procedures (bougienage), orally inserted stents, radiation therapy, laser photocoagulation, and photodynamic therapy. In some cases, cervical esophagostomy with feeding jejunostomy is required.

Relief provided by esophageal dilation rarely lasts more than a few days. Flexible metal mesh stents are more effective at maintaining esophageal patency. Some plastic-coated models can also be used to occlude tracheoesophageal fistulas, and some are available with a valve that prevents reflux when the stent must be placed near the lower esophageal sphincter.

Endoscopic laser therapy can palliate dysphagia by burning a central channel through the tumor and can be repeated if needed. Photodynamic therapy uses an injection of porfimer sodium, a hematoporphyrin derivative that is taken up by tissues and acts as a photosensitizer. When activated by a laser beam directed on the tumor, this substance releases cytotoxic oxygen singlets that destroy tumor cells. Patients receiving this treatment must avoid sun exposure for 6 wk after treatment because the skin also is sensitized to light.

Supportive care: Nutritional support by enteral or parenteral supplementation enhances the tolerability and feasibility of all treatments. An endoscopically or surgically placed feeding tube provides a more distal route for feeding when the esophagus is obstructed.

Because nearly all cases of esophageal cancer are fatal, end-of-life care should always aim to control symptoms, especially pain and inability to swallow secretions (see also p. 2764). At some point, many patients need substantial doses of opioids. Patients should be advised to make end-of-life care decisions early in the course of disease and to record their wishes in an advance directive.

STOMACH CANCER

Etiology of stomach cancer is multifactorial, but *Helicobacter pylori* plays a significant role. Symptoms include early satiety, obstruction, and bleeding but tend to occur late in the disease. Diagnosis is by endoscopy, followed by CT and endoscopic ultrasound for staging. Treatment is mainly surgery; chemotherapy may provide a temporary response. Long-term survival is poor except for those with local disease.

Stomach cancer accounts for about 21,000 cases and 12,000 deaths in the US annually. Gastric adenocarcinoma accounts for 95% of malignant tumors of the stomach; less common are localized gastric lymphomas (see p. 1116) and leiomyosarcomas. Stomach cancer is the 2nd most common cancer worldwide, but the incidence varies widely; it is extremely high in Japan, Chile, and Iceland. In the US, incidence has declined in recent decades to the 7th most common cause of death from cancer. In the US, it is most common in blacks, Hispanics, and American Indians. Its incidence increases with age; >75% of patients are >50 yr.

Etiology and Pathophysiology

H. pylori infection is the cause of most stomach cancer. Autoimmune atrophic gastritis (see p. 120) and various genetic factors (see GIST tumors on p. 172) are also risk factors.

Gastric polyps can be precursors of cancer. Inflammatory polyps may develop in patients taking NSAIDs, and fundic foveolar polyps are common in patients taking proton pump inhibitors. Adenomatous polyps, particularly multiple ones, although rare, are the most likely to develop malignancy. Malignancy is particularly likely if an adenomatous polyp is >2 cm in diameter or has a villous histology. Because malignant transformation cannot be detected by inspection, all polyps seen at endoscopy should be removed. The incidence of stomach cancer is generally decreased in patients with duodenal ulcer.

Gastric adenocarcinomas can be classified by gross appearance: (1) Protruding—the tumor is polypoid or fungating. (2) Penetrating—the tumor is ulcerated. (3) Superficial spreading—the tumor spreads along the mucosa or infiltrates superficially within the wall of the stomach. (4) Linitis plastica—the tumor infiltrates the stomach wall with an associated fibrous reaction that produces a rigid "leather bottle" stomach. (5) Miscellaneous—the tumor demonstrates characteristics of two or more of the other types; this classification is the largest. Protruding tumors have a better prognosis than spreading tumors because they become symptomatic earlier.

Symptoms and Signs

Initial symptoms are nonspecific, often consisting of dyspepsia suggestive of peptic ulcer. Patients and physicians alike tend to dismiss symptoms or treat the patient for acid disease. Later, early satiety (fullness after ingesting a small amount of food) may occur if the cancer obstructs the pyloric region or if the stomach becomes nondistensible secondary to linitis plastica. Dysphagia may result if cancer in the cardiac region of the stomach obstructs the esophageal outlet. Loss of weight or strength, usually resulting from dietary restriction, is common. Massive hematemesis or melena is uncommon, but secondary anemia may follow occult blood loss. Occasionally, the first symptoms are caused by metastasis (eg, jaundice, ascites, fractures).

Physical findings may be unremarkable or limited to heme-positive stools. Late in the course, abnormalities include an epigastric mass; umbilical, left supraclavicular or left axillary lymph nodes; hepatomegaly; and an ovarian or rectal mass. Pulmonary, CNS, and bone lesions may occur.

Diagnosis

Differential diagnosis commonly includes peptic ulcer and its complications.

Patients suspected of having stomach cancer should have endoscopy with multiple biopsies and brush cytology. Occasionally, a biopsy limited to the mucosa misses tumor tissue in the submucosa. X-rays, particularly double-contrast barium studies, may demonstrate lesions, but rarely obviate the need for subsequent endoscopy.

Patients in whom cancer is identified require CT of the chest and abdomen to determine extent of tumor spread. If CT is negative for metastasis, endoscopic ultrasound should be performed to determine the depth of the tumor and regional lymph node involvement. Findings guide therapy and help determine prognosis.

Basic blood tests, including CBC, electrolytes, and liver function tests, should be performed to assess anemia, hydration, general condition, and possible liver metastases. Carcinoembryonic antigen (CEA) should be measured before and after surgery.

Screening with endoscopy is used in high-risk populations (eg, Japanese) but is not recommended in the US. Follow-up screening for recurrence in treated patients consists of endoscopy and CT of the chest, abdomen, and pelvis. If an elevated CEA dropped after surgery, follow-up should include CEA levels; a rise signifies recurrence.

Prognosis

Prognosis depends greatly on stage but overall is poor (5-yr survival: < 5 to 15%) because most patients present with advanced disease. If tumor is limited to the mucosa or submucosa, 5-yr survival may be as high as 80%. For tumors involving local lymph nodes, survival is 20 to 40%. More widespread disease is almost always fatal within 1 yr. Gastric lymphomas have a better prognosis and are discussed in Ch. 143 (see p. 1116).

Treatment

Treatment decisions depend on tumor staging and the patient's wishes (some may choose to forgo aggressive treatment—see p. 2768).

Curative surgery involves removal of most or all of the stomach and adjacent lymph nodes and is reasonable in patients with disease limited to the stomach and perhaps the regional lymph nodes (< 50% of patients). Adjuvant chemotherapy or combined chemotherapy and radiation therapy after surgery is of uncertain benefit.

Resection of locally advanced regional disease results in a 10-mo median survival (vs. 3 to 4 mo without resection).

Metastasis or extensive nodal involvement precludes curative surgery, and at most, palliative procedures should be undertaken. However, the true extent of tumor spread often is not recognized until curative surgery is attempted. Palliative surgery typically consists of a gastroenterostomy to bypass a pyloric obstruction and should be performed only if the patient's quality of life can be improved. In patients not undergoing surgery, combination chemotherapy regimens (5-fluorouracil, doxorubicin, mitomycin, cisplatin, or leucovorin in various combinations) may produce temporary response but little improvement in 5-yr survival. Radiation therapy is of limited benefit.

GASTROINTESTINAL STROMAL TUMORS

Gastrointestinal stromal tumors (GIST) are tumors of the GI tract derived from mesenchymal precursor cells in the gut wall. They result from mutations of a growth factor receptor gene, *C-KIT*. Some are caused by previous radiation therapy to the abdomen for other tumors.

Tumors are slow growing, and malignant potential varies from minimal to significant. Most (60 to 70%) occur in the stomach, 20 to 25% in the small bowel, and a small number in the esophagus, colon, and rectum. Average age at presentation is 50 to 60.

Symptoms vary with location but include bleeding, dyspepsia, and obstruction. Diagnosis is usually by endoscopy, with biopsy and endoscopic ultrasound for staging. Treatment is surgical removal. The role of radiation and chemotherapy is unclear, but the tyrosine kinase inhibitor imatinib has been beneficial.

SMALL-BOWEL TUMORS

Small-bowel tumors account for 1 to 5% of GI tumors.

Benign tumors include leiomyomas, lipomas, neurofibromas, and fibromas. All may cause abdominal distention, pain, bleeding, diarrhea or, if obstruction develops, vomiting. Polyps are not as common as in the colon.

Adenocarcinoma, a malignant tumor, is uncommon. Usually it arises in the duodenum or proximal jejunum and causes minimal symptoms. In patients with Crohn's disease, the tumors tend to occur distally and in bypassed or inflamed loops of bowel; adenocarcinoma occurs more often in Crohn's disease of the small bowel than in Crohn's disease of the colon.

Primary malignant lymphoma (see p. 1116) arising in the ileum may produce a long, rigid segment. Small-bowel lymphomas arise often in long-standing untreated celiac sprue.

Carcinoid tumors (see p. 1312) occur most often in the small bowel, particularly the ileum, and the appendix, and in these locations are often malignant. Multiple tumors occur in 50% of cases. Of those > 2 cm in diameter, 80% have metastasized locally or to the liver by the time of operation. About 30%

of small-bowel carcinoids cause obstruction, pain, bleeding, or the carcinoid syndrome. Treatment is surgical resection; repeat operations may be required.

Kaposi's sarcoma (see p. 1024), first described as a disease of elderly Jewish and Italian men, occurs in an aggressive form in Africans, transplant recipients, and AIDS patients, who have GI tract involvement 40 to 60% of the time. Lesions may occur anywhere in the GI tract but usually in the stomach, small bowel, or distal colon. GI lesions usually are asymptomatic, but bleeding, diarrhea, protein-losing enteropathy, and intussusception may occur. A second primary intestinal malignancy occurs in ≤ 20% of patients; most often it is lymphocytic leukemia, non-Hodgkin's lymphoma, Hodgkin's disease, or adenocarcinoma of the GI tract. Treatment depends on the cell type and location and extent of the lesions.

Diagnosis and Treatment

Enteroclysis is probably the most common study for mass lesions of the small bowel. Push endoscopy of the small bowel with an enteroscope may be used to visualize and biopsy tumors. Capsule video endoscopy can help identify small-bowel lesions, particularly bleeding sites; a swallowed capsule transmits 2 images/sec to an external recorder. The capsule is not useful in the stomach or colon because it tumbles in these larger organs.

Treatment is surgical resection. Electrocautery, thermal obliteration, or laser phototherapy at the time of enteroscopy or surgery may be an alternative to resection.

POLYPS OF THE COLON AND RECTUM

An intestinal polyp is any mass of tissue that arises from the bowel wall and protrudes into the lumen. Most are asymptomatic except for minor bleeding, which is usually occult. The main concern is malignant transformation; most colon cancers arise in a previously benign adenomatous polyp. Diagnosis is by endoscopy. Treatment is endoscopic removal.

Polyps may be sessile or pedunculated and vary considerably in size. Incidence of polyps ranges from 7 to 50%; the higher figure includes very small polyps (usually hyperplastic polyps or adenomas) found at autopsy. Polyps, often multiple, occur most commonly in the rectum and sigmoid and decrease in frequency toward the cecum. Multiple polyps may represent familial adenomatous polyposis (see p. 174). About 25% of patients with cancer of the large bowel also have satellite adenomatous polyps.

Adenomatous (neoplastic) polyps are of greatest concern. Such lesions are classified histologically as tubular adenomas, tubulovillous adenomas (villoglandular polyps), or villous adenomas. The likelihood of malignancy in an adenomatous polyp at the time of discovery is related to size, histologic type, and degree of dysplasia; a 1.5-cm tubular adenoma has a 2% risk of containing a malignancy, vs. 35% risk in 3-cm villous adenomas.

Non-adenomatous (non-neoplastic) polyps include hyperplastic polyps, hamartomas, juvenile polyps, pseudopolyps, lipomas, leiomyomas, and other rarer tumors. **Peutz-Jeghers syndrome** is an autosomal dominant disease with multiple hamartomatous polyps in the stomach, small bowel, and colon. Symptoms include melanotic pigmentation of the skin and mucous membranes, especially of the lips and gums. Juvenile polyps occur in children, typically outgrow their blood supply and autoamputate some time during or after puberty. Treatment is required only for uncontrollable bleeding or intussusception. Inflammatory polyps and pseudopolyps occur in chronic ulcerative colitis and in Crohn's disease of the colon. Multiple juvenile polyps (but not sporadic ones) convey an increased cancer risk. The specific number of polyps resulting in increased risk is not known.

Symptoms, Signs, and Diagnosis

Most polyps are asymptomatic. Rectal bleeding, usually occult and rarely massive, is the most frequent complaint. Cramps, abdominal pain, or obstruction may occur with a large lesion. Rectal polyps may be palpable by digital examination. Occasionally, a polyp on a long pedicle may prolapse through the anus. Large villous adenomas may rarely cause watery diarrhea that may result in hypokalemia.

Diagnosis is usually made by colonoscopy. Barium enema, particularly double-contrast examination, is effective, but colonoscopy is preferred because polyps also may be removed during that procedure. Because rectal polyps are often multiple and may coexist with cancer, complete colonoscopy to the cecum is mandatory even if a distal lesion is found by flexible sigmoidoscopy.

Prevention and Treatment

Aspirin and COX-2 inhibitors may help prevent formation of new polyps in patients with polyps or colon cancer.

Polyps should be removed completely with a snare or electrosurgical biopsy forceps during total colonoscopy; complete excision is particularly important for large villous adenomas, which have a high potential for malignancy. If colonoscopic removal is unsuccessful, laparotomy should be performed.

Subsequent treatment depends on the histology of the polyp. If dysplastic epithelium does not invade the muscularis mucosa, the line of resection in the polyp's stalk is clear, and the lesion is well differentiated, endoscopic excision and close endoscopic follow-up should suffice. Patients with deeper invasion, an unclear resection line, or a poorly differentiated lesion should have segmental resection of the colon. Because invasion through the muscularis mucosa provides access to lymphatics and increases the potential for lymph node metastasis, such patients should have further evaluation (as in colon cancer, below).

The scheduling of follow-up examinations after polypectomy is controversial. Most authorities recommend total colonoscopy annually for 2 yr (or barium enema if total colonoscopy is impossible), with removal of newly discovered lesions. If two annual examinations are negative for new lesions, colonoscopy is recommended every 2 to 3 yr.

Familial Adenomatous Polyposis

Familial adenomatous polyposis is a hereditary disorder causing numerous colonic polyps and resulting in colon carcinoma by age 40. Patients are usually asymptomatic but may have heme-positive stool. Diagnosis is by colonoscopy and genetic testing. Treatment is colectomy.

Familial adenomatous polyposis (FAP) is an autosomal dominant disease in which ≥ 100 adenomatous polyps carpet the colon and rectum. The disorder occurs in 1 in 8,000 to 14,000 people. Polyps are present in 50% of patients by age 15, and 95% by 35. Malignancy develops before age 40 in nearly all untreated patients.

Patients also can develop various extracolonic manifestations (previously termed Gardner's syndrome), both benign and malignant. Benign manifestations include desmoid tumors, osteomas of the skull or mandible, sebaceous cysts, and adenomas in other parts of the GI tract. Patients are at increased risk for malignancy in the duodenum (5 to 11%), pancreas (2%), thyroid (2%), brain (medulloblastoma in < 1%), and liver (hepatoblastoma in 0.7% of children < 5).

Symptoms, Signs, and Diagnosis

Many patients are asymptomatic, but rectal bleeding, typically occult, occurs. Diagnosis is made by finding > 100 polyps on colonoscopy. Diagnosed patients should have genetic testing to identify the specific mutation, which should then be sought for in 1st-degree relatives. If genetic testing is unavailable, relatives should be screened with annual sigmoidoscopy beginning at age 12, reducing frequency with each decade. If no polyps are evident by age 50, screening frequency is then the same as for average-risk patients.

Children of parents with FAP should be screened for hepatoblastoma from birth to age 5 yr with annual serum fetoprotein levels and possibly liver ultrasound.

Treatment

Colectomy should be performed at the time of diagnosis. Total proctocolectomy, either with ileostomy or mucosal proctectomy and ileoanal pouch, eliminates the risk of cancer. If subtotal colectomy (removal of most of the colon, leaving the rectum) with ileorectal anastomosis is performed, the rectal remnant must be inspected every 3 to 6 mo; new polyps must be excised or fulgurated. Aspirin or COX-2 inhibitors may inhibit new polyp formation. If new ones appear too rapidly or prolifically to remove, excision of the rectum and permanent ileostomy are needed.

After colectomy, patients should have upper endoscopy every 6 mo to 4 yr, depending on the number of polyps (if any) in the stomach and duodenum. Annual physical examination of the thyroid, and possibly ultrasound, also is recommended.

COLORECTAL CANCER

Colorectal cancer is extremely common. Symptoms include blood in the stool or

change in bowel habits. Screening is with fecal occult blood testing. Diagnosis is by colonoscopy. Treatment is surgical resection and chemotherapy for nodal involvement.

Colorectal cancer accounts for about 130,000 cases and 57,000 deaths in the US annually. In Western countries, the colon and rectum account for more new cases of cancer per year than any anatomic site except the lung. Incidence begins to rise at age 40 and peaks at age 60 to 75. Overall, 70% of cases occur in the rectum and sigmoid, and 95% are adenocarcinomas. Colon cancer is more common in women; rectal cancer is more common in men. Synchronous cancers (more than one) occur in 5% of patients.

Etiology and Epidemiology

Colorectal cancer most often occurs as transformation within adenomatous polyps. About 80% of cases are sporadic, and 20% have an inheritable component. Predisposing factors include chronic ulcerative colitis and granulomatous colitis; the risk of cancer increases with the duration of these disorders.

Populations with a high incidence of colorectal cancer eat low-fiber diets that are high in animal protein, fat, and refined carbohydrates. Carcinogens may be ingested in the diet but are more likely produced by bacterial action on dietary substances or biliary or intestinal secretions. The exact mechanism is unknown.

Colorectal cancer spreads by direct extension through the bowel wall, hematogenous metastasis, regional lymph node metastasis, perineural spread, and intraluminal metastasis.

Symptoms and Signs

Colorectal adenocarcinoma grows slowly, and a long interval elapses before it is large enough to produce symptoms. Symptoms depend on lesion's location, type, extent, and complications.

The right colon has a large caliber, thin wall and its contents are liquid; thus, obstruction is a late event. Bleeding is usually occult. Fatigue and weakness caused by severe anemia may be the only complaints. Tumors sometimes grow large enough to be palpable through the abdominal wall before other symptoms appear.

The left colon has a smaller lumen, the feces are semisolid, and cancer tends to encircle the bowel, causing alternating constipation and increased stool frequency or diarrhea. Partial obstruction with colicky abdominal pain or complete obstruction may be the presenting picture. The stool may be streaked or mixed with blood. Some patients present with symptoms of perforation, usually walled off (focal pain and tenderness), or rarely with diffuse peritonitis.

In rectal cancer, the most common presenting symptom is bleeding with defecation. Whenever rectal bleeding occurs, even with obvious hemorrhoids or known diverticular disease, coexisting cancer must be ruled out. Tenesmus or a sensation of incomplete evacuation may be present. Pain is common with perirectal involvement.

Some patients first present with signs and symptoms of metastatic disease (eg, hepatomegaly, ascites, supraclavicular lymph node enlargement).

Screening and Diagnosis

Screening: Early diagnosis depends on routine examination, particularly fecal occult blood (FOB) testing. Cancer detected by this method tends to be at an earlier stage and hence more curable. For average-risk patients, FOB testing should be performed annually after age 50, with flexible sigmoidoscopy every 5 yr. Some authorities recommend colonoscopy every 10 yr instead of sigmoidoscopy. Colonoscopy every 3 yr may be even better. Screening of patients with high-risk conditions (eg, ulcerative colitis) is discussed under the specific condition.

Diagnosis: Patients with positive FOB tests require colonoscopy, as do those with lesions seen on sigmoidoscopy or barium study. All lesions should be completely removed for histologic examination. If a lesion is sessile or not removable at colonoscopy, surgical excision should be strongly considered.

Barium enema x-ray, particularly a double-contrast study, can detect many lesions but is somewhat less accurate than colonoscopy and is not preferred as an initial diagnostic test.

Once cancer is diagnosed, patients should have abdominal CT, chest x-ray, and routine laboratory tests to seek metastatic disease, anemia, and evaluate overall condition.

Elevated serum carcinoembryonic antigen (CEA) levels are present in 70% of patients with colorectal cancer, but this test is not specific and therefore not recommended for screening. However, if CEA is high preoperatively and low after removal of a colon tumor, monitoring CEA may help to detect recurrence earlier. CA 19-9 and CA 125 are other tumor markers that may be similarly used.

Prognosis and Treatment

Prognosis depends greatly on stage (see TABLE 21–2). The 10-yr survival rate for cancer limited to the mucosa approaches 90%; with extension through the bowel wall, 70 to 80%; with positive lymph nodes, 30 to 50%; with metastatic disease < 20%.

Surgery: Surgery for cure can be attempted in the 70% of patients presenting without metastatic disease. Attempt to cure consists of wide resection of the tumor and its regional lymphatic drainage with reanastomosis of bowel segments. If there is ≤ 5 cm of normal bowel present between the lesion and the anal verge, an abdominoperineal resection is performed, with permanent colostomy.

Resection of a limited number (1 to 3) of liver metastases is recommended in select nondebilitated patients as a subsequent procedure. Criteria include those whose primary tumor has been resected, whose liver metastases are in one hepatic lobe, and who have no extrahepatic metastases. Only a small number of patients with liver metastases meet these criteria, but 5-yr postoperative survival is 25%.

Adjuvant therapy: Chemotherapy (typically 5-fluorouracil and leucovorin) improves survival by 10 to 30% in colon cancer patients with positive lymph nodes. Rectal cancer patients with 1 to 4 positive lymph nodes benefit from combined radiation and chemotherapy; when > 4 positive lymph nodes are found, combined modalities are less effective. Preoperative radiation therapy and chemotherapy to improve the resectability rate of rectal cancer or decrease the incidence of lymph node metastasis are gaining favor.

Follow-up: Postoperatively, colonoscopy should be performed annually for 5 yr, and every 3 yr thereafter if no polyps or tumors are found. If preoperative colonoscopy was incomplete because of an obstructing cancer, a "completion" colonoscopy should be performed 3 mo after surgery.

Additional screening for recurrence should include history, physical examination, and laboratory tests (CBC, liver function tests) every 3 mo for 3 yr and then every 6 mo for 2 yr. Imaging studies (CT or MRI) are often recommended at 1-yr intervals but are of uncertain benefit for routine follow-up in the absence of abnormalities on examination or blood tests.

Palliation: When curative surgery is not possible or the patient is an unacceptable surgical risk, limited palliative surgery (eg, to relieve obstruction or resect a perforated area) may be indicated; median survival is 7 mo. Some obstructing tumors can be debulked by endoscopic laser treatment or electrocoagulation or held open by stents. Chemotherapy may shrink tumors and prolong life for several months.

Other drugs, such as irinotecan (camptosar), oxaliplatin, levamisole, methotrexate, folinic acid, celecoxib, thalidomide, and capecitabine (a 5-fluorouracil precursor),

TABLE 21–2. STAGING COLORECTAL CANCER

STAGE	TUMOR (Maximum Penetration)	REGIONAL LYMPH NODE METASTASIS	DISTANT METASTASIS
0	Tis	N0	M0
I	T1 or T2	N0	M0
II	T3	N0	M0
III	Any T or	Any N	M0
	T4	N0	M0
IV	Any T	Any N	M1

TNM classification: Tis = carcinoma in situ; T1 = submucosa; T2 = muscularis propria; T3 = penetrates all layers (for rectal cancer, includes perirectal tissue); T4 = adjacent organs or peritoneum.

N0 = none; N1 = 1 to 3 regional nodes; N2 = ≥ 4 regional nodes; N3 = apical or vascular trunk nodes.

M0 = none; M1 = present.

have been investigated. No regimen is clearly more effective for metastatic colorectal cancer. Chemotherapy for advanced colon cancer should be managed by an experienced chemotherapist who has access to investigational drugs.

When metastases are confined to the liver, ambulatory hepatic artery infusion with floxuridine or radioactive microspheres via an implantable subcutaneous pump or an external pump worn on the belt may offer more benefit than systemic chemotherapy; however, these therapies are of uncertain benefit. When metastases are also extrahepatic, intrahepatic arterial chemotherapy offers no advantage over systemic chemotherapy.

Anorectal Cancer

The most common anorectal cancer is adenocarcinoma. Squamous cell (nonkeratinizing squamous cell or basaloid) carcinoma of the anorectum accounts for 3 to 5% of distal large-bowel cancers. Basal cell carcinoma, Bowen's disease (intradermal carcinoma), extramammary Paget's disease, cloacogenic carcinoma, and malignant melanoma are less common. Other tumors include lymphoma and various sarcomas. Metastasis occurs along the lymphatics of the rectum and into the inguinal lymph nodes.

Risk factors include infection with human papillomavirus (HPV), chronic fistulas, irradiated anal skin, leukoplakia, lymphogranuloma venereum, and condyloma acuminatum. Gay men practicing receptive anal intercourse are at increased risk. Patients with HPV infection may manifest dysplasia in slightly abnormal or normal-appearing anal epithelium ("anal intraepithelial neoplasia," histologically graded I, II, or III). These changes are more common in HIV-infected patients, particularly gay men. Higher grades may progress to invasive carcinoma. It is unclear whether early recognition and eradication improve long-term outcome; hence, screening recommendations are unclear.

Wide local excision is often satisfactory treatment of perianal carcinomas. Combination chemotherapy and radiation therapy result in a high rate of cure when used for anal squamous and cloacogenic tumors. Abdominoperineal resection is indicated when radiation and chemotherapy do not result in complete regression of tumor and there are no metastases outside of the radiation field.

Hereditary Nonpolyposis Colorectal Carcinoma

Hereditary nonpolyposis colorectal carcinoma (HNPCC) is an autosomal dominant disorder responsible for 3 to 5% of cases of colorectal cancer. Symptoms, initial diagnosis, and treatment are similar to other forms of colorectal cancer. HNPCC is suspected by history and confirmed by genetic testing. Patients also require surveillance for other malignancies, particularly endometrial and ovarian cancer.

Patients with one of several known mutations have a 70 to 80% lifetime risk of developing colorectal cancer (CRC). Compared to sporadic forms of colon cancer, HNPCC occurs at a younger age (mid 40s), and the lesion is more likely to be proximal to the splenic flexure. The precursor lesion is usually a single colonic adenoma, unlike the multiple adenomas present in patients with familial adenomatous polyposis (FAP), the other main hereditary form of CRC.

However, similar to FAP, numerous extracolonic manifestations occur. Nonmalignant disorders include café au lait spots, sebaceous gland tumors, and keratoacanthomas. Common associated malignancies include endometrial and ovarian tumors (39% and 9% risk, respectively, by age 70). Patients also have an elevated risk of cancer of the ureter, renal pelvis, stomach, biliary tree, and small bowel.

Symptoms, Signs, and Diagnosis

Symptoms and signs are similar to other forms of colorectal cancer, and diagnosis and management of the tumor itself are the same. The specific diagnosis of HNPCC is confirmed by genetic testing. However, deciding who to test is difficult because (unlike FAP) there is no typical clinical appearance. Thus, suspicion of HNPCC requires a detailed family history, which should be obtained in all younger patients identified with CRC.

To meet the Amsterdam II criteria for HNPCC, all three of the following historical elements must be present: (1) three or more relatives with CRC or an HNPCC-associated malignancy, (2) colorectal cancer involving at least two generations, and (3) at least one case of CRC before age 50.

Patients meeting these criteria should have their tumor tissue tested for a DNA abnormality termed microsatellite instability (MSI). If

MSI is present, genetic testing for specific HNPCC mutations is indicated. Other authorities use additional criteria (eg, Bethesda criteria) to initiate MSI testing. If MSI testing is not available locally, the patient should be referred to a center where it is.

Patients with confirmed HNPCC require ongoing screening for other malignancies. For endometrial cancer, annual endometrial aspiration or transvaginal ultrasound is recommended. For ovarian cancer, options include annual transvaginal ultrasound and serum CA 125 levels. Prophylactic hysterectomy and oophorectomy are also an option. Urinalysis may be used to screen for renal tumors.

First-degree relatives of patients with HNPCC should have colonoscopy every 1 to 2 yr beginning in their 20s, and annually after age 40. Female 1st-degree relatives should be tested annually for endometrial and ovarian cancer. More distant blood relatives should have genetic testing; if results are negative, they should have colonoscopy at the frequency for average-risk patients.

PANCREATIC CANCER

Pancreatic cancer, primarily ductal adenocarcinoma, accounts for about 30,500 cases and 29,700 deaths in the US annually. Symptoms include weight loss, abdominal pain, and jaundice. Diagnosis is by CT. Treatment is surgical resection and adjuvant chemotherapy and radiation therapy. Prognosis is poor because disease is often advanced at the time of diagnosis.

Most pancreatic cancers are exocrine tumors that develop from ductal and acinar cells. Pancreatic endocrine tumors are discussed below.

Adenocarcinomas of the exocrine pancreas arise from duct cells 9 times more often than from acinar cells; 80% occur in the head of the gland. Adenocarcinomas appear at the mean age of 55 yr and occur 1.5 to 2 times more often in men. Prominent risk factors include smoking, a history of chronic pancreatitis, and possibly long-standing diabetes mellitus (primarily in women). Heredity plays some role. Alcohol and caffeine consumption do not appear to be risk factors.

Symptoms and Signs

Symptoms occur late; by diagnosis, 90% of patients have locally advanced tumors that have involved retroperitoneal structures, spread to regional lymph nodes, or metastasized to the liver or lung.

Most patients have severe upper abdominal pain, which usually radiates to the back. The pain may be relieved by bending forward or assuming the fetal position. Weight loss is common. Adenocarcinomas of the head of the pancreas produce obstructive jaundice (often causing pruritus) in 80 to 90% of patients. Cancer in the body and tail may cause splenic vein obstruction, resulting in splenomegaly, gastric and esophageal varices, and GI hemorrhage. The cancer causes diabetes in 25 to 50% of patients, leading to symptoms of glucose intolerance (eg, polyuria and polydipsia).

Diagnosis

The preferred tests are an abdominal helical CT or MRI of the pancreas (MRCP). If CT or MRCP demonstrates unresectable or metastatic disease, a percutaneous needle aspiration of an accessible lesion might be considered to obtain a tissue diagnosis. If CT demonstrates a potentially resectable tumor or no tumor, MRCP or endoscopic ultrasound may be used to stage disease or detect small tumors not visible with CT. Patients with obstructive jaundice may have ERCP as the first diagnostic procedure.

Routine laboratory tests should be obtained. Elevation of alkaline phosphatase and bilirubin indicate bile duct obstruction or liver metastases. Pancreas-associated antigen CA 19-9 may be used to follow patients diagnosed with pancreatic carcinoma and screen those at high risk. However, this test is not sensitive or specific enough to be used for population screening. Elevated levels should drop with successful treatment; subsequent increases indicate progression. Amylase and lipase levels are usually normal.

Prognosis and Treatment

Prognosis varies with stage, but overall is poor (5-yr survival: < 2%) because many patients have advanced disease at the time of diagnosis.

About 80 to 90% of patients are considered surgically unresectable at time of diagnosis because of metastases or invasion of major blood vessels. Depending on location of the tumor, the procedure of choice is most commonly a Whipple's operation (pancreaticoduodenectomy). Adjuvant therapy with 5-fluorouracil (5-FU) and external beam radiation therapy is typically given, resulting in about 40% 2-yr and 25% 5-yr survival. This combination is also used for patients with localized but unresectable tumors and results in median survival of about 1 yr. Newer drugs (eg, gemcitabine) may be more effective than 5-FU–based chemotherapy, but no drug, singly or in combination, is clearly superior. Patients with hepatic or distant metastases may be offered chemotherapy as part of an investigational program, but the outlook is dismal with or without such treatment and some patients may choose to forego it.

If an unresectable tumor is found at operation and gastroduodenal or bile duct obstruction is present or pending, a double gastric and biliary bypass operation is usually performed to relieve obstruction. In patients with inoperable lesions and jaundice, endoscopic placement of a bile duct stent relieves jaundice. However, surgical bypass should be considered in patients with unresectable lesions if life expectancy is > 6 to 7 mo because of complications associated with stents.

Symptomatic treatment: Ultimately, most patients experience pain and die. Thus, symptomatic treatment is as important as controlling disease. Appropriate end-of-life care should be discussed (see also p. 2762).

Patients with moderate to severe pain should receive an oral opioid in doses adequate to provide relief. Concern about addiction should not be a barrier to effective pain control. For chronic pain, long-acting preparations (eg, transdermal fentanyl, oxycodone, oxymorphone) are usually best. Percutaneous or operative splanchnic (celiac) block effectively controls pain in most patients. In cases of intolerable pain, opioids administered subcutaneously or by IV, epidural, or intrathecal infusion provide additional relief.

If palliative surgery or endoscopic placement of a biliary stent fails to relieve pruritus secondary to obstructive jaundice, the patient can be managed with cholestyramine (4 g po once/day to qid). Phenobarbital 30 to 60 mg po tid to qid may be helpful.

Exocrine pancreatic insufficiency is treated with tablets of porcine pancreatic enzymes (pancrelipase). The patient should take enough to supply 16,000 to 20,000 lipase units before each meal or snack. If a meal is prolonged (as in a restaurant) some of the tablets should be taken during the meal. Optimal intraluminal pH for the enzymes is 8; thus, some clinicians give a proton pump inhibitor or H_2 blocker bid. Diabetes mellitus should be closely monitored and controlled.

Cystadenocarcinoma

Cystadenocarcinoma is a rare adenomatous pancreatic cancer that arises as a malignant degeneration of a mucous cystadenoma and presents as upper abdominal pain and a palpable abdominal mass. Diagnosis is made by abdominal CT or MRI, which typically shows a cystic mass containing debris; the mass may be misinterpreted as necrotic adenocarcinoma or pancreatic pseudocyst. Unlike ductal adenocarcinoma, cystadenocarcinoma has a relatively good prognosis. Only 20% of patients have metastasis at the time of operation; complete excision of the tumor by distal or total pancreatectomy or by Whipple's operation results in a 65% 5-yr survival.

Intraductal Papillary-Mucinous Tumor

Intraductal papillary-mucinous tumor (IPMT) is a rare cancer resulting in mucus hypersecretion and ductal obstruction. Histology may be benign, borderline, or malignant. Most (80%) occur in women and in the tail of the pancreas (66%).

Symptoms consist of pain and recurrent bouts of pancreatitis. Diagnosis is made by CT, sometimes along with endoscopic ultrasound, MRCP, or ERCP. Benign and malignant disease cannot be differentiated without surgical removal, which is the treatment of choice. With surgery, 5-yr survival is > 95% for benign or borderline cases, but 50 to 75% for malignant tumors.

PANCREATIC ENDOCRINE TUMORS

Pancreatic endocrine tumors arise from islet and gastrin-producing cells and often produce many hormones. They have two general presentations. Nonfunctioning tumors may cause obstructive symptoms of the biliary tract or duodenum, bleeding into the GI tract, or abdominal masses. Functioning tumors hypersecrete a particular hormone, causing various syndromes (see Table 21–3). These clinical syndromes can also occur in multiple endocrine neoplasia, in which tumors or hyperplasia affects two or more endocrine glands, usually the parathyroid, pituitary, thyroid, or adrenals (see p. 1314).

TABLE 21–3. PANCREATIC ENDOCRINE TUMORS

TUMOR	HORMONE	TUMOR LOCATION	SYMPTOMS AND SIGNS
ACTHoma	ACTH	Pancreas	Cushing's syndrome
Gastrinoma	Gastrin	Pancreas (60%) Duodenum (30%) Other (10%)	Abdominal pain, peptic ulcer, diarrhea
Glucagonoma	Glucagon	Pancreas	Glucose intolerance, rash, weight loss, anemia
GRFoma	Growth hormone releasing factor	Lung (54%) Pancreas (30%) Jejunum (7%) Other (13%)	Acromegaly
Insulinoma	Insulin	Pancreas	Fasting hypoglycemia
Somatostatinoma	Somatostatin	Pancreas (56%) Duodenum/jejunum (44%)	Glucose intolerance, diarrhea, gallstones
Vipoma	Vasoactive intestinal peptidase	Pancreas (90%) Other (10%)	Severe watery diarrhea, hypokalemia, flushing

Treatment for functioning and nonfunctioning tumors is surgical resection. If metastases preclude curative surgery, various antihormone treatments may be tried for functioning tumors. Because of tumor rarity, chemotherapy trials have not identified definitive treatment. However, streptozotocin has selective activity against pancreatic islet cells and is commonly used, either alone or in combination with 5-fluorouracil or doxorubicin. Some centers use chlorozotocin and interferon.

INSULINOMA

An insulinoma is a rare pancreatic β-cell tumor that hypersecretes insulin. The main symptom is fasting hypoglycemia. Diagnosis is by a 48- or 72-h fast with measurement of glucose and insulin levels, followed by endoscopic ultrasound. Treatment is surgery when possible. Drugs that block insulin secretion (eg, diazoxide, octreotide, Ca channel blockers, β-blockers, phenytoin) are used for patients not responding to surgery.

Of all insulinomas, 80% are single and may be curatively resected if identified. Only 10% of insulinomas are malignant. Insulinoma occurs in 1/250,000 at a median age of 50 yr, except in multiple endocrine neoplasia (MEN) type I (about 10% of insulinomas), when it occurs in the 20s. Insulinomas associated with MEN type I are more likely to be multiple.

Surreptitious administration of exogenous insulin can cause episodic hypoglycemia mimicking insulinoma.

Symptoms and Signs

Hypoglycemia secondary to an insulinoma occurs during fasting. Symptoms are insidious and may mimic various psychiatric and neurologic disorders. CNS disturbances include headache, confusion, visual disturbances, motor weakness, palsy, ataxia, marked personality changes, and possible progression to loss of consciousness, seizures, and coma. Symptoms of sympathetic stimulation (faintness, weakness, tremulousness, palpitation, sweating, hunger, nervousness) are often absent.

Diagnosis

Serum glucose should be measured during symptoms. If hypoglycemia is present (glucose < 40 mg/dL [2.78 mmol/L]), an insulin level should be measured on a simultaneous sample. Hyperinsulinemia of > 6 μU/mL (42 pmol/L) suggests an insulin-mediated cause, as does a serum insulin to serum glucose ratio > 0.3 (μU/mL)/(mg/dL).

Insulin is secreted as proinsulin, consisting of an α chain and β chain connected by a C-peptide. Because pharmaceutical insulin consists only of the β chain, surreptitious insulin administration can be detected by measuring C-peptide and proinsulin levels. In patients with insulinoma, C-peptide is ≥ 0.2 nmol/L and proinsulin ≥ 5 pmol/L. These levels are normal or low in patients with surreptitious insulin administration.

Because many patients have no symptoms (and hence no hypoglycemia) at the time of evaluation, diagnosis requires admission to the hospital for a 48- or 72-h fast. Nearly all (98%) with insulinoma develop symptoms within 48 h of fasting; 70 to 80% within 24 h. Hypoglycemia as the cause of the symptoms is established by Whipple's triad: (1) Symptoms occur during the fast; (2) symptoms occur in the presence of hypoglycemia; (3) ingestion of carbohydrates relieves the symptoms. Hormone levels are obtained as described above when the patient is having symptoms.

If Whipple's triad is not observed after prolonged fasting and the plasma glucose after an overnight fast is > 50 mg/dL (> 2.78 mmol/L), a C-peptide suppression test can be performed. During insulin infusion (0.1 U/kg/h), patients with insulinoma fail to suppress C peptide to normal levels (≤ 1.2 ng/ mL [≤ 0.40 nmol/L]).

Endoscopic ultrasound has > 90% sensitivity and helps localize the tumor. CT has not proven useful, and arteriography or selective portal and splenic vein catheterization is generally unnecessary.

Treatment

Overall surgical cure rates approach 90%. A small, single insulinoma at or near the surface of the pancreas can usually be enucleated surgically. If a single large or deep adenoma is within the pancreatic body or tail, if there are multiple lesions of the body or tail (or both), or if no insulinoma is found (an unusual circumstance), a distal, subtotal pancreatectomy is performed. In < 1% of cases, the insulinoma is ectopically located in peripancreatic sites of the duodenal wall or periduodenal area and can be found only by diligent search during surgery. Pancreaticoduodenectomy (Whipple's operation) is performed for resectable malignant insulinomas of the proximal pancreas. Total pancreatectomy is performed if a previous subtotal pancreatectomy proves inadequate.

If hypoglycemia continues, diazoxide starting at 1.5 mg/kg po bid with a natriuretic can be used. Doses can be increased up to 4 mg/kg. A somatostatin analog, octreotide (100 to 500 μg sc bid to tid), is variably effective and should be considered for patients with continuing hypoglycemia refractory to diazoxide. Patients who respond may be converted to a long-acting octreotide formulation administered 20 to 30 mg IM once/mo. Patients using octreotide may also need to take supplemental pancreatic enzymes because octreotide suppresses pancreatic enzyme secretion. Other drugs that have modest and variable effect on insulin secretion include verapamil, diltiazem, and phenytoin.

If symptoms are not controlled, chemotherapy may be tried, but response is limited. Streptozotocin has a 30 to 40% response rate, and when combined with 5-fluorouracil, a 60% response rate lasting up to 2 yr. Other agents include doxorubicin, chlorozotocin, and interferon.

Zollinger-Ellison Syndrome

(Z-E Syndrome; Gastrinoma)

Zollinger-Ellison syndrome is caused by a gastrin-producing tumor usually located in the pancreas or the duodenal wall. Gastric acid hypersecretion and peptic ulceration result. Diagnosis is by measuring serum gastrin levels. Treatment is proton pump inhibitors and surgical removal.

Gastrinomas occur in the pancreas or duodenal wall 80 to 90% of the time. The remainder occur in the splenic hilum, mesentery, stomach, lymph node, or ovary. About 50% of patients have multiple tumors. Gastrinomas usually are small (< 1 cm in diameter) and grow slowly. About 50% are malignant. About 40 to 60% of patients with gastrinoma have multiple endocrine neoplasia (see p. 1314).

Symptoms and Signs

Zollinger-Ellison syndrome typically presents as aggressive peptic ulcer disease, with ulcers occurring in atypical locations (up to 25% are located distal to the duodenal bulb). However, as many as 25% do not have an ulcer at diagnosis. Typical ulcer symptoms and complications (eg, perforation, bleeding, obstruction) can occur. Diarrhea is the initial symptom in 25 to 40% of patients.

Diagnosis

The syndrome is suspected by history, particularly when symptoms are refractory to standard acid suppressant therapy.

The most reliable test is serum gastrin. All patients have levels > 150 pg/mL; markedly elevated levels of > 1000 pg/mL in a patient with compatible clinical features and gastric acid hypersecretion of > 15 mEq/h establish the diagnosis. However, moderate hypergastrinemia can occur with hypochlorhydric states (eg, pernicious anemia, chronic gastritis, use of proton pump inhibitors), in renal insufficiency with decreased clearance of gastrins, in massive intestinal resection, and in pheochromocytoma.

A secretin provocative test may be useful in patients with gastrin levels < 1000 pg/mL. An IV bolus of secretin 2 μg/kg is given with serial measurements of serum gastrin (10 and 1 min before, and 2, 5, 10, 15, 20 and 30 min after injection). The characteristic response in gastrinoma is an increase in gastrin levels, the opposite of what occurs in those with antral G-cell hyperplasia or typical peptic ulcer disease. Patients also should be evaluated for *Helicobacter pylori* infection, which commonly results in peptic ulceration and moderate excess gastrin secretion.

Once the diagnosis has been established, the tumor(s) must be localized. The first test is abdominal CT or somatostatin receptor scintigraphy, which may identify the primary tumor and metastatic disease. Selective arteriography with magnification and subtraction is also helpful. If no signs of metastases are present and the primary is uncertain, endoscopic ultrasound should be performed. Selective arterial secretin injection is an alternative.

Prognosis and Treatment

Five- and 10-yr survival is > 90% when an isolated tumor is removed surgically, versus 43% and 25% respectively with incomplete removal.

Acid suppression: Proton pump inhibitors are the drugs of choice: omeprazole or esomeprazole 40 mg po bid. The dose may be decreased gradually once symptoms resolve and acid output declines. A maintenance dose is needed; patients need to take these drugs indefinitely unless they undergo surgery.

Octreotide injections, 100 to 500 μg sc bid to tid, may also decrease gastric acid production and may be palliative in patients not responding well to proton pump inhibitors. A long-acting form of octreotide can be used 20 to 30 mg IM once/mo.

Surgery: Surgical removal should be attempted in patients without apparent metastases. At surgery, duodenotomy and intraoperative endoscopic transillumination or ultrasound help localize tumors. Surgical cure is possible in 20% of patients if the gastrinoma is not part of a multiple endocrine neoplasia syndrome.

Chemotherapy: In patients with metastatic disease, streptozocin in combination with 5-fluorouracil or doxorubicin is the preferred chemotherapy for islet cell tumors. It may reduce tumor mass (in 50 to 60%) and serum gastrin levels and is a useful adjunct to omeprazole. Patients with metastatic disease are not cured by chemotherapy.

VIPOMA

A vipoma is a non-β pancreatic islet cell tumor secreting vasoactive intestinal peptide (VIP), resulting in a syndrome of watery diarrhea, hypokalemia, and achlorhydria (WDHA syndrome). Diagnosis is by serum VIP levels, and tumor is localized with CT and endoscopic ultrasound. Treatment is surgical resection.

Of these tumors, 50 to 75% are malignant, and some may be quite large (7 cm) at diagnosis. In about 6%, vipoma occurs as part of multiple endocrine neoplasia (see p. 1314).

Symptoms and Signs

The major symptoms are prolonged massive watery diarrhea (fasting stool volume > 750 to 1000 mL/day and nonfasting volumes of > 3000 mL/day) and symptoms of hypokalemia, acidosis, and dehydration. In half, diarrhea is constant; in the rest, diarrhea severity varies over time. 33% have diarrhea < 1 yr before diagnosis, but 25% have diarrhea ≥ 5 yr before diagnosis. Lethargy, muscular weakness, nausea, vomiting, and crampy abdominal pain occur frequently. Flushing similar to the carcinoid syndrome occurs in 20% of patients during attacks of diarrhea.

Diagnosis

Diagnosis requires demonstration of secretory diarrhea (stool osmolality is close to plasma osmolality, and twice the sum of Na and K concentration in the stool accounts for all measured stool osmolality). Other causes of secretory diarrhea and, in particular, laxative abuse must be excluded (see p. 77). In such patients, serum VIP levels should be measured (ideally during a bout of diarrhea). Markedly elevated levels establish the diagnosis, but mild elevations may occur with short bowel syndrome and inflammatory diseases. Patients with elevated VIP levels should have tumor localization studies, such as endoscopic ultrasound and octreotide scintigraphy or arteriography to localize metastases.

Electrolytes and CBC should be measured. Hyperglycemia and impaired glucose tolerance occur in ≤ 50% of patients. Hypercalcemia occurs in half of patients.

Treatment

Initially, fluids and electrolytes must be replaced. Bicarbonate must be given to replace fecal loss and avoid acidosis. Because fecal losses of water and electrolytes increase as rehydration is achieved, continual IV replacement may become difficult.

Octreotide usually controls diarrhea, but large doses may be needed. Responders may benefit from a long-acting octreotide formulation administered 20 to 30 mg IM once/mo. Patients using octreotide may also need to take supplemental pancreatic enzymes because octreotide suppresses pancreatic enzyme secretion.

Tumor resection is curative in 50% of patients with a localized tumor. In those with metastatic tumor, resection of all visible tumor may provide temporary relief of symptoms. The combination of streptozocin and doxorubicin may reduce diarrhea and tumor mass if objective response occurs (in 50 to 60%). Chemotherapy is not curative.

GLUCAGONOMA

A glucagonoma is a pancreatic α-cell tumor that secretes glucagon, producing hyperglycemia and a characteristic skin rash. Diagnosis is by elevated glucagon levels and imaging studies. Tumor is localized with CT and endoscopic ultrasound. Treatment is surgical resection.

Glucagonomas are very rare but similar to other islet cell tumors in that the primary and metastatic lesions are slow-growing: 15-yr survival is common. Eighty percent of glucagonomas are malignant. The average age at symptom onset is 50 yr; 80% of patients are women. A few patients have multiple endocrine neoplasia type I.

Symptoms and Signs

Because glucagonomas produce glucagon, the symptoms are the same as those of diabetes. Frequently, weight loss, normochromic anemia, hypoaminoacidemia, and hypolipidemia are present, but the most distinctive clinical feature is a chronic eruption involving the extremities, often associated with a smooth, shiny, vermilion tongue and cheilitis. The exfoliating, brownish red, erythematous lesion with superficial necrolysis is termed necrolytic migratory erythema.

Diagnosis

Most patients with glucagonoma have glucagon levels > 1000 pg/mL (normal < 200). However, moderate elevations occur in renal insufficiency, acute pancreatitis, severe stress, and fasting. Correlation with symptoms is required. Patients should have abdominal CT followed by endoscopic ultrasound; MRI may be used if CT is unrevealing.

Treatment

Resection of the tumor alleviates all symptoms. Unresectable, metastatic, or recurrent tumors are treated with combination streptozocin and doxorubicin, which may decrease levels of circulating immunoreactive glucagon, lessen symptoms, and improve response rates (50%) but are unlikely to improve survival. Octreotide injections partially suppress glucagon production and relieve the erythema, but glucose tolerance may also decrease because octreotide decreases insulin secretion. Octreotide may quickly reverse anorexia and weight loss caused by the catabolic effect of glucagon excess. Patients who respond may be converted to a long-acting octreotide formulation administered 20 to 30 mg IM once/mo. Patients using octreotide may also need to take supplemental pancreatic enzymes because octreotide suppresses pancreatic enzyme secretion.

Locally applied, oral, or parenteral zinc may cause the erythema to disappear, but resolution may occur after simple hydration or IV administration of amino or fatty acids, suggesting that the erythema is not solely caused by zinc deficiency.

SECTION 3 HEPATIC AND BILIARY DISORDERS

22 APPROACH TO THE PATIENT WITH LIVER DISEASE

The liver is the most metabolically complex organ. Hepatocytes (liver parenchymal cells) perform the liver's metabolic functions: formation and excretion of bile; regulation of carbohydrate homeostasis; lipid synthesis and secretion of plasma lipoproteins; control of cholesterol metabolism; formation of urea, serum albumin, clotting factors, enzymes, and numerous other proteins; and metabolism or detoxification of drugs and other foreign substances.

At the cellular level, the portal triads consist of adjacent and parallel terminal branches of bile ducts, portal veins, and hepatic arteries that border the hepatocytes (see FIG. 22–1). Terminal branches of the hepatic veins are in the center of hepatic lobules. Because blood flows from the portal triads

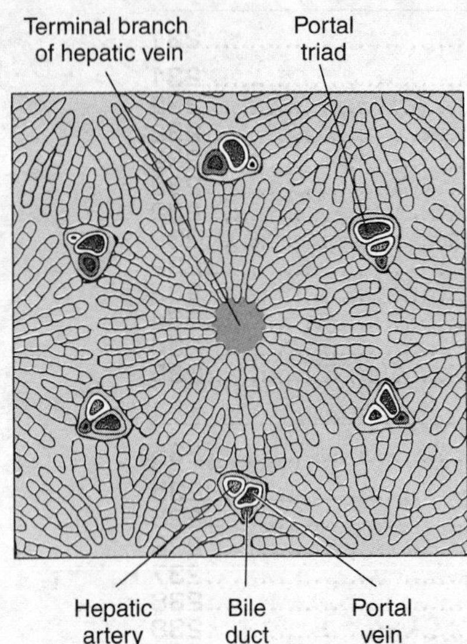

Fig. 22–1. Organization of the liver. The liver is organized into lobules around terminal branches of the hepatic vein. Between the lobules are portal triads. Each triad consists of branches of a bile duct, portal vein, and hepatic artery.

past the hepatocytes and drains via vein branches in the center of the lobule, the center of the lobule is the area most susceptible to ischemia.

Liver disorders can result from a wide variety of insults, including infections, drugs, toxins, ischemia, and autoimmune disorders. Occasionally, liver disorders occur postoperatively (see sidebar 22–1). Most liver disorders produce some degree of hepatocellular injury and necrosis, resulting in various abnormal laboratory test results and, sometimes, symptoms. Symptoms may be due to liver disease itself (eg, jaundice due to acute hepatitis) or to complications of liver disease (eg, acute GI bleeding due to cirrhosis and portal hypertension).

Despite necrosis, the liver can regenerate itself. Even extensive patchy necrosis can resolve completely (eg, in acute viral hepatitis). Incomplete regeneration and fibrosis, however, may result from injury that bridges entire lobules or from less pronounced but ongoing damage.

Specific diseases preferentially affect certain parts of the hepatobiliary system (eg, acute viral hepatitis is primarily manifested by damage to hepatocytes or hepatocellular injury; primary biliary cirrhosis, by impairment of biliary secretion; and cryptogenic cirrhosis, by liver fibrosis and resultant portal venous hypertension). The part of the hepatobiliary system affected determines the symptoms, signs, and laboratory abnormalities (see also Ch. 23 on p. 201). Some disorders (eg, severe alcoholic liver disease) affect multiple liver structures, resulting in a combination of patterns of symptoms, signs, and laboratory abnormalities.

The prognosis of serious complications is worse in older adults, who have less capacity to recover from severe physiologic stresses and inability to tolerate toxic accumulations.

History

Nonspecific symptoms include fatigue, anorexia, nausea, and, occasionally, vomiting, particularly in severe disorders. Loose, fatty stools (steatorrhea) can occur when cholestasis prevents sufficient bile from reaching the intestines. Fever can develop in viral or alcoholic hepatitis.

Jaundice, occurring in both hepatocellular dysfunction and cholestatic disorders, is the most specific symptom. It is often accompanied by dark urine and light stools. Right upper quadrant pain due to liver disorders usually suggests distention or inflammation of the liver capsule (eg, by passive venous congestion, inflammation, or tumor). Occasionally, erectile dysfunction and feminization develop; these may reflect the effects of alcohol more than liver disorders.

Risk factors for liver disorders include use of alcohol, certain drugs (prescription and nonprescription) and herbal products, and other liver toxins. Risk factors for hepatitis include these factors, as well as infectious exposure, shellfish, needle sticks, parenteral drug use, tattoos, body piercing, and, particularly before 1992, blood transfusions. Family history can indicate disorders such as hemochromatosis, Wilson's disease, and α_1-antitrypsin deficiency.

Sidebar 22–1. POSTOPERATIVE LIVER DYSFUNCTION

Mild liver dysfunction sometimes occurs after major surgery even in the absence of pre-existing liver disorders. This dysfunction usually results from hepatic ischemia or poorly understood effects of anesthesia. Patients with pre-existing well-compensated liver disease (eg, cirrhosis with normal liver function) usually tolerate surgery well. However, surgery can increase the severity of some pre-existing liver disorders; eg, laparotomy may precipitate acute liver failure in a patient with viral or alcoholic hepatitis.

Postoperative jaundice: Diagnosis of postoperative jaundice requires liver laboratory tests. Timing of symptoms also aids in diagnosis.

Multifactorial mixed hyperbilirubinemia is the most common reason for postoperative jaundice. It is caused by increased formation of bilirubin and decreased hepatic clearance. This most often occurs after major surgery or trauma requiring multiple transfusions. Hemolysis, sepsis, resorption of hematomas, and blood transfusions can increase the bilirubin load; simultaneously, hypoxemia, hepatic ischemia, and other poorly understood factors impair hepatic function. This condition is usually maximal within a few days of operation. Hepatic insufficiency is rare, and hyperbilirubinemia typically resolves slowly but completely. Liver laboratory tests can often differentiate multifactorial mixed hyperbilirubinemia from hepatitis; in multifactorial mixed hyperbilirubinemia, severe hyperbilirubinemia with mild aminotransferase and alkaline phosphatase elevations are common. In hepatitis, aminotransferase levels are usually very high.

Ischemic postoperative "hepatitis" results from insufficient liver perfusion, not inflammation. The cause is transient perioperative hypotension or hypoxia. Typically, aminotransferase levels increase rapidly (often > 1000 units/L), but bilirubin is only mildly elevated. Ischemic hepatitis is usually maximal within a few days of operation and resolves within a few days.

Halothane-related hepatitis can result from use of anesthetics containing halothane or related agents. It usually develops within 2 wk, is often preceded by fever, and is sometimes accompanied by a skin rash and eosinophilia.

True postoperative hepatitis is now rare. It used to result mainly from transmission of the hepatitis C virus during blood transfusion.

Postoperative cholestasis: The most common cause of postoperative cholestasis is biliary obstruction due to intra-abdominal complications or drugs given postoperatively. Intrahepatic cholestasis occasionally develops after major surgery, especially after abdominal or cardiovascular procedures (benign postoperative intrahepatic cholestasis). The pathogenesis is unknown, but the condition usually resolves slowly and spontaneously. Occasionally, postoperative cholestasis results from acute acalculous cholecystitis or pancreatitis.

Physical Examination

Abnormalities detectable on a physical examination usually do not develop until late during the course.

Liver abnormalities: Palpation may reveal hepatomegaly (liver enlargement) when liver size is large for the person's body mass. It suggests acute hepatitis, fatty liver, alcoholic liver disease, passive venous congestion, liver hemorrhage (into a cyst or the parenchyma), metastatic cancer, or biliary obstruction. Palpable lumps suggest cancer. In cirrhosis, the liver is firm, irregularly shaped, and with blunt edges; individual nodules are rarely palpable.

Tenderness occurs in acute hepatitis, passive congestion, liver hemorrhage, and cancer. Because of patient anxiety, liver tenderness is overdiagnosed. True liver tenderness (a deep-seated ache) is best elicited by percussion or compression of the rib cage. Occasionally, severe pain and tenderness mimic peritonitis.

Auscultation of friction rubs or bruits over the liver, although rare, suggests tumor.

Other abnormalities: Abdominal distention, shifting dullness, and a fluid wave suggest ascites. Visibly dilated abdominal veins and splenomegaly can suggest portal hypertension. Asterixis, drowsiness, confusion, and fetor hepaticus suggest portal-systemic encephalopathy. A cirrhotic habitus (ie, wasted extremities, protuberant abdomen) often signals advanced cirrhosis. In men, testicular atrophy, gynecomastia, erectile dysfunction, and female habitus are common, particularly in alcoholic cirrhosis, and may be caused more by alcohol use than by liver dysfunction.

Skin abnormalities include spider angiomas (vascular spiders) and palmar erythema. In cirrhotic patients, clubbing suggests advanced portal-systemic venous shunting. Muddy skin pigmentation, excoriations from constant pruritus, and cutaneous lipid deposits (xanthelasmas or xanthomas) may suggest chronic cholestasis. Slate gray or bronze skin suggests hemochromatosis with deposition of iron and melanin.

ASCITES

Ascites is the condition in which there is free fluid in the peritoneal cavity. The most common cause is portal hypertension. Symptoms usually result from abdominal distention. Diagnosis is based on physical examination, ultrasound, or CT. Treatments include bed rest, dietary Na restriction, diuretics, and therapeutic paracentesis. Ascitic fluid can become infected (spontaneous bacterial peritonitis), often with pain and fever. Diagnosis of infection involves analysis and culture of ascitic fluid. Infection is treated with antibiotics.

Etiology

Ascites can result from chronic, but not acute, liver diseases. More than 90% of hepatic cases result from portal hypertension, usually due to cirrhosis. Other hepatic causes, which are uncommon, include chronic hepatitis, severe alcoholic hepatitis without cirrhosis, and hepatic vein obstruction (Budd-Chiari syndrome). Portal vein thrombosis does not usually cause ascites unless hepatocellular damage is also present.

Nonhepatic causes include generalized fluid retention associated with systemic diseases (eg, heart failure, nephrotic syndrome, severe hypoalbuminemia, constrictive pericarditis) and peritoneal disorders (eg, carcinomatous or infectious peritonitis, biliary leak due to surgery or another medical procedure). Less common causes include renal dialysis, pancreatitis, SLE, and endocrine disorders (eg, myxedema).

Pathophysiology

Mechanisms are complex and incompletely understood. Factors include altered Starling's forces in the portal vessels (low oncotic pressure due to hypoalbuminemia plus increased portal venous pressure), avid renal Na retention (urinary Na concentration is typically < 5 mEq/L), and possibly increased hepatic lymph formation.

Mechanisms that appear to contribute to renal Na retention include activation of the renin-angiotensin-aldosterone system; increased sympathetic tone; intrarenal shunting of blood away from the cortex; increased formation of nitric oxide; and altered formation or metabolism of ADH, kinins, prostaglandins, and atrial natriuretic factor. Vasodilation in the splanchnic arterial circulation may be a trigger, but the specific roles and interrelationships of these abnormalities remain uncertain.

Spontaneous bacterial peritonitis (SBP) is infection of ascitic fluid without an apparent source. SBP is particularly common in cirrhotic ascites, especially in alcoholics. It can produce serious sequelae or death. The most common bacteria causing SBP are the gram-negative *Escherichia coli* and *Klebsiella pneumoniae* and the gram-positive *Streptococcus pneumoniae;* usually only a single organism is involved.

Symptoms and Signs

Small amounts of ascitic fluid cause no symptoms. Moderate amounts cause increased abdominal girth and weight gain. Massive amounts may cause nonspecific diffuse abdominal pressure, but actual pain is uncommon. If ascites results in elevation of the diaphragm, dyspnea may occur. Symptoms of SBP may include new abdominal discomfort and fever.

Signs include shifting dullness on abdominal percussion and a fluid wave. Volumes <1500 mL may not produce physical findings. Massive ascites produces tautness of the abdominal wall and flattening of the umbilicus. In liver diseases or peritoneal disorders, ascites is usually isolated or disproportionate to peripheral edema; in systemic diseases (eg, heart failure), the reverse is usually true.

Signs of SBP may include fever, malaise, encephalopathy, worsening hepatic failure, and unexplained clinical deterioration. Peritoneal signs (eg, abdominal tenderness and rebound) are present but may be somewhat diminished by the presence of ascitic fluid.

Diagnosis

Diagnosis may be based on physical examination if there is a large amount of fluid, but imaging tests are more sensitive. Ultrasound and CT reveal much smaller volumes of fluid (100 to 200 mL) than does physical examination. SBP is suspected in a patient with ascites who also has abdominal pain, fever, or unexplained deterioration.

Diagnostic paracentesis (see p. 89) should be performed if ascites is newly diagnosed, if its cause is unknown, or if SBP is suspected. About 50 to 100 mL of fluid is removed and analyzed for gross appearance, protein content, cell count and differential, cytology, culture, and, as clinically indicated, acid-fast stain and/or amylase. In contrast to ascites due to inflammation or infection, ascites due to portal hypertension produces fluid that is clear and straw-colored, has a low protein concentration (usually < 3 g/dL, but occasionally > 4 g/dL), a low PMN count (< 250 cells/μL), and, most reliably, a high serum-to-ascites albumin concentration, which is the serum albumin concentration minus the ascitic albumin concentration. Gradients > 1.1 g/dL suggest ascites due to portal hypertension. In ascitic fluid, turbidity and a PMN count > 500 cells/μL suggest infection, whereas bloody fluid usually signals a tumor or TB. The rare milky (chylous) ascites is most common with lymphoma.

Clinical diagnosis of SBP can be difficult; its diagnosis requires a high index of suspicion and liberal use of diagnostic paracentesis, including culture. Blood cultures are also indicated. Transferring ascitic fluid to blood culture media before incubation increases the sensitivity of culture to almost 70%. Because SBP usually results from a single organism, obtaining mixed flora on culture suggests a perforated abdominal viscus or contaminated specimen.

Treatment

Bed rest and dietary Na restriction (20 to 40 mEq/day) are the first, and least risky, treatments for ascites due to portal hypertension. Diuretics should be used if rigid Na restriction fails to initiate diuresis within a few days. Spironolactone is usually effective (in oral doses ranging from 50 to 200 mg bid). A loop diuretic (eg, furosemide 20 to 160 mg po usually once/day, or 20 to 80 mg po bid) should be added if spironolactone is insufficient. Because spironolactone can cause K retention and furosemide K depletion, the combination of these drugs often provides optimal diuresis with a lower risk of K abnormalities. Fluid restriction is helpful only if serum Na is < 130 mEq/L. Changes in body weight and urinary Na determinations reflect response to treatment. Weight loss of about 0.5 kg/day is optimal, because the ascitic compartment cannot be mobilized much more rapidly. More aggressive diuresis depletes fluid from the intravascular compartment, especially when peripheral edema is absent; this may cause renal failure or electrolyte imbalance (eg, hypokalemia) that may precipitate portal-systemic encephalopathy. Inadequate dietary Na restriction is the usual cause of persistent ascites.

Therapeutic paracentesis is an alternative. Removal of 4 L/day is safe, provided that salt-poor albumin (about 40 g/paracentesis) is concomitantly infused IV as needed to prevent intravascular volume depletion. Even single total paracentesis may be safe. Therapeutic paracentesis shortens the hospital stay with relatively little risk of electrolyte imbalance or renal failure; nevertheless, patients require ongoing diuretics and tend to reaccumulate fluid more rapidly than those treated without paracentesis.

Techniques for the autologous infusion of ascitic fluid (eg, the LeVeen peritoneovenous shunt) often produce complications and are generally no longer used. Transjugular intrahepatic portal-systemic shunting (TIPS) can lower portal pressure and successfully treat ascites resistant to other treatments, but TIPS is invasive and may produce complications, including portal-systemic encephalopathy and worsening hepatocellular function.

If SBP is suspected and > 500 PMNs/μL of ascitic fluid are found, an antibiotic such as cefotaxime 2 g IV q 4 to 8 h (pending Gram stain and culture results) is given for at least 5 days, until ascitic fluid shows < 250 PMNs/μL. Antibiotics increase the chance of survival. Because SBP recurs within a year in up to 70% of patients, prophylactic antibiotics are indicated; quinolones (eg, norfloxacin 400 mg po once/day) are most widely used. Prophylaxis in ascitic patients with variceal hemorrhage decreases the risk of SBP.

FATTY LIVER

Fatty liver (hepatic steatosis) is excessive accumulation of lipid in hepatocytes, the most common liver response to injury.

Fatty liver develops for many reasons, involves many different biochemical mechanisms, and causes different types of liver damage. Clinically, it is most useful to distinguish between fatty liver due to pregnancy, that due to alcoholic liver disease (see p. 211), and that developing in the absence of pregnancy and alcoholism (nonalcoholic fatty liver disease [NAFLD]). The latter includes simple fatty infiltration (a benign condition) and nonalcoholic steatohepatitis, a less common but more important variant.

Nonalcoholic Steatohepatitis

Nonalcoholic steatohepatitis is a syndrome that develops in patients who are not alcoholic and produces liver damage that is histologically indistinguishable from alcoholic hepatitis. It develops most often in middle-aged women, many of whom are overweight or have increased blood sugar or lipids. Pathogenesis is poorly understood but appears to be linked to insulin resistance (eg, as in obesity or the metabolic syndrome). Most patients are asymptomatic. Laboratory findings include elevations in aminotransferase levels. Biopsy is required to confirm the diagnosis. Treatment includes elimination of causes and risk factors.

Nonalcoholic steatohepatitis (NASH—sometimes called steatonecrosis) is diagnosed most often in women between 40 and 60, many of whom have obesity, type 2 diabetes mellitus, or hyperlipidemia, but can occur in all ages and both sexes.

Pathophysiology involves fat accumulation (steatosis), inflammation, and, variably, fibrosis. Steatosis results from hepatic triglyceride accumulation. Possible mechanisms for steatosis include reduced synthesis of very low density lipoprotein (VLDL) and increased hepatic triglyceride synthesis (possibly due to decreased oxidation of fatty acids or increased free fatty acids being delivered to the liver). Inflammation may result from lipid peroxidative damage to cell membranes. These changes can stimulate hepatic stellate cells, resulting in fibrosis. If advanced, NASH can cause cirrhosis and portal hypertension.

Most patients are asymptomatic. However, some have fatigue, malaise, or right upper quadrant abdominal discomfort. Hepatomegaly develops in about 75% of patients. Splenomegaly may develop if advanced hepatic fibrosis is present and is usually the first indication that portal hypertension has developed. Patients with cirrhosis due to NASH are often asymptomatic and may lack the usual signs of chronic liver disease.

Diagnosis

The most common laboratory abnormalities are elevations in aminotransferase levels. Unlike alcoholic liver disease, the ratio of AST/ALT in NASH is usually < 1. Alkaline phosphatase and γ-glutamyl transpeptidase (GGT) occasionally increase. Hyperbilirubinemia, prolongation of PT, and hypoalbuminemia are uncommon.

For diagnosis, strong evidence (such as a history corroborated by friends and relatives) should confirm that alcohol intake is not excessive (eg, < 20 g/day). Serology should demonstrate absence of hepatitis B and C infection (ie, hepatitis B surface antigen and hepatitis C virus antibody should be negative). Liver biopsy should reveal damage similar to that seen in alcoholic hepatitis, usually including large fat droplets (macrovesicular fatty infiltration). Indications for biopsy include unexplained signs of portal hypertension (including splenomegaly or cytopenia) and unexplained elevations in aminotransferase levels that persist for > 6 mo in a patient with diabetes, obesity, or hyperlipidemia. Imaging tests, including ultrasound, CT, and, particularly, MRI, may identify hepatic steatosis. However, these tests cannot identify the inflammation typical of NASH and cannot differentiate NASH from other causes of hepatic steatosis.

Prognosis and Treatment

Prognosis is controversial. Probably, most patients do not develop hepatic insufficiency or cirrhosis. However, some drugs (eg, cytotoxic drugs) and metabolic disorders are associated with acceleration of NASH. Prognosis is often good unless complications (eg, variceal hemorrhage) develop.

The only widely accepted treatment goal is to eliminate potential causes and risk factors. Such a goal may include discontinuation of drugs or toxins, weight loss, and treatment for hyperlipidemia or hyperglycemia. Many other treatments (eg, ursodeoxycholic acid, vitamin E, metronidazole, metformin, betaine, glucagon, glutamine infusion) have not been proven effective.

JAUNDICE

(See also Hyperbilirubinemia on p. 2275.)

Jaundice is yellowing of the skin, sclerae, and other tissues caused by excess circulating bilirubin.

Overview of Bilirubin Metabolism

The breakdown of heme produces bilirubin (an insoluble waste product) and other bile pigments. Bilirubin must be made water-soluble to be excreted. This transformation occurs in five steps: formation, plasma transport, liver uptake, conjugation, and biliary excretion.

Formation: About 250 to 350 mg of unconjugated bilirubin forms daily; 70 to 80% derives from the breakdown of degenerating RBCs, and 20 to 30% (early-labeled bilirubin) derives primarily from other heme proteins in the bone marrow and liver. Hb is degraded to iron and biliverdin, which is converted to bilirubin.

Plasma transport: Unconjugated (indirect-reacting) bilirubin is not water-soluble and so is transported in the plasma bound to albumin. It cannot pass through the glomerular membrane into the urine. Albumin binding weakens under certain conditions (eg, acidosis), and some substances (eg, salicylates, certain antibiotics) compete for the binding sites.

Liver uptake: The liver takes up bilirubin rapidly but does not take up the attached serum albumin.

Conjugation: Unconjugated bilirubin in the liver is conjugated to form mainly bilirubin diglucuronide, or conjugated (direct-reacting) bilirubin. This reaction, catalyzed by the microsomal enzyme glucuronyl transferase, renders the bilirubin water-soluble.

Biliary excretion: Tiny canaliculi formed by adjacent hepatocytes progressively coalesce into ductules, interlobular bile ducts, and larger hepatic ducts. Outside the porta hepatis, the main hepatic duct joins the cystic duct from the gallbladder to form the common bile duct, which drains into the duodenum at the ampulla of Vater.

Conjugated bilirubin is secreted into the bile canaliculus with other bile constituents. In the intestine, bacteria metabolize bilirubin to form urobilinogen, much of which is further metabolized to stercobilins, which render the stool brown. In complete biliary obstruction, stools lose their normal color and become light gray (clay-colored stool). Some urobilinogen is reabsorbed, extracted by hepatocytes, and re-excreted in the bile (enterohepatic circulation). A small amount is excreted in the urine.

Because conjugated bilirubin is excreted in urine and unconjugated bilirubin is not, only conjugated hyperbilirubinemia (eg, due to hepatocellular or cholestatic jaundice) causes bilirubinuria.

Etiology

Jaundice can result from increased formation of bilirubin or hepatobiliary disease (hepatobiliary jaundice). Hepatobiliary jaundice can result from hepatocellular dysfunction or cholestasis. Cholestasis can be intrahepatic or extrahepatic.

Increased formation and hepatocellular diseases that impair liver uptake or decrease conjugation cause unconjugated hyperbilirubinemia. Impaired biliary excretion produces conjugated hyperbilirubinemia. Although these mechanisms seem distinct, in clinical practice, jaundice, particularly jaundice due to hepatobiliary disease, almost always produces multiple defects; the result is both unconjugated and conjugated hyperbilirubinemia (mixed hyperbilirubinemia).

Rarely, certain disorders produce predominantly unconjugated or conjugated hyperbilirubinemia. Unconjugated hyperbilirubinemia due to increased bilirubin formation can result from hemolytic disorders; those due to decreased conjugation can result from Gilbert syndrome (mild) and Crigler-Najjar syndrome (severe).

Conjugated hyperbilirubinemia due to impaired excretion can result from Dubin-Johnson syndrome. Conjugated hyperbilirubinemia due to intrahepatic cholestasis can result from hepatitis, drug toxicity, and alcoholic liver disease. Less common causes include primary biliary cirrhosis, cholestasis of pregnancy, and metastatic cancer. Conjugated hyperbilirubinemia due to extrahepatic cholestasis can result from a common bile duct stone or pancreatic cancer. Less common causes include benign stricture of the common duct (usually related to prior surgery), ductal carcinoma, pancreatitis or pancreatic pseudocyst, and sclerosing cholangitis.

Liver disease and biliary obstruction usually cause multiple defects, increasing both conjugated and unconjugated bilirubin.

Evaluation

Evaluation of jaundice should first address whether hepatobiliary disease is present. Hepatobiliary jaundice can result from cholestasis or hepatocellular dysfunction. Cholestasis can be intrahepatic or extrahepatic. Determining the cause of jaundice indicates diagnosis (eg, hemolysis or Gilbert syndrome if there is no hepatobiliary disease; viruses, toxins, hepatic manifestations of systemic diseases, or primary liver diseases in hepatocellular dysfunction; gallstones in extrahepatic cholestasis). Although laboratory and imaging tests are essential, most errors result from inadequate clinical data and overreliance on test results.

History: Nausea or vomiting preceding jaundice often indicates acute hepatitis or common bile duct obstruction by a stone; abdominal pain or rigors favors the latter. Gradual development of anorexia and malaise is common in alcoholic liver disease, chronic hepatitis, and cancer.

Because urine can darken from hyperbilirubinemia before jaundice is visible, the onset of dark urine indicates the onset of hyperbilirubinemia more accurately than the onset of jaundice.

Physical examination: Mild jaundice is best seen by examining the sclerae in natural light; it is usually detectable when serum bilirubin reaches 2 to 2.5 mg/dL (34 to 43 μmol/L). Mild jaundice without dark urine suggests unconjugated hyperbilirubinemia (most often caused by hemolysis or Gilbert syndrome); more severe jaundice or jaundice accompanied by dark urine suggests hepatobiliary disease. Signs of portal hypertension or portal-systemic encephalopathy, or skin or endocrine changes, suggest chronic liver disease.

In patients with hepatomegaly and ascites, distended jugular veins suggest heart failure or constrictive pericarditis. Cachexia and an unusually hard or lumpy liver more often indicate metastases than cirrhosis. Diffuse lymphadenopathy suggests infectious mononucleosis in acute jaundice, and lymphoma or leukemia in chronic jaundice. Hepatosplenomegaly without other signs of chronic liver disease may be caused by an infiltrative disorder (eg, lymphoma, amyloidosis, or, in endemic areas, schistosomiasis or malaria), although jaundice is usually minimal or absent in such disorders.

Testing: (see also p. 201) Aminotransferases and alkaline phosphatase levels should be measured. Mild hyperbilirubinemia (eg, bilirubin < 3 mg/dL [< 51 μmol/L]) with normal aminotransferase and alkaline phosphatase levels is often unconjugated (eg, due to hemolysis or Gilbert syndrome rather than hepatobiliary disease). Moderate or severe hyperbilirubinemia, bilirubinuria, high alkaline phosphatase levels, or high aminotransferase levels suggest hepatobiliary disease. Unconjugated hyperbilirubinemia is usually confirmed by bilirubin fractionation. However, because hyperbilirubinemia produced by any hepatobiliary disease is largely conjugated, bilirubin fractionation is unwarranted if test results reflect hepatobiliary disease.

Other blood tests should be performed selectively. For example, hepatitis serology should be obtained (see p. 225) for suspected acute or chronic hepatitis, PT or INR for suspected hepatic insufficiency, albumin and globulin levels for suspected chronic liver disease, and antimitochondrial antibody levels for suspected primary biliary cirrhosis. In cases of isolated elevation of alkaline phosphatase, γ-glutamyl transpeptidase (GGT) should be obtained; levels are elevated in hepatobiliary disease but not if the high alkaline phosphatase level is due to a bone disorder.

In hepatobiliary disease, neither bilirubin fractionation nor the degree of bilirubin elevation helps differentiate hepatocellular from cholestatic jaundice. Aminotransferase elevations > 500 units suggest a hepatocellular cause such as hepatitis or acute liver hypoxia; disproportionate increases of alkaline phosphatase (eg, alkaline phosphatase > 3 times normal and aminotransferase < 200 units) suggest cholestasis. Liver infiltration can also increase alkaline phosphatase disproportionately to aminotransferases but usually increases bilirubin only slightly or not at all.

Because hepatobiliary disease alone rarely causes bilirubin levels > 30 mg/dL (> 513 μmol/L), higher levels usually reflect a combination of severe hepatobiliary disease and hemolysis or renal dysfunction. Low albumin and high globulin levels suggest chronic rather than acute liver disease. An elevated PT or INR that decreases after giving vitamin K (5 to 10 mg IM for 2 to 3 days) favors cholestasis over hepatocellular disease but is not conclusive.

Imaging is best for diagnosing infiltrative and cholestatic causes of jaundice. Abdominal ultrasound, CT, or MRI is usually performed first. These tests can detect abnormalities within the biliary tree and focal liver lesions but are less accurate in diagnosing diffuse hepatocellular disorders (eg, hepatitis, cirrhosis). In extrahepatic cholestasis, endoscopic or magnetic resonance cholangiopancreatography (ERCP, MRCP) provides a more accurate assessment of the biliary tree; ERCP also permits treatment of the obstruction (eg, stone removal, stenting of strictures).

Liver biopsy is seldom required for diagnosing jaundice but can help in intrahepatic cholestasis and in some kinds of hepatitis. Laparoscopy (peritoneoscopy) permits direct inspection of the liver and gallbladder without the trauma of a full laparotomy. Unexplained cholestatic jaundice warrants laparoscopy occasionally and diagnostic laparotomy rarely.

Cholestatic Conjugated Hyperbilirubinemia

Cholestasis (obstructive jaundice) can cause conjugated hyperbilirubinemia. Cholestasis results when bile flow is impaired. The term cholestasis is preferred to obstructive jaundice because mechanical obstruction is not always present. Cholestasis in infants differs from cholestasis in other age groups (see p. 2288).

Etiology

Bile flow may be impaired at any point, from the liver cell canaliculus to the ampulla of Vater.

Intrahepatic causes include hepatitis, drug toxicity, and alcoholic liver disease. Less common causes include primary biliary cirrhosis, cholestasis of pregnancy, and metastatic cancer.

Extrahepatic causes include a common duct stone and pancreatic cancer. Less common causes include benign stricture of the common duct (usually related to prior surgery), ductal carcinoma, pancreatitis or pancreatic pseudocyst, and sclerosing cholangitis.

Pathophysiology

Mechanisms are complex, even in mechanical obstruction. The pathophysiologic effects reflect absence of bile constituents (most importantly, bilirubin, bile salts, and lipids) in the intestines, and their backup, which causes spillage into the systemic circulation. Stools are often pale because less bilirubin reaches the intestine. Absence of bile salts can produce malabsorption, leading to steatorrhea and deficiencies of fat-soluble vitamins (particularly A, K, and D); vitamin K deficiency can reduce prothrombin levels. In long-standing cholestasis, concomitant vitamin D and Ca malabsorption can cause osteoporosis or osteomalacia.

Bilirubin retention produces mixed hyperbilirubinemia. Some conjugated bilirubin reaches and darkens the urine. High levels of circulating bile salts are associated with, but may not cause, pruritus. Cholesterol and phospholipid retention produces hyperlipidemia despite fat malabsorption (although increased liver synthesis and decreased plasma esterification of cholesterol also contribute); triglyceride levels are largely unaffected. The lipids circulate as a unique, abnormal, low-density lipoprotein called lipoprotein X.

Evaluation

Evaluation consists of history, physical examination, and diagnostic tests. Distinguishing between intrahepatic and extrahepatic causes is crucial.

History: Cholestasis produces jaundice, dark urine, pale stools, and generalized pruritus. If chronic, cholestasis may produce bleeding (due to vitamin K malabsorption) or bone pain (due to osteoporosis from vitamin D and Ca malabsorption). Abdominal pain and systemic symptoms (eg, anorexia, vomiting, fever) reflect the underlying cause rather than cholestasis itself. Symptoms of hepatitis, heavy alcohol ingestion, or recent use of potentially cholestatic drugs suggest intrahepatic cholestasis. Rigors, biliary colic, or pain typical of pancreatic disorders (eg, pancreatic cancer) suggests extrahepatic cholestasis.

Physical examination: If chronic, cholestasis may produce muddy skin pigmentation, excoriations (from pruritus), or cutaneous lipid deposits (xanthelasmas or xanthomas). Signs of chronic hepatocellular disease (eg, spider angiomas, splenomegaly, ascites) suggest intrahepatic cholestasis. Signs of cholecystitis (see p. 242) suggest extrahepatic cholestasis.

Testing: Regardless of etiology, alkaline phosphatase levels characteristically increase, more from increased synthesis than from impaired excretion. Aminotransferase levels are usually only moderately elevated. Bilirubin levels are variable. To help confirm hepatic origin of high levels of alkaline phosphatase if other liver tests are normal, γ-glutamyl transpeptidase (GGT) is measured. If hepatic insufficiency is suspected, PT (usually reported as the INR) is measured. Neither alkaline phosphatase, GGT, nor bilirubin levels, however, indicate the cause of cholestasis.

Other laboratory tests may reveal the cause of cholestasis, but only occasionally. Marked elevations in aminotransferase levels suggest a hepatocellular cause but occasionally occur in extrahepatic cholestasis, especially with acute obstruction by a common duct stone. High serum amylase levels are uncommon but suggest common bile duct obstruction. Correction of a prolonged PT or INR after administration of vitamin K suggests extrahepatic obstruction, but hepatocellular disorders may also respond. Presence of antimitochondrial antibodies strongly suggests primary biliary cirrhosis.

Imaging tests of the biliary tract are essential (see p. 204). Ultrasound, CT, and MRI reliably detect bile duct dilation, which usually occurs after the first several hours of symptoms due to mechanical obstruction. The underlying cause of obstruction may also be shown; in general, gallstones are more reliably seen on ultrasound and pancreatic lesions on CT. Ultrasound is usually preferred because of its lower cost and lack of ionizing radiation. If ultrasound demonstrates extrahepatic obstruction but not its cause, a more definitive study, usually endoscopic or magnetic resonance cholangiopancreatography (ERCP, MRCP), is indicated. Diagnostic laparoscopy or laparotomy is rarely indicated if extrahepatic obstruction is progressive and no cause can be found with imaging tests.

Liver biopsy is indicated for suspected intrahepatic cholestasis if the diagnosis is not clear from noninvasive studies. Because it predisposes to puncture of the biliary tree, which can cause peritonitis, ductal dilation should be ruled out (by ultrasound or CT) before biopsy.

Treatment

Extrahepatic biliary obstruction requires mechanical decompression. Other goals include treatment of the underlying cause, symptoms, and complications (eg, vitamin malabsorption).

Decompression of extrahepatic biliary obstruction usually requires laparotomy, endoscopy (eg, for removal of ductal stones) or, for strictures or partially obstructed areas, insertion of stents and drainage catheters. For obstruction due to inoperable cancers, stents can usually be placed transhepatically or endoscopically to provide drainage.

Pruritus usually subsides with correction of the underlying disorder or with cholestyramine 2 to 8 g po bid, which binds bile salts in the intestine. However, cholestyramine is ineffective in complete biliary obstruction. Unless severe hepatocellular damage is present, hypoprothrombinemia usually subsides after use of phytonadione (vitamin K_1) 5 to 10 mg sc once/day for 2 to 3 days. Ca and vitamin D supplements, with or without a bisphosphonate, slow the progression of osteoporosis only slightly in long-standing irreversible cholestasis. Vitamin A supplements prevent deficiency, and severe steatorrhea can be minimized by replacing some dietary fat with medium-chain triglycerides.

Noncholestatic Conjugated Hyperbilirubinemia

Disorders of bilirubin metabolism causing conjugated hyperbilirubinemia without cholestasis produce no symptoms or sequelae other than jaundice. In contrast to unconjugated hyperbilirubinemia in Gilbert syndrome, bilirubin may appear in the urine. Aminotransferase and alkaline phosphatase levels are usually normal. Treatment is unnecessary.

Dubin-Johnson syndrome: This rare autosomal recessive disorder involves impaired excretion of bilirubin glucuronides. It is usually diagnosed by liver biopsy; the liver is deeply pigmented as a result of an intracellular melanin-like substance but is otherwise histologically normal.

Rotor's syndrome: This rare disorder is clinically similar to Dubin-Johnson syndrome, but the liver is not pigmented, and other subtle metabolic differences are present.

Unconjugated Hyperbilirubinemia

Unconjugated hyperbilirubinemia is a disorder of bilirubin metabolism consisting of overproduction or defective conjugation of bilirubin.

Hemolysis: RBC hemolysis is the most frequent clinically important cause of increased bilirubin formation. Although the normal liver can conjugate excess bilirubin, hemolysis may increase bilirubin to an unmanageable amount. Still, even in brisk hemolysis, serum bilirubin is rarely > 5 mg/dL (> 86 μmol/L). However, hemolysis combined with liver disease may cause higher levels; in these cases, canalicular bile excretion also becomes impaired, producing some conjugated hyperbilirubinemia. (See discussion of hemolytic anemia on p. 1045.)

Gilbert syndrome: Gilbert syndrome is a presumably lifelong disorder whose only significant abnormality is asymptomatic, mild, unconjugated hyperbilirubinemia. It can be mistaken for chronic hepatitis or other liver disorders. Gilbert syndrome may affect as many as 5% of people. Although family members may be affected, a clear genetic pattern is difficult to establish.

Pathogenesis may involve complex defects in the liver's uptake of bilirubin. Glucuronyl transferase activity is low, though not as low as in Crigler-Najjar syndrome type II. In many patients, RBC destruction is also slightly accelerated, but this acceleration does not explain hyperbilirubinemia. Liver histology is normal.

Gilbert syndrome is most often detected in young adults serendipitously by finding an elevated bilirubin level, which usually fluctuates between 2 and 5 mg/dL (34 and 86 μmol/L) and tends to increase with fasting and other stresses.

Gilbert syndrome is differentiated from hepatitis by fractionation that shows predominantly unconjugated bilirubin, otherwise normal liver function test results, and absence of urinary bilirubin. It is differentiated from hemolysis by the absence of anemia and reticulocytosis. Treatment is unnecessary. Patients should be reassured that they do not have liver disease.

Crigler-Najjar syndrome: This rare inherited disorder is caused by deficiency of the enzyme glucuronyl transferase. Patients with autosomal recessive type I (complete) disease have severe hyperbilirubinemia. They usually die of kernicterus by age 1 yr but may survive into adulthood. Treatment may include phototherapy and liver transplantation. Patients with autosomal dominant type II (partial) disease (which has variable penetrance) often have less severe hyperbilirubinemia (< 20 mg/dL [< 342 μmol/L]) and usually live into adulthood without neurologic damage. Phenobarbital 1.5 to 2 mg/kg po tid, which induces the partially deficient glucuronyl transferase, may be effective.

Primary shunt hyperbilirubinemia: This rare, familial, benign condition is associated with overproduction of early-labeled bilirubin.

PORTAL HYPERTENSION

Portal hypertension is caused most often by cirrhosis (in developed countries), schistosomiasis (in endemic areas), or hepatic vascular abnormalities. Consequences include esophageal varices and portal-systemic encephalopathy. Diagnosis is based on clinical criteria, often in conjunction with imaging studies and endoscopy. Treatment involves prevention of GI bleeding with endoscopy, drugs, or both, and sometimes with portocaval shunting.

The portal vein, formed by the superior mesenteric and splenic veins, drains blood from the abdominal GI tract, spleen, and pancreas into the liver. Within reticuloendothelium-lined blood channels (sinusoids), blood from the terminal portal venules merges with hepatic arterial blood. Blood flows out of the sinusoids via the hepatic veins into the inferior vena cava.

Normal portal pressure is 5 to 10 mm Hg (7 to 14 cm H_2O), which exceeds inferior vena caval pressure by 4 to 5 mm Hg (portal venous gradient). Higher values are defined as portal hypertension.

Etiology and Pathophysiology

Portal hypertension results mainly from increased resistance to flow, which commonly arises from disease within the liver itself or uncommonly from blockage of the splenic or portal vein or impaired hepatic venous outflow (see TABLE 22–1). Increased flow volume is a rare cause, although it often contributes to portal hypertension in cirrhosis and in hematologic disorders that produce massive splenomegaly.

In cirrhosis, tissue fibrosis and regeneration increase resistance in the sinusoids and terminal portal venules. However, other, potentially reversible, factors contribute, such as contractility of sinusoidal lining cells, production of vasoactive substances (eg, endothelins, nitric oxide), various systemic mediators of arteriolar resistance, and, possibly, swelling of hepatocytes.

Over time, portal hypertension creates portal-systemic venous collaterals. These may slightly decrease portal vein pressure but

TABLE 22–1. CLASSIFICATION AND MOST COMMON CAUSES OF PORTAL HYPERTENSION

CLASSIFICATION	CAUSE
Prehepatic	Portal or splenic vein thrombosis Increased portal flow: arteriovenous fistula, massive splenomegaly from primary hematologic disease
Hepatic	Presinusoidal: schistosomiasis, other periportal disorders (eg, primary biliary cirrhosis, sarcoidosis, congenital hepatic fibrosis), idiopathic portal hypertension Sinusoidal: cirrhosis (all etiologies) Postsinusoidal: veno-occlusive disease
Posthepatic	Hepatic vein thrombosis (Budd-Chiari syndrome) Obstruction of the inferior vena cava Resistance to right heart filling (eg, constrictive pericarditis, restrictive cardiomyopathy)

can produce complications. Engorged serpentine submucosal vessels (varices) in the distal esophagus and sometimes in the gastric fundus can rupture, causing sudden, catastrophic GI bleeding. Bleeding rarely occurs unless the portal pressure gradient is > 12 mm Hg. Gastric mucosal vascular congestion (portal hypertensive gastropathy) can cause acute or chronic bleeding independent of varices. Visible abdominal wall collaterals are common; veins radiating from the umbilicus (caput medusae) are much rarer and indicate extensive flow in the umbilical and periumbilical veins. Collaterals around the rectum can produce rectal varices that can bleed.

Portal-systemic collaterals shunt blood away from the liver. Thus, less blood reaches the liver when portal flow increases (diminished hepatic reserve). In addition, toxic substances from the intestine are shunted directly to the systemic circulation, contributing to portal-systemic encephalopathy (see p. 197). Venous congestion within visceral organs due to portal hypertension contributes to ascites via altered Starling's forces. Splenomegaly and hypersplenism (see p. 1090) commonly occur as a result of increased splenic vein pressure. Thrombocytopenia, leukopenia, and, less commonly, hemolytic anemia may result.

Portal hypertension is often associated with a hyperdynamic circulation. Mechanisms are complex and appear to involve altered sympathetic tone, production of nitric oxide and other endogenous vasodilators, and enhanced activity of humoral factors (eg, glucagon).

Symptoms, Signs, and Diagnosis

Portal hypertension is asymptomatic; symptoms and signs result from its complications. The most dangerous is acute variceal bleeding (see p. 92). Patients typically present with sudden painless upper GI bleeding, often massive. Bleeding from portal hypertensive gastropathy is often subacute or chronic. Ascites, splenomegaly, or portal-systemic encephalopathy may be present.

Portal hypertension is inferred in a patient with chronic liver disease by the presence of collateral circulation, splenomegaly, ascites, or portal-systemic encephalopathy. Proof requires direct portal pressure measurement by a transjugular catheter, which is invasive and usually not performed. Imaging may help when cirrhosis is suspected. Ultrasound or CT often reveals dilated intra-abdominal collaterals, and Doppler ultrasound can determine portal vein patency and flow.

Esophagogastric varices and portal hypertensive gastropathy are best diagnosed by endoscopy, which may also identify predictors of esophagogastric variceal bleeding (eg, red markings on a varix).

Prognosis and Treatment

Mortality during acute variceal hemorrhage may exceed 50%. Prognosis is predicted by the degree of hepatic reserve and the degree of bleeding. For survivors, the bleeding risk within the next 1 to 2 yr is 50 to 75%. Ongoing endoscopic or drug therapy lowers the bleeding risk but decreases long-term mortality only marginally. Treatment of acute bleeding is discussed on p. 93.

When possible, the underlying disorder is treated. Long-term treatment of esophagogastric varices that have bled is a series of endoscopic banding or sclerotherapy sessions to obliterate residual varices, then surveillance endoscopy every few months for recurrent varices. Banding is generally preferable to sclerotherapy because of lower risks.

Long-term drug therapy for varices that have bled involves β-blockers; these drugs lower portal pressure primarily by diminishing portal flow, although the effects vary. Propranolol (40 to 80 mg po bid) or nadolol (40 to 160 mg po once/day) is preferred, with dosage titrated to decrease heart rate by about 25%. Adding isosorbide mononitrate 10 to 20 mg po bid may further reduce portal pressure. Combined long-term endoscopic and drug therapy may be slightly more effective than either alone. Patients who do not adequately respond to either treatment should be considered for transjugular intrahepatic portal-systemic shunting (TIPS) or a surgical portocaval shunt. TIPS creates a stent between the portal and hepatic venous circulation within the liver. Although TIPS may result in fewer immediate deaths than surgical shunting, particularly during acute bleeding, it often needs to be repeated because the stent becomes stenosed or occluded with time. Long-term benefits are unknown. Liver transplantation may help some patients.

For patients with varices that have not yet bled, β-blockers lower the risk of bleeding.

For bleeding from portal hypertensive gastropathy, drugs can be used to decrease portal pressure. A shunt should be considered if drugs fail, but results may be less successful than for esophageal variceal bleeding.

Because it rarely causes clinical problems, hypersplenism requires no specific treatment, and splenectomy should be avoided.

PORTAL–SYSTEMIC ENCEPHALOPATHY

Portal-systemic encephalopathy is a neuropsychiatric syndrome. It most often results from high gut protein or acute metabolic stress (eg, GI bleeding, infection, electrolyte abnormality) in a patient with portal-systemic shunting. Symptoms are mainly neuropsychiatric (eg, confusion, flapping tremor, coma). Diagnosis is based on clinical findings. Treatment usually is correction of the acute cause, restriction of dietary protein, and administration of oral lactulose.

Portal-systemic encephalopathy better describes the pathophysiology than hepatic encephalopathy or hepatic coma, but all three terms are used interchangeably.

Etiology

Portal-systemic encephalopathy may occur in fulminant hepatitis caused by viruses, drugs, or toxins, but it more commonly occurs in cirrhosis or other chronic disorders when extensive portal-systemic collaterals have developed as a result of portal hypertension. Encephalopathy also follows portal-systemic anastomoses, such as surgically created anastomoses connecting the portal vein and vena cava (portacaval shunts, or transjugular intrahepatic portal-systemic shunting [TIPS]).

In patients with chronic liver disease, acute episodes of encephalopathy are usually precipitated by reversible causes. The most common are metabolic stress (eg, infection; electrolyte imbalance, especially hypokalemia; dehydration; use of diuretic drugs), disorders that increase gut protein (eg, GI bleeding, high-protein diet), and nonspecific cerebral depressants (eg, alcohol, sedatives, analgesics).

Pathophysiology

Portal-systemic shunting causes absorbed products that would otherwise be detoxified by the liver to enter the systemic circulation, where they may be toxic to the brain, particularly the cerebral cortex. The substances causing brain toxicity are not precisely known. Ammonia, a product of protein digestion, is an important cause, but other factors (eg, alterations in cerebral benzodiazepine receptors and neurotransmission by γ-aminobutyric acid [GABA]) may also contribute. Aromatic amino acid levels in serum are usually high and branched-chain levels low, but these levels probably do not cause encephalopathy.

Symptoms and Signs

Symptoms and signs of encephalopathy tend to develop in progressive stages (see TABLE 22–2). Symptoms usually do not become apparent until brain function is moderately impaired. Constructional apraxia, in which the patient cannot reproduce simple designs (eg, a star), develops early. Agitation and mania can develop but are uncommon. A characteristic flapping tremor (asterixis) is elicited when the patient holds his

TABLE 22–2. CLINICAL STAGES OF PORTAL-SYSTEMIC ENCEPHALOPATHY

STAGE	COGNITION AND BEHAVIOR	NEUROMUSCULAR FUNCTION
0 (subclinical)	Asymptomatic loss of cognitive abilities	None
1	Sleep disturbances; impaired concentration; depression, anxiety, or irritability	Monotone voice; tremor; poor handwriting; constructional apraxia
2	Drowsiness; disorientation; poor short-term memory; disinhibited behavior	Ataxia; dysarthria; asterixis; automatisms (yawning, blinking, sucking)
3	Somnolence; confusion; amnesia; anger, paranoia, or other bizarre behavior	Nystagmus; muscular rigidity; hyper- or hyporeflexia
4	Coma	Dilated pupils; oculocephalic or oculovestibular reflexes; decerebrate posturing

arms outstretched with wrists dorsiflexed. Neurologic deficits are symmetric. Neurologic signs in coma usually reflect bilateral diffuse hemispheric dysfunction. Signs of brain stem dysfunction develop only in advanced coma, often during the hours or days before death. A musty, sweet breath odor (fetor hepaticus) can occur regardless of the stage of encephalopathy

Diagnosis

Diagnosis ultimately is based on clinical findings, but testing may help. Psychometric testing may reveal subtle neuropsychiatric deficits, which can help confirm early encephalopathy. Ammonia levels generally serve as a laboratory marker for encephalopathy but are neither specific nor highly sensitive and do not indicate the severity of encephalopathy. An EEG usually shows diffuse slow-wave activity, even in mild cases, and may be sensitive but is not specific for early encephalopathy. CSF examination is not routinely necessary; the only usual abnormality is mild protein elevation.

Other potentially reversible disorders that could cause similar manifestations (eg, infection, subdural hematoma, hypoglycemia, intoxication) should be ruled out. If portal-systemic encephalopathy is confirmed, the precipitating cause should be sought.

Prognosis

In chronic liver disease, correction of the precipitating cause usually causes encephalopathy to regress without permanent neurologic sequelae. Some patients, especially those with portacaval shunts or TIPS, require continuous therapy, and irreversible extrapyramidal signs or spastic paraparesis rarely develops. Coma (stage 4 encephalopathy) associated with fulminant hepatitis is fatal in up to 80% of patients despite intensive therapy; the combination of advanced chronic liver failure and portal-systemic encephalopathy is often fatal.

Treatment

Treating the cause usually reverses mild cases. Eliminating toxic enteric products is the other goal and is accomplished using several methods. The bowels should be cleared using enemas or, more often, oral lactulose syrup, which can be tube-fed to comatose patients. This synthetic disaccharide is an osmotic cathartic. It also lowers colonic pH, decreasing fecal ammonia production. The initial dosage, 30 to 45 mL po tid, should be adjusted to produce two or three soft stools daily. Dietary protein should also be eliminated (20 to 40 g/day may be allowed in mild cases) and lost calories replaced with oral or IV carbohydrate.

Sedation deepens encephalopathy and should be avoided whenever possible. For coma caused by fulminant hepatitis, meticulous supportive and nursing care coupled with prevention and treatment of complications increase the chance of survival. High-dose corticosteroids, exchange transfusion, and other complex procedures designed to remove circulating toxins generally do not improve outcome. Patients deteriorating because of fulminant hepatic failure may be saved by liver transplantation.

Other potential therapies, including levodopa, bromocriptine, flumazenil, sodium benzoate, infusions of branched-chain amino acids, keto-analogs of essential amino acids, and prostaglandins, have not proven effective. Complex plasma filtering systems (artificial liver) show some promise but require much more study.

SYSTEMIC ABNORMALITIES IN LIVER DISEASE

Liver disease often produces systemic symptoms and abnormalities (see Portal-Systemic Encephalopathy on p. 197).

Circulatory Abnormalities

Hypotension in advanced liver failure may contribute to renal dysfunction. The pathogenesis of the hyperdynamic circulation (increased cardiac output and heart rate) and hypotension that develop in advanced liver failure or cirrhosis is poorly understood. However, peripheral arterial vasodilation probably contributes to both.

For specific disorders of hepatic circulation (eg, Budd-Chiari syndrome), see Ch. 28 on p. 231.

Endocrine Abnormalities

Glucose intolerance, hyperinsulinism, insulin resistance, and hyperglucagonemia are often present in patients with cirrhosis; the elevated insulin levels reflect decreased hepatic degradation rather than increased secretion, whereas the opposite is true for hyperglucagonemia. Abnormal thyroid function tests may reflect altered hepatic handling of thyroid hormones and changes in plasma binding proteins rather than thyroid abnormalities.

Chronic liver disease commonly impairs menstruation and fertility. Males with cirrhosis, especially alcoholics, often have both hypogonadism (including testicular atrophy, erectile dysfunction, decreased spermatogenesis) and feminization (gynecomastia, female habitus). The biochemical basis is not fully understood. Gonadotropin reserve of the hypothalamic-pituitary axis is often blunted. Circulating testosterone levels are low, resulting mainly from decreased synthesis but also from increased peripheral conversion to estrogens. The levels of estrogens other than estradiol are usually increased, but the relationship between estrogens and feminization is complex. These changes are more prevalent in alcoholic liver disease than in cirrhosis of other etiologies, suggesting that alcohol, rather than liver disease, may be the cause. In fact, evidence indicates that alcohol itself is toxic to the testes.

Hematologic Abnormalities

Anemia is common in patients with liver disease. Contributing factors may include blood loss, folic acid deficiency, hemolysis, marrow suppression by alcohol, and a direct effect of chronic liver disease. Leukopenia and thrombocytopenia often accompany splenomegaly in advanced portal hypertension.

Coagulation abnormalities are common and complex. Hepatocellular dysfunction and inadequate absorption of vitamin K may impair liver synthesis of clotting factors. An abnormal PT or INR results and, depending on the severity of hepatocellular dysfunction, may respond to parenteral phytonadione (vitamin K_1) 5 to 10 mg once/day for 2 to 3 days. Thrombocytopenia, disseminated intravascular coagulation, and fibrinogen abnormalities also contribute to clotting disturbances in many patients.

Renal and Electrolyte Abnormalities

Renal and electrolyte abnormalities are common, especially in patients with ascites.

Hypokalemia may result from excess urinary K loss due to increased circulating aldosterone, renal retention of ammonium ion in exchange for K, secondary renal tubular acidosis, or diuretic therapy. Management consists of giving oral KCl supplements and withholding K-wasting diuretics.

Hyponatremia is common even though the kidney may avidly retain Na (see Ascites on p. 188); it usually occurs with advanced hepatocellular disease and is difficult to correct. Relative water overload is much more often responsible than total body Na depletion;

K depletion may also contribute. Water restriction and K supplements may help; use of diuretics that increase free water clearance is controversial. Saline solution IV is indicated only if profound hyponatremia causes seizures or if total body Na depletion is suspected; it should be avoided in patients with cirrhosis who have fluid retention, because it worsens ascites and only temporarily increases serum Na levels.

Advanced liver failure can alter acid-base balance, usually producing metabolic alkalosis. Blood urea concentrations are often low because of impaired liver synthesis; GI bleeding causes elevations because of an increased enteric load rather than renal impairment. In the latter case, normal creatinine values tend to confirm normal kidney function.

Renal failure in liver disease may reflect rare disorders that directly affect both the kidneys and the liver (eg, carbon tetrachloride toxicity); circulatory failure with decreased renal perfusion, with or without frank acute tubular necrosis; or functional renal failure, often called hepatorenal syndrome. Hepatorenal syndrome is progressive oliguria and azotemia in the absence of structural damage to the kidney; it usually occurs in patients with fulminant hepatitis or advanced cirrhosis with ascites. Its unknown pathogenesis probably involves extreme vasodilation of the splanchnic arterial circulation, leading to decreased central arterial volume. Neural or humoral reductions in renocortical blood flow follow, resulting in a diminished glomerular filtration rate. Low urinary Na concentration and benign sediment usually distinguish it from tubular necrosis, but prerenal azotemia may be more difficult to distinguish; in equivocal cases, response to a volume load should be assessed. Once established, renal failure due to the hepatorenal syndrome is usually rapidly progressive and fatal (type 1 hepatorenal syndrome), although some cases are less severe, with stable low-grade renal insufficiency (type 2). Liver transplantation is the only accepted treatment for type 1 hepatorenal syndrome; transjugular intrahepatic portal-systemic shunting (TIPS) and vasoconstrictors show some promise, but more study is needed.

THE ASYMPTOMATIC PATIENT WITH ABNORMAL LABORATORY TEST RESULTS

Because aminotransferases and alkaline phosphatase are included in commonly obtained laboratory test panels, abnormalities are often detected in patients without signs or symptoms of liver disease. In such patients, the physician should obtain a history of exposure to possible liver toxins, including alcohol; prescription and nonprescription drugs, herbal teas, and remedies; and occupational or other chemical exposures. Mild isolated elevations of ALT or AST (< 2 times normal) may require only repeat testing; they resolve in about ⅓ of cases. If abnormalities occur in other laboratory tests, are severe, or persist on subsequent testing, further evaluation is indicated.

Further evaluation of aminotransferase elevations includes consideration of fatty liver, which can often be suspected clinically. If fatty liver is not apparent, the patient should be screened for hepatitis B and C. Patients > 40 should be screened for hemochromatosis (see p. 1132); patients < 30 should be screened for Wilson's disease (see p. 51), and most patients, especially young or middle-aged women, should be screened for autoimmune disorders. Patients at risk should be screened for malaria and schistosomiasis. If at this point the results are negative, screening for α_1-antitrypsin deficiency (see p. 410) is indicated. If the entire evaluation reveals no cause, liver biopsy may be warranted.

Isolated elevation of alkaline phosphatase levels in an asymptomatic patient requires confirmation of hepatic origin by demonstrating elevation of 5′-nucleotidase or γ-glutamyl transpeptidase. If hepatic origin is confirmed, liver imaging, usually with ultrasound or magnetic resonance cholangiopancreatography, is indicated. If no structural abnormality is found on imaging, intrahepatic cholestasis is possible and may be suggested by a history of exposure to drugs or toxins. Infiltrative diseases and liver metastases (eg, due to colon cancer) should also be considered. In women, antimitochondrial antibody should be obtained. Persistent unexplained elevations or suspicion of intrahepatic cholestasis warrants consideration of liver biopsy.

23 TESTING FOR HEPATIC AND BILIARY DISORDERS

Diagnosis of liver and biliary system disorders may include laboratory tests, imaging tests, and liver biopsy. Individual tests, particularly those of liver biochemistry and excretion, often have limited sensitivity and specificity. Therefore, combined and serial testing are used to better diagnose and assess the cause and severity of disease.

LABORATORY TESTS

Laboratory tests generally are effective in detecting hepatic dysfunction, assessing the severity of liver injury, refining the diagnosis concerning any identified abnormalities, monitoring the course of liver disease, and evaluating the response to treatment. Many tests of liver biochemistry and excretory performance are called liver function tests. However, some of these tests, rather than assessing liver function, assess liver necrosis or injury by measuring liver enzymes released into the bloodstream (eg, aminotransferases). Only some liver function tests actually assess liver function by evaluating hepatobiliary excretion (eg, bilirubin) or the liver's synthetic capability (eg, PT [usually reported as the INR]). Tests that detect liver inflammation, altered immunoregulation, or viral hepatitis include hepatitis serology (see p. 225), immunoglobulins, antibodies, and autoantibodies. These tests reflect B lymphocyte rather than hepatocyte function. Other laboratory tests may reflect specific disorders, such as α-fetoprotein in hepatocellular carcinoma.

The most useful laboratory tests, particularly for screening for evidence of liver disease, are serum aminotransferases, bilirubin, and alkaline phosphatase. Certain patterns of liver biochemical abnormalities help distinguish hepatocellular injury from impaired bile excretion (cholestasis—see TABLE 23–1). A few laboratory tests are diagnostic by themselves (eg, hepatitis B surface antigen [HBsAg] for hepatitis B virus, serum copper and ceruloplasmin for suspected Wilson's disease, serum α_1-antitrypsin for α_1-antitrypsin deficiency).

TABLE 23–1. COMMON PATTERNS OF LABORATORY TEST ABNORMALITIES

PATTERN	AMINOTRANSFERASE ELEVATIONS	ALKALINE PHOSPHATASE ELEVATIONS	PROLONGATION OF PROTHROMBIN TIME
Acute necrosis or injury	Usually severe	Often present but may be mild	Prolonged if hepatic insufficiency develops
Chronic hepatocellular disease	Usually moderate to severe	Often present but may be mild	Prolonged if hepatic insufficiency develops
Cholestasis	Often present but may be mild	Usually moderate to severe	Prolonged if chronic steatorrhea causes vitamin K malabsorption
Infiltration	Often present but may be mild	Often present but may be mild	Not usually prolonged
Insufficiency (failure)	Depends on underlying cause	Depends on underlying cause	Often present but may be mild

Tests for Liver Injury

Aminotransferases: Alanine aminotransferase (ALT) and aspartate aminotransferase (AST) leak from damaged cells, making them sensitive indicators of liver injury. Acute hepatocellular necrosis or injury (eg, hepatitis) typically results in high values (500 to > 2000 IU/L; normal, ≤ 40 IU/L), usually for days or, in viral hepatitis, weeks. Serial measurements better reflect severity and prognosis than do single values: a fall to normal indicates recovery unless accompanied by a rise in bilirubin and PT or INR (which may predict massive liver failure). Modest elevations (100 to 300 IU/L) persist in chronic liver diseases. In biliary obstruction, values usually are < 300 IU/L, except where passage of a common duct stone transiently increases levels to the thousands. Values < 100 IU/L are nonspecific.

Although ALT is somewhat specific for liver disease, AST may be elevated because of rhabdomyolysis or damage to heart or brain tissue. In most liver diseases, the ratio of AST to ALT is < 1, but in alcohol-related liver damage, the ratio characteristically is > 2; pyridoxine, which is deficient in most alcoholic patients, is required for ALT synthesis but is less essential for AST synthesis.

Lactate dehydrogenase: LDH, commonly included in routine analysis, is insensitive for hepatocellular injury but sensitive for cancers involving the liver. Elevations may also indicate hemolysis, MI, or pulmonary embolism.

Tests for Cholestasis

Bilirubin: Bilirubin is the pigment in bile produced from the breakdown of heme proteins. Unconjugated bilirubin is lipid-soluble and is transported in plasma bound to albumin. It is conjugated in the liver to form water-soluble conjugated bilirubin. Conjugated bilirubin is then excreted through the biliary system into the duodenum, where it undergoes metabolism to form unconjugated bilirubin, colorless urobilinogens, and then orange-colored urobilins, most of which are eliminated in feces.

Hyperbilirubinemia results from increased bilirubin production, decreased liver uptake or conjugation, or decreased biliary excretion (see p. 191). Total bilirubin normally is mostly unconjugated, with values of < 1.2 mg/dL (< 20 μmol/L). Fractionation can measure the proportion of bilirubin that is conjugated (or direct, ie, measured directly). Fractionation is required only in neonatal jaundice or if bilirubin is elevated, but other liver test results are normal, suggesting that hepatobiliary disease is not the cause.

Unconjugated hyperbilirubinemia (indirect bilirubin fraction > 85%) reflects increased bilirubin production (eg, hemolysis) or defective liver uptake or conjugation (eg, Gilbert syndrome). Such increases in unconjugated bilirubin are generally less than 5-fold (< 6 mg/dL [< 100 μmol/L]) unless concurrent liver disease exists.

Conjugated hyperbilirubinemia (direct bilirubin fraction > 50%) results from decreased bile formation or excretion (cholestasis). Serum bilirubin is insensitive for liver dysfunction and does not distinguish cholestasis from hepatocellular disease. Severe hyperbilirubinemia, however, may predict a poor prognosis in primary biliary cirrhosis, alcoholic hepatitis, and acute liver failure.

Unconjugated bilirubin, because it is water-insoluble and bound to albumin, cannot be excreted in urine. Thus, bilirubinuria generally indicates high serum conjugated bilirubin and hepatobiliary disease. Bilirubinuria can be detected at the bedside with commercial urine test strips in acute viral hepatitis or other hepatobiliary disorders before jaundice appears. However, the urine test strip has limited value because it may be falsely negative with prolonged storage of the urine specimen, vitamin C ingestion, or nitrates in the urine (eg, from UTIs). Similarly, increases in urobilinogen have limited value; they are neither specific nor sensitive.

Alkaline phosphatase: Increases in levels of this hepatocyte enzyme suggest cholestasis. However, alkaline phosphatase consists of several isoenzymes and originates in various tissues, particularly in bone.

Alkaline phosphatase levels increase 4-fold or higher 1 to 2 days after the onset of biliary obstruction, regardless of the site of obstruction. Levels may remain elevated for several days after the obstruction resolves because the half-life of alkaline phosphatase is about 7 days. Increases of up to 3 times normal occur in many liver disorders, including hepatitis, cirrhosis, space-occupying lesions, and infiltrative disorders. Isolated elevations (ie, when other liver test results are normal) occur often in focal liver lesions (eg, abscess, tumor) or in partial or intermittent bile duct obstruction. Isolated elevations also occur in the absence of liver or biliary disease, such as some malignancies without apparent liver involvement (eg, bronchogenic carcinoma, Hodgkin's lymphoma, renal cell carcinoma), after fatty meals (originating in the small intestine), in pregnancy (from placenta), in growing children and adolescents (from bone growth), and in chronic renal failure (from intestine and bone). Fractionating these alkaline phosphatases is technically difficult. Elevation of enzymes more specific to the liver, 5′ nucleotidase or γ-glutamyl transpeptidase (GGT), can differentiate hepatic from extrahepatic sources of alkaline phosphatase. An isolated alkaline phosphatase elevation in an otherwise asymptomatic elderly person usually originates from bone (eg, Paget's disease) and does not require further investigation.

5′-Nucleotidase: Increases in levels of this enzyme are as sensitive as alkaline phosphatase for detecting cholestasis and biliary obstruction but are more specific, almost always indicating hepatobiliary disease. Because levels of alkaline phosphatase and 5′-nucleotidase do not always correlate, one can be normal while the other is increased.

γ-Glutamyl transpeptidase (GGT): Levels of this enzyme rise in hepatobiliary disease, especially cholestasis, and correlate loosely with levels of alkaline phosphatase and 5′-nucleotidase. Levels do not increase with bone lesions, during childhood, or during pregnancy. However, levels increase with induction of microsomal enzymes (eg, by ingesting certain drugs, such as anticonvulsants, and particularly in alcoholics), limiting its specificity.

Tests of Hepatic Synthetic Capacity

PT and INR: PT may be expressed in time (sec) or, preferably, as a ratio of measured PT vs control PT, termed the INR (see p. 1077). The INR is the more accurate laboratory reference with which to monitor patients taking anticoagulants. The PT or INR is a valuable measure of the liver's ability to synthesize vitamin K–dependent clotting factors: factors II (prothrombin), V, VII, and X. Changes can occur rapidly, because some of the involved clotting factors have short biologic half-lives (eg, 6 h for factor VII). Abnormalities indicate severe hepatocellular dysfunction, an ominous sign in acute liver disease. In chronic liver disease, a rising PT or INR indicates progression to advanced cirrhosis. The PT or INR does not increase in mild hepatocellular dysfunction and is often normal in cirrhosis.

A prolonged PT and abnormal INR can result from other coagulation disorders, such as a consumptive coagulopathy or a deficiency of vitamin K. Fat malabsorption, including cholestasis, can cause vitamin K deficiency. In chronic cholestasis, marked hepatocellular dysfunction can be ruled out if vitamin K replacement (10 mg sc) corrects the PT within 2 days.

Serum proteins: Hepatocytes synthesize most serum proteins, including α- and β-globulins, albumin, and clotting factors (but not γ-globulin, which is produced by B lymphocytes). Hepatocytes also make proteins that aid in the diagnosis of specific disorders: α_1-antitrypsin (absent in α_1-antitrypsin deficiency), ceruloplasmin (reduced in Wilson's disease), transferrin (saturated with iron in hemochromatosis), and ferritin (greatly increased in hemochromatosis). Because levels of these proteins increase in response to tissue damage (eg, inflammation), elevations are not specific for liver disorders.

Serum albumin commonly decreases in chronic liver disease because of an increase in volume of distribution (eg, due to ascites), a decrease in hepatic synthesis, or both. Values < 3 g/dL (< 30 g/L) suggest advanced cirrhosis. Alcoholism, chronic inflammation, and protein malnutrition also depress albumin synthesis. Hypoalbuminemia can also result from excess albumin loss from the kidney (ie, nephrotic syndrome), gut (eg, protein-losing gastroenteropathies), and skin (eg, burns or exfoliative dermatitis). Because albumin has a half-life of about 20 days, serum levels take weeks to increase or decrease.

Other Laboratory Tests

Ammonia: Ammonia is produced by colonic bacteria and metabolism of glutamine. The liver metabolizes ammonia to urea. Ammonia levels increase during portal-systemic (hepatic) encephalopathy. In advanced disease, levels may also increase because of high-protein meals, GI bleeding, hypokalemia or metabolic alkalosis, or metabolic diseases involving urea metabolism. Because the degree of elevation in ammonia correlates poorly with the severity of hepatic encephalopathy, the ammonia level has limited accuracy in monitoring therapy.

Serum immunoglobulins: In chronic liver disease, serum immunoglobulins often increase. However, elevations are not specific and usually are not helpful clinically. Levels increase slightly in acute hepatitis, moderately in chronic active hepatitis, and markedly in autoimmune hepatitis. The pattern of immunoglobulin increase adds little, although generally IgM is quite high in primary biliary cirrhosis; IgA, in alcoholic liver disease; and IgG, in chronic active hepatitis.

Antibodies: Specific antibodies and antigens may be diagnostic (eg, viral antigens and antibodies in hepatitis).

Antimitochondrial antibodies: These heterogeneous antibodies are positive, usually in high titers, in > 95% of patients with primary biliary cirrhosis. They also are occasionally present in autoimmune chronic active hepatitis, in drug-induced hepatitis, and in other autoimmune disorders, such as connective tissue disorders, myasthenia gravis, autoimmune thyroiditis, Addison's disease, and autoimmune hemolytic anemia. Antimitochondrial antibodies can help determine the cause of cholestasis because they are usually absent in extrahepatic biliary obstruction and primary sclerosing cholangitis.

Other antibodies: Other antibodies often present in autoimmune hepatitis include smooth muscle antibodies against actin, antinuclear antibodies (ANA) providing a homogenous (diffuse) fluorescence, and antibodies to liver/kidney microsome type 1 (anti-LKM1). Isolated abnormalities of any of these antibodies are never diagnostic and do not reveal pathogenesis.

α-Fetoprotein (AFP): AFP, a glycoprotein normally synthesized by the yolk sac in the embryo and then the fetal liver, is elevated in the newborn and hence the pregnant mother. AFP decreases rapidly during the first year of life, reaching adult values (normally < 20 ng/mL) by the age of 1 yr. Marked elevations (> 500 ng/mL) in a high-risk patient (eg, with a liver mass detected on ultrasound) is diagnostic of primary hepatocellular carcinoma (HCC), although not all HCCs produce AFP. Because small tumors can have low levels of AFP, rising values suggest the presence of HCC. The degree of AFP elevation, however, is not prognostic. In populations in which chronic hepatitis B infection and HCC are common (eg, sub-Saharan Africans, ethnic Chinese), AFP may reach levels as high as 100,000 ng/mL, whereas regions with lower frequencies of the tumor have more modest levels (about 3000 ng/mL).

A few other conditions (eg, embryonic teratocarcinomas, hepatoblastomas, some hepatic metastases from GI tract cancers, some cholangiocarcinomas) cause levels ≥ 500 ng/mL. In fulminant hepatitis, AFP can occasionally rise to 500 ng/mL; lesser elevations occur in acute and chronic hepatitis. These levels probably reflect liver regeneration. Thus, sensitivity and specificity of AFP vary according to population, but values ≥ 20 ng/mL range from 39 to 64% and from 76 to 91%, respectively. Because values ≤ 500 ng/mL are nonspecific, 500 ng/mL has been suggested as the diagnostic cutoff level.

IMAGING TESTS

Imaging is essential for accurately diagnosing biliary tract disease and is important for diagnosing focal liver lesions (eg, abscess, tumor), but it is limited in diagnosing diffuse hepatocellular disease (eg, hepatitis, cirrhosis).

Ultrasound: Ultrasound, traditionally performed transabdominally and requiring a period of fasting, provides structural, but not functional, information. It is the least expensive, safest, and most sensitive technique for imaging the biliary system, especially the gallbladder. Ultrasound is the procedure of choice in screening for biliary tract abnormalities, differentiating intrahepatic from extrahepatic causes of jaundice, and detecting liver masses. The kidney, pancreas, and blood vessels are also often visible on hepatobiliary ultrasound. Ultrasound can be difficult in the presence of intestinal gas or obesity and is operator-dependent. Endoscopic ultrasonography incorporates an ultrasound transducer into the tip of an endoscope, which allows for greater image resolution even if intestinal gas is present.

Gallstones cast intense echoes with distal acoustic shadowing that move with gravity. Diagnostic accuracy on transabdominal ultrasound is extremely high (sensitivity > 95%) for gallstones > 2 mm in diameter. Endoscopic ultrasound can detect stones as small as 0.5 mm (microlithiasis) in the gallbladder or biliary system. Transabdominal and endoscopic ultrasound also can detect biliary sludge (a mixture of particulate material and bile) as low-level echoes that layer in the dependent portion of the gallbladder, without acoustic shadowing. Cholecystitis produces a thickened gallbladder wall (>3 mm), pericholecystic fluid, an impacted stone in the gallbladder neck, and tenderness on palpation of the gallbladder with the ultrasound probe (ultrasonographic Murphy's sign).

On transabdominal and endoscopic ultrasound, bile ducts stand out as echo-free tubular structures. The diameter of the common duct is normally < 6 mm, increases slightly with age, and can reach 10 mm after cholecystectomy. Dilated ducts are virtually pathognomonic for extrahepatic obstruction in the appropriate clinical setting. Ultrasound can miss early or intermittent obstruction without dilated ducts. Transabdominal ultrasound may not reveal the level or cause of biliary obstruction (eg, sensitivity for common duct stones is < 40%). Endoscopic ultrasound has a better yield.

Transabdominal ultrasound detects focal liver lesions (> 1 cm in diameter) more accurately than diffuse diseases (eg, fatty liver, cirrhosis). In general, cysts are echo-free; solid lesions (eg, tumors, abscesses) tend to be echogenic. Carcinoma appears as a nonspecific solid mass. Ultrasound has been used to screen for hepatocellular carcinoma in those at high risk (eg, with chronic hepatitis B). The ability to localize focal lesions permits ultrasound-guided aspiration and biopsy. The advent of endoscopic ultrasound may further refine several of these diagnostic approaches.

Doppler ultrasound is a noninvasive method with which to assess direction of blood flow and patency of blood vessels around the liver, particularly the portal vein. Doppler ultrasound can reveal evidence of portal hypertension with collateral flow, assess the patency of liver shunts (eg, surgical portocaval, percutaneous transhepatic), and reveal hepatic artery thrombosis after liver transplantation. It also can detect unusual vascular structures, such as cavernous transformation of the portal vein.

CT: CT is commonly used to identify hepatic masses, particularly small metastases, with an accuracy of about 80%. CT with IV contrast is accurate for diagnosing cavernous hemangiomas of the liver as well as differentiating them from other abdominal masses. Neither obesity nor intestinal gas obscures CT images. CT can detect fatty liver and the increased hepatic density associated with iron overload. CT is less helpful than ultrasound in diagnosing biliary obstruction but often provides the best assessment of the pancreas.

Cholescintigraphy: In this procedure, IV technetium-labeled iminodiacetic compounds (eg, hydroxy or diisopropyl iminodiacetic acid [HIDA or DISIDA]) are given which are taken up by the liver and excreted in the bile, thus outlining the path of bile excretion, particularly the cystic duct.

In calculous cholecystitis, which usually is caused by impaction of a stone in the cystic duct, the gallbladder is not visible. The test has a sensitivity of 95% and a specificity of 90% but is infrequently needed to diagnose acute cholecystitis. False-positive results are common in critically ill patients.

In suspected acalculous cholecystitis, the gallbladder is scanned before and after administration of cholecystokinin (which causes the gallbladder to contract). The difference in scintigraphic count, termed the gallbladder ejection fraction, is below normal in acalculous cholecystitis.

Cholescintigraphy also detects bile leaks (eg, after surgery or trauma) and anatomic abnormalities (eg, congenital choledochal cysts, choledochoenteric anastomoses). After cholecystectomy, cholescintigraphy can quantitate biliary drainage and assist in defining sphincter of Oddi dysfunction.

Radionuclide liver scanning: Ultrasound and CT have largely supplanted radionuclide scanning, which has been used to diagnose diffuse parenchymal disease and mass lesions of the liver. Radionuclide scanning demonstrates the distribution of an injected radioactive tracer, usually technetium (^{99m}Tc-sulfur colloid), which distributes uniformly within the normal liver. Space-occupying lesions >4 cm, such as liver cysts, abscesses, metastases, and tumors, appear as defects. Generalized liver disease (eg, cirrhosis, hepatitis) decreases the liver uptake of the tracer, with more appearing in the spleen and bone marrow. In hepatic vein obstruction, liver uptake is decreased except in the caudate lobe because of its drainage into the inferior vena cava.

Oral cholecystography: The oral cholecystogram (OCG) was once the procedure of choice for diagnosing gallstones and suspected cholecystitis. Unlike ultrasound, OCG measures the concentrating function of the gallbladder. OCG has been replaced by ultrasound, however, because OCG is less accurate, can take up to 48 h to complete, and can cause diarrhea and, rarely, a hypersensitivity reaction with kidney damage.

Plain x-ray of the abdomen: The plain x-ray is an inaccurate tool for diagnosing hepatobiliary disease, even gallstones. Rarely, it can help in gravely ill patients by revealing air in the biliary tree, which suggests emphysematous cholangitis.

MRI: MRI images blood vessels (without using contrast) and hepatic tissues. Although expensive, its indications are still evolving. MRI is superior to CT and ultrasound for diagnosing diffuse liver diseases (eg, fatty liver, hemochromatosis), and for clarifying some focal defects (eg, hemangiomas). MRI also reveals blood flow and therefore can complement Doppler ultrasound and CT angiography in diagnosing vascular abnormalities and in performing vascular mapping before liver transplantation.

MRI of the biliary tree is magnetic resonance cholangiopancreatography (MRCP). MRCP is more sensitive than CT or ultrasound in diagnosing common bile duct abnormalities, particularly stones. Its images are comparable to those from ERCP and percutaneous transhepatic cholangiography, which are more invasive. MRCP, therefore, is a useful screening tool when biliary obstruction is suspected and before proceeding to therapeutic ERCP (eg, for simultaneous imaging and stone removal).

ERCP: ERCP combines endoscopy through the second portion of the duodenum with contrast imaging of the biliary and pancreatic ducts. First, an endoscope is placed in the descending duodenum, then the papilla of Vater is cannulated, and the pancreatic and biliary ducts are injected with contrast. ERCP is the procedure of choice when bile duct stones are suspected but have not been found on less invasive tests. The test is especially valuable for diagnosing correctable biliary tract lesions causing persistent jaundice (eg, stone, stricture, sphincter of Oddi dysfunction). Besides providing excellent images of the biliary tract and pancreas, ERCP reveals some of the upper GI tract and the periampullary area. Biopsies and interventional procedures may be performed (eg, sphincterotomy, biliary stone extraction, placement of a biliary stent in a stricture—see Ch. 30 on p. 240). Its sensitivity and specificity for common bile duct stones are about 95%. The morbidity from a diagnostic ERCP with only injection of contrast material is about 1%. The addition of sphincterotomy raises morbidity to 4 to 9% (mainly pancreatitis and bleeding). ERCP with manometry to measure sphincter of Oddi pressure causes pancreatitis in up to 25%.

Percutaneous transhepatic cholangiography (PTC): PTC involves puncture of the liver with a needle under fluoroscopic or ultrasound guidance to cannulate the peripheral intrahepatic bile duct system above the common hepatic duct into which contrast material is injected. PTC is highly diagnostic for biliary disease and can be therapeutic (eg, for decompression of the biliary system, insertion of an endoprosthesis). However, ERCP is generally preferred because PTC causes more complications (eg, sepsis, bleeding, bile leaks).

Operative cholangiography: This is direct injection of a contrast agent at laparotomy for visualization of the cystic duct or common bile duct. Operative cholangiography is indicated when jaundice occurs and noninvasive studies are equivocal, leading to suspicion of common duct stones. It then can be followed by common duct exploration for removal of biliary stones. Technical difficulties have limited its use, particularly during laparoscopic cholecystectomy.

LIVER BIOPSY

Liver biopsy can provide histologic and other information that otherwise would not be obtained (see TABLE 23–2). Although only a small core of tissue is obtained, it is usually representative, even with focal lesions. Ultrasound- or CT-guided biopsies improve the yield. For example, biopsy performed under ultrasound guidance is 66% sensitive for metastatic cancer. Biopsy is especially valuable in detecting TB or other granulomatous infiltrations and in clarifying graft problems (ischemic injury, rejection, biliary tract disease, viral hepatitis) after liver transplantation. Serial biopsies, commonly performed over years, may be necessary for monitoring disease progression.

Gross examination and histopathology are often definitive. Cytology, frozen section, and culture may be useful in selected cases. Metal content can be measured in the biopsy specimen: copper in suspected Wilson's disease and iron in hemochromatosis.

Limitations of liver biopsy include (1) sampling error; (2) occasional errors or uncertainty in cases of cholestasis; and (3) the need for a skilled histopathologist (many pathologists have little experience with needle specimens).

Liver biopsy can be performed percutaneously at the bedside or with ultrasound guidance. The latter is preferred because of its slightly lower complication rate plus the opportunity to visualize the liver and target focal lesions. Absolute contraindications include inability to remain still and maintain expiration for the procedure, a bleeding tendency (INR > 1.2 despite receiving vitamin K, bleeding time > 10 min), and severe thrombocytopenia (< 50,000/mL). Relative contraindications include profound anemia, peritonitis, marked ascites, high-grade biliary obstruction, and a subphrenic or right pleural infection or effusion. Nonetheless, percutaneous liver biopsy is sufficiently safe to be performed on an outpatient basis. Mortality is 0.01%. Major complications (eg, intra-abdominal hemorrhage, bile peritonitis, lacerated liver) develop in about 2% of cases. Complications usually become evident within 3 to 4 h, the recommended period for monitoring the patient.

Transjugular venous biopsy of the liver is reserved for patients with a severe coagulopathy. The procedure involves cannulating the right internal jugular vein and passing a catheter through the inferior vena cava into the hepatic vein. A fine needle is advanced through the hepatic vein into the liver. A successful biopsy is obtained in > 95% of cases, with a low complication rate: 0.2% bleed from puncture of the liver capsule.

TABLE 23–2. INDICATIONS FOR LIVER BIOPSY

Unexplained liver enzyme abnormalities
Alcoholic liver disease or nonalcoholic steatosis (diagnose and stage)
Chronic hepatitis (diagnose and stage)
Suspected rejection after liver transplantation that cannot be diagnosed by less invasive methods
Hepatosplenomegaly of unknown cause
Unexplained intrahepatic cholestasis
Suspected malignancy (focal lesions)
Unexplained liver enzyme abnormalities
Unexplained systemic illness–eg, fever of unknown origin, inflammatory or granulomatous diseases (culture is performed with biopsy)

24 DRUGS AND THE LIVER

Interaction between drugs and the liver can be categorized as (1) effects of liver disease on drug metabolism, (2) liver damage caused by drugs, and (3) hepatic drug metabolism (see p. 2526). The number of possible interactions is vast.

EFFECTS OF LIVER DISEASE ON DRUG METABOLISM

Liver disease may have complex effects on drug clearance, biotransformation, and pharmacokinetics. Pathogenetic factors include alterations in intestinal absorption, plasma protein binding, hepatic extraction ratio, liver blood flow and portal-systemic shunting, biliary excretion, enterohepatic circulation, and renal clearance. Net results for an individual drug are unpredictable and do not correlate well with the type of liver damage, its severity, or liver laboratory test results. Thus, no general rules are available for modifying drug dosage in patients with liver disease.

Clinical effects can vary independent of drug bioavailability, especially in chronic liver disease; eg, cerebral sensitivity to opioids and sedatives is often enhanced in a patient with chronic liver disease. Thus, seemingly small doses of these drugs given to cirrhotic patients may precipitate encephalopathy. The mechanism of this effect probably involves alterations in cerebral drug receptors.

LIVER DAMAGE CAUSED BY DRUGS

The mechanisms by which drugs damage the liver are variable, complex, and often poorly understood. Some drugs are directly toxic: with these, injury is generally characteristic for the drug, begins within hours of exposure, and is dose-related. Other drugs produce damage only rarely and only in susceptible people; the injury generally first occurs within a few weeks but occasionally may be delayed for several months after drug exposure. This injury is not dose-related. These reactions are rarely allergic; they are more accurately described as idiosyncratic. The distinction between direct toxicity and idiosyncrasy may not always be clear; eg, some drugs whose injury appears idiosyncratic probably damage cell membranes directly with toxic intermediate metabolites.

Although there is no perfect system for classifying liver damage caused by drugs, damage can be categorized as acute reactions (which consist of hepatocellular necrosis), cholestasis (with or without inflammation), and miscellaneous reactions (see TABLE 24–1). Some drugs can cause chronic damage, which rarely leads to tumor growth.

Diagnosis and Treatment

Drug-induced hepatotoxicity is suspected when patients have unusual patterns of liver disease (eg, mixed or atypical patterns of cholestasis and hepatitis); in hepatitis or cholestasis for which common causes have been excluded; during administration of a drug with known hepatotoxicity (see TABLE 24–1), even in the absence of symptoms or signs; or if a liver biopsy reveals histologic features suggesting a drug etiology. Jaundice due to drug-induced hemolysis may at first suggest hepatotoxicity, but in such cases, bilirubin is unconjugated and other liver function test results are normal.

No diagnostic tests can confirm that a drug caused hepatotoxicity. Diagnosis requires exclusion of other possible causes (eg, imaging tests to exclude obstruction if cholestasis is present; viral serology if hepatitis is present) and a temporal relationship between the drug and hepatotoxicity. A pattern of repeated, reversible hepatotoxicity after repeated doses is the most conclusive evidence, but because of the risk of serious liver damage, rechallenging a patient with a suspected hepatotoxic drug generally is not done. Biopsy is sometimes necessary, generally to exclude other treatable conditions. If the diagnosis is still unclear after testing, a trial of drug withdrawal may be indicated for diagnosis as well as treatment.

For a few drugs that cause direct hepatotoxicity (eg, acetaminophen), blood levels can be used to assess the probability of liver damage. However, drug levels may fall if tests are delayed. Many nonprescription herbal products cause liver toxicity; patients with unexplained liver injury should be asked whether they are taking such products.

Treatment for drug-induced hepatotoxicity generally consists of withdrawing the drug and providing supportive therapy.

Hepatocellular Necrosis

Hepatocellular necrosis is conceptually divided into direct toxicity and idiosyncrasy, although this distinction may be artificial. The hallmark is elevated aminotransferase levels, often to a striking degree. Patients with mild or moderate hepatocellular necrosis may develop manifestations of hepatitis (eg, jaundice, malaise). Patients with severe necrosis may develop manifestations of fulminant hepatitis (eg, hepatic insufficiency, portal-systemic encephalopathy).

Direct toxicity: Most direct hepatotoxins produce dose-related hepatic necrosis and often affect other organs (eg, kidneys).

Direct hepatotoxic damage from prescribed drugs can generally be prevented or minimized by following recommendations regarding maximum drug dosing and patient monitoring. Poisoning with direct hepatotoxins (eg, acetaminophen, iron, *Amanita* mushrooms) often produces gastroenteritis within hours. However, manifestations of liver damage may develop after only 1 to 4 days. Cocaine use occasionally causes acute hepatocellular necrosis, perhaps by inducing hepatocellular ischemia.

Idiosyncrasy: Drugs can produce acute hepatocellular necrosis that is indistinguishable, even histologically, from viral hepatitis. The mechanisms are uncertain and probably vary with individual drugs. Isoniazid and halothane have been most thoroughly studied.

The mechanism of the rare halothane-related hepatitis is unclear but may include formation of reactive intermediates, cellular hypoxia, lipid peroxidation, and autoimmune-mediated damage. Risk factors include

TABLE 24–1. COMMON HEPATOTOXIC DRUG REACTIONS

DRUG	REACTION
Acetaminophen	Acute, direct hepatocellular toxicity; chronic toxicity
Allopurinol	Miscellaneous acute reactions
Amanita mushrooms	Acute, direct hepatocellular toxicity
Aminosalicylic acid	Miscellaneous acute reactions
Amiodarone	Chronic toxicity
Antibiotics, various	Miscellaneous acute reactions
Antineoplastics, various	Miscellaneous acute reactions
Arsenic compounds	Chronic toxicity
Aspirin	Miscellaneous acute reactions
C-17 alkylated steroids	Acute cholestasis, steroid type
Chlorpropamide	Acute cholestasis, phenothiazine type
Diclofenac	Acute, idiosyncratic hepatocellular toxicity
Erythromycin estolate	Acute cholestasis, phenothiazine type
Halothane-related anesthetics	Acute, idiosyncratic hepatocellular toxicity
Hepatic intra-arterial antineoplastics	Chronic toxicity
HMG-CoA reductase inhibitors (statins)	Miscellaneous acute reactions
Hydrocarbons	Acute, direct hepatocellular toxicity
Indomethacin	Acute, idiosyncratic hepatocellular toxicity
Iron	Acute, direct hepatocellular toxicity
Isoniazid	Acute, idiosyncratic hepatocellular toxicity; chronic toxicity
Methotrexate	Chronic toxicity
Methyldopa	Acute, idiosyncratic hepatocellular toxicity; chronic toxicity
Methyltestosterone	Acute cholestasis, steroid type
Monoamine oxidase inhibitors	Acute, idiosyncratic hepatocellular toxicity
Niacin	Chronic toxicity
Nitrofurantoin	Chronic toxicity
Oral contraceptives	Acute cholestasis, steroid type
Phenothiazines (eg, chlorpromazine)	Acute cholestasis, phenothiazine type; chronic toxicity
Phenylbutazone	Acute cholestasis, phenothiazine type
Phenytoin	Acute, idiosyncratic hepatocellular toxicity
Phosphorus	Acute, direct hepatocellular toxicity
Propylthiouracil	Acute, idiosyncratic hepatocellular toxicity
Quinidine	Miscellaneous acute reactions
Sulfonamides	Miscellaneous acute reactions
Tetracycline, high-dose IV	Acute, direct hepatocellular toxicity
Tricyclic antidepressants	Acute cholestasis, phenothiazine type
Valproate	Miscellaneous acute reactions
Vitamin A	Chronic toxicity

obesity (possibly because halothane metabolites are stored in adipose tissue) and repeated exposures to the anesthetic at relatively short intervals. Hepatitis typically develops within a few days to 2 wk after exposure, is heralded by fever, and is often severe. Occasionally, eosinophilia or a skin rash develops. Mortality is 20 to 40% if severe jaundice is present, but survivors usually recover completely. Methoxyflurane and enflurane, which are related anesthetics, can produce the same syndrome.

CHOLESTASIS

Many drugs can produce a primarily cholestatic reaction. Usually the pathogenesis is poorly understood, but at least two forms of cholestatic injury—phenothiazine- and steroid-type—are clinically and histologically distinct. Diagnostic testing often includes noninvasive imaging to exclude biliary obstruction. Further testing (eg, magnetic resonance cholangiopancreatography, ERCP, liver biopsy) is necessary only if cholestasis persists after the drug is stopped.

Phenothiazine-type cholestasis is a periportal inflammatory reaction. Immunologic mechanisms are suggested by some evidence, such as occasional eosinophilia or other signs of hypersensitivity reactions, but direct toxicity to hepatic canaliculi is also possible. This type of cholestasis occurs in about 1% of patients given chlorpromazine and less often in those given other phenothiazines. Cholestasis is often acute and is accompanied by fever and high levels of aminotransferases and alkaline phosphatase. Differentiation from extrahepatic obstruction may be difficult, even by liver biopsy. If the drug is stopped, complete resolution is typical, although progression to chronic cholestasis with fibrosis occurs rarely. Cholestasis produced by tricyclic antidepressants, chlorpropamide, phenylbutazone, erythromycin estolate, and many other drugs is clinically similar; however, progression to chronic liver damage from these drugs has not been clearly established.

Steroid-type cholestasis appears to be an exaggeration of the physiologic effect of sex hormones on bile formation rather than an immunologic sensitivity or membrane cytotoxicity. Impaired canalicular water flow, microfilament dysfunction, altered membrane fluidity, and genetic factors may be responsible. Little or no hepatocellular inflammation exists. Although the incidence varies worldwide, it occurs in 1 to 2% of women taking oral contraceptives. Gradual onset of cholestasis without systemic symptoms is characteristic. Alkaline phosphatase is elevated, but aminotransferase levels are usually not very high, and liver biopsy shows only centrizonal bile stasis with little portal or hepatocellular damage. Complete resolution follows drug withdrawal in most cases but may be prolonged.

Cholestasis of pregnancy (see p. 2180) is closely related to steroid-related cholestasis. Women with cholestasis of pregnancy may develop cholestasis with subsequent oral contraceptive use and vice versa.

MISCELLANEOUS ACUTE REACTIONS

Some drugs cause mixed forms of hepatic dysfunction, granulomatous reactions (eg, quinidine, allopurinol, sulfonamides), or variants of liver injury that are difficult to classify. HMG-CoA reductase inhibitors (statins) produce subclinical aminotransferase elevations in 1 to 2% of patients, although clinically important liver injury is infrequent. Many antineoplastic drugs also cause liver damage; the mechanisms vary.

CHRONIC LIVER DISEASE

Certain drugs can cause chronic liver disease. Isoniazid, methyldopa, and nitrofurantoin can produce chronic hepatitis. Resolution usually occurs if fibrosis is not present. The illness may begin acutely or insidiously. Progression to cirrhosis may occur. Chronic hepatitis-like histology with scarring occurs rarely in patients using acetaminophen long-term in doses as low as 3 g/day, although higher doses are usually required. Alcoholics appear to be more susceptible, and the disorder is suspected in alcoholics found incidentally to have unusually high aminotransferase levels, especially AST (values rarely exceed 300 IU in alcoholic hepatitis alone). Amiodarone occasionally produces chronic liver injury with Mallory bodies and histologic features otherwise similar to alcoholic liver disease; membrane phospholipidosis is a factor in pathogenesis.

A sclerosing cholangitis–like syndrome can develop from hepatic intra-arterial chemotherapy, especially with floxuridine. Patients receiving methotrexate long-term (usually for psoriasis or RA) can develop insidiously progressive hepatic fibrosis, particularly in the case of alcoholics or if the drug is given daily; liver function tests are often unremarkable, and liver biopsy is needed. Although fibrosis caused by methotrexate is rarely clinically important, most authorities recommend biopsy when the cumulative drug dose reaches 1.5 to 2 g and occasionally thereafter. Noncirrhotic hepatic fibrosis that can produce portal hypertension can result from use of arsenical compounds or excessive amounts of vitamin A (eg, > 15,000 U/day for months) or niacin (see p. 32). In many tropical and subtropical countries, chronic liver disease and hepatocellular carcinoma are believed to result from ingesting foods containing fungal aflatoxins.

Besides causing cholestasis, oral contraceptives may also occasionally cause benign hepatic adenomas and, very rarely, hepatocellular carcinoma. Adenomas are usually subclinical but may present with sudden intraperitoneal rupture and hemorrhage, requiring emergency laparotomy. Most adenomas do not cause symptoms and are found incidentally during imaging tests. Because oral contraceptives increase clotting generally, they increase the risk of hepatic vein thrombosis (Budd-Chiari syndrome). Use of these drugs also increases the risk of gallstones because they enhance bile lithogenicity.

25 ALCOHOLIC LIVER DISEASE

Alcohol causes a spectrum of liver injury that can progress from fatty liver to alcoholic hepatitis (often considered an intermediate stage) to cirrhosis.

Alcohol consumption is high in most Western countries. In the US, annual ingestion is estimated at 10 L of pure ethanol equivalent per person; 15 million people abuse or are dependent on alcohol. The male:female ratio is 11 : 4.

Risk Factors

The major causative factors in alcoholic liver disease are quantity of alcohol consumed, duration of alcohol abuse (usually > 8 yr), nutritional status, and genetic and metabolic traits. Among susceptible people, a linear correlation generally exists between the amount and duration of alcohol use and the development of liver disease. As little as 20 g of alcohol in women or 60 g in men can cause serious liver damage when consumed daily for several years. Consuming more than 60 g/day for 2 to 4 wk produces fatty liver even in otherwise healthy men; 80 g/day may lead to alcoholic hepatitis; and 160 g/day over a decade can lead to cirrhosis. Alcohol content is estimated to be the beverage volume (in mL) multiplied by its percentage of alcohol. For example, 16 mL of alcohol is contained in roughly 40 mL of an 80-proof (40% alcohol) beverage. Each mL of alcohol contains about 0.79 g. Although values can vary, the percentage of alcohol is about 2 to 7% for most beers and 10 to 15% for most wines.

Only 10 to 20% of alcoholics develop cirrhosis. Women are more susceptible than men (even when adjusting for smaller body size), probably because women have less alcohol dehydrogenase in their gastric mucosa, which lessens the first-pass oxidation of alcohol. Alcoholic liver disease often runs in families, suggesting genetic factors (eg, deficiency of cytoplasmic enzymes that eliminate alcohol). Malnutrition, particularly protein-energy malnutrition, increases susceptibility. Other risk factors include a diet high in unsaturated fat, iron deposition in the liver, and concomitant hepatitis C virus infection.

Pathophysiology

Alcohol is readily absorbed from the stomach and small intestine. It cannot be stored; > 90% is metabolized through oxidation. The first breakdown product is acetaldehyde, which is produced by three enzymatic pathways: alcohol dehydrogenase (responsible for about 80% of metabolism), cytochrome P-450 2E1 (CYP2E1), and catalase.

Acetaldehyde is converted to acetate by mitochondrial aldehyde dehydrogenase. Chronic alcohol consumption enhances acetate formation. The processes generate hydrogen, which converts nicotinamide-adenine dinucleotide (NAD) to its reduced form (NADH), increasing the redox potential in the liver. This replaces fatty acids as a fuel, lowers fatty acid oxidation, and allows triglycerides to accumulate, causing fatty liver and hyperlipidemia. The excess hydrogen also converts pyruvate to lactate, which decreases glucose production (hypoglycemia can result), causing renal acidosis, reduced urate excretion, hyperuricemia, and thus gout.

Alcohol metabolism may also make the liver hypermetabolic, causing hypoxia and free radical–induced lipid peroxidative damage. Alcohol and undernutrition deplete antioxidants, such as glutathione and vitamins A and E, which predispose to such damage.

Acetaldehyde initiates much of the inflammation and fibrosis of alcoholic hepatitis. It transforms the stellate (Ito) cells lining liver blood channels (sinusoids) into fibroblasts that develop myocontractile elements and actively produce collagen. The sinusoids narrow and fill, limiting transport and blood flow. Gut endotoxins, which the impaired liver can no longer detoxify, lead to production of inflammatory cytokines. Acetaldehyde and lipid peroxidation products recruit leukocytes, resulting in production of more inflammatory cytokines. This elicits a vicious circle of inflammation that culminates in fibrosis and loss of hepatocytes.

Fat is deposited throughout the hepatocytes, a result of increased input from peripheral adipose tissue, elevated triglyceride synthesis, decreased lipid oxidation, and reduced lipoprotein production that impairs fat export from the liver.

Pathology

Fatty liver, alcoholic hepatitis, and cirrhosis often are considered separate, progressive manifestations of alcoholic liver disease. Their features, however, often overlap.

Fatty liver (steatosis) is the initial and most common consequence of excessive alcohol ingestion. It is potentially reversible. Fatty liver is the accumulation of macrovesicular fat as large droplets of triglyceride that displaces the hepatocyte nucleus. Less often, fat appears in a microvesicular form as small droplets that do not displace the nucleus. Microvesicular fat represents mitochondrial damage. The liver enlarges, and the cut surface is yellow.

Alcoholic hepatitis (steatohepatitis) is a combination of fatty liver, diffuse liver inflammation, and liver necrosis (often focal), all in various degrees of severity. Cirrhosis may be present as well. The damaged hepatocytes either are swollen with a granular cytoplasm (balloon degeneration) or contain fibrillar protein in the cytoplasm (Mallory or alcoholic hyaline bodies). Severely damaged hepatocytes become necrotic. Collagen accumulation and fibrosis of the terminal hepatic venules compromise hepatic perfusion and contribute to portal hypertension. Histologic features that predict progression to cirrhosis include perivenular fibrosis, microvesicular fat, and giant mitochondria.

Cirrhosis is advanced liver disease characterized by extensive fibrosis that disrupts the normal liver architecture. The amount of fat present varies. Alcoholic hepatitis may coexist. The feeble compensatory attempt at hepatic regeneration produces relatively small nodules (micronodular cirrhosis), shrinking the liver. In time, particularly with abstinence, this can progress to macronodular cirrhosis (see p. 216).

Iron accumulation in the liver occurs in up to 10% of alcoholics with normal, fatty, or cirrhotic livers. Accumulation is not predicted by iron intake or body iron stores.

Symptoms and Signs

Symptoms match the stage and severity of disease. Symptoms generally become apparent in patients during their 30s; severe problems appear about a decade later.

Fatty liver usually causes no symptoms. In ⅓ of patients, the liver is enlarged, smooth, and occasionally tender.

Alcoholic hepatitis ranges from a mild, reversible illness to a life-threatening disease. In moderate cases, patients usually are malnourished and present with fatigue, fever, jaundice, right upper quadrant pain, tender hepatomegaly, and, sometimes, a hepatic bruit. Their condition often deteriorates in the first few weeks of hospitalization. Severe cases may involve jaundice, ascites, hypoglycemia, electrolyte abnormalities, hepatic insufficiency with coagulopathy or portal-systemic encephalopathy, or other manifestations of cirrhosis. If severe hyperbilirubinemia > 20 mg/dL (> 360 μmol/L), prolonged PT or INR (unresponsive to vitamin K sc), and encephalopathy are present, the risk of death is 20 to 50%, and the risk of cirrhosis is 50%.

Cirrhosis may cause symptoms ranging from minimal to those of alcoholic hepatitis or the complications of end-stage liver disease. Commonly, portal hypertension (often with esophageal varices and upper GI bleeding, ascites, portal-systemic encephalopathy), hepatorenal syndrome, or even hepatocellular carcinoma is present.

In any chronic alcoholic liver disease, Dupuytren's contracture of the palmar fascia, vascular spiders, peripheral neuropathy, Wernicke's encephalopathy, Korsakoff's psychosis, and, in men, signs of hypogonadism and feminization (eg, smooth skin, lack of male-pattern baldness, gynecomastia, testicular atrophy) may be present. These manifestations more likely reflect the effect of alcoholism than of liver disease. Malnutrition may lead to enlarged parotid glands. Hepatitis C virus infection occurs in about 25% of alcoholics, a combination that markedly worsens the progression of liver disease.

Diagnosis

Alcohol is suspected as the cause of liver disease in any patient whose consumption exceeds 80 g/day. If the diagnosis is suspected, liver function tests, CBC, and hepatitis serology are performed. No specific test exists for alcoholic liver disease.

Elevations of aminotransferases are moderate (< 300 IU/L) and do not reflect the extent of the liver damage. Further, AST exceeds ALT by a ratio of > 2. The basis for the low ALT is a dietary deficiency of pyridoxal phosphate (vitamin B_6), which is needed for the enzyme to function. Its effect on AST is less pronounced. Serum γ-glutamyl transpeptidase (GGT) increases as a result of ethanol-induced enzyme induction as well as from use of other drugs, cholestasis, and liver injury. Macrocytosis with an MCV > 100 fL reflects the direct effect of alcohol on the bone marrow as well as the macrocytic anemia resulting from folate deficiency, which is common among malnourished alcoholics. Indices of the severity of liver disease are serum bilirubin, which represents secretory function, and PT or INR, which reflects synthetic ability. Thrombocytopenia can result from the direct toxic effects of alcohol on the bone marrow or from hypersplenism that occurs in portal hypertension.

Imaging tests are not routinely needed for diagnosis. If performed for other reasons, abdominal ultrasound or CT may suggest fatty liver or show evidence of splenomegaly, portal hypertension, or ascites.

Patients with abnormalities suggesting alcoholic liver disease should undergo screening tests for other treatable forms of liver disease, especially viral hepatitis. Because features of fatty liver, alcoholic hepatitis, and cirrhosis overlap, describing the precise findings is more useful than assigning the patient to a specific category, which can only be determined by liver biopsy. Liver biopsy is performed to stage the severity of liver disease (see p. 206). In addition to confirming liver disease, biopsy also helps identify excessive alcohol use as the likely cause and establishes the stage of liver injury. If iron accumulation is observed, quantitation of the iron content and genetic testing can eliminate hereditary hemochromatosis as the cause.

Prognosis and Treatment

The prognosis for alcoholic liver disease is determined by the degree of hepatic fibrosis and inflammation. Fatty liver and alcoholic hepatitis without fibrosis are reversible if alcohol is avoided; with abstinence, complete resolution of fatty liver occurs within 6 wk. Fibrosis and cirrhosis are irreversible. Once cirrhosis and its complications (ascites, bleeding) develop, the 5-yr survival rate is about 50%: the rate is higher with abstinence and lower if drinking continues. Alcoholic liver disease, particularly with coexisting chronic hepatitis C infection, predisposes to hepatocellular carcinoma.

Abstinence is the mainstay of treatment; it can prevent further damage from alcoholic liver disease and thus prolong life. Because compliance is problematic, a compassionate team approach is essential. Excellent results can come from support groups such as Alcoholics Anonymous as long as the patient is motivated (see p. 1687).

General management emphasizes supportive care. A nutritious diet and vitamin supplements (especially B vitamins) are provided, especially during the first few days of abstinence. However, supplements have not proved to affect outcomes, even in hospitalized patients with alcoholic hepatitis. Alcohol withdrawal requires benzodiazepines (eg, diazepam). Excessive sedation in patients with marked alcoholic liver disease can precipitate hepatic encephalopathy.

Management of specific complications (eg, infection, bleeding from esophageal varices, specific nutritional deficiencies, Wernicke's encephalopathy, Korsakoff's psychosis, electrolyte abnormalities, portal hypertension, ascites, portal-systemic encephalopathy) are discussed elsewhere in THE MANUAL.

Few specific treatments exist for alcoholic liver disease. The value of corticosteroids in alcoholic hepatitis is controversial, but these drugs may help patients with the most severe disease. Drugs used to decrease fibrosis (eg, colchicine, penicillamine) or inflammation (eg, pentoxifylline) have not proved effective. Propylthiouracil may provide some benefit in treating the putative hypermetabolic state of the alcoholic liver but has never gained acceptance. Antioxidants (eg, *S*-adenosyl-L-methionine, polyunsaturated phosphatidylcholine) show promise in ameliorating liver injury but require further study. Antioxidant remedies, such as silymarin (milk thistle) and vitamins A and E, are unproven.

Liver transplantation can produce 5-yr survival rates comparable to those for nonalcoholic liver disease—as high as 80% in the absence of active liver disease and 50% with acute alcoholic hepatitis. Because up to 50% of patients resume drinking after transplantation, most programs require 6 mo of abstinence before transplantation is performed.

26 FIBROSIS AND CIRRHOSIS

Hepatic fibrosis is accumulation of excessive extracellular matrix (a type of scar) in response to a wide variety of chronic liver injuries (see TABLE 26–1). Hepatic fibrosis can regress if the insult is reversible (eg, viral clearance). More commonly, however, injury is chronic or repeated, leading to progressive distortion and dysfunction of liver architecture and, ultimately, cirrhosis.

Cirrhosis is fibrosis that progresses to produce diffuse disorganization of normal hepatic structure with attempts at hepatic regeneration. Development usually requires >6 mo of liver disease but can occur more rapidly if biliary atresia is present in infancy or after liver transplantation for cirrhosis secondary to hepatitis B or C virus infection.

Although advanced liver fibrosis and cirrhosis have been considered irreversible, improvement is sometimes possible (eg, with antiviral therapy in chronic viral hepatitis).

FIBROSIS

Hepatic fibrosis is an accumulation in the liver of connective tissue in response to hepatocellular damage of nearly any cause. It results from excessive production or deficient degradation of the extracellular matrix. Fibrosis itself causes no symptoms but can lead to portal hypertension or cirrhosis. Diagnosis is based on liver biopsy. Treatment involves correcting the underlying cause when possible. Treatments aimed at reversing fibrosis itself are under study.

Activation of the hepatic perivascular stellate cells (Ito cells, fat-storing cells) initiates fibrosis. These and adjacent cells proliferate, becoming contractile cells, termed myofibroblasts. These cells enhance the degradation of the normal matrix and, partly because of alterations in metalloproteinase enzymes that regulate matrix collagen metabolism, produce excess abnormal matrix. Kupffer cells (resident macrophages), injured hepatocytes, platelets, and leukocytes aggregate, releasing reactive O_2 species and inflammatory mediators (eg, platelet-derived growth factor, transforming growth factors, and connective tissue growth factor), which accelerate fibrosis.

Myofibroblasts, stimulated by endothelin-1, also contribute to increased portal vein resistance, which increases the density of the abnormal matrix. Fibrous tracts join branches of afferent portal veins and efferent hepatic veins, bypassing the hepatocytes and limiting their blood supply. Hence, fibrosis contributes both to hepatocyte ischemia (and hepatocellular dysfunction) and portal hypertension. The extent to which these processes contribute determines how the liver is affected. For example, congenital hepatic fibrosis affects portal vein branches, largely sparing the parenchyma. The result is portal hypertension with sparing of hepatocellular function.

Symptoms, Signs, and Diagnosis

Hepatic fibrosis itself does not cause symptoms. Symptoms may develop secondary to the primary disorder or to portal hypertension. However, portal hypertension is often asymptomatic until cirrhosis develops.

Liver biopsy is the only means of diagnosing or detecting hepatic fibrosis. The diagnosis is usually made when a liver biopsy is performed for another reason. Special stains (eg, aniline blue, trichrome, silver stains) may highlight the fibrous tissue.

Treatment

Because fibrosis is a sign of hepatic damage, treatment usually is directed toward the underlying cause. Treatments aimed at reversing the fibrosis itself are under study and target such strategies as (1) decreasing inflammation (eg, ursodeoxycholic acid, corticosteroids), (2) inhibiting hepatic stellate cell activation (eg, γ-interferon, vitamin E as an antioxidant, peroxisome peroxidase reductase [PPAR]-γ ligands such as thiazolidinediones to down-regulate activation), (3) inhibiting collagen synthesis or metabolism (eg, penicillamine, colchicine, corticosteroids), (4) inhibiting stellate cell contraction (eg, endothelin antagonists or nitric oxide donors), and (5) enhancing extracellular matrix degradation (eg, transforming growth factor-β or metalloproteinase-mediated degradation with several experimental drugs). Unfortunately, many drugs usually are too toxic for long-term use (eg, corticosteroids, penicillamine) or have no proven efficacy (eg, colchicine). Multiple antifibrotic drug therapy may prove most beneficial.

TABLE 26–1. DISEASES AND DRUGS THAT CAN CAUSE FIBROSIS

Diseases with direct hepatic effects
- Certain storage diseases and inborn errors of metabolism
  - α_1-Antitrypsin deficiency
  - Copper storage diseases (Wilson's disease)
  - Fructosemia
  - Galactosemia
  - Glycogen storage diseases (especially types III, IV, VI, IX, and X)
  - Iron-overload syndromes (hemochromatosis)
  - Lipid abnormalities (eg, Gaucher's disease)
  - Peroxisomal disorders (eg, Zellweger syndrome)
  - Tyrosinemia
- Congenital hepatic fibrosis
- Infections
  - Bacterial (eg, brucellosis)
  - Parasitic (eg, echinococcosis)
  - Viral (eg, chronic hepatitis B or C)

Disorders affecting hepatic blood flow
- Budd-Chiari syndrome
- Heart failure
- Hepatic veno-occlusive disease
- Portal vein thrombosis

Drugs and chemicals
- Alcohol
- Amiodarone
- Chlorpromazine
- Isoniazid
- Methotrexate
- Methyldopa
- Oxyphenisatin
- Tolbutamide
- Toxins (eg, iron, copper)

CIRRHOSIS

Cirrhosis is fibrosis that progresses to produce diffuse disorganization of normal hepatic structure, characterized by regenerative nodules surrounded by dense fibrotic tissue. Symptoms may not develop for years and are often nonspecific, such as anorexia, fatigue, and weight loss. Late manifestations include portal hypertension, ascites, and liver failure. Diagnosis requires liver biopsy. Treatment generally is supportive.

Cirrhosis is a leading cause of death worldwide. The causes of cirrhosis are the same as those for fibrosis (see TABLE 26–1). In developed countries, most cases result from chronic alcohol abuse or chronic hepatitis C virus infection. In many parts of Asia and Africa, cirrhosis results from chronic hepatitis B infection. Cirrhosis of unknown etiology (cryptogenic cirrhosis) is becoming less common as many specific causes (eg, chronic hepatitis C, steatohepatitis) are being identified. Primary biliary cirrhosis is discussed on p. 218, and primary sclerosing cholangitis is discussed on p. 246.

Pathophysiology

Variation exists among individuals regarding the rate of the progression of fibrosis to cirrhosis and the morphology of the cirrhosis, even in response to the same stimulus. The reasons for such differences are unknown.

In response to injury, growth regulators induce hepatocellular hyperplasia (producing regenerating nodules) and arterial growth (angiogenesis). Among the growth regulators are cytokines and hepatic growth factors (eg, epithelial growth factor, hepatocyte growth factor, transforming growth factor-α, tumor necrosis factor). Insulin, glucagon, and patterns of intrahepatic blood flow also determine how and where nodules develop.

Angiogenesis produces new vessels within the fibrous sheath that surrounds nodules; these "bridges" connect the hepatic artery and portal vein to the hepatic venules, restoring the intrahepatic circulatory pathway. Such interconnecting vessels provide relatively low-volume, high-pressure venous drainage that cannot accommodate as much blood volume as normal, which increases portal vein pressure. Such distortions in blood flow to the nodules along with compression of hepatic venules by regenerating nodules contribute to portal hypertension.

Cirrhosis can cause intrapulmonary right-to-left shunting and ventilation/perfusion mismatch, resulting in hypoxia. Progressive loss of hepatic function leads to liver failure and ascites. Hepatocellular carcinoma frequently complicates cirrhosis, particularly cirrhosis resulting from chronic hepatitis B and C viruses, hemochromatosis, alcohol-related liver disease, α_1-antitrypsin deficiency, and glycogen storage disease.

Histopathology: Cirrhosis involves both regenerating nodules and fibrosis. Incompletely formed liver nodules, nodules without fibrosis (nodular regenerative hyperplasia), and congenital hepatic fibrosis (ie, widespread fibrosis without regenerating nodules) are not true cirrhosis. Cirrhosis can be micronodular or macronodular. Micronodular cirrhosis is characterized by uniformly small nodules (< 3 mm in diameter) and thick regular bands of connective tissue. Typically, nodules lack lobular organization; terminal (central) hepatic venules and portal triads are distorted. With time, macronodular cirrhosis often develops, in which nodules vary in size (3 mm to 5 cm in diameter) and contain some rather normal lobular organization of portal triads and terminal hepatic venules. Broad fibrous bands of varying thickness surround the large nodules. Collapse of the normal liver architecture is suggested by the concentration of portal triads within the fibrous scars. Mixed cirrhosis (incomplete septal cirrhosis) combines elements of micronodular and macronodular cirrhosis.

Symptoms and Signs

Cirrhosis may be asymptomatic for years. Often, the first symptoms are nonspecific, such as generalized weakness, anorexia, malaise, and weight loss. The liver is typically palpable and firm, with a blunt edge, but is sometimes small and difficult to palpate. Nodules usually are not palpable.

Malnutrition is common, secondary to anorexia with poor food intake, especially when insufficient bile excretion causes malabsorption of fats and fat-soluble vitamins. Commonly, patients with cirrhosis due to alcoholic liver disease also have pancreatic insufficiency, which contributes to malabsorption.

If cholestasis is present (eg, in primary biliary cirrhosis), jaundice, pruritus, and xanthelasmas may result. Portal hypertension is complicated by GI bleeding from esophagogastric varices, portal hypertensive gastropathy, or rectal varices; splenomegaly with possible hypersplenism; portal-systemic encephalopathy; and ascites. Hepatic insufficiency eventually may develop, leading to a coagulopathy, possibly the hepatorenal syndrome (see p. 200), and contributing to jaundice and hepatic encephalopathy.

Other clinical signs may suggest chronic liver disease or chronic alcohol use but are not specific for cirrhosis: muscle wasting, palmar erythema, parotid gland enlargement, white nails, Dupuytren's contractures, vascular spiders (< 10 may be normal), gynecomastia, axillary hair loss, testicular atrophy, and peripheral neuropathy.

Diagnosis

Cirrhosis is suspected in patients with manifestations of portal hypertension. Occasionally, it may be suspected in those with earlier nonspecific symptoms, particularly in those with known risk factors.

Diagnostic testing begins with liver function tests and a CBC. Laboratory tests may increase suspicion for cirrhosis but cannot exclude it. If laboratory tests and clinical data suggest cirrhosis, the diagnosis is confirmed with liver biopsy.

Laboratory test results may be normal or may reveal nonspecific abnormalities due to complications of cirrhosis or alcoholism. Aminotransferase levels are often modestly elevated, whereas alkaline phosphatase may be normal or, particularly with biliary obstruction, increased. Bilirubin usually is normal. Decreased serum albumin and a prolonged PT directly reflect impaired hepatic function. Serum globulin increases in cirrhosis or other chronic liver diseases. Anemia is common and usually normocytic, but it may be microcytic and hypochromic from chronic GI bleeding, macrocytic from folate deficiency (in alcoholism), or hemolytic from hypersplenism. Alcohol directly suppresses the bone marrow, sometimes causing pancytopenia. Hypersplenism also can lead to leukopenia and thrombocytopenia.

Imaging tests may be performed to diagnose other conditions or specific causes of cirrhosis but are not indicated for the diagnosis of cirrhosis itself. However, they may show abnormalities that suggest cirrhosis. CT may reveal a nodular texture. Liver scans using technetium-99m sulfur colloid may show irregular liver uptake and increased spleen and bone marrow uptake. Doppler ultrasound may reveal changes in hepatic vessels indicative of portal hypertension.

Patients with cirrhosis do not require routine endoscopy to screen for esophageal varices unless upper GI bleeding occurs. Patients with cirrhosis and chronic viral hepatitis B or C or hemochromatosis should be screened for hepatocellular carcinoma (eg, with measurement of α-fetoprotein and ultrasound every 6 to 12 mo—see p. 237).

Prognosis and Treatment

Prognosis often is unpredictable. It depends on factors such as etiology, severity, presence of complications, comorbid conditions, host factors, and effectiveness of therapy. Patients who continue to drink alcohol, even small amounts, have a very poor prognosis. The Child-Turcotte-Pugh scoring system (see TABLE 26–2) uses clinical and laboratory information to stratify disease severity, surgical risk, and overall prognosis.

TABLE 26–2. CHILD-TURCOTTE-PUGH SCORING SYSTEM

CLINICAL AND LABORATORY MEASUREMENTS	POINTS SCORED FOR INCREASING ABNORMALITY*		
	1	2	3
Encephalopathy (grade†)	None	1–2	3–4
Ascites	None	Mild (or controlled by diuretics)	At least moderate despite diuretic treatment
PT (seconds prolonged)	< 4	4–6	> 6
[or INR]	< 1.7	1.7–2.3	> 2.3
Albumin (g/dL)	> 3.5	2.8–3.5	< 2.8
Bilirubin (mg/dL)	< 2	2–3	> 3

*Scoring system: 5–6 points, grade A (lowest risk); 7–9 points, grade B; 10–15 points, grade C (highest risk)

†Grade 1: Sleep disturbances; impaired concentration; depression, anxiety, or irritability.
Grade 2: Drowsiness; disorientation; poor short-term memory; disinhibited behavior.
Grade 3: Somnolence; confusion; amnesia; anger, paranoia, or other bizarre behavior.
Grade 4: Coma.

In general, treatment is supportive and includes withdrawal of injurious drugs, provision of nutrition (including supplemental vitamins), and treatment of underlying causes and complications. All alcohol and hepatotoxic drugs must be avoided. Doses of drugs metabolized in the liver must be reduced.

Patients with varices need therapy to prevent bleeding (see p. 196). Further benefit arises from treatments that can retard hepatic fibrosis (see p. 215). Liver transplantation should be performed in end-stage liver failure in suitable candidates.

Some people with cirrhosis continue to abuse alcohol. Physicians should prepare for withdrawal symptoms during hospitalization.

PRIMARY BILIARY CIRRHOSIS

Primary biliary cirrhosis is an autoimmune liver disease characterized by the progressive destruction of intrahepatic bile ducts, leading to cholestasis, cirrhosis, and liver failure. Patients usually are asymptomatic at presentation but may experience fatigue or may have symptoms of cholestasis (eg, pruritus, steatorrhea) or cirrhosis (eg, portal hypertension, ascites). Laboratory tests reveal cholestasis, increased IgM, and, characteristically, antimitochondrial antibodies in the serum. Liver biopsy usually is necessary for diagnosis and staging. Treatment includes ursodeoxycholic acid, cholestyramine (for pruritus), supplementary fat-soluble vitamins, and, for advanced disease, liver transplantation.

Etiology and Pathophysiology

Primary biliary cirrhosis (PBC) is the most common chronic cholestatic liver disease in adults. More than 90% of cases develop in women aged 35 to 70. The disease clusters in families. Its cause is unknown, but an autoimmune mechanism is suspected because antibodies to antigens located on the inner mitochondrial membranes occur in > 95% of cases. These antimitochondrial antibodies are not cytotoxic and are not involved in bile duct damage. PBC commonly is associated with other autoimmune disorders, such as RA, systemic sclerosis, Sjögren's syndrome, CREST syndrome, autoimmune thyroiditis, and renal tubular acidosis, which also suggests an autoimmune mechanism.

CD4 and CD8 T lymphocytes characteristically mediate inflammation of the epithelial cells lining small bile ducts. Bile ducts proliferate. Bile acids are retained and inflame the liver parenchyma, leading to fibrosis in periportal areas. Eventually, hepatic inflammation decreases, and hepatic fibrosis progresses to cirrhosis.

Symptoms and Signs

About 30 to 50% of patients present without symptoms; PBC is detected incidentally by abnormalities in liver function tests, typically an elevated alkaline phosphatase. Symptoms or signs may develop during any stage of the disease and may include fatigue or reflect cholestasis (and the resulting fat malabsorption, which may produce vitamin deficiencies and osteoporosis), hepatocellular dysfunction, or cirrhosis. Symptoms usually develop insidiously. Pruritus, fatigue, or both are the initial symptoms in > 50% of patients and can precede other symptoms by months or years. Other common features at presentation include an enlarged, firm, nontender liver (in 25%); splenomegaly (15%); hyperpigmentation (25%); xanthelasmas (10%); and jaundice (10%). Eventually, all the features and complications of cirrhosis occur. Peripheral neuropathy and other autoimmune disorders associated with PBC may also develop.

Diagnosis

PBC is suspected in middle-aged women with classic symptoms or cholestatic liver biochemistry: elevated alkaline phosphatase and γ-glutamyl transpeptidase but minimally abnormal aminotransferases (ALT and AST). Serum bilirubin is usually normal in the early stages; elevation indicates disease progression and a worsening prognosis. Serum IgM is markedly high. A positive serum antimitochondrial antibody (sometimes also positive at low titers in type 1 autoimmune hepatitis) strongly suggests the diagnosis. Other autoantibodies in patients with PBC include rheumatoid factor (66%), anti-smooth muscle antibody (66%), antithyroid antibody (40%), and antinuclear antibody (35%). Liver biopsy is usually done to confirm the diagnosis and may reveal pathognomonic bile duct lesions early during the course. However, PBC has four stages, and as fibrosis progresses, PBC becomes morphologically indistinguishable from other forms of cirrhosis.

Extrahepatic biliary obstruction should be ruled out by imaging tests (ie, ultrasound, magnetic resonance cholangiopancreatography, and, sometimes, ERCP) if necessary.

Prognosis

PBC usually progresses to terminal stages over 15 to 20 yr, although the rate of progression varies. It may not diminish quality of life for many years. Patients who present without symptoms tend to develop symptoms over 2 to 7 yr but may not do so for 10 to 15 yr. Once symptoms develop, the median life expectancy is 10 yr. Predictors of rapid progression include rapid progression of symptoms, advanced histologic changes, advanced patient age, presence of edema, presence of associated autoimmune disorders, and abnormalities in bilirubin, albumin, or PT or INR. The prognosis is ominous when pruritus disappears, xanthomas shrink, and serum cholesterol decreases.

Treatment

Treatment goals include arresting or reversing liver damage, treating complications (chronic cholestasis and liver failure), and, eventually, liver transplantation. All alcohol use and any hepatotoxic drugs should be stopped. Ursodeoxycholic acid (4.3 to 5 mg/kg po tid or 3.25 to 3.75 mg/kg po qid with meals) decreases liver damage, prolongs survival, and delays the need for liver transplantation. About 20% of patients do not show biochemical improvement after ≥ 4 mo; these patients may have advanced disease and require liver transplantation in a few years. Other drugs proposed to decrease liver damage have not improved overall clinical outcomes or are controversial. These drugs include corticosteroids, penicillamine, colchicine, methotrexate, azathioprine, cyclosporine, and chlorambucil.

Pruritus may be controlled with cholestyramine 6 to 8 g po bid. Some patients with pruritus respond to ursodeoxycholic acid and ultraviolet light; others may warrant a trial of rifampin or an opioid antagonist, such as naltrexone. Fat malabsorption may require supplemental Ca and vitamins A, D, E, and K. Osteoporosis may require, in addition to Ca and vitamin D supplements, weight-bearing exercises, bisphosphonates, estrogens, or raloxifene. In later stages, treatment for associated portal hypertension (see p. 195) or cirrhosis (see p. 215) becomes necessary.

Liver transplantation yields excellent results. The general indication is decompensated liver disease: uncontrolled variceal bleeding, refractory ascites, intractable pruritus, and hepatic encephalopathy. The 1-yr survival rate after liver transplantation is > 90%; 5-yr survival rate, > 80%. PBC recurs in about 15% of patients in the first few years, although this finding has not been clinically important.

27 HEPATITIS

Hepatitis is an inflammation of the liver characterized by diffuse or patchy necrosis. Major causes are specific hepatitis viruses, alcohol, and drugs. Less common causes include other viruses (eg, infectious mononucleosis, yellow fever, cytomegalovirus) and leptospirosis. Parasitic infections (eg, schistosomiasis, malaria, amebiasis), pyogenic infections, and abscesses affect the liver but are not considered hepatitis. Liver involvement with TB and other granulomatous infiltrations is sometimes called granulomatous hepatitis, but the clinical, biochemical, and histologic features differ from those of diffuse hepatitis.

Various systemic infections and other illnesses may produce small focal areas of hepatic inflammation or necrosis. This nonspecific reactive hepatitis can cause minor liver function abnormalities but is usually asymptomatic.

Some types of noninfectious liver inflammation and hepatic infections are summarized in TABLE 27–1.

ACUTE VIRAL HEPATITIS

Acute viral hepatitis is diffuse liver inflammation caused by specific hepatotropic viruses that have diverse modes of transmission and epidemiologies. A nonspecific viral prodrome is followed by anorexia, nausea, and often fever or right upper quadrant pain. Jaundice often develops, typically as

TABLE 27–1. SELECTED DISEASES OR ORGANISMS ASSOCIATED WITH LIVER INFLAMMATION

DISEASE OR ORGANISM	MANIFESTATIONS
Viruses	
Cytomegalovirus	In neonates: hepatomegaly, jaundice, congenital defects. In adults: mononucleosis-like illness with hepatitis; may occur posttransfusion
Epstein-Barr	Infectious mononucleosis. Clinical hepatitis with jaundice in 5–10%; subclinical liver involvement in 90–95%. Acute hepatitis in young adults (important)
Yellow fever	Jaundice with systemic toxicity, bleeding. Liver necrosis with little inflammatory reaction
Other	Hepatitis occasionally from herpes simplex, echo-, coxsackie, rubeola, rubella, or varicella virus
Bacteria	
Actinomycosis	Granulomatous reaction of liver with progressive necrotizing abscesses
Pyogenic abscess	Serious infection acquired via portal pyemia, cholangitis, or hematogenous or direct spread. Various organisms, especially gram-negative and anaerobic. Illness and toxicity, yet only mild liver dysfunction. Differentiate from amebiasis
Tuberculosis	Hepatic involvement common. Granulomatous infiltration. Usually subclinical; jaundice rare. Disproportionately increased alkaline phosphatase
Other	Minor focal hepatitis in numerous systemic infections (common, usually subclinical)
Fungi	
Histoplasmosis	Granulomas in liver and spleen (usually subclinical) that heal with calcification
Other	Granulomatous infiltration sometimes in cryptococcosis, coccidioidomycosis, blastomycosis, and others
Protozoa	
Amebiasis	Important disease, often without obvious dysentery. Usually large single abscess with liquefaction. Illness, tender hepatomegaly, surprisingly mild liver dysfunction. Differentiate from pyogenic abscess
Malaria	Hepatosplenomegaly in endemic areas (major cause). Jaundice absent or mild unless active hemolysis
Toxoplasmosis	Transplacental infection. In neonates: jaundice, CNS and other systemic manifestations
Visceral leishmaniasis	Infiltration of reticuloendothelial system by parasite. Hepatosplenomegaly
Helminths	
Ascariasis	Biliary obstruction by adult worms, parenchymal granulomas from larvae
Clonorchiasis	Biliary tract infestation; cholangitis, stones, cholangiocarcinoma
Echinococcosis	One or more hydatid cysts, usually calcified rim. May be large but often asymptomatic; liver function preserved. Can rupture into peritoneum or biliary tract

TABLE 27–1. SELECTED DISEASES OR ORGANISMS ASSOCIATED WITH LIVER INFLAMMATION—Continued

DISEASE OR ORGANISM	MANIFESTATIONS
Fascioliasis	Acute: tender hepatomegaly, fever, eosinophilia. Chronic: biliary fibrosis, cholangitis
Schistosomiasis	Periportal granulomatous reaction to ova with progressive hepatosplenomegaly, pipestem fibrosis, portal hypertension, varices. Hepatocellular function preserved; not true cirrhosis
Toxocariasis	Visceral larva migrans syndrome. Hepatomegaly with granulomas, eosinophilia
Spirochetes	
Leptospirosis	Acute fever, prostration, jaundice, bleeding, renal injury. Liver necrosis (often mild despite severe jaundice)
Syphilis	Congenital: neonatal hepatosplenomegaly, fibrosis. Acquired: variable hepatitis in secondary stage, gummas with irregular scarring in tertiary stage
Relapsing fever	*Borrelia* infection. Systemic symptoms, hepatomegaly, sometimes jaundice
Unknown	
Idiopathic granulomatous hepatitis	Active chronic granulomatous inflammation not resulting from known causes (sarcoid variant?). Systemic symptoms (possibly dominate) with fever, malaise
Sarcoidosis	Granulomatous infiltration (common, usually subclinical); jaundice rare. Occasionally progressive inflammation with scarring, portal hypertension
Ulcerative colitis, Crohn's disease	Spectrum of hepatic disease, especially in ulcerative colitis. Includes periportal inflammation (pericholangitis), sclerosing cholangitis, cholangiocarcinoma, autoimmune hepatitis. Poor correlation with activity or treatment of bowel disorder

other symptoms begin to resolve. Most cases resolve spontaneously, but some progress to chronic hepatitis. Occasionally, acute viral hepatitis progresses to acute hepatic failure (fulminant hepatitis). Good hygiene can prevent acute viral hepatitis. Depending on the specific virus, preexposure and postexposure prophylaxis may be possible using vaccines or serum globulins. Treatment is usually supportive.

(See also Neonatal Hepatitis B Virus Infection on p. 2327.)

Acute viral hepatitis is a common, important worldwide disease that has different causes; each type shares clinical, biochemical, and morphologic features. Liver infections caused by nonhepatitis viruses (eg, Epstein-Barr, yellow fever, cytomegalovirus) generally are not termed acute viral hepatitis.

Etiology and Epidemiology

At least five specific viruses appear to be responsible (see TABLE 27–2). Other unidentified viruses probably also cause acute viral hepatitis.

Hepatitis A virus (HAV): HAV is a single-stranded RNA picornavirus. It is the most common cause of acute viral hepatitis and is particularly common in children and young adults. In some countries, > 75% of adults have been exposed. HAV spreads primarily by fecal-oral contact and thus may occur in areas of poor hygiene. Waterborne and food-borne epidemics occur, especially in underdeveloped countries. Eating contaminated raw shellfish is sometimes responsible. Sporadic cases are also common, usually as a result of person-to-person contact. Fecal shedding of the virus occurs before symptoms develop and usually ceases a few days after

TABLE 27–2. CHARACTERISTICS OF HEPATITIS VIRUSES

	HEPATITIS A VIRUS	HEPATITIS B VIRUS	HEPATITIS C VIRUS	HEPATITIS D VIRUS	HEPATITIS E VIRUS
Nucleic acid	RNA	DNA	RNA	*	RNA
Serologic diagnosis	IgM anti-HA	HBsAg	Anti-HCV	Anti-HDV	Anti-HEV
Major transmission	Fecal–oral	Blood	Blood	Needle	Water
Incubation period (days)	15–45	40–180	20–120	30–180	14–60
Epidemics	Yes	No	No	No	Yes
Chronicity	No	Yes	Yes	Yes	No
Liver cancer	No	Yes	Yes	Yes	No

HBsAg = hepatitis B surface antigen.
*Incomplete RNA, requires presence of hepatitis B virus for replication.

symptoms begin; thus, infectivity often has already ceased when hepatitis becomes clinically evident. HAV has no known chronic carrier state and does not produce chronic hepatitis or cirrhosis.

Hepatitis B virus (HBV): HBV is the most thoroughly characterized and complex hepatitis virus. The infective particle consists of a viral core plus an outer surface coat. The core contains circular double-stranded DNA and DNA polymerase, and it replicates within the nuclei of infected hepatocytes. Surface coat is added in the cytoplasm and, for unknown reasons, is produced in great excess.

HBV is the second most common cause of acute viral hepatitis. Prior unrecognized infection is common but is much less widespread than with HAV. HBV is often transmitted parenterally, typically by contaminated blood or blood products. Routine screening of donor blood for hepatitis B surface antigen (HBsAg) has nearly eliminated the previously common posttransfusion transmission, but transmission through needles shared by drug users remains common. Risk of HBV is increased for patients in renal dialysis and oncology units and for hospital personnel in contact with blood. Nonparenteral spread occurs between sex partners, both heterosexual and homosexual, and in closed institutions, such as mental health institutions and prisons, but infectivity is far lower than for HAV, and the means of transmission is often unknown. The role of insect bites in transmission is unclear. Many cases of acute hepatitis B occur sporadically without a known source.

HBV, for unknown reasons, is sometimes associated with several primarily extrahepatic disorders, including polyarteritis nodosa and other connective tissue diseases, membranous glomerulonephritis, and essential mixed cryoglobulinemia. The pathogenic role of HBV in these disorders is unclear, but autoimmune mechanisms are suggested.

Chronic HBV carriers provide a worldwide reservoir of infection. Prevalence varies widely according to several factors, including geography (eg, < 0.5% in North America and northern Europe, > 10% in some regions of the Far East). Vertical transmission from mother to infant is common (see p. 2180).

Hepatitis C virus (HCV): HCV is a single-stranded RNA flavivirus. Six major HCV subtypes exist with varying amino acid sequences (genotypes); these subtypes vary geographically and in virulence and response to therapy. HCV can also alter its amino acid pattern over time in an infected person (quasi-species).

Infection is most commonly transmitted through blood, primarily when parenteral drug users share needles, but also through tattoos or body piercing. Sexual transmission and vertical transmission from mother to infant are relatively rare. Transmission through blood transfusion has become very rare since the advent of screening tests on donated blood. Some sporadic cases occur in patients without apparent risk factors. HCV prevalence varies with geography and other risk factors.

HCV sometimes occurs simultaneously with specific systemic disorders, including essential mixed cryoglobulinemia, porphyria cutanea tarda (about 60 to 80% of porphyria patients have HCV, but only a few HCV patients develop porphyria), and glomerulonephritis; the mechanisms are uncertain. In addition, up to 20% of patients with alcoholic liver disease harbor HCV. The reasons for this high association are unclear, because concomitant alcohol and drug use accounts for only a portion of cases. In these patients, HCV and alcohol act synergistically to exacerbate liver damage.

Hepatitis D virus (HDV): HDV, or delta agent, is a defective RNA virus that can replicate only in the presence of HBV. It occurs uncommonly as a co-infection with acute hepatitis B or as a superinfection in chronic hepatitis B. Infected hepatocytes contain delta particles coated with HBsAg. Prevalence of HDV varies widely geographically, with endemic pockets in several countries. Parenteral drug users are at relatively high risk, but HDV (unlike HBV) has not widely permeated the homosexual community.

Hepatitis E virus (HEV): HEV is an enterically transmitted RNA virus. Outbreaks of acute HEV hepatitis, often waterborne and linked to fecal contamination of the water supply, have occurred in China, India, Mexico, Pakistan, Peru, Russia, and central and northern Africa. These outbreaks have epidemiologic characteristics similar to HAV epidemics. Sporadic cases also occur. No outbreaks have occurred in the US or in Western Europe. Like hepatitis A, HEV does not produce chronic hepatitis or cirrhosis, and there is no chronic carrier state.

Symptoms and Signs

Acute infection tends to develop in predictable phases. Infection begins with an incubation period (see TABLE 27–2), during which the virus multiplies and spreads without symptoms. The prodromal, or pre-icteric, phase follows, producing nonspecific symptoms, such as profound anorexia, malaise, nausea and vomiting, and, often, fever or right upper quadrant abdominal pain. Urticaria and arthralgias occasionally occur, especially in HBV infection. After 3 to 10 days, the urine darkens, followed by jaundice (the icteric phase). Systemic symptoms often regress, and the patient feels better despite worsening jaundice. During the icteric phase, the liver is usually enlarged and tender, but the edge of the liver remains soft and smooth. Mild splenomegaly occurs in 15 to 20% of patients. Jaundice usually peaks within 1 to 2 wk and then fades during a 2- to 4-wk recovery phase. Appetite usually returns after the first week. Acute viral hepatitis usually resolves spontaneously after 4 to 8 wk.

Sometimes anicteric hepatitis, a minor flulike illness without jaundice, is the only manifestation. It occurs more often than icteric hepatitis in HCV infection and in children with HAV infection.

Recrudescent hepatitis occurs in a few patients and is characterized by recurrent manifestations during the recovery phase. Manifestations of cholestasis may develop during the icteric phase (cholestatic hepatitis) but usually resolve. When they persist, despite general regression of inflammation, they cause prolonged jaundice, elevated alkaline phosphatase, and pruritus.

HAV often does not produce jaundice and may not produce any symptoms. It almost invariably resolves after the acute infection, although there can be early recrudescence.

HBV produces a wide spectrum of liver diseases, from a subclinical carrier state to severe or fulminant acute hepatitis, particularly in the elderly, in whom mortality can reach 10 to 15%. Hepatocellular carcinoma can ultimately develop in chronic HBV infection, even without being preceded by cirrhosis.

HCV may be asymptomatic during the acute infection. Its severity often fluctuates, sometimes with recrudescent hepatitis and roller-coaster aminotransferase levels for many years or even decades. HCV has the highest rate of chronicity (about 75%). The resultant chronic hepatitis is usually asymptomatic or benign but progresses to cirrhosis in 20 to 30% of patients; cirrhosis often takes decades to appear. Hepatocellular carcinoma can result from HCV-induced cirrhosis but results only rarely from chronic infection without cirrhosis (unlike HBV infection).

Acute HDV infection typically presents as unusually severe acute HBV infection (co-infection), an acute exacerbation in chronic HBV carriers (superinfection), or a relatively aggressive course of chronic HBV infection.

HEV may be severe, especially in pregnant women.

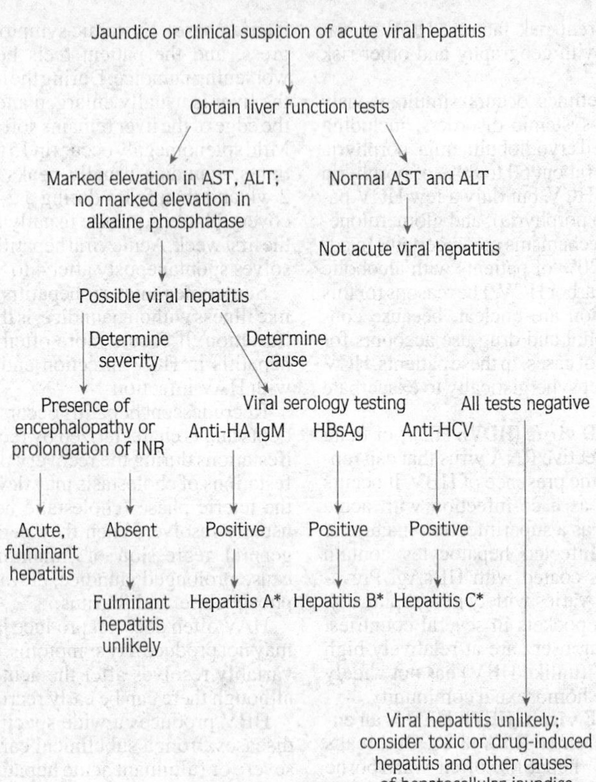

Fig. 27–1. Simplified diagnostic approach to possible acute viral hepatitis.

Diagnosis

In the prodromal phase, hepatitis mimics various nonspecific viral illnesses and is difficult to diagnose. Anicteric patients suspected of having hepatitis based on risk factors are tested initially with nonspecific liver function tests, including aminotransferases, bilirubin, and alkaline phosphatase. Usually, acute hepatitis is suspected only during the icteric phase. Thus, acute hepatitis should be differentiated from other disorders causing jaundice (see FIG. 27–1 and p. 191).

Acute hepatitis can usually be differentiated from other causes of jaundice by its marked elevations of AST and ALT (typically ≥400 IU/L). ALT is typically higher than AST, but absolute levels correlate poorly with clinical severity. Values increase early in the prodromal phase, peak before jaundice is maximal, and fall slowly during the recovery phase. Urinary bilirubin usually precedes jaundice. Hyperbilirubinemia in acute viral hepatitis is of variable severity, and fractionation is of no clinical value. Alkaline phosphatase is usually only moderately raised; marked elevation suggests extrahepatic cholestasis and prompts imaging tests (eg, ultrasound). Liver biopsy generally is not needed unless the diagnosis is uncertain. If laboratory results suggest acute hepatitis, particularly if ALT and AST are > 1000 IU/L, INR is obtained. Manifestations of portal-systemic encephalopathy, bleeding diathesis, or prolongation of INR suggest fulminant hepatitis (see p. 227).

If acute hepatitis is suspected, efforts are next directed toward identifying its cause. A history of exposure may provide the only clue of drug or toxic hepatitis. The history should also elicit risk factors for viral hepatitis. Prodromal sore throat and diffuse adenopathy suggest infectious mononucleosis rather than viral hepatitis. Alcoholic hepatitis is suggested by a history of drinking, more gradual onset of symptoms, and presence of vascular spiders or signs of chronic alcohol use or chronic liver disease (see also p. 211). Aminotransferase levels rarely exceed 300 IU/L, even in severe cases. Also, unlike in viral hepatitis, AST is typically higher than ALT, although this difference by itself does not reliably differentiate the two. In uncertain cases, liver biopsy usually distinguishes alcoholic from viral hepatitis.

In patients with suggestive findings, the following studies are performed to screen for hepatitis viruses A, B, and C: IgM anti-HA, HBsAg, IgM antibody to hepatitis B core (IgM anti-HBc), and anti-HCV. If any are positive, further serology testing may be necessary to differentiate acute from past or chronic infection (see TABLES 27–3, 27–4, and 27–5). If serology suggests hepatitis B, testing for hepatitis B e-antigen (HBeAg) and anti-HBe is usually performed to help determine the prognosis and to guide antiviral therapy. If serologically confirmed HBV is severe, anti-HDV is obtained. If the patient has recently traveled to an endemic area, IgM anti-HEV should be obtained if available.

HAV is present in serum only during acute infection and cannot be detected by clinically available tests. IgM antibody typically develops early in the infection and peaks about 1 to 2 wk after the development of jaundice. It diminishes within several weeks, followed by the development of protective IgG antibody (anti-HA), which persists usually for life. Thus, IgM antibody is a marker of acute infection, whereas IgG anti-HA merely indicates previous exposure to HAV and immunity to recurrent infection.

HBV has at least three distinct antigen-antibody systems that can be tested: HBsAg, HBcAg, and HBeAg. Viral DNA (HBV DNA) can also be tested. HBV surface coat can be detected in serum as HBsAg. HBsAg characteristically appears during the incubation period, usually 1 to 6 wk before clinical or biochemical illness develops, and implies infectivity of the blood. It disappears during convalescence. However, HBsAg is occasionally transient. The corresponding protective antibody (anti-HBs) appears weeks or months later, after clinical recovery, and usually persists for life; thus, its detection indicates past HBV infection and relative immunity. In 5 to 10% of patients, HBsAg persists and antibodies do not develop: These patients become asymptomatic carriers of the virus or develop chronic hepatitis.

HBcAg reflects the viral core. It is detectable in infected liver cells but is not detectable in serum except by special techniques. Antibody to HBcAg (anti-HBc) generally appears at the onset of clinical illness; thereafter, titers gradually diminish, usually over years or life. Its presence with anti-HBs indicates recovery from previous HBV infection. Anti-HBc is also present in chronic HBsAg carriers, who do not mount an anti-HBs response. In acute infection, anti-HBc is mainly of the IgM class, whereas in chronic infection, IgG anti-HBc predominates. IgM anti-HBc is a sensitive marker of acute HBV infection and occasionally is the only marker of recent infection, reflecting a window between disappearance of HBsAg and appearance of anti-HBs.

TABLE 27–3. HEPATITIS A SEROLOGY

	ACUTE HAV	PRIOR HAV*
IgM anti-HA	+	–
IgG anti-HA	–	+

HAV = Hepatitis A virus.

*Previous HAV infection; no chronic HAV exists

TABLE 27–4. HEPATITIS B SEROLOGY*

	ACUTE HBV	CHRONIC HBV	PRIOR HBV†
HBsAg	+	+	–
Anti-HBs	–	–	+‡
IgM anti-HBc	+	–	–
IgG anti-HBc	–	+	±
HBeAg	±	±	–
Anti-HBe	–	±	±
HBV DNA	+	+	–

HBV = Hepatitis B virus; HBsAg = hepatitis B surface antigen; HBcAg = hepatitis B core antigen; HBeAg = hepatitis B e-antigen.

*Anti-HDV antibody levels should be obtained if serology confirms HBV and infection is severe.

†Previous HBV infection with recovery.

‡Anti-HBs is also seen as the sole serologic marker after HBV vaccination.

TABLE 27–5. HEPATITIS C SEROLOGY

	ACUTE HCV	CHRONIC HCV	PRIOR HCV*
Anti-HCV	+	+	+
HCV RNA	+	+	–

HCV = Hepatitis C virus.
*Previous HCV infection with spontaneous recovery or successful therapy.

HBeAg is a protein derived from the viral core (not to be confused with hepatitis E virus). Present only in HBsAg-positive serum, HBeAg tends to suggest more active viral replication and greater infectivity. In contrast, presence of the corresponding antibody (anti-HBe) suggests lower infectivity. Thus, e-antigen markers are more helpful in prognosis than in diagnosis. Chronic liver disease develops more often among patients with HBeAg and less often among patients with anti-HBe.

In patients with active HBV infection, viral DNA (HBV-DNA) can be detected in the serum with special testing, although this test is not routinely available.

In HCV, serum antibody (anti-HCV) almost always implies active infection; it is not protective. Anti-HCV usually appears within 2 wk of acute infection but is sometimes delayed. In a small proportion of patients, anti-HCV merely reflects prior exposure with clearance of the virus rather than active infection. ALT and AST levels are normal. In unclear cases, HCV-RNA is measured.

In HDV, anti-HDV implies active infection. It may not be detectable until weeks after the acute illness.

In HEV, IgM anti-HEV is not routinely available for measurement. In a patient with endemic exposure and compatible clinical findings, anti-HEV suggests acute HEV infection.

Biopsy, if performed, usually reveals similar histopathology regardless of the specific virus: patchy cell dropout, acidophilic hepatocellular necrosis, mononuclear inflammatory infiltrate, histologic evidence of regeneration, and preservation of the reticulin framework. HBV can occasionally be diagnosed by the presence of ground-glass hepatocytes (caused by HBsAg-packed cytoplasm) and by special immunologic stains for the viral components. However, these findings are unusual in acute HBV and are much more common in chronic HBV infection. HCV causation can sometimes be inferred from subtle morphologic clues. Liver biopsy may help predict prognosis in acute hepatitis but is rarely performed solely for this purpose. Complete histologic recovery occurs unless extensive necrosis bridges entire acini (bridging necrosis). Most patients with bridging necrosis recover fully. However, some cases progress to chronic hepatitis.

Treatment

No treatments attenuate acute viral hepatitis except, occasionally, postexposure immunoprophylaxis. Alcohol should be avoided because it can increase liver damage. Restrictions on diet or activity, including commonly prescribed bed rest, have no scientific basis. Most patients may safely return to work after jaundice resolves, even if AST or ALT levels are slightly elevated. For cholestatic hepatitis, cholestyramine 8 g po once/day or bid can relieve itching. Viral hepatitis should be reported to the local or state health department.

Prevention

Because treatments have limited efficacy, prevention of viral hepatitis is very important. Personal hygiene helps prevent transmission, particularly fecal-oral transmission, as occurs with HAV and HEV. Blood and other body fluids (eg, saliva, semen) of patients with acute HBV and HCV and stool of patients with HAV are considered infectious. Barrier protection is recommended, but isolation of patients does little to prevent spread of HAV and is of no value in HBV or HCV disease. Posttransfusion infection is minimized by avoiding unnecessary transfusions and screening all donors for HBsAg and anti-HCV. Screening has decreased the incidence of posttransfusion hepatitis to 1/100,000 units of blood component transfused.

Immunoprophylaxis can involve active immunization using vaccines and passive immunization.

HAV: Preexposure HAV prophylaxis should be provided for travelers to highly endemic areas. It should also be considered for military personnel, day-care center employees, diagnostic laboratory workers, and, because they have an increased risk of fulminant hepatitis from HAV, patients with chronic liver disorders. Several vaccines against HAV are available, each with different doses and schedules; they are safe, provide protection within about 4 wk, and provide prolonged protection (probably for > 20 yr).

Standard immune globulin, formerly immune serum globulin, prevents or decreases the severity of HAV and should be given for postexposure prophylaxis; 0.02 mL/kg IM is generally recommended, but some experts advise 0.06 mL/kg (3 to 5 mL for adults).

HBV: Vaccination in endemic areas has dramatically reduced local prevalence. Preexposure immunization has long been recommended for people at high risk. However, selective vaccination of high-risk groups in the US and other nonendemic areas has not substantially decreased the incidence of HBV; thus vaccination is now recommended for all US residents < 18 beginning at birth. Universal worldwide vaccination is desirable but is too expensive to be feasible.

Two recombinant vaccines are available; both are safe, even during pregnancy. Three IM deltoid injections are given at baseline, at 1 mo, and at 6 mo. Children are given lower doses, and immunosuppressed patients or those on hemodialysis are given higher doses.

After vaccination, levels of anti-HBs remain protective in immunocompetent recipients for 5 yr in 80 to 90% and 10 yr in 60 to 80%. Booster doses of vaccine are recommended for hemodialysis or immunosuppressed patients whose anti-HBs is < 10 mIU/mL.

HBV postexposure immunoprophylaxis combines vaccination with hepatitis B immune globulin (HBIG), a product with high titers of anti-HBs. HBIG probably does not prevent infection but prevents or attenuates clinical illness. For infants born to HBsAg-positive mothers, an initial dose of vaccine plus 0.5 mL of HBIG is given IM in the thigh immediately after birth. For anyone having sexual contact with an HBsAg-positive person or percutaneous or mucous membrane exposure to HBsAg-positive blood, 0.06 mL/kg of HBIG is given IM within days, along with vaccine. Any previously vaccinated patient sustaining a percutaneous HBsAg-positive exposure is tested for anti-HBs; if titers are < 10 mIU/mL, a booster dose of vaccine is given.

HDV, HCV, HEV: No product exists for immunoprophylaxis of HDV, HCV, or HEV. However, prevention of HBV prevents HDV. The propensity of HCV for changing its genome hampers vaccine development.

Fulminant Hepatitis

Fulminant hepatitis is a rare syndrome of massive necrosis of liver parenchyma and a decrease in liver size (acute yellow atrophy) that usually occurs in infection with certain hepatitis viruses or with toxic agents or in drug-induced injury.

HBV is sometimes responsible, and up to 50% of cases of fulminant hepatitis B involve HDV co-infection. Fulminant hepatitis with HAV is rare but may be more likely in people with pre-existing liver disorders. The role of HCV remains uncertain.

Patients rapidly deteriorate from portal-systemic encephalopathy often followed by coma within hours or a few days, sometimes with cerebral edema. Bleeding commonly results from hepatic failure or disseminated intravascular coagulation, and functional renal failure (hepatorenal syndrome—see p. 200) may develop. Increasing PT, portal-systemic encephalopathy, and, particularly, renal failure are ominous.

Meticulous nursing care and aggressive treatment of complications improve the outcome. However, emergency liver transplantation provides the best hope for survival. Survival in adults is uncommon without transplantation; children tend to do better. Patients who survive usually recover fully.

CHRONIC HEPATITIS

Chronic hepatitis is hepatitis that lasts > 6 mo. Common causes include hepatitis B and C viruses, autoimmune mechanisms (autoimmune hepatitis), and drugs. Many patients have no history of acute hepatitis, and the first indication is discovery of asymptomatic aminotransferase elevations. Some patients first present with cirrhosis or its complications (eg, portal hypertension). Biopsy is necessary to confirm the diagnosis and to grade and stage the disease. Treatment is directed toward complications and the underlying cause (eg, corticosteroids for autoimmune hepatitis, antiviral therapy for viral hepatitis). Liver transplantation is often indicated for end-stage disease.

Etiology and Classification

Hepatitis lasting > 6 mo is generally defined as chronic, although this duration is arbitrary. Hepatitis B virus (HBV) and hepatitis C virus (HCV) are frequent causes of chronic hepatitis; 5 to 10% of cases of HBV (with or without hepatitis D virus co-infection) and about 75% of cases of HCV become chronic.

Hepatitis A and E viruses are not causes. Although the mechanism of chronicity is uncertain, liver injury is mostly determined by the patient's immune reaction to the infection.

Many cases are idiopathic. A high proportion of these idiopathic cases have prominent features of immune-mediated hepatocellular injury (autoimmune hepatitis), including the presence of serologic immune markers; an association with histocompatibility haplotypes common in autoimmune diseases (eg, HLA-B1, HLA-B8, HLA-DR3, HLA–DR4); a predominance of T lymphocytes and plasma cells in liver histologic lesions; complex in vitro defects in cellular immunity and immunoregulatory functions; an association with other autoimmune disorders (eg, RA, autoimmune hemolytic anemia, proliferative glomerulonephritis); and response to therapy with corticosteroids or immunosuppressants. Sometimes chronic hepatitis has features of both autoimmune hepatitis and another chronic liver disorder (eg, primary biliary cirrhosis, chronic viral hepatitis). These conditions are called overlap syndromes.

Many drugs, including isoniazid, methyldopa, nitrofurantoin, and, rarely, acetaminophen, can cause chronic hepatitis. The mechanism varies with the drug and may involve altered immune responses, cytotoxic intermediate metabolites, or genetically determined metabolic defects.

Other causes of chronic hepatitis include alcoholic hepatitis and nonalcoholic steatohepatitis. Less often, chronic hepatitis results from α_1-antitrypsin deficiency or Wilson's disease.

Cases were once classified histologically as chronic persistent, chronic lobular, or chronic active hepatitis. A more useful recent classification system specifies the etiology, the intensity of histologic inflammation and necrosis (grade), and the degree of histologic fibrosis (stage). Inflammation and necrosis are potentially reversible; fibrosis generally is not.

Symptoms and Signs

Clinical features vary. About ⅓ of cases develop after acute hepatitis, but most develop insidiously de novo. Many patients are asymptomatic, especially in chronic HCV. However, malaise, anorexia, and fatigue are common, sometimes with low-grade fever and nonspecific upper abdominal discomfort. Jaundice is usually absent. Often, particularly with HCV, the first findings are signs of chronic liver disease (eg, splenomegaly, spider nevi, palmar erythema). A few patients with chronic hepatitis develop manifestations of cholestasis. In the autoimmune variant, especially in young women, manifestations may involve virtually any body system and can include acne, amenorrhea, arthralgia, ulcerative colitis, pulmonary fibrosis, thyroiditis, nephritis, and hemolytic anemia.

Chronic HCV is occasionally associated with lichen planus, mucocutaneous vasculitis, glomerulonephritis, porphyria cutanea tarda, and, perhaps, non-Hodgkin's B-cell lymphoma. About 1% of patients develop symptomatic cryoglobulinemia with fatigue, myalgias, arthralgias, neuropathy, glomerulonephritis, and skin rashes (urticaria, purpura, or leukocytoclastic vasculitis); asymptomatic cryoglobulinemia is more common.

Diagnosis

The diagnosis is suspected in patients with suggestive symptoms and signs, incidentally noted elevations in aminotransferase levels, or previously diagnosed acute hepatitis. Liver function tests are obtained if not previously performed and include serum ALT, AST, alkaline phosphatase, and bilirubin. Aminotransferase elevations are the most characteristic laboratory abnormalities. Although levels can vary, they are typically 100 to 500 IU/L. ALT is usually higher than AST. Aminotransferase levels can be normal during chronic hepatitis if the disease is quiescent, particularly with HCV. Alkaline phosphatase is usually normal or only slightly elevated but occasionally may be markedly high. Bilirubin is usually normal unless the disease is severe or advanced. However, abnormalities in these laboratory tests are not specific and can result from other disorders, such as alcoholic liver disease, recrudescent acute viral hepatitis, and primary biliary cirrhosis.

If laboratory results are compatible with hepatitis, viral serology is obtained to exclude HBV and HCV (see FIG. 27–1 and TABLES 27–3, 27–4, and 27–5). Unless these studies indicate viral etiology, further testing is required. The first tests obtained include autoantibodies, immunoglobulins, and α_1-antitrypsin level. Children and young adults are screened for Wilson's disease with a ceruloplasmin level. Marked elevations in serum immunoglobulins suggest chronic autoimmune hepatitis but are not conclusive. Autoimmune hepatitis is normally diagnosed by the presence of antibodies at titers of ≥ 1:80 (in adults) or 1:20 (in children) of the antinuclear (ANA), anti-smooth muscle, or anti-liver-kidney microsomal 1 (anti-LKM1) types.

Unlike with acute hepatitis, biopsy is necessary. Mild cases may have only minor hepatocellular necrosis and inflammatory cell infiltration, usually in portal regions, with normal acinar architecture and little or no fibrosis. Such cases rarely develop clinically important liver disease or cirrhosis. In more severe cases, biopsy typically shows periportal necrosis with mononuclear cell infiltrates (piecemeal necrosis) accompanied by variable periportal fibrosis and bile duct proliferation. The acinar architecture may be distorted by zones of collapse and fibrosis, and frank cirrhosis sometimes coexists with signs of ongoing hepatitis. Biopsy is also used to grade and stage the disease.

In most cases, the specific cause of chronic hepatitis cannot be discerned on biopsy, although cases caused by HBV can be distinguished by the presence of ground-glass hepatocytes and special stains for HBV components. Autoimmune cases usually have a more pronounced infiltration by lymphocytes and plasma cells. Patients with histologic, but not serologic, criteria for chronic autoimmune hepatitis are diagnosed with variant autoimmune hepatitis; many have overlap syndromes.

Serum albumin and PT should be obtained to determine severity; hepatic insufficiency is suggested by low serum albumin or prolonged PT. If symptoms or signs of cryoglobulinemia develop during chronic hepatitis, particularly with HCV, cryoglobulin levels and rheumatoid factor should be obtained; high levels of rheumatoid factor and low levels of complement also suggest cryoglobulinemia.

Patients with chronic HBV should be screened annually for hepatocellular cancer by ultrasound and serum α-fetoprotein measurement, although the cost-effectiveness of this practice is debated. Patients with chronic HCV should be similarly screened only if cirrhosis is present.

Prognosis

Prognosis is highly variable. Chronic hepatitis caused by a drug often regresses completely when the offending drug is withdrawn. Without treatment, cases caused by HBV can resolve (uncommon), progress rapidly, or progress slowly to cirrhosis over decades. Resolution often begins with a transient increase in disease severity and results in seroconversion from hepatitis B e-antigen (HBeAg) to anti-HBe. Co-infection with HDV causes the most severe form of chronic HBV; without treatment, cirrhosis develops in up to 70% of patients. Untreated chronic hepatitis due to HCV produces cirrhosis in 20 to 30% of patients, although development may take decades. Chronic autoimmune hepatitis usually responds to therapy but sometimes produces progressive fibrosis and eventual cirrhosis.

Chronic HBV increases the risk of hepatocellular cancer; the risk is also increased in chronic HCV, but only if cirrhosis has already developed (see p. 236).

Treatment

Treatment goals include management of complications (eg, ascites, encephalopathy) and treatment of the underlying cause. Drugs that cause hepatitis should be stopped. Underlying disorders, such as Wilson's disease, should be treated. In chronic viral hepatitis due to HBV, prophylaxis of contacts may be helpful (see p. 226); corticosteroids and immunosuppressive drugs should be avoided, because they enhance viral replication. No prophylactic measures are required for contacts of HCV.

Autoimmune hepatitis: Corticosteroids, with or without azathioprine, prolong survival. Prednisone is usually started at 30 to 40 mg po once/day, then tapered to the lowest dose that maintains aminotransferase at normal or near-normal levels. Some experts give concomitant azathioprine 1 to 1.5 mg/kg po once/day; others add azathioprine only if low-dose prednisone fails to maintain suppression. Most patients require long-term, low-dose maintenance treatment. Liver transplantation may be required for end-stage disease.

HBV: Treatment is indicated in HBeAg-positive patients with elevated aminotransferase levels. Therapy aims to eliminate HBV DNA and convert the patient from HBeAg to anti-HBe; loss of HBsAg occurs in about 10% of patients. Interferon (IFN—usually IFN-α2b) or lamivudine is used.

IFN is given 5 million IU sc once/day or 10 million IU sc 3 times/wk for 4 mo. In about 40% of patients, this regimen eliminates HBV DNA and causes seroconversion to anti-HBe; a successful response is usually presaged by a temporary increase in aminotransferase levels. IFN must be given by injection and is often poorly tolerated. The first 1 to 2 doses produce an influenza-like syndrome. Later, IFN can produce fatigue, malaise, depression, bone marrow suppression, and, rarely, bacterial infections or autoimmune disorders. In patients with advanced cirrhosis, IFN can precipitate hepatic failure and is therefore contraindicated. Other contraindications include renal failure, immunosuppression, solid organ transplantation, cytopenia, and substance abuse. HBV patients co-infected with hepatitis D virus usually respond poorly to therapy. Unlike in HCV, use of pegylated IFN has not been adequately studied in chronic HBV, but initial reports appear favorable.

Alternatively, lamivudine 100 mg po once/day is given. Although it has few adverse effects, unlike IFN, it requires prolonged therapy, often for years. Lamivudine suppresses HBV DNA and aminotransferase levels in almost all patients, but relapse occurs if the drug is discontinued before seroconversion of HBeAg to anti-HBe. Seroconversion occurs in about 15 to 20% of patients after 1 yr of treatment, rising to about 40% after 3 yr. Development of resistance to the drug is common after prolonged therapy. Unlike IFN, lamivudine can be given safely to patients with advanced HBV cirrhosis, because it does not precipitate liver failure. Combined treatment with IFN and lamivudine does not appear to be more successful than therapy with either drug alone.

Adefovir (given orally) will probably become standard treatment for chronic HBV but requires further study. It is generally safe, and drug resistance appears to be uncommon.

Liver transplantation should be considered for end-stage liver disease caused by HBV, but the infection aggressively attacks the graft, and prognosis is less favorable than for liver transplants performed for other indications. Long-term posttransplant therapy with lamivudine improves the outcome.

HCV: For chronic hepatitis due to HCV, treatment is indicated if aminotransferase levels are elevated and biopsy shows active inflammatory disease with evolving fibrosis. Therapy aims to permanently eliminate HCV RNA (sustained response), which is associated with permanent normalization of aminotransferase and cessation of histologic progression.

Combination therapy with pegylated IFN-α plus ribavirin gives the best results. Pegylated IFN-α2b, given as 1.5 μg/kg sc once/wk, and pegylated IFN-α2a, given as 180 μg sc once/wk, give comparable results. Ribavirin is usually given at 500 to 600 mg po bid, though 400 mg bid may be sufficient for viral genotypes 2 and 3.

HCV genotype and viral load are measured before treatment, because results influence therapy. Genotype 1 is the most common type but is relatively resistant to treatment. Combination therapy is given for 1 yr; a sustained response rate of about 45 to 50% overall occurs. Results are more favorable in patients with early disease and less favorable in those who already have cirrhosis. HCV viral load should be measured at 3 mo and treatment abandoned if RNA has not declined by at least 2 log levels compared to pretreatment values.

Less common genotypes 2 and 3 respond more favorably. Combination therapy is required for only 6 mo and gives an overall sustained response rate of about 75%. Longer treatment does not improve the results.

Adverse effects of pegylated IFN-α are the same as those of standard IFN but may be marginally less severe. In a few patients, treatment needs to be abandoned due to intolerable adverse effects. The drug should be given cautiously or not at all to patients with ongoing substance abuse or major psychiatric disorders. Ribavirin is usually well tolerated but commonly produces anemia due to hemolysis; dosage should be decreased if hemoglobin falls to < 10 g/dL. Ribavirin is teratogenic for both men and women, necessitating contraception until 6 mo after completion of treatment. Patients who cannot tolerate ribavirin should be given pegylated IFN-α, but results are not as good as with combination treatment. Ribavirin monotherapy is of no value.

In most adult transplant centers, advanced cirrhosis due to HCV is now the most common indication for liver transplantation. Although HCV recurs in the graft, the course is usually indolent, and long-term survival rates are relatively high.

28 VASCULAR DISORDERS

Hepatic blood supply is about ⅔ from the portal vein (rich in nutrients) and ⅓ from the hepatic artery (rich in oxygen). The hepatic vein drains the liver. When portal vein blood flow increases, hepatic artery flow decreases and vice versa (the hepatic arterial buffer response). These dual, reciprocally compensatory blood supplies provide some protection from hepatic ischemia in healthy people.

Despite its dual blood supplies, the liver can sustain injury from ischemia, insufficient venous drainage, and vascular insults. Insufficient venous drainage may involve focal or diffuse obstruction. Manifestations of focal venous obstruction depend on the location of the occlusion. Diffuse venous congestion causes congestive hepatopathy. Specific vascular lesions can involve the hepatic artery, hepatic vein, or portal vein. In peliosis hepatis, a vascular lesion involves the sinusoids (microvascular anastomoses between the portal and hepatic veins).

HEPATIC ISCHEMIA

Diffuse ischemia can cause ischemic hepatitis, whereas focal ischemia can cause hepatic infarction or ischemic cholangiopathy.

Ischemic Hepatitis

(Acute Hepatic Infarction; Hypoxic Hepatitis; Shock Liver)

Ischemic hepatitis is diffuse liver injury secondary to generalized hepatic ischemia from any cause.

The most common causes of ischemic hepatitis are reduced cardiac output, systemic hypotension, and systemic hypoxia. Centrizonal necrosis develops without liver inflammation. A high aminotransferase level is the only suggestion of hepatitis.

Ischemic hepatitis is suspected in patients with systemic hypoperfusion. Serum aminotransferase rises (up to 200-fold) within hours along with LDH. Serum bilirubin increases only 4-fold. If perfusion is restored, aminotransferase falls over 1 to 2 wk.

Treatment is directed at the underlying cause. In most cases, liver function is fully recovered. Fulminant liver failure, however, can occur in patients with preexisting cirrhosis.

Hepatic Infarction

Hepatic infarction is focal hepatocellular necrosis due to focal hepatic ischemia from any cause.

The most common cause of hepatic infarction is hepatic artery occlusion (see p. 232). Most hepatic infarcts are asymptomatic and undiagnosed. Some patients experience right upper quadrant pain, fever, and nausea and vomiting. Jaundice and high transient elevations of aminotransferase may occur.

Abdominal CT scan can detect a hepatic infarct as a focal, often wedge-shaped lesion of low attenuation. Recognition of hepatic infarction prompts evaluation of the patency of the hepatic artery. Treatment of hepatic infarction is directed at its cause.

Ischemic Cholangiopathy

Ischemic cholangiopathy is focal ischemia of the biliary tree due to any process that disrupts the peribiliary arterial plexus.

Common causes of ischemic cholangiopathy include orthotopic liver transplantation (because of hepatic artery thrombosis or graft-rejection injury to the peribiliary plexus), chemoembolization, radiation therapy, iatrogenic hepatic artery injury or ligation at laparoscopic cholecystectomy, and thrombosis resulting from hypercoagulable states. The result is cholestasis, sometimes with bile duct necrosis, cholangitis, or biliary stricture.

Symptoms and laboratory and imaging tests reflect cholestasis (see p. 193). If ischemia is suspected, liver function tests and ultrasonography (frequently negative) are obtained. If ischemic cholangiopathy is suspected after orthotopic liver transplantation, cholangiography is performed by MRI or endoscopy. If transplantation is the cause, multiple strictures are present.

Treatment of ischemic cholangiopathy is directed at its cause. After liver transplantation, treatment includes antirejection therapy and possibly endoscopic balloon dilation of biliary strictures or retransplantation.

CONGESTIVE HEPATOPATHY

(Passive Hepatic Congestion)

Congestive hepatopathy is diffuse venous congestion within the liver that results from right-sided heart failure.

Moderate or severe right-sided heart failure increases central venous pressure, which is transmitted to the liver via the inferior vena cava and hepatic veins. Hepatic dysfunction is usually mild and asymptomatic, but severe congestion produces right upper quadrant discomfort (from stretching of the liver capsule), hepatomegaly, ascites, splenomegaly, and jaundice. Chronic congestion leads to atrophy of hepatocytes, distention of sinusoids, and centrilobular fibrosis, which, if severe, produces cirrhosis (cardiac cirrhosis). The basis is probably sinusoidal thrombosis that propagates to the central veins and branches of the portal vein, causing ischemia.

Liver function tests and analysis of ascitic fluid are obtained. Mild hepatic venous congestion produces mild unconjugated hyperbilirubinemia. Profound congestion often produces disproportionate elevation of bilirubin; serum aminotransferase may be mildly elevated (twofold to threefold), and PT/INR may be prolonged. Ascitic fluid shows a high albumin content and serum ascites/albumin gradient. Treatment is directed at the underlying heart failure.

HEPATIC ARTERY DISORDERS

HEPATIC ARTERY OCCLUSION

Causes of hepatic artery occlusion include thrombosis (eg, due to hypercoagulable states, severe arteriosclerosis, vasculitis), embolus (eg, due to endocarditis, tumors, therapeutic embolization, chemoembolization), iatrogenic causes (eg, ligation at surgery), vasculitis, hepatic artery aneurysm, toxemia of pregnancy, cocaine use, and sickle cell crisis. The result usually is a hepatic infarct. In a patient with liver transplantation or preexisting portal vein thrombosis, hepatic artery thrombosis produces ischemic hepatitis.

Diagnosis is confirmed by imaging with Doppler ultrasound and celiac arteriography.

Treatment addresses the underlying cause, such as structural arterial abnormalities, emboli (eg, endocarditis, tumors), coagulopathy, or vasculitis.

ANEURYSMS

Aneurysms of the hepatic artery tend to be saccular and multiple. Common causes are infection, arteriosclerosis, trauma, and vasculitis. Untreated, aneurysms may cause death by rupturing into the common bile duct (producing hemobilia), peritoneum (producing peritonitis), or adjacent hollow viscera. Hemobilia may produce jaundice, upper GI bleeding, and abdominal pain in the right upper quadrant.

Diagnosis is made by CT with radiopaque dye. Treatment is embolization or surgical ligation.

CONGENITAL ANOMALIES

Although congenital anomalies of the hepatic artery are common, they are rarely clinically important; they may be noted during vascular imaging tests or surgery.

HEPATIC VEIN DISORDERS

Obstruction of hepatic venous outflow can occur in the extrahepatic vessels (Budd-Chiari syndrome) or intrahepatic vessels (veno-occlusive disease) but often occurs in both.

BUDD-CHIARI SYNDROME

Budd-Chiari syndrome is obstruction of hepatic venous outflow that originates anywhere from the right atrium to the small radicles of the hepatic vein. Manifestations range from no symptoms to fulminant liver failure. Diagnosis is based on ultrasound. Treatment includes supportive medical therapy and measures to establish and

maintain venous patency, such as thrombolysis, decompression with shunts, and long-term anticoagulation.

Etiology and Pathophysiology

Obstruction that originates in the small radicles of the hepatic vein overlaps with veno-occlusive disease. In the Western world, the most common cause of Budd-Chiari syndrome is a clot at the junction of the hepatic veins and inferior vena cava. Common causes include thrombotic coagulopathies (eg, protein C or S deficiency, antithrombin III deficiency, pregnancy, oral contraceptive use), hematologic diseases (eg, polycythemia, paroxysmal nocturnal hemoglobinopathy, myeloproliferative disorder), inflammatory bowel disease, connective tissue disease, and trauma. Other causes are infection (eg, hydatid cyst, ameba) and tumor invasion of the hepatic vein (eg, hepatocellular or renal cell carcinoma). The cause of obstruction is often unknown. In Asia and South Africa, the cause is often a membranous obstruction (webs) of the inferior vena cava above the liver, likely representing recanalization of a prior thrombus in adults or a developmental defect (eg, venous stenosis) in children.

Consequences of venous obstruction include ascites, portal hypertension, and hypersplenism.

Symptoms and Signs

Manifestations range from asymptomatic to fulminant liver failure or cirrhosis. Acute obstruction (classic Budd-Chiari syndrome) causes right upper quadrant pain, nausea and vomiting, mild jaundice, tender hepatomegaly, and ascites. With complete inferior vena cava obstruction, patients have edema of the abdominal wall and legs plus visibly tortuous superficial abdominal veins from the pelvis to the costal margin. Fulminant liver failure and encephalopathy occur rarely and sporadically during pregnancy. A more subacute course (< 6 mo) manifests as hepatomegaly, coagulopathy, ascites, splenomegaly, variceal bleeding, and the hepatorenal syndrome. Most presentations are chronic (>6 mo) and include fatigue, tortuous superficial abdominal veins, and, in some patients, variceal bleeding, ascites, and decompensated cirrhosis.

Diagnosis

Budd-Chiari syndrome is suspected when hepatomegaly, ascites, liver failure, or cirrhosis is present or when abnormal liver function test results coincide with risk factors for thrombosis. Abdominal Doppler ultrasound results show the direction of blood flow and the site of obstruction. CT and MRI are useful if ultrasound is not diagnostic. Angiography is necessary if surgery is planned. Laboratory tests, though not diagnostic, help evaluate liver function.

Prognosis and Treatment

Most patients with complete venous obstruction die of liver failure within 3 yr. Those with incomplete obstruction have a variable course.

Treatment includes supportive medical therapy for complications (eg, ascites, liver failure) and decompression. Thrombolysis may dissolve acute clots and relieve hepatic congestion. For caval webs or hepatic venous stenosis, percutaneous transluminal balloon angioplasty with intraluminal stents maintains outflow. Transjugular intrahepatic stents and many surgical shunts also provide decompression. Shunts generally are not used if hepatic encephalopathy is present and hepatic synthetic function is impaired, because shunts often worsen liver function. Also, shunts tend to thrombose, especially with hematologic disorders. Long-term anticoagulation is often necessary to prevent recurrence. Liver transplantation may be lifesaving in cases of fulminant disease or decompensated cirrhosis.

VENO-OCCLUSIVE DISEASE

(Sinusoidal Obstruction Syndrome)

Hepatic veno-occlusive disease is caused by occlusion of the terminal hepatic venules and hepatic sinusoids rather than of the hepatic veins or inferior vena cava.

Venous congestion produces ischemic necrosis that can lead to cirrhosis and portal hypertension. Common causes include irradiation, graft-vs-host disease resulting from bone marrow (or hematopoietic cell) transplantation, pyrrolizidine alkaloids from Crotalaria and Senecio plants (eg, medicinal bush teas), and other hepatotoxins (eg, dimethylnitrosamine, aflatoxin, azathioprine, some anticancer drugs).

Initial manifestations of veno-occlusive disease include sudden jaundice, ascites, and tender, smooth hepatomegaly. Onset is within the first 2 wk of transplantation in bone marrow recipients, who either recover spontaneously within a few weeks (patients with mild cases may respond to an increase in immunosuppression) or die of fulminant liver failure. Others with veno-occlusive disease have recurrent ascites, portal hypertension, and, eventually, cirrhosis.

The diagnosis is suspected in patients, particularly recipients of bone marrow transplantation, with typical symptoms. Liver function tests, ultrasound, and PT/INR are obtained. Typical results include elevations in aminotransferase levels, conjugated bilirubin, and, if disease is severe, PT/INR. Ultrasound shows retrograde flow in the portal vein. In a patient with typical clinical, laboratory, and ultrasound findings, particularly in bone marrow transplant recipients, further testing may not be necessary. However, if the diagnosis is unclear, liver biopsy or calculation of the difference between measured hepatic venous and portal venous pressures is necessary. A difference in pressures of > 10 mm Hg suggests veno-occlusive disease.

Treatment includes withdrawal of the causative agent, supportive therapy, and transjugular intrahepatic stents for relief of portal hypertension. Liver transplantation is a last resort. Ursodeoxycholic acid helps prevent graft-vs-host disease in bone marrow transplant recipients.

PORTAL VEIN DISORDERS

Nearly all portal vein disorders obstruct portal vein blood flow and cause portal hypertension (see p. 195). Obstruction can be extrahepatic (eg, portal vein thrombosis, congenital atresia of the portal vein) or intrahepatic (eg, microvascular portal vein obstruction in schistosomiasis).

PORTAL VEIN THROMBOSIS

Portal vein thrombosis produces portal hypertension and consequent GI bleeding. Diagnosis is based on ultrasound. Treatment involves control of GI bleeding (usually with endoscopy or IV octreotide), sometimes surgical shunts or β-blockers, and, for acute thrombosis, possibly thrombolysis.

Etiology

Portal vein thrombosis in neonates commonly results from umbilical stump infection that spreads via the umbilical vein to the portal vein. In older children, the culprit is acute appendicitis, in which infection sometimes enters the portal system, causing vascular infection (pylephlebitis), which can trigger thrombosis. Congenital anomalies of the portal vein causing portal vein thrombosis usually accompany congenital defects elsewhere. In adults, common causes are surgery (eg, splenectomy), hypercoaguable states (eg, myeloproliferative disorder, protein C or S deficiency), cancer (eg, hepatocellular or pancreatic carcinoma), cirrhosis, and pregnancy. The cause is unknown in about 50% of cases.

Symptoms, Signs, and Diagnosis

Symptoms rarely develop acutely unless mesenteric venous thrombosis occurs simultaneously, which causes significant abdominal pain. Most symptoms and signs develop chronically secondary to portal hypertension and include splenomegaly (especially in children) and GI bleeding. Ascites is rarely due to portal hypertension alone and, if present, indicates hepatocellular dysfunction from a separate disorder.

Portal vein thrombosis is suspected in patients with manifestations of portal hypertension without cirrhosis and in patients with even mild abnormalities in liver function or enzymes who have risk factors such as neonatal umbilical infection, childhood appendicitis, or a hypercoagulable state. Doppler ultrasound is usually diagnostic, revealing diminished or absent portal vein flow and sometimes the thrombus. Difficult cases may require MRI or CT with contrast. Angiography may be required to guide shunt surgery.

Treatment

In acute cases, anticoagulation sometimes prevents clot propagation but does not dissolve existing clots. In neonates and children, treatment is directed at the cause (eg, omphalitis, appendicitis). Otherwise, treatment is directed at portal hypertension (see p. 195) and variceal bleeding (see p. 92). Endoscopic banding is usually used to control variceal bleeding. Octreotide IV, a synthetic analog of somatostatin, may also help. These therapies have decreased the use of surgical shunts (eg, mesocaval, splenorenal), which have problems with occlusion and operative mortality (5 to 50%). β-Blockade (often combined with nitrates) is predicted to be as effective for preventing bleeding as in portal hypertension from cirrhosis but has not been tested.

PELIOSIS HEPATIS

Peliosis hepatis is a typically asymptomatic disorder in which multiple blood-filled cystic spaces are distributed randomly in the liver.

Measuring a few millimeters to about 3 cm in diameter, the cysts of peliosis hepatis often lack a cell lining and are surrounded by hepatocytes. Some, however, have an endothelial cell lining and occur with dilated hepatic sinusoids. The cause is likely damaged sinusoidal lining cells. Peliosis hepatis is associated with hormones (anabolic steroids, oral contraceptives, glucocorticoids), tamoxifen, vinyl chloride, vitamin A, and, particularly in kidney transplantation patients, azathioprine.

Peliosis hepatis is usually asymptomatic but occasionally causes rupture with hemorrhage (sometimes fatal) or overt liver disease, characterized by jaundice, hepatomegaly, and liver failure. Mild cases may be detected only incidentally when liver function test results are mildly abnormal and when cysts are seen on ultrasound.

29 LIVER MASSES AND GRANULOMAS

Liver masses include cysts, benign tumors, primary liver cancers, and metastatic liver cancer.

HEPATIC CYSTS

Isolated cysts are commonly detected incidentally on abdominal ultrasound or CT. These cysts are usually asymptomatic and have no clinical significance. The rare congenital polycystic liver is commonly associated with polycystic disease of the kidneys (see p. 1978) and other organs. It produces progressive lumpy hepatomegaly (sometimes massive) in adults. Nevertheless, hepatocellular function is remarkably well preserved, and portal hypertension does not develop.

Other hepatic cysts include hydatid (echinococcal) cysts (see p. 1561); the rare autosomal-recessive Caroli's disease, characterized by segmental cystic dilation of intrahepatic bile ducts (often becoming symptomatic in adulthood, with stone formation, cholangitis, and sometimes cholangiocarcinoma); and true cystic tumors (rare).

BENIGN LIVER TUMORS

Benign liver tumors are relatively common. Most are asymptomatic, but some cause hepatomegaly, right upper quadrant discomfort, or intraperitoneal hemorrhage. Most are detected incidentally on ultrasound or other scans. Liver function tests are usually normal or only slightly abnormal. Diagnosis is usually possible with imaging tests but may require biopsy. Treatment is not routinely needed.

Hepatocellular adenoma is the most important benign tumor to recognize. It occurs primarily in women of childbearing age, particularly those taking oral contraceptives. Most adenomas are asymptomatic, but larger ones may cause right upper quadrant discomfort. Rarely, adenomas present as peritonitis and shock due to rupture and intraperitoneal hemorrhage. Rarely, they undergo malignant transformation. Diagnosis is often suspected on the basis of ultrasound or CT results, but biopsy is usually needed for confirmation. Adenomas due to contraceptive use often regress if the drug is stopped. Some authorities recommend resecting subcapsular adenomas.

Focal nodular hyperplasia is a localized hamartoma that histologically may resemble macronodular cirrhosis. Diagnosis is usually based on MRI or CT with contrast, but biopsy may be necessary. Treatment is rarely needed.

Other benign tumors include hemangiomas, which are usually small and asymptomatic and occur in 1 to 5% of adults. They often have a characteristic highly vascular appearance and are found incidentally on ultrasound, CT, or MRI. Rupture is rare, even in large tumors, and treatment generally is not indicated. In infants, large hemangiomas occasionally cause arteriovenous shunting sufficient to produce heart failure and sometimes consumption coagulopathy. Benign bile duct adenomas and various rare mesenchymal tumors can also affect the hepatobiliary system.

PRIMARY LIVER CANCER

Primary liver cancer is usually hepatocellular carcinoma. Most liver cancers present with nonspecific manifestations, delaying the diagnosis. Prognosis is usually poor.

Hepatocellular Carcinoma

Hepatocellular carcinoma (hepatoma) usually occurs in patients with cirrhosis and is common in areas where infection with hepatitis B and C viruses is prevalent. Symptoms and signs usually are nonspecific. Diagnosis is based on α-fetoprotein (AFP) levels, imaging tests, and sometimes liver biopsy. Screening with periodic AFP measurement and ultrasound is sometimes recommended for high-risk patients. Prognosis is grim, but small localized tumors can sometimes be cured by surgical resection or liver transplantation.

Etiology and Epidemiology

Hepatocellular carcinoma is usually a complication of cirrhosis. It is the most common type of primary liver cancer and results in about 14,000 deaths annually in the US. The disease is more common outside the US, particularly in Southeast Asia, Japan, Korea, and sub-Saharan Africa. Incidence generally parallels geographic prevalence of chronic hepatitis B virus (HBV) infection; the risk increases > 100-fold among HBV carriers. Incorporation of HBV DNA into the host's genome may initiate malignant transformation, even in the absence of chronic hepatitis or cirrhosis. Other disorders that cause hepatocellular carcinoma include cirrhosis from chronic hepatitis C virus (HCV) infection, hemochromatosis, and alcoholic cirrhosis. Patients with cirrhosis due to other causes are also at increased risk. Environmental carcinogens may play a role; eg, ingestion of food contaminated with fungal aflatoxins is believed to contribute to the high incidence of hepatoma in subtropical regions.

Symptoms and Signs

Abdominal pain, weight loss, right upper quadrant mass, and unexplained deterioration in a previously stable patient with cirrhosis are the most common clinical presentations. Fever may occur. Occasionally, hemorrhage of the tumor causes bloody ascites, shock, or peritonitis, which may be the first manifestation of hepatocellular carcinoma. Occasionally, a hepatic friction rub or bruit develops. Systemic metabolic complications occasionally occur, including hypoglycemia, erythrocytosis, hypercalcemia, and hyperlipidemia. These complications may manifest clinically.

Diagnosis

Diagnosis is based on AFP measurement and an imaging study. Presence of AFP in an adult signifies dedifferentiation of hepatocytes, which most often indicates hepatocellular carcinoma; high AFP levels are present in 60 to 90% of patients. Values of > 400 μg/L are otherwise rare except in teratocarcinoma of the testis, a much less common tumor. Lower values are less specific and can occur with hepatocellular regeneration (eg, in hepatitis). The roles of other blood tests, such as des-γ-carboxyprothrombin and α-L-fucosidase, are evolving.

Depending on local preferences and capabilities, the first imaging study may be contrast-enhanced CT, ultrasound, or MRI. Hepatic arteriography is occasionally helpful in the diagnosis of equivocal cases and can also be used to outline the vascular anatomy when surgery is planned.

If imaging demonstrates characteristic findings and AFP is elevated, the diagnosis is clear. Liver biopsy, preferably guided by ultrasound, is indicated for definitive diagnosis.

Prognosis and Treatment

Unless the tumor is < 2 cm and localized to one lobe of the liver, 2-yr survival is < 5%. Surgical resection provides the best hope but is suitable only for the few cases in which the tumor is small and localized. Other treatments include hepatic arterial chemoembolization, intratumoral ethanol injection, cryoablation, and radiofrequency ablation, but none gives very good results. Radiation and systemic chemotherapy generally do not help. If the tumor is small, extrahepatic disease is nonexistent, and hepatic reserve is poor, liver transplantation instead of surgical resection can be considered and generally gives better results.

Prevention and Screening

Use of vaccine against HBV eventually decreases the incidence, especially in endemic areas. Preventing the development of cirrhosis of any cause can also have a significant effect (eg, via therapy of chronic HCV, detection of early hemochromatosis, management of alcoholism).

Screening of patients with cirrhosis is reasonable, although this measure is controversial and has not been clearly shown to decrease mortality. One commonly used protocol is to measure AFP and perform an ultrasound at 6- or 12-mo intervals. Many experts also advise screening patients with long-standing HBV even in the absence of cirrhosis.

Other Primary Liver Cancers

Fibrolamellar carcinoma, cholangiocarcinoma, hepatoblastoma, and angiosarcoma are uncommon or rare. Diagnosis usually requires biopsy. Prognosis is usually poor. Some cancers, if localized, can be resected. With resection or liver transplantation, survival may be prolonged.

Fibrolamellar carcinoma is a distinct variant of hepatocellular carcinoma with a characteristic morphology of malignant hepatocytes enmeshed in lamellar fibrous tissue. It usually occurs in young adults and has no association with preexisting cirrhosis, hepatitis B or C virus (HBV or HCV), or other known risk factors. AFP levels are rarely elevated. Prognosis is better than for hepatocellular carcinoma, and many patients survive several years after tumor resection.

Cholangiocarcinoma, a tumor arising from biliary epithelium, is common in China, where underlying infestation with liver flukes is believed to be partially responsible. Elsewhere, it is less common than hepatocellular carcinoma. Histologic overlap between the two may occur. Patients with long-standing ulcerative colitis and sclerosing cholangitis have an increased risk of cholangiocarcinoma.

Hepatoblastoma, although rare, is one of the most common primary liver cancers in infants, particularly when familial adenomatous polyposis (see p. 174) is present in the family. It can also develop in children. Hepatoblastoma occasionally presents with precocious puberty caused by ectopic gonadotropin production, but it is usually detected because of failing systemic health and a right upper quadrant mass. An elevated AFP level and abnormal imaging test results may help in diagnosis.

Angiosarcoma is rare and is associated with specific chemical carcinogens, including industrial vinyl chloride.

METASTATIC LIVER CANCER

Liver metastases are common in many types of cancer, especially those of the GI tract, breast, lung, and pancreas. The first symptoms usually are nonspecific (eg, weight loss, right upper quadrant discomfort) but are sometimes the presenting symptoms of the primary cancer. Liver metastases are suspected in patients with weight loss and hepatomegaly and in those with primary tumors at high risk of hepatic spread. Diagnosis is usually supported by an imaging test, most often ultrasound or spiral CT with contrast. Treatment usually involves palliative chemotherapy.

Metastatic liver cancer is more common than primary hepatic malignancy and is sometimes the initial clinical manifestation of cancer originating in the GI tract, breast, lung, or pancreas.

Symptoms and Signs

Early liver metastases may be asymptomatic. Nonspecific symptoms of malignancy (eg, weight loss, anorexia, fever) often develop first. The liver may be enlarged, hard, or tender; massive hepatomegaly with easily palpable lumps signifies advanced disease. Hepatic bruits and pleuritic-type pain with an overlying friction rub are uncommon but characteristic. Splenomegaly is occasionally present, especially when the primary cancer is pancreatic. Concomitant peritoneal tumor seeding may produce ascites, but jaundice is usually absent or mild initially unless a tumor causes biliary obstruction. In the terminal stages, progressive jaundice and hepatic encephalopathy presage death.

Diagnosis

In suspected cases, liver function tests often are obtained but usually are not specific for the diagnosis. Alkaline phosphatase, γ-glutamyl transpeptidase, and sometimes LDH typically increase earlier or to a greater degree than do other test results; aminotransferase levels vary. Imaging tests have good sensitivity and specificity. Ultrasound is usually helpful, but spiral CT with contrast often gives more accurate results. MRI is comparably accurate.

Liver biopsy provides the definitive diagnosis and is performed if other studies are equivocal or if histologic information (eg, cell type of the liver metastasis) may determine the treatment plan. Ultrasound- or CT-guided biopsy is preferable to blind biopsy.

Treatment

Treatment depends on the extent of metastasis. With solitary or very few metastases due to colorectal cancer, surgical resection may prolong survival. Depending on characteristics of the primary tumor, systemic chemotherapy may shrink tumors and prolong life but is not curative; hepatic intra-arterial chemotherapy sometimes achieves the same ends with fewer or milder adverse systemic effects. Radiation therapy to the liver occasionally alleviates severe pain due to advanced metastases but does not prolong life. Extensive disease is fatal and is best managed by palliation for the patient and support for the family (see p. 2762).

Hematologic Malignancies and the Liver

Hepatic involvement in advanced leukemia and related blood disorders is exceedingly common. Liver biopsy is not needed. In hepatic lymphoma, especially Hodgkin's disease, the extent of liver involvement determines staging and treatment but, unfortunately, may be difficult to assess. Hepatomegaly and abnormal liver function tests may reflect a systemic reaction to Hodgkin's disease rather than spread to the liver, and biopsy often shows nonspecific focal mononuclear infiltrates or granulomas of uncertain significance.

HEPATIC GRANULOMAS

Hepatic granulomas have numerous possible causes and are usually asymptomatic. However, the disorder causing the granulomas may produce extrahepatic manifestations and/or hepatic inflammation, fibrosis, and portal hypertension. Diagnosis is based on liver biopsy, but biopsy is necessary only if a treatable underlying cause (eg, infection) is suspected or other liver disorders are ruled out. Treatment is determined by the underlying disorder.

Hepatic granulomas may be insignificant but more often reflect clinically relevant disease. The term granulomatous hepatitis is often used to describe the condition, but the disorder is not true hepatitis, and the presence of granulomas does not imply hepatocellular inflammation.

Etiology and Pathophysiology

A granuloma is a localized collection of chronic inflammatory cells with epithelioid cells and giant multinucleated cells. Caseation necrosis or foreign body tissue (eg, schistosome eggs) may be present. Most granulomas are in the parenchyma, but granulomas may occur in the triads in primary biliary cirrhosis.

Granuloma formation is incompletely understood. Granulomas may develop in response to poorly soluble exogenous or endogenous irritants. Immunologic mechanisms are involved.

Hepatic granulomas have many causes (see TABLE 29–1), more often drugs and systemic disorders (often infections) than primary liver disorders. The infections are important to recognize because they require specific treatments. TB and schistosomiasis are the most important infectious causes worldwide; viral causes are less common. Sarcoidosis is the most important noninfectious cause; the liver is involved in about ⅔ of patients and occasionally is the dominant clinical manifestation.

Granulomas are much less common in primary liver diseases, of which primary biliary cirrhosis is the only important cause. Small granulomas occasionally occur in other liver diseases but are of no clinical significance.

Idiopathic granulomatous hepatitis is a rare syndrome of hepatic granulomas and recurrent fever, myalgias, fatigue, and other systemic symptoms often occurring intermittently for years. Some experts believe it is a variant of sarcoidosis.

Hepatic granulomas rarely affect hepatocellular function. However, when granulomas are part of a broader inflammatory reaction involving the liver (eg, drug reactions, infectious mononucleosis), hepatocellular dysfunction is present. Sometimes inflammation causes progressive hepatic fibrosis and portal hypertension, typically with schistosomiasis and occasionally with extensive sarcoidal infiltration.

Symptoms, Signs, and Diagnosis

Granulomas themselves are typically asymptomatic; even extensive infiltration usually produces only minor hepatomegaly and little or no jaundice. Symptoms, if they occur, reflect the underlying cause (eg, constitutional symptoms in infections, hepatosplenomegaly in schistosomiasis).

When hepatic granulomas are suspected, liver function tests are generally obtained, but results are nonspecific and are rarely helpful in diagnosis. Alkaline phosphatase (and γ–glutamyl transferase) is often mildly elevated but occasionally may be markedly elevated. Other test results may be normal or may reveal abnormalities that reflect additional hepatic damage (eg, widespread hepatic inflammation due to a drug reaction). Imaging tests, such as ultrasound, CT, or MRI, usually are not diagnostic; they may show calcification (if chronic) or filling defects, particularly with confluent lesions.

Diagnosis is based on liver biopsy. However, biopsy is usually indicated only to diagnose treatable causes (eg, infections) or to differentiate from nongranulomatous disorders (eg, chronic viral hepatitis). Biopsy sometimes reveals evidence of the specific cause (eg, schistosomal ova, caseation of TB, fungal organisms). However, other studies (eg, cultures, skin tests, laboratory tests, x-rays, other tissue specimens) are often needed.

In patients with constitutional or other symptoms suggesting infection (eg, FUO), specific measures are taken to increase the diagnostic sensitivity of biopsy for infections (eg, sending a portion of the fresh biopsy specimen for culture and performing special stains for acid-fast bacilli, fungi, and other organisms). Often, cause cannot be established.

TABLE 29–1. CAUSES OF HEPATIC GRANULOMAS

Drugs (eg, allopurinol, phenylbutazone, quinidine, sulfonamides)

Infections

- Bacterial (actinomycosis, brucellosis, cat-scratch fever, syphilis, TB* and other mycobacteria, tularemia)
- Fungal (blastomycosis, cryptococcosis, histoplasmosis)
- Parasitic (schistosomiasis*, toxoplasmosis, visceral larva migrans)
- Viral (cytomegalovirus, infectious mononucleosis, Q fever)

Liver disorders (primary biliary cirrhosis)

Systemic disorders (Hodgkin's lymphoma, polymyalgia rheumatica and other connective tissue disorders, sarcoidosis*)

* Most common causes

Prognosis and Treatment

Hepatic granulomas caused by drugs or infection regress completely after treatment. Sarcoid granulomas may disappear spontaneously or persist for years, usually without clinically important liver disease. Progressive fibrosis and portal hypertension rarely develop (sarcoidal cirrhosis). In schistosomiasis, progressive portal scarring is typical (pipestem fibrosis); liver function is usually preserved, but marked splenomegaly and variceal hemorrhage can occur.

Treatment is directed at the underlying cause. When cause is unknown, treatment is usually withheld and follow-up instituted with periodic liver function tests. However, if symptoms of TB (eg, prolonged fever) and deteriorating health occur, empiric antituberculous therapy may be justified. Patients with progressive hepatic sarcoidosis may improve with corticosteroids, although whether these drugs prevent hepatic fibrosis is unclear. Corticosteroids, however, are not indicated for most patients with sarcoidosis and are warranted only if TB and other infections can be excluded confidently.

30 GALLBLADDER AND BILE DUCT DISORDERS

Bile Formation

The liver produces about 500 to 600 mL of bile each day. Bile is isosmotic with plasma and consists primarily of water, electrolytes, bile salts, phospholipids (mostly lecithin), cholesterol, bilirubin, and other endogenously produced or ingested compounds, such as proteins that regulate GI function and drugs or their metabolites. Bilirubin is a degradation product of heme compounds from worn-out RBCs. The formation of bile salts, also called bile acids, induces the secretion of other bile constituents, particularly Na and water. The functions of bile salts include excretion of potentially toxic compounds (eg, bilirubin, drug metabolites); solubilization of intestinal fats and fat-soluble vitamins, facilitating their absorption; and induction of osmotic catharsis.

Bile formation and secretion require active transport as well as processes such as endocytosis and passive diffusion. Bile forms in the canaliculus between adjacent hepatocytes. Bile acid secretion at the canaliculus is the rate-limiting step in bile formation. Secretion and absorption also occur in the bile ducts.

In the liver, bile flows from the intrahepatic collecting system into the proximal, or common, hepatic duct. About 50% of bile secreted in the fasting state passes from the common hepatic duct into the gallbladder via the cystic duct; the rest flows directly into the common bile duct formed by the junction of the common hepatic and cystic ducts. During fasting, little bile flows from the liver. Meanwhile, the gallbladder absorbs up to 90% of bile water, concentrating and storing bile.

Bile empties from the gallbladder into the common bile duct. The common bile duct joins with the pancreatic duct to form the ampulla of Vater, which empties into the duodenum. Before joining the pancreatic duct, the common bile duct tapers to a diameter of ≤ 0.6 cm. The sphincter of Oddi surrounds both pancreatic and common bile ducts; each duct has its own sphincter. Bile does not normally flow retrograde into the pancreatic duct. These sphincters are highly sensitive to cholecystokinin and other gut hormones (eg, gastrin-releasing peptide) and to alterations in cholinergic tone (eg, by anticholinergics).

With the average meal, release of gut hormones and cholinergic stimulation initiate gallbladder contraction and biliary sphincter relaxation, promoting the passage of about 75% of the gallbladder's contents into the duodenum. Conversely, during fasting, an increase in sphincter tone facilitates gallbladder filling. Bile salts are poorly absorbed by passive diffusion in the proximal small intestine; most intestinal bile acids reach the terminal ileum, which actively absorbs 90% into the portal venous circulation. Returned to the liver, bile salts are efficiently extracted, promptly modified (eg, conjugated if they arrive in the "free" form), and secreted back into bile. Bile salts circulate through this pathway—the enterohepatic circulation—10 to 12 times/day.

CHOLELITHIASIS

Cholelithiasis is the presence of one or more calculi (gallstones) in the gallbladder. In the US, 20% of people > 65 yr have gallstones, and most disorders of the extrahepatic biliary tract arise from gallstones. Gallstones may be asymptomatic or cause biliary colic but do not cause dyspepsia. Other common consequences of gallstones include cholecystitis; biliary tract obstruction (usually as a result of bile duct stones), sometimes with infection (cholangitis); and gallstone pancreatitis. Diagnosis is usually based on ultrasound. If cholelithiasis causes symptoms or complications, cholecystectomy becomes necessary.

Risk factors for gallstones include female sex, obesity, increased age, American Indian ethnicity, a Western diet, and a family history.

Pathophysiology

Gallstones and biliary sludge form from different types of material.

Cholesterol stones account for > 85% of gallstones in the Western world. For cholesterol gallstones to form, three events must transpire. (1) Bile must be supersaturated with cholesterol. Normally, water-insoluble cholesterol is made water-soluble by combining with bile salts and lecithin to form mixed micelles. Supersaturation of bile with cholesterol can result from excessive cholesterol secretion (as in diabetes), a decrease in bile salt secretion (eg, in fat malabsorption), or a lecithin deficiency (eg, as occurs in a genetic disorder that causes a form of progressive intrahepatic familial cholestasis). (2) The excess cholesterol must precipitate from solution as solid microcrystals. The precipitation is accelerated by mucin, fibronectin, α_1-globulin, or immunoglobulin. Apolipoprotein A-I and A-II may slow the process. (3) Microcrystals must aggregate. This aggregation is facilitated by mucin, impaired gallbladder contractility (which results from excess cholesterol in bile itself), and slowed intestinal transit that allows the bacterial transformation of cholic acid to deoxycholic acid.

Biliary sludge consists of Ca bilirubinate, cholesterol microcrystals, and mucin. Sludge develops during gallbladder stasis, as occurs during pregnancy or while receiving TPN. Most sludge is asymptomatic and disappears when the primary condition resolves. Alternatively, sludge can produce biliary colic, gallstones, or pancreatitis.

Black pigment stones are small, hard gallstones composed of Ca bilirubinate and inorganic Ca salts (eg, Ca carbonate, Ca phosphate). Factors that accelerate their development include alcoholism, chronic hemolysis, and older age.

Brown pigment stones are soft and greasy, consisting of bilirubinate and fatty acids (Ca palmitate or stearate). They form during infection, parasitic infestation (eg, liver flukes in Asia), and inflammation.

Gallstones grow at about 1 to 2 mm/yr, taking 5 to 20 yr before becoming large enough to cause problems. Most gallstones form within the gallbladder, but brown pigment stones form in the ducts. Gallstones may migrate to the bile duct after cholecystectomy or, particularly in the case of brown pigment stones, develop behind strictures as a result of stasis.

Symptoms and Signs

Eighty percent of gallstones are asymptomatic; in the remainder, symptoms range from biliary colic to cholecystitis to life-threatening cholangitis. Diabetics are predisposed to severe manifestations. Stones may traverse the cystic duct without symptoms. However, transient cystic duct obstruction characteristically causes pain (biliary colic). Pain may occur in the right upper quadrant but is often poorly localized or occurs elsewhere in the abdomen, particularly among diabetics and the elderly. It may radiate into the back or down the arm. It begins suddenly, becomes intense within 15 min to 1 h, remains steady for 1 to 6 h, then gradually disappears over 30 to 90 min, leaving a dull ache. The pain is usually severe. Nausea and some vomiting often occur, but fever and chills do not. Mild right upper quadrant or epigastric tenderness may be present, but peritoneal findings are absent, and laboratory tests are normal. Between episodes, the patient feels well.

Although biliary-type pain can follow a heavy meal, fatty food is not a specific precipitating factor. Symptoms of dyspepsia, such as belching, bloating, fullness, and nausea, have been inaccurately ascribed to gallbladder disease. These symptoms are common, having about equal prevalence in cholelithiasis, peptic ulcer disease, and functional GI diseases.

Little correlation exists between the severity and frequency of biliary colic and the pathologic changes in the gallbladder. Biliary colic can occur in the absence of cholecystitis. However, if colic lasts > 6 h with vomiting or fever, acute cholecystitis or pancreatitis is likely.

Diagnosis

Gallstones are suspected in patients with biliary colic. Laboratory tests usually are not helpful. Abdominal ultrasonography is the method of choice for detecting gallbladder stones, with 95% sensitivity and specificity. Sludge may also be detectable. CT and MRI scans and oral cholecystography (rarely available now, though quite accurate) are alternatives (see p. 205). Endoscopic ultrasound is particularly accurate for detecting gallstones < 3 mm and may be needed if other studies are equivocal. Asymptomatic gallstones often are detected incidentally during imaging studies performed for other reasons (eg, 10 to 15% are noncholesterol calcified stones visible on plain x-rays).

Prognosis and Treatment

Asymptomatic gallstones: Asymptomatic gallstones become symptomatic at a rate of about 2%/yr. Most patients with asymptomatic stones decide that the discomfort, expense, and risk of elective surgery are not worth removing an organ that may never cause clinical illness, despite the potential complications of untreated gallstones. However, in diabetics, asymptomatic gallstones must be removed.

Symptomatic gallstones: Although most biliary colic resolves spontaneously, symptoms recur in 20 to 40% of patients/yr, and complications such as cholecystitis, choledocholithiasis, cholangitis, and gallstone pancreatitis occur in 1 to 2% of patients/yr. Thus, gallbladder removal (cholecystectomy) is indicated.

Open cholecystectomy, which involves laparotomy, is safe and effective. When this procedure is performed electively during a period free of complications, the overall mortality rate is 0.1 to 0.5%. However, laparoscopic cholecystectomy has become the treatment of choice. It offers a far shorter convalescence, decreased postoperative discomfort, improved cosmetic results, and no increase in morbidity or mortality. Laparoscopic cholecystectomy is converted to an open procedure in about 5% of cases, usually because of an inability to identify the anatomy of the gallbladder or to manage a complication. Older age generally increases the risks of any type of surgery.

In patients who have had biliary colic, the episodes of biliary pain typically disappear after cholecystectomy. For reasons that are unclear, some patients who also have dyspepsia and fatty food intolerance find that these symptoms also resolve. Cholecystectomy does not result in nutritional problems, and no dietary limitations are required after surgery. Some patients develop diarrhea, often an unmasking of bile salt malabsorption.

For patients who decline surgical treatment or for whom surgical risks are high (eg, because of concomitant medical disorders or advanced age), gallbladder stones can sometimes be dissolved by giving bile acids orally for many months. Stones must be made of cholesterol (best determined by their radiolucency on plain abdominal films), and the gallbladder should be free of obstruction as determined by filling on cholescintigraphy or, if available, oral cholecystography. However, some clinicians assume that stones in the neck of the cystic duct are nonobstructing; thus they do not perform cholescintigraphy or oral cholecystography. Ursodiol (ursodeoxycholic acid) 8 to 10 mg/kg/day po in 2 to 3 divided doses, with the major portion (eg, ⅔ to ¾) of the dose given in the evening, reduces biliary secretion of cholesterol and decreases the cholesterol saturation of bile. Because of their higher surface area:volume ratio, small gallstones dissolve more quickly (eg, 80% of stones < 0.5 cm dissolve within 6 mo). Large stones have a much poorer success rate even when higher doses of ursodeoxycholic acid are given (10 to 12 mg/kg/day). About 15 to 20% of patients are candidates for dissolution, having stones < 1 cm, with success rates of up to 40% after 2 yr of treatment. However, even after successful dissolution, stones recur in 50% by 5 yr. Ursodeoxycholic acid can prevent stone formation in morbidly obese patients undergoing rapid weight reduction either after gastric bypass surgery or while on a very low calorie diet. Alternative methods of stone dissolution (insertion of methyl-*tert*-butyl ether directly into the gallbladder) or stone fragmentation (extracorporeal shock wave lithotripsy) are now largely unavailable because of overwhelming patient acceptance of laparoscopic cholecystectomy.

CHOLECYSTITIS

Cholecystitis, which is inflammation of the gallbladder, can be acute or chronic.

Acute Cholecystitis

Acute cholecystitis is inflammation of the gallbladder that develops over hours, usually as a result of cystic duct obstruction by a gallstone. Symptoms include right upper quadrant pain and tenderness, sometimes accompanied by fever, chills, nausea, and vomiting. Abdominal ultrasound detects the gallstone and sometimes the associated inflammation. Treatment usually involves antibiotics and cholecystectomy.

Acute cholecystitis is the most common complication of cholelithiasis. Conversely, ≥ 95% of patients with acute cholecystitis have cholelithiasis. When a stone becomes impacted in the cystic duct and causes persistent obstruction, acute inflammation results. Bile stasis releases inflammatory enzymes (eg, phospholipase A, converting lecithin to lysolecithin, which may mediate inflammation). The damaged mucosa secretes more fluid into the gallbladder. The resulting distention releases more inflammatory mediators (eg, prostaglandins), worsening mucosal damage and causing ischemia, which perpetuates inflammation. Bacterial infection can develop, and necrosis and perforation can occur. If resolution occurs, the gallbladder becomes fibrotic and contracted and fails to concentrate bile or to empty properly.

Acute acalculous cholecystitis (ie, cholecystitis without stones) accounts for 5 to 10% of cholecystectomies performed for acute cholecystitis. Risk factors include critical illness (often surgery, burns, sepsis, or major trauma), prolonged fasting or TPN (which predispose to bile stasis), shock, and vasculitis (eg, SLE, polyarteritis nodosa). The mechanism probably involves inflammatory mediators released because of ischemia, infection, or bile stasis. Sometimes an infecting organism can be identified (eg, *Salmonella* or cytomegalovirus in immunodeficient patients). In young children, acute acalculous cholecystitis tends to follow a febrile illness without an identifiable infecting organism.

Symptoms and Signs

Most patients have had prior attacks of biliary colic or acute cholecystitis. The pain of cholecystitis has a quality and location similar to that of biliary colic but with longer duration (ie, > 6 h) and greater severity. Vomiting is common, as is right subcostal tenderness. Within a few hours, Murphy's sign (deep inspiration exacerbates the pain during palpation of the right upper quadrant and halts inspiration) develops with involuntary guarding of right-sided abdominal muscles. Fever, usually low grade, is common. In the elderly, fever may not develop, and the first or only symptoms may be systemic and nonspecific (eg, anorexia, vomiting, malaise, weakness, fever).

If the disease is untreated, 10% of patients develop localized perforation, and 1% develop free perforation and peritonitis. Increasing abdominal pain, high fever, and rigors with rebound tenderness or ileus suggest empyema (pus in the gallbladder), gangrene, or perforation. If acute cholecystitis is accompanied by jaundice or cholestasis, partial common duct obstruction is possible, usually due to stones or inflammation. Common duct stones passed from the gallbladder may block, narrow, or inflame the pancreatic duct, producing pancreatitis (gallstone pancreatitis). Mirizzi's syndrome is a rare complication in which a gallstone impacted in the cystic duct or Hartman's pouch compresses and obstructs the common duct. Rarely, a large stone erodes the gallbladder wall, creating a cholecystoenteric fistula; the stone may pass freely or obstruct the small intestine (gallstone ileus). Acute cholecystitis usually begins to subside in 2 to 3 days and resolves within 1 wk.

Acute acalculous cholecystitis tends to cause the same symptoms as calculous cholecystitis, but the symptoms may be masked in severely ill patients who cannot communicate clearly. The only clue may be abdominal distention or unexplained fever. Untreated, the disease can rapidly progress to gallbladder gangrene and perforation, leading to sepsis, shock, and peritonitis, with a mortality of 65%. Choledocholithiasis and cholangitis can also develop (see p. 245).

Diagnosis

Acute cholecystitis is suspected in patients with suggestive symptoms and signs. Diagnosis is usually based on ultrasound, which can detect gallstones as well as focal tenderness over the gallbladder (ultrasonographic Murphy's sign). Pericholecystic fluid or thickening of the gallbladder wall indicates acute inflammation. If results are equivocal, cholescintigraphy is used; failure of radioactivity to fill the gallbladder suggests an obstructed cystic duct. False positives can occur in critically ill or fasting patients receiving TPN, patients with severe liver disease, or those with a previous sphincterotomy. Abdominal CT may reveal cholecystitis as well as gallbladder perforation or pancreatitis. Magnetic resonance cholangiography is accurate but is more costly than ultrasound. CBC, liver function tests, amylase, and lipase are usually obtained but are rarely diagnostic. Leukocytosis with a left shift is common. In uncomplicated acute cholecystitis, there should be no marked biochemical liver function abnormalities or lipase elevations.

In acute acalculous cholecystitis, laboratory tests are not specific. Leukocytosis and abnormal liver biochemistries are common. A cholestatic pattern may result from sepsis itself, choledocholithiasis, or cholangitis. Ultrasonography can be performed at the bedside. Gallstones are absent. A sonographic Murphy's sign and pericholecystic fluid accumulation suggest gallbladder disease, whereas a distended gallbladder, biliary sludge, and a thickened gallbladder wall (from low albumin or ascites) may result simply from being critically ill. CT is also accurate and may identify extrabiliary abnormalities. Cholescintigraphy is more helpful; absence of filling may indicate edematous cystic duct obstruction. However, gallbladder stasis may itself prevent filling. Giving morphine, which increases tone in the sphincter of Oddi and enhances filling, can eliminate such a false-positive result.

Treatment

Management includes hospital admission, IV fluids, and opioids. No oral feedings are given, and nasogastric suction is instituted if vomiting is a problem. Parenteral antibiotics are usually initiated to treat possible infection, but evidence of benefit is lacking. Empiric coverage is directed at gram-negative enteric organisms such as *Escherichia coli, Enterococcus, Klebsiella*, and *Enterobacter* and can be accomplished with regimens such as piperacillin/tazobactam 4 g IV q 6 h, ampicillin/sulbactam 3 g IV q 6 h, or ticarcillin/clavulanate 4 g IV q 6 h.

Cholecystectomy cures acute cholecystitis and relieves biliary pain. When the diagnosis is clear and the patient is at low surgical risk, cholecystectomy is best performed during the initial 24 to 48 h. For high-risk patients with severe chronic disease (eg, cardiopulmonary), cholecystectomy should be deferred until such conditions improve with medical therapy or until cholecystitis subsides. If cholecystitis subsides, cholecystectomy may be performed ≥ 6 wk later. Empyema, gangrene, perforation, and acalculous cholecystitis require urgent surgical management. In patients at very high surgical risk, percutaneous cholecystostomy may be an alternative to cholecystectomy.

Chronic Cholecystitis

Chronic cholecystitis is long-standing gallbladder inflammation almost always due to gallstones.

Damage in chronic cholecystitis ranges from mild infiltration to thick-walled, fibrotic gallbladder contraction. Gallstones are almost always the cause. Acute cholecystitis is another contributory factor.

Symptoms and Signs

Inflammation in chronic cholecystitis, sometimes with extensive damage, can occur without producing biliary colic. Thus, the absence of biliary colic does not exclude chronic cholecystitis. However, most patients have recurrent biliary colic. There may be upper abdominal tenderness but usually not fever. Once symptoms begin, they are likely to recur.

Diagnosis and Treatment

Chronic cholecystitis is suspected in patients who have recurrent biliary colic or gallstones noted incidentally on plain abdominal x-rays. Ultrasound or another imaging test usually reveals gallstones. Ultrasound may not reveal gallbladder fibrosis. Cholescintigraphy may demonstrate nonvisualization.

Laparoscopic cholecystectomy is indicated to prevent both symptom recurrence and further tissue damage.

ACALCULOUS BILIARY PAIN

Acalculous biliary pain is biliary colic occurring without gallstones resulting from structural or functional disorders, sometimes treated with laparoscopic cholecystectomy.

Biliary colic can occur in the absence of gallstones, particularly in young women. It accounts for up to 15% of laparoscopic cholecystectomies performed. Common causes include microscopic stones, abnormal gallbladder motility, an overly sensitive biliary tract, sphincter of Oddi dysfunction, hypersensitivity of the adjacent duodenum, and, possibly, gallstones that have spontaneously passed. Some patients eventually develop other functional GI disorders.

Acalculous biliary pain is suspected in patients with biliary colic whose test results reveal no gallstones. Testing includes ultrasound and endoscopic ultrasound. To measure gallbladder emptying (ejection fraction), cholescintigraphy is performed after cholecystokinin infusion (while avoiding use of potentially interfering drugs such as Ca channel blockers and anticholinergics). To detect sphincter of Oddi dysfunction, ERCP with biliary manometry is performed. To detect duodenal hypersensitivity, endoscopic barostat testing is performed but may be available only at research centers. Laparoscopic cholecystectomy improves outcomes for microscopic stones and possibly abnormal gallbladder motility. Whether abnormalities on other tests warrant laparoscopic cholecystectomy is under investigation.

POSTCHOLECYSTECTOMY SYNDROME

Postcholecystectomy syndrome is the occurrence of abdominal symptoms after cholecystectomy.

Postcholecystectomy syndrome occurs in 5 to 40% of patients; however, most symptoms are dyspepsia or otherwise nonspecific rather than true biliary colic. Some cases have another cause (eg, retained bile duct stone, pancreatitis, gastroesophageal reflux). In about 10%, biliary colic appears to result from functional or structural abnormalities of the sphincter of Oddi. Papillary stenosis, which is rare, is a fibrotic narrowing around the sphincter, perhaps caused by trauma and inflammation from pancreatitis, instrumentation (eg, ERCP), or prior passage of a stone.

Patients with postcholecystectomy pain should be evaluated as indicated for extrabiliary as well as biliary causes. If the pain suggests biliary colic, alkaline phosphatase, bilirubin, ALT, amylase, and lipase should be measured and ERCP with biliary manometry or biliary nuclear medicine scan obtained. Elevated liver biochemistries suggest sphincter of Oddi dysfunction, whereas elevated amylase and lipase suggest dysfunction of the sphincter's pancreatic portion. Dysfunction is best detected by biliary manometry, which shows increased pressure in the biliary tract with reproduction of the pain, although ERCP has a risk of inducing pancreatitis. A slowed hepatic hilum-duodenal transit time on scan also suggests sphincter of Oddi dysfunction. Diagnosis of papillary stenosis is based on ERCP. Endoscopic sphincterotomy can relieve recurrent pain due to sphincter of Oddi dysfunction and especially due to papillary stenosis but is controversial for patients who have postcholecystectomy pain and no objective abnormalities.

CHOLEDOCHOLITHIASIS AND CHOLANGITIS

Choledocholithiasis is the formation or presence of stones in the bile ducts. It can cause biliary colic, biliary obstruction, gallstone pancreatitis, or bile duct infection (cholangitis). Diagnosis usually requires visualization by magnetic resonance cholangiopancreatography or ERCP. Early endoscopic or surgical decompression is indicated.

Primary stones (usually pigment stones) form in the bile ducts. Secondary stones (usually cholesterol) form in the gallbladder but migrate to the bile ducts. Residual stones are those missed at the time of cholecystectomy. Recurrent stones develop in the ducts > 3 yr after surgery. In developed countries, over 85% of common duct stones are secondary; affected patients also have stones still located in the gallbladder. Conversely, up to 10% of patients with symptomatic gallstones have associated common duct stones. After cholecystectomy, brown pigment stones may occur from stasis (eg, a postoperative stricture) and infection. The proportion of ductal stones that are pigmented increases with time after cholecystectomy.

Bile duct stones may pass into the duodenum asymptomatically. Biliary colic occurs if they become partially obstructed. More complete obstruction causes duct dilatation, jaundice, and, eventually, bacterial infection (cholangitis). Stones that obstruct the ampulla of Vater can induce gallstone pancreatitis. Some patients (usually the elderly) present with biliary obstruction due to stones that have caused no symptoms previously.

In **acute cholangitis,** bile duct obstruction permits bacteria to ascend from the duodenum. Although most (85%) cases result from common bile duct stones, bile duct obstruction can result from tumor or other conditions (see TABLE 30–1). Common infecting organisms include gram negatives (eg, *Escherichia coli, Klebsiella, Enterobacter*); less common are gram positives (eg, *Enterococcus* sp) and mixed anaerobes (eg, *Bacteroides, Clostridia*). Symptoms include abdominal pain, jaundice, and fever or chills (Charcot's triad). The abdomen is tender, and often the liver is tender and enlarged (often containing abscesses). Confusion and hypotension predict about a 50% mortality rate and high morbidity.

Diagnosis

Common duct stones should be suspected in patients with jaundice and biliary colic. Liver function tests and an imaging study should be obtained. Elevated levels of bilirubin, alkaline phosphatase, ALT, and γ-glutaryl-transferase, consistent with extrahepatic obstruction, are suggestive, particu-

TABLE 30–1. CAUSES OF BILE DUCT OBSTRUCTION OTHER THAN STONES OR TUMORS

- Duct trauma as a result of surgery (common)
- Scarring as a result of chronic pancreatitis
- Ductal obstruction from external compression by a cyst or hernia of the common bile duct (choledochocele) or by a pancreatic pseudocyst (rare)
- Extrahepatic or intrahepatic strictures as a result of primary sclerosing cholangitis
- AIDS-related cholangiopathy or cholangitis; direct cholangiography may show results similar to primary sclerosing cholangitis or papillary stenosis; etiology is probably infection, most likely with cytomegalovirus, *Cryptosporidium*, or *Microsporidia*
- *Clonorchis sinensis* can cause obstructive jaundice with intrahepatic ductal inflammation, proximal stasis, stone formation, and cholangitis (in Southeast Asia)
- Migration of *Ascaris lumbricoides* into the common bile duct (rare)

larly in patients with symptoms of acute cholecystitis.

Ultrasound may reveal stones in the gallbladder and occasionally in the common duct. The common duct is dilated (> 6 mm in diameter if the gallbladder is intact; > 10 mm after a cholecystectomy). If the ducts are not dilated early in the presentation (eg, first day), then stones have probably passed. If doubt exists, magnetic resonance cholangiopancreatography (MRCP) is highly accurate for retained stones. ERCP is performed if MRCP is equivocal; it can be therapeutic as well as diagnostic. CT scan is less accurate than ultrasound.

For suspected acute cholangitis, CBC and blood cultures should also be obtained. Leukocytosis is common, and aminotransferases may reach 1000 IU/L, suggesting acute hepatic necrosis, often due to microabscesses. Blood cultures guide antibacterial therapy.

Treatment

For suspected biliary obstruction, ERCP and sphincterotomy are necessary to remove the stone. Laparoscopic cholecystectomy, which is not as well suited for operative cholangiography or common duct exploration, can be undertaken electively after the ERCP and sphincterotomy. Open cholecystectomy with common duct exploration has a higher mortality and morbidity. In patients at high risk for cholecystectomy, such as the elderly, sphincterotomy alone is an alternative.

Acute cholangitis is an emergency requiring aggressive supportive care and urgent removal of the stones endoscopically or surgically. Antibiotics are given, similar to those used for acute cholecystitis (see p. 244). Alternatives, in order of preference, are imipenem and ciprofloxacin; metronidazole is given to very ill patients to cover anaerobes.

PRIMARY SCLEROSING CHOLANGITIS

Primary sclerosing cholangitis is a chronic cholestatic syndrome characterized by patchy inflammation, fibrosis, and strictures of the intrahepatic and extrahepatic bile ducts. Eighty percent of patients have inflammatory bowel disease, often ulcerative colitis. Symptoms of fatigue and pruritus develop late. Diagnosis is based on contrast cholangiography (with ERCP) or magnetic resonance cholangiopancreatography. Disease leads to eventual obliteration of the bile ducts with cirrhosis, hepatic failure, and sometimes cholangiocarcinoma. Liver transplantation is indicated for advanced disease.

Etiology

The cause of is unknown. However, primary sclerosing cholangitis (PSC) is strongly associated with inflammatory bowel disease, occurring in about 5% of patients with ulcerative colitis and in about 1% with Crohn's disease. This association and the presence of several autoantibodies (eg, anti-smooth muscle and perinuclear antineutrophilic antibodies [p-ANCA]) suggest immune-mediated mechanisms. T lymphocytes appear to be involved with the destruction of the bile ducts, suggesting disordered cellular immunity. A genetic predisposition is suggested by a tendency for the disease to develop in multiple family members and higher incidence in those with HLA-B8 and HLA-DR3, which are often correlated with autoimmune diseases. An unknown trigger (eg, bacterial infection or ischemic duct injury) probably causes PSC to develop in genetically predisposed patients. Sclerosing cholangitis in HIV-infected patients may be due to cryptosporidiosis or cytomegalovirus.

Symptoms and Signs

Mean age at diagnosis is 40 yr; 70% of patients are men. The onset is usually insidious, with progressive fatigue and pruritus. Jaundice tends to develop later. Repeated episodes of right upper quadrant pain and fever, possibly due to ascending bacterial cholangitis, occur in 10 to 15% of patients at presentation. Steatorrhea and deficiencies of fat-soluble vitamins can develop. Persistent jaundice harbingers advanced disease. Symptomatic gallstones and choledocholithiasis tend to develop in about ⅓ of patients. Some patients are asymptomatic until late in the course of the disease, first presenting with hepatosplenomegaly or cirrhosis. The terminal phase involves decompensated cirrhosis, portal hypertension, ascites, and liver failure.

Despite the association between PSC and inflammatory bowel disease, the two diseases tend to run separate courses. Ulcerative colitis may appear years before PSC, yet tends to have a milder course when associated with PSC. The presence of both diseases increases the risk of colorectal carcinoma, regardless of whether a liver transplantation has been performed for PSC. Similarly, total colectomy does not change the course of PSC. Cholangiocarcinoma develops in 10 to 15% of patients with PSC.

Diagnosis

PSC is suspected in patients with unexplained abnormal liver biochemistry tests; if the patient has inflammatory bowel disease, suspicion is even higher. A cholestatic pattern in liver biochemistries is typical, with alkaline phosphatase and γ-glutaryl-transferase usually elevated more than aminotransferases. Gamma globulin and IgM levels tend to be elevated, and antismooth muscle and p-ANCA are usually positive. Antimitochondrial antibody, positive in primary biliary cirrhosis, is characteristically negative.

Imaging of the hepatobiliary system usually begins with ultrasound to exclude extrahepatic biliary obstruction. The diagnosis of PSC necessitates demonstration of multiple strictures and dilations involving the intrahepatic and extrahepatic bile ducts, which requires cholangiography (ultrasound can only suggest such damage). Direct cholangiography (eg, by ERCP) has been the gold standard; however, magnetic resonance cholangiopancreatography (MRCP) provides excellent images and is becoming a first-choice noninvasive alternative. Liver biopsy is generally not required for diagnosis. When performed for another reason, it reveals bile duct proliferation, periductal fibrosis, inflammation, and loss of bile ducts. As the disease progresses, fibrosis extends from the portal regions and eventually leads to biliary cirrhosis.

Surveillance using ERCP with brush cytology may help predict development of cholangiocarcinoma.

Prognosis and Treatment

Some patients may be asymptomatic for many years, but the disorder tends to progress. The time from diagnosis to hepatic failure is about 12 yr.

Asymptomatic patients generally require only monitoring (eg, physical examination and liver function tests twice/yr). Ursodeoxycholic acid may reduce itching and improve biochemical markers. Chronic cholestasis (see p. 193) and cirrhosis may require treatment. Recurrent bacterial cholangitis is treated with antibiotics and ERCP as needed.

If one dominant stricture exists (in about 20%), endoscopic dilation is necessary to relieve symptoms and exclude tumor development by brushings. Any underlying infection (eg, cryptosporidiosis, cytomegalovirus) is treated.

Liver transplantation is the only treatment that improves life expectancy in idiopathic PSC; it may be curative. Recurrent bacterial cholangitis or complications of end-stage liver disease, such as intractable ascites, portal-systemic encephalopathy, or bleeding esophageal varices, are reasonable indications for liver transplantation.

TUMORS OF THE GALLBLADDER AND BILE DUCTS

Gallbladder and bile duct tumors are a frequent cause of extrahepatic biliary obstruction. Symptoms may be absent but often are constitutional or reflect biliary obstruction. Diagnosis is based on ultrasound, CT, or cholangiography. Prognosis is usually poor. Mechanical bile drainage can often relieve pruritus, recurrent sepsis, and pain due to biliary obstruction.

Cholangiocarcinomas and other bile duct tumors, which are rare, are usually malignant. Cholangiocarcinomas occur predominantly in the extrahepatic bile ducts: 60 to 80% in the perihilar region (Klatskin tumors) and 10 to 30% in the distal ducts. Risk factors include older age, primary sclerosing cholangitis, infestation with liver flukes, and a choledochal cyst.

Gallbladder carcinoma has an incidence of 2.5/100,000 and is most common in South America and Asia. The median survival is 3 mo.

Gallbladder polyps are asymptomatic mucosal projections of cholesterol ester and lipid < 10 mm in diameter that develop in the lumen of the gallbladder. They result from cholesterolosis and are found in about 5% of people undergoing ultrasound. True adenomas are rare and benign.

Symptoms and Signs

Patients with cholangiocarcinomas most commonly present with pruritus and painless obstructive jaundice (typical age, 50 to 70 yr). Early perihilar tumors may produce only vague abdominal pain, anorexia, and weight loss. Other features may include acholic stool, palpable mass, hepatomegaly, or distended gallbladder (Courvoisier's sign, with distal cholangiocarcinoma). Pain may resemble that of biliary colic (reflecting biliary obstruction) or may be constant and progressive. Sepsis is unusual but may be induced by ERCP.

Patients with gallbladder carcinoma present with symptoms ranging from an incidental finding at cholecystectomy done for biliary pain and cholelithiasis (70 to 90% have stones) to advanced disease with constant pain, weight loss, and an abdominal mass.

Diagnosis

Cholangiocarcinomas are suspected when extrahepatic biliary obstruction is unexplained. Laboratory tests reflect the degree of cholestasis. Diagnosis is based on ultrasound or CT. If these methods are inconclusive, magnetic resonance cholangiopancreatography (MRCP) or ERCP with percutaneous transhepatic cholangiography may be necessary. In some cases, ERCP not only detects the tumor, but also, with brushings, provides a tissue diagnosis, making ultrasound- or CT-guided needle biopsy unnecessary. Contrast-enhanced CT assists in staging.

Gallbladder carcinomas are better defined by CT than by ultrasound. Open laparotomy is necessary to determine disease extent, which guides therapy.

Treatment

Stenting or surgically bypassing the obstruction relieves pruritus, jaundice, and perhaps fatigue.

Hilar cholangiocarcinomas with CT evidence of spread are stented percutaneously or via ERCP. Distal duct cholangiocarcinomas are stented endoscopically. If cholangiocarcinoma appears localized, surgical exploration determines resectability by hilar resection or pancreaticoduodenectomy. Adjuvant chemotherapy and radiation therapy are showing promising results for cholangiocarcinomas.

Many gallbladder carcinomas are treated symptomatically.

SECTION 4

MUSCULOSKELETAL AND CONNECTIVE TISSUE DISORDERS

31 APPROACH TO THE PATIENT WITH JOINT DISEASE

Some musculoskeletal disorders affect primarily the joints, causing arthritis. Others affect primarily the bones (eg, fractures, Paget's disease, tumors), muscles or other extra-articular soft tissues (eg, polymyalgia rheumatica, fibromyalgia), or periarticular soft tissues (eg, bursitis, tendinitis, sprain). Arthritis has myriad possible causes, including infection, autoimmune disease, crystal-induced inflammation, other kinds of inflammation, and noninflammatory tissue degeneration; systemic diseases may be involved. Arthritis may affect single or multiple joints, in either a symmetric or asymmetric manner.

History

The physician should ask about systemic and extra-articular symptoms as well as joint symptoms. Many symptoms, including fever, chills, malaise, weight loss, Raynaud's phenomenon, mucocutaneous symptoms (eg, rash, eye irritation or pain, photosensitivity), and GI or cardiopulmonary symptoms, can be associated with joint disorders.

Pain is the most common symptom of many joint disorders. The history should address the location, severity, character, and factors that aggravate or relieve pain. The clinician must determine whether pain is worse upon first moving a joint or after prolonged use and whether it is present upon wakening or develops during the day. Usually, pain originating from superficial structures is better localized than pain originating from deeper structures. Pain originating in small distal joints tends to be better localized than pain originating in large proximal joints.

Joint pain can be referred from extra-articular structures or from other joints. Arthritis often produces "aching" pain, whereas neuropathies often produce "burning" pain.

"Stiffness" may mean weakness, fatigue, or fixed limitation of motion to patients. The clinician must separate an inability to move a joint from reluctance to move a joint because of pain. Stiffness of importance to rheumatic disease is difficulty in motion that develops when attempting to move a joint after a period of rest. The duration of stiffness after beginning joint motion reflects its severity. Stiffness is more severe in inflammatory joint disorders. Morning stiffness can be an important early symptom of RA.

Fatigue is a desire to rest that reflects exhaustion. It differs from weakness, inability to move, and reluctance to move due to pain with movement.

Instability, or buckling of a joint, may suggest weakness of the ligaments or other structures that stabilize the joint, which are assessed by stress testing. Buckling occurs most often in the knee and most often results from an internal joint derangement.

Physical Examination

Each involved joint is inspected and palpated, and the range of motion is estimated. With polyarticular disease, certain nonarticular signs (eg, fever, wasting, rash) may reflect systemic disorders.

The rest position of joints is noted, along with any erythema, swelling, deformity, and skin abrasions or punctures. Involved joints are compared with their uninvolved opposites or with those of the examiner.

Joints are gently palpated, noting the presence and location of warmth and tenderness. Determining whether tenderness is present along the joint line or over tendon insertions or bursae is particularly important. Soft masses, bulges, or tissues that fill normal concavities or spaces (representing joint effusion or synovial proliferation) are noted. Palpation of swollen joints can sometimes differentiate among joint effusion, synovial thickening, and capsular or bony enlargement. Small joints (eg, the acromioclavicular, tibiofibular, radioulnar) can be the source of pain that was initially believed to arise from a nearby major joint. Bony enlargement (often due to osteophytes) is noted.

Active range of motion (the maximum range through which the patient can move the joint) is recorded first; limitation may reflect weakness, pain, or stiffness as well as mechanical abnormalities. Then passive range of motion (the maximum range through which the examiner can move the joint) is assessed; passive limitation generally reflects mechanical abnormalities (eg, scarring, swelling, deformities) rather than weakness or pain.

Crepitus, a palpable or audible grinding produced by motion, is noted. It may be caused by roughened articular cartilage or from tendons; crepitus-producing motions should be determined and may suggest which structures are involved.

There are specific features that should be sought at various joints.

Elbow: Synovial swelling and thickening caused by joint disease occur in the lateral aspect between the radial head and olecranon, producing a bulge. Full 180° extension of the joint should be attempted. Although full extension is possible with nonarthritic or extra-articular lesions, its loss is an early change in arthritis. The area around the joint is examined for swellings. Rheumatoid nodules are firm, occurring especially along the extensor surface of the forearm. Tophi are sometimes visible under the skin as cream-colored aggregates and indicate gout. Swelling of the olecranon bursa occurs over the tip of the olecranon, is cystic, and does not limit joint motion; infection, trauma, gout, and RA are possible causes. Epitrochlear nodes occur above the medial epicondyle; they can result from inflammation in the hand but can also suggest sarcoidosis or lymphoma.

Shoulder: Because pain can be referred between areas around the shoulder, shoulder palpation should include the glenohumeral, acromioclavicular, and sternoclavicular joints, the coracoid process, clavicle, acromion process, subacromial bursa, biceps tendon, and greater and lesser tuberosities of the humerus, as well as the neck. Glenohumeral joint effusions may produce a bulge between the coracoid process and the humeral head. Possible causes include RA, osteoarthritis, septic arthritis, Milwaukee shoulder (see p. 304), and other arthropathies.

Limited motion, weakness, pain, and other disturbed mobility from rotator cuff impairment can be quickly screened by having the patient attempt to abduct and raise both arms above the head and then to slowly lower them. Muscle atrophy and neurologic changes should be sought.

Knee: At the knee, gross deformities such as swelling (eg, joint effusion, popliteal cysts), quadriceps muscle atrophy, and joint instability may be obvious when the patient stands and walks. With the patient supine, the examiner should palpate the knee, identifying the patella, femoral condyles, tibial tuberosity, tibial plateau, fibular head, medial and lateral joint lines, popliteal fossa, and quadriceps and patellar tendons. The medial and lateral joint lines correspond to locations of the medial and lateral menisci and can be located by palpation while slowly flexing and extending the knee. Tender extra-articular bursae such as the anserine bursa below the medial joint line should be differentiated from true intra-articular disturbances.

Detection of small knee effusions is often difficult and is best accomplished using the "bulge sign." The knee is fully extended and the leg slightly externally rotated while the patient is supine with muscles relaxed. The medial aspect of the knee is stroked to express any fluid away from this area. Placement of one hand on the suprapatellar pouch and gentle stroking or pressing on the lateral aspect of the knee can create a fluid wave or bulge, visible medially when an effusion is present. Larger effusions can be identified visually or by balloting the patella. Joint effusion can result from many joint diseases, including RA, osteoarthritis, gout, and trauma.

Full 180° extension of the knee is attempted to detect flexion contractures. The patella is tested for free, painless motion.

Hip: Examination begins with gait evaluation. A limp is common in patients with significant hip arthritis. It may be caused by pain, leg shortening, flexion contracture, or muscle weakness. Loss of internal rotation (often the earliest change in hip osteoarthritis or any hip synovitis), flexion, extension, or abduction can usually be demonstrated. Placement of one hand on the patient's iliac crest detects pelvic movement that might be mistaken for hip movement. Flexion contracture can be identified by attempting leg extension with the opposite hip maximally flexed to stabilize the pelvis. Tenderness over the femoral greater trochanter indicates bursitis (which is extra-articular) rather than an intra-articular disorder. Pain with passive range of motion (assessed by internal and external rotation with the patient supine and the hip and knee flexed to 90°) suggests intra-articular origin.

Other: Hand examination is discussed further on p. 329 and under polyarticular pain on p. 259. Foot and ankle examination is discussed throughout Ch. 43 on p. 337. Examination of the neck and back is discussed on p. 323.

Testing

Laboratory testing and imaging studies often provide less information than the history and physical examination. While some testing may be warranted in some patients, extensive testing is often not.

Blood tests: Some tests, although not specific, can be helpful in supporting the possibility of certain systemic rheumatic diseases. These include antinuclear antibodies (ANA) and complement in SLE, rheumatoid factor and anti-citrullinated peptide (CCP) in RA, and antineutrophil cytoplasmic antibodies (ANCA) in the vasculitides. Tests such as WBC count, ESR, and C-reactive protein may help determine the likelihood that arthritis is inflammatory due to infectious or other systemic diseases, but these tests are not highly specific or sensitive. For example, an elevated ESR or C-reactive protein level suggests inflammation or may be due to aging or a large number of nonarticular inflammatory conditions. Also, elevation may not occur in all inflammatory disorders.

Imaging studies: Imaging studies are often unnecessary. Plain x-rays in particular reveal mainly bony abnormalities, and most joint disorders do not affect bone primarily. However, imaging may help in the initial evaluation of relatively localized, unexplained persistent or severe joint and particularly spine abnormalities; they may reveal primary or metastatic tumors, osteomyelitis, bone infarctions, periarticular calcifications (as in calcific tendinitis), or other changes in deep structures that may escape physical examination. If chronic RA, gout, or osteoarthritis is suspected, erosions, cysts, and joint space narrowing with osteophytes may be visible. In pseudogout, Ca pyrophosphate deposition may be visible in intra-articular cartilage.

For musculoskeletal imaging, plain x-rays may be obtained first, but these are often less accurate than CT or MRI. MRI is the most accurate study for fractures not visible on plain x-rays, particularly in the hip and pelvis, and for soft tissues and internal derangements of the knee. CT is useful if MRI is contraindicated or unavailable. Ultrasound, arthrography, and bone scanning may help in certain conditions, as can biopsy of bone, synovium, or other tissues.

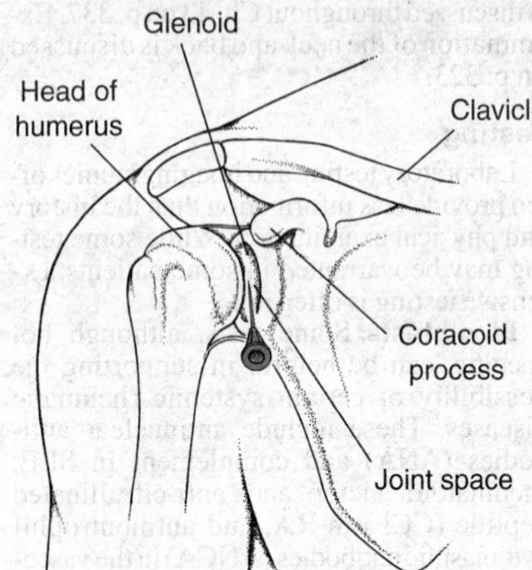

Fig. 31–1. Arthrocentesis of the shoulder. The glenohumeral joint is punctured while the patient sits with the arm at the side and hand on the lap. The needle is inserted anteriorly, slightly inferior and lateral to the coracoid process, aiming posteriorly toward the glenoid fossa. A posterior approach is also possible.

Arthrocentesis: Arthrocentesis is the process of puncturing the joint with a needle. If there is an effusion and arthrocentesis is performed correctly, fluid can generally be withdrawn. Examination of synovial fluid is the most accurate way to determine the cause of joint effusions and is indicated in all patients with severe or unexplained monarticular joint effusions and in patients with unexplained polyarticular effusions.

Arthrocentesis is performed using strictly sterile technique. Infection or other rash over the site used to enter the joint is a contraindication. Preparations for collecting samples should be made before performing the procedure. Local anesthesia, with lidocaine or difluoroethane spray, is often used. To avoid nerves, arteries, and veins, which are usually on the joint's flexor surface, many joints are punctured on the extensor surface. A 20-gauge needle can be used for most joints, removing as much fluid as possible. Specific anatomic landmarks are used (see FIGS. 31–1 to 31–3).

Metacarpophalangeal joints, metatarsophalangeal joints, and interphalangeal joints of the hands and feet are punctured similarly to each other, using a 20- or 22-gauge needle. The needle is inserted dorsally, to either side of the extensor tendon.

Synovial fluid examination: At the bedside, gross characteristics of the fluid are assessed, such as its color, turbidity, and viscosity. Viscosity can be assessed using the "string" sign. The length of a viscous string of joint fluid dropped from the syringe is normally > 3 cm. Inflammation decreases viscosity, decreasing the length of the string.

Gross characteristics allow many effusions to be tentatively classified as noninflammatory, inflammatory, or infectious (see TABLE 31–1). Effusions can also be hemorrhagic. Each type of effusion suggests certain joint diseases (see TABLE 31–2). So-called noninflammatory effusions are actually mildly inflammatory but tend to suggest diseases such as osteoarthritis, in which inflammation is not severe.

Laboratory tests commonly performed on joint fluid include cell count, leukocyte differential, culture (if infection is a concern—see p. 312), and wet drop examination for cells and crystals. However, the exact tests often depend upon what diagnoses are suspected.

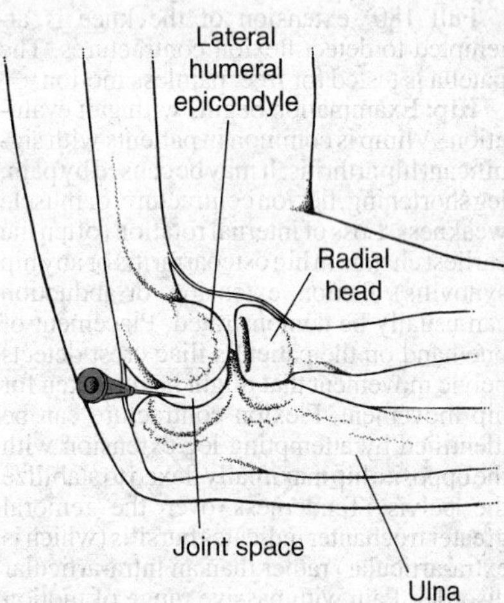

Fig. 31–2. Arthrocentesis of the elbow. The ulnohumeral joint is entered while the patient's elbow is flexed at 60° and the wrist is pronated. The needle enters the joint's lateral surface, between the lateral humeral epicondyle and the ulna.

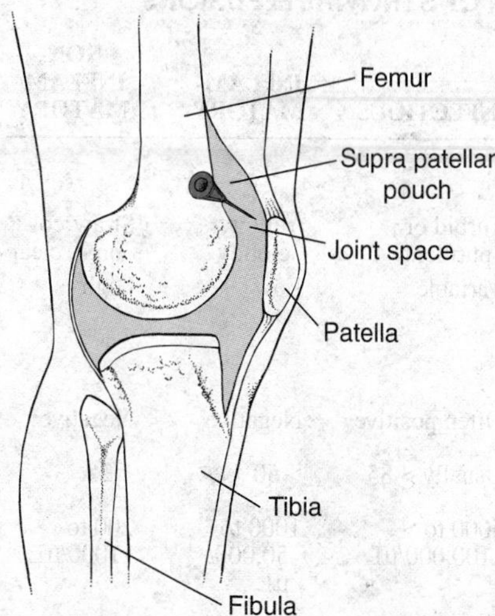

Fig. 31–3. Arthrocentesis of the knee. The knee and connecting suprapatellar pouch can be punctured while the patient is supine and knee is extended. The needle, usually 20-gauge, can be inserted laterally, just under the cephalad edge of the patella. Alternatively, the needle can be inserted medially, under the cephalad half of the patella.

Microscopic examination of a wet drop preparation of synovial fluid for crystals (only a few drops of fluid from a joint are needed), using polarized light, is essential for definitive diagnosis of gout, pseudogout, and other crystal-induced arthritides (see p. 299). A polarizer over the light source and another between the specimen and the examiner's eye allow visualization of crystals with a shiny white birefringence. Compensated polarized light is provided by inserting a first-order red plate, as is found in commercially available microscopes. The effects of a compensator can be reproduced by placing two strips of clear adhesive tape on a glass slide and placing this slide over the lower polarizer. Such a homemade system should be tested against a commercial polarizing microscope. If a wet drop reveals crystals that are not typical of monosodium urate (gout) or Ca pyrophosphate (pseudogout), several less common crystals (cholesterol, liquid lipid crystals, oxalate, cryoglobulins) or artifacts (eg, depot corticosteroid crystals) should be considered.

Other synovial fluid findings that occasionally make or suggest a specific diagnosis include the presence of specific organisms (identifiable by Gram or acid-fast stain); LE cells; marrow spicules or fat globules (caused by fracture); "Reiter's cells" (monocytes on Wright's stained smears that have phagocytized PMNs), present most often in reactive arthritis; amyloid fragments (identifiable by Congo red stain); and sickled RBCs (caused by sickle cell hemoglobinopathies).

Measurements of rheumatoid factor in synovial fluid can give false-positive or false-negative results and, thus, should not be performed. Extremely low synovial fluid glucose levels in specimens carefully handled in fluoride tubes may suggest infection.

MONARTICULAR JOINT PAIN

Monarticular pain may originate in a joint, be referred, or originate from periarticular structures (eg, bursitis or tendinitis). Pain from intra-articular structures is often inflammatory arthritis but may be noninflammatory (eg, osteoarthritis, internal derangement).

Acute monarticular joint pain requires particularly rapid diagnosis because some of its causes, particularly infectious (septic) arthritis and crystal-induced arthritis, require rapid treatment. Both of these disorders are inflammatory and cause joint effusions. Crystal-induced arthritis is usually caused by monosodium urate (gout) or Ca pyrophosphate dihydrate crystal deposition disease (pseudogout). Acute monarticular arthritis may occasionally be the initial presentation of psoriatic arthritis or various types of polyarticular inflammatory arthritis. Less common causes of acute monarticular arthritis are disorders such as adjacent osteomyelitis, bone infarcts, foreign bodies, hemarthroses (eg, in hemophilia or coagulopathies), and tumors.

Evaluation

Evaluation should determine whether the joint or periarticular structures are the cause of symptoms and whether there is inflammation. If inflammation is present or the diagnosis is unclear, signs and

TABLE 31–1. CLASSIFICATION OF SYNOVIAL EFFUSIONS

	NORMAL	HEMOR-RHAGIC	INFECTIOUS	INFLAM-MATORY	NON-INFLAM-MATORY
Gross examination					
Appearance	Clear	Bloody	Turbid or purulent	Yellow, cloudy	Straw-colored, clear
Viscosity	High	Variable	Variable	Low	High
Routine laboratory examination					
Culture	Negative	Negative	Often positive	Negative	Negative
PMN %*	< 25	—	Usually > 85	> 50	< 25
WBC count*	< 200/μL	Affected by amount of blood	5000 to > 100,000/μL	1000 to 50,000/μL	200 to 1000/μL

*WBC count and PMN % in infectious arthritis are lower if organism is less virulent (eg, gonococcal, Lyme, tuberculous, or fungal arthritis) or partially treated. Some effusions in SLE and other connective tissue diseases are only equivocally inflammatory, with a WBC count of 500 to 2000/μL. Noninfectious effusions rarely have up to 100,000 WBC/μL.

symptoms of polyarticular and systemic disorders should be sought and all joints examined.

History: Severe joint pain that develops over hours suggests crystal-induced (or less often infectious) arthritis. A previous attack of crystal-induced arthritis with development of similar symptoms suggests recurrence. Risk factors for gout include male sex, older age, and use of diuretics or other drugs that increase uric acid (urate) levels. Risk factors for infection include immunosuppressive or corticosteroid therapy, diabetes, IV drug use, extra-articular foci of infection, tick bite or residence in a Lyme-endemic area, previous intra-articular corticosteroids, and joint prostheses. Urethritis can suggest reactive arthritis or a gonococcal infection, but gonococcal arthritis often develops in patients without symptoms of urethritis.

Pain during rest and on initiating activity suggests inflammatory arthritis, whereas pain worsened by movement and relieved by rest suggests mechanical disorders (eg, osteoarthritis). Gradual onset of pain is typical of RA or noninfectious arthritis but can result from certain infectious arthritides (eg, tuberculous, fungal).

Physical examination: Pain aggravated by passive motion of another structure (eg, passive hip rotation worsening knee pain) suggests referred pain. Pain worse with active than with passive joint motion may indicate tendinitis or bursitis; joint inflammation generally restricts active and passive range of joint motion severely. Tenderness or swelling at only one side of a joint suggests an extra-articular origin (eg, in ligaments, tendons, or bursae); findings on several aspects of the joint suggest an intra-articular cause.

Increased heat and erythema suggest inflammation, but erythema is often absent during inflammation. Although gout can involve many different single joints or combinations of joints, acute, painful monarticular arthritis of the metatarsophalangeal joint of a great toe (podagra) is especially suggestive.

Testing: Bursitis and tendinitis can often be diagnosed without further testing. In severe or unexplained acute monarticular arthritis or bursitis with swelling, synovial fluid

TABLE 31–2. DIFFERENTIAL DIAGNOSIS BASED ON SYNOVIAL FLUID CLASSIFICATION*†

HEMORRHAGIC	INFECTIOUS	INFLAMMATORY	NONINFLAMMATORY
Anticoagulant treatment Hemangioma Coagulopathy Neurogenic (neuropathic) arthropathy Pigmented villonodular synovitis Scurvy Thrombocytopenia Trauma with or without fracture Tumor	Various organisms depending on patient characteristics (see TABLE 39–2 on p. 314)	Acute crystal synovitis (gout and pseudogout) Ankylosing spondylitis Crohn's disease Lyme disease Partially treated or less virulent bacterial infections Progressive systemic sclerosis Psoriatic arthritis Reactive arthritis Reiter's syndrome RA Rheumatic fever SLE Ulcerative colitis	Amyloidosis Ehlers-Danlos syndrome Hypertrophic pulmonary osteoarthropathy Metabolic diseases causing osteoarthritis Neurogenic (neuropathic) arthropathy Osteoarthritis Osteochondritis dissecans Osteochondromatosis Progressive systemic sclerosis Rheumatic fever Sickle cell disease SLE Subsiding or early inflammation Trauma

*See TABLE 31–1 for classification. This differential diagnosis is only a partial listing.
†Some disorders span classifications (eg, neuropathic arthropathy can be hemorrhagic or noninflammatory; progressive systemic sclerosis can be inflammatory or noninflammatory).

examination is essential; arthrocentesis or bursal aspiration confirms effusion and may provide a specific diagnosis (eg, culture of an organism in synovial fluid in infectious arthritis). Finding crystals in synovial fluid confirms crystal-induced arthritis but does not rule out coexisting infection. X-rays should generally be obtained if bone abnormalities (such as fracture or infection) or Ca pyrophosphate deposition (chondrocalcinosis) or calcific periarthritis is suspected. Other tests are only adjunctive but are obtained depending on what diagnoses are being considered. Blood tests (eg, ESR, antinuclear antibodies, rheumatoid factor) may help determine the cause of noninfectious inflammatory arthritis as described elsewhere in THE MANUAL.

Treatment

The underlying disorder is treated. Joint inflammation is usually treated symptomatically with NSAIDs. Pain without inflammation is usually more safely treated with acetaminophen. Joint immobilization with a splint or sling can sometimes relieve pain. Heat therapy may relieve muscle spasm around joints, and cold therapy may be analgesic in inflammatory joint diseases.

POLYARTICULAR PAIN

Polyarticular arthralgia can originate from arthritis, or from extra-articular disorders (eg, polymyalgia rheumatica, fibromyalgia).

Arthritis can be inflammatory or noninflammatory (eg, osteoarthritis). Inflammatory arthritis may involve peripheral joints only, or both peripheral and axial joints. Inflammatory arthritis involving ≤4 joints is termed peripheral oligo- or pauciarticular arthritis. Involvement of > 4 joints is called peripheral polyarticular arthritis. Each of these types has specific, likely causes (see TABLE 31–3).

Often, arthritis is transient and resolves without diagnosis or may not fulfill the criteria for any defined rheumatic disease; a tentative

TABLE 31–3. COMMON CAUSES OF POLYARTICULAR ARTHRITIS

Peripheral polyarticular
RA
SLE
Viral arthritis
Serum sickness
Psoriatic arthritis
Peripheral oligoarticular
Behçet's disease
Enteropathic arthritis
Infective endocarditis
Gout (or pseudogout)
Psoriatic arthritis
Reactive arthritis
Rheumatic fever
Lyme disease arthritis
Peripheral with axial involvement
Ankylosing spondylitis
Enteropathic arthritis
Psoriatic arthritis
Reactive arthritis

diagnosis may be made so that treatment can proceed. Systemic disease should be considered in all atypical and undiagnosed conditions.

Evaluation

Clinical data, particularly the history, are the most powerful diagnostic tools.

History: The location of symptoms may reveal whether pain originates in joints or other structures such as bones, tendons, bursae, muscles, other soft-tissue structures, or nerves. In arthritis, an inflammatory disorder is suggested by prominent morning stiffness, nontraumatic joint swelling, and fever or weight loss. Pain that is diffuse and described inconsistently or vaguely may result from fibromyalgia or functional disorders.

Back pain with arthritis suggests a spondyloarthropathy such as ankylosing spondylitis. Arthritis with urethral or GI symptoms suggests reactive arthritis. Recurrent diarrhea or abdominal pain suggests arthritis complicating inflammatory bowel disease.

Physical examination: Fever, wasting, or rashes may reflect systemic rheumatic or nonrheumatic disorders. Musculoskeletal examination should first determine whether the problem is intra-articular and, if so, whether it is inflammatory. Long-standing arthritis can restrict passive joint motion.

TABLE 31–4. DIFFERENTIAL FEATURES OF THE HAND IN RHEUMATOID ARTHRITIS AND OSTEOARTHRITIS

CRITERIA	RHEUMATOID ARTHRITIS	OSTEOARTHRITIS
Character of swelling	Synovial, capsular, soft tissue; bony only in late stages	Bony with irregular spurs; occasional soft cysts
Tenderness	Usual	None or mild except during occasional acute onset
Distal interphalangeal involvement	Not usual, except in thumb	Usual
Proximal interphalangeal involvement	Usual	Frequent
Metacarpophalangeal involvement	Usual	Unusual
Wrist involvement	Usual or common	Rare, except in base of thumb metacarpal-carpal joint

Adapted from Bilka PJ: Physical examination of the arthritic patient. *Bulletin on the Rheumatic Diseases* 20:596–599, copyright 1970. Used by permission of The Arthritis Foundation.

Periarticular findings may help differentiate among disorders. For example, coexisting tendinitis is common in gonococcal arthritis, RA, and other systemic diseases; bone tenderness may be prominent in sickle cell disease and hypertrophic pulmonary osteoarthropathy. Other extra-articular findings may also suggest a specific type of arthritis (eg, tophi in gout, rheumatoid nodules in RA).

Examination of the hand may help differentiate between arthritides. The main differential features of the hand in osteoarthritis and RA are outlined in TABLE 31–4. Swan-neck or boutonnière deformities may result from chronic RA. Distal interphalangeal (DIP) joint involvement with pitting in the adjacent nail and slightly asymmetric involvement of other joints may suggest psoriatic arthritis. Asymmetric involvement of the fingers may represent reactive arthritis, and asymmetric DIP joint involvement plus tophi suggests chronic gout. Thickening of the skin and flexion contractures may indicate progressive systemic sclerosis. Raynaud's phenomenon suggests progressive systemic sclerosis, SLE, or mixed connective tissue disease. Clubbing of the fingertips and bony tenderness of the distal radius and ulna caused by underlying periostitis can occur in hypertrophic pulmonary osteoarthropathy. Sore, painful hands with few objective abnormalities often represent SLE and, less often, dermatomyositis, although in these disorders there may also be joint synovitis similar to that in RA. Scaling erythema over the extensor joint surfaces, especially over the knuckles, may indicate dermatomyositis.

Testing: If the specific diagnosis cannot be established clinically and if determining whether arthritis is inflammatory will help determine the diagnosis, ESR and C-reactive protein may help. Elevated results suggest inflammation but are very nonspecific, particularly in older adults. Other tests may be needed for diagnostic dilemmas.

32 AUTOIMMUNE RHEUMATIC DISORDERS

Autoimmune rheumatic disorders include eosinophilic fasciitis, mixed connective tissue disease, polymyositis and dermatomyositis, relapsing polychondritis, Sjögren's syndrome, SLE, and systemic sclerosis. RA and the spondyloarthropathies and their variants (see in Ch. 34 on p. 283) are probably also immune mediated. The triggers and precise pathophysiology remain unknown for all these disorders, although many aspects of pathogenesis are becoming clearer.

EOSINOPHILIC FASCIITIS

Eosinophilic fasciitis is an uncommon disorder characterized by symmetric and painful inflammation, swelling, and induration of the arms and legs. Diagnosis is by biopsy of skin and fascia. Treatment is with corticosteroids.

The cause of eosinophilic fasciitis (EF) is unknown. The disorder occurs mostly in middle-aged men but can occur in women and children.

Symptoms and Signs

The disease often begins in a relatively sedentary person who performs strenuous physical activity (eg, chopping wood). The initial features are pain, swelling, and inflammation of the skin and subcutaneous tissues, followed by induration, creating a characteristic orange-peel configuration most evident over the anterior surfaces of the extremities. The face and trunk are occasionally involved. Restriction of arm and leg movement usually develops insidiously. Contractures commonly evolve, secondary to induration and thickening of the fascia, but the process may also involve tendons, synovial membranes, and muscle. Typically, EF does not involve the fingers and toes (acral areas). Muscle strength is unimpaired, but myalgia and arthritis may occur. Carpal tunnel syndrome may also occur.

Fatigue and weight loss are common. Rarely, aplastic anemia, thrombocytopenia, and lymphoproliferative processes develop.

Diagnosis

EF should be suspected in patients with typical symptoms. The cutaneous manifestations may suggest systemic sclerosis; however, systemic sclerosis usually also has Raynaud's phenomenon, acral involvement, telangiectasia, and visceral changes (eg, esophageal dysmotility), all of which are absent in EF.

Diagnosis is confirmed by en bloc biopsy of affected skin and fascia deep enough to include adjacent muscle fibers. Characteristic findings are inflammation of the fascia, with or without eosinophils.

Blood tests are not diagnostic, but CBC shows eosinophilia (in early active disease), and serum protein electrophoresis shows polyclonal hypergammaglobulinemia. Autoantibodies are usually absent. MRI, although not specific, can demonstrate thickened fascia, the increased signal intensity in the superficial muscle fibers correlating with the inflammation.

Prognosis and Treatment

Most patients respond rapidly to high doses of prednisone (40 to 60 mg po once/day followed by gradual reduction to 5 to 10 mg/day as soon as the fascitis resolves). Continued low doses may be required for 2 to 5 yr. Although the long-term outcome varies, EF is often self-limited and uncomplicated. Monitoring with CBCs is advised because of the occasional hematologic complications.

MIXED CONNECTIVE TISSUE DISEASE

Mixed connective tissue disease is an uncommon syndrome characterized by clinical features of SLE, systemic sclerosis, polymyositis or dermatomyositis, and RA and by very high titers of circulating antinuclear antibody to a ribonucleoprotein (RNP) antigen. Hand swelling, Raynaud's phenomenon, polyarthralgia, inflammatory myopathy, esophageal hypomotility, and pulmonary dysfunction are common. Diagnosis is by the combination of clinical features, antibodies to RNP, and absence of antibodies specific for other autoimmune diseases. Treatment is similar to that for SLE, with corticosteroids if disease is moderate or severe.

Mixed connective tissue disease (MCTD) occurs worldwide and in all races, with a peak incidence in the teens and 20s. The cause is unknown. In some patients, the disorder evolves into classic systemic sclerosis or SLE.

Symptoms and Signs

Raynaud's phenomenon may precede other manifestations by years. Frequently, the first manifestations resemble early SLE, scleroderma, polymyositis or dermatomyositis, or RA. Whatever the initial presentation, limited disease tends to progress and become widespread, and the clinical pattern changes over time.

The most frequent finding is swelling of the hands that eventually produces a sausagelike appearance of the fingers. Skin findings include lupus or dermatomyositis-like rashes. Diffuse scleroderma-like skin changes and ischemic necrosis or ulceration of the fingertips are much less frequent in MCTD.

Almost all patients have polyarthralgias, and 75% have frank arthritis. Often the arthritis is nondeforming, but erosive changes and deformities similar to those in RA may be present. Proximal muscle weakness with or without tenderness is common.

Renal disease occurs in about 10% and is often mild but occasionally causes morbidity or mortality. A trigeminal sensory neuropathy develops more frequently in MCTD than in other connective tissue diseases.

Diagnosis

MCTD should be suspected when additional overlapping features are present in patients appearing to have SLE, scleroderma, polymyositis, or RA. Patients should first be tested for antinuclear antibodies (ANA) and antibody to extractable nuclear antigen (ENA) and RNP antigen. If results of these tests are compatible with MCTD (eg, RNP antibodies very high), γ-globulin level, serum complement levels, rheumatoid factors, anti Jo-1 (anti histidyl t-RNA synthetase), and antibodies to the ribonuclease-resistant Smith (Sm) component of ENA, and double-stranded DNA should be tested to exclude other possible diagnoses. Further workup depends on symptoms and signs; manifestations of myositis, renal involvement, or pulmonary involvement prompt tests of those organs (eg, CPK, MRI, electromyogram, or muscle biopsy for diagnosis of myositis).

Almost all patients have high titers (often >1:1000) of fluorescent ANA that produce a speckled pattern. Antibodies to ENA are usually present at very high titers (>1:100,000). Antibody to RNP is present, whereas antibody to the ribonuclease-resistant Sm component of ENA is absent.

Rheumatoid factors are frequently positive, and titers are often high. The ESR is frequently elevated.

Prognosis and Treatment

The overall 10-yr survival rate is 80%, but prognosis depends largely on which manifestations predominate. Causes of death include pulmonary hypertension, renal failure, MI, colonic perforation, disseminated infection, and cerebral hemorrhage. Some patients have sustained remissions for many years without treatment.

General management and initial drug therapy are similar to those of SLE. Most patients with moderate or severe disease respond to corticosteroids, particularly if treated early. Mild disease is often controlled by salicylates, other NSAIDs, antimalarials, or sometimes low-dose corticosteroids. Severe major organ involvement usually requires higher doses of corticosteroids (eg, prednisone 1 mg/kg po once/day) or immunosuppressants. If patients develop features of myositis or systemic sclerosis, treatment is as for those diseases.

POLYMYOSITIS AND DERMATOMYOSITIS

Polymyositis and dermatomyositis are uncommon systemic rheumatic diseases characterized by inflammatory and degenerative changes in the muscles (polymyositis) and in the skin and muscles (dermatomyositis). The most specific skin sign is a heliotropic rash. Manifestations include symmetric weakness, some tenderness, and later atrophy, principally of the proximal limb girdle muscles. Complications can include visceral involvement and malignancy. Diagnosis is by clinical findings and abnormalities on muscle tests, which may include muscle enzymes, MRI, electromyography, and muscle biopsy. Treatment is with corticosteroids, sometimes combined with immunosuppressants or IV immunoglobulin.

The female:male ratio is 2:1. These diseases may appear at any age but occur most commonly from age 40 to 60 or, in children, from age 5 to 15.

Etiology

The cause appears to be an autoimmune reaction to muscle tissue in genetically susceptible people. Familial clustering occurs, and HLA subtypes DR3, DR52, DR6 appear to predispose. Possible inciting events include viral myositis and underlying malignancy. Picornavirus-like structures have been found in muscle cells, and viruses can trigger similar disorders in animals. The association of malignancy with dermatomyositis (much less so with polymyositis) suggests that a tumor may incite myositis as the result of an autoimmune reaction against a common antigen in muscle and tumor.

Deposits of IgM, IgG, and the third component of complement occur in the blood vessel walls of skeletal muscle, particularly in childhood dermatomyositis. Other autoimmune disorders may also develop in patients with polymyositis.

Pathophysiology

Pathologic changes include cellular damage and atrophy, with variable degrees of inflammation. Muscles in the hands, feet, and face are affected less than other skeletal muscles. Involvement of visceral muscles in the pharynx and upper esophagus and occasionally the heart, stomach, or intestines can impair the functions of those organs. High blood levels of myoglobin from rhabdomyolysis can damage the kidneys. Inflammation may occur in joints and lung, especially in patients with antisynthetase antibodies.

Classification

There are 5 subtypes of polymyositis: (1) Primary idiopathic polymyositis can occur at any age and does not involve the skin. (2) Primary idiopathic dermatomyositis is similar to primary idiopathic polymyositis but also involves the skin. (3) Polymyositis or dermatomyositis associated with malignant tumors can occur at any age but is most common in older adults and in patients with an associated connective tissue disease; the malignancy can develop up to 2 yr before or after the myositis. (4) Childhood polymyositis or dermatomyositis is associated with systemic vasculitis. (5) Polymyositis or dermatomyositis can occur with an associated connective tissue disorder, most often progressive systemic sclerosis, mixed connective tissue disease, and SLE.

Inclusion body myositis is often incorrectly grouped with polymyositis. It is a separate disorder that has clinical manifestations similar to chronic idiopathic polymyositis; however, it develops at an older age, frequently involves distal muscles (eg, hand and feet muscles), has a longer duration, responds poorly to therapy, and has a different histologic appearance.

Symptoms and Signs

Onset of polymyositis may be acute (particularly in children) or insidious (particularly in adults). Acute viral infections occasionally precede or incite the initial symptoms—usually proximal muscle weakness or rash. Muscle tenderness and pain are usually less dramatic than weakness. Polyarthralgias, Raynaud's phenomenon, dysphagia, pulmonary symptoms, and constitutional complaints, notably fever, fatigue, and weight loss, may also occur. Raynaud's phenomenon is very common in patients who also have other connective tissue disorders.

Muscle weakness may progress over weeks to months. However, it takes destruction of 50% of muscle fibers to cause symptomatic weakness (ie, muscle weakness indicates advanced myositis). Patients may have difficulty raising their arms above their shoulders, climbing steps, or rising from a sitting position. Patients may become wheelchair-bound or bedridden because of weakness of pelvic and shoulder girdle muscles. The flexors of the neck may be severely affected, causing an inability to raise the head from the pillow. Involvement of pharyngeal and upper esophageal muscles may impair swallowing and cause regurgitation. Muscles of the hands, feet, and face escape involvement. Limb contractures may eventually develop.

Skin rash, which occurs in dermatomyositis, tends to be dusky and erythematous. Periorbital edema with a purplish appearance (heliotropic rash) is specific for dermatomyositis. The skin rash may be slightly elevated and smooth or scaly; it may appear on the forehead, V of the neck and shoulders, chest and back, forearms and lower legs, elbows and knees, medial malleoli, and radiodorsal aspects of the proximal interphalangeal and metacarpophalangeal joints (Gottron's papules). The base and sides of the fingernails may be hyperemic. Desquamating dermatitis with splitting of the skin may evolve over the radial aspects of the fingers. The primary skin lesions frequently fade completely but may be followed by secondary changes (brownish pigmentation, atrophy, scarring, or vitiligo). Subcutaneous calcification may occur, particularly in children.

Polyarthralgia or polyarthritis, often with swelling, effusions, and other manifestations of nondeforming arthritis, occurs in about 30% of patients. However, joint manifestations tend to be mild. They occur more often in a subset with Jo-1 or other antisynthetase antibodies.

Visceral involvement (except that of the pharynx and upper esophagus) is less common in polymyositis than in some other rheumatic disorders (eg, SLE, systemic sclerosis). Occasionally, and especially in patients with antisynthetase antibodies, interstitial pneumonitis (manifested by dyspnea and cough) is the most prominent manifestation. Cardiac dysrhythmias (arrhythmias, conduction disturbances, abnormal systolic time intervals) can occur but are often asymptomatic. GI symptoms, more common in children with associated vasculitis, may include hematemesis, melena, and manifestations of bowel perforation.

Diagnosis

Polymyositis should be suspected in patients with proximal muscle weakness with or without muscle tenderness. Dermatomyositis should be suspected in patients with a heliotropic rash or Gottron's papules and in patients with symptoms of polymyositis and any skin findings compatible with dermatomyositis. Polymyositis and dermatomyositis share certain clinical findings with systemic sclerosis or, less frequently, with SLE or vasculitis. Establishing the diagnosis requires as many as possible of the following 5 criteria: (1) proximal muscle weakness; (2) characteristic skin rash; (3) elevated serum muscle enzymes (CK, or if this is not elevated, aminotransferases or aldolase); (4) characteristic electromyographic or MRI abnormalities; and (5) muscle biopsy changes (the definitive test).

Muscle biopsy excludes some similar conditions such as inclusion body myositis and postviral rhabdomyolysis. Biopsy findings can be variable, but chronic inflammation and muscle degeneration and regeneration are typical. A definitive (usually tissue) diagnosis is needed to justify potentially toxic treatments. By identifying regions of muscle edema and inflammation, MRI can help select a biopsy site.

Laboratory studies can increase or decrease suspicion for the disorder, assess its severity, identify overlaps, and help detect complications. Antinuclear antibodies are positive in a few patients, most often those with another connective tissue disorder. About 60% of patients have antibodies to thymic nuclear antigen (PM-1) or whole thymus and Jo-1. The relationship between these autoantibodies and disease pathogenesis remains unclear, although antibody to Jo-1 is a significant marker for fibrosing alveolitis, pulmonary fibrosis, arthritis, and Raynaud's phenomenon.

Periodic measurement of CK is helpful in monitoring treatment. However, in patients with widespread muscle atrophy, levels are occasionally normal despite chronic, active myositis. Muscle biopsy, MRI, or high CK levels can often differentiate a relapse of polymyositis from corticosteroid-induced myopathy.

Because patients often have unsuspected malignancies, some authorities recommend screening any adult who has dermatomyositis or those ≥ 60 who have polymyositis with the following: physical examination that includes breast, pelvis, and rectum (with occult blood testing); CBC; biochemical profile; mammogram; carcinoembryonic antigen; urinalysis; and chest x-ray. Younger patients without symptoms of malignancy need not undergo screening.

Prognosis

Long remissions (even apparent recovery) occur in up to half of treated patients within 5 yr, more often in children. Relapse, however, may still occur at any time. Overall 5-yr survival rate is 75%, higher in children. Death in adults is preceded by severe and progressive muscle weakness, dysphagia, malnutrition, aspiration pneumonia, or respiratory failure with superimposed pulmonary infection. Polymyositis tends to be more severe and resistant to treatment in patients with cardiac or pulmonary involvement. Death in children may be a result of bowel vasculitis. Malignancy, if present, generally determines the overall prognosis.

Treatment

Physical activities should be curtailed until the inflammation subsides. Corticosteroids are the drugs of choice initially. For acute disease, adults receive prednisone ≥ 40 to 60 mg po once/day. Serial measurements of CK provide the best early guide of therapeutic effectiveness, falling toward or reaching normal in most patients in 6 to 12 wk, followed by improved muscle strength. Once enzyme levels have returned to normal, prednisone is reduced initially by about 2.5 mg/day q wk, and then more gradually; if muscle enzyme levels rise, the dose is increased. Patients who appear to recover can have treatment gradually withdrawn with close monitoring, but most adults require chronic maintenance with prednisone (up to 10 to 15 mg/day). Children require initial doses of prednisone of 30 to 60 mg/m^2 once/day. In children, it may be possible to discontinue prednisone after ≥ 1 yr of remission.

Occasionally, patients treated chronically with high-dose corticosteroids become increasingly weak because of a superimposed corticosteroid myopathy.

If a patient fails to respond to corticosteroids or develops a corticosteroid myopathy or another complication that necessitates discontinuation or decrease of prednisone, immunosuppressants (methotrexate, cyclophosphamide, azathioprine, cyclosporine) should be tried. Some patients have received only methotrexate (generally in higher doses than used for RA) for ≥ 5 yr. IV immunoglobulins can be effective in some patients refractory to drug treatment, but the prohibitive cost has precluded comparative trials.

Myositis associated with tumors, metastatic disease, or inclusion body myositis usually is more refractory to corticosteroids. Malignancy-associated myositis may remit if the tumor is removed.

RELAPSING POLYCHONDRITIS

Relapsing polychondritis is an episodic, inflammatory, and destructive disorder involving primarily cartilage of the ear and nose but also potentially affecting the eyes, tracheobronchial tree, heart valves, kidneys, joints, skin, and blood vessels. Diagnosis is clinical. Treatment requires prednisone and sometimes immunosuppressants.

Relapsing polychondritis affects men and women equally; onset typically is in middle age. An association with RA, systemic vasculitis, SLE, and other connective tissue diseases suggests an autoimmune etiology.

Symptoms and Signs

Acute pain, erythema, and swelling most commonly affect the pinna cartilage. Nasal cartilage inflammation is the next most common, followed by arthritis that varies from arthralgias to symmetric or asymmetric nondeforming arthritis involving large and small joints, with a predilection for the costochondral joints. The next most common manifestations, in decreasing order of frequency, are inflammation of the eye (conjunctivitis, scleritis, iritis, keratitis, chorioretinitis); cartilaginous tissue of the larynx, trachea, or bronchi (causing hoarseness, cough, and tenderness); internal ear; cardiovascular system (aortic regurgitation, pericarditis, myocarditis, aortic aneurysms, aortitis); kidney; and skin. Bouts of acute inflammation heal over weeks to months, with recurrences over several years.

Advanced disease can lead to destruction of supporting cartilage, producing floppy ears, saddle nose, pectus excavatum, and visual, auditory, and vestibular abnormalities. Tracheal narrowing can lead to pneumonia or even tracheal collapse. Systemic vasculitis (leukocytoclastic vasculitis or polyarteritis nodosa), myelodysplastic syndrome, or malignancy occasionally develops.

Diagnosis

Diagnosis is established if the patient develops at least 3 of the following: bilateral chondritis of the external ears, inflammatory polyarthritis, nasal chondritis, ocular inflammation, respiratory tract chondritis, or auditory or vestibular dysfunction. Biopsy of involved cartilage is helpful if clinical diagnosis is not clear-cut.

Laboratory tests are not necessary but may help decrease the likelihood of other disorders. Synovial fluid is usually mildly inflammatory, if at all. Blood tests may show normocytic-normochromic anemia, leukocytosis, elevated ESR or γ-globulin levels, and occasionally positive rheumatoid factor, antinuclear antibodies (ANA), or in up to 25%, antineutrophil cytoplasmic antibodies (ANCA). Abnormal renal function may indicate an associated vasculitis. A positive c-ANCA test (ANCA that are reactive mainly to proteinase-3) suggests Wegener's granulomatosis, which can cause similar findings (see p. 281).

Patients need close monitoring, usually with CT, for evidence of tracheal narrowing.

Prognosis and Treatment

Mortality after 5 yr is 30%, from collapse of laryngeal and tracheal structures or from cardiovascular complications such as large-vessel aneurysm, cardiac valvular insufficiency, or systemic vasculitis.

Mild disease may respond to NSAIDs in anti-inflammatory doses. However, most patients are treated with prednisone 30 to 60 mg po once/day, with tapering of the dose as soon as there is a clinical response. Some patients require chronic use. In such patients, methotrexate 7.5 to 20 mg po once/wk can reduce the requirement for corticosteroids. Very severe cases may require other immunosuppressants, such as cyclosporine, cyclophosphamide, or azathioprine (see p. 288). None of these therapies have been tested in controlled trials or been shown to decrease mortality. If tracheal narrowing causes stridor, a tracheostomy or stent may be needed.

SJÖGREN'S SYNDROME

Sjögren's syndrome is a chronic, probably autoimmune, systemic inflammatory disorder of unknown cause characterized by dryness of the mouth, eyes, and other mucous membranes. It can be primary or secondary to other autoimmune disorders. Sjögren's syndrome may also cause rheumatoid-like arthritis or affect various exocrine glands or other organs. Diagnosis is by specific criteria relating to eye, mouth, and salivary gland involvement, autoantibodies, and histopathology. Treatment is symptomatic.

Sjögren's syndrome (SS) is a relatively common autoimmune connective tissue disorder. It is most frequent in middle-aged women. About 30% of patients with autoimmune disorders such as RA, SLE, scleroderma, vasculitis, mixed connective tissue disease, Hashimoto's thyroiditis, primary biliary cirrhosis, or chronic autoimmune hepatitis develop SS. Genetic associations have been found (eg, HLA-DR3 antigens in whites with primary SS).

Pathophysiology

Salivary, lacrimal, and other exocrine glands become infiltrated with $CD4^+$ T cells and with some B cells. The T cells produce inflammatory cytokines (eg, IL-2, γ-interferon). Salivary duct cells also produce cytokines, eventually damaging the secretory ducts. Atrophy of the secretory epithelium of the lacrimal glands causes desiccation of the cornea and conjunctiva (keratoconjunctivitis sicca—see p. 899). Lymphocytic infiltration and intraductal cellular proliferation in the parotid gland cause luminal narrowing and in some cases formation of compact cellular structures termed myoepithelial islands; atrophy of the gland can result. Dryness and GI mucosal or submucosal atrophy and diffuse infiltration by plasma cells and lymphocytes may cause symptoms (eg, dysphagia).

Symptoms and Signs

SS often affects the eyes or mouth initially and sometimes exclusively. Dry eyes can produce irritation and photosensitivity. In advanced cases, the cornea is severely damaged, epithelial strands hang from the corneal surface (keratitis filiformis), and vision can be impaired. Diminished saliva (xerostomia) results in difficulty chewing, swallowing, secondary *Candida* infection, tooth decay, and calculi in the salivary ducts. Taste and smell may be diminished. Dryness may also develop in the skin and in mucous membranes of the nose, throat, larynx, bronchi, vulva, and vagina. Dryness of the respiratory tract may produce cough or lung infections. Alopecia may occur. Parotid glands enlarge in ⅓ of patients and are usually firm, smooth, and mildly tender. Chronic salivary gland enlargement is rarely painful.

Arthritis occurs in about ⅓ of patients and is similar in distribution and character to RA.

Other common extraglandular manifestations include generalized lymphadenopathy, Raynaud's phenomenon, parenchymal lung involvement (which is common but infrequently serious), and vasculitis that can occasionally affect the peripheral nerves or CNS or cause skin rashes (including purpura), glomerulonephritis, or mononeuritis multiplex. Kidney involvement can produce renal tubular acidosis, impaired concentrating ability, kidney stones, or interstitial nephritis. Pseudolymphoma, malignant lymphoma, or Waldenström's macroglobulinemia can develop; patients develop non-Hodgkin lymphoma at 40 times the normal rate and require careful follow-up. Chronic hepatobiliary disease, pancreatitis (exocrine pancreatic tissue is similar to that of salivary glands), and fibrinous pericarditis may also occur.

Diagnosis

SS should be suspected in patients with scratchy or dry eyes or dry mouth, enlarged salivary glands, purpura, or renal tubular acidosis. Such patients should receive diagnostic tests that can include evaluation of the eyes and salivary glands and serologic tests. Diagnosis is based on 6 criteria: eye symptoms, oral symptoms, eye tests, salivary gland involvement, autoantibodies, and histopathology. SS is probable if ≥ 3 criteria (including objective criteria) are positive and definite if ≥ 4 criteria are positive.

Eye symptoms consist of ≥ 3 mo of either dry eyes or use of tear substitutes ≥ 3 times/day; slit-lamp examination may also confirm dry eyes. Oral symptoms consist of > 3 mo of daily dry mouth sensation, daily use of liquids to aid in swallowing, or swollen salivary glands.

The Schirmer test measures the quantity of tears secreted in 5 min after irritation from a filter paper strip placed under each lower eyelid. A young person normally moistens 15 mm of each paper strip. Most people with SS moisten < 5 mm, although about 15% of test results are false-positive and 15% are false-negative. Ocular staining with an eyedrop of rose bengal or lissamine green solution is highly specific. Slit-lamp examination showing a fluorescein tear breakup in < 10 sec is also suggestive.

Salivary gland involvement can be confirmed by abnormally low saliva production (≤ 1.5 mL/15 min) as measured by salivary flow, sialography, or salivary scintiscanning, although these tests are less often used.

Serologic criteria have limited sensitivity and specificity. They include antibodies to Ro (SS-A autoantibodies—see SLE on p. 266) or to nuclear antigens (termed La or SS-B autoantibodies), antinuclear antibodies, or an elevated level of antibodies against γ-globulin. Rheumatoid factor is present in > 70% of patients. ESR is elevated in 70%, 33% have anemia, and up to 25% have leukopenia.

Biopsy of minor salivary glands in the buccal mucosa should be performed if diagnosis is not clear. Histopathologic involvement is confirmed if labial minor salivary glands show multiple large foci of lymphocytes with atrophy of acinar tissue.

Prognosis and Treatment

The disease is chronic, and death may occasionally result from pulmonary infection and, rarely, from renal failure or lymphoma. Other connective tissue disorders usually worsen prognosis. There is no specific treatment for the basic process.

Dry eyes should be treated with OTC lubricating eyedrops qid and prn. Skin and vaginal dryness can be treated with lubricants.

Mouth dryness may be avoided by sipping fluids throughout the day, chewing sugarless gum, and using a saliva substitute containing carboxymethylcellulose as a mouthwash. Drugs that decrease salivary secretion (eg, antihistamines, antidepressants, other anticholinergics) should be avoided. Fastidious oral hygiene and regular dental visits are essential. Stones must be promptly removed, preserving viable salivary tissue. The pain of suddenly enlarged salivary glands is generally best treated with warm compresses and analgesics. Pilocarpine, 5 mg po tid to qid, or cevimeline HCl, 30 mg po tid, can stimulate salivary production but should be avoided in patients with bronchospasm and closed-angle glaucoma.

Treatment is occasionally indicated for connective tissue involvement (eg, severe vasculitis or visceral involvement); corticosteroids (eg, prednisone 1 mg/kg po once/day) or cyclophosphamide 5 mg/kg po once/day may be used. Arthralgias may improve with hydroxychloroquine 200 to 400 mg po once/day.

SYSTEMIC LUPUS ERYTHEMATOSUS

(Disseminated Lupus Erythematosus)

Systemic lupus erythematosus is a chronic, multisystem, inflammatory disorder of probable autoimmune etiology, occurring predominantly in young women. Common manifestations include arthralgias and arthritis; malar and other skin rashes; pleuritis or pericarditis; renal or CNS involvement; and hematologic cytopenia. Diagnosis requires clinical and serologic criteria. Treatment of severe ongoing active disease requires corticosteroids, often hydroxychloroquine, and sometimes immunosuppressants.

Of all cases, 70 to 90% occur in women (usually of child-bearing age). SLE is more common in blacks than whites. It can affect patients of any age, including neonates. Increased awareness of mild forms has resulted in a worldwide rise in reported cases. In some countries, the prevalence of SLE rivals that of RA. SLE is probably precipitated by yet unknown environmental triggers that produce autoimmune reactions in genetically predisposed people. Some drugs (eg, hydralazine, procainamide) produce a lupus-like syndrome.

Symptoms and Signs

Clinical findings vary greatly. SLE may develop abruptly with fever or insidiously over months or years with episodes of arthralgias and malaise. Vascular headaches, epilepsy, or psychoses may be initial findings. Manifestations referable to any organ system may appear. Periodic exacerbations (flares) may occur.

Joint symptoms, ranging from intermittent arthralgias to acute polyarthritis, occur in about 90% of patients and may precede other manifestations by years. Most lupus polyarthritis is nondestructive and nondeforming. However, in long-standing disease, deformities may develop (eg, the metacarpophalangeal and interphalangeal joints may develop ulnar drift or swan-neck deformities without bony or cartilaginous erosions [Jaccoud's arthritis]).

Skin lesions include malar butterfly erythema (flat or raised) that generally spares the nasolabial folds. The absence of papules and pustules helps distinguish this from rosacea. A variety of other erythematous, firm, maculopapular lesions can occur elsewhere, including exposed areas of the face and neck, upper chest, and elbows. Skin blistering and ulceration are rare, although recurrent ulcers on mucous membranes (particularly the central portion of the hard palate near the junction of the hard and soft palate, the buccal and gum mucosa, and the anterior nasal septum) are common. Generalized or focal alopecia is common during active phases of SLE. Panniculitis can produce subcutaneous nodular lesions. Vasculitic skin lesions may include mottled erythema on the palms and fingers, periungual erythema, nail-fold infarcts, urticaria, and palpable purpura. Petechiae may develop secondary to thrombocytopenia. Photosensitivity occurs in 40% of patients.

Cardiopulmonary symptoms commonly include recurrent pleurisy, with or without pleural effusion. Pneumonitis is rare, although minor impairments in pulmonary function are common. Severe pulmonary hemorrhage occasionally occurs and has a 50% mortality. Other complications include pulmonary emboli, pulmonary hypertension, and shrinking lung syndrome. Cardiac complications include pericarditis (most commonly), pericardial effusion, and myocarditis. Serious, rare complications are coronary artery vasculitis and Libman-Sacks endocarditis. Accelerated atherosclerosis is an increasing cause of morbidity and mortality. Congenital heart block can develop in neonates.

Generalized adenopathy is common, particularly in children, young adults, and blacks. Splenomegaly occurs in 10% of patients. The spleen may develop periarterial fibrosis.

Neurologic symptoms can result from involvement of any part of the central or peripheral nervous system or meninges. Mild cognitive impairment is common. There may also be headaches, personality changes, ischemic stroke, subarachnoid hemorrhage, seizures, psychoses, organic brain syndrome, aseptic meningitis, peripheral neuropathies, transverse myelitis, or cerebellar dysfunction.

Renal involvement can develop at any time and may be the only manifestation of SLE. It may be benign and asymptomatic or progressive and fatal. Renal lesions can range in severity from a focal, usually benign, glomerulitis to a diffuse, potentially fatal, membranoproliferative glomerulonephritis. Common manifestations include proteinuria (most often), an abnormal urinary sediment manifested by RBC casts and leukocytes, hypertension, and edema.

Obstetric manifestations include early and late fetal loss. However, pregnancy can be successful (see p. 2169), particularly after 6 to 12 mo of remission.

Hematologic manifestations include anemia (often autoimmune hemolytic), leukopenia (including lymphopenia, with < 1500 cells/μL,), and thrombocytopenia (sometimes life-threatening autoimmune thrombocytopenia). Recurrent arterial or venous thrombosis, thrombocytopenia, and a high probability of obstetric complications occur in patients with antiphospholipid antibodies. Thromboses probably account for many of the complications of SLE, including obstetric complications.

GI manifestations can result from bowel vasculitis or impaired bowel motility. In addition, pancreatitis can result from SLE or from treatment with corticosteroids or azathioprine. Manifestations may include abdominal pain from serositis, nausea, vomiting, manifestations of bowel perforation, and pseudo-obstruction. SLE rarely causes parenchymal liver disease.

Diagnosis

SLE should be suspected in patients, particularly young women, with any of the symptoms and signs. However, early-stage SLE can mimic other connective (or nonconnective) tissue disorders, including RA if arthritic symptoms predominate. Mixed connective tissue disease can mimic SLE but also may involve features of systemic sclerosis, rheumatoid-like polyarthritis, and polymyositis or dermatomyositis. Infections that develop as a result of treatment-caused immunosuppression can mimic SLE also.

Laboratory testing differentiates SLE from other connective tissue disorders; antinuclear antibodies (ANA), CBC, urinalysis, and chemistry profile including renal and liver function tests should be obtained. The diagnosis is especially likely if ≥ 4 of the criteria in TABLE 32–1 are present at any time but is still possible if < 4 criteria are present. If the diagnosis is suspected but not established, additional testing for autoantibodies can be useful. Establishing the diagnosis may require repeated evaluations over months or years.

The fluorescent test for ANA is the best screen for SLE; positive ANA tests (usually in high titer: > 1:80) occur in > 98%. However, positive ANA tests can also occur in RA, other connective tissue diseases, malignancies, and

TABLE 32–1. CRITERIA FOR THE CLASSIFICATION OF SLE*

At least 4 of the following are required to classify patients as having SLE in reports of clinical research.

- Malar rash
- Discoid rash
- Photosensitivity
- Oral ulcers
- Arthritis
- Serositis
- Renal disorder
- Leukopenia (< 4000/μL), lymphopenia (< 1500/μL), hemolytic anemia, or thrombocytopenia (< 100,000/μL)
- Neurologic disorder
- Positive anti-DNA or anti-Sm antibody, or positive test for antiphospholipid antibodies
- Antinuclear antibodies in raised titer

*These 11 criteria are from the American College of Rheumatology and are also often used as aids in diagnosis. Although at least 4 criteria are not needed to make a diagnosis of SLE, the criteria help in recognizing manifestations of SLE.

even in 1% of normal individuals. Drugs such as hydralazine, procainamide, β-blockers, and tumor necrosis factor (TNF)-α antagonists can produce positive ANA results as well as a lupus-like syndrome; the ANA eventually becomes negative if the drug is discontinued. Positive ANA should prompt testing for anti-double-stranded DNA antibodies; high titers are highly specific for SLE but occur in only 25 to 30% of people with SLE.

Other ANA and anticytoplasmic antibodies (eg, Ro [SSA], La [SSB], Sm, RNP, Jo-1) should be obtained if the diagnosis of SLE is not otherwise clear. Ro is predominantly cytoplasmic; anti-Ro antibodies are occasionally present in ANA-negative SLE patients presenting with chronic cutaneous lupus. Anti-Ro is the causal antibody for neonatal lupus and congenital heart block. Anti-Sm is highly specific for SLE but, like anti-double-stranded DNA, is not sensitive.

Leukopenia is common, and lymphopenia occurs if the disorder is active. Hemolytic anemia may occur. Thrombocytopenia in SLE may be difficult or impossible to differentiate from idiopathic thrombocytopenic purpura except that patients will be ANA-positive. False-positive serologic tests for syphilis occur in 5 to 10% of SLE patients. They may be associated with the lupus anticoagulant and a prolonged PTT. Abnormal values in one or more of these assays indicate the presence of antiphospholipid antibodies (eg, anticardiolipin antibodies), which should then be measured directly by ELISA (*e*nzyme-*l*inked *i*mmuno*s*orbent *a*ssay). Antibodies to β_2-glycoprotein I are possibly more sensitive. Antiphospholipid antibodies predict arterial or venous thrombosis, thrombocytopenia, and, during pregnancy, spontaneous abortion or late fetal death.

Other tests help monitor disease severity and determine the need for treatment. Serum complement levels (C3, C4) are often depressed in active disease and are usually lowest in patients with active nephritis. ESR is elevated almost uniformly during active disease. C-reactive protein levels are not necessary: they may be strikingly low in SLE, even with ESR > 100 mm/h.

Screening for renal involvement begins with urinalysis. RBC and granular casts suggest active nephritis. Urinalysis should be performed at regular intervals, perhaps every 6 mo, even for patients in apparent remission. However, urinalysis may be repeatedly normal despite biopsy-documented renal involvement. Renal biopsy is usually not necessary for diagnosis of SLE or to confirm renal involvement but may help evaluate the status of renal disease (ie, active inflammation vs postinflammatory scarring) and guide therapy. Patients with chronic renal insufficiency and mostly sclerotic glomeruli are not likely to benefit from aggressive immunosuppressive therapy.

Prognosis

The course is usually chronic, relapsing, and unpredictable. Remissions may last for years. If the initial acute phase is controlled, even if very severe (eg, with cerebral thrombosis or severe nephritis), the long-term prognosis is usually good. The 10-yr survival in most developed countries is > 95%. Improved prognosis is in part due to earlier diagnosis and more effective therapies. More severe disease requires more toxic therapies, which increase risk of mortality. Examples of such complications include infection from immunosuppression and coronary artery disease or osteoporosis from chronic corticosteroids.

Treatment

To simplify therapy, SLE should be classified as mild (eg, fever, arthritis, pleurisy, pericarditis, headache, rash) or severe (eg, hemolytic anemia, thrombocytopenic purpura, massive pleural and pericardial involvement, significant renal damage, acute vasculitis of the extremities or GI tract, florid CNS involvement).

Mild or remittent disease: Little or no therapy may be needed. Arthralgias are usually controlled with NSAIDs. Aspirin (80 to 325 mg once/day) is useful in patients with the thrombotic tendency that accompanies anticardiolipin antibodies and who have never had a thrombotic event, but high doses in SLE may cause liver toxicity. Antimalarials help, particularly when joint and skin manifestations are prominent. Hydroxychloroquine 200 mg po once/day or bid is preferred. Alternatives include chloroquine 250 mg po once/day and quinacrine 50 to 100 mg po once/day. Combinations of these drugs are sometimes used. Hydroxychloroquine can produce retinal toxicity. The eyes should be examined at 6-mo intervals.

Severe disease: Corticosteroids are first-line therapy. A combination of prednisone and immunosuppressants is recommended in active, serious CNS lupus, vasculitis especially affecting viscera or nerves, or active reversible lupus nephritis. Prednisone is usually given in doses of 40 to 60 mg po once/day, but the dose may vary according to the manifestation of SLE. Oral azathioprine 1 to 2.5 mg/kg once/day or oral cyclophosphamide 1 to 4 mg/kg once/day can be used as an immunosuppressant. For renal involvement, cyclophosphamide is usually given in intermittent IV "pulses" instead of daily oral doses; eg, about 500 mg to 1 g/m^2 IV (together with mesna and fluid loading to protect the bladder) monthly for 6 mo and then once q 3 mo for 18 mo (less frequently if there is renal or hematologic toxicity (see TABLE 32–2).

In CNS lupus or other critical crises, methylprednisolone 1 g by slow (1-h) IV infusion on 3 successive days is often the initial treatment, followed by IV cyclophosphamide, as above. Mycophenolate mofetil 500 to 1000 mg po once/day or bid is an alternative to cyclophosphamide for renal SLE. Immunoglobulin G (IgG) 400 mg/kg IV once/day for 5 consecutive days may be useful for refractory thrombocytopenia. Stem cell transplantation after mobilization of stem cells with cyclophosphamide 2 g/m^2 IV is being tested for refractory SLE. Transplantation can be used for end-stage renal disease.

Improvement of severe SLE often takes 4 to 12 wk and may not be evident until corticosteroids are reduced. Thrombosis or embolism of cerebral, pulmonary, or placental vessels requires short-term treatment with heparin and longer treatment with warfarin, aiming for an INR of 3 (sometimes lifelong).

Suppressive therapy: For most patients, the risk of flares can be decreased without prolonged high-dose corticosteroids. Chronic disease should be treated with the lowest dose of corticosteroids and other drugs that control inflammation (eg, antimalarials, low-dose immunosuppressants). Treatment should be guided by clinical features primarily, although anti-double-stranded DNA antibody titers or low serum complement levels may be followed. If a patient needs long-term high-dose corticosteroids, alternative oral immunosuppressants should be considered. Ca, vitamin D, and bisphosphonate therapy should be considered in patients on chronic corticosteroids.

Focal complications and coexisting medical conditions: Long-term anticoagulation is vital in patients with antiphospholipid antibodies and recurrent thrombosis (see p. 759).

TABLE 32–2. PROTOCOL FOR CHEMOTHERAPY WITH CYCLOPHOSPHAMIDE AND IV MESNA

Use constant supervision regarding tolerance throughout entire procedure.

1. Using 50 mL of normal saline, mix ondansetron 10 mg and dexamethasone 10 mg and infuse over 10 to 30 min.
2. Using 250 mL of normal saline, mix in mesna 250 mg (used to bind acrolein, a metabolite of cyclophosphamide that is a bladder irritant) and infuse over 1 h.
3. Using 250 mL of normal saline, mix in cyclophosphamide 8 to 20 mg/kg and infuse over 1 h. Patient must wait 2 h before starting second dose of mesna.
4. Using 250 mL of normal saline, mix in mesna 250 mg and infuse along with 500 mL of normal saline using different IV site (ie, 500 mL of saline used as a flush). Patient must take ondansetron 8 mg po the next morning.

If a pregnant patient has antiphospholipid antibodies, thrombotic complications can be avoided with corticosteroids (prednisone ≤ 30 mg once/day), low-dose aspirin, or anticoagulation with heparin. Daily heparin given subcutaneously with or without one baby aspirin throughout the 2nd and 3rd trimesters may be the most successful prophylactic measure.

VARIANT FORMS OF LUPUS

Discoid lupus erythematosus (DLE): DLE, also sometimes called chronic cutaneous lupus erythematosus, is a set of skin changes that can occur as part of lupus, with or without systemic involvement. Skin lesions begin as erythematous plaques and progress to atrophic scars. They cluster in light-exposed areas of the skin, such as the face, scalp, and ears. Untreated, lesions extend and develop central atrophy and scarring. There may be widespread, scarring alopecia. Mucous membrane involvement may be prominent, especially in the mouth.

Patients presenting with typical discoid lesions should be evaluated for SLE. Antibodies against double-stranded DNA are almost invariably absent in DLE. Biopsy from the active margin of a skin lesion, although it does not differentiate DLE from SLE, can rule out other disorders (eg, lymphoma or sarcoidosis).

Early treatment can prevent permanent atrophy. Exposure to sunlight or ultraviolet light should be minimized (eg, using potent sunscreens when outdoors). Topical corticosteroid ointments (particularly for dry skin) or creams (less greasy than ointments) tid to qid (eg, triamcinolone acetonide 0.1 or 0.5%, fluocinolone 0.025 or 0.2%, flurandrenolide 0.05%, betamethasone valerate 0.1%, and, particularly betamethasone dipropionate 0.05%) usually cause involution of small lesions; they should not be used excessively or on the face (where they cause skin atrophy). Resistant lesions can be covered with plastic tape coated with flurandrenolide. Alternatively, intradermal injection with triamcinolone acetonide 0.1% suspension (< 0.1 mL per site) may resolve lesions, but secondary atrophy frequently follows. Antimalarials (eg, hydroxychloroquine 200 mg po once/day or bid) can help. In resistant cases, combinations (eg, hydroxychloroquine 200 mg/day plus quinacrine 50 to 100 mg po once/day) may be required for months to years.

Subacute cutaneous lupus erythematosus (SCLE): SCLE is a variant form of SLE in which skin involvement is prominent. Patients with SCLE develop extensive recurring skin rashes. Annular or papulosquamous lesions may develop on the face, arms, and trunk. Lesions are usually photosensitive and can develop hypopigmentation but rarely scar. Arthritis and fatigue are common in SCLE, but neurologic and renal manifestations are not. Patients may be ANA-positive or ANA-negative. Most have antibodies to Ro (SSA). Infants whose mothers have Ro antibodies may have congenital SCLE or congenital heart block. SCLE should be treated similarly to SLE.

SYSTEMIC SCLEROSIS

(Scleroderma)

Systemic sclerosis is a chronic disease of unknown cause characterized by diffuse fibrosis, degenerative changes, and vascular abnormalities in the skin, joints, and internal organs (especially the esophagus, lower GI tract, lung, heart, and kidney). Common symptoms include Raynaud's phenomenon, polyarthralgia, dysphagia, heartburn, and swelling and eventually skin tightening and contractures of the fingers. Lung, heart, and kidney involvement accounts for most deaths. Diagnosis is clinical, but laboratory tests help. Specific treatment is difficult, and emphasis is often on treatment of complications.

Systemic sclerosis (SSc) is about 4 times more common in women than men. It is most common in the 3rd to 5th decades of life and is rare in children. SSc can develop as part of mixed connective tissue disease.

Etiology and Pathophysiology

Immunologic mechanisms and heredity (certain HLA subtypes) play a role in etiology. SSc-like syndromes can result from exposure to vinyl chloride, bleomycin, pentazocine, epoxy and aromatic hydrocarbons, contaminated rapeseed oil, or L-tryptophan.

Pathophysiology involves vascular damage and activation of fibroblasts; collagen and other extracellular proteins in various tissues are overproduced.

In SSc, the skin develops more compact collagen fibers in the reticular dermis, epidermal thinning, loss of rete pegs, and atrophy of dermal appendages. T lymphocytes may accumulate, and extensive fibrosis in the dermal and subcutaneous layers develops. In the nail folds, capillary loops dilate and some microvascular loops are lost. In the extremities, chronic inflammation and fibrosis of the synovial membrane and surfaces and periarticular soft tissues occur.

Esophageal motility becomes impaired, and the lower esophageal sphincter becomes incompetent; gastroesophageal reflux and secondary strictures can develop. The intestinal muscularis mucosa degenerates, leading to pseudodiverticula in the colon and ileum. Interstitial and peribronchial fibrosis or intimal hyperplasia of small pulmonary arteries can develop; if long-standing, pulmonary hypertension can result. Diffuse myocardial fibrosis or cardiac conduction abnormalities occur. Intimal hyperplasia of interlobular and arcuate arteries can develop within the kidneys, causing renal ischemia and hypertension.

SSc varies in severity and progression, ranging from generalized skin thickening with rapidly progressive and often fatal visceral involvement (SSc with diffuse scleroderma) to isolated skin involvement (often just the fingers and face) and slow progression (often several decades) before serious visceral disease. The latter form is termed limited cutaneous scleroderma or CREST syndrome (*C*alcinosis cutis, *R*aynaud's phenomenon, *E*sophageal dysmotility, *S*clerodactyly, *T*elangiectasias). In addition, SSc can overlap with other connective tissue disorders—eg, sclerodermatomyositis (tight skin and muscle weakness indistinguishable from polymyositis) and mixed connective tissue disease.

Symptoms and Signs

The most common initial symptoms and signs are Raynaud's phenomenon and insidious swelling of the distal extremities with gradual thickening of the skin of the fingers. Polyarthralgia is also prominent. GI disturbances (eg, heartburn, dysphagia) or respiratory complaints (eg, dyspnea) are occasionally the first manifestations.

Swelling of the skin is usually symmetric and progresses to induration. It may be confined to the fingers (sclerodactyly) and hands, or it may affect most or all of the body. The skin eventually becomes taut, shiny, and hypo- or hyperpigmented; the face becomes masklike; and telangiectases may appear on the fingers, chest, face, lips, and tongue. Subcutaneous calcifications may develop, usually on the fingertips (pulps) and over bony eminences. Trophic ulcers are common, especially on the fingertips, overlying the finger joints, or over calcinotic nodules. Abnormal capillary and microvascular loops in the nails can be seen with an ophthalmoscope or dissecting microscope.

Polyarthralgias or mild arthritis can be prominent. Flexion contractures may develop in the fingers, wrists, and elbows. Friction rubs may develop over the joints, tendon sheaths, and large bursae.

Esophageal dysfunction is the most frequent visceral disturbance and occurs in most patients. Dysphagia (usually retrosternal) usually develops first. Later, acid reflux can cause heartburn and stricture. Barrett's esophagus occurs in ⅓ of patients and predisposes to complications (eg, stricture, adenocarcinoma). Hypomotility of the small bowel produces anaerobic bacterial overgrowth that can lead to malabsorption. Air may penetrate the damaged bowel wall and be visible on x-rays (pneumatosis intestinalis). Leakage of bowel contents into the peritoneal cavity can produce peritonitis. Distinctive wide-mouthed diverticula can develop in the colon. Biliary cirrhosis may develop in patients with CREST syndrome.

Lung involvement generally progresses indolently, with substantial individual variability, but is a common cause of death. Lung fibrosis can impair gas exchange, leading to exertional dyspnea and restrictive disease with eventual respiratory failure. Acute alveolitis (potentially responsive to therapy) can develop. Esophageal dysfunction can lead to aspiration pneumonia. Pulmonary hypertension may develop, as can heart failure, both of which are poor prognostic findings. Pericarditis with effusion or pleurisy can occur. Cardiac arrhythmias are common.

Severe, often sudden renal disease (renal crisis) may occur, most commonly in the first 4 to 5 yr and in patients with diffuse scleroderma. It is usually heralded by sudden, severe hypertension.

Diagnosis

SSc should be considered in patients with Raynaud's phenomenon, typical musculoskeletal or skin manifestations, or unexplained dysphagia, malabsorption, pulmonary fibrosis, pulmonary hypertension, cardiomyopathies, or conduction disturbances. Diagnosis can be obvious in patients with combinations of classic manifestations, such as Raynaud's phenomenon, dysphagia, and tight skin. However, in some patients, the diagnosis cannot be made clinically, and confirmatory laboratory tests can increase the probability of disease but do not rule it out.

Serum antinuclear antibodies (ANA) and SCL-70 antibody (topoisomerase I) should be obtained. ANA are present in ≥ 90%, often with an antinucleolar pattern. Antibody to centromeric protein (anticentromere antibody) occurs in the serum of a high proportion of patients with CREST syndrome and is detectable on the ANA. SCL-70 antigen is a DNA-binding protein sensitive to nucleases. Patients with diffuse scleroderma are more likely than those with CREST to have anti-SCL-70 antibodies. Rheumatoid factor also is positive in 33% of patients.

If lung involvement is suspected, pulmonary function testing, chest CT, and echocardiography can begin to define its severity. Acute alveolitis is often detected by high-resolution chest CT.

Prognosis

The course depends on the type of SSc but is often unpredictable. Typically, progression is slow. Overall 10-yr survival is about 65%. Most patients with diffuse skin disease eventually develop visceral complications, which are the usual causes of death. Prognosis is poor if cardiac, pulmonary, or renal manifestations are present early. Heart failure may be intractable. Ventricular ectopy, even if asymptomatic, increases the risk of sudden death. Acute renal insufficiency, if untreated, progresses rapidly and causes death within months. Patients with CREST syndrome may have disease that is limited and nonprogressive for long periods; visceral changes (eg, pulmonary hypertension caused by vascular disease of the lung, a peculiar form of biliary cirrhosis) eventually develop, but the course is often remarkably benign.

Treatment

No drug significantly influences the natural history of SSc overall, but various drugs are of value in treating specific symptoms or organ systems. NSAIDs can help arthritis. Corticosteroids may be helpful if there is overt myositis or mixed connective tissue disease. Penicillamine, long used for treatment of skin thickening, has been shown to be ineffective in recent trials.

Various immunosuppressants, including methotrexate, azathioprine, and cyclophosphamide, may help pulmonary alveolitis. Successful lung transplantation has been reported. Epoprostenol (prostacyclin) and bosentan may be helpful for pulmonary hypertension. Ca channel blockers, such as nifedipine 20 mg po tid or as an extended-release formulation, or angiotensin receptor blockers, such as losartan 50 mg po once/day, may help Raynaud's phenomenon. Patients should dress warmly. IV infusions of prostaglandin E_1 (alprostadil) or epoprostenol or sympathetic blockers can be used for digital ischemia. Reflux esophagitis is relieved by frequent small feedings, high-dose proton pump inhibitors, and sleeping with the head of the bed elevated. Esophageal strictures may require periodic dilation; gastroesophageal reflux may possibly require gastroplasty. Tetracycline 500 mg po bid or another broad-spectrum antibiotic can suppress overgrowth of intestinal flora and may alleviate malabsorption symptoms. Physiotherapy may help preserve muscle strength but is ineffective in preventing joint contractures. No treatment affects calcinosis.

For acute renal crisis, prompt treatment with an ACE inhibitor can dramatically prolong survival. Blood pressure is usually, but not always, controlled. If end-stage renal disease develops, dialysis and transplantation can be used, although the mortality rate remains high.

33 VASCULITIS

Vasculitis is inflammation of blood vessels, which may be generalized or localized. It can be a component of a number of systemic diseases.

Etiology and Pathophysiology

Vasculitis can be primary (the cause is unknown) or secondary to a drug, toxin, infection, other antigen, or another disorder. It can be confined to a single organ or organ system (eg, the skin) or can affect multiple systems.

The pathophysiology of most vasculitic disorders is poorly understood but can involve deposition of immune complexes in vessel walls and other immune-mediated mechanisms. It probably develops in response to some trigger. There is sometimes a genetic predisposition.

Vasculitis can affect any blood vessel—artery, arteriole, vein, venule, or capillary. Most damage results when inflammation narrows arteries and causes tissue necrosis.

Histologic changes tend to be similar. In many acute lesions, the predominant inflammatory cells are PMNs; in chronic lesions, lymphocytes. Inflammation may be segmental or involve the entire vessel. Variable degrees of cellular infiltration and necrosis or scarring within one or more layers of the vessel wall occur at sites of inflammation. Inflammation within the media of a muscular artery tends to destroy the internal elastic lamina. Inflammation at any point in the vessel wall tends to resolve with fibrosis and intimal hypertrophy. Intimal hypertrophy or secondary clot formation can narrow the arterial lumen and accounts for tissue ischemia or necrosis. Once the vessel wall integrity is breached, RBCs and fibrin may leak into the surrounding connective tissue. Histologic changes that are relatively specific to a disorder may occur (eg, numerous giant cells and destruction of internal elastica in giant cell arteritis).

Classification

Vasculitic disorders can be classified according to the size and depth of the predominant vessel involved. However, substantial overlap often exists. Vasculitis contributes to the pathophysiology of many other diseases, such as RA, SLE, and childhood polymyositis and dermatomyositis.

Systemic necrotizing vasculitis is a class of systemic vasculitic disorders of medium-sized vessels capable of producing infarction in various organs. The conditions include polyarteritis nodosa, microscopic polyangiitis, Churg-Strauss disease, Wegener's granulomatosis, and occasional isolated vasculitis in single organs or polyangiitis overlap syndromes.

Diagnosis

Because some vasculitic disorders have potentially toxic treatments, tissue biopsy should be obtained to confirm the diagnosis whenever possible. Clinical and other data may suggest vessels likely to be affected. For example, if clinical and electromyographic (EMG) findings of mononeuritis multiplex suggest infarction of a specific peripheral nerve, the artery supplying that nerve would be chosen for biopsy. If a suspected vasculitic disorder preferentially affects a certain artery, angiography of that artery may indicate whether and where the artery is affected. In temporal arteritis, symptoms may suggest the likely site of arterial involvement. Blind biopsies should usually be avoided.

Because vasculitis is often segmental or focal, biopsy may not show inflammation even within an involved vessel. Sampling from multiple areas or long segments within a vessel may increase diagnostic sensitivity. Also, intimal hypertrophy and fibrosis or perivasculitis may suggest an adjacent area of vasculitis. Most laboratory tests are nonspecific, but serum tests for antineutrophil cytoplasmic antibodies are especially useful in Wegener's granulomatosis and microscopic polyangiitis.

If secondary vasculitis is suspected and the primary cause is known or suspected, tissue biopsy is not always necessary. If the suspected cause is a drug or other antigen, withdrawing the antigen may produce a response. If vasculitis is secondary to another disorder, that disorder may be treatable directly. If symptoms and signs resolve, no further action may be necessary.

BEHÇET'S SYNDROME

Behçet's syndrome is a multisystem, inflammatory, relapsing, chronic vasculitic disorder. Common manifestations include recurrent oral ulcers, ocular inflammation, genital ulcers, and skin lesions. Blindness, neurologic or GI involvement, venous thromboses, and arterial aneurysms are the most serious manifestations. Diagnosis is clinical using international criteria. Treatment is mainly symptomatic but may involve corticosteroids for acute severe ocular or neurologic involvement or immunosuppressants for severe chronic features.

The cause is unknown. Immunologic (including autoimmune) and viral or bacterial triggers have been suggested, and HLA-B51 is associated with cases from the Mediterranean area of Turkey and Iran to China, Korea, and Japan. Behçet's syndrome is uncommon in the US.

Histopathologic vasculitic changes and thromboses are common to all involved organs. The syndrome generally begins in the 20s and occurs nearly equally in men and women. Some cases have been reported in children.

Symptoms and Signs

Almost all patients have recurrent painful oral ulcers resembling those of aphthous stomatitis; in most, these ulcers are the first manifestations. Similar ulcers occur on the penis and scrotum, on the vulva where they are painful, or in the vagina where they may cause little or no pain.

Ocular disease usually occurs only after years of ulcers; the most common is a relapsing iridocyclitis that often presents as pain, photophobia, and hazy vision; hypopyon with a layer of pus visible in the anterior chamber is specific but unusual. The posterior segment may also be involved, with choroiditis, retinal vasculitis, and papillitis that can diminish visual acuity. Untreated posterior uveitis may cause blindness.

Various skin lesions (papules, pustules, vesicles, folliculitis) occur in 80% of cases. Particularly suggestive are erythema nodosum–like lesions and, in about 40% of patients, pustular inflammatory reactions to minor trauma (eg, needle punctures). Relatively mild, self-limiting, and nondestructive arthralgias or neutrophil-mediated arthritis especially involving the knees and other large joints occurs in 50% of patients. Recurrent superficial or deep migratory thrombophlebitis develops in about 25% and may lead to vena caval obstruction. CNS involvement is less common but may present as chronic meningoencephalitis, small-vessel disease with a multiple sclerosis–like pattern, or paralyzing or life-threatening brain stem and spinal cord lesions. GI manifestations vary from nonspecific abdominal discomfort to abdominal pain and diarrhea with intestinal ulcers resembling Crohn's disease. Generalized vasculitis may cause arterial aneurysms or thromboses at various sites including the lungs. Focal glomerulonephritis is infrequent and usually asymptomatic.

Diagnosis

Behçet's syndrome should be suspected in young adults with recurrent oral aphthous ulcers, unexplained ocular findings, or genital ulcers. Diagnosis is clinical and may require months. International criteria for diagnosis include recurrent oral ulcers and two of the following: recurrent genital ulcers, eye lesions, skin lesions, or a positive pathergy test in the absence of any other clinical explanation. The latter is a papular or pustular reaction to skin puncture with a 20-gauge needle.

Differential diagnosis includes reactive arthritis, Stevens-Johnson syndrome, SLE, Crohn's disease, ulcerative colitis, ankylosing spondylitis, and herpes simplex infection (especially with recurrent aseptic meningitis). Behçet's syndrome has no specific findings that exclude all other possibilities but is often distinguished by its relapsing course and multiple organ involvement. Laboratory abnormalities are nonspecific but characteristic of inflammatory disease (elevated ESR and α_2- and γ-globulins, mild leukocytosis).

Prognosis and Treatment

Behçet's syndrome is generally chronic but controllable; symptoms tend to abate over time. Remission and relapse may last from weeks to years and even extend over decades. However, blindness, vena caval obstruction, and paralysis may complicate the course; the occasional deaths usually are associated with neurologic, vascular (eg, aneurysmal), and GI involvement.

Treatment is symptomatic. Needle punctures provoke inflammatory skin lesions and should be avoided when possible. Colchicine 0.5 mg po bid may decrease the frequency and severity of oral and genital ulcers. Topical corticosteroids may temporarily relieve ocular and most oral disease. However, topical or systemic corticosteroids do not alter the frequency of relapses.

Occasional patients with severe uveitis or CNS involvement respond to high-dose systemic corticosteroids (eg, prednisone 60 to 80 mg po once/day). Patients with posterior uveitis that does not respond to prednisone can be treated with azathioprine 50 to 150 mg po once/day or cyclosporine 5 mg/kg po once/day, increased incrementally if needed to 10 mg/kg once/day until a therapeutic effect is observed; trough levels of cyclosporine should be maintained between 50 and 200 ng/mL (42 and 166 nmol/L). Cyclophosphamide and chlorambucil have been used in refractory disease. Other reported but still incompletely evaluated therapies include interferon-α, thalidomide (in patients with no possibility for pregnancy), pentoxifylline, etanercept, and infliximab.

CHURG-STRAUS DISEASE

(Allergic Angiitis and Granulomatosis)

Churg-Straus disease is a systemic necrotizing vasculitis with granulomas and often affects the lungs. Symptoms may be similar to those of classic polyarteritis nodosa plus pulmonary symptoms. Diagnosis is by biopsy. Treatment is similar to that of polyarteritis nodosa.

Churg-Straus disease (CSD) differs from polyarteritis nodosa in that it frequently involves the lungs, may involve small and large vessels, causes granulomas, and is strongly associated with asthma and eosinophilia. The cause is unknown, but CSD has been precipitated by lowering the dose of corticosteroids in patients taking leukotriene receptor antagonists for asthma. However, eosinophilia and association with asthma suggest that hypersensitivity is involved in its pathophysiology. CSD is uncommon, with about 3 cases/million population. Mean age at onset is 44 yr.

In CSD, granulomas form in vessels and tissues. Eosinophils accumulate in tissues and the blood. Organs and organ systems commonly affected include the lungs, skin, cardiovascular system (eg, coronary artery vasculitis, hypertension), kidneys, peripheral nervous system, and GI tract.

Symptoms, Signs, and Diagnosis

Clinical manifestations are similar to those of polyarteritis nodosa except that lung involvement is often the predominant abnormality. Wheezing is common, dyspnea and cough may occur, and chest x-rays show pulmonary infiltrates.

The diagnosis should be suspected in patients who have wheezing or pulmonary infiltrates and symptoms or signs suggesting vasculitis in other organ systems. CBC with differential and antineutrophil cytoplasmic antibodies (ANCA) should be obtained. More than 80% of patients with CSD have eosinophils ≥ 1000 cells/μL. Some patients have a positive p-ANCA (ANCA that is reactive mainly to myeloperoxidase). ANCA testing can help differentiate CSD from Wegener's granulomatosis, as c-ANCA (ANCA that is reactive mainly to proteinase-3) is typically negative in CSD. The diagnosis of vasculitis is made by biopsy. Prognosis and treatment are similar to those of polyarteritis nodosa, although CSD is generally more responsive to corticosteroids.

HENOCH-SCHÖNLEIN PURPURA

(Allergic or Anaphylactoid Purpura)

Henoch-Schönlein purpura is a vasculitis affecting primarily small vessels that occurs most often in children. Common manifestations include palpable purpura, arthralgias, GI symptoms and signs, and glomerulonephritis. Diagnosis is clinical. Disease is usually self-limited. Corticosteroids can relieve arthralgias and GI symptoms but do not alter the course of the disease. Progressive glomerulonephritis may require high-dose corticosteroids and cyclophosphamide.

Henoch-Schönlein purpura (HSP) is caused by deposition of IgA-containing immune complexes in small arteries of skin and other sites, with consequent activation of complement. Possible inciting antigens include URI viruses, drugs, foods, insect bites, and immunizations. The typical renal lesion is focal, segmental proliferative glomerulonephritis.

Symptoms and Signs

The disease begins with a sudden palpable purpuric rash that typically involves the extensor surfaces of the feet, legs, and arms and a strip across the buttocks. The purpura may start as small areas of urticaria that become indurated and palpable. Crops of new lesions may appear over days to several weeks. Many patients also have fever and polyarthralgia with associated periarticular tenderness and swelling of the ankles, knees, hips, wrists, and elbows. GI manifestations are common and include colicky abdominal pain, abdominal tenderness, and melena. Intussusception occasionally develops. Stool may test positive for occult blood. Symptoms usually remit after about 4 wk but often recur at least once after a disease-free interval of several weeks. In most patients, the disorder subsides without serious sequelae; however, some patients develop chronic renal failure.

Diagnosis, Prognosis, and Treatment

HSP should be suspected in patients, particularly children, with typical skin findings. The clinical diagnosis is confirmed by biopsy of skin lesions, with identification of leukocytoclastic vasculitis with IgA in the vessel walls. Hematuria, proteinuria, and RBC casts indicate kidney involvement. Renal biopsy should be obtained if renal function is deteriorating and may help define the prognosis. Diffuse glomerular involvement or crescentic changes in most glomeruli predict progressive renal failure.

Treatment, except for the elimination of a possible offending drug, is primarily symptomatic. Corticosteroids (eg, prednisone 2 mg/kg up to a total of 50 mg po once/day) may help to control edema, joint pain, and abdominal pain, but their effect on renal involvement is not clear. Nevertheless, immunosuppressive therapy (pulse IV methylprednisolone followed by oral prednisone and cyclophosphamide) can be given to attempt to control inflammation in patients who develop severe renal disease.

MICROSCOPIC POLYANGIITIS

Microscopic polyangiitis is a pauci-immune systemic necrotizing vasculitis that may involve small vessels and may affect the

lungs and kidneys. Diagnosis is by biopsy and measurement of antineutrophil cytoplasmic antibodies. Treatment is similar to that of polyarteritis nodosa.

Microscopic polyangiitis affects arteries but also arterioles, capillaries, and venules. Immune complexes are not involved. Microscopic polyangiitis is more common than polyarteritis nodosa (PAN) but is still uncommon (about 2.4 cases/million). Unlike PAN, microscopic polyangiitis can affect the pulmonary capillaries and commonly produces glomerulonephritis.

Symptoms, Signs, and Diagnosis

Symptoms and signs are similar to classic PAN except that cough and dyspnea are more common. Microscopic polyangiitis is suspected in patients with evidence of systemic necrotizing vasculitis with pulmonary or renal involvement. The presence of vasculitis is diagnosed by biopsy. Microscopic polyangiitis can be distinguished from classic PAN by the absence of immune complex deposition and the additional involvement of small vessels, particular pulmonary capillaries, or glomerulonephritis on biopsy.

Laboratory testing for antineutrophil cytoplasmic antibodies (ANCA) helps differentiate microscopic polyangiitis from PAN and from Wegener's granulomatosis, which can also cause pulmonary and renal vasculitis. ANCA that are based on the reaction to myeloperoxidase and that have staining concentrated around and in neutrophilic nuclei (p-ANCA) are most common in microscopic polyangiitis.

Prognosis and Treatment

Prognosis and treatment are similar to PAN. In critically ill patients, such as those with pulmonary hemorrhage, high-dose IV or oral corticosteroids and IV cyclophosphamide 500 to 750 mg/m^2 once/mo for 6 mo have been used.

POLYARTERITIS NODOSA

(Polyarteritis; Periarteritis Nodosa)

Polyarteritis nodosa, a systemic necrotizing vasculitis, consists of segmental inflammation and necrosis of medium-sized muscular arteries, with secondary tissue ischemia. Symptoms and signs are nonspecific (eg, fever, weight loss, abdominal pain, mononeuritis multiplex, hypertension, edema) and may be acute or chronic. Unusual combinations of symptoms can be a clue. Diagnosis requires biopsy or arteriography. Treatment with corticosteroids and immunosuppressants is often effective.

Polyarteritis nodosa (PAN) is rare; onset is most common between ages 40 and 50 but can occur at any age. It is more common in men.

Etiology and Pathophysiology

The cause is unknown, but immune mechanisms appear to be involved. The variety of clinical and pathologic features suggests multiple pathogenic mechanisms. About 20% of patients have hepatitis B infection. Drugs may be a cause. Usually, no predisposing antigen is incriminated. A systemic vasculitis similar to PAN develops in some patients with certain lymphomas and leukemias.

The characteristic lesion is segmental, necrotizing inflammation of medial and adventitial layers of medium-sized arteries, most commonly at points of vessel bifurcation. Lesions are usually present in all stages of development and healing. Early lesions contain PMNs and occasionally eosinophils; later lesions contain lymphocytes and plasma cells. Intimal proliferation with secondary thrombosis and occlusion leads to organ and tissue infarction. Weakening of the muscular vessel wall may cause small aneurysms and arterial dissection. Healing can result in nodular fibrosis of the adventitia.

Cutaneous, peripheral nerve, hepatic, cardiac, and GI involvement is most frequent. The pulmonary arteries are not involved. Renal lesions are primarily glomerular ischemia and infarction rather than glomerulonephritis. Massive hepatic infarction can develop but is rare; when hepatic infarction develops, PAN is the cause in about 50% of cases. Focal areas of hepatic capsular vasculitis are more common.

Symptoms and Signs

PAN mimics many diseases. The course may be acute and prolonged; subacute and fatal after several months; or insidious, presenting as a chronic debilitating disease. The location and severity of the arteritis and the extent of secondary circulatory impairment largely determine what symptoms develop. Manifestations of PAN commonly predominate in one organ or organ system in any given person.

The most common initial complaints are fever (85%); abdominal pain (65%); symptoms of peripheral neuropathy, often a mononeuritis multiplex (50%); weakness (45%); and weight loss (45%). Hypertension (60%), edema (50%), and oliguria and uremia (15%) may be present in patients with renal involvement. Right upper quadrant abdominal tenderness is common. Diffuse or localized abdominal pain, nausea, vomiting, and bloody diarrhea may reflect organ ischemia, perforation of the bowel or gallbladder, peritonitis, or intussusception. Hemorrhage from the GI tract or into the retroperitoneal space may occur. Angina occurs in 25% of patients, although asymptomatic coronary disease is more common. CNS involvement can produce headache (30%) and seizures (10%). Myalgias with areas of focal ischemic myositis and arthralgias are common; frank arthritis of large joints may occur. Skin lesions, including palpable purpura, palpable subcutaneous nodules along the course of the affected artery, and irregular areas of necrosis, occur in a few patients. Testicular pain is also possible.

Diagnosis

PAN is suspected in patients with unexplained fever, abdominal pain, renal failure, or hypertension; unexplained arthralgia, muscle tenderness or weakness, subcutaneous nodules, purpuric skin rashes, pain in the abdomen or extremities; or rapidly developing hypertension. The diagnosis is usually suggested by the combination of clinical and laboratory features, after other causes have been excluded, and particularly if the illness is multisystem. A systemic illness associated with peripheral, usually multiple, neuritis involving major nerve trunks (eg, radial, peroneal, sciatic) in a bilaterally asymmetric or symmetric fashion (mononeuritis multiplex) also suggests PAN.

Diagnosis requires demonstration of necrotizing arteritis on biopsy or the typical aneurysms in medium-sized arteries on angiography. Blind biopsy is usually futile because of the disease's focal nature; biopsy should target clinical sites of disease. Skin, subcutaneous tissue, sural nerve, and muscle, if suspected of being involved, are preferred to the kidney and liver. Electromyography and nerve conduction studies may help select the site of muscle or nerve biopsy if clinical findings are absent or minimal. The gastrocnemius muscle should not be biopsied unless it is the only symptomatic muscle because of the risk of postoperative venous thrombosis. Testicular biopsy, sometimes advocated because microscopic lesions at this site are frequent, has such a low yield that it should be avoided if other suspected sites are accessible. Renal biopsy in patients with evidence of renal disease and liver biopsy in patients with grossly abnormal liver function tests may only be appropriate if other sites fail to provide diagnostic material. Even without a firm tissue diagnosis, abdominal angiography is diagnostic if typical aneurysms are seen in renal, hepatic, and celiac vessels.

Laboratory tests are nonspecific and not diagnostic. Leukocytosis of 20,000 to 40,000/μL (80% of patients), proteinuria (60%), and microscopic hematuria (40%) are the most frequent abnormalities. Thrombocytosis, markedly elevated ESR, anemia caused by blood loss or renal failure, hypoalbuminemia, and elevated serum immunoglobulins can occur. Measurement of autoantibodies may be necessary to differentiate other connective tissue diseases, but autoantibodies are rarely present in PAN. Liver enzymes are often mildly elevated.

Prognosis and Treatment

Untreated disease (acute or chronic) is usually fatal, often ending in failure of the heart, kidneys, or other vital organs or in GI catastrophe or ruptured aneurysm. Without therapy, 67% of patients die within 1 yr; 88% die within 5 yr. Oliguria and hypertension are ominous findings; renal failure is the cause of death in 65%. Potentially fatal nosocomial or opportunistic infections are common.

Many patients achieve long-term remission with aggressive treatment. Therapy must be vigorous and multifaceted. Any suspected offending agents (including drugs) should be sought and avoided and associated infections treated.

High-dose corticosteroids (eg, prednisone 60 mg po once/day) may prevent progression and induce partial or near-complete remission in about 30% of patients. Because long-term therapy is necessary, adverse effects, including hypertension, which may accelerate preexisting renal damage, often intervene, and the risk of infection is enhanced. The daily dose should be reduced if there is improvement (eg, reduced fever, decreased ESR, improved cardiac and renal function, improved neuropathy, disappearance of cutaneous lesions, or diminished pain).

Long-term hyperadrenocorticism can be minimized by giving corticosteroids in a single morning dose every other day; this may suffice as maintenance therapy but is rarely successful as early treatment.

Immunosuppressants are very commonly used if a patient does not respond to corticosteroids during the first few weeks of therapy or if prohibitively high doses of corticosteroids appear necessary to control disease (by these criteria, most patients qualify). Cyclophosphamide 2 to 3 mg/kg po once/day may be given. Supervision by physicians familiar with its use is important. The dose should generally be adjusted to maintain the peripheral blood WBC count at > 3000/μL. Careful hydration is needed to decrease risks of bladder hemorrhage, cystitis, or bladder cancer. Pulse IV cyclophosphamide may be less toxic but may also be less effective.

Treatment of symptoms and complications may include antihypertensive therapy, careful fluid management, and treatment of renal insufficiency and anemia. Surgical intervention is required if GI involvement leads to intussusception or to mesenteric artery thrombosis and bowel or visceral infarction. In patients with hepatitis B- or C-associated vasculitis, interferon-α and newer antiviral drugs such as lamivudine offer some promise.

POLYMYALGIA RHEUMATICA

Polymyalgia rheumatica is a syndrome closely associated with temporal arteritis. It affects older adults, typically causing severe pain and stiffness in proximal muscles, without weakness or atrophy, and nonspecific systemic symptoms. ESR is usually markedly elevated. Diagnosis is clinical. Treatment with low-dose corticosteroids usually is effective.

Etiology and pathogenesis are unknown. Since polymyalgia rheumatica (PMR) is closely associated with temporal arteritis (TA), some authorities consider the two disorders to be different phases of the same process. PMR appears to be more common than TA. A few patients with PMR develop TA, but 40 to 60% of patients with TA have PMR. Whether the symptoms of PMR result from vasculitis is unclear; they more likely come from low-grade synovitis. PMR usually occurs in patients > 60; the female:male ratio is 2:1.

Symptoms, Signs, and Diagnosis

Onset may be acute or subacute. PMR is characterized by severe pain and stiffness of the neck and pectoral and pelvic girdles; stiffness is particularly severe in the morning or after inactivity. Pain is most often localized to the proximal muscles rather than the joints; symptoms are usually bilateral. Systemic symptoms, such as weight loss, malaise, fever, and depression, are common. PMR does not cause muscle weakness, although pain may limit muscular effort.

PMR should be suspected in older adults with typical symptoms. Establishing the diagnosis requires characteristic symptoms and signs and the exclusion of alternative diagnoses. ESR, CBC, thyroid-stimulating hormone, and CK are usually obtained. In most, the ESR is elevated, often > 100 mm/h, usually > 50 mm/h (Westergren method). Normochromic-normocytic anemia may be present. Electromyography, biopsy, and other tests (eg, rheumatoid factor) are normal in PMR but are sometimes obtained to rule out alternative diagnoses.

PMR is distinguished from RA by the absence of chronic small joint synovitis (although some joint swelling may be present), erosive or destructive lesions, rheumatoid factor, and rheumatoid nodules. PMR is differentiated from polymyositis by normal muscle enzymes, electromyography, and muscle biopsy and by the prominence of pain over weakness. PMR is differentiated from hypothyroidism by normal thyroid function tests and normal muscle enzyme levels. PMR is differentiated from multiple myeloma by the absence of monoclonal gammopathy, and from fibromyalgia by more localized symptoms and a typically elevated ESR.

Because patients with PMR may develop TA, they should be warned to immediately report headache, muscle pain when chewing, and, particularly, visual disturbances.

Treatment

PMR usually responds dramatically to prednisone initiated at 15 to 20 mg po once/day. Patients with suspicion of TA should be given higher doses and undergo temporal artery biopsy. As symptoms subside, corticosteroids are tapered to the lowest effective dose, regardless of ESR. Some patients are able to stop corticosteroids in ≤ 2 yr, whereas others require small amounts for years. NSAIDs are rarely sufficient. In older patients, it is especially important to watch for and treat corticosteroid adverse effects such as diabetes and hypertension. Patients on chronic prednisone should receive a bisphosphonate to prevent osteoporosis.

PREDOMINANTLY CUTANEOUS VASCULITIS

(Leukocytoclastic Vasculitis; Hypersensitivity Vasculitis)

Primarily cutaneous vasculitis is vasculitis that affects mainly small cutaneous vessels, causing skin lesions.

Common causes of predominantly cutaneous vasculitis include serum sickness, infections (eg, hepatitis C), cancers, rheumatologic or other autoimmune disorders, and hypersensitivity to drugs. Systemic vasculitis is possible but generally less severe than with the systemic necrotizing forms of vasculitis. Immune complex deposition probably mediates vessel inflammation. Often, neutrophils fragment (leukocytoclasis) within small vessels, causing leukocytoclastic vasculitis.

Predominantly cutaneous vasculitis can cause a variety of skin lesions, most commonly palpable purpura. There are often systemic symptoms, such as polyarthralgia and fever. Diagnosis is by skin biopsy. Treatment is determined by the underlying cause of the vasculitis. If no cause is identified and severe systemic vasculitis develops, the patient should receive corticosteroids and sometimes immunosuppressants, similar to polyarteritis nodosa.

TAKAYASU'S ARTERITIS

(Pulseless Disease; Occlusive Thromboaortopathy; Aortic Arch Syndrome)

Takayasu's arteritis is an inflammatory disease of unknown cause affecting the aorta and its branches, occurring most often in adolescents and young women. It causes asymmetry of pulses and symptoms and signs of arterial obstruction. Diagnosis is by aortic arteriography or magnetic resonance angiography. Treatment involves corticosteroids and, if tissues are ischemic, vascular interventions such as angioplasty or stenting.

Takayasu's arteritis is uncommon. Although it has been reported worldwide, it shows a predilection for Asians. Female:male ratio is 8:1, and the age of onset is typically between 15 and 30. Inflammation narrows the vessel lumen and can result in thrombosis. In the late stage, weakness of the arterial walls may give rise to aneurysms. Takayasu's arteritis occasionally affects the pulmonary and coronary arteries as well as the aorta and its branches.

Symptoms and Signs

About ½ of patients initially develop malaise, fever, night sweats, weight loss, arthralgias, and fatigue. This phase gradually subsides and is followed by a more chronic stage characterized by focal symptoms resulting from ischemia of aortic branches, usually in its arch and thoracic regions. The other ½ of patients present with only focal symptoms.

Focal symptoms include syncope and transient visual disturbances caused by ischemic attacks in the carotid and vertebrobasilar arteries, along with pain with use of the arms. Muscle atrophy may affect the face and arms. Obstruction in the descending thoracic aorta sometimes produces signs of aortic coarctation. If the abdominal aorta (particularly the renal arteries) is affected, the patient may have renovascular hypertension, which may be severe. Takayasu's arteritis can cause coronary artery inflammation (producing angina or MI), or, infrequently, aortic insufficiency; these sequelae or hypertension can result in heart failure. Rarely, pulmonary artery obstruction leads to pulmonary hypertension.

Signs of arterial obstruction may be absent until blockage becomes severe. When blockage is severe, pulses may be diminished or absent and BP low or unmeasurable in the involved arteries arising from the aortic arch. Unless an acquired coarctation is present, these pulses contrast sharply with the generally brisk pulses and normal BP in the legs. If the arms are severely affected, systemic BP is accurately measured only in the legs. Bruits may be heard over partially narrowed arteries.

Diagnosis

The diagnosis should be suspected in patients who develop symptoms that suggest ischemia of organs supplied by the aorta or its branches or who have decreased or absent peripheral pulses, especially in young Asian women. Arterial bruits and right-left or upper extremity–lower extremity discrepancies in pulses or BP are also suggestive.

Confirmation requires aortic arteriography or magnetic resonance angiography to evaluate all vessel branches. Characteristic findings include stenosis, obstruction, irregularities in vessel lumens, poststenotic dilation, collateral pathways around obstructed vessels, and aneurysms. Laboratory tests are nonspecific and are not necessary; if there is an initial systemic illness, anemia and marked elevation of the ESR are often present.

Prognosis and Treatment

Takayasu's arteritis may rarely spontaneously remit or stabilize. However, major complications (eg, stroke, MI, severe hypertension, heart failure, aneurysm) occur in about 50%. Accelerated atherosclerosis may be a late complication. With treatment, 95% of patients without major complications survive > 5 yr.

Corticosteroids, required for all patients, often dramatically relieve symptoms and may lessen long-term vascular complications. Prednisone 60 mg po once/day is continued until symptoms subside and then tapered 5 mg/day q 2 wk until the dose is 10 mg/day. Treatment may be necessary for many months or years; duration is guided by symptoms, signs, vascular imaging, and ESR, although active disease can be present despite a normal ESR. Methotrexate or other cytotoxic drugs can be added in corticosteroid-resistant cases, but their efficacy is questionable. A platelet inhibitor (eg, aspirin 325 mg once/day) may be helpful. Hypertension should be treated aggressively; ACE inhibitors may be effective because hypertension is frequently renovascular.

Vascular intervention is important in reestablishing blood flow to ischemic tissues. Angioplasty, stenting, or surgery may be effective. Arterial and aortic aneurysms may require surgery.

TEMPORAL ARTERITIS

(Giant Cell Arteritis; Cranial Arteritis)

Temporal arteritis is a chronic inflammatory disease of large blood vessels, particularly the carotid artery and its branches, occurring primarily in older adults. Simultaneous polymyalgia rheumatica is common. Focal symptoms and signs may include headaches, visual disturbances, temporal artery tenderness, and pain in the jaw muscles while chewing. Fever, weight loss, malaise, and fatigue are also common. ESR is typically very high. Diagnosis is most often by biopsy. Treatment with high-dose corticosteroids is usually highly effective and prevents visual loss.

Etiology and pathogenesis of temporal arteritis (TA) are unknown. It is rare in patients < 55 and is slightly more common in women. The prevalence is highest in people of northern European origin and can reach 15 to 25 cases/100,000 population.

Pathology

Vasculitis may be localized, multifocal, or widespread, most often involving temporal, cranial, or other carotid system arteries. Segments of the aorta, its branches, the coronary arteries, and the peripheral arteries may also rarely be affected. The disease tends to affect arteries containing elastic tissue, with granulomatous inflammation primarily of the media; lymphocytes, epithelioid cells, and often giant cells predominate. The elastica is disrupted and the intimal layer is markedly thickened, with narrowing and occlusion of the lumen that can produce ischemia.

Symptoms and Signs

Presentations are diverse, depending on the distribution of the arteritis, but typically include severe, sometimes throbbing headache (especially temporal and occipital), visual disturbances (amaurosis fugax, diplopia, scotomata, ptosis, blurred vision), and pain in the masseter and temporalis muscles on chewing (jaw claudication). Patients may report scalp pain with combing their hair. Systemic symptoms may include fever, fatigue, malaise, unexplained weight loss, and sweats. Patients may also present with symptoms of polymyalgia rheumatica (PMR), carpal tunnel syndrome, radiculopathy, and, rarely, pulse deficits similar to those in Takayasu's arteritis. Blindness caused by ischemic optic neuropathy occurs in ≤ 10% of patients but can occur suddenly and irreversibly. Physical examination may reveal swelling and tenderness with nodularity over the temporal arteries and, rarely, bruits over the large vessels.

Diagnosis

TA should be suspected in patients > 55 with almost any new symptoms or signs compatible with ischemia of an artery above the neck or with jaw pain on chewing, new-onset headaches, or tender temporal arteries. Symptoms of PMR increase suspicion. If the diagnosis is suspected, ESR (or C-reactive protein) and CBC should be obtained. ESR is usually markedly elevated (often > 100 mm/h, Westergren method) during the active phase but is normal in about 1% of patients. C-reactive protein may also be elevated. Normochromic-normocytic anemia is often present. Leukocytosis is common but nonspecific.

TA can be diagnosed clinically on a provisional basis, but the diagnosis should be verified by temporal artery biopsy. A temporal artery that has no tenderness or swelling may be abnormal on biopsy. However, because vasculitis may involve only small segments of the temporal artery, bilateral biopsy with removal of segments of ≥ 2 cm is often recommended to maximize the diagnostic yield. Findings of TA may still be evident even after ≥ 3 days of high-dose corticosteroid treatment, but neither treatment nor biopsy should be delayed.

In patients with pulse deficits, angiography may identify areas of arterial narrowing. If obtained for other reasons, serum alkaline phosphatase may be elevated, and there may be a polyclonal hyperglobulinemia.

Treatment

Treatment should be started as soon as TA is suspected, even if biopsy must be delayed for several days. Treatment almost always prevents blindness. Most patients respond to prednisone 60 mg po once/day for 2 to 4 wk. If symptoms improve, prednisone can be tapered gradually according to individual patient response, usually by 5 to 10 mg/day per wk until reaching 40 mg po once/day, then by 2 to 5 mg/day per wk until reaching 10 to 20 mg po once/day, then by 1 mg/day per wk thereafter.

Although ESR tends to decrease during treatment, normalization is not necessary. Doses of prednisone should not be increased simply based on the ESR. If symptoms flare with tapering, the dose is slightly increased. Some patients can be weaned from prednisone within 1 yr, but many require low doses for years. Azathioprine and methotrexate have occasionally been used in patients with unacceptable corticosteroid adverse effects, although evidence of efficacy is sparse.

WEGENER'S GRANULOMATOSIS

Wegener's granulomatosis is an uncommon disease that usually begins as a localized granulomatous inflammation of upper or lower respiratory tract mucosa and may progress to generalized necrotizing granulomatous vasculitis and glomerulonephritis. Patients may have recurrent nasal discharge or bleeding, lung infiltrates or nodules, hypertension, glomerulonephritis, and manifestations of systemic vasculitis. Diagnosis requires biopsy. Treatment is with cyclophosphamide and corticosteroids.

The cause is unknown, although immunologic mechanisms may play a role. Wegener's granulomatosis occurs in about 1 in 25,000 people, is most common in whites, but can occur in all ethnic groups and at any age. The mean age at onset is 40 yr.

Pathophysiology

Wegener's granulomatosis tends to produce necrotizing vasculitis of small arteries and veins and intravascular and extravascular granulomas. Multinucleated giant cells are present, particularly in the lungs. Although the respiratory tract and kidneys are affected most often, almost any organ can be involved. The nose and nasopharynx can develop inflammation, granulomatous tissue, and necrosis. The lungs typically develop infiltrates and can develop multiple cavities. Kidney involvement usually begins as focal glomerulitis that can progress to crescentic glomerulonephritis. Necrotizing renal vasculitis is possible, but kidney granulomas are uncommon.

Symptoms and Signs

Onset may be insidious or acute, and the full spectrum of the disease may take years to evolve. Presenting complaints, usually referable to the upper respiratory tract, include purulent or bloody nasal discharge, paranasal sinus pain, nasal mucosal ulcerations (with consequent secondary bacterial infection), serous or purulent otitis media, cough, and hemoptysis. Nasal granulomas, which can resemble chronic paranasal sinusitis, can give the nasal mucous membrane a red, raised granular appearance and friable texture. Nasal perforation may occur. Other presenting symptoms include fever, malaise, anorexia, weight loss, migratory polyarthritis, granulomatous or leukocytoclastic vasculitis skin lesions, nasolacrimal duct obstruction, retrobulbar granulomas with proptosis, and episcleritis. Chondritis of the ear pinna and MI from coronary artery vasculitis may occur.

A disseminated vasculitis may develop with constitutional symptoms, pulmonary symptoms such as dyspnea or hemoptysis, necrotizing inflammatory skin lesions, renovascular hypertension, and kidney failure. Occasionally, the disease remains limited to the lungs. Renal involvement is the hallmark of generalized disease. Profound anemia can produce weakness and fatigue.

Diagnosis

Wegener's granulomatosis should be suspected in patients with chronic, unexplained respiratory symptoms and signs, particularly if there are suggestive manifestations in other organ systems, especially the kidney.

Antineutrophilic cytoplasmic antibodies (ANCA) testing and biopsy are most helpful. ANCA with a predominant reaction to proteinase-3 (c-ANCA) are present in about 90% of patients with kidney and respiratory involvement but in only about 70% of patients without kidney involvement. Specificity of c-ANCA for Wegener's granulomatosis is high, but c-ANCA is not diagnostic. Confirmation ideally requires histologic demonstration of necrotizing granulomatous vasculitis in a patient with respiratory manifestations and glomerulonephritis. Nasal and sinus tissues are most accessible but may not yield diagnostic material. Very suspicious lesions may merit first biopsy, but lung biopsy is most likely to show characteristic findings. Lung biopsy should not be long delayed if there is pulmonary involvement; open thoracotomy provides the best access to affected tissue. To assess kidney involvement, urinalysis is obtained to look for proteinuria, hematuria, and RBC casts. Renal biopsy may be necessary if glomerulonephritis is suspected because of hematuria and proteinuria, especially if there is elevation of serum creatinine. However, renal biopsy will not show granulomas, so is less diagnostic than are other biopsies.

Leukocytosis is common. Anemia is common and may be profound. Eosinophilia is uncommon. ESR is elevated when there is active inflammation. Mild hypergammaglobulinemia may be present.

Differential diagnosis includes polyarteritis nodosa, Churg-Strauss disease, microscopic polyangiitis, the vascular renal phase of infective endocarditis, and SLE. Polyarteritis nodosa is unlikely if lung involvement is prominent and ruled out by granulomatous findings on biopsy. Churg-Strauss disease and microscopic polyangiitis are differentiated by their absence of nasal involvement and ANCA that is reactive mainly to myeloperoxidase (p-ANCA). In Churg-Strauss disease, there is also more prominent eosinophilia. Blood cultures and clinical manifestations distinguish infective endocarditis. SLE can usually be differentiated by the presence of antinuclear antibodies and in some cases low serum complement.

Prognosis and Treatment

Patients with relatively limited disease may have nasal and pulmonary lesions with little or no systemic involvement. Pulmonary manifestations may improve or worsen spontaneously. The complete syndrome usually progresses rapidly to renal failure once the diffuse vasculitis begins. Untreated, diffuse vasculitis is rapidly fatal.

Prognosis has been dramatically improved by treatment with immunosuppressants. Early diagnosis and treatment are crucial, because a high remission rate is now possible and renal complications can be avoided or reduced.

Cyclophosphamide (about 2 mg/kg po once/day) is the drug of choice. Careful hydration is needed to decrease risks of bladder hemorrhage, cystitis, and bladder cancer. Corticosteroids, which reduce the vasculitic edema, are given concurrently (prednisone 1 mg/kg po once/day). After 2 to 3 mo, prednisone is tapered until the patient is maintained solely on oral cyclophosphamide (long-term IV dosing of cyclophosphamide appears to be less effective in maintaining remissions). Cyclophosphamide is given for ≥ 1 yr after clinical remission. Daily dose is then decreased by 25 mg q 2 to 3 mo. Disease activity can be assessed by symptoms, signs, chest x-rays, urinalysis, and renal function. C-ANCA may normalize but is not the most important measure to follow. Patients who achieve remission on cyclophosphamide may be maintained on treatment with methotrexate ≤ 20 to 25 mg po once/wk. Azathioprine is a less effective alternative.

To prevent secondary *Pneumocystis* pneumonia, many clinicians use long-term prophylactic trimethoprim-sulfamethoxazole (160/800 mg po once/day).

Long-term complete remission can be achieved, even with advanced active disease.

Kidney transplantation has been successful in renal failure, although a patient who received a cadaver kidney implant developed renal lesions typical of Wegener's granulomatosis. An increased incidence of solid tumors and bladder cancer after many years may reflect high-dose cyclophosphamide use.

34 JOINT DISORDERS

Joint disorders may be inflammatory (rheumatoid arthritis, juvenile rheumatoid arthritis, spondyloarthropathies) or relatively less inflammatory (osteoarthritis, neurogenic arthropathy). Crystal-induced and infectious joint disorders are discussed in Chs. 35 and 39, respectively.

RHEUMATOID ARTHRITIS

Rheumatoid arthritis is a chronic autoimmune disease, producing damage mediated by cytokines, chemokines, and metalloproteases. Peripheral joints (eg, wrists, metacarpophalangeal joints) are symmetrically inflamed, often resulting in progressive destruction of articular structures, usually accompanied by systemic symptoms. Diagnosis requires specific clinical, laboratory, and radiologic criteria. Treatment involves drugs, physical measures, and sometimes surgery. Drug therapy combines NSAIDs, which help reduce symptoms, and disease-modifying antirheumatic drugs, which slow disease progression.

Rheumatoid arthritis (RA) affects about 1% of the population. Women are affected 2 to 3 times more often than men. Onset may be at any age, most often between 35 and 50 yr. Children (see JRA on p. 289) or the elderly can be affected.

Etiology and Pathophysiology

Although RA involves autoimmune reactions, the precise cause is unknown; many factors may contribute. A genetic predisposition has been identified and, in white populations, localized to a shared epitope in the HLA-DR β_1 locus of class II histocompatibility antigens. Unknown environmental factors (eg, viral infections) are thought to play a role, as is cigarette smoking.

Prominent immunologic abnormalities include immune complexes produced by synovial lining cells and in inflamed blood vessels. Plasma cells produce antibodies (eg, rheumatoid factor [RF]) that contribute to these complexes. Macrophages also migrate to diseased synovium in early disease; increased macrophage-derived lining cells are prominent along with vessel inflammation. Lymphocytes that infiltrate the synovial tissue are primarily CD4+ T cells. Macrophages and lymphocytes produce pro-inflammatory cytokines and chemokines (eg, tumor necrosis factors [TNF], granulocyte-macrophage colony-stimulating factor, various interleukins [IL], interferon-γ) in the synovium. Release of inflammatory mediators probably contributes to the systemic and joint manifestations of RA.

In chronically affected joints, the normally thin, delicate synovium thickens and develops many villous folds. The synovial lining cells produce various materials, including collagenase and stromelysin, which contribute to cartilage destruction; IL-1 and TNF-α, which stimulate cartilage destruction, osteoclast-mediated bone absorption, synovial inflammation, and prostaglandins (which potentiate inflammation). Fibrin deposition, fibrosis, and necrosis are also present. Through these inflammatory mediators, hyperplastic synovial tissue (pannus) erodes cartilage, subchondral bone, articular capsule, and ligaments. PMNs often predominate in the synovial fluid.

Rheumatoid nodules develop in about 30% of patients with RA. They are granulomas consisting of a central necrotic area surrounded by palisaded histiocytic macrophages, all enveloped by lymphocytes, plasma cells, and fibroblasts. Nodules and vasculitis can also develop in many visceral organs.

Symptoms and Signs

Onset is usually insidious, beginning with systemic symptoms and progressing to joint symptoms, but symptoms can occur

TABLE 34–1. DIAGNOSING RHEUMATOID ARTHRITIS*

Any 4 criteria must be present to classify patients as having rheumatoid arthritis:

- Morning stiffness for ≥ 1 h†
- Arthritis of ≥ 3 joints†
- Arthritis of hand joints (wrist, metacarpophalangeal, or proximal interphalangeal joints)†
- Symmetric arthritis†
- Rheumatoid nodules
- Serum rheumatoid factor (positive in < 5% of normal control subjects)
- Radiographic changes (hand x-ray changes typical of rheumatoid arthritis must include erosions or unequivocal bony decalcification)

*Based on criteria from the American Rheumatism Association (now the American College of Rheumatology).
†Must be present for ≥ 6 wk.

simultaneously. Systemic symptoms include early morning stiffness of affected joints, generalized afternoon fatigue and malaise, anorexia, generalized weakness, and low-grade fever. Joint symptoms include pain and stiffness.

Joint symptoms are characteristically symmetric. Typically, stiffness lasts > 60 min on rising in the morning but may occur after any prolonged inactivity. Involved joints become quite tender, with erythema, warmth, swelling, and limitation of motion. The wrists and the index and middle metacarpophalangeal joints are most commonly involved. Others include the proximal interphalangeal [PIP], metatarsophalangeal, elbows, and ankles; however, any joint may be involved. The axial skeleton is rarely involved except for the upper cervical spine. Synovial thickening is detectable. Joints are often held in flexion to minimize pain, which results from joint capsular distention.

Fixed deformities, particularly flexion contractures, may develop rapidly; ulnar deviation of the fingers with an ulnar slippage of the extensor tendons off the metacarpophalangeal joints is typical, as are swan-neck and boutonnière deformities (see FIG. 42–2 on p. 331). Joint instability can also occur. Carpal tunnel syndrome can result from wrist synovitis pressing on the median nerve. Ruptured popliteal (Baker's) cysts can develop, producing calf swelling and tenderness suggestive of deep venous thrombosis.

Subcutaneous rheumatoid nodules are not usually an early sign but eventually develop in up to 30% of patients, usually at sites of pressure and chronic irritation (eg, the extensor surface of the forearm). Visceral nodules, usually asymptomatic, are common in severe RA. Other extra-articular signs include vasculitis causing leg ulcers or mononeuritis multiplex, pleural or pericardial effusions, pulmonary nodules, pulmonary fibrosis, pericarditis, myocarditis, lymphadenopathy, Felty's syndrome, Sjögren's syndrome, and episcleritis. Involvement of the cervical spine can produce atlantoaxial subluxation (see p. 328) and spinal cord compression (see p. 1913); it may worsen with extension of the neck (eg, during endotracheal intubation).

The course is unpredictable. The disease progresses most rapidly during the first 6 yr, particularly the first year; 80% of patients develop some permanent joint abnormalities within 10 yr.

Diagnosis

RA should be suspected in patients with polyarticular, symmetric arthritis. Criteria for the diagnosis of RA are listed in TABLE 34–1; presence of ≥ 4 criteria establishes the diagnosis. Patients should have a RF test, hand and wrist x-rays, and baseline x-rays of affected joints to document future erosive changes.

RFs, antibodies to human γ-globulin, are present in about 70% of RA patients. However, RF, often in low titers, occurs in patients with other diseases, including other connective tissue diseases (eg, SLE), granulomatous diseases, chronic infections (eg, viral hepatitis, subacute bacterial endocarditis, TB), and malignancies. Low RF titers can also occur in 3% of the general population and 20% of the elderly. A RF titer measured by latex agglutination of > 1:80 helps confirm RA. RF is now most often measured by nephelometry, with normal ranges that vary according to laboratory.

Anti-citrullinated peptide (anti-CCP) antibodies have high specificity (90%) and sensitivity (96%) for RA. Anti-CCP antibodies are useful in the differential diagnosis of early polyarthritis.

X-rays show only soft-tissue swelling during the first months of disease. Subsequently, periarticular osteoporosis, joint space (articular cartilage) narrowing, and marginal erosions may become visible. Erosions often develop within the first year but may occur any time. MRI appears to be more sensitive and detects earlier articular inflammation and erosions.

If RA is diagnosed, additional tests help detect complications and unexpected abnormalities. CBC with differential should be obtained. A normochromic (or slightly hypochromic)-normocytic anemia occurs in 80%; Hb is usually > 10 g/dL. If Hb is ≤ 10 g/dL, superimposed iron deficiency or other causes of anemia should be considered. Neutropenia occurs in 1 to 2% of cases, often with splenomegaly (Felty's syndrome). Acute-phase reactants (eg, thrombocytosis, elevated ESR, elevated C-reactive protein) reflect disease activity. A mild polyclonal hypergammaglobulinemia often occurs. ESR is elevated in 90% of patients with active disease. Serum complement is normal or elevated.

Synovial fluid examination is necessary in any new onset arthritis or synovial effusion to rule out other disorders and differentiate RA from other inflammatory arthritides (eg, septic and crystal-induced arthritis). In RA, during active joint inflammation, synovial fluid is turbid, yellow, and sterile, with reduced viscosity and usually 10,000 to 50,000 WBCs/μL; PMNs typically predominate, but > 50% may be lymphocytes and other mononuclear cells. WBC cytoplasmic inclusions may be seen on a wet smear but are also present in other inflammatory effusions. Crystals are absent.

Differential diagnosis: Many disorders can simulate RA. Some patients with crystal-induced arthritis may even meet criteria for RA; however, synovial fluid examination should clarify the diagnosis. The presence of crystals makes RA unlikely. Joint involvement and subcutaneous nodules can result from gout, cholesterol, and amyloidosis as well as RA; aspiration or biopsy of the nodules may be needed.

SLE usually can be distinguished if there are skin lesions on light-exposed areas, hair loss, oral and nasal mucosal lesions, absence of joint erosions in even long-standing arthritis, joint fluid that often has < 2000 WBCs/μL (predominantly mononuclear cells), antibodies to double-stranded DNA, renal disease, and low serum complement levels. Arthritis similar to RA can also occur in other connective tissue disorders (eg, polyarteritis, scleroderma, dermatomyositis, or polymyositis), or there can be features of more than one disease, which suggests an overlapping syndrome or mixed connective tissue disease.

Sarcoidosis, Whipple's disease, multicentric reticulohistiocytosis, and other systemic diseases may involve joints; other clinical features and tissue biopsy sometimes help differentiate these conditions. Acute rheumatic fever has a migratory pattern of joint involvement and evidence of antecedent streptococcal infection (culture or changing antistreptolysin-O titer); in contrast, RA has an additive arthritis.

Reactive arthritis (see p. 292) can be differentiated by antecedent GI or GU symptoms; asymmetric involvement of the heel, sacroiliac joints, and large joints of the leg; conjunctivitis; iritis; painless buccal ulcers; balanitis circinata; or keratoderma blennorrhagicum on the soles and elsewhere. Also, serum and joint fluid complement levels are often elevated.

Psoriatic arthritis (see p. 294) tends to be asymmetric and is not usually associated with RF, but differentiation may be difficult in the absence of nail or skin lesions. Distal interphalangeal (DIP) joint involvement and severely mutilating arthritis (arthritis mutilans) can be suggestive. Ankylosing spondylitis (see p. 290) may be differentiated by spinal and axial joint involvement, absence of subcutaneous nodules, and negative RF test.

Osteoarthritis (see p. 294) can be differentiated by the joints involved; the absence of rheumatoid nodules, systemic manifestations, or significant amounts of RF; and synovial fluid WBC counts < 2000/μL.

Prognosis

RA decreases life expectancy by 3 to 7 yr, with heart disease, infection, and GI bleeding accounting for most excess mortality; drug treatment, malignancy, as well as the underlying disease may be responsible.

At least 10% are eventually severely disabled despite full treatment. Whites and women have a poorer prognosis, as do those with subcutaneous nodules, advanced age at disease onset, inflammation in ≥ 20 joints, continued cigarette smoking, high ESR, and high levels of RF.

Treatment

Treatment involves a balance of rest and exercise, adequate nutrition, physical measures, drugs (see p. 286), and sometimes surgery.

Rest and nutrition: Complete bed rest is rarely indicated, even for a short time; however, regular rest should be prescribed. An ordinary nutritious diet is generally sufficient.

Rarely, patients have food-associated exacerbations; no specific foods have been noted to exacerbate RA. Food and diet quackery is common and should be discouraged. Substituting ω-3 fatty acids (in fish oils) for dietary ω-6 fatty acids (in meats) may partially and transiently relieve symptoms by transiently decreasing production of inflammatory prostaglandins.

Physical measures: Joint splinting reduces local inflammation and may relieve severe symptoms. Orthopedic or athletic shoes with good heel and arch support are frequently helpful; metatarsal supports placed posteriorly to painful metatarsophalangeal joints decrease the pain of weight bearing. Molded shoes may be needed for severe deformities. Self-help devices enable many patients with debilitating RA to perform activities of daily living.

Exercise should proceed as tolerated. During acute inflammation, passive range-of-motion exercise helps prevent flexion contractures. However, contractures can be prevented and muscle strength restored more successfully after inflammation begins to subside; active exercise (including walking and specific exercises for involved joints) to restore muscle mass and preserve range of joint motion should not be fatiguing. Flexion contractures may require intensive exercise, casting, or immobilization in progressively more stretched-open positions. Paraffin baths may warm digits and facilitate finger exercise.

Surgery: Surgery must always be considered in terms of the total disease. For example, deformed hands and arms limit crutch use during rehabilitation; seriously affected knees and feet limit benefit from hip surgery. Reasonable objectives for each patient must be determined, and function must be considered. Surgery may be performed while the disease is active.

Arthroplasty with prosthetic joint replacement is indicated if damage severely limits function; total hip and knee replacements are most consistently successful. Prosthetic hips and knees cannot tolerate vigorous activity (eg, competitive athletics). Excision of subluxed painful metatarsophalangeal joints may greatly aid walking. Thumb fusions may provide stability for pinch. Neck fusion may be needed for C1-2 subluxation with severe pain or potential for spinal cord compression. Arthroscopic or open synovectomy can relieve joint inflammation, but only temporarily.

Drugs for Rheumatoid Arthritis

The goal is to reduce inflammation as a means of preventing erosions and progressive deformity. Disease-modifying antirheumatic drugs (DMARDs) are used early, often in combination. Many promising new drugs that appear to slow the progression of RA are available. NSAIDs are of some help for the pain of RA but do not prevent erosions or disease progression. Sometimes, systemic corticosteroids are added to control severe polyarticular symptoms. Intra-articular depot corticosteroids can control severe monarticular or even oligoarticular symptoms.

NSAIDs: Aspirin is no longer used for RA, as effective doses are often toxic. Only one NSAID should be given at a time (see TABLE 34–2), although patients may also take aspirin at ≤ 325 mg/day for its antiplatelet cardioprotective effect. Because the maximal response for NSAIDs can take up to 2 wk, doses should be increased no more frequently than this. Doses of drugs with flexible dosing can be increased until response is maximal or maximum dosage is reached.

NSAIDs can cause peptic ulcer disease and GI bleeding. They should be avoided in patients with symptoms or signs of peptic ulcer disease. Other possible adverse effects include headache, confusion and other CNS symptoms, worsening of hypertension, edema, and decreased platelet adhesiveness. Creatinine levels can rise because of inhibited renal prostaglandins; less frequently, interstitial nephritis can occur. Patients with urticaria, rhinitis, or asthma from aspirin can have the same problems with these other NSAIDs. Agranulocytosis has been reported.

NSAIDs inhibit cyclooxygenase enzymes and thus decrease production of prostaglandins. Some prostaglandins under cyclooxygenase-1 (COX-1) control have important effects in many parts of the body (eg, they protect gastric mucosa and inhibit platelet adhesiveness). Other prostaglandins are induced by inflammation and are produced by cyclooxygenase-2 (COX-2). COX-2 inhibitors, or coxibs (eg, celecoxib), appear to have efficacy comparable to nonselective NSAIDs and are less likely to cause GI toxicity. There is no apparent renal-sparing effect of coxibs. However, recent evidence indicates that some, if not all, coxibs increase the risk of cardiovascular events (eg, MI, stroke) with long-term use. Use of coxibs for long periods or in patients with cardivascular risk factors should be approached cautiously.

Disease-modifying antirheumatic drugs (DMARDs): These agents appear to slow the progression of RA and are indicated

TABLE 34–2. NONSTEROIDAL ANTI-INFLAMMATORY DRUG TREATMENT OF RHEUMATOID ARTHRITIS

DRUG	USUAL DOSAGE	MAXIMUM RECOMMENDED DAILY DOSE
Nonselective		
Diclofenac	75 mg bid or 50 mg tid, 100 mg once/day sustained-release	150 mg
Etodolac	300–500 mg po bid	1200 mg
Fenoprofen	300–600 mg qid	3200 mg
Flurbiprofen	100 mg bid or tid	300 mg
Ibuprofen	400–800 mg qid	3200 mg
Indomethacin	25 mg tid to qid, 75 mg bid sustained-release	200 mg
Ketoprofen	50–75 mg qid, 200 mg once/day sustained-release	300 mg
Meclofenamate	50 mg tid or qid	400 mg
Nabumetone	1000–2000 mg/day in one dose or divided doses	2000 mg
Naproxen	250–500 mg bid	1500 mg
Oxaprozin	1200 mg once/day	1800 mg
Piroxicam	20 mg once/day	20 mg
Sulindac	150–200 mg bid	400 mg
Tolmetin	400 mg tid	1800 mg
COX-2 specific		
Celecoxib	200 mg once/day or bid	400 mg
Meloxicam	7.5 mg once/day	15 mg

in nearly all patients with RA. They differ from each other chemically and pharmacologically. Most take weeks or months to have an effect. About ⅔ of patients improve overall, but complete remissions are uncommon. Many result in evidence of decreased disease activity (eg, decreases in ESR or in erosions on x-ray). They have minimal immediate analgesic effects, so NSAIDs must often be continued. Patients should be fully apprised of the risks of DMARDs and monitored carefully for evidence of toxicity.

Combinations of DMARDs may be more effective than single drugs. For example, hydroxychloroquine, sulfasalazine, and methotrexate together are more effective that methotrexate alone or the other two together.

Methotrexate is a folate antagonist with immunosuppressive effects at high dose. It is anti-inflammatory at doses used in RA. It is very effective and has a relatively rapid onset (clinical benefit often within 3 to 4 wk). It is most often administered as a single oral dose once/wk, starting at 7.5 mg and gradually increased as needed, to a maximum dose of 25 mg. Doses of > 20 mg/wk are best given subcutaneously. Methotrexate should be used with caution in patients with hepatic dysfunction and those with diabetes. Alcohol should be avoided. Dose-related liver fibrosis can develop insidiously and is most often reversible. Bone marrow suppression is possible. Pneumonitis is rare but potentially fatal. Stomatitis and nausea can also develop. Supplemental folate, 1 mg po once/day, may reduce the toxicity of methotrexate. CBC, AST, ALT, alkaline phosphatase, albumin, and creatinine level should be obtained every 6 to 8 wk. A liver biopsy may be needed if liver function tests are persistently twice the upper limit of normal and the patient needs to continue to use methotrexate. Severe relapses of arthritis can occur after withdrawal of methotrexate.

Hydroxychloroquine can also control symptoms of mild or moderate RA. Toxic effects are usually mild and include dermatitis, myopathy, and generally reversible corneal opacity. However, irreversible retinal degeneration has been reported. Funduscopic examination and visual fields should be assessed before and every 6 to 12 mo during treatment. The initial dosage of 400 mg po once/day (eg, with breakfast or dinner) is continued for about 4 to 12 wk and then reduced to 200 mg once/day. The drug should be stopped if no improvement occurs after 9 mo. If improvement is achieved, the dosage is usually maintained at 200 to 400 mg once/day, which can be continued as long as effective.

Sulfasalazine can improve symptoms and slow development of joint damage. It is usually given as enteric-coated tablets, starting with 500 mg as an evening dose and increasing to 500 mg in the morning and 1000 mg in the evening, then increasing to 1000 to 1500 mg bid. Benefit should occur within 3 mo. Toxic effects may include gastric symptoms, neutropenia, hemolysis, hepatitis, and rash. Enteric coating or dose reduction may increase tolerability. CBCs should be obtained after 2 to 4 wk and then about every 12 wk during therapy. AST and ALT should be obtained at about 6-mo intervals and whenever the dose is increased.

Parenteral gold compounds can slow progression of RA. Their use has decreased in recent years because of their toxicity and the availability of more effective drugs. Gold compounds can be given as gold sodium thiomalate IM at weekly intervals: 10 mg the first week, 25 mg the second, and 25 to 50 mg/wk thereafter until a total of 1 g has been given or significant improvement is apparent. When maximum improvement is achieved, dosage is gradually decreased to 50 mg every 2 to 4 wk. Relapse commonly occurs in 3 to 6 mo if no gold is given after remission. Improvement can often be sustained for several years with prolonged maintenance therapy. Auranofin is an oral gold preparation administered as 3 mg bid or 6 mg once/day.

Gold compounds are contraindicated in patients with significant hepatic or renal disease or blood dyscrasia. Common toxic reactions to gold include pruritus, dermatitis, stomatitis, albuminuria with or without a nephrotic syndrome, and bone marrow suppression. Oral gold may induce loose bowel movements. A toxic reaction mandates withholding the drug temporarily or permanently, and sometimes the use of a corticosteroid or chelating drug.

Oral penicillamine improves symptoms and may slow progression. However, it is rarely used because of toxicity and lack of effect.

Corticosteroids: Systemic corticosteroids decrease symptoms more rapidly and to a greater degree than other drugs. They also appear to slow bone erosion. However, they do not prevent joint destruction, and their clinical benefit often diminishes with time. Furthermore, severe rebound follows the withdrawal of corticosteroids in active disease. Because of their long-term adverse effects, many doctors recommend that corticosteroids be given to maintain function only until another DMARD has taken effect.

Corticosteroids may be used for severe joint or systemic manifestations of RA (eg, vasculitis, pleurisy, pericarditis). In general, prednisone should not exceed 7.5 mg po once/day, except in patients with severe systemic manifestations. Large loading doses followed by rapid dose reduction are not generally recommended, nor is alternate-day therapy, because RA is usually too symptomatic on the days corticosteroids are not given. Relative contraindications include peptic ulcer disease, hypertension, untreated infections, diabetes mellitus, and glaucoma. The risk of TB should be considered before corticosteroid therapy is begun.

Intra-articular injections of depot corticosteroids may temporarily help control pain and swelling in one or two particularly painful joints. Triamcinolone hexacetonide may suppress inflammation for the longest time; the dose is adjusted for the joint injected (eg, 10 to 40 mg in a knee). Triamcinolone acetonide and methylprednisolone acetate are also effective. Any single joint should not be injected with a corticosteroid more than 3 to 4 times a year, as too-frequent injections may accelerate joint destruction. Because injectable corticosteroid esters are crystalline, local inflammation transiently increases within a few hours in < 2% of injections. Although infection occurs in only 1:40,000, it must be considered if pain occurs > 24 h after injection.

Cytotoxic or immunosuppressive drugs: Treatment with azathioprine, cyclosporine, or cyclophosphamide provides efficacy similar to DMARDs. However, immunosuppressants are more toxic, particularly cyclophosphamide (for dosing, see p. 278), which can cause bone marrow suppression and increase risk of cancer. Thus, these drugs are used only for patients in whom treatment with DMARDs has failed or to decrease the need for corticosteroids. Azathioprine should be initiated at about 1 mg/kg (50 to 100 mg) po once/day or bid; dosage can be increased by 0.5 mg/kg/day after 6 to 8 wk while monitoring CBC, AST, and ALT, and thereafter at 4-wk intervals to a maximum of 2.5 mg/kg/day. Maintenance should be at the lowest effective dose. Low-dose cyclosporine may also be effective alone or when combined with methotrexate. It may be less toxic than azathioprine and cyclophosphamide. Doses are commonly 50 mg po bid but, to minimize toxic effects on BP, renal function, and the GI tract, should generally not exceed 1.75 mg/kg po bid.

New drugs: Leflunomide interferes with an enzyme involved with pyrimidine metabolism. It is about as effective as methotrexate but is less likely to suppress bone marrow or cause pneumonitis. It can be used with methotrexate. Dose is 20 mg once/day (10 mg once/day if adverse effects occur). The major adverse effects are skin reactions and hepatic dysfunction.

Anakinra is a recombinant IL-1 receptor antagonist. IL-1 is heavily involved in the pathogenesis of RA. Anakinra is administered as a single daily injection 100 mg sc. Injection site reactions are the most common; infection and leukopenia have been reported.

TNF-α antagonists can also retard RA, reducing the progression of erosions and reducing the number of new erosions. Although not all patients respond, many have a feeling of well being, sometimes with the first injection. Inflammation is often dramatically reduced. Etanercept is administered 25 mg sc twice/wk. Infliximab is administered as a 3 mg/kg IV infusion in saline at baseline, 2 wk, and 6 wk; subsequent injections are at 8-wk intervals. Adalimumab is administered as 40 mg sc once every 2 wk. Although there are some differences among agents, the most serious problem is infection, particularly with reactivated TB. Patients should be screened for TB with a chest x-ray or PPD. Other potential problems include abnormal liver function tests, lymphoma, development of antinuclear antibodies with or without SLE, cytopenias, and demyelinating neurologic disorders. They should not be used in patients with coronary artery disease or heart failure. Etanercept, infliximab, and adalimumab can and probably should be used with methotrexate.

JUVENILE RHEUMATOID ARTHRITIS

Juvenile rheumatoid arthritis is a rheumatic disease that begins at or before age 16. Arthritis, fever, rash, adenopathy, splenomegaly, and iridocyclitis are typical of some forms. Diagnosis is clinical. Treatment involves NSAIDs and often disease-modifying antirheumatic drugs.

Juvenile rheumatoid arthritis (JRA) is uncommon. The cause is unknown, but there appears to be a genetic predisposition and an autoimmune pathophysiology. JRA may be similar to adult RA (see p. 283).

Symptoms and Signs

Patients with JRA can have joint stiffness, swelling, effusion, pain, and tenderness. JRA may interfere with growth and development. Micrognathia (receded chin) due to early closure of mandibular epiphyses may occur. Iridocyclitis may develop, which may cause conjunctival injection, pain, and photophobia but can be asymptomatic; scarring and glaucoma with band keratopathy can result. Symptoms and signs of JRA tend to fall into 3 possible patterns.

Systemic onset (Still's disease) occurs in about 20% of patients. High fever, rash, splenomegaly, generalized adenopathy, and serositis with pericarditis or pleuritis are common. These may precede the development of arthritis. Fever (quotidian) is often highest in the afternoon or evening and may persist for up to 2 wk. A transient rash often appears with the fever or may be diffuse and migratory, with urticarial or macular lesions.

Pauciarticular onset is characterized by involvement of ≤ 4 joints. It occurs in about 40% of patients, usually young girls. Iridocyclitis is most common in pauciarticular JRA, developing in nearly 20%. Many affected older boys have the HLA-B27 allele. Most of these boys subsequently develop classic features of one of the spondyloarthropathies (eg, ankylosing spondylitis, psoriatic arthritis, reactive arthritis).

Polyarticular onset involves ≥ 5 joints, often ≥ 20. It occurs in the remaining 40% of patients and is often similar to adult RA. Arthritis tends to be symmetric and develop slowly.

Diagnosis

JRA should be suspected in children with symptoms of arthritis, signs of iridocyclitis, generalized adenopathy, splenomegaly, or unexplained fever lasting more than a few days, or rash. Diagnosis is primarily clinical. Patients suspected of having JRA should be tested for rheumatoid factor (RF), antinuclear antibodies (ANA), and ESR as these tests may be helpful in diagnosing JRA and distinguishing its subtypes. In Still's disease, RF and ANA are absent. In pauciarticular-onset JRA, ANA are present in up to 75%. In polyarticular-onset JRA, RF usually is negative, but in some patients, mostly adolescent girls, it can be positive.

To diagnose iridocyclitis, *slit-lamp examination should be performed, even in the absence of eye symptoms*. A recently diagnosed patient with pauciarticular onset should have an eye examination every 3 to 4 mo, a patient with polyarticular onset about every 6 mo.

Prognosis and Treatment

Complete remissions occur in 50 to 75% of treated patients. Patients with polyarticular onset and a positive RF have a less favorable prognosis.

Similar to the therapy of adult RA patients, disease-modifying antirheumatic drugs (DMARDs), particularly the biologic agents, have dramatically changed the therapeutic approach.

Symptoms may be reduced with NSAIDs. Naproxen 5 to 10 mg/kg po bid, ibuprofen 5 to 10 mg/kg po qid, and indomethacin 0.5 to 1.0 mg/kg po tid are among the most useful. Salicylates are rarely used because of their possible role in causing Reye's syndrome (see p. 2401).

Except for severe systemic disease, systemic corticosteroids can usually be avoided. When necessary, the lowest possible dose is used (eg, oral prednisone, 0.0125 to 0.5 mg/kg qid, or the same daily dose given once or twice per day). Growth retardation, osteoporosis, and osteonecrosis are the major hazards of prolonged corticosteroid use in children. Intra-articular depot corticosteroids can be given, the dosage for children adjusted to their smaller joints.

Methotrexate and hydroxychloroquine are useful DMARDs for polyarticular disease. Adverse effects are monitored as with adults. Bone marrow depression and hepatic toxicity are monitored with CBC, AST, ALT, and albumin. Visual field examinations are necessary with hydroxychloroquine. Occasionally, sulfasalazine is used, especially in cases of suspected spondyloarthropathy. IM gold and penicillamine are rarely used.

Etanercept, used as in adults, blocks tumor necrosis factor (TNF)-α and is often effective; 0.4 mg/kg sc (up to a maximum of 25 mg) is given twice/wk.

Physical therapy, exercises, splints, and other supportive measures help prevent flexion contractures. Adaptive devices can improve function and minimize unnecessary stresses on inflamed joints. Iridocyclitis is treated with ophthalmic corticosteroid drops and mydriatics (see p. 913).

SPONDYLOARTHROPATHIES

Spondyloarthropathies share certain clinical characteristics (eg, back pain, uveitis, GI symptoms, rashes). Some are strongly associated with the HLA-B27 allele. Clinical and genetic similarities suggest that they also share similar causes or pathophysiologies. Rheumatoid factor is negative in the spondyloarthropathies (hence, they are also called the seronegative spondyloarthropathies). They include ankylosing spondylitis, reactive arthritis, psoriatic arthritis, and other disorders.

Ankylosing Spondylitis

Ankylosing spondylitis is a systemic disorder characterized by inflammation of the axial skeleton and large peripheral joints, nocturnal back pain, back stiffness, accentuated kyphosis, constitutional symptoms, and anterior uveitis. Diagnosis requires demonstrating sacroiliitis on x-ray. Treatment is with NSAIDs or tumor necrosis factor antagonists and physical measures that maintain joint flexibility.

Ankylosing spondylitis (AS) is 3 times more frequent in men than in women and begins most often between ages 20 and 40. It is 10 to 20 times more common in 1st-degree relatives of AS patients than in the general population. The risk of AS in 1st-degree relatives with the HLA-B27 allele is about 20%. Increased prevalence of HLA-B27 in whites or HLA-B7 in blacks supports a genetic predisposition. However, the concordance rate in identical twins is only about 50%, suggesting that environmental factors contribute. The pathophysiology probably involves immune-mediated inflammation.

Symptoms and Signs

The most frequent presentation is back pain, but disease can begin in peripheral joints, especially in children and women, and rarely with acute iridocyclitis (iritis or anterior uveitis). Other early symptoms and signs are diminished chest expansion from diffuse costovertebral involvement, low-grade fever, fatigue, anorexia, weight loss, and anemia.

Back pain—often nocturnal and of varying intensity—eventually becomes recurrent. Morning stiffness, typically relieved by activity, and paraspinal muscle spasm develop. A flexed or bent-over posture eases back pain and paraspinal muscle spasm; thus, kyphosis is common in untreated patients. Severe hip arthritis can eventually develop. In late stages, the patient has accentuated kyphosis, loss of lumbar lordosis, and a fixed bent forward posturing, with compromised pulmonary function and inability to lie flat. There may be peripheral potentially deforming joint involvement. Achilles tendinitis can occur.

Systemic manifestations occur in ⅓ of patients. Recurrent, acute anterior uveitis is common but usually self-limited; uncommonly it becomes protracted and severe enough to impair vision. Neurologic signs occasionally result from compression radiculitis or sciatica, vertebral fracture or subluxation, or cauda equina syndrome (see p. 1910). Cardiovascular manifestations can include aortic insufficiency, aortitis, angina, pericarditis, and cardiac conduction abnormalities (which may be asymptomatic). Dyspnea, cough, or hemoptysis can result from nontuberculous fibrosis or cavitation of an upper lobe of the lung; secondary infection with *Aspergillus* can develop. Rarely, AS results in secondary amyloidosis. Subcutaneous nodules do not develop.

Diagnosis

AS should be suspected in patients, particularly young men, with nocturnal back pain and kyphosis, diminished chest expansion, Achilles tendinitis, or unexplained anterior uveitis. A 1st-degree relative with AS should heighten suspicion. Patients should generally be tested with ESR, C-reactive protein, and CBC. IgM, rheumatoid factor (RF), and antinuclear antibodies are only needed if peripheral arthritis suggests other diagnoses. No laboratory test is diagnostic, but results can increase suspicion for the disorder or rule out other disorders than can simulate AS. If, after these tests, AS is still suspected, patients should undergo imaging of the lumbosacral spine; demonstration of sacroiliitis on x-ray confirms the diagnosis.

Alternatively, AS can be diagnosed by the modified New York criteria. Using these criteria, the patient must have radiographic evidence of sacroiliitis and one of the following: (1) restriction of lumbar spinal motion in both the sagittal (looking from the side) and frontal (looking from the back) planes, (2) restriction of chest expansion, adjusted for age, and (3) a history of inflammatory back pain. Historical features that distinguish inflammatory back pain from noninflammatory back pain include onset at ≤ 40 yr, gradual onset, morning stiffness, improvement with activity, and duration ≥ 3 mo before seeking medical attention.

ESR and other acute-phase reactants (eg, C-reactive protein) are inconsistently elevated in patients with active AS. Tests for RF and antinuclear antibodies are negative. The HLA-B27 genetic marker is not of diagnostic value.

The earliest x-ray abnormalities are pseudowidening from subchondral erosions, followed by sclerosis or later narrowing and eventually fusion in the sacroiliac joints. Changes are symmetric. Early changes in the spine are upper lumbar vertebral squaring with sclerosis at the corners, spotty ligamentous calcification; and one or two evolving syndesmophytes. Late changes result in a "bamboo spine" appearance, resulting from prominent syndesmophytes, diffuse paraspinal ligamentous calcification, and osteoporosis; these changes develop in some patients on average over 10 yr.

Changes typical of AS may not become visible on plain x-rays for years. CT and MRI show changes earlier, but there is no consensus regarding their role in routine diagnosis.

A herniated intervertebral disk can cause back pain and radiculopathy similar to AS, but the pain is limited to the spine, usually causes more sudden symptoms, and produces no systemic manifestations or laboratory test abnormalities. If necessary, CT or MRI can differentiate it from AS. Involvement of a single sacroiliac joint suggests a different spondyloarthropathy, possibly infection. Tuberculous spondylitis can simulate AS (see p. 1517).

Diffuse idiopathic skeletal hyperostosis (DISH) occurs primarily in men > 50 yr and may resemble AS clinically and on x-ray. Patients may have some spinal pain, stiffness, and insidious loss of motion. X-ray findings in DISH include large ossifications anterior to spinal ligaments (the calcification appears as if someone poured candle wax in front and on the sides of the vertebrae), bridging several vertebrae and usually affecting the cervical and lower thoracic spine. However, the anterior spinal ligament is intact and frequently bulging, and sacroiliac and spinal apophyseal joints are not eroded. Additional differentiating features are stiffness that is not accentuated in the morning and a normal ESR.

Prognosis and Treatment

AS is characterized by mild or moderate flares of active inflammation alternating with periods of little or no inflammation. Proper treatment in most patients results in minimal or no disability and in full, productive lives despite back stiffness. Occasionally, the course is severe and progressive, resulting in pronounced incapacitating deformities. Prognosis is bleak for patients with refractory uveitis and for the rare patient with secondary amyloidosis.

The goals of treatment are relieving pain, maintaining joint range of motion, and preventing end-organ damage.

NSAIDs reduce pain and suppress joint inflammation and muscle spasm, thereby increasing range of motion, which facilitates exercise and prevents contractures. Most NSAIDs work in AS, and tolerance and toxicity dictate drug choice. The daily dose of NSAIDs should be as low as possible, but maximum doses may be needed with active disease. Drug withdrawal should be attempted only slowly, after systemic and joint signs of active disease have been suppressed for several months.

Sulfasalazine may help reduce peripheral joint symptoms and laboratory markers of inflammation. Dosage should be started at 500 mg/day and increased by 500 mg/day at 1-wk intervals to 1 to 1.5 g bid maintenance. Peripheral joint symptoms may also improve with methotrexate (see under RA on p. 287). Systemic corticosteroids, immunosuppressants, and most disease-modifying antirheumatic drugs have no proven benefit and should generally not be used. There is increasing evidence that the biologic agents (eg, etanercept, infliximab, adalimumab) are effective in the presence of inflammatory back pain.

For proper posture and joint motion, daily exercise and other supportive measures (eg, postural training, therapeutic exercise) are vital to strengthen muscle groups that oppose the direction of potential deformities (ie, the extensor rather than flexor muscles). Reading while lying prone pushing up on the elbows or pillows and thus extending the back may help keep the back flexible.

Intra-articular depot corticosteroids may be beneficial, particularly when one or two peripheral joints are more severely inflamed than others, thereby compromising exercise and rehabilitation. They may also help if systemic drugs are ineffective. Corticosteroids injected into the sacroiliac joints may occasionally help severe sacroiliitis.

For acute uveitis, topical corticosteroids and mydriatics are usually adequate. If severe hip arthritis develops, total hip arthroplasty may improve pain and flexibility dramatically.

REACTIVE ARTHRITIS

Reactive arthritis is an acute spondyloarthropathy that is often related to an infection, usually GU or GI. Common manifestations include asymmetric arthritis of variable severity that tends to affect the lower extremities, constitutional symptoms, enthesitis, tendinitis, and mucocutaneous ulcers, including hyperkeratotic or crusted vesicular lesions (keratoderma blennorrhagicum). Diagnosis is clinical. Treatment involves NSAIDs and sometimes sulfasalazine or immunosuppressants.

Spondyloarthropathy associated with urethritis or cervicitis, conjunctivitis, and mucocutaneous lesions (previously called Reiter's syndrome) is one type of reactive arthritis.

Etiology and Epidemiology

Two forms of reactive arthritis are common: sexually transmitted and dysenteric. The sexually transmitted form occurs primarily in men aged 20 to 40. Genital infections with *Chlamydia trachomatis* are most often implicated. Men or women can acquire the dysenteric form after enteric infections, primarily *Shigella, Salmonella, Yersinia,* or *Campylobacter*. Reactive arthritis probably results from joint infection or postinfectious inflammation. Although there is evidence of microbial antigens in the synovium, organisms cannot be cultured from joint fluid.

The prevalence of the HLA-B27 allele is 63 to 96% vs 6 to 15% in healthy white controls, thus supporting a genetic predisposition.

Symptoms and Signs

Reactive arthritis can range from transient monarticular arthritis to a severe, multisystem disorder. Constitutional symptoms may include fever, fatigue, and weight loss. Arthritis may be mild or severe. Joint involvement is generally asymmetric and oligoarticular or polyarticular, occurring predominantly in the large joints of the lower extremities and in the toes. Back pain may occur, usually with severe disease. Enthesopathy (inflammation at tendinous insertion into bone—eg, plantar fasciitis, digital periostitis, Achilles tendinitis) is common and characteristic. Mucocutaneous lesions—small, transient, painless superficial ulcers—commonly occur on the oral mucosa, tongue, and glans penis (balanitis circinata). Particularly characteristic are vesicles (sometimes identical to pustular psoriasis) of the palms and soles and around the nails that become hyperkeratotic and form crusts (keratoderma blennorrhagicum). Rarely, cardiovascular complications (aortitis, aortic insufficiency, cardiac conduction defects), pleuritis, and CNS or peripheral nervous system symptoms develop.

In reactive arthritis, urethritis develops 7 to 14 days after sexual contact (or occasionally dysentery); low-grade fever, conjunctivitis, and arthritis develop over the next few weeks. Not all features may occur, so incomplete forms need to be considered. In men, the urethritis is less painful and productive of purulent discharge than acute gonococcal urethritis and may be associated with hemorrhagic cystitis or prostatitis. In women, urethritis and cervicitis may be mild (with dysuria or slight vaginal discharge) or asymptomatic. Conjunctivitis is the most common eye lesion. It usually causes eye redness and grittiness, but keratitis and anterior uveitis can develop also, causing eye pain, photophobia, and tearing.

Diagnosis

Reactive arthritis should be suspected in patients with acute, asymmetric arthritis affecting the large joints of the lower extremities or toes, particularly if there is tendinitis or a history of an antecedent diarrhea or dysuria. Diagnosis is ultimately clinical and requires the typical peripheral arthritis with symptoms of GU or GI infection or one of the other extra-articular features. Because these may manifest at different times, definitive diagnosis may require several months. Serum and synovial fluid complement levels are high, but these findings are not usually diagnostic and need not be measured except to rule out other disorders.

Disseminated gonococcal infection can closely simulate reactive arthritis (see p. 1653). Arthrocentesis may fail to differentiate them, owing to inflammatory characteristics of synovial fluid in both disorders and the difficulty of culturing gonococci from this fluid. Clinical characteristics may help; disseminated gonococcal infection tends to involve upper and lower extremities equally, be more migratory, tends not to produce back pain, and vesicles tend not to be hyperkeratotic. A positive gonococcal culture from blood or skin lesions helps differentiate the two disorders, but a positive culture from the urethra or cervix does not. If differentiation is still difficult, ceftriaxone may be required for simultaneous diagnosis and treatment.

Psoriatic arthritis can simulate reactive arthritis, producing similar skin lesions, uveitis, and asymmetric arthritis. Psoriatic arthritis, however, often affects mostly the upper extremities and especially the distal interphalangeal joints, may be abrupt in onset but may also develop gradually, produces less enthesopathy, and tends not to produce mouth ulcers or symptoms of GU or GI infection.

Prognosis and Treatment

Reactive arthritis often resolves in 3 to 4 mo, but up to 50% of patients experience recurrent or prolonged symptoms over several years. Joint, spinal, or sacroiliac inflammation or deformity may occur with chronic or recurrent disease. Some patients are disabled.

NSAIDs (eg, indomethacin 25 to 50 mg po tid) usually help relieve symptoms. If induced by infection with *C. trachomatis*, doxycycline 100 mg po bid for up to 3 mo may accelerate recovery, but this is controversial. Sulfasalazine as used to treat RA may also be helpful (see p. 288). If symptoms are severe despite NSAIDs and sulfasalazine, azathioprine or methotrexate may be considered. Systemic corticosteroids have no proven value.

Local injection of depot corticosteroids for enthesopathy or resistant oligoarthritis may relieve symptoms. Physical therapy aimed at maintaining joint mobility is helpful during the recovery phase. Anterior uveitis is treated as usual, with corticosteroid and mydriatic eye drops. Conjunctivitis and mucocutaneous lesions require only symptomatic treatment.

Psoriatic Arthritis

Psoriatic arthritis is a chronic inflammatory arthritis that occurs in people with psoriasis of the skin or nails. The arthritis is often asymmetric, and some forms involve the distal interphalangeal joints. Diagnosis is clinical. Treatment is usually similar to that of RA but can also involve etretinate or phototherapy.

Psoriatic arthritis develops in 5 to 40% of psoriasis patients. Prevalence is increased in AIDS patients. Risk for some involvement is increased in patients with HLA-B27 or some other specific alleles and in family members. Etiology and pathophysiology are unknown.

Symptoms and Signs

Psoriasis of the skin or nails may precede or follow joint involvement. Skin lesions may be hidden in the scalp, gluteal folds, or umbilicus and go unrecognized by the patient.

The distal interphalangeal (DIP) joints of fingers and toes are especially affected. Asymmetric involvement of large and small joints, including the sacroiliacs and spine, is common. Joint and skin symptoms may improve or worsen simultaneously. Rheumatoid nodules are absent. Arthritic remissions tend to be more frequent, rapid, and complete than in RA, but progression to chronic arthritis and crippling may occur. There may be arthritis mutilans (destruction of multiple hand joints with telescoping of the digits).

Back pain may be present. It is often accompanied by asymmetric syndesmophytes of the spine.

Diagnosis

Psoriatic arthritis should be suspected in patients with both psoriasis and arthritis. Because psoriasis may be overlooked or hidden or develop only after arthritis occurs, psoriatic arthritis should be considered in any patient with seronegative inflammatory arthritis; these patients should be examined for psoriasis and nail pitting and should be questioned about a family history of psoriasis. Patients suspected of having psoriatic arthritis should be tested for rheumatoid factor, which can coexist. Psoriatic arthritis is diagnosed clinically and by excluding other disorders that can cause such similar manifestations. X-ray findings common in psoriatic arthritis include DIP involvement, resorption of terminal phalanges, arthritis mutilans, and extensive destruction and dislocation of large and small joints.

Treatment

Treatment is directed at control of skin lesions (see p. 966) and at joint inflammation. Drug therapy is similar to that for RA, particularly methotrexate. Hydroxychloroquine is inconsistently of benefit and may cause exfoliative dermatitis or aggravate underlying psoriasis. Benefit may be gained from NSAIDs, cyclosporine and gold, TNF antagonists (see p. 289 under Drugs for RA) have been particularly effective.

Phototherapy using long-wave ultraviolet-A light with psoralen (PUVA) combined with oral methoxsalen 600 μg/kg po 2 h before PUVA twice/wk appears to be highly effective for psoriatic lesions and somewhat effective for peripheral arthritis, but not for spine involvement.

Other Spondyloarthropathies

Spondyloarthropathy can develop in association with GI conditions (sometimes called enteropathic arthritis), such as inflammatory bowel disease, intestinal bypass surgery, or Whipple's disease. Juvenile-onset spondyloarthropathy is an asymmetric, mostly lower extremity spondyloarthropathy that begins most commonly in boys aged 7 to 16. Spondyloarthropathy can also develop in people without characteristics of other specific spondyloarthropathies (undifferentiated spondyloarthropathy). Treatment of the arthritis of these other spondyloarthropathies is similar to that of treatment of reactive arthritis (see p. 293).

OSTEOARTHRITIS

(Degenerative Joint Disease; Osteoarthrosis; Hypertrophic Osteoarthritis)

Osteoarthritis is a chronic arthropathy of an entire joint characterized by disruption and potential loss of joint cartilage along with other joint changes, including bone hypertrophy (osteophyte formation). Symptoms include gradually developing pain aggravated or triggered by activity, stiffness relieved < 30 min after activity, and occasional

joint swelling. Diagnosis is confirmed by x-rays. Treatment involves physical measures (including rehabilitation), drugs, and surgery.

Osteoarthritis (OA), the most common joint disorder, often becomes symptomatic in the 40s and 50s and is nearly universal by age 80. Only half of those with pathologic changes of OA have symptoms. Below age 40, most OA is in men and results from trauma. Women predominate from age 40 to 70, after which men and women are equally affected.

Classification

OA is classified as primary (idiopathic) or secondary to some known cause. Primary OA may be localized to certain joints (eg, chondromalacia patellae is a mild OA that occurs in young people). If primary OA involves multiple joints, it is classified as primary generalized OA. Primary OA is usually subdivided by the site of involvement (eg, hands and feet, knee, hip). Secondary OA appears to result from conditions that change the microenvironment of the cartilage. These include significant trauma; congenital joint abnormalities; metabolic defects (eg, hemochromatosis, Wilson's disease); postinfectious arthritis, endocrine, and neuropathic diseases; and disorders that alter the normal structure and function of hyaline cartilage (eg, RA, gout, chondrocalcinosis).

Pathophysiology

Normal joints have little friction with movement and do not wear out with typical use, overuse, or trauma. Hyaline cartilage is avascular, aneural, and alymphatic. It is 95% water and extracellular cartilage matrix and only 5% chondrocytes. Chondrocytes have the longest cell cycle in the body (similar to CNS and muscle cells). Cartilage health and function depend on compression and release of weight bearing and use (ie, compression pumps fluid from the cartilage into the joint space and into capillaries and venules, whereas release allows the cartilage to reexpand, hyperhydrate, and absorb necessary nutrients).

OA begins with tissue damage from mechanical injury (eg, torn meniscus), transmission of inflammatory mediators from the synovium into cartilage, or defects in cartilage metabolism. The tissue damage stimulates chondrocytes to attempt repair, which increases production of proteoglycans and collagen. However, production of the enzymes that degrade cartilage, as well as inflammatory cytokines, which are normally present in small amounts, also increases. Inflammatory mediators trigger an inflammatory cycle that further stimulates the chondrocytes and synovial lining cells, eventually breaking down the cartilage. Chondrocytes undergo programmed cell death (apoptosis). Once cartilage is destroyed, exposed bone becomes eburnated and sclerotic.

All joint tissues become involved in OA. Subchondral bone stiffens, then undergoes infarction, becomes osteoporotic, and develops subchondral cysts. Attempts at bony repair produce subchondral sclerosis and osteophytes at the joint margins. The osteophytes seem to develop in an attempt to stabilize the joint. The synovium becomes inflamed and thickened and produces synovial fluid with less viscosity and greater volume. Periarticular tendons and ligaments become stressed, resulting in tendinitis and contractures. As the joint becomes less mobile, surrounding muscles thin and become less supportive. Menisci fissure and may fragment.

OA of the spine can, at the disk level, produce marked thickening and proliferation of the posterior longitudinal ligaments, resulting in transverse bars that encroach on the anterior spinal cord; hypertrophy and hyperplasia of the ligamenta flava often compress the posterior cord. In contrast, the anterior and posterior nerve roots, ganglia, and common spinal nerve are relatively well protected in the intervertebral foramina, where they occupy only 25% of the available and well-cushioned space.

Symptoms and Signs

Onset is most often gradual, usually beginning with one or a few joints. Pain is the earliest symptom, sometimes described as a deep ache. Pain is usually worsened by weight bearing and relieved by rest but can eventually become constant. Stiffness follows awakening or inactivity but lasts < 30 min and lessens with movement. As OA progresses, joint motion becomes restricted, and tenderness and crepitus or grating sensations appear. Proliferation of cartilage, bone, ligament, tendon, capsules, and synovium, along with varying amounts of joint effusion, ultimately produce the joint enlargement characteristic of OA. Flexion contractures may eventually develop. Acute and severe synovitis is uncommon.

The joints most often affected in generalized OA include the distal interphalangeal (DIP) and proximal interphalangeal (PIP) (joints) (producing Heberden's and Bouchard's nodes), thumb carpometacarpal joint, intervertebral disks and zygapophyseal joints in the cervical and lumbar vertebrae, 1st metatarsophalangeal joint, hip, and knee.

Cervical and lumbar spinal OA may lead to myelopathy or radiculopathy. However, the clinical signs of myelopathy are usually mild. Radiculopathy can be prominent but is less common because the nerve roots and ganglia are well protected. Insufficiency of the vertebral arteries, infarction of the spinal cord, and esophageal compression by osteophytes occasionally occur. Symptoms and signs may also derive from subchondral bone, ligamentous structures, synovium, periarticular bursae, capsules, muscles, tendons, disks, and periosteum, all of which are pain sensitive. Venous pressure may increase within the subchondral bone marrow and cause pain (sometimes called "bone angina").

Hip OA causes gradual loss of range of motion. Pain may be felt in the inguinal area or trochanter or referred to the knee. As cartilage is lost in knee OA (medial loss occurs in 70% of cases), the ligaments become lax and the joint becomes less stable, with local pain arising from the ligaments and tendons.

Tenderness on palpation and pain on passive motion are relatively late signs. Muscle spasm and contracture add to the pain. Mechanical block by intra-articular loose bodies or abnormally placed menisci can occur and cause locking or catching. Deformity and subluxations can also develop.

Erosive OA produces synovitis and cysts in the hand. It primarily affects the DIP or PIP joints. The thumb carpometacarpal joints are involved in 20% of hand OA, but the metacarpophalangeal joints and wrists are usually spared.

Diagnosis

OA should be suspected in patients with gradual onset of symptoms and signs, particularly in older adults. If OA is suspected, plain x-rays should be obtained of the most symptomatic joints. X-rays generally reveal marginal osteophytes, narrowing of the joint space, increased density of the subchondral bone, subchondral cyst formation, bony remodeling, and joint effusions. Standing x-rays of knees are more sensitive to joint space narrowing.

Laboratory studies are normal in OA but may be required to rule out other disorders (eg, RA) or to diagnose an underlying disorder causing secondary OA. If OA causes joint effusions, synovial fluid analysis can sometimes differentiate it from inflammatory arthritides; in OA, synovial fluid is usually clear, viscous, and has ≤ 2000 WBC/μL.

OA involvement outside the usual joints suggests secondary OA; further evaluation may be required to determine the underlying primary disorder (eg, endocrine, metabolic, neoplastic, biomechanical disorders).

Prognosis and Treatment

OA is usually sporadically progressive but occasionally, with no predictability, stops or reverses. Treatment goals are relieving pain, maintaining joint flexibility, and optimizing joint and overall function. Primary treatments include physical measures that involve rehabilitation; support devices; exercise for strength, flexibility, and endurance; and modifications in activities of daily living. Adjunctive therapies include drug treatment and surgery.

Rehabilitation techniques are best begun before disability develops. Exercises (range of motion, isometric, isotonic, isokinetic, postural, strengthening—see p. 2749) maintain healthy cartilage and range of motion and increase the capacity for tendons and muscles to absorb stress during joint motion. Exercise can sometimes arrest or even reverse hip and knee OA. Stretching exercises should be performed daily. Immobilization for any prolonged period of time can promote contractures and worsen the clinical course. However, a few minutes of rest (q 4 to 6 h in the daytime) can help if balanced with exercise and use.

Modifying activities of daily living can help. For example, a patient with lumbar spine, hip, or knee OA should avoid soft deep chairs and recliners from which posture is poor and rising is difficult. The regular use of pillows under the knees encourages contractures and should also be avoided. Patients should sit in straight-back chairs without slumping, sleep on a firm bed, perhaps with a bed board, use a car seat shifted forward and designed for comfort, perform postural exercises, wear well-supported shoes or athletic shoes, and continue employment and physical activity.

Drug therapy is an adjunct to the physical program. Acetaminophen in doses of up to 1 g po qid may relieve pain and is safe. More potent analgesia may be required.

NSAIDs, including cyclooxygenase-2 (COX-2) inhibitors or coxibs, may be considered if patients have refractory pain or signs of inflammation (eg, redness, warmth). NSAIDs may be used simultaneously with other analgesics (eg, tramadol, opioids) to provide better relief of symptoms.

Muscle relaxants (usually in low doses) occasionally relieve pain that arises from muscles strained by attempting to support OA joints. In the elderly, however, they tend to cause more adverse effects than relief.

Oral corticosteroids have no role. However, intra-articular depot corticosteroids help relieve pain and increase joint flexibility when effusions or signs of inflammation are present; these drugs should not be used more than 4 times a year in any given joint.

Synthetic hyaluronans (similar to hyaluronic acid, a normal component of the joint) can be injected into the knee, with pain relief for prolonged periods of time (up to a year). The treatment is a series of 3 to 5 weekly injections.

In OA of the spine, knee, or thumb carpometacarpal joint, various supports can relieve pain and increase function, but to preserve flexibility, they should be accompanied by specific exercise programs. In erosive OA, range-of-motion exercises performed in warm water can help prevent contractures. Other adjunctive measures can relieve pain, including acupuncture, transcutaneous electrical nerve stimulation, and local rubs (eg, with capsaicin). Laminectomy, osteotomy, and total joint replacement should be considered if all nonsurgical approaches fail.

Glucosamine sulfate 1500 mg once/day has been suggested to relieve pain and slow joint deterioration; chondroitin sulfate 1200 mg once/day has also been suggested for pain relief. They are under evaluation. Experimental therapies that may preserve cartilage or allow chondrocyte grafting are being studied.

NEUROGENIC ARTHROPATHY

(Neuropathic Arthropathy; Charcot's Joints)

Neurogenic arthropathy is a rapidly destructive arthropathy due to impaired pain perception and position sense, which can result from various underlying disorders, most commonly diabetes and stroke. Common manifestations include joint swelling, effusion, deformity, and instability. Pain may be disproportionately mild due to the underlying neuropathy. Diagnosis requires x-ray confirmation. Treatment consists of joint immobilization, which slows disease progression, and sometimes surgery, if the disease is advanced.

Pathophysiology

TABLE 34–3 lists conditions that predispose to neurogenic arthropathy. Impaired deep pain sensation or proprioception affects the joint's normal protective reflexes, often allowing trauma (especially repeated minor episodes) and small periarticular fractures to pass unrecognized. Increased bone blood flow from reflex vasodilation, resulting in active bone resorption, contributes to bone and joint damage. Each new injury sustained by the joint causes more distortion as it heals. Hemorrhagic joint effusions and multiple small fractures can occur, accelerating disease progression. Ligamentous laxity, muscular hypotonia, and rapid destruction of joint cartilage are common, predisposing to joint dislocations, which also accelerate disease progression. Advanced neurogenic arthropathy can cause hypertrophic changes, destructive changes, or both.

Symptoms and Signs

Arthropathy does not usually develop until years after onset of the neurologic condition but can then progress rapidly and lead to complete joint disorganization in a few months. Pain is a common early symptom. However, because the ability to sense pain is commonly impaired, the degree of pain is often unexpectedly mild for the degree of joint damage. A prominent, often hemorrhagic, effusion and subluxation and instability of the joint are usually present during early stages. Acute joint dislocation sometimes occurs also.

During later stages, pain may be more severe if the disease has caused rapid joint destruction (eg, periarticular fractures or tense hematomas). During advanced stages, the joint is swollen from bony overgrowth and massive synovial effusion. Deformity results from dislocations and displaced fractures. Fractures and bony healing may produce many loose pieces of cartilage or bone that can slough into the joint, producing a coarse, grating, often audible crepitus usually more unpleasant for

TABLE 34–3. CONDITIONS UNDERLYING NEUROGENIC ARTHROPATHY

Condition
Amyloid neuropathy (secondary amyloidosis)
Arnold-Chiari malformation
Congenital insensitivity to pain
Degenerative spinal disease with nerve root compression
Diabetes mellitus
Familial-hereditary neuropathies:
Familial amyloid polyneuropathy
Familial dysautonomia (Riley-Day syndrome)
Hereditary sensory neuropathy
Hypertrophic interstitial neuropathy (Dejerine-Sottas disease)
Peroneal muscular atrophy (Charcot-Marie-Tooth disease)
Gigantism with hypertrophic neuropathy
Leprosy
Spina bifida with meningomyelocele (in children)
Subacute combined degeneration of the spinal cord
Syringomyelia
Tabes dorsalis
Tumors and injuries of the peripheral nerves and spinal cord

the observer than for the patient. The joint may feel like a "bag of bones."

Although many joints can be involved, the knee and the ankle are most often affected. Distribution depends largely on the underlying disease. Thus, tabes dorsalis affects the knee and hip, and diabetes mellitus affects the foot and ankle. Syringomyelia commonly affects the spine and upper limb joints, especially the elbow and shoulder. Frequently, only one joint is affected and usually no more than two or three (except for the small joints of the feet), in an asymmetric distribution.

Infectious arthritis may develop with or without systemic symptoms (eg, fever, malaise), particularly with diabetes. Structures such as blood vessels, nerves, and the spinal cord can become compressed due to the tissue overgrowth.

Diagnosis

The diagnosis should be considered in a patient with a predisposing neurologic disorder who develops a destructive but unexpectedly painless arthropathy, usually several years after the onset of the underlying neurologic condition. If neurogenic arthropathy is suspected, x-rays should be obtained. Diagnosis is established by characteristic x-ray abnormalities in a patient with a predisposing condition and typical symptoms and signs.

X-ray abnormalities in early neurogenic arthropathy are often similar to those in OA. The cardinal signs are bone fragmentation, bone destruction, new bone growth, and loss of joint space. There may also be synovial effusion and joint subluxation. Later, the bones are deformed, and new bone forms adjacent to the cortex, starting within the joint capsule and often extending up the shaft, particularly in long bones. Rarely, calcification and ossification occur in the soft tissues. Large, bizarrely shaped osteophytes may be present at the joint margins or within joints. Large curved ("parrot's beak") osteophytes frequently develop in the spine in the absence of clinical spinal disease.

In its early stages, neurogenic arthropathy can simulate OA. However, neurogenic arthropathy progresses more rapidly than OA and frequently causes proportionately less pain.

Prevention and Treatment

Prevention of arthropathy may be possible in a patient at risk. Early diagnosis of asymptomatic or minimally symptomatic fractures facilitates early treatment; immobilization (with splints, special boots, or calipers) protects the joint from further injury, possibly stopping disease evolution. Treatment of the underlying neurologic condition may slow progression of the arthropathy and, if joint destruction is still in the early stages, partially reverse the process. For a grossly disorganized joint, arthrodesis using internal fixation, compression, and an adequate bone graft may be successful. For grossly disorganized hip and knee joints, if neurogenic arthropathy is not expected to be progressive, good results can be obtained with total hip and knee replacements. However, loosening and dislocation of the prosthesis are major hazards.

35 CRYSTAL-INDUCED ARTHRITIDES

Arthritis can result from intra-articular deposition of crystals: monosodium urate, Ca pyrophosphate dihydrate, apatite (basic Ca phosphate), and, rarely, others such as Ca oxalate crystals. Diagnosis requires synovial fluid analysis (see p. 254). Polarized light microscopy is used to specifically identify most crystals; basic Ca phosphate crystals are of ultramicroscopic size and require other methods. Crystals may be engulfed in WBCs or may be extracellular. The presence of crystals does not exclude the possibility of simultaneous infectious or other inflammatory forms of arthritis.

GOUT

Gout is precipitation of monosodium urate crystals into tissue, usually in and around joints, most often causing recurrent acute or chronic arthritis. Acute arthritis is initially monarticular and often involves the first metatarsophalangeal joint; symptoms include acute pain, tenderness, warmth, redness, and swelling. Diagnosis requires identification of crystals in synovial fluid. Treatment of acute attacks is with anti-inflammatory drugs. Attacks are prevented with NSAIDs and/or colchicine, and, for persistent hyperuricemia, allopurinol or uricosuric drugs.

Etiology and Pathophysiology

The greater the degree and duration of hyperuricemia, the greater is the likelihood and the more severe are the symptoms. Urate levels can be elevated because of decreased excretion, increased production, or increased purine intake. Why only some people with elevated serum uric acid (urate) levels develop gout is not known.

Decreased renal excretion is by far the most common cause of hyperuricemia. It may be hereditary and also occurs in patients receiving chronic diuretics and in those with diseases that decrease GFR. Ethanol increases purine catabolism in the liver and increases the formation of lactic acid, which blocks urate secretion by the renal tubules. Cyclosporine, usually given to transplant patients, irreversibly damages renal tubules, leading to urate retention.

Increased urate production may be caused by increased nucleoprotein turnover in hematologic conditions (eg, lymphoma, leukemia, hemolytic anemia) and in conditions with increased rates of cellular proliferation and cell death (eg, psoriasis, cytotoxic cancer therapy). Increased urate production may also occur as a primary hereditary abnormality. In most cases, the cause is unknown, but a few cases are attributable to enzyme abnormalities; deficiency of hypoxanthine-guanine phosphoribosyltransferase (complete deficiency is Lesch-Nyhan syndrome) is a possible cause, as is overactivity of phosphoribosylpyrophosphate synthetase.

Increased intake of purine-rich foods (eg, liver, kidney, anchovies) can contribute to hyperuricemia. However, a strict low-purine diet lowers plasma urate by only about 1 mg/dL.

Urate precipitates as needle-shaped monosodium urate (MSU) crystals, which are deposited extracellularly in avascular tissues (eg, cartilage) or in relatively avascular tissues (eg, tendons, tendon sheaths, ligaments, walls of bursae) around cooler distal joints and tissues (eg, ears). In severe, long-standing hyperuricemia, MSU crystals may be deposited in larger central joints and in the parenchyma of organs such as the kidney. At the acid pH of urine, urate precipitates readily as small platelike or irregular crystals that may aggregate to form gravel or stones, which may cause obstruction. Tophi are MSU crystal aggregates that most often develop in joint and cutaneous tissue.

Acute gouty arthritis may follow medical stress (eg, infection, vascular occlusion, minor trauma, surgery), fatigue, emotional stress, use of thiazide diuretics or drugs with uricosuric activity (eg, allopurinol), or indulgence in purine-rich food or alcohol. Attacks are often precipitated by a sudden increase or, more commonly, a sudden decrease in plasma urate levels. Tophi in and around joints can limit motion and cause deformities, producing chronic tophaceous gouty arthritis.

Symptoms and Signs

Acute gouty arthritis usually begins with sudden onset of pain (often nocturnal). The metatarsophalangeal joint of a great toe is most often involved (podagra), but the instep, ankle, knee, wrist, and elbow are also common sites. Rarely, the hip, shoulder, sacroiliac, sternoclavicular, or cervical spine joints are involved. The pain becomes progressively more severe, usually over a few hours, and is often excruciating. Swelling, warmth, redness, and exquisite tenderness may suggest infection. The overlying skin may become tense, warm, shiny, and red or purplish. Fever, tachycardia, chills, and malaise sometimes occur.

The first few attacks usually affect only a single joint and last only a few days. Later attacks may affect several joints simultaneously or sequentially and persist up to 3 wk if untreated. Subsequent attacks develop after progressively shorter symptom-free intervals. Eventually, several attacks may occur each year.

Tophi develop most often in patients with chronic gout, but they can occur in patients who have never had acute gouty arthritis. They are usually firm yellow or white papules or nodules, single or multiple. They can develop in various locations, commonly the fingers, hands, feet, and around the olecranon or Achilles tendon. Patients with osteoarthritic Heberden's nodes often develop tophi in the nodes. This occurs often in elderly women taking diuretics. Normally painless, tophi, especially in the olecranon bursae, can become acutely inflamed and painful. Tophi may even erupt through the skin, discharging chalky masses of urate crystals. Tophi may eventually cause deformities.

Chronic gouty arthritis can cause pain, deformity, and limited joint motion similar to RA. However, in RA, all affected joints flare and subside together, whereas in gout, inflammation can be flaring in some joints while subsiding in others. About 20% of patients with gout develop urolithiasis with uric acid stones or Ca oxalate stones. Complications include obstruction and infection, with secondary tubulointerstitial disease. Untreated progressive renal dysfunction, most often related to coexisting hypertension or, less often, some other cause of nephropathy, further impairs excretion of urate, accelerating crystal deposition in tissues.

Diagnosis

Gout should be suspected in patients with acute monarticular or oligoarthritis, particularly older adults or those with other risk factors. Podagra is particularly suggestive. Similar symptoms can result from infectious arthritis (see p. 312) and Ca pyrophosphate dihydrate (CPPD) crystal deposition disease (see p. 303). CPPD generally attacks larger joints and its clinical course is usually milder. Acute rheumatic fever with joint involvement and juvenile RA may simulate gout but occur mostly in young people, who rarely get gout. Acute fracture in patients unable to provide a history of injury also may be confused with gout.

Patients suspected of acute gouty arthritis should have arthrocentesis and synovial fluid analysis on initial presentation. A typical recurrence in a patient with known gout does not mandate arthrocentesis, but it should be performed if there is any question of the diagnosis. Synovial fluid analysis can confirm the diagnosis by identifying needle-shaped, strongly negatively birefringent urate crystals that are free in the fluid or engulfed by phagocytes. Synovial fluid during attacks has inflammatory characteristics (see TABLE 35–1), usually 2,000 to 100,000 WBCs/μL, with > 50% polymorphonuclear WBCs; these findings overlap considerably with infectious arthritis, which must be excluded by Gram stain and culture.

An elevated serum urate level supports the diagnosis of gout but is neither specific nor sensitive; at least 30% of patients have normal serum urate at the time of an acute attack. However, the serum urate level reflects the size of the extracellular miscible urate pool. The level should be measured on 2 or 3 occasions in patients with newly proven gout to establish a baseline; if elevated (> 7 mg/dL [> 0.41 mmol/L]), 24-h urinary urate excretion can also be measured. Normal 24-h excretion is about 600 to 900 mg on a regular diet. Quantification of urinary uric acid can indicate whether hyperuricemia results from impaired excretion or increased production and help guide any serum urate–lowering therapy.

X-rays of the affected joint may be obtained to look for bony tophi but are probably unnecessary if the diagnosis has been established by synovial fluid analysis. In CPPD, radiopaque deposits are present in

TABLE 35–1. MICROSCOPIC EXAMINATION OF CRYSTALS IN JOINTS

CRYSTAL TYPE	BIREFRINGENCE	ELONGATION*	SHAPE	LENGTH (μm)
Monosodium urate	Strong	Negative	Needle- or rod-shaped	2–15
Ca pyrophosphate dihydrate	Weak	Positive	Rhomboid- or rod-shaped	2–15
Ca oxalate†	Weak or strong	Positive or indeterminate	Bipyramidal	5–30
Basic Ca phosphate	Not birefringent with polarized light	—	Shiny, coinlike, or slightly irregular	3–65

*Crystals that have negative elongation are yellow parallel to the axis of slow vibration marked on the compensator; positive elongation appears blue in the same direction.
†Occur primarily in patients with renal failure.

fibrocartilage and/or hyaline articular cartilage (particularly the knee).

Chronic gouty arthritis should be suspected in patients with persistent joint disease or subcutaneous or bony tophi. Plain x-rays of the first metatarsophalangeal or other affected joint may be useful. These may show "punched-out" lesions of subchondral bone with overhanging bony margins, most commonly in the first metatarsophalangeal joint; these must be ≥5 mm in diameter before becoming visible on x-ray. Bony lesions are not specific or diagnostic but nearly always precede the appearance of subcutaneous tophi.

Palindromic rheumatism (acute attacks of inflammation in or near one or occasionally several joints) can simulate gout. Its onset is often even more sudden than in gout, and the pain and erythema can be as severe. Attacks subside spontaneously and completely in 1 to 3 days. Such attacks may herald the onset of RA, and rheumatoid factor tests can help in differentiation; they are positive in about 50% of patients (these tests are positive in 10% of gouty patients also). The inflammation in palindromic rheumatism is nearly always periarticular but may appear to be intra-articular.

Prognosis

With early diagnosis, therapy enables most patients to live a normal life. For many patients with advanced disease, tophi can be resolved, joint function improved, and renal dysfunction arrested. Gout is generally more severe in patients whose initial symptoms appear before age 30. Renal failure is the most likely cause of death from gout.

Some patients do not improve sufficiently with treatment. The usual reasons include noncompliance, alcoholism, and undertreatment by physicians.

Treatment

Objectives are (1) termination of an acute attack with NSAIDs or corticosteroids, (2) prevention of recurrent acute attacks with daily colchicine or an NSAID, and (3) prevention of further deposition of MSU crystals and resolution of existing tophi by lowering the serum urate level. Coexisting hypertension, hyperlipidemia, and obesity are common and should be treated.

Treatment of acute attacks: NSAIDs are effective in treating acute attacks and are generally well tolerated. However, they can still cause adverse effects, including GI upset, hyperkalemia, increases in creatinine, and fluid retention. Elderly and dehydrated patients are at particular risk, especially if there is a history of renal disease. COX-2 inhibitors, or coxibs, produce less GI toxicity but not necessarily less renal toxicity and appear to increase the risk of cardiovascular events (eg, MI, stroke) with long-term use. Use of coxibs for long pariods or in patients with cardiovascular risk factors should be approached cautiously. For any NSAID, anti-inflammatory (high) doses (see TABLE 34–2 on p. 287) are necessary for several days.

Colchicine, a traditional therapy, often produces a dramatic response if begun soon after the onset of symptoms. Joint pain generally begins to subside after 12 to 24 h of treatment and ceases within 3 to 7 days. One regimen is colchicine 0.6 mg po q 1 h until symptoms improve to a maximum total dose of 4 to 5 mg or until diarrhea or vomiting occurs. However, diarrhea, sometimes severe, develops in up to 80% of patients given oral colchicine in this schedule for an acute attack. If treatment is started very early, regimens such as 0.6 to 1.2 mg bid to tid for 1 to 2 days may be effective and better tolerated. If acute colchicine is tolerated, 0.5 to 1.2 mg once/day can be continued as the attack subsides.

IV colchicine is much less likely to cause GI symptoms and is an attractive alternative, particularly for postoperative patients. Colchicine 1 mg is diluted with 0.9% saline to 20 mL and injected slowly (over 2 to 5 min); a second 1-mg dose can be given in 12 h if needed; no more than 2 mg is given in 24 h (and no more than 4 mg over 7 days). *IV colchicine should not be given to patients receiving prophylactic oral colchicine, as severe bone marrow suppression, shock, and death may occur.* IV colchicine is also locally irritating, particularly if extravasated.

Acute attacks may also be treated with corticosteroids. Aspiration of affected joints, followed by instillation of corticosteroid ester crystal suspension, is very effective, particularly for monarticular symptoms; prednisolone tebutate 4 to 40 mg or prednisolone acetate 5 to 25 mg can be used, with dose depending on the size of the affected joint. Single-dose ACTH 80 U IM (now difficult to obtain) is very effective, particularly if multiple joints are involved. IM or intra-articular corticosteroids may be especially useful in treating gouty attacks in patients who cannot take oral drugs. Oral prednisone is occasionally used in short courses, eg, 30 to 50 mg once/day for polyarticular attacks.

In addition to NSAIDs or corticosteroid drugs, supplementary analgesics, rest, and splinting of the inflamed joint may be helpful. Drugs that lower the serum urate level should not be initiated until acute symptoms have been completely controlled.

Prevention of recurrent attacks: The frequency of acute attacks is reduced by taking one to two 0.6-mg tablets of colchicine daily (depending on tolerance and severity). An extra two or three 0.6-mg tablets of colchicine taken at the first suggestion of an attack usually aborts flares. A (reversible) neuropathy or myopathy can develop during chronic colchicine ingestion. Attack frequency can also be decreased with daily low-dose NSAIDs.

Lowering the serum urate level: Neither colchicine, NSAIDs, nor corticosteroids retard the progressive joint damage produced by tophi. Such damage can be prevented and, if present, reversed with urate-lowering drugs. Tophaceous deposits are resorbed by lowering serum urate to 4 mg/dL, which is below the level of saturation (> 7.0 mg/dL [> 0.41 mmol/L] at normal core body temperature and pH, and 4.5 mg/dL [0.26 mmol/L] the saturation level at the normal temperature [31° C] of the bunion joint), and maintaining it there indefinitely. This is accomplished by increasing urate excretion with a uricosuric drug or by blocking urate production with allopurinol or, in severe tophaceous gout, with both types of drugs used together. Hypouricemic therapy is indicated for patients with tophaceous deposits, more than 2 attacks/year despite prophylactic colchicine and/or an NSAID no matter what the serum urate, gout with persistent serum urate ≥ 9 mg/L, or urolithiasis. Hyperuricemia is not treated in the absence of gout.

Drugs are extremely effective in lowering serum urate; dietary restriction of purines is less effective, but high intake of high-purine food should be avoided. Carbohydrate restriction can lower serum urate in patients with insulin resistance because high insulin levels suppress urate excretion. Because acute attacks tend to develop during the first months of hypouricemic therapy, such therapy should be started in conjunction with daily colchicine or NSAIDs and during a symptom-free period. The goal is to keep serum urate ≤ 4.5 mg/dL (≤ 0.026 mmol/L). Resolution of tophi may take many months even with maintenance of serum urate at this level. Serum urate should be measured periodically, usually monthly while determining required drug dosage and then yearly to confirm the effectiveness of therapy.

Allopurinol, which inhibits urate synthesis, is the most commonly prescribed hypouricemic therapy. It is especially helpful in treating patients who repeatedly pass uric acid or Ca oxalate stones or who have severe renal dysfunction. Uric acid stones or gravel may dissolve during allopurinol treatment. Treatment begins with 100 mg po once/day and can be increased, up to 300 to 600 mg po once/day to achieve target urate levels; however, the dose must be decreased in patients with renal insufficiency. Adverse effects include mild GI distress and skin rash, which can be a harbinger of life-threatening hepatitis, vasculitis, or leukopenia. Adverse effects are most common in patients with renal dysfunction.

Uricosuric therapy is preferred to allopurinol as initial therapy for patients ≤ 60 yr with normal renal function, no history of urolithiasis, and decreased renal urate excretion. Probenecid and sulfinpyrazone are both available in the US. Probenecid treatment begins with 250 mg po bid, with doses increased as needed, to a maximum of 1 g po tid. Sulfinpyrazone treatment begins with 50 to 100 mg po bid, with doses increased as needed, to a maximum of 100 mg po qid. Sulfinpyrazone is more potent than probenecid but is more toxic. Salicylates antagonize both drugs and should be avoided. Acetaminophen provides comparable analgesia without interfering with drug efficacy.

Other treatments: Fluid intake ≥ 3 L/day is desirable for all patients, especially those who chronically pass urate gravel or stones. Alkalinization of urine (with K citrate, 20 to 40 mEq po bid, or acetazolamide, 500 mg po at bedtime) is also occasionally effective for those with persistent uric acid urolithiasis despite hypouricemic therapy and adequate hydration. However, excessive urine alkalinization may produce deposition of Ca oxalate crystals. Extracorporeal shock wave lithotripsy may be needed to disintegrate renal stones. Large tophi in areas with healthy skin may be removed surgically; all others should slowly resolve under adequate hypouricemic therapy.

Asymptomatic Hyperuricemia

Asymptomatic hyperuricemia is elevation of serum urate > 7 mg/dL (> 0.42 mmol/L) in the absence of clinical gout. Generally, treatment is not required. However, patients with overexcretion of urate who are at risk of urolithiasis may receive allopurinol.

CALCIUM PYROPHOSPHATE DIHYDRATE CRYSTAL DEPOSITION DISEASE

(Pseudogout)

Calcium pyrophosphate dihydrate (CPPD) crystal deposition disease involves intra-articular and/or extra-articular deposition of CPPD crystals. Manifestations are protean and may be minimal or include intermittent attacks of acute arthritis and a degenerative arthropathy that is often severe. Diagnosis requires identification of CPPD crystals in synovial fluid. Treatment is with intra-articular corticosteroids or oral NSAIDs or colchicine.

Etiology and Incidence

The cause is unknown. Frequent association with other conditions, such as trauma (including surgery), amyloidosis, myxedema, hypomagnesemia, hyperparathyroidism, gout, hemochromatosis, and old age, suggests that CPPD crystal deposits are secondary to degenerative or metabolic changes in the affected tissues. Some cases are familial, usually transmitted in an autosomal dominant pattern, with complete penetration by age 40. Both symptomatic and asymptomatic CPPD crystal deposition (chondrocalcinosis) are common with aging.

The incidence of radiologic (usually asymptomatic) chondrocalcinosis in patients aged 70 is about 3%, reaching nearly 50% in patients aged 90. Asymptomatic chondrocalcinosis is common in the knee, hip, anulus fibrosus, and symphysis pubis. Men and women are affected equally.

Symptoms and Signs

Acute, subacute, or chronic arthritis can occur, usually in the knee or other large peripheral joints, which can mimic many other forms of arthritis. Attacks are sometimes similar to gout but are usually less severe. There may be no symptoms between attacks or continuous low-grade symptoms in multiple joints, similar to RA or osteoarthritis. These patterns tend to persist for life.

Diagnosis

CPPD deposition disease should be suspected in older patients with arthritis, particularly inflammatory arthritis. Diagnosis is established by identifying rhomboid or rod-shaped, weakly positively birefringent crystals on polarized light microscopy of synovial fluid (see TABLE 35–1). Coincident infectious arthritis must be ruled out by Gram stain and culture. X-rays are indicated if synovial fluid cannot be obtained for analysis; findings of multiple linear or punctate calcification in articular cartilage, especially fibrocartilages, support the diagnosis.

Prognosis and Treatment

The prognosis for individual attacks is usually excellent. However, chronic arthritis can occur, and severe destructive arthropathy resembling neuropathic (Charcot's) joints occasionally occurs.

Symptoms of acute synovial effusion abate with synovial fluid drainage and instillation of a microcrystalline corticosteroid ester suspension into the joint space (eg, 40 mg prednisolone acetate or prednisolone tertiary butylacetate into a knee). Indomethacin, naproxen, or another NSAID given at anti-inflammatory doses (see TABLE 34–2 on p. 287) often stops acute attacks promptly. IV colchicine may also be effective in patients who cannot take oral drugs (see p. 302). Colchicine 0.6 mg po once/day or bid can prevent acute attacks.

APATITE AND CALCIUM OXALATE CRYSTAL DEPOSITION DISEASES

Apatite and calcium oxalate crystal disorders tend to cause clinical manifestations similar to other crystal-induced arthritides.

Apatite (basic calcium phosphate) crystal deposition disease: Most pathologic calcifications throughout the body contain mixtures of carbonate-substituted hydroxyapatite and octacalcium phosphate. Because these ultramicroscopic crystals are nonacidic Ca phosphates, the term "basic calcium phosphate" (BCP) is much more precise than "apatite." These ultramicroscopic crystals occur in snowball-like clumps in rheumatic conditions (eg, calcific tendinitis, calcific periarthritis, some cases of progressive systemic sclerosis and dermatomyositis). They also occur in joint fluids of patients with all degenerative arthropathies sufficiently advanced to produce joint space narrowing on x-ray.

BCP crystals can destroy joints and can cause severe intra-articular or periarticular inflammation. The Milwaukee shoulder syndrome is one example, a profoundly destructive arthropathy affecting predominantly elderly women that usually develops in the shoulders and (often) knees.

Acute podagra due to periarticular BCP deposition can mimic gout; it occurs as a discrete syndrome in young women (less often in young men) and is treated the same as acute gout.

Besides synovial fluid analysis, x-rays should be obtained of symptomatic joints. On x-ray, BCP crystals may be visible as periarticular cloudlike opacities. Definitive assay for BCP crystals in synovial fluid is not readily available. Clumped crystals can be identified only with transmission electron microscopy. The clumps are not birefringent under polarized light.

Treatment with oral or IV colchicine, an NSAID, or, if a large joint is involved, intra-articular corticosteroid ester crystal suspension is helpful. Such treatment is described above for acute gout.

Ca oxalate crystal deposition disease: Ca oxalate crystal deposition occurs most often in azotemic patients receiving hemodialysis or peritoneal dialysis, particularly those treated with ascorbic acid (vitamin C), which is metabolized to oxalate. Crystals may deposit in blood vessel walls and skin, as well as joints. The crystals appear as birefringent bipyramidal structures (see TABLE 35–1). Synovial fluid may have > 2000 WBC/μL. On x-ray, Ca oxalate crystals are indistinguishable from BCP periarticular calcifications or CPPD crystal deposits in cartilage. Treatment is the same as for CPPD crystals.

36

OSTEOPOROSIS

Osteoporosis is a progressive metabolic bone disease that decreases bone density (bone mass per unit volume), with deterioration of bone structure. Skeletal weakness leads to fractures with minor or inapparent trauma, particularly in the thoracic and lumbar spine, wrist, and hip. Acute or chronic back pain is common. Diagnosis is by dual-energy x-ray absorptiometry. Prevention and treatment involve Ca and vitamin D supplements, exercises to maximize bone and muscle strength and minimize the risk of falls, and drug therapy to preserve bone mass or stimulate new bone formation.

Pathophysiology and Classification

Normally, bone formation and resorption are closely coupled. Osteoblasts (cells that make the organic matrix of bone and then mineralize bone) and osteoclasts (cells that resorb bone) are regulated by parathyroid hormone (PTH), calcitonin, estrogen, vitamin D, cytokines (eg, interleukin-1, tumor necrosis factor-α, granulocyte-macrophage colony-stimulating factor, interleukin-6), and other local factors such as prostaglandins.

Peak bone mass in men and women occurs by the mid 20s. Blacks reach higher bone mass than whites and Asians, while Hispanics have intermediate values. Men have higher bone mass than women. Bone mass plateaus for about 10 yr, during which time bone formation approximately equals bone resorption. After this, bone loss occurs at a rate of about 0.3 to 0.5%/yr. Beginning with menopause, bone loss accelerates in women to about 3 to 5%/yr for about 5 to 7 yr.

Osteoporotic bone loss affects cortical and trabecular (cancellous) bone. Cortical thickness and the number and size of trabeculae decrease, resulting in increased porosity. Trabeculae may be disrupted or entirely absent.

Osteoporosis can develop as a primary disorder or secondarily due to some other factor.

Primary osteoporosis: More than 95% of osteoporosis is primary; there are three types.

Idiopathic osteoporosis is uncommon but occurs in children and young adults of both sexes with normal gonadal function.

Type I osteoporosis (postmenopausal osteoporosis) results from increased osteoclast activity and affects primarily trabecular bone. It occurs between ages 51 and 75 and is 6 times more common in women than in men. Estrogen loss may elevate levels of cytokines, which are thought to increase recruitment and activity of osteoclasts in trabecular bone, resulting in increased bone resorption. Late menarche, early menopause, and nulliparity increase the risk. Although calcitonin levels are decreased in women compared with men, calcitonin deficiency does not appear to be important. In men, prematurely low levels of serum testosterone can increase osteoclast activity, causing type I osteoporosis. Type I is largely responsible for fractures affecting predominantly trabecular bone, such as vertebral compression fractures and Colles' (distal radius) fractures.

Type II osteoporosis (involutional or senile osteoporosis) results from the normal gradual decline in the number and activity of osteoblasts that occurs with aging and affects both trabecular and cortical bone. It typically affects patients > 60 and is twice as common in women as in men. In older women, types I and II often occur together. Estrogen deficiency is probably an important factor in both men and women, but reduction in Ca or vitamin D intake or vitamin D synthesis or resistance to vitamin D activity—resulting in secondary hyperparathyroidism—may contribute. Vertebral compression fractures and fractures of the femoral neck, proximal humerus, proximal tibia, and pelvis can result.

Secondary osteoporosis: Secondary osteoporosis accounts for < 5% of osteoporosis cases. The causes (see TABLE 36–1) may also aggravate bone loss and increase fracture risk in patients with primary osteoporosis.

Risk Factors

Because stress, including weight bearing, is necessary for bone growth, immobilization or extended sedentary periods result in bone loss. Being thin predisposes to decreased bone mass. Insufficient dietary intake of Ca, P, and vitamin D predisposes to bone loss, as does endogenous acidosis (eg, high-protein diets). Cigarette smoking and excessive caffeine or alcohol use also adversely affect bone mass. Whites and Asians are at higher risk. A family history of osteoporosis also increases risk. Other risk factors (eg, decreasing amounts of sex

TABLE 36–1. CAUSES OF SECONDARY OSTEOPOROSIS

Chronic renal failure
COPD
Drugs (eg, corticosteroids, ethanol, phenytoin, tobacco, barbiturates, heparin)
Endocrine disease (eg, glucocorticoid excess, hyperparathyroidism, hyperthyroidism, hypogonadism, hyperprolactinemia, diabetes mellitus)
Hypervitaminosis A
Immobilization
Liver disease
Malabsorption syndromes
Malignancy
Prolonged weightlessness (as found in space flight)
RA
Sarcoidosis

hormones) predispose to specific types of osteoporosis.

Symptoms and Signs

Most of the chronic pain typical of osteoporosis results from fractures, which may develop after minimal, inapparent, or no trauma. Patients may be asymptomatic for years, until fractures begin to occur. Eventually, patients often develop pain in the bones or muscles, particularly of the back. Vertebral compression fractures are common, usually in weight-bearing vertebrae (T6 and below). The pain begins acutely, usually does not radiate, is aggravated by weight bearing, may produce local tenderness, and generally begins to subside in 1 wk. However, residual pain may last for months or be constant.

Multiple thoracic compression fractures eventually cause dorsal kyphosis, with exaggerated cervical lordosis (dowager's hump). Abnormal stress on the spinal muscles and ligaments may cause chronic, dull, aching pain, particularly in the lower back. Fractures can develop at other sites, commonly the hip or wrist, usually from falls.

Screening and Diagnosis

Dual-energy x-ray absorptiometry (DEXA) screening is recommended for all women > 65. Bone density should also be measured in women between 50 and 65 who have risk factors, including a family history of osteoporosis, a history of fragility fractures, and low body weight. Screening is also recommended for both men and women who have had fragility fractures, even at younger ages.

Osteoporosis should be suspected in patients who sustain fractures after only mild or trivial trauma; older adults, particularly those with risk factors and unexplained back pain; patients with decreased bone density that is incidentally noted on radiographic studies; and patients at risk of secondary osteoporosis. If radiographic studies have been obtained or are necessary to evaluate symptoms (eg, back pain), osteoporosis may be obvious. However, radiographic studies are often equivocal, and the diagnosis should be established by DEXA.

Plain x-rays: Bones show decreased radiodensity and loss of trabecular structure, but not until about 30% of bone has been lost. A loss of horizontally oriented trabeculae increases the prominence of the cortical end plates and of vertically oriented, weight-bearing trabeculae. Loss of height and increased biconcavity characterize vertebral compression fractures. Thoracic vertebral fractures may produce anterior wedging. In long bones, although the cortices may be thin, the periosteal surface remains smooth. Vertebral fractures at T4 or above suggest malignancy rather than osteoporosis.

Corticosteroid-induced osteoporosis is likely to produce rib fractures and exuberant callus formation at sites of healing fractures. Osteomalacia may produce x-ray and DEXA abnormalities similar to those of osteoporosis (see sidebar 36–1). Hyperparathyroidism can be differentiated when it produces subperiosteal resorption or cystic bone lesions, but these are uncommon.

DEXA scanning: In addition to its use in screening, DEXA is diagnostic for osteoporosis, predicts the risk of fracture, and can be used to follow treatment response. Bone density of the lumbar spine, hip, distal radius or ulna, or the entire body can be measured. (Quantitative CT scanning can produce similar measurements in the spine or hip.) Measurement at the spine may show osteoporosis earlier than at the hip, but the hip is a better indicator in elderly patients because osteoarthritis of the spine may mask the presence of osteoporosis. A DEXA result of > 1 standard deviation from the average value in 25-yr-old sex- and race-matched controls is defined as osteopenia and suggests an increased risk for osteoporosis; > 2.5 is diagnostic for osteoporosis.

Sidebar 36–1. OSTEOPENIA: DIFFERENTIATING OSTEOPOROSIS AND OSTEOMALACIA

Osteopenia is decreased bone mass. Two metabolic bone diseases decrease bone mass: osteoporosis and osteomalacia. In osteoporosis, there is a decrease in bone mass with a normal ratio of bone mineral to bone matrix. In osteomalacia, the ratio of bone mineral to bone matrix is high.

Osteoporosis results from a combination of low peak bone mass, increased bone resorption, and impaired bone formation. Osteomalacia is due to impaired mineralization, usually because of severe vitamin D deficiency or abnormal vitamin D metabolism (see p. 41). Osteoporosis is much more common than osteomalacia in the US. The two disorders may coexist, and their clinical expression is similar; moreover, mild to moderate vitamin D deficiency can occur in osteoporosis.

Other testing: Once osteoporosis is diagnosed, patients should be checked for causes of secondary osteoporosis. Serum Ca should be measured to rule out asymptomatic hyperparathyroidism. PTH levels may be increased in type II patients with decreased Ca absorption or hypercalciuria. Other tests such as thyroid-stimulating hormone or free thyroxine to check for hyperthyroidism, vitamin D levels, measurements of urinary free cortisol, and blood counts and other tests to rule out malignancy, especially myeloma (eg, serum protein electrophoresis), should be considered depending on the clinical presentation. Serum alkaline phosphatase is usually normal but may be elevated by recent fracture.

Patients with weight loss should be screened for GI disorders as well as malignancy. Bone biopsy is reserved for unusual cases (eg, young patients with pathologic fractures and no apparent cause). Levels of serum or urine N-telopeptide crosslinks (NTX) or free deoxypyridinoline (DPYR) may reflect increased breakdown of collagen. These tests are not sufficiently accurate for routine clinical use but may be used to assess the effectiveness of therapy.

Prevention and Treatment

The goals are to preserve bone mass, prevent fractures, decrease pain, and maintain function. Treatment and preventive measures are appropriate for patients with documented osteoporosis, patients taking long-term systemic corticosteroids, and patients at high risk (eg, osteopenia with multiple risk factors).

Preserving bone mass: The rate of bone loss can be slowed with drugs and, when possible, modification of risk factors. Ca and vitamin D intake and physical activity must be adequate for drug treatment to be effective.

Risk factor modification can include maintaining adequate body weight, increasing weight-bearing exercise, minimizing caffeine and alcohol intake, and stopping smoking. The optimal amount of weight-bearing exercise is not established, but an average of 30 min/day is recommended. A physical therapist can develop a safe exercise program.

All men and women should consume at least 1000 mg of elemental Ca daily. An intake of 1200 to 1500 mg/day is recommended for postmenopausal women and older men and for periods of increased requirements, such as pubertal growth, pregnancy, and lactation. Diet alone is rarely adequate; Ca supplements are needed, most commonly as Ca carbonate or Ca citrate. Supplements differ in their elemental Ca concentration. Ca citrate is better absorbed in patients with achlorhydria, but both are well absorbed when taken with meals. Ca should be taken in divided doses of 500 to 600 mg bid or tid.

Vitamin D in doses of 400 U once/day is generally recommended, but up to 1000 U/day is safe and may be helpful in osteoporotic patients. Patients with vitamin D deficiency may need high doses.

Bisphosphonates are first-line drug therapy. By inhibiting bone resorption, bisphosphonates preserve bone mass and can decrease vertebral and hip fractures by 50%. In postmenopausal patients without osteoporosis, alendronate 5 mg po once/day or 35 mg once/wk or risedronate 5 mg po once/day or 35 mg once/wk prevents bone loss. To treat osteoporosis, alendronate can be given at doses of 10 mg po once/day or 70 mg po once/wk or risedronate at 5 mg po once/day or 35 mg once/wk. Oral bisphosphonates must be taken on an empty stomach with a full glass of water, and the patient must remain upright for ≥ 30 min. Weekly therapy is generally preferred for its greater convenience and probably fewer adverse effects. If a patient cannot tolerate oral bisphosphonates, pamidronate or zoledronic acid can be given by IV infusion. However, these have not yet been shown to prevent fractures.

Salmon calcitonin is less effective than bisphosphonates for treating osteoporosis. The subcutaneous dose is 100 IU/day or every other day; the nasal spray dose is 200 U/day in alternating nostrils (one spray). Salmon calcitonin may provide short-term analgesia after an acute fracture.

Estrogen can preserve bone density and prevent fractures. Most effective if started within 4 to 6 yr of menopause, estrogen may slow bone loss and possibly reduce fractures even when started much later. It is usually given as conjugated estrogen 0.625 to 1.25 mg po once/day. However, 0.3 mg po once/day may be as effective. Use of estrogen increases the risk of thromboembolism and endometrial cancer and may increase the risk of breast cancer. The risk of endometrial cancer can be reduced in women with an intact uterus by taking a progestin with estrogen (see p. 2082). However, taking a combination of a progestin and estrogen increases the risk of breast cancer, coronary artery disease, stroke, and biliary disease.

Raloxifene is a selective estrogen receptor modulator (SERM) that may be appropriate for prevention and treatment of osteoporosis in women who cannot take bisphosphonates. It reduces vertebral fractures by about 50% but has not been shown to reduce nonvertebral fractures. Raloxifene does not stimulate the uterus and antagonizes estrogen effects in the breast, probably reducing the risk of breast cancer.

Parathyroid hormone, which stimulates new bone formation, is generally reserved for patients who fail to respond to antiresorptive drugs, as well as Ca, vitamin D, and exercise. When given daily by injection for an average of 20 mo, synthetic parathyroid hormone (PTH 1-34; teriparatide) increased bone mass and reduced fractures.

Preventing fractures: Many elderly patients are at risk for falls because of poor coordination, poor vision, muscle weakness, confusion, and use of drugs that cause postural hypotension or alter the sensorium. Educating patients about the risks of falls and fractures and developing individualized programs to increase physical stability and attenuate risk can help. Strengthening exercises may increase stability. Hip pads can reduce the incidence of hip fracture despite continued falls.

Treating pain and maintaining function: Acute back pain from a vertebral compression fracture should be treated with orthopedic support, analgesics, and (when muscle spasm is prominent) heat and massage (see p. 2752). Chronic backache may be relieved by an orthopedic garment and exercises to strengthen paravertebral muscles. Avoiding heavy lifting can help. Bed rest should be minimized, and consistent, carefully designed weight-bearing exercise encouraged.

37 PAGET'S DISEASE OF BONE

(Osteitis Deformans)

Paget's disease of bone is a chronic disorder of the adult skeleton in which bone turnover is accelerated in localized areas. Normal matrix is replaced with softened and enlarged bone. The disease may be asymptomatic or cause gradual onset of bone pain or deformity. Diagnosis is by x-ray. Treatment includes symptomatic measures and often drugs, usually bisphosphonates.

Etiology is unknown. Appearance of involved bone on electron microscopy suggests a viral infection, but a viral cause has not been established. Paget's disease is sometimes familial, but a specific genetic pattern has been suggested. About 1% of adults in the US >40 have Paget's disease, with a 3:2 male predominance. The disease is most common in Europe (except Scandinavia), Australia, and New Zealand.

Pathophysiology

Any bone can be involved. The bones most commonly affected are, in decreasing order, the pelvis, femur, skull, tibia, vertebrae, clavicle, and humerus. Bone turnover is accelerated at involved sites. Pagetic lesions are metabolically active and highly vascular. Excessively active osteoclasts are often large and contain many nuclei. Osteoblastic repair is also hyperactive, producing coarsely woven, thickened lamellae and trabeculae. This abnormal structure weakens the bone, despite bony enlargement and heavy calcification. Overgrown bone may compress nerves and other structures passing through small foramina. Osteoarthritis may develop in joints adjacent to involved bone.

Symptoms and Signs

There are usually no symptoms for a prolonged period. If symptoms occur, they develop insidiously, with pain, stiffness, fatigue, and bone deformity. Bone pain is aching, deep, and occasionally severe, sometimes worse at night. Pain also may arise from compression neuropathy or osteoarthritis. If the skull is involved, there may be headaches and hearing impairment.

Signs may include skull enlargement bitemporally and frontally (frontal "bossing"); dilated scalp veins; nerve deafness in one or both ears; angioid streaks in the fundus of the eye; a short kyphotic trunk with simian appearance; hobbling gait; and anterolateral angulation (bowing) of the thigh or leg, often with warmth and tenderness. Spinal stenosis or spinal cord compression may develop. Large or numerous lesions may lead to high-output heart failure. Deformities may develop from bowing of the long bones or osteoarthritis. Pathologic fractures may be the presenting manifestation. Sarcomatous degeneration develops in < 1% and is often suggested by increasingly severe pain.

Hypercalcemia (see p. 1254) occasionally develops in patients who are immobile. It also occurs in the 10 to 15% of patients with Paget's disease who develop secondary hyperparathyroidism.

Diagnosis

Paget's disease should be suspected in patients with unexplained bone pain or deformity. It should also be suspected in patients who have suggestive findings on x-ray, in patients who have an unexplained elevation of serum alkaline phosphatase on laboratory tests performed for other reasons, or in older patients who develop hypercalcemia during bed rest.

If Paget's disease is suspected, plain x-rays and serum alkaline phosphatase, Ca, and PO_4 levels should be obtained. Characteristic x-ray findings include increased bone density, abnormal architecture with coarse cortical trabeculation or cortical thickening, bowing, and bony enlargement. There may be stress microfractures of the tibia or femur. Characteristic laboratory findings include elevated serum alkaline phosphatase (increased anabolic activity of bone) but usually normal serum PO_4 levels. Serum Ca is usually normal but can increase due to immobilization or hyperparathyroidism. If alkaline phosphatase is not elevated or it is unclear if the increased serum alkaline phosphatase is of bony origin, a bone-specific fraction can be measured.

Occasionally, increased catabolic activity of bone, measured by urine markers of bone collagen turnover (eg, pyridinoline crosslinks), supplements the findings. Radionuclide bone scan using technetium-labeled phosphonates should be performed at baseline to determine the extent of bony involvement. To establish the diagnosis, there must be confirmation on x-ray.

Treatment

Localized, asymptomatic disease requires no treatment. Symptomatic treatment includes analgesics or NSAIDs for pain. Orthotics help correct abnormal gait caused by bowed lower extremities. Some patients require orthopedic surgery (eg, hip or knee replacement, decompression of the spinal cord). Weight bearing should be encouraged and bed rest avoided.

Drug therapy suppresses osteoclast activity. It is indicated (1) to prevent or reduce bleeding during orthopedic surgery; (2) to prevent or retard progression of complications (eg, hearing loss, deformity, osteoarthritis, paraparesis or paraplegia related to vertebral Paget's disease, or other neurologic deficits, particularly in a poor surgical candidate); and (3) to treat pain that is clearly related to the pagetic process and not to another source (eg, osteoarthritis). Although disease progression can be retarded, existing deficits

TABLE 37–1. DRUG THERAPY FOR PAGET'S DISEASE

DRUG	DOSAGE	COMMENTS
Alendronate	40 mg po once/day for 6 mo	Taken as a single dose on rising in the morning, at least 30 min before eating
Etidronate disodium	5–10 mg/kg po once/day for 6 mo; higher doses (20 mg/kg po once/day for 3 mo) may be needed in markedly active disease	Taken as a single dose on an empty stomach at least 2 h before or after eating. Can be repeated after a 3- to 6-mo interim if needed
Pamidronate	30–90 mg IV once/day given as a 4-h infusion for 3 consecutive days or once/mo for 3 mo	For patients intolerant of oral bisphosphonates; more frequent doses can be used in patients with resistant disease
Risedronate	30 mg po once/day for 2 mo	Taken same as alendronate
Tiludronate	400 mg po once/day for 3 mo	Taken same as alendronate
Synthetic salmon calcitonin	50–100 IU (0.25–0.5 mL) sc or IM once/day	The dose may be tapered to 50 IU every other day and perhaps to twice or once weekly after a favorable initial response (often after 1 mo)

(eg, deformity, osteoarthritis, hearing loss, neural impingement) are not reversed. Generally, most people with an alkaline phosphatase level twice the upper limit of the normal range should be treated.

Several bisphosphonates are available and are the drugs of choice (see TABLE 37–1). Synthetic salmon calcitonin is an alternative to bisphosphonates for patients intolerant or resistant to them.

38 AVASCULAR NECROSIS

(Osteonecrosis; Ischemic Necrosis of Bone; Aseptic Necrosis; Osteochondritis Dissecans)

Avascular necrosis is focal bone infarction, which may be secondary to various conditions or idiopathic. Severe osteoarthritis can result. Symptoms include bone or joint pain. Early diagnosis is best made by MRI. Treatment includes rest, analgesics, range-of-motion exercises, and, in some cases, surgery.

In the US, avascular necrosis (AVN) affects about 20,000 new patients annually and causes 5% of cases of osteoarthritis of the hip. The femoral head (hip) is most commonly involved; the distal femur and proximal tibia (knee) and the humeral head (shoulder) are frequently involved; the body of the talus, carpal, scaphoid, and navicular bone are less commonly involved. In 33 to 72% of patients with nontraumatic AVN, disease is bilateral. Idiopathic AVN of the hip affects men 4 to 5 times more often than women, with a peak incidence between ages 30 and 60. AVN of the knee is most common in elderly women.

Etiology

AVN involves ischemic death of osteocytes and other bone marrow components, producing subchondral bone infarction. Of the many conditions associated with AVN, some are more clearly causative (see TABLE 38–1).

Posttraumatic AVN develops when blood supply is impaired. Susceptible bone is usually intra-articular and has a limited attachment of soft tissue and accompanying vasculature. The hips, shoulders, body of the talus, and carpal scaphoid are commonly affected.

AVN after hip dislocation or fracture results from tears of the ligamentum teres and joint capsule that compromise blood vessels. Posterior dislocations are especially likely to result in AVN. AVN develops in 52% of hips that remain dislocated > 12 h but in only 22% of those reduced within 12 h. AVN after hip fractures is common with transcervical or subcapital fractures but is rare with intertrochanteric or other extracapsular fractures. The incidence does not seem related to the surgeon's skill or type of fixation device.

The most common risk factors for nontraumatic AVN are alcohol consumption, use of > 25 mg/day of prednisone for several months or more, and sickle cell disease. Less common risk factors include decompression sickness, Gaucher's disease, tumors (lymphomas, leukemias, metastatic bone tumors), vascular disease (including vasculitis), and radiation therapy.

About 25% of cases occur in patients with no detectable risk factors and are considered idiopathic. However, some patients have clotting abnormalities due to protein C or S deficiencies, hyperhomocystinemia, or anticardiolipin antibodies (see Ch. 135 on p. 1080).

Symptoms and Signs

Although pain may develop insidiously, many patients remember the hour when they first felt incapacitating pain. As the bone progressively collapses, almost all patients develop pain aggravated by mechanical stresses (eg, in the hip; standing, moving, walking) and eased by rest. Eventually, 67% of patients have pain at rest and 40% have pain at night, which may be accompanied by prolonged morning pain and stiffness.

AVN of the hip produces groin pain that intermittently radiates down the anteromedial thigh. Some patients note increased pain and a distinct clicking with motion, particularly when rising from sitting. They have limited motion (particularly flexion, abduction, and internal rotation) and adopt an antalgic gait. A click may be elicited by externally rotating the flexed abducted hip (Figure 4 sign).

TABLE 38–1. CAUSES OF AVASCULAR NECROSIS

Definite
- Alcohol abuse
- Coagulation disorders
- Corticosteroids (high dose)
- Decompression sickness
- Fatty liver
- Fracture of the femoral neck
- Gaucher's disease
- Hip dislocation
- Radiation therapy
- Sickle cell disease
- Tumors

Possible
- Atherosclerosis
- Cushing's syndrome
- Diabetes mellitus
- Gout
- Legg-Calvé-Perthes disease
- Lipid disturbances
- Pancreatitis
- SLE
- Smoking

AVN of the knee usually produces sudden pain without preceding trauma. It is usually localized to the medial side of the knee. There is tenderness over the medial femoral condyle and, in ⅓ of patients, mild to moderate effusion.

AVN of the shoulder may produce only transient and minimal symptoms until advanced disease develops. The major complaints are pain and limited motion, particularly active motion. Passive motion is preserved. It is unusual for AVN to involve just the shoulder.

Diagnosis

After fractures, increased pain and limp or deterioration of joint function suggests AVN. Early diagnosis requires a high index of suspicion in patients with conditions associated with AVN who develop pain in their hips, knees, or shoulders.

Diagnosis is made by an imaging study. Plain x-ray is usually performed first but is insensitive and can be normal for months or even years after the onset of symptoms. Early x-ray changes include subtle osteosclerosis and osteoporosis. The femoral head may develop subchondral lucency (the crescentic signal). Next, bone collapses and degenerative joint changes occur.

MRI is the most sensitive and specific test. Bone scans also are sensitive and accurate and can screen multiple joints simultaneously. A CT scan may be needed to gauge the degree of bone collapse, which may predict the response to treatments such as surgical core decompression.

Prevention and Treatment

To minimize AVN from corticosteroid use, patients should be given as low a dose as needed for effect and for as short a duration as acceptable. To prevent AVN from decompression sickness, patients should adhere to decompression tables during deep-sea diving.

Conservative measures often include analgesics, range-of-motion exercises, and restriction of weight bearing (if knees or hips are affected), in an attempt to prevent or minimize bone collapse. Failure of conservative treatment is usually apparent within 2 yr. Patients should be followed for at least this long.

Early conservative surgical intervention with core decompression or cortical bone grafts may best prevent serious joint dysfunction in the hips and knees, but surgery is less often necessary in the shoulder. Surgery is most successful if done before the bone collapses. Core decompression involves drilling a core of bone out, which reduces intraosseous pressure and promotes revascularization. Electrical stimulation (subthreshold) has been used in conjunction with core decompression in order to stimulate new bone formation and prevent collapse. If performed before radiographically detectable collapse, up to 75% of patients avoid joint replacement. Cortical bone grafts may provide mechanical support to prevent collapse as the bone revascularizes. Because this is a more extensive procedure than core decompression, crutches must be used for 4 to 6 mo as compared to 2 to 3 mo for core decompression. Osteotomy might also be used to alter mechanics of the joint and redistribute the maximal load-bearing forces to prevent collapse and deformation. Crutch walking is required for 6 to 12 mo.

If joint abnormalities develop, severe degenerative changes are inevitable. If the pain becomes severe and is not relieved by nonopioids, total joint replacement is indicated. Because prosthetic hips and knees last 15 or 20 yr, total joint replacement is often the procedure of choice for patients > 65, whose prosthesis may last for the rest of their life. Younger patients, especially those who persist in vigorous physical activities, will likely need a second procedure.

39 INFECTIONS OF JOINTS AND BONES

ACUTE INFECTIOUS ARTHRITIS

Acute infectious arthritis is a joint infection that evolves over hours or days. The infection resides in synovial or periarticular tissues and is usually bacterial—in younger adults, typically *Neisseria gonorrhoeae*. However, nongonococcal bacterial infections can also occur and can rapidly destroy joint structures. Symptoms include rapid onset of pain, effusion, and restriction of both active and passive range of motion, usually within a single joint. Diagnosis requires synovial fluid analysis and culture. Treatment is IV antibiotics and drainage of pus from joints.

Acute infectious arthritis often develops in children. About 50% of children with joint infection are < 3 yr. However, routine childhood vaccination for *Haemophilus influenzae* and *Streptococcus pneumoniae* is decreasing the incidence in this age group.

Risk factors are listed in TABLE 39–1. Risk is substantially increased in patients with RA, a past history of joint infection, IV drug abuse, or a prosthetic joint (see p. 317). RA patients are at particular risk for bacterial arthritis (prevalence 0.3 to 3.0%; annual incidence 0.5%). Most children who develop infectious arthritis do not have risk factors.

Etiology

Infectious organisms reach joints by direct penetration (eg, trauma, surgery, arthrocentesis, bites), extension from an adjacent infection (eg, osteomyelitis, a soft-tissue abscess, an infected wound), or hematogenous spread from a remote site of infection.

Common organisms are listed in TABLE 39–2. In adults, most cases result from bacteria and are classified as gonococcal or nongonococcal. *Neisseria gonorrhoeae* is the most common cause in young adults and adolescents and results when *N. gonorrhoeae* spreads from infected mucosal surfaces (cervix, urethra, rectum, pharynx) via the bloodstream. Affected patients often have simultaneous genital infections with *Chlamydia trachomatis* (see p. 1651).

TABLE 39–1. RISK FACTORS FOR INFECTIOUS ARTHRITIS

Advanced age (50% of adult cases are > 60 yr)
Alcoholism
Anemia
Arthrocentesis or surgery
Chronic medical illness (eg, lung or liver disease)
Diabetes
Hemophilia
History of previous joint infection
Immunodeficiency, including HIV
Immunosuppressive therapy, including corticosteroids
IV drug abuse
Malignancy
Prosthetic joint implant
Hemodialysis
RA
Risk factors for sexually transmitted diseases (eg, multiple sex partners, absence of barrier precautions)
Sickle cell disease
Skin infections
SLE

Pathophysiology

Infecting organisms multiply in the synovial fluid and synovial lining. Some bacteria (eg, *Staphylococcus aureus*) produce virulence factors (adhesins), which allow bacteria to penetrate, remain within, and infect joint tissues. Other bacterial products (eg, endotoxin from gram-negative organisms, cell wall fragments, exotoxins from gram-positive organisms, immune complexes formed by bacterial antigens and host antibodies) augment the inflammatory reaction.

PMNs migrate into the joint and phagocytose the infecting organisms. Phagocytosis of bacteria also results in PMN autolysis with release of lysosomal enzymes into the joint, which damage synovia, ligaments, and cartilage. Therefore, PMNs are both the major host defense system and the cause of joint damage. Articular cartilage can be destroyed within hours or days. Inflammatory synovitis may occasionally persist even after the infection has been eradicated by antibiotics. Persistent antigen debris from bacteria or infection may alter cartilage, causing it to become antigenic and—together with the adjuvant effects of bacterial components—immune-mediated, "sterile" chronic inflammatory synovitis results.

Symptoms and Signs

Over a few hours to a few days, patients develop moderate to severe joint pain, warmth, tenderness, effusion, restricted active and passive motion, and sometimes redness. Systemic symptoms may be absent. Infants and children may present with limited spontaneous movement of a limb (pseudoparalysis), irritability, feeding disturbances, and high, low-grade, or no fever.

Gonococcal arthritis most often causes a distinctive dermatitis-polyarthritis-tenosynovitis syndrome. Classic manifestations are fever (for 5 to 7 days); shaking chills; multiple skin lesions (petechiae, papules, pustules, hemorrhagic vesicles or bullae, necrotic lesions) on mucosal surfaces and on the skin of the trunk, hands, or lower extremities; migratory arthralgias, arthritis, and tenosynovitis, which evolves into persistent inflammatory arthritis in one or more rarely a few joints, most often the small joints of the hands, wrists, elbows, knees, and ankles, and rarely the axial skeletal joints. Symptoms of the original mucosal infection (eg, urethritis, cervicitis) may not be present.

Nongonococcal bacterial arthritis causes progressive moderate to severe joint pain that is markedly worsened by movement or palpation. Most infected joints are swollen, red, and warm. Fever is absent or low grade in up to 50% of patients; 20% of patients report a shaking chill. Gram-negative joint infections tend

TABLE 39–2. ORGANISMS THAT COMMONLY CAUSE ACUTE INFECTIOUS ARTHRITIS

PATIENT GROUPS	ORGANISM	TYPICAL SOURCES
Adults and adolescents	Gonococci, nongonococcal bacteria (*Staphylococcus aureus*, streptococci), *Neisseria meningitidis* in unusual cases	Cervical, urethral, rectal, or pharyngeal infection with bacteremic dissemination (for gonococci)
Newborns	Group B streptococci, *Escherichia coli* (and other gram-negative enteric bacteria), *S. aureus*	Maternal-fetal transmission; IV punctures or catheters with bacteremic dissemination
Children ≤ 3 yr	*Streptococcus pyogenes, S. pneumoniae, S. aureus*	Bacteremia (eg, otitis media, URIs, skin infections, meningitis)
Age 3 yr to adolescence	*S. aureus*, streptococci, *Neisseria gonorrhoeae, Pseudomonas aeruginosa, Kingella kingae*	Bacteremia or contiguous spread
Children with meningitis, bacteremia, palpable purpura	*N. meningitidis* (uncommon)	Bacteremia
All ages	Viruses (eg, parvovirus B19; hepatitis B; hepatitis C; rubella virus [active infection and after immunization]; togavirus; varicella; mumps [in adults]; adenovirus; coxsackie viruses A9, B2, B3, B4, and B6; retroviruses, including HIV; Epstein-Barr virus)	Viremia or immune complex deposition
Patients with possible tick exposure	*Borrelia burgdorferi* (causing Lyme disease)	Bacteremia
Patients with bite wounds	Often polymicrobial	Direct joint penetration, usually the small joints of the hands
Human	*Eikenella corrodens*, group B streptococci, *S. aureus*, oral anaerobes (eg, *Fusobacterium* sp, peptostreptococci, *Bacteroides* sp)	
Dogs or cats	*S. aureus, Pasteurella multocida, Pseudomonas* sp, *Moraxella* sp, *Haemophilus* sp	
Rats	*S. aureus, Streptobacillus moniliformis, Spirillum minus*	
Elderly; patients with severe joint trauma; serious disease (immunosuppression, hemodialysis, SLE, RA, diabetes, malignancy)	Gram-negative bacteria (eg, *Enterobacter, P. aeruginosa, Serratia marcescens*)	Urinary tract, skin

TABLE 39–2. ORGANISMS THAT COMMONLY CAUSE ACUTE INFECTIOUS ARTHRITIS—Continued

PATIENT GROUPS	ORGANISM	TYPICAL SOURCES
Patients with joint penetration (by injury, arthrocentesis, or arthrotomy), contiguous infection, diabetes, malignancy	Anaerobes (eg, *Propionibacterium acnes, Peptostreptococcus magnus, Fusobacterium* sp, *Clostridium* sp, *Bacteroides* sp); often as mixed infections with facultative or aerobic bacteria such as *S. aureus, S. epidermidis, E. coli*	Abdomen, genitals, odontogenic infections, sinuses, ischemic limbs, decubitus ulcers
HIV-infected patients	*S. aureus*, streptococci, *Salmonella* sp, mycobacteria	Skin, mucous membranes, catheters
IV drug abusers	Gram-negative bacteria, *S. aureus*, streptococci	Bacteremia

to be indolent and subtle, unlike staphylococcal joint infections, which are more fulminant. In 80% of adults, nongonococcal bacterial arthritis is monarticular and usually occurs in a peripheral joint: knee, hip, shoulder, wrist, ankle, elbow. In children, ≥90% is monarticular: knee (39%), hip (26%), ankle (13%). Polyarticular involvement is somewhat more common in patients who are immunosuppressed or have an underlying chronic arthritis (eg, RA, osteoarthritis). In IV drug abusers, axial joints are often involved (eg, sternoclavicular, costochondral, hip, shoulder, vertebrae, symphysis pubis, sacroiliac joints).

Infection due to human, dog, or cat bites usually develops within 48 h. Rat bites produce systemic symptoms such as fever, rash, and joint pain or true arthritis with regional adenopathy within about 2 to 10 days.

Viral infectious arthritis sometimes produces symptoms similar to acute nongonococcal bacterial arthritis and is more likely than bacterial to be polyarticular.

Patients with *Borrelia burgdorferi* arthritis may have other symptoms of Lyme disease (see p. 1479) or present only with acute monarthritis or oligoarthritis.

Diagnosis

Infectious arthritis is suspected in patients with acute monarticular arthritis and in patients with other combinations of symptoms characteristic of particular infectious arthritis syndromes (eg, migratory polyarthritis, tenosynovitis and skin lesions typical of disseminated gonococcal infection; erythema migrans or other symptoms and signs of Lyme disease). Even mild joint symptoms should arouse suspicion in patients with risk factors, such as RA, a prosthetic joint, or an extra-articular infection capable of spreading to a joint (eg, genital gonococcal infection, bacteremia, any anaerobic infection).

Patients suspected of having acute infectious arthritis should have arthrocentesis with synovial fluid examination and culture and usually imaging and blood studies.

Synovial fluid examination is the cornerstone of diagnosis. Fluid is examined grossly and sent for cell count and differential, Gram stain, aerobic and anaerobic culture, and crystals. Foul-smelling synovial fluid suggests anaerobic infection. Fluid from an acutely infected joint usually reveals a WBC count > 20,000/μL (often > 100,000/μL) consisting of > 95% PMNs. WBC counts tend to be higher in nongonococcal bacterial than in gonococcal infectious arthritis. WBC counts may also be lower in early or partially treated infections. Gram stain reveals organisms in 50 to 75% of joints with acute bacterial arthritis, most often with staphylococci. If positive, Gram stain can be virtually diagnostic, but cultures are definitive. The presence of crystals does not exclude infectious arthritis. Sometimes synovial fluid analysis cannot differentiate between infectious and other inflammatory synovial fluid. If differentiation is impossible by clinical means or synovial fluid, infectious arthritis is assumed, pending culture results.

Plain x-rays of the involved joint are not diagnostic but can exclude other conditions (eg, fractures, chondrocalcinosis). Abnormalities in early acute bacterial arthritis are limited to soft-tissue swelling and signs of synovial effusions. After 10 to 14 days of untreated bacterial infection, destructive changes of joint space narrowing (reflecting cartilage destruction) and erosions or foci of subchondral osteomyelitis may appear. Gas visible within the joints suggests infection with *Escherichia coli* or anaerobes.

MRI is considered if the joint is not easily accessible for examination and aspiration (eg, an axial joint). MRI or ultrasound can identify sites of effusion or abscess that can be aspirated or drained for both diagnosis and therapy. MRI can provide early suggestion of associated osteomyelitis. Bone scans using technetium-99m can be falsely negative in infectious arthritis. Also, because they show increased uptake with increased blood flow in inflamed synovial membranes and in metabolically active bone, they can be falsely positive in noninfectious inflammatory arthritis.

Blood cultures, CBC, and ESR (or C-reactive protein) are usually obtained. However, normal results do not exclude infection.

If gonococcal arthritis is suspected, blood and synovial fluid samples should be *immediately* plated on nonselective chocolate agar, and specimens from the urethra, endocervix, rectum, and pharynx on selective Thayer Martin medium. Genital chlamydial cultures are also obtained. Blood cultures are positive in 60 to 75% of cases during the first week and may be the only method by which to identify the organism; cultures from joints with early tenosynovitis or arthritis are often negative. Synovial fluid cultures from joints with frank purulent arthritis are usually positive, and fluid from skin lesions may be positive. If disseminated gonococcal infection is suspected based on clinical criteria, it is assumed to be present even if all gonococcal cultures are negative.

Diagnosis of Lyme disease is discussed on p. 1479.

Prognosis and Treatment

Acute nongonococcal bacterial arthritis can destroy articular cartilage, permanently damaging the joint within hours or days. Gonococcal arthritis does not usually damage joints permanently. Factors that increase susceptibility to infectious arthritis may also increase disease severity. In patients with RA, functional outcome is particularly poor, and the mortality rate is increased.

Treatment consists of IV antibiotics and, for acute nongonococcal bacterial arthritis or any septic arthritis with persistent effusion, drainage of pus from infected joints. Initial antibiotic selection is directed at the most likely pathogens. The regimen is adjusted based on the results of culture and susceptibility testing.

Gonococcal arthritis is treated with ceftriaxone 1 g IV once/day until at least 24 h after symptoms and signs resolve, followed by ciprofloxacin 500 mg po bid for 7 days. Joint drainage and debridement may be unnecessary. Coexisting genital infection with *C. trachomatis* is also treated, often with doxycycline 100 mg bid for 7 days, and sexual contacts of the patient are treated as necessary (see p. 1652).

If nongonococcal gram-positive infection is suspected in an adult, the empiric choice is one of the following: a semisynthetic penicillin (eg, nafcillin 2 g IV q 4 h), a cephalosporin (eg, ceftriaxone 1 g IV once/day), vancomycin 1 g IV q 12 h (if methicillin resistance is common [eg, with *S. aureus*]), or clindamycin 600 to 900 mg IV q 8 h. If gram-negative infection is suspected, empiric treatment includes a parenteral 3rd-generation cephalosporin and, if infection is severe, an aminoglycoside.

Parenteral antibiotics are continued until clinical improvement is clear (usually 2 wk), and oral antibiotics should be given at high doses for another 2 to 6 wk according to the clinical response. Infections caused by streptococci and *Haemophilus* are usually eradicated after 2 wk of oral antibiotics following IV treatment. Staphylococcal infections require at least 3 wk and often 6 wk or longer, especially in patients with prior arthritis.

In addition to antibiotics, acute nongonococcal bacterial arthritis requires large-bore needle aspiration of intra-articular pus at least once/day, or tidal irrigation lavage, arthroscopic lavage, or arthrotomy for debridement. Infected RA joints should generally undergo even earlier and more aggressive surgical debridement and drainage. Acute bacterial arthritis requires joint splinting for the first few days to reduce pain, followed by passive and active range-of-motion exercises to limit contractures, with muscle strengthening as soon as tolerated.

Viral arthritis is treated supportively. Bite wounds are treated with antibiotics and surgical drainage as necessary (see p. 2638).

CHRONIC INFECTIOUS ARTHRITIS

Chronic infectious arthritis develops over weeks and is usually caused by mycobacteria, fungi, or bacteria with low pathogenicity.

Chronic infectious arthritis accounts for 5% of infectious arthritis and is most likely to develop in patients with RA, HIV infection, immunosuppression, or prosthetic joints (see below); however, it can occur in otherwise normal individuals. Examples of possible causes are *Mycobacterium tuberculosis, M. marinum, M. kansasii, Candida* sp, *Coccidioides immitis, Histoplasma capsulatum, Cryptococcus neoformans, Blastomyces dermatitidis, Sporothrix schenckii, Aspergillus fumigatus, Actinomyces israelii,* and *Brucella* sp. The arthritis of Lyme disease is usually acute but may be chronic. Unusual opportunistic organisms are possible in HIV-infected patients. In chronic infectious arthritis, the synovial membrane can proliferate and can erode articular cartilage and subchondral bone.

Onset is indolent, with gradual swelling, mild warmth, minimal or no redness of the joint area, and aching pain that may be mild. Usually a single joint is involved. A prolonged duration and lack of response to conventional antibiotics suggest a mycobacterial or fungal cause.

Patients should have fungal and mycobacterial cultures of synovial fluid or synovial tissue, as well as routine studies. Plain x-ray findings may differ from acute infectious arthritis in that joint space is preserved longer, and marginal erosions and bony sclerosis may occur. Mycobacterial and fungal joint infections require prolonged treatment, usually with multiple antibiotics, depending on sensitivity testing results.

PROSTHETIC JOINT INFECTIOUS ARTHRITIS

Prosthetic joints are at risk for acute and chronic infection, which can produce morbidity or mortality.

Infections are more common in prosthetic joints. They are frequently caused by intraoperative inoculations of bacteria into the joint or by postoperative bacteremia resulting from skin infection, pneumonia, dental procedures, invasive instrumentation, UTI, or possibly falls. They develop within 1 yr of surgery in ⅔ of cases. During the first few months after surgery, the causes are *Staphylococcus aureus* in 50% of cases, mixed flora in 35%, gram-negative organisms in 10%, and anaerobes in 5%.

There is a history of a fall within 2 wk of symptom onset in about 25% of patients and of prior surgical revisions in about 20%. Some have had a postoperative wound infection that appeared to resolve, satisfactory postoperative recovery for many months, and then development of persistent joint pain at rest and on weight bearing. Symptoms and signs may include prosthesis loosening, pain, swelling, and limited motion; temperature may be normal. Sepsis may occur and produce significant morbidity or mortality.

Treatment must be prolonged. Options include long-term antibiotics in patients not fit for surgery; excision arthroplasty with or without fusion (in patients with uncontrolled infection and insufficient bone stock); arthrotomy for prosthesis removal, with meticulous debridement of all cement, abscesses, and devitalized tissues, followed by prolonged antibiotics; and immediate or delayed (1 to 3 mo) implantation of a new prosthesis using antibiotic-impregnated cement. Infection develops in 38% of new implants, whether replaced immediately or after delay.

OSTEOMYELITIS

Osteomyelitis is inflammation and destruction of bone caused by bacteria, mycobacteria, or fungi. Common symptoms are localized bone pain and tenderness with constitutional symptoms (in acute osteomyelitis) or without constitutional symptoms (in chronic osteomyelitis). Diagnosis is by radiography and cultures. Treatment is with antibiotics and sometimes surgery.

Etiology and Pathophysiology

Osteomyelitis is produced by bloodborne organisms (hematogenous osteomyelitis), by contiguous spread (from infected tissue or an infected prosthetic joint), or by open wounds (from contaminated open fractures or bone surgery). Trauma, ischemia, and foreign bodies predispose to osteomyelitis. Osteomyelitis may form under deep decubitus ulcers.

About 80% of osteomyelitis results from contiguous spread or from open wounds; it is often polymicrobial. *Staphylococcus aureus* is present in ≥ 50%; other common bacteria include streptococci, gram-negative enteric organisms, and anaerobic bacteria. Osteomyelitis that results from contiguous spread is common in the feet (in patients with diabetes or peripheral vascular disease), at sites of bone penetrated by trauma or surgery, and in bones contiguous to decubitus ulcers, such as the hips and sacrum.

Hematogenously spread osteomyelitis usually results from a single organism. In children, gram-positive bacteria are most common, usually affecting the metaphyses of the tibia, femur, or humerus. Hematogenously spread osteomyelitis in adults usually affects the vertebrae. Risk factors in adults are older age, debilitation, hemodialysis, sickle cell disease, and IV drug use. Common infecting organisms include *S. aureus* and enteric gram-negative bacteria (in adults who are older, debilitated, or receiving hemodialysis); *S. aureus, Pseudomonas aeruginosa,* and *Serratia* sp (in IV drug users); and *Salmonella* sp (in patients with sickle cell disease). Fungi and mycobacteria can cause hematogenous osteomyelitis, usually in immunocompromised patients or in areas of endemic infection with histoplasmosis, blastomycosis, or coccidioidomycosis. The vertebrae are often involved.

Osteomyelitis tends to occlude local blood vessels, which causes bone necrosis and local spread of infection. Infection may expand through the bone cortex and spread under the periosteum, with formation of subcutaneous abscesses that may drain spontaneously through the skin.

If treatment of acute osteomyelitis is only partially successful, low-grade chronic osteomyelitis develops.

Symptoms and Signs

Patients with acute osteomyelitis of peripheral bones usually experience weight loss, fatigue, fever, and localized warmth, swelling, erythema, and tenderness.

Vertebral osteomyelitis produces localized back pain and tenderness with paravertebral muscle spasm that is unresponsive to conservative treatment. Patients are usually afebrile.

Chronic osteomyelitis produces intermittent (months to many years) bone pain, tenderness, and draining sinuses.

Diagnosis

Acute osteomyelitis is suspected in patients with localized peripheral bone pain, fever, and malaise; or localized refractory vertebral pain. Chronic osteomyelitis is suspected in patients with persistent localized bone pain, particularly if they have risk factors.

If osteomyelitis is suspected, CBC and ESR or C-reactive protein, as well as plain x-rays of the affected bone, are obtained. The WBC count may not be elevated, but the ESR and C-reactive protein usually are. X-rays become abnormal after 2 to 4 wk, showing periosteal elevation, bone destruction, soft-tissue swelling, and, in the vertebrae, loss of vertebral body height or narrowing of the adjacent infected intervertebral disk space and destruction of the end plates above and below the disk.

If x-rays are equivocal or symptoms are acute, CT or MRI can define abnormalities and reveal abscesses (eg, paravertebral abscesses). Alternatively, a radioisotope bone scan can be performed. It is abnormal earlier than plain x-rays but does not distinguish among infection, fractures, and tumors. Bacteriologic diagnosis is necessary for optimal therapy of osteomyelitis; bone biopsy with a needle or surgical excision and aspiration or debridement of abscesses provides tissue for culture and antibiotic sensitivity testing. Culture of sinus drainage does not necessarily reveal the bone pathogen.

Treatment

Antibiotics are selected to cover both gram-positive and gram-negative organisms until culture results and sensitivities are available. In children and adults, initial antibiotic treatment should include a penicillinase-resistant semisynthetic penicillin (eg, nafcillin or oxacillin 2 g IV q 4 h) and a 3rd- or 4th-generation cephalosporin (such as ceftriaxone 1 g IV q 12 to 24 h or cefepime 2 g IV q 8 h). Antibiotics must be given parenterally for 4 to 8 wk. If any constitutional findings (eg, fever, malaise, weight loss) persist or if large areas of bone are destroyed, necrotic tissue is debrided surgically. Surgery may also be needed to drain coexisting paravertebral or epidural abscesses or to stabilize the spine to prevent injury. Skin or pedicle grafts may be needed to close large surgical defects. Broad-spectrum antibiotics should be continued for > 3 wk after surgery. In chronic osteomyelitis, long-term suppressive antibiotic therapy may be needed.

40 BURSITIS, TENDINITIS, AND FIBROMYALGIA

BURSITIS

Bursitis is acute or chronic inflammation of a bursa. The cause is usually unknown, but trauma, either repetitive or acute, may play a role, as may infection and crystal-induced disease. Symptoms include pain, particularly with motion, swelling, and tenderness. Diagnosis is usually clinical; however, diagnosis of infection and crystal-induced disease requires analysis of bursal fluid. Treatment includes splinting, NSAIDs, sometimes corticosteroid injections, and treatment of any underlying cause.

Bursae are sac-like cavities or potential cavities that contain fluid and are located where friction occurs (eg, where tendons or muscles pass over bony prominences). Bursae minimize friction between moving parts and facilitate movement. They may communicate with joints.

Bursitis may occur in the shoulder (subacromial or subdeltoid bursitis) secondary to rotator cuff tendinitis, which is usually the primary lesion in the shoulder. Other commonly affected bursae include the olecranon (miners' elbow), prepatellar (housemaid's knee) or suprapatellar, retrocalcaneal (Achilles), iliopectineal (iliopsoas), ischial (tailor's or weaver's bottom), greater trochanteric, anserine, and first metatarsal head (bunion) bursae.

Etiology

Bursitis may be caused by injury, chronic overuse, inflammatory arthritis (eg, gout, RA), or acute or chronic infection (eg, pyogenic organisms, particularly *Staphylococcus aureus*). Infection is most common in the olecranon and prepatellar bursae. Acute bursitis may follow unusual exercise or strain and usually causes bursal effusion. Chronic bursitis may follow previous attacks of bursitis or repeated trauma. The bursal wall is thickened, with proliferation of its synovial lining; bursal adhesions, villus formation, tags, and chalky deposits may develop. Bursitis occasionally causes inflammation in a communicating joint.

Symptoms and Signs

Acute bursitis causes pain, particularly with motion, and localized tenderness. Swelling, sometimes with other signs of inflammation, is frequent if the bursa is superficial (eg, prepatellar, olecranon). Crystal-induced or bacterial-induced bursitis is usually erythematous as well as painful and warm.

Chronic bursitis may last for several months and may have multiple recurrences. If inflammation persists near a joint, the patient may have joint fibrosis with limited range of motion.

Diagnosis

Bursitis should be suspected in patients with swelling or signs of inflammation over bursae. It can generally be diagnosed clinically. If the swelling is particularly painful, red, or warm, or if bursitis involves the olecranon or prepatellar bursa, then infection and crystal-induced disease should be excluded by bursal puncture. Using local anesthesia and sterile technique, fluid is withdrawn from the bursa and analyzed for cell count, gram stain and culture, and microscopic search for crystals. Gram stain is not sensitive, and WBC counts in infection can be lower than in septic joints. Urate crystals are easily seen with polarized light, but the apatite crystals typical of calcific tendinitis appear only as shiny, non-birefringent chunks. X-rays should be obtained if the bursitis is persistent or if infection or calcification is suspected.

Hemorrhage into a bursa can cause manifestations similar to acute bursitis, as blood is inflammatory. Cellulitis can cause signs of inflammation but does not normally cause bursal effusion; cellulitis overlying the bursa is a relative contraindication to bursal puncture through the cellulitis, but aspiration must occasionally be done if septic bursitis is strongly suspected.

Treatment

Crystal-induced disease (see p. 299), infection, or an underlying chronic repetitive irritation should be treated if present. In infection, the choice of antibiotic is determined by results of Gram stain and culture. Empiric antibiotics should cover *S. aureus*. Infectious bursitis requires drainage or excision in addition to antibiotics.

Acute nonseptic bursitis is treated with temporary rest or immobilization and high-dose NSAIDs, sometimes with opioids. Voluntary movement should be increased as pain subsides. Pendulum exercises are helpful for the shoulder joint. If oral drugs and rest are inadequate, then aspiration and intrabursal injection of depot corticosteroids 0.5 to 1 mL (eg, triamcinolone acetonide 40 mg/mL) are the treatment of choice. About 1 mL of local anesthetic (eg, 0.5% bupivacaine, 1% lidocaine) may be mixed with the corticosteroid and injected with the same needle, or local anesthesia can be provided before the corticosteroid injection with 1% lidocaine. The dose and volume of corticosteroid can vary according to the size of the bursa. Infrequently, a flare occurs within several hours of injection of a depot corticosteroid; this is probably a form of crystal-induced synovitis. It usually lasts ≤ 24 h and responds to cold compresses plus analgesics. Repeat aspiration and injection may be required.

Chronic bursitis is treated the same as acute bursitis, except that splinting and rest are less likely to help and range-of-motion exercises are especially important. Rarely, the bursa needs to be excised.

TENDINITIS AND TENOSYNOVITIS

These conditions are degeneration (tendinopathy) and associated inflammation (tendinitis) of a tendon or inflammation of the tendon sheath lining (tenosynovitis). Symptoms usually include pain with motion and tenderness on palpation. Chronic tendon deterioration or inflammation can cause scars that restrict motion. Diagnosis is clinical. Treatment includes rest, NSAIDs, and sometimes corticosteroid injections.

A tendinopathy involves tearing or degenerative changes (sometimes with a Ca deposit) in the tendon. Tendinitis and tenosynovitis involve inflammation; the most common site is the synovial-lined sheath that surrounds the tendon (the tendon sheath).

The most common sites are the shoulder and associated tendons (rotator cuff), the tendon of the long head of the biceps muscle, flexor carpi radialis or ulnaris, flexor digitorum, popliteus tendon, Achilles tendon (see p. 2637), and the abductor pollicis longus and extensor pollicis brevis, which share a common fibrous sheath (de Quervain's syndrome—see p. 336).

Etiology

The cause is often unknown. Most cases occur in people who are middle-aged or older as the vascularity of tendons decreases; repetitive microtrauma may contribute. Repeated or extreme trauma (short of rupture), strain, or excessive (unaccustomed) exercise probably also contribute. Tendinitis may also be related to systemic disease (most commonly RA, systemic sclerosis, gout, reactive arthritis, diabetes, and, very rarely amyloidosis or markedly elevated blood cholesterol levels). In younger adults, particularly women, disseminated gonococcal infection may cause acute migratory tenosynovitis.

Symptoms, Signs, and Diagnosis

Involved tendons are usually painful on motion; their sheaths may become swollen and accumulate fluid. Swelling may be only palpable or can also be visible. In systemic sclerosis, the tendon sheath may remain dry but causes friction, which can be felt or heard with a stethoscope when the tendon moves within its sheath. Along the tendon, localized tenderness of variable severity is present on palpation.

Rotator cuff tendinitis (see also p. 2632) is the most common cause of shoulder pain. Active abduction in an arc of 40 to 120° and internal rotation produce pain. Passive abduction produces less pain. Ca deposits in the tendon are sometimes visible on x-ray.

In bicipital tendinitis, pain in the biceps tendon is aggravated by shoulder flexion or resisted supination of the forearm. Tenderness can be elicited proximally over the bicipital groove of the humerus by "flipping" (rolling) the bicipital tendon (under the examiner's thumb).

Volar flexor tenosynovitis (digital tendinitis—see also p. 336) is one of the most common musculoskeletal entities and is often overlooked. Pain occurs in the palm on the volar aspect of the thumb or other digits and may radiate distally. The diagnosis is made by eliciting tenderness on palpation of the tendon and sheath and by noting swelling and possibly a nodule. In later stages, triggering or snapping of the digit occurs on flexion (trigger finger).

Trochanteric bursitis, in reality, is gluteus medius tendinitis. It occurs over the lateral prominence of the greater trochanter of the femur and is usually associated with chronic pressure, trauma, or inflammation at this site (eg, in RA). Localized tenderness is characteristic.

Treatment

Symptoms are relieved by rest or immobilization (splint or sling) of the tendon, application of heat (for chronic inflammation) or cold (for acute inflammation), and high-dose NSAIDs (see TABLE 34–2 on p. 287) for 7 to 10 days. Indomethacin or colchicine may be helpful if gout is responsible (see p. 299). After inflammation is controlled, exercises that gradually increase range-of-motion should be performed several times/day, especially in the shoulder, which can develop contractures rapidly.

Injection of the tendon sheath with a sustained-release corticosteroid (eg, dexamethasone acetate 8 mg/mL or methylprednisolone acetate 20 to 40 mg/mL, depending on the site) may be helpful. An injection through the same needle of an equal or double volume of local anesthetic (eg, 0.5% bupivacaine) can confirm the diagnosis if immediate pain relief is obtained. Care should be taken not to inject the tendon per se (which can be recognized by marked resistance to injection) because the tendon can be weakened, increasing the risk of rupture. Rest of the injected part diminishes the slight risk of rupture. Infrequently, symptoms can worsen for up to 24 h after the injection.

Repeat injections and symptomatic therapy may be required. Surgical exploration and removal of Ca deposits or rotator cuff repair, followed by graded physical therapy, are needed rarely for persistent cases. Surgery is occasionally required for release of occasional function-limiting scars or, as in RA, for tenosynovectomy of chronic inflammation.

FIBROMYALGIA

(Myofascial Pain Syndrome; Fibrositis; Fibromyositis)

Fibromyalgia is a common nonarticular disorder of unknown cause characterized by achy pain, tenderness, and stiffness of muscles, areas of tendon insertions, and adjacent soft tissues. Diagnosis is clinical. Treatment includes exercise, local heat, and drugs for pain and sleep.

Any fibromuscular tissues may be involved, especially those of the occiput, neck, shoulders, thorax, low back, and thighs.

Localized soft-tissue pain and tenderness (ie, myofascial pain syndrome [see also p. 865], is often related to overuse or microtrauma). In fibromyalgia, symptoms and signs are more generalized, and there is no specific histologic abnormality. It sometimes occurs in patients with systemic rheumatic disorders, which complicates the diagnosis. Fibromyalgia is common, occurring most often in women; it can occur even in children or adolescents. The cause is unknown, but disruption of stage 4 sleep may contribute, as can emotional stress. Fibromyalgia may be precipitated by a viral or other systemic infection (eg, Lyme disease).

Symptoms, Signs, and Diagnosis

Stiffness and pain in fibromyalgia frequently begin gradually, diffusely, and with an achy quality. Symptoms can be exacerbated by environmental or emotional stress, poor sleep, trauma, exposure to dampness or cold, or by a physician who gives the patient the incorrect message that it is "all in the head." Patients tend to be stressed, tense, anxious, fatigued, striving, and sometimes depressed. Many patients also have irritable bowel symptoms or tension headaches.

Fibromyalgia is suspected in patients with generalized pain and tenderness, especially disproportionate to the physical findings; with negative laboratory results despite widespread symptoms; or when fatigue is the predominant symptom. Tests should include ESR or C-reactive protein, CK, and probably screens for hypothyroidism and hepatitis C (which can cause similar symptoms). The diagnosis is supported by explicit tender points and other findings, which comprise diagnostic criteria (see FIG. 40–1). Patients meeting some, but not all, criteria may still have fibromyalgia. Chronic fatigue syndrome (see p. 2740) can cause similar generalized myalgias. Polymyalgia rheumatica (see p. 278) can cause generalized myalgias, particularly in older adults but tends to affect proximal muscles selectively and produce a high ESR.

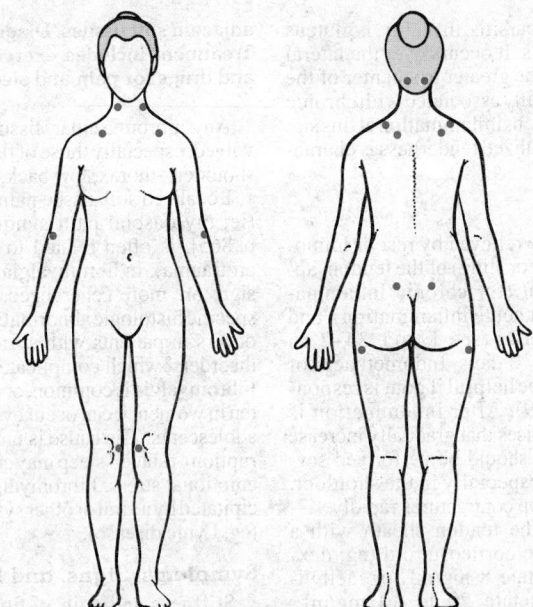

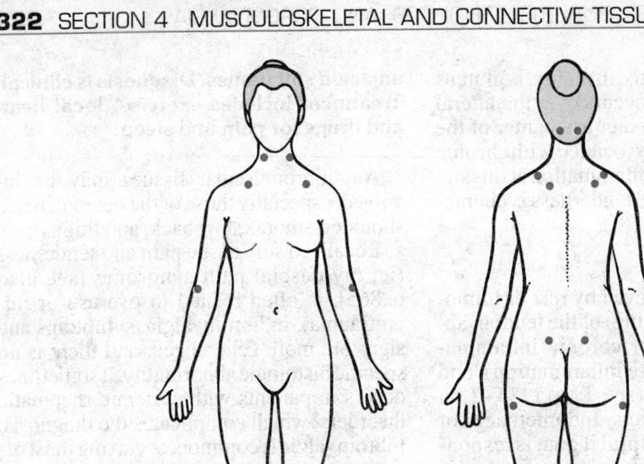

Fig. 40–1. Diagnosing fibromyalgia. For diagnosis, patients tend to have the following features: (1) Pain on palpation of at least 11 of the 18 tender points. Digital palpation should be performed with a force of about 4 kg. For a tender point to be considered positive, palpation must be painful. (2) A history of widespread pain for at least 3 mo. Pain is considered widespread when the patient has pain in the left and right side of the body, above and below the waist, and in the axial skeleton (cervical spine or anterior chest or thoracic spine or low back.)

Prognosis and Treatment

Fibromyalgia may remit spontaneously if stress decreases but can recur at frequent intervals or become chronic. Functional prognosis is usually favorable with a comprehensive, supportive program, although some degree of symptoms tends to persist.

Relief may be obtained from stretching exercises, aerobic exercises, sufficient sound sleep, local applications of heat, and gentle massage. Overall stress management is important.

The involved muscles should undergo daily gentle and prolonged stretches, lasting for about 30 sec and repeated about 5 times. Aerobic exercise (eg, fast walking, swimming, exercise bicycle) can improve symptoms.

Improving sleep is critical. Low-dose oral tricyclic antidepressants at bedtime (eg, amitriptyline 10 to 50 mg, trazodone 50 to 150 mg, doxepin 10 to 25 mg) or the pharmacologically similar cyclobenzaprine 10 to 40 mg may promote deeper sleep and decrease muscle pain. The lowest effective dose should be used. Drowsiness, dry mouth, and other adverse effects may make one or more of these drugs intolerable, particularly in older adults.

Nonopioid analgesics may help individual patients but have not generally been shown to be effective. Opioids should be avoided. Incapacitating areas of focal tenderness may rarely be injected with 0.5% bupivacaine or 1% lidocaine 1 to 5 mL, but this should not be a primary focus of therapy. Caution must be taken not to aggravate sleep problems with drugs that may cause insomnia. Anxiety or depression, if present, may require treatment.

41 NECK AND BACK PAIN

Neck and back pain are common, particularly with aging. Low back pain affects 50% of adults > 60. Symptoms may simply be local pain, which can be sharp or dull, continuous or intermittent, depending on the cause and the degree of concomitant muscle spasms. The reflex tightening of paraspinal muscles in response to a painful vertebral column disorder may be more excruciating than the primary condition. If the spinal cord or nerve roots are affected, a variety of neurologic symptoms may result, including paresthesias and weakness. Pain may radiate distally along the distribution of affected nerve roots (radicular pain or, in the low back, sciatica).

Etiology

Many conditions produce neck and back pain (see TABLE 41–1); most can involve both areas, only a few are specific to one location. Nerve compression, including herniated disk and spinal cord compression, is discussed on p. 1913. Arthritides and ankylosing spondylitis are discussed on p. 290. Nonvertebral disorders are discussed in various other chapters in THE MANUAL.

Most often, neck or back pain derives from benign, self-limited musculoskeletal derangements, such as muscle strain, and ligament sprain. Other common causes include fibromyalgia (see p. 321) and osteoarthritis (see p. 294).

Serious causes include infections (eg, infectious arthritis, osteomyelitis, diskitis, spinal epidural abscess), tumors (primary tumors of vertebrae or spinal cord), metastatic vertebral tumors (most often from breast, lung, or prostate), injuries (eg, fractures, dislocations, subluxations), and spinal cord compression. Causes of spinal cord compression include injuries, herniated intervertebral disks including the cauda equina syndrome, tumors, and subluxation of the first cervical vertebrae on the second (atlantoaxial subluxation).

Evaluation

The history and physical examination often suggest the cause of neck and back pain. Neurologic symptoms and signs are particularly important to elicit. Tests are obtained based on findings during examination.

History: The nature of the pain, including location, exacerbating and relieving factors, and surrounding events, is elicited.

Pain, numbness, paresthesias, or weakness along a nerve root distribution suggests nerve root compression. Weakness or loss of sensation at a spinal level, incontinence, or urinary retention may suggest spinal cord compression.

Onset with injury is usually apparent, but some patients do not connect painful spasm with an apparently minor strain the previous day. Pain from injury is localized, relieved by rest, and worsened by motion. Pain from infection and malignancy is constant, unrelieved by rest, and progressive. Pain and stiffness that are worse upon awakening and last > 45 min suggest ankylosing spondylitis or RA. Pain that is diffuse or changes locations, particularly if unrelated to other factors or associated with poor sleep, suggests fibromyalgia. Morning stiffness of the spine and muscles of the proximal extremities, particularly in an older person, suggests polymyalgia rheumatica.

Associated symptoms and history are important. Fever and IV drug use or known immunosuppression suggests an infectious cause. Weight loss or a history of cancer suggests a malignant etiology, either metastases or pathologic fracture.

Physical examination: A general examination is performed, with particular attention to the spine, as well as careful neurologic examination.

Spinal examination begins with inspection. If possible, the patient should also be observed moving (eg, walking into the office or exam room, undressing) when unaware he is being scrutinized. The neck and back are normally slightly lordotic. Contorted posture suggests muscle spasm, which can be enough to cause scoliosis. Focal erythema may indicate infection, overuse of local heat or irritant creams, or, in certain populations, use of ethnic remedies such as coining or cupping.

Systematic palpation of the spinal column and adjacent areas is performed. Focal bony tenderness suggests infection, tumor, or fracture. Symmetric trigger points (areas that when palpated reproduce neck or back pain) over the back, chest, elbows, and knees suggest fibromyalgia. Trapezius trigger

TABLE 41–1. CAUSES OF NECK AND BACK PAIN

LOCATION	CONDITION
Neck only	Atlantoaxial subluxation Referred pain from carotid or vertebral artery dissection, angina, MI, meningitis, esophageal disease, thyroiditis Herpes zoster Temporomandibular joint disorder Torticollis
Lower back only	Lumbar spinal stenosis Osteitis condensans ilii Osteoporotic fractures (can also be thoracic and occasionally cervical) Referred pain from hip, buttock, or pelvic disorders Referred visceral pain from aortic dissection or aneurysm, renal colic, pancreatitis, retroperitoneal tumor, pleural effusion, pyelonephritis Sacroiliac osteoarthritis Sacroiliitis Spondylolisthesis
Either neck or lower back	Ankylosing spondylitis (usually lower back and can also be thoracic) Arthritis (osteoarthritis, rheumatoid; rheumatoid rarely affects the lower back) Congenital abnormalities (eg, spina bifida, lumbarization of S1) Fibromyalgia Intervertebral disk disease Infection (eg, osteomyelitis, diskitis, spinal epidural abscess, infectious arthritis) Injury (eg, dislocation, subluxation, fracture) Muscle or ligament strain Paget's disease Polymyalgia rheumatica Tumor (primary or metastatic) Spinal cord compression

points may be from cervical disk disease or cervical osteoarthritis affecting the facet joints.

Active and passive range of motion of the neck and back are ascertained. Decreased active range of motion often indicates pain or muscle spasm; intervertebral disk disease is a particularly common cause. Decreased passive range of motion indicates structural spinal abnormalities, most often due to osteoarthritis or multiple osteoporotic fractures, but possibly from other causes such as injuries, ankylosing spondylitis, or diffuse idiopathic skeletal hyperostosis (DISH—see p. 291). An electrical sensation that radiates down the spine with trunk flexion (Lhermitte's sign) suggests spinal cord compression.

Complete neurologic examination is required. Signs that suggest spinal cord compression include bilateral reflex, motor, and sensory abnormalities that occur at a spinal level or that involve the anal sphincter (ie, poor rectal tone, decreased bulbocavernosus reflex or anal wink). Spinal nerve root compression may produce ipsilateral reflex, motor, or sensory deficits confined to the distribution of the affected root. In general, among reflex, motor, and sensory findings, reflex findings are the most objective, and sensory findings are the most subjective.

Extra-axial joint abnormalities may suggest inflammatory arthritis, osteoarthritis, or other systemic musculoskeletal disorders that can affect the spine.

Testing: If symptoms or signs suggest a serious medical condition (eg, MI, leaking or ruptured aortic aneurysm), appropriate tests should be obtained. Patients with possible spinal cord compression or spinal epidural abscess require immediate MRI; if unavailable, CT or myelography (rarely used) can be performed. For suspected osteomyelitis, imaging, usually an MRI, is performed within hours. Plain x-rays are indicated for bony injuries such as fractures, dislocations, and subluxations. Plain x-rays may demonstrate bony changes that can suggest disorders such as osteoarthritis, RA, osteoporosis, vertebral metastases, some infections, and others. However, plain x-rays also identify many abnormalities that are unrelated to symptoms. Testing for the diagnosis of most disorders in TABLE 41–1 is discussed elsewhere in THE MANUAL.

A patient with a clear-cut episode of minor trauma (eg, lifting a box), no neurologic signs and symptoms, and no risk factors for pathologic fracture or subluxation may be treated symptomatically without testing.

Treatment

Acute musculoskeletal neck or back pain is usually treated with oral analgesics (eg, acetaminophen, NSAIDs). Acute muscle spasms may be relieved by ice or heat. Oral muscle relaxants (eg, cyclobenzaprine, methocarbamol, metaxalone) are controversial; because of their CNS adverse effects, these drugs should generally be avoided in elderly patients. Opioids may occasionally be necessary for severe pain.

Spinal manipulation may help pain caused by muscle spasm or after an acute back injury; however, some forms of manipulation may pose risks in patients with disk disease and osteoporosis. Prolonged bed rest and spinal traction are not beneficial. Diathermy may help reduce muscle spasm and pain after the acute stage.

Neck Pain

The most common causes of neck pain are listed above. Patients with RA, juvenile RA, or ankylosing spondylitis may have atlantoaxial subluxation (see p. 328). Causes of referred neck pain include angina, MI, arterial dissection, meningitis, esophageal obstruction, esophageal mass or inflammation, and thyroiditis. On examination, reproduction of radicular pain with neck extension and lateral rotation (Spurling's sign) suggests cervical disk disease. Signs of stroke in the presence of neck pain, particularly with pulse deficits, suggest aortic, carotid, or vertebral arterial dissection. Symptomatic treatment of musculoskeletal neck pain may require a cervical collar and contour pillow for 10 to 14 days to decrease spasm, then a cervical posture and stabilization and stretching program.

Back Pain

The most common causes of back pain are listed above. Osteoporotic fractures are a common cause of back pain in elderly women. Causes of referred pain include ruptured abdominal aortic aneurysm, renal colic, pleural effusion, aortic dissection, and retroperitoneal inflammation (eg, pancreatitis, pyelonephritis) or infiltration (eg, tumor). However, the etiology is often multifactorial, with an underlying condition exacerbated by fatigue, physical deconditioning, and sometimes psychosocial stress or psychiatric abnormality. Certain congenital abnormalities of the spine (eg, facet abnormalities) that were formerly thought responsible for back pain are just as common in patients without pain.

Pain from osteoporotic fractures is constant but usually not progressive, may improve when supine, and usually improves over 4 to 12 wk; it can occur without a history of trauma (see Ch. 36 on p. 305). Pain and stiffness in the morning in a young man suggests ankylosing spondylitis or other spondyloarthropathy. Worsening with back flexion suggests intervertebral disk disease. Worsening with extension suggests spinal stenosis, facet arthritis, or retroperitoneal inflammation or infiltration. Aggravation of lumbar and posterior thigh pain with walking suggests spinal stenosis.

On examination, kyphosis (dowager's hump) suggests osteoporosis. Muscle spasm induced by straight leg raising suggests intervertebral disk disease; pain induced by straight leg raising may also suggest this but is less specific. A pulsatile abdominal mass, particularly with signs of shock, suggests ruptured abdominal aortic aneurysm. Flank tenderness suggests pyelonephritis.

Diagnostic studies may be deferred in patients with no signs or symptoms of concern if the patient is < 50, has no motor or reflex neurologic deficits, no sphincter complaints, no history of cancer, and no fever or weight loss. However, if pain persists for > 6 wk, an imaging study (if the etiology is not clear) or other diagnostic workup (directed at a specific etiology if one is clinically suspected) should be considered. The choice may depend on causes suspected. For example, if osteoporotic fracture is likely, x-ray may be adequate. Whether imaging studies should begin with plain x-rays or MRI if no specific etiology is suspected is not clear. A definitive diagnosis cannot be established in many patients.

In most people with a single acute attack of low back pain, the cause is a self-limited musculoskeletal condition or is nonspecific and multifactorial, and recovery usually occurs over several days to 1 wk. In these patients, attacks may recur or symptoms may become chronic, especially if patients engage in activities beyond their physical capacities. Chronic pain (see full discussion on p. 1776) is a complex phenomenon often involving peripheral and central sensitization and neurologic remodeling, as well as depression and sometimes secondary gain (eg, litigation).

Initial symptomatic treatment of acute nonspecific musculoskeletal back pain usually includes 1 to 2 days of rest (only if needed to minimize pain) and a subsequent lumbar stabilization program. More prolonged bed rest, traction, and corsets are generally not indicated. Exercises that strengthen abdominal and lower back muscles, along with instruction in work posture, are indicated when symptoms permit, to strengthen the supporting structures of the back and decrease the likelihood of the condition becoming chronic or recurrent.

Reassurance about the benign prognosis of acute nonspecific musculoskeletal back pain can relieve anxiety. The physician should be thorough, kind, firm, and nonjudgmental. A low-dose tricyclic antidepressant may improve disturbed sleep and relieve chronic muscle pain. If depression or secondary gain persists for several months, psychological evaluation should be considered.

SPASMODIC TORTICOLLIS

Spasmodic torticollis is characterized by involuntary tonic contractions or intermittent spasms of neck muscles. The cause is unknown, and diagnosis is clinical. Treatment can include physical therapy, drugs, and selective denervation of neck muscles with surgery or locally injected botulinum toxin.

In torticollis, contraction of the neck muscles causes the neck to turn from its usual position. Torticollis is caused most often by a dystonic reaction to drugs. Spasmodic, or adult-onset, torticollis is idiopathic. It is the most common dystonia (see p. 1880). About 5% of patients with spasmodic torticollis have a family history. One third of patients have other dystonias (eg, eyelids, face, jaw, hand). Torticollis can also be congenital or secondary to other conditions such as lesions of the brain stem and basal ganglia.

Symptoms and Signs

Symptoms may begin at any age but usually begin between the 3rd and 6th decades, with a peak in the 4th to 5th decades. Symptoms usually begin gradually but may be sudden. Painful tonic contractions or intermittent spasms of the sternocleidomastoid, trapezius, and other neck muscles occur, usually unilaterally, and cause abnormal head position. Sternocleidomastoid muscle contraction causes rotation of the head to the opposite side and lateral flexion of the neck to the same side. Rotation may involve any plane but almost always has a horizontal component. Besides rotational tilting (torticollis), the head can tilt laterally (laterocollis), forward (anterocollis), or backward (retrocollis). During sleep, muscle spasms disappear.

Spasmodic torticollis ranges from mild to severe. Usually, it progresses slowly for 1 to 5 yr, then plateaus. About 10 to 20% of patients recover spontaneously within 5 yr of onset (usually milder cases of younger onset). However, it may persist for life and can result in restricted movement and postural deformity.

Diagnosis

The diagnosis is made by the characteristic symptoms and signs and by excluding alternative diagnoses. Tardive dyskinesia can produce torticollis but can usually be distinguished by a history of chronic antipsychotic use and involuntary movements in muscles outside of the neck. Basal ganglia disease and occasionally CNS infections can produce movement disorders but usually involve muscles besides those in the neck. CNS infections are also usually acute and produce other symptoms. Neck infections or tumors are usually differentiated by features of the primary process. Antipsychotics and other drugs can cause acute torticollis, but the symptoms usually develop in hours and resolve within days.

Treatment

Spasms can sometimes be temporarily inhibited by physical therapy and massage (eg, slight tactile pressure to the jaw on the same side toward which the head is rotated [sensory biofeedback techniques], or any light touch).

Injections of botulinum toxin type A into the dystonic muscles can reduce painful spasms for 1 to 3 mo in about 70% of patients, restoring a more neutral position of the head. However, this treatment can lose effectiveness with repeated injections because antibodies develop against the toxin. Drugs can usually relieve pain but suppress dystonic movements in only about 25 to 33% of patients. Anticholinergics such as trihexyphenidyl 10 to 25 mg po once/day or bid may help, but adverse effects may limit their use; benzodiazepines (particularly clonazepam 0.5 mg po bid) and baclofen and carbamazepine may help. All drugs should be started in low doses: Doses should be increased until symptoms are controlled or intolerable adverse effects (particularly likely in older patients) develop.

Surgery is controversial. The most successful surgical approach selectively severs nerves to affected neck muscles, permanently weakening or paralyzing them. Results are favorable when performed at centers with extensive experience.

Rarely, an emotional problem contributes to spasmodic torticollis; it should be treated psychiatrically. The psychiatric prognosis is best if symptom onset coincided with exogenous stress.

SCIATICA

Sciatica is pain along the sciatic nerve. It usually results from compression of nerve roots in the lower back. Common causes include disk disease, osteophytes, and narrowing of the spinal canal (spinal stenosis). Symptoms include pain radiating from the buttocks down the leg. Diagnosis is by MRI or CT. Electromyography and nerve conduction studies help confirm the affected level. Treatment includes symptomatic measures and sometimes surgery, particularly if there is a neurologic deficit.

Etiology

Sciatica is generally caused by nerve root compression, usually from intervertebral disk protrusion (see p. 1913), bony irregularities (eg, osteoarthritic osteophytes, spondylolisthesis), or intraspinal tumor or abscess. Compression may occur within the spinal canal or intervertebral foramen. The nerves can also be compressed outside the vertebral column, in the pelvis or buttocks. The L5-S1, L4-L5, and L3-L4 nerve roots are most often affected (see TABLE 224–1 on p. 1910).

Symptoms and Signs

Pain radiates along the course of the sciatic nerve, most often down the buttocks and the posterior aspect of the leg to below the knee. The pain is typically burning, lancinating, or stabbing. It may occur with or without low back pain. Valsalva maneuver may worsen the pain.

Nerve root compression can produce sensory, motor, or, the most objective finding, reflex deficits (see also p. 1901). L5-S1 disk herniation may affect the ankle jerk reflex, whereas L3-L4 herniation may affect the knee jerk. Straight leg raising may produce pain radiating down the leg when the leg is raised above 60° and sometimes less. This is sensitive for sciatica; pain radiating down the involved leg with lifting of the contralateral leg (crossed straight leg raising) is more specific for sciatica.

Diagnosis

Sciatica is suspected by the characteristic pain. If suspected, sensation, strength, and reflexes should be tested. If there are neurologic deficits, or if symptoms persist for > 6 wk, imaging and electrodiagnostic studies should be performed. Structural abnormalities causing sciatica (including spinal stenosis) are most accurately diagnosed by MRI or CT. Electrodiagnostic studies can confirm the presence and degree of nerve root compression and can exclude conditions that may mimic sciatica, such as polyneuropathy and nerve entrapment. These studies may help determine whether the lesion involves single or multiple nerve levels and whether the clinical findings correlate with MRI abnormalities (especially valuable before surgery).

Treatment

Acute pain relief can come from 24 to 48 h of bed rest in a recumbent position with the head of the bed elevated about 30° (semi-Fowler's position). Treatment begins with 6 wk of the measures used to treat low back pain, including nonopioid analgesics such as NSAIDs and acetaminophen. In addition, symptoms may improve with drugs that decrease neuropathic pain (see p. 1779), such as gabapentin or other anticonvulsants or low-dose tricyclic antidepressants (no tricyclic is superior to another). Gabapentin should start at 100 to 300 mg po at bedtime, but doses typically have to be much higher, up to 3600 mg/day. As with all sedating drugs, care should be taken in the elderly, those at risk for falls, and those with arrhythmias.

Muscle spasm may be relieved with therapeutic heat or cold (see p. 2753), and physical therapy may be useful. Controversy exists concerning the use of corticosteroids for acute radicular pain. Given epidurally, corticosteroids may accelerate pain relief, but they probably should not be used unless pain is severe or persistent.

Indications for surgery are unequivocal disk herniation, with muscular weakness or progressive neurologic deficit, and intolerable and intractable pain that interferes with job or personal functions in an emotionally stable patient and that has not improved with 6 wk of conservative treatment. Alternatively, in some patients, epidural corticosteroids are helpful.

Classic diskectomy with limited laminotomy for intervertebral disk herniation is the standard procedure. If herniation is localized, microdiskectomy may be performed, which allows a smaller skin incision and laminotomy. Chemonucleolysis, using intradiskal injection of chymopapain, has fallen out of favor.

Predictions of poor surgical outcome include prominent psychiatric factors, persistence of symptoms for more than 6 mo, heavy manual labor, prominence of back pain (nonradicular), and secondary gain (ie, litigation and compensability).

LUMBAR SPINAL STENOSIS

Lumbar spinal stenosis is narrowing of the lumbar spinal canal, which produces pressure on the sciatic nerve roots (or sometimes the cord) before their exit from the foramina, causing positional back pain and symptoms of nerve root compression.

Spinal stenosis can be congenital or acquired. It may involve the cervical or lumbar spine. Acquired lumbar spinal stenosis (LSS) is a common mechanism for sciatica in middle-aged or elderly patients. Its most common causes are degenerative, such as osteoarthritis, disk disease, and spondylolisthesis with compression of the cauda equina. Other causes may include Paget's disease, RA, and ankylosing spondylitis.

LSS produces pain in the buttocks, thighs, or calves on walking, running, climbing stairs, or even standing. The pain is not relieved by standing still but by flexing the back or by sitting (although paresthesias may continue). Walking up hills is less painful than walking down because the back is slightly flexed. Pain, paresthesias, weakness, and diminished reflexes may occur in the affected nerve root distribution. Rarely, spinal cord compression may produce cauda equina syndrome (see p. 1910).

Spinal stenosis is suspected by characteristic symptoms. Diagnostic studies are obtained as in sciatica. Symptoms involving the calves may simulate intermittent claudication. Claudication can be differentiated by skin atrophy and by abnormalities in pulses, capillary refill, and vascular tests.

Conservative treatments and indications for surgery are similar to those for sciatica. Surgery for advanced spinal stenosis involves decompression of nerve root entrapment by vertebral canal and foraminal encroachments, which sometimes requires laminectomy at two or three levels and foraminotomies. Spinal stability must be preserved. Spinal fusion is indicated if there is instability or severe, well-localized arthritic changes in one or two interspaces.

NONTRAUMATIC SUBLUXATION

Spinal dislocation and subluxation (partial dislocation) are usually due to obvious trauma. However, atlantoaxial subluxation and spondylolisthesis can occur with minimal or unrecognized trauma. Rarely, cervical disk disease can also produce nontraumatic spinal subluxation.

ATLANTOAXIAL SUBLUXATION

(C1–C2 subluxation)

Atlantoaxial subluxation is misalignment between the 1st and 2nd cervical vertebrae, which may occur only with neck flexion.

Atlantoaxial subluxation can result from major trauma such as a high-speed deceleration injury; however, it can occur without trauma in patients with RA, juvenile RA, or ankylosing spondylitis. Atlantoaxial subluxation is usually asymptomatic but may cause vague neck pain, occipital headache, or occasionally intermittent (and potentially fatal) cervical spinal cord compression.

It is usually diagnosed with plain cervical x-rays; however, plain x-rays may not demonstrate subluxation that is intermittent unless flexion views are obtained. Flexion, done by the patient, shows dynamic instability of the entire cervical spine. If x-rays are normal and subluxation is strongly suspected, an MRI, which is more sensitive, should be performed. MRI also provides the most sensitive evaluation of spinal cord compression and is obtained immediately if cord compression is suspected.

Indications for treatment include pain, neurologic deficits, and potential spinal instability. Treatment includes symptomatic measures and cervical immobilization, usually beginning with a rigid cervical collar. Surgery may be needed to stabilize the spine.

SPONDYLOLISTHESIS

Spondylolisthesis is subluxation of lumbar vertebrae, usually occurring in adolescence. It often occurs because of a congenital defect in the pars interarticularis (spondylolysis).

Spondylolisthesis is usually fixed. It usually involves the L3-L4, L4-L5, or L5-S1 vertebrae. It can result from major trauma such as high-speed deceleration injuries. Patients with spondylolisthesis due to major trauma may have spinal cord compression or other neurologic deficits (see p. 1913), but this occurs rarely. Spondylolisthesis often occurs in adolescents or young adults who are athletes or who have sustained only minimal trauma; the reason is that a lumbar vertebra is weakened because the pars interarticularis has an underlying congenital defect. This defect is easily fractured; separation of the fracture fragments produces the subluxation. Spondylolisthesis can also occur with minimal trauma in patients > 60 yr who have underlying osteoarthritis.

Spondylolisthesis is staged according to the degree of subluxation of adjacent vertebral bodies. Stage I spondylolisthesis corresponds to subluxation of 0 to 25%; stage II to 25 to 50%; stage III to 50 to 75%; and stage IV to 75 to 100%. Spondylolisthesis of stages I or II, particularly in the young, may cause no or only minimal pain. Spondylolisthesis can predispose to later development of spinal stenosis. Spondylolisthesis is evident on plain lumbar x-rays. Treatment is usually symptomatic, as for other causes of musculoskeletal low back pain.

42 HAND DISORDERS

Common hand disorders include a variety of deformities, ganglia, infections, Kienböck's disease, nerve compression syndromes, and noninfectious tenosynovitis. Complex regional pain syndrome (reflex sympathetic dystrophy) is discussed on p. 1780, and hand injuries are discussed in Ch. 369 on p. 2557.

Evaluation

History and physical examination findings are often diagnostic in hand disorders.

History: The history should include information about the trauma or other events that may be associated with symptoms. The presence and duration of deformity and difficulty with motion are noted. The presence, duration, severity, and factors that exacerbate or relieve pain are elicited. Associated symptoms, such as fever, swelling, rashes, Raynaud's phenomenon (see p. 751), paresthesias, and weakness, are also recorded.

Physical examination: Examination should include inspection and palpation for tenderness and swelling. Active range of motion should be tested for any possible tendon injury. Passive range of motion can assess whether specific motions aggravate pain. Sensation is tested most accurately by two-point discrimination, using two ends of a paper clip. Motor function testing involves muscles innervated by the radial, median, and ulnar nerves. Vascular examination should include evaluation of capillary refill, radial and ulnar pulses, and Allen's test (see p. 370). Stress testing is helpful when specific ligament injuries are suspected (eg, ulnar collateral ligament in gamekeeper's thumb—see p. 2570).

Laboratory testing: Laboratory testing has a limited role. Plain x-rays and MRI are helpful for injuries, arthritis, and Kienböck's disease or to rule out hidden foreign bodies that could be sources of infections. Nerve conduction testing can help diagnose nerve compression syndromes. Bone scans may assist in diagnosing occult fractures and reflex sympathetic dystrophy.

DEFORMITIES

Deformities can result from generalized disorders (eg, arthritis) or dislocations, fractures, and other localized disorders. Most nontraumatic localized disorders can be diagnosed by physical examination. Once a hand deformity becomes firmly established, it cannot be significantly altered by splinting, exercise, or other nonsurgical treatment.

MALLET FINGER

Mallet finger is a flexion deformity of the distal interphalangeal joint preventing extension (see FIG. 42–1).

This deformity results from an extensor tendon rupture or an avulsion fracture of the distal phalanx. Closed injuries may be treated with splinting that holds the distal interphalangeal (DIP) joint in extension and leaves the proximal interphalangeal (PIP) joint free. Avulsion fractures are usually united after 6 wk, but pure tendon injuries require an additional 2 to 4 wk of night-time splinting. Surgery may be required if there is a fracture that involves a large proportion of the articular surface or if the joint is subluxated.

SWAN-NECK DEFORMITY

A swan-neck deformity consists of hyperextension of the PIP joint, flexion of the DIP joint, and, sometimes flexion of the metacarpophalangeal joint (see FIG. 42–2).

Although characteristic in RA, swan-neck deformity has several causes, including untreated mallet finger, laxity of the ligaments of the volar aspect of the PIP joint, spasticity of intrinsic hand muscles, rupture of the flexor tendon of the PIP joint, and malunion of a fracture of the middle or proximal phalanx. The inability to correct or compensate for hyperextension of the PIP joint makes finger closure impossible and can cause severe disability. Treatment is aimed at correcting the underlying cause when possible (eg, correcting the mallet finger or any bony malalignment, releasing spastic intrinsic muscles). Mild deformities in patients with RA may be treated with a functional ring splint.

True swan-neck deformity does not affect the thumb, which has only one interphalangeal joint. However, severe hyperextension of the interphalangeal joint of the thumb with flexion of the metacarpophalangeal (MCP) joint can occur; this is called a duck bill, Z (zigzag) type, or 90°-angle deformity. With simultaneous thumb instability, pinch is greatly impaired. This deformity can usually be corrected by interphalangeal arthrodesis along with tendon reconstruction at the MCP joint.

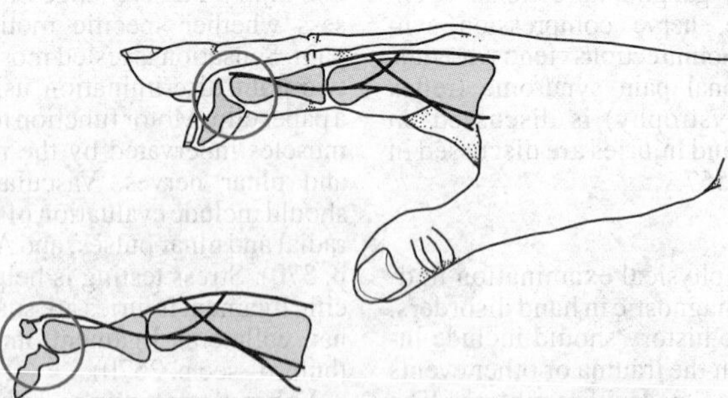

Fig. 42–1. Mallet finger. Impaired flexion at the distal interphalangeal joint can result from a tendon injury or bony avulsion.

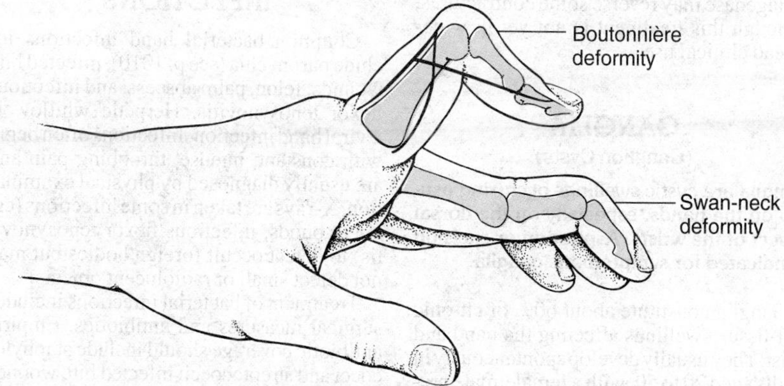

Fig. 42–2. Boutonnière and swan-neck deformities.

BOUTONNIÈRE DEFORMITY

(Buttonhole Deformity)

A boutonnière deformity consists of flexion of the PIP joint accompanied by hyperextension of the DIP joint (see FIG. 42–2).

This deformity can result from tendon laceration, dislocation, fracture, osteoarthritis, or RA. Classically, the deformity is caused by disruption of the central slip attachment of the extensor tendon to the base of the middle phalanx, allowing the proximal phalanx to protrude ("buttonhole") between the lateral bands of the extensor tendon. Initial treatment consists of splinting, but it must occur before scarring and fixed deformities develop. Surgical reconstruction often cannot restore normal motion but may decrease the deformity and improve hand function.

DUPUYTREN'S CONTRACTURE

(Palmar Fibromatosis)

Dupuytren's contracture is progressive contracture of the palmar fascial bands, producing flexion deformities of the fingers.

This is one of the more common hand deformities; the incidence is higher in men and increases after age 45. This autosomal dominant condition with variable penetrance occurs more commonly in patients with diabetes, alcoholism, or epilepsy. However, the specific factor that causes the palmar fascia to thicken and contract is unknown.

Symptoms and Signs

The earliest manifestation is usually a tender nodule in the palm, most often near the middle or ring finger; it gradually becomes painless. Next, a superficial cord forms and contracts the MCP joints and interphalangeal joints of the fingers. The hand eventually becomes arched. The disease is occasionally associated with fibrous thickening of the dorsum of the PIP joints (Garrod's pads), Peyronie's disease (penile fibromatosis) in about 7 to 10% of patients, and rarely nodules on the plantar surface of the feet (plantar fibromatosis). Other types of flexion deformities of the fingers can also occur in diabetes, systemic sclerosis, and chronic reflex sympathetic dystrophy, which need to be differentiated.

Treatment

Injection of a corticosteroid suspension into the nodule can relieve local tenderness if begun before contractures develop. If the hand cannot be placed flat on a table or, especially, when significant contracture develops at the PIP joints, surgery is usually indicated. Excision of the diseased fascia must be meticulous because it surrounds neurovascular bundles and tendons. Incomplete excision or new disease results in recurrent contracture, especially in patients who are young at disease onset or who have a family history, Garrod's pads, Peyronie's disease, or plantar foot involvement. Injectable collagenase may reverse some contractures, although this treatment is not yet in widespread clinical use.

GANGLIA

(Ganglion Cysts)

Ganglia are cystic swellings occurring usually on the hands, especially on the dorsal aspect of the wrists. Aspiration or excision is indicated for symptomatic ganglia.

Ganglia constitute about 60% of chronic soft-tissue swellings affecting the hand and wrist. They usually develop spontaneously in adults aged 20 to 50, with a female:male preponderance of 3:1.

Etiology, Pathogenesis, and Diagnosis

The cause of most ganglia is unknown. The cystic structures are near or attached (often by a pedicle) to tendon sheaths and joint capsules. The wall of the ganglion is smooth, fibrous, and of variable thickness. The cyst is filled with clear gelatinous, sticky, or mucoid fluid of high density. The fluid in the cyst is sometimes almost pure hyaluronic acid.

Most ganglia are isolated abnormalities. The dorsal wrist ganglion arises from the scapholunate joint and constitutes about 65% of ganglia of the wrist and hand. The volar wrist ganglion arises over the distal aspect of the radius and constitutes about 20 to 25% of ganglia. Flexor tendon sheath ganglia and mucous cysts (arising from dorsal distal interphalangeal joint) make up the remaining 10 to 15%. Ganglia may spontaneously regress.

Another type of ganglion on the dorsal wrist occurs in patients with RA; it is easily differentiated by its soft irregular appearance and association with proliferative rheumatoid extensor tenosynovitis.

Treatment

Most ganglia do not require treatment. However, if the patient is disturbed by its appearance or if the ganglion is painful or tender, a single aspiration is effective in up to 70% of patients. Attempting to rupture the ganglion by hitting it with a hard object risks local injury without likely benefit. Nonsurgical treatment fails in about 15 to 30%, necessitating surgical excision. Recurrence rates after surgical removal are about 10 to 15%.

INFECTIONS

Common bacterial hand infections include paronychia (see p. 1010), infected bite wounds, felon, palm abscess, and infectious flexor tenosynovitis. Herpetic whitlow is a viral hand infection. Infections often begin with constant, intense, throbbing pain and are usually diagnosed by physical examination. X-rays are taken in some infections (eg, bite wounds, infectious flexor tenosynovitis) to detect occult foreign bodies but may not detect small or radiolucent objects.

Treatment of bacterial infections includes surgical measures and antibiotics. Empiric antibiotic coverage should include staphylococci and streptococci; infected bite wounds require coverage for additional organisms.

INFECTED BITE WOUNDS

A small puncture wound, particularly from a human or cat bite, may involve significant injury to the tendon, joint capsule, or articular cartilage. The most common cause of human bites is a tooth-induced injury to the metacarpophalangeal joint as a result of a punch to the mouth (clenched fist injury). The oral flora of humans includes *Eikenella corrodens,* staphylococci, streptococci, and anaerobes. Patients with clenched fist injuries tend to wait hours or days after the wound occurs before seeking medical attention, which increases the severity of the infection. Animal bites usually contain multiple potential pathogens, including *Pasteurella multocida* (particularly in cat bites), staphylococci, streptococci, and anaerobes. Serious complications include infectious arthritis and osteomyelitis.

Symptoms, Signs, and Diagnosis

Erythema and pain localized to the bite suggest infection. Tenderness along the course of a tendon suggests spread to the tendon sheath. Pain worsening significantly with motion suggests infection of a joint or tendon sheath.

The diagnosis is clinical, but if the skin is broken, x-rays should be obtained to detect fracture or teeth or other foreign bodies that could be a nidus of continuing infection.

Treatment

Treatment includes surgical debridement, with the wound left open, and antibiotics. For outpatient treatment, empiric antibiotics usually include monotherapy with amoxicillin/clavulanate 500 mg po tid or combined therapy with a penicillin 500 mg po qid (for *E. corrodens, P. multocida,* streptococci, and anaerobes) plus a cephalosporin (eg, cephalexin 500 mg po qid) or semisynthetic penicillin (eg, dicloxacillin 500 mg po qid) for staphylococci. If the patient is allergic to penicillin, clindamycin 300 mg po q 6 h can be used. The hand should be splinted in the functional position and elevated (see FIG. 42–3).

Noninfected bites may require surgical debridement and prophylaxis with 50% of the dose of antibiotic used to treat infected wounds.

FELON

A felon is an infection of the pulp space of the fingertip, usually with staphylococci and streptococci.

The most common site is the distal pulp, which may be involved centrally, laterally, or apically. The septa between pulp spaces ordinarily limit the spread of infection, resulting in an abscess, which creates pressure and necrosis of adjacent tissues. The underlying bone, joint, or flexor tendons may become infected. There is intense throbbing pain and a swollen, warm, extremely tender pulp. Treatment involves prompt incision and drainage (using a midlateral incision that adequately divides the fibrous septa) and administration of oral antibiotics. Empiric treatment with a cephalosporin is adequate.

PALM ABSCESS

A palm abscess is a purulent infection of deep spaces in the palm, typically with staphylococci or streptococci.

Palm abscesses can include collar-button abscesses, thenar space abscesses, and midpalmar space abscesses. An abscess can occur in any of the deep palmar compartments and spread between the metacarpals, from the midpalmar space to the dorsum, presenting as an infection on the dorsum of the hand. Intense throbbing pain occurs with swelling and severe tenderness on palpation. X-rays should be obtained to detect occult foreign bodies. Incision and drainage in the operating room (with cultures), with care to avoid the many important anatomic structures, and antibiotics (eg, a cephalosporin) are required.

INFECTIOUS FLEXOR TENOSYNOVITIS

Infectious flexor tenosynovitis is an acute infection within the flexor tendon sheath.

The usual cause is a penetration and bacterial inoculation of the sheath. Infectious flexor tenosynovitis produces Kanavel's signs: flexed resting position of the digit, fusiform swelling, tenderness along the flexor tendon sheath, and pain with passive extension of the digit. X-rays should be obtained to detect occult foreign bodies. Acute calcific tendinitis and RA can restrict motion and produce pain in the tendon sheath but can usually be differentiated from infectious flexor tenosynovitis by a more gradual

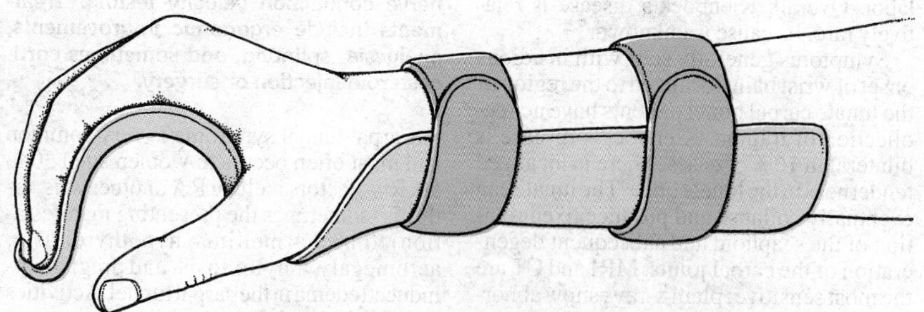

Fig. 42–3. Splint in the functional position (20° wrist extension, 60° metacarpophalangeal joint flexion, slight interphalangeal joint flexion).

onset and the absence of some of Kanavel's signs.

Treatment is surgical drainage (eg, irrigation of the tendon sheath by inserting a cannula into one end and allowing the irrigating fluid to pass along the tendon sheath to the other end). Antibiotic therapy (beginning empirically with a cephalosporin) and cultures are also required.

Herpetic Whitlow

Herpetic whitlow is a cutaneous infection of the distal aspect of the finger caused by herpes simplex virus.

Herpetic whitlow may cause intense pain. The digital pulp is not very tense. Vesicles develop on the volar or dorsal distal phalanx but often not until 2 to 3 days after pain begins. The intense pain can simulate a felon, but herpetic whitlow can usually be differentiated by the absence of tenseness in the pulp or the presence of vesicles.

The condition is self-limited but may recur. Incision and drainage are contraindicated. Topical acyclovir 5% can shorten the duration of a first episode. Oral acyclovir (800 mg po bid) may prevent recurrences if given immediately after onset of recurrent symptoms. Open or draining vesicles should be covered to prevent transmission.

KIENBÖCK'S DISEASE

Kienböck's disease is avascular necrosis of the lunate bone.

Kienböck's disease occurs most commonly in the dominant hand of men aged 20 to 45, usually in workers doing heavy manual labor. Overall, Kienböck's disease is relatively rare. Its cause is unknown.

Symptoms generally start with insidious onset of wrist pain, localized to the region of the lunate carpal bone; patients have no recollection of trauma. Kienböck's disease is bilateral in 10% of cases. There is localized tenderness in the lunate bone. The lunate can eventually collapse and produce fixed rotation of the scaphoid and subsequent degeneration of the carpal joints. MRI and CT are the most sensitive; plain x-rays show abnormalities later, usually beginning with a sclerotic lunate, then later cystic changes, fragmentation, and collapse.

Treatment is aimed at relieving pressure on the lunate by surgically shortening the radius or lengthening the ulna. Alternative treatments attempt to revascularize the lunate (eg, implanting a blood vessel or bone graft on a vascular pedicle). Salvage procedures (eg, proximal row carpectomy or intercarpal fusions) may help preserve some wrist function if the carpal joints have degenerated. Total wrist arthrodesis can be performed as a last resort to relieve pain.

NERVE COMPRESSION SYNDROMES

Common nerve compression syndromes include carpal tunnel syndrome, cubital tunnel syndrome, and radial tunnel syndrome. Compression of nerves often causes paresthesias; these paresthesias can often be reproduced by tapping the compressed nerve, usually with the examiner's fingertip (Tinel's sign). Suspected nerve compression can be confirmed by testing nerve conduction velocity and distal latencies, which accurately measure motor and sensory nerve conduction. Initial treatment is usually conservative, but surgical decompression may be necessary if conservative measures fail or if there are significant motor or sensory deficits.

Carpal Tunnel Syndrome

Carpal tunnel syndrome is compression of the median nerve as it passes through the carpal tunnel in the wrist. Symptoms include pain and paresthesias in the median nerve distribution. Diagnosis is suggested by symptoms and signs and confirmed by nerve conduction velocity testing. Treatments include ergonomic improvements, analgesia, splinting, and sometimes corticosteroid injection or surgery.

Carpal tunnel syndrome is very common and most often occurs in women aged 30 to 50. Risk factors include RA or other wrist arthritis (sometimes the presenting manifestation), diabetes mellitus, hypothyroidism, acromegaly, amyloidosis, and pregnancy-induced edema in the carpal tunnel. Activities or jobs that require repetitive flexion and extension of the wrist may contribute. Most cases are idiopathic.

Symptoms, Signs, and Diagnosis

Symptoms include pain of the hand and wrist associated with tingling and numbness, classically distributed along the median nerve (the palmar side of the thumb, the index and middle fingers, and the radial half of the ring finger) but possibly involving the entire hand. Typically, the patient wakes at night with burning or aching pain and with numbness and tingling and shakes the hand to obtain relief and restore sensation. Thenar atrophy and weakness of thumb opposition and abduction may develop late.

The diagnosis is strongly suggested by Tinel's sign, in which median nerve paresthesias are reproduced by tapping at the volar surface of the wrist over the site of the median nerve in the carpal tunnel. Reproduction of tingling with wrist flexion (Phalen's sign) is also suggestive. However, clinical differentiation from other types of peripheral neuropathy may sometimes be difficult. If symptoms are severe or the diagnosis is uncertain, conduction testing should be performed on the median nerve.

Treatment

Changing the position of computer keyboards and making other ergonomic corrections may provide relief. Otherwise, treatment includes wearing a lightweight neutral wrist splint (see FIG. 42–4), especially at night, and using mild analgesics (eg, acetaminophen, NSAIDs). If these measures fail to control symptoms, a corticosteroid (eg, 2 to 3 mL dexamethasone, 4 mg/mL) should be injected into the carpal tunnel at a site just ulnar to the palmaris longus tendon and proximal to the distal crease at the wrist. If bothersome symptoms persist or recur or if hand weakness and thenar wasting progress, the carpal tunnel can be surgically decompressed using an open or endoscopic technique.

CUBITAL TUNNEL SYNDROME

(Ulnar Neuropathy)

Cubital tunnel syndrome is compression or traction of the ulnar nerve at the elbow.

The ulnar nerve is commonly irritated at the elbow or, rarely, the wrist. Cubital tunnel syndrome is most often caused by leaning on the elbow or by prolonged and excessive elbow flexion. It is less common than carpal tunnel syndrome. Baseball pitching, which can injure the medial elbow ligaments, confers risk.

Symptoms, Signs, and Diagnosis

Symptoms include numbness and paresthesia along the ulnar nerve distribution (in the ring and little fingers and the ulnar aspect of the hand) and elbow pain. In advanced stages, weakness of the intrinsic muscles of the hand and the flexors of the ring and little fingers may develop. Weakness interferes with pinch between the thumb and index finger and with hand grip.

Cubital tunnel syndrome is differentiated from ulnar nerve entrapment at the wrist (in Guyon's canal) by the presence of sensory deficits (on sensory testing or with Tinel's sign) over the ulnar dorsal hand, and the presence of ulnar nerve deficits proximal to the wrist on muscle testing or nerve conduction velocity testing.

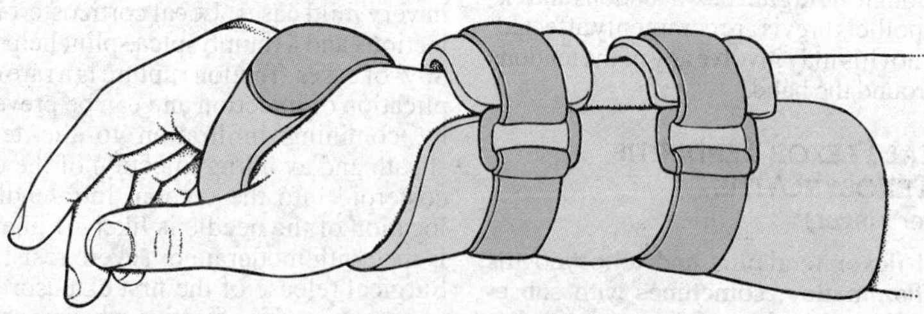

Fig. 42–4. Neutral wrist splint.

Treatment

Treatment involves splinting at night, with the elbow extended at 45°, and use of an elbow pad during the day. Surgical decompression can help if conservative treatment fails.

RADIAL TUNNEL SYNDROME
(Posterior Interosseous Nerve Syndrome)

Radial tunnel syndrome is compression of the radial nerve in the proximal forearm.

Compression at the elbow can result from trauma, ganglia, lipomas, bone tumors, or radiocapitellar ("elbow") synovitis.

Symptoms, Signs, and Diagnosis

Symptoms include lancinating pain in the dorsum of the forearm and lateral elbow. Pain is precipitated by attempted extension of the wrist and fingers and forearm supination. Sensory loss is rare because the radial nerve is principally a motor nerve at this level. When weakness of the extensor muscles is the primary finding, the condition is posterior interosseus nerve palsy. Lateral epicondylitis can cause similar tenderness around the lateral epicondyle but does not produce Tinel's sign or tenderness along the course of the radial nerve.

Treatment

Splinting allows avoidance of the forceful or repeated motion of supination or wrist dorsiflexion, reducing pressure on the nerve. If wristdrop or weakened digital extension develops, or conservative treatment fails to produce relief after 3 mo, surgical decompression may be needed.

NONINFECTIOUS TENOSYNOVITIS

(See also p. 320.)

Although the digital flexor tendons and extensor pollicis brevis are commonly affected, tenosynovitis may involve any of the tendons in or around the hand.

DIGITAL FLEXOR TENDINITIS AND TENOSYNOVITIS
(Trigger Finger)

Digital flexor tendinitis and tenosynovitis are inflammation, sometimes with subsequent fibrosis, of tendons and tendon sheaths of the digits.

These conditions are idiopathic but are common in patients with RA or diabetes mellitus. In diabetes, they often coexist with carpal tunnel syndrome and occasionally with fibrosis of the palmar fascia. Pathologic changes begin with a thickening or nodule within the tendon; when located at the site of the tight first annular pulley, the thickening or nodule blocks smooth extension or flexion of the finger. The finger may lock in flexion, or "trigger," suddenly extending with a snap.

Treatment of acute inflammation and pain includes splinting, moist heat, and anti-inflammatory doses of NSAIDs (see p. 286). If these measures fail, injection of a corticosteroid suspension into the flexor tendon sheath may provide safe, rapid relief of pain and triggering. Operative release can be performed if corticosteroid therapy fails.

DE QUERVAIN'S SYNDROME
(Washerwoman's Sprain)

De Quervain's syndrome is stenosing tenosynovitis of the short extensor (extensor pollicis brevis) and long abductor tendon (abductor pollicis longus) of the thumb within the first extensor compartment.

De Quervain's syndrome usually occurs after repetitive use (especially wringing) of the wrist, although it occasionally occurs in association with RA. The major symptom is aching pain at the wrist and thumb, aggravated by motion. Tenderness can be elicited just proximal to the radial styloid process over the site of the involved tendon sheaths. Diagnosis is highly suggested by the Finkelstein test. The patient adducts the involved thumb into the palm and wraps the fingers over the thumb. The test is positive if passive ulnar deviation of the wrist provokes severe pain at the affected tendon sheaths.

Rest, warm soaks, and NSAIDs may help in very mild cases. Local corticosteroid injections and a thumb spica splint help 70 to 80% of cases. Tendon rupture is a rare complication of injection and can be prevented by confining infiltration to the tendon sheath and avoiding injection of the corticosteroid into the tendon. Intratendinous location of the needle is likely if injection is met with moderate or severe resistance. Surgical release of the first extensor compartment is very effective when conservative therapy fails.

43 FOOT AND ANKLE DISORDERS

Most foot problems result from anatomic disorders or abnormal function of articular or extra-articular structures (see FIG. 43–1). Less commonly, foot problems reflect a systemic disorder (see TABLE 43–1). In diabetics and people with peripheral vascular disease, careful examination of the feet, with evaluation of vascular sufficiency and neurologic integrity, should be performed at least twice/year.

The feet are also common sites for corns and calluses (see p. 951) and infections by fungus (see p. 992), bacteria (see p. 980), and viruses (see p. 998).

TABLE 43–2 lists foot and ankle disorders according to anatomic site. TABLE 43–3 lists common causes of heel pain according to location.

TIBIALIS POSTERIOR TENDINOSIS

Tibialis posterior tendinosis, degeneration of the tibialis posterior tendon, is the most common cause of pain behind the medial malleolus.

The posterior tibial tendon lies immediately behind the medial malleolus. Degeneration results from long-standing biomechanical problems, such as excessive pronation usually in obese people.

Early on, patients experience occasional pain behind the inner ankle. Over time, the pain becomes severe, with painful swelling behind the medial malleolus. Normal standing and walking become difficult.

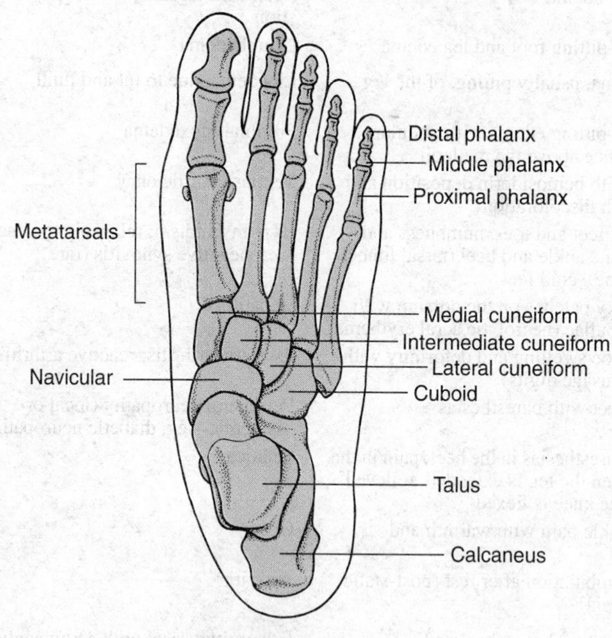

Fig. 43–1. Bones of the foot.

TABLE 43–1. FOOT MANIFESTATIONS OF SYSTEMIC DISORDERS

FOOT SYMPTOMS	POSSIBLE CAUSE
Pain at rest (feet elevated), relieved by dependency	End-stage peripheral arterial disease
Cold, red or cyanotic feet	Advanced arterial ischemia
Episodically red, hot, very painful feet	Erythromelalgia—idiopathic (most commonly) or secondary to various medical conditions
Foot pain that becomes severe within seconds or possibly minutes, particularly in patients with atrial fibrillation	Embolic arterial occlusion
Cyanosis of a single toe (blue toe syndrome)	Anticoagulation therapy; thromboembolic disease due to aortic-iliac stenosis, or cholesterol embolization (following coronary artery bypass or catheterization)
Bilateral episodic digital pallor and cyanosis	Raynaud's disease or phenomenon
Bilateral resting peripheral cyanosis	Heart failure, especially if peripheral pulses are palpable
Bilateral permanent painless cyanosis (in a young female)	Acrocyanosis
Bilateral edema	Renal, hepatic, or cardiac disease; drugs (eg, Ca channel blockers)
Unilateral edema	Deep vein thrombosis; lymphatic obstruction
Firm non-pitting foot and leg edema	Lymphedema
Firm edema, usually pitting, of the leg only	Lipedema, due to fat and fluid
Firm non-pitting edema with nodular appearance above the malleoli	Pretibial myxedema
Edema with hemosiderin deposition and brownish discoloration	Venous insufficiency
Edema of feet and toes, numbness and pain at the ankle and heel (tarsal tunnel syndrome), cold feet	Hypothyroidism; relapsing symmetric seronegative synovitis (rare)
Red, dusky patches on the dorsum with flaccid bullae (necrolytic acral erythema)	Hepatitis C
Isolated toe swelling and deformity with pain (sausage digits)	Psoriatic arthritis; reactive arthritis
Painful feet with paresthesias	Peripheral neuropathy (local or systemic—eg, diabetic neuropathy)
Pain or paresthesias in the heel; pain in the foot when the leg is extended, relieved when the knee is flexed	Sciatica
Toe or ankle pain with warmth and redness	Gout
Painful ambulation after rest (post-static dyskinesia)	Arthritis
Thickened (> 22 mm) heel pad	Hyperpituitarism with acromegaly

Palpation of the tendon in an inverted-plantar flexed position usually elicits pain. Standing on the toes is usually painful and may not be possible if the tendon is ruptured. Pain and swelling behind the medial malleolus, especially with tibialis posterior tendon pain on palpation, are highly suggestive. MRI confirms injury to the tendon and its extent.

Complete rupture requires surgery if normal function is the goal. Surgery is especially important in young active patients with acute tears. Conservative therapy consists of mechanically off-loading the tendon using orthotics and ankle braces. Corticosteroid injections exacerbate the degenerative process (see sidebar 43–1).

TABLE 43–2. FOOT AND ANKLE DISORDERS BY ANATOMIC SITE

Ankle (anterolateral)
- Meniscoid body
- Neuralgia of the intermediate dorsal cutaneous nerve
- Peroneal tenosynovitis

Ankle (medial)
- Tarsal tunnel syndrome
- Tibialis posterior tendinosis

Ball of the foot
- Corns and calluses
- Interdigital nerve pain (Morton's neuroma)
- Metatarsalgia
- Metatarsophalangeal joint pain
- Sesamoiditis

Heel (plantar)
- Inferior calcaneal bursitis
- Plantar fasciosis

Heel (posterior)
- Achilles tendon enthesopathy
- Anterior Achilles tendon bursitis
- Posterior Achilles tendon bursitis

Heel (sides)
- Epiphysitis of the calcaneus (Sever's disease)
- Medial plantar nerve entrapment

Plantar arch (sole)
- Plantar fascial sprain
- Plantar fibromatosis

Toe
- Bunion
- Hammer toe
- Ingrown toe nail
- Onychomycosis
- Paronychia

TARSAL TUNNEL SYNDROME

(Posterior Tibial Nerve Neuralgia)

Posterior tibial nerve neuralgia is pain along the course of the posterior tibial nerve, usually resulting from nerve compression.

At the level of the ankle, the posterior tibial nerve passes through a fibro-osseous canal and divides into the medial and lateral plantar nerves. Tarsal tunnel syndrome refers to compression of the nerve within this canal, but the term has been loosely applied to neuralgia of the posterior tibial nerve resulting from any cause. Synovitis of the flexor tendons of the ankle caused by abnormal foot function, inflammatory arthritis (eg, RA), fracture, and ankle venous stasis edema are contributing factors. Patients with hypothyroidism may develop tarsal tunnel-like symptoms as a result of perineural mucin deposition.

Symptoms and Signs

Pain (occasionally burning and tingling) is usually retromalleolar and sometimes in the plantar medial heel and may extend along the plantar surface as far as the toes. While the pain is worse during standing and walking, pain at rest may occur as the disorder progresses. Recalcitrant symptoms may result from fibro-osseus compression.

Diagnosis and Treatment

Tapping or palpating the posterior tibial nerve below the medial malleolus at a site of compression or injury often produces distal tingling (Tinel's sign). False-negative results on electrodiagnostic tests are common. The cause of any swelling near the nerve should be determined.

Strapping the foot in a neutral or slightly inverted position or wearing an orthotic that keeps the foot inverted reduces nerve tension. Local infiltration of an insoluble corticosteroid/anesthetic may be effective if the cause is inflammation or fibrosis. Surgical decompression may be necessary to relieve suspected fibro-osseus compression with recalcitrant symptoms.

TABLE 43–3. DISORDERS ASSOCIATED WITH HEEL PAIN ACCORDING TO LOCATION

LOCATION OF PAIN	ASSOCIATED DISORDER
Plantar surface of the heel	Plantar fasciosis (plantar fascitis, calcaneal spur syndrome)
Medial and lateral margins of the heel	Epiphysitis of the calcaneus (Sever's disease, in children), medial plantar nerve entrapment
Anterior to the Achilles tendon at the retromalleolar space	Fracture of the posterolateral talar tubercle, tibialis posterior tendinosis, anterior Achilles tendon bursitis, tarsal tunnel syndrome
Posterior to the Achilles tendon	Posterior Achilles tendon bursitis
Calcaneal insertion of the Achilles tendon	Achilles tendon enthesopathy

METATARSALGIA

Metatarsalgia is a general term for pain in the area of the metatarsophalangeal joints (ball of the foot). Most common causes include interdigital nerve pain (Morton's neuroma), metatarsophalangeal joint pain, and sesamoiditis.

INTERDIGITAL NERVE PAIN

(Morton's Neuroma/Neuralgia)

Interdigital nerve irritation (neuralgia) or persistent benign enlargement of the perineurium (neuroma) can produce pain, which may be nonspecific, burning, or lancinating, or produce a foreign body sensation. Diagnosis is usually clinical. Treatment may involve correction of footwear, local injection, or sometimes surgical excision.

The interdigital nerves of the foot travel beneath and between the metatarsals, extending distally to innervate the toes. Neuralgia of the interdigital nerve along its distal innervation near the ball of the foot develops primarily as a result of improper or constrictive foot wear or, less commonly, nerve traction resulting from abnormal foot structure. As a result of chronic repetitive trauma, a benign thickening of the nerve develops (Morton's neuroma).

Symptoms and Signs

Interdigital neuralgia is characterized by pain around the metatarsal heads or the toes. Early interdigital neuralgia often produces an occasional mild ache or discomfort in the ball of the foot, usually when wearing a specific shoe. Neuralgia is usually unilateral. As the condition progresses, the nerve thickens (Morton's neuroma). The pain becomes worse, often with a burning or lancinating quality or paresthesias. In time, patients are unable to wear most shoes. While walking, patients often falsely sense a pebble in their shoes, which they take off for relief. Neuroma most frequently affects the 3rd interspace. Only slightly less common is involvement of the 2nd interspace. Sometimes both interspaces or feet are involved simultaneously.

Diagnosis and Treatment

The symptoms are often specific, and the diagnosis is confirmed by tenderness on plantar palpation of the interdigital space. While MRI does not usually confirm neuroma, it may be useful to rule out other interspace lesions or arthritis causing similar symptoms.

Neuralgia of recent onset usually resolves quickly with properly fitting shoes and insoles or with local anesthetic injection. In contrast, neuromas may require one or more perineural infiltrations of long-acting corticosteroids with a local anesthetic. Injection is at a 45° angle to the foot, into the interspace at the level of the dorsal aspect of the metatarsophalangeal joints. An appropriate orthotic often relieves symptoms. If conservative therapy is ineffective, excision often brings complete relief. However, another neuroma occasionally develops at the site of nerve excision (amputation neuroma).

Metatarsophalangeal Joint Pain

Metatarsophalangeal joint pain usually results from tissue changes due to aberrant foot biomechanics. Symptoms and signs include pain with walking and tenderness. Diagnosis is clinical; however, infection or systemic rheumatic diseases such as RA may need to be excluded by testing. Treatment includes orthotics, sometimes local injection, and occasionally surgery.

Metatarsophalangeal joint pain most commonly results from misalignment of the joint surfaces with altered foot biomechanics, causing joint subluxations, capsular impingement, and joint cartilage destruction (osteoarthrosis). Synovial impingement by misaligned joints may develop, causing mild heat and swelling (osteoarthritic synovitis). Hammertoe deformities may result in subluxation of the metatarsal heads downward, causing metatarsalgia.

Metatarsophalangeal joint subluxations also occur as a result of inflammatory arthropathy, particularly RA. Inflammatory synovitis and interosseous muscle atrophy in RA lead to subluxations of the lesser metatarsophalangeal joints as well, resulting in hammer toe deformities. Consequently, the metatarsal fat pad, which usually cushions the stress between the metatarsals and interdigital nerves during walking, moves distally under the toes; interdigital neuralgia or Morton's neuroma may result. To compensate for the loss of cushioning, adventitial bursae may develop.

Symptoms, Signs, and Diagnosis

Symptoms include pain on walking. Dorsal and plantar joint tenderness is usually present on palpation and during passive range of motion. Mild swelling with minimal heat occurs in osteoarthritic synovitis. Significant warmth, swelling, and redness suggest inflammatory arthropathies; their absence makes inflammatory arthropathies unlikely. Monarticular heat, redness, and swelling indicate infection until proven otherwise. When warmth, redness, and swelling involve multiple joints, a rheumatic disease work-up is indicated, eg, antinuclear antibodies, rheumatoid factor, ESR. Metatarsophalangeal joint pain can usually be differentiated from neuralgia or neuroma of the interdigital nerves by the absence of burning, numbness, and tingling and interspace pain, although these symptoms may develop from joint inflammation; if so, palpation can help in differentiation.

Treatment

Orthotics redistribute and relieve pressure from the noninflamed joints. If inflammation is present (synovitis), a local corticosteroid/anesthetic injection may be useful. With excess subtalar eversion or when the feet are highly arched, an orthotic that corrects these abnormal motions should be prescribed. Surgery may be needed if conservative therapy is ineffective.

Sesamoiditis

Sesamoiditis is pain at the sesamoid bones beneath the head of the 1st metatarsal, with or without inflammation or fracture. Diagnosis is usually clinical. Treatment is usually modification of footwear.

Sidebar 43–1. CONSIDERATIONS FOR USING CORTICOSTEROID INJECTIONS

Corticosteroid injections should be used judiciously to avoid adverse effects. Injectable corticosteroids should be reserved for inflammation, which is not present in most foot disorders, or symptoms due to scar tissue. Because the dorsum of the toes, tarsus, ankle, and retrocalcaneal space have little connective tissue between the skin and underlying bone, injection of insoluble corticosteroids into these structures may cause depigmentation, atrophy, or ulceration, especially in elderly patients with peripheral arterial disease.

Insoluble corticosteroids can be given deeply with greater safety, eg, in the heel pad, tarsal canal, or metatarsal interspaces. The foot should be immobilized for a few days after tendon sheaths are injected. Unusual resistance to injection suggests injection into a tendon, which, if it occurs repeatedly, weakens the tendon, predisposing to subsequent rupture, and should be avoided.

The two semilunar shaped sesamoid bones aid the foot in locomotion. The medial bone is the tibial sesamoid, and the lateral bone is the fibular sesamoid. Direct trauma or positional change of the sesamoids due to alterations in foot structure (eg, lateral displacement of a sesamoid due to lateral deviation of the great toe) can make the sesamoids painful.

Symptoms and Signs

The pain of sesamoiditis is beneath the head of the 1st metatarsal, usually made worse by walking, and may be worse when wearing certain shoes. Occasionally, inflammation occurs, producing mild warmth and swelling or occasionally redness that may extend medially and appear to involve the 1st metatarsophalangeal joint. Sesamoid fracture can also cause pain, moderate swelling, and possibly inflammation.

Diagnosis and Treatment

With the foot and big toe dorsiflexed, the examiner inspects the metatarsal head and palpates each sesamoid. Tenderness is localized to a sesamoid, usually the tibial sesamoid. Hyperkeratotic tissue may indicate that a wart or corn is causing pain. If inflammation produces swelling around the 1st metatarsophalangeal joint, arthrocentesis may be necessary to exclude gout and infectious arthritis. If fracture, osteoarthritis, or displacement is suspected, x-rays are obtained. Sesamoids separated by cartilage or fibrous tissue (bipartite sesamoids) may appear fractured on x-rays. If plain x-rays are equivocal, MRI may be ordered.

Simply not wearing shoes that cause pain may be sufficient. If symptoms persist, shoes with a thick sole and orthotics are prescribed and help by reducing sesamoid pressure. If fracture without displacement is present, conservative therapy may be sufficient and may also involve immobilization of the joint with the use of a flat rigid surgical shoe. While surgery may help in recalcitrant cases, it is controversial because of the potential for disturbing biomechanics and locomotion of the foot. If inflammation is present, treatment includes conservative measures plus local infiltration of a corticosteroid/anesthetic solution to help reduce symptoms.

PLANTAR FASCIOSIS

(Plantar Fascitis)

Plantar fasciosis is pain at the site of the attachment of the plantar fascia and the calcaneus, with or without accompanying pain along the medial border of the plantar fascia. Diagnosis is mainly clinical. Treatment involves calf muscle and plantar soft-tissue foot–stretching exercises, night splints, and orthotics.

Syndromes of pain in the plantar fascia have been called plantar fascitis; however, because there is generally no inflammation, planter fasciosis is more correct. Other terms used include calcaneal enthesopathy pain or calcaneal spur syndrome; however, there may be no bone spurs on the calcaneus. The usual cause is shortening or contracture of the calf muscles and plantar fascia. Risk factors for such shortening include a sedentary lifestyle, occupations requiring sitting, and wearing high-heel shoes. The disorder may involve acute or chronic stretching, tearing, and degeneration of the fascia at its attachment site. Multiple injections of corticosteroids may contribute.

Symptoms and Signs

Plantar fasciosis is characterized by pain on weight bearing at the bottom of the heel, particularly when first arising in the morning, which usually improves within 5 to 10 min, only to return later in the day. Acute severe heel pain, especially with mild local puffiness, may indicate an acute tear. Some patients have burning or sticking pain along the plantar medial border of the foot when walking.

Diagnosis

Other disorders causing heel pain can mimic plantar fasciosis. Throbbing heel pain, particularly when the shoes are removed or with mild heat and puffiness, is more suggestive of calcaneal bursitis (see p. 343). Acute severe heel pain with redness and heat may indicate gout. Pain that radiates from the low back to the heel may be an S1 radiculopathy due to an L5 disk herniation.

Plantar fasciosis is confirmed if firm thumb pressure applied to the calcaneus when the foot is dorsiflexed elicits pain. Fascial pain along the plantar medial border of the fascia may also be present. If findings are equivocal, demonstration of a heel spur on x-ray may support the diagnosis; however, absence does not rule out the diagnosis, and visible spurs may not be the cause of symptoms. Also, infrequently, calcaneal spurs appear ill defined on x-ray, exhibiting fluffy new bone formation, suggesting spondyloarthropathy (eg, ankylosing spondylitis, reactive arthritis). If an acute fascial tear is suspected, MRI is performed.

Treatment

The most effective treatments include calf-stretching exercises and night splinting (Royce night splint) that stretches the calf and plantar fascia. However, compliance is usually poor. OTC or custom-made foot orthotics may also alleviate fascial tension and symptoms. Immediate relief can be provided by a 0.5-inch soft, flexible heel support or injection of a local anesthetic without a corticosteroid. For acute fascial tears, treatment is immobilization.

INFERIOR CALCANEAL BURSITIS

Bursitis can also develop at the inferior calcaneus, near the insertion of the plantar fascia. Symptoms and signs include throbbing heel pain, particularly when the shoes are removed, mild warmth, and swelling. Diagnosis is clinical. Treatment is injection of a local anesthetic/corticosteroid mixture.

ACHILLES TENDON ENTHESOPATHY

Achilles tendon enthesopathy is pain at the insertion of the Achilles tendon at the posterosuperior aspect of the calcaneus.

The cause is chronic traction of the Achilles tendon on the calcaneus. Contracted or shortened calf muscles resulting from a sedentary lifestyle and obesity or athletic overuse are factors.

Pain at the posterior heel below the top of the shoe counter during ambulation is characteristic. Palpation of the tendon at its insertion is diagnostic. Manual dorsiflexion of the ankle during palpation usually exacerbates the pain.

Physical therapy aimed at calf muscle stretching should be prescribed 10 min tid. The patient can exert pressure posteriorly to stretch the calf muscle while facing a wall at arms' length, with knees extended and foot dorsiflexed. Royce night splints should be prescribed. Heel lifts may temporarily relieve pain.

ANTERIOR ACHILLES TENDON BURSITIS

(Albert's Disease; Retromalleolar Bursitis)

Anterior Achilles tendon bursitis is inflammation of the retromalleolar (retrocalcaneal) bursa, located anterior (deep) to the attachment of the Achilles tendon to the calcaneus.

Bursitis is due to trauma (eg, from rigid or poorly filling shoes) or inflammatory arthritis (eg, RA). On occasion, small calcaneal erosions may develop from severe inflammation.

Symptoms caused by trauma develop rapidly; those caused by systemic disease develop gradually. Pain, swelling, and warmth around the heel are common, as are difficulty walking and wearing shoes. The bursa is tender. Initially, the swelling is localized anterior to the Achilles tendon but in time extends medially and laterally.

Using the thumb and index finger, side-to-side compression anterior to the Achilles tendon produces pain. Fracture of the posterolateral talar tubercle also produces tenderness anterior to the insertion of the Achilles tendon. Bursitis is often differentiated from the fracture by the localization of warmth and swelling contiguous to the tendon and pain localized primarily in the soft tissue. Also, x-rays are taken to rule out fracture as well as erosive calcaneal changes characteristic of RA or other rheumatic disorders.

Intrabursal injection of a soluble corticosteroid/anesthetic and warm compresses may be effective.

POSTERIOR ACHILLES TENDON BURSITIS

Posterior Achilles tendon bursitis is inflammation of a bursa that forms in response to shoe pressure and is located at the top edge of the posterior shoe counter between the skin and Achilles tendon.

Symptoms and Signs

Symptoms and signs develop at the top edge of the posterior shoe counter. Early symptoms may be limited to redness and pain. Later, superficial skin erosion may occur. After months or longer, a fluctuant, tender, cystic nodule 1- to 3-cm in diameter develops. It is red or flesh colored. In chronic cases, the bursa becomes fibrotic.

Diagnosis and Treatment

The presence of the small, tender, flesh-colored or red nodule is diagnostic. Rarely, Achilles tendon xanthoma develops at the top edge of the posterior shoe counter but tends to be pink and asymptomatic. Achilles tendon enthesopathy causes pain mainly at the tendon's insertion but may also cause pain at the top edge of the posterior shoe counter. Enthesopathy is differentiated by the absence of a soft-tissue lesion.

Properly fitting shoes with low heels are essential. A foam rubber or felt heel pad may be needed to lift the heel high enough so that the bursa does not hit the shoe counter. Padding around the bursa or the wearing of a backless shoe until inflammation subsides is indicated. Intrabursal injection of a local anesthetic/corticosteroid offers temporary relief; the Achilles tendon itself must be avoided. Surgical removal of a portion of the underlying bone may be necessary to reduce soft-tissue impingement.

EPIPHYSITIS OF THE CALCANEUS

(Sever's Disease)

Epiphysitis of the calcaneus is painful disruption between the calcaneal apophysis and the body of the heel that occurs before calcaneal ossification is complete.

The calcaneus develops from two centers of ossification: one begins at birth, the other usually after age 8. Ossification is usually complete by age 15. The cartilaginous disruption in calcaneal epiphysitis may result from an excessive pull on the apophysis by contracted or shortened calf muscles. Bone growth spurts without adaptive calf muscle lengthening may play a role.

Pain develops in a patient (usually aged 9 to 14) with a history of athletic activity; it affects the sides or margins of the heel and is aggravated by standing on tip toes or running. Warmth and swelling are occasionally present. The diagnosis is clinical. X-rays are not helpful.

Heel pads relieve symptoms by reducing the pull of the Achilles tendon on the heel. Casting is also used to relieve pain and stretch the gastro-soleus complex. Royce night splints may be used. Reassurance is important, as symptoms may last several months.

MEDIAL PLANTAR NERVE ENTRAPMENT

Medial plantar nerve entrapment is symptomatic compression of the medial branch of the posterior tibial nerve at the medial heel.

Symptoms include almost constant pain, off and on weight bearing. Simple standing is often difficult. Burning, numbness, and paresthesias are usually absent. On physical examination, symptoms can be reproduced by palpation over the proximal aspect of the abductor hallucis and/or the origin of the plantar fascia at the medial tubercle of the calcaneus.

Treatment is unrewarding. Conservative and surgical treatments often yield frustrating results. Immobilization and foot orthoses to prevent movement may be helpful.

PLANTAR FIBROMATOSIS

Plantar fibromatosis is a benign proliferative neoplasia of the plantar fascia.

In plantar fibromatosis, nodules are displayed most easily when the foot is dorsiflexed against the leg. Most patients have palmar nodules, usually located at the 4th metacarpophalangeal joint. Reported associations with diabetes, epilepsy, and alcoholism may be anecdotal. Treatment is usually not indicated. Surgery usually results in recurrence and may also result in unintentional instability of the foot when fascial removal is excessive.

HAMMER TOE DEFORMITY

Hammer toe is a C-shaped deformity due to dorsal subluxation at the metatarsophalangeal joint.

The usual cause is misalignment of the joint surfaces due to a genetic predisposition toward aberrant foot biomechanics and tendon contractures. RA and neurologic disorders such as Charcot-Marie-Tooth disease are other causes. Toes two and five are the most common to develop hammer toe. Second toe hammer toes commonly result from pressure due to an excessively abducted great toe (hallux valgus deformity) causing a bunion (see p. 345). Painful corns (see p. 951) often develop in hammer toe deformity, particularly of the 5th toe. Reactive adventitial bursas often develop beneath corns, which may become inflamed.

Symptoms include pain while wearing shoes, especially shoes with low and narrow toe boxes, and sometimes metatarsalgia. Diagnosis is clinical. Joints are examined for coexistent arthritis (eg, RA).

Shoes should have a wide toe box. Toe pads sold in pharmacies also help by shielding the affected toes from the overlying shoe. If these measures are ineffective, surgical correction of the deformity often relieves symptoms. If there is metatarsalgia, orthotics are prescribed.

BUNION

Bunion is a prominence of the medial portion of the head of the 1st metatarsal bone. The cause is often variations in position of the 1st metatarsal bone or great toe, such as lateral angulation of the great toe (hallux valgus). Secondary osteoarthritis and spur formation are common. Symptoms may include pain and redness, bursitis medial to the joint, and synovitis. Diagnosis is usually clinical. Treatment is usually a shoe with a wide toe box, protective pads, and orthotics. For bursitis or synovitis, corticosteroid injection is helpful.

Contributing factors may include excessive turning in (pronation) of the ankles and occasionally trauma. Joint misalignment causes osteoarthritis with cartilage erosion and exostosis formation, resulting in joint motion being limited (hallux limitus) or eliminated (hallux rigidus). In late stages, synovitis occurs, causing joint swelling. In reaction to pressure from tight shoes, an adventitious bursa can develop medial to the joint prominence, which can become painful, swollen, and inflamed.

Symptoms and Signs

The initial symptom may be pain at the joint prominence when wearing certain shoes. The joint capsule may be tender at any stage. Later symptoms may include a painful, warm, red, cystic, movable, fluctuant swelling located medially (adventitial bursitis) and swelling and mild inflammation affecting the entire joint (osteoarthritic synovitis), which is more circumferential. With hallux limitus or rigidus, there is restriction of passive joint motion, tenderness of the lateral aspect of the joint, and increased dorsiflexion of the distal phalanx.

Diagnosis

The diagnosis is clinical. Acute circumferential intense pain, warmth, swelling, and redness suggest gouty arthritis or infectious arthritis, often mandating examination of synovial fluid. If multiple joints are affected, systemic rheumatic disease should be considered. If clinical diagnosis of osteoarthritic synovitis is equivocal, x-rays are obtained. Suggestive findings include joint space narrowing and bony spurs extending from the metatarsal head or sometimes from the base of the proximal phalanx. Radiographic periarticular erosions (Martel's sign) suggest gout.

Treatment

Mild discomfort may improve by wearing a shoe with a wide toe box. If not, bunion pads purchased in most pharmacies can shield the painful area. Orthotics can also be prescribed to redistribute and relieve pressure from the affected articulation. If conservative therapy fails or if the patient is unwilling to wear large, wide shoes and orthotics because they are unattractive, surgery aimed at correcting abnormal bony alignments and restoring joint mobility should be strongly considered. For bursitis, bursal aspiration and injection of a corticosteroid are indicated. For osteoarthritic synovitis, oral NSAIDs or an intra-articular corticosteroid/anesthetic mixture reduces symptoms. For hallux limitus or hallux rigidus, treatment aims to preserve joint mobility using passive stretching exercises, which occasionally require injection of a local anesthetic to relieve muscle spasm. Sometimes surgical release of contractures is necessary.

INGROWN TOENAIL

(Onychocryptosis)

An ingrown toenail is incurvation or impingement of a nail border into its adjacent nail fold, causing pain.

Causes include tight shoes, abnormal gait (eg, toe-walking), bulbous toe shape, or congenital variations in nail contour (pincer nails). Sometimes an underlying osteochondroma is responsible, especially in the young.

In the elderly, peripheral edema is a risk factor. Eventually, infection can occur along the nail margin (paronychia—see p. 1010).

Pain occurs at the corner of the nail fold, or less commonly, along its entire lateral margin. Initially only mild discomfort may be present, especially when wearing certain shoes. In chronic cases, granulation tissue develops, more often in the young.

Diagnosis is clinical. Redness, swelling, and pain suggest paronychia. In young patients with ingrown toenails, x-rays are obtained to exclude underlying osteochondroma. In the elderly, apparent granulation tissue around the toe suggests the possibility of amelanotic melanoma, which is often overlooked; biopsy is necessary.

In mild cases, inserting cotton between the ingrown nail plate and painful fold (using a thin toothpick) may provide immediate relief and, if continued, correct the problem. If the shoes are too tight, a larger toe box is indicated. In most cases, however, particularly with paronychia, excision of the ingrown toenail using local anesthesia is the only effective treatment. If ingrown toenails recur, permanent destruction of the nail matrix by application of phenol or surgical excision is indicated. Phenol should not be used if there is arterial insufficiency.

44 TUMORS OF BONES AND JOINTS

In children, most bone tumors are primary and some are malignant; metastatic tumors are rare. In adults, metastatic tumors are about 20 times more common than primary malignant tumors. Joint tumors are extremely rare in both children and adults.

Symptoms, Signs, and Diagnosis

Bone tumors typically cause pain and swelling. The most common problem in diagnosing bone tumors is failure to suspect them. Persistent or progressive unexplained pain of the trunk or extremities, particularly if associated with a mass, is suspicious. Plain x-rays are the first test, but lesions suggestive of tumors usually require biopsy. Some tumors have characteristic x-ray findings and can be diagnosed without biopsy.

Certain x-ray signs (eg, symmetry, sclerosis of tumor borders, lysis, mineralization) may help distinguish benign from malignant tumors. X-ray signs that suggest malignancy include a lytic appearance; irregular tumor borders; areas, especially multiple areas, of bone destruction ("moth-eaten appearance"); cortical destruction; soft-tissue extension; and pathologic fracture. Certain tumors have a characteristic appearance (eg, Ewing's tumor has a lytic, destructive appearance; giant cell tumor has a cystic appearance). The tumor's location may narrow diagnostic possibilities (eg, Ewing's tumor commonly appears first in the shaft of a long bone; osteosarcoma usually appears in the metaphysis toward the end of a long bone; giant cell tumor usually affects the epiphysis).

Heterotopic ossification (myositis ossificans) and exuberant callus formation after fracture can cause mineralization around bony cortices and in adjacent soft tissues, mimicking malignant tumors. Langerhans' cell histiocytosis (histiocytosis X, Letterer-Siwe disease, Hand-Schüller-Christian disease, eosinophilic granuloma) can cause solitary or multiple bone lesions that are usually distinguishable on x-ray. In solitary lesions, there may be periosteal new bone formation, suggesting a malignant bone tumor. Osteopoikilosis ("spotted bones") is an asymptomatic condition of no clinical consequence that can simulate bone metastases. It is characterized by multiple small round or oval foci of bony sclerosis, usually in the tarsal, carpal, or pelvic bones or the metaepiphyseal regions of tubular bones.

CT and MRI may help define the location and extent of a bone tumor and sometimes suggest a specific diagnosis. If tumors are suspected of being metastatic or involving multiple foci (multicentric), then radioisotopic bone scanning should be performed to search for all tumors.

Biopsy is usually essential for diagnosis. The pathologist should be given pertinent details of the clinical history and x-ray findings.

Histopathologic diagnosis may be difficult and requires sufficient tissue from a representative portion of the tumor (usually the soft portion). The best results are obtained in centers with extensive experience in bone biopsies. Immediate, accurate, definitive diagnosis is possible in > 90% of cases.

BENIGN BONE TUMORS

Osteochondroma: Osteochondromas (osteocartilaginous exostoses), the most common benign bone tumors, may arise from any bone but tend to occur near the ends of long bones. They occur most often in people aged 10 to 20 and may be single or multiple. Multiple osteochondromas tend to run in families. Secondary malignant chondrosarcoma develops in about 10% of patients with multiple osteochondromas and in < 1% of those with single lesions.

Excision or other treatment is needed if the tumor is near a nerve, causes pain (particularly if the bone fractures), or disturbs growth, or its appearance on x-ray suggests transformation into malignant chondrosarcoma (see p. 348).

Chondroma: Chondromas may occur at any age but tend to occur in adults. They are usually located within the bone marrow cavity. These tumors are usually asymptomatic but may enlarge and become painful. They are often found when x-rays are taken for another reason. On x-ray, the tumors may appear lytic, with areas of stippled calcification. They are usually visible on a bone scan and thus may raise concern of a malignancy. X-ray findings may be diagnostic; if they are not, or if the tumor is painful, the diagnosis should be confirmed by biopsy.

An asymptomatic chondroma does not need excision or other treatment; however, follow-up x-rays are indicated to rule out disease progression. These are performed 6 mo and 1 yr later or whenever symptoms develop.

Chondroblastoma: Chondroblastoma is rare, occurring most commonly in people aged 10 to 20. Arising in the epiphysis, this tumor may continue to grow and destroy bone. On x-ray, it appears as a cyst containing spots of calcification. It must be surgically excised.

Chondromyxofibroma: Chondromyxofibroma is very rare and occurs before age 30. Its x-ray appearance (usually eccentric, sharply circumscribed, lytic, and located near the end of long bones) suggests the diagnosis. Treatment is surgical excision or curettage.

Osteoid osteoma: Osteoid osteoma, which tends to affect young adults, can occur in any bone but is most common in long bones. It can cause pain (usually worse at night) that is typically relieved by mild analgesics, particularly aspirin. Physical examination may reveal atrophy of regional muscles. Characteristic appearance on x-ray is a small radiolucent zone surrounded by a larger sclerotic zone. If a tumor is suspected, a technetium-99m bone scan should be performed; an osteoid osteoma appears as an area of increased uptake. Permanent relief is obtained if the small radiolucent zone is removed surgically or with percutaneous radiofrequency ablation.

Benign giant cell tumor: These tumors, which most commonly affect people in their 20s and 30s, occur in the epiphyses and may erode the rest of the bone and extend into the soft tissues. Giant cell tumors are notorious for their tendency to recur. Rarely, a giant cell tumor may metastasize, even though it remains histologically benign. Benign giant cell tumors appear lytic on x-ray. Most benign giant cell tumors are treated by curettage and packing with methyl methacrylate. If a tumor is very large, complete excision may be necessary.

PRIMARY MALIGNANT BONE TUMORS

(See also Ch. 142 on p. 1105.)

Multiple myeloma: Multiple myeloma is the most common primary malignant bone tumor and is of hematopoietic derivation (see also p. 1129). It occurs mostly in older adults. The neoplastic process is usually multicentric and often involves the bone marrow so diffusely that bone marrow aspiration is diagnostic. X-rays usually show sharply circumscribed lytic lesions or diffuse demineralization.

Osteosarcoma: Osteosarcoma (osteogenic sarcoma) is the second most common primary bone tumor and is highly malignant. It is most common in people aged 10 to 20, although it can occur at any age. Osteosarcoma usually develops around the knee or in other long bones, particularly the metaphyses. It can metastasize, usually to lung or bone. Pain and swelling are the usual symptoms. X-ray findings vary and may include sclerotic or lytic features. Diagnosis requires biopsy. Patients need a chest x-ray and CT scan to detect lung metastases and a bone scan to detect bone metastases.

Treatment with adjuvant chemotherapy increases survival from 20% at 2 yr to > 75% at 5 yr. Treatment usually begins prior to any surgery. Decreased tumor size on x-ray, decreased pain level, and decreased serum alkaline phosphatase indicate response. After several courses of chemotherapy, limb-sparing surgery (ie, in which the tumor is resected and the limb reconstructed) can proceed. Continuation of chemotherapy after surgery is usually necessary.

Fibrosarcoma: Fibrosarcomas have the same characteristics as osteosarcomas, affect the same age group, and pose the same problems.

Malignant fibrous histiocytoma: This tumor is clinically similar to osteosarcoma and fibrosarcoma. It tends to occur in children and teenagers. Treatment is the same as for osteosarcoma.

Chondrosarcoma: Chondrosarcomas are malignant tumors of cartilage. They differ from osteosarcomas clinically, therapeutically, and prognostically. Of chondrosarcomas, 90% are primary tumors. Rarely, chondrosarcomas arise in other, pre-existing conditions, particularly multiple osteochondromas. Chondrosarcomas tend to occur in older adults. They often develop in flat bones (eg, pelvis, scapula) but can develop in any portion of any bone and can implant in surrounding soft tissues.

Plain x-rays often reveal punctate calcifications. Primary chondrosarcomas often also exhibit cortical bone destruction and loss of normal bone trabeculae. Secondary chondrosarcoma may be suggested by the appearance of punctate calcifications or an increase in size of an osteochondroma. Technetium-99m bone scintigraphy is an accurate screening study. Biopsy is required for diagnosis and can also determine the tumor's grade (probability of metastasizing).

Regardless of grade, the treatment is total surgical resection. When surgical resection with maintenance of function is impossible, amputation may be necessary. Because of the potential to implant, meticulous care must be taken to avoid spillage of tumor cells into the soft tissues when performing a biopsy or surgery. Recurrence is inevitable if tumor cells spill. If no spillage occurs, the cure rate depends on the tumor grade. Low-grade tumors are nearly all cured with adequate treatment. Neither radiation nor chemotherapy is effective as primary or adjunctive treatment.

Ewing's tumor: Ewing's tumor (Ewing's sarcoma) is a round-cell bone tumor with a peak incidence between 10 and 20 yr. Most develop in the extremities, but any bone may be involved. Ewing's tumor tends to be extensive, sometimes involving the entire bone shaft. Pain and swelling are the most common symptoms. Lytic destruction is the most common x-ray finding, but multiple layers of subperiosteal reactive new bone formation may give an "onion-skin" appearance. Plain x-rays do not usually reveal the full extent of bone involvement. CT and MRI better define disease extent, which can help guide treatment. Many other benign and malignant tumors can appear identical, so diagnosis is made by biopsy.

Treatment includes various combinations of surgery, chemotherapy, and radiation therapy. Currently, > 60% of patients with primary localized Ewing's tumor may be cured by this multimodal approach. Cure is sometimes possible even with metastatic disease.

Malignant lymphoma of bone: Malignant lymphoma of bone (reticulum cell sarcoma) affects adults, usually in their 40s and 50s. It may arise in any bone. The tumor consists of small round cells, often with a mixture of reticulum cells, lymphoblasts, and lymphocytes. It can develop as an isolated primary bone tumor, in association with similar tumors in other tissues, or as a metastasis from known soft tissue lymphomatous disease. Pain and swelling are the usual symptoms. Pathologic fracture is common. X-rays reveal bone destruction, which may be mottled or patchy depending on the stage. In advanced disease, the entire outline of the affected bone may be lost.

In isolated primary bone lymphoma, the 5-yr survival rate is ≥ 50%. Combination radiation and chemotherapy is as curative as amputation or other extensive ablative surgery. Amputation is indicated only rarely, when function is lost because of pathologic fracture or extensive soft-tissue involvement that cannot be otherwise managed.

Malignant giant cell tumor: Malignant giant cell tumor, which is rare, is usually located at the extreme end of a long bone. X-ray reveals classic features of malignant destruction (predominantly lytic destruction, cortical destruction, soft-tissue extension, and pathologic fracture). A malignant giant cell tumor that develops in a previously benign giant cell tumor is characteristically radioresistant. The same principles of treatment apply as in osteosarcoma, but the cure rate is low.

Chordoma: Chordoma, which is rare, develops from the remnants of the primitive notochord. It tends to occur at the ends of the spinal column, usually in the sacrum or near the base of the skull. A chordoma in the sacrococcygeal region produces nearly constant pain. A chordoma in the base of the skull can produce deficits in any cranial nerve, most commonly in those to the eye.

Symptoms may exist for months to several years before diagnosis. A chordoma appears on x-ray as an expansive, destructive bone lesion that may be associated with a soft-tissue mass. Metastasis is unusual, but local recurrence is not. Chordomas in the sacrococcygeal region may be cured by radical en bloc excision. Chordomas in the base of the skull are usually inaccessible to surgery but may respond to radiation therapy.

METASTATIC BONE TUMORS

Any cancer may metastasize to bone, but metastases from carcinomas are the most common, particularly those arising in the breast, lung, prostate, kidney, and thyroid. Any bone may be involved, but bones distal to the knees and elbows are involved less often. Bone metastases may produce symptoms before a primary tumor is suspected.

X-rays often detect metastatic bone lesions. However, whole-body radioisotopic bone scanning may be more sensitive to early metastases than plain x-rays and is helpful in defining the full extent of metastases. Biopsy is necessary if the primary tumor has not been otherwise diagnosed, as biopsy may give clues to the location of the primary tumor.

Treatment depends on the type of primary tissue involved and the organ of origin. Radiation therapy, combined with selected chemotherapeutic or hormonal agents, is the most common modality. If bone destruction is extensive, resulting in imminent or actual pathologic fracture, surgical fixation may be required to provide stabilization. When the primary cancer has been removed and only a single bone metastasis remains, excision combined with radiation, chemotherapy, or both may occasionally be curative.

OTHER BONE MASSES

Many non-neoplastic conditions of bone may clinically or radiologically mimic solitary bone tumors.

Unicameral bone cyst: Simple unicameral bone cysts occur in the long bones in children. They predispose to pathologic fractures, which is usually how they present. Cysts < 5 cm heal and may disappear as the fracture heals. Cysts > 5 cm, particularly in children, may require excision and bone grafting; however, many respond to injections of corticosteroids.

Fibrous dysplasia: Fibrous dysplasia involves abnormal bone development during childhood. It may affect one or several bones. Cutaneous pigmentation and endocrine abnormalities may be present (Albright's syndrome). The abnormal bone lesions of fibrous dysplasia commonly stop developing at puberty. They rarely undergo malignant degeneration. On x-ray, the lesions appear cystic and may be extensive and deforming. Calcitonin may help relieve pain. Progressive deformities, fractures that do not heal with immobilization, or intractable pain may improve with orthopedic surgery.

Aneurysmal bone cyst: An aneurysmal bone cyst is idiopathic and usually develops before age 20. This cystic lesion usually occurs in the metaphyseal region of the long bones, but almost any bone may be affected. It tends to grow slowly. Periosteal new bone formation tends to limit the periphery of the mass. Pain and swelling are common. The lesion may be present for a few weeks to a few years before diagnosis. The appearance on x-ray is often characteristic: The rarefied area is usually well circumscribed and eccentric; its periosteum bulges, extending into the soft tissues, and may be surrounded by new bone formation.

Surgical removal of the entire lesion is the most successful treatment; regression after incomplete removal sometimes occurs. Radiation should be avoided when possible because sarcomas occasionally develop. However, radiation is the treatment of choice in surgically inaccessible vertebral lesions that are compressing the spinal cord.

JOINT TUMORS

Tumors rarely affect joints, unless by direct extension of an adjacent bone or soft-tissue tumor. However, two conditions—osteochondromatosis and pigmented villonodular synovitis—occur in the lining (synovium) of joints. These are benign but locally aggressive. Both disorders usually affect one joint, most often the knee, and are treated by synovectomy and removal of any intra-articular foreign bodies.

Synovial osteochondromatosis: Synovial osteochondromatosis is characterized by numerous calcified cartilaginous loose bodies, each of which may be no larger than a grain of rice, in a swollen, painful joint.

Pigmented villonodular synovitis: In pigmented villonodular synovitis, the synovium becomes thickened and contains hemosiderin, which gives the tissue its blood-stained appearance. This tissue tends to invade adjacent bone, causing cystic destruction. The painful process is difficult to control.

SECTION 5 PULMONARY DISORDERS

45 APPROACH TO THE PATIENT WITH PULMONARY SYMPTOMS

Key components in the evaluation of patients with pulmonary symptoms are the history, physical examination, and, in most cases, a chest x-ray. These components establish the need for subsequent testing, including pulmonary function testing and ABG analysis (see p. 364), CT scan and other imaging tests (see p. 374), and bronchoscopy (see p. 375).

History

The history can often establish whether symptoms of dyspnea, chest pain, wheezing, stridor, hemoptysis, and cough are likely to be pulmonary in origin. The history should focus on which symptom is primary when more than one occurs concurrently and whether constitutional symptoms, such as fever, weight loss, and night sweats, also occur. Other important information includes occupational and environmental exposures; family, travel, and contact history; previous illnesses and use of medications or illicit drugs; and previous test results (eg, tuberculin skin test, chest x-rays).

Physical Examination

Physical examination starts with assessment of general appearance. Discomfort and anxiety, habitus, and the effect of talking or movement on symptoms all can be assessed while greeting the patient and taking a history and may provide useful information relevant to pulmonary status. Next comes inspection, auscultation, and chest percussion and palpation.

Inspection: Inspection should focus on signs of respiratory difficulty and hypoxemia, such as restlessness, cyanosis, and accessory muscle use, and of possible chronic pulmonary disease, such as clubbing or pedal edema.

Cyanosis is bluish discoloration of the lips, face, or nail beds, signifying low arterial O_2 saturation (< 85%).

Accessory muscle use is defined as use of intercostal, sternocleidomastoid, and/or scalene muscles to breathe. Intercostal retractions (inward movement of the rib interspaces) are common in infants and in patients with severe airflow limitation; paradoxical breathing (inward motion of the abdomen during inspiration) signifies respiratory muscle fatigue or weakness.

Clubbing is enlargement of the fingertips (or toes) due to proliferation of connective tissue between the fingernail and the bone. Diagnosis is based on an increase in the profile angle of the nail as it exits the finger (to > 176°) or on an increase in the phalangeal depth ratio (to > 1) (see FIG. 45–1). "Sponginess" of the nail bed beneath the cuticle also suggests clubbing. Clubbing is most commonly observed in lung cancer but is an important sign of chronic pulmonary disease, such as cystic fibrosis and idiopathic pulmonary fibrosis; it occurs less commonly in cyanotic heart disease, chronic infection (eg, infective endocarditis), stroke, inflammatory bowel disease, and cirrhosis. Clubbing occasionally occurs with osteoarthropathy and periostitis (primary or hereditary hypertrophic osteoarthropathy); in this instance, clubbing may be accompanied by skin changes, such as hypertrophied skin on the dorsa of the hands (pachydermoperiostosis), seborrhea, and coarse facial features. Digital clubbing can also occur as a benign hereditary abnormality; benign clubbing can be distinguished from pathologic clubbing by the absence of pulmonary symptoms or disease and by patient report of clubbing from an early age.

Chest wall deformities, such as pectus excavatum and kyphoscoliosis, may restrict respirations and exacerbate symptoms of preexisting pulmonary disease.

Respiratory rate should be assessed and counted for 1 min to account for fluctuations in rate attributable to abnormal breathing patterns.

Cheyne-Stokes respiration (periodic breathing) is a cyclic fluctuation of respiratory rate and depth. From periods of brief apnea, patients breathe progressively faster and deeper (hyperpnea), then slower and less deeply until they become apneic and repeat the cycle. Cheyne-Stokes respiration is most often caused by heart failure, neurologic disease (eg, stroke, advanced dementia), or medications. The pattern in heart failure is probably attributable to delays in cerebral circulation; respiratory centers lag in recognition of systemic acidosis/hypoxia (causing hyperpnea) and of alkalosis/hypocapnia (causing apnea).

Biot's respiration is an uncommon variant of Cheyne-Stokes respiration in which irregular periods of apnea alternate with periods in which 4 or 5 deep, equal breaths are taken. It differs from Cheyne-Stokes respiration in that it is characterized by abrupt starts and stops and lacks periodicity. It results from injury to the CNS and occurs in such disorders as meningitis.

Kussmaul's respirations are deep, regular respirations caused by metabolic acidosis.

Jugular venous distention is usually a sign of volume overload or right heart failure (see p. 574).

Auscultation: Auscultation is arguably the most important component of the physical

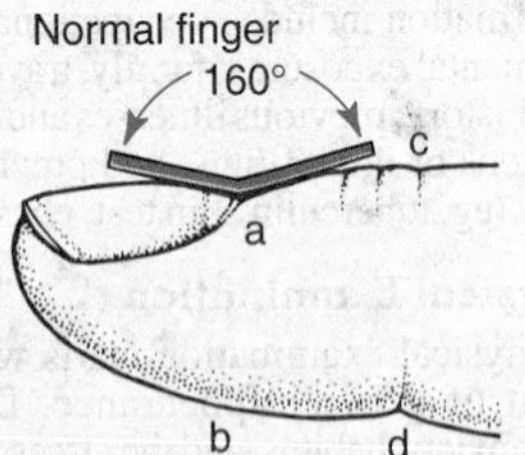

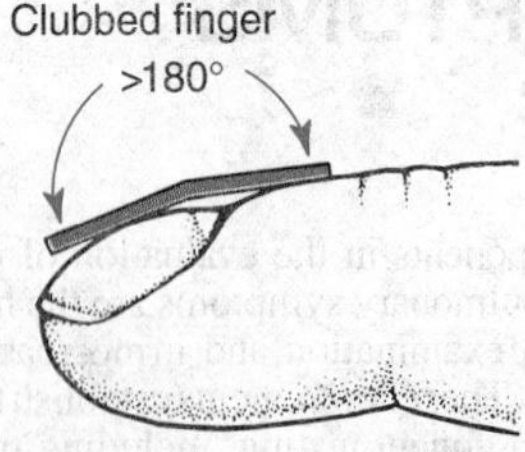

Fig. 45–1. Measuring finger clubbing. The ratio of the anteroposterior diameter of the finger at the nail bed (a–b) to that at the distal interphalangeal joint (c–d) is a simple measurement of finger clubbing. It can be obtained readily and reproducibly with calipers. If the ratio is > 1, clubbing is present. Finger clubbing is also characterized by loss of the normal angle at the nail bed.

examination. All fields of the chest should be listened to, including the flanks, to detect abnormalities associated with each lobe of the lung. Features to listen for include the character and volume of breath sounds, the presence or absence of vocal sounds, pleural friction rubs, and ratio of inspiration to expiration (I:E ratio).

Vesicular breath sounds are the normal sounds heard over most lung fields. Bronchial breath sounds are slightly louder, harsher, and higher pitched. They normally can be heard over the trachea and over areas of lung consolidation, such as pneumonia. Adventitious sounds are abnormal sounds, such as crackles, rhonchi, wheezes, and stridor.

Crackles, previously called rales, are discontinuous adventitious breath sounds. Fine crackles are short high-pitched sounds; coarse crackles are longer-lasting low-pitched sounds. Crackles have been compared to the sound of crinkling plastic wrap and can be simulated by rubbing strands of hair together between 2 fingers near one's ear. They occur most commonly with atelectasis and alveolar filling processes, such as pulmonary edema, and interstitial lung disease; they signify distention of fibrotic lung tissue or opening of collapsed alveoli.

Rhonchi are low-pitched respiratory sounds that can be heard during inspiration or expiration. They occur in a variety of conditions, including chronic bronchitis. The mechanism may relate to variations in obstruction as airways distend with inhalation.

Wheezes are a whistling, musical breath sound worse during expiration than inspiration. Wheezing can be a physical finding or a symptom usually associated with dyspnea.

Stridor is a high-pitched, predominantly inspiratory sound formed by extrathoracic upper airway obstruction. It usually can be heard without a stethoscope. Stridor is usually louder than wheezing, is predominantly inspiratory, and is heard loudly over the larynx. It should trigger a concern for life-threatening upper airway obstruction.

Decreased breath sounds signify poor air movement in airways, as occurs with asthma and COPD where bronchospasm or other mechanisms limit airflow. Breath sounds may also be decreased in the presence of a pleural effusion or pneumothorax.

Bronchophony is clear transmission of the patient's spoken voice through the chest wall. It results from alveolar consolidation, such as in pneumonia.

Egophony is said to occur when a patient says the letter "e" and the examiner hears the letter "a" on auscultation. It is heard in any condition that results in pulmonary consolidation, such as pneumonia.

Whispered pectoriloquy is transmission of the patient's whispered voice through the chest wall at an increased volume. It is most often heard in pneumonia.

Friction rubs are grating or creaking sounds that fluctuate with the respiratory cycle and sound like skin rubbing against wet leather. They are a sign of pleural inflammation and are heard in pleurisy, after thoracotomy, and with empyema.

I:E ratio is normally 1:2 but is prolonged to ≥1:3 when airflow is limited, such as in asthma and COPD, even in the absence of wheezing.

Cardiac auscultation may reveal signs of pulmonary hypertension, such as a loud P_2 (pulmonic 2nd heart sound), and of right heart failure, such as a right ventricular S_4 (4th heart sound—see p. 578) and tricuspid regurgitation.

Percussion and palpation: Percussion is the primary physical maneuver used to detect the presence and level of pleural effusion. Findings on percussion of areas of dullness signify underlying fluid or, less commonly, consolidation. Palpation includes tactile fremitus, vibration of the chest wall felt when a patient is asked to speak; it is decreased in pleural effusion and pneumothorax and increased in pulmonary consolidation. Point tenderness on palpation may signal underlying rib fracture or pleural inflammation.

In cor pulmonale (see p. 664), a right ventricular impulse at the left lower sternal border may become evident and may be increased in amplitude and duration (right ventricular heave).

CHEST PAIN

Pulmonary and pleural diseases cause chest pain; examples include pneumonia, pulmonary embolism, pleuritis, lung cancer, and rib fractures. Cardiac causes of chest pain require urgent evaluation and treatment (see p. 580).

COUGH

Cough is an explosive expiratory maneuver that is reflexively or deliberately intended to clear the airways. Coughing is a normal response to the presence of mucus or other foreign material in the airway or upper airway, but persistent coughing is annoying and generally indicates irritation of the pulmonary airways. It is the 5th most common symptom prompting patients to visit their physician. Awareness of cough varies considerably. A cough that appears suddenly, interferes with sleep, or causes musculoskeletal chest wall pain can be distressing. A cough that develops over decades (eg, in a smoker with mild chronic bronchitis) may be hardly noticeable or may be considered normal by the patient.

Etiology

Likely etiologies of cough differ depending on whether the symptom is acute (< 3 wk) or chronic.

Acute cough is most often caused by a URI, especially the common cold. Other causes include pneumonia; postnasal drip resulting from rhinitis or sinusitis that can be allergic, viral, or bacterial in origin; and COPD exacerbations. Cough may rarely be the only presenting symptom of pulmonary embolus. In the elderly, acute cough may signify aspiration or heart failure.

Chronic cough in smokers is most often caused by chronic bronchitis, defined as the presence of productive cough over ≥ 3 mo for > 2 yr consecutively. Compression of upper airways by tumor is much less common but should always be considered. The most common causes regardless of smoking history include postnasal drip syndrome, gastroesophageal reflux disease (GERD), asthma (cough-variant asthma), and use of ACE inhibitors. Less common causes include eosinophilic bronchitis (characterized by sputum eosinophilia without airway hyperresponsiveness) and bronchiectasis. The causes of chronic cough in children are similar to those of adults, but aspiration and pertussis must also be considered. Tracheobronchitis after a URI is a common cause of cough but rarely lasts > 3 mo after the infection. Rarely, impacted cerumen or a foreign body in the external auditory canal triggers reflex cough through stimulation of the auricular branch of the vagus nerve. Psychogenic cough is even rarer and is a diagnosis of exclusion.

Evaluation

History: URI and sinus symptoms suggest postnasal drip syndrome, but postnasal drip often causes cough without other symptoms. Heartburn, hoarseness, and chronic nocturnal or early morning cough, especially if no other symptoms are present, suggests GERD. Cough after exposure to dusts or allergens suggests cough-variant asthma. Chronic cough with production of purulent sputum in smokers suggests chronic bronchitis. A change in cough in these patients may, however, be an early manifestation of lung cancer. Cough productive of gritty sputum may signify broncholithiasis. Copious volumes of sputum suggest alveolar cell carcinoma.

Physical examination: Physical examination should focus on signs of sinusitis, rhinitis, and postnasal drip. Lung auscultation during cough may help detect lung sounds suggestive of asthma (wheezing) or bronchiectasis (rhonchi). Examination of the ears can detect triggers of reflex cough.

Testing: Most patients with acute or chronic cough without clear etiology by history and examination can be treated empirically for postnasal drip syndrome, GERD, or asthma based on clinical judgment; an adequate response to these therapeutic interventions precludes the need for further testing. A chest x-ray can be performed but usually is not helpful. Patients with chronic cough and inadequate responses to interventions can undergo more extensive testing for asthma (pulmonary function tests with methacholine challenge, sinus disease [sinus CT], or GERD [esophageal pH monitoring]). Bronchoscopy should be performed in selected patients in whom lung cancer or other bronchial tumor is suspected.

Treatment

Treatment is management of the underlying cause. Little evidence exists to support the use of cough suppressants or mucolytic agents for cough, but patients often expect or request such treatment, and multiple options exist. Coughing is an important mechanism for clearing secretions from the airways and can assist in treating respiratory infections. Therefore, cough suppression in infectious conditions should be done with caution. Nonspecific treatments for cough should be reserved as much as possible for patients with a URI and for those receiving therapy for the underlying cause but for whom cough is still troubling.

Antitussives depress the medullary cough center (dextromethorphan and codeine) or anesthetize stretch receptors of vagal afferent fibers in bronchi and alveoli (benzonatate). Dextromethorphan, a congener of the narcotic levorphanol, is effective as a tablet or syrup at a dose of 15 to 30 mg 1 to 4 times/day for adults or 0.25 mg/kg qid for children. Codeine has antitussive, analgesic, and sedative effects, but dependence is a potential problem, and nausea, vomiting, constipation, and tolerance are common adverse effects. Usual doses are 10 to 20 mg po q 4 to 6 h as needed for adults and 0.25 to 0.5 mg/kg qid for children. Other opioids (eg, hydrocodone, hydromorphone, methadone, morphine) have antitussive properties but are avoided because of high potential for dependence and abuse. Benzonatate, a congener of tetracaine in liquid-filled capsules, is effective at a dose of 100 to 200 mg po tid. Inhaled ipratropium is not generally considered an antitussive but may be of use in some patients with acute cough due to URI.

Expectorants are thought to decrease viscosity and facilitate expectoration, or coughing up, of secretions, but are of limited benefit. Guaifenesin (200 to 400 mg po q 4 h in syrup or tablet form) is most commonly used because it has no serious adverse effects, but multiple expectorants exist, including bromhexine, ipecac, saturated solution of potassium iodide (SSKI), and domiodol. Aerosolized expectorants, which include isoproterenol, beclomethasone, N-acetylcysteine, and deoxyribonuclease (DNase), are generally reserved for hospital-based treatment of cough in patients with bronchiectasis or cystic fibrosis. Ensuring adequate hydration may facilitate expectoration, as may inhalation of steam, although neither has been rigorously tested.

Topical treatments, such as acacia, licorice, glycerin, honey, and wild cherry cough drops or syrups (demulcents), are locally and perhaps emotionally soothing but are not supported by scientific evidence.

Protussives, which stimulate cough, are indicated for such disorders as cystic fibrosis and bronchiectasis, in which a productive cough is thought to be important for airway clearance and preservation of pulmonary function. DNase or hypertonic saline is given in conjunction with chest physical therapy and postural drainage to promote cough and expectoration. This approach seems to be beneficial in cystic fibrosis but not in most other causes of chronic cough.

Bronchodilators, such as albuterol and ipratropium or inhaled corticosteroids, can be effective for cough after URI and in cough-variant asthma.

DYSPNEA

Dyspnea is unpleasant or uncomfortable breathing. It has multiple components and is experienced and described differently depending on the cause.

Dyspnea has multiple pulmonary, cardiac, and other causes (see TABLE 45–1). Often, more than one mechanism underlies the sensation.

The basis for the sensation of discomfort of dyspnea is unclear but may be a centrally perceived discrepancy between respiratory muscle tension (the need to take a deep breath) and length (the ability to take a deep breath). This mechanism partially explains why some forms of breathlessness and hyperpnea, such as with metabolic acidosis (Kussmaul's respirations), in CNS disease (Biot's and Cheyne-Stokes respirations), and during

TABLE 45–1. CAUSES OF DYSPNEA

Acute onset (within minutes)

- Pulmonary
  - Pneumothorax
  - Pulmonary embolism
  - Bronchospasm
    - Asthma (with previous history)
    - Reactive airway disease (with previous exposure)
  - Foreign body
  - Toxic inhalation (eg, chlorine, hydrogen sulfide)
- Cardiac
  - Acute myocardial ischemia or infarction
    - Papillary muscle dysfunction or rupture
    - Ventricular dysfunction
  - Cardiogenic pulmonary edema
- Other
  - Diaphragmatic paralysis
  - Anxiety disorder—hyperventilation

Subacute onset (within hours or days)

- Same as acute onset, with addition of:
  - Pneumonia
  - Acute bronchitis
  - Poisoning
    - Salicylate
    - Ethylene glycol

Nonacute onset (hours–years)

- Pulmonary
  - Obstructive lung disease
  - Restrictive lung disease
  - Interstitial lung disease
  - Pleural effusion
- Cardiac
  - Ventricular dysfunction
  - Pericardial effusion and tamponade
- Other
  - Anemia
  - Physical deconditioning

exercise among trained athletes, are not experienced as dyspnea.

Evaluation

History: Reports of shortness of breath or of being unable to take a deep breath are more common among patients with COPD exacerbation. Chest tightness or increased effort to breathe suggests asthma or an obstructive ventilatory disorder. A feeling of suffocation is characteristic of pulmonary edema. Heavy breathing on exertion is common in physical deconditioning, whereas air hunger, or an urgent sense of a need to breathe in more air, has been linked to hypercapnia, restricted chest wall excursions, and pulmonary edema. Phrases such as "out of breath" and "hard to breathe" are nonspecific.

Abrupt onset of dyspnea with or without sharp chest pain suggests spontaneous pneumothorax or pulmonary embolism; concomitant leg pain and swelling or recent immobility support pulmonary embolism. Abrupt onset of productive cough and fever suggests bacterial pneumonia, particularly that caused by *Streptococcus pneumoniae* if it is accompanied by pleuritic chest pain. Severe dyspnea that appears 1 to 2 h after falling asleep (paroxysmal nocturnal dyspnea) is pathognomonic for left ventricular dysfunction, but it must be distinguished from nocturnal awakening by cough from asthma or mucus hypersecretion. Dyspnea while recumbent (orthopnea) also implies left ventricular dysfunction or, less commonly, pericardial effusion, respiratory muscle weakness, or diaphragmatic paralysis. Dyspnea that worsens when sitting upright and resolves when recumbent (platypnea) is unusual and suggests pulmonary arteriovenous malformation or the hepatopulmonary syndrome; it may also occur after pneumonectomy, in recurrent pulmonary embolism, and in chronic pulmonary diseases that preferentially affect the lower lobes, such as aspiration pneumonia and α_1-antitrypsin deficiency. Dyspnea accompanied by paresthesias in the fingers or around the mouth suggests hyperventilation. Exertional dyspnea in the absence of objective findings on examination or testing may indicate anemia, primary pulmonary hypertension (if it occurs in a young woman), or, more likely, physical deconditioning.

Physical examination: Absent or markedly diminished breath sounds on only one side suggest pneumothorax or pleural effusion; these can be distinguished by increased resonance and dullness to percussion, respectively. Wheezing (see p. 363) suggests asthma or COPD. Stridor (see p. 363) suggests extrathoracic airway obstruction (eg, foreign body, epiglottitis, vocal cord dysfunction). Crackles in the dyspneic patient suggest left heart failure or interstitial lung disease. Rhonchi suggest COPD.

Testing: A chest x-ray should be taken in most patients. Acute dyspnea also warrants pulse oximetry, which provides a noninvasive measure of O_2 saturation. An ECG to detect cardiac ischemia is mandatory unless cardiac ischemia can be excluded clinically. In patients with severe or deteriorating respiratory status, an ABG should be performed to more precisely quantify hypoxemia, measure P_{CO_2}, and measure any acid-base disorders stimulating hyperventilation and to calculate the alveolar-arterial gradient (see p. 370). Patients suspected of having pulmonary embolism should undergo ventilation/perfusion scanning or CT angiography.

Chronic dyspnea may warrant additional tests, such as CT scan, pulmonary function tests, echocardiography, and bronchoscopy.

Treatment

Treatment is correction of the underlying cause. Hypoxemia is addressed with supplemental O_2 as needed to maintain $Sa_{O_2} \geq 88\%$ or $Pa_{O_2} > 55$ mm Hg as levels above these thresholds provide adequate O_2 delivery to tissues. Levels below these thresholds are on the steep portion of the O_2-Hb dissociation curve, in which small declines in arterial O_2 tension result in large declines in Hb saturation (see FIG. 46–4 on p. 371). O_2 saturation should be maintained at > 93% if myocardial or cerebral ischemia is a concern. Morphine 0.5 to 5 mg IV helps reduce anxiety and the discomfort of dyspnea in various conditions, including MI, pulmonary embolism, and the dyspnea that commonly accompanies terminal illnesses (see p. 2765). However, opioids can be deleterious in patients with acute airflow limitation (eg, asthma, COPD) because they suppress the ventilatory drive and worsen respiratory acidemia.

HYPERVENTILATION SYNDROME

Hyperventilation syndrome is anxiety-related dyspnea and tachypnea often accompanied by systemic symptoms.

Hyperventilation syndrome is common in young women but can affect either sex at any age. It is sometimes precipitated by emotionally stressful events. Hyperventilation syndrome is separate from panic disorder (see p. 1674), although the 2 conditions overlap; about ½ of patients with panic disorder have hyperventilation syndrome and ¼ of patients with hyperventilation syndrome have panic disorder.

History: Patients with acute hyperventilation syndrome present with dyspnea sometimes so severe as to feel like suffocation. It is accompanied by agitation and a sense of terror or by somatic symptoms of chest pain, paresthesias (peripheral and perioral), peripheral tetany, and presyncope or syncope or sometimes by a combination of all of these. Tetany occurs because respiratory alkalosis causes both hypophosphatemia and hypocalcemia. Patients with chronic hyperventilation syndrome present far less dramatically and often escape detection; they sigh deeply and frequently and often have nonspecific somatic symptoms in the context of mood and anxiety disorders and emotional stress.

Physical examination: Physical examination is normal in both acute and chronic hyperventilation syndrome, although patients may be tachypneic and appear anxious or agitated.

Testing: Hyperventilation syndrome is a diagnosis of exclusion; the challenge is to use tests and resources judiciously to distinguish this syndrome from more serious diagnoses. Basic testing includes pulse oximetry, chest x-ray, and ECG. Pulse oximetry in hyperventilation syndrome shows O_2 saturation at or close to 100%. Chest x-ray is normal. ECG is performed to detect cardiac ischemia, although hyperventilation syndrome itself can cause ST-segment depressions, T-wave inversions, and prolonged QT intervals. ABGs are needed when other causes of hyperventilation are suspected, such as metabolic acidosis. Occasionally, acute hyperventilation syndrome is indistinguishable from acute pulmonary embolism, and tests for pulmonary embolism (eg, D-dimer, ventilation/perfusion scan, helical CT) may be necessary.

Treatment

Treatment is reassurance. Some physicians advocate teaching the patient maximal exhalation and diaphragmatic breathing. Most patients require treatment for underlying mood or anxiety disorders that includes cognitive therapy, stress reduction techniques, and/or drugs (anxiolytics, antidepressants, or lithium).

HEMOPTYSIS

Hemoptysis is coughing up of blood from the respiratory tract. Most of the lung's blood (95%) circulates through low-pressure pulmonary arteries and ends up in the pulmonary capillary bed, where gas is exchanged; about 5% of the blood supply circulates through high-pressure bronchial arteries, which originate at the aorta and supply major airways and supporting structures. The blood in hemoptysis generally arises from this bronchial circulation, except when pulmonary arteries are damaged by trauma, by erosion of a granulomatous or calcified lymph node or tumor, or, rarely, by pulmonary arterial catheterization or when pulmonary capillaries are affected by inflammation. Blood-streaked sputum is common in many minor respiratory illnesses, such as URI and viral bronchitis. Massive hemoptysis is production of 600 mL of blood (about a full kidney basin's worth) within 24 h.

The differential diagnosis is broad (see TABLE 45–2). Bronchitis, bronchiectasis, TB, and necrotizing pneumonia or lung abscess account for 70 to 90% of cases. Cavitary *Aspergillus* infection is being increasingly recognized as a cause but is not as common as malignancy; hemoptysis in smokers ≥ 40 yr triggers suspicion of primary lung cancer. Metastatic cancer rarely causes hemoptysis. Pulmonary-renal and diffuse alveolar hemorrhage syndromes (see p. 485), pulmonary embolism and infarction (see p. 412), and left ventricular failure (especially secondary to mitral stenosis) are less common causes of hemoptysis. Hemoptysis in heart failure is unusual but occurs as a result of pulmonary venous hypertension from left ventricular failure. Primary bronchial adenoma and arteriovenous malformations are rare but tend to cause severe bleeding. Rarely, hemoptysis occurs during menstruation (catamenial hemoptysis) because of intrathoracic endometriosis.

Evaluation

History: A key objective is to distinguish hemoptysis from hematemesis and from nasopharyngeal or oropharyngeal bleeding. This distinction can generally be accomplished with history and physical examination. An

TABLE 45-2. DIFFERENTIAL DIAGNOSIS OF HEMOPTYSIS

Larynx and pharynx
Carcinoma
Lymphoma
Tuberculous ulceration

Trachea and large bronchi
Benign or malignant primary tumor (carcinoma and adenoma)
Bronchogenic cyst
Broncholithiasis
Erosion by an aortic aneurysm
Erosion by a caseocalcific node
Erosion by a tumor from nodes, esophagus, or other mediastinal structures
Severe acute bronchitis
Telangiectasia
Trauma

Smaller bronchial structures
Acute bronchitis
Adenoma (carcinoid or cylindromatous)
Bronchiectasis
Bronchopulmonary sequestration
Carcinoma
Chronic bronchitis
Trauma

Pulmonary parenchyma
Abscess
Active granulomatous disease (tuberculous, fungal, parasitic, syphilitic)
Acute pneumonia
Fungus ball (aspergilloma) in an old cavity
Goodpasture's syndrome or variants
Idiopathic hemosiderosis
Infarct
Primary or metastatic tumor
Trauma

Heart and blood vessels
Aortic aneurysm with leakage into the pulmonary parenchyma
Atrial myxoma
Fibrous mediastinitis with pulmonary vein obstruction
Left ventricular failure
Mitral stenosis
Pulmonary arteriovenous malformation
Pulmonary embolism/infarct
Primary pulmonary hypertension

Bleeding diathesis
Anticoagulant therapy
Deficiency of vitamin K–dependent factors: prothrombin (II), Stuart factor (X), factor VII, Christmas factor (IX)
Disseminated intravascular coaulation
Fibrinolytic therapy: urokinase, streptokinase
Miscellaneous congenital coagulation defects
Thrombocytopenia

extensive smoking history suggests malignancy. A patient's sensation of where the bleeding may be coming from may help identify its origin if it is emanating from one of the upper lobes.

Physical examination: Examination focuses on ruling out upper airway sites of bleeding and on listening over the lungs for focal abnormalities that may indicate the area where bleeding may be occurring. Unfortunately, blood originating from any area can be aspirated throughout the lung.

Testing: Patients with minor hemoptysis can undergo testing on an outpatient basis. A chest x-ray is mandatory. Patients with normal results, a consistent history, and nonmassive hemoptysis can undergo empirical treatment for bronchitis. Those with abnormal results and those without a supporting history should undergo CT and bronchoscopy. CT may reveal pulmonary lesions that are not apparent on the chest x-ray and can help locate lesions in anticipation of bronchoscopy and biopsy. A ventilation/perfusion scan or CT angiogram can confirm the diagnosis of pulmonary embolism; CTs and pulmonary angiography can also detect pulmonary arteriovenous fistulas. When the etiology is obscure, fiberoptic inspection of the pharynx, larynx, esophagus, and/or airways may be indicated to distinguish hemoptysis from hematemesis and from nasopharyngeal or oropharyngeal bleeding.

Patients with massive hemoptysis require treatment and stabilization before testing. The cause of hemoptysis remains unknown in 30 to 40% of cases. The prognosis for patients with cryptogenic hemoptysis is generally favorable, usually with resolution of bleeding within 6 mo of evaluation.

Treatment

The two objectives of treatment are to prevent aspiration of blood to the uninvolved lung (which can cause asphyxiation) and to prevent exsanguination from ongoing bleeding.

Protection of the uninvolved lung can be difficult because the site of bleeding often is unclear. Strategies include positioning maneuvers (eg, having the patient lie with the bleeding lung in a dependent position) and selective intubation and obstruction of the bronchus going to the bleeding lung.

Prevention of exsanguination involves reversal of any bleeding diathesis and direct efforts to stop the bleeding. Clotting deficiencies can be reversed with fresh-frozen plasma and factor-specific or platelet transfusions. Laser therapy, cauterization, or direct injection with epinephrine or vasopressin can be performed bronchoscopically.

Massive hemoptysis is one of the few indications for rigid bronchoscopy, which provides control of the airway, allows for a larger field of view than flexible bronchoscopy, allows better suctioning, and is more suited to therapeutic interventions, such as laser therapy. Embolization of a pulmonary segment is becoming the preferred method with which to stop massive hemoptysis, with reported success rates of up to 90%. Emergency surgery is indicated for massive hemoptysis not controlled by rigid bronchoscopy or embolization and is generally considered a last resort.

Early resection may be indicated for bronchial adenoma or carcinoma. Broncholithiasis (erosion of a calcified lymph into an adjacent bronchus) may require pulmonary resection if endobronchial removal of the stone via rigid bronchoscopy cannot be performed. Bleeding secondary to heart failure or mitral stenosis usually responds to specific therapy for heart failure, but in rare cases, emergency mitral valvulotomy is necessary for life-threatening hemoptysis due to mitral stenosis. Bleeding from a pulmonary embolism is rarely massive and almost always stops spontaneously. If emboli recur and bleeding persists, anticoagulation may be contraindicated, and placement of an inferior vena cava filter is the treatment of choice.

Because bleeding from bronchiectatic areas usually results from infection, treatment of the infection with appropriate antibiotics and postural drainage is essential.

Sedatives and opioids suppress the ventilatory drive and should be avoided.

SOLITARY PULMONARY NODULE

A solitary pulmonary nodule is defined as a discrete lesion < 3 cm in diameter that is completely surrounded by lung parenchyma, does not touch the hilum or mediastinum, and is without associated atelectasis or pleural effusion (for evaluation of a mediastinal mass, see p. 505).

Solitary pulmonary nodules are most often detected incidentally when a chest x-ray is taken for other reasons.

The differential diagnosis of a solitary pulmonary nodule is extensive. Malignant causes are primary lung cancer (usually adenocarcinoma or small cell carcinoma) and metastatic cancer (breast melanoma; colon, renal, and testicular carcinoma; sarcoma; and head and neck cancer). The likelihood of malignancy increases with age.

Nonmalignant causes are granulomatous infection (TB, atypical mycobacterial infection, histoplasmosis, coccidioidomycosis, blastomycosis), benign tumors (hamartoma, lipoma), connective tissue disease (RA, Wegener's granulomatosis), parasitic infection (dirofilariasis [dog heartworm]), ascariasis, infection with *Pneumocystis jiroveci* (formerly called *P. carinii*), and pulmonary arteriovenous malformations. Nonpulmonary soft-tissue densities caused by nipple shadows, warts, cutaneous nodules, and bone abnormalities are often confused for a nodule on chest x-ray.

Evaluation

The primary goal of evaluation is to detect malignancy and active infection.

History: Older age, current or past cigarette smoking, and a history of malignancy all increase the probability of malignancy. These risk factors (plus nodule size) have been used to estimate likelihood ratios for malignant disease (see TABLE 45–3). History may reveal other information that suggests an underlying etiology (eg, a history of treated colon, breast, or renal cell carcinoma) but, in general, is not helpful in determining a cause when the major risk factors have been excluded.

Physical examination: A thorough physical examination may uncover findings that suggest an underlying etiology for a pulmonary nodule but usually does not help determine a cause.

TABLE 45–3. ESTIMATING THE PROBABILITY OF MALIGNANCY OF A SOLITARY PULMONARY NODULE

I. Establish likelihood ratios (LRs)* for malignancy with the following table:

Finding	Likelihood Ratio for Malignancy	Finding	Likelihood Ratio for Malignancy
Diameter of nodule (cm)		Current smoker or quit within past 9 yr	
< 1.5	0.1	Average number of cigarettes per day:	
1.5–2.2	0.5	1–9	0.3
2.3–3.2	1.7	10–20	1.0
3.3–4.2	4.3	21–40	2.0
4.3–5.2	6.6	≥ 41	3.9
5.3–6.0	29.4		
Patient's age (yr)		Quit smoking (yr)	
≤ 35	0.1	≤ 3	1.4
36–44	0.3	4–6	1.0
45–49	0.7	7–12	0.5
50–59	1.5	≥ 13	0.1
60–69	2.1		
70–83	5.7		
Smoking history		Overall prevalence	
Never smoked	0.15	Clinical settings	0.7
Pipe or cigar only	0.3	Community surveys	0.1
Ex-cigarette smoker	1.5		

II. Multiply the LRs for nodule diameter, patient's age, smoking history, and cancer prevalence to obtain an estimate of the odds of malignancy in a solitary pulmonary nodule (Odds CA);

That is, OddsCA = LR Size × LR Age × LR Smoking × LR Prev

III. Convert the odds into a probability of cancer:

Probability of cancer (PCA) = OddsCA / (1 + OddsCA)

So for a 65-yr-old patient who smokes a pack of cigarettes (20) daily and who has a 2.0 cm nodule:

I. LR Size = 1.5; LR Age = 2.1; LR Smoking = 1.0; LR Prev = 0.7

II. OddsCA = (1.5 × 2.1 × 1.0 × 0.7) / 1 = 2.21:1

III. PCA (as %) = 2.21/(1+ 2.21) × 100 = 69%

*The LR is a measure of how predictive a finding is of disease and is defined as the probability of the finding being present in a patient with disease divided by the probability of the finding being present in a patient without disease; ie, it is the ratio of true positives to false positives or of sensitivity to 1- specificity.

Adapted from Cummings, SR, Lillington, GA, Richard, RJ: Estimating the probability of malignancy in solitary pulmonary nodules. A Bayesian approach. *The American Review of Respiratory Disease* 134(3):449–452, 1986.

Testing: Four radiographic characteristics help narrow the differential diagnosis of a solitary pulmonary nodule: growth rate; pattern of calcification, if present; margins; and size. These characteristics are sometimes evident on the original plain film but usually require a CT scan. CT can also distinguish pulmonary from pleural radiopacities. CT has a sensitivity of 70% and a specificity of 60% for detecting malignancy.

Growth rate is determined by comparison with previous chest x-ray or CT, if available. A lesion that has not enlarged in ≥ 2 yr suggests a benign etiology. Tumors that have volume doubling times from 21 to 400 days are likely to be malignant. Small nodules should be monitored every year for 2 yr.

Calcification suggests benign disease, particularly if it is central (tuberculoma, histoplasmoma), concentric (healed histoplasmosis), or in popcorn configuration (hamartoma). CT scanning is often necessary to detect these patterns. Margin patterns are also suggestive. Spiculated or irregular (scalloped) margins are more indicative of malignancy. Diameter < 1.5 cm strongly suggests a benign etiology; diameter > 5.3 cm strongly suggests malignancy.

PET scanning has an uncertain role in evaluation. It has a sensitivity > 90% and a specificity of about 78% for detecting malignancy, but it is relatively new, and its role in evaluating pulmonary nodules is still being developed. False-negative PET scans can result from metabolically inactive tumors, and false-positive results can occur in a variety of infectious and inflammatory conditions.

When historical information or radiographic appearance is not diagnostic, biopsy and culture may be useful, but usually only when history supports TB or coccidioidomycosis as possible diagnoses. Although cancers can be diagnosed by biopsy, definitive treatment is resection, and so invasive testing should be reserved for patients in whom nonmalignant causes are a possibility.

Treatment

If the suspicion of malignancy is very low, the lesions are very small (< 1 cm), or the patient refuses or is not a candidate for surgical intervention, observation is reasonable. Monitoring with follow-up at 3 mo, 6 mo, and then yearly for 2 yr is recommended. If the lesion has not grown for > 2 yr, it is likely benign. When cancer is the most likely cause or when nonmalignant causes are unlikely, patients should undergo resection unless surgery is contraindicated due to poor pulmonary function, comorbidities, or withholding of consent.

STRIDOR

Stridor is a high-pitched, predominantly inspiratory sound formed by extrathoracic upper airway obstruction. The most common cause in children is epiglottitis, croup, or foreign body aspiration. Common causes in adults include vocal cord dysfunction, postextubation vocal cord edema or paralysis, laryngeal tumors, allergic reactions, aspirated foreign body, and retropharyngeal abscess.

Evaluation

History: Sore throat and fever suggest abscess; sore throat, fever, and drooling suggest epiglottitis. Preceding URI symptoms and cough suggest croup. Dysphonia suggests laryngeal tumor. Abrupt onset suggests acute allergic reaction or aspirated foreign body.

Physical examination: Examination focuses initially on determining the patency of the airway. Examination includes measuring vital signs and determining if the patient is in acute distress as evidenced by use of accessory muscles and intercostal retractions. Inspiratory stridor suggests obstruction of the trachea, larynx, or epiglottis and is usually a medical emergency, whereas expiratory stridor suggests bronchial obstruction.

Testing: Testing should include pulse oximetry and chest and neck x-rays. Lateral soft-tissue x-rays of the neck can be diagnostic of epiglottitis. X-rays can also identify foreign objects in the neck or chest. Confirmation of the cause of stridor may require direct laryngoscopy to detect vocal cord abnormalities and tumors. In more chronic cases of stridor, flow-volume loops can help distinguish extrathoracic from intrathoracic causes.

Treatment

Definitive treatment of stridor is treatment of the underlying cause. Helium-O_2 (heliox) improves airflow and reduces stridor in disorders of the large airways, such as postextubation laryngeal edema, croup, and laryngeal tumors; mechanism of action is thought to be reduced flow turbulence as a result of lower density of helium compared with O_2.

Vocal Cord Dysfunction

Paradoxical movement of the vocal cords is adduction of the true vocal cords on inspiration and abduction on expiration; it causes inspiratory functional airway obstruction and stridor that is often mistaken for asthma. This disorder commonly occurs in patients with mental disease. Diagnosis is made by observing inspiratory closure of the vocal cords with direct laryngoscopy. Treatment involves educating the patient about the nature of the problem; counseling from a speech therapist on special breathing techniques, such as panting, which can relieve episodes of stridor and obstruction; and avoidance of asthma misdiagnosis and treatment.

WHEEZING

Wheezing is a symptom as well as a physical finding. Wheezing occurs as a result of airway narrowing. Asthma is the most classic cause of wheezing, but wheezing may be part of COPD, heart failure exacerbation (cardiac asthma), bronchiolitis in children, anaphylaxis, toxic inhalation, foreign body aspiration, tracheomalacia, or vocal cord dysfunction.

Evaluation

History: Wheezing in a patient with known asthma or COPD is usually presumed to represent an exacerbation. A history of cough, postnasal drip, exposure to allergens, or toxic or irritant gases may suggest a trigger. Acute onset without a history of lung disease suggests allergic reaction or impending anaphylaxis. Worsening with cold air, dust, tobacco smoke, perfumes, or other factors suggests asthma.

Physical examination: Localized wheezing suggests focal bronchial obstruction by tumor or foreign body. Diffuse wheezing indicates that all airways are involved or that the site of airway narrowing is in the trachea or at the level of the vocal cords. Urticaria or angioedema suggests an allergic reaction. Fever and URI symptoms suggest infection, especially bronchiolitis in children < 2 yr. Crackles, distended neck veins, and peripheral edema suggest heart failure.

Testing: A pulse oximetry reading and a chest x-ray should be taken. Segmental or subsegmental atelectasis or infiltrate suggests an obstructing endobronchial lesion. Radio-opacity in the airways or focal areas of hyperinflation suggests a foreign body.

Spirometry (see Ch. 46, below) can confirm airflow limitation and quantify its reversibility and severity. Flow-volume loops can help diagnose large airway obstructions, such as those caused by tumors or vocal cord dysfunction, and can differentiate extrathoracic from intrathoracic sites of obstruction. Extrathoracic variable obstruction causes flattening of the inspiratory limb of the flow-volume loop, whereas intrathoracic variable obstructions cause flattening of the expiratory limb (see FIG. 46–3E and 3F on p. 369). Fixed lesions affect both limbs.

Treatment

Definitive treatment of wheezing is treatment of underlying causes. Wheezing itself can be relieved with inhaled bronchodilators (eg, albuterol 2.5 mg nebulized solution or 180 µg metered dose inhalation) except in the case of foreign body or vocal cord abnormalities.

46 TESTS OF PULMONARY FUNCTION

Pulmonary function tests provide measures of flow rates, lung volumes, gas exchange, and respiratory muscle function. Basic pulmonary function tests available in the ambulatory setting include spirometry and pulse oximetry; these tests provide physiologic measures of pulmonary function and can be used to quickly narrow a differential diagnosis and suggest a subsequent strategy of additional testing or therapy. More complicated testing includes esophageal pressure measurement to determine pressure-volume relationships and exercise testing. These provide a more detailed description of physiologic abnormalities and the likely underlying pathology. The choice and sequence of testing are guided by information from the history and physical examination.

FLOW RATES, LUNG VOLUMES, AND FLOW-VOLUME LOOPS

Flow rate and lung volume measurements can be used to differentiate obstructive from restrictive pulmonary disorders, to characterize disease severity, and to measure responses to therapy. Measurements are typically reported as absolute flows and volumes and as percentages of predicted values derived from large populations of people presumed to have normal lung function. Variables that help predict normal values include age, sex, ethnicity, and height.

Flow rates: Quantitative measures of inspiratory and expiratory flow are obtained by forced spirometry. Nose clips are used to occlude the nares.

In assessments of expiratory flow, the patient inhales as deeply as possible, seals his lips around a mouthpiece, and exhales as forcefully and completely as possible into an apparatus that records the exhaled volume (forced vital capacity [FVC]) and the volume exhaled in the first second (the forced expiratory volume in 1 sec [FEV_1]—see FIG. 46–1). Newer instruments measure flow and integrate time in order to estimate volumes. In assessments of inspiratory flow and volume, the patient exhales as completely as possible, then forcibly inhales. These maneuvers provide several measures. The FVC is the maximal amount of air that the patient can forcibly exhale after taking a maximal inhalation. The FEV_1 is the most reproducible flow parameter and is especially useful in diagnosing and monitoring patients with obstructive pulmonary disease.

The forced expiratory flow measured during exhalation of 25 to 75% of the FVC may be a more sensitive marker of mild small airway obstruction than the FEV_1, but reproducibility is poor. The peak expiratory flow (PEF) is the peak flow occurring during exhalation and is used primarily for home monitoring of patients with asthma and for determining diurnal variations in airflow.

Interpretation of these measures depends on good patient effort, which is often improved by coaching during the actual maneuver. Acceptable spirograms demonstrate good test initiation (eg, a quick and forceful onset of exhalation), no coughing, smooth curves, and absence of early termination of expiration (eg, minimum exhalation time of 6 sec with no change in volume for the last 1 sec). Reproducible efforts agree within 5% or 100 mL with other efforts. Results not meeting these minimum acceptable criteria should be interpreted with caution.

Lung volumes: Lung volumes (see FIG. 46–2) are measured by determining functional residual capacity (FRC) and with spirometry.

FRC is measured using gas dilution techniques or body-box plethysmography. Gas dilution techniques include nitrogen washout and helium equilibration. With nitrogen washout, the patient exhales to FRC and then breathes from a spirometer containing 100% O_2. The test ends when the exhaled nitrogen concentration is zero. The collected volume of exhaled nitrogen is equal to 81% of the initial FRC. With helium equilibration, the patient exhales to FRC and then connects to a closed system containing known volumes of helium and O_2. Helium concentration is measured until it is the same on inhalation and exhalation, indicating it has equilibrated with the volume of gas in the lung, which is estimated by helium dilution. Both of these techniques may underestimate FRC because they measure only the lung volume that communicates with the upper airways, and in patients with severe airflow limitation, a considerable volume of trapped gas may communicate very poorly or not at all.

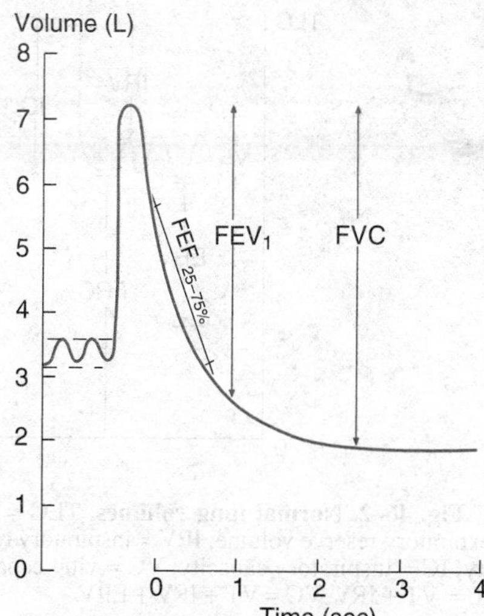

Fig. 46–1. Normal spirogram. FEV_1 = forced expiratory volume in the 1st second of forced vital capacity maneuver; $FEF_{25-75\%}$ = forced expiratory flow during expiration of 25 to 75% of the FVC; FVC = forced vital capacity (the maximum amount of air forcibly expired after maximum inspiration).

Body-box plethysmography uses Boyle's law to measure the compressible gas volume within the thorax and is more accurate than gas dilution techniques. While sitting in an airtight box, the patient tries to inhale against a closed mouthpiece from FRC. As the chest wall expands, the pressure in the closed box rises. Knowing the pre-inspiratory box volume and the pressure in the box before and after the inspiratory effort allows for a calculation

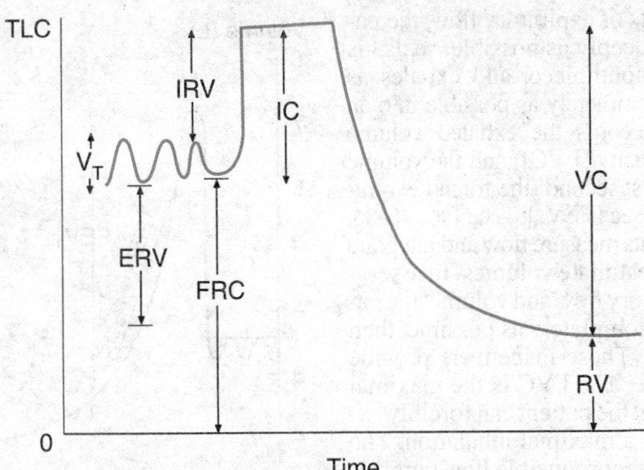

Fig. 46–2. Normal lung volumes. TLC = total lung capacity; VT = tidal volume; ERV = expiratory reserve volume; IRV = inspiratory reserve volume; FRC = functional residual capacity; IC = inspiratory capacity; VC = vital capacity; RV = residual volume; FRC = RV + ERV; IC = VT + IRV; VC = VT + IRV + ERV.

of the change in box volume, which must equal the change in lung volume.

Knowing FRC allows the lung to be divided into subvolumes that are either measured with spirometry or calculated (see FIG. 46–2). Normally the FRC represents about 40% of total lung capacity (TLC).

Flow-volume loop: In contrast to the spirogram, which displays flow (in L) over time (in sec), the flow-volume loop (see FIG. 46–3) displays flow (in L/sec) as it relates to lung volume (in L) during maximal inspiration from complete exhalation (residual volume [RV]) and during maximum expiration from complete inhalation (TLC). The principal advantage of the flow-volume loop is that it can show whether flows are appropriate for a particular lung volume. For example, flow is normally slower at low lung volumes. Because patients with pulmonary fibrosis have low lung volumes, flow appears to be decreased if measured alone. However, when flow is measured against lung volumes, it becomes apparent that flow is actually higher than normal because of the increased elastic recoil characteristic of fibrotic lungs.

Flow-volume loops require that absolute lung volumes be measured. Unfortunately, many laboratories simply plot flow against the FVC; the flow-FVC loop does not have an inspiratory limb and therefore does not provide as much information.

Patterns of Abnormalities

Most common respiratory disorders can be categorized as obstructive or restrictive on the basis of flow rates and lung volumes (see TABLE 46–1).

Obstructive disease: Obstructive disease is a reduction in flow rates, particularly the FEV_1 and the FEV_1 as a percentage of the FVC (FEV_1/FVC). The reduction in FEV_1 determines the degree of the obstructive defect (see TABLE 46–2). Obstructive defects are caused by increased resistance to flow from abnormalities within the airway lumen (eg, tumors, secretions, mucosal thickening); changes in the wall of the airway (eg, contraction of smooth muscle, edema); or elastic recoil (eg, the parenchymal destruction that occurs in emphysema). With decreased flow rates, expiratory times are longer than usual, and air may become trapped in the lungs from incomplete emptying and increased lung volumes (eg, TLC, RV).

Improvement of FEV_1 and FEV_1/FVC by ≥ 12% or 200 mL with the administration of a bronchodilator confirms the diagnosis of asthma or airway hyperresponsiveness. However, some patients with asthma can have normal pulmonary function and normal spirometric parameters between exacerbations. When suspicion of asthma remains high despite normal spirometry, provocative testing with methacholine, a synthetic analog of acetylcholine that is a nonspecific bron-

TABLE 46–1. CHARACTERISTIC PHYSIOLOGIC CHANGES ASSOCIATED WITH PULMONARY DISORDERS

MEASURE	OBSTRUCTIVE DISORDERS	RESTRICTIVE DISORDERS	MIXED DISORDERS
FEV_1/FVC	Decreased	Normal or increased	Decreased
FEV_1	Decreased	Decreased, normal, or increased	Decreased
FVC	Decreased or normal	Decreased	Decreased
TLC	Normal or increased	Decreased	Decreased
RV	Normal or increased	Decreased	Decreased, normal, or increased

FEV_1 = forced expiratory volume in 1 sec; FVC = forced vital capacity; TLC = total lung capacity; RV = residual volume.

chial irritant, is indicated to detect or exclude bronchoconstriction. In a methacholine challenge test, spirometric parameters are measured at baseline and after inhalation of increasing concentrations of methacholine. Laboratories have different definitions of airway hyperreactivity, but in general a provocative concentration of methacholine that causes a 20% drop in FEV_1 from baseline (PC_{20}) of < 1 mg/mL is considered diagnostic of asthma, whereas a PC_{20} > 16 mg/mL excludes the diagnosis. PC_{20} values between 1 and 16 mg/mL are inconclusive.

Exercise testing may be used to detect exercise-induced bronchoconstriction but is less sensitive than methacholine challenge testing for detecting general airway hyperresponsiveness. The patient performs a constant level of work on a treadmill or cycle ergometer for 6 to 8 min at an intensity selected to produce a heart rate of 80% of predicted maximum heart rate. The FEV_1 and FVC are measured before and 5, 15, and 30 min after exercise. Exercise-induced bronchospasm reduces FEV_1 or FVC ≥ 15% after exercise.

Restrictive disease: Restrictive disease is a reduction in lung volume, specifically, a TLC < 80% of the predicted value. The decrease in TLC determines the severity of

TABLE 46–2. SEVERITY OF OBSTRUCTIVE AND RESTRICTIVE LUNG DISEASES

SEVERITY*	OBSTRUCTIVE FEV_1/FVC (% predicted)	OBSTRUCTIVE FEV_1 (% predicted)	RESTRICTIVE TLC (% predicted)
Normal	≥ 70	≥ 80	≥ 80
Mild	< 70	≥ 80	70–79
Moderate	< 70	$50 \le FEV_1 < 80$	50–69
Severe	< 70	$30 \le FEV_1 < 50$	< 50
Very severe	< 70	< 30 *or* < 50 with chronic respiratory failure	—

*Criteria vary by guideline.

FEV_1 = forced expiratory volume in 1 sec.

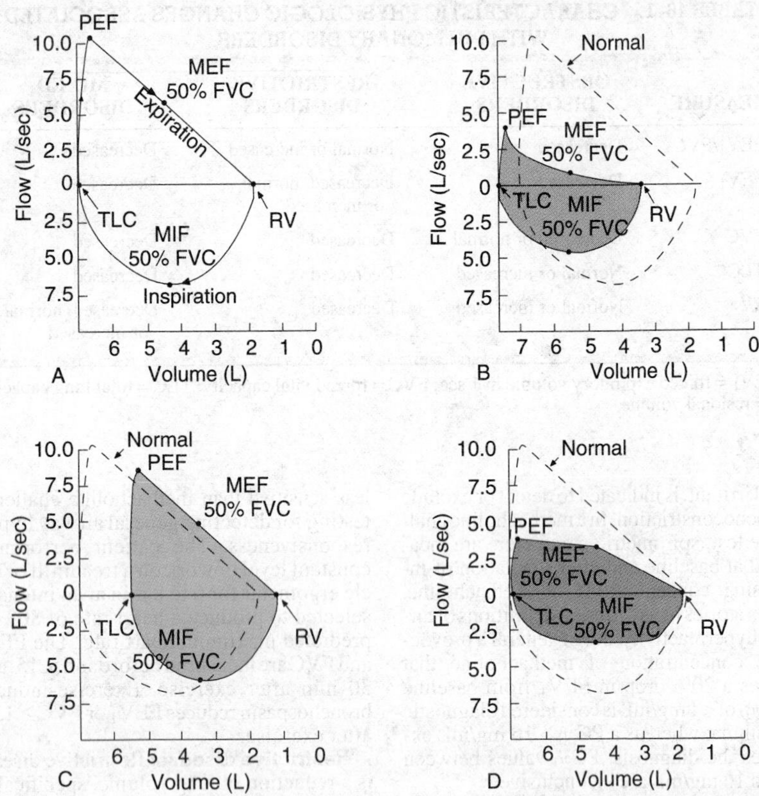

Fig. 46–3. Flow-volume loops. (A) Normal. Inspiratory limb of loop is symmetric and convex. Expiratory limb is linear. Flow rates at the midpoint of the inspiratory and expiratory capacity are often measured. Maximal inspiratory flow at 50% of forced vital capacity (MIF 50%FVC) is greater than maximal expiratory flow at 50% FVC (MEF 50%FVC) because dynamic compression of the airways occurs during exhalation. **(B) Obstructive disease** (eg, emphysema, asthma). Although all flow rates are diminished, expiratory prolongation predominates, and MEF < MIF. Peak expiratory flow is sometimes used to estimate degree of airway obstruction but is dependent on patient effort. **(C) Restrictive disease** (eg, interstitial lung disease, kyphoscoliosis). The loop is narrowed because of diminished lung volumes, but the shape is generally the same as in normal volume. Flow rates are greater than normal at comparable lung volumes because the increased elastic recoil of lungs holds the airways open. **(D) Fixed obstruction of the upper airway** (eg, tracheal stenosis, goiter). The top and bottom of the loops are flattened so that the configuration approaches that of a rectangle. Fixed obstruction limits flow equally during inspiration and expiration, and MEF = MIF. **(E) Variable extrathoracic obstruction** (eg, unilateral vocal cord paralysis, vocal cord dysfunction). When a single vocal cord is paralyzed, it moves passively with pressure gradients across the glottis. During forced inspiration, it is drawn inward, resulting in a plateau of decreased inspiratory flow. During forced expiration, it is passively blown aside, and expiratory flow is unimpaired. Therefore, MIF 50%FVC < MEF 50%FVC. **(F) Variable intrathoracic obstruction** (eg, tracheomalacia). During a forced inspiration, negative pleural pressure holds the "floppy" trachea open. With forced expiration, loss of structural support results in tracheal narrowing of the trachea and a plateau of diminished flow. Flow is maintained briefly before airway compression occurs.

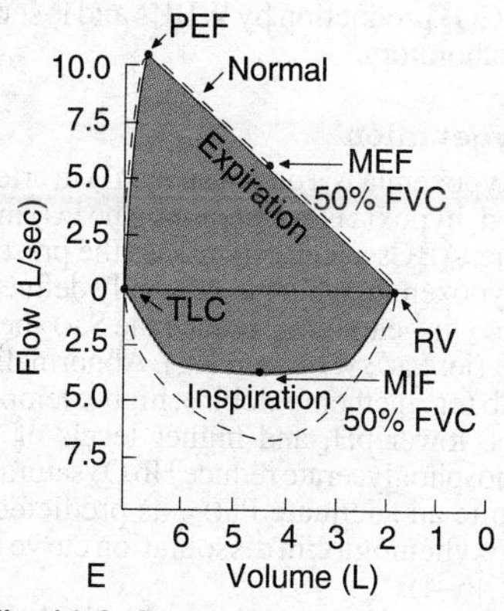

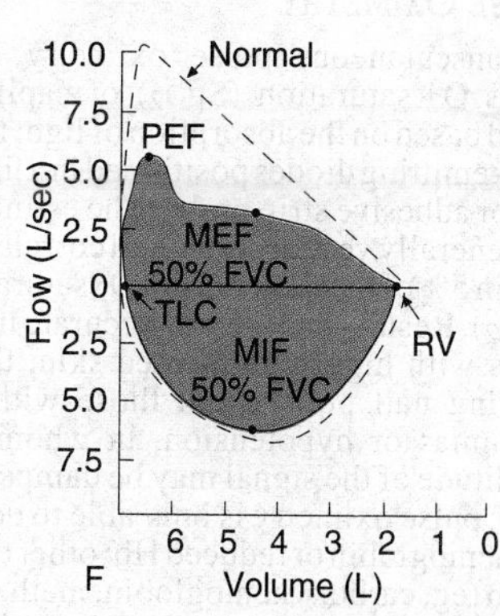

Fig. 46–3. Continued.

restriction (see TABLE 46–2). The decrease in lung volumes produces a decrease in flow rates (reduced FEV_1 and FVC—see FIG. 46–3B). However, the airflow relative to the specific volume is increased, so the FEV_1/FVC ratio is normal or increased. Restrictive defects are caused by a loss in lung volume (eg, lobectomy), abnormalities of structures surrounding the lung (eg, pleural disease, kyphosis, obesity), weakness of the inspiratory muscles of respiration (eg, neuromuscular disease), or abnormalities of the lung parenchyma (eg, pulmonary fibrosis). The feature common to all is a decrease in the compliance of the lungs, the chest wall, or both.

MEASUREMENT OF GAS EXCHANGE

The diffusing capacity for carbon monoxide (DL_{CO}) is a measure of the ability of gas to transfer from alveoli to RBCs across the alveolar epithelium and the capillary endothelium. The DL_{CO} depends not only on the area and thickness of the blood-gas barrier but also on the volume of blood in the pulmonary capillaries. The distribution of alveolar volume and ventilation also affects the measurement. DL_{CO} is measured by sampling end-expiratory gas for carbon monoxide (CO) after a patient inspires a small amount of CO, holds his breath, and exhales. Measured DL_{CO} should be adjusted for alveolar volume (which is estimated from dilution of helium) and the patient's Hct. DL_{CO} is reported as mL/min/mm Hg and as a percentage of a predicted value.

Conditions that primarily affect the pulmonary vasculature, such as primary pulmonary hypertension and pulmonary embolism, decrease DL_{CO}. Conditions that affect the lung diffusely, such as emphysema and pulmonary fibrosis, decrease both DL_{CO} and alveolar ventilation (V_A). Reduced DL_{CO} also occurs in patients with past lung resection because total lung volume is smaller, but DL_{CO} corrects to or even exceeds normal when adjusted for V_A because increased additional vascular surface area is recruited in the remaining lung. Anemic patients often have lower DL_{CO} values that correct when adjusted for Hb. DL_{CO} may be higher than predicted in patients with heart failure, presumably because the increased pulmonary venous and arterial pressure results in recruitment of additional pulmonary microvessels. DL_{CO} is also increased in patients with polycythemia, in part because of increased Hct and because of the vascular recruitment that occurs with increased pulmonary pressures due to increased viscosity. DL_{CO} is increased in patients with alveolar hemorrhage because RBCs in the alveolar space can also bind CO. DL_{CO} is also increased in patients with asthma. Although this increase is attributed to presumed vascular recruitment, the actual mechanism is unknown.

Pulse Oximetry

Transcutaneous pulse oximetry estimates O_2 saturation (SpO_2) of capillary blood based on the absorption of light from light-emitting diodes positioned in a finger clip or adhesive strip probe. The estimates are generally very accurate and correlate to within 5% of measured atrial O_2 saturation (SaO_2). Results may be less accurate in patients with highly pigmented skin, those wearing nail polish, and those with arrhythmias or hypotension, in whom the amplitude of the signal may be dampened. Also, pulse oximetry is only able to detect oxyhemoglobin or reduced Hb; other types of Hb (eg, carboxyhemoglobin, methemoglobin) are assumed to be oxyhemoglobin and falsely elevate the SpO_2 measurement.

Arterial Blood Gas Sampling

ABG sampling is performed to obtain accurate measures of PaO_2, $PaCO_2$, and blood pH; these variables combined with the patient's temperature allow for calculation of HCO_3 level (which can also be measured directly from venous blood) and SaO_2. ABG sampling can also accurately measure carboxyhemoglobin and methemoglobin.

The radial artery is usually used. Because arterial puncture in rare cases leads to thrombosis and impaired perfusion of distal tissue, Allen's test is first performed to ensure adequate collateral circulation. With this maneuver, the radial and ulnar pulses are simultaneously occluded until the hand becomes pale. The ulnar pulse is then released while the pressure on the radial pulse is maintained. A blush across the entire hand within 7 sec of release of the ulnar pulse suggests adequate flow through the ulnar artery.

Under sterile conditions, a 22- to 25-gauge needle attached to a heparinized syringe is inserted just proximal to the maximal impulse of the radial arterial pulse and advanced slightly distally into the artery until pulsatile blood is returned. Systolic BP often pushes back the syringe plunger. After 3 to 5 mL of blood is collected, the needle is quickly withdrawn, and firm pressure is applied to the puncture site to facilitate hemostasis. Simultaneously, the ABG specimen is placed on ice to reduce O_2 consumption and CO_2 production by WBCs and is sent to the laboratory.

Oxygenation

Hypoxemia is a decrease in PO_2 in arterial blood; hypoxia is a decrease in the PO_2 in the tissue. ABGs accurately assess the presence of hypoxemia, which is generally defined as a PaO_2 low enough to reduce the SaO_2 below 90% (ie, $PaO_2 < 60$ mm Hg). Abnormalities in Hb (eg, methemoglobin), higher temperatures, lower pH, and higher levels of 2,3-diphosphoglycerate reduce Hb O_2 saturation despite an adequate PaO_2, as predicted by the oxyhemoglobin dissociation curve (see FIG. 46–4).

Causes of hypoxemia can be divided into those with elevated or normal alveolar-arterial PO_2 gradients [$(A\text{-}a)DO_2$], defined as the difference between alveolar O_2 tension (PAO_2) and PaO_2. PAO_2 is calculated as follows:

$$PAO_2 = \left[FIO_2 \times \left(P_{atm} - P_{H_2O}\right)\right] - PaCO_2/R,$$

where FIO_2 is the fraction of inspired O_2 (eg, 0.21 at room air), P_{atm} is the ambient barometric pressure (eg, 760 mm Hg at sea level), P_{H_2O} is the partial pressure of water vapor (eg, usually 47 mm Hg), $PaCO_2$ is the measured partial pressure of arterial CO_2, and R is the respiratory quotient, which is assumed to be 0.8 in a resting patient on a normal diet.

At sea level and on room air, $FIO_2 = 0.21$, and the $(A\text{-}a)DO_2$ can be simplified as follows:

$$(A - a)DO_2 = 150 - PaCO_2/0.8 - PaO_2,$$

where $(A\text{-}a)DO_2$ is typically <20 but increases with age (because of age-related decline in pulmonary function) and with increasing FIO_2 (because, although Hb becomes 100% saturated at a PaO_2 of about 150 mm Hg, O_2 is soluble in blood, and the O_2 content of plasma continues to increase at increasing FIO_2). Estimations of normal $(A\text{-}a)DO_2$ values as $< (2.5 + [FIO_2 \times \text{age in years}])$ or as less than the absolute value of the FIO_2 (eg, < 21 on room air; < 30 on 30% FIO_2) correct for these effects.

Hypoxemia with increased $(A\text{-}a)DO_2$ is caused by ventilation-perfusion (V/Q) mismatch, right-to-left shunting, and impaired

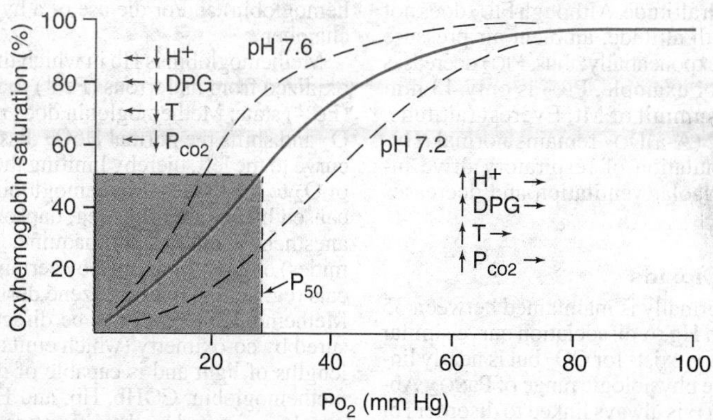

Fig. 46–4. Oxyhemoglobin dissociation curve. Arterial oxyhemoglobin saturation is related to partial pressure of O_2 (PO_2). PO_2 at 50% saturation (P_{50}) is normally 27 mm Hg. The dissociation curve is shifted to the right by increased hydrogen ion (H^+) concentration, increased RBC 2,3-diphosphoglycerate (DPG), increased temperature (T), and increased partial pressure of carbon dioxide (PCO_2). Decreased levels of H^+, DPG, temperature, and PCO_2 shift the curve to the left. Hb characterized by a rightward shifting of the curve has a decreased affinity for O_2, and that characterized by a leftward shifting of the curve has an increased affinity for O_2.

diffusing capacity. Hypoxemia with normal (A-a)DO_2 is caused by hypoventilation and low partial pressures of inspired O_2 (PIO_2). Hypoxemia due to all causes except right-to-left shunting responds to supplemental O_2.

V/Q mismatch is one of the more common reasons for hypoxemia and contributes to the hypoxemia occurring with COPD and asthma. In the normal lung, regional perfusion closely matches regional ventilation because of the arteriolar vasoconstriction that occurs in response to alveolar hypoxia. In disease states, dysregulation leads to perfusion of alveolar units that are receiving less than complete ventilation (V/Q mismatch). As a result, systemic venous blood passes through the pulmonary capillaries without achieving normal levels of PaO_2. Supplemental O_2 can correct hypoxemia due to V/Q mismatch by increasing the PAO_2, although the increased (A-a)DO_2 persists.

Right-to-left shunting is an extreme example of V/Q mismatch. With shunting, deoxygenated pulmonary arterial blood arrives at the left side of the heart without having passed through ventilated lung segments. Shunting may occur through lung parenchyma, through abnormal connections between the pulmonary arterial and venous circulations, or through intracardiac communications (eg, patent foramen ovale).

Impaired diffusing capacity only rarely occurs in isolation; usually it is accompanied by significant V/Q mismatch. Because O_2 completely saturates Hb after only a fraction of the time that blood is in contact with alveolar gas, hypoxemia due to impaired diffusing capacity occurs only when cardiac output is increased (eg, with exercise), when barometric pressure is low (eg, at high altitudes), or when > 50% of the pulmonary parenchyma is destroyed. As with V/Q mismatch, the (A-a)DO_2 is increased, but PaO_2 can be rapidly increased by increasing the FIO_2.

Hypoventilation (reduced alveolar ventilation) decreases the PAO_2 and increases the $PaCO_2$, thereby decreasing PaO_2. In cases of pure hypoventilation, the (A-a)DO_2 is normal. Causes of hypoventilation include decreased respiratory rate or depth (eg, neuromuscular disease, severe obesity, drug overdose) or an increase in the fraction of dead space ventilation in patients already at their maximal ventilatory limit (eg, an exacerbation of severe COPD). Hypoventilatory hypoxemia responds to supplemental O_2.

Decreased FIO_2 is a final uncommon cause of hypoxemia that in most cases occurs only at high altitude. Although FIO_2 does not change with altitude, ambient air pressure decreases exponentially; thus, PIO_2 decreases as well. For example, PIO_2 is only 43 mm Hg at the summit of Mt. Everest (altitude, 29,028 ft). $(A-a)DO_2$ remains normal. Hypoxic stimulation of respiratory drive increases alveolar ventilation and decreases $PaCO_2$ level.

Carbon Dioxide

PCO_2 normally is maintained between 35 and 45 mm Hg. A dissociation curve similar to that for O_2 exists for CO_2 but is nearly linear over the physiologic range of $PaCO_2$. Abnormal PCO_2 is always linked to disorders of ventilation and is always associated with acid-base changes.

Hypercapnia is $PCO_2 > 45$ mg Hg. Causes of hypercapnia are the same as those of hypoventilation (see p. 371). Hypocapnia is $PCO_2 < 35$ mm Hg. Hypocapnia is always caused by hyperventilation due to pulmonary (eg, pulmonary edema or embolism), cardiac (eg, heart failure), metabolic (eg, acidosis), drug-induced (eg, aspirin, progesterone), CNS (eg, infection, tumor, bleeding, increased intracranial pressure) or physiologic (eg, pain, pregnancy) disorders or conditions. Hypocapnia is thought to directly increase bronchoconstriction and lower the threshold for cerebral and myocardial ischemia, perhaps through its effects on acid-base status.

Carboxyhemoglobinemia and Methemoglobinemia

CO binds to Hb with an affinity 210 times that of O_2 and prevents O_2 transport. Clinically toxic carboxyhemoglobin levels are most often the result of exposure to exhaust fumes or from smoke inhalation, although cigarette smokers have detectable levels. Patients with CO poisoning may present with nonspecific symptoms such as malaise, headache, and nausea. Because poisoning often occurs during colder months (because of indoor use of combustible fuel heaters), symptoms may be confused with a viral syndrome such as influenza. Clinicians must be alert to the possibility of CO poisoning and measure levels of carboxyhemoglobin when indicated; COHb can be directly measured from an arterial sample.

Treatment is the administration of 100% O_2 (which shortens the half-life of carboxyhemoglobin) and/or the use of a hyperbaric chamber.

Methemoglobin is Hb in which the iron is oxidized from its ferrous (Fe^{2+}) to its ferric (Fe^{3+}) state. Methemoglobin does not carry O_2 and shifts the normal HbO_2 dissociation curve to the left, thereby limiting the release of O_2 to the tissues. Methemoglobinemia is caused by certain drugs (eg, dapsone, local anesthetics, nitrates, primaquine, sulfonamides) or, less commonly, by certain chemicals (eg, aniline dyes, benzene derivatives). Methemoglobin level can be directly measured by co-oximetry (which emits 4 wavelengths of light and is capable of detecting methemoglobin, COHb, Hb, and HbO_2) or may be estimated by the difference between the O_2 saturation calculated from the measured PaO_2 and the directly measured SaO_2. Patients with methemoglobinemia most often have asymptomatic cyanosis. In severe cases, O_2 delivery is reduced to such a degree that symptoms of tissue hypoxia result, such as confusion, angina, and myalgias. Stopping the causative drug or chemical exposure is often sufficient. Rarely, methylene blue (a reducing agent) or exchange transfusion is needed.

TESTS OF RESPIRATORY MUSCLE FUNCTION

Maximal inspiratory pressure (MIP) and maximal expiratory pressure (MEP) measurements may aid in evaluating respiratory muscle weakness. MIP is the pressure generated during maximal inspiratory effort against a closed system. It is usually measured at residual volume (RV) because inspiratory muscle strength is inversely related to lung volume. MEP is measured during a similar maneuver at total lung capacity (TLC) because expiratory muscle strength is directly related to lung volume. The information available from these maneuvers is nonspecific, however, and cannot distinguish between insufficient effort, muscle weakness, and neurologic disease.

The maximal voluntary ventilation (MVV) is another combined measure of the neuromuscular and respiratory systems. The MVV is the total volume of air exhaled during 12 sec of rapid, deep breathing. It can also be estimated as the forced expiratory volume in

1 sec (FEV_1) × 35 or 40. A significant difference between the predicted and measured MVV may indicate insufficient neuromuscular reserve, abnormal respiratory mechanics, or an inadequate effort. Progressive reduction of tidal volumes during the test is suggestive, but rarely diagnostic, of neuromuscular abnormalities.

The sniff test is sometimes used in suspected cases of diaphragmatic paralysis or paresis. During continuous fluoroscopic examination, the patient makes a quick, short, strong inspiratory effort ("sniff"). This maneuver minimizes the contribution of the other muscles of respiration (eg, intercostals). A weakened hemidiaphragm may have decreased excursion compared with the contralateral diaphragm or may move upward paradoxically. Occasionally, electromyographic interrogation of the diaphragm and phrenic nerve is performed but is of uncertain diagnostic accuracy. Muscle and nerve biopsies may be helpful in selected cases.

EXERCISE TESTING

The two most common forms of exercise testing used to evaluate pulmonary disease are the 6-min walk test and full cardiopulmonary exercise testing.

Six-minute walk test: This simple test measures the maximal distance that a patient can walk at his own pace in 6 min. The test globally assesses functional capacity but does not provide specific information on the multiple systems (cardiac, pulmonary, hematologic, musculoskeletal) involved in exercise, nor does it assess patient effort. This test is used for preoperative and postoperative evaluation of lung transplantation and lung volume reduction surgery, to monitor response to therapeutic interventions and pulmonary rehabilitation, and to predict mortality and morbidity in patients with cardiac and pulmonary vascular disease.

Cardiopulmonary exercise testing (CPET): This computerized test provides a breath-by-breath analysis of respiratory gas exchange at rest and during a period of exercise, the intensity of which is increased incrementally until symptoms limit testing or the patient reaches maximal levels. Information on airflow, O_2 consumption, CO_2 production, and heart rate are collected and used for computation of other variables; ABGs may also be sampled. Exercise is performed on a treadmill or on a bicycle ergometer; the ergometer may be preferable because work rate can be directly measured.

CPET primarily determines if the patient has normal or reduced maximal exercise capacity (VO_2max). Reduced VO_2max can further suggest probable causes. CPET is used to define which organ systems contribute to a patient's symptoms of exertional dyspnea and exercise intolerance and to what extent. The test is also more sensitive for detecting early or subclinical disease than are less comprehensive tests that are done at rest. Examples of applications include assessment of exercise capacity for disability evaluation, preoperative assessment, determining whether symptoms of dyspnea are the result of cardiac or pulmonary problems in patients who have disorders of both organ systems, selection of candidates for cardiac transplantation, and assessing prognosis in selected diseases, such as heart disease, pulmonary vascular disease, and cystic fibrosis. CPET can also help gauge responses to therapeutic interventions and guide prescription of exercise in rehabilitation programs. In following the response to therapy or disease progression, a steady-state CPET involving at least 6 min of constant work at 50 to 70% of the maximal work rate achieved during a maximal CPET may be more useful than an incremental, maximal CPET. Repeated evaluation at this work rate over time provides comparable data and is sensitive to improvement or decline in cardiopulmonary function.

Multiple variables are assessed during CPET, and no single one is diagnostic of a cause for exercise limitation. Instead, an integrative approach using clinical data, trends during exercise, and recognition of underlying patterns of physiologic responses is used.

47 DIAGNOSTIC AND THERAPEUTIC PULMONARY PROCEDURES

Diagnostic tests besides pulmonary function testing (see p. 364) include a variety of types of chest imaging, electrocardiography, and ventilation/perfusion (V/Q) scanning. Diagnostic procedures include bronchoscopy, mediastinoscopy and mediastinotomy, pleural biopsy, thoracentesis, thoracoscopy and video-assisted thoracoscopic surgery (VATS), thoracotomy, transthoracic needle biopsy, and tube thoracostomy; pulmonary artery catheterization is discussed in CRC01. Therapeutic procedures include chest physiotherapy and pulmonary rehabilitation.

CHEST IMAGING

There are no absolute contraindications to undergoing noninvasive imaging procedures.

Chest x-ray: Plain chest x-rays provide images of structures in and around the thorax and are most useful for identifying abnormalities in the heart, lung parenchyma, pleurae, chest wall, diaphragm, mediastinum, and hilum. They are usually the initial test performed to evaluate the lungs. The standard chest x-ray is taken from back to front (posteroanterior view) to minimize x-ray scatter that could artifactually enlarge the cardiac silhouette and from the side of the thorax (lateral view). Lordotic or oblique views can be obtained to evaluate pulmonary nodules or to clarify abnormalities that may be due to superimposed structures, though chest CT provides more information and has largely superseded these views. Lateral decubitus views may be used to distinguish free-flowing from loculated pleural effusion, but again, CT provides more information. End-expiratory views are used to detect pneumothoraces.

Screening chest x-rays are often performed but are almost never indicated; one exception is in the asymptomatic patient with a positive tuberculin skin test, in whom a single posteroanterior chest x-ray without a lateral view is used to make decisions regarding treatment for pulmonary TB. Portable (usually anteroposterior) chest x-rays are almost always suboptimal and should be used only when a patient is too ill to be transported to the radiology department.

Chest fluoroscopy is the use of a continuous x-ray beam to image movement. It is useful for detecting unilateral diaphragmatic paralysis. During a sniff test, in which the patient is instructed to forcibly inhale through the nose (or sniff), a paralyzed hemidiaphragm moves cranially (paradoxically) while the unaffected hemidiaphragm moves caudally.

Computed tomography: CT defines intrathoracic structures and abnormalities more clearly than does a chest x-ray. Conventional (planar) CT provides multiple 10 mm-thick cross-sectional images of the chest. Its main advantage is wide availability. Disadvantages are motion artifact and limited detail from volume averaging of tissue within each 10-mm slice.

High-resolution CT (HRCT) provides 1-mm-thick cross-sectional images; this is particularly helpful in evaluation of interstitial lung diseases (eg, lymphangitic carcinomatosis, sarcoid, fibrosing alveolitis) and bronchiectasis.

Helical (spiral) CT provides multiplanar images of the entire chest as patients hold their breath for 8 to 10 sec while being moved continuously through the CT gantry. Helical CT is thought to be at least equivalent to conventional CT for most purposes. Its main advantages are speed, less radiation exposure, and an ability to construct 3-dimensional images. Software can also generate images of bronchial mucosa (virtual bronchoscopy). Its main disadvantages are less availability and the requirement for breath-holding, which can be difficult for patients with symptomatic pulmonary disease.

CT angiography uses a bolus of IV contrast to highlight the pulmonary arteries, which is useful in diagnosis of pulmonary embolism. Dye load is comparable to conventional angiography, but the test is quicker and less invasive.

Magnetic resonance imaging: MRI has a relatively limited role in pulmonary imaging but is preferred over CT in specific circumstances (eg, for assessment of superior sulcus and other tumors that abut the chest wall). In patients with suspected pulmonary embolism in whom IV contrast cannot be used, MRI can sometimes identify large proximal emboli but usually is limited in this disorder.

Advantages include absence of radiation exposure, excellent visualization of vascular structures, lack of artifact from bone, and excellent soft-tissue contrast. Disadvantages include respiratory and cardiac motion and the time it takes to do the procedure.

Ultrasonography: Ultrasonography is primarily used to facilitate such procedures as thoracentesis and central venous catheter insertion. Endobronchial ultrasound is sometimes used in conjunction with fiberoptic bronchoscopy.

V/Q scanning: V/Q scanning uses radionuclides to detect areas of the lung where supply of O_2 (ventilation) and blood (perfusion) are mismatched. Areas of ventilation without perfusion, perfusion without ventilation, or matched increases and decreases in both can be detected with 6 to 8 views of the lung. V/Q scanning is used almost exclusively for diagnosis of pulmonary embolism. Split-function ventilation scanning, in which the degree of ventilation is quantified for each lobe, is used to predict the effect of lobar or lung resection on pulmonary function; postsurgical forced expiratory volume in 1 sec (FEV_1) is the percentage of uptake of ventilation tracer in the healthy fraction of the lungs multiplied by preoperative FEV_1 (in liters). A value of < 0.8 L (or < 40% of that predicted for the patient) indicates limited pulmonary reserve and the likelihood of unacceptably high perioperative morbidity and mortality.

Positron emission tomography scanning: PET scanning uses radioactively labeled glucose (fluorodeoxyglucose) to measure metabolic activity in tissues. It is used in pulmonary medicine to determine if lung nodules and mediastinal lymph nodes harbor tumor (metabolic staging) and if cancer is recurrent in previously irradiated, scarred areas of the lung. PET is superior to CT scanning for mediastinal evaluation for staging because PET can identify tumor in normal-sized lymph nodes and at extrathoracic sites, thereby decreasing the need for invasive procedures such as mediastinoscopy and needle biopsy. Current spatial resolution of PET is 7 to 8 mm; thus the test is not useful for lesions < 1 cm. PET reveals metastatic disease in up to 14% of patients in whom it would not otherwise be suspected. The sensitivity of PET (80 to 95%) is comparable to that of histologic tissue examination. False-positive results have been reported; slowly growing tumors (eg, bronchoalveolar carcinoma, carcinoid tumor, some metastatic malignancies) may cause false-negative results. A new generation of combined CT-PET scanners may become the most cost-effective technology for lung cancer diagnosis and staging.

ELECTROCARDIOGRAPHY

Electrocardiography is a useful adjunct to other pulmonary tests because it provides information about the right heart (see also p. 593).

Chronic pulmonary hypertension leading to chronic right atrial and ventricular hypertrophy may manifest as prominent P waves (P pulmonale) and ST-segment depression in leads II, III, and aVF; rightward shift in QRS axis; and decreased progression of R waves in precordial leads. COPD patients commonly have low voltage due to interposition of hyperexpanded lungs between the heart and ECG electrodes.

Acute right ventricle overload or failure, as occurs in submassive or massive pulmonary embolism, manifests as right axis deviation (R > S in V_1), with S-wave deepening in lead I, Q-wave deepening in lead III, and ST-segment elevation and T-wave inversion in lead III and the precordial leads ($S_1Q_3T_3$ pattern). Right bundle branch block also sometimes occurs.

BRONCHOSCOPY

Bronchoscopy is introduction of an endoscope into the airways. Flexible fiberoptic bronchoscopy has replaced rigid bronchoscopy for virtually all diagnostic and most therapeutic indications. Rigid bronchoscopy is now used only when a wider aperture and channels are required for better visualization and instrumentation. Examples include active vigorous pulmonary hemorrhage, in which the rigid bronchoscope can better identify the bleeding source and, with its larger suction channel, can better suction blood and prevent asphyxiation; aspirated foreign bodies in young children; and obstructive endobronchial lesions that require laser debulking or stent placement. Nearly all flexible bronchoscopes are color video–compatible, facilitating airway visualization and documentation of findings.

Diagnostically, flexible fiberoptic bronchoscopy allows for direct airway visualization down to and including subsegmental bronchi; sampling of respiratory secretions and cells via bronchial washings, brushings, and lavage of peripheral airways and alveoli; and biopsy of endobronchial, parenchymal, and mediastinal structures. Therapeutic uses include suctioning of retained secretions.

Absolute contraindications include untreatable life-threatening arrhythmia, inability to adequately oxygenate the patient during the procedure, and acute respiratory failure with hypercapnia (unless the patient is endotracheally intubated and ventilated). Relative contraindications include an uncooperative patient, recent MI, high-grade tracheal obstruction, and uncorrectable coagulopathy. Transbronchial biopsy should be performed with caution in patients with uremia, superior vena cava obstruction, or pulmonary hypertension because of increased risk of bleeding and pneumothorax. Inspection of the airways is safe in these patients, however.

Bronchoscopy should be performed only by a pulmonologist or trained surgeon in a monitored setting, typically a bronchoscopy suite, operating room, or ICU (for ventilated patients).

The patient should receive nothing by mouth for at least 4 h before bronchoscopy and have IV access, intermittent BP monitoring, continuous pulse oximetry, and cardiac monitoring; supplemental O_2 should be available. Premedication with atropine 0.01 mg/kg IM or IV to decrease secretions and vagal tone is common, although this practice has been questioned in recent studies. Short-acting benzodiazepines, opioids, or both may be given to patients before the procedure to decrease anxiety, discomfort, and cough.

The pharynx and vocal cords are anesthetized with nebulized or aerosolized (1 or 2%) lidocaine (maximum, 250 to 300 mg for a 70-kg patient). The bronchoscope is lubricated with lidocaine jelly and passed through the nostril or through the mouth with an oral airway or bite block. After inspection of the nasopharynx and larynx, the scope is passed through the vocal cords during inspiration and into the trachea and upper airways.

Several ancillary procedures can be performed as needed with or without fluoroscopic guidance. In bronchial washing, saline is sprayed in and aspirated from the airways. In bronchial brushing, a brush is advanced through the bronchoscope and used to abrade suspicious lesions to obtain cells. In bronchoalveolar lavage, 50 to 200 mL of sterile saline is infused into the distal bronchoalveolar tree; aspiration of the fluid retrieves cells, protein, and microorganisms located at the alveolar level. Local areas of pulmonary edema created by lavage may cause transient hypoxemia. In transbronchial biopsy, forceps are advanced through the bronchoscope and airway to biopsy one or more sites in the lung parenchyma. Transbronchial biopsy can be performed without x-ray guidance, but evidence supports increased diagnostic yields and lower incidence of pneumothorax when fluoroscopic guidance is used.

Patients are typically observed 2 to 4 h after the procedure on supplemental O_2. Return of a gag reflex and maintenance of O_2 saturation off O_2 are the two primary indices of recovery. Standard practice is to obtain an expiratory posteroanterior chest x-ray after transbronchial lung biopsy to exclude pneumothorax.

Serious complications are uncommon; minor bleeding from a biopsy site and fever occur in 10 to 15%. Premedication can cause oversedation with respiratory depression, hypotension, and cardiac arrhythmias. Rarely, topical anesthesia causes laryngospasm, bronchospasm, seizures, methemoglobinemia with refractory cyanosis, or cardiac arrhythmias or arrest. Bronchoscopy itself may cause minor laryngeal edema or injury with hoarseness, hypoxemia in patients with compromised gas exchange, arrhythmias (most commonly premature atrial contractions, ventricular premature beats, or bradycardia), and, very rarely, transmission of infection from suboptimally sterilized equipment. Transbronchial biopsy can cause pneumothorax (2 to 5%) and significant hemorrhage (1 to 1.5%). Mortality is 1 to 4/10,000 patients. The elderly and others with serious comorbidities (severe COPD, coronary artery disease, pneumonia with hypoxemia, advanced neoplasia, mental dysfunction) are at greatest risk. Transbronchial biopsy increases mortality to 12/10,000 patients but can preclude the need for thoracotomy.

MEDIASTINOSCOPY AND MEDIASTINOTOMY

Mediastinoscopy is introduction of an endoscope into the mediastinum. Mediastinotomy is surgical opening of the mediastinum. The two are complementary procedures; mediastinotomy gives direct access to aortopulmonary window lymph nodes, which are inaccessible to mediastinoscopy. Both procedures are performed to evaluate or excise mediastinal lymphadenopathy or masses and to stage cancers (eg, lung and esophageal cancer), though PET scan is decreasing the need for the procedures in the latter indication.

Contraindications include superior vena cava syndrome; previous mediastinal irradiation, mediastinoscopy, median sternotomy, or tracheostomy; and aneurysm of the aortic arch.

Mediastinoscopy and mediastinotomy are performed by surgeons in an operating room using general anesthesia. For mediastinoscopy, neck soft tissue is bluntly dissected down to the trachea and distally to the carina through an incision in the suprasternal notch. A mediastinoscope is inserted into the space, allowing access to paratracheal, tracheobronchial, azygous, and subcarinal nodes and to the superior posterior mediastinum. Anterior mediastinotomy (Chamberlain procedure) is surgical entry to the mediastinum through a parasternal 2nd left intercostal space incision, allowing access to anterior mediastinal and aortopulmonary window lymph nodes, common sites of metastases for left upper lobe lung cancers.

Complications occur in < 1% of patients and include bleeding, infection, vocal cord paralysis from recurrent laryngeal nerve damage, chylothorax from duct injury, and pneumothorax.

PHYSIOTHERAPY

Chest physiotherapy consists of external mechanical maneuvers, such as chest percussion, postural drainage, and vibration, to augment mobilization and clearance of airway secretions. It is indicated for patients in whom cough is insufficient to clear thick, tenacious, or loculated secretions. Examples include cystic fibrosis, bronchiectasis, lung abscess, neuromuscular diseases, and pneumonias in dependent lung regions.

Contraindications are relative and include discomfort from physical positions or manipulations, anticoagulation, rib or vertebral fractures or osteoporosis, and recent hemoptysis.

Chest physiotherapy may be administered by a respiratory therapist, although the techniques can often be taught to family members of patients. The most common procedures used are postural drainage and chest percussion, in which the patient is rotated to facilitate drainage of secretions from a specific lobe or segment while being clapped with cupped hands to loosen and mobilize retained secretions that can then be expectorated or drained. The procedure is somewhat uncomfortable and tiring for the patient. Alternatives to chest percussion, the benefits of which remain unproven, include mechanical vibrators, inflatable vests, controlled patterns of breathing, positive expiratory pressure devices to maintain airway patency, and ultra-low-frequency airway oscillation devices to mobilize sputum.

Complications are unusual but include position-related hypoxia and aspiration of secretions in other lung regions.

PLEURAL BIOPSY

Pleural biopsy is performed to determine the underlying cause of an exudative pleural effusion when repeated thoracenteses are nondiagnostic. Improved laboratory techniques, newer diagnostic tests for pleural fluid (eg, adenosine deaminase levels, interferon-γ, PCR studies for suspected tuberculosis), and more widespread availability of thoracoscopy have made the procedure less necessary.

Percutaneous pleural biopsy should be done only by a pulmonologist or surgeon trained in the procedure. Technique is essentially the same as that for thoracentesis and can be done at the bedside; no specific patient preparation is necessary. At least 3 specimens obtained from one skin location, with 3, 6, and 9 o'clock positioning of the needle-cutting chamber, are needed for histology and culture.

Chest x-ray should be performed after biopsy because of increased risk of complications, which are the same as those for thoracentesis but with higher incidence of pneumothorax and hemorrhage.

PULMONARY REHABILITATION

Pulmonary rehabilitation is the use of exercise, education, and behavioral intervention to enhance quality of life. It is indicated for any condition in which respiratory symptoms cause activity restriction—eg, COPD, interstitial lung disease, neuromuscular disease causing chest wall weakness—and for respiratory retraining after prolonged ventilator dependence. Contraindications are relative and include comorbidities that could complicate attempts to increase a patient's level of exercise, such as untreated angina or left ventricular dysfunction. These do not preclude application of other components of pulmonary rehabilitation programs, however.

For many patients with chronic respiratory disease, medical therapy only partially allays the symptoms and complications of their illness. A comprehensive program of pulmonary rehabilitation may lead to significant clinical improvement by reducing shortness of breath, increasing exercise tolerance, and, to a lesser extent, decreasing the number of hospitalizations. However, these programs do not improve survival.

Pulmonary rehabilitation is best administered as part of an integrated program of exercise training, education, and psychosocial and behavioral intervention by a team of physicians, nurses, respiratory therapists, physical and occupational therapists, and psychologists or social workers. Exercise training involves aerobic exercise and respiratory muscle and extremity strength training; lower extremity strength training may be particularly important for patients with COPD. Education involves smoking cessation; teaching breathing strategies (such as pursed-lip breathing, in which exhalations are begun against closed lips to splint open airways before breathing out); principles of conserving physical energy; treatment options, including drug therapy; and advanced-care planning. Psychosocial interventions involve counseling and feedback for the depression, anxieties, and fear that obstruct the patient's full participation in activities.

THORACENTESIS

Thoracentesis is chest wall puncture for aspiration of pleural fluid. It is used to determine the etiology of a pleural effusion (diagnostic thoracentesis), to relieve dyspnea caused by pleural fluid (therapeutic thoracentesis), and, occasionally, to perform pleurodesis.

Relative contraindications include uncertain fluid location by examination; minimal fluid volume; altered chest wall anatomy; pulmonary disease severe enough to make complications life threatening (see p. 379); bleeding diatheses; uncontrolled coughing; and coagulopathy. No absolute contraindications to thoracentesis exist except refusal or inability to consent to the procedure.

Thoracentesis can be safely performed at the patient's bedside or in an outpatient setting. Presence and location of pleural fluid is verified by physical examination (chest percussion) or by imaging techniques. Ultrasonography, CT, or both may be useful if chest x-rays are equivocal, if prior thoracentesis attempts were unsuccessful, or if the fluid is loculated.

Thoracentesis is best performed with the patient sitting upright and leaning slightly forward with arm support. Recumbent or supine thoracentesis (eg, in a ventilated patient) is possible but best done with ultrasound or CT guidance. Only unstable patients and those at high risk of decompensation from complications require monitoring (eg, pulse oximeter, ECG).

Under sterile conditions, 1 to 2% lidocaine is injected with a 25-gauge needle to anesthetize the skin. A larger (20- or 22-gauge) needle with anesthetic is then inserted at the upper border of the rib one intercostal space below the fluid level in the midscapular line. The needle is advanced with periodic aspiration (to avoid inadvertent insertion into a blood vessel and intravascular injection), and anesthetic is injected at progressively deeper levels. The most painful level after the skin is the parietal pleura, which should be infiltrated the most. The needle is then advanced beyond the parietal pleura until pleural fluid is aspirated, at which point the depth of the needle should be noted. A large-bore (16- to 19-gauge) thoracentesis needle-catheter device is then attached to a 3-way stopcock, which is connected to a 30- to 50-mL syringe and tubing that drains into a container. The thoracentesis needle is passed through the skin and subcutaneous tissue along the upper border of the rib into the effusion at about the same depth noted during anesthesia. The catheter is inserted through the needle, and the needle is withdrawn to decrease the risk of pneumothorax. Pleural fluid can then be aspirated and, with a turn of the stopcock, collected in tubes or bags for further evaluation.

Fluid should be removed in stages not to exceed 1.5 L/day; hypotension and pulmonary edema may occur with removal of > 1.5 L of fluid at one sitting or with rapid evacuation of the pleural space using a vacuum or suction bottle. When large volumes of fluid must be removed, blood pressure should be monitored continuously.

It has been standard practice to obtain a chest x-ray after thoracentesis to rule out pneumothorax, document the extent of fluid removal, and view lung fields previously obscured by fluid, but evidence suggests that routine chest x-ray is not necessary in asymptomatic patients.

Coughing is common as the lung re-expands; it does not signify pneumothorax. If the pleural process is inflammatory, pleuritic pain, an audible pleural rub, or both may develop as fluid is removed because of approximation of inflamed visceral and parietal pleura. When substantial volumes of fluid are removed from the pleural space, the plunger on the syringe should be released periodically midway during an aspiration. If the fluid in the syringe is drawn back into the pleural space when negative pressure on the syringe is decreased, pleural pressure may be too negative, and the lung may be restricted from re-expanding because of enveloping adhesions or tumor.

Complications include pneumothorax, hemoptysis from lung puncture, re-expansion pulmonary edema or hypotension after rapid removal of large volumes of fluid, hemothorax from damage to intercostal vessels, puncture of the spleen or liver, and vasovagal syncope. Bloody fluid that does not clot in a collecting tube indicates that blood in the pleural space was not iatrogenic, because free blood in the pleural space rapidly defibrinates.

THORACOSCOPY AND VIDEO-ASSISTED THORACOSCOPIC SURGERY

Thoracoscopy is introduction of an endoscope into the pleural space. Thoracoscopy can be used for visualization (pleuroscopy) or for surgical procedures. Surgical thoracoscopy is more commonly referred to as video-assisted thoracoscopic surgery (VATS). Pleuroscopy can be performed with conscious sedation in an endoscopy suite, whereas VATS requires general anesthesia and is usually performed in the operating room. Both procedures induce a pneumothorax to create a clear view.

Thoracoscopy is used to evaluate exudative effusions and various pleural and lung lesions when noninvasive testing is inconclusive. The diagnostic accuracy for malignant and tuberculous disease of the pleura is 95%. The procedure is also used for pleurodesis in patients with recurrent malignant effusions and to break up loculations in patients with empyema.

Indications for VATS include correction of spontaneous primary pneumothorax, bullectomy and lung volume reduction surgery in emphysema, wedge resection, and, in some medical centers, lobectomy and even pneumonectomy. Less common indications are excision of benign mediastinal masses, biopsy and staging of esophageal cancer, sympathectomy for severe hyperhidrosis or causalgia, and repair of traumatic injuries to the lung, pleura, and diaphragm.

Contraindications are the same as those for thoracentesis; adhesive obliteration of the pleural space is an absolute contraindication. Biopsy is contraindicated in patients with highly vascular cancers, severe pulmonary hypertension, and severe bullous lung disease.

Though some pulmonologists perform pleuroscopy, VATS is performed by thoracic surgeons. Both procedures are similar to chest tube insertion; a trocar is inserted into an intercostal space through a skin incision, through which a thoracoscope is inserted. Additional incisions permit the use of video cameras and accessory instruments.

After thoracoscopy, a chest tube is usually required for 1 to 2 days. Complications are similar to those of thoracentesis. Postprocedural fever is common (16%); pleural tears causing air leak and/or subcutaneous emphysema are less common (2% each). Hemorrhage, lung perforation, and gas embolism are serious but rare.

THORACOTOMY

Thoracotomy is surgical opening of the chest. It is performed to evaluate and treat pulmonary problems when noninvasive procedures are nondiagnostic or unlikely to be definitive.

Contraindications are those general to surgery and include coagulopathy that cannot be corrected and instability or insufficiency of major organ systems.

Three basic approaches are used. In limited anterior or lateral thoracotomy, a 6- to 8-cm intercostal incision is made to approach anterior structures. A posterolateral thoracotomy gives access to pleurae, hilum, mediastinum, and the entire lung. When access to both lungs is desired, as in lung volume reduction surgery, a sternal splitting incision (median sternotomy) may be used.

Patients undergoing limited thoracotomy require a chest tube for 1 to 2 days and in many cases can leave the hospital in 3 to 4 days. The principal indications for thoracotomy today are lobectomy and pneumonectomy (eg, lung cancer surgery). Video-assisted thoracoscopic surgery has replaced thoracotomy for open pleural and lung biopsies.

Complications are greater than those for any other pulmonary biopsy procedure because of the risks of general anesthesia, surgical trauma, and a longer hospital stay with more postoperative discomfort. Hemorrhage, infection, pneumothorax, bronchopleural fistula, and reactions to anesthetics are the greatest hazards. Mortality for exploratory thoracotomy ranges from 0.5 to 1.8%.

TRANSTHORACIC NEEDLE BIOPSY

Transthoracic needle biopsy of thoracic or mediastinal structures uses a cutting needle to aspirate a core of tissue for histologic analysis. Transthoracic needle biopsy is performed to evaluate peripheral lung nodules or masses; hilar, mediastinal, and pleural abnormalities; and undiagnosed infiltrates or pneumonias when bronchoscopy is contraindicated or nondiagnostic. When performed with CT guidance and with a skilled cytopathologist in attendance, transthoracic needle biopsy confirms the diagnosis of malignancy with > 95% accuracy. Needle biopsy yields an accurate diagnosis in benign processes only 50 to 60% of the time.

Contraindications are similar to those of thoracentesis. Additional contraindications include mechanical ventilation, contralateral pneumonectomy, suspected vascular lesions, putrid lung abscess, hydatid cyst, pulmonary hypertension, bullous lung disease, intractable coughing, coagulopathy, and platelet count < 50,000/μL and other bleeding diatheses.

Transthoracic needle biopsy is usually performed by an interventional radiologist, often with a cytopathologist present. Under sterile conditions, local anesthesia, and imaging guidance—usually CT but sometimes ultrasound for pleural-based lesions—a biopsy needle is passed into the suspected lesion while the patient holds his breath. The lesion is aspirated with or without saline; 2 or 3 samples are collected for cytologic and bacteriologic processing. After the procedure, fluoroscopy and chest x-rays are used to rule out pneumothorax and hemorrhage. Core needle biopsies are used to obtain a cylinder of tissue suitable for histologic examination.

Complications include pneumothorax (10 to 37%), hemoptysis (10 to 25%), parenchymal hemorrhage, air embolism, and subcutaneous emphysema.

TUBE THORACOSTOMY

Tube thoracostomy is insertion of a tube into the pleural space. It is used to drain air or fluid from the chest (eg, for large or recurrent effusion refractory to thoracentesis, pneumothorax, complicated parapneumonic effusions, empyema, and hemothorax) and to perform pleurodesis or fibrinolytic adhesiolysis.

Chest tube insertion is best performed by a physician trained in the procedure. Other physicians can handle emergency situations using a needle and syringe. Tube insertion requires one or two hemostats or Kelly clamps, a silk suture, gauze dressing, and a chest tube. Recommended tube sizes are 16 to 24 French (F) for pneumothorax; 20 to 24 F for malignant pleural effusion; 28 to 36 F for bronchopleural fistula, complicated parapneumonic effusions, and empyema; and 32 to 40 F for hemothorax.

The insertion site and patient position depend on whether air or fluid is being drained. For pneumothorax, the tube is usually inserted in the 4th intercostal space and for other indications in the 5th or 6th intercostal space, in the midaxillary line with the ipsilateral arm abducted above the head.

No specific patient preparation is necessary except, in some cases, conscious sedation. Under sterile conditions, the skin, subcutaneous tissue, rib periosteum, and parietal pleura are locally anesthetized, more generously than with thoracentesis (see p. 378). Proper location is confirmed by return of air or fluid in the anesthetic syringe. A purse-string suture can be placed but not yet tied around the site while the anesthetic takes effect. A 2-cm skin incision is made, and the intercostal soft tissue down to the pleura is then bluntly dissected by advancing a clamped hemostat or Kelly clamp and opening it; the pleura is then perforated with the clamped instrument and opened in the same way. A finger can be used to widen the tract and confirm entry into the pleural space. The chest tube, with a clamp grasping the tip, is inserted through the tract and directed inferoposteriorly for effusions or apically for pneumothorax until all of the tube's holes are inside the chest wall. The purse-string suture is closed, the tube is sutured to the chest wall, and a sterile dressing with petroleum gauze to help seal the wound is placed over the site.

The tube is connected to water seal to prevent air from entering the chest through the tube and to allow drainage without suction (for effusions or empyema) or with suction (for pneumothorax). A posteroanterior and lateral chest x-ray is obtained after insertion to check the tube's position.

The tube is removed when the condition for which it was placed resolves. In the case of pneumothorax, suction is stopped and the tube is placed on water seal for several hours to ensure that the air leak has stopped and that the lung remains expanded. At the moment of removal, the patient is asked to take a deep breath and then to forcibly exhale; the tube is removed during exhalation and the site is covered with petroleum gauze, a sequence that reduces the chance of pneumothorax during removal. For effusions or hemothorax, the tube is typically removed when the drainage is < 100 mL/day.

Complications include malpositioning of the tube in the lung parenchyma, in the lobar fissure, under the diaphragm, or subcutaneously; clotting, kinking, or dislodgement of the tube, requiring replacement; re-expansion pulmonary edema; subcutaneous emphysema; infection of residual pleural fluid or recurrent effusion; pulmonary or diaphragmatic laceration; and, rarely, perforation of other structures.

48 ASTHMA

Asthma is a disease of diffuse airway inflammation caused by a variety of triggering stimuli resulting in partially or completely reversible bronchoconstriction. Symptoms and signs include dyspnea, chest tightness, and wheezing. The diagnosis is based on history, physical examination, and pulmonary function tests. Treatment involves controlling triggering factors and drug therapy, most commonly with inhaled β-agonists and inhaled corticosteroids. Prognosis is good with treatment.

Epidemiology

The prevalence of asthma appears to have increased continuously since the 1970s, and asthma now affects an estimated 4 to 7% of people worldwide. About 12 to 17 million people in the US have asthma; from 1982 to 1992, the prevalence increased from 34.7 to 49.4 per 1000. Prevalence is higher for people < 18 yr (6.1%) than for those 18 to 64 yr (4.1%) and is higher in males before puberty and in females after puberty. It is also higher in urban populations and among blacks and some Hispanic groups. Asthma mortality has also increased, and about 5000 deaths occur from asthma annually in the US. The death rate is 5 times higher for blacks than for whites. Asthma is the leading cause of hospitalization for children and is the number one chronic condition causing elementary school absenteeism. In 2002, the total cost of asthma care was $14 billion.

Etiology

Development of asthma is multifactorial and depends on interactions between multiple susceptibility genes and environmental factors.

Susceptibility genes are thought to include those for T-helper 2 (T_H2) cells and their cytokines (IL-4, -5, -9, and -13) and the recently identified *ADAM33* gene, which may stimulate airway smooth muscle and fibroblast proliferation or regulate cytokine production.

Evidence clearly implicates household (dust mite, cockroach, pet) and other environmental (pollen) allergens in disease development in older children and adults. Endotoxin infection or exposure early in life can induce tolerance and may be protective. Air pollution is not definitively linked to disease development, though it may trigger exacerbations. Diets low in vitamins C and E and in ω–3 fatty acids have been linked to asthma, as has obesity. Asthma has also been linked to perinatal factors, such as young maternal age, poor maternal nutrition, prematurity, low birthweight, and lack of breastfeeding. The role of childhood exposure to cigarette smoke is controversial, with some studies finding a contributory and some a protective effect.

Indoor exposures to nitrogen oxide and volatile organic compounds are implicated in the development of the reactive airways dysfunction syndrome (RADS), a syndrome of persistent reversible airway obstruction in people with no history of asthma (see also p. 476). Whether RADS is separate from asthma or a form of occupational asthma is controversial, but the two conditions have many similarities (eg, wheezing, dyspnea, cough) and respond to corticosteroids.

Pathophysiology and Classification

Genetic and environmental components may interact by determining the balance between T-helper 1 (T_H1) and T_H2 cell lineages. Experts believe that infants are born with a disposition toward pro-allergic and pro-inflammatory T_H2 immune responses, characterized by growth and activation of eosinophils and IgE production, but that early childhood exposure to bacterial and viral infections and endotoxins shifts the body to T_H1 responses, which suppresses T_H2 cells and induces tolerance. Trends in developed countries toward smaller families with fewer children, cleaner indoor environments, and early use of vaccinations and antibiotics may deprive children of these T_H2-suppressing, tolerance-inducing exposures and may partly explain the continuous increase in asthma prevalence in developed countries (the hygiene hypothesis).

In asthmatics, these T_H2 cells and other cell types—notably, eosinophils and mast cells, but also other $CD4^+$ subtypes and neutrophils—form an extensive inflammatory infiltrate in airway epithelium and smooth muscle, leading to desquamation, subepithelial fibrosis, and smooth muscle hypertrophy. Hypertrophy of smooth muscle narrows the airway and increases reactivity to allergens, infections, irritants, parasympathetic stimulation (which causes release of pro-inflammatory neuropeptides, such as substance P, neurokinin A, and calcitonin gene-related peptide), and other bronchoconstrictive triggers. Additional contributors to airway hyperreactivity include loss of inhibitors of bronchoconstriction (epithelium-derived relaxing factor, prostaglandin E_2) and other substances that metabolize endogenous bronchoconstrictors (endopeptidases) as a result of desquamated epithelium and mucosal edema. Mucus plugging and peripheral blood eosinophilia are additional classic findings in asthma and may be epiphenomena of airway inflammation.

Common triggers of an asthma attack include environmental and occupational allergens; infections (respiratory syncytial virus and parainfluenza infection in young children, URIs and pneumonia in older children and adults); exercise, especially in cold or dry environments; inhaled irritants (air pollution); and anxiety, anger, and excitement. Aspirin is a trigger in up to 30% of older or more severe asthmatics and is typically accompanied by nasal polyps with nasal and sinus congestion. Gastroesophageal reflux disease (GERD) has recently been recognized as a common trigger of asthma, possibly via esophageal acid-induced reflex bronchoconstriction or by microaspiration of acid. Allergic rhinitis often coexists with asthma; it is unclear whether the two are different manifestations of the same allergic process or whether rhinitis is a discrete asthma trigger.

In the presence of triggers, the pathophysiologic changes characteristic of asthma cause reversible airway obstruction and nonuniform lung ventilation. Relative perfusion exceeds relative ventilation in obstructed areas, and alveolar O_2 tensions fall and alveolar CO_2 tensions rise as a result. Most patients can compensate by hyperventilating, thereby maintaining Pa_{CO_2} below normal levels. But in severe exacerbations, diffuse bronchoconstriction causes severe gas trapping, the respiratory muscles are put at a profound mechanical disadvantage and become incapable of generating inspiratory force, and the work of breathing increases. Under these conditions, hypoxemia and hyperexertion worsen and Pa_{CO_2} rises. Respiratory and metabolic acidosis may result and, if left untreated, result in respiratory and cardiac arrest.

Asthma is classified into 4 categories—mild intermittent, mild persistent, moderate persistent, and severe persistent—according to symptoms (see TABLE 48–1). Because the course of asthma varies, a patient may move among categories. Regardless of the category, a patient may have mild, moderate, or severe exacerbations. For example, some patients with mild intermittent asthma have severe, life-threatening exacerbations separated by long periods of no or mild symptoms and normal pulmonary function. The term status asthmaticus describes severe, intense, prolonged bronchospasm that is resistant to treatment.

Asthma and COPD are sometimes easily confused; they cause similar symptoms and similar results on pulmonary function tests but differ in important biologic ways that are not always clinically apparent.

Symptoms and Signs

Patients with mild intermittent or mild persistent asthma are typically asymptomatic between exacerbations. Those with more severe disease or those with exacerbations experience dyspnea, chest tightness, audible wheezing, and coughing; coughing may be the only symptom in some patients (cough-variant asthma). Symptoms can follow a circadian rhythm and worsen during sleep, often around 4 AM. Many patients with more severe disease suffer nocturnal awakenings (nocturnal asthma).

Signs are wheezing, pulsus paradoxus (fall of systolic BP > 10 mm Hg during inspiration—see p. 573), tachypnea, tachycardia, and visible efforts to breathe (use of neck and suprasternal [accessory] muscles, upright posture, pursed lips, inability to speak). The expiratory phase of respiration is prolonged, with an inspiratory:expiratory ratio of at least 1:3. Wheezes can be present through both phases or just on expiration. A patient with severe bronchoconstriction may have no audible wheezing because of markedly limited airflow.

A patient with a severe exacerbation and impending respiratory failure typically has some combination of altered consciousness; cyanosis; pulsus paradoxus > 15 mm Hg; O_2 saturation (O_{2sat}) < 90%; $PaCO_2$ > 45 mm Hg (sea level); and hyperinflation. Rarely, pneumothorax or pneumomediastinum is seen on chest x-ray.

Symptoms and signs disappear between acute asthma attacks, although soft wheezes may be audible during forced expiration, after exercise, and at rest in some asymptomatic patients. Hyperinflation of the lungs may alter the chest wall in patients with long-standing uncontrolled asthma, producing a barrel-shaped thorax.

All symptoms and signs are nonspecific, are reversible with timely treatment, and typically are brought on by exposure to one or more triggers.

Diagnosis

Diagnosis is based on history and physical examination and is confirmed with pulmonary function tests. Diagnosis of underlying causes and the exclusion of diseases that cause wheezing are also important.

Pulmonary function tests: Patients suspected of having asthma should undergo pulmonary function testing to confirm and quantify the severity and reversibility of airway obstruction. Pulmonary function data quality is effort-dependent and requires patient education before the test. If it is safe to do so, bronchodilators should be stopped before the test: 6 h for short-acting β-agonists, such as albuterol; 8 h for ipratropium; 12 to 36 h for theophylline; 24 h for long-acting β-agonists, such as salmeterol and formoterol; and 48 h for tiotropium.

Spirometry (see Ch. 46 on p. 364) should be obtained before and after inhalation of a short-acting bronchodilator. Signs of airway obstruction before bronchodilator inhalation include reduced forced expiratory volume in the first second (FEV_1) and a reduced ratio of FEV_1 to forced vital capacity (FEV_1/FVC). The FVC may also be decreased. Lung volume measurements may show an increase in the residual volume and/or the functional residual capacity because of air trapping. An improvement in FEV_1 of > 12% or > 0.2 L in response to bronchodilator treatment confirms reversible airway obstruction, although absence of this finding should not preclude a therapeutic trial of bronchodilators. Spirometry should be repeated at least yearly in known asthmatics to monitor disease progression.

Flow-volume loops should also be reviewed to diagnose or exclude vocal cord dysfunction, a common cause of upper airway obstruction that mimics asthma.

Provocative testing, in which inhaled methacholine (or alternatives, such as inhaled histamine, adenosine, bradykinin, or exercise testing) is used to provoke bronchoconstriction, is indicated for suspected asthmatics with normal findings on spirometry

TABLE 48–1. CLASSIFICATION AND MANAGEMENT OF CHRONIC ASTHMA

CATEGORY	SYMPTOMS*	PULMONARY FUNCTION*	TREATMENT
Mild intermittent	Daytime symptoms ≤ 2 days/wk or no symptoms and normal PEF between exacerbations Nighttime symptoms ≤ 2 times/mo Exacerbations brief (from a few hours to a few days); intensity may vary	FEV_1 ≥ 80% predicted PEF ≥ 80% personal best PEF variability < 20%	***All patients:*** No daily drugs required; rescue β-agonist as needed for symptoms; systemic corticosteroids if needed for exacerbations
Mild persistent	Daytime symptoms > 2 times/wk but not daily Nighttime symptoms > 2 times/mo Exacerbations that sometimes limit activity	FEV_1 ≥ 80% predicted PEF ≥ 80% personal best PEF variability 20–30%	***Children ≤ 5 yr:*** Preferred: Low-dose ICS via nebulizer, MDI with holding chamber, or DPI Alternative: Mast cell stabilizers or leukotriene receptor antagonist ***Children > 5 yr and adults:*** Preferred: Low-dose ICS Alternative: Mast cell stabilizers, leukotriene modifiers (≥ 12 yr), or theophylline AND Rescue β-agonist
Moderate persistent	Daily daytime symptoms Nighttime symptoms > 1 time/wk Daily use of inhaled short-acting β-agonist Exacerbations that limit activity Exacerbations ≥ 2 times/wk; may last days	FEV_1 60–80% predicted PEF 60–80% personal best PEF variability > 30%	***Children ≤ 5 yr:*** Preferred: Low-to-medium-dose ICS plus long-acting β-agonist, or medium-dose ICS Alternatives: Low-dose ICS plus either leukotriene receptor antagonist or theophylline ***If needed (eg, for patients with recurring severe exacerbations):*** Preferred: Medium-dose ICS plus long-acting β-agonist Alternatives: Medium-dose ICS plus either leukotriene receptor antagonist or theophylline ***Children > 5 yr and adults:*** Preferred: Low-to-medium-dose ICS plus long-acting β-agonist

TABLE 48–1. CLASSIFICATION AND MANAGEMENT OF CHRONIC ASTHMA—Continued

CATEGORY	SYMPTOMS*	PULMONARY FUNCTION*	TREATMENT
			Alternatives: Low-to-medium-dose ICS plus either leukotriene modifier or theophylline; increase ICS within medium-dose range AND Rescue β-agonist ***If needed (eg, for patients with recurring severe exacerbations):*** Preferred: Increase ICS within medium-dose range and add long-acting β-agonist Alternatives: Increase ICS within medium-dose range and add either leukotriene modifier or theophylline
Severe persistent	Continual symptoms Frequent nighttime symptoms Limited physical activity Frequent exacerbations	$FEV_1 \leq 60\%$ predicted PEF ≤ 60% personal best PEF variability > 30%	***All patients:*** Preferred: High-dose ICS plus long-acting β-agonist and, if needed, corticosteroid tablets or syrup (1–2 mg/kg/day, not to exceed 60 mg/day)
Symptom relief	All patients: Short-acting β-agonist, 2–4 puffs		

PEF = peak expiratory flow; FEV_1 = forced expiratory volume in 1 sec; ICS = inhaled corticosteroid; MDI = metered dose inhaler; DPI = dry-powder inhaler.

*Patient is assigned to most severe category in which any feature occurs; pulmonary function typically not available for children < 5 yr.

Modified from the National Asthma Education and Prevention Program, Expert Panel Report II, National Heart, Lung, & Blood Institute, 1997.

and flow-volume testing, suspected cough-variant asthma and no contraindications. Contraindications include FEV_1 < 1 L or < 50%, recent MI or stroke, and severe hypertension (systolic BP > 200 mm Hg; diastolic BP > 100 mm Hg). A decline in FEV_1 of > 20% supports the diagnosis of asthma. However, FEV_1 may decline in response to these drugs in other diseases, such as COPD.

Other tests: Other tests may be helpful in some circumstances.

Diffusing capacity for carbon monoxide (DL_{CO}) testing can help distinguish asthma from COPD. Values are normal or elevated in asthma and usually reduced in COPD, particularly in the setting of emphysema.

A chest x-ray may help exclude underlying causes of asthma or alternative diagnoses, such as heart failure or pneumonia. The chest x-ray in asthma is usually normal but may show hyperinflation or segmental atelectasis, a sign of mucous plugging. Infiltrates, especially those that come and go and that are associated with findings of central bronchiectasis, suggest allergic bronchopulmonary aspergillosis (see p. 398).

Allergy testing is indicated for all children whose history suggests allergic triggers (because all children are potentially eligible for immunotherapy). It should be considered for adults whose history indicates relief of symptoms with allergen avoidance and for those in whom a trial of therapeutic anti-IgE antibody therapy (see p. 393) is being considered. Skin testing and measurement of allergen-specific IgE via radioallergosorbent testing (RAST) can identify specific allergic triggers (see pp. 1354–1355). Elevated blood eosinophils (>400 cells/μL) and nonspecific IgE (>150 IU) are suggestive but not diagnostic of allergic asthma because they can be elevated in a variety of other conditions.

Sputum evaluation for eosinophils is not commonly practiced; finding large numbers of eosinophils is suggestive of asthma but is neither sensitive nor specific.

Peak expiratory flow (PEF) measurements with inexpensive handheld flow meters are recommended for home monitoring of disease severity and for guiding therapy.

Evaluation of exacerbations: Known asthmatics with an acute exacerbation should have pulse oximetry and either PEF or FEV_1 measurement. All 3 measures help establish the severity of an exacerbation and document treatment response. PEF values are interpreted in light of the patient's personal best, which may vary widely among patients who are equally well controlled. A 15 to 20% reduction from this baseline indicates a significant exacerbation. When baseline values are not known, the percent predicted value gives a general idea of airflow limitation but not the individual patient's degree of worsening.

Chest x-ray is not necessary for most exacerbations but should be obtained in patients with symptoms suggestive of pneumonia or pneumothorax.

ABG measurements should be obtained in patients with marked respiratory distress or signs and symptoms of impending respiratory failure.

Prognosis

Asthma resolves in most children with the disease, but for as many as one in four, wheezing persists into adulthood or relapse occurs in later years. Female sex, smoking, earlier age of onset, sensitization to household dust mites, and airway hyperresponsiveness are risk factors for persistence and relapse.

About 5000 deaths/yr are attributable to asthma in the US, most of which are preventable with treatment. Thus, the prognosis is good with adequate access and adherence to treatment. Risk factors for death include increasing requirements for oral corticosteroids before hospitalization, previous hospitalization for acute exacerbations, and lower peak flows at presentation. Several studies show that use of inhaled corticosteroids decreases hospital admission and mortality rates.

Over time, the airways in some asthmatic patients undergo permanent structural changes (remodeling) that prevent return to normal lung functioning. Early aggressive use of anti-inflammatory drugs may help prevent this remodeling.

Treatment

Treatment of asthma—both chronic disease and acute exacerbations—involves control of triggering factors, drug treatment tailored to severity of disease, monitoring of response to treatment and disease progression, and patient education to maximize self-management of disease. Objectives are to prevent exacerbations and chronic symptoms, including nocturnal awakenings; minimize the need for emergency department visits or hospitalizations; maintain baseline (normal) pulmonary function and activity levels; and avoid adverse treatment effects.

Control of triggering factors: Triggering factors may in some patients be controlled with use of synthetic fiber pillows and impermeable mattress covers and frequent washing of bedsheets, pillowcases, and blankets in hot water. Upholstered furniture, soft toys, carpets, and pets should be removed (dust mites, animal dander), and dehumidifiers should be used in basements and in other poorly aerated, damp rooms (molds). Steam treatment of homes diminishes dust mite allergens. The fact that control of triggering factors is more difficult in urban environments does not diminish the importance of these measures; elimination of cockroach exposure by way of house cleaning and extermination is especially important. High-efficiency particulate air (HEPA) vacuums and filters may relieve symptoms, but their effects on pulmonary function and on the need for drugs are unproven. Sulfite-sensitive patients should avoid red wine. Nonallergenic triggers, such as cigarette smoke, strong odors, irritant fumes, cold temperatures, high humidity, and exercise, should also be avoided or controlled when possible. Patients with aspirin-induced asthma can use acetaminophen, choline magnesium salicylate, or cyclooxygenase (COX)-2 inhibitors in place of NSAIDs. Asthma is a relative contraindication to the use of nonselective β-blockers, including topical formulations, but cardioselective drugs (eg metoprolol, atenolol) probably have no adverse effects.

Drug therapy: Major drug classes commonly used in the treatment of chronic asthma and asthma exacerbations include bronchodilators (β-agonists, anticholinergics), corticosteroids, mast cell stabilizers, leukotriene modifiers, and methylxanthines (see TABLE 48–2). Drugs in these classes are inhaled or taken orally; inhaled drugs come in aerosolized and powdered forms. Use of aerosolized forms with a spacer or holding chamber facilitates deposition of the drug in the airways rather than the pharynx; patients should be advised to wash and dry their spacers after each use to prevent bacterial contamination. In addition, use of aerosolized forms requires coordination between actuation of the inhaler (drug delivery) and inhalation; powdered forms reduce the need for coordination, because drug is delivered only when the patient inhales. In addition, powdered forms reduce the release of fluorocarbon propellants into the environment.

β-Agonists (β-adrenergics) relax bronchial smooth muscle, decrease mast cell degranulation and histamine release, inhibit microvascular leakage into the airways, and increase mucociliary clearance. β-Agonists come in short- and long-acting preparations (see TABLE 48–2). Short-acting β-agonists (eg, albuterol) inhaled 2 to 8 puffs as needed are the drug of choice for relieving acute bronchoconstriction and preventing exercise-induced bronchoconstriction. They take effect within minutes and are active for up to 6 to 8 h, depending on the drug. Long-acting drugs, inhaled at bedtime or bid and active for up to 12 h, are used for moderate and severe asthma as well as for mild asthma that causes nocturnal awakening. Long-acting β-agonists also interact synergistically with inhaled corticosteroids and permit lower dosing of corticosteroids. Oral β-agonists have more systemic effects and generally should be avoided. Tachycardia and tremor are the most common acute adverse effects of inhaled β-agonists and are dose-related. Hypokalemia occurs uncommonly and to only a mild extent. The safety of regular long-term use of β-agonists is controversial; regular, possibly excessive use is associated with increased mortality, but it is unclear whether this is an adverse effect or if regular use reflects suboptimal treatment of the disease with other drugs. Daily use of β-agonists, increased dosing or diminishing effects, or use of one or more canisters a month suggests inadequate control of disease and the need to begin or intensify other therapies. Use of levalbuterol (a solution containing the R-isomer of albuterol) theoretically minimizes adverse effects, but its long-term efficacy and safety is unproven.

Anticholinergics relax bronchial smooth muscle through competitive inhibition of muscarinic (M_3) cholinergic receptors. Ipratropium has minimal effect when used alone for asthma but may have an additive effect when combined with short-acting β-agonists. Adverse effects include pupillary dilation, blurred vision, and dry mouth. Tiotropium is a 24-h inhaled anticholinergic that has not been adequately evaluated for asthma use.

Corticosteroids inhibit airway inflammation, reverse β-receptor down-regulation, block leukotriene synthesis, and inhibit cytokine production and adhesion protein activation. They block the late response (but not the early response) to inhaled allergens. Routes of administration include oral, IV, and inhaled. In acute asthma exacerbation, early use of systemic corticosteroids often aborts the exacerbation, decreases the need for hospitalization, prevents relapse, and speeds recovery. Oral and IV routes are equally effective. Inhaled corticosteroids have no role in acute exacerbation but are indicated for long-term suppression, control, and reversal of inflammation and symptoms. They substantially reduce the need for maintenance oral corticosteroid therapy and are considered disease-modifying drugs because they slow or halt the deterioration of pulmonary function characteristic of untreated asthma. Adverse local effects of inhaled corticosteroids include dysphonia and oral candidiasis, which can be prevented or minimized by having the patient use a spacer and/or gargle with water after corticosteroid inhalation. Systemic effects are all dose-related, can occur with oral or inhaled forms, and occur mainly with inhaled doses > 800 μg/day. They include suppression of the adrenal-pituitary axis, osteoporosis, cataracts, skin atrophy, hyperphagia, and easy bruisability. Whether inhaled corticosteroids suppress growth in children is controversial: Most children reach their predicted adult height. Quiescent TB may be reactivated by systemic corticosteroid use.

Text continues on page 392.

TABLE 48–2. DRUG TREATMENT OF CHRONIC ASTHMA

DRUG	FORM	DOSAGE Child	DOSAGE Adult	COMMENTS
Short-acting β-agonists				
Albuterol	*MDI:* 90 µg/puff	2 puffs tid to qid and 5 min before exercise prn	2 puffs tid to qid and 5 min before exercise prn	Used mainly as rescue drug; not recommended for maintenance treatment. Regular use indicates diminishing asthma control and need for additional drug. Double MDI/DPI dose for mild and nebulized dose for severe exacerbations. MDI/DPI as effective as nebulized therapy if patient can coordinate inhalation maneuver using spacer/holding chamber. Nebulized albuterol can be mixed with other nebulizer solutions
	DPI: 200 µg/capsule	1 capsule q 4–6 h and before exercise	1–2 capsules q 4–6 h and before exercise	
	Nebulized solution: 2.5 and 5 mg/mL 0.63 and 1.25 mg/3 mL	0.05 mg/kg (minimum 1.25 mg, maximum 2.5 mg) in 3 mL saline q 4–6 h	1.25–5 mg in 3 mL saline q 4–8 h	
Bitolterol	*MDI:* 370 µg/puff *Nebulized solution:* 2 mg/mL (0.2%)	Not established	0.5–3.5 mg (0.25–1 mL) in 2–3 mL saline q 4–8 h	Cannot mix with other nebulizer solutions
Levalbuterol	*Nebulized solution:* 0.31, 0.63, and 1.25 mg/3 mL	0.025 mg/kg (minimum 0.63 mg, maximum 1.25 mg) q 4–8 h	0.63–2.5 mg q 4–8 h	R-isomer of albuterol. 0.63 mg is equivalent to 1.25 mg racemic albuterol. May have fewer adverse effects
Pirbuterol	*MDI:* 200 µg/puff	Same as albuterol	Same as albuterol	
Long-acting β-agonists				
Formoterol	*DPI:* 12 µg/capsule	1 capsule q 12 h	1 capsule q 12 h	May be used for acute symptom relief in an exacerbation. Efficacy and safety unstudied in children < 5 yr. Capsules for single use; patients should be educated to avoid swallowing

TABLE 48–2. DRUG TREATMENT OF CHRONIC ASTHMA—Continued

DRUG	FORM	DOSAGE Child	DOSAGE Adult	COMMENTS
Salmeterol	*MDI:* 21 μg/ puff *DPI:* 50 μg/ discus	1–2 puffs q 12 h 1 actuation q 12 h	2 puffs q 12 h 1 actuation q 12 h	Duration of action 12 h. One dose nightly is helpful for nocturnal asthma. Not to be used for acute symptom relief in an exacerbation. DPI can be used in children > 4 yr, MDI in patients > 12 yr
Anticholinergics				
Ipratropium	*MDI:* 18 μg/ puff *Nebulized solution:* 0.25 mg/μL (0.025%)	1–2 puffs q 6 h 0.25–0.5 mg q 6 h	2–3 puffs q 6 h 0.25 mg q 6 h	May mix in same nebulizer as albuterol. Should not be used as first-line therapy, and no clear benefits when added to β-agonists in long-term maintenance therapy
Corticosteroids (inhaled)				
Beclomethasone	*MDI CFC:* 42 or 84 μg/ puff	Low: 84–336 μg Medium: 336–672 μg High: > 672 μg	Low: 168–504 μg Medium: 504–840 μg High: > 840 μg	Doses depend on severity and range from 1–2 puffs to whatever dose is needed to control disease. All may have systemic effects when used long term (see text); high-dose threshold is that above which hypothalamic-pituitary-adrenal suppression is produced
	MDI HFA: 40 or 80 μg/ puff	Low: 80–160 μg Medium: 160–320 μg High: > 320 μg	Low: 80–240 μg Medium: 240–480 μg High: > 480 μg	
Budesonide	*DPI:* 200 μg/ inhalation	Low: 200–400 μg Medium: 400–800 μg High: < 800 μg	Low: 200–600 μg Medium: 600–1200 μg High: > 1200 μg	
	Nebulized solution: 0.5 mg in suspension	Low: 0.5 mg Medium: 1.0 mg High: 2.0 mg	Not indicated for adults	

Table continues on the following page.

TABLE 48–2. DRUG TREATMENT OF CHRONIC ASTHMA—Continued

DRUG	FORM	DOSAGE: Child	DOSAGE: Adult	COMMENTS
Flunisolide	*MDI:* 250 μg/ puff	Low: 500–750 μg Medium: 750–1250 μg High: > 1250 μg	Low: 500–1000 μg Medium: 1000–2000 μg High: > 2000 μg	
Fluticasone	*MDI:* 44, 100, or 220 μg/puff	Low: 88–176 μg Medium: 176–440 μg High: > 440 μg	Low: 88–264 μg Medium: 264–660 μg High: < 660 μg	
	DPI: 50, 100, or 250 μg/ inhalation	Low: 100–200 μg Medium: 200–400 μg High: > 400 μg	Low: 100–300 μg Medium: 300–600 μg High: > 600 μg	
Triamcinolone	*MDI:* 100 μg/ puff	Low: 400–800 μg Medium: 800–1200 μg High: > 1200 μg	Low: 400–1000 μg Medium: 1000–1200 μg High: > 2000 μg	
Systemic corticosteroids				
Methylprednisolone	*Tablets:* 2, 4, 8, 32 mg	Maintenance: 0.25–2 mg/kg/day Short-course burst: 1–2 mg/kg/day, max 60 mg/ day for 3 to 10 days	Maintenance: 7.5–60 mg/day Short-course burst: 40–60 mg/day as single or 2 divided doses for 3–10 days	Maintenance doses should be given in a single dose in the morning or every other day as needed for control. Some evidence suggests clinical effectiveness increases with no increase in adrenal suppression when dose given at 3 PM. Short-course burst doses are effective for establishing control when initiating therapy or during a period of gradual deterioration. The burst should be continued until the patient achieves 80% PEF personal best or symptoms resolve; may require longer than 3–10 days of therapy
Prednisolone	*Tablets:* 5 mg *Solution:* 5 or 15 mg/5 mL			
Prednisone	*Tablets:* 1, 2.5, 5, 10, 20, 50 mg *Solution:* 5 mg/mL, 5 mg/5mL			

TABLE 48–2. DRUG TREATMENT OF CHRONIC ASTHMA—Continued

DRUG	FORM	DOSAGE Child	DOSAGE Adult	COMMENTS
Combination drugs				
Ipratropium and albuterol	*MDI:* 18 μg/puff ipratropium and 90 μg/puff albuterol	1–2 puffs q 8 h	2–3 puffs q 6 h	Ipratropium prolongs bronchodilator effect of albuterol
	Nebulized solution: 0.5 mg ipratropium and 2.5 mg albuterol in a 3-mL vial	1.5–3 mL q 8 h	3 mL q 4–6 h	
Fluticasone and salmeterol	*DPI:* 100, 250, or 500 μg fluticasone and 50 μg salmeterol	1 inhalation bid; dose depends on severity of asthma	1 inhalation bid; dose depends on severity of asthma	100/50 dose indicated for patients not controlled on low-to-medium dose inhaled corticosteroids 250/50 dose indicated for patients not controlled on medium-to-high dose inhaled corticosteroids
Mast cell stabilizers				
Cromolyn	*MDI:* 1 mg/puff	1–2 puffs tid to qid	2–4 puffs tid to qid	Should be taken before exercise or allergen exposure; one dose provides effective anaphylaxis for 1–2 h
	Nebulized solution: 20 mg/ampule	1 ampule tid to qid	1 ampule tid to qid	
Nedocromil	*MDI:* 1.75 mg/puff	1–2 puffs bid to qid	2–4 puffs bid to qid	Nedocromil has an unpleasant taste
Leukotriene modifiers				
Montelukast	*Tablet:* 4, 5, or 10 mg	4 mg at bedtime (2–5 yr); 5 mg at bedtime (6–14 yr); 10 mg at bedtime (> 14 yr)	10 mg at bedtime	Leukotriene receptor antagonist; competitive inhibitor of leukotriene D_4 and E_4. Should not be used in children < 2 yr
Zafirlukast	*Tablet:* 10 or 20 mg	10 mg bid (7–11 yr); 20 mg bid (≥ 12 yr)	20 mg bid	Leukotriene receptor antagonist. Competitive inhibitor of LTD_4 and LTE_4. Must be taken at 1 h before or 2 h after meals. Should not be used in children < 7 yr

Table continues on the following page.

TABLE 48–2. DRUG TREATMENT OF CHRONIC ASTHMA—Continued

DRUG	FORM	DOSAGE Child	DOSAGE Adult	COMMENTS
Zileuton	*Tablet:* 300 or 600 mg	600 mg qid (> 12 yr)	600 mg qid	5-Lipoxygenase inhibitor. Dosing may limit adherence. May cause liver enzyme elevations and inhibit metabolism of drugs processed by CYP3A4, including theophylline. Should not be used in children < 12 yr
Methylxanthines				
Theophylline	*Tablet:* 100, 200, 300, 400, or 600 mg	Initial dose 10 mg/kg/day up to 300 mg, then adjust dose to achieve serum concentration of 5–15 μg/mL at steady state Maximum usually 800 mg/day	Initial dose 10 mg/kg/day, then adjust dose to achieve serum concentration of 5–15 μg/mL at steady state Maximum (< 1 yr): 0.2 (age in wk) + 5 = mg/kg/day Maximum (≥ 1 yr): 16 mg/kg/day	Wide interpatient variability in metabolic clearance, drug interactions, potential for adverse effects mandate routine serum level monitoring. Availability of safer alternatives has led to declining use of this drug

MDI = metered dose inhaler; DPI = dry-powder inhaler; CFC = chlorofluorocarbon; HFA = hydrofluroalkane; PEF = peak expiratory flow.

Adapted from NAEPP Expert Panel Report, Guidelines for the Diagnosis and Management of Asthma.

Mast cell stabilizers inhibit histamine release from mast cells, reduce airway hyperresponsiveness, and block the early and late responses to allergens. They are given by inhalation prophylactically to patients with exercise- and allergen-induced asthma; they are ineffective once symptoms have occurred. They are the safest of all antiasthmatic drugs but the least effective.

Leukotriene modifiers are taken orally and can be used for long-term control and prevention of symptoms in patients with mild persistent to severe persistent asthma. The main adverse effect is liver enzyme elevation; extremely rarely, patients develop a clinical syndrome resembling Churg-Strauss syndrome.

Methylxanthines relax bronchial smooth muscle (probably by nonselectively inhibiting phosphodiesterase) and may improve myocardial and diaphragmatic contractility through unknown mechanisms. Methylxanthines appear to inhibit intracellular release of Ca, decrease microvascular leakage into the airway mucosa, and inhibit the late response to allergens. They decrease the infiltration of eosinophils into bronchial mucosa and of T lymphocytes into epithelium. Methylxanthines are used for long-term control as an adjunct to β-agonists; extended-release theophylline helps manage nocturnal asthma. The drug is falling into disuse because of its many adverse effects and interactions compared with other drugs. Adverse effects include headache, vomiting, cardiac arrhythmias, and seizures. Methylxanthines have a narrow therapeutic index; multiple drugs (any metabolized by the cytochrome P450 pathway, eg, macrolide antibiotics) and conditions (eg, fever, liver disease, heart failure) alter methylxanthine metabolism and elimination. Serum theophylline levels should be monitored periodically and maintained between 5 and 15 μg/mL (28 and 83 μmol/L).

Other drugs are used uncommonly in specific circumstances. Immunotherapy may be indicated when symptoms are triggered by allergy, as suggested by history and confirmed by allergy testing. Immunotherapy is more successful in children than adults. If symptoms are not significantly relieved by 24 mo, then therapy is stopped. If symptoms are relieved, therapy should continue for ≥ 3 yr, although the optimum duration is unknown. Corticosteroid-sparing drugs are occasionally prescribed to reduce dependence on high-dose oral corticosteroids. All carry significant toxicities. Low-dose methotrexate (5 to 15 mg/wk) can lead to modest improvements in FEV_1 and modest decreases (3.3 mg/day) in daily oral corticosteroid use. Gold and cyclosporine are also modestly effective, but toxicity and need for monitoring limit their use. Omalizumab is an anti-IgE antibody developed for use in severely allergic asthmatic patients with elevated IgE levels. It decreases oral corticosteroid requirements and relieves symptoms. Dose is determined by a dosing chart based on the patient's weight and IgE levels; the drug is administered sc every 2 wk. Other therapies for management of chronic asthma include nebulized lidocaine, nebulized heparin, colchicine, and high-dose IV immune globulin. Limited evidence supports the use of these therapies, and their benefits are unproven, so none can yet be recommended for clinical use.

Monitoring response to treatment: Peak expiratory flow (PEF) testing, a measure of airflow and airway obstruction, helps establish the severity of an asthma exacerbation by documenting response to treatments and monitoring trends in disease severity in real-world settings through patient-kept diaries. Home PEF monitoring is especially useful for charting disease progression and responses to treatment in patients with moderate to severe persistent asthma. When asthma is quiescent, one PEF measurement in the morning suffices. If the patient's PEF falls below 80% of his personal best, then twice-a-day monitoring to assess circadian variation is useful. Circadian variation of > 20% indicates airway instability and the need to re-evaluate the therapeutic regimen.

Patient education: The importance of patient education cannot be overemphasized. Patients do better the more they know about asthma—what triggers an attack, what drug to use when, proper inhaler technique, how to use a spacer with a metered-dose inhaler (MDI), and the importance of early use of corticosteroids in exacerbations. Every patient should have a written action plan for day-to-day management, especially for management of acute attacks, that is based on the patient's best personal peak flow rather than on predicted normal value. Such a plan leads to much better asthma control, largely attributable to improved adherence to therapies.

Treatment of acute exacerbation: The goal of asthma exacerbation treatment is to relieve symptoms and return patients to their personal best PEF. Patients should be instructed to self-administer inhaled albuterol or a similar short-acting β-agonist for an acute exacerbation and measure PEF if possible. Patients who feel better after 2 to 4 puffs from an MDI administered up to 3 times up to 20 min apart and who have a PEF > 80% of baseline can manage the acute exacerbation at home. Patients who do not respond, have severe symptoms, or have a PEF < 80% should follow a treatment management program outlined by the physician or should go to the emergency department for drug intervention (see TABLE 48–3 for specific dosing information).

Inhaled bronchodilators (β-agonists and anticholinergics) are the mainstay of asthma treatment in the emergency department. In adults and older children, albuterol given by an MDI and spacer is as effective as that given by nebulizer. Nebulized treatment is preferred for younger children because of difficulties coordinating MDIs and spacers; recent evidence suggests that bronchodilator response improves when the nebulizer is powered with helium-O_2 (heliox) rather than with O_2. Subcutaneous epinephrine 1:1000 solution or terbutaline is an alternative for

TABLE 48–3. DRUG TREATMENT OF ASTHMA EXACERBATIONS

DRUG	FORM	DOSAGE Child	DOSAGE Adult	COMMENTS
Systemic β-agonists				
Epinephrine	*Solution:* 1 mg/mL (1:1000)	0.01 mg/kg up to 0.5 mg sc q 20 min for 3 doses	0.3–0.5 mg sc q 20 min for 3 doses	Subcutaneous administration is no more effective than inhalation and is associated with more adverse effects. Use in adults controversial and may be contraindicated
Terbutaline	*Solution:* 1 mg/mL	0.01 mg/kg q 20 min for 3 doses, then q 2–6 h sc prn	0.25 mg q 20 min sc for 3 doses	
Short-acting β-agonists				
Albuterol	*MDI*: 90 μg/puff	4–8 puffs q 20 min for 3 doses, then q 1–4 h prn	4–8 puffs q 20 min for up to 4 h, then q 1–4 h prn	MDI as effective as nebulized solution if patient can coordinate inhalation maneuver using spacer/holding chamber
	Nebulized solution: 5 mg/mL and 0.63, 1.25, and 2.5 mg/3 mL	0.15 mg/kg (minimum 2.5 mg) q 20 min for 3 doses, then 0.15–0.3 mg/kg up to 10 mg q 1–4 h prn, or 0.5 mg/kg/h continuous nebulization	2.5–5 mg q 20 min for 3 doses, then 2.5–10 mg q 1–4 h prn, or 10–15 mg/h continuous nebulization	
Bitolterol	*MDI*: 370 μg/puff	Same as albuterol	Same as albuterol	Has not been studied in severe asthma exacerbations. Cannot mix with other nebulizer solutions. Thought to be half as potent as albuterol on a mg basis
	Nebulized solution: 2 mg/mL (0.2%)	Same as albuterol	Same as albuterol	
Levalbuterol	*Nebulized solution*: 0.63 and 1.25 mg/3 mL	0.075 mg/kg (minimum 1.25 mg) q 20 min for 3 doses, then 0.075–0.15 mg/kg up to 5 mg q 1–4 h prn, or 0.25 mg/kg/h continuous nebulization	1.25–2 mg q 20 min for 3 doses, then 1.25–5 mg q 1–4 h prn, or 5–7.5 mg/h continuous nebulization	R-isomer of albuterol. 0.63 mg is equivalent to 1.25 mg racemic albuterol. May have fewer adverse effects
Pirbuterol	*MDI*: 200 μg/puff	Same as albuterol	Same as albuterol	Thought to be half as potent as albuterol on a per-mg basis

TABLE 48–3. DRUG TREATMENT OF ASTHMA EXACERBATIONS—Continued

DRUG	FORM	DOSAGE Child	DOSAGE Adult	COMMENTS
Anticholinergics				
Ipratroprium	*MDI:* 18 μg/puff	4–8 puffs prn	4–8 puffs prn	Should be added to β-agonists and not used as first-line therapy. May be mixed in same nebulizer as albuterol. Dose delivered from MDI is low and has not been studied in exacerbations
	Nebulized solution: 0.25 mg/mL (0.025%)	0.25 mg q 20 min for 3 doses, then q 2–4 h prn	0.5 mg q 30 min for 3 doses, then q 2–4 h prn	
Combination drugs				
Ipratroprium and albuterol	*MDI:* 18 μg/puff ipratroprium and 90 μg/puff albuterol	4–8 puffs prn	4–8 puffs prn	Ipratropium prolongs bronchodilator effect of albuterol
	Nebulized solution: 0.5 mg ipratroprium and 2.5 mg albuterol in a 3 mL vial	1.5 mL q 20 min for 3 doses, then q 2–4 h	3 mL q 30 m for 3 doses, then q 2–4 h prn	
Systemic corticosteroids				
Methylprednisolone	*Tablets:* 2, 4, 8, 32 mg	*Inpatient:* 1 mg/kg q 6 h for 48 h, then 0.5–1.0 mg/kg bid (maximum, 60 mg/day) until PEF = 70% of predicted or personal best *Outpatient burst:* 0.5–1.0 mg/kg bid, maximum 60 mg/day for 3–10 days	*Inpatient:* 40–60 mg q 6 h or q 8 h for 48 h, then 60–80 mg/day until PEF reaches 70% of predicted or personal best *Outpatient burst:* 40 to 60 mg in single or 2 divided doses for 3–10 days	No advantage to IV over oral administration if GI function is normal. No advantage to higher doses in severe exacerbations. Usual regimen is to continue frequent multiple daily dose until the patient achieves an FEV_1 or PEF of 50% of predicted or personal best and then lower the dose to bid, usually within 48 h. Therapy following a hospitalization or ED visit may last 3–10 days. No need to taper does if patients are also given inhaled corticosteroids
Prednisolone	*Tablets:* 5 mg *Solution:* 5 or 15 mg/5 mL			
Prednisone	*Tablets:* 1, 2.5, 5, 10, 20, 50 mg *Solution:* 5 mg/mL, 5 mg/5mL			

MDI = metered dose inhaler; PEF = peak expiratory flow; ED = emergency department.
Adapted from NAEPP Expert Panel Report, Guidelines for the Diagnosis and Management of Asthma.

children. Terbutaline may be preferable to epinephrine because of its lesser cardiovascular effect and longer duration of action, but it is no longer produced in large quantities and is expensive. Subcutaneous administration of β-agonists is theoretically problematic for adults because of adverse cardiostimulatory effects. However, clinically demonstrable ill effects are few, and subcutaneous administration may benefit patients unresponsive to maximal inhaled therapy or those unable to receive effective nebulized treatment (eg, those who cough excessively, have poor ventilation, or are uncooperative). Nebulized ipratropium can be co-administered with nebulized albuterol for patients who do not respond optimally to albuterol alone; some evidence favors simultaneous high-dose β-agonist and ipratropium as first-line treatment, but no data favor continuous β-agonist nebulization over intermittent administration. Theophylline has very little role in treatment.

Systemic corticosteroids (prednisone, prednisolone, methylprednisolone) should be given for all but the mildest acute exacerbation; they are unnecessary for patients whose PEF normalizes after 1 or 2 bronchodilator doses. IV and oral routes of administration are equally effective. IV methylprednisolone can be given if an IV line is already in place and can be switched to oral dosing whenever necessary or convenient. Tapering usually starts after 7 to 10 days and should last 2 to 3 wk.

Antibiotics are indicated only when history, examination, or chest x-ray suggests underlying bacterial infection; most infections underlying asthma exacerbations are viral in origin, but mycoplasma and chlamydia have been demonstrated in recent study populations.

O_2 is indicated when patients with asthma exacerbation have an O_{2sat} < 90% as measured by pulse oximetry or ABG measurements; O_2 should be given by nasal cannula or face mask at a flow rate or concentration sufficient to correct hypoxemia.

Reassurance is the best approach when anxiety is the cause of asthma exacerbation. Anxiolytics and morphine are relatively contraindicated because they are associated with increased mortality and the need for mechanical ventilation.

Hospitalization generally is required if patients have not returned to their baseline within 4 h. Criteria for hospitalization vary, but definite indications are failure to improve, worsening fatigue, relapse after repeated β-agonist therapy, and significant decrease in Pa_{O_2} (< 50 mm Hg) or increase in Pa_{CO_2} (> 40 mm Hg), indicating progression to respiratory failure.

Patients who continue to deteriorate despite aggressive treatment are candidates for noninvasive positive pressure ventilation or, for severely affected patients and those failing to respond, endotracheal intubation and mechanical ventilation (see p. 544). Patients requiring intubation may benefit from sedation, but paralytics should be avoided because of possible interactions with corticosteroids that can cause prolonged neuromuscular weakness.

Generally, volume-cycled ventilation in assist-control mode is used because it provides constant alveolar ventilation when airway resistance is high and changing. The ventilator should be set to a rate of 8 to 14 breaths/min with a rapid inspiratory flow rate (> 60 to 80 L/min) to prolong exhalation and to minimize auto-PEEP (positive end-expiratory pressure).

Initial tidal volumes can be set to 10 to 12 mL/kg. High peak airway pressures can generally be ignored, because they result from high airway resistance and inspiratory flow rates and do not reflect the degree of lung distention produced by alveolar pressure. However, if plateau pressures exceed 30 to 35 cm H_2O, then tidal volume should be reduced to between 5 and 7 mL/kg to limit the risk of pneumothorax. An exception is when decreased compliance of the chest wall (eg, obesity) or abdomen (eg, ascites) may substantially contribute to the elevated pressures. When reduced tidal volumes are necessary, a moderate degree of hypercapnia is acceptable, but if arterial pH falls below 7.10, a slow sodium bicarbonate infusion is indicated to maintain pH between 7.20 and 7.25. Once airflow obstruction is relieved and Pa_{CO_2} and arterial pH normalize, patients can usually be quickly weaned from the ventilator.

Other therapies are reported effective for asthma exacerbation, but none have been thoroughly studied. Heliox is used to decrease the work of breathing and improve ventilation through a decrease in turbulent flow attributable to helium, a gas less dense than O_2. Despite the theoretical benefits of heliox, studies have reported conflicting results concerning its efficacy; lack of ready availability also limits its use. Magnesium sulfate relaxes smooth muscle, but efficacy in management of asthma exacerbation in the emergency department is controversial. General anesthesia in patients with status asthmaticus causes bronchodilation by an unclear mechanism, perhaps by a direct relaxant effect on airway smooth muscle or attenuation of cholinergic tone.

Treatment of chronic asthma: Appropriate drug use keeps most chronic asthmatics out of the emergency department and hospital. Many drugs are available, and selection and sequence of drugs are based on asthma severity (see TABLE 48–2). "Step-down" therapy—a reduction in drug dose to the minimal amount needed for control of symptoms—is indicated for all asthma severities.

Patients with mild intermittent asthma do not need drugs daily. A short-acting β-agonist (eg, 2 inhalations of albuterol as a rescue drug) is sufficient for acute symptoms; use for more than 2 times/wk, use of ≥ 2 canisters a year, or decreasing response to the drug may indicate the need for long-term control therapy. Regardless of the severity of the asthma, the frequent need for a rescue β-agonist indicates that the asthma is not well-controlled.

Patients with mild persistent asthma (adults and children) should receive anti-inflammatory therapy. Low-dose inhaled corticosteroids are the treatment of choice, but some patients may be controlled with mast cell stabilizers, leukotriene modifiers, or extended-release theophylline. A short-acting rescue β-agonist (eg, albuterol, 2 to 4 puffs) is indicated as rescue therapy for breakthrough symptoms. Patients who require rescue therapy daily require medium-dose inhaled corticosteroids or combination therapy (see below).

Patients with moderate persistent asthma should be treated with inhaled corticosteroids in a dose adjusted to response combined with a long-acting inhaled β-agonist (salmeterol, 2 puffs bid). A long-acting inhaled β-agonist alone is insufficient treatment but in combined therapy allows for a lower inhaled corticosteroid dosage and is more effective for nocturnal symptoms. Alternatives to this approach include inhaled corticosteroids alone in medium dose range or substitution of leukotriene receptor antagonists or extended-release theophylline for long-acting β-agonists in combination with low-to-medium-dose inhaled corticosteroids. In patients with GERD and moderate persistent asthma, anti-reflux treatment may reduce the frequency and dose of drugs needed for symptom control. In patients with allergic rhinitis and moderate persistent asthma, nasal corticosteroids may reduce the frequency of asthma exacerbations requiring emergency department visits.

Patients with severe persistent asthma are a minority who require several drugs in high doses. Options include a combination high-dose inhaled corticosteroid combined with long-acting β-agonist (salmeterol) or a combination of an inhaled corticosteroid, long-acting β-agonist, and leukotriene modifier. Short-acting inhaled β-agonists are indicated in both cases for rescue of breakthrough symptoms. Systemic corticosteroids are indicated for patients inadequately managed on these regimens; alternate-day dosing helps minimize adverse effects associated with a daily dosing.

Exercise-induced asthma: Exercise-induced asthma can generally be prevented by inhalation of a short-acting β-agonist or mast cell stabilizers before starting the exercise. If β-agonists are not effective or if exercise-induced asthma is frequent or severe, in most cases the patient has more severe asthma than is recognized and requires long-term therapy aimed at control.

Aspirin-sensitive asthma: The primary treatment for aspirin-sensitive asthma is avoidance of NSAIDs. Cyclooxygenase-2 (COX-2) inhibitors do not appear to be triggers. Leukotriene modifiers can blunt the response to NSAIDs. Alternatively, inpatient desensitization has been successful in small series of patients.

Future therapies: Multiple therapies are being developed to target specific components of the inflammatory cascade. Therapies directed at IL-4 and IL-13 are under investigation.

Special Populations

Infants, children, and adolescents: Asthma is difficult to diagnose in infants, thus underrecognition and undertreatment are common. Empiric trials of inhaled bronchodilators and anti-inflammatory drugs may be helpful for both. Drugs may be given by nebulizer or MDI with a holding chamber with or without a face mask. Infants and children < 5 yr requiring treatment more than 2 times/wk should be given daily anti-inflammatory therapy with inhaled corticosteroids (preferred), leukotriene receptor antagonists, or cromolyn.

Children > 5 yr and adolescents with asthma can be treated similar to adults but should be encouraged to maintain physical activities, exercise, and sports. Predicted norms for pulmonary function tests in adolescents are closer to childhood (not adult) standards. Adolescents and mature younger children should participate in developing their own asthma management plans and establishing their own goals for therapy to improve compliance. The action plan should be understood by teachers and school nurses to ensure reliable and prompt access to rescue drugs. Cromolyn and nedocromil are often tried in this group but are not as beneficial as inhaled corticosteroids; long-acting drugs prevent the embarrassment of having to take drugs at school.

Pregnant women: About ⅓ of female asthmatics who become pregnant notice relief of symptoms; ⅓ notice worsening (at times to a severe degree); and ⅓ notice no change. GERD may be an important contributor to symptomatic disease in pregnancy. Asthma control during pregnancy is crucial (see p. 2168), because poorly controlled maternal disease can result in increased prenatal mortality, premature delivery, and low birth weight. Asthma drugs have not been shown to have adverse fetal effects, but no large well-controlled studies have been conducted to truly document safety for the developing fetus.

ALLERGIC BRONCHOPULMONARY ASPERGILLOSIS

Allergic bronchopulmonary aspergillosis is a hypersensitivity reaction to *Aspergillus fumigatus* that occurs almost exclusively in patients with asthma or, less commonly, cystic fibrosis. Immune responses to *Aspergillus* antigens cause airway obstruction and, if untreated, bronchiectasis and pulmonary fibrosis. Symptoms and signs are those of asthma with the addition of productive cough and, occasionally, fever and anorexia. Diagnosis is suspected based on history and imaging tests and confirmed by *Aspergillus* skin testing and measurement of IgE levels, circulating precipitins, and *A. fumigatus*–specific antibodies. Treatment is with corticosteroids and, in patients with refractory disease, itraconazole.

Etiology and Pathophysiology

Allergic bronchopulmonary aspergillosis (ABPA) develops when airways of patients with asthma or cystic fibrosis become colonized with *Aspergillus fumigatus* (a ubiquitous fungus in the soil). For unclear reasons, colonization in these patients prompts vigorous antibody (IgE and IgG) and cell-mediated immune responses (type I, III, and IV hypersensitivity reactions) to *Aspergillus* antigens, leading to frequent, recurrent asthma exacerbations. Over time, the immune reactions, combined with direct toxic effects of the fungus, lead to airway damage with dilatation and, ultimately, bronchiectasis and fibrosis. The disease is characterized histologically by mucoid impaction of airways, eosinophilic pneumonia, infiltration of alveolar septa with plasma and mononuclear cells, and an increase in the number of bronchiolar mucous glands and goblet cells. Rarely, other fungi, such as *Penicillium, Candida, Curvularia, Helminthosporium,* and/or *Drechslera* spp, cause an identical syndrome called allergic bronchopulmonary mycosis in the absence of underlying asthma or cystic fibrosis.

Aspergillus is present intraluminally but is not invasive. Thus, allergic bronchopulmonary aspergillosis must be distinguished from invasive aspergillosis, which occurs exclusively in immunocompromised patients; from aspergillomas, which are collections of *Aspergillus* in patients with established cavitary lesions or cystic airspaces; and from the rare *Aspergillus* pneumonia, which occurs in patients who take low doses of prednisone long term (eg, those with COPD).

Symptoms and Signs

Symptoms are those of asthma or pulmonary cystic fibrosis exacerbation, with the addition of cough productive of dirty-green or brown plugs and, occasionally, hemoptysis. Fever, headache, and anorexia are common systemic symptoms in severe disease. Signs are those of airway obstruction, specifically, wheezing and prolonged expiration, which are indistinguishable from asthma exacerbation.

Diagnosis

The diagnosis is suspected in asthmatic patients with any combination of recurrent asthma exacerbations, migratory or nonresolving infiltrates on chest x-ray (often due to atelectasis from mucoid plugging and bronchial obstruction), evidence of bronchiectasis on imaging studies (see p. 441), sputum cultures positive for *A. fumigatus*, and/or notable peripheral eosinophilia. Other x-ray findings include gloved finger infiltrates from mucous plugging and tram line shadows indicative of edematous bronchial walls. These findings may also be seen in bronchiectasis from other causes, but the signet ring sign of enlarged airways adjacent to pulmonary vasculature distinguishes bronchiectasis from ABPA on high-resolution CT.

Several criteria have been proposed for the diagnosis (see TABLE 48–4), but in practice 4 essential criteria are generally assessed. An immediate wheal-and-flare reaction to an initial skin prick test with *Aspergillus* antigen should prompt measurement of serum IgE and *Aspergillus* precipitins, although up to 25% of asthmatic patients without allergic bronchopulmonary aspergillosis may have a positive skin test. An IgE level > 1000 ng/mL and positive precipitins should prompt measurement of specific anti-*Aspergillus* immunoglobulins, although up to 10% of healthy patients have circulating precipitins. A finding of *A. fumigatus*–specific IgG and IgE antibodies in concentrations at least twice those found in patients without ABPA establishes the diagnosis. Whenever test results diverge, such as with an IgE > 1000 ng/mL but negative *A. fumigatus*–specific immunoglobulins, testing should be repeated and/or the patient should be followed over time to definitively establish or exclude the diagnosis.

Findings suggestive of but nonspecific for the disease include presence in sputum of *A. mycelia*, eosinophils, and/or Charcot-Leyden crystals (elongated eosinophilic bodies formed from eosinophilic granules) and late-onset skin reactivity (erythema, edema, and tenderness at 6 to 8 h) to *Aspergillus* antigen.

Treatment

Treatment is based on disease stage (see TABLE 48–5). Stage I is treated with prednisone 0.5 to 0.75 mg/kg once/day for 2 to 4 wk, then tapered over 4 to 6 mo. Chest x-ray, blood eosinophils, and IgE levels should be checked quarterly for improvement, defined as resolution of infiltrates, ≥ 50% decline in eosinophils, and 33% decline in IgE. Patients who achieve stage II disease require annual monitoring only. Stage II patients who relapse (Stage III) are given another trial of prednisone. Stage I or III patients who do not improve with prednisone (Stage IV) are candidates for antifungal treatment. Itraconazole 200 mg po bid for 4 to 6 mo with a 6-mo taper is recommended as a substitute for prednisone and as a corticosteroid-sparing drug. Itraconazole therapy requires checking drug levels and monitoring liver enzymes and triglyceride and K levels.

All patients should be optimally treated for their underlying asthma or cystic fibrosis. In addition, patients taking long-term corticosteroids should be monitored for complications, such as cataracts, hyperglycemia, and osteoporosis, and possibly prescribed treatments to prevent bone demineralization and *Pneumocystis jiroveci* (formerly *P. carinii*) lung infection.

TABLE 48–4. DIAGNOSTIC CRITERIA FOR ALLERGIC BRONCHOPULMONARY ASPERGILLOSIS

Asthma or cystic fibrosis*
Elevated *Aspergillus*-specific IgE and IgG*
Elevated serum IgE (> 1000 ng/mL)*
Proximal bronchiectasis*
Wheal-and-flare skin reaction to *Aspergillus* antigen*
Blood eosinophilia (> 1×10^9)
Serum precipitins to *Aspergillus* antigen
Transient or fixed pulmonary infiltrates

*Indicates minimal essential criteria. Inclusion of proximal bronchiectasis is controversial and may not be necessary for diagnosis.

TABLE 48–5. STAGES OF ALLERGIC BRONCHOPULMONARY ASPERGILLOSIS*

	STAGE	CRITERIA
I	Acute	All diagnostic criteria present
II	Remission	Symptoms resolved for > 6 mo
III	Relapse	Recurrence of one or more of the diagnostic criteria
IV	Refractory	Corticosteroid-dependent or refractory to treatment
V	Fibrosis	Diffuse fibrosis and bronchiectasis

*Stages do not progress sequentially.

49 CHRONIC OBSTRUCTIVE PULMONARY DISEASE

Chronic obstructive pulmonary disease is partially reversible airflow obstruction caused by an abnormal inflammatory response to toxins, often cigarette smoke. α_1-Antitrypsin deficiency and a variety of occupational exposures are less common causes in nonsmokers. Symptoms are productive cough and dyspnea that develop over years; common signs include decreased breath sounds and wheezing. Severe cases may be complicated by weight loss, pneumothorax, right heart failure, and respiratory failure. Diagnosis is based on history, physical examination, chest x-ray, and pulmonary function tests. Treatment is with bronchodilators, corticosteroids, and, when necessary, O_2. About 50% of patients die within 10 yr of initial diagnosis.

Chronic obstructive pulmonary disease (COPD) comprises chronic obstructive bronchitis and emphysema. Many patients have features of both.

Chronic obstructive bronchitis is chronic bronchitis with airflow obstruction. Chronic bronchitis (also called chronic mucous hypersecretion syndrome) is defined as productive cough for at least 3 mo in 2 successive years. Chronic bronchitis becomes chronic obstructive bronchitis if spirometric evidence of airflow obstruction develops. Chronic asthmatic bronchitis is a similar, overlapping condition characterized by chronic productive cough, wheezing, and partially reversible airflow obstruction in smokers with a history of asthma. In some cases, the distinction between chronic obstructive bronchitis and asthmatic bronchitis is unclear.

Emphysema is destruction of lung parenchyma leading to loss of elastic recoil and loss of alveolar septa and radial airway traction, which increases the tendency for airway collapse. Lung hyperinflation, airflow limitation, and air trapping follow. Airspaces enlarge and may eventually develop bullae.

Epidemiology

In 2000, an estimated 24 million people in the US had COPD, of whom only 10 million were diagnosed. In the same year, COPD was the 4th leading cause of death, resulting in 119,054 deaths—compared with 52,193 deaths in 1980. From 1980 to 2000, the COPD mortality rate increased 64% (from 40.7 to 66.9/100,000).

Prevalence, incidence, and mortality rates increase with age. Prevalence is higher in males, but total mortality is similar in both sexes. Incidence and mortality are generally higher in whites, blue-collar workers, and people with fewer years of formal education, probably because these groups have a higher prevalence of smoking. COPD seems to aggregate in families independent of α_1-antitrypsin (α_1-antiprotease inhibitor) deficiency (see p. 410).

COPD is increasing worldwide because of the increase in smoking in nonindustrialized countries, the reduction in mortality due to infectious diseases, and the widespread use of biomass fuels. It caused an estimated 2.74 million deaths worldwide in 2000 and is projected to become 1 of the top 5 causes of disease burden globally by the year 2020.

Etiology and Pathophysiology

Cigarette smoking is the primary risk factor in most countries, although only about 15% of smokers develop clinically apparent COPD; an exposure history of 40 or more pack-years is especially predictive. Smoke from burning biomass fuels for indoor cooking and heating is an important contributing factor in underdeveloped countries. Smokers with preexisting airway reactivity (defined by increased sensitivity to inhaled methacholine), even in the absence of clinical asthma, are at greater risk of developing COPD than are those without. Low body weight, childhood respiratory diseases, passive cigarette smoke exposure, air pollution, and occupational dust (eg, mineral or cotton dust) or chemical (eg, cadmium) exposure contribute to the risk of COPD but are of minor importance compared with cigarette smoking.

Genetic factors also contribute. The best-defined genetic disorder is α_1-antitrypsin deficiency (see p. 410), which is a significant cause of emphysema in nonsmokers and influences susceptibility to disease in smokers. Polymorphisms in microsomal epoxide hydrolase, vitamin D–binding protein, IL-1β, and IL-1 receptor antagonist genes are all associated with rapid decline in forced expiratory volume in 1 sec (FEV_1) in selected populations.

In genetically susceptible people, inhalational exposures trigger an inflammatory response in airways and alveoli that leads to disease. The process is thought to be mediated by an increase in protease activity and a decrease in antiprotease activity (see p. 410). Lung proteases, such as neutrophil elastase, matrix metalloproteinases, and cathepsins, break down elastin and connective tissue in the normal process of tissue repair. Their activity is balanced by antiproteases, such as α_1-antitrypsin, airway epithelium–derived secretory leukoproteinase inhibitor, elafin, and matrix metalloproteinase tissue inhibitor. In people with COPD, activated neutrophils and other inflammatory cells release proteases as part of the inflammatory process; protease activity exceeds antiprotease activity, and tissue destruction and mucus hypersecretion result. Neutrophil and macrophage activation also leads to accumulation of free radicals, superoxide anions, and hydrogen peroxide, which inhibit antiproteases and cause bronchoconstriction, mucosal edema, and mucous hypersecretion. Neutrophil-induced oxidative damage, release of profibrotic neuropeptides (eg, bombesin), and reduced levels of vascular endothelial growth factor may also play a role, as does infection.

Bacteria, especially *Haemophilus influenzae,* colonize the normally sterile lower airways of about 30% of patients with active COPD. In more severely affected patients (eg, those with previous hospitalizations), *Pseudomonas aeruginosa* is common. Some experts postulate that smoking and airflow obstruction lead to impaired mucus clearance in lower airways, which predisposes to infection. The repeated bouts of infection lead to increased inflammatory burden that hastens disease progression. There is no evidence, however, that long-term use of antibiotics slows the progression of COPD in susceptible smokers.

The cardinal pathophysiologic feature of COPD is airflow limitation caused by emphysema and/or airflow obstruction caused by mucus hypersecretion, mucus plugging, and/or bronchospasm. Increased airway resistance increases the work of respiration, as does lung hyperinflation. Increased work of breathing may lead to alveolar hypoventilation with hypoxia and hypercapnia, although hypoxia is also caused by ventilation/perfusion (V/Q) mismatch. Some patients with advanced disease develop chronic hypoxemia and hypercapnia. Chronic hypoxemia increases pulmonary vascular tone which, if diffuse, causes pulmonary hypertension and cor pulmonale. O_2 administration may then worsen hypercapnia in some patients by decreasing hypoxic ventilatory drive, leading to alveolar hypoventilation.

Histologic changes include peribronchiolar inflammatory infiltrates, bronchial smooth muscle hypertrophy, and airspace distortion due to loss of alveolar attachments and alveolar septal destruction. Enlarged alveolar spaces sometimes consolidate into bullae, defined as airspaces ≥ 1 cm in diameter. Bullae may be entirely empty or have strands of lung tissue traversing them in areas of locally severe emphysema; they occasionally occupy the entire hemithorax.

Symptoms and Signs

COPD takes years to develop and progress. Productive cough usually is the initial sign in patients in their 40s and 50s who have smoked ≥ 20 cigarettes/day for > 20 yr. Dyspnea that is progressive, persistent, exertional, or worse during respiratory infection eventually appears by the time patients reach their late 50s. Symptoms usually progress quickly in patients who continue to smoke and who have higher lifetime tobacco exposure. Morning headache develops in more advanced disease and signals nocturnal hypercapnia or hypoxemia.

Acute exacerbations occur sporadically during the course of COPD and are heralded by increased symptom severity. The specific cause of any exacerbation is almost always impossible to determine, but exacerbations are often attributed to viral URIs or acute bacterial bronchitis. As COPD progresses, acute exacerbations tend to become more frequent, averaging about 3 episodes/yr. Those who suffer acute exacerbations are much more likely to have recurrent exacerbations.

Signs include wheezing, lung hyperinflation manifest as decreased heart and lung sounds, and increased anteroposterior diameter of the thorax (barrel chest). Patients with advanced emphysema lose weight and experience muscle wasting because of immobility;

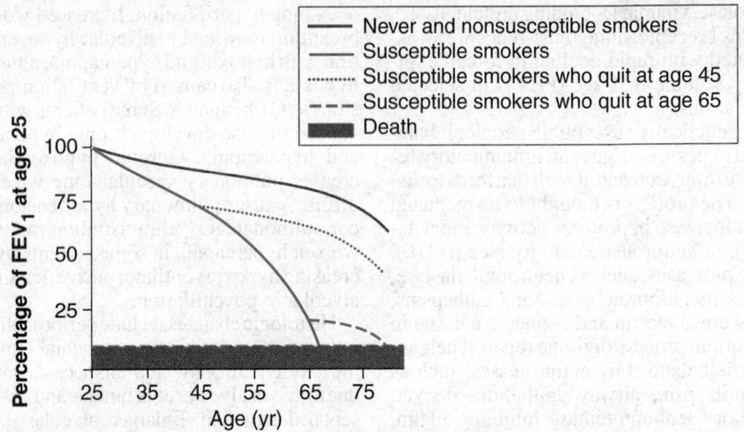

Fig. 49–1. Effect of smoking status on decline in FEV_1 with age. FEV_1 declines with age, but the decline is steeper in smokers who are susceptible to smoking effects and thus more likely to develop COPD. Quitting smoking alters the rate of decline, delaying the age at which disability and death occur. FEV_1 = Forced expiratory volume in 1 sec. Data from Fletcher C, Peto R: The natural history of chronic airflow obstruction. *British Medical Journal* 1:1645–1648, 1977.

hypoxia; release of systemic inflammatory mediators, such as tumor necrosis factor (TNF)-α; and increased metabolic rate. Signs of advanced disease include pursed-lip breathing, accessory muscle use with paradoxical indrawing of the lower intercostal interspaces (Hoover's sign), and cyanosis. Signs of cor pulmonale include neck vein distention; splitting of the 2nd heart sound with an accentuated pulmonic component; tricuspid insufficiency murmur; and peripheral edema. Right ventricular heaves are uncommon in COPD because of hyperinflated lungs.

Spontaneous pneumothorax is also common as a result of rupture of bullae and is suspected in any patient with COPD whose pulmonary status abruptly worsens.

Systemic disorders that may have a component of emphysema and/or airflow limitation suggesting the presence of COPD include HIV infection, sarcoidosis, Sjögren's syndrome, bronchiolitis obliterans, lymphangioleiomyomatosis, and eosinophilic granuloma.

Diagnosis

Diagnosis is suggested by history, physical examination, and chest imaging and is confirmed by pulmonary function tests. Differential diagnosis includes asthma, heart failure, and bronchiectasis. COPD and asthma are sometimes easily confused. Asthma (see also p. 381) and COPD are distinguished by history and by the presence of reversibility of airflow obstruction on pulmonary function testing.

Pulmonary function tests: Patients suspected of having COPD should undergo pulmonary function testing to confirm airway obstruction and to quantify its severity and reversibility (see also Ch. 46 on p. 364). Pulmonary function testing is also useful for following disease progression and monitoring response to treatment. The primary diagnostic tests are FEV_1, which is the volume of air forcefully expired during the first second after a full breath; forced vital capacity (FVC), which is the total volume of air expired with maximal force; and flow-volume loops, which are simultaneous spirometric recording of airflow and volume during forced maximal expiration and inspiration.

Reduction of FEV_1, FVC, and the ratio of FEV_1/FVC are the hallmark of airway obstruction. Flow-volume loops show a concave pattern in the expiratory tracing (see FIG. 46–3F on p. 369). FEV_1 declines up to 60 mL/yr in smokers, compared with a less steep decline of 25 to 30 mL/yr in nonsmokers, beginning at about age 30 (see FIG. 49–1).

In middle-aged smokers who already have a low FEV_1, the decline occurs at a more rapid rate. When the FEV_1 falls below about 1 L, patients develop dyspnea with activities of daily living; when the FEV_1 falls below about 0.8 L, they are at risk of hypoxemia, hypercapnia, and cor pulmonale. FEV_1 and FVC are easily measured with office spirometry and define severity of disease (see TABLE 49–1) because they correlate with symptoms and mortality. Normal reference values are determined by patient age, sex, and height.

TABLE 49–1. SEVERITY AND TREATMENT OF COPD

STAGE	CHARACTERISTICS	RECOMMENDED TREATMENT	ADDITIONAL TREATMENT
All		Avoidance of risk factors Influenza vaccination	
0: At risk	Chronic symptoms (cough, sputum) Exposure to risk factors Normal spirometry		
I: Mild COPD	$FEV_1/FVC < 70\%$ $FEV_1 \geq 80\%$ predicted With or without symptoms	Short-acting bronchodilator when needed	
II: Moderate COPD	IIA $FEV_1/FVC < 70\%$ $50\% \leq FEV_1 < 80\%$ predicted With or without symptoms	Regular treatment with one or more bronchodilators Rehabilitation	
	IIB $FEV_1/FVC < 70\%$ $30\% \leq FEV_1 > 50\%$ predicted With or without symptoms	Regular treatment with one or more bronchodilators Rehabilitation	Inhaled corticosteroids for recurrent exacerbations
III: Severe COPD	$FEV_1/FVC < 70\%$ $FEV_1 < 30\%$ predicted or presence of respiratory failure or right heart failure	Regular treatment with one or more bronchodilators Inhaled corticosteroids for recurrent exacerbations Treatment of complications Rehabilitation Long-term oxygen therapy if respiratory failure Consider surgical treatments	

FEV_1 = Forced expiratory volume in 1 sec; FVC = forced vital capacity.

Modified from Pauwels RA, Buist AS, Calverley PM, Jenkins CR, Hurd SS. Global strategy for the diagnosis, management, and prevention of chronic obstructive pulmonary disease. NHLBI/WHO Global Initiative for Chronic Obstructive Lung Disease (GOLD) Workshop summary. *American Journal of Respiratory and Critical Care Medicine* 163:1256–1276, 2001.

Additional pulmonary function testing is necessary only in specific circumstances, such as before lung volume reduction surgery (see p. 408). Other test abnormalities may include an increased total lung capacity, functional residual capacity, and residual volume, which can help distinguish COPD from restrictive pulmonary disease, in which these measures are diminished; decreased vital capacity; and decreased single-breath diffusing capacity for carbon monoxide (DL_{CO}). Decreased DL_{CO} is nonspecific and is reduced in other disorders that affect the pulmonary vascular bed, such as interstitial lung disease, but can help distinguish COPD from asthma, in which DL_{CO} is normal or elevated.

Imaging tests: The chest x-ray has characteristic, though not diagnostic, findings. Changes with emphysema include lung hyperinflation manifested as a flat diaphragm, narrow heart, rapid tapering of hilar vessels (anteroposterior view), and widening of the retrosternal airspace. The flattening of the diaphragm due to hyperinflation causes an increase in the angle formed by the sternum and anterior diaphragm on a lateral film from the normal value of 45° to > 90°. Bullae—radiolucencies > 1 cm surrounded by arcuate hairline shadows—reflect locally severe disease. Emphysematous changes predominantly in the lung bases indicate α_1-antitrypsin deficiency (see p. 410). The lungs may look normal or have increased lucency secondary to loss of parenchyma. The chest x-rays of patients with chronic obstructive bronchitis may be normal or may demonstrate a bi-basilar increase in bronchovascular markings.

Prominent hila may suggest large central pulmonary arteries seen with pulmonary hypertension. Right ventricular enlargement seen in cor pulmonale may be masked by lung hyperinflation or may manifest as encroachment of the heart shadow on the retrosternal space or by widening of the transverse cardiac shadow in comparison with previous chest x-rays.

CT scans may clarify abnormalities seen on chest x-ray suggestive of coexisting or complicating diseases, such as pneumonia, pneumoconiosis, or lung cancer. CT helps assess the extent and distribution of emphysema, estimated either by visual scoring or with analysis of the distribution of lung density. These parameters may be useful in preparation for lung volume reduction surgery.

Adjunctive tests: α_1-Antitrypsin levels should be measured in patients < 50 yr with symptomatic COPD and in nonsmokers of any age with COPD to detect α_1-antitrypsin deficiency (see p. 410). Other indications of α_1-antitrypsin deficiency include a family history of premature COPD or infantile liver disease, lower-lobe distribution of emphysema, and COPD associated with antineutrophil cytoplasmic antibody (ANCA)-positive vasculitis. Low levels of α_1-antitrypsin should be confirmed by phenotyping.

The ECG, often performed to exclude cardiac causes of dyspnea, typically demonstrates diffusely low QRS voltage with a vertical heart axis caused by lung hyperinflation and increased P-wave voltage or rightward shifts of the P-wave vector caused by right atrial enlargement in patients with advanced emphysema. Findings of right ventricular hypertrophy include an R or R′ wave as tall as or taller than the S wave in lead V_1; an R wave smaller than the S wave in lead V_6; and/or right-axis deviation > 110° without right bundle branch block. Multifocal atrial tachycardia, an arrhythmia that can accompany COPD, manifests as a tachyarrhythmia with polymorphic P waves and variable PR intervals.

Echocardiography is occasionally useful for assessing right ventricular function and pulmonary hypertension, although it is technically difficult in COPD patients. It is most often indicated when coexistent left ventricular or valvular heart disease is suspected.

CBC is of little diagnostic value in the evaluation of COPD but may show erythrocythemia (Hct > 48%) as a reflection of chronic hypoxemia.

Evaluation of exacerbations: Patients with acute exacerbations who display increased work of breathing, somnolence, and low O_2 saturations on oximetry should undergo ABG sampling to quantify hypoxemia and hypercapnia. Hypercapnia may exist with hypoxemia. In such patients, the hypoxemia often provides more respiratory stimulation than hypercapnia (which is the norm), and O_2 therapy may worsen hypercapnia by attenuating hypoxic ventilatory drive and worsening hypoventilation.

Findings of partial pressure of arterial O_2 (PaO_2) < 50 mm Hg or partial pressure of arterial CO_2 ($PaCO_2$) > 50 mm Hg in the setting of respiratory acidemia define acute respiratory failure (see p. 544). However, some patients with chronic COPD survive at such levels for prolonged periods.

A chest x-ray is often obtained to check for pneumonia or pneumothorax. Rarely, infiltrates in patients receiving chronic systemic corticosteroids may represent *Aspergillus* pneumonia.

Yellow or green sputum is a reliable indicator of sputum neutrophils and suggests bacterial colonization or infection. Gram stain usually shows neutrophils with a mixture of organisms, often gram-positive diplococci (*Streptococcus pneumoniae*) and/or gram-negative rods (*H. influenzae*). Other oropharyngeal commensal flora, such as *Moraxella* (*Branhamella*) *catarrhalis*, occasionally cause exacerbations. In hospitalized patients, Gram stains and cultures may demonstrate resistant gram-negative organisms (eg, *Pseudomonas*) or, rarely, gram-positive infection with *Staphylococcus*.

Prognosis

Severity of airway obstruction predicts survival in patients with COPD. The mortality rate in patients with an $FEV_1 \geq 50\%$ of predicted is slightly greater than that of the general population. If the FEV_1 is 0.75 to 1.25 L, 5-yr survival is about 40 to 60%; if < 0.75 L, about 30 to 40%. Cardiac disease, low body weight, resting tachycardia, hypercapnia, and hypoxemia decrease survival, whereas a significant response to bronchodilators is associated with improved survival. Risk factors for death in patients with acute exacerbation requiring hospitalization include older age, higher Pa_{CO_2}, and use of maintenance oral corticosteroids.

Mortality in COPD often results from intercurrent illnesses rather than from progression of the underlying disease in those who have stopped smoking. Death is generally caused by acute respiratory failure, pneumonia, lung cancer, cardiac disease, or pulmonary embolism.

Treatment of Stable COPD

Treatment of cor pulmonale, a common complication of long-standing, severe COPD, is discussed on p. 664.

Treatment of chronic stable COPD aims to prevent exacerbations and provide long-term improvement in lung and physical function through drug and O_2 therapy, smoking cessation, exercise, enhancement of nutrition, and pulmonary rehabilitation. Surgical treatment of COPD is indicated for selected patients. COPD management involves treatment of both chronic stable disease and of exacerbations.

Drug therapy: Recommended drug therapy is summarized in TABLE 49–1. Bronchodilators are the mainstay of COPD management; drugs include inhaled β-agonists and anticholinergics. Any patient with symptomatic COPD should be taking 1 or both of these classes of drugs, which are equally effective. For initial therapy, the choice between short-acting β-agonists, long-acting β-agonists, anticholinergics (which have a greater bronchodilating effect), or combination β-agonist and anticholinergic therapy is often a matter of tailoring cost and convenience to the patient's preferences and symptoms. There is no evidence that regular bronchodilator use slows deterioration of pulmonary function, but the drugs acutely relieve symptoms and increase pulmonary function and exercise capacity.

In treatment of chronic stable disease, administration by metered-dose inhaler or dry-powder inhaler is preferred over nebulized home treatment; home nebulizers are prone to contamination from incomplete cleaning and drying. Patients should be taught to exhale to functional residual capacity, inhale the aerosol slowly to total lung capacity, and hold the inhalation for 3 to 4 sec before exhaling. Spacers help ensure optimal delivery of drug to the distal airways and reduce the importance of coordinating activation of the inhaler with inhalation. Some spacers alert the patient if they are inhaling too rapidly.

β-Agonists relax bronchial smooth muscle and increase mucociliary clearance. Albuterol aerosol, 2 puffs (100 μg/puff) inhaled from a metered-dose inhaler 4 to 6 times/day prn, is usually the drug of choice because of low cost; regular dosing offers no advantages over as-needed use and causes more adverse effects. Long-acting β-agonists are preferable for patients with nocturnal symptoms or for those who find frequent dosing inconvenient; options include salmeterol powder, 1 puff (50 μg) inhaled bid; or formoterol powder (12 μg) inhaled bid. The dry-powder formulations may be more effective for patients who have trouble coordinating use of a metered-dose inhaler. Patients should be taught the difference between short- and long-acting drugs, because long-acting drugs that are used as needed or more than twice/day increase the risk of cardiac arrhythmias. Adverse effects commonly result from use of any β-agonist and include tremor, anxiety, tachycardia, and mild hypokalemia.

Anticholinergics relax bronchial smooth muscle through competitive inhibition of muscarinic receptors (M_1, M_2, and M_3). Ipratropium is most commonly used because of low cost and availability; dose is 2 to 4 puffs q 4 to 6 h. Ipratropium has a slower onset of action (within 30 min; peak effect in 1 to 2 h), so a β_2-agonist is often prescribed with it in a single combination inhaler or as a separate as-needed rescue drug. Tiotropium, a long-acting quaternary anticholinergic, is M_1 and M_3 selective and may therefore have an advantage over ipratropium, because M_2 receptor blockade (as occurs with ipratropium) may limit bronchodilation. Dose is 18 μg once/day. Tiotropium is not available worldwide, however, and additional studies are needed before its precise role can be clarified. Adverse effects of all anticholinergics are pupillary dilation, blurred vision, and dry mouth.

Inhaled corticosteroids inhibit airway inflammation, reverse β-receptor down-regulation, and inhibit leukotriene and cytokine production. They do not alter the course of pulmonary function decline in COPD patients who continue to smoke, but they do improve short-term pulmonary function in some patients, are additive to the effect of bronchodilators, and may diminish the frequency of COPD exacerbations. Dose depends on the drug; examples include fluticasone 500 to 1000 μg/day and beclomethasone 400 to 2000 μg/day. The long-term risks of inhaled corticosteroids in older populations are not proven but probably include osteoporosis and cataract formation. Long-term users therefore should undergo periodic ophthalmologic and bone densitometry screening and should possibly receive supplemental calcium, vitamin D, and a bisphosphonate as indicated.

Combinations of a long-acting β-agonist (eg, salmeterol) and an inhaled corticosteroid (eg, fluticasone) are more effective than either drug alone in the treatment of chronic stable disease.

Oral or systemic corticosteroids can be used to treat chronic stable COPD but seem to benefit only 10 to 20% of patients, and long-term risks may exceed benefits. Formal comparisons between oral and inhaled corticosteroids have not been performed. Oral dosing should start at 30 mg prednisone once/day, and response to treatment should be monitored by spirometry. If the FEV_1 improves ≥ 20%, then the dose should be tapered at a rate of a 5-mg equivalent of prednisone per week to the lowest amount that maintains the improvement. If exacerbation occurs during tapering, inhaled corticosteroids may be helpful, but a resumption of higher dosing is likely to provide more rapid symptom relief and improvement in FEV_1. By contrast, if initial FEV_1 improvement is < 20%, then corticosteroids should be tapered rapidly and stopped. Alternate-day dosing is an option if it reduces adverse effects while sustaining daily improvement.

Theophylline plays a small role in the treatment of chronic stable COPD and of acute COPD exacerbations now that safer, more effective drugs are available. Theophylline decreases smooth muscle spasm, enhances mucociliary clearance, improves right ventricular function, and decreases pulmonary vascular resistance and arterial pressure. Its mode of action is poorly understood but appears to differ from that of β_2-agonists and anticholinergics. Its role in improving diaphragmatic function and dyspnea during exercise is controversial. Low-dose theophylline (300 to 400 mg/day) has anti-inflammatory properties and may enhance the effects of inhaled corticosteroids.

Theophylline can be used for patients who have not adequately responded to inhaled agents and who have shown symptomatic benefit from a trial of the drug. Serum levels need not be monitored unless the patient does not respond to the drug, develops symptoms of toxicity, or is questionably adherent; slowly absorbed oral theophylline preparations, which require less frequent dosing, enhance compliance. Toxicity is common and includes sleeplessness and GI upset, even at low blood levels. More serious adverse effects, such as supraventricular and ventricular arrhythmias and seizures, tend to occur at blood levels > 20 mg/L. Hepatic metabolism of theophylline varies greatly and is influenced by genetic factors, age, cigarette smoking, hepatic dysfunction, and some drugs, such as macrolide and fluoroquinolone antibiotics and nonsedating histamine$_2$ blockers.

Phosphodiesterase-4 antagonists and antioxidants are under investigation for anti-inflammatory effects in the treatment of COPD.

Oxygen therapy: Long-term O_2 therapy prolongs life in COPD patients whose Pa_{O_2}

is chronically <55 mm Hg. Continual 24-h use is more effective than a 12-h nocturnal regimen. O_2 therapy brings Hct toward normal levels; moderately improves neuropsychologic factors, possibly by facilitating sleep; and ameliorates pulmonary hemodynamic abnormalities. O_2 therapy also increases exercise tolerance in many patients.

A sleep study should be considered for patients with advanced COPD who do not meet the criteria for long-term O_2 therapy (see TABLE 49–2) but whose clinical assessment suggests pulmonary hypertension in the absence of daytime hypoxemia. Nocturnal O_2 may be prescribed if a sleep study shows episodic desaturation to ≤ 88%. Such treatment prevents progression of pulmonary hypertension, but its effects on survival are unknown.

O_2 is administered by nasal cannula at a flow rate sufficient to achieve a $PaO_2 > 60$ mm Hg ($SaO_2 > 90\%$), usually ≤ 3 L/min at rest. O_2 is supplied by electrically driven O_2 concentrators, liquid O_2 systems, or cylinders of compressed gas. Concentrators, which limit mobility but are the least expensive, are preferable for patients who spend most of their time at home. Such patients require small O_2 tanks for backup in case of an electrical failure and for portable use.

A liquid system is preferable for patients who spend much time out of their homes. Portable canisters of liquid O_2 are easier to carry and have more capacity than portable cylinders of compressed gas. Large compressed-air cylinders are the most expensive way of providing O_2 and should be used only if no other source is available. All patients must be taught the dangers of smoking during O_2 use.

Various devices can conserve the amount of O_2 used by the patient, either by using a reservoir system or by permitting O_2 flow only during inspiration. These devices correct hypoxemia as effectively as do continuous flow systems.

Some patients need supplemental O_2 during air travel, because flight cabin pressure in commercial airliners is low. Eucapnic COPD patients with a sea level $PaO_2 > 68$ mm Hg generally have an in-flight $PaO_2 > 50$ mm Hg and do not require supplemental O_2. All COPD patients with hypercapnia, significant anemia (Hct < 30), or coexisting heart or cerebrovascular disease should use supplemental O_2 during long flights and should notify the airline when making their reservation. Patients are not permitted to transport or use their own O_2. The airline provides its own O_2 system, and most require a minimum notice of 24 h, a physician's statement of necessity, and an O_2 prescription before the flight. Patients should bring their own nasal cannulas, because some airlines provide only face masks. Arrangements for O_2 equipment in the destination city, if required, should be made in advance so that the supplier can meet the traveler at the airport.

TABLE 49–2. INDICATIONS FOR LONG-TERM O_2 THERAPY IN COPD

$PaO_2 \le 55$ mm Hg or $SaO_2 \le 88\%$* in patients receiving optimal medical regimen for at least 30 days†

$PaO_2 = 55$ to 59 mm Hg or $SaO_2 \le 89\%$* for patients with cor pulmonale or erythrocytosis (Hct > 55%)

Can be considered for
- $PaO_2 \ge 60$ mm Hg or $SaO_2 \ge 90\%$* for patients whose room-air PaO_2 is ≤ 55 mm Hg or $SaO_2 \le 88\%$ during exercise or sleep

PaO_2 = partial pressure of arterial O_2; SaO_2 = arterial O_2 saturation.

*Arterial O_2 levels measured at rest during air breathing.

†Patients who are recovering from an acute respiratory illness and who meet the listed criteria should be given O_2 and rechecked on room air in 30 days.

Smoking cessation: Smoking cessation (see p. 2733) is both extremely difficult and extremely important; it slows but does not altogether halt the progression of airway inflammation (see FIG. 49–1). Simultaneous use of multiple strategies is most effective: establishment of a quit date, behavior modification techniques, group sessions, nicotine replacement therapy (by gum, transdermal patch, inhaler, lozenge, or nasal spray), bupropion, and physician encouragement. Quit rates are about 30% at 1 yr even with bupropion combined with nicotine replacement, the most effective intervention.

Vaccinations: All patients with COPD should be given annual influenza vaccinations. If a patient is unable to receive an influenza vaccination or if the prevailing influenza strain is not included in the annual vaccine formulation, prophylactic treatment (amantadine, rimantadine, oseltamivir, or zanamivir) is appropriate during community influenza outbreaks. Pneumococcal polysaccharide vaccine, although of unproven efficacy in COPD, has minimal adverse effects and should probably also be administered.

Physical activity: Skeletal muscle deconditioning resulting from inactivity or prolonged hospitalization for respiratory failure can be ameliorated with a program of graded exercise. Specific training of respiratory muscles is less helpful than general aerobic conditioning. A typical training program begins with slow walking on a treadmill or unloaded cycling on an ergometer for a few minutes. Duration and exercise load is progressively increased over 4 to 6 wk until the patient can exercise for 20 to 30 min nonstop with manageable dyspnea. Patients with very severe COPD can usually achieve an exercise regimen of walking for 30 min at 1 to 2 mph. Maintenance exercise should be performed 3 to 4 times/wk to maintain fitness levels. O_2 saturation is monitored and supplemental O_2 provided as needed. Upper extremity resistance training is helpful in performing daily tasks such as bathing, dressing, and housecleaning. COPD patients should be taught ways to conserve energy during activities of daily living and pace their activities. Difficulties in sexual function should be discussed and advice given on using energy-conserving techniques for sexual gratification.

Nutrition: COPD patients are at risk of weight loss and nutritional deficiencies because of a 15 to 25% increase in resting energy expenditure from breathing; a larger postprandial increase in metabolism and heat production (ie, the thermal effect of feeding), perhaps because a distended stomach interferes with descent of the already flattened diaphragm and increases the work of breathing; a higher energy cost of daily activities; reduced caloric intake relative to need; and the catabolic effect of inflammatory cytokines such as TNF-α. Generalized muscle strength and efficiency of O_2 use are impaired. Patients with poorer nutritional status have a worse prognosis, so it is prudent to recommend a balanced diet with adequate caloric intake in conjunction with exercise to prevent or reverse malnutrition and muscle atrophy. However, excessive weight gain should be avoided, and obese patients should strive to achieve more normal body mass index. Studies of nutritional supplementation alone have not resulted in improvement in pulmonary function or exercise capacity. The roles of anabolic steroids (eg, megace, oxandrolone), growth hormone supplementation, and TNF antagonists in reversing malnutrition and improving functional status and prognosis in COPD are not well defined.

Pulmonary rehabilitation: Pulmonary rehabilitation programs serve as adjuncts to drug treatment to improve physical function; many hospitals and health care organizations offer formal multidisciplinary rehabilitation programs. Pulmonary rehabilitation includes exercise, education, and behavioral intervention. Treatment should be individualized; patients and family members are taught about COPD and medical treatments, and the patient is encouraged to take as much responsibility for personal care as possible. A carefully integrated rehabilitation program helps patients with severe COPD accommodate to physiologic limitations while providing realistic expectations for improvement.

The benefits of rehabilitation are greater independence and improved quality of life and exercise capacity. Modest increases are seen in lower extremity strength, endurance, and maximum O_2 consumption. Pulmonary rehabilitation typically does not improve pulmonary function or increase longevity, however. Patients with severe disease require a minimum of 3 mo of rehabilitation to benefit and should continue with maintenance programs.

Specialized programs are available for patients who remain ventilator-bound after acute respiratory failure. Some patients can be liberated from the ventilator entirely, whereas others can remain off the ventilator during the day. For patients with adequate home support, training of family members can permit some patients to be sent home with ventilators.

Surgery: Surgical options for treatment of severe COPD include lung volume reduction and transplantation.

Lung volume reduction by resection of nonfunctioning emphysematous areas improves exercise tolerance and 2-yr mortality in patients with severe, predominantly upper-lung emphysema who have low baseline exercise capacity after pulmonary rehabilitation. Other patients may experience symptom relief and improved exercise capacity after surgery, but mortality has been shown to be the same or increased compared with that for drug therapy. Long-term effects of the procedure are unknown. Improvement is less than that with lung transplantation. The mechanism of improvement is believed to be enhanced lung recoil and improved diaphragmatic function and V/Q relationships. Operative mortality is about 5%. The best candidates for lung volume reduction are those with an FEV_1 20 to 40% of predicted, a DL_{CO} > 20% of predicted, significantly impaired exercise capacity, heterogeneous pulmonary disease on CT with an upper-lobe predominance, $Paco_2$ < 50 mm Hg, and absence of severe pulmonary hypertension and coronary artery disease.

Rarely, patients have extremely large bullae that compress the functional lung. These patients can be helped by surgical resection of these bullae, with resulting relief of symptoms and improved pulmonary function. In general, resection is most beneficial for patients with bullae affecting > ⅓ of a hemithorax and an FEV_1 about ½ the predicted normal value. Improved pulmonary function is related to the amount of normal or minimally diseased lung tissue that was compressed by the resected bullae. Serial chest x-rays and CT are the most useful procedures for determining whether a patient's functional status is due to compression of viable lung by bullae or to generalized emphysema. A markedly reduced DL_{CO} (< 40% predicted) indicates widespread emphysema and suggests a poorer outcome from surgical resection.

Since 1989, single-lung transplantation has largely replaced double-lung transplantation in COPD patients. Candidates for transplantation are patients < 60 yr with an FEV_1 < 25% predicted or with severe pulmonary hypertension. The goal of lung transplantation is to improve quality of life, because survival time is rarely increased. The 5-yr survival after transplantation for emphysema is 45 to 60%. Lifelong immunosuppression is required, with the attendant risk of opportunistic infections.

Treatment of Acute COPD Exacerbation

The immediate objectives are to ensure adequate oxygenation, reverse airway obstruction, and treat underlying causes.

The cause is usually unknown, although some acute exacerbations result from bacterial or viral infections. Smoking, irritative inhalational exposure, and high levels of air pollution also contribute. Mild exacerbations often can be treated on an outpatient basis in patients with adequate home support. Elderly frail patients and patients with comorbidities, a history of respiratory failure, or acute changes in ABG measurements are admitted to the hospital for observation and treatment. Patients with life-threatening exacerbations manifested by uncorrected hypoxemia, acute respiratory acidosis, new arrhythmias, or deteriorating respiratory function despite hospital treatment and those who require sedation for management should be admitted to the ICU and their respiratory status monitored frequently.

Oxygen: Most patients require O_2 supplementation, even those who do not need it chronically. O_2 administration may worsen hypercapnia by attenuating hypoxic respiratory drive. After 30 days, room-air Pao_2 should be reassessed to determine if the patient still requires supplemental O_2.

Ventilatory assistance: Noninvasive positive-pressure ventilation (eg, pressure support or bi-level positive airway pressure ventilation by face mask [see p. 547]) is an alternative to full mechanical ventilation. Noninvasive ventilation appears to decrease the need for intubation, reduce hospital stay, and reduce mortality in patients with severe exacerbations (defined as a pH < 7.30 in hemodynamically stable patients not at immediate risk of respiratory arrest). Noninvasive ventilation appears to have no effect in patients with less severe exacerbation. However, it may be indicated for patients in this group whose ABGs worsen despite initial drug therapy or who appear to be imminent candidates for full mechanical ventilation but who do not require intubation for control of the airway or sedation for agitation. Deterioration on noninvasive ventilation should prompt conversion to invasive mechanical ventilation.

Deteriorating ABG levels and mental status and progressive respiratory fatigue are indications for endotracheal intubation and mechanical ventilation. Ventilator settings, management strategies, and complications are discussed in Ch. 65 on p. 544. Risk factors for ventilatory dependence include an FEV_1 < 0.5 L, stable ABGs with a Pao_2 < 50 mm Hg and/or $Paco_2$ > 60 mm Hg, severe exercise limitation, and poor nutritional status. Therefore, a discussion of the patient's wishes regarding intubation and mechanical ventilation should be initiated and documented (see p. 2768).

If a patient requires prolonged intubation (eg, > 2 wk), a tracheostomy is indicated to facilitate comfort, communication, and eating. With a good multidisciplinary rehabilitation program, including nutritional and psychologic support (see p. 378), many patients requiring prolonged mechanical ventilation can be successfully weaned and can return to their former level of function.

Drug therapy: β-agonists, anticholinergics, and/or corticosteroids should be started concurrently with O_2 therapy (regardless of how O_2 is administered) with the aim of reversing airway obstruction.

β-agonists are the cornerstone of drug therapy for acute exacerbations. The most widely used drug is albuterol, 2.5 mg by nebulizer or 2 to 4 inhalations (100 µg/puff) by metered-dose inhaler q 2 to 6 h. Inhalation using a metered-dose inhaler produces rapid bronchodilation; there are no data indicating that nebulizers are more effective than metered-dose inhalers.

Ipratropium, the most commonly used anticholinergic, is proven effective in acute COPD exacerbation and should be given concurrently or alternating with β-agonists using a metered-dose inhaler. Dosage is 0.25 to 0.5 mg by nebulizer or 2 to 4 inhalations (21 µg/puff) by metered-dose inhaler q 4 to 6 h. Ipratropium generally provides bronchodilating effect similar to β-agonists. The role of the longer-acting anticholinergic tiotropium in treating acute exacerbations has not been defined.

Corticosteroids should be begun immediately for all but mild exacerbations. Options include prednisone, 60 mg once/day po tapered over 7 to 14 days, and methylprednisolone, 60 mg once/day IV tapered over 7 to 14 days. These drugs are equivalent in their acute effects; inhaled corticosteroids have no role in the treatment of acute exacerbation.

Methylxanthines, once considered essential to treatment of acute COPD exacerbation, are no longer used. Toxicities exceeded benefit.

Antibiotics are recommended for exacerbations in patients with purulent sputum. Some physicians give antibiotics empirically for change in sputum color or for nonspecific chest x-ray abnormalities. Routine cultures and Gram stains are not necessary before treatment unless an unusual or resistant organism is suspected. Trimethoprim-sulfamethoxazole 160 mg/800 mg bid, amoxicillin 250 to 500 mg tid, tetracycline 250 mg qid, and doxycycline 50 to 100 bid given for 7 to 14 days are all effective and inexpensive first-line drugs. The choice of drug should be dictated by local patterns of bacterial sensitivity and patient history. In most cases, treatment should be initiated with oral drugs if tolerated. If the patient is seriously ill or if clinical evidence suggests that the infectious organisms are resistant, more expensive second-line drugs can be used. These drugs include amoxicillin-clavulanate 250 to 500 mg tid; fluoroquinolones, such as ciprofloxacin, levofloxacin, or gatifloxacin; 2nd-generation cephalosporins, such as cefuroxime or cefaclor; and extended-spectrum macrolides, such as azithromycin, clarithromycin, or telithromycin. These drugs are effective against β-lactamase–producing strains of *H. influenzae* and *M. catarrhalis* but have not been shown to be more effective than first-line drugs for most patients. Patients can be taught to recognize a change in sputum from normal to purulent as a sign of impending exacerbation and to start a 10- to 14-day course of antibiotic therapy. Long-term antibiotic prophylaxis is recommended only for patients with underlying structural changes in the lung, such as bronchiectasis or infected bullae.

α_1-ANTITRYPSIN DEFICIENCY

α_1-Antitrypsin deficiency is congenital lack of a primary lung antiprotease—α_1-antitrypsin—leading to increased protease tissue destruction and emphysema in adults. Hepatic accumulation of abnormal α_1-antitrypsin can cause liver disease in both children and adults. Serum α_1-antitrypsin level < 11 µmol/L (80 mg/dL) confirms the diagnosis. Treatment is smoking cessation, bronchodilators, early treatment of infection, and, in selected cases, α_1-antitrypsin replacement. Severe liver disease may require transplantation. Prognosis is related mainly to degree of lung impairment.

α_1-Antitrypsin is a neutrophil elastase inhibitor (an antiprotease), the major function of which is to protect the lungs from protease-mediated tissue destruction. Most α_1-antitrypsin is synthesized by liver cells and monocytes and passively diffuses through the circulation into the lungs; some is secondarily produced by alveolar macrophages and epithelial cells. The protein conformation (and, hence, functionality) and quantity of circulating α_1-antitrypsin is determined by codominant expression of parental alleles; > 90 different alleles have been identified and described by protease inhibitor (PI*) phenotype.

Inheritance of some variant alleles causes a change in conformation of the α_1-antitrypsin molecule, leading to polymerization and retention within hepatocytes. The hepatic accumulation of aberrant α_1-antitrypsin molecules causes neonatal cholestatic jaundice in 10 to 20% of patients; the remainder are probably able to degrade the abnormal protein, although the exact protective mechanism is unclear. About 20% of cases of neonatal hepatic involvement result in development of cirrhosis in childhood. About 10% without childhood liver disease develop cirrhosis as adults. Liver involvement increases the risk of liver cancer.

In the lung, α_1-antitrypsin deficiency increases neutrophil elastase activity, which facilitates tissue destruction leading to emphysema (especially in smokers, because cigarette smoke also increases protease activity). α_1-Antitrypsin deficiency is estimated to account for 1 to 2% of all cases of COPD.

Other disorders possibly associated with α_1-antitrypsin variants include panniculitis, life-threatening hemorrhage (through a mutation that converts α_1-antitrypsin from a neutrophil elastase to a coagulation factor inhibitor), aneurysms, ulcerative colitis, and glomerular disease.

Epidemiology and Classification

More than 95% of people with severe α_1-antitrypsin deficiency and emphysema are homozygous for the Z allele (PI*ZZ) and have α_1-antitrypsin levels of about 30 to 40 mg/dL (5 to 6 μmol/L). Prevalence in the normal population is 1/1500 to 5000. Most are whites of Northern European descent; the Z allele is rare in Asians and blacks. Though emphysema is common in PI*ZZ patients, many nonsmoking homozygotes do not develop emphysema; those who do typically have a family history of COPD. PI*ZZ smokers have a lower life expectancy than PI*ZZ nonsmokers, who have a lower life expectancy than PI*MM nonsmokers and smokers. Nonsmoking PI*MZ heterozygotes may be at increased risk of developing a more rapid fall in FEV_1 over time than do normal subjects.

Other rare phenotypes include PI*SZ and two types with nonexpressing alleles, PI*Z-null and PI*null-null (see TABLE 49–3). The null phenotype leads to undetectable serum levels of α_1-antitrypsin. Normal serum levels of malfunctioning α_1-antitrypsin may be seen with rare mutations.

TABLE 49–3. EXPRESSION OF PHENOTYPE IN α_1-ANTITRYPSIN DEFICIENCY

PHENOTYPE	α_1-ANTITRYPSIN SERUM LEVEL	RISK OF EMPHYSEMA
PI*ZZ	2.5–7 μmol/L	High
PI*MZ	17–33 μmol/L	Minimally increased
PI*SZ	8–16 μmol/L	Slightly increased
PI*SS	15–33 μmol/L	Minimally increased
PI*null-null	0	High
PI*Z-null	0–5 μmol/L	High
PI*MM	20–48 μmol/L	Normal

Symptoms and Signs

Infants with hepatic involvement present with cholestatic jaundice and hepatomagaly during the first week of life; jaundice usually resolves by 2 to 4 mo of age. Cirrhosis may develop in childhood or adulthood (symptoms and signs of cirrhosis and hepatocellular carcinoma are discussed elsewhere in THE MANUAL).

α_1-Antitrypsin deficiency most commonly causes early emphysema; symptoms and signs are those of COPD (see p. 401). Lung involvement occurs earlier in smokers than in nonsmokers but in both cases is rare before age 25. Severity of pulmonary disease varies greatly; pulmonary function is well preserved in some PI*ZZ smokers and can be severely impaired in some PI*ZZ nonsmokers. PI*ZZ people identified in population surveys (ie, those without symptoms or pulmonary disease) tend to have better pulmonary function, whether they smoke or not, than do index people (those identified because they have pulmonary disease). As a group, nonindex people with severe α_1-antitrypsin deficiency who have never smoked have a normal life expectancy and only moderate impairment of pulmonary function. Airflow obstruction occurs more frequently in men and in people with asthma, recurrent respiratory infections, occupational dust exposure, and a family history of pulmonary disease. The most common cause of death in α_1-antitrypsin deficiency is emphysema, followed by cirrhosis, often with hepatic carcinoma.

Panniculitis, an inflammatory disease of subcutaneous soft tissue, manifests as indurated, tender, discolored plaques or nodules, typically on the lower abdomen, buttocks, and thighs (see p. 976).

Diagnosis

α_1-Antitrypsin deficiency is suspected in smokers who develop emphysema before age 45; in nonsmokers without occupational exposures who develop emphysema at any age; in patients with predominately lower lung emphysema (as shown on chest x-ray); in patients with a family history of emphysema or unexplained cirrhosis; in patients with panniculitis; in newborns with jaundice or liver enzyme elevations; and in any patient with unexplained liver disease. Diagnosis is confirmed by serum α_1-antitrypsin levels < 80 mg/dL (< 11 μmol/L).

Treatment

Treatment of pulmonary disease is with purified human α_1-antitrypsin (60 mg/kg IV over 45 to 60 min given once weekly, or 250 mg/kg over 4 to 6 h given once monthly [pooled only]), which can maintain the serum α_1-antitrypsin level above a target protective level of 80 mg/dL (35% of normal). Because emphysema produces permanent structural change, therapy cannot improve damaged lung structure or function but is given to halt progression. Treatment is extremely expensive and is therefore reserved for nonsmoking patients with mild to moderately abnormal pulmonary function and serum α_1-antitrypsin < 80 mg/dL (< 11 μmol/L). It is not indicated for patients who have severe disease or for patients with normal or heterozygous phenotypes.

Smoking cessation, use of bronchodilators, and early treatment of respiratory infections are particularly important for α_1-antitrypsin–deficient patients with emphysema. Experimental treatments, such as phenylbutyric acid that can reverse the misfolding of the abnormal α_1-antitrypsin proteins in the hepatocytes, thereby stimulating protein release, are being investigated. For severely impaired people < 60 yr, lung transplantation should be considered. Lung volume reduction in treating the emphysema of α_1-antitrypsin deficiency is controversial. Gene therapy is under study.

Treatment of liver disease is supportive. Enzyme replacement does not help because the disease is caused by abnormal processing rather than by enzyme deficiency. Liver transplantation may be used for patients with liver failure.

Treatment of panniculitis is not well defined. Corticosteroids, antimalarials, and tetracyclines have been used.

50 PULMONARY EMBOLISM

Pulmonary embolism is the occlusion of one or more pulmonary arteries by thrombi that originate elsewhere, typically in the large veins of the lower extremities or pelvis. Risk factors are conditions that impair venous return and that cause endothelial injury or dysfunction, especially in patients with an underlying hypercoagulable state. Symptoms include dyspnea, pleuritic chest pain, cough, and, in severe cases, syncope or cardiorespiratory arrest. Signs are nonspecific and may include tachypnea, tachycardia, hypotension, and loud pulmonic component of the 2nd heart sound. Diagnosis is based on a ventilation/perfusion scan, a CT angiogram, or a pulmonary arteriogram. Treatment is with anticoagulants, thrombolytics, and, occasionally, surgery to remove the clot.

Pulmonary embolism (PE) affects an estimated 650,000 people and causes up to 200,000 deaths/yr, accounting for an estimated 15% of all hospital deaths/yr. The incidence of PE in children is about 5/10,000 admissions.

Etiology and Pathophysiology

Nearly all PEs arise from thrombi in the lower extremity or pelvic veins (deep venous thrombosis [DVT]—see p. 754). Thrombi in either system may be occult. Thromboemboli can also originate in upper extremity veins or in right cardiac chambers. Risk factors for DVT and PE are similar in children and adults and include conditions that impair venous return or that cause endothelial injury or dysfunction particularly in patients with an underlying baseline hypercoagulable state (see TABLE 50–1). Bed rest and confinement without walking, even for a few hours, are common precipitators.

Once DVT develops, the clot may dislodge and travel through the venous system and right heart to lodge in the pulmonary arteries, where it partially or completely occludes one or more vessels. The consequences depend on the size and number of emboli, the pulmonary reaction, and the ability of the body's intrinsic thrombolytic system to dissolve the clot.

Small emboli may have no acute physiologic effects; many begin to lyse immediately and resolve within hours or days. Larger emboli can cause a reflex increase in ventilation (tachypnea); hypoxemia from ventilation/perfusion (V/Q) mismatch and shunting; atelectasis from alveolar hypocapnia and abnormalities in surfactant; and an increase in pulmonary vascular resistance caused by mechanical obstruction and vasoconstriction. Endogenous lysis reduces most emboli, even those of moderate size, without treatment, and physiologic alterations decrease over hours or days. Some emboli resist lysis and may organize and persist. Occasionally, chronic residual obstruction leads to pulmonary hypertension (chronic thromboembolic pulmonary hypertension) that may develop over years and result in chronic right heart failure. When large emboli occlude major arteries, or when many small emboli occlude > 50% of the distal arterial system, right ventricular pressure increases, causing acute right ventricular failure, failure with shock (massive PE), or sudden death in severe cases. The risk of death depends on the degree and rate of rise of right-sided pressures and on the patient's underlying cardiopulmonary status; higher pressures more commonly occur in patients with preexisting cardiopulmonary disease. Healthy patients may survive a PE that occludes > 50% of the pulmonary vascular bed.

Pulmonary infarction occurs in < 10% of patients diagnosed with PE. This low rate has been attributed to the dual blood supply to the lung (ie, bronchial and pulmonary). Infarction is typically characterized by a radiographic infiltrate, chest pain, fever, and, occasionally, hemoptysis.

Nonthrombotic PE: PE from a variety of nonthrombotic sources causes clinical syndromes that differ from thrombotic PE.

TABLE 50–1. RISK FACTORS FOR DEEP VENOUS THROMBOSIS AND PULMONARY EMBOLISM

- Age > 60 yr
- Atrial fibrillation
- Cigarette smoking (including passive smoke)
- Estrogen receptor modulators (raloxifene, tamoxifen)
- Extremity trauma
- Heart failure*
- Hypercoagulability disorders*
  - Antiphospholipid antibody syndrome
  - Antithrombin III deficiency
  - Factor V Leiden mutation (activated protein C resistance)
  - Heparin-induced thrombocytopenia and thrombosis
  - Hereditary fibrinolytic defects
  - Hyperhomocystinemia
  - Increase in factor VIII
  - Increase in factor XI
  - Increase in von Willebrand's factor
  - Paroxysmal nocturnal hemoglobinuria
  - Protein C deficiency
  - Protein S deficiency
  - Prothrombin G-A gene variant
  - Tissue factor pathway inhibitor
- Immobilization*
- Indwelling venous catheters
- Malignancy*
- Myeloproliferative disease (hyperviscosity)
- Nephrotic syndrome
- Obesity
- Oral contraceptives/estrogen replacement
- Pregnancy and postpartum*
- Prior venous thromboembolism
- Sickle cell anemia
- Surgery within past 3 mo*

*One of the most common risk factors.

Air embolism is caused by introduction of large amounts of air into systemic veins or into the right heart, which then move to the pulmonary arterial system. Causes include surgery, blunt or barometric trauma (such as from mechanical ventilation), defective or uncapped venous catheters, and rapid decompression after underwater diving. Microbubble formation in the pulmonary circulation may cause endothelial damage, hypoxemia, and diffuse infiltrates. In large volume air embolism, pulmonary outflow tract obstruction may occur, which can be rapidly fatal.

Fat embolism is caused by introduction of fat or bone marrow particles into the systemic venous system and then to pulmonary arteries. Causes include long bone fractures, orthopedic procedures, microvascular occlusion or necrosis of bone marrow in patients with sickle cell crisis, and, rarely, toxic modification of native or parenteral serum lipids. Fat embolism causes a pulmonary syndrome similar to the acute respiratory distress syndrome, with severe hypoxemia of rapid onset often accompanied by neurologic changes and a petechial rash.

Amniotic fluid embolism is a rare syndrome caused by introduction of amniotic fluid into the maternal venous and then pulmonary arterial system associated with labor (see p. 2205). The syndrome can occasionally occur during prepartum uterine manipulations. Patients can have cardiac and respiratory distress due to anaphylaxis, vasoconstriction causing acute severe pulmonary hypertension, and direct pulmonary microvascular toxicity.

Septic embolism occurs when infected material embolizes to the lung. Causes include drug use, right-sided infective endocarditis, and septic thrombophlebitis. Septic embolism causes symptoms and signs of pneumonia or sepsis and is initially associated with nodular opacities on the chest x-ray, which may progress to peripheral infiltrates and may cavitate.

Foreign body embolism is caused by introduction of particulate matter into the pulmonary arterial system, usually by IV injection of inorganic substances such as talc by heroin users or elemental mercury by patients with mental disorders.

Tumor embolism is a rare complication of malignancy (usually adenocarcinomas) in which neoplastic cells from an organ enter the systemic venous and pulmonary arterial system, where they lodge, proliferate, and obstruct flow. Patients typically present with symptoms of dyspnea and pleuritic chest pain and signs of cor pulmonale that develop over weeks to months. Diagnosis, which is suggested by micronodules or diffuse pulmonary infiltrates, can be confirmed by biopsy or occasionally by cytologic aspiration and histologic study of pulmonary capillary blood.

Systemic gas embolism is a rare syndrome that occurs when barotrauma during mechanical ventilation with high airway pressure leads to air dissection from lung parenchyma in the pulmonary venous and then systemic arterial system. Gas emboli cause CNS changes (including stroke), cardiac injury, and shoulder or anterior chest livedo reticularis. Diagnosis is based on exclusion of other vascular processes in the setting of recognized barotrauma.

Symptoms and Signs

Most PEs are small, physiologically insignificant, and asymptomatic. Even when present, symptoms are nonspecific and vary in frequency and intensity, depending on the extent of pulmonary vascular occlusion and preexisting cardiopulmonary function.

Larger emboli cause acute dyspnea and pleuritic chest pain and, less commonly, cough and/or hemoptysis. Massive PE presents with hypotension, tachycardia, syncope, or cardiac arrest.

The most common signs of PE are tachycardia and tachypnea. Less commonly, patients have hypotension, a loud 2nd heart sound (S_2) due to a loud pulmonic component (P_2), and/or crackles or wheezing. In the presence of right ventricular failure, distended internal jugular veins and a right ventricular heave may be evident, and right ventricular gallop (3rd and 4th heart sounds [S_3 and S_4]), with or without tricuspid regurgitation, may be audible. Fever can occur; DVT and PE are often overlooked causes of fever.

Chronic thromboembolic pulmonary hypertension causes symptoms and signs of right heart failure, including exertional dyspnea, easy fatigue, and peripheral edema that develops over months to years.

Diagnosis

Diagnosis is challenging, because symptoms and signs are nonspecific and diagnostic tests are either imperfect or invasive. Diagnosis starts by including PE in the differential diagnosis of a large number of conditions with similar symptoms, including cardiac ischemia, heart failure, COPD exacerbation, pneumothorax, pneumonia, sepsis, acute chest syndrome (in sickle cell patients), and acute anxiety with hyperventilation. Initial evaluation should include pulse oximetry, ECG, and chest x-ray. The chest x-ray usually is nonspecific but may show atelectasis, focal infiltrates, an elevated hemidiaphragm, and/or a pleural effusion. The classic findings of focal loss of vascular markings (Westermark's sign), a peripheral wedge-shaped density (Hampton's hump), or enlargement of the right descending pulmonary artery (Palla's sign) are suggestive but very insensitive.

Pulse oximetry provides a quick way to assess oxygenation; hypoxemia is one sign of PE, and other significant disorders must be investigated.

ECG most often shows tachycardia and various ST-T wave abnormalities, which are not specific for PE (see FIG. 50–1). An $S_1Q_3T_3$ or a new right bundle branch block may indicate the effect of abrupt rise in right ventricular pressure on right ventricular conduction; these are specific but insensitive, occurring in only about 5% of patients. Right axis deviation ($R > S$ in V_1) and P-pulmonale may be present. T-wave inversion in leads V_1 to V_4 also occurs.

Clinical probability of PE can be assessed by combining ECG and chest x-ray findings with those from the history and physical examination (see TABLE 50–2). Patients with a low clinical probability of PE may need no or only minimal additional testing. Patients with an intermediate clinical probability need additional testing. Patients with a high probability may be candidates for immediate treatment pending confirmation with additional testing.

Noninvasive testing: Noninvasive testing typically can be obtained more quickly and carries less morbidity than invasive testing. Tests most useful for diagnosing or excluding PE are D-dimer testing, V/Q scanning, duplex ultrasonography, helical CT scanning, and echocardiography.

There is no universally accepted algorithm for the best choice and sequence of tests, but one common approach is to screen with the D-dimer, obtain lower extremity ultrasonography when the D-dimer is positive, and progress to CT or V/Q if the duplex is negative. Patients with moderate to high probability of disease based on clinical criteria who have low or intermediate probability V/Q scans usually require pulmonary arteriography or helical CT to make or exclude the diagnosis. A positive lower extremity ultrasound establishes the need for anticoagulation and obviates the need for further diagnostic testing. A negative ultrasound study does not negate the need for additional studies. Positive D-dimers, ECG, ABG measurements, chest x-ray, and echocardiograms are adjunctive tests that lack sufficient specificity to be diagnostic alone.

D-dimer is a by-product of intrinsic fibrinolysis; thus elevated levels suggest recent presence of a thrombus. The test is extremely sensitive; > 90% of patients with DVT/PE have elevated levels. However, a positive result is not specific for venous thrombus because many patients without DVT/PE also have elevated levels. In contrast, a low D-dimer has a negative predictive value of > 90%, making it useful for excluding DVT/PE, especially when initial estimates of likelihood of disease are < 50%. Documented cases of PE have occurred in the context of negative D-dimers using older enzyme-linked immunosorbent assays, but newer highly specific and rapid assays make a negative D-dimer sufficiently reliable for excluding the diagnosis of PE in routine practice.

V/Q scans detect areas of lung that are ventilated but not perfused, as occurs in PE; results are reported as low, intermediate, or high probability of PE based on patterns of V/Q mismatch. A completely normal scan essentially excludes PE with nearly 100% accuracy, but a low-probability scan still carries a 15% likelihood of PE. Perfusion deficits may occur in many other lung conditions, including pleural effusion, chest mass, pulmonary hypertension, pneumonia, and COPD.

Duplex ultrasonography is a safe, noninvasive, portable technique for detecting lower extremity (primarily femoral vein) thrombi. A clot can be detected in up to 3 ways: by visualizing the lining of the vein, by demonstrating incompressibility of the vein, and by demonstrating reduced flow by Doppler. The test has a sensitivity of > 90% and a specificity of > 95% for thrombus. It cannot reliably detect a clot in calf or iliac veins. Absence of thrombi in the femoral veins does not exclude the possibility of thrombus from other sources, but patients with negative duplex test results have > 95% event-free survival, because thrombi from other sources are so much less common. Ultrasonography has been incorporated into many diagnostic algorithms, because an ultrasound positive for femoral vein thrombosis indicates the need for anticoagulation, which may make further testing for PE or other thrombi unnecessary.

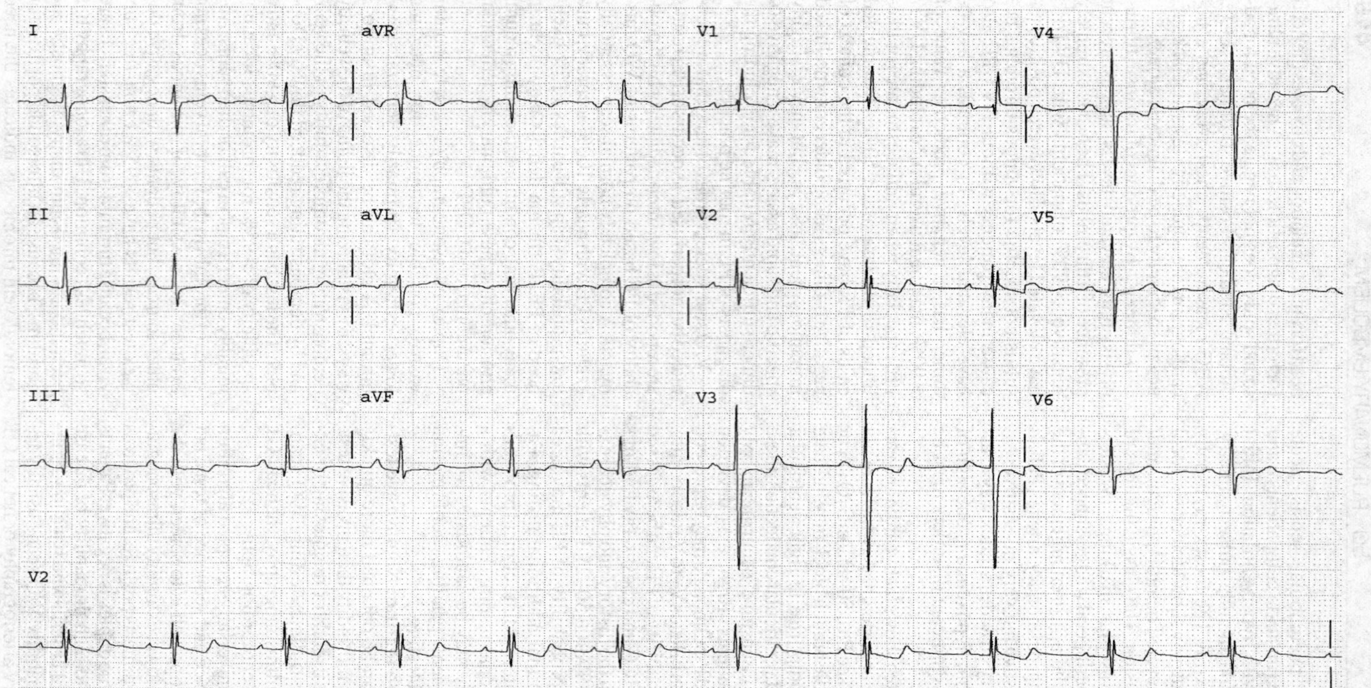

Fig. 50–1. ECG in pulmonary embolism. ECG shows sinus rhythm at a rate of 75 beats/min; S wave in lead I with Q-wave, T-wave inversion, and ST-segment elevation in lead III ($S_1Q_3T_3$); and QRS right axis deviation with R-wave amplitude greater than S-wave amplitude in lead V_1. There are peaked P waves in lead II.

TABLE 50–2. CLINICAL PREDICTION RULE FOR DIAGNOSING PULMONARY EMBOLISM

I. Establish clinical probability—add risks to determine probability

CLINICAL RISK	POINTS
Clinical signs and symptoms of DVT (objective leg swelling, pain with palpation)	3
PE as or more likely than alternative diagnosis	3
Heart rate > 100 beats/min	1.5
Immobilization ≥ 3 days	1.5
Surgery in previous 4 wk	1.5
Previous DVT or PE	1.5
Hemoptysis	1
Malignancy (including those stopping cancer treatment within 6 mo)	1
High probability: > 6	
Moderate probability: 2–6	
Low probability: < 2	

II. Use pretest probability to determine testing

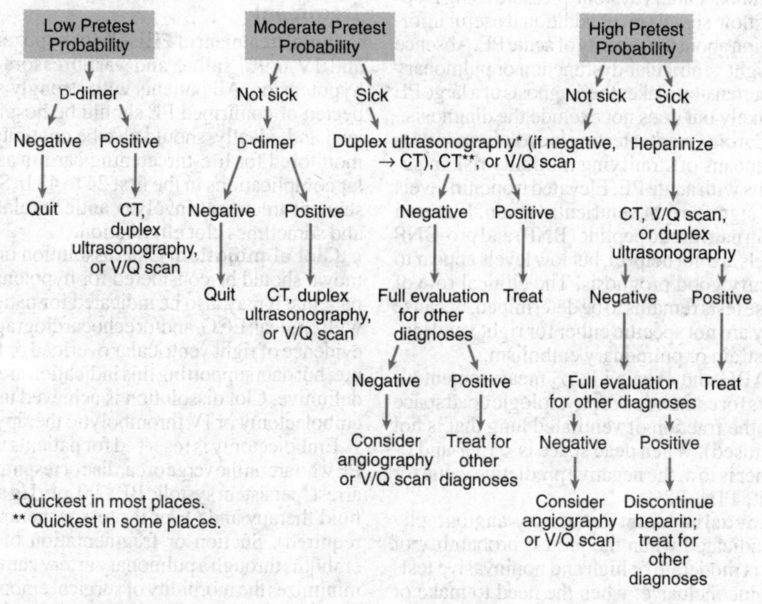

DVT = Deep venous thrombosis; PE = pulmonary embolism; V/Q = ventilation/perfusion.

Contrast helical (spiral) CT scanning is an alternative to V/Q scanning and pulmonary arteriography in many settings because it is fast, available, and noninvasive and gives more information about other lung pathology. However, the patient must be able to hold his breath for several seconds. The sensitivity of CT is highest for PE in lobar and segmental vessels and lowest for emboli in smaller subsegmental vessels (about 30% of all PEs) and thus is less sensitive than perfusion scans (60% vs > 99%). It is also less specific than pulmonary arteriograms (90% vs > 95%), because visual artifacts can result from incomplete mixing of contrast. A positive scan may be diagnostic of PE, but a negative scan does not necessarily exclude subsegmental disease, though the clinical significance of emboli in smaller subsegmental vessels remains to be determined. New scanners with higher resolution are likely to improve the diagnostic accuracy, thereby replacing perfusion scans and arteriograms.

Echocardiography as a diagnostic test for PE is controversial. Its sensitivity is > 80% for detecting right ventricular dysfunction (eg, dilation and hypokinesis, which occur where pulmonary artery pressure exceeds 40 mm Hg). This is a useful measure of hemodynamic severity in acute PE, but right ventricular dysfunction is present in multiple conditions, including COPD, heart failure, and sleep apnea and is therefore a nonspecific finding. Estimation of pulmonary artery systolic pressure using Doppler flow signals gives additional useful information about the severity of acute PE. Absence of right ventricular dysfunction or pulmonary hypertension makes the diagnosis of a large PE unlikely but does not exclude the diagnosis.

Cardiac marker testing is evolving as a useful means of stratifying mortality risk in patients with acute PE. Elevated troponin levels can signify right ventricular strain. Elevated brain natriuretic peptide (BNP) and pro-BNP levels are not helpful, but low levels appear to signify good prognosis. The clinical role of these tests remains to be determined, because they are not specific either for right ventricular strain or pulmonary embolism.

ABG and exhaled P_{CO_2} measurement allows for estimation of physiologic dead space (ie, the fraction of ventilated lung that is not perfused). When dead space is < 15% and D-dimer is low, the negative predictive value for acute PE is 98%.

Invasive tests: Pulmonary angiography is indicated when the pretest probability of PE is moderate or high and noninvasive tests are inconclusive; when the need to make or exclude the diagnosis is urgent, such as in an acutely ill patient; and when anticoagulation is contraindicated.

Pulmonary arteriography is still the most accurate test for diagnosing PE, but it is needed much less often because of the sensitivity of ultrasonography and helical CT. An arteriogram with intraluminal filling defects or abrupt cut-off of flow is positive. Findings suggestive but not diagnostic of PE include partial occlusion of pulmonary arterial branches with increased proximal and decreased distal caliber, oligemic zones, and persistence of dye in the proximal artery during the late (venous) phase of the arteriogram. In lung segments with obstructed arteries, venous filling with contrast medium is delayed or absent.

Prognosis

An estimated 10% of patients with PE die within 1 h. Of those who survive the 1st hour, only about 30% are diagnosed and receive treatment; > 95% of these patients survive. Thus, most mortality from PE occurs in patients who are never diagnosed, and the best prospects for reducing mortality lie in improving diagnosis, not in improving treatment. Patients with chronic thromboembolic disease represent a tiny fraction of patients with PE who survive. Anticoagulant therapy reduces the rate of recurrence of PE to about 5% in all patients.

Treatment

Initial treatment of PE is O_2 for hypoxemia and IV 0.9% saline and vasopressors for hypotension. All patients with strongly suspected or confirmed PE should be hospitalized and, ideally, should also be continually monitored for life-threatening cardiovascular complications in the first 24 to 48 h. Subsequent treatment involves anticoagulation and sometimes clot elimination.

Clot elimination: Clot dissolution or removal should be considered for hypotensive patients. It may also be indicated for patients with clinical, ECG, and/or echocardiographic evidence of right ventricular overload or failure, but data supporting this indication are not definitive. Clot dissolution is achieved using embolectomy or IV thrombolytic therapy.

Embolectomy is reserved for patients with PE who are on the verge of cardiac or respiratory arrest (persistent systolic BP ≤ 90 mm Hg after fluid therapy and O_2 or if pressor therapy is required). Suction or fragmentation of the embolus through a pulmonary artery catheter minimizes the morbidity of surgical embolectomy but with undocumented advantages in efficacy. Surgical embolectomy appears to improve survival in patients with massive PE but is not widely available and is associated with substantial mortality. The decision to proceed with embolectomy and the choice of technique depends on local resources and expertise.

Thrombolytic therapy with tissue plasminogen activator (tPA), streptokinase, or urokinase offers a noninvasive way to rapidly restore pulmonary blood flow but is controversial, because long-term benefits do not clearly outweigh the risk of hemorrhage. Thrombolytics speed the resolution of radiographic abnormalities and hemodynamic function (heart rate and right ventricular function) and prevent cardiopulmonary deterioration in patients with submassive PE but have not been shown to improve survival. Thrombolytics are recommended by some for normotensive PE patients with echocardiographic evidence of proximal pulmonary artery (large) embolism or of right ventricular dysfunction due to PE or preexisting disease. Others reserve thrombolytic therapy for patients with massive PE (hypotension, hypoxemia, or obstruction of 2 or more lobar arteries). Absolute contraindications to thrombolytics include prior hemorrhagic stroke; active bleeding from any source; intracranial trauma or surgery within 2 mo; recent femoral or large arterial puncture; GI bleeding, including guaiac-positive stools (< 6 mo); and CPR. Relative contraindications include recent surgery (≤ 10 days), hemorrhagic diathesis (as in hepatic insufficiency), pregnancy, and severe hypertension (systolic BP > 180 or diastolic BP > 110 mm Hg).

Options for thrombolysis include streptokinase, urokinase, and alteplase (recombinant tPA). No agent is proven superior. Standard IV regimens are streptokinase 250,000 units over 30 min followed by continuous infusion of 100,000 units/h for 24 h; urokinase 4400 units/kg over 10 min followed by 4400 units/kg/h for 12 h; or alteplase 100 mg continuous infusion over 2 h followed by an additional 40 mg over another 4 h (10 mg/h) if clinical presentation and repeat pulmonary angiogram suggests failure of clot lysis and initial dosing does not cause bleeding. Streptokinase is now rarely used because it is associated with allergic and pyrogenic reactions and requires constant infusion.

An initial loading dose of heparin should be given concurrently, but the activated PTT should be allowed to fall to 1.5 to 2.5 times the baseline value before beginning continuous infusion. Direct delivery of thrombolytics to the clot via a pulmonary artery catheter is occasionally used for patients with massive PE or for those with relative contraindications to systemic thrombolytics, but this approach does not prevent systemic thrombolysis. Bleeding, if it occurs, can be reversed with cryoprecipitate or fresh frozen plasma and compression of vascular access sites.

Anticoagulation: Because venous thromboses rarely embolize completely, anticoagulation is required acutely to prevent residual clots from extending and embolizing. Patients in whom anticoagulants are contraindicated or those who have thromboemboli despite therapeutic anticoagulation should have placement of a percutaneous inferior vena cava filter.

Heparin, either unfractionated or low mol wt, is the mainstay of treatment of acute DVT and PE and should be given immediately on diagnosis or sooner if clinical suspicion is high; inadequate anticoagulation in the first 24 h is linked to increased risk of recurrent PE for up to 3 mo. Heparin accelerates the action of antithrombin III, an inhibitor of coagulation factors; unfractionated heparin also has antithrombin III–mediated anti-inflammatory properties, which may facilitate clot organization and reduce thrombophlebitis. Unfractionated heparin should be given as a bolus and infusion by protocol (see TABLE 50–3) to achieve an activated PTT 1.5 to 2.5 times that of normal control. Subcutaneous low mol wt heparin (LMWH) is as efficacious as unfractionated heparin and may cause less thrombocytopenia. Because of its long half-life, it is useful in out-

TABLE 50–3. WEIGHT-BASED NOMOGRAM FOR HEPARIN

1. Heparin bolus 80 units/kg, followed by
2. Heparin infusion 18 units/kg/h*
3. Check PTT 6 h after bolus
4. Adjust heparin as needed:

PTT (sec)	Infusion Rate Change (mL/h)*
< 35	Repeat 80 units/kg bolus, increase rate by 4 units/kg/h
35–45	Repeat 80 units/kg bolus, increase rate by 2 units/kg/h
46–70	No change
71–90	Reduce rate by 2 units/kg/h
> 90	Hold infusion for 1 h, reduce rate by 3 units/kg/h

5. Check PTT 6 h after dosage change; when two consecutive PTTs are therapeutic, check q 24 h.

*Heparin concentration = 40 units/mL, usually as 20,000 units/500 mL.

Adapted from Raschke RA et al. *Annals of Internal Medicine* 119:874–881, 1993.

patient treatment of DVT and to facilitate earlier discharge of patients who have not achieved therapeutic anticoagulation with warfarin.

All heparins can cause bleeding, thrombocytopenia, urticaria, and, rarely, thrombosis or anaphylaxis. Long-term heparin administration may cause hypokalemia, liver enzyme elevations, and osteoporosis. Patients should be screened for bleeding with serial CBCs and tests for occult blood in stool. Bleeding caused by overheparinization can be stopped with a maximum of 50 mg of protamine per 5000 units unfractionated heparin (or 1 mg in 20 mL normal saline infused over 10 to 20 min for LMWH, though the precise dose is undefined because protamine only partially neutralizes LMWH inactivation of factor Xa). Treatment with heparin or LMWH is continued until full anticoagulation has been achieved with oral warfarin. The use of LMWH in long-term anticoagulation after acute PE has not been studied but will likely be limited by cost and ease of administration compared with oral warfarin.

Warfarin is the oral drug of choice for long-term anticoagulation in all patients except pregnant women and patients with new or worsening venous thromboembolism during warfarin treatment. Five to 10 mg po once/day should be started within 48 h of onset of effective heparinization or, in the rare patient with protein C deficiency, only after therapeutic anticoagulation is achieved. The therapeutic goal is usually an INR of 2 to 3.

Physicians prescribing warfarin should be wary of multiple drug interactions, including interactions with nonprescription medicinal herbs. Patients with transient risk factors for DVT or PE (eg, fracture or surgery) can stop the drug after 3 to 6 mo. Patients with nontransient risk factors (eg, hypercoagulability), no known risk factors, or recurrent DVT or PE should take warfarin for at least 6 mo and possibly for life unless complications of therapy intervene. In low-risk patients, low-intensity warfarin (to maintain INR at 1.5 to 2.0) may be safe and effective for at least 2 to 4 yr, but this regimen requires further proof of safety before it can be routinely recommended. Bleeding is the most common complication of warfarin treatment; patients > 65 and those with comorbidities (especially diabetes, recent MI, Hct < 30%, creatinine > 1.5 mg/dL) and a history of stroke or GI bleeding appear to be at greatest risk. Bleeding can be reversed with 2.5 to 10 mg of vitamin K sc or po and, in an emergency, with fresh frozen plasma. Vitamin K may cause flushing, local pain, and, rarely, anaphylaxis.

Inferior vena cava filter (IVCF) placement is reserved for patients with contraindications to anticoagulation and thrombolysis, with recurrent emboli on adequate anticoagulation, or after pulmonary embolectomy. Several kinds of filters are available, differing in size and retrievability. The filter is placed via catheterization of the internal jugular or femoral veins; optimum location is just below the entry of the renal veins. Filters reduce acute and subacute thrombotic complications but are associated with longer term complications; for example, venous collaterals can develop and provide a pathway by which PE can still occur around the filter. Patients with recurrent DVT or chronic risks for DVT may therefore still require anticoagulation; the filters provide some protection until contraindications to anticoagulation subside or resolve. Despite widespread use of filters, efficacy in preventing PE is unstudied and unproven.

Prevention

Prevention of PE means prevention of DVT; the need depends on the patient's risks. Bed-bound patients and those undergoing surgical, especially orthopedic, procedures especially benefit, and most of these patients can be identified before a thrombus forms (see TABLE 50–4). Preventive drugs include low-dose unfractionated heparin (LDUH), LMWH, warfarin, newer anticoagulants, compression devices, and stockings.

Choice of drug or device depends on duration of treatment, contraindications, relative costs, and ease of use.

LDUH is given in doses of 5000 units sc 2 h preoperatively and q 8 to 12 h thereafter for 7 to 10 days or until the patient is fully ambulatory. Immobilized patients not undergoing surgery should receive 5000 units sc q 12 h indefinitely or until reversal of risk.

LMWH dosing depends on the drug; enoxaparin 30 mg sc q 12 h, dalteparin 2500 units once/day, and tinzaparin 3500 units once/day are 3 of many equally effective LMWHs that are as efficacious as LDUH for preventing DVT and PE.

Warfarin is usually effective and safe at a dose of 2 to 5 mg once/day or at a dose adjusted to maintain an INR of 1.5 to 2.

Newer anticoagulants, including hirudin, a subcutaneous direct thrombin inhibitor; ximelagatran (melagatran), an oral direct thrombin inhibitor; and danaparoid and fondaparinux, which are selective factor Xa

TABLE 50–4. RISK OF DEEP VENOUS THROMBOSIS AND PULMONARY EMBOLISM IN SURGICAL PATIENTS

RISK CATEGORY	EXAMPLES	PREVENTIVE MEASURES	RISK OF DVT/PE (%)			
			Calf	Proximal	PE	Fatal PE
Low	Minor surgery* in patients < 40 yr with no clinical risk factors	None except early and aggressive ambulation	2	0.4	0.2	0.002
Moderate	Minor surgery in patients with risk factors; minor surgery in patients 40–60 yr with no clinical risk factors; major surgery in patients < 40 yr with no other clinical risk factors	LDUH q 12 h, LMWH, IPC, or elastic stockings	10–20	2–4	1–2	0.1–0.4
High	Minor surgery in patients > 60 yr or 40–60 with risk factors; major surgery in patients > 40 yr or with other clinical risk factors	LDUH q 8 h, LMWH, or IPC	20–40	4–8	2–4	0.4–1.0
Very high	Major surgery in patients > 40 yr with previous venous thromboembolic, malignant, or hypercoagulable condition; hip or knee arthroplasty or hip fracture surgery; major trauma; spinal cord injury	LMWH, oral anticoagulation, IPC/elastic stockings plus either LDUH q 8 h or LMWH	40–80	10–20	4–10	0.2–5

DVT = Deep venous thrombosis; PE = pulmonary embolism; LDUH = low-dose unfractionated heparin; LMWH = low mol wt heparin; IPC = intermittent pneumatic compression.

*Minor surgery is defined here as an operation that does not involve general anesthesia or respiratory assistance.

Adapted with permission from Geerts WH, Heit JA, Clagett GP, et al: Prevention of venous thromboembolism. *Chest* 119:132S–175S, 2001.

inhibitors, have demonstrated efficacy in DVT and PE prevention but warrant further study to determine their cost-effectiveness and safety relative to heparins and warfarin. Aspirin is better than placebo but worse than all other available drugs for preventing DVT and PE (see also TABLE 50–5).

Intermittent pneumatic compression (IPC) provides rhythmic external compression to the legs or to the legs and thighs. It is more effective for preventing calf than proximal DVT and thus is considered inadequate after hip or knee surgery. IPC is contraindicated in obese patients and can theoretically trigger PE in immobilized patients who have developed occult DVT while not undergoing preventive treatment.

Graded elastic stockings are of questionable benefit except in low-risk surgical patients. However, combining stockings with other prophylactic measures may be more protective than any single approach.

For surgical procedures with a high incidence of venous thromboembolism, such as hip and lower extremity orthopedic surgery

TABLE 50–5. ANTICOAGULATION OPTIONS IN THROMBOEMBOLIC DISEASE

CATEGORY	DOSE	COMMENTS
Heparins		
Unfractionated heparin	See TABLE 50–3	
Low mol wt		
Ardeparin	50 units/kg sc q 12 h	Not for IM or IV use—not indicated for PE
Certoparin	3000 units sc daily	
Dalteparin	2500 units IV bolus	200 units/kg sc daily
Danaparoid	2000 unit IV bolus, then 750 units sc q 12 h	Heparinoid; monitor using antifactor Xa assay
Enoxaparin	1 mg/kg sc q 12 h or 1.5 mg/kg sc daily	
Nadroparin	200 units/kg sc q 12 h	
Parnaparin	3200 to 4250 units sc daily	Prophylaxis dose
Reviparin	1750 units sc daily	Prophylaxis dose
Tinzaparin	175 units/kg sc daily	
Vitamin K inhibitor		
Warfarin	5 mg daily initially, then titrate to desired INR	
Thrombin inhibitors		
Hirudin	0.75 mg/kg sc q 12 h	
Lepirudin	1.25 mg/kg sc q 12 h	
Argatroban	2 µg/kg/min IV infusion (for HIT) or 350 µg/kg IV bolus, then 25 µg/kg/min (for PCI)	
Ximelagatran (melagatran)	24 µg po q 12 h	
Factor Xa inhibitor		
Fondaparinux	2.5 mg sc daily	

PE = pulmonary embolism; HIT = heparin-induced thrombocytopenia; PCI = percutaneous coronary intervention.

(see TABLE 50–4), both LDUH and aspirin are inadequate; LMWH or adjusted-dose warfarin is recommended. For total knee replacement, risk reductions provided by LMWH and IPC are comparable, and the combination should be considered for patients with concomitant clinical risks. The regimens for orthopedic surgery may be initiated preoperatively and should be continued for at least 7 days postoperatively. In selected patients at very high risk of both venous thromboembolism and bleeding, placement of an IVCF is a prophylactic option.

A high incidence of venous thromboembolism is also associated with elective neurosurgery, acute spinal cord injury, and multiple trauma. Although physical methods (IPC, elastic stockings) have been used in neurosurgical patients because of concern about intracranial bleeding, LMWH appears to be an acceptable alternative. The combination of IPC and LMWH may be more effective than either alone in high-risk patients. Limited data support the combination of IPC, elastic stockings, and LMWH in spinal cord injury or in multiple trauma. For very high risk patients, an IVCF may be considered.

The most common nonsurgical conditions in which DVT prophylaxis is indicated are acute MI and ischemic stroke. For MI patients, LDUH is effective; IPC, elastic stockings, or both may be used when anticoagulants are contraindicated. For stroke patients, LDUH or LMWH can be used; IPC, elastic stockings, or both may be beneficial.

Recommendations for some other nonsurgical conditions include LDUH for patients with heart failure; adjusted-dose warfarin (INR 1.3 to 1.9) for patients with metastatic breast cancer; and warfarin 1 mg/day for cancer patients with an indwelling central venous catheter.

51 ACUTE BRONCHITIS

Acute bronchitis is inflammation of the upper airways, commonly following a URI. The cause is usually a viral infection though it is sometimes a bacterial infection; the pathogen is rarely identified. The most common symptom is cough with or without fever and/or sputum production. In patients with COPD, hemoptysis, burning chest pain, and hypoxemia may also occur. Diagnosis is clinical. Treatment is supportive; antibiotics are necessary only for patients with chronic lung disease. Prognosis is excellent in patients without lung disease, but in patients with COPD, acute respiratory failure may result.

Acute bronchitis is frequently a component of a URI caused by rhinovirus, parainfluenza, influenza A or B, respiratory syncytial virus, coronavirus, or other viral infection. Less common causes may be *Mycoplasma pneumoniae, Bordetella pertussis,* and *Chlamydia pneumoniae.* Patients at risk include those who smoke and those with COPD and other diseases that impair bronchial clearance mechanisms, such as cystic fibrosis or conditions leading to bronchiectasis (see p. 439).

Symptoms, Signs, and Diagnosis

Symptoms are a nonproductive or minimally productive cough accompanied or preceded by URI symptoms. Subjective dyspnea results from chest pain with breathing, not hypoxia, except in those with underlying lung disease. Signs are often absent but may include scattered rhonchi and wheezing. Sputum may be clear, purulent, or, occasionally, bloody. Sputum characteristics do not correspond with a particular etiology (ie, viral vs bacterial).

Diagnosis is based on clinical presentation. Chest x-ray is only necessary if fever, dyspnea, or other symptoms and signs suggest pneumonia. Sputum gram stain and culture have no role.

Treatment and Prognosis

Acute bronchitis in otherwise healthy subjects is a major reason that antibiotics are overused. Nearly all patients require only symptomatic treatment, such as acetaminophen and hydration. Antitussives should only be used to facilitate sleep (see p. 356). Patients with wheezing may benefit from an inhaled β-agonist (eg, albuterol) or an anticholinergic (eg, ipratropium) for ≤ 7 days. Oral antibiotics (eg, 7 days of amoxicillin 500 mg tid, doxycycline 100 mg bid, or trimethoprim-sulfamethoxazole 160/800 mg bid) are presumed to be beneficial for patients with COPD (see p. 400) or other serious pulmonary disease who have at least 2 of the following: increased cough, increased dyspnea, increase in sputum purulence.

Cough resolves within 2 wk in 75% of patients. Patients with persistent cough should undergo a chest x-ray and be evaluated for pertussis (whooping cough) and noninfectious etiologies, such as postnasal drip, allergic rhinitis, and cough-variant asthma. Some patients benefit from inhaled corticosteroids for a few days if cough persists because of airway irritation.

52 PNEUMONIA

(See also Neonatal Pneumonia on p. 2332.)

Pneumonia is acute inflammation of the lungs caused by infection. Initial diagnosis is usually based on chest x-ray. Causes, symptoms, treatment, preventive measures, and prognosis differ depending on whether the infection is bacterial, viral, fungal, or parasitic; whether it is acquired in the community, hospital, or nursing home; and whether it develops in a patient who is immunocompetent or immunocompromised.

An estimated 2 to 3 million people in the US develop pneumonia each year, of whom about 45,000 die. Pneumonia is the most common fatal hospital-acquired infection and the most common overall cause of death in developing countries.

Bacteria are the most common cause of pneumonia in adults > 30 yr, *Streptococcus pneumoniae* infection being the most common pathogen across all age groups, settings, and geographic regions. However, pathogens of every sort, from viruses to parasites, cause pneumonia.

The airways and lungs are constantly exposed to pathogens in the external environment; the upper airways and oropharynx in particular are colonized with so-called normal flora rendered harmless by host defenses. Infection develops when pathogens overcome multiple host defenses.

Upper airway defenses include salivary IgA, proteases, and lysozymes; growth inhibitors produced by normal flora; and fibronectin, which coats the mucosae and inhibits adherence. Nonspecific lower airway defenses include cough, mucociliary clearance, and airway angulation preventing infection in airspaces. Specific lower airway defenses include a variety of pathogen-specific immune mechanisms, including IgA and IgG opsonization, anti-inflammatory effects of surfactant, phagocytosis by alveolar macrophages, and T-cell–mediated immune responses. These mechanisms protect most people against infection. But numerous conditions alter normal flora (eg, systemic illness, malnutrition, hospital or nursing home exposure, antibiotic exposure), increase virulence (eg, antibiotic exposure), or impair these defenses (eg, cigarette smoking, nasogastric or endotracheal intubation). Pathogens that then reach airspaces by inhalation, contiguous or hematogenous spread, or aspiration can multiply and cause pneumonia.

Specific pathogens causing pneumonia cannot be found in > ½ of patients, even with extensive diagnostic investigation. But because pathogens and outcomes tend to be similar by setting and host risk factors, categorization of pneumonias as community-acquired, hospital-acquired (including ventilator-acquired and postoperative), nursing home–acquired, and those that occur in the immunocompromised host allows treatment to be established empirically.

The term interstitial pneumonia refers to a variety of unrelated conditions of unknown cause characterized by inflammation and fibrosis of the pulmonary interstitium. These conditions bear little resemblance to infectious pneumonia and are discussed in Ch. 55 on p. 443.

COMMUNITY-ACQUIRED PNEUMONIA

Community-acquired pneumonia develops in people with limited or no contact with medical institutions or settings. The most commonly identified pathogens are *Streptococcus pneumoniae, Haemophilus influenzae,* and atypical organisms (ie, *Chlamydia pneumoniae, Mycoplasma pneumoniae, Legionella* sp). Symptoms and signs are fever, cough, dyspnea, tachypnea, and tachycardia. Diagnosis is based on clinical presentation and chest x-ray. Treatment is with empirically chosen antibiotics. Prognosis is excellent for relatively young and/or healthy patients, but many pneumonias, especially when caused by *S. pneumoniae* and influenza virus, are fatal in older, sicker patients.

Etiology

Many organisms cause community-acquired pneumonia, including bacteria, viruses, and fungi. Pathogens vary by patient age and other factors (see TABLES 52–1 and 52–2), but the relative importance of each as a cause of community-acquired pneumonia is uncertain, because most patients do not undergo thorough testing, and because even with testing, specific agents are identified in < 50% of cases.

S. pneumoniae, H. influenzae, C. pneumoniae, and *M. pneumoniae* are the most common bacterial causes. Chlamydia and mycoplasma are clinically indistinguishable from other causes. Common viral agents include respiratory syncytial virus (RSV), adenovirus, influenza, metapneumovirus, and parainfluenza virus in children and influenza in the elderly. Bacterial superinfection can make distinguishing viral from bacterial infection difficult.

C. pneumoniae accounts for 5 to 10% of community-acquired pneumonia and is the 2nd most common cause of lung infections in healthy people aged 5 to 35 yr. *C. pneumoniae* is commonly responsible for outbreaks of respiratory infection within families, in college dormitories, and in military training camps. It causes a relatively benign form of pneumonia that infrequently requires hospitalization.

TABLE 52–1. COMMUNITY-ACQUIRED PNEUMONIA IN CHILDREN

AGE	ORGANISMS	TREATMENT
Birth to 3 wk	Group B streptococci, *Listeria monocytogenes*, gram-negative bacilli, cytomegalovirus	Ampicillin (or nafcillin) *and* Gentamicin (or cefotaxime)*
3 wk to 3 mo	*Streptococcus pneumoniae,* viral infection (RSV, parainfluenza, metapneumovirus), *Bordetella pertussis, Staphylococcus aureus, Chlamydia trachomatis* (transnatal exposure)	***Outpatient:*** Erythromycin 10 mg/kg IV q 6 h for 10–14 days ***Inpatient non-ICU:*** Cefuroxime 50 mg/kg IV q 8–12 h ***Inpatient ICU:*** Cefotaxime 66 mg/kg IV tid *and* Cloxacillin 50 mg/kg IV q 6 h
4 mo to 4 yr	*S. pneumoniae,* viral infection (RSV, parainfluenza, influenza, adenovirus, rhinovirus, metapneumovirus), *Mycoplasma pneumoniae* (in older children), group A streptococci	***Outpatient:*** Erythromycin 10 mg/kg po qid ***Inpatient:*** Erythromycin 10 mg/kg po qid *and* Cefuroxime 50 mg/kg IV q 8 h
5 to 15 yr	*S. pneumoniae, M. pneumoniae, Chlamydia pneumoniae*	***Outpatient:*** Clarithromycin 500 mg po bid ***Inpatient:*** Ceftriaxone 50 mg/kg once/day IV (maximum 2 g) *and* Azithromycin 10 mg/kg once/day (maximum 500 mg)

RSV = respiratory syncytial virus.

*For doses and discussion of neonatal pneumonia, see p. 2332.

Data from McIntosh K: Community-acquired pneumonia in children. *The New England Journal of Medicine* 346:429–437, 2002.

Chlamydia psittaci pneumonia (psittacosis) occurs in patients who own birds.

A host of other organisms cause lung infection in immunocompetent patients, although the term community-acquired pneumonia is usually reserved for the more common bacterial and viral etiologies.

Q fever, tularemia, anthrax, and plague are uncommon bacterial syndromes in which pneumonia may be a prominent feature; the latter three should raise the suspicion of bioterrorism.

Adenovirus, Epstein-Barr virus, and coxsackievirus are common viruses that rarely cause pneumonia. Varicella virus and hantavirus cause lung infection as part of adult chickenpox and hantavirus pulmonary syndrome; a novel coronavirus causes severe acute respiratory syndrome (SARS—see p.1600).

The most common fungal pathogens are *Histoplasma capsulatum* (histoplasmosis) and *Coccidioides immitis* (coccidioidomycosis). Less common fungi include *Blastomyces dermatitidis* (blastomycosis) and *Paracoccidioides braziliensis* (paracoccidioidomycosis).

Parasites causing lung infection in developed countries include *Plasmodium* sp (malaria), *Toxocara canis* or *catis* (visceral larva migrans), *Dirofilaria immitis* (dirofilariasis), and *Paragonimus westermani* (paragonimiasis). (For a discussion of pulmonary TB or of specific microorganisms, see p. 1508.)

Symptoms and Signs

Symptoms include malaise, cough, dyspnea, and chest pain. Cough typically is productive in older children and adults and dry

TABLE 52–2. COMMUNITY-ACQUIRED PNEUMONIA IN ADULTS

GROUP	LIKELY ORGANISMS	EMPIRIC TREATMENT
I. Outpatients—No modifying factors present*	*Streptococcus pneumoniae, Mycoplasma pneumoniae, Chlamydia pneumoniae, Haemophilus influenzae,* respiratory viruses, miscellaneous (*Legionella* sp, *Mycobacterium tuberculosis,* endemic fungi)	Macrolide (azithromycin 500 mg po once, then 250 mg once/day; clarithromycin 250 to 500 mg po bid); or extended-release clarithromycin 1 g once/day *or* Doxycycline 100 mg po bid (if allergic to macrolide)
II. Outpatients—Modifying factors present	*S. pneumoniae,* including drug-resistant forms; *M. pneumoniae; C. pneumoniae;* mixed infection (bacteria + atypical pathogen or virus); *H. influenzae;* enteric gram negatives; respiratory viruses; miscellaneous (*Moraxella catarrhalis, Legionella* sp, anaerobes [aspiration], *M. tuberculosis,* endemic fungi)	β-lactam (cefpodoxime 200 mg po q 12 h; cefuroxime 500 mg po q 12 h; amoxicillin 1 g q 8 h; amoxicillin/clavulanate 875/125 mg q 12 h) *plus* Macrolide or doxycycline (if allergic to macrolide) po *or* Antipneumococcal fluoroquinolone† po
IIIA. Inpatient—Not in ICU, no modifying factors	*S. pneumoniae, H. influenzae; M. pneumoniae; C. pneumoniae;* mixed infection (bacteria + atypical pathogen or virus); respiratory viruses; *Legionella* sp, miscellaneous *(M. tuberculosis,* endemic fungi, *Pneumocystis jiroveci* (formerly *P. carinii*)	Azithromycin 500 mg IV q 24 h, *or* Doxycycline 100 mg po bid *plus* β-lactam (see Group II for choices) if macrolide allergic or intolerant *or* Antipneumococcal fluoroquinolone† IV
IIIB. Inpatient—Not in ICU, modifying factors	*S. pneumoniae,* including drug-resistant forms; *H. influenzae; M. pneumoniae; C. pneumoniae;* mixed infection (bacteria + atypical pathogen or virus); enteric gram-negatives; anaerobes (aspiration); respiratory viruses; *Legionella* sp, miscellaneous *(M. tuberculosis,* endemic fungi, *P. jiroveci)*	β-lactam‡ IV (cefotaxime 1 to 2 g IV q 8 to 12 h; ceftriaxone 1 g IV q 24 h) *plus* Macrolide (erythromycin 4–5 mg/kg po qid, azithromycin 500 mg IV or po q 24 h, or clarithromycin 250 to 500 mg po bid, or extended-release clarithromycin 1 g once/day), or doxycycline 100 mg po bid *or* Antipneumococcal fluoroquinolone† IV
IVA. ICU patient—no *Pseudomonas* risk factors	*S. pneumoniae,* including drug-resistant forms, *Legionella* sp, *H. influenzae,* enteric gram-negatives, *S. aureus, M. pneumoniae,* respiratory viruses, miscellaneous (*C. pneumoniae, M. tuberculosis,* endemic fungi)	β-lactam IV (cefotaxime 1 to 2 g IV q 8 to 12 h; ceftriaxone 1 g IV q 24 h) *plus either* Antipneumococcal fluoroquinolone† IV *or* Azithromycin 500 mg IV q 24 h

TABLE 52–2. COMMUNITY-ACQUIRED PNEUMONIA IN ADULTS—Continued

GROUP	LIKELY ORGANISMS	EMPIRIC TREATMENT
IVB. ICU patient—*Pseudomonas* risk factors present	Same as previous plus *Pseudomonas* sp	Antipseudomonal β-lactam§ or if β-lactam allergic or intolerant, aztreonam 1 to 2 g q 8 h, an aminoglycoside *plus* Ciprofloxacin 400 mg IV q 12 h *or* Antipseudomonal β-lactam§ *plus* an aminoglycoside *plus* azithromycin or a nonpseudomonal fluoroquinolone*

*Modifying factors:

Increased risk of drug-resistant pneumococcus: Age > 65, alcoholism, β-lactam antibiotic within 3 mo, exposure to child in day care center, immunosuppression (including corticosteroid use; HIV infection considered separately), multiple coexisting illnesses.

Increased risk of enteric gram-negatives: Antibiotic use within 3 mo, cardiopulmonary disease (including COPD and heart failure), multiple coexisting illnesses, nursing home residence.

Increased risk of Pseudomonas aeruginosa: Broad spectrum antibiotics > 7 days in past month, corticosteroid use, malnutrition, structural pulmonary disease.

† Antipneumococcal fluoroquinolones = levofloxacin 500 to 750 mg po or IV q 24 h, trovafloxacin 200 mg po or IV once/day (300 mg initial loading dose for hospital-acquired pneumonia), gemifloxacin 320 mg po once/day.

‡ Antipseudomonal fluoroquinolones = levofloxacin 500 mg po or IV q 24 h, gatifloxacin 400 mg po or IV q 24 h.

§ Antipseudomonal β-lactams = cefepime 1 to 2 g IV q 12 h, imipenem 500 mg IV q 6 h, meropenem 500 mg to 1 g IV q 8 h, piperacillin/ tazobactam 3.375 g IV q 4 h.

Data from Niederman MS, Mandell LA, Anzueto A, et al: Guidelines for the management of adults with community-acquired pneumonia: Diagnosis, assessment of severity, antimicrobial therapy, and prevention. *American Journal of Respiratory and Critical Care Medicine* 163:1730–1754, 2001.

in infants, young children, and the elderly. Dyspnea usually is mild and exertional and is rarely present at rest. Chest pain is pleuritic and is adjacent to the infected area. Pneumonia may manifest as upper abdominal pain when lower lobe infection irritates the diaphragm. Symptoms become variable at the extremes of age; infection in infants may manifest as nonspecific irritability and restlessness; in the elderly, as confusion and obtundation.

Signs include fever, tachypnea, tachycardia, crackles, bronchial breath sounds, egophony, and dullness to percussion. Signs of pleural effusion may also be present (see p. 493). Nasal flaring, use of accessory muscles, and cyanosis are common in infants.

Symptoms and signs were previously thought to differ by type of pathogen, but presentations overlap considerably. In addition, no single symptom or sign is sensitive or specific enough to predict the organism. Symptoms are even similar for noninfective lung diseases such as pulmonary embolism, pulmonary malignancy, and other inflammatory lung diseases.

Diagnosis

Diagnosis is suspected on the basis of clinical presentation and is confirmed by chest x-ray (see TABLE 52–3). The most serious condition misdiagnosed as pneumonia is pulmonary embolism, which may be more likely in patients with minimal sputum production, no accompanying URI or systemic symptoms, and risk factors for thromboembolism (see TABLE 50–1 on p. 413).

Chest x-ray almost always demonstrates some degree of infiltrate; rarely, an infiltrate is absent in the first 24 to 48 h of illness. In general, no specific findings distinguish one type of infection from another, though multilobar infiltrates suggest *S. pneumoniae* or *Legionella pneumophila* infection, and

TABLE 52–3. PROBABILITY OF PNEUMONIA GIVEN CHEST X-RAY INFILTRATE

Assign 1 point each for:

- Temperature > 37.8°C
- Heart rate > 100 beats/min
- Crackles on auscultation
- Decreased breath sounds
- Absence of asthma

Score	Likelihood Ratio	Probability of Pneumonia*
0–1	0.3	≤ 1%
2–3	—	3–10%
4–5	8.2	25–50%

*Based on baseline prevalence (pretest probability) of 5%.

Data from Heckerling PS, Tape TG, Wigton RS, et al: Clinical prediction rule for pulmonary infiltrates. *Annals of Internal Medicine* 113: 664–670, 1990.

interstitial pneumonia suggests viral or mycoplasma etiology.

Hospitalized patients (see p. 430) should undergo WBC count and electrolytes, BUN, and creatinine testing to classify risk and hydration status. Two sets of blood cultures are often obtained to detect pneumococcal bacteremia and sepsis, because about 12% of all patients hospitalized with pneumonia have bacteremia; *S. pneumoniae* accounts for ⅔ of these cases. Whether the results of blood cultures actually alter therapy commonly enough to warrant the expense is under study. Pulse oximetry or ABG should also be performed.

Attempts to identify a pathogen are not routinely indicated; exceptions may be made for critically ill patients, patients in whom a drug-resistant or unusual organism is suspected (eg, TB), and patients who are deteriorating or not responding to treatment within 72 h. Sputum Gram stain and culture are controversial, because specimens often are contaminated and because overall diagnostic yield is low. Samples can be obtained noninvasively by simple expectoration or after hypertonic saline nebulization for those unable to produce sputum. Alternatively, patients can undergo bronchoscopy or endotracheal suctioning, either of which can be easily performed through an endotracheal tube in mechanically ventilated patients. Testing should include mycobacterial and fungal stains and cultures in deteriorating patients and in those unresponsive to broad-spectrum antibiotics.

Additional tests are indicated in some circumstances. Patients at risk of *Legionella* pneumonia (eg, patients who smoke, have chronic pulmonary disease, are > 40, receive chemotherapy, or take immunosuppressants for organ transplantation) should undergo urinary *Legionella* antigen testing, which stays positive long after treatment is initiated but detects only *L. pneumophila* serogroup 1 (70% of cases). A 4-fold rise in antibody titers to ≥ 1 : 128 (or a single convalescent serum of ≥ 1 : 256) is also considered diagnostic. These tests are specific (95 to 100%) but are not very sensitive (40 to 60%); thus, a positive test indicates infection, but a negative test does not exclude it.

Infants and young children with possible RSV infection should undergo rapid antigen testing of nasal or throat swabs. No other tests for viral pneumonias exist; viral culture and serologic tests are rarely clinically warranted.

PCR testing for mycoplasma and chlamydia species, although not widely available, holds promise as a highly sensitive and specific rapid diagnostic test and is likely to play a greater role as PCR technologies are refined.

A test for SARS-associated coronavirus exists, but its role in clinical practice is unknown, and its application is limited outside of known outbreaks (see p. 1600). In rare situations, anthrax should be considered (see p. 1449).

Prognosis

Candidates for outpatient treatment usually improve over 24 to 72 h. Hospitalized patients may improve or deteriorate depending on comorbidities. Aspiration is a major risk factor for death, as is older age, number and type of comorbidities, and certain infectious agents. Death may be caused by pneumonia itself, progression to sepsis syndrome affecting other organs, or exacerbation of underlying comorbidities.

Pneumococcal infection still accounts for about 66% of all fatal cases of community-acquired pneumonia in which an etiologic agent is known. The overall mortality rate in hospitalized patients is about 12%. Poor prognostic factors include age < 1 or > 60 yr; involvement of more than one lobe; peripheral WBC count < 5000/μL; comorbidities (heart failure, alcoholism, hepatic and renal insufficiency), immunosuppression (agammaglobulinemia, anatomic or functional asplenia), infection with serotypes 3 and 8; and hematogenous spread with either positive blood cultures or extrapulmonary complications (arthritis, meningitis, or endocarditis). Infants and children are at special risk of pneumococcal otitis media, bacteremia, and meningitis.

Mortality in *Legionella* infection is 10 to 20% among community-acquired cases and is higher among immunosuppressed or hospitalized patients. Patients who respond do so slowly, and x-ray abnormalities usually persist for ≥ 1 mo. Most patients require hospitalization, many require ventilator support, and 10 to 20% die despite appropriate antibiotic therapy.

Prognosis in mycoplasma pneumonia is excellent; nearly all patients recover. Chlamydial pneumoniae responds slower to treatment than mycoplasma and tends to recur if therapy is stopped prematurely. Young adults usually do well, but the elderly have a mortality rate of 5 to 10%.

Treatment

A prediction rule may be used to identify those patients who can be safely treated as outpatients and those who require hospitalization because of high risk of complications (see TABLE 52–4). The rule should supplement, not replace, clinical judgment, because many unrepresented factors, such as likelihood of adherence, ability to care for self, and wishes to avoid hospitalization, should also influence triage decisions. ICU admission is required for patients who need mechanical ventilation and for those with hypotension (systolic BP < 90 mm Hg). Other criteria for ICU admission include respiratory rate > 30/min, PaO_2/inspired O_2 (FIO_2) < 250, multilobar pneumonia, diastolic BP < 60 mm Hg, confusion, and BUN > 19.6 mg/dL. Appropriate treatment involves starting antibiotics as soon as possible, preferably ≤ 8 h after presentation. Supportive care includes fluids, antipyretics, analgesics, and O_2 for patients with hypoxemia.

Because organisms are difficult to identify, antibiotics are selected based on likely pathogens and severity of illness. Consensus guidelines have been developed by many professional organizations; one widely used set is detailed in TABLE 52–2. Guidelines should be adapted to local susceptibility patterns, drug formularies, and individual patient circumstances. Importantly, none provide recommendations for treatment of viral pneumonia.

TABLE 52–4. RISK STRATIFICATION FOR COMMUNITY-ACQUIRED PNEUMONIA

FACTOR	POINTS
Age	
Men	Age (yr)
Women	Age (yr) −10
Nursing home resident	10
Coexisting illness	
Malignancy	30
Liver disease	20
Heart failure	10
Cerebrovascular disease	10
Renal disease	10
Physical examination	
Altered mental status	20
Respiratory rate ≥ 30	20
Systolic BP < 90 mm Hg	20
Temperature ≥ 40° or < 35°C	15
Heart rate ≥ 125 beats/min	10
Test results	
Arterial pH < 7.35	30
BUN ≥ 30 mg/dL (11 mmol/L)	20
Na <130 mmol/L	20
Glucose ≥ 250 mg/dL (14 mmol/L)	10
Hematocrit < 30%	10
PaO_2 < 60 mm Hg or O_{2sat} < 90%*	10
Pleural effusion	10

POINTS	MORTALITY	RECOMMENDATION
≤ 70	<1%	Outpatient treatment†
71–90	<5%	Outpatient treatment†
91–130	5–15%	Admit
>130	>15%	Admit

*Many consider hypoxemia an absolute indication for admission.

†Consider acute care admission, subacute care admission, observation period, home IV antibiotics, or home nursing visits for patients who are frail, isolated, or living in unstable environments.

Adapted from Pneumonia: New prediction model proves promising (AHCPR Publication No. 97-R031).

Ribavirin and RSV Ig have been used alone and in combination for RSV bronchiolitis in children, but their effectiveness is controversial, and neither is standard practice. Ribavirin is not used in adults with RSV infection. Amantadine or rimantadine 200 mg po once/day started within 48 h of symptom onset reduces the duration and severity of symptoms in patients who develop presumed influenza A infection as part of an outbreak, but efficacy for preventing adverse outcomes of influenza pneumonia is unknown. Zanamivir (10 mg inhaled bid) and oseltamivir (75 mg po bid) are similarly effective in reducing the duration of symptoms caused by influenza A or B if started within 48 h of symptom onset, though zanamivir may be contraindicated in patients with asthma. Acyclovir 5 to 10 mg/kg IV q 8 h for adults or 250 to 500 mg/m^2 body surface area IV q 8 h for children is advocated for varicella lung infections. Some patients with viral pneumonia, especially those with influenza, develop superimposed bacterial infections and require antibiotics directed against *S. pneumoniae*, *H. influenzae*, and *Staphylococcus aureus*.

With empiric treatment, 90% of patients with bacterial pneumonia improve, manifested by decreased cough and dyspnea, defervescence, relief of chest pain, and decline in WBC count. Failure to improve should trigger suspicion of an unusual organism, antibiotic resistance with inadequate coverage, co-infection or superinfection with a 2nd infectious agent, an obstructive endobronchial lesion, immunosuppression, metastatic focus of infection with reseeding (in the case of pneumococcal infection), or nonadherence to treatment (in the case of outpatients). If none of these can be proven, treatment failure is likely due to inadequate host defenses.

Most viral pneumonias resolve without specific treatment.

Follow-up x-rays should be obtained 6 wk after treatment in patients > 35; persistence of an infiltrate at ≤ 6 wk raises suspicions of an underlying, possibly malignant endobronchial lesion or of TB.

Prevention

Some forms of community-acquired pneumonia are preventable with pneumococcal conjugate vaccine (for patients < 2 yr), *H. influenzae* B (HIB) vaccine (for patients < 2 yr), and influenza vaccine (for patients > 65 yr)—see p. 1399 and FIG. 266–3 on p. 2235. *Pneumococcus,* HIB, and influenza vaccines are also recommended for high-risk patients. High-risk patients not vaccinated against influenza may be given amantadine, rimantadine, or oseltamivir during influenza epidemics.

HOSPITAL-ACQUIRED PNEUMONIA

Hospital-acquired pneumonia develops at least 48 h after hospitalization. The most common pathogens are gram-negative bacilli and *Staphylococcus aureus*; drug-resistant organisms are an important concern. Symptoms and signs are the same as those for community-acquired pneumonia, but in ventilated patients, pneumonia may also manifest as worsening oxygenation and increased tracheal secretions. Diagnosis is suspected on the basis of clinical presentation and chest x-ray and is confirmed by blood culture or bronchoscopic sampling of the lower respiratory tract. Treatment is with antibiotics. Overall prognosis is poor, due in part to comorbidities.

Hospital-acquired pneumonia includes ventilator-associated pneumonia, postoperative pneumonia, and pneumonia that develops in unventilated but otherwise moderately or critically ill hospitalized inpatients.

Etiology

The most common cause is microaspiration of bacteria that colonize the oropharynx and upper airways in seriously ill patients.

Risk factors: Endotracheal intubation with mechanical ventilation poses the greatest overall risk; ventilator-associated pneumonia constitutes > 85% of all cases, with pneumonia occurring in 17 to 23% of ventilated patients. Endotracheal intubation breaches airway defenses, impairs cough and mucociliary clearance, and facilitates microaspiration of bacteria-laden secretions that pool above the inflated endotracheal tube cuff. In addition, bacteria form a biofilm on and within the endotracheal tube that protects them from antibiotics and host defenses.

In nonintubated patients, risk factors include previous antibiotic treatment, high gastric pH (from stress ulcer prophylaxis therapy), and coexisting cardiac, pulmonary, hepatic, and renal insufficiency. Major risk factors for postoperative pneumonia are age > 70, abdominal or thoracic surgery, and dependent functional status.

Pathogens: Pathogens and antibiotic resistance patterns vary significantly among institutions and can vary within institutions over short periods (eg, month to month). In general, the most important pathogen is *Pseudomonas aeruginosa*, which is especially common in pneumonias acquired in intensive care settings and in patients with cystic fibrosis, neutropenia, advanced AIDS, and bronchiectasis. Other important pathogens include enteric gram-negative bacteria (*Enterobacter* sp, *Klebsiella pneumoniae, Escherichia coli, Serratia marcescens, Proteus* sp, *Acinetobacter* sp) and both methicillin-sensitive and methicillin-resistant *Staphylococcus aureus*.

S. aureus, pneumococcus, and *Haemophilus influenzae* are most commonly implicated when pneumonia develops within 4 to 7 days of hospitalization, whereas enteric gram-negative organisms become more common with increasing duration of intubation.

Prior antibiotic treatment greatly increases the likelihood of polymicrobial infection; resistant organisms, particularly methicillin-resistant *S. aureus*; and *Pseudomonas* infection. Infection with a resistant organism markedly worsens mortality and morbidity.

High-dose corticosteroids increase the risk of *Legionella* and *Pseudomonas* infections.

Symptoms, Signs, and Diagnosis

Symptoms and signs in nonintubated patients are generally the same as those for community-acquired pneumonia (see p. 425). Pneumonia in critically ill, mechanically ventilated patients more typically causes fever and increased respiratory and/or heart rate or changes in respiratory parameters, such as an increase in purulent secretions or worsening hypoxemia. Noninfectious causes of pulmonary deterioration, such as acute respiratory distress syndrome (ARDS), pneumothorax, and pulmonary edema, must be excluded.

Diagnosis is imperfect. In practice, hospital-acquired pneumonia is often suspected on the basis of the appearance of a new infiltrate on a chest x-ray that is taken for evaluation of new symptoms or signs or of leucocytosis. However, no symptom, sign, or x-ray finding is sensitive or specific for the diagnosis, because all can be caused by atelectasis, pulmonary embolism, or pulmonary edema and may be part of the clinical findings in ARDS.

Gram stain and culture of endotracheal aspirates are controversial, because specimens are likely to be contaminated with bacteria that are colonizers as well as pathogens, and a positive culture may or may not indicate infection. Bronchoscopic sampling of lower airway secretions for quantitative culture seems to yield more reliable specimens, but the effect of this approach on outcomes is controversial. Measurement of inflammatory mediators in bronchoalveolar lavage fluid may play a future role in diagnosis; eg, a concentration of soluble triggering receptor expressed on myeloid cells (a protein expressed and shed by immune cells during infection) > 5 pg/mL may help distinguish bacterial and fungal pneumonia from noninfectious causes of clinical and radiographic changes in ventilated patients. However, this approach requires further investigation, and the only finding that reliably identifies both pneumonia and the responsible organism is a blood or pleural fluid culture that is positive for a respiratory pathogen.

Prognosis

The mortality associated with hospital-acquired pneumonia due to gram-negative infection is about 25 to 50% despite the availability of effective antibiotics. Whether death is due to underlying illness or to the pneumonia itself is uncertain. Women may be at greater risk of death. The mortality rate associated with *S. aureus* pneumonia is 10 to 40%, in part due to the serious conditions with which it is associated (eg, need for a ventilator, advanced age, cancer chemotherapy, chronic pulmonary disease).

Treatment

A few patients may have a pneumonia risk score (see TABLE 52–5) low enough to suggest that alternative diagnoses should be sought. Otherwise, treatment is with antibiotics that are chosen empirically based on local sensitivity patterns, specific patient risk factors, and the conditions noted in TABLE 52–2.

Indiscriminate use of antibiotics is a major contributor to development of antimicrobial resistance. Therefore, treatment may begin with initial use of broad-spectrum drugs, which are replaced by the most specific drug available for the pathogens identified by culture. Alternative strategies for limiting resistance that has not proven effective include stopping antibiotics after 72 h in patients whose pulmonary infection scores (see TABLE 52–5)

TABLE 52–5. HOSPITAL-ACQUIRED PNEUMONIA RISK INDEX

FACTOR	POINTS
Temperature (°C)	
≥ 36.5 and ≤ 38.4	0
≥ 38.5 and ≤ 38.9	1
≥ 39 and ≤ 36	2
Blood leukocytes, μL	
≥ 4,000 and ≤ 11, 000	0
< 4,000 or > 11,000	1
Band forms ≥ 50%	1
Tracheal secretions	
None	0
Nonpurulent	1
Purulent	2
Oxygenation: PaO_2/FIO_2, mm Hg	
> 240 or ARDS	0
≤ 240 and no ARDS	2
Pulmonary radiography	
No infiltrate	0
Diffuse (or patchy) infiltrate	1
Localized infiltrate	2
Progression of infiltrate*	
None	0
Progression (heart failure and ARDS excluded)	2
Growth of pathogenic bacteria on tracheal aspirate culture*	
No, rare, or light growth	0
Moderate or heavy growth	1
Same bacteria as on Gram stain	1

PaO_2/FIO_2 = ratio of arterial O_2 pressure to fraction of inspired O_2; ARDS = acute respiratory distress syndrome.

*Criteria applicable 72 h after initial diagnosis. Score > 6 suggests hospital-acquired pneumonia. Score < 6 suggests alternative process.

Adapted from Singh N, Rogers P, Atwood CW, et al: Short-course empiric antibiotic therapy for patients with pulmonary infiltrates in the intensive care unit. *American Journal of Respiratory and Critical Care Medicine* 162:505–511, 2000.

improve to < 6 and regularly rotating empirically chosen antibiotics (eg, q 3 to 6 mo).

Initial antibiotics: Multiple regimens exist, but all should include antibiotics that cover both resistant gram-negative and gram-positive organisms. Options include a carbapenem (imipenem-cilastatin 500 mg IV q 6 h or meropenem 1 to 2 g IV q 8 h), monobactam (aztreonam 1 to 2 g IV q 8 h), or antipseudomonal β-lactam (ticarcillin 3 g IV with or without clavulanic acid q 4 h, piperacillin 3 g IV with or without tazobactam q 4 to 6 h, ceftazidime 2 g IV q 8 h, or cefepime 1 to 2 g q 12 h), given alone or combined with an aminoglycoside (gentamicin or tobramycin 1.7 mg/kg IV q 8 h or 5 to 6 mg/kg once/day or amikacin 5 mg/kg q 8 h) and/or vancomycin 1 g q 12 h. Linezolid may be used for some pulmonary infections involving methicillin-resistant *S. aureus*, especially in patients who cannot take vancomycin. Daptomycin should not be used for pulmonary infections.

Prevention

Noninvasive ventilation using continuous positive airway pressure (CPAP) or bi-level positive airway pressure (BiPAP) prevents the breach in airway defense that occurs with endotracheal intubation and eliminates the need for intubation in some patients. Semi-upright or upright positioning reduces risk of aspiration and pneumonia compared with recumbent positioning.

Continuous aspiration of subglottic secretions using a specially designed endotracheal tube attached to a suction device seems to reduce the risk of aspiration.

Selective decontamination of the oropharynx (using topical gentamicin, colistin, and vancomycin cream) or of the entire GI tract (using polymyxin, an aminoglycoside or quinolone, and either nystatin or amphotericin) also seems to be effective, although it may increase the risk of colonization with resistant organisms.

Surveillance cultures and routinely changing ventilator circuits or endotracheal tubes have not been shown to decrease ventilator-associated pneumonia.

NURSING HOME–ACQUIRED PNEUMONIA

Common nursing home–acquired pneumonia pathogens are usually gram-negative bacilli, *Staphylococcus aureus, Streptococcus pneumoniae, Haemophilus influenzae,* anaerobes, and influenza. Symptoms and signs are similar to those of pneumonia in other settings, except many elderly patients have less prominent changes in vital signs. Diagnosis is based on clinical presentation

and chest x-ray, which are often not available in nursing homes immediately. Treatment is with antibiotics provided in the nursing home for less severe illness and in the hospital for more severe infection. Mortality is moderately high but may be due in part to comorbidities.

Nursing home–acquired pneumonia falls between community- and hospital-acquired pneumonia in etiology and management. *S. pneumoniae* and gram-negative bacilli may be roughly equally responsible for most infections, though there is debate over whether gram-negative bacilli are pathogens or merely colonizers. *H. influenzae* and *Moraxella catarrhalis* are next most common; *Chlamydia, Mycoplasma,* and *Legionella* spp are rarely identified. Risk factors are those common among debilitated nursing home residents, such as poor functional status; impaired mood, mental status, and swallowing; and presence of a tracheostomy tube.

Symptoms, Signs, and Diagnosis

Symptoms often resemble those of community- or hospital-acquired pneumonia but may be more subtle; cough and altered mental status are common, as are nonspecific symptoms of anorexia, weakness, restlessness and agitation, falling, and incontinence. Subjective dyspnea occurs but is less common. Signs include diminished or absent responsiveness, fever, tachycardia, tachypnea, wheezes or crackles, and stentorous, wet breathing.

Diagnosis is based on clinical presentation and chest x-ray. X-rays are often difficult to obtain in nursing home patients, so it may be necessary to transfer them to a hospital at least for initial evaluation. In some cases, treatment may be started without x-ray confirmation. Nursing home residents may initially lack a radiographic infiltrate, presumably because of the dehydration that commonly accompanies febrile pneumonia in the elderly and/or a blunted immune response, although the phenomenon is not proven to occur. Because detection of physical changes may be delayed in a nursing home setting and because residents are at greater risk of complications, evaluation for hypoxemia with pulse oximetry and for decreased intravascular volume with serum BUN and creatinine should also be performed.

Prognosis

Mortality rate for patients requiring admission for treatment is 13 to 41%, whereas that

TABLE 52–6. NURSING HOME–ACQUIRED PNEUMONIA RISK INDEX

VARIABLE AND VALUE	POINTS ASSIGNED
Serum urea nitrogen (mg/dL)*	
≤ 16	0
16.1–27	1
27.1–38	2
38.1–49	3
49.1–60	4
60.1–71	5
> 71	6
WBC count (10^3/μL)	
≤ 14	0
14.1–24	1
>24	2
Absolute lymphocyte count	
> 800/μL (0.8×10^9/L)	0
≤ 800/μL (0.8×10^9/L)	1
Pulse (beats/min)	
≤72	0
73–102	1
> 132	3
Sex	
Female	0
Male	1
Body mass index (kg/m^2)	
> 31	0
25.1–31	1
19.1–25	2
13.1–19	3
≤ 13	4
Activities of daily living†	
0	0
1–2	1
3–4	2
Mood deterioration over last 90 days	
No	0
Yes	2

*To convert to mmol/L, multiply by 0.357; to convert a value in mmol/L to mg/dL, multiply by 6.

†Based on grooming, using the toilet, locomotion, and eating. Each is assigned a zero if the resident is independent, requires supervision, or requires limited assistance or 1 if the resident requires extensive assistance or is totally dependent. The 4 scores are summed to derive a score of zero to 4 and assigned points as shown.

Score	Mortality
1–4	Low (2–3%)
5–6	Relatively low (6–7%)
7–8	Moderate (15–16%)
9–10	High (34–36%)
11–17	Very high (60–62%)

for patients treated in the nursing home is 7 to 19%. Mortality rate exceeds 30% in patients with more than 2 of the following findings: respiratory rate > 30 breaths/min, heart rate > 125 beats/min, acute mental status change, and history of dementia. An alternative predictive index incorporates laboratory data (see TABLE 52–6). Physicians should follow all medical directives, because pneumonia is often a terminal event in debilitated nursing home patients.

Treatment

Few data are available to guide decisions about where treatment should take place, but in general, patients should be hospitalized if they have 2 or more unstable vital signs and if the nursing home cannot administer acute care. Some nursing home residents are not candidates for hospital transfer. One dose of antibiotics to cover *S. pneumoniae, H. influenzae,* common gram-negative bacilli, and *S. aureus* should be given before transfer; a common regimen is an oral antipneumococcal quinolone (eg, levofloxacin 750 mg once/day, moxifloxacin 400 mg once/day, or gemifloxacin 400 mg once/day).

PNEUMONIA IN THE IMMUNOCOMPROMISED HOST

Pneumonia in the immunocompromised host is often caused by unusual pathogens. Symptoms and signs depend on the pathogen. Diagnosis is based on blood cultures and bronchoscopic sampling of respiratory secretions, sometimes with quantitative cultures. Treatment depends on the host defect and pathogen.

The potential pathogens in patients with compromised defenses are legion. Likely pathogens based on the type of defect in host defenses are listed in TABLE 52–7. However, respiratory symptoms and changes on chest x-rays in immunocompromised hosts may be due to a variety of processes other than infection, such as pulmonary hemorrhage, pulmonary edema, radiation injury, pulmonary toxicity due to cytotoxic drugs, and tumor infiltrates.

Symptoms, Signs, and Diagnosis

Symptoms and signs may be the same as those found with community-acquired pneumonia or hospital-acquired pneumonia in immunocompetent patients, though immunocompromised patients may have no fever or respiratory signs and are less likely to have purulent sputum if they are neutropenic. In some patients, the only sign is fever.

An immunocompromised patient with respiratory symptoms, signs, or fever should undergo chest x-ray. If an infiltrate is present, diagnostic studies should include sputum Gram stain and culture and blood cultures. Optimally, firm diagnosis is made with induced sputum and/or bronchoscopy, especially in patients with chronic pneumonia, atypical presentation, severe defects in immune function, and failure to respond to broad-spectrum antibiotics.

Likely pathogens can often be predicted on the basis of symptoms, x-ray changes, and the type of immunodeficiency. In patients with acute symptoms, likely diagnoses are bacterial infection, hemorrhage, pulmonary edema, a leukocyte agglutinin reaction, and pulmonary emboli. A subacute or chronic presentation is more suggestive of a fungal or mycobacterial infection, an opportunistic viral infection, *Pneumocystis jiroveci* (formerly *P. carinii*) pneumonia, tumor, a cytotoxic drug reaction, or radiation injury.

X-rays showing localized consolidation usually indicate an infection involving bacteria, mycobacteria, fungi, or *Nocardia* sp. A diffuse interstitial pattern is more likely to represent a viral infection, *P. jiroveci* pneumonia, drug or radiation injury, or pulmonary edema. Diffuse nodular lesions suggest mycobacteria, *Nocardia* sp, fungi, or tumor. Cavitary disease suggests mycobacteria, *Nocardia* sp, fungi, or bacteria.

In organ or marrow transplantation recipients with bilateral interstitial pneumonia, the usual cause is cytomegalovirus, or the disease is idiopathic. A pleural-based consolidation is usually aspergillosis. In AIDS patients, bilateral pneumonia is usually *P. jiroveci* pneumonia. About 30% of patients with HIV infection have *P. jiroveci* pneumonia as the initial AIDS-defining diagnosis, and > 80% of AIDS patients have this infection at some time if prophylaxis is not given (see p. 1640). Patients with HIV infection become vulnerable to *P. jiroveci* pneumonia when the $CD4^+$ helper cell count is < 200/μL.

Treatment

In neutropenic patients, empiric treatment depends on the host defect, x-ray, and severity of illness. Generally, broad-spectrum drugs are needed to cover gram-negative bacilli,

TABLE 52–7. PNEUMONIA IN THE IMMUNOCOMPROMISED HOST

HOST DEFECT	DISORDERS OR THERAPY ASSOCIATED WITH DEFECT*	LIKELY PATHOGENS
Defective polymorphonuclear neutrophils		
Neutropenia	Acute leukemia, aplastic anemia, cancer chemotherapy	Gram-negative bacteria, *Staphylococcus aureus, Aspergillus* sp, *Candida* sp
Defective chemotaxis	Diabetes mellitus	*S. aureus,* gram-negative aerobes
Defective intracellular killing	Chronic granulomatous disease	*S. aureus*
Defective alternative pathway	Sickle cell disease	*Streptococcus pneumoniae, Haemophilus influenzae*
C5 deficiency	Congenital disorder	*S. pneumoniae, S. aureus,* gram-negative bacteria
Cell-mediated immunodeficiency		
(T-cell deficiency/dysfunction)	Hodgkin lymphoma, cancer chemotherapy, corticosteroid therapy	Mycobacteria, viruses (herpes simplex, cytomegalovirus), *Strongyloides* sp, opportunistic fungi (*Aspergillus, Mucor, Cryptococcus* spp), *Nocardia* sp, *Toxoplasma* sp
	AIDS	*Pneumocystis jiroveci* (formerly *P. carinii*), *Toxoplasma* sp, cytomegalovirus, herpes simplex virus, opportunistic fungi (*Aspergillus, Mucor, Cryptococcus* spp), mycobacteria
Humoral immunodeficiency		
(B-cell deficiency/dysfunction)	Multiple myeloma, agammaglobulinemia	*S. pneumoniae, H. influenzae, Neisseria meningitidis*
	Selective deficiency: IgA, IgG, IgM	*S. pneumoniae, H. influenzae*
	Hypogammaglobulinemia	*P. jiroveci,* cytomegalovirus, *S. pneumoniae, H. influenzae*

*Examples.

Staphylococcus aureus, and anaerobes, as for hospital-acquired pneumonia (see p. 431).

PNEUMOCYSTIS JIROVECI PNEUMONIA

***P. jiroveci* (formerly *P. carinii*) is a common cause of pneumonia in immunosuppressed patients, especially in those infected with HIV. Symptoms include fever, dyspnea, and cough. Diagnosis requires demonstration of the organism in a sputum specimen. Treatment is with antibiotics, usually trimethoprim-sulfamethoxazole or pentamidine, and corticosteroids for patients with Pa_{O_2} < 70 mm Hg. Prognosis is generally good with timely treatment.**

P. jiroveci is a ubiquitous organism transmitted by aerosol route and causes no disease in immunocompetent patients. Patients with HIV infection and $CD4^+$ counts < 200/μL, organ transplant recipients, those who have hematologic malignancies, and patients taking corticosteroids are at risk of developing *P. jiroveci* pneumonia. Most have fever, dyspnea, and a dry, nonproductive cough that evolves subacutely over several weeks (HIV infection) or acutely over several days (other causes of compromised cell-mediated immunity). The chest x-ray characteristically shows diffuse, bilateral perihilar infiltrates, but 20 to 30% of patients have normal x-rays. ABGs show hypoxemia, with an increase in the alveolar-arterial O_2 gradient, and pulmonary function tests show altered diffusing capacity (although this is rarely done as a diagnostic test). Diagnosis requires histopathologic demonstration of the organism with methenamine silver, Giemsa, Wright-Giemsa, modified Grocott, Weigert-Gram, or monoclonal antibody stain. Sputum specimens are usually obtained by induced sputum or bronchoscopy. Sensitivity ranges from 30 to 80% for induced sputum and is > 95% for bronchoscopy with bronchoalveolar lavage.

Treatment is with trimethoprim-sulfamethoxazole (TMP-SMX) 4 to 5 mg/kg IV or po tid for 14 to 21 days. Treatment can be started before diagnosis is confirmed because *P. jiroveci* cysts persist in the lungs for weeks. Adverse effects more common in patients with AIDS include skin rash, neutropenia, hepatitis, and fever. Alternative regimens are pentamidine 4 mg/kg IV once/day, atovaquone 750 mg po bid, TMP-SMX 5 mg/kg po qid with dapsone 100 mg po once/day, or clindamycin 300 to 900 mg IV q 6 to 8 h with primaquine base 15 to 30 mg/day po, also for 21 days. The major limitation of pentamidine is the high frequency of toxic adverse effects, including renal failure, hypotension, and hypoglycemia. Adjunctive therapy with corticosteroids is advocated for those with a Pa_{O_2} < 70 mm Hg. The suggested regimen is prednisone 40 mg bid (or its equivalent) for the first 5 days, 40 mg/day for the next 5 days (as a single dose or as 20 mg bid), and then 20 mg once/day for the duration of treatment.

HIV-infected patients who have had *P. jiroveci* pneumonia or who have a $CD4^+$ count < 200/μL should receive prophylaxis with TMP-SMX 80/400 mg once/day; if this treatment is not tolerated, dapsone 100 mg po once/day or aerosolized pentamidine 300 mg once/month can be used. These prophylactic regimens are also probably indicated for non-HIV-infected patients at risk of *P. jiroveci* pneumonia.

Overall mortality for *P. jiroveci* pneumonia in hospitalized patients is 15 to 20%. Risk factors for death may include previous history of *P. jiroveci* pneumonia, older age, and, in HIV-infected patients, $CD4^+$ cell count < 50/μL.

ASPIRATION PNEUMONITIS AND PNEUMONIA

Aspiration pneumonitis and pneumonia are caused by inhaling toxic substances, usually gastric contents into the lungs. The result may be undetectable or chemical pneumonitis, bacterial pneumonia, or airway obstruction. Symptoms include cough and dyspnea. Diagnosis is based on clinical presentation and x-ray. Treatment and prognosis differ by aspirated substance.

Aspiration can cause lung inflammation (chemical pneumonitis), infection (bacterial pneumonia or abscess), or airway obstruction. Drowning is discussed on p. 2617; airway obstruction, on p. 524. Most episodes of aspiration cause minor symptoms or pneumonitis rather than infection or obstruction.

Risks for aspiration include impaired cognition, impaired swallowing, vomiting, GI and respiratory devices and procedures (eg, nasogastric or endotracheal tube), and gastroesophageal reflux disease.

Chemical pneumonitis: Multiple substances are either directly toxic to the lung or stimulate an inflammatory response when aspirated; gastric acid is the prototype, but others include petroleum products (such as petroleum jelly) and laxative oils (such as mineral, castor, and paraffin oil), all of which cause lipoid pneumonia. Aspirated gasoline and kerosene also cause a chemical pneumonitis.

Gastric contents produce damage mainly from gastric acid, although food and other ingested material (eg, activated charcoal as in treatment of overdose) are injurious in quantity. Gastric acid causes a chemical burn of the airways and lung leading to rapid bronchoconstriction, atelectasis, edema, and alveolar hemorrhage. Symptoms include acute dyspnea with cough, sometimes productive of pink frothy sputum; tachypnea; tachycardia; fever; diffuse crackles; and wheezing. Chest x-ray shows diffuse infiltrates frequently but not exclusively in dependent segments, while pulse-oximetry and ABGs demonstrate hypoxemia. Treatment is supportive, often involving mechanical ventilation. Antibiotics often are given to patients with witnessed or known gastric aspiration. The syndrome may resolve spontaneously, usually within a few days; may progress to acute respiratory distress syndrome; and/or may be complicated by bacterial superinfection.

Aspiration of oils or petroleum jelly causes exogenous lipoid pneumonia, which is characterized histologically by chronic granulomatous inflammation with fibrosis. It is often asymptomatic and is detected incidentally on chest x-ray or may present with low-grade fever, gradual weight loss, and crackles. Chest x-ray findings vary; consolidation, cavitation, interstitial or nodular infiltrates, pleural effusion, and other changes may be slowly progressive. Treatment is avoidance of the toxic substance.

Aspiration pneumonia: Healthy people commonly aspirate small amounts of oral secretions, but normal defense mechanisms usually clear the inoculum without sequelae. Aspiration of larger amounts, or aspiration in a patient with impaired pulmonary defenses, often causes pneumonia and/or abscess (see also Ch. 53, below).

Symptoms and signs of pneumonia and abscess are similar and include chronic low-grade dyspnea, fever, weight loss, and cough productive of putrid, foul-tasting sputum. Patients may have signs of poor oral hygiene. Chest x-ray shows an infiltrate, frequently but not exclusively, in the dependent lung segments, ie, the superior segment of a lower lobe or the posterior segment of an upper lobe. Anaerobes often can be cultured from sputum, but it is unclear whether they are primary infecting organisms to which treatment should be directed or whether they are simply one of several organisms causing infection.

Treatment is with clindamycin 450 to 900 mg IV q 8 h followed by 300 mg po qid once fever and clinical symptoms subside. Penicillin (either penicillin G 1 to 2 million units q 4 to 6 h or amoxicillin 0.5 to 1 g po tid) plus either metronidazole 500 mg po tid, amoxicillin-clavulanate 875/125 mg po tid, or imipenem is an acceptable alternative to clindamycin. Duration of treatment is usually 1 to 2 wk unless the pneumonia is complicated by lung abscess formation, in which case treatment may be required for 6 wk, and up to 3 mo. Empyema is another common complication.

Airway obstruction: Airway obstruction by fluid (eg, near-drowning) or solid food has a range of consequences, from atelectasis to hypoxemia and death. Diagnosis is obvious from history; treatment is suction aspiration (fluid) or bronchoscopic removal of food if possible. Corticosteroids are sometimes used when food cannot be completely retrieved, but efficacy is unproven.

53 LUNG ABSCESS

Lung abscess is a necrotizing infection characterized by localized pus. It is almost always caused by aspiration of oral secretions by patients who have impaired consciousness. Symptoms are persistent cough, fever, sweats, and weight loss. Diagnosis is based on history, physical examination, and chest x-ray. Treatment usually is with clindamycin or combination β-lactam/β-lactamase inhibitors.

Etiology and Pathophysiology

Most lung abscesses develop after aspiration of oral secretions by patients with gingivitis or poor oral hygiene who are unconscious or obtunded from alcohol, illicit drugs, anesthesia, sedatives, or opioids. Older patients and those unable to handle their oral secretions, often because of neurologic disease, are also at risk. Lung abscess less commonly complicates necrotizing pneumonia that may develop from hematogenous seeding of the lungs due to septic embolism from IV drug use or suppurative thromboembolism. In contrast to aspiration, these conditions typically cause multiple rather than isolated lung abscesses.

The most common pathogens are anaerobic bacteria, but about ½ of all cases involve both anaerobic and aerobic organisms (see TABLE 53–1). The most common aerobic pathogens are streptococci. Immunocompromised patients with lung abscess are more

TABLE 53–1. CAUSES OF CAVITARY LUNG LESIONS

Lung abscess
- Anaerobic bacteria
  - Gram-negative bacilli
    - *Fusobacterium* sp
    - *Prevotella* sp
    - *Bacteroides* sp
  - Gram-positive cocci
    - *Peptostreptococcus* sp
  - Gram-positive bacilli
    - *Clostridium* sp
    - *Actinomyces* sp
- Aerobic bacteria
  - Gram-positive cocci
    - *Streptococcus milleri* and other streptococci
    - *Staphylococcus aureus*
  - Gram-negative bacilli
    - *Klebsiella pneumoniae*
    - *Pseudomonas aeruginosa*
    - *Burkholderia pseudomallei*
  - Gram-positive bacilli
    - *Nocardia*
- Mycobacteria
  - *Mycobacterium tuberculosis*
  - *Mycobacterium avium-cellulare*
  - *Mycobacterium kansasii*
- Fungi
  - Histoplasmosis
  - Aspergillosis
  - Coccidioidomycosis
  - Blastomycosis
  - Cryptococcal infection
  - Mucormycosis
  - Sporotrichosis
  - *Pneumocystis jiroveci* (formerly *P. carinii*) infection
- Parasites
  - Paragonimiasis
  - Echinococcal infection
  - Amebic infection

Bronchiectasis

Noninfectious causes
- Lung cancer
- Bullae with air-fluid level
- Pulmonary sequestration
- Pulmonary embolism
- Wegener's granulomatosis
- Nodular silicosis nodule with central necrosis

likely to have infection with *Nocardia, mycobacteria,* or fungi. People from developing countries are at risk of abscess due to *Mycobacterium tuberculosis*, amebic infection (*Entamoeba histolytica*), paragonimiasis, or *Burkholderia pseudomallei*.

Introduction of these pathogens into the lungs first causes inflammation, which leads to tissue necrosis and then abscess formation. Most commonly, the abscess ruptures into a bronchus, and its contents are expectorated, leaving an air- and fluid-filled cavity. In about ⅓ of cases, direct or indirect extension (via bronchopleural fistula) into the pleural cavity results in empyema. Cavitary pulmonary lesions are not always abscesses (see TABLE 53–1).

Symptoms and Signs

Symptoms of abscess due to anaerobic bacteria or mixed anaerobic/aerobic bacteria are usually chronic (eg, over weeks or months) and include productive cough, fever, sweats, and weight loss. Severe prostration may occur. Sputum may be purulent or blood-streaked and classically smells or tastes foul. Symptoms of abscess due to aerobic bacteria develop more acutely and resemble bacterial pneumonia. Abscesses due to organisms other than anaerobes (eg, *Mycobacteria, Nocardia*) lack putrid respiratory secretions, may be more likely to occur in nondependent lung regions, and do not respond to standard antibiotics.

Signs of lung abscess, when present, are nonspecific and resemble those of pneumonia: decreased breath sounds indicating consolidation or effusion, temperature ≥ 39.4° C, crackles over the affected area, egophony, and dullness to percussion in the presence of effusion. Patients typically have signs of periodontal disease and a history of a problem or condition causing impaired consciousness.

Diagnosis

Lung abscess is suspected based on history, physical examination, and chest x-ray. In anaerobic infection due to aspiration, chest x-ray classically shows consolidation, with a single cavity containing an air-fluid level in portions of the lung that are dependent when the patient is recumbent (eg, posterior segment upper lobe or superior segment lower lobe). This pattern helps distinguish anaerobic abscess from other causes of cavitary pulmonary disease, such as diffuse or embolic pulmonary disease, which may cause multiple cavitations, or TB, which involves the apices. CT scan is not routinely needed but may be useful when the x-ray suggests a cavitating lesion or when an underlying pulmonary mass obstructing the drainage of a lung segment is suspected. Anaerobic bacteria are rarely identifiable on culture because uncontaminated specimens are difficult to obtain and because most laboratories do not culture anaerobes well or often. If sputum is putrid, then anaerobic infection is assumed to be the cause. Bronchoscopy is sometimes indicated to exclude malignancy.

When anaerobic infection is less likely, then aerobic, fungal, or mycobacterial infection is suspected, and attempts are made to identify a pathogen. Cultures of sputum, bronchoscopic aspirates, or both are helpful.

Treatment

Treatment is with antibiotics. Clindamycin 600 mg IV q 6 to 8 h is usually the drug of choice given its excellent anaerobic and streptococcal coverage. The primary alternative is a combination β-lactam/β-lactamase inhibitor (eg, ampicillin/sulbactam 1 to 2 g IV q 6 h, ticarcillin/clavulanate 3 to 6 g IV q 6 h, piperacillin/tazobactam 3 g IV q 6 h). Metronidazole 500 mg q 8 h may be used but must be combined with penicillin 2 million units q 6 h IV. Less seriously ill patients may be given oral antibiotics such as clindamycin 300 mg po q 6 h or amoxicillin/clavulanate 875/125 mg po q 12 h. IV regimens can be converted to oral ones when the patient defervesces.

Optimal duration of treatment is unknown, but common practice is to treat for 3 to 6 wk unless the chest x-ray shows complete resolution sooner. In general, the larger the abscess, the longer it will take to resolve on x-ray. Larger abscesses, therefore, typically require several weeks or months of treatment.

Most authorities do not recommend chest physical therapy and postural drainage because they may cause spillage of infection into other bronchi with extension of the infection or acute obstruction. If the patient is weak or paralyzed or has respiratory failure, tracheostomy and suctioning may be necessary. Rarely, bronchoscopic aspiration helps facilitate drainage. An accompanying empyema must be drained; fluid provides a good source for anaerobic culture. Percutaneous or surgical drainage of lung abscesses is necessary in the roughly 10% of patients in whom lesions do not respond to antibiotics. Resistance to antibiotic treatment is most common with large cavities and with infections that complicate obstructions.

When surgery is necessary, lobectomy is the most common procedure; segmental resection may suffice for small lesions. Pneumonectomy may be necessary for multiple abscesses or for pulmonary gangrene unresponsive to drug therapy.

54 BRONCHIECTASIS

Bronchiectasis is dilation and destruction of larger bronchi caused by chronic infection and inflammation. Common causes are cystic fibrosis, immune defects, and infections, though some cases appear to be idiopathic. Symptoms are chronic cough and purulent sputum expectoration; some patients may also have fever and dyspnea. Diagnosis is based on history and imaging, usually involving high-resolution CT, though standard chest x-rays may be diagnostic. Treatment and prevention of acute exacerbations are with antibiotics, drainage of secretions, and management of complications, such as superinfection and hemoptysis. Treatment of underlying causes is important whenever possible.

Etiology and Pathophysiology

Diffuse bronchiectasis develops in patients with genetic, immune, or anatomic defects that affect the airways. Cystic fibrosis is the most common cause; ciliary dyskinesia and severe α_1-antitrypsin deficiency are less common genetic causes. Hypogammaglobulinemia and immune deficiencies may also cause diffuse disease, as may rare abnormalities in airway structure (eg, tracheobronchomegaly [Mounier-Kuhn syndrome], cartilage deficiency [Williams-Campbell syndrome]). Diffuse bronchiectasis is an uncommon complication of more common conditions, such as RA, Sjögren's syndrome, and allergic bronchopulmonary aspergillosis, probably via multiple mechanisms.

TABLE 54–1. FACTORS PREDISPOSING TO BRONCHIECTASIS

CATEGORY	EXAMPLES AND COMMENTS
Infections	
Bacterial	*Pseudomonas aeruginosa, Haemophilus influenzae, Moraxella catarrhalis, Klebsiella* sp, *Staphylococcus aureus*
Fungal	*Histoplasma capsulatum*
Mycobacterial	Non-TB mycobacteria
Viral	Adenovirus, influenza, herpes simplex, measles, pertussis
Congenital diseases	
α_1-Antitrypsin deficiency	Bronchiectasis only seen in some patients with severe deficiency
Ciliary defects	Prevalence of 1/15,000–40,000 patients. Bronchiectasis, sinusitis, ± infertility, ± situs inversus (Kartagener's syndrome = clinical triad of dextrocardia, sinus disease, and situs inversus. Triad may catch only 50% of patients with ciliary defects; cilia beat during embryogenesis to place internal organs in anatomic position, thus patients with ciliary defects are equally likely to have their organs located on the right or left)
Cystic fibrosis	Most common (prevalence 1/3300). Defect in Na and Cl transport causes viscous secretions. Often complicated by *P. aeruginosa* or *S. aureus* infection
Immunodeficiencies	
Primary	Hypogammaglobulinemia, including IgG subclass deficiencies (IgG_2, IgG_4); chronic granulomatous disease; complement deficiencies
Secondary	Immunosuppressive drug regimens, HIV infection
Airway obstruction	
Extrinsic compression	From tumor mass or lymphadenopathy
Foreign body	Aspirated or intrinsic (eg, broncholith)
Malignancy	Endobronchial lesion
Mucoid impaction	Allergic bronchopulmonary aspergillosis
Postoperative	After lobar resection, remaining lobes may kink or twist with repositioning
Connective tissue diseases	Prevalence 1 to 3%. Bronchiectasis secondary to chronic aspiration
RA	
Sjögren's syndrome	
SLE	
Relapsing polychondritis	
Congenital structural defects	
Lymphatic	Yellow nail syndrome
Tracheobronchial	Tracheobronchomegaly (Meunier-Kuhn syndrome), cartilage deficiency (Williams-Campbell syndrome)
Vascular	Pulmonary sequestration
Toxic inhalation	Direct airway damage alters structure and function
Ammonia	
Chlorine	
Nitrogen dioxide	

TABLE 54–1. FACTORS PREDISPOSING TO BRONCHIECTASIS—Continued

CATEGORY	EXAMPLES AND COMMENTS
Miscellaneous	
Inflammatory bowel disease	Usually chronic ulcerative colitis; bowel resection may exacerbate pulmonary disease
Transplantation	May be secondary to frequent infection from immunosuppression

Data from Barker, AF: Bronchiectasis. *The New England Journal of Medicine* 346:1383–1393, 2002.

Focal bronchiectasis develops from untreated pneumonia or obstruction (eg, from foreign bodies and tumors, extrinsic compression, or shifts in anatomy after lobar resection). Other disorders are listed in TABLE 54–1; some cases have no readily apparent cause.

All of these conditions impair airway clearance mechanisms and host defenses, conferring an inability to clear secretions and predisposing to infection and chronic inflammation. As a result of frequent infection, most commonly with *Haemophilus influenzae* (35%), *Pseudomonas aeruginosa* (31%), *Moraxella catarrhalis* (20%), *Staphylococcus aureus* (14%), and *Streptococcus pneumoniae* (13%), airways become inspissated with viscous mucous containing inflammatory mediators and pathogens and slowly become dilated, scarred, and distorted. Histologically, bronchial walls are thickened by edema, inflammation, and neovascularization. Destruction of surrounding interstitium and alveoli causes fibrosis, emphysema, or both.

Mycobacteria other than TB can cause bronchiectasis as well as colonize the lungs of patients with bronchiectasis from other causes.

Symptoms and Signs

The primary symptom of bronchiectasis is chronic cough that may produce large volumes of thick, tenacious, purulent sputum. Dyspnea and wheezing are common. Hemoptysis, which can be massive, is due to neovascularization of the airways from the bronchial (as opposed to pulmonary) arteries. Low-grade fever occurs with acute exacerbations of disease, during which the extent of cough and the volume and purulence of sputum production increase. Chronic bronchitis (see p. 400) may mimic bronchiectasis clinically, but bronchiectasis is distinguished by more voluminous production of purulent sputum on a daily basis and typical CT scan abnormalities.

Halitosis and abnormal breath sounds, including crackles, rhonchi, and wheezing, are typical signs of disease. Finger clubbing may also be present.

Symptoms characteristically begin insidiously and recur increasingly, worsening gradually over years. In advanced cases, hypoxemia, pulmonary hypertension, and right heart failure can occur.

Superinfection with multidrug-resistant organisms including mycobacteria other than TB should be considered a possible underlying cause of symptoms in patients with recurrent exacerbations or worsening airflow limitation on pulmonary function tests.

Diagnosis

Diagnosis is based on a history, physical examination, and radiologic testing, beginning with a chest x-ray. X-ray findings suggestive of bronchiectasis include scattered irregular opacities caused by mucous plugs, honeycombing, and rings and "tram lines" caused by thickened, dilated airways facing into or perpendicular to the x-ray beam, respectively. Radiographic patterns may differ by underlying disease: Bronchiectasis due to cystic fibrosis develops predominantly in upper lobes, whereas that due to other causes is more diffuse or predominates in the lower lobes. High-resolution CT is the test of choice for defining the extent of bronchiectasis. The test is nearly 100% sensitive and specific. CT typically shows bronchial varicosities and cysts (sometimes appearing as grapelike clusters), scattered mucous plugs, and airways that are dilated > 1.5 times the diameter of nearby blood vessels. Dilated medium-sized bronchi may extend almost to the pleurae. Atelectasis, consolidation, and decreased vascularity are nonspecific findings.

A differential diagnosis of dilated airways includes bronchitis and "traction bronchiectasis" that occurs when pulmonary fibrosis pulls airways open.

Pulmonary function tests should be obtained for purposes of documenting baseline function and for following the progression of disease over time. Bronchiectasis is associated with airflow limitation (reduced forced expiratory volume in 1 sec [FEV_1], forced vital capacity [FVC], and FEV_1/FVC); the FEV_1 can improve in response to β-agonist bronchodilators. Lung volume measurements and diffusing capacity for carbon monoxide (DL_{CO}) may be decreased.

Tests to help diagnose an underlying cause include sputum evaluation, including staining and cultures for bacterial, mycobacterial (*Mycobacterium avium* complex and *Mycobacterium tuberculosis*), and fungal (*Aspergillus*) infection. Mycobacterial superinfection is diagnosed by repeatedly culturing mycobacteria other than TB in high colony counts and by finding granulomas on biopsy with concurrent radiologic evidence of disease. Additional tests may include sweat chloride testing to diagnose cystic fibrosis, which should be performed even in older patients; rheumatoid factor and other serologic tests to look for connective tissue disease; immunoglobulins including IgG subclasses to document some immunodeficiencies; *Aspergillus* precipitins, IgE, and eosinophilia to rule out allergic bronchopulmonary aspergillosis; and α_1-antitrypsin levels to document α_1-antitrypsin deficiency. When the clinical presentation suggests ciliary dyskinesia (by concurrent sinus disease and middle and lower lobe bronchiectasis with or without infertility), a nasal or bronchial epithelial biopsy should be obtained and examined by transmission electron microscopy for abnormal ciliary structure. A less invasive alternative is examination of sperm motility. The diagnosis of ciliary dyskinesia should be made cautiously by an experienced physician trained in specialized techniques, because nonspecific structural defects can be present in up to 10% of cilia in healthy patients and in those with pulmonary disease; infection can cause transient dyskinesia; and ciliary ultrastructure may be normal in patients with primary ciliary dyskinesia syndromes characterized by abnormal ciliary function.

Bronchoscopy is indicated when an anatomic or an obstructing object or lesion is suspected.

Prognosis and Prevention

Overall, prognosis is thought to be good, with about 80% of patients having no further deterioration of lung function on the basis of bronchiectasis alone. However, cystic fibrosis patients have a median survival of 32 yr, and most patients continue to have intermittent acute exacerbations.

Prevention of bronchiectasis requires timely recognition and treatment of underlying causes. Unfortunately, most patients seek medical attention because the disease is already established.

Treatment

Treatment involves preventing exacerbations, treating underlying causes, aggressively managing acute exacerbations, and controlling complications.

There is no consensus on the best approach to prevent or limit acute exacerbations. Options include daily prophylactic oral antibiotics (eg, ciprofloxacin 500 mg bid) and, in patients with cystic fibrosis who are colonized with *P. aeruginosa,* inhaled tobramycin (300 mg bid every other month). In patients with diffuse bronchiectasis due to other causes, aerosolized gentamicin (40 mg bid) may also be effective.

As with all chronic pulmonary disease, annual vaccination against influenza and against pneumococcus is recommended.

Various techniques can facilitate clearance of secretions, including postural drainage and chest percussion, positive expiratory pressure devices, intrapulmonary percussive ventilators, pneumatic vests, and autogenic drainage (a breathing technique thought to help move secretions from peripheral to central airways). A mucolytic (rhDNase) has been shown to have clinical utility in patients with cystic fibrosis. Patients should be introduced to these techniques by a respiratory therapist and should use whichever technique is most effective; no evidence favors one technique over another.

Additional treatment depends on the underlying cause. For cystic fibrosis, see p. 2308. Allergic bronchopulmonary aspergillosis is treated with corticosteroids and possibly with azole antifungals (see p. 398). Patients with immunoglobulin deficiencies should receive replacement therapy. Those with α_1-antitrypsin deficiency should receive replacement therapy.

Treatment of acute exacerbations is with antibiotics that will cover *H. influenzae, P. aeruginosa, M. catarrhalis, S. aureus,* and *S. pneumoniae* (eg, ciprofloxacin 500 mg po bid or levofloxacin 500 mg po once/day for 7 to 14 days). Azithromycin 500 mg 3 times/wk has demonstrated efficacy in cystic fibrosis bronchiectasis, but it is unclear whether macrolides are useful in other forms of the disorder. Antibiotic treatment should be accompanied by increased efforts to facilitate clearance of sputum from the airway.

Control of acute complications includes treating mycobacterial superinfection and hemorrhage.

An empirical multidrug regimen for *M. avium* complex may include clarithromycin 500 mg po bid or azithromycin 250 mg once/day; rifampin 600 mg po once/day or rifabutin 300 mg po once/day; and ethambutol 25 mg/kg po once/day for 2 mo followed by 15 mg/kg once/day. All drugs should be taken on a continuous maintenance basis until sputum cultures are negative for 12 mo. Surgical resection is rarely necessary but should be considered when antibiotic treatment is inadequate and the disease is sufficiently localized.

Massive hemorrhage is generally treated with bronchial artery embolization along with antibiotic treatment for an acute exacerbation.

55 INTERSTITIAL LUNG DISEASES

(Diffuse Interstitial Lung Diseases)

Interstitial lung diseases are characterized by alveolar septal thickening, fibroblast proliferation, collagen deposition, and, if the process remains unchecked, pulmonary fibrosis. Numerous conditions and agents, including most connective tissue diseases and occupational lung exposures, and many drugs cause similar interstitial changes (see Ch. 57 on p. 469 and TABLE 55–1). But in up to 30% of patients, no clear cause can be found; the term idiopathic interstitial pneumonia refers to these patients. Other idiopathic interstitial diseases differ in histology, clinical features, and presentation and thus are considered unique diseases; these include eosinophilic pulmonary diseases, hypersensitivity pneumonitis, pulmonary Langerhans' cell granulomatosis, lymphangioleiomyomatosis, pulmonary alveolar proteinosis, and sarcoidosis.

IDIOPATHIC INTERSTITIAL PNEUMONIAS

Idiopathic interstitial pneumonias are interstitial lung diseases of unknown etiology that share similar clinical features. Classified into 6 histologic subtypes, all are characterized by varying degrees of inflammation and fibrosis and all cause dyspnea and typical radiographic abnormalities. Diagnosis is based on history, physical examination, imaging, pulmonary function tests, and lung biopsy. Treatment varies by subtype but typically involves corticosteroids, cytotoxic drugs, or both; treatment is frequently ineffective. Prognosis varies by subtype and ranges from excellent to nearly always fatal.

The 6 histologic subtypes of idiopathic interstitial pneumonia (IIP) in decreasing order of frequency are usual interstitial pneumonia (UIP), known clinically as idiopathic pulmonary fibrosis; nonspecific interstitial pneumonia; bronchiolitis obliterans organizing pneumonia; respiratory bronchiolitis-associated interstitial lung disease (ILD); desquamative interstitial pneumonia; and acute interstitial pneumonia. Lymphoid interstitial pneumonia, although still considered a subtype of IIP, is now thought to be part of the lymphoproliferative disease spectrum rather than primary ILD (see p. 459). These subtypes are characterized by varying degrees of interstitial inflammation and fibrosis, and all cause dyspnea; diffuse, usually reticular opacities on chest x-ray; and inflammation and/or fibrosis on biopsy. The subtypes are important to distinguish, however, because they have different clinical features and responses to treatment (see TABLE 55–2).

Diagnosis

Known causes of ILD must be excluded. Chest x-ray is always obtained as well as pulmonary function tests (see p. 364) and high-resolution CT (HRCT), which distinguishes

TABLE 55–1. CAUSES OF INTERSTITIAL LUNG DISEASE*

CAUSE	DIFFERENTIAL DIAGNOSIS
Circulatory disorders	Pulmonary edema Pulmonary veno-occlusive disease
Connective tissue disease	Ankylosing spondylitis Behçet's syndrome Dermatomyositis Goodpasture's syndrome Mixed connective tissue disease Polymyositis RA Sjögren's syndrome SLE
Environmental pulmonary disease	Inorganic:* Aluminum oxide fibrosis, asbestosis, baritosis, berylliosis, coal worker's lung, metal polisher's lung/hard metal fibrosis, siderosis, silicosis, stannosis, talc pneumoconiosis Organic:* Bagassosis, bird fancier's lung, coffee worker's lung, farmer's lung, humidifier's lung, hot tub lung, malt worker's lung, maple bark stripper's lung, mushroom worker's lung, tea grower's lung
Infections	Aspergillosis Histoplasmosis Parasitic infection TB Viral infection
Vasculitis	Churg-Strauss syndrome Giant cell arteritis Wegener's granulomatosis
Miscellaneous diseases	Alveolar proteinosis Amyloidosis Chronic aspiration Eosinophilic granuloma Eosinophilic pneumonia Gaucher's disease Lipoid pneumonia Lymphangioleiomyomatosis Microlithiasis Neurofibromatosis Niemann-Pick disease Pulmonary lymphoma Sarcoidosis Tuberous sclerosis

*For drug causes, see TABLE 55–3.

airspace from interstitial disease, provides better assessment of the extent and distribution of disease, and is more likely to detect underlying or coexisting disease (eg, occult mediastinal adenopathy, carcinoma, emphysema). HRCT is best performed with the patient prone to reduce dependent lung atelectasis.

Lung biopsy is usually needed to confirm the diagnosis except when HRCT demonstrates a diagnostic pattern. Bronchoscopic transbronchial biopsy can rule out ILD by detecting other diseases but does not yield enough tissue to diagnose ILD. Biopsy of multiple sites with an open or video-assisted thoracoscopic surgery (VATS) procedure is required.

Bronchoalveolar lavage helps narrow the differential diagnosis in selected patients and can provide information about disease progression and response to therapy. The usefulness of this procedure in the initial clinical assessment and follow-up of most patients with these diseases has not been established, however.

IDIOPATHIC PULMONARY FIBROSIS

(Cryptogenic Fibrosing Alveolitis)

Idiopathic pulmonary fibrosis, the most common form of IIP, causes progressive pulmonary fibrosis predominantly in male smokers. Symptoms and signs develop over months to years and include exertional dyspnea, cough, and fine (Velcro) crackles. Diagnosis is based on history, physical examination, chest x-ray, and pulmonary function tests and is confirmed with HRCT, lung biopsy, or both if necessary. No specific treatment has proven effective, but corticosteroids, cyclophosphamide, azathioprine, or a combination are often given. Most patients deteriorate even with treatment; median survival is < 3 yr from diagnosis.

Etiology and Pathophysiology

Idiopathic pulmonary fibrosis (IPF), identified histologically as UIP, accounts for 50% of cases of IIP. IPF affects men and women in their 50s and 60s in a ratio of 2 : 1. Current or former cigarette smoking is most strongly associated with the disease. There is some genetic predisposition; familial clustering occurs in up to 3% of cases.

Although IPF is called a pneumonia, inflammation seems to play a relatively minor role. Environmental, genetic, or other unknown factors are thought to initially trigger alveolar epithelial cell injury, but self-perpetuating and aberrant interstitial fibroblast and mesenchymal cell proliferation (with collagen deposition and fibrosis) are thought to account for development of clinical disease. The key histologic findings are subpleural fibrosis with sites of fibroblast proliferation (fibroblast foci) and dense scarring, alternating with areas of normal lung tissue (heterogeneity). Scattered interstitial inflammation occurs with lymphocyte, plasma cell, and histiocyte infiltration. Cystic dilatation of peripheral alveoli (honeycombing) is found in all patients and increases with advanced disease. A similar histologic pattern uncommonly occurs in cases of ILD of known etiology (see TABLE 55–1); the term UIP is reserved for idiopathic lesions not associated with known conditions.

Symptoms and Signs

Symptoms and signs typically develop over 6 mo to several years and include dyspnea on exertion and nonproductive cough. Constitutional symptoms, such as low-grade fever and myalgias, are uncommon. The classic sign of IPF is fine, dry, bibasilar inspiratory crackles (Velcro crackles). Clubbing is present in about 50% of cases. The remainder of the examination is normal until disease is advanced; in advanced disease, signs of pulmonary hypertension and right ventricular systolic dysfunction may develop.

Diagnosis

Diagnosis is based on history, imaging tests, pulmonary function tests, and biopsy. IPF is commonly overlooked at first because of clinical similarities to other diseases, such as bronchitis, asthma, and heart failure.

Chest x-ray typically shows diffuse reticular opacities in the lower and peripheral lung zones. Small cystic lesions (honeycombing) and dilated airways due to traction bronchiectasis are additional findings.

Pulmonary function tests typically reveal a restrictive pattern (see Ch. 46 on p. 364). Diffusing capacity for carbon monoxide (DL_{CO}) is also reduced. ABGs show hypoxemia, which is often exaggerated or elicited by exercise and low arterial CO_2 levels.

HRCT shows diffuse, patchy, subpleural, reticular opacities with irregularly thickened interlobular septa and intralobular lines; subpleural honeycombing; and traction bronchiectasis. Ground-glass opacities affecting > 30% of the lung suggest an alternative diagnosis.

Laboratory testing plays little role in diagnosis. Elevated ESR, C-reactive protein, and hypergammaglobulinemia are common. Antinuclear antibody or rheumatoid factor is elevated in up to 30% of patients and, depending on the titer, may not imply underlying connective tissue disease.

Prognosis

Most patients have moderate to advanced clinical disease at the time of diagnosis and deteriorate despite treatment. Normal PaO_2 at presentation and fewer fibroblastic foci on biopsy improve the prognosis. Prognosis is worse with advanced age, poor pulmonary function at presentation, and severe dyspnea. Median survival is < 3 yr from time of diagnosis. An increase in the frequency of hospitalization for unexpected respiratory infection and insufficiency indicates the approach of the patient's end of life and should prompt discussions about advance care planning (see p. 2768). Lung cancer occurs more frequently in patients with IPF, but cause of death is usually respiration failure, respiratory infection, or heart failure with ischemia and arrhythmia.

Treatment

No specific treatment has proven effective. Supportive therapy consists of O_2 for hypoxemia and antibiotics for pneumonias. End-stage disease may qualify selected patients for lung transplantation. Corticosteroids and cytotoxic drugs (cyclophosphamide, azathioprine) have traditionally been given to IPF patients empirically in an attempt to halt the progression of inflammation, but limited data support their efficacy. Nevertheless, it is common practice to attempt treatment with prednisone (0.5 to 1.0 mg/kg po once/day for 3 mo, tapered to 0.25 mg/kg once/day over the next 3 to 6 mo) combined with cyclophosphamide or azathioprine (1 to 2 mg/kg po once/day). Every 3 mo for 1 yr, clinical, radiographic, and physiologic responses are assessed, and drug doses are increased or decreased accordingly. Therapy is stopped if there is no objective response.

Pirfenidone, an antifibrotic agent, may stabilize pulmonary function and reduce exacerbations. Antifibrotics that inhibit collagen synthesis (relaxin), profibrotic growth factors (suramin), and endothelin-1 (an angiotensin receptor blocker) have only been demonstrated effective in vitro.

TABLE 55–2. KEY FEATURES OF IDIOPATHIC INTERSTITIAL PNEUMONIAS

KEY FEATURE	IPF/CFA	NSIP	DIP	RBILD	AIP	COP	LIP*
Age at onset (yr)	> 60	40–60	40–50	40–50	Any age	40–50	Any age
M:F ratio	Male predominance	Equal	Male predominance	Slight male predominance	Equal	Equal	Female predominance
Prodrome	Chronic (> 12 mo)	Subacute to chronic (months to years)	Subacute (weeks to months)	Subacute (weeks to months)	Abrupt (1–2 wk)	Subacute (< 3 mo)	Chronic (> 12 mo)
History of cigarette smoking	> 60%	> 40%	> 90%	> 90%	Unknown	< 50%	Unknown
Chest x-ray findings	Basal-predominant reticular abnormality with volume loss	Ground-glass and reticular opacity	Ground-glass opacity	Bronchial wall thickening; ground-glass opacity	Progressive diffuse ground-glass density/consolidation	Patchy bilateral consolidation	Reticular opacities, nodules
High-resolution CT findings	Peripheral, subpleural, basal; reticular; honeycombing; traction bronchiectasis/bronchiolectasis; architectural distortion; focal ground glass	Peripheral, subpleural, basal, symmetric; ground-glass attenuation; irregular lines; consolidation	Lower zone, peripheral predominance in most; ground-glass attenuation; reticular lines	Diffuse pattern; bronchial wall thickening; centrilobular nodules; patchy ground-glass opacity	Diffuse consolidation and ground-glass opacity, often with lobular sparing; traction bronchiectasis later	Subpleural/peribronchial; patchy consolidation and/or nodules	Diffuse pattern. Centrilobular nodules; ground-glass attenuation; septal and bronchovascular thickening; thin-walled cysts

Histologic pattern	Usual interstitial pneumonia	NSIP	DIP	RB	Diffuse alveolar damage	Organizing pneumonia	LIP
Treatment	Poor response to corticosteroid or cytotoxic agents	Corticosteroid responsiveness	Smoking cessation; corticosteroid responsiveness	Smoking cessation; corticosteroid responsiveness	Mechanical ventilation; corticosteroid responsiveness unknown	Corticosteroid responsiveness	Corticosteroid responsiveness
Prognosis	50–70% mortality in 5 yr	Unclear; <10% mortality in 5 yr	5% mortality in 5 yr	Rare deaths	60% mortality in < 6 mo	Complete recovery in 2/3; relapse is common	Not well defined
CT differential diagnosis	Asbestosis; connective tissue disease; hypersensitivity pneumonitis; sarcoidosis	Usual interstitial pneumonia; DIP; COP; hypersensitivity pneumonitis	RBILD; hypersensitivity pneumonitis; sarcoidosis; *Pneumocystis jiroveci* (formerly *P. carinii*) pneumonia	DIP; NSIP; hypersensitivity pneumonitis	Hydrostatic edema; pneumonia; acute eosinophilic pneumonia	Infection; vasculitis; sarcoidosis; alveolar carcinoma; lymphoma; eosinophilic pneumonia; NSIP	Sarcoidosis; lymphangitic carcinoma; Langerhans' cell granulomatosis

*Lymphoid interstitial pneumonia, once considered a subtype of IIP, is now thought to be part of the lymphoproliferative disease spectrum rather than primary ILD.

IPF = idiopathic pulmonary fibrosis; CFA = cryptogenic fibrosing alveolitis; NSIP = nonspecific interstitial pneumonia; DIP = desquamative interstitial pneumonia; RBILD = respiratory bronchiolitis-associated interstitial lung disease; AIP = acute interstitial pneumonia; COP = cryptogenic organizing pneumonia; LIP = lymphoid interstitial pneumonia.

Interferon-γ-1b has shown promise when combined with prednisone in a small group of patients, but a larger double-blind multinational randomized trial found no effect on progression-free survival time, pulmonary function, or quality of life.

Lung transplantation is successful for otherwise healthy IPF patients < 55 yr with end-stage pulmonary disease (< 40% of all IPF patients).

Desquamative Interstitial Pneumonia

Desquamative interstitial pneumonia is chronic lung inflammation characterized by mononuclear cell infiltration of the airspaces.

Over 90% of patients with desquamative interstitial pneumonia are smokers, who tend to develop the disease in their 30s or 40s. The disease tends to affect the lung parenchyma uniformly. The alveolar walls are lined with plump cuboidal pneumocytes; there is moderate infiltration of the alveolar septum by lymphocytes, plasma cells, and, occasionally, eosinophils, and alveolar septal fibrosis is mild at worst. The most striking feature is the presence of numerous pigmented macrophages within distal airspaces, mistaken as desquamated pneumocytes when the disease was first described. Honeycombing is rare. Similar but much less extensive findings are seen in respiratory bronchiolitis-associated ILD (RBILD), leading to the suggestion that desquamative interstitial pneumonia and RBILD are different manifestations of the same disease caused by cigarette smoking.

The symptoms, signs, pulmonary function test findings, and approach to diagnosis are otherwise the same as for idiopathic pulmonary fibrosis (IPF).

Chest x-ray abnormalities are less severe than in IPF; findings may be normal in up to 20% of cases. HRCT shows patchy, subpleural ground-glass opacities, usually without reticular opacities.

Treatment with smoking cessation results in clinical improvement in an estimated 75% of patients; those who do not improve may respond to corticosteroid or cytotoxic drugs. Prognosis is good, with about 70% survival at 10 yr.

Respiratory Bronchiolitis-Associated Interstitial Lung Disease

Respiratory bronchiolitis-associated ILD is a syndrome of small airway inflammation and interstitial lung disease occurring in smokers.

Most smokers develop a subclinical bronchiolitis characterized by mild or moderate inflammation of the small airways. The few patients who develop more severe inflammation with clinically significant interstitial disease are said to have respiratory bronchiolitis-associated ILD (RBILD). Male-to-female ratio is 2:1. RBILD is characterized histologically by submucosal inflammation of the membranous and respiratory bronchioles manifested by the presence of tan-brown pigmented macrophages (resulting from increased iron content, as is seen in smokers), mucus stasis, and metaplastic cuboidal epithelium in bronchioles and alveoli. Alveolar septal scarring always occurs. These findings, however, occur in some hypersensitivity reactions, occupational lung exposures (usually due to mineral dusts), viral infections, and drug reactions. RBILD also resembles desquamative interstitial pneumonia histologically, but in RBILD inflammation is patchier and less extensive. The similarity of the 2 conditions has led to the suggestion that they are different manifestations of the same disease caused by cigarette smoking.

Symptoms of cough and breathlessness with exertion resemble those of other ILDs, especially IPF, but are milder. Crackles on examination are the only physical finding.

Diagnosis is based on history, imaging tests, pulmonary function tests, and biopsy. Chest x-ray findings include diffuse, fine reticular or nodular opacities; bronchial wall thickening; prominent peribronchovascular interstitium; small regular and irregular opacities; and small peripheral ring shadows. HRCT scanning often shows hazy ground-glass opacities. A mixed obstructive-restrictive pattern is common on pulmonary function tests, although results may be normal or show an isolated increase in residual volume. ABG measurements show mild hypoxemia. Routine laboratory tests are not helpful.

Treatment of RBILD is smoking cessation; evidence of efficacy of corticosteroids is anecdotal. The natural clinical course of the disease is unknown, but prognosis is good with smoking cessation.

Acute Interstitial Pneumonia

(Accelerated Interstitial Pneumonia; Hamman-Rich Syndrome)

Acute interstitial pneumonia is an idiopathic version of the acute respiratory distress syndrome (ARDS—see p. 556).

Acute interstitial pneumonia (AIP) affects apparently healthy men and women usually > 40 yr equally.

AIP is defined histologically by organizing diffuse alveolar damage, a nonspecific pattern seen in other causes of lung injury unrelated to IIP. The hallmark of organizing diffuse alveolar damage is diffuse, marked alveolar septal edema with inflammatory cell infiltration; fibroblast proliferation; occasional hyaline membranes; and thickening. Septa are lined with atypical, hyperplastic type II pneumocytes, and airspaces are collapsed. Thrombi develop in small arteries but are nonspecific.

Symptoms are abrupt onset of fever, cough, and shortness of breath and last 7 to 14 days, quickly progressing in most patients to respiratory failure.

Diagnosis is based on history, imaging tests, pulmonary function tests, and biopsy. Chest x-ray findings are similar to those in ARDS and show diffuse bilateral airspace opacification. HRCT scan shows bilateral patchy symmetric areas of ground-glass attenuation and sometimes bilateral areas of airspace consolidation in a predominantly subpleural distribution. Mild honeycombing, usually affecting < 10% of the lung, may be seen. Routine laboratory tests are nonspecific and generally not helpful.

Diagnosis is confirmed by biopsy showing diffuse alveolar damage in the absence of known causes of ARDS and diffuse alveolar damage (eg, sepsis, drugs, toxins, radiation, and viral infection). The disease must also be distinguished from diffuse alveolar hemorrhage syndrome, acute eosinophilic pneumonia, and idiopathic bronchiolitis obliterans organizing pneumonia.

Treatment is supportive and usually requires mechanical ventilation. Corticosteroid therapy is generally used, but efficacy has not been established.

Mortality is > 60%; most patients die within 6 mo of presentation, and death is usually due to respiratory failure. In patients who survive the initial acute episode, recovery of pulmonary function is complete, although the disease may recur.

Bronchiolitis Obliterans Organizing Pneumonia

(Cryptogenic Organizing Pneumonia)

Bronchiolitis obliterans organizing pneumonia is an idiopathic condition in which granulation tissue obstructs bronchioles and alveolar ducts with chronic inflammation and organizing pneumonia in adjacent alveoli.

Idiopathic bronchiolitis obliterans organizing pneumonia (BOOP) affects men and women equally, usually in their 40s or 50s. Cigarette smoking does not appear to be a risk factor.

About ½ the patients recall having a community-acquired pneumonia-like syndrome (ie, a nonresolving flu-like illness characterized by cough, fever, malaise, fatigue, and weight loss). Progressive cough and exertional dyspnea are what usually prompt the patient to seek medical attention. Examination demonstrates inspiratory crackles.

Diagnosis is based on history, physical examination, imaging tests, pulmonary function tests, and biopsy. Chest x-ray shows bilateral, diffuse, peripherally distributed alveolar opacities with normal lung volumes; a peripheral distribution similar to that seen in chronic eosinophilic pneumonia may occur. Rarely, alveolar opacities are unilateral. Recurrent and migratory pulmonary opacities are common. Rarely, irregular linear or nodular interstitial opacities or honeycombing are seen at presentation. HRCT scans of the lung show patchy airspace consolidation, ground-glass opacities, small nodular opacities, and bronchial wall thickening and dilatation. The patchy opacities are more common in the periphery of the lung, often in the lower lung zone. CT scans may show much more extensive disease than is expected from review of the chest x-ray.

Pulmonary function tests usually show a restrictive defect, although an obstructive defect ([FEV_1/FVC] < 70%) is found in 21% of patients, and pulmonary function is occasionally normal.

Routine laboratory tests are nonspecific. Leukocytosis without an increase in eosinophils occurs in about ½ of patients. The initial ESR often is elevated. Rest and exercise hypoxemia is common.

Lung biopsy shows excessive proliferation of granulation tissue within small airways and alveolar ducts, with chronic inflammation in the surrounding alveoli. Foci of organizing pneumonia (ie, a BOOP pattern) are nonspecific and can occur secondary to other pathologic processes, including infections, Wegener's granulomatosis, lymphoma, hypersensitivity pneumonitis, and eosinophilic pneumonia.

Treatment is similar to that for idiopathic pulmonary fibrosis. Clinical recovery occurs in ⅔ of treated patients, often within 2 wk. Relapses occur in up to 50% of patients, but these patients are responsive to additional courses of corticosteroids.

Nonspecific Interstitial Pneumonia

Nonspecific interstitial pneumonia refers to a histologic appearance in ILD that does not conform to the other more specific histologic patterns.

Nonspecific interstitial pneumonia appears to be a discrete entity. Its incidence and prevalence are unknown, but it appears to be the 2nd most common form of IIP (14 to 36% of reported cases). Most cases occur in patients who have connective-tissue disease, drug-induced ILD, or chronic hypersensitivity pneumonitis as an underlying feature. Some cases have no identified etiology and are not associated with another disease.

Clinical presentation is similar to that of IPF. Most patients are between 40 and 60 yr. Cough and dyspnea are present for months to years.

Chest x-ray primarily demonstrates lower-zone reticular opacities. Bilateral patchy opacities can also be seen. HRCT scan findings include bilateral patchy ground-glass attenuation, bilateral areas of consolidation, irregular lines, and bronchial dilatation. Ground-glass attenuation is the predominant finding in most cases and is the sole abnormality in about ⅓ of cases.

The main histologic feature of nonspecific interstitial pneumonia is homogenous inflammation and fibrosis, as opposed to the heterogeneity in usual interstitial pneumonia. The changes are temporally uniform, but the process may be patchy, with intervening areas of unaffected lung. Honeycomb areas are rare.

Most patients have a good prognosis after treatment with corticosteroids. Relapse may occur. The disease progresses in a few patients, who die 5 to 10 yr after diagnosis. The estimated 10-yr mortality is < 15 to 20%.

DRUG-INDUCED PULMONARY DISEASE

Drug-induced pulmonary disease is not a single disorder, but rather, a common clinical problem in which a patient without previous pulmonary disease develops respiratory symptoms, chest x-ray changes, deterioration of pulmonary function, and/or histologic changes while receiving drug therapy. Over 150 drugs or categories of drugs have been reported to cause pulmonary disease; the mechanism is rarely known, but many drugs are thought to provoke a hypersensitivity response.

Depending on the drug, drug-induced syndromes can resemble interstitial fibrosis, bronchiolitis obliterans organizing pneumonia, asthma, noncardiogenic pulmonary edema, pleural effusions, pulmonary eosinophilia, pulmonary hemorrhage, or veno-occlusive disease (see TABLE 55–3), with corresponding chest x-ray, CT, and pulmonary function test findings.

Diagnosis is based on observation of responses to withdrawal from and, if practical, reintroduction to the suspected drug.

Treatment is drug discontinuation. A screening pulmonary function test is commonly obtained in patients about to begin or already taking drugs with pulmonary toxicities, but the benefits of screening for prediction or early detection of toxicity is unproven.

EOSINOPHILIC PULMONARY DISEASES

Eosinophilic pulmonary diseases are a group of diseases characterized by the accumulation of eosinophils in alveolar spaces, the interstitium, or both. Peripheral blood eosinophilia is also common. Known causes of eosinophilic pulmonary disease include infections (especially helminthic infections),

TABLE 55–3. DRUGS CAUSING SPECIFIC CLINICAL PRESENTATIONS OF PULMONARY TOXICITY

CONDITION	DRUG OR AGENT
Asthma	Aspirin, β-blockers (timolol), cocaine, dipyridamole, hydrocortisone, IL-2, methylphenidate, nitrofurantoin, protamine, sulfasalazine, vinca alkaloids (with mitomycin)
Bronchiolitis obliterans organizing pneumonia	Amiodarone, bleomycin, cocaine, cyclophosphamide, methotrexate, minocycline, mitomycin-C, penicillamine, sulfasalazine, tetracycline
Hypersensitivity pneumonitis	Azathioprine plus 6-mercaptopurine, busulfan, fluoxetine, radiation
Interstitial pneumonia or fibrosis	Amphotericin B, bleomycin, busulfan, carbamazepine, chlorambucil, cocaine, cyclophosphamide, diphenylhydantoin, flecainide, heroin, melphalan, methadone, methotrexate, methylphenidate, methysergide, mineral oil, nitrofurantoin, nitrosoureas, procarbazine, silicone, tocainide, vinca alkaloids (with mitomycin)
Noncardiac pulmonary edema	Beta mimetics (terbutaline, ritodrine), chlordiazepoxide, cocaine, cytarabine, ethiodized oil, gemcitabine, heroin, hydrochlorothiazide, methadone, mitomycin-C, phenothiazines, protamine, sulfasalazine, tocolytic agents, tricyclics, tumor necrosis factor, vinca alkaloids (with mitomycin)
Parenchymal hemorrhage	Anticoagulants, azathioprine plus 6-mercaptopurine, cocaine, mineral oil, nitrofurantoin, radiation
Pleural effusion	Amiodarone, anticoagulants, bleomycin, bromocriptine, busulfan, granulocyte-macrophage colony-stimulating factor, IL-2, methotrexate, methysergide, mitomycin-C, nitrofurantoin, para-aminosalicylic acid, procarbazine, radiation, tocolytic agents
Pulmonary infiltrate with eosinophilia	Amiodarone, amphotericin B, bleomycin, carbamazepine, diphenylhydantoin, ethambutol, etoposide, granulocyte-macrophage colony-stimulating factor, isoniazid, methotrexate, minocycline, mitomycin-C, nitrofurantoin, para-aminosalicylic acid, procarbazine, radiation, sulfasalazine, sulfonamides, tetracycline, trazodone
Pulmonary vascular disease	Appetite suppressants (dexfenfluramine, fenfluramine, phentermine), busulfan, cocaine, heroin, methadone, methylphenidate, nitrosoureas, radiation

drug-induced pneumonitis (eg, antibiotics, phenytoin, L-tryptophan), inhaled toxins (eg, cocaine), systemic diseases (eg, Churg-Strauss), and allergic bronchopulmonary aspergillosis, but often the cause is unknown.

Diagnosis is based on demonstration of opacities on chest x-ray and identification of eosinophilia (>450/μL) in peripheral blood, bronchoalveolar lavage fluid, or lung biopsy tissue. Pulmonary opacities on chest x-ray associated with blood eosinophilia are sometimes called the PIE (pulmonary infiltrates with eosinophilia) syndrome.

Eosinophils are primarily tissue-dwelling and are several hundred–fold more abundant in tissues than in blood. Consequently, blood eosinophil numbers do not necessarily indicate the extent of eosinophilic involvement in affected tissues. Eosinophils are most numerous in tissues with a mucosal epithelial interface with the environment, such as the respiratory, GI, and lower GU tracts. Eosinophils are not found in the lungs of healthy people, so their presence in tissue or bronchoalveolar lavage (> 5% of differential count) identifies a pathologic process. Pulmonary eosinophilia may occur in the absence of peripheral eosinophilia.

Eosinophils are exquisitely sensitive to corticosteroids and completely disappear from the bloodstream within a few hours after administration of corticosteroids. This rapid disappearance from the blood may obscure the diagnosis in patients who receive corticosteroids before the diagnostic assessment is instituted.

The 2 primary eosinophilic pulmonary diseases of unknown etiology are chronic and acute eosinophilic pneumonia. Hypereosinophilia syndrome, a systemic disease affecting multiple organs, is discussed on p. 1095.

Chronic Eosinophilic Pneumonia

Chronic eosinophilic pneumonia is an abnormal, chronic accumulation of eosinophils in the lung.

Prevalence and incidence of chronic eosinophilic pneumonia (CEP) are unknown. Etiology is suspected to be an allergic diathesis. Most patients are nonsmokers.

Symptoms, Signs, and Diagnosis

Patients often present with fulminant illness characterized by cough, fever, progressive breathlessness, weight loss, wheezing, and night sweats. Asthma accompanies or precedes the illness in > 50% of cases.

Diagnosis requires exclusion of infectious causes and is based on clinical presentation, blood tests, and chest x-ray. Peripheral blood eosinophilia, a very high ESR, iron deficiency anemia, and thrombocytosis are all frequently found. Chest x-ray findings of bilateral peripheral or pleural-based opacities (present in about 60% of cases), most commonly in the middle and upper lung zones, is described as the "photographic negative" of pulmonary edema and is virtually pathognomonic (although seen in < 25% of patients). A similar pattern is identified on CT in virtually all cases. Bronchoalveolar lavage eosinophilia > 40% is suggestive of CEP; serial bronchoalveolar lavage examinations may help document the course of disease. Biopsy demonstrates interstitial and alveolar eosinophils and histiocytes, including multinucleated giant cells, and bronchiolitis obliterans organizing pneumonia. Fibrosis is minimal.

Treatment

Patients with CEP are uniformly responsive to IV or oral corticosteroids; failure to respond indicates another diagnosis. Initial treatment is prednisone 40 to 60 mg once/day. Clinical improvement is often striking and rapid, often occurring within 48 h. Complete resolution of symptoms and x-ray abnormalities occurs within 14 days in most patients and by 1 mo in almost all. Symptoms and plain chest x-rays are both reliable and efficient guides to therapy. Although CT scanning is more sensitive for the detection of radiographic abnormalities, there is no benefit gained by repeating it. Peripheral eosinophil counts, ESR, and IgE levels can also be used to follow the clinical course during treatment. However, not all patients have abnormal laboratory test results.

Symptomatic or radiographic relapse occurs in 50 to 80% of cases either after cessation of therapy or, less commonly, with tapering of the corticosteroid dose. Relapse can occur months to years after the initial presenting episode. Thus, corticosteroid therapy is occasionally continued indefinitely. Inhaled corticosteroids (eg, fluticasone or beclomethasone 500 to 750 μg bid) appear to be effective, especially in reducing the maintenance dose of oral corticosteroid.

CEP occasionally leads to physiologically important, irreversible fibrosis, although death is extremely unusual. Relapse does not appear to indicate treatment failure, a worse prognosis, or greater morbidity. Patients continue to respond to corticosteroids similar to those before relapse. Fixed airflow obstruction can occur in some patients who recover, but the abnormalities are usually of borderline clinical significance.

Acute Eosinophilic Pneumonia

Acute eosinophilic pneumonia is characterized by rapid eosinophilic infiltration of the lung interstitium.

Incidence and prevalence of acute eosinophilic pneumonia (AEP) are unknown. AEP can occur at any age but most often affects patients between 20 and 40 yr, with a male-to-female ratio of 21 : 1. The cause is unknown, but AEP may be an acute hypersensitivity reaction to an unidentified inhaled antigen in an otherwise healthy person. Cigarette or other smoke exposure may be involved.

Symptoms and Signs

AEP causes an acute febrile illness of short duration (usually < 7 days). Symptoms are nonproductive cough, dyspnea, malaise, myalgias, night sweats, and pleuritic chest pain. Signs include tachypnea, fever (often > 38.5°C), and bibasilar inspiratory crackles and, occasionally, rhonchi on forced exhalation. AEP frequently presents as acute respiratory failure requiring mechanical ventilation. Rarely, hyperdynamic shock can occur.

Diagnosis

The diagnosis is based on clinical presentation and findings from routine testing and is confirmed by bronchoscopy. AEP is a diagnosis of exclusion and requires the absence of known causes of eosinophilic pneumonia and of respiratory failure. The CBC in most patients demonstrates markedly elevated eosinophil counts. ESR and IgE levels are high but are nonspecific.

The chest x-ray initially may show only subtle reticular or ground-glass opacities, often with Kerley B lines. Isolated alveolar (about 25% of cases) or reticular (about 25% of cases) opacities may also be seen on presentation. The pattern is unlike that seen in chronic eosinophilic pneumonia, in which the opacities are localized to the lung periphery. Small pleural effusions occur in ⅔ of patients and are frequently bilateral. High-resolution CT is always abnormal with bilateral, random, patchy ground-glass or reticular opacities. Pleural fluid examination shows marked eosinophilia with high pH. Pulmonary function tests often demonstrate a restrictive process with reduced diffusing capacity for carbon monoxide (DL_{CO}).

Bronchoscopy should be performed for lavage and, occasionally, biopsy. Bronchoalveolar lavage fluid often shows a high number and percentage (> 25%) of eosinophils. The most common histopathologic features on biopsy include eosinophilic infiltration with acute and organizing diffuse alveolar damage, but few cases have undergone lung biopsy.

Treatment and Prognosis

Some patients improve spontaneously. Most are treated with prednisone 40 to 60 mg po once/day. In the setting of respiratory failure, methylprednisolone 60 to 125 mg q 6 h is preferred. The prognosis is excellent; response to corticosteroids and complete recovery without recurrence is almost universal. Pleural effusions resolve more slowly than parenchymal opacities.

LÖFFLER'S SYNDROME

Löffler's syndrome is characterized by absent or mild respiratory symptoms, fleeting migratory pulmonary opacities, and peripheral blood eosinophilia. Parasitic infections, especially *Ascaris lumbricoides,* may be the cause, but an identifiable etiologic agent is not found in up to ⅓ of patients. The disease usually resolves within 1 mo.

HYPERSENSITIVITY PNEUMONITIS

(Extrinsic Allergic Alveolitis)

Hypersensitivity pneumonitis is a syndrome of cough, dyspnea, and fatigue caused by sensitization and subsequent hypersensitivity to environmental (frequently occupational) antigens. Acute, subacute, and chronic forms exist; all are characterized by acute interstitial inflammation and development of granulomas and fibrosis with long-term exposure. Diagnosis is based on a combination of history, physical examination, imaging tests, bronchoalveolar lavage, and biopsy. Short-term treatment is with corticosteroids; long-term treatment is antigen avoidance.

Etiology and Pathophysiology

Over 300 antigens have been identified as triggers for hypersensitivity pneumonitis, although 8 account for about 75% of cases. Antigens are commonly categorized by type and occupation (see TABLE 55–4); farmer's lung, caused by inhalation of hay dust containing thermophilic actinomycetes, is the prototype. Substantial overlap exists between hypersensitivity pneumonitis and chronic bronchitis in farmers, in whom chronic bronchitis is far more common, occurs independent of smoking status, is linked to thermophilic actinomycete exposure, and leads to findings similar to those of hypersensitivity pneumonitis on diagnostic testing.

TABLE 55–4. EXAMPLES OF HYPERSENSITIVITY PNEUMONITIS

ASSOCIATION	DISEASE	ANTIGEN	SOURCE
Farming	Farmer's lung	Thermophilic actinomycetes; fungi, especially *Aspergillus* sp	Vegetable compost (moldy grain, hay, silage)
	Tobacco grower's lung	*Aspergillus* sp, *Scopulariopsis brevicaulis*	Tobacco plants
	Mushroom worker's lung	Thermophilic actinomycetes, *Hypsizigus marumoreus*	Mushroom compost
	Potato riddler's lung	Thermophilic actinomycetes, *Aspergillus* sp	Moldy hay around potatoes
	Cheese washer's lung	*Penicillium casei, Aspergillus clavatus*	Moldy cheese
	Bagassosis	Thermophilic actinomycetes	Moldy bagasse (sugar cane)
	Compost lung	*Aspergillus* sp	Compost
	Wine grower's lung	*Botrytis cincrea*	Moldy grapes
	Coffee worker's lung	Coffee bean dust	Coffee beans
Water	Sewer worker's lung	*Cephalosporium* sp	Contaminated basement (sewage)
	Tap water lung	Unknown	Contaminated tap water
	Humidifier lung	*Aureobasidium* sp, *Candida albicans,* thermophilic actinomycetes	Contaminated water in humidification or air-conditioning systems
	Hot tub lung	*Cladosporium* sp, *Mycobacterium avium* complex	Contaminated mist and mold on ceilings and around tub
	Sauna taker's lung	*Aureobasidium* sp	Contaminated sauna water
Birds	Bird fancier's lung	Parakeet, pigeon, chicken, turkey, and duck proteins	Avian droppings or feathers
Animals	Sausage worker's lung	*Penicillium nalgiovense*	Dry sausage mold
	Pituitary snuff taker's lung	Animal proteins	Heterologous (bovine, porcine) pituitary snuff
	Furrier's lung	Animal fur dust	Animal pelts
	Laboratory worker's hypersensitivity pneumonitis	Rodent proteins	Male rat urine and fur
	Fish food lung	Unknown	Fish food
	Fish meal worker's lung	Fish meal dust	Fish meal dust
	Mummy handler's lung	Unknown	Cloth mummy wrappings
Grains	Miller's lung	*Sitophilus granarius* (wheat weevil)	Infested wheat flour
	Malt worker's lung	*Aspergillus* sp	Moldy barley

TABLE 55–4. EXAMPLES OF HYPERSENSITIVITY PNEUMONITIS—Continued

ASSOCIATION	DISEASE	ANTIGEN	SOURCE
Milling and construction	Woodworker's lung	Wood dust, *Alternaria* sp, *Baccilus subtilis*	Oak, cedar, pine, spruce, and mahogany dusts
	Wood trimmer's disease	*Rhizopus, Mucor* spp	Contaminated wood trimmings
	Wood pulp worker's disease	*Penicillium* sp	Oak and maple tree pulp
	Sequoiosis	*Aureobasidium, Graphium* spp	Redwood sawdust
	Thatched-roof worker's disease	*Sacchoromonospora viridis*	Dried grass and leaves
Industry	Detergent worker's lung	*Bacillus subtilis*	*Bacillus subtilus* enzymes in detergent
	Chemical worker's lung	Isocyanates	Polyurethane foam, varnishes, lacquer
	Vineyard sprayer's lung	Copper sulfate	Copper sulfate use
Textiles	Byssinosis (brown lung)	Mill dust	Cotton, flax, and hemp dust
	Lycoperdonosis	Puffball spores	Folk medicine

The disease seems to represent a type IV hypersensitivity reaction, in which repeated exposure to antigen in genetically susceptible people leads to acute neutrophilic and mononuclear alveolitis, followed by interstitial lymphocytic infiltration and granulomatous reaction. Fibrosis with bronchiolar obliteration occurs with continued exposure.

Circulating precipitins (antibodies sensitized to antigen) seem not to have a primary etiologic role, and clinical history of allergy (such as asthma and seasonal allergies) is not a predisposing factor. Cigarette smoking seems to delay or prevent development, perhaps through down-regulation of the lung's immune response to inhaled antigens. However, smoking may exacerbate the disease once established.

Hypersensitivity pneumonitis must be distinguished from disorders that are clinically similar but that have different pathophysiologies. Organic dust toxic syndrome (pulmonary mycotoxicosis, grain fever), for example, is a syndrome consisting of fever, chills, myalgias, and dyspnea that does not require prior sensitization and is thought to be caused by inhalation of toxins produced by fungi or other contaminants of organic dust. Silo filler's disease may lead to respiratory failure, acute respiratory distress syndrome (ARDS), and bronchiolitis obliterans or bronchitis but is caused by inhalation of toxic nitrogen oxides produced by freshly fermented corn or alfalfa silage. Occupational asthma causes dyspnea in people previously sensitized to an inhaled antigen, but features such as airflow obstruction, airway eosinophilia, and differences in triggering antigens distinguish it from hypersensitivity pneumonitis (see p. 476).

Symptoms and Signs

Symptoms and signs tend to depend on whether onset is acute, subacute, or chronic. Only a small proportion of exposed people develop symptoms and in most cases only after weeks to months of exposure and sensitization.

Acute disease occurs in previously sensitized people with acute high-level antigen exposure and manifests as fever, chills, cough, chest tightness, and dyspnea 4 to 8 h after exposure. Anorexia, nausea, and vomiting may also be present. Physical examination shows

TABLE 55–5. DIAGNOSTIC CRITERIA FOR HYPERSENSITIVITY PNEUMONITIS

DIAGNOSTIC CATEGORY	CRITERIA
Definite HP	1, 2, and 3
	1, 2, and 4a
	1, 2a, 3, and 5
	2, 3, and 5
Probable HP	1, 2a, and 3
Subclinical HP	1 and 3a
Sensitized	1 only

Criteria

1. Known exposure to antigen
   a. History of exposure
   b. Confirmation of presence of antigen in environment by investigation
   c. Presence of elevated, specific IgG serum precipitins
2. Clinical, chest x-ray, and pulmonary function test findings
   a. Characteristic symptoms and signs (especially after antigen exposure)
   b. Characteristic chest x-ray or high-resolution CT findings
   c. Abnormal pulmonary function test results
3. Lymphocytosis on bronchoalveolar lavage
   a. $CD4^+/CD8^+$ ratio < 1
   b. Positive response to lymphocyte transformation testing
4. Recurrence of clinical and pulmonary function test findings with antigen challenge testing
   a. Environmental exposure
   b. Controlled exposure to antigen extract
5. Histology
   a. Noncaseating granulomas
   b. Mononuclear cell infiltrate

HP = Hypersensitivity pneumonitis.

tachypnea, diffuse fine-to-medium inspiratory rales, and, in almost all cases, absence of wheezing.

Chronic disease occurs in people with chronic low-level antigen exposure (such as owners of birds) and manifests as onset over months to years of exertional dyspnea, productive cough, fatigue, and weight loss. There are few physical findings; clubbing uncommonly occurs and fever is absent. In advanced cases, pulmonary fibrosis produces signs and symptoms of right heart failure, respiratory failure, or both.

Subacute disease falls between the acute and chronic forms and manifests either as cough, dyspnea, fatigue, and anorexia that develops over days to weeks or as acute superimposed on chronic symptoms.

Diagnosis

Diagnosis is based on a combination of history, physical examination, imaging tests, pulmonary function tests, bronchoalveolar lavage, and biopsy (see TABLE 55–5). The differential diagnosis is broad and includes environmental pulmonary diseases (see Ch. 57 on p. 469), sarcoidosis, bronchiolitis obliterans, connective tissue–associated pulmonary disease, and other ILDs.

Clues in the history include atypical pneumonias recurring at roughly regular intervals; symptom onset after moving to a new job or home; a hot tub, a sauna, a swimming pool, or other sources of standing water or water damage in the home or regular exposure to them elsewhere; having birds as pets; and exacerbation and relief of symptoms in and away from specific settings, respectively.

Examination often is not useful in making the diagnosis, although abnormal lung sounds and clubbing may be present.

Imaging tests typically are obtained for patients with the above history, signs, and symptoms. Chest x-ray is neither sensitive nor specific for detecting disease and is frequently normal in patients with acute and subacute forms. It may demonstrate reticular or nodular opacities, usually when symptoms are present. Chest x-rays of patients with chronic disease are more likely to show reticular or nodular opacities in the upper lobes with reduced lung volumes and honeycombing, similar to that of idiopathic pulmonary fibrosis. Abnormalities are far more commonly detected by high-resolution CT (HRCT), and HRCT is considered standard for evaluating parenchymal changes in hypersensitivity pneumonitis. The most typical HRCT finding is the presence of profuse poorly defined centrilobular micronodules. These micronodules may be found in patients with acute, subacute, or chronic disease and, in the correct clinical context, strongly suggest hypersensitivity pneumonitis. Occasionally, ground-glass attenuation is the predominant or only finding. It is usually diffuse but sometimes spares the periphery of the secondary lobule. Focal areas of hyperlucency, similar to those seen in obliterative bronchiolitis, may be a prominent feature in some patients (eg, mosaic attenuation with air trapping on expiratory HRCT). In chronic hypersensitivity pneumonitis, there are signs of lung fibrosis (eg, lobar volume loss, linear/reticular opacities, or honeycombing). Some nonsmoking patients with chronic hypersensitivity pneumonitis have findings of upper lobe emphysema. Mediastinal lymphadenopathy is uncommon, thereby distinguishing hypersensitivity pneumonitis from sarcoidosis.

Pulmonary function tests should be obtained as part of the standard evaluation of suspected cases of hypersensitivity pneumonitis. The disease can produce obstructive, restrictive, or a mixed pattern of airway changes. Advanced disease most commonly produces a restrictive defect (decreased lung volumes), a decreased diffusing capacity for carbon monoxide (DL_{CO}), and hypoxemia. Airway obstruction is unusual in acute disease but may develop in chronic disease.

Bronchoalveolar lavage is rarely specific for the diagnosis but is often a component of the diagnostic assessment for chronic respiratory symptoms and pulmonary function abnormalities. A lymphocytosis in lavage fluid (> 60%) with $CD4^+/CD8^+$ ratio < 1.0 is characteristic of disease; by contrast, lymphocytosis with $CD4^+$ predominance (ratio > 1.0) is more characteristic of sarcoidosis. Other findings may include mast cells > 1% (after acute exposure) and increased neutrophils and eosinophils.

Lung biopsy is indicated when noninvasive testing is inconclusive. Transbronchial biopsy performed through a bronchoscope is sufficient as long as multiple specimens are taken from areas of active disease and multiple sequential sections of tissue are examined histologically. Findings vary but include lymphocytic alveolitis, noncaseating granulomas, and granulomatosis. Interstitial fibrosis may be seen but is usually mild in the absence of advanced radiographic changes.

Additional testing is indicated when additional support for the diagnosis is required or to detect other causes of ILD. Circulating precipitins (specific precipitating antibodies to the suspected antigen) are suggestive but are neither sensitive nor specific and thus are not helpful. Identification of a specific precipitating antigen may require detailed aerobiologic and/or microbiologic assessment of the workplace by industrial hygiene specialists but usually are guided by known sources of inciting antigens (eg, *Bacillus subtilis* in detergent factories). Skin tests are not helpful, and eosinophilia is absent. Tests helpful in detecting other diseases include serologies and cultures (for psittacosis and other pneumonias) and autoantibodies (for collagen-vascular disease). Elevated eosinophils may suggest chronic eosinophilic pneumonias, and hilar and paratracheal lymph node enlargement is more characteristic of sarcoidosis.

Prognosis, Treatment, and Prevention

Pathologic changes are completely reversible if detected early and if antigen exposure is eliminated. Acute disease is self-limiting with antigen avoidance; symptoms usually lessen within hours. Chronic disease has a more complicated prognosis: once fibrosis has been established, patients usually have irreversible pathophysiology, although these changes often stabilize if the patient is no longer exposed to the offending environment.

Treatment of acute or subacute hypersensitivity pneumonitis is with corticosteroids, usually prednisone 60 mg once/day for 1 to 2 wk, then tapered over the next 2 to 4 wk to 20 mg once/day, followed by weekly decrements of 2.5 mg until the drug is stopped. This regimen relieves initial symptoms but does not appear to alter long-term outcome.

The most important long-term treatment is avoidance of exposure to antigens. A complete change of environment is rarely realistic, especially for farmers and other workers, in which case dust control measures (such as wetting down compost before disturbing it) or using air filters or protective masks may be effective. Fungicides may be used to prevent the growth of antigenic microorganisms (eg, in hay or on sugar cane), but the long-term safety of this approach is unproven. Extensive cleaning of wet ventilation systems, removal of moist carpets, and maintenance of low humidity are also effective in some settings. Patients must be told, however, that these measures may be inadequate in the presence of continued exposure.

LYMPHANGIOLEIOMYOMATOSIS

Lymphangioleiomyomatosis is nonmalignant growth of smooth muscle cells throughout the lung, pulmonary blood vessels,

lymphatics, and pleurae. It is rare and occurs exclusively in young women. The cause is unknown. Symptoms are dyspnea, cough, chest pain, and hemoptysis; spontaneous pneumothorax is common. Diagnosis is suspected on the basis of symptoms and chest x-ray and is confirmed by high-resolution CT. Prognosis is uncertain, but the disease is slowly progressive and over years often leads to respiratory failure and death. Primary treatment is lung transplantation.

Epidemiology, Etiology, and Pathophysiology

Lymphangioleiomyomatosis (LAM) is a disease exclusive to women, affecting most between 20 and 40 yr. Whites are at greatest risk. LAM affects < 1 in 1 million people. It is characterized by nonmalignant proliferation of atypical smooth muscle cells throughout the chest, including lung parenchyma, vasculature, lymphatics, and pleurae, leading to distortion of lung architecture, cystic emphysema, and progressive deterioration of lung function. It is included in the current chapter because patients with LAM are occasionally misdiagnosed as having ILD.

The cause of LAM is unknown. The tempting hypothesis that female sex hormones play a role in pathogenesis remains unproven. The disease usually arises spontaneously, but LAM bears many similarities to the pulmonary findings of tuberous sclerosis (TS—see p. 2379); LAM occurs in some patients with TS and is thought by some to be a forme fruste of TS. Mutations in the tuberous sclerosis complex-2 gene (*TSC-2*) have been described in LAM cells and angiomyolipomas. These observations suggest 1 of 2 possibilities: (1) somatic mosaicism for *TSC-2* mutations within the lungs and kidneys results in foci of disease superimposed against a background of normal cells within these tissues (although multiple discrete sites of disease might be expected) or (2) LAM represents dissemination of angiomyolipoma tissue to the lung in a fashion analogous to the syndrome of benign metastasizing leiomyoma.

Symptoms and Signs

Initial symptoms are dyspnea and, less commonly, cough, chest pain, and hemoptysis. There are few signs of disease, but some women have crackles and rhonchi. Many patients present with spontaneous pneumothorax. They may also present with manifestations of lymphatic obstruction, including chylothorax, chylous ascites, and chyluria. Symptoms are thought to worsen during pregnancy and possibly during air travel; air travel is especially contraindicated in women with new or worsening respiratory symptoms; history of a pneumothorax or hemoptysis; or evidence of extensive subpleural bullous or cystic changes on high-resolution CT (HRCT) scans. Renal angiomyolipomas (hamartomas made of smooth muscle, blood vessels, and adipose) occur in up to 50% of patients and, although usually asymptomatic, can cause bleeding, which usually presents as hematuria or flank pain if they grow large.

Diagnosis

Diagnosis is suspected in young women with dyspnea, interstitial changes with normal or increased lung volumes on chest x-ray, spontaneous pneumothorax, and/or chylous effusion. Diagnosis is confirmed by biopsy, but HRCT is performed in all patients suspected of having the disease. Findings of multiple, small, diffusely distributed cysts are generally pathognomonic for LAM.

Biopsy is indicated only when HRCT findings are nondiagnostic. Findings of an abnormal proliferation of smooth muscle cells (LAM cells) associated with cystic changes on histologic examination confirm disease.

Pulmonary function tests support the diagnosis and are especially useful for monitoring. Typical findings are of an obstructive or mixed obstructive/restrictive pattern. The lungs are usually hyperinflated with an increase in the total lung capacity (TLC) and thoracic gas volume. Gas trapping (an increase in residual volume [RV] and RV/TLC ratio) is commonly present. The PaO_2 and diffusing capacity for carbon monoxide (DL_{CO}) are commonly reduced. Diminished exercise performance is found in most patients.

Prognosis and Treatment

Prognosis is unclear because the disease is so rare and because the clinical course of patients with LAM is variable. In general, the disease is slowly progressive, leading eventually to respiratory failure and death, but the time to death varies widely among reports. Women should be advised that progression may accelerate during pregnancy. Median survival is likely > 8 yr from diagnosis.

Standard treatment is lung transplantation, but disease can recur in grafted lungs. Alternative treatments, such as hormonal manipulation with progestins, tamoxifen, and oophorectomy, are largely ineffective. Pneumothoraces may be difficult to manage because they are often recurrent, bilateral, and less responsive to standard measures. Recurrent pneumothorax requires pleural abrasion, talc or chemical pleurodesis, or pleurectomy. Patients can receive psychologic support from the LAM Foundation in the US.

LYMPHOID INTERSTITIAL PNEUMONIA

(Lymphocytic Interstitial Pneumonitis)

Lymphoid interstitial pneumonia is lymphocytic infiltration of the alveolar interstitium and air spaces. The cause is unknown. It most often occurs in children with HIV infection and in people of any age with autoimmune disease. Symptoms and signs are cough, progressive dyspnea, and crackles. Diagnosis is based on history, physical examination, imaging tests, pulmonary function tests, and lung biopsy. Treatment is with corticosteroids, cytotoxic drugs, or both, although efficacy is unknown. Five-year survival is 50 to 66%.

Lymphoid interstitial pneumonia (LIP) is a rare disease characterized by infiltration of alveoli and alveolar septa with small lymphocytes and varying numbers of plasma cells. Noncaseating granulomas may be present but are usually rare and inconspicuous.

LIP is the most common cause of pulmonary disease after *Pneumocystis* infection in HIV-positive children and is an AIDS-defining illness in up to ½ of HIV-positive children. LIP affects < 1% of adults with or without HIV infection. Females are affected more commonly.

The cause is postulated to be an autoimmune disease or a nonspecific response to infection with Epstein-Barr virus, HIV, or other viruses. Evidence of an autoimmune etiology includes its frequent association with Sjögren's syndrome (25% of cases) and other diseases (eg, SLE, RA, Hashimoto's disease—14% of cases). Evidence of an indirect viral etiology includes frequent association with immunodeficient states (HIV/AIDS, combined variable immunodeficiency, agammaglobulinemia—14% of cases) and findings of Epstein-Barr virus DNA and HIV RNA in lung tissue of LIP patients. According to this theory, LIP is an extreme manifestation of the normal ability of lymphoid tissue in the lung to respond to inhaled and circulating antigen.

Symptoms and Signs

In adults, LIP causes symptoms of progressive dyspnea and cough. These manifestations progress over months or, in some cases, years and appear at a mean age of 54. Weight loss, fever, arthralgias, and night sweats occur but are less common.

In children, LIP causes bronchospasm, cough, and/or respiratory distress and failure to thrive, usually at age 2 or 3 yr.

Examination may reveal crackles. Findings such as hepatosplenomegaly, arthritis, and lymphadenopathy are uncommon and suggest an accompanying or alternative diagnosis.

Diagnosis

Diagnosis is based on history, physical examination, imaging tests, and pulmonary function tests and is confirmed by lung biopsy.

Chest x-ray shows bibasilar linear reticular or nodular opacities, a nonspecific finding that is seen in a number of pulmonary infections. Alveolar opacities, honeycombing, or both may be present in more advanced disease. High-resolution CT of the chest helps establish the extent of disease, define the hilar anatomy, and identify pleural involvement. Characteristic findings are centrilobular and subpleural nodules, thickened bronchovascular bundles, ground-glass opacities, and, rarely, diffuse cystic structures.

Pulmonary function tests show restrictive defects with reduced lung volumes and diffusing capacity for carbon monoxide (DL_{CO}) and preserved airflow. Marked hypoxemia may occur. Bronchoalveolar lavage should be performed to rule out infection and may reveal an increased number of lymphocytes.

About 80% of patients have a serum protein abnormality, most commonly a polyclonal gammopathy and, especially in children, hypogammaglobulinemia, the significance of which is unknown. These elements are sufficient to confirm the diagnosis in HIV-positive children. In adults, diagnosis requires demonstration of expansion of the alveolar septae with lymphocytic and other immune cell (plasma cell, immunoblastic, and histiocytic) infiltrates. Germinal centers and multinucleated giant cells with noncaseating granulomas are also seen. Infiltrates appear occasionally along bronchi and vessels but most commonly along alveolar septa. Immunohistochemical staining and flow cytometry must be performed on the tissue to distinguish LIP from primary lymphomas; in LIP, the infiltrate is polyclonal (both

T and B cells), whereas other lymphomas produce monoclonal infiltrates.

Prognosis and Treatment

The natural history and prognosis of LIP are poorly understood. Good prognosis may be linked to severity of radiographic abnormalities, which may indicate a more vigorous immune response. Spontaneous resolution, resolution after treatment with corticosteroids or other immunosuppressive drugs, progression to lymphoma, or development of pulmonary fibrosis with respiratory insufficiency may ensue. Five-year survival is 50 to 66%. Common causes of death are infection, development of malignant lymphoma (5%), and progressive fibrosis.

Treatment is with corticosteroids, cytotoxic drugs, or both, but, as with many other causes of ILD, the efficacy of this approach is unknown.

PULMONARY ALVEOLAR PROTEINOSIS

Pulmonary alveolar proteinosis is accumulation of surfactant in alveoli. Etiology is almost always unknown. Symptoms are dyspnea, fatigue, and malaise. Diagnosis is based on bronchoalveolar lavage, although characteristic x-ray and laboratory test abnormalities occur. Treatment is with whole lung lavage. Prognosis is generally good with treatment.

Etiology and Pathophysiology

Pulmonary alveolar proteinosis is most often idiopathic and occurs in otherwise healthy men and women between 30 and 50 yr. Rare secondary forms occur in patients with acute silicosis, *Pneumocystis jiroveci* (formerly *P. carinii*) infection, hematologic malignancies, or immunosuppression and in those with significant inhalation exposures to aluminum, titanium, cement, and cellulose dusts. Rare congenital forms causing neonatal respiratory failure also exist. It is unclear whether idiopathic and secondary cases share a common pathophysiology. Impaired alveolar macrophage processing of surfactant due to abnormal granulocyte-macrophage colony-stimulating factor (GM-CSF) signaling is thought to contribute to the disorder, perhaps due to reduced or absent function of the common β chain of the GM-CSF/IL-13/IL-5 receptor on mononuclear cells (seen in some children but not in adults with the disorder). Anti–GM-CSF antibodies have also been found in most patients. Toxic lung injury is suspected but not proven in secondary inhalation causes.

Alveoli are filled with acellular PAS-positive lipoproteinacious surfactant. Alveolar and interstitial cells remain normal. Posterobasal lung segments are mostly affected. The pleura and mediastinum are unaffected.

Symptoms, Signs, and Diagnosis

Most patients present with progressive exertional dyspnea and weight loss, fatigue, malaise, or low-grade fever. Cough, occasionally producing chunky or gummy sputum, occurs but is less common. Clubbing and cyanosis are uncommon. Inspiratory crackles are rare because alveoli are fluid-filled; when crackles are present, they suggest infection.

Pulmonary alveolar proteinosis is usually first suspected when a chest x-ray is taken for nonspecific respiratory symptoms. The x-ray shows bilateral mid- and lower-lung field opacities in a butterfly distribution with normal hila.

Diagnosis requires bronchoalveolar lavage, with or without transbronchial biopsy. Lavage fluid is milky or opaque, stains PAS-positive, and is characterized by scattered surfactant-engorged macrophages, an increase in T lymphocytes, and high levels of surfactant apoprotein-A. Thoracoscopic or open lung biopsy is performed when bronchoscopy is contraindicated or when specimens from lavage fluid are nondiagnostic. Tests typically ordered before treatment begins include high-resolution CT (HRCT), pulmonary function tests, ABGs, and laboratory tests.

HRCT shows ground-glass opacification, thickened intralobular structures, and interlobular septa in typical polygonal shapes (crazy-paving). This finding is not specific, however, as it may also be seen in patients with lipoid pneumonia, bronchoalveolar cell carcinoma, and *Pneumocystis jiroveci* pneumonia.

Pulmonary function tests show reduction in diffusing capacity for carbon monoxide (DL_{CO}) that is disproportionate to the decreases in vital capacity, residual volume, functional residual capacity, and total lung capacity.

Laboratory abnormalities include polycythemia, hypergammaglobulinemia, increased serum LDH levels, and increased serum surfactant proteins A and D: All are suggestive but nondiagnostic. ABGs may show hypoxemia with mild to moderate exercise or at rest if disease is more severe.

Prognosis

Without treatment, pulmonary alveolar proteinosis remits spontaneously in up to 10% of patients. A single whole lung lavage is curative in up to 40%; other patients require lavage every 6 to 12 mo for many years. Five-year survival is about 80%; the most common cause of death is respiratory failure, typically occurring within the 1st yr after diagnosis. Secondary pulmonary infections with bacterial (*Mycobacteria, Nocardia*) and other organisms (*Aspergillus, Cryptococcus,* and other opportunistic fungi) occasionally develop because of impaired macrophage function; these infections require treatment.

Treatment

Treatment is unnecessary for patients without symptoms or for those with only mild symptoms. Whole lung lavage is performed in patients with troubling dyspnea using general anesthesia and a double-lumen endotracheal tube. One lung is lavaged up to 15 times with 1 to 2 L saline while the other lung is ventilated. The process is then reversed. Lung transplantation is not performed because the disorder recurs in the grafted lung.

Systemic corticosteroids play no role in management and may increase the risk of secondary infection. The role of GM-CSF (IV or sc) in management remains to be determined. An open-label study showed clinical improvement in 57% of the patients studied.

PULMONARY LANGERHANS' CELL GRANULOMATOSIS

(Eosinophilic Granuloma, Pulmonary Granulomatosis X, Histiocytosis X)

Pulmonary Langerhans' cell granulomatosis (histiocytosis) is proliferation of monoclonal Langerhans' cells in lung interstitium and airspaces. Etiology is unknown, but cigarette smoking plays a primary role. Symptoms are dyspnea, cough, fatigue, and/or pleuritic chest pain. Diagnosis is based on history with imaging tests or bronchoalveolar lavage and biopsy. Treatment is smoking cessation. Corticosteroids are given in many cases, but efficacy is unknown. Lung transplantation is curative when combined with smoking cessation. Prognosis is good overall, although patients are at increased risk of malignancy.

Pulmonary Langerhans' cell granulomatosis (PLCG) is a disease in which monoclonal CD1a-positive Langerhans' cells (a type of histiocyte) infiltrate the bronchioles and alveolar interstitium, accompanied by lymphocytes, plasma cells, neutrophils, and eosinophils. PLCG is one manifestation of Langerhans' cell histiocytosis (see p. 1096), which can affect organs in isolation (most notably the lungs, skin, bones, pituitary, and lymph nodes) or simultaneously. PLCG occurs in isolation ≥ 85% of the time.

The etiology of PLCG is unknown, but the disease occurs almost exclusively in whites 20 to 40 yr who smoke. Men and women are affected equally. Women develop disease later, but any differences in disease presentation by sex may represent differences in smoking behavior. Pathophysiology may involve recruitment and proliferation of Langerhans' cells in response to cytokines and growth factors secreted by alveolar macrophages in response to cigarette smoke.

Symptoms and Signs

Typical symptoms and signs of PLCG are dyspnea, nonproductive cough, fatigue, and/or pleuritic chest pain, and 10 to 25% of patients have sudden, spontaneous pneumothorax (see p. 496). About 15% of patients are asymptomatic, with disease noted incidentally on a chest x-ray taken for another reason. Bone pain from bone cysts (18%), skin rash (13%), and polyuria from diabetes insipidus (5%) are the most common manifestations of extrapulmonary involvement and occur in up to 15% of patients, rarely being the presenting symptoms of PLCG. There are few signs of PLCG; the physical examination results are usually normal.

Diagnosis

PLCG is suspected based on history, physical examination, and chest x-ray and is confirmed by high-resolution CT (HRCT) and bronchoscopy with biopsy and bronchoalveolar lavage.

Chest x-ray classically demonstrates bilaterally symmetric nodular opacities in the middle and upper lung fields with cystic changes and normal or increased lung volumes. The lung bases are often spared. Appearance may mimic COPD or lymphangioleiomyomatosis (see p. 457). Confirmation on HRCT of middle and upper lobe cysts (often with bizarre shapes) and/or nodules with interstitial thickening is considered diagnostic of PLCG. Pulmonary function test findings are normal, restrictive, obstructive, or mixed depending on when the test is performed during the course of the disease. Most commonly, the diffusing capacity for carbon monoxide (DL_{CO}) is reduced and exercise is impaired.

Bronchoscopy and biopsy are indicated when imaging and pulmonary function tests are inconclusive. Finding > 5% of CD1a cells in bronchoalveolar lavage fluid is highly suggestive of the disease. Biopsy shows proliferation of Langerhans' cells with occasional clustering of eosinophils (the origin of the outdated term eosinophilic granuloma) in the midst of cellular and fibrotic nodules that may take on a stellate configuration. Immunohistochemical staining is positive for CD1a, S-100 protein, and HLA-DR antigens.

Treatment

The main treatment is smoking cessation, which leads to symptom resolution in up to ⅓ of patients. As with other ILDs, empiric use of corticosteroids and cytotoxic drugs is common practice even though their effectiveness is unproven. Lung transplantation is an option for otherwise healthy patients with accelerating respiratory insufficiency, but the disease may recur in the transplanted lung if the patient continues or resumes smoking.

Spontaneous resolution of symptoms occurs in some patients with minimally symptomatic disease; 5-yr survival is about 75%, and median survival is 12 yr. However, some patients develop slowly progressive disease, for which the clinical markers include continued smoking, age extremes, multiorgan involvement, persistent constitutional symptoms, numerous cysts on chest x-ray, reduced DL_{CO}, low FEV1/FVC (< 66%), high residual volume (RV)/total lung capacity (TLC) ratio (> 33%), and need for prolonged corticosteroids. Cause of death is respiratory insufficiency or malignancy. Lung cancer risk is increased because of cigarette smoking.

56 SARCOIDOSIS

Sarcoidosis is characterized by noncaseating granulomas in one or more organs and tissues; etiology is unknown. The lungs and lymphatic system are most often affected, but sarcoidosis may affect any organ. Pulmonary symptoms range from none (limited disease) to exertional dyspnea and, rarely, respiratory or other organ failure (advanced disease). Diagnosis usually is first suspected because of pulmonary involvement and is confirmed by chest x-ray, biopsy, and exclusion of other causes of granulomatous inflammation. First-line treatment is corticosteroids. Prognosis is excellent for limited disease but poor for more advanced disease.

Sarcoidosis primarily affects people aged 20 to 40 but occasionally affects children and older adults. Worldwide, prevalence is greatest in black Americans and northern Europeans, especially Scandinavians. Disease presentation varies widely by racial and ethnic background, with black Americans and Puerto Ricans demonstrating more frequent extrathoracic manifestations. Sarcoidosis is slightly more prevalent in women. Incidence increases in winter and early spring, for unknown reasons.

Etiology and Pathophysiology

Sarcoidosis is thought to be due to an inflammatory response to an environmental exposure in a genetically susceptible person. Although uncertain, proposed triggers include viral, bacterial, and mycobacterial infections and inhalation of inorganic (eg, aluminum, zirconium, talc) or organic (eg, pine tree pollen, clay) agents. The unknown antigen triggers a cell-mediated immune response characterized by the accumulation of T lymphocytes and macrophages, release of cytokines and chemokines, and organization of responding cells into granulomas. Clusters of disease in families and communities suggest a genetic predisposition, shared exposures, or, less likely, person-to-person transmission.

The result of the inflammatory process is formation of noncaseating granulomas, the hallmark of sarcoidosis. Granulomas are collections of mononuclear cells and macrophages that are differentiated into epithelioid and multinucleated giant cells, surrounded by lymphocytes, plasma cells, mast cells, fibroblasts, and collagen. Granulomas occur most commonly in the lung and lymph nodes but can involve many other sites, including the liver, spleen, eyes (see p. 914), sinuses, skin, bones, joints, skeletal muscle, kidney, reproductive organs, heart, salivary glands, and nervous system. The granulomas in the lung are distributed along lymphatics, with most found in peribronchiolar, subpleural, and perilobular regions.

Symptoms and Signs

Symptoms and signs depend on the site and degree of involvement and vary over time, ranging from spontaneous remission to chronic indolent illness. Therefore, frequent reassessment for new symptoms in different organs is needed. Most cases are probably asymptomatic and thus go undetected. Pulmonary disease occurs in > 90% of adult patients.

Symptoms and signs may include dyspnea, cough, chest discomfort, and crackles on examination. Fatigue, malaise, weakness, anorexia, weight loss, and low-grade fever are also common; sarcoidosis is an unusual cause of fever of unknown origin. Nontender lymphadenopathy is often the only sign. Systemic involvement causes various symptoms (see TABLE 56–1), which vary by race, sex, and age. Blacks are more likely than whites to have involvement of the eye, liver, bone marrow, peripheral lymph nodes, and skin other than erythema nodosum. Women are more likely to have erythema nodosum and eye or nervous system involvement. Men and older patients are more likely to be hypercalcemic.

In children < 4 yr, arthritis, rash, and uveitis are the most common presentations. Sarcoidosis may be confused with juvenile RA in this age group.

Diagnosis

Sarcoidosis is most often suspected when hilar adenopathy is incidentally detected on chest x-ray. These changes are the most common abnormality, and x-ray appearance is roughly predictive of the likelihood of spontaneous remission (see TABLE 56–2) in patients with pulmonary involvement. Therefore, a chest x-ray should be the first test if it has not already been obtained in patients suspected of having sarcoidosis.

Because pulmonary involvement is so frequent, a normal chest x-ray generally excludes the diagnosis. In cases in which the disease is highly suspected despite a normal chest x-ray, high-resolution chest CT is more sensitive for detecting hilar and mediastinal lymphadenopathy; CT findings in more advanced stages (II to IV) include thickening of the bronchovascular bundles and bronchial walls; beading of the interlobular septa; ground-glass opacification; parenchymal nodules, cysts, or cavities; and/or traction bronchiectasis.

When imaging suggests sarcoidosis, the diagnosis is confirmed by demonstration of noncaseating granulomas on biopsy and exclusion of alternative causes of granulomatous disease (see TABLE 56–3). The diagnostic evaluation, therefore, requires selection of a biopsy site; exclusion of other causes of granulomatous disease; and assessment of the severity and extent of disease to determine if therapy is indicated.

Sites for biopsy may be obvious from physical examination and initial assessment: peripheral lymph nodes, skin lesions, and conjunctivae are all easily accessible. However, bronchoscopic transbronchial biopsy is the diagnostic procedure of choice in patients with intrathoracic involvement, because the sensitivity is as high as 90% in experienced hands. Video-assisted thoracoscopy can provide access to lung tissue when bronchoscopic transbronchial biopsy is nondiagnostic. Mediastinoscopy is sometimes performed when hilar or mediastinal lymphadenopathy exists in the absence of pulmonary infiltrates, especially if lymphoma is in the differential diagnosis. However, even in patients with only mediastinal adenopathy on x-ray or CT, transbronchial biopsies are often diagnostic. Open lung biopsy provides another way to obtain tissue but requires general anesthesia and is now rarely necessary. Clinical and x-ray findings may be accurate enough for diagnosis in stage I disease or in stage II disease when biopsy is not possible.

Exclusion of other diagnoses is critical, especially when symptoms and x-ray signs are minimal, because many other diseases and processes can cause granulomatous inflammation (see TABLE 56–3). Biopsy tissue

TABLE 56–1. SYSTEMIC INVOLVEMENT IN SARCOIDOSIS

SYSTEM	ESTIMATED FREQUENCY	COMMENTS
Pleuropulmonary		
Pulmonary	> 90%	Granulomas form in alveolar septa, bronchiolar, and bronchial walls, causing diffuse pulmonary disease; pulmonary arteries and veins are also involved
		Often asymptomatic. Spontaneously resolves in many patients but can cause progressive pulmonary dysfunction leading to limitations in physical function, respiratory failure, and death in a few
Pleural	Rare	Produces lymphocytic exudative effusions, usually bilateral
Lymphatic	90%	Hilar or mediastinal involvement incidentally detected by chest x-ray in most patients. Others display nontender peripheral or cervical lymphadenopathy
GI		
Hepatic	40–75%	Usually asymptomatic; manifests as mild elevations in liver function test results, hypolucencies on CT scans with radiopaque dye
		Rarely causes clinically significant cholestasis, cirrhosis
		Unclear distinction between sarcoidosis and granulomatous hepatitis when sarcoidosis affects liver only
Splenic	10%	Usually asymptomatic, manifests with left upper quadrant pain, thrombocytopenia, incidental finding on x-ray or CT
Other	Rare	Rare reports of gastric granulomas, rare intestinal involvement; mesenteric lymphadenopathy may cause abdominal pain
Ocular	25%	Uveitis most common, causing blurred vision, photophobia, and tearing. Can cause blindness, but spontaneously resolves in most
		Conjunctivitis, iridocyclitis, chorioretinitis, dacryocystitis, lacrimal gland infiltration causing dry eyes, optic neuritis, glaucoma, and cataracts also reported
		Ocular involvement more common in black Americans and Japanese
		Annual or biannual screening indicated for early disease detection
Musculoskeletal		
Muscle	50–80%	Asymptomatic disease with or without enzyme elevations in most; sometimes insidious or acute myopathy with muscle weakness
Joint	25–50%	Ankle, knee, wrist, elbow arthritis most common; may cause chronic arthritis with Jaccoud's deformities or dactylitis
		Löfgren's syndrome is triad of acute polyarthritis, erythema nodosum, and hilar adenopathy. Has distinct features; more common in Scandinavian and Irish women, often responsive to NSAIDs, and often self-limited; low rate of relapse
Bone	5%	Osteolytic or cystic lesions; osteopenia

TABLE 56–1. SYSTEMIC INVOLVEMENT IN SARCOIDOSIS—Continued

SYSTEM	ESTIMATED FREQUENCY	COMMENTS
Dermatologic	25%	Erythema nodosum: red indurated tender nodules on anterior legs; more common in Europeans, Puerto Ricans, and Mexicans; usually remits in 1–2 mo; surrounding joints often arthritic (Löfgren's syndrome—see under Joint on p. 464); may be good prognostic sign
		Nonspecific skin lesions; plaques, macules and papules, subcutaneous nodules, and hypopigmentation and hyperpigmentation also common
		Lupus pernio: Violaceous plaques on nose, cheeks, lips, and ears; more common in black Americans and Puerto Ricans; often associated with lung fibrosis; poor prognostic sign
Neurologic	< 10%	Cranial neuropathy, especially 7th (causing facial nerve palsy) and 8th (causing hearing loss). Optic and peripheral neuropathy also common. Any cranial nerve can be affected
		CNS involvement, with nodular lesions or diffuse meningeal inflammation typically in cerebellar and brain stem regions
		Hypothalamic diabetes insipidus, polyphagia and obesity, thermoregulatory and libidinal changes
Renal	10%	Asymptomatic hypercalciuria most common; interstitial nephritis; chronic renal failure caused by nephrolithiasis and nephrocalcinosis requires renal replacement (dialysis or transplantation) in some
Cardiac	5%	Conduction blocks and arrhythmias most common and may cause sudden death; heart failure from restrictive cardiomyopathy (primary) or pulmonary hypertension (secondary) also occurs
		Transient papillary muscle dysfunction and pericarditis rare
		More common in Japanese, in whom cardiomyopathy is most frequent cause of sarcoidosis-related death
Reproductive	Rare	Case reports of endometrial, ovarian, epididymal, and testicular involvement. No effect on fertility. Disease may subside during pregnancy and relapse postpartum
Oral	< 5%	Asymptomatic parotid swelling most common; also causes parotitis with xerostomia; may be a component of keratoconjunctivitis sicca
		Heerfordt's syndrome (also called uveoparotid fever): uveitis, bilateral parotid swelling, facial palsy, and chronic fever
		Oral lupus pernio may disfigure hard palate and may involve cheek, tongue, and gums
Nasal sinus	< 10%	Acute and chronic granulomatous inflammation of sinus mucosa produces symptoms indistinguishable from common allergic and infectious sinusitis. Biopsy confirms diagnosis. Increased in patients with lupus pernio

Table continues on the following page.

TABLE 56–1. SYSTEMIC INVOLVEMENT IN SARCOIDOSIS—Continued

SYSTEM	ESTIMATED FREQUENCY	COMMENTS
Endocrine	Rare	Hypothalamic and pituitary stalk infiltration may cause panhypopituitarism; may cause thyroid infiltration without dysfunction; secondary hypoparathyroidism from hypercalcemia
Psychiatric	10%	Depression common, uncertain if a primary manifestation of sarcoidosis or a response to prolonged course of disease and frequent recurrences
Hematologic	< 5–30%	Lymphopenia; anemia of chronic disease; anemia due to granulomatous infiltration of bone marrow sometimes producing pancytopenia; splenic sequestration producing thrombocytopenia; leukopenia

should be cultured for fungi and mycobacteria. Exposure history to occupational (silicates, beryllium), environmental (moldy hay, birds, and other antigenic triggers of hypersensitivity pneumonitis), and infectious (TB, coccidioidomycosis, histoplasmosis) antigens should be explored. PPD skin testing should be performed early in the assessment along with anergy controls.

Pulmonary function tests and exercise pulse-oximetry assess disease severity. Pulmonary function test results are often normal in early stages but demonstrate restriction and reduced diffusing capacity for carbon monoxide (DL_{CO}) in advanced disease. Airflow obstruction also occurs and may suggest involvement of the bronchial mucosae. Pulse oximetry is often normal when measured at rest but may show effort desaturation with more extensive lung involvement. ABG analysis at rest and during exercise is more sensitive than pulse oximetry.

Recommended screening tests for extrapulmonary disease include ECG, slit-lamp ophthalmologic examination, and routine renal and liver function testing. Echocardiography, neuroimaging, lumbar puncture, bone films or MRI, and electromyography may be appropriate when symptoms suggest cardiac, neurologic, or rheumatologic disease. Abdominal CT with radiopaque dye is not routinely recommended but can provide evidence of hepatic or splenic involvement with enlargement and hyperlucent lesions.

Laboratory testing plays an adjunctive role in establishing the diagnosis and extent of organ involvement. CBC, electrolytes (including calcium), BUN, creatinine, and liver function tests generally provide useful information in screening for extrathoracic involvement. CBC may show anemia, eosinophilia, or leukopenia. Serum Ca may be elevated because of production of vitamin D analogs by activated macrophages. BUN, creatinine, and liver function tests may be elevated in renal and hepatic sarcoidosis. Total protein may be elevated because of hypergammaglobulinemia. Elevated ESR is nonspecific. Measurement of Ca in a urine specimen collected over 24 h is recommended to exclude hypercalciuria, even in patients with normal serum Ca levels. Elevated serum ACE levels also suggest sarcoidosis but are nonspecific and may be low in patients taking ACE inhibitors or elevated in patients with a variety of other conditions (eg, hyperthyroidism, Gaucher's disease, silicosis, mycobacterial disease, hypersensitivity pneumonitis). ACE levels may be useful for following disease activity and therapeutic response in patients with confirmed sarcoidosis. Increased ACE levels in CSF may be useful for diagnosing CNS sarcoidosis.

Other adjunctive tests include bronchoalveolar lavage and gallium scanning. The findings on bronchoalveolar lavage vary considerably, but lymphocytosis (lymphocytes > 10%) and/or a $CD4^+/CD8^+$ ratio of > 3.5 in the lavage fluid cell differential suggests the diagnosis in the proper clinical context. Absence of these findings does not exclude sarcoidosis, however.

Whole-body gallium scanning may provide useful supportive evidence in the absence of tissue confirmation. Symmetrical increased uptake in mediastinal and hilar nodes (lambda sign) and in lacrimal, parotid, and salivary glands (panda sign) are patterns highly suggestive of sarcoidosis. A negative result in patients taking prednisone is unreliable.

Prognosis

Although spontaneous improvement is common, the severity and manifestations of disease are highly variable, and many patients require courses of corticosteroids some time during the course of their disease. Thus, serial monitoring for evidence of relapse is imperative. About 90% of patients who have spontaneous remission do so within the first 2 yr after diagnosis; < 10% of these patients have relapses after 2 yr. Those patients who do not experience remission within 2 yr are likely to have chronic disease.

Sarcoidosis is thought to be chronic in up to 30% of patients, and 10 to 20% experience permanent sequelae. The disease is fatal in 1 to 5% of patients. Pulmonary fibrosis with respiratory failure is the most common cause of death worldwide, followed by pulmonary hemorrhage from aspergilloma. In Japan, however, infiltrative cardiomyopathy causing heart failure and arrhythmias is the most common cause of death.

Prognosis is worse for patients with extrapulmonary sarcoidosis and for blacks. Recovery occurs in 89% of whites and 76% of blacks with no extrathoracic disease and in 70% of whites and 46% of blacks with extrathoracic disease. The presence of erythema nodosum and acute arthritis are good prognostic signs. Uveitis, lupus pernio, chronic hypercalcemia, neurosarcoidosis, nephrocalcinosis, myocardial disease, and extensive pulmonary involvement are all poor prognostic signs. However, little difference is demonstrable in long-term outcome between treated and untreated patients, and relapse is common when treatment ends.

Treatment

Because sarcoidosis often spontaneously resolves, asymptomatic patients and those with mild symptoms do not require treatment, although they should be monitored for signs of deterioration. These patients can be followed with serial x-rays, pulmonary function tests (including diffusing capacity), and markers of extrathoracic involvement (eg, routine renal and liver function testing). Patients who require treatment regardless of stage include those with worsening symptoms; limitation of activity; markedly abnormal or deteriorating lung function; worrisome x-ray changes (cavitation, fibrosis, conglomerate masses, signs of pulmonary hypertension); heart, nervous system, or eye involvement; renal or hepatic insufficiency or failure; or disfiguring skin and joint disease.

Treatment is with corticosteroids. A standard protocol is prednisone 0.3 to 1 mg/kg po once/day depending on symptoms and severity

TABLE 56–2. STAGING SARCOIDOSIS

STAGE	DEFINITION	INCIDENCE OF SPONTANEOUS REMISSION
0	Normal chest x-ray	Usually remits; no correlation with prognosis
I	Bilateral hilar, paratracheal, and mediastinal lymphadenopathy without parenchymal infiltrates	60–80%
II	Bilateral hilar/mediastinal adenopathy with interstitial infiltrates (usually upper lung fields)	50–65%
III	Diffuse interstitial infiltrates without hilar adenopathy	< 30%
IV	Diffuse fibrosis, often associated with fibrotic-appearing conglomerate masses, traction bronchiectasis, traction cysts	0%

TABLE 56–3. DIFFERENTIAL DIAGNOSIS OF SARCOIDOSIS

Infectious
- Mycobacterial
  - TB
  - Atypical mycobacteria
- Fungal
  - Aspergillosis
  - Blastomycosis
  - Coccidioidomycosis
  - Cryptococcal infection
  - Histoplasmosis
- Other
  - Brucellosis
  - Cat-scratch disease (lymph nodes only)
  - Mycoplasmal infection
  - *Pneumocystis jiroveci* (formerly *P. carinii*) infection
  - Syphilis

Rheumatologic
- Juvenile RA
- Kikuchi's lymphadenitis (lymph nodes only)
- Necrotizing sarcoid granulomatosis
- RA
- Sjögren's syndrome
- Wegener's granulomatosis

Hematologic malignancy
- Hodgkin lymphoma
- Non-Hodgkin lymphoma
- Splenic lymphoma

Hypersensitivity
- Occupational metals
  - Aluminum
  - Berylliosis
  - Titanium
  - Zirconium
- Organic antigens producing hypersensitivity pneumonitis
  - Actinomycetes
  - Atypical mycobacterial antigens
  - Fungi
  - Mushroom spores
  - Other bioaerosols
- Inorganic antigens producing hypersensitivity pneumonitis
  - Isocyanates
  - Pyrethrins
- Drug reaction

Other
- Inflammatory bowel disease
- Foreign body aspiration or inoculation
- Granulomatous hepatitis
- Granulomatous lesion of unknown significance
- Lymphoid interstitial pneumonia

of findings. Alternate-day regimens are also used (eg, prednisone 40 to 60 mg po once every other day). It is rare to exceed 40 mg/day; however, higher doses may be needed to reduce complications in patients with ocular, myocardial, or neurologic disease. Response usually occurs within 2 to 4 wk, so symptoms and results of chest x-ray and pulmonary function tests may be reassessed between 4 and 12 wk. Chronic, insidious cases may respond more slowly. The drug is tapered to a maintenance dose (eg, prednisone ≤ 10 mg every other day if possible) after evidence of response and is continued for a minimum of 12 mo if improvement occurs. The optimal duration of treatment is unknown. Premature taper can result in relapse. The drug is slowly stopped if response is absent or equivocal. Corticosteroids can ultimately be stopped in most patients, but because relapse occurs up to 50% of the time, monitoring should be repeated, usually every 3 to 6 mo. Corticosteroid treatment should be resumed for recurrence of symptoms and signs, including dyspnea, arthralgia, fever, hepatic insufficiency, cardiac arrhythmia, CNS involvement, hypercalcemia, ocular disease uncontrolled by local drugs, and disfiguring skin lesions.

Data on use of inhaled corticosteroids for pulmonary sarcoidosis are not definitive, but some evidence suggests that this route of administration can relieve cough in patients with endobronchial involvement. Topical corticosteroids may be useful in some cases of dermatologic and ocular disease.

About 10% of patients requiring therapy are unresponsive to tolerable doses of a corticosteroid and should be given a 6-mo trial of methotrexate starting at 2.5 mg po once/wk and increasing in increments of 2.5 mg/wk to a total of 10 to 15 mg/wk as tolerated to keep WBC > 3000/μL. Initially, methotrexate and corticosteroids are both given; over 8 wk, the corticosteroid dose can be tapered and, in many cases, stopped. The maximal response to methotrexate, however, may take 6 to 12 mo. In such cases, prednisone must be tapered more slowly. Serial blood counts and liver enzyme tests should be performed every 1 to 2 wk initially and then every 4 to 6 wk once a stable dose is achieved. Folic acid (1 mg po once/day) is recommended for patients treated with methotrexate.

Other drugs reported to be effective in small numbers of patients who are corticosteroid-resistant or who experience complicating adverse effects include azathioprine, cyclophosphamide, chlorambucil, chloroquine or hydroxychloroquine, thalidomide, pentoxifylline, and infliximab.

Hydroxychloroquine 200 mg po bid to tid can be as effective as corticosteroids for treatment of disfiguring skin sarcoidosis and in treatment of hypercalciuria. Although immunosuppressants are often more effective in refractory cases, relapse is common after cessation.

No available drugs have consistently prevented pulmonary fibrosis.

Lung transplantation is an option for patients with end-stage pulmonary involvement, although disease may recur in the transplanted organ.

57 ENVIRONMENTAL PULMONARY DISEASES

Environmental pulmonary diseases result from inhalation of dusts, allergens, chemicals, gases, and environmental pollutants. The lungs are continually exposed to the external environment and are susceptible to a host of environmental diseases. Pathologic processes can involve any part of the lung, including the airways (eg, occupational asthma, reactive airways dysfunction syndrome, toxic inhalations), interstitium (eg, pneumoconioses, hypersensitivity pneumonitis), and pleurae (eg, asbestos-related diseases).

Prevention of occupational and environmental respiratory disease centers on reducing exposure (primary prevention). This includes administrative controls (eg, limiting the number of people placed in hazardous conditions), engineering controls (eg, enclosures, ventilation systems, safe clean-up procedures), product substitution (eg, using safer, less toxic materials), and use of respiratory protection devices.

Many clinicians erroneously assume that a patient who has used a respirator or respiratory protection device (dust mask or gas mask) has been well protected. While respirators do afford a degree of protection, especially in situations in which fresh air is provided by tank or air hose, the benefit is limited and idiosyncratic. When recommending use of a respirator, clinicians should consider several factors. Workers with cardiovascular disease may be unable to perform jobs that require strenuous work, especially if they must wear a self-contained breathing apparatus (tank). Respirators that are tight-fitting and that require the wearer to draw air through filter cartridges can increase the work of breathing, especially troublesome for patients with asthma, COPD, or interstitial lung disorders.

Medical surveillance is a form of secondary prevention. Workers can be offered medical tests that identify disease at early states when medical treatment might help reduce long-term consequences.

AIR POLLUTION–RELATED ILLNESS

The major components of air pollution in developed countries are nitrogen dioxide (from combustion of fossil fuels), ozone (from the effect of sunlight on nitrogen dioxide and hydrocarbons), and suspended solid or liquid particles. Burning of biomass fuel is an additional important source of particulate matter indoors in developing countries. Passive smoking can be considered as related.

The effect of air pollution on lung disease can be substantial at high pollution levels, which can trigger asthma and COPD exacerbations. People living in areas with high traffic, especially when stagnant air is created by thermal inversions, are at particular risk. Of the so-called criteria air pollutants (oxides of nitrogen, oxides of sulfur, ozone, carbon monoxide, lead, and particulates), only CO and lead do not affect airways hyperreactivity. Long-term exposure may increase respiratory infections and symptoms in the general population, especially children.

Ozone, which is the major component of smog, is a strong respiratory irritant and oxidant. Levels tend to be highest in the summer, late morning, and early afternoon. Short-term exposures can produce dyspnea, chest pain, and airways reactivity. Children who participate in outdoor sports during high ozone pollution days are more likely to develop asthma. Long-term exposure to ozone produces a small, permanent decrease in lung function.

Oxides of sulfur, resulting from combustion of fossil fuels that are high in sulfur content, can create acid aerosols with high solubility, resulting in upper airway deposition. Sulfur oxides can induce airways inflammation, possibly increasing the risk for chronic bronchitis as well as inducing bronchoconstriction.

Particulate air pollution is a complex mixture, derived from fossil fuel combustion (especially diesel). The particles can have both local and systemic inflammatory effects, suggesting an explanation for their impact on both respiratory and cardiovascular health. Ultrafine particles (< 2.5 μm) produce a greater inflammatory response per mass than do larger particles. Data to date suggest that particulate air pollution increases death rates from all causes, especially cardiovascular and respiratory illness.

ASBESTOS-RELATED DISORDERS

Asbestos-related disorders are caused by inhalation of asbestos fibers. The disorders include asbestosis; lung carcinoma; nonmalignant pleural plaque formation and thickening; benign pleural effusions; and malignant mesothelioma. Asbestosis and mesothelioma both cause progressive dyspnea. Diagnosis is based on history and chest x-ray or CT and, in the case of malignancy, tissue biopsy. Treatment is supportive, except for malignancies, which may require surgery and/or chemotherapy.

Asbestos is a naturally occurring silicate whose heat-resistant and structural properties made it useful for inclusion in construction and shipbuilding materials, automobile brakes, and some textiles. Chrysotile (a serpentine fiber), crocidolite, and amosite (amphibole, or straight, fibers) are the 3 main types of asbestos that cause disease. Asbestos can affect the lung and/or the pleura.

Pulmonary Disease

Pulmonary disease can be nonmalignant or malignant.

Asbestosis: Asbestosis, a form of interstitial pulmonary fibrosis, is much more common than malignant disease. Shipbuilders, textile and construction workers, home remodelers, workers who do asbestos abatement, and miners exposed to asbestos fibers are among the many categories of workers at risk of the disease. Secondhand exposure may occur among family members of exposed workers and among those who live close to mines. Pathophysiology is similar to that of other pneumoconioses—alveolar macrophages attempting to engulf inhaled fibers release cytokines and growth factors that stimulate inflammation, collagen deposition, and ultimately fibrosis—except that asbestos fibers themselves may also be directly toxic to lung tissue. Risk of disease is generally related to duration and intensity of exposure and type, length, and thickness of inhaled fibers.

Asbestosis is initially asymptomatic but can cause progressive dyspnea, nonproductive cough, and fatigue; the disease progresses in > 10% of patients after cessation of exposure. Advanced asbestosis may cause clubbing, dry bibasilar crackles, and, in severe cases, symptoms and signs of right ventricular failure (cor pulmonale).

Diagnosis is based on history of exposure and chest x-ray or chest CT. Chest x-ray shows linear reticular or nodular opacities signifying fibrosis, usually in the peripheral lower lobes, often accompanied by pleural changes (see p. 471). Honeycombing signifies more advanced disease, which may involve the mid lung fields. As with silicosis, severity is graded on the International Labor Organization scale based on size, shape, location, and profusion of opacities. In contrast to silicosis, asbestosis produces reticular opacities with a lower lobe predominance. Hilar and mediastinal adenopathy are uncharacteristic and suggest a different diagnosis. Chest x-ray is insensitive; high-resolution chest CT (HRCT) is useful when asbestosis is a likely diagnosis. HRCT is also superior to the chest x-ray in identifying the pleural abnormalities. Pulmonary function tests, which may show reduced lung volumes and DLco, are nonspecific but help characterize changes in lung function over time after the diagnosis is made. Bronchoalveolar lavage or lung biopsy is indicated only when noninvasive measures fail to provide conclusive diagnosis; demonstration of asbestos fibers indicates asbestosis in people with pulmonary fibrosis, although such fibers can occasionally be found in lungs of exposed people without disease.

No specific treatment exists. Early detection of hypoxemia and right ventricular failure leads to use of supplemental O_2 and treatment of heart failure. Pulmonary rehabilitation can be helpful for patients with impairment. Preventive measures include eliminating exposure, asbestos abatement in nonoccupational settings, smoking cessation, and pneumococcal and influenza vaccination. Smoking cessation is particularly important in light of the multiplicative risk of lung cancer in those who have both tobacco smoke and asbestos exposures. Prognosis varies; many patients do well with no or mild symptoms, whereas some develop progressive dyspnea and a few develop respiratory failure, right ventricular failure, and malignancy.

Lung carcinoma (nonsmall cell) develops in patients with asbestosis at 8 to 10 times the rate of those without asbestosis and is especially common in workers exposed to amphibole fibers, although all forms of inhaled asbestos have been associated with an elevated cancer risk. Asbestos and smoking have a synergistic effect on lung cancer risk (see p. 503).

Pleural Disease

Pleural disease, a hallmark of asbestos exposure, includes formation of pleural plaques, calcification, thickening, adhesions, effusion, and mesothelioma. Pleural disease produces effusion and malignancy but few symptoms. All pleural changes are diagnosed by chest x-ray or HRCT, though chest CT is more sensitive than chest x-ray for detecting pleural disorders. Treatment is rarely needed except in the case of malignant mesothelioma.

Discrete plaques, which occur in up to 60% of workers exposed to asbestos, typically affect the bilateral parietal pleurae between the 5th and 9th ribs and adjacent to the diaphragm. Plaque calcification is common and can lead to misdiagnosis of severe pulmonary disease when radiographically superimposed on lung fields. HRCT can distinguish pleural from parenchymal disease in this setting.

Diffuse thickening affects visceral as well as parietal pleurae. It may be an extension of pulmonary fibrosis from parenchyma to the pleurae or a nonspecific reaction to pleural effusion. With or without calcification, pleural thickening can cause a restrictive defect. Rounded atelectasis is a manifestation of pleural thickening in which invagination of pleura into the parenchyma can entrap lung tissue, causing atelectasis. On chest x-ray and CT, it typically appears as a curvilinear cicatricial mass, often in the lower lung zones, and can be confused radiographically with a pulmonary malignancy.

Pleural effusions occur but are less common than the other pleural changes they accompany. Effusions are exudative, often hemorrhagic, and typically resolve spontaneously (see p. 490).

Pleural mesothelioma: Pleural mesothelioma is the only known pleural malignancy and is caused by asbestos exposure in nearly all cases. Asbestos workers have up to a 10% lifetime risk of developing the disease, with an average latency of 30 yr. Risk is independent of smoking. Mesothelioma can spread locally or metastasize to the pericardium, diaphragm, peritoneum, and, rarely, the tunica vaginalis of the testis. Patients most often present with dyspnea and nonpleuritic chest pain. Constitutional symptoms are uncommon at time of clinical presentation. Invasion of the chest wall and other adjacent structures may cause severe pain, hoarseness, dysphagia, Horner's syndrome, brachial plexopathy, or ascites. Extrathoracic spread occurs in up to 80% of patients, most commonly including the hilar and mediastinal lymph nodes, liver, adrenals, and kidneys.

The pleural form of mesothelioma, which represents more than 90% of all cases, presents on x-ray as diffuse unilateral or bilateral pleural thickening that appears to encase the lungs, usually producing blunting of the costophrenic angles. Pleural effusions are present in 95% of cases and are typically unilateral, massive effusions. Diagnosis is based on pleural fluid cytology or pleural biopsy and, if these are nondiagnostic, biopsy by video-assisted thoracoscopic surgery (VATS) or thoracotomy. Staging is done with chest CT, mediastinoscopy, and MRI. Sensitivity and specificity of MRI and CT are comparable, although MRI is helpful in determining tumor extension into the spine or spinal cord. PET may have better sensitivity and specificity for distinguishing benign from malignant pleural thickening. Bronchoscopy rules out coexisting endobronchial malignancies. Increased hyaluronidase levels in pleural fluid are suggestive but not diagnostic of disease.

Soluble mesothelin-related proteins released into the serum by mesothelial cells are being studied as possible tumor markers for disease detection and monitoring.

Mesothelioma remains an incurable cancer. Surgery to remove the pleura; ipsilateral lung, phrenic nerve, and hemidiaphragm; and pericardium combined with chemotherapy or radiation therapy may be considered, although it does not substantially change prognosis or survival time, and long-term survival is uncommon. Moreover, complete surgical resection is not feasible in most patients. Combination pemetrexed (an antifolate antimetabolite) and cisplatin shows promise but warrants further study.

The major focus of supportive care is on relief of pain and dyspnea. Given the diffuse nature of the disease, radiation therapy is usually unsuitable except as a tool for treating localized pain and for needle-tract metastases but should be avoided for treatment of nerve root pain. To help reduce dyspnea caused by pleural effusions, pleurodesis or pleurectomy can be used. Adequate analgesia is difficult but important to achieve, usually requiring opioids, with both transcutaneous and indwelling epidural catheters being used in pain management. Chemotherapy using cisplatin with gemcitabine has relieved symptoms in most cases and has demonstrated tumor shrinkage in ½ of patients studied. Multimodality therapies are advocated by some authorities. Intrapleural injection of granulocyte-macrophage colony-stimulating factor or interferon-γ; IV ranpirnase (a ribonuclease); and gene therapies are under study.

No treatment has been shown to substantially prolong survival. Survival from time of diagnosis averages 8 to 15 mo depending on the location and cell type. A small number of patients, usually younger patients with shorter duration of symptoms, have a more favorable prognosis, sometimes surviving for several years after diagnosis.

BERYLLIUM DISEASE

(Berylliosis)

Acute beryllium disease (ABD) and chronic beryllium disease (CBD) are caused by inhalation of dust or fumes from beryllium compounds and products. ABD is now rare; CBD is characterized by formation of granulomas throughout the body, especially the lungs, intrathoracic lymph nodes, and skin. CBD causes progressive dyspnea, cough, and fatigue. Diagnosis is by history, beryllium lymphocyte proliferation test, and biopsy. Treatment is with corticosteroids.

Etiology and Pathophysiology

Beryllium exposure is a common but underrecognized cause of illness in many industries, including beryllium mining and extraction, alloy production, metal alloy machining, electronics, telecommunications, nuclear weapons, defense, aircraft, automotive, aerospace, and computers and electronics recycling.

ABD is a chemical pneumonitis causing diffuse parenchymal inflammatory infiltrates and nonspecific intra-alveolar edema. Other tissues (eg, skin and conjunctivae) may be affected. ABD is now rare because most industries have reduced exposure levels, but cases were common between 1940 and 1970, and many progressed from ABD to CBD.

CBD remains a common illness in industries that use beryllium and beryllium alloy. It differs from most pneumoconioses in that it is a cell-mediated hypersensitivity disease. Beryllium is presented to $CD4^+$ T lymphocytes by antigen-presenting cells, principally in the context of HLA-DP molecules. T cells in the blood, lung, or other organs, in turn, recognize the beryllium, proliferate, and form T-cell clones. These clones then release proinflammatory cytokines, such as tumor necrosis factor-α, IL-2, and interferon-γ. These amplify the immune response, resulting in formation of mononuclear cell infiltrates and noncaseating granulomas in target organs where beryllium has deposited. On average, 2 to 6% of beryllium-exposed people develop beryllium sensitization (defined by positive blood lymphocyte proliferation to beryllium salts in vitro), with most progressing to disease. Certain high-risk populations, such as beryllium metal and alloy machinists, have CBD prevalence > 17%. Workers with bystander exposures, such as secretaries and security guards, also develop sensitization and disease but at lower rates. The typical pathologic consequence is a diffuse pulmonary, hilar, and mediastinal lymph node granulomatous reaction histologically indistinguishable from sarcoidosis. Early granuloma formation with mononuclear and giant cells can also occur. Many lymphocytes are found when cells are washed from the lungs (bronchoalveolar lavage [BAL]) during bronchoscopy. These T cells proliferate when exposed to beryllium in vitro, much as the blood cells do (beryllium lymphocyte proliferation test [BeLPT]).

Symptoms, Signs, and Diagnosis

Patients with CBD often have dyspnea, cough, weight loss, and a highly variable chest x-ray pattern, usually showing diffuse interstitial consolidation. Patients complain of insidious and progressive exertional dyspnea, cough, chest pain, weight loss, night sweats, and fatigue. Symptoms may develop within months of 1st exposure or > 40 yr after exposure has ceased. Some people remain asymptomatic. The chest x-ray may be normal or show diffuse infiltrates that can be nodular, reticular, or have a hazy ground-glass appearance, often with hilar adenopathy resembling the pattern seen in sarcoidosis. A miliary pattern also occurs. High-resolution chest x-ray is more sensitive than x-ray, although cases of biopsy-proven disease occur even in people with normal imaging tests.

Diagnosis depends on a history of exposure, the appropriate clinical manifestations, and an abnormal blood and/or BAL BeLPT. BAL BeLPT is highly sensitive and specific, helping to distinguish CBD from sarcoidosis and other forms of diffuse pulmonary disease.

Prognosis

ABD can be fatal, but prognosis is usually excellent if patients do not progress to CBD. CBD often results in progressive loss of respiratory function. Early abnormalities include air flow obstruction and decreased oxygenation on ABG at rest and during exercise testing. Decreased diffusing capacity for carbon monoxide (DL_{CO}) and restriction appear later. Pulmonary hypertension and right heart failure develop in about 10% of cases, with death from cor pulmonale. Beryllium sensitization progresses to CBD at a rate of about 8%/yr after initial detection through workplace medical surveillance programs. Subcutaneous granulomatous nodules caused by inoculation with beryllium splinters or dust usually persist until excised.

Treatment

Some CBD patients never require treatment because of the relatively slow rate of disease progression. Treatment is with corticosteroids, which result in symptomatic improvement and better oxygenation. Treatment is generally started only in those patients with significant symptoms and evidence of abnormal gas exchange or evidence of an accelerated decline in lung function or oxygenation. In symptomatic patients with abnormal pulmonary function, prednisone 40 to 60 mg po once/day or every other day is given for 3 to 6 mo, after which measures of pulmonary physiology and gas exchange are repeated to document a response to therapy. The dose is then gradually tapered to the lowest that maintains symptomatic and objective improvement (usually about 10 to 15 mg once/day or every other day). Lifelong treatment with corticosteroids is usually required. There is anecdotal evidence that the addition of methotrexate (10 to 25 mg po once/wk) has a corticosteroid-sparing effect in CBD, similar to that observed in sarcoidosis.

In ABD, the lungs often become edematous and hemorrhagic. Mechanical ventilation is necessary in severely affected patients.

Unlike many cases of sarcoidosis, spontaneous remission of CBD is rare. In patients with end-stage CBD, lung transplantation can be lifesaving. Other supportive measures, such as supplemental O_2 therapy, pulmonary rehabilitation, and drugs for treatment of right heart failure, are used as needed.

Prevention

Industrial dust suppression is the basis for preventing beryllium exposure. Exposures must be reduced to levels that are as low as reasonably achievable—preferably more than 10-fold below current OSHA standards—to reduce the risk of sensitization and CBD. Medical surveillance, using the blood BeLPT and chest x-ray, is recommended for all exposed workers, including those with direct or indirect contact. The disease (both acute and chronic) must be promptly recognized and affected workers removed from further beryllium exposure.

BUILDING-RELATED ILLNESSES

Building-related illnesses (BRIs) are a heterogeneous group of disorders whose etiology is linked to the environment of modern airtight buildings. Such buildings are characterized by sealed windows and dependence on heating, ventilation, and air conditioning systems for circulation of air. Most cases occur in nonindustrial office buildings but can occur in apartment buildings, single family dwellings, schools, museums, and libraries.

BRIs can be specific or nonspecific.

Specific BRIs: Specific BRIs are those for which a link between building-related exposure and illness is proven. Examples include *Legionella* infection (see p. 1464), occupational asthma (see p. 476), hypersensitivity pneumonitis (see p. 453), and inhalational fever.

Inhalational fever is a febrile reaction caused by exposures to organic aerosols or dusts. Names used to describe this type of BRI include humidifier fever, grain fever, swine confinement fever, and mycotoxicosis. Metal fumes and polymer fumes can also produce febrile illness. The term organic dust toxic syndrome (ODTS) has been used to encompass the reaction to any organic dust, although the term toxic pneumonitis has also entered common parlance.

In nonindustrial building settings, the BRI called humidifier fever occurs as a consequence of humidifiers or other types of ventilation units serving as a reservoir for the growth of microbes (bacteria, fungi) and as a method of aerosolizing these contaminants. The disorder usually manifests as low-grade fever, malaise, cough, and dyspnea. Improvement with removal from exposure (eg, weekend away from the office building) is often one of the 1st indications of etiology. The condition has an acute onset and is self-limiting (usually 2 to 3 days). Physical signs may be absent or subtle. Clusters of cases are common. Unlike immunologically mediated conditions, such as hypersensitivity pneumonitis and building-related asthma, inhalational fevers do not require a period of sensitization. Disease can occur on 1st exposure. Acute episodes do not generally require treatment apart from removal from the contaminated environment and antipyretics. If symptoms persist, further investigation may be required to rule out infection, hypersensitivity pneumonitis, or other conditions. Biologic sampling (to detect airborne microbials in the work environment) can be costly and time consuming but is necessary in some cases to document the source of contaminated air. Inhalational fevers of all types are usually prevented by good maintenance of ventilation systems.

Nonspecific BRIs: Nonspecific BRIs are those for which a link between building-related exposure and illness are more difficult to prove. The term sick building syndrome has been used to refer to illnesses that occur in clusters within a building for which the symptoms are often nonspecific, including itchy, irritated, dry or watery eyes; rhinorrhea or nasal congestion; throat soreness or tightness; dry itchy skin or unexplained skin rashes; and headache, lethargy, and difficulty concentrating.

Some building-related factors appear to account for symptoms in some instances; these include higher building temperature, higher humidity, and poor ventilation, typically with a failure to incorporate sufficient fresh air from outdoors. But patient factors, including female sex, history of atopy, increased attention to body sensations, worry about the meaning of symptoms, anxiety, depression, and occasionally mass hysteria, also seem to underlie experience of symptoms.

BYSSINOSIS

Byssinosis is a form of reactive airway disease characterized by bronchoconstriction in cotton, flax, and hemp workers. The etiologic agent is unknown. Symptoms are chest tightness and dyspnea that worsen on the 1st day of the work week and subside as the week progresses. Diagnosis is based on history and pulmonary function tests. Treatment includes avoidance of exposure and use of asthma drugs.

Byssinosis occurs almost entirely in workers who contact unprocessed, raw cotton, especially those exposed to open bales or who work in cotton spinning or in the card room. Byssinosis can occur after acute exposure but usually occurs in workers with a history of chronic exposure. Evidence suggests that some agent in the cotton bract leads to bronchoconstriction. Although bacterial endotoxin is a likely cause, the absence of similar symptoms in other settings in which workers are exposed to endotoxin leaves some uncertainty. Prolonged exposure to cotton dust was once thought to cause emphysema, a theory not disproved. Chronic bronchitis symptoms are common among those exposed to cotton dust.

Symptoms and Signs

Symptoms are chest tightness and dyspnea that lessen with repeated exposure. Symptoms develop on the 1st day of work after a weekend or vacation and diminish or disappear by the end of the week. With repeated exposure over a period of years, chest tightness tends to return and persist through midweek and occasionally to the end of the week or as long as the person continues to work. This typical temporal pattern distinguishes byssinosis from asthma.

Signs of acute exposure are tachypnea and wheezing. Patients with more chronic exposure may have crackles.

Diagnosis and Treatment

Diagnosis is based on history and pulmonary function tests that show typical airflow obstruction and a reduction in ventilatory capacity, especially if measured at the start and end of a 1st work shift. Hyperresponsiveness to methacholine is also often observed. Surveillance measures, including symptom reporting and spirometry in textile workers, can aid in early detection.

Treatment includes avoidance or reduction of exposure and use of asthma drugs.

COAL WORKERS' PNEUMOCONIOSIS

(Anthracosis; Black Lung Disease; Coal Miner's Pneumoconiosis)

Coal workers' pneumoconiosis (CWP) is caused by inhalation of coal dust. Deposition of dust produces dust-laden macrophages around bronchioles (coal macules), occasionally causing focal bronchiolar emphysema. CWP usually causes no symptoms but can progress to progressive massive fibrosis with impaired lung function. Diagnosis is based on history and chest x-ray. Treatment is generally supportive.

Etiology and Pathophysiology

CWP is caused by chronic inhalation of dust from high-carbon coal (anthracite and bituminous), typically over ≥ 20 yr. Inhalation of silica contained in coal may also contribute to clinical disease. Alveolar macrophages engulf the dust, release cytokines that stimulate inflammation, and collect in lung interstitium around bronchioles and alveoli (coal macules). Coal nodules develop as collagen accumulates, and focal emphysema develops as bronchiole walls weaken and dilate. Fibrosis can occur but is usually limited to areas adjacent to coal macules. Distortion of lung architecture, airflow obstruction, and functional impairment are usually mild but can be highly destructive in a subset of patients.

Two forms are described: simple, with individual coal macules, and complicated, with coalescence of macules and progressive massive fibrosis (PMF). Patients with simple CWP develop PMF at a rate of about 1 to 2%. In this condition, nodules coalesce to form black, rubbery parenchymal masses usually in the upper posterior fields. The masses may encroach on and destroy vascular supply and airways or may cavitate. PMF can develop and progress even after exposure to coal dust has ceased. Despite the similarity of coal-induced PMF and conglomerate silicosis, the development of PMF in coal workers is unrelated to silica content of the coal.

An association between CWP and features of RA is well-described. It is unclear whether CWP predisposes miners to developing RA, whether RA takes on a unique form in patients with CWP, or whether RA alters the response of miners to coal dust. Multiple rounded nodules in the lung appearing over a relatively short time (Caplan's syndrome) represent an immunopathologic response related to rheumatoid diathesis. Histologically, they resemble rheumatoid nodules but have a peripheral region of more acute inflammation. Patients with CWP are at a slightly increased risk of developing active TB and non-TB mycobacterial infections. The same principles of TB surveillance and treatment apply to CWP as for silicosis. Weak associations have been reported between CWP and progressive systemic sclerosis and stomach cancer.

Symptoms and Signs

CWP does not usually cause symptoms. Most chronic pulmonary symptoms in coal miners are caused by other conditions, such as industrial bronchitis from coal dust or coincident emphysema from smoking. Cough can be chronic and problematic in patients even after they leave the workplace, even in those who do not smoke.

PMF causes progressive dyspnea. Black sputum (melanoptysis) is rare and is caused by rupture of PMF lesions into the airways. PMF often progresses to pulmonary hypertension with right ventricular and respiratory failure.

Diagnosis

Diagnosis depends on a history of exposure and chest x-ray or thoracic CT appearance of diffuse, small rounded opacities or nodules (CWP) or of at least one opacity > 10 mm against a background of CWP (PMF). The specificity of the chest x-ray for PMF is low, because up to ⅓ of lesions identified as being PMF turn out to be malignancies, scars, or other lesions. Chest CT is also more sensitive than chest x-ray for detecting coalescing nodules, early PMF, and cavitation. Pulmonary function tests are nondiagnostic but are useful for characterizing lung function in patients in whom obstructive, restrictive, or mixed defects may develop. Because abnormalities of gas exchange are observed in some patients with extensive simple CWP and in those with complicated CWP, baseline and periodic measures of diffusing capacity for carbon monoxide (DL_{CO}) and ABG at rest and during exercise are recommended.

Treatment and Prevention

Treatment is rarely necessary in simple CWP, although smoking cessation and TB surveillance are recommended. Patients with pulmonary hypertension and/or hypoxemia are given supplemental O_2 therapy. Pulmonary rehabilitation can help the more severely affected workers perform activities of daily living. Preventive measures include eliminating exposure, smoking cessation, and pneumococcal and influenza vaccination. Workers with CWP, especially those with PMF, should be restricted from further exposure, especially to high concentrations of dust. TB is treated in accordance with current recommendations (see p. 1511).

CWP can be prevented by suppressing coal dust at the coal face. Despite long-standing regulations, exposures continue to occur in the mining trade. Respiratory masks provide only limited protection.

OCCUPATIONAL ASTHMA

Occupational asthma is reversible airway obstruction that develops after months to years of sensitization to an allergen encountered in the workplace. Symptoms are dyspnea, wheezing, cough, and, occasionally, upper respiratory allergic symptoms. Diagnosis is based on occupational history, including assessment of job activities, allergens in the work environment, and a temporal association between work and symptoms. Allergen skin testing and provocative inhalational challenge may be used in specialized centers but are usually unnecessary. Treatment involves removing the person from the environment and using asthma drugs as needed (see also p. 387).

Occupational asthma is development of asthma in a worker who has no previous history of asthma; symptoms typically develop over months to years from sensitization to an allergen encountered in the workplace. Once sensitized, the worker invariably responds to much lower concentrations of the allergen than that which initiated the response. Occupational asthma differs from occupationally aggravated asthma, which is an exacerbation or worsening of asthma in workers with previously existing clinical or subclinical disease as a result of single or repeated workplace exposures to pulmonary irritants such as dusts and fumes. Occupationally aggravated asthma, which is more common than occupational asthma, generally subsides with reduction of exposure and appropriate asthma treatment. It has a better prognosis and does not require the same level of clinical investigation of specific triggering allergens.

Several other airway diseases caused by inhalational workplace exposures can be distinguished from occupational and occupationally aggravated asthma.

In reactive airways dysfunction syndrome (RADS), which is nonallergenic, people with no history of asthma develop persistent, reversible airway obstruction after acute overexposure to irritant dust, fume, or gas. Airway inflammation persists even after removal of the acute irritant, and the syndrome is indistinguishable from asthma.

In reactive upper airways syndrome, upper airway (ie, nasal, pharyngeal) mucosal symptoms develop after acute or repeated exposure to airways irritants.

In irritant-associated vocal cord dysfunction, which mimics asthma, abnormal apposition and closure of the vocal cords, especially during inspiration, occurs after acute irritant inhalation.

In industrial bronchitis (irritant-induced chronic bronchitis), bronchial inflammation causes cough after acute or chronic inhalational exposures to irritants.

In bronchiolitis obliterans, bronchiolar damage occurs after acute inhalational exposure to gases (eg, anhydrous ammonia). The 2 major forms are proliferative and constrictive. The constrictive form is more common and may or may not be associated with other forms of diffuse lung injury.

Etiology

Occupational asthma is caused by both immune- and non–immune-mediated mechanisms. Immune mechanisms involve IgE- and non–IgE-mediated hypersensitivity to workplace allergens. Hundreds of occupational allergens exist, ranging from low mol wt chemicals to large proteins. Examples include grain dust, proteolytic enzymes used in detergent manufacturing, red cedar wood, isocyanates, formalin (rarely), antibiotics (eg, ampicillin, spiramycin), epoxy resins, and tea.

Non–immune-mediated inflammatory mechanisms, responsible for occupational airways disease, cause direct irritation of the respiratory epithelium and upper airway mucosae.

Symptoms and Signs

Symptoms include shortness of breath, chest tightness, wheezing, and cough, often with upper respiratory symptoms such as sneezing, rhinorrhea, and tearing. Upper airway and conjunctival symptoms may precede the typical asthmatic symptoms by months or years. Symptoms may develop during work hours after specific dust or vapor exposure but often do not become apparent until several hours after leaving work, thereby making the association with occupational exposure less obvious. Nocturnal wheezing may be the only symptom. Often, the symptoms disappear on weekends or during vacations, although with ongoing exposure temporal exacerbations and relief become less apparent.

Diagnosis

Diagnosis depends on recognizing the link between workplace allergens and clinical asthma. Diagnosis is suspected on the basis of an occupational history of allergen exposures. A materials safety data sheet can be used to list potential allergens and confirm when immunologic tests (eg, skin prick, puddle, or patch testing), through use of suspected antigens, demonstrate that a causative agent in the workplace is affecting a person. An increase in bronchial hyperresponsiveness after exposure to the suspected antigen is also helpful in making the diagnosis.

In difficult cases, a carefully controlled inhalation challenge test performed in the laboratory confirms the cause of the airway obstruction. Such procedures should be reserved for clinical centers experienced in inhalation challenge testing and capable of monitoring the sometimes severe reactions that can occur. Pulmonary function tests or peak expiratory flow measurements that show decreasing airflow during work are further evidence that occupational exposure is causative. Methacholine challenge tests can be used to establish the degree of airway hyperreactivity. Sensitivity to methacholine may decrease after exposure to the occupational allergen has ceased.

Differentiation from idiopathic asthma is generally based on the pattern of symptoms, demonstration that allergens are present in the workplace, and the relationship between exposure to allergens and symptoms and physiologic worsening.

Treatment and Prevention

Treatment is the same as for idiopathic asthma, including inhaled bronchodilators and corticosteroids (see p. 387).

Dust suppression is essential. However, elimination of all instances of sensitization and clinical disease may not be possible. Once sensitized, patients with occupational asthma may react to extremely low levels of airborne allergen. Those who return to environments in which the allergen persists generally have a poorer prognosis, with more respiratory symptoms, more abnormal lung physiology, a greater need for drugs, and more frequent and severe exacerbations. Whenever possible, a symptomatic person should be removed from a setting known to produce symptoms. If exposure continues, symptoms tend to persist. Occupational asthma can sometimes be cured if it is diagnosed early and exposure ceases.

SILICOSIS

Silicosis is caused by inhalation of crystalline-free silica dust and is characterized by nodular pulmonary fibrosis. Chronic silicosis initially causes no symptoms or only mild dyspnea but over years can advance to involve most of the lung and cause dyspnea, hypoxemia, pulmonary hypertension, and respiratory impairment. Diagnosis is based on history and chest x-ray. No effective treatment exists except supportive care and, for severe cases, lung transplantation.

Etiology

Silicosis, the oldest known occupational pulmonary disease, is caused by inhalation of tiny particles of silicon in the form of crystalline "free" silica (usually quartz) or, less commonly, by inhalation of silicates, minerals containing silicon dioxide bound to other elements, such as talc. Workers at greatest risk are those who move or blast rock and sand (miners, quarry workers, stonecutters) or who use silica-containing rock or sand abrasives (sand blasters; glass makers; foundry, gemstone, and ceramic workers; potters). Coal miners are at risk of mixed silicosis and coal workers' pneumoconiosis (see p. 475).

Chronic silicosis is the most common form and generally develops only after exposure over decades. Accelerated silicosis (rare) and acute silicosis may develop after more intense exposures over several years or months. Silica is also a cause of lung cancer.

Factors that influence the likelihood of progression to silicosis include duration and intensity of exposure, the form of silicon (exposure to crystalline form poses greater risk than bound form), surface characteristics (exposure to uncoated form poses greater risk than coated form), and rapidity of inhalation after the dust is fractured and becomes airborne (exposure immediately after fracturing poses greater risk than delayed exposure). The current limit for free silica in the industrial atmosphere is 100 $\mu g/m^3$, an 8-h time-weighted average based on the percentage of silica in the dust.

Pathophysiology

Alveolar macrophages engulf inhaled free silica particles and enter lymphatics and interstitial tissue. The macrophages cause release of cytokines (tumor necrosis factor-α, IL-1), growth factors (tumor growth factor-β), and oxidants, stimulating parenchymal inflammation, collagen synthesis, and, ultimately, fibrosis.

When the macrophages die, they release the silica into interstitial tissue around the small bronchioles, causing formation of the pathognomonic silicotic nodule. These nodules initially contain macrophages, lymphocytes, mast cells, fibroblasts with disorganized patches of collagen, and scattered birefringent particles that are best seen by polarized light microscopy. As they mature, the nodule centers become a dense ball of fibrotic scar with a classic onion-skin appearance, surrounded by an outer layer of inflammatory cells. In low-intensity or short-term exposures, these nodules remain discrete and cause no compromise of lung function (simple chronic silicosis). But, with higher-intensity or more prolonged exposures (complicated chronic silicosis), these nodules coalesce and cause progressive fibrosis and reduction of lung volumes (TLC, VC) on pulmonary function tests, or they coalesce, sometimes forming large conglomerate masses (also called progressive massive fibrosis).

In acute silicosis, which is caused by intense silica dust exposure over short periods, alveolar spaces fill with a PAS-positive staining proteinaceous material similar to that found in pulmonary alveolar proteinosis (silicoproteinosis—see p. 460). Mononuclear cells infiltrate alveolar septa. The occupational history of acute exposure is needed to distinguish silicoproteinosis from the idiopathic variety.

Symptoms, Signs, and Complications

Chronic silicosis patients are often asymptomatic but many eventually develop dyspnea on exertion that progresses to dyspnea at rest. Productive cough, when present, may be due to silicosis, coexisting chronic occupational (industrial) bronchitis, or smoking. Breath sounds diminish as the disease advances, and pulmonary consolidation, pulmonary hypertension, and respiratory failure with or without right ventricular failure may develop in advanced disease.

Accelerated silicosis patients experience the same symptoms as those with chronic silicosis but over a shorter period. Similar pathologic lesions and radiographic abnormalities often develop over months to years.

Acute silicosis patients experience rapid progression of dyspnea, weight loss, and fatigue, with diffuse bilateral crackles. Respiratory failure often develops within 2 yr.

Conglomerate (complicated) silicosis, the advanced form of chronic or accelerated disease characterized by widespread masses of fibrosis, typically occurs in the upper lung zones. It causes severe, chronic respiratory symptoms.

All patients with silicosis are at increased risk of pulmonary TB or nontubercular mycobacterial disease, possibly from impaired macrophage function and an increased risk of activation of latent infection. Other complications include spontaneous pneumothorax, broncholithiasis, and tracheobronchial obstruction. Emphysema is a common finding in areas immediately peripheral to conglomerate nodules and in areas of progressive massive fibrosis. Silica exposure and silicosis are risk factors for lung cancer.

Diagnosis

Diagnosis is based on x-ray findings in conjunction with exposure history. Biopsy plays a confirmatory role when x-ray findings are unclear. Adjunctive tests are performed to distinguish silicosis from other diseases.

Chronic silicosis is recognized by multiple 1- to 3-mm rounded opacities or nodules on chest x-ray or CT, usually in upper lung fields. CT is more sensitive than x-ray, especially when spiral and high-resolution algorithms are used. Severity is graded on a standardized scale developed by the International Labor Organization, in which specially trained readers examine the chest x-ray for size and shape of opacities; concentration of opacities (profusion); and pleural changes. An equivalent scale does not exist for CT appearance. Calcified hilar and mediastinal lymph nodes are common and occasionally take on an eggshell appearance. Pleural thickening is uncommon unless a severe parenchymal disease abuts the pleura. Rarely, calcified pleural thickening is seen in patients with little parenchymal involvement. Bullae commonly form around the conglomerate masses. Tracheal deviation may occur when the masses become large and cause volume loss. True cavities may indicate TB. Numerous diseases resemble chronic silicosis on x-ray, including welders' siderosis, hemosiderosis, sarcoidosis, chronic beryllium disease, hypersensitivity pneumonitis, coal workers' pneumoconiosis, miliary TB, fungal pulmonary diseases, and metastatic malignancy. Eggshell calcifications in hilar and mediastinal lymph nodes may help distinguish silicosis from other pulmonary diseases but are not a pathognomonic finding and are not commonly present.

Accelerated silicosis looks like chronic silicosis on x-ray but develops more rapidly.

Acute silicosis is recognized by rapid progression of symptoms and by diffuse alveolar bibasilar opacities on x-ray because of the filling of the alveoli with fluid. On CT, areas of ground-glass density consisting of reticular infiltration and areas of patchy increased attenuation and inhomogeneity occur. The multiple rounded opacities of chronic and accelerated silicosis are not characteristic of acute silicosis.

Conglomerate silicosis is recognizable by confluent opacities > 10 mm in diameter against a background of chronic silicosis.

Adjunctive tests: Chest CT may be used to distinguish asbestosis from silicosis, although this differentiation can usually be made on the basis of chest x-ray and exposure history. CT is better at detecting the transition from simple to conglomerate silicosis.

Tuberculin skin testing, sputum culture and cytology, CT scan, PET scan, and bronchoscopy all may assist in distinguishing silicosis from disseminated TB or malignancy.

Pulmonary function tests (PFTs) and measures of gas exchange (diffusing capacity for carbon monoxide [DL_{CO}], ABG) are not diagnostic but help monitor disease. Early chronic silicosis may manifest with reduced lung volumes that are at the lower end of the predicted range and with normal functional residual capacity and residual volume. PFTs in conglomerate silicosis reveal decreased lung volumes, DL_{CO}, and airway obstruction. ABGs show hypoxemia usually without CO_2 retention. Measurements of gas exchange during exercise, using pulse oximetry or preferably indwelling arterial catheter, is one of the most sensitive measures of pulmonary impairment.

Antinuclear antibodies and elevated rheumatoid factor are detectable in some patients and are suggestive but not diagnostic of coexisting connective tissue disease. There is an excess risk of progressive systemic sclerosis (scleroderma) in patients with silicosis, and some patients with silicosis develop RA associated with 3- to 5-mm pulmonary rheumatoid nodules on chest x-ray or CT.

Treatment

Whole lung lavage may be useful in some cases of acute silicosis. Whole lung lavage can reduce the total mineral dust load in the lungs of patients with chronic silicosis. Case series have shown short-term reduction in symptoms after lavage, but controlled trials have not been performed. Anecdotal evidence supports the use of oral corticosteroids in acute and accelerated silicosis. Lung transplantation is a last-resort therapy.

Patients with obstruction may be treated empirically with bronchodilators and inhaled corticosteroids. Patients should be monitored and treated for hypoxemia to forestall pulmonary hypertension. Pulmonary rehabilitation may help patients perform activities of daily living. Workers who develop silicosis should be removed from further exposure. Other preventive measures include smoking cessation and pneumococcal and influenza vaccination.

Prevention

The most effective preventive interventions occur at an industrial rather than clinical level and include dust suppression, process isolation, ventilation, and use of non–silica–containing abrasives. Respiratory masks provide imperfect protection and, although helpful, are not an adequate solution. Surveillance of exposed workers with respiratory questionnaires, spirometry, and chest x-rays is recommended. Frequency of surveillance depends to some degree on the expected intensity of the exposure. Physicians must be alert to the risk of TB and nontuberculous mycobacterial infections in silica-exposed patients, especially miners. People exposed to silica but without silicosis have 3 times the risk of developing TB compared with the nonexposed general population. Miners with silicosis have a > 20-fold risk of TB and non-TB mycobacterial infection compared with the general population and are more likely to develop both pulmonary and extrapulmonary manifestations. Patients exposed to silica with a positive tuberculin test and negative sputum TB cultures should be given isoniazid chemoprophylaxis in keeping with guidelines for other tuberculin reactors. Recommendations for treatment are the same as for other patients with TB. Relapse is more common in patients with silicotuberculosis, sometimes necessitating longer courses than are usually recommended.

TOXIC INHALATION INJURY

The effect of inhaling toxic gases depends on the extent and duration of exposure and on the specific irritant. Toxic exposures predominantly affect the airways, causing tracheitis, bronchitis, and bronchiolitis.

Acute Exposure

Acute exposure to high concentrations of toxic gas over a short time is characteristic of industrial accidents resulting from a faulty valve or pump in a gas tank or during gas transport. Many people may be exposed and affected. Chlorine, phosgene, sulfur dioxide, hydrogen chloride or sulfide, nitrogen dioxide, ozone, and ammonia are among the most important irritant gases.

Respiratory damage is related to the size of inhaled particles and the solubility of the gas. More water-soluble gases (eg, chlorine, ammonia, sulfur dioxide, hydrogen chloride) immediately cause mucous membrane irritation, which may alert the victims to the need to escape the exposure. Permanent damage to the upper respiratory tract, distal airways, and lung parenchyma occurs only if the victim's escape from the gas source is impeded. Less soluble gases (eg, nitrogen dioxide, phosgene, ozone) do not produce early warning signs and are more likely to cause severe bronchiolitis, with or without pulmonary edema. In nitrogen dioxide intoxication (as occurs in silo fillers and welders), a lag of up to 12 h may occur before symptoms of pulmonary edema develop.

Symptoms, Signs, and Diagnosis

Soluble irritant gases cause severe burning and other manifestations of irritation of the eyes, nose, throat, trachea, and major bronchi. Marked cough, hemoptysis, wheezing, retching, and dyspnea are common. Severity is generally dose-related. Nonsoluble gases cause fewer immediate symptoms but can present with dyspnea or cough.

Diagnosis is usually obvious from the history; management does not differ by specific inhaled agent but rather by symptoms. The upper airway may be obstructed by edema, secretions, and/or laryngospasm. Chest x-ray findings of patchy or confluent alveolar consolidation usually indicates pulmonary edema. Evidence of any of these indicates a need for prophylactic endotracheal intubation.

Prognosis

Most people recover fully. Bacterial infections, which are common, are the most serious complication. A few develop acute respiratory distress syndrome (ARDS), usually within 24 h. Bronchiolitis obliterans progressing to respiratory failure can develop 10 to 14 days after acute exposure to ammonia, nitrogen oxides, sulfur dioxide, and mercury. This pattern of injury is associated with airflow obstruction mixed with restriction and is seen on CT as a pattern of bronchiolar thickening and a patchy mosaic of hyperinflation. Bronchiolitis obliterans with organized pneumonia can ensue when granulation tissue accumulates in the terminal airways and alveolar ducts during the body's reparative process. ARDS without or with late pulmonary fibrosis may develop in a minority of cases.

Occasionally, heavy exposures lead to reversible airway obstruction (reactive airways dysfunction syndrome) persistent for ≥ 1 yr, resolving slowly in some cases. Smokers may be more susceptible to persistent toxin-related lung injury. Injuries to the lower airways can obstruct airflow long-term, especially after exposures to ammonia, ozone, chlorine, and gas mixtures.

Treatment

Immediate management includes removal from exposure, observation, and supportive care. If possible, the victim should be moved into fresh air and given supplemental O_2. Treatment is directed toward maintaining sufficient gas exchange by ensuring adequate oxygenation and alveolar ventilation. Severe airflow obstruction is managed with inhaled racemic epinephrine, endotracheal intubation or tracheostomy, and mechanical ventilation, if necessary. Bronchodilators and O_2 therapy may suffice in less severe cases. The efficacy of corticosteroid therapy (eg, prednisone 45 to 60 mg once/day for 1 to 2 wk) is difficult to prove but is frequently used empirically.

After the acute phase has been managed, physicians must remain alert to the development of reactive airways dysfunction syndrome, bronchiolitis obliterans with or without organized pneumonia, pulmonary fibrosis, and delayed-onset ARDS. Because of the risk of ARDS, any patient with acute upper airway injury after inhalation of toxic aerosols or gases should be observed for 24 h.

Prevention

Care in handling gases and chemicals is the most important preventive measure. The availability of adequate respiratory protection (eg, gas masks with self-contained air supply) is also very important if accidental exposure occurs; rescuers without protective gear who rush in to extricate a victim often succumb themselves or develop acute and chronic airways disease.

Chronic Exposure

Low-level continuous or intermittent exposure to irritant gases or chemical vapors may lead to chronic bronchitis, although the role of such exposure is especially difficult to substantiate in smokers.

Chronic inhalational exposure to some agents (eg, bis[chloromethyl]ether or certain metals) causes lung and other cancers (eg, liver angiosarcomas after vinyl chloride monomer exposure, mesothelioma with asbestos).

58 PULMONARY HYPERTENSION

Pulmonary hypertension is increased pressure in the pulmonary circulation. It has many secondary causes; when the cause is unknown it is called primary pulmonary hypertension (PPH). In PPH, pulmonary vessels become constricted, hypertrophied, and fibrosed. Pulmonary hypertension leads to right ventricular overload and failure. Symptoms are fatigue, exertional dyspnea, and, occasionally, chest discomfort and syncope. Diagnosis is by measuring pulmonary artery pressure. Treatment is with vasodilators and, in selected advanced cases, lung transplantation. Prognosis is poor overall if a treatable secondary cause is not found.

Epidemiology, Etiology, and Pathophysiology

Pulmonary hypertension is defined as a mean pulmonary arterial pressure ≥ 25 mm Hg at rest or ≥ 35 mm Hg during exercise. Many conditions and drugs cause pulmonary hypertension (see TABLE 58–1). PPH is pulmonary hypertension in the absence of such causes. However, the end result can be similar. PPH is rare, affecting 1 or 2 per million people.

PPH affects women about twice as often as men. The mean age at diagnosis is 35 yr. The disease can be familial or sporadic; sporadic cases are about 10 times more common. Most familial cases have mutations in the gene for the bone morphogenetic protein receptor type 2 (*BMPR2*), part of the transforming growth factor (TGF)-β family of receptors. About 20% of sporadic cases also have *BMPR2* mutations. Many people with PPH

TABLE 58–1. CAUSES OF SECONDARY PULMONARY HYPERTENSION

- Pulmonary
  - Chronic high altitude exposure
  - Chronic thromboembolic disease
  - Congenital pulmonary arteriovenous shunts
  - COPD
  - Hypoventilation syndromes
  - Interstitial lung disease/pulmonary fibrosis
  - Obstructive sleep apnea
  - Pulmonary capillary hemangiomatosis (rare)
- Cardiac
  - Congenital heart disease
  - High-output heart failure
  - Left ventricular diastolic dysfunction (multiple causes)
  - Left-to-right shunt with Eisenmenger's complex
  - Patent ductus arteriosus
- Connective tissue diseases
  - Mixed connective tissue disease
  - RA
  - Scleroderma and CREST (calcinosis cutis, Raynaud's phenomenon, esophageal dysmotility, sclerodactyly, telangiectasias) syndrome
  - SLE
  - Vasculitis
- Portal hypertension/liver failure
- Infectious disease
  - HIV
  - Parasitic disease (schistosomiasis, filariasis, helminthiasis)
- Drugs and toxins
  - Amphetamines
  - Anorexigens (fenfluramine, dexfenfluramine)
  - Cocaine
  - L-tryptophan (contaminated)
  - Toxic rapeseed oil ingestion
- Hematologic
  - Polycythemia vera
  - Sickle cell anemia
- Persistent pulmonary hypertension of the newborn

have increased levels of angiopoietin-1; angiopoietin-1 appears to down-regulate *BMPR1A*, a sister receptor to *BMPR2*, and may stimulate serotonin production and endothelial smooth muscle proliferation. Other possible contributing factors include abnormalities in serotonin transport and previous infection with human herpesvirus 8.

PPH is characterized by variable vasoconstriction, smooth muscle hypertrophy, and vascular wall remodeling. Vasoconstriction is thought to be due in part to enhanced activity of thromboxane and endothelin-1 (both vasoconstrictors) and reduced activity of prostacyclin and nitric oxide (both vasodilators). The increased pulmonary vascular pressure that results from vascular obstruction further injures the endothelium. Injury activates coagulation at the intimal surface, which may worsen the hypertension. Thrombotic coagulopathy from increased plasminogen activator inhibitor type 1 and fibrinopeptide A and decreased tissue plasminogen activator activity may also contribute. Focal coagulation at the endothelial surface should not be confused with chronic thromboembolic pulmonary hypertension, which is pulmonary hypertension caused by organized pulmonary emboli.

In most patients, PPH eventually leads to right ventricular hypertrophy followed by dilatation and right ventricular failure.

Symptoms and Signs

Progressive exertional dyspnea and easy fatigability occur in almost all cases. Atypical chest discomfort and exertional lightheadedness or presyncope may accompany dyspnea. These symptoms are due primarily to insufficient cardiac output. Raynaud's phenomenon occurs in about 10% of PPH patients. Of this 10%, 99% are women. Hemoptysis is rare but may be fatal; hoarseness due to recurrent laryngeal nerve compression by an enlarged pulmonary artery (Ortner's syndrome) also occurs rarely.

In advanced disease, signs may include right ventricular heave, widely split second heart sound (S_2), accentuated pulmonic component of S_2 (P_2), pulmonary ejection click, right ventricular third heart sound (S_3), and jugular vein distention. Liver congestion and peripheral edema are common late manifestations.

Diagnosis

The diagnosis of PPH is suspected in patients with significant exertional dyspnea who are otherwise relatively healthy and have no history or signs of other diseases known to cause pulmonary hypertension (see TABLE 58–1).

Patients initially undergo chest x-ray, spirometry, and ECG to identify more common causes of dyspnea, followed by Doppler echocardiography to assess right ventricular and pulmonary artery pressures as well as to detect structural heart disease causing secondary pulmonary hypertension.

The most common x-ray result in PPH is enlarged hilar vessels that rapidly prune into the periphery. Spirometry and lung volumes may be normal or show mild restriction, but diffusing capacity for carbon monoxide (DL_{CO}) is usually reduced. Common ECG findings include right axis deviation, R > S in V_1, $S_1Q_3T_3$, and peaked P waves.

Additional tests are obtained as indicated to diagnose secondary causes not apparent clinically. These include ventilation-perfusion scanning to detect thromboembolic disease; pulmonary function tests to identify obstructive or restrictive lung disease; and serum serologic tests to gather evidence for or against rheumatologic disease. Chronic thromboembolic pulmonary hypertension is suggested by CT or lung scan and is diagnosed by arteriography. Other tests, such as HIV testing, liver function tests, and polysomnography, are performed in the appropriate clinical context.

When initial evaluation reveals no conditions associated with secondary pulmonary hypertension, pulmonary artery catheterization is necessary to measure right atrial and ventricular, pulmonary artery, and pulmonary capillary wedge pressures and cardiac output. Right-sided O_2 saturation should be measured to exclude atrial septal defect. Mean pulmonary arterial pressure > 25 mm Hg in the absence of an underlying cause defines PPH. However, most patients with PPH present with significantly higher pressure (eg, 60 mm Hg). Vasodilating drugs (eg, inhaled nitric oxide, IV epoprostenol, adenosine) are often administered during the procedure; decrease in right-sided pressures in response to these drugs helps in the selection of drugs for treatment. Biopsy, once widely performed, is neither needed nor recommended because of high morbidity and mortality.

Once PPH is diagnosed, the patient's family history is reviewed to detect possible genetic transmission, which is suggested by premature deaths in otherwise healthy members of the extended family. In familial PPH, genetic counseling is needed to advise family members of the risk of disease (about 20%) and to advocate serial screening with echocardiograms. Testing for mutations in the *BMPR2* gene in familial PPH may play a future role.

Prognosis

Untreated patients have a median survival of 2.5 yr. Cause of death is usually sudden death in the context of right ventricular failure. Five-year survival for epoprostenol-treated patients is 54%, whereas that for the minority of patients who respond to Ca channel blockers is > 90%. Signs predictive of poor survival include low cardiac output, higher pulmonary artery and right atrial pressures, lack of response to vasodilators, heart failure, hypoxemia, and reduced overall physical functioning.

Treatment

Secondary pulmonary hypertension: Treatment of secondary pulmonary hypertension involves management of the underlying disorder. Patients with severe pulmonary hypertension secondary to chronic thromboembolic disease should undergo pulmonary thromboendarterectomy. Under cardiopulmonary bypass, organized endothelialized thrombus is dissected along the pulmonary trunk in a procedure more complex than acute surgical embolectomy. This procedure cures pulmonary hypertension in a substantial percentage of patients and restores cardiopulmonary function; operative mortality is < 10% in experienced centers.

Primary pulmonary hypertension: Treatment of PPH is rapidly evolving. Oral Ca channel blockers sustain reduction in pulmonary artery pressure or pulmonary vascular resistance in about 10 to 15% of patients and are the first drugs used. No differences in efficacy exist by Ca channel blocker type, though most specialists avoid verapamil because of its negative inotropic effects. Response to Ca channel blockers is a favorable prognostic sign, and patients who respond should continue this treatment. Those who do not respond are given other drugs.

IV epoprostenol, a prostacyclin analog, improves function and lengthens survival even in patients who are unresponsive to a vasodilator during catheterization. Disadvantages are the need for continuous central catheter infusion and significant adverse effects, including flushing, diarrhea, and bacteremia due to the indwelling central catheter. Inhaled (iloprost), oral (beraprost), and subcutaneous (treprostinil) prostacyclin analogs are under study as alternatives.

Bosentan, an oral endothelin-receptor antagonist, is also useful in some patients, generally those with milder disease who are not vasodilator-responsive. Oral sildenafil and L-arginine are also under study.

Lung transplantation offers the only hope of cure but has high morbidity due to the problems of rejection and infection and a 60% 5-yr survival rate related to bronchiolitis obliterans. Lung transplantation is reserved for patients with New York Heart Association class IV disease (defined as dyspnea associated with minimal activity, leading to bed to chair limitations) who have not been helped by prostacyclin analogs.

Many patients require adjunctive therapies to treat heart failure, including diuretics, and should receive warfarin to prevent thromboembolism.

PORTOPULMONARY HYPERTENSION

Portopulmonary hypertension is severe pulmonary hypertension with portal hypertension in patients without other secondary causes.

Pulmonary hypertension occurs in patients with a variety of conditions leading to portal hypertension with or without cirrhosis. Portopulmonary hypertension occurs less commonly than the hepatopulmonary syndrome in patients with chronic liver disease (3.5 to 12%).

Presenting symptoms are dyspnea and fatigue. Chest pain and hemoptysis can also occur. Patients have physical findings and ECG abnormalities consistent with pulmonary hypertension and may develop evidence of cor pulmonale (elevated jugular venous pulse, edema). Tricuspid regurgitation is common. The diagnosis is suspected by echocardiography and confirmed by right heart catheterization. Treatment is that of primary pulmonary hypertension except for avoidance of hepatotoxic drugs. Some patients have benefitted from vasodilator therapy. The underlying liver disease is a major determinant of outcome. Portopulmonary hypertension is a relative contraindication to liver transplantation because of increased morbidity and mortality. Some patients with mild pulmonary hypertension regress after transplantation.

HEPATOPULMONARY SYNDROME

Hepatopulmonary syndrome is hypoxemia caused by vasodilation in patients with portal hypertension; dyspnea and hypoxemia are worse in the upright position.

The hepatopulmonary syndrome results from the formation of microscopic intrapulmonary arteriovenous dilatations in patients with chronic liver disease. The mechanism is unknown but is thought to be due to increased hepatic production or decreased hepatic clearance of vasodilators, possibly involving nitric oxide. The vascular dilatations cause overperfusion relative to ventilation, leading to hypoxemia. Because the lesions frequently are more numerous at the lung bases, the hepatopulmonary syndrome causes platypnea (dyspnea) and orthodeoxia (hypoxemia) in the seated or upright position that subside with recumbency. Most patients also have stigmata of chronic liver disease, such as spider angiomas. About 20% of patients, however, present with pulmonary symptoms alone.

The hepatopulmonary syndrome is suspected in any patient with known liver disease who reports dyspnea (particularly platypnea). Patients with clinically significant symptoms should undergo pulse oximetry. If the syndrome is advanced, ABGs should be measured on air and on 100% O_2 to determine shunt fraction.

A useful diagnostic test is contrast echocardiography. IV microbubbles from agitated saline that are normally obstructed by pulmonary capillaries rapidly transit the lung and appear in the left atrium within 7 beats. Similarly, IV technetium-99m–labeled albumin may transit the lungs and appear in the kidney and brain. Pulmonary angiography may reveal diffusely fine or blotchy vascular configuration. Angiography is generally not needed unless thromboembolism is suspected.

The main treatment is supplemental O_2 for symptoms. Other therapies, such as somatostatin to inhibit vasodilation, are of modest benefit in only some patients. Coil embolization is virtually impossible because of the number and size of the lesions. Inhaled nitric oxide synthesis inhibitors may be a future treatment option. Hepatopulmonary syndrome may regress after liver transplantation or if the underlying liver disease subsides. Prognosis is poor without treatment (survival < 2 yr).

59 DIFFUSE ALVEOLAR HEMORRHAGE AND PULMONARY-RENAL SYNDROMES

DIFFUSE ALVEOLAR HEMORRHAGE SYNDROME

Diffuse alveolar hemorrhage syndrome is persistent or recurrent pulmonary hemorrhage.

Diffuse alveolar hemorrhage syndrome is an independent diagnostic entity because it suggests a differential diagnosis and a specific sequence of tests and treatments. The differential diagnosis is broad and includes autoimmune diseases, including systemic vasculitides and Goodpasture's syndrome; antiphospholipid antibody syndrome; pulmonary infections; toxic exposures; drug reactions; bone marrow and solid organ transplantation; cardiac disorders such as mitral stenosis; coagulation disorders caused by diseases or anticoagulant drugs; isolated pauci-immune pulmonary capillaritis; and idiopathic pulmonary hemosiderosis.

Isolated pauci-immune pulmonary capillaritis is a small-vessel vasculitis limited to the lung; its only manifestation is alveolar hemorrhage affecting people aged 18 to 35 yr.

Idiopathic pulmonary hemosiderosis is diffuse alveolar hemorrhage syndrome with no detectable underlying disease. It occurs mainly in children < 10 yr and is thought to be due to a defect in the alveolar capillary endothelium, possibly from autoimmune injury.

Some of these diseases can also cause glomerulonephritis, in which case the patient is said to have pulmonary-renal syndrome (see p. 486).

Symptoms, Signs, and Diagnosis

Symptoms and signs of milder diffuse alveolar hemorrhage syndrome are dyspnea, cough, and fever; however, many patients present with acute respiratory failure. Hemoptysis is common but may be absent in up to ⅓ of patients. Children with idiopathic pulmonary hemosiderosis may have failure to thrive. There are no specific physical examination findings.

Diagnosis is often suggested by chest x-ray findings of diffuse bilateral alveolar infiltrates. Urinalysis is indicated to exclude glomerulonephritis and pulmonary-renal syndrome. Others tests include CBC, coagulation studies, platelet counts, and serologic tests (antinuclear antibody, anti-dsDNA, anti-glomerular basement membrane [anti-GBM] antibodies, antineutrophil cytoplasmic antibodies [ANCA], antiphospholipid antibody) to look for underlying causes; p-ANCA titers are elevated in some cases of isolated pauci-immune pulmonary capillaritis. Diagnosis of idiopathic pulmonary hemosiderosis involves demonstration of iron-deficiency anemia and hemosiderin-laden macrophages on bronchoalveolar lavage or lung biopsy in the absence of evidence of small-vessel vasculitis (pulmonary capillaritis) or of other diagnoses.

Other tests depend on clinical context. Pulmonary function tests may be performed to document lung function; increased diffusing capacity for carbon monoxide (DL_{CO}) due to increased uptake of carbon monoxide by intra-alveolar Hb is consistent with hemorrhage. Echocardiography may be indicated to exclude mitral stenosis. Bronchoalveolar lavage typically returns lavage fluid that remains hemorrhagic even after sequential sampling. Lung biopsy is frequently needed when an underlying cause remains unclear.

Prognosis and Treatment

Recurrent diffuse alveolar hemorrhage syndrome causes pulmonary hemosiderosis and fibrosis, both of which develop when ferritin aggregates within alveoli and exerts toxic effects. COPD occurs in some patients with recurrent diffuse alveolar hemorrhage secondary to microscopic polyarteritis.

Treatment involves correcting the cause. Corticosteroids and possibly cyclophosphamide are used to treat vasculitides, connective tissue diseases, and Goodpasture's syndrome. Corticosteroids are also used to treat idiopathic pulmonary hemosiderosis; immunosuppressants are added for nonresponders.

TABLE 59–1. DIFFERENTIAL DIAGNOSIS OF PULMONARY-RENAL SYNDROME

Connective tissue disease
- Polymyositis or dermatomyositis
- Progressive systemic sclerosis
- RA
- SLE

Goodpasture's syndrome

Renal disease
- Idiopathic immune complex glomerulonephritis
- IgA nephropathy
- Rapidly progressive glomerulonephritis with heart failure

Systemic vasculitis
- Behçet's syndrome
- Churg-Strauss syndrome
- Cryoglobulinemia
- Henoch-Schönlein purpura
- Microscopic polyarteritis
- Wegener's granulomatosis

Other
- Drugs (penicillamine)
- Heart failure

PULMONARY-RENAL SYNDROME

Pulmonary-renal syndrome (PRS) is diffuse alveolar hemorrhage and glomerulonephritis occurring simultaneously. PRS is always a manifestation of underlying autoimmune disease but is gaining recognition as a diagnostic entity because it suggests a differential diagnosis and a specific sequence of tests and treatments. Goodpasture's syndrome is the prototype cause, but PRS can also be caused by SLE, Wegener's granulomatosis, microscopic polyangiitis, and, less commonly, by other vasculitides and connective tissue disease (see TABLE 59–1). The number of cases of PRS caused by these latter diseases is probably greater than those caused by Goodpasture's syndrome, but patients with those diseases more commonly present in other ways; only a few present with PRS.

PRS is less commonly a manifestation of IgA-mediated disease, such as IgA nephropathy and Henoch-Schönlein purpura, and of immune complex–mediated renal disease, such as essential mixed cryoglobulinemia. Rarely, rapidly progressive glomerulonephritis alone can cause PRS through a mechanism of renal failure, volume overload, and pulmonary edema with hemoptysis.

PRS is suspected in patients with hemoptysis not obviously attributable to other causes (such as pneumonia, carcinoma, or bronchiectasis), particularly when hemoptysis is accompanied by diffuse parenchymal infiltrates. Initial testing includes urinalysis for evidence of hematuria, serum creatinine for renal function assessment, and CBC for evidence of anemia. Pulmonary function tests are not diagnostic, but the finding of an increased diffusing capacity for carbon monoxide (DL_{CO}) suggests pulmonary hemorrhage and is due to the increased uptake of carbon monoxide by intra-alveolar Hb.

Serum antibody testing may help distinguish some causes. Antiglomerular basement membrane (anti-GBM) antibodies are pathognomonic for Goodpasture's syndrome, although they also occur in patients with Alport's syndrome after kidney transplantation. Antibodies to double-stranded DNA and reduced serum complements are typical of SLE. Antineutrophil cytoplasmic antibodies (ANCA) directed against proteinase-3 (PR3-ANCA or cytoplasmic ANCA [c-ANCA]) are present in Wegener's granulomatosis. Antineutrophil cytoplasmic antibodies directed against myeloperoxidase (MPO-ANCA, or perinuclear ANCA [p-ANCA]) suggest microscopic polyangiitis.

GOODPASTURE'S SYNDROME

(Anti-GBM Antibody Disease)

Goodpasture's syndrome is an autoimmune syndrome of alveolar hemorrhage and glomerulonephritis caused by circulating anti-GBM antibodies. Goodpasture's syndrome most often develops in genetically susceptible people who smoke cigarettes, but hydrocarbon exposure and viral respiratory infections are additional possible triggers. Symptoms are dyspnea, cough, fatigue, hemoptysis, and/or hematuria. Goodpasture's syndrome is suspected in patients with hemoptysis or hematuria and is confirmed by the presence of anti-GBM antibodies in the blood. Treatment includes plasmapheresis, corticosteroids, and immunosuppressants, such as cyclophosphamide. Prognosis is good when treatment is begun before onset of respiratory or renal failure.

Goodpasture's syndrome is the combination of glomerulonephritis with alveolar hemorrhage in the presence of anti-GBM antibodies. Goodpasture's syndrome most often manifests as diffuse alveolar hemorrhage and glomerulonephritis together but can occasionally cause glomerulonephritis (10 to 20%) or pulmonary disease (10%) alone. Men are affected more often than women.

Anti-GBM antibodies are directed against the noncollagenous (NC-1) domain of the α3 chain of type IV collagen, which is found in highest concentration in the basement membranes of renal and pulmonary capillaries. Environmental exposures—cigarette smoking, viral URI, and hydrocarbon solvent inhalation most commonly and pneumonia less commonly—expose alveolar capillary antigens to circulating antibody in genetically susceptible people, most notably those with HLA-DRw15, -DR4, and -DRB1 alleles. Circulating anti-GBM antibodies bind to basement membranes, fix complement, and trigger a cell-mediated inflammatory response, causing glomerulonephritis and/or pulmonary capillaritis.

Symptoms and Signs

Hemoptysis is the most prominent symptom; however, hemoptysis may be absent in the presence of hemorrhage, and the patient may present with only chest x-ray infiltrates or infiltrates and respiratory distress and/or failure. Dyspnea, cough, fatigue, fever, and weight loss are common. Up to 40% of patients have gross hematuria, although pulmonary hemorrhage may precede renal manifestations by weeks to years.

Signs vary over time and range from clear lungs on auscultation to crackles and rhonchi. Some patients have peripheral edema and pallor from anemia.

Diagnosis

If initial testing supports the diagnosis of PRS, additional tests are required. Diagnosis of Goodpasture's syndrome requires demonstration of serum anti-GBM antibodies by indirect immunofluorescence testing or, when available, direct enzyme-linked immunosorbent assay (ELISA) testing with recombinant or human NC-1 α3. Other serologic tests are obtained, such as an antinuclear antibody (ANA) to detect SLE and antistreptolysin-O titer to detect poststreptococcal glomerulonephritis, which may be associated with many of the causes of PRS. ANCA testing is positive (in peripheral pattern) in 25% of Goodpasture's cases. In the presence of glomerulonephritis (hematuria, proteinuria, red cell casts on urinalysis, and/or renal insufficiency), renal biopsy may be indicated. A rapidly progressive focal segmental necrotizing glomerulonephritis with crescent formation is found on biopsy in Goodpasture's syndrome and all other causes of PRS. Immunofluorescence staining of renal or lung tissue classically demonstrates linear IgG deposition along the glomerular or alveolar capillaries. This also occurs in the diabetic kidney and in fibrillary glomerulonephritis, a rare disorder causing PRS, but GBM binding of antibodies in these disorders is nonspecific.

Pulmonary function tests and bronchoalveolar lavage are not diagnostic of Goodpasture's syndrome but can be used to help confirm diffuse alveolar hemorrhage in patients with glomerulonephritis and pulmonary infiltrates but without hemoptysis. Lavage fluid that remains hemorrhagic after sequential sampling establishes diffuse alveolar hemorrhage, especially in the context of falling Hct.

Prognosis and Treatment

Goodpasture's syndrome is often rapidly progressive and can be fatal if prompt recognition and treatment are delayed; prognosis is good when treatment is begun before onset of respiratory or renal failure.

Immediate survival in the face of pulmonary hemorrhage and respiratory failure is linked to airway control; endotracheal intubation and mechanical ventilation are recommended for patients with borderline ABGs and impending respiratory failure.

Treatment is daily or every-other-day plasmapheresis for 2 to 3 wk using 4-L exchanges to remove anti-GBM antibodies, combined with an IV corticosteroid (usually methylprednisolone 1 g over 20 min every other day for 3 doses followed by 1 mg/kg prednisone once/day) and cyclophosphamide (2 mg/kg once/day) for 6 to 12 mo to prevent formation of new antibodies. Therapy can be tapered when pulmonary and renal function stop improving. Long-term morbidity is related to the degree of renal impairment at presentation; patients requiring dialysis at presentation and those with >50% crescents on biopsy have <2-yr survival and often require dialysis unless kidney transplantation is performed. Hemoptysis may be a good prognostic sign because it leads to earlier detection of disease; the minority of patients who are ANCA-positive respond better to treatment. Relapse occurs in a small number and is linked to continued tobacco use and respiratory infection. In patients with end-stage renal disease who receive kidney transplantation, disease can recur in the graft.

60 MEDIASTINAL AND PLEURAL DISORDERS

Mediastinal and pleural disorders include masses, mediastinitis, pleural effusion, pleural fibrosis and calcification, pneumomediastinum, pneumothorax, and viral pleuritis.

MEDIASTINAL MASSES

Mediastinal masses are caused by a variety of cysts and tumors; likely causes differ by patient age and by whether the mass occurs in the anterior, middle, or posterior mediastinum. The masses may be asymptomatic (in adults) or cause obstructive respiratory symptoms (in children). Testing involves CT scan with biopsy and adjunctive tests as needed. Treatment differs by cause.

Classification and Etiology

Mediastinal masses are divided into those that occur in the anterior, middle, and posterior mediastinum. Each compartment has characteristic lesions (see FIG. 60–1). The anterior mediastinum extends from the sternum to the pericardium and brachiocephalic vessels posteriorly. The middle mediastinum lies between the anterior and posterior mediastinum. The posterior mediastinum is bounded by the pericardium and trachea anteriorly and the vertebral column posteriorly.

The most common mediastinal masses in children are neurogenic tumors and cysts. In adults, neurogenic tumors and thymoma are the most common anterior lesions; lymphomas (both Hodgkin and non-Hodgkin) occur most frequently between ages 20 and 40 in the anterior mediastinum.

Symptoms and Signs

Symptoms and signs of mediastinal masses depend on location. Many are asymptomatic. In general, malignant lesions are much more likely to produce symptoms than are benign lesions. The most common symptoms are chest pain and weight loss. In children, mediastinal masses are more likely to cause tracheobronchial compression and stridor or symptoms of recurrent bronchitis or pneumonia. Large anterior mediastinal masses may cause dyspnea on lying supine. Lesions in the middle mediastinum may compress blood vessels or airways, producing the superior vena cava syndrome or airway obstruction. Lesions in the posterior mediastinum may encroach on the esophagus, producing dysphagia or odynophagia.

Diagnosis

Mediastinal masses are most often incidentally discovered on chest x-ray or other imaging tests during an examination for chest symptoms. Additional diagnostic testing, usually imaging and biopsy, is indicated to determine etiology.

CT scanning with IV contrast is the most valuable imaging technique. With thoracic CT, normal variants and benign tumors, such as fat- and fluid-filled cysts, can be distinguished from other processes. A definitive diagnosis can be obtained for many mediastinal masses with needle aspiration or needle biopsy. Fine-needle aspiration techniques usually suffice for carcinomatous lesions, but a cutting-needle biopsy should be performed whenever lymphoma, thymoma, or a neural mass is suspected (see TABLE 60–1). If TB is a concern, a PPD is performed. If ectopic thyroid is considered, thyroid-stimulating hormone is measured.

Treatment

Treatment depends on etiology. Some benign lesions, such as pericardial cysts, can be observed. Most malignant tumors should be removed surgically, but some, such as lymphomas, are best treated with chemotherapy. Granulomatous disease should be treated with the appropriate antimicrobial drug.

MEDIASTINITIS

Mediastinitis is acute inflammation of the mediastinum.

The two most common causes of mediastinitis are esophageal perforation and median sternotomy.

Esophageal perforation may complicate esophagoscopy or insertion of a Sengstaken-Blakemore or Minnesota tube (for esophageal

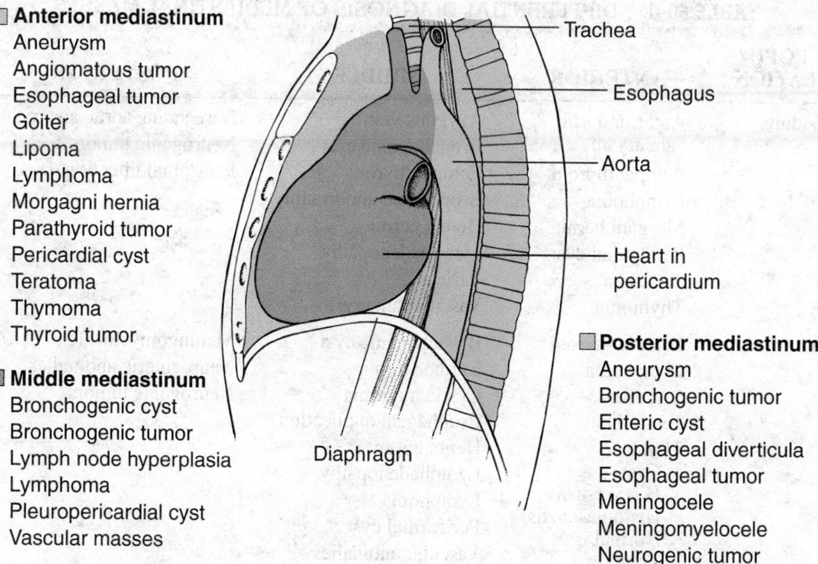

Fig. 60–1. Common diagnostic possibilities of mediastinal masses by compartment.

variceal bleeding). It may occur with vomiting (Boerhaave's syndrome). Patients with esophageal perforation are generally acutely ill, with severe chest pain and dyspnea due to mediastinal infection and inflammation. Diagnosis usually is obvious from clinical presentation but is confirmed by chest x-ray or CT showing air in the mediastinum. Treatment is with parenteral antibiotics selected to cover oral and GI flora, eg, clindamycin 450 mg IV q 6 h plus ceftriaxone 2 g once/day, for at least 2 wk. Many patients require emergency exploration of the mediastinum with primary repair of the esophageal tear and drainage of the pleural space and mediastinum.

Median sternotomy is complicated by mediastinitis in about 1% of cases. These patients most commonly present with wound drainage or sepsis. Diagnosis is based on finding infected fluid from a needle aspiration through the sternum. Treatment consists of immediate surgical drainage, debridement, and parenteral broad-spectrum antibiotics. Mortality approaches 50% in some series.

Chronic fibrosing mediastinitis usually is due to TB or histoplasmosis but can be due to sarcoidosis, silicosis, or other fungal diseases. Patients develop an intense fibrotic process that leads to compression of mediastinal structures that can lead to the superior vena cava syndrome, tracheal stenosis, or obstruction of the pulmonary arteries or veins.

Diagnosis is based on demonstration of enlarged mediastinal lymph nodes by chest x-ray or CT scan. If the cause is TB, anti-TB therapy is indicated. Otherwise, no known treatment is beneficial, but some physicians have begun inserting vascular stents in an attempt to limit compression of selected central vessels.

PLEURAL EFFUSION

Pleural effusions are accumulations of fluid within the pleural space. They have multiple causes and usually are classified as transudates or exudates. Detection is by physical examination and chest x-ray; thoracentesis and pleural fluid analysis are often required to determine cause. Asymptomatic transudates require no treatment. Symptomatic transudates and almost all exudates require

TABLE 60–1. DIFFERENTIAL DIAGNOSIS OF MEDIASTINAL MASSES

POPULATION	ANTERIOR	MIDDLE	POSTERIOR
Adults	Anterior aortic aneurysm Ectopic thyroid Lymphoma Morgani hernia Pericardial cyst Teratoma Thymoma	Azygous vein Bronchogenic cyst Ectopic thyroid Esophageal abnormality Hiatus hernia Lymphadenopathy Varices Vascular aneurysm	Descending aortic aneurysm Neurogenic tumors Paraspinal infection
Children	Ectopic thyroid Lymphoma Sarcoma Teratoma Thymus Cyst Histiocytosis Histoplasmosis Normal Thymoma	Bronchogenic cyst Cardiac tumor Cystic hygroma Esophageal duplication Hemangioma Lymphadenopathy Lymphoma Pericardial cyst Vascular anomalies	Meningomyelocele Neuroenteric anomalies Neurogenic tumors

thoracentesis, chest tube drainage, pleurodesis, and/or pleurectomy.

Normally, 10 to 20 mL of pleural fluid similar in composition to plasma but lower in protein (< 1.5 g/dL) is spread thinly over visceral and parietal pleurae, facilitating movement between the lung and chest wall. The fluid enters the pleural space from systemic capillaries in the parietal pleurae and exits via parietal pleural stomas and lymphatics. Pleural fluid accumulates when too much fluid enters or too little exits the pleural space.

Classification and Etiology

Pleural effusions have numerous causes (see TABLE 60–2) and usually are categorized as transudates or exudates based on laboratory characteristics of the fluid (see TABLE 60–3). A transudate can usually be treated without extensive evaluation, whereas the cause of an exudate requires investigation. Bilateral effusions usually share the same characteristics.

Transudative effusions are caused by some combination of increased hydrostatic pressure and decreased oncotic pressure in the pulmonary or systemic circulation. Heart failure is the most common cause, followed by cirrhosis with ascites and hypoalbuminemia, usually from the nephrotic syndrome.

Exudative effusions are caused by local processes leading to increased capillary permeability resulting in exudation of fluid, protein, cells, and other serum constituents. Causes are numerous, the most common being pneumonia, malignancy, pulmonary embolism, viral infection, and TB. Yellow nail syndrome is a rare disorder causing chronic exudative pleural effusions, lymphedema, and dystrophic yellow nails, all thought to be the result of impaired lymphatic drainage.

Chylous effusion (chylothorax) is a milky white effusion high in triglycerides caused by traumatic or neoplastic (most often lymphomatous) damage to the thoracic duct.

Chyliform (cholesterol or pseudochylous) effusions resemble chylous effusions but are low in triglycerides and high in cholesterol. Chyliform effusions are thought to be due to release of cholesterol from lysed

TABLE 60–2. CAUSES OF PLEURAL EFFUSION

TYPE	CAUSE	COMMENTS
Transudate	Heart failure	Bilateral, 81%; right-sided, 12%; left-sided, 7% Left ventricular failure increases interstitial pressure, leading to fluid transudation and pleural effusion
	Cirrhosis with ascites (hepatic hydrothorax)	Right-sided, 70%; left-sided, 15%; bilateral, 15% Ascitic fluid migrates to the pleural space through diaphragmatic defects; occurs in about 5% of patients with clinically apparent ascites
	Hypoalbuminemia	Uncommon. Bilateral in > 90%; decreased intravascular oncotic pressure causes transudation into pleural space; associated with edema or anasarca elsewhere
	Nephrosis	Usually bilateral, subpulmonic common; decreased intravascular oncotic pressure plus hypervolemia causes transudation into pleural space
	Hydronephrosis	Urine dissects retroperitoneally into pleural space and produces urinothorax
	Superior vena cava syndrome	Malignancy or thrombosed central catheter blocks intrathoracic lymphatic flow
	Constrictive pericarditis	Increases IV hydrostatic pressure; in some cases with massive anasarca, mechanism similar to hepatic hydrothorax
	Atelectasis	Increases negative intrapleural pressure
	Peritoneal dialysis	Mechanism similar to hepatic hydrothorax; pleural fluid has characteristics similar to dialysate
	Trapped lung	Encasement with fibrous peel increases negative intrapleural pressure
	Systemic capillary leak syndrome	Rare, occurs with anasarca and pericardial effusion
	Myxedema	Occurs in about 5%; transudate if pericardial effusion also present; either transudate or exudate if isolated pleural effusion
Exudate	Pneumonia (parapneumonic effusion)	May be uncomplicated or loculated and/or purulent (empyema); thoracentesis necessary to differentiate
	Malignancy	Lung, pleural, and breast cancers most common, but effusion can occur with any tumor metastatic to pleurae; chest pain is typically dull and aching
	Pulmonary embolism	Present in about 30% of cases; almost always exudative; bloody in < 50%; pulmonary embolism suspected when dyspnea is disproportionate to size of effusion
	Viral infection	Effusion usually small with or without parenchymal infiltrate; systemic rather than pulmonary symptoms predominate
	Coronary artery bypass surgery	Left-sided or larger on the left, 73%; bilateral and equal, 20%; right-sided or larger on the right, 7%. 10% have > 25% hemithorax filled with fluid 30 days postoperatively; bloody effusions related to postoperative bleeding and resolve; nonbloody effusions recur, and cause often remains unknown
	TB	Effusion usually unilateral or ipsilateral to parenchymal infiltrates; effusion due to hypersensitivity reaction to TB protein; TB cultures positive < 20%

Table continues on the following page.

TABLE 60–2. CAUSES OF PLEURAL EFFUSION—Continued

TYPE	CAUSE	COMMENTS
	Sarcoidosis	Effusion in 1–2%; patients have extensive parenchymal sarcoid and often extrathoracic sarcoid; pleural fluid is predominantly lymphocytic
	Uremia	Effusion in about 3%; > 50% have chest symptoms, most commonly fever (50%), chest pain (30%), cough (35%), and dyspnea (20%); diagnosis of exclusion
	Infradiaphragmatic abscess	Causes "sympathetic" subpulmonic effusion; neutrophils predominant in pleural fluid, but pH and glucose normal
	HIV infection	Effusion multifactorial: parapneumonic, TB, pulmonary Kaposi's sarcoma, *Pneumocystis jiroveci* (formerly called *P. carinii)* pneumonia, and other opportunistic infections
	Rheumatoid disease	Patient is typically an elderly man with rheumatoid nodules and deforming arthritis; must differentiate from parapneumonic effusion
	Lupus erythematosus	May be first manifestation of SLE; common with drug-induced SLE; diagnosis established by serologic tests of blood, not of pleural fluid
	Drugs	Many drugs, most notably bromocriptine, dantrolene nitrofurantoin, IL-2 (for treatment of renal cell cancer and melanoma), and methysergide. Also seen with drug-induced lupus
	Ovarian hyperstimulation syndrome	Complicates ovulation induction with human chorionic gonadotropin (hCG) and occasionally clomiphene; effusion develops 7–14 days after hCG injection; 52% right-sided, 27% bilateral
	Pancreatitis	Acute: Present in about 50%; bilateral, 77%; left-sided, 16%; right-sided, 8%. Due to transdiaphragmatic transfer of the exudative inflammatory fluid and diaphragmatic inflammation Chronic: Due to sinus tract from pancreatic pseudocyst through diaphragm into pleural space, chest symptoms rather than abdominal symptoms dominant, patients look like they have cancer
	Esophageal rupture	Patients extremely sick, medical emergency, morbidity and mortality due to infection of the mediastinum and pleural space
	Benign asbestos pleural effusion	Occurs > 30 yr after initial exposure; frequently asymptomatic, tends to come and go, must rule out mesothelioma
	Ovarian tumor (Meige's disease)	Mechanism similar to hepatic hydrothorax; not all patients with ovarian mass, ascites, and pleural effusion are inoperable; diagnosis requires disappearance of ascites and effusion postoperatively
	Yellow nail syndrome	Triad of pleural effusion, lymphedema, and yellow nails; elements may appear decades apart; pleural fluid has relatively high protein but low LDH; effusion tends to recur, and there is no pleuritic chest pain

TABLE 60–3. CRITERIA FOR IDENTIFYING EXUDATIVE PLEURAL EFFUSIONS

TEST	EXUDATE	SENSITIVITY	SPECIFICITY
Light's criteria (1 or more of the following 3)		98	83
Fluid LDH*	≥ 2/3 ULN for serum LDH	82	89
Pleural fluid: serum total protein ratio	≥ 0.5	86	84
Pleural fluid: serum LDH ratio	≥ 0.6	90	82
Fluid total protein	≥ 3 g/dL	90	90
Fluid cholesterol	≥ 60 mg/dL ≥ 43 mg/dL	54 75	92 80
Pleural fluid: Serum cholesterol ratio	≥ 0.3	89	81
Serum–pleural fluid protein†	≤ 3.1 g/dL	87	92

ULN = upper limit of normal.

*Correction for increase in LDH from RBC lysis = measured LDH − 0.0012 × RBC count/μL.

†Preferred test for patients prescribed diuretics after development of effusion if Light's exudative criteria are met.

Data from Light RW: Pleural effusion. *New England Journal of Medicine* 346:1971–1977, 2002.

RBCs and neutrophils in long-standing effusions when absorption is blocked by the thickened pleura.

Hemothorax is bloody fluid (pleural fluid hematocrit > 50% peripheral hematocrit) in the pleural space due to trauma or, rarely, as a result of coagulopathy or after rupture of a major blood vessel, such as the aorta or pulmonary artery.

Empyema is pus in the pleural space. It can occur as a complication of pneumonia, thoracotomy, abscesses (lung, hepatic, or subdiaphragmatic), or penetrating trauma. Empyema necessitans is soft-tissue extension of empyema leading to chest wall infection and external drainage.

Trapped lung is lung encased by a fibrous peel caused by empyema or tumor. Because the lung cannot expand, the pleural pressure becomes more negative than normal, increasing transudation of fluid from parietal pleural capillaries. The fluid characteristically is borderline between a transudate and an exudate, ie, the biochemical values are within 15% of the cutoff levels for Light's criteria (see TABLE 60–3).

Iatrogenic effusions can be caused by migration or misplacement of a feeding tube or central venous catheter, leading to infusion of tube feedings or IV solution into the pleural space.

Effusions with no obvious cause are often due to occult pulmonary emboli, TB, or malignancy. Etiology is unknown for about 15% of effusions even after extensive study; many of these effusions are thought to be due to viral infection.

Symptoms and Signs

Some pleural effusions are asymptomatic and are discovered incidentally on physical examination or chest x-ray. Many cause dyspnea, pleuritic chest pain, or both. Pleuritic chest pain, a vague discomfort or sharp pain that worsens on inspiration, indicates inflammation of the parietal pleura. Pain is usually felt over the inflamed site, but the posterior and peripheral portions of the diaphragmatic pleura are supplied by the lower 6 intercostal nerves, and irritation there may cause pain in the lower chest wall or abdomen that may simulate intra-abdominal disease. Irritation of the central portion of the diaphragmatic pleura, innervated by the phrenic nerves, causes pain referred to the neck and shoulder.

Physical examination reveals absent tactile fremitus, dullness to percussion, and decreased breath sounds on the side of the effusion. These findings can also be produced by pleural thickening. With large-volume effusions, respiration is usually rapid and shallow. A pleural friction rub, although infrequent, is the classic physical sign. The friction rub varies from a few intermittent sounds that may simulate crackles to a fully developed harsh grating, creaking, or leathery sound synchronous with respiration, heard on inspiration and expiration. Friction sounds adjacent to the heart (pleuropericardial rub) may vary with the heartbeat and may be confused with the friction rub of pericarditis. Pericardial rub is best heard over the left border of the sternum in the 3rd and 4th intercostal spaces, is characteristically a to-and-fro sound synchronous with the heartbeat, and is not influenced significantly by respiration. Sensitivity and specificity of the physical examination for detecting effusion are probably low.

Diagnosis

Diagnostic tests are indicated to document the presence of pleural fluid and to determine its cause.

Chest x-ray is the first test performed to confirm the presence of pleural fluid. The lateral upright chest x-ray should be examined when a pleural effusion is suspected. In an upright film, 75 mL of fluid blunts the posterior costophrenic angle. Larger pleural effusions opacify portions of the hemithorax; effusions > 4 L may cause complete opacification and even mediastinal shift.

Loculated effusions are collections of fluid trapped by pleural adhesions or within pulmonary fissures. Lateral decubitus x-rays, chest CT, or ultrasound should be performed if it is unclear whether an x-ray density represents fluid or whether suspected fluid is loculated or free-flowing; these tests are more sensitive than upright films and can detect fluid volumes < 10 mL. Loculated effusions, particularly those in the horizontal or oblique fissure, can be confused with a solid pulmonary mass (pseudotumor). They may change shape and size with changes in the patient's position and amount of pleural fluid.

CT scan is not routinely indicated but is valuable for evaluating the underlying lung parenchyma for infiltrates or masses when the lung is obscured by the effusion and for distinguishing loculated fluid from solid mass.

Thoracentesis (see p. 378) should be performed on almost all patients who have pleural fluid that is ≥10 mm in thickness on lateral decubitus x-ray or ultrasound that is new or of uncertain etiology. Despite common practice, chest x-ray need not be repeated after thoracentesis unless the patient develops symptoms suggestive of pneumothorax (dyspnea or chest pain) or unless air may have entered the pleural space during the procedure. Thoracentesis and subsequent pleural fluid analysis (see below) often are not necessary for pleural effusions that are chronic, have a known cause, and cause no symptoms.

Ultrasonography is helpful for identifying pleural fluid collections for thoracentesis when blind thoracentesis is unsuccessful.

Pleural fluid analysis is performed to diagnose the cause of pleural effusion. Analysis begins with visual inspection, which can distinguish bloody and chylous (or chyliform) from other effusions; can identify purulent effusions strongly suggestive of empyema; and can identify viscous fluid, which is characteristic of some mesotheliomas. Fluid should always be sent for total protein, LDH, cell count and cell differential, Gram stain, and aerobic and anaerobic bacterial cultures. Other tests (glucose, cytology, TB fluid markers [adenosine deaminase or interferon-γ], amylase, mycobacterial, and fungal stains and cultures) are used in appropriate clinical settings.

Fluid chemistries help distinguish transudates from exudates; multiple criteria exist, not one of which perfectly discriminates between the two. When Light's criteria are used (see TABLE 60–3), the serum LDH and total protein for comparison with pleural fluid should be obtained as close as possible to the time of thoracentesis. Light's criteria correctly identify almost all exudates but misidentify about 20% of transudates as exudates. If transudative effusion is suspected (eg, due to heart failure or cirrhosis) and none of the biochemical measurements are > 15% above the cutoff levels for Light's criteria, then the difference between the serum and the pleural fluid protein is measured. If the difference is > 3.1 g/dL, then the patient probably has a transudative effusion.

If the diagnosis remains unclear after pleural fluid analysis, a spiral CT scan is indicated to look for pulmonary emboli, pulmonary infiltrates, or mediastinal lesions. Findings of pulmonary emboli indicate the need for long-term anticoagulation; parenchymal infiltrates, the need for bronchoscopy; and mediastinal lesions, the need for transthoracic needle aspiration or mediastinoscopy. However, spiral CT requires a patient to hold his breath for ≥ 24 sec, and not all patients can comply. If spiral CT is unrevealing, observation is the best course unless the patient has a history of malignancy, weight loss, persistent fever, or other findings suggestive of malignancy or TB, in which case thoracoscopy may be indicated. Needle biopsy of the pleura can be performed when thoracoscopy is unavailable. When thoracoscopy is unrevealing, an open thoracotomy must sometimes be performed. Most patients with exudative effusions should have a PPD placed with controls.

Treatment

The underlying cause is treated; the effusion itself generally does not require treatment if it is asymptomatic, because many resorb spontaneously, especially those due to uncomplicated pneumonias, pulmonary embolism, and surgery. Pleuritic pain can usually be managed with oral analgesics, though a short course of oral opioids is sometimes necessary.

Thoracentesis is sufficient treatment for many symptomatic effusions and can be repeated for effusions that reaccumulate. Removal of > 1.5 L of pleural fluid at a time should be avoided, because it can lead to pulmonary edema due to rapid re-expansion of alveoli previously compressed by fluid.

Effusions that are chronic, recurrent, and causing symptoms can be treated with pleurodesis or with an indwelling catheter (see p. 498). Effusions caused by pneumonia and malignancy may require additional specific measures.

Parapneumonic effusion: In the presence of adverse prognostic factors (pH < 7.20, glucose < 60 mg/dL, positive Gram stain or culture, loculations), the effusion should be completely drained via thoracentesis or tube thoracostomy. If complete drainage is impossible, fibrinolytics (urokinase 100,000 units in 100 mL saline solution) should be administered intrapleurally. If this is ineffective, thoracoscopy should be performed to lyse adhesions and facilitate drainage. If thoracoscopy is unsuccessful, thoracotomy with surgical decortication (eg, removal of scar, clot, or fibrous membrane surrounding the lung) should be performed.

Malignant pleural effusion: If dyspnea caused by malignant pleural effusion is relieved by thoracentesis but fluid reaccumulates (with dyspnea) more than once, chronic drainage or pleurodesis is indicated; asymptomatic effusions and those unresponsive to thoracentesis do not require additional procedures.

Indwelling catheter drainage is the preferred approach for ambulatory patients, because the catheter can be inserted on an outpatient basis and the pleural fluid drained intermittently into vacuum bottles. Shunting of pleural fluid to the peritoneum (pleuroperitoneal shunt) is useful for patients with malignant effusion who fail pleurodesis or who have trapped lung.

Pleurodesis is created by instilling a sclerosing agent into the pleural space to fuse the visceral and parietal pleura and eliminate the space. The most effective and commonly used sclerosing agents are talc, doxycycline, and bleomycin delivered via chest tube or thoracoscopy. Pleurodesis is contraindicated if the mediastinum has shifted toward the side of the effusion or if the lung does not expand after a chest tube is inserted.

PLEURAL FIBROSIS AND CALCIFICATION

Pleural fibrosis and calcification are usually benign sequelae of pleural inflammation or asbestos exposure.

Pleural fibrosis and calcification can be either postinflammatory or asbestos related.

Postinflammatory: Pleural inflammation commonly causes acute pleural thickening. In most cases, the thickening resolves almost completely. Some patients are left with minor degrees of pleural thickening, which usually produces no symptoms or impairment of lung function. Occasionally, the lung becomes encased with a thick, fibrous pleural peel that limits expansion, pulls the mediastinum toward the side of disease, and impairs pulmonary function. Chest x-ray shows asymmetry of the lungs with thickened pleura (trapped lung). Differentiating localized pleural thickening from loculated pleural fluid may be difficult on x-ray, but the entire pleural surface may be seen on a CT scan.

Pleural fibrosis after inflammation can, on occasion, calcify. Calcification produces a dense image on the chest x-ray and almost always involves the visceral pleura. Postinflammatory calcifications are invariably unilateral.

Asbestos related: Exposure to asbestos can lead to focal, plaquelike pleural fibrosis, at times with calcification, occurring ≥ 20 yr after the initial exposure. Any pleural or pericardial surface can be affected, but asbestos-related pleural plaques are usually in the lower ⅔ of the thorax and are bilateral. Calcification most often affects the parietal diaphragmatic pleura and may be the only evidence of exposure. Dense pleural fibrosis can also follow asbestos exposure.

PNEUMOMEDIASTINUM

Pneumomediastinum is air in mediastinal interstices.

The three main causes of pneumomediastinum are alveolar rupture with dissection of air into the mediastinum, esophageal perforation, and esophageal or bowel rupture with dissection of air from the neck or the abdomen into the mediastinum. The primary symptom is substernal chest pain which can, on occasion, be severe. Physical examination shows subcutaneous emphysema, usually in the suprasternal notch, along with a crunching or clicking noise synchronous with the heartbeat which is best heard over the heart when the patient is in the left lateral decubitus position (Hamman's sign). The diagnosis is confirmed by chest x-ray, which shows air in the mediastinum. Treatment usually is not necessary, although tension pneumomediastinum with compression of mediastinal structures (rare) can be relieved with needle aspiration, leaving the needle open to the atmosphere as is done with tension pneumothorax.

PNEUMOTHORAX

Pneumothorax is air in the pleural space causing partial or complete lung collapse. Pneumothorax can occur spontaneously or from underlying pulmonary disease, trauma, or medical procedures. Diagnosis is based on physical examination and chest x-ray. Most pneumothoraces require transcatheter aspiration or tube thoracostomy.

Intrapleural pressure is normally negative (less than atmospheric pressure) because of inward lung and outward chest wall recoil. In pneumothorax, air enters the pleural space from outside the chest or from the lung itself via mediastinal tissue planes or direct pleural perforation. Intrapleural pressure rises, and lung volume decreases.

Classification and Etiology

Primary spontaneous pneumothorax occurs in patients without underlying pulmonary disease, typically in tall, thin young men in their teens and 20s. It is thought to be due to spontaneous rupture of subpleural apical blebs or bullae that result from smoking or that are inherited. It generally occurs at rest, although some cases occur with activities involving reaching or stretching. Primary spontaneous pneumothorax also occurs during diving and high-altitude flying because of unequally transmitted pressure changes in the lung.

Secondary spontaneous pneumothorax occurs in patients with underlying pulmonary disease. It most often results from rupture of a bleb or bulla in patients with severe COPD (forced expiratory volume in 1 sec [FEV_1] < 1 L), HIV-related *Pneumocystis jiroveci* (formerly called *P. carinii*) infection, cystic fibrosis, or any underlying pulmonary parenchymal disease (see TABLE 60–4). Secondary spontaneous pneumothorax is typically more serious than primary spontaneous pneumothorax because it occurs in older patients who have less pulmonary and cardiac reserve. Catamenial pneumothorax is a rare form of secondary spontaneous pneumothorax that occurs within 48 h of the onset of menstruation in premenopausal women and sometimes in postmenopausal women taking estrogen. The cause is intrathoracic endometriosis, possibly from migration of peritoneal endometrial tissue through diaphragmatic defects or embolization through pelvic veins. With menstruation, a hole develops in the pleura as the endometrial tissue is shed.

Traumatic pneumothorax is a common complication of blunt and penetrating chest injuries.

Tension pneumothorax is a pneumothorax causing progressive rise in intrapleural pressure to levels that become positive throughout the respiratory cycle and collapse the lung, shift the mediastinum, and impair venous return to the heart. Air continues to get into the pleural space but cannot exit. Without proper treatment, the impaired venous return can cause systemic hypotension and respiratory and cardiac arrest within minutes. Tension pneumothorax most commonly occurs in patients receiving positive-pressure mechanical ventilation (particularly during resuscitation). It is rarely a complication of traumatic pneumothorax, when a chest wound acts as a one-way valve that traps increasing volumes of air in the pleural space with inspiration.

Iatrogenic pneumothorax is caused by medical interventions, including transthoracic needle aspiration, thoracentesis, central venous catheter placement, mechanical ventilation, and cardiopulmonary resuscitation.

Symptoms and Signs

Nontraumatic pneumothoraces are sometimes asymptomatic. Symptoms include dyspnea, pleuritic chest pain, and anxiety. Dyspnea may be sudden or gradual in onset depending on the rate of development and size of the pneumothorax. Pain can simulate cardiac ischemia, musculoskeletal injury (when referred to the shoulder), or an intra-abdominal process (when referred to the abdomen).

Physical findings classically consist of absent tactile fremitus, hyperresonance to percussion, and decreased breath sounds on the side with the pneumothorax. If the pneumothorax is large, the side with the pneumothorax may be enlarged with the trachea visibly shifted to the opposite side.

Diagnosis

Diagnosis is made with upright inspiratory chest x-ray. Radiolucent air and the absence of lung markings juxtaposed between a shrunken lobe or lung and the parietal pleura are diagnostic of pneumothorax. Tracheal deviation and mediastinal shift occur with large pneumothoraces.

TABLE 60–4. CAUSES OF SPONTANEOUS PNEUMOTHORAX

Primary
- Subpleural blebs attributed to smoking

Secondary
- More common
  - Asthma
  - COPD
  - Cystic fibrosis
  - Necrotizing pneumonia
  - *Pneumocystic jiroveci* (formerly *P. carinii*) infection
  - TB
- Less common
  - Pulmonary
    - Idiopathic pulmonary fibrosis
    - Langerhans' cell granulomatosis
    - Lung cancer
    - Lymphangioleiomyomatosis
    - Sarcoidosis
    - Connective-tissue disease
    - Ankylosing spondylitis
    - Ehlers-Danlos syndrome
    - Marfan's syndrome
    - Polymyositis/dermatomyositis
    - RA
    - Sarcoma
    - Scleroderma
- Other
  - Thoracic endometriosis
  - Tuberous sclerosis

The size of a pneumothorax is defined as the percentage of the hemithorax that is vacant. This is determined by taking 1 minus the ratio of the cubes of the width of the lung and hemithorax. For example, if the width of the hemithorax is 10 cm and the width of the lung is 5 cm, the ratio is $5^3/10^3 = 0.125$. Thus the size of the pneumothorax is 1 minus 0.125, or 87.5%. If adhesions are present between the lung and the chest wall, the lung will not collapse symmetrically, the pneumothorax may appear atypical or loculated, and the calculation will not hold.

Small pneumothoraces are sometimes overlooked on chest x-ray. Conditions that mimic pneumothorax radiographically include emphysematous bullae, skin folds, and overlap of stomach or bowel markings on lung fields.

Treatment

Patients should receive supplemental O_2 until the chest x-ray is available; O_2 accelerates pleural reabsorption of air. Treatment then depends on the type, size, and effects of pneumothorax. Primary spontaneous pneumothorax that is < 20% and that does not cause respiratory or cardiac symptoms can be safely observed without treatment if follow-up chest x-rays obtained at about 6 and 48 h show no progression. Larger or symptomatic primary spontaneous pneumothoraces should be evacuated by catheter drainage.

Catheter drainage is accomplished by insertion of a small-bore IV or pigtail catheter into the chest in the 2nd intercostal space at the mid-clavicular line. The catheter is attached to a three-way stopcock and syringe. Air is withdrawn from the pleural space through the stopcock into the syringe and expelled into the room. The process is repeated until the lung re-expands or until 4 L of air are removed. If the lung expands, the catheter can be removed or kept in place attached to a one-way Heimlich valve (thus permitting ambulation). If the lung does not expand, a chest tube should be inserted; in either approach, patients are usually hospitalized for observation. Primary spontaneous pneumothoraces can also be managed initially with a chest tube attached to a water seal without or with suction. Patients with primary spontaneous pneumothoraces should also undergo smoking cessation counseling, because smoking is a primary risk.

Secondary and traumatic pneumothoraces are generally treated with tube thoracostomy (see p. 380), although hospitalization and observation may not be needed for some patients with a small pneumothorax. Symptomatic patients with iatrogenic pneumothoraces are best managed initially with aspiration.

Tension pneumothorax is a medical emergency. It should be treated immediately by inserting a 14- or 16-gauge needle with catheter through the chest wall in the 2nd intercostal space at the mid-clavicular line. The sound of high-pressure air escaping confirms diagnosis. The catheter can be left open to air or attached to a Heimlich valve. Emergency decompression must be followed immediately by tube thoracostomy, after which the catheter is removed.

Complications

The three main problems encountered when treating pneumothorax are air leaks, failure of the lung to expand, and re-expansion pulmonary edema.

Air leaks are usually due to the primary defect—ie, continued leakage of air from the lung into the pleural space—but can be due to air leaking around the chest tube insertion site if the site is not properly sutured and sealed. Air leaks are more common in secondary than in primary spontaneous pneumothorax. Most resolve spontaneously in < 1 wk.

Failure of the lung to re-expand is usually due to a persistent air leak, an endobronchial obstruction, a trapped lung, or a malpositioned chest tube. If an air leak or an incompletely expanded lung persists beyond 1 wk, the patient should be evaluated for thoracoscopy or thoracotomy.

Re-expansion pulmonary edema occurs when the lung is rapidly expanded, as occurs when a chest tube is connected to negative pressure after having been collapsed for > 2 days. Treatment is supportive with O_2, diuretics, and cardiopulmonary support as needed.

Prevention

Recurrence approaches 50% in the 3 yr after initial spontaneous pneumothorax; the best preventive procedure is a video-assisted thoracic surgery (VATS) procedure in which blebs are stapled and a pleurodesis is created with pleural abrasion, parietal pleurectomy, or talc insufflation; in some medical centers thoracotomy is still used. These procedures are recommended when catheter drainage fails with spontaneous pneumothorax, when there is a recurrent pneumothorax, or in patients with secondary spontaneous pneumothorax. Recurrence after these procedures is < 5%. Patients who cannot undergo thoracoscopy may undergo chemical pleurodesis through a chest tube (see p. 495), a procedure that, though much less invasive, reduces the recurrence rate to only about 25%.

VIRAL PLEURITIS

Viral pleuritis is a viral infection of the pleurae.

Viral pleuritis is most commonly caused by infection with coxsackie B virus. Occasionally, echovirus causes a rare condition known as epidemic or Bornholm's pleurodynia, manifesting as pleuritis, fever, and chest muscle spasms; the condition occurs in the late summer and affects adolescents and young adults. The primary symptom is pleuritic pain; pleural friction rub may be a sign (see p. 494). Diagnosis is made clinically, and treatment is symptomatic, with oral NSAIDs or a short course of oral opioids if needed.

61 SLEEP APNEA

Breathing disorders that occur during sleep include obstructive sleep apnea and central sleep apnea. Less severe forms include snoring and upper airway resistance syndrome. The term sleep-disordered breathing is used to encompass all such disorders. (See also Ch. 215 on p. 1834.)

OBSTRUCTIVE SLEEP APNEA

Obstructive sleep apnea comprises episodes of partial and/or complete closure of the upper airway during sleep leading to breathing cessation, defined as > 10 sec. Symptoms include restlessness, snoring, recurrent awakening, morning headache, and excessive daytime sleepiness. Diagnosis is based on sleep history, physical examination, and polysomnography. Treatment is with nasal continuous positive airway pressure, oral appliances, and, in refractory cases, surgery. Prognosis is good with treatment, but most cases are undiagnosed and untreated, resulting in hypertension, heart failure, and injury and death from motor vehicle and other accidents resulting from hypersomnolence.

In at-risk patients, sleep destabilizes the upper airway, causing partial or complete obstruction of the nasopharynx, oropharynx, or both. When breathing is diminished but not absent, the condition is called obstructive sleep hypopnea.

The prevalence of obstructive sleep apnea (OSA) in developed countries is 2 to 4%; the condition is underrecognized and often undiagnosed even in symptomatic patients. OSA is up to 4 times more common in men, perhaps because it is underdiagnosed in women, because women may be more reluctant to report symptoms of snoring, or because of gender bias in referral.

Etiology

Anatomic risk factors include obesity (body mass index > 30); an oropharynx "crowded" by a short or retracted mandible and prominent tongue, tonsils, lateral pharyngeal walls, or lateral parapharyngeal fat pads; a rounded head; and a shirt collar size > 18 inches. Other identified risk factors include postmenopausal status and alcohol or sedative use. Family history of sleep apnea is present in 25 to 40% of cases, perhaps reflective of intrinsic ventilatory drive or pharyngeal structure; the likelihood of the disease increases progressively as more family members have it. OSA is also often found in association with chronic disease, such as hypertension, stroke, diabetes, gastroesophageal reflux disease, nocturnal angina, heart failure, and hypothyroidism.

Because obesity is a common risk factor for both OSA and the obesity-hypoventilation syndrome (see p. 57), the two conditions may coexist.

Airway obstruction causes paroxysms of inspiratory effort, reductions in gas exchange, disruption of normal sleep architecture, and partial or complete arousals from sleep. Hypoxia and/or hypercapnia and sleep fragmentation interact to produce characteristic symptoms and signs.

OSA is an extreme form of sleep-related upper airway resistance. Less severe forms do not produce O_2 desaturation and include primary snoring; pharyngeal airflow resistance causing noisy inspiration but without sleep arousals; and the upper airway resistance syndrome, which is more severe pharyngeal airflow resistance causing snoring and transient sleep arousals. People with upper airway resistance syndrome are typically younger and less obese than those with OSA and complain of daytime sleepiness more than do those with primary snoring. But the symptoms, diagnostic evaluation, and treatment of snoring and upper airway resistance syndrome are otherwise the same as for OSA.

Symptoms and Signs

Symptoms include loud disruptive snoring, which is reported by 80 to 85% of OSA patients. However, most people who snore do not have OSA, and few need extensive evaluation. Other symptoms include choking, gasping, or snorting during sleep, restless sleep, and difficulty staying asleep (see TABLE 61–1). Most patients are unaware of symptoms during sleep but are informed by bed partners or roommates. Daytime symptoms include fatigue, hypersomnolence, and impaired concentration. The frequency of sleep complaints and degree of daytime sleepiness roughly correlate with the number and length of nocturnal arousals. Hypertension and diabetes are twice as common among people who snore, even after age and obesity are accounted for. OSA can be associated with cardiac arrhythmias (eg, bradycardia, asystole) and heart failure.

Diagnosis

The diagnosis is suspected in patients with identifiable risk factors and/or symptoms. The patient and sleeping partner should be interviewed. The differential diagnosis of excessive daytime sleepiness is broad (see p. 1839) and includes reduced quantity or quality of sleep due to poor sleep hygiene; narcolepsy; sedation or mental status changes from drugs; chronic diseases, including cardiovascular, respiratory, or metabolic disturbances and accompanying therapies (eg, diuretics, insulin); depression; alcohol or drug abuse; and other primary sleep disorders (eg, periodic limb movement disorder, restless legs syndrome). A sleep history should be taken in all older patients; in patients with symptoms of daytime fatigue, sleepiness, and lack of energy; in overweight or obese patients; and in patients with chronic medical conditions such as hypertension (which may be caused by OSA), heart failure (which may cause and be caused by OSA), and stroke. Most patients who report only snoring, without other symptoms or cardiovascular risk, however, do not need an extensive evaluation for OSA.

The physical examination should include evaluation for nasal obstruction, tonsillar hypertrophy, signs of poor control of hypertension, and measurement of neck size.

The diagnosis is confirmed with polysomnography (see p. 1837), which comprises continuous measures of breathing effort by plethysmography; airflow at the nose and mouth by flow sensors; O_2 saturation by oximetry; sleep architecture by EEG (for sleep stages), chin electromyography (for hypotonia), and electro-oculograms for rapid eye movements. Also, the patient is observed by video. ECG is useful for determining whether arrhythmias occur with apneic episodes. Other variables evaluated include limb muscle activity (to assess nonrespiratory causes of sleep arousal, such as restless legs syndrome and periodic limb movements disorder) and body position (apnea may occur only in the supine position).

Some facilities use portable monitors that measure only heart rate, pulse oximetry, and nasal airflow to diagnose OSA. Although some studies show excellent correlation between these monitors and polysomnography, controversy over their routine use persists, because coexisting sleep disorders (eg, restless legs syndrome) may go unrecognized.

The common summary measure used to describe respiratory disturbances during sleep is the apnea-hypopnea index (AHI)—the total number of episodes of apnea and hy-

TABLE 61–1. DEFINITION OF OBSTRUCTIVE SLEEP APNEA

Excessive daytime sleepiness unexplained by other factors and ≥ 2 of the following:

- Loud disruptive snoring
- Nocturnal choking/gasping/snorting
- Recurrent nocturnal awakening
- Unrefreshing sleep
- Daytime fatigue
- Impaired concentration

and

Sleep monitoring documenting > 5 episodes of hypopnea and apnea per hour popnea during sleep divided by the hours of sleep time. AHI values can be computed for different sleep stages. The respiratory disturbance index (RDI) is a similar measure, which refers to the number of times per hour that blood O_2 saturation falls > 3%. With an EEG, an arousal index (AI) can be computed, which is the number of arousals per hour of sleep. The AI may be correlated with AHI or RDI, but about 20% of apneas and desaturation episodes are not accompanied by arousals, or other causes of arousals are present. An AHI > 5 is required for the diagnosis of OSA; values > 15 and > 30 indicate moderate and severe levels of sleep apnea, respectively. Snoring confers a 7-fold increase in the likelihood of having AHI > 5. The AI and RDI correlate only moderately with a patient's symptoms.

Adjunctive testing may include upper airway imaging, thyroid-stimulating hormone, and other tests as appropriate to assess chronic medical conditions associated with OSA.

Prognosis

Prognosis is excellent with proper treatment. However, untreated OSA, which is common because it is so frequently undiagnosed, can have long-term sequelae, including poorly controlled hypertension and heart failure. The adverse effects of hypersomnolence, such as loss of employment and sexual dysfunction, can affect families considerably.

Perhaps most importantly, excessive daytime sleepiness is a major risk factor for serious injury and death from accidents, especially motor vehicle accidents. Sleepy patients should therefore be warned of the risk of operating a motor vehicle or engaging in activities during which sleep attacks would be hazardous. In addition, perioperative cardiac arrest has been attributed to OSA, probably due to the effects of anesthesia on the condition after removal of a mechanical airway. Patients should therefore inform an anesthesiologist of the diagnosis before undergoing surgery and should expect to receive continuous positive airway pressure (CPAP) during hospitalization.

Treatment

Initial treatment addresses underlying risk factors. Modifiable risk factors include obesity, alcohol and sedative use, and poor control of chronic disease. Weight loss is an important component of OSA treatment but is extremely difficult for most people, especially those fatigued or sleepy.

Surgical correction of upper airway obstruction caused by enlarged tonsils and nasal polyps should be considered; surgery for macroglossia or micrognathia is also an option.

The aim of treatment specific to OSA is to reduce episodes of hypoxia and sleep fragmentation; treatment is tailored to the patient and to the degree of impairment. Cure is defined as a resolution of symptoms with AHI reduction below a threshold, usually 10/h. Moderate and severe levels of sleepiness are predictors of treatment success.

CPAP: Nasal CPAP is the treatment of choice for most patients with subjective sleepiness; it is of questionable benefit for patients who deny sleepiness. CPAP improves upper airway patency by application of positive pressure to the collapsible upper airway. Effective pressures typically range from 3 to 15 cm H_2O. Disease severity does not correlate with pressure requirements. If clinical improvement is not apparent, pressure can be titrated by repeat polysomnography. Regardless of AHI, CPAP can also reduce neurocognitive impairments and blood pressure. If CPAP is withdrawn, symptoms recur over several days, though short interruptions of therapy for acute medical conditions are usually well tolerated. Duration of therapy is indefinite.

Failures of nasal CPAP commonly occur because of limited patient adherence. Adverse effects include sore throat, which can be alleviated in some cases with the use of warm humidified air, and discomfort resulting from a poorly fitting mask.

CPAP can be augmented with inspiratory assistance (bi-level positive airway pressure) for patients with obesity-hypoventilation syndrome (see p. 57).

Oral appliances: Oral appliances are designed to advance the mandible or, at the very least, prevent mandible retrusion with sleep. Some are also designed to pull the tongue forward. Use of these appliances to treat both snoring and OSA is gaining acceptance. Comparisons of appliances to CPAP are limited, and specific indications and cost-effectiveness have not been established.

Surgery: Surgery is reserved for patients refractory to noninvasive therapies. Uvulopalatopharyngoplasty (UPPP) is the most common procedure. It involves a submucosal resection of tissue from the tonsillar pillars to the arytenoepiglottic folds, including resection of the adenoids, to enlarge the upper airway. Equivalence with CPAP was demonstrated in one study using CPAP as a bridge to surgery, but the two interventions have not been directly compared. Patients who are morbidly obese or who have anatomic narrowing of the airway may not realize success with UPPP. Moreover, recognition of sleep apnea after UPPP is obscured because snoring is absent. These silent obstructions may be as severe as apneic episodes before surgical intervention.

Adjunctive surgical procedures include midline glossectomy and mandibulomaxillary advancement. The latter is often offered as a 2nd-stage procedure if UPPP is not curative. Studies of this 2-stage approach across centers in unselected patients are not available.

Tracheostomy is the most effective therapeutic maneuver for obstructive apnea but is a procedure of last resort. It bypasses the site of obstruction during sleep. It is indicated for patients who are most severely affected by OSA and/or obstructive sleep hypopnea (eg, those with cor pulmonale). It may take ≥ 1 yr before the stoma is healed.

Laser-assisted uvuloplasty has been promoted as a treatment for loud snoring along with radiofrequency tissue ablation. It provides 2- to 6-mo reductions of 70 to 80% in snoring loudness; however, efficacy declines after 1 yr. Sleep apnea syndrome should be considered in these evaluations so as not to delay more appropriate treatment.

Adjunctive treatments: Adjunctive treatments are commonly used but have no proven role as first-line treatment.

O_2 may provoke respiratory acidosis and morning headache in some patients, and it is impossible to predict who will respond favorably.

A number of drugs have been used as ventilatory drive stimulants (eg, tricyclic antidepressants, theophylline) but cannot be routinely advocated because of limited efficacy and/or a low therapeutic index.

Nasal dilatory devices and throat sprays sold OTC for snoring have no proven benefits.

Patient education and support: An informed patient and family are better able to cope with a treatment strategy, including tracheostomy in patients refractory to other treatment. Patient support groups are effective in providing information and in supporting timely and effective treatment.

CENTRAL SLEEP APNEA

Central sleep apnea is a heterogenous group of conditions characterized by changes in ventilatory drive or decreased ability to breathe without airway obstruction; most of these conditions cause asymptomatic changes in breathing pattern during sleep.

Patients with central sleep apnea (CSA) fall into two categories. One group presents with hypercapnia with decreased ventilatory drive or a decreased ability to breathe. Causes include central lesions, such as brain stem infarctions, encephalitis, and Arnold-Chiari malformation; neuromuscular diseases, such as muscular dystrophy, amyotrophic lateral sclerosis, and postpolio syndrome; and chest wall abnormalities, notably, kyphoscoliosis. The other group presents with eucapnia or hypocapnia with increased ventilatory drive but sleep-induced apnea and periodic breathing. Cheyne-Stokes breathing is a discrete pattern of this form of CSA thought to be caused by delays in cerebral circulation that, in turn, cause a lag in recognition by respiratory centers of acidosis/hypoxia (causing hyperpnea) and of alkalosis/hypocapnia (causing apnea). Causes include heart failure, high altitude, pain, and anxiety.

Congenital central hypoventilation (Ondine's curse) is a rare disorder of idiopathic CSA in newborns and may be associated with Hirschsprung's disease. It may be related to an inborn error in neurogenesis.

CSA is mostly asymptomatic and is detected by caretakers or bed partners who notice long respiratory pauses, shallow breaths, or restless sleep. Patients with hypercapnic forms may experience daytime somnolence, lethargy, and morning headache.

Diagnosis is suspected on the basis of history and confirmed by polysomnography. Testing may not be necessary, however, if CSA causes no symptoms or is clearly related to an identifiable disorder. Additional testing may involve brain or brain stem imaging to evaluate central causes.

Primary treatment is correction of underlying conditions and avoidance of sedatives. Secondary treatment is provision of supplemental O_2 or, in patients with hypercapnic CSA, noninvasive continuous or bi-level positive airway pressure. Acetazolamide is effective in CSA caused by high altitude. Phrenic nerve pacing is an option for children > 2 yr with congenital CSA.

62 TUMORS OF THE LUNGS

Lung tumors may be malignant or benign, primary or metastatic (see TABLE 62–1). Lung carcinoma, also called bronchogenic carcinoma or lung cancer, is the most common nondermatologic cancer and the most common lung tumor.

LUNG CARCINOMA

Lung carcinoma is a malignant lung tumor usually categorized as small cell or non–small cell. Cigarette smoking is the major risk factor for most types. Symptoms include cough, chest discomfort, and, less commonly, hemoptysis, but many patients are asymptomatic and some present with metastatic disease. Diagnosis is suspected by chest x-ray or CT scan and confirmed by biopsy. Treatment is with surgery, chemotherapy, and/or radiation therapy. Despite advances in treatment, the prognosis is poor, and attention is focused on early detection and prevention.

Epidemiology, Pathophysiology, and Classification

An estimated 171,900 new cases of lung carcinoma are diagnosed each year in the US, and the disease causes 157,200 deaths annually. The incidence is rising in women and appears to be leveling off in men. Black men are at especially high risk.

Cigarette smoking, including passive (secondhand) smoking, is the most important cause. Risk differs by age and smoking intensity and duration; risk after smoking cessation declines but probably never returns to baseline. Exposure to radon, a breakdown product of naturally occurring radium and uranium, is the most important environmental risk factor in nonsmokers. Occupational exposure to radon (in uranium miners); asbestos (in construction and demolition workers, pipefitters, shipbuilders, and automotive mechanics); silica (in miners and sandblasters); arsenic (in workers in copper smelting, pesticide manufacturing, and wood-treatment plants); chromates (in stainless steel and pigment manufacturing plants); nickel (in battery and stainless steel manufacturing plants); chloromethyl ethers; beryllium; and coke oven emissions (in steel workers) accounts for a small number of cases per year (see Ch. 57 on p. 469). The risk of cancer is greater with combined exposure to occupational toxins and cigarette smoking than with either one alone. COPD and pulmonary fibrosis may increase susceptibility; β-carotene supplementation may increase susceptibility

TABLE 62–1. CLASSIFICATION OF PRIMARY LUNG TUMORS

- **Malignant**
  - Carcinoma
    - Small cell
      - Oat cell
      - Intermediate cell
      - Combined
    - Non–small cell
      - Adenocarcinoma
        - Acinar
        - Bronchioloalveolar
        - Papillary
        - Solid
      - Adenosquamous
      - Large cell
        - Clear cell
        - Giant cell
      - Squamous cell
        - Spindle cell
  - Other
    - Bronchial gland carcinoma
      - Adenoid cystic
      - Mucoepidermoid
    - Carcinoid
    - Lymphoma
      - Primary pulmonary Hodgkin
      - Primary pulmonary non-Hodgkin
- **Benign**
  - Laryngotracheobronchial
    - Adenoma
    - Hamartoma
    - Myoblastoma
    - Papilloma
  - Parenchymal
    - Fibroma
    - Hamartoma
    - Leiomyoma
    - Lipoma
    - Neurofibroma/schwannoma
    - Sclerosing hemangioma

TABLE 62–2. FEATURES OF LUNG CARCINOMA

FEATURE	SMALL CELL	NON–SMALL CELL Adenocarcinoma	Squamous Cell	Large Cell
% of lung cancers	15%	25–35%	30–35%	10–15%
Location	Submucosa of airways, perihilar mass	Peripheral nodule or mass	Central, endobronchial	Peripheral nodule or mass
Risks	Smoking (100%)	Smoking, occupational exposure (asbestos, radon)		
Treatment	Etoposide or irinotecan or topotecan + carboplatin or cisplatin; concurrent radiation therapy in limited-stage disease; no role for surgery	Stage I and II: Surgery with or without adjurant chemotherapy Stage IIIA: Surgery with or without adjuvant therapy or concurrent chemoradiation Stage IIIB: Radiation with or without chemotherapy Stage IV: Chemotherapy with or without palliative radiation		
Complications	Common cause of SVC syndrome, paraneoplastic syndromes	Hemoptysis, airway obstruction, pneumonia, pleuritic involvement with pain, pleural effusion, SVC syndrome, Pancoast's tumor (shoulder or arm pain), hoarseness (laryngeal nerve involvement), neurologic symptoms from brain metastasis, pathologic fractures from bone metastasis, jaundice from liver metastasis		
5-yr survival with treatment	Limited: 20% Extensive: < 5%	Stage I: 57–67% Stage II: 39–55% Stage III: 5–25% Stage IV: < 1%		

SVC = superior vena cava.

in smokers. Air pollution and cigar smoke contain carcinogens but have never been shown to cause lung carcinoma.

Respiratory epithelial cells require prolonged exposure to cancer-promoting agents and accumulation of multiple genetic mutations before becoming neoplastic. Mutations in genes that stimulate cell growth (*K-RAS, MYC*), code for growth factor receptors (*EGFR, HER2/neu*), and inhibit apoptosis (*BCL-2*) contribute to proliferation of abnormal cells. So do mutations that inhibit tumor-suppressor genes (*p53, APC*). When enough of these mutations accumulate, lung carcinoma results.

Lung carcinoma is generally classified as small cell (SCLC) and non–small cell (NSCLC). SCLC is a highly aggressive cancer almost always occurring in smokers and causing widespread metastatic disease in 60% of patients by the time of diagnosis. Clinical behavior of NSCLC is more variable and depends on histologic type (see TABLE 62–2).

Symptoms and Signs

About 25% of lung carcinomas are asymptomatic and are detected incidentally with chest imaging. Symptoms and signs develop from local tumor, regional spread, and metastasis. Paraneoplastic syndromes and constitutional symptoms may occur at any stage.

Local tumor causes cough and, less commonly, dyspnea because of airway obstruction, postobstructive atelectasis, and lymphangitic spread. Fever may occur with postobstructive pneumonia. Up to ½ of patients report vague or localized chest pain. Hemoptysis is less common, and blood loss is minimal, except in rare instances when tumor erodes a major artery, causing massive hemorrhage and death by asphyxiation.

Regional spread may cause pleuritic chest pain or dyspnea from pleural effusion, hoarseness due to tumor encroachment on the recurrent laryngeal nerve, and dyspnea and hypoxia from diaphragmatic paralysis due to involvement of the phrenic nerve.

Compression or invasion of the superior vena cava (SVC syndrome) can produce headache or a sensation of head fullness, facial or upper extremity swelling, and supine breathlessness and flushing (plethora). Signs of SVC syndrome are facial and upper extremity edema, dilated neck and subcutaneous veins over the face and upper trunk, and facial and truncal plethora. SVC syndrome is more common in patients with SCLC.

Apical tumors, usually NSCLC, can invade the brachial plexus, pleura, or ribs, causing shoulder and upper extremity pain and weakness or atrophy of the ipsilateral hand (Pancoast's tumor). Horner's syndrome (ptosis, miosis, enophthalmos, and anhidrosis) results when the paravertebral sympathetic chain or cervical stellate ganglion is involved. Spread of tumor to pericardium may be asymptomatic or lead to constrictive pericarditis or cardiac tamponade (see p. 732). Rarely, esophageal compression causes dysphagia.

Metastases always eventually cause symptoms that vary by location. Metastases to the liver cause GI symptoms and ultimately hepatic insufficiency. Metastases to the brain cause behavioral changes, confusion, aphasia, seizures, paresis or paralysis, nausea and vomiting, and, ultimately, coma and death. Bone metastases cause severe pain and pathologic fractures. Lung carcinoma commonly metastasizes to the adrenal glands but rarely leads to adrenal insufficiency.

Paraneoplastic syndromes are not caused by cancer directly (see p. 1150). Common paraneoplastic syndromes in patients with lung carcinoma include hypercalcemia (caused by tumor production of parathyroid hormone-related protein), syndrome of inappropriate antidiuretic hormone secretion (SIADH), finger clubbing with or without hypertrophic osteoarthropathy, hypercoagulability with migratory superficial thrombophlebitis (Trousseau's syndrome), myasthenia (Eaton-Lambert syndrome), and a variety of neurologic syndromes, including neuropathies, encephalopathies, encephalitides, myelopathies, and cerebellar disease. Mechanisms for neuromuscular syndromes involve tumor expression of autoantigens with production of autoantibodies, but the cause of most others is unknown.

Constitutional symptoms most commonly include weight loss and fatigue and are sometimes the first indication of underlying malignancy.

Diagnosis

Chest x-ray is the initial test. It may show clearly defined abnormalities, such as a single mass or multifocal masses or a solitary pulmonary nodule (see p. 361), or more subtle changes, such as an enlarged hilum, widened mediastinum, tracheobronchial narrowing, atelectasis, nonresolving parenchymal infiltrate, cavitary lesion, or unexplained pleural thickening or effusion. These findings are suggestive but not diagnostic of lung carcinoma and require follow-up with high-resolution CT (HRCT) and cytopathologic confirmation.

CT demonstrates many characteristic patterns and appearances that may confirm the diagnosis. CT also can guide needle biopsy of accessible lesions and is useful for staging.

The method used to obtain cells or tissue for confirmation depends on the accessibility of tissue and the location of suspect lesions. Sputum or pleural fluid cytology is the least invasive method. In patients with productive cough, sputum specimens obtained on awakening may contain high concentrations of malignant cells, but yield for this method is about 50% overall. Pleural fluid is another convenient source of cells, but effusions accompany ≤ ⅓ of all lung carcinomas; nevertheless, a malignant effusion immediately stages a cancer as at least stage IIIB (see TABLE 62–3) and is a poor prognostic sign. In general, false-negative cytology readings can be minimized by obtaining as large a volume of sputum or fluid as possible early in the day and sending the sample to the pathology laboratory immediately to minimize delays in processing, which lead to cell breakdown. Percutaneous biopsy is the next least invasive procedure. It is more useful for metastatic sites (supraclavicular or other peripheral lymph nodes, pleura, liver, and adrenals) than for lung lesions because of a 20 to 25% risk of pneumothorax and the risk of false-negative results unlikely to change the perceived need for treatment.

Bronchoscopy is the procedure most often used for diagnosing lung carcinoma. In theory, the procedure of choice for obtaining tissue is the one that is least invasive. In practice,

TABLE 62–3. INTERNATIONAL STAGING SYSTEM FOR LUNG CANCER

Primary tumor (T)	
Tis	Carcinoma in situ
T1	Tumor ≤ 3 cm without invasion more proximal than the lobar bronchus (ie, not in the main bronchus)
T2	Tumor with any one of the following features: > 3 cm Involves main bronchus ≥ 2 cm distal to carina Invades the visceral pleura Atelectasis or obstructive pneumonitis that extends to the hilar region but does not involve the entire lung
T3	Tumor of any size with any one of the following features: Invades chest wall (including superior sulcus tumors), diaphragm, mediastinal pleura, or parietal pericardium Involves main bronchus < 2 cm distal to carina but without carinal involvement Atelectasis or obstructive pneumonitis of the entire lung
T4	Tumor of any size with any of the following features: Invades mediastinum, heart, great vessels, trachea, esophagus, vertebral body, carina Malignant pleural or pericardial effusion Satellite tumor nodule(s) within the same lobe as primary tumor
Regional lymph nodes (N)	
N0	No regional lymph node metastasis
N1	Metastasis to ipsilateral peribronchial and/or ipsilateral hilar lymph nodes, and intrapulmonary nodes involved by direct extension of the primary tumor
N2	Metastasis to ipsilateral mediastinal and/or subcarinal lymph node(s)
N3	Metastasis to contralateral mediastinal, contralateral hilar, ipsilateral or contralateral scalene, or supraclavicular lymph node(s)
Distant metastasis (M)	
M0	No distant metastasis
M1	Distant metastasis present [includes metastatic tumor nodule(s) in a lobe(s) ipsilateral to but different from the primary tumor]

Stage 0 Tis	Stage IIB T2 N1 M0 *or* T3 N0 M0
Stage IA TI N0 M0	Stage IIIA T3 N1 M0 *or* T1-3 N2 M0
Stage IB T2 N0 M0	Stage IIIB Any T N3 M0 *or* T4 Any N M0
Stage IIA T1 N1 M0	Stage IV Any T Any N M1

Adapted with permission from Mountain, CF: Revisions in the international system for staging lung cancer. *Chest* 111(6):1710–1717, 1997.

bronchoscopy is often performed in addition to or instead of less invasive procedures, because diagnostic yields are greater and because bronchoscopy is important for staging. A combination of washings, brushings, and fine-needle aspiration of visible endobronchial lesions and of paratracheal, subcarinal, mediastinal, and hilar lymph nodes yields a tissue diagnosis in 90 to 100% of cases. Mediastinoscopy is a higher-risk procedure and is usually used before surgery to confirm or exclude the presence of tumor in enlarged mediastinal lymph nodes of undetermined significance (see p. 507).

Open lung biopsy, performed via open thoracotomy or using video assistance (VATS—see p. 379), is indicated when less invasive methods do not provide a diagnosis in patients whose clinical characteristics and radiographic features strongly suggest resectable tumor.

Staging

SCLC is categorized as limited-stage and extensive-stage disease. Limited-stage disease is cancer confined to one hemithorax (including ipsilateral lymph nodes) that can be encompassed within one tolerable radiation therapy port, excluding the presence of pleural or pericardial effusion. Extensive-stage disease is cancer outside a single hemithorax and presence of malignant pleural or pericardial effusion. About ⅓ of patients with SCLC have limited-stage disease; the remainder often have extensive distant metastases.

NSCLC staging involves determining tumor size, tumor and lymph node location, and the presence or absence of distant metastases (see TABLES 62–2 and 62–3).

Thin-section CT from the neck to upper abdomen (to detect cervical and supraclavicular and hepatic and adrenal metastases) is the first staging test for both SCLC and NSCLC. However, CT often cannot distinguish postinflammatory from malignant intrathoracic lymph node enlargement or benign from malignant hepatic or adrenal lesions (distinctions that determine stage). Thus, other tests are usually performed when CT abnormalities are present in these areas. PET scanning is an accurate, noninvasive test used to identify malignant mediastinal lymph nodes and other distant metastases (metabolic staging). Integrated PET-CT, in which PET and CT images are combined into a single image by scanners in a single gantry, is more accurate for NSCLC staging than CT or PET alone or than visual correlation of the two tests. The use of PET and PET-CT is limited by cost and availability. When a PET scan is unavailable, bronchoscopy and, less commonly, mediastinoscopy or video-assisted thoracoscopy can be used to biopsy questionable mediastinal lymph nodes. Without PET scanning, suspect hepatic or adrenal lesions must be evaluated by needle biopsy.

MRI of the chest is slightly more accurate than high-chest HRCT for staging apical tumors and cancers close to the diaphragm.

Patients with headache or neurologic abnormalities should undergo head CT or MRI and evaluation for SVC syndrome. Patients with bone pain or elevated serum Ca or alkaline phosphatase should undergo a radionuclide bone scan. These imaging tests are not indicated in the absence of suspicious symptoms, signs, or laboratory test abnormalities. Other blood tests, such as CBC, serum albumin, and creatinine, play no role in staging but provide important prognostic information about the patient's ability to tolerate treatment.

Prognosis

Prognosis is poor, even with newer treatments. On average, untreated patients with advanced NSCLC survive 6 mo, whereas 5-yr survival for treated patients is about 9 mo. Patients with extensive-stage SCLC do especially poorly, with a 5-yr survival rate < 1%. The median survival time for limited-stage disease is 20 mo, with a 5-yr survival rate of 20%. In many patients with SCLC, chemotherapy prolongs life and improves quality of life enough to warrant its use. The 5-yr survival rate of patients with NSCLC varies by stage, from 60 to 70% for patients with stage I to virtually 0% for those with stage IV disease; recent evidence suggests improved survival in early-stage disease with a platinum-based chemotherapy regimen. Given the disappointing results in late-stage disease, efforts at reducing mortality have increasingly focused on early detection and active interventions to prevent disease.

A screening chest x-ray in high-risk patients detects lung carcinomas at early stages but does not decrease mortality. A screening CT is more sensitive for detecting tumors, but more false-positive readings increase the number of unnecessary invasive diagnostic procedures needed to verify CT findings. Such procedures are costly and risk complications. A strategy of yearly CT screening of smokers with follow-up PET scan or HRCT to evaluate indeterminate lesions is being studied. So far, this strategy does not seem to lessen mortality and cannot be recommended as routine practice. The future of screening may lie in a combination of molecular analysis for genetic markers (such as *K-RAS, p53, EGFR*), sputum cytometry, and detection of cancer-related volatile organic compounds (eg, alkane, benzene) in exhaled breath.

Treatment

Treatment generally involves assessment of eligibility for surgery followed by choice of surgery, chemotherapy, and/or radiation as appropriate, depending on tumor type and stage. Many nontumor-related factors affect eligibility. Poor cardiopulmonary reserve; malnutrition; frailty or poor physical performance status; comorbidities, including cytopenias; and psychiatric or cognitive illness all may lead to a decision for palliative over curative treatment or for no treatment at all, even though cure might technically be possible.

Surgery is performed only on patients who will have adequate pulmonary reserve once a lobe or lung is resected. Patients with preoperative forced expiratory volume in 1 sec (FEV_1) > 2 L generally tolerate pneumonectomy. Those with FEV_1 < 2 L should undergo a quantitative radionuclide perfusion scan to determine the proportion of function the patient can expect to lose from resection. Postoperative FEV_1 can be predicted by multiplying percent perfusion of the nonresected lung by the preoperative FEV_1. A predicted FEV_1 > 800 mL or > 40% of the predicted normal FEV_1 suggests adequate postoperative lung function, though studies of lung volume reduction surgery in COPD patients suggest that patients with FEV_1 < 800 mL can tolerate resection if the cancer is located in poorly functional bullous (generally apical) lung regions. Patients undergoing resection at hospitals that perform more resections have fewer complications and are more likely to survive than those who undergo surgery at low-volume hospitals.

Multiple chemotherapy regimens exist for treatment of lung carcinoma; no one regimen is proven superior. Choice of regimen, therefore, often depends on local practice, contraindications, and toxicities. Treatment options for disease that recurs after treatment vary by location and include repeat chemotherapy for local recurrence, radiation therapy for metastases, and brachytherapy for endobronchial disease when additional external radiation cannot be tolerated.

Radiation treatment carries the risk of radiation pneumonitis when large areas of lung are exposed to high doses of radiation over time. Radiation pneumonitis can occur up to 3 mo after treatment. Cough, dyspnea, low-grade fever, or pleuritic chest pain may signal the condition, as may rales or pleural friction rub. Chest x-rays may be nonspecific; CTs may show nonspecific infiltration without discrete mass. The diagnosis is often one of exclusion. Radiation pneumonitis is treated with 60 mg prednisone for 2 to 4 wk followed by a gradual taper.

Because many patients with lung carcinoma die, the need for end-of-life care should be anticipated. Symptoms of breathlessness, pain, anxiety, nausea, and anorexia are especially common and can be treated with parenteral morphine; oral, transdermal, or parenteral opioids; and antiemetics (see p. 2764).

SCLC: SCLC of any stage is typically initially responsive to treatment, but responses are usually short-lived. Surgery generally plays no role in treatment of SCLC, although it may be curative in the rare patient who has a small focal tumor without spread (such as a solitary pulmonary nodule).

In limited-stage disease, a combination of etoposide and a platinum compound (either cisplatin or carboplatin) in 4 to 6 cycles is thought to be most effective, although combinations with other drugs—including vinca alkaloids (vinblastine, vincristine, vinorelbine), alkylating drugs (cyclophosphamide, ifosfamide), doxorubicin, taxanes (docetaxel, paclitaxel), and gemcitabine—are also commonly used. Radiation further improves response; the very definition of limited-stage disease as disease confined to a hemithorax is based on the significant improvement in survival observed with radiation. The use of cranial radiation to prevent brain metastases is advocated by some experts; micrometastases are common in SCLC, and chemotherapy does not cross the blood-brain barrier.

In extensive-stage disease, treatment is the same as with limited-stage disease but without concurrent radiation. Replacing etoposide with topoisomerase inhibitors (irinotecan or topotecan) may improve survival. These drugs alone or in combination with other drugs are also commonly used in refractory disease and in cancer of either stage that has recurred. Radiation is often used as palliative treatment for metastases to bone or brain.

In general, recurrent SCLC carries a poor prognosis, although patients who maintain a good performance status should be offered a clinical trial.

NSCLC: Treatment of NSCLC depends on the stage. For stage I and II disease, the standard is surgical resection with either lobectomy or pneumonectomy combined with mediastinal lymph node sampling or complete dissection. Lesser resections, including segmentectomy and wedge resection, are considered for patients with poor pulmonary reserve. Surgery is curative in about 55 to 75% of patients with stage I and in 35 to 55% of patients with stage II disease. Adjuvant chemotherapy is probably helpful in early-stage disease (stages Ib and II). An increase in 5-yr overall survival (69% vs 54%) and disease-free survival (61% vs 49%) occurs with cisplatin plus vinorelbine. Because the improvement is small, the decision for adjuvant chemotherapy should be made on an individual basis. The role of neoadjuvant chemotherapy in early-stage NSCLC is under investigation.

Stage III disease is one or more locally advanced tumors with regional nodal involvement but no distant metastases. For stage IIIA tumors with occult mediastinal nodal metastases discovered at the time of surgery, resection results in 20 to 25% 5-yr survival. Radiation therapy with or without concurrent chemotherapy is considered standard for unresectable clinically staged IIIA disease, but survival is poor (median survival, 10 to 14 mo). Recent trials suggest slightly better results with preoperative chemotherapy plus radiation followed by surgery and subsequent chemotherapy. This remains an area of investigation.

Stage IIIB patients with contralateral mediastinal nodal disease, supraclavicular nodal disease, or malignant pleural effusions are offered radiation or chemotherapy or both. The addition of radiation-sensitizing chemotherapeutic drugs, such as cisplatin, paclitaxel, vincristine, and cyclophosphamide, improves survival slightly. Patients with locally advanced tumors invading the heart, great vessels, mediastinum, or spine usually receive radiation. In select cases (T4N0M0 tumors), surgical resection with either neoadjuvant or adjuvant chemoradiation may be feasible. The 5-yr survival rate for treated stage IIIB patients is 5%.

In stage IV disease, palliation of symptoms is the goal. Chemotherapy and radiation may be used to reduce tumor burden, treat symptoms, and improve quality of life. However, median survival is only 9 mo; < 25% of patients survive 1 yr. Surgical palliative procedures may be required and may include thoracentesis and pleurodesis of recurrent effusions, placement of indwelling pleural drainage catheters, bronchoscopic fulguration of tumors involving the trachea and mainstem bronchi, placement of stents to prevent airway occlusion, and, in some cases, spinal stabilization for impending spinal cord compression.

Several novel biologic agents specifically target lung tumors. Gefitinib, an epidermal growth factor receptor (EGFR) tyrosine kinase inhibitor, may be used in patients who have not responded to platinum and docetaxel therapy. Other biologic agents under investigation include other EGFR inhibitors, antisense oligonucleotides to EGFR mRNA (messenger RNA), and farnesyl transferase inhibitors.

It is important to distinguish between recurrent NSCLC, an independent 2nd primary tumor, locally recurrent NSCLC, and distant metastatic NSCLC. The treatment of an independent 2nd primary tumor and locally recurrent NSCLC follows the same guidelines as for primary tumor stages I to III. If surgery was used initially, radiation therapy is the main modality. If recurrence manifests as distant metastases, patients are treated as stage IV with a focus on palliation.

Complications: Initial treatment of malignant pleural effusion is with thoracentesis. Asymptomatic effusions require no treatment; symptomatic effusions that recur despite multiple thoracenteses are drained through a chest tube. Infusion of talc (or occasionally, tetracycline or bleomycin) into the pleural space (a procedure called pleurodesis) scars the pleura, eliminates the pleural space, and is effective in > 90% of cases (see p. 495).

Treatment of SVC syndrome is the same as treatment of lung carcinoma: with chemotherapy (SCLC), radiation therapy (NSCLC), or both (NSCLC). Corticosteroids are commonly used but are of unproven benefit. Treatment of apical tumors is with surgery with or without preoperative radiation or with radiation with or without adjuvant chemotherapy. Treatment of paraneoplastic syndromes varies by syndrome (see p. 1150).

Prevention

No active interventions are proven effective except for smoking cessation. Remediation of high radon levels in private residences removes known cancer-promoting radiation, but a reduction in lung cancer incidence is unproven. Increasing dietary intake of fruits and vegetables high in retinoids and β-carotene appears to have no effect on lung carcinoma incidence. Vitamin supplementation is either unproven (vitamin E) or harmful (β-carotene) in smokers. Preliminary evidence hinting that NSAIDs and vitamin E supplementation may protect former smokers from lung carcinoma requires confirmation. New molecular approaches targeting cell signaling and cell cycle pathways and tumor-associated antigens are under investigation.

AIRWAY TUMORS

Airway tumors can arise from primary tracheobronchial tumors, adjacent primary tumors with airway invasion, or metastatic disease to the airway.

Primary tracheal tumors are rare (0.1/100,000 people). They are often malignant and found at a locally advanced stage. The most common malignant tracheal tumors include adenoid cystic carcinoma, squamous cell carcinoma, carcinoid, and mucoepidermoid carcinomas. The most common benign airway tumor is a squamous papilloma, although pleomorphic adenomas and granular cell and benign cartilaginous tumors also occur.

Symptoms, Signs, and Diagnosis

Patients often present with dyspnea, cough, wheezing, hemoptysis, and stridor. Hemoptysis occurs with squamous cell carcinoma and can lead to earlier diagnosis, whereas wheezing or stridor occurs more often with the adenoid cystic variant. Dysphagia and hoarseness can also be present initially and usually indicate advanced disease.

Symptoms of airway narrowing can herald life-threatening airway obstruction and require immediate hospitalization and evaluation with bronchoscopy. Bronchoscopy can both stabilize the airways and obtain specimens for diagnosis. If a malignancy is found, more extensive testing for metastases is done.

Prognosis and Treatment

Prognosis depends on the histology. Squamous cell carcinomas tend to metastasize to regional lymph nodes and directly invade mediastinal structures, leading to high local and regional recurrence rates. Even with definitive surgical resection, the 5-yr survival is 20 to 40%. Adenoid cystic carcinomas are typically indolent but tend to metastasize to the lungs and to spread perineurally, leading to high recurrence rates after resection. However, these patients have a higher 5-yr survival of 60 to 75% because of the slow rate of growth.

Primary airway tumors should be treated definitively with surgical resection if possible. Tracheal, laryngotracheal, or carinal resections are the most common procedures. Up to 50% of the length of the trachea can be safely resected with primary re-anastomosis. If a lung or thyroid cancer invades the airway, surgery is sometimes still feasible if assessment indicates sufficient tissue available for airway reconstruction. Adjuvant radiation is recommended if adequate surgical margins cannot be obtained.

Most primary airway tumors are not resectable because of metastasis, locally advanced stage, or patient comorbidities. In cases of endoluminal tumors, a therapeutic bronchoscopy can mechanically core-out the tumor. Other techniques to eliminate obstruction include laser vaporization, photodynamic therapy, cryotherapy, and endobronchial brachytherapy. Tumors that compress the trachea are treated with airway stenting, radiotherapy, or both.

BRONCHIAL CARCINOID

Bronchial carcinoids are rare, slow-growing neuroendocrine tumors arising from bronchial mucosa that affect patients in their 40s to 60s.

Half of patients are asymptomatic, and ½ present with symptoms of airway obstruction, including dyspnea, wheezing, and cough, which often leads to a misdiagnosis of asthma. Recurrent pneumonia, hemoptysis, and chest pain are also common. Paraneoplastic syndromes, including Cushing's syndrome due to ectopic ACTH, acromegaly due to ectopic growth hormone–releasing factor, and Zollinger-Ellison due to ectopic gastrin production, are more common than carcinoid syndrome (see p. 1313), which occurs in <3% of patients with the tumor. A left-sided heart murmur (mitral stenosis or regurgitation) occurs rarely due to serotonin-induced valvular damage (as opposed to the right-sided valvular lesions of GI carcinoid).

Diagnosis is based on bronchoscopic biopsy, but evaluation often initially involves chest CT, which reveals tumor calcifications in up to ⅓ of patients. Indium-111–labeled octreotide scans are useful for determining regional and metastatic spread. Increased urinary serotonin and 5-hydroxyindoleacetic acid levels support the diagnosis but are not commonly present.

Treatment is with surgical removal with or without adjuvant chemotherapy. Prognosis depends on tumor type. Five-year survival for typical (well-differentiated) carcinoids is > 90%; for atypical tumors, 50 to 70%.

CHEST WALL TUMORS

Primary chest wall tumors consist of 5% of all thoracic tumors and 1 to 2% of all primary tumors. Almost ½ are benign, the most common of which are osteochondroma, chondroma, and fibrous dysplasia. A wide range of malignant chest wall tumors exist. Over ½ are metastases from distant organs or direct invasions from adjacent structures (breast, lung, pleura, mediastinum). The most common malignant primary tumors arising from the chest wall are sarcomas; about 45% originate from soft tissue and 55% from cartilaginous or bony tissue. Chondrosarcomas are the most common primary bone chest wall sarcoma and arise in the anterior tract of ribs and less commonly from the sternum, scapula, or clavicle. Other bony tumors include osteosarcoma and small-cell malignant tumors (Ewing's sarcoma, Askin's tumor). The most common soft-tissue primary malignant tumors are fibrosarcomas (desmoids, neurofibrosarcomas) and malignant fibrous histiocytomas. Other primary tumors include chondroblastomas, osteoblastomas, melanomas, lymphomas, rhabdomyosarcomas, lymphangiosarcomas, multiple myeloma, and plasmacytomas.

Symptoms, Signs, and Diagnosis

Soft-tissue chest wall tumors often present as a localized mass without other symptoms; some patients have fever. Patients usually do not experience pain until the tumor is more advanced. In contrast, primary cartilaginous and bone tumors are often painful.

Patients with chest wall tumors require chest x-ray, CT, and sometimes an MRI to determine the original site and extent of the tumor and whether it is a primary chest wall tumor or a metastasis. Biopsy confirms the diagnosis.

Prognosis and Treatment

Prognosis varies by cell type and stage; firm conclusions are limited by the low incidence of any given tumor. Sarcomas have been the most well studied, and primary chest wall sarcomas have a reported 5-yr survival of 16.7%. Survival is better with early-stage disease.

Most chest wall tumors are treated with surgical resection and reconstruction as the primary modality. Reconstruction often utilizes a combination of myocutaneous flaps and prosthetic materials. The presence of a malignant pleural effusion is a contraindication for surgical resection. Also, in cases of multiple myeloma or isolated plasmacytoma, chemotherapy and radiation should be the primary therapy. Small-cell malignant tumors such as Ewing's sarcoma and Askin's tumor should be treated with a multimodality approach combining chemotherapy, radiation, and surgery. In cases of chest wall metastasis from distant tumors, a palliative chest wall resection is recommended only when nonsurgical options do not alleviate symptoms.

SECTION 6

CRITICAL CARE MEDICINE

63 APPROACH TO THE CRITICALLY ILL PATIENT

Critical care medicine specializes in caring for the most seriously ill patients. These patients are best treated in an ICU with experienced personnel. Some hospitals maintain separate units for special populations (eg, cardiac, surgical, neurologic, pediatric, or neonatal patients). ICUs have a high nurse:patient ratio to provide the necessary high intensity of service, including treatment and monitoring of physiologic parameters.

Supportive care for the ICU patient includes provision of adequate nutrition (see p. 22) and prevention of infection, stress ulcers and gastritis (see p. 118), and pulmonary embolism (see p. 420). Because 15 to 25% of patients admitted to ICUs die there, physicians should know how to minimize suffering and help dying patients maintain dignity (see p. 2762).

PATIENT MONITORING AND TESTING

Some monitoring is manual (ie, by direct observation and physical examination) and intermittent, with the frequency depending on the patient's illness. This monitoring usually includes measurement of vital signs (temperature, BP, pulse, and respiration rate), quantification of all fluid intake and output, and often daily weight. BP may be recorded by an automated sphygmomanometer; many of these devices also incorporate a transcutaneous sensor for pulse oximetry, which is monitored as well.

Other monitoring is ongoing and continuous, provided by complex devices that require special training and experience. Most such devices generate an alarm if certain physiologic parameters are exceeded. Every ICU should strictly follow protocols for investigating alarms.

Blood Tests

Although frequent blood draws can destroy veins, cause pain, and lead to anemia, ICU patients typically have routine daily blood tests to help detect problems early. Generally, patients need a daily set of electrolytes and a CBC. Patients with arrhythmias should also have Mg, phosphate, and Ca levels. Patients on TPN need weekly liver enzymes and coagulation profiles. Other tests are done as needed (eg, blood culture for fever, CBC after bleeding episode).

Point-of-care testing uses miniaturized, highly automated devices to perform certain blood tests at the patient's bedside or unit (particularly ICU, emergency department, and operating room). Commonly available tests include blood chemistries, glucose, ABGs, CBC, cardiac markers, and coagulation tests. Many are performed in < 2 min and require < 0.5 mL blood.

Cardiac Monitoring

Most critical care patients have cardiac activity monitored by a 3-lead system; signals are usually sent to a central monitoring station by a small radio transmitter worn by the patient. Automated systems generate alarms for abnormal rates and rhythms and store abnormal tracings for subsequent review.

Some specialized cardiac monitors track advanced parameters associated with coronary ischemia, although their clinical benefit is unclear. These include continuous ST segment monitoring and heart rate variability. Loss of normal beat-to-beat variability signals a reduction in autonomic activity and possibly coronary ischemia and increased risk of death.

Pulmonary Artery Catheter Monitoring

Use of a pulmonary artery catheter (PAC) is common in ICU patients. This device is a balloon-tipped, flow-directed catheter that is inserted via central veins through the right side of the heart into the pulmonary artery. The catheter typically contains several ports that can monitor pressure or inject fluids. Some PACs also include a sensor to measure central (mixed) venous O_2 saturation. Data from PACs are used mainly to determine cardiac output and preload. Preload is most commonly estimated by the pulmonary artery occlusion pressure (PAOP—see p. 515). However, preload may be more accurately determined by right ventricular end-diastolic volume, which is measured through the use

TABLE 63–1. POTENTIAL INDICATIONS FOR PULMONARY ARTERY CATHETERIZATION

Cardiac disorders
- Acute valvular regurgitation
- Cardiac tamponade
- Complicated heart failure
- Complicated MI
- Ventricular septal rupture

Hemodynamic instability*
- Assessment of volume status
- Shock

Hemodynamic monitoring
- Cardiac surgery
- Postoperative care in critically ill patients
- Surgery and postoperative care in patients with significant heart disease

Pulmonary disorders
- Complicated pulmonary embolism
- Pulmonary hypertension

*Particularly if inotropic drugs required.

of fast-response thermistors gated to heart rate.

Despite widespread use, PACs have not been shown to reduce morbidity and mortality. Indeed, PAC use has been associated with excess mortality. This finding may be explained by complications of PAC use and misinterpretation of the data obtained. Nevertheless, most physicians believe PACs aid in the management of certain critically ill patients when combined with other objective and clinical data. As with many physiologic measurements, a changing trend is typically more significant than a single abnormal value. Possible indications for PACs are listed in TABLE 63–1.

Procedure: The PAC is inserted through the subclavian or internal jugular vein with the balloon deflated. Once the catheter tip reaches the superior vena cava, partial inflation of the balloon permits blood flow to guide the catheter. The position of the catheter tip is usually determined by pressure monitoring (see TABLE 63–2 for intracardiac and great vessel pressures) or occasionally by fluoroscopy. Entry into the right ventricle is indicated by a sudden increase in systolic pressure to about 30 mm Hg; diastolic pressure remains unchanged from right atrial or vena caval pressure. When the catheter enters the pulmonary artery, the systolic pressure does not change, but diastolic pressure rises above right ventricular end-diastolic pressure or central venous pressure (CVP), ie, the pulse pressure narrows. Further movement of the catheter wedges the balloon in a distal pulmonary artery. A chest x-ray confirms proper placement.

The systolic pressure (normal, 15 to 30 mm Hg) and diastolic pressure (normal, 5 to 13 mm Hg) are recorded with the catheter balloon deflated. The diastolic pressure corresponds well to the occlusion pressure, although diastolic pressure can exceed occlusion pressure when pulmonary vascular resistance is elevated secondary to primary pulmonary disease (eg, pulmonary fibrosis, pulmonary hypertension).

TABLE 63–2. NORMAL PRESSURES IN THE HEART AND GREAT VESSELS

TYPE OF PRESSURE	AVERAGE (mm Hg)	RANGE (mm Hg)
Right atrium	3	0–8
Right ventricle		
Peak-systolic	25	15–30
End-diastolic	4	0–8
Pulmonary artery		
Mean	15	9–16
Peak-systolic	25	15–30
End-diastolic	9	4–14
Pulmonary artery occlusion		
Mean	9	2–12
Left atrium		
Mean	8	2–12
A wave	10	4–16
V wave	13	6–12
Left ventricle		
Peak-systolic	130	90–140
End-diastolic	9	5–12
Brachial artery		
Mean	85	70–150
Peak-systolic	130	90–140
End-diastolic	70	60–90

Adapted from Fowler NO: *Cardiac Diagnosis and Treatment*, ed 3. Philadelphia, JB Lippincott, 1980, p. 11.

Pulmonary artery occlusion pressure (PAOP): With the balloon inflated, pressure at the tip of the catheter reflects the static back pressure of the pulmonary veins. The balloon must not remain inflated for > 30 sec to prevent pulmonary infarction. Normally, PAOP approximates left atrial pressure, which in turn approximates left ventricular end-diastolic pressure (LVEDP), which itself reflects left ventricular end-diastolic volume (LVEDV). The LVEDV represents preload, which is the actual target parameter. Many factors cause PAOP to reflect LVEDV inaccurately. These factors include mitral stenosis, high levels of positive end-expiratory pressure (> 10 cm H_2O), and changes in left ventricular compliance (eg, due to MI, pericardial effusion, or increased afterload). Technical difficulties result from excessive balloon inflation, improper catheter position, alveolar pressure exceeding pulmonary venous pressure, or severe pulmonary hypertension (which may make the balloon difficult to wedge).

Elevated PAOP occurs in left-sided heart failure. Decreased PAOP occurs in hypovolemia or decreased preload.

Mixed venous oxygenation: Mixed venous blood comprises blood from the superior and inferior vena cava that has passed through the right heart to the pulmonary artery. The blood may be sampled from the distal port of the PAC, but some catheters have embedded fiberoptic sensors that directly measure O_2 saturation. Causes of low mixed venous O_2 content ($SmvO_2$) include anemia, pulmonary disease, carboxyhemoglobin, low cardiac output, and increased tissue metabolic needs. The ratio of SaO_2 to (SaO_2 minus $SmvO_2$) determines the adequacy of O_2 delivery. The ideal ratio is 4:1, whereas 2:1 is the minimum acceptable ratio to maintain aerobic metabolic needs.

Cardiac output: Cardiac output (CO) is measured either by intermittent bolus injection of ice water or, in new catheters, continuous warm thermodilution. The cardiac index divides the CO by body surface area to correct for patient size (see TABLE 63–3).

Other variables can be calculated from the CO. These include systemic and pulmonary vascular resistance and right and left ventricular stroke work (RVSW, LVSW).

Complications and precautions: PACs may be difficult to insert. Cardiac arrhythmias are the most common complication. Pulmonary infarction secondary to overinflated or permanently wedged balloons, pulmonary artery perforation, intracardiac perforation, valvular injury, and endocarditis may occur. Rarely, the catheter may curl into a knot within the right ventricle (especially in patients with heart failure, cardiomyopathy, or increased pulmonary pressure).

TABLE 63–3. NORMAL VALUES FOR CARDIAC INDEX AND RELATED MEASUREMENTS

MEASUREMENT	UNITS ± SD
O_2 uptake	143 ± 14.3 mL/min/m^2
Arteriovenous O_2 difference	4.1 ± 0.6 dL
Cardiac index	3.5 ± 0.7 L/min/m^2
Stroke index	46 ± 8.1 mL/beat/m^2
Total systemic resistance	1130 ± 178 dynes-sec-cm^{-5}
Total pulmonary resistance	205 ± 51 dynes-sec-cm^{-5}
Pulmonary arteriolar resistance	67 ± 23 dynes-sec-cm^{-5}

SD = standard deviation.

Adapted from Barratt-Boyes BG, Wood EH: Cardiac output and related measurements and pressure values in the right heart and associated vessels, together with an analysis of the hemodynamic response to the inhalation of high oxygen mixtures in healthy subjects. *Journal of Laboratory and Clinical Medicine* 51:72–90, 1958.

Pulmonary artery rupture occurs in < 0.1% of PAC insertions. This catastrophic complication is often fatal and occurs immediately upon wedging the catheter—either initially or on subsequent occlusion pressure check. Because of this, many physicians prefer to monitor pulmonary artery diastolic pressures rather than occlusion pressures.

Noninvasive Cardiac Output

To avoid the complications of PACs, other methods of determining CO are being developed.

Thoracic bioimpedance systems use topical electrodes on the anterior chest and neck to measure electrical impedance of the thorax. This value varies with beat-to-beat changes in thoracic blood volume and hence can estimate

CO. The system is harmless and provides values quickly (within 2 to 5 min); however, the technique is very sensitive to alteration of the electrode contact with the patient. Thoracic bioimpedance is more valuable in recognizing changes in a given patient than in precisely measuring CO.

The esophageal Doppler monitor (EDM) device is a soft 6-mm catheter that is passed nasopharyngeally into the esophagus and positioned behind the heart. A Doppler flow probe at its tip allows continuous monitoring of CO and stroke volume. Unlike the invasive PAC, the EDM does not cause pneumothorax, arrhythmia, or infection. An EDM may actually be more accurate than a PAC in patients with cardiac valvular lesions, septal defects, arrhythmias, or pulmonary hypertension. However, the EDM may lose its waveform with only a slight positional change and produce dampened, inaccurate readings.

Consequently, while thoracic bioimpedance and EDM are potentially useful, neither is yet as reliable as a PAC.

Intracranial Pressure Monitoring

Intracranial pressure (ICP) monitoring is standard for patients with severe closed head injury. These devices are used to optimize cerebral perfusion pressure (mean arterial pressure minus intracranial pressure). Typically, the cerebral perfusion pressure should be kept > 70 mm Hg.

Several types of ICP monitors are available. The most useful method places a catheter through the skull into a cerebral ventricle ("ventriculostomy" catheter). This device is preferred because the catheter can also drain CSF and hence decrease ICP. However, the ventriculostomy is also the most invasive method, has the highest infection rate, and is the most difficult to place. Occasionally, the ventriculostomy becomes occluded due to severe brain edema.

Other types of intracranial devices include an intraparenchymal monitor and an epidural bolt. Of these, the intraparenchymal monitor is more commonly used. All ICP devices should generally be changed or removed after 5 to 7 days due to the risk of infection.

Other Types of Monitoring

Gastric tonometry determines the gastric intramucosal pH (pH_i) and tissue CO_2 through a special nasogastric tube with a semipermeable liquid- or gas-filled balloon at the tip. Both a decreased pH_i and an elevated tissue CO_2 to arterial CO_2 ratio occur with decreased splanchnic perfusion and therefore are markers of systemic hypoperfusion. The liquid-filled balloon requires intermittent sampling. The gas-filled balloon has an infrared sensor at the tip that provides a constant readout; however, this model has not proved very reliable. Although able to diagnose hypoperfusion, the readings are slow to normalize after successful resuscitation.

Sublingual capnometry uses a similar correlation between elevated sublingual pCO_2 and systemic hypoperfusion to monitor shock states using a noninvasive sensor placed under the tongue. This is easier to use than gastric tonometry and responds quickly to perfusion changes with resuscitation.

Tissue spectroscopy uses a noninvasive near infrared (NIR) sensor generally placed on the skin above the target tissue to monitor mitochondrial cytochrome a,a redox states, which reflect tissue perfusion. NIR may help diagnose acute compartment syndromes (eg, in trauma) or ischemia after free tissue transfer, and may be helpful in postoperative monitoring of lower extremity vascular bypass grafts. NIR monitoring of small-bowel pH may be used to gauge the adequacy of resuscitation.

SCORING SYSTEMS

Several scoring systems have been developed to grade the severity of illness in critically ill patients. These systems are moderately accurate in predicting individual survival but are more valuable for monitoring quality of care by enabling comparison of outcomes among groups of critically ill patients with similar illness severity.

The most common system is the 2nd version of the Acute Physiologic Assessment and Chronic Health Evaluation (APACHE II) score introduced in 1985. It generates a point score ranging from 0 to 71 based on 12 physiologic variables, age, and underlying health (see TABLE 63–4). The APACHE III system was developed in 1991 and is more complex than the APACHE II system, having 17 physiologic variables, and is somewhat less used. Many other systems exist, including the 2nd Simplified Acute Physiology Score (SAPS II) and several Mortality Probability Models.

VASCULAR ACCESS

A number of procedures are used to gain vascular access.

TABLE 63–4. APACHE II SCORING SYSTEM*

PHYSIOLOGIC VARIABLE†	POINT SCORE								
	+4	+3	+2	+1	0	+1	+2	+3	+4
1 Temperature, core (°C)	≥ 41°	39–40.9°	—	38.5–38.9°	36–38.4°	34–35.9°	32–33.9°	30–31.9°	≤ 29.9°
2 Mean arterial pressure (mm Hg)	≥ 160	130–159	110–129	—	70–109	—	50–69	—	≤ 49
3 Heart rate	≥ 180	140–179	110–139	—	70–109	—	55–69	40–54	≤ 39
4 Respiratory rate (non-ventilated or ventilated)	≥ 50	35–49	—	25–34	12–24	10–11	6–9	—	≤ 5
5 Oxygenation: a) $FIO_2 \geq 0.5$: use $A\text{-}aDO_2$	≥ 500	350–499	200–349	—	< 200	—	—		
b) $FIO_2 < 0.5$: use PaO_2 (mm Hg)	—	—	—	—	> 70	61–70	—	55–60	< 55
6 Arterial pH	≥ 7.7	7.6–7.69	—	7.5–7.59	7.33–7.49	—	7.25–7.32	7.15–7.24	< 7.15
7 Serum Na (mMol/L)	≥ 180	160–179	155–159	150–154	130–149	—	120–129	111–119	≤ 110
8 Serum K (mMol/L)	≥ 7	6–6.9	—	5.5–5.9	3.5–5.4	3–3.4	2.5–2.9	—	< 2.5
9 Serum creatinine (mg/dL); double point score for **acute** renal failure	≥ 3.5	2–3.4	1.5–1.9	—	0.6–1.4	—	< 0.6	—	—
10 Hct (%)	≥ 60	—	50–59.9	46–49.9	30–45.9	—	20–29.9	—	< 20
11 WBC (in 1000s)	≥ 40	—	20–39.9	15–19.9	3–14.9	—	1–2.9	—	< 1
12 Glasgow coma score (GCS)	Score = 15 minus actual GCS (see TABLE 212–2 on p. 1803)								

Acute physiology score is the sum of the 12 individual variable points.
Add 0 points for age < 44; 2 points, 45–54 yr; 3 points, 55–64 yr; 5 points, 65–74 yr; 6 points ≥ 75 yr.
Add chronic health status points: 2 points if elective postoperative patient with immunocompromise or history of severe organ insufficiency; 5 points for nonoperative patient or emergency postoperative patient with immunocompromise or severe organ insufficiency.‡

	+4	+3	+2	+1	0	+1	+2	+3	+4
(13)§ Serum HCO_3 (venous-mMol/L) use only if no ABGs	≥ 52	41–51.9	—	32–40.9	22–31.9	—	18–21.9	15–17.9	< 15

*APACHE II Score = acute physiology score + age points + chronic health points. Minimum score = 0; maximum score = 71. Increasing score is associated with increasing risk of hospital death.
†Choose worst value in the past 24 h.
‡Chronic health status: Organ insufficiency (eg, hepatic, cardiovascular, renal, pulmonary) or immunocompromised state must have preceded current admission.
§Optional variable; use only if no ABGs.

Adapted from Knaus WA, Draper EA, Wagner DP, Zimmerman JE: APACHE II: A severity of disease classification system. *Critical Care Medicine* 13:818–829, 1985.

Peripheral Vein Catheterization

Most patients' needs for IV fluid and drugs can be met with a percutaneous peripheral venous catheter. Venous cutdown can be used when percutaneous catheter insertion is not feasible. Typical cutdown sites are the cephalic vein in the arm and the saphenous vein at the ankle.

Common complications (eg, local infection, venous thrombosis, thrombophlebitis, interstitial fluid extravasation) can be reduced by meticulous sterile technique during insertion and by replacing or removing the catheters within 72 h.

Central Venous Catheterization

Patients needing secure or long-term vascular access (eg, for administration of antibiotics, chemotherapy, or TPN) are best treated with a central venous catheter (CVC). CVCs allow infusion of solutions that are too concentrated or irritating for peripheral veins and also allow monitoring of central venous pressure (CVP—see p. 565).

Procedure: CVCs are inserted using sterile technique and local anesthesia (eg, 1% lidocaine). The superior vena cava is entered via percutaneous puncture of the subclavian or the internal or external jugular vein or by venous cutdown on the basilic vein. The inferior vena cava may be entered through the common femoral vein percutaneously or by cutdown on the saphenous vein. The choice of site depends on operator preference and patient habitus and ambulatory status. However, femoral venous catheters have a slightly higher rate of complications than those above the waist. Also, during cardiac arrest, fluid and drugs administered through a femoral or saphenous vein CVC often fail to circulate above the diaphragm because of the increased intrathoracic pressure generated by CPR. In this case, a subclavian or internal jugular approach may be preferred.

If possible, the patient's coagulation status and platelet count should be normalized before CVC insertion. Percutaneous femoral lines must be inserted below the inguinal ligament. Otherwise, laceration of the external iliac vein or artery above the inguinal ligament may result in retroperitoneal hemorrhage; external compression of these vessels is nearly impossible. The subclavian vein also is not compressible with external pressure, and thus hemorrhage can be serious. A cutdown decreases the risk of bleeding-associated complications, particularly if coagulopathy is present.

After a subclavian or internal jugular catheter is inserted, a chest x-ray is taken to locate the catheter tip and to exclude a pneumothorax. To prevent cardiac arrhythmias, catheters in the right atrium or ventricle should be withdrawn until the tip is within the superior vena cava.

To reduce the risk of venous thrombosis and catheter sepsis, CVCs should be removed as soon as possible. The skin entry site must be cleansed and inspected daily for local infection; the catheter must be replaced if local or systemic infection occurs. Some clinicians feel it is beneficial to change CVC catheters at regular intervals (eg, q 5 to 7 days) in patients with sepsis who remain febrile; this may reduce the risk of bacterial colonization of the catheter.

Complications: CVCs can cause many complications (see TABLE 63–5). Pneumothorax occurs in 1% of patients after CVC insertion. Atrial or ventricular arrhythmias frequently occur during catheter insertion but are generally self-limited and subside when the guide wire or catheter is withdrawn from within the heart. The incidence of catheter bacterial colonization without systemic infection may be as high as 35%, whereas that of true sepsis is 2 to 8%. Accidental arterial catheterization may rarely require surgical repair of the artery. Hydrothorax and hydromediastinum may occur when catheters are positioned extravascularly. Catheter damage to the tricuspid valve, bacterial endocarditis, and air and catheter embolism occur rarely.

Arterial Catheterization

The use of automated noninvasive BP devices has diminished the use of arterial lines simply for pressure monitoring. However, they are beneficial in unstable patients who require minute-to-minute pressure measurement and in those requiring frequent ABG sampling. Indications include refractory shock and respiratory failure. The BP is frequently somewhat higher when measured by an arterial catheter than by sphygmomanometry. Initial upstroke, maximum systolic pressure, and pulse pressure increase the more distal the point of measurement, while the diastolic and mean arterial pressures decline. Vessel calcification, atherosclerosis, proximal occlusion, and extremity position can all affect the value of arterial catheter measurements.

Procedure: Arterial catheters are inserted using sterile technique and local anesthesia (eg, 1% lidocaine). They are typically inserted percutaneously into the radial, femoral, axillary, brachial, dorsalis pedis, and (in children) temporal arteries. The radial artery is most frequently used; insertion into the femoral artery has fewer complications but should be avoided after vascular bypass surgery (due to potential injury to the bypass graft) or if distal vascular insufficiency is present (to avoid precipitating ischemia). When percutaneous insertion is unsuccessful, a cutdown may be performed.

Before radial artery catheterization, Allen's test (digital compression of both ulnar and radial arteries causes palmar blanching followed by hyperemia when either artery is released) can determine if there is sufficient ulnar collateral flow to perfuse the hand in the event of radial artery occlusion. If reperfusion does not occur within 8 sec of releasing the compressed ulnar artery, arterial catheterization should not be performed.

Complications: At all sites, bleeding, infection, thrombosis, and distal embolism may occur. Catheters should be removed if signs of local or systemic infection are present.

Radial arterial complications include ischemia of the hand and forearm due to thrombosis or embolism, intimal dissection, or spasm at the site of catheterization. The risk of arterial thrombosis is higher in small arteries (explaining the greater incidence in women) and with increased duration of catheterization. Occluded arteries nearly always recanalize after catheter removal.

Femoral arterial complications include atheroembolism during guide wire insertion. The incidence of thrombosis and distal ischemia is much lower than for radial arterial catheterization.

Axillary arterial complications include hematomas, which are infrequent but may require urgent care because brachial plexus compression can result in permanent peripheral neuropathy. Flushing the axillary arterial catheter may introduce air or a clot. To avoid neurologic sequelae of these emboli, the left axillary artery should be selected for catheterization (the left axillary artery branches further distal to the carotid vessels than does the right).

Intraosseous Infusion

Any fluid or substance routinely administered IV (including blood products) may be given via a sturdy needle inserted in the medullary cavity of select long bones. Fluids reach the central circulation as quickly as with venous infusion. This technique is used almost exclusively in infants and young children, whose bony cortices are thin and easily penetrated and in whom peripheral and central venous access can be quite difficult, particularly in shock or cardiac arrest, but it can be used in older patients.

Procedure: A special-purpose intraosseous needle with stylet is used. The preferred insertion sites in children are the proximal tibia and distal femur; both areas are given a sterile preparation and included in the operative field. For tibial insertion, the needle is placed on the broad, flat anteromedial surface 1 to 2 cm distal to the tibial tubercle. For the femur, the

TABLE 63–5. COMPLICATIONS ASSOCIATED WITH CENTRAL VENOUS LINES

COMPLICATION	POSSIBLE SEQUELAE
Common	
Carotid injury	Bleeding, respiratory compromise, a neurologic event
Puncture of pleura or lung	Pneumothorax
Puncture of vein	Bleeding, extravasation of fluid, hemodynamic compromise
Subclavian artery injury	Bleeding, vascular compromise of the extremity, hemothorax, hemodynamic compromise
Less common	
Air embolism	Cardiac arrest
Arrhythmias	Cardiac arrest
Brachial plexus injury	Compromise of an extremity
Erosion of catheter	Bleeding, extravasation of fluid, hemodynamic compromise
Infection	Sepsis
Injury to clavicle, rib, or vertebra	Osteomyelitis
Lymphatic injury	Chylothorax
Valvular injury	Endocarditis

site is 3 cm above the lateral condyle in the midline. For older children, the medial surface of the distal tibia 2 cm above the medial malleolus may be easier.

For all sites, the needle is inserted with a rotary, coring motion. Stabilizing the needle shaft at the skin surface with a gloved fingertip aids control, allowing advancement to be stopped once the cortex is penetrated. On entering the medullary cavity, the stylet is removed and infusion begun.

Complications: Poor control during insertion may result in the needle exiting the opposite cortex; subsequent infusion will largely enter the soft tissues, so a site on another bone should be tried. Osteomyelitis may occur, but is uncommon (eg, < 2 to 3%). Growth plate damage has not been reported. Other complications include bleeding and compartment syndrome.

OXYGEN DESATURATION

(Hypoxia)

ICU (and other) patients without respiratory disorders may develop hypoxia (O_2 saturation < 90%) during a hospital stay. Hypoxia in patients with known respiratory conditions is discussed under those disorders.

Etiology

Numerous disorders cause hypoxia (eg, dyspnea, respiratory failure); however, acute hypoxia developing in a patient hospitalized with a nonrespiratory illness usually has a more limited set of causes. These can be divided into disorders of ventilation and oxygenation.

Ventilation: Decreased ventilatory drive typically results from oversedation, fatigue, deterioration of mental status from an underlying condition (eg, head injury, sepsis, stroke), or shock of any etiology. Severe pain (eg, from rib fractures, thoracic or abdominal surgery) occasionally limits ventilation enough to cause hypoxia.

Obstruction to ventilation can result from mucus plugging of airways or endotracheal tube, bronchospasm, and endotracheal tube dislodgement.

Oxygenation: Common pulmonary causes include atelectasis, pneumonia, pneumothorax, pulmonary embolus (PE), pulmonary contusion, and aspiration pneumonitis. Acute respiratory distress syndrome (ARDS—see p. 556) may develop following sepsis, trauma, pancreatitis, or disseminated intravascular coagulation. Fat emboli syndrome may occur following major bony injury (eg, pelvis or femur fracture).

Nonpulmonary causes are primarily iatrogenic fluid overload and heart failure (either an exacerbation of underlying disease or from an acute MI during hospitalization).

Evaluation

Total fluid administration over the hospital stay and, in particular, the previous 24 h should be ascertained to identify volume overload. Drugs should be reviewed for sedative administration and dosage. In significant hypoxia (O_2 saturation < 85%), treatment begins simultaneously with evaluation.

History: Very sudden onset dyspnea and hypoxia suggests PE or pneumothorax (mainly in a patient on positive pressure ventilation). Fever, chills, and productive cough (or increased secretions) suggest pneumonia. A history of cardiopulmonary disease (eg, asthma, COPD, heart failure) may indicate an exacerbation thereof. Unilateral extremity pain suggests deep venous thrombosis (DVT) and hence possible PE.

Physical examination: Patency of the airway and strength and adequacy of respirations should be immediately assessed. For patients on mechanical ventilation, it is important to determine that the endotracheal tube is not obstructed or dislodged. Unilateral decreased breath sounds with clear lung fields suggests pneumothorax or right mainstem bronchus intubation; with crackles and fever, pneumonia is more likely. Distended neck veins with bilateral lung crackles suggests volume overload; distention with clear lungs and tracheal deviation suggests tension pneumothorax. Bilateral lower extremity edema suggests heart failure, but unilateral edema suggests DVT and hence possible PE. Wheezing represents bronchospasm (typically asthma or allergic reaction, but it may rarely occur with PE or heart failure). Decreased mental status suggests hypoventilation.

Testing: Hypoxia is generally recognized initially by pulse oximetry. Patients should have a chest x-ray, ECG, and an ABG (to confirm hypoxia and evaluate adequacy of ventilation). If diagnosis remains unclear after this, testing for PE (see p. 414) should be considered. Bronchoscopy may be performed in the intubated patient to rule out (and remove) a tracheobronchial plug. Pulmonary artery catheterization may be needed to rule out heart failure if volume status is unclear.

Treatment

Identified causes are treated as discussed elsewhere in THE MANUAL. If hypoventilation persists, mechanical ventilation via noninvasive positive pressure ventilation or endotracheal intubation is necessary (see p. 544). Persistent hypoxia requires supplemental O_2.

O_2 therapy: The amount of O_2 administered is guided by ABG or pulse oximetry to maintain PaO_2 between 60 and 80 mm Hg (ie, 92 to 100% saturation) without causing O_2 toxicity. This level provides satisfactory tissue O_2 delivery; because the oxyhemoglobin dissociation curve is sigmoidal, increasing PaO_2 to > 80 mm Hg increases O_2 delivery very little and is not necessary. The lowest fractional inspired O_2 (FIO_2) that provides an acceptable PaO_2 should be provided. O_2 toxicity is both concentration- and time-dependent. Sustained elevations in FIO_2 > 60% result in inflammatory changes, alveolar infiltration, and, eventually, pulmonary fibrosis. An FIO_2 > 60% should be avoided unless necessary for survival. An FIO_2 < 60% is well tolerated for long periods.

An FIO_2 < 40% can be given via nasal cannula or simple face mask. Nasal cannulas use an O_2 flow of 1 to 6 L/min. Because 6 L/min is sufficient to fill the nasopharynx, higher flow rates are of no benefit. Simple face masks and nasal cannulas do not deliver a precise FIO_2 because of admixture of O_2 with room air from leakage and mouth breathing. However, Venturi-type masks can deliver very accurate O_2 concentrations.

An FIO_2 > 40% requires use of an O_2 mask with a reservoir that is inflated by O_2 from the supply. In the typical non-rebreather mask, the patient inhales 100% O_2 from the reservoir, but on exhalation a rubber flap valve diverts exhaled breath to the environment, preventing admixture of CO_2 and water vapor with the inspired O_2. Because of leakage, such masks deliver FIO_2 of at most 80 to 90%.

OLIGURIA

Oliguria is urine output < 500 mL in 24 h in an adult or < 0.5 mL/kg/h in an adult or child (< 1 mL/kg/h in neonates).

Etiology

Oliguria can have prerenal (blood-flow related), renal (intrinsic kidney disorders), or postrenal (outlet obstruction) causes. There are numerous such entities (see p. 1980), but a limited number cause most cases of acute oliguria in the hospitalized patient.

Prerenal oliguria results from renal hypoperfusion. The most common causes are hypovolemia, low cardiac output, and decreased systemic vascular resistance (eg, sepsis). These conditions often coexist and rapidly (ie, < 1 h) reduce urine output.

Renal causes are primarily acute tubular necrosis (ATN), the most common causes of which include prolonged hypoperfusion (> 4 h), x-ray contrast dye, rhabdomyolysis, and nephrotoxic drugs (eg, aminoglycosides and other antibiotics and NSAIDs).

Postrenal causes are obstructive, from prostatic hypertrophy, stones, Foley catheter obstruction, and neurogenic bladder.

Evaluation

History: In communicative patients, marked urge to void suggests outlet obstruction, whereas thirst and no urge to void suggest volume depletion. In obtunded (and presumably catheterized) patients, a sudden decrease in urine flow in a normotensive patient suggests catheter occlusion or displacement, whereas a gradual decrease is more likely ATN or a prerenal cause.

Recent medical events are helpful, including review of recent BP readings, surgical procedures, and drug and x-ray contrast administration. Recent surgery or trauma may be consistent with hypovolemia. A severe crush injury, deep electrical burn, or heatstroke suggests rhabdomyolysis.

Physical examination: Signs of hypovolemia, sepsis, and cardiac failure should be sought. Palpable bladder distention indicates an outlet obstruction. Dark brown urine suggests myoglobinuria.

Testing: In all catheterized patients (and those with an ileal conduit), patency should be ascertained by irrigation before further testing; this may solve the problem. In many remaining patients, etiology is clinically apparent (eg, shock, sepsis). In others, particularly those with multiple disorders, testing is needed to differentiate prerenal from renal (ATN) causes. If a central venous or pulmonary artery catheter is in place, volume status (and with a pulmonary artery catheter, cardiac output) can be determined. However, many physicians would not insert such a line for acute oliguria unless other indications were present. An alternative in the patient without signs of volume overload is to rapidly administer a test bolus of IV fluid, 500 mL

0.9% saline (20 mL/kg in children); an increase in output suggests a prerenal cause.

Laboratory tests should be obtained. Serum electrolytes, BUN, and creatinine are standard; often urine Na and creatinine concentration are also obtained. Prerenal conditions generally result in BUN/creatinine ratio > 20, vs ≤ 10 in both normal states and ATN. In prerenal conditions, urine Na is < 20 mEq/L as the kidney attempts to retain maximum Na to preserve intravascular volume. In ATN, urine Na is usually > 40 mEq/L. The fractional Na excretion (FE_{NA}) is a more accurate representation of the kidney's ability to retain Na and is defined as:

$$\frac{\text{urine Na/plasma Na}}{\text{urine creatinine/plasma creatinine}}$$

A ratio < 1 indicates the kidney is able to reabsorb Na, and hence the problem is prerenal. A ratio > 1 indicates a probable renal cause.

Treatment

Identified causes are treated; outflow obstruction is corrected, volume is replaced, cardiac output is normalized. Nephrotoxic drugs are stopped, and another drug is substituted. Hypotension should be avoided to prevent further renal insults. Patients with renal failure that cannot be reversed may require renal replacement therapy (eg, continuous venovenous hemofiltration or hemodialysis).

AGITATION, CONFUSION, AND NEUROMUSCULAR BLOCKADE

ICU patients are often agitated, confused, and uncomfortable. They can become frankly psychotic (ICU psychosis). These symptoms are unpleasant for the patient and often interfere with care and safety. At worst they may be life threatening (eg, the patient dislodges his endotracheal tube or IV lines).

Etiology

In a critically ill patient, the original medical condition (eg, head injury, toxin ingestion, hypoxia, or shock) often causes agitation and confusion. Pain from injuries, surgical procedures, and even "routine" measures such as venipuncture and nasogastric intubation contributes. Subsequent complications such as pulmonary embolism, sepsis, and organ failure may initiate or worsen agitation. Underlying disorders play a role; patients with drug or alcohol dependency may go into withdrawal; patients with liver disease may develop hepatic encephalopathy. Patients who are endotracheally intubated tend to be particularly at risk for agitation and pose the most difficulty. Certain commonly used drugs (eg, H_2 blockers, antihistamines, opioids, benzodiazepines) can cause delirium.

The ICU environment itself exacerbates the problem. High noise level, constant bright lights, and round-the-clock medical interventions typically result in sleep deprivation both in terms of total sleep time and the length of any single period of sleep. The elderly are particularly prone to this. In addition, patients with relatively normal mentation commonly experience fear, both of death and of unpleasant medical procedures.

Evaluation

The chart should be reviewed and the patient examined before sedatives are ordered for "agitation."

History: The presenting injury or illness is a prime causative suspect. Nursing notes and discussion with personnel may identify dysfunctional sleep patterns or inadequate analgesia. Underlying liver disease suggests possible hepatic encephalopathy. Known substance dependency or abuse suggests a withdrawal syndrome. Awake, coherent patients are asked what is troubling them.

Physical examination: O_2 saturation < 90% suggests a hypoxic etiology. Low BP and urine output suggest CNS hypoperfusion. Fever and tachycardia suggest sepsis or delirium tremens. Neck stiffness suggests meningitis, although this finding may be difficult to demonstrate in an agitated patient. Focal findings on neurologic examination suggest stroke, hemorrhage, or increased intracranial pressure (ICP).

The degree of agitation can be quantified using a scale such as the Riker Sedation-Agitation Scale (see TABLE 63–6) or the Ramsay Sedation Scale. Use of such scales allows better consistency between observers and the identification of trends. Patients who are under neuromuscular blockade are difficult to evaluate because they may be highly agitated and uncomfortable despite appearing motionless. It is typically necessary to allow paralysis to wear off periodically (eg, daily) so that the patient can be assessed.

TABLE 63–6. RIKER SEDATION-AGITATION SCALE

SCORE	EXPLANATION
7 Dangerous agitation	Tries to remove monitors and devices or climb out of bed; tosses and turns; lashes out at staff
6 Very agitated	Remains restless despite frequent verbal reassurance; bites endotracheal tube; requires restraint
5 Agitated	Anxious or restless; attempts to move; calms down with reassurance
4 Calm and cooperative	Calm; easy to arouse; able to follow instructions
3 Sedated	Difficult to awaken; responds to verbal prompts or gentle shaking but drifts off again
2 Very sedated	Incommunicative; responds to physical stimuli but not verbal instructions; may move spontaneously
1 Unarousable	Incommunicative; little or no response to painful stimuli

Testing: Identified abnormalities (eg, hypoxia) should be further clarified with appropriate testing. Head CT need not routinely be performed unless focal neurologic findings are present or no other etiology is found. The Bispectral Index may be helpful in determining the level of sedation/agitation of patients under neuromuscular blockade.

Treatment

Underlying causes (eg, hypoxia, shock, drugs) should be addressed. The environment should be optimized (eg, darkness, quiet, and minimal sleep interruption at night) as much as is compatible with medical care. Clocks, calendars, outside windows, and TV or radio programs also help connect the patient with the world, lessening confusion. Family presence and consistent nursing personnel may be calming.

Pharmacologic treatment is dictated by the most vexing symptoms. Pain is treated with analgesics; anxiety and insomnia, with sedatives; and psychosis and delirium, with small doses of an antipsychotic drug. Intubation may be needed when sedative and analgesic requirements are high enough to jeopardize the airway or respiratory drive. Many agents are available; generally short-acting drugs are preferred for patients who need frequent neurologic examination or who are being weaned to extubation.

Analgesia: Pain should be treated with appropriate doses of IV opioids; conscious patients with painful conditions (eg, fractures, surgical incisions) who are unable to communicate should be assumed to have pain and receive analgesics accordingly. Mechanical ventilation is itself somewhat uncomfortable, and patients generally should receive a combination of opioid and amnestic sedative agents. Fentanyl is the opioid of choice because of its potency, short duration of action, and minimal cardiovascular effects. A common regimen can be 30 to 100 mg/h of fentanyl; individual requirements are highly variable.

Sedation: Despite analgesia, many patients remain sufficiently agitated to require sedation. A sedative also can provide patient comfort at a lower dose of analgesic. Benzodiazepines (eg, lorazepam, midazolam) are most common, but propofol, a sedative-hypnotic agent may be used. A common regimen for sedation is lorazepam 1 to 2 mg IV q 1 to 2 h or a continuous infusion at 1 to 2 mg/h. These drugs pose risks of respiratory depression, hypotension, delirium, and prolonged physiologic effects in some patients. Long-acting benzodiazepines such as diazepam, flurazepam, and chlordiazepoxide should be avoided in the elderly. Antipsychotics with less anticholinergic effect, such as haloperidol 1 to 3 mg IV, may work best when combined with benzodiazepines.

Neuromuscular blockade: For intubated patients, neuromuscular blockade is *not* a substitute for sedation; it only removes visible manifestations of the problem (agitation) without correcting it. However, neuromuscular blockade may be required during tests (eg CT, MRI) or procedures (eg, central line placement) that require the patient to be motionless, or when unable to ventilate the patient despite adequate analgesia and sedation.

Prolonged neuromuscular blockade should be avoided unless the patient has severe lung injury and cannot perform any work of breathing safely. Use for > 1 to 2 days may lead to prolonged weakness, particularly when corticosteroids are concomitantly given. Common regimens include vecuronium (continuous infusion as directed by stimulation).

64 RESPIRATORY AND CARDIAC ARREST

Respiratory and cardiac arrest are distinct, but inevitably one leads to the other if untreated. (See also respiratory failure in Ch. 65 on p. 544, dyspnea on p. 357, and hypoxia on p. 520.)

RESPIRATORY ARREST

Interruption of pulmonary gas exchange for > 5 min may irreversibly damage vital organs, especially the brain. Cardiac arrest almost always follows unless respiratory function is immediately restored.

Etiology

Respiratory arrest can be caused by airway obstruction, decreased respiratory effort from neurologic or muscular disorders, or drug overdose.

Airway obstruction may involve the upper or lower airway. Infants < 3 mo are usually nose breathers and thus may have upper airway obstruction secondary to nasal blockage. At all ages, loss of muscular tone with decreased consciousness may cause upper airway obstruction as the posterior tongue displaces into the oropharynx. Other causes of upper airway obstruction include blood, mucus, vomitus, or foreign body; spasm or edema of the vocal cords; and pharyngolaryngeal tracheal inflammation (eg, epiglottitis, croup), tumor, or trauma. Patients with congenital developmental disorders often have abnormal upper airways that are more easily obstructed.

Lower airway obstruction may occur from aspiration, bronchospasm, airspace filling disorders (eg, pneumonia, pulmonary edema, pulmonary hemorrhage), and drowning.

Decreased respiratory effort due to CNS impairment may result from drug overdose, carbon monoxide or cyanide poisoning, CNS infection, brain stem infarct or hemorrhage, and intracranial hypertension (due to mass lesions, hydrocephalus, or brain injury). Respiratory muscle weakness may be secondary to spinal cord injury, neuromuscular diseases (eg, myasthenia gravis, botulism, poliomyelitis, Guillain-Barré syndrome), neuromuscular blocking drugs, and metabolic disturbances.

Symptoms and Signs

With respiratory arrest, the patient is unconscious, or about to become so, and cyanotic (unless markedly anemic). If uncorrected, cardiac arrest follows within minutes from onset of hypoxemia.

Before complete respiratory arrest, patients with intact neurologic function may be agitated, confused, and struggling to breathe. Tachycardia and diaphoresis are present; there may be intercostal or sternoclavicular retractions. Patients with CNS impairment or respiratory muscle weakness exhibit feeble, gasping, or irregular respirations and paradoxical breathing movements. Patients with a foreign body in the airway may choke and point to their necks.

Infants, especially if < 3 mo old, may develop acute apnea without warning, secondary to overwhelming infection, metabolic disorders, or respiratory fatigue.

Diagnosis and Treatment

Respiratory arrest is usually clinically obvious; treatment begins simultaneously with diagnosis. The first consideration is to identify a foreign body obstructing the airway. If present, there will be marked resistance to ventilation during mouth-to-mouth or bag-valve-mask ventilation. Foreign material may be discovered during laryngoscopy for endotracheal intubation (see p. 525 for removal).

Treatment is to clear the airway, establish an alternate airway, and provide mechanical ventilation (see below and p. 544).

AIRWAY ESTABLISHMENT AND CONTROL

Airway management consists of clearing the upper airway, maintaining an open air passage with a mechanical device, and/or assisting respirations. There are many indications for airway control (see TABLE 64–1). In most situations, a manual resuscitation bag and mask provides adequate temporary ventilation, allowing time to systematically achieve definitive airway control. When equipment is not available, mouth-to-mouth (or mouth-to-mouth-and-nose in infants) ventilation is effective if properly performed.

Clearing and Opening the Upper Airway

Obstruction caused by relaxation of the soft tissues of the oropharynx may be relieved temporarily by neck extension (head tilt), chin lift, and thrusting the jaw forward (see FIG. 64–1); these maneuvers stretch the anterior neck structures, lifting and drawing the tongue away from the posterior pharyngeal wall. Obstruction from dentures and oropharyngeal foreign material (eg, blood, secretions) may be removed by finger sweep of the oropharynx and suction, taking care not to push the material deeper (more likely in infants and young children, in whom a blind

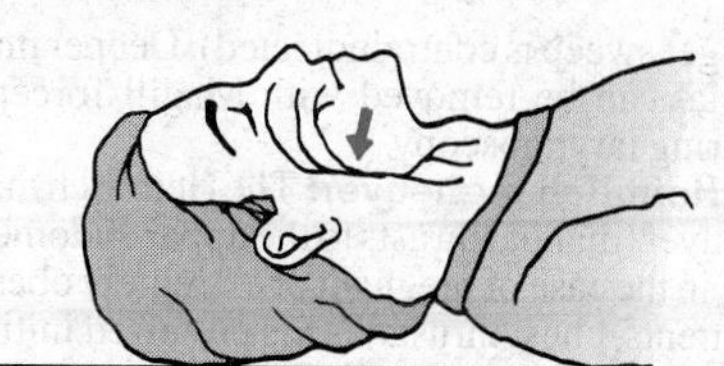

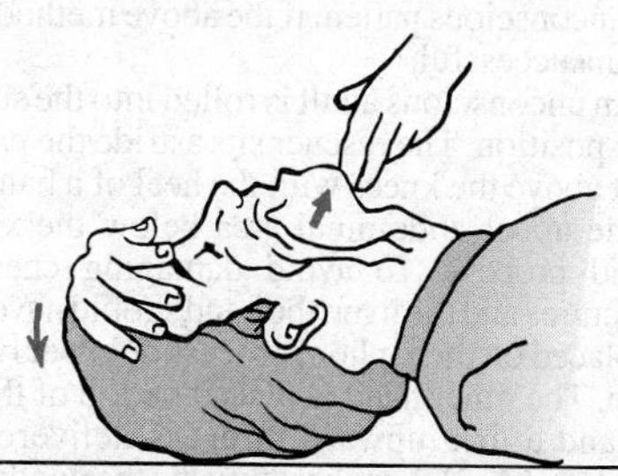

Fig. 64–1. Expired air ventilation—adult. Position to open airway alone. (Adapted from "Standards and Guidelines for Cardiopulmonary Resuscitation [CPR] and Emergency Cardiac Care [ECC]," in *Journal of the American Medical Association* 25:2956 and 2959, June 6, 1986. Copyright 1986, American Medical Association.)

TABLE 64–1. SITUATIONS REQUIRING AIRWAY CONTROL

EMERGENCIES	URGENCIES
Cardiac arrest	Respiratory failure
Respiratory arrest or apnea (eg, from CNS disease, drugs, hypoxia)	Need for ventilatory support (eg, in acute respiratory distress syndrome, exacerbations of COPD or asthma, diffuse infectious or other parenchymal lung problems, neuromuscular diseases, respiratory center depression, extreme respiratory muscle fatigue)
Deep coma, when the tongue relaxes to occlude the glottis	Need to relieve the work of breathing in patients in shock, with low cardiac output, or with myocardial stress that must be decreased
Acute laryngeal edema	Before gastric lavage in patients with an oral drug overdose and altered consciousness
Laryngospasm	Very high O_2 consumption (eg, in peritonitis, with limited respiratory reserves)
Foreign body at the larynx (eg, the "cafe coronary")	Before bronchoscopy in patients with marginal respiratory status
Drowning	Before radiologic procedures in patients with altered sensorium, particularly if sedation is required
Smoke or toxic chemical inhalation	
Respiratory burn (heat or chemical)	
Aspiration of gastric contents	
Upper airway trauma	
Head or high spinal cord injuries	

finger sweep is contraindicated). Deeper material can be removed with Magill forceps during laryngoscopy.

Heimlich maneuver: The Heimlich maneuver (manual thrusts to the upper abdomen or, in the case of pregnant or extremely obese patients, chest thrusts) is the preferred initial method in the awake, choking patient and in the unconscious patient if the above methods are unsuccessful.

An unconscious adult is rolled into the supine position. The rescuer sits astride the patient above the knees with the heel of a hand in the upper abdominal area below the xiphoid process. To avoid damaging chest structures and the liver, the hand should never be placed on the xiphoid process or lower rib cage. The other hand is placed on top of the 1st and a firm upward thrust is delivered (see FIG. 64–2). For chest thrusts, the hand is placed over the sternum similar to the position used for cardiac compression. With both techniques, 6 to 10 quick, firm thrusts may be necessary to dislodge a foreign body.

In conscious adults, the rescuer stands behind the patient with arms encircling his midsection. One fist is clenched and placed midway between the umbilicus and xiphoid. The other hand grabs the fist, and a firm inward and upward thrust is delivered by pulling with both arms (see FIG. 64–3).

In older children, the Heimlich maneuver may be performed. However, in children < 20 kg (typically < 5 yr), very moderate pressure should be applied, and the rescuer should kneel at the child's feet rather than astride.

Infants < 1 yr should not have a Heimlich maneuver but should be held in a prone, head-down position, supporting the head with the fingers of one hand, while the rescuer delivers 5 back blows (see FIG. 64–4). Five chest thrusts should then be delivered with the infant in a head-down position with his back on the rescuer's thigh (supine). This sequence of back blows and chest thrusts is repeated until the airway is cleared.

Airway and Respiratory Devices

If there is no spontaneous respiration after airway opening, and no respiratory devices are available, rescue breathing (mouth-to-mouth or mouth-to-mouth-and-nose) is started. Exhaled air contains 16 to 18% O_2 and 4 to 5% CO_2, which is adequate to maintain blood O_2 and CO_2 values close to normal. Larger-than-necessary volumes of air may produce gastric distention with associated risk of aspiration.

Bag-valve-mask devices (BVMs) consist of a self-inflating bag (resuscitator bag) with a nonrebreathing valve mechanism. These devices do not maintain airway patency, so

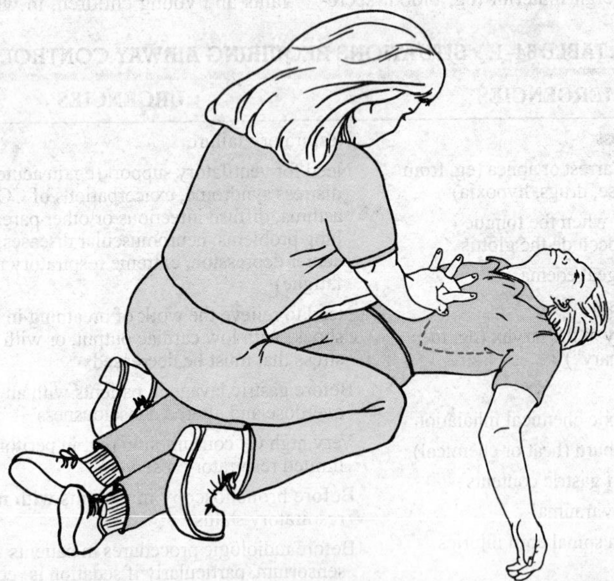

Fig. 64–2. Abdominal thrusts with victim lying (conscious or unconscious).

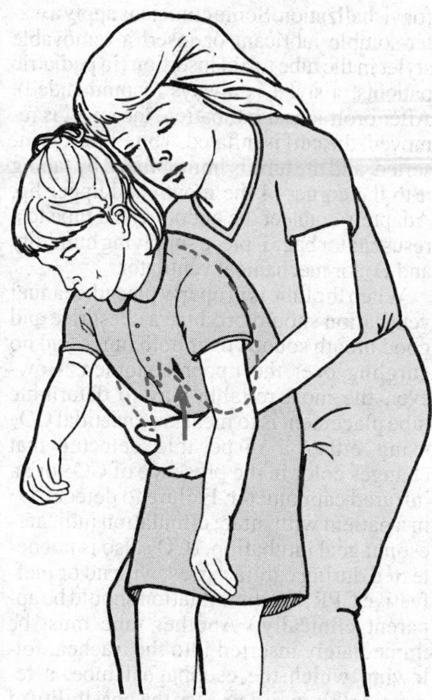

Fig. 64–3. Abdominal thrusts with victim standing or sitting (conscious).

patients with soft-tissue relaxation require additional devices to keep the airway open. Supplemental O_2 delivers from 60 to 100% inspired O_2. Ventilation may be maintained for prolonged periods with a BVM, allowing time for careful nasotracheal or orotracheal intubation. However, if BVM ventilation is used for > 5 min, anterior cricoid pressure should be applied to prevent gastric insufflation and a nasogastric tube should be inserted to evacuate air, which is invariably introduced into the stomach during BVM ventilation. BVMs are also used with artificial airways, including endotracheal tubes and laryngeal mask airways. Pediatric bags have an adjustable pressure relief valve that limits peak airway pressures (usually at 35 to 45 cm H_2O); this valve must be closed when used with a mask to optimize ventilation.

An oropharyngeal airway or a nasal trumpet keeps soft tissues of the oropharynx from collapsing and blocking the airway. These devices facilitate BVM ventilation, although they produce gagging in fully conscious patients. The proper oropharyngeal airway size should be equal to the distance between the corner of the patient's mouth and the angle of the jaw.

A laryngeal mask airway can be inserted into the lower oropharynx to prevent airway obstruction by soft tissues; it contains a passage to allow easy BVM ventilation. Some models also have a channel that can guide an endotracheal tube into the trachea. This device causes minimal complications and has gained popularity because laryngoscopy is not needed for insertion, allowing use by minimally trained rescuers. Because it causes gagging, use is limited to obtunded patients and for short periods (hours).

A double-lumen esophageal/tracheal airway device with proximal and distal balloons (Combitube) may be used to occlude the pharynx and esophagus. It is inserted blindly, usually ending up in the esophagus, in which case ventilation is accomplished through one lumen. If it passes into the trachea, the patient is ventilated via the other lumen. Thus, insertion technique is easy to master, and the device is helpful for minimally trained rescuers. The device is not satisfactory for prolonged use and should be changed for an endotracheal tube as soon as practical. Use is limited to prehospital cases where endotracheal intubation is unavailable or in the emergency department following failed intubation.

An endotracheal tube is the definitive method to secure a compromised airway, prevent aspiration, and initiate mechanical ventilation and should replace BVM ventilation

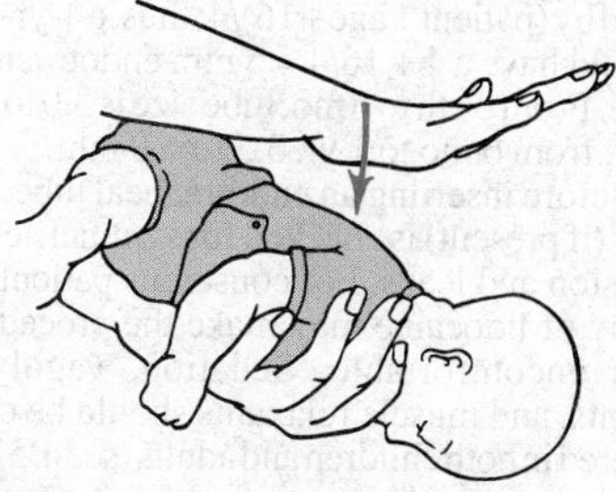

Fig. 64–4. Expired air ventilation—child. Head-down position: dislodgment of foreign bodies from tracheobronchial tube. (Adapted from "Standards and Guidelines for Cardiopulmonary Resuscitation [CPR] and Emergency Cardiac Care [ECC]," in *Journal of the American Medical Association* 25:2956 and 2959, June 6, 1986. Copyright 1986, American Medical Association.)

as soon as possible. It also permits suctioning of the lower respiratory tract. Placement typically requires laryngoscopy. It is indicated in comatose patients and others who need prolonged mechanical ventilation.

Airway Techniques

Most patients requiring an artificial airway can be managed with endotracheal intubation; a few require a surgical airway (eg, cricothyrotomy or tracheostomy).

Endotracheal intubation: Manual airway control, ventilation, and oxygenation are always indicated before attempting tracheal intubation. Orotracheal intubation is preferred in apneic and critically ill patients because it can usually be performed faster than nasotracheal intubation, which is reserved for awake, spontaneously breathing patients, in whom comfort has higher priority.

Larger endotracheal tubes have high-volume, low-pressure balloon cuffs that minimize risk of aspiration. Cuffed tubes are typically used only in adults and children > 8 yr, although cuffed tubes may be appropriate for selected infants and younger children. Most adults can accept tubes with an internal diameter ≥ 8 mm; these are preferable to smaller tubes because they have lower airflow resistance (reducing the work of breathing), facilitate suctioning of secretions, allow passage of a bronchoscope, and may aid in liberation from mechanical ventilation. The balloon cuff is inflated with air using a 10-mL syringe, and a manometer is used to verify that balloon pressure is < 30 cm H_2O. For infants and children ≥ 1 yr, tube size is calculated by (patient's age + 16)/4; thus, a 4-yr-old should have a 4 + 16/4 = 5 mm endotracheal tube. From birth to 6 mo, tube size is 3.0 to 3.5 mm; from 6 mo to 1 yr, 3.5 to 4.0 mm.

Before inserting an endotracheal tube, the cuff (if present) is checked for symmetric expansion and leaks. For conscious patients, a spray of lidocaine may make the procedure less uncomfortable. Sedation, vagolytic agents, and muscle relaxants should be considered in both children and adults (see p. 530). Either a straight or curved laryngoscope blade can be used depending on the experience and preference of the operator; straight blades are preferred for children < 8 yr. Technique for exposing the glottis and vocal cords differs slightly for each blade, but in all cases the cords must be clearly visualized, or esophageal intubation is likely. Anterior cricoid or laryngeal pressure is often required for visualization. Some clinicians apply a water-soluble lubricant or insert a removable stylet in the tube to aid insertion (in pediatric patients, a stylet is always recommended). After orotracheal intubation, the stylet is removed, the cuff is inflated, a bite-block is inserted, and the tube is immobilized by taping it to the corner of the mouth and upper lip. Adapters connect the endotracheal tube to a resuscitator bag, T-piece supplying humidity and O_2, or mechanical ventilator.

When the tube is properly placed, manual ventilation should produce a chest rise and good breath sounds over both lungs and no gurgling over the upper abdomen. However, the most reliable way to determine tube placement is to measure end-tidal CO_2 using either a disposable detector that changes color in the presence of CO_2 or an infrared capnometer. Failure to detect CO_2 in a patient with intact circulation indicates esophageal intubation. (CO_2 also is not detected during cardiac arrest with no or ineffective CPR, but this situation should be apparent clinically.) Another tube must be immediately inserted into the trachea, following which the esophageal tube is removed (this may decrease the possibility of aspiration if the patient regurgitates following removal of the tube from the esophagus). If breath sounds are diminished or absent over one lung (usually the left), the cuff should be deflated and the tube carefully pulled back 1 to 2 cm (0.5 to 1 cm in infants) while listening over the chest for breath sounds to reposition it into the trachea. A rule of thumb for proper placement is that the centimeter mark of the tube at the gums or teeth is usually equal to 3 times the inner diameter of the tube (eg, for a 5.0 tube, the 15-cm mark should be at the teeth). A chest x-ray taken after tube insertion confirms tip position, optimally in the mid-third of the trachea with the balloon at least 2 cm below the vocal cords but above the carina. Some clinicians recommend daily chest x-rays to confirm proper tube position. In all patients, auscultation of both lung fields should be performed at regular intervals to exclude migration of the tube distally into a bronchus or cephalad.

Mechanical aids may assist in difficult cases (eg, patients with cervical spine injury or disease, massive facial trauma, airway abnormality). A lighted stylet is available; when the tube is properly positioned in the trachea, the skin overlying the larynx is illuminated.

Alternatively, a guidewire may be inserted percutaneously through the cricothyroid membrane and passed retrograde out through the mouth. An endotracheal tube is then guided over the wire into the trachea. In another method, the endotracheal tube is slipped over a fiberoptic bronchoscope, which is inserted transorally or transnasally and then through the glottis, following which the tube is advanced over the scope into the trachea.

Nasotracheal intubation can be performed in spontaneously breathing patients typically without laryngoscopy, which may cause it to be preferred in patients with cervical spine injury. The tube is inserted through a nostril anesthetized with a topical agent (eg, benzocaine, lidocaine) and advanced slowly to a position just above the larynx. As the patient breathes in, opening the vocal cords, the tube is promptly passed into the trachea. Because of airway anatomy, this technique is very difficult in children and is not recommended.

Surgical airway: If the upper airway is obstructed because of foreign body or massive trauma or if ventilation cannot be accomplished by other means, surgical entry into the trachea is required.

Cricothyrotomy can establish an emergency airway (see FIG. 64–5). The patient lies supine, shoulders raised by pillows or sheets, and neck extended. After sterile preparation, the larynx is grasped with one hand while a blade is used to incise the skin, subcutaneous tissue, and cricothyroid membrane precisely in the midline. An appropriately sized tracheostomy tube is advanced through the opening into the trachea. In an out-of-hospital, immediately life-threatening airway obstruction, a knife handle, disposable pen barrel, or other hollow object can be used to keep the airway open. If other equipment is unavailable, a 12- to 14-gauge IV catheter can be passed into the trachea through the cricothyroid membrane. The larynx is grasped with one hand while the sterile needle-catheter is inserted percutaneously through the precise midline of the cricothyroid membrane, pointing the needle tip slightly inferiorly, aspirating while advancing, and taking care not to perforate the posterior tracheal wall or to stray out of the midline into large vessels. Once tracheal position is confirmed by aspiration of air, the catheter is advanced into the trachea. A 3-way stopcock and an O_2 pressure source provide oxygenation but limited ventilation. Complications include hemorrhage, subcutaneous emphysema, and pneumomediastinum.

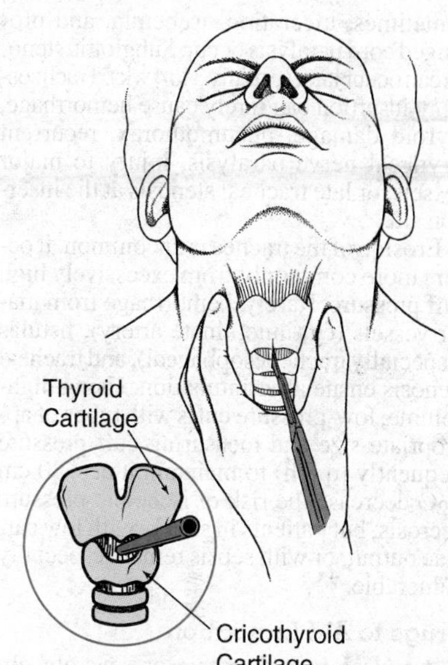

Fig. 64–5. Emergency cricothyrotomy. The patient lies supine with the neck extended. After sterile preparation, the larynx is grasped with one hand while a blade is used to incise the skin, subcutaneous tissue, and cricothyroid membrane precisely in the midline, accessing the trachea. A hollow tube is used to keep the airway open.

Tracheostomy is a more complex procedure involving surgical exposure and opening of the trachea. It is preferably performed in an operating room by a surgeon. In emergencies, the procedure has a higher rate of complications than cricothyrotomy and offers no advantage. It is, however, the preferred procedure for a long-term (>48 h) surgical airway. Percutaneous tracheostomy is an attractive alternative for critically ill patients who should not be moved to the operating room. This bedside technique uses a simple skin puncture and single or multiple dilators to insert a tracheostomy tube.

Complications: Intubation can damage lips, teeth, tongue, and supraglottic and subglottic areas. Inappropriate tube placement in the esophagus results in a fatal failure to ventilate and also can cause gastric distention (rarely rupture) and aspiration of regurgitated gastric contents. Any translaryngeal tube injures the vocal cords somewhat;

sometimes, ulceration, ischemia, and prolonged cord paralysis occur. Subglottic stenosis can occur later (usually 3 to 4 wk). Tracheostomy insertion can rarely cause hemorrhage, thyroid damage, pneumothorax, recurrent laryngeal nerve paralysis, injury to major vessels, or late tracheal stenosis at the insertion site.

Erosion of the trachea is uncommon. It occurs more commonly from excessively high cuff pressure. Rarely, hemorrhage from major vessels (eg, innominate artery), fistulas (especially tracheoesophageal), and tracheal stenosis ensue after intubation. Using high-volume, low-pressure cuffs with tubes of appropriate size and measuring cuff pressure frequently (q 8 h) to maintain it at < 30 cm H_2O decrease the risk of ischemic pressure necrosis, but patients in shock, with low cardiac output, or with sepsis remain especially vulnerable.

Drugs to Aid Intubation

A pulseless and apneic or severely obtunded patient can (and should) be intubated without pharmacologic assistance. Other patients receive pretreatment with sedating and paralytic drugs to facilitate intubation and minimize discomfort (termed rapid sequence intubation).

Pretreatment: If time permits, the patient prebreathes 100% O_2 for 3 to 5 min; this can maintain satisfactory oxygenation up to 4 or 5 min of apnea.

Laryngoscopy causes a sympathetic-mediated pressor response with an increase in heart rate, BP, and possibly intracranial pressure. To blunt this response, when time permits, some practitioners give lidocaine 1.5 mg/kg IV 1 to 2 min before sedation and paralysis. Children and adolescents often have a vagal response (marked bradycardia) in response to intubation and are given atropine 0.02 mg/kg IV (minimum 0.1 mg in infants, 0.5 mg in children and adolescents) at the same time. Some physicians include a small dose of a neuromuscular blocker (NMB), such as vecuronium 0.01 mg/kg IV, in patients > 4 yr to prevent muscle fasciculations caused by full doses of succinylcholine. Fasciculations may result in muscle pain on awakening and cause transient hyperkalemia; however, the actual benefit of such pretreatment is unclear.

Sedation and analgesia: Laryngoscopy and intubation are uncomfortable; thus, a short-acting IV drug with sedative or combined sedative and analgesic properties is mandatory immediately before the procedure. At this point, an assistant applies pressure over the cricoid cartilage (Sellick maneuver) to occlude the esophagus and prevent regurgitation and aspiration.

Etomidate 0.3 mg/kg, a nonbarbiturate hypnotic, may be the preferred agent. Fentanyl 5 µg/kg (2 to 5 µg/kg in children; NOTE: this is higher than the analgesic dose), an opioid (and thus with analgesic as well as sedative properties), also works well and causes no cardiovascular depression. However, at higher doses chest wall rigidity may occur. Ketamine 1 to 2 mg/kg is a dissociative anesthetic with cardiostimulatory properties. It is generally safe but may cause hallucinations or bizarre behavior on awakening. Thiopental 3 to 4 mg/kg and methohexital 1 to 2 mg/kg are effective but tend to cause hypotension.

Paralysis: Skeletal muscle relaxation with an IV NMB markedly facilitates intubation.

Succinylcholine (1.5 mg/kg IV, 2.0 mg/kg for infants), a depolarizing NMB, has the most rapid onset (30 sec to 1 min) and shortest duration (3 to 5 min). It should be avoided in patients with burns, muscle crush injuries > 1 to 2 days old, spinal cord injury, neuromuscular disease, renal failure, and possibly penetrating eye injury. About 1/15,000 children (and fewer adults) have a genetic susceptibility to malignant hyperthermia from succinylcholine. Succinylcholine should always be given with atropine in children since pronounced bradycardia may occur.

Alternative nondepolarizing NMBs have longer duration of action (> 30 min) but also have slower onset unless used in high doses that prolong paralysis significantly. Drugs include atracurium 0.5 mg/kg, mivacurium 0.15 mg/kg, rocuronium 1.0 mg/kg, and vecuronium 0.1 to 0.2 mg/kg injected over 60 sec.

Topical anesthesia: Intubation of an awake patient (typically not done in children) requires anesthesia of the nose and pharynx. A commercial aerosol preparation of benzocaine, tetracaine, butyl aminobenzoate (butamben), and benzalkonium is commonly used. Alternatively, 4% lidocaine can be nebulized and inhaled via face mask.

CARDIAC ARREST

Cardiac arrest is the terminal event in any fatal disorder. It also may occur suddenly (defined as within 24 h of onset of symptoms in a previously functioning person), and as such occurs outside the hospital in about 400,000 people/yr in the US, with a 90% mortality.

Etiology

In adults, sudden cardiac arrest results primarily from cardiac disease (of all types, but especially coronary artery disease). In a significant percentage, sudden cardiac arrest is the first manifestation of heart disease. Other causes include circulatory shock from noncardiac disorders (especially pulmonary embolism, GI hemorrhage, trauma), ventilatory failure, and metabolic disturbance (including drug overdose).

In children, cardiac causes of sudden cardiac arrest are much less common (< 15 to 20%). Instead, predominant causes include trauma, poisoning, and various respiratory disorders (eg, airway obstruction, smoke inhalation, drowning, infection, sudden infant death syndrome).

Pathophysiology

Cardiac arrest produces global ischemia with consequences at the cellular level that adversely affect patients following resuscitation. The main consequences involve direct cellular damage and edema formation. Edema is particularly harmful in the brain, which has no room to expand, resulting in increased intracranial pressure and corresponding decrease in cerebral perfusion post-resuscitation. A number of successfully resuscitated patients have short- or long-term cerebral dysfunction.

Decreased ATP production leads to loss of membrane integrity with efflux of K and influx of Na and Ca. Excess Na produces cellular edema. Excess Ca damages mitochondria (depressing ATP production), increases nitric oxide production (leading to formation of damaging free radicals), and in certain circumstances, activates proteases that damage cellular contents.

In neurons, the abnormal ion flux additionally causes depolarization, releasing neurotransmitters. A particularly damaging neurotransmitter is glutamate, which activates a specific Ca channel, worsening intracellular Ca overload.

Inflammatory mediators (eg, IL-1B, tumor necrosis factor-α) are elaborated, some of which lead to microvascular thrombosis and loss of vascular integrity with further edema formation. Apoptosis is activated in severe ischemia by numerous mediators, resulting in accelerated cell death.

Symptoms and Signs

In critically or terminally ill patients, cardiac arrest is often preceded by a period of clinical deterioration with rapid, shallow breathing, arterial hypotension, and a progressive decrease in mental alertness. In other cases of cardiac arrest, collapse occurs without warning, occasionally accompanied by a brief (< 5 sec) seizure.

Diagnosis and Treatment

Diagnosis is by clinical findings of apnea, pulselessness, and unconsciousness. Arterial pressure is not measurable. A cardiac monitor may indicate ventricular fibrillation, ventricular tachycardia, or asystole. Sometimes a perfusing rhythm (eg, sinus bradycardia) is present; this may represent true pulseless electrical activity (electromechanical dissociation) or extreme hypotension with failure to detect a pulse.

In children, the presenting rhythm is typically bradyarrhythmia followed by asystole; however, about 15 to 20% of children present with ventricular tachycardia or fibrillation. Thus, the need for rapid defibrillation should be considered in any child with sudden cardiac arrest not preceded by respiratory symptoms.

The patient is evaluated for potentially treatable causes, such as hypoxia, massive volume loss, cardiac tamponade, tension pneumothorax, or massive pulmonary embolus. Unfortunately, many causes will not be identified during CPR. Clinical examination and chest x-ray can detect tension pneumothorax. If available, immediate cardiac ultrasound can detect cardiac contractions and also recognize cardiac tamponade, extreme hypovolemia (empty heart), right ventricular overload suggestive of pulmonary embolism, and focal wall motion abnormalities suggestive of MI. Primary causes must be promptly treated. If no treatable conditions are present but cardiac motion is detected or pulses are present by Doppler, severe circulatory shock is identified and IV pressors (eg, norepinephrine, dopamine, or epinephrine) are given in addition to volume infusion.

Further treatment is with cardiopulmonary resuscitation. Rapid intervention is essential.

CARDIOPULMONARY RESUSCITATION

(For neonatal resuscitation, see p. 2258.)

Cardiopulmonary resuscitation (CPR) is an organized, sequential response to cardiac arrest, including recognition of absent breathing and circulation, basic life support (BLS) with chest compressions and rescue breathing, advanced cardiac life support (ACLS) with definitive airway and rhythm control, and post-resuscitative care. Rapid initiation of chest compression and early defibrillation (if indicated) are the keys to success. Speed, efficiency, and proper application of CPR directly determine successful neurologic outcome; the rare exception is in profound hypothermia from cold water immersion, in which successful resuscitation may be accomplished even after prolonged arrest (up to 60 min).

After establishing unresponsiveness (tap, shake, or shout) and absence of breathing, the rescuer calls for help (including a defibrillator) and begins basic life support following the mnemonic ABC (Airway, Breathing, Circulation, see FIG. 64–6). Next, defibrillation (D) with a manual or automated defibrillator is used to try to convert ventricular fibrillation (VF) or pulseless ventricular tachycardia (VT) to a perfusing rhythm.

The techniques used in basic 1- and 2-rescuer CPR are listed in TABLE 64–2; their mastery is best acquired by hands-on training such as that provided in the US under the auspices of the American Heart Association (1-800-AHA-USA1) or similar organizations in other countries.

Airway and Breathing

Except in witnessed cardiac arrest when a defibrillator is available in < 3 min, opening the airway is the first priority (see p. 525).

Mouth-to-mouth (adults and children) or combined mouth-to-mouth-and-nose (infants) rescue breathing is begun. Cricoid pressure may be applied continuously by a 2nd rescuer until airway control is achieved by endotracheal intubation. Firm pressure on the rigid cartilaginous rings of the trachea occludes the esophagus, minimizing the chance of gastric inflation from ventilations and blocking the exit of gastric contents if regurgitation occurs; pressure must be much lighter in young children to avoid collapsing the trachea. If abdominal distention develops, the airway is rechecked for patency and the amount of air delivered during rescue breathing is reduced. Nasogastric intubation to relieve gastric distention is delayed until suction equipment is available because regurgitation with aspiration of gastric contents may occur during insertion. If marked gastric distention interferes with ventilation and cannot be corrected by the above methods, the patient is positioned on his side, the epigastrium compressed, and the airway cleared.

TABLE 64–2. TECHNIQUES OF CPR FOR HEALTH CARE PROFESSIONALS

	ONE-RESCUER CPR	TWO-RESCUER CPR	BREATH SIZE
Adults	2 breaths (1 sec each) after every 30 chest compressions at 100/min	2 breaths (1 sec) after every 30 chest compressions at 100/min*	Each breath about 500 mL (caution against hyperventilation)
Children (1 to 8)	2 breaths (1 sec duration) after every 30 chest compressions at 100/min	2 breaths (1 sec duration) after every 15 chest compressions at 100/min*	Smaller breaths than for adults (enough to make chest rise)
Infants (< 1 yr)	2 breaths (1 sec duration) after every 30 chest compressions at 100/min	2 breaths (1 sec duration) after every 15 chest compressions at 100/min*	Only small puffs from rescuer's cheeks

*With an advanced airway in place, give 8 to 10 breaths/min without pause of chest compressions.

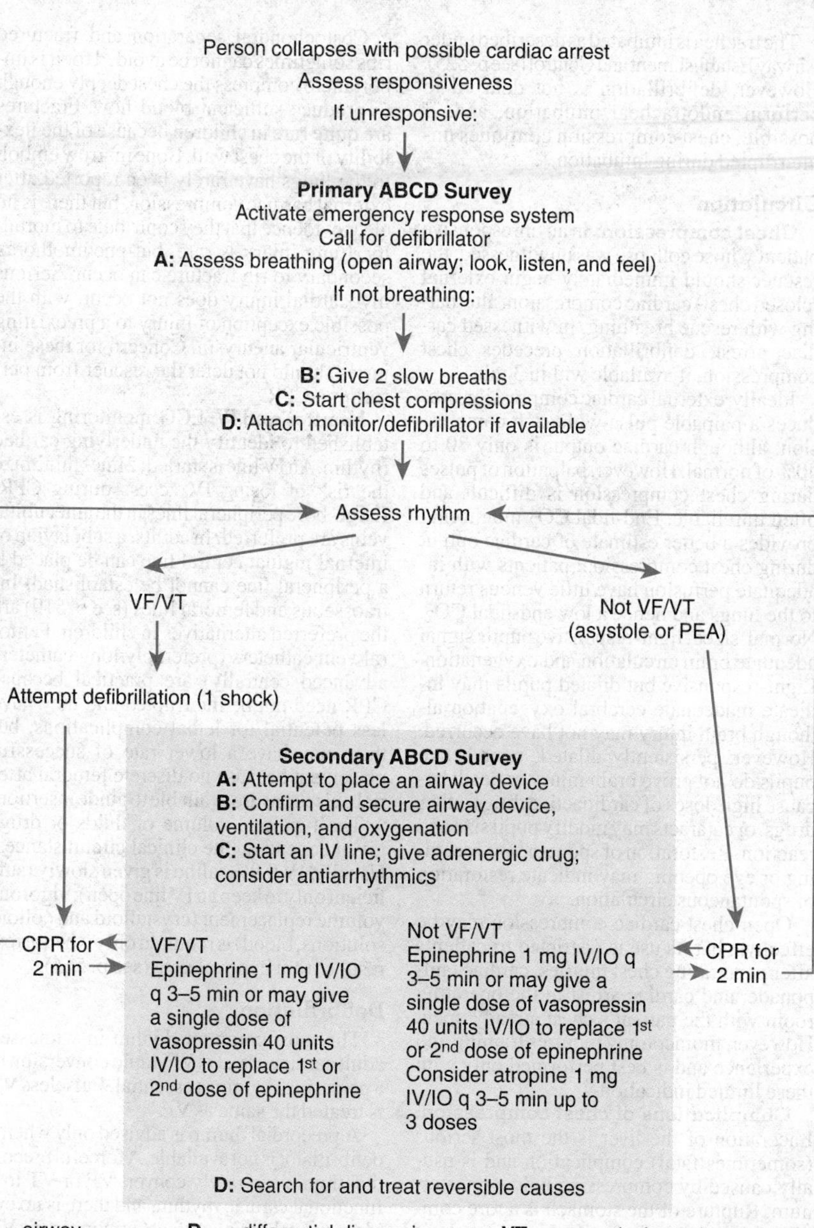
Person collapses with possible cardiac arrest
Assess responsiveness
If unresponsive:
Primary ABCD Survey
Activate emergency response system
Call for defibrillator
A: Assess breathing (open airway; look, listen, and feel)
If not breathing:
B: Give 2 slow breaths
C: Start chest compressions
D: Attach monitor/defibrillator if available
Assess rhythm
VF/VT
Not VF/VT (asystole or PEA)
Attempt defibrillation (1 shock)
Secondary ABCD Survey
A: Attempt to place an airway device
B: Confirm and secure airway device, ventilation, and oxygenation
C: Start an IV line; give adrenergic drug; consider antiarrhythmics
CPR for 2 min
VF/VT
Epinephrine 1 mg IV/IO q 3–5 min or may give a single dose of vasopressin 40 units IV/IO to replace 1st or 2nd dose of epinephrine
Not VF/VT
Epinephrine 1 mg IV/IO q 3–5 min or may give a single dose of vasopressin 40 units IV/IO to replace 1st or 2nd dose of epinephrine
Consider atropine 1 mg IV/IO q 3–5 min up to 3 doses
CPR for 2 min
D: Search for and treat reversible causes

A = airway
B = breathing
C = circulation
D = differential diagnosis
VF = ventricular fibrillation
IO = intraosseously
VT = ventricular tachycardia
PEA = pulseless electrical activity

Based on Comprehensive Emergency Cardiac Care Algorithm from the American Heart Association.

Fig. 64–6. Adult comprehensive emergency cardiac care.

The trachea is intubated as described under Airway Establishment and Control (see p. 525). However, defibrillation is not delayed to perform endotracheal intubation, and, if possible, chest compression continues uninterrupted during intubation.

Circulation

Chest compression: In an unresponsive patient whose collapse was unwitnessed, the rescuer should immediately begin external (closed chest) cardiac compression, alternating with rescue breathing. In witnessed cardiac arrest, defibrillation precedes chest compression, if available within 3 min.

Ideally, external cardiac compression produces a palpable pulse with each compression, although cardiac output is only 30 to 40% of normal. However, palpation of pulses during chest compression is difficult and often unreliable. End-tidal CO_2 monitoring provides a better estimate of cardiac output during chest compression; patients with inadequate perfusion have little venous return to the lungs and hence a low end-tidal CO_2. Normal-sized, light-responsive pupils signal adequate brain circulation and oxygenation. Light-responsive but dilated pupils may indicate inadequate cerebral oxygenation although brain injury may not have occurred. However, persistently dilated, nonreactive pupils do not prove brain injury or death because high doses of cardioactive drugs, other drugs, or cataracts may modify pupil size and reaction. Restoration of spontaneous breathing or eye opening may indicate restoration of spontaneous circulation.

Open-chest cardiac compression may be effective, but its use is restricted to patients after penetrating chest injuries, cardiac tamponade, and cardiac arrest in the operating room with the patient's chest already open. However, thoracotomy requires training and experience and is best performed only with these limited indications.

Complications of chest compression: Laceration of the liver is the most serious (sometimes fatal) complication and is usually caused by compressing below the sternum. Rupture of the stomach is a rare complication (particularly if the stomach is distended with air). Delayed rupture of the spleen is very rare. A more frequent complication is regurgitation followed by aspiration of gastric contents, producing aspiration pneumonia that may be fatal.

Costochondral separation and fractured ribs sometimes cannot be avoided for it is important to compress the chest deeply enough to produce sufficient blood flow. Fractures are quite rare in children because of the flexibility of the chest wall. Bone marrow emboli to the lungs have rarely been reported after external cardiac compression, but there is no clear evidence that they contribute to mortality. Lung injury is rare, but pneumothorax secondary to rib fracture can occur. Serious myocardial injury does not occur, with the possible exception of injury to a preexisting ventricular aneurysm. Concern for these injuries should not deter the rescuer from performing CPR.

Monitor and IV: ECG monitoring is established to identify the underlying cardiac rhythm. An IV line is started; 2 lines minimize the risk of losing IV access during CPR. Large-bore peripheral lines in the antecubital veins are preferred. In adults, a subclavian or internal jugular central line can be placed if a peripheral line cannot be established. Intraosseous and femoral lines (see p. 519) are the preferred alternatives in children. Femoral vein catheters (preferably long catheters advanced centrally) are practical because CPR need not be interrupted and they have less potential for lethal complications, but they may have a lower rate of successful placement because no discrete femoral arterial pulsations are available to guide insertion.

The type and volume of fluids or drugs given depend on the clinical circumstances. Usually, IV 0.9% saline is given slowly (sufficient only to keep an IV line open); vigorous volume replacement (crystalloid and colloid solutions, blood) is required only when arrest results from hypovolemia (see p. 564).

Defibrillation

The most common rhythm in witnessed adult cardiac arrest is VF; rapid conversion to a perfusing rhythm is essential. Pulseless VT is treated the same as VF.

A precordial thump is advised only when a defibrillator is not available. A forceful precordial thump can rarely convert VF or VT to a functional cardiac rhythm, and there is no evidence of deleterious effect (eg, converting VT to VF) in the cardiac arrest setting. However, it is not recommended in children. One or 2 blows can be delivered to the junction of the middle and lower third of the sternum with a clenched fist held 20 to 25 cm above the chest.

Prompt direct current (DC) cardioversion is more effective than antiarrhythmic drugs; however, the success of defibrillation is time dependent, with about a 10% decline in success after each minute of VF (or pulseless VT). Automated external defibrillators (AEDs) allow minimally trained rescuers to treat VT or VF. Their placement with 1st responders (police and fire vehicles) and in public locations appears to increase the rate of resuscitation.

Defibrillating paddles or AED pads are placed between the clavicle and the 2nd intercostal space along the right sternal border, and over the 5th or 6th intercostal space at the apex of the heart. Conventional defibrillators are used with conducting paste or gel pads; the conducting material is incorporated into AED pads. Only 1 initial countershock is given (previously recommended 3 stacked shocks). Energy level for biphasic defibrillators is between 120 and 200 joules (2 joules/kg in children); monophasic defibrillators are set at 360 joules. CPR resumes immediately. Postshock rhythm is not checked until after 2 min of CPR; this may be done earlier in continuously monitored patients. Any subsequent shocks are delivered at the same or higher energy level (maximum 360 joules, 2 to 4 joules/kg in children). Patients remaining in VF or VT are given drug therapy as described below.

Special Circumstances

In accidental electrical shock, the rescuer must be certain that the patient is no longer in contact with the electrical source to avoid shock to himself. Use of nonmetallic grapples or rods and grounding of the rescuer allows for safe removal of the patient before starting CPR.

In near-drowning, rescue breathing may be started in shallow water, although chest compression cannot be effectively performed until the patient is horizontal on a firm surface. Placing the patient on a surfboard or float may help.

If cardiac arrest follows traumatic injury, airway opening maneuvers and a brief period of external ventilation after clearing the airway take priority to exclude airway obstruction as the cause of arrest. To minimize cervical spine movement, only jaw thrust, not head tilt and chin lift, is used. However, because most patients with traumatic cardiac arrest have marked hypovolemia due to blood loss, or nonsurvivable brain injury, chest compressions will be ineffective. The main survivable causes of traumatic cardiac arrest include cardiac tamponade and tension pneumothorax, which require immediate needle decompression; if this is unavailable or ineffective, BLS measures are futile.

Drugs for ACLS

Despite widespread and long-standing use, no drug has definitively been shown to increase survival to hospital discharge in patients with cardiac arrest. Some drugs do appear to improve the return of spontaneous circulation and thus may reasonably be given (for dosing, including pediatric, see TABLE 64–3).

In a patient with a peripheral IV line, drug administration is followed by a fluid bolus ("wide open" IV in adults; 3 to 5 mL in young children) to flush the agent into the central circulation. In a patient without IV or intraosseous access, atropine and epinephrine, when indicated, may be given via the endotracheal tube at 2 to 2.5 times the IV dose.

First-line drugs: Epinephrine is the main drug used in cardiac arrest although its benefit is increasingly challenged. It is given q 3 to 5 min. Epinephrine has combined α- and β-adrenergic effects. The α-adrenergic effects may augment coronary diastolic pressure, thereby increasing subendocardial perfusion during chest compressions. Epinephrine also increases the likelihood of successful defibrillation. However, β-adrenergic effects may be detrimental because they increase O_2 requirements (especially of the heart) and cause vasodilation. Intracardiac injection of epinephrine is not recommended because pneumothorax, coronary artery laceration, and cardiac tamponade may occur.

A single dose of vasopressin 40 units is an alternative to epinephrine (adults only); it is not proven superior to epinephrine.

Atropine sulfate is a parasympatholytic drug that increases heart rate and conduction through the atrioventricular node. It is given for asystole (except in children), bradyarrhythmias, and high-degree atrioventricular nodal block, although no survival benefit has been demonstrated.

Amiodarone can be given once if defibrillation is unsuccessful following epinephrine or vasopressin. It is also of potential value if VT or VF recurs following successful defibrillation; a lower dose is given over 10 min followed by a continuous infusion.

TABLE 64–3. DRUGS FOR RESUSCITATION*

DRUG†	ADULT DOSE	PEDIATRIC DOSE	COMMENTS
Adenosine	6 mg initial, then 12 mg × 2	0.1 mg/kg initial, then 0.2 mg/kg × 2	Rapid IV push followed by flush; max dose 12 mg
Amiodarone			
For VF/ pulseless VT	300 mg	5 mg/kg	Give IV push over 2 min
For perfusing VT	Load: 150 mg Infusion: drip 1 mg/min × 6 h, then 0.5 mg/ min × 24 h	5 mg/kg over 20–60 min, repeat to max 15 mg/kg/day	Give initial dose IV push over 10 min
Amrinone	Load: 0.75 mg/kg over 2–3 min Infusion: drip 5–10 μg/kg/min	Load: 0.75–1 mg/kg over 5 min, may repeat up to 3 mg/kg Infusion: 5–10 μg/kg/min	500 mg in 250 mL 0.9% saline gives 2 mg/mL
Atropine	0.5–1 mg	0.02 mg/kg	Repeat q 3–5 min to effect or total dose 0.04 mg/kg; minimum dose 0.1 mg
Endotracheal	1–2 mg		
Ca chloride	1 g	20 mg/kg	10% solution has 100 mg/mL
Ca gluceptate	0.66 g	N/A	22% solution, 220 mg/mL
Ca gluconate	0.6 g	60–100 mg/kg	10% solution, 100 mg/mL
Dobutamine	2–20 μg/kg/min start 2–5 μg/kg/ min	Same	500 mg in 250 mL 5% D/W gives 2000 μg/mL
Dopamine	2–20 μg/kg/min start 2–5 μg/kg/ min	Same	400 mg in 250 mL 5% D/W gives 1600 μg/mL
Epinephrine			
Bolus	1 mg	0.01 mg/kg	Repeat q 3 to 5 min as needed
Endotracheal	2–2.5 mg	0.1 mg/kg	8 mg in 250 mL 5% D/W gives 32 μg/mL
Infusion	2–10 μg/min	0.1–1.0 μg/kg/min	
Glucose	25 g 50% D/W	0.5–1 g/kg	Avoid high concentrations 5% D/W: give 10–20 mL/kg 10% D/W: give 5–10 mL/kg 25% D/W: give 2–4 mL/kg (older children, large vein)

TABLE 64–3. DRUGS FOR RESUSCITATION*—Continued

DRUG†	ADULT DOSE	PEDIATRIC DOSE	COMMENTS
Mg sulfate	1–2 g	25–50 mg/kg to maximum 2 g	Give over 2–5 min
Milrinone	Load: 50 μg/kg over 10 min Infusion: 0.5 μg/kg/min	Load: 50–75 μg/kg over 10 min Infusion: 0.5–0.75 μg/kg/min	50 mg in 250 mL 5% D/W gives 200 μg/mL
Naloxone	2 mg	0.1 mg/kg if < 20 kg or < 5 yr	Repeat as needed
Norepinephrine	Infusion: 2–16 μg/min	Infusion: start 0.05–0.1 μg/kg/min, maximum 2 μg/kg/min	8 mg in 250 mL 5% D/W gives 32 μg/mL
Phenylephrine	Infusion: 0.1–1.5 μg/kg/min	Infusion: 0.1–0.5 μg/kg/min	10 mg in 250 mL 5% D/W gives 40 μg/mL
Procainamide	30 mg/min to effect or max 17 mg/kg	Same	Not recommended for pulseless arrest in pediatric patients
$NaHCO_3$	50 mEq	1 mEq/kg	Infuse slowly and only when ventilation adequate 4.2% contains 0.5 mEq/mL 8.4% contains 1 mEq/mL
Vasopressin	40 units × 1	Not recommended	Single dose

*For indications and use, see text.
†IV or intraosseous.
VF = ventricular fibrillation; VT = ventricular tachycardia.

Other drugs: Ca chloride is recommended for patients with hyperkalemia, hypermagnesemia, hypocalcemia, or Ca channel blocker toxicity. In others, because intracellular Ca is already higher than normal, additional Ca is likely to be detrimental. Because cardiac arrest in patients on renal dialysis is often a result of or accompanied by hyperkalemia, these patients may benefit from a trial of Ca if bedside K determination is unavailable. Caution is necessary because Ca exacerbates digitalis toxicity and can of itself cause cardiac arrest.

Mg sulfate has not been shown to improve outcome in randomized clinical studies. However, it may be helpful in patients with torsades de pointes or known or suspected Mg deficiency (ie, alcoholics, protracted diarrhea).

Procainamide is a 2nd-line drug for treatment of refractory VF or VT. However, procainamide is not recommended in pulseless arrest in pediatric patients.

Phenytoin may rarely be used to treat VF or VT, but only when it is due to digitalis toxicity and is refractory to other drugs. Dose is 50 mg/min given until rhythm improves or total dose reaches 18 mg/kg.

$NaHCO_3$ is no longer recommended unless cardiac arrest is caused by hyperkalemia, hypermagnesemia, or tricyclic antidepressant overdose with complex ventricular arrhythmias. In pediatric patients, $NaHCO_3$ should be considered when cardiac arrest is prolonged (> 10 min); it is administered only if there is good ventilation. When $NaHCO_3$ is used, arterial pH should be monitored before infusion and after each 50-mEq dose (1 to 2 mEq/kg in children).

Lidocaine and bretylium are no longer used during CPR.

Dysrhythmia Treatment

VF/pulseless VT is treated with one DC shock, preferably with biphasic waveform; chest compression is interrupted as little as possible. Recommended energy levels vary: 120 to 200 joules for biphasic waveform and 360 joules for monophasic. If this is unsuccessful, epinephrine 1 mg IV is administered and repeated q 3 to 5 min. Alternatively, vasopressin 40 U IV can be given only once (not in pediatric patients). Cardioversion at the same energy level is attempted 1 min after each drug administration (the role of escalating biphasic energy levels is unclear). If VF persists, amiodarone 300 mg IV is given. Then, if VF/VT recurs, 150 mg is given followed by infusion of 1 mg/min q 6 h, then 0.5 mg/min. (For pediatric energy levels, see TABLE 64–4; for drug doses, see TABLE 64–3.)

Asystole can be mimicked by a loose or disconnected monitor lead; thus, monitor connections should be checked and rhythm viewed in an alternative lead. If asystole is confirmed and heart block is suspected, transcutaneous pacing is performed and the patient is given epinephrine 1 mg IV repeated q 3 to 5 min, and atropine 1 mg IV repeated q 3 to 5 min to a total dose of 0.04 mg/kg. Electrical pacing is rarely successful, but if it is to work it must be instituted early. Note, atropine and pacing are contraindicated in pediatric patients with asystole. Defibrillation of apparent asystole (because it "might be fine VF") is discouraged because electrical shocks injure the nonperfused heart.

Pulseless electrical activity is circulatory collapse that occurs despite satisfactory electrical complexes on the ECG. Patients with pulseless electrical activity receive 500- to 1000-mL (20 mL/kg) infusion of 0.9% saline and epinephrine 0.5 to 1.0 mg IV, repeated q 3 to 5 min. If the heart rate is < 60/min, atropine 0.5 to 1 mg IV is given. Cardiac tamponade can cause pulseless electrical activity, but this usually occurs in patients with known pericardial effusion or major chest trauma. In such settings, immediate pericardiocentesis is performed (see FIG. 78–2 on p. 737). Tamponade is rarely an occult cause of cardiac arrest but, if suspected, can be confirmed by pericardiocentesis or, if immediately available, ultrasound.

Termination of Resuscitation

CPR must be continued until the cardiopulmonary system is stabilized, the patient is pronounced dead, or a lone rescuer is physically unable to continue. If cardiac arrest occurs in hypothermic patients, CPR should be continued until the body is rewarmed to 34° C.

Decision to pronounce death is somewhat subjective, taking into account duration of arrest before treatment, age, prior medical conditions, and other factors, but typically is made following failure to establish spontaneous circulation after 30 to 45 min of CPR and ACLS measures.

POST-RESUSCITATIVE CARE

Return of spontaneous circulation (ROSC) is only an intermediate goal in resuscitation. Only 3 to 8% of patients with ROSC survive to hospital discharge. To maximize the likelihood of good outcome, physiologic parameters must be optimized and underlying conditions addressed. In adults, it is particularly important to recognize MI (see p. 635) and institute reperfusion therapy (eg, thrombolysis, percutaneous transluminal coronary angioplasty) rapidly. CAUTION: *Thrombolysis following aggressive CPR sometimes causes cardiac tamponade.*

Post-resuscitation laboratory studies include ABG, CBC, and blood chemistries, including electrolytes, glucose, BUN, creatinine, and cardiac markers. (Creatine phosphokinase will usually be elevated due to skeletal muscle damage from CPR.) Arterial PaO_2 should be kept near normal values (80 to 100 mm Hg). Hct should be maintained ≥ 30, glucose at 80 to 120 mg/dL, and electrolytes, especially K, should be within the normal range.

BP support: Mean arterial pressure (MAP) should be maintained > 80 mm Hg in older adults, or > 60 mm Hg in younger and previously healthy patients. In patients known to be hypertensive, a reasonable target is systolic BP 30 mm Hg below pre-arrest level.

Patients with low MAP or signs of left ventricular failure may benefit from pulmonary artery catheter monitoring (see p. 513) to measure cardiac output, pulmonary artery occlusion pressure (PAOP), and mixed venous O_2 saturation (a measure of peripheral perfusion) allowing optimal titration of therapy. Mixed venous O_2 saturation should be > 60%.

Patients with low MAP and low central venous pressure or PAOP should have IV fluid challenge with 0.9% saline infused in 250-mL increments. Older adults with moderately low MAP (70 to 80 mm Hg) and normal or high central venous pressure/PAOP may receive infusion of an inotrope, dobutamine started at 2 to 5 µg/kg/min. Alternatively, amrinone or milrinone is used (see TABLE 64–3). If this is ineffective, the inotrope and vasoconstrictor dopamine should be considered. Alternatives are epinephrine and the peripheral vasoconstrictors norepinephrine and phenylephrine (see TABLE 64–3). Vasoactive drugs should be used in the minimal dose necessary to achieve low-normal MAP because they may increase vascular resistance and decrease organ perfusion, especially in the mesenteric bed. They also increase the workload on the heart at a time when its capability is decreased due to post-resuscitation myocardial dysfunction. If MAP remains < 70 mm Hg in patients who may have sustained MI, intra-aortic balloon counterpulsation should be considered. Patients with normal MAP and high central venous pressure/PAOP may improve with either inotropic therapy or afterload reduction with nitroprusside or nitroglycerin.

Intra-aortic balloon counterpulsation can assist low-output circulatory states due to left ventricular pump failure refractory to drugs. A balloon catheter is introduced via the femoral artery, percutaneously or by arteriotomy, retrograde into the thoracic aorta just distal to the left subclavian artery. The balloon inflates during each diastole, augmenting coronary artery perfusion, and deflates during systole, decreasing afterload. Its primary value is as a temporizing measure when the cause of shock is potentially correctable by surgery or percutaneous intervention (eg, acute MI with major coronary obstruction, acute mitral insufficiency, or ventricular septal defect).

Dysrhythmia treatment: Although VF or VT may recur after resuscitation, prophylactic antiarrhythmic drugs do not improve survival and are no longer indicated. However, patients manifesting such rhythms may be treated with procainamide or amiodarone as described above.

Post-resuscitation rapid supraventricular tachycardias occur frequently due to high levels of β-adrenergic catecholamines (both endogenous and exogenous) associated with cardiac arrest and resuscitation. These rhythms should be treated if extreme, prolonged, or associated with hypotension or signs of coronary ischemia. An esmolol IV infusion is given, beginning at 50 µg/kg/min.

Patients who had arrest from VF or VT not associated with an acute MI are candidates for an implantable cardioverter-defibrillator (ICD). Current devices are implanted similar to pacemakers and have intracardiac leads and sometimes subcutaneous electrodes. They can sense arrhythmias and deliver either cardioversion or cardiac pacing as indicated.

Neurologic support: Between 8 and 20% of adults have some degree of CNS dysfunction following resuscitation from cardiac arrest. Hypoxic brain injury is a result of direct neuronal ischemic damage and cerebral edema (see also Pathophysiology on p. 531). Damage may evolve over 48 to 72 h after resuscitation.

Maintenance of oxygenation and cerebral perfusion pressure (avoiding hypotension) can reduce cerebral complications. Also, because hyperglycemia may damage the post-ischemic brain, it should be treated vigorously and glucose administration should be avoided except for documented hypoglycemia.

Additionally, there is now persuasive evidence of the benefits of inducing mild hypothermia. Surface cooling with ice packs can reduce core body temperature to between 30° and 34° C. Alternative methods of cooling include cardiopulmonary bypass or newly available intravascular cooling devices.

Numerous pharmacologic treatments, including free radical scavengers, antioxidants, glutamate inhibitors, and Ca channel blockers, are of theoretic benefit; many have been successful in animal models, but none have proven effective in human trials.

CPR in Infants and Children

Despite the use of CPR, mortality rates for cardiac arrest are 80 to 97% for infants and children. The mortality rate is almost 25% for respiratory arrest alone. Neurologic outcome is often severely compromised.

About 50 to 65% of children requiring CPR are < 1 yr; of these, most are < 6 mo. About 6% of neonates require resuscitation at delivery (see p. 2258); the incidence increases significantly if birth weight is < 1500 g.

Standardized outcome guidelines should be followed in reporting outcomes of CPR in children; eg, the modified Pittsburgh Outcome Categories Scale reflects cerebral and overall performance (see TABLE 64–5).

TABLE 64–4. GUIDE TO PEDIATRIC RESUSCITATION—MECHANICAL MEASURES

AGE (YR)	TERM NB	< 1 MO	1	2	3	4	5	6	7	8	9	10	11	12	13	14	15	16
Weight (kg)	3.5	< 10	10	12	14	16	18	20	22	25	28	30	35	40	45	50	55	60
Ventilation (V) rate/min	30–60	20	20	20	20	20	20	20	20	20	16	16	16	16	16	16	16	16
Compression (C) rate/min	120*	100	100	100	100	100	100	100	100	100	100	100	100	100	100	100	100	100
Compression: ventilation ratio	← 3:1 →	← 5:1 →								← 15:2 (1 or 2 rescuers, unprotected airway) → ← 5:1 (2 rescuers, protected airway) →								
Compression techniques	Thumb compression, hands around chest (preferred) or 2 fingers		← 1 hand →							← 2 hands →								
Airway size (Portex) in cm	000 3.5	00 5	00 5	0 6	0 6	7	7	7	7	7	7	7	7	7	8	8	8	8
Masks in Laerdal sizes or equivalent	Circular 0/1	Rendell-Baker type # 1		Rendell-Baker type # 2			← Dome cuff mask # 3 →					← Dome cuff mask # 4 →						
Ventilation bag with reservoir for 100% O_2 delivery	Infant 240 mL	← Child 400–500 mL →									← Adult 1600 mL →							

Laryngoscope blade size		Miller 0	1	1	1	2	2	2	2	2	2	2	3	3	3	3	3	3	3
		Straight blade	← Straight blade (preferred) or curved blade →								← Curved or straight blade →								
ETT size (Portex) in mm		3	3.5	4	4.5	4.5	5	5	5.5	5.5	6	6	6	6	6.5	6.5	6.5	6.5	7
		Uncuffed	← Uncuffed →									← Cuffed →							
Suction catheter	Direct oro-pharyngeal	10 F	← Pediatric tonsil suction →				← Adult tonsil suction →												
	Through ETT	← 8 Fr →					← 10 Fr →												
Defibrillation (joules)	Dose (2 joules/kg)	7	10	20	20	30	30	30	50	50	50	50	70	70	70	100	100	200	200
		Pediatric paddles		← Adult paddles →															
	Frequency	← If no response, give maximum dose × 2 →																	
	Maximum dose (4 joules/kg)	20	30	50	50	50	70	70	100	100	100	100	100	150	150	200	200	300	300
Cardioversion (joules)	Synchro-nized shock (0.5 joules/kg)	2	3	5	5	7	7	10	10	10	10	10	20	20	20	20	30	30	30
	Frequency	← Increase dose slowly at subsequent attempt to maximum →																	
	Maximum dose (1 joule/kg)	5	5	10	10	10	20	20	20	20	20	30	30	30	50	50	50s	50	70

*Pause for ventilation.

ETT = endotracheal tube; Fr = French.

Courtesy of Dr. B. Paes and Dr. M. Sullivan, the Departments of Pediatrics and Medicine, St. Joseph's Hospital, The Children's Hospital, Hamilton Health Sciences Corporation, McMaster University Hamilton, Ontario, Canada.

TABLE 64–5. PEDIATRIC CEREBRAL PERFORMANCE CATEGORY SCALE*

SCORE	CATEGORY	DESCRIPTION
1	Normal	Age-appropriate level of functioning; preschool-aged child developmentally appropriate; school-aged child attends regular classes
2	Mild disability	Can interact at an age-appropriate level; minor neurologic disease that is controlled and does not interfere with daily functioning (eg, seizure disorder); preschool-aged child may have minor developmental delays, but more than 75% of all daily living developmental milestones are above the 10th percentile; school-aged child attends regular school, but grade is not appropriate for age, or child is failing appropriate grade because of cognitive difficulties
3	Moderate disability	Below age-appropriate functioning; neurologic disease that is not controlled and severely limits activities; most activities of preschool-aged child's daily living developmental milestones are below the 10th percentile; school-aged child can perform activities of daily living but attends special classes because of cognitive difficulties or a learning deficit
4	Severe disability	Preschool-aged child's activities of daily living milestones are below the 10th percentile, and child is excessively dependent on others for provision of activities of daily living; school-aged child may be so impaired as to be unable to attend school; school-aged child is dependent on others for provision of activities of daily living; abnormal motor movements for preschool- and school-aged children may include nonpurposeful, decorticate, or decerebrate responses to pain
5	Coma or vegetative state	Unawareness
6	Death	

*Worst level of performance for any single criterion is used for categorizing. Deficits are scored only if they result from a neurologic disorder. Assessments are made on the basis of medical records or interview with caretaker.

From *Recommended Guidelines for Uniform Reporting of Pediatric Advanced Life Support: The Pediatric Utstein Style; Statement for Health Care Professionals* from the Task Force of the American Academy of Pediatrics, the American Heart Association, and the European Resuscitation Council; *Pediatrics* 96(4):765–779, 1995.

Major Differences Between Pediatric and Adult CPR

Pre-arrest: *Bradycardia in a distressed child is a sign of impending cardiac arrest.* Neonates, infants, and young children are more likely to develop bradycardia from hypoxemia, whereas older children initially tend to have tachycardia. An infant or child with a heart rate < 60/min and signs of poor perfusion that do not rise with ventilatory support should have cardiac compressions (see FIG. 64–7). Bradycardia secondary to heart block is unusual, although it may occur.

After adequate oxygenation and ventilation, epinephrine is the drug of choice.

BP should be measured with an appropriate-sized cuff, but direct invasive arterial BP monitoring is mandatory in severely compromised children.

Since BP varies with age, an easy guideline to remember the lower limits of normal (< 5th percentile) by age is as follows: < 1 mo,

60 mm Hg; 1 mo to 1 yr, 70 mm Hg; > 1 yr, 70 + 2 × age in yr. Thus, in a 5 yr old, hypotension would be defined by a BP of < 80 mmHg [70 + 2 × 5]). Of significant importance is that children maintain BP longer because of stronger compensatory mechanisms (increased heart rate, increased systemic vascular resistance). Once hypotension occurs, cardiorespiratory arrest may rapidly follow. All effort should be made to treat signs of shock (increased heart rate, cool extremities, capillary refill > 2 sec, poor peripheral pulses) before hypotension develops.

Equipment and environment: Equipment size, drug dosage, and CPR parameters vary with patient age and weight (see TABLES 64–3 and 64–4). Size-variable equipment includes defibrillator paddles or electrode pads, masks, ventilation bags, airways, laryngoscope blades, endotracheal tubes, suction catheters. Weight should be measured rather than guessed; alternatively, commercially

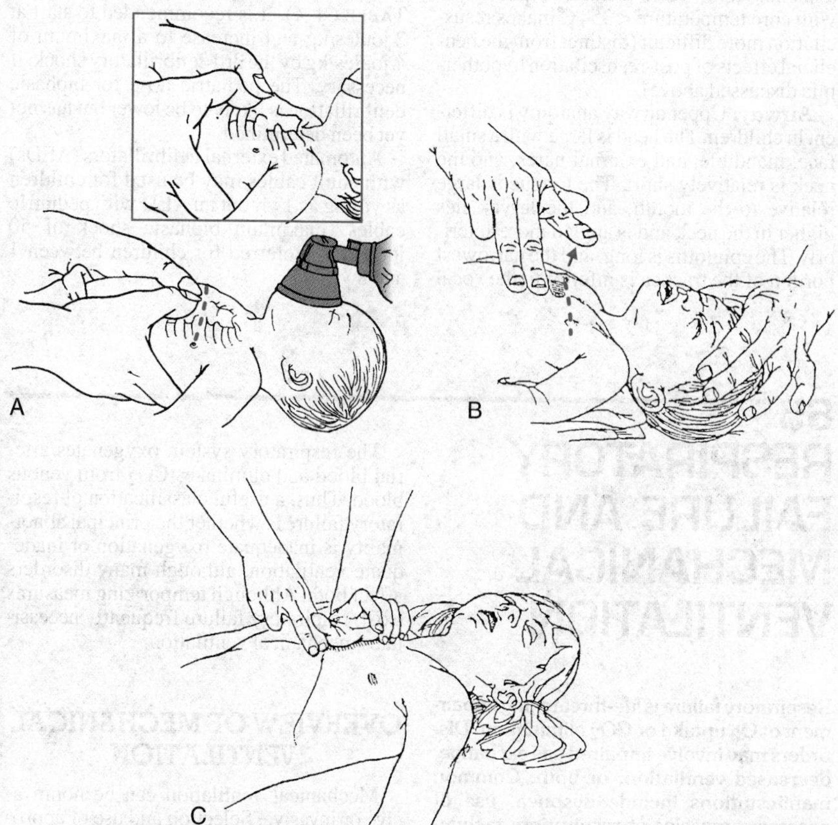

Fig. 64–7. Chest compression. A: Side-by-side thumb placement for chest compressions is preferred for neonates and small infants whose chest can be encircled. Thumbs should overlap if used in very small neonates. B: Two fingers are used for infants. Fingers should be maintained in the upright position during compression. For neonates, this technique will result in too low a position, ie, at or below the xiphoid; the correct position is just below the nipple line. C: Hand position for chest compression for a child. (Adapted from American Heart Association: Standards and Guidelines for CPR. *Journal of the American Medical Association* 1992; 268:2251–2281. Copyright 1992, American Medical Association.)

available measuring tapes that are calibrated to read standard patient weight based on body length can be used. Some tapes are printed with the recommended drug dose and equipment size for each weight. Dosages should be rounded down; eg, a 2 ½ yr old should receive the dose for a 2 yr old.

Susceptibility to heat loss is greater in infants and children because of a large surface area relative to body mass and less subcutaneous tissue. A neutral external thermal environment is crucial during CPR and post-resuscitation and may range from 36.5° C in a neonate to 35° C in a child. Hypothermia with core temperature < 35° C makes resuscitation more difficult (distinct from the beneficial effects of post-resuscitation hypothermia discussed above).

Airway: Upper airway anatomy is different in children. The head is large with a small face, mandible, and external nares, and the neck is relatively short. The tongue is large relative to the mouth, and the larynx lies higher in the neck and is angled more anteriorly. The epiglottis is long, and the narrowest portion of the trachea is inferior to the vocal cords at the cricoid ring, allowing the use of uncuffed endotracheal tubes. In younger children, a straight laryngoscope blade generally allows better visualization of the vocal cords than a curved blade, since the larynx is more anterior and the epiglottis is more floppy and redundant.

Rhythm disturbances: In asystole, atropine and pacing are not used.

VF and pulseless VT occur in only about 15 to 20% of cardiac arrests. Vasopressin is not indicated. When cardioversion is used, the absolute energy dose is less than for adults, and should be 2 to 4 joules/kg monophasic (see TABLE 64–4). It is recommended to start at 2 joules/kg and increase to a maximum of 4 joules/kg by the 3rd defibrillatory shock, if necessary. The pediatric dose for biphasic defibrillation is likely to be lower but has not yet been determined.

Automated external defibrillators (AEDs) with adult cables may be used for children as young as 1 yr, but an AED with pediatric cables (maximum biphasic shock of 50 joules) is preferred for children between 1 and 8 yr.

65 RESPIRATORY FAILURE AND MECHANICAL VENTILATION

The respiratory system oxygenates arterial blood and eliminates CO_2 from venous blood. Thus, a useful classification of respiratory failure is whether the principal abnormality is inadequate oxygenation or inadequate ventilation, although many disorders affect both. Although temporizing measures exist, respiratory failure frequently necessitates mechanical ventilation.

Respiratory failure is life-threatening impairment of O_2 uptake or CO_2 elimination. Disorders may involve impaired gas exchange, decreased ventilation, or both. Common manifestations include dyspnea, use of accessory muscles of respiration, tachypnea, tachycardia, diaphoresis, cyanosis, altered consciousness, and eventually obtundation. Diagnosis is clinical, supplemented by ABGs and chest x-ray. Treatment is in an ICU and involves correction of the underlying cause, supplemental O_2, control of secretions, and ventilatory assistance if needed.

OVERVIEW OF MECHANICAL VENTILATION

Mechanical ventilation can be noninvasive or invasive. Selection and use of appropriate techniques require understanding of respiratory mechanics.

Respiratory Mechanics

Normal inspiration generates negative intrapleural pressure, which creates a pressure gradient between outside air and the lung, resulting in airflow. In mechanical ventilation,

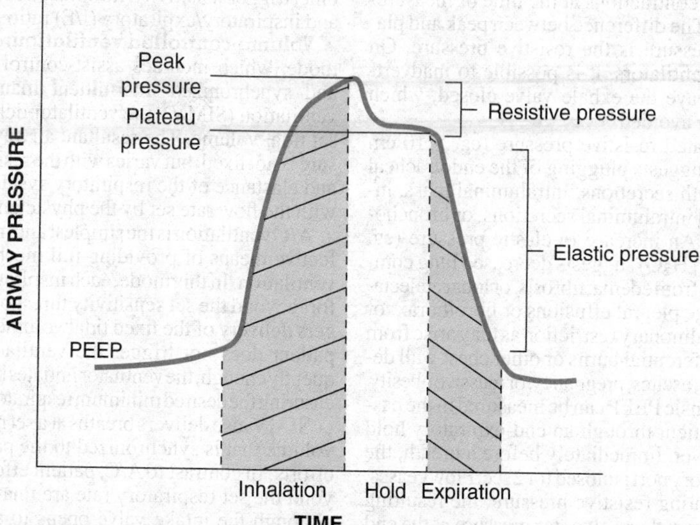

Fig. 65–1. Components of airway pressure during mechanical ventilation, illustrated by an inspiratory-hold maneuver. PEEP = positive end-expiratory pressure.

the pressure gradient is the result of increased (positive) pressure of the air source.

Peak airway pressure is measured at the airway opening (P_{ao}) and is routinely displayed by mechanical ventilators. It represents the total pressure needed to overcome the inspiratory flow resistance (resistive pressure), the elastic recoil of the lung and chest wall (elastic pressure), and the alveolar pressure present at the beginning of the breath (positive end-expiratory pressure [PEEP]). Thus (see also FIG. 65–1):

Peak airway pressure =
resistive pressure +
elastic pressure + PEEP

Resistive pressure is the product of circuit resistance and airflow. In the mechanically ventilated patient, resistance to airflow occurs in the ventilator circuit, the endotracheal tube, and most importantly, in the patient's airways. Note that even when these factors are constant, an increase in airflow increases resistive pressure.

Elastic pressure is the product of the elastic recoil of the lungs and chest wall (elastance) and the volume of gas delivered. For a given volume, elastic pressure is increased by increased lung stiffness (as in pulmonary fibrosis) or restricted excursion of the chest wall or diaphragm (eg, tense ascites). Because elastance is the inverse of compliance, high elastance is the same as low compliance.

End-expiratory pressure in the alveoli is normally the same as atmospheric pressure. However, when the alveoli fail to empty completely because of airway obstruction, airflow limitation, or shortened expiratory time, end-expiratory pressure may be positive relative to the atmosphere. This pressure is called intrinsic PEEP or autoPEEP to differentiate it from externally applied (therapeutic) PEEP, which is set by adjusting the mechanical ventilator or by adding a mask to the airway that applies positive pressure throughout the respiratory cycle.

Any elevation in peak airway pressure (eg, >25 cm H_2O) should prompt measurement of the end-inspiratory pressure (plateau pressure) by an end-inspiratory hold maneuver to determine the relative contributions of resistive and elastic pressures. The maneuver keeps the exhale valve closed for an additional 0.3 to 0.5 sec after inspiration, delaying exhalation. During this time, P_{ao} falls from its peak value as airflow ceases. The resulting end-inspiratory pressure represents the elastic pressure once PEEP is subtracted (assuming the patient is not making active inspiratory or expiratory muscle contractions at the time of measurement). The difference between peak and plateau pressure is the resistive pressure. On some ventilators, it is possible to inadvertently leave the exhale valve closed, which must be avoided.

Elevated resistive pressure (eg, > 10 cm H_2O) suggests plugging of the endotracheal tube with secretions, intraluminal mass, increased intraluminal secretions, or bronchospasm. An increase in elastic pressure (eg, > 10 cm H_2O) suggests decreased lung compliance from edema, fibrosis, or lobar atelectasis; large pleural effusions or fibrothorax; or extrapulmonary restriction as may arise from circumferential burns or other chest wall deformity, ascites, pregnancy, or massive obesity.

Intrinsic PEEP can be measured in the passive patient through an end-expiratory hold maneuver. Immediately before a breath, the expiratory port is closed for 2 sec. Flow ceases, eliminating resistive pressure; the resulting pressure reflects alveolar pressure at the end of expiration (intrinsic PEEP). A nonquantitative method of identifying intrinsic PEEP is to inspect the expiratory flow tracing. If expiratory flow continues until the next breath, or the patient's chest fails to come to rest before the next breath, intrinsic PEEP is present. The consequences of elevated intrinsic PEEP include increased inspiratory work of breathing and decreased venous return.

The demonstration of intrinsic PEEP should prompt a search for causes of airflow obstruction (eg, airway secretions, bronchospasm), although a high minute ventilation (> 20 L/min) alone can result in intrinsic PEEP in a patient with no airflow obstruction. If the cause is airflow limitation, intrinsic PEEP can be reduced by shortening inspiratory time (ie, increasing inspiratory flow) or reducing the respiratory rate, thereby allowing a greater fraction of the respiratory cycle to be spent in exhalation.

Means and Modes of Mechanical Ventilation

Mechanical ventilators are typically volume or pressure controlled; some newer models combine features of both. Because pressures and volumes are directly linked by the pressure-volume curve, any given volume will correspond to a specific pressure, and vice versa, regardless of whether the ventilator is pressure or volume controlled.

Adjustable ventilator settings differ with mode, but include respiratory rate, tidal volume, trigger sensitivity, flow rate, waveform, and inspiratory/expiratory (I/E) ratio.

Volume-controlled ventilation: In this mode, which includes assist-control (A/C) and synchronized intermittent mandatory ventilation (SIMV), the ventilator delivers a set tidal volume. The resultant airway pressure is not fixed, but varies with the resistance and elastance of the respiratory system, and with the flow rate set by the physician.

A/C ventilation is the simplest and most effective means of providing full mechanical ventilation. In this mode, each inspiratory effort beyond the set sensitivity threshold triggers delivery of the fixed tidal volume. If the patient does not trigger the ventilator frequently enough, the ventilator initiates breaths, ensuring the desired minimum respiratory rate.

SIMV also delivers breaths at a set rate and volume that is synchronized to the patient's efforts. In contrast to A/C, patient efforts beyond the set respiratory rate are unassisted, although the intake valve opens to allow a breath. This mode remains popular, despite the fact that it neither provides full ventilator support as does A/C nor is an effective means of liberating the patient from mechanical ventilation.

Pressure-cycled ventilation: This mode includes pressure control ventilation (PCV), pressure support ventilation (PSV), and several noninvasive modalities applied via a tight-fitting face mask. In all of these, the ventilator delivers a set inspiratory pressure. Hence, tidal volume varies depending on the resistance and elastance of the respiratory system. In this mode, changes in respiratory system mechanics can result in unrecognized changes in minute ventilation. Because it limits the distending pressure of the lung, this mode can theoretically benefit patients with acute respiratory distress syndrome (ARDS), although no clear clinical advantage over A/C has been demonstrated.

PCV is similar to A/C; each inspiratory effort beyond the set sensitivity threshold delivers full pressure support maintained for a fixed inspiratory time. A minimum respiratory rate is maintained.

In **PSV,** a minimum rate is not set; all breaths are triggered by the patient. Pressure is typically cut off when back-pressure causes flow to drop below a certain point. Thus, a longer or deeper inspiratory effort by the patient results in a larger tidal volume. This mode is commonly used to liberate the patient from mechanical ventilation by letting him assume more of the work of breathing. A similar mode is continuous positive airway pressure (CPAP), in which a constant pressure is maintained throughout the respiratory cycle. In contrast to PSV, in which different inspiratory and expiratory pressures are possible, CPAP applies the same pressure.

Noninvasive positive pressure ventilation (NIPPV) is the delivery of positive pressure ventilation via a tight-fitting mask that covers the nose or both the nose and mouth. Because of its use in spontaneously breathing patients, it is primarily applied as a form of PSV, although volume control can be used. The physician sets both the expiratory positive airway pressure (EPAP) and the inspiratory positive airway pressure (IPAP), with respirations triggered by the patient. Because the airway is unprotected, aspiration is possible, so patients must have adequate mentation and airway protective reflexes and no imminent indication for surgery or transport off the floor for prolonged procedures. NIPPV should be avoided in patients who are hemodynamically unstable or those with evidence of impaired gastric emptying, such as occurs with ileus, bowel obstruction, or pregnancy. In such circumstances, the swallowing of significant quantities of air may result in life-threatening aspiration. Indications for conversion to endotracheal intubation and conventional mechanical ventilation include the development of shock or frequent arrhythmias, ongoing myocardial ischemia, and transport to a cardiac catheterization laboratory or surgical suite where control of the airway and full ventilatory support are desired. Obtunded patients and those with copious secretions are not good candidates. Also, IPAP must be set below esophageal opening pressure (20 cm H_2O) to avoid gastric insufflation.

Ventilator settings: Ventilator settings are tailored to the underlying condition, but the basic principles are as follows.

Tidal volume and respiratory rate set the minute ventilation. Too high a volume risks overinflation. Too high a rate risks inadequate expiratory time. A tidal volume of 8 to 9 mL/kg ideal body weight (see p. 551) is usually appropriate, although some patients with normal lung mechanics (particularly those with neuromuscular disease) may benefit from a somewhat higher tidal volume to prevent atelectasis. Certain disorders (eg, ARDS) may require lower volumes (see p. 550).

Sensitivity adjusts the level of inspiratory effort required to trigger the ventilator. A typical setting is −2 cm H_2O. Too high a setting will cause weak patients to be unable to trigger a breath. Too low a setting may lead to overventilation by causing the machine to auto-cycle.

I:E ratio can be adjusted in some modes. Initial settings for patients with normal mechanics are generally 1:3. Patients with asthma or COPD exacerbations should have ratios of 1:4 or even more.

Inspiratory flow rate is adjusted in other modes (ie, either the flow rate or the I:E ratio is adjusted, not both). The inspiratory flow should generally be set at about 60 L/min but can be increased up to 120 L/min for patients with airflow limitation.

PEEP can be applied in any ventilator mode. PEEP increases end-expired lung volume and prevents airspace closure at the end of expiration. Most patients undergoing mechanical ventilation may benefit from the application of PEEP at 5 cm H_2O to limit the atelectasis that frequently accompanies endotracheal intubation and the supine position. Higher levels of PEEP improve oxygenation in alveolar filling disorders, such as cardiogenic pulmonary edema and ARDS, by redistributing pulmonary edema fluid from the alveoli to the interstitium and opening collapsed alveoli. PEEP permits lower levels of fractional inspired O_2 (FIO_2) to be used while preserving adequate arterial oxygenation. This is important in limiting the lung injury that may result from prolonged exposure to a high FIO_2 (≥ 0.6). PEEP increases intrathoracic pressure and thus may impede venous return, provoking hypotension in the hypovolemic patient. PEEP that is too low may allow cyclic opening and closing of alveoli, causing alveolar damage from the resultant repetitive shear forces.

Complications of Mechanical Ventilation

Complications can be divided into those resulting from endotracheal intubation and those from mechanical ventilation itself. The former include sinusitis, ventilator-associated pneumonia (see p. 430), tracheal stenosis, vocal cord injury, and tracheal-esophageal or tracheal-vascular fistula. Complications of mechanical ventilation itself include pneumothorax, hypotension, and ventilator-associated lung injury (VALI), with airway and/or parenchymal damage occurring as a result of cyclical air space opening and closing, lung overdistention, or both.

If acute hypotension develops in the mechanically ventilated patient, tension pneumothorax must always be considered. More commonly, however, hypotension is a result of decreased venous return caused by high intrathoracic pressure, as occurs in patients receiving high levels of PEEP or in those with high levels of intrinsic PEEP from asthma or COPD, particularly when hypovolemia is present. Hypotension may also be due to sympathetic lysis from sedatives used to facilitate intubation and ventilation. If there are no physical findings suggestive of tension pneumothorax, and ventilation-related causes are a possible etiology, pending a portable chest x-ray, the patient may be disconnected from the ventilator and gently bagged manually at 2 to 3 breaths/min with 100% O_2 while volume is infused (eg, 500 to 1000 mL of 0.9% saline in adults, 20 mL/kg in children); an immediate improvement suggests a ventilation-related cause, and ventilator settings should be adjusted accordingly.

As with other critically ill patients, GI bleeding and venous thromboembolic disease may occur. All patients receiving mechanical ventilation should receive deep venous thrombosis prophylaxis, either heparin 5000 units sc bid or sequential compression devices. To prevent GI bleeding, patients should receive an H_2 blocker (eg, famotidine 20 mg enterally or IV bid) or sucralfate (1 g enterally qid). Proton pump inhibitors should be reserved for patients with a preexisting indication or active bleeding.

The most effective way to reduce complications of mechanical ventilation is to limit its duration.

ACUTE HYPOXEMIC RESPIRATORY FAILURE

Acute hypoxemic respiratory failure is severe arterial hypoxemia that is refractory to supplemental O_2. It is caused by intrapulmonary shunting of blood secondary to airspace flooding. Findings include dyspnea and tachypnea. Diagnosis is by ABGs and chest x-ray. Treatment usually requires mechanical ventilation.

Etiology and Pathophysiology

TABLE 65–1 lists the causes of acute hypoxemic respiratory failure (AHRF). Most common are pulmonary edema, severe pneumonia, and acute respiratory distress syndrome (ARDS—see p. 556). Pulmonary edema may occur when capillary hydrostatic pressures are elevated, as in left ventricular failure or hypervolemia, or when capillary permeability is increased, as occurs in acute lung injury. Such injury may be direct (eg, pneumonia, acid aspiration) or indirect (eg, sepsis, pancreatitis, massive blood transfusion). In all forms of acute lung injury, alveoli are flooded by proteinaceous edema fluid, and abnormalities in surfactant promote airspace collapse, further decreasing the volume of aerated lung and worsening intrapulmonary shunting.

Flooded airspaces allow no inspired gas to enter, so the blood perfusing those alveoli remains at the mixed venous O_2 content no matter how high the fractional inspired O_2 (FIO_2). This ensures constant admixture of deoxygenated blood into the pulmonary vein and hence arterial hypoxemia. In contrast, hypoxemia that is the result of mismatching of ventilation and perfusion (as occurs in asthma or COPD) is readily corrected by supplemental O_2 and is not considered AHRF. This is because airspaces with ventilation/perfusion mismatch allow some inhaled gas to enter, so giving high concentrations of O_2 will raise PaO_2.

Symptoms, Signs, and Diagnosis

Acute hypoxemia (see also p. 520) may produce dyspnea, restlessness, and anxiety. Signs include confusion or alteration of consciousness, cyanosis, tachypnea, tachycardia, and diaphoresis. Cardiac arrhythmia and coma can result. Airway flooding produces crackles on chest auscultation, which are typically diffuse but sometimes worse at the lung bases. Jugular venous distention occurs with severe ventricular failure.

Hypoxemia is usually first recognized by pulse oximetry. Patients with low O_2 saturation should have an ABG and chest x-ray. Symptomatic patients should be treated with supplemental O_2 while awaiting test results.

If supplemental O_2 does not improve the O_2 saturation to >90%, right-to-left shunting of blood should be suspected. An obvious alveolar infiltrate on chest x-ray implicates alveolar flooding as the cause, rather than an intracardiac shunt.

Once AHRF is diagnosed, the cause must be determined, considering both pulmonary and extrapulmonary causes. Sometimes a known ongoing disorder (eg, acute MI, pancreatitis, sepsis) is an obvious cause. In other cases, history is suggestive; pneumonia should be suspected in an immunocompromised patient, and alveolar hemorrhage is suspected after bone marrow transplant or in a patient with a connective tissue disease. Frequently, however, critically ill patients have received a large volume of IV fluids for resuscitation, and high-pressure AHRF (eg, ventricular failure, fluid overload) resulting from treatment must be distinguished from an underlying low-pressure AHRF (eg, ARDS, pneumonia).

High-pressure pulmonary edema is suggested by a 3rd heart sound, jugular venous distention, and peripheral edema on examination and by diffuse central infiltrates, cardiomegaly, and an abnormally wide vascular pedicle seen on chest x-ray. The diffuse infiltrates of ARDS are generally more peripheral. Focal infiltrates are typically caused by lobar pneumonia, atelectasis, or lung contusion. Although echocardiography may demonstrate left ventricular dysfunction, implying a cardiac origin, this finding is not specific because heart disease is common in critically ill patients. Although controversial, insertion of a pulmonary artery catheter (see p. 513) may help confirm the diagnosis, particularly when overlapping diagnoses are possible.

Treatment

Underlying causes must be addressed as discussed elsewhere in THE MANUAL. AHRF is initially treated with high flows of 70 to 100% O_2 by a non-rebreather face mask. If O_2 saturation > 90% is not obtained, mechanical ventilation probably should be instituted. Specific management varies by condition.

Mechanical ventilation in cardiogenic pulmonary edema: Mechanical ventilation benefits the failing left ventricle in several ways. Positive inspiratory pressure reduces ventricular preload and afterload and unloads the respiratory muscles, reducing the work of breathing. Reducing the work of breathing redistributes cardiac output away from overworked respiratory muscles toward vital organs (eg, brain, gut, kidneys). Expiratory pressure

TABLE 65–1. CAUSES OF ACUTE HYPOXEMIC RESPIRATORY FAILURE

- Diffuse lung lesions
  - Cardiogenic (hydrostatic or high-pressure) edema
    - Left ventricular failure (from ischemic heart disease, cardiomyopathy, valvular disease)
    - Volume overload (particularly with coexisting renal or cardiac disease)
  - Permeability (low-pressure) edema (ARDS)
    - Most common
      - Sepsis and systemic inflammatory response syndrome
      - Acid aspiration
      - Multiple transfusions for hypovolemic shock
    - Less common
      - Near drowning
      - Pancreatitis
      - Air or fat embolism
      - Cardiopulmonary bypass
      - Drug reaction or overdose
      - Leukoagglutination
      - Inhalation injury
      - Infusion of biologics (eg, IL-2)
  - Edema of unclear or mixed etiology
    - Reexpansion
    - Neurogenic, postictal
    - Tocolysis-associated
    - High-altitude
  - Alveolar hemorrhage
    - Connective tissue disease
    - Thrombocytopenia
    - Bone marrow transplantation
    - Infection in immunocompromised patients
- Focal lung lesions
  - Lobar pneumonia
  - Lung contusion
  - Lobar atelectasis

ARDS = acute respiratory distress syndrome.

Modified from: O'Connor MF, Hall JB, Schmidt GA, Wood LDH: Acute hypoxemic respiratory failure. In Hall JB, Schmidt GA, Wood LDH: *Principles of Critical Care,* 2nd ed. New York, McGraw-Hill, 1998, p. 537–564.

(expiratory positive airway [EPAP] or positive end-expiratory [PEEP]) redistributes pulmonary edema and opens collapsed alveoli.

Noninvasive positive pressure ventilation (NIPPV) is useful in averting endotracheal intubation in many patients because drug therapy often gives rapid improvement. Typical settings are inspiratory positive airway pressure (IPAP) of 10 to 15 cm H_2O and EPAP of 5 to 8 cm H_2O, while the least FIO_2 necessary to achieve arterial O_2 saturation ≥ 90% is administered.

Conventional mechanical ventilation can use several ventilator modes. Most often, assist-control (A/C) is used in the acute setting, when full ventilatory support is desired. Initial settings are tidal volume of 6 mL/kg ideal body weight (see p. 551), respiratory rate of 25/min, FIO_2 of 1.0, and PEEP of 5 to 8 cm H_2O. PEEP may then be titrated upward in 2.5-cm H_2O increments while the FIO_2 is decreased to nontoxic levels. Pressure support ventilation also can be used (with similar levels of PEEP). The initial pressure delivered should be sufficient to fully rest the respiratory muscles as judged by subjective patient assessment, respiratory rate, and accessory muscle use. Typically, a pressure support level of 10 to 20 cm H_2O over PEEP is required.

Mechanical ventilation in ARDS: Nearly all patients require mechanical ventilation, which, in addition to improving oxygenation, reduces O_2 demand by resting respiratory muscles. Goals include keeping the plateau airway pressures < 30 cm H_2O and the tidal volume equal to 6 mL/kg predicted body weight to minimize further lung injury from alveolar overdistention. Ideally, the FIO_2 should be kept < 0.7 to minimize possible O_2 toxicity.

NIPPV is occasionally useful with ARDS. However, compared to cardiogenic pulmonary edema, higher levels of support for a longer duration are often required, and EPAP of 8 to 12 cm H_2O is often necessary to maintain adequate oxygenation. This requires inspiratory pressures > 18 to 20 cm H_2O, which are poorly tolerated; maintaining an adequate seal becomes difficult, the mask becomes more uncomfortable, and skin necrosis and gastric insufflation may occur. Also, NIPPV-treated patients who subsequently need intubation have generally progressed to a more advanced condition than if they had been intubated earlier; thus, critical desaturation is possible at the time of intubation. Intensive monitoring and careful selection of patients (see p. 547) are required.

Conventional mechanical ventilation in ARDS previously focused on normalizing ABG values and ignored the mechanical effects of lung insufflation. It is now clear that alveolar overdistention can perpetuate lung injury, and that such overdistention occurs readily in patients with ARDS when historical tidal volumes of 10 to 12 mL/kg are used, because many fewer alveoli are available to accept a given tidal volume. ARDS patients have lower mortality when ventilated with a tidal volume of 6 mL/kg ideal body weight (see Equation on p. 551). This necessitates an increase in respiratory rate, even up to 35/min, to counteract the hypercapnia caused by small tidal volumes. Nonetheless, significant respiratory acidosis often develops, which is accepted for the greater good of limiting ventilator-associated lung injury and is generally well tolerated. Tolerance of increased PCO_2 is called permissive hypercapnia. Because hypercapnia may produce dyspnea and cause the patient to be discoordinated with the ventilator, patients should receive analgesics (eg, morphine) and high doses of sedatives (eg, propofol initiated at 5 μg/kg/min and increasing to effect up to 50 μg/kg/min; because of the risk of hypertriglyceridemia, triglyceride levels should be checked every 48 h). This regimen is preferred to neuromuscular blockade, which does not increase patient comfort and may cause residual weakness after prolonged use.

PEEP improves oxygenation in ARDS by increasing the volume of aerated lung through alveolar recruitment, permitting the use of a lower FIO_2. Some investigators titrate PEEP to both arterial O_2 saturation and lung compliance as determined at the bedside; however, this approach is not demonstrably better than using the least amount of PEEP that results in an adequate arterial O_2 saturation on a nontoxic FIO_2. This is often a PEEP of 8 to 15 cm H_2O, although the occasional patient with severe ARDS may require levels > 20 cm H_2O. In these cases, close attention must be paid to other means of optimizing O_2 delivery and minimizing O_2 consumption (see p. 558).

The best indicator of alveolar overdistention is measurement of a plateau pressure through an end-inspiratory hold maneuver as outlined above; it should be checked every 4 h and after each change in PEEP or tidal volume. The target plateau pressure is < 30 cm

H_2O. If the plateau pressure exceeds this value, the physician should reduce the tidal volume in 0.5- to 1.0-mL/kg increments as tolerated to a minimum of 4 mL/kg, raising the respiratory rate to compensate for the reduction in minute ventilation and inspecting the ventilator waveform display to ensure that full exhalation occurs. The respiratory rate may often be raised as high as 35/min before overt gas trapping from incomplete exhalation results. If plateau pressure is < 25 cm H_2O and tidal volume is < 6 mL/kg, tidal volume may be increased to 6 mL/kg or until plateau pressure is > 25 cm H_2O. Some investigators believe pressure control ventilation protects the lungs better, although supportive data are lacking.

Generally, the following approach is recommended for ventilator management in ARDS: Initially use A/C mode with tidal volume 6 mL/kg ideal body weight, respiratory rate 25/min, flow rate 60 L/min, FIO_2 1.0, and PEEP 15 cm H_2O. Once O_2 saturation is > 90%, FIO_2 is decreased to nontoxic levels (≤ 0.6). Then, PEEP is decreased in 2.5-cm H_2O increments as tolerated to find the least PEEP associated with an arterial O_2 saturation of 90% on an FIO_2 of ≤ 0.6. The respiratory rate is increased up to 35/min to achieve a pH > 7.15, or until the expiratory flow tracing demonstrates end-expiratory flow.

Ideal body weight (IBW) rather than actual body weight is used to determine the appropriate tidal volume for patients with lung disease receiving mechanical ventilation:

IBW (kg) Males:

$$50 + 2.3(\text{height in inches} - 60)$$
$$or\ \ 50 + 0.91(\text{height in cm} - 152.4)$$

IBW (kg) Females:

$$45.5 + 2.3(\text{height in inches} - 60)$$
$$or\ \ 45.5 + 0.91(\text{height in cm} - 152.4)$$

VENTILATORY FAILURE

Ventilatory failure is a rise in $PaCO_2$ (hypercapnia) that occurs when the respiratory load can no longer be supported by the strength of the system. The most common causes are acute exacerbations of asthma and COPD. Findings include dyspnea, tachypnea, and confusion. Death can result. Diagnosis is by ABGs and patient observation; chest x-ray and clinical evaluation may help delineate cause. Treatment varies by condition but often includes mechanical ventilation.

Etiology and Pathophysiology

Hypercapnia occurs when alveolar ventilation either falls or fails to rise adequately in response to increased CO_2 production.

A fall in alveolar ventilation is the result of a decrease in minute ventilation or an increase in dead space ventilation.

Minute ventilation decreases when there is an imbalance between the load on the respiratory system (including resistive loads, lung and chest wall elastic loads, and minute ventilation loads) and the neuromuscular competence for an effective inspiratory effort (see FIG. 65–2 for causes).

Physiologic dead space is that part of the respiratory tree that does not participate in gas exchange. This includes the anatomic dead space (oropharynx, trachea, and airways), and the alveolar dead space (ie, alveoli that are ventilated but not perfused). The physiologic dead space normally comprises 30 to 40% of tidal volume but increases to 50% in endotracheally intubated patients and to > 70% in massive pulmonary embolism, severe emphysema, and status asthmaticus. Thus, for any given minute ventilation, the greater the dead space, the poorer the CO_2 elimination.

Increased CO_2 production is usually only a contributory cause of ventilatory failure. It increases with fever, sepsis, trauma, burns, hyperthyroidism, malignant hyperthermia, and an increase in the work of breathing.

Hypercapnia lowers arterial pH (respiratory acidosis). Severe acidemia (pH < 7.2) contributes to pulmonary arteriolar vasoconstriction, systemic vascular dilation, reduced myocardial contractility, hyperkalemia, hypotension, and cardiac irritability, with the potential for life-threatening arrhythmias. Acute hypercapnia also causes cerebral vasodilation and increased intracranial pressure, a major problem in patients with acute head injury. Over time, tissue buffering and renal compensation can largely correct the acidemia. However, sudden increases in $PaCO_2$ can occur faster than compensatory changes ($PaCO_2$ rises 3 to 6 mm Hg/min in a totally apneic patient).

Symptoms and Signs

Symptoms are mainly dyspnea. Signs include vigorous use of accessory ventilatory

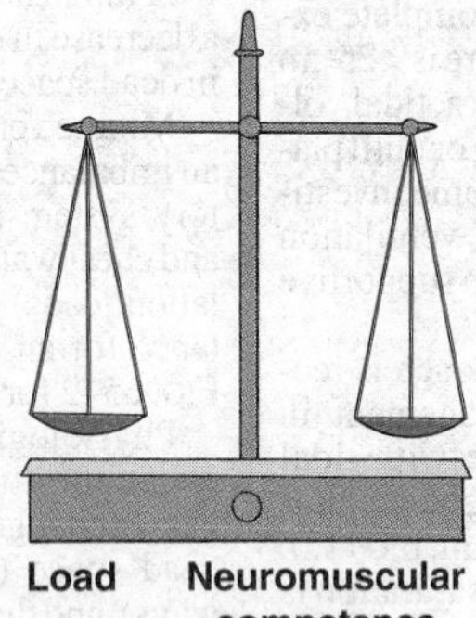

Chest wall elastic loads
Abdominal distention
Ascites
Obesity
Pleural effusion
Pneumothorax
Rib fracture
Tumor
Lung elastic loads
Alveolar edema
Atelectasis
Infection
Intrinsic PEEP
Minute ventilation loads
Excess calories
Hypovolemia
Pulmonary embolus
Sepsis
Resistive loads
Bronchospasm (eg, asthma, bronchiolitis, COPD)
Edema, secretions, or scarring of airway
Obstructive sleep apnea
Upper airway obstruction (eg, croup, epiglottitis)
Load
Neuromuscular competence
Impaired respiratory drive
Brainstem lesion
Drug overdose
Hypothyroidism
Sleep-disordered breathing
Impaired neurotransmission
Aminoglycosides
Amyotrophic lateral sclerosis
Botulism
Spinal cord lesion
Guillain-Barré syndrome
Myasthenia gravis
Neuromuscular blockers
Phrenic nerve injury
Muscle weakness
Electrolyte abnormalities
Fatigue
Hypoperfusion states
Hypoxemia
Myopathy
Undernutrition

Fig. 65–2. The balance between load (resistive, elastic, and minute ventilation) and neuromuscular competence (drive, transmission, and muscle strength) determines the ability to sustain alveolar ventilation. PEEP = positive end-expiratory pressure.

muscles, tachypnea, tachycardia, diaphoresis, anxiety, declining tidal volume, irregular or gasping breathing patterns, and paradoxical abdominal motion.

CNS manifestations range from subtle personality changes to marked confusion, obtundation, or coma. Chronic hypercapnia is better tolerated than acute, with fewer symptoms.

Diagnosis

Ventilatory failure should be suspected in patients with respiratory distress, visible ventilatory fatigue or cyanosis, changes in sensorium, and in those with disorders causing neuromuscular weakness. Tachypnea is also a concern; respiratory rates > 28 to 30/min cannot be sustained for very long, particularly in elderly or weakened patients.

Patients suspected of ventilatory failure should have ABG analysis, continuous pulse oximetry, and chest x-ray. Respiratory acidosis on the ABG (eg, pH < 7.35 and P_{CO_2} > 50) confirms the diagnosis. Patients with chronic ventilatory failure often have quite elevated P_{CO_2} (eg, 60 to 90 mm Hg) at baseline, typically with a pH that is only slightly acidemic; in such patients, the degree of acidemia must serve as the primary marker for acute hypoventilation.

Because ABGs can be normal in incipient ventilatory failure, certain bedside pulmonary function tests can help predict ventilatory failure, particularly in those patients with neuromuscular weakness who may succumb to ventilatory failure without exhibiting respiratory distress. Vital capacity < 10 to 15 mL/kg and a maximum negative inspiratory force of 15 cm H_2O suggest imminent ventilatory failure.

Once ventilatory failure is diagnosed, the cause must be identified. Sometimes a known ongoing disorder (eg, acute asthma, COPD, myasthenia gravis) is an obvious cause. In other cases, history is suggestive; sudden onset of tachypnea and hypotension following surgery suggests pulmonary embolism; focal neurologic findings suggest a CNS or neuromuscular cause. Neuromuscular competence may be assessed through measurement of inspiratory muscle strength (negative inspiratory force and positive expiratory force), neuromuscular transmission (nerve conduction tests and electromyography), and investigations into causes of diminished drive (toxicology screens, brain imaging, sleep studies, and thyroid function tests).

Treatment

Treatment aims to correct the imbalance between the strength of the respiratory system and its load and varies with underlying etiology. Obvious precipitants (eg, bronchospasm, mucus plugging, foreign bodies) should be reversed if possible.

The 2 most common causes are acute exacerbation of asthma (ie, status asthmaticus [SA]) and COPD. Respiratory failure from COPD is termed acute-on-chronic respiratory failure (ACRF).

Status asthmaticus: Patients should be treated in an ICU with personnel skilled in airway management available.

Noninvasive positive pressure ventilation (NIPPV) can immediately reduce the work of breathing and may forestall endotracheal intubation while awaiting improvement from drug therapy. In contrast to patients with COPD, who often welcome NIPPV, the mask often increases the perception of dyspnea in asthmatic patients, so introduction must be careful. After an explanation of its benefit, the patient holds the mask against his face while modest amounts of pressure are applied (continuous positive airway pressure [CPAP] 3 to 5 cm H_2O). Once tolerated, the mask is strapped in place while pressures are increased to patient comfort and reduced work of breathing as assessed by respiratory rate and accessory muscle use. Final settings are typically inspiratory positive airway pressure (IPAP) 10 to 15 cm H_2O and expiratory positive airway pressure (EPAP) 5 to 8 cm H_2O. Patients should be selected carefully (see p. 547).

Conventional mechanical ventilation via endotracheal intubation is indicated for impending respiratory failure as indicated clinically by obtundation, monosyllabic speech, slumped posture, and shallow breathing. ABGs showing worsening hypercapnia are also an indication, although blood-gas confirmation is not required and should not replace the physician's judgment. Oral intubation is preferred over nasal because it allows use of a larger endotracheal tube, which decreases airway resistance and permits easier suctioning.

Hypotension and pneumothorax occasionally occur after intubation for SA (see under Complications of Mechanical Ventilation on p. 547 for management). These complications and their corresponding mortality have declined significantly because of a ventilator strategy that emphasizes limiting dynamic hyperinflation over achieving eucapnia. In SA, ventilation sufficient to achieve a normal pH typically causes severe hyperinflation. To avoid this, initial ventilator settings include a tidal volume of 5 to 7 mL/kg and a respiratory rate of 10 to 18 /min. Inspiratory flows can be quite high (eg, 120 L/min) with a square wave pattern. This strategy reduces minute ventilation and increases the time available for exhalation. Dangerous dynamic hyperinflation is unlikely so long as the measured plateau pressure is < 30 to 35 cm H_2O and intrinsic positive end-expiratory pressure (PEEP) is < 15 cm H_2O. Plateau pressure > 35 cm H_2O is addressed by reducing the tidal volume (assuming that clinical evaluation does not indicate that the high pressures are the result of decreased compliance of the chest wall or abdomen) or the respiratory rate.

Although it is possible to reduce peak airway pressure by reducing peak flow rate or by changing the waveform to a descending profile, this should *not* be done. Although high flow rates require a high pressure to overcome the high airway resistance of SA, this pressure is dissipated across robust, cartilage-containing airways. Lower flow rates reduce time available for exhalation, thereby increasing the end-expiratory volume (and the resultant intrinsic PEEP) and allowing a greater inspiratory volume during the next breath.

Using low tidal volumes often results in hypercapnia, which is permitted for the greater good of reducing dynamic hyperinflation. An arterial pH > 7.15 is generally well tolerated but often requires large doses of sedatives and opioids. Neuromuscular blockers should be avoided after the peri-intubation period, as the use of these agents in combination with corticosteroids can cause a severe and occasionally irreversible myopathy, particularly after 24 h of combined use. Patient agitation should be addressed with sedation rather than paralysis.

Most patients with SA improve to the point of liberation from mechanical ventilation within 2 to 5 days, although a minority experience protracted severe airflow obstruction. The general approach to liberation is discussed on p. 555.

ACRF: In patients with ACRF from COPD, the O_2 cost of breathing is several times that of patients without underlying lung disease. This increased respiratory load is balanced by a barely adequate neuromuscular competence, so the patient easily becomes too tired to maintain ventilation. These patients are vulnerable to respiratory failure from seemingly trivial insults, and recovery requires systematic identification and correction of these precipitants (see also p. 400). To restore the balance between neuromuscular competence and load, airflow obstruction and dynamic hyperinflation are reduced with bronchodilators and corticosteroids, and infection is treated with antibiotics. Low serum levels of K, phosphorus, and Mg may exacerbate muscle weakness, frustrating recovery, and must be identified and treated.

NIPPV is the preferred initial treatment for many patients with ACRF, resulting in decreased rates of ventilator-associated pneumonia, length of stay, and mortality versus endotracheal intubation. Perhaps 75% of patients managed with NIPPV do not require endotracheal intubation. Advantages include the ease of application and removal; once initial stabilization has occurred, NIPPV may be stopped temporarily to allow oral intake in selected patients. Trials of unassisted breathing are easily performed, and NIPPV is reapplied as indicated.

Typical settings are IPAP of 10 to 15 cm H_2O and EPAP of 5 to 8 cm H_2O, titrated to the work of breathing as assessed by patient report, respiratory rate and tidal volume, and accessory muscle use. The same concerns regarding the potential effect of excessive IPAP on total lung capacity as discussed above exist in these patients as well.

Deterioration (and need for endotracheal intubation) is best assessed clinically; ABGs may be misleading. Although worsening hypercapnia typically indicates treatment failure, patients differ markedly in tolerance of hypercapnia. Some with $Paco_2$ > 100 mm Hg are alert and conversant on NIPPV, whereas others require intubation at much lower levels.

Conventional mechanical ventilation in ACRF aims to minimize dynamic hyperinflation and intrinsic PEEP while resting the fatigued respiratory muscles. Initial recommended settings are assist-control (A/C) with a tidal volume of 5 to 7 mL/kg and a respiratory rate of 20 to 24/min, although some patients need lower initial rates to limit intrinsic PEEP. This intrinsic PEEP represents an inspiratory threshold load that must be overcome by the patient to trigger the ventilator, further increasing the work of breathing and preventing full rest on the ventilator. To counterbalance the effect of intrinsic PEEP, external PEEP should be applied to a level ≤ 85% of intrinsic PEEP (typical setting 5 to 10 cm H_2O). This decreases the work of breathing and rarely worsens dynamic hyperinflation. To maximize the time for expiration, high inspiratory flow rates should be used. These settings minimize the risk of alkalemia that follows overly vigorous initial ventilation. Hypotension also may occur immediately after intubation (see p. 548).

Most patients should be rested on full ventilator support for 24 to 48 h before spontaneous breathing trials are considered. The patient often sleeps heavily during this time and, in contrast to SA, typically requires little sedation. Adequate rest is often not achieved unless sufficient attention is paid to ongoing patient effort. This effort may manifest as accessory muscle use, inappropriately low airway pressures at the onset or throughout inspiration, or frequent failures to trigger the ventilator, indicating high intrinsic PEEP and/or weakness. Ventilator settings must be adjusted to relieve these phenomena primarily by lengthening expiratory time; failure to liberate the patient from the ventilator is hardly surprising if the respiratory muscles are never adequately rested. However, distinguishing weakened respiratory muscles from fatigue vs the reduced respiratory muscle strength that occurs near total lung capacity is impossible.

OTHER TYPES OF RESPIRATORY FAILURE

Perioperative respiratory failure is usually caused by atelectasis in the perioperative period. Effective means of preventing or treating atelectasis include incentive spirometry, ensuring adequate analgesia for chest and abdominal incisions, and upright positioning and early mobilization. Atelectasis caused by abdominal distention should be alleviated according to the cause (eg, nasogastric suction for excessive intraluminal air, paracentesis to evacuate tense ascites).

Hypoperfusion from any cause may result in respiratory failure through inadequate delivery of O_2 to respiratory muscles coupled to excess respiratory muscle load (eg, acidosis, sepsis). Mechanical ventilation is useful at diverting blood flow from overworked respiratory muscles to critical organs such as the brain, kidney, and gut.

LIBERATION FROM MECHANICAL VENTILATION

The discontinuation of ventilatory support is best achieved not by gradually reducing the level of ventilatory support ("weaning") but by systematically identifying and eliminating the precipitants of respiratory failure. Once this has been achieved, the ventilator is no longer necessary. However, if precipitants are still present or recovery is incomplete, reducing needed ventilatory support is more likely to delay recovery. It is now clear that daily spontaneous breathing trials on a T-piece reduce the duration of mechanical ventilation compared with gradual reduction of the respiratory rate using synchronized intermittent mandatory ventilation, and, in some studies, versus pressure support trials as well.

Once the patient is no longer in shock, has an adequate arterial saturation on a fractional inspired O_2 (FIO_2) ≤ 0.5 with a positive end-expiratory pressure (PEEP) ≤ 7.5 cm H_2O, and does not have an obviously unsustainable respiratory load (eg, minute ventilation > 20 L/min), a daily spontaneous breathing trial is performed using a T-piece or continuous positive airway pressure (CPAP) of 5 cm H_2O. Patients capable of sustaining spontaneous breathing generally breathe slowly and deeply, instead of rapidly and shallowly. This observation has been formalized as the rapid shallow breathing (RSB) index, determined by dividing the patient's unassisted respiratory rate (in breaths/min) by the tidal volume (in L). A value < 105 suggests that spontaneous breathing is likely to be successful, although a single isolated measurement is not perfectly predictive of success. The decision to extubate is a separate one from the decision to stop ventilatory support and requires evaluation of the patient's mentation and airway protective reflexes, as well as the patency of the airway.

Although sedatives and opioids are essential for ensuring comfort, rest, and synchrony with the ventilator, their use may prolong mechanical ventilation. Such drugs may accumulate and cause protracted sedation, frustrating attempts to perform spontaneous breathing trials even when the cause of respiratory failure has been corrected. The level of sedation should be continually assessed, and progressive sedative withdrawal should be begun as soon as possible. Formal protocols can be used, or simple daily interruption can be carried out. The infusion is stopped until the patient is either awake and following commands or needs re-sedation for agitation, ventilator discoordination, or physiologic derangements. If sedation is still needed, it is restarted at ½ the previous dose and titrated as necessary.

66 ACUTE LUNG INJURY AND ACUTE RESPIRATORY DISTRESS SYNDROME

Acute lung injury (ALI) and acute respiratory distress syndrome (ARDS) are inflammatory disorders of the lung most commonly caused by sepsis, pneumonia, trauma, and/or aspiration. ALI and ARDS are characterized by hypoxemia and diffuse infiltrates on chest x-ray in the absence of elevated left atrial pressure. ALI and ARDS differ only in the degree of hypoxemia. Diagnosis is by clinical presentation, ABGs, and imaging studies. Treatment is with lung-protective, low tidal volume mechanical ventilation, supportive therapy, and treatment of underlying causes. Mortality is still high (30 to 40%) and worsens with age and comorbidities, although overall mortality rates have declined in the past decade.

ALI and ARDS are syndromes of widespread lung inflammation and increased pulmonary vascular permeability. ALI and ARDS are the same clinical disorder, differing only in severity of hypoxemia (see TABLE 66–1). Distinguishing between these two forms is arbitrary given that PaO_2 correlates poorly with lung pathology and clinical course.

TABLE 66–1. CONSENSUS DEFINITION OF ALI/ARDS

- Acute onset of respiratory failure
- Diffuse bilateral infiltrates on chest radiograph
- Absence of left atrial hypertension (pulmonary artery occlusive pressure* [PAOP] ≤ 18 mm Hg) or no clinical evidence of left atrial hypertension
- Hypoxemia, defined as $PaO_2/FIO_2 \le 300$ (ALI) or ≤ 200 (ARDS)†

*If available. There is no consensus mandating pulmonary artery catheter insertion in suspected ALI/ARDS unless otherwise clinically indicated.

†PaO_2 in mm Hg, FIO_2 in decimal fraction (eg, 0.5).

FIO_2 = fraction of inspired O_2.

Etiology and Pathophysiology

ALI/ARDS is caused by a multitude of disorders that directly or indirectly injure the lungs (see TABLE 66–2); sepsis and pneumonia are the most common, causing about 60% of cases. Alcoholics are at increased risk. Because definitions were only recently standardized, the incidence of ALI/ARDS is uncertain. However, recent estimates indicate that about 190,000 cases/yr occur in the US.

ALI/ARDS is thought to develop when pulmonary or systemic inflammation leads to systemic release of cytokines and other proinflammatory molecules. The cytokines activate alveolar macrophages and recruit neutrophils to the lungs, which in turn release leukotrienes, oxidants, platelet-activating factor, and proteases. These substances damage capillary endothelium and alveolar epithelium, disrupting the barriers between capillaries and airspaces. Edema fluid, protein, and cellular debris flood the airspaces and interstitium, causing disruption of surfactant, airspace collapse, ventilation-perfusion mismatch, shunting, stiffening of the lungs with decreased compliance, and pulmonary hypertension. The injury is distributed heterogeneously but mainly affects dependent lung zones. Histopathologically, diffuse alveolar damage results with intra-alveolar neutrophils, RBCs, and cellular debris and denuded epithelial basement membranes with formation of hyaline membranes.

ALI/ARDS resolves spontaneously for many patients through active clearance of alveolar edema, passive clearance of soluble protein, alveolar reepithelialization, and possibly neutrophilic apoptosis. Proliferation of interstitial fibroblasts and myofibroblasts with early collagen deposition may also occur at this stage without diffuse fibrosis. However, some patients later develop diffuse fibrosis and loss of normal architecture (fibrosing alveolitis, or late diffuse alveolar damage).

Symptoms and Signs

Symptoms and signs are nonspecific and typically develop within 24 to 48 h of initial injury or illness. Dyspnea is the primary symptom, occasionally accompanied by cough or chest pain. Signs invariably include tachypnea and tachycardia. Accessory muscle use, cyanotic or mottled skin, and abnormal breath sounds (crackles, rhonchi, and/or wheezes) may be present.

Diagnosis

ALI/ARDS is primarily a clinical diagnosis. Once diagnosed, testing may be required to identify a cause.

ALI/ARDS is suspected when dyspnea and respiratory insufficiency rapidly develop in settings that predispose to ARDS. A similar clinical presentation can result from acute heart failure and from pulmonary infections. All patients should have ABGs and chest x-ray; diagnosis is confirmed by demonstration of hypoxemia and widespread chest x-ray infiltrates in the absence of clinical or manometric signs of left atrial hypertension (see TABLE 66–1).

ABGs initially show a low Pa_{O_2}, a normal or low Pa_{CO_2}, and an elevated pH (acute uncompensated respiratory alkalosis), unless metabolic acidosis is present secondary to sepsis. The low Pa_{O_2} is only partially responsive to O_2 supplementation because the pathophysiology involves shunting of blood through areas of unventilated lung.

Chest x-ray shows bilateral, symmetrical or asymmetrical, fluffy alveolar infiltrates. At the onset of illness, radiographic changes may lag behind physiologic changes, making hypoxemia seem more severe than x-ray findings would suggest. CT in the acute phase usually shows filling of airspaces in dependent lung fields (dorsal caudal in supine patients) with interlobular septal thickening, and often small pleural effusions. Late in the course, if fibrosing alveolitis develops, reticulonodular and ground-glass opacities with honeycombing and/or bullae are apparent on chest x-ray and CT.

If left atrial filling pressures are in doubt after clinical evaluation, a measurement of pulmonary artery occlusion pressure (PAOP) by right heart catheterization can clarify the diagnosis. A PAOP < 18 mm Hg in combination with the above findings is diagnostic of ALI/ARDS. A PAOP > 20 mm Hg suggests heart failure or hypervolemia.

Underlying causes: The cause of ALI/ARDS is often obvious. When it is not, a review of drugs and recent diagnostic tests, procedures, and treatments may suggest an unrecognized cause, such as use of radiographic contrast, air embolism, or transfusion. When the cause is still uncertain, bronchoscopy with bronchoalveolar lavage (BAL) and biopsy for detection of aspiration, infection, hemorrhage, malignancy, or other disorders should be considered.

Complications: Tachycardia, hypotension, and/or a sudden increase in the peak inspiratory pressure required for mechanical ventilation suggests possible pneumothorax; patients with such findings should have a chest x-ray immediately. Fever and an elevated WBC count with purulent tracheal aspirate suggest bacterial superinfection of the lungs (eg, hospital-acquired pneumonia); such patients should have 2 sets of blood cultures and culture of the tracheal aspirate.

TABLE 66–2. CLINICAL DISORDERS THAT CAUSE ARDS

DIRECT LUNG INJURY	INDIRECT LUNG INJURY
Common causes	Common causes
Aspiration	Sepsis
Pneumonia	Severe trauma
Less common causes	Less common causes
Diffuse alveolar hemorrhage	Bone marrow transplantation
Fat embolism	Burns
Lung transplantation	Cardiopulmonary bypass
Near-drowning	Drug overdose (eg, aspirin, cocaine, opioids, phenothiazines, tricyclics)
Pulmonary contusion	Massive blood transfusion (>15 U)
Toxic gas inhalation	Pancreatitis
	Radiographic contrast (rare)
	Stroke or seizure (neurogenic pulmonary edema)

Adapted from Ware LB and Matthay MA: The acute respiratory distress syndrome. *N Engl J Med* 2000; 342(18):1334–1349.

Prognosis

Mortality in ALI/ARDS until recently was very high (40 to 60%) but has declined in recent years to 30 to 40%, probably because of improvements in mechanical ventilation and in treatment of sepsis. Most often, death is not caused by respiratory dysfunction but rather is related to sepsis and multiorgan dysfunction. Persistence of neutrophils and high cytokine levels in BAL fluid predict a poor prognosis. Mortality otherwise increases with age, presence of sepsis, and severity of preexisting organ insufficiency or coexisting organ dysfunction.

Pulmonary function returns close to normal in 6 to 12 mo in most ALI/ARDS patients who survive; however, patients with a protracted clinical course or severe disease may have residual pulmonary symptoms and many have persistent neuromuscular weakness.

Treatment

Treatment of ALI/ARDS includes mechanical ventilation, supportive care, and treatment of underlying causes. Treatment of underlying causes is discussed elsewhere in THE MANUAL.

Mechanical ventilation: Nearly all ALI/ARDS patients require endotracheal intubation and mechanical ventilation during the acute phase of their illness. A few patients with ALI can be managed with high fractional inspired O_2 (FIO_2) delivered by face mask alone, or with noninvasive positive pressure ventilation (NIPPV) delivered by face mask, which effectively delivers positive end-expiratory pressure (PEEP).

Endotracheal intubation and mechanical ventilation should be considered when the respiratory rate approaches 30/min, when an $FIO_2 > 0.60$ cannot maintain arterial O_2 saturation > 90% for more than a few hours, or when the patient's breathing appears to be failing or tiring. Intubation should not be delayed until the patient is in extremis.

Mechanical ventilation carries the potential risk of O_2 toxicity and may be associated with barotrauma and ventilator-induced lung injury. Recommendations for ventilator settings are designed to reduce these risks. The goal is to keep inspired O_2 < 50 to 60% and plateau airway pressures < 30 cm H_2O. The patient should be ventilated in assist-control mode with tidal volume set at 5 to 6 mL/kg predicted body weight. Mild to moderate respiratory acidosis is acceptable. This tidal volume–plateau pressure limited ventilator strategy reduces mortality in ARDS. (See full discussion on ventilator management of ARDS in Ch. 65 on p. 550.)

Prone positioning improves oxygenation in some patients, by allowing recruitment of nonventilating lung regions. However, there is no evidence for improved survival. Prone positioning is contraindicated in pregnant patients and in those with shock, spinal instability, and increased intracranial pressure.

Readiness for liberation from mechanical ventilation (see p. 555), sometimes termed weaning, is based on improved lung function (ie, a decreasing need for O_2 and PEEP), improvement of chest radiographic appearance, and resolution of tachypnea.

Fluid management: There is no consensus on fluid management. A lower preload (with limited fluids and perhaps even diuretics) limits transudation of fluid in the lungs, but a higher preload optimizes cardiac output and maintains end-organ perfusion. It is not currently clear which approach maximizes survival. Pulmonary artery catheterization can be used to assess volume status and guide infusions when necessary, but the effect on mortality is unclear. Studies of the utility of pulmonary arterial catheterization and the 2 types of fluid management are underway.

In addition to intravascular volume and arterial oxygenation, O_2 delivery is influenced by the amount of Hb and the cardiac output. If an anemic patient is difficult to oxygenate on a nontoxic FIO_2 (eg, requires PEEP ≥ 15 cm H_2O), RBCs should be transfused to a Hb of 10 to 12 g/dL. Persistent hypotension despite adequate intravascular volume should usually be managed with inotropes, not more fluid; dobutamine 2.5 to 10 μg/kg/min can raise cardiac output and improve O_2 delivery. A central venous saturation ≥ 70% generally indicates adequate cardiac output.

Supportive treatment: Supportive treatment involves prompt recognition and treatment of acquired pneumonias; management of organ system failure, especially renal failure; stress ulcer prophylaxis with H_2 blockers or sucralfate; and deep vein thrombosis prophylaxis. Nutrition must be maintained, via an enteral route if possible.

Experimental treatments: A definitive pharmacologic treatment for ALI/ARDS that reduces morbidity and mortality remains elusive. Inhaled nitric oxide, surfactant replacement, and many other agents directed at modulating the inflammatory response have been studied and found not to reduce morbidity or mortality. Some small studies suggest that systemic corticosteroids may be beneficial in late-stage ALI/ARDS, but a larger, prospective randomized trial found no reduction in mortality. Corticosteroids may be deleterious when given early in the course of the condition.

67 SHOCK AND FLUID RESUSCITATION

(See also Ch. 68 on p. 566.)

The fundamental defect in shock is reduced perfusion of vital tissues. Definitive treatment restores adequate tissue perfusion, usually by administering IV fluids.

SHOCK

Shock is a state of organ hypoperfusion with resultant cellular dysfunction and death. Mechanisms may involve decreased circulating volume, decreased cardiac output, and vasodilation sometimes with shunting of blood to bypass capillary exchange beds. Symptoms include altered mental status, tachycardia, hypotension, and oliguria. Diagnosis is clinical, including BP measurement. Treatment is with IV fluids, correction of underlying cause, and sometimes vasopressors.

Pathophysiology

The fundamental defect in shock is reduced perfusion of vital tissues. Once perfusion declines so that O_2 is inadequate for aerobic metabolism, cells shift to anaerobic metabolism with increased production of CO_2 and accumulation of lactic acid. Cellular function declines, and if shock persists, irreversible cell damage and death occur.

During shock, both the inflammatory and clotting cascades may be triggered in areas of hypoperfusion. Hypoxic vascular endothelial cells activate WBCs, which bind to the endothelium and release directly damaging substances (reactive O_2 species, proteolytic enzymes) and inflammatory mediators (eg, cytokines, leukotrienes, tumor necrosis factor [TNF]). Some of these mediators bind to cell surface receptors and activate nuclear factor kappa B (NFκB), which leads to production of additional cytokines and also nitric oxide (NO), a potent vasodilator. Septic shock (see p. 566) may be more proinflammatory than other forms because of the actions of bacterial toxins, especially endotoxin.

Vasodilation of capacitance vessels leads to pooling of blood and hypotension because of "relative" hypovolemia (ie, too much volume to be filled by the existing amount of blood). Localized vasodilation may shunt blood past the capillary exchange beds, causing focal hypoperfusion despite normal cardiac output and BP. Additionally, excess NO is converted to peroxynitrite, a free radical that damages mitochondria and decreases ATP production.

Mechanical microvascular obstruction occurs in shock, limiting substrate delivery. Leukocytes and platelets adhere to the endothelium, and the clotting system is activated with fibrin deposition.

Multiple mediators, along with endothelial cell dysfunction, markedly increase microvascular permeability, allowing fluid and sometimes plasma proteins to escape into the interstitial space. In the GI tract, increased permeability possibly allows translocation of the enteric bacteria from the lumen to the blood stream, potentially leading to sepsis or metastatic infection.

Neutrophil apoptosis may be inhibited, enhancing the release of inflammatory mediators. In other cells, apoptosis may be augmented, increasing cell death and thus worsening organ function.

BP is not always low in the early stages of shock (although hypotension eventually occurs if shock is not reversed). Similarly, not all patients with "low" BP have shock. The degree and consequences of hypotension vary with the adequacy of physiologic compensation and the patient's underlying diseases. Thus, a modest degree of hypotension that is well tolerated by a young, relatively healthy person might result in severe cerebral, cardiac, or renal dysfunction in a patient with significant arteriosclerosis.

Compensation: Initially, when O_2 delivery (DO_2) is decreased, tissues compensate by extracting a greater percentage of delivered O_2 (the practical maximum is to a mixed-venous O_2 saturation of 30%). Additionally, low arterial pressure triggers an adrenergic response with sympathetic-mediated vasoconstriction and often increased heart rate. Initially, vasoconstriction is selective, shunting blood to the heart and brain. Circulating β-adrenergic amines (epinephrine, norepinephrine) also increase cardiac contractility and trigger release of corticosteroids from the adrenal gland, renin from the kidney, and glucose from the liver. Increased glucose may overwhelm ailing mitochondria, causing further lactate production.

Reperfusion: Reperfusion of ischemic cells can cause further injury. As substrate is reintroduced, neutrophil activity may heighten, increasing production of damaging superoxide and hydroxyl radicals. After blood flow is restored, inflammatory mediators may be circulated to other organs.

Multiple organ dysfunction syndrome (MODS): The combination of direct and reperfusion injury may cause MODS—progressive dysfunction of 2 or more organs consequent to life-threatening illness or injury. MODS can follow any type of shock but is most common when infection is involved; organ failure is one of the defining features of septic shock (see p. 566). MODS also occurs in > 10% of patients with severe traumatic injury and is the primary cause of death in those surviving > 24 h.

Any organ system can be affected, but the most frequent target organ is the lung, in which increased membrane permeability leads to flooding of alveoli due to capillary leaks. Progressive hypoxia may be increasingly resistant to supplemental O_2 therapy. This condition is termed acute lung injury or, if severe, acute respiratory distress syndrome (ARDS—see p. 556).

The kidneys are injured when renal perfusion is critically reduced, leading to acute tubular necrosis and renal insufficiency manifested by oliguria and progressive rise in serum creatinine.

In the heart, reduced coronary perfusion and mediators (including TNF and IL-1) may depress contractility, worsen myocardial compliance, and down-regulate β-receptors. These factors decrease cardiac output, further worsening both myocardial and systemic perfusion and causing a vicious circle often culminating in death.

The GI tract can develop ileus and submucosal hemorrhage. Liver hypoperfusion can produce focal or extensive hepatocellular necrosis, transaminase elevation, and decreased clotting factors.

Etiology and Classification

There are several mechanisms of organ hypoperfusion and shock. Shock may be due to low circulating volume (hypovolemic shock), vasodilation (distributive shock), primary decrease in cardiac output (both cardiogenic and obstructive shock), or a combination.

Hypovolemic shock: Hypovolemic shock is caused by a critical decrease in intravascular volume. Diminished venous return (preload) results in decreased ventricular filling and reduced stroke volume. Unless compensated for by increased heart rate, cardiac output decreases.

A common cause is bleeding (hemorrhagic shock), typically from trauma, surgical interventions, peptic ulcer, esophageal varices, or aortic aneurysm. Bleeding may be overt (eg, hematemesis or melena) or concealed (eg, ruptured ectopic pregnancy).

Hypovolemic shock may also follow increased losses of body fluids other than blood (see TABLE 67–1).

Hypovolemic shock may be due to inadequate fluid intake (with or without increased fluid loss). Water may be unavailable, neurologic disability may impair the thirst mechanism, or physical disability may impair access.

In hospitalized patients, hypovolemia can be compounded if early signs of circulatory insufficiency are incorrectly ascribed to heart failure and fluids are withheld or diuretics given.

Distributive shock: Distributive shock results from a relative inadequacy of intravascular volume caused by arterial or venous vasodilation; circulating blood volume is normal. In some cases, cardiac output (and DO_2) is high, but increased blood flow through arteriovenous shunts bypasses capillary beds, causing cellular hypoperfusion (demonstrated by decreased O_2 consumption). In other situations, blood pools in venous capacitance beds and cardiac output falls.

Distributive shock may be caused by anaphylaxis (anaphylactic shock—see p. 1360); bacterial infection with endotoxin release (septic shock—see p. 566); severe injury to the brain or spinal cord (neurogenic shock); and ingestion of certain drugs or poisons, such as nitrates, opioids, and adrenergic blockers. Anaphylactic and septic shock often have a component of hypovolemia as well.

Cardiogenic and obstructive shock: Cardiogenic shock is a relative or absolute reduction in cardiac output due to a primary cardiac disorder. Mechanical factors that interfere with filling or emptying of the heart or great vessels explain obstructive shock. Causes are listed in TABLE 67–2.

Symptoms and Signs

Lethargy, confusion, and somnolence are common. The hands and feet are pale, cool, clammy, and often cyanotic, as are the earlobes, nose, and nailbeds. Capillary filling time is prolonged, and except in distributive shock, the skin appears grayish or dusky and moist. Overt diaphoresis may occur. Peripheral pulses are weak and typically rapid; often, only femoral or carotid pulses are palpable. Tachypnea and hyperventilation may be present. BP tends to be low (< 90 mm Hg systolic) or unobtainable; direct measurement by intra-arterial catheter, if performed, often gives higher, more accurate, values. Urine output is low.

Distributive shock produces similar symptoms, except the skin may appear warm or flushed. The pulse may be bounding rather than weak. In septic shock, fever, usually preceded by chills, is generally present. Some patients with anaphylactic shock have urticaria or wheezing.

Numerous other symptoms (eg, chest pain, dyspnea, abdominal pain) may occur due to the underlying disease or secondary organ failure.

TABLE 67–1. HYPOVOLEMIC SHOCK CAUSED BY BODY FLUID LOSS

SITE OF FLUID LOSS	MECHANISM OF LOSS
Skin	Thermal or chemical burn, sweating from excessive heat exposure
GI tract	Vomiting or diarrhea
Kidneys	Diabetes mellitus or insipidus, adrenal insufficiency, "salt-losing" nephritis, the polyuric phase after acute tubular damage, and use of potent diuretics
Intravascular fluid lost to the extravascular space	Increased capillary permeability secondary to anoxia, cardiac arrest, sepsis, bowel ischemia, acute pancreatitis

Diagnosis

Diagnosis is mostly clinical, based on evidence of insufficient tissue perfusion (obtundation, oliguria, peripheral cyanosis) and signs of compensatory mechanisms (tachycardia, tachypnea, diaphoresis). Specific criteria include obtundation, heart rate > 100, respiratory rate > 22, hypotension (systolic BP < 90 mm Hg) or a 30 mm Hg fall in baseline BP, and urine output < 0.5 mL/kg/h. Laboratory findings that support the diagnosis include lactate > 3 mmol/L, base deficit < −5 mEq/L, and $PaCO_2$ < 32 mm Hg. However, none of these findings alone is diagnostic, and each is evaluated in the overall clinical context, including physical signs.

Diagnosis of cause: Recognizing the underlying cause of shock is more important than categorizing the type. Often, the cause is obvious or can be recognized quickly by history and physical examination, aided by simple testing.

Chest pain (with or without dyspnea) suggests MI, aortic dissection, or pulmonary embolism. A systolic murmur may indicate ventricular septal rupture or mitral insufficiency from acute MI. A diastolic murmur may indicate aortic regurgitation from aortic dissection involving the root. Cardiac tamponade is suggested by jugular venous distention, muffled heart sounds, and a paradoxical pulse. Pulmonary embolism severe enough to produce shock typically produces decreased O_2 saturation. Tests include ECG, chest x-ray, ABG measurements, lung scan, helical CT, and/or echocardiography.

Abdominal or back pain or a tender abdomen suggests pancreatitis, ruptured abdominal aortic aneurysm, peritonitis, and in women of childbearing age, ruptured ectopic pregnancy. A pulsatile midline mass suggests ruptured abdominal aortic aneurysm. A tender adnexal mass suggests ectopic pregnancy. Testing typically includes abdominal CT (if the patient is unstable, bedside ultrasound can be helpful), CBC, amylase, and lipase, and for women of childbearing age, urine pregnancy test.

Fever, chills, and focal signs of infection suggest septic shock, particularly in immunocompromised patients. Isolated fever, contingent on history and clinical settings, may point to heat stroke. Tests include chest x-ray; urinalysis; CBC; and cultures of blood, urine, and other relevant body fluids.

In a few patients, the cause is occult. Patients with no focal signs or symptoms indicative of cause should have ECG, chest x-ray, and ABG. If results of these tests are normal, the most likely causes include drug overdose, occult infection (including toxic shock), and obstructive shock.

Ancillary testing: If not already obtained, ECG, chest x-ray, CBC, serum electrolytes,

TABLE 67–2. MECHANISMS OF CARDIOGENIC AND OBSTRUCTIVE SHOCK

TYPE	MECHANISM	CAUSE
Obstructive	Mechanical interference with ventricular filling	Tension pneumothorax, cardiac tamponade, atrial tumor or clot
	Interference with ventricular emptying	Pulmonary embolism
Cardiogenic	Impaired myocardial contractility	Myocardial ischemia or MI, myocarditis, drugs
	Abnormalities of cardiac rhythm	Tachycardia, bradycardia
	Cardiac structural disorder	Acute mitral or aortic regurgitation, ruptured interventricular septum, prosthetic valve malfunction

BUN, creatinine, PT, PTT, liver function tests, and fibrinogen and fibrin split products are performed to monitor patient status and serve as a baseline. If the patient's volume status is difficult to determine, monitoring of central venous pressure (CVP) or pulmonary artery occlusion pressure (PAOP) may be useful. CVP < 5 mm Hg (< 7 cm H_2O) or PAOP < 8 mm Hg may indicate hypovolemia, although CVP may be greater in hypovolemic patients with preexisting pulmonary hypertension.

Prognosis and Treatment

Untreated shock is usually fatal. Even when treated, mortality from cardiogenic shock after MI and from septic shock is high (60 to 65%). Prognosis depends on the cause, preexisting or complicating illness, time between onset and diagnosis, and promptness and adequacy of therapy.

First aid involves keeping the patient warm. Hemorrhage is controlled, airway and ventilation checked, and respiratory assistance given if necessary. Nothing is given by mouth, and the patient's head is turned to one side to avoid aspiration if emesis occurs.

Treatment begins simultaneously with evaluation. Supplemental O_2 by face mask is provided. In severe shock or if ventilation is inadequate, endotracheal intubation with mechanical ventilation is necessary. Two large (16- to 18-gauge) IV catheters are inserted into separate peripheral veins. A central venous line or, in children, an intraosseous needle provides an alternative when peripheral veins cannot promptly be accessed (see also p. 519).

Typically, 1 L (or 20 mL/kg in children) of 0.9% saline is infused over 15 min. In major hemorrhage, Ringer's lactate is commonly used. Unless clinical parameters return to normal, the infusion is repeated. Smaller volumes (eg, 250 to 500 mL) are used for patients with signs of high right-sided pressure (eg, distention of neck veins) or acute MI. A fluid challenge should probably not be given to a patient with signs of pulmonary edema. Further fluid therapy is based on the underlying condition and may require monitoring of CVP or PAOP.

Patients in shock are critically ill and should be admitted to an ICU. Monitoring includes ECG; systolic, diastolic, and mean BP, preferably by intra-arterial catheter; respiratory rate and depth; pulse oximetry; urine flow by indwelling bladder catheter; body temperature; and clinical status, including sensorium (eg, Glasgow Coma Scale—see TABLE 212–2 on p. 1803), pulse volume, skin temperature, and color. Measurement of CVP, PAOP, and thermodilution cardiac output using a balloon-tipped pulmonary arterial catheter may be helpful for diagnosis and initial management of patients with shock of uncertain or mixed etiology or with severe shock, especially when accompanied by oliguria or pulmonary edema. Echocardiography (bedside or transesophageal) is a less invasive alternative. Serial measurements of ABGs, Hct, electrolytes, serum creatinine, and plasma lactate are obtained. Sublingual CO_2 measurement (see p. 516), if available, is a noninvasive monitor of visceral perfusion. A well-designed flow sheet is helpful.

Because tissue hypoperfusion makes intramuscular absorption unreliable, all parenteral drugs are given IV. Opioids generally are avoided because they may cause vasodilation, but severe pain may be treated with morphine 1 to 4 mg IV given over 2 min and repeated q10 to 15 min if necessary. Although cerebral hypoperfusion may cause anxiety, sedatives or tranquilizers are not routinely given.

After initial resuscitation, specific treatment is directed at the underlying condition. Additional supportive care is guided by the type of shock.

In hemorrhagic shock, surgical control of bleeding is primary. Vigorous volume replacement (see also p. 564) accompanies rather than precedes surgical control. Blood transfusion is used for hemorrhagic shock unresponsive to 2 L (or 40 mL/kg in children) of crystalloid. Failure to respond usually indicates insufficient volume administration or unrecognized ongoing hemorrhage. Vasopressor agents are not indicated for treatment of hemorrhagic shock unless cardiogenic, obstructive, or distributive causes are also present.

Distributive shock with profound hypotension after initial fluid replacement with 0.9% saline may be treated with inotropic or vasopressor agents (eg, dopamine, norepinephrine—see TABLE 67–3). Patients with septic shock also receive broad-spectrum antibiotics (see p. 569). Patients with anaphylactic shock unresponsive to fluid challenge (especially if accompanied by bronchoconstriction) receive epinephrine 0.05 to 0.1 mg IV, followed by epinephrine infusion of 5 mg in 500 mL 5% D/W at 10 mL/h or 0.02 (μg/kg/min (see also p. 1360).

In cardiogenic shock, structural disorders (eg, valvular dysfunction, septal rupture) are repaired surgically. Coronary thrombosis is treated either by percutaneous interventions (angioplasty, stenting), coronary artery bypass surgery, or thrombolysis (see also Ch. 73 on p. 626). Tachydysrhythmia (eg, rapid atrial fibrillation, ventricular tachycardia) is slowed by cardioversion or with drugs. Bradycardia is treated with a transcutaneous or transvenous pacemaker; atropine 0.5 mg IV up to 4 doses q 5 min may be given pending pacemaker placement. Isoproterenol (2 mg/500 mL 5% D/W at 1 to 4 μg/min [0.25 to 1 mL/min]) may occasionally be useful if atropine is ineffective, but it is not advised in patients with coronary ischemia.

Shock after acute MI is treated with volume expansion if PAOP is low or normal; 15 to 18 mm Hg is considered optimal. If a pulmonary artery catheter is not in place, cautious volume infusion (250- to 500-mL bolus of 0.9% saline) may be tried while auscultating the chest frequently for signs of fluid overload. Shock after right ventricular MI will usually respond partially to volume expansion; however, vasopressor agents may be needed.

TABLE 67–3. INOTROPIC AND VASOACTIVE CATECHOLAMINES

DRUG	DOSAGE	HEMODYNAMIC ACTIONS
Norepinephrine	4 mg/250 mL or 500 mL 5% D/W continuous IV infusion at 8–12 μg/min initially, then at 2–4 μg/min as maintenance, with wide variations	α-Adrenergic: vasoconstriction β-Adrenergic: inotropic and chronotropic effects*
Dopamine	400 mg/500 mL 5% D/W continuous IV infusion at 0.3 mL (0.25 mg)–1.25 mL (1 mg)/min 2–10 μg/kg/min for low dose 20 μg/kg/min for high dose	α-Adrenergic: vasoconstriction† β-Adrenergic: inotropic and chronotropic effects and vasodilation† Nonadrenergic: renal and splanchnic vasodilation
Dobutamine	250 mg/250 mL 5% D/W continuous IV infusions at 2.5–10 μg/kg/min	β-Adrenergic: inotropic effects‡

*Effects not apparent if arterial pressure is elevated too much.
†Effects depend on dosage and underlying pathophysiology.
‡Chronotropic, arrhythmogenic, and direct vascular effects are minimal at lower doses.

If hypotension is moderate (eg, mean arterial pressure [MAP] 70 to 90 mm Hg), dobutamine infusion, amrinone (0.75 mg/kg IV over 2 to 3 min followed by infusions of 5 to 10 μg/kg/min) or milrinone (50 μg/kg IV, followed by 0.5 μg/kg/min) may be used to improve cardiac output and reduce left ventricular filling pressure. Tachycardia and arrhythmias occasionally occur during dobutamine administration, particularly at higher doses, necessitating dose reduction. Vasodilators (eg, nitroprusside, nitroglycerin), which increase venous capacitance or lower systemic vascular resistance, reduce the workload on the damaged myocardium and may increase cardiac output in patients without severe hypotension. Combination therapy (eg, dopamine or dobutamine with nitroprusside or nitroglycerin) may be particularly useful but requires close ECG and pulmonary and systemic hemodynamic monitoring.

For more serious hypotension (MAP < 70 mm Hg), norepinephrine or dopamine may be given, with a target systolic pressure of 80 to 90 mm Hg (and not > 110 mm Hg). Intra-aortic balloon counterpulsation appears to be valuable for temporarily reversing shock in patients with acute MI, and it should be considered as a bridge to surgical intervention in patients with acute MI complicated by ventricular septal rupture or with severe acute mitral regurgitation who require vasopressor support for > 30 min.

In obstructive shock, cardiac tamponade requires immediate pericardiocentesis, which can be performed at the bedside. Tension pneumothorax should be immediately decompressed with a needle in the second intercostal space, midclavicular line. Massive pulmonary embolism resulting in shock is treated with thrombolysis or surgical embolectomy.

INTRAVENOUS FLUID RESUSCITATION

Almost all circulatory shock states require large-volume IV fluid replacement, as does severe intravascular volume depletion (eg, from diarrhea or heat stroke). Intravascular volume deficiency is acutely compensated by vasoconstriction, followed over hours by migration of fluid from the extravascular compartment to the intravascular, maintaining circulating volume at the expense of total body water. However, this compensation is overwhelmed following major losses. Maintenance fluid requirements and mild dehydration are discussed in Ch. 156 on p. 1233 and Ch. 276 on p. 2289.

Fluids

Choice of resuscitation fluid depends on the cause of the deficit.

Hemorrhage: Loss of RBCs diminishes O_2-carrying capacity. However, the body increases cardiac output to maintain oxygen delivery (DO_2) and also increases O_2 extraction. These factors provide a safety margin of about 9 times the resting O_2 requirement. Thus, non–O_2-carrying fluids (eg, crystalloid or colloid solutions) may be used to restore intravascular volume in mild to moderate blood loss. However, once Hb declines to < 8 g/dL, O_2-carrying capacity must be restored by infusion of blood (or in the future by blood substitutes). Patients with coronary or cerebral vascular disease require blood for Hb < 10 g/dL.

Crystalloid solutions for intravascular volume replenishment are typically isotonic (eg, 0.9% saline or Ringer's lactate [RL]). H_2O freely travels outside the vasculature, so as little as 10% of isotonic fluid remains in the intravascular space. With hypotonic fluid (eg, 0.45% saline), even less remains in the vasculature and thus is not used for resuscitation. Both 0.9% saline and RL are equally effective; RL may be preferred in hemorrhagic shock because it somewhat minimizes acidosis. However, the Ca in RL may trigger clotting in transfused blood unless the ratio of blood:RL is > 2:1. For patients with acute brain injury and hemorrhagic shock, 0.9% saline is preferred. Hypertonic saline (7.5%) is also an effective crystalloid; it shifts more volume from the extravascular space and therefore requires lower absolute volume, which has practical advantages in a pre-hospital setting.

Colloid solutions (eg, hydroxyethyl starch, albumin, dextrans) are also effective for volume replacement during major hemorrhage. Despite theoretical benefits over crystalloid, no differences in survival have been proven. Albumin is the colloid of choice, although it may have a negative inotropic effect. Both dextrans and hydroxyethyl starch adversely affect coagulation when > 1.5 L is given.

Blood typically is administered as packed RBCs, which should be cross-matched, but in an urgent situation, 1 to 2 units of type O Rh-negative blood is an acceptable alternative. When > 1 to 2 units are transfused (eg, in major trauma), blood is warmed to 37° C. Patients receiving > 8 to 10 units may require replacement of clotting factors with infusion of fresh frozen plasma or cryoprecipitate and platelet transfusion (see also p. 1136).

Blood substitutes are O_2-carrying fluids that can be Hb-based or perfluorocarbons. Hb-based fluids may contain free Hb that is liposome-encapsulated or modified (eg, by surface modification or cross-linking with other molecules) to limit renal excretion and toxicity. Because the antigen-bearing RBC membrane is not present, these substances do not require cross-matching. They also can be stored > 1 yr, providing a more stable source than banked blood. Perfluorocarbons are IV carbon-fluorine emulsions that carry large amounts of O_2. However, they have not been proven to increase survival and cannot be given in amounts sufficient to compensate for critical RBC losses.

Nonhemorrhagic hypovolemia: Isotonic crystalloid solutions are typically given for intravascular repletion during shock and hypovolemia. Colloid solutions are generally not used. Patients with dehydration and adequate circulatory volume typically have a free water deficit, and hypotonic solutions (eg, D5 0.45% saline) are used.

Route and Rate of Administration

Standard, large (eg, 14- to 16-gauge) peripheral IV catheters are adequate for most fluid resuscitation. With infusion pump they typically allow infusion of 1 L of crystalloid in 10 to 15 min and 1 unit of packed RBCs in 20 min. For patients at risk of exsanguination, a large (eg, 8.5 French) central venous catheter provides more rapid infusion rates; a pressure infusion device can infuse 1 unit packed RBCs in < 5 min.

Patients in shock typically require and tolerate infusion at the maximum rate. Adults are given 1 L of crystalloid (20 mL/kg in children) or, in hemorrhagic shock, 5 to 10 mL/kg of colloid or packed RBCs, and the patient is reassessed. An exception is a patient with cardiogenic shock who typically does not require large volume infusion.

Patients with intravascular volume depletion without shock can receive infusion at a controlled rate, typically 500 mL/h. Children should have fluid deficit calculated (see p. 2290) and replacement given over 24 h (½ in the first 8 h).

Endpoint and Monitoring

The actual endpoint of fluid administration in shock is normalization of DO_2. However, this parameter is not often measured directly. Surrogate endpoints include clinical indicators of end organ perfusion and measurements of preload.

Adequate end organ perfusion is best indicated by urine output of > 0.5 to 1 mL/kg/h. Heart rate, mental status, and capillary refill may be affected by the underlying disease process and are less reliable markers. Because of compensatory vasoconstriction, mean arterial pressure (MAP) is only a rough guideline; organ hypoperfusion may be present despite apparently normal values. An elevated serum lactate level reflects hypoperfusion; however, levels do not decline for several hours after successful resuscitation; sublingual CO_2 levels respond more rapidly (eg, within minutes) and may be a more useful indicator.

Because urine output does not provide a minute-to-minute indication, measures of preload may be helpful in guiding fluid resuscitation for critically ill patients. Central venous pressure (CVP) is the mean pressure in the superior vena cava, reflecting right ventricular end-diastolic pressure or preload. Normal CVP ranges from 2 to 7 mm Hg (3 to 9 cm H_20). A sick or injured patient with a CVP < 3 mm Hg is presumed to be volume depleted and may be given fluids with relative safety. When the CVP is within the normal range, volume depletion cannot be excluded, and the response to 100- to 200-mL fluid boluses should be assessed; a modest increase in CVP in response to fluid generally indicates hypovolemia. An increase of > 3 to 5 mm Hg in response to a 100-mL fluid bolus suggests limited cardiac reserve. A CVP > 12 to 15 mm Hg casts doubt on hypovolemia as the sole etiology of hypoperfusion, and fluid administration risks fluid overload.

Because the CVP may be unreliable in assessing volume status or left ventricular function, pulmonary artery catheterization (see p. 513) may be considered for diagnosis or for more precise titration of fluid administration if there is no cardiovascular improvement after initial therapy. Care must be taken when interpreting filling pressures in patients during mechanical ventilation, particularly when positive end-expiratory pressure (PEEP) levels exceeding 10 cm H_2O are being used or during respiratory distress when pleural pressures fluctuate widely. Measurements are made at the end of expiration, and the transducer is referenced to atrial zero levels (mid chest) and carefully calibrated.

Traumatic hemorrhagic shock: These patients may require a slightly different approach. Experimental and clinical evidence indicates that internal hemorrhage (eg, from visceral or vascular laceration or crush) may be worsened by resuscitation to normal or supranormal MAP. Some physicians advocate an MAP of 60 to 80 mm Hg as the resuscitation endpoint in such patients pending surgical control of bleeding.

After blood loss is controlled, the Hct is used to guide the need for further transfusion. To minimize the use of blood products, a target Hct of 23 to 28% is suggested. Patients who may have difficulty tolerating moderate anemia (eg, those with coronary or cerebral artery disease) are kept above 30%. A higher Hct does not improve outcome and, by causing increased blood viscosity, may impair perfusion of capillary beds.

Complications

Overly rapid infusion of any type of fluid may precipitate pulmonary edema.

Hemodilution from crystalloid infusion is not of itself injurious, although Hct must be monitored to note whether threshold values for transfusion are met.

RBC transfusion has a low risk of directly transmitting infection but in critically ill patients it appears to cause a slightly higher rate of hospital-acquired infection. This may be minimized by using blood < 12 days old; such RBCs are more plastic and less likely to cause sludging in the microvasculature. Other complications of massive transfusion are discussed on p. 1137.

68 SEPSIS AND SEPTIC SHOCK

(See also Ch. 67 on p. 559.)

Sepsis, severe sepsis, and septic shock are inflammatory states resulting from systemic bacterial infection. In severe sepsis and septic shock, there is critical reduction in tissue perfusion. Common causes include gram-negative organisms, staphylococci, and meningococci. Symptoms often begin with shaking chills and include fever, hypotension, oliguria, and confusion. Acute failure of multiple organs can occur, including the lungs, kidneys, and liver. Treatment is aggressive fluid resuscitation, antibiotics, supportive care, and sometimes intensive control of blood glucose and administration of corticosteroids and activated protein C.

A spectrum of severity exists (see TABLE 68–1).

Sepsis is systemic infection accompanied by a reaction that has been termed the systemic inflammatory response syndrome (SIRS). SIRS represents an acute inflammatory reaction with systemic manifestations caused by release into the bloodstream of numerous endogenous mediators of inflammation. SIRS can also be caused by acute pancreatitis and major trauma, including burns. It has previously been defined by 2 or more of the following:

- Temperature > 38° C or < 36° C
- Heart rate > 90 beats/min
- Respiratory rate > 20 breaths/min or Pa_{CO_2} < 32 mm Hg
- WBC count > 12,000 cells/μL or < 4000 cells/μL, or > 10% immature forms

However, these criteria are now viewed as suggestive but not sufficiently precise to be diagnostic.

Severe sepsis is sepsis accompanied by signs of failure of at least one organ. Cardiovascular failure is typically manifested by hypotension, respiratory failure by hypoxemia, renal failure by oliguria, and hematologic failure by coagulopathy.

Septic shock is severe sepsis with organ hypoperfusion and hypotension that are poorly responsive to initial fluid resuscitation.

Etiology

Most cases of septic shock are caused by hospital-acquired gram-negative bacilli or gram-positive cocci and often occur in immunocompromised patients and those with chronic and debilitating diseases. Rarely, it is caused by *Candida* or other fungi. A unique form of shock caused by staphylococcal and streptococcal toxins is called toxic shock (see p. 1448).

TABLE 68–1. SEPSIS IN THE UNITED STATES

CATEGORY	NUMBER OF CASES	CRUDE MORTALITY (%)	NUMBER OF DEATHS ANNUALLY
Sepsis	400,000	15	60,000
Severe sepsis (sepsis plus organ failure)	300,000	20	60,000
Septic shock (severe sepsis plus refractory hypotension)	200,000	45	90,000

Sepsis = systemic inflammatory response syndrome including ≥ 2 of the following: temperature > 38° C or < 36° C; pulse > 90/min; respirations > 20/min; WBCs > 12,000, < 4,000/mm^3, or > 10% band forms.

Data from Wenzel RP: Treating sepsis. *N Engl J Med* 2002; 347(13): 966–967.

Septic shock occurs more often in neonates (see p. 2333), patients > 35 yr, and pregnant women. Predisposing factors include diabetes mellitus; cirrhosis; leukopenia, especially that associated with cancer or treatment with cytotoxic drugs; invasive devices, including endotracheal tubes, vascular or urinary catheters, drainage tubes, and other foreign materials; and prior treatment with antibiotics or corticosteroids. Common causative sites of infection include the lungs and the urinary, biliary, and GI tracts.

Pathophysiology

The pathogenesis of septic shock is not completely understood. An inflammatory stimulus (eg, a bacterial toxin) triggers production of proinflammatory mediators, including tumor necrosis factor and IL-1. These cytokines cause neutrophil-endothelial cell adhesion, activate the clotting mechanism, and generate microthrombi. They also release numerous other mediators, including leukotrienes, lipoxygenase, histamine, bradykinin, serotonin, and IL-2. These are opposed by anti-inflammatory mediators, such as IL-4 and IL-10, resulting in a negative feedback mechanism.

Initially, arteries and arterioles dilate, decreasing peripheral arterial resistance; cardiac output typically increases. This stage has been referred to as "warm shock." Later, cardiac output may decrease, BP falls (with or without an increase in peripheral resistance), and typical features of shock appear.

Even in the stage of increased cardiac output, vasoactive mediators cause blood flow to bypass capillary exchange vessels (a distributive defect). Poor capillary flow from this shunting along with capillary obstruction by microthrombi decreases delivery of O_2 and impairs removal of CO_2 and waste products. Decreased perfusion causes dysfunction and sometimes failure of one or more organs, including the kidneys, lungs, liver, brain, and heart.

Coagulopathy may develop because of intravascular coagulation with consumption of major clotting factors, excessive fibrinolysis in reaction thereto, and more often a combination of both.

Symptoms, Signs, and Diagnosis

With sepsis, the patient typically has fever, tachycardia, and tachypnea; BP remains normal. Other signs of the causative infection are generally present. As severe sepsis or septic shock develops, the first sign may be confusion or decreased alertness. BP generally falls, yet the skin is paradoxically warm. Oliguria (< 0.5 mL/kg/h) is present. Later, extremities become cool and pale, with peripheral cyanosis and mottling. Organ failure produces additional signs and symptoms specific to the organ involved.

Sepsis is suspected in a patient with a known infection who develops systemic signs of inflammation or organ dysfunction. Similarly, a patient with otherwise unexplained signs of systemic inflammation should be evaluated for infection by history, physical examination, and tests, including urinalysis and urine culture (particularly in patients who have indwelling catheters), serial blood cultures, and cultures of other suspect body fluids. Blood levels of procalcitonin and C-reactive protein are elevated in severe sepsis and may facilitate diagnosis, but these are not specific. Ultimately, diagnosis is clinical.

Other causes of shock (eg, hypovolemia, MI) should be sought by history, physical examination, ECG, and serum cardiac markers. Even without MI, hypoperfusion may result in ECG findings of ischemia including nonspecific ST-T wave abnormalities, T-wave inversions, and supraventricular and ventricular arrhythmias.

CBC, ABG, chest x-ray, serum electrolytes, lactate levels or sublingual PCO_2, and liver function are followed. At the onset of septic shock, the WBC count may initially decrease to < 4,000/μL, and PMNs may be as low as 20%. However, this situation reverses within 1 to 4 h, and a significant increase in both the total WBC count to > 15,000/μL and PMNs to > 80% (with predominantly juvenile forms) usually occurs. A sharp decrease in platelet count to ≤ 50,000/μL is often present early.

Hyperventilation with respiratory alkalosis (low $PaCO_2$ and increased arterial pH) occurs early, in part as compensation for lactic acidemia. Serum HCO_3 is usually low, and serum and blood lactate increase. As shock progresses, metabolic acidosis worsens, and serum pH decreases. Early respiratory failure leads to hypoxemia with $PaO_2 < 70$ mm Hg. Diffuse infiltrates may appear on the chest x-ray (see ARDS on p. 556). BUN and creatinine usually increase progressively as a result of renal insufficiency. Bilirubin and transaminases may rise, although overt hepatic failure is uncommon.

Up to 50% of patients with severe sepsis develop relative adrenal insufficiency (ie, normal or slightly elevated baseline cortisol levels that do not increase significantly in response to further stress or exogenous ACTH). Adrenal function may be tested by measuring serum cortisol at 8 AM; a level < 5 mg/dL is inadequate. Alternatively, cortisol can be measured before and after injection of 250 μg of synthetic ACTH; a rise of < 9 μg/dL is considered insufficient. However, most physicians simply administer replacement doses of corticosteroids without testing.

Hemodynamic measurements with a pulmonary artery catheter can be used when the specific type of shock is unclear or when large fluid volumes (eg, > 4 to 5 L 0.9% saline over 6 to 8 h) are needed. Unlike in hypovolemic shock, cardiac output during septic shock is more likely to be normal or increased and peripheral resistance decreased. Neither central venous pressure (CVP) nor pulmonary artery occlusive pressure (PAOP) is likely to be abnormal, unlike in hypovolemic, obstructive, or cardiogenic shock (see p. 560). Echocardiography (including transesophageal echocardiography) is a useful alternative for evaluating cardiac performance.

Prognosis and Treatment

Overall mortality in patients with septic shock is decreasing and now averages 40% (range 10 to 90%, depending on patient characteristics). Poor outcomes often follow failure to institute early aggressive therapy (eg, within 6 h of suspected diagnosis). Once severe lactic acidosis with decompensated metabolic acidosis becomes established, especially in conjunction with multiorgan failure, septic shock is likely to be irreversible and fatal.

Patients with septic shock should be treated in an ICU. The following should be monitored frequently (see also p. 513): systemic pressure; CVP; pulse oximetry; ABGs; blood glucose, lactate, and electrolyte levels; renal function, and possibly sublingual PCO_2. Urine output, a good indicator of renal perfusion, should be measured, usually with an indwelling catheter.

Fluid resuscitation with 0.9% saline should be given until CVP reaches 8 mm Hg (10 cm H_2O) or PAOP reaches 12 to 15 mm Hg. Oliguria with hypotension is not a contraindication to vigorous fluid resuscitation. The quantity of fluid required often far exceeds the normal blood volume and may reach 10 L over 4 to 12 h. PAOP or echocardiography can identify limitations in left ventricular function and incipient pulmonary edema due to fluid overload.

If a patient with septic shock remains hypotensive after CVP or PAOP has been raised to target levels, dopamine may be administered to increase mean BP to at least 60 mm Hg. If dopamine dose exceeds 20 μg/kg/min, another vasopressor, typically norepinephrine, may be added. However, vasoconstriction produced by higher doses of dopamine and norepinephrine poses risks of organ hypoperfusion and acidosis, and these drugs have not been proven to improve survival.

O_2 is given by mask or nasal prongs. Tracheal intubation and mechanical ventilation may subsequently be needed for respiratory failure (see p. 544).

Parenteral antibiotics should be given after specimens of blood, body fluids, and wound sites have been taken for Gram stain and culture. Prompt empiric therapy is essential and may be lifesaving; antibiotic selection requires an educated guess based on the suspected source, clinical setting, knowledge of organisms and sensitivity patterns common to that specific inpatient unit, and previous culture results.

One regimen for septic shock of unknown cause is gentamicin or tobramycin 5.1 mg/kg IV once/day plus a 3rd-generation cephalosporin (cefotaxime 2 g q 6 to 8 h or ceftriaxone 2 g once/day, or, if *Pseudomonas* is suspected, ceftazidime 2 g IV q 8 h). Alternatively, ceftazidime plus a fluoroquinolone (eg, ciprofloxacin) may be used. Monotherapy with maximal therapeutic doses of ceftazidime (2 g IV q 8 h) or imipenem (1 g IV q 6 h) may be effective but is not recommended.

Vancomycin must be added if resistant staphylococci or enterococci are suspected. If there is an abdominal source, a drug effective against anaerobes should be included (eg, metronidazole). When culture and sensitivity results are available, the antibiotic regimen is changed accordingly. Antibiotics are continued for several days after shock resolves and evidence of infection subsides.

Abscesses must be drained and necrotic tissues (eg, infarcted bowel, gangrenous gallbladder, abscessed uterus) surgically excised. The patient's condition will continue to deteriorate despite antibiotic therapy unless septic foci are eliminated.

Strict normalization of blood glucose improves outcome in critically ill patients, even those not known to be diabetic. A continuous IV insulin infusion (crystalline zinc 1 to 4 U/h) is titrated to maintain glucose between 80 to 110 mg/dL (4.4 to 6.1 mmol/L). This approach necessitates frequent (eg, q 1 to 4 h) glucose measurement.

Corticosteroid therapy appears beneficial. Treatment is with replacement, rather than pharmacologic, doses. One regimen consists of hydrocortisone 50 mg IV q 6 h (or 100 mg q 8 h) plus fludrocortisone 50 μg po once/day during hemodynamic instability and for 3 days thereafter.

Activated protein C (drotrecogin alfa), a recombinant drug with fibrinolytic and anti-inflammatory activity, appears beneficial for severe sepsis and septic shock if begun early; benefit has been demonstrated only in patients with significant risk of death as defined by APACHE II score > 25 (see TABLE 63–4 on p. 517). Dosage is 24 μg/kg/h by continuous IV infusion for 96 h. Bleeding is the most common complication; thus contraindications include hemorrhagic stroke within 3 mo, spinal or intracranial surgery within 2 mo, acute trauma with a risk of bleeding, and intracranial neoplasm. Risk-benefit assessment is required in other patients with increased risk of serious bleeding (eg, with thrombocytopenia or recent GI bleeding, receiving concurrent heparin, or with recent aspirin or other anticoagulant use).

Other therapies for severe sepsis include cooling for hyperthermia and early treatment of renal failure (eg, with continuous venovenous hemofiltration).

Trials of monoclonal antibodies to the lipid A fraction of endotoxin, antileukotrienes, and antibodies to tumor necrosis factor have been unsuccessful.

SECTION 7
CARDIOVASCULAR DISORDERS

69 APPROACH TO THE CARDIAC PATIENT

Symptoms or the physical examination may suggest a cardiovascular disorder. For confirmation, selected noninvasive and invasive tests are usually done (see Ch. 70 on p. 589).

History

A thorough history is fundamental; it cannot be replaced by testing. A family history is taken because many cardiac disorders (eg, coronary artery disease, systemic hypertension, bicuspid aortic valve, hypertrophic cardiomyopathy, mitral valve prolapse) have a heritable basis.

Major cardiac symptoms include chest pain or discomfort, dyspnea (see p. 357), weakness, fatigue, palpitations, light-headedness, sense of an impending faint, and syncope. These symptoms commonly occur in more than one cardiac disorder and in noncardiac disorders.

Physical Examination

Complete examination of all systems is essential to detect peripheral and systemic effects of cardiac disorders and evidence of noncardiac disorders that might affect the heart.

Vital signs: BP is measured in both arms and, for suspected congenital cardiac disorders or peripheral vascular disorders, in both legs. The bladder of an appropriately sized cuff encircles 80% of the limb's circumference, and the bladder's width is 40% of the circumference. The 1st sound heard as the Hg column falls is systolic pressure; disappearance of the sound is diastolic pressure (5th-phase Korotkoff sound). Up to a 15 mm Hg pressure differential between the right and left arms is normal; a greater differential suggests a vascular abnormality (eg, dissecting thoracic aorta) or a peripheral vascular disorder. Leg pressure is usually 20 mm Hg higher than arm pressure. Ankle-brachial index (ratio of ankle to arm systolic BP) is normally > 1.

Heart rate and rhythm are assessed by palpating the carotid or radial pulse.

BP and heart rate are measured with the patient supine, seated, and standing, with 1 min between each change in position. A difference of ≤ 10 mm Hg is normal; the difference tends to be a little greater in the elderly.

Respiratory rate, if abnormal, may indicate cardiac decompensation or a primary lung disorder. The rate increases in patients with heart failure or anxiety and decreases in the moribund. Shallow, rapid respirations may indicate pleuritic pain.

Temperature may be elevated by acute rheumatic fever or cardiac infection (eg, endocarditis). After MI, fever is very common, and other causes are sought only if fever persists > 72 h.

Pulsus paradoxus: Normally during inspiration, systolic arterial BP can decrease up to 10 mm Hg, and pulse rate increases to compensate. A greater decrease in systolic BP or weakening of the pulse during inspiration is considered pulsus paradoxus. It occurs commonly in cardiac tamponade; occasionally in constrictive pericarditis, severe asthma, or COPD; and rarely in restrictive cardiomyopathy, severe pulmonary embolism, or hypovolemic shock.

BP decreases during inspiration because negative intrathoracic pressure increases venous return and hence right ventricular (RV) filling; as a result, the interventricular septum bulges slightly into the left ventricular (LV) outflow tract, decreasing cardiac output and thus BP. This mechanism (and the drop in systolic BP) is exaggerated in disorders that cause high negative intrathoracic pressure (eg, asthma) or that restrict RV filling (eg, cardiac tamponade, cardiomyopathy) or outflow (eg, pulmonary embolism).

Pulsus paradoxus is quantified by inflating a BP cuff to just above systolic BP and deflating it very slowly (eg, ≤ 2 mm Hg/heartbeat). The pressure is noted when Korotkoff sounds are first heard (at first, only during expiration) and when Korotkoff sounds are heard continuously. The difference between the pressures is the "amount" of pulsus paradoxus.

Pulses: Major peripheral pulses in the arms and legs are palpated for symmetry and volume (intensity); elasticity of the arterial wall is noted. Absence of pulses may suggest an arterial disorder (eg, atherosclerosis) or systemic embolism. However, peripheral pulses may be difficult to feel in obese or muscular people. The pulse has a rapid upstroke, then collapses in disorders with a rapid runoff of arterial blood (eg, arteriovenous communication, aortic regurgitation). The pulse is rapid and bounding in thyrotoxicosis and hypermetabolic states; it is slow and sluggish in myxedema. If pulses are asymmetric, auscultation over peripheral vessels may detect a bruit due to stenosis.

Observation, palpation, and auscultation of both carotid pulses may suggest a specific disorder (see TABLE 69–1). Aging and arteriosclerosis lead to vessel rigidity, which tends to eliminate the characteristic findings. In very young children, the carotid pulse may be normal, even when severe aortic stenosis is present.

Auscultation over the carotid arteries can distinguish murmurs from bruits. Murmurs originate in the heart or great vessels and are usually louder over the upper precordium and diminish toward the neck. Bruits are

TABLE 69–1. CAROTID PULSE AMPLITUDE AND ASSOCIATED DISORDERS

CAROTID PULSE AMPLITUDE	ASSOCIATED DISORDER
Bounding and prominent	Hypertension, hypermetabolic states, disorders with a rapid rise and fall of pressure (eg, patent ductus arteriosus)
Jerky, with full expansion followed by sudden collapse (Corrigan's or water-hammer pulse)	Aortic valve regurgitation
Low in amplitude and volume with a delayed peak	Aortic stenosis (obstructing left ventricular outflow)
Double-peaked (bifid) with a rapid rise	Hypertrophic cardiomyopathy
Bifid with normal or delayed rise	Combined aortic stenosis and regurgitation
Diminished unilaterally or bilaterally, often with a systolic bruit	Extracranial carotid stenosis due to atherosclerosis

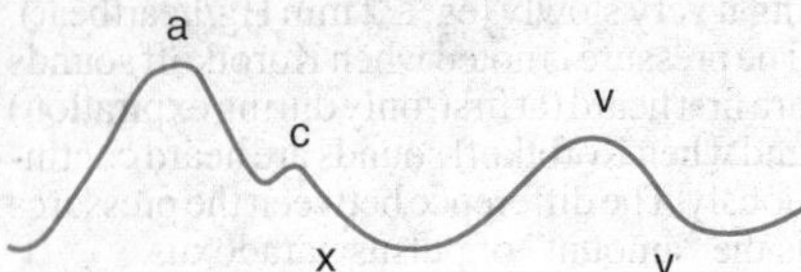

Fig. 69–1. Normal jugular vein waves. The *a* wave is caused by right atrial contraction (systole) and is followed by the *x* descent, which is caused by atrial relaxation The *c* wave, an interruption of the *x* descent, is caused by the transmitted carotid pulse; it is seldom discerned clinically. The *v* wave is caused by right atrial filling during ventricular systole (tricuspid valve is closed). The *y* descent is caused by rapid filling of the right ventricle during ventricular diastole before atrial contraction.

higher-pitched, are heard only over the arteries, and seem more superficial. An arterial bruit must be distinguished from a venous hum. Unlike an arterial bruit, a venous hum is usually continuous, heard best with the patient sitting or standing, and is eliminated by compression of the ipsilateral internal jugular vein.

Veins: The peripheral veins are observed for varicosities, arteriovenous malformations (AVMs) and shunts, and overlying inflammation and tenderness due to thrombophlebitis. An AVM or a shunt produces a continuous murmur (heard on auscultation) and often a palpable thrill (because resistance is always lower in the vein than in the artery during systole and diastole).

The neck veins are examined to estimate venous wave height and waveform. Height is proportional to right atrial pressure, and waveform reflects events in the cardiac cycle; both are best observed in the internal jugular vein.

The jugular veins are usually examined with the patient reclining at 45°. Then the top of the venous column is normally just below the clavicles (upper limit of normal: 4 cm above the sternal notch in a vertical plane). The venous column is elevated in heart failure, volume overload, constrictive pericarditis, tricuspid stenosis, superior vena cava obstruction, or reduced compliance of the RV. If such conditions are severe, the venous column can extend to jaw level, and its top can be detected only when the patient sits upright or stands. The venous column is low in hypovolemia.

Normally, the venous column can be briefly elevated by firm hand pressure on the abdomen (hepatojugular reflux); the column falls back in a few seconds despite continued abdominal pressure (because a compliant RV increases its stroke volume via the Frank-Starling mechanism). However, the column remains elevated during abdominal pressure in disorders that cause a dilated and poorly compliant RV or in obstruction of RV filling by tricuspid stenosis or right atrial tumor.

Normally, the venous column falls slightly during inspiration as lowered intrathoracic pressure draws blood from the periphery into the vena cava. A rise in the venous column during inspiration (Kussmaul's sign) occurs typically in chronic constrictive pericarditis, right ventricular MI, and COPD, and usually in heart failure and tricuspid stenosis.

Jugular vein waves (see FIG. 69–1) can usually be discerned clinically but are better seen on the screen during central venous pressure monitoring.

The *a* waves are increased in pulmonary hypertension. Giant *a* waves (cannon waves) are seen in atrioventricular dissociation when the atrium contracts while the tricuspid valve is closed. The *a* waves disappear in atrial fibrillation and are accentuated when RV compliance is poor (eg, in pulmonary hypertension or pulmonic stenosis). The *v* waves are very prominent in tricuspid regurgitation. The *x* descent is steep in cardiac tamponade. When RV compliance is poor, the *y* descent is very abrupt because the elevated column of venous blood rushes into the RV when the tricuspid valve opens, only to be stopped abruptly by the rigid RV wall (in restrictive myopathy) or the pericardium (in constrictive pericarditis).

Chest observation and palpation: Chest contour and any visible cardiac impulses are inspected. The precordium is palpated for pulsations (determining apical impulse and thus cardiac situs), thrills, and atrial and ventricular gallop. Location of thrills suggests the cause (see TABLE 69–2).

Chest deformities, such as shield chest and pectus carinatum (a prominent birdlike sternum), may be associated with hereditary disorders involving congenital cardiac defects (eg, Turner's syndrome). Rarely, a localized upper chest bulge indicates aortic aneurysm due to syphilis. Pectus excavatum (depressed sternum) with a narrow anteroposterior chest diameter and an abnormally straight thoracic spine may suggest myxomatous degeneration of valves or chordae (particularly mitral).

TABLE 69–2. LOCATION OF THRILLS AND ASSOCIATED DISORDERS

LOCATION OF THRILL	ASSOCIATED DISORDER
Over the base of the heart at the 2nd intercostal space, just to the right of the sternum, during systole	Aortic stenosis
At the apex during systole	Mitral regurgitation
To the left of the sternum at the 2nd intercostal space	Pulmonic stenosis
At the 4th intercostal space	Small muscular ventricular septal defect (Roger's disease)

A central precordial heave that can be seen and palpated as a lifting sensation under the sternum and anterior chest wall to the left of the sternum suggests severe RV hypertrophy (RVH). Occasionally, in congenital disorders that produce severe RVH, the precordium bulges asymmetrically to the left of the sternum.

A sustained thrust at the apex (easily differentiated from the less focal, somewhat diffuse precordial heave of RVH) suggests LV hypertrophy (LVH). Abnormal focal systolic impulses in the precordium can sometimes be felt in patients with a dyskinetic ventricular aneurysm. An abnormal diffuse systolic impulse lifts the precordium in patients with severe mitral regurgitation. The lift occurs because the left atrium expands, causing anterior cardiac displacement. A diffuse and inferolaterally displaced apical impulse is found when the LV is dilated and hypertrophied (eg, in mitral regurgitation).

A sharp impulse at the 2nd intercostal space to the left of the sternum may result from exaggerated pulmonic valve closure in pulmonary hypertension. A similar early systolic impulse at the cardiac apex may represent closure of a stenotic mitral valve; opening of the stenotic valve sometimes can be felt at the beginning of diastole. These findings coincide with an augmented 1st heart sound (S_1) and an opening snap of mitral stenosis, heard on auscultation.

Cardiac Auscultation

Auscultation of the heart requires excellent hearing and the ability to distinguish subtle differences in pitch and timing. Hearing-impaired health care practitioners can use amplified stethoscopes. High-pitched sounds are best heard with the diaphragm of the stethoscope. Low-pitched sounds are best heard with the bell. Very little pressure should be exerted when using the bell. Excessive pressure converts the underlying skin into a diaphragm and eliminates very low pitched sounds.

The entire precordium is examined systematically, typically beginning over the apical impulse with the patient in left lateral decubitus position. The patient rolls supine, and auscultation continues at the lower left sternal border, proceeds cephalad with auscultation of each interspace, then caudad from the right upper sternal border. The clinician also listens over the left axilla and above the clavicles. The patient sits upright for auscultation of the back, then leans forward to aid auscultation of aortic and pulmonic diastolic murmurs or pericardial friction rub.

Major auscultatory findings include heart sounds, murmurs, and rubs. Heart sounds are brief, transient sounds produced by valve opening and closure; they are divided into systolic and diastolic sounds.

Murmurs are produced by blood flow turbulence and are more prolonged than heart sounds; they may be systolic, diastolic, or continuous. They are graded by intensity (see TABLE 69–3). Timing of the murmur in the cardiac cycle correlates with the cause (see TABLE 69–4); auscultatory findings correlate with specific heart valve disorders. Various maneuvers (eg, inspiration, Valsalva,

TABLE 69–3. HEART MURMUR INTENSITY

GRADE	DESCRIPTION
1	Barely audible
2	Soft but easily heard
3	Loud without a thrill
4	Loud with a thrill
5	Loud with minimal contact between stethoscope and chest
6	Loud with no contact between stethoscope and chest

TABLE 69–4. ETIOLOGY OF MURMURS BY TIMING

TIMING	ASSOCIATED DISORDERS
Mid systolic (ejection)	Aortic obstruction (supravalvular stenosis, coarctation of the aorta, aortic stenosis, aortic sclerosis, hypertrophic cardiomyopathy, subvalvular stenosis)
	Increased blood flow across the aortic valve (hyperkinetic states, aortic regurgitation)
	Dilation of ascending aorta (atheroma, aortitis, aneurysm of aorta)
	Pulmonic obstruction (supravalvular pulmonary artery stenosis, pulmonic stenosis, infundibular stenosis)
	Increased blood flow across the pulmonic valve (hyperkinetic states, left-to-right shunt from atrial septal defect, ventricular septal defect)
	Dilation of pulmonary artery
Holosystolic	Mitral regurgitation, tricuspid regurgitation, ventricular septal defect
Early diastolic (regurgitant)	Aortic regurgitation: acquired or congenital valve abnormality (myxomatous or calcific degeneration, rheumatic fever, endocarditis), dilation of valve ring (aortic dissection, annuloaortic ectasia, cystic medial necrosis, or hypertension), widening of commissures (syphilis); congenital bicuspid valve with ventricular septal defect
	Pulmonic regurgitation: acquired or congenital valve abnormality, dilation of valve ring (pulmonary hypertension, Marfan syndrome), tetralogy of Fallot, ventricular septal defect
Mid diastolic	Mitral stenosis (rheumatic fever, congenital stenosis, cor triatriatum)
	Increased blood flow across nonstenotic mitral valve (mitral regurgitation, ventricular septal defect, patent ductus arteriosus, high-output states, complete heart block)
	Tricuspid stenosis
	Increased blood flow across nonstenotic tricuspid valve (tricuspid regurgitation, atrial septal defect, anomalous pulmonary venous return)
	Left or right atrial tumors, atrial ball-valve thrombi
Continuous	Patent ductus arteriosus, coarctation of the pulmonary artery, coronary or intercostal arteriovenous fistula, ruptured aneurysm of sinus of Valsalva, aortic septal defect, cervical venous hum, anomalous left coronary artery, proximal coronary artery stenosis, mammary souffle (venous hum from engorged breast vessels during pregnancy), pulmonary artery branch stenosis, bronchial collateral circulation, small (restrictive) atrial septal defect with mitral stenosis, coronary cameral fistula, aortic–right ventricular or atrial fistula

handgrip, squatting, amyl nitrate inhalation) can modify cardiac physiology slightly, making differentiation of causes of heart murmur possible (see TABLE 69–5).

All heart murmurs are evaluated by chest x-ray and ECG. Most require echocardiography to confirm the diagnosis and determine severity, usually followed by a cardiac consultation if significant disease is suspected.

Rubs are high-pitched scratchy sounds often with 2 or 3 separate components; during tachycardia, the sound may be almost continuous.

The clinician focuses attention sequentially on each phase of the cardiac cycle, noting each heart sound and murmur. Intensity, pitch, duration, and timing of the sounds and the intervals between them are analyzed, often providing an accurate diagnosis. A diagram of the major auscultatory and palpatory findings of the precordium should be routinely drawn in the patient's chart each time the patient's cardiovascular system is examined (see FIG. 69–2). With such diagrams, findings from each examination can be compared.

Systolic heart sounds: Systolic sounds include the 1st heart sound (S_1) and clicks. S_1 and the 2nd heart sound (S_2) are normal components of the cardiac cycle, the familiar "lub-dub" sounds.

S_1 occurs just after the beginning of systole and is predominantly due to mitral closure but may also include tricuspid closure components. It is often split and has a high pitch. S_1 is loud in mitral stenosis. It is soft or absent in mitral regurgitation due to valve leaflet sclerosis and rigidity but is often distinctly heard in mitral regurgitation due to myxomatous degeneration of the mitral apparatus or due to ventricular myocardial abnormality (eg, papillary muscle dysfunction, ventricular dilation).

Clicks occur only during systole; they are distinguished from S_1 and S_2 by their higher pitch and briefer duration. Some clicks occur at different times during systole as hemodynamics change. Clicks may be single or multiple.

Clicks in congenital aortic or pulmonic stenosis are thought to result from abnormal ventricular wall tension. These clicks occur early in systole (very near S_1) and are not affected by hemodynamic changes. Similar clicks occur in severe pulmonary hypertension. Clicks in mitral or tricuspid valve

TABLE 69–5. MANEUVERS THAT AID IN DIAGNOSIS OF MURMURS

MANEUVER	EFFECT ON BLOOD FLOW	EFFECT ON HEART SOUNDS
Inspiration	Simultaneously increases venous flow into the right heart, decreases venous flow into the left heart	Augments right heart sounds (eg, murmurs of tricuspid stenosis and regurgitation, those of pulmonic stenosis* [immediately] and regurgitation [usually]); reduces left heart sounds
Valsalva maneuver	Reduces size of left ventricle (LV); decreases venous return to the right heart and subsequently to the left heart	Augments murmur of hypertrophic obstructive cardiomyopathy and diastolic murmur of mitral stenosis; reduces murmurs of aortic stenosis, mitral regurgitation, and tricuspid stenosis
Release of Valsalva maneuver	Increases volume of LV	Augments murmur of aortic stenosis, that of aortic regurgitation (after 4 or 5 beats), and those of pulmonic regurgitation or pulmonic stenosis* (immediately); reduces murmur of tricuspid stenosis
Isometric handgrip	Increases afterload and peripheral arterial resistance	Reduces murmurs of aortic stenosis and hypertrophic obstructive cardiomyopathy; augments murmurs of mitral regurgitation and aortic regurgitation and diastolic murmur of mitral stenosis
Squatting	Simultaneously decreases venous return to the right heart and increases afterload and peripheral resistance	Augments murmurs of aortic regurgitation, aortic stenosis, mitral valve prolapse, and mitral regurgitation and diastolic murmur of mitral stenosis; reduces murmur of hypertrophic obstructive cardiomyopathy
Amyl nitrite	Causes intense venodilation, which reduces venous return to the right heart	Augments murmurs of hypertrophic obstructive cardiomyopathy and mitral valve prolapse; reduces murmur of aortic stenosis

*Patient may need to be standing for effect on pulmonic stenosis to be heard.

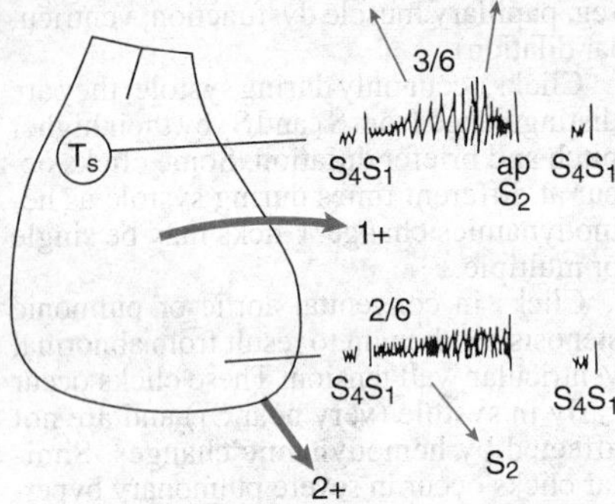

Fig. 69–2. Diagram of physical findings in a patient with aortic stenosis and mitral regurgitation. Murmur, character, intensity, and radiation are depicted. Sound of pulmonic closure exceeds that of aortic closure. Left ventricular (LV) thrust and right ventricular (RV) lift (heavy arrows) are identified. A 4th heart sound (S_4) and systolic thrill (T_S) are present. a = aortic closure sound; p = pulmonic closure sound; S_1 = 1st heart sound; S_2 = 2nd heart sound; 3/6 = grade of crescendo-diminuendo murmur (radiates to both sides of neck); 2/6 = grade of pansystolic apical crescendo murmur; 1+ = mild precordial lift of RV hypertrophy (arrow shows direction of lift); 2+ = moderate LV thrust (arrow shows direction of thrust).

prolapse, typically occurring in mid to late systole, are thought to result from abnormal tension on redundant and elongated chordae tendineae or valve leaflets.

Clicks due to myxomatous degeneration of valves may occur any time during systole but move toward S_1 during maneuvers that transiently decrease ventricular filling volume (eg, standing, Valsalva maneuver). If ventricular filling volume is increased (eg, by lying supine), clicks move toward S_2, particularly in mitral valve prolapse. For unknown reasons, characteristics of the clicks may vary greatly between examinations, and clicks may come and go.

Diastolic heart sounds: Diastolic sounds include the 2nd, 3rd, and 4th heart sounds (S_2, S_3, and S_4), diastolic knocks, and mitral valve sounds. Unlike systolic sounds, diastolic sounds are low-pitched; they are softer in intensity and longer in duration. Except for S_2, these sounds are always abnormal in adults.

S_2 occurs at the beginning of diastole, due to aortic and pulmonic valve closure. Aortic valve closure normally precedes pulmonic valve closure unless the former is late or the latter is early. Aortic valve closure is late in left bundle branch block or aortic stenosis; pulmonic valve closure is early in some forms of preexcitation phenomena. Delayed pulmonic valve closure may result from increased blood flow through the RV (eg, in atrial septal defect of the common secundum variety) or complete right bundle branch block. Increased RV flow in atrial septal defect also abolishes the normal respiratory variation in aortic and pulmonic valve closure, producing a fixed split S_2. Left-to-right shunts with normal RV volume flow (eg, in membranous ventricular septal defects) do not cause fixed splitting. A single S_2 may occur when the aortic valve is regurgitant, severely stenotic, or atretic (in truncus arteriosus when there is a common valve).

S_3 occurs in early diastole, when the ventricle is dilated and noncompliant. It occurs during passive diastolic ventricular filling and indicates serious ventricular dysfunction in adults; in children, it can be normal. RV S_3 is heard best (sometimes only) during inspiration (because negative intrathoracic pressure augments RV filling volume) with the patient supine. LV S_3 is best heard during expiration (because the heart is nearer the chest wall) with the patient in the left lateral decubitus position.

S_4 is produced by augmented ventricular filling, caused by atrial contraction, near the end of diastole. It is similar to S_3 and heard best or only with the bell of the stethoscope. During inspiration, RV S_4 increases and LV S_4 decreases. S_4 is heard much more often than S_3 and indicates a lesser degree of ventricular dysfunction, usually diastolic. S_4 is absent in atrial fibrillation (because the atria do not contract) but is almost always present in active myocardial ischemia or soon after MI. S_3, with or without S_4, is usual in significant systolic LV dysfunction; S_4 without S_3 is usual in diastolic LV dysfunction.

A summation gallop occurs when S_3 and S_4 are present in a patient with tachycardia, which shortens diastole so that the 2 sounds merge. Loud S_3 and S_4 may be palpable at the apex with the patient in the left lateral decubitus position.

A diastolic knock occurs at the same time as S_3, in early diastole. It is not accompanied by S_4 and is a louder, thudding sound, which indicates abrupt arrest of ventricular filling by a noncompliant, constricting pericardium.

An opening snap may occur in early diastole in mitral stenosis or, rarely, in tricuspid stenosis. Mitral opening snap is very high pitched, brief, and heard best with the diaphragm of the stethoscope. The more severe mitral stenosis is (ie, the higher the left atrial pressure), the closer the opening snap is to the pulmonic component of S_2. Intensity is related to the compliance of the valve leaflets: The snap sounds loud when leaflets remain elastic, but it gradually softens and ultimately disappears as sclerosis, fibrosis, and calcification of the valve develop. Mitral opening snap, although sometimes heard at the apex, is often heard best or only at the lower left sternal border.

Systolic murmurs: Systolic murmurs may be normal or abnormal. They may be early, mid, or late systolic, or holosystolic (pansystolic). Systolic murmurs may be divided into ejection, regurgitant, and shunt murmurs.

Ejection murmurs are due to turbulent forward flow through narrowed or irregular valves or outflow tracts (eg, due to aortic or pulmonic stenosis). They are typically mid systolic and have a crescendo-diminuendo character that usually becomes louder and longer as flow becomes more obstructed. The greater the stenosis and turbulence, the longer the crescendo phase and the shorter the diminuendo phase.

Systolic ejection murmurs may occur without hemodynamically significant outflow tract obstruction and thus do not indicate a disorder. In normal infants and children, flow is often mildly turbulent, producing soft ejection murmurs. The elderly often have ejection murmurs due to valve and vessel sclerosis.

During pregnancy, many women have soft ejection murmurs at the 2nd intercostal space to the left or right of the sternum. The murmurs occur because a physiologic increase in blood volume and cardiac output increases flow velocity through normal structures. The murmurs may be greatly exaggerated if severe anemia complicates the pregnancy.

Regurgitant murmurs represent retrograde or abnormal flow (eg, due to mitral regurgitation, tricuspid regurgitation, or ventricular septal defects) into chambers that are at lower resistance. They are typically holosystolic and tend to be louder with high-velocity, low-volume regurgitation or shunts and softer with high-volume regurgitation or shunts.

Shunt murmurs may originate at the site of the shunt (eg, patent ductus arteriosus, ventricular septal defects) or result from altered hemodynamics remote from the shunt (eg, pulmonic systolic flow murmur due to an atrial septal defect with left-to-right shunt).

Diastolic murmurs: Diastolic murmurs are always abnormal; most are early or mid diastolic but may be late diastolic (presystolic). Early diastolic murmurs are typically due to aortic or pulmonic regurgitation. Mid diastolic (or early to mid diastolic) murmurs are typically due to mitral or tricuspid stenosis. A late diastolic murmur may be due to rheumatic mitral stenosis in a patient in sinus rhythm.

A mitral or tricuspid murmur due to an atrial tumor or thrombus may be evanescent and may vary with position and from one examination to the next because the position of the intracardiac mass changes.

Continuous murmurs: Continuous murmurs occur throughout the cardiac cycle. They are always abnormal, indicating a constant shunt flow throughout systole and diastole. They may be due to various cardiac defects (see TABLE 69–4). Some defects produce a thrill; many are associated with signs of RVH and LVH. As pulmonary artery resistance increases in shunt lesions, the diastolic component gradually decreases. When pulmonary and systemic resistance equalize, the murmur may disappear.

Patent ductus arteriosus murmurs are loudest at the 2nd intercostal space just below the medial end of the left clavicle. Aorticopulmonary window murmurs are central and heard at the 3rd intercostal space level. Murmurs of systemic arteriovenous fistulas are best heard directly over the lesions; those of pulmonic arteriovenous fistulas and pulmonary artery branch stenosis are more diffuse and heard throughout the chest.

During pregnancy, a continuous venous hum from breast vessels (mammary souffle) may be mistaken for a continuous cardiac murmur.

Pericardial friction rub: A pericardial friction rub is caused by movement of inflammatory adhesions between visceral and parietal pericardial layers. It is a high-pitched or squeaking sound; it may be systolic, diastolic and systolic, or triphasic (when atrial contraction accentuates the diastolic component during late diastole). The rub sounds like pieces of leather squeaking as they are rubbed together. Rubs are best heard with the patient leaning forward or on hands and knees with breath held in expiration.

CHEST PAIN

The heart, lungs, esophagus, and great vessels provide afferent visceral input through the same thoracic autonomic ganglia. A painful stimulus in these organs is typically perceived as originating in the chest, but because afferent nerve fibers overlap in the dorsal ganglia, thoracic pain may be felt anywhere between the epigastrium and the jaw, including the arms or shoulders (as referred pain). Painful stimuli from thoracic organs can produce discomfort described as pressure, gas, burning, aching, and sometimes sharp pain. Because the sensation is visceral in origin, many patients deny they are having pain and insist it is merely discomfort.

Etiology

Many disorders produce chest pain or discomfort. Some (eg, acute MI, unstable angina, thoracic aortic dissection, tension pneumothorax, esophageal rupture, pulmonary embolism) are immediately life threatening. Some (eg, angina pectoris, pericarditis, myocarditis, pneumothorax, pneumonia, pancreatitis, various thoracic malignancies) are potentially life threatening. Others (eg, gastroesophageal reflux disease [GERD], peptic ulcer, esophageal motility disorders, costochondritis, chest trauma, biliary tract disease, herpes zoster) are uncomfortable but usually not dangerous.

Chest pain in children and young adults (< 30 yr) is less likely to result from myocardial ischemia, although MI can occur in people in their 20s. Musculoskeletal or pulmonary disorders are more common causes in these age groups.

Evaluation

History: Location, duration, character, and quality of the pain and triggering and relieving factors are important. Past cardiac disorders, use of drugs that can trigger coronary artery spasm (eg, cocaine, triptans, phosphodiesterase inhibitors), and presence of risk factors for coronary artery disease (CAD) or pulmonary embolism (eg, leg pain or injury, recent immobilization, travel, pregnancy) may be important. The presence or absence of risk factors for CAD (eg, hypertension, hypercholesterolemia, smoking, positive family history) alters the probability of underlying CAD but does not help diagnose the cause of acute chest pain.

Symptoms due to serious thoracic disorders overlap and vary greatly, but distinctions can sometimes be made. Crushing pain radiating to the jaw or arm suggests acute ischemia or MI. Patients often ascribe myocardial ischemic pain to indigestion. Exertional pain relieved by rest indicates angina pectoris. Tearing pain radiating to the back suggests thoracic aortic dissection. Burning pain radiating from epigastrium to throat, exacerbated by lying down and relieved by antacids, suggests GERD. Fever, chills, and cough suggest pneumonia. Significant dyspnea suggests pulmonary embolism or pneumonia.

Pain can be exacerbated by respiration, movement, or both in serious or minor disorders; these triggers are not specific. Brief (< 5 sec), sharp, intermittent pains rarely result from serious disorders.

Physical examination: Although not specific, tachycardia, bradycardia, tachypnea, hypotension, or signs of hypoperfusion (eg, confusion, ashen color, diaphoresis) increase the likelihood of a serious underlying disorder.

Unilateral absence of breath sounds suggests pneumothorax; resonance to percussion and dilated neck veins suggest tension pneumothorax. Fever and rales suggest pneumonia. Fever alone may be due to pulmonary embolism, pericarditis, acute MI, or esophageal rupture. Pericardial rub suggests pericarditis. The 4th heart sound (S_4), late systolic murmur of papillary muscle dysfunction, or both suggest MI. Focal CNS abnormalities, an aortic regurgitant murmur, or marked asymmetry in pulse or BP between arms suggests thoracic aortic dissection. Leg swelling and tenderness suggest deep venous thrombosis and thus possible pulmonary embolism. Tenderness of the chest to palpation, present in about 15% of patients with acute MI, is not specific for origin of pain in chest wall.

Testing: For anyone with chest pain, minimal testing includes pulse oximetry, ECG, and chest x-ray. For adults, blood tests for cardiac markers are often done. Results of these tests should be integrated with findings from the history and physical examination, and specific diagnoses should be pursued. Blood tests are not valuable as a primary screen. In particular, a single normal set of cardiac markers should not be used to rule out a cardiac cause. If myocardial ischemia is likely, tests should include serial measurement of cardiac markers and ECGs and possibly stress ECG or a stress imaging test (see p. 630).

A diagnostic trial of sublingual nitroglycerin or an oral liquid antacid does not adequately differentiate myocardial ischemia from GERD or gastritis. Either drug may relieve symptoms of either disorder.

Treatment: Specific identified disorders are treated. If etiology is not clearly benign, patients are usually admitted to the hospital or an observation unit for cardiac monitoring and more extensive evaluation. Symptoms are treated with acetaminophen or opioids as needed, pending a diagnosis.

PALPITATIONS

Palpitations are the perception of cardiac activity by the patient. They may be described as a fluttering, racing, or skipping sensation. Sinus rhythm at a normal rate is not ordinarily perceived. Associated symptoms vary with etiology.

Etiology

Causes range from benign to life threatening. Some patients simply have heightened awareness of normal cardiac activity, particularly when exercise, febrile illness, or anxiety increases heart rate. However, in most cases, palpitations result from arrhythmia (see Ch. 75 on p. 673).

The most common arrhythmias are premature atrial contractions (PACs) or ventricular contractions (PVCs), which usually are harmless. Other arrhythmias include paroxysmal supraventricular tachycardia (PSVT), atrial fibrillation or flutter, and ventricular tachycardia. Some arrhythmias (eg, PACs, PVCs, PSVT) often occur spontaneously without serious disease, but others are often caused by an underlying cardiac disorder, such as myocardial ischemia, valvular heart disease, or conduction system disturbances. Disorders that increase myocardial contractility (eg, thyrotoxicosis, pheochromocytoma) may produce palpitations. Some drugs, including caffeine, alcohol, and sympathomimetics (eg, epinephrine, ephedrine, theophylline), frequently produce palpitations. Anemia, hypoxia, and electrolyte abnormalities (eg, diuretic-induced hypokalemia) can trigger or exacerbate palpitations.

Evaluation

History: PACs and PVCs are often described as occasional skipped beats; other symptoms are uncommon. Atrial fibrillation is identified as a sustained irregularity. Supraventricular or ventricular tachycardia is often perceived as a rapid, regular heartbeat with sudden onset and termination; previous similar episodes are common. Sometimes asking the patient to tap out the beat of palpitations is better than a verbal description.

The patient is asked about weakness, dyspnea, light-headedness, and syncope, which suggest coronary artery disease (CAD) or another serious underlying disorder. Chronic fatigue and weakness suggest anemia or heart failure. Palpitations in patients with CAD may be accompanied by ischemic chest pain due to decreased diastolic coronary flow during tachycardia or bradycardia.

The patient is asked about use of caffeine, alcohol, or other drugs (eg, cocaine, methamphetamine, other illegal stimulants, OTC diet aids, dietary supplements).

Physical examination: Palpation of the arterial pulse and cardiac auscultation may reveal a rhythm disturbance, which, except for the unique irregular irregularity in some cases of rapid atrial fibrillation, is rarely diagnostic. Thyroid enlargement or tenderness with exophthalmos suggests thyrotoxicosis. Marked hypertension and regular tachycardia suggest pheochromocytoma.

Testing: ECG is done; however, unless done during symptoms, it usually does not provide a diagnosis because most cardiac arrhythmias are intermittent. A patient in the emergency department may be placed on a cardiac monitor for 1 or 2 h. If no diagnosis is apparent, a 24-h Holter monitor or, if intermittent symptoms occur infrequently, an event recorder triggered by the patient is useful.

When a serious disorder is suspected, a pulse oximetry reading is taken. Serum electrolytes are measured in patients at risk of electrolyte abnormalities; a CBC is obtained when symptoms suggest anemia. Thyroid function tests are indicated when atrial fibrillation is newly diagnosed.

Treatment

For isolated PACs and PVCs, simple reassurance is usually sufficient. Identified rhythm disturbances and underlying disorders are treated. Precipitating drugs and substances are withdrawn or changed.

ORTHOSTATIC HYPOTENSION

Orthostatic (postural) hypotension is an excessive fall in BP (typically > 20/10 mm Hg) when an upright position is assumed.

Faintness, light-headedness, dizziness, confusion, or blurred vision occurs within seconds of standing. Some patients experience syncope (see p. 584) or even generalized seizures. Exercise or a heavy meal may exacerbate symptoms. Most other associated symptoms and signs relate to the cause. Orthostatic hypotension is a manifestation of abnormal BP regulation due to various conditions, not a specific disorder.

Orthostatic hypotension occurs in about 20% of the elderly; it is more common among those with coexisting disorders, especially hypertension, and among residents of long-term care facilities. Many falls may result from unrecognized orthostatic hypotension. Symptoms tend to be more severe shortly after eating and after vagal stimulation (eg, urination, defecation).

Postural orthostatic tachycardia syndrome (POTS): POTS (also called postural autonomic tachycardia or chronic or idiopathic orthostatic intolerance) is a syndrome of orthostatic intolerance in younger patients. Although tachycardia and various symptoms (eg, fatigue, light-headedness, exercise intolerance, cognitive impairment) occur with standing, there is little or no fall in BP. The reason for symptoms is unclear.

Pathophysiology

Normally, the gravitational stress of suddenly standing causes blood (½ to 1 L) to pool in the capacitance veins of the legs and trunk. The subsequent transient decrease in venous return reduces cardiac output and thus BP. The first effects are those of cerebral hypoperfusion; however, decreased BP does not always produce cerebral hypoperfusion.

Baroreceptors in the aortic arch and carotid bodies respond to hypotension by activating autonomic reflexes to rapidly normalize BP. The sympathetic system increases heart rate and contractility. Then, vasomotor tone of the capacitance vessels increases. Simultaneous parasympathetic (vagal) inhibition also increases heart rate. With continued standing, activation of the renin-angiotensin-aldosterone system and ADH secretion cause Na and water retention and increase circulating blood volume.

Etiology

Homeostatic mechanisms may be inadequate to restore low BP if afferent, central, or efferent portions of the autonomic reflex arc are impaired by disorders or drugs, if myocardial contractility or vascular responsiveness is depressed, if hypovolemia is present, or if hormonal responses are faulty (see TABLE 69–6).

The most common cause in the elderly is decreased baroreceptor responsiveness plus decreased arterial compliance. Decreased baroreceptor responsiveness delays cardioacceleration in response to standing. Paradoxically, hypertension may contribute to poor baroreceptor sensitivity, increasing vulnerability to orthostatic hypotension. Postprandial orthostatic hypotension is also common. It may be caused by the insulin response to high-carbohydrate meals and blood pooling in the GI tract; this condition is worsened by alcohol intake.

Evaluation

Orthostatic hypotension is diagnosed when a marked fall in measured BP and symptoms suggesting hypotension are provoked by standing and relieved by lying down. A cause must be sought.

History: The patient is asked about known triggers (eg, drugs, bed rest, fluid loss) and symptoms of autonomic insufficiency (eg, visual impairment [due to mydriasis and loss of accommodation], incontinence, constipation, heat intolerance [due to impaired sweating], impotence). Other symptoms of neurologic, cardiovascular, and malignant disorders are noted.

Physical examination: BP and heart rate are measured after 5 min supine and at 1 and 3 min after standing; patients unable to stand may be assessed while sitting upright. Hypotension without a compensatory increase in heart rate (< 10 beats/min) suggests autonomic impairment; marked increase (to > 100 beats/min) suggests hypovolemia or, if symptoms develop without hypotension, POTS. Other findings suggesting autonomic impairment include parkinsonism.

Testing: ECG and serum electrolytes and glucose are routinely checked. However, these and other tests are usually of little benefit unless suggested by specific symptoms.

Autonomic function can be evaluated. With an intact autonomic system, heart rate increases in response to inspiration. The heart is monitored as the patient breathes slowly and deeply (about 5 sec inspiration and 7 sec expiration) for 1 min. The longest interbeat (R-R) interval during expiration is normally at least 1.15 times the minimum R-R interval during inspiration; a shorter interval suggests

TABLE 69–6. CAUSES OF ORTHOSTATIC HYPOTENSION

CAUSE	EXAMPLES
Neurologic (involving autonomic dysfunction)	
Central	Multiple system atrophy (previously Shy-Drager syndrome) Parkinson's disease Strokes (multiple)
Spinal cord	Tabes dorsalis Transverse myelitis Tumors
Peripheral	Amyloidosis Diabetic, alcoholic, or nutritional neuropathy Familial dysautonomia (Riley-Day syndrome) Guillain-Barré syndrome Paraneoplastic syndromes Pure autonomic failure (formerly called idiopathic orthostatic hypotension) Surgical sympathectomy
Cardiovascular	
Hypovolemia	Adrenal insufficiency Dehydration Hemorrhage
Impaired vasomotor tone	Bed rest (prolonged) Hypokalemia
Impaired cardiac output	Aortic stenosis Constrictive pericarditis Heart failure MI Tachyarrhythmias or bradyarrhythmias
Other	Hyperaldosteronism* Peripheral venous insufficiency Pheochromocytoma*
Drugs	
Vasodilators	Ca channel blockers Nitrates
Autonomically active	α-Blockers (prazosin, phenoxybenzamine) Antihypertensives (clonidine, methyldopa, reserpine, [rarely] β-blockers)† Antipsychotics (particularly phenothiazines) Monoamine oxidase inhibitors (MAOIs) Tricyclic or tetracyclic antidepressants
Other	Alcohol Barbiturates Levodopa (in Parkinson's [rarely]) Loop diuretics (eg, furosemide) Quinidine Vincristine (neurotoxic)

*Causes supine hypertension.
†Symptoms are more common when treatment is begun.

autonomic dysfunction. A similar variation in R-R interval should exist between rest and a 10- to 15-sec Valsalva maneuver. Patients with abnormal R-R intervals or with autonomic symptoms or signs require further evaluation for diabetes, Parkinson's disease, and possibly multiple system atrophy (see p. 1768) and pure autonomic failure (see p. 1769); the last may require plasma norepinephrine or vasopressin measurements with the patient supine and upright.

Tilt table testing (see p. 603) varies less than supine and upright BP assessment and eliminates augmentation of venous return by leg muscle contraction. The patient may remain upright for 30 to 45 min of BP assessment. It may be done when autonomic dysfunction is suspected. The dose of a suspected drug may be reduced or the drug withdrawn to confirm the drug as the cause.

Prevention and Treatment

Patients requiring prolonged bed rest should sit up each day and exercise in bed when possible. Patients should rise slowly from a recumbent or sitting position, consume adequate fluids, limit or avoid alcohol, and exercise regularly when feasible. Regular modest-intensity exercise promotes overall vascular tone and reduces venous pooling. Elderly patients should avoid prolonged standing. Sleeping with the head of the bed raised may relieve symptoms by promoting Na retention and reducing nocturnal diuresis.

Postprandial hypotension can often be prevented by reducing the size and carbohydrate content of meals, minimizing alcohol intake, and avoiding sudden standing after meals.

Waist-high fitted elastic hose may increase venous return, cardiac output, and BP after standing. In severe cases, inflatable aviator-type antigravity suits, although often poorly tolerated, may be needed to produce adequate leg and abdominal counterpressure.

Increasing Na intake may expand intravascular volume and lessen symptoms. In the absence of heart failure or hypertension, Na intake can be increased 5 to 10 g above the usual dietary level by liberally salting food or taking NaCl tablets. This approach risks heart failure, particularly in elderly patients and patients with impaired myocardial function; development of dependent edema without heart failure does not contraindicate continuing this approach.

Fludrocortisone, a mineralocorticoid, causes Na retention, which expands plasma volume, and often lessens symptoms but is effective only when Na intake is adequate. Dosage is 0.1 mg po at bedtime, increased weekly to 1 mg or until peripheral edema occurs. This drug may also improve the peripheral vasoconstrictor response to sympathetic stimulation. Supine hypertension, heart failure, and hypokalemia may occur; K supplements may be needed.

Midodrine, a peripheral α-agonist that is both an arterial and venous constrictor, is often effective. Dosage is 2.5 mg to 10 mg po tid. Adverse effects include paresthesias and itching (probably secondary to piloerection). This drug is not recommended for patients with coronary artery or peripheral arterial disease.

NSAIDs (eg, indomethacin 25 to 50 mg po tid) may inhibit prostaglandin-induced vasodilation, increasing peripheral vascular resistance. However, NSAIDs may cause GI symptoms and unwanted vasopressor reactions (reported with concurrent use of indomethacin and sympathomimetic drugs).

L-dihydroxyphenylserine, a norepinephrine precursor, may be beneficial for autonomic dysfunction (reported in limited trials).

Propranolol or other β-blockers may enhance the beneficial effects of Na and mineralocorticoid therapy. β-Blockade with propranolol leads to unopposed α-adrenergic peripheral vascular vasoconstriction, preventing the vasodilation that occurs when some patients stand.

SYNCOPE

Syncope is a sudden, brief loss of consciousness (LOC) with loss of postural tone followed, by definition, by spontaneous revival. Typically, the patient is pale, motionless, diaphoretic, and hypotensive, with cool extremities, a weak pulse, and shallow rapid breathing. Light-headedness and a sense of an impending faint without LOC (near-syncope) are usually considered with syncope because the causes are the same; when the patient is upright, syncope often follows (in orthostatic hypotension). Syncope and near-syncope are fairly common and recur in up to ⅓ of people. Although the cause is often benign, identifying the occasional life-threatening cause (eg, tachyarrhythmia, heart block) is important.

Pathophysiology and Etiology

Syncope results from global CNS dysfunction, which may have many causes. Typically,

CNS dysfunction results from cerebral hypoperfusion. Cerebral hypoperfusion most commonly results from disorders that decrease cardiac output (CO). CO can be impaired by primary cardiac disorders or conditions that decrease venous return (eg, reflex-mediated vasomotor instability). Occasionally, cerebrovascular disorders cause hypoperfusion. In the elderly, syncope often has more than one cause.

Primary cardiac disorders: Mechanisms for decreased CO include outflow obstruction, diastolic filling disorders, arrhythmias, and less commonly, pump failure. Cardiac causes of syncope, unlike other causes, have a significant risk of sudden death. The risk is from the underlying disorder, not from syncope itself.

Cardiac outflow may be obstructed because of valvular stenosis (particularly aortic), hypertrophic cardiomyopathy, a defective prosthetic valve, or a pulmonary embolus. Intracardiac tumors (eg, atrial myxoma) or ball-valve thrombi can intermittently obstruct blood flow through the heart, sometimes only with certain changes in position. Exercise and hypovolemia exacerbate outflow obstruction (particularly in aortic stenosis and hypertrophic cardiomyopathy) and may precipitate syncope. Inotropic drugs also may trigger syncope in patients with hypertrophic cardiomyopathy.

Arrhythmias cause syncope when heart rate is too fast to allow adequate ventricular filling (eg > 150 to 180 beats/min) or too slow to provide adequate output (eg, < 30 to 35 beats/min). When other cardiovascular (eg, obstructive) disorders are present, less extreme heart rate changes may cause syncope.

Bradyarrhythmias that can cause syncope include sick sinus syndrome (with or without tachyarrhythmias) and high-grade atrioventricular block, especially when onset is abrupt. Although bradyarrhythmias develop at all ages, they are most common among the elderly, usually because of fibrosis of the conduction system (due to ischemia or age-related degeneration). Digoxin, β-blockers (including ophthalmic drops), Ca channel blockers, and other drugs may cause bradyarrhythmias and syncope.

Tachyarrhythmias may be of supraventricular or ventricular origin; they may result from ischemia, heart failure, cardiomyopathy, drug toxicity (quinidine syncope is best known), electrolyte abnormalities (eg, hypokalemia, hypomagnesemia), preexcitation, or other disorders.

Systolic or diastolic ventricular dysfunction (eg, in acute MI, myocarditis, or cardiac tamponade) may decrease CO, rarely causing syncope. Acute MI causes syncope usually only if arrhythmia or heart block (particularly common with inferior MI) is also present; syncope rarely results from ischemic ventricular dysfunction alone. However, syncope is the presenting symptom of MI in a few patients, particularly in the elderly.

Reflex-mediated vasomotor instability: Several stimuli can trigger a reflex-mediated withdrawal of sympathetic tone and increase in vagal tone, leading to neurally mediated (neurogenic) syncope. Predisposing factors may be involved.

Increased intrathoracic pressure (due to cough, straining to void or defecate, or another Valsalva maneuver) can limit venous return and increase vagal tone, resulting in decreased CO and syncope.

Strong emotion, pain, fear, sight of blood, or injury can produce strong vagal stimulation, causing vasovagal syncope. An initial increase in BP and heart rate is followed by an abrupt decrease in BP and sometimes heart rate. This form of syncope is common and benign; assuming a horizontal position results in complete recovery.

Carotid sinus pressure (due to inadvertent pressure on the neck or constricting clothing) can activate one or both carotid sinuses, causing peripheral vasodilation, hypotension, and syncope in people whose carotid sinuses are abnormally sensitive.

Swallowing sometimes produces syncope, usually in patients with an esophageal disorder (particularly structural abnormalities) and usually due to vasovagal reflex mechanisms inducing bradycardia and vasodilation.

Orthostatic hypotension: Orthostatic hypotension (see also p. 581) results from failure of normal mechanisms to compensate for the temporary decrease in venous return after standing. Orthostatic hypotension is a common benign cause of syncope. Causes include autonomic dysfunction, cardiovascular disorders, and many drugs (see TABLE 69–6). Assuming a horizontal position results in complete recovery from syncope due to orthostatic hypotension.

Cerebrovascular disorders: Cerebral hypoperfusion may be caused by vascular insufficiency, especially in the posterior circulation. Because hypoperfusion must affect centrencephalic structures to cause LOC, most cerebrovascular disorders do not result in syncope. However, basilar artery ischemia, due to transient ischemic attack or migraine, can produce syncope, as can hyperventilation-induced CNS vasoconstriction. Rarely, vertebrobasilar insufficiency due to severe cervical arthritis or spondylosis causes syncope when the head is moved in certain positions.

Other causes: Patients with a conversion disorder may have hysterical fainting. Patients with an anxiety disorder may faint because of hyperventilation, in which hypocapnia-induced vasoconstriction reduces cerebral blood flow.

Severe anemia may result in inadequate oxygenation and syncope, as may Takayasu's arteritis (by impairing blood flow through the carotid arteries or vertebrobasilar system).

In the subclavian steal syndrome, subclavian artery stenosis proximal to the origin of the vertebral artery "steals" flow from the vertebral artery to supply the arm during exertion, causing syncope with an orthostatic component on standing.

Weight lifter's syncope, which is benign, involves several mechanisms. Hyperventilation before lifting causes hypocapnia, cerebral vasoconstriction, and peripheral vasodilation. The Valsalva maneuver of lifting decreases venous return and CO; squatting further impedes venous return and potentiates systemic vasodilation and decreased BP.

Standing for long periods without moving can cause venous pooling (with decreased venous return and inadequate cardiac filling), leading to syncope (parade ground syncope). This type of syncope occurs in healthy people and is benign.

Breath-holding spells in infants can cause syncope. In early pregnancy, syncope is common because of hormonal changes; it is somewhat less common later, occurring if the gravid uterus presses on the inferior vena cava and impairs venous return. Seizures, including febrile seizures in children, can cause LOC that may mimic syncope.

Evaluation

History and physical examination, with particular attention to cardiovascular abnormalities, suggest a cause in 40 to 50% of cases. Identification of syncope due to cardiac causes is important because sudden death is a risk.

LOC also occurs during seizures; these episodes are not considered syncope, although many patients who have had unwitnessed seizures are brought to the hospital for apparent syncope. Conversely, patients with syncope due to hypoperfusion often have brief (eg, < 5 sec) seizure activity, which should not be mistakenly attributed to a seizure disorder. Narcolepsy also may be mistaken for syncope, particularly at initial presentation.

History: Drugs used (particularly antihypertensives, diuretics, vasodilators, and antiarrhythmics with proarrhythmic or atrioventricular conduction-altering actions) must be identified.

The patient is asked to describe associated events and symptoms, which may aid diagnosis (see TABLE 69–7). Syncope that begins and ends suddenly and spontaneously is typical of cardiac causes, most commonly an arrhythmia. Syncope precipitated by unpleasant physical or emotional stimuli (eg, pain, fright), usually occurring in the upright position, and often preceded by vagally mediated warning symptoms (eg, nausea, weakness, yawning, apprehension, blurred vision, diaphoresis) suggests vasovagal syncope. Syncope that occurs most often when assuming an upright position (particularly in elderly patients after prolonged bed rest, in patients with severe varicose veins, or in patients taking certain drug classes) suggests orthostatic syncope. Syncope that occurs after standing for long periods without moving is usually due to venous pooling.

Syncope associated with dyspnea, tachypnea, chest discomfort, cyanosis, and hypotension may be due to pulmonary embolism and usually indicates massive pulmonary vascular obstruction. It may also be due to tension pneumothorax.

Syncope that begins gradually (with warning symptoms), resolves slowly, and is often preceded by paresthesias and chest discomfort suggests hyperventilation.

LOC that is abrupt in onset; is associated with muscular jerking or convulsions, incontinence, and tongue biting; and is followed by postictal confusion or somnolence suggests a seizure.

Physical examination: Postural changes in heart rate and BP suggest hypovolemia or other causes of orthostatic hypotension. A carotid bruit or diminished carotid pulse suggests cerebral ischemia. A harsh, late-peaking, basal murmur radiating to the carotid arteries suggests aortic stenosis; a systolic murmur

TABLE 69–7. DIFFERENTIATING SYNCOPE BY CAUSE

FEATURE	NEURALLY MEDIATED HYPOTENSION	ARRHYTHMIAS	OUTFLOW OBSTRUCTION	SEIZURES
Sex	Females more than males	Males more than females	Equal	Equal
Age	< 55 yr	> 54 yr	Any age	< 45 yr
Frequency of episodes	> 2	< 3	> 1	> 1
Triggers	Standing, warm room, emotional upset	Any setting	Exercise	Any setting
Premonitory symptoms	Palpitations, blurred vision, nausea, warmth, diaphoresis, light-headedness	Usually none; sometimes palpitations, vertigo, or light-headedness	Usually none; sometimes angina or dyspnea	Sudden onset or brief aura (déjà vu, olfactory, gustatory, visual)
Duration of loss of consciousness	> 5 sec	< 6 sec	Brief (occasionally cardiac arrest and death)	Longer: 1–5 min
Observations during the event	Pallor, diaphoresis, dilated pupils, slow pulse, low BP, sometimes incontinence, sometimes brief clonic movements	Blue skin tone (no pallor); sometimes incontinence, brief clonic movements, or stertorous breathing	Blue skin tone (no pallor), sometimes incontinence, sometimes brief clonic movements	Blue face (no pallor), tonic/clonic movements, incontinence (common), frothing at the mouth, tongue biting, horizontal eye deviation, elevated pulse and BP
Observations after the event	Residual symptoms common (eg, prolonged fatigue in > 90%); quick, complete recovery of orientation	Residual symptoms uncommon (unless unconsciousness is prolonged); quick, complete recovery of orientation	Residual symptoms uncommon (unless unconsciousness is prolonged); quick, complete recovery of orientation	Postictal state with prolonged confusion and somnolence; often aching muscles and headache

that increases with the Valsalva maneuver and disappears with squatting suggests hypertrophic cardiomyopathy. A click and murmur heard earlier in systole and more prominently during standing indicate mitral valve prolapse, suggesting the cause is an arrhythmia. Further evaluation is needed for suspected hemorrhage, other causes of hypovolemia, or a focal CNS disorder.

Asking the patient to hyperventilate or applying carotid sinus pressure (to detect carotid sinus hypersensitivity) may reproduce symptoms. Carotid sinus pressure requires ECG monitoring and should not be applied bilaterally.

If observed by the clinician, hysterical fainting can be distinguished from syncope because consciousness is not lost (although some patients are excellent mimics), heart rate and BP remain normal, and pallor and diaphoresis are absent.

Testing: Resting ECG is done for all patients. The ECG may reveal arrhythmia, a conduction abnormality, ventricular hypertrophy, preexcitation, QT prolongation, pacemaker malfunction, myocardial ischemia, or

MI. If there are no clinical clues, measuring cardiac markers and obtaining ECGs to rule out MI in older patients plus Holter ECG monitoring for at least 24 h is prudent. Any detected arrhythmia must be associated with altered consciousness to be implicated as the cause, but most patients do not experience syncope during monitoring. An event recorder may be useful if warning symptoms precede syncope.

If possible, pulse oximetry should be done during or immediately after an episode to identify hypoxemia (which may indicate pulmonary embolism). If hypoxemia is present, a lung scan or other test for pulmonary embolism is indicated (see p. 414). Other laboratory tests are done based on clinical suspicion; reflexively obtained laboratory panels are of little use. Hct is measured if anemia is suspected; electrolytes are measured, particularly if hypokalemia or hypomagnesemia is suspected. Cardiac markers (eg, serum troponin, CPK-MB) are measured if acute MI is suspected.

In general, if syncope results in an injury or is recurrent, more intensive evaluation for the cause is warranted. Injury is less likely when the cause of syncope is benign, because LOC is slightly slower than when the cause is cardiac.

Patients with arrhythmia, myocarditis, or ischemia should be evaluated as inpatients. Others may be evaluated as outpatients.

Echocardiography is indicated for patients with exercise-induced syncope, cardiac murmurs, or suspected intracardiac tumors.

Exercise or pharmacologic stress testing is done when intermittent myocardial ischemia is suspected. A signal-averaged ECG may identify predisposition to ventricular arrhythmias in patients with ischemic heart disease or post-MI patients.

Tilt table testing is done if history and physical examination indicate vasodepressor or other reflex-induced syncope (see p. 603). It is also used to evaluate exercise-induced syncope if echocardiography or exercise stress testing is negative.

Invasive electrophysiologic testing is considered if noninvasive testing does not identify arrhythmia in patients with unexplained recurrent syncope; a negative response defines a low-risk subgroup with a high rate of remission of syncope. The role of electrophysiologic testing is controversial in other patients. Exercise testing is less valuable, unless physical activity precipitated syncope.

EEG is warranted if a seizure disorder is suspected; CT and MRI of the head and brain are indicated only if signs and symptoms suggest a focal CNS disorder or an intracranial process.

Prognosis and Treatment

For young people who have syncope of unknown cause but no cardiovascular disorder, the prognosis is favorable; elaborate evaluation is rarely required. Syncope is more likely to be due to a significant disorder in elderly than in younger patients. For patients with coronary artery disease, myocarditis, hypertrophic cardiomyopathy, aortic stenosis, or known ventricular arrhythmias, syncope denotes a poor prognosis.

Placing the patient in a horizontal position with legs elevated typically ends the syncopal episode. If the patient sits upright too rapidly, syncope may recur; propping the patient upright or transporting the patient in an upright position may prolong cerebral hypoperfusion and prevent recovery.

Further treatment depends on the cause. Hypertrophic cardiomyopathy causing obstruction is treated with β-blockers, verapamil, or septal myomectomy; these treatments and amiodarone may alleviate associated arrhythmias.

Bradyarrhythmias may require pacemaker implantation; tachyarrhythmias require specific drug therapy, radioablation, or surgical correction. Ventricular arrhythmias may require implantable defibrillators. Carotid sinus hypersensitivity may require pacemaker insertion for bradyarrhythmias or carotid sinus radiation to alleviate the vasodepressor component. Hypovolemia, anemia, an electrolyte abnormality, and drug toxicity are treated. For aortic stenosis, aortic valve surgery may be done. It is not contraindicated by older age.

70 CARDIOVASCULAR TESTS AND PROCEDURES

Many noninvasive and invasive tests can delineate cardiac structure and function (see TABLE 70–1). Also, treatments can be administered during certain invasive diagnostic tests (eg, percutaneous coronary intervention during cardiac catheterization, radiofrequency ablation during electrophysiologic testing).

CARDIAC CATHETERIZATION

Cardiac catheterization is the passage of a catheter through peripheral arteries or veins into cardiac chambers and coronary arteries. Cardiac catheterization can be used to perform various tests, including angiography, intravascular ultrasonography, measurement of cardiac output (CO), endomyocardial biopsy, and measurements of myocardial metabolism. These tests define coronary artery anatomy, cardiac anatomy, and cardiac function to establish diagnoses and help select treatment. Cardiac catheterization is also the basis for several therapeutic interventions.

Procedure

Patients must be npo for 4 to 6 h before cardiac catheterization. Most patients do not require overnight hospitalization.

Left heart catheterization is most commonly used to assess coronary artery anatomy; it is also useful for assessing aortic BP and systemic vascular resistance, aortic and mitral valve function, and left ventricular (LV) pressure and function. The procedure is done by percutaneous femoral, radial, or brachial artery puncture, and a catheter is passed into the coronary artery ostia or across the aortic valve into the LV. Catheterization of the left atrium (LA) and LV is occasionally done using transseptal perforation during right heart catheterization.

Right heart catheterization is most commonly used to assess right atrial (RA), right ventricular (RV), and pulmonary artery pressure and pulmonary artery occlusion pressure (PAOP)—see FIG. 70–1 and p. 515; PAOP approximates LA and, LV end-diastolic pressure. In seriously ill patients, PAOP helps assess volume status and, with simultaneous measurements of CO, can help guide therapy. Right heart catheterization is also useful for assessing pulmonary vascular resistance, tricuspid or pulmonic valve function, and RV pressure; RV pressure may help in the diagnosis of cardiomyopathy, constrictive pericarditis, and cardiac tamponade when noninvasive testing is nondiagnostic. The procedure is done by femoral, subclavian,

TABLE 70–1. TESTS FOR ASSESSING CARDIAC ANATOMY AND FUNCTION

APPLICATION	TESTS
Left ventricular function	Echocardiography Multiple-gated acquisition (MUGA) radionuclide imaging Gated MRI Contrast ventriculography
Coronary artery disease diagnosis and prognosis	Exercise or pharmacologic stress testing with ECG, myocardial perfusion imaging, or echocardiography Magnetic resonance angiography Coronary angiography Intravascular ultrasonography
Myocardial viability	Resting single-photon emission computed tomography (SPECT) myocardial perfusion imaging Stress testing (using low-dose dobutamine) with echocardiography Positron emission tomography (PET)

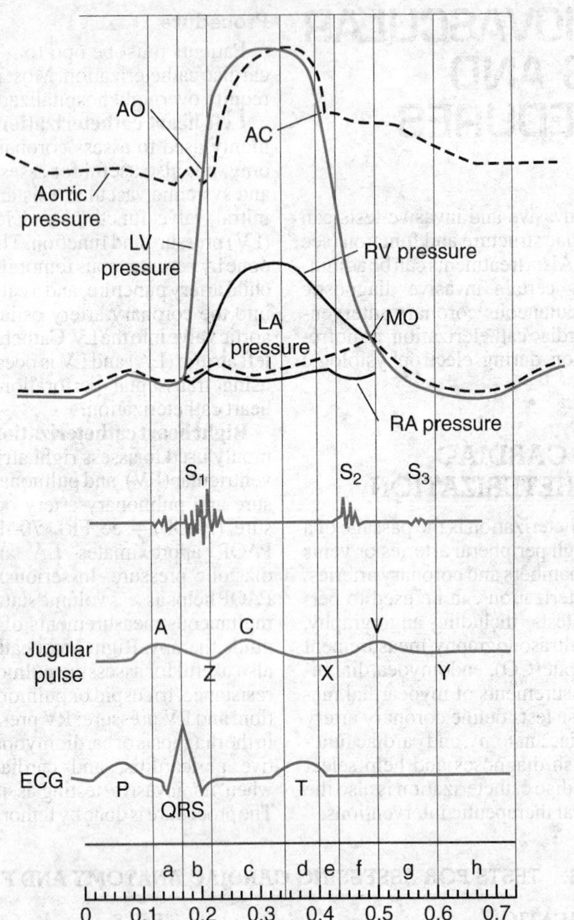

Fig. 70–1. Diagram of the cardiac cycle, showing pressure curves of the cardiac chambers, heart sounds, jugular pulse wave, and the ECG. AO = aortic valve opening; AC = aortic valve closing; LV = left ventricle; LA = left atrium; RV = right ventricle; RA = right atrium; MO = mitral valve opening. The phases of the cardiac cycle are atrial systole (a), isometric contraction (b), maximal ejection (c), reduced ejection (d), protodiastolic phase (e), isometric relaxation (f), rapid inflow (g), and diastasis, or slow LV filling (h). For illustrative purposes, time intervals between valvular events have been modified, and the z point has been prolonged.

internal jugular, or antecubital vein puncture; a catheter is passed into the RA, through the tricuspid valve, into the RV, and across the pulmonary valve into the pulmonary artery (see p. 514). Selective catheterization of the coronary sinus can also be done.

Specific Tests

Angiography: Injection of radiopaque dye into coronary or pulmonary arteries, the aorta, and cardiac chambers is useful in certain circumstances. Digital subtraction angiography is used for nonmoving arteries and for chamber cineangiography.

Coronary angiography via left heart catheterization is used to evaluate coronary artery anatomy in various clinical situations, as in patients with unstable angina, atypical chest pain, valvular disorders before valvular replacement, or unexplained heart failure.

Pulmonary angiography via right heart catheterization is used to diagnose pulmonary embolism; intraluminal filling defects or arterial cutoffs are diagnostic. Radiopaque dye is usually selectively injected into one or both pulmonary arteries and their segments.

Aortic angiography via left heart catheterization is used to assess aortic regurgitation, coarctation, patent ductus arteriosus, and dissection.

Ventriculography is used to visualize ventricular wall motion and ventricular outflow tracts, including subvalvular, valvular, and supravalvular regions. After LV mass and volume are determined from single planar or biplanar ventricular angiograms, end-systolic and end-diastolic volumes and ejection fraction can be calculated.

Intravascular ultrasonography: Miniature ultrasound transducers on the end of coronary artery catheters can produce images of coronary vessel lumina and walls and delineate blood flow. This technique is being increasingly used at the same time as coronary angiography.

Tests for cardiac shunts: Measuring blood O_2 content at successive levels in the heart and great vessels can help determine the presence, direction, and volume of central shunts. The maximal normal difference in O_2 content is 0.5 mL/dL between the pulmonary artery and RV, 0.9 mL/dL between the RV and RA, and 1.9 mL/dL between the RA and superior vena cava. If the blood O_2 content in a chamber exceeds that of the more proximal chamber by more than these values, a left-to-right shunt at that level is probable. Right-to-left shunts are strongly suspected when LA, LV, or arterial O_2 saturation is low (≤92%) and does not improve with pure O_2 (fractional inspirational O_2 = 1.0). Left heart or arterial desaturation plus increased O_2 content in blood samples drawn beyond the shunt site on the right side of circulation suggests a bidirectional shunt.

Measurement of cardiac output and flow: CO is the volume of blood ejected by the heart per minute (normal at rest: 4 to 8 L/min). Techniques used to calculate CO include the Fick, indicator-dilution, and thermodilution techniques (see TABLE 70–2).

With the Fick technique, CO is proportional to O_2 consumption divided by arteriovenous O_2 difference.

Dilution techniques rely on the assumption that after an indicator is injected into the circulation, it appears and disappears proportionately to CO.

TABLE 70–2. CARDIAC OUTPUT EQUATIONS

Fick technique

$$CO = \frac{\text{Ambient } O_2 - \text{expired } O_2 \text{ (mL/min)}}{(1.36)\ (\text{Hb g/dL}) \times (SaO_2 - SvO_2)}$$

Numerator is O_2 absorbed by lungs (mL/min).

Indicator-dilution technique

$$CO = \frac{\text{Injectate mass (mg)}}{\int_{\infty} C(t)\,dt}$$

Denominator is the sum of dye concentrations (C) at each time interval (t).

Thermodilution technique

$$CO = \frac{(T_B - T_I) \times \text{injectate volume (mL)} \times 53.5}{\int_{\infty} T_B(t)\,dt}$$

$T_B - T_I$ is the difference between body and injectate temperatures; injectate is usually dextrose or saline. Denominator is the sum of changes in temperature at each time interval (t).

SaO_2 = arterial O_2 saturation (%); SvO_2 = mixed venous O_2 saturation (%), measured in the pulmonary artery.

Usually, CO is expressed in relation to BSA as the cardiac index (CI) in L/min/m^2 (ie, CI = CO/BSA—see TABLE 70–3). BSA is calculated using DuBois' height (ht)-weight (wt) equation:

$$\text{BSA in m}^2 = (\text{wt in kg})^{0.425} \times (\text{ht in cm})^{0.725} \times 0.007184$$

Endomyocardial biopsy: This procedure helps assess transplant rejection and myocardial disorders due to infection. The biopsy catheter (biotome) can be passed into either ventricle, usually the right. Three to 5 samples of myocardial tissue are removed from the septal endocardium. The main complication, cardiac perforation, occurs in 0.3 to 0.5% of patients; it may cause hemopericardium leading to cardiac tamponade.

Contraindications and Complications

Relative contraindications to cardiac catheterization include renal insufficiency, coagulopathy, fever, systemic infection, uncontrolled arrhythmia or hypertension,

TABLE 70–3. NORMAL VALUES FOR CARDIAC INDEX AND RELATED MEASUREMENTS

MEASUREMENT	NORMAL VALUE	SD
O_2 uptake	143 mL/min/m^2*	14.3
Arterio-venous O_2 difference	4.1 dL	0.6
Cardiac index	3.5 L/min/m^2	0.7
Stroke index	46 mL/beat/m^2	8.1
Total systemic resistance	1130 dynes-sec-cm^{-5}	178
Total pulmonary resistance	205 dynes-sec-cm^{-5}	51
Pulmonary arteriolar resistance	67 dynes-sec-cm^{-5}	23

SD = standard deviation.

*Varies with BMI.

Adapted from Barratt-Boyes BG, Wood EH: "Cardiac output and related measurements and pressure values in the right heart and associated vessels, together with an analysis of the hemodynamic response to the inhalation of high oxygen mixtures in healthy subjects." *Journal of Laboratory and Clinical Medicine* 51:72–90, 1958.

uncompensated heart failure, and radiopaque dye allergies in patients who have not been appropriately premedicated (see p. 2718).

Injection of radiopaque dye produces a transient sense of warmth throughout the body in many patients. Tachycardia, a slight fall in systemic pressure, an increase in CO, nausea, vomiting, and coughing may occur. Serious complications (eg, cardiac arrest, anaphylactic reactions, shock, seizures, cyanosis, renal toxicity) are rare. Rarely, bradycardia occurs when a large amount of dye is injected; asking the patient to cough often restores normal rhythm. Patients with a high Hct are susceptible to thrombosis; the Hct should be < 65% before angiography is done. Allergic reactions may include urticaria and conjunctivitis, which usually respond to diphenhydramine 50 mg IV. Bronchospasm, laryngeal edema, and dyspnea are rare reactions, treated with salbutamol or epinephrine. Anaphylactic shock is treated with adrenaline and other supportive measures. If the catheter tip contacts the ventricular endocardium, ventricular arrhythmias commonly occur, but ventricular fibrillation is rare. If it occurs, direct current (DC) cardioversion is administered immediately (see p. 535). Radiopaque dyes, all hypertonic, are excreted by the kidneys.

Mortality rate is 0.1 to 0.2%. MI (0.1%) and stroke (0.1%) may result in significant morbidity. Local vascular injury at the site of catheterization can cause hemorrhage or formation of pseudoaneurysms or arteriovenous fistulas.

CORONARY ARTERY BYPASS GRAFTING

Coronary artery bypass grafting (see also p. 634) involves bypassing native coronary arteries with high-grade stenosis or occlusion not amenable to angioplasty with stenting. Indications are changing as percutaneous interventions (see p. 598) are being increasingly used.

The procedure involves thoracotomy via a midline sternotomy. A heart-lung machine is usually used to establish cardiopulmonary bypass, although new techniques avoid it by directly revascularizing the beating heart. The left internal mammary artery is typically used as a pedicled graft to the left anterior descending coronary artery. Other grafts consist of segments of saphenous vein removed from the leg. Occasionally, the right internal mammary artery or radial artery from the nondominant arm can be used.

Common complications include bleeding, infection, and atrial fibrillation but can involve any system (eg, pulmonary, renal, brain, GI). Typically, hospital stays are 4 to 5 days but may be prolonged by complications.

ECHOCARDIOGRAPHY

Echocardiography uses ultrasound waves to produce an image of the heart and great vessels. It helps assess heart wall thickness (eg, in hypertrophy or atrophy) and motion and provides information about ischemia and infarction. It can be used to assess diastolic filling patterns of the left ventricle, which can help in the diagnosis of left ventricular hypertrophy, hypertrophic or restrictive cardiomyopathy, severe heart failure, constrictive pericarditis, and severe aortic regurgitation.

In transthoracic echocardiography (TTE), a transducer is placed along the left or right sternal border, at the cardiac apex, at the suprasternal notch (to visualize the aortic valve, left ventricular outflow tract, and descending aorta), or over the subcostal region. In transesophageal echocardiography (TEE), a transducer on the tip of an endoscope visualizes the heart via the esophagus.

TTE, the most common technique, provides 2-dimensional tomographic images of most major cardiac structures. TEE is used to assess posterior cardiac structures (eg, left atrium, left atrial appendage, interatrial septum) because they are closer to the esophagus than to the anterior chest wall. TEE can also produce images of the ascending aorta, which arises behind the 3rd costal cartilage; of structures < 3 mm (eg, thrombi, vegetations); and of prosthetic valves.

Two-dimensional (cross-sectional) echocardiography is most commonly used; contrast and spectral Doppler echocardiography provide additional information.

Contrast echocardiography is 2-dimensional TTE done while agitated saline is rapidly injected into the cardiac circulation. Agitated saline develops microbubbles, which produce a cloud of echoes in the right cardiac chambers and which, if a septal defect is present, appear on the left side of the heart. Usually, the microbubbles do not traverse the pulmonary capillary bed; however, one agent, sonicated albumin microbubbles, can do so and can enter left heart structures after IV injection.

Spectral Doppler echocardiography can record velocity, direction, and type of blood flow. This technique is useful for detecting abnormal blood flow (eg, due to regurgitant lesions) or velocity (eg, due to stenotic lesions). Spectral Doppler echocardiography does not provide spatial information about the size or shape of the heart or its structures.

Color Doppler echocardiography combines 2-dimensional and spectral Doppler echocardiography to provide information about the size and shape of the heart and its structures as well as the velocity of and direction of blood flow around the valves and outflow tracts. Color is used to code blood flow information; by convention, red is toward and blue away from the transducer.

Stress echocardiography is TTE done during and after exercise or pharmacologic stress. Stress echocardiography shows regional wall motion abnormalities that result from an imbalance in blood flow in epicardial blood vessels during stress. Computer programs can provide side-by-side assessment of ventricular contraction during systole and diastole at rest and under stress. Exercise and pharmacologic protocols are the same as those used in radionuclide stress testing. Stress echocardiography and radionuclide stress testing detect ischemia about equally well. The choice between tests is often based on availability, the provider's experience, and cost.

ELECTROCARDIOGRAPHY

The standard ECG provides 12 different vector views of the heart's electrical activity as reflected by electrical potential differences between positive and negative electrodes placed on the limbs and chest wall. Six of these views are vertical (using frontal leads I, II, and III and limb leads aVR, aVL, and aVF), and 6 are horizontal (using precordial leads V_1, V_2, V_3, V_4, V_5, and V_6). The 12-lead ECG is crucial for establishing many cardiac diagnoses, especially arrhythmias and myocardial ischemia (see TABLE 70–4). It can also identify atrial enlargement, ventricular hypertrophy (see TABLE 70–5), and conditions that predispose to syncope or sudden death (eg, Wolff-Parkinson-White syndrome, long QT syndrome, Brugada syndrome).

Standard ECG Components

By convention, the ECG tracing is divided into the P wave, PR interval, QRS complex, QT interval, ST segment, T wave, and U wave (see FIG. 70–2).

The **P wave** represents atrial depolarization. It is upright in most leads except aVR. It may be biphasic in leads II and V_1; the initial component represents right atrial activity, and the 2nd component represents left atrial activity. An increase in amplitude of either or both components occurs with atrial enlargement. Right atrial enlargement produces a P wave > 2 mm in leads II, III, and aVF (P pulmonale); left atrial enlargement produces a P wave that is broad and double-peaked in lead II (P mitrale). Normally, the P axis is between 0° and 75°.

The **PR interval** is the time between onset of atrial depolarization and onset of ventricular depolarization. Normally, it is 0.10 to 0.20 sec; prolongation defines 1st-degree atrioventricular block.

TABLE 70–4. INTERPRETATION OF ABNORMAL ECGs

ABNORMAL COMPONENT	POSSIBLE CAUSES
P waves (abnormal)	Left or right atrial hypertrophy, atrial escape (ectopic) beats
P waves (absent)	Atrial fibrillation, sinus node exit block, hyperkalemia (severe)
P-P interval (varying)	Sinus arrhythmia
PR interval (long)	First-degree atrioventricular block, Mobitz type I atrioventricular block, multifocal atrial tachycardia
QRS complex (wide)	Right or left bundle branch block, ventricular flutter or fibrillation, hyperkalemia
QT interval (long)	MI, myocarditis, hypocalcemia, hypokalemia, hypomagnesemia, hypothyroidism, subarachnoid or intracerebral hemorrhage, stroke, antiarrhythmics (eg, sotalol, amiodarone), tricyclic antidepressants, other drugs
QT interval (short)	Hypercalcemia, hypermagnesemia, Graves' disease, digoxin
ST segment (depression)	Myocardial ischemia; acute posterior MI; digoxin; ventricular hypertrophy; pulmonary embolism; left bundle branch block; right bundle branch block in leads V_1–V_3 +/– II, III, and aVF; hyperventilation; hypokalemia
ST segment (elevation)	Myocardial ischemia, acute MI, left bundle branch block, acute pericarditis, left ventricular hypertrophy, hyperkalemia, pulmonary embolism, digoxin, normal variation (eg, athletic heart syndrome), hypothermia
T wave (tall)	Hyperkalemia, acute MI, left bundle branch block, stroke, ventricular hypertrophy
T wave (small, flattened, or inverted)	Myocardial ischemia, age, race, hyperventilation, anxiety, drinking hot or cold beverages, left ventricular hypertrophy, certain drugs (eg, digoxin), pericarditis, pulmonary embolism, conduction disturbances (eg, right bundle branch block), electrolyte disturbances (eg, hypokalemia)
U wave (prominent)	Hypokalemia, hypomagnesemia, ischemia

The **QRS complex** represents ventricular depolarization. The Q wave is the initial downward deflection; normal Q waves last < 0.05 sec in all leads except $V_{1\text{-}3}$, in which any Q wave is considered abnormal, indicating past or current infarction. The R wave is the 1st upward deflection; criteria for normal height or size are not absolute, but taller R waves may be caused by ventricular hypertrophy. A 2nd upward deflection in a QRS complex is designated R′. The S wave is the 2nd downward deflection if there is a Q wave and the 1st downward deflection if not. The QRS complex may be R alone, QS (no R), QR (no S), RS (no Q), or RSR′, depending on the ECG lead, vector, and presence of heart disorders. Normally, the QRS interval is 0.07 to 0.10 sec. An interval of 0.10 and 0.11 sec is considered incomplete bundle branch block or a nonspecific intraventricular conduction delay, depending on QRS morphology; ≥ 0.12 sec is considered complete bundle branch block or an intraventricular conduction delay. Normally, the QRS axis is 90° to –30°. An axis of –30° to –90° is considered left axis deviation and occurs in left anterior fascicular block (–60°) and inferior MI. An axis of 90° to 180° is considered right axis deviation; it occurs in any condition that increases pulmonary pressures and causes right ventricular hypertrophy (cor pulmonale, acute pulmonary embolism, pulmonary hypertension), and it sometimes occurs in right bundle branch block or left posterior fascicular block.

The **QT interval** is the time between onset of ventricular depolarization and end of ventricular repolarization. The QT interval must be corrected for heart rate using the formula:

$$QTc = \frac{QT}{\sqrt{RR}}$$

where QT_c is the corrected QT interval; R-R interval is the time between 2 QRS complexes. All intervals are recorded in seconds. QT_c prolongation is strongly implicated in development of torsades de pointe ventricular tachycardia (see p. 707). QT_c is often difficult to calculate because the end of the T wave is often unclear.

The **ST segment** represents completed ventricular myocardial depolarization. Normally, it is horizontal along the baseline of the PR (or TP) intervals or slightly off baseline. Myocardial ischemia and infarction, pericarditis, hyperkalemia, left ventricular hypertrophy, pulmonary embolism, and digoxin cause more extreme elevation from baseline.

The **T wave** reflects ventricular repolarization. It usually takes the same direction as the QRS complex (concordance); opposite polarity (discordance) may indicate past or current infarction. The T wave is usually smooth and rounded but may be of low amplitude in hypokalemia and hypomagnesemia and may be peaked in hyperkalemia and hypocalcemia.

The **U wave** appears uncommonly in patients who have hypokalemia, hypomagnesemia, or ischemia.

Specialized ECG Tests

A standard 12-lead ECG represents only a single brief period of cardiac activity; enhanced techniques can provide additional information.

Additional precordial leads are used to help diagnose right ventricular and posterior wall MI. Right-sided leads are placed across the right side of the chest to mirror standard left-sided leads. They are labeled V_1R to V_6R; sometimes only V_4R is used, because it is the most sensitive for right ventricular MI. Posterior leads V_8 and V_9 are placed on the left posterior hemithorax at the 5th intercostal space.

TABLE 70–5. CRITERIA FOR ECG DIAGNOSIS OF LEFT VENTRICULAR HYPERTROPHY

CRITERION	FINDING	POINTS
Romhilt-Estes (5 points = definite LVH; 4 points = probable LVH)	R or S wave ≥ 20 mm in any limb lead **or** S wave in V_1 or V_2 ≥ 30 mm **or** R wave in V_5 or V_6 ≥ 30 mm	3
	ST-T changes typical of LVH	
	Digitalis	1
	No digitalis	3
	Left atrial changes: P terminal wave in V_1, amplitude ≥ 1 mm, and duration ≥ 0.04 sec	3
	Left axis deviation ≥ –30°	2
	QRS duration ≥ 90 msec	1
	Interval between QRS and R-wave peak in V_5 or V_6 ≥ 0.05 sec	1
Sokolow-Lyon	V_1 S wave + V_5 or V_6 R wave ≥ 35 mm **or** aVL R wave ≥ 11 mm	
Cornell	Men: V_3 S wave + aVL R wave > 28 mm Women: V_3 S wave + aVL R wave > 20 mm	

LVH = left ventricular hypertrophy.

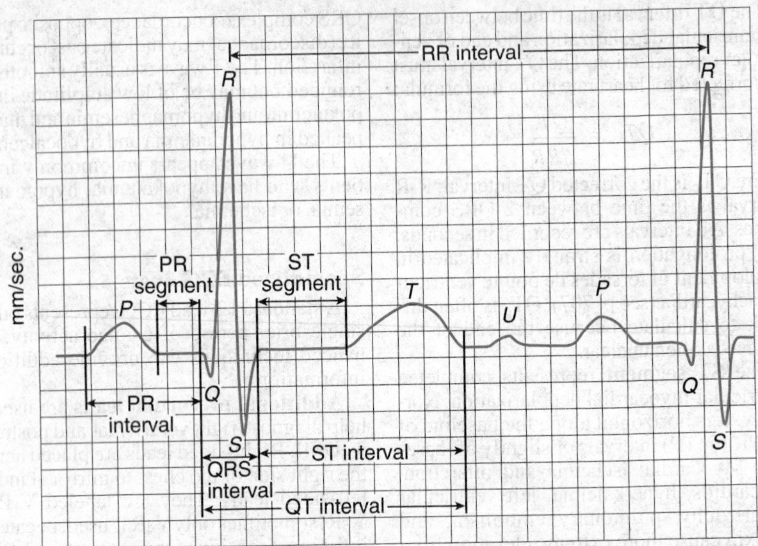

Fig. 70–2. ECG waves. P wave = activation (depolarization) of atria. QRS complex = depolarization of ventricles, consisting of the Q, R, and S waves. T wave = ventricular repolarization. ST segment plus T wave (ST-T) = ventricular repolarization. PR interval = time interval between onset of atrial depolarization and onset of ventricular depolarization. QT interval = time interval between onset of ventricular depolarization and end of ventricular repolarization. U wave = probably after-depolarization (relaxation) of ventricles. R-R interval = time interval between 2 QRS complexes.

An esophageal lead is much closer to the atria than surface leads; it is an option when the presence of P waves on a standard recording is uncertain and when detecting atrial electrical activity is important, as when atrial or ventricular origin of wide-complex tachycardia must be differentiated or when atrioventricular dissociation is suspected. An esophageal lead may also be used to monitor intraoperative myocardial ischemia or to detect atrial activity during cardioplegia. The lead is placed by having the patient swallow an electrode, which is then connected to a standard ECG machine, often in the lead II port.

Signal-averaging of QRS waveforms creates a digital composite of several hundred cardiac cycles to detect high-frequency, low-amplitude potentials and microcurrents at the terminal part of the QRS complex. These findings represent areas of slow conduction through abnormal myocardium, indicating increased risk of reentrant ventricular tachycardia. Signal-averaged ECG is still largely a research technique but is occasionally used to assess risk of sudden cardiac death (eg, in post-MI patients without evidence of conduction delay, patients with myocardial ischemia and unexplained syncope, and those with nonischemic cardiomyopathy) and to assess efficacy of surgery to correct the arrhythmia. This technique may also be useful for assessing the proarrhythmic effects of antiarrhythmic drugs and for detecting rejection of heart transplants. Signal averaging of P waves is being studied as a way to identify patients at risk of atrial fibrillation.

Continuous ST-segment monitoring is used for early detection of ischemia and serious arrhythmias. Monitoring can be automated (dedicated electronic monitoring units are available) or done clinically using serial ECGs. Applications include emergency department monitoring of patients with crescendo angina, evaluation after percutaneous intervention, intraoperative monitoring, and postoperative care.

QT dispersion (the difference between the longest and shortest QT intervals on a

12-lead ECG) has been proposed as a measure of myocardial repolarization heterogeneity. Increased dispersion suggests electrically heterogeneous myocardium caused by ischemia or fibrosis, with increased risk of reentrant arrhythmias and sudden death. QT dispersion predicts mortality risk but is not widely measured because measurement error is common, values in patients with and without disease overlap substantially, there is no reference standard, and other validated risk predictors are available.

Heart rate variability reflects the balance between sympathetic and parasympathetic (vagal) input to the heart. Decreased variability suggests decreased vagal input and increased sympathetic input, which predict increased risk of arrhythmias and mortality. The most common measure of variability is the mean of the standard deviations of all normal R-R intervals in a 24-h ECG recording. Heart rate variability is used primarily in research, but evidence suggests that it provides useful information about left ventricular dysfunction after MI, heart failure, and hypertrophic cardiomyopathy. Most Holter monitors have software that measures and analyzes heart rate variability.

Holter monitoring is continuous monitoring and recording of the ECG, BP, or both for 24 or 48 h. It is useful for evaluating intermittent arrhythmias and, secondarily, for detecting hypertension. The Holter monitor is portable, enabling patients to participate in normal daily activities; it may also be used for sedentary hospitalized patients if automated monitoring is unavailable. Patients are asked to record symptoms and activities so that they may be correlated with events on the monitor. The Holter monitor does not automatically analyze the ECG data; a physician does so at a later date.

Event recorders are worn for up to 30 days and can detect infrequent rhythm disturbances that 24-h Holter monitoring may miss. The recorder does not operate continuously but is activated by the patient when symptoms occur. A memory loop enables information to be stored for seconds or minutes before and after activation. The patient can transmit ECG data by telephone to be read by a physician. If patients have serious events (eg, syncope) at intervals of > 30 days, an event recorder may be placed subcutaneously; it can be activated by a small magnet. Battery life for subcutaneous recorders is 14 mo.

ELECTROPHYSIOLOGIC STUDIES

In electrophysiologic studies, recording and stimulating electrodes are inserted via right- or left-sided cardiac catheterization into all 4 cardiac chambers. Atria are paced from the right or left atrium, ventricles are paced from the right ventricular apex or right ventricular out-flow tract, and cardiac conduction is recorded. Programmed stimulation techniques may be used to trigger and terminate a reentrant arrhythmia.

Electrophysiologic studies are indicated primarily for evaluation and treatment of arrhythmias that are difficult to capture, serious, or sustained. These studies may be used to make a primary diagnosis, to evaluate the efficacy of antiarrhythmic drugs, or to map arrhythmia foci before radiofrequency catheter ablation (see p. 691); various mapping techniques are available.

IMAGING TESTS

Standard imaging tests include chest x-ray, CT, and MRI. Standard CT and MRI have limited application because the heart constantly beats, but faster CT and MR techniques can provide useful cardiac images.

Chest x-rays: Chest x-rays are often useful as a starting point in a cardiac diagnosis. Posteroanterior and lateral views provide a gross view of atrial and ventricular size and shape and pulmonary vasculature, but additional tests are almost always required for precise characterization of cardiac structure and function.

CT: Spiral (helical) CT may be used to evaluate pericarditis, congenital cardiac disorders (especially abnormal arteriovenous connections), disorders of the great vessels (eg, aortic aneurysm, aortic dissection), cardiac tumors, acute pulmonary embolism, chronic pulmonary thromboembolic disease, and arrhythmogenic right ventricular dysplasia. However, CT requires a radiopaque dye, which may limit its use in patients with renal impairment.

Electron beam CT, formerly called ultrafast CT or cine CT, is used primarily to detect and quantify coronary artery calcification, an early sign of atherosclerosis.

MRI: Standard MRI is useful for evaluating areas around the heart, particularly the mediastinum and great vessels (eg, for studying aneurysms, dissections, and stenoses). With ECG-gated data acquisition, image resolution can approach that of CT or echocardiography, clearly delineating myocardial wall thickness and motion, chamber volumes, intraluminal masses or clot, and valve planes. Sequential MRI after injecting a paramagnetic contrast agent (gadolinium-diethylenetriamine pentaacetic acid [Gd-DTPA]) produces higher resolution of myocardial perfusion patterns than does radionuclide imaging. Blood flow velocities in cardiac chambers can be measured. MRI can assess tissue viability by assessing the contractile response to inotropic stimulation with dobutamine or by using a contrast agent (eg, Gd-DTPA, which is excluded from cells with intact membranes).

Magnetic resonance angiography (MRA) is used to assess blood volumes of interest (eg, blood vessels in the chest or abdomen); all blood flow can be assessed simultaneously. MRA can be used to detect aneurysms, stenosis, or occlusions in the carotid, coronary, renal, or peripheral arteries. Use of this technique to detect deep venous thrombosis is being studied.

PET: Positron emission tomography (PET) can demonstrate myocardial perfusion and metabolism.

Perfusion agents include carbon-11 (^{11}C) CO_2, oxygen-15 (^{15}O) water, nitrogen-13 (^{13}N) ammonia, and rubidium-82 (^{82}Rb). Only ^{82}Rb does not require an on-site cyclotron.

Metabolic agents include fluorine-18 (^{18}F)-labeled deoxyglucose (FDG) and ^{11}C acetate. FDG detects the enhancement of glucose metabolism under ischemic conditions, and can thus distinguish ischemic but still viable myocardium from scar tissue. Sensitivity is greater than with myocardial perfusion imaging, possibly making FDG imaging useful for selecting patients for revascularization and for avoiding such procedures when only scar tissue is present. This use may justify the greater expense of PET. Half-life of ^{18}F is long enough (110 min) that FDG can often be produced off-site. Techniques that enable FDG imaging to be used with conventional SPECT cameras may make this type of imaging widely available.

Uptake of ^{11}C acetate appears to reflect overall O_2 metabolism by myocytes. Uptake does not depend on such potentially variable factors as blood glucose levels, which can affect FDG distribution. ^{11}C acetate imaging may better predict postintervention recovery of myocardial function than FDG imaging. However, because of a 20-min half-life, ^{11}C must be produced by an on-site cyclotron.

PERCUTANEOUS CORONARY INTERVENTIONS

Percutaneous coronary interventions (PCI) include percutaneous transluminal coronary angioplasty (PTCA) with or without stenting. Primary indications are treatment of angina pectoris (stable or unstable), myocardial ischemia, and acute MI (particularly in patients with developing or established cardiogenic shock). Elective PCI may be appropriate for post-MI patients who have recurrent or inducible angina before hospital discharge and for patients who have angina and remain symptomatic despite medical treatment. Percutaneous transluminal angioplasty (PTA) is used to treat peripheral arterial disease (see p. 750).

PTCA is done via percutaneous femoral, radial, or brachial artery puncture. A guiding catheter is inserted into a large peripheral artery and threaded to the appropriate coronary ostium. A balloon-tipped catheter, guided by fluoroscopy or intravascular ultrasonography, is aligned within the stenosis, then inflated to disrupt the atherosclerotic plaque and dilate the artery. Angiography is repeated after the procedure to document any changes. The procedure is commonly done in 2 or 3 vessels as needed.

Restenosis requiring repeat PTCA or coronary artery bypass grafting (CABG) is the most common complication of PTCA. Restenosis rate is highest (up to 35%) in the first 6 mo after angioplasty but can be reduced by stent insertion and anticoagulation during PTCA.

Stents are most useful for short lesions in large native coronary arteries not previously treated with PTCA, for focal lesions in saphenous vein grafts, and for treatment of abrupt closure during PTCA. The role of stenting in acute MI, ostial or left main disease, chronic total occlusions, and bifurcation lesions is still evolving. Some stents elute drugs (eg, sirolimus, paclitaxel) that limit neointimal proliferation to reduce the risk of restenosis. In intracoronary brachytherapy, the site of stenosis is exposed to radiation in the form of small pellets embedded in a nylon ribbon temporarily (eg, 30 min) placed in the coronary artery prior to stenting. This appears to decrease the risk of early restenosis, but it is unclear whether later stenosis is slightly increased; trials are ongoing. Radioactive stents have not proven effective at limiting restenosis. Stenting is not risk-free; complications include stent thrombosis, restenosis, bleeding secondary to aggressive adjunctive anticoagulation, side branch occlusion, and stent embolism.

Various anticoagulation regimens are used during and after angioplasty to reduce the incidence of thrombosis at the site of balloon dilation; clopidogrel and glycoprotein IIb/IIIa inhibitors are the standard of care for patients with unstable non-ST-segment elevation MI. Clopidogrel (often in combination with aspirin) is continued for 9 to 12 mo after PCI. Ca channel blockers and nitrates may also reduce risk of coronary spasm.

Contraindications and Complications

Absolute contraindications include lack of cardiac surgical support and significant obstruction of the left main coronary artery without a nonobstructed bypass graft to the left anterior descending or left circumflex arteries. Relative contraindications include coagulopathy, hypercoagulable states, diffusely diseased vessels without focal stenoses, a single diseased vessel providing all perfusion to the myocardium, total occlusion of a coronary artery, and $< 50\%$ stenosis.

Significant complications occur in 2 to 3% of patients within 30 days of PCI. Complications besides restenosis are similar to those of coronary angiography, although risk of death, MI, and stroke is greater. Abrupt coronary artery closure secondary to spasm, dissection, or thrombus formation occurs in up to 4%, sometimes causing silent infarction. Treatment consists of drugs (for the disorder causing closure), stents, or, in extreme circumstances, intra-aortic balloon pumps or emergency CABG. Of all angiographic procedures, PCI has the highest risk of contrast nephropathy; this risk can be reduced by preprocedural hydration and use of a nonionic contrast agent, acetylcysteine, or hemofiltration in patients with preexisting renal insufficiency.

RADIONUCLIDE IMAGING

Radionuclide imaging uses a special detector (gamma camera) to create an image following injection of radioactive material. This is performed to evaluate coronary artery disease (CAD), valvular or congenital cardiac disorders, cardiomyopathy, and other cardiac disorders. Radionuclide imaging exposes patients to less radiation than do comparable x-ray studies. However, because the radioactive material is retained in the patient briefly, sophisticated radiation alarms (eg, in airports) may be triggered by the patient for several days following such testing.

Planar techniques, which produce a 2-dimensional image, are rarely used; single-photon emission computed tomography (SPECT), which uses a rotating camera system and tomographic reconstruction to produce a 3-dimensional image, is more common in the US. With multihead SPECT systems, imaging can often be completed in ≤ 10 min. Visual comparison of stress and delayed images can be supplemented by quantitative displays. With SPECT, inferior and posterior abnormalities and small areas of infarction and the vessels responsible for infarction can be identified. The mass of infarcted and viable myocardium can be quantified, helping determine prognosis.

Myocardial Perfusion Imaging

In myocardial perfusion imaging, IV radionuclides are taken up by cardiac tissues in rough proportion to perfusion; thus, areas of decreased uptake represent areas of relative or absolute ischemia. For this reason, myocardial perfusion imaging is used with stress testing to evaluate patients with chest pain of uncertain origin, to determine the functional significance of coronary artery stenosis or collateral vessels seen on angiography, and to evaluate the success of reperfusion interventions (eg, coronary artery bypass grafting [CABG], percutaneous intervention, thrombolysis). After acute MI, myocardial perfusion imaging can help estimate prognosis because it can show extent of the perfusion abnormality due to acute MI, extent of scarring due to previous infarcts, and residual peri-infarct or other areas of reversible ischemia.

Radioactive thallium-201 (^{201}Tl), which acts as a K analog, was the original tracer used in stress testing. It is injected at peak stress and imaged with SPECT, followed 4 h later by injection of $\frac{1}{2}$ the original dose during rest and by repeat SPECT. The goal of this protocol is to evaluate reversible perfusion defects that may warrant intervention. After stress testing, the perfusion imbalance between normal coronary arteries and those distal to a stenosis appears as a relative decrease in ^{201}Tl uptake in the areas perfused by the stenosed arteries. Sensitivity of stress testing with ^{201}Tl for CAD is similar whether imaging is done after exercise or pharmacologic stress.

Because the imaging characteristics of ^{201}Tl are not ideal for the gamma camera, several technetium-99m (^{99m}Tc) myocardial perfusion markers have been developed: sestamibi (commonly used), tetrofosmin, and teboroxime (see TABLE 70–6). Protocols include 2-day stress-rest, 1-day rest-stress, and 1-day stress-rest. Some protocols use dual isotopes (^{201}Tl and ^{99m}Tc), although this approach is expensive. With either of these markers, sensitivity is about 90%, and specificity is about 71%.

For 2-day protocols, imaging at rest may be omitted if the initial stress test shows no evidence of abnormal perfusion. When higher doses of ^{99m}Tc (> 30 mCi) are used, 1st-transit function studies (with ventriculography) may be used with perfusion imaging.

Other radionuclides include iodine-123 (^{123}I)-labeled fatty acids, which produces cold spots where myocardium is ischemic; gallium citrate-67 (^{67}Ga), which accumulates in sites of active inflammation (eg, in acute inflammatory cardiomyopathy); and iodine-123 (^{123}I) metaiodobenzylguanidine, a neurotransmitter analog taken up and stored in neurons of the sympathetic nervous system and used in research to evaluate heart failure, diabetes, certain arrhythmias, and arrhythmogenic right ventricular dysplasia.

Attenuation of myocardial activity by overlying soft tissue may cause false-positives. Attenuation by breast tissue in women is especially common. Attenuation by the diaphragm and abdominal contents may produce spurious inferior wall defects in both sexes but is more common among men. Attenuation is more likely with ^{99m}Tc than with ^{201}Tl.

Infarct Avid Imaging

Infarct avid imaging uses radiolabeled markers that accumulate in areas of damaged myocardium, such as ^{99m}Tc pyrophosphate and antimyosin (indium 111 [^{111}In]-labeled antibodies to cardiac myosin). Images usually become positive 12 to 24 h after acute MI and remain positive for about 1 wk; they may remain positive if myocardial necrosis continues post-MI or if aneurysms develop. This technique is rarely used now because other diagnostic tests for MI (eg, biomarkers) are more readily available and less expensive and because it provides no prognostic information other than infarct size.

Radionuclide Ventriculography

Radionuclide ventriculography is used to evaluate ventricular function. It is useful for

TABLE 70–6. TECHNETIUM-99m MYOCARDIAL PERFUSION MARKERS

MARKER	CHARACTERISTICS
^{99m}Tc sestamibi	Myocardial uptake is slower than that with thallium, but there is little myocardial washout, allowing timing flexibility; patients with acute symptoms can be injected with sestamibi immediately and imaged several hours later. Uptake depends more on blood flow than on viable myocardium; viable regions with low blood flow may be misclassified as scar. Studies may be done on a single or on separate days, with a low initial dose during stress followed by a much higher dose at rest. With ECG-gated imaging, ventricular wall motion, wall thickening, and ejection fraction can be estimated.
^{99m}Tc tetrofosmin	Similar to sestamibi.
^{99m}Tc teboroxime	First-pass extraction from the myocardium is high, with rapid washout; ½ of peak myocardial activity is gone by 10 min. Because of its rapid dynamics, use with treadmill exercise is difficult. Preliminary studies suggest that stress-redistribution testing may be completed within 15 min of pharmacologic stress. Coronary artery disease may be detectable by analysis of myocardial washout of the tracer after injection at rest, without the need for stress.

measuring resting and exercise ejection fraction in CAD, valvular heart disease, and congenital heart disease. Some clinicians prefer it for serial assessment of ventricular function in patients taking cardiotoxic cancer chemotherapy (eg, anthracyclines). However, radionuclide ventriculography has been largely replaced by echocardiography, which is less expensive, does not require radiation exposure, and theoretically can measure ejection fractions as accurately.

^{99m}Tc-labeled RBCs are injected into the ventricles. Left ventricular (LV) and right ventricular (RV) function can be evaluated by 1st-transit studies (a type of beat-to-beat evaluation) or by gated (ECG-synchronized) blood pool imaging done over several minutes (multiple-gated acquisition [MUGA]). Either study can be done during rest or after exercise. First-transit studies are rapid and relatively easy, but MUGA provides better images and is more widely used.

In 1st-transit studies, 8 to 10 cardiac cycles are imaged as the marker mixes with blood and passes through the central circulation. First-transit studies are ideal for assessing RV function and intracardiac shunts.

In MUGA, imaging is synchronized with the R wave of the ECG. Multiple images are taken of short, sequential portions of each cardiac cycle for 5 to 10 min. Computer analysis generates an average blood pool configuration for each portion of the cardiac cycle and synthesizes the configurations into a continuous cinematic loop resembling a beating heart.

MUGA can quantitate numerous indexes of ventricular function, including regional wall motion, ejection fraction (EF); ratio of stroke volume to end-diastolic volume, ejection and filling rates, LV volume, and indexes of relative volume overload (eg, LV:RV stroke volume ratios). EF is used most commonly.

MUGA during rest has virtually no risk. It is used for serially evaluating RV and LV function in various disorders (eg, valvular heart disorders); for monitoring patients taking potentially cardiotoxic drugs (eg, doxorubicin); and for assessing the effects of angioplasty, CABG, thrombolysis, and other procedures in patients with CAD or MI. Arrhythmias are a relative contraindication because there may be few normal cardiac cycles.

LV: MUGA is useful for detecting LV aneurysms; sensitivity and specificity are > 90% for typical anterior or anteroapical true aneurysms. Conventional gated blood pool imaging shows inferoposterior LV aneurysms less well than it shows anterior and lateral aneurysms; additional views are required. Gated SPECT imaging takes longer (about 20 to 25 min with a multihead camera) than a single planar gated view (5 to 10 min) but shows all portions of the ventricles.

RV: MUGA is used to assess RV function in patients who have a lung disorder or an inferior LV infarct that may involve the RV. Normally, RVEF (40 to 55% with most techniques) is lower than LVEF. RVEF is subnormal in many patients with pulmonary hypertension and in patients with RV infarction or cardiomyopathy affecting the RV. Idiopathic cardiomyopathy is usually characterized by biventricular dysfunction, unlike typical CAD, which usually causes more LV than RV dysfunction.

Valves: MUGA can be used with rest-stress protocols to assess valvular disorders that result in LV volume overload. In aortic regurgitation, a reduction in resting EF or no increase in EF with exercise is a sign of deteriorating cardiac function and may indicate a need for valvular repair. MUGA also can be used to calculate the regurgitant fraction in regurgitation of any valve. Normally, the stroke volume of the 2 ventricles is equal. However, in patients with left-sided valvular regurgitation, LV stroke volume exceeds that of the RV by an amount proportional to the regurgitant fraction. Thus, if the RV is normal, the regurgitant fraction of the LV can be calculated from the LV:RV stroke volume ratio.

Shunts: With MUGA and commercially available computer programs, size of a congenital shunt can be quantified by the stroke volume ratio or, during the 1st transit of the marker, by the ratio of abnormal early pulmonary recirculation of radioactivity to total pulmonary radioactivity.

STRESS TESTING

In stress testing, the heart is monitored by ECG and often imaging studies during an induced episode of increased cardiac demand so that ischemic areas potentially at risk of infarction can be identified. Heart rate is increased to 85% of age-predicted maximum (target heart rate) or until symptoms develop, whichever occurs first.

Stress testing is used for diagnosis of coronary artery disease (CAD) and for risk stratification and monitoring of patients with known CAD. In patients with CAD, a blood supply that is adequate at rest may be inadequate when cardiac demands are increased by exercise or other forms of stress. Stress testing is less invasive and less expensive than cardiac catheterization, and it detects pathophysiologic abnormalities of blood flow; however, it is less accurate for diagnosis in patients with a low pretest likelihood of CAD. It can define the functional significance of abnormalities in coronary artery anatomy identified with coronary angiography during catheterization.

Risks of stress testing include infarction and sudden death, which occur in about 1/1000 patients tested. Stress testing has several contraindications (see TABLE 70–7). Patients must be npo for 4 to 6 h before the test.

Stress Methodology

Cardiac demand can be increased by exercise or drugs.

Exercise stress testing: Exercise is preferred to drugs for increasing cardiac demand because it more closely replicates ischemia-inducing stressors. Usually, a patient walks on a conventional treadmill, following the Bruce protocol or a similar exercise schedule, until the target heart rate is reached or symptoms occur. The Bruce protocol increases treadmill speed and slope incrementally at roughly 3-min intervals.

Pharmacologic stress testing: Pharmacologic stress testing is usually used when patients cannot walk on a treadmill long enough to reach their target heart rate because of deconditioning, musculoskeletal disorders, obesity, peripheral arterial disease, or other disorders. Drugs used include IV dipyridamole, adenosine, and dobutamine.

Dipyridamole augments endogenous adenosine, causing coronary artery vasodilation. It increases myocardial blood flow in normal coronary arteries but not in arteries distal to a stenosis, creating a "steal" phenomenon from stenosed arteries and an imbalance in perfusion. Dipyridamole-induced ischemia or other adverse effects (eg, nausea, vomiting, headache, bronchospasm) occur in about 10% of patients, but these effects can be reversed by IV aminophylline. Severe reactions occur in < 1% of patients. Contraindications include asthma, acute phase MI, unstable angina pectoris, critical aortic stenosis, and systemic hypotension (systolic BP < 90 mm Hg).

Adenosine has the same effect as dipyridamole but must be given in continuous IV infusion because it is rapidly degraded in the plasma. Adverse effects include transient flushing and chest pain, which can be reversed by terminating the infusion.

Dobutamine is an inotrope, chronotrope, and vasodilator used mainly when dipyridamole and adenosine are contraindicated (eg, in patients with asthma or 2nd-degree atrioventricular block) and when echocar-

TABLE 70–7. CONTRAINDICATIONS TO EXERCISE STRESS TESTING

ABSOLUTE CONTRAINDICATIONS	RELATIVE CONTRAINDICATIONS
Acute coronary syndrome (MI within 48 h or uncontrolled unstable angina)	Atrioventricular block if high-degree
Aortic dissection (acute)	Bradyarrhythmias
Aortic stenosis if symptomatic or severe	Electrolyte imbalance
Arrhythmias if symptomatic or hemodynamically significant	Hypertension (systolic > 200 mm Hg or diastolic > 110 mm Hg)
Heart failure if decompensated	Hypertrophic obstructive cardiomyopathy
Myocarditis or pericarditis if acute	Inability to exercise adequately due to mental or physical impairment
Pulmonary embolism or pulmonary infarction if acute	Stenosis of heart valve if moderate or severe
	Stenosis of left main coronary artery
	Systemic illness
	Tachyarrhythmias

diography is used to image the heart. Dobutamine must be used with caution in patients who have severe hypertension or arrhythmia, left ventricular outflow tract obstruction, multiple previous MIs, or acute MI.

Xanthine compounds (eg, aminophylline, theophylline, caffeine) may produce a false-negative result during stress testing with dipyridamole, so such substances (including tea and coffee) should be avoided for 24 h before testing.

Diagnostic Methodology

Several imaging tests can detect ischemia after exercise or pharmacologic stress.

ECG is always used with stress testing to diagnose CAD and help determine prognosis. ECG is most useful in patients with intermediate likelihood of CAD based on age and sex and with a normal ECG at rest. Diagnosis involves assessment of ST-segment response (a measure of global subendocardial ischemia), BP response, and the patient's symptoms. Average sensitivity is 67%; average specificity is 72%. Sensitivity and specificity are lower in women partly because incidence of CAD is lower in young and middle-aged women. Prognosis worsens with depth of ST depression.

Radionuclide myocardial perfusion imaging (see p. 599) is more sensitive (85 to 90%) and specific (70 to 80%) than ECG stress testing; combining findings from both tests increases sensitivity for CAD. Myocardial perfusion imaging is particularly useful for patients with baseline ECG abnormalities that may interfere with interpretation of ECG changes during a stress test (eg, patients with bundle branch block, those with fixed-rate pacemakers, those taking digitalis). It is also useful for groups with a high probability of false-positives on exercise ECGs (eg, premenopausal women, patients with mitral valve prolapse). This imaging test can help determine the functional significance of coronary artery stenosis, identified by coronary angiography, when surgeons are choosing lesions to bypass or dilate via percutaneous transluminal coronary angioplasty.

Echocardiography is useful when information about more than just perfusion is needed; echocardiography detects wall motion abnormalities that are a sign of regional ischemia and, using Doppler techniques, helps evaluate valvular disorders that may contribute to or result from ischemia (see p. 592). The echocardiogram is typically obtained immediately before and after an exercise treadmill test or during dobutamine infusion. Echocardiography is relatively portable, does not use ionizing radiation, has a rapid acquisition time, and is inexpensive, but it is difficult to perform in obese patients and in patients with COPD and lung hyperinflation. Done by experts, stress echocardiography has a predictive value similar to that of stress myocardial radionuclide perfusion testing.

Radionuclide ventriculography is occasionally used with exercise stress testing instead of echocardiography to assess exercise ejection fraction (EF), the best prognostic indicator in patients with CAD. Normally, EF is ≥ 5 percentage points higher during exercise than at rest. Ventricular dysfunction (eg, due to valvular heart disorders, cardiomyopathy, or CAD) can decrease exercise EF below baseline or prevent it from increasing. In patients with CAD, the 8-yr survival rate is 80% with an exercise EF of 40 to 49%, 75% with an exercise EF of 30 to 39%, and 40% with an exercise EF of < 30%.

TILT TABLE TESTING

Tilt table testing is used to evaluate syncope in younger, apparently healthy patients and, when cardiac and other tests have not provided a diagnosis, in elderly patients. Tilt table testing produces maximal venous pooling, which can trigger vasovagal (neurocardiogenic) syncope and reproduce the symptoms and signs that accompany it (nausea, light-headedness, pallor, hypotension, bradycardia).

After an overnight fast, a patient is placed on a motorized table with a foot board at one end and is held in place by a single strap over the stomach; an IV line is inserted. After the patient remains supine for 15 min, the table is tilted nearly upright to 60 to 80° for 45 min. If vasovagal symptoms develop, vasovagal syncope is confirmed. If they do not occur, a drug (eg, isoproterenol) may be given to induce them. Sensitivity varies from 30 to 80% depending on the protocol used. The false-positive rate is 10 to 15%.

With vasovagal syncope, heart rate and BP usually decrease. Some patients have only a decrease in heart rate (cardioinhibitory); others have only a decrease in BP (vasodepressor). Other responses include a gradual decrease in systolic and diastolic BP with little change in heart rate (dysautonomic pattern), significant increase in heart rate (> 30 beats/min) with little change in BP (postural orthostatic tachycardia syndrome), and report of syncope with no hemodynamic changes (psychogenic syncope).

Relative contraindications include severe aortic or mitral stenosis, hypertrophic cardiomyopathy, and severe coronary artery disease (CAD). In particular, isoproterenol should not be used in patients with hypertrophic cardiomyopathy or severe CAD.

71 ARTERIAL HYPERTENSION

Hypertension is sustained elevation of resting systolic BP (≥ 140 mm Hg), diastolic BP (≥ 90 mm Hg), or both. Hypertension with no known cause (primary; formerly, essential hypertension) is most common; hypertension with an identified cause (secondary hypertension) is usually due to a renal disorder. Usually, no symptoms develop unless hypertension is severe or long-standing. Diagnosis is by sphygmomanometry. Tests may be done to determine cause, assess damage, and identify other cardiovascular risk factors. Treatment involves lifestyle changes and drugs, including diuretics, β-blockers, ACE inhibitors, angiotensin II receptor blockers, and Ca channel blockers.

In the US, about 50 million people have hypertension. Only about 70% of these people are aware that they have hypertension, only 59% are being treated, and only 34% have adequately controlled BP. In adults, hypertension occurs more often in blacks (32%) than in whites (23%) or Mexican Americans (23%), and morbidity and mortality are greater in blacks.

BP increases with age. About ⅔ of people > 65 have hypertension, and people with a normal BP at age 55 have a 90% lifetime risk of developing hypertension. Because hypertension becomes so common with age, the age-related increase in BP may seem innocuous, but higher BP increases morbidity and mortality risk. Hypertension may develop during pregnancy (see p. 2180 and Preeclampsia and Eclampsia on p. 2197).

Etiology

Hypertension may be primary (85 to 95% of cases) or secondary.

Primary hypertension: Hemodynamics and physiologic components (eg, plasma volume, plasma renin activity) vary, indicating that primary hypertension is unlikely to have a single cause. Even if one factor is initially responsible, multiple factors are probably involved in sustaining elevated BP (the mosaic theory). In afferent systemic arterioles, malfunction of ion pumps on sarcolemmal membranes of smooth muscle cells may lead to chronically increased vascular tone. Heredity is a predisposing factor, but the exact mechanism is unclear. Environmental factors (eg, dietary Na, obesity, stress) seem to affect only genetically susceptible people.

Secondary hypertension: Causes include renal parenchymal disease (eg, chronic glomerulonephritis or pyelonephritis, polycystic renal disease, connective tissue disorders, obstructive uropathy), renovascular disease (see below), pheochromocytoma, Cushing's syndrome, primary aldosteronism, hyperthyroidism, myxedema, and coarctation of the aorta. Excessive alcohol intake and use of oral contraceptives are common causes of curable hypertension. Use of sympathomimetics, corticosteroids, cocaine, or licorice commonly contributes to hypertension.

Pathophysiology

Because BP equals cardiac output (CO) × total peripheral vascular resistance (TPR), pathogenic mechanisms must involve increased CO, increased TPR, or both.

In most patients, CO is normal or slightly increased, and TPR is increased. This pattern is typical of primary hypertension and hypertension due to pheochromocytoma, primary aldosteronism, renovascular disease, and renal parenchymal disease.

In other patients, CO is increased (possibly because of venoconstriction in large veins), and TPR is inappropriately normal for the level of CO; later in the disorder, TPR increases and CO returns to normal, probably because of autoregulation. Some disorders that increase CO (thyrotoxicosis, arteriovenous fistula, aortic regurgitation), particularly when stroke volume is increased, produce isolated systolic hypertension. Some elderly patients have isolated systolic hypertension with normal or low CO, probably due to inelasticity of the aorta and its major branches. Patients with high, fixed diastolic pressures often have decreased CO.

Plasma volume tends to decrease as BP increases; rarely, plasma volume remains normal or increases. Plasma volume tends to be high in hypertension due to primary aldosteronism or renal parenchymal disease and may be quite low in hypertension due to pheochromocytoma. Renal blood flow gradually decreases as diastolic BP increases and arteriolar sclerosis begins. GFR remains normal until late in the disorder; as a result, the filtration fraction is increased. Coronary, cerebral, and muscle blood flow is maintained unless severe atherosclerosis coexists in these vascular beds.

Abnormal Na transport: In some cases of hypertension, Na transport across the cell wall is abnormal, because the Na-K pump (Na^+, K^+-ATPase) is defective or inhibited or because permeability to Na^+ is increased. The result is increased intracellular Na, which makes the cell more sensitive to sympathetic stimulation. Ca follows Na, so accumulation of intracellular Ca may be responsible for the increased sensitivity. Because Na^+, K^+-ATPase may pump norepinephrine back into sympathetic neurons (thus inactivating this neurotransmitter), inhibition of this mechanism could also enhance the effect of norepinephrine, increasing BP. Defects in Na transport may occur in normotensive children of hypertensive parents.

Sympathetic nervous system: Sympathetic stimulation increases BP, usually more in patients with prehypertension (BP 120 to 139/80 to 89 mm Hg) or hypertension (systolic BP $\geq$ 140 mm Hg, diastolic BP $\geq$ 90 mm Hg, or both) than in normotensive patients. Whether this hyperresponsiveness resides in the sympathetic nervous system or in the myocardium and vascular smooth muscle is unknown. A high resting pulse rate, which may result from increased sympathetic nervous activity, is a well-known predictor of hypertension. In some hypertensive patients, circulating plasma catecholamine levels during rest are higher than normal.

Renin-angiotensin-aldosterone system: This system helps regulate blood volume and therefore BP. Renin, an enzyme formed in the juxtaglomerular apparatus, catalyzes conversion of angiotensinogen to angiotensin I. This inactive product is cleaved by ACE, mainly in the lungs but also in the kidneys and brain, to angiotensin II, a potent vasoconstrictor that also stimulates autonomic centers in the brain to increase sympathetic discharge and stimulates release of aldosterone and ADH. Aldosterone and ADH cause Na and water retention, elevating BP. Aldosterone also enhances K excretion; low plasma K (< 3.5 mEq/L) increases vasoconstriction through closure of K channels. Angiotensin III, present in the circulation, stimulates aldosterone release as actively as angiotensin II but has much less pressor activity. Because chymase enzymes also convert angiotensin I to angiotensin II, drugs that inhibit ACE do not fully suppress angiotensin II production.

Renin secretion is controlled by at least 4 mechanisms, which are not mutually exclusive: (1) A renal vascular receptor responds to changes in tension in the afferent arteriolar wall; (2) a macula densa receptor detects changes in the delivery rate or concentration of NaCl in the distal tubule; (3) circulating angiotensin has a negative feedback effect on renin secretion; and (4) via the renal nerve, the sympathetic nervous system stimulates renin secretion mediated by β-receptors.

Angiotensin is generally acknowledged to be responsible for renovascular hypertension, at least in the early phase, but the role of the renin-angiotensin-aldosterone system in primary hypertension is not established. However, in black and elderly patients with hypertension, renin levels tend to be low. The elderly also tend to have low angiotensin II levels.

Hypertension due to chronic renal parenchymal disease (renoprival hypertension) results from combination of a renin-dependent mechanism and a volume-dependent mechanism. In most cases, increased renin activity is not evident in peripheral blood. Hypertension is typically moderate and sensitive to Na and water balance.

Vasodilator deficiency: Deficiency of a vasodilator (eg, bradykinin, nitric oxide) rather than excess of a vasoconstrictor (eg, angiotensin, norepinephrine) may cause hypertension. If the kidneys do not produce adequate amounts of vasodilators (because of renal parenchymal disease or bilateral nephrectomy), BP can increase. Vasodilators and vasoconstrictors (mainly endothelin) are also produced in endothelial cells. Therefore, endothelial dysfunction greatly affects BP.

Pathology and complications: No pathologic changes occur early in hypertension. Severe or prolonged hypertension damages target organs (primarily the cardiovascular system, brain, and kidneys), increasing risk of coronary artery disease (CAD), MI, stroke (particularly hemorrhagic), and renal failure. The mechanism involves development of generalized arteriolosclerosis and acceleration of atherogenesis (see p. 620). Arteriolosclerosis is characterized by medial hypertrophy, hyperplasia, and hyalinization; it is particularly apparent in small arterioles, notably in the eyes and the kidneys. In the kidneys, the changes narrow the arteriolar lumen, increasing TPR; thus, hypertension leads to more hypertension. Furthermore, once arteries are narrowed, any slight additional shortening of already hypertrophied smooth muscle reduces the lumen to a greater extent than in normal-diameter arteries. These effects may explain why the longer hypertension has existed, the less likely specific treatment (eg, renovascular surgery) for secondary causes is to restore BP to normal.

Because of increased afterload, the left ventricle gradually hypertrophies, causing diastolic dysfunction. The ventricle eventually dilates, causing dilated cardiomyopathy and heart failure (HF) due to systolic dysfunction. Thoracic aortic dissection is typically a consequence of hypertension; almost all patients with abdominal aortic aneurysms have hypertension.

Symptoms and Signs

Hypertension is usually asymptomatic until complications develop in target organs. Dizziness, flushed facies, headache, fatigue, epistaxis, and nervousness are not caused by uncomplicated hypertension. Severe hypertension (hypertensive emergencies—see p. 617) can cause severe cardiovascular, neurologic, renal, and retinal symptoms (eg, symptomatic coronary atherosclerosis, HF, hypertensive encephalopathy, renal failure).

A 4th heart sound is one of the earliest signs of hypertensive heart disease.

Retinal changes may include arteriolar narrowing, hemorrhages, exudates, and, with encephalopathy, papilledema (see p. 919). Changes are classified (according to the Keith, Wagener, and Barker classification) into 4 groups with increasingly worse prognosis: constriction of arterioles only (grade 1), constriction and sclerosis of arterioles (grade 2), hemorrhages and exudates in addition to vascular changes (grade 3), and papilledema (grade 4).

Diagnosis

Hypertension is diagnosed and classified by sphygmomanometry. History, physical examination, and other tests help identify etiology and determine whether target organs are damaged.

BP must be measured twice—first with the patient supine or seated, then after the patient has been standing for ≥ 2 min—on 3 separate days. The average of these measurements is used for diagnosis. BP is classified as normal, prehypertension, or stage 1 (mild) or stage 2 hypertension (see TABLE 71–1). Normal BP is much lower for infants and children (see p. 2231).

Ideally, BP is measured after the patient rests > 5 min and at different times of day. A BP cuff is applied to the upper arm. An appropriately sized cuff covers ⅔ of the biceps; the bladder is long enough to encircle > 80% of the arm, and bladder width equals at least 40% of the arm's circumference. Thus, obese patients require large cuffs. The health care practitioner inflates the cuff above the expected systolic pressure and gradually releases the air while listening over the brachial artery. The pressure at which the 1st heartbeat is heard as the pressure falls is systolic BP. Disappearance of the sound marks diastolic BP. The same principles are followed to measure BP in a forearm (radial artery) and thigh (popliteal artery). Sphygmomanometers that contain mercury are most accurate. Mechanical devices should be calibrated periodically; automated readers are often inaccurate.

BP is measured in both arms; if BP in one arm is much higher, the higher value is used. BP is also measured in a thigh (with a much larger cuff) to rule out coarctation of the aorta, particularly in patients with diminished or delayed femoral pulses; with coarctation, BP is significantly lower in the legs. If BP is in the low hypertensive range or is markedly labile, more BP measurements are desirable. BP measurements may be sporadically high before hypertension becomes sustained; this phenomenon probably accounts for "white coat hypertension," in which BP is elevated when measured in the physician's office but normal when measured at home or by ambulatory BP monitoring. However, extreme BP elevation alternating with normal readings is unusual and possibly suggests pheochromocytoma or unacknowledged drug use.

History: The history includes the known duration of hypertension and previously recorded levels; any history or symptoms of CAD, HF, or other relevant coexisting disorders (eg, stroke, renal dysfunction, peripheral arterial disease, dyslipidemia, diabetes, gout); and a family history of any of these disorders. Social history includes exercise levels and use of tobacco, alcohol, and stimulant drugs (prescribed and illicit). A dietary history focuses on intake of salt and stimulants (eg, tea, coffee, dark sodas).

Physical examination: The physical examination includes measurement of height, weight, and waist circumference; funduscopic examination (see p. 919) for retinopathy; auscultation for bruits in the neck or abdomen; and a full cardiac, respiratory, and neurologic examination. The abdomen is palpated for kidney enlargement and abdominal masses. Peripheral arterial pulses are evaluated; diminished or delayed femoral pulses suggest aortic coarctation, particularly in patients < 30.

Testing: The more severe the hypertension and the younger the patient, the more extensive the evaluation. Generally, when hypertension is newly diagnosed, routine testing to detect target-organ damage and cardiovascular risk factors is done. Tests include urinalysis, spot urine albumin:creatinine ratio, blood tests (creatinine, K, Na, fasting plasma glucose, lipid profile), and ECG. Thyroid-stimulating hormone is often measured. Ambulatory BP monitoring, renal radionuclide imaging, chest x-ray, screening tests for pheochromocytoma, and renin-Na profiling are not routinely necessary. Peripheral plasma renin activity is not helpful in diagnosis or drug selection.

Depending on results of initial tests and examination, other tests may be needed. If urinalysis detects albuminuria (proteinuria), cylindruria, or microhematuria or if serum creatinine is elevated (≥ 1.4 mg/dL in men; ≥ 1.2 mg/dL in women), renal ultrasonography to evaluate kidney size may provide useful information. Patients with hypokalemia unrelated to diuretic use are evaluated for primary aldosteronism (see p. 1214) and high salt intake.

TABLE 71–1. JNC 7 CLASSIFICATION OF BLOOD PRESSURE IN ADULTS

CLASSIFICATION	BP (mm Hg)
Normal	< 120/80
Prehypertension	120–139/80–89
Stage 1	140–159 (systolic) or 90–99 (diastolic)
Stage 2	≥ 160 (systolic) or ≥ 100 (diastolic)

JNC = Joint National Committee on Prevention, Detection, Evaluation, and Treatment of High Blood Pressure.

On ECG, a broad, notched P-wave indicates atrial hypertrophy and, although nonspecific, may be one of the earliest signs of hypertensive heart disease. Left ventricular hypertrophy, indicated by a sustained apical thrust and abnormal QRS voltage with or without evidence of ischemia, may occur later. If either of these findings is present, echocardiography is often done. In patients with an abnormal lipid profile or symptoms of CAD, tests for other cardiovascular risk factors (eg, C-reactive protein) may be useful.

If coarctation of the aorta is suspected, chest x-ray, echocardiography, CT, or MRI helps confirm the diagnosis.

Patients with labile, significantly elevated BP and symptoms such as headache, palpitations, tachycardia, excessive perspiration, tremor, and pallor are screened for pheochromocytoma (eg, by measuring plasma free metanephrines—see p. 1217).

Patients with symptoms suggesting Cushing's syndrome, a connective tissue disorder, eclampsia, acute porphyria, hyperthyroidism, myxedema, acromegaly, or CNS disorders are evaluated (see elsewhere in THE MANUAL).

Prognosis

The higher the BP and the more severe the retinal changes and other evidence of target-organ involvement, the worse the prognosis. Systolic BP predicts fatal and nonfatal cardiovascular events better than diastolic BP. Without treatment, 1-yr survival is < 10% in patients with retinal sclerosis, cotton-wool exudates, arteriolar narrowing, and hemorrhage

TABLE 71–2. CHOICE OF ANTIHYPERTENSIVE DRUG CLASS

DRUGS	INDICATIONS
Diuretics*	Old age Black race Heart failure Obesity
β-Blockers*	Youth White race Angina pectoris Atrial fibrillation (to control ventricular rate)† Essential tremor Hyperkinetic circulation Migraine headaches† Paroxysmal supraventricular tachycardia† Post-MI (cardioprotective effect)*†
Long-acting Ca channel blockers	Old age Black race Angina pectoris Arrhythmias (eg, atrial fibrillation, paroxysmal supraventricular tachycardia) Isolated systolic hypertension in elderly patients (dihydropyridines)* High CAD risk (nondihydropyridines)*
ACE inhibitors‡	Youth White race Left ventricular failure due to systolic dysfunction* Type I diabetes with nephropathy* Severe proteinuria in chronic renal disorders or diabetic glomerulosclerosis Impotence due to other drugs
Angiotensin II receptor blockers‡	Youth White race Conditions for which ACE inhibitors are indicated but not tolerated because of cough Type 2 diabetes with nephropathy

*Reduced morbidity and mortality rates in randomized studies.

†β-Blockers without intrinsic sympathomimetic activity.

‡Contraindicated in pregnancy.

(grade 3 retinopathy), and <5% in patients with the same changes plus papilledema (grade 4 retinopathy). CAD is the most common cause of death among treated hypertensive patients. Ischemic or hemorrhagic stroke is a common consequence of inadequately treated hypertension. However, effective control of hypertension prevents most complications and prolongs life.

General Treatment

Primary hypertension has no cure, but some causes of secondary hypertension can be corrected. In all cases, control of BP can significantly limit adverse consequences. Despite the theoretical efficacy of treatment, BP is lowered to the desired level in only ⅓ of hypertensive patients in the US.

For all patients, treatment aims to reduce BP to < 140/90 mm Hg; for those with a kidney disorder or diabetes, the goal is < 130/80 mm Hg or as near this level as tolerated. Even the elderly and frail elderly can tolerate a diastolic BP as low as 60 to 65 mm Hg well and without an increase in cardiovascular events. Ideally, patients or family members measure BP at home, provided they have been trained to do so, they are closely monitored, and the sphygmomanometer is regularly calibrated. Treatment of hypertension during pregnancy requires special considerations because some antihypertensive drugs can harm the fetus (see p. 2181).

Lifestyle modifications: Recommendations include regular aerobic physical activity at least 30 min/day most days of the week; weight loss to a body mass index of 18.5 to 24.9; smoking cessation; a diet rich in fruits, vegetables, and low-fat dairy products with reduced saturated and total fat content; dietary Na of < 2.4 g/day (< 6 g NaCl); and alcohol consumption of ≤ 1 oz/day in men and ≤ 0.5 oz/day in women. In stage 1 (mild) hypertension with no signs of target-organ damage, lifestyle changes may make drugs unnecessary. Patients with uncomplicated hypertension do not need to restrict their activities as long as BP is controlled. Dietary modifications can also help control diabetes, obesity, and dyslipidemias. Patients with prehypertension are encouraged to follow these lifestyle recommendations.

Drugs: If systolic BP remains > 140 mm Hg or diastolic BP remains > 90 mm Hg after 6 mo of lifestyle modifications, antihypertensive drugs are required. Unless hypertension is severe, drugs are usually started at low doses. Drugs are initiated simultaneously with lifestyle changes for all patients with prehypertension or hypertension plus diabetes, a kidney disorder, target-organ damage, or cardiovascular risk factors and for those with an initial BP of > 160/100 mm Hg. Signs of hypertensive emergencies require immediate BP reduction with parenteral antihypertensives.

For most hypertensive patients, one drug, usually a thiazide diuretic, is given initially. Depending on the patient's characteristics and coexisting disorders, other drugs can be used initially or added to the thiazide. Low-dose aspirin (81 mg once/day) appears to reduce incidence of cardiac events in hypertensive patients and is recommended when tolerated and not contraindicated.

Some antihypertensives are contraindicated in certain disorders (eg, β-blockers in asthma) or are indicated particularly for certain disorders (eg, β-blockers or Ca channel blockers for angina pectoris, ACE inhibitors for diabetes or proteinuria—see TABLES 71–2 and 71–3). When a single drug is used, black men may respond best to a Ca channel blocker (eg, diltiazem). Thiazides appear to be particularly effective in people > 60 and in blacks.

If the initial drug is ineffective or has intolerable adverse effects, another drug can be substituted. If the initial drug is only partly effective but well tolerated, the dose can be increased or a second drug with a different mechanism added.

If initial systolic BP is > 160 mm Hg, 2 drugs are often used. Options include combining a diuretic with a β-blocker, an ACE inhibitor, or an angiotensin II receptor blocker and combining a Ca channel blocker with an ACE inhibitor. An appropriate combination and dose are determined; many are available as single tablets, which improve compliance (see TABLE 71–4). For severe or refractory hypertension, 3 or 4 drugs may be necessary.

Achieving adequate control often requires several evaluations and changes in drug therapy. Reluctance to titrate or add drugs until BP is at an acceptable level must be overcome. Lack of patient compliance, particularly because lifelong treatment is required, can interfere with adequate BP control. Education, with empathy and support, is essential for success.

TABLE 71–3. ANTIHYPERTENSIVES FOR HIGH-RISK PATIENTS

COEXISTING CONDITION	DRUG CLASSES
Heart failure	ACE inhibitors Angiotensin II receptor blockers β-Blockers K-sparing diuretics Other diuretics
Post-MI	β-Blockers ACE inhibitors K-sparing diuretics
Cardiovascular risk factors	β-Blockers ACE inhibitors Diuretics Ca channel blockers
Diabetes	Diuretics β-Blockers ACE inhibitors Angiotensin II receptor blockers Ca channel blockers
Chronic kidney disorders	ACE inhibitors Angiotensin II receptor blockers
Risk of recurrent stroke	ACE inhibitors Diuretics

Drugs for Hypertension

Diuretics: Main classes (see TABLE 71–5) are thiazides, loop diuretics, and K-sparing diuretics. Loop diuretics are used to treat hypertension only in patients who have lost > 50% of kidney function; these diuretics are given twice/day. Diuretics modestly reduce plasma volume and reduce vascular resistance, possibly via shifts in Na from intracellular to extracellular loci. These drugs are the least expensive initial therapy, and the dose needed is small, especially for the elderly (eg, for most people > 60 hydrochlorothiazide 12.5 mg is sufficient). Thiazides are most commonly used. In addition to other antihypertensive effects, they cause vasodilation as long as intravascular volume is normal. All thiazides are equally effective in equivalent doses.

All diuretics except the K-sparing distal tubular diuretics cause significant K loss, so serum K is measured q 1 mo until the level stabilizes. Unless serum K is normalized, K channels in the arterial walls close; the resulting vasoconstriction makes achieving the BP goal difficult. Patients with K levels < 3.5 mEq/L are given K supplements. Supple-

TABLE 71–4. COMBINATION DRUGS USED FOR HYPERTENSION

CLASSES	DRUGS	AVAILABLE STRENGTHS (mg/mg)
Diuretic/diuretic	Triamterene/hydrochlorothiazide	37.5/25, 50/25, 75/50
	Spironolactone/hydrochlorothiazide	25/25, 50/50
	Amiloride/hydrochlorothiazide	5/50
β-Blocker/diuretic	Propranolol/hydrochlorothiazide	40/25, 80/25
	Metoprolol/hydrochlorothiazide	50/25, 100/25
	Atenolol/chlorthalidone	50/25, 100/25
	Nadolol/bendroflumethiazide	40/5, 80/5
	Timolol/hydrochlorothiazide	10/25
	Propranolol LA (long acting)/ hydrochlorothiazide	80/50, 120/50, 160/50
	Bisoprolol/hydrochlorothiazide	2.5/6.25, 5/6.25, 10/6.25
Adrenergic inhibitor/ diuretic	Guanethidine/hydrochlorothiazide	10/25
	Methyldopa/hydrochlorothiazide	250/15, 250/25, 500/30, 500/50
	Methyldopa/chlorothiazide	250/150, 250/250
	Reserpine/chlorothiazide	0.125/250, 0.25/500
	Reserpine/chlorthalidone	0.125/25, 0.25/50
	Reserpine/hydrochlorothiazide	0.125/25, 0.125/50
	Clonidine/chlorthalidone	0.1/15, 0.2/15, 0.3/15
ACE inhibitor/diuretic	Captopril/hydrochlorothiazide	25/15, 25/25, 50/15, 50/25
	Enalapril/hydrochlorothiazide	5/12.5, 10/25
	Lisinopril/hydrochlorothiazide	10/12.5, 20/12.5, 20/25
	Fosinopril/hydrochlorothiazide	10/12.5, 20/12.5
	Quinapril/hydrochlorothiazide	10/12.5, 20/12.5, 20/25
	Benazepril/hydrochlorothiazide	5/6.25, 10/12.5, 20/12.5, 20/25
	Moexipril/hydrochlorothiazide	7.5/12.5, 15/25
Angiotensin II receptor blocker/diuretic	Losartan/hydrochlorothiazide	50/12.5, 100/25
	Valsartan/hydrochlorothiazide	80/12.5, 160/12.5
	Irbesartan/hydrochlorothiazide	75/12.5, 150/12.5, 300/12.5
	Candesartan/hydrochlorothiazide	16/12.5, 32/12.5
	Telmisartan/hydrochlorothiazide	40/12.5, 80/12.5
Ca channel blocker/ ACE inhibitor	Amlodipine/benazepril	2.5/10, 5/10, 5/20, 10/20
	Verapamil (extended-release)/ trandolapril	180/2, 240/1, 240/2, 240/4
	Felodipine (extended-release)/ enalapril	5/5
Vasodilator/diuretic	Hydralazine/hydrochlorothiazide	25/25, 50/25, 100/25
	Prazosin/polythiazide	1/0.5, 2/0.5, 5/0.5
Triple combination	Reserpine/hydralazine/hydrochlorothiazide	0.10/25/15

ments may be continued long-term at a lower dose, or a K-sparing diuretic (eg, daily spironolactone 25 to 100 mg, triamterene 50 to 150 mg, amiloride 5 to 10 mg) may be added. Supplements or addition of a K-sparing diuretic is also recommended for any patients who are also taking digitalis, have a known heart disorder, have an abnormal ECG, have ectopy or arrhythmias, or develop ectopy or arrhythmias while taking a diuretic. Although the K-sparing diuretics do not cause hypokalemia, hyperuricemia, or hyperglycemia, they are not as effective as thiazides in controlling hypertension and thus are not used for initial treatment. K-sparing diuretics or supplements are not needed when an ACE inhibitor or angiotensin II receptor blocker is used because these drugs increase serum K.

In most patients with diabetes, thiazides do not affect control of diabetes. Uncommonly, diuretics precipitate or worsen type 2 diabetes in patients with metabolic syndrome.

Thiazide and related diuretics can mildly increase serum cholesterol (mostly low density lipoprotein) and triglyceride levels, although this effect may not persist > 1 yr. Furthermore, levels seem to increase only in a few patients; the increase is apparent within 4 wk of treatment and can be ameliorated by a low-fat diet. The possibility of a slight increase in lipid levels does not contraindicate diuretics in hyperlipidemic patients.

A hereditary predisposition probably explains the few cases of gout due to diuretic-induced hyperuricemia. Diuretic-induced hyperuricemia without gout does not require treatment or discontinuation of the diuretic.

β-Blockers: These drugs (see TABLE 71–6) slow heart rate and reduce myocardial contractility, thus reducing BP. All β-blockers are similar in antihypertensive efficacy. In patients with diabetes, chronic peripheral arterial disease, or COPD, a cardioselective β-blocker (acebutolol, atenolol, betaxolol, bisoprolol, metoprolol) may be preferable,

TABLE 71–5. ORAL DIURETICS FOR HYPERTENSION

DRUG	USUAL DOSE* (mg)	SELECTED ADVERSE EFFECTS
Thiazide and related diuretics		
Bendroflumethiazide	2.5–5 once/day (maximum: 20)	Hypokalemia (which increases digitalis toxicity), hyperuricemia, glucose intolerance, hypercholesterolemia, hypertriglyceridemia, hypercalcemia, sexual dysfunction in men, weakness, rash; possibly increased blood levels of lithium
Chlorothiazide	62.5–500 bid (maximum: 1000)	
Chlorthalidone	12.5–50 once/day	
Hydrochlorothiazide	12.5–50 once/day	
Hydroflumethiazide	12.5–50 once/day	
Indapamide	1.25–5 once/day	
Methyclothiazide	2.5–5 once/day	
Metolazone (immediate release)	0.5–1 once/day	
Metolazone (extended release)	2.5–5 once/day	
K-sparing diuretics		
Amiloride	5–20 once/day	Hyperkalemia (particularly in patients with renal failure and in patients treated with an ACE inhibitor, angiotensin II receptor blocker, or NSAID), nausea, GI distress, gynecomastia, menstrual irregularities (spironolactone); possibly increased blood levels of lithium
Eplerenone†	25–100 once/day	
Spironolactone†	25–100 once/day	
Triamterene	25–100 once/day	

*Larger doses may be required in patients with renal failure.
†Aldosterone receptor blockers.

TABLE 71–6. β-BLOCKERS FOR HYPERTENSION

DRUG	DAILY DOSE (mg)	SELECTED ADVERSE EFFECTS	COMMENTS
Acebutolol*†	200–800 once/day	Bronchospasm, fatigue, insomnia, sexual dysfunction, exacerbation of heart failure, masking of symptoms of hypoglycemia, triglyceridemia, increased total cholesterol and decreased high density lipoprotein cholesterol (except for pindolol, acebutolol, penbutolol, carteolol, and labetalol)	Contraindicated in patients with asthma, greater than 1st-degree atrioventricular block, or sick sinus syndrome; should be used cautiously in patients with heart failure or insulin-treated diabetes; should not be stopped abruptly in patients with coronary artery disease; carvedilol approved for treating heart failure
Atenolol*	25–100 once/day		
Betaxolol*	5–20 once/day		
Bisoprolol*	2.5–20 once/day		
Carteolol†	2.5–10 once/day		
Carvedilol‡	6.25–25 bid		
Labetalol‡	100–900 bid		
Metoprolol*	25–150 bid		
Metoprolol (extended release)	50–400 once/day		
Nadolol	40–320 once/day		
Penbutolol†	10–20 once/day		
Pindolol†	5–30 bid		
Propranolol	20–160 bid		
Propranolol, long acting	60–320 once/day		
Timolol	10–30 bid		

*Cardioselective.
†With intrinsic sympathomimetic activity.
‡An α-β-blocker. Labetalol can be given IV for hypertensive emergencies. For IV administration, start as 20 mg up to a maximum 300 mg.

although cardioselectivity is only relative and decreases as dose increases. Even cardioselective β-blockers are contraindicated by asthma or by COPD with a prominent bronchospastic component.

β-Blockers are particularly useful in patients who have angina, who have had an MI, or who have HF. These drugs are no longer considered problematic for the elderly.

β-Blockers with intrinsic sympathomimetic activity (eg, acebutolol, carteolol, penbutolol, pindolol) do not adversely affect serum lipids; they are less likely to produce severe bradycardia.

β-Blockers have CNS adverse effects (sleep disturbances, fatigue, lethargy) and exacerbate depression; nadolol affects the CNS the least and may be best when CNS effects must be avoided. β-Blockers are contraindicated in patients with 2nd- or 3rd-degree atrioventricular block, asthma, or sick sinus syndrome.

Ca channel blockers: Dihydropyridines (see TABLE 71–7) are potent peripheral vasodilators and reduce BP by decreasing TPR; they sometimes cause reflexive tachycardia. The nondihydropyridines verapamil and diltiazem slow the heart rate, decrease atrioventricular conduction, and decrease myocardial contractility; these drugs should not be prescribed for patients with 2nd- or 3rd-degree atrioventricular block or with left ventricular failure.

Long-acting nifedipine, verapamil, or diltiazem is used to treat hypertension, but short-acting nifedipine and diltiazem are associated with a high rate of MI and are not recommended.

A Ca channel blocker is preferred to a β-blocker in patients with angina pectoris and a bronchospastic disorder, with coronary spasms, or with Raynaud's disease.

ACE inhibitors: These drugs (see TABLE 71–8) reduce BP by interfering with the conversion of angiotensin I to angiotensin II and by inhibiting the degradation of bradykinin, thereby decreasing peripheral vascular resistance without causing reflex tachycardia.

These drugs reduce BP in many hypertensive patients, regardless of plasma renin activity. Because these drugs provide renal protection, they are the drugs of choice for diabetics and may be preferred for blacks.

A dry, irritating cough is the most common adverse effect, but angioedema is the most serious and, if it affects the oropharynx, can be fatal. Angioedema is most common among blacks and smokers. ACE inhibitors may increase serum K and creatinine levels, especially in patients with chronic renal failure and those taking K-sparing diuretics, K supplements, or NSAIDs. ACE inhibitors are the least likely of the antihypertensives to cause erectile dysfunction. ACE inhibitors are contraindicated during pregnancy. In patients with a renal disorder, serum creatinine and K levels are monitored at least q 3 mo. Patients who have renal insufficiency (serum creatinine ≥ 1.4 mg/dL) and are given ACE inhibitors can usually tolerate up to a 30 to 35% increase in serum creatinine above baseline. ACE inhibitors can cause acute renal failure in patients who are hypovolemic or who have severe HF, severe bilateral renal artery stenosis, or severe stenosis in the artery to a solitary kidney.

Thiazide diuretics enhance the antihypertensive activity of ACE inhibitors more than that of other classes of antihypertensives.

Angiotensin II receptor blockers: These drugs (see TABLE 71–8) block angiotensin II receptors and therefore interfere with the renin-angiotensin system. Angiotensin II receptor blockers and ACE inhibitors are equally effective as antihypertensives; angiotensin II receptor blockers may provide added benefits via tissue ACE blockade. The 2 classes have the same beneficial

TABLE 71–7. CALCIUM CHANNEL BLOCKERS FOR HYPERTENSION

DRUG	USUAL DOSE (mg)	SELECTED ADVERSE EFFECTS	COMMENTS
Benzothiazepine derivatives			
Diltiazem, sustained release	60–180 bid	Headache, dizziness, asthenia, flushing, edema, negative inotropic effect; possibly liver dysfunction	Contraindicated in heart failure due to systolic dysfunction, sick sinus syndrome, or greater than 1st-degree atrioventricular block
Diltiazem, extended release	120–360 once/day		
Diphenylalkylamine derivatives			
Verapamil	40–120 tid	Same as for benzothiazepine derivatives, plus constipation	Same as for benzothiazepine derivatives
Verapamil, sustained release	120–480 once/day		
Dihydropyridines			
Amlodipine	2.5–10 once/day	Dizziness, flushing, headache, weakness, nausea, heartburn, pedal edema, tachycardia	Contraindicated in heart failure, possibly except for amlodipine; use of short-acting nifedipine possibly associated with higher MI rate
Felodipine	2.5–20 once/day		
Isradipine	2.5–10 bid		
Nicardipine	20–40 tid		
Nicardipine, sustained release	30–60 bid		
Nifedipine, extended release	30–90 once/day		
Nisoldipine	10–60 once/day		

TABLE 71–8. ACE INHIBITORS AND ANGIOTENSIN II RECEPTOR BLOCKERS FOR HYPERTENSION

DRUG	USUAL DOSE (mg)	SELECTED ADVERSE EFFECTS
ACE inhibitors*		
Benazepril	5–40 once/day	Rash, cough, angioedema, hyperkalemia (particularly in patients with renal insufficiency or taking NSAIDs, K-sparing diuretics, or K supplements), dysgeusia, reversible acute renal failure if stenosis affecting one or both kidneys threatens renal function, proteinuria (rare at recommended doses), neutropenia (rarely), hypotension with initiation of treatment (particularly in patients with high plasma renin activity or with hypovolemia due to diuretics or other conditions)
Captopril	12.5–150 bid	
Enalapril	2.5–40 once/day	
Fosinopril	10–80 once/day	
Lisinopril	5–40 once/day	
Moexipril	7.5–60 once/day	
Quinapril	5–80 once/day	
Ramipril	1.25–20 once/day	
Trandolapril	1–4 once/day	
Angiotensin II receptor blockers		
Candesartan	8–32 once/day	Dizziness, angioedema (very rare); theoretically, same adverse effects as ACE inhibitors on renal function (except proteinuria and neutropenia), serum K, and BP
Eprosartan	400–1200 once/day	
Irbesartan	75–300 once/day	
Losartan	25–100 once/day	
Olmesartan	20–40 once/day	
Telmisartan	20–80 once/day	
Valsartan	80–320 once/day	

*All ACE inhibitors and angiotensin II receptor blockers are contraindicated in pregnancy (category C during 1st trimester; category D during 2nd and 3rd trimesters).

effects in patients with left ventricular failure or with nephropathy due to type 1 diabetes. An angiotensin II receptor blocker used with an ACE inhibitor or a β-blocker reduces the hospitalization rate for patients with HF. Angiotensin II receptor blockers may be safely started in people < 60 with initial serum creatinine of ≤ 3 mg/dL.

Incidence of adverse events is low; angioedema occurs but much less frequently than with ACE inhibitors. Precautions for use of angiotensin II receptor blockers in patients with renovascular hypertension, hypovolemia, and severe HF are the same as those for ACE inhibitors. Angiotensin II receptor blockers are contraindicated during pregnancy.

Adrenergic modifiers: This class (see TABLE 71–9) includes central α_2-agonists, postsynaptic α_1-blockers, and peripheral-acting adrenergic blockers.

α_2-Agonists (eg, methyldopa, clonidine, guanabenz, guanfacine) stimulate α_2-adrenergic receptors in the brain stem and reduce sympathetic nervous activity, lowering BP. Because they have a central action, they are more likely than other antihypertensives to produce drowsiness, lethargy, and depression; they are no longer widely used. Clonidine can be applied transdermally once/wk as a patch; thus, it may be useful for noncompliant patients (eg, those with dementia).

Postsynaptic α_1-blockers (eg, prazosin, terazosin, doxazosin) are no longer used for primary treatment of hypertension because evidence suggests no mortality benefit. Also, doxazosin used alone or with antihypertensives other than diuretics increases risk of HF.

Peripheral-acting adrenergic blockers (eg, reserpine, guanethidine, guanadrel) deplete tissue stores of norepinephrine. Reserpine also depletes the brain of norepinephrine and serotonin. Guanethidine and guanadrel block sympathetic transmission at the neuroeffector junction. Guanethidine, in particular, is potent but difficult to titrate, so it is rarely used. Guanadrel is shorter acting and has fewer adverse effects. These 3 adrenergic blockers are not routinely recommended for initial therapy; they are used as 3rd or 4th drugs if required.

Direct vasodilators: These drugs (including minoxidil and hydralazine—see TABLE 71–10) work directly on vessels, independently of the autonomic nervous system. Minoxidil is more potent than hydralazine but has more adverse effects, including Na and water retention and hypertrichosis, which is poorly tolerated by women; minoxidil should be reserved for severe, refractory hypertension. Hydralazine is used during pregnancy (eg, for preeclampsia) and as an adjunct antihypertensive. Long-term, high-dose (> 300 mg/day) hydralazine has been associated with a drug-induced lupus syndrome, which resolves when the drug is stopped.

TABLE 71–9. ADRENERGIC MODIFIERS FOR HYPERTENSION

DRUG	USUAL DOSE (mg)	SELECTED ADVERSE EFFECTS	COMMENTS
α_2-Agonists (central acting)			
Clonidine	0.05–0.3 bid	Drowsiness, sedation, dry mouth, fatigue, sexual dysfunction, rebound hypertension with abrupt discontinuance (particularly if doses were high doses or concomitant β-blockers are continued), localized skin reaction to clonidine patch; possibly liver damage, Coombs'-positive hemolytic anemia with methyldopa	Should be used cautiously in elderly patients because of orthostatic hypotension; interferes with measurements of urinary catecholamine levels by fluorometric methods
Clonidine TTS (patch)	0.1–0.3 once/wk		
Guanabenz	2–16 bid		
Guanfacine	0.5–3 once/day		
Methyldopa	250–1000 bid		
α-Blockers			
Doxazosin	1–16 once/day	"First-dose" syncope, orthostatic hypotension, weakness, palpitations, headache	Should be used cautiously in elderly patients because of orthostatic hypotension; relieves symptoms of benign prostatic hyperplasia
Prazosin	1–10 bid		
Terazosin	1–20 once/day		
Peripheral-acting adrenergic blockers			
Guanadrel sulfate	5–50 bid	Diarrhea, sexual dysfunction, orthostatic hypotension with guanadrel sulfate or guanethidine, lethargy, nasal congestion, depression, activation of peptic ulcer with Rauwolfia alkaloids or reserpine	For reserpine, contraindicated in patients with history of depression and should be used cautiously in patients with history of peptic ulcer For guanadrel sulfate or guanethidine, should be used cautiously because orthostatic hypotension is a risk
Guanethidine	10–50 once/day		
Rauwolfia alkaloids	50–100 once/day		
Reserpine	0.05–0.25 once/day		

TABLE 71–10. DIRECT VASODILATORS FOR HYPERTENSION

DRUG	USUAL DOSE (mg)	SELECTED ADVERSE EFFECTS*	COMMENTS
Hydralazine	10–50 qid	Positive antinuclear antibody test, drug-induced lupus (rare at recommended doses)	Augments vasodilating effects of other vasodilating drugs
Minoxidil	1.25–40 bid	Na and water retention, hypertrichosis; possibly new or worsening pleural and pericardial effusions	Reserved for severe, refractory hypertension

*Both drugs may cause headache, tachycardia, and fluid retention and may precipitate angina in patients with coronary artery disease.

RENOVASCULAR HYPERTENSION

Renovascular hypertension is BP elevation due to partial or complete occlusion of one or more renal arteries or their branches. It is usually asymptomatic unless longstanding. A bruit can be heard over one or both renal arteries in < 50% of patients. Diagnosis is by physical examination and renal imaging with duplex ultrasonography, radionuclide imaging, or magnetic resonance angiography. Angiography is done before definitive treatment with surgery or angioplasty.

Renovascular disease is one of the most common causes of curable hypertension but accounts for < 2% of all cases of hypertension. Stenosis or occlusion of one or both main renal arteries, an accessory renal artery, or any of their branches can cause hypertension by stimulating release of renin from juxtaglomerular cells of the affected kidney. The area of the arterial lumen must be decreased by ≥ 70% before stenosis is likely to cause hypertension. For unknown reasons, renovascular hypertension is much less common among blacks than among whites.

Overall, about ⅔ of cases are caused by atherosclerosis and ⅓ by fibromuscular dysplasia. Atherosclerosis is more common among men > 50 and affects mainly the proximal ⅓ of the renal artery. Fibromuscular dysplasia is more common among younger patients (usually women) and usually affects the distal ⅔ of the main renal artery and the branches of the renal arteries. Rarer causes include emboli, trauma, inadvertent ligation during surgery, and extrinsic compression of the renal pedicle by tumors.

Renovascular hypertension is characterized by high cardiac output and high peripheral resistance.

Symptoms, Signs, and Diagnosis

Renovascular hypertension is usually asymptomatic. A systolic-diastolic bruit in the epigastrium, usually transmitted to one or both upper quadrants and sometimes to the back, is almost pathognomonic, but it is present in only about 50% of patients with fibromuscular dysplasia and is rare in patients with renal atherosclerosis.

Renovascular hypertension should be suspected if diastolic hypertension develops abruptly in a patient < 30 or > 50; if new or previously stable hypertension rapidly worsens within 6 mo; or if hypertension is initially very severe, associated with worsening renal function, or highly refractory to drug treatment. A history of trauma to the back or flank or acute pain in this region with or without hematuria suggests renovascular hypertension (possibly due to arterial injury), but these historical findings are rare. Asymmetric renal size (discovered incidentally during imaging tests) and recurrent episodes of unexplained acute pulmonary edema or heart failure also suggest it.

If renovascular hypertension is suspected, ultrasonography, magnetic resonance angiography (MRA), or radionuclide imaging may be done to identify patients who should have renal angiography, the definitive test.

Duplex Doppler ultrasonography can assess renal blood flow and is a reliable noninvasive method for identifying significant stenosis (eg, > 60%) in the main renal arteries. Sensitivity and specificity approach 90% with experienced technicians. It is less accurate with branch stenosis.

MRA is a more accurate and specific noninvasive test to assess the renal arteries.

Radionuclide imaging is often done before and after an oral dose of captopril 50 mg. The ACE inhibitor causes the affected artery to narrow, producing decreased perfusion on the scintiscan. Narrowing also causes an increase in serum renin, which is measured before and after captopril. This test may be less reliable in blacks and in patients with decreased renal function.

Renal angiography is done if MRA indicates a lesion amenable to angioplasty or stenting or if other screening tests are positive. Digital subtraction angiography with selective injection of the renal arteries can also confirm the diagnosis, but angioplasty or stent placement cannot be done in the same procedure.

Measurements of renal vein renin activity are sometimes misleading and, unless surgery is being considered, are not necessary. However, in unilateral disease, a renal vein renin activity ratio of > 1.5 (affected to unaffected side) usually predicts a good outcome with revascularization. The test is done when patients are depleted of Na, stimulating the release of renin.

Treatment

Opening the obstructed renal artery using angioplasty with or without a stent usually relieves hypertension if the renal vein renin activity ratio is > 1.5:1. Even when the ratio is lower, revascularization or removal of the affected kidney often cures hypertension.

Percutaneous transluminal angioplasty (PTA) is recommended for most patients, including younger patients with fibromuscular dysplasia of the renal artery. Placement of a stent reduces the risk of restenosis; antiplatelet drugs (aspirin, clopidogrel) are given afterward. Saphenous vein bypass grafting is recommended only when extensive disease in the renal artery branches makes PTA technically unfeasible. Sometimes complete surgical revascularization requires microvascular techniques that can only be done ex vivo with autotransplantation of the kidney. Cure rate is 90% in appropriately selected patients; surgical mortality rate is < 1%. Medical treatment is always preferable to nephrectomy in young patients whose kidneys cannot be revascularized for technical reasons.

Atherosclerotic lesions respond less well to surgery and angioplasty than do lesions due to fibromuscular dysplasia, presumably because patients are older and vascular disease is more extensive. Hypertension may persist, and surgical complications are more common. Surgical mortality rate is higher than that in young patients with fibromuscular dysplasia. Restenosis occurs within 2 yr after PTA in up to 50% of patients with renovascular atherosclerosis, especially when the lesion is located at the ostium of the renal artery, and, with stenting, in about 25%.

Without treatment, the prognosis is similar to that for patients with untreated primary hypertension. Medical treatment is inadequate without intervention to alleviate the stenosis, but aggressive medical treatment in compliant patients usually ameliorates and sometimes controls hypertension.

HYPERTENSIVE EMERGENCIES

A hypertensive emergency is severe hypertension with signs of damage to target organs (primarily the brain, cardiovascular system, and kidneys). Diagnosis is by BP measurement, ECG, urinalysis, and serum BUN and creatinine measurements. Treatment is immediate BP reduction with IV drugs (eg, nitroprusside, β-blockers, hydralazine).

Target-organ damage includes hypertensive encephalopathy, preeclampsia and eclampsia, acute left ventricular failure with pulmonary edema, myocardial ischemia, acute aortic dissection, and renal failure. Damage is rapidly progressive and often fatal.

Hypertensive encephalopathy may involve a failure of cerebral autoregulation of blood flow. Normally, as BP increases, cerebral vessels constrict to maintain constant cerebral perfusion. Above a mean arterial pressure (MAP) of about 160 mm Hg (lower for normotensive people whose BP suddenly increases), the cerebral vessels begin to dilate rather than remain constricted. As a result, the very high BP is transmitted directly to the capillary bed with transudation and exudation of plasma into the brain, causing cerebral edema, including papilledema. Pathophysiology of other target-organ manifestations is discussed elsewhere in THE MANUAL.

Although many patients with stroke and intracranial hemorrhage present with elevated BP, elevated BP is often a consequence rather than a cause of the condition. Whether rapidly lowering BP is beneficial in these conditions is unclear; it may even be harmful.

Hypertensive urgencies: Very high blood pressure (eg, diastolic > 120 to 130 mm Hg) without target-organ damage (except perhaps grades 1 to 3 retinopathy—see p. 606) may be considered a hypertensive urgency. BP at these levels often worries the physician; however, acute complications are unlikely, so immediate BP reduction is not required. However, patients should be started on a 2-drug oral combination (see p. 609), and close evaluation (with evaluation of treatment efficacy) should be continued on an outpatient basis.

Symptoms, Signs, and Diagnosis

BP is elevated, often markedly (diastolic > 120 mm Hg). CNS symptoms include rapidly changing neurologic abnormalities (eg, confusion, transient cortical blindness, hemiparesis, hemisensory defects, seizures). Cardiovascular symptoms include chest pain and dyspnea. Renal involvement may be asymptomatic, although severe azotemia due to advanced renal failure may produce lethargy or nausea.

Physical examination focuses on target organs, with neurologic examination, funduscopy, and cardiovascular examination. Global cerebral deficits (eg, confusion, obtundation, coma) with or without focal deficits suggest encephalopathy; normal mental status with focal deficits suggests stroke. Severe retinopathy (sclerosis, cotton-wool spots, arteriolar narrowing, hemorrhage, papilledema) is usually present with hypertensive encephalopathy, and some degree of retinopathy is present in many other hypertensive emergencies. Jugular venous distention, basilar lung crackles, and a 3rd heart sound suggest pulmonary edema. Asymmetry of pulses between arms suggests aortic dissection.

Testing typically includes ECG, urinalysis, and serum BUN and creatinine. Patients with neurologic findings require head CT to diagnose intracranial bleeding, edema, or infarction. Patients with chest pain or dyspnea require chest x-ray. ECG abnormalities suggesting target-organ damage include signs of left ventricular hypertrophy or acute ischemia. Urinalysis abnormalities typical of renal involvement include RBCs, RBC casts, and proteinuria.

Diagnosis is based on the presence of a very high BP and findings of target-organ involvement.

Treatment

Hypertensive emergencies are treated in an ICU; BP is progressively (although not abruptly) reduced using a short-acting, titratable IV drug. Choice of drug and speed and degree of reduction vary somewhat with the target organ involved, but generally a 20 to 25% reduction in MAP over an hour or so is appropriate, with further titration based on symptoms. Achieving "normal" BP urgently is not necessary. Typical 1st-line drugs include nitroprusside, fenoldopam, nicardipine, and labetalol (see TABLE 71–11). Nitroglycerin alone is less potent.

Oral drugs are not indicated because onset is variable and the drugs are difficult to titrate. Short-acting oral nifedipine, although it reduces BP rapidly, may lead to acute cardiovascular and cerebrovascular events (sometimes fatal) and is therefore not recommended.

Nitroprusside is a venous and arterial dilator, reducing preload and afterload; thus, it is the most useful for hypertensive patients with heart failure. It is also used for hypertensive encephalopathy and, with β-blockers, for aortic dissection. Starting dose is 0.25 to 1.0 μg/kg/min titrated in increments of 0.5 μg/kg to a maximum of 8 to 10 μg/kg/min; maximum dose is given for ≤ 10 min to minimize risk of cyanide toxicity. The drug is rapidly broken down into cyanide and nitric oxide (the active moiety). Cyanide is detoxified to thiocyanate. However, administration of > 2 μg/kg/min can lead to cyanide accumulation with toxicity to the CNS and heart; manifestations include agitation, seizures, cardiac instability, and an anion gap metabolic acidosis. Prolonged administration (> 1 wk or, in patients with renal insufficiency, 3 to 6 days) leads to accumulation of thiocyanate, with lethargy, tremor, abdominal pain, and vomiting. Other adverse effects include transitory elevation of hair follicles (cutis anserina) if BP is reduced too rapidly. Thiocyanate levels should be monitored daily after 3 consecutive days of therapy, and the drug should be stopped if the serum thiocyanate level is > 12 mg/dL (> 2 mmol/L). Because the drug is broken down by ultraviolet light, the IV bag and tubing are wrapped in an opaque covering.

TABLE 71–11. PARENTERAL DRUGS FOR HYPERTENSIVE EMERGENCIES

DRUG	DOSE	ADVERSE EFFECTS*	SPECIAL INDICATIONS
Sodium nitroprusside	0.25–10 μg/kg/min IV infusion† (maximum dose for 10 min only)	Nausea, vomiting, agitation, muscle twitching, sweating, cutis anserina (if BP is reduced too rapidly), thiocyanate and cyanide toxicity	Most hypertensive emergencies; should be used cautiously in patients with high intracranial pressure or azotemia
Nicardipine	5–15 mg/h IV	Tachycardia, headache, flushing, local phlebitis	Most hypertensive emergencies, except acute heart failure; should be used cautiously in patients with myocardial ischemia
Fenoldopam	0.1–0.3 μg/kg/min IV infusion; maximum dose 1.6 μg/kg/min	Tachycardia, headache, nausea, flushing, hypokalemia, elevation of intraocular pressure in patients with glaucoma	Most hypertensive emergencies; should be used cautiously in patients with myocardial ischemia
Nitroglycerin	5–100 μg/min IV infusion†	Headache, tachycardia, nausea, vomiting, apprehension, restlessness, muscular twitching, palpitations, methemoglobinemia, tolerance with prolonged use	Myocardial ischemia, heart failure
Enalaprilat	0.625–5 mg q 6 h IV	Precipitous fall in BP in high-renin states, variable response	Acute left ventricular failure; should be avoided in acute MI
Hydralazine	10–40 mg IV 10–20 mg IM	Tachycardia, flushing, headache, vomiting, aggravation of angina	Eclampsia
Labetalol	20 mg IV bolus over 2 min, followed q 10 min by 40 mg, then up to 3 doses of 80 mg; or 0.5–2 mg/min IV infusion	Vomiting, scalp tingling, burning in throat, dizziness, nausea, heart block, orthostatic hypotension	Most hypertensive emergencies, except acute left ventricular failure; should be avoided in patients with asthma
Esmolol	250–500 μg/kg/min for 1 min, then 50–100 μg/kg/min for 4 min; may repeat sequence	Hypotension, nausea	Aortic dissection perioperatively
Phentolamine	5–15 mg IV	Tachycardia, flushing, headache	Catecholamine excess

*Hypotension may occur with all drugs.
†Requires a special delivery system (eg, infusion pump for nitroprusside, non–polyvinyl chloride tubing for nitroglycerin).

Fenoldopam is a peripheral dopamine-1 agonist that causes systemic and renal vasodilation and natriuresis. Onset is rapid and half-life is brief, making it an effective alternative to nitroprusside, with the added benefit that it does not cross the blood-brain barrier. Initial dosage is 0.1 μg/kg/min IV infusion, titrated upward by 0.1 μg/kg q 15 min to a maximum of 1.6 μg/kg/min.

Nitroglycerin is a vasodilator that affects veins more than arterioles. It can be used to manage hypertension during and after coronary artery bypass graft surgery, acute MI, unstable angina pectoris, and acute pulmonary edema. IV nitroglycerin is preferable to nitroprusside for patients with severe coronary artery disease because nitroglycerin increases coronary flow, whereas Na nitroprusside tends to decrease coronary flow to ischemic areas, possibly because of a "steal" mechanism. Starting dose is 10 to 20 μg/min titrated upward by 10 μg/min q 5 min to maximum antihypertensive effect. For long-term BP control, nitroglycerin must be used with other drugs. The most common adverse effect is headache (in about 2%); others include tachycardia, nausea, vomiting, apprehension, restlessness, muscular twitching, and palpitations.

Nicardipine, a dihydropyridine Ca channel blocker with less negative inotropic effects than nifedipine, acts primarily as a vasodilator. It is most often used for postoperative hypertension and during pregnancy. Dosage is 5 mg/h IV, increased q 15 min to a maximum of 15 mg/h. It may cause flushing, headache, and tachycardia; it can decrease GFR in patients with renal insufficiency.

Labetalol is a β-blocker with some α_1-blocking effects, thus producing vasodilation without the typical accompanying reflex tachycardia. It can be given as a constant infusion or as frequent boluses; use of boluses has not been shown to produce significant hypotension. Labetalol is used during pregnancy, for intracranial disorders requiring BP control, and after MI. Infusion is 0.5 to 2 mg/min, titrated upward to a maximum of 4 to 5 mg/min. Boluses begin with 20 mg IV followed q 10 min by 40 mg, then 80 mg (up to 3 doses) to a maximum total of 300 mg. Adverse effects are minimal, but because of its β-blocking activity, labetalol should not be used for hypertensive emergencies in patients with asthma. Low doses may be used for left ventricular failure if nitroglycerin is given simultaneously.

72 ARTERIOSCLEROSIS

Arteriosclerosis is a general term for several disorders that cause thickening and loss of elasticity in the arterial wall. Atherosclerosis, the most common form, is also the most serious because it causes coronary artery disease and cerebrovascular disease. Nonatheromatous forms of arteriosclerosis include arteriolosclerosis and Mönckeberg's arteriosclerosis.

ATHEROSCLEROSIS

Atherosclerosis is patchy intimal plaques (atheromas) in medium and large arteries; the plaques contain lipids, inflammatory cells, smooth muscle cells, and connective tissue. Risk factors include dyslipidemia, diabetes, cigarette smoking, family history, sedentary lifestyle, obesity, and hypertension. Symptoms develop when growth or rupture of the plaque reduces or obstructs blood flow; symptoms vary by artery affected. Diagnosis is clinical and confirmed by angiography, ultrasonography, or other imaging tests. Treatment includes risk factor and dietary modification, physical activity, and antiplatelet drugs.

Atherosclerosis can affect all large and medium-sized arteries, including the coronary, carotid, and cerebral arteries, the aorta, its branches, and major arteries of the extremities. It is the leading cause of morbidity and mortality in the US and in most Western countries. In recent years, age-related mortality attributable to atherosclerosis has been decreasing, but in 2001, coronary and cerebrovascular atherosclerosis still caused > 650,000 deaths in the US (more than cancer and almost 6 times more than accidents). Atherosclerosis is rapidly increasing in prevalence in developing countries, and as people in developed countries live longer, incidence will increase. By 2020, atherosclerosis is expected to be the leading cause of death worldwide.

Etiology and Pathophysiology

The hallmark of atherosclerosis is the atherosclerotic plaque, which contains lipids (intracellular and extracellular cholesterol and phospholipids), inflammatory cells (eg, macrophages, T cells), smooth muscle cells, connective tissue (eg, collagen, glycosaminoglycans, elastic fibers), thrombi, and Ca deposits. All stages of atherosclerosis—from initiation and growth to complication of the plaque—are considered an inflammatory response to injury. Endothelial injury is thought to have a primary role.

Atherosclerosis preferentially affects certain areas of the arterial tree. Nonlaminar or turbulent blood flow (eg, at branch points in the arterial tree) leads to endothelial dysfunction and inhibits endothelial production of nitric oxide, a potent vasodilator and anti-inflammatory molecule. Such blood flow also stimulates endothelial cells to produce adhesion molecules, which recruit and bind inflammatory cells. Risk factors for atherosclerosis (eg, dyslipidemia, diabetes, cigarette smoking, hypertension), oxidative stressors (eg, superoxide radicals), angiotensin II, and systemic infection and inflammation also inhibit nitric oxide production and stimulate production of adhesion molecules, proinflammatory cytokines, chemotactic proteins, and vasoconstrictors; exact mechanisms are unknown. The net effect is endothelial binding of monocytes and T cells, migration of these cells to the subendothelial space, and initiation and perpetuation of a local vascular inflammatory response. Monocytes in the subendothelium transform into macrophages. Lipids in the blood, particularly low density lipoprotein (LDL) and very low density lipoprotein (VLDL), also bind to endothelial cells and are oxidized in the subendothelium. Uptake of oxidized lipids and macrophage transformation into lipid-laden foam cells result in the typical early atherosclerotic lesions called fatty streaks. Degraded erythrocyte membranes that result from rupture of vasa vasorum and intraplaque hemorrhage may be an important additional source of lipids within plaques.

Macrophages elaborate proinflammatory cytokines that recruit smooth muscle cell migration from the media and that further attract and stimulate growth of macrophages. Various factors promote smooth muscle cell replication and increase production of dense extracellular matrix. The result is a subendothelial fibrous plaque with a fibrous cap, made of intimal smooth muscle cells surrounded by connective tissue and intracellular and extracellular lipids. A process similar to bone formation causes calcification within the plaque.

Atherosclerotic plaques may be stable or unstable. Stable plaques regress, remain static, or grow slowly over several decades until they may cause stenosis or occlusion. Unstable plaques are vulnerable to spontaneous erosion, fissure, or rupture, causing acute thrombosis, occlusion, and infarction long before they cause stenosis. Most clinical events result from unstable plaques, which do not appear severe on angiography; thus, plaque stabilization may be a way to reduce morbidity and mortality.

The strength of the fibrous cap and its resistance to rupture depend on the relative balance of collagen deposition and degradation. Plaque rupture involves secretion of metalloproteinases, cathepsins, and collagenases by activated macrophages in the plaque. These enzymes digest the fibrous cap, particularly at the edges, causing the cap to thin and ultimately rupture. T cells in the plaque contribute by secreting cytokines. Cytokines inhibit smooth muscle cells from synthesizing and depositing collagen, which normally reinforces the plaque.

Once the plaque ruptures, plaque contents are exposed to circulating blood, triggering thrombosis; macrophages also stimulate thrombosis because they contain tissue factor, which promotes thrombin generation in vivo. One of 5 outcomes may occur: The resultant thrombus may organize and be incorporated into the plaque, changing the plaque's shape and causing its rapid growth; the thrombus may rapidly occlude the vascular lumen and precipitate an acute ischemic event; the thrombus may embolize; the plaque may fill with blood, balloon out, and immediately occlude the artery; or plaque contents (rather than thrombus) may embolize, occluding vessels downstream.

Plaque stability depends on multiple factors, including plaque composition (relative proportion of lipids, inflammatory cells, smooth muscle cells, connective tissue, and thrombus); wall stress (cap fatigue); size and location of the core; and configuration of the plaque in relation to blood flow. By contributing to rapid growth and lipid deposition, intraplaque hemorrhage may play an important role in transforming stable into unstable plaques. In general, unstable coronary artery plaques have a high macrophage content, a thick lipid core, and a thin fibrous cap; they narrow the vessel lumen by < 50% and tend to rupture unpredictably. Unstable carotid artery plaques have the same composition but typically cause problems through severe stenosis and occlusion, not rupture. Low-risk plaques have a thicker cap and contain fewer lipids; they often narrow the vessel lumen by > 50% and produce predictable exercise-induced stable angina.

Clinical consequences of plaque rupture depend not only on plaque anatomy but also on relative balance of procoagulant and anticoagulant activity in the blood and on the vulnerability of the myocardium to arrhythmias.

A link between infection and atherosclerosis has been suggested to explain the serologic associations between infections (eg, *Chlamydia pneumoniae*, cytomegalovirus) and coronary artery disease. Putative mechanisms include indirect effects of chronic inflammation in the bloodstream, cross-reactive antibodies, and inflammatory effects of infectious pathogens on the arterial wall.

TABLE 72–1. RISK FACTORS FOR ATHEROSCLEROSIS

Nonmodifiable
- Age
- Family history of premature atherosclerosis*
- Male sex

Modifiable, established
- Certain dyslipidemias (high total or LDL level, low HDL level)
- Cigarette smoking
- Diabetes mellitus
- Hypertension

Modifiable, under study
- *Chlamydia pneumoniae* infection
- High CRP level
- High level of small, dense LDL
- High lipoprotein(a) level
- Hyperhomocysteinemia
- Hyperinsulinemia
- Hypertriglyceridemia
- 5-Lipoxygenase polymorphisms
- Obesity†
- Prothrombotic states (eg, hyperfibrinogenemia, high plasminogen activator inhibitor level)
- Renal insufficiency
- Sedentary lifestyle†

LDL = low density lipoprotein, HDL = high density lipoprotein, CRP = C-reactive protein.

*Premature atherosclerosis is disease in a 1st-degree relative before age 55 for men and before age 65 for women.

†It is unclear how much these factors contribute independent of other frequently-associated risk factors (eg, diabetes, dyslipidemia).

Risk Factors

There are numerous risk factors (see TABLE 72–1). Certain factors tend to cluster as the metabolic syndrome, which is becoming increasingly prevalent. This syndrome includes abdominal obesity, atherogenic dyslipidemia, hypertension, insulin resistance, a prothrombotic state, and a proinflammatory state (see also p. 61). Insulin resistance is not synonymous with the metabolic syndrome but may be key in its etiology.

Dyslipidemia (high total, high LDL, or low high density lipoprotein [HDL] cholesterol), hypertension, and diabetes promote atherosclerosis by amplifying or augmenting endothelial dysfunction and inflammatory pathways in vascular endothelium.

In dyslipidemia, subendothelial uptake and oxidation of LDL increases; oxidized lipids stimulate production of adhesion molecules and inflammatory cytokines and may be antigenic, inciting a T cell–mediated immune response and inflammation in the arterial wall. HDL protects against atherosclerosis via reverse cholesterol transport (see p. 1295); it may also protect by transporting antioxidant enzymes, which can break down and neutralize oxidized lipids. The role of hypertriglyceridemia in atherogenesis is complex, and whether it has an effect independent of other lipid abnormalities is unclear.

Hypertension may lead to vascular inflammation via angiotensin II–mediated mechanisms. Angiotensin II stimulates endothelial cells, vascular smooth muscle cells, and macrophages to produce proatherogenic mediators, including proinflammatory cytokines; superoxide anions; prothrombotic factors; growth factors; and lectin-like oxidized LDL receptors.

Diabetes leads to the formation of advanced glycation end products, which increase the production of proinflammatory cytokines from endothelial cells. Oxidative stress and reactive oxygen radicals, generated in diabetes, directly injure the endothelium and promote atherogenesis.

Cigarette smoke contains nicotine and other chemicals that are toxic to vascular endothelium. Smoking, including passive smoking, increases platelet reactivity (possibly promoting platelet thrombosis) and plasma fibrinogen levels and Hct (increasing blood viscosity). Smoking increases LDL and decreases HDL; it also promotes vasoconstriction, which is particularly dangerous in arteries already narrowed by atherosclerosis. HDL increases by about 6 to 8 mg/dL within 1 mo of smoking cessation.

Hyperhomocysteinemia increases risk of atherosclerosis, although not as much as the above risk factors. It may result from folate deficiency or a genetic metabolic defect. The pathophysiologic mechanism is unknown but may involve direct endothelial injury, stimulation of monocyte and T-cell recruitment, LDL uptake by macrophages, and smooth muscle cell proliferation.

Lipoprotein(a) is a modified version of LDL that has a cysteine-rich region homologous with plasminogen. High levels may predispose to atherothrombosis, but mechanism is unclear.

A high level of small, dense LDL, characteristic of diabetes, is highly atherogenic. Mechanism may include increased susceptibility to oxidation and nonspecific endothelial binding (see p. 1296).

A high CRP level does not reliably predict extent of atherosclerosis but can predict likelihood of ischemic events. It may indicate increased risk of atherosclerotic plaque rupture, ongoing ulceration or thrombosis, or increased activity of lymphocytes and macrophages. CRP may have a direct role in atherogenesis through multiple mechanisms, including downregulation of nitric oxide synthesis and upregulation of angiotensin type 1 receptors, chemoattractant proteins, and adhesion molecules.

C. pneumoniae infection or other infections (eg, viral, HIV, *Helicobacter pylori*) may cause endothelial dysfunction through direct infection, exposure to endotoxin, or stimulation of systemic or subendothelial inflammation.

Renal insufficiency promotes development of atherosclerosis via several pathways, including worsening hypertension and insulin resistance, decreased apolipoprotein A-I levels, and increased lipoprotein(a), homocysteine, fibrinogen, and CRP levels.

Prothrombotic states increase likelihood of atherothrombosis (see p. 1080).

5-Lipoxygenase polymorphisms (deletion or addition of alleles) may promote atherosclerosis by increasing leukotriene production within plaques, which causes vascular permeability and monocyte-macrophage migration, thus increasing subendothelial inflammation and dysfunction.

Symptoms and Signs

Atherosclerosis is initially asymptomatic, often for decades. Symptoms and signs develop when lesions impede blood flow. Transient ischemic symptoms (eg, stable exertional angina, transient ischemic attacks, intermittent claudication) may develop when stable plaques grow and reduce the arterial lumen by > 70%. Symptoms of unstable angina or infarction, ischemic stroke, or rest pain in the limbs may develop when unstable plaques rupture and acutely occlude a major artery, with superimposition of thrombosis or embolism. Atherosclerosis may also cause sudden death without preceding stable or unstable angina pectoris.

Atherosclerotic involvement of the arterial wall can lead to aneurysms and arterial dissection, which can manifest as pain, a pulsatile mass, absent pulses, or sudden death.

Diagnosis and Screening

Approach depends on the presence or absence of symptoms.

Symptomatic patients: Patients with symptoms and signs of ischemia are evaluated for the amount and location of vascular occlusion by various invasive and noninvasive tests, depending on the organ involved (see elsewhere in THE MANUAL). Such patients also should be evaluated for atherosclerosis risk factors by history and physical examination, fasting lipid profile and blood sugar, Hb A1c level, and homocysteine level.

Because atherosclerosis is a systemic disease, patients with documented disease at one site (eg, peripheral arteries) should be evaluated for disease at other sites (eg, coronary and carotid arteries).

Because not all atherosclerotic plaques have similar risk, various imaging technologies are being studied as a way to identify plaques especially vulnerable to rupture. Most technologies are catheter-based; they include intravascular ultrasonography (which uses an ultrasound transducer on the tip of a catheter to produce images of the arterial lumen), angioscopy, plaque thermography (to detect the increased temperature in plaques with active inflammation), optical coherence tomography (which uses infrared laser light for imaging), and elastography (to identify soft, lipid-rich plaques). Immunoscintigraphy is a noninvasive alternative using radioactive tracers that localize in vulnerable plaque.

Some clinicians measure serum markers of inflammation. CRP levels > 3 mg/dL are highly predictive of cardiovascular events. High levels of lipoprotein-associated phospholipase A2 appear to predict cardiovascular events in patients with a normal or low LDL level.

Asymptomatic patients: In patients with risk factors for atherosclerosis but no symptoms or signs of ischemia, the role of additional testing is unclear. Although imaging studies such as electron beam or multidetector row CT, MRI, and ultrasound (see Ch. 329 on p. 2715) can detect atherosclerotic plaque, they probably do not improve prediction of ischemic events over assessment of risk factors or established prediction tools (eg, Framingham risk index—see TABLES 159–6 and 159–7 on pp. 1305–1306) and are not routinely recommended.

Urinary microalbuminuria (> 30 mg albumin/24 h) is a marker for renal disorders and their progression, as well as a strong predictor of cardiovascular and noncardiovascular morbidity and mortality; however, the direct relationship between microalbuminuria and atherosclerosis has not been established.

Treatment

Treatment involves aggressive modification of risk factors to slow progression and induce regression of existing plaques. Recent evidence suggests that LDL should be < 70 mg/dL in those with disease or at high risk for cardiovascular events. Lifestyle changes include diet, smoking cessation, and regular physical activity. Drugs to treat dyslipidemia, hypertension, and diabetes are often required. These lifestyle changes and drugs directly or indirectly improve endothelial function, reduce inflammation, and improve clinical outcome. Antiplatelet drugs help all patients.

Diet: Substantial decreases in saturated fat and simple carbohydrate intake and increases in fruit, vegetable, and fiber intake are recommended; these dietary changes are a prerequisite for lipid control and are essential for all patients. Calorie intake should be limited to keep weight within the normal range.

Small decreases in fat intake do not appear to lessen or stabilize atherosclerosis. Effective change requires limiting fat intake to 20 g/day, consisting of 6 to 10 g of polyunsaturated fat with ω-6 (linoleic acid) and ω-3 (eicosapentaenoic acid, docosahexaenoic acid) fatty acids in equal proportion, ≤ 2 g of saturated fat, and the rest as monounsaturated fat. Trans fatty acids, which are highly atherogenic, should be avoided.

Increasing carbohydrates to compensate for decreasing saturated fats in the diet increases plasma triglyceride levels and reduces HDL levels. Thus, any caloric deficiency should be made up with proteins and unsaturated fats rather than carbohydrates. Excessive sugar intake should be avoided, although sugar intake has not been directly related to cardiovascular risk. Instead, consumption of complex carbohydrates (eg, vegetables, whole grains) is encouraged.

Fruits and vegetables (5 daily servings) seem to decrease risk of coronary atherosclerosis, but whether this effect is due to phytochemicals or to a proportional decrease in saturated fat intake and increase in fiber and vitamin intake is unclear. Phytochemicals called flavonoids (in red and purple grapes, red wine, black teas, and dark beers) appear especially protective; high concentrations in red wine may help explain why incidence of coronary atherosclerosis in the French is relatively low, even though they use more tobacco and consume more fat than Americans do. But no clinical data indicate that eating flavonoid-rich foods or using supplements instead of foods prevents atherosclerosis.

Increased fiber intake decreases total cholesterol and may have a beneficial effect on glucose and insulin levels. Daily intake of at least 5 to 10 g of soluble fiber (eg, oat bran, beans, soy products, psyllium) is recommended; this amount decreases LDL by about 5%. Insoluble fiber (eg, cellulose, lignin) does not appear to affect cholesterol but may confer additional health benefits (eg, reduced risk of colon cancer, possibly by stimulating bowel movement or reducing contact time with dietary carcinogens). However, excessive fiber interferes with the absorption of certain minerals and vitamins. In general, foods rich in phytochemicals and vitamins are also rich in fiber.

Alcohol increases HDL and has poorly defined antithrombotic, antioxidant, and anti-inflammatory properties. These effects appear to be the same for wine, beer, and hard liquor, and occur at moderate levels of consumption; 1 oz 5 to 6 times/wk protects against coronary atherosclerosis. However, at higher doses, alcohol can cause significant health problems. Thus, the relationship between alcohol and total mortality rate is J-shaped; mortality rate is lowest for men who consume < 14 drinks/wk and women who consume < 9 drinks/wk.

There is little evidence that dietary supplementation with vitamins, phytochemicals, and trace minerals reduces risk of atherosclerosis. The one exception is fish oil supplements (see p. 1308).

Physical activity: Regular physical activity (eg, 30 to 45 min of walking, running, swimming, or cycling 3 to 5 times/wk) reduces incidence of some risk factors (hypertension, dyslipidemia, diabetes), coronary artery disease (eg, MI), and death attributable to atherosclerosis in patients with and without previous ischemic events. Whether the association is causal or merely indicates that healthier people are more likely to exercise regularly is unclear. Optimal intensity, duration, frequency, and type of exercise have not been established, but most evidence suggests an inverse linear relationship between aerobic physical activity and risk. Walking regularly increases the distance patients with peripheral vascular disease can walk without pain.

An exercise program that involves aerobic exercise has a clear role in prevention of atherosclerosis and promoting weight loss (see p. 2628). Before starting a new exercise program, the elderly and people who have risk factors for atherosclerosis or who have had recent ischemic events should probably be evaluated by a physician; evaluation includes history, physical examination, and assessment of risk factor control.

Antiplatelet drugs: Oral antiplatelet drugs are essential because most complications result from plaque fissure or rupture with platelet activation and thrombosis.

Aspirin is most widely used. It is indicated for secondary prevention and recommended for primary prevention of coronary atherosclerosis in patients at high risk (eg, diabetics with or without atherosclerosis, patients with ≥ 20% risk of cardiac events within 10 yr). Optimal dose and duration are unknown, but 70 to 160 mg po once/day indefinitely is commonly used for primary prevention because it is effective while minimizing risk of bleeding. For secondary prevention and for patients with poorly controlled risk factors, 325 mg is a proven option. In about 10 to 20% of patients taking aspirin for secondary prevention, ischemic events recur. The reason may be aspirin resistance; assays to detect lack of thromboxane suppression (indicated by elevated urinary 11-dehydro thromboxane B_2) are being studied for clinical use. Some evidence suggests that ibuprofen can interfere with aspirin's antithrombotic effect, so other NSAIDs are recommended for patients taking aspirin for prevention.

Clopidogrel (usually 75 mg/day) is substituted for aspirin when ischemic events recur in patients taking aspirin. Clopidogrel is used with aspirin to treat acute non-ST-segment elevation MI (see p. 637); the combination is also given for 9 to 12 mo after percutaneous intervention (PCI) to reduce risk of ischemic events.

Ticlopidine is no longer widely used because it causes severe neutropenia in 1% of users and has severe GI adverse effects.

Other drugs: ACE inhibitors, angiotensin II receptor blockers, statins, and thiazolidinediones (eg, rosiglitazone, pioglitazone) have anti-inflammatory properties that reduce risk of atherosclerosis independent of their effects on BP, lipids, and glucose. ACE inhibitors inhibit the contributions of angiotensin to endothelial dysfunction and inflammation. Statins enhance endothelial nitric oxide production, stabilize atherosclerotic plaques, reduce lipid accumulation in the arterial wall, and induce regression of plaques. Thiazolidinediones may control expression of proinflammatory genes. Routine use of statins for primary prevention of ischemic events is controversial. However, several well-controlled studies support their use in high-risk patients (eg, diabetics with normal BP and lipid levels and patients with multiple risk factors, including hyperlipidemia and/or hypertension). Statins are sometimes recommended for patients with normal LDL and high CRP; few data now support this practice, but it is under study.

Folic acid 0.8 mg po bid is used to treat and prevent hyperhomocysteinemia, but whether it reduces the risk of coronary atherosclerosis has not been established. Vitamins B_6 and B_{12} also lower homocysteine levels, but few data justify their use; both are under study. Ca 500 mg po bid may help normalize BP in certain people. Macrolide and other antibiotics are being studied to determine whether treating chronic occult *C. pneumoniae* infections can suppress inflammation and alter the course and manifestations of atherosclerosis.

NONATHEROMATOUS ARTERIOSCLEROSIS

Nonatheromatous arteriosclerosis is age-related fibrosis in the aorta and its major branches.

Nonatheromatous arteriosclerosis causes intimal thickening and weakens and disrupts the elastic lamellae. The smooth muscle (media) layer atrophies, and the lumen of the affected artery widens (becomes ectatic), predisposing to aneurysm or dissection. Hypertension is a major factor in development of aortic arteriosclerosis and aneurysm. Intimal injury, ectasia, and ulceration may lead to thrombosis, embolism, or complete arterial occlusion.

Arteriolosclerosis affects distal arteries in patients with diabetes or hypertension. Hyaline arteriolosclerosis affects small arteries and arterioles in patients with diabetes; typically, hyaline thickening occurs, the arteriolar wall degenerates, and the lumen narrows, causing diffuse ischemia, especially in the kidneys. Hyperplastic arteriolosclerosis occurs more often in patients with hypertension; typically, laminated, concentric thickening and luminal narrowing occur, sometimes with fibrinoid deposits and vessel wall necrosis (necrotizing arteriolitis). Hypertension promotes these changes, and arteriolosclerosis, by increasing arteriolar rigidity and increasing peripheral resistance, may help sustain the hypertension.

Mönckeberg's arteriosclerosis (medial calcific sclerosis) affects patients > 50; age-related medial degeneration occurs with focal calcification and even bone formation within the arterial wall. Segments of the artery may become a rigid calcified tube without luminal narrowing. The diagnosis is usually obvious by plain x-ray. This disorder is clinically important only because it can greatly reduce arterial compressibility, causing extremely but falsely elevated BP readings.

73 CORONARY ARTERY DISEASE

Coronary artery disease involves impairment of blood flow through the coronary arteries, most commonly by atheromas. Clinical presentations include silent ischemia, angina pectoris, acute coronary syndromes (unstable angina, MI), and sudden cardiac death. Diagnosis is by symptoms, ECG, stress testing, and sometimes coronary angiography. Prevention consists of modifying reversible risk factors (eg, hypercholesterolemia, physical inactivity, smoking). Treatment includes drugs and procedures to reduce ischemia and restore or improve coronary blood flow.

In the US, coronary artery disease (CAD) is the leading cause of death in both sexes, accounting for about ⅓ of all deaths. Mortality rate among white men is about 1/10,000 at ages 25 to 34 and nearly 1/100 at ages 55 to 64. Mortality rate among white men aged 35 to 44 is 6.1 times that among age-matched white women. For unknown reasons, the sex difference is less marked in nonwhites. Mortality rate among women increases after menopause and, by age 75, equals or even exceeds that of men.

Etiology and Pathophysiology

Usually, CAD is due to subintimal deposition of atheromas in large and medium-sized coronary arteries (atherosclerosis—see p. 620). Less often, CAD is due to coronary spasm. Rare causes include coronary artery embolism, dissection, aneurysm (eg, in Kawasaki disease), and vasculitis (eg, in SLE, syphilis).

Coronary atherosclerosis is often irregularly distributed in different vessels but typically occurs at points of turbulence (eg, vessel bifurcations). The arterial lumen progressively narrows, resulting in ischemia (causing angina pectoris). The degree of stenosis required to produce ischemia varies with O_2 demand.

Occasionally, an atheromatous plaque ruptures or splits. Reasons are unclear but probably relate to an inflammatory process that softens the plaque. Rupture exposes thrombogenic material, which activates platelets and the coagulation cascade, resulting in an acute thrombus and ischemia. The consequences of acute ischemia, collectively referred to as acute coronary syndromes (ACS), depend on the location and degree of obstruction and range from unstable angina to transmural infarction.

Coronary artery spasm is a transient, focal increase in vascular tone, markedly narrowing the lumen and reducing blood flow; symptomatic ischemia (variant angina—see p. 634) may result. Marked narrowing can trigger thrombus formation, causing infarction. Spasm can occur in arteries with or without atheroma. In arteries without atheroma, basal coronary artery tone is probably increased, and response to vasoconstricting stimuli is probably exaggerated. The exact mechanism is unclear but may involve abnormalities of nitric oxide production or an imbalance between endothelium-derived contracting and relaxing factors. In arteries with atheroma, the atheroma may cause local hypercontractility; proposed mechanisms include loss of sensitivity to intrinsic vasodilators (eg, acetylcholine) and increased production of vasoconstrictors (eg, angiotensin II, endothelin, leukotrienes, serotonin, thromboxane) in the area of the atheroma. Recurrent spasm may damage the intima, leading to atheroma formation. Use of vasoconstricting drugs (eg, cocaine, nicotine) can trigger coronary spasm.

Risk Factors

Risk factors for CAD are the same as those for atherosclerosis: high blood levels of low-density lipoprotein (LDL) cholesterol and lipoprotein a, low blood levels of high-density lipoprotein (HDL) cholesterol, diabetes mellitus (particularly type 2), smoking, obesity, and physical inactivity. Smoking may be a stronger predictor of MI in women (especially those < 45). Genetic factors play a role, and several systemic disorders (eg, hypertension, hypothyroidism) contribute to risk. A high level of apoprotein B (apo B) is an important risk factor; it may identify increased risk when total cholesterol or LDL level is normal.

High blood levels of C-reactive protein indicate plaque instability and inflammation and may be a stronger predictor of risk of ischemic events than high levels of LDL. High blood levels of triglycerides and insulin (reflecting insulin resistance) may be risk factors, but data are less clear. CAD risk is increased by smoking; a diet high in fat and calories and low in phytochemicals (found in fruits and vegetables), fiber, and vitamins C and E; a diet relatively low in ω-3 (n-3) polyunsaturated fatty acids (PUFAs), at least in some people; and poor stress management.

Anatomy

The right and left coronary arteries arise from the right and left coronary sinuses in the root of the aorta just above the aortic valve orifice. The coronary arteries divide into large and medium arteries that run along the heart's surface (epicardial coronary arteries) and subsequently send smaller arterioles into the myocardium. The left coronary artery begins as the left main artery and quickly divides into the left anterior descending (LAD) and circumflex arteries. The LAD artery usually follows the anterior interventricular groove and, in some people, continues over the apex. This artery supplies the anterior septum (including the proximal conduction system) and anterior free wall of the left ventricle (LV). The circumflex artery, which is usually smaller than the LAD artery, supplies the lateral LV free wall. Most people have right dominance: The right coronary artery passes along the atrioventricular (AV) groove over the right side of the heart; it supplies the sinus node (in 55%), right ventricle, and usually the AV node and inferior myocardial wall. About 10 to 15% of people have left dominance: The circumflex artery is larger and continues along the posterior AV groove to supply the posterior wall and AV node.

Prevention

Prevention of CAD involves modifying atherosclerosis risk factors (see p. 624): smoking cessation, weight loss, a healthful diet, regular exercise, modification of serum lipids (particularly with HMG-CoA reductase inhibitors [statins]), and control of hypertension and diabetes.

ANGINA PECTORIS

Angina pectoris is a clinical syndrome of precordial discomfort or pressure due to transient myocardial ischemia. It is typically

precipitated by exertion and relieved by rest or sublingual nitroglycerin. Diagnosis is by symptoms, ECG, and myocardial imaging. Treatment may include nitrates, β-blockers, Ca channel blockers, and coronary angioplasty or coronary artery bypass graft surgery.

Etiology and Pathophysiology

Angina pectoris occurs when cardiac workload and resultant myocardial O_2 demand exceed the ability of coronary arteries to supply an adequate amount of oxygenated blood, as can occur when the arteries are narrowed. Narrowing usually results from atherosclerosis but may result from coronary artery spasm or, rarely, coronary artery embolism. Acute coronary thrombosis can cause angina if obstruction is partial or transient, but it usually causes MI.

Because myocardial O_2 demand is determined mainly by heart rate, systolic wall tension, and contractility, narrowing of a coronary artery typically results in angina that occurs during exertion and is relieved by rest.

In addition to exertion, cardiac workload can be increased by disorders such as hypertension, aortic stenosis, aortic regurgitation, or hypertrophic cardiomyopathy. In such cases, angina can result whether atherosclerosis is present or not. These disorders can also decrease relative myocardial perfusion because myocardial mass is increased (causing decreased diastolic flow).

A decreased O_2 supply, as in severe anemia or hypoxia, can precipitate or aggravate angina.

In stable angina, the relationship between workload or demand and ischemia is usually relatively predictable. However, atherosclerotic arterial narrowing is not entirely fixed; it varies with the normal fluctuations in arterial tone that occur in all people. Thus, more people have angina in the morning, when arterial tone is relatively high. Also, abnormal endothelial function may contribute to variations in arterial tone; eg, in endothelium damaged by atheromas, stress of a catecholamine surge causes vasoconstriction rather than dilation (normal response).

As the myocardium becomes ischemic, coronary sinus blood pH falls, cellular K is lost, lactate accumulates, ECG abnormalities appear, and ventricular function deteriorates. Left ventricular (LV) diastolic pressure frequently increases during angina, sometimes inducing pulmonary congestion and dyspnea. The exact mechanism by which ischemia produces discomfort is unclear but may involve nerve stimulation by hypoxic metabolites.

Symptoms and Signs

Angina may be a vague, barely troublesome ache or may rapidly become a severe, intense precordial crushing sensation. It is rarely described as pain. Discomfort is most commonly felt beneath the sternum, although location varies. Discomfort may radiate to the left shoulder and down the inside of the left arm, even to the fingers; straight through to the back; into the throat, jaws, and teeth; and, occasionally, down the inside of the right arm. It may also be felt in the upper abdomen.

Some patients have atypical angina (eg, bloating, gas, abdominal distress) often ascribing symptoms to indigestion; belching may even seem to relieve the symptoms. Others have dyspnea due to the sharp, reversible increase in LV filling pressure that often accompanies ischemia. Frequently, the patient's description is imprecise, and whether the problem is angina, dyspnea, or both may be difficult to determine. Because ischemic symptoms require a minute or more to resolve, brief, fleeting sensations rarely represent angina.

Between and even during attacks of angina, physical findings may be normal. However, during the attack, heart rate may increase modestly, BP is often elevated, heart sounds become more distant, and the apical impulse is more diffuse. Palpation of the precordium may reveal localized systolic bulging or paradoxical movement, reflecting segmental myocardial ischemia and regional dyskinesia. The 2nd heart sound may become paradoxical because LV ejection is more prolonged during an ischemic attack. A 4th heart sound is common. A mid or late systolic apical murmur—shrill but not especially loud—may occur if ischemia causes localized papillary muscle dysfunction, producing mitral regurgitation.

Angina pectoris is typically triggered by exertion or strong emotion, usually persists no more than a few minutes, and subsides with rest. Response to exertion is usually predictable, but in some patients, exercise that is tolerated one day may precipitate angina the next because of variations in arterial tone. Symptoms are exaggerated when exertion follows a meal or occurs in cold weather; walking into the wind or first contact with cold air after leaving a warm room may precipitate an attack. Symptom severity is often classified by the degree of exertion resulting in angina (see TABLE 73–1).

Attacks may vary from several a day to symptom-free intervals of weeks, months, or years. They may increase in frequency (called crescendo angina) to a fatal outcome or gradually decrease or disappear if adequate collateral coronary circulation develops, if the ischemic area infarcts, or if heart failure or intermittent claudication supervenes and limits activity.

Nocturnal angina may occur if a dream causes striking changes in respiration, pulse rate, and BP. Nocturnal angina may also be a sign of recurrent LV failure, an equivalent of nocturnal dyspnea.

Angina may occur spontaneously during rest (called angina decubitus). It is usually accompanied by a modestly increased heart rate and a sometimes markedly higher BP, which increase O_2 demand. These increases may be the cause of rest angina or the result of ischemia induced by plaque rupture and thrombus formation. If angina is not relieved, unmet myocardial O_2 demand increases further, making MI more likely.

Because angina characteristics are usually predictable for a given patient, any changes (ie, rest angina, new-onset angina, increasing angina) should be considered serious. Such changes are termed unstable angina (see p. 637).

TABLE 73–1. CANADIAN CARDIOVASCULAR CLASSIFICATION SYSTEM OF ANGINA PECTORIS

CLASS	ACTIVITIES TRIGGERING CHEST PAIN
1	Strenuous, rapid, or prolonged exertion Not usual physical activities (eg, walking, climbing stairs)
2	Walking rapidly Walking uphill Climbing stairs rapidly Walking or climbing stairs after meals Cold Wind Emotional stress
3	Walking, even 1 or 2 blocks at usual pace and on level ground Climbing stairs, even 1 flight
4	Any physical activity Sometimes rest

Adapted from Braunwald E, Antman EM, Beasley JW, et al: ACC/AHA Guidelines for the management of patients with unstable angina and non-ST segment elevation myocardial infarction: A report of the American College of Cardiology/American Heart Association Task Force on Practice Guidelines (Committee on the management of patients with unstable angina). *Journal of American College of Cardiology* 36:970–1062, 2000.

Diagnosis

Diagnosis is suspected if chest discomfort is typical and is precipitated by exertion and relieved by rest. Patients whose chest discomfort lasts > 20 min or occurs during rest or who have syncope or heart failure are evaluated for an acute coronary syndrome (see p. 635). Chest discomfort may also be caused by GI disorders (eg, reflux, esophageal spasm, indigestion—see p. 65), costochondritis, anxiety, panic attacks, hyperventilation, and other cardiac disorders (eg, pericarditis, mitral valve prolapse, supraventricular tachycardia, atrial fibrillation), even when coronary blood flow is not compromised (see p. 580).

Testing: If typical exertional symptoms are present, ECG is indicated. Because angina resolves quickly with rest, ECG rarely can be done during an attack except during stress testing. If done during an attack, ECG is likely to show reversible ischemic changes: ST-segment depression (typically), ST-segment elevation, decreased R-wave height, intraventricular or bundle branch conduction disturbances, and arrhythmia (usually ventricular extrasystoles). Between attacks, the ECG (and usually LV function) at rest is normal in about 30% of patients with a typical history of angina pectoris, even those with extensive 3-vessel disease. In the remaining 70%, the ECG shows evidence of previous infarction, hypertrophy, or nonspecific ST-segment and T-wave (ST-T) abnormalities. An abnormal resting ECG alone does not establish or refute the diagnosis.

More specific tests include stress testing with ECG or with myocardial imaging (eg, echocardiography, radionuclide imaging) and coronary angiography. Further testing is needed to confirm the diagnosis, evaluate disease severity, determine appropriate exercise levels for the patient, and help predict prognosis.

Noninvasive tests are considered first. For CAD, the most accurate are stress echocardiography and myocardial perfusion imaging with single-photon emission computed tomography (SPECT) or PET. However, these tests are more expensive than simple stress testing with ECG.

If a patient has a normal resting ECG and can exercise, exercise stress testing with ECG is done. In men with chest discomfort suggesting angina, stress ECG testing has a specificity of 70%; sensitivity is 90%. Sensitivity is similar in women, but specificity is lower, particularly in women < 55 (< 70%). However, women are more likely than men to have an abnormal resting ECG when CAD is present (32% vs 23%). Although sensitivity is reasonably high, exercise ECG can miss severe CAD (even left main or 3-vessel disease). In patients with atypical symptoms, a negative stress ECG usually rules out angina pectoris and CAD; a positive result may or may not represent coronary ischemia and indicates need for further testing.

When the resting ECG is abnormal, false-positive ST-segment shifts are common on the stress ECG, so patients should have stress testing with myocardial imaging. Exercise or pharmacologic stress (eg, with dobutamine or dipyridamole infusion) may be used. The choice of imaging modality depends on institutional availability and expertise. Imaging tests can help assess LV function and response to stress; identify areas of ischemia, infarction, and viable tissue; and determine the site and extent of myocardium at risk. Stress echocardiography can also detect ischemia-induced mitral regurgitation.

Coronary angiography (see also p. 590) is the standard for diagnosing CAD but is not always necessary to confirm the diagnosis. It is indicated primarily to locate and assess severity of coronary artery lesions when revascularization (percutaneous intervention [PCI] or coronary artery bypass graft [CABG] surgery) is being considered. Angiography may also be indicated when knowledge of coronary anatomy is necessary to advise about work or lifestyle needs (eg, discontinuing job or sports activities). Obstruction is assumed to be physiologically significant when the luminal diameter is reduced > 70%. This reduction correlates well with the presence of angina pectoris unless spasm or thrombosis is superimposed.

Intravascular ultrasonography provides images of coronary artery structure. An ultrasound probe on the tip of a catheter is inserted in the coronary arteries during angiography. This test can provide more information about coronary anatomy than other tests; it is indicated when the nature of lesions is unclear or when apparent disease severity does not match symptom severity. Used with angioplasty, it can help ensure optimal placement of stents.

Prognosis

The main adverse outcomes are unstable angina, MI, and sudden death due to arrhythmias. Annual mortality rate is about 1.4% in patients with angina, no history of MI, a normal resting ECG, and normal BP. However, women with CAD tend to have a worse prognosis. Mortality rate is about 7.5% when systolic hypertension is present, 8.4% when the ECG is abnormal, and 12% when both are present. Type 2 diabetes about doubles the mortality rate for each scenario.

Prognosis worsens with increasing age, increasingly severe anginal symptoms, presence of anatomic lesions, and poor ventricular function. Lesions in the left main coronary artery or proximal left anterior descending artery indicate particularly high risk. Although prognosis correlates with number and severity of coronary arteries affected, prognosis is surprisingly good for patients with stable angina, even those with 3-vessel disease, if ventricular function is normal.

Treatment

Reversible risk factors are modified as much as possible (see also p. 624). Smokers should stop smoking; ≥ 2 yr after stopping smoking, risk of MI is reduced to that for people who never smoked. Hypertension is treated diligently because even mild hypertension increases cardiac workload. Weight loss alone often reduces the severity of angina. Sometimes treatment of mild LV failure markedly lessens angina. Paradoxically, digitalis occasionally intensifies angina, presumably because increased myocardial contractility increases O_2 demand or because arterial tone is increased or both. Aggressive reduction of total and LDL cholesterol (via diet plus drugs as necessary) slows the progression of CAD, may cause some lesions to regress (see p. 1302), and improves endothelial function and thus arterial response to stress. An exercise program emphasizing walking often improves the sense of well-being, reduces CAD risk, and improves exercise tolerance.

Drugs: The main goals are to relieve acute symptoms and prevent or reduce ischemia (see TABLE 73–2).

For an acute attack, sublingual nitroglycerin is the most effective drug.

To prevent ischemia, all patients diagnosed with CAD or at high risk of developing CAD should take an antiplatelet drug daily. β-Blockers, unless contraindicated or not tolerated, are given to most patients. For some patients, prevention requires Ca channel blockers or long-acting nitrates.

Antiplatelet drugs inhibit platelet aggregation. Aspirin binds irreversibly to platelets and inhibits cyclooxygenase and platelet aggregation. Clopidogrel blocks adenosine diphosphate–induced platelet aggregation. Either drug can reduce risk of ischemic events (MI, sudden death) but are most effective when given together; patients unable to tolerate one should receive the other drug alone.

β-Blockers limit symptoms and prevent infarction and sudden death better than other drugs. β-Blockers block sympathetic stimulation of the heart and reduce systolic BP, heart rate, contractility, and cardiac output, thus decreasing myocardial O_2 demand and increasing exercise tolerance. They also increase the threshold for ventricular fibrillation. Most patients tolerate these drugs well. Many β-blockers are available and effective. Dose is titrated upward as needed until limited by bradycardia or adverse effects. Patients who cannot tolerate β-blockers (eg, those with asthma) are given a Ca channel blocker with negative chronotropic effects (eg, diltiazem, verapamil).

Nitroglycerin is a potent smooth-muscle relaxant and vasodilator. Its main sites of action are in the peripheral vascular tree, especially in the venous or capacitance system, and in coronary blood vessels. Even severely atherosclerotic vessels may dilate in areas without atheroma. Nitroglycerin lowers systolic BP and dilates systemic veins, thus reducing myocardial wall tension, a major determinant of myocardial O_2 need. Sublingual nitroglycerin is given for an acute attack or for prevention before exertion. Dramatic relief usually occurs within 1.5 to 3 min, is complete by about 5 min, and lasts up to 30 min. The dose may be repeated q 4 to 5 min up to 3 times if relief is incomplete. Patients should always carry nitroglycerin tablets or aerosol spray to use promptly at the onset of an angina attack. Patients should store tablets in a tightly sealed, light-resistant glass container, so that potency is not lost. Because the drug deteriorates quickly, small amounts should be obtained frequently.

Long-acting nitrates (oral or transdermal) are used if symptoms persist after the β-blocker dose is maximized. If angina occurs at predictable times, a nitrate is given to cover those times. Oral nitrates include isosorbide dinitrate and mononitrate (the active metabolite of the dinitrate). They are effective within 1 to 2 h; their effect lasts 4 to 6 h. Sustained-release formulations of isosorbide mononitrate appear to be effective throughout the day. For transdermal use, cutaneous nitroglycerin patches have largely replaced nitroglycerin ointments primarily because ointments are inconvenient and messy. Patches slowly release the drug for a prolonged effect; exercise capacity improves 4 h after patch application and wanes in 18 to 24 h. Nitrate tolerance may occur, especially when plasma concentrations are kept constant. Because MI risk is highest in early morning, an afternoon or early evening respite period from nitrates is reasonable unless a patient commonly has angina at that time. For nitroglycerin, an 8- to 10-h respite period seems sufficient. Isosorbide may require a 12-h respite period. Sustained-release isosorbide mononitrate does not appear to elicit tolerance.

Ca channel blockers may be used if symptoms persist despite use of nitrates or if nitrates are not tolerated. Ca channel blockers are particularly useful if hypertension or coronary spasm is also present. Different types of Ca channel blockers have different effects. Dihydropyridines (eg, nifedipine, amlodipine, felodipine) have no chronotropic effects and vary substantially in their negative inotropic effects. Shorter-acting dihydropyridines may cause reflex tachycardia and are associated with increased mortality in CAD patients; they should not be used to treat stable angina. Longer-acting formulations of dihydropyridines have fewer tachycardic effects; they are most commonly used with a β-blocker. In this group, amlodipine has the weakest negative inotropic effects; it may be used in

TABLE 73–2. DRUGS FOR CORONARY ARTERY DISEASE

DRUG	DOSAGE	USE
Antiplatelet Drugs		
Aspirin	**For stable angina:** 81 mg po once/day (enteric-coated) **For ACS:** 160–325 mg po chewed (not enteric-coated) on arrival at emergency department and once/day thereafter during hospitalization 81 mg* po once/day long-term after discharge	All patients with CAD or at high risk of developing CAD, unless aspirin is not tolerated or is contraindicated; used long-term
Clopidogrel (preferred) or	75 mg po once/day	Used with aspirin or, in patients who cannot tolerate aspirin, alone
Ticlopidine	250 mg po bid	
Glycoprotein IIb/IIIa inhibitors	IV for 24–36 h	Some patients with ACS, particularly those who are having PCI with stent placement and high-risk patients with unstable angina or NSTEMI
Abciximab	0.25 mg/kg bolus, then 10 μg/min	
Eptifibatide	180 μg/kg bolus, then 2 μg/kg/min	
Tirofiban	0.4 μg/kg/min for 30 min, then 0.1 μg/kg/min	
β-Blockers		
Atenolol	50 mg po q 12 h acutely 50–100 mg po bid long-term	All patients with ACS, unless a β-blocker is not tolerated or is contraindicated, especially high-risk patients; used long-term
Metoprolol	1–3 boluses of 5 mg given 2–5 min apart as tolerated (up to 15 mg), then 25–50 mg po q 6 h, beginning 15 min after last IV dose and continued for 48 h; then 100 mg bid or 200 mg once/day given indefinitely	
Opioids		
Morphine	2–4 mg IV, repeated as needed	All patients with chest pain due to ACS
Nitrates: Short Acting		
Sublingual nitroglycerin (tablet or spray)	0.3–0.6 mg q 4–5 min up to 3 doses	All patients for immediate relief of chest pain; used as needed
Nitroglycerin as continuous IV drip	Started at 5 μg/min and increased 2.5–5.0 μg every few minutes until required response occurs	Selected patients with ACS: during the first 24–48 h, those with heart failure (unless hypotension is present), large anterior MI, or persistent angina, or hypertension (BP is reduced by 10–20 mm Hg but not to < 80–90 mm Hg systolic); for longer use, those with recurrent angina or persistent pulmonary congestion

TABLE 73–2. DRUGS FOR CORONARY ARTERY DISEASE—Continued

DRUG	DOSAGE	USE
Nitrates: Long Acting		
Isosorbide dinitrate	10–20 mg po qid; can be increased to 40 mg qid	Patients who have unstable angina and continue to have anginal symptoms after the β-blocker dose is maximized
Isosorbide mononitrate	20 mg po bid, with 7 h between 1st and 2nd doses	
Isosorbide mononitrate (sustained-release)	30 or 60 mg once/day, increased to 120 mg or, rarely, 240 mg	
Nitroglycerin patches	0.2–0.8 mg/h applied between 6:00 and 9:00 AM and removed 12 to 14 h later to avoid tolerance	
Nitroglycerin ointment 2% preparation (15 mg/2.5 cm)	1.25 cm spread evenly over upper torso or arms q 6 to 8 h and covered with plastic, increased to 7.5 cm as tolerated, and removed for 8 to 12 h each day to avoid tolerance	
Antithrombotics		
Enoxaparin†	30 mg IV (bolus) followed by 1 mg/kg sc q 12 h (maximum, 100 mg)	Patients with unstable angina or NSTEMI Patients < 75 yr receiving tenecteplase Almost all patients with STEMI (unless PCI is indicated and can be done in < 90 min); drug is continued until PCI or CABG is done or patient is discharged
Unfractionated heparin	60–70 units/kg IV (maximum, 5000 units; bolus), followed by 12–15 units/kg/h (maximum 1000 units/h) for 3 to 4 days	Patients with unstable angina or NSTEMI as alternative to enoxaparin
	60 units/kg IV (maximum, 4000 units; bolus) given when alteplase, reteplase, or tenecteplase is started, then followed by 12 units/kg/h (maximum, 1000 units/h) for 48–72 h	Patients with STEMI as alternative to enoxaparin, particularly patients > 75 yr (because enoxaparin with tenecteplase appears to increase risk of intracerebral bleeding)
Warfarin	Dose adjusted to maintain INR of 2.5–3.5	May be useful long-term

*Higher doses of aspirin do not provide greater protection and increase risk of adverse effects.
†Of low mol wt heparins (LMWHs), enoxaparin is preferred.

ACS = acute coronary syndromes; CABG = coronary artery bypass graft; NSTEMI = non-ST-segment elevation MI; PCI = percutaneous intervention; STEMI = ST-segment elevation MI.

patients with LV systolic dysfunction. Diltiazem and verapamil, other types of Ca channel blockers, have negative chronotropic and inotropic effects. They can be used alone in patients with β-blocker intolerance and normal LV systolic function but may increase cardiovascular mortality in patients with LV systolic dysfunction.

Percutaneous intervention (PCI): PCI (eg, angioplasty, stenting) should be considered if angina persists despite drug therapy and worsens quality of life or if anatomic lesions (noted during angiography) put a patient at high risk of mortality. The choice between PCI and CABG surgery depends on extent and location of anatomic lesions, the experience of the surgeon and medical center, and, to some extent, patient preference. PCI is usually preferred for 1- or 2-vessel disease with suitable anatomic lesions. Lesions that are long or near bifurcation points are often not amenable to PCI. Most PCI is done with stenting rather than balloon angioplasty alone, and as stent technology improves, PCI is being used for more complicated cases. Risk is comparable with that for CABG. Mortality rate is 1 to 3%; MI rate is 3 to 5%. In < 3%, intimal dissection causes obstruction requiring emergency CABG. After stenting, aspirin is supplemented with clopidogrel for at least 1 mo, but preferably 6 to 17 mo, and a statin is added if not already being used. About 5 to 15% of stents reocclude in a few days or weeks, requiring placement of a new stent inside the original or CABG. Occasionally, occluded stents are asymptomatic. Angiography 1 yr later shows an apparently normal lumen in about 30% of affected vessels. Patients may quickly return to work and usual activities, but strenuous activities should be avoided for 6 wk.

Coronary artery bypass graft (CABG) surgery: CABG uses sections of autologous veins (eg, saphenous) or, preferably, arteries to bypass diseased segments. At 1 yr, about 85% of venous bypass grafts are patent, but after 10 yr, as many as 97% of internal mammary artery grafts are patent. Arteries also hypertrophy to accommodate increased flow. CABG is preferred for patients with left main artery disease, 3-vessel disease, or diabetes mellitus.

CABG is typically performed during cardiopulmonary bypass with the heart stopped; a bypass machine pumps and oxygenates blood. Risks of the procedure include stroke and MI. For patients with a normal-sized heart, no history of MI, good ventricular function, and no additional risk factors, risk is < 5% for perioperative MI, 2 to 3% for stroke, and ≤ 1% for mortality; risk increases with age and presence of underlying disease. Operative mortality rate is 3 to 5 times higher for a second bypass than for the first; thus, timing of the first bypass should be optimal.

After cardiopulmonary bypass, about 25 to 30% of patients develop cognitive dysfunction, possibly caused by microemboli originating in the bypass machine. Dysfunction ranges from mild to severe and may persist for weeks to years. To minimize this risk, some centers use a "beating heart" technique (ie, no cardiopulmonary bypass), in which a device mechanically stabilizes the part of the heart being worked on.

CABG is very effective in selected patients with angina. The ideal candidate has severe angina pectoris and localized disease, with an otherwise healthy heart. About 85% of patients have complete or dramatic symptom relief. Exercise stress testing shows positive correlation between graft patency and improved exercise tolerance, but exercise tolerance sometimes remains improved despite graft closure.

CAD may progress despite bypass surgery. Postoperatively, the rate of proximal obstruction of bypassed vessels increases. Vein grafts become obstructed early if thrombi form and later (several years) if atherosclerosis causes slow degeneration of the intima and media. Aspirin prolongs vein graft patency; continued smoking has a profound adverse effect on patency.

CABG improves survival for patients with left main disease, those with 3-vessel disease and poor LV function, and some patients with 2-vessel disease. However, for patients with mild or moderate angina (class I or II) or 3-vessel disease and good ventricular function, CABG appears to only marginally improve survival. For patients with 1-vessel disease, outcomes with drug therapy, PCI, and CABG are similar; exceptions are left main disease and proximal left anterior descending disease, for which revascularization appears advantageous. Patients with type 2 diabetes also do better with CABG than with PCI.

Variant Angina

Variant angina is angina pectoris secondary to epicardial coronary artery spasm (Prinzmetal's angina).

Most patients have significant fixed proximal obstruction of at least one major coronary artery. Spasm usually occurs within 1 cm of the obstruction (often accompanied by ventricular arrhythmia).

Symptoms are anginal discomfort occurring mainly during rest and only rarely and inconsistently during exertion (unless significant coronary artery obstruction is also present). Attacks tend to occur regularly at certain times of day.

Diagnosis is suspected if ST-segment elevation occurs during the attack. Between anginal attacks, the ECG may be normal or show a stable abnormal pattern. Confirmation is by provocative testing with ergonovine or acetylcholine, which may precipitate coronary artery spasm, identified by significant ST-elevation or by observation of a reversible spasm during cardiac catheterization. Testing is done most commonly in a cardiac catheterization laboratory and occasionally in a coronary care unit.

Average survival at 5 yr is 89 to 97%, but mortality risk is greater for patients with both variant angina and atherosclerotic coronary artery obstruction. Usually, sublingual nitroglycerin promptly relieves variant angina; Ca channel blockers may effectively prevent symptoms. Theoretically, β-blockers may exacerbate spasm by allowing unopposed α-adrenergic vasoconstriction, but this effect has not been proved clinically. Oral drugs most commonly used are sustained-release diltiazem 120 to 540 mg once/day, sustained-release verapamil 120 to 480 mg once/day (dose must be reduced in patients with renal or hepatic dysfunction), or amlodipine 15 to 20 mg once/day (dose must be reduced in elderly patients and patients with hepatic dysfunction). In refractory cases, amiodarone may be useful. Although these drugs relieve symptoms, they do not appear to alter prognosis.

SYNDROME X

Syndrome X is cardiac microvascular dysfunction or constriction causing angina (microvascular angina).

Some patients with typical angina that is relieved by rest or nitroglycerin have normal coronary arteriograms (eg, no atherosclerosis, embolism, or inducible arterial spasm). Some of these patients have ischemia detected during stress testing; others do not. In some patients, the cause of ischemia seems to be reflex intramyocardial coronary constriction and reduced coronary flow reserve. Other patients have microvascular dysfunction within the myocardium: The abnormal vessels do not dilate in response to exercise or other cardiovascular stressors; sensitivity to cardiac pain may also be increased. Prognosis is good, although symptoms of ischemia may recur for years. In many patients, β-blockers relieve symptoms. This disorder should not be confused with variant angina due to epicardial coronary spasm or with another disorder called syndrome X, which refers to the metabolic syndrome (see p. 61).

SILENT ISCHEMIA

Patients with CAD (particularly diabetics) may have ischemia without symptoms. Ischemia is evidenced by transient asymptomatic ST-T abnormalities seen during 24-h Holter monitoring. Radionuclide studies can sometimes document asymptomatic myocardial ischemia during physical or mental stress (eg, mental arithmetic). Silent ischemia and angina pectoris may coexist, occurring at different times. Prognosis depends on severity of CAD.

ACUTE CORONARY SYNDROMES

(Unstable Angina; Acute MI)

Acute coronary syndromes result from acute obstruction of a coronary artery. Consequences depend on degree of obstruction and range from unstable angina to non-ST-segment elevation MI (NSTEMI), ST-segment elevation MI (STEMI), and sudden cardiac death. Symptoms are similar in each of these syndromes (except sudden death) and include chest discomfort with or without dyspnea, nausea, and diaphoresis. Diagnosis is by ECG and the presence or absence of serologic markers. Treatment is antiplatelet drugs, anticoagulants, nitrates, β-blockers, and, for STEMI, emergency reperfusion via fibrinolytic drugs, percutaneous intervention, or, occasionally, coronary artery bypass graft surgery.

In the US, about 1.5 million MIs occur annually; MI results in death for 400,000 to 500,000 people, with about half dying before they reach the hospital (see Cardiac Arrest on p. 530).

Etiology

Acute coronary syndromes (ACS) usually occur when an acute thrombus forms in an atherosclerotic coronary artery. Atheromatous plaque sometimes becomes unstable or inflamed, causing it to rupture or split, exposing thrombogenic material, which activates platelets and the coagulation cascade and produces an acute thrombus. Platelet activation involves a conformational change in membrane glycoprotein IIb/IIIa receptors, allowing cross-linking (and thus aggregation) of platelets. Even atheromas causing minimal obstruction can rupture and result in thrombosis; in > 50% of cases, stenosis is < 40%. The resultant thrombus abruptly interferes with blood flow to parts of the myocardium. Spontaneous thrombolysis occurs in about ⅔ of patients; 24 h later, thrombotic obstruction is found in only about 30%. However, in virtually all cases, obstruction lasts long enough to produce tissue necrosis.

Rarely, these syndromes are caused by arterial embolism (eg, in mitral or aortic stenosis, infective endocarditis, or marantic endocarditis). Cocaine use and other causes of coronary spasm can sometimes result in MI. Spasm-induced MI may occur in normal or atherosclerotic coronary arteries.

Pathophysiology

Initial consequences vary with size, location, and duration of obstruction and range from transient ischemia to infarction. Measurement of newer, more sensitive markers indicate that some cell necrosis probably occurs even in mild forms; thus, ischemic events occur on a continuum, and classification into subgroups, although useful, is somewhat arbitrary. Sequelae of the acute event depend primarily on the mass and type of cardiac tissue infarcted.

Myocardial dysfunction: Ischemic (but not infarcted) tissue has impaired contractility, resulting in hypokinetic or akinetic segments; these segments may expand or bulge during systole (called paradoxical motion). The size of the affected area determines effects, which range from minimal to mild heart failure to cardiogenic shock. Some degree of heart failure occurs in about ⅔ of hospitalized patients with acute MI. It is termed ischemic cardiomyopathy if low cardiac output and heart failure persist. Ischemia involving the papillary muscle may lead to mitral valve regurgitation.

MI: MI is myocardial necrosis resulting from abrupt reduction in coronary blood flow to part of the myocardium. Infarcted tissue is permanently dysfunctional; however, there is a zone of potentially reversible ischemia adjacent to infarcted tissue.

MI affects predominantly the LV, but damage may extend into the right ventricle (RV) or the atria. RV infarction usually results from obstruction of the right coronary or a dominant left circumflex artery; it is characterized by high RV filling pressure, often with severe tricuspid regurgitation and reduced cardiac output. An inferoposterior infarction causes some degree of RV dysfunction in about ½ of patients and produces hemodynamic abnormality in 10 to 15%. RV dysfunction should be considered in any patient who has inferoposterior infarction and elevated jugular venous pressure with hypotension or shock. RV infarction complicating LV infarction may significantly increase mortality risk.

Anterior infarcts tend to be larger and result in a worse prognosis than inferoposterior infarcts. They are usually due to left coronary artery obstruction, especially in the anterior descending artery; inferoposterior infarcts reflect right coronary or dominant left circumflex artery obstruction.

Transmural infarcts involve the whole thickness of myocardium from epicardium to endocardium and are usually characterized by abnormal Q waves on ECG. Nontransmural or subendocardial infarcts do not extend through the ventricular wall and cause only ST-segment and T-wave (ST-T) abnormalities. Subendocardial infarcts usually involve the inner ⅓ of myocardium, where wall tension is highest and myocardial blood flow is most vulnerable to circulatory changes. These infarcts may follow prolonged hypotension. Because the transmural depth of necrosis cannot be precisely determined clinically, infarcts are usually classified by the presence or absence of ST-segment elevation or Q waves on the ECG. Volume of myocardium destroyed can be roughly estimated by the extent and duration of CK elevation.

Electrical dysfunction: Ischemic and necrotic cells are incapable of normal electrical activity, resulting in various ECG changes (predominantly ST-T abnormalities), arrhythmias, and conduction disturbances. ST-T abnormalities of ischemia include ST-segment depression (often downsloping from the J point), T-wave inversion, ST-segment elevation (often referred to as injury current), and peaked T waves in the hyperacute phase of infarction. Conduction disturbances can reflect damage to the sinus node, the atrioventricular (AV) node, or specialized conduction tissues. Most changes are transient; some are permanent.

Classification

Classification is based on ECG changes and presence or absence of cardiac markers in blood. Distinguishing NSTEMI and STEMI is useful because prognosis and treatment are different.

Unstable angina (acute coronary insufficiency, preinfarction angina, intermediate syndrome) is defined as

- Rest angina that is prolonged (usually > 20 min)
- New-onset angina of at least Canadian Cardiovascular Society (CCS) class III severity
- Increasing angina; previously diagnosed angina that has become distinctly more frequent, more severe, longer in duration, or lower in threshold (eg, increased by ≥ 1 CCS class or to at least CCS class III)

Also, ECG changes such as ST-segment depression, ST-segment elevation, or T-wave inversion may occur during unstable angina but are transient. Of cardiac markers, CPK is not elevated but troponin-I may be slightly increased. Unstable angina is clinically unstable and a prelude often to MI or arrhythmias or, less commonly, to sudden death.

Non-ST-segment elevation MI (NSTEMI, subendocardial MI) is myocardial necrosis (evidenced by cardiac markers in blood) without acute ST-segment elevation or Q waves. ECG changes such as ST-segment depression, T-wave inversion, or both may be present.

ST-segment elevation MI (STEMI, transmural MI) is myocardial necrosis with ECG changes showing ST-segment elevation that is not quickly reversed by nitroglycerin or showing new left bundle branch block. Q waves may be present.

Symptoms and Signs

Symptoms of ACS depend somewhat on the extent and location of obstruction and are quite variable. Except when infarction is massive, recognizing the amount of ischemia by symptoms alone is difficult.

After the acute event, many complications can occur. They usually involve electrical dysfunction (eg, conduction defects, arrhythmias), myocardial dysfunction (eg, heart failure, interventricular septum or free wall rupture, ventricular aneurysm, pseudoaneurysm, cardiogenic shock), or valvular dysfunction (typically mitral regurgitation). Electrical dysfunction can be significant in any form of ACS, but usually, large parts of myocardium must be ischemic to cause significant myocardial dysfunction. Other complications of ACS include recurrent ischemia, mural thrombosis, pericarditis, and post-MI syndrome (Dressler's syndrome).

Unstable angina: Symptoms are those of angina pectoris (see p. 628), except that the pain or discomfort of unstable angina usually is more intense, lasts longer, is precipitated by less exertion, occurs spontaneously at rest (as angina decubitus), is progressive (crescendo) in nature, or involves any combination of these features.

NSTEMI and STEMI: Symptoms of NSTEMI and STEMI are the same. Days to weeks before the event, about ⅔ of patients experience prodromal symptoms, including unstable or crescendo angina, shortness of breath, and fatigue. Usually, the first symptom of infarction is deep, substernal, visceral pain described as aching or pressure, often radiating to the back, jaw, left arm, right arm, shoulders, or all of these areas. The pain is similar to angina pectoris but is usually more severe and long-lasting; more often accompanied by dyspnea, diaphoresis, nausea, and vomiting; and relieved little or only temporarily by rest or nitroglycerin. However, discomfort may be mild; about 20% of acute MIs are silent (ie, asymptomatic or producing vague symptoms not recognized as illness by the patient) more commonly in diabetics. Some patients present with syncope. Patients often interpret their discomfort as indigestion, particularly because spontaneous relief may be falsely attributed to belching or antacid consumption. Women are more likely to present with atypical chest discomfort. Elderly patients may report dyspnea more than ischemic-type chest pain. In severe ischemic episodes, the patient often has significant pain and feels restless and apprehensive. Nausea and vomiting may occur, especially with inferior MI. Dyspnea and weakness due to LV failure, pulmonary edema, shock, or significant arrhythmia may dominate.

Skin may be pale, cool, and diaphoretic. Peripheral or central cyanosis may be present. Pulse may be thready, and BP is variable, although many patients initially have some degree of hypertension during pain.

Heart sounds are usually somewhat distant; a 4th heart sound is almost universally present. A soft systolic blowing apical murmur (reflecting papillary muscle dysfunction) may occur. During initial examination, a friction rub or more striking murmurs suggest a preexisting heart disorder or another diagnosis. Detection of a friction rub within a few hours after onset of MI symptoms suggests acute pericarditis rather than MI. However, friction rubs, usually evanescent, are common on days 2 and 3 post-STEMI. The chest wall is tender when palpated in about 15% of patients.

In RV infarction, signs include elevated RV filling pressure, distended jugular veins (often with Kussmaul's sign—see p. 574), clear lung fields, and hypotension.

Diagnosis

ACS should be considered in men > 30 yr and women > 40 yr (younger in diabetics) whose main symptom is chest pain or discomfort. Pain must be differentiated from the pain of pneumonia, pulmonary embolism, pericarditis, rib fracture, costochondral separation, esophageal spasm, acute aortic dissection, renal calculus, splenic infarction, or various abdominal disorders (see Chest Pain on p. 580). In patients with previously diagnosed hiatus hernia, peptic ulcer, or a gallbladder disorder, the clinician must be wary of attributing new symptoms to these disorders.

The approach is the same when any ACS is suspected: initial and serial ECG and serial cardiac marker measurements, which distinguish among unstable angina, NSTEMI, and STEMI. Every emergency department should have a triage system to immediately identify patients with chest pain for rapid assessment and ECG. Pulse oximetry and chest x-ray (particularly to look for mediastinal widening, which suggests aortic dissection) is also done.

ECG: ECG is the most important test and should be done within 10 min of presentation. It is the center of the decision pathway because fibrinolytics benefit patients with STEMI but may increase risk for those with NSTEMI.

For STEMI, initial ECG is usually diagnostic, showing ST-segment elevation ≥ 1 mm in 2 or more contiguous leads subtending the damaged area (see FIGS. 73–1 to 73–6). Pathologic Q waves are not necessary for the diagnosis. The ECG must be read carefully because ST-segment elevation may be subtle, particularly in the inferior leads (II, III, aVF); sometimes the reader's attention is mistakenly focused on leads with ST-segment depression. If symptoms are characteristic, ST-segment elevation on ECG has a specificity of 90% and a sensitivity of 45% for diagnosing MI. Serial tracings (obtained q 8 h for 1 day, then daily) showing a gradual evolution toward a stable, more normal pattern or development of abnormal Q waves over a few days tends to confirm the diagnosis.

Because nontransmural (non–Q-wave) infarcts are usually in the subendocardial or midmyocardial layers, they do not produce diagnostic Q waves or distinct ST-segment elevation on the ECG. Instead, they commonly produce only varying degrees of ST-T abnormalities that are less striking, variable, or nonspecific and sometimes difficult to interpret (NSTEMI). If such abnormalities resolve (or worsen) on repeat ECGs, ischemia is very likely. However, when repeat ECGs are unchanged, acute MI is unlikely and, if still suspected clinically, requires other evidence to make the diagnosis. A normal ECG taken when a patient is painfree does not rule out unstable angina; a normal ECG taken during pain, although it does not rule out angina, suggests that the pain is not ischemic.

If RV infarction is suspected, a 15-lead ECG is usually recorded; additional leads are placed at V_4R, and, to detect posterior infarction, V_8 and V_9.

ECG diagnosis of MI is more difficult when a left bundle branch block configuration is present because it resembles STEMI changes. ST-segment elevation concordant with the QRS complex strongly suggests MI as does > 5-mm ST-segment elevation in at least 2 precordial leads. But generally, any patient with suspect symptoms and new-onset (or not known to be old) left bundle branch block is treated as for STEMI.

Cardiac markers: Cardiac markers are cardiac enzymes (eg, CPK-MB) and cell contents (eg, troponin I, troponin T, myoglobin) that are released into the bloodstream after myocardial cell necrosis. The markers appear at different times after injury and decrease at different rates (see FIG. 73–7). Usually, several different markers are measured at regular intervals, typically q 6 to 8 h for 1 day. Newer bedside tests, which are more convenient, can be just as sensitive when done at shorter intervals (eg, time 0, 1, 3, and 6 h after presentation).

Troponins are most specific for MI but can also be elevated by ischemia without infarction; elevated levels (actual number varies with assay used) are considered diagnostic. Borderline elevated troponin levels in patients with unstable angina indicate increased risk of adverse events and thus the need for further evaluation and treatment. False positives sometimes occur in heart failure and renal failure. CPK-MB is slightly less specific. False positives occur with renal failure, hypothyroidism, and skeletal muscle injury. Myoglobin is not specific for MI but, because it increases earlier than other markers, may be an early warning sign to assist in triage of patients with nondiagnostic ECGs.

Other tests: Routine laboratory tests are nondiagnostic but, if obtained, show nonspecific abnormalities compatible with tissue necrosis (eg, increased ESR, moderately elevated WBC with a shift to the left).

Myocardial imaging (see also p. 597) is not needed to make the diagnosis if cardiac markers or ECG is positive. However, in patients with MI, bedside echocardiography is invaluable for detecting mechanical complications. Before or shortly after discharge, patients with symptoms suggesting an ACS but nondiagnostic ECGs and normal cardiac markers should have a stress imaging test (radionuclide or echocardiographic imaging with pharmacologic or exercise stress). Imaging abnormalities in such patients indicate increased risk of complications in the next 3 to 6 mo.

Right heart catheterization using a balloon-tipped pulmonary artery catheter (see p. 513) can be used to measure right heart, pulmonary artery, and pulmonary artery occlusion pressures and cardiac output. This test is usually done only if patients have significant complications (eg, severe heart failure, hypoxia, hypotension).

Coronary angiography most often combines diagnosis with treatment (eg, angioplasty, stenting). However, it may be used diagnostically in patients with evidence of ongoing ischemia (ECG findings or symptoms), hemodynamic instability, recurrent ventricular tachyarrhythmias, and other abnormalities that suggest recurrence of ischemic events.

Prognosis

Unstable angina: About 30% of patients with unstable angina have an MI within 3 mo of onset; sudden death is less common. Marked ECG changes with chest pain indicate higher risk of subsequent MI or death.

NSTEMI and STEMI: Overall mortality rate is about 30%, with 50 to 60% of these patients dying before reaching the hospital (typically due to ventricular fibrillation). In-hospital mortality rate is about 10% (typically due to cardiogenic shock) but varies significantly with severity of LV failure (see TABLE 73–3). Most patients who die of cardiogenic shock have an infarct or a combination of scar and new infarct affecting ≥ 50% of LV mass. Five clinical characteristics predict 90% of the mortality in patients who present with STEMI (see TABLE 73–4): older age (31% of total mortality), lower systolic BP (24%), Killip class > 1 (15%), faster heart rate (12%), and anterior location (6%). Mortality rate of diabetics and women tends to be higher.

Mortality rate of patients who survive initial hospitalization is 8 to 10% in the year after acute MI. Most fatalities occur in the first 3 to 4 mo. Persistent ventricular arrhythmia, heart failure, poor ventricular function, and recurrent ischemia indicate high risk. Many authorities recommend stress ECG before hospital discharge or within 6 wk. Good exercise performance without ECG abnormalities is associated with a favorable prognosis; further evaluation is usually not required. Poor exercise performance is associated with a poor prognosis.

Cardiac performance after recovery depends largely on how much functioning myocardium survives the acute attack. Scars from previous infarcts add to the acute damage. When > 50% of LV mass is damaged, prolonged survival is unusual.

General Treatment

Treatment is designed to relieve distress, reverse ischemia, limit infarct size, reduce cardiac workload, and prevent and treat complications. An ACS is a medical emergency; outcome is greatly influenced by rapid diagnosis and treatment.

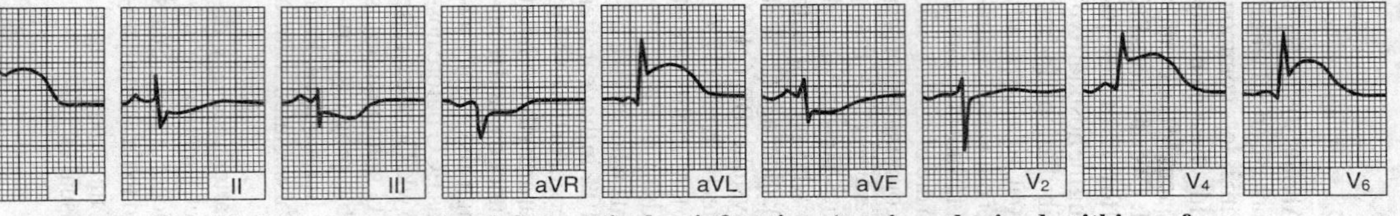

Fig. 73–1. Acute anterior left ventricular infarction (tracing obtained within a few hours of onset of illness). There is striking hyperacute ST-segment elevation in leads I, aVL, V_4, and V_6 and reciprocal depression in other leads.

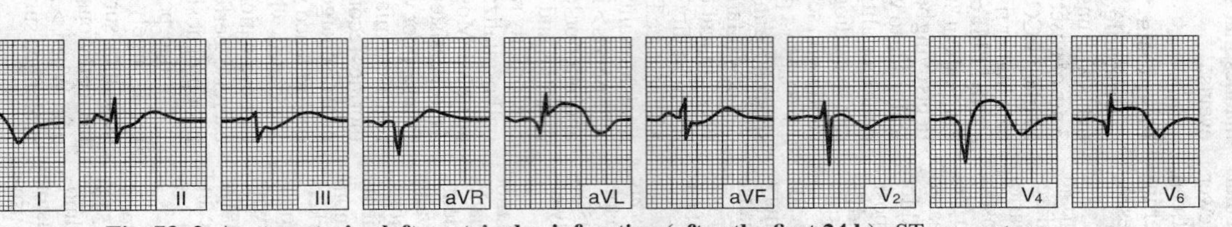

Fig. 73–2. Acute anterior left ventricular infarction (after the first 24 h). ST segments are less elevated; significant Q waves develop and R waves are lost in leads I, aVL, V_4, and V_6.

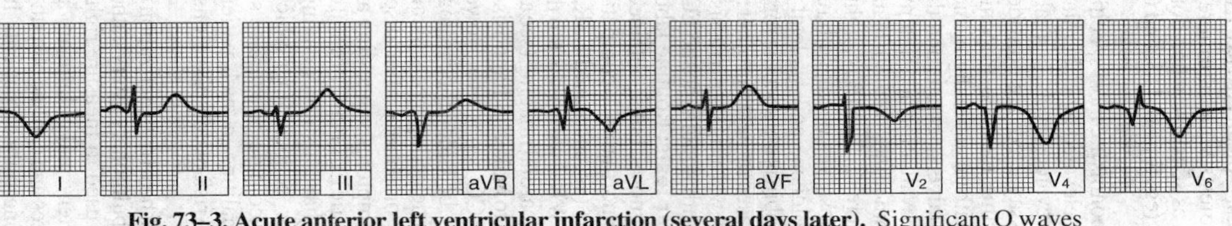

Fig. 73–3. Acute anterior left ventricular infarction (several days later). Significant Q waves and loss of R-wave voltage persist. ST segments are now essentially isoelectric. The ECG will probably change only slowly over the next several months.

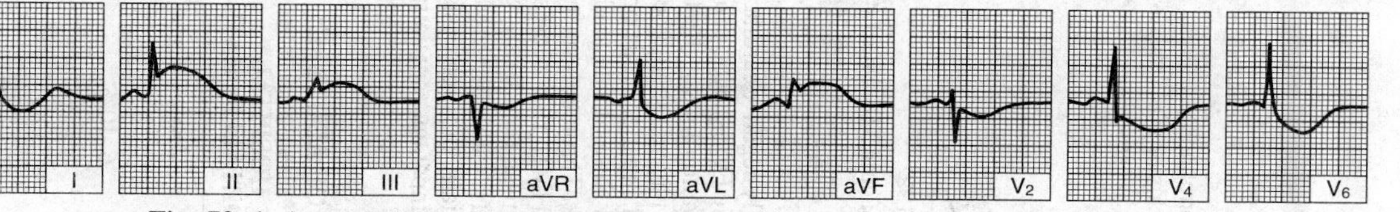

Fig. 73–4. Acute inferior diaphragmatic left ventricular infarction (tracing obtained within a few hours of onset of illness). There is hyperacute ST-segment elevation in leads II, III, and aVF and reciprocal depression in other leads.

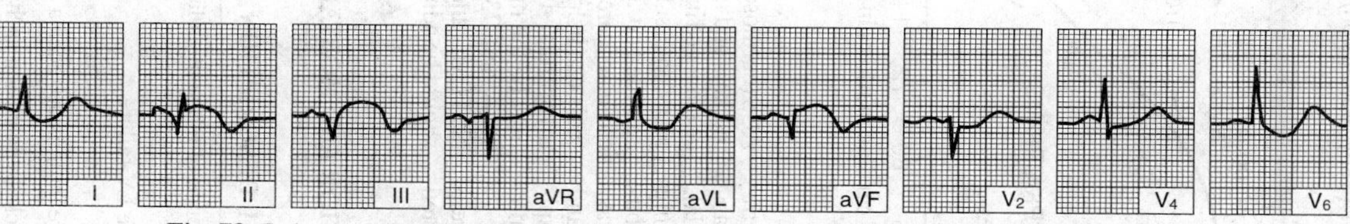

Fig. 73–5. Acute inferior diaphragmatic left ventricular infarction (after the first 24 h). Significant Q waves develop with decreasing ST-segment elevation in leads II, III, and aVF.

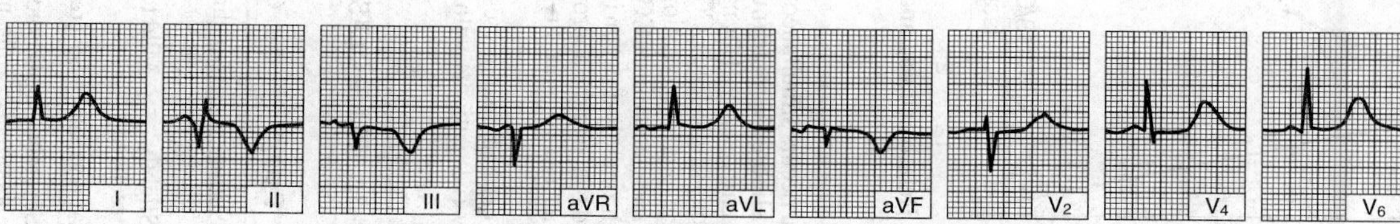

Fig. 73–6. Acute inferior diaphragmatic left ventricular infarction (several days later). ST segments are now isoelectric. Abnormal Q waves in leads II, III, and aVF indicate that myocardial scars persist.

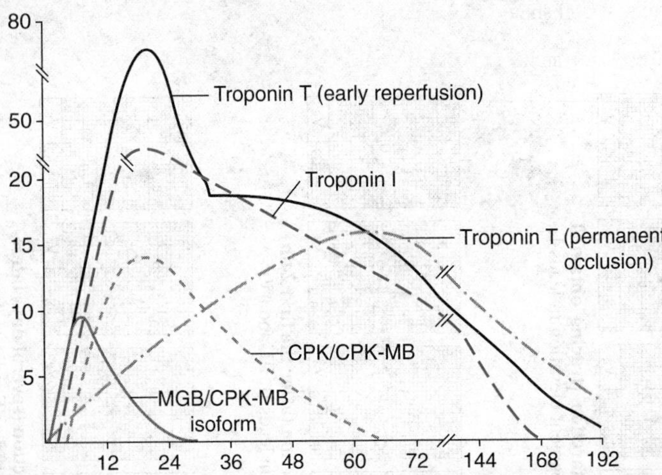

Fig. 73–7. Relative timing and levels of cardiac markers in blood after acute MI. MGB = myoglobulin.

Treatment occurs simultaneously with diagnosis. A reliable IV route must be established, O_2 given (typically 2 L by nasal cannula), and continuous single-lead ECG monitoring started. Prehospital interventions by ambulance personnel (including ECG, chewed aspirin, early thrombolysis when indicated and possible, and triage to the appropriate hospital) can reduce risk of mortality and complications.

Bedside cardiac marker tests can help identify low-risk patients with a suspected ACS (eg, those with initially negative cardiac markers and nondiagnostic ECGs), who can be managed in 24-h observation units or chest pain centers. Higher-risk patients should be admitted to a monitored inpatient unit or coronary care unit (CCU). Several validated tools can help stratify risk. Thrombolysis in myocardial infarction (TIMI) risk scores may be the most widely used (see TABLES 73–4 and 73–5). Patients with suspected NSTEMI and intermediate or high risk should be admitted to an inpatient care unit.

TABLE 73–3. KILLIP CLASSIFICATION AND MORTALITY RATE OF ACUTE MI*

CLASS	PAO_2†	CLINICAL DESCRIPTION	HOSPITAL MORTALITY RATE
1	Normal	No clinical evidence of left ventricular (LV) failure	3–5%
2	Slightly reduced	Mild to moderate LV failure	6–10%
3	Abnormal	Severe LV failure, pulmonary edema	20–30%
4	Severely abnormal	Cardiogenic shock: hypotension, tachycardia, mental obtundation, cool extremities, oliguria, hypoxia	> 80%

*Determined by repeated examination of the patient during the course of illness.
†Determined while the patient is breathing room air.

Modified from Killip T, Kimball JT: Treatment of myocardial infarction in a coronary care unit. A two-year experience with 250 patients. *The American Journal of Cardiology* 20:457–464, 1967.

Those with STEMI should be admitted to a CCU.

Only heart rate and rhythm recorded by single-lead ECG are consistently useful for routine, continuous monitoring. However, some clinicians recommend routine multilead monitoring with continuous ST-segment recording to identify transient, recurrent ST-segment elevations or depressions. Such findings, even in patients without symptoms, suggest ischemia and identify higher-risk patients who may require more aggressive evaluation and treatment.

Qualified nurses can interpret the ECG for arrhythmia and initiate protocols for its treatment. All staff members should know how to do CPR.

Contributing disorders (eg, anemia, heart failure) are aggressively treated.

The care unit should be a quiet, calm, restful area. Single rooms are preferred; privacy consistent with monitoring should be ensured. Usually, visitors and telephone calls are restricted to family members during the first few days. A wall clock, a calendar, and an outside window help orient the patient and prevent a sense of isolation, as can access to a radio, television, and newspaper.

Bed rest is mandatory for the first 24 h. On day 1, patients without complications (eg, hemodynamic instability, ongoing ischemia), including those in whom reperfusion with fibrinolytics or PCI is successful, can sit in a chair, begin passive exercises, and use a commode. Walking to the bathroom and doing nonstressful paperwork is allowed shortly thereafter. If reperfusion is not successful or complications are present, patients require bed rest longer, but they (particularly elderly patients) are mobilized as soon as possible. Prolonged bed rest results in rapid physical deconditioning, with development of orthostatic hypotension, decreased work capacity, increased heart rate during exertion, and increased risk of deep venous thrombosis. Prolonged bed rest also intensifies feelings of depression and helplessness.

Anxiety, mood changes, and denial are common. A mild tranquilizer (usually a benzodiazepine) is often given, but many experts believe such drugs are rarely needed.

Depression is common by the 3rd day of illness and is almost universal at some time during recovery. After the acute phase of illness, the most important tasks are often management of depression, rehabilitation, and institution of long-term preventive programs.

TABLE 73–4. MORTALITY RISK AT 30 DAYS IN STEMI

Scoring

RISK FACTOR	POINTS
Age ≥ 75	3
Age 65–74	2
Diabetes mellitus, hypertension, or angina	1
Systolic BP < 100 mm Hg	3
Heart rate > 100 beat/min	2
Killip class II–IV	2
Weight < 67 kg	1
Anterior ST-elevation or left branch bundle block	1
Time to treatment > 4 h	1
Total points possible	**0–14**

Risk

TOTAL POINTS	MORTALITY RATE AT 30 DAYS (%)
0	0.8
1	1.6
2	2.2
3	4.4
4	7.3
5	12.4
6	16.1
7	23.4
8	26.8
> 8	35.9

STEMI = ST-segment elevation MI.

Based on data from Morrow DA et al: TIMI risk score for ST-elevation myocardial infarction: a convenient, bedside, clinical score for risk assessment at presentation. *Circulation* 102 (17):2031–2037, 2000 and ACC/AHA guidelines for the management of patients with acute myocardial infarction.

Overemphasis on bed rest, inactivity, and the seriousness of the disorder reinforces depressive tendencies, so patients are encouraged to sit up, get out of bed, and engage in appropriate activities as soon as possible. The effects of the disorder, prognosis, and individualized

TABLE 73–5. RISK OF ADVERSE EVENTS* AT 14 DAYS IN NSTEMI

Scoring

RISK FACTOR	POINTS
Age > 65	1
CAD risk factors (must have ≥ 3 for 1 point) Family history Hypertension Current smoker High cholesterol Diabetes mellitus	1
Known CAD (stenosis ≥ 50%)	1
Previous chronic use of aspirin	1
Two episodes of rest angina in past 24 h	1
Elevated cardiac markers	1

Risk level is based on total points: 1–2 = low; 3–4 = intermediate; 5–7 = high.

Absolute Risk

TOTAL POINTS	RISK OF EVENTS AT 14 DAYS (%)*
0 or 1	4.7
2	8.3
3	13.2
4	19.9
5	26.2
6 or 7	40.9

*Events include all-cause mortality, MI, and recurrent ischemia requiring urgent revascularization.

NSTEMI = non-ST-segment elevation MI.

Based on data from Antman EM et al: The TIMI risk score for unstable angina/non-ST elevation MI: A method of prognostication and therapeutic decision making. *JAMA* 284:835–42, 2000.

rehabilitation program should be explained to the patient.

Maintaining normal bowel function with stool softeners (eg, bisacodyl) to prevent straining is important. Urinary retention is common among elderly patients, especially after several days of bed rest or if atropine was given. A catheter may be required but can usually be removed when the patient can stand or sit to void.

Because smoking is prohibited, a hospital stay may encourage smoking cessation. All caregivers should devote considerable effort to making smoking cessation permanent.

Although acutely ill patients have little appetite, tasty food in modest amounts is good for morale. Patients are usually offered a soft diet of 1500 to 1800 kcal/day with Na reduction to 2 to 3 g. Na reduction is not required after the first 2 or 3 days if there is no evidence of heart failure. Patients are given a diet low in cholesterol and saturated fats, which is used to teach healthy eating.

Because the chest pain of MI usually subsides within 12 to 24 h, any chest pain that remains or recurs later is investigated. It may indicate such complications as recurrent ischemia, pericarditis, pulmonary embolism, pneumonia, gastritis, or ulcer.

Drugs

Antiplatelet and antithrombotic drugs, which stop clots from forming, are used routinely. Anti-ischemic drugs (eg, β-blockers, IV nitroglycerin) are frequently added, particularly when chest pain or hypertension is present (see TABLE 73–2). Fibrinolytics (see TABLE 73–6) are sometimes used for STEMI but worsen outcome for unstable angina or NSTEMI.

Chest pain can be treated with morphine or nitroglycerin. Morphine 2 to 4 mg IV, repeated q 15 min as needed, is highly effective but can depress respiration, can reduce myocardial contractility, and is a potent venous vasodilator. Hypotension and bradycardia secondary to morphine can usually be overcome by prompt elevation of the lower extremities. Nitroglycerin is initially given sublingually, followed by continuous IV drip if needed.

BP is normal or slightly elevated in most patients on arrival at the emergency department; BP gradually falls over the next several hours. Continued hypertension requires treatment with antihypertensives, preferably IV nitroglycerin, to lower BP and reduce cardiac workload. Severe hypotension or other signs of shock are ominous and must be treated aggressively with IV fluids and sometimes vasopressors (see p. 562).

Antiplatelet drugs: Aspirin, clopidogrel, ticlopidine, and glycoprotein (GP) IIb/IIIa inhibitors are examples. All patients are given aspirin 160 to 325 mg (not enteric-coated), if not contraindicated, at presentation and

81 mg once/day indefinitely thereafter. Chewing the first dose before swallowing quickens absorption. Aspirin reduces short- and long-term mortality risk. If aspirin cannot be taken, clopidogrel 75 mg once/day or ticlopidine 250 mg bid may be used. Clopidogrel has largely replaced ticlopidine for routine use because neutropenia is a risk with ticlopidine and WBC must be monitored regularly. In patients with unstable angina or NSTEMI for whom an early noninterventional approach is planned, both aspirin and clopidogrel are given for at least 1 mo.

GP IIb/IIIa inhibitors (abciximab, tirofiban, eptifibatide) are potent antiplatelet drugs that must be given IV. They are most commonly used with PCI, particularly when a stent has been placed; results appear to be better if the drugs are initiated at least 6 h before PCI. If PCI is not being done, a GP IIb/IIIa inhibitor

TABLE 73–6. IV FIBRINOLYTIC DRUGS AVAILABLE IN THE US

CHARACTERISTIC	STREPTOKINASE	ANISTREPLASE	ALTEPLASE	RETEPLASE	TENECTEPLASE
Dosage (IV)	1.5×10^6 U over 30–60 min	30 mg over 5 min	15 mg bolus, then 0.75 mg/kg over next 30 min (maximum 50 mg), followed by 0.50 mg/kg over 60 min (maximum 35 mg) for total dose of 100 mg	10 units in 2-min bolus repeated once after 30 min	Weight-adjusted single bolus over 5 sec < 60 kg: 30 mg 60–69 kg: 35 mg 70–79 kg: 40 mg 80–89 kg: 45 mg ≥ 90 kg: 50 mg
Circulating half-life (min)	20	100	6	13–16	Initial half-life of 20–24 min; terminal phase half-life of 90–130 min
Concurrent heparin	No	No	Yes	Yes	Yes
Allergic reactions	Yes	Yes	Rare	Rare	Rare
Systemic fibrinogen depletion	Severe	Severe	Moderate	Moderate	Moderate
Intracerebral hemorrhage rate	≈ 0.3%	≈ 0.6%	≈ 0.6%	≈ 0.8%	0.5–0.7%
Recanalization rate, 90 min	≈ 40%	≈ 63%	≈ 79%	≈ 80%	≈ 80%
Lives saved per 100 treated	≈ 2.5	≈ 2.5	≈ 3.5	≈ 3.0	≈ 3.5
Cost per dose	Least expensive	Expensive	Most expensive	Most expensive	Most expensive

Adapted from ACC/AHA guidelines for the management of patients with acute myocardial infarction. *Journal of American College of Cardiology* 28:1328–1419, 1996.

is given to high-risk patients, especially those with elevated cardiac markers, symptoms that persist despite adequate drug therapy, or both. The GP IIb/IIIa inhibitor is continued for 24 to 36 h, and angiography is done before the infusion period is over. Routine use of GP IIb/IIIa inhibitors with fibrinolytics is not recommended at this time.

Antithrombotic drugs: Either a low mol wt heparin (LMWH) or unfractionated heparin is given routinely unless contraindicated (eg, by active bleeding or use of streptokinase or anistreplase). For unstable angina and NSTEMI, either drug can be used. For STEMI, choice of drug depends on mode of reperfusion. If unfractionated heparin is used, activated PTT (aPTT) is monitored at 6 h, then q 6 h thereafter until it is 1.5 to 2 times the control value; with LMWH, measurement of aPTT is unnecessary.

Enoxaparin is the LMWH of choice; it is most effective when started at admission. Nadroparin and dalteparin are also effective. The usefulness of hirudin and bivalirudin, new direct antithrombotic drugs, requires further clinical study.

β-Blockers: These drugs are recommended unless contraindicated (eg, by bradycardia, heart block, hypotension, or asthma), especially for high-risk patients. β-Blockers reduce heart rate, arterial pressure, and contractility, thereby reducing cardiac workload and O_2 demand. IV β-blockers given within the first few hours improve prognosis by reducing infarct size, recurrence rate, incidence of ventricular fibrillation, and mortality risk. Infarct size largely determines cardiac performance after recovery.

Heart rate and BP must be carefully monitored during treatment with β-blockers. Dosage is reduced if bradycardia or hypotension develops. Excessive adverse effects may be reversed by infusion of the β-adrenergic agonist isoproterenol 1 to 5 μg/min.

Nitrates: A short-acting nitrate, nitroglycerin, is used to reduce cardiac workload in selected patients. Nitroglycerin dilates veins, arteries, and arterioles, reducing LV preload and afterload. As a result, myocardial O_2 demand is reduced, lessening ischemia. IV nitroglycerin is recommended during the first 24 to 48 h for patients with heart failure, large anterior MI, persistent chest discomfort, or hypertension. BP can be reduced by 10 to 20 mm Hg but not to < 80 to 90 mm Hg systolic. Longer use may benefit patients with recurrent chest pain or persistent pulmonary congestion. In high-risk patients, nitroglycerin given in the first few hours reduces infarct size and short-term and possibly long-term mortality risk. Nitroglycerin is not routinely given to low-risk patients with uncomplicated MI.

Other drugs: ACE inhibitors appear to reduce mortality risk in MI patients, especially in those with anterior infarction, heart failure, or tachycardia. The greatest benefit occurs in the highest-risk patients early during convalescence. ACE inhibitors are given > 24 h after thrombolysis stabilization and, because of continued beneficial effect, may be prescribed long-term.

Angiotensin II receptor blockers may be an effective alternative for patients who cannot tolerate ACE inhibitors (eg, because of cough). Currently, they are not 1st-line treatment after MI. Contraindications include hypotension, renal failure, bilateral renal artery stenosis, and known allergy.

Treatment of Unstable Angina and NSTEMI

Drugs are given as described above. Either LMWH or unfractionated heparin can be used. In selected patients, PCI (or sometimes CABG) may also be used. Fibrinolytics are not indicated for unstable angina or NSTEMI. Risk outweighs potential benefit.

PCI: Emergency PCI is not routinely indicated for unstable angina or NSTEMI. However, early angiography with PCI (within 72 h of admission if possible) is indicated for high-risk patients (see TABLE 73–4), particularly for those with hemodynamic instability, markedly elevated cardiac markers, or both and for those who have symptoms despite maximal drug therapy. This approach improves outcome, particularly when GP IIb/IIIa inhibitors are also used. For intermediate-risk patients and for those who have evidence of continuing myocardial ischemia, early angiography is indicated to identify the causative lesion and to evaluate the extent of other lesions and LV function. Thus, the potential benefit of PCI or CABG can be determined.

Treatment of STEMI

Aspirin, β-blockers, and nitrates are given as described above. Heparin or LMWH is almost always used; choice of drug depends on mode of reperfusion.

In STEMI, rapidly restoring blood flow to the affected myocardium by PCI or fibrinolytics dramatically reduces mortality risk.

Emergency CABG may be best for about 3 to 5% of patients who have complex coronary anatomy (noted during emergency angiography). CABG must also be considered when PCI is unsuccessful or cannot be used (eg, in acute coronary artery dissection). Done by experienced surgeons, CABG for acute STEMI has about a 4 to 12% mortality and a 20 to 43% morbidity rate.

PCI: If done within 3 h of MI onset by experienced personnel, PCI is more effective than fibrinolytics and is the preferred mode of reperfusion. However, if PCI is not available within that interval or is contraindicated, an IV fibrinolytic drug is used. In facilitated PCI, a patient is given a fibrinolytic before PCI. The precise time window in which fibrinolytic should be given before PCI is not yet known.

Indications for doing PCI later include hemodynamic instability, contraindications to fibrinolytics, malignant arrhythmias requiring or pending transvenous pacing or requiring repeated cardioversion, and age > 75. PCI should be considered after fibrinolytics if chest pain or ST-segment elevation persists ≥ 60 min after initiation of fibrinolytics or if pain and ST-segment elevation recur, but only if PCI can be initiated < 90 min after onset of recurrence. If PCI is unavailable, fibrinolytics can be repeated.

After PCI, especially if a stent is used, adjunctive therapy with abciximab (the preferred GP IIb/IIIa inhibitor) is begun and continued for 18 to 24 h thereafter.

Fibrinolytics (thrombolytics): Reperfusion using fibrinolytics is most effective if given in the first few minutes to hours after onset of MI. The earlier a fibrinolytic is begun, the better. The goal is a "door-to-needle" time of 30 to 60 min. Greatest benefit occurs within 3 h, but the drugs may be effective up to 12 h. Although controversial, prehospital use of fibrinolytics by trained paramedics can significantly reduce time to treatment; outcome is being evaluated. Used with aspirin, fibrinolytics reduce hospital mortality rate by 30 to 50% and improve ventricular function.

ECG criteria for fibrinolytics include ST-segment elevation in 2 or more contiguous leads, typical symptoms and left bundle branch block (not known to be old), and strictly posterior MI (a large R wave in V_1 and ST-segment depression in leads V_1–V_4, confirmed with a 15-lead ECG). A few patients present in the hyperacute phase of MI with giant T waves. This finding does not meet current criteria for fibrinolytics; ECG is repeated in 20 to 30 min to see if ST-segment elevation has developed.

Absolute contraindications to fibrinolytics include aortic dissection, pericarditis, previous hemorrhagic stroke (at any time), previous ischemic stroke within 1 yr, active internal bleeding (not menses), and intracranial tumor. Relative contraindications include blood pressure > 180/110 mm Hg (after initial antihypertensive therapy), trauma or major surgery within 4 wk, active peptic ulcer, pregnancy, bleeding diathesis, noncompressible vascular punctures, and current anticoagulation (INR > 2). Patients who previously received streptokinase or anistreplase are not given that drug.

Tenecteplase (TNK), alteplase (rTPA), reteplase (rPA), streptokinase, and anistreplase (anisoylated plasminogen activator complex—APSAC), all given IV, are plasminogen activators. They convert single chain plasminogen to double chain plasminogen, which has fibrinolytic activity. They have different characteristics and dosing regimens (see TABLE 73–6).

Tenecteplase and reteplase are recommended most often because tenecteplase is given as a single bolus over 5 sec and reteplase as a double bolus. Administration time and drug errors are reduced compared with other fibrinolytics, which have a more complicated dosing regimen. Tenecteplase, like alteplase, has an intermediate risk of intracranial hemorrhage, has a higher rate of recanalization than other fibrinolytics, and is expensive. Reteplase has the highest risk of intracranial hemorrhage and a recanalization rate similar to that of tenecteplase, and it is expensive.

Streptokinase may induce allergic reactions, especially if it has been used previously, and must be given by infusion over 30 to 60 min; however, it has a low incidence of intracerebral hemorrhage and is relatively inexpensive. Anistreplase, related to streptokinase, is similarly allergenic and slightly more expensive but can be given as a single bolus. Neither requires concomitant heparin. For both, recanalization rate is lower than that with other plasminogen activators.

Alteplase is given in an accelerated or front-loaded dosage over 90 min. Alteplase with concomitant IV heparin improves patency, is nonallergenic, has a higher recanalization rate than other fibrinolytics, and is expensive.

Antithrombotic drugs: Unfractionated IV heparin or LMWH is given to all patients with STEMI unless streptokinase or anistreplase is given or other contraindications exist.

If heparin is used, aPTT is monitored at 6 h, then q 6 h thereafter until it is 1.5 to 2 times the control value; LMWH does not require measurement of aPTT. Antithrombotics may be continued > 72 h if patients are at high risk of thromboembolic events.

The LMWH enoxaparin used with tenecteplase appears to be as effective as unfractionated heparin and is cost-effective. Enoxaparin has not been adequately studied with alteplase, reteplase, or PCI. The first sc dose is given immediately after the IV dose; sc dosing is continued until revascularization is done or the patient is discharged. In patients > 75 yr, enoxaparin given with tenecteplase appears to increase risk of intracerebral bleeding. For these patients, unfractionated heparin in a weight-adjusted dose is preferred.

Use of IV heparin with streptokinase or anistreplase is not currently recommended. The potential advantages of sc heparin vs no antithrombotic drug are unclear. However, in patients at high risk of systemic emboli (ie, with large anterior MI, known LV thrombus, or atrial fibrillation [AF]), heparin IV reduces incidence of subsequent thromboembolic events.

Complications

Electrical dysfunction occurs in > 90% of MI patients (see also p. 673). Electrical dysfunction that commonly causes mortality in the first 72 h includes tachycardia (from any focus) rapid enough to reduce cardiac output and lower BP, Mobitz type II block (2nd degree) or complete (3rd degree) AV block, ventricular tachycardia (VT), and ventricular fibrillation (VF). Asystole is uncommon, except as a terminal manifestation of progressive LV failure and shock. Patients with disturbances of cardiac rhythm are checked for hypoxia and electrolyte abnormalities, which can be causative or contributory.

Sinus node disturbances: If the artery supplying the sinus node is affected, sinus node disturbances can occur; they are more likely if there is a preexisting sinus node disorder (common among the elderly). Sinus bradycardia, the most common sinus node disturbance, is usually not treated unless there is hypotension or the heart rate is < 50 beats/min. A lower heart rate, if not extreme, means reduced cardiac workload and possibly reduced infarct size. For bradycardia with hypotension (which may reduce myocardial perfusion), atropine sulfate 0.5 to 1 mg IV is used; it can be repeated after several minutes if response is inadequate. Several small doses are best because high doses may induce tachycardia. Occasionally, a temporary transvenous pacemaker must be inserted.

Persistent sinus tachycardia is usually ominous, often reflecting LV failure and low cardiac output. Without heart failure or another evident cause, this arrhythmia may respond to a β-blocker, given po or IV depending on degree of urgency.

Atrial arrhythmias: Atrial arrhythmias (atrial ectopic beats, AF, and, less commonly, atrial flutter) occur in about 10% of MI patients and may reflect LV failure or right atrial infarction. Paroxysmal atrial tachycardia is uncommon and usually occurs in patients who have had previous episodes of it. Atrial ectopy is usually benign, but if frequency increases, causes, particularly heart failure, are sought. Frequent atrial ectopic beats may respond to a β-blocker.

AF is usually transient if it occurs within the first 24 h. Risk factors include age > 70, heart failure, previous history of MI, large anterior infarct, atrial infarction, pericarditis, hypokalemia, hypomagnesemia, a chronic lung disorder, and hypoxia. Fibrinolytics reduce incidence. Recurrent paroxysmal AF is a poor prognostic sign and increases risk of systemic emboli.

For AF, heparin is usually used because systemic emboli are a risk (see p. 696). IV β-blockers (eg, atenolol 2.5 to 5.0 mg over 2 min to total dose of 10 mg in 10 to 15 min, metoprolol 2 to 5 mg q 2 to 5 min to a total dose of 15 mg in 10 to 15 min) slow the ventricular rate. Heart rate and BP are closely monitored. Treatment is withheld when ventricular rate decreases satisfactorily or systolic BP is < 100 mm Hg. IV digoxin, which is not as effective as β-blockers, is used cautiously and only in patients with AF and LV systolic dysfunction. Usually, digoxin takes at least 2 h to effectively slow heart rate. For patients without evident LV systolic dysfunction or conduction delay manifested by a wide QRS complex, IV verapamil or IV diltiazem may be considered. Diltiazem may be given as an IV infusion to control heart rate for long periods.

If AF compromises circulatory status (eg, causing LV failure, hypotension, or chest pain), urgent electrical cardioversion is done. If AF returns after cardioversion, IV amiodarone should be considered.

For atrial flutter, rate is controlled as for AF, but heparin is not required.

Conduction defects: Mobitz type I block (Wenckebach block, progressive prolongation of PR interval) is relatively common with an inferior-diaphragmatic infarction; it is usually self-limited and rarely progresses to higher grade block. Mobitz type II block (dropped beats) usually indicates massive anterior MI, as does complete heart block with wide QRS complexes (atrial impulses do not reach the ventricle); both are uncommon. Frequency of complete (3rd degree) AV block depends on site of infarction. Complete AV block occurs in 5 to 10% of patients with inferior infarction and is usually transient. It occurs in < 5% with uncomplicated anterior infarction but in up to 26% of those with right bundle branch block and left posterior hemiblock.

Mobitz type I block usually does not warrant treatment. For true Mobitz type II block with dropped beats or for AV block with slow, wide QRS complexes, temporary transvenous pacing is the treatment of choice. External pacing can be used until a temporary transvenous pacemaker can be placed. Although isoproterenol infusion may restore rhythm and rate temporarily, it is not used because it increases O_2 demand and risk of rhythm abnormalities. Atropine 0.5 mg q 3 to 5 min to a total dose of 2.5 mg may be useful for narrow-complex AV block with a slow ventricular rate but is not recommended for new wide-complex AV block.

Ventricular arrhythmias: These arrhythmias are common and may result from hypoxia, electrolyte imbalance (hypokalemia, possibly hypomagnesemia), or sympathetic overactivity in ischemic cells adjacent to infarcted tissue (which is not electrically active). Treatable causes of ventricular arrhythmias are sought and corrected. Serum K should be kept above 4.0 mEq/L. IV KCl is recommended; usually, 10 mEq/h can be infused, but for severe hypokalemia (K < 2.5 mEq/L), 20 to 40 mEq/h can be infused through a central venous line.

Ventricular ectopic beats, which are common after MI, do not warrant specific treatment.

Nonsustained VT (< 30 sec) and even sustained slow VT (accelerated idioventricular rhythm) without hemodynamic instability do not usually require treatment in the first 24 to 48 h. Polymorphic VT, sustained (≥ 30 sec) monomorphic VT, or any VT with symptoms of instability (eg, heart failure, hypotension, chest pain) is treated with synchronized cardioversion. VT without hemodynamic instability may be treated with IV lidocaine, procainamide, or amiodarone. Some clinicians also treat complex ventricular arrhythmias with Mg sulfate 2 g IV over 5 min whether or not serum Mg is low. VT may occur months after MI. Late VT is more likely to occur in patients with transmural infarction and to be sustained.

VF occurs in 5 to 12% of patients during the first 24 h after MI, usually within 6 h. Late VF usually indicates continued or recurrent myocardial ischemia and, when accompanied by hemodynamic deterioration, is a poor prognostic sign. VF is treated with immediate unsynchronized cardioversion (see p. 538).

An IV β-blocker early in MI followed by continued oral β-blockers reduces the incidence of ventricular arrhythmias (including VF) and mortality in patients who do not have heart failure or hypotension. Prophylaxis with other drugs (eg, lidocaine) increases mortality risk and is not recommended.

After the acute phase, the presence of complex ventricular arrhythmias or nonsustained VT, especially with significant LV systolic dysfunction, increases mortality risk. An implantable cardioverter-defibrillator (ICD) should be considered. Programmed endocardial stimulation can help select the most effective antiarrhythmics or determine the need for an ICD. Before treatment with an antiarrhythmic or ICD, coronary angiography and other tests are done to look for recurrent myocardial ischemia, which may require PCI or CABG.

Heart failure: Patients with large infarctions (by ECG or serum markers) and those with mechanical complications, hypertension, or diastolic dysfunction are more likely to develop heart failure. Clinical findings depend on infarct size, elevation of LV filling pressure, and degree of reduction in cardiac output. Dyspnea, inspiratory rales at the lung bases, and hypoxemia are common.

Treatment depends on severity. For mild cases, a loop diuretic (eg, furosemide 20 to 40 mg IV once/day or bid) to reduce ventricular filling pressure is often sufficient. For severe cases, vasodilators (eg, IV nitroglycerin) are often used to reduce preload and afterload; during treatment, pulmonary artery occlusion pressure is often measured via right heart (Swan-Ganz) catheterization. ACE inhibitors are used as long as systolic BP remains > 100 mm Hg. A short-acting ACE inhibitor given in low doses (eg, captopril 3.125 to 6.25 mg po q 4 to 6 h, increasing doses as tolerated) is best for initial treatment. Once the maximum dose is reached (maximum for captopril, 50 mg tid), a longer-acting

ACE inhibitor (eg, fosinopril, lisinopril, ramipril) is substituted for the long-term. If heart failure remains in New York Heart Association class II or worse (see TABLE 74–1 on p. 657), an aldosterone inhibitor (eg, eplerenone, spironolactone) should be added. For severe heart failure, an intra-arterial counterpulsation balloon pump may provide temporary hemodynamic support. When revascularization or surgical repair is not feasible, heart transplantation is considered. Long-term LV or biventricular implantable assist devices may be used as a bridge to transplantation; if transplantation is impossible, the LV assist device is occasionally used as permanent treatment. Occasionally, use of such a device results in recovery and can be removed in 3 to 6 mo.

If heart failure causes hypoxemia, O_2 is given by nasal prongs (to maintain PaO_2 at about 100 mg Hg). It may help oxygenate myocardium and limit the ischemic zone.

Papillary muscle disorders: Functional papillary muscle insufficiency occurs in about 35% of patients during the first few hours of infarction. Papillary muscle ischemia causes incomplete coaptation of the mitral valve leaflets, which is transient in most patients. But in some patients, papillary muscle or free wall scarring causes permanent mitral regurgitation. Functional papillary muscle insufficiency is characterized by an apical late systolic murmur and typically resolves without treatment.

Papillary muscle rupture occurs most often after an inferoposterior infarct due to right coronary artery occlusion. It produces acute, severe mitral regurgitation. Papillary muscle rupture is characterized by the sudden appearance of a loud apical holosystolic murmur and thrill, usually with pulmonary edema. Occasionally, when severe regurgitation is silent but suspected clinically, echocardiography is done. Mitral valve repair or replacement is effective.

Myocardial rupture: Interventricular septum or free wall rupture occurs in 1% of patients with acute MI. It causes 15% of hospital mortality.

Interventricular septum rupture, although rare, is 8 to 10 times more common than papillary muscle rupture. Intraventricular septum rupture is characterized by the sudden appearance of a loud systolic murmur and thrill medial to the apex along the left sternal border in the 3rd or 4th intercostal space, accompanied by hypotension with or without signs of LV failure. Diagnosis may be confirmed using a balloon-tipped catheter and comparing blood O_2 saturation or PO_2 of right atrial, RV, and pulmonary artery samples. A significant increase in RV PO_2 is diagnostic, as is Doppler echocardiography. Treatment is surgery, which should be delayed for up to 6 wk after MI so that infarcted myocardium can heal maximally; if hemodynamic instability persists, earlier surgery is indicated despite a high mortality risk.

Free wall rupture increases in incidence with age and is more common among women. It is characterized by sudden loss of arterial pressure with momentary persistence of sinus rhythm and often by signs of cardiac tamponade. Surgery is rarely successful. Rupture of a free wall is almost always fatal.

Ventricular aneurysm: A localized bulge in the ventricular wall, usually the LV wall, can occur at the site of a large infarction. Ventricular aneurysms are common, especially with a large transmural infarct (usually anterior). Aneurysms may develop in a few days, weeks, or months. They are unlikely to rupture but may lead to recurrent ventricular arrhythmias, low cardiac output, and mural thrombosis with systemic embolism. A ventricular aneurysm may be suspected when paradoxical precordial movements are seen or felt. ECG shows persistent ST-segment elevation, and chest x-ray shows a characteristic bulge of the cardiac shadow. Echocardiography is done to confirm the diagnosis and determine whether a thrombus is present. Surgical excision may be indicated when LV failure or arrhythmia persists. Use of ACE inhibitors during acute MI modifies LV remodeling and may reduce the incidence of aneurysm.

Pseudoaneurysm is incomplete rupture of the free LV wall; it is limited by the pericardium. Pseudoaneurysms almost always contain a thrombus and often rupture completely. They are repaired surgically.

Hypotension and cardiogenic shock: Hypotension may be due to decreased ventricular filling or loss of contractile force secondary to massive MI. Marked hypotension (eg, systolic BP < 90 mm Hg) with tachycardia and symptoms of end-organ hypoperfusion (reduced urine output, mental confusion, diaphoresis, cold extremities) is termed cardiogenic shock (see also p. 560). Pulmonary congestion develops rapidly in cardiogenic shock.

Decreased LV filling is most often caused by reduced venous return secondary to hypovolemia, especially in patients receiving intensive loop diuretic therapy, but it may reflect RV infarction. Marked pulmonary congestion suggests loss of LV contractile force (LV failure) as the cause. Treatment depends on the cause. In some patients, determining the cause requires use of a pulmonary artery catheter to measure intracardiac pressures. If pulmonary artery occlusion pressure is < 18 mm Hg, decreased filling, usually due to hypovolemia, is likely; if pressure is > 18 mm Hg, LV failure is likely. For hypotension due to hypovolemia, cautious fluid replacement with 0.9% saline is usually possible without left heart overload (excessive rise in left atrial pressure). However, sometimes LV function is so compromised that adequate fluid replacement sharply increases pulmonary artery occlusion pressure to levels associated with pulmonary edema (> 25 mm Hg). If left atrial pressure is high, hypotension is probably due to LV failure, and if diuretics are ineffective, inotropic therapy or circulatory support may be required.

In cardiogenic shock, an α- or β-agonist may be temporarily effective. Dopamine, a catecholamine with α and β_1 effects, is given at 0.5 to 1 μg/kg/min, increased until response is satisfactory or dose is about 10 μg/kg/min. Higher doses induce vasoconstriction and atrial and ventricular arrhythmias. Dobutamine, a β-agonist, may be given IV at 2.5 to 10 μg/kg/min or in higher doses. It often causes or exacerbates hypotension; it is most effective when hypotension is secondary to low cardiac output with increased peripheral vascular resistance. Dopamine may be more effective than dobutamine when a vasopressor effect is also required. In refractory cases, dobutamine and dopamine may be combined. An intra-aortic counterpulsation balloon pump can often temporarily support the patient. Direct lysis of the clot, angioplasty, or emergency CABG may greatly improve ventricular function. PCI or CABG may be considered for persistent ischemia, refractory ventricular arrhythmia, hemodynamic instability, or shock if coronary anatomy is suitable.

RV ischemia or infarction: RV infarction rarely occurs in isolation; it usually accompanies inferior LV infarction, and the first sign may be hypotension developing in a previously stable patient. Right-sided ECG leads may show ST-segment changes. Volume loading with 1 to 2 L of 0.9% saline is often effective. Dobutamine may help. Nitrates and diuretics are not used; they reduce preload (and hence cardiac output), producing severe hypotension.

Recurrent ischemia: Any chest pain that remains or recurs 12 to 24 h post-MI may represent recurrent ischemia. Post-MI ischemic pain indicates that more myocardium is at risk of infarction. Usually, recurrent ischemia can be identified by reversible ST-T changes on the ECG; BP may be elevated. However, because recurrent ischemia may be silent (ECG changes without pain) in up to ⅓ of patients, serial ECGs are routinely obtained q 8 h for 1 day and then daily. Recurrent ischemia is treated similarly to unstable angina. Sublingual or IV nitroglycerin is usually effective. Coronary angiography and PCI or CABG should be considered to salvage ischemic myocardium.

Mural thrombosis: Mural thrombosis occurs in about 20% of patients with acute MI. Systemic embolism occurs in about 10% of patients with LV thrombosis; risk is highest in the first 10 days but persists at least 3 mo. Risk is highest (≈60%) for patients with large anterior infarctions (especially involving the distal septum and apex), a dilated and diffusely hypokinetic LV, or chronic AF. Anticoagulants are given to reduce risk of emboli. If not contraindicated, full-dose IV heparin followed by warfarin for 3 to 6 mo is given to maintain INR between 2 and 3. Anticoagulants are continued indefinitely when a dilated diffusely hypokinetic LV, LV aneurysm, or chronic AF is present. Aspirin may also be given indefinitely.

Pericarditis: Pericarditis (see p. 732) results from extension of myocardial necrosis through the wall to the epicardium; it develops in about ⅓ of patients with acute transmural MI. A friction rub usually begins 24 to 96 h after MI onset. Earlier onset of the friction rub is unusual, although hemorrhagic pericarditis occasionally complicates the early phase of MI. Acute tamponade is rare. Pericarditis is diagnosed by ECG, which shows diffuse ST-segment elevation and sometimes PR-interval depression. Echocardiography is frequently done but is usually normal. Occasionally, small pericardial effusions and even unsuspected tamponade are detected. Aspirin or another NSAID usually relieves symptoms. High doses or prolonged use of NSAIDs or corticosteroids may impair infarct healing and should be avoided.

Post-MI syndrome (Dressler's syndrome): Post-MI syndrome develops in a few patients several days to weeks or even months after acute MI; incidence appears to have decreased in recent years. It is characterized by fever, pericarditis with a friction rub, pericardial effusion, pleurisy, pleural effusions, pulmonary infiltrates, and joint pain. This syndrome is caused by an autoimmune reaction to material from necrotic myocytes. It may recur. Differentiating post-MI syndrome from extension or recurrence of infarction may be difficult. However, in post-MI syndrome, cardiac markers do not increase significantly, and ECG changes are nonspecific. NSAIDs are usually effective, but the syndrome can recur several times. In severe cases, a short, intensive course of another NSAID or a corticosteroid may be necessary. High doses of an NSAID or a corticosteroid are not used for more than a few days because they may interfere with early ventricular healing after an acute MI.

Rehabilitation and Postdischarge Treatment

Physical activity is gradually increased during the first 3 to 6 wk after discharge. Resumption of sexual activity, often of great concern to the patient, and other moderate physical activities may be encouraged. If good cardiac function is maintained 6 wk after acute MI, most patients can return to all their normal activities. A regular exercise program consistent with lifestyle, age, and cardiac status reduces risk of ischemic events and enhances general well-being.

The acute illness and treatment of ACS should be used to strongly motivate the patient to modify risk factors. Evaluating the patient's physical and emotional status and discussing them with the patient, advising about lifestyle (eg, smoking, diet, work and play habits, exercise), and aggressively managing risk factors may improve prognosis.

Drugs: Several drugs clearly reduce mortality risk post-MI and are used unless contraindicated or not tolerated.

Aspirin reduces mortality and reinfarction rates in post-MI patients by 15 to 30%. Enteric-coated aspirin 81 mg once/day is recommended long-term. Data suggest that warfarin with or without aspirin reduces mortality and reinfarction rates.

β-Blockers are considered standard therapy. Most available β-blockers (eg, acebutolol, atenolol, metoprolol, propranolol, timolol) reduce post-MI mortality rate by about 25% for at least 7 yr.

ACE inhibitors are given to all post-MI patients. These drugs may provide long-term cardioprotection by improving endothelial function. If an ACE inhibitor is not tolerated because of cough or rash (but not angioedema or renal dysfunction), an angiotensin II receptor blocker may be substituted.

HMG-CoA reductase inhibitors (statins) are prescribed. Reducing cholesterol levels after MI reduces rates of recurrent ischemic events and mortality in patients with elevated or normal cholesterol levels. Statins appear to benefit post-MI patients regardless of their initial cholesterol level. Post-MI patients whose primary problem is low HDL or elevated triglycerides may benefit from a fibrate, but evidence of benefit is less clear. A lipid-lowering drug should be continued indefinitely, unless significant adverse effects occur.

74 HEART FAILURE AND CARDIOMYOPATHIES

Heart failure is generally defined as a change in the pumping function of the heart accompanied by typical signs or symptoms, such as shortness of breath or fatigue. Cardiomyopathy is a general term for disease of heart muscle. There are several types—ischemic, hypertensive, dilated, hypertrophic, infiltrative, and restrictive—any of these may result in heart failure.

HEART FAILURE

(Congestive Heart Failure)

(For heart failure in children, see p. 2405.)

Heart failure is a syndrome of ventricular dysfunction. Left ventricular failure causes shortness of breath and fatigue, and right ventricular failure causes peripheral and abdominal fluid accumulation; both ventricles are usually involved to some extent.

Diagnosis is clinical, supported by chest x-ray and echocardiography. Treatment includes diuretics, ACE inhibitors, β-blockers, and correction of the underlying disorder.

Heart failure (HF) affects about 5 million people in the US; > 500,000 new cases occur each year.

Physiology

Cardiac contractility (force and velocity of contraction), ventricular performance, and myocardial O_2 requirements are determined by preload, afterload, substrate availability (eg, O_2, fatty acids, glucose), heart rate and rhythm, and amount of viable myocardium. Cardiac output (CO) equals stroke volume times heart rate; it is also affected by venous return, peripheral vascular tone, and neurohumoral factors.

Preload is the loading condition of the heart at the end of its relaxation phase (diastole) just before contraction (systole). Preload represents the degree of end-diastolic fiber stretch and end-diastolic volume, which is influenced by ventricular diastolic pressure and the composition of the myocardial wall. Typically, left ventricular (LV) end-diastolic pressure, especially if above normal, is a reasonable measure of preload. LV dilation, hypertrophy, and changes in myocardial distensibility (compliance) modify preload.

Afterload is the force resisting myocardial fiber contraction at the start of systole; it is determined by chamber pressure, volume, and wall thickness at the time the aortic valve opens. Clinically, systemic BP at or shortly after the aortic valve opens represents peak systolic wall stress and approximates afterload.

The Frank-Starling principle describes the relationship between preload and cardiac performance. It states that, normally, systolic contractile performance (represented by stroke volume or CO) is proportional to preload within the normal physiologic range (see FIG. 74–1). Contractility is difficult to measure without cardiac catheterization but is reasonably reflected by the ejection fraction (EF), which is the percentage of end-diastolic volume ejected with each contraction (LV stroke volume/end-diastolic volume).

Cardiac reserve is the ability of the heart to increase its performance above resting levels in response to emotional or physical stress; body O_2 consumption may increase from 250 to ≥ 1500 mL/min during maximal exertion. Mechanisms include increasing heart rate,

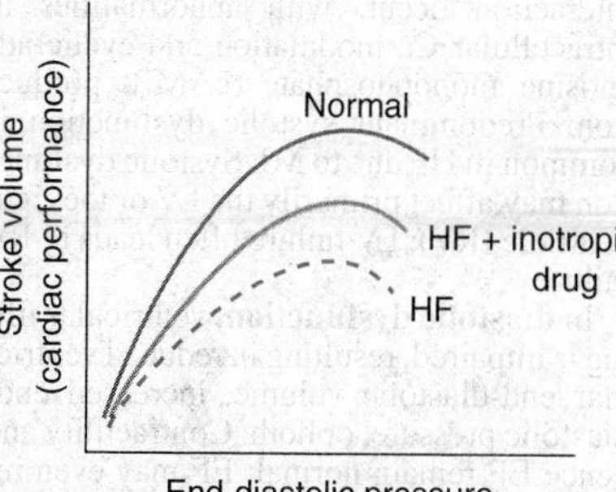

Fig. 74–1. Frank-Starling principle. Normally (top curve), as preload increases, cardiac performance also increases. However at a certain point, performance plateaus, then declines. In heart failure (HF) due to systolic dysfunction (bottom curve), the overall curve shifts downward, reflecting reduced cardiac performance at a given preload, and as preload increases, cardiac performance increases less. With treatment (middle curve), performance is improved, although not normalized.

systolic and diastolic volume, stroke volume, and tissue extraction of O_2 (the difference between O_2 content in arterial blood and mixed venous or pulmonary artery blood). In well-trained young adults during maximal exercise, heart rate may increase from 55 to 70 beats/min at rest to 180 beats/min, and CO may increase from 6 to ≥ 25 L/min. At rest, arterial blood contains about 18 mL O_2/dL of blood, and mixed venous or pulmonary artery blood contains about 14 mL/dL. O_2 extraction is thus about 4.0 mL/dL, but when demand is increased, it may increase to 12 to 14 mL/dL. These mechanisms also help compensate for HF.

Pathophysiology

In HF, the heart may not provide tissues with adequate blood for metabolic needs, and cardiac-related elevation of pulmonary or systemic venous pressures may result in organ congestion. This condition can result from abnormalities of systolic or diastolic function or, commonly, both.

In **systolic dysfunction,** the ventricle contracts poorly and empties inadequately, leading initially to increased diastolic volume and pressure. Later, EF falls. Many defects in energy utilization, energy supply, electrophysiologic functions, and contractile element interaction occur, with abnormalities in intracellular Ca modulation and cyclic adenosine monophosphate (cAMP) production. Predominant systolic dysfunction is common in HF due to MI. Systolic dysfunction may affect primarily the LV or the right ventricle (RV); LV failure often leads to RV failure.

In **diastolic dysfunction,** ventricular filling is impaired, resulting in reduced ventricular end-diastolic volume, increased end-diastolic pressure, or both. Contractility and hence EF remain normal; EF may even increase as the poorly filled LV empties more completely to maintain CO. Markedly reduced LV filling can produce low CO and systemic symptoms. Elevated left atrial pressures can produce pulmonary congestion. Diastolic dysfunction usually results from impaired ventricular relaxation (an active process), increased ventricular stiffness, constrictive pericarditis, or atrioventricular valve stenosis. Resistance to filling increases with age, probably reflecting myocyte loss and increased interstitial collagen deposition; thus, diastolic dysfunction is particularly common among the elderly. Diastolic dysfunction is presumed to be predominant in hypertrophic cardiomyopathy, disorders with ventricular hypertrophy (eg, hypertension, significant aortic stenosis), and amyloid infiltration of the myocardium. LV filling and function may also be impaired if marked increases in RV pressure shift the interventricular septum to the left.

In **LV failure,** CO decreases and pulmonary venous pressure increases. As pulmonary capillary pressure exceeds the oncotic pressure of plasma proteins (about 24 mm Hg), fluid extravasates from the capillaries into the interstitial space and alveoli, reducing pulmonary compliance and increasing the work of breathing. Lymphatic drainage increases but cannot compensate for the increase in pulmonary fluid. Marked fluid accumulation in alveoli (pulmonary edema) significantly alters ventilation-perfusion (V/Q) relationships: Deoxygenated pulmonary arterial blood passes through poorly ventilated alveoli, decreasing systemic arterial oxygenation (PaO_2) and causing dyspnea. However, dyspnea may occur before V/Q abnormalities, probably because of elevated pulmonary venous pressure and increased work of breathing; the precise mechanism is unclear. In severe or chronic LV failure, pleural effusions characteristically develop in the right hemithorax and later bilaterally, further aggravating dyspnea. Minute ventilation increases; thus, $PaCO_2$ decreases and blood pH increases (respiratory alkalosis). Marked interstitial edema of the small airways may interfere with ventilation, elevating $PaCO_2$—a sign of impending respiratory failure.

In **RV failure,** systemic venous pressure increases, causing fluid extravasation and consequent edema, primarily in dependent tissues (feet and ankles of ambulatory patients) and abdominal viscera. The liver is affected most, but stomach and intestine also become congested; fluid accumulation in the peritoneal cavity (ascites) can occur. RV failure commonly causes moderate hepatic dysfunction, with usually modest increases in conjugated and unconjugated bilirubin, PT, and hepatic enzymes (eg, alkaline phosphatase, AST, ALT). The impaired liver breaks down less aldosterone, further contributing to fluid accumulation. Chronic venous congestion in the viscera can cause anorexia, malabsorption and protein-losing enteropathy (characterized by diarrhea and marked hypoalbuminemia), chronic GI blood loss, and rarely ischemic bowel infarction.

Cardiac response: If ventricular function is impaired, a higher preload is required to maintain CO. As a result, the LV is remodeled over time: It becomes less ovoid and more spherical, dilates, and hypertrophies. Initially compensatory, these changes eventually increase diastolic stiffness and wall tension, compromising cardiac performance, especially during physical stress. Increased wall stress raises O_2 demand and accelerates apoptosis (programmed cell death) of myocardial cells.

Hemodynamic responses: With reduced CO, tissue O_2 delivery is maintained by increasing O_2 extraction and sometimes shifting the oxyhemoglobin dissociation curve (see FIG. 46–4 on p. 371) to the right to favor O_2 release.

Reduced CO with lower systemic BP activates arterial baroreflexes, increasing sympathetic tone and decreasing parasympathetic tone. As a result, heart rate and myocardial contractility increase, arterioles in selected vascular beds constrict, venoconstriction occurs, and Na and water are retained; these changes compensate for reduced ventricular performance and help maintain hemodynamic homeostasis in the early stages of HF. However, these compensatory changes increase cardiac work, preload, and afterload;

reduce coronary and renal perfusion; cause fluid accumulation resulting in congestion; increase K excretion; and may cause myocyte necrosis and arrhythmias.

Renal responses: As cardiac function deteriorates, renal blood flow and GFR decrease, and blood flow within the kidneys is redistributed. The filtration fraction and filtered Na decrease, but tubular resorption increases, leading to Na and water retention. Blood flow is further redistributed away from the kidneys during exercise but improves during rest, possibly contributing to nocturia.

Decreased perfusion of the kidneys (and possibly decreased arterial systolic stretch secondary to declining ventricular function) activates the renin-angiotensin-aldosterone system (see also p. 605), increasing Na and water retention and renal and peripheral vascular tone. These effects are amplified by the intense sympathetic activation accompanying HF.

The renin-angiotensin-aldosterone-vasopressin (antidiuretic hormone [ADH]) system produces a cascade of potentially deleterious effects. Angiotensin II worsens HF by causing vasoconstriction, including efferent renal vasoconstriction, and by enhancing aldosterone production, which not only enhances Na reabsorption in the distal nephron but also produces myocardial and vascular collagen deposition and fibrosis. Angiotensin II increases norepinephrine release, stimulates release of ADH, and triggers apoptosis. Angiotensin II may be involved in vascular and myocardial hypertrophy, thus contributing to the remodeling of the heart and peripheral vasculature, potentially worsening HF. Aldosterone can be synthesized in the heart and vasculature independently of angiotensin II (perhaps mediated by corticotropin, nitric oxide, free radicals, and other stimuli) and may have deleterious effects in these organs.

Neurohumoral responses: In conditions of stress, neurohumoral responses help increase heart function and maintain BP and organ perfusion, but chronic activation of these responses is detrimental to the normal balance between myocardial-stimulating and vasoconstricting hormones and between myocardial-relaxing and vasodilating hormones.

The heart contains many neurohumoral receptors (α_1, β_1, β_2, β_3, angiotensin II type 1 [AT_1] and type 2 [AT_2], muscarinic, endothelin, serotonin, adenosine, cytokine); the role of these receptors is not yet fully defined. In patients with HF, β_1 receptors (which constitute 70% of cardiac β receptors) are downregulated, probably in response to intense sympathetic activation; the effect of downregulation is to impair myocyte contractility.

Plasma norepinephrine levels are increased, largely reflecting sympathetic nerve stimulation since plasma epinephrine levels are not increased. Detrimental effects include vasoconstriction with increased preload and afterload, direct myocardial damage including apoptosis, reduced renal blood flow, and activation of other neurohumoral systems including the renin-angiotensin-aldosterone-ADH cascade.

ADH is released in response to a fall in BP via various neurohormonal stimuli. Increased ADH decreases renal excretion of free water, possibly contributing to hyponatremia in HF. ADH levels in HF with normal BP vary.

Atrial natriuretic peptide is released in response to increased atrial volume and pressure; brain (B-type) natriuretic peptide (BNP) is released from the ventricle in response to ventricular stretching. These peptides enhance renal excretion of Na, but in patients with HF, the effect is blunted by decreased renal perfusion pressure, receptor downregulation, and perhaps enhanced enzymatic degradation.

Because endothelial dysfunction occurs in HF, fewer endogenous vasodilators (eg, nitric oxide, prostaglandins) are produced, and more endogenous vasoconstrictors (eg, endothelin) are produced.

The failing heart and other organs produce tumor necrosis factor (TNF)-α. This cytokine increases catabolism and is possibly responsible for cardiac cachexia (loss of lean tissue ≥ 10%), which may accompany severely symptomatic HF, and for other detrimental changes.

Classification and Etiology

Both cardiac and systemic factors can impair cardiac performance and produce HF. Cardiac factors include myocardial damage (eg, acute in MI or myocarditis, chronic in fibrosis due to various disorders), valvular disorders, arrhythmias (tachyarrhythmias or bradyarrhythmias), and reduced substrate availability (ie, ischemia). Systemic factors include any disorder that increases demand for CO (causing high-output HF) or resistance to output (afterload), such as systemic hypertension.

The traditional distinction of left and right ventricular failure is somewhat misleading because the heart is an integrated pump, and changes in one chamber ultimately affect the whole heart. However, these terms indicate the major site of pathology leading to HF and can be useful for initial evaluation and treatment.

LV failure characteristically develops in ischemic heart disease, hypertension, aortic stenosis, most forms of cardiomyopathy, acquired mitral or aortic valvular regurgitation, and congenital heart disorders (eg, ventricular septal defect, patent ductus arteriosus with large shunts).

RV failure is most commonly caused by previous LV failure (which increases pulmonary venous pressure and leads to pulmonary arterial hypertension, thus overloading the RV) or by a severe lung disorder (when it is called cor pulmonale—see p. 664). Other causes are multiple pulmonary emboli, pulmonary venous occlusive disease, RV infarction, primary pulmonary hypertension, tricuspid regurgitation or stenosis, mitral stenosis, and pulmonary artery or valve stenosis. Some conditions mimic RV failure, except cardiac function may be normal; they include volume overload and increased systemic venous pressure in polycythemia or overtransfusion, acute renal failure with Na and H_2O retention–induced overhydration, and obstruction of either vena cava.

Biventricular failure results from disorders that affect the whole myocardium (eg, viral myocarditis, amyloidosis, Chagas' disease).

High-output HF results from a persistent need for a high CO, which may eventually result in an inability of a normal heart to maintain adequate output. Conditions that may increase CO include severe anemia, beriberi, thyrotoxicosis, advanced Paget's disease, arteriovenous fistula, and persistent tachycardia. CO is high in various forms of cirrhosis, but much of the observed fluid retention is due to hepatic mechanisms.

Cardiomyopathy is a general term reflecting disease of the myocardium and is sometimes used to reflect etiology (eg, ischemic vs hypertensive cardiomyopathy). Most commonly, the term refers to a primary disorder of the ventricular myocardium that is not caused by congenital anatomic defects; valvular, systemic, or pulmonary vascular disorders; isolated pericardial, nodal, or conduction system disorders; or epicardial coronary artery disease (CAD). Cardiomyopathy does not always lead to symptomatic HF. It is often idiopathic and is classified as dilated congestive, hypertrophic, or infiltrative-restrictive cardiomyopathy.

Symptoms and Signs

Presentation differs depending on the extent to which the RV and LV are initially affected. Severity varies significantly and is usually classified by the New York Heart Association system (see TABLE 74–1). Severe LV failure may produce pulmonary edema (see p. 663).

In LV failure, the most common symptoms are dyspnea, reflecting pulmonary congestion, and fatigue, reflecting low CO. Dyspnea usually occurs during exertion and is relieved by rest. As HF worsens, dyspnea can occur during rest and at night, sometimes causing nocturnal cough. Dyspnea occurring immediately or soon after lying flat and relieved promptly by sitting up (orthopnea) is common. In paroxysmal nocturnal dyspnea (PND), dyspnea awakens patients several hours after they lie down and is relieved only after they sit up for 15 to 20 min. In severe HF, periodic cycling of breathing (Cheyne-Stokes respiration—see p. 354)—a brief period of increased breathing (hyperpnea) followed by a brief period of no breathing (apnea)—can occur during the day or night; the sudden hyperpneic phase may awaken the patient from sleep. This breathing differs from PND in that the hyperpneic phase is short, lasting only a few seconds and resolving in < 1 min. PND is associated with pulmonary congestion, and Cheyne-Stokes respiration with low CO. Sleep-related breathing disorders, such as sleep apnea (see p. 499), are common in HF and may aggravate HF. Severely reduced cerebral blood flow and hypoxemia can cause chronic irritability and impair mental performance.

In RV failure, the most common symptoms are ankle swelling and fatigue. Sometimes patients feel a sensation of fullness in the abdomen or neck. Hepatic congestion can cause right upper quadrant abdominal discomfort, and stomach and intestinal congestion can cause anorexia and abdominal bloating.

Less specific HF symptoms include cool peripheries, postural light-headedness, nocturia, and decreased daytime micturition. Skeletal muscle wasting can occur in severe biventricular failure and may reflect some disuse but also increased catabolism associated with increased cytokine production. Significant weight loss (cardiac cachexia) is an ominous sign associated with high mortality.

TABLE 74–1. NEW YORK HEART ASSOCIATION (NYHA) CLASSIFICATION OF HEART FAILURE

NYHA CLASS	DEFINITION	LIMITATION	EXAMPLE
I	Ordinary physical activity does not cause undue fatigue, dyspnea, palpitation, or angina	None	Can complete any activity requiring ≤ 7 mets: carry 11 kg up 8 steps; carry objects weighing 36 kg; shovel snow; spade soil; ski; play squash, handball or basketball; jog/walk 8 km/h
II	Ordinary physical activity causes fatigue, dyspnea, palpitation, or angina	Slight	Can complete any activity requiring ≤ 5 mets: sexual intercourse without stopping, garden, roller skate, walk 7 km/h on level ground
III	Comfortable at rest; less than ordinary physical activity causes fatigue, dyspnea, palpitation, or angina	Moderate	Can complete any activity requiring ≤ 2 mets: shower or dress without stopping, strip and make bed, clean windows, play golf, walk 4 km/h
IV	Symptoms at rest; any physical activity increases discomfort	Severe	Cannot do or cannot complete any activity requiring ≥ 2 mets; cannot do any of the above activities

General examination may detect signs of systemic disorders that cause or aggravate HF (eg, anemia, hyperthyroidism, alcoholism, hemochromatosis).

In LV failure, tachycardia and tachypnea may occur; patients with severe LV failure may appear visibly dyspneic or cyanotic, hypotensive, and confused or agitated because of hypoxia and poor cerebral perfusion. Central cyanosis (affecting all of the body, including warm areas such as the tongue and mucous membranes) reflects severe hypoxemia. Peripheral cyanosis of the lips, fingers, and toes reflects low blood flow with increased O_2 extraction. If vigorous massage improves nail bed color, cyanosis may be peripheral; increasing local blood flow does not improve color if cyanosis is central.

Cardiac findings in LV systolic dysfunction include a diffuse, sustained, and laterally displaced apical impulse; audible and occasionally palpable 3rd (S_3) and 4th (S_4) heart sounds, and an accentuated pulmonic component (P_2) of the 2nd heart sound (S_2). A pansystolic murmur of mitral regurgitation at the apex may occur. Pulmonary findings include inspiratory basilar crackles and, if pleural effusion is present, dullness to percussion and diminished breath sounds at lung bases.

Signs of RV failure include nontender peripheral pitting edema (digital pressure leaves visible and palpable imprints, sometimes quite deep) in the feet and ankles; an enlarged and sometimes pulsatile liver palpable below the right costal margin; abdominal swelling and ascites; and visible elevation of the jugular venous pressure, sometimes with large *a* or *v* waves that are visible even when the patient is seated or standing (see p. 574 and FIG. 69–1). In severe cases, peripheral edema can extend to the thighs or even the sacrum, scrotum, lower abdominal wall, and occasionally even higher. Severe edema in multiple areas is termed anasarca. Edema may be asymmetric if patients lie predominantly on one side.

With hepatic congestion, the liver may be palpably enlarged or tender, and hepatojugular or abdominal-jugular reflux may be detected (see p. 574). Precordial palpation may detect the left parasternal lift of RV enlargement, and auscultation may detect the murmur of tricuspid regurgitation or the RV S_3 along the left sternal border.

Diagnosis

Clinical findings (eg, exertional dyspnea, orthopnea, edema, tachycardia, pulmonary rales, S_3, jugular venous distention) suggest HF but are not apparent early. Similar symptoms may result from COPD or recurrent pneumonia or may be erroneously attributed to old age. Suspicion for HF should be high in patients with a history of MI, hypertension, or valvular disorders or murmurs and should be moderate in any elderly or diabetic patient.

Chest x-ray, ECG, and an objective test of cardiac function, typically echocardiography, should be done. Blood tests, except for B-type natriuretic peptide, are not used for diagnosis but are useful for identifying cause and systemic effects.

Chest x-ray findings suggesting HF include an enlarged cardiac silhouette, pleural effusion, fluid in the major fissure, and horizontal lines in the periphery of lower posterior lung fields (Kerley B lines). These findings reflect chronic elevation of left atrial pressure and chronic thickening of the intralobular septa due to edema. Upper lobe pulmonary venous congestion and interstitial or alveolar edema may also be present. Careful examination of the cardiac silhouette on a lateral projection can identify specific ventricular and atrial chamber enlargement. The x-ray may also suggest alternative diagnoses (eg, COPD, interstitial pulmonary fibrosis, lung cancer).

ECG findings are not diagnostic, but an abnormal ECG, especially showing previous MI, LV hypertrophy, left bundle branch block, or tachyarrhythmia (eg, rapid atrial fibrillation), increases suspicion for HF and may help identify the cause.

Echocardiography can help evaluate chamber dimensions, valve function, EF, wall motion abnormalities, LV hypertrophy, and pericardial effusion. Intracardiac thrombi, tumors, and calcifications within the heart valves, mitral annulus, and aortic wall abnormalities can be detected. Localized or segmental wall motion abnormalities strongly suggest underlying CAD but can also be present with patchy myocarditis. Doppler or color Doppler echocardiography accurately detects valvular disorders and shunts. Doppler studies of mitral and pulmonary venous inflow often help identify and quantify LV diastolic dysfunction. Measuring LVEF can distinguish between predominant diastolic dysfunction (EF > 0.40) and systolic dysfunction (EF < 0.40), which may require different treatment. Three-dimensional echocardiography may become important but currently is available only in specialized centers.

Radionuclide imaging also can help assess systolic and diastolic function, previous MI, and inducible ischemia or myocardial hibernation. Cardiac MRI provides accurate images of cardiac structures but is not always available and is more expensive.

Recommended blood tests include CBC, blood creatinine, BUN, electrolytes (including Mg and Ca), glucose, albumin, and liver function tests. Thyroid function tests are recommended for patients with atrial fibrillation and for selected, especially elderly, patients. Serum BNP levels are high in HF; this finding may help when clinical findings are unclear or other diagnoses (eg, COPD) need to be excluded. It may be particularly useful for patients with a history of both pulmonary and cardiac disorders.

Cardiac catheterization and coronary angiography are indicated when CAD is suspected or when the diagnosis and etiology are uncertain.

Endocardial biopsy is usually done only when an infiltrative cardiomyopathy is strongly suspected.

Prognosis

Generally, patients with HF have a poor prognosis unless the cause is correctable. Mortality rate at 1 yr from 1st hospitalization for HF is about 30%. In chronic HF, mortality depends on severity of symptoms and ventricular dysfunction and can range from 10 to 40%/yr.

HF usually involves gradual deterioration, interrupted by bouts of severe decompensation, and ultimately death. However, death can also be sudden and unexpected, without prior worsening of symptoms.

End-of-life care: All patients and family members should be taught about disease progression. For some patients, improving quality of life is as important as increasing quantity of life. Thus, determining patients' wishes about resuscitation (eg, endotracheal intubation, CPR) if their condition deteriorates is important, especially when HF is severe. All patients should be reassured that symptoms will be relieved, and they should be encouraged to seek medical attention early if their symptoms change significantly. Involvement of pharmacists, nurses, social workers, and clergy, who may be part of an interdisciplinary team or disease management program already in place, is particularly important in end-of-life care.

Treatment

Immediate inpatient treatment is required for patients with HF due to certain disorders (eg, acute MI, atrial fibrillation with a rapid ventricular rate, severe hypertension, acute valvular regurgitation), as well as for patients with pulmonary edema (see p. 663), severe symptoms, new-onset HF, or HF unresponsive to outpatient treatment. Patients with mild exacerbations of previously diagnosed HF can be treated at home. The primary goal is to diagnose and to correct or treat the disorder that led to HF.

Short-term goals include improving symptoms and hemodynamics; avoiding hypokalemia, renal dysfunction, and symptomatic hypotension; and correcting neurohumoral activation. Long-term goals include correcting hypertension, preventing MI and atherosclerosis, reducing hospitalizations, and improving survival and quality of life. Treatment involves dietary and lifestyle changes, drugs (see p. 660), and sometimes surgery.

Dietary Na restriction helps limit fluid retention. All patients should eliminate salt in cooking and at the table and avoid salted foods; the most severely ill should limit Na to < 1 g/day by consuming only low-Na foods. Monitoring daily morning weight helps detect Na and water accumulation early; if weight increases > 4.4 kg, patients may be able to adjust their diuretic dose themselves, but if weight gain continues or symptoms occur, they should seek medical attention. Patients with atherosclerosis or diabetes should strictly follow a diet appropriate for their disorder. Obesity may cause and always aggravates the symptoms of HF; patients should attain a BMI of 21 to 25.

Regular light activity (eg, walking), tailored to symptoms, is generally encouraged. Activity prevents skeletal muscle deconditioning, which worsens functional status; whether this measure improves survival is under study. Rest is appropriate during acute exacerbations.

Treatment is tailored to the patient, considering causes, symptoms, and response to drugs, including adverse effects. Treatment of systolic and diastolic dysfunction differs somewhat, although there is overlap. The patient and family should be involved in treatment choices. They should be taught the importance of drug compliance, warning signs of decompensation, and use of supplemental drug doses for symptom relief. Intensive case management, particularly by monitoring drug compliance and frequency of unscheduled visits to the physician or emergency department and hospitalizations, can identify when intervention is needed. Specialized HF nurses are valuable in education, follow-up, and dosage adjustment according to predefined protocols. Many centers (eg, specialized outpatient clinics) have integrated health care practitioners from different disciplines (eg, HF nurses, pharmacists, social workers, rehabilitation specialists) into multidisciplinary teams or outpatient HF management programs. These approaches can improve outcomes and reduce hospitalizations and are most effective in the sickest patients.

If hypertension, severe anemia, hemochromatosis, uncontrolled diabetes, thyrotoxicosis, beriberi, alcoholism, Chagas' disease, or toxoplasmosis is successfully treated, patients may dramatically improve. Management of extensive ventricular infiltration (eg, in amyloidosis) remains unsatisfactory.

Surgery: Surgery may be appropriate when certain underlying disorders are present. Usually, surgery in HF patients should be performed in a specialized center. Surgical closure of congenital or acquired intracardiac shunts can be curative. Coronary artery bypass grafting to reduce ischemia may help some patients with ischemic cardiomyopathy. If HF is primarily due to a valvular disorder, valve repair or replacement is considered (see in Ch. 76 on p. 708). Patients with primary mitral regurgitation are more likely to benefit than patients with mitral regurgitation secondary to LV dilation, in whom myocardial function is likely to continue to be poor postoperatively. Surgery done before myocardial dilation and damage become irreversible is preferable.

Heart transplantation (see p. 1370) is the treatment of choice for patients < 60 who have severe, refractory HF and no other life-threatening conditions. Survival is 82% at 1 yr and 75% at 3 yr; however, mortality rate while waiting for a donor is 12 to 15%. Human organ donation remains low. LV assist devices can be a bridge to transplantation or, in a few selected patients, permanent. Artificial hearts are not yet a viable alternative. Surgical options under study include implantation of restraining devices to reduce progressive dilation and a modified aneurysmectomy called surgical ventricular restoration. Dynamic cardiomyoplasty and excision of segments of dilated myocardium (Batista procedure) are no longer recommended.

Arrhythmias (see also p. 673): Sinus tachycardia, a common compensatory change in HF, usually subsides when HF treatment is effective. If it does not, associated causes (eg, hyperthyroidism, pulmonary emboli, fever, anemia) should be sought. If it persists despite correction of causes, a β-blocker, given in gradually increasing doses, should be considered.

Atrial fibrillation with an uncontrolled ventricular rate must be treated. β-Blockers are the treatment of choice although rate-limiting Ca channel blockers, used cautiously, may be used if systolic function is preserved. Adding digoxin or low-dose amiodarone may help some patients. If HF is mild, conversion to sinus rhythm may be no better than rate control, but some patients with HF benefit from being in sinus rhythm. If rapid atrial fibrillation does not respond to drugs, permanent pacemaker insertion with complete or partial ablation of the atrioventricular node may be considered in selected patients.

Isolated ventricular premature beats, which are common in HF, do not require specific treatment. Sustained ventricular tachycardia that persists despite optimal medical treatment of HF may require an antiarrhythmic drug. Amiodarone and β-blockers are the drugs of choice because other antiarrhythmics have adverse proarrhythmic effects when LV systolic dysfunction is present. Because amiodarone increases digoxin levels, the digoxin dose should be decreased by ½. Because long-term use of amiodarone can cause adverse effects, a low-dose (200 to 300 mg po once/day) is used when possible; blood tests for liver function and thyroid-stimulating hormone are done q 6 mo, and if chest x-ray is abnormal or dyspnea worsens significantly, chest x-ray and pulmonary function tests are done yearly to check for pulmonary fibrosis. For sustained ventricular arrhythmias, amiodarone 400 mg po once/day may be required.

An implantable cardioverter-defibrillator (ICD) is recommended for patients with an otherwise good life expectancy if they have symptomatic sustained ventricular tachycardia (especially if it causes syncope), ventricular fibrillation, or an LVEF < 0.30 after MI.

Refractory HF: After treatment, symptoms often persist. Reasons include persistence of the underlying disorder (eg, hypertension, ischemia, valvular regurgitation) despite treatment, suboptimal treatment of HF, drug noncompliance, excess intake of dietary Na or alcohol, and presence of an undiagnosed thyroid disorder, anemia, or supervening arrhythmia (eg, atrial fibrillation with rapid ventricular response, intermittent ventricular tachycardia). Also, drugs used to treat other disorders may interfere with HF treatment; NSAIDs, thiazolidinediones (eg, pioglitazone) for diabetes, and short-acting dihydropyridine or nondihydropyridine Ca channel blockers can worsen HF and usually should not be used. Biventricular pacing relieves symptoms for patients who have HF, severe systolic dysfunction, and a widened QRS complex.

Drugs

Drugs for symptom relief include diuretics, nitrates, and digoxin. ACE inhibitors, β-blockers, aldosterone receptor blockers, and angiotensin II receptor blockers are effective for long-term management and improve survival. Different strategies are used for systolic and diastolic dysfunction. In patients with severe diastolic dysfunction, diuretics and nitrates should be used in lower doses because these patients do not tolerate reduced BP or plasma volume well. In patients with hypertrophic cardiomyopathy (see p. 669), digoxin is not effective and may be harmful.

Diuretics: Diuretics (see TABLE 71–5 on p. 611) are given to all patients with symptomatic systolic dysfunction; dose is adjusted to the lowest dose that stabilizes weight and relieves symptoms. Loop diuretics are preferred. Furosemide is used most often, starting at 20 to 40 mg po once/day, increased to 120 mg once/day (or 60 mg bid) if needed based on response and renal function. Bumetanide is an alternative. In refractory cases, furosemide 40 to 160 mg IV, ethacrynic acid 50 to 100 mg IV, bumetanide 0.5 to 2 mg po or 0.5 to 1.0 mg IV, or metolazone 2.5 to 10 mg po may have an additive effect. Loop diuretics (particularly when used with metolazone) may cause hypovolemia with hypotension, hyponatremia, hypomagnesemia, and severe hypokalemia.

Serum electrolytes are monitored, initially daily (when diuretics are given IV) and subsequently as needed, particularly after a dose increase. The K-sparing diuretics spironolactone or eplerenone (which are also aldosterone receptor blockers) can be added to offset the K-losing effects of higher-dose loop diuretics; hyperkalemia may result, especially when ACE inhibitors or angiotensin II receptor blockers are also taken, so electrolytes must still be monitored. Thiazide diuretics are not normally used unless hypertension is present.

Reliable patients are taught to take additional diuretic doses as needed when weight or peripheral edema increases. They should seek medical attention promptly if weight gain persists.

Experimental ADH blockers increase water excretion and serum Na levels and may cause less hypokalemia and renal dysfunction. They may become useful adjuncts to current diuretic therapy.

ACE inhibitors: All patients with systolic dysfunction are given oral ACE inhibitors unless contraindicated (eg, by plasma creatinine > 2.8 mg/dL [250 μmol/L], bilateral renal artery stenosis, renal artery stenosis in a solitary kidney, or previous angioedema due to ACE inhibitors).

ACE inhibitors reduce production of angiotensin II and breakdown of bradykinin, mediators that affect the sympathetic nervous system, endothelial function, vascular tone, and myocardial performance. Hemodynamic effects include arterial and venous vasodilation, sustained decreases in LV filling pressure during rest and exercise, decreased systemic vascular resistance, and favorable effects on ventricular remodeling. ACE inhibitors prolong survival and reduce HF hospitalizations. For patients with atherosclerosis and a vascular disorder, these drugs may reduce MI and stroke risk. For diabetics, they delay onset of nephropathy. Thus, ACE inhibitors may be used in patients with diastolic dysfunction and any of these disorders.

The starting dose should be low ($^1/_4$ to $^1/_2$ target dose depending on BP and renal function); the dose is gradually adjusted upward over 2 to 4 wk as tolerated, then continued indefinitely. Usual target doses of representative drugs include enalapril 10 to 20 mg bid, lisinopril 20 to 30 mg once/day, ramipril 5 mg bid, and captopril 50 mg bid.

If the hypotensive effect (more marked in patients with hyponatremia or volume depletion) is troublesome, it can often be minimized by reducing the dose of concomitant diuretics. ACE inhibitors often cause moderate reversible renal insufficiency due to vasodilation of the efferent glomerular arteriole. An initial 20 to 30% increase in creatinine is no reason to stop the drug but does require slower increases in dose, reduction in diuretic dose, or avoidance of NSAIDs. K retention may result because aldosterone's effect is reduced, especially in patients receiving K supplements. Cough occurs in 5 to 15% of patients, probably because bradykinin accumulates, but other causes of cough should also be considered. Occasionally, rash or dysgeusia occurs. Angioneurotic edema is rare but can be life threatening and is a contraindication to this class of drugs. Alternatively, angiotensin II receptor blockers can be used, although rarely cross-reactivity is reported. Both are contraindicated in pregnancy.

Plasma electrolytes and renal function should be measured before an ACE inhibitor is started, at 1 mo, and after each significant increase in dose or change in clinical condition. If dehydration or poor renal function due to acute illness develops, an ACE inhibitor may need to be stopped temporarily.

Angiotensin II receptor blockers (ARBs): These drugs are not demonstrably superior to ACE inhibitors but are less likely to cause cough and angioedema; they may be used when these adverse effects prohibit ACE inhibitor use. Whether ACE inhibitors and ARBs are equally effective in chronic HF is unclear, and the best dose is still under study. Usual oral target doses are valsartan 160 mg bid, candesartan 32 mg once/day, and losartan 50 to 100 mg once/day. Introduction, upward titration, and monitoring of ARBs and ACE inhibitors are similar. Like ACE inhibitors, ARBs can cause reversible renal dysfunction. If dehydration or poor renal function due to acute illness develops, an ARB may need to be stopped temporarily.

Adding ARBs to ACE inhibitors, β-blockers, and diuretics should be considered for HF patients with persistent symptoms and repeated hospitalizations. Such combination therapy requires increased monitoring of BP, plasma electrolytes, and renal function.

Aldosterone receptor blockers: Because aldosterone can be produced independently of the renin-angiotensin system, its adverse effects are not inhibited completely even by maximal use of ACE inhibitors and ARBs. Thus, the aldosterone receptor blockers spironolactone and eplerenone can reduce mortality, including from sudden death. Generally, spironolactone 25 to 50 mg po once/day is given to patients with severe chronic HF, and eplerenone 10 mg po once/day to patients who have acute HF with LVEF < 30% after MI. K supplements should be stopped. Serum K and creatinine should be checked q 1 to 2 wk for the 1st 4 to 6 wk and after dosage changes; dose is lowered if K is between 5.5 and 6.0 mEq/L and stopped if K is > 6.0 mEq/L, if creatinine increases above 2.5 mg/dL (220 μmol/L), or if ECG changes of hyperkalemia are present.

β-Blockers: β-Blockers, unless otherwise contraindicated (by asthma, 2nd- or 3rd-degree atrioventricular block, or previous intolerance), are an important addition to ACE inhibitors for chronic systolic dysfunction in most patients, including the elderly, and for diastolic dysfunction in hypertension and hypertrophic cardiomyopathy. Some of these drugs improve LVEF, survival, and other major cardiovascular outcomes in patients with chronic systolic dysfunction, including those with severe symptoms. β-Blockers are particularly useful for diastolic dysfunction because they reduce heart rate, prolonging diastolic filling time, and possibly improve ventricular relaxation.

During acute decompensation, β-blockers must be used with caution. They are not started until patients are stabilized and have little evidence of fluid retention; for patients already taking a β-blocker, the dose is temporarily withheld or reduced.

The starting dose should be low ($\frac{1}{8}$ to $\frac{1}{4}$ of the target daily dose), then gradually increased over 6 to 8 wk as tolerated. Usual oral target doses are carvedilol 25 mg bid (50 mg bid for patients ≥ 85 kg), bisoprolol 10 mg once/day, metoprolol 50 to 75 mg bid (tartrate) or 200 mg once/day (succinate extended-release). Carvedilol, a 3rd-generation nonselective β-blocker, is also a vasodilator with α-blocking and antioxidant effects; it is the preferred β-blocker but is more expensive in many countries. Some β-blockers (eg, bucindolol, xamoterol) do not appear beneficial and may be harmful.

After initial treatment, heart rate and myocardial O_2 consumption decrease, and stroke volume and filling pressure are unchanged. With the slower heart rate, diastolic function improves. Ventricular filling returns to a more normal pattern (increasing in early diastole), which appears less restrictive. Improved myocardial function is measurable in many patients after 6 to 12 mo; EF and CO increase, and LV filling pressure decreases. Exercise capacity improves.

When started, β-blockers may require a temporary increase in diuretic dose if the acute negative inotropic effects of β-blockade cause cardiac depression and fluid retention. In such cases, slower upward titration of the β-blocker dose is warranted.

Vasodilators: Hydralazine plus isosorbide dinitrate may help patients truly intolerant of ACE inhibitors or ARBs (usually because of significant renal dysfunction), although long-term benefit of this combination is limited. As vasodilators, these drugs improve hemodynamics, reduce valvular regurgitation, and increase exercise capacity without causing significant renal impairment. Hydralazine is started at 25 mg po qid and increased q 3 to 5 days to a target total dose of 300 mg/day, although many patients cannot tolerate > 200 mg/day because of hypotension. Isosorbide dinitrate is started at 20 mg po tid (with a 12-h nitrate-free interval) and increased to a target of 40 to 50 mg tid. Whether lower doses (frequently used in clinical practice) provide long-term benefit is unknown. In general, vasodilators have been replaced by ACE inhibitors, which are easier to use, are usually better tolerated, and have greater proven benefit.

Nitrates alone can relieve HF symptoms; patients can be taught to use nitroglycerin spray as needed for acute symptoms and a patch for nocturnal dyspnea. In patients with HF and angina, nitrates are safe, effective, and well tolerated.

Other vasodilators such as Ca channel blockers are not used to treat systolic dysfunction. Short-acting dihydropyridines (eg, nifedipine) and nondihydropyridines (eg, diltiazem, verapamil) are deleterious. However, amlodipine and felodipine are well tolerated and may be useful for patients with HF and associated angina or hypertension. Both drugs may cause peripheral edema; rarely, amlodipine causes pulmonary edema. Felodipine should not be taken with grapefruit juice, which significantly increases plasma levels and adverse effects by inhibiting cytochrome P-450 metabolism. In patients with diastolic dysfunction, Ca channel blockers may be used as needed to treat hypertension or ischemia or to control ventricular rate in atrial fibrillation. Verapamil is used in hypertrophic cardiomyopathy.

Digitalis preparations: These drugs inhibit the Na-K pump (Na^+, K^+-ATPase). As a result, they cause weak positive inotropism, reduce sympathetic activity, block the atrioventricular node (slowing the ventricular rate in atrial fibrillation or prolonging PR interval in sinus rhythm), reduce vasoconstriction, and improve renal blood flow. Digoxin is the most commonly prescribed digitalis preparation. It is excreted by the kidneys; elimination half-life is 36 to 40 h in patients with normal renal function. Digitoxin is largely excreted in the bile. It is an alternative for patients with poor renal function but is infrequently prescribed.

Digoxin has no proven survival benefit but, when used with diuretics and an ACE inhibitor, may help control symptoms. Digoxin is most effective in patients with large LV end-diastolic volumes and an S_3. Acute withdrawal of digoxin may increase the hospitalization rate and worsen symptoms. Toxicity is a concern, especially in patients with renal dysfunction and perhaps in women. These patients may need a lower oral dose, as may the elderly, patients with a low lean body mass, and patients also taking amiodarone; patients > 80 kg may need a higher dose. In general, lower doses are used than in the past, and a trough (8 to 12 h postdose) digoxin level of 1 to 1.2 ng/mL is acceptable. Prescription patterns vary widely by physician and by country.

In patients with normal renal function, digoxin (0.125 to 0.375 mg po once/day depending on age, sex, and body size) achieves full digitalization in about 1 wk (5 half-lives). More rapid digitalization can be achieved with digoxin 0.5 mg IV followed by 0.25 mg at 8 and 16 h or with 0.5 mg po followed by 0.25 mg at 8, 16, and 24 h.

Digoxin (and all digitalis glycosides) has a narrow therapeutic window. The most important toxic effects are life-threatening arrhythmias (eg, ventricular fibrillation, ventricular tachycardia, complete atrioventricular block). Bidirectional ventricular tachycardia, nonparoxysmal junctional tachycardia in the presence of atrial fibrillation, and hyperkalemia are serious signs of digitalis toxicity. Nausea, vomiting, anorexia, diarrhea, confusion, amblyopia, and, rarely, xerophthalmia may occur. If hypokalemia or hypomagnesemia (often due to diuretic use) is present, lower doses and serum levels can cause toxicity. Electrolyte levels must be monitored frequently in patients taking diuretics and digoxin, so that abnormalities can be prevented if possible; K-sparing diuretics may be helpful.

When digitalis toxicity occurs, the drug should be stopped; electrolyte abnormalities should be corrected (IV if abnormalities are severe and toxicity is acute). Patients with severe toxicity are admitted to a monitored unit, and digoxin immune Fab (ovine antidigoxin antibody fragments) is given if arrhythmias are present or if significant overingestion is accompanied by a serum K of > 5 mEq/L. This drug is also useful for glycoside toxicity due to plant ingestion. Dose is based on the steady-state serum digoxin level or total amount ingested. Ventricular arrhythmias are treated with lidocaine or phenytoin. Atrioventricular block with a slow ventricular rate may require a temporary transvenous pacemaker; isoproterenol is contraindicated because it increases risk of ventricular arrhythmia.

Other drugs: Various positive inotropic drugs have been evaluated in HF, but except for digoxin, they increase mortality risk. Regular outpatient IV infusions of inotropes (eg, dobutamine) increase mortality and are no longer recommended. Drugs under study include Ca sensitizers, cytokine blockers, endothelin blockers, matrix metalloproteinase (MMP) inhibitors, and immune modulators.

PULMONARY EDEMA

Pulmonary edema is acute, severe left ventricular failure with pulmonary venous hypertension and alveolar flooding. Findings are severe dyspnea, diaphoresis, wheezing, and sometimes blood-tinged frothy sputum. Diagnosis is clinical and by chest x-ray. Treatment is with O_2, IV nitrates, diuretics, morphine, and sometimes endotracheal intubation and mechanical ventilation.

If LV filling pressure increases suddenly, plasma fluid moves rapidly from pulmonary capillaries into interstitial spaces and alveoli, causing pulmonary edema. About $\frac{1}{2}$ of cases result from acute coronary ischemia; $\frac{1}{4}$ from decompensation of significant underlying HF, including diastolic dysfunction HF due to hypertension; and the rest from arrhythmia, an acute valvular disorder, or acute volume overload often due to IV fluids. Drug or dietary noncompliance is often involved.

Symptoms and Signs

Patients present with extreme dyspnea, restlessness, and anxiety with a sense of suffocation. Cough producing blood-tinged sputum, pallor, cyanosis, and marked diaphoresis are common; some patients froth at the mouth. Frank hemoptysis is uncommon. The pulse is rapid and low volume, and BP is variable. Marked hypertension indicates significant cardiac reserve; hypotension is ominous. Inspiratory fine crackles are widely dispersed anteriorly and posteriorly over both lung fields. Marked wheezing (cardiac asthma) may occur. Noisy respiratory efforts often make cardiac auscultation difficult; a summation gallop—merger of 3rd (S_3) and 4th (S_4) heart sounds)—may be present. Signs of RV failure (eg, neck vein distention, peripheral edema) may be present.

Diagnosis and Treatment

A COPD exacerbation can mimic pulmonary edema due to LV failure or even that due to biventricular failure if cor pulmonale (see below) is present. Pulmonary edema may be the presenting symptom in patients without a history of cardiac disorders, but COPD patients with such severe manifestations have a known history of COPD, although they may be too dyspneic to relate it. A chest x-ray, done immediately, is usually diagnostic, showing marked interstitial edema. Bedside measurement of serum brain (B-type) natriuretic peptide (BNP) levels (elevated in pulmonary edema; normal in COPD exacerbation) is helpful. ECG, pulse oximetry, and blood tests (cardiac markers, electrolytes, BUN, creatinine, and, for severely ill patients, ABGs) are done. Hypoxemia can be severe. CO_2 retention is a late, ominous sign of secondary hypoventilation.

Initial treatment includes 100% O_2 by nonrebreather mask; upright position; furosemide 0.5 to 1.0 mg/kg IV; nitroglycerin 0.4 mg sublingually q 5 min, followed by an IV drip at 10 to 20 μg/min, titrated upward at 10 μg/min q 5 min as needed to a maximum 300 μg/min or systolic BP of 90 mm Hg; and morphine 1 to 5 mg IV once or twice. If hypoxia is significant, noninvasive ventilatory assistance with bilevel positive airway pressure (BiPAP) is helpful, but if CO_2 retention is present or the patient is obtunded, tracheal intubation and assisted ventilation are required.

Specific additional treatment depends on etiology: thrombolysis or direct percutaneous coronary angioplasty with or without a stent for acute MI or another acute coronary syndrome; a vasodilator for severe hypertension; direct-current cardioversion for supraventricular or ventricular tachycardia; and an IV β-blocker, IV digoxin, or cautious use of an IV Ca channel blocker to slow the ventricular rate for rapid atrial fibrillation (cardioversion is preferred). Other treatments, such as IV BNP (nesiritide) and new inotropic drugs, are under study. Because fluid status before onset of pulmonary edema is usually normal in patients with acute MI, diuretics are less useful than in patients with chronic HF and may precipitate hypotension. If BP falls or shock develops, IV dobutamine and an intra-aortic balloon pump (counterpulsation) may be required (see p. 564).

Once patients are stabilized, long-term HF treatment is as described above.

COR PULMONALE

Cor pulmonale is right ventricular enlargement secondary to a lung disorder that produces pulmonary artery hypertension. Right ventricular failure follows. Findings include peripheral edema, neck vein distention, hepatomegaly, and a parasternal lift. Diagnosis is clinical and by echocardiography. Treatment is directed at the cause.

Cor pulmonale results from a lung disorder; it does not refer to right ventricular (RV) enlargement secondary to left ventricular (LV) failure, a congenital heart disorder, or an acquired valvular disorder. Cor pulmonale is usually chronic but may be acute and reversible. Primary pulmonary hypertension (ie, not caused by a pulmonary or cardiac disorder) is discussed on p. 481.

Pathophysiology and Etiology

Lung disorders cause pulmonary hypertension by several mechanisms: loss of capillary beds (eg, due to bullous changes in COPD or thrombosis in pulmonary embolism); vasoconstriction caused by hypoxia, hypercapnia, or both; increased alveolar pressure (eg, in COPD, during mechanical ventilation); and medial hypertrophy in arterioles (often a response to pulmonary hypertension due to other mechanisms).

Pulmonary hypertension increases afterload on the RV, resulting in the same cascade of events that occurs in HF, including elevated end-diastolic and central venous pressure and ventricular hypertrophy and dilation. Demands on the RV may be intensified by increased blood viscosity due to hypoxia-induced polycythemia. Rarely, RV failure affects the LV if a dysfunctional septum bulges into the LV, interfering with filling and thus producing diastolic dysfunction.

Acute cor pulmonale usually results from massive pulmonary embolization or from injury due to mechanical ventilation for acute respiratory distress syndrome (see p. 556).

Chronic cor pulmonale is caused usually by COPD (chronic bronchitis, emphysema) and less often by extensive loss of lung tissue due to surgery or trauma, chronic unresolved pulmonary emboli, pulmonary veno-occlusive disease, scleroderma, pulmonary interstitial fibrosis, kyphoscoliosis, obesity with alveolar hypoventilation, neuromuscular disorders involving respiratory muscles, or idiopathic alveolar hypoventilation. In patients with COPD, an acute exacerbation or pulmonary infection may trigger RV overload. In chronic cor pulmonale, risk of venous thromboembolism is increased.

Symptoms, Signs, and Diagnosis

Initially, cor pulmonale is asymptomatic, although patients usually have significant symptoms due to the underlying lung disorder (eg, dyspnea, exertional fatigue). Later, as RV pressures increase, physical signs commonly include a left parasternal systolic lift, a loud pulmonic component of the 2nd heart sound (S_2), and murmurs of functional tricuspid and pulmonic insufficiency. Later, an RV gallop rhythm (3rd [S_3] and 4th [S_4] heart sounds) augmented during inspiration, distended jugular veins (with a dominant *a* wave unless tricuspid regurgitation is present), hepatomegaly, and lower-extremity edema may occur.

Cor pulmonale should be suspected in all patients with one of its causes. Chest x-rays show RV and proximal pulmonary artery enlargement with distal arterial attenuation. ECG evidence of RV hypertrophy (eg, right axis deviation, QR wave in lead V_1, and dominant R wave in leads V_1 to V_3) correlates well with degree of pulmonary hypertension. However, because pulmonary hyperinflation and bullae in COPD cause realignment of the heart, physical examination, x-rays, and ECG may be relatively insensitive. Echocardiography or radionuclide imaging is done to evaluate LV and RV function; echocardiography can assess RV systolic pressure but is often technically limited by the lung disorder. Right heart catheterization may be required for confirmation.

Treatment

Treatment is difficult; it focuses on the cause (see elsewhere in THE MANUAL), particularly alleviation or moderation of hypoxia.

If peripheral edema is present, diuretics may seem appropriate, but they are helpful only if LV failure and pulmonary fluid overload are also present; they may be harmful because small decreases in preload often worsen cor pulmonale. Pulmonary vasodilators (eg, hydralazine, Ca channel blockers, nitrous oxide, prostacyclin), although beneficial in primary pulmonary hypertension, are not effective. Digoxin is effective only if patients have concomitant LV dysfunction; caution is required because patients with COPD are sensitive to digoxin's effects. Phlebotomy during hypoxic cor pulmonale has been suggested, but the benefits of decreasing blood viscosity are not likely to offset the harm of reducing O_2-carrying capacity unless significant polycythemia is present. For patients with chronic cor pulmonale, long-term anticoagulants reduce risk of venous thromboembolism.

DILATED CONGESTIVE CARDIOMYOPATHY

Dilated cardiomyopathy is myocardial dysfunction producing heart failure in which ventricular dilation and systolic dysfunction predominate. Symptoms include dyspnea, fatigue, and peripheral edema. Diagnosis is clinical and by chest x-ray and echocardiography. Treatment is directed at the cause; heart transplantation may be needed.

Etiology and Pathophysiology

Dilated cardiomyopathy (DCM) has many known and probably many unidentified causes (see TABLE 74–2). The most common cause in temperate zones is diffuse coronary artery disease (CAD) with diffuse ischemic myopathy. More than 20 viruses can cause DCM; in temperate zones, coxsackievirus B is most common. In Central and South America, Chagas' disease due to *Trypanosoma cruzi* is the most common infectious cause. DCM is becoming increasingly common among patients with AIDS. Other causes include toxoplasmosis, thyrotoxicosis, and beriberi. Many toxic substances, particularly alcohol, various organic solvents, and certain chemotherapeutic drugs (eg, doxorubicin), damage the heart.

In some patients, DCM is believed to start with acute myocarditis (probably viral in most cases), followed by a variable latent phase, a phase with diffuse necrosis of myocardial myocytes (due to an autoimmune reaction to virus-altered myocytes), and chronic fibrosis. Regardless of the cause, the remaining myocardium dilates, thins, and hypertrophies in

TABLE 74–2. ETIOLOGY OF CARDIOMYOPATHY

FORM	ETIOLOGY
Dilated congestive cardiomyopathy (acute or chronic)	Chronic diffuse myocardial ischemia (coronary artery disease)
	Infections (acute or chronic): bacteria, spirochetes, rickettsia, viruses (including HIV), fungi, protozoa, helminths
	Granulomatous diseases: sarcoidosis, granulomatous or giant cell myocarditis, Wegener's granulomatosis
	Metabolic disorders: nutritional disorders (beriberi, selenium deficiency, carnitine deficiency, kwashiorkor), familial storage disorders, uremia, hypokalemia, hypomagnesemia, hypophosphatemia, diabetes mellitus, hyperthyroidism, hypothyroidism, pheochromocytoma, acromegaly, morbid obesity
	Drugs and toxins: ethanol, cocaine, anthracyclines, cobalt, psychotherapeutic drugs (tricyclic and quadricyclic antidepressants, phenothiazine), catecholamines, cyclophosphamide, radiation
	Tumors
	Connective tissue disorders
	Isolated familial (mendelian dominant)
	Hereditary neuromuscular and neurologic disorders (Friedreich's ataxia)
	Pregnancy (peripartum period)
Hypertrophic cardiomyopathy	Autosomal dominant inheritance, pheochromocytoma, acromegaly, neurofibromatosis
Restrictive cardiomyopathy	Amyloidosis, diffuse systemic sclerosis, endocardial fibrosis, Fabry's disease, fibroelastosis, Gaucher's disease, hemochromatosis, Löffler's syndrome, sarcoidosis, hypereosinophilia syndrome, tumors

compensation (see FIG. 74–2), often leading to functional mitral or tricuspid regurgitation and atrial dilation.

The disorder affects both ventricles in most patients, only the left ventricle (LV) in a few, and only the right ventricle (RV) rarely.

Mural thrombi frequently form once chamber dilation is significant, especially during the acute myocarditis phase. Cardiac arrhythmias often complicate the acute myocarditis and late chronic dilated phases as may atrioventricular (AV) block. Atrial fibrillation commonly occurs as the left atrium dilates.

Symptoms, Signs, and Diagnosis

Onset is usually gradual except in acute myocarditis. Symptoms depend on which ventricle is affected. LV dysfunction causes exertional dyspnea and fatigue due to elevated LV diastolic pressure and low cardiac output. RV failure causes peripheral edema and neck vein distention. When only the RV is affected, atrial arrhythmias and sudden death due to malignant ventricular tachyarrhythmias are typical. About 25% of all patients with DCM have atypical chest pain.

Diagnosis is by history, physical examination, and exclusion of other causes of ventricular failure (eg, systemic hypertension, primary valvular disorders, MI—see TABLE 74–3). Thus, chest x-ray, ECG, and echocardiography are required. If acute symptoms or chest pain is present, serum cardiac markers are measured; although typically indicative of coronary ischemia, troponin levels can be elevated in heart failure, especially if renal function is decreased. Specific causes suspected clinically are diagnosed (see elsewhere in THE MANUAL). If no specific cause is apparent, serum ferritin and iron-binding capacity and thyroid-stimulating hormone levels are measured and serologic tests for *Toxoplasma,* coxsackievirus, and echovirus are done to rule out treatable causes.

The ECG may show sinus tachycardia, low-voltage QRS complexes, and nonspecific ST-segment depression with low voltage or inverted T waves. Sometimes pathologic Q waves are present in the precordial leads, simulating previous MI. Left bundle branch block is common.

Chest x-ray shows cardiomegaly usually of all chambers. Pleural effusion, particularly on the right, often accompanies increased pulmonary venous pressure and interstitial edema. Echocardiography shows dilated, hypokinetic cardiac chambers and rules out primary valvular disorders. Segmental wall motion abnormalities, typical of MI, can also occur in DCM because the process may be patchy. Echocardiography may also show a mural thrombus. MRI is not routinely done but may be useful when detailed imaging of myocardial structure or function is needed. In cardiomyopathy, MRI may show abnormal myocardial tissue texture.

Coronary angiography is required when the diagnosis is in doubt after noninvasive tests, particularly for patients with chest pain or elderly patients, who are more likely to have CAD. However, nonobstructive coronary artery lesions detected by angiography may not be the cause of DCM. Either ventricle can be biopsied during catheterization, but biopsy is not usually done because the yield can be low, the disease process can be patchy, and results may not change treatment.

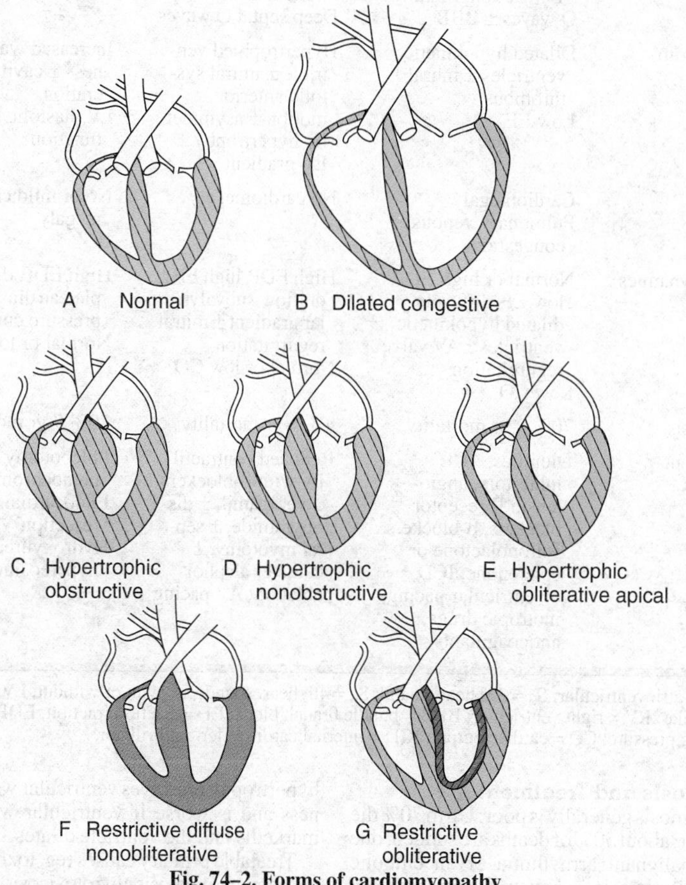

Fig. 74–2. Forms of cardiomyopathy.

TABLE 74–3. DIAGNOSIS AND TREATMENT OF CARDIOMYOPATHIES

FEATURE OR METHOD	DILATED CONGESTIVE	HYPERTROPHIC	RESTRICTIVE
Pathophysiology	Systolic dysfunction	Diastolic dysfunction ± outflow obstruction	Diastolic dysfunction
Clinical examination	LV and RV failure Cardiomegaly Functional AV valve regurgitation S_3 and S_4	Angina, exertional dyspnea, syncope, sudden death Ejection ± mitral regurgitation murmurs S_4 Bifid carotid pulse with a brisk upstroke and rapid downstroke	Exertional dyspnea and fatigue LV ± RV failure Functional AV valve regurgitation
ECG	Nonspecific ST- and T-wave abnormalities Q waves ± BBB	LV hypertrophy and ischemia Deep septal Q waves	LV hypertrophy or low voltage
Echocardiography	Dilated hypokinetic ventricles ± mural thrombus Low EF	Hypertrophied ventricle ± mitral systolic anterior motion ± asymmetric hypertrophy ± LV gradient	Increased wall thickness ± cavity obliteration LV diastolic dysfunction
X-ray	Cardiomegaly Pulmonary venous congestion	No cardiomegaly	No or mild cardiomegaly
Hemodynamics	Normal or high EDP, low EF, diffusely dilated hypokinetic ventricles ± AV valve regurgitation Low CO	High EDP, high EF ± outflow subvalvular gradient ± mitral regurgitation Normal or low CO	High EDP, dip and plateau diastolic LV pressure curve Normal or low CO
Prognosis	70% 5-yr mortality	4% 1-yr mortality	70% 5-yr mortality
Treatment	Diuretics, ACE inhibitors, angiotensin II receptor blockers, β-blockers, spironolactone or eplerenone, ICD, biventricular pacing, inotropic drugs, anticoagulants	Reduced contractility with β-blockers ± verapamil, ± disopyramide, ± septal myotomy, ± catheter alcohol ablation; AV pacing	Phlebotomy for hemochromatosis Endocardial resection Hydroxyurea for hypereosinophilia

AV = atrioventricular; S_3 = 3rd heart sound; S_4 = 4th heart sound; ± = with or without; LV = left ventricular; RV = right ventricular; BBB = bundle branch block; EF = ejection fraction; EDP = end-diastolic pressure; CO = cardiac output; ICD = internal cardioverter-defibrillator.

Prognosis and Treatment

Prognosis generally is poor: Up to 70% die in < 5 yr; about 50% of deaths are sudden, due to a malignant arrhythmia or an embolic event. Prognosis is better if compensatory hypertrophy preserves ventricular wall thickness and is worse if ventricular walls thin markedly and the ventricle dilates.

Treatable primary causes (eg, toxoplasmosis, hemochromatosis, thyrotoxicosis, beriberi) are corrected. Otherwise, treatment is the same as for heart failure (see p. 658): ACE inhibitors, β-blockers, aldosterone receptor blockers, angiotensin II receptor blockers, diuretics, digoxin, and nitrates. Corticosteroids, azathioprine, and equine antithymocyte globulin are no longer used; although they may shorten the acute phase of certain inflammatory myocarditic myopathies (eg, acute postviral or sarcoid myocarditis), they do not improve long-term outcome. Antivirals are not helpful.

Because mural thrombi may form, prophylactic oral anticoagulants (see p. 759) are often given to help prevent systemic or pulmonary emboli, although no controlled trials support this treatment. Significant cardiac arrhythmias are treated with antiarrhythmic drugs, although aggressive treatment of heart failure reduces risk of arrhythmia. Permanent pacemakers may be required if AV block occurs during the chronic dilated phase; however, AV block during acute myocarditis often resolves, so permanent pacemakers are usually not needed. If patients have a widened QRS interval and severe symptoms, biventricular pacing can be considered.

Because prognosis is poor, patients with DCM are often candidates for heart transplantation. Selection criteria include absence of associated systemic disorders, psychologic disorders, and high, irreversible pulmonary vascular resistance; because hearts are scarce, younger patients (usually < 60) are given higher priority.

HYPERTROPHIC CARDIOMYOPATHY

Hypertrophic cardiomyopathy is a congenital or acquired disorder characterized by marked ventricular hypertrophy with diastolic dysfunction but without increased afterload (eg, valvular aortic stenosis, coarctation of the aorta, systemic hypertension). Symptoms include chest pain, dyspnea, syncope, and sudden death. A systolic murmur, increased by Valsalva maneuver, is typically present in the hypertrophic obstructive type. Diagnosis is by echocardiography. Treatment is with β-blockers, verapamil, disopyramide, and sometimes chemical reduction or surgical removal of outflow tract obstruction.

Hypertrophic cardiomyopathy (HCM) is a common cause of sudden death in young athletes. It may cause unexplained syncope and may not be diagnosed before autopsy.

Etiology and Pathophysiology

Most cases of HCM are inherited (see TABLE 74–2). At least 50 different mutations that are inherited in an autosomally dominant pattern have been identified; spontaneous mutations are common. Perhaps 1 in 500 people is affected; phenotypic expression varies markedly.

The myocardium is abnormal with cellular and myofibrillar disarray, although this finding is not specific for HCM. In the most common form, the upper interventricular septum below the aortic valve is markedly hypertrophied and thickened, with little or no hypertrophy of the left ventricular (LV) posterior wall; this pattern is called asymmetric septal hypertrophy. During systole, the septum thickens, and sometimes the anterior leaflet of the mitral valve, already abnormally oriented because of the abnormally shaped ventricle, is sucked toward the septum by a Venturi effect of high velocity blood flow, further obstructing the outflow tract and decreasing cardiac output. The resulting disorder may be termed hypertrophic obstructive cardiomyopathy. Less commonly, midventricular hypertrophy leads to an intracavitary gradient at the papillary muscle level. In both forms, the distal LV may ultimately thin and dilate. Apical hypertrophy can also occur but does not obstruct outflow, although it may obliterate the apical portion of the LV during systole.

Contractility is grossly normal, resulting in a normal ejection fraction (EF). Later, EF is elevated because the ventricle has a small volume and empties nearly completely to maintain cardiac output.

Hypertrophy results in a stiff, noncompliant chamber (usually the LV) that resists diastolic filling, elevating end-diastolic pressure and thus increasing pulmonary venous pressure. As resistance to filling increases, cardiac output decreases, an effect worsened by any outflow tract gradient present. Because tachycardia allows less time for filling, symptoms tend to appear mainly during exercise or tachyarrhythmias.

Coronary blood flow may be impaired, causing angina pectoris, syncope, or arrhythmias in the absence of epicardial coronary artery disease (CAD). Flow may be impaired because capillary density relative to myocyte size is inadequate (capillary/myocyte imbalance) or lumen diameter of intramyocardial coronary arteries is narrowed by intimal and medial hyperplasia and hypertrophy. Also, exercise lowers peripheral vascular resistance and aortic root diastolic pressure, thus reducing coronary perfusion pressure.

In some cases, myocytes gradually die, probably because capillary/myocyte imbalance causes chronic diffuse ischemia. As myocytes die, they are replaced by diffuse fibrosis. Then, the hypertrophied ventricle with diastolic dysfunction gradually dilates and systolic dysfunction also develops.

Infective endocarditis can complicate HCM because of the mitral valve abnormality and because of rapid blood flow through the outflow tract during early systole. Atrioventricular block is sometimes a late complication.

Symptoms and Signs

Typically, symptoms appear between age 20 and 40 and are exertional. They include chest pain (usually resembling typical angina—see p. 627), dyspnea, palpitations, and syncope. Patients may have one or several symptoms. Syncope usually occurs without warning during exertion, is due to nonsustained ventricular or atrial arrhythmia, and is a marker of increased risk of sudden death. Sudden death due to HCM is thought to result from ventricular tachycardia or fibrillation. Because systolic function is preserved, fatigability is seldom reported.

BP and heart rate are usually normal, and signs of increased venous pressure are rare. When the outflow tract is obstructed, the carotid pulse has a brisk upstroke, bifid peak, and rapid downstroke. The apex beat may have a sustained thrust due to LV hypertrophy. A 4th heart sound (S_4) is often present and is associated with a forceful atrial contraction against a poorly compliant LV in late diastole.

Septal hypertrophy produces a systolic ejection-type murmur that does not radiate to the neck and may be heard at the left sternal edge in the 3rd or 4th intercostal space. A mitral regurgitation murmur due to distortion of the mitral apparatus may be heard at the apex. When the right ventricular outflow tract is narrowed, a systolic ejection murmur is sometimes heard in the 2nd interspace at the left sternal border. The LV outflow ejection murmur of HCM can be increased by a Valsalva maneuver (which reduces venous return and LV diastolic volume), by measures to lower aortic pressure (eg, nitroglycerin), or by a postextrasystolic contraction (which increases the outflow tract pressure gradient). Handgrip increases aortic pressure, thereby reducing the murmur's intensity.

Diagnosis

Diagnosis is suspected based on a typical murmur and symptoms. Unexplained syncope in young athletes should always raise suspicion. HCM must be distinguished from aortic stenosis and CAD, which produce similar symptoms. ECG and 2-dimensional echocardiography (the best noninvasive confirmatory test) are done. Chest x-ray is often taken but is usually normal because the ventricles are not dilated (although the left atrium may be enlarged). Patients with syncope or sustained arrhythmias should be evaluated as inpatients. Exercise testing and Holter monitoring may be helpful for patients considered at high risk, although identifying such patients is difficult.

The ECG usually shows voltage criteria for LV hypertrophy (eg, S wave in lead V_1 plus R wave in lead V_5 or $V_6 > 35$ mm). Very deep septal Q waves in leads I, aVL, V_5, and V_6 are often present with asymmetric septal hypertrophy; HCM sometimes produces a QRS complex in V_1 and V_2, simulating previous septal infarction. T waves are usually abnormal; the most common finding is deep symmetric T-wave inversion in leads I, aVL, V_5, and V_6. ST-segment depression in the same leads is common. The P wave is often broad and notched in leads II, III, and aVF, with a biphasic P wave in leads V_1 and V_2, indicating left atrial hypertrophy. Incidence of preexcitation phenomenon of the Wolff-Parkinson-White syndrome type, which may cause palpitations, is increased.

Two-dimensional Doppler echocardiography can differentiate the forms of cardiomyopathy (see FIG. 74–2) and quantify degree of outflow tract obstruction, including pressure gradient and area of the stenotic segment. These measurements are particularly useful for monitoring the effect of medical or surgical treatment. Midsystolic closure of the aortic valve sometimes occurs when outflow tract obstruction is severe.

Cardiac catheterization is usually done only when invasive therapy is considered. Usually, no significant stenoses are present in the coronary arteries, but metabolic tests may detect myocardial ischemia due to intramyocardial artery lumen reduction, capillary/myocyte imbalance, or abnormal ventricular wall stress. Elderly patients may also have CAD.

Prognosis and Treatment

Overall, annual mortality is 1 to 3% for adults but is higher for children. Mortality rate is inversely proportional to the age at which symptoms appear and is highest in patients who have frequent nonsustained ventricular tachycardia or syncope or have been resuscitated after sudden cardiac arrest. Prognosis is worse for young patients with a family history of sudden death and for patients > 45 yr with angina or exertional dyspnea. Death is usually sudden, and sudden death is the most common sequelae; chronic heart failure occurs less often. Genetic counseling is appropriate for patients with asymmetric septal hypertrophy, which appears to accelerate during puberty.

Treatment is directed primarily at abnormal diastolic compliance. β-Blockers and rate-limiting Ca channel blockers with a lower arterial dilation capacity (eg, verapamil), alone or combined, are the mainstays. By decreasing myocardial contractility, these drugs dilate the heart. By slowing the heart rate, they prolong the diastolic filling period. Both effects decrease outflow obstruction, thus improving ventricular diastolic function. In severe cases, disopyramide may be added for its negative inotropic effect.

Drugs that reduce preload (eg, nitrates, diuretics, ACE inhibitors, angiotensin II receptor blockers) decrease chamber size and worsen symptoms and signs. Vasodilators increase the outflow tract gradient and produce a reflex tachycardia that further worsens ventricular diastolic function. Inotropic drugs (eg, digitalis glycosides, catecholamines) worsen outflow tract obstruction, do not relieve the high end-diastolic pressure, and may induce arrhythmias.

If syncope or sudden cardiac arrest has occurred or if arrhythmia is confirmed by ECG or 24-h ambulatory monitoring, an internal cardioverter-defibrillator or antiarrhythmics should be considered. Antibiotic prophylaxis for infective endocarditis is recommended for patients with HCM (see p. 729). Competitive sports should be avoided because many sudden deaths occur during increased exertion.

Treatment of the dilated congestive phase of HCM is the same as that of dilated cardiomyopathy with predominant systolic dysfunction.

If septal hypertrophy and outflow tract obstruction cause significant symptoms despite medical therapy, surgery is needed. Catheter alcohol ablation is variably effective but is becoming more widely used; surgical septal myotomy or myomectomy reduces symptoms more reliably but does not prolong life.

RESTRICTIVE CARDIOMYOPATHY

Restrictive cardiomyopathy is characterized by noncompliant ventricular walls that resist diastolic filling; one or both ventricles, most commonly the left, may be affected. Symptoms include fatigue and exertional dyspnea. Diagnosis is by echocardiography. Treatment is often unsatisfactory and is best directed at the cause. Surgery is sometimes useful.

Restrictive cardiomyopathy (RCM) is the least prevalent form of cardiomyopathy. It is classified as nonobliterative (myocardial infiltration by an abnormal substance) or obliterative (fibrosis of the endocardium and subendocardium). Either type may be diffuse or nondiffuse (when the disorder affects only one ventricle or part of one ventricle unevenly).

Etiology and Pathophysiology

The cause is usually unknown; identified causes are listed in TABLE 74–2. Some disorders that cause RCM also affect other tissues. Infiltration of the myocardium by amyloid (amyloidosis) or iron (hemochromatosis) usually also affects other organs; rarely, amyloidosis affects coronary arteries. Sarcoidosis and Fabry's disease may also affect nodal conduction tissue. Löffler's syndrome (a subcategory of hypereosinophilic syndrome with primary cardiac involvement), which occurs in the tropics, begins as an acute arteritis with eosinophilia, followed by thrombus formation on the endocardium, chordae, and atrioventricular (AV) valves, progressing to fibrosis. Endocardial fibroelastosis, which occurs in temperate zones, affects only the left ventricle.

Endocardial thickening or myocardial infiltration (sometimes with death of myocytes, papillary muscle infiltration, compensatory myocardial hypertrophy, and fibrosis) may occur in one, typically the left, or both ventricles. As a result, the mitral or tricuspid valves may malfunction, leading to regurgitation. Functional AV valve regurgitation may result from myocardial infiltration or endocardial thickening. If nodal and conduction tissues are affected, the sinoatrial node malfunctions, sometimes causing various grades of AV block.

The main hemodynamic consequence is diastolic dysfunction with a rigid, noncompliant ventricle, impaired diastolic filling, and high filling pressure, leading to pulmonary venous hypertension. Systolic function may deteriorate if compensatory hypertrophy of infiltrated or fibrosed ventricles is inadequate. Mural thrombi can form, resulting in systemic emboli.

Symptoms, Signs, and Diagnosis

Symptoms are exertional dyspnea, orthopnea, and, when the right ventricle is affected, peripheral edema. Fatigue results from a fixed cardiac output due to resistance to ventricular filling. Atrial and ventricular arrhythmias and AV block are common; angina and syncope are uncommon. Symptoms and signs closely mimic those of constrictive pericarditis (see p. 732).

Physical examination detects a quiet precordium, a low-volume and rapid carotid pulse, pulmonary crackles, and pronounced neck vein distention with a rapid *y* descent (see FIG. 69–1 on p. 574). A 4th heart sound (S_4) is almost always present; a 3rd heart sound (S_3) may occur and must be differentiated from the precordial knock of constrictive pericarditis. In some cases, a murmur of functional mitral or tricuspid regurgitation results because myocardial or endocardial infiltration or fibrosis changes chordae or ventricular geometry. Pulsus paradoxus does not occur.

ECG, chest x-ray, and echocardiography are required. The ECG is usually nonspecifically abnormal, showing ST-segment and T-wave abnormalities and sometimes low voltage. Pathologic Q waves, not due to previous MI, sometimes occur. Left ventricular hypertrophy due to compensatory myocardial hypertrophy sometimes occurs. On chest x-ray, the heart size is often normal or small but can be enlarged in late-stage amyloidosis or hemochromatosis.

Echocardiography shows normal systolic function. Common findings include dilated atria and myocardial hypertrophy. RCM due to amyloidosis has an unusually bright echo pattern from the myocardium. Echocardiography helps differentiate constrictive pericarditis with its thickened pericardium, but paradoxical septal motion can occur in either disorder. If the diagnosis is still in doubt, CT may be more sensitive in showing whether the pericardium is normal, and MRI can show abnormal myocardial texture in disorders with myocardial infiltration (eg, by amyloid or iron).

Cardiac catheterization and myocardial biopsy are not often necessary. If done, catheterization detects high atrial pressure in RCM, with a prominent *y* descent and an early diastolic dip followed by a high diastolic plateau in the ventricular pressure curve. In contrast to constrictive pericarditis findings, diastolic pressure is usually a few mm of Hg higher in the left ventricle than in the right. Angiography detects normal-sized ventricular cavities with normal or decreased systolic shortening. AV valve regurgitation may be present. Biopsy can detect endocardial fibrosis and thickening, myocardial infiltration by iron or amyloid, and chronic myocardial fibrosis. Coronary angiography is normal, except when amyloidosis affects epicardial coronary arteries. Occasionally, cardiac catheterization is not diagnostic, and rarely, thoracotomy is required to explore the pericardium.

Tests for the most common causes of RCM (eg, rectal biopsy for amyloidosis, iron tests or liver biopsy for hemochromatosis) should be done.

Prognosis and Treatment

Prognosis is poor (see TABLE 74–3), similar to that with dilated congestive cardiomyopathy, because the diagnosis is often made at a late stage. No treatment is available for most patients; symptomatic, supportive care can be provided.

Diuretics must be used with caution because they can lower preload; the noncompliant ventricles depend on preload to maintain cardiac output. Digitalis does little to alter hemodynamic abnormalities and may be dangerous in cardiomyopathy due to amyloidosis, in which extreme digitalis sensitivity is common. Afterload reducers (eg, nitrates) may cause profound hypotension and usually are not useful.

If the diagnosis is made at an early stage, specific treatment of hemochromatosis, sarcoidosis, and Loëffler's syndrome may help.

75 ARRHYTHMIAS AND CONDUCTION DISORDERS

The normal heart beats in a regular, coordinated way because electrical impulses generated and spread by myocytes with unique electrical properties trigger a sequence of organized myocardial contractions. Arrhythmias and conduction disorders are caused by abnormalities in the generation or conduction of these electrical impulses or both.

Any heart disorder, including congenital abnormalities of structure (eg, accessory AV connection) or function (eg, hereditary ion channelopathies), can disturb rhythm. Systemic factors that can cause or contribute to a rhythm disturbance include electrolyte abnormalities (particularly low K or Mg), hypoxia, hormonal imbalances (eg, hypothyroidism, hyperthyroidism), and drugs and toxins (eg, alcohol, caffeine).

Anatomy and Physiology

At the junction of the superior vena cava and high lateral right atrium is a cluster of cells that generates the initial electrical impulse of each normal heart beat, called the sinoatrial (SA) or sinus node. Electrical discharge of these pacemaker cells stimulates adjacent cells, leading to stimulation of successive regions of the heart in an orderly sequence. Impulses are transmitted through the atria to the atrioventricular (AV) node via preferentially conducting internodal tracts and unspecialized atrial myocytes. The AV node is located on the right side of the interatrial septum. It has a slow conduction velocity and thus delays impulse transmission. AV nodal transmission time is heart-rate dependent and is modulated by autonomic tone and circulating catecholamines to maximize cardiac output at any given atrial rate.

The atria are electrically insulated from the ventricles by the annulus fibrosus except in the anteroseptal region. There, the bundle of His, the continuation of the AV node, enters the top of the interventricular septum, where it bifurcates into the left and right bundle branches, which terminate in Purkinje fibers. The right bundle branch conducts impulses to the anterior and apical endocardial regions of the right ventricle. The left bundle branch fans out over the left side of the interventricular septum. Its anterior portion (left anterior hemifascicle) and its posterior portion (left posterior hemifascicle) stimulate the left side of the interventricular septum, which is the 1st part of the ventricles to be electrically activated. Thus, the interventricular septum depolarizes left to right, followed by near-simultaneous activation of both ventricles from the endocardial surface through the ventricular walls to the epicardial surface.

Electrophysiology: The passage of ions across the myocyte cell membrane is regulated through specific ion channels that produce cyclical depolarization and repolarization of the cell, called an action potential. The action potential of a working myocyte begins when the cell is depolarized from its diastolic −90 mV transmembrane potential to a potential of about −50 mV. At this threshold potential, voltage-dependent fast Na channels open, causing rapid depolarization mediated by Na influx down its steep concentration gradient. The fast Na channel is rapidly inactivated and Na influx stops, but other time- and voltage-dependent ion channels open, allowing Ca to enter through slow Ca channels (a depolarizing event) and K to leave through K channels (a repolarizing event). At first, these 2 processes are balanced, maintaining a positive transmembrane potential, prolonging the plateau phase of the action potential. During this phase, Ca entering the cell is responsible for electromechanical coupling and myocyte contraction. Eventually, Ca influx ceases, and K efflux increases, causing rapid repolarization of the cell back to the −90 mV resting transmembrane potential. While depolarized, the cell is resistant (refractory) to a subsequent depolarizing event; initially, a subsequent depolarization is not possible (absolute refractory period), and after partial but incomplete repolarization, a subsequent depolarization is possible but occurs slowly (relative refractory period).

There are 2 general types of cardiac tissue. Fast-channel tissues (working atrial and ventricular myocytes, His-Purkinje system) have a high density of fast Na channels and action potentials characterized by little or no spontaneous diastolic depolarization (and thus very slow rates of pacemaker activity), very rapid initial depolarization rates (and thus rapid conduction velocity), and loss of refractoriness coincident with repolarization (and thus short refractory periods and the ability to conduct repetitive impulses at high frequencies). Slow-channel tissues (SA and AV nodes) have a low density of fast Na channels and action potentials characterized by more rapid spontaneous diastolic depolarization (and thus more rapid rates of pacemaker activity), slow initial depolarization rates (and thus slow conduction velocity), and loss of refractoriness that is delayed after repolarization (and thus long refractory periods and the inability to conduct repetitive impulses at high frequencies).

Normally, the SA node has the most rapid rate of spontaneous diastolic depolarization, so its cells produce spontaneous action potentials at a higher frequency than other tissues. Thus, the SA node is the dominant automatic tissue (pacemaker) in a normal heart. If the SA node does not produce impulses, tissue with the next highest automaticity rate, typically the AV node, functions as the pacemaker. Sympathetic stimulation increases the discharge frequency of pacemaker tissue, and parasympathetic stimulation decreases it.

Normal rhythm: The resting sinus heart rate in adults is usually 60 to 100 beats/min. Slower rates (sinus bradycardia) occur in young people, particularly athletes (see p. 768), and during sleep. Faster rates (sinus tachycardia) occur with exercise, illness, or emotion through sympathetic neural and circulating catecholamine drive. Normally, a marked diurnal variation in heart rate occurs, with lowest rates just before early morning awakening. A slight increase in rate during inspiration with a decrease in rate during expiration (respiratory sinus arrhythmia) is also normal; it is mediated by oscillations in vagal tone and is particularly common among healthy young people. The oscillations lessen but do not entirely disappear with age. Absolute regularity of the sinus rhythm rate is pathologic and occurs in patients with autonomic denervation (eg, in advanced diabetes) or with severe heart failure.

Most cardiac electrical activity is represented on the ECG (see FIG. 70–1 on p. 590), although SA node, AV node, and His-Purkinje depolarization does not involve enough tissue to be detected. The P wave represents atrial depolarization. The QRS complex represents ventricular depolarization, and the T wave represents ventricular repolarization.

The PR interval (from the beginning of the P wave to the beginning of the QRS complex) is the time from the beginning of atrial activation to the beginning of ventricular activation. Much of this interval reflects slowing of impulse transmission in the AV node. The R-R interval (time between 2 QRS complexes) represents the ventricular rate. The QT interval (from the beginning of the QRS complex to the end of the T wave) represents the duration of ventricular depolarization. Normal values for the QT interval are slightly longer in women; they are also longer with a slower heart rate. The QT interval is corrected (QTc) for influence of heart rate. The most common formula (all intervals in sec) is:

$$QTc = \frac{QT}{\sqrt{RR}}$$

Pathophysiology

Rhythm disturbances result from abnormalities of impulse formation, impulse conduction, or both. Bradyarrhythmias result from decreased intrinsic pacemaker function or blocks in conduction, principally within the AV node or the His-Purkinje system. Most tachyarrhythmias are caused by reentry; some result from enhanced normal automaticity or from abnormal mechanisms of automaticity.

Reentry is the circular propagation of an impulse around 2 interconnected pathways with different conduction characteristics and refractory periods (see FIG. 75–1). Under certain conditions, typically precipitated by a premature beat, reentry can produce continuous circulation of an activation wavefront producing a tachyarrhythmia (see FIG. 75–2). Normally, reentry is prevented by tissue refractoriness following stimulation. However, 3 conditions favor reentry: shortening of tissue refractoriness (eg, by sympathetic stimulation), lengthening of the conduction pathway (eg, by hypertrophy or abnormal conduction pathways), and slowing of impulse conduction (eg, by ischemia).

Symptoms and Signs

Arrhythmia and conduction disturbances may be asymptomatic or cause palpitations (sensation of skipped beats or rapid or forceful beats—see p. 581), symptoms of hemodynamic compromise (eg, dyspnea, chest discomfort, presyncope, syncope), or cardiac arrest. Occasionally, polyuria results from release of atrial natriuretic peptide during prolonged supraventricular tachycardias (SVTs).

Palpation of pulse and cardiac auscultation can determine ventricular rate and its regularity or irregularity. Examination of the

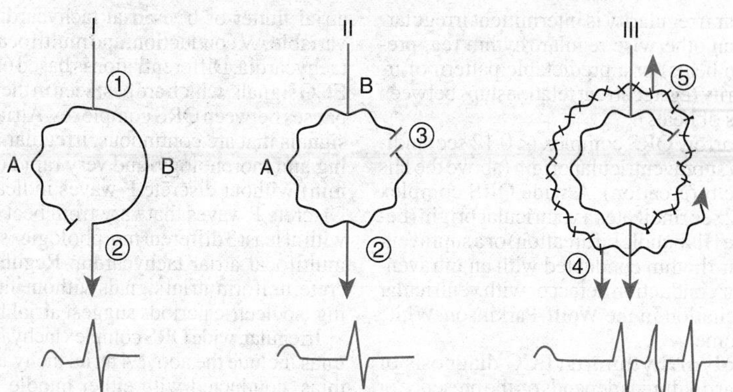

Fig. 75–1. Mechanism of typical reentry. Two pathways connect the same points. Pathway A has slower conduction and a shorter refractory period. Pathway B conducts normally and has a longer refractory period.

I. A normal impulse arriving at I goes down both A and B pathways. Conduction through pathway A is slower and finds tissue at 2 already depolarized and thus refractory. A normal sinus beat results.

II. A premature impulse finds pathway B refractory and is blocked, but it can be conducted on pathway A because its refractory period is shorter. On arriving at 2, the impulse continues forward and retrograde up pathway B, where it is blocked by refractory tissue at 3. A sinus beat with an increased PR interval results.

III. If conduction over pathway A is sufficiently slow, a premature impulse may continue retrograde all the way up pathway B, which is now past its refractory period. If pathway A is also past its refractory period, the impulse may reenter pathway A and continue to circle, sending an impulse each cycle to the ventricle (4) and retrograde to the atrium (5), producing a sustained reentrant tachycardia.

jugular venous pulse waves may help in the diagnosis of AV blocks and atrial tachyarrhythmias. For example, in complete AV block, the atria intermittently contract when the AV valves are closed, producing large *a* (cannon) waves in the jugular venous pulse (see p. 574). Other physical findings of arrhythmias are few.

Diagnosis

History and physical examination may detect an arrhythmia and suggest possible causes, but diagnosis requires a 12-lead ECG or, less reliably, a rhythm strip, preferably obtained during symptoms to establish the relationship between symptoms and rhythm.

The ECG is approached systematically; calipers measure intervals and identify subtle irregularities. The key diagnostic features are rate of atrial activation, rate and regularity of ventricular activation, and the relationship between the two. Irregular activation signals are classified as regularly irregular or irregularly irregular (no detectible pattern).

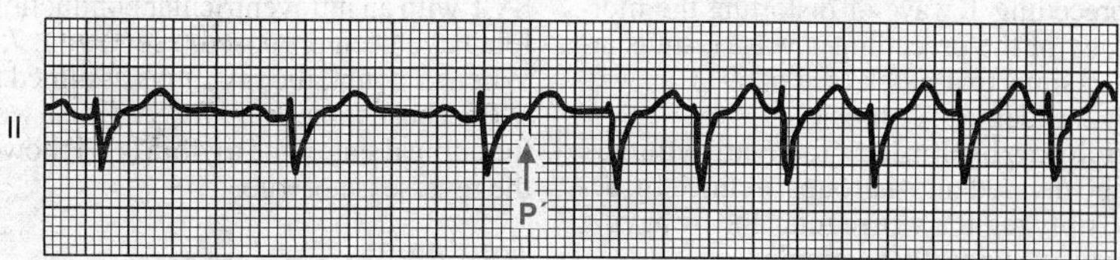

Fig. 75–2. Initiation of an atrioventricular nodal reentry tachycardia. There is an abnormal P wave (P′) and atrioventricular nodal delay (long P′R) before onset of the tachycardia.

Regular irregularity is intermittent irregularity in an otherwise regular rhythm (eg, premature beats) or a predictable pattern of irregularity (eg, recurrent relationships between groups of beats).

A narrow QRS complex (< 0.12 sec) indicates a supraventricular origin (above the His bundle bifurcation). A wide QRS complex (≥ 0.12 sec) indicates a ventricular origin (below the His bundle bifurcation) or a supraventricular rhythm conducted with an intraventricular conduction defect or with ventricular preexcitation in the Wolff-Parkinson-White syndrome.

Bradyarrhythmias: ECG diagnosis of bradyarrhythmias depends on the presence or absence of P waves, morphology of the P waves, and the relationship between P waves and QRS complexes.

A bradyarrhythmia with no relationship between P waves and QRS complexes indicates AV dissociation; the escape rhythm can be junctional (narrow QRS complex) or ventricular (wide QRS complex).

A regular QRS rhythm with a 1:1 relationship between P waves and QRS complexes indicates absence of AV block. P waves preceding QRS complexes indicate sinus bradycardia (if P waves are normal) or sinus arrest with an escape atrial bradycardia (if P waves are abnormal). P waves after QRS complexes indicate sinus arrest with a ventricular escape rhythm and retrograde ventriculoatrial conduction. In this case, the QRS complex is wide.

When the QRS rhythm is irregular, P waves usually outnumber QRS complexes; some P waves produce QRS complexes, but some do not (indicating 2nd-degree AV block—see p. 695). An irregular QRS rhythm with a 1:1 relationship between P waves and the following QRS complexes usually indicates sinus arrhythmia with gradual acceleration and deceleration of the sinus rate (if P waves are normal).

Pauses in an otherwise regular QRS rhythm may be caused by blocked P waves (an abnormal P wave can usually be discerned just after the preceding T wave or distorting the morphology of the preceding T wave), sinus arrest, or sinus exit block (see p. 691), as well as by 2nd-degree AV block.

Tachyarrhythmias: Tachyarrhythmias may be divided into 4 groups, defined by being visibly regular vs irregular and by having a narrow vs wide QRS complex.

Irregular, narrow QRS complex tachyarrhythmias include atrial fibrillation (AF), atrial flutter or true atrial tachycardia with variable AV conduction, and multifocal atrial tachycardia. Differentiation is based on atrial ECG signals, which are best seen in the longer pauses between QRS complexes. Atrial ECG signals that are continuous, irregular in timing and morphology, and very rapid (> 300/min) without discrete P waves indicate AF. Discrete P waves that vary from beat to beat with at least 3 different morphologies suggest multifocal atrial tachycardia. Regular, discrete, uniform atrial signals without intervening isoelectric periods suggest atrial flutter.

Irregular, wide QRS complex tachyarrhythmias include the above 4 atrial tachyarrhythmias, conducted with either bundle branch block or ventricular preexcitation, and polymorphic ventricular tachycardia (VT). Differentiation is based on atrial ECG signals and the presence in polymorphic VT of a very rapid rate (> 250/min).

Regular, narrow QRS complex tachyarrhythmias include sinus tachycardia, atrial flutter or true atrial tachycardia with a consistent AV conduction ratio, and paroxysmal SVTs (AV nodal reentrant SVT, orthodromic reciprocating AV tachycardia in the presence of an accessory AV connection, and SA nodal reentrant SVT). Vagal maneuvers or pharmacologic AV nodal blockade can help distinguish among these tachycardias. With these maneuvers, sinus tachycardia is not terminated, but it slows or AV block develops, disclosing normal P waves. Similarly, atrial flutter and true atrial tachycardia are usually not terminated, but AV block discloses flutter waves or abnormal P waves. The most common forms of paroxysmal SVT (AV nodal reentry and orthodromic reciprocating tachycardia) must terminate if AV block occurs.

Regular, wide QRS complex tachyarrhythmias include those listed for a regular, narrow QRS complex tachyarrhythmia, each with bundle branch block or ventricular preexcitation, and monomorphic VT. Vagal maneuvers can help distinguish among them. ECG criteria to distinguish between VT and SVT with an intraventricular conduction defect have been proposed (see TABLE 75–1). When in doubt, the rhythm is assumed to be VT because some drugs for SVTs can worsen the clinical state if the rhythm is VT; however, the reverse is not true.

Treatment

The need for treatment varies; it is guided by symptoms and risks of the arrhythmia.

Asymptomatic arrhythmias without serious risks do not require treatment even if they worsen. Symptomatic arrhythmias may require treatment to improve quality of life. Potentially life-threatening arrhythmias require treatment.

Treatment is directed at causes. If necessary, direct antiarrhythmic therapy, including antiarrhythmic drugs, cardioversion-defibrillation, pacemakers, or a combination, is used. Patients with arrhythmias that have caused or are likely to cause symptoms of hemodynamic compromise may have to be restricted from driving until response to treatment has been assessed.

TABLE 75–1. MODIFIED BRUGADA CRITERIA FOR VENTRICULAR TACHYCARDIA

Criterion		
Is there AV dissociation (independent P/QRS, capture beats, fusion beats)?	No	Yes = VT
Is there an RS in any precordial lead?	Yes	No = VT
Is QRS onset to nadir of S wave > 100 msec in any precordial lead?	No	Yes = VT
Are there morphologic criteria* for VT in both V_1 and V_6?	No	Yes = VT
Diagnosis of supraventricular tachycardia with aberrant conduction		

*Morphologic criteria
With RBBB QRS: In V_1, monophasic R, or QR, or RS
In V_6, R/S < 1 or monophasic R or QR
With LBBB QRS: In V_1, R > 30 msec wide or RS > 60 msec wide
In V_6, QR or QS

VT = ventricular tachycardia; AV = atrioventricular; RBBB = right bundle branch block; LBBB = left bundle branch block.

Drugs for Arrhythmias

Most antiarrhythmic drugs are grouped into 4 main classes (Vaughan Williams classification) based on their dominant cellular electrophysiologic effect (see TABLE 75–2). Digoxin and adenosine are not included in the Vaughan Williams classification. Digoxin shortens atrial and ventricular refractory periods and is vagotonic, thereby prolonging AV nodal conduction and AV nodal refractory periods. Adenosine slows or blocks AV nodal conduction and can terminate tachyarrhythmias that rely upon AV nodal conduction for their perpetuation.

Class I: Na channel blockers (membrane-stabilizing drugs) block fast Na channels, slowing conduction in fast-channel tissues (working atrial and ventricular myocytes, His-Purkinje system). In the ECG, this effect may be reflected as widening of the P wave, widening of the QRS complex, prolongation of the PR interval, or a combination.

Class I drugs are subdivided based on the kinetics of the Na channel effects. Class Ib drugs have fast kinetics, class Ic drugs have slow kinetics, and class Ia drugs have intermediate kinetics. The kinetics of Na channel blockade determine the heart rates at which their electrophysiologic effects become manifest. Because class Ib drugs have fast kinetics, they express their electrophysiologic effects only at fast heart rates. Thus, an ECG obtained during normal rhythm at normal rates usually shows no evidence of fast-channel tissue conduction slowing. Class Ib drugs are not very potent antiarrhythmics and have minimal effects on atrial tissue. Because class Ic drugs have slow kinetics, they express their electrophysiologic effects at all heart rates. Thus, an ECG obtained during normal rhythm at normal heart rates usually shows fast-channel tissue conduction slowing. Class Ic drugs are more potent antiarrhythmics. Because class Ia drugs have intermediate kinetics, their fast-channel tissue conduction slowing effects may or may not be evident on an ECG obtained during normal rhythm at normal rates. Class Ia drugs also block repolarizing K channels, prolonging the refractory periods of fast-channel tissues. On the ECG, this effect is reflected as QT-interval prolongation even at normal rates. Class Ib drugs and class Ic drugs do not block K channels directly.

The primary indications are SVTs for class Ia and Ic drugs and VTs for all class I drugs. The most worrisome adverse effect is proarrhythmia, a drug-related arrhythmia worse than the arrhythmia being treated. Class Ia drugs may produce torsades de pointes VT; class Ia and class Ic drugs may organize and slow atrial tachyarrhythmias enough to permit 1:1 AV conduction with marked acceleration of the ventricular response rate. All class I drugs may worsen VTs. They also tend to depress ventricular

Text continues on page 683.

TABLE 75–2. ANTIARRHYTHMIC DRUGS (VAUGHAN-WILLIAMS CLASSIFICATION)

DRUG	DOSAGE	TARGET LEVELS	ADVERSE EFFECTS	COMMENTS
Class Ia	Uses: APB and VPB suppression, SVT and VT suppression, AF or atrial flutter, and VF suppression			
Disopyramide	IV: Initially, 1.5 mg/kg over > 5 min followed by an infusion of 0.4 mg/kg/h Oral immediate-release: 100 or 150 mg q 6 h Oral controlled-release: 200 or 300 mg q 12 h	2–7.5 μg/mL	Anticholinergic effects (urinary retention, glaucoma, dry mouth, blurred vision, intestinal upset), hypoglycemia, torsades de pointes, ventricular tachycardia	Drug should be used cautiously in patients with impaired LV function Dosage should be decreased in patients with renal insufficiency Adverse effects may contribute to noncompliance If QRS interval widens (> 50% if initially < 120 msec or > 25% if initially > 120 msec) or if QTc interval is prolonged > 550 msec, infusion rate or dosage should be decreased or drug stopped IV form is not available in the US
Procainamide	IV: 10–15 mg/kg bolus at 25–50 mg/min followed by a constant IV infusion of 1–4 mg/min Oral: 250–625 mg (rarely, up to 1 g) q 3 or 4 h	4–8 g/mL	Hypotension (with IV infusion), serologic abnormalities (especially ANA) in almost 100% taking > 12 mo, drug-induced lupus (arthralgia, fever, pleural effusions) in 15–20%, agranulocytosis in < 1%, torsades de pointes, ventricular tachycardia	Sustained-release preparations obviate the need for frequent dosing If QRS interval widens (> 50% if initially < 120 msec or > 25% if initially >120 msec) or if QTc interval is prolonged > 550 msec, infusion rate or dosage should be decreased or drug stopped

TABLE 75–2. ANTIARRHYTHMIC DRUGS (VAUGHAN-WILLIAMS CLASSIFICATION)—Continued

DRUG	DOSAGE	TARGET LEVELS	ADVERSE EFFECTS	COMMENTS
Quinidine	Oral: 200–400 mg q 4–6 h	2–6 μg/mL	Diarrhea, colic, and flatulence; fever; thrombocytopenia; liver function abnormalities; torsades de pointes; ventricular tachycardia; overall adverse effect rate of 30%	If QRS interval widens (> 50% if initially < 120 msec or > 25% if initially >120 msec) or if QTc interval is prolonged > 550 msec, infusion rate or dosage should be decreased or drug stopped
Class Ib	Uses: Suppression of ventricular arrhythmias (VPB, VT, VF)			
Lidocaine	IV: 100 mg over 2 min followed by continuous infusion of 4 mg/min (2 mg/min in patients > 65); 5 min after 1st dose, a 2nd 50-mg bolus is given	2–5 μg/L	Tremor, seizures; if administration is too rapid, drowsiness, delirium, paresthesias	To reduce toxicity risk, dosage or infusion rate should be reduced to 2 mg/min after 24 h Extensive 1st-pass hepatic metabolism occurs
Mexiletine	Oral immediate-release: 100–250 mg po q 8 h Oral slow-release: 360 mg po q 12 h IV: 2 mg/kg at 25 mg/min followed by 250-mg infusion over 1 h, 250-mg infusion over next 2 h, and maintenance infusion of 0.5 mg/min	0.5–2 μg/mL	Nausea, vomiting, tremor, seizures	Oral slow-release and IV forms are not available in the US
Class Ic	Uses: APB and VPB suppression, SVT and VT suppression, AF or atrial flutter, and ventricular fibrillation suppression			
Flecainide	Oral: 100 mg q 8 or 12 h IV: 1–2 mg/kg over 10 min	0.2–1 μg/mL	Occasionally, blurred vision and paresthesias; increased mortality in post-MI patients with asymptomatic or minimally symptomatic VPBs	IV form is not available in US If QRS complex widens (> 50% if initially < 120 msec and > 25% if initially > 120 msec), dose must be decreased or drug stopped

Table continues on the following page.

TABLE 75–2. ANTIARRHYTHMIC DRUGS (VAUGHAN-WILLIAMS CLASSIFICATION)—Continued

DRUG	DOSAGE	TARGET LEVELS	ADVERSE EFFECTS	COMMENTS
Propafenone	Oral: Initially, 150 mg tid, titrated up to 150–300 mg tid IV: 2-mg/kg bolus, followed by 2 mg/min infusion	0.1–1.0 μg/mL	Has β-blocking activity and can worsen reactive airway disorders; occasionally GI upset	Pharmacokinetics is nonlinear; increases in dose should not exceed 50% of previous dose Bioavailability and protein binding vary; drug has saturable 1st-pass metabolism IV form is not available in the US
Class II β-blockers	Uses: Supraventricular tachyarrhythmias (APB, ST, SVT, AF, atrial flutter), and ventricular arrhythmias (often in a supportive role)			
Atenolol	Oral: 50–100 mg once/day	Drug levels not measured; dose adjusted to reduce heart rate by > 25%	GI disturbances, insomnia, nightmares, lethargy, erectile dysfunction	These drugs are contraindicated in bronchospastic airway disorders
Carvedilol	Oral: Initially, 6.25 mg bid, followed by titration to 25 mg bid			
Acebutolol	Oral: 200 mg bid			
Betaxolol	Oral: 20 mg once/day			
Bisoprolol	5 mg once/day			
Esmolol	IV: 50–200 μg/kg/min			
Metoprolol	Oral: 50–100 mg bid IV: 5 mg q 5 min up to 15 mg			
Nadolol	Oral: 60–80 mg once/day			
Propranolol	Oral: 10–30 mg tid or qid IV: 1–3 mg (may repeat once after 5 min if needed)			

TABLE 75–2. ANTIARRHYTHMIC DRUGS (VAUGHAN-WILLIAMS CLASSIFICATION)—Continued

DRUG	DOSAGE	TARGET LEVELS	ADVERSE EFFECTS	COMMENTS
Class III Membrane-stabilizing drugs	Uses: Any tachyarrhythmia except torsades de pointes VT			
Amiodarone	Oral: 600–1200 mg/day for 7–10 days, then 400 mg/day for 3 wk, followed by a maintenance dose (ideally, ≤ 200 mg/day) IV: 150–450 mg over 1–6 h (depending on urgency) followed by a maintenance dose of 0.5–2.0 mg/min	1–2.5 μg/mL	Pulmonary fibrosis (in up to 5% of patients treated for > 5 yr), which may be fatal; QTc prolongation; torsades de pointes (rare); bradycardia; gray or blue discoloration of sun-exposed skin; hepatic abnormalities; peripheral neuropathy; corneal microdeposits (in almost all treated patients), usually without serious visual effects and reversed by stopping the drug; changes in thyroid function	Drug has noncompetitive β-blocking, Ca channel blocking, and Na channel blocking effects, with a long delay in onset of action By prolonging refractoriness, drug may produce homogeneous conditions of repolarization throughout the heart IV form can be used for conversion
Azimilide	Oral: 100–200 mg once/day	200–1000 ng/mL	Torsades de pointes VT	
Bretylium*	IV: Initially, 5 mg/kg, followed by 1–2 mg/min as a constant infusion IM: Initially, 5–10 mg/kg, which may be repeated to a total dose of 30 mg/kg IM maintenance dose of 5 mg/kg q 6–8 h	0.8–2.4 μg/mL	Hypotension	Drug has class II properties Effects may be delayed 10–20 min Drug is used to treat potentially lethal refractory ventricular tachyarrhythmias (intractable VT, recurrent VF), for which it is usually effective within 30 min of injection

Table continues on the following page.

TABLE 75–2. ANTIARRHYTHMIC DRUGS (VAUGHAN-WILLIAMS CLASSIFICATION)—Continued

DRUG	DOSAGE	TARGET LEVELS	ADVERSE EFFECTS	COMMENTS
Dofetilide	IV: 2.5–4 μg/mL Oral: 500 μg bid if CrCl > 60 mL/min; 250 μg bid if CrCl is 40–60 mL/min; 125 μg bid if CrCl is 20–40 mL/min	—	Torsades de pointes VT	Drug is contraindicated if QTc > 440 msec or if CrCl < 20 mL/min
Ibutilide	IV: For patients ≥ 60 kg, 1 mg IV infusion or, for patients < 60 kg, 0.01 mg/kg over 10 min, with dose repeated after 10 min if the first infusion is unsuccessful	N/A	Torsades de pointes ventricular tachycardia (in 2%)	Drug is used to terminate AF (success rate, about 40%) and atrial flutter (success rate, about 65%)
Sotalol	Oral: 80–160 mg q 12 h IV: 10 mg over 1–2 min	0.5–4 μg/mL	Similar to class II; possibly depressed left ventricular function and torsades de pointes VT	Drug is a β-blocker; racemic [D-L] form has class II properties, with most of class III activity in D-isomer. Only racemic sotalol is available for clinical use Drug should not be used in patients with renal insufficiency
Class IV Ca channel blockers	Uses: Termination of SVT and slowing of rapid AF or atrial flutter			
Diltiazem	Oral slow-release (diltiazem CD): 120 mg to 360 mg once/day IV: 5–15 mg/h for up to 24 h	0.1–0.4 μg/mL	Can precipitate VF in patients with VT; negative inotropy	IV form is most commonly used to slow ventricular response rate to AF or atrial flutter
Verapamil	Oral: 40–120 mg tid or, for sustained-release form, 180 mg once/day to 240 mg bid IV: 5–15 mg over 10 min Oral prophylaxis: 40–120 mg tid	N/A	Can precipitate VF in patients with VT; negative inotropy	IV form is used to terminate narrow-complex tachycardias involving the AV node (success rate, almost 100% with 5–10 mg IV over 10 min)

TABLE 75–2. ANTIARRHYTHMIC DRUGS (VAUGHAN-WILLIAMS CLASSIFICATION)—Continued

DRUG	DOSAGE	TARGET LEVELS	ADVERSE EFFECTS	COMMENTS
Other antiarrhythmics				
Adenosine	6 mg rapid IV bolus, repeated twice at 12 mg if needed. Flush bolus with additional 20 mL saline	N/A	Transient dyspnea, chest discomfort, and flushing (in 30–60%); bronchospasm	Drug slows or blocks AV nodal conduction Duration of action is extremely short Contraindications include asthma and high-grade heart block Dipyridamole potentiates effects
Digoxin	IV loading dose: 0.5 mg Oral maintenance dose: 0.125–0.25 mg/day	0.8–1.6 µg/mL	Anorexia, nausea, vomiting, and often serious arrhythmias (VPBs, VT, APBs, atrial tachycardia, 2nd-degree or 3rd-degree AV block, and combinations of these arrhythmias)	Contraindications include antegrade conduction over an accessory AV connection pathway (manifest Wolff-Parkinson-White syndrome) because if AF occurs, ventricular responses may be excessive (digoxin shortens refractory periods of the accessory connection)

AF = atrial fibrillation; ANA = antinuclear antibody; APB = atrial premature beat; AV = atrioventricular; CrCl = creatinine clearance; VF = ventricular fibrillation; LV = left ventricular; QTc = QT interval corrected for heart rate; SVT = supraventricular tachycardia; VPB = ventricular premature beat; VT = ventricular tachycardia.

*Availability uncertain.

Text continued from page 677.

contractility. Because these adverse effects of class I drugs are more likely to occur in patients with a structural heart disorder, class I drugs are not generally recommended for such patients. Thus, these drugs are usually used only in patients who do not have a structural heart disorder or in patients who have a structural heart disorder but who have no other therapeutic alternatives.

Class II: Class II drugs are β-blockers, which affect predominantly slow-channel tissues (SA and AV nodes), where they decrease rate of automaticity, slow conduction velocity, and prolong refractoriness. Thus, heart rate is slowed, the PR interval is lengthened, and the AV node transmits rapid atrial depolarizations at a lower frequency. Class II drugs are used primarily to treat SVTs, including sinus tachycardia, AV nodal reentry, AF, and atrial flutter. These drugs are also used to treat VTs to raise the threshold for ventricular fibrillation (VF) and reduce the ventricular proarrhythmic effects of β-adrenoceptor stimulation. β-Blockers are generally well tolerated; adverse effects include lassitude, sleep disturbance, and GI upset. These drugs are contraindicated in patients with asthma.

Class III: Class III drugs are primarily K channel blockers, which prolong action potential duration and refractoriness in slow- and fast-channel tissues. Thus, the capacity of all cardiac tissues to transmit impulses at high frequencies is reduced, but conduction velocity is not significantly affected. Because the action potential is prolonged, rate of automaticity is reduced. The predominant effect on the ECG is QT-interval prolongation. These drugs are used to treat SVTs and VTs. Class III drugs have a risk of ventricular proarrhythmia, particularly torsades de pointes VT.

Class IV: Class IV drugs are the nondihydropyridine Ca channel blockers, which depress Ca-dependent action potentials in slow channel tissues and thus decrease rate of automaticity, slow conduction velocity, and prolong refractoriness. Heart rate is slowed, the PR interval is lengthened, and the AV node transmits rapid atrial depolarizations at a lower frequency. These drugs are used primarily to treat SVTs.

Devices and Procedures

Direct-current (DC) cardioversion-defibrillation: A transthoracic DC shock of sufficient magnitude depolarizes the entire myocardium, rendering the entire heart momentarily refractory to repeat depolarization. Thereafter, the most rapid intrinsic pacemaker, usually the SA node, reassumes control of heart rhythm. Thus, DC cardioversion-defibrillation very effectively terminates tachyarrhythmias that result from reentry. However, it is less effective for terminating tachyarrhythmias that result from automaticity because the return rhythm is likely to be the automatic tachyarrhythmia. For tachyarrhythmias other than VF, the DC shock must be synchronized to the QRS complex (called DC cardioversion) because a shock that falls during the vulnerable period (near the peak of the T wave) can induce VF. In VF, synchronization of a shock to the QRS complex is neither necessary nor possible. A DC shock applied without synchronization to a QRS complex is DC defibrillation.

When DC cardioversion is elective, patients should fast for 6 to 8 h to avoid the possibility of aspiration. Because the procedure is frightening and painful, brief general anesthesia or IV analgesia and sedation (eg, fentanyl 1 μg/kg, then midazolam 1 to 2 mg q 2 min to a maximum of 5 mg) is necessary. Equipment and personnel to maintain the airways must be present.

The electrodes (pads or paddles) used for cardioversion may be placed anteroposteriorly (along the left sternal border over the 3rd and 4th intercostal spaces and in the left infrascapular region) or anterolaterally (between the clavicle and the 2nd intercostal space along the right sternal border and over the 5th and 6th intercostal spaces at the apex of the heart). After synchronization to the QRS complex is confirmed on the monitor, a shock is given. The most appropriate energy level varies with the tachyarrhythmia being treated. Cardioversion efficacy increases with use of biphasic shocks, in which the current polarity is reversed part way through the shock waveform. Complications are usually minor and include atrial and ventricular premature beats and muscle soreness. Less commonly, but more likely if patients have marginal left ventricular function or multiple shocks are used, cardioversion precipitates myocyte damage and electromechanical dissociation.

DC cardioversion-defibrillation can also be applied directly to the heart during a thoracotomy or through use of an intracardiac electrode catheter; then, much lower energy levels are required.

Pacemakers: Pacemakers sense electrical events and respond when necessary by delivering electrical stimuli to the heart. Permanent pacemaker leads are placed via thoracotomy or transvenously, but some temporary emergency pacemaker leads can be placed on the chest wall.

Indications are numerous (see TABLE 75–3) but generally involve symptomatic bradycardia or high-grade AV block. Some tachyarrhythmias may be terminated by overdrive pacing, which captures the ventricle by providing a brief period of pacing at a faster rate; the pacemaker is then slowed to the desired rate. Nevertheless, ventricular tachyarrhythmias are better treated with devices that can cardiovert and defibrillate as well as pace (implantable cardioverter defibrillators).

Types of pacemakers are designated by 3 to 5 letters (see TABLE 75–4), representing which cardiac chambers are paced; which chambers are sensed; how the pacemaker responds to a sensed event (inhibits or triggers pacing); whether it can increase heart rate during exercise (rate-modulating); and whether pacing is multisite (in both atria, both ventricles, or more than one pacing lead

Text continues on page 690.

TABLE 75–3. INDICATIONS FOR PERMANENT PACEMAKERS

ARRHYTHMIA	INDICATED (ESTABLISHED BY EVIDENCE)	POSSIBLY INDICATED AND SUPPORTED BY BULK OF EVIDENCE	POSSIBLY INDICATED BUT LESS WELL SUPPORTED BY EVIDENCE	NOT INDICATED
Sinus node dysfunction	Symptomatic bradycardia, including symptomatic frequent sinus pauses and bradycardia due to essential drugs (alternatives contraindicated) Symptomatic chronotropic incompetence (heart rate cannot meet physiologic demands; ie, it is too slow for activity)	Heart rate of < 40 beats/min when symptoms have not been clearly associated with the bradycardia Syncope of unexplained origin with significant sinus node dysfunction seen on ECG or triggered in an electrophysiologic study	Heart rate of < 40 beats/min in minimally symptomatic patients	Asymptomatic bradycardia Symptoms consistent with bradycardia but clearly shown not to be associated with it Symptomatic bradycardia due to nonessential drugs
AV block	Any 2nd-degree AV block associated symptomatic bradycardia Third-degree or high-grade 2nd-degree AV block at any anatomic level if associated with one of the following: Symptomatic bradycardia (including with heart failure) thought due to the block Arrhythmias and other disorders requiring drugs that cause symptomatic bradycardia Documented asystole ≥ 3.0 sec or any escape rate of < 40 beats/min in awake, asymptomatic patients Catheter ablation of the AV junction Postoperative block not expected to resolve after surgery	Asymptomatic 3rd-degree AV block at any anatomic level when average ventricular rates during waking are ≥ 40 beats/min, especially with cardiomegaly or LV dysfunction Asymptomatic type II 2nd-degree AV block with narrow QRS complex (pacemaker is indicated if QRS complex is wide) Asymptomatic type I 2nd-degree AV block within or below His bundle levels, detected during an electrophysiologic study done for other reasons First- or 2nd-degree AV block with symptoms suggesting pacemaker syndrome	First-degree AV block of > 0.30 sec with LV dysfunction and symptoms of heart failure when a shorter AV interval would improve hemodynamics, probably by reducing left atrial filling pressure AV block of any degree (including 1st) associated with neuromuscular disorders in which conduction abnormalities may progress unpredictably (eg, myotonic muscular dystrophy, Kearns-Sayre syndrome, Erb's [limb-girdle] dystrophy, Charcot-Marie-Tooth disease [peroneal atrophy] with or without symptoms)	Asymptomatic 1st-degree AV block Asymptomatic type I 2nd-degree AV block at the AV node level or not known to be within or below His bundle levels AV block expected to resolve or unlikely to recur (eg, due to drug toxicity or Lyme disease or occurring asymptomatically during hypoxia in sleep apnea syndrome)

Table continues on the following page.

TABLE 75–3. INDICATIONS FOR PERMANENT PACEMAKERS—Continued

ARRHYTHMIA	INDICATED (ESTABLISHED BY EVIDENCE)	POSSIBLY INDICATED AND SUPPORTED BY BULK OF EVIDENCE	POSSIBLY INDICATED BUT LESS WELL SUPPORTED BY EVIDENCE	NOT INDICATED
	Neuromuscular disorders in which conduction abnormalities may progress unpredictably (eg, myotonic muscular dystrophy, Kearns-Sayre syndrome, Erb's [limb-girdle] dystrophy, Charcot-Marie-Tooth disease [peroneal atrophy] with or without symptoms)			
Tachyarrhythmias	Sustained, pause-dependent VT, with or without prolonged QT interval, when pacing has been documented as effective	High-risk patients with congenital long QT syndrome	AV reentrant or AV node reentrant supraventricular tachycardia refractory to drugs or ablation Prevention of symptomatic, recurrent atrial fibrillation refractory to drugs when sinus node dysfunction coexists	Frequent or complex ventricular ectopy without sustained VT when long QT syndrome is absent Torsades de pointes VT with reversible causes
After acute MI	Persistent 2nd-degree AV block in the His-Purkinje system with bilateral BBB or 3rd-degree AV block within or below the His-Purkinje system Transient 2nd- or 3rd-degree AV block at the AV node level and associated with BBB Persistent symptomatic 2nd- or 3rd-degree AV block	None	Persistent 2nd- or 3rd-degree AV block at the AV node level	Transient AV block without intraventricular conduction defects Transient AV block with isolated left anterior fascicular block Acquired left anterior fascicular block without AV block Persistent 1st-degree AV block with BBB of long or unknown duration

Multifascicular block	Intermittent 3rd-degree AV block Type II 2nd-degree AV block Alternating BBB	Syncope not shown to be due to AV block after other likely causes (especially ventricular tachycardia) are excluded Very prolonged HV interval (≥100 msec) in asymptomatic patients, detected incidentally during a electrophysiologic study Nonphysiologic, infra-His block induced by pacing, detected incidentally during a electrophysiologic study	Neuromuscular disorders in which conduction abnormalities may progress unpredictably (eg, myotonic muscular dystrophy, Kearns-Sayre syndrome, Erb's [limb-girdle] dystrophy, Charcot-Marie-Tooth disease [peroneal atrophy] with or without symptoms)	Fascicular block without AV block or symptoms Fascicular block with 1st-degree AV block and without symptoms
Congenital heart disorders	Advanced 2nd- or 3rd-degree AV block causing symptomatic bradycardia, ventricular dysfunction, or low cardiac output Sinus node dysfunction correlated with symptoms during age-inappropriate bradycardia Postoperative high-grade 2nd- or 3rd-degree AV block that is not expected to resolve or that persists ≥ 7 days after surgery Congenital 3rd-degree AV block with a wide QRS escape rhythm, complex ventricular ectopy, or ventricular dysfunction	Bradycardia-tachycardia syndrome requiring long-term antiarrhythmic treatment other than digitalis Congenital 3rd-degree AV block persisting after age 1 yr if average heart rate is < 50 beats/min, ventricular rate pauses abruptly for 2 or 3 times the basic cycle length, or associated symptoms due to chronotropic incompetence occur Long QT syndrome with 2:1 2nd-degree AV block or 3rd-degree AV block	Transient postoperative 3rd-degree AV block that converts to sinus rhythm with residual bifascicular block Congenital 3rd-degree AV block in asymptomatic infants, children, adolescents, or young adults with an acceptable ventricular rate, a narrow QRS complex, and normal ventricular function Asymptomatic sinus bradycardia in adolescents with a congenital heart disorder and resting heart rate of < 40	Transient postoperative AV block when AV conduction returns to normal Asymptomatic postoperative bifascicular block with or without 1st-degree AV block Asymptomatic type I 2nd-degree AV block Asymptomatic sinus bradycardia in adolescents when the longest RR interval is < 3 sec and minimum heart rate is > 40 beats/min

Table continues on the following page.

TABLE 75–3. INDICATIONS FOR PERMANENT PACEMAKERS—Continued

ARRHYTHMIA	INDICATED (ESTABLISHED BY EVIDENCE)	POSSIBLY INDICATED AND SUPPORTED BY BULK OF EVIDENCE	POSSIBLY INDICATED BUT LESS WELL SUPPORTED BY EVIDENCE	NOT INDICATED
	Congenital 3rd-degree AV block in infants with a ventricular rate of < 50 beats/min or with a congenital heart disorder and a ventricular rate of < 70 beats/min Sustained pause-dependent VT, with or without prolonged QT, when pacing has been documented as effective	Asymptomatic sinus bradycardia in children with a complex congenital heart disorder and resting heart rate of < 40 beats/min or pauses in ventricular rate of > 3 sec Patients with a congenital heart disorder and impaired hemodynamics due to sinus bradycardia or loss of AV synchrony	beats/min or pauses in ventricular rate of > 3 sec Neuromuscular disorders with AV block of any degree (including 1st) with or without symptoms, because an AV conduction disorder may progress unpredictably	
Hypersensitive carotid sinus syndrome and neurocardiogenic syncope	Recurrent syncope due to carotid sinus stimulation Ventricular asystole of > 3 sec due to carotid sinus pressure in patients not taking drugs that depress sinus node or AV conduction	Recurrent syncope without obvious triggering events and with a hypersensitive cardioinhibitory response Significantly symptomatic recurrent neurocardiogenic syncope associated with bradycardia documented clinically or during tilt table testing	None	Hyperactive cardioinhibitory response to carotid sinus stimulation without symptoms or with vague symptoms (eg, dizziness, lightheadedness) Recurrent syncope, lightheadedness, or dizziness without a hyperactive cardioinhibitory response Situational vasovagal syncope that can be averted by avoidance

Post-cardiac transplantation	Symptomatic bradyarrhythmias or chronotropic incompetence expected to persist and other established indications for permanent pacing	None	Transient symptomatic bradyarrhythmias or chronotropic incompetence that may persist for months and require treatment	Asymptomatic bradyarrhythmias that develop after cardiac transplantation
Hypertrophic cardiomyopathy	Same as established indications for sinus node dysfunction or AV block	None	Medically refractory, symptomatic hypertrophic cardiomyopathy when resting or induced LV outflow is significantly obstructed	Asymptomatic or medically controlled hypertrophic cardiomyopathy Symptomatic hypertrophic cardiomyopathy with no evidence of LV outflow obstruction
Dilated cardiomyopathy	Same as established indications for sinus node dysfunction or AV block	Medically refractory, symptomatic New York Heart Association class III or IV idiopathic dilated or ischemic cardiomyopathy with a prolonged QRS interval (≥ 130 msec), LV end-diastolic dimension of ≥ 55 mm and LV ejection fraction of ≤ 35% (biventricular pacing)	None	Asymptomatic dilated cardiomyopathy Symptomatic dilated cardiomyopathy when symptoms are controlled with drugs Symptomatic ischemic cardiomyopathy when the ischemia can be effectively treated

AV = atrioventricular; BBB = bundle branch block; HV interval = interval from the start of the HIS signal to the beginning of the 1st ventricular signal; LV = left ventricular; VT = ventricular tachycardia.

Data from Gregoratos G et al: "ACC/AHA/NASPE 2002 Guideline update for implantation of cardiac pacemakers and antiarrhythmia devices." *Circulation* 106(16):2145–2161, 2002.

TABLE 75–4. PACEMAKER CODES

I	II	III	IV	V
CHAMBER PACED	**CHAMBER SENSED**	**RESPONSE TO SENSED EVENT**	**RATE MODULATION**	**MULTISITE PACING**
A = Atrium V = Ventricle D = Dual (both)	A = Atrium V = Ventricle D = Dual (both)	O = None I = Inhibits pacemaker T = Triggers pacemaker to stimulate ventricles D = Dual (both): For events sensed in ventricles, inhibits; for events sensed in atria, triggers	O = Not programmable R = Rate-modulated	O = None A = Atrium V = Ventricle D = Dual (both)

Text continued from page 684.

in a single chamber). For example, a VVIR pacemaker paces (V) and senses (V) events in the ventricle, inhibits pacing in response to sensed event (I), and can increase its rate during exercise (R).

VVI and DDD pacemakers are the devices most commonly used. They offer equivalent survival benefits, but compared with VVI pacemakers, physiologic pacemakers (AAI, DDD, VDD) appear to reduce risk of AF and heart failure and slightly improve quality of life.

Advances in pacemaker design include lower-energy circuitry, new battery designs, and corticosteroid-eluting leads (which reduce pacing threshold), all of which increase pacemaker longevity. Mode switching refers to an automatic change in the mode of pacing in response to sensed events (eg, from DDDR to VVIR during AF).

Pacemakers may malfunction by oversensing or undersensing events, failing to pace or capture, or pacing at an abnormal rate. Tachycardias are an especially common complication. Rate-modulating pacemakers may increase stimuli in response to vibration, muscle activity, or voltage induced by magnetic fields during MRI. In pacemaker-mediated tachycardia, a normally functioning dual-chamber pacemaker senses a ventricular premature or paced beat transmitted to the atrium through the AV node or a retrograde-conducting accessory pathway, which triggers ventricular stimulation in a rapid, repeating cycle. Additional complications associated with normally functioning devices include cross-talk inhibition, in which sensing of the atrial pacing impulse by the ventricular channel of a dual-chamber pacemaker leads to inhibition of ventricular pacing, and pacemaker syndrome, in which AV asynchrony induced by ventricular pacing causes fluctuating, vague cerebral (eg, lightheadedness), cervical (eg, neck pulsations), or respiratory (eg, dyspnea) symptoms.

Environmental interference comes from electromagnetic sources such as surgical electrocautery and MRI, although MRI may be safe when the pacemaker generator and leads are not inside the magnet. Cellular telephones and electronic security devices are a potential source of interference; telephones should not be placed close to the device but are not a problem when used normally for talking. Walking through metal detectors does not cause pacemaker malfunction as long as patients do not linger.

Complications during implantation are uncommon but may include myocardial perforation, bleeding, and pneumothorax. Postoperative complications include infection, lead migration, and impulse generator migration.

Implantable cardioverter-defibrillators (ICDs): ICDs cardiovert or defibrillate the heart in response to VT or VF. Contemporary tiered-therapy ICDs also provide antibradycardia pacing and antitachycardia pacing (to terminate responsive atrial or ventricular tachycardias) and store intracardiac electrograms. ICDs are implanted subcutaneously or subpectorally, with electrodes inserted transvenously or, rarely, via thoracotomy.

ICDs are the preferred treatment for patients who have had an episode of VF or hemodynamically significant VT not due to reversible or transient conditions (eg, electrolyte disturbance, antiarrhythmic drug proarrhythmia, acute MI). ICDs may also be indicated for patients with VT or VF inducible during an electrophysiologic study and for patients with idiopathic or ischemic cardiomyopathy, a left ventricular ejection fraction of < 35%, and a high risk of VT or VF. Other indications are less clear (see TABLE 75–5). Because ICDs treat rather than prevent VT or VF, patients prone to these arrhythmias may require an ICD and antiarrhythmic drugs to reduce the number of episodes and need for uncomfortable shocks; this approach also prolongs the life of the ICD.

Impulse generators for ICDs typically last about 5 yr. ICDs may malfunction by delivering inappropriate pacing or shocks in response to sinus rhythm or SVTs or by not delivering appropriate pacing or shocks when needed. Causes include lead or impulse generator migration, undersensing and an increase in pacing threshold due to epicardial fibrosis at the site of prior shocks, and battery depletion. If a patient reports that the ICD has discharged, it can be electronically interrogated to determine the reason.

Radiofrequency (RF) ablation: If a tachyarrhythmia depends on a specific pathway or ectopic site of automaticity, the site can be ablated by low-voltage, high-frequency (300 to 750 MHz) electrical energy, applied through an electrode catheter. This energy heats and necroses an area < 1 cm in diameter and up to 1 cm deep. Before energy can be applied, the target site or sites must be mapped at an electrophysiologic study (see p. 597).

Success rate is > 90% for reentrant tachycardias (via the AV node or an accessory pathway), focal atrial tachycardia and flutter, and focal idiopathic VTs (right ventricular outflow tract, left septal, or bundle branch reentrant VT). Because AF often originates or is maintained by an arrhythmogenic site in the pulmonary veins, this site can be ablated directly or, more commonly, electrically isolated by ablations at the pulmonary vein–left atrial junction or in the left atrium. Alternatively, in patients with refractory AF and rapid ventricular rates, the AV node may be ablated after permanent pacemaker implantation. RF ablation is sometimes successful in patients with VT refractory to drugs and with ischemic heart disease.

RF ablation is safe; mortality is < 1/2000. Complications include valvular damage, embolism, cardiac perforation, tamponade (1%), and unintended AV node ablation.

Surgery: Surgery to remove a focus of a tachyarrhythmia is becoming less necessary as the less invasive RF ablation techniques evolve. But it is still indicated when an arrhythmia is refractory to RF ablation or when another indication requires a cardiac surgical procedure, most commonly when patients with AF require valve replacement or repair or when patients with VT require revascularization or resection of a left ventricular aneurysm.

SINUS NODE DYSFUNCTION

(Sick Sinus Syndrome)

Sinus node dysfunction refers to a number of conditions producing physiologically inappropriate atrial rates. Symptoms may be minimal or include weakness, palpitations, and syncope. Diagnosis is by ECG. Symptomatic patients require a pacemaker.

Sinus node dysfunction includes inappropriate sinus bradycardia, alternating bradycardia and atrial tachyarrhythmias (bradycardia-tachycardia syndrome), sinus pause or arrest, and sinoatrial (SA) exit block. Sinus node dysfunction affects mainly the elderly, especially those with another cardiac disorder or diabetes.

Sinus pause is temporary cessation of sinus node activity, seen on ECG as disappearance of P waves for seconds to minutes. The pause usually triggers escape activity in lower pacemakers (eg, atrial or junctional), preserving heart rate and function, but long pauses cause dizziness and syncope.

In sinoatrial exit block, the SA node depolarizes, but conduction of impulses to atrial tissue is impaired. In 1st-degree SA block, the SA node impulse is merely slowed, and ECG is normal. In type I 2nd-degree SA (SA Wenckebach) block, impulse conduction slows before blocking, seen on the ECG as a P-P interval that decreases progressively until the P wave drops altogether, creating a pause and the appearance of grouped beats; the duration of the pause is less than 2 P-P cycles. In type II 2nd-degree SA block, conduction of impulses is blocked without slowing beforehand, producing a pause that is a multiple (usually twice) of the P-P interval and the appearance of grouped beats. In 3rd-degree SA block, conduction is blocked; P waves are absent, giving the appearance of sinus arrest.

TABLE 75–5. INDICATIONS FOR IMPLANTABLE CARDIOVERTER-DEFIBRILLATORS IN VENTRICULAR TACHYCARDIA AND VENTRICULAR FIBRILLATION

INDICATED (ESTABLISHED BY EVIDENCE)	POSSIBLY INDICATED AND SUPPORTED BY BULK OF EVIDENCE	POSSIBLY INDICATED BUT LESS WELL SUPPORTED BY EVIDENCE	NOT INDICATED
VT or VF causing cardiac arrest when there is no transient or reversible cause Spontaneous sustained VT in patients with a structural heart disorder Syncope of undetermined etiology with hemodynamically significant sustained VT or VF induced by an electrophysiologic study when drugs are ineffective or not tolerated Sustained VT not responsive to drugs or other treatments in patients with structurally normal hearts Patients with CAD and LV ejection fraction ≤ 0.3 measured at least 1 mo post-MI and 3 mo after CABG surgery or PCI Patients with idiopathic CCM, NYHA functional class II/III heart failure symptoms, and LV ejection fraction ≤ 0.35	Patients with CAD and LV ejection fraction 0.3–0.35 measured at least 1 mo post-MI or 3 mo after CABG surgery or PCI with inducible VT/AF at electrophysiologic study or QRS duration > 120 msec	Cardiac arrest presumed due to VF when an electrophysiologic study is contraindicated Severe symptoms attributable to VT in patients awaiting cardiac transplantation Genetic conditions with high risk of life-threatening VT or VF (eg, long QT syndrome, hypertrophic cardiomyopathy) Syncope of unknown etiology or family history of unexplained sudden cardiac death in patients with Brugada syndrome Syncope of unknown etiology in patients with an advanced structural heart disorder	Syncope of unknown etiology in absence of inducible VT or VF or a structural heart disorder Incessant VT or VF VT or VF with mechanisms amenable to catheter or surgical ablation VT or VF due to transient or reversible disorders when correction is feasible and likely to reduce risk Psychiatric disorders that may worsen with ICD implantation or that preclude follow-up Life expectancy < 6 mo Drug-refractory end-stage heart failure in patients ineligible for heart transplantation

CABG = coronary artery bypass graft; CAD = coronary artery disease; CCM = congestive cardiomyopathy; ICD = implantable cardioverter defibrillator; LV = left ventricular; NYHA = New York Heart Association; PCI = percutaneous coronary intervention; VF = ventricular fibrillation; VT = ventricular tachycardia.

Data modified from Gregoratos G et al: ACC/AHA/NASPE 2002 Guideline update for implantation of cardiac pacemakers and antiarrhythmia devices. *Circulation* 106(16):2145–2161, 2002.

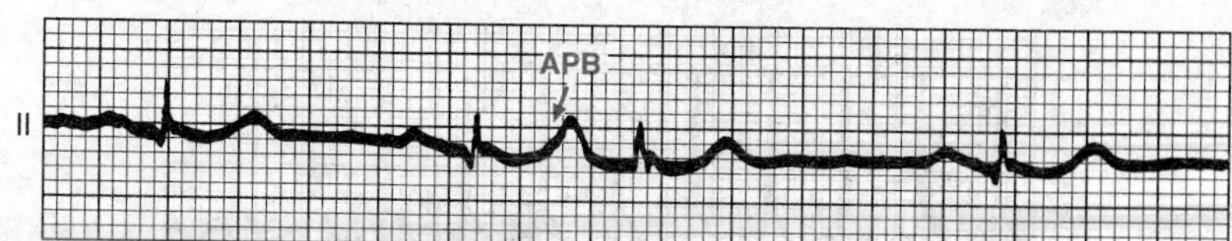

Fig. 75–3. Atrial premature beat (APB). In lead II, after the 2nd beat of sinus origin, the T wave is deformed by an APB. Because the APB occurs relatively early during the sinus cycle, the sinus node pacemaker is reset, and a pause—less than fully compensatory—precedes the next sinus beat.

The most common cause of sinus node dysfunction is idiopathic SA node fibrosis, which may be accompanied by degeneration of lower elements of the conducting system. Other causes include drugs, excessive vagal tone, and many ischemic, inflammatory, and infiltrative disorders.

Symptoms, Signs, and Diagnosis

Many patients are asymptomatic, but depending on the heart rate, all the symptoms of bradycardias and tachycardias can occur (see p. 674). A slow, irregular pulse suggests the diagnosis, which is confirmed by ECG, rhythm strip, or continuous 24-h ECG recording. Some patients present with atrial fibrillation (AF), and the underlying sinus node dysfunction manifests only after conversion to sinus rhythm.

Prognosis and Treatment

Prognosis is mixed; without treatment, mortality is about 2%/yr, primarily resulting from an underlying structural heart disorder. Each year, about 5% of patients develop AF with its risks of heart failure and stroke.

Treatment is pacemaker implantation. Risk of AF is greatly reduced when a physiologic (atrial or atrial and ventricular) pacemaker rather than a ventricular pacemaker is used. Antiarrhythmic drugs may prevent paroxysmal tachyarrhythmias after pacemaker insertion. Theophylline and hydralazine are options to increase heart rate in healthy, younger patients who have bradycardia without syncope.

ECTOPIC SUPRAVENTRICULAR RHYTHMS

Various rhythms result from supraventricular foci (usually in the atria); many are asymptomatic and require no treatment.

Atrial premature beats (APBs), or premature atrial contractions (PACs), are common episodic impulses. They may occur in normal hearts with or without precipitating factors (eg, coffee, tea, alcohol, pseudoephedrine) or may be a sign of a cardiopulmonary disorder. They occasionally cause palpitations. Diagnosis is by ECG (see FIG. 75–3). APBs may be normally, aberrantly, or not conducted. Normally conducted APBs are usually followed by a noncompensatory pause; aberrantly conducted APBs (usually with right bundle branch block morphology) must be distinguished from premature beats of ventricular origin.

Atrial escape beats are ectopic atrial beats that emerge after long sinus pauses or sinus arrest. They may be single or multiple; escape beats from a single focus may produce a continuous rhythm (called ectopic atrial rhythm). Heart rate is typically slower, the P wave morphology is typically different, and PR interval is slightly shorter than in sinus rhythm.

Wandering atrial pacemaker (multifocal atrial rhythm) is an irregularly irregular rhythm caused by the random discharge of multiple ectopic atrial foci. By definition, heart rate is ≤ 100 beats/min. This arrhythmia most typically occurs in patients who have a pulmonary disorder and are hypoxic, acidotic, theophylline-intoxicated, or a combination. On ECG, P-wave morphology differs from beat to beat and there are 3 or more distinct P-wave morphologies. The presence of P waves distinguishes wandering atrial pacemaker from atrial fibrillation.

Multifocal atrial tachycardia (chaotic atrial tachycardia) is an irregularly irregular rhythm caused by the random discharge of multiple ectopic atrial foci. By definition, heart rate is > 100 beats/min. Except for the rate, features are the same as those of wandering atrial pacemaker. Symptoms, when they occur, are those of rapid tachycardia. Treatment is directed at the underlying pulmonary disorder.

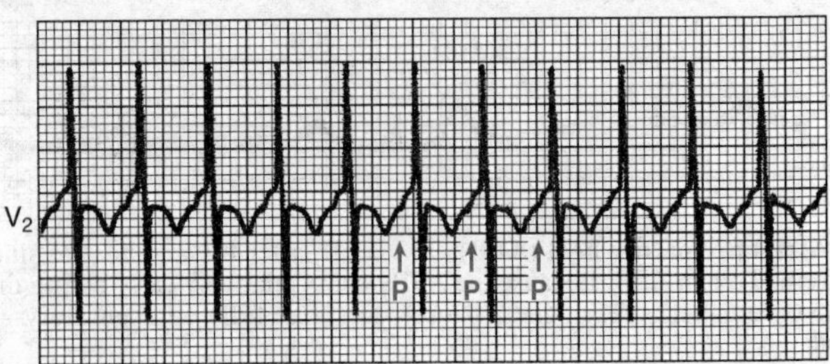

Fig. 75–4. True atrial tachycardia. This rare narrow QRS tachycardia arises from an abnormal automatic focus or localized intra-atrial reentry. P waves precede the QRS complexes; it is a long RP tachycardia (PR < RP).

Atrial tachycardia is a regular rhythm caused by the consistent, rapid atrial activation from a single atrial focus. Heart rate is usually 150 to 200 beats/min; however, with a very rapid atrial rate, nodal dysfunction, or digitalis toxicity, atrioventricular (AV) block may be present, and ventricular rate may be slower. Mechanisms include enhanced atrial automaticity and intra-atrial reentry. Atrial tachycardia is the least common form (5%) of supraventricular tachycardia and usually occurs in patients with a structural heart disorder. Other causes include atrial irritation (eg, pericarditis), drugs (eg, digoxin), alcohol, and toxic gas inhalation. Symptoms are those of other tachycardias. Diagnosis is by ECG; P waves, which differ in morphology from normal sinus P waves, precede QRS complexes but may be hidden within the preceding T wave (see FIG. 75–4). Vagal maneuvers may be used to slow the heart rate, allowing visualization of P waves when they are hidden, but these maneuvers do not usually terminate the arrhythmia (demonstrating that the AV node is not an obligate part of the arrhythmia circuit). Treatment involves managing causes and slowing ventricular response rate using a β-blocker or Ca channel blocker. An episode may be terminated by direct-current cardioversion. Pharmacologic approaches to termination and prevention of atrial tachycardia include antiarrhythmic drugs in class Ia, Ic, and III. If these noninvasive measures are ineffective, alternatives include overdrive pacing and radiofrequency ablation of the ectopic focus.

Nonparoxysmal junctional tachycardia is caused by abnormal automaticity in the AV node or adjacent tissue, which typically follows open heart surgery, acute inferior MI, myocarditis, or digitalis toxicity. Heart rate is 60 to 120 beats/min; thus, symptoms are usually absent. ECG shows regular, normal-appearing QRS complexes without identifiable P waves or with retrograde P waves (inverted in the inferior leads) that occur shortly before (< 0.1 sec) or after the QRS complex. The rhythm is distinguished from paroxysmal supraventricular tachycardia by the lower heart rate and gradual onset and offset. Treatment is directed at causes.

ATRIOVENTRICULAR BLOCK

Atrioventricular (AV) block is partial or complete interruption of impulse transmission from the atria to the ventricles. The most common cause is idiopathic fibrosis and sclerosis of the conduction system. Diagnosis is by ECG; symptoms and treatment depend on degree of block, but treatment, when necessary, usually involves pacing.

AV block is caused by idiopathic fibrosis and sclerosis of the conduction system in about 50% of patients and by ischemic heart disease in 40%; the rest are due to drugs (eg, β-blockers, Ca channel blockers, digoxin, amiodarone); increased vagal tone; valvulopathy; or congenital heart, genetic, or other disorders.

First-degree AV block: All normal P waves are followed by QRS complexes, but the PR interval is longer than normal (> 0.20 sec—see FIG. 75–5). First-degree AV block may be physiologic in younger patients with high vagal tone and in well-trained athletes. First-degree AV block is always asymptomatic and no treatment is required, but further investigation may be indicated when it accompanies another heart disorder or appears to be caused by drugs.

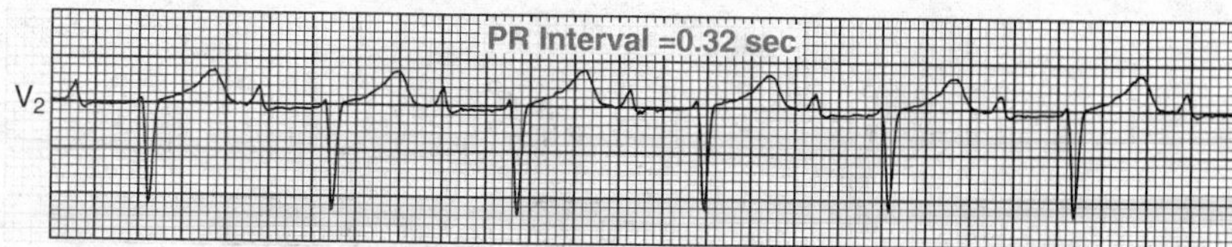

Fig. 75–5. Atrioventricular block. For 1st-degree block, conduction is slowed without skipped beats. All normal P waves are followed by QRS complexes, but the PR interval is longer than normal (> 0.2 sec). For 3rd-degree block, there is no relationship between P waves and QRS complexes, and the P wave rate is greater than the QRS rate.

Second-degree AV block: Some normal P waves are followed by QRS complexes, but some are not. Three types exist:

In Mobitz type I 2nd-degree AV block, the PR interval progressively lengthens with each beat until the atrial impulse is not conducted and the QRS complex is dropped (Wenckebach phenomenon); AV nodal conduction resumes with the next beat, and the sequence is repeated (see FIG. 75–6). Mobitz type I 2nd-degree AV block may be physiologic in younger and more athletic patients. The block occurs at the AV node in about 75% of patients with a narrow QRS complex and at infranodal sites (His bundle, bundle branches, or fascicles) in the rest. If the block becomes complete, a reliable junctional escape rhythm typically develops. Treatment is therefore unnecessary unless the block causes symptomatic bradycardia and transient or reversible causes have been excluded. Treatment is pacemaker insertion, which may also benefit asymptomatic patients with Mobitz type I 2nd-degree AV block at infranodal sites detected by electrophysiologic studies done for other reasons.

In Mobitz type II 2nd-degree AV block, the PR interval remains constant. Beats are intermittently nonconducted and QRS complexes dropped, usually in a repeating cycle of every 3rd (3:1 block) or 4th (4:1 block) P wave (see FIG. 75–7). Mobitz type II 2nd-degree AV block is always pathologic; the block occurs at the His bundle in 20% of patients and in the bundle branches in the rest. Patients may be asymptomatic or experience light-headedness, presyncope, and syncope, depending on the ratio of conducted to blocked beats. Patients are at risk of developing symptomatic high-grade or complete AV block, in which the escape rhythm is likely to be ventricular and thus too slow and unreliable to maintain systemic perfusion; therefore, a pacemaker is indicated.

In high-grade 2nd-degree AV block, every 2nd (or more) P wave is blocked (see FIG. 75–8). The distinction between Mobitz type I and Mobitz type II block is difficult to make because 2 P waves are never conducted in a row. Risk of complete AV block is difficult to predict, and a pacemaker is indicated.

Patients with any form of 2nd-degree AV block and a structural heart disorder should be considered candidates for permanent pacing unless there is a transient or reversible cause.

Third-degree AV block: Heart block is complete (see FIG. 75–9): There is no electrical communication between the atria and ventricles and no relationship between P waves and QRS complexes (AV dissociation). Cardiac function is maintained by an escape junctional or ventricular pacemaker. Escape rhythms originating above the bifurcation of

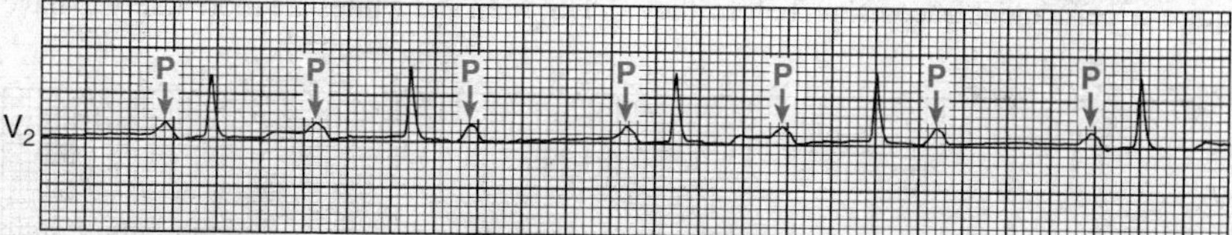

Fig. 75–6. Mobitz type I 2nd-degree atrioventricular block. The PR interval progressively lengthens with each beat until the atrial impulse is not conducted and the QRS complex is dropped (Wenckebach phenomenon); AV nodal conduction resumes with the next beat, and the sequence is repeated.

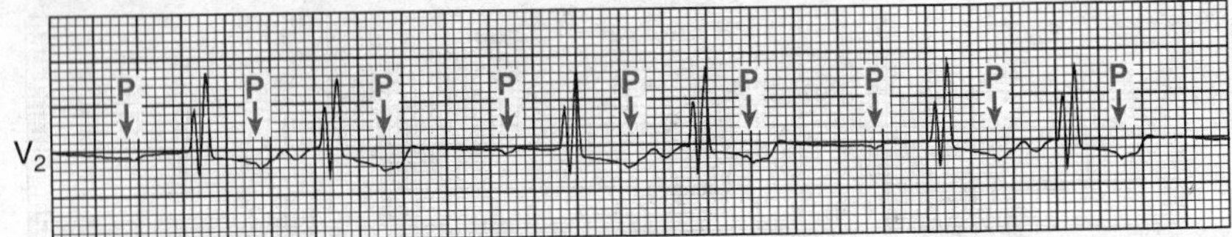

Fig. 75–7. Mobitz type II 2nd-degree atrioventricular block. The PR interval remains constant. Beats are intermittently nonconducted, and QRS complexes dropped, usually in a repeating cycle of every 3rd (3:1 block) or 4th (4:1 block) P wave.

the His bundle produce narrow QRS complexes, relatively rapid (> 40 beats/min) and reliable heart rates, and mild symptoms (eg, fatigue, postural light-headedness, effort intolerance). Escape rhythms originating below the bifurcation produce wider QRS complexes, slower and unreliable heart rates, and more severe symptoms (eg, presyncope, syncope, heart failure). Signs include those of AV dissociation, such as cannon *a* waves, BP fluctuations, and changes in loudness of the 1st heart sound (S_1). Risk of asystole-related syncope and sudden death is greater if low escape rhythms are present.

Most patients require a pacemaker (see TABLE 75–4). If the block is caused by antiarrhythmic drugs, stopping the drug may be effective, although temporary pacing may be needed. Block caused by acute inferior MI usually reflects AV nodal dysfunction and may respond to atropine or resolve spontaneously over several days. Block caused by anterior MI usually reflects extensive myocardial necrosis involving the His-Purkinje system and requires immediate transvenous pacemaker insertion with interim external pacing as necessary. Spontaneous resolution may occur but warrants evaluation of AV nodal and infranodal conduction (eg, electrophysiologic study, exercise testing, 24-h ECG).

Most patients with congenital 3rd-degree AV block have a junctional escape rhythm that maintains a reasonable rate, but they require a permanent pacemaker before they reach middle age. Less commonly, patients with congenital AV block have a slow escape rhythm and require a permanent pacemaker at a young age, perhaps even during infancy.

ATRIAL FIBRILLATION

Atrial fibrillation is a rapid, irregularly irregular atrial rhythm. Symptoms include palpitations and sometimes weakness, dyspnea, and presyncope. Atrial thrombi often form, causing a significant risk of embolic stroke. Diagnosis is by ECG. Treatment involves rate control with drugs, prevention of thromboembolism with anticoagulation, and sometimes conversion to sinus rhythm by drugs or cardioversion.

Atrial fibrillation (AF) has been attributed to multiple wavelets with chaotic reentry within the atria. However, in many cases, firing of an ectopic focus within venous structures adjacent to the atria (usually the pulmonary veins) is responsible for initiation and perhaps maintenance of AF. In AF, the atria do not contract, and the atrioventricular (AV) conduction system is bombarded with many electrical stimuli, causing inconsistent impulse transmission and an irregularly irregular ventricular rate, which is usually in the tachycardia rate range.

AF is one of the most common arrhythmias, affecting about 2.3 million adults in the US. Men and whites are more likely to have

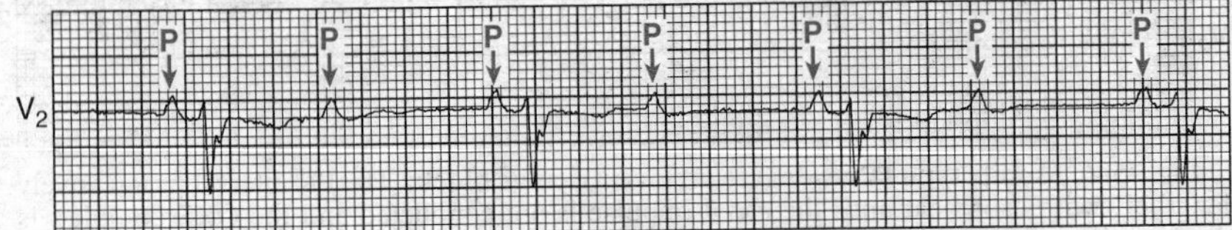

Fig. 75–8. Second-degree atrioventricular block (high grade).

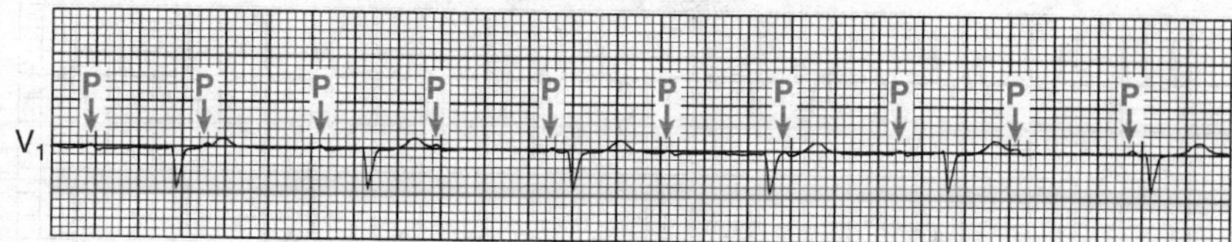

Fig. 75–9. Third-degree atrioventricular block.

it than women and blacks. Prevalence increases with age; almost 10% of people > 80 yr are affected. It tends to occur in patients with a heart disorder, sometimes precipitating heart failure because cardiac output decreases in the absence of atrial contraction. The absent atrial contractions also predispose to thrombus formation; annual risk of cerebrovascular embolic events is about 7%. Risk of stroke is higher in patients with a rheumatic valvular disorder, hyperthyroidism, hypertension, diabetes, left ventricular systolic dysfunction, or previous thromboembolic events. Systemic emboli can also cause malfunction or necrosis of other organs (eg, heart, kidneys, GI tract, eye) or a limb.

Etiology and Classification

The most common causes are hypertension, cardiomyopathy, mitral or tricuspid valvular disorders, hyperthyroidism, and binge alcohol drinking (holiday heart). Less common causes include pulmonary embolism, atrial septal and other congenital heart defects, COPD, myocarditis, and pericarditis. AF without an identifiable cause in patients < 60 yr is called lone AF.

Acute AF is new-onset AF lasting < 48 h.

Paroxysmal AF is recurrent AF that typically lasts < 48 h and that converts spontaneously to normal sinus rhythm.

Persistent AF lasts > 1 wk and requires treatment to convert to normal sinus rhythm.

Permanent AF cannot be converted to sinus rhythm. The longer AF is present, the less likely is spontaneous conversion and the more difficult is cardioversion because of atrial remodeling.

Symptoms and Signs

AF is often asymptomatic, but many patients have palpitations, vague chest discomfort, or symptoms of heart failure (eg, weakness, lightheadedness, dyspnea), particularly when the ventricular rate is very rapid (often 140 to 160 beats/min). Patients may also present with symptoms and signs of acute stroke or of other organ damage due to systemic emboli.

The pulse is irregularly irregular with loss of *a* waves in the jugular venous pulse. A pulse deficit (the apical ventricular rate is faster than the rate palpated at the wrist) may be present because left ventricular stroke volume is not always sufficient to produce a peripheral pressure wave at fast ventricular rates.

Diagnosis

Diagnosis is by ECG. Findings include absence of P waves, f (fibrillatory) waves between QRS complexes (irregular in timing, irregular in morphology; baseline undulations at rates > 300/min not always apparent in all leads), and irregularly irregular R-R intervals (see FIG. 75–10). Other irregular rhythms may resemble AF on ECG but can be distinguished by the presence of discrete P or flutter waves, which can sometimes be made more visible with vagal maneuvers. Muscle tremor or electrical interference may resemble f waves, but the underlying rhythm is regular. AF may also produce a phenomenon that mimics ventricular extrasystoles or ventricular tachycardia (Ashman phenomenon). This phenomenon typically occurs when a short R-R interval follows a long R-R interval; the longer interval lengthens the refractory period of the infra-Hisian conduction system, and subsequent QRS complexes are conducted aberrantly, typically with right bundle branch morphology.

Echocardiography and thyroid function tests are important in the initial evaluation. Echocardiography is done to assess structural heart defects (eg, left atrial enlargement, left ventricular wall motion abnormalities suggesting past or present ischemia, valvular disorders, cardiomyopathy) and to identify additional risk factors for stroke (eg, atrial blood stasis or thrombus, complex aortic plaque). Atrial thrombi are most likely in the atrial appendages, where they are best detected by transesophageal rather than transthoracic echocardiography.

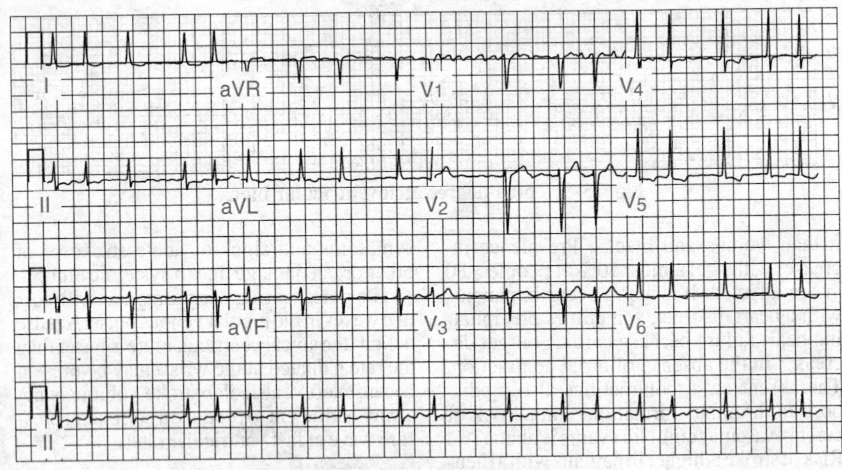

Fig. 75–10. Atrial fibrillation.

Treatment

If a significant underlying disorder is suspected, patients with new-onset AF may benefit from hospitalization, but those with recurrent episodes do not require it unless other symptoms suggest it. Once causes have been managed, treatment of AF focuses on ventricular rate control, rhythm control, and prevention of thromboembolism.

Ventricular rate control: Patients with AF of any duration require rate control (typically to < 80 beats/min at rest) to control symptoms and prevent tachycardia-induced cardiomyopathy.

For acute paroxysms of rapid rate (eg, 140 to 160 beats/min), IV AV node blockers are used (for doses, see TABLE 75–2). CAUTION: *AV node blockers should not be used in patients with Wolff-Parkinson-White syndrome when an accessory AV pathway is involved (indicated by wide QRS duration); these drugs increase frequency of conduction via the bypass tract, possibly causing ventricular fibrillation.* β-Blockers (eg, metoprolol, esmolol) are preferred if excess catecholamines are suspected (eg, in thyroid disorders, exercise-triggered cases); nondihydropyridine Ca channel blockers (eg, verapamil, diltiazem) are also effective. Digoxin is the least effective but may be preferred if heart failure is present. These drugs may be used orally for long-term rate control. When β-blockers, nondihydropyridine Ca channel blockers, and digoxin—separately or in combination—are ineffective, amiodarone may be required.

For patients who do not respond to or cannot take rate-controlling drugs, radiofrequency ablation of the AV node may be done to produce complete heart block; insertion of a permanent pacemaker is then necessary. Ablation of only one AV nodal pathway (AV node modification) reduces the number of atrial impulses reaching the ventricles and eliminates the need for a pacemaker, but this approach is considered less effective than complete ablation.

Rhythm control: In patients with heart failure or other hemodynamic compromise directly attributable to new-onset AF, restoration of normal sinus rhythm is indicated to improve cardiac output. In other cases, conversion of AF to normal sinus rhythm is optimal, but the antiarrhythmic drugs that are capable of doing so (class Ia, Ic, III) have a risk of adverse effects and may increase mortality. Conversion to sinus rhythm does not necessarily eliminate the need for chronic anticoagulation.

For acute conversion, synchronized cardioversion or drugs can be used. Before conversion is attempted, the ventricular rate should be controlled to < 120 beats/min, and, if AF has been present > 48 h, patients should be anticoagulated (conversion, regardless of method used, increases risk of thromboembolism). Anticoagulation with warfarin (see p. 699) should be maintained for > 3 wk before conversion when possible and continued indefinitely because AF may recur. Alternatively, the patient can be anticoagulated with heparin, and transesophageal echocardiography done; if there is no intra-atrial clot, cardioversion can be done immediately.

Synchronized cardioversion (100 joules, followed by 200 and 360 joules as needed) converts AF to normal sinus rhythm in 75 to 90% of patients, although recurrence rate is high. Efficacy and maintenance of sinus rhythm after the procedure is improved with use of class Ia, Ic, or III drugs 24 to 48 h before the procedure. Cardioversion is more effective in patients with shorter duration of AF, lone AF, or AF with a reversible cause; it is less effective when the left atrium is enlarged (> 5 cm), atrial appendage flow is low, or a significant underlying structural heart disorder is present.

Drugs for conversion to sinus rhythm include class Ia (procainamide, quinidine, disopyramide), Ic (flecainide, propafenone), and III (amiodarone, dofetilide, ibutilide, sotalol) antiarrhythmics (see TABLE 75–2). All are effective in about 50 to 60% of patients, but adverse effects differ. These drugs should not be used until rate has been controlled by a β-blocker or nondihydropyridine Ca channel blocker. These converting drugs are also used for long-term maintenance of sinus rhythm (with or without previous cardioversion). Choice depends on patient tolerance. However, for paroxysmal AF that occurs only or almost only at rest or during sleep when vagal tone is high, drugs with vagolytic effects (eg, disopyramide) may be particularly effective, and exercise-induced AF may be better prevented with a β-blocker.

ACE inhibitors and angiotensin II receptor blockers may attenuate the myocardial fibrosis that provides a substrate for AF in patients with heart failure, but the role of these drugs in routine AF treatment has yet to be defined.

Prevention of thromboembolism: Measures to prevent thromboembolism are necessary at the time of cardioversion and during long-term treatment of most patients.

Warfarin titrated to an INR of 2 to 3 should be given for ≥ 3 wk before elective cardioversion of lone AF present for > 48 h and continued for 4 wk after successful cardioversion. Anticoagulants should be continued indefinitely for patients with recurrent paroxysmal, persistent, or permanent AF in the presence of risk factors for thromboembolism. Healthy patients with a single episode of lone AF are anticoagulated for 4 wk.

Aspirin is less effective than warfarin but is used for patients with no risk factors for thromboembolism or those with contraindications to warfarin. Ximelagatran (36 mg po bid), a direct thrombin inhibitor that does not require INR monitoring, may be equivalent to warfarin for stroke prevention in high-risk patients but requires further study before it can be recommended over warfarin. The left atrial appendage may be surgically ligated or closed with a transcatheter device when warfarin and antiplatelet drugs are absolutely contraindicated.

ATRIAL FLUTTER

Atrial flutter is a rapid regular atrial rhythm due to an atrial reentrant circuit. Symptoms are mainly palpitations. Atrial thrombi may form and embolize. Diagnosis is by ECG. Treatment involves rate control with drugs, prevention of thromboembolism with anticoagulants, and often conversion to sinus rhythm with drugs or cardioversion.

Atrial flutter is much less common than atrial fibrillation, but its causes and hemodynamic consequences are similar. Many patients with atrial flutter also have periods of atrial fibrillation.

Classical atrial flutter is due to a large reentrant circuit (several cm) in the right atrium. The atria depolarize at a rate of 250 to 350/min (typically 300/min). Because the atrioventricular (AV) node cannot usually conduct at this rate, typically ½ of the impulses get through (2:1 block), resulting in a regular ventricular rate of 150 beats/min. Sometimes block varies from moment to moment, causing an irregular ventricular rhythm. Less commonly, a fixed 3:1, 4:1, or 5:1 block may be present.

The probability of a thromboembolic event, once considered rare in atrial flutter, is now thought to be about ½ of that in atrial fibrillation.

Symptoms and Signs

Symptoms depend primarily on ventricular rate and the nature of any underlying heart disorder. If ventricular rate is < 120 beats/min and regular, there are likely to be few or no symptoms. Faster rates and variable AV conduction usually produce palpitations, and decreased cardiac output may produce symptoms of hemodynamic compromise (eg, chest discomfort, dyspnea, weakness, syncope). Close inspection of the jugular venous pulse reveals flutter *a* waves.

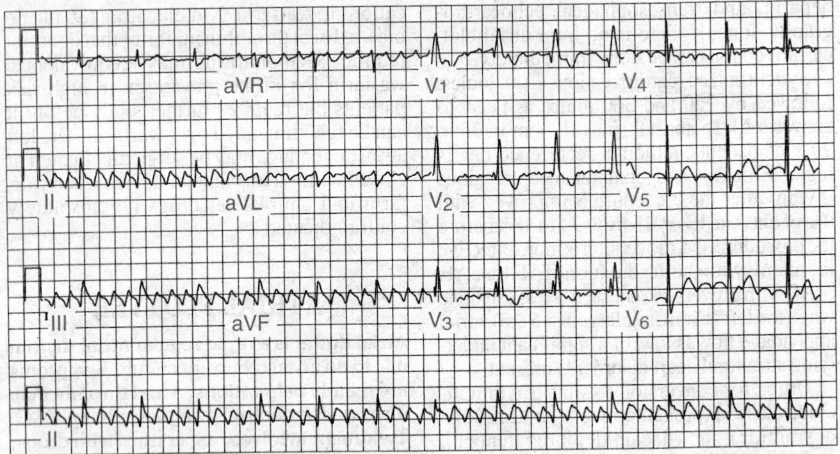

Fig. 75–11. Atrial flutter with variable atrioventricular block. (NOTE: Conducted with right bundle branch block).

Diagnosis

The diagnosis is by ECG, which shows continuous and regular atrial activation with a sawtooth pattern, most obvious in leads II, III, and aVF (see FIG. 75–11). Carotid sinus massage can increase AV block and better expose the typical flutter waves. A similar response may follow pharmacologic AV nodal blockade (eg, with adenosine), but such therapy does not terminate atrial flutter.

Treatment

As for atrial fibrillation, treatment focuses on ventricular rate control, rhythm control, and prevention of thromboembolism. However, pharmacologic rate control is more difficult to achieve in atrial flutter than in atrial fibrillation. Thus for most patients, electrical conversion (using synchronized cardioversion or overdrive pacing) is the treatment of choice for an initial episode and is mandatory with 1:1 AV conduction or hemodynamic compromise. Typically, low-energy (50 joules) conversion is effective. Anticoagulation, as in atrial fibrillation, is necessary before cardioversion.

If drugs are used to restore sinus rhythm, rate must first be controlled with β-blockers or nondihydropyridine Ca channel blockers. Many of the antiarrhythmics that can restore sinus rhythm (especially class Ia and Ic) can slow atrial flutter, shorten AV nodal refractoriness (by their vagolytic effects), or do both enough to allow 1:1 conduction with paradoxical increase in ventricular rate and hemodynamic compromise. These drugs may be used for long-term maintenance as required to prevent recurrence.

An antitachycardia pacing system is an alternative to chronic antiarrhythmics in selected patients. Also, ablation procedures designed to interrupt the atrial reentrant circuit may effectively prevent atrial flutter, particularly classic atrial flutter.

Patients with chronic or recurrent atrial flutter require warfarin (to maintain an INR of 2 to 3) or aspirin therapy long-term. The choice between the 2 therapies is based on the same considerations as for atrial fibrillation.

REENTRANT SUPRAVENTRICULAR TACHYCARDIAS

Reentrant supraventricular tachycardias involve reentrant pathways with a component above the bifurcation of the His bundle. Patients have sudden episodes of palpitations that begin and terminate abruptly; some have dyspnea or chest discomfort. Diagnosis is clinical and by ECG. Treatment is with vagotonic maneuvers and, if they are ineffective, with IV adenosine or nondihydropyridine Ca channel blockers for narrow QRS rhythms, procainamide or amiodarone for wide QRS rhythms, or synchronized cardioversion for all cases.

Pathophysiology and Etiology

The reentry pathway (see FIG. 75–1) in supraventricular tachycardia (SVT) is within the atrioventricular (AV) node in about 50%, involves an accessory bypass tract in 40%, and is within the atria or sinoatrial (SA) node in 10%.

AV nodal reentrant tachycardia occurs most often in otherwise healthy patients. It is most commonly triggered by an atrial premature beat.

Accessory pathway reentrant tachycardia involves tracts of conducting tissue that partially or totally bypass normal AV connections (bypass tracts). They run most commonly from the atria directly to the ventricles and less commonly from the atrium to a portion of the conduction system or from a portion of the conduction system to the ventricle. They can be triggered by atrial premature beats or ventricular premature beats.

Wolff-Parkinson-White (WPW) syndrome: WPW (preexcitation) syndrome is the most common accessory pathway SVT, occurring in about 1 to 3/1000 people. WPW syndrome is mainly idiopathic, although it is more common among patients with hypertrophic or other forms of cardiomyopathy, transposition of the great vessels, or Epstein's anomaly.

In classic (or manifest) WPW syndrome, antegrade conduction occurs over both the accessory pathway and the normal conducting system during sinus rhythm. The accessory pathway, being faster, depolarizes some of the ventricle early, resulting in a short PR interval and a slurred upstroke to the QRS complex (delta wave—see FIG. 75–12). The delta wave prolongs QRS duration to > 0.1 sec, although the overall configuration, apart from the delta wave, may appear normal. Depending on the orientation of the delta wave, a pseudoinfarction pattern Q-wave may be present. Because the early depolarized parts of the ventricle also repolarize early, the T-wave vector may be abnormal.

In concealed WPW syndrome, the accessory pathway does not conduct in an antegrade direction; consequently, the above ECG abnormalities do not appear. However, it conducts in a retrograde direction and thus can participate in reentrant tachycardia.

In the most common form of reentrant tachycardia (called orthodromic reciprocating tachycardia), the circuit uses the normal AV conduction pathway to activate the ventricles, returning to the atrium via the accessory AV connection. The resultant QRS complex is thus narrow (unless bundle branch block coexists) and without a delta wave. Orthodromic reciprocating tachycardia is typically a short RP tachycardia with the retrograde P wave in the ST segment.

Rarely, the reentrant circuit revolves in the opposite direction, from the atrium to the ventricle via the accessory AV connection, and returns from the ventricle retrogradely up the normal AV conduction system (called antidromic reciprocating tachycardia). The QRS complex is wide because the ventricles are activated abnormally. In patients with 2 accessory AV connections (not uncommon), a reciprocating tachycardia using one accessory connection in the antegrade direction and the other in the retrograde direction may occur.

Tachycardias in WPW syndrome may begin as or degenerate into atrial fibrillation (AF), which can be very dangerous (see p. 703). Enlarged atria due to hypertrophic and other forms of cardiomyopathy makes patients with WPW syndrome more prone to AF.

Symptoms and Signs

Most patients present during young adulthood or middle age. They typically have episodes of sudden-onset, sudden-offset, rapid, regular palpitations often associated with symptoms of hemodynamic compromise (eg, dyspnea, chest discomfort, light-headedness).

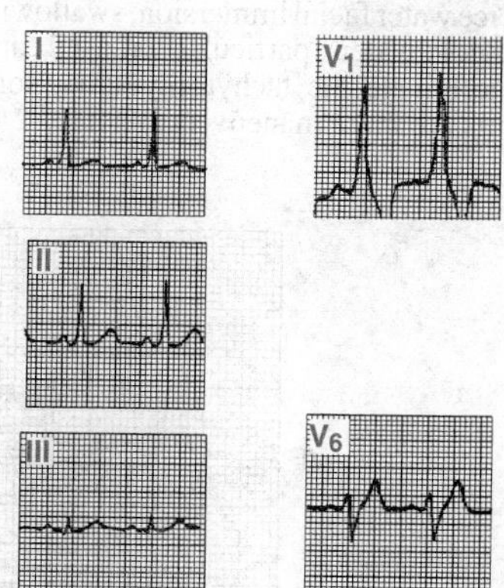

Fig. 75–12. Classic Wolff-Parkinson-White (WPW) syndrome. Leads I, II, III, V_1, and V_6 show classic features of WPW syndrome, with a short PR interval and a delta wave during sinus rhythm.

Attacks may last only a few seconds or persist for several hours (rarely, > 12 h).

Infants present with episodic breathlessness, lethargy, feeding problems, or rapid precordial pulsations. If the episode of tachycardia is protracted, they may present with heart failure.

Examination is usually unremarkable except for a heart rate of 160 to 240 beats/min.

Diagnosis

Diagnosis is by ECG showing rapid, regular tachycardia. Previous tracings, if available, are reviewed for signs of manifest WPW syndrome.

P waves vary. In most cases of AV node reentry, retrograde P waves are in the terminal portion of the QRS complex (often producing a pseudo-R′ deflection in lead V_1); about ⅓ occur just after the QRS complex, and very few occur before. P waves always follow the QRS complex in orthodromic reciprocating tachycardia of WPW syndrome.

QRS complex is narrow except with coexisting bundle branch block, antidromic tachycardia, or dual accessory connection reciprocating tachycardia. Wide-complex tachycardia must be distinguished from ventricular tachycardia (see TABLE 75–5 and FIGS. 75–12 and 75–13).

Treatment

Many episodes stop spontaneously before treatment. Vagotonic maneuvers (eg, Valsalva maneuver, unilateral carotid sinus massage, ice water facial immersion, swallowing of ice-cold water), particularly if used early, may terminate the tachyarrhythmia; some patients use these maneuvers at home.

If these maneuvers are ineffective and the QRS complex is narrow (indicating orthodromic conduction), AV node blockers are used; blocking conduction through the AV node for one beat interrupts the reentrant cycle. Adenosine is the 1st choice. Dose is 6 mg by rapid IV bolus (0.05 to 0.1 mg/kg in children), followed by a 20-mL saline bolus. If this dosage is ineffective, 2 subsequent 12-mg doses are given q 5 min. Adenosine sometimes causes a brief (2- to 3-sec) period of cardiac standstill, which may distress patient and physician. Verapamil 5 mg IV or diltiazem 0.25 to 0.35 mg/kg IV are alternatives.

For a regular, wide QRS complex tachycardia known to be an antidromic reciprocating tachycardia not involving double accessory pathways (which must be identified by the history; they cannot be established acutely), AV nodal blockers may also be effective. However, if the mechanism of the tachycardia is unknown, ventricular tachycardia has not been excluded, and AV nodal blockers should be avoided because they may worsen ventricular tachycardias. In such cases (or those in which drugs are ineffective), IV procainamide or amiodarone can be used. Alternatively, synchronized cardioversion with 50 joules (0.5 to 2 joules/kg for children) is quick and safe and may be preferred to these more toxic drugs.

When episodes of AV nodal reentrant tachycardia are frequent or bothersome, options include long-term antiarrhythmics or transvenous catheter radiofrequency ablation. Generally, ablation is recommended, but if it is not acceptable, drug prophylaxis usually begins with digoxin and proceeds, as required, to β-blockers, Ca channel blockers,

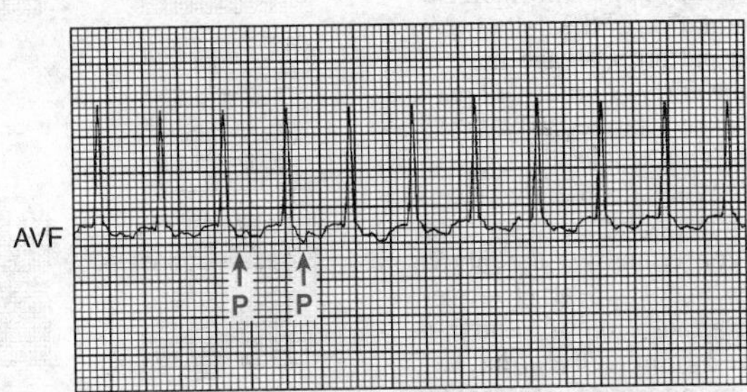

Fig. 75–13. Narrow QRS tachycardia: Orthodromic reciprocating tachycardia using an accessory pathway in Wolff-Parkinson-White syndrome. Activation is as follows: atrioventricular node, His-Purkinje system, ventricle, accessory pathway, atria. The P wave closely follows the QRS complex; it is a short RP tachycardia (PR > RP).

or both, then to one or more class Ia, class Ic, or class III antiarrhythmics.

ATRIAL FIBRILLATION AND WOLFF-PARKINSON-WHITE SYNDROME

Atrial fibrillation is a medical emergency in the setting of antegrade conduction over an accessory pathway in Wolff-Parkinson-White syndrome.

In manifest WPW syndrome, antegrade conduction occurs over the accessory pathway. If AF develops, the normal rate-limiting effects of the AV node are bypassed, and the resultant excessive ventricular rates (sometimes 200 to 240 beats/min) may lead to ventricular fibrillation (see FIG. 75–14) and sudden death. Patients with concealed WPW syndrome are not at risk because in them, antegrade conduction does not occur over the accessory connection.

The treatment of choice is direct-current cardioversion. The usual rate-slowing drugs used in AF are not effective, and digoxin and the nondihydropyridine Ca channel blockers are contraindicated because they may increase the ventricular rate and cause ventricular fibrillation. If cardioversion is impossible, drugs that prolong the refractory period of the accessory connection should be used. IV procainamide or amiodarone is preferred, but any class Ia, class Ic, or class III antiarrhythmic can be used.

BUNDLE BRANCH AND FASCICULAR BLOCK

Bundle branch block is partial or complete interruption of impulse conduction in a bundle branch; fascicular block is similar interruption in a hemifascicle of the bundle. The 2 disorders often coexist. There are usually no symptoms, but presence of either suggests a heart disorder. Diagnosis is by ECG. No specific treatment is indicated.

Conduction blocks can be caused by many heart disorders, including intrinsic degeneration without another associated heart disorder.

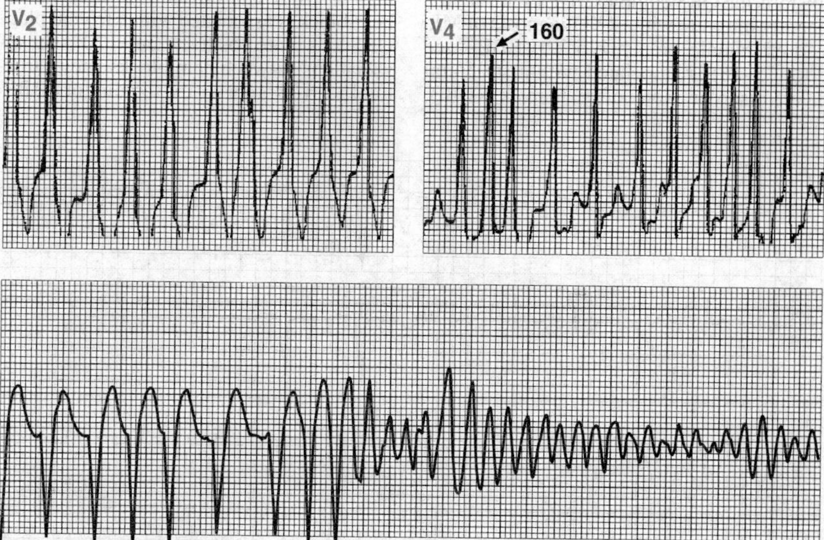

Fig. 75–14. Atrial fibrillation in Wolff-Parkinson-White syndrome. Ventricular response is very fast (RR intervals minimum of 160 msec). Shortly thereafter, ventricular fibrillation develops (lead II continuous rhythm strip at bottom).

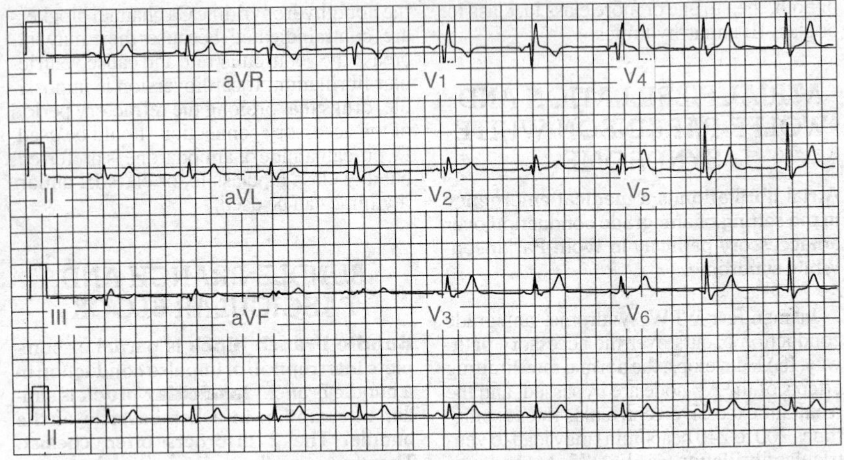

Fig. 75–15. Right bundle branch block.

Right bundle branch block (RBBB—see FIG. 75–15) can occur in apparently normal people. It may also occur with anterior MI, indicating substantial myocardial injury. New appearance of RBBB should prompt a search for underlying cardiac pathology, but often, none is found. Transient RBBB may occur after pulmonary embolism. Although RBBB distorts the QRS complex, it does not significantly interfere with ECG diagnosis of MI.

Left bundle branch block (LBBB—see FIG. 75–16) is associated with a structural heart disorder more often than is RBBB. LBBB usually precludes use of ECG for diagnosis of MI.

Fascicular block involves the anterior or posterior fascicle of the left bundle branch. Interruption of the left anterior fascicle produces left anterior hemiblock characterized by modest QRS prolongation (< 120 msec) and a frontal plane QRS axis more negative than −30° (left axis deviation). Left posterior hemiblock is associated with a frontal plane QRS axis more positive than +120°. The associations between hemiblocks and a structural heart disorder are the same as for LBBB.

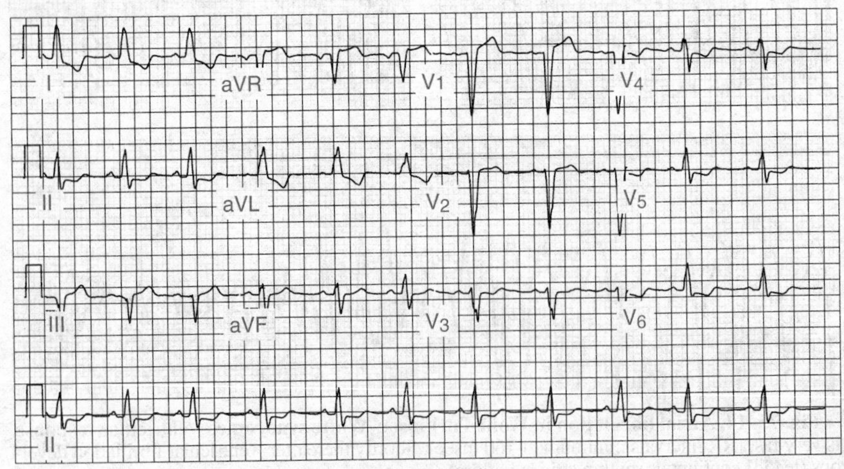

Fig. 75–16. Left bundle branch block.

Hemiblocks may coexist with other conduction disturbances: RBBB and left anterior or posterior hemiblock (bifascicular block); and left anterior or posterior hemiblock, RBBB, and 1st-degree AV block (incorrectly called trifascicular block; 1st-degree block is usually AV nodal in origin). Trifascicular block refers to RBBB with alternating left anterior and left posterior hemiblock or alternating LBBB and RBBB. Presence of bifascicular or trifascicular block after MI implies extensive cardiac damage. Bifascicular blocks require no direct treatment unless intermittent 2nd- or 3rd-degree AV block is present. True trifascicular blocks require immediate, then permanent pacing.

Nonspecific intraventricular conduction defects are diagnosed when the QRS complex is prolonged (> 120 msec), but the QRS pattern is not typical of LBBB or RBBB. The conduction delay may occur beyond the Purkinje fibers and result from slow cell-to-cell myocyte conduction. No specific treatment is indicated.

VENTRICULAR PREMATURE BEATS

Ventricular premature beats (VPBs) are single ventricular impulses caused by reentry within the ventricle or abnormal automaticity of ventricular cells. They are extremely common in healthy patients and in patients with a heart disorder. VPBs may be asymptomatic or cause palpitations. Diagnosis is by ECG. Treatment is usually not required.

Ventricular premature beats (VPBs), also called premature ventricular contractions (PVCs), may occur erratically or at predictable intervals (eg, every 3rd [trigeminy] or 2nd [bigeminy] beat). VPBs may increase with stimulants (eg, anxiety, stress, alcohol, caffeine, sympathomimetic drugs), hypoxia, or electrolyte abnormalities.

VPBs may be experienced as missed or skipped beats; the VPB itself is not sensed but rather the following augmented sinus beat. When VPBs are very frequent, particularly when they represent every 2nd heart beat, mild hemodynamic symptoms are possible because the sinus rate has been effectively halved. Existing ejection murmurs may be accentuated because of increased cardiac filling and augmented contractility after the compensatory pause.

Diagnosis is by ECG showing a wide QRS complex without a preceding P wave, typically followed by a fully compensatory pause.

Prognosis and Treatment

VPBs are not significant in patients without a heart disorder, and no treatment is required beyond avoiding obvious triggers. β-Blockers are offered only if symptoms are intolerable. Other antiarrhythmics that suppress VPBs increase risk of more serious arrhythmias.

In patients with a structural heart disorder (eg, aortic stenosis, post MI), treatment is controversial even though frequent VPBs (> 10/h) correlate with increased mortality, because no studies have shown that pharmacologic suppression reduces mortality. In post-MI patients, mortality rate is higher with class I antiarrhythmics than with placebo. This finding probably reflects adverse effects of the antiarrhythmics. β-Blockers are beneficial in symptomatic heart failure and post MI. If VPBs increase during exercise in a patient with coronary artery disease, evaluation for the possible need of percutaneous transluminal coronary angioplasty or coronary artery bypass graft surgery should be considered.

VENTRICULAR TACHYCARDIA

Ventricular tachycardia is ≥ 3 consecutive ventricular beats at a rate ≥ 120 beats/min. Symptoms depend on duration and vary from none to palpitations to hemodynamic collapse and death. Diagnosis is by ECG. Treatment of more than brief episodes is with cardioversion or antiarrhythmics depending on symptoms. If necessary, long-term treatment is with an implantable cardioverter defibrillator.

Some experts use a cutoff rate of ≥ 100 beats/min for ventricular tachycardia (VT). Repetitive ventricular rhythms at slower rates are called accelerated idioventricular rhythms or slow VT; they are usually benign and are not treated unless associated with hemodynamic symptoms.

Most patients with VT have a significant heart disorder, particularly prior MI or a cardiomyopathy. Electrolyte abnormalities (particularly hypokalemia or hypomagnesemia), acidemia, hypoxemia, and adverse drug effects contribute. The long QT syndrome (congenital or acquired) is associated with a particular form of VT, torsades de pointes.

VT may be monomorphic or polymorphic and nonsustained or sustained. Monomorphic VT results from a single abnormal focus or reentrant pathway and has regular, identical-appearing QRS complexes. Polymorphic VT results from several different foci or pathways and is thus irregular, with varying QRS complexes. Nonsustained VT lasts < 30 sec; sustained VT lasts ≥ 30 sec or is terminated sooner because of hemodynamic collapse. VT frequently deteriorates to ventricular fibrillation and thus cardiac arrest (see p. 530).

Symptoms, Signs, and Diagnosis

VT of short duration or slow rate may be asymptomatic. Sustained VT is almost always symptomatic, causing palpitations, symptoms of hemodynamic compromise, or sudden cardiac death.

Diagnosis is by ECG (see FIG. 75–17). Any wide QRS complex tachycardia (QRS ≥ 0.12 sec) should be considered VT until proved otherwise. Diagnosis is supported by ECG findings of dissociated P-wave activity, fusion or capture beats, uniformity of QRS vectors in the V leads (concordance) with discordant T-wave vector (opposite QRS vectors), and a frontal-plane QRS axis in the northwest quadrant. Differential diagnosis includes supraventricular tachycardia conducted with bundle branch block or via an accessory pathway (see TABLE 75–1). However, because some patients tolerate VT surprisingly well, concluding that a well-tolerated wide QRS complex tachycardia must be of supraventricular origin is a mistake. Using drugs appropriate for supraventricular tachycardia (eg, verapamil, diltiazem) in patients with VT may cause hemodynamic collapse and death.

Treatment

Acute: Treatment depends on symptoms and duration of VT. Hypotensive VT requires synchronized direct-current cardioversion with ≥ 100 joules. Stable sustained VT can be treated with IV drugs, usually lidocaine (see TABLE 75–2), which acts quickly but is frequently ineffective. If lidocaine is ineffective, IV procainamide may be given, but it may take up to 1 h to work. Failure of IV procainamide is an indication for cardioversion.

Nonsustained VT does not require immediate treatment unless the runs are frequent or long enough to produce symptoms. In such cases, antiarrhythmic drugs are used as for sustained VT.

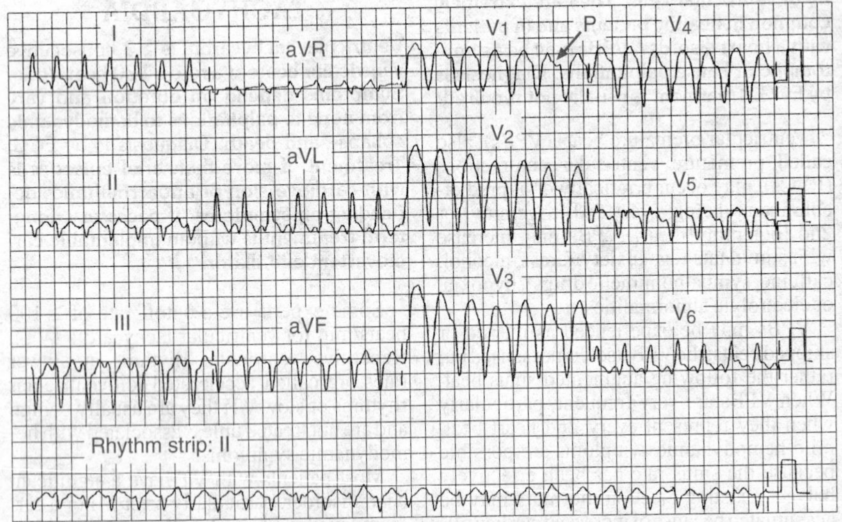

Fig. 75–17. Broad QRS ventricular tachycardia. The QRS duration is 160 msec. An independent P wave can be seen in V_1 (*arrow*). There is an extreme mean frontal axis shift.

Long-term: The primary goal is preventing sudden death, rather than simply suppressing the arrhythmia. It is best accomplished by use of an implantable cardioverter-defibrillator (ICD—see p. 690). However, the decision about whom to treat is complex and depends on the estimated probability of life-threatening VTs and the severity of underlying heart disorders (see TABLE 75–5).

Long-term treatment is not required when the index episode of VT resulted from a transient cause (eg, during the 48 h after onset of MI) or a reversible cause (acid-base disturbances, electrolyte abnormalities, proarrhythmic drug effect).

In the absence of a transient or reversible cause, patients who have had an episode of sustained VT typically require an ICD. Most patients with sustained VT and a significant structural heart disorder should also receive a β-blocker. If an ICD cannot be used, amiodarone may be the preferred antiarrhythmic for prevention of sudden death.

Because nonsustained VT is a marker for increased risk of sudden death in patients with a structural heart disorder, such patients (particularly those with an ejection fraction < 0.35) require further evaluation. Emerging data suggest such patients should receive ICD.

When prevention of VTs is important (usually in patients who have an ICD and are having frequent episodes of VT), antiarrhythmics or transcatheter radiofrequency or surgical ablation of the arrhythmogenic substrate is required. Any class Ia, Ib, Ic, II, or III drug can be used. Because β-blockers are safe, they are the 1st choice unless contraindicated. If an additional drug is required, sotalol is commonly used, then amiodarone.

Transcatheter radiofrequency ablation is used most commonly in patients who have VT with well-defined syndromes (eg, right ventricular outflow tract VT or left septal VT [Belhassen VT, verapamil-sensitive VT]) and otherwise healthy hearts.

TORSADES DE POINTES VENTRICULAR TACHYCARDIA

Torsades de pointes is a specific form of polymorphic VT in patients with a long QT interval. It is characterized by rapid, irregular QRS complexes, which appear to be twisting around the ECG baseline. This arrhythmia may cease spontaneously or degenerate into ventricular fibrillation. It causes significant hemodynamic compromise and often death. Diagnosis is by ECG. Treatment is with IV Mg, measures to shorten QT interval, and unsynchronized cardioversion when ventricular fibrillation is precipitated.

The long QT interval responsible for torsades de pointes can be congenital or drug-induced.

Two established congenital long QT-interval syndromes are Jervell and Lange-Nielsen syndrome (autosomal recessive with associated deafness) and Romano-Ward syndrome (autosomal dominant with no deafness). However, at least 6 subforms of long QT-interval syndrome that result from defects in genes that encode specific transmembrane K or Na channels have been identified.

More commonly, torsades de pointes results from a drug, usually a class Ia, Ic, or III antiarrhythmic; other drugs include tricyclic antidepressants, phenothiazines, and certain antivirals and antifungals (see www.torsades.org for an up-to-date list).

QT-interval prolongation predisposes to arrhythmia by prolonging repolarization, which induces early after-depolarizations and spatial dispersion of refractoriness.

Symptoms, Diagnosis, and Treatment

Patients often present with syncope because the underlying rate (200 to 250 beats/min) is nonperfusing. Palpitations are common among conscious patients. Sometimes the long QT interval is detected after resuscitation.

Diagnosis is by ECG showing an undulating QRS axis, with the polarity of complexes shifting around the baseline (see FIG. 75–18). ECG between episodes shows a long QT interval after correction for heart rate (QTc). Normal values average about 0.44 sec, although they vary among individuals and by sex. A family history may suggest a congenital syndrome.

An acute episode prolonged enough to cause hemodynamic compromise is treated with unsynchronized cardioversion, beginning with 100 joules. Nevertheless, early recurrence is the rule. Patients often respond to Mg: $MgSO_4$ 2 g IV over 1 to 2 min. If this treatment is unsuccessful, a 2nd bolus is given in 5 to 10 min, and an Mg infusion of 3 to 20 mg/min may be started in patients without renal

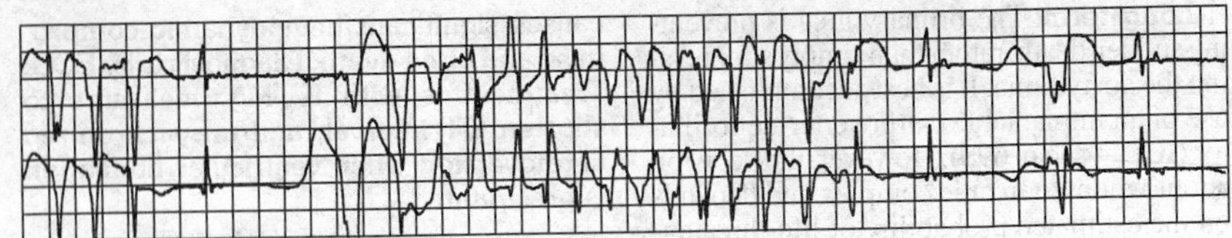

Fig. 75–18. Torsades de pointes ventricular tachycardia.

insufficiency. Lidocaine (class Ib) shortens the QT interval and may be effective especially for drug-induced torsades de pointes. Class Ia, Ic, and III antiarrhythmics are avoided.

If a drug is the cause, it is stopped, but until drug clearance is complete, patients with frequent or long runs of torsades de pointes require treatment to shorten the QT interval. Because increasing the heart rate shortens the QT interval, temporary pacing, IV isoproterenol, or both are often effective. Long-term treatment is required for patients with a congenital long QT-interval syndrome. Treatment choices include β-blockers, permanent pacing, ICD, or a combination. Family members should be evaluated by ECG.

VENTRICULAR FIBRILLATION

Ventricular fibrillation produces uncoordinated quivering of the ventricle with no useful contractions. It causes immediate syncope and death within minutes. Treatment is with cardiopulmonary resuscitation, including immediate defibrillation.

Ventricular fibrillation (VF) is due to multiple wavelet reentrant electrical activity and is manifested on ECG by ultrarapid baseline undulations that are irregular in timing and morphology (see FIG. 75–14).

VF is the presenting rhythm for about 70% of patients in cardiac arrest and is thus the terminal event in many disorders. Overall, most patients with VF have an underlying heart disorder (typically ischemic, but also hypertrophic or dilated cardiomyopathies, arrhythmogenic right ventricular dysplasia [ARVD], or Brugada syndrome). Risk of VF in any disorder is increased by electrolyte abnormalities, acidosis, hypoxemia, or ischemia.

VF is much less common among infants and children, in whom asystole is the more common presentation of cardiac arrest.

Treatment is with cardiopulmonary resuscitation, including defibrillation (see p. 534). The success rate for immediate (within 3 min) defibrillation is about 95%, provided that overwhelming pump failure does not preexist. When it does, even immediate defibrillation is only 30% successful, and most resuscitated patients die of pump failure before hospital discharge.

Patients who have VF without a reversible or transient cause are at high risk of future VF events and of sudden death. Most of these patients require an implantable cardioverter-defibrillator; many require concomitant antiarrhythmics to reduce the frequency of subsequent episodes of ventricular tachycardia and VF.

76 VALVULAR DISORDERS

Any heart valve can become stenotic or insufficient, causing hemodynamic changes long before symptoms. Most often, valvular stenosis or insufficiency occurs in isolation in individual valves, but multiple valvular disorders may coexist.

Treatment depends on severity of disease but usually involves catheter-based valvuloplasty (eg, percutaneous balloon commissurotomy, valvotomy) or surgery (eg, surgical commissurotomy, valve repair, valve replacement). Two kinds of valve prosthesis are used: bioprosthetic (porcine) and mechanical (metal).

Traditionally, a mechanical valve has been used in patients < 65 and in older patients with a long life expectancy, because bioprosthetic valves deteriorate over 10 to 12 yr. Patients with a mechanical valve require lifelong anticoagulation to an INR of 2.5 to 3.5 (to prevent thromboembolism) and antibiotics before some medical or dental procedures (to prevent endocarditis). A bioprosthetic valve, which does not require anticoagulation, has been used in patients > 65, younger patients with a life expectancy < 10 yr, and those with some right-sided lesions. However, newer bioprosthetic valves may be more durable than 1st-generation valves; thus, patient preference regarding valve type can now be considered.

Women of childbearing age who require valve replacement and plan to become pregnant must balance the increased risk of teratogenicity from warfarin with mechanical valves against that of accelerated valve deterioration with bioprosthetic valves. These risks can be reduced by use of heparin instead of warfarin in the first 12 wk and last 2 wk of the pregnancy or by frequent echocardiographic screening.

Endocarditis prophylaxis is also indicated for nearly all patients with valvular heart disorders (see TABLE 77–3 on p. 730).

AORTIC REGURGITATION

Aortic regurgitation is incompetency of the aortic valve causing flow from the aorta into the left ventricle during diastole. Causes include idiopathic valvular degeneration, rheumatic fever, endocarditis, myxomatous degeneration, congenital bicuspid aortic valve, syphilitic aortitis, and connective tissue or rheumatologic disorders. Symptoms include exertional dyspnea, orthopnea, paroxysmal nocturnal dyspnea, palpitations, and chest pain. Signs include widened pulse pressure and a holodiastolic murmur. Diagnosis is by physical examination and echocardiography. Treatment is aortic valve replacement and, in some cases, vasodilating drugs.

Etiology and Pathophysiology

Aortic regurgitation (AR) may be acute or chronic. The primary causes of acute AR are infective endocarditis and dissection of the ascending aorta. Mild chronic AR in adults is most often caused by a bicuspid or fenestrated aortic valve (2% of men and 1% of women), especially when severe diastolic hypertension (pressure ≥ 110 mm Hg) is present. Moderate to severe chronic AR in adults is most often caused by idiopathic degeneration of the aortic valves or root, rheumatic fever, infective endocarditis, myxomatous degeneration, or trauma. In children, the most common cause is a ventricular septal defect with aortic valve prolapse. Rarely, AR is caused by seronegative spondyloarthropathies (ankylosing spondylitis, reactive arthritis, psoriatic arthritis), RA, SLE, arthritis associated with ulcerative colitis, luetic (syphilitic) aortitis, osteogenesis imperfecta, thoracic aortic aneurysm, aortic dissection, supravalvular aortic stenosis, Takayasu's arteritis, rupture of a sinus of Valsalva, acromegaly, and temporal (giant cell) arteritis. AR due to myxomatous degeneration may develop in patients with Marfan or Ehlers-Danlos syndromes.

In chronic AR, left ventricular (LV) volume and LV stroke volume gradually increase because the LV receives aortic blood regurgitated in diastole in addition to blood from the pulmonary veins and left atrium. LV hypertrophy compensates for the increase in LV volume over years, but decompensation eventually develops. These changes may ultimately cause arrhythmias, heart failure (HF), or cardiogenic shock.

Symptoms and Signs

Acute AR causes symptoms of HF and cardiogenic shock. Chronic AR is typically asymptomatic for years; progressive exertional dyspnea, orthopnea, paroxysmal nocturnal dyspnea, and palpitations develop insidiously. Symptoms of HF correlate poorly with objective measures of LV function. Chest pain (angina pectoris) affects only about 5% of patients who do not have coexisting coronary artery disease (CAD) and, when it occurs, is especially common at night. Patients may present with endocarditis (eg, fever, anemia, weight loss, embolic phenomena) because the abnormal aortic valve is predisposed to bacterial seeding.

Signs vary by severity. As chronic disease progresses, systolic BP increases while diastolic BP decreases, creating a widened pulse pressure. With time, the LV impulse may become enlarged, sustained, increased in amplitude, and displaced downward and laterally, with systolic depression of the entire left parasternal area, giving a rocking motion to the left chest.

A systolic apical or carotid thrill may become palpable in later stages of AR; it is caused by large forward stroke volumes and low aortic diastolic pressure.

Auscultatory findings include a normal 1st heart sound (S_1) and a nonsplit, loud, sharp or slapping 2nd heart sound (S_2) caused by increased elastic aortic recoil. The murmur of AR is blowing, high-pitched, diastolic, and decrescendo, beginning soon after the aortic component of S_2 (A_2); it is loudest at the 3rd or 4th left parasternal intercostal space. The murmur is heard best with the diaphragm of the stethoscope when the patient is leaning forward, with breath held at end-expiration. It increases in volume in response to maneuvers that increase afterload (eg, squatting, isometric handgrip). If AR is slight, the murmur may occur only in early diastole. If LV diastolic pressure is very high, the murmur is shorter because aortic and LV diastolic pressures equalize earlier in diastole.

Other abnormal sounds include a forward ejection and backward regurgitant flow (to-and-fro) murmur, an ejection click soon after the S_1, and an aortic ejection flow murmur. A diastolic murmur heard near the axilla or mid left thorax (Cole-Cecil murmur) is caused by fusion of the aortic murmur with the 3rd heart sound (S_3), which is due to simultaneous filling of LV from the left atrium and AR. A mid-to-late diastolic rumble heard at the apex (Austin Flint murmur) may result from rapid regurgitant flow into the LV, causing mitral valve leaflet vibration at the peak of atrial flow; this murmur mimics the diastolic murmur of mitral stenosis.

Other signs are unusual; sensitivity and specificity are low or unknown. Visible signs include head bobbing (Musset's sign) and pulsation of the fingernail capillaries (Quincke's sign, best seen with slight pressure) or uvula (Müller's sign). Palpable signs include a large-volume pulse with rapid rise and fall (slapping, water-hammer, or collapsing pulse) and pulsation of the carotid arteries (Corrigan's sign), retinal arteries (Becker's sign), liver (Rosenbach's sign), or spleen (Gerhard's sign). BP findings may include popliteal systolic pressure ≥ 60 mm Hg higher than brachial pressure (Hill's sign) and a fall in diastolic BP of > 15 mm Hg with arm elevation (Mayne's sign). Auscultatory signs include a sharp sound heard over the femoral pulse (pistol-shot sound, or Traube's sign) and a femoral systolic bruit distal and a diastolic bruit proximal to arterial compression (Duroziez's murmur).

Diagnosis

Diagnosis is suspected based on history and physical examination and confirmed by echocardiography. Doppler echocardiography is the test of choice to detect and quantify the magnitude of regurgitant blood flow. Two-dimensional echocardiography can quantify aortic root size and anatomy and LV function. An end-systolic LV volume > 60 mL/m^2, end-systolic LV diameter > 50 mm, and LVEF < 50% suggest decompensation. Echocardiography can also assess severity of pulmonary hypertension secondary to LV failure, detect vegetations or pericardial effusions (eg, in aortic dissection), and provide information about prognosis.

Radionuclide imaging may be used to determine LVEF if echocardiographic results are borderline abnormal or if echocardiography is technically difficult.

An ECG and chest x-ray should be obtained. ECG may show repolarization abnormalities with or without QRS voltage criteria of LV hypertrophy, left atrial enlargement, and T-wave inversion with ST-segment depression in precordial leads. Chest x-ray may show cardiomegaly and a prominent aortic root in patients with chronic progressive AR. If AR is severe, signs of pulmonary edema and HF may also be present. Exercise testing may help assess functional capacity and symptoms in patients with documented AR and equivocal symptoms.

Coronary angiography is usually not necessary for diagnosis but should be done before surgery, even if no angina is present, because about 20% of patients with severe AR have significant CAD, which may need concomitant coronary artery bypass graft surgery.

Prognosis and Treatment

With treatment, the 10-yr survival for patients with mild to moderate AR is 80 to 95%. With appropriately timed valve replacement (ie, before HF and using criteria below), long-term prognosis for patients with moderate to severe AR is good. However, the prognosis for those with severe AR and HF is considerably poorer.

Treatment of acute AR is aortic valve replacement. Treatment of chronic AR varies by symptoms and degree of LV dysfunction. Patients with symptoms precipitated by normal daily activity or during exercise testing require aortic valve replacement; patients who prefer to avoid surgery may be treated with vasodilators (eg, long-acting nifedipine 30 to 90 mg po once/day or ACE inhibitors); also, diuretics or nitrates to reduce preload may be beneficial for severe AR. Asymptomatic patients with LVEF < 55%, an end-systolic diameter ≥ 55 mm ("55 rule"), or an end-diastolic diameter > 75 mm also require surgery; oral drugs are a 2nd-best option for this group. Additional surgical criteria include fractional shortening < 25 to 29%, end-diastolic radius to myocardial wall thickness ratio > 4.0, and cardiac index < 2.2 to 2.5 L/min/m^2.

Patients who do not meet these criteria should be reevaluated by physical examination, echocardiography, and possibly rest-exercise radionuclide cineangiography to measure LV contractility q 6 to 12 mo.

Antibiotic prophylaxis against endocarditis is indicated before procedures that can result in bacteremia (see TABLE 77–3 on p. 730).

AORTIC STENOSIS

Aortic stenosis (AS) is narrowing of the aortic valve obstructing blood flow from the left ventricle to the ascending aorta during systole. Causes include a congenital bicuspid valve, idiopathic degenerative sclerosis with calcification, and rheumatic fever. Progressive untreated AS ultimately results in the classic triad of syncope, angina, and exertional dyspnea; heart failure and arrhythmias may develop. A carotid pulse with small amplitude and delayed upstroke and a crescendo-decrescendo ejection murmur are characteristic. Diagnosis is by physical examination and echocardiography. Asymptomatic AS often requires no treatment. For progressive severe or symptomatic AS in children, balloon valvotomy is used; adults require valve replacement.

Etiology and Pathophysiology

Aortic sclerosis, thickening of aortic valve structures by fibrosis and calcification initially without stenosis, is the most common cause of AS in elderly patients; over years, aortic sclerosis progresses to stenosis in as many as 15% of patients. Aortic sclerosis is also the most common overall cause of AS requiring surgery. Aortic sclerosis resembles atherosclerosis, with deposition of lipoproteins, active inflammation, and calcification of the valves; risk factors are similar (see p. 622).

The most common cause of AS in patients < 70 yr is a congenital bicuspid aortic valve. Congenital AS occurs in 3 to 5/1000 live births and affects more men.

In developing countries, rheumatic fever is the most common cause in all age groups. Supravalvular AS caused by a discrete, congenital membrane or hypoplastic constriction just above the sinuses of Valsalva is uncommon. A sporadic form of supravalvular AS is associated with a characteristic facies (high and broad forehead, hypertelorism, strabismus, upturned nose, long philtrum, wide mouth, dental abnormalities, puffy cheeks, micrognathia, low-set ears). When associated with idiopathic hypercalcemia of infancy, this form is known as Williams syndrome. Subvalvular AS caused by a congenital membrane or fibrous ring just beneath the aortic valve is uncommon.

Aortic regurgitation may accompany AS, and about 60% of patients > 60 yr with significant AS also have mitral annular calcification, which may lead to significant mitral regurgitation.

The left ventricle (LV) gradually hypertrophies in response to AS. Significant LV hypertrophy causes diastolic dysfunction and, with progression, may lead to decreased contractility, ischemia, or fibrosis, any of which may cause systolic dysfunction and heart failure (HF). LV chamber enlargement occurs only if the myocardium is damaged (eg, by infarction). Patients with AS have a higher incidence of GI and other bleeding (called Heyde's syndrome) because the high shear stress of stenotic valves makes multimeric von Willebrand factor more susceptible to cleavage by a plasma metalloprotease and may increase platelet clearance. GI bleeding may also be due to angiodysplasia. Hemolysis and aortic dissection are also more common.

Symptoms and Signs

Congenital AS is usually asymptomatic until at least age 10 or 20 yr, when symptoms may begin to develop insidiously. In all forms, progressive untreated AS ultimately results in exertional syncope, angina, and dyspnea (SAD triad). Other symptoms and signs may include those of HF and arrhythmias, including ventricular fibrillation leading to sudden death.

Exertional syncope occurs because cardiac output cannot increase enough to meet demands of physical activity. Nonexertional syncope may result from altered baroreceptor responses or ventricular fibrillation. Exertional angina pectoris affects about ⅔ of patients; about ½ have significant coronary artery atherosclerosis, and ½ have normal coronary arteries but have ischemia induced by LV hypertrophy.

There are no visible signs of AS. Palpable signs include carotid and peripheral pulses that are reduced in amplitude and delayed compared with LV contraction (pulsus parvus et tardus) and an LV impulse that is sustained (thrusts with the 1st heart sound [S_1] and relaxes with the 2nd heart sound [S_2]) because of LV hypertrophy. The LV impulse does not become displaced unless systolic dysfunction HF develops. A palpable 4th heart sound (S_4), felt best at the apex, and a systolic thrill, corresponding with the murmur of AS and felt best at the left upper sternal border, are occasionally present in severe cases. Systolic BP may be high with mild or moderate AS and fall as AS becomes more severe.

On auscultation, S_1 is normal and S_2 is single because aortic valve closing is delayed with merger of the aortic (A_2) and pulmonic (P_2) components of S_2 or, in severe cases, because A_2 is absent. As the severity increases, S_1 and S_2 diminish and may ultimately disappear. An S_4 may be audible. An ejection click may be audible early after S_1 in patients with congenital bicuspid AS when valve leaflets are stiff but not completely immobile. The click does not change with dynamic maneuvers.

The hallmark finding is a crescendo-decrescendo ejection murmur, heard best with the diaphragm of the stethoscope at the left upper sternal border when a patient who is sitting upright leans forward. The murmur typically radiates to the right clavicle and both carotid arteries (left often louder than right) and has a harsh or grating quality. But in elderly patients, vibration of the unfused cusps of calcified aortic valve leaflets may transmit a louder, more high-pitched, "cooing" or musical sound to the cardiac apex, with softening or absence of the murmur parasternally (Gallavardin's phenomenon), thereby mimicking mitral regurgitation. The murmur is soft when stenosis is less severe, grows louder as stenosis progresses, and becomes longer and peaks in volume later in systole (ie, crescendo phase becomes longer and decrescendo phase becomes shorter) as stenosis becomes more severe. As LV contractility decreases in critical AS, the murmur diminishes and may disappear before death.

The murmur of AS typically increases with maneuvers that increase LV volume (eg, leg-raising, squatting, Valsalva release, after a ventricular premature beat) and decreases with maneuvers that decrease LV volume (Valsalva maneuver) or increase afterload (isometric handgrip). These dynamic maneuvers have the opposite effect on a hypertrophic cardiomyopathy murmur, which can otherwise resemble that of AS.

Diagnosis

Diagnosis is suspected clinically and confirmed by echocardiography. Two-dimensional transthoracic echocardiography is used to identify a stenotic aortic valve and possible causes, to quantify LV hypertrophy and degree of diastolic or systolic dysfunction, and to detect coexisting valvular heart disorders (aortic regurgitation, mitral valve disorders) and complications (eg, endocarditis). Doppler echocardiography is used to quantify degree of stenosis by measuring aortic valve area, jet velocity, and transvalvular systolic pressure gradient.

A valve area of 0.5 to 1.0 cm^2 or a gradient > 45 to 50 mm Hg represents severe stenosis; an area < 0.5 cm^2 and a gradient > 50 mm Hg represent critical stenosis. The gradient may be overestimated in aortic regurgitation and underestimated in LV systolic dysfunction. Aortic valve outflow velocity < 2 to 2.5 m/sec with valvular calcifications may indicate aortic sclerosis rather than mild AS. Aortic valve sclerosis often progresses to AS and should be monitored closely.

Cardiac catheterization is necessary to determine whether coronary artery disease (CAD) is the cause of angina or to resolve differences between clinical and echocardiographic findings.

An ECG and chest x-ray are obtained. ECG typically shows changes of LV hypertrophy with or without an ischemic ST- and T-wave pattern. Chest x-ray findings may include calcification of the aortic cusps and evidence of HF. LV size is usually normal unless terminal systolic dysfunction has occurred.

Prognosis

AS may progress slowly or quickly and thus requires regular follow-up to detect progression, particularly in sedentary elderly patients. In such patients, flow may become significantly compromised without triggering symptoms.

Overall, about 3 to 6% of asymptomatic patients with normal systolic function develop symptoms or LVEF depression within a year. Predictors of adverse outcome (death or symptoms requiring surgery) include valve area < 0.5 cm^2, peak aortic velocity > 4 m/sec, rapid rate of increase in peak aortic velocity (> 0.3 m/sec/yr), and moderate to severe valvular calcification. Mean survival in untreated patients is about 5 yr after angina develops, 4 yr after syncope develops, and 3 yr after HF develops. Aortic valve replacement relieves symptoms and improves survival. Risk with surgery increases for patients who require simultaneous coronary artery bypass graft (CABG) and for those with depressed systolic LV function.

About 50% of deaths occur suddenly. Therefore, while awaiting surgery, patients with a critical gradient across the aortic valve should restrict activity to avoid sudden death.

Aortic sclerosis appears to increase risk of MI by 40% and may increase risk of angina, HF, and stroke, The reason may be progression to AS or coexistence of dyslipidemia, endothelial dysfunction, or underlying systemic or local inflammation that causes valvular sclerosis and CAD.

Treatment

Asymptomatic patients with a peak systolic gradient ≤ 25 mm Hg and a valve area > 1.0 cm^2 have a low mortality and low overall risk of requiring surgery in the next 2 yr; annual evaluation for symptom progression by echocardiography to determine gradient and valve area is appropriate.

Asymptomatic patients with gradients of 25 to 50 mm Hg or valve area < 1.0 cm^2 are at higher risk of developing symptoms in the next 2 yr; management is controversial, but most patients should have elective valve replacement. Valve replacement is indicated for patients who have severe asymptomatic AS and primarily require CABG. Surgery may be indicated for patients who become hypotensive during exercise treadmill testing; those with LV ejection fraction < 50%; and those with moderate to severe valvular calcification, peak aortic velocity > 4 m/sec, and a rapid progression rate for peak aortic velocity (> 0.3 m/sec/yr). Patients with ventricular arrhythmias and severe LV hypertrophy are also often referred for surgery, but benefits are less clear. Recommendations for patients without any of these qualifying conditions include more frequent monitoring for progression of symptoms, LV hypertrophy, gradients, and valve area with medical management as needed. Medical management is largely limited to β-blockers, which slow heart rate and thereby improve coronary artery blood flow and diastolic filling in patients with angina or diastolic dysfunction, and, for older patients, statins, which halt progression of AS due to aortic sclerosis. Other drugs may be detrimental. Use of preload reducers (eg, diuretics) can reduce LV filling and cardiac output; afterload reducers (eg, ACE inhibitors) can cause hypotension and decrease coronary artery perfusion. Nitrates are an option for angina, but rapid-acting nitrates can precipitate orthostatic hypotension and, rarely, syncope because the greatly obstructed ventricle cannot compensate for a sudden fall in BP. Nitroprusside has been used as a temporizing measure to reduce afterload in patients with decompensated HF in the hours before valve replacement, but because this drug can have the same effect as rapid-acting nitrates, it must be used cautiously and monitoring is required.

Symptomatic patients should undergo valve replacement or balloon valvotomy. Valve replacement is indicated for virtually all who can tolerate surgery. Sometimes the patient's own pulmonic valve can be used, providing optimal function and durability; the pulmonic valve is then replaced with a bioprosthesis (called the Ross procedure). The aortic valve can sometimes be repaired, rather than replaced, in patients with coexisting prominent aortic regurgitation in a bicuspid valve. Preoperative evaluation for CAD is indicated so that CABG and valve replacement, if indicated, can be performed during the same procedure.

Balloon valvotomy is used primarily in children and very young adults with congenital AS. In older patients, balloon valvuloplasty results in high rates of restenosis, aortic regurgitation, stroke, and death but may be indicated as a transitional intervention in hemodynamically unstable patients awaiting surgery and in patients who cannot tolerate surgery.

MITRAL VALVE PROLAPSE

Mitral valve prolapse (MVP) is a billowing of mitral valve leaflets into the left atrium during systole. The most common cause is idiopathic myxomatous degeneration. MVP is usually benign, but complications include mitral regurgitation, endocarditis, valve rupture, and possibly thromboembolism. MVP is usually asymptomatic, although some patients experience chest pain, dyspnea, and symptoms of sympathetic excess (eg, palpitations, dizziness, near syncope, migraines, anxiety). Signs include a crisp mid-systolic click, followed by a late systolic murmur if regurgitation is present. Diagnosis is by physical examination and echocardiography. Prognosis is excellent. No specific treatment is necessary unless mitral regurgitation is present, although patients with sympathetic symptoms may benefit from β-blockers.

MVP is common; prevalence is 1 to 5% in otherwise normal populations. Women and men are affected equally; onset usually follows the adolescent growth spurt.

Etiology

MVP is most often caused by myxomatous degeneration of the mitral valve and chordae tendineae. Degeneration is usually idiopathic, although it may be inherited in an autosomal dominant or, rarely, in an X-linked recessive fashion. Myxomatous degeneration may also be caused by connective tissue disorders (eg, Marfan syndrome, Ehlers-Danlos syndrome, adult polycystic kidney disease, osteogenesis imperfecta, pseudoxanthoma elasticum, SLE, polyarteritis nodosa), and muscular dystrophies. MVP is more common among patients with Graves' disease, hypomastia, von Willebrand's syndrome, sickle cell disease, and rheumatic heart disease. Myxomatous degeneration may also affect the aortic or tricuspid valve, resulting in aortic or tricuspid prolapse; tricuspid regurgitation is uncommon.

Normal (ie, nonmyxomatous) mitral valve leaflets may prolapse if papillary muscle dysfunction is present or the mitral annulus is dilated (eg, in dilated cardiomyopathy) or narrowed (eg, in hypertrophic cardiomyopathy or by atrial septal [secundum] defects). Transient MVP may occur when intravascular volume decreases significantly, as in severe dehydration or sometimes during pregnancy (when the woman is recumbent and the gravid uterus compresses the inferior vena cava, reducing venous return).

Mitral regurgitation (MR) is the most common complication of MVP. MR may be acute (due to ruptured chordae tendineae or flail mitral valve leaflets) or chronic; sequelae of chronic MR include heart failure and atrial fibrillation (AF) with thromboembolism. Whether MVP causes stroke independent of MR and AF is unclear. In addition, MR increases relative risk of infective endocarditis, as do thickened, redundant mitral valve leaflets.

Symptoms and Signs

Most are asymptomatic. Some experience nonspecific symptoms (eg, chest pain, dyspnea, palpitations, dizziness, near syncope, migraines, anxiety), thought to be associated with poorly defined abnormalities in adrenergic signaling and sensitivity rather than with mitral valve pathology. In about ⅓ of patients, emotional stress precipitates palpitations, which may be a symptom of benign arrhythmias (atrial premature beats, paroxysmal atrial tachycardia, ventricular premature beats, complex ventricular ectopy).

Occasionally, patients present with MR. Rarely, patients present with endocarditis (eg, fever, weight loss, thromboembolic phenomena) or stroke. Sudden death occurs in < 1%, most often resulting from ruptured chordae tendineae and flail mitral valve leaflets. Death due to a fatal arrhythmia is rare.

Typically, MVP causes no visible or palpable cardiac signs. MVP alone causes a crisp mid-systolic click heard best with the diaphragm of the stethoscope over the left apex when the patient is in the left lateral decubitus position. MVP with MR causes a click with a late-systolic MR murmur. The click becomes audible or moves closer to the 1st heart sound (S_1) and becomes louder with maneuvers that decrease left ventricle (LV) size (eg, sitting, standing, Valsalva maneuver); the same maneuvers cause an MR murmur to appear or become louder and last longer. These effects occur because decreasing LV size causes papillary muscles and chordae tendineae to pull together more centrally beneath the valve, resulting in quicker, more forceful prolapse with earlier, more severe regurgitation. Conversely, squatting or isometric handgrip delays the S_1 click and shortens the MR murmur. The systolic click may be confused with the click of congenital aortic stenosis, which can be distinguished because it occurs very early in systole and does not move with postural or LV volume changes. Other findings include a systolic honk or whoop, thought to be caused by valvular leaflet vibration; these findings are usually transient and may vary with respiratory phase. An early diastolic opening snap caused by return of the prolapsed valve to its normal position is rarely heard.

Other physical findings associated with but not diagnostic of MVP include hypomastia, pectus excavatum, straight back syndrome, and a narrow anteroposterior chest diameter.

Diagnosis

Diagnosis is suggested clinically and confirmed by 2-dimensional echocardiography. Holosystolic displacement of ≥ 3 mm or late systolic displacement of ≥ 2 mm identifies 95% of patients with MVP; the percentage is slightly higher if echocardiography is done while the patient is standing. Thickened, redundant mitral valve leaflets and displacement of ≥ 5 mm are thought to indicate more extensive myxomatous degeneration and greater risk of endocarditis and mitral regurgitation.

Holter monitoring and 12-lead ECG may be useful for documenting arrhythmias in patients with palpitations.

Prognosis and Treatment

MVP is usually benign, but severe myxomatous degeneration of the valve can lead to MR. In patients with severe MR, incidence of LV or left atrium enlargement, arrhythmias (eg, AF), infective endocarditis, stroke, need for valve replacement, and death is about 2 to 4%/yr.

MVP does not usually require treatment. β-blockers may be used to relieve symptoms of excess sympathetic tone (eg, palpitations, migraines, dizziness) and to reduce risk of dangerous tachycardias, although no data support this practice. A typical regimen is atenolol 25 to 50 mg po once/day or propranolol 20 to 40 mg po bid. AF may require additional treatment (see p. 698).

Treatment of MR depends on severity and associated left atrial and LV changes.

Antibiotic prophylaxis against endocarditis is recommended before high-risk procedures (see TABLE 77–3 on p. 730) only when MR or thickened, redundant valves are present. Anticoagulants to prevent thromboembolism are recommended only for patients with AF or prior transient ischemic attack or stroke.

MITRAL REGURGITATION

Mitral regurgitation (MR) is incompetency of the mitral valve causing flow from the left ventricle (LV) into the left atrium during systole. Common causes include mitral valve prolapse, ischemic papillary muscle dysfunction, rheumatic fever, and annular dilation secondary to LV systolic dysfunction and dilation. Complications include progressive heart failure, arrhythmias, and endocarditis. Symptoms and signs include palpitations, dyspnea, and a holosystolic apical murmur. Diagnosis is by physical examination and echocardiography. Prognosis depends on LV function and severity and duration of MR. Patients with mild, asymptomatic MR may be monitored, but progressive or symptomatic MR requires mitral valve repair or replacement.

Etiology and Pathophysiology

MR may be acute or chronic. Causes of acute MR include ischemic papillary muscle dysfunction or rupture; infective endocarditis; acute rheumatic fever; spontaneous, traumatic, or ischemic tears or rupture of the mitral valve leaflets or subvalvular apparatus; acute dilation of the LV due to myocarditis or ischemia; and mechanical failure of a prosthetic mitral valve.

Common causes of chronic MR include those of acute MR plus mitral valve prolapse (MVP), mitral annular enlargement, and nonischemic papillary muscle dysfunction (eg, due to LV enlargement). Uncommon causes of chronic MR include atrial myxoma, a congenital endocardial cushion defect with a cleft anterior leaflet, SLE, acromegaly, and calcification of the mitral annulus (mainly in elderly women).

In infants, the most likely causes of MR are papillary muscle dysfunction, endocardial fibroelastosis, acute myocarditis, cleft mitral valve with or without an endocardial cushion defect, and myxomatous degeneration of the mitral valve. MR may coexist with mitral stenosis when thickened valvular leaflets do not close.

Acute MR may cause acute pulmonary edema and biventricular failure with cardiogenic shock, respiratory arrest, or sudden cardiac death. Complications of chronic MR include gradual enlargement of the left atrium (LA); LV enlargement and hypertrophy, which initially compensates for regurgitant flow (preserving forward stroke volume) but eventually decompensates (reducing forward stroke volume); atrial fibrillation (AF) with thromboembolism; and infective endocarditis.

Symptoms and Signs

Acute MR causes the same symptoms and signs as acute heart failure and cardiogenic shock (see p. 650). Most patients with chronic MR are initially asymptomatic and develop symptoms insidiously as the LA enlarges, pulmonary BP increases, and LV remodeling occurs. Symptoms include dyspnea, fatigue (due to heart failure), and palpitations (often due to AF); rarely, patients present with endocarditis (eg, fever, weight loss, embolic phenomena).

Signs develop only when MR becomes moderate to severe. Inspection and palpation may detect a brisk apical impulse and sustained left parasternal movement due to expansion of an enlarged LA. An LV impulse that is sustained, enlarged, and displaced downward and to the left suggests LV hypertrophy and dilation. A diffuse precordial lift occurs with severe MR because the LA enlarges, causing anterior cardiac displacement. A regurgitant murmur (or thrill) may also be palpable in severe cases.

On auscultation, the 1st heart sound (S_1) may be soft or absent if valve leaflets are rigid (eg, in combined mitral stenosis and MR due to rheumatic fever) but is usually present if the leaflets are not rigid. The 2nd heart sound (S_2) may be widely split unless severe pulmonary hypertension has developed. A 3rd heart sound (S_3), loud at the apex in proportion to the degree of MR, reflects a greatly dilated LV. A 4th heart sound (S_4) is characteristic of recent ruptured chordae, when the LV has not had enough time to dilate.

The cardinal sign of MR is a holosystolic (pansystolic) murmur, heard best at the apex with the diaphragm of the stethoscope when the patient is in the left lateral decubitus position. In mild MR, the systolic murmur is high-pitched or blowing, but as flow increases, it becomes low- or medium-pitched. The murmur begins with S_1 in conditions causing leaflet incompetency throughout systole (eg, destruction), but it often begins after S_1 (eg, when chamber dilation during systole distorts the valve apparatus or when myocardial ischemia or fibrosis alters dynamics). When the murmur begins after S_1, it always continues to S_2. The murmur radiates toward the left axilla; intensity may remain the same or vary. If intensity varies, the murmur tends to crescendo in volume up to S_2. MR murmurs increase in intensity with handgrip or squatting because peripheral vascular resistance to ventricular ejection increases, augmenting regurgitation into the LA; murmurs decrease in intensity with standing or the Valsalva maneuver. A short rumbling mid-diastolic inflow murmur due to torrential mitral diastolic flow may follow or seem to prolong S_3.

MR murmurs may be confused with tricuspid regurgitation, which can be distinguished because its murmur is augmented during inspiration.

Diagnosis

Diagnosis is suspected clinically and confirmed by echocardiography. Doppler echocardiography is used to detect regurgitant flow and help quantify its severity; 2-dimensional echocardiography is used to determine the cause of MR and to detect pulmonary hypertension.

If endocarditis or valvular thrombi are suspected, transesophageal echocardiography (TEE) can provide a more detailed view of the mitral valve and LA. TEE is also indicated when mitral valve repair instead of replacement is being considered to confirm the absence of severe fibrosis and calcification.

An ECG and chest x-ray are usually obtained initially. ECG may show LA enlargement and LV hypertrophy with or without ischemia. Sinus rhythm is usually present when MR is acute because the atria have not had time to stretch and remodel.

Chest x-ray in acute MR may show pulmonary edema; abnormalities in cardiac silhouette are not evident unless an underlying chronic disorder is also present. Chest x-ray in chronic MR may show LA and LV enlargement. It may also show pulmonary vascular congestion and pulmonary edema with heart failure. Pulmonary vascular congestion is confined to the right upper lobe in about 10% of patients; such congestion is probably caused by dilation of the right superior and central pulmonary veins secondary to selective regurgitation into these veins.

Cardiac catheterization is done before surgery, mainly to determine whether coronary artery disease (CAD) is present. A prominent atrial systolic *v* wave is seen on pulmonary artery occlusion pressure (pulmonary capillary wedge pressure) tracings during ventricular systole. Ventriculography can be used to quantify MR.

Prognosis and Treatment

Prognosis varies by acuity and cause of MR. Once MR becomes severe, about 10% of asymptomatic patients become symptomatic per year thereafter. About 10% of patients with chronic MR caused by MVP require surgical intervention.

Acute MR requires emergency mitral valve repair or replacement; patients with ischemic papillary muscle rupture may also require coronary revascularization. Pending surgery, nitroprusside or nitroglycerin infusion may be used to reduce afterload, thus improving forward stroke volume and reducing ventricular and regurgitant volume.

Definitive treatment of chronic MR is also mitral valve repair or replacement, but patients with asymptomatic or mild chronic MR and no pulmonary hypertension or AF may do well with periodic monitoring. The ideal timing for surgery is uncertain, but intervention before ventricular decompensation (defined as echocardiographic end-diastolic dimension > 7 cm, end-systolic dimension > 4.5 cm, and ejection fraction < 60%) improves outcomes and decreases the chance of worsening LV function. After decompensation, ventricular function becomes dependent on the afterload reduction of MR, and in about 50% of decompensated patients, valve replacement causes a markedly depressed ejection fraction. For patients with moderate MR and significant CAD, perioperative mortality rate is 1.5% with bypass surgery alone and 25% with concomitant valve replacement. If technically feasible, valve repair instead of replacement is preferred; perioperative mortality rate is 2 to 4% (compared with 5 to 10% for replacement), and long-term prognosis is good (80 to 94% survival rate at 5 to 10 yr, compared with 40 to 60% for replacement).

Antibiotic prophylaxis is indicated before procedures that can cause bacteremia (see TABLE 77–3 on p. 730). For rheumatic MR that is at least moderately severe, daily penicillin until about age 30 is recommended to prevent recurrent acute rheumatic fever. In most Western countries, rheumatic fever is too rare after age 30 to require prophylaxis. Because long-term antibiotic treatment may induce resistance in microorganisms that can cause endocarditis, patients taking daily penicillin may require addition of other antibiotics for endocarditis prophylaxis.

Anticoagulants are used to prevent thromboemboli (see p. 420) in patients with heart failure or AF. Although severe MR tends to flush out atrial thrombi and is thus somewhat protective against thrombosis, most cardiologists still recommend anticoagulants.

MITRAL STENOSIS

Mitral stenosis (MS) is narrowing of the mitral orifice impeding blood flow from the left atrium to the left ventricle. The most common cause is rheumatic fever. Common complications are pulmonary hypertension, atrial fibrillation, and thromboembolism. Symptoms are those of heart failure; signs include an opening snap and a diastolic murmur. Diagnosis is by physical examination and echocardiography. Prognosis is good. Medical treatment includes diuretics, β-blockers or rate-limiting Ca channel blockers, and anticoagulants; surgical treatment for more severe disease consists of balloon valvotomy, commissurotomy, or valve replacement.

In MS, mitral valve leaflets become thickened and immobile and the mitral orifice becomes narrowed due to fusion of the commissures. The most common cause is rheumatic fever (see p. 2358), even though most patients do not recall the disorder. Less common causes include congenital MS, bacterial endocarditis, SLE, atrial myxoma, RA, malignant carcinoid syndrome with an atrial right-to-left shunt, and methysergide. If the valve cannot close completely, mitral regurgitation (MR) may coexist with MS. Many patients with MS due to rheumatic fever also have aortic regurgitation.

The normal area of the mitral valve orifice is 4 to 6 cm^2. An area of 1 to 2 cm^2 reflects moderate to severe MS and often causes exertional symptoms. An area < 1 cm^2 represents critical stenosis and may cause symptoms during rest. Left atrial (LA) size and pressure increase progressively to compensate for MS; pulmonary venous and capillary pressures also increase and may cause secondary pulmonary hypertension, leading to right ventricular (RV) heart failure and tricuspid and pulmonic regurgitation. Rate of progression varies.

Valvular change with LA enlargement predisposes to atrial fibrillation (AF), a risk factor for thromboembolism.

Symptoms and Signs

Symptoms correlate poorly with disease severity because the disease often progresses insidiously and patients reduce their activity without being aware of it; many patients are asymptomatic until they become pregnant or AF develops. Initial symptoms are usually those of heart failure (eg, exertional dyspnea, orthopnea, paroxysmal nocturnal dyspnea, fatigue). They typically do not appear until 15 to 40 yr after an episode of rheumatic fever, but in developing countries, much younger children may become symptomatic. Paroxysmal or chronic AF exacerbates existing diastolic dysfunction, precipitating pulmonary edema and acute dyspnea when ventricular rate is poorly controlled. AF may also cause palpitations; in up to 15% of un-anticoagulated patients, it causes systemic embolism with symptoms of stroke or leg ischemia.

Less common symptoms include hemoptysis due to rupture of small pulmonary vessels and pulmonary edema, particularly during pregnancy when blood volume increases; hoarseness due to compression of the left recurrent laryngeal nerve by a dilated LA or pulmonary artery (Ortner's syndrome); and symptoms of pulmonary hypertension (see p. 481) and RV failure (see p. 654).

Inspection and palpation may detect a palpable 1st (S_1) and 2nd heart sound (S_2). S_1 is best palpated at the apex, and S_2 at the upper left sternal border. The pulmonic component of S_2(P_2) is responsible for the impulse and results from pulmonary hypertension. An RV impulse (heave) palpable at the left sternal border may accompany jugular venous distention when pulmonary hypertension is present and RV diastolic dysfunction develops.

Auscultatory findings include a loud S_1 caused by the leaflets of a stenotic mitral valve closing abruptly (M_1), like a sail on "coming about"; it is heard best at the apex. A normally split S_2 with an exaggerated P_2 due to pulmonary hypertension is also heard. Most prominent is an early diastolic opening snap as the leaflets billow into the left ventricle (LV), which is loudest close to left lower sternal border; it is followed by a low-pitched decrescendo-crescendo rumbling diastolic murmur, heard best with the bell of the stethoscope at the apex (or over the palpable apex beat) at end-expiration when the patient is in the left lateral decubitus position. The opening snap may be soft or absent if the mitral valve is sclerosed, fibrosed, or calcified; the snap moves closer to P_2 (increasing duration of the murmur) as MS becomes more severe and LA pressure increases. The diastolic murmur increases after a Valsalva maneuver (when blood pours into the LA), after exercise, and in response to squatting and handgrip; it may be softer or absent when an enlarged RV displaces the LV posteriorly and when other disorders (pulmonary hypertension, right-sided valve abnormalities, AF with fast ventricular rate) decrease blood flow across the mitral valve. The presystolic crescendo is caused by narrowing of the mitral valve orifice during LV contraction and so remains in AF, but only at the end of short diastoles when LA pressure is still high.

Diastolic murmurs that may coexist with the MS murmur are Graham Steell's murmur (a soft decrescendo diastolic murmur heard best along the left sternal border and caused by pulmonic regurgitation secondary to severe pulmonary hypertension) and, when rheumatic carditis has affected both the mitral and aortic valves, the Austin Flint murmur (a mid-to-late diastolic rumble heard at the apex and caused by the effects of aortic valvular regurgitant flow on the mitral leaflets). Disorders that cause diastolic murmurs mimicking the murmur of MS include MR (because of large volume flow across the mitral orifice), aortic regurgitation (which causes an Austin Flint murmur), and atrial myxoma (which causes a murmur typically varying in loudness and position from beat to beat).

MS may cause signs of cor pulmonale (see p. 664). The classic mitral facies, a plum-colored malar flush, occurs only when cardiac output is low and pulmonary hypertension is severe; cause is cutaneous vasodilation and chronic hypoxemia.

Occasionally, the first symptoms and signs of MS are those of an embolic stroke or of endocarditis; endocarditis is rare in MS unless MR is also present.

Diagnosis

Diagnosis is suspected clinically and confirmed by echocardiography. Two-dimensional echocardiography provides information about the degree of valvular calcification and stenosis and LA size; Doppler echocardiography provides information about the transvalvular gradient and pulmonary artery pressure. Transesophageal echocardiography can be used to detect or exclude small LA thrombi, especially those in the LA appendage, which often cannot be seen transthoracically.

An ECG and chest x-ray are usually obtained. The ECG may show LA enlargement, manifest as a P wave lasting > 0.12 msec with prominent negative deflection of its terminal component (duration: > 0.04 msec; amplitude: > 0.10 mV) in V_1; broad, notched P waves in lead II; or both. Low voltage in V_1, right axis QRS deviation, and tall R waves in V_1 suggest RV hypertrophy.

Chest x-ray usually shows straightening of the left cardiac border due to a dilated LA appendage. The main pulmonary artery (trunk) may be prominent; the descending right pulmonary artery diameter is ≥ 16 mm if pulmonary hypertension is significant. The upper lobe pulmonary veins may be dilated because the lower lobe veins are compressed, forcing more blood into upper lobes. A double shadow of an enlarged LA may be seen along the right cardiac border. Horizontal lines in the lower posterior lung fields (Kerley's B lines) indicate interstitial edema associated with high LA pressure.

Cardiac catheterization, indicated only for perioperative assessment of coronary artery disease (CAD) before surgical repair, can confirm elevated LA and pulmonary artery pressures and size of valve area.

Prognosis and Treatment

The natural history of MS varies, but the interval between onset of symptoms and severe disability is about 7 to 9 yr. Outcome is affected by the patient's preprocedural age and functional status, pulmonary hypertension, and degree of MR. Results of valvotomy and commissurotomy are equivalent; both restore valvular function in 95% of patients. However, function deteriorates in most patients, and many require repeat procedures. Risk factors for death are AF and pulmonary hypertension; cause of death is most commonly heart failure or pulmonary or cerebrovascular embolism.

Asymptomatic patients require only prophylaxis against recurrent rheumatic fever (eg, with IM injections of benzathine penicillin G 1.2 million units q 3 or 4 wk) until age 25 to 30 and prophylaxis against endocarditis before high-risk procedures (see TABLE 77–3).

Mildly symptomatic patients usually respond to diuretics and, if sinus tachycardia or AF is present, to β-blockers or Ca channel blockers, which can control ventricular rate. Anticoagulants are indicated to prevent thromboembolism in AF. All patients should be encouraged to continue at least low levels of physical exercise despite exertional dyspnea.

More severely symptomatic patients and patients with evidence of pulmonary hypertension require valvotomy, commissurotomy, or valve replacement.

Percutaneous balloon valvotomy is the procedure of choice for younger patients; older patients who cannot tolerate more invasive procedures; and patients without heavily calcified valves, subvalvular distortion, LA thrombi, or significant MR. In this echocardiographic-guided procedure, a balloon is passed transseptally from the right atrium to the LA and inflated to separate fused mitral valve leaflets. Outcomes are equivalent to those of more invasive procedures. Complications are uncommon and include MR, embolism, LV perforation, and atrial septal defect, which is likely to persist only if the pressure difference between the 2 atria is high.

Patients with severe subvalvular disease, valvular calcification, or LA thrombi may be candidates for commissurotomy, in which fused mitral valve leaflets are separated using a dilator passed through the LA or LV (closed commissurotomy) or manually (open commissurotomy); both procedures require a thoracotomy. Choice of procedure is based on surgeon's experience and on severity of fibrosis and calcification.

Valve replacement is a last resort but is indicated for patients with a mitral valve area ≤ 1.5 cm^2, moderate to severe symptoms, and valvular pathology (eg, fibrotic cusps) that precludes use of other procedures.

PULMONIC REGURGITATION

Pulmonic (pulmonary) regurgitation (PR) is incompetency of the pulmonic valve causing blood flow from the pulmonary artery into the right ventricle during diastole. The most common cause is pulmonary hypertension. PR is usually asymptomatic. Signs include a decrescendo diastolic murmur.

Diagnosis is by echocardiography. Usually, no specific treatment is necessary except for management of conditions causing pulmonary hypertension.

Secondary pulmonary hypertension (see TABLE 58–1 on p. 482) is by far the most common cause of PR. Less common causes are infective endocarditis, surgical repair of tetralogy of Fallot, idiopathic pulmonary artery dilation, and congenital valvular heart disease. Carcinoid syndrome, rheumatic fever, syphilis, and catheter-induced trauma are rare causes. Severe PR is rare and most often results from an isolated congenital defect involving dilation of the pulmonary artery and pulmonary valve annulus.

PR may contribute to development of right ventricular (RV) hypertrophy and eventually RV dysfunction–induced heart failure (HF), but in most cases, pulmonary hypertension contributes to this complication much more significantly. Rarely, acute RV dysfunction–induced HF develops when endocarditis causes acute PR.

Symptoms and Signs

PR is usually asymptomatic. A few patients develop symptoms and signs of RV dysfunction–induced HF (see p. 656).

Palpable signs are attributable to pulmonary hypertension and RV hypertrophy. They include a palpable pulmonic component (P_2) of the 2nd heart sound (S_2) at the left upper sternal border and a sustained RV impulse that is increased in amplitude at the left middle and lower sternal border.

On auscultation, the 1st heart sound (S_1) is normal. The S_2 may be split or single. When split, P_2 may be loud and audible shortly after the aortic component of S_2 (A_2) because of pulmonary hypertension, or P_2 may be delayed because of increased RV stroke volume. S_2 may be single because of prompt pulmonic valve closing with a merged A_2-P_2 or, rarely, because of congenital absence of the pulmonic valve. An RV 3rd heart sound (S_3), 4th heart sound (S_4), or both may be audible with RV dysfunction–induced HF or RV hypertrophy; these sounds can be distinguished from left ventricular heart sounds because they are located at the left parasternal 4th intercostal space and because they grow louder with inspiration.

The murmur of PR due to pulmonary hypertension is a high-pitched, early diastolic decrescendo murmur that begins with P_2 and ends before S_1 and that radiates toward the mid-right sternal edge (Graham Steell's murmur); it is heard best at left upper sternal border with the diaphragm of the stethoscope while the patient holds the breath at end-expiration and sits upright. The murmur of PR without pulmonary hypertension is shorter, lower-pitched (rougher in quality), and begins after P_2. Both murmurs may resemble the murmur of aortic regurgitation but can be distinguished by inspiration (which makes the PR murmur louder) and by Valsalva release. After Valsalva release, the PR murmur immediately becomes loud (because of immediate venous return to the right side of the heart), but the AR murmur requires 4 or 5 beats to do so. Also, a soft PR murmur may sometimes become even softer during inspiration because this murmur is usually best heard at the 2nd left intercostal space, where inspiration pushes the stethoscope away from the heart.

Diagnosis and Treatment

PR is usually incidentally detected during a physical examination or Doppler echocardiography done for other reasons. An ECG and chest x-ray are obtained. Either may show signs of RV hypertrophy; chest x-ray typically shows evidence of conditions underlying pulmonary hypertension.

Treatment is management of the condition causing PR. Pulmonary valve replacement is an option if symptoms and signs of RV dysfunction–induced HF develop, but outcomes and risks are unclear because the need for replacement is so infrequent.

PULMONIC STENOSIS

Pulmonic stenosis is narrowing of the pulmonary outflow tract causing obstruction of blood flow from the right ventricle to the pulmonary artery during systole.

Pulmonic stenosis (PS) is most often congenital and affects predominantly children; stenosis may be valvular or just below the valve in the outflow tract (infundibular). Less common causes are Noonan's syndrome (a familial syndrome similar to Turner's syndrome but with no chromosomal defect) and carcinoid syndrome in adults.

Many children remain asymptomatic for years and do not present to a physician until adulthood. When symptoms develop, they resemble those of aortic stenosis (syncope, angina, dyspnea). Visible and palpable signs reflect the effects of right ventricular (RV) hypertrophy and include a prominent jugular venous *a* wave (due to forceful atrial contraction against a hypertrophied RV), an RV precordial lift or heave, and a left parasternal systolic thrill at the 2nd intercostal space. On auscultation, the 1st heart sound (S_1) is normal and the 2nd heart sound (S_2) splitting is widened because of prolonged pulmonic ejection (pulmonic component of S_2 [P_2] is delayed). In RV failure and hypertrophy, the 3rd and 4th heart sounds (S_3 and S_4) are rarely audible at the left parasternal 4th intercostal space. A click in congenital PS is thought to result from abnormal ventricular wall tension. The click occurs early in systole (very near S_1) and is not affected by hemodynamic changes. A harsh crescendo-decrescendo ejection murmur is audible and is heard best at the left parasternal 2nd (valvular stenosis) or 4th (infundibular stenosis) intercostal space with the diaphragm of the stethoscope when the patient leans forward. Unlike the aortic stenosis murmur, a PS murmur does not radiate, and the crescendo component lengthens as stenosis progresses. The murmur grows louder immediately with Valsalva release and with inspiration; the patient may need to be standing for this effect to be heard.

Diagnosis is by Doppler echocardiography, which can characterize the stenosis as mild (≤ 40 mm Hg peak gradient), moderate (41 to 79 mm Hg), or severe (≥ 80 mm Hg). ECG is often part of the evaluation; it may be normal or show RV hypertrophy or right bundle branch block. Right heart catheterization is indicated only when 2 levels of obstruction are suspected (valvular and infundibular), when clinical and echocardiographic findings differ, or before intervention is done.

Prognosis without treatment is generally good and improves with appropriate intervention. Treatment is balloon valvuloplasty, indicated for symptomatic patients and asymptomatic patients with normal systolic function and a peak gradient > 40 to 50 mm Hg.

TRICUSPID REGURGITATION

Tricuspid regurgitation (TR) is insufficiency of the tricuspid valve causing blood flow from the right ventricle to the right atrium during systole. The most common cause is dilation of the right ventricle. Symptoms and signs are usually absent, but severe TR can cause neck pulsations, a holosystolic murmur, and right ventricular–induced heart failure or atrial fibrillation. Diagnosis is by physical examination and echocardiography. TR is usually benign and does not require treatment, but some patients require annuloplasty, valve repair or replacement, or excision.

Etiology

TR is most commonly caused by dilation of the right ventricle (RV) with malfunction of a normal valve, as occurs in pulmonary hypertension, RV dysfunction–induced heart failure (HF), and pulmonary outflow tract obstruction. TR results less commonly from infective endocarditis in IV drug abusers, carcinoid syndrome, rheumatic fever, idiopathic myxomatous degeneration, ischemic papillary muscle dysfunction, congenital defects (eg, cleft tricuspid valve, endocardial cushion defects), Ebstein's anomaly (downward displacement of a distorted tricuspid cusp into the RV), Marfan syndrome, and use of certain drugs (eg, ergotamine, fenfluramine, phentermine).

Long-standing severe TR may lead to RV dysfunction–induced HF and atrial fibrillation (AF).

Symptoms and Signs

TR usually causes no symptoms, but some patients experience neck pulsations due to elevated jugular pressures. Acute or severe TR may cause symptoms of RV dysfunction–induced HF. Patients may also develop symptoms of AF or atrial flutter.

The only visible sign of moderate to severe TR is jugular venous distention, with a prominent merged *c-v* (or *s*) wave and a steep *y* descent. In severe TR, a right jugular venous thrill may be palpable, as may systolic hepatic pulsation and an RV impulse at the left lower sternal border. On auscultation, the 1st heart sound (S_1) may be normal or barely audible if a TR murmur is present; the 2nd heart sound (S_2) may be split (with a loud pulmonic component [P_2] in pulmonary hypertension) or single because of prompt pulmonic valve closing with merger of P_2 and the aortic component (A_2). An RV 3rd heart sound (S_3), 4th heart sound (S_4), or both may be audible with RV dysfunction–induced HF or RV hypertrophy; these sounds can be distinguished from left ventricular heart sounds because they are located at the left parasternal 4th intercostal space and because they become louder with inspiration.

The murmur of TR is a holosystolic murmur heard best at the right or left middle or lower sternal border or at the epigastrium with the diaphragm of the stethoscope when the patient is sitting upright or standing. The murmur may be high-pitched if TR is trivial and due to pulmonary hypertension, or it may be medium-pitched if TR is severe and has other causes. The murmur varies with respiration, becoming louder with inspiration (Carvallo's sign) and other maneuvers that increase venous return (leg raising, hepatic pressure, after a ventricular premature beat). The murmur does not typically radiate but is sometimes audible over the liver.

Diagnosis

Mild TR is most often detected on echocardiography done for other reasons. More moderate or severe TR may be suggested by history and physical examination and confirmed by Doppler echocardiography. An ECG and chest x-ray are also often obtained. ECG is usually normal but, in advanced cases, may show tall peaked P waves caused by right atrial enlargement, a tall R or QR wave in V_1 characteristic of RV hypertrophy, or AF. Chest x-ray is usually normal but, in advanced cases with RV hypertrophy or RV dysfunction–induced HF, may show an enlarged superior vena cava, an enlarged right atrial or RV silhouette (behind the upper sternum in the lateral projection), or pleural effusion.

Cardiac catheterization is rarely indicated for evaluation of TR. When catheterization is indicated (eg, to evaluate coronary anatomy), findings include a prominent atrial systolic *v* wave during ventricular systole and normal or elevated atrial systolic pressures.

Prognosis and Treatment

Few reliable data about prognosis exist because so few patients develop severe TR in isolation.

TR is usually well tolerated and does not require treatment. Medical treatment of causes (eg, HF, endocarditis) is indicated. Surgical interventions are reserved for patients who have moderate to severe TR and a left-sided valve disorder (eg, mitral stenosis) causing pulmonary hypertension and high RV pressures and who also require mitral valve repair. For these patients, intervention can prevent death due to low cardiac output. Surgery may also be indicated for symptomatic patients with severe TR when left atrial pressure is < 60 mm Hg.

Surgical options include annuloplasty, valve repair, and valve replacement. Annuloplasty, in which the tricuspid valve annulus is sutured to a prosthetic ring or a tailored reduction in annulus circumferential size is performed, is indicated when TR is due to annular dilation. Valve repair or replacement is indicated when TR is due to primary valve abnormalities or when annuloplasty is not technically feasible. Tricuspid valve replacement is indicated when TR is due to carcinoid syndrome or Ebstein's anomaly. A porcine valve is used to reduce the risk of thromboembolism associated with the low flow and pressures of the right heart; in the right heart, unlike the left heart, porcine valves last > 10 yr.

If endocarditis has damaged the tricuspid valve and cannot be cured with antibiotics, the valve may be totally excised and not replaced until 6 to 9 m later; this procedure is well tolerated.

TRICUSPID STENOSIS

Tricuspid stenosis (TS) is narrowing of the tricuspid orifice that obstructs blood flow from the right atrium to the right ventricle. Almost all cases result from rheumatic fever. Symptoms include a fluttering discomfort in the neck, fatigue, cold skin, and right upper quadrant abdominal discomfort. Jugular pulsations are prominent, and a presystolic murmur is often heard at the left sternal edge in the 4th intercostal space and is increased during inspiration. Diagnosis is by echocardiography. TS is usually benign, requiring no specific treatment, but symptomatic patients may benefit from surgery.

TS is almost always due to rheumatic fever; tricuspid regurgitation is almost always also present, as is a mitral valve disorder (usually mitral stenosis). Rare causes of TS include SLE, carcinoid syndrome, right atrial (RA) myxoma, congenital malformations, primary or metastatic tumor, and localized constrictive pericarditis. The RA becomes hypertrophied and distended, and sequelae of right heart disease–induced heart failure develop but without RV dysfunction; the RV remains underfilled and small. Uncommonly, atrial fibrillation occurs.

Symptoms and Signs

The only symptoms of severe TS are fluttering discomfort in the neck (due to giant *a* waves in the jugular pulse), fatigue and cold skin (due to low cardiac output), and right upper quadrant abdominal discomfort (due to an enlarged liver).

The primary visible sign is a giant flickering *a* wave with gradual *y* descent in the jugular veins. With atrial fibrillation, a *v* wave becomes prominent in the jugular pulse. Jugular venous distention may occur, increasing with inspiration (Kussmaul's sign). The face may become dusky and scalp veins may dilate when the patient is recumbent (suffusion sign). Hepatic pulsation may be palpable just before systole. Peripheral edema is common.

On auscultation, TS may produce a soft opening snap. A mid-diastolic rumble is rare. TS produces a short, scratchy, crescendo-decrescendo presystolic murmur heard best with the diaphragm of the stethoscope at the left parasternal 4th or 5th interspace or at the epigastrium when the patient is sitting upright and leaning forward (moving the heart against the chest wall) or in the right lateral decubitus position (increasing flow across the valve). The murmur becomes louder and longer with maneuvers that increase venous return (exercise, inspiration, leg-raising, Mueller maneuver) and softer and shorter with maneuvers that decrease venous return (standing, Valsalva maneuver).

Findings of TS often coexist with those of mitral stenosis and are less prominent. The murmurs can be distinguished clinically (see TABLE 76–1).

TABLE 76–1. DISTINGUISHING MURMURS OF TRICUSPID AND MITRAL STENOSIS

FEATURE	TRICUSPID STENOSIS	MITRAL STENOSIS
Character	Scratchy	Rumbling, low-pitched
Duration	Short	Long
Timing	Starts in early diastole and does not increase up to S_1	Increases through diastole
Augmenting factor	Inspiration	Exercise
Site	Lower right and left parasternal borders	Cardiac apex with patient in left lateral decubitus position

S_1 = 1st heart sound.

Diagnosis

Diagnosis is suspected based on history and physical examination and confirmed by Doppler echocardiography showing a pressure gradient > 2 mm Hg across the tricuspid valve with high velocity turbulent flow and slowed atrial filling. Two-dimensional echocardiography may show RA enlargement. An ECG and chest x-ray are often obtained. ECG may show RA enlargement out of proportion to RV hypertrophy and tall, peaked P waves in inferior leads and V_1. Chest x-ray may show a dilated superior vena cava and RA enlargement, indicated by an enlarged right heart border. Liver enzymes are elevated because of passive hepatic congestion.

Cardiac catheterization (see p. 589) is rarely indicated for evaluation of TR. When catheterization is indicated (eg, to evaluate coronary anatomy), findings include elevated RA pressure with a slow fall in early diastole and a diastolic pressure gradient across the tricuspid valve.

Treatment

Evidence to guide treatment is scarce. For all symptomatic patients, treatment should include a low-salt diet, diuretics, and ACE inhibitors. Patients with transvalvular pressure gradients as low as 3 mm Hg and valve areas < 1.5 cm^2 may benefit from interventions. Options include balloon valvotomy and, for patients with a poor response who can tolerate surgery, open valve repair or replacement. Comparative outcomes are unstudied. Correction of TS without treatment of coexisting mitral stenosis can precipitate left ventricular heart failure.

77 ENDOCARDITIS

Endocarditis usually refers to infection of the endocardium (ie, infective endocarditis). The term can also include noninfective endocarditis, in which sterile platelet and fibrin thrombi form on cardiac valves and adjacent endocardium. Noninfective endocarditis sometimes leads to infective endocarditis. Both can result in embolization and impaired cardiac function.

INFECTIVE ENDOCARDITIS

Infective endocarditis is infection of the endocardium, usually with bacteria (commonly, streptococci and staphylococci) or fungi. It produces fever, heart murmurs, petechiae, anemia, embolic phenomena, and endocardial vegetations. Vegetations may result in valvular incompetence or obstruction, myocardial abscess, or mycotic aneurysm. Diagnosis requires demonstration of microorganisms in blood and usually echocardiography. Treatment consists of prolonged antimicrobial treatment and sometimes surgery.

Endocarditis can occur at any age. Men are affected about twice as often. IV drug abusers and immunocompromised patients are at highest risk.

Pathophysiology and Etiology

The normal heart is relatively resistant to infection. Bacteria and fungi do not easily adhere to the endocardial surface, and constant blood flow helps prevent them from settling on endocardial structures. Thus, 2 factors are generally required for endocarditis: a predisposing abnormality of the endocardium and microorganisms in the bloodstream (bacteremia). Rarely, massive bacteremia or particularly virulent microorganisms cause endocarditis on normal valves.

Endocardial factors: Endocarditis usually involves the heart valves. Major predisposing factors are congenital heart defects, rheumatic valvular disease, bicuspid or calcific aortic valves, mitral valve prolapse, and hypertrophic cardiomyopathy. Prosthetic valves are a particular risk. Occasionally, mural thrombi, ventricular-septal defects, and patent ductus arteriosus sites become infected. The actual nidus for infection is usually a sterile fibrin-platelet vegetation formed when damaged endothelial cells release tissue factor.

Infective endocarditis occurs most often on the left side (eg, mitral or aortic valve). About 10 to 20% of cases are right-sided (tricuspid or pulmonic valve). IV drug abusers have a much higher incidence of right-sided endocarditis (about 30 to 70%).

Microorganisms: Microorganisms that infect the endocardium may originate from distant infected sites (eg, cutaneous abscess, UTI) or have obvious portals of entry such as a central venous catheter or a drug injection site. Almost any implanted foreign material (eg, ventricular or peritoneal shunt, prosthetic device) is at risk of bacterial colonization, thus becoming a source of bacteremia and hence endocarditis. Endocarditis also may result from asymptomatic bacteremia, such as typically occurs during invasive dental, medical, or surgical procedures. Even toothbrushing and chewing can cause bacteremia (usually due to viridans streptococci) in patients with gingivitis.

Causative microorganisms vary by site of infection, source of bacteremia, and host risk factors (eg, IV drug abuse), but overall, streptococci and *Staphylococcus aureus* cause 80 to 90% cases. Enterococci, gram-negative bacilli, HACEK organisms (see p. 1463 and footnote in TABLE 77–2), and fungi cause most of the rest. Why streptococci and staphylococci frequently adhere to vegetations and why gram-negative aerobic bacilli seldom adhere are unclear. However, the ability of *S. aureus* to adhere to fibronectin may play a role, as may dextran production by viridans streptococci.

After colonizing vegetations, microorganisms are covered by a layer of fibrin and platelets, which prevents access by neutrophils, Ig, and complement and thus blocks host defenses.

Consequences: Endocarditis has local and systemic consequences.

Local consequences include formation of myocardial abscesses with tissue destruction and sometimes conduction system abnormalities (usually with low septal abscesses). Severe valvular regurgitation may develop suddenly, causing heart failure and death (usually due to mitral or aortic valve lesions).

Aortitis may result from contiguous spread of infection. Prosthetic valve infections are particularly likely to involve valve ring abscesses, obstructing vegetations, myocardial abscesses, and mycotic aneurysms manifested by valve obstruction, dehiscence, and conduction disturbances.

Systemic consequences are primarily due to embolization of infected material from the heart valve and, primarily in chronic infection, immune-mediated phenomena. Right-sided lesions typically produce septic pulmonary emboli, which may result in pulmonary infarction, pneumonia, or empyema. Left-sided lesions may embolize to any organ, particularly the kidneys, spleen, and CNS. Mycotic aneurysms can form in any major artery. Cutaneous and retinal emboli are common. Diffuse glomerulonephritis may result from immune complex deposition.

Classification

Infective endocarditis may have an indolent, subacute course or a more acute, fulminant course with greater potential for rapid decompensation.

Subacute bacterial endocarditis (SBE), although aggressive, usually develops insidiously and progresses slowly (ie, over weeks to months). Often, no source of infection or portal of entry is evident. SBE is caused most commonly by streptococci (especially viridans, microaerophilic, anaerobic, and nonenterococcal group D streptococci and enterococci) and less commonly by *S. aureus, Staphylococcus epidermidis*, and fastidious *Haemophilus* sp. SBE often develops on abnormal valves after asymptomatic bacteremia due to periodontal, GI, or GU infections.

Acute bacterial endocarditis (ABE) usually develops abruptly and progresses rapidly (ie, over days). A source of infection or portal of entry is often evident. When bacteria are virulent or bacterial exposure is massive, ABE can affect normal valves. It is usually caused by *S. aureus*, group A hemolytic streptococci, pneumococci, or gonococci.

Prosthetic valvular endocarditis (PVE) develops in 2 to 3% of patients within 1 yr after valve replacement and in 0.5%/yr thereafter. It is more common after aortic than after mitral valve replacement and equally affects mechanical and bioprosthetic valves. Early-onset infections (< 2 mo after surgery) are caused mainly by contamination during surgery with antimicrobial-resistant bacteria (eg, *S. epidermidis*, diphtheroids, coliform bacilli, *Candida* sp, *Aspergillus* sp). Late-onset infections are caused mainly by contamination with low-virulence organisms during surgery or by transient asymptomatic bacteremias, most often with streptococci; *S. epidermidis*; diphtheroids; and the fastidious gram-negative bacilli, *Haemophilus* sp, *Actinobacillus actinomycetemcomitans*, and *Cardiobacterium hominis*.

Symptoms and Signs

SBE: Initially, symptoms are vague: low-grade fever (< 39° C), night sweats, fatigability, malaise, and weight loss. Chills and arthralgias may occur. Symptoms and signs of valvular insufficiency may be a first clue. Initially, ≤ 15% of patients have fever or a murmur, but eventually almost all develop both. Physical examination may be normal or include pallor, fever, change in a preexisting murmur or development of a new regurgitant murmur, and tachycardia.

Retinal emboli can cause round or oval hemorrhagic retinal lesions with small white centers (Roth's spots). Cutaneous manifestations include petechiae (on the upper trunk, conjunctivae, mucous membranes, and distal extremities), painful erythematous subcutaneous nodules on the tips of digits (Osler's nodes), nontender hemorrhagic macules on the palms or soles (Janeway lesions), and splinter hemorrhages under the nails. About 35% of patients have CNS effects, including transient ischemic attacks, stroke, toxic encephalopathy, and, if a mycotic CNS aneurysm ruptures, brain abscess and subarachnoid hemorrhage. Renal emboli may cause flank pain and, rarely, gross hematuria. Splenic emboli may cause left upper quadrant pain. Prolonged infection may cause splenomegaly or clubbing of fingers and toes.

ABE and PVE: Symptoms and signs are similar to those of SBE, but the course is more rapid. Fever is almost always present initially, and patients appear toxic; sometimes septic shock develops. Heart murmur is present initially in about 50 to 80% and eventually in > 90%. Rarely, purulent meningitis occurs.

Right-sided endocarditis: Septic pulmonary emboli may cause cough, pleuritic chest pain, and sometimes hemoptysis. A murmur of tricuspid regurgitation is typical.

Diagnosis

Because symptoms and signs are nonspecific, vary greatly, and may develop insidiously, diagnosis requires a high index of suspicion. Endocarditis should be suspected in patients with fever and no obvious source of infection, particularly if a heart murmur is present. Suspicion of endocarditis should be very high if blood cultures are positive in patients who have a history of a heart valve disorder, who have had certain recent invasive procedures, or who abuse IV drugs. Patients with documented bacteremia should be examined thoroughly and repeatedly for new valvular murmurs and signs of emboli.

If endocarditis is suspected, 3 blood cultures (20 mL each) should be obtained within 24 h (if presentation suggests ABE, 2 cultures within the first 1 to 2 h). When endocarditis is present and no prior antibiotic therapy was given, all 3 blood cultures usually are positive because the bacteremia is continuous; at least 1 culture is positive in 99%. If prior antimicrobial therapy was given, blood cultures should still be obtained, but they may be negative.

Echocardiography, typically transthoracic (TTE) rather than transesophageal (TEE), should be done. Although TEE is somewhat more accurate, it is invasive and more costly. TEE should be done when endocarditis is suspected in patients with prosthetic valves, when TTE is nondiagnostic, and when diagnosis of infective endocarditis has been established clinically.

Other than positive blood cultures, there are no specific laboratory findings. Established infections often cause a normocytic-normochromic anemia, elevated WBC count, increased ESR, increased Igs, circulating immune complexes, and rheumatoid factor, but these findings are not diagnostically helpful. Urinalysis often shows microscopic hematuria and, occasionally, RBC casts, pyuria, or bacteriuria.

Identification of the organism and its antimicrobial susceptibility is vital to guide treatment. Blood cultures may require 3 to 4 wk incubation for certain organisms. Other organisms (eg, *Aspergillus* sp) may not produce positive cultures. Some organisms (eg, *Coxiella burnetii, Bartonellosis* sp, *Chlamydia psittaci, Brucella* sp) require serodiagnosis; others (eg, *Legionella pneumophila*) require special culture media. Negative blood culture results may indicate suppression due to prior antimicrobial therapy, infection with organisms that do not grow in standard culture media, or another diagnosis (eg, noninfective endocarditis, atrial myxoma with embolic phenomena, vasculitis).

Infective endocarditis is definitively diagnosed when microorganisms are seen histologically in (or cultured from) endocardial vegetations obtained during cardiac surgery, embolectomy, or autopsy. Because vegetations are not usually available for examination, clinical criteria for establishing a diagnosis (with a sensitivity and specificity > 90%) have been developed (see TABLE 77–1).

Prognosis

Untreated, infective endocarditis is always fatal. Even with treatment, death is more likely and the prognosis is generally poorer for older people and people who have infection with resistant organisms, an underlying disorder, or a long delay in treatment. The prognosis is also poorer for people with aortic or multiple valve involvement, large vegetations, polymicrobial bacteremia, prosthetic valve infections, mycotic aneurysms, valve ring abscess, and major embolic events. The mortality rate for viridans streptococcal endocarditis without major complications is < 10% but is virtually 100% for *Aspergillus* endocarditis after prosthetic valve surgery.

The prognosis is better with right-sided than left-sided endocarditis because tricuspid valve dysfunction is tolerated better, systemic emboli are absent, and right-sided *S. aureus* endocarditis responds better to antimicrobial therapy.

Treatment

Treatment consists of a prolonged course of antimicrobial therapy. Surgery may be needed for mechanical complications or resistant organisms. Typically, antimicrobials are given IV. Because they must be given for 2 to 8 wk, home IV therapy is often used.

Any apparent source of bacteremia must be managed: necrotic tissue debrided, abscesses drained, and foreign material and infected devices removed. Existing IV catheters (particularly central venous ones) should be changed. If endocarditis persists in a patient with a newly inserted central venous catheter, that catheter should also be removed. Organisms within biofilms adherent to catheters and other devices may not respond to antimicrobial therapy, leading to treatment failure or relapse. If continuous infu-

TABLE 77–1. REVISED DUKE CLINICAL DIAGNOSTIC CRITERIA FOR INFECTIVE ENDOCARDITIS

MAJOR CRITERIA	MINOR CRITERIA
Two positive blood cultures for organisms typical of endocarditis	Predisposing heart disorder
Three positive blood cultures for organisms consistent with endocarditis	IV drug abuse
Serologic evidence of *Coxiella burnetii*	Fever ≥ 38°C
Echocardiographic evidence of endocardial involvement:	Vascular phenomena: arterial embolism, septic pulmonary embolism, mycotic aneurysm, intracranial hemorrhage, conjunctival petechiae, or Janeway lesions
Oscillating intracardiac mass on a heart valve, on supporting structures, in the path of regurgitant jets, or on implanted material without another anatomic explanation	Immunologic phenomena: glomerulonephritis, Osler's nodes, Roth's spots, or rheumatoid factor
Cardiac abscess	Microbiologic evidence of infection consistent with but not meeting major criteria
New dehiscence of prosthetic valve	Serologic evidence of infection with organism consistent with endocarditis
New valvular regurgitation	

For definite clinical diagnosis: 2 major criteria or 1 major and 3 minor criteria or 5 minor criteria.
For possible clinical diagnosis: 1 major and 1 minor criteria or 3 minor criteria.
For rejection of diagnosis: Firm alternative diagnosis explaining the findings of infective endocarditis, resolution of symptoms and signs after antimicrobial therapy for ≤ 4 days, no pathologic evidence of infective endocarditis found during surgery or autopsy, or failure to meet the clinical criteria for possible endocarditis.

Adapted from Li, JS, Sexton DJ, Mick N et al: Proposed modifications to the Duke criteria for the diagnosis of infective endocarditis. *Clinical Infectious Diseases* 2000:30:633–8.

sions are used instead of intermittent boluses, infusions should not be interrupted for long periods.

Antibiotic regimens: Drugs and dosages depend on the microorganism and its antimicrobial susceptibility (for typical regimens, see TABLE 77–2). Initial therapy before organism identification should be broad spectrum to cover all likely organisms. Typically, patients with native valves and no IV drug abuse receive ampicillin 500 mg/h continuous IV infusion plus nafcillin 2 g IV q 4 h plus gentamicin 1 mg/kg IV q 8 h. Patients with a prosthetic valve receive vancomycin 15 mg/kg IV q 12 h plus gentamicin 1 mg/kg q 8 h plus rifampin 300 po q 8 h. IV drug abusers receive nafcillin 2 g IV q 4 h. In all regimens, penicillin-allergic patients require substitution of vancomycin 15 mg/kg IV q 12 h.

IV drug abusers frequently do not adhere to treatment, abuse IV access lines, and tend to leave the hospital too soon. For such patients, short-course IV or (less preferably) oral therapy may be used. For right-sided endocarditis caused by methicillin-sensitive *S. aureus*, nafcillin 2 g IV q 4 h plus gentamicin 1 mg/kg IV q 8 h for 2 wk is effective, as is an oral regimen of ciprofloxacin 750 mg po bid plus rifampin 300 mg po bid. Left-sided endocarditis does not respond to 2-wk courses.

Cardiac valve surgery: Surgery (debridement, valve repair or replacement) is frequently required for abscess, persistent infection despite antimicrobial therapy (ie, persistent positive blood cultures or recurrent emboli), or severe valvular regurgitation.

Timing of surgery requires experienced clinical judgment. If heart failure caused by a correctable lesion is worsening (particularly when the organism is *S. aureus*, a gram-negative bacillus, or a fungus), surgery may be required after only 24 to 72 h of antimicrobial therapy. In patients with prosthetic valves, surgery may be required when TEE shows valve dehiscence on a paravalvular abscess, when valve dysfunction precipitates heart failure, when recurrent emboli are detected, or when the infection is caused by an antimicrobial-resistant organism.

Response to treatment: After starting therapy, patients with penicillin-susceptible

TABLE 77–2. ANTIBIOTIC REGIMENS FOR ENDOCARDITIS

TYPE	DRUG AND DOSAGE FOR ADULTS	DRUG AND DOSAGE FOR ADULTS ALLERGIC TO PENICILLIN
Penicillin-susceptible streptococci (penicillin G MIC ≤ 0.1 μg/mL), including most viridans streptococci	Penicillin G 12–18 million units/day IV continuously or 2–3 million units q 4 h for 4 wk or, if gentamicin 1 mg/kg* IV (up to 80 mg) q 8 h is given concurrently, for 2 wk	Ceftriaxone 2 g once/day IV for 4 wk or, if gentamicin 1 mg/kg* IV (up to 80 mg) q 8 h is given concurrently, for 2 wk through a central venous catheter (can be given on outpatient basis) if there is no history of penicillin anaphylaxis Vancomycin† 15 mg/kg IV q 12 h for 4 wk
Streptococci relatively resistant to penicillin (penicillin G MIC > 0.1 μg/mL), including enterococci and some other streptococcal strains	Gentamicin 1 mg/kg* IV q 8 h plus penicillin G 18 to 30 million units/day IV or ampicillin 12 g/day IV continuously or 2 g q 4 h for 4–6 wk‡	Desensitization to penicillin Vancomycin† 15 mg/kg IV (up to 1 g) q 12 h plus gentamicin 1mg/kg* IV q 8 h for 4–6 wk
Pneumococci or group A streptococci	Penicillin G 12 to 18 million units/day IV continuously for 4 wk if susceptible to penicillin Vancomycin† 15 mg/kg IV q 12 h for 4 wk for pneumococci with penicillin G MIC ≥ 2 μg/mL	Ceftriaxone 2 g once/day IV for 4 wk through a central venous catheter (can be given on outpatient basis) if there is no history of penicillin anaphylaxis Vancomycin† 15 mg/kg IV q 12 h for 4 wk
Penicillin-resistant *Staphylococcus aureus* strains	For patients with a left-sided native valve: Oxacillin or nafcillin 2 g IV q 4 h for 4–6 wk§ For patients with a right-sided native valve: Oxacillin or nafcillin 2 g IV q 4 h for 2–4 wk plus gentamicin 1 mg/kg* IV q 8 h for 2 wk For patients with a prosthetic valve: Oxacillin or nafcillin 2 g IV q 4 h for 6–8 wk plus gentamicin 1 mg/kg* IV q 8 h for 2 wk plus rifampin 300 mg po q 8 h for 6–8 wk	Cefazolin 2 g IV q 8 h for 4–6 wk if staphylococci are susceptible to oxacillin or nafcillin and if there is no history of penicillin anaphylaxis Cefazolin 2 g IV q 8 h for 2–4 wk plus gentamicin 1 mg/kg* IV q 8 h for 2 wk Cefazolin 2 g IV q 8 h for 4–6 wk plus gentamicin 1 mg/kg* IV q 8 h for 2 wk plus rifampin 300 mg po q 8 h for 6–8 wk Vancomycin† 15 mg/kg IV q 12 h alone if native valve, plus gentamicin 1 mg/kg* IV q 8 h for 2 wk, plus rifampin 300 mg po q 8 h if prosthetic valve for 4–6 wk
Oxacillin and nafcillin-resistant *S. aureus* strains	Vancomycin† 15 mg/kg IV q 12 h alone if native valve, plus gentamicin 1 mg/kg IV* q 8 h for 2 wk, plus rifampin 300 mg po q 8 h if prosthetic valve for 6–8 wk	

TABLE 77–2. ANTIBIOTIC REGIMENS FOR ENDOCARDITIS—Continued

TYPE	DRUG AND DOSAGE FOR ADULTS	DRUG AND DOSAGE FOR ADULTS ALLERGIC TO PENICILLIN
HACEK microorganisms	Ceftriaxone 2 g once/day IV for 4 wk Ampicillin 12 g/day IV continuously or 2 g q 4 h plus gentamicin 1 mg/kg* IV q 8 h for 4 wk	Ceftriaxone 2 g once/day IV for 4 wk or, if gentamicin 1 mg/kg* IV (up to 80 mg) q 8 h is given concurrently, for 2 wk if there is no history of penicillin anaphylaxis
Coliform bacilli	Sensitivity-proven β-lactam antimicrobial (eg, ceftriaxone 2 g IV q 12–24 h or ceftazidime 2 g IV q 8 h) plus an aminoglycoside (eg, gentamicin 2 mg/kg* IV q 8 h) for 4–6 wk	
Pseudomonas aeruginosa	Ceftazidime 2 g IV q 8 h or cefepime 2 g IV q 8 h or imipenem 500 mg IV q 6 h plus tobramycin 2.5 mg/kg q 8 h for 6–8 wk; amikacin 5 mg/kg q 12 h substituted for tobramycin if bacteria are susceptible	Ceftazidime 2 g IV q 8 h or cefepime 2 g IV q 8 h plus tobramycin 2.5 mg/kg q 8 h for 6–8 wk; amikacin 5 mg/kg q 12 h substituted for tobramycin if bacteria are susceptible only to amikacin

*Based on ideal rather than actual weight in obese patients.

†With vancomycin, serum levels must be monitored if doses > 2 g/24 h are administered.

‡If enterococcal endocarditis lasts > 3 mo and involves large vegetations or vegetations on prosthetic valves, treatment should last for 6 wk.

§Some clinicians add gentamicin 1 mg/kg IV q 8 h for 3–5 days in patients with a native valve.

HACEK microorganisms: *Haemophilus parainfluenzae, H. aphrophilus, Actinobacillus actinomycetemcomitans, Cardiobacterium hominis, Eikenella corrodens*, and *Kingella kingae*.

streptococcal endocarditis usually feel better, and fever is reduced within 3 to 7 days. Fever may continue for reasons other than persistent infection (eg, drug allergy, phlebitis, infarction due to emboli). Patients with staphylococcal endocarditis tend to respond more slowly.

Relapse usually occurs within 4 wk. Antibiotic retreatment may be effective, but surgery may also be required. In patients without prosthetic valves, recrudescence of endocarditis after 6 wk usually results from a new infection rather than a relapse. Even after successful antimicrobial therapy, sterile emboli and valve rupture may occur up to 1 yr later.

Prevention

Antimicrobial prophylaxis is recommended for patients at high to moderate risk of infective endocarditis before procedures associated with bacteremias and subsequent infective endocarditis (see TABLES 77–3, 77–4, and 77–5). For most patients and procedures, a single dose shortly before the procedure is effective.

NONINFECTIVE ENDOCARDITIS

Noninfective endocarditis (nonbacterial thrombotic endocarditis) refers to formation of sterile platelet and fibrin thrombi on cardiac valves and adjacent endocardium in response to trauma, circulating immune complexes, vasculitis, or a hypercoagulable state. Symptoms are those of systemic arterial embolism. Diagnosis is by echocardiography and negative blood cultures. Treatment consists of anticoagulants.

TABLE 77–3. PROCEDURES REQUIRING ANTIMICROBIAL ENDOCARDITIS PROPHYLAXIS

ORAL-DENTAL PROCEDURES	MEDICAL OR SURGICAL PROCEDURES
Dental extractions	Biliary tract surgery
Dental implant placement and reimplantation of avulsed teeth	Bronchoscopy with a rigid bronchoscope
Intraligamentary local anesthetic injections	Cystoscopy
Periodontal procedures, including surgery, scaling, root planing, and probing	ERCP with biliary obstruction
Prophylactic cleaning of teeth or implants when bleeding is anticipated	Esophageal stricture dilation
Root canal instrumentation or surgery beyond the apex	Intestinal mucosa surgery
Subgingival placement of orthodontic bands but not brackets	Prostatic surgery
	Respiratory mucosa surgery
	Sclerotherapy for esophageal varices
	Tonsillectomy or adenoidectomy
	Urethral dilation

Adapted from Dajani AS, Taubert KS, Wilson W, et al: Prevention of bacterial endocarditis. *JAMA* 277:1794–1801, 1997.

Etiology and Pathophysiology

Vegetations are caused by physical trauma, not infection. They may be clinically undetectable or become a nidus for infection (leading to infective endocarditis), produce emboli, or impair valvular function.

Catheters passed through the right heart may injure the tricuspid and pulmonic valves, resulting in platelet and fibrin attachment at the site of injury. In disorders such as SLE, circulating immune complexes may result in friable platelet and fibrin vegetations along a valve leaflet closure (Libman-Sacks lesions). These lesions do not usually cause significant valvular obstruction or regurgitation. Antiphospholipid syndrome (lupus anticoagulants, recurrent venous thrombosis, stroke, spontaneous abortions, livedo reticularis)

TABLE 77–4. RECOMMENDED ENDOCARDITIS PROPHYLAXIS DURING ORAL-DENTAL, RESPIRATORY TRACT, OR ESOPHAGEAL PROCEDURES*

ROUTE	DRUG AND DOSAGE IN ADULTS (AND CHILDREN)	DRUG AND DOSAGE IN ADULTS (AND CHILDREN) ALLERGIC TO PENICILLIN
Oral (given 1 h before procedure)	Amoxicillin 2 g (50 mg/kg) po	Clindamycin 600 mg (20 mg/kg) po Cephalexin or cefadroxil 2 g (50 mg/kg) po Azithromycin or clarithromycin 500 mg (15 mg/kg) po
Parenteral (given ½ h before procedure)	Ampicillin 2 g (50 mg/kg) IM or IV	Clindamycin 600 mg (20 mg/kg) IV Cefazolin 1 g (25 mg/kg) IM or IV

*For patients with moderate to high risk.

Adapted from Dajani AS, Taubert KS, Wilson W, et al: Prevention of bacterial endocarditis. *JAMA* 277:1794–1801, 1997

TABLE 77–5. RECOMMENDED ENDOCARDITIS PROPHYLAXIS DURING GI OR GU PROCEDURES

RISK LEVEL*	DRUG AND DOSAGE IN ADULTS (AND CHILDREN)	DRUG AND DOSAGE IN ADULTS (AND CHILDREN) ALLERGIC TO PENICILLIN
High	Ampicillin 2 g (50 mg/kg) IM or IV and gentamicin 1.5 mg/kg (1.5 mg/kg)—not to exceed 120 mg—IV or IM ½ h before the procedure; ampicillin 1 g (25 mg/kg) IM or IV or amoxicillin 1 g (25 mg/kg) po 6 h after the procedure	Vancomycin 1 g (20 mg/kg) IV over 1–2 h and gentamicin 1.5 mg/kg (1.5 mg/kg)—not to exceed 120 mg—IV or IM within ½ h of the procedure
Moderate	Amoxicillin 2 g (50 mg/kg) po 1 h before the procedure or ampicillin 2 g (50 mg/kg) IM or IV within ½ h of starting the procedure	Vancomycin 1 g (20 mg/kg) IV over 1–2 h within ½ h of the procedure

*Risk level is based on concomitant conditions.

High: Prosthetic heart valve (bioprosthetic or homograft), history of endocarditis, complex cyanotic congenital heart disease, or surgically constructed systemic pulmonary shunts or conduits

Moderate: Congenital cardiac malformation, acquired valvular insufficiency, hypertrophic cardiomyopathy, or mitral valve prolapse with murmur or thickened valve leaflets

Adapted from Dajani AS, Taubert KS, Wilson W, et al: Prevention of bacterial endocarditis. *JAMA* 277:1794–1801, 1997.

also can lead to sterile endocardial vegetations and systemic emboli. Rarely, Wegener's granulomatosis leads to noninfective endocarditis.

Marantic endocarditis: In patients with chronic wasting diseases, disseminated intravascular coagulation, mucin-producing metastatic carcinomas (of lung, stomach, or pancreas), or chronic infections (eg, TB, pneumonia, osteomyelitis), large thrombotic vegetations may form on valves and produce significant emboli to the brain, kidneys, spleen, mesentery, extremities, and coronary arteries. These vegetations tend to form on congenitally abnormal cardiac valves or those damaged by rheumatic fever.

Symptoms, Signs, and Diagnosis

Vegetations themselves do not cause symptoms. Symptoms result from embolization and depend on the organ affected (eg, brain, kidney, spleen). Fever and a heart murmur are sometimes present.

Noninfective endocarditis should be suspected when chronically ill patients develop symptoms suggesting arterial embolism. Serial blood cultures (see p. 726) and echocardiography should be done. Negative blood cultures and valvular vegetations (but not atrial myxoma) suggest the diagnosis. Examination of embolic fragments after embolectomy can help make the diagnosis. Differentiation from culture-negative infective endocarditis may be difficult but is important. An anticoagulant is often needed in noninfective endocarditis but is contraindicated in infective endocarditis.

Prognosis and Treatment

Prognosis is generally poor, more because of the seriousness of predisposing disorders than the cardiac lesion. Treatment consists of anticoagulation with heparin or warfarin, although results of such treatment have not been evaluated. Predisposing disorders should be treated whenever possible.

78 PERICARDITIS

Pericarditis is inflammation of the pericardium, often with fluid accumulation. Pericarditis may be caused by many disorders (eg, infection, MI, trauma, tumors, metabolic disorders) but is often idiopathic. Symptoms include chest pain or tightness, often worsened by deep breathing. Cardiac output may be greatly reduced. Diagnosis is based on symptoms, a friction rub, ECG changes, and evidence of pericardial fluid accumulation on x-ray or echocardiogram. Finding the cause requires further evaluation. Treatment depends on the cause, but general measures include analgesics, anti-inflammatory drugs, and sometimes surgery.

Pericarditis is the most common pericardial disorder. Congenital pericardial disorders are rare.

Anatomy and Pathophysiology

The pericardium has 2 layers. The visceral pericardium is a single layer of mesothelial cells that is attached to the myocardium, folds back (reflects) on itself over the origin of the great vessels, and joins with a tough, fibrous layer to envelop the heart as the parietal pericardium. The sac created by these layers contains a small amount of fluid (< 25 to 50 mL), composed mostly of an ultrafiltrate of plasma. The pericardium limits distention of the cardiac chambers and increases the heart's efficiency.

The pericardium is richly innervated with sympathetic and somatic afferents. Stretch-sensitive mechanoreceptors sense changes in cardiac volume and tension and may be responsible for transmitting pericardial pain. The phrenic nerves are embedded in the parietal pericardium and are vulnerable to injury during surgery on the pericardium.

Pericarditis may be acute or chronic. Acute pericarditis develops quickly, producing an inflammatory reaction. Chronic pericarditis (defined as persisting > 6 mo) develops more slowly; its prominent feature is effusion. Acute disease may become chronic. Adverse hemodynamic effects and rhythm disturbance are rare, although cardiac tamponade is possible. Occasionally, pericarditis produces a marked thickening and stiffening of the pericardium (constrictive pericarditis). Pericarditis can lead to inflammation of the epicardial myocardium.

Pericardial effusion is accumulation of fluid in the pericardium. The fluid may be serous fluid (sometimes with fibrin strands), serosanguineous fluid, blood, pus, or chyle.

Cardiac tamponade occurs when a large pericardial effusion impairs cardiac filling, leading to low cardiac output and sometimes shock and death. If fluid (usually blood) accumulates rapidly, even small amounts (eg, 150 mL) may produce tamponade because the pericardium cannot stretch quickly enough to accommodate. Slow accumulation of up to 1500 mL may not produce tamponade. Loculated effusion may produce localized tamponade on the right or left side of the heart.

Constrictive pericarditis, which is uncommon, results from marked inflammatory, fibrotic thickening of the pericardium. Sometimes the visceral and parietal layers adhere to each other or to the myocardium. The fibrotic tissue often contains Ca deposits. The stiff, thickened pericardium markedly impairs ventricular filling, decreasing stroke volume and cardiac output. Significant pericardial fluid accumulation is rare. Rhythm disturbance is common. The diastolic pressures in the ventricles, atria, and venous beds become virtually the same. Systemic venous congestion occurs, causing considerable transudation of fluid from systemic capillaries, with dependent edema and, later, ascites. Chronic elevation of systemic venous and hepatic venous pressure may lead to cardiac cirrhosis.

Etiology

Acute pericarditis may result from infection, connective tissue disorders, uremia, trauma, MI, or certain drugs (see TABLE 78–1). Infectious pericarditis is most often viral. Purulent bacterial pericarditis is uncommon but may follow infective endocarditis, pneumonia, septicemia, penetrating trauma, or cardiac surgery. Often, the cause cannot be identified (called nonspecific or idiopathic pericarditis), but many of these cases are probably viral. Overall, the most common causes are viral and idiopathic. Acute MI causes 10 to 15% of cases of acute pericarditis. Post-MI syndrome (Dressler's syndrome) is a less common cause occurring when reperfusion with percutaneous transluminal coronary angioplasty (PTCA) or thrombolytic drugs is ineffective. Pericarditis occurs after pericardiotomy (called postpericardiotomy syndrome) in 5 to 30% of cardiac operations.

Chronic pericardial effusion or constrictive pericarditis may follow almost any disorder that causes acute pericarditis, as well as TB, tumor, irradiation, and cardiac surgery. Sometimes no cause of chronic pericarditis is identified. Pericarditis with large effusion (serous, serosanguineous, or bloody) is most commonly caused by metastatic tumors, most often by lung or breast carcinoma, sarcoma (especially melanoma), leukemia, or lymphoma.

Fibrosis of the pericardium may follow purulent pericarditis or myocardial infection (myocarditis—a common cause in young people) or accompany a connective tissue disorder. In elderly patients, common causes are malignant tumors, MI, and TB. Hemopericardium (accumulation of blood within the pericardium) may lead to pericarditis or pericardial fibrosis; common causes include chest trauma, iatrogenic injury (eg, from cardiac catheterization, pacemaker insertion, or central venous line placement), and rupture of a thoracic aortic aneurysm.

Symptoms, Signs, and Diagnosis

Some patients present with symptoms and signs of inflammation (acute pericarditis); others present with those of fluid accumulation (pericardial effusion). Symptoms and signs vary depending on the severity of inflammation and the amount and rate of fluid accumulation. Even a large amount of pericardial fluid may be asymptomatic if it develops slowly (eg, over months).

Acute pericarditis: Acute pericarditis tends to cause chest pain and a pericardial rub, sometimes with dyspnea. The first evidence can be tamponade, with hypotension, shock, or pulmonary edema.

Because the innervation of the pericardium and myocardium is the same, the chest pain of pericarditis is sometimes similar to that of myocardial inflammation or ischemia: Dull or sharp precordial or substernal pain may radiate to the neck, trapezius ridge (especially the left), or shoulders. Pain ranges from mild to severe. Unlike ischemic chest pain, pain due to pericarditis is usually aggravated by thoracic motion, cough, and breathing; it may be relieved by sitting up and leaning forward. Tachypnea and nonproductive cough may be present; fever, chills, and weakness are common. In 15 to 25% of patients with idiopathic pericarditis, symptoms recur intermittently for months or years.

TABLE 78–1. CAUSES OF ACUTE PERICARDITIS

- Idiopathic
- Infectious
  - Viral (echovirus, influenza virus, coxsackie B virus, HIV*)
  - Bacterial† (streptococci; staphylococci; gram-negative bacilli; in children, *Haemophilus influenzae*)
  - Fungal (histoplasmosis, coccidioidomycosis, candidiasis, blastomycosis)
  - Parasitic (toxoplasmosis, amebiasis, echinococcosis)
- Autoimmune (RA, SLE, scleroderma)
- Inflammatory (amyloidosis, inflammatory bowel disease, sarcoidosis)
- Uremia
- Trauma
- MI
- Post-MI (Dressler's) syndrome
- Drugs (eg, hydralazine, isoniazid, methysergide, phenytoin, procainamide)

*If patients with AIDS develop lymphoma, Kaposi's sarcoma, or certain infections (ie, *Mycobacterium avium*, *M. tuberculosis*, *Nocardia*, other fungal or viral infections), pericarditis may follow.

†Tuberculous pericarditis accounts for < 5% of cases of acute or subacute pericarditis in the US but the majority of cases in some areas of India and Africa.

The most important physical finding is a triphasic or a systolic and diastolic precordial friction rub. However, the rub is often intermittent and evanescent; it may be present only during systole or, less frequently, only during diastole. Considerable amounts of pericardial fluid may muffle heart sounds, increase the area of cardiac dullness, and change the size and shape of the cardiac silhouette.

If acute pericarditis is suspected, hospitalization is sometimes required for initial evaluation. ECG and chest x-ray are done. If symptoms or signs of elevated right-sided pressure, tamponade, or an enlarged cardiac silhouette are present, echocardiography to check for effusion and cardiac filling abnormalities is also done. Blood tests may detect leukocytosis and an elevated ESR, but these findings are nonspecific.

The diagnosis is based on the presence of typical clinical findings and ECG abnormalities. Serial ECGs may be needed to show abnormalities.

The ECG in acute pericarditis may show abnormalities confined to ST segments and T waves, usually in most leads (see FIG. 78–1). The ST segments in 2 or 3 of the standard leads become elevated but subsequently return to baseline. Unlike MI, acute pericarditis does not cause reciprocal depression in ST segments (except in leads aVR and V_1), and there are no pathologic Q waves. The PR segment may be depressed. After several days or longer, T waves may become flattened and then inverted throughout the ECG, except in lead aVR; T-wave inversion occurs after the ST segment has returned to baseline and thus differs from the pattern of acute ischemia or MI.

Because the pain of pericarditis may resemble that of acute MI and pulmonary infarction, additional tests (eg, serum cardiac marker measurement, lung scan) may be required if the history and ECG findings are atypical for pericarditis.

Postpericardiotomy and post-MI syndrome may be difficult to identify and must be distinguished from recent MI, pulmonary embolism, and pericardial infection after surgery. Pain, friction rub, and fever appearing 2 wk to several months after surgery and a rapid response to aspirin, NSAIDs, or corticosteroids aid diagnosis.

Pericardial effusion: Pericardial effusion is often painless, but when it occurs with acute pericarditis, pain may be present. Typically, heart sounds are muffled. A pericardial rub may be heard. With large effusions, compression of the base of the left lung can decrease breath sounds (heard near the left scapula) and produce crackles (rales). Arterial pulse, jugular venous pulse, and BP are normal unless intrapericardial pressure increases substantially, causing tamponade.

In the post-MI syndrome, pericardial effusion can occur with fever, friction rub, effusion, pleurisy, pleural effusions, and joint pain. This syndrome usually occurs within 10 days to 2 mo after MI. It is usually mild but may be severe. Occasionally, the heart ruptures post-MI, causing hemopericardium and tamponade, usually 1 to 10 days post-MI and more commonly in women.

Diagnosis is suggested by clinical findings but often is suspected only after finding an enlarged cardiac silhouette on chest x-ray. On ECG, QRS voltage is often decreased, and sinus rhythm remains in about 90% of patients. With large, chronic effusions, the ECG may show electrical alternans (ie, P, QRS, or T

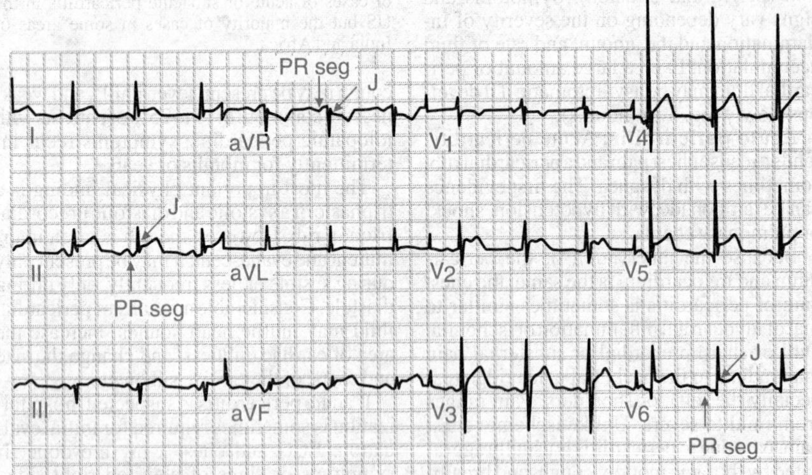

Fig. 78–1. Acute pericarditis: Stage 1 ECG. J points, except aVR and V_1, are elevated. T waves are essentially normal. PR segments, except aVR and V_1, are depressed. PR deviations are commonly absent in one limb lead (here, aVL).

wave amplitude increases and decreases on alternate beats). Electrical alternans is associated with variation in cardiac position (swinging heart). Echocardiography has a high degree of sensitivity and specificity for detecting pericardial fluid.

Patients with a normal ECG, small ($< \frac{1}{2}$ L) effusion, and no suspicious findings from the history and examination may be observed with serial examination and echocardiography. Other patients must be evaluated further to determine etiology.

Cardiac tamponade: The clinical findings are similar to those of cardiogenic shock: decreased cardiac output, low systemic arterial pressure, tachycardia, and dyspnea. Neck veins are markedly dilated. Severe cardiac tamponade is nearly always accompanied by a fall of > 10 mm Hg in systolic BP during inspiration (pulsus paradoxus—see p. 573). In advanced cases, pulse may disappear during inspiration. (However, pulsus paradoxus can also occur in COPD, bronchial asthma, pulmonary embolism, right ventricular infarction, and noncardiogenic shock.) Heart sounds are muffled unless the effusion is small.

Low voltage and electrical alternans on the ECG suggest cardiac tamponade, but these findings lack sensitivity and specificity. When tamponade is suspected, echocardiography is done unless even a brief delay might be life threatening. Then pericardiocentesis is done immediately for diagnosis and treatment. On an echocardiogram, respiratory variation of transvalvular and venous flows and compression or collapse of right cardiac chambers in the presence of a pericardial effusion support the diagnosis.

If tamponade is suspected, right heart (Swan-Ganz) catheterization may be done. In cardiac tamponade, there is no early diastolic dip in the ventricular pressure record. In the atrial pressure curve, *x* descent is preserved and *y* descent is lost. In contrast, in severe congestive states due to dilated cardiomyopathy, pulmonary artery occlusion or left ventricular diastolic pressure usually exceeds right atrial mean pressure and right ventricular diastolic pressure by ≥ 4 mm Hg.

Constrictive pericarditis: Fibrosis or calcification rarely produces symptoms unless constrictive pericarditis develops. The only early abnormalities may be elevated ventricular diastolic, atrial, pulmonary, and systemic venous pressures. Symptoms and signs of peripheral venous congestion (eg, peripheral edema, neck vein distention, hepatomegaly) may appear with an early diastolic sound (pericardial knock), often best heard during inspiration. This sound is due to abrupt slowing of diastolic ventricular filling by the rigid pericardium. Ventricular systolic function (based on ejection fraction) is usually preserved. Prolonged elevation of pulmonary venous pressure results in dyspnea (particularly during exertion) and orthopnea. Fatigue may be severe. Distention of neck veins with a rise in venous pressure during inspiration (Kussmaul's sign) is present; it is absent in tamponade. Pulsus paradoxus is rare and is usually less severe than in tamponade. Lungs are not congested unless severe left ventricular constriction develops.

Diagnosis may be suspected based on ECG, chest x-ray, and Doppler echocardiography findings, but cardiac catheterization and CT (or MRI) are usually required. Because ventricular filling is restricted, ventricular pressure tracings show a sudden dip followed by a plateau (resembling a square root sign) in early diastole. Rarely, right heart biopsy is needed to exclude restrictive cardiomyopathy.

ECG changes are nonspecific. QRS voltage is usually low. T waves are usually nonspecifically abnormal. Atrial fibrillation occurs in about $\frac{1}{3}$ of patients; atrial flutter is less common.

Lateral chest x-rays often show pericardial calcification best, but the finding is nonspecific.

The changes on echocardiogram are also nonspecific. When the right and left ventricular filling pressures are equally elevated, Doppler echocardiography helps distinguish constrictive pericarditis from restrictive cardiomyopathy. During inspiration, mitral diastolic flow velocity usually falls > 25% in constrictive pericarditis but < 15% in restrictive cardiomyopathy. In constrictive pericarditis, inspiratory tricuspid flow velocity increases more than it normally does, but it does not do so in restrictive cardiomyopathy. Determining tissue velocities at the mitral annulus may be helpful when excessively high left atrial pressure blunts respiratory variation in transvalvular velocities.

If clinical and echocardiographic findings suggest constrictive pericarditis, cardiac catheterization is done. It helps confirm and quantify the abnormal hemodynamics that define constrictive pericarditis: Mean pulmonary artery occlusion pressure (pulmonary capillary wedge pressure), pulmonary artery diastolic pressure, right ventricular end-diastolic pressure, and mean right atrial pressure are all at about 10 to 30 mm Hg. The pulmonary artery and right ventricular systolic pressures are normal or modestly elevated, so that pulse pressures are small. In the atrial pressure curve, *x* and *y* descents are typically accentuated; in the ventricular pressure curve, a diastolic dip occurs at the time of rapid ventricular filling. These changes almost always occur with significant constrictive pericarditis.

Right ventricular systolic pressure of > 50 mm Hg often occurs in restrictive cardiomyopathy but less often in constrictive pericarditis. When the pulmonary artery occlusion pressure equals the right atrial mean pressure and an early diastolic dip in the ventricular pressure curve occurs with large *x* and *y* waves in the right atrial curve, either disorder may be present.

CT or MRI can identify pericardial thickening > 5 mm. Such thickening with typical hemodynamic changes can confirm a diagnosis of constrictive pericarditis. When no pericardial thickening or fluid is seen, the diagnosis of restrictive cardiomyopathy is favored but not proved.

Diagnosis of cause: After pericarditis is diagnosed, tests to determine etiology and the effect on cardiac function are done. In a young, previously healthy adult who presents with a viral infection and pericarditis, an extensive evaluation is usually unnecessary. Differentiating viral from idiopathic pericarditis is difficult, expensive, and generally of little practical importance.

A biopsy of pericardial tissue or aspiration of pericardial fluid may be needed to establish a diagnosis. Acid-fast stains and cultures of pericardial fluid help identify infectious causes. Samples are examined for malignant cells. However, complete drainage of a newly identified pericardial effusion is usually unnecessary for diagnosis. Persistent (usually > 3 mo) or progressive effusion, particularly when the etiology is uncertain, also warrants pericardiocentesis.

The choice between needle pericardiocentesis and surgical drainage depends on institutional resources and physician experience, the etiology of the effusion, the need for diagnostic tissue samples, and the prognosis of the patient. Needle pericardiocentesis is often best when the etiology is known or the presence of tamponade is in question. Surgical drainage is best when the presence of tamponade is certain but the etiology is unclear.

Laboratory tests of pericardial fluid other than culture and cytology are usually nonspecific. But specific diagnoses are sometimes possible using newer visual, cytologic, and immunologic analysis of fluid obtained via pericardioscopic-guided biopsy.

Cardiac catheterization is useful for evaluating pericarditis and identifying the cause of reduced cardiac function.

CT or MRI can help identify metastases, although echocardiography is usually sufficient.

Other tests include CBC, acute-phase reactants, routine chemistries, cultures, autoimmune tests, and, when appropriate, tests for HIV, histoplasmosis complement fixation (in endemic areas), streptozyme, and neutralizing antibodies for coxsackievirus, influenza virus, and echovirus. Anti-DNA and anti-RNA antibody tests may be useful. A PPD skin test is done.

Treatment

Hospitalization to watch for complications is usually advisable. Possible causative drugs (eg, anticoagulants, procainamide, phenytoin) are stopped. For cardiac tamponade, immediate pericardiocentesis (see FIG. 78–2) is done; removal of even a small volume of fluid may be lifesaving.

Pain can usually be controlled with aspirin 325 to 650 mg po q 4 to 6 h or other NSAIDs (eg, ibuprofen 600 to 800 mg po q 6 to 8 h) for 1 to 4 days. Colchicine 1 mg/day, added to NSAIDs or given alone, is effective for the initial episode of pericarditis and helps prevent recurrences. The intensity of therapy is dictated by the patient's distress. Severe pain may require opioids and corticosteroids (eg, prednisone 60 to 80 mg po once/day for 1 wk, followed by rapid tapering of the dose). Corticosteroids are particularly useful in acute pericarditis due to uremia or a connective tissue disorder. Anticoagulants are usually contraindicated in acute pericarditis because they may cause intrapericardial bleeding and even fatal tamponade; however, they can be given in early pericarditis complicating acute MI. Uncommonly, pericardial resection is required.

Infections are treated with specific antimicrobial drugs. Complete drainage is often necessary.

In postpericardiotomy syndrome, post-MI syndrome, or idiopathic pericarditis, antibiotics are not indicated. An NSAID at full doses may control pain and effusion. When required

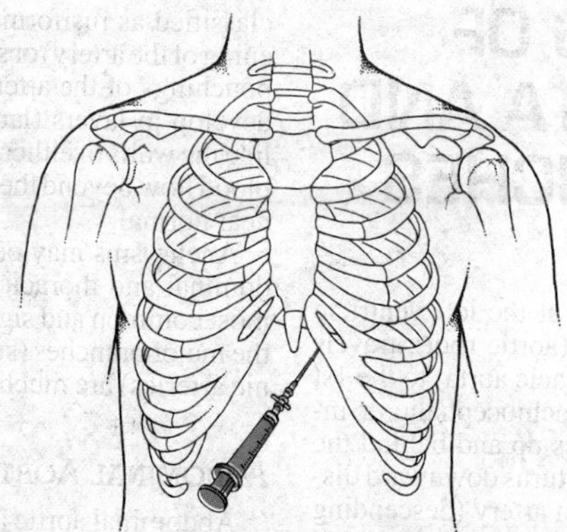

Fig. 78–2. Pericardiocentesis. Except in emergencies (eg, cardiac tamponade), pericardiocentesis, a potentially lethal procedure, should be done using echocardiographic guidance in a cardiac catheterization laboratory and should be supervised by a cardiologist or thoracic surgeon if possible. Resuscitation equipment must be at hand. IV sedation (eg, morphine 0.1 mg/kg or meperidine 1 mg/kg plus midazolam 3 to 5 mg) is desirable. The patient should be recumbent, with the head elevated 30° from the horizontal. Under aseptic conditions, the skin and subcutaneous tissues are infiltrated with lidocaine. A 75-mm short-beveled, 16-gauge needle is attached via a 3-way stopcock to a 30- or 50-mL syringe. The pericardium may be entered via the right or left xiphocostal angle or from the tip of the xiphoid process with the needle directed inward, upward, and close to the chest wall. The needle is advanced with constant suction applied to the syringe. Echocardiography may be used to guide the needle as agitated saline is injected through it. Once in place, the needle should be clamped next to the skin to prevent it from entering further than necessary and possibly puncturing the heart or injuring a coronary vessel. ECG monitoring is essential for detecting arrhythmias produced when the myocardium is touched or punctured. As a rule, right atrial pressure and pulmonary artery occlusion pressure (pulmonary capillary wedge pressure) are monitored. Fluid is withdrawn until intrapericardial pressure falls below right atrial pressure, usually to subatmospheric levels. If continued drainage is needed, a plastic catheter may be passed through the needle into the pericardium and the needle withdrawn. The catheter may be left in place for 2 to 4 days.

to control pain, fever, and effusion, prednisone 20 to 60 mg po once/day may be given for 3 to 4 days. If the response is satisfactory, the dose is gradually reduced, and the drug may be stopped in 7 to 14 days. But sometimes many months of treatment are needed.

For pericarditis due to rheumatic fever, another connective tissue disorder, or tumor, therapy is directed at the underlying process.

For pericardial effusion due to trauma, surgery is sometimes required to repair the injury and evacuate blood from the pericardium.

Pericarditis due to uremia may respond to increased frequency of hemodialysis, aspiration, or systemic or intrapericardial adrenal corticosteroids. Intrapericardial triamcinolone may be useful.

Chronic effusions are best treated by treating the cause, if known. Recurrent or persistent symptomatic effusions may be treated with balloon pericardiotomy, a surgical pericardial window, or sclerosing drugs (eg, tetracycline). Recurrent effusion due to malignant tumor invasion may be treated with sclerosing drugs. Asymptomatic effusions of unknown cause may require only observation.

Congestion in chronic constrictive pericarditis may be alleviated with bed rest, salt restriction, and diuretics. Digoxin is indicated only if atrial arrhythmias or ventricular systolic dysfunction is present. Symptomatic constrictive pericarditis usually requires pericardial resection. However, patients with mild symptoms, heavy calcification, or extensive myocardial damage may be poor surgical candidates. The mortality rate for pericardial resection may approach 40% in New York Heart Association (NYHA) functional class IV patients. Patients who have constrictive pericarditis due to irradiation or a connective tissue disorder are especially likely to have severe myocardial damage and may not benefit from pericardial resection.

79 DISEASES OF THE AORTA AND ITS BRANCHES

The aorta originates at the left ventricle above the aortic valve (aortic root), travels upward (ascending thoracic aorta) to the 1st branch of the aorta (brachiocephalic or innominate artery), arches up and behind the heart (aortic arch), then turns downward distal to the left subclavian artery (descending aorta) through the thorax (thoracic aorta) and abdomen (abdominal aorta). The abdominal aorta ends by dividing into the 2 common iliac arteries.

ANEURYSMS

Aneurysms are abnormal dilations of arteries caused by weakening of the arterial wall. Common causes include hypertension, atherosclerosis, infection, trauma, and hereditary or acquired connective tissue disorders. Aneurysms are usually asymptomatic but can cause pain and lead to ischemia, thromboembolism, spontaneous dissection, and rupture, which may be fatal. Diagnosis is by imaging tests (eg, ultrasonography, CT angiography, magnetic resonance angiography, aortography). Treatment of unruptured aneurysms is with risk factor modification (eg, strict BP control) plus surveillance imaging or with surgery, depending on size and location of the aneurysm and presence of symptoms. Treatment of ruptured aneurysms is immediate surgical repair and placement of a synthetic graft or endograft.

Aneurysms, defined as a ≥ 50% increase in arterial diameter compared with normal segments, result from localized weakening of an arterial wall. True aneurysms involve all 3 layers of the artery (intima, media, and adventitia). A pseudoaneurysm (false aneurysm) is a communication between the arterial lumen and overlying connective tissue resulting from arterial rupture; a blood-filled cavity forms outside the vessel wall and seals the leak as it thromboses. Aneurysms are classified as fusiform (circumferential widening of the artery) or saccular (localized outpouchings of the artery wall). Thrombi that develop in layers (laminated thrombi) may line the walls of either type and are a sign that blood flow beyond the aneurysm is normal or near normal.

Aneurysms may occur in any artery. Abdominal and thoracic aortic aneurysms are most common and significant; aneurysms of the major branches (subclavian and splanchnic arteries) are much less common.

Abdominal Aortic Aneurysms

Abdominal aortic aneurysms (AAAs) account for 3/4 of aortic aneurysms and affect 0.5 to 3.2% of the population. Prevalence is 3 times greater in men. AAAs typically begin below the renal arteries but may include renal arterial ostia; about 50% involve the iliac arteries. Generally, aortic diameter ≥ 3 cm constitutes an AAA. Most AAAs are fusiform; some are saccular. Many are lined with laminated thrombi. AAAs involve all layers of the aorta and do not involve dissection; however, a thoracic aortic dissection may extend to the distal abdominal aorta.

Etiology

The most common cause is weakening of the arterial wall, usually associated with atherosclerosis. Other causes include trauma, vasculitis, cystic medial necrosis, and postsurgical anastomotic disruption. Uncommonly, syphilis and localized bacterial or fungal infection, typically due to sepsis or infective endocarditis, weaken the arterial wall and cause infected (mycotic) aneurysms.

Smoking is the strongest risk factor. Other risk factors include hypertension, older age (peak incidence at age 70 to 80), family history (in 15 to 25%), Caucasian race, and male sex.

Symptoms and Signs

Most AAAs are asymptomatic; symptoms and signs, when they do occur, may not be specific. As AAAs expand, they may cause pain, which is steady, deep, boring, visceral, and felt most prominently in the lumbosacral region; patients may be aware of an abnormally prominent abdominal pulsation. Rapidly enlarging aneurysms that are about to rupture are frequently tender, but most aneurysms grow slowly without symptoms.

The aneurysm may or may not be palpable as a pulsatile mass, depending on its size and patient habitus. The probability that a patient with a pulsatile palpable mass has an aneurysm > 3 cm is about 40% (positive predictive value). A systolic bruit may be audible over the aneurysm. Patients who do not die immediately from a ruptured AAA typically present with abdominal or back pain, hypotension, and tachycardia. They may have a history of recent upper abdominal trauma.

Patients with an occult AAA sometimes present with symptoms of complications (eg, extremity pain due to embolization of mural thrombi) or of the cause (eg, fever, malaise, or weight loss due to infection or vasculitis). Uncommonly, large AAAs cause disseminated intravascular coagulation, perhaps because large areas of abnormal endothelial surface trigger rapid thrombosis and consumption of coagulation factors.

Diagnosis

Most AAAs are diagnosed incidentally when they are detected during physical examination or when abdominal ultrasonography, CT, or MRI is done for other reasons. An AAA should be considered in elderly patients who present with acute abdominal or back pain whether a palpable pulsatile mass is present or not.

When symptoms or physical examination findings suggest AAA, abdominal ultrasonography or CT is usually the test of choice. For hemodynamically unstable patients with presumed rupture, ultrasonography provides bedside results more rapidly, but intestinal gas and distention may limit its accuracy. Laboratory tests, including CBC, electrolytes, BUN, creatinine, PT, PTT, blood typing, and compatibility testing, are done in preparation for possible surgery.

If rupture is not suspected, CT angiography (CTA) or magnetic resonance angiography (MRA) can more precisely characterize aneurysm size and anatomy. If thrombi line the aneurysm wall, CTA may underestimate true size; noncontrast CT may provide a more accurate estimate. Aortography is essential if renal artery or aortoiliac disease is suspected or if correction with endovascular stent-grafts (endografts) is being considered.

Plain abdominal x-rays are neither sensitive nor specific; however, if obtained for other purposes, aortic calcification may outline the aneurysm wall. If a mycotic aneurysm is suspected, bacterial and fungal blood cultures should be obtained.

Treatment

Some AAAs enlarge at a steady rate (2 to 3 mm/yr), some enlarge exponentially, and, for unknown reasons, about 20% remain the same size indefinitely. The need for treatment is related to size, which is linked to risk of rupture (see TABLE 79–1).

Ruptured AAAs require immediate surgery. Without treatment, mortality rate approaches 100%. With treatment, mortality rate is about 50%; the figure is not lower because many patients have coexisting coronary, cerebrovascular, and peripheral atherosclerosis. Patients who present in hemorrhagic shock require fluid resuscitation (see p. 564) and blood transfusions, but mean arterial pressure should not be elevated to > 70 to 80 mm Hg because bleeding may increase. Preoperative control of hypertension is important.

Elective surgical repair is recommended for aneurysms > 5 to 5.5 cm (when risk of rupture increases to > 5 to 10%/yr), unless coexisting medical conditions contraindicate surgery. Additional indications for elective surgery include increase in aneurysm size by > 0.5 cm within 6 mo regardless of size, chronic abdominal pain, thromboembolic complications, or an iliac or femoral artery aneurysm that causes lower-limb ischemia. Before elective repair, screening for coronary artery disease (CAD) is essential (see TABLE 70–1 on p. 589) because many patients with an AAA have generalized atherosclerosis and surgical repair poses a major risk for cardiovascular events. Good medical treatment of CAD

TABLE 79–1. ABDOMINAL AORTIC ANEURYSM SIZE AND RUPTURE RISK*

AAA DIAMETER (cm)	RUPTURE RISK (%/yr)
< 4	0
4–4.9	1%
5–5.9*	5–10%
6–6.9	10–20%
7–7.9	20–40%
> 8	30–50%

*Elective surgical repair should be considered for aneurysms > 5.0–5.5 cm.

or revascularization is essential for reducing morbidity and mortality due to AAA repair.

Surgical repair consists of replacing the aneurysmal portion of the abdominal aorta with a synthetic graft. If the iliac arteries are involved, the graft must be extended to include them. If the aneurysm extends above the renal arteries, the renal arteries must be reimplanted into the graft, or bypass grafts must be created.

Placement of an endograft within the aneurysmal lumen via the femoral artery is a less invasive alternative and is indicated when risk of perioperative complications is high. This procedure excludes the aneurysm from systemic blood flow and reduces risk of rupture. The aneurysm eventually thromboses, and 50% of aneurysms decrease in diameter. Short-term results are good, but long-term results are unknown. Complications include angulation, kinking, thrombosis, migration of the endograft, and endoleak (persistent flow of blood into the aneurysm sac after endograft placement). Thus, follow-ups must be more frequent after endograft placement than after a traditional repair. If no complications occur, imaging tests are recommended at 1 mo, 6 mo, 12 mo, and every year thereafter. Complex anatomy (eg, short aneurysm neck below renal arteries, severe arterial tortuosity) makes endograft placement inappropriate in 30 to 50% of patients.

Repair of aneurysms < 5 cm does not appear to improve survival. These aneurysms should be monitored with ultrasonography or CT q 6 to 12 mo for expansion that warrants treatment. Duration for monitoring of incidentally detected, asymptomatic aneurysms has not been established. Control of atherosclerotic risk factors, especially smoking cessation and use of antihypertensives as appropriate, is important. If a small or moderate-sized aneurysm becomes > 5.5 cm and if risk of perioperative complications is lower than estimated risk of rupture, surgery is indicated; risk of rupture vs that of perioperative complications should be discussed frankly with the patient.

Treatment of a mycotic aneurysm consists of vigorous antimicrobial therapy directed at the pathogen, followed by excision of the aneurysm. Early diagnosis and treatment improve outcome.

Thoracic Aortic Aneurysms

Thoracic aortic aneurysms (TAAs) account for $\frac{1}{4}$ of aortic aneurysms. Men and women are affected equally. About 40% of TAAs occur in the ascending thoracic aorta (between the aortic valve and brachiocephalic, or innominate, artery), 10% occur in the aortic arch (including the brachiocephalic, carotid, and subclavian arteries), 35% occur in the descending thoracic aorta (distal to the left subclavian artery), and 15% occur in the upper abdomen (as thoracoabdominal aneurysms).

Etiology and Pathophysiology

Most TAAs result from atherosclerosis. Risk factors for both include prolonged hypertension, dyslipidemia, and smoking; additional risk factors for TAAs include presence of aneurysms elsewhere and older age (peak incidence at age 65 to 70).

Congenital connective tissue disorders (eg, Marfan syndrome, Ehlers-Danlos syndrome) cause cystic medial necrosis, a degenerative change that leads to TAAs complicated by aortic dissection (see p. 742) and by widening of the proximal aorta and aortic valve (annuloaortic ectasia), which causes aortic regurgitation. Marfan syndrome causes 50% of cases of annuloaortic ectasia, but cystic medial necrosis and its complications can occur in young people even if no congenital connective tissue disorder is present.

Infected (mycotic) TAAs result from hematogenous spread in systemic or local infections (eg, sepsis, pneumonia), lymphangitic spread (eg, in TB), or direct extension (eg, in osteomyelitis or pericarditis). Bacterial endocarditis and tertiary syphilis are uncommon causes. TAAs occur in some connective tissue diseases (eg, temporal arteritis, Takayasu's arteritis, Wegener's granulomatosis).

Blunt chest trauma causes pseudoaneurysms (extramural hematomas due to blood that has leaked through the torn aortic wall).

TAAs may dissect, compress or erode into adjacent structures, lead to thromboembolism, leak, or rupture.

Symptoms and Signs

Most TAAs are asymptomatic until complications (eg, aortic regurgitation, dissection) develop. Compression of adjacent structures can cause chest or back pain, cough, wheezing, dysphagia, hoarseness (due to left recurrent laryngeal or vagus nerve compression), chest pain (due to coronary artery compression), and superior vena cava syndrome. Erosion of aneurysms into the lungs causes hemoptysis or pneumonitis. Thromboembolism may cause stroke, abdominal pain (due to mesenteric embolism), or extremity pain. Patients who do not immediately die of a ruptured TAA present with severe chest or back pain, hypotension, or shock; exsanguination most commonly occurs into the pleural or pericardial space. When erosion into the esophagus (aortoesophageal fistula) precedes rupture, patients may present with massive hematemesis.

Additional signs include Horner's syndrome due to compression of sympathetic ganglia, palpable downward pull of the trachea with each cardiac contraction (tracheal tug), and tracheal deviation. Visible or palpable chest wall pulsations, occasionally more prominent than the left ventricular apical impulse, are unusual but may occur.

Syphilitic aneurysms of the aortic root classically lead to aortic regurgitation and inflammatory stenosis of the coronary artery ostia, which may manifest as chest pain due to myocardial ischemia. Syphilitic aneurysms do not dissect.

Diagnosis

TAAs are usually first suspected when a chest x-ray incidentally shows a widened mediastinum or enlargement of the aortic knob. These findings or symptoms and signs suggesting an aneurysm should be followed up with a 3-dimensional imaging test. CTA can delineate aneurysm size and proximal or distant extent, detect leakage, and identify coincident pathology. MRA may provide similar detail. Transesophageal echocardiography (TEE) can delineate size and extent and detect leakage of aneurysms of the ascending but not descending aorta; TEE is especially useful for detecting aortic dissection. Contrast angiography provides the best image of the arterial lumen but no information on extraluminal structures, is invasive, and has a significant risk of renal and extremity atheroembolism and contrast nephropathy. Choice of imaging test is based on availability and local experience; however, if rupture is suspected, TEE or CTA, depending on availability, is done immediately.

Aortic root dilation or unexplained ascending aorta aneurysms warrant serologic testing for syphilis. If a mycotic aneurysm is suspected, bacterial and fungal blood cultures are obtained.

Prognosis and Treatment

TAAs enlarge an average of 5 mm/yr; risk factors for rapid enlargement include larger size of aneurysm, location in the descending aorta, and presence of mural thrombi. Median diameter at aneurysm rupture is 6 cm for ascending aneurysms and 7 cm for descending aneurysms, but rupture of smaller aneurysms may occur in patients with Marfan syndrome. Survival rate of patients with untreated large TAAs is 65% at 1 yr and 20% at 5 yr.

Treatment is surgical repair and control of hypertension if present.

Ruptured TAAs, if untreated, are universally fatal; they require immediate intervention, as do leaking aneurysms and those that cause acute dissection or acute valvular regurgitation. Surgery involves a median sternotomy (for ascending and aortic arch aneurysms) or left thoracotomy (for descending and thoracoabdominal aneurysms) and subsequent excision of the aneurysm and replacement with a synthetic graft. Transcatheter-placed endovascular stent-grafts (endografts) for descending TAAs are being studied as a less invasive alternative to open surgery. With emergency surgery, 1-mo mortality rate is about 40 to 50%. In patients who survive, incidence of serious complications (eg, renal failure, respiratory failure, severe neurologic damage) is high.

Elective surgery is indicated for large aneurysms (diameter > 5 to 6 cm in the ascending aorta, > 6 to 7 cm in the descending aorta, and, for patients with Marfan syndrome, > 5 cm in any location) and also for those that rapidly enlarge (> 1 cm/yr). Elective surgery is also indicated for symptomatic, traumatic, or syphilitic aneurysms. For syphilitic aneurysms, benzathine penicillin 2.4 million units/wk IM is given for 3 wk afterward. For patients allergic to penicillin, tetracycline or erythromycin 500 mg po qid for 30 days is acceptable.

Although surgical repair of an intact TAA improves outcome, mortality rate may still exceed 5 to 10% at 30 days and is 40 to 50% at 10 yr. Risk of death increases greatly if aneurysms are complicated (eg, in the aortic arch or thoracoabdominal aorta) or if patients have CAD, are older, are symptomatic, or have preexisting renal insufficiency. Perioperative complications (eg, stroke, spinal injury, renal failure) occur in about 10 to 20%.

Asymptomatic aneurysms that do not meet criteria for elective surgical repair are treated with aggressive BP control using a β-blocker and other antihypertensives if necessary, serial CT q 6 to 12 mo, and frequent follow-ups to check for symptoms. Smoking cessation is essential.

Aortic Branch Aneurysms

Aneurysms may occur in any major aortic branch; such aneurysms are much less common than abdominal or thoracic aortic aneurysms. Risk factors include atherosclerosis, hypertension, cigarette smoking, and older age. Localized infection can cause mycotic aneurysms.

Subclavian artery aneurysms are sometimes associated with cervical ribs or thoracic outlet syndrome.

Splanchnic artery aneurysms are uncommon. About 60% occur in the splenic artery, 20% in the hepatic artery, and 5.5% in the superior mesenteric artery. Splenic artery aneurysms occur in more women than men (4:1). Causes include medial fibromuscular dysplasia, portal hypertension, multiple pregnancies, penetrating or blunt abdominal trauma, pancreatitis, and infection. Hepatic artery aneurysms occur in more men than women (2:1). They may result from previous abdominal trauma, illicit IV drug use, medial degeneration of the arterial wall, or periarterial inflammation. Renal artery aneurysms may dissect or rupture, causing acute occlusion (see p. 2030).

Symptoms and Signs

Symptoms vary. Subclavian aneurysms can cause local pain, a pulsating sensation, venous thrombosis or edema (due to compression of adjacent veins), distal ischemic symptoms, transient ischemic attacks, stroke, or hoarseness or impaired motor and sensory function (due to compression of the recurrent laryngeal nerve or brachial plexus). Superior mesenteric aneurysms may cause abdominal pain and ischemic colitis.

Regardless of location, mycotic or inflammatory aneurysms may cause local pain and sequelae of systemic infection (eg, fever, malaise, weight loss).

Diagnosis and Treatment

Most aortic branch aneurysms are not diagnosed before rupture, although calcified asymptomatic or occult aneurysms may be seen on x-rays or other imaging tests done for other reasons. Ultrasonography or CT is typically used to detect or confirm aortic branch aneurysms; angiography can be used as needed to evaluate distal symptoms thought to be due to the aneurysm or embolism.

Treatment is surgical removal and replacement with a graft. The decision to repair asymptomatic aneurysms is based on risk of rupture, extent and location of the aneurysm, and perioperative risk.

Surgery for subclavian artery aneurysms may involve removal of a cervical rib (if present) before repair and replacement.

For splanchnic aneurysms, risk of rupture and death is as high as 10% and is particularly high for women of childbearing age and for patients with hepatic aneurysms (> 35%). Elective repair of splanchnic aneurysms is therefore indicated for women of childbearing age, for symptomatic aneurysms in other age groups, and for hepatic aneurysms. For splenic aneurysms, repair may consist of ligation without arterial reconstruction or aneurysm exclusion and vascular reconstruction. Depending on location of the aneurysm, splenectomy may be necessary.

Treatment of mycotic aneurysms is aggressive antibiotic therapy directed at the specific pathogen. Generally, these aneurysms must also be surgically repaired.

AORTIC DISSECTION

Aortic dissection is the surging of blood through a tear in the aortic intima with separation of the intima and media and creation of a false lumen. The intimal tear may be a primary event or secondary to hemorrhage within the media. The dissection may occur anywhere along the aorta and extend proximally or distally into other arteries. Hypertension is an important contributor. Symptoms and signs include abrupt onset of tearing chest or back pain, and dissection may result in aortic regurgitation and compromised circulation in branch arteries. Diagnosis is by imaging tests (eg, transesophageal echocardiography, CT angiography, MRI, contrast aortography). Treatment always involves aggressive BP control and serial imaging to monitor progression of dissection; surgical repair of the aorta and placement of a synthetic graft is needed for ascending aortic dissection and for certain descending aortic dissections. One fifth of patients die before reaching the hospital, and up to 1/3 die of operative or perioperative complications.

Evidence of dissection is found in 1 to 3% of all autopsies. Blacks, men, the elderly, and people with hypertension are especially at risk. Peak incidence occurs at age 50 to 65 or, for patients with congenital connective tissue disorders (eg, Marfan syndrome), at age 20 to 40.

Aortic dissections are classified anatomically. The DeBakey classification system, which is most widely used, distinguishes dissections starting in the ascending aorta and extending at least to the aortic arch and sometimes beyond (type I; 50%); those starting in and confined to the ascending aorta (type II; 35%); and those starting in the descending thoracic aorta just beyond the left subclavian artery origin and extending distally or, less commonly, proximally (type III; 15%). In the simpler Stanford system, dissection involving the ascending aorta (type A) is distinguished from dissection confined to the descending thoracic aorta (type B). Although dissection may originate anywhere along the aorta, it occurs most commonly at the proximal ascending aorta (within 5 cm of the aortic valve) or the descending thoracic aorta (just beyond the origin of the left subclavian artery). Rarely, dissection is confined to individual arteries (eg, coronary or carotid arteries), typically in pregnant or postpartum women.

Etiology and Pathophysiology

Aortic dissection always occurs in the setting of preexisting degeneration of the aortic media. Causes include connective tissue disorders and injury (see TABLE 79–2). Atherosclerotic risk factors, notably hypertension, contribute in > ⅔ of patients. After intimal rupture, which is a primary event in some patients and secondary to hemorrhage within the media in others, blood flows into the media, creating a false channel that extends distally or, less commonly, proximally along the artery.

Dissections may communicate back with the true aortic lumen through intimal rupture at a distal site, maintaining systemic blood flow. But serious consequences are common: compromise of the blood supply of tributary arteries (including coronary arteries), aortic valvular dilation and regurgitation, heart failure, and fatal rupture of the aorta through the adventitia into the pericardium or left pleural space. Acute dissections and those present < 2 wk are most likely to cause these complications; risk decreases at ≥ 2 wk if evidence indicates thrombosis of the false lumen and loss of communication between the true and false lumina.

TABLE 79–2. CONDITIONS CONTRIBUTING TO AORTIC DISSECTION

CATEGORY	EXAMPLES
Atherosclerotic risk factors	Cocaine Dyslipidemia Hypertension Smoking
Connective tissue disorders, acquired	Behçet's syndrome Giant cell arteritis Syphilis Takayasu's arteritis
Connective tissue disorders, congenital or hereditary	Bicuspid aortic valve Coarctation of the aorta Cystic medial necrosis Ehlers-Danlos syndrome Marfan syndrome Turner's syndrome Familial thoracic aortic aneurysm
Iatrogenic	Aortic catheterization Aortic valve surgery
Trauma	Deceleration injuries

Variants of aortic dissection include separation of the intima and media by intramural hematoma without a clear intimal tear or flap, intimal tear and bulge without hematoma or false lumen, and dissection or hematoma caused by ulceration of atherosclerotic plaque. These variants are thought to be precursors of classic aortic dissection.

Symptoms and Signs

Typically, excruciating precordial or interscapular pain, often described as tearing or ripping, occurs abruptly. The pain frequently migrates from the original location as the dissection extends along the aorta. Up to 20% of patients present with syncope due to severe pain, aortic baroreceptor activation, extracranial cerebral artery obstruction, or cardiac tamponade.

Occasionally, patients present with symptoms of stroke, MI, intestinal infarction, paraparesis or paraplegia due to interruption of the blood supply to the spinal cord, or ischemic limb due to acute distal arterial occlusion.

About 20% of patients have partial or complete deficits of major arterial pulses, which may wax and wane. Limb BPs may differ, sometimes by > 30 mm Hg; this finding suggests a poor prognosis. A murmur of aortic regurgitation is heard in about 50% of patients with proximal dissection. Peripheral signs of aortic regurgitation may be present. Rarely, heart failure results from severe acute aortic regurgitation. Leakage of blood or inflammatory serous fluid into the left pleural space may lead to signs of pleural effusion; occlusion of a limb artery may cause signs of peripheral ischemia or neuropathy. Renal artery occlusion may cause oliguria or anuria. Cardiac tamponade may cause pulsus paradoxus and jugular venous distention.

Diagnosis

Aortic dissection must be considered in any patient with chest pain, thoracic back pain, unexplained syncope or abdominal pain, stroke, or acute-onset heart failure, especially when pulses or BPs in the limbs are unequal. Such patients require a chest x-ray; in 60 to 90%, the mediastinal shadow is widened, usually with a localized bulge signifying the site of origin. Left pleural effusion is common.

If chest x-ray suggests dissection, transesophageal echocardiography (TEE), CT angiography (CTA), or magnetic resonance angiography (MRA) is done immediately after the patient is stabilized. Findings of an intimal flap and double lumina confirm dissection.

Multiplanar TEE is 97 to 99% sensitive and, with M-mode echocardiography, is nearly 100% specific. It can be done at the bedside in < 20 min and does not require contrast agents. If TEE is unavailable, CTA is recommended; it has a positive predictive value of 100% and a negative predictive value of 86%.

MRA has nearly 100% sensitivity and specificity for aortic dissection. But it is time-consuming and ill-suited for emergencies. It is probably best used for stable patients with subacute or chronic chest pain when dissection is suspected.

Contrast aortography is an option if surgery is being considered. In addition to identifying the origin and extent of dissection, severity of aortic regurgitation, and extent of involvement of the aorta's major branches, aortography helps determine whether simultaneous coronary artery bypass surgery is needed. Echocardiography should also be done to check for aortic regurgitation and thus determine whether the aortic valve should be repaired or replaced concomitantly.

ECG is nearly universally done. However, findings range from normal to markedly abnormal (in acute coronary artery occlusion or aortic regurgitation), so the test is not diagnostically helpful. Assays for soluble elastin compounds and smooth-muscle myosin heavy-chain protein are being studied; they look promising but are not routinely available. Serum CPK-MB and troponin may help distinguish aortic dissection from MI, except when dissection causes MI.

Routine laboratory tests may detect slight leukocytosis and anemia if blood has leaked from the aorta. Increased LDH may be a nonspecific sign of celiac or mesenteric arterial trunk involvement.

A cardiothoracic surgeon should be consulted early during the diagnostic evaluation.

Prognosis

About 20% of patients with aortic dissection die before reaching the hospital. Without treatment, mortality rate is 1 to 3%/h during the first 24 h, 30% at 1 wk, 80% at 2 wk, and 90% at 1 yr.

Hospital mortality rate for treated patients is about 30% for proximal dissection and 10% for distal. For treated patients who survive the acute episode, survival rate is about 60% at 5 yr and 40% at 10 yr. About 1/3 of late deaths are due to complications of the dissection; the rest are due to other disorders.

Treatment

Patients who do not immediately die of aortic dissection should be admitted to an ICU with intra-arterial BP monitoring; an indwelling urethral catheter is used to monitor urine output. Blood should be typed and cross-matched for 4 to 6 units of packed RBCs when surgery is likely. Hemodynamically unstable patients should be intubated.

Drugs to decrease arterial pressure, arterial shear stress, ventricular contractility, and pain are started immediately to maintain systolic BP at ≤ 110 mm Hg or the lowest level compatible with adequate cerebral, coronary, and renal perfusion. A β-blocker is usually used first. Propranolol 0.5 mg IV is followed by 1 to 2 mg q 3 to 5 min until the pulse slows to 60 to 70 beats/min or until a total dose of 0.15 mg/kg is given over 30 to 60 min; this dosage decreases ventricular contractility and counters the reflex chronotropic effects of nitroprusside. This dose can be repeated IV q 2 to 4 h to maintain β-blockade. Patients with COPD or asthma may be given a more cardioselective β-blocker. Options include metoprolol 5 mg IV up to 4 doses 15 min apart or esmolol 50 to 200 μg/kg/min in a constant IV infusion, or labetalol (an α- and β-adrenergic blocker) 1 to 2 mg/min in a constant IV infusion or 5 to 20 mg IV initial bolus with additional doses of 20 to 40 mg given q 10 to 20 min until BP is controlled or a total of 300 mg has been given, followed by additional 20- to 40-mg doses q 4 to 8 h prn. Alternatives to β-blockers include Ca channel blockers (eg, verapamil 0.05 to 0.1 mg/kg IV bolus or diltiazem 0.25 mg/kg [up to 25 mg] IV bolus or 5 to 10 mg/h by continuous infusion).

If systolic BP remains > 110 mm Hg despite use of β-blockers, nitroprusside in a constant IV infusion can be started at 0.2 to 0.3 μg/kg/min and titrated upward (often to 200 to 300 μg/min) as necessary to control BP. Nitroprusside should not be given without a β-blocker or Ca channel blocker, because reflex sympathetic activation in response to vasodilation can increase ventricular inotropy and aortic shear stress, worsening the dissection.

A trial of drug therapy alone is appropriate for uncomplicated, stable dissection confined to the descending aorta (type B) and for stable, isolated dissection of the aortic arch. Surgery is virtually always indicated if dissection involves the proximal aorta. Surgery is also indicated for limb or visceral ischemia, uncontrolled hypertension, continued aortic enlargement, extension of the dissection, and evidence of aortic rupture, regardless of dissection type. Surgery may also be best for acute distal dissections in patients with Marfan syndrome.

The goal of surgery is to obliterate entry into the false channel, and reconstitute the aorta with a synthetic graft. If present, significant aortic regurgitation must be treated by resuspending the aortic leaflets or replacing the valve. Surgical outcomes are best with early, aggressive intervention; mortality rate ranges from 7 to 36%. Predictors of poor outcome include hypotension, renal failure, age > 70, abrupt onset of chest pain, pulse deficit, and ST-segment elevation on ECG.

Stent-grafts that seal entry to the false lumen and improve patency of the true lumen, balloon fenestration (in which an opening is made in the dissection flap that separates the true and false lumina), or both may be noninvasive alternatives for patients with type A dissection and persistent postoperative peripheral ischemia and for patients with type B dissection if peripheral ischemic complications develop.

All patients, including those treated surgically, are given long-term antihypertensive drug therapy, usually including β-blockers, Ca channel blockers, and ACE inhibitors. Almost any combination of antihypertensives is acceptable; exceptions are those that act mainly by vasodilation (eg, hydralazine, minoxidil) and β-blockers that have intrinsic sympathomimetic action (eg, acebutolol, pindolol). Avoidance of strenuous physical activity is often recommended. MRI is done before discharge and repeated at 6 mo and 1 yr, then q 1 to 2 yr.

The most important late complications include redissection, formation of localized aneurysms in the weakened aorta, and progressive aortic regurgitation. These complications may require surgical repair.

AORTITIS

Aortitis is inflammation of the aorta, sometimes causing aneurysm or occlusion.

Aortitis is caused by several connective tissue disorders (eg, Takayasu's arteritis, temporal arteritis, ankylosing spondylitis, relapsing polychondritis) and infections (eg, bacterial endocarditis, syphilis, Rocky Mountain spotted fever, fungal infections). It is also a feature of Cogan's syndrome (inflammatory keratitis, vestibular and auditory dysfunction, and aortitis). Inflammation usually involves all layers of the aorta (intima, media, adventitia) and may lead to occlusion of the aorta or its branches or weakening of the arterial wall, resulting in aneurysms. Pathogenesis, symptoms and signs, diagnosis, and treatment differ by etiology.

ABDOMINAL AORTIC BRANCH OCCLUSION

Various branches of the aorta can be occluded by atherosclerosis, fibromuscular dysplasia, or other conditions, producing symptoms and signs of ischemia or infarction. Diagnosis is by imaging tests. Treatment

is with embolectomy, angioplasty, or sometimes surgical bypass grafting.

Acute occlusion of branches of the abdominal aorta may result from embolism, atherothrombosis, or dissection; chronic occlusion may result from atherosclerosis, fibromuscular dysplasia, or external compression by mass lesions. Common sites of occlusion include the splanchnic arteries (eg, superior mesenteric arteries, celiac axis, renal arteries) and the aortic bifurcation. Chronic occlusion of the celiac axis is more common among women for unclear reasons.

Symptoms and signs (eg, pain, organ failure, necrosis) result from ischemia or infarction. Acute mesenteric occlusion causes intestinal ischemia and infarction, resulting in severe, diffuse abdominal pain—an abdominal catastrophe (see p. 98). Acute occlusion of the celiac axis may cause liver or spleen infarction. Chronic mesenteric vascular insufficiency rarely causes symptoms unless both the superior mesenteric artery and celiac axis are substantially narrowed or occluded, because collateral circulation between the major splanchnic trunks is extensive. Symptoms of chronic mesenteric vascular insufficiency typically occur postprandially (as intestinal angina) because digestion requires increased mesenteric blood flow; pain begins about 30 min to 1 h after eating and is steady, severe, usually periumbilical, and may be relieved by sublingual nitroglycerin. Patients become fearful of eating; weight loss, often extreme, is common. Rarely, malabsorption develops and contributes to weight loss. Patients may have an abdominal bruit, nausea, vomiting, diarrhea or constipation, and dark stools.

Acute occlusion due to renal artery embolism causes sudden flank pain, followed by hematuria (see p. 2030). Chronic occlusion may be asymptomatic or result in new or hard-to-control hypertension and other sequelae of renal insufficiency or failure.

Acute occlusion of the aortic bifurcation or distal branches can cause sudden onset of pain at rest, pallor, paralysis, absence of peripheral pulses, and coldness in the legs (see p. 751). Chronic occlusion can cause intermittent claudication in the legs and buttocks and erectile dysfunction (Leriche syndrome). Femoral pulses are absent. A limb may be jeopardized.

Diagnosis and Treatment

Diagnosis is based primarily on history and physical examination and is confirmed by duplex ultrasonography, CT angiography, magnetic resonance angiography, or traditional angiography. Acute occlusion is a surgical emergency requiring embolectomy or percutaneous transluminal angioplasty (PTA) with or without stenting. Chronic occlusion, if symptomatic, may require surgery or angioplasty. Risk factor modification and antiplatelet drugs may help.

Acute mesenteric occlusion (eg, in the superior mesenteric artery), which causes significant morbidity and mortality, requires prompt revascularization. Prognosis is poor if the intestine is not revascularized within 4 to 6 h.

For chronic occlusion of the superior mesenteric artery and celiac axis, nitroglycerin may temporarily relieve symptoms. If symptoms are severe, surgical bypass from the aorta to the splanchnic arteries distal to the occlusion usually results in revascularization. Long-term patency of the grafts exceeds 90%. In appropriately selected patients (particularly among older patients who may be poor candidates for surgery), revascularization by PTA with or without stenting may be successful. Symptoms may resolve rapidly, and weight may be regained.

Acute renal artery occlusion requires embolectomy; sometimes PTA can be done. Initial treatment of chronic occlusion involves antihypertensives. If BP is not controlled adequately or if renal function deteriorates, PTA with stenting or, when PTA is impossible, open surgical bypass or embolectomy can improve blood flow.

Occlusion of the aortic bifurcation requires urgent embolectomy, usually done transfemorally. If chronic occlusion of the aortic bifurcation causes claudication, an aortoiliac or aortofemoral graft can be used to surgically bypass the occlusion. PTA is an alternative for selected patients.

80 PERIPHERAL ARTERIAL DISORDERS

Peripheral arterial disorders include acrocynanosis, erythromelalgia, fibromuscular dysplasia, peripheral arterial aneurysms, peripheral arterial disease (caused by atherosclerosis), Raynaud's phenomenon, and thromboangiitis obliterans.

ACROCYANOSIS

Acrocyanosis is persistent, painless, symmetric cyanosis of the hands, feet, or face caused by vasospasm of the small vessels of the skin in response to cold.

Acrocyanosis usually occurs in women and is not associated with occlusive arterial disease. The digits and hands or feet are persistently cold and bluish, sweat profusely, and may swell. In acrocyanosis, unlike Raynaud's phenomenon, cyanosis persists and is not easily reversed, trophic changes and ulcers do not occur, and pain is absent. Pulses are normal.

Treatment, other than reassurance and avoidance of cold, is usually unnecessary. Vasodilators may be tried but are usually ineffective.

ERYTHROMELALGIA

Erythromelalgia is distressing paroxysmal vasodilation of small arteries in the feet and hands and, less commonly, in the face, ears, or knees; it causes burning pain, increased skin temperature, and redness.

This rare disorder may be primary (cause unknown) or secondary to myeloproliferative disorders (eg, polycythemia vera, thrombocythemia), hypertension, venous insufficiency, diabetes mellitus, SLE, RA, lichen sclerosus, gout, spinal cord disorders, or multiple sclerosis.

Burning pain, heat, and redness in the feet or hands last a few minutes to several hours. In most patients, symptoms are triggered by warmth (temperatures of 29 to 32° C) and are typically relieved by immersion in ice water. Trophic changes do not occur. Symptoms may remain mild for years or become severe enough to cause total disability. Generalized vasomotor dysfunction is common, and Raynaud's phenomenon may occur.

Diagnosis is clinical. Testing is done to detect causes. Because erythromelalgia may precede a myeloproliferative disorder by several years, repeated blood counts may be indicated. Differential diagnosis includes posttraumatic reflex dystrophies, shoulder-hand syndrome, peripheral neuropathy, causalgia, Fabry's disease, and bacterial cellulitis.

Treatment is warmth avoidance, rest, elevation of the extremity, and application of cold. For primary erythromelalgia, gabapentin or a prostaglandin analog (eg, misoprostol) may be of benefit. For secondary erythromelalgia, the underlying disorder is treated; aspirin may be helpful when a myeloproliferative disorder is involved.

FIBROMUSCULAR DYSPLASIA

Fibromuscular dysplasia includes a heterogenous group of nonatherosclerotic, noninflammatory arterial changes, causing some degree of vascular stenosis, occlusion, or aneurysm.

Fibromuscular dysplasia usually occurs in women aged 40 to 60. The cause is unknown. However, there may be a genetic component, and smoking may be a risk factor. Fibromuscular dysplasia is more common among people with certain connective tissue disorders (eg, Ehlers-Danlos syndrome type 4, cystic medial necrosis, hereditary nephritis, neurofibromatosis).

Medial dysplasia, the most common type, is characterized by alternating regions of thick and thin fibromuscular ridges containing collagen along the media (medial dysplasia) or by extensive collagen deposition in the outer half (perimedial dysplasia). Fibromuscular dysplasia may affect the renal arteries (60 to 75%), carotid and intracranial arteries (25 to 30%), intra-abdominal arteries (9%), or external iliac arteries (5%).

Fibromuscular dysplasia is usually asymptomatic regardless of location. Symptoms, when they occur, vary by location: claudication in the thighs and calves, femoral bruits, and decreased femoral pulses when leg arteries are affected; secondary hypertension when renal arteries are affected; transient ischemic attack or stroke symptoms when carotid arteries are affected; aneurysmal symptoms when intracranial arteries are affected, and, rarely, mesenteric ischemic symptoms when intra-abdominal arteries are affected.

Definitive diagnosis is made by angiography showing a beaded appearance (in medial or perimedial dysplasia) or a concentric band or long smooth narrowing (in other forms).

Treatment varies by location. It may involve percutaneous transluminal angioplasty, bypass surgery, or aneurysm repair. Smoking cessation is important. Control of other risk factors for atherosclerosis (hypertension, dyslipidemia, diabetes) helps prevent accelerated development of arterial stenoses.

PERIPHERAL ARTERIAL ANEURYSMS

Peripheral arterial aneurysms are abnormal dilations of the peripheral arteries caused by weakening of the arterial wall (see also p. 738).

About 70% of peripheral arterial aneurysms are popliteal aneurysms; 20% are iliofemoral aneurysms. Aneurysms at these locations frequently accompany abdominal aortic aneurysms, and > 50% are bilateral. Rupture is relatively infrequent, but these aneurysms may lead to thromboembolism. They occur in men much more often than women (> 20:1); mean age at presentation is 65. Aneurysms in arm arteries are relatively rare; they may cause limb ischemia, distal embolism, and stroke.

Infectious (mycotic) aneurysms may occur in any artery but are most common in the femoral. They are usually due to salmonellae, staphylococci, or *Treponema pallidum* (which causes syphilis).

Common causes include atherosclerosis, popliteal artery entrapment, and septic emboli.

Peripheral arterial aneurysms are usually asymptomatic at the time of detection. Extremities may be painful, cold, pale, paresthetic, or pulseless because of thromboemboli or, rarely, aneurysm rupture. Infectious aneurysms may cause local pain, fever, malaise, and weight loss.

Diagnosis is by ultrasonography, magnetic resonance angiography, or CT. Popliteal aneurysms may be suspected when physical examination detects an enlarged, pulsatile artery; the diagnosis is confirmed by imaging tests.

Risk of rupture of extremity aneurysms is low (< 5% for popliteal and 1 to 14% for iliofemoral aneurysms). For leg artery aneurysms, surgical repair is therefore often elective; it is indicated when the arteries are twice normal size or when the patient is symptomatic. However, surgical repair is indicated for all arm artery aneurysms because serious complications (eg, thromboembolism) are a risk. The affected segment of artery is excised and replaced with a graft. Limb salvage rate after surgical repair is 90 to 98% for asymptomatic patients and 70 to 80% for symptomatic patients.

PERIPHERAL ARTERIAL DISEASE

Peripheral arterial disease (PAD), also called peripheral vascular disease, is atherosclerosis of the lower extremities causing ischemia. Mild PAD may be asymptomatic or cause intermittent claudication; severe PAD may cause rest pain with skin atrophy, hair loss, cyanosis, ischemic ulcers, and gangrene. Diagnosis is by history, physical examination, and measurement of the ankle-brachial index. Treatment of mild PAD includes risk factor modification, exercise, antiplatelet drugs, and cilostazol or possibly pentoxifylline as needed for symptoms. Severe PAD usually requires angioplasty or surgical bypass and may require amputation. Prognosis is generally good with treatment, although mortality rate is relatively high because coronary artery or cerebrovascular disease often coexists.

Etiology

PAD affects about 12% of people in the US; men are affected more commonly. Risk factors are the same as those for atherosclerosis: hypertension, dyslipidemia (high low density lipoprotein [LDL] cholesterol, low high density lipoprotein [HDL] cholesterol), cigarette smoking (including passive smoking), diabetes, and a family history of atherosclerosis. Obesity, male sex, and a high homocysteine level are also risk factors. Atherosclerosis is a systemic disorder; 50 to 75% of patients with PAD also have clinically significant coronary artery disease (CAD) or cerebrovascular disease. However, CAD may be silent because PAD prevents patients from exerting themselves enough to trigger angina.

Symptoms and Signs

Typically, PAD causes intermittent claudication, which is a painful, aching, cramping, uncomfortable, or tired feeling in the legs that occurs during walking and is relieved by rest. Claudication usually occurs in the calves but can occur in the feet, thighs, hips, buttocks, or, rarely, arms. Claudication is a manifestation of exercise-induced reversible ischemia, similar to angina pectoris. As PAD progresses, the distance that can be walked without symptoms may decrease, and patients with severe PAD may experience pain during rest, reflecting irreversible ischemia. Rest pain is usually worse distally, is aggravated by leg elevation (often causing pain at night), and lessens when the leg is below heart level. The pain may feel like burning, although this finding is nonspecific. About 20% of patients with PAD are asymptomatic, sometimes because they are not active enough to trigger leg ischemia. Some patients have atypical symptoms (eg, nonspecific exercise intolerance, hip or other joint pain).

Mild PAD often causes no signs. Moderate to severe PAD commonly causes diminished or absent peripheral (popliteal, tibialis posterior, dorsalis pedis) pulses; Doppler ultrasonography can often detect these pulses when they cannot be palpated.

When below heart level, the foot may appear dusky red (called dependent rubor). In some patients, elevating the foot causes loss of color and worsens ischemic pain; when the foot is lowered, venous filling is prolonged (> 15 sec). Edema is usually not present unless the patient has kept the leg immobile and in a dependent position to relieve pain. Patients with chronic PAD may have thin, pale (atrophic) skin with hair thinning or loss. Distal legs and feet may feel cool. The affected leg may sweat excessively and become cyanotic, probably because of sympathetic nerve overactivity.

As ischemia worsens, ulcers may appear (typically on the toes or heel, occasionally on the leg or foot), especially after local trauma. The ulcers tend to be surrounded by black, necrotic tissue (dry gangrene). They are usually painful, but people with peripheral neuropathy due to diabetes or alcoholism may not feel them. Infection of ischemic ulcers (wet gangrene) occurs readily, producing rapidly progressive cellulitis.

The level of arterial occlusion influences location of symptoms. Aortoiliac PAD may cause buttock, thigh, or calf claudication; hip pain; and, in men, erectile dysfunction (Leriche syndrome). In femoropopliteal PAD, claudication typically occurs in the calf; pulses below the femoral artery are weak or absent. In PAD of more distal arteries, femoropopliteal pulses may be present, but foot pulses are absent.

Diagnosis

PAD is suspected clinically but is underrecognized because many patients have atypical symptoms or are not active enough to have symptoms. Spinal stenosis may also cause leg pain during walking but can be distinguished because the pain (called pseudoclaudication) requires sitting, not just rest, for relief, and distal pulses remain intact.

Diagnosis is confirmed by noninvasive testing. First, bilateral arm and ankle systolic BP is measured; because ankle pulses may be difficult to palpate, a Doppler probe may be placed over the dorsalis pedis or posterior tibial arteries. Doppler ultrasonography is often used, because pressure gradients and pulse volume waveforms can help distinguish isolated aortoiliac PAD from femoropopliteal PAD and below-the-knee PAD.

A low (≤ 0.90) ankle-brachial index (ratio of ankle to arm systolic BP) indicates PAD, which can be classified as mild (0.71 to 0.90), moderate (0.41 to 0.70), or severe (≤ 0.40). If the index is normal (0.91 to 1.30) but suspicion of PAD remains high, the index is determined after exercise stress testing. A high index (> 1.30) may indicate noncompressible leg vessels (as occurs in Mönckeberg's arteriosclerosis with calcification of the arterial wall). If index is > 1.30 but suspicion of PAD remains high, additional tests (eg, Doppler ultrasonography, measurement of BP in the 1st toe using toe cuffs) are done to check for arterial stenoses or occlusions. Ischemic lesions are unlikely to heal when systolic BP is < 55 mm Hg in patients without diabetes or < 70 mm Hg in patients with diabetes; below-the-knee amputations usually heal if BP is ≥ 70 mm Hg.

Angiography provides details of the location and extent of arterial stenoses or occlusion; it is a prerequisite for surgical correction or percutaneous transluminal angioplasty (PTA). It is not a substitute for noninvasive testing because it provides no information about the functional significance of abnormal findings. Magnetic resonance angiography and CT angiography are noninvasive tests that may eventually supplant contrast angiography.

Treatment

All patients require aggressive risk factor modification, including smoking cessation and control of diabetes, dyslipidemia, hypertension, and hyperhomocysteinemia. β-Blockers are safe unless PAD is very severe.

Exercise—35 to 50 min of treadmill or track walking in an exercise-rest-exercise pattern 3 to 4 times/wk—is an important but underrecognized treatment. It can increase symptom-free walking distance and improve quality of life. Mechanisms probably include increased collateral circulation, improved endothelial function with microvascular vasodilation, decreased blood viscosity, improved RBC filterability, decreased ischemia-induced inflammation, and improved O_2 extraction.

Patients are advised to keep the legs below heart level. For pain relief at night, the head of the bed can be elevated 4 to 6 inches to improve blood flow to the feet.

Patients are also advised to avoid cold and drugs that cause vasoconstriction (eg, pseudoephedrine, contained in many headache and cold remedies).

Preventive foot care is crucial, especially for patients with diabetes. It includes daily foot inspection for injuries and lesions; treatment of calluses and corns by a podiatrist; daily washing of the feet in lukewarm water with mild soap, followed by gentle, thorough drying; and avoidance of thermal, chemical, and mechanical injury, especially that due to poorly fitting footwear. For foot ulcer management, see also p. 1014.

Antiplatelet drugs may modestly lessen symptoms and improve walking distance; more importantly, these drugs modify atherogenesis and help prevent acute coronary syndromes and transient ischemic attacks (see also p. 644). Options include aspirin 81 mg once/day, aspirin 25 mg plus dipyridamole 200 mg once/day, and clopidogrel 75 mg po once/day or ticlopidine 250 mg po bid with or without aspirin. Aspirin is typically used alone first, followed by addition or substitution of other drugs if PAD progresses.

For relief of claudication, pentoxifylline 400 mg po tid with meals or cilostazol 100 mg po bid may be used to relieve intermittent claudication by improving blood flow and enhancing tissue oxygenation in affected areas; however, these drugs are no substitute for risk factor modification and exercise. Use of pentoxifylline is controversial because evidence of its effectiveness is mixed. A trial of ≥ 2 mo may be warranted, because adverse effects are uncommon and mild. The most common adverse effects of cilostazol are headache and diarrhea. Cilostazol is contraindicated by severe heart failure.

Other drugs that may relieve claudication are being studied; they include L-arginine (the precursor of endothelium-dependent vasodilator), nitric oxide, vasodilator prostaglandins, and angiogenic growth factors (eg, vascular endothelial growth factor [VEGF], basic fibroblast growth factor [bFGF]). Gene therapy for PAD is also being studied. In patients with severe limb ischemia, long-term parenteral use of vasodilator prostaglandins may decrease pain and facilitate ulcer healing, and intramuscular gene transfer of DNA encoding VEGF may promote collateral blood vessel growth.

Percutaneous intervention: PTA with or without stenting is the primary nonsurgical method for dilating vascular occlusions. PTA with stenting may keep the artery open better than balloon compression alone, with a lower rate of reocclusion. Stents work best in large arteries with high flow (iliac and renal); they are less useful for smaller arteries and for long occlusions.

Indications for PTA are similar to those for surgery: intermittent claudication that inhibits daily activities, rest pain, and gangrene. Suitable lesions are flow-limiting, short iliac stenoses (< 3 cm) and short, single or multiple stenoses of the superficial femoropopliteal segment. Complete occlusions (up to 10 or 12 cm long) of the superficial femoral artery can be successfully dilated, but results are better for occlusions ≤ 5 cm. PTA is also useful for localized iliac stenosis proximal to a bypass of the femoropopliteal artery.

PTA is less useful for diffuse disease, long occlusions, and eccentric calcified plaques. Such lesions are particularly common in diabetes, often affecting small arteries.

Complications of PTA include thrombosis at the site of dilation, distal embolization, intimal dissection with occlusion by a flap, and complications related to heparin use.

With appropriate patient selection (based on complete and adequate angiography), the initial success rate approaches 85 to 95% for iliac arteries and 50 to 70% for thigh and calf arteries. Recurrence rates are relatively high (25 to 35% at ≤3 yr); repeat PTA may be successful.

Surgery: Surgery is indicated for patients who can safely tolerate a major vascular procedure and whose severe symptoms do not respond to noninvasive treatments. The goal is to relieve symptoms, heal ulcers, and avoid amputation. Because many patients have underlying CAD, which places them at risk of acute coronary syndromes during surgical procedures for PAD, patients usually undergo cardiac evaluation prior to surgery.

Thromboendarterectomy (surgical removal of an occlusive lesion) is used for short, localized lesions in the aortoiliac, common femoral, or deep femoral arteries.

Revascularization (eg, femoropopliteal bypass grafting) uses synthetic or natural materials (often the saphenous or another vein) to bypass occlusive lesions. Revascularization helps prevent limb amputation and relieve claudication.

In patients who cannot undergo major vascular surgery, sympathectomy may be effective when a distal occlusion causes severe ischemic pain. Chemical sympathetic blocks are as effective surgical sympathectomy, so the latter is rarely done.

Amputation is a procedure of last resort, indicated for uncontrolled infection, unrelenting rest pain, and progressive gangrene. Amputation should be as distal as possible, preserving the knee for optimal use with a prosthesis.

External compression therapy: External pneumatic compression of the lower limb to increase distal blood flow is an option for limb salvage in patients who have severe PAD and are not candidates for surgery. Theoretically, it controls edema and improves arterial flow, venous return, and tissue oxygenation, but data supporting its use are lacking. Pneumatic cuffs or stockings are placed on the lower leg and inflated rhythmically during diastole, systole, or part of both periods for 1 to 2 h several times/wk.

Acute Peripheral Arterial Occlusion

Peripheral arteries may be acutely occluded by a thrombus, an embolus, aortic dissection, or acute compartment syndrome.

Acute peripheral arterial occlusion may result from rupture and thrombosis of an atherosclerotic plaque, an embolus from the heart or thoracic or abdominal aorta, an aortic dissection, or acute compartment syndrome (see p. 2567).

Symptoms and signs are sudden onset of the 5 P's: severe pain, polar sensation (coldness), paresthesias (or anesthesias), pallor in an extremity, and pulselessness. The occlusion can be roughly localized to the arterial bifurcation just distal to the last palpable pulse (eg, at the common femoral bifurcation when the femoral pulse is palpable; at the popliteal bifurcation when the popliteal pulse is palpable). Severe cases may cause loss of motor function. After 6 to 8 h, muscles may be tender when palpated.

Diagnosis is clinical. Immediate angiography is required to confirm location of the occlusion, identify collateral flow, and guide therapy. Treatment consists of embolectomy (catheter or surgical), thrombolysis, or bypass surgery.

A thrombolytic drug, especially when given by regional catheter infusion, is most effective for acute arterial occlusions of <2 wk. Tissue plasminogen activator and urokinase are most commonly used. A catheter is threaded to the occluded area, and the thrombolytic drug is given at a rate appropriate for the patient's size and the extent of thrombosis. Treatment is usually continued for 4 to 24 h, depending on severity of ischemia and signs of thrombolysis (relief of symptoms and return of pulses or improved blood flow shown by Doppler ultrasonography). About 20 to 30% of patients with acute arterial occlusion require amputation within the first 30 days.

RAYNAUD'S PHENOMENON

Raynaud's phenomenon (Raynaud's disease) is vasospasm of parts of the hand in response to cold or emotional stress, causing reversible discomfort and color changes (pallor, cyanosis, erythema, or a combination) in one or more digits. Occasionally, other acral parts (eg, nose, tongue) are affected. The disorder may be primary or secondary. Diagnosis is clinical; testing focuses on distinguishing primary from secondary disease. Treatment of uncomplicated cases includes avoidance of cold, biofeedback, smoking cessation, and, as needed, vasodilating Ca channel blockers (eg, nifedipine) or prazosin.

Primary Raynaud's phenomenon is much more common (>80% of cases) than secondary;

TABLE 80–1. CAUSES OF SECONDARY RAYNAUD'S PHENOMENON

CAUSE	EXAMPLES
Connective tissue disorders	Giant cell arteritis Mixed or undifferentiated connective tissue disease Polymyositis/dermatomyositis RA Scleroderma Sjögren's syndrome SLE Takayasu's arteritis
Endocrine disorders	Hypothyroidism Pheochromocytoma
Hematologic disorders	Cold agglutinin disease Cryofibrinogenemia Cryoglobulinemia Paraproteinemia Polycythemia vera
Infections	*Helicobacter pylori* infection Parvovirus B19 infection
Neoplastic disorders	Angiocentric lymphoma Carcinoid syndrome Ovarian carcinoma Paraneoplastic syndrome
Neurologic disorders	Carpal tunnel syndrome
Mechanical conditions	Frost bite Trauma Vibration
Vascular disorders	Atherosclerosis (severe) Atheroembolism Axillary crutch pressure (chronic) Thoracic outlet syndrome Thromboangiitis obliterans
Drugs	Amphetamines Antineoplastic drugs (eg, bleomycin, cisplatin, vinblastine) β-Blockers Clonidine Cocaine Ergot preparations Interferon-α and -β Methysergide Nicotine Polyvinyl chloride Sympathomimetic drugs

it occurs without symptoms or signs of other disorders. It is sporadic in about 75% of cases but may be familial. About 15 to 20% of people with primary Raynaud's phenomenon develop a more serious systemic disorder.

Secondary Raynaud's phenomenon accompanies various disorders and conditions, mostly connective tissue disorders (see TABLE 80–1). Nicotine commonly contributes to it but is often overlooked. Raynaud's phenomenon may accompany migraine headaches, variant angina, and pulmonary hypertension, suggesting that these disorders share a common vasospastic mechanism.

Overall prevalence is about 3 to 5%; women are affected more, and younger people are affected more than older. Raynaud's phenomenon is probably due to an exaggerated α_2-adrenergic response that triggers vasospasm; the mechanism is not defined.

Symptoms and Signs

Sensations of coldness, burning pain, paresthesias, or intermittent color changes of one or more digits are precipitated by exposure to cold, emotional stress, or vibration. All can be reversed by removing the stimulus. Rewarming the hands accelerates restoration of normal color and sensation.

Color changes are clearly demarcated across the digit. They may be triphasic (pallor, followed by cyanosis and after warming by erythema due to reactive hyperemia), biphasic (cyanosis, erythema), or uniphasic (pallor or cyanosis only). Changes are often symmetric. Raynaud's phenomenon does not occur proximal to the metacarpophalangeal joints; it most commonly affects the middle 3 fingers and rarely affects the thumb. Vasospasm may last minutes to hours but is rarely severe enough to cause tissue loss.

Raynaud's phenomenon secondary to a connective tissue disorder may progress to painful digital gangrene; Raynaud's phenomenon secondary to scleroderma tends to cause extremely painful, infected ulcers on the fingertips.

Diagnosis

Diagnosis is made and primary and secondary forms are distinguished clinically, supported by nail fold capillaroscopy and blood testing. For nail fold capillaroscopy, a drop of immersion oil is placed at the fingernail base; nail fold capillaries are magnified and examined using an ophthalmoscope set at 10 to 40 diopters. Distorted or dilated capillary loops suggest a connective tissue disorder as the cause. Blood tests (eg, measurement of ESR, antinuclear antibodies, rheumatoid factor, anticentromere antibody, anti-SCL-70 antibody) are done to detect accompanying disorders.

Diagnostic criteria for primary Raynaud's phenomenon are age at onset < 40 (in ⅔ of cases), mild symmetric attacks affecting both hands, no tissue necrosis or gangrene, no history or physical findings suggesting another cause, and normal nail fold capillaries, ESR, and blood test results.

Diagnostic criteria for secondary Raynaud's phenomenon are age at onset > 30, severe painful attacks that may be asymmetric and unilateral, ischemic lesions, history and findings suggesting an accompanying disorder, enlarged and tortuous nail fold capillaries, and abnormal ESR and blood test results.

Raynaud's phenomenon differs from acrocyanosis, which causes persistent cyanosis that is not easily reversed and does not cause trophic changes, ulcers, or pain.

Treatment

Treatment of the primary form involves avoidance of cold, smoking cessation, and, if stress is a triggering factor, relaxation techniques (eg, biofeedback) or counseling. Drugs are used more often than behavioral treatments because of convenience. Vasodilating Ca channel blockers (extended-release nifedipine 60 to 90 mg po once/day, amlodipine 5 to 20 mg po once/day, felodipine 2.5 to 10 mg po bid, or isradipine 2.5 to 5 mg po bid) are most effective, followed by prazosin 1 to 5 mg po once/day or bid. Topical nitroglycerine paste, pentoxifylline 400 mg po bid or tid with meals, or both may be effective, but no evidence supports routine use. β-Blockers, clonidine, and ergot preparations are contraindicated because they cause vasoconstriction and may trigger or worsen symptoms.

Treatment of the secondary form focuses on the underlying disorder. Ca channel blockers or prazosin is also indicated. Antibiotics, analgesics, and, occasionally, surgical debridement may be necessary for ischemic ulcers. Low-dose aspirin may prevent thrombosis but theoretically may worsen vasospasm via prostaglandin inhibition. IV prostaglandins (alprostadil, epoprostenol, iloprost) appear to be effective and may be an option for patients with ischemic digits. However, these drugs are not yet widely available, and their role is yet to be defined. Cervical or local sympathectomy is controversial; it is reserved for patients with progressive disability unresponsive to all other measures, including treatment of underlying disorders. Sympathectomy often abolishes the symptoms, but relief may last only 1 to 2 yr.

THROMBOANGIITIS OBLITERANS

(Buerger's disease)

Thromboangiitis obliterans is inflammatory thrombosis of small and medium-sized arteries and some superficial veins, causing arterial ischemia in distal extremities and superficial thrombophlebitis. Tobacco use is the primary risk factor. Symptoms and signs include claudication, nonhealing foot ulcers, rest pain, and gangrene. Diagnosis is by clinical findings, noninvasive vascular testing, angiography, and exclusion of other causes. Treatment is cessation of tobacco use; prognosis is excellent when tobacco use is stopped, but when it is not, the disorder inevitably progresses, often requiring amputation.

Thromboangiitis obliterans occurs almost exclusively in tobacco users (nearly all of them smokers) and predominantly affects men aged 20 to 40; only about 5% of cases occur in women. It occurs more commonly in people with HLA-A9 and HLA-B5 genotypes. Prevalence is highest in Asia and the Far and Middle East.

Thromboangiitis obliterans produces segmental inflammation in small and medium-sized arteries and, frequently, in superficial veins of the extremities. In acute thromboangiitis obliterans, occlusive thrombi accompany neutrophilic and lymphocytic infiltration of the intima; endothelial cells proliferate, but the internal elastic lamina remains intact. In an intermediate phase, thrombi organize and recanalize incompletely; the media is preserved but may be infiltrated with fibroblasts. In older lesions, periarterial fibrosis may occur, sometimes affecting the adjacent vein and nerve.

The cause is unknown, although cigarette smoking is a primary risk factor. The mechanism may involve delayed hypersensitivity or toxic angiitis. According to another theory, thromboangiitis obliterans may be an autoimmune disorder caused by cell-mediated sensitivity to types I and III human collagen, which are constituents of blood vessels.

Symptoms and Signs

Symptoms and signs are those of arterial ischemia and superficial thrombophlebitis. About 40% of patients have a history of migratory phlebitis, usually in the superficial veins of a foot or leg. Onset is gradual, starting in the most distal vessels of the upper and lower extremities and progressing proximally, culminating in distal gangrene and persistent pain. Coldness, numbness, tingling, or burning may develop before objective evidence of disease. Raynaud's phenomenon is common. Intermittent claudication occurs in the affected extremity (usually in the arch of the foot or in the leg; rarely in the hand, arm, or thigh) and may progress to rest pain. Frequently, if pain is severe and persistent, the affected leg feels cold, sweats excessively, and becomes cyanotic, probably because of sympathetic nerve overactivity. Ischemic ulcers develop in most patients and may progress to gangrene.

Pulses are impaired or absent in one or more pedal arteries and often at the wrist. In young men who smoke and have extremity ulcers, a positive Allen's test (the hand remains pale after the examiner simultaneously compresses the radial and ulnar arteries, then alternately releases them) suggests the disorder. Pallor with elevation and rubor with dependency frequently occur in affected hands, feet, or digits. Ischemic ulceration and gangrene, usually of one or more digits, may occur early in the disorder but not acutely. Noninvasive tests show greatly decreased blood flow and pressure in the affected toes, feet, and fingers.

Diagnosis

History and physical examination suggest the diagnosis. It is confirmed when the ankle-brachial index (ratio of ankle to arm systolic BP) for legs or segmental pressures for arms indicates distal ischemia, when echocardiography excludes cardiac emboli, when blood tests (eg, measurement of antinuclear antibody, rheumatoid factor, complement, anticentromere antibody, anti-SCL-70 antibody) exclude vasculitis, when tests for antiphospholipid antibodies exclude antiphospholipid antibody syndrome (although these levels may be slightly elevated in thromboangiitis obliterans), and when angiography shows characteristic findings (segmental occlusions of the distal arteries in the hands and feet, tortuous, corkscrew collateral vessels around occlusions, and no atherosclerosis).

Treatment

Treatment is cessation of tobacco use (see p. 2733). Continuing to use tobacco inevitably leads to disease progression and severe ischemia, often requiring amputation.

Other measures include avoiding cold; drugs that can cause vasoconstriction; and thermal, chemical, and mechanical injury, especially that due to poorly fitting footwear. For patients in the 1st phase of smoking cessation, iloprost 0.5 to 3 ng/kg/min IV infusion over 6 h may help prevent amputation. Pentoxifylline, Ca channel blockers, and thromboxane inhibitors may be tried empirically, but no data support their use. Use of antiendothelial cell antibody measurements to follow the course of disease is being studied.

81 PERIPHERAL VENOUS AND LYMPHATIC DISORDERS

Venous and lymphatic disorders usually involve impairment of flow, abnormal vessel dilation, or both.

DEEP VENOUS THROMBOSIS

Deep venous thrombosis (DVT) is clotting of blood in a deep vein of an extremity (usually calf or thigh) or the pelvis. DVT is the primary cause of pulmonary embolism. DVT results from conditions that impair venous return, lead to endothelial injury or dysfunction, or cause hypercoagulability. DVT may be asymptomatic or cause pain and swelling in an extremity. Diagnosis is by history, physical examination, and duplex ultrasonography, with D-dimer or other testing as necessary. Treatment is with

anticoagulants. Prognosis is generally good with prompt, adequate treatment; common long-term complications include venous insufficiency with or without postphlebitic syndrome.

DVT can develop in deep veins of the upper extremities (4 to 13% of DVT cases), lower extremities, or pelvis (see FIG. 81–1). Lower extremity DVT is much more likely to cause pulmonary embolism (PE), possibly because of the higher clot burden. The superficial femoral and popliteal veins in the thighs and the posterior tibial veins in the calves are most commonly affected. Calf vein DVT is less likely to be a source of large emboli but can cause repeated showers of small emboli or propagate to the proximal thigh veins and from there cause PE. About 50% of patients with DVT have occult PE, and about 20% with PE have demonstrable DVT.

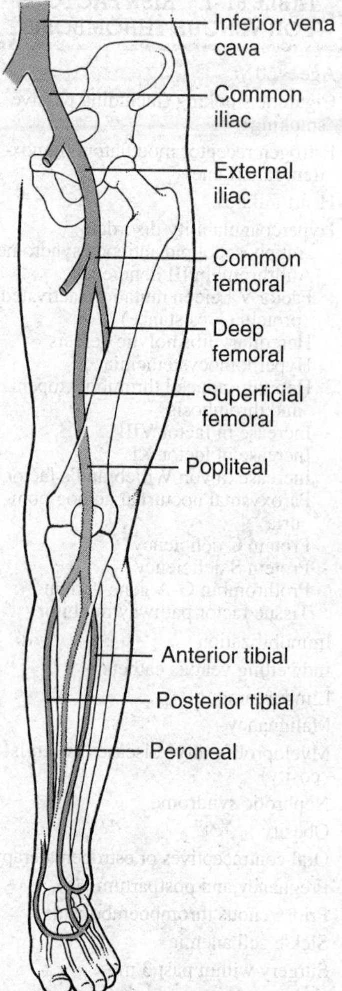

Fig. 81–1. Deep veins.

Etiology and Pathophysiology

Many factors can contribute to DVT (see TABLE 81–1). Lower extremity DVT most often results from impaired venous return (eg, in immobilized patients), endothelial injury or dysfunction (eg, after leg fractures), or hypercoagulability.

Upper extremity DVT most often results from endothelial injury due to central venous catheters, pacemakers, or injection drug use. Upper extremity DVT occasionally occurs as part of superior vena cava (SVC) syndrome or results from a hypercoagulable state or subclavian vein compression at the thoracic outlet; the compression may be due to a normal or an accessory 1st rib or fibrous band (thoracic outlet syndrome) or occur during strenuous arm activity (effort thrombosis, or Paget Schroetter syndrome, which accounts for 1 to 4% of upper extremity DVT cases).

Many malignancies predispose to DVT, and DVT is a known harbinger of some occult cancers. However, 85 to 90% of patients with DVT have no underlying malignancy.

DVT usually begins in venous valve cusps. Thrombi consist of thrombin, fibrin, and RBCs with relatively few platelets (red thrombi); without treatment, thrombi may propagate proximally, embolize within days, or both.

Common complications include chronic venous insufficiency and postphlebitic syndrome, as well as PE. Much less commonly, acute DVT leads to phlegmasia alba dolens or phlegmasia cerulea dolens, both of which, unless promptly diagnosed and treated, can result in venous (wet) gangrene.

In phlegmasia alba dolens, a rare complication of DVT during pregnancy, the leg turns milky white. Pathophysiology is unclear, but edema may increase soft-tissue pressure beyond capillary perfusion pressures. Ischemia develops only if capillary flow becomes impaired; the result is wet gangrene.

In phlegmasia cerulea dolens, massive iliofemoral venous thrombosis causes near total venous occlusion; the leg becomes

TABLE 81–1. RISK FACTORS FOR VENOUS THROMBOSIS

Age > 60 yr
Cigarette smoking (including passive smoking)
Estrogen receptor modulators (tamoxifen, raloxifene)
Heart failure
Hypercoagulability disorders
- Antiphospholipid antibody syndrome
- Antithrombin III deficiency
- Factor V Leiden mutation (activated protein C resistance)
- Hereditary fibrinolytic defects
- Hyperhomocysteinemia
- Heparin-induced thrombocytopenia and thrombosis
- Increase in factor VIII
- Increase in factor XI
- Increase in von Willebrand's factor
- Paroxysmal nocturnal hemoglobinuria
- Protein C deficiency
- Protein S deficiency
- Prothrombin G-A gene variant
- Tissue factor pathway inhibitor

Immobilization
Indwelling venous catheters
Limb trauma
Malignancy
Myeloproliferative disease (hyperviscosity)
Nephrotic syndrome
Obesity
Oral contraceptives or estrogen therapy
Pregnancy and postpartum
Prior venous thromboembolism
Sickle cell anemia
Surgery within past 3 mo

ischemic, extremely painful, and cyanotic. Pathophysiology may involve complete stasis of venous and arterial blood flow in the lower extremity because venous return is occluded or massive edema cuts off arterial blood flow. Wet gangrene may result.

DVT variants are uncommon. Suppurative (septic) thrombophlebitis, a bacterial infection of a superficial peripheral vein, is usually caused by venous catheterization that leads to infection and clotting. Jugular vein suppurative thrombophlebitis (Lemierre's syndrome), a bacterial (usually anaerobic) infection of the internal jugular vein and surrounding soft tissues, may follow tonsillopharyngitis and is often complicated by bacteremia and sepsis. In septic pelvic thrombophlebitis, pelvic thromboses develop postpartum, causing periodic fever.

Thrombophlebitis without DVT is most commonly caused by IV catheterization or infusion or injection drug use.

Symptoms and Signs

Most deep vein thrombi occur in the small calf veins and are asymptomatic and never detected. When present, symptoms and signs (eg, vague aching pain, tenderness along the distribution of the veins, edema, erythema) are nonspecific, vary in frequency and severity, and are similar in arms and legs. Dilated collateral superficial veins may become visible or palpable. Calf discomfort elicited by ankle dorsiflexion with the knee extended (Homans' sign) occasionally occurs with distal leg DVT but is neither sensitive nor specific. Leg tenderness, swelling of the whole leg, > 3 cm difference in circumference between calves, pitting edema, and collateral superficial veins may be most predictive; DVT is likely with a combination of 3 or more in the absence of another likely diagnosis (see TABLE 81–2). Low-grade fever may be present; DVT may be the cause of FUO, especially in postoperative patients. If PE occurs, symptoms include shortness of breath and pleuritic chest pain (see p. 414).

Common causes of asymmetric leg swelling that mimic DVT are superficial phlebitis, soft-tissue trauma, cellulitis, pelvic venous or lymphatic obstruction, and popliteal bursitis (Baker's cyst) that obstructs venous return. Abdominal or pelvic tumors are less common causes. Use of drugs that cause dependent edema (eg, dihydropyridine Ca channel blockers, estrogen, high-dose opioids), venous hypertension (usually due to right heart failure), and hypoalbuminemia cause symmetric bilateral leg swelling; swelling may be asymmetric if venous insufficiency coexists and is worse in one leg.

Common causes of calf pain that mimic acute DVT include venous insufficiency and postphlebitic syndrome; cellulitis that causes painful erythema of the calf; ruptured popliteal (Baker's) cyst, which causes calf swelling, pain, and sometimes bruising in the region of the medial malleolus (pseudo-DVT); and partial or complete tears of the gastrocnemius or plantaris tendon.

Diagnosis

History and physical examination help determine probability of DVT before testing (see TABLE 81–2). Diagnosis is by ultrasonography with Doppler flow studies (duplex ultrasonography). The need for additional tests (eg, D-dimer testing) and their choice and sequence depend on ultrasonography results plus pretest probability . No single testing protocol is best.

Ultrasonography identifies thrombi by directly visualizing the venous lining and by demonstrating abnormal vein compressibility or, with Doppler flow studies, impaired venous flow. The test is > 90% sensitive and > 95% specific for femoral and popliteal vein thrombosis but is less accurate for iliac or calf vein thrombosis.

If pretest probability of DVT is moderate or high, D-dimer testing should be done at the same time as duplex ultrasonography. D-dimer is a by-product of fibrinolysis; elevated levels suggest recent presence and lysis of thrombi. The test is > 90% sensitive but only 5% specific; thus, elevated levels do not assist with diagnosis, but absence of circulating D-dimer helps exclude DVT, especially when initial estimates of likelihood of DVT are < 50% and duplex ultrasonography results are negative. DVT and PE have occurred when D-dimer levels using enzyme-linked immunosorbent assays (ELISA) were negative; however, newer latex- or whole blood-agglutination assays, which are more specific and rapid, are likely to make D-dimer testing reliable enough for routine use to exclude DVT when probability of DVT is low or moderate.

Contrast venography is rarely used because the radiopaque dye can cause venous thrombosis and allergic reactions and because ultrasonography is noninvasive, more readily available, and almost equally accurate for detecting DVT. Venography may be indicated when ultrasonography results are normal but pretest suspicion for DVT is high or when ultrasonography results are abnormal and suspicion for DVT is low. The complication rate is 2%, mostly because of contrast dye allergy.

Noninvasive alternatives to contrast venography are being studied. They include magnetic resonance venography and direct MRI of thrombi using T1-weighted gradient-echo sequencing and a water-excitation radiofrequency pulse; theoretically, the latter can provide simultaneous views of thrombi in deep veins and subsegmental pulmonary arteries.

Patients with confirmed DVT and an obvious cause (eg, immobilization, surgical procedure, leg trauma) need no further testing. If symptoms and signs suggest PE, additional imaging (eg, ventilation/perfusion [V/Q] scanning or helical CT) is required.

Testing to detect hypercoagulability is controversial but is sometimes done in patients who have idiopathic recurrent DVT, in patients who have DVT and a personal or family history of other thromboses, and in young patients with no obvious predisposing factors. Some evidence suggests that presence of hypercoagulability does not predict DVT recurrence as well as clinical risk factors. Screening patients with DVT for malignancy has a low yield. Routine preventive screening, with a complete history and physical examination aimed at detecting malignancy and organ-specific testing as indicated by examination, is probably adequate.

TABLE 81–2. PROBABILITY OF DEEP VENOUS THROMBOSIS BASED ON CLINICAL FACTORS

Factors

Tenderness along distribution of the veins in calf or thigh

Swelling of entire leg

Calf swelling (> 3 cm difference in circumference between calves, measured 10 cm below tibial tuberosity)

Pitting edema greater in affected leg

Dilated collateral superficial veins

Malignancy (including cases in which treatment was stopped within 6 mo)

Immobilization of lower extremity (eg, due to paralysis, paresis, casting)

Surgery leading to immobility for > 3 days within past 4 wk

Another diagnosis as likely as or more likely than deep venous thrombosis

Probability

Probability equals the number of factors, subtracting 2 if another diagnosis is as likely as or more likely than DVT.

High probability:	≥ 3 points
Moderate probability:	1–2 points
Low probability:	≤ 0 points

Based on data from Anand SS Well, PS, Hunt, D et al: *JAMA* 279(14):1094–1099,1998.

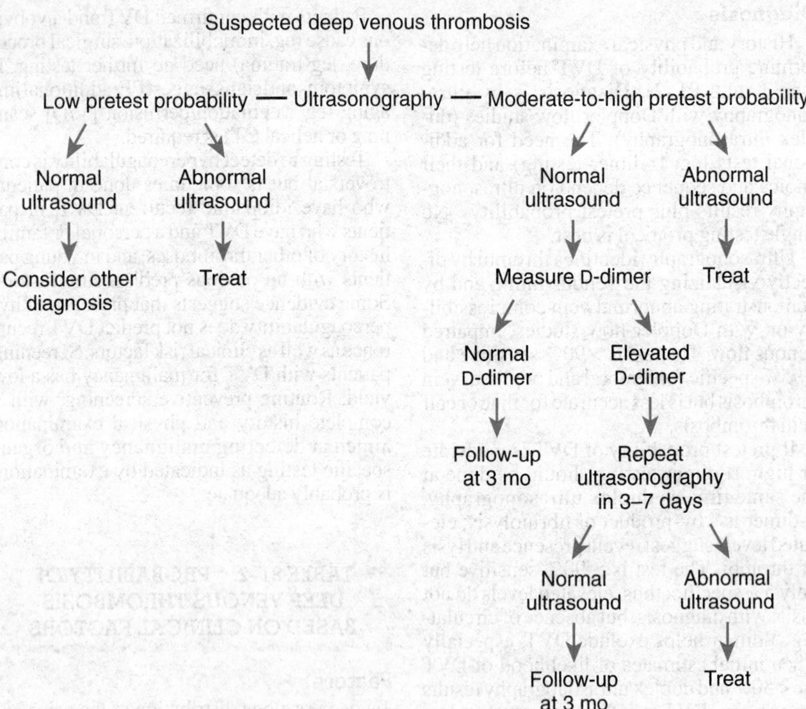

Fig. 81–2. One approach to testing for suspected deep venous thrombosis.

Prognosis

Without adequate treatment, lower extremity DVT has a 3% risk of fatal PE; death due to upper extremity DVT is very rare. Risk of recurrent DVT is least for patients with transient risk factors (eg, surgery, trauma, temporary immobility) and greatest for patients with persistent risk factors (eg, heart failure, malignancy), idiopathic DVT, or incomplete resolution of past DVT (residual thrombus). A D-dimer level of < 250 ng/mL after warfarin is stopped may help predict a relatively low risk of DVT or PE recurrence. Risk of venous insufficiency is impossible to predict. Risk factors for postphlebitic syndrome include proximal thrombosis, recurrent ipsilateral DVT, overweight (BMI 22 to 30 kg/m^2), and obesity (BMI > 30 kg/m^2).

Treatment

Treatment is aimed primarily at PE prevention (see also p. 420) and secondarily at symptom relief and prevention of chronic venous insufficiency and postphlebitic syndrome. Treatment of lower and upper extremity DVT is generally the same.

All patients with DVT are given anticoagulants, initially an injectable heparin (unfractionated or low mol wt), followed by warfarin started within 24 to 48 h. Inadequate anticoagulation in the first 24 h may increase risk of PE. Acute DVT can be treated on an outpatient basis unless PE is suspected, severe symptoms require parenteral analgesics, other disorders preclude safe outpatient discharge, or other factors (eg, functional, socioeconomic) might prevent the patient from adhering to prescribed treatments. General supportive measures include pain control with analgesics other than aspirin and NSAIDS (because of their antiplatelet effects) and, during periods of inactivity, elevation of legs (supported by a pillow or other soft surface to avoid venous compression). Patients may be as physically active as they can tolerate; there is no evidence that early activity increases risk of clot dislodgement and PE.

Anticoagulants: Low mol wt heparins (LMWH; eg, enoxaparin, dalteparin, reviparin, tinzaparin—see TABLE 50–5 on p. 422) are the initial treatment of choice because they can be given on an outpatient basis. LMWHs are as effective as unfractionated heparin (UFH) for reducing DVT recurrence, thrombus extension, and risk of death due to PE. Like UFH, LMWHs accelerate the action of antithrombin III (which inhibits coagulation factor proteases), leading to inactivation of coagulation factor Xa and, to a lesser degree, IIa. LMWHs also have some antithrombin III–mediated anti-inflammatory properties, which facilitate clot organization and resolution of symptoms and inflammation.

LMWHs are typically given sc in a standard weight-based dose (eg, enoxaparin 1.5 mg/kg sc once/day or 1 mg/kg sc q 2 h to a maximum of 200 mg/day or dalteparin 200 units/kg sc once/day). Obese patients may require higher doses; cachectic patients require lower doses. Patients with renal failure are best treated with UFH. Monitoring is unnecessary because LMWHs do not significantly prolong the activated partial thromboplastin time (aPTT), responses are predictable, and there is no clear relationship between LMWH overdose and bleeding. Treatment is continued until full anticoagulation is achieved with warfarin. However, early evidence suggests that LMWH is effective for long-term DVT treatment in high-risk patients, and thus, LMWH may become an acceptable alternative to warfarin for some patients, although warfarin is likely to be the treatment of choice because of its low cost and ease of administration.

UFH may be used instead of LMWH for hospitalized patients and for patients who have renal insufficiency or failure (creatinine clearance 10 to 50 mL/min) because UFH is not cleared by the kidneys. UFH is given as a bolus and infusion (see TABLE 50–3 on p. 419) to achieve full anticoagulation, defined as aPTT 1.5 to 2.5 times that of the reference range (or a minimum serum heparin level of 0.2 to 0.4 units/mL measured by protamine titration assay). UFH 3500 to 5000 units sc q 8 to 12 h can be substituted for parenteral UFH to facilitate patient mobility; the dose can be adjusted based on aPTT, measured before dosing. Treatment is continued until full anticoagulation has been achieved with warfarin.

Complications of heparin include bleeding, thrombocytopenia (rare with LMWHs), urticaria, and, rarely, thrombosis and anaphylaxis. Long-term use of UFH causes hypokalemia, liver enzyme elevations, and osteoporosis. Rarely, UFH given sc causes skin necrosis. Inpatients and possibly outpatients should be screened for bleeding with serial CBCs and tests for occult blood in stool. Bleeding due to overheparinization can be stopped with protamine sulfate. The dose is 1 mg protamine for each mg LMWH given as 1 mg in 20 mL normal saline infused slowly over 10 to 20 min. If a 2nd dose is required, it should be at ½ the 1st dose. However, the precise dose is undefined because protamine only partially neutralizes LMWH inactivation of factor Xa. With all infusions, the patient should be observed for hypotension and a reaction similar to an anaphylactic-like reaction.

Warfarin is the drug of choice for long-term anticoagulation for all patients except pregnant women (who should continue to take heparin) and patients who have had new or worsening venous thromboembolism during warfarin treatment (who may be candidates for an inferior vena cava filter). Warfarin 5 to 10 mg can be started immediately with heparin, except in patients with protein C deficiency in whom full anticoagulation with heparin (aPTT: 1.5 to 2.5 times the reference range) should be achieved before warfarin is started. The elderly and patients with a liver disorder typically require lower warfarin doses. Therapeutic goal is an INR of 2.0 to 3.0. INR is monitored weekly for the first 1 to 2 mo of warfarin treatment and monthly thereafter; the dose is increased or decreased by 0.5 to 3 mg to maintain the INR within this range. Patients taking warfarin should be informed of possible drug interactions, including interactions with nonprescription medicinal herbs.

Patients with transient risk factors for DVT (eg, immobilization, surgery) can discontinue warfarin after 3 to 6 mo. Patients with nonmodifiable risk factors (eg, hypercoagulability), spontaneous DVT with no known risk factors, or recurrent DVT and patients who have had PE should take warfarin for at least 6 mo and probably for life unless complications occur. In low-risk patients, low-intensity warfarin (to maintain INR at 1.5 to 2.0) may be safe and effective for at least 2 to 4 yr, but this treatment requires further proof of safety before it can be routinely recommended.

Bleeding is the most common complication. Risk factors for major bleeding (defined as life-threatening hemorrhage or loss of ≥ 2 units of blood in ≤ 7 days) include age ≥ 65; history of prior GI bleeding or stroke; recent MI; and coexisting anemia (Hct < 30%), renal insufficiency (serum creatinine > 1.5 mg/dL), or diabetes. Anticoagulation can be reversed with vitamin K; the dose is 1 to 4 mg po if INR is 5 to 9, 5 mg po if INR is > 9, and 10 mg IV (given slowly to avoid anaphylaxis) if hemorrhage occurs. If hemorrhage is severe, a transfusion of coagulation factors, fresh frozen plasma, or prothrombin complex concentrate should also be given. Overanticoagulation (INR > 3 or 4) without bleeding can be managed by omitting several doses and more frequent INR monitoring, then giving warfarin at a lower dose. Rarely, warfarin causes skin necrosis in patients with protein C or S deficiency or factor V Leiden mutations.

Other anticoagulants, such as direct thrombin inhibitors (eg, hirudin given sc, lepirudin, bivalirudin, desirudin, argatroban, ximelagatran) and selective factor Xa inhibitors (eg, fondaparinux), are being studied for treatment of acute DVT. Ximelagatran is an oral prodrug that is metabolized to melagatran (a direct thrombin inhibitor that is difficult to administer); ximelagatran requires no patient monitoring and appears comparable in efficacy to LMWH and warfarin.

Inferior vena cava filter (IVCF): An IVCF may help prevent PE in patients with lower extremity DVT and contraindications to anticoagulants or with recurrent DVT (or emboli) despite adequate anticoagulation. An IVCF is placed in the inferior vena cava just below the renal veins via catheterization of an internal jugular or femoral vein. IVCFs reduce risk of acute and subacute thrombotic complications but can have longer-term complications (eg, venous collaterals can develop, providing a pathway for emboli to circumvent the IVCF). Also, IVCFs can dislodge. Thus, patients with recurrent DVT or nonmodifiable risk factors for DVT may still require anticoagulation; IVCFs provide some protection until contraindications to anticoagulation subside or resolve. Despite widespread use of IVCFs, efficacy in preventing PE is unstudied and unproved.

Thrombolytic drugs: Streptokinase, urokinase, and alteplase lyse clots and appear to more effectively prevent postphlebitic syndrome than heparin alone, but risk of bleeding is higher. Their use is under study. Thrombolytics may be indicated for large proximal thrombi, especially those in the iliofemoral veins, and for phlegmasia alba or cerulea dolens. Local perfusion with an indwelling catheter may be preferable to IV administration.

Surgery: Surgery is rarely needed. However, thrombectomy, fasciotomy, or both are mandatory for phlegmasia alba or cerulea dolens unresponsive to thrombolytics to try to prevent limb-threatening gangrene.

Prevention

Patients at low risk of DVT (eg, those who are undergoing minor surgery but have no clinical risk factors for DVT; those who must be temporarily inactive for long periods, as during an airplane flight) should be encouraged to walk or otherwise move their legs periodically; no medical treatment is needed. Dorsiflexion 10 times/h is probably sufficient.

Patients at higher risk of DVT (eg, those undergoing minor surgery if they have clinical risk factors for DVT; those undergoing major surgery, especially orthopedic surgery, even without risk factors; bedbound patients) require additional preventive treatment (see Table 50–4 on p. 421). Most of these patients can be identified and treated before a thrombus forms. After surgery, elevating the legs and avoiding sitting in chairs (which, by placing the legs in a dependent position, impedes venous return) can help. Additional treatment may involve low-dose UFH, LMWH, warfarin, newer anticoagulants, compression devices or stockings, or a combination, depending on patient's risk level, type of surgery (if applicable), projected duration of preventive treatment, contraindications, adverse effects, relative cost, ease of use, and local practice.

Low-dose UFH 5000 units sc is given 2 h before surgery and q 8 to 12 h thereafter for 7 to 10 days or until patients are fully ambulatory. Bedbound patients who are not undergoing surgery are given 5000 units sc q 12 h indefinitely or until risk factors are reversed.

LMWHs are more effective than low-dose UFH for preventing DVT and PE, but widespread use is limited by cost. Enoxaparin 30 mg sc q 12 h, dalteparin 2500 units once/day, and tinzaparin 3500 units once/day are equally effective.

Warfarin 2 to 5 mg once/day or at a dose adjusted to maintain an INR of 1.5 to 2 is given routinely, but efficacy and safety are unproved.

Newer anticoagulants (eg, hirudin, ximelagatran, danaparoid, fondaparinux) are effective for preventing DVT and PE, but their cost-effectiveness and safety compared with heparin and warfarin require further study. Aspirin is better than placebo but worse than all other available drugs for preventing DVT and PE (see TABLE 50–5 on p. 422).

Intermittent pneumatic compression (IPC) uses a pump to cyclically inflate and deflate hollow plastic leggings, providing external compression to the lower legs and sometimes thighs. Intermittent pneumatic compression (IPC) may be used instead of or with anticoagulants before and during surgery. IPC is more effective for preventing calf than proximal DVT and is thus considered inadequate after hip or knee surgery. IPC is usually contraindicated in obese patients and can theoretically trigger PE in immobilized patients who, without preventive treatment, develop occult DVT.

The benefit of graded compression stockings is questionable except for low-risk surgical patients. However, combining stockings with other preventive measures may be more protective than any single approach.

For surgical procedures or disorders with a high incidence of venous thromboembolism (eg, orthopedic surgery, elective neurosurgery, spinal cord injury, multiple trauma), neither low-dose UFH nor aspirin is adequate. For hip and lower-extremity orthopedic surgery, LMWH or adjusted-dose warfarin is recommended. For total knee replacement, LMWH and IPC are comparable, and the combination should be considered for patients with clinical risk factors. For orthopedic surgery, preventive treatment should be started before surgery and continued for at least 7 days afterward. For neurosurgery, physical measures (IPC, elastic stockings) have been used because intracranial bleeding is a concern; however, LMWH appears to be an acceptable alternative. The combination of IPC and LMWH may be more effective than either alone in high-risk patients. Limited data support the combination of IPC, elastic stockings, and LMWH in patients with spinal cord injury or multiple trauma.

For patients who are at very high risk of venous thromboembolism and bleeding and are taking anticoagulants, IVCF placement is an option.

Preventive treatment is also indicated for patients who have had an acute MI or ischemic stroke. Low-dose UFH is effective in patients who are not already receiving IV heparin or thrombolytics; IPC, elastic stockings, or both may be used when anticoagulants are contraindicated. After a stroke, low-dose UFH or LMWH can be used; IPC, elastic stockings, or both may be beneficial. Other recommendations include low-dose UFH for patients with heart failure, adjusted-dose warfarin (INR 1.3 to 1.9) for those with metastatic breast cancer, and warfarin 1 mg once/day for those with cancer and an indwelling central venous catheter.

Primary prevention of venous insufficiency and postphlebitic syndrome is knee-high compression stockings providing 30 to 40 mm Hg pressure.

CHRONIC VENOUS INSUFFICIENCY AND POSTPHLEBITIC SYNDROME

Chronic venous insufficiency is impaired venous return, sometimes causing lower extremity discomfort, edema, and skin changes. Postphlebitic (postthrombotic) syndrome is symptomatic chronic venous insufficiency. Causes are disorders that result in venous hypertension, usually through venous damage or incompetence of venous valves, as occurs after deep venous thrombosis (DVT). Diagnosis is by history, physical examination, and duplex ultrasonography. Treatment is compression, wound care, and, rarely, surgery. Prevention requires adequate treatment of DVT and compression stockings.

Chronic venous insufficiency affects up to 5% of people in the US. Postphlebitic syndrome may affect $\frac{1}{5}$ to $\frac{2}{3}$ of patients with DVT, usually within 1 to 2 yr after acute DVT.

Etiology and Pathophysiology

Venous return from the lower extremities relies on contraction of calf muscles to push blood from intramuscular (soleal) sinusoids and gastrocnemius veins into and through deep veins. Venous valves direct blood proximally to the heart. Chronic venous insufficiency occurs when venous obstruction (eg, in DVT), venous valvular insufficiency, or decreased contraction of muscles surrounding the veins (eg, due to immobility) decrease forward venous flow and increase venous pressure (venous hypertension). Prolonged venous hypertension causes tissue edema, inflammation, and hypoxia, leading to

TABLE 81–3. CLINICAL CLASSIFICATION OF CHRONIC VENOUS INSUFFICIENCY

CLASS	SIGNS
0	No signs of venous disease
1	Ectatic or reticular veins*
2	Varicose veins*
3	Edema
4	Skin changes due to venous stasis (pigmentation, stasis dermatitis, lipodermatoclerosis)
5	Skin changes due to venous stasis and healed ulceration
6	Skin changes due to venous stasis and active ulceration

*May occur idiopathically without chronic venous insufficiency.

symptoms. Pressure may be transmitted to superficial veins if valves in perforator veins, which connect deep and superficial veins, are ineffective.

DVT is the most common identifiable risk factor for chronic venous insufficiency, followed by trauma, age, and obesity. Idiopathic cases are often attributed to a past history of occult DVT.

Symptomatic chronic venous insufficiency that follows DVT is referred to as postphlebitic (or postthrombotic) syndrome. Risk factors for postphlebitic syndrome in patients with DVT include proximal thrombosis, recurrent ipsilateral DVT, overweight (BMI 22 to 30 kg/m^2), and obesity (BMI > 30 kg/m^2). Age, female sex, and estrogen therapy are also associated with the syndrome but are probably nonspecific. Use of compression stockings after DVT decreases risk.

Symptoms and Signs

Chronic venous insufficiency may not cause any symptoms but always causes signs; postphlebitic syndrome always causes symptoms but may not cause signs. Both disorders are a concern because their symptoms can mimic those of acute DVT and both can lead to substantial reductions in physical activity and quality of life.

Symptoms include a sense of fullness, heaviness, aching, cramps, tiredness, and paresthesias in the legs; these symptoms worsen with standing or walking and are relieved by rest and elevation. Pruritus may accompany skin changes. Signs occur along a continuum: no changes to varicose veins (rare) to stasis dermatitis on the lower legs and at the ankles, with or without ulceration (see TABLE 81–3).

Venous stasis dermatitis consists of reddish brown hyperpigmentation, induration, venous ectasia, lipodermatosclerosis (fibrosing subcutaneous panniculitis), and venous stasis ulcers; all of these effects indicate longer-standing disease or more severe venous hypertension.

Venous stasis ulcers may develop spontaneously or after affected skin is scratched or injured. They typically occur around the medial malleolus, tend to be shallow and moist, and may be malodorous (especially when poorly cared for) or painful. They do not penetrate the deep fascia. In contrast, ulcers due to peripheral arterial disease eventually expose tendons or bone.

Leg edema tends to be unilateral or asymmetric; bilateral symmetric edema is more likely to result from a systemic disorder (eg, heart failure, hypoalbuminemia) or certain drugs (eg, Ca blockers).

In general, unless the lower extremities are adequately cared for, patients with any manifestation of chronic venous insufficiency or postphlebitic syndrome are at risk of progression to more advanced forms.

Diagnosis

Diagnosis is usually based on history and physical examination. A clinical scoring system that ranks 5 symptoms (pain, cramps, heaviness, pruritus, paresthesia) and 6 signs (edema, hyperpigmentation, induration, venous ectasia, redness, pain with calf compression) on a scale of 0 (absent or minimal) to 3 (severe) is increasingly recognized as a standard diagnostic tool. Scores of 5 to 14 on 2 visits separated by ≥ 6 mo indicate mild-to-moderate disease, and scores of ≥ 15 indicate severe disease.

Lower-extremity duplex ultrasonography helps exclude DVT. Absence of edema and a reduced ankle-brachial index help distinguish peripheral arterial disease from chronic venous insufficiency and postphlebitic syndrome. Absence of ankle pulses suggests peripheral arterial disease.

Prevention and Treatment

Primary prevention involves adequate anticoagulation after DVT and use of compression stockings for up to 2 yr after DVT or lower extremity venous trauma. Lifestyle changes (eg, weight loss, regular exercise, reduction of dietary NaCl) are also important.

Treatment involves leg elevation; compression using bandages, stockings, and pneumatic devices; topical wound care; and surgery, depending on the disorder's severity. Drugs have no role in routine treatment of chronic venous insufficiency, although many patients are given aspirin, topical corticosteroids, diuretics for edema, or antibiotics. Some experts believe that weight loss, regular exercise, and reduction of dietary NaCl may benefit patients with bilateral chronic venous insufficiency. However, all interventions are difficult for many patients to implement.

Elevating the leg above the level of the right atrium decreases venous hypertension and edema, is appropriate for all patients, and should be done a minimum of 3 times/day for ≥ 30 min. However, most patients cannot adhere to this schedule during the day.

Compression is effective for treatment and prevention of the effects of chronic venous insufficiency and postphlebitic syndrome and is indicated for all patients. Elastic bandages are used initially until edema and ulcers resolve and leg size stabilizes; commercial compression stockings are then used. Stockings that provide 20 to 30 mm Hg of distal circumferential pressure are indicated for smaller varicose veins and mild chronic venous insufficiency; 30 to 40 mm Hg is indicated for larger varicose veins and moderate disease; and 40 to > 60 mm Hg is indicated for severe disease. Stockings should be put on when patients awaken, before leg edema worsens with activity, and should exert maximal pressure at the ankles and gradually less pressure proximally. Adherence to this treatment varies; many younger or more active patients consider stockings irritating, restricting, or cosmetically undesirable; older patients may have difficulty putting them on.

Intermittent pneumatic compression (IPC) uses a pump to cyclically inflate and deflate hollow plastic leggings. IPC provides external compression, squeezing blood and fluid out of the lower legs. It effectively treats severe postphlebitic syndrome and venous stasis ulcers but may be no more effective than compression stockings alone.

Topical wound care is important in venous stasis ulcer management (see full discussion on p. 1014). When an Unna boot (zinc oxide–impregnated bandages) is properly applied, covered by compression bandages, and changed weekly, almost all ulcers heal. Occlusive interactive dressings (eg, hydrocolloids such as aluminum chloride [DuoDERM]) provide a moist environment for wound healing and promote growth of new tissue; they may be used for ulcers with light to moderate exudate, but they probably add little to simple Unna bandaging and are expensive. Passive dressings are absorptive, making them most appropriate for heavier exudate.

Drugs have no role in routine treatment of chronic venous insufficiency, although many patients are given aspirin, topical corticosteroids, diuretics for edema, or antibiotics. Surgery (eg, venous ligation, stripping, valve reconstruction) is also generally ineffective. Grafting autologous skin or skin created from epidermal keratinocytes or dermal fibroblasts may be an option for patients with refractory stasis ulcers when all other measures are ineffective, but the graft will reulcerate unless underlying venous hypertension is managed.

SUPERFICIAL VENOUS THROMBOSIS

Superficial venous thrombosis is a blood clot in a superficial vein of the upper or lower extremities or, less commonly, in one or more veins of the chest or breast (Mondor's disease).

Superficial venous thrombosis in the upper extremity most commonly results from IV catheterization; varicose veins seem to be the main risk factor for the lower extremity, especially among women. Superficial venous thrombi rarely cause serious complications and rarely embolize.

Typically, patients present with a superficial, often painful or tender indurated cord contiguous with a palpable normal superficial vein. The overlying skin is usually warm and erythematous. Migratory superficial venous thrombosis, which develops, resolves, and recurs in normal veins of the arms, legs, and torso at various times, is a possible harbinger of pancreatic cancer and other adenocarcinomas (Trousseau's syndrome).

Diagnosis is based on history and physical examination. Treatment traditionally involves warm compresses and NSAIDs, but local thrombectomy with a local anesthetic is very effective.

VARICOSE VEINS

Varicose veins are dilated superficial veins in the lower extremities. Usually, no cause is obvious. Varicose veins are typically asymptomatic but may cause a sense of fullness, pressure, and pain or hyperesthesia in the legs. Diagnosis is by physical examination. Treatment is compression, wound care, sclerotherapy, and surgery.

Varicose veins may occur alone or with chronic venous insufficiency.

Etiology is usually unknown, but varicose veins may result from primary venous valvular insufficiency with reflux or from primary dilation of the vein wall due to structural weakness. In some people, varicose veins result from chronic venous insufficiency and venous hypertension. Most people have no obvious risk factors. Varicose veins are common within families, suggesting a genetic component. Varicose veins are more common among women because estrogen affects venous structure, pregnancy increases pelvic and leg venous pressures, or both. Rarely, varicose veins are part of Klippel-Trénaunay-Weber syndrome, which includes congenital arteriovenous fistulas and diffuse cutaneous capillary angiomas.

Symptoms, Signs, and Diagnosis

Varicose veins may initially be tense and palpable but are not necessarily visible. Later, they may progressively enlarge, protrude, and become obvious; they can cause a sense of fullness, fatigue, pressure, and superficial pain or hyperesthesia in the legs. Varicose veins are most visible when the patient stands. For unclear reasons, stasis dermatitis and venous stasis ulcers are uncommon. When skin changes (eg, induration, pigmentation, eczema) occur, they typically affect the medial malleolar region. Ulcers may develop after minimal trauma to an affected area; they are usually small, superficial, and painful. Varicose veins occasionally thrombose, causing pain. Superficial varicose veins may produce thin venous bullae in the skin, which may rupture and bleed after minimal trauma. Very rarely, such bleeding, if undetected during sleep, is fatal.

Diagnosis is usually obvious from the physical examination. Trendelenburg's test (comparing venous filling before and after release of a thigh tourniquet) is no longer used to identify retrograde blood flow past incompetent saphenous valves, partly because sensitivity, specificity, and observer variability for this maneuver have not been determined.

Treatment

Treatment aims to relieve symptoms, improve the leg's appearance, and, in some cases, prevent complications. Treatment includes compression stockings and local wound care as needed.

Injection therapy (sclerotherapy) and surgery are indicated for prevention of recurrent variceal thrombosis and for skin changes; these procedures are also commonly used for cosmetic reasons. Sclerotherapy uses an irritant (eg, sodium tetradecyl sulfate) to induce a thrombophlebitic reaction that fibroses and occludes the vein; however, many varicose veins recannulate. Surgery involves ligation or stripping of the long and sometimes the short saphenous veins. These procedures provide good short-term symptom relief, but long-term efficacy is poor.

Regardless of treatment, new varicose veins develop, and treatment often must be maintained indefinitely.

IDIOPATHIC TELANGIECTASIAS

Idiopathic telangiectasias are fine, dilated intracutaneous veins that are not clinically significant but may be extensive and unsightly.

Telangiectasias are usually asymptomatic. However, some patients report a burning sensation or pain, and many women consider even the smallest telangiectasias cosmetically unacceptable.

Telangiectasias can usually be eliminated by intracapillary injections of 0.3% solution of sodium tetradecyl sulfate through a fine-bore needle. Hypertonic saline 23.4% is sometimes used but causes fairly severe, temporary, localized pain; therefore, large areas of spider veins may require several treatments. Pigmentation may develop but usually subsides, often completely. Skin ulceration may result if the injection is extravascular or too large. Laser treatment is effective, but large areas require several treatments. Small telangiectasias may persist or recur after initial treatment.

ARTERIOVENOUS FISTULA

An arteriovenous fistula is an abnormal communication between an artery and a vein.

An arteriovenous fistula may be congenital (usually affecting smaller vessels) or acquired as a result of trauma (eg, a bullet or stab wound) or erosion of an arterial aneurysm into an adjacent vein.

The fistula may cause symptoms and signs of arterial insufficiency (eg, extremity ulceration due to reduced arterial flow, embolization, or ischemia) or chronic venous insufficiency due to high-pressure arterial flow in the affected veins (eg, peripheral edema, varicose veins, stasis pigmentation). If the fistula is near the surface, a mass can be felt, and the affected area is usually swollen and warm with distended, often pulsating superficial veins. A thrill can be palpated over the fistula, and a continuous loud, to-and-fro (machinery) murmur with accentuation during systole can be heard during auscultation. Rarely, if a significant portion of cardiac output is diverted through the fistula to the right heart, high-output heart failure develops.

Congenital fistulas need no treatment unless significant complications develop (eg, leg lengthening in a growing child). When necessary, percutaneous vascular techniques can be used to place coils or plugs into the vessels to occlude the fistula. Treatment is seldom completely successful, but complications are often controlled. Acquired fistulas usually have a single large connection and can be effectively treated by surgery.

LYMPHEDEMA

Lymphedema is edema of a limb due to lymphatic hypoplasia (primary) or to obstruction or disruption (secondary) of lymphatic vessels. Symptoms and signs are brawny, fibrous, nonpitting edema in one or more limbs. Diagnosis is by physical examination. Treatment consists of exercise, pressure gradient dressings, massage, and sometimes surgery. Cure is unusual, but treatment may lessen symptoms and slow or halt progression. Patients are at risk of cellulitis, lymphangitis, and, rarely, lymphangiosarcoma.

Classification and Etiology

Lymphedema may be primary (due to lymphatic hypoplasia) or secondary (due to obstruction or disruption of lymphatic vessels).

Primary lymphedemas: Primary lymphedemas are inherited and uncommon. They vary in phenotype and patient age at presentation.

Congenital lymphedema appears before age 2 and is due to lymphatic aplasia or hypoplasia. Milroy's disease is an autosomal dominant familial form of congenital lymphedema attributed to *VEGF3* mutations and sometimes associated with cholestatic jaundice and edema or diarrhea due to a protein-losing enteropathy caused by intestinal lymphangiectasia.

Lymphedema praecox appears between ages 2 and 35, typically in women at the onset of menses or pregnancy. Meige's disease is an autosomal dominant familial form of lymphedema praecox attributed to mutations in a transcription factor gene (*FOXC2*) and associated with extra eyelashes (distichiasis); cleft palate; and leg, arm, and sometimes facial edema.

Lymphedema tarda occurs after age 35. Familial and sporadic forms exist; the genetic basis of both is unknown. Clinical findings are similar to those of lymphedema praecox but may be less severe.

Lymphedema is prominent in other genetic syndromes, including Turner's syndrome; yellow nail syndrome, characterized by pleural effusions and yellow nails; and Hennekam syndrome, a rare congenital syndrome of intestinal and other lymphangiectases, facial anomalies, and mental retardation.

Secondary lymphedema: Secondary lymphedema is far more common than primary. It is most commonly caused by surgery (especially lymph node dissection, typically for breast cancer), radiation therapy (especially axillary or inguinal), trauma, lymphatic obstruction by a tumor, and, in developing countries, lymphatic filariasis. Mild lymphedema may also result from leakage of lymph into interstitial tissues in patients with chronic venous insufficiency.

Symptoms and Signs

Symptoms of secondary lymphedema include aching discomfort and a sensation of heaviness or fullness.

The cardinal sign is soft-tissue edema, graded in 3 stages. In stage 1, the edema is pitting, and the affected area often returns to normal by morning. In stage 2, the edema is nonpitting, and chronic soft-tissue inflammation causes early fibrosis. In stage 3, the edema is brawny and irreversible, largely because of soft-tissue fibrosis. The swelling is most often unilateral and may worsen during warm weather, before menstruation, and after a long time with the limb in a dependent position. It can affect any part of the limb (isolated proximal or distal) or the entire extremity; it can restrict range of motion when swelling is periarticular. Disability and emotional distress can be significant, especially when lymphedema results from medical or surgical treatment.

Skin changes are common and include hyperkeratosis, hyperpigmentation, verrucae, papillomas, and fungal infections.

Lymphangitis (see p. 985) may develop, most often when bacteria enter through skin cracks between the toes as a result of fungal infections or through cuts to the hand. Lymphangitis is almost always streptococcal, causing erysipelas; sometimes it is staphylococcal. The affected limb becomes red and feels hot; red streaks may extend proximally from the point of entry, and lymphadenopathy may develop. Rarely, the skin breaks down.

Diagnosis

Diagnosis is usually obvious from physical examination. Additional tests are indicated when secondary lymphedema is suspected. CT and MRI can identify sites of lymphatic obstruction; radionuclide lymphoscintigraphy can identify lymphatic hypoplasia or sluggish flow. Progression can be monitored by measuring limb circumference, measuring water volume displaced by the submerged limb, or using skin or soft-tissue tonometry; these tests have not been validated. In developing countries, tests for lymphatic filariasis should be done (see p. 1548).

Prognosis and Treatment

Cure is unusual once lymphedema occurs. Meticulous treatment and possibly preventive measures can lessen symptoms and slow or halt disease progression. Rarely, long-standing lymphedema leads to lymphangiosarcoma (Stewart-Treves syndrome), usually in postmastectomy patients and in patients with filariasis.

Treatment of primary lymphedema may include soft-tissue reduction and reconstruction if quality of life is significantly reduced.

Treatment of secondary lymphedema involves managing its cause. For lymphedema itself, several interventions to mobilize fluid (complex decongestive therapy) can be used. They include manual lymphatic drainage, in which the limb is elevated and "milked" toward the heart; gradient pressure bandages or sleeves; limb exercises; and limb massage, including intermittent pneumatic compression. Surgical soft-tissue reduction, lymphatic reanastomoses, and formation of drainage channels are sometimes tried but have not been rigorously studied.

Preventive measures include avoiding heat, vigorous exercise, and constrictive garments (including blood pressure cuffs) around the affected limb. Skin and nail care require meticulous attention; vaccination, phlebotomy, and IV catheterization in the affected limb should be avoided.

Lymphangitis is treated with β-lactamase–resistant antibiotics with gram-positive coverage (eg, oxacillin, cloxacillin, dicloxacillin).

82 SPORTS AND THE HEART

Exercise and athletic training are of significant overall cardiovascular benefit, but occasionally they have adverse consequences.

SUDDEN CARDIAC DEATH IN ATHLETES

An estimated 1/200,000 apparently healthy young athletes develops abrupt-onset ventricular tachycardia or fibrillation and dies suddenly during exercise. Males are affected 9 times more often; basketball and football players in the US and soccer players in Europe may be at highest risk.

Sudden cardiac death in young athletes has many causes (see TABLE 82–1), but the most common is undetected hypertrophic cardiomyopathy. Athletes with thin, compliant chest walls are at risk of commotio cordis (sudden ventricular tachycardia or fibrillation after a blow to the precordium) even when no cardiovascular disorder is present. The blow may involve a moderate-force projectile (eg, baseball, hockey puck, lacrosse ball) or impact with another player during a vulnerable phase of myocardial repolarization. Some young athletes die of aortic aneurysm rupture (in Marfan syndrome).

Sudden cardiac death in older athletes is generally caused by coronary artery disease. Occasionally, hypertrophic cardiomyopathy, mitral valve prolapse, or acquired valvular disease is involved.

In other conditions underlying sudden death in athletes (eg, asthma, heat stroke, illicit or performance-enhancing drug-related complications), ventricular tachycardia or fibrillation is a terminal, not a primary event.

Symptoms and signs are those of cardiovascular collapse; diagnosis is obvious. Immediate treatment with advanced cardiac life support is successful in < 20%; the percentage may increase as distribution of community-based, automated external defibrillators expands. For survivors, treatment is management of the underlying condition.

Screening

Before participation in sports, athletes are commonly screened to identify risk. Screening recommendations for all children, adolescents, and college-age young adults include a medical and family history and physical examination (including BP and supine and standing cardiac auscultation). Family history or symptoms or signs of hypertrophic cardiomyopathy or of Marfan syndrome require further evaluation; confirmation of either disorder may preclude sports participation. Athletes with presyncope or syncope should be evaluated for anomalous coronary arteries. Athletes should be counseled against use of illicit and performance-enhancing drugs. History and examination are neither sensitive nor specific; false-negative and false-positive findings are common because prevalence of cardiac disorders in an apparently healthy population is very low. Use of screening ECG or echocardiography would improve disease detection but would produce even more false-positive diagnoses and is impractical at a population level.

TABLE 82–1. CAUSES OF SUDDEN CARDIAC DEATH IN YOUNG ATHLETES*

Obstructive hypertrophic cardiomyopathy
Commotio cordis
Coronary artery anomalies (eg, anomalous left main coronary artery origin, anomalous right coronary artery origin, coronary arterial hypoplasia)
Increased cardiac mass
Myocarditis
Ruptured aortic aneurysm
Arrhythmogenic right ventricular dysplasia
Tunneled left anterior descending coronary artery
Aortic stenosis
Premature atherosclerotic coronary artery disease
Dilated cardiomyopathy
Myxomatous degeneration of mitral valve
Long QT syndrome
Brugada syndrome
Wolff-Parkinson-White syndrome (anterograde conduction only)
Catecholaminergic polymorphic tachycardia
Right ventricular outflow tract tachycardia
Coronary vasospasm
Cardiac sarcoidosis
Cardiac trauma
Ruptured cerebral artery aneurysm

*Causes are listed in approximate order of frequency.

ATHLETIC HEART SYNDROME

Athletic heart syndrome is a constellation of structural and functional changes that occur in the heart of people who train for > 1 h most days. The syndrome is asymptomatic; signs include bradycardia, a systolic murmur, and extra heart sounds. ECG abnormalities are common. Diagnosis is clinical or by echocardiography. No treatment is necessary. The syndrome is significant because it must be distinguished from serious cardiac disorders.

Intensive, prolonged endurance and strength training produces many physiologic adaptations. Volume and pressure loads in the left ventricle (LV) increase, which, over time, increase LV muscle mass, wall thickness, and chamber size. Maximal stroke volume and cardiac output increase, contributing to a lower resting heart rate and longer diastolic filling time. Lower heart rate results primarily from increased vagal tone, but decreased sympathetic activation and other nonautonomic factors that decrease intrinsic sinus node activity may play a role. Bradycardia decreases myocardial O_2 demand; at the same time, increases in total Hb and blood volume enhance O_2 transport. Despite these changes, systolic and diastolic function remains normal. Structural changes in women are typically less than those in men of the same age, body size, and training.

Symptoms and Signs

There are no symptoms. Signs vary but may include bradycardia; an LV impulse that is laterally displaced, enlarged, and increased in amplitude; a systolic ejection (flow) murmur at the left lower sternal border; a 3rd heart sound (S_3) due to early, rapid diastolic ventricular filling; a 4th heart sound (S_4), heard best during resting bradycardia because diastolic filling time is increased; and hyperdynamic carotid pulses. These signs reflect structural cardiac changes that are adaptive for intense exercise.

Diagnosis

Findings are typically detected during routine screening or during evaluation of unrelated symptoms. Most athletes do not require extensive testing, although ECG is often warranted. If symptoms suggest a cardiac disorder, ECG, echocardiography, and exercise stress testing are done.

Athletic heart syndrome is a diagnosis of exclusion; it must be distinguished from disorders that cause similar findings but are life threatening (eg, hypertrophic or dilated cardiomyopathies, ischemic heart disease, arrhythmogenic right ventricular dysplasia).

ECG typically shows sinus bradycardia; rarely, heart rate is < 40 beats/min. Sinus arrhythmia often accompanies the slow heart rate. Resting bradycardia may predispose to increased atrial or ventricular ectopy, including wandering supraventricular pacemaker and, uncommonly, atrial fibrillation, but pauses after ectopic beats do not exceed 4 sec. First-degree atrioventricular (AV) block is detected in up to $\frac{1}{3}$ of athletes; 2nd-degree AV block (mainly type 1) that occurs during rest but disappears with exercise is less common. Third-degree AV block is abnormal and should be investigated thoroughly. Waveform changes include high voltage QRS complexes with inferolateral T-wave changes or strain pattern, which reflect LV hypertrophy, and early depolarization changes with biphasic T waves in anterior leads, which reflect inhomogeneous repolarization from reduced resting sympathetic tone. Both resolve with exercise. Deep anterolateral T-wave inversion and incomplete right bundle branch block may also occur. ECG changes correlate poorly with level of training and cardiovascular performance.

Echocardiography can distinguish athletic heart syndrome from cardiomyopathies (see TABLE 82–2), but because there is a contin-

TABLE 82–2. FEATURES DISTINGUISHING ATHLETIC HEART SYNDROME FROM CARDIOMYOPATHY

FEATURE	ATHLETIC HEART SYNDROME	CARDIOMYOPATHY
Left ventricular hypertrophy*	< 13 mm	> 15 mm
Left ventricular end-diastolic diameter†	< 60 mm	> 70 mm
Diastolic function	Normal (E:A ratio > 1)	Abnormal (E:A ratio < 1)
Septal hypertrophy	Symmetric	Asymmetric (in hypertrophic cardiomyopathy)
Family history	None	May be present
BP response to exercise	Normal	Normal or reduced systolic BP response
Deconditioning	Left ventricular hypertrophy regression	No left ventricular hypertrophy regression

*A value of 13 to 15 mm is indeterminate.

†A value of 60 to 70 mm is indeterminate.

E:A ratio = ratio of early to late atrial transmitral flow velocity.

uum from physiologic to pathologic cardiac enlargement, the distinction is not always clear. In general, echocardiographic changes correlate poorly with level of training and cardiovascular performance. Trace mitral regurgitation and tricuspid regurgitation are commonly detected.

During exercise stress testing, heart rate remains lower than normal at submaximal stress and increases appropriately and comparably to nonathletes at maximal stress; it rapidly recovers after exercise. BP response is normal: Systolic BP increases, diastolic BP falls, and mean BP stays relatively constant. Many resting ECG changes decrease or disappear during exercise; this finding is unique to athletic heart syndrome, distinguishing it from pathologic conditions. However, pseudonormalization of T-wave inversions could reflect myocardial ischemia and thus warrants further investigation in older athletes.

Prognosis and Treatment

Although gross structural changes resemble those in some cardiac disorders, no adverse effects are apparent. In most cases, structural changes and bradycardia regress with detraining, although up to 20% of elite athletes have residual chamber enlargement, raising questions, in the absence of long-term data, about whether the athletic heart syndrome is truly benign.

No treatment is required, although 3 mo of deconditioning may be needed to monitor LV regression as a way of distinguishing this syndrome from cardiomyopathy. Such deconditioning can greatly interfere with an athlete's life and may meet with resistance.

83 CARDIAC TUMORS

Cardiac tumors may be primary (benign or malignant) or metastatic (malignant). Myxoma, a benign primary tumor, is the most common type. Cardiac tumors may occur in any cardiac tissue; they can cause valvular or inflow-outflow tract obstruction, thromboembolism, arrhythmias, or pericardial disorders. Diagnosis is by echocardiography followed by biopsy. Treatment of benign tumors is usually surgical resection; recurrence is common. Treatment of metastatic malignancy depends on tumor type and origin; prognosis is generally poor.

Primary cardiac tumors are found in < 1/2000 people at autopsy; metastatic tumors are 30 to 40 times more common. Usually, primary cardiac tumors originate in the myocardium or endocardium; they may also originate in valve tissue, cardiac connective tissue, or the pericardium.

Classification

Benign primary tumors: Examples are myxomas, papillary fibroelastomas, rhabdomyomas, fibromas, hemangiomas, teratomas, lipomas, paragangliomas, and pericardial cysts.

Myxoma is most common, accounting for 50% of all primary cardiac tumors. Incidence in women is 2 to 4 times that in men; in uncommon familial forms (Carney complex), men are affected more often. About 75% of myxomas occur in the left atrium; the rest occur in the other chambers as a solitary tumor or, less commonly, at several sites. About 75% are pedunculated and may prolapse through the mitral valve and obstruct ventricular filling during diastole; the remainder are broad-based and sessile. Myxomas may be myxoid and gelatinous; smooth, firm, and lobular; or friable and irregular. Friable irregular myxomas increase risk of systemic embolism.

Carney complex is a familial, autosomal dominant syndrome of recurrent cardiac myxomas with some combination of cutaneous myxomas, myxoid mammary fibroadenomas, pigmented skin lesions (lentigines, ephelides, blue nevi), multiple endocrine neoplasia (primary pigmented nodular adrenocortical disease causing Cushing's syndrome, growth hormone and prolactin-producing pituitary adenoma, testicular tumors, thyroid adenoma or carcinoma, and ovarian cysts), psammomatous melanotic schwannoma, breast ductal adenoma, and osteochondromyxoma. Patients are often younger at presentation (median age, 20 yr), have multiple myxomas (particularly in the ventricles), and have a higher risk of myxoma recurrence.

Papillary fibroelastomas are the 2nd most common benign primary tumor. They are avascular papillomas that predominantly occur on the aortic and mitral valves. Men and women are affected equally. They have papillary fronds branching from a central core, resembling sea anemones. About 45% are pedunculated. They do not cause valvular dysfunction but increase risk of embolism.

Rhabdomyomas account for 20% of all primary cardiac tumors and 90% of those in children. Rhabdomyomas affect mainly infants and children, 50% of whom also have tuberous sclerosis. Rhabdomyomas are usually multiple and located intramurally in the septum or free wall of the left ventricle, where they affect the cardiac conduction system. They are firm white lobules that typically regress with age; a minority of patients develop tachyarrhythmias and heart failure due to left ventricular outflow tract obstruction.

Fibromas also affect mainly children; they are associated with adenoma sebaceum of the skin and kidney tumors. They occur primarily on valve tissue and may develop in response to inflammation. They can compress or invade the cardiac conduction system, causing arrhythmias and sudden death. Some fibromas occur as part of a syndrome with generalized body overgrowth, jaw keratocytes, skeletal abnormalities, and various benign and malignant tumors (Gorlin's or basal cell nevus syndrome).

Hemangiomas account for 5 to 10% of benign tumors. They cause symptoms in a minority of patients. Most often, they are incidentally detected during examinations done for other reasons.

Teratomas of the pericardium affect mainly infants and children; they are often attached to the base of the great vessels. About 90% are located in the anterior mediastinum; the rest, mainly in the posterior mediastinum.

Lipomas can develop at a wide range of ages. They originate in the endocardium or epicardium and have a large pedunculated base. Many are asymptomatic, but some obstruct flow or cause arrhythmias.

Paragangliomas, including pheochromocytomas, rarely occur in the heart; when they do, they are usually localized to the base of the heart near vagus nerve endings. They may manifest with symptoms due to catecholamine secretion.

Pericardial cysts may resemble a cardiac tumor or pericardial effusion on chest x-ray. They are usually asymptomatic, although some cause compressive symptoms (eg, chest pain, dyspnea, cough).

Malignant primary tumors: Malignant primary tumors include sarcomas, pericardial mesothelioma, and primary lymphomas.

Sarcoma is the most common malignant and 2nd most common primary cardiac tumor (after myxoma). Sarcomas affect mainly middle-aged adults (mean, 41 yr). Almost 40% are angiosarcomas, most of which originate in the right atrium and involve the pericardium, causing right ventricular inflow tract obstruction, pericardial tamponade, and lung metastasis. Other types include undifferentiated sarcoma (25%), malignant fibrous histiocytoma (11 to 24%), leiomyosarcoma (8 to 9%), fibrosarcoma, rhabdomyosarcoma, liposarcoma, and osteosarcoma; these types are more likely to originate in the left atrium, causing mitral valve obstruction and heart failure.

Pericardial mesothelioma is rare; it affects all ages, males more than females. It causes tamponade and can metastasize to the spine, adjacent soft tissues, and brain.

Primary lymphoma is extremely rare; it usually occurs in AIDS patients or other people with immunodeficiency. These tumors grow rapidly and cause heart failure, arrhythmias, tamponade, and superior vena cava (SVC) syndrome.

Metastatic tumors: Lung and breast carcinoma, soft-tissue sarcoma, and renal cancer are the most common sources of metastases to the heart. Malignant melanoma, leukemia, and lymphoma often metastasize to the heart, but the metastases may not be clinically significant. When Kaposi's sarcoma spreads systemically in immunodeficient (usually AIDS) patients, it may spread to the heart, but clinical cardiac complications are uncommon.

Symptoms and Signs

Cardiac tumors cause symptoms and signs typical of much more common disorders (eg, heart failure, stroke, coronary artery disease). Symptoms and signs of benign primary cardiac tumors depend on tumor type, location, size, and friability and can be classified as extracardiac, intramyocardial, or intracavitary.

Extracardiac symptoms and signs may be constitutional or mechanical. Constitutional symptoms of fever, chills, lethargy, arthralgias, and weight loss are caused exclusively by myxomas, perhaps as a result of cytokine (eg, IL-6) release; petechiae may also occur. These and other findings may erroneously suggest bacterial endocarditis, connective tissue disorders, and occult malignancy. Mechanical symptoms (eg, dyspnea, chest discomfort) result from compression of cardiac chambers or coronary arteries or from pericardial irritation or tamponade caused by growth or hemorrhage within the pericardium. Pericardial tumors may produce pericardial friction rubs.

Intramyocardial symptoms and signs are caused by arrhythmias, usually atrioventricular or intraventricular block or paroxysmal supraventricular or ventricular tachycardias. The cause is tumors that compress or encroach on the conduction system (notably rhabdomyomas and fibromas).

Intracavitary symptoms and signs are due to tumors that obstruct valvular function, blood flow, or both (causing valvular stenosis, valvular insufficiency, or heart failure) or to tumors (especially gelatinous myxomas) that cause thrombus or tumor fragments to embolize into the systemic circulation (brain, coronary arteries, kidneys, spleen, extremities) or the lungs. Intracavitary symptoms and signs may vary with body position, which can alter hemodynamics and physical forces associated with the tumor.

Myxomas usually cause some combination of constitutional and intracavitary symptoms and signs. Myxomas may cause a diastolic murmur that mimics that of mitral stenosis but whose loudness and location vary from beat to beat with body position. About 15% of pedunculated left atrial myxomas produce an audible "tumor plop" as they drop into the mitral orifice during diastole. Myxomas may also cause arrhythmias. Raynaud's phenomenon and finger clubbing are less typical but may occur.

Fibroelastomas, often discovered incidentally at autopsy, are usually asymptomatic; however, they may be a source of systemic emboli. Rhabdomyomas are usually asymptomatic. Fibromas cause arrhythmias and sudden death. Hemangiomas are usually asymptomatic but may cause any of the extracardiac, intramyocardial, or intracavitary symptoms. Teratomas cause respiratory distress and cyanosis due to compression of the aortic and pulmonary artery or SVC syndrome.

Symptoms and signs of malignant cardiac tumors are more acute in onset and progress more rapidly. Cardiac sarcomas most commonly cause symptoms of ventricular inflow tract obstruction and pericardial tamponade. Mesothelioma causes symptoms of pericarditis or tamponade. Primary lymphoma causes refractory progressive heart failure, tamponade, arrhythmias, and SVC syndrome. Metastatic cardiac tumors may manifest as sudden cardiac enlargement, tamponade (due to rapid accumulation of hemorrhagic pericardial effusion), heart block, other arrhythmias, or sudden unexplained heart failure. Fever, malaise, weight loss, night sweats, and loss of appetite may also be present.

Diagnosis

Diagnosis, which is often delayed because symptoms and signs mimic those of much more common disorders, is confirmed by echocardiography and is tissue-typed by biopsy. Transesophageal echocardiography is better for visualizing atrial tumors; transthoracic echocardiography is better for ventricular tumors. If results are equivocal, gated radionuclide imaging, CT, or MRI is used; infrequently, contrast ventriculography during cardiac catheterization is required. Biopsy is done during catheterization or open thoracotomy.

Extensive testing often precedes echocardiography in patients with myxomas because their symptoms are nonspecific. Anemia, thrombocytopenia, and elevation of WBC count, ESR, C-reactive protein, and γ-globulins are common. ECG may show left atrial enlargement. Routine chest x-ray may show Ca deposits in right atrial myxomas or in teratomas seen as anterior mediastinal masses. Myxomas are sometimes diagnosed when tumor cells are found in a surgically removed embolus.

Arrhythmias and heart failure with features of tuberous sclerosis suggest rhabdomyomas or fibromas. New cardiac symptoms and signs in a patient with a known extracardiac malignancy suggest cardiac metastases; chest x-ray may show bizarre changes in the cardiac silhouette.

Treatment and Prognosis

Treatment of benign primary tumors is surgical excision followed by serial echocardiography over 5 to 6 yr to monitor for recurrence; tumors are excised unless another disorder (eg, dementia) contraindicates surgery.

Surgery is usually curative (95% survival at 3 yr). Exceptions are rhabdomyomas, most of which regress spontaneously and do not require treatment, and pericardial teratoma, which may require urgent pericardiocentesis. Patients with fibroelastoma may also require valvular repair or replacement. When rhabdomyomas or fibromas are multifocal, surgical excision is usually ineffective, and prognosis is poor after the 1st year of life; survival at 5 yr may be as low as 15%.

Treatment of malignant primary tumors is usually palliative (eg, radiation therapy, chemotherapy, management of complications) because prognosis is poor.

Treatment of metastatic cardiac tumors depends on tumor origin; it may include systemic chemotherapy or palliation.

SECTION 8

EAR, NOSE, THROAT, AND DENTAL DISORDERS

84 APPROACH TO THE PATIENT WITH EAR PROBLEMS

Earache, hearing loss, otorrhea, tinnitus, and vertigo are the principal symptoms of ear problems. Hearing loss is discussed in Ch. 95 on p. 781.

In addition to the ears, nose, nasopharynx, and paranasal sinuses, the teeth, tongue, tonsils, hypopharynx, larynx, salivary glands, and temporomandibular joint are examined; pain and discomfort may be referred from them to the ears. It is important to examine cranial nerve function (see pp. 1750 and 1867) and to perform bedside tests of hearing (see p. 785) and of the vestibular apparatus. The patient is also examined for nystagmus (a rhythmic movement of the eyes—see sidebar 84–1).

Testing

Patients with abnormal hearing on history or physical examination or with tinnitus or vertigo undergo an audiogram (see p. 785). Patients with nystagmus or altered vestibular function may benefit from computerized

Sidebar 84–1. NYSTAGMUS

Nystagmus is a rhythmic movement of the eyes that can have various causes. Vestibular disorders can result in nystagmus because of the interconnection of the vestibular system and the oculomotor nuclei. The presence of vestibular nystagmus helps identify vestibular disorders and sometimes distinguishes central from peripheral vertigo. Vestibular nystagmus has a slow component caused by the vestibular input and a quick, corrective component that causes movement in the opposite direction. The direction of the nystagmus is defined by the direction of the quick component because it is easier to see. Nystagmus may be rotary, vertical, or horizontal and may occur spontaneously, with gaze, or with head motion.

Initial inspection for nystagmus is done with the patient lying supine with unfocused gaze (+30 diopter or Frenzel's lenses can be used to prevent gaze fixation). The patient is then slowly rotated to a left and then to a right lateral position. The direction and duration of nystagmus are noted. If nystagmus is not detected, then the Dix-Hallpike (or Barany) maneuver is performed. In this maneuver, the patient sits erect on a stretcher so that when lying back his head extends beyond the end. With support, he is rapidly lowered to horizontal with his head extended back 45° below horizontal and rotated 45° to the left. Direction and duration of nystagmus and development of vertigo are noted. The patient is returned to upright and the maneuver repeated with rotation to the right. Any position or maneuver that produces nystagmus should be repeated to see if it fatigues. Nystagmus secondary to peripheral nervous system disorders has a latency period of 3 to 10 sec and fatigues rapidly, whereas nystagmus secondary to CNS causes has no latency period and does not fatigue. During induced nystagmus, the patient is instructed to focus on an object. Nystagmus from peripheral disorders is inhibited by visual fixation.

Caloric stimulation of the ear canal induces nystagmus in a person with an intact vestibular system. Failure to induce nystagmus or > 20% difference in duration between sides suggests a lesion on the side of the decreased response. With the patient supine and the head elevated 30°, each ear is irrigated sequentially with 3 mL of ice water. Alternatively, 240 mL of warm water (40 to 44°C) may be used, taking care not to burn the patient with overly hot water. Cold water produces nystagmus to the opposite side; warm water produces nystagmus to the same side. A mnemonic device is COWS (Cold to the Opposite and Warm to the Same).

electronystagmography (ENG), which quantifies spontaneous, gaze, or positional nystagmus that might not be visually detectable. Computerized ENG caloric testing quantitates the strength of response of the vestibular system to cool and warm irrigations in each ear, enabling the physician to discriminate unilateral weakness. Different components of the vestibular system can be tested by varying head and body position or by presenting visual stimuli.

Primary imaging tests include CT of the temporal bone with or without radiopaque dye and gadolinium-enhanced MRI of the brain, with attention paid to the internal auditory canals to rule out an acoustic neuroma. These tests may be indicated in cases of trauma to the ear and/or head, chronic infection, hearing loss, vertigo, facial paralysis, and otalgia of obscure origin.

EARACHE

(Otalgia)

Earache occurs from otologic causes (involving the external or middle ear) or from nonotologic causes referred to the ear from remote disease processes (see TABLE 84–1). With chronic pain (eg, > 2 to 3 wk), a tumor must be considered, particularly in older patients.

Eustachian tube obstruction inhibits equilibration between middle ear pressure and atmospheric pressure, causing pain with change in ambient pressure. Otitis media produces painful inflammation of the mucous membrane and pain from increased middle ear pressure, with bulging of the tympanic membrane.

Evaluation

History and physical examination: If results of an ear examination are normal, a

TABLE 84–1. CAUSES OF EARACHE

LOCATION	CONDITION	HISTORY	PHYSICAL EXAMINATION
Otologic Causes			
Middle ear or mastoid process	Otitis media, acute otitis media, chronic otitis media	Preceding URI	Bulging, red tympanic membrane
	Acute barotitis media (barotrauma)	Rapid change in air pressure as in air travel or scuba diving	Hemorrhage on or behind the tympanic membrane
	Acute eustachian tube obstruction	Gurgling, crackling, or popping noises, with or without nasal congestion	Unilateral conductive hearing loss and decreased tympanic membrane mobility
	Acute mastoiditis	Fever, postauricular pain, otorrhea. Previous URI, incompletely or inadequately treated otitis media	Fever, postauricular swelling and tenderness to palpitation. Sometimes, downward or lateral pinna displacement, edema of posterior portion of external canal
External ear	Otitis externa	Earache localized to the canal, particularly in a swimmer, diabetic, or patient with seborrheic dermatitis	Erythematous, edematous ear canal; exquisite tenderness with movement of the tragus, and thick white otorrhea
	Bullous myringitis	Sudden pain, sometimes history of herpes	Small blebs on the tympanic membrane, sometimes herpetic lesions adjacent to tragus
	Cerumen, impacted or foreign body	Vague pain accompanied by hearing loss and without other symptoms	Visualization
Nonotologic Causes			
Cancer	Nasopharynx, pharynx, tonsil, base of tongue, larynx	Often tobacco and/or alcohol use	Varies; sometimes unilateral or remitting middle ear effusion
Infection	Tonsillopharyngitis, peritonsillar, or other oropharyngeal abscess	Pain with swallowing	Pharyngeal erythema and sometimes swelling
Neurologic	Neuralgia (trigeminal, sphenopalatine, glossopharyngeal, geniculate)	Severe, lancinating pain episodes	None
Other	Post-tonsillectomy or adenoidectomy	History of surgery	Varies
	Temporomandibular joint disorder	Pain with jaw movement	Lack of smooth temporomandibular joint movement; trismus

source of referred pain is sought in areas innervated by cranial nerves responsible for sensation in the external and middle ear (5th, 9th, and 10th). Specific areas include the nose, paranasal sinuses, nasopharynx, teeth, gingiva, temporomandibular joint, mandible, parotid glands, tongue, palatine tonsils, pharynx, larynx, trachea, and esophagus.

Testing: Otologic causes are usually diagnosed during otoscopic examination. Depending on clinical findings, nonotologic causes may require testing, including audiometry; vestibular function testing; dental films; CT of the head, temporal bone, neck, and sinuses; and MRI.

Treatment

Underlying causes are treated. Pain may be treated with oral analgesics (eg, NSAIDs, acetaminophen). Patients with temporomandibular disorder should see a dentist experienced in its treatment and should avoid chewing gum and hard foods when experiencing symptoms.

Earache is often caused by trauma resulting from ear irrigations. Patients should not perform ear irrigations unless instructed by a physician to do so, and then only gently. An oral irrigator should never be used to irrigate the ear.

OTORRHEA

Otorrhea is drainage exiting the ear. It may be serous, serosanguineous, or purulent. Drainage may originate from the ear canal, the middle ear, or the cranial vault. Associated symptoms may include otalgia, fever, pruritus, vertigo, tinnitus, and hearing loss.

Etiology

Causes of acute (< 6 wk) otorrhea include acute otitis media with perforation of the tympanic membrane, otitis externa, drainage through a patent tympanostomy tube, recent trauma (causing CSF leak), and surgery.

Causes of chronic otorrhea (which may also present acutely) include chronic purulent otitis media, cholesteatoma, foreign body, Wegener's granulomatosis, necrotizing otitis externa (frequently associated with immunodeficiency and diabetes), mastoiditis, and osteomyelitis (bacterial, fungal, or TB).

Evaluation and Treatment

History: Acute otalgia with relief after appearance of otorrhea suggests acute otitis media with perforation. A history of swimming or seborrheic dermatitis suggests otitis externa. Recent head trauma or surgery suggests CSF leakage. A history of tympanic membrane perforation or chronic eustachian tube dysfunction suggests cholesteatoma. A history of untreated or poorly treated acute otitis media suggests mastoiditis.

Physical examination: Otoscopic examination can usually diagnose perforated tympanic membrane, external otitis media, foreign body, or other uncomplicated sources of otorrhea. Crystal clear fluid is usually CSF, although with trauma fluid may be bloody. Flaky debris littering the ear canal suggests cholesteatoma. Periauricular swelling and intense tenderness, granulation tissue within the canal, and facial nerve paralysis suggest necrotizing otitis externa. Redness and tenderness over the mastoid suggest mastoiditis.

Testing: If CSF leakage is in question, discharge can be tested for glucose or β_2-transferrin. Patients without an obvious etiology on examination require audiogram, CT scan of the temporal bone or gadolinium MRI scan, or pathologic examination of granulation tissue in the auditory canal. Most physicians will not treat a suspected CSF leak with antibiotics without a definitive diagnosis so as not to mask the onset of meningitis.

Treatment: Treatment depends on the final diagnosis. Antibiotics are administered, as appropriate, for infectious causes.

TINNITUS

Tinnitus is a noise in the ears; it is experienced by 10 to 15% of the population. Subjective tinnitus is perception of sound in the absence of an acoustic stimulus and is heard only by the patient. Objective tinnitus results from noise generated by vascular tissue near the ear and, in some cases, is heard by the examiner.

Tinnitus may be described as buzzing, ringing, roaring, whistling, or hissing and is sometimes variable and complex. It may be intermittent, continuous, or pulsatile (synchronous with the heartbeat). Continuous tinnitus is at best annoying and is often quite distressing. Some patients adapt to its presence better than others; depression occasionally results. Stress generally exacerbates tinnitus.

Etiology

Subjective tinnitus may occur with almost any ear disorder. Common causes include acoustic trauma (noise-induced sensorineural hearing loss), sensorineural hearing loss from other causes, obstruction of the ear canal by cerumen or a foreign body, infections (external otitis, myringitis, otitis media, labyrinthitis, petrositis, syphilis, meningitis), and eustachian tube obstruction. Salicylates in high dosages may cause reversible tinnitus. Aminoglycoside antibiotics and some chemotherapeutic drugs (eg, cisplatin) can cause hearing loss that may be accompanied by tinnitus.

Objective tinnitus, an uncommon occurrence involving an audible, pulsatile hum, can be caused by turbulent flow through the carotid artery or jugular vein. Highly vascular middle ear tumors (eg, glomus tympanicum and glomus jugulare tumors) and dural arteriovenous malformations (AVMs) may also cause objective tinnitus.

Evaluation

History: Exposure to loud noise or to certain drugs before onset suggests acoustic trauma or ototoxicity, respectively. Unilateral tinnitus, particularly with hearing loss, may suggest acoustic neuroma. Acute unilateral hearing loss and vertigo, particularly after barotrauma, may suggest a perilymphatic fistula. Episodic tinnitus, fullness in the ear, severe vertigo, and fluctuating or permanent hearing loss in the same ear suggest Meniere's disease (see p. 794).

Physical examination: Bruit or venous hum on auscultation of the neck suggests a vascular etiology. Bruit only on auscultation of the ear with use of an olive-tipped or electronic stethoscope suggests a dural AVM.

Testing: An audiogram is performed, and if hearing loss is found, tests are done to differentiate conductive, sensory, and neural hearing losses (see p. 785). Gadolinium-enhanced MRI rules out acoustic neuroma in cases of unilateral tinnitus, particularly in the presence of hearing loss. Other testing depends on patient presentation. Unilateral pulsatile and objective tinnitus may require investigation of the carotid and vertebral system with an arteriogram. In such cases, the risk of arteriogram must be weighed against the potential benefit of detecting and treating (with embolization) a potential dural AVM. Magnetic resonance angiography probably is not sensitive enough to detect most dural AVMs.

Treatment

Treatment of the underlying disease may lessen tinnitus. Correcting hearing loss (eg, with a hearing aid) relieves tinnitus in about 50% of patients. In some cases, recognizing and treating depression relieves tinnitus, suggesting a psychologic component. However, a psychologic cause should not be assumed.

Although no specific medical or surgical therapy is available, many patients find that background sound masks the tinnitus and may help them fall asleep. Some patients benefit from a tinnitus masker, a device worn like a hearing aid that provides a low-level sound that can suppress tinnitus. Electrical stimulation of the inner ear, as with a cochlear implant, occasionally reduces the tinnitus but is appropriate only for patients who are profoundly deaf.

VERTIGO

Vertigo is a false sensation of movement associated with difficulty in balance or gait. Typically, the perceived motion is rotary—a spinning or whirling sensation—but some patients simply feel they are being pulled to one side. The patient may feel as though he or the environment is moving. Symptoms may be acute and severe, causing nausea and vomiting, and may occur episodically.

Pathophysiology and Etiology

Perception of stability, motion, and orientation to gravity originates in the vestibular system, which consists of the 3 semicircular canals and 2 otolith organs—the saccule and utricle. Rotary motion causes flow of endolymph in the semicircular canal oriented in the plane of motion. Depending on the direction of flow, endolymph movement either stimulates or inhibits neuronal output from hair cells lining the canal. Similar hair cells in the saccule and utricle are embedded in a matrix of Ca carbonate crystals (otoliths). Deflection of the otoliths by gravity stimulates or inhibits neuronal output from the attached hair cells. Nerve impulses from the vestibular system are transmitted along the 8th cranial nerve to vestibular nuclei in the brain stem and cerebellum. From there, connections are made to the oculomotor system, spinal cord, and cerebral cortex, which integrate the information to produce the perception of motion.

Vertigo results from lesions or disturbances anywhere along this pathway (see TABLE 84–2). Vertigo secondary to disorders of the inner ear or 8th cranial nerve is considered

TABLE 84–2. CAUSES OF VERTIGO

- Benign positional vertigo
- Drugs
  - Aminoglycosides
  - Chloroquine
  - Furosemide
  - Quinine
- Infection
  - Herpes zoster oticus
  - Labyrinthitis
  - Neurosyphilis
  - Otitis media
  - Vestibular neuronitis
- Meniere's disease
- Multiple sclerosis
- Panic attack
- Trauma
  - Labyrinthine contusion
  - Perilymphatic fistula
  - Temporal bone fracture
  - Tympanic membrane rupture
- Tumors
  - Acoustic neuroma
  - Cerebellopontine angle tumor
- Vascular
  - Basilar artery migraine
  - Cerebellar artery infarction
  - Cerebellar hemorrhage
  - Vasculitis
  - Vertebrobasilar insufficiency
- Rare
  - Autoimmune ear disease
  - Cholesteatoma

peripheral vertigo, whereas vertigo secondary to disorders of the vestibular nuclei and their pathways in the brain stem and cerebellum is considered central vertigo. Occasionally, vertigo may be psychogenic. Elderly patients may have multifactorial dizziness secondary to drug adverse effects or to age-diminished visual, vestibular, and proprioceptive abilities.

Evaluation

Along with a general ENT examination, neurologic examination (see p. 1748) is important, particularly of the 8th cranial nerve (vestibular system and hearing) and cerebellum.

History: Severe episodic vertigo is usually peripheral in origin.

Benign paroxysmal positional vertigo (BPPV—the most common type of vertigo—see p. 791) is suggested by severe spinning spells of < 1 min initiated a few seconds after lying down and turning to the affected side or turning in bed toward the affected side. Although BPPV sometimes persists, it is generally self-limited.

Viral neuronitis is suggested by acute onset of incapacitating vertigo with no hearing loss that lasts for up to 1 wk. Symptoms gradually abate, although motion-provoked vertigo may persist 2 to 3 mo.

Acute labyrinthitis (secondary to either viral infection or vascular occlusion) is suggested by hearing loss and tinnitus and no evidence of bacterial infection.

Meniere's disease is suggested by recurrent, severe episodes of vertigo and unilateral tinnitus, ear fullness, pressure, and (initially) low-frequency hearing loss (see p. 794). Individual episodes of Meniere's disease typically last from 20 min to several hours. In the early stages, hearing loss generally returns to baseline after each episode, but in later stages hearing loss persists and progresses. Meniere's disease cannot be diagnosed after only one episode, because its symptoms are similar to mild vestibular neuronitis.

Physical examination: A physical examination of the ears and head and neck is indicated to rule out ear infection or other abnormalities. A clinical vestibular examination is done, including a Dix-Hallpike maneuver and examination of extraocular movements and nystagmus (see sidebar 84–1). A positive response to the Dix-Hallpike maneuver that fatigues rapidly suggests positional vertigo. Nystagmus that does not extinguish with visual fixation and vertical nystagmus suggests a central etiology.

Testing: Gadolinium-enhanced MRI is indicated for patients with vertigo only when other neurologic abnormalities or headache is present or if history and physical examination suggest a CNS etiology, such as a cerebellopontine angle tumor (in which case 8th nerve cuts are obtained). For patients with chronic vertigo, CT or MRI is performed to look for evidence of stroke, multiple sclerosis, or other CNS lesions.

Patients for whom results of bedside tests of hearing and vestibular function are abnormal or equivocal should undergo formal testing with audiometry and electronystagmography.

Laboratory tests are rarely helpful, except for patients with chronic vertigo and bilateral hearing loss, for whom a test should be obtained to rule out syphilis.

Patients with chronic dizziness should be examined to rule out cardiac, neurologic, and metabolic causes.

Treatment

Any identified disorders are treated. Symptom relief is important; the most effective vestibular nerve suppressants are diazepam (2 to 5 mg po q 6 to 8 h, with higher doses given under supervision for severe vertigo) and oral antihistamine/anticholinergic drugs (eg, meclizine 25 to 50 mg po tid). All of these drugs can cause drowsiness, thereby limiting their use for certain patients. Nausea can be treated with prochlorperazine 10 mg IM qid or 25 mg rectally bid. Patients with recurrent or positional vertigo secondary to unilateral vestibular weakness usually benefit greatly from vestibular rehabilitation therapy prescribed by an experienced physical therapist. The goal is to enhance the brain's ability to compensate for the loss of vestibular function in one ear. Most patients compensate well, although some, especially the elderly, have more difficulty. Patients with BPPV generally respond well to either vestibular adaptation exercises or to canalith repositioning maneuvers (eg, Epley or Semont maneuver—see p. 791).

85 HEARING LOSS

Nearly 10% of people in the US have some degree of hearing loss. About 1/800 to 1/1000 newborns are born with severe to profound hearing loss. Two to 3 times as many are born with lesser hearing loss. During childhood, another 2 to 3/1000 children acquire moderate to severe hearing loss. Adolescents are at risk from excessive exposure to noise and/or head trauma. Older adults typically experience a progressive decrease in hearing (presbycusis—see p. 783), which is probably related to aging and noise exposure. The prevalence of hearing impairment in people > 65 is 25 to 40%; in those > 75, 40 to 66%.

Hearing deficits in early childhood can result in lifelong impairments in receptive and expressive language skills. The severity of the handicap is determined by the age at which the hearing loss occurred; the nature of the loss—its duration, the frequencies affected, and the degree; and the susceptibilities of the individual child (eg, coexisting visual impairment, mental retardation, primary language deficits, inadequate linguistic environment). Children who have other sensory, linguistic, or cognitive deficiencies are affected most severely.

Hearing loss can be classified as conductive, sensorineural, or both (mixed loss). Conductive hearing loss occurs secondary to lesions in the external auditory canal, tympanic membrane, or middle ear. These lesions prevent sound from being effectively conducted to the inner ear. Sensorineural hearing loss is caused by lesions of either the inner ear (sensory) or the auditory (8th) nerve (neural—see TABLE 85–1). This distinction is important,

TABLE 85–1. DIFFERENCES BETWEEN SENSORY AND NEURAL HEARING LOSSES

TEST	SENSORY HEARING LOSS	NEURAL HEARING LOSS
Speech discrimination	Moderate decrement	Severe decrement
Discrimination with increasing intensity	Improves	Deteriorates
Recruitment	Present	Absent
Acoustic reflex decay	Absent or mild	Present
Tone decay	Absent or mild	Marked
Waveforms in auditory brain stem responses	Well formed, with normal latencies	Absent or with abnormally long latencies
Otoacoustic emissions	Absent	Present

TABLE 85–2. CONGENITAL CAUSES OF HEARING LOSS

TYPE OF LOSS*	ANATOMIC AREA AFFECTED	ETIOLOGY†
Conductive	External and middle ear	Genetic Idiopathic (unknown) malformation Drug-induced malformation (thalidomide)
Sensory	Inner ear	Genetic Idiopathic (unknown) malformation Congenital infection (eg, rubella, cytomegalovirus, toxoplasmosis, syphilis) Rh incompatibility Anoxia Maternal ingestion of ototoxic drugs (eg, for TB or severe infection) Drug-induced malformation (thalidomide)
Neural	CNS	Anoxia Idiopathic (unknown) malformation Genetic Congenital infection (eg, rubella, cytomegalovirus, toxoplasmosis, syphilis) Rh incompatibility

*A number of the congenital hearing losses may be mixed losses—a combination of conductive and sensory and/or neural.

†Listed in approximate order of greatest frequency first.

because sensory hearing loss is sometimes reversible and is seldom life threatening. A neural hearing loss is rarely recoverable and may be due to a potentially life-threatening brain tumor—commonly a cerebellopontine angle tumor. Mixed loss may be caused by severe head injury with or without fracture of the skull or temporal bone, by chronic infection, or by one of many genetic disorders. It may also occur when a transient conductive hearing loss, commonly from otitis media, is superimposed on a sensorineural hearing loss.

Etiology

Hearing loss can be congenital (see TABLE 85–2) or acquired (see TABLE 85–3), progressive or sudden (see also Sudden Deafness on p. 789), temporary or permanent, unilateral or bilateral, and mild or profound. Drug-induced ototoxicity is discussed on p.792.

Cerumen (earwax) accumulation is the most common cause of treatable hearing loss, especially in the elderly. Foreign bodies obstructing the canal are sometimes a problem in children.

Infections, particularly otitis media and its sequelae, are common causes of conductive hearing loss, especially in children. Almost every child experiences mild to moderate transient hearing loss due to otitis media. However, repeated or severe infections can destroy the ossicles, particularly the long process of the incus, causing permanent deficits. Untreated otitis media may lead to development of a cholesteatoma, a benign tumor that can cause conductive hearing loss. Residual middle ear fluid (secretory otitis media) after infection commonly causes temporary hearing loss. Sensorineural hearing loss can result from various other infections, both congenital and acquired.

Acoustic trauma (noise-induced sensorineural hearing loss) may result from a single, extreme noise exposure (eg, a nearby gunshot or explosion) or may develop over time from chronic exposure to noise > 85 decibels (dB—see sidebar 85–1). Although people vary greatly in susceptibility to noise-induced hearing loss, nearly everyone loses some hearing if exposed to sufficiently intense noise for an adequate time. The loss is usually temporary, typically lasting several hours or a day after prolonged loud exposure; some experience tinnitus as well. However, repeated exposure to loud noise ultimately results in loss of hair cells in the organ of Corti. Hearing loss typically occurs first at 4 kHz and gradually spreads to the lower and higher frequencies as exposure continues. In contrast to most other causes of sensorineural hearing losses, noise-induced hearing loss may be less severe at 8 kHz than at 4 kHz.

Autoimmune disease can cause sensorineural hearing loss at all ages and other signs and symptoms as well.

Presbycusis is sensorineural hearing loss that occurs with aging. It probably results from age-related changes and the chronic effects of noise exposure. Progressive deterioration and cell death of the sensory hair cells, stria vascularis, ganglion cells, and cochlear nuclei play a role. The hearing loss usually affects the highest frequencies (18 to 20 kHz) early on and gradually affects the lower frequencies; it usually becomes clinically significant when it affects the critical 4- to 8-kHz range around age 55 to 65 (sometimes sooner). The loss of high-frequency hearing significantly affects speech comprehension. Although the loudness of speech seems normal, certain consonant sounds (eg, C, D, K, P, S, T) become hard

TABLE 85–3. ACQUIRED CAUSES OF HEARING LOSS

TYPE OF LOSS	ANATOMIC AREA AFFECTED	ETIOLOGY*
Conductive	External ear	Cerumen Otitis externa Foreign body (eg, nuts, crayons, cotton swabs) Allergic reactions Tumors—benign Tumors—malignant Trauma Amputation Burns
	Middle ear	Otitis media Allergy Physical trauma (eg, tympanic membrane perforation, destruction of one or more of the 3 small bones in the inner ear, blood in the middle ear) Genetic disease (eg, otosclerosis, Paget's disease, mucopolysaccharidoses) Tumors, benign (cholesteatoma, glomus jugulare) Tumors, malignant (most commonly metastatic)
Sensory	Inner ear	Genetic Sound trauma Idiopathic (presbycusis) Ototoxic drugs—reversible (eg, aspirin)
		Infection (eg, meningitis, viral labyrinthitis) Autoimmune disease (eg, RA, SLE) Ototoxic drugs, irreversible (eg, aminoglycosides), and antimetabolites (eg, cisplatinum) Barotrauma resulting in perilymphatic fistula Physical trauma—skull fracture involving the inner ear
Neural	CNS	Tumors, benign (eg, neurofibroma, meningioma) Demyelinating diseases (eg, multiple sclerosis) Tumors, malignant (rare)
Mixed	Middle and inner ear	Genetic disorders (otosclerosis, Paget's disease, and a number of other genetically determined bony abnormalities) Otitis media Trauma—physical Trauma—barotrauma

*Listed in approximate order of greatest frequency first.

Sidebar 85–1. SOUND LEVELS

Loudness is measured in decibels (dB). A dB is a unitless figure that compares 2 values and is defined as the logarithm of the ratio of a measured value to a reference value, multiplied by a constant:

$$dB = k \log (V_{measured}/V_{ref}).$$

By convention, the reference value for loudness is taken as the quietest 1000 Hz sound detectable by young, healthy human ears. * The sound may be measured in terms of sound pressure level (N/m^2), sound intensity (watts/m^2), or other units.

Because sound intensity equals the square of sound pressure, the constant (k) for sound pressure level is 20; for sound intensity, 10. Thus, each 20-dB increase represents a 10-fold increase in sound pressure level but a 100-fold increase in sound intensity.

Db	Example
0	Faintest sound heard by human ear
30	Whisper, quiet library
60	Normal conversation, sewing machine, typewriter
90	Lawnmower, shop tools, truck traffic (8 h/day is the maximum exposure without protection†)
100	Chainsaw, pneumatic drill, snowmobile (2 h/day is the maximum exposure without protection)
115	Sandblasting, loud rock concert, automobile horn (15 min/day is the maximum exposure without protection)
140	Gun muzzle blast, jet engine (noise causes pain and even brief exposure injures unprotected ears; injury may occur even with hearing protectors)
180	Rocket launching pad

*In audiometric testing, because human ears respond differently at different frequencies, the reference value changes for each frequency tested. Threshold values reported on audiograms take this into account; the normal threshold is always 0 dB, regardless of the actual sound pressure level.

†Mandatory federal standard, but protection is recommended for more than brief exposure to sound levels > 85 db.

to hear; affected people often think the speaker is mumbling. A speaker attempting to speak more loudly usually accentuates vowel sounds (which are low frequency), doing little to improve speech recognition.

Evaluation

Evaluation consists of detecting and quantifying hearing loss and determining etiology (particularly reversible causes).

Screening: Although most adults and older children notice a sudden hearing loss, progressive losses and all losses in infants and young children must be detected by screening. Screening should begin in infancy (see p. 2234) so that linguistic input can allow optimal language development. Suspected hearing loss at any time should prompt referral to a specialist. If screening is not performed, severe bilateral losses may not be recognized until age 2 yr, and mild to moderate or severe unilateral losses often are not recognized until the child reaches school age.

History: Caregivers may suspect that a newborn has a severe hearing loss within the 1st week of life when the newborn does not respond to voices or other sounds. Any child with delays in speech or language development or difficulty in school should undergo evaluation for hearing loss. Mental retardation, aphasia, and autism also must be considered. Delayed motor development may signal vestibular deficit, which is often associated with a sensorineural hearing loss.

Older adults typically complain that other people are not speaking clearly rather than that their own hearing is decreased; often, family members prompt evaluation for hearing loss. Speech comprehension is particularly difficult when background noise is present. Screening in adults can be successfully carried out using the questionnaire from the Hearing Handicap Inventory for the Elderly—Screening Version. In this test, the patient is asked the following questions:

- Does a hearing problem cause you to feel embarrassed when you meet people?
- Does a hearing problem cause you to feel frustrated when talking to a family member?
- Do you have difficulty hearing when someone whispers?
- Do you feel handicapped by a hearing problem?
- Does a hearing problem cause you difficulty when visiting friends, relatives, or neighbors?
- Does a hearing problem cause you to attend religious services less often than you would like?
- Does a hearing problem cause you to have arguments with family members?
- Does a hearing problem cause you difficulty when listening to television or radio?
- Do you feel that any difficulty with your hearing hampers your personal or social life?
- Does a hearing problem cause you difficulty when in a restaurant with relatives or friends?

The patient responds to each question with "no" (0 points), "sometimes" (2 points), or "yes" (4 points). The points are then tallied, with higher scores suggesting a greater degree of hearing impairment. Scores > 10 suggest significant hearing impairment and necessitate follow-up.

Accompanying symptoms, particularly neurologic ones (eg, dizziness, vertigo, nystagmus, headache, facial palsy), should trigger an immediate otologic evaluation, including a hearing test. History of CNS or ear infection, use of ototoxic drugs, exposure to loud noise, head trauma, sudden loss of hearing, ear pain (otalgia), and/or a family history of hearing loss may suggest a cause of hearing loss. Examples are a history of disorientation in the dark (loss of vestibular function), episodes of vertigo (the subjective feeling of rotation or movement in space), development of weakness or asymmetry of the face, and an abnormal sense of taste.

Physical examination: The physician evaluates the external ear for obstruction, infection, and congenital malformations and the tympanic membrane for perforation, otitis media, and cholesteatoma. In the neurologic examination, cranial nerve function, particularly balance, facial weakness, and taste functions, is important (see p. 1750).

Weber's and Rinne's tests use a tuning fork to differentiate conductive from sensorineural hearing loss. In Weber's test, the stem of a vibrating 512-Hz and/or 1024-Hz tuning fork is placed on the midline of the head, and the patient indicates in which ear the tone is louder. In unilateral conductive hearing loss, the tone is louder in the ear with hearing loss. In unilateral sensorineural hearing loss, the tone is louder in the normal ear, because the tuning fork stimulates both inner ears equally and the patient perceives the stimulus with the unaffected ear. In Rinne's test, hearing by bone and by air conduction is compared. Bone conduction bypasses the external and middle ear and tests the integrity of the inner ear, 8th cranial nerve, and central auditory pathways. The stem of a vibrating tuning fork is held against the mastoid (for bone conduction); as soon as the sound is no longer perceived, the fork is removed from the mastoid, and the still vibrating tines are held close to the pinna (for air conduction). Normally, the fork can once more be heard, indicating that air conduction is better than bone conduction. With a conductive hearing loss, the relationship is reversed; bone conduction is louder than air conduction. With a sensorineural hearing loss, both air and bone conduction are reduced, but air conduction remains louder.

Audiologic tests: Typical audiologic tests include measurement of pure-tone thresholds with air and bone conduction, speech reception threshold, speech discrimination, tympanometry, acoustic reflex testing, and, occasionally, reflex decay testing. Information gained from these tests helps determine whether more definitive differentiation of sensory from neural hearing loss is needed.

Pure-tone audiometry quantifies hearing loss. An audiometer delivers sounds of specific frequencies (pure tones) at different intensities to determine the patient's hearing threshold (how loud a sound must be to be perceived) for each frequency. Hearing in each ear is tested from 125 or 250 to 8000 Hz by both air conduction (using earphones) and bone conduction (using an oscillator in contact with the mastoid process or forehead). Test results are plotted on graphs called audiograms (see FIG. 85–1), which show the difference between the patient's hearing threshold and normal hearing at each frequency. The difference is measured in dB (see sidebar 85–1). The normal threshold is considered 0 dB hearing level (Hl); hearing loss is considered present if the patient's threshold is > 25 dB Hl. When hearing loss is such as to require loud test tones, intense tones presented to one ear may be heard in the other ear. In such cases, a masking sound, usually narrow band noise, is presented to the non–test ear to isolate it.

Speech audiometry includes the speech reception threshold (SRT) and the word recognition score. The SRT is a measure of the intensity at which speech is recognized. To determine the SRT, the examiner presents the patient with a list of words at specific sound intensities. These words usually have two equally accented syllables (spondees), such as railroad, staircase, and baseball. The examiner notes the intensity at which the patient repeats 50% of the words correctly. The SRT approximates the average hearing level at speech frequencies (eg, 500 Hz, 1000 Hz, 2000 Hz).

The word recognition score tests the ability to discriminate among the various speech sounds or phonemes. It is determined by presenting 50 phonetically balanced one-syllable words at an intensity of 35 to 40 dB

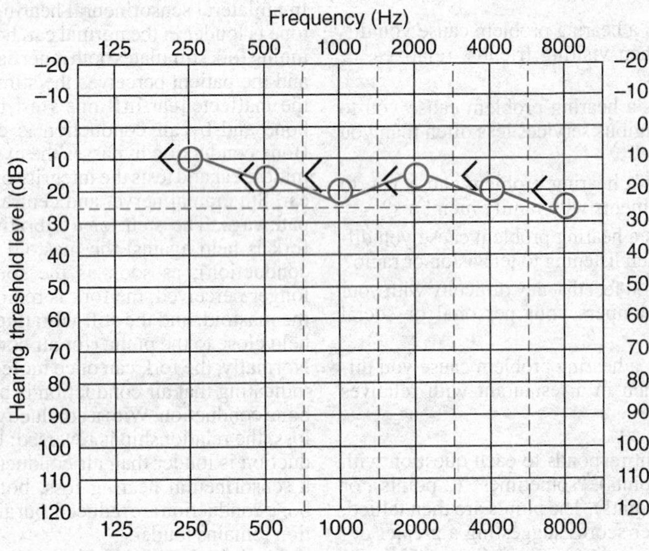

Fig. 85–1. Audiogram of right ear in a patient with normal hearing. Normal audiogram of the right ear. The vertical lines represent the frequencies that are tested from 125 to 8000 Hz. The horizontal lines record the threshold at which the patient states that the sound is heard. Normal thresholds are 0 dB +/– 10 dB. Patients with a hearing threshold ≤ 20 dB are considered to have average or better-than-average hearing. The greater the dB, the louder the sound and the worse the hearing. O is the standard symbol for air conduction of the right ear; X is the standard for air conduction for the left ear. The < is the standard symbol for unmasked bone condition for the right ear; > is the standard symbol for unmasked bone conduction of the left ear.

above the patient's SRT. The word list contains phonemes in the same relative frequency found in conversational English. The score is the percentage of words correctly repeated by the patient and reflects the ability to understand speech under optimal listening conditions. A normal score ranges from 90 to 100%. The word recognition score is normal with conductive hearing loss, albeit at a higher intensity level, but can be reduced at all intensity levels with sensorineural hearing loss. Discrimination is even poorer in neural than in sensory hearing loss.

Tympanometry measures the impedance of the middle ear to acoustic energy and does not require patient participation. It is commonly used to screen children for middle ear effusions. A probe containing a sound source, microphone, and air pressure regulator is placed snugly with an airtight seal into the ear canal. The probe microphone records the reflected sound from the tympanic membrane while pressure in the canal is varied. Normally, maximal compliance of the middle ear occurs when the pressure in the ear canal equals atmospheric pressure. Abnormal compliance patterns suggest specific anatomic disruptions. In eustachian tube obstruction and middle ear effusion, maximal compliance occurs with a negative pressure in the ear canal. When the ossicular chain is disrupted, as in necrosis or dislocation of the long process of the incus, the middle ear is excessively compliant. When the ossicular chain is fixed, as in stapedial ankylosis in otosclerosis, compliance may be normal or reduced.

The acoustic reflex is contraction of the stapedius muscle in response to loud sounds, which changes the compliance of the tympanic membrane, protecting the middle ear from acoustic trauma. The reflex is tested by presenting a tone and measuring what intensity provokes a change in middle ear impedance as noted by movement of the tympanic membrane. An absent reflex could indicate a tumor of the auditory nerve.

Advanced testing: Gadolinium-enhanced MRI of the head to detect lesions of the cerebellopontine angle may be needed in patients with poor word recognition, asymmetric sensorineural hearing loss, and/or abnormal neurologic examination in whom the etiology is not clear.

The auditory brain stem response uses surface electrodes to monitor brain wave response to acoustic stimulation in people who cannot otherwise respond.

Electrocochleography measures the activity of the cochlea and the auditory nerve with an electrode placed on or through the eardrum. It can be used to assess and monitor patients with dizziness, in intraoperative monitoring, and in awake patients. Otoacoustic emissions testing measures sounds produced by outer hair cells of the cochlea in response to a sound stimulus usually placed in the ear canal. It is used to screen newborns and infants for hearing loss and to monitor the hearing of patients who are using ototoxic drugs (eg, gentamicin, cisplatin).

Certain patients, such as children with a reading or other learning problem and elderly people who appear to hear but not comprehend, should undergo a central auditory evaluation. It measures discrimination of degraded or distorted speech, discrimination in the presence of a competing message in the opposite ear, the ability to fuse incomplete or partial messages delivered to each ear into a meaningful message, and the capacity to localize sound in space when acoustic stimuli are delivered simultaneously to both ears.

Treatment

The underlying causes of a hearing loss should be determined and treated. Ototoxic drugs should be discontinued or their dose lowered. Blood levels of some ototoxic antibiotics (eg, gentamicin) can be measured.

Fluid from middle ear effusion can be drained by myringotomy and prevented with the insertion of a tympanostomy tube. Tumors (benign and malignant) blocking the eustachian tube or ear canal can be removed. Hearing loss caused by autoimmune disorders may respond to corticosteroids.

Damage to the tympanic membrane or ossicles or otosclerosis may require reconstructive surgery. Brain tumors causing hearing loss may in some cases be removed and hearing preserved.

Many causes of hearing loss have no cure, and treatment involves compensating for the hearing loss. Most patients with moderate to severe loss benefit from hearing aids. Those with severe to profound loss may benefit from a cochlear implant.

Hearing aids: Amplification of sound with a hearing aid helps many people. Although hearing aids do not restore hearing to normal, they can significantly improve communication. Physicians should encourage hearing aid use and help patients overcome a sense of social stigma that continues to obstruct use of these devices, perhaps by making the analogy that a hearing aid is to hearing as eye glasses are to vision.

All hearing aids have a microphone, amplifier, speaker, earpiece, and volume control, although they differ in the location of these components. An audiologist should be involved in selection and fitting of a hearing aid.

The best models are adjusted to a person's particular pattern of hearing loss. People with mainly high-frequency hearing loss do not benefit from simple amplification, which merely makes the garbled speech they hear sound louder. They generally need a hearing aid that selectively amplifies the high frequencies. Some hearing aids contain vents in the ear mold, which facilitate the passage of high-frequency sound waves. Some use digital sound processing with multiple frequency channels so that amplification more precisely matches hearing loss as measured on the audiogram.

Telephone use can be difficult for people with hearing aids. Typical hearing aids cause squealing when the ear is placed next to the phone handle. Some hearing aids have a phone coil with a switch that turns the microphone off and links the phone coil directly to the speaker magnet in the phone.

For moderate to severe hearing loss, a postauricular (ear-level) aid, which fits behind the pinna and is coupled to the ear mold with flexible tubing, is appropriate. An in-the-ear aid is contained entirely within the ear mold and fits less conspicuously into the concha and ear canal; it is appropriate for mild to moderate hearing loss. Canal aids are contained entirely within the ear canal and are cosmetically acceptable to many people who would otherwise refuse to use a hearing aid, but they are difficult for some people (especially the elderly) to manipulate. The CROS aid (*C*ontralateral *R*outing *O*f *S*ignals) is used for severe unilateral hearing loss; a hearing-aid microphone is placed in the nonfunctioning ear, and sound is routed to the functioning ear through a wire or radio transmitter. This device enables the wearer to hear sounds from the nonfunctioning side, allowing for some limited capacity to localize sound. If the better ear also has some hearing loss, the sound from both sides can be amplified with the bineural CROS (BiCROS) aid. The body aid type is appropriate for profound hearing loss. It is worn in a shirt pocket or a body harness and connected by a wire to the earpiece (the receiver), which is coupled to the ear canal by a plastic insert (ear mold).

A bone conduction aid may be used when an ear mold or tube cannot be used, as in atresia of the ear canal or persistent otorrhea. An oscillator is held against the head, usually over the mastoid, with a spring band, and sound is conducted through the skull to the cochlea. Bone conduction hearing aids require more power, introduce more distortion, and are less comfortable to wear than air conduction hearing aids. Some bone conduction aids (bone-anchored aids) are surgically implanted in the mastoid process, avoiding the discomfort and prominence of the spring band.

Cochlear implants: Profoundly deaf patients who cannot hear important environmental sounds (eg, doorbells, ringing telephones, alarms) even with a hearing aid may benefit from a cochlear implant. This device provides electrical signals directly into the auditory nerve via multiple electrodes implanted in the cochlea. An external microphone and processor convert sound waves to electrical impulses, which are transmitted through the skin electromagnetically from an external induction coil to an internal coil implanted in the skull above and behind the ear. The internal coil connects to electrodes inserted in the scala tympani.

Cochlear implants help with speech reading by providing information about the intonation of words and the rhythm of speech. Some people with cochlear implants can discriminate words without visual clues, allowing them to talk on the telephone. Cochlear implants enable deaf people to hear and distinguish environmental sounds and warning signals. They also help deaf people modulate their voices and make their speech more intelligible.

Coping mechanisms: Light alerting systems enable people to know when the doorbell is ringing or a baby is crying. Special sound systems help people hear in theaters, churches, or other places where competing noise exists. Many television programs carry closed captioning. Telephone communication devices are also available.

Lip reading (speech reading) is particularly important for people who can hear but have trouble discriminating sounds. Many people learn to read lips even without formal training. To be useful, the listener must be able to see the speaker's mouth. Health care personnel should be sensitive to this issue and always position themselves appropriately when speaking to the hearing impaired. Observing the position of a speaker's lips allows recognition of the consonant being spoken, thereby improving speech comprehension in patients with high-frequency hearing loss.

Patients can gain control over their listening environment by modifying or avoiding difficult situations. For example, people can visit a restaurant during off-peak hours, when it is quieter. They can ask for a booth, which blocks out some extraneous sounds. In direct conversations, people may ask the speaker to face them. At the beginning of a telephone conversation, people can identify themselves as being hearing-impaired. At a conference, the speaker can be asked to use an assistive listening system, which makes use of either inductive loop, infrared, or FM technology that sends sound through the microphone to the patient's hearing aid.

People with profound hearing loss often communicate using sign language. American Sign Language (ASL) is the most common version in the US. Other forms include Signed English, Signing Exact English, and Cued Speech.

Treatment in Children

In addition to treatment of underlying cause and provision of hearing aids, children with hearing loss require support of language development with appropriate therapy. Because children must hear language to learn it spontaneously, deaf children develop language only with special training, ideally beginning as soon as the hearing loss is identified. Deaf infants must be provided with a form of language input. For example, a visually based sign language can provide a foundation for later development of oral language.

Children ≥ 1 yr with profound bilateral hearing loss who cannot benefit from hearing aids may be candidates for a cochlear implant. Although cochlear implants allow auditory communication in many children with either congenital or acquired deafness, they appear to be more effective in those who already have developed language. Children who have postmeningitic deafness develop an ossified inner ear; they should receive cochlear implants early to maximize effectiveness. Children whose acoustic nerves have been destroyed by a tumor may be helped by implantation of brain stem auditory stimulating electrodes. Children with cochlear implants may have a slightly greater risk of meningitis than either children without cochlear implants or adults with cochlear implants.

Children with unilateral deafness should be allowed to use a special system in the classroom, such as an FM auditory trainer. With these systems, the teacher speaks into a microphone that sends signals to a hearing aid in the child's good ear, improving the child's ability to hear speech against a noisy background.

Prevention

Prevention of hearing loss consists mainly of limiting duration and intensity of noise exposure. People required to expose themselves to loud noise must wear ear protectors, eg, plastic plugs in the ear canals or glycerin-filled muffs over the ears. The Occupational Safety and Health Administration (OSHA) of the US Department of Labor and similar agencies in many countries have standards regarding the length of time that a person can be exposed to a noise. The greater the noise, the lesser the time of exposure.

SUDDEN DEAFNESS

Sudden deafness is severe sensorineural hearing loss that develops within a few hours. It affects about 1/5000 people/yr.

Sudden deafness has causes that differ from chronic hearing loss and must be addressed urgently.

Mechanical causes include blunt head trauma with fracture or hemorrhage involving the cochlea. Large ambient pressure changes or strenuous activities, such as weight lifting, can induce a perilymphatic fistula between the middle and inner ear.

Infectious causes include mumps and measles. Other causative viruses include influenza, varicella, adenoviruses, and Epstein-Barr virus. Lyme disease is a rare cause.

Vascular disorders involving the terminal branch of the anterior inferior cerebellar artery cause ischemia of the 8th cranial nerve in rare cases. Diseases include Waldenström's macroglobulinemia, sickle cell disease, and some forms of leukemia.

Ototoxic drugs (see p. 792) can result in hearing loss occurring within a day, especially if with overdose, systemically or when applied to a large wound area, such as a burn. There is a rare genetic disorder that increases the susceptibility to aminoglycoside ototoxicity.

Idiopathic sudden deafness may involve occult viral or bacterial infections; head trauma;

autoimmune disorders, such as Cogan's syndrome; toxic causes, such as snake bites; ototoxic drugs; circulatory problems; neurologic causes, such as multiple sclerosis; increased intracranial pressure; brain tumors; hyperlipidemia; and Meniere's disease.

Symptoms and Signs

Initial hearing loss is usually profound. A patient with perilymphatic fistula may hear an explosive sound in the affected ear when the fistula occurs and experience vertigo, nystagmus, and tinnitus. Viral infections may manifest only as hearing loss but can be associated with vertigo, nausea, or vomiting.

Diagnosis

Traumatic, ototoxic, and some infectious causes are usually apparent clinically. A perilymphatic fistula may be confirmed by tympanometry and electronystagmography (ENG). Other causes require a complete medical history. All patients should undergo an initial examination of the ear canal. Unless the diagnosis is determined from the history and physical examination, the patient should undergo an audiogram. Additional tests that may be needed include MRI, CBC with differential, ESR, antinuclear antibody, and tests for hypercoagulability.

The fistula may be demonstrated by combining the pressure changes in the ear canal used in tympanometry with ENG. Nystagmus resulting from pressure changes in the ear canal can be detected by ENG and suggests a perilymphatic fistula.

Treatment

Treatment addresses the underlying condition. Perilymphatic fistulas require surgical exploration and repair of the defect; hematologic abnormalities require correction.

In viral and idiopathic cases, the deficit returns to normal in most patients and is partially recovered in others. In those patients who recover their hearing, improvement usually occurs within 10 to 14 days. Mainly in patients with autoimmune disorders such as Cogan's syndrome, glucocorticoids are used. Glucocorticoids may also be helpful for patients with an idiopathic sudden sensorineural hearing loss.

86 INNER EAR DISORDERS

(See also Ch. 85.)

The inner ear is in the petrous area of the temporal bone. Within the bone is the osseous labyrinth, which encases the membranous labyrinth. The osseous labyrinth includes the vestibular system (made up of the semicircular canals and the vestibule) and the cochlea. The vestibular system is responsible for balance and posture, the cochlea for hearing.

ACOUSTIC NEUROMA

(Acoustic Neurinoma; 8th Nerve Tumor; Vestibular Schwannoma)

An acoustic neuroma is a Schwann cell–derived tumor of the 8th cranial nerve. Symptoms include unilateral hearing loss. Diagnosis is based on audiology and confirmed by MRI. Treatment is surgical removal.

Acoustic neuromas almost always arise from the vestibular division of the 8th cranial nerve and account for about 7% of all intracranial tumors. As the tumor expands, it projects from the internal auditory meatus into the cerebellopontine angle and compresses the cerebellum and brain stem. The 5th cranial nerve and later the 7th are affected. Acoustic neuroma is common in neurofibromatosis type 2.

Symptoms, Signs, and Diagnosis

Slowly progressive unilateral sensorineural hearing loss is the hallmark symptom. However, the onset of hearing loss may be abrupt, and the degree of impairment may fluctuate. Other early symptoms include unilateral tinnitus, dizziness and dysequilibrium, headache, sensation of pressure or fullness in the ear, otalgia, trigeminal neuralgia, and numbness or weakness of the facial nerve.

An audiogram is the first test performed (see p. 785). It usually reveals an asymmetric sensorineural hearing loss and a greater impairment of speech discrimination than would be expected for the degree of the hearing loss. Acoustic reflex decay, the absence of waveforms, and increased latency of the 5th waveform in auditory brain stem response testing are further evidence of a neural lesion. Although not usually required in the routine evaluation of a patient with asymmetric sensorineural hearing loss, caloric testing demonstrates marked vestibular hypoactivity (canal paresis). Such findings indicate the need for imaging tests, preferably gadolinium-enhanced MRI.

Treatment

Small tumors may be removed with microsurgery that preserves the facial nerve. A middle cranial fossa or retrosigmoid approach may preserve remaining hearing; a translabyrinthine route may be used if no useful hearing remains. Large tumors are removed with the translabyrinthine approach regardless of the remaining hearing. Stereotactic radiation as the sole treatment modality is used predominantly in the management of small tumors in older patients; its long-term efficacy and adverse effects are under study.

BENIGN PAROXYSMAL POSITIONAL VERTIGO

(Benign Postural or Positional Vertigo)

In benign paroxysmal positional vertigo, short (< 60 sec) episodes of vertigo occur with certain head positions. Nausea and nystagmus develop. Diagnosis is clinical. Treatment involves canalith repositioning maneuvers. Drugs and surgery are rarely, if ever, indicated.

Benign paroxysmal positional vertigo (BPPV) is the most common cause of relapsing otogenic vertigo. It affects people increasingly as they age and can severely affect balance in the elderly, leading to potentially injurious falls. The condition is thought to be caused by displacement of otoconial crystals (Ca carbonate crystals normally embedded in the saccule and utricle). This displaced material stimulates hair cells in the posterior semicircular canal, creating the illusion of motion. Etiologic factors include spontaneous degeneration of the utricular otolithic membranes, labyrinthine concussion, otitis media, ear surgery, recent viral infection (such as viral neuronitis), head trauma, prolonged anesthesia or bed rest, previous vestibular disorders (eg, Meniere's disease), and occlusion of the anterior vestibular artery.

Symptoms, Signs, and Diagnosis

Vertigo is triggered when the patient's head moves (eg, when rolling over in bed or bending over to pick something up). Acute vertigo lasts only a few seconds to minutes; episodes tend to peak in the morning and abate throughout the day. Nausea and vomiting may occur, but hearing loss and tinnitus do not.

Diagnosis is based on characteristic symptoms, on nystagmus as determined by the Dix-Hallpike maneuver (a provocative test for positional nystagmus—see sidebar 84–1 on p. 776), and on absence of other abnormalities on neurologic examination. Such patients require no further testing. Patients with nystagmus suggesting a CNS lesion undergo gadolinium-enhanced MRI. Unlike the positional nystagmus of BPPV, the positional nystagmus of CNS lesions lacks latency, fatigability, and severe subjective sensation and may continue for as long as the position is maintained. Nystagmus due to a CNS lesion may be vertical or change direction and, if rotary, is likely to be in the unexpected direction.

Treatment

BPPV usually subsides spontaneously in several weeks or months but may continue for months or years. Because the condition can be long-lasting, drug treatment (like that used in Meniere's disease [see p. 794]) is not recommended. Often, the adverse effects of drugs worsen dysequilibrium.

Because BPPV is fatigable, one therapy is to have the patient perform provocative maneuvers early in the day in a safe environment. Symptoms are then minimal for the rest of the day.

Canalith repositioning maneuvers (Epley—see FIG. 86–1—and Semont maneuvers) involve moving the head through a series of specific positions intended to return the errant canalith to the utricle. After performing these maneuvers, the patient should remain erect or semi-erect for 1 to 2 days. Both maneuvers can be repeated as necessary.

For the Semont maneuver, the patient is seated upright in the middle of a stretcher. The

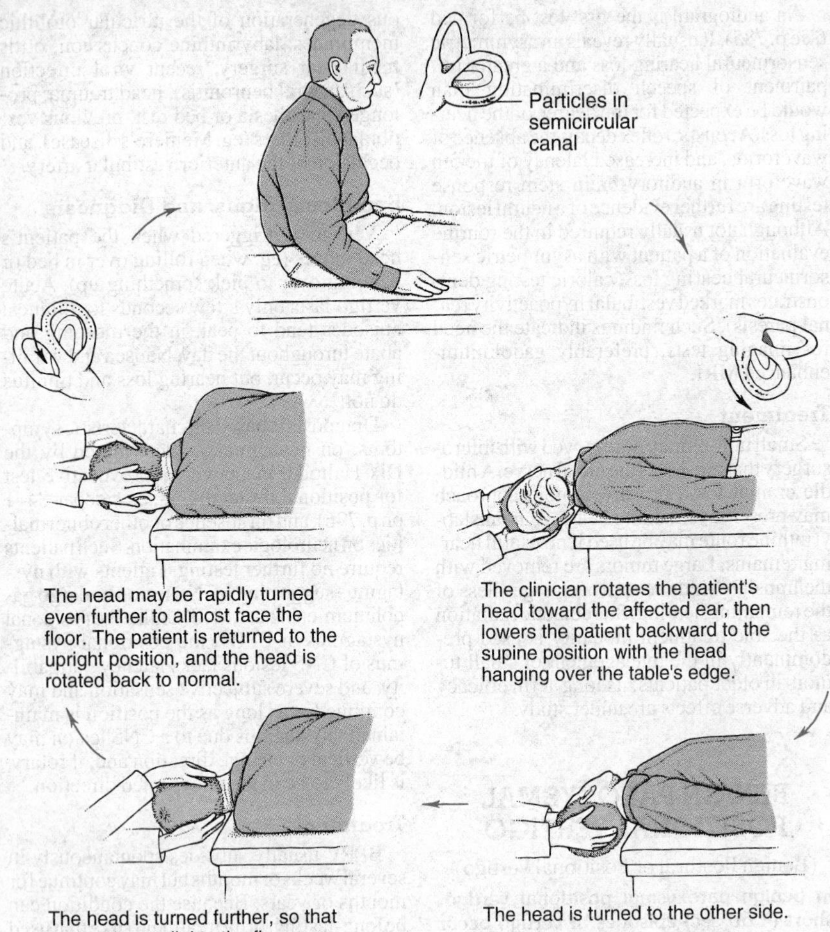

Particles in semicircular canal
The head may be rapidly turned even further to almost face the floor. The patient is returned to the upright position, and the head is rotated back to normal.
The clinician rotates the patient's head toward the affected ear, then lowers the patient backward to the supine position with the head hanging over the table's edge.
The head is turned further, so that the ear is parallel to the floor.
The head is turned to the other side.

Fig. 86–1. The Epley maneuver. This maneuver is used to treat benign positional vertigo by returning displaced otoliths to the utricle. If vertigo occurs during any of the positions, that position is held until the vertigo subsides.

patient's head is rotated toward the unaffected ear; this rotation is maintained throughout the maneuver. Next, the torso is lowered laterally onto the stretcher so that the patient is lying on the side of the affected ear with the nose pointed up. After 3 min in this position, the patient is quickly moved through the upright position without straightening the head and is lowered laterally to the other side now with the nose pointed down. After 3 min in this position, the patient is slowly returned to the upright position, and the head is rotated back to normal.

DRUG-INDUCED OTOTOXICITY

A wide variety of drugs can be ototoxic, including aminoglycoside antibiotics, vancomycin, salicylates, quinine and its synthetic substitutes, antineoplastics (particularly cisplatin), and diuretics (ethacrynic acid and furosemide).

Factors affecting ototoxicity include dose, duration of therapy, concurrent renal failure, infusion rate, lifetime dose, co-administration with other drugs having ototoxic potential, and genetic susceptibility. Ototoxic drugs should not be used for otic topical application when the tympanic membrane is perforated, lest the drugs enter the inner ear.

Streptomycin tends to cause more damage to the vestibular portion than to the auditory portion of the inner ear. Although vertigo and difficulty maintaining balance tend to be temporary, severe loss of vestibular sensitivity may persist, sometimes permanently. Loss of vestibular sensitivity causes difficulty walking, especially in the dark, and oscillopsia (a sensation of bouncing of the environment with each step). About 4 to 15% of patients who receive 1 g/day for > 1 wk develop measurable hearing loss, which usually occurs after a short latent period (7 to 10 days) and slowly worsens if treatment is continued. Complete, permanent deafness may follow.

Neomycin has the greatest cochleotoxic effect of all antibiotics. When large doses are given orally or by colonic irrigation for intestinal sterilization, enough may be absorbed to affect hearing, particularly if mucosal lesions are present. Neomycin should not be used for wound irrigation or for intrapleural or intraperitoneal irrigation, because massive amounts of the drug may be retained and absorbed, causing deafness. Kanamycin and amikacin are close to neomycin in cochleotoxic potential and are both capable of causing profound, permanent hearing loss while sparing balance. Viomycin has both cochlear and vestibular toxicity. Vancomycin causes hearing loss, especially in the presence of renal insufficiency. Gentamicin and tobramycin have vestibular and cochlear toxicity, causing impairment in balance and hearing.

Antineoplastic drugs, particularly those containing platinum (cisplatin and carboplatin), can cause tinnitus and hearing loss. Hearing loss can be profound and permanent, occurring immediately after the first dose, or can be delayed until several months after completion of treatment. Sensorineural hearing loss strikes bilaterally, progresses decrementally, and is permanent.

Ethacrynic acid and furosemide given IV have caused profound, permanent hearing loss in patients with renal failure who were receiving aminoglycoside antibiotics.

Salicylates in high doses (> 12 325-mg tablets of aspirin per day) cause temporary hearing loss and tinnitus. Quinine and its synthetic substitutes can also cause temporary hearing loss.

Prevention

Ototoxic antibiotics should be avoided in pregnancy. The elderly and people with preexisting hearing loss should not be treated with ototoxic drugs if other effective drugs are available. The lowest effective dosage of ototoxic drugs should be used and levels should be closely monitored. If possible before treatment with an ototoxic drug, hearing should be measured and then monitored during treatment; symptoms are not reliable warning signs.

HERPES ZOSTER OTICUS

(Geniculate Herpes; Ramsay Hunt Syndrome; Viral Neuronitis)

Herpes zoster oticus is infection of the 8th cranial nerve ganglia and the geniculate ganglion of the facial nerve by the herpes zoster virus.

Risk factors for herpes infection include immunodeficiency secondary to cancer, chemotherapy, radiation therapy, or HIV infection.

Symptoms, Signs, and Diagnosis

Symptoms include severe ear pain, transient or permanent facial paralysis (resembling Bell's palsy), vertigo lasting days to weeks, and hearing loss (which may be permanent or which may resolve partially or completely). Vesicles occur on the pinna and in the external auditory canal along the distribution of the sensory branch of the facial nerve. Symptoms of meningoencephalitis (eg, headache, confusion, stiff neck) are uncommon. Sometimes other cranial nerves are involved.

Diagnosis usually is clinical. If there is any question about viral etiology, vesicular scrapings may be collected for direct immunofluorescence or for viral cultures, and MRI is performed.

Treatment

Although there is no reliable evidence that corticosteroids, antiviral drugs, or surgical decompression makes a difference, they are the only possibly useful treatments.

Corticosteroids are started with prednisone 40 mg po once/day for 2 days, followed by gradual tapering of the dose over the next week. Acyclovir 800 mg po q 4 h 5 times/day or valacyclovir 1 g po bid for 10 days may shorten the clinical course. Vertigo is effectively suppressed with diazepam 2 to 5 mg po q 4 to 6 h. Pain may require oral opioids. Postherpetic neuralgia may be treated with amitriptyline. Surgical decompression of the fallopian canal may be indicated if the facial palsy is complete (no visible facial movement). Before surgery, however, electroneurography is performed and should demonstrate a > 90% decrement.

MENIERE'S DISEASE

(Endolymphatic Hydrops)

Meniere's disease is an inner ear disorder that produces vertigo, fluctuating sensorineural hearing loss, and tinnitus. There is no diagnostic test. Vertigo and nausea are treated with anticholinergics or benzodiazepines. Diuretics and a low-salt diet may decrease frequency and severity of episodes. For severe cases, the vestibular system can be ablated with topical gentamicin or surgery.

In Meniere's disease, pressure and volume changes of the labyrinthine endolymph affect inner ear function. The etiology of endolymphatic fluid buildup is unknown. Risk factors include a family history of Meniere's disease, preexisting autoimmune disorders, allergies, trauma to the head or ear, and, rarely, syphilis (even several decades previously). Peak incidence is between ages 20 and 50.

Symptoms and Signs

Patients have sudden attacks of vertigo lasting up to 24 h, usually with nausea and vomiting. Accompanying symptoms include diaphoresis, diarrhea, and gait unsteadiness. Tinnitus may be constant or intermittent, buzzing or roaring; it is not related to position or motion. Hearing impairment, typically affecting low frequencies, may follow. Before an episode, most patients sense fullness or pressure in the affected ear. In 50% of patients, only one ear is affected.

During the early stages, symptoms remit between episodes; symptom-free interludes may last > 1 yr. As the disease progresses, however, hearing impairment persists and gradually worsens, and tinnitus may be constant.

Diagnosis

The diagnosis, made clinically, is primarily one of exclusion. Similar symptoms can result from viral labyrinthitis or neuritis, a cerebellopontine angle tumor (eg, acoustic neuroma), or a brain stem stroke. Patients with suggestive symptoms should have an audiogram and an MRI (with gadolinium enhancement) of the CNS with attention to the internal auditory canals to exclude other causes. Audiogram typically demonstrates a low-frequency sensorineural hearing loss in the affected ear.

On examination during an acute attack, the patient has nystagmus and falls to the affected side. Between attacks, the Fukada stepping test (marching in place with eyes closed) can be used; the patient with Meniere's disease often turns away from the affected ear, consistent with a unilateral labyrinthine lesion. Additionally, Rinne's and Weber's tuning fork testing may indicate sensorineural hearing loss (see p. 785).

Treatment

Meniere's disease tends to be self-limited. Treatment of an acute attack is aimed at symptom relief. Anticholinergics (eg, prochlorperazine or promethazine 25 mg rectally or 10 mg po q 6 to 8 h) can minimize vagal-mediated GI symptoms, and antihistamines (eg, diphenhydramine, meclizine, or cyclizine 50 mg po q 6 h) or benzodiazepines (eg, diazepam 5 mg po q 6 to 8 h) are used to sedate the vestibular system. Some physicians also use a corticosteroid burst (eg, prednisone 60 mg once/day for 1 wk, tapered over another wk) for an acute episode.

A low-salt (< 1.5 g/day) diet, avoidance of alcohol and caffeine, and a diuretic (eg, hydrochlorothiazide 25 mg po once/day) may help prevent vertigo.

Intratympanic gentamicin (chemical labyrinthectomy) may be used when drugs are unsuccessful. Typical dose is 1 mL (at a 30 mg/mL concentration, made by diluting the commercial 40 mg/mL preparation with bicarbonate) injected through the tympanic membrane. Follow-up with serial audiometry is recommended to distinguish hearing loss from cochleotoxicity. The injection can be repeated in 4 wk if vertigo persists without hearing loss.

Surgery is reserved for patients with frequent, severely debilitating episodes who are unresponsive to other modalities. Endolymphatic sac decompression relieves vertigo in some patients and poses minimal risk of hearing loss. Vestibular neurectomy (an intracranial procedure) relieves vertigo in about 95% of patients and usually preserves hearing. A surgical labyrinthectomy is performed only if preexisting hearing loss is profound.

Unfortunately, there is no known way to prevent the natural progression of hearing loss. Most patients sustain moderate to severe sensorineural hearing loss in the affected ear within 10 to 15 yr.

PURULENT LABYRINTHITIS

Purulent (suppurative) labyrinthitis is bacterial infection of the inner ear, often causing deafness and loss of vestibular function.

Purulent labyrinthitis usually occurs when bacteria spread to the inner ear during the course of severe acute otitis media, purulent meningitis, or an enlarging cholesteatoma.

Symptoms include severe vertigo and nystagmus, nausea and vomiting, tinnitus, and varying degrees of hearing loss. Pain and fever are common.

Purulent labyrinthitis is suspected if vertigo, nystagmus, and/or sensorineural hearing loss occur during an episode of acute otitis media. CT of the temporal bones is done to identify erosion of the otic capsule bone or other complications of acute otitis media, such as coalescent mastoiditis. MRI may be indicated if symptoms of meningitis or brain abscess, such as altered mental status, meningismus, or high fever, are present; in such cases, a lumbar puncture and blood cultures also are performed.

Treatment is with IV antibiotics appropriate for meningitis (eg, ceftriaxone 50 to 100 mg/kg IV once/day to maximum 2 g) adjusted according to results of culture and sensitivity testing. A myringotomy (and sometimes tympanostomy tube placement) is done to drain the middle ear. Mastoidectomy may be required.

VESTIBULAR NEURONITIS

Vestibular neuronitis causes a self-limited episode of vertigo, presumably due to inflammation of the vestibular division of the 8th cranial nerve; some vestibular dysfunction may persist.

Although etiology is unclear, a viral cause is suspected.

Symptoms, Signs, and Diagnosis

Symptoms include a single attack of severe vertigo, with nausea and vomiting and persistent nystagmus toward the affected side, which lasts 7 to 10 days. The nystagmus is unidirectional, horizontal, and spontaneous, with fast-beat oscillations in the direction of the unaffected ear. The absence of concomitant tinnitus or hearing loss is a hallmark of vestibular neuronitis. The condition slowly subsides after this initial episode. Some patients have residual disequilibrium, especially with rapid head movements, probably due to permanent vestibular injury.

Patients undergo an audiologic assessment, electronystagmography with caloric testing, and gadolinium-enhanced MRI of the head, with attention to the internal auditory canals to exclude other diagnoses, such as cerebellopontine angle tumor, brain stem hemorrhage, or infarction. MRI may show enhancement of the vestibular nerves, consistent with inflammatory neuritis.

Treatment

Symptoms are addressed as in Meniere's disease (see p. 794), ie, with anticholinergics, antihistamines or benzodiazepines, and a corticosteroid burst with rapid taper. If vomiting is prolonged, IV fluids and electrolytes may be required. Vestibular rehabilitation (usually administered by a physical therapist) helps compensate for any residual vestibular deficit.

87 MIDDLE EAR AND TYMPANIC MEMBRANE DISORDERS

(See also Otic Tumors on p. 843.)

Middle ear disorders may be secondary to infection, eustachian tube obstruction, or trauma. Information about objects placed in the ear and symptoms such as rhinorrhea, nasal obstruction, sore throat, URI, allergies, headache, systemic symptoms, and fever aid diagnosis. The appearance of the external auditory canal and tympanic membrane (see FIG. 87–1) often yields a diagnosis. The nose, nasopharynx, and oropharynx are examined for signs of infection and allergy and for evidence of masses. Middle ear function is evaluated with use of pneumatic otoscopy, Weber's and Rinne's tuning fork tests, tympanometry, and audiologic tests (see p. 785).

MASTOIDITIS

Mastoiditis is a bacterial infection of the mastoid air cells typically following acute otitis media. Symptoms include redness, tenderness, swelling, and fluctuation over the mastoid process, with displacement of the pinna. Diagnosis is clinical. Treatment is with antibiotics, such as ceftriaxone, and sometimes mastoidectomy.

In acute purulent otitis media, inflammation often extends into the mastoid antrum and air cells, resulting in fluid accumulation. In a few patients, bacterial infection develops in the collected fluid, typically with the same organism causing the otitis media; pneumococcus is most common. Mastoid infection can produce osteitis of the septae, leading to coalescence of the air cells. The infection may decompress through a perforation in the tympanic membrane or extend through the lateral mastoid cortex, forming a postauricular subperiosteal abscess. Rarely, it extends centrally, causing a temporal lobe abscess or septic thrombosis of the lateral sinus.

Symptoms, Signs, and Diagnosis

Symptoms begin days to weeks after onset of acute otitis media and include fever and persistent, throbbing otalgia. Nearly all patients have signs of otitis media (see p. 797) and purulent otorrhea. Redness, swelling, tenderness, and fluctuation may develop over the mastoid process; the pinna is displaced laterally and inferiorly.

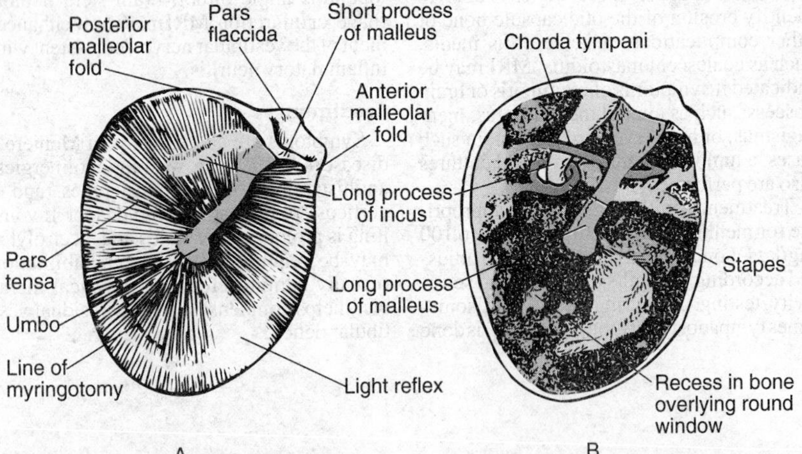

Fig. 87–1. Tympanic membrane of right ear (A); tympanic cavity with tympanic membrane removed (B).

Diagnosis is clinical. CT is rarely necessary but may confirm the diagnosis and monitor for extension and complications. Any middle ear drainage is sent for culture and sensitivity. Tympanocentesis for culture purposes can be performed if no spontaneous drainage occurs. CBC and ESR may be abnormal but are neither sensitive nor specific and add little to the diagnosis.

Treatment

IV antibiotic treatment is initiated immediately with a drug that provides CNS penetration, such as ceftriaxone 1 to 2 g (children, 50 to 75 mg/kg) once/day continued for ≥ 2 wk. Oral treatment with a quinolone may be acceptable. Subsequent antibiotic choice is guided by culture and sensitivity test results.

A subperiosteal abscess requires mastoidectomy (complete removal of mastoid air cells).

MYRINGITIS

(Bullous Myringitis)

Myringitis is a form of acute otitis media in which vesicles develop on the tympanic membrane.

Myringitis can develop with viral, bacterial (particularly *Streptococcus pneumoniae*), or mycoplasmal otitis media. Pain occurs suddenly and persists for 24 to 48 h. Hearing loss and fever suggest a bacterial origin. Diagnosis is based on otoscopic visualization of vesicles on the tympanic membrane.

Because differentiation between a viral, bacterial, and mycoplasmal cause is difficult, antibiotics effective against organisms causing otitis media are prescribed (see TABLE 87–1). Severe, continued pain may be relieved by rupturing the vesicles with a myringotomy knife or by oral analgesics (eg, oxycodone with acetaminophen). Topical analgesics (eg, benzocaine, antipyrine) may also be beneficial.

OTITIS MEDIA

Otitis media is infection of the middle ear. It generally causes pain and may result in hearing loss. Three forms exist: acute, secretory, and chronic.

ACUTE OTITIS MEDIA

Acute otitis media is a bacterial or viral infection of the middle ear, usually accompanying a URI. Symptoms include otalgia, often with systemic symptoms (fever, nausea, vomiting, diarrhea), especially in the very young. Diagnosis is based on otoscopy. Treatment is with analgesics and sometimes antibiotics.

Although acute otitis media (AOM) can occur at any age, it is most common between ages 3 mo and 3 yr. At this age, the eustachian tube is structurally and functionally immature; the angle of the eustachian tube is more horizontal; and the angle of the tensor veli palatini muscle and the cartilaginous eustachian tube renders the opening mechanism less efficient.

The etiology may be viral or bacterial. Viral infections are often complicated by secondary bacterial infection. In newborns, gram-negative enteric bacilli, particularly *Escherichia coli,* and *Staphylococcus aureus* cause AOM. In older infants and children < 14 yr, the most common organisms are *Streptococcus pneumoniae, Moraxella (Branhamella) catarrhalis,* and nontypeable *Haemophilus influenzae;* less common causes are group A β-hemolytic streptococci and *S. aureus.* In patients > 14 yr, *S. pneumoniae,* group A β-hemolytic streptococci, and *S. aureus* are most common, followed by *H. influenzae.*

Bacterial middle ear infection in rare cases spreads locally, resulting in acute mastoiditis, petrositis, or labyrinthitis. Intracranial spread is extremely rare and usually causes meningitis, but brain abscess, subdural empyema, epidural abscess, lateral sinus thrombosis, or otitic hydrocephalus may occur. Even with antibiotic treatment, intracranial complications are slow to resolve, especially in immunocompromised patients.

Symptoms and Signs

The usual initial symptom is earache, often with hearing loss. Infants may simply be cranky or have difficulty sleeping. Fever, nausea, vomiting, and diarrhea often occur in young children. Otoscopic examination reveals a bulging, erythematous tympanic membrane (TM) with indistinct landmarks and displacement of the light reflex. Air insufflation (pneumatic otoscopy) shows poor mobility of the TM. Spontaneous perforation

TABLE 87–1. ANTIBIOTICS FOR OTITIS MEDIA

TREATMENT GROUP	DRUG	DOSE* (by age)	COMMENTS
Initial treatment	Amoxicillin	< 14 yr: 40 to 45 mg/kg q 12 h > 14 yr: 500 mg q 8 h	Preferred High-dose regimen for possible resistant organisms
	Penicillin-allergic		
	Erythromycin/sulfisoxazole	< 14 yr: 10 to 12.5 mg/kg qid	Dose based on the sulfisoxazole component Sulfonamides contraindicated in infants < 2 mo
	Erythromycin	≥ 14 yr: 250 mg po q 6 h	
	Azithromycin	< 14 yr: 10 mg/kg day 1, then 5 mg/kg once/day for 4 days > 14 yr: 500 mg day 1, then 250 mg once/day for 4 days	Shorter course, once-daily dosing, more expensive
	Trimethoprim-sulfamethoxazole	> 2 mo: 4/20 mg/kg q 12 h ≥ 14 yr: 160/800 mg q 12 h	Sulfonamides contraindicated in infants < 2 mo
Resistant cases† (no improvement after 72 h treatment)	Cefaclor	< 14 yr: 10 to 20 mg/kg q 12 h ≥ 14 yr: 250 mg q 8 h	
	Cefuroxime	< 14 yr: 15 mg/kg q 12 h > 14 yr: 500 mg q 12 h	Maximum 1000 mg/day
	Amoxicillin-clavulanate	< 14 yr: 40 to 45 mg/kg q 12 h ≥ 14 yr: 500 mg q 12 h	Dose based on amoxicillin component Use new formulation to limit clavulanate to maximum 10 mg/kg/day
	Clarithromycin	< 14 yr: 7.5 mg/kg q 12 h ≥ 14 yr: 250 mg q 12 h	
Parenteral	Ceftriaxone	50 mg/kg IM once Repeat at 24 and 48 h if resistant case	Consider if compliance likely to be poor

*Treatment duration typically 10 to 12 days unless otherwise specified. Drugs are given orally unless otherwise specified.

†Other agents include cefdinir, cefpodoxime, ceftibuten, and clindamycin.

of the TM produces serosanguineous or purulent otorrhea.

Severe headache, confusion, or focal neurologic signs may occur with intracranial spread of infection. Facial paralysis or vertigo suggests local extension to the fallopian canal or labyrinth.

Diagnosis and Treatment

Diagnosis usually is clinical. Except for fluid obtained during myringotomy, cultures are not generally obtained.

Although 80% of cases resolve spontaneously, in the US, antibiotics are often given (see TABLE 87–1). Antibiotics relieve symptoms quicker (although results after 1 to 2 wk are similar) and may reduce the chance of residual hearing loss and labyrinthine or intracranial sequelae. However, with the recent emergence of resistant organisms, pediatric organizations have strongly recommended initial antibiotics only for those at highest risk (eg, those who are younger or more severely ill—see TABLE 87–2) or for those with recurrent AOM (eg, ≥ 4 episodes in 6 mo). Others can safely be observed for up to 72 h and antibiotics given only if no improvement is seen; if follow-up by phone is planned, a prescription can be given at the initial visit to save time and expense.

All patients receive analgesics (eg, acetaminophen, ibuprofen). In adults, topical vasoconstrictors, such as phenylephrine 0.25% 3 drops q 3 h, improve eustachian tube function. To avoid rebound congestion, these preparations should not be used > 4 days. Systemic decongestants (eg, pseudoephedrine 30 to 60 mg po q 6 h prn) may be helpful. Antihistamines (eg, chlorpheniramine 4 mg po q 4 to 6 h for 7 to 10 days) may improve eustachian tube function in people with allergies but should be reserved for the truly allergic. For children, neither vasoconstrictors nor antihistamines are of benefit.

Myringotomy may be performed for a bulging TM, particularly if severe or persistent pain, fever, vomiting, or diarrhea is present. The patient's hearing, tympanometry, and TM appearance and movement are monitored until normal.

Prevention

Routine childhood vaccination against pneumococci (with pneumococcal conjugate vaccine), *H influenzae* type B, and influenza decreases the incidence of AOM. Infants should not sleep with a bottle, and elimination of household smoking may decrease incidence.

TABLE 87–2. GUIDELINES FOR USING ANTIBIOTICS IN ACUTE OTITIS MEDIA

AGE	DIAGNOSIS CERTAIN	DIAGNOSIS UNCERTAIN
< 6 mo	Antibiotics	Antibiotics
6 mo to 2 yr	Antibiotics	Antibiotics if illness severe* Observe 72 h if illness not severe†
≥ 2 yr	Antibiotics if illness severe Observe 72 h if illness not severe	Observe 72 h

*Temperature ≥ 39.5°C rectally any time within previous 24 h; moderate to severe otalgia; or physician's judgment that child is seriously ill.

†Appropriate only if phone or office follow-up assured within 72 h. Antibiotics are started if no improvement.

Modified from: Rosenfeld RM, Observation option toolkit for acute otitis media. *Int J Pediatr Otorhinolaryngol* 2001;58:1–8.

Secretory Otitis Media

(Serous Otitis Media)

Secretory otitis media is an effusion in the middle ear resulting from incomplete resolution of acute otitis media or obstruction of the eustachian tube without infection. Symptoms include hearing loss and a sense of fullness or pressure in the ear. Diagnosis is based on appearance of the tympanic membrane and sometimes on tympanometry. Treatment may include a trial of systemic antibiotics, decongestants, antihistamines if allergies are present, and myringotomy for persistent cases.

Normally, the middle ear is ventilated 3 to 4 times/min as the eustachian tube opens during swallowing, and O_2 is absorbed by blood in the vessels of the middle ear mucous membrane. If patency of the eustachian tube is impaired, a relative negative pressure develops within the middle ear, which can lead to fluid accumulation. This fluid may cause hearing loss.

Secretory otitis media is a common sequelae to AOM in children (often identified on routine ear recheck) and may persist for weeks to months. In other cases, eustachian tube obstruction may be secondary to inflammatory processes in the nasopharynx, allergies, hypertrophic adenoids or other obstructive lymphoid aggregations on the torus of the eustachian tube and in Rosenmüller's fossa, or benign or malignant tumors. The effusion may be sterile or (more commonly) contain pathogenic bacteria, although overt inflammation is absent.

Symptoms, Signs, and Diagnosis

Many patients report no symptoms, but some (or their family members) note hearing loss. Patients may experience a feeling of fullness, pressure, or popping in the ear with swallowing. Otalgia is rare.

The TM is amber or gray, and the light reflex is displaced. It is mildly retracted and the landmarks accentuated. On air insufflation, the TM is immobile. An air-fluid level or bubbles of air may be visible through the TM.

Diagnosis is clinical. Tympanometry may be performed to confirm middle ear effusion. Adults must undergo nasopharyngeal examination to exclude malignancy.

Treatment

For most patients, watchful waiting is all that is required. Antibiotics and decongestants are not proved to be of value. For patients in whom allergies are clearly involved, antihistamines and topical corticosteroids may be helpful.

If no improvement occurs in 1 to 3 mo, myringotomy may be performed for aspiration of fluid and insertion of a tympanostomy tube, which allows ventilation of the middle ear and temporarily ameliorates eustachian tube obstruction, regardless of cause. Tympanostomy tubes may be inserted for persistent conductive hearing loss or to help prevent recurrence of AOM.

Occasionally, the middle ear is temporarily ventilated with the Valsalva maneuver or politzerization. To perform the Valsalva maneuver, the patient keeps his mouth closed and tries to forcibly blow air out through his pinched nostrils (ie, popping the ear). To perform politzerization, the physician blows air with a special syringe (middle ear inflator) into one of the patient's nostrils and blocks the other while the patient swallows. This forces the air into the eustachian tube and middle ear. Neither procedure should be performed if the patient has a cold and rhinorrhea.

Persistent, recurrent secretory otitis media may require correction of underlying nasopharyngeal conditions. Children may benefit from adenoidectomy, including the removal of the central adenoid mass as well as lymphoid aggregations on the torus of the eustachian tube and in Rosenmüller's fossa. Antibiotics should be administered for bacterial rhinitis, sinusitis, and nasopharyngitis. Demonstrated allergens should be eliminated from the patient's environment and immunotherapy considered.

Chronic Otitis Media

Chronic otitis media is a persistent, chronically draining (> 6 wk), suppurative perforation of the tympanic membrane. Symptoms include painless otorrhea with conductive hearing loss. Complications include development of aural polyps, cholesteatoma, and other infections. Treatment requires complete cleaning of the ear canal several times daily, careful removal of granulation tissue, and application of topical corticosteroids and antibiotics. Systemic antibiotics and surgery are reserved for severe cases.

Chronic otitis media can result from AOM, eustachian tube obstruction, mechanical trauma, thermal or chemical burns, blast injuries, or iatrogenic causes (eg, after tympanostomy tube placement). Further, patients with craniofacial abnormalities, Down syndrome, cri du chat syndrome, cleft lip, choanal atresia, or microcephaly have an increased risk.

Chronic otitis media may become exacerbated after a URI or when water enters the middle ear during bathing or swimming. Infections often are caused by gram-negative bacilli or *Staphylococcus aureus,* resulting in painless, purulent, sometimes foul-smelling otorrhea. Persistent chronic otitis media may result in destructive changes in the middle ear (such as necrosis of the long process of the incus) or aural polyps (granulation tissue prolapsing into the ear canal through the TM perforation). Aural polyps are a serious sign, almost invariably suggesting cholesteatoma.

A cholesteatoma is an epithelial cell growth that forms in the middle ear, mastoid, or epitympanum after chronic otitis media. Lytic enzymes, such as collagenases, produced by the cholesteatoma can destroy adjacent bone and soft tissue. The cholesteatoma is also a nidus for infection; purulent labyrinthitis, facial paralysis, or intracranial abscess may develop.

Symptoms, Signs, and Diagnosis

Chronic otitis media usually presents with conductive hearing loss and otorrhea. Pain is uncommon unless an associated osteitis of the temporal bone occurs. The TM is perforated and draining, and the auditory canal is macerated and littered with granulation tissue.

A patient with cholesteatoma has white debris in the middle ear, a draining polypoid mass protruding through the TM perforation, and an ear canal that appears clogged with mucopurulent granulation tissue.

Diagnosis is usually clinical. Drainage is cultured. When cholesteatoma or other complications are suspected (as in a febrile patient or one with vertigo or otalgia), CT or MRI is performed. These tests may reveal intratemporal or intracranial processes (labyrinthitis, ossicular or temporal erosion, abscesses).

Treatment

The ear canal is irrigated with a bulb syringe 3 times/day with a slightly warmed solution of half peroxide and half sterile water. After the ear drains, topical neomycin/polymyxin B suspension is instilled, 5 to 10 drops tid for 7 to 10 days.

Granulation tissue is removed with microinstruments or cauterized with silver nitrate sticks. A solution of 2% acetic acid with hydrocortisone 1% is then instilled into the ear. As aural toilet improves and granulation tissue resolves, penetration of topical antibiotics improves.

Severe exacerbations require systemic antibiotic therapy with amoxicillin 250 to 500 mg po q 8 h for 10 days or a 3rd-generation cephalosporin, subsequently modified by culture results and response to therapy.

Tympanoplasty is indicated for patients with marginal or attic perforations and chronic central TM perforations. A disrupted ossicular chain may be repaired during tympanoplasty as well. Cholesteatomas must be removed surgically; because recurrence is common, reconstruction of the middle ear is usually deferred until a 2nd-look operation is performed 6 to 8 mo later.

OTIC BAROTRAUMA

(Barotitis or Aerotitis Media)

Otic barotrauma is ear pain or damage to the tympanic membrane caused by rapid changes in pressure.

To maintain equal pressure on both sides of the tympanic membrane (TM), gas must move freely between the nasopharynx and middle ear. When a URI, allergy, or other mechanism interferes with eustachian tube functioning during changes in environmental pressure, the pressure in the middle ear either falls below ambient pressure, causing retraction of the TM, or rises above it, causing bulging. With negative middle ear pressure, a transudate of fluid may form in the middle ear. As the pressure differential increases, ecchymosis and subepithelial hematoma may develop in the mucous membrane of the middle ear and the TM. A very large pressure differential may cause bleeding into the middle ear, TM rupture, and the development of a perilymph fistula through the oval or round window.

Symptoms are severe pain and conductive hearing loss. Symptoms usually worsen during rapid ascent (eg, during scuba diving) or descent (eg, during air travel). Sensorineural hearing loss or vertigo during descent suggests the development of a perilymph fistula; the same symptoms during ascent from a deep-sea dive suggest bubble formation in the inner ear.

Prevention and Treatment

A person with nasal congestion due to URI or allergies should avoid flying and diving. When these activities are unavoidable, a topical nasal vasoconstrictor (eg, phenylephrine 0.25 to 1.0%) is applied 30 to 60 min before descent or ascent.

Routine self-treatment of pain associated with changing pressure in an aircraft includes chewing gum, attempting to yawn and swallow, blowing against closed nostrils, and using decongestant nasal sprays.

If hearing loss is sensorineural and vertigo is present, a perilymph fistula is suspected and middle ear exploration to close a fistula is considered. If pain is severe and loss is found to be conductive, a myringotomy is helpful.

OTOSCLEROSIS

Otosclerosis is a disease of the bone of the otic capsule that produces an abnormal accumulation of new bone within the oval window.

In otosclerosis, the new bone traps and restricts the movement of the stapes, causing conductive hearing loss (see p. 781). Otosclerosis also may produce a sensorineural hearing loss, particularly when the foci of otosclerotic bone are adjacent to the scala media. Half of all cases are inherited. The measles virus may play an inciting role in patients with a genetic predisposition for otosclerosis.

Although about 10% of white adults have some otosclerosis (compared with 1% of blacks), only about 10% of affected people develop conductive hearing loss. Hearing loss from otosclerosis may manifest as early as age 7 or 8, but most cases do not become evident until the late teen or early adult years, when slowly progressive, asymmetric hearing loss is diagnosed. Fixation of the stapes may progress rapidly during pregnancy.

A hearing aid may restore hearing. Alternatively, microsurgery to remove some or all of the stapes and to replace it with a prosthesis may be beneficial.

TRAUMATIC PERFORATION OF THE TYMPANIC MEMBRANE

Traumatic perforation of the tympanic membrane can cause pain, bleeding, hearing loss, tinnitus, and vertigo. Diagnosis is based on otoscopy. Treatment often is unnecessary. Antibiotics may be needed for infection; surgery may be needed for perforations persisting > 2 mo, disruption of the ossicular chain, or injuries affecting the inner ear.

Traumatic causes of tympanic membrane (TM) perforation include:

- Insertion of objects into the ear canal purposely (eg, cotton swabs) or accidentally
- Concussion from an explosion or open-handed slap across the ear
- Head trauma (with or without basilar fracture)
- Sudden negative pressure (eg, strong suction applied to the ear canal)
- Barotrauma (eg, during air travel or scuba diving)
- Iatrogenic perforation during irrigation or foreign body removal

Penetrating injuries of the TM may result in dislocations of the ossicular chain, fracture of the stapedial footplate, displacement of fragments of the ossicles, bleeding, a perilymph fistula from the oval or round window resulting in leakage of perilymph into the middle ear space, or facial nerve injury.

Symptoms, Signs, and Diagnosis

Traumatic perforation of the TM causes sudden severe pain sometimes followed by bleeding from the ear, hearing loss, and tinnitus. Hearing loss is more severe if the ossicular chain is disrupted or the inner ear is injured. Vertigo suggests injury to the inner ear. Purulent otorrhea may begin in 24 to 48 h, particularly if water enters the middle ear.

Perforation is generally evident on otoscopy. Any blood obscuring the ear canal is carefully suctioned. Irrigation and pneumatic otoscopy are avoided. Extremely small perforations may require otomicroscopy or middle ear impedance studies for definitive diagnosis. If possible, audiometric studies are performed before and after treatment to avoid confusion between trauma-induced and treatment-induced hearing loss.

Patients with marked hearing loss or severe vertigo are evaluated by an otolaryngologist as soon as possible. Exploratory tympanotomy may be needed to assess and repair damage. Patients with a large TM defect should also be evaluated, because the displaced flaps may need to be repositioned.

Treatment

Often, no specific treatment is needed. The ear should be kept dry; routine antibiotic eardrops are unnecessary. However, prophylaxis with an oral broad-spectrum antibiotic or antibiotic eardrops is necessary if contaminants may have entered through the perforation as occurs in dirty injuries.

If the ear becomes infected, amoxicillin 250 mg po q 8 h is administered for 7 days.

Although most perforations close spontaneously, surgery is indicated for a perforation persisting > 2 mo. Persistent conductive hearing loss suggests disruption of the ossicular chain, necessitating surgical exploration and repair.

88 EXTERNAL EAR DISORDERS

The external ear (pinna and external auditory canal) can be affected by congenital, dermatologic, infectious, neoplastic, obstructive, and traumatic disorders. Congenital defects are discussed on p. 2424.

DERMATITIS

Dermatitis is inflammation of the ear canal involving itching and skin changes either from exposure to allergens (contact dermatitis) or spontaneous occurrences (aural eczematoid dermatitis).

Common contact allergens include nickel-containing earrings and numerous beauty products (eg, hairsprays, lotions, hair dye). Aural eczematoid dermatitis is more common in people with a predisposition toward atopy and with other similar dermatitides (eg, seborrhea, psoriasis).

Both contact dermatitis and aural eczematoid dermatitis produce itching, redness, discharge, desquamation, hyperpigmentation, and, sometimes, fissuring. A secondary infection can occur.

Contact dermatitis requires avoidance or withdrawal of allergic triggers. Trial and error may be needed to identify the offending agent. Topical corticosteroids (eg, 1% hydrocortisone cream) can decrease inflammation and itching.

Aural eczematoid dermatitis can be treated with dilute aluminum acetate solution (Burow's solution), which can be applied as often as required for comfort. Itching and inflammation can be reduced with topical corticosteroids. If diffuse external otitis ensues, antibiotic therapy may be required (see p. 804).

EXTERNAL OTITIS

External otitis is infection of the ear canal, typically by bacteria. Symptoms include itching, pain, and discharge. Diagnosis is based on inspection. Treatment is with topical drugs, including antibiotics, corticosteroids, and/or acetic acid.

External otitis may manifest as a localized furuncle or as a diffuse infection of the entire canal (generalized or diffuse external otitis). This condition is often called swimmer's ear because it sometimes afflicts people who swim in fresh water. Malignant external otitis (see p. 804) is a severe *Pseudomonas* infection of the temporal bone.

Etiology

Diffuse external otitis is usually caused by bacteria, such as *Pseudomonas aeruginosa, Proteus vulgaris, Staphylococcus aureus,* or *Escherichia coli.* Fungal external otitis (otomycosis), typically caused by *Aspergillus niger* or *Candida albicans,* is less common. Furuncles usually are due to *S. aureus*.

Predisposing conditions include allergies, psoriasis, eczema, seborrheic dermatitis, decreased canal acidity (possibly due to the repeated presence of water from a lake or swimming pool), irritants (eg, hair spray, hair dye), and inadvertent injury to the canal caused by excessive cleaning with cotton swabs or other objects. Attempts to clean the ear canal may push debris and cerumen deeper into the canal; these accumulated substances tend to trap water, resulting in skin maceration that sets the stage for bacterial infection.

Symptoms and Signs

Patients experience itching and pain. Sometimes, a foul-smelling discharge and hearing loss occur if the canal becomes swollen or filled with purulent debris. Exquisite tenderness accompanies traction of the pinna or pressure over the tragus. Otoscopic examination is painful and difficult to conduct. It shows the ear canal to be red, swollen, and littered with moist, purulent debris. Otomycosis caused by *A. niger* usually presents with grayish black or yellow dots (fungal conidiophores) surrounded by a cottonlike material (fungal hyphae). Infection caused by *C. albicans* does not show any visible evidence of fungi but usually contains a thickened, creamy white exudate.

Furuncles cause severe pain and may drain sanguineous, purulent material. They appear as a focal, erythematous swelling.

Diagnosis, Prevention, and Treatment

Diagnosis is based on inspection. When discharge is copious, external otitis can be difficult to differentiate from perforated otitis media; pain with pulling on the pinna indicates external otitis. Fungal infection is diagnosed by appearance.

External otitis often can be prevented by irrigating the ears with a 1:1 mixture of rubbing alcohol and vinegar immediately after swimming. The alcohol helps remove water, and the vinegar alters the pH of the canal.

In diffuse external otitis, topical antibiotics and corticosteroids are effective. First, the infected debris should be gently and thoroughly removed from the canal with suction or dry cotton wipes. Mild external otitis can be treated by altering the ear canal's pH with 2% acetic acid and by relieving inflammation with topical hydrocortisone; these are administered 5 drops tid for 7 days. Moderate external otitis requires the addition of an antibacterial solution or suspension, such as neomycin, polymyxin, bacitracin, or ciprofloxacin. When inflammation of the ear canal is relatively severe, a cotton wick should be placed into the ear canal and wetted with the necessary drugs 4 times/day. The wick is left in place for 24 to 72 h, after which time the swelling may have receded enough to allow the instillation of drops directly into the canal.

Severe external otitis or the presence of cellulitis extending beyond the ear canal may require systemic antibiotics, such as cephalexin 250 mg po qid to 500 mg po bid or ciprofloxacin 500 mg po bid. If the patient is allergic to penicillin, erythromycin in the same dose can be used. An analgesic, such as an NSAID or even an oral opioid, may be necessary for the first 24 to 48 h. Fungal external otitis requires thorough cleaning of the ear canal and application of an antimycotic solution (eg, gentian violet, cresylate acetate, nystatin, clotrimazole). Repeated cleanings and treatments may be needed.

A furuncle, if obviously pointing, should be incised and drained. Incision is of little value, however, if the patient is seen at an early stage. Topical antibiotics are ineffective; oral antistaphylococcal antibiotics should be administered. Analgesics, such as oxycodone with acetaminophen, may be necessary for pain relief. Dry heat can also lessen pain and hasten resolution.

MALIGNANT EXTERNAL OTITIS

Malignant external otitis is typically a *Pseudomonas* osteomyelitis of the temporal bone.

Soft tissue, cartilage, and bone are all affected. The osteomyelitis spreads along the base of the skull and may cross the midline.

Malignant external otitis occurs mainly in elderly patients with diabetes or in immunocompromised patients and is often initiated by *Pseudomonas* external otitis. It is characterized by persistent and severe earache, foul-smelling purulent otorrhea, and granulation tissue in the ear canal (usually the external ear canal at the junction of the bony and cartilaginous portions). Varying degrees of conductive hearing loss may occur. In severe cases, facial nerve paralysis may ensue.

Diagnosis is based on a CT scan of the temporal bone, which may show increased radiodensity in the air-cell system and middle ear radiolucency (demineralization) in some areas. Cultures are obtained, and the ear canal is biopsied to differentiate the granulation tissue of this disorder from a malignant tumor.

Treatment is with a 6-wk IV course of a fluoroquinolone or an aminoglycoside-semisynthetic penicillin combination. Extensive bone disease may require more prolonged antibiotic therapy. Careful control of diabetes is essential. Surgery usually is not necessary.

OBSTRUCTIONS

The ear canal may be obstructed by cerumen (earwax), insertion of a foreign object, or an insect. Itching, pain, and temporary conductive hearing loss may result. Most causes of obstruction are readily apparent during otoscopic examination. Treatment is manual removal.

Cerumen may get pushed further into the ear canal and accumulate during ill-advised attempts to clean the ear canal with cotton swabs, resulting in obstruction. Cerumen solvents (hydrogen peroxide, carbamide peroxide, glycerin, triethanolamine) may be used to soften very hard wax before irrigation or direct removal. However, the prolonged use of these agents may lead to canal skin irritation or allergic reactions. Although cerumen may be removed by irrigation, rolling the cerumen out of the ear canal with a blunt curet or loop or removing it with a suction tip (eg, Baron, size 7 French) is quicker, neater, safer, and more comfortable for the patient. Irrigation is contraindicated if the patient has a history of otorrhea or perforation of the tympanic membrane; water entering the middle ear through a perforation may exacerbate chronic otitis media.

Foreign bodies are common, particularly in children, who often insert objects, particularly beads, erasers, and beans, into the ear canal. Foreign bodies may remain unnoticed until they provoke an inflammatory response, causing pain, itching, infection, and foul-smelling, purulent drainage. A foreign body in the ear canal is best removed by reaching behind it and rolling it out with a blunt hook. Forceps tend to push smooth objects deeper into the canal. Unfortunately, a foreign body lying medial to the isthmus is difficult to remove without injuring the tympanic membrane and ossicular chain. Metal and glass beads can sometimes be removed by irrigation, but hygroscopic foreign bodies (eg, beans or other vegetable matter) swell when water is added, complicating removal. A general anesthetic may be needed when a child cannot remain still or when removal is difficult, threatening injury to the tympanic membrane or ossicles. Further, if manipulating a presumed foreign object results in bleeding, immediate otolaryngologic consultation should be sought. Bleeding may indicate a mucosal polyp originating in the middle ear, which may be attached to the ossicles or facial nerve.

Insects in the canal are most annoying while alive. Filling the canal with viscous lidocaine kills the insect, which provides immediate relief and allows the immobilized insect to be removed with forceps.

PERICHONDRITIS

Perichondritis is infection of the perichondrium of the pinna in which pus accumulates between the cartilage and the perichondrium.

Causes of perichondritis include trauma, insect bites, body piercings, and incision of superficial infections of the pinna. Because the cartilage's blood supply is provided by the perichondrium, separation of the perichondrium from both sides of the cartilage may lead to avascular necrosis and a deformed pinna. Septic necrosis may also ensue, often with infection by gram-negative bacilli. Symptoms include redness, pain, and swelling. The course of perichondritis tends to be indolent, long-term, and destructive.

The affected area is incised, and a drain is left in place for 24 to 72 h. Systemic antibiotics are initiated with an aminoglycoside and semisynthetic penicillin. Subsequent antibiotic choice is guided by culture and sensitivity tests. Warm compresses may help.

89 APPROACH TO THE PATIENT WITH NASAL, ORAL, AND PHARYNGEAL SYMPTOMS

The nose, mouth, and pharynx (consisting of the nasopharynx, oropharynx, and hypopharynx) may be affected by inflammation, infection, trauma, tumors, and several miscellaneous conditions. In addition, clues suggesting systemic disease may be found in the mouth and adjacent structures (see TABLE 89–1). Dental symptoms are discussed in Ch. 94 on p. 844.

Anatomy and Physiology

Mouth: Normally, keratinized epithelium occurs on the facial aspect of the lips, dorsum of the tongue, hard palate, and gingiva around the teeth. Nonkeratinized mucosa occurs over alveolar bone further from the teeth, inside the lips and cheeks, on the sides and undersurface of the tongue, on the soft palate, and covering the floor of the mouth. The skin and mucosa of the lips are demarcated by the vermilion border.

The buccal mucosa, including the vestibule and nonkeratinized alveolar mucosa, is usually smooth, moist, and pink. Innocuous entities in this region include linea alba (a thin

TABLE 89–1. ORAL FINDINGS IN SYSTEMIC DISORDERS

ORAL MANIFESTATION	POSSIBLE INDICATION
Candidiasis	Diabetes, AIDS, other causes of immunosuppression (eg, agranulocytosis, neutropenia, leukemia, immunoglobulin defects, disorders of leukocyte function), antibiotic use
Atrophic glossitis (a smooth tongue caused by atrophy of filiform papillae)	Iron deficiency
Painful atrophy of the oral mucosa and surface of the tongue, sometimes with aphthous ulcers	Megaloblastic anemias
Magenta tongue	Vitamin B_{12} deficiency
Darkly pigmented areas (if not a racial characteristic)	Hemochromatosis; Addison's disease; Peutz-Jeghers syndrome; melanoma (rare, but may be seen on the palate)
Linear, grayish discoloration (lead line) in the gingiva adjacent to teeth	Lead, silver, or bismuth poisoning
Violaceous patches	Kaposi's sarcoma, AIDS
Keratotic lichenoid patches, sometimes with painful mucosal atrophy	Graft-vs-host disease if in the mouth of an organ -transplant recipient
Reddish discoloration of the teeth	Congenital erythropoietic porphyria
High, arched soft palate	Marfan syndrome
Notched incisors, domed or "mulberry" molars	Congenital syphilis
No or minimal tooth decay	Hereditary fructose intolerance (rare)
Multiple impacted supernumerary teeth and osteomas	Gardner's syndrome

white line, typically bilateral, on the level of the occlusal plane, where the cheek is bitten), Fordyce's granules (aberrant sebaceous glands appearing as < 1 mm light yellow spots that may also occur on the lips), and white sponge nevus (bilateral thick white folds over most of the buccal mucosa). Recognizing these entities avoids needless biopsy and apprehension. The orifices of the parotid (Stensen's) ducts are opposite the maxillary 1st molar on each side.

The dorsal surface of the tongue is covered with numerous whitish elevations, the filiform papillae. Interspersed among them are isolated reddish prominences, the fungiform papillae, occurring mostly on the anterior part of the tongue. The circumvallate papillae, numbering 8 to 12, are considerably larger and lie posteriorly in a "V" pattern. They do not project from the tongue but instead are surrounded by a trench. The foliate papillae appear as a series of parallel, slitlike folds on the lateral borders of the tongue, near the anterior pillars of the fauces. They vary in length and can easily be confused with lesions, as may the foramen cecum, median rhomboid glossitis, and, rarely, a lingual thyroid nodule. Lingual tonsils may be considered components of Waldeyer's ring, are at the back of the tongue, and may also be mistaken for lesions.

Innervation is supplied by the lingual nerves (branches of the 5th cranial nerves), which supply general sensory innervation, and the chorda tympani fibers (of the 7th cranial nerve), which innervate the taste buds of the anterior ⅔ of the tongue. Behind the circumvallate papillae, the glossopharyngeal nerves (9th cranial nerves) provide the sensations of touch and taste. Sweet and salty taste receptors are located at and near the tip; sour, on the sides; and bitter, on the most posterior part of the tongue. The hypoglossal nerves (12th cranial nerves) control movement of the tongue.

The major salivary glands are the paired parotid, submandibular, and sublingual glands. Most oral mucosal surfaces contain many minor mucus-secreting salivary glands. Anteriorly and near the midline on each side of the floor of the mouth are the openings of Wharton's ducts, which drain the ipsilateral submandibular and sublingual glands. The parotid glands drain into the cheeks via Stensen's ducts.

Throat: The uvula hangs in the midline at the far end of the soft palate. It varies greatly in length. A long uvula and loose or excess velopharyngeal tissue may cause snoring and occasionally contribute to obstructive sleep apnea.

Tonsils and adenoids are patches of lymphoid tissue surrounding the posterior pharynx in an area termed Waldeyer's ring. Their role is to combat infection.

The larynx is discussed in Ch. 92 on p. 834.

Nose: The nasal cavity is covered with a highly vascular mucosa that warms and humidifies incoming air. On each lateral wall of the cavity are 3 turbinates, which are bony shelves that increase the surface area, thereby allowing more effective heat and moisture exchange. Nasal mucus traps incoming particulate matter. The space between the middle and inferior turbinate is the middle meatus, into which the maxillary and most of the ethmoid sinuses drain. Polyps may develop between the turbinates, often in association with asthma, allergy, aspirin use, and cystic fibrosis.

Sinuses: The paranasal sinuses are mucus-lined bony cavities that connect to the nasopharynx. The 4 types are maxillary, frontal, ethmoid, and sphenoid sinuses. They are located in the facial and cranial bones (see FIG. 89–1). The physiologic role of the sinuses is unclear.

Evaluation

Examination of the nose, mouth, and pharynx is part of every general physical examination. Oral findings in many systemic diseases are unique, sometimes pathognomonic, and may be the first sign of disease, and oral cancer may be detected at an early stage.

History: General information includes use of alcohol or tobacco (both major risk factors for head and neck cancer) and systemic symptoms, such as fever and weight loss.

A dental history may indicate a particular dental problem or neglect of dental care. Difficulty chewing food suggests insufficient teeth for proper mastication, loose or painful teeth, poorly fitting dental appliances, or disorders of the temporomandibular joint (TMJ) or the masticatory muscles. Slight bleeding after brushing suggests mild gingivitis; frequent, spontaneous, or profuse bleeding may indicate a blood dyscrasia.

Oropharyngeal symptoms include pain, presence of ulcers, and difficulty swallowing or speaking. Nasal and sinus symptoms include presence and duration of congestion, discharge, or bleeding.

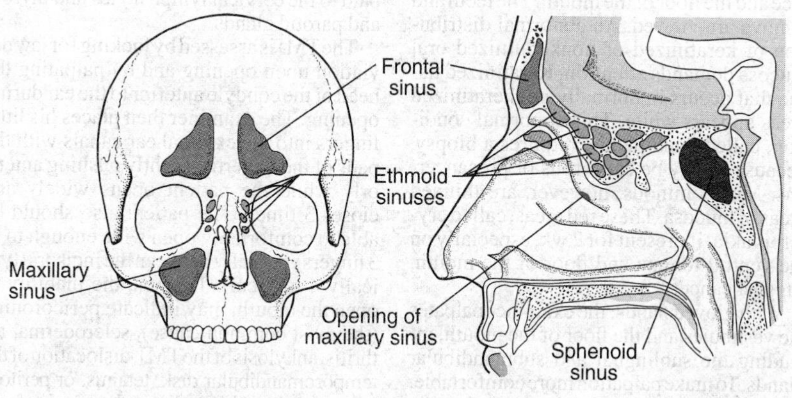

Fig. 89–1. Paranasal sinuses.

Physical examination: A thorough inspection requires good illumination, a tongue blade, gloves, and a gauze pad. Complete or partial dentures are removed so that underlying soft tissues can be seen.

Most physicians use a head-mounted light. However, because the light cannot be precisely aligned on the axis of vision, it is difficult to avoid shadowing in narrow areas (eg, nasal cavity). Better illumination results with a head-mounted convex mirror; the physician looks through a hole in the center of the mirror, so the illumination is always on-axis. The head mirror reflects light from a source (any incandescent light) placed behind the patient and slightly to one side and requires practice to use effectively.

The examiner initially looks at the face for asymmetry, masses, and skin lesions. Slight facial asymmetry is universal, but more marked asymmetry may indicate an underlying disorder, either congenital or acquired (see TABLE 89–2).

The lips are palpated. With the patient's mouth open, the buccal mucosa and vestibules are examined with a tongue blade; then the hard and soft palates, uvula, and oropharynx are viewed. The patient is asked to extend the tongue as far as possible, exposing the dorsum, and to move the extended tongue as far as possible to each side, so that its posterolateral surfaces can be seen. If a patient does not extend the tongue far enough to expose the circumvallate papillae, the examiner grasps the tip of the tongue with a gauze pad and extends it. The tongue is then raised to view the ventral surface and the floor of the mouth. The teeth and gingiva are viewed. An abnormal distribution of keratinized or nonkeratinized oral mucosa demands attention. Keratinized tissue that occurs in normally nonkeratinized areas appears white. This abnormal condition, called leukoplakia, requires a biopsy, because it may be cancerous or precancerous. More ominous, however, are thinned areas of mucosa. These red areas, called erythroplakia, if present for 2 wk, especially on the ventral tongue and floor of the mouth, suggest cancer.

With gloved hands, the examiner palpates the vestibules and the floor of the mouth, including the sublingual and submandibular glands. To make palpation more comfortable, the examiner asks the patient to relax the mouth, keeping it open just wide enough to allow access.

The nose is examined using a nasal speculum, which is held so that the 2 blades open in an anteroposterior (or slightly oblique) direction and do not press against the septum. The physician notes crusting, discharge, septal deviation or perforation; whether mucosa is erythematous, boggy, or swollen; and presence of polyps. The skin over the frontal and maxillary sinuses is examined for erythema and tenderness, suggesting sinus inflammation.

If necessary, the nasopharynx and hypopharynx can be examined with mirrors, which should be warmed before use to avoid fogging. A small mirror is used for the nasopharynx. It is held just below the uvula, angling upward; the tongue is pushed down with a tongue blade. A larger mirror is used for the hypopharynx and larynx. The tongue is retracted with a gauze pad as described above, and the mirror is placed against the soft palate, angling downward. If patients do not tolerate mirror examination, a flexible fiberoptic nasopharyngoscope is helpful. A topical anesthetic (eg, lidocaine 4%) is sprayed in the nose and throat, and the nose is also sprayed with a decongestant (eg, phenylephrine 0.5%). After several minutes, the scope is gently passed through the nares, and the nasal cavity, hypopharynx, and larynx are inspected.

Neck examination consists of inspection and palpation for masses. If masses are found, the physician notes whether they are tender; fluctuant, firm, or stony hard; and movable or fixed. Masses caused by infection are tender and mobile; malignancies tend to be nontender, hard, and fixed. Particular attention is paid to the cervical lymph nodes and thyroid and parotid glands.

The TMJ is assessed by looking for jaw deviation upon opening and by palpating the head of the condyle anterior to the ear during opening. The examiner then places his little fingers into the external ear canals with the pads of the fingertips lightly pushing anteriorly while the patient opens widely and closes 3 times. The patient also should be able to comfortably open wide enough to fit 3 fingers vertically between the incisors (typically 4 to 5 cm). Trismus, the inability to open the mouth, may indicate pericoronitis (the most common cause), scleroderma, arthritis, ankylosis of the TMJ, dislocation of the temporomandibular disk, tetanus, or peritonsillar abscess. Unusually wide opening suggests subluxation or type III Ehlers-Danlos syndrome.

TABLE 89–2. SOME DISORDERS OF THE ORAL REGION BY PREDOMINANT SITE OF INVOLVEMENT

SITE	DISORDER OR LESION	DESCRIPTION
Lips	Actinic atrophy	Thin atrophic mucosa with erosive areas; predisposes to neoplasia
	Angioedema	Acute swelling
	Angular cheilitis (cheilosis)	Fissuring at corners of mouth, often with maceration
	Cheilitis glandularis	Enlarged, nodular labial glands with inflamed, dilated secretory ducts; sometimes everted, hypertrophic lips
	Cheilitis granulomatosa	Diffusely swollen lips, primarily the lower
	Erythema multiforme	Multiple bullae that rupture quickly, leaving hemorrhagic ulcers; includes Stevens-Johnson syndrome
	Exfoliative cheilitis	Chronic desquamation of superficial mucosal cells
	Keratoacanthoma	A benign, locally destructive epithelial tumor resembling squamous cell carcinoma; regresses spontaneously in about 6 mo
	Peutz-Jeghers syndrome	Brownish black melanin spots, with GI polyposis
	Secondary herpes simplex (cold sore)	Short-lived vesicle followed by small painful ulcer at the vermillion border (common)
	Verruca vulgaris (wart)	Pebbly surface
Buccal mucosa	Aspirin burn	Painful white area; when wiped off, exposes an inflamed area
	Fordyce's granules	Cream-colored macules about 1 mm in diameter; benign
	Hand-foot-and-mouth disease	Small ulcerated vesicles
	Herpangina	Vesicles in posterior of mouth
	Irritation fibroma	Smooth-surfaced, dome-shaped, sessile
	Koplik's spots	Tiny, grayish white macules with red margins near orifice of parotid duct
	Linea alba	Thin white line, typically bilateral, on the level of the occlusal plane; benign
	Smokeless tobacco lesion	White or gray corrugated; usually behind lower lip; tends toward malignancy
	Verrucous carcinoma	Slow-growing, exophytic, usually well differentiated; at site of snuff application; metastasis unusual, occurring late
	White sponge nevus	Thick white folds over most of buccal mucosa except gingivae; benign
Palate	Infectious mononucleosis	Petechiae at junction of hard and soft palate
	Kaposi's sarcoma	Red to purple painless macules progressing to painful papules
	Necrotizing sialometaplasia	Large, rapidly developing ulcer, often painless; appears grossly malignant; heals spontaneously in 1–3 mo

Table continues on the following page.

TABLE 89–2. SOME DISORDERS OF THE ORAL REGION BY PREDOMINANT SITE OF INVOLVEMENT—Continued

SITE	DISORDER OR LESION	DESCRIPTION
	Papillary inflammatory hyperplasia	Red, spongy tissue, succeeded by fibrous tissue folds; velvety texture; benign; occurs in the area under poorly fitting dentures
	Pipe smoker's palate (nicotine stomatitis)	Red punctate areas at ducts of minor salivary glands, often with severe, usually benign leukoplakia
	Secondary herpes simplex	Small papules quickly coalescing into series of ulcers (uncommon)
	Torus palatinus	Overgrowth of bone in midline; benign
	Wegener's granulomatosis	Lethal midline granuloma, with bone destruction, sequestration, and perforation
Tongue and floor of mouth	Ankyloglossia	Tongue unable to protrude; speech difficulty
	Benign lymphoepithelial cyst	Yellowish nodule on ventral part of tongue or anterior floor of mouth
	Benign migratory glossitis (geographic tongue, erythema migrans)	Changing patterns of hyperkeratosis and erythema on dorsum and edges; desquamated filiform papillae in irregular circinate pattern, often with an inflamed center and a white or yellow border
	Dermoid cyst	Swollen floor of mouth
	Enlargement of tongue	Localized or generalized depending on how many teeth are missing; adjacent teeth may indent tongue
	Fissured (scrotal) tongue	Deep furrows in lateral and dorsal areas
	Glossitis	Red, painful tongue; often secondary to another condition, allergic, or idiopathic
	Hairy tongue	Dark, elongated filiform papillae
	Linea alba	Thin white line on edges of tongue, usually bilateral
	Lingual thyroid nodule	Smooth-surfaced nodular mass of thyroid tissue follicles, on the far posterior dorsum of tongue, usually at the midline
	Ludwig's angina	Can compromise the airway by forcing the tongue superiorly and posteriorly
	Median rhomboid glossitis	Red (usually) patch in midline of tongue, without papillae; asymptomatic
	Neurilemoma	Persistent swelling, sometimes at site of prior trauma
	Pernicious anemia	Smooth, pale tongue, often with glossodynia or glossopyrosis
	Ranula	Large mucocele penetrating the mylohyoid muscle; may plunge deep into the neck; swollen floor of mouth
	Thyroglossal duct cyst	Midline swelling that moves upward when tongue protrudes
	TB	Ulcers on dorsum, cervical adenopathy

TABLE 89–2. SOME DISORDERS OF THE ORAL REGION BY PREDOMINANT SITE OF INVOLVEMENT—Continued

SITE	DISORDER OR LESION	DESCRIPTION
Salivary glands	Benign lymphoepithelial lesion (Mikulicz's disease)	Unilateral or bilateral enlargement of salivary glands; often with dry mouth and eyes
	Sialadenitis	Swelling, often painful; benign
	Sialolithiasis	Swelling (eg, of floor of mouth) that increases at mealtime or after eating a pickle
	Sjögren's syndrome	Systemic disease causing dry mucous membranes
	Xerostomia	Dry mouth; usually secondary to medication
Various	Acute herpetic gingivostomatitis	Widespread ulcerating vesicular lesions; always present on gingiva; other locations may be involved
	Behçet's syndrome	Multiple oral ulcers similar to those of aphthous stomatitis; also includes dry eyes
	Cicatricial pemphigoid	Bullae that rupture quickly, leaving ulcers; ocular lesions develop after oral lesions; found on alveolar mucosa and vestibules
	Condyloma acuminatum	Venereally transmitted wart forming cauliflower-like clumps
	Dyskeratosis	Occurs with erythroplakia, leukoplakia (white patch on mucous membrane that does not rub off), and mixed red and white lesions; precancerous
	Hemangioma	Purple to dark red lesions, similar to port wine stain; benign
	Hereditary hemorrhagic telangiectasia	Localized dilated blood vessels
	Lichen planus	Lacy pattern (Wickham's striae), sometimes erosive; may become malignant; most common on buccal mucosa, lateral tongue
	Lymphangioma	Localized swelling or discoloration; benign; most common on tongue
	Mucocele (mucous retention cyst)	Soft nodule; if superficial, covered by thin epithelium; appears bluish; most common on lips and floor of mouth
	Noma	Small vesicle or ulcer that rapidly enlarges and becomes necrotic
	Pemphigoid	Small yellow or hemorrhagic, tense bullae; may last several days before rupture; most common on vestibules and alveolar mucosa
	Pemphigus	Bullae that rupture quickly, leaving ulcers
	Recurrent aphthous stomatitis (canker sores)	Small painful ulcers or large, painful scarring ulcers
	Syphilis	Chancre (red papule rapidly developing into a painless ulcer with a serosanguineous crust), mucous patch, gumma

Oral Changes in the Elderly

With aging, resting salivary secretion diminishes and can be further diminished by drugs, although meal-stimulated salivary flow is usually adequate. The flattened cusps of worn teeth and weakness of the masticatory muscles may make chewing tiresome, impairing food intake. Loss of bone mass in the jaws (particularly the alveolar portion), dryness of the mouth, thinning of the oral mucosa, and impaired coordination of lip, cheek, and tongue movements may make denture retention difficult. The taste buds become less sensitive, so the elderly may add abundant seasonings, particularly salt (which is harmful for some), or they may desire very hot foods for more taste, sometimes burning the often atrophic oral mucosa. Gingival recession and xerostomia contribute to development of root caries. Despite these changes, improved dental hygiene has greatly decreased the prevalence of tooth loss, and most older people can expect to retain their teeth.

Poor oral health contributes to poor nutritional intake, which impairs general health. Dental disease (particularly periodontitis) is associated with a 2-fold increased risk of coronary artery disease and a 3- to 5-fold increased risk of having a low-birth-weight infant. Edentulous patients cannot have periodontitis (because they do not have a periodontium), although periodontitis may have resulted in endentulousness. Aspiration pneumonia in patients with periodontitis can involve anaerobic organisms and have a high mortality rate. Bacteremias secondary to acute or chronic dental infection, particularly periodontitis, may contribute to brain abscesses, cavernous sinus thrombosis, endocarditis, prosthetic joint infections, and unexplained fevers.

HALITOSIS

(Fetor Oris; Oral Malodor)

Halitosis is a frequent or persistent unpleasant odor to the breath.

About 85% of cases result from oral conditions. A variety of systemic and extra-oral conditions account for the remainder.

Halitosis most often results from fermentation of food particles by anaerobic gram-negative bacteria in the mouth, producing such volatile sulfur compounds as hydrogen sulfide and methyl mercaptan. Causative bacteria may be present in areas of gingival or periodontal disease, particularly when ulceration or necrosis is present. In patients with healthy periodontal tissue, these bacteria deposit on the dorsal posterior tongue. Factors contributing to the overgrowth of causative bacteria include decreased salivary flow (eg, due to parotid disease or Sjögren's syndrome), salivary stagnation, and increased salivary pH.

Necrotic oral or nasopharyngeal cancer is a rare cause of halitosis.

Certain ingested substances (tobacco, alcohol) and foods (onions, garlic, some spices) contain volatile compounds that are released into exhaled air after systemic absorption.

Rarely, sinus or pulmonary infection produces malodor of exhaled breath. This is more common if infection is caused by a nasal or pulmonary foreign body or with bronchiectasis or anaerobic lung abscess. Food trapped in a Zenker's diverticulum also causes halitosis.

Several systemic diseases produce volatile substances detectable on the breath, although not the particularly foul, pungent odors typically considered halitosis. Diabetic ketoacidosis produces a sweet or fruity odor of acetone; liver failure, a "mousy" or sometimes faintly sulfurous odor; and renal failure, an odor of urine or ammonia. GI disorders do not generally cause halitosis because the esophagus is normally collapsed. It is a fallacy that breath odor reflects the state of digestion and bowel function.

Psychogenic halitosis is a patient's belief that he has bad breath despite the fact that others do not perceive it. This occurs in various mental disorders and may be reported by the hypochondriacal patient who commonly amplifies normal body sensations.

Evaluation and Treatment

While obtaining the history, the physician should particularly seek symptoms of focal infection or systemic illness.

During the physical examination, the nose and oropharynx are examined for signs of infection, foreign body, or gingival disease. A sniff test of exhaled air is conducted. In general, oral causes result in the most putrefying, pungent smell, whereas systemic conditions result in a more subtle, abnormal odor. Ideally, for 48 h before the examination, the patient avoids eating garlic or onions, and for 2 h before, the patient abstains from eating, chewing, drinking, gargling, rinsing, or smoking. During the test, the patient exhales 10 cm from the examiner's nose, first through the mouth and then with the mouth closed. A worse odor through the mouth suggests an oral etiology. A worse odor through the nose suggests nasal or sinus etiology. Similar odor through both nose and mouth suggests a systemic or pulmonary cause. If site of origin is unclear, the posterior tongue is scraped with a plastic spoon. After 5 sec, the spoon is sniffed 5 cm from the examiner's nose.

Extensive diagnostic evaluation should not be undertaken unless the history and physical examination suggest an underlying disease. Portable sulfur monitors, gas chromatography, and chemical tests of tongue scrapings are best left to research protocols.

Underlying diseases are treated. If the cause is oral, the patient should see a dentist for professional cleaning and treatment of gingival disease and caries. Home treatment involves enhanced oral hygiene, including thorough flossing, tooth brushing, and brushing of the tongue with the toothbrush. Mouthwashes are of little benefit except to mask odor for about 20 min. Psychogenic halitosis may require psychiatric consultation.

NASAL CONGESTION AND RHINORRHEA

The most common causes of nasal congestion and rhinorrhea are viral and allergic. Dry air may provoke congestion. Acute sinusitis is slightly less common, and a nasal foreign body is unusual (and occurs predominantly in children).

Patients who use topical decongestants > 1 day often experience significant rebound congestion when the effects of the drug wear off, causing them to continue using the decongestant. This situation (rhinitis medicamentosa) may persist for some time and be misinterpreted as continuation of the original problem rather than a consequence of treatment.

Evaluation

History includes the nature of the discharge, including relation to patient location and season, and associated symptoms (eg, fever, pain). Examination focuses on the nose, throat, and area over the sinuses.

Sore throat, malaise, and erythematous nasal mucosa suggest a URI. Watery, itchy eyes and pale, boggy nasal mucosa suggest allergy, particularly if symptoms are seasonal or if they recur with exposure to possible triggers (eg, animal dander, down pillows). Mucopurulent discharge (sometimes with a foul or metallic taste), focal facial pain or headache, and sometimes erythema or tenderness over the maxillary or frontal sinus suggest sinusitis. Unilateral foul-smelling discharge in a child suggests a nasal foreign body. Testing is generally not indicated for acute nasal symptoms unless invasive sinusitis (see p. 831) is suspected in a diabetic or immunocompromised patient.

Treatment

Specific conditions are treated. Symptomatic relief of congestion can be achieved with topical or oral decongestants (eg, phenylephrine or pseudoephedrine, respectively). Prolonged use should be avoided. Viral rhinorrhea can be treated with oral antihistamines because of their anticholinergic properties unrelated to their histamine-blocking properties. Allergic congestion and rhinorrhea can be treated with antihistamines; in such cases, nonanticholinergic antihistamines provoke fewer adverse effects. Nasal corticosteroids also help allergic conditions.

NECK MASS

A palpable mass in the neck may be infectious, inflammatory, congenital, traumatic, or neoplastic. Salivary gland enlargement has similar causes (see TABLE 193–1 on p. 1646).

Infections, both viral and bacterial, anywhere in the oropharynx may cause reactive cervical lymphadenitis. Less commonly, a primary bacterial infection of the lymph node occurs. Some systemic infections (eg, mononucleosis, HIV, TB) cause cervical lymph node enlargement—usually generalized rather than isolated.

Tumors include primary cancers and lymph node metastases from many different malignancies, including the upper respiratory or upper alimentary tract; lymphoma, including Hodgkin lymphoma; thyroid or salivary gland carcinoma; and distant primary sites, such as the lung, prostate, breast, stomach, colon, or kidney. About 60% of supraclavicular triangle masses are metastases from distant primary sites. Elsewhere in the neck, 80% of cancerous cervical adenopathy originates in the upper respiratory or alimentary tract. Likely sites of origin are the posterior-lateral border of the tongue and the floor of the mouth followed by the nasopharynx, palatine tonsil, laryngeal surface of the epiglottis, and hypopharynx, including the pyriform sinuses.

Evaluation

History: A new mass following symptoms of URI or pharyngitis and enlarging over only a few days suggests benign reactive lymphadenopathy. Risk factors for malignancy are assessed, including consumption of alcohol or tobacco (particularly snuff or chewing tobacco), ill-fitting dental appliances, and chronic oral candidiasis. Poor oral hygiene may correlate with risk. A persisting mass in patients with risk factors suggests malignancy. Pain in the mass suggests an inflammatory cause, whereas a painless mass suggests a cyst or tumor. Persistent nonspecific signs and symptoms mandate a thorough evaluation.

Physical examination: The scalp, ears, nasal cavities, oral cavity, nasopharynx, oropharynx, hypopharynx, and larynx are closely inspected (see p. 808) for signs of infection or visible lesions. Red and white mucosal patches (erythroplakia and leukoplakia) may be premalignant or malignant.

The neck mass, base of the tongue, and thyroid and salivary glands are palpated. Tenderness suggests inflammation (particularly infectious). A hard, fixed, nontender mass suggests malignancy, whereas mobility suggests otherwise.

The spleen and other lymph nodes are palpated. Generalized adenopathy and splenomegaly suggest infectious mononucleosis or a lymphoreticular malignancy.

Testing: If the nature of the mass is readily apparent (eg, lymphadenopathy from recent pharyngitis) or is in a healthy young patient with a recent, tender swelling, then no immediate testing is required. However, the patient is reexamined regularly; if the mass fails to resolve, further evaluation is needed.

Most other patients should have a CBC and chest x-ray. If examination reveals an oral or nasopharyngeal lesion that fails to begin resolving within 2 wk, then testing may include x-rays, CT, MRI, or fine-needle biopsy. Then, if indicated, that site should be biopsied. In young patients without risk factors for head and neck cancer, the neck mass may be biopsied. Older patients, particularly those with risk factors for cancer, should first undergo further testing to identify the primary site; biopsy of the neck mass may simply reveal undifferentiated squamous cell carcinoma without illuminating the source. Such patients should have direct laryngoscopy, bronchoscopy, and esophagoscopy with biopsy of all suspicious areas. CT of the head, neck, and chest and possibly a thyroid scan are performed. If a primary tumor is not found, then the neck mass should undergo excisional biopsy, which is preferable to an incisional biopsy because it does not leave a transected mass in the neck. The excisional biopsy should be performed in anticipation of further regional surgery in case the mass is malignant. If a primary tumor is still not identified, random biopsy of the nasopharynx, palatine tonsils, and base of the tongue should be considered.

PHARYNGITIS

Pharyngitis, sore throat, is pain in the posterior pharynx, with or without swallowing. Pain can be severe; many patients refuse oral intake.

Most causes are infectious. The most common by far is tonsillopharyngitis, either viral or bacterial. Less common causes are an abscess (peritonsillar, parapharyngeal, and, in children, retropharyngeal) and epiglottitis. Epiglottitis is more common in children but can occur in adults.

Because some patients consider the anterior neck their throat, they may complain of "sore throat" with nonpharyngeal disorders (eg, thyroiditis, lymphadenitis).

Evaluation

Epiglottitis and, less commonly, pharyngeal abscess, pose a threat to the airway and must be differentiated from simple tonsillopharyngitis, which is usually self-limited.

Copious coryza suggests viral tonsillopharyngitis; throat culture is the only reliable way to differentiate viral from bacterial causes. A muffled "hot-potato" voice (speaking as if one were holding a hot object in one's mouth) suggests a peritonsillar abscess (see p. 822). Stridor and sitting upright leaning forward suggest epiglottitis (see p. 820). Pharyngeal examination should not be performed if epiglottitis is suspected, because it may trigger complete airway obstruction. Otherwise, pharyngeal inflammation, exudate, or both may be present with tonsillopharyngitis or abscess; the pharynx almost always appears normal in epiglottitis. Focal swelling is usually apparent with abscess.

If etiology is unclear from examination, lateral neck x-ray may demonstrate an edematous epiglottis or enlargement of the retropharyngeal space. CT of the neck may demonstrate the location and extent of an abscess.

Treatment

Specific conditions are treated, most notably, streptococcal pharyngitis (see p. 1447). Local treatments with warm saltwater gargles and topical anesthetics (eg, benzocaine, lidocaine, dyclonine) may help temporarily in tonsillopharyngitis (see p. 825). Patients in severe pain (even from tonsillopharyngitis) may require short-term use of opioids.

SMELL AND TASTE ABNORMALITIES

Because flavors are distinguished by aroma, smell and taste are interdependent. Dysfunction of one often disturbs the other. Disorders of smell and taste are rarely incapacitating or life threatening, so they often do not receive close medical attention, although their effect on quality of life can be severe.

Taste: Although abnormal taste sensations may be due to mental disorders, local causes should always be sought. Glossopharyngeal and facial nerve integrity can be determined by testing taste on both sides of the dorsum of the tongue with sugar, salt, vinegar (acid), and quinine (bitter).

Drying of the oral mucosa from heavy smoking, Sjögren's syndrome, radiation therapy of the head and neck, or desquamation of the tongue can impair taste, and various drugs (eg, those with anticholinergic properties and vincristine) alter taste. In all instances, the gustatory receptors are diffusely involved. When limited to one side of the tongue (eg, in Bell's palsy), ageusia (loss of the sense of taste) is rarely noticed.

Smell: The inability to detect certain odors, such as gas or smoke, may be dangerous, and several systemic and intracranial disorders should be excluded before dismissing symptoms as harmless. Whether brain stem disease (involvement of the nucleus solitarius) can cause disorders of smell and taste is uncertain, because other neurologic manifestations usually take precedence.

Anosmia (loss of the sense of smell) is probably the most common abnormality (see p. 833). Hyperosmia (increased sensitivity to odors) usually reflects a neurotic or histrionic personality but can occur intermittently with seizure disorders. Dysosmia (disagreeable or distorted sense of smell) may occur with infection of the nasal sinuses, partial damage to the olfactory bulbs, or mental depression. Some cases, accompanied by a disagreeable taste, result from poor dental hygiene. Uncinate epilepsy can produce brief, vivid, unpleasant olfactory hallucinations. Hyposmia (diminished sense of smell) and hypogeusia (diminished sense of taste) can follow acute influenza, usually temporarily.

Rarely, idiopathic dysgeusia (distorted sense of taste), hypogeusia, and dysosmia respond to zinc supplementation.

STOMATITIS

Oral inflammation and ulcers, known as stomatitis, may be mild and localized or severe, widespread, and painful. Symptoms are caused by inflammation of the oral mucosa. Stomatitis may involve swelling and redness of the oral mucosa or discrete, painful ulcers (single or multiple). Less commonly, whitish lesions are produced, and, rarely, the mouth appears normal (burning mouth syndrome) despite significant symptoms. Symptoms hinder eating, sometimes leading to dehydration and malnutrition. Secondary infection occasionally occurs. Some conditions are recurrent.

Stomatitis may be caused by infection, systemic disease, a physical or chemical irritant, or an allergic reaction; many cases are idiopathic (see Recurrent Aphthous Stomatitis on p. 817). Because the normal flow of saliva protects the mucosa against many insults, xerostomia (see p. 818) predisposes the mouth to stomatitis of any cause.

Infections: Viral causes are most common, but bacteria and fungi are sometimes involved. Oral infections can be clinically significant in immunocompromised patients.

Primary herpes simplex infection produces multiple vesicular lesions on the intraoral mucosa on both keratinized and nonkeratinized surfaces and always includes the gingiva. These lesions rapidly ulcerate. Clinical manifestation occurs most often in children. Subsequent reactivations (secondary herpes simplex, "cold sore"), however, usually appear on the lip at the vermilion border and, rarely, on the hard palate.

Primary varicella zoster infection (chickenpox) often produces vesicles on the oral mucosa. Reactivation (shingles) produces similar lesions in the distribution of a nerve root; if the trigeminal nerve is involved, unilateral oral ulcers may result.

Many other viruses are involved. Coxsackievirus can produce hand-foot-and-mouth disease in young children, with both cutaneous and intraoral lesions, or herpangina, with isolated oral ulcers. Other infections include Epstein-Barr virus, influenza, cytomegalovirus, and HIV.

Acute necrotizing ulcerative gingivitis (see p. 855) is a nonspecific, mainly fusospirochetal bacterial infection producing inflammation and punched-out ulcers on the dental papillae and marginal gingivae. A severe variant, termed noma (gangrenous stomatitis), can produce full-thickness tissue destruction (sometimes involving the lips or cheek), typically in a debilitated patient. It begins as a gingival, buccal, or palatal (midline lethal granuloma) ulcer that becomes necrotic and spreads rapidly. Tissue sloughing may occur.

Sexually transmitted diseases can produce stomatitis. Gonorrhea very rarely produces burning ulcers and erythema of the gingiva and tongue as well as the more common pharyngitis. Primary syphilis chancres may appear in the mouth, and about 20% of patients with secondary syphilis develop painless, shallow oral mucosal ulcers (mucous patch), typically with a yellow or gray base and slight surrounding erythema. Tertiary syphilis may produce oral gummas or a generalized glossitis and mucosal atrophy. The site of a gumma is the only time that squamous cell carcinoma will develop on the dorsum of the tongue.

Rare bacterial causes include *Mycobacterium tuberculosis,* inoculated by sputum from the lungs. Cervicofacial bacterial actinomycosis (lumpy jaw) may resemble a fungal infection and may contain pathognomonic yellow (sulfur) granules in purulent exudate.

Candida albicans and related species, which are normal oral flora, can overgrow in people who have taken antibiotics or corticosteroids or who are debilitated, such as patients with AIDS. Overgrowth may produce a pseudomembrane with a cheesy substance on friable mucosa. The chronic erythematous and erosive forms are more common but are also more difficult to recognize. Oral and perioral lesions occur infrequently in blastomycosis, histoplasmosis, coccidioidomycosis, cryptococcosis (mainly in debilitated patients), and mucormycosis (particularly in people with diabetes).

Systemic diseases: Behçet's syndrome, Stevens-Johnson syndrome, and inflammatory bowel disease can produce bullous or ulcerative oral mucosal lesions. Pemphigoid and pemphigus vulgaris cause oral vesicles and ulcers. Sprue (gluten-sensitive enteropathy) may produce oral ulcers. Hemorrhagic oral lesions may occur in erythema multiforme, scurvy, leukemia, thrombocytopenic purpura, and platelet disorders. Unprovoked bleeding, xerostomia, and an ammonia-like odor accompany uremia. The mucocutaneous lymph node syndrome (Kawasaki disease) affects children, causing erythema of the lips and oral mucosa. Stomatitis may result from hypovitaminosis (particularly B vitamins or vitamin C), iron-deficiency anemia with dysphagia (as in Plummer-Vinson syndrome), or agranulocytosis. Pellagra produces a smooth, fiery red tongue; painful mouth; and mucosal ulcers.

Cyclic neutropenia is a rare condition probably caused by a defect in neutrophil maturation, resulting in regular, cyclic bouts of neutropenia (< 500/μL) with fever, malaise, lymphadenopathy, and oral ulcers. It usually presents in childhood.

Irritants and allergies: Physical irritation is frequently involved. Cheek biting, mouth breathing, jagged teeth, orthodontic appliances, ill-fitting dentures, and nursing bottles with nipples that are hard or too long may cause stomatitis. Other contributors are excessive use of alcohol, tobacco, hot foods, and spices.

Drugs and chemicals may be sensitizing (typically resulting in a type IV hypersensitivity reaction) or directly irritating (ie, triggering inflammatory mediator release without involvement of memory T cells or IgE). Common substances include ingredients in toothpaste, mouthwash, candy, gum (especially if made from chicle), dyes, lipstick, and, rarely, dental materials. Stomatitis also may result from occupational exposure to dyes, heavy metals, acid fumes, or metal or mineral dust. Many drugs are implicated in stomatitis. The most common are cytotoxic cancer chemotherapy drugs, and gold salts. Nicorandil (K channel blocker), iodides, barbiturates, and NSAIDs are rare causes. Some foods, especially highly acidic ones, may produce oral ulcers.

Evaluation

History: Occasionally, causes are obvious in the history (eg, cytotoxic chemotherapy). Relation of symptoms to food, drugs, and other substances is sought. Recurrent GI symptoms suggest inflammatory bowel disease or sprue. Ocular symptoms suggest Behçet's syndrome. Nonspecific symptoms suggesting chronic illness (weight loss, malaise, fever) and risk factors for HIV infection are important.

Physical examination: Cutaneous bullae suggest Stevens-Johnson syndrome, pemphigus vulgaris, or pemphigoid. Cutaneous vesicles suggest chickenpox or herpes zoster. Other cutaneous lesions may implicate erythema multiforme, hand-foot-and-mouth disease, or secondary syphilis.

Location of oral lesions may help; interdental ulcers occur with herpes simplex or acute necrotizing ulcerative gingivitis. Lesions on keratinized surfaces suggest herpes simplex, recurrent aphthous stomatitis, or physical injury. Unilateral lesions suggest herpes zoster.

Testing: Clues suggesting specific diseases are pursued, as discussed elsewhere in THE MANUAL. Patients with acute stomatitis and no symptoms, signs, or risk factors for systemic illness probably require no testing. If stomatitis is recurrent, viral and bacterial cultures, CBC, serum iron, ferritin, vitamin B_{12}, folate, zinc, and endomysial antibody (for sprue) are obtained. Biopsy at the periphery of normal and abnormal tissue can be done for persistent lesions that do not have an obvious etiology. Systematically eliminating foods from the diet can be useful, as can changing brands of toothpaste or mouthwash.

Treatment

Underlying disorders are treated. Meticulous oral hygiene (using a soft toothbrush) may help prevent secondary infection. A soft diet that does not include acidic or salty foods is followed.

Numerous topical treatments, alone or in combination, are used to ease symptoms. These treatments include anesthetics, protective coatings, corticosteroids, antibiotics, antihistamines, and physical measures such as cautery.

For topical anesthesia, 5 mL of 2% viscous lidocaine is diluted in 10 mL water and used as a rinse and then expectorated q 3 h. A carboxymethylcellulose paste with or without 1% triamcinolone qid reduces irritation of painful local lesions. Other topical drugs include sucralfate and aluminum-magnesium liquid antacids; 30 mL of these drugs may be used alone but are often mixed with 2% viscous lidocaine 5 mL and diphenhydramine (an antihistamine with mild local anesthetic properties) and, often, kaolin, 12.5 mg to rinse and expectorate. Some physicians add tetracycline or nystatin suspension. If an infectious etiology is unlikely, fluocinonide gel may be applied to each ulcer. Amlexanox 5% paste can be applied qid ($^1/_4$ on tip of finger, wiped across ulcer).

Chemical or physical cautery can ease pain. Silver nitrate sticks are not as effective as low-power (2- to 3-watt), defocused, pulsed-mode CO_2 laser treatments, after which pain relief is immediate and lesions tend not to recur locally.

RECURRENT APHTHOUS STOMATITIS

Recurrent aphthous stomatitis is a common condition in which round or ovoid painful ulcers recur on the oral mucosa. Etiology is unclear. Diagnosis is clinical. Treatment is symptomatic and usually includes topical corticosteroids.

Recurrent aphthous stomatitis (RAS) affects 20 to 30% of adults and a greater percentage of children at some time in their lives. Etiology is unclear, but RAS tends to run in families. The damage is predominately cell-mediated. Cytokines, such as IL-2, IL-10, and, particularly, tumor necrosis factor-α, play a role.

Predisposing factors include oral trauma, stress, and foods, particularly chocolate, coffee, peanuts, eggs, cereals, almonds, strawberries, cheese, and tomatoes, although allergy does not appear to be involved. Factors that may, for unknown reasons, be protective include oral contraceptives, pregnancy, and tobacco, including smokeless tobacco and nicotine-containing tablets.

Symptoms and Signs

Symptoms and signs usually begin in childhood (80% of patients are < 30 yr) and decrease in frequency and severity with aging. Symptoms may involve as few as one ulcer 2 to 4 times/yr or almost continuous disease, with new ulcers forming as old ones heal. Pain or burning for 1 to 2 days precedes ulcers, but there are no antecedent vesicles or bullae. Severe pain, disproportional to the size of the lesion, can last from 4 to 7 days.

Ulcers are well-demarcated, shallow, ovoid, or round and have a necrotic center with a yellow-gray pseudomembrane, a red halo, and slightly raised red margins.

Minor aphthae (Mikulicz's) account for 85% of cases. They occur on the floor of the mouth, lateral and ventral tongue, buccal mucosa, and pharynx; are < 8 mm (typically 2 to 3 mm); and heal in 10 days without scarring.

Major aphthae (Sutton's disease, periadenitis mucosa necrotica recurrens) constitute 10% of cases. Appearing after puberty, the prodrome is more intense and the ulcers deeper, larger (> 1 cm), and longer lasting (weeks to months) than minor aphthae. They appear in the lips, soft palate, and throat. Fever, dysphagia, malaise, and scarring may occur.

Herpetiform ulcers (morphologically resembling but unrelated to herpesvirus) account for 5% of cases. They begin as multiple (up to 100) 1- to 3-mm crops of small, painful clusters of ulcers on an erythematous base. They coalesce to form larger ulcers that last 2 wk. They tend to occur in women and at a later age of onset than do other forms of RAS.

Diagnosis

Evaluation proceeds as described above under stomatitis. Diagnosis is based on appearance and on exclusion, because there are no definitive histologic features or laboratory tests.

Primary oral herpes simplex may mimic RAS but usually occurs in younger children, always involves the gingiva and may affect any keratinized mucosa (hard palate, attached gingiva, dorsum of tongue), and is associated with systemic symptoms. Viral culture can be performed to identify herpes simplex. Recurrent herpetic lesions are usually unilateral.

Similar recurrent episodes can occur with Behçet's syndrome, inflammatory bowel disease, sprue, HIV infection, and nutritional deficiencies; these conditions generally have systemic symptoms and signs. Isolated recurrent oral ulcers can occur with herpes infection, HIV, and, rarely, nutritional deficiency. Viral testing and serum hematologic tests can identify these conditions.

Drug reactions may mimic RAS but are usually temporally related to ingestion. However, reactions to foods or dental products may be difficult to identify; sequential elimination may be necessary.

Treatment

General treatments for stomatitis (see p. 817) may help patients with RAS. Chlorhexidine gluconate mouthwashes and topical corticosteroids, the mainstays of therapy, should be used during the prodrome, if possible. The corticosteroid can be dexamethasone 0.5 mg/5 mL tid used as a rinse and then expectorated or clobetasol ointment 0.05% or fluocinonide ointment 0.05% in carbymethylcellulose mucosal protective paste (1:1) applied tid. Patients using these corticosteroids should be monitored for candidiasis. If topical corticosteroids are ineffective, prednisone (eg, 40 mg po once/day) may be needed for ≤ 5 days. Continuous or particularly severe RAS is best treated by a specialist in oral medicine. Treatment may require prolonged systemic corticosteroids, azathioprine or other immunosuppressants, pentoxifylline, or thalidomide. Intralesional injections can be done with betamethasone, dexamethasone, or triamcinolone. Supplemental B_1, B_2, B_6, B_{12}, folic acid, or iron lessens RAS in some patients.

XEROSTOMIA

Xerostomia is dry mouth. Many patients notice that their mouth is dry; others may not be conscious of it but carry water bottles to constantly sip from. Most patients with xerostomia have definite signs of reduced salivary flow (eg, dry and sticky mucosa, foamy or stringy saliva). Xerostomia interferes with speech and swallowing, causes fetid breath, and, because the reduced salivary flow no longer washes away bacteria, impairs oral hygiene. In long-standing xerostomia, tooth decay can be severe. Caries may develop at the margins of restorations or in unusual places (eg, at the neck or tip of the tooth). *Candida albicans* infection is common, producing either erythema and atrophy of the dorsum of the tongue or a white, cheesy curd that bleeds when wiped off.

Etiology

Xerostomia is usually caused by medical treatment but sometimes results from disease processes or aging.

Xerostomia is most often due to drugs, most commonly anticholinergics (including drugs for motion sickness, anxiolytics, antihistamines, antidepressants, antipsychotics, and decongestants), antiparkinsonians, and, to a lesser degree, opioids, particularly meperidine. Severe xerostomia can follow radiation to the salivary glands during treatment for head and neck cancer (5200 cGy causes severe, permanent dryness, but even low doses can cause temporary drying).

Xerostomia is common in Sjögren's syndrome and occasionally occurs in sarcoidosis, amyloidosis, and HIV infection. Less commonly, salivary gland involvement in TB or leprosy results in xerostomia. Temporary drying may also be caused by viral infections, dehydration, and fear.

Evaluation

Diagnosis is based on symptoms, appearance, and absence of salivary flow when massaging the salivary glands. Cause is often apparent, but if sarcoid is considered possible, biopsy of a labial salivary gland is recommended.

Salivary flow rates can be measured to monitor therapy. Saliva is stimulated with citric acid or by chewing paraffin and is collected by devices placed over the major duct orifices. Normal parotid flow is 0.4 to 1.5 mL/min/gland. Diagnosis may be achieved easily by holding a tongue blade against the buccal mucosa for 5 sec. If the tongue blade falls off when released, then salivary flow is normal. The more difficult it is to remove the tongue blade, the more severe the xerostomia.

Treatment

Patients with xerostomia and functional salivary gland tissue should avoid decongestants and antihistamines and maintain meticulous oral hygiene (including application of fluoride rinses or gels). Sipping sugarless fluids frequently, chewing xylitol-containing gum, and using a saliva substitute containing carboxymethylcellulose or hydroxyethylcellulose may help.

Drug therapy includes cevimeline or pilocarpine, both cholinergic agonists. Cevimeline (30 mg po tid) has less M2 (cardiac) receptor activity than pilocarpine and a longer half-life. The main adverse effect is nausea. Pilocarpine (5 mg po tid) may be given after ophthalmologic and cardiorespiratory contraindications are excluded; adverse effects include sweating, flushing, and polyuria.

If drugs that cause xerostomia are given before bedtime, xerostomia occurring during sleep may seem less troubling but is more likely to lead to caries than is daytime xerostomia. A few drops of water should be sipped before taking nitroglycerin, because xerostomia may prevent the dissolution. The most effective way to prevent caries is to sleep with individually fitted carriers containing 1.1% fluoride. If 2 carriers cannot be worn at once, then each arch should be covered every other night.

90 OROPHARYNGEAL DISORDERS

Oropharyngeal disorders include adenoid disorders, epiglottitis, parapharyngeal abscess, peritonsillar abscess and cellulitis, retropharyngeal abscess, salivary stones, sialadenitis, submandibular space infection, tonsillopharyngitis, Tornwaldt's cyst, and velopharyngeal insufficiency. Oral, pharyngeal, and salivary gland tumors are discussed in Ch. 93 on p. 838.

ADENOID DISORDERS

Hypertrophy or inflammation of the adenoids is common in children. Symptoms include nasal obstruction, sleep disturbances, and middle ear effusions with hearing loss. Diagnosis is enhanced by flexible fiberoptic nasopharyngoscopy. Treatment often includes intranasal corticosteroids, antibiotics, and, for significant nasal obstruction or persistent middle ear effusion, adenoidectomy.

The adenoids are a rectangular mass of lymphatic tissue in the posterior nasopharynx. They are largest in children 2 to 6 yr, who most frequently develop adenoid hypertrophy or chronic adenoiditis. Enlargement may be physiologic or secondary to viral or bacterial infection; allergy; irritants, including secondary tobacco smoke; and, possibly, gastroesophageal reflux. Other risk factors include exposure to multiple children at day care. Severe hypertrophy can obstruct the eustachian tubes (causing otitis media), posterior choanae (causing sinusitis), or both.

Symptoms, Signs, and Diagnosis

Although patients with adenoid hypertrophy may not complain of symptoms, they usually have chronic mouth breathing, snoring, possibly sleep disturbance, halitosis, conductive hearing loss (secondary to recurrent otitis media or persistent middle ear effusions), and a hyponasal voice quality. Chronic adenoiditis can also produce chronic or recurrent nasopharyngitis, rhinosinusitis, epistaxis, halitosis, and cough.

Adenoid hypertrophy is suspected in children and adolescents with characteristic symptoms, persistent middle ear effusions, or recurrent acute otitis media or rhinosinusitis. Although the gold standard for office assessment of the nasopharynx is flexible nasopharyngoscopy, x-ray imaging and sleep tape recording are also often used. A sleep study may help estimate the severity of any sleep disturbance.

Treatment

Underlying allergy or infection is treated with intranasal corticosteroids and antibiotics, respectively. In children with persistent middle ear effusions or frequent otitis media, adenoidectomy often limits recurrence. Children > 4 yr who require tympanostomy tubes often undergo adenoidectomy when tubes are placed. Surgery is also recommended for younger children with recurrent epistaxis or significant nasal obstruction (eg, sleep disturbance, voice change). Children with recurrent or persistent rhinosinusitis despite adequate drug therapy require irrigation and culture of the maxillary sinuses, investigation of allergic causes and reflux, and sometimes adenoidectomy. Although it requires general anesthesia, adenoidectomy can usually be performed on an outpatient basis with recovery in 48 to 72 h.

EPIGLOTTITIS

(Supraglottitis)

Epiglottitis is a rapidly progressive bacterial infection of the epiglottis and surrounding tissues that may lead to sudden respiratory obstruction and death. Symptoms include severe sore throat, dysphagia, high fever, drooling, and inspiratory stridor. Diagnosis requires direct visualization of the supraglottic structures, which is not to be performed until full respiratory support is available. Treatment includes airway protection and antibiotics.

Epiglottitis used to be primarily a disease of children and usually caused by *Haemophilus influenzae* type B. Now, because of widespread vaccination, it has been almost eradicated in children (more cases occur in adults). Causal organisms in children and adults include *Streptococcus pneumoniae, Staphylococcus aureus,* nontypeable *H. influenzae, H. parainfluenzae,* β-hemolytic streptococci, *Branhamella catarrhalis,* and *Klebsiella pneumoniae*. *H. influenzae* type B is still a cause in adults and unvaccinated children.

Bacteria that have colonized the nasopharynx spread locally to produce supraglottic cellulitis with marked inflammation of the epiglottis, vallecula, aryepiglottic folds, arytenoids, and laryngeal ventricles. With *H. influenzae* type B, infection may spread hematogenously.

The inflamed supraglottic structures mechanically obstruct the airway, increasing the work of breathing, ultimately causing respiratory failure. Clearance of inflammatory secretions is also impaired.

Symptoms and Signs

In children, sore throat, odynophagia, and dysphagia develop abruptly. Fatal asphyxia may occur within a few hours of onset. Drooling is very common. Additionally, the child has signs of toxicity (poor or absent eye contact, failure to recognize parents, signs of poor perfusion, cyanosis, irritability, inability to be consoled or distracted) and is febrile and anxious. Dyspnea, tachypnea, and inspiratory stridor may be present, often causing the child to sit upright, lean forward, and hyperextend the neck with the jaw thrust forward and mouth open in an effort to enhance air exchange (tripod position). Relinquishing this position may herald respiratory failure. Suprasternal, supraclavicular, and subcostal inspiratory retractions may be present.

In adults, symptoms are similar to those of children, including sore throat, fever, dysphagia, and drooling, but peak symptoms usually take > 24 h to develop. Because of the larger diameter of the adult airway, obstruction is less common and less fulminant. Often, there is no visible oropharyngeal inflammation. However, severe throat pain with a normal-appearing pharynx raises suspicion of epiglottitis.

Diagnosis

Epiglottitis is suspected in patients with severe sore throat and no pharyngitis and also in patients with sore throat and inspiratory stridor. Stridor in children may also result from croup (viral laryngotracheal bronchitis see TABLE 90–1 and p. 2307), bacterial tracheitis, and airway foreign body. The tripod position may also occur with peritonsillar or retropharyngeal abscess.

The patient is hospitalized if epiglottitis is suspected. Diagnosis requires direct examination, usually with flexible fiberoptic laryngoscopy. (CAUTION: *Examination of the pharynx and larynx may precipitate complete respiratory obstruction in children, and the pharynx and larynx should not be directly examined except in the operating room, where the most advanced airway intervention is available.*) Although plain x-rays may be helpful, a child with stridor should not be transported to the x-ray suite. Direct laryngoscopy that reveals a beefy-red, stiff, edematous epiglottis is diagnostic. Cultures from the supraglottic tissues and blood can then be performed to search for the causative organism.

Adults can usually safely undergo flexible fiberoptic laryngoscopy.

Treatment and Prevention

In children, the airway must be secured immediately, preferably by nasotracheal intubation. An endotracheal tube is usually required until the patient has been stabilized for 24 to 48 h (usual total intubation time is < 60 h). Alternatively, a tracheotomy is performed. If respiratory arrest occurs before an airway is established, bag-mask ventilation may be a life-saving temporary measure. For emergency care of children with epiglottitis, each institution should have a protocol that involves critical care, otolaryngology, anesthesia, and pediatrics.

Adults whose airway is severely obstructed can be endotracheally intubated during flexible fiberoptic laryngoscopy. Other adults may not require immediate intubation but should be observed for airway compromise in an ICU with an intubation set and cricothyrotomy tray at the bedside.

A β-lactamase–resistant antibiotic, such as ceftriaxone 50 to 75 mg/kg IV once/day (maximum 2 g), should be used empirically, pending culture and sensitivity test results.

TABLE 90–1. DIFFERENTIATING EPIGLOTTITIS FROM CROUP

EPIGLOTTITIS	CROUP*
Onset is acute and fulminant	Onset is more gradual
Common age is 2–8 yr (if not vaccinated against *Haemophilus influenzae* type B) and adults	Common age is 6–36 mo
Barking cough is uncommon	Barking cough is characteristic
Epiglottis is markedly edematous and cherry red	Epiglottis may be erythematous
Neck x-ray shows an enlarged epiglottis (thumb sign) and distention of the hypopharynx	Neck x-ray shows subepiglottic narrowing (steeple sign) and a normal-sized epiglottis

*Also called viral laryngotracheal bronchitis.

Epiglottitis caused by *H. influenzae* type B can be effectively prevented with the *H. influenzae* type B (Hib) conjugate vaccine.

PARAPHARYNGEAL ABSCESS

A parapharyngeal abscess is a deep neck abscess treated with antibiotics and surgical drainage.

The parapharyngeal (pharyngomaxillary) space is lateral to the superior pharyngeal constrictor. This space connects to every other major fascial neck space and is divided into anterior and posterior compartments by the styloid process. The posterior compartment contains the carotid artery, internal jugular vein, and numerous nerves. Infections in the parapharyngeal space usually originate in the tonsils or pharynx, although local spread from odontogenic sources and lymph nodes may occur.

Abscess swelling can compromise the airway. Posterior space abscess can erode into the carotid artery or cause septic thrombophlebitis of the internal jugular vein (Lemierre syndrome).

Symptoms, Signs, and Diagnosis

Most patients have fever, sore throat, odynophagia, and swelling in the neck down to the hyoid bone. Anterior space abscesses produce trismus and induration along the angle of the mandible, with medial bulging of the tonsil and lateral pharyngeal wall. Posterior space abscesses produce swelling that is more prominent in the posterior pharyngeal wall. Trismus is minimal. Posterior abscesses may involve structures within the carotid sheath, possibly causing rigors, high fever, bacteremia, neurologic deficits, and, possibly, massive hemorrhage from carotid artery rupture. Diagnosis is suspected in patients with poorly defined deep neck infection or other typical symptoms and is confirmed using contrast-enhanced CT.

Treatment

Treatment may require airway control. Parenteral broad-spectrum antibiotics (eg, ceftriaxone, clindamycin) and surgical drainage are generally needed. Posterior abscesses are drained externally through the submaxillary fossa. Anterior abscesses can often be drained through an intra-oral incision. Several days of parenteral culture-determined antibiotics are required after drainage, followed by 10 to 14 days of oral antibiotics. Occasionally, small abscesses can be treated with IV antibiotics alone.

PERITONSILLAR ABSCESS AND CELLULITIS

Peritonsillar abscess and cellulitis are acute pharyngeal infections most common in adolescents and young adults. Symptoms are severe sore throat, trismus, "hot-potato" voice, and uvular deviation. Diagnosis requires needle aspiration. Treatment includes broad-spectrum antibiotics, drainage of any pus, hydration, analgesics, and, occasionally, acute tonsillectomy.

Etiology and Pathophysiology

Abscess (quinsy) and cellulitis probably represent a spectrum of the same process in which bacterial infection of the tonsils and pharynx spreads to the soft tissues. Infection is virtually always unilateral and is located between the tonsil and the superior pharyngeal constrictor muscle. It usually involves multiple bacteria. *Streptococcus* and *Staphylococcus* are the most frequent aerobic pathogens, whereas *Bacteroides* sp is the predominant anaerobic pathogen.

Symptoms, Signs, and Diagnosis

Symptoms include gradual onset of severe unilateral sore throat, dysphagia, fever, otalgia, and asymmetric cervical adenopathy. Trismus, "hot-potato" voice (speaking as if one were holding a hot object in one's mouth), a toxic appearance (see Epiglottitis on p. 820), drooling, severe halitosis, tonsillar erythema, and exudates are common. Abscess and cellulitis both have swelling above the affected tonsil, but with abscess there is more of a discrete bulge, with deviation of the soft palate and uvula.

Peritonsillar cellulitis is recognized in patients with severe sore throat who have trismus, "hot-potato" voice, and uvular deviation. All such patients require needle aspiration of the tonsillar mass and cultures. Aspiration of pus differentiates abscess from cellulitis. CT or ultrasound of the neck can help confirm the diagnosis when the physical examination is difficult or the diagnosis is in doubt, particularly when the condition must be differentiated from a parapharyngeal or other deep neck infection.

Treatment

Cellulitis subsides, usually within 48 h, with hydration and high-dose penicillin (eg, 2 million units IV q 4 h or 1 g po qid); alternative drugs include a 1st-generation cephalosporin or clindamycin. Culture-directed antibiotics are then prescribed for 10 days. Abscesses are incised and drained in the emergency department using thorough local anesthesia and sometimes conscious sedation; many clinicians believe needle aspiration alone provides adequate drainage. Although most patients can be treated as outpatients, some need brief hospitalization for parenteral antibiotics, IV hydration, and airway monitoring. Rarely, an immediate tonsillectomy is performed, particularly in a young or uncooperative patient who has other indications for elective tonsillectomy (eg, history of frequently recurrent tonsillitis or obstructive sleep apnea).

RETROPHARYNGEAL ABSCESS

Retropharyngeal abscesses, most common in young children, can cause sore throat, fever, neck stiffness, and stridor. Diagnosis requires lateral neck x-ray or CT. Treatment

is with endotracheal intubation, drainage, and antibiotics.

Retropharyngeal abscesses develop in the retropharyngeal lymph nodes at the back of the pharynx, adjacent to the vertebrae. They can be seeded by infection of the pharynx, sinuses, adenoids, or nose. They occur mainly in children 1 to 8 yr, because the retropharyngeal lymph nodes begin to recede by 4 to 5 yr. However, adults may develop infection from foreign body ingestion or after instrumentation. Common organisms include aerobic (*Streptococcus* and *Staphylococcus* sp) and anaerobic (*Bacteroides* and *Fusobacterium*) bacteria and, increasingly in adults and children, HIV and TB.

The most serious consequences include airway obstruction, septic shock, rupture of the abscess into the airway resulting in aspiration pneumonia or asphyxia, mediastinitis, carotid rupture, and suppurative thrombophlebitis of the internal jugular veins.

Symptoms, Signs, and Diagnosis

Symptoms and signs are usually preceded in children by an acute URI and in adults by foreign body ingestion or instrumentation. Children may have odynophagia, dysphagia, fever, cervical lymphadenopathy, nuchal rigidity, stridor, dyspnea, snoring or noisy breathing, and torticollis. Adults may have severe neck pain but less often have stridor. The posterior pharyngeal wall may bulge to one side.

Diagnosis is suspected in patients with severe, unexplained sore throat and neck stiffness; stridor; or noisy breathing. Lateral soft-tissue x-rays of the neck, taken in the maximum possible hyperextension and during inspiration, may show focal widening of the prevertebral soft tissues, reversal of normal cervical lordosis, air in the prevertebral soft tissues, or erosion of the adjacent vertebral body. CT can help diagnose questionable cases, help differentiate cellulitis from an abscess, and assess extent of the abscess.

Treatment

Antibiotics, such as a broad-spectrum cephalosporin (eg, ceftriaxone 50 to 75 mg/kg IV once/day) or clindamycin, may occasionally be sufficient for children with small abscesses. However, most patients also require drainage through an incision in the posterior pharyngeal wall. Endotracheal intubation is performed preoperatively and maintained for 24 to 48 h.

SALIVARY STONES

(Sialolithiasis)

Stones composed of Ca salts often obstruct salivary glands, causing pain, swelling, and sometimes infection. Diagnosis is made clinically or with CT, ultrasound, or sialogram. Treatment involves stone expression with saliva stimulants, manual manipulation, a probe, or surgery.

Etiology and Pathophysiology

The major salivary glands are the paired parotid, submandibular, and sublingual glands. Stones in the salivary glands are most common in adults. Eighty percent of stones originate in the submandibular glands and obstruct Wharton's duct. Most of the rest originate in the parotid glands and block Stensen's duct. Only about 1% originate in the sublingual glands. Multiple stones occur in about 25% of cases.

Most salivary stones are composed of Ca phosphate with small amounts of Mg and carbonate. Patients with gout may have uric acid stones. Stone formation requires a nidus on which salts can precipitate plus salivary stasis. Stasis occurs in patients who are debilitated, dehydrated, have reduced food intake, or take anticholinergics. Persisting or recurrent stones predispose to infection of the involved gland (sialadenitis—see p. 824).

Symptoms, Signs, and Diagnosis

Obstructing stones cause glandular swelling and pain, particularly after eating, which stimulates saliva flow. Symptoms may subside after a few hours. Relief may coincide with a gush of saliva. Some stones cause intermittent or no symptoms. If a stone is lodged distally, it may be visible or palpable at the duct's outlet.

If a stone is not apparent on examination, the patient can be given a sialagogue (eg, lemon juice, hard candy, or some other substance that triggers saliva flow). Reproduction of symptoms is almost always diagnostic of a stone. CT, ultrasound, and sialography are highly sensitive and are used if clinical diagnosis is equivocal. Contrast sialography may be performed through a catheter inserted into the duct and can differentiate between stone, stenosis, and tumor. This technique is occasionally therapeutic. Because 90% of submandibular calculi are radiopaque and 90% of parotid calculi are radiolucent, plain x-rays are not always accurate. MRI is not indicated.

Treatment

Analgesics, hydration, and massage can relieve symptoms. Antistaphylococcal antibiotics can be used to prevent acute sialadenitis if started early. Stones may pass spontaneously or when salivary flow is stimulated by sialagogues; patients are encouraged to suck a lemon wedge or sour candy every 2 to 3 h. Stones right at the duct orifice can sometimes be expressed manually by squeezing with the fingertips. Dilation of the duct with a small probe may facilitate expulsion. Surgical removal of stones succeeds if other methods fail. Stones at or near the orifice of the duct may be removed transorally, whereas those in the hilum of the gland often require complete excision of the salivary gland.

SIALADENITIS

Sialadenitis is bacterial infection of a salivary gland, usually due to an obstructing stone or gland hyposecretion. Symptoms are swelling, pain, redness, and tenderness. Diagnosis is clinical. CT, ultrasound, and MRI may help identify the cause. Treatment is with antibiotics.

Etiology

Sialadenitis usually occurs after hyposecretion or duct obstruction but may develop without an obvious cause. The major salivary glands are the parotid, submandibular, and sublingual glands. Sialadenitis is most common in the parotid gland and typically occurs in patients in their 50s and 60s, in chronically ill patients with xerostomia, and in those who have had radiation therapy to the oral cavity. Teenagers and young adults with anorexia are also prone to this disorder. The most common causative organism is *Staphylococcus aureus;* others include streptococci, coliforms, and various anaerobic bacteria.

Symptoms, Signs, and Diagnosis

Fever, chills, and unilateral pain and swelling develop. The gland is firm and diffusely tender, with erythema and edema of the overlying skin. Pus can often be expressed from the duct on compressing the affected gland and should be cultured. Focal enlargement may indicate an abscess. CT, ultrasound, and MRI can confirm sialadenitis or abscess that is not obvious clinically, though MRI may miss an obstructing stone.

Treatment

Initial treatment is with antibiotics active against *S. aureus* (eg, dicloxacillin, 250 mg po qid, a 1st-generation cephalosporin, or clindamycin), modified according to culture results. With the increasing prevalence of methicillin-resistant *S. aureus,* especially among the elderly living in extended-care nursing facilities, vancomycin is often required. Hydration, sialagogues (eg, lemon juice, hard candy, or some other substance that triggers saliva flow), warm compresses, gland massage, and good oral hygiene are also important. Abscesses require drainage. Occasionally, a superficial parotidectomy or submandibular gland excision is indicated for patients with chronic or relapsing sialadenitis.

Other Salivary Gland Infections

Mumps often cause parotid swelling (see also Table 193–1 on p. 1646). Patients with HIV infection often have parotid enlargement secondary to one or more lymphoepithelial cysts. Cat scratch disease from *Bartonella* infection often invades periparotid lymph nodes and may infect the parotid glands by contiguous spread. Although cat scratch disease is self-limited, antibiotic therapy is often provided, and incision and drainage are necessary if an abscess develops.

Atypical mycobacterial infections in the tonsils or teeth may spread contiguously to the major salivary glands. The PPD may be negative, and the diagnosis may require biopsy and tissue culture for acid-fast bacteria. Treatment recommendations are controversial. Options include surgical debridement with curettage, complete excision of the infected tissue, and use of anti-TB drug therapy (rarely necessary).

SUBMANDIBULAR SPACE INFECTION

(Ludwig's Angina)

Submandibular space infection is acute cellulitis of the soft tissues below the mouth. Symptoms include pain, dysphagia, and potentially fatal airway obstruction. Diagnosis usually is clinical. Treatment includes airway management, surgical drainage, and IV antibiotics.

Submandibular space infection is a rapidly spreading, bilateral, indurated cellulitis occurring in the suprahyoid soft tissues, the floor of the mouth, and both sublingual and submaxillary spaces without abscess formation. Although not a true abscess, it resembles one clinically and is treated similarly.

The condition usually develops from an odontogenic infection, especially of the 2nd and 3rd mandibular molars, or as an extension of peritonsillar cellulitis. Contributing factors may include poor dental hygiene, tooth extractions, and trauma (eg, fractures of the mandible, lacerations of the floor of the mouth).

Symptoms, Signs, and Diagnosis

Early manifestations are pain in any involved teeth with severe tender localized submental and sublingual induration. Boardlike firmness of the floor of the mouth and brawny induration of the suprahyoid soft tissues may develop rapidly. Drooling, trismus, dysphagia, stridor from laryngeal edema, and elevation of the posterior tongue against the palate may be present. Fever, chills, and tachycardia are usually present as well. The condition can cause airway obstruction within hours and does so more often than do other neck infections.

The diagnosis usually is obvious. If not, CT is performed.

Treatment

Maintaining airway patency is of the highest priority. Because swelling makes oral endotracheal intubation difficult, fiberoptic nasotracheal intubation performed with topical anesthesia in the operating room or ICU with the patient awake is preferable. Patients without immediate need for intubation require intense observation and may benefit temporarily from a nasal trumpet.

Incision and drainage with placement of drains deep into the mylohyoid muscles relieve the pressure. Antibiotics should be chosen to cover both oral anaerobes and aerobes (eg, clindamycin, ampicillin-sulbactam, high-dose penicillin).

TONSILLOPHARYNGITIS

(See also p. 1446 for streptococcal pharyngitis.)

Tonsillopharyngitis is acute infection of the pharynx or palatine tonsils or both. Symptoms may include sore throat, dysphagia, cervical lymphadenopathy, and fever. Diagnosis is clinical, supplemented by culture or rapid antigen test. Treatment is dependent on symptoms and, in the case of GABHS, involves antibiotics.

Etiology and Pathophysiology

The tonsils participate in systemic immune surveillance. In addition, local tonsillar defenses include a lining of antigen-processing squamous epithelium that involves B- and T-cell responses.

Tonsillopharyngitis is usually viral, most often caused by the common cold viruses (adenovirus, rhinovirus, influenza, coronavirus, respiratory syncytial virus), but occasionally by Epstein-Barr virus, herpes simplex virus, cytomegalovirus, or HIV. In about 30% of cases, the cause is bacterial. Group A β-hemolytic streptococcus (GABHS) is most common (see p. 1446), but *Staphylococcus aureus, Streptococcus pneumoniae, Mycoplasma pneumoniae,* and *Chlamydia pneumoniae* are sometimes involved. Rare causes include pertussis, *Fusobacterium,* diphtheria, syphilis, and gonorrhea.

Tonsillopharyngitis of all varieties constitutes about 15% of all office visits to primary care physicians. GABHS occurs most commonly between ages 5 and 15 and is uncommon before age 3.

Symptoms and Signs

Pain with swallowing is the hallmark and is often referred to the ears. Very young children who are not able to complain of sore throat often refuse to eat. High fever, malaise, headache, and GI upset are common, as are halitosis and a muffled voice. A scarlatiniform or nonspecific rash may also be present. The tonsils are swollen and red and often have purulent exudates. Tender cervical lymphadenopathy may be present. Fever, adenopathy, palatal petechiae, and exudates are somewhat more common with GABHS than with viral tonsillopharyngitis, but there is much overlap. GABHS usually resolves within 7 days. Untreated GABHS may lead to local suppurative complications (eg, peritonsillar abscess or cellulitis) and sometimes to rheumatic fever or glomerulonephritis.

Diagnosis

Pharyngitis itself is easily recognized clinically. However, its cause is not. Rhinorrhea and cough usually indicate a viral cause. Infectious mononucleosis is suggested by posterior cervical or generalized adenopathy, hepatosplenomegaly, fatigue, and malaise for > 1 wk; a full neck with petechiae of the soft palate; and thick tonsillar exudates. A dirty gray, thick, tough membrane that bleeds if peeled away indicates diphtheria (rare in the US).

Because GABHS requires antibiotics, it must be diagnosed. Criteria for testing are controversial. Many authorities recommend testing with a rapid antigen test or culture for all children. Rapid antigen tests are specific but not sensitive and may need to be followed by a culture, which is about 90% specific and 90% sensitive. In adults, many authorities recommend using 4 criteria: history of fever, tonsillar exudates, absence of cough, and tender anterior cervical lymphadenopathy. Patients who meet 1 or no criteria are unlikely to have GABHS and should not be tested. Patients who meet 2 criteria can be tested. Patients who meet 3 or 4 criteria can be tested or treated empirically for GABHS.

Treatment

Supportive treatments include analgesia, hydration, and rest. Penicillin V is usually considered the drug of choice for GABHS tonsillopharyngitis; dose is 250 mg po bid for 10 days for patients < 27 kg and 500 mg for those > 27 kg (see also p. 1447). Amoxicillin is effective and more palatable if a liquid preparation is required. If compliance is a concern, a single dose of benzathine penicillin 1.2 million units IM (600,000 units for children ≤ 27 kg) is effective. Other oral drugs include macrolides for patients allergic to penicillin, a 1st-generation cephalosporin, and clindamycin.

Treatment may be started immediately or delayed until culture results are back. If treatment is started presumptively, it should be stopped if cultures are negative. Follow-up throat cultures are not routinely performed. They are useful in patients with multiple GABHS recurrences or if pharyngitis spreads to close contacts at home or school.

Tonsillectomy should be considered if GABHS tonsillitis recurs repeatedly (> 6 episodes/yr, > 4 episodes/yr for 2 yr, > 3 episodes/yr for 3 yr) or if acute infection is severe and persistent despite antibiotics. Other criteria for tonsillectomy include obstructive sleep disorder, recurrent peritonsillar abscess, and suspicion of malignancy.

Numerous effective surgical techniques are used to perform tonsillectomy, including electrocautery, microdebrider, radiofrequency coblation, and sharp dissection. Significant intraoperative or postoperative bleeding occurs in < 2% of patients, usually within 24 h of surgery or after 7 days, when the eschar detaches. Patients with bleeding should go to the hospital. If bleeding continues on arrival, patients generally are examined in the operating room and hemostasis is obtained. If a clot is present in the tonsillar fossa, patients are observed for 24 h. Postoperative IV rehydration is necessary in ≤ 3% of patients, possibly in fewer patients with use of optimal preoperative hydration, perioperative antibiotics, analgesics, and corticosteroids. Postoperative airway obstruction occurs most frequently in children < 2 yr who have preexisting severe obstructive sleep disorders and in patients who are morbidly obese, have neurologic disorders, have craniofacial anomalies, or have significant preoperative obstructive sleep apnea. Complications are generally more common and serious in adults.

TORNWALDT'S CYST

(Pharyngeal Bursa)

Tornwaldt's cyst is a rare cyst in the midline of the nasopharynx that may become infected.

Tornwaldt's cyst is a remnant of the embryonal notochord superficial to the superior constrictor muscle of the pharynx and covered by the mucous membrane of the nasopharynx. It may become infected, causing persistent purulent drainage with a foul taste and odor, eustachian tube obstruction, and sore throat.

Purulent exudate may be seen at the opening of the cyst. Diagnosis is based on nasopharyngoscopy supplemented by CT or MRI when the diagnosis is in doubt. Treatment consists of marsupialization or excision.

VELOPHARYNGEAL INSUFFICIENCY

Velopharyngeal insufficiency is incomplete closure of a sphincter between the oropharynx and nasopharynx, often resulting from anatomic abnormalities of the palate and causing hypernasal speech. Treatment is with speech therapy and surgery.

Velopharyngeal insufficiency is incomplete closure of the velopharyngeal sphincter between the oropharynx and the nasopharynx. Closure, normally achieved by the sphincteric action of the soft palate and the superior constrictor muscle, is impaired in patients with cleft palate, repaired cleft palate, congenitally short palate, submucous cleft palate, palatal paralysis, and, sometimes, enlarged tonsils. The condition may also result when adenoidectomy or uvulopalatopharyngoplasty is performed in a patient with a congenital underdevelopment (submucous cleft) or paralysis of the palate.

Symptoms, Signs, and Diagnosis

Speech in a patient with velopharyngeal insufficiency is characterized by hypernasal resonant voice, nasal emission of air, nasal turbulence, and inability to produce sounds requiring oral pressure (plosives). Severe velopharyngeal insufficiency results in regurgitation of solid foods and fluids through the nose. Inspection of the palate during phonation may reveal palatal paralysis.

The diagnosis is suspected in patients with the typical speech abnormalities. Palpation of the midline of the soft palate may reveal a cleft. Direct inspection with a fiberoptic nasoendoscope is the primary diagnostic technique. Multiview videofluoroscopy during connected speech and swallowing (modified barium swallow), performed in conjunction with a speech pathologist, can also be used.

Treatment

Treatment consists of speech therapy and surgical correction by a palatal elongation pushback procedure, posterior pharyngeal wall implant, pharyngeal flap, or pharyngoplasty, depending on the mobility of the lateral pharyngeal walls, the degree of velar elevation, and the size of the defect.

91 NOSE AND PARANASAL SINUS DISORDERS

(See Ch. 89 for a detailed description of the anatomy of the nose and sinuses.)

BACTERIAL INFECTIONS

Nasal vestibulitis is bacterial infection of the nasal vestibule, typically with *Staphylococcus aureus.* It may result from nose picking or excessive nose blowing and causes annoying crusts and bleeding when the crusts slough off. Bacitracin or mupirocin ointment applied topically bid for 14 days is effective.

Furuncles of the nasal vestibule are usually staphylococcal; they may develop into spreading cellulitis of the tip of the nose. Systemic antistaphylococcal antibiotics (eg, cephalexin 500 mg po qid) are given and warm compresses and topical mupirocin applied. Furuncles are incised and drained to prevent local thrombophlebitis and subsequent cavernous sinus thrombosis.

EPISTAXIS

Epistaxis is nose bleeding, which occurs from the anterior or posterior portion of the nasal septum. Diagnosis is by direct visualization. Treatment varies by site of bleeding but includes cautery and various types of packing.

Most nasal bleeding is anterior, originating from a plexus of vessels in the anteroinferior septum (Kiesselbach's area). Less common but more serious are posterior nosebleeds, which tend to occur in patients with preexisting atherosclerotic vessels or bleeding disorders who have undergone nasal or sinus surgery. In Rendu-Osler-Weber syndrome, multiple severe nosebleeds may result from arteriovenous aneurysms in the mucous membrane. Severe epistaxis is often caused by coagulopathy from liver disease.

Most epistaxes occur secondary to local trauma (including nose blowing and picking) and drying of the nasal mucous membrane. Less common causes include local infections, such as vestibulitis, rhinitis, and sinusitis; systemic infections, such as AIDS; foreign bodies (particularly in children); arteriosclerosis; hypertension (when poorly controlled); a benign or malignant tumor in a paranasal sinus or in the nasopharynx; and septal perforations. Epistaxis of any cause is common in patients with bleeding tendencies (eg, thrombocytopenia, liver disease, coagulopathies, anticoagulant use).

Symptoms, Signs, and Diagnosis

Bleeding ranges from a trickle to a strong flow. Although major epistaxis quickly involves both nares, most patients can localize the initial flow to one side, which focuses the clinical examination.

Anterior bleeding sites are usually apparent on direct examination with a nasal speculum and a bright light. If no site is apparent and bleeding is severe or recurrent, fiberoptic endoscopy may be necessary.

Routine laboratory testing is not required. Patients with symptoms or signs of bleeding from other sites (eg, melena, petechiae) and those with severe or recurrent epistaxis undergo CBC, PT, and PTT. CT may be performed if a foreign body, a tumor, a fracture, or sinusitis is suspected.

Treatment

Presumptive treatment for actively bleeding patients is that for anterior bleeding. The need for blood replacement is determined by the Hb level, symptoms of anemia, and vital signs.

Anterior epistaxis: Bleeding can usually be controlled by pinching the nasal alae together for 10 min. If this maneuver fails, a cotton pledget impregnated with a vasoconstrictor (eg, phenylephrine 0.25%) and a topical anesthetic (eg, lidocaine 2%) is inserted and the nose pinched for another 10 min. The bleeding point may then be cauterized with electrocautery or silver nitrate on an applicator stick. Cauterizing 4 quadrants immediately adjacent to the bleeding vessel is most effective. Care must be taken to avoid burning the mucous membrane too deeply. Alternatively, a nasal tampon of expandable foam may be inserted. Coating the tampon with a topical ointment, such as bacitracin or mupirocin, may help. If these methods are ineffective, various commercial nasal balloons can be used to tamponade bleeding sites. Alternatively, an anterior nasal pack consisting of ½-in petrolatum gauze may be inserted; up to 72 in may be required. This procedure is painful, and analgesics usually are needed.

Posterior epistaxis: Posterior bleeding may be difficult to control. Commercial nasal balloons are quick and convenient; a gauze posterior pack is effective but more difficult to position. Both are very uncomfortable; IV sedation and analgesia may be needed, and hospitalization is required.

The posterior gauze pack consists of 4-in gauze squares folded, rolled, tied into a tight bundle with 2 strands of heavy silk suture, and coated with antibiotic ointment. The ends of 1 suture are tied to a catheter that has been introduced through the nasal cavity on the side of the bleeding and brought out through the mouth. As the catheter is withdrawn from the nose, the postnasal pack is pulled into place above the soft palate in the nasopharynx. The 2nd suture hangs down the back of the throat and is trimmed below the level of the soft palate so that it can be used to remove the pack. This oral suture prevents aspiration into the larynx if the pack falls from the nasopharynx into the airway. The nasal cavity anterior to this pack is firmly packed with ½-in petrolatum gauze, and the 1st suture is tied over a roll of gauze at the anterior nares to secure the postnasal pack. The packing remains in place for 4 to 5 days. An antibiotic (eg, amoxicillin/clavulanate 875 mg po bid for 7 to 10 days) is given to prevent sinusitis and otitis media. Postnasal packing lowers the arterial Po_2, and supplementary O_2 is given while the packing is in place.

Rarely, the internal maxillary artery and its branches must be ligated to control the bleeding. The arteries may be ligated with clips using microscopic guidance and a surgical approach through the maxillary sinus. Alternatively, embolization by angiography may be used.

Bleeding disorders: In Rendu-Osler-Weber syndrome, a split-thickness skin graft (septal dermatoplasty) reduces the number of nosebleeds and allows the anemia to be corrected. Laser (Nd:YAG) photocoagulation, another coagulation technique, is performed in the operating room. Selective embolization is very effective, particularly in patients who cannot tolerate general anesthesia or for whom surgical intervention has not been successful. New endoscopic sinus devices have made transnasal surgery more effective.

In patients with liver disease, blood may be swallowed in large amounts and should be eliminated promptly with enemas and cathartics to prevent hepatic encephalopathy. The

GI tract should be sterilized with nonabsorbable antibiotics (eg, neomycin 1 g po qid) to prevent the breakdown of blood and the absorption of ammonia.

FOREIGN BODIES

Nasal foreign bodies are found occasionally in young children, the mentally retarded, and psychiatric patients. Common objects pushed into the nose include beads, beans, seeds, nuts, insects, and button batteries (which may cause chemical burns). When mineral salts are deposited on a long-retained foreign body, the object is called a rhinolith.

A nasal foreign body is suspected in any patient with a unilateral, foul-smelling, bloody, purulent rhinorrhea. Diagnosis is often made through another party's observation of the item being pushed into the nose or through visualization with a nasal speculum.

Nasal foreign bodies can sometimes be removed in the office with a nasal speculum and Hartmann's nasal forceps. Pretreatment with topical phenylephrine may aid visualization and removal. To avoid pushing a slippery, round object deeper, it is better to reach behind the object with the bent tip of a blunt probe and pull it forward. Sometimes, general anesthesia is necessary if a rhinolith has formed or if the foreign body may be displaced dorsally and then aspirated, resulting in airway obstruction.

POLYPS

Nasal polyps are fleshy outgrowths of the nasal mucosa that form at the site of dependent edema in the lamina propria of the mucous membrane, usually around the ostia of the maxillary sinuses.

Allergic rhinitis, acute and chronic infections, and cystic fibrosis all predispose to the formation of polyps. Bleeding polyps occur in rhinosporidiosis. Unilateral polyps occasionally occur in association with or represent benign or malignant tumors of the nose or paranasal sinuses. They can also occur in response to a foreign body. Nasal polyps are strongly associated with aspirin allergy, sinus infections, and asthma.

Symptoms, Signs, and Diagnosis

Symptoms include obstruction and postnasal drainage, congestion, sneezing, rhinorrhea, anosmia, hyposmia, facial pain, and ocular itching.

Diagnosis generally is based on physical examination. A developing polyp is teardrop-shaped; when mature, it resembles a peeled seedless grape.

Treatment

Corticosteroids, such as beclomethasone (42 μg/spray) or flunisolide (25 μg/spray) aerosols, given as 1 or 2 sprays in each nasal cavity bid, may shrink or eliminate polyps, as may a 1-wk tapered course of oral corticosteroids. Surgical removal is still required in many cases. Polyps that obstruct the airway or promote sinusitis are removed, as are unilateral polyps that may be obscuring benign or malignant tumors. However, polyps tend to recur unless the underlying allergy or infection is controlled. After removal of nasal polyps, topical beclomethasone or flunisolide therapy tends to retard recurrence. In severe recurrent cases, maxillary sinusotomy or ethmoidectomy may be indicated. These procedures are usually performed endoscopically.

RHINITIS

(See also Allergic Rhinitis on p. 1357.)

Rhinitis is inflammation of the nasal mucous membrane, with resultant nasal congestion, rhinorrhea, and variable associated symptoms depending on etiology (eg, itching, sneezing, purulence, anosmia, ozena). The cause is usually viral, although irritants can cause it. Diagnosis is usually clinical. Treatment includes humidification of room air, sympathomimetic amines, and antihistamines. Bacterial superinfection requires appropriate antibiotic treatment.

Acute rhinitis (edema and vasodilation of the nasal mucous membrane, rhinorrhea, and obstruction) is the usual manifestation of a common cold (see p. 1595); other causes include streptococcal, pneumococcal, and staphylococcal infections.

Chronic rhinitis is generally a prolongation of subacute inflammatory or infectious rhinitis but may also occur in syphilis, TB, rhinoscleroma, rhinosporidiosis, leishmaniasis, blastomycosis, histoplasmosis, and leprosy—all of which are characterized by granuloma formation and destruction of soft tissue, cartilage, and bone. Nasal obstruction, purulent rhinorrhea, and frequent bleeding result. Rhinoscleroma causes progressive nasal obstruction from indurated inflammatory tissue in the lamina propria. Rhinosporidiosis is characterized by bleeding polyps. Both low humidity and airborne irritants can result in chronic rhinitis. Low humidity—eg, the desert or too much time on an airplane—can cause or exacerbate epistaxis from minor nasal septal deformities.

Atrophic rhinitis results in atrophy and sclerosis of mucous membrane; the mucous membrane changes from ciliated pseudostratified columnar epithelium to stratified squamous epithelium, and the lamina propria is reduced in amount and vascularity. Atrophic rhinitis is associated with advanced age, Wegener's granulomatosis, and iatrogenically induced excessive nasal tissue extirpation. Although the exact etiology is unknown, bacterial infection frequently plays a role. Nasal mucosal atrophy often occurs in the elderly.

Vasomotor rhinitis is a chronic condition in which intermittent vascular engorgement of the nasal mucous membrane leads to watery rhinorrhea and sneezing. Etiology is uncertain, and no allergy can be identified. A dry atmosphere appears to aggravate the condition.

Symptoms and Signs

Acute rhinitis results in itching, nasal congestion, rhinorrhea, and sneezing. Symptoms and signs of chronic rhinitis are similar but may include purulent rhinorrhea and bleeding.

Atrophic rhinitis results in abnormal patency of the nasal cavities, crust formation, anosmia, and epistaxis that may be recurrent and severe.

Vasomotor rhinitis results in sneezing and watery rhinorrhea. The turgescent mucous membrane varies from bright red to purple. The condition is marked by periods of remission and exacerbation. Vasomotor rhinitis is differentiated from specific viral and bacterial infections of the nose by the lack of purulent exudate and crusting. It is differentiated from allergic rhinitis by the absence of an identifiable allergen.

Diagnosis and Treatment

Acute viral rhinitis is diagnosed clinically. It may be treated symptomatically with decongestants (either topical vasoconstriction with a sympathomimetic amine, such as phenylephrine 0.25% q 3 to 4 h for not more than 7 days; or systemic sympathomimetic amines, such as pseudoephedrine 30 mg po q 4 to 6 h). Antihistamines may be helpful. Those with anticholinergic properties dry mucous membranes and therefore may increase irritation. Decongestants may also relieve symptoms of acute bacterial rhinitis and chronic rhinitis, whereas an underlying bacterial infection requires culture or biopsy, pathogen identification, antibiotic sensitivities, and appropriate antimicrobial treatment.

Treatment of atrophic rhinitis is directed at reducing the crusting and eliminating the odor with topical antibiotics (eg, bacitracin), topical or systemic estrogens, and vitamins A and D. Occluding or reducing the patency of the nasal cavities surgically decreases the crusting caused by the drying effect of air flowing over the atrophic mucous membrane.

Treatment of vasomotor rhinitis is by trial and error and is not always satisfactory. Patients benefit from humidified air, as may be provided by a humidified central heating system or a vaporizer in the workroom or bedroom. Systemic sympathomimetic amines (eg, for adults, pseudoephedrine 30 mg po q 4 to 6 h prn) relieve symptoms but are not recommended for long-term use. Topical vasoconstrictors are avoided because they cause the vasculature of the nasal mucous membrane to lose its sensitivity to other vasoconstrictive stimuli—eg, the humidity and temperature of inspired air.

SEPTAL DEVIATION AND PERFORATION

Deviations of the nasal septum due to developmental abnormalities or trauma are common but often are asymptomatic and require no treatment. Symptomatic septal deviation causes nasal obstruction and predisposes the patient to sinusitis (particularly if the deviation obstructs the ostium of a paranasal sinus) and to epistaxis due to drying air currents. Other symptoms may include facial pain, headaches, and noisy night breathing. Septal deviation is usually evident on examination, although a flashlight and examination of the anterior nasal passage may not be sufficient. Treatment consists of septoplasty (septal reconstruction).

Septal ulcers and perforations may result from nasal surgery; repeated trauma, such as chronic nose picking; cosmetic piercing; toxic exposures (eg, acids, chromium, phosphorus, copper vapor); chronic cocaine use; chronic nasal spray use (including corticosteroids and OTC phenylephrine sprays); transnasal O_2 use; or diseases such as TB, syphilis, leprosy, SLE, and Wegener's granulomatosis. Crusting around the margins and repeated epistaxis, which can be severe, may result. Small perforations may whistle. Anterior rhinoscopy or fiberoptic endoscopy can be used to view septal perforations. Topical bacitracin or mupirocin ointment reduces crusting, as may saline nasal spray. Symptomatic septal perforations are occasionally repaired with buccal or septal mucous membrane flaps; closing the perforation with a silicone septal button is a reliable option.

SINUSITIS

Sinusitis is inflammation of the paranasal sinuses due to viral, bacterial, or fungal infections or allergic reactions. Symptoms include nasal obstruction and congestion, purulent rhinorrhea, cough, facial pain, malaise, and sometimes fever. Treatment is with antibiotics, such as amoxicillin, penicillin, erythromycin, or trimethoprim-sulfamethoxazole, given for 12 to 14 days for acute sinusitis and for up to 6 wk for chronic sinusitis. Decongestants and application of heat and humidity may help relieve symptoms and improve sinus drainage. Recurrent sinusitis may require surgery to improve sinus drainage.

Sinusitis may be classified as acute (completely resolved in < 30 days); subacute (completely resolved in 30 to 90 days); recurrent (multiple discrete acute episodes, each completely resolved in < 30 days but recurring in cycles, with at least 10 days between complete resolution of symptoms and initiation of a new episode); and chronic (lasting > 90 days).

Etiology

Acute sinusitis is usually precipitated by viral URI, followed by secondary bacterial colonization with streptococci, pneumococci, *Haemophilus influenzae,* or staphylococci. In a URI, the swollen nasal mucous membrane obstructs the ostium of a paranasal sinus, and the O_2 in the sinus is absorbed into the blood vessels of the mucous membrane. The resulting relative negative pressure in the sinus (vacuum sinusitis) is painful. If the vacuum is maintained, a transudate from the mucous membrane develops and fills the sinus; the transudate serves as a medium for bacteria that enter the sinus through the ostium or through a spreading cellulitis or thrombophlebitis in the lamina propria of the mucous membrane. An outpouring of serum and leukocytes to combat the infection results, and painful positive pressure develops in the obstructed sinus. The mucous membrane becomes hyperemic and edematous.

Chronic sinusitis may be exacerbated by gram-negative bacilli or anaerobic microorganisms. In a few cases, chronic maxillary sinusitis is secondary to dental infection. Fungal infections (*Aspergillus, Sporothrix, Pseudoallescheria*) tend to strike the immunocompromised patient, whereas hospital-acquired infections complicate cystic fibrosis, nasogastric and nasotracheal intubation, and debilitated patients. Typical organisms include *Staphylococcus aureus, Klebsiella pneumoniae, Pseudomonas aeruginosa, Proteus mirabilis,* and *Enterobacter.* Allergic fungal sinusitis is characterized by diffuse nasal congestion, markedly viscid nasal secretions, and, often, nasal polyps. It is an allergic response to the presence of topical fungi, often *Aspergillus,* and is not caused by an invasive infection.

Symptoms, Signs, and Diagnosis

Acute and chronic sinusitis produce similar symptoms and signs, including purulent rhinorrhea, pressure and pain in the face, nasal congestion and obstruction, hyposmia, halitosis, and productive cough (especially at night). The area over the affected sinus may be tender, swollen, and erythematous. Maxillary sinusitis causes pain in the maxillary area, toothache, and frontal headache. Frontal sinusitis produces pain in the frontal area and frontal headache. Ethmoid sinusitis causes pain behind and between the eyes, frontal headache often described as splitting, periorbital cellulitis, and tearing. Pain from sphenoid sinusitis is less well localized and is referred to the frontal or occipital area. Malaise may be present. Fever and chills suggest an extension of the infection beyond the sinuses.

The nasal mucous membrane is red and turgescent; yellow or green purulent rhinorrhea may be present. Seropurulent or mucopurulent exudate may be seen in the middle meatus with maxillary, anterior ethmoid, or frontal sinusitis and in the area medial to the middle turbinate with posterior ethmoid or sphenoid sinusitis.

Sinus infections are usually diagnosed clinically. Absence or dullness of light on transillumination may suggest fluid-filled maxillary or frontal sinuses. In acute and chronic sinusitis, the swollen mucous membranes and retained exudate cause the affected sinus to appear opaque on 4-view x-rays. Plain x-rays are not as valuable as CT, which provides better definition of the extent and degree of sinusitis. X-rays of the apices of the teeth may be required in chronic maxillary sinusitis to exclude a periapical abscess. When questions persist (eg, regarding intracranial extension, treatment failure, or hospital-acquired causes of sinusitis), culture and sensitivity tests can be done on sinus secretions obtained through endoscopy or sinus puncture and aspiration.

Sinusitis in children is suspected when purulent rhinorrhea persists for > 10 days along with fatigue and cough. Fever is uncommon. Local facial pain or discomfort may be present. Nasal examination discloses purulent drainage; CT is confirmatory. The CT scan is of limited cuts in the coronal projection to limit radiation exposure.

Treatment

In acute sinusitis, improved drainage and control of infection are the aims of therapy. Steam inhalation; hot, wet towels over the affected sinuses; and hot beverages improve nasal vasoconstriction and promote drainage. Topical vasoconstrictors, such as phenylephrine 0.25% spray q 3 h, are effective but should be used for a maximum of 5 days or for a repeating cycle of 3 days on and 3 days off until the sinusitis is resolved; systemic vasoconstrictors, such as pseudoephedrine 30 mg po (for adults) q 4 to 6 h, are less effective.

In acute and chronic sinusitis, antibiotics are given for at least 10 days and often for 14 days. In acute sinusitis, amoxicillin 500 mg po q 8 h with or without clavulanate is primary therapy. Erythromycin 250 mg po q 6 h with trimethoprim-sulfamethoxazole 80/400 mg q 6 h can be given to patients allergic to penicillin. Second-line therapy includes cefuroxime 500 mg q 12 h or moxifloxacin 400 mg once/day. For children, similar antibiotics are used, adjusted for the patient's weight. Fluoroquinolones, however, are not used in children because of concerns of premature epiphyseal growth plate closure.

In exacerbations of chronic sinusitis in children or adults, a broad-spectrum antibiotic, such as amoxicillin/clavulanate 875 mg q 12 h (12.5 to 25 mg/kg q 12 h in children), cefuroxime, or, in adults, moxifloxacin, is used. In chronic sinusitis, prolonged antibiotic therapy for 4 to 6 wk often brings complete resolution. The sensitivities of pathogens isolated from the sinus exudate and the patient's response guide subsequent therapy.

Sinusitis unresponsive to antibiotic therapy may require surgery (maxillary sinusotomy, ethmoidectomy, or sphenoid sinusotomy) to improve ventilation and drainage and to remove inspissated mucopurulent material, epithelial debris, and hypertrophic mucous membrane. These procedures are usually performed intranasally with the aid of an endoscope. Chronic frontal sinusitis may be managed either with osteoplastic obliteration of the frontal sinuses or endoscopically in selected patients. The use of intraoperative computer-aided surgery to localize disease and prevent injury to surrounding contiguous structures (such as the eye and brain) has become common.

Sinusitis in Immunocompromised Patients

Aggressive and even fatal fungal or bacterial sinusitis can occur in patients who are immunocompromised because of poorly controlled diabetes, neutropenia, or HIV infection.

Mucormycosis (phycomycosis)—a mycosis due to fungi of the order Mucorales, including species of *Mucor, Absidia,* and *Rhizopus*—may develop in patients with poorly controlled diabetes. It is characterized by black, devitalized tissue in the nasal cavity and neurologic signs secondary to retrograde thromboarteritis in the carotid arterial system. Diagnosis is based on histopathologic demonstration of mycelia in the avascularized tissue. Treatment requires control of the underlying condition (such as reversal of ketoacidosis in diabetes) and IV administration of amphotericin B. Prompt biopsy of intranasal tissue for histology and culture is warranted.

Aspergillosis and **candidiasis** of the paranasal sinuses strike patients who are immunocompromised secondary to therapy with cytotoxic drugs or to immunosuppressive diseases, such as leukemia, lymphoma, multiple myeloma, and AIDS. These infections can appear as polypoid tissue in the nose as well as thickened mucosa; tissue is required for diagnosis. Aggressive paranasal sinus surgery and IV amphotericin B therapy are used to control these often-fatal infections.

SMELL AND TASTE DISORDERS

Because distinct flavors depend on aromas to stimulate the olfactory chemoreceptors, smell and taste are physiologically interdependent. Dysfunction of one often disturbs the other. Disorders of smell and taste are rarely incapacitating or life threatening, so they often do not receive close medical attention, although their effect on quality of life can be severe. Loss of olfaction and/or gustation in the elderly leads to reduced oral intake and can add to the debilitation of the patient. The inability to detect certain odors, such as gas or smoke, may be dangerous, and several systemic and intracranial disorders should be excluded before dismissing symptoms as harmless. Whether brain stem disease (involvement of the nucleus solitarius) can cause disorders of smell and taste is uncertain, because other neurologic manifestations usually take precedence.

Anosmia (loss of the sense of smell) is probably the most common abnormality (see below). Hyperosmia (increased sensitivity to odors) usually reflects a neurotic or histrionic personality but can occur intermittently with seizure disorders. Dysosmia (disagreeable or distorted sense of smell) may occur with infection of the nasal sinuses, partial damage to the olfactory bulbs, or psychologic depression. Some cases of dysosmia, accompanied by a disagreeable taste, result from poor dental hygiene. Uncinate epilepsy can produce brief, vivid, unpleasant olfactory hallucinations. Hyposmia (diminished sense of smell) and hypogeusia (diminished sense of taste) can follow acute influenza, usually temporarily.

Drying of the oral mucosa from heavy smoking, Sjögren's syndrome, radiation therapy of the head and neck, or desquamation of the tongue can impair taste, and various drugs (eg, those with anticholinergic properties and vincristine) alter taste. In all instances, the gustatory receptors are diffusely involved. When limited to one side of the tongue (eg, in Bell's palsy), ageusia (loss of the sense of taste) is rarely noticed.

Rarely, idiopathic dysgeusia (distorted sense of taste), hypogeusia, and dysosmia respond to zinc supplementation.

ANOSMIA

Anosmia is the complete loss of smell.

Anosmia occurs when intranasal swelling or other obstruction prevents odors from gaining access to the olfactory area; when the olfactory neuroepithelium is destroyed (as occurs in viral infections, atrophic rhinitis, or the chronic rhinitis of granulomatous diseases and tumors); or when the olfactory nerve fila, bulbs, tracts, or central connections are destroyed (eg, by head trauma, intracranial surgery, infections, or tumors). Head trauma is a major cause of anosmia in young adults; viral infections and Alzheimer's, in older adults. Prior URI, especially influenza infection, is implicated in 14 to 26% of all presenting cases of hyposmia or anosmia.

Most patients with anosmia have normal perception of salty, sweet, sour, and bitter substances but lack flavor discrimination, which is largely dependent on olfaction. Therefore, they often complain of losing the sense of taste (ageusia). If unilateral, anosmia is often unrecognized.

Diagnosis, if the cause is not apparent, requires thorough evaluation for intranasal and intracranial diseases and examination of the cranial nerves (see p. 1750) and of the upper respiratory tract (particularly the nose and nasopharynx). CT, with radiopaque dye, of the head to rule out tumors and unsuspected fractures of the floor of the anterior cranial fossa is obtained. A psychophysical assessment of odor and taste identification and threshold detection is performed as well.

Treatment of allergic or bacterial rhinitis and sinusitis or removal of nasal polyps and benign tumors may recover olfaction. Conditions causing destruction of the olfactory neuroepithelium or its central pathways do not lend themselves to effective treatment, although spontaneous recovery may follow regeneration of the olfactory neuroepithelium and its central pathways.

92 LARYNGEAL DISORDERS

The larynx contains the vocal cords and serves as the opening to the tracheobronchial tree. Laryngeal disorders include various benign tumors, contact ulcers, granulomas, laryngitis, laryngoceles, spasmodic dysphonia, vocal cord paralysis, and vocal cord polyps and nodules. For acute laryngotracheobronchitis, see Croup on p. 2307.

Laryngeal cancer is discussed on p. 840.

Most laryngeal disorders cause dysphonia, which is impairment of the voice. A persistent change in the voice (eg, > 3 wk) requires visualization of the vocal cords, including their mobility. Although the voice changes with age, becoming breathy and aperiodic, acute or prominent changes in the elderly should not be presumed to result from aging, and evaluation is required.

The voice should be assessed and recorded, particularly if surgical procedures are planned. Examination of the larynx includes external inspection and palpation and internal visualization of the epiglottis, false cords, true cords, arytenoids, pyriform sinuses, and subglottic region below the cords. Internal visualization is accomplished by either indirect mirror examination or direct flexible fiberoptic laryngoscopy in an outpatient setting with a topical anesthetic. Rigid laryngoscopy with the patient under general anesthesia allows for biopsy when necessary or assessment of passive mobility of the vocal cords when immobilized by either paralysis or fixation (see sidebar 92–1).

BENIGN TUMORS

Benign laryngeal tumors include juvenile papillomas hemangiomas, fibromas, chondromas, myxomas, and neurofibromas. They may appear in any part of the larynx. Symptoms include hoarseness, breathy voice, dyspnea, aspiration, dysphagia, pain, otalgia (pain referred to the ear), and hemoptysis. Diagnosis is based on direct or indirect visualization of the larynx, supplemented by CT. Removal restores the voice, the functional integrity of the laryngeal sphincter, and the airway. Smaller lesions may be excised endoscopically using the CO_2 laser and general anesthesia. Larger lesions extending beyond the laryngeal framework often require pharyngotomy or laryngofissure.

Cancerous tumors are discussed in Ch. 93 on p. 838.

CONTACT ULCERS

Contact ulcers are unilateral or bilateral erosions of the mucous membrane over the vocal process of the arytenoid cartilage.

Contact ulcers are usually due to voice abuse in the form of repeated sharp glottal attacks (abrupt loudness at the onset of phonation), often experienced by singers. They may also occur after endotracheal intubation if an oversized tube erodes the mucosa overlying the cartilaginous vocal processes. Gastroesophageal reflux may also cause or aggravate contact ulcers. Symptoms include varying degrees of hoarseness and mild pain with phonation and swallowing. Biopsy to exclude carcinoma or TB is important. Prolonged ulceration leads to nonspecific granulomas that also produce varying degrees of hoarseness.

Treatment consists of ≥ 6 wk of voice rest. Patients must recognize the limitations of their voice and learn to adjust their postrecovery vocal activities to avoid recurrence. Granulomas tend to recur after surgical removal. Risk of recurrence is reduced through vigorous treatment of gastroesophageal reflux (see p. 112). Suppression of bacterial flora by antibiotics during postoperative healing is also recommended.

LARYNGITIS

Laryngitis is inflammation of the larynx, usually due to a virus or overuse. The result is acute change in the voice, with decreased volume and hoarseness. Diagnosis is based on clinical findings. Laryngoscopy is required for symptoms > 3 wk. Viral laryngitis is self-limited. Other infectious or irritating causes may require specific treatment.

The most common cause of acute laryngitis is a viral URI. Coughing-induced laryngitis may also occur in bronchitis, pneumonia, influenza, pertussis, measles, and diphtheria.

Excessive use of the voice (especially with loud speaking or singing), allergic reactions, gastroesophageal reflux, bulimia, or inhalation of irritating substances, such as cigarette smoke or certain aerosolized drugs, can cause acute or chronic laryngitis.

Symptoms, Signs, and Diagnosis

An unnatural change of voice is usually the most prominent symptom. Volume is typically greatly decreased; some patients have aphonia. Hoarseness, a sensation of tickling, rawness, and a constant urge to clear the throat may occur. Symptoms vary with the severity of the inflammation. Fever, malaise, dysphagia, and throat pain may occur in more severe infections. Laryngeal edema, although rare, may cause dyspnea.

Indirect or direct flexible laryngoscopy, recommended for symptoms persisting > 3 wk, discloses mild to marked erythema of the mucous membrane, which may also be edematous. If a pseudomembrane is present, diphtheria is suspected.

Treatment

No specific treatment is available for viral laryngitis. Cough suppressants, voice rest, and steam inhalations relieve symptoms and promote resolution of acute laryngitis. Smoking cessation and treatment of acute or chronic bronchitis may relieve laryngitis. Depending on the presumed cause, specific treatments to control gastroesophageal reflux, bulimia, or drug-induced laryngitis may be beneficial.

LARYNGOCELES

Laryngoceles are evaginations of the mucous membrane of the laryngeal ventricle.

Internal laryngoceles displace and enlarge the false vocal cords, resulting in hoarseness and airway obstruction. External laryngoceles extend through the thyrohyoid membrane, producing a mass in the neck. Laryngoceles tend to occur in musicians who play wind instruments. Laryngoceles are filled with air and can be expanded by the Valsalva maneuver. They appear on CT as smooth, ovoid, low-density masses. Laryngoceles may become infected (laryngopyocele) or filled with mucoid fluid. Treatment is excision.

Sidebar 92–1. THE PROFESSIONAL VOICE

People who use their voice professionally for public speaking and singing often experience voice disorders presenting as hoarseness/breathiness, lowered vocal pitch, vocal fatigue, nonproductive cough, persistent throat clearing, and/or throat ache. These symptoms often have benign causes, such as vocal nodules, vocal fold edema, polyps, or granulomas. Such disorders are usually caused by vocal fold hyperfunction (excessive laryngeal muscular tension when speaking) and possibly laryngopharyngeal reflux.

Treatment in most cases includes the following:

- Voice evaluation using a computer-assisted program to assess pitch and intensity and to determine parameters of vocal acoustics
- Behavioral treatment (decreasing musculoskeletal laryngeal tension when speaking) using the same computer program for visual and auditory biofeedback
- A vocal hygiene program to eliminate vocally abusive behaviors, such as excessive loudness, long duration, vocal tension, and habitual throat clearing
- An antireflux regimen, when appropriate
- Adequate hydration to promote an adequate glottal mucosal wave
- Diet modification before vocal performances, which may include avoidance of dairy products, caffeine, and ambient tobacco smoke and other inhaled irritants.

SPASMODIC DYSPHONIA

Spasmodic dysphonia (vocal cord spasms) is intermittent spasm of laryngeal muscles that causes an abnormal voice.

Cause is unknown, but usually spasmodic dysphonia follows a URI, a period of excessive voice use, or occupational or emotional stress. Onset is between ages 30 and 50, and about 60% of patients are women.

In the adductor type of spasmodic dysphonia, patients attempt to speak through the spasmodic closure with a voice that appears squeezed, effortful, or strained. These spasmodic episodes usually occur when vowel sounds are being formed, particularly at the beginning of words. The less common abductor form results in sudden interruptions of sound caused by momentary abduction of the vocal cords accompanied by audible escape of air during connected speech.

Surgery has been more successful than other approaches for adductor spasmodic dysphonia. The use of botulinum toxin injection has restored a normal voice in 70% of patients for up to 3 mo. Because the effect is temporary, injections may be repeated. There is no known temporary alleviation of the abductor form of this disorder.

VOCAL CORD PARALYSIS

Vocal cord paralysis has numerous causes and can affect speaking, breathing, and swallowing. The left vocal cord is affected twice as often as the right and in females more often than males (3:2). Diagnosis is based on direct visualization. An extensive assessment may be necessary to determine the cause. Several direct surgical approaches are available if treating the cause is not curative.

Vocal cord paralysis may result from lesions at the nucleus ambiguus, its supranuclear tracts, the main trunk of the vagus, or the recurrent laryngeal nerves.

Paralysis is usually unilateral. About ⅓ of unilateral vocal cord paralyses are neoplastic in origin, ⅓ are traumatic, and ⅓ are idiopathic. Intracranial tumors, vascular accidents, and demyelinating diseases cause nucleus ambiguus paralysis. Tumors at the base of the skull and trauma to the neck cause vagus paralysis. Recurrent laryngeal nerve paralysis is caused by neck or thoracic lesions (eg, aortic aneurysm; mitral stenosis; mediastinal tuberculous adenitis; tumors of the thyroid gland, esophagus, lung, or mediastinal structures), trauma, thyroidectomy, neurotoxins (eg, lead), neurotoxic infections (eg, diphtheria), cervical spine injury or surgery, Lyme disease, and viral illness. Viral neuronitis probably accounts for most idiopathic cases.

Bilateral vocal cord paralysis is a life-threatening disorder caused by thyroid and cervical surgery, tracheal intubation, trauma, and neurodegenerative and neuromuscular diseases.

Symptoms and Signs

Vocal cord paralysis results in loss of vocal cord abduction and adduction. Paralysis may affect phonation, respiration, and deglutition, and food and fluids may be aspirated into the trachea. The paralyzed cord generally lies 2 to 3 mm lateral to the midline. In recurrent laryngeal nerve paralysis, the cord may move with phonation but not with inspiration. In unilateral paralysis, the voice may be hoarse and breathy, but the airway is usually not obstructed because the normal cord abducts sufficiently. In bilateral paralysis, both cords generally lie within 2 to 3 mm of the midline, and the voice is of good quality but of limited intensity. The airway, however, is inadequate, resulting in stridor and dyspnea with moderate exertion as each cord is drawn to the midline glottis by an inspiratory Bernoulli effect. Aspiration is also a danger.

Diagnosis

Diagnosis is based on laryngoscopy. The cause must always be sought. Evaluation is guided by abnormalities identified on history and physical examination. During the history, the physician asks about all possible causes of peripheral neuropathy, including chronic heavy metal exposure (arsenic, lead, mercury), drug effects from phenytoin and vincristine, and history of connective tissue disorders, Lyme disease, sarcoidosis, diabetes, and alcoholism. Further evaluation may include enhanced CT of the head, neck, and chest; thyroid scan; barium swallow or bronchoscopy, and esophagoscopy. Cricoarytenoid arthritis, which may cause fixation of the cricoarytenoid joint, must be differentiated from a neuromuscular etiology. Fixation is best documented by absence of passive mobility during rigid laryngoscopy under general anesthesia. Cricoarytenoid arthritis may complicate such conditions as RA, external blunt trauma, and prolonged endotracheal intubation.

Treatment

In unilateral paralysis, treatment is directed at improving voice quality through augmentation, medialization, or reinnervation.

Augmentation involves injecting a paste of plasticized particles, collagen, micronized dermis, or autologous fat into the paralyzed cord, bringing the cords closer together to improve the voice and prevent aspiration.

Medialization is shifting the vocal cord toward the midline by inserting an adjustable spacer laterally to the affected cord. This can be performed with a local anesthetic, allowing the position of the spacer to be "tuned" to the patient's voice. Unlike augmentation with plasticized particles, which permanently fixes the cord, the spacer is both adjustable and removable.

Reinnervation has only rarely been successful.

In bilateral paralysis, an adequate airway must be reestablished. Tracheotomy may be needed permanently or temporarily during a URI. An arytenoidectomy with lateralization of the true vocal cord opens the glottis and improves the airway but may adversely affect voice quality. Posterior laser cordectomy opens the posterior glottis and may be preferred to endoscopic or open arytenoidectomy. Successful laser establishment of a posterior glottic airway usually obviates the need for long-term tracheotomy while preserving a serviceable voice quality.

VOCAL CORD POLYPS AND NODULES

Chronic irritation causes changes in the vocal cords that can lead to polyps or nodules. Both produce hoarseness and a breathy voice. Persistence of these symptoms for > 3 wk dictates visualization of the vocal cords. Diagnosis is based on laryngoscopy and on biopsy to rule out cancer. Surgical removal restores the voice, and removal of the irritating source prevents recurrence.

Etiology and Pathophysiology

Polyps and nodules result from injury to the lamina propria of the true vocal cords. Polyps may occur at the mid third of the membranous cords and are more often unilateral. They frequently result from an initiating acute phonatory injury. Nodules usually occur bilaterally at the junction of the anterior and middle third of the cords. Their main cause is chronic voice abuse—yelling, shouting, singing loudly, or using an unnaturally low frequency. Polyps may have several other causes, including gastric reflux, untreated hypothyroid states, chronic laryngeal allergic reactions, or chronic inhalation of irritants, such as industrial fumes or cigarette smoke. Polyps tend to be larger and more protuberant than nodules and often have a dominant surface blood vessel.

Symptoms, Signs, and Diagnosis

Both result in slowly developing hoarseness and a breathy voice. Diagnosis is based on direct or indirect visualization of the larynx with a mirror or laryngoscope. Biopsy of discrete lesions to exclude carcinoma is performed by microlaryngoscopy.

Treatment

Correction of the underlying cause cures most nodules and prevents recurrence. Removal of the offending irritants allows healing, and voice therapy with a speech therapist reduces the trauma to the vocal cords from improper singing or protracted loud speaking. Nodules usually regress with voice therapy alone.

Most polyps must be surgically removed to restore a normal voice. Cold-knife microsurgical excision during direct microlaryngoscopy is preferable to laser excision, which is more likely to cause collateral thermal injury if improperly applied.

In microlaryngoscopy, an operating microscope is used to examine, biopsy, and operate on the larynx. Images can be recorded on video as well. The patient is anesthetized, and the airway is secured by high-pressure jet ventilation through the laryngoscope, endotracheal intubation, or, for an inadequate upper airway, tracheotomy. Because the microscope allows observation with magnification, tissue can be removed precisely and accurately, minimizing damage (possibly permanent) to the vocal mechanism. Laser surgery can be performed through the optical system of the microscope to allow for precise cuts. Microlaryngoscopy is preferred for almost all laryngeal biopsies, for procedures involving benign tumors, and for many forms of phonosurgery.

93 TUMORS OF THE HEAD AND NECK

The most common noncutaneous tumor of the head and neck is squamous cell carcinoma of the larynx, followed by squamous cell carcinomas of the palatine tonsil, tongue, and floor of the mouth. Somewhat less common are tumors of the salivary gland, jaw, nose and paranasal sinuses, and ear. Tumors of the thyroid gland, eye, and skin are discussed elsewhere in THE MANUAL.

Excluding the skin and thyroid gland, > 90% of head and neck cancers are squamous cell (epidermoid) carcinomas, and 5% are melanomas, lymphomas, and sarcomas. Patients with sarcomas or carcinomas of the salivary glands, thyroid, or paranasal sinuses are usually < 59 yr, and patients with squamous cell carcinoma are generally > 59 yr.

Etiology

About 85% of patients with cancer of the head and neck have a history of alcohol use, smoking, or both. Other suspected causes include use of snuff or chewing tobacco, ill-fitting dental appliances, chronic candidiasis, and poor oral hygiene. In India, oral cancer is extremely common, probably because of chewing betel quid (a mixture of substances, also called paan).

Long-term exposure to sunlight and the use of tobacco products are the primary causes of squamous cell carcinoma of the lower lip.

The Epstein-Barr virus plays a role in the pathogenesis of nasopharyngeal cancer. Patients who in the past were treated with radiation for acne, excess facial hair, enlarged thymus, or hypertrophic tonsils and adenoids are predisposed to thyroid and salivary gland cancers and benign salivary tumors.

Symptoms, Signs, and Diagnosis

Most head and neck cancers first manifest as an asymptomatic lump, ulceration, or visible mucosal lesion (eg, leukoplakia, erythroplakia). Subsequent symptoms depend on location and extent of the tumor and include pain, paresthesia, nerve palsies, trismus, and halitosis.

Definitive diagnosis usually requires a combination of imaging tests, endoscopy, and fine-needle aspiration, supplemented by excisional biopsy (see Neck Mass on p. 813). Routine physical examination (including a thorough oral examination) is the best way to detect cancers early.

Staging

Head and neck cancers may remain localized for months to years. Local tissue invasion is eventually followed by metastasis to regional lymph nodes. Distant lymphatic metastases tend to occur late. Hematogenous metastases are usually associated with large or persistent tumors and occur more commonly in immunocompromised patients. Common sites of distant metastases are the lungs, liver, bone, and brain.

Head and neck cancers are staged (see TABLE 93–1) according to size and site of the

TABLE 93–1. STAGING OF HEAD AND NECK CANCER

STAGE	TUMOR (MAXIMUM PENETRATION)	REGIONAL LYMPH NODE METASTASIS	DISTANT METASTASIS
I	T1	N0	M0
II	T2	N0	M0
III	T3 or	N0	M0
	T1-3	N1	M0
IV	T4	Any N	M0
	Any T	Any N	M1

TNM classification: T1 ≤ 2 cm in greatest dimension; T2 = 2–4 cm or affects 2 areas within a specific site; T3 > 4 cm or affects 3 areas within a specific site; T4 = invades specific structures.
N0 = none; N1 = one node ≤ 3 cm; N2 = node between 3 and 6 cm; N3 = node > 6 cm.
M0 = none; M1 = present.

primary tumor (T), number and size of metastases to the cervical lymph nodes (N), and evidence of distant metastases (M). Staging usually requires imaging with CT, MRI, or both.

Prognosis and Treatment

Prognosis is favorable if diagnosis is early and treatment is timely and appropriate. Exophytic or verrucous tumors generally respond better than do invasive, infiltrative, or ulcerative tumors. In general, the more poorly differentiated the cancer, the greater the chance of regional and distant metastases. With invasion of muscle, bone, or cartilage, cure rates are significantly decreased. Perineural spread, as evidenced by pain, paralysis, or numbness, indicates a highly aggressive tumor that is unlikely to be cured. Cervical or distant metastasis greatly reduces survival rate.

With appropriate treatment, 5-yr survival approaches 90% for stage I, 75% for stage II, 45 to 75% for stage III, and < 35% for stage IV. Patients > 70 yr often have longer disease-free intervals and better survival rates.

Many stage I tumors, regardless of location, respond similarly to surgery and to radiation therapy; other factors determine the choice of therapy. If radiation therapy is chosen for primary therapy, it is delivered to the primary site and sometimes bilaterally to the cervical lymph nodes. In some cases, surgical procedures are needed to achieve the expected 90% cure rate.

Tumors > 2 cm or with bone or cartilage invasion (with or without regional neck metastasis) require surgical resection of the primary site and usually regional lymph nodes. If lymph node metastases are found or deemed very likely to be present (estimated by physical examination, imaging tests, fine-needle aspiration, and biopsy), then postoperative radiation to the primary site and cervical lymph nodes bilaterally is generally recommended. For patients who are not surgical candidates, radiation therapy—with or without chemotherapy—may be chosen.

In advanced (most stage II and all stage III and IV) squamous cell carcinoma, a combination of surgery and radiation therapy offers a better chance of cure. Surgery is more effective in controlling the gross tumor, whereas radiation is more effective in controlling inapparent tumor at the periphery of the primary lesion and microscopic or non-palpable metastases. Postoperative radiation is usually preferred over preoperative radiation, because radiated tissues heal poorly.

Primary chemotherapy is reserved for chemosensitive tumors, such as Burkitt's lymphoma, or for patients who have widespread metastases (eg, hepatic or pulmonary involvement). Whether chemotherapy combined with surgery or radiation therapy increases the cure rate is not known, but combined therapy prolongs the cancer-free interval. Several drugs—cisplatin, fluorouracil, bleomycin, and methotrexate—provide palliation for pain and shrink the tumor in patients who cannot be treated with surgery or radiation therapy.

Adverse effects of treatment: Surgery requires rehabilitation for swallowing and speaking. Reconstruction procedures, including grafts, regional pedicle flaps, and complex free flaps, are used to restore function and appearance.

Toxic effects of chemotherapy include malaise, severe nausea and vomiting, mucositis, transient hair loss, gastroenteritis, hematopoietic and immune suppression, and infection.

Therapeutic radiation for head and neck cancers has several undesirable adverse effects. The function of any salivary gland within the beam is permanently destroyed by a dose of about 40 Gy, resulting in xerostomia, which markedly increases the risk of dental caries. The blood supply of bone, particularly in the mandible, is compromised by doses of > 60 Gy, and osteoradionecrosis may occur (see also p. 849). In this condition, tooth extraction sites break down, sloughing bone and soft tissue. Therefore, any needed dental treatment, including scaling, fillings, and extractions, should be done before receiving radiation. Any teeth in poor condition that cannot be rehabilitated should be extracted. Radiation therapy may also cause oral mucositis and dermatitis in the overlying skin, which may result in dermal fibrosis. Loss of taste (ageusia) and impaired smell (dysosmia) may occur.

A palpable mass or ulcerated lesion with edema or pain at the primary site after therapy strongly suggests a persistent tumor. Such patients require CT (with thin cuts) or MRI.

For local recurrence after surgical treatment, all scar planes and reconstructive flaps are excised along with residual cancer. Radiation, chemotherapy, or both may be given but have limited effectiveness.

Patients with recurrence after radiation therapy should not receive additional radiation and are best treated with surgery.

Palliative surgery or radiation may temporarily alleviate pain, and in 30 to 50% of patients, chemotherapy can produce improvement that lasts a mean of 3 mo. Median survival for recurrent or metastatic disease is 6 mo.

Care of people with incurable head and neck cancers is challenging. Pain, difficulty eating, choking on secretions, and other problems make adequate symptomatic treatment essential. Patient directives regarding such care should be clarified early (see p. 2768).

Prevention

Removing risk factors is critical. All patients should cease tobacco use and limit alcohol consumption. This also helps prevent disease recurrence in those treated for cancer. A new primary cancer develops in 30% of patients who continue to use tobacco and alcohol but in only 13% of those who stop. Cancer of the lower lip may be prevented by sunscreen use and tobacco cessation.

Because 60% of head and neck cancers are well advanced (Stage III or IV) at the time of diagnosis, the most promising strategy for reducing morbidity and mortality is diligent routine examination of the oral cavity.

JAW TUMORS

Numerous tumor types, both benign and malignant, originate in the jaw. Symptoms are swelling, pain, tenderness, and unexplained tooth mobility; some tumors are discovered on routine dental x-rays. Treatment depends on location and tumor type. Benign tumors may not need surgical excision.

Bony outgrowths (torus palatinus, torus mandibularis) may develop on the maxilla and mandible; they are benign and of concern only if they interfere with dental care. Multiple osteomas seen on dental x-ray may suggest Gardner's syndrome.

If not initially detected on x-ray, jaw tumors are diagnosed clinically because their growth causes swelling of the face, palate, or alveolar ridge (the part of the jaw supporting the teeth). They can also cause bone tenderness and severe pain.

Ameloblastoma, the most common epithelial odontogenic tumor, usually arises in the posterior mandible. It is slowly invasive and rarely metastatic. On x-ray, it typically appears as multiloculated or soap-bubble radiolucency. Treatment is wide surgical excision.

Odontoma, the most common odontogenic tumor, affects the dental follicle or the dental tissues and usually appears in the mandibles of young people. Odontomas include fibrous odontomas and cementomas. A clinically absent molar tooth suggests a composite odontoma. Typically, no treatment is indicated. These tumors may be excised when the diagnosis is in doubt.

Osteosarcoma, giant cell tumor, Ewing's tumor, multiple myeloma, and metastatic tumors may affect the jaw. Treatment is the same as for those tumors in other bony sites.

LARYNGEAL CANCER

Ninety percent of laryngeal cancer is squamous cell carcinoma. Smoking, alcohol abuse, and being black, male, and > 60 yr increase risk. Early diagnosis is common because vocal, swallowing, or respiratory symptoms develop early. Diagnosis is based on laryngoscopy and biopsy. Treatment is with surgery and sometimes radiation. Reestablishment of speaking ability is generally needed.

Squamous cell carcinoma is the most common malignancy of the larynx. In the US, it is 4 times more common in men and is more common among blacks than whites. Over 95% of patients are smokers; 15 pack-years of smoking increases the risk 30-fold. Sixty percent of patients present with localized disease alone, 25% with local disease and regional nodal metastatic disease, and 15% with advanced disease, distant metastases, or both. Common sites of origin are the true vocal cords (glottis) particularly the anterior portion, supraglottic larynx (epiglottis), hypopharynx (pyriform sinus), and postcricoid area.

Verrucous carcinoma, a rare variant of squamous cell carcinoma, usually arises in the glottic area.

Symptoms, Signs, and Diagnosis

Carcinoma of the epiglottis or pyriform sinus is often asymptomatic until it presents as a mass. However, these and postcricoid carcinomas may cause pain and dysphagia. Such patients should undergo indirect laryngoscopy without delay.

Cordal or glottic carcinoma produces hoarseness early; all patients with hoarseness lasting > 2 wk should be examined by indirect laryngoscopy. Any lesions should undergo biopsy by direct laryngoscopy.

Patients with carcinoma on biopsy should have further endoscopic evaluation of the upper airway and GI tract for coexisting cancers and a metastatic assessment with CT or MRI of the neck, chest, and abdomen. Distant metastases most frequently occur in the lungs and liver.

Treatment and Prognosis

For early-stage glottic carcinoma, laser excision, radiation therapy, or sometimes cordectomy results in a 5-yr survival rate of 85 to 95%; laser excision and radiation therapy usually preserve a normal voice. For advanced carcinoma with anterior commissure involvement, impaired vocal cord mobility, thyroid cartilage invasion, or subglottic extension, surgery is necessary. A hemilaryngectomy, which preserves laryngeal phonation and sphincteric functions, is often possible with lesions limited to one vocal cord. More advanced carcinoma requires total laryngectomy.

Early supraglottic carcinoma can be effectively treated with radiation therapy. Laser ablation has also shown considerable success on superficial squamous cell carcinomas in the head and neck region. If the carcinoma is more advanced but does not affect the true vocal cords, a supraglottic partial laryngectomy can be performed to preserve the voice and glottic sphincter. If the true vocal cords are also affected, a total laryngectomy is required.

Early hypopharyngeal carcinoma may be managed by an extended partial laryngectomy. More advanced lesions require a total laryngectomy. In advanced supraglottic and hypopharyngeal carcinoma, a combination of radiation therapy and surgery may be more successful than surgery alone because of the possibility of undetected residual tumor.

Postcricoid carcinoma requires total laryngopharyngectomy and replacement of the hypopharynx and cervical esophagus with a free jejunal graft with microvascular anastomoses. For metastasis to the cervical lymph nodes, laryngeal surgery is combined with radical or modified radical neck dissection.

Verrucous carcinoma is treated surgically.

Five-yr survival rates are > 80% for lesions on the true cords but 50% for supraglottic lesions.

Retinoic acid derivatives have been used to prevent development of subsequent cancers.

Rehabilitation: After total laryngectomy, the patient requires creation of a new voice by way of esophageal speech, a tracheoesophageal fistula, or an electrolarynx. In all 3 techniques, sound is articulated into speech by the pharynx, palate, tongue, teeth, and lips.

Esophageal speech involves taking air into the esophagus during inspiration and gradually eructating the air through the pharyngoesophageal junction to produce a sound.

If tracheotomy results in loss of voice, postsurgical management may include the placement of a one-way valve, or tracheoesophageal fistula, to facilitate phonation. This valve forces air into the esophagus during expiration to produce a sound. Patients receive physical rehabilitation, speech therapy, and appropriate training in the maintenance and use of this valve and must be cautioned against the possible aspiration of food, fluids, and secretions.

An electrolarynx is a battery-powered sound source that is held against the neck to produce sound.

NASOPHARYNGEAL CANCER

Nasopharyngeal cancers are rare in the US but common in the South China Sea region. Symptoms develop late, including unilateral bloody nasal discharge, obstruction, facial swelling, and numbness. Diagnosis is based on inspection and biopsy, with MRI to evaluate extent. Treatment is with radiation, chemotherapy, and, rarely, surgery.

Squamous cell carcinoma is the most common malignant tumor of the nose and paranasal sinuses. It occurs in children and young adults. Rare in North America, it is one of the most common cancers among people of Chinese, especially southern Chinese, and Southeast Asian ancestry, including Chinese immigrants to North America. It is slightly less prevalent in 1st-generation Chinese-Americans. Epstein-Barr virus is a significant risk factor, and there is hereditary predisposition.

Other nasopharyngeal cancers include adenoid cystic and mucoepidermoid carcinomas, malignant mixed tumors, adenocarcinomas, lymphomas, fibrosarcomas, osteosarcomas, chondrosarcomas, and melanomas.

Hypernephroma is the most common metastatic tumor in the paranasal sinuses.

Symptoms, Signs, and Diagnosis

The first symptom is often nasal or eustachian tube obstruction causing middle ear effusion. Other symptoms include purulent bloody rhinorrhea, frank epistaxis, cranial nerve paralysis, and cervical lymphadenopathy. Because lymphatics of the nasopharynx communicate across the midline, bilateral metastases are common.

Patients suspected of having nasopharyngeal cancer undergo examination with a nasopharyngeal mirror or endoscope, and lesions are biopsied. Cervical node biopsy should not be performed as the initial procedure (see Neck Mass on p. 813). MRI (gadolinium enhanced, with fat suppression) of the head with attention to the nasopharynx and skull base is obtained—the skull base is involved in about 25%.

Treatment and Prognosis

Because of the location and extent of involvement, nasopharyngeal cancers often are not amenable to surgical resection. They are typically treated with radiation therapy and chemotherapy.

ORAL SQUAMOUS CELL CARCINOMA

Oral squamous cell carcinoma affects about 30,000 Americans each year. Ninety percent are smokers. Alcohol is also a risk factor. Early, curable lesions are rarely symptomatic; thus, preventing fatal disease requires early detection by screening. Treatment is with surgery, radiation, or both. The overall 5-yr survival rate is 52%.

In the US, 3% of cancers in men and 2% in women are oral squamous cell carcinomas, most of which occur after age 50. Oral squamous cell carcinoma is the most common oral or pharyngeal cancer.

The chief risk factors for oral squamous cell carcinoma are smoking (especially > 2 packs/day) and alcohol use. Risk increases dramatically when alcohol use exceeds 6 oz of distilled liquor, 6 oz of wine, or 12 oz of beer/day. The combination of heavy smoking and alcohol abuse is estimated to raise the risk 100-fold in women and 38-fold in men. Squamous cell carcinoma of the tongue may also result from Plummer-Vinson syndrome, syphilis, or chronic trauma.

About 40% of intraoral squamous cell carcinomas begin on the floor of the mouth or on the lateral and ventral surfaces of the tongue. About 38% of all oral squamous cell carcinomas occur on the lower lip, and about 11% begin in the palate and tonsillar area. Squamous cell carcinoma of the tonsil, 2nd in frequency only to carcinoma of the larynx among malignancies of the upper respiratory tract, occurs predominantly in males.

Symptoms, Signs, and Diagnosis

Oral lesions are asymptomatic initially. They may appear in areas of erythroplakia or leukoplakia and may be exophytic or ulcerated. Both variants are indurated and firm with a rolled border. Tonsillar carcinoma usually presents as an asymmetric swelling and sore throat; pain often radiates to the ipsilateral ear. A metastatic mass in the neck may be the first symptom.

Biopsy of suspect areas is obtained, particularly where the lesion is speckled. Direct laryngoscopy, bronchoscopy, and esophagoscopy are performed to exclude a simultaneous 2nd primary cancer. CT of the head and neck is usually performed. Chest x-ray is obtained; chest CT is performed if an advanced stage is suspected or confirmed.

Prognosis

If carcinoma of the tongue is localized (no lymph node involvement), 5-yr survival is about 50%. For localized carcinoma of the floor of the mouth, 5-yr survival is 65%. With lymph node metastasis, the 5-yr survival is 20%. For lower lip lesions, 5-yr survival is 90%, and metastases are rare. Carcinoma of the upper lip tends to be more aggressive and metastatic. For carcinoma of the palate and tonsillar area, 5-yr survival is 68% if patients are treated before lymph node involvement but only 17% after involvement. Metastases reach the regional lymph nodes first and later the lungs.

Treatment

Surgery and radiation therapy are the treatments of choice. Regional or distant disease necessitates a more radical treatment approach.

For tongue lesions, radiation therapy is often the treatment of choice because surgery is extensive, disfiguring, and associated with poor quality of life. In addition, patients with cancer of the floor of the mouth are often medically compromised and are not good candidates for surgery. Rarely, distant metastases are found in sites where chemotherapy may be of some palliative value (eg, lung, bone, heart, pericardium).

Treatment of squamous cell carcinoma of the lip is surgical excision. When large areas of the lip exhibit premalignant change, the lip can be surgically shaved, or a laser can remove all affected mucosa. Thereafter, appropriate sunscreen application is recommended.

Treatment of tonsillar carcinoma combines radiation therapy and surgery, which consists of radical resection of the tonsillar fossa, sometimes with partial mandibulectomy and radical neck dissection.

OTIC TUMORS

A number of malignant and benign otic tumors occur, usually presenting with hearing loss.

Malignant otic tumors: Basal cell and squamous cell carcinomas may arise in the ear canal. Persistent inflammation from chronic otitis media may predispose to the development of squamous cell carcinoma. Extensive resection is indicated, followed by radiation therapy. En bloc resection of the ear canal with sparing of the facial nerve is performed when lesions are limited to the canal and have not invaded the middle ear.

Rarely, squamous cell carcinoma originates in the middle ear. The persistent otorrhea of chronic otitis media may be a predisposing factor. Radiation therapy and resection of the temporal bone are necessary.

Nonchromaffin paragangliomas (chemodectomas) arise in the temporal bone from glomus bodies in the jugular bulb (glomus jugulare tumors) or the medial wall of the middle ear (glomus tympanicum tumors). They produce a pulsatile red mass in the middle ear. The first symptom often is tinnitus that is synchronous with the pulse. Hearing loss develops, followed by vertigo. Excision is the treatment of choice. For tumors too large to excise, radiation therapy is used.

Benign otic tumors: Sebaceous cysts, osteomas, and keloids may arise in and occlude the ear canal, causing retention of cerumen and conductive hearing loss. Excision is the treatment of choice.

Ceruminomas arise in the outer third of the ear canal. These tumors appear benign histologically and do not metastasize regionally or distantly, but they are locally invasive and potentially destructive and should be excised widely.

SALIVARY GLAND TUMORS

Most salivary gland tumors are benign, arising in the parotid glands. A painless salivary mass is evaluated by fine-needle aspiration or biopsy. Imaging with CT and MRI can be helpful. For malignant tumors, treatment with excision and radiation results in 50% cure, even with the highest grade malignancies.

About 85% of salivary gland tumors occur in the parotid glands, occasionally in the submandibular and minor glands, and about 1% in the sublingual glands. About 75 to 80% are benign, slow-growing, movable, painless, usually solitary nodules beneath normal skin or mucosa. Occasionally, when cystic, they are firm.

Benign tumors: The most common type of tumor is a benign pleomorphic adenoma (mixed tumor), occurring primarily in women >40 yr. Malignant transformation is possible, resulting in carcinoma ex mixed tumor. Other benign tumors include monomorphic adenoma, oncocytoma, and papillary cystadenoma lymphomatosum (previously known as cylindroma). These tumors rarely recur and rarely become malignant.

Malignant salivary gland tumors: Malignant tumors are less common and are characterized by rapid growth or a sudden growth spurt. They are firm, nodular, and usually fixed to adjacent tissue, often with a poorly defined periphery. Pain and neural involvement are common. Eventually, the overlying skin or mucosa may become ulcerated.

Mucoepidermoid carcinoma is the most common salivary gland cancer, typically occurring in people in their 20s to 50s. It commonly occurs in a minor salivary gland of the palate. Any unexplained persistent retromolar swelling is considered to be mucoepidermoid carcinoma until proved otherwise by biopsy. It may occur deep within the bone, often in the wall of a dentigerous cyst. All types of mucoepidermoid carcinoma may metastasize.

Adenoid cystic carcinoma is the most common malignant tumor of minor salivary glands (and of the trachea). It is a slowly growing malignant transformation of a much more common benign cylindroma. Its peak incidence is between ages 40 and 60, and symptoms include severe pain and, often, facial nerve paralysis.

Acinic cell carcinoma, a common parotid tumor, occurs in people in their 40s and 50s.

Carcinoma ex mixed tumor is adenocarcinoma arising in a preexisting benign carcinoma ex mixed tumor. Only the carcinomatous element metastasizes.

Symptoms, Signs, and Diagnosis

Most benign and malignant tumors present as a painless mass. However, malignant tumors may invade nerves, causing localized or regional pain, numbness, paresthesia, causalgia, or a loss of motor function. CT and MRI locate the tumor and describe its extent. Biopsy confirms the cell type. A search for spread to regional nodes or distant metastases in the lung, liver, bone, or brain may be indicated before treatment is selected.

Treatment and Prognosis

Treatment of benign tumors is surgery. The recurrence rate is high when excision is incomplete. Treatment of mucoepidermoid carcinoma consists of wide excision and postoperative radiation. The 5-yr survival rate is 95% with the low-grade type, primarily affecting mucus cells, and 50% with the high-grade type, primarily affecting epidermoid cells. Treatment of adenoid cystic carcinoma is wide surgical excision, but local recurrence is common. Lung metastases and death are likely. The prognosis for acinic cell carcinoma is favorable after wide excision.

94 APPROACH TO THE DENTAL PATIENT

A physician should always examine the mouth and be able to recognize oral pathology. However, consultation with a dentist is needed for patients with tooth problems and for those with xerostomia (see p. 818) or unexplained swelling or pain in the mouth, face, or neck. Children with abnormal facies (who may also have dental malformations requiring correction) should also be evaluated by a dentist. In FUO or a systemic infection of unknown cause, a dental disorder should be considered. A dental consultation is necessary before head and neck radiation therapy and is advisable before chemotherapy.

A dentist should consult a physician when a systemic disorder is suspected, when the patient is taking certain drugs (eg, warfarin), and when a patient's ability to withstand general anesthesia or extensive oral surgery must be evaluated. Patients with heart valve abnormalities typically require antibiotic prophylaxis before undergoing certain dental procedures.

Common dental disorders are discussed in Ch. 95 on p. 851. Dental emergencies, including toothache, are discussed in Ch. 96 on p. 858.

Anatomy and Development

Teeth: The teeth are categorized as incisors, canines, premolars, and molars and conventionally are numbered beginning with the maxillary right 3rd molar (see FIG. 94–1).

Each tooth has a crown and a root. The canines have the largest and strongest roots. An inner pulp contains blood vessels, lymphatics, and nerves, surrounded by the hard but porous dentin, a very hard enamel coating above the root, and the bonelike cementum over the root, which is usually covered by gingiva (see FIG. 94–2). Twenty deciduous teeth normally begin appearing at close to age 6 mo and should all be in place by age 30 mo (see TABLE 269–1 on p. 2249). These teeth are followed by 32 permanent teeth that begin to appear by about age 6. The period from age 6 to 11 is called the mixed dentition stage, in which both deciduous and permanent teeth are present. Timing of tooth eruption is one indicator of skeletal age and may identify growth retardation or establish age for forensic purposes.

Supporting tissues: The gingiva surrounds the teeth at the base of their crowns. The alveolar ridges are trabecular bone containing sockets for the teeth. The periodontium consists of the tissues that support the

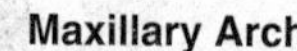

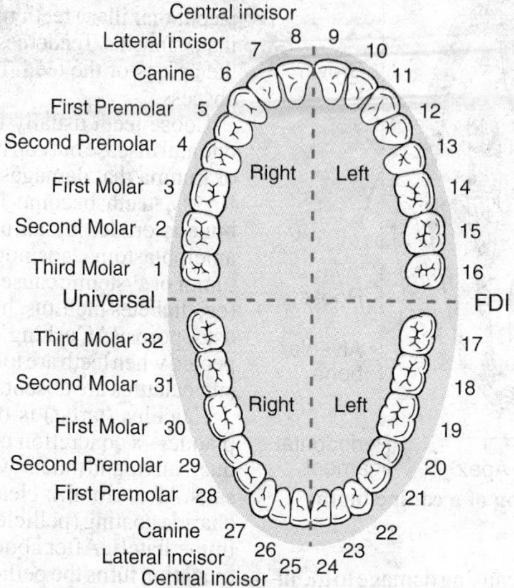

Fig. 94–1. Identifying the teeth. The numbering system shown is the one most commonly used in the US.

teeth—the gingiva, epithelial attachment, connective tissue attachment, periodontal ligament, and alveolar bone. The mandible and maxilla support the alveolar ridges and house the teeth. Saliva from the salivary glands bathes and protects the teeth. The tongue directs food between the grinding surfaces and helps clean the teeth. The maxilla receives innervation from the maxillary nerve, the 2nd division of the trigeminal nerve (the 5th cranial nerve). The mandibular nerve, which is the 3rd and most inferior division of the trigeminal nerve, innervates the mandible.

In the elderly, or in the case of some periodontal diseases, gingival recession exposes the dental root adjacent to the crown, making root caries common. If tooth destruction results, the mechanical stimulation necessary for maintaining bone integrity ceases. Consequently, atrophy of the alveolar ridge (senile atrophy) begins as soon as teeth are lost.

Evaluation

The first routine dental examination should take place by age 1 yr or when the first tooth erupts. Subsequent evaluations should take place at 6-mo intervals or whenever symptoms develop.

History: Important dental symptoms include bleeding, pain, malocclusion, new growths, and chewing problems.

Bleeding or pain with brushing usually suggests localized periodontal problems, such as gingivitis or, rarely, acute necrotizing ulcerative gingivitis. However, easily induced gingival hemorrhaging may also indicate a bleeding diathesis or leukemia.

Face, head, or neck pain can indicate infection, malocclusion, poorly fitting dental appliances, temporomandibular disorders, Eagle's syndrome (elongation of the styloid process or ossification of the stylohyoid ligament causing pain when the head is turned), spasm of the masticatory muscles (see Myofascial Pain Syndrome on p. 865), or occult lesions with low-grade anaerobic infections spreading to the bone. Pain referred to the ear may arise from an inflamed gingival flap around a partly erupted mandibular 3rd molar (pericoronitis) or from a localized osteitis (dry socket) after a lower molar is extracted.

Facial numbness or paresthesias may be due to a tumor of the antrum or nasopharynx, stroke, tumors involving the brain stem, viral infection, or multiple sclerosis. Paresthesia of the lower lip may result from extraction of

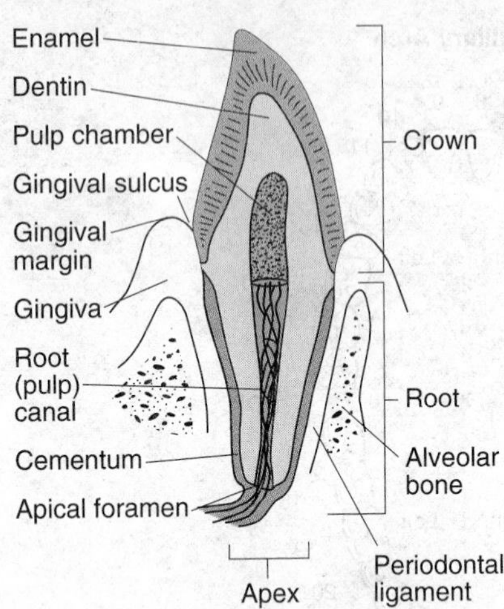

Fig. 94–2. Section of a canine tooth.

a mandibular molar causing damage to the inferior alveolar nerve. Rarely, it indicates an oral tumor.

Masticatory fatigue may be caused by a congenital muscular or neuromuscular disorder in younger people or by poorly occluding artificial dentures in older people. It is a cardinal symptom of myasthenia gravis. Pain with mastication (jaw claudication) may indicate polymyalgia rheumatica or giant cell (temporal) arteritis.

Weight loss can result from an oral or dental problem. For example, a person may be unable to chew food well because of too loose, too few, or painful teeth; poorly fitting dental appliances; stomatitis; or a temporomandibular disorder.

Physical examination: Inspection of soft tissues in the mouth (see p. 808), including gingiva and mucous membranes, may reveal inflammation, exudates, vesicles, tumors, ulcers, or red or white patches as evidence of local or systemic disease.

Teeth are inspected for shape, alignment, defects, mobility, color, and presence of adherent plaque, materia alba (dead bacteria, food debris, desquamated epithelial cells), and calculus. They are gently tapped with a tongue depressor or mirror handle to assess tenderness (percussion sensitivity).

Tenderness to percussion suggests deep caries that has caused a necrotic pulp with periapical abscess or severe periodontal disease. Percussion sensitivity or pain on biting can also indicate an incomplete fracture of a tooth. Percussion tenderness in multiple adjacent maxillary teeth may result from maxillary sinusitis. Tenderness to palpation around the apices of the teeth may also indicate an abscess.

Loose teeth usually indicate severe periodontal disease but can be caused by bruxism or trauma that damages periodontal tissues. Rarely, teeth become loose when alveolar bone is eroded by an underlying mass (eg, ameloblastoma, eosinophilic granuloma). A tumor or systemic cause of alveolar bone loss (eg, diabetes mellitus, hyperparathyroidism, osteoporosis, Cushing's syndrome) is suspected when teeth are loose and heavy plaque and calculus are absent.

Calculus (tartar) is mineralized bacterial plaque—a concretion of bacteria, food residue, saliva, and mucus with Ca and phosphate salts. After a tooth is cleaned, a mucopolysaccharide coating (pellicle) is deposited almost immediately. After about 24 h, bacterial colonization turns the pellicle into plaque. After about 72 h, the plaque calcifies, becoming calculus. When present, calculus is deposited most heavily on the lingual (inner, or tongue) surfaces of the mandibular anterior teeth near the submandibular and sublingual duct orifices (Wharton's ducts) and on the buccal (cheek) surfaces of the maxillary molars near the parotid duct orifices (Stensen's ducts).

Caries (tooth decay—see p. 851) appears as defects in the tooth enamel. Caries first appears as white spots, later becoming brown.

Attrition (wearing of biting surfaces) can result from chewing abrasive foods or tobacco or from the wear that accompanies aging, but it usually indicates bruxism (clenching or grinding of teeth—see p. 849). Another common cause is abrasion of a porcelain crown against adjacent enamel. Attrition makes chewing less effective and causes noncarious teeth to become painful when the eroding enamel exposes the underlying dentin. Dentin is sensitive to touch and to temperature changes. A dentist can desensitize such teeth or restore the dental anatomy by placing crowns or onlays over badly worn teeth.

Deformed teeth may indicate a developmental or endocrine disorder. In Down syndrome, teeth are small. In congenital syphilis, the incisors may be small at the incisal third, producing a pegged or screwdriver shape with a notch in the center of the incisal edge (Hutchinson's incisors), and the 1st molar is small, with a small occlusal surface and roughened, lobulated, often hypoplastic enamel (mulberry molar). In ectodermal dysplasia, teeth are absent or conical, so that dentures are needed from childhood. Dentinogenesis imperfecta, an autosomal dominant disorder, produces abnormal dentin that is dull bluish brown and opalescent and does not cushion the overlying enamel adequately. Such teeth cannot withstand occlusal stresses and rapidly become worn. People with pituitary dwarfism or with congenital hypoparathyroidism have small dental roots; people with gigantism have large ones. Acromegaly produces excess cementum in the roots as well as enlargement of the jaws, so teeth may become widely spaced. Congenitally narrow lateral incisors occur in the absence of systemic disease. The most commonly congenitally absent teeth are the 3rd molars, followed in frequency by the maxillary lateral incisors and 2nd mandibular premolars.

Defects in tooth color must be differentiated from the darkening or yellowing that occurs from food pigments, with aging, and, most prominently, with smoking. A tooth may appear gray because of pulpal necrosis, usually due to extensive caries penetrating the pulp or because of hemosiderin deposited in the dentin after trauma, with or without pulpal necrosis. Children's teeth darken appreciably and permanently after even short-term use of tetracyclines by the mother during the 2nd half of pregnancy or by the child during odontogenesis (tooth development), specifically calcification of the crowns, which lasts until age 9. Tetracyclines rarely cause permanent discoloration of fully formed teeth in adults. However, minocycline darkens bone, which can be seen in the mouth when the overlying gingiva and mucosa are thin. Affected teeth fluoresce with distinctive colors under ultraviolet light corresponding to the specific tetracycline taken. In congenital porphyria, both the deciduous and permanent teeth may have red or brownish discoloration but always fluoresce red from the pigment deposited in the dentin. Congenital hyperbilirubinemia causes a yellowish tooth discoloration. Teeth can be whitened (see TABLE 94–1).

Defects in tooth enamel may be caused by rickets, which results in a rough, irregular band in the enamel. Any prolonged febrile illness during odontogenesis can produce a permanent narrow zone of chalky, pitted enamel or simply white discoloration visible after the tooth erupts. Thus, the age at which the disease occurred and its duration can be estimated from the location and height of the band. Amelogenesis imperfecta, an autosomal dominant disease, causes severe enamel hypoplasia. Chronic vomiting and esophageal

TABLE 94–1. TOOTH WHITENING PROCEDURES

WHO PERFORMED BY	INGREDIENTS	COMMENTS
Dentist		
In office	Concentrated hydrogen peroxide is applied to teeth, to which a light or laser is applied	Very effective. Gingiva, skin, and eyes must be protected
At home	Custom-made trays are used, to which the patient adds 6% carbamide peroxide (becomes 3% hydrogen peroxide when applied) and a thickening agent containing copolymers of acrylic acid cross-linked with a polyalkenyl polyether	Very effective
Patient (OTC products)		
Commercial whitening strips	Composed of carbamide peroxide	Very effective
Whitening toothpaste	Usually contain carbamide or hydrogen peroxide	Moderately effective
Paint-on whitening	Usually composed of titanium dioxide	Not very effective

reflux decalcify the dental crowns, primarily the lingual surfaces of the maxillary anterior teeth. Chronic snorting of cocaine can result in widespread decalcification of teeth, because the drug dissociates in saliva into a base and hydrochloride.

Swimmers who spend a lot of time in overchlorinated pools lose considerable amounts of enamel from the outer facial (buccal) sides of the teeth, especially the maxillary incisors, canines, and 1st premolars. If Na carbonate has been added to the pool water to correct pH, then brown calculus deposits form but can be removed by dental cleanings.

Fluorosis is mottled enamel that may develop in children who drink water containing > 1 ppm of fluoride during tooth development. Fluorosis depends on the amount of fluoride ingested. Enamel changes range from irregular whitish opaque areas to severe brown discoloration of the entire crown with a roughened surface. Such teeth are highly resistant to dental caries.

Testing: For a new patient or for someone who requires extensive care, a full mouth x-ray series is taken. This series consists of 14 to 16 periapical films to show the roots and bone plus 4 to 7 bite-wing films to check for caries between teeth. Modern techniques reduce radiation exposure to a near-negligible level. Patients at high risk of caries (ie, those who have had caries detected during the clinical examination, have many restorations, or have recurrent caries on teeth previously restored) should undergo bite-wing x-rays q 12 to 18 mo. Otherwise, bite-wings are indicated q 2 to 3 yr. A panoramic x-ray can yield useful information about tooth development, cysts or tumors of the jaws, supernumerary or congenitally absent teeth, 3rd molar impaction, Eagle's syndrome (less frequently), and, incidentally, carotid plaques.

Dental Care of Patients With Systemic Disorders

Certain medical conditions (and their treatment) predispose patients to dental problems or affect dental care.

Hematologic disorders: People who have disorders that interfere with coagulation (eg, hemophilia, acute leukemia, thrombocytopenia) require medical consultation before undergoing dental procedures that might cause bleeding (eg, extraction, mandibular block). Hemophiliacs should have clotting factors administered before, during, and after an extraction. Such oral surgery should be performed in the hospital in consultation with a hematologist. All patients with bleeding disorders should maintain a lifelong routine of regular dental visits, which includes cleanings, fillings, topical fluoride, and preventative sealants, to avoid extractions.

Cardiovascular disorders: After an MI, dental procedures should be avoided for 6 mo, if possible. Patients with pulmonary or cardiac disease who require inhalation anesthesia for dental procedures should be hospitalized.

Endocarditis prophylaxis is required for dental procedures in patients with congenital defects of the heart or great vessels, valvular disease (including mitral valve prolapse), hypertrophic cardiomyopathy, or a prosthetic cardiac valve. The heart is better protected against low-grade bacteremias, which occur in chronic dental conditions, when dental treatment is received (with prophylaxis) than when it is not received. Although probably of marginal benefit, antibiotic prophylaxis is sometimes recommended for patients with hemodialysis shunts and within 2 yr of receipt of a major prosthetic joint (hip, knee, shoulder, elbow).

Epinephrine and levonordefrin are added to local anesthetics to increase the duration of anesthesia. In some cardiovascular patients, these drugs cause arrhythmias, myocardial ischemia, or hypertension. Plain anesthetic is used for procedures lasting < 60 min, but in longer procedures or where hemostasis is needed, up to 0.04 mg epinephrine (2 dental cartridges with 1:100,000 epinephrine) is considered safe. Generally, no healthy patient should receive > 0.2 mg epinephrine at any one appointment. Absolute contraindications to epinephrine (any dose) are uncontrolled hyperthyroidism, pheochromocytoma, blood pressure > 200 systolic or > 115 diastolic, uncontrolled arrhythmias despite drug therapy, and unstable angina, MI, or stroke within 6 mo.

Some electrical dental equipment, such as an electrosurgical cautery, a pulp tester, or an ultrasonic scaler, can interfere with early-generation pacemakers.

Cancer: Extracting a tooth adjacent to a carcinoma of the gingiva, palate, or antrum facilitates invasion of the alveolus (tooth socket) by the tumor. Therefore, a tooth should be extracted only during the course of definitive treatment. In patients with leukemia or agranulocytosis, infection may follow an extraction despite the use of antibiotics.

Immunosuppression: People with impaired immunity are prone to severe mucosal and periodontal infections by fungi, herpes and other viruses, and, less commonly, bacteria. The infections may produce hemorrhage, delayed healing, or sepsis. Dysplastic or neoplastic oral lesions may develop after a few years of immunosuppression. People with AIDS may develop Kaposi's sarcoma, non-Hodgkin lymphoma, hairy leukoplakia, candidiasis, aphthous ulcers, or a rapidly progressive form of periodontal disease.

Endocrine disorders: Dental treatment may be complicated by the presence of some endocrine disorders. For example, people with hyperthyroidism may develop tachycardia and excessive anxiety as well as thyroid storm if given epinephrine. Insulin requirements may be reduced upon elimination of oral infection in diabetics; insulin dose may require reduction when food intake is limited because of pain after oral surgery. In people with diabetes, hyperglycemia with resultant polyuria may lead to dehydration, resulting in decreased salivary flow (xerostomia), which, along with elevated salivary glucose levels, contributes to caries.

Patients receiving corticosteroids and those with adrenocortical insufficiency may require supplemental corticosteroids during major dental procedures. Patients with Cushing's syndrome or who are taking corticosteroids may have alveolar bone loss, delayed wound healing, and increased capillary fragility.

Neurologic disorders: Patients with seizures who require dental appliances should have nonremovable appliances that cannot be swallowed or aspirated. Patients unable to brush or floss effectively may use chlorhexidine rinses in the morning and at bedtime.

Drugs: Certain drugs, such as corticosteroids, immunosuppressants, and antineoplastics, compromise healing and host defenses. When possible, dental procedures should not be performed while these drugs are being given.

Some antineoplastics (eg, doxorubicin, 5-fluorouracil, bleomycin, dactinomycin, cytosine, arabinoside, methotrexate) cause stomatitis, which is worse in patients with preexisting periodontal disease. Before such drugs are prescribed, oral prophylaxis should be completed, and patients should be instructed in proper tooth brushing and flossing.

Drugs that interfere with clotting may need to be reduced or stopped before surgery. Patients taking aspirin, NSAIDs, or clopidogrel should stop doing so 4 days before undergoing dental surgery and can resume taking these drugs the day after bleeding stops. Warfarin should be stopped 2 to 3 days before oral surgery. PT is obtained; INR of 1.5 is considered safe for surgery. For people receiving hemodialysis, dental procedures should be performed the day after dialysis, when heparinization has subsided.

Radiation therapy: CAUTION: *Extraction of teeth from irradiated tissues (particularly if the total dose was > 65 Gy, especially in the mandible) is commonly followed by osteoradionecrosis of the jaw. This is a catastrophic complication in which extraction sites break down, frequently sloughing bone and soft tissue.* Thus, if possible, patients should have any necessary dental treatment completed before undergoing radiation therapy of the head and neck region, with time allowed for healing. Teeth that may not survive should be extracted. Necessary sealants and topical fluoride should be applied. After radiation, extraction should be avoided, if possible, with the use of dental restorations and root canal treatment.

Head and neck radiation often damages salivary glands, causing xerostomia, which promotes caries. Patients must therefore practice lifelong good oral hygiene. A fluoride gel and fluoride mouth rinse should be used daily. Rinsing with 0.12% chlorhexidine for 30 to 60 sec, if tolerated, can be done in the morning and at bedtime. Viscous lidocaine may enable a patient with sensitive oral tissues to brush and floss the teeth and eat. A dentist must be seen at 3-, 4-, or 6-mo intervals, depending on findings at the last examination. Irradiated tissue under dentures is likely to break down, so dentures should be checked and adjusted whenever discomfort is noted. Irradiated patients may develop oral mucosal inflammation and diminished taste as well as trismus due to fibrosis of the masticatory muscles. Trismus may be minimized by such exercises as opening and closing the mouth widely 20 times 3 or 4 times/day. If extraction is required after radiation, 10 to 20 treatments in a hyperbaric oxygen chamber may forestall or prevent osteoradionecrosis.

BRUXISM

Bruxism is clenching or grinding of teeth. Bruxism can abrade and eventually wear down dental crowns, loosen teeth, and cause headaches. Most grinding and clenching occurs during sleep, so the patient may be oblivious to it, but family members may notice.

Treatment requires that the patient consciously try to reduce bruxism while awake. Plastic mouthpieces (night guards) that prevent occlusal contact by fitting between the teeth can be used at night and during the day if needed. Such devices, including a heat-moldable type, are available OTC and in some sporting goods stores. Mild anxiolytics, particularly benzodiazepines, may help but should not be used for extended periods.

MALOCCLUSION

Malocclusion is abnormal contact between the maxillary and mandibular teeth.

Normally, each dental arch consists of teeth in side-by-side contact, forming a smooth curve, with the maxillary anterior teeth overlying the upper third of the mandibular anterior teeth. The buccal (outer) cusps of the maxillary posterior teeth are external to the corresponding cusps of the mandibular posterior teeth. On each side of the mouth, the anterior buccal cusp of the maxillary 1st permanent molar fits into the anterior buccal groove of the mandibular 1st molar. Because the outer parts of all maxillary teeth are normally external to the mandibular teeth, the lips and cheeks are displaced from between the teeth so that they are not bitten. The lingual (inner) surfaces of the lower teeth form a smaller arc than those of the upper teeth, confining the tongue and minimizing the likelihood of its being bitten. All the maxillary teeth should contact the corresponding mandibular teeth, so that the masticatory forces (which may be > 150 lb in the molar region and 250 lb when clenched during sleep) are widely distributed. If these forces are applied to only a few teeth, those teeth will eventually loosen.

Etiology

Malocclusion often results from jaw and tooth size discrepancies (ie, the jaw is too small or the teeth are too large for the jaw to accommodate them in proper alignment) but may be caused by a number of congenital deformities and disorders or by tooth loss. When permanent teeth are lost, adjacent teeth shift and opposing teeth extrude, causing malocclusion unless a bridge, implant, or partial denture is worn to prevent these movements. When children lose deciduous teeth prematurely, the teeth more posterior in the arch or the permanent 1st molars often drift forward, leaving insufficient space for other permanent teeth to erupt. In cleidocranial dysostosis, deciduous teeth are retained too long, and many permanent teeth fail to erupt. Malocclusion after facial trauma may indicate tooth displacement or jaw fracture. In ectodermal dysplasia, malocclusion results from having too few teeth.

Evaluation

Occlusion is checked on both sides of the mouth by retracting each cheek with a tongue depressor while telling the patient to close on the back teeth. Malocclusion sometimes is identified as early as the first dental visit. Early identification may make later treatment easier and more effective.

Treatment

Malocclusions are corrected primarily for aesthetic and psychologic reasons. However, in some cases, treatment may increase resistance to caries (in specific teeth), to anterior tooth fracture, and, possibly, to periodontal disease or stripping of the gingiva on the palate. Treatment may improve speech and mastication as well. Occlusion can be improved by aligning teeth properly, by selectively grinding teeth and restorations that contact prematurely, and by inserting crowns or onlays to build up tooth surfaces that are below the plane of occlusion.

Orthodontic appliances (braces) apply a continuous mild force to teeth to gradually remodel the surrounding alveolar bone. Extraction of one or more permanent teeth (usually a 1st premolar) may be needed to allow other teeth to be repositioned or to erupt into a stable alignment. After the teeth are properly aligned, the patient wears a plastic-and-wire retainer 24 h/day initially, then only at night for 2 to 3 yr.

When orthodontic treatment alone is insufficient, surgical correction of jaw abnormalities contributing to malocclusion (orthognathic surgery) may be indicated.

DENTAL APPLIANCES

Teeth may be lost to trauma or be removed when treatment fails. Missing teeth cause cosmetic, phonation, and occlusion problems and may allow movement of remaining teeth.

Dental appliances include fixed bridges, removable partial or complete dentures, and bone-integrated implants.

A **bridge** (fixed partial denture) is composed of false teeth cast or soldered to each other and, at each end, to a crown that is cemented to adjacent natural (abutment) teeth, which bear all stress of biting. A bridge is not removed. A bridge is smaller than a removable partial denture, but one or multiple bridges can be made to replace many of the teeth in a dental arch.

A removable **partial denture,** typically an appliance with clasps that snap over abutment teeth, may be removed for cleaning and during sleep. Part of the occlusal stress may be borne by the soft tissues under the denture, often on both sides of the jaw. This appliance is usually used when many teeth have to be replaced and bridges are not feasible or affordable.

Complete dentures are removable appliances used when no teeth remain. They help a patient chew and improve speech and appearance but do not provide the efficiency or sensation of natural dentition. When teeth are absent, the mandible resorbs, causing ill-fitting dentures that require revision (called reline or rebase) or replacement. Alternatives are oral surgical procedures to enlarge the alveolar ridge or dental implants to replace missing teeth.

An **implant** is typically a titanium shaft that replaces a tooth root. One or more implants are placed into the alveolar bone, where they ankylose. After 4 to 6 mo, artificial teeth are attached to the implants. Implants are not readily removable, although the prostheses they support can be. The potential for infection at these sites warrants scrupulous attention to oral hygiene.

Dental appliances and surgery: Generally, all removable dental appliances are removed before general anesthesia, throat surgery, or convulsive therapy to prevent their breakage or aspiration. They are stored in water to prevent changes in shape. However, some anesthesiologists believe that leaving appliances in place aids the passage of an airway tube, keeps the face in a more normal shape so that the anesthetic mask fits better, prevents natural teeth from injuring the opposing gingiva of a completely edentulous jaw, and does not interfere with laryngoscopy.

Denture problems: Occasionally, the mucosa beneath a denture becomes inflamed (denture sore mouth, inflammatory papillary hyperplasia). Contributing factors to this usually painless condition include candidal infections, poor denture fit, poor hygiene, excessive movement of the denture, and, most frequently, wearing a denture 24 h/day. The mucosa appears red and velvety. Candidal overgrowth may be indicated by adherent cottonlike patches or, more commonly, erosive lesions on the mucosa. The presence of *Candida* can be confirmed by the microscopic appearance of typical branching hyphae. Without *Candida,* inflammatory papillary hyperplasia is unlikely.

A new well-made denture almost always improves the situation. Other treatments consist of improving oral and denture hygiene, refitting the existing denture, removing the denture for extended periods, and using antifungal therapy (nystatin rinses for the mouth and overnight nystatin soaks for the denture). Soaking the denture in a commercial cleanser is sometimes helpful. Other options are applying nystatin suspension to the tissue surface of the denture and clotrimazole troches 10 mg 5 times/day. Ketoconazole 200 mg po once/day may be required. If inflammation persists, biopsy is indicated, and systemic conditions should be ruled out.

95 COMMON DENTAL DISORDERS

Common dental disorders include caries, gingivitis, peridontitis, and pulpitis. Dental emergencies, such as toothache, fractured or avulsed teeth, and postextraction problems, are discussed in Ch. 96 on p. 858.

CARIES

Caries is tooth decay, commonly called cavities. The symptoms—tender, painful teeth—appear late. Diagnosis is based on inspection, probing of the enamel surface with a fine metal instrument, and dental x-rays. Treatment involves removing affected tooth

structure and restoring it with various materials. Fluoride, diligent dental hygiene, sealants, and proper diet can prevent virtually all caries.

Etiology and Pathophysiology

Caries is caused by acids produced by bacteria retained within dental plaque. Plaque is, at first, a soft, thin film of food debris, mucin, dead epithelial cells, and bacteria that develops on the tooth surface within about 24 h after the tooth is cleaned. *Mutans streptococci* is a group of related bacteria causing caries. Some strains are more cariogenic than others. Eventually, the soft plaque becomes hard with Ca and other minerals (hard plaque), which cannot easily be removed with a toothbrush.

Many teeth have open enamel pits, fissures, and grooves, which may extend from the surface to the dentin. These defects may be wide enough to harbor bacteria but too narrow to clean effectively. They predispose teeth to caries.

A tooth surface is more susceptible to caries when it is poorly calcified or in an acidic environment. Typically, decalcification begins when the pH at the tooth falls below 5.5 (as occurs with colonization by acid-producing bacteria and/or with the drinking of cola beverages, which contain phosphoric acid).

Rampant caries in deciduous teeth suggests prolonged contact with infant formula, milk, or juice, typically when an infant goes to bed with a bottle (baby or nursing bottle caries).

The elderly often take drugs that reduce salivary flow, predisposing to caries. The elderly also have a higher incidence of root caries because of gingival recession and exposure of root surfaces.

Untreated caries leads to tooth destruction, infections, and the need for extractions and replacement prostheses. Premature loss of deciduous teeth may shift the adjacent teeth, hindering eruption of their permanent successors.

Symptoms, Signs, and Diagnosis

Caries initially involves only the enamel and produces no symptoms. A cavity that invades the dentin causes pain, first when hot, cold, or sweet foods or beverages contact the involved tooth, and later with chewing or percussion. Pain can be intense and persistent when the pulp is severely involved (see Pulpitis on p. 857).

Routine, frequent (q 6 to 12 mo) clinical evaluation identifies early caries at a time when minimal intervention prevents its progression. A thin probe, sometimes special dyes, and transillumination by fiberoptic lights are used, frequently supplemented by new devices that detect caries by changes in electrical conductivity, as well as laser reflectivity. However, x-rays are still important for detecting caries, determining the depth of involvement, and identifying caries under existing restorations.

Treatment

Incipient caries should be remineralized, if possible, through cleanings and multiple fluoride applications.

The primary treatment of caries is removal by drilling, followed by filling of the resultant defect. For very deep cavities, a temporary filling may be left in place 6 to 10 wk in the hope that a tooth will deposit reparative dentin, preventing exposure of the pulp, which necessitates root canal treatment. Fillings for occlusal surfaces of posterior teeth, which bear the brunt of mastication, must be composed of strong materials. The most common material has been silver amalgam, a combination of silver, mercury, copper, tin, and, occasionally, zinc, palladium, or indium. Amalgam is inexpensive and lasts an average of 14 yr. However, with good oral hygiene and if placed with use of a rubber dam for isolation from saliva, many amalgam fillings last > 40 yr. Although concern has been raised about mercury poisoning, the number of amalgam fillings a person has bears no relationship to blood mercury levels. Replacing amalgam is expensive, damages tooth structure, and is not recommended.

Composite resins, which have a more acceptable appearance, have long been used in anterior teeth, where aesthetics is primary and the forces of chewing are minimal. Some patients request them in posterior teeth as well. However, composite resins under high occlusal stress generally last less than half as long as amalgam and tend to develop recurrent decay. This occurs because the material shrinks when it hardens and also expands and contracts with heat and cold more than tooth or other filling materials. Newer porcelain or ceramic inlays resemble enamel, but long-term results are not yet known.

If decay leaves too little dentin to hold a restoration, a dentist replaces the missing dentin with cement, amalgam, composite, or other materials. Sometimes a post must be inserted into one or more roots to support a gold, silver, or composite core, which replaces the coronal dentin. This may necessitate a root canal filling. The outer tooth surfaces (what would have been the enamel) are then reduced so that an artificial crown, usually made of gold, porcelain, or both, can be placed. Crowns for anterior teeth consist of, or are covered with, porcelain.

Prevention

For most people, caries is preventable. Removal of plaque at least q 24 h, usually by brushing and flossing, helps prevent dental caries. The gingival third of the tooth is the most important area to clean but is the area most often neglected. Electric and electronic toothbrushes are excellent, but a manual soft toothbrush, used for an average of 3 to 4 min, suffices. Using excess toothpaste, particularly an abrasive type, may erode the teeth. Dental floss is placed between each of the teeth, curved against the side of each tooth, and moved up and down 3 times, going just beneath the gingival margin. Flosses that are very thin (dental tape) or coated with wax or polytetraethylene can be used for exceptionally tight contacts between teeth or rough filling margins.

Teeth with fluoride incorporated into their enamel are more resistant to acidic decalcification and more readily recalcify when pH increases. If drinking water is not adequately fluoridated, fluoride supplements are recommended for children from shortly after birth through age 8 yr and for pregnant women beginning at 3 mo gestation (when teeth are forming in the fetus). The dose must be selected according to the amount of fluoride present in the drinking water and the age of the child. The total dose should not be so high as to cause dental fluorosis. Fluoridated toothpaste should also be used by people of all ages.

Fluoridation offers less protection against caries in pits and fissures compared with those on smooth surfaces. Pits and fissures require use of sealants (plastic materials that adhere tightly to the surface of the enamel) to prevent nutrients from reaching bacteria, reducing their growth and acid production.

Cavities first form on permanent teeth in the early teens to late 20s. A caries-prone subset typically has a low fluoride exposure and a relatively cariogenic microflora acquired from the mother. Maintaining good oral hygiene and minimizing sugar intake are especially needed.

If these measures do not decrease cavity formation, more intensive therapy aims at changing the flora. After cavities are treated, pits and fissures, which can harbor *M. streptococci* are sealed. This treatment is followed by 60-sec mouth rinses using 0.12% chlorhexidine bid for 2 wk, which may reduce the cariogenic bacteria in plaque and allow repopulation with less cariogenic strains of *M. streptococci*. To encourage repopulation, xylitol in the form of hard candy or chewing gum is used for 5 min tid. Additionally, topical fluoride may be applied by a dentist or used at night in a custom-made fluoride carrier.

For pregnant women with a history of severe caries, the above regimen may be used before the child's teeth erupt. If this is not feasible, the mother can use xylitol, as mentioned above, from the time of the baby's birth to the age at which the mother no longer samples the child's food (the hypothesized mode of transfer).

For prevention of caries in deciduous teeth (once they have erupted) in infants, bedtime bottles should contain only water.

GINGIVITIS

Gingivitis is inflammation of the gingiva, producing bleeding with swelling, redness, exudate, a change of normal contours, and, occasionally, discomfort. Diagnosis is based on inspection. Treatment involves professional teeth cleaning and intensified home dental hygiene. Advanced cases may require antibiotics or surgery.

Normally, the gingiva are firm, tightly adapted to the teeth, and contoured to a point. Keratinized gingiva near the crowns is pink stippled tissue. It should fill the entire space between the crowns. The gingiva farther from the crowns, called alveolar mucosa, is nonkeratinized, highly vascular, red, movable, and continuous with the buccal mucosa. A tongue depressor should express no blood or pus from normal gingiva.

Inflammation, or gingivitis, the most common gingival problem, may evolve into periodontitis.

Etiology

The most common cause of gingivitis is poor oral hygiene. Poor oral hygiene allows plaque to accumulate between the gingiva and the teeth (gingivitis does not occur in edentulous areas). Irritation from plaque deepens the normal crevice between the tooth and gingiva, creating gingival pockets. These pockets contain bacteria that may cause both gingivitis and (root) caries. Other local factors, such as malocclusion, dental calculus, food impaction, faulty dental restorations, and xerostomia, play a secondary role.

Gingivitis also commonly occurs at puberty, during menstruation and pregnancy, and at menopause, presumably because of hormonal changes. Similarly, oral contraceptives may exacerbate inflammation.

Gingivitis may be an early sign of a systemic disorder, particularly those that affect the response to infection (eg, diabetes, AIDS, vitamin deficiency, leukopenia), particularly if it occurs in patients with minimal dental plaque. Some patients with Crohn's disease have a cobblestone area of granulomatous gingival hypertrophy when intestinal flare-ups occur. Exposure to heavy metals (eg, lead, bismuth) may cause gingivitis and a dark line at the gingival margin. Severe deficiency of niacin or vitamin C can cause gingivitis.

Symptoms and Signs

Simple gingivitis first causes a deepening of the sulcus (gingival crevice) between the tooth and the gingiva, followed by a band of red, inflamed gingiva along one or more teeth, with swelling of the interdental papillae and easy bleeding. Pain is usually absent. It may resolve, remain superficial for years, or occasionally progress to periodontitis.

Pericoronitis is acute, painful inflammation of the gingival flap over a partly erupted tooth, usually around mandibular 3rd molars (wisdom teeth). Infection is common, and an abscess may develop. Pericoronitis often recurs as food gets trapped beneath the flap. The gingival flap disappears when the tooth is fully erupted.

Desquamative gingivitis may occur during menopause. It is characterized by deep red, painful gingival tissue that bleeds easily. Vesicles may precede desquamation. The gingiva is soft because the keratinized cells that resist abrasion by food particles are absent. A similar gingival lesion may be associated with pemphigus vulgaris, bullous pemphigoid, benign mucous membrane pemphigoid, or atrophic lichen planus.

During pregnancy, swelling, especially of the interdental papillae, is likely to occur. Pedunculated gingival growths often arise in the interdental papillae during the 1st trimester, may persist throughout pregnancy, and may or may not subside after delivery. Pregnancy tumors are soft reddish masses that are, histologically, pyogenic granulomas. They develop rapidly and then remain static. An underlying irritant is common, such as calculus or a restoration with a rough margin.

Uncontrolled diabetes can exaggerate the effects of gingival irritants, making secondary infections and acute gingival abscesses common.

In leukemia, the gingiva may become engorged with a leukemic infiltrate, exhibiting clinical symptoms of edema, pain, and easily induced bleeding.

In scurvy (vitamin C deficiency), the gingiva are inflamed, hyperplastic, and engorged, bleeding easily. Petechiae and ecchymoses may appear throughout the mouth.

In pellagra (niacin deficiency), the gingiva are inflamed, bleed easily, and are susceptible to secondary infection. Additionally, the lips are reddened and cracked, the mouth feels scalded, the tongue is smooth and bright red, and the tongue and mucosa may have ulcerations.

Diagnosis and Treatment

Finding erythematous, friable tissue at the gum lines confirms the diagnosis. To detect early gingival disease, some dentists frequently measure the depth of the pocket around each tooth. Depths < 3 mm are normal; deeper pockets are at high risk of gingivitis and periodontitis.

Simple gingivitis is controlled by proper oral hygiene with or without an antibacterial mouth rinse. Thorough scaling (professional scraping with a sharp instrument) should be performed. If appropriate, poorly contoured restorations are reshaped or replaced and local irritants removed. Excess gingiva, if present, can be excised. Drugs causing gingival hyperplasia should be stopped if possible. Pregnancy tumors are excised.

Treatment of pericoronitis consists of removal of debris from under the gingival flap; irrigation with saline, 1.5% hydrogen peroxide, or 0.12% chlorhexidine; and, particularly when episodes recur, extraction. If severe infection develops, antibiotics may be given for a day before extraction and continued during healing. A common regimen is penicillin VK 500 mg po q 6 h for 10 days (or until 3 days after all inflammation has subsided). Abscesses associated with pericoronitis require localized incision and drainage, a periodontal flap and root debridement, or extraction.

In gingivitis from systemic disorders, treatment is directed at the underlying cause. In desquamative gingivitis during menopause, sequential administration of estrogens and progestins may be beneficial, but adverse effects of this therapy (see p. 2082) limit recommendations for its use. Gingivitis from pemphigus vulgaris (see p. 949) and similar mucocutaneous conditions may require systemic corticosteroid therapy.

Prevention

Daily removal of plaque with dental floss and a toothbrush and routine cleaning by a dentist or hygienist at 6-mo to 1-yr intervals can help prevent gingivitis. Patients with systemic disorders predisposing to gingivitis require more frequent professional cleanings (from q 2 wk to 4 times/yr).

ACUTE NECROTIZING ULCERATIVE GINGIVITIS

(Fusospirochetosis; Trench Mouth; Vincent's Infection or Angina)

Acute necrotizing ulcerative gingivitis is a painful infection of the gums. Symptoms are acute pain, bleeding, and foul breath. Diagnosis is based on clinical findings. Treatment is gentle debridement, oral hygiene, mouth rinses, supportive care, and, if debridement must be delayed, antibiotics.

Acute necrotizing ulcerative gingivitis occurs most frequently in smokers and debilitated patients who are under stress. Other risk factors are poor oral hygiene, nutritional deficiencies, and sleep deprivation.

Symptoms, Signs, and Diagnosis

The usually abrupt onset may be accompanied by malaise or fever. The chief manifestations are acutely painful, bleeding gingiva; excessive salivation; and overwhelming foul breath (fetor oris). Ulcerations, which are pathognomonic, are present on the dental papillae and marginal gingiva; these have a characteristically punched-out appearance and are covered by a gray pseudomembrane. Similar lesions on the buccal mucosa and tonsils are rare. Swallowing and talking may be painful. Regional lymphadenopathy often is present.

Rarely, tonsillary or pharyngeal tissues are affected, and diphtheria or infection due to agranulocytosis must be ruled out.

Treatment

Treatment consists of gentle debridement with a hand scaler or ultrasonic device. Debridement is performed over several days. The patient uses a soft toothbrush to wipe the teeth. Rinses at hourly intervals with warm normal saline or twice/day with 1.5% hydrogen peroxide or 0.12% chlorhexidine may help during the first few days after initial debridement. Essential supportive measures include improved oral hygiene (performed gently at first), adequate nutrition, high fluid intake, rest, analgesics as needed, and avoiding irritation (eg, from smoking or from hot or spicy foods). Marked improvement usually occurs within 24 to 48 h, after which debridement can be completed. If debridement is delayed (eg, if a dentist or the instruments necessary for debridement are unavailable), oral antibiotics (eg, penicillin VK 500 mg, erythromycin 250 mg, or tetracycline 250 mg q 6 h) provide rapid relief and can be continued until 72 h after symptoms resolve. If the gingival contour inverts (ie, if the tips of papillae are lost) during the acute phase, surgery is eventually required to prevent subsequent periodontitis.

OTHER GINGIVAL DISORDERS

Hyperplasia of gingival tissues may occur without inflammation in response to various drugs, particularly phenytoin, cyclosporine, and nifedipine or, less commonly, other Ca channel blockers. Hyperplasia is characterized by diffuse, relatively avascular smooth or nodular enlargement of the gingiva, which may almost cover some teeth. The hypertrophied tissue is often excised. If possible, substitutions are made for the offending drugs. Scrupulous oral hygiene may minimize recurrence.

Carcinoma can also originate in the gingiva and spread to regional lymph nodes.

PERIODONTITIS

Periodontitis is inflammation of the periodontium—the periodontal ligament, gingiva, cementum, and alveolar bone. It usually

presents as a worsening of gingivitis. Symptoms are rare except with HIV or when abscesses develop, in which pain and swelling are common. Diagnosis is based on inspection, periodontal probing, and x-rays. Treatment involves dental cleaning that extends under the gums and a vigorous home hygiene program. Advanced cases may require antibiotics and surgery.

Etiology and Pathophysiology

Periodontitis usually develops when gingivitis, usually with abundant calculus beneath the gingival margin, has not been adequately treated. In periodontitis, the deep pockets can harbor anaerobic organisms that do more damage than those usually present in simple gingivitis. The gingiva progressively loses its attachment to the teeth, periodontal pockets deepen, and bone loss begins. With progressive bone loss, teeth may loosen and gingiva recedes. Tooth migration is common in later stages.

Systemic diseases that predispose patients to periodontitis include diabetes (especially type 1); acquired, familial, and cyclic neutropenia; leukemia; Down syndrome; leukocyte adhesion deficiency syndromes; Papillon-Lefèvre syndrome; Crohn's disease; histiocytosis syndromes; agranulocytosis; lazy leukocyte syndrome; hypogammaglobulinemia; Chédiak-Higashi syndrome; glycogen storage disease; infantile genetic agranulocytosis; Ehlers-Danlos syndrome (types IV and VIII); vitamin C deficiency (scurvy); and hypophosphatasia. Faulty occlusion, causing an excessive functional load on teeth, may contribute to progression of a particular type of periodontitis characterized by angular bony defects.

Periodontitis is usually chronic. Chronic periodontitis occurs in localized and generalized forms, and people with significant disease tend to be > 35 yr.

Aggressive periodontitis: Several more rapidly progressive subtypes of chronic periodontitis exist, collectively known as aggressive periodontitis. Aggressive periodontitis may develop as early as childhood, sometimes before age 3. Patients may have severe bone loss, even tooth loss, by age 20. Neutrophil function may be defective in aggressive periodontitis; its clinical significance is unknown.

In one type of aggressive periodontitis that occurs in healthy adolescents (formerly called localized juvenile periodontitis or periodontosis), patients often have significant colonization of *Actinobacillus actinomycetemcomitans*. Typically, the signs of inflammation are minor. The disease is detected by periodontal probing or x-rays, which show localized, deep (vertical) bone loss, commonly limited to the first molars and incisors. Bone loss progresses faster than in adult periodontitis, often at a rate of 3 to 4 µm/day.

Another, uncommon, type of aggressive periodontitis (formerly called prepubertal periodontitis) affects deciduous teeth usually shortly after eruption. Generalized acute proliferative gingivitis and rapid alveolar bone destruction are its hallmarks. Patients also have frequent bouts of otitis media and are usually diagnosed by age 4. In some patients, the disease resolves before the permanent teeth erupt. Treatment regimens are under study.

The prototypical aggressive periodontitis (formerly called rapidly progressive periodontitis) occurs in patients aged 20 to 35. It is often associated with *A. actinomycetemcomitans, Porphyromonas gingivalis, Eikenella corrodens,* and many gram-negative bacilli, but cause and effect are not clear. Some cases result from undiagnosed localized juvenile periodontitis or prepubertal periodontitis, but others appear independently.

HIV-associated periodontitis is a particularly virulent, rapidly progressing disease. Clinically, it resembles acute necrotizing ulcerative gingivitis (see p. 855) combined with rapidly progressive periodontitis. Patients may lose 9 to 12 mm of attachment in as little as 6 mo.

Symptoms, Signs, and Diagnosis

Pain is usually absent unless an acute infection forms in one or more periodontal pockets or if HIV-associated periodontitis is present. Impaction of food in the pockets can cause pain at meals. Abundant plaque along with redness, swelling, and exudate are characteristic. Gums may be tender and bleed easily, and the breath may be foul.

Inspection of the teeth and gingiva combined with probing of the pockets and measurement of their depth are usually sufficient for diagnosis. Pockets deeper than 4 mm indicate periodontitis. Dental x-rays reveal alveolar bone loss adjacent to the periodontal pockets.

Treatment

For all forms of periodontitis, the 1st phase of treatment consists of thorough scaling and root planing (ie, removal of diseased or toxin-affected dentin followed by smoothening of the root) to remove plaque and calculus deposits. Thorough home oral hygiene is necessary. The patient is reevaluated at 2 wk and at 3 mo. If pockets are no deeper than 4 mm at this point, the only treatment needed is regular cleanings.

If deeper pockets persist, systemic antibiotics can be used. A common regimen is tetracycline 250 mg po qid for 10 days. Tetracyclines concentrate in the gingival sulcus and diminish bone destruction by inhibiting collagenase. In addition, a filament containing tetracycline, a gel containing doxycycline, or chips of chlorhexidine can be placed into recalcitrant pockets. The gel and chips are resorbed, whereas the filament is removed in 7 to 10 days.

Another approach is to surgically eliminate the pocket and recontour the bone so that the patient can clean the depth of the sulcus (pocket reduction/elimination surgery). In selected situations, regenerative surgery and bone grafting are done to encourage alveolar bone growth. Splinting of loose teeth and selective reshaping of tooth surfaces to eliminate traumatic occlusion may be necessary. Extractions are often necessary in advanced disease. Contributing systemic factors should be controlled before initiating periodontal therapy.

Ninety percent of patients with HIV-associated periodontitis respond to irrigation of the sulcus with povidone-iodine (which the dentist applies with a syringe), regular use of chlorhexidine mouth rinses, and systemic antibiotics, usually metronidazole 250 mg po tid for 14 days.

Localized juvenile periodontitis requires periodontal surgery plus oral antibiotics (eg, a tetracycline 250 mg qid or metronidazole 250 mg tid for 14 days).

PULPITIS

Pulpitis is inflammation of the dental pulp resulting from untreated caries, trauma, or multiple restorations. Its principal symptom is pain. Diagnosis is based on clinical findings and is confirmed by x-ray. Treatment involves removing decay, restoring the damaged tooth, and, sometimes, performing root canal therapy or extracting the tooth.

Pulpitis can occur when caries progresses deeply into the dentin, when a tooth requires multiple invasive procedures, or when trauma disrupts the lymphatic and blood supply to the pulp. It begins as a reversible condition in which the tooth can be saved by a simple filling. It becomes irreversible as swelling inside the rigid encasement of the dentin compromises circulation, making the pulp necrotic, which predisposes to infection.

Infectious sequelae of pulpitis include apical periodontitis, periapical abscess, cellulitis, and osteomyelitis of the jaw. Spread from maxillary teeth may cause purulent sinusitis, meningitis, brain abscess, orbital cellulitis, and cavernous sinus thrombosis. Spread from mandibular teeth may cause Ludwig's angina, parapharyngeal abscess, mediastinitis, pericarditis, empyema, and jugular thrombophlebitis.

Symptoms, Signs, and Diagnosis

In reversible pulpitis, pain occurs when a stimulus (usually cold or sweets) is applied to the tooth. When the stimulus is removed, the pain ceases within 1 to 2 sec.

In irreversible pulpitis, pain occurs spontaneously or lingers minutes after the stimulus is removed. A patient may have difficulty locating the tooth from which the pain originates, even confusing the maxillary and mandibular arches (but not the left and right sides of the mouth). The pain may then cease for several days because of pulpal necrosis. As infection develops and extends through the apical foramen, the tooth becomes exquisitely sensitive to pressure and percussion. A periapical (dentoalveolar) abscess elevates the tooth from its socket and feels "high" when the patient bites down.

Diagnosis is based on the history and physical examination, which makes use of provoking stimuli (application of heat, cold, percussion). X-rays help determine whether inflammation has extended beyond the tooth apex and help exclude other conditions.

Treatment

In reversible pulpitis, pulp vitality can be maintained if the tooth is treated, usually by caries removal, and then restored.

Irreversible pulpitis and its sequelae require endodontic (root canal) therapy or tooth extraction. In endodontic therapy, an opening is made in the tooth and the pulp is removed. The root canal system is thoroughly debrided, shaped, and then filled with gutta-percha. After root canal therapy, adequate healing is manifested clinically by resolution of symptoms and radiographically by bone filling in the radiolucent area at the root apex over a period of months. If the patient has systemic signs of infection, such as fever, an oral antibiotic is prescribed (penicillin VK 500 mg q 6 h or, for patients allergic to penicillin, clindamycin 150 mg or 300 mg q 6 h). If symptoms persist or worsen, root canal therapy is usually repeated in case a root canal was missed, but alternative diagnoses (eg, temporomandibular disorder, occult tooth fracture, neurologic disorder) should be considered.

Very rarely, subcutaneous or mediastinal emphysema develops after compressed air or a high-speed air turbine dental drill has been used during root canal therapy or extraction. These devices can force air into the tissues around the tooth socket that dissects along fascial planes. Acute onset of jaw and cervical swelling with characteristic crepitus of the swollen skin on palpation is diagnostic. Treatment usually is not required, although prophylactic antibiotics are sometimes prescribed.

96 DENTAL EMERGENCIES

Emergency dental treatment by a physician is sometimes required when a dentist is unavailable.

Oral analgesics effective for most dental problems include acetaminophen 650 to 1000 mg q 6 h and NSAIDS such as ibuprofen 400 to 800 mg q 6 h. For severe pain, these drugs may be combined with opioids, such as codeine 60 mg; hydrocodone 5 mg, 7.5 mg, or 10 mg; or oxycodone 5 mg.

Antibiotics for dental infections include penicillin VK 500 mg po q 6 h, erythromycin 500 mg po q 6 h, and clindamycin 300 mg po q 8 h. Amoxicillin 2 g is typically given 1 h prior to certain dental procedures (anything that could cause bacteremia, usually from gum bleeding and root canal treatments) as prophylaxis in patients with valvular heart disease and others at risk for endocarditis. For those who cannot tolerate penicillins, clindamycin 600 mg can be given 1 h before as prophylaxis.

FRACTURED AND AVULSED TEETH

If a tooth is fractured without exposing the dental pulp, the patient is given a mild analgesic and referred to a dentist. If the pulp is exposed (indicated by bleeding from the tooth) or if the tooth is mobile, dental referral is urgent.

Avulsed primary teeth are not replaced because they typically become necrotic, then infected. They may also become ankylosed and do not exfoliate, thereby interfering with the eruption of the permanent tooth.

If a secondary tooth is avulsed, the patient should replace it in its socket immediately and seek dental care to stabilize it. If this cannot be done, the tooth should be kept moist in milk until professionally cleaned in 0.9% saline solution, replaced, and stabilized. The tooth should not be scrubbed, because scrubbing may remove viable periodontal ligament fibers, which aid in reattachment. A patient with an avulsed tooth should take an antibiotic for several days. If the avulsed tooth cannot be found, it may have been aspirated, embedded in soft tissue, or swallowed. A chest x-ray may be needed to rule out aspiration, but a swallowed tooth is harmless.

A partially avulsed tooth that is repositioned and stabilized quickly usually is permanently retained. A completely avulsed tooth may be permanently retained if replaced in the socket with minimal handling within 1 h. When replacement is delayed, the long-term retention rate drops, and root resorption eventually occurs. Nevertheless, a patient may be able to use the tooth for several years.

MANDIBULAR DISLOCATION

Spontaneous mandibular dislocation usually occurs in people with a history of such dislocations. Although a dislocated mandible is occasionally caused by trauma, the initiat-

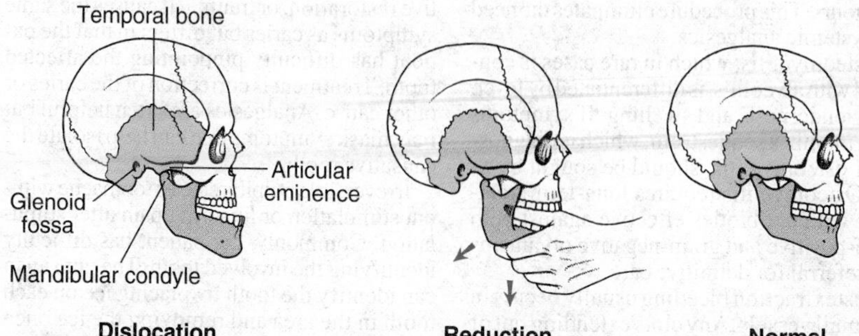

Fig. 96–1. Mandibular reduction. The patient's head is stabilized. The operator places his thumbs on the external oblique line of the mandible (lateral to the 3rd molar area) or, after wrapping his thumbs in gauze, on the occlusal surface of the lower molars. The other fingers are curled under the mandible. The patient is asked to open wide, as if yawning, and the operator then applies downward force on the molars while applying upward force over the chin until the mandible reduces.

ing episode is usually a wide opening followed by biting pressure (eg, biting into a large sandwich with hard bread), a wide yawn, or a dental procedure. People prone to dislocation may have naturally loose temporomandibular joint (TMJ) ligaments.

The patient presents with a wide-open mouth which he is unable to close. Pain is secondary to the patient's attempt to close the mouth. If the mandibular midline deviates to one side, the dislocation is unilateral. Although rarely used, a local anesthetic (eg, 2% lidocaine 2 to 5 mL) injected into the ipsilateral joint and into the adjacent area of insertion of the lateral pterygoid muscle may allow the mandible to reduce spontaneously.

Manual reduction may be necessary (see FIG. 96–1). Premedication may be used (eg, diazepam 5 to 10 mg IV at 5 mg/min or midazolam 3 to 5 mg IV at 2 mg/min and an opioid such as meperidine 25 mg IV or fentanyl 0.5 to 1 µg/kg IV) but is not necessary, especially if time will be lost preparing the IV. The longer the mandible is dislocated, the more difficult it is to reduce and the greater the likelihood that dislocation will recur.

Barton's bandage may be needed for 2 or 3 days. Most importantly, the patient must avoid opening the mouth wide for at least 6 wk. When anticipating a yawn, the patient should place a fist under the chin to prevent wide opening. Food must be cut into small pieces. If the patient suffers from chronic dislocations and more conservative treatment modalities have been exhausted, an oral-maxillofacial surgeon may be consulted. As a treatment of last resort, the ligaments around the TMJ can be surgically tightened (shortened) in an attempt to stabilize the joint, or the articular eminence can be reduced (eminectomy).

POSTEXTRACTION PROBLEMS

Swelling is normal after oral surgery and is proportional to the degree of manipulation and trauma. If swelling does not begin to subside by the 3rd postoperative day, infection is likely and an antibiotic is given.

Postoperative pain varies from moderate to severe and is treated with analgesics.

Postextraction alveolitis (dry socket) is pain emanating from bare bone if the socket's clot lyses. Although assumed to be due to bacterial action, it is much more common in smokers and oral contraceptive users. It is peculiar to the removal of mandibular molars, usually wisdom teeth. Typically, the pain begins on the 2nd or 3rd postoperative day, is referred to the ear, and lasts from a few days to many weeks. Alveolitis is best treated with topical analgesics: a 1- to 2-in iodoform gauze strip saturated in eugenol or coated with an anesthetic ointment, such as lidocaine 2.5% or tetracaine 0.5%, is placed in the socket. The gauze is changed every 1 to 3 days until symptoms do not return if the gauze is left out for a few hours. This procedure eliminates the need for systemic analgesics.

Osteomyelitis, which in rare cases is confused with alveolitis, is differentiated by fever, local tenderness, and swelling. If symptoms last a month, a sequestrum, which is diagnostic of osteomyelitis, should be sought by x-ray. Osteomyelitis requires long-term treatment with antibiotics effective against both gram-positive and gram-negative organisms and referral for definitive care.

Postextraction bleeding usually occurs in the small vessels. Any clots extending out of the socket are removed with gauze, and then a 4-in gauze pad (folded) or a tea bag is placed over the socket and the patient is instructed to apply continuous pressure by biting for 1 h. The procedure may have to be repeated 2 or 3 times. Patients are told to wait at least 1 h before checking the site so as not to disrupt clot formation. They are also informed that a few drops of blood diluted in a mouth full of saliva appear to be more blood than is actually present. If bleeding continues, the site may be anesthetized by nerve block or local infiltration with 2% lidocaine containing 1:100,000 epinephrine. The socket is then curetted to remove existing clot and to freshen the bone and is irrigated with normal saline. Then the area is sutured under gentle tension. Local hemostatic agents, such as oxidized cellulose, topical thrombin on a gelatin sponge, or microfibrillar collagen may be placed in the socket before suturing.

If these measures fail, a systemic cause (eg, bleeding diathesis) is sought. If possible, patients taking low-dose aspirin should discontinue this practice 4 days before an extraction to minimize bleeding.

TOOTHACHE AND INFECTION

Caries extending through the enamel into dentin causes pain with stimulation (eg, heat, cold, sweet food or drink). Pain is isolated to a single tooth and usually stops when the stimulus is removed. The patient should avoid the provoking stimuli and seek dental treatment. A simple restoration (filling) usually is curative.

Reversible pulpitis is inflammation of the pulp, typically due to caries, minor pulp damage from previous large restorations, a defective restoration, or trauma. It causes the same symptoms as caries but differs in that the patient has difficulty pinpointing the affected tooth. Treatment is correction of the caries or other cause. Analgesics are often helpful but may mask symptoms that can help isolate the causative tooth.

Irreversible pulpitis causes toothache without stimulation or lingering pain after stimulation. Commonly, the patient has difficulty identifying the involved tooth. The physician can identify the tooth by placing ice on each tooth in the area and removing the ice once the patient feels pain. In healthy teeth, the pain stops almost immediately. Pain lingering more than a few seconds indicates irreversible pulpitis. Uncommonly, cold actually lessens symptoms (suppurative pulpitis), and the patient may present with a glass of ice water from which he regularly sips. Analgesics are needed until a dentist can perform root canal therapy or extraction. A patient who is seen frequently for emergencies but who never obtains definitive dental treatment may be seeking opioids.

Pressure necrosis frequently results from pulpitis, because the pulp is encased in a rigid compartment. Typically, once inflamed pulp becomes necrotic, the previously noted types of pain end. This symptom-free period may last hours to weeks. Subsequently, periapical inflammation and/or infection (apical periodontitis) develops. Infection is usually caused by resident oral bacteria. Apical periodontitis causes pain when chewing or biting. Normally, the patient can indicate the involved tooth. If not, the physician identifies it by tapping the teeth with a metal probe or tongue blade until the pain is reproduced. Antibiotics and analgesics are appropriate if dental care is delayed.

Periapical abscess may follow untreated caries or pulpitis. If the abscess is associated with well-developed (soft) fluctuance, it is drained through incision of the most dependent point of the swelling with a #15 scalpel blade. Rarely, extraoral drainage is used. Infections of < 3 days' duration respond better to penicillin, whereas those lasting > 3 days respond better to clindamycin.

Cellulitis can follow untreated dental infections. Rarely, cavernous sinus thrombosis (see p. 925) or Ludwig's angina (see p. 824) develops. The latter 2 conditions are life threatening and require immediate hospitalization, removal of the infected tooth, and culture-guided parenteral antibiotics.

Sinusitis is suspected if many or all maxillary posterior teeth on one side are sensitive to percussion or if the patient reports pain on bending over with the head down.

Erupting or impacted molars, particularly 3rd molars, can be painful and may cause inflammation of adjacent soft tissue (pericoronitis) that can progress to serious infection. Treatment is with chlorhexidine rinses or hypertonic saltwater soaks (a tablespoon of salt mixed in a glass of hot water—no hotter than the coffee or tea a patient normally drinks). The salt water is held in the mouth on the affected side until it cools and then is expectorated and immediately replaced with another mouthful. Three or 4 glasses of salt water gargle a day usually controls inflammation and pain until the tooth can be removed. Antibiotics are appropriate if dental care is delayed.

Less common causes of acute perioral swelling include periodontal abscess, infected cysts, antritis, allergy, salivary gland obstruction or infection, and peritonsillar infection. Teething pain in young children may be accompanied by excess salivation and fever. Acetaminophen, appropriate for the weight of the child, helps relieve symptoms.

97 TEMPOROMANDIBULAR DISORDERS

(See also Mandibular Dislocation on p. 858, Temporal Bone Fractures on p. 2585, and Jaw Tumors on p. 840.)

The term temporomandibular disorders is an umbrella term for conditions producing dysfunction of the jaw joint or pain in the jaw and face, often in or around the temporomandibular joint (TMJ), including masticatory and other muscles of the head and neck, the fascia, or both. A person is considered to have a temporomandibular disorder only if pain or limitation of motion is severe enough to require professional care.

Temporomandibular disorders typically are multifactorial, but most are related to disturbed movement of the mandibular condyle in the glenoid fossa or against the cartilaginous articular disk (see FIG. 97–1). This disk, shaped like a donut with a closed hole or like a mature red blood cell, serves as a cushion between joint surfaces. Causes for this disturbed movement include clenching and grinding of the teeth, trauma, arthritis, and malocclusion and missing teeth. Even the trauma of persistent gum chewing can be enough to damage the joint.

Diagnosis

Disorders of the TMJ itself must be distinguished from the many conditions that mimic them (see TABLE 97–1). Pain exacerbated by finger pressure on the joint when the mouth is opened implicates the TMJ.

The patient is asked to describe the pain and designate painful areas. The occipital muscles and each of the major muscle groups involved in mastication are palpated for general tenderness and trigger points (spots that radiate pain to another area). The patient is observed opening the mouth as wide as is comfortable. When the patient opens and closes his mouth with the junction of the

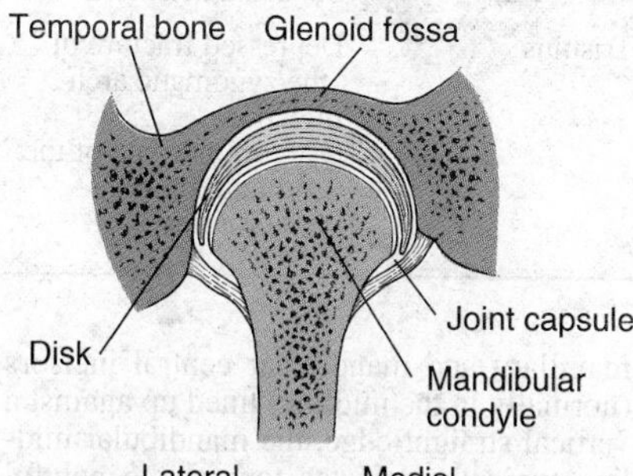

Fig. 97–1. The temporomandibular joint. The joint is formed by the mandibular condyle and the glenoid fossa of the temporal bone; a cartilaginous articular disk functions as a cushion between the joint surfaces.

TABLE 97–1. SOME CONDITIONS THAT MIMIC TEMPOROMANDIBULAR DISORDERS

SYMPTOM	CONDITION
Headaches	Sinusitis Temporal arteritis Tension, migraine, and cluster headaches
Pain	Postherpetic neuralgia Reflex sympathetic dystrophy or traumatic neuroma after head or neck surgery Toothache Trigeminal neuralgia
Pain accompanied by hearing problems	Obstruction of the ear canals or eustachian tube Otitis media
Pain in the head, neck, and other areas of the body	Fibromyalgia Generalized myofascial pain
Pain, numbness	Intracranial aneurysm Metastatic tumors
Pain that radiates to the temporomandibular joint region	Whiplash injuries affecting muscle or cervical spine
Pain that worsens when the patient swallows or turns the head	Cervical spine or muscle disorders Eagle syndrome (calcified styloid process) Glossopharyngeal neuralgia Subacute thyroiditis
Trismus	Depressed fracture of the zygomatic arch Infection Osteochondroma of the coronoid process Pericoronitis

maxillary and mandibular central incisors (normally in the midline) lined up against a vertical straight edge, the mandibular midline typically deviates toward the painful side. Palpation and auscultation of the joint during opening and closing may reveal tenderness, catching, clicking, or popping. Condylar motion can best be palpated by placing the 5th fingers into the external ear canals and exerting very gentle forward pressure as the patient moves the jaw.

ANKYLOSIS OF THE TEMPOROMANDIBULAR JOINT

Ankylosis of the temporomandibular joint is immobility or fusion of the joint.

Ankylosis of the temporomandibular joint (TMJ) most often results from trauma or infection, but it may be congenital or a result of RA. Chronic, painless limitation of motion occurs. When ankylosis leads to arrest of condylar growth, facial asymmetry is common (see Condylar Hypoplasia on p. 864). Intra-articular (true) ankylosis must be distinguished from extra-articular (false) ankylosis, which may be caused by enlargement of the coronoid process, depressed fracture of the zygomatic arch, or scarring from surgery, irradiation, or infection. In most cases of true ankylosis, x-rays of the TMJ show loss of normal bony architecture.

Treatment may include a condylectomy if the ankylosis is intra-articular or an ostectomy of part of the ramus if the coronoid process and zygomatic arch are also affected. Jaw-opening exercises must be performed for months to years to maintain the surgical correction, but forced opening of the jaws without surgery is generally ineffective because of bony fusion.

ARTHRITIS OF THE TEMPOROMANDIBULAR JOINT

Infectious arthritis, traumatic arthritis, osteoarthritis, RA, and secondary degenerative arthritis can affect the temporomandibular joint.

Infectious arthritis: Infection of the temporomandibular joint (TMJ) may result from direct extension of adjacent infection or hematogenous spread of bloodborne organisms (see also Acute Infectious Arthritis on p. 312). The area is inflamed, and jaw movement is limited. Local signs of infection associated with evidence of a systemic disease or with an adjacent infection suggest the diagnosis. X-ray results are negative in the early stages but may show bone destruction later. If suppurative arthritis is suspected, the joint is aspirated to confirm the diagnosis and to identify the causative organism. Diagnosis must be made rapidly to prevent permanent joint damage.

Treatment includes antibiotics, proper hydration, pain control, and motion restriction. Parenteral penicillin G is the drug of choice until a specific bacteriologic diagnosis can be made on the basis of culture and sensitivity testing. Suppurative infections are aspirated or incised. Once the infection is controlled, jaw-opening exercises help prevent scarring and limitation of motion.

Traumatic arthritis: Rarely, acute injury (eg, due to difficult tooth extraction or endotracheal intubation) may lead to arthritis of the TMJ. Pain, tenderness, and limitation of motion occur. Diagnosis is based primarily on history. X-ray results are negative except when intra-articular edema or hemorrhage widens the joint space. Treatment includes NSAIDs, application of heat, a soft diet, and restriction of jaw movement.

Osteoarthritis: The TMJ may be affected, usually in people > 50 yr. Occasionally, patients complain of stiffness, grating, or mild pain. Crepitation results from a hole worn through the disk, causing bone to grate on bone. Joint involvement is generally bilateral. X-rays may show flattening and lipping of the condyle, suggestive of dysfunctional change. Treatment is symptomatic.

Rheumatoid arthritis: The TMJ is affected in > 50% of adults and children with RA, but it is usually among the last joints affected. Pain, swelling, and limited movement are the most common findings. In children, destruction of the condyle results in mandibular growth disturbance and facial deformity. Ankylosis may follow. X-rays of the TMJ are usually negative in early stages but later show bone destruction, which may result in an anterior open-bite deformity. The diagnosis is suggested by TMJ inflammation associated with polyarthritis and is confirmed by other findings typical of the disease.

Treatment is similar to that of RA in other joints. In the acute stage, NSAIDs may be given, and jaw function should be restricted. A night guard or splint is often helpful. When symptoms subside, mild jaw exercises help prevent excessive loss of motion. Surgery is necessary if ankylosis develops but should not be performed until the condition is quiescent.

Secondary degenerative arthritis: This type of arthritis usually develops in people aged 20 to 40 after trauma or in people with persistent myofascial pain syndrome (see p. 865). It is characterized by limited opening of the mouth, unilateral pain during jaw movement, joint tenderness, and crepitation. When it is associated with the myofascial pain syndrome, symptoms wax and wane. Diagnosis is based on x-rays, which generally show condylar flattening, lipping, spurring, or erosion. Unilateral joint involvement helps distinguish secondary degenerative arthritis from osteoarthritis.

Treatment is conservative, as it is for myofascial pain syndrome, although arthroplasty or high condylectomy may be necessary. An occlusal splint (mouth guard) usually relieves symptoms. The splint is worn constantly, except during meals, oral hygiene, and appliance cleaning. When symptoms resolve, the length of time that the splint is worn each day is gradually reduced. Intra-articular injection of corticosteroids may relieve symptoms but may harm the joint if repeated often.

CONDYLAR HYPERPLASIA

Condylar hyperplasia is a disorder of unknown etiology characterized by persistent or accelerated growth of the condyle when growth should be slowing or ended. Growth eventually stops on its own.

Slowly progressive unilateral enlargement of the head and neck of the condyle causes crossbite malocclusion, facial asymmetry, and shifting of the midpoint of the chin to the unaffected side. The patient may appear prognathic. The lower border of the mandible is often convex on the affected side. Chondroma and osteochondroma may produce similar symptoms and signs, but they grow more rapidly and may cause even greater asymmetric condylar enlargement.

On x-ray, the temporomandibular joint may appear normal, or the condyle may be proportionally enlarged and the mandibular neck elongated. CT is usually performed to determine if bone growth is generalized, which confirms the diagnosis, or localized to part of the condylar head. If growth is localized, a biopsy may be necessary to distinguish between tumor and hyperplasia.

Treatment

Treatment usually includes condylectomy during the period of active growth. If growth has stopped, orthodontics and surgical mandibular repositioning are indicated. If the height of the mandibular body is greatly increased, facial symmetry can be further improved by reducing the inferior border.

CONDYLAR HYPOPLASIA

Condylar hypoplasia is facial deformity caused by a short mandibular ramus.

This condition usually results from trauma, infection, or irradiation occurring during the growth period but may be idiopathic. The deformity involves fullness of the face, deviation of the chin to the affected side, an elongated mandible, and flatness of the face on the unaffected side. Mandibular deviation causes malocclusion.

Diagnosis is based on a history of progressive facial asymmetry during the growth period, x-ray evidence of condylar deformity and antegonial notching (a depression in the inferior border of the mandible just anterior to the angle of the mandible), and, frequently, a causative history.

Treatment consists of surgical shortening of the unaffected side of the mandible or lengthening of the affected side. Presurgical orthodontic therapy helps optimize results.

INTERNAL JOINT DERANGEMENT

Internal joint derangement is anterior misalignment of the articular disk above the condyle. Symptoms are localized joint pain and popping on jaw movement. Diagnosis is based on history and physical examination. Treatment is with analgesics, jaw rest, muscle relaxation, physical therapy, and bite splinting. If these methods fail, surgery may be necessary. Early treatment greatly improves results.

The superior head of the lateral pterygoid muscle may pull the articular disk out of place when abnormal jaw mechanics place unusual stress on the joint. Abnormal jaw mechanics can be due to congenital or acquired asymmetries or to the sequelae of trauma or arthritis. If the disk remains anterior, the derangement is said to be without reduction. Restricted jaw opening (locked jaw) and pain in the ear and around the TMJ result. If at some point in the joint's excursion the disk returns to the head of the condyle, it is said to be with reduction. Derangement with reduction occurs in about ⅓ of the population at some point. All types of derangement can cause capsulitis (or synovitis), which is inflammation of the tissues surrounding the joint (eg, tendons, ligaments, connective tissue, synovium). Capsulitis can also occur spontaneously or result from arthritis, trauma, or infection.

Symptoms and Signs

Derangement with reduction often causes a clicking or popping sound when the mouth is opened. Pain may be present, particularly when chewing hard foods. Patients are often embarrassed because they think others can hear noise when they chew. Indeed, although the sound seems louder to the patient, others can sometimes hear it.

Derangement without reduction usually produces no sound, but maximum opening between the tips of the upper and lower incisors is reduced from the normal 40 to 45 mm to ≤ 30 mm. Pain and a change in the patient's perception of his bite generally result.

Capsulitis results in localized joint pain, tenderness, and, sometimes, restricted opening.

Diagnosis

Diagnosis of derangement with reduction requires observation of the jaw when the mouth is opened. When the jaw is opened > 10 mm, a click or pop is heard or a catch is felt as the disk pops back over the head of the condyle. The condyle remains on the disk during further opening. Usually, another click is heard during closing when the condyle slips over the posterior rim of the disk and the disk slips forward (reciprocal clicking).

Diagnosis of derangement without reduction requires that the patient open as wide as possible. The opening is measured, and gentle pressure is then exerted to open the mouth a little wider. Normally, the jaw opens about 45 to 50 mm; if the disk is deranged, it will open about 20 mm. Closing or protruding the jaw against resistance worsens the pain.

Capsulitis is often diagnosed based on a history of injury or infection along with exquisite tenderness over the joint and by exclusion when pain remains after treatment for myofascial pain syndrome, disk derangement, arthritis, and structural asymmetries. However, capsulitis may be present with any of the above.

Treatment

Derangement with reduction does not require treatment if the patient can open reasonably wide (about 40 mm or the width of the index, middle, and ring fingers) without discomfort. If pain occurs, mild analgesics, such as NSAIDs (ibuprofen 400 mg po q 6 h), can be used. If onset is < 6 mo, an anterior repositioning splint may be used to position the mandible forward and on the disk. The splint is a horseshoe-shaped appliance of hard, transparent acrylic (plastic) made to fit snugly over the teeth of one arch. Its chewing surface is designed to hold the mandible forward when the patient closes on the splint. In this position, the disk is always on the head of the condyle. The splint is gradually adjusted to allow the mandible to move posteriorly. If the disk stays with the condyle as the superior head of the external pterygoid stretches, the disk is said to be captured. The longer the disk is displaced, the more deformed it becomes and the less likely repositioning will succeed. Surgical plication of the disk may be performed, with variable success.

Derangement without reduction may not require treatment other than analgesics. Splints may help if the articular disk has not been significantly deformed, but long-term use may result in irreversible changes in oral architecture. In some cases, the patient is instructed to slowly stretch the disk out of position, which allows the jaw to open normally. Various arthroscopic and open surgical procedures are available when conservative treatment fails.

Capsulitis is initially treated with NSAIDs, jaw rest, and muscle relaxation. If these treatments are unsuccessful, corticosteroids may be injected into the joint, or arthroscopic joint lavage and debridement are used.

MYOFASCIAL PAIN SYNDROME

Myofascial pain syndrome can occur in patients with a normal temporomandibular joint. It is caused by tension, fatigue, or spasm in the masticatory muscles (medial or internal and lateral or external pterygoids, temporalis, and masseter). Symptoms include bruxism, pain and tenderness in and around the masticatory apparatus or referred to other locations in the head and neck, and, often, abnormalities of jaw mobility. Diagnosis is based on history and physical examination. Conservative treatment, including analgesics, muscle relaxation, habit modification, and bite splinting, usually is effective.

This syndrome is the most common disorder affecting the temporomandibular region. It is more common among women and has a bimodal age distribution in the early 20s and around menopause. The muscle spasm causing the disorder usually is the result of nocturnal bruxism (clenching or grinding of the teeth). Whether bruxism is caused by irregular tooth contacts, emotional stress, or sleep disorders is controversial. Bruxism usually has a multifactorial etiology. Myofascial pain syndrome is not limited to the muscles of mastication. It can occur anywhere in the body, most commonly involving muscles in the neck and back.

Symptoms, Signs, and Diagnosis

Symptoms include pain and tenderness of the masticatory muscles and often pain and limitation of jaw excursion. Nocturnal bruxism may lead to headache that is more severe on awakening and that gradually subsides during the day. Such pain should be distinguished from temporal arteritis. Daytime symptoms, including headache, may worsen if bruxism continues throughout the day.

The jaw deviates when the mouth opens but usually not as suddenly or always at the same point of opening as it does with internal joint derangement. Exerting gentle pressure, the examiner can open the patient's mouth another 1 to 3 mm beyond unaided maximum opening.

A simple test may aid the diagnosis: Tongue blades of 2 or 3 thicknesses are placed between the rear molars on each side, and the patient is asked to bite down gently. The distraction produced in the joint space may ease the symptoms. X-rays usually do not help except to rule out arthritis. If temporal arteritis is suspected, ESR is measured.

Treatment

A plastic splint or mouth guard from the dentist can keep teeth from contacting each other and prevent the damages of bruxism. Comfortable, heat moldable splints are available from many sporting goods stores or drugstores. Low doses of a benzodiazepine at bedtime are often effective for acute exacerbations and temporary relief of symptoms. Mild analgesics, such as NSAIDs or acetaminophen, are indicated. Because the condition is chronic, opioids should not be used, except perhaps briefly for acute exacerbations. The patient must learn to stop clenching the jaw and grinding the teeth. Hard-to-chew foods and chewing gum should be avoided. Physical therapy, biofeedback to encourage relaxation, and counseling help some patients. Physical modalities include transcutaneous electric nerve stimulation and "spray and stretch," in which the jaw is stretched open after the skin over the painful area has been chilled with ice or sprayed with a skin refrigerant, such as ethyl chloride. Botulinum toxin has recently been used successfully to relieve muscle spasm in myofascial pain syndrome. Most patients, even if untreated, stop having significant symptoms within 2 to 3 yr.

SECTION 9
EYE DISORDERS

98 APPROACH TO THE OPHTHALMOLOGIC PATIENT

Examination of the eye can be undertaken with routine equipment, including a standard ophthalmoscope; thorough examination requires special equipment and evaluation by an ophthalmologist. (See FIG. 98–1 for a cross-section of the eye.)

History

History provides information on the location, speed of onset, duration, and history of previous ocular symptoms; the presence and nature of pain, discharge, or redness; and changes in visual acuity. Worrisome symptoms besides vision loss and eye pain include flashing lights, showers of floaters (both of which are symptoms of retinal detachment), diplopia, and loss of peripheral vision.

Physical Examination

Visual acuity: The first step is to record visual acuity. Patients who require corrective lenses should wear them during testing. However, testing can be performed in patients who are not wearing or who do not require corrective lenses by having them look through a pinhole device (a paddle with multiple pinholes or an index card with an array of 18-gauge needle punctures); these holes focus light rays and compensate for refractive error. Visual acuity in each eye is tested as the opposite eye is covered. Vision is tested by having the patient look at an eye chart 20 ft (6 m) away. Normal and abnormal vision is quantified by

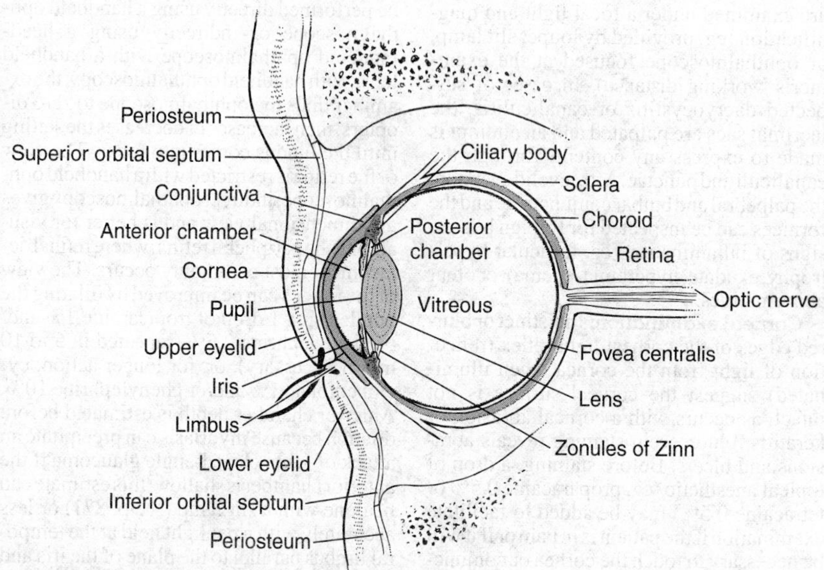

Fig. 98–1. Cross-section of the eye. The zonules of Zinn keep the lens suspended, and the muscles of the ciliary body focus the lens. The ciliary body also secretes aqueous humor, which fills the anterior and posterior chambers, passes through the pupil into the anterior chamber, and drains primarily via Schlemm's canal (see FIG. 103–1 on p. 905). The iris regulates light entering the eye by adjusting the size of its central opening, the pupil. Visual images are focused on the retina. The fovea centralis is the area of sharpest visual acuity. The conjunctiva covers the eyeball and lines the upper and lower lids; it ends at the limbus. The cornea is covered with an epithelium that differs in many respects from the conjunctival epithelium.

Snellen notation. A Snellen notation of 20/40 (6/12) indicates that the smallest letter that can be read by someone with normal vision at 40 ft (12 m) has to be brought to 20 ft (6 m) before it is recognized by the patient. Near vision is checked by asking the patient to read a standard "near card" or newsprint at 14 in (35 cm); patients > 40 yr who require corrective lenses (reading glasses) should wear them during near vision testing.

Refractive error can be roughly estimated with a handheld ophthalmoscope by noting the lens necessary for the examiner to focus on the retina; this procedure requires the examiner to use his own corrective lenses and is never a substitute for a comprehensive assessment of refraction. More commonly, refractive error is measured with a standard phoropter or an automated refractor (a device that measures changes in light projected and reflected by the patient's eye). These devices also measure astigmatism (see p. 881).

Eyelid and conjunctival examination: Eyelid margins and subcutaneous tissues are examined under a focal light and magnification (eg, provided by loupe, slit lamp, or ophthalmoscope focused at the examiner's working distance). In cases of suspected dacryocystitis or canaliculitis, the lacrimal sacs are palpated and an attempt is made to express any contents through the canaliculi and punctae. After eyelid eversion, the palpebral and bulbar conjunctivae and the fornices can be inspected for foreign bodies, signs of inflammation (eg, follicular hypertrophy, exudate, hyperemia, edema), or other abnormalities.

Corneal examination: Indistinct or blurred edges of the corneal light reflex (reflection of light from the cornea when illuminated) suggest the corneal surface is not intact, as occurs with a corneal abrasion or keratitis. Fluorescein staining reveals abrasions and ulcers. Before staining, a drop of topical anesthetic (eg, proparacaine 0.5% or tetracaine 0.5%) may be added to facilitate examination if the patient is in pain or if it will be necessary to touch the cornea or conjunctiva (eg, to remove a foreign body or measure intraocular pressure). A sterile, individually packaged fluorescein strip is moistened with 1 drop of sterile saline or topical anesthetic and, with the patient's eye turned upward, is touched momentarily to the inside of the lower eyelid. The patient blinks several times to spread the dye into the tear film, and then the eye is examined under magnification and cobalt blue illumination. Areas where corneal or conjunctival epithelium is absent (abraded or ulcerated) fluoresce green.

Pupil examination: The size and shape of the pupils are noted, and pupillary reaction to light is tested by quickly moving a penlight back and forth by each eye (swinging flashlight test). Normal response under illumination is bilateral (consensual) pupillary constriction; pupillary enlargement without consensual constriction is a sign of afferent papillary defect (Marcus Gunn pupil), indicating ipsilateral optic nerve dysfunction or extensive retinal disease.

Extraocular muscles: The examiner guides the patient to look in 8 directions (up, up and right, right, down and right, down, down and left, left, left and up) with a moving finger, observing for gaze deviation, limitation of movement, and/or dysconjugate gaze consistent with cranial nerve palsy, orbital disease, or other abnormalities that restrict movement.

Ophthalmoscopy: Ophthalmoscopy can be performed directly using a handheld ophthalmoscope or indirectly using a head-mounted ophthalmoscope with a handheld lens. With handheld ophthalmoscopy, the examiner dials the ophthalmoscope to zero diopters, then increases or decreases the setting until the fundus comes into focus. The view of the retina is restricted with a handheld ophthalmoscope; indirect ophthalmoscopy gives a 3-dimensional view and is better for visualizing the peripheral retina, where retinal detachment most commonly occurs. The view of the fundus can be improved by dilating the pupils using 1 drop of tropicamide 1% and/or phenylephrine 2.5% (repeated in 5 to 10 min if necessary), or, for longer action, cyclopentolate 1% and/or phenylephrine 10%. Anterior chamber depth is estimated before dilation because mydriasis can precipitate an attack of acute closed-angle glaucoma if the anterior chamber is shallow; this estimate can be done with a slit lamp (see p. 871) or less accurately with a penlight held at the temporal limbus parallel to the plane of the iris and pointed toward the nose. If the medial iris is in shadow, then the chamber is shallow and dilation should be avoided. Other contraindications to dilation include head trauma, suspicion of a ruptured globe, a narrow angle, or closed-angle glaucoma.

Ophthalmoscopy can detect lens or vitreous opacities, assess the optic cup-to-disk ratio, and identify retinal and vascular changes.

The optic cup is the central depression and the optic disk is the entire area of the optic nerve; an increase in the ratio of the cup-to-nerve areas signifies loss of ganglion cells and is increased in glaucoma. Retinal changes include hemorrhage, manifested as small or large areas of blood, and drusen (small subretinal yellow-white spots that signify dry age-related macular degeneration). Vascular changes include arteriovenous nicking, a sign of chronic hypertension in which retinal veins are compressed by arteries where the two cross; copper wiring, a sign of arteriosclerosis in which thickened arteriolar walls increase the thickness of the light reflex; silver wiring, a sign of hypertension in which thin, fibrotic arteriolar walls decrease the thickness of the light reflex; and loss of venous pulsations, a sign of increased intracranial pressure in patients known to have had pulsations previously.

Slit-lamp examination: A slit lamp focuses the height and width of a beam of light for a precise stereoscopic view of the eyelids, conjunctivae, cornea, anterior chamber, iris, lens, and anterior vitreous. It is especially useful for identifying corneal foreign bodies and abrasions and for measuring the depth of and identifying inflammation or cells in the anterior chamber. It can also identify ciliary flush, inflammation localized to the limbal region over the ciliary body seen with uveitis; and scleral edema, seen as a bowing forward of the slit beam when it is focused beneath the conjunctiva and usually a sign of scleritis. Tonometry (see below) and gonioscopy, which quantifies the iridocorneal angle and requires the use of a special lens, may be performed.

Visual field testing: Visual fields may be impaired by lesions anywhere in the neural visual pathways from the optic nerves to the occipital lobes (see TABLE 98–1 and FIG. 107–1 on p. 922). Glaucoma causes loss of peripheral vision. Fields can be assessed by direct confrontation testing or more formal methods. In direct confrontation, the patient maintains a fixed gaze at the examiner's eye or nose. The examiner brings a small target (eg, a match or a finger) from the patient's visual periphery into each of the 4 visual quadrants and asks the patient to indicate when he first sees the object. Each eye is tested separately. Abnormalities in target detection should prompt formal testing with more precise instruments. More formal methods include use of a "tangent screen," Goldmann perimeter, or computerized automated perimetry (in which the visual field is constructed quickly by a computer based on the patient's response to flashing lights). The Amsler grid is used to test central vision. Findings of distortion of the grid (metamorphopsia) may indicate choroidal neovascularization.

Color vision testing: Twelve to 24 Ishihara color plates, which have numbers or symbols hidden in a field of colored dots, are commonly used to test color vision. Color-blind patients or those with acquired color deficiency (eg, in optic nerve diseases) cannot see some or all of the hidden numbers. Most congenital color blindness is red-green; most acquired (eg, from glaucoma or optic nerve disease) is blue-yellow.

Testing

Tonometry: Tonometry measures intraocular pressure by determining the amount of force needed to indent the cornea. Handheld pen-type tonometers are used for screening. It requires topical anesthesia (eg, proparacaine 0.5%). Office-based screening with noncontact "air-puff" tonometry can also be used; it requires less training because it makes no direct corneal contact. Goldmann applanation tonometry is the most accurate method but requires more training and is typically used only by ophthalmologists. Measurement of intraocular pressure is not adequate screening for glaucoma.

Fluorescein angiography: After IV injection of fluorescein solution, the retinal, choroidal, optic disk, or iris vasculature is photographed in rapid sequence. Fluorescein angiography is used to investigate underperfusion and neovascularization in conditions such as diabetes, age-related macular degeneration, retinal vascular occlusion, and ocular histoplasmosis. It is also useful in preoperative assessment for retinal laser procedures.

Electroretinography: Electrodes are placed on each cornea and on the surrounding skin, and electrical activity in the retina is recorded. This technique determines retinal function in patients with retinal degeneration. It does not evaluate vision.

Ultrasonography: B-mode ultrasonography provides 2-dimensional structural information even in the presence of opacities of the cornea and lens. Examples of ophthalmologic applications include assessment of retinal tumors, detachments, and vitreous hemorrhages; location of foreign bodies; detection of posterior scleral edema characteristic of

TABLE 98–1. TYPES OF FIELD DEFECTS

TYPE	DESCRIPTION	CAUSES
Altitudinal field defect	Loss of all or part of the superior or inferior half of the visual field, but in no case does the defect cross the horizontal median	*More common*: Ischemic optic neuropathy, hemibranch retinal artery occlusion, retinal detachment *Less common*: Glaucoma, optic nerve or chiasmal lesion, optic nerve coloboma
Arcuate scotoma	A small, arcuate-shaped field loss due to damage to the ganglion cells that feed into a particular part of the optic nerve head, which follows the arcuate shape of the nerve fiber pattern; the defect does not cross the horizontal median	*More common*: Glaucoma *Less common*: Ischemic optic neuropathy (especially nonarteritic), optic disk drusen, high myopia
Binasal field defect (uncommon)	Loss of all or part of the medial half of both visual fields; the defect does not cross the vertical median	*More common*: Glaucoma, bitemporal retinal disease (eg, retinitis pigmentosa) *Rare*: Bilateral occipital disease, tumor or aneurysm compressing both optic nerves
Bitemporal hemianopia	Loss of all or part of the lateral half of both visual fields; the defect does not cross the vertical median	*More common*: Chiasmal lesion (eg, pituitary adenoma, meningioma, craniopharyngioma, aneurysm, glioma) *Less common*: Tilted optic disks *Rare*: Nasal retinitis pigmentosa
Blind-spot enlargement	Enlargement of the normal blind spot at the optic nerve head	Papilledema, optic nerve drusen, optic nerve coloboma, myelinated nerve fibers at the optic disk, drugs, myopic disk with a crescent
Central scotoma	A loss of visual function in the middle of the visual field, typically affecting the fovea centralis	Macular disease; optic neuropathy (eg, ischemic, Leber's hereditary, optic neuritis); optic atrophy (eg, from tumor compressing the nerve, toxic/metabolic disease); rarely, an occipital cortex lesion
Homonymous hemianopia	Loss of part or all of the left half or right half of both visual fields; the defect does not cross the vertical median	Optic tract or lateral geniculate body lesion; temporal, parietal, or occipital lobe lesion of the brain (stroke and tumor more common; aneurysm and trauma less common). Migraine may cause a transient homonymous hemianopia
Constriction of the peripheral fields leaving only a small residual central field	Loss of the outer part of the entire visual field in one or both eyes	Glaucoma; retinitis pigmentosa or some other peripheral retinal disorder; chronic papilledema; after panretinal photocoagulation; central retinal artery occlusion with cilioretinal artery sparing; bilateral occipital lobe infarction with macular sparing; nonphysiologic vision loss; carcinoma-associated retinopathy; rarely, drugs

Adapted from *The Wills Eye Manual*, Douglas J. Rhee, M.D. and Mark F. Pyfer, M.D.© 1999 by Lippincott Williams & Wilkins.

posterior scleritis; and distinction of choroidal melanoma from metastatic carcinoma and subretinal hemorrhage. A-mode ultrasonography is 1-dimensional ultrasound used to determine the axial length of the eye, a measurement needed to calculate the power of an intraocular lens before it is implanted. Ultrasonic pachymetry is use of ultrasound to measure the thickness of the cornea before refractive surgery (eg, LASIK) and in patients with corneal dystrophies.

CT and MRI: These imaging techniques are most often used for evaluation of ocular trauma, particularly if an intraocular foreign body is suspected, and in the evaluation of orbital tumors, optic neuritis, and optic nerve tumors. MRI should not be performed when there is suspicion of intraocular foreign body.

Electronystagmography: See p. 775.

ACUTE VISION LOSS

Vision loss may be acute or gradual; gradual vision loss is caused by multiple processes, including cataracts, glaucoma, and atrophic age-related macular degeneration. Vision loss may also be partial or complete; partial vision loss presents as visual field defects and has a variety of manifestations and causes (see TABLE 98–1).

Acute vision loss may be due to central retinal artery or vein occlusion (including artery occlusion caused by temporal arteritis), optic neuritis or neuropathy, vitreous hemorrhage, retinal detachment, neovascular age-related macular degeneration, stroke, or functional disorders (eg, hysterical conversion reactions or malingering). In some instances, acute vision loss may last only minutes to hours (amaurosis fugax); causes include ocular migraine, emboli to retinal arteries, and transient ischemic attacks.

Sudden, unilateral, painless complete vision loss suggests central retinal artery or vein occlusion, embolus, ischemic optic neuropathy, vitreous hemorrhage, retinal detachment, or optic neuritis, although optic neuritis may cause pain on eye movement. Painful loss may be due to acute closed-angle glaucoma, uveitis, or, rarely, corneal hydrops. A unilateral curtain or window shade being drawn down suggests retinal detachment or a progressive vasculature problem, such as branch retinal artery occlusion. Complex, continuous, shimmering or flashing lights (scintillating scotoma) or kaleidoscopic phenomena that obscure vision in both eyes but that clear after about 20 min suggest migraine headache. Bilateral visual field loss, sometimes with additional neurologic symptoms and duration of < 24 h, suggests a transient ischemic attack of the visual cortex.

The patient requires a complete ophthalmologic examination, including tests of visual acuity, peripheral vision and the presence and shape of any field defects, slit-lamp examination, and gonioscopy (if angle closure is suspected). A specific field defect can indicate the location of a visual pathway lesion (see FIG. 98–1). Flare and cells in the anterior chamber suggest uveitis; a swollen and opacified cornea suggests corneal hydrops; high intraocular pressure with a mid-dilated pupil suggests acute closed-angle glaucoma. On dilated fundus examination, localized retinal whitening suggests branch retinal vein occlusion; whitening of the entire retina suggests central retinal vein occlusion and may be accompanied by a macular cherry-red spot. A swollen optic nerve with or without surrounding flame-shaped hemorrhage signifies optic neuritis. Findings of vitreous hemorrhage or retinal detachment are diagnostic.

Additional testing may be necessary depending on examination findings; ESR should be performed to exclude temporal arteritis, and fluorescein angiography may be indicated to document retinal vein occlusion.

Treatment is management of the underlying condition.

ANISOCORIA

(Unequal Pupils)

Anisocoria is usually physiologic, causes no symptoms, and does not impair normal pupillary light response. Abnormal causes include Horner's syndrome (congenital, traumatic, postsurgical, or due to migraine, stroke, lung tumors, or demyelinating diseases), Adie's pupil (idiopathic impaired constriction), 3rd cranial nerve palsy, uveitis (idiopathic or due to systemic disease), syphilis (Argyll Robertson pupil), and mydriatic drugs. Anticholinergic drugs used in sea-sickness patches (eg, scopolamine) or animal flea collars or sprays can cause mydriasis if they contact the eye, as can insecticides.

Physical examination of patients with anisocoria should be performed in lighted and dark rooms. If the difference in size is greater in light, the larger pupil is abnormal;

causes include Adie's pupil, traumatic damage to the iris, 3rd cranial nerve palsy, and drugs. If the difference in size is greater in the dark, the smaller pupil is abnormal and likely to be physiologic or a sign of Horner's syndrome. The cause of either can be distinguished by an ophthalmologist using miotic or sympathomimetic drops and by measuring pupillary reaction to accommodation.

BLURRED VISION

Blurred vision is the most common ophthalmologic complaint and can mean general visual dimming (which in an extreme form becomes blindness), reduced field of vision, or distortion of vision.

The most common causes are refractive error, cataracts, glaucoma, diabetic retinopathy, and age-related macular degeneration; less common causes include retinal detachment, optic neuritis or neuropathy, stroke, retinal vascular occlusion, uveitis, and keratitis.

It is important to determine if blurred vision affects one or both eyes, if pupils are normal or an afferent pupillary defect (APD) is present, and if corrective lenses (or pinhole visual acuity testing) improves vision. Monocular blurring with an APD suggests optic neuritis, neuropathy, or atrophy. Binocular blurring with improvement of visual acuity with pinhole testing suggests refractive error. Other variants (monocular blurring with normal pupils, binocular blurring without pinhole improvement) suggest other causes.

Follow-up testing may include tonometry (for glaucoma), fluorescein angiography (for age-related macular degeneration, branch retinal vein occlusion/central retinal vein occlusion, diabetic retinopathy), and MRI (for optic neuritis, stroke).

Most patients have some measure of refractive error and respond to corrective lenses, but other underlying causes must also be treated.

DIPLOPIA

(Double Vision)

Combination of images from each eye into a single image (fusion) requires intact, bilaterally coordinated extraocular movements. Diplopia, or double vision, may be monocular or binocular. Monocular diplopia is present with only one eye open; binocular diplopia disappears when either eye is closed. Causes of monocular diplopia include cataract, refractive error (most often astigmatism), corneal scarring, dislocated lens, keratoconus, and retinal detachment. Binocular diplopia almost always suggests dysconjugate alignment of the eyes. Causes of intermittent binocular diplopia include myasthenia gravis and latent eye deviation (phoria) that becomes uncompensated. Causes of constant binocular diplopia include palsy of the 3rd, 4th, or 6th cranial nerves; orbital disease (eg, thyroid eye disease, tumor, pseudotumor); or CNS abnormalities (vertebrobasilar insufficiency, internuclear ophthalmoplegia).

History should determine if diplopia involves one or both eyes intermittently or constantly and if the images are separated vertically, horizontally, or a combination of both. Diplopia must also be distinguished from blurriness.

Vision in each eye should be checked with the other eye covered to determine if the diplopia is monocular or binocular. Examination should note presence of eyelid droop, pupillary abnormalities, or dysconjugate eye movement during extraocular muscle testing.

Ocular motility is checked by having the patient hold his head steady and having the patient track the examiner's finger, which is moved to extreme gaze to the right, left, upward, downward, diagonally to either side, and finally inward toward the patient's nose. Mild paresis of ocular motility sufficient to cause diplopia may escape detection by such examination. If diplopia occurs in one direction of gaze, the eye that produces each image can be determined by repeating the examination with a red glass placed over one of the patient's eyes. The image that is more peripheral originates in the paretic eye; eg, if the more peripheral image is red, the red glass is covering the paretic eye. If a red glass is not available, the paretic eye can sometimes be identified by having the patient close each eye; the eye that, when closed, eliminates the more peripheral image, is paretic. If the paretic eye is recognized but it is unclear whether the eye is esotropic (crossed in) or exotropic (crossed out), a red glass can be placed in front of the paretic eye. If the paretic eye is esotropic, the red light appears to the right of the white light. If the paretic eye is exotropic, the red light appears to the left of the white light.

Specific maneuvers (eg Park's 3-step, which compares eye alignment in different positions; the Hess screen and Lancaster red-green tests, which assess patient responses to dissimilar images produced by special glasses; and double Maddox rod testing, which assesses degree of rotation of striated lenses necessary to make lens lines appear parallel) can be performed to identify the involved muscle(s) and/or cranial nerve(s).

Follow-up testing may include corneal topography (measurement of corneal shape) to identify keratoconus; phorometry (testing of ocular muscle balance) to detect phoria; exophthalmometry (measurement of the amount of protrusion of the eyeball) to measure exophthalmos; CT or MRI to detect orbital disease or CNS abnormalities; and blood testing for thyroid dysfunction and diabetes, which underlie some cranial nerve palsies.

Treatment is management of the underlying cause.

EYELID SWELLING

The most common causes of eyelid swelling are allergy, which may be local (contact sensitivity) or systemic (eg, angioedema or accompanying allergic rhinitis), and chalazia. Less common inflammatory and infectious causes include blepharitis, conjunctivitis, preseptal or orbital cellulitis, cavernous sinus thrombosis, dacryoadenitis and canaliculitis, trauma and burns, and trichiasis. Less common noninflammatory causes include prolapse of orbital fat, eyelid laxity, hypothyroidism, and fluid retention (eg, with pregnancy and cardiac and renal disease).

History of atopy, acute onset, and/or itching suggests an allergic cause. Foreign body sensation suggests blepharitis. Fever and pain suggest preseptal or orbital cellulitis. Physicians should elicit information about systemic illnesses, recent eye injury or surgery, and drug use (especially ACE inhibitors).

Examination should determine if warmth, erythema, and pain are present and if swelling is unilateral or bilateral. Bilateral painless swelling without erythema suggests allergy, systemic disease, or orbital fat herniation. Bilateral painless swelling with erythema suggests blepharitis, conjunctivitis, or burns, although these disorders may cause unilateral swelling too. Unilateral painless swelling with erythema suggests an insect bite, preseptal cellulitis, or disorder of the lacrimal system (eg, canaliculitis or dacryoadenitis). Unilateral painful swelling with erythema suggests orbital cellulitis.

In most cases, diagnosis can be established clinically, and no testing is necessary. Exceptions include trauma, cellulitis, cavernous sinus thrombosis, and systemic diseases, for which imaging and laboratory tests may be necessary.

For allergic eyelid edema, avoidance of the allergen combined, if needed, with cold compresses and topical corticosteroids (eg, fluorometholone 0.1% ointment tid for not more than 7 days) or systemic antihistamines is often the only treatment needed. Treatment of other underlying causes is discussed elsewhere in THE MANUAL.

EYE PAIN

Surface pain is experienced as scratchiness or a foreign body sensation and is most often caused by disorders of the eyelids, conjunctivae, or cornea. Deeper pain, often described as aching or throbbing, may be serious and demands investigation. Causes of deep eye pain include glaucoma, uveitis, scleritis, endophthalmitis, orbital cellulitis, and orbital pseudotumor. Rarely, uncorrected refractive error and accommodative dysfunction cause dull pain. Migraine and sinusitis occasionally cause referred eye pain.

Pain associated with headache, nausea or vomiting, and halos suggests closed-angle glaucoma. Pain associated with photophobia and ciliary flush suggests uveitis. A boring pain that awakens a patient from sleep suggests scleritis. Pain with markedly reduced vision and a history of recent eye surgery suggests endophthalmitis.

A cloudy (eg, translucent) cornea with a pupil dilated to 5 to 6 mm and high intraocular pressure suggest closed-angle glaucoma. Findings of anterior chamber cell and flare on slit-lamp examination are diagnostic of uveitis. Scleral edema is suggestive of scleritis. Purulent discharge, WBCs in the anterior chamber (hypopyon), and vitreal inflammation with history of recent eye surgery suggest endophthalmitis. Pain, exophthalmos, and intraorbital inflammation on CT suggest orbital pseudotumor.

Patients should undergo tonometry and gonioscopy if appropriate. Slit-lamp examination can demonstrate anterior scleral edema (anterior scleritis), whereas B-mode ultrasound can demonstrate posterior scleral edema (posterior scleritis). CT is indicated to investigate suspected orbital pseudotumor.

Aspiration and culture of vitreous fluid is used to diagnose endophthalmitis.

Treatment is management of underlying conditions, but mild analgesics (eg, NSAIDs, acetaminophen) may be useful. When diagnostic testing excludes serious disorders, patients with refractive errors or accommodative dysfunction may respond to corrective lenses.

EXOPHTHALMOS

(Proptosis)

Exophthalmos is protrusion of the eyeball. The most common cause is Graves' disease, which causes edema and lymphoid infiltration of the orbital tissues. Other causes are orbital tumors (eg, lymphoma, hemangioma, vascular malformations), inflammatory conditions (eg, orbital cellulitis), carotid-cavernous sinus or dural-cavernous sinus fistula, cavernous sinus thrombosis, trauma, eyeball enlargement (as in congenital glaucoma and unilateral high myopia), retrobulbar hemorrhage, and spheno-orbital meningioma. Hyperthyroidism without infiltrative eye disease, Cushing's disease, severe obesity, and orbital diseases may cause changes in the appearance of the face and eyes that resemble exophthalmos but are not.

Symptoms of Graves' eye disease may include pain, lacrimation, dry eyes, irritation, photophobia, ocular muscle weakness causing diplopia, and vision loss caused by optic nerve compression; systemic symptoms include palpitations, anxiety, increased appetite, weight loss, and insomnia (see p. 1195).

Sudden unilateral onset suggests intraorbital hemorrhage (which can occur after surgery, retrobulbar injection, or trauma) or inflammation of the orbit or paranasal sinuses. A 2- to 3-wk onset suggests chronic inflammation or orbital inflammatory pseudotumor (non-neoplastic cellular infiltration and proliferation); slower onset suggests an orbital tumor.

Findings typical of hyperthyroidism but unrelated to infiltrative eye disease include eyelid retraction, eyelid lag, temporal flare of the upper eyelid, and staring. Other signs include eyelid erythema and conjunctival infection. Prolonged exposure causes corneal drying and can lead to infection and ulceration. Fever suggests orbital cellulitis or cavernous sinus thrombosis. Pulsating exophthalmos with an orbital bruit suggests a carotid-cavernous sinus or dural-cavernous sinus fistula. Unilateral disease suggests a nonthyroid cause, although Graves' disease occasionally causes unilateral exophthalmos.

Exophthalmos can be confirmed with exophthalmometry, which measures the distance between the lateral angle of the bony orbit and the cornea; normal values are < 20 mm in whites and < 22 mm in blacks. CT or MRI is often useful to confirm the diagnosis and to identify structural causes of unilateral exophthalmos. Thyroid function testing is indicated when Graves' disease is suspected.

Lubrication to protect the cornea is required in severe cases. When lubrication is not sufficient, surgery to provide better coverage of the eye surface or to reduce the exophthalmos may be required. Systemic corticosteroids (eg, prednisone 1 mg/kg po once/day for 1 wk, tapered over ≥ 1 mo) are often helpful in controlling edema and orbital congestion from both thyroid eye disease and inflammatory orbital pseudotumor. Other interventions vary by etiology. Graves' exophthalmos is not affected by treatment of the thyroid condition but may lessen over time. Tumors must be surgically removed. Selective embolization or, rarely, trapping procedures may be effective in cases of arteriovenous fistulas involving the cavernous sinus.

FLOATERS

Floaters are opaque shapes, often cell- or strand-like, that move across the visual field. They may be unilateral or bilateral. They may shift or maintain their relative position with eye movement and are typically most noticeable against a plain background (eg, a wall or window or the sky).

Chronic stable floaters are common and are caused by idiopathic condensation of vitreous protein and collagen. These floaters tend to become less noticeable and less bothersome with time. They rarely indicate disease. Acute showers of floaters occur with vitreous hemorrhage or detachment or with retinal tears or detachment. Floaters that fall between chronic stable and acute in number and frequency may result from cellular debris in the vitreous caused by vitritis (inflammation in the vitreous), uveitis, or tumor (masquerade syndrome).

Showers of "sparks" or lightning flashes (photopsia) that accompany a shower of floaters suggest retinal detachment, as does perception of a curtain of visual loss moving across the visual field.

Floaters, flashes of light, or changes in the visual field of recent onset or those that increase in severity or frequency warrant meticulous examination of the entire retina after dilation; indirect ophthalmoscopy is used to look for posterior vitreous detachment, retinal tears or detachment, or vitreous hemorrhage.

Indirect ophthalmoscopy is usually adequate for detecting or excluding a serious underlying cause, but in cases where vitreous hemorrhage obscures the view of part of the retina, B-mode ultrasound can exclude retinal detachment.

Chronic stable floaters are of no clinical significance, require no treatment, and eventually become less noticeable. Treatment of retinal tears and detachment is described on p. 920.

RED EYE

(Pink Eye)

Red eye is caused by dilated conjunctival vessels or subconjunctival hemorrhage. The most common cause is infectious or allergic conjunctivitis; the most serious cause is closed-angle glaucoma, followed by uveitis, corneal ulcers, and scleritis (see TABLE 98–2). Other causes include foreign bodies, trauma, episcleritis, keratitis, retrobulbar processes (often also causing exophthalmos), hordeola, and subconjunctival hemorrhage.

Red eye usually coexists with pain, headache, or nausea and vomiting when caused by closed-angle glaucoma. It often coexists with discharge and crusting when caused by infectious conjunctivitis. Abrupt onset of red eye alone suggests trauma or direct eye irritation. Preauricular lymphadenopathy suggests viral conjunctivitis. Itching and watery discharge suggest allergic conjunctivitis. Scratchiness or a foreign body sensation suggests corneal abrasion, conjunctivitis, or keratoconjunctivitis sicca. A deep ache may also indicate scleritis. Halos or rainbow-like fringes suggest corneal edema. Photophobia suggests a corneal abrasion, corneal ulcer, or uveitis.

Diminished visual acuity suggests significant pathology, including glaucoma, corneal ulcer, hyphema from trauma, and uveitis. Discharge suggests allergic or viral (watery) or bacterial (purulent) conjunctivitis. Exophthalmos suggests a retrobulbar process, such as an abscess, orbital tumor, or Graves' disease. An irregular corneal light reflex suggests corneal edema, possibly due to acute closed-angle glaucoma, or a damaged corneal surface, possibly due to abrasion or keratitis. Ciliary flush suggests uveitis, glaucoma, or keratitis. Elevated intraocular pressure is diagnostic of glaucoma. Pupil irregularity or a midpoint fixed pupil may be due to uveitis or glaucoma (or to a neuro-ophthalmic problem).

No tests are necessary for patients with features strongly suggestive of allergic or viral conjunctivitis or subconjunctival hemorrhage. Others should generally undergo slit-lamp examination, tonometry, and fluorescein staining. CT or ultrasound is indicated to evaluate a suspected foreign body or, more rarely, to identify intraocular or orbital pathology.

Treatment is management of the underlying condition. Redness itself is rarely treated (eg, with vasoconstrictors) without a specific diagnosis.

TEARING

(Epiphora)

Tearing may be caused by excess production or decreased drainage of tears (see TABLE 98–3 and FIG. 98–2).

Excess production occurs most commonly with irritation, such as from a foreign body (including inturned eyelashes) or corneal epithelial defect; with allergic rhinitis or conjunctivitis; as a reflex reaction to the sensation of irritation caused by dry eyes; and with the common cold. In newborns, congenital glaucoma and congenital nasolacrimal duct obstruction are causes.

Decreased drainage has multiple causes; primary categories are nasolacrimal obstruction, punctal stenosis, and eyelid abnormalities.

Nasolacrimal obstruction may be congenital or acquired. In congenital obstruction, a membrane at the distal end of the nasolacrimal duct persists, causing tearing and purulent discharge; the condition may present as chronic conjunctivitis.

Acquired nasolacrimal duct obstruction is most often a result of age-related stenosis of the nasolacrimal duct. Other causes include past nasal or facial bone fractures or sinus surgery, which disrupt the nasolacrimal duct; inflammatory diseases (eg, sarcoidosis, Wegener's granulomatosis); and dacryocystitis (see p. 880).

TABLE 98–2. DIFFERENTIAL DIAGNOSIS OF RED EYE

DIAGNOSTIC FEATURE	INFECTIOUS KERATITIS OR CONJUNCTIVITIS	UVEITIS	CORNEAL ULCER	CLOSED-ANGLE GLAUCOMA	EPISCLERITIS/ SCLERITIS	TRAUMA
Pain	Burning but not severe	Moderately severe ache; photophobia	Can be severe	Very severe ache; associated with nausea and emesis	Episcleritis: irritation Scleritis: severe ache	Usually severe ache or foreign body sensation
Vision	Normal	Moderately decreased	Can be severely decreased	Considerably decreased	Usually normal; can be decreased in posterior scleritis	Usually markedly blurred
Intraocular pressure	Normal	Usually normal or low, occasionally increased	Usually normal	Increased	Normal	May be normal, increased, or decreased
Lacrimation or discharge	Mucous or mucopurulent	Lacrimation	Purulent	Lacrimation	Lacrimation	Lacrimation
Hyperemia	Superficial conjunctival hyperemia of globe and eyelids	Circumcorneal	Diffuse	Circumcorneal and episcleral	Large patch (20–100%) of bulbar hyperemia	Diffuse (hemorrhagic)
Appearance of cornea	Normal	Transparent precipitates may be present on posterior surface	Infiltrate with overlying epithelial defect	Cloudy	Normal	If corneal injury, may be hazy
Anterior chamber	Normal depth	Normal depth	May have sterile hypopyon	Very shallow	Normal depth	Normal depth, may contain blood
Appearance of iris	Normal	Dull and swollen	May have vascular congestion	Congested and bulging	Normal	May be obscured by blood or lacerated
Pupils	Normal	Small, irregular	Normal	Mid-dilated, unreactive	Normal	May be large, normal, small, or irregular
Pupillary response to light	Normal	Minimal	Normal	Minimal	Normal	Usually minimal

Punctal or canalicular stenosis physically prevents tears from entering the canalicular system, causing tears to drain down the cheek. Causes include chronic conjunctivitis, especially herpetic; certain types of chemotherapy; adverse reactions to eyedrops (especially topical echothiophate iodide); and radiation.

Ectropion and entropion are eyelid disorders that cause tearing; with both, the punctum inverts or everts with the eyelid and no longer properly drains tears. In addition, with entropion, the eyelashes rub against the cornea, stimulating excessive tear production. Ectropion and entropion may also cause dry eyes (see p. 887).

Symptoms and Signs

Symptoms that accompany tearing may help narrow the differential diagnosis. Itching suggests an allergic cause; nasal pain suggests dacryocystitis; constant foreign body sensation suggests a corneal foreign body, corneal abrasion, corneal ulcer, or trichiasis; intermittent foreign body sensation suggests dry eyes; other symptoms (eg, photophobia) suggest uveitis or keratitis. In newborns, conjunctivitis causes onset of signs and symptoms at a much earlier age (ie, hours to 2 wk old) than does nasolacrimal duct obstruction (ie, > 2 wk old).

Diagnosis

Diagnosis is most often obvious from history and physical examination. The examiner should look for signs of underlying causes, such as foreign bodies, sinus pain, canthal swelling or mass, and eyelid abnormalities. The Schirmer test (see p. 900) may be used to quantify tear production. An adjunctive test performed by ophthalmologists that may be indicated to diagnose specific causes of tearing is probing and saline irrigation of the lacrimal drainage system with and without fluorescein dye. Reflux through the opposite punctum/canaliculus signals fixed obstruction; reflux and nasal drainage signify stenosis. Imaging tests and procedures (dacryocystography, CT, nasal endoscopy) are sometimes useful to delineate abnormal anatomy when surgery is being considered or occasionally to detect an abscess when infection is suspected.

Treatment

Foreign bodies should be removed and underlying allergies treated. The use of artificial tears lessens tearing when dry eyes or corneal epithelial defects are the cause. Congenital nasolacrimal duct obstruction often resolves spontaneously; before 1 yr, manual compression of the lacrimal sac 4 or 5 times/day may relieve the distal obstruction. After 1 yr, the nasolacrimal duct may need probing with the patient under general anesthesia; if obstruction is recurrent, a temporary drainage tube may be inserted.

In acquired nasolacrimal duct obstruction, irrigation of the nasolacrimal duct may be therapeutic when underlying causes do not respond to treatment. As a last resort, a passage between the lacrimal sac and the nasal cavity can be created surgically (dacryocystorhinostomy [DCR]).

For the treatment of congenital glaucoma, see p. 2446.

Ectropion and entropion typically require surgery (see p. 887). In cases of punctal or canalicular stenosis, dilation is usually curative. If canalicular stenosis is severe and

TABLE 98–3. CAUSES OF TEARING

Increased production
- Foreign body (including trichiasis, distichiasis)
- Allergies
- Conjunctivitis
- Reflex tearing from dry eye
- Keratitis
- Corneal abrasion
- Uveitis

Decreased drainage
- Nasolacrimal obstruction
  - Congenital
  - Acquired
    - Idiopathic
    - Sarcoidosis
    - Wegener's granulomatosis
    - Dacryocystitis
    - Canaliculitis
      - Idiopathic
      - Infectious (*Staphylococcus aureus*, varicella zoster, herpes simplex, Stevens-Johnson syndrome)
      - Drugs (echothiophate iodide, epinephrine)
      - Radiation
    - Trauma
    - Foreign body
    - Tumor
- Eyelid abnormalities
    - Ectropion
    - Entropion
- Punctal stenosis

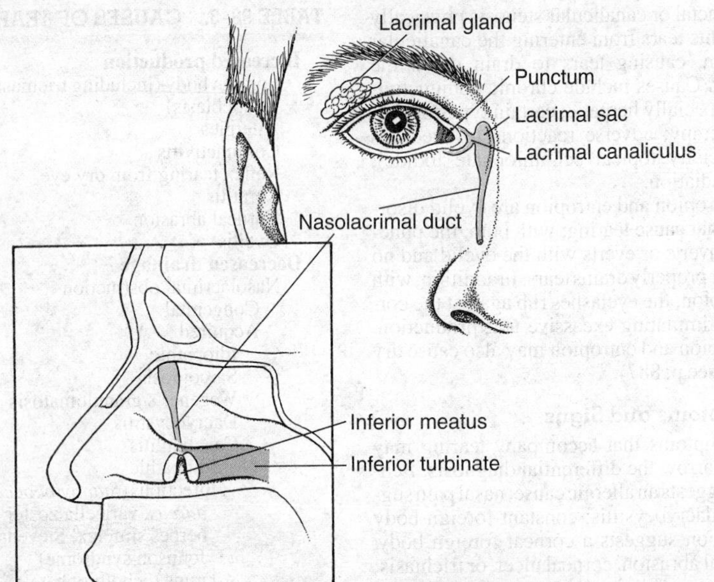

Fig. 98–2. Anatomy of the lacrimal system.

bothersome, a surgical procedure that places a glass tube leading from the caruncle into the nasal cavity can be considered.

DACRYOCYSTITIS

Dacryocystitis is infection of the lacrimal sac, usually with staphyloccocal or streptococcal species and usually as a consequence of nasolacrimal duct obstruction.

In acute dacryocystitis, the patient presents with pain, redness, and edema around the lacrimal sac. Diagnosis is suspected on the basis of symptoms and signs and when pressure over the lacrimal sac causes reflux of mucoid material through the puncta. Initial treatment is with warm compresses and either oral antibiotics for mild cases (cephalexin 500 mg q 6 h) or IV antibiotics (cefazolin 1 g q 6 h) for more severe cases. The abscess can be drained and the antibiotics changed based on culture results if the initial antibiotic proves ineffective.

Patients with chronic dacryocystitis usually present with a mass under the medial canthal tendon and chronic conjunctivitis. Definitive treatment for a resolved acute dacryocystitis or a chronic conjunctivitis is usually with surgery (DCR).

CANALICULITIS

Canaliculitis is infection of the canaliculus (see FIG. 98–2).

The most common cause is infection with *Actinomyces israelii*, a gram-positive bacillus with fine branching filaments, but other bacteria, fungi (eg, *Candida albicans*), and viruses (eg, herpes simplex) may be causative. Symptoms and signs are tearing, discharge, red eye (especially nasally), and mild tenderness over the involved side. Diagnosis is suspected on the basis of symptoms and signs, expression of turbid secretions with pressure over the lacrimal sac, and a gritty sensation that can be felt during probing of the lacrimal system caused by necrotic material. Treatment is warm compresses, irrigation of the canaliculus with antibiotic solution, and removal of any concretions, which usually requires surgery. Antibiotic selection is usually empiric but may be guided by irrigation samples.

OTHER EYE SYMPTOMS

Discharge usually accompanies red eye and is commonly caused by allergic or infectious conjunctivitis, blepharitis, and, in infants; ophthalmia neonatorum. Infectious discharge may be purulent in bacterial infection, such as staphylococcal conjunctivitis or gonorrhea. Less common causes include dacryocystitis and canaliculitis.

Halos around light may result from cataracts; acute closed-angle glaucoma; conditions that result in corneal edema, such as corneal endothelial dystrophy or bullous keratopathy; corneal haziness; mucus on the cornea; or drugs, such as digoxin or chloroquine.

Photophobia (light sensitivity or intolerance) may be normal, especially in lightly pigmented people or in those with lightly pigmented irises, and is relieved by dark glasses. It may also be a nonspecific symptom of corneal disease (eg, corneal epithelial abrasions and erosions, keratitis), dry eyes, uveitis, optic neuritis, or acute closed-angle glaucoma. When eye examination is normal, nonocular causes, including migraine and meningitis, should be considered.

Scotomata are visual field deficits. Negative scotomata are blind spots; positive scotomata are light spots or scintillating flashes. Negative scotomata may not be noticed by the patient unless they involve central vision and interfere significantly with visual acuity; they are caused by retinal hemorrhage, edema, or detachment. Negative scotomata can also result from optic nerve dysfunction (eg, glaucoma with a central visual field defect, optic neuritis, ischemic optic neuropathy). A scotoma found in the same visual field area in each eye is usually a quadrantic or hemianoptic defect resulting from a lesion in the optic pathways. Positive scotomata represent a response to abnormal stimulation of some portion of the visual system, as occurs in migraines. Examination of the eyes, including visual field testing, is mandatory; bilateral scotomata, if not caused by bilateral retinal lesions, demand detailed visual field examination and a neurologic evaluation.

Dry eyes (see p. 899) are most often idiopathic or associated with older age but can also be caused by connective tissue diseases. Tear deficiency is quantified using Schirmer's test; treatment is artificial tears.

99 REFRACTIVE ERROR

In the emmetropic (normally refracted) eye, entering light rays are focused on the retina by the cornea and the lens, creating a sharp image to transmit to the brain. The lens is elastic, more so in younger people. During accommodation, the ciliary muscles adjust lens shape to properly focus images. Refractive errors are a failure of the eye to focus images sharply on the retina, causing blurred vision (see FIG. 99–1).

In **myopia,** or nearsightedness, the point of focus is in front of the retina because the cornea is too steeply curved or the axial length of the eye is too long. Distant objects are blurred, but near objects can be seen clearly. To correct this, a concave (minus) lens is used. Myopic refractive errors in children frequently increase until the child stops growing.

In **hyperopia,** or farsightedness, the point of focus is behind the retina because the cornea is too flatly curved or the axial length is too short. Both distant and near objects are blurred. To correct this, a convex (plus) lens is used.

In **astigmatism,** nonspherical curvature of the cornea or lens causes light rays to focus at different points. To correct astigmatism, a cylindric lens (a segment cut from a cylinder) is used. Cylindric lenses have no refractive power along one axis and are concave or convex along the other axis.

Presbyopia is loss of the lens' ability to change shape to focus on near objects due to aging. Typically, presbyopia becomes noticeable by the time a person reaches his 40s. A convex (plus) lens is used for correction when viewing near objects. These may be supplied as separate glasses or built into a lens as bifocals or variable focus lenses.

Anisometropia is a significant difference between the refractive errors of the 2 eyes (usually > 2 diopters). When corrected with eyeglasses, differences in image size (aniseikonia) are produced that can lead to difficulties in

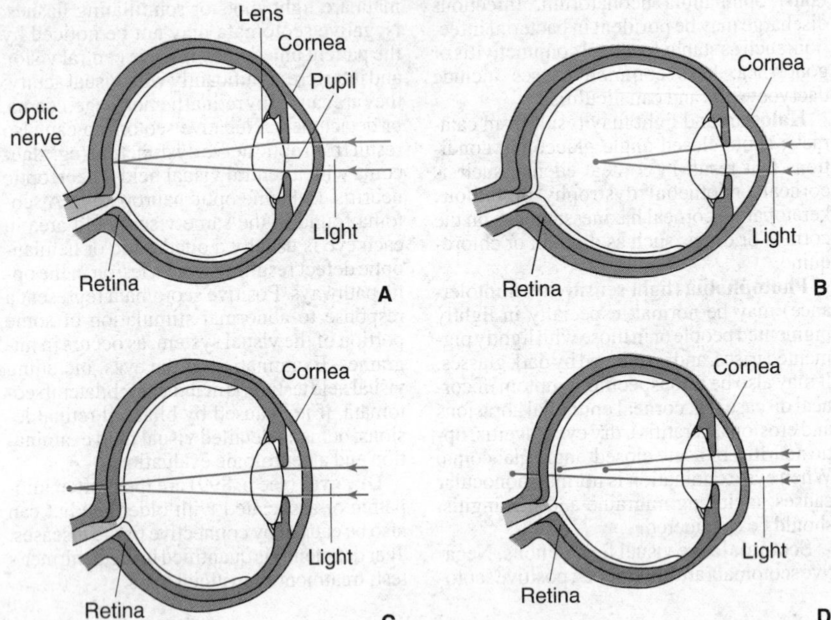

Fig. 99–1. Errors of refraction. (A) Emmetropia; (B) myopia; (C) hyperopia; (D) astigmatism.

fusion and even to suppression of one of the images.

Symptoms, Signs, and Diagnosis

The primary symptom of refractive errors is blurred vision for distant and/or near objects. Sometimes, the excessive ciliary muscle tone can cause headaches. Occasionally, excessive staring can lead to ocular surface desiccation, causing eye irritation, itching, visual fatigue, foreign body sensation, and redness. Frowning when reading and excessive blinking or rubbing of the eyes are symptoms in children.

Refraction should be checked once q 1 or 2 yr. Screening children helps detect refractive errors before they interfere with learning. A comprehensive eye examination (see p. 869) should accompany refraction, whether done by an ophthalmologist or an optometrist.

CONTACT LENSES

Contact lenses often provide better visual acuity and peripheral vision than do eyeglasses and are prescribed to correct myopia, hyperopia, astigmatism, anisometropia, aniseikonia, aphakia (absence of the lens) after cataract removal, and keratoconus (a conical cornea). Either soft or rigid lenses are used to correct myopia and hyperopia. Rigid and toric soft contact lenses are used to correct significant astigmatism; they are satisfactory in many cases but require expert fitting.

Presbyopia can also be corrected with contact lenses. In one approach, the nondominant eye is corrected for reading and the dominant eye for distant vision (monovision). Rigid and soft bifocal and multifocal contact lenses can also be successful, but the fitting procedure is time-consuming because precise alignment is essential.

Neither rigid nor soft contact lenses offer the eyes the protection against blunt or sharp injury that eyeglasses do. Contact lenses occasionally cause superficial corneal changes (which may be painless) or abrasions accompanied by pain, photophobia, and anxiety. Discomfort may also be caused by poorly fitting lenses; by changes (eg, swelling) in the cornea; by wearing lenses in a harmful (eg, O_2-poor, smoky, windy) environment; by improperly inserting or removing lenses; by small foreign particles (eg, soot, dust) trapped between the lens and the cornea; or after removing the lenses, especially after prolonged use (overwear syndrome). With overwear syndrome, spontaneous healing may occur in a day or so if lenses are not worn. In some cases, treatment is required—eg, topical antibiotic eyedrops or ointments and dilation of the pupil with a mydriatic to ease photophobia. (Mydriatics work by paralyzing the muscles of the iris and ciliary body, because movement of the inflamed muscles causes pain.) Recovery is usually rapid, complete, and without vision impairment. An ophthalmologist should be consulted before lenses are worn again.

Care and Complications

Instructions for hygiene and handling lenses must be strictly observed. Poor contact lens hygiene may lead to persistent inflammation or infection of the cornea.

Risk factors for contact lens–related corneal infection (keratitis) include poor lens hygiene, overnight or extended wear, use of tap water in the cleaning regimen, and eyes with a compromised ocular surface (eg, dryness, poor corneal sensation). Infections require rapid management by an ophthalmologist.

A corneal ulcer is suspected when a contact lens wearer experiences intense eye pain, redness, photophobia, and tearing (see also p. 896). Diagnosis is by slit-lamp examination and fluorescein staining. A corneal infiltrate (collection of WBCs in the corneal stroma) and an overlying epithelial defect occur. At times, the corneal infiltrate is large and dense enough to be seen with the naked eye as a white spot on the cornea. Microbiologic analysis of cultures and smears of the corneal infiltrate, contact lens, and contact lens case is indicated. Treatment includes cessation of contact lens wear and antibiotic drops as dictated by culture results. Initial therapy includes broad-spectrum antibiotic coverage using a fluoroquinolone antibiotic drop q 15 to 60 min around the clock for 24 to 72 h, then at gradually longer intervals. An additional antibiotic, such as cefazolin or vancomycin, is used if the ulcer is large or close to the visual axis. Neglected cases may respond poorly or not at all to treatment, and severe vision loss may result.

Rigid Corneal Contact Lenses

Older polymethyl methacrylate rigid contact lenses have been replaced by gas-permeable contact lenses (GPCLs) made of fluorocarbon and polymethyl methacrylate admixtures. GPCLs are 6.5 to 10 mm in diameter and cover part of the cornea, floating on the tear layer overlying it.

Rigid contact lenses can improve vision for people with myopia, hyperopia, and astigmatism. If the corneal surface is irregular, rigid lenses often provide a smooth refracting surface and thus improve visual acuity.

For complete wearing comfort, rigid contact lenses require an adaptation period, sometimes as long as 1 wk. During this time, the wearer gradually increases the number of hours the lenses are worn each day. Wearers usually experience temporary (< 2 h) blurred vision (spectacle blur) when wearing eyeglasses after removing contact lenses. *No pain should occur at any time. Pain is a sign of an ill-fitting contact lens or corneal irritation.*

Soft Hydrophilic Contact Lenses

Soft contact lenses are made of poly-2-hydroxyethyl methacrylate and other flexible plastics and are 30 to 79% water. They are 13 to 15 mm in diameter and cover the entire cornea. Soft contact lenses can improve vision for people with myopia and hyperopia. Because soft contact lenses mold to the existing corneal curvature, anything greater than minimal astigmatism cannot be treated unless a special toric lens, which has different curvatures molded onto the front lens surface, is used. Weighting the lower aspect of the lens maintains its orientation.

Soft contact lenses are also prescribed for treatment of recurrent corneal erosions and other corneal disorders (bandage lenses). Prophylactic antibiotic eyedrops (eg, fluoroquinolone qid) may be advisable with a bandage lens. Extended wearing of contact lenses, especially in aphakia after cataract surgery, is practical, but an ophthalmologist should examine the patient at least 4 times/yr. The patient should clean the lenses once/wk.

Because of their larger size, soft contact lenses are easier to handle, are not as likely as rigid lenses to eject spontaneously, and are less likely to allow foreign bodies to lodge beneath them. Immediate wearing comfort allows a brief adaptation period.

Soft contact lenses have a higher incidence of corneal infections, which increases for every night a person wears them during sleep. When dry, soft contact lenses are brittle and break easily. They require a certain amount of moisture (based on the water content) from the tear film to retain adequate shape and pliability.

Therefore, patients with dry eye generally are more comfortable wearing lenses with low water content.

REFRACTIVE SURGERY

The goal of refractive surgery is to decrease dependence on eyeglasses or contact lenses. Most people who undergo refractive surgery achieve this goal; about 95% do not need corrective lenses for distance vision. Corneal refractive surgery alters the curvature of the cornea to focus light more precisely on the retina.

Ideal candidates for refractive surgery are people with healthy eyes who are not satisfied wearing eyeglasses or contact lenses for their daily and/or recreational activities. Preoperative examination excludes people with active ocular diseases, including severe dry eye. Candidates should not have a history of autoimmune or connective tissue disease because of potential problems with wound healing. Latent herpes simplex virus may be reactivated after surgery; patients should be advised accordingly. Refraction should be stable for at least 1 yr, and candidates should be > 18 yr.

Adverse effects include temporary foreign body sensation, glare, halos, and dryness; occasionally, these symptoms persist. Potential complications include overcorrection and undercorrection, infection, and irregular astigmatism. In excimer laser procedures performed on the superficial corneal stroma, haze formation is possible. If infection, irregular astigmatism, or haze formation causes permanent changes in the central cornea, best-corrected acuity could be lost. The complication rate is low; chance of vision loss is < 1% if the patient was considered to be a good candidate for refractive surgery.

Laser In Situ Keratomileusis

In laser in situ keratomileusis (LASIK), a flap of corneal tissue is created with a microkeratome and turned back, the underlying stromal bed is sculpted with the excimer laser, and the flap is replaced without suturing. Because surface epithelium is not disrupted centrally, vision returns rapidly. Most people notice a significant improvement the next day. LASIK can be used to treat myopia, astigmatism, and hyperopia.

Advantages of LASIK over photorefractive keratectomy are the desirable lack of healing response (the central corneal epithelium is not removed, thereby decreasing the risk of central haze formation), the larger range of refractive errors that can be treated effectively, the shorter visual rehabilitation period, and minimal postoperative pain. Disadvantages include possible flap-related complications, such as flap dislocation, and the need for adequate corneal thickness to prevent long-term corneal ectasia. Ectasia occurs when the corneal thickness has been reduced to a level at which intraocular pressure causes instability and bulging of the weakened corneal stroma, causing blurring, increasing myopia, and irregular astigmatism.

Photorefractive Keratectomy

Photorefractive keratectomy (PRK) is used mainly in patients with thin corneas and in military pilots (LASIK is not yet approved by the armed forces). Photoablation with the excimer laser is used to flatten the central corneal tissue. Corneal epithelium is removed before photoablation and generally takes 3 days to regenerate, during which time a bandage contact lens is worn. More than 95% of patients see 20/40 or better without eyeglasses after surgery.

Laser Epithelial Keratomileusis

Laser epithelial keratomileusis (LASEK) is a variation of PRK in which corneal epithelium is not discarded, but rather removed carefully and then replaced after photoablation is completed. An alcohol solution is used to loosen the epithelial attachments to the corneal stroma, and then special instruments are used to fold it back out of the way of the laser ablation. After laser sculpting of the corneal stroma, the epithelial layer is smoothed back to its original location and a bandage contact lens is applied. Healing is generally similar to PRK; however, less corneal haze reportedly occurs. Patients who are otherwise good refractive surgery candidates but who have corneas too thin to safely undergo LASIK are considered for LASEK. Some surgeons prefer surface laser procedures (PRK and LASEK) even in patients with adequate corneal thickness for LASIK.

Radial and Astigmatic Keratotomy

Radial and astigmatic keratotomy procedures change the shape of the cornea by making deep corneal incisions using a diamond blade. Radial keratotomy has been replaced by laser vision correction and is rarely used because it offers no clear advantages over laser vision correction and has a higher retreatment rate. Astigmatic keratotomy is used to treat astigmatism at the time of cataract surgery or after corneal transplant.

Intracorneal Ring Segments

Intracorneal ring segments (INTACS) are thin arc-shaped segments of biocompatible plastic that are inserted in pairs through a small radial corneal incision into the peripheral corneal stroma at $^2/_3$ depth. After INTACS are inserted, the central corneal curvature is flattened, and myopia is reduced. INTACS are approved for mild myopia (< 3 diopters) and minimal astigmatism (< 1 diopter). INTACS maintain a central clear optical zone because the 2 segments are placed in the corneal periphery. INTACS can be replaced or even removed if desired. Risks include induced astigmatism, undercorrection and overcorrection, infection, glare, halo, and incorrect depth placement. Vision results are very good; in US clinical studies, 97% of patients saw 20/40 or better and 74% of patients saw 20/20 or better.

100 EYELID DISORDERS

Common eyelid disorders include blepharitis, blepharospasm, chalazion and hordeolum, entropion and ectropion, trichiasis, and tumors.

BLEPHARITIS

Blepharitis is inflammation of the eyelid margins that may be acute or chronic. Symptoms and signs include itching and burning of the lid margins with redness and edema. Diagnosis is by history and examination. Acute ulcerative blepharitis is usually treated with topical antibiotics or systemic antivirals. Acute nonulcerative blepharitis is occasionally treated with topical corticosteroids. Chronic disease is treated with eyelid hygiene (seborrheic blepharitis), warm compresses (meibomian gland dysfunction), and tear supplements (seborrheic blepharitis, meibomian gland dysfunction).

Etiology

Blepharitis may be acute (ulcerative or nonulcerative) or chronic (seborrheic blepharitis or meibomian gland dysfunction). Acute ulcerative blepharitis is usually caused by bacterial infection (usually staphylococcal) of the eyelid margin at the origins of the eyelashes involving the lash follicles and the meibomian glands. It may also be due to a virus (eg, herpes simplex, varicella zoster). Acute nonulcerative blepharitis is usually caused by an allergic reaction involving the same area (eg, atopic blepharodermatitis, seasonal allergic blepharoconjunctivitis, contact sensitivity dermatoblepharoconjunctivitis).

Chronic blepharitis is noninfectious inflammation of unknown cause. Seborrheic blepharitis is often associated with seborrheic dermatitis of the face and scalp (see p. 960). Secondary bacterial colonization often occurs on the scales that develop on the eyelid margin.

Meibomian glands in the eyelid produce lipids (meibum) that stabilize tears by forming a lipid layer on top of the aqueous tear layer, reducing evaporation. In meibomian gland dysfunction, the lipid composition is abnormal and gland ducts and orifices become inspissated with hard, waxy plugs, and most patients have increased tear evaporation and keratoconjunctivitis sicca. The disorder is often associated with rosacea (see p. 946) and a history of recurrent hordeola or chalazia.

Symptoms and Signs

Symptoms common to all forms of blepharitis include itching and burning of the eyelid margins and conjunctival irritation with lacrimation and photophobia.

In acute ulcerative blepharitis, small pustules develop in eyelash follicles and eventually break down to form shallow marginal ulcers. Tenacious adherent crusts leave a bleeding surface when removed. Eyelids become glued together by dried secretions during sleep. Recurrent ulcerative blepharitis can cause loss of eyelashes and eyelid scarring.

In acute nonulcerative blepharitis, eyelid margins become edematous and erythematous; eyelashes may become crusted with dried serous fluid.

In seborrheic blepharitis, greasy, easily removable scales develop on lid margins. In meibomian gland dysfunction, examination reveals dilated, inspissated gland orifices that exude a waxy, thick, yellowish secretion with pressure. Most patients with seborrheic blepharitis and meibomian gland dysfunction have secondary keratoconjunctivitis sicca, which also causes a foreign body sensation, grittiness, eye strain and fatigue, and blurring with prolonged visual effort.

Diagnosis and Treatment

Diagnosis is usually by slit-lamp examination. Chronic blepharitis that does not respond to treatment requires biopsy to exclude eyelid tumors that can simulate the condition.

Acute ulcerative blepharitis is treated with an antibiotic ointment (eg, bacitracin/polymyxin B or gentamicin 0.3% qid for 7 to 10 days). Acute viral ulcerative blepharitis is treated with systemic antivirals (eg, for herpes simplex, acyclovir 400 mg po tid for 7 days; for varicella zoster, acyclovir 800 mg po 5 times/day for 7 days).

Treatment of acute nonulcerative blepharitis begins with avoiding the offending action (eg, rubbing) or substance (eg, new eye drops). Cold compresses over the closed eyelid may speed resolution. If swelling persists > 24 h, topical corticosteroids (eg, fluorometholone ophthalmic ointment 0.1% tid for 7 days) can be used.

The initial treatment for both seborrheic blepharitis and meibomian gland dysfunction is directed toward the secondary keratoconjunctivitis sicca (see p. 899). Tear supplements, bland ointments at night, and punctal plugs are effective in most patients. If needed, additional treatment for seborrheic blepharitis includes gentle cleansing of the lid margin bid with a cotton swab dipped in a dilute solution of baby shampoo (2 to 3 drops in ½ cup of warm water). A topical antibiotic ointment (bacitracin/polymyxin B or sulfacetamide 10% bid for up to 3 mo) may be added when cases are unresponsive over weeks to lid hygiene. If needed, additional treatment for meibomian gland dysfunction includes warm compresses to melt the waxy plugs and occasionally eyelid massage to extrude trapped secretions to coat the ocular surface. Tetracycline (eg, doxycycline 100 mg po bid tapered over 3 to 4 mo) may also be effective. Isotretinoin can also be used for meibomian gland dysfunction, but it can lead to dryness.

Prognosis

Acute blepharitis most often responds to treatment but may recur and/or develop into chronic blepharitis. Chronic blepharitis is by definition indolent, recurrent, and resistant to treatment. Exacerbations are inconvenient, uncomfortable, and cosmetically unappealing but do not usually result in corneal scarring or vision loss.

BLEPHAROSPASM

Blepharospasm is spasm of muscles around the eye causing involuntary blinking and eye closing.

Blepharospasm can occur as a result of other eye diseases, but its cause is most often unknown. It affects women more than men and tends to occur within families. Secondary blepharospasm may also occur in people with ocular irritation (eg, trichiasis, corneal foreign body, keratoconjunctivitis sicca) and with systemic neurologic diseases that cause spasm (eg, Parkinson's disease).

Symptoms are involuntary blinking and closing of the eyes; in severe cases, people cannot open their eyes. Spasms may be made worse by fatigue, bright light, and anxiety. Treatment involves injecting botulinum toxin into the eyelid muscles; treatment must be repeated in most instances; it can cause permanent ptosis. Anxiolytics may help. Surgery to cut the periorbital muscles is also effective but, because of potential complications, is considered only if botulinum toxin fails. Sunglasses help decrease the light sensitivity that may cause or accompany blepharospasm.

CHALAZION AND HORDEOLUM

Chalazia and hordeola are sudden onset of localized swellings of the eyelid; a chalazion is caused by noninfectious meibomian gland occlusion, whereas a hordeolum is caused by infection. Both conditions initially cause lid hyperemia and edema, swelling, and pain; with time, a chalazion becomes a small

nontender nodule in the eyelid center, whereas a hordeolum remains painful and localizes to a lid margin. Diagnosis is clinical. Treatment is with hot compresses. Both conditions improve spontaneously, but incision or, for chalazia, intralesional corticosteroids may be used to hasten resolution.

A chalazion is noninfectious occlusion of a meibomian gland causing extravasation of irritating lipid material in the eyelid soft tissues and focal inflammatory response.

A hordeolum, or stye, is an acute localized pyogenic (usually staphylococcal) infection or abscess of the eyelid that may be external or internal.

An external hordeolum results from infection and obstruction of an eyelash follicle and adjacent glands of Zeis or Moll. It frequently develops in association with blepharitis. Symptoms are pain, redness, and tenderness of the eyelid margin, occasionally with tearing, photophobia, and a foreign body sensation. Signs are tenderness and a small yellowish spot (pointing) at the base of the eyelashes, indicative of suppuration, surrounded by hyperemia, induration, and diffuse edema. Within 2 to 4 days, the lesion ruptures, with discharge of pus and relief of pain.

Chalazia and hordeola are initially clinically indistinguishable; both cause lid hyperemia and edema, swelling, and pain. After 1 to 2 days, an external hordeolum becomes localized to the lid margin, whereas a chalazion centers in the body of the eyelid; a small nontender nodule or lump then develops and points toward the inner surface of the lid, or rarely, the outer surface. A chalazion usually drains or absorbs spontaneously over 2 to 8 wk but can persist longer.

An internal hordeolum, which is much rarer, results from infection of a meibomian gland. Symptoms are the same as those of a chalazion, with pain, redness, and edema localized to the posterior tarsal conjunctival surface. Inspection of the tarsal conjunctivae shows a small elevation or yellow area at the site of the affected gland. Later, an abscess forms, pointing on the conjunctival side of the lid; it sometimes points through the skin. Spontaneous rupture is rare, and recurrence is common.

Diagnosis of chalazion and both kinds of hordeola is clinical; an internal hordeolum is very rare and could be considered when inflammation is severe or when systemic signs of infection are present. If the chalazion or hordeolum lies near the inner canthus of the lower lid, it must be differentiated from dacryocystitis (see p. 880), the diagnosis of which can usually be excluded by noting the location of maximum induration and tenderness (eg, eyelid for a chalazion, the side of the nose for dacryocystitis). In addition, successful lacrimal duct irrigation would rule out dacryocystitis. Chronic chalazia that do not respond to treatment require biopsy to exclude tumor of the eyelid.

Most chalazia disappear gradually after 1 to 2 mo, and external hordeola usually rupture on their own after 2 to 4 days. Hot compresses for 5 to 10 min bid or tid can be used to hasten resolution. An external hordeolum can also be incised with a sharp, fine-tipped blade as soon as pointing occurs. Incision and curettage or intrachalazion corticosteroid administration (0.05 to 0.2 mL triamcinolone 25 mg/mL) may be indicated if chalazia are large, unsightly, and persist for more than several weeks despite conservative therapy. Antibiotics (eg, dicloxacillin or erythromycin 250 mg po qid) are indicated when cellulitis accompanies a hordeolum.

Treatment of internal hordeola is oral antibiotics and incision and drainage if needed. Topical antibiotics are usually ineffective.

ENTROPION AND ECTROPION

Entropion is inversion of an eyelid; ectropion is eversion of the lower eyelid.

Entropion, inversion of an eyelid, is caused by age-related tissue relaxation, postinfectious or posttraumatic change, and blepharospasm. Eyelashes rub against the eyeball and may lead to corneal ulceration and scarring. Diagnosis is clinical. Definitive treatment is surgery.

Ectropion, eversion of the lower eyelid, is caused by age-related tissue relaxation; cranial nerve VII palsy; and posttraumatic, postsurgical, and orbital changes. Symptoms are tearing (due to poor drainage of tears through the nasolacrimal system, which no longer contacts the eyeball) and symptoms of dry eyes with superficial keratitis (see p. 899), possibly due to exposure with inadequate blinking. Diagnosis is clinical, but significant causes (eg, orbital tumor) and sequelae (eg, keratitis) should be excluded. Symptomatic treatment is artificial tears; definitive treatment is surgery.

TRICHIASIS

Trichiasis is an anatomic misalignment of eyelashes, which rub against the eyeball.

Trichiasis is most often idiopathic, but known causes include blepharitis, posttraumatic and postsurgical changes, conjunctival scarring (eg, secondary to cicatricial pemphigoid, atopic keratoconjunctivitis, Stevens-Johnson syndrome, postchemical injury), epiblepharon (an extra lower eyelid skin fold that directs lashes into a vertical position), and distichiasis (a congenital extra row of eyelashes). Symptoms are foreign body sensation, tearing, and red eye. Diagnosis is usually clinical. Evaluation includes fluorescein staining to exclude corneal abrasion or ulceration. Treatment is eyelash removal with forceps or, in frequently recurring cases, with electrolysis or cryosurgery.

TUMORS

The skin of the eyelids is a common site for growth of benign and malignant tumors.

Xanthelasma is a common, benign deposit of yellow-white flat plaques of lipid material that occur subcutaneously on the upper and lower eyelids. Although xanthelasmas may be associated with dyslipidemias, most are not. Diagnosis is by appearance. No treatment is necessary, although xanthelasmas can be removed for cosmetic reasons, and underlying dyslipidemias should be treated.

Basal cell carcinoma frequently occurs at the eyelid margins, at the inner canthus, and on the upper cheek (see also p. 1023). Biopsy establishes the diagnosis. Treatment is surgical excision or radiation therapy. Mohs' surgery may be needed to preserve eyelid function.

Other malignant tumors are less common; they include squamous cell or meibomian gland carcinoma and melanomas. Eyelid tumors simulating chronic blepharitis or chronic chalazion occur. Therefore, chronic blepharitis, chronic chalazion, or similar lesions should be biopsied if unresponsive to initial treatment.

101 CONJUNCTIVAL AND SCLERAL DISORDERS

The conjunctiva lines the back of the eyelids (palpebral or tarsal conjunctiva), extends into the space between the lid and the globe (forniceal conjunctiva), then folds back on itself as it spreads over the sclera to the cornea (bulbar conjunctiva). The conjunctiva helps maintain the tear film and protect the eye from foreign objects and infection.

The sclera is the thick white sphere of dense connective tissue that encloses the eye and maintains its shape. Anteriorly, the sclera fuses with the cornea, and posteriorly it blends with the meninges where the optic nerve penetrates the globe.

The episclera is a thin vascular membrane between the conjunctiva and the sclera.

The most common disorders are inflammatory (conjunctivitis, episcleritis, scleritis). Conjunctivitis can be acute or chronic and is infectious, allergic, or irritant in origin, whereas episcleritis and scleritis usually result from immune-mediated disease. Episcleritis usually does not threaten vision, but scleritis can destroy vision and the eye. Major symptoms of conjunctivitides are similar (eg, conjunctival hyperemia); early, accurate diagnosis is important.

CICATRICIAL PEMPHIGOID

(Benign Mucous Membrane Pemphigoid; Ocular Cicatricial Pemphigoid)

Cicatricial pemphigoid is a chronic, bilateral, progressive scarring and shrinkage of the conjunctiva with opacification of the cornea. Early symptoms are hyperemia, discomfort, itching, and discharge; progression leads to both eyelid and corneal damage and sometimes blindness. Diagnosis is confirmed

by biopsy. Treatment may require systemic immunosuppression.

Cicatricial pemphigoid is an autoimmune disease in which binding of anticonjunctival basement membrane antibodies results in conjunctival inflammation. It is unrelated to bullous pemphigoid.

Symptoms and Signs

Usually beginning as a chronic conjunctivitis, the condition progresses to symblepharon (scarring of the palpebral conjunctiva to the globe); trichiasis (in-turning eyelashes); keratoconjunctivitis sicca; corneal neovascularization, opacification, and keratinization; and conjunctival shrinkage and keratinization. Chronic corneal epithelial defects can lead to secondary bacterial ulceration, scarring, and blindness. Oral mucous membrane involvement with ulceration and scarring is common, but skin involvement, characterized by scarring bullae and erythematous plaques, is uncommon.

Diagnosis and Treatment

Diagnosis is suspected clinically by the presence of symblepharon without a history of local radiation or severe perennial allergic conjunctivitis. It is confirmed by conjunctival biopsy demonstrating antibody deposition on the basement membrane.

Tear substitutes and cryoepilation or electroepilation of the in-turning eyelashes may increase patient comfort and reduce the risk of ocular infection. For progressive scarring or corneal opacification, systemic immunosuppression with dapsone or cyclophosphamide is indicated.

CONJUNCTIVITIS

Conjunctival inflammation typically occurs from infection, allergy, or irritation. Symptoms are conjunctival hyperemia and ocular discharge and, depending on the etiology, discomfort and itching. Diagnosis is clinical; sometimes cultures are indicated. Treatment depends on etiology and may include topical antibiotics, antihistamines, mast cell stabilizers, and corticosteroids.

Infectious conjunctivitis is most commonly viral or bacterial and is contagious. Rarely, mixed or unidentifiable pathogens are present. Numerous substances can produce allergic conjunctivitis (see p. 893). Nonallergic conjunctival irritation can result from foreign bodies; wind, dust, smoke, fumes, chemical vapors, and other types of air pollution; and intense ultraviolet light of electric arcs, sunlamps, and reflection from snow.

Conjunctivitis is typically acute, but both infectious and allergic conditions can be chronic. Conditions that cause chronic conjunctivitis include ectropion, entropion, blepharitis, and chronic dacryocystitis.

Symptoms, Signs, and Diagnosis

Any source of inflammation causes conjunctival vascular dilation and lacrimation or discharge. Thick discharge may blur vision.

Itching and watery discharge predominate in allergic conjunctivitis. Chemosis and papillary hyperplasia also suggest allergic conjunctivitis. Irritation or foreign body sensation, photophobia, or purulent discharge suggests infectious conjunctivitis. Severe eye pain suggests scleritis (see p. 895).

Usually, history and examination suggest the diagnosis (see also TABLE 101–1). However,

TABLE 101–1. DIFFERENTIATING FEATURES IN ACUTE CONJUNCTIVITIS

ETIOLOGY	DISCHARGE; CELL TYPE	EYELID EDEMA	NODE INVOLVEMENT	ITCHING
Bacterial	Purulent; polymorphonuclear leukocytes	Moderate	Usually none	None
Viral	Clear; mononuclear cells	Minimal	Usually	None
Allergic	Clear, mucoid, ropy; eosinophils	Moderate to severe	None	Intense

cultures are indicated for severe symptoms, in immunocompromised patients, in the vulnerable eye (eg, after a corneal transplant, in exophthalmos due to Graves' disease), and if initial therapy fails.

Treatment

Most infectious conjunctivitis is highly contagious and spreads by droplet, fomites, and hand-to-eye inoculation. To avoid transmitting infection, the physician must wash his hands thoroughly and disinfect equipment after examining the patient. The patient should wash his hands thoroughly after touching his eyes or nasal secretions, avoid touching the noninfected eye after touching the infected eye, avoid sharing towels or pillows, and not swim in pools. Eyes should be kept free of discharge and should not be patched. Small children with conjunctivitis should be kept home from school to avoid spread.

VIRAL CONJUNCTIVITIS

Viral conjunctivitis is a highly contagious acute conjunctival infection usually caused by adenovirus. Symptoms include irritation, lacrimation, photophobia, and mucoid or purulent discharge. Diagnosis is clinical. Infection is self-limited, but severe cases sometimes require topical corticosteroids.

Etiology

Conjunctivitis may accompany the common cold and other systemic viral infections (especially measles, but also chickenpox, rubella, and mumps). Isolated viral conjunctivitis usually results from adenoviruses and sometimes enteroviruses.

Epidemic keratoconjunctivitis usually results from adenovirus serotypes Ad 5, 8, 11, 13, 19, and 37. Pharyngoconjunctival fever usually results from serotypes Ad 3, 4, and 7. Outbreaks of acute hemorrhagic conjunctivitis, a rare conjunctivitis associated with infection by enterovirus type 70, have occurred in Africa and Asia.

Symptoms, Signs, and Diagnosis

After an incubation period of about 5 to 12 days, conjunctival hyperemia, watery discharge, and ocular irritation usually begin in one eye and spread rapidly to the other. Follicles are present on the palpebral conjunctiva. A preauricular lymph node is often enlarged and painful. Many patients have had contact with someone with conjunctivitis and/or a recent URI.

In severe adenoviral conjunctivitis, patients may have significant photophobia and foreign body sensation. Pseudomembranes of fibrin and inflammatory cells on the tarsal conjunctiva and/or focal corneal inflammation may blur vision. Even after conjunctivitis has resolved, residual corneal subepithelial opacities (multiple, coin-shaped, 0.5 to 1.0 mm in diameter) may be visible with a slit lamp for up to 2 yr. Corneal opacities occasionally result in decreased vision and significant glare.

Diagnosis is usually clinical; special tissue cultures are necessary for growth of the virus but are rarely indicated. Secondary bacterial infection is rare. However, if any signs are consistent with bacterial conjunctivitis (eg, purulent discharge), smears from the eye should be examined microscopically and cultured for bacteria.

Treatment

Viral conjunctivitis is highly contagious, and transmission precautions must be followed (as above). Children should generally be kept out of school until resolution.

Viral conjunctivitis is self-limiting, lasting 1 wk in mild cases to up to 3 wk in severe cases. It requires only cool compresses for symptomatic relief. However, patients with severe photophobia or whose vision is affected may benefit from topical corticosteroids (eg, 1% prednisolone acetate q 6 to 8 h). Herpes simplex keratitis (see p. 897) must be ruled out first because corticosteroids can exacerbate it.

ACUTE BACTERIAL CONJUNCTIVITIS

Bacterial conjunctivitis is caused by numerous bacteria. Symptoms are hyperemia, lacrimation, irritation, and discharge. Diagnosis is clinical. Treatment is with topical antibiotics, augmented by systemic antibiotics in more serious cases.

Most bacterial conjunctivitis is acute; chronic bacterial conjunctivitis is due to *Chlamydia* (which includes trachoma and adult inclusion conjunctivitis) and rarely *Moraxella*.

Etiology

Bacterial conjunctivitis is usually due to *Staphylococcus aureus, Streptococcus pneumoniae, Haemophilus* sp, or, less commonly, *Chlamydia trachomatis* (see Adult Inclusion

Conjunctivitis, below). *Neisseria gonorrhoeae* causes gonococcal conjunctivitis, which usually results from sexual contact with a person with a genital infection.

Ophthalmia neonatorum (see also p. 2325) is conjunctivitis that occurs in 20 to 40% of newborns delivered through an infected birth canal. It can be due to maternal gonococcal or chlamydial infection.

Symptoms, Signs, and Diagnosis

Symptoms are typically unilateral but frequently spread to the opposite eye within a few days. Discharge is purulent.

The bulbar and tarsal conjunctivae are intensely hyperemic and edematous. Petechial subconjunctival hemorrhages, chemosis, eyelid edema, and an enlarged preauricular lymph node are typically absent.

With adult gonococcal conjunctivitis, symptoms develop 12 to 48 h after exposure. Severe eyelid edema, chemosis, and a profuse purulent exudate are present. Rare complications include corneal ulceration, abscess, perforation, panophthalmitis, and blindness.

Ophthalmia neonatorum from gonococcal infection appears 2 to 5 days after delivery. With ophthalmia neonatorum from a chlamydial infection, symptoms appear within 5 to 14 days. Symptoms are bilateral, intense papillary conjunctivitis, with lid edema, chemosis, and mucopurulent discharge.

Smears and bacterial cultures should be obtained when symptoms are severe, in immunocompromised patients, if initial therapy fails, and in a vulnerable eye (eg, after a corneal transplant, in exophthalmos due to Graves' disease). Smears and conjunctival scrapings should be examined microscopically and stained with Gram stain to identify bacteria and with Giemsa stain to identify the characteristic epithelial cell basophilic cytoplasmic inclusion bodies of chlamydial conjunctivitis.

Treatment

Bacterial conjunctivitis is very contagious, and standard infection control measures (see p. 890) should be followed.

If neither gonococcal nor chlamydial infection is suspected, most clinicians treat presumptively for 7 to 10 days with moxifloxacin 0.5% drops tid or other fluoroquinolone or trimethoprim/polymyxin B qid. A poor clinical response after 2 or 3 days indicates that the cause is a resistant bacterium, a virus, or an allergy. Culture and sensitivity studies determine subsequent treatment.

Adult gonococcal conjunctivitis requires a single dose of ceftriaxone 1 g IM or ciprofloxacin 500 mg po bid for 5 days. Bacitracin 500 units/g or gentamicin 0.3% ophthalmic ointment instilled into the affected eye q 2 h may be used in addition to systemic treatment. Sex partners should also be treated. Because chlamydial genital infection is often present in patients with gonorrhea, patients should also receive a single dose of azithromycin 1 g or doxycycline 100 mg po bid for 7 days.

Ophthalmia neonatorum is prevented by the routine use of silver nitrate or erythromycin drops at birth. Infections that escape this treatment require systemic treatment. For gonococcal infection, ceftriaxone 25 to 50 mg/kg IV or IM is given once/day for 7 days. Chlamydial infection is treated with erythromycin 12.5 mg/kg po or IV qid for 14 days. The parents should also be treated.

ADULT INCLUSION CONJUNCTIVITIS

(Adult Chlamydial Conjunctivitis; Swimming Pool Conjunctivitis)

Adult inclusion conjunctivitis is caused by sexually transmitted *Chlamydia trachomatis*. Symptoms include chronic unilateral hyperemia and mucopurulent discharge. Diagnosis is clinical. Treatment is with systemic antibiotics.

Adult inclusion conjunctivitis is caused by *Chlamydia trachomatis* serotypes D through K. In most instances, adult inclusion conjunctivitis results from sexual contact with a person with a genital infection. Usually, patients have acquired a new sex partner in the preceding 2 mo. Rarely, adult inclusion conjunctivitis is acquired from contaminated swimming pool water.

Symptoms, Signs, and Diagnosis

Adult inclusion conjunctivitis has an incubation period of 2 to 19 days. It is usually characterized by a unilateral mucopurulent discharge. The tarsal conjunctiva is often more hyperemic than the bulbar conjunctiva. Characteristically, there is a marked tarsal follicular response. Occasionally, superior corneal opacities and vascularization occur. Preauricular lymph nodes may be swollen on the side of the involved eye. Often, symptoms have been present for many weeks or months and have not responded to topical antibiotics.

Chronicity, mucopurulent discharge, marked tarsal follicular response, and failure of topical antibiotics differentiate adult inclusion conjunctivitis from bacterial conjunctivitis. Smears, bacterial cultures, and chlamydial studies should be obtained. Immunofluorescent staining techniques, PCR, and special cultures are used to detect *Chlamydia trachomatis*. Smears and conjunctival scrapings should be examined microscopically and stained with Gram stain to identify bacteria and with Giemsa stain to identify the characteristic epithelial cell basophilic cytoplasmic inclusion bodies of chlamydial conjunctivitis.

Treatment

Azithromycin 1 g po once only or either doxycycline 100 mg po bid or erythromycin 500 mg po qid for 1 wk cures the conjunctivitis and concomitant genital infection. Sex partners also require treatment.

TRACHOMA

(Egyptian Ophthalmia; Granular Conjunctivitis)

Trachoma is a chronic conjunctivitis caused by *Chlamydia trachomatis* and characterized by progressive exacerbations and remissions. It is the leading cause of preventable blindness worldwide. Initial symptoms are conjunctival hyperemia, eyelid edema, photophobia, and lacrimation. Later, corneal neovascularization and scarring of the conjunctiva, cornea, and eyelids occur. Diagnosis is usually clinical. Treatment is with topical or systemic antibiotics.

Trachoma is endemic in poverty-stricken parts of North Africa, the Middle East, the Indian subcontinent, Australia, and Southeast Asia. The causative organism is *Chlamydia trachomatis* (serotypes A, B, Ba, and C). It is highly contagious in its early stages and is transmitted by eye-to-eye contact, hand-to-eye contact, eye-seeking flies, or the sharing of contaminated articles (eg, towels, handkerchiefs, eye makeup—see Adult Inclusion Conjunctivitis on p. 891).

Symptoms and Signs

After an incubation period of about 7 days, conjunctival hyperemia, eyelid edema, photophobia, and lacrimation gradually appear, usually bilaterally. Small follicles develop in the upper tarsal conjunctiva 7 to 10 days later and gradually increase in size and number for 3 or 4 wk. Inflammatory papillae appear on the upper tarsal conjunctiva, and corneal neovascularization begins during this stage, with invasion of the upper half of the cornea by loops of vessels from the limbus, a finding known as pannus. The stage of follicular/papillary hypertrophy and corneal neovascularization may last from several months to > 1 yr, depending on response to therapy. The entire cornea may ultimately be involved, reducing vision.

Without treatment, a cicatricial (scarring) stage follows. The follicles and papillae gradually shrink and are replaced by scar tissue that often causes entropion and lacrimal duct obstruction. Entropion leads to further corneal scarring and neovascularization. Secondary bacterial infection is common, contributing to scarring and disease progression. The corneal epithelium becomes dull and thickened, and lacrimation is decreased. Small corneal ulcers may appear at the site of peripheral corneal infiltrates, stimulating further neovascularization.

Diagnosis

Diagnosis is usually clinical because testing is rarely available in endemic areas. Lymphoid follicles on the tarsal plate or along the corneal limbus, linear conjunctival scarring, and corneal pannus are considered diagnostic in the proper clinical setting. If diagnosis is uncertain, *C. trachomatis* can be isolated in culture or identified by PCR and immunofluorescence techniques. In the early stage, minute basophilic cytoplasmic inclusion bodies within conjunctival epithelial cells in Giemsa-stained conjunctival scrapings differentiate trachoma from nonchlamydial conjunctivitis. Inclusion bodies are also found in adult inclusion conjunctivitis (see p. 891), but the setting and developing clinical picture distinguish it from trachoma. Palpebral vernal conjunctivitis appears similar to trachoma in its follicular hypertrophic stage, but symptoms are different and milky flat-topped papillae are present, whereas eosinophils, not basophilic inclusion bodies, are found in the scrapings.

Prognosis and Treatment

For individual or sporadic cases, azithromycin 20 mg/kg (maximum 1 g) po as a single dose is 78% effective. Alternatives are doxycycline 100 mg bid or tetracycline 250 mg qid for 4 wk. In hyperendemic areas, tetracycline or erythromycin ophthalmic ointment applied bid for 5 consecutive days each month for 6 mo has been effective. Dramatic reductions in endemic trachoma have been made using community-wide oral azithromycin in a single dose or in repeated doses. Reinfection due to re-exposure is common in endemic areas. Better personal hygiene and environmental measures (eg, access to potable water) can reduce reinfection.

Eyelid deformities (eg, entropion) should be treated surgically.

On healing, the conjunctiva is smooth and grayish white. The extent of residual corneal opacity and vision loss varies. Rarely, corneal neovascularization regresses completely, and corneal transparency is restored without treatment.

ALLERGIC CONJUNCTIVITIS

(Atopic Conjunctivitis; Atopic Keratoconjunctivitis; Hay Fever Conjunctivitis; Perennial Allergic Conjunctivitis; Seasonal Allergic Conjunctivitis; Vernal Keratoconjunctivitis)

Allergic conjunctivitis is an acute, intermittent, or chronic conjunctival inflammation usually caused by airborne allergens. Symptoms include itching, lacrimation, discharge, and conjunctival hyperemia. Diagnosis is clinical. Treatment is with topical antihistamines and mast cell stabilizers.

Etiology

Allergic conjunctivitis is due to a type I hypersensitivity reaction to a specific antigen.

Seasonal allergic conjunctivitis (hay fever conjunctivitis) is due to airborne pollen of trees, grasses, or weeds. It tends to peak during the spring, late summer, or early fall and disappear during the winter months—corresponding to the life cycle of the causative plant.

Perennial allergic conjunctivitis (atopic conjunctivitis, atopic keratoconjunctivitis) is due to dust mites, animal dander, and other nonseasonal allergens. These allergens, particularly those in the home, tend to cause symptoms year-round.

Vernal keratoconjunctivitis is a more severe type of conjunctivitis most likely allergic in origin. It is most common in males aged 5 to 20 who also have eczema, asthma, or seasonal allergies. Vernal conjunctivitis typically reappears each spring and subsides in the fall and winter. Many children outgrow the condition by early adulthood.

Symptoms and Signs

Patients complain of bilateral intense ocular itching, conjunctival hyperemia, photophobia, eyelid edema, and watery or stringy discharge. Concomitant rhinitis is common. Many patients have other atopic diseases, such as eczema, allergic rhinitis, or asthma.

Findings characteristically include conjunctival edema and hyperemia and an often tenacious mucoid discharge containing numerous eosinophils. The bulbar conjunctiva may appear translucent, bluish, and thickened. Chemosis and a characteristic boggy blepharedema of the lower eyelid are common. In seasonal and perennial allergic conjunctivitis, fine papillae on the upper tarsal conjunctiva give a velvety appearance. Chronic itching can lead to chronic eyelid rubbing, periocular hyperpigmentation, and dermatitis.

In more severe forms of perennial allergic conjunctivitis, larger tarsal conjunctival papillae, conjunctival scarring, corneal neovascularization, and corneal scarring with variable loss of visual acuity can occur.

In vernal keratoconjunctivitis, usually the palpebral conjunctiva of the upper eyelid is involved, but the bulbar conjunctiva is sometimes affected. In the palpebral form, square, hard, flattened, closely packed, pale pink to grayish "cobblestone" papillae are present, chiefly in the upper tarsal conjunctiva. The uninvolved tarsal conjunctiva is milky white. In the bulbar ("limbal") form, the circumcorneal conjunctiva becomes hypertrophied and grayish. Occasionally, a small, circumscribed loss of corneal epithelium occurs, causing pain and increased photophobia. Symptoms usually disappear during the cold months and become milder over the years.

Diagnosis and Treatment

The diagnosis is usually clinical. Eosinophils are present in conjunctival scrapings, which may be taken from the lower or upper tarsal conjunctiva; however, such testing is rarely indicated.

Avoidance of known allergens and use of tear supplements can reduce symptoms; antigen desensitization is occasionally helpful. Topical OTC antihistamine/vasoconstrictors (eg, naphazoline/pheniramine) are useful for mild cases. If these drugs are insufficient, topical prescription antihistamines (eg, olopatadine, ketotifen), NSAIDs (eg, ketorolac), or mast cell stabilizers (eg, pemirolast, nedocromil) can be used separately or in combination.

Topical corticosteroids (eg, loteprednol, fluorometholone 0.1%, prednisolone acetate 0.12% to 1% drops tid) can be useful in recalcitrant cases. Because topical corticosteroids can exacerbate ocular herpes simplex virus infections, possibly leading to corneal ulceration and perforation and, with long-term use, to glaucoma and possibly cataracts, their use should be initiated and monitored by an ophthalmologist. Topical cyclosporine may be indicated where corticosteroids are needed but cannot be used.

Seasonal allergic conjunctivitis is less likely to require multiple drugs or intermittent topical corticosteroids.

OTHER CONJUNCTIVAL DISORDERS

Pinguecula and ptergyium are benign growths of the conjunctiva that can result from chronic actinic irritation. Both typically appear adjacent to the cornea at the 3- and/or 9-o'clock position. A pinguecula is a raised yellowish white mass on the bulbar conjunctiva, adjacent to the cornea. It does not tend to grow onto the cornea. However, it may cause irritation or cosmetic blemish and, although rarely necessary, can easily be removed. A pterygium is a fleshy triangular growth of bulbar conjunctiva that may spread across and distort the cornea, induce astigmatism, and change the refractive power of the eye. Symptoms may include decreased vision and foreign body sensation. It is more common in hot, dry climates. Removal is often indicated for cosmesis, to reduce irritation, and to improve or preserve vision.

Subconjunctival hemorrhages are extravasations of blood beneath the conjunctiva usually resulting from minor trauma, straining, sneezing, or coughing; rarely, they occur spontaneously. The extent and location of hyperemia can help determine etiology. Diffuse hyperemia of both the bulbar and tarsal conjunctivae is typical of conjunctivitis. Subconjunctival hemorrhages alarm the patient but are of no pathologic significance except when associated with blood dyscrasia, which is rare. They are absorbed spontaneously, usually within 2 wk. Topical corticosteroids, antibiotics, vasoconstrictors, and compresses do not speed reabsorption; reassurance is adequate therapy.

Circumcorneal conjunctival hyperemia produced by dilated, fine, straight, deep vessels that radiate 1 to 3 mm out from the limbus, without significant hyperemia of the bulbar and tarsal conjunctivae, occurs with iritis, acute glaucoma, and some types of keratitis. A large patch of deep hyperemia involving 20 to 100% of the bulbar conjunctiva without hyperemia of the tarsal conjunctiva is typical of episcleritis and scleritis (see also Red Eye on p. 877).

Edema of the bulbar conjunctiva results in a translucent, bluish, thickened conjunctiva. Gross edema with ballooning of the conjunctiva, often leading to prolapse of conjunctiva, is known as chemosis.

Edema of the tarsal conjunctiva (typical of allergic conjunctivitis) results in fine, minute projections (papillae), giving the conjunctiva a velvety appearance.

Hyperplasia of lymphoid follicles in the conjunctiva can occur in viral or chlamydial conjunctivitis. It appears as small bumps with pale centers, giving a cobblestone appearance. It occurs most commonly in the inferior tarsal conjunctiva. Treatment is for viral or chlamydial conjunctivitis.

EPISCLERITIS

Episcleritis is recurring inflammation of the episcleral tissue of unknown etiology that is self-limiting and does not threaten vision. Symptoms are a localized area of hyperemia of the globe, irritation, and lacrimation. Diagnosis is clinical. Treatment is symptomatic.

Episcleritis occurs in young adults, more commonly in women. It is usually idiopathic but can be associated with connective tissue diseases.

Mild irritation occurs. Additionally, a bright red patch is present just under the bulbar conjunctiva (simple episcleritis). A hyperemic, edematous, raised nodule may also be present (nodular episcleritis). The palpebral conjunctiva is normal.

Episcleritis is distinguished from conjunctivitis because hyperemia is localized to a limited area of the globe and lacrimation is much less. It is distinguished from scleritis by lack of severe pain.

The condition is self-limited and is rarely associated with serious systemic disease. A topical corticosteroid (eg, prednisolone acetate, 1% drops qid for 5 days and gradually reduced over 3 wk) or an oral NSAID usually shortens the attack. Topical vasoconstrictors (eg, tetrahydrozoline) to improve the appearance are optional.

SCLERITIS

Scleritis is a severe, destructive, vision-threatening inflammation involving the deep episclera and sclera. Symptoms are moderate to marked pain, hyperemia of the globe, lacrimation, and photophobia. Diagnosis is clinical. Treatment is with systemic corticosteroids and possibly immunosuppressants.

Scleritis is most common in women aged 30 to 50 yr, and many have connective tissue diseases, such as RA, SLE, polyarteritis nodosa, Wegener's granulomatosis, or relapsing polychondritis. A few cases are infectious in origin. Scleritis most commonly involves the anterior segment and occurs in 3 types—diffuse, nodular, and necrotizing (scleromalacia perforans).

Symptoms, Signs, and Diagnosis

Pain (often characterized as a deep, boring ache) is severe enough to interfere with sleep and appetite. Photophobia and lacrimation may occur. Hyperemic patches develop deep beneath the bulbar conjunctiva and are more violaceous than those of episcleritis. The palpebral conjunctiva is normal. The involved area may be focal (ie, one quadrant of the globe) or involve the entire globe and may contain a hyperemic, edematous, raised nodule (nodular scleritis) or an avascular area (necrotizing scleritis).

In severe cases of necrotizing scleritis, perforation of the globe and loss of the eye may result. Connective tissue disease occurs in 20% of patients with diffuse or nodular scleritis and in 50% of patients with necrotizing scleritis. Necrotizing scleritis in patients with connective tissue disease signals an underlying systemic vasculitis. Diagnosis is made clinically and with a slit lamp. Smears or biopsies are necessary to confirm infectious scleritis. CT or ultrasound may be needed for posterior scleritis.

Prognosis and Treatment

Of patients with scleritis, 14% lose significant visual acuity within 1 yr and 30% in 3 yr. Patients with necrotizing scleritis and underlying systemic vasculitis have a mortality rate of up to 50% in 10 yr (mostly from MI).

A systemic corticosteroid (eg, prednisone 1 mg/kg po once/day) is the initial therapy. If scleritis is unresponsive to or intolerant of systemic corticosteroids or the patient has necrotizing scleritis and connective tissue disease, systemic immunosuppression with cyclophosphamide or azathioprine is indicated, but only in consultation with a rheumatologist. Scleral grafts may be indicated for threatened perforation.

102 CORNEAL DISORDERS

The cornea is subject to infection, noninfectious inflammation, ulceration, mechanical damage, and environmental injury. Infection (keratitis), frequently with accompanying secondary conjunctivitis, can be due to viruses, bacteria, *Acanthamoeba*, or fungi. Ulceration usually represents progression of keratitis. Evaluation of the cornea requires slit-lamp examination and, sometimes, microbial studies.

BULLOUS KERATOPATHY

Bullous keratopathy is the presence of corneal epithelial bullae, resulting from corneal endothelial disease.

Bullous keratopathy is caused by edema of the cornea, resulting from failure of the corneal endothelium to maintain the normally dehydrated state of the cornea. Most frequently it is due to Fuchs' corneal endothelial dystrophy or corneal endothelial trauma. Corneal endothelial trauma can occur during intraocular surgery (eg, cataract removal) or after placement of a poorly designed or malpositioned intraocular lens implant, promoting the development of bullous keratopathy. Fuchs' dystrophy causes bilateral, progressive corneal endothelial cell loss, sometimes leading to bullous keratopathy by age 50 to 60.

Subepithelial fluid-filled bullae form on the corneal surface and the corneal stroma swells, leading to eye discomfort, decreased visual acuity, loss of contrast, glare, and photophobia. Some bullae rupture, and bacteria can invade a ruptured bulla, leading to a corneal ulcer. The main symptom of rupture is moderate to severe pain.

The bullae and swelling of the corneal stroma can be seen on slit-lamp examination.

Treatment should be by an ophthalmologist and includes the use of dehydrating agents (eg, hypertonic saline), intraocular pressure–lowering agents, and soft contact lenses for some mild to moderate cases; corneal transplantation is usually successful.

CORNEAL ULCER

A corneal ulcer is local necrosis of corneal tissue due to invasion by bacteria, fungi, viruses, or *Acanthamoeba*. It can be initiated by mechanical trauma or nutritional deficiencies. Symptoms are progressive redness, foreign body sensation, ache, photophobia, and lacrimation. Diagnosis is by slit-lamp examination, fluorescein stain, and microbial studies. Treatment, with topical anti-infectives and often dilating drops, is urgent and requires an ophthalmologist.

Etiology and Pathophysiology

Corneal ulcers occur as complications of herpes simplex keratitis, neurotrophic keratitis, chronic blepharitis, trachoma, bullous keratopathy, and cicatricial pemphigoid. Inadequate contact lens sterilization may be a source of infection (see p. 883). Mechanical irritation may predispose to bacterial infection after sleeping with contact lenses in place, corneal trauma, or a corneal foreign body. Ulcers can also be caused by eyelid abnormalities such as entropion, trichiasis, and corneal exposure due to incomplete eyelid closure (eg, lagophthalmos, Bell's palsy, eyelid defects after trauma, exophthalmos). Ulcers may occur secondary to vitamin A deficiency or protein malnutrition.

Ulcers may be a rare stage of recurrent herpes simplex keratitis and may be particularly refractory to treatment. Ulcers caused by *Acanthamoeba* and fungi are indolent but progressive; those caused by *Pseudomonas aeruginosa* rapidly develop deep and extensive corneal necrosis.

Corneal ulcers tend to heal with scar tissue, causing opacification of the cornea and decreased visual acuity. Uveitis, corneal perforation with iris prolapse, pus in the anterior chamber (hypopyon), panophthalmitis, and destruction of the eye may occur with or without treatment. The deeper the ulcer, the more severe the symptoms and complications.

Symptoms, Signs, and Diagnosis

Eye ache, foreign body sensation, photophobia, and lacrimation may be minimal initially.

A corneal ulcer begins as a dull, grayish, circumscribed superficial opacity and subsequently necroses and suppurates to form an excavated ulcer. An epithelial defect is present and stains with fluorescein. Considerable circumcorneal hyperemia is usual. In long-standing cases, blood vessels may grow in from the limbus (corneal neovascularization). The ulcer may spread to involve the width of the cornea and/or may penetrate deeply. Hypopyon (layered WBCs in the anterior chamber) may occur.

Corneal ulcers due to *Acanthamoeba* are intensely painful and may demonstrate transient corneal epithelial defects, multiple corneal stromal infiltrates, and, later, a large ring-shaped infiltrate. Fungal ulcers are more chronic than bacterial ulcers, are densely infiltrated, and show occasional discrete islands of infiltrate (satellite lesions) at the periphery.

Diagnosis is made by finding a corneal infiltrate with an epithelial defect that stains with fluorescein. All but small ulcers should be cultured by scraping with a sterile platinum spatula (typically by an ophthalmologist).

Treatment

Treatment for corneal ulcers from any cause begins with moxifloxacin 0.5% or gatifloxacin 0.3% for small ulcers and fortified (higher than stock concentration) antibiotic drops, such as tobramycin 15 mg/mL and cefazolin 50 mg/mL, for more significant ulcers. Frequent dosing (eg, q 15 min for 4 doses, followed by q 1 h around the clock) is necessary initially. Patching is contraindicated because it produces a dark, warm environment that favors bacterial growth and interferes with administration of topical drugs.

Herpes simplex (see p.897) is treated with trifluridine 1% drops q 2 h while awake or acyclovir 400 mg po 5 times/day for 10 days. A cycloplegic may be added.

Fungal infections are treated with one of many topical antifungal drops (eg, natamycin 5% or amphotericin B 0.15%), initially q 1 h during the day and q 2 h overnight. Deep infections may require additional oral ketoconazole, fluconazole, or itraconazole. If *Acanthamoeba* is identified, traditional therapy is propamidine and neomycin supplemented with miconazole, clotrimazole, or oral ketoconazole. A newer treatment is polyhexamethylene biguanide 0.02% or chlorhexidine 0.02% q 1 to 2 h until clinical improvement is evident, then gradually reduced to 4 times/day and continued for a number of months until all inflammation has resolved. Polyhexamethylene biguanide and chlorhexidine are not available as ocular agents but can be prepared by a pharmacy.

In severe cases, debridement of the infected epithelium or even penetrating keratoplasty may be required. Patients who are poorly compliant or who have large, central, or refractory ulcers may be hospitalized.

HERPES SIMPLEX KERATITIS

(Herpes Simplex Keratoconjunctivitis)

Herpes simplex keratitis is corneal infection with herpes simplex virus (see also p. 1606). It may involve the iris and frequently recurs. Symptoms and signs include foreign body sensation, lacrimation, photophobia, and conjunctival hyperemia. Recurrences may lead to corneal hypoesthesia, ulceration, and permanent scarring. Diagnosis is based on the characteristic dendritic corneal ulcer and sometimes viral culture. Treatment is with topical and perhaps systemic antiviral agents.

Symptoms, Signs, and Diagnosis

The initial (primary) infection is usually an undistinguished self-limiting conjunctivitis. Foreign body sensation, lacrimation, photophobia, and conjunctival hyperemia are early symptoms. Vesicular blepharitis (blisters on the eyelid) follows, symptoms worsen, vision blurs, and blisters break down and ulcerate, then clear without scarring in about a week. Herpes simplex keratitis is slow to heal, frequently taking several weeks. Recurrences usually take the form of epithelial keratitis (also called dendritic keratitis) with the same symptoms plus a characteristic branched lesion of the corneal epithelium that resembles a branching tree with knoblike terminals, all of which stain with fluorescein. Multiple recurrences may result in corneal hypesthesia or anesthesia, ulceration, and permanent scarring.

Diskiform keratitis, involving the corneal stroma, is a deeper, disk-shaped, localized area of corneal edema and haze with accompanying anterior uveitis. It may cause pain and vision loss and occurs in patients who have had epithelial keratitis. It is probably an immunologic response to the virus.

The slit-lamp finding of a dendrite is characteristic enough for the diagnosis in most cases. When the appearance is not conclusive, definitive diagnosis can be made by viral culture of the lesion.

Treatment

Topical therapy (eg, trifluridine 1% drops 9 times/day) is usually effective. Occasionally, acyclovir is indicated 400 mg po 5 times/day for the initial infection or 400 mg po tid for recurrent infection. Immunocompromised patients usually require IV antivirals (eg, acyclovir 5 mg/kg IV q 8 h for 7 days). If the epithelium surrounding the dendrite is loose and edematous, debridement by gentle swabbing with a cotton-tipped applicator before beginning drug therapy may speed healing. *Topical corticosteroids are contraindicated in epithelial keratitis* but may be effective when used with an antiviral drug in later stage stromal (diskiform keratitis) involvement or uveitis. Atropine 1% instilled tid is useful if uveitis is present. A slit lamp is required to manage patients with viral epithelial keratitis. If one is not available or if stromal or uveal involvement occurs, referral to an ophthalmologist is necessary.

HERPES ZOSTER OPHTHALMICUS

(Herpes Zoster Virus Ophthalmicus; Ophthalmic Herpes Zoster; Varicella-Zoster Virus Ophthalmicus)

Herpes zoster ophthalmicus is varicella-zoster virus infection (see also p. 1609) involving the eye. Symptoms and signs, which may be intense, include dermatomal forehead rash and painful inflammation of all the tissues of the anterior and, rarely, posterior segments of the eye. Diagnosis is by characteristic appearance of the anterior eye when accompanied by zoster dermatitis of the 1st branch of the trigeminal nerve. Treatment is with oral antiviral drugs, mydriatics, and topical corticosteroids.

Varicella-zoster of the forehead involves the globe in 3/4 of cases when the nasociliary nerve is affected (as indicated by a lesion on the tip of the nose) and in 1/3 of cases not involving the tip of the nose. Overall, the globe is involved in 1/2 of patients.

Symptoms and Signs

During acute disease, in addition to the forehead rash, marked eyelid edema; conjunctival, episcleral, and circumcorneal hyperemia; corneal edema; epithelial and stromal keratitis; uveitis; glaucoma; and pain may be present. Keratitis accompanied by uveitis may be severe and is followed by scarring. Late sequelae—glaucoma, cataract, chronic or recurrent uveitis, corneal scarring, neovascularization, and hypesthesia—are common and threaten vision.

Diagnosis

Diagnosis is based on a typical acute herpes zoster rash on the forehead or on an appropriate history and a late atrophic forehead lesion. Herpetic lesions in this distribution that do not yet involve the eye suggest significant risk and should stimulate an ophthalmologic consultation before the eye becomes involved. Culture and immunologic or PCR studies of skin acutely or serial serologic tests are performed only when lesions are atypical and the diagnosis uncertain.

Treatment

Early treatment with acyclovir 800 mg po 5 times/day or famciclovir 500 mg or valacyclovir 1 g po tid for 7 days reduces ocular complications. Unlike patients with herpes simplex virus infection, patients with keratitis or uveitis from herpes zoster ophthalmicus require topical corticosteroids (eg, dexamethasone 0.1% instilled q 2 h initially, lengthening the interval to q 4 to 8 h as symptoms improve). The pupil should be kept dilated with atropine 1% or scopolamine 0.25% 1 drop tid. Intraocular pressure must be monitored and treated if it rises above normal values.

Use of a brief course of high-dose oral corticosteroids to prevent postherpetic neuralgia in patients > 60 yr who are in good general health remains controversial.

INTERSTITIAL KERATITIS

(Parenchymatous Keratitis)

Interstitial keratitis is chronic, nonulcerative inflammation of the middle layers of the cornea (ie, mid-stroma) that is sometimes associated with uveitis. The cause is usually infectious. Symptoms are photophobia, pain, lacrimation, and gradual vision blurring. Diagnosis is by slit-lamp examination and serologic tests to determine the cause. Treatment is directed at the cause and may require topical corticosteroids.

Interstitial keratitis, another manifestation of certain corneal infections, is rare in the US. Most cases occur in children as a late complication of congenital syphilis (see p. 2322). Ultimately, both eyes may be involved. A similar but less dramatic bilateral keratitis occurs in Cogan's syndrome, Lyme disease, and Epstein-Barr virus infection. Rarely, acquired syphilis or TB may cause a unilateral form in adults.

Symptoms, Signs, and Diagnosis

Photophobia, pain, lacrimation, and gradual vision blurring are common. The lesion begins as patches of inflammation in the middle corneal layers (ie, stroma). Typically with syphilis and occasionally with other causes, the entire cornea develops a ground-glass appearance, obscuring the iris. New blood vessels grow in from the limbus and produce orange-red areas (salmon patches). Anterior uveitis and choroiditis are common in syphilitic interstitial keratitis. Inflammation and neovascularization usually begin to subside after 1 to 2 mo. Some corneal opacity usually remains, causing mild to moderate vision impairment.

The specific etiology must be determined. The stigmas of congenital syphilis, vestibuloauditory symptoms, history of an expanding rash, and tick exposure support a specific etiology. However, all patients should have serologic testing, including fluorescent treponemal antibody absorption test or the microhemagglutination assay for *Treponema pallidum*, Lyme titer, and Epstein-Barr panel. Patients with negative serologic test results may have Cogan's syndrome. To prevent permanent vestibuloauditory damage, symptoms of hearing loss, tinnitus, or vertigo require referral to an otolaryngologist.

Treatment

Treatment of the underlying condition may resolve the keratitis. Additional topical treatment with a corticosteroid, such as prednisolone 1% qid, is often advisable. An ophthalmologist should be consulted.

Cogan's Syndrome

Cogan's syndrome is a rare autoimmune disease involving the eye and the inner ear.

Cogan's syndrome affects young adults, with 80% of patients between 14 and 47 yr. The disease appears to result from an autoimmune reaction directed against an unknown common autoantigen in the cornea and inner ear. About 10 to 30% of patients also have a severe systemic vasculitis, which may include life-threatening aortitis.

Ocular involvement includes bilateral interstitial keratitis, other corneal stromal keratitis, episcleritis, scleritis, uveitis, papillitis, or orbital inflammation. Ocular symptoms include irritation, photophobia, and decreased vision. Vestibuloauditory symptoms include sensorineural hearing loss, tinnitus, and vertigo. The presenting symptoms involve the ocular system in 38%, the vestibuloauditory system in 46%, and both in 15%. By 5 mo, 75% of patients have both ocular and vestibuloauditory symptoms. Nonspecific systemic complaints include fever, headache, joint pain, and myalgia. Ocular examination shows typical findings of interstitial keratitis (see p. 898) or inflammation of other layers of the corneal stroma, ocular redness, intraocular inflammation, optic nerve edema, and/or exophthalmos. A diastolic heart murmur may be present with significant aortitis.

Diagnosis is by clinical findings and exclusion of other causes (eg, syphilis, Lyme disease). Evaluation by an ophthalmologist and otolaryngologist is important. Untreated disease may lead to corneal scarring and visual loss and, in 60 to 80%, permanent hearing loss.

Treatment must be initiated expeditiously with high-dose corticosteroids. Prednisone 1 mg/kg po once/day is used for 2 to 6 mo. Some clinicians add cyclophosphamide, methotrexate, or cyclosporine for recalcitrant cases.

KERATOCONJUNCTIVITIS SICCA

(Dry Eyes; Keratitis Sicca)

Keratoconjunctivitis sicca is chronic, bilateral desiccation of the conjunctiva and cornea due to an inadequate tear film. Symptoms include itching, burning, irritation, and photophobia. Diagnosis is clinical; the Schirmer test may be helpful. Treatment is with topical tear supplements, blockage of the nasolacrimal openings, and sometimes oral tetracyclines and/or topical antibiotics or topical cyclosporine.

Etiology

This condition may be caused by inadequate tear volume (aqueous tear-deficient keratoconjunctivitis sicca) or, more commonly, by accelerated tear evaporation because of poor tear quality (evaporative keratoconjunctivitis sicca).

Aqueous tear-deficient keratoconjunctivitis sicca is most commonly an isolated idiopathic condition in postmenopausal women. It is also commonly part of Sjögren's syndrome (see p. 264). Less commonly, it is secondary to other conditions that scar the lacrimal ducts (eg, cicatricial pemphigoid, Stevens-Johnson syndrome, trachoma). It may result from a damaged or malfunctioning lacrimal gland due to graft-vs-host disease, HIV (diffuse infiltrative lymphocytosis syndrome), local radiation therapy, or familial dysautonomia.

Evaporative keratoconjunctivitis sicca is caused by loss of the tear film due to abnormally rapid evaporation from an inadequate oil layer on the surface of the aqueous layer of tears. Symptoms may result from abnormal oil quality (ie, meibomian gland dysfunction) or a degraded normal oil layer (ie, seborrheic blepharitis). Patients frequently have acne rosacea.

Symptoms and Signs

Patients report itching, burning, photophobia, pressure behind the eye, or a gritty, pulling, or foreign body sensation. A sharp stabbing pain, eye strain or fatigue, and blurred vision may also occur. Some patients note a flood of tears after severe irritation. Typically, symptoms fluctuate in intensity and may be intermittent, aggravated by prolonged visual efforts (eg, reading, working on the computer, driving, watching television). Local environments that are dry, dusty, or smoky can also aggravate symptoms. Certain systemic drugs, including isotretinoin, sedatives, diuretics, antihypertensives, oral contraceptives, and all anticholinergics (including antihistamines and many GI drugs), can aggravate symptoms. Symptoms lessen on cool, rainy, or foggy days or in other high-humidity environments, such as in the shower. Although keratoconjunctivitis sicca rarely decreases vision, irritation can be intense.

With both forms, the conjunctiva is hyperemic, and there is often scattered, fine, punctate loss of corneal (superficial punctate keratitis) and/or conjunctival epithelium. When the condition is severe, the involved areas, mainly between the eyelids (the intrapalpebral or exposure zone), stain with fluorescein. Patients often blink at an accelerated rate because of irritation. Rarely, an insufficient blink rate can also cause exposure and drying.

With the aqueous tear-deficient form, the conjunctiva can appear dry and lusterless with redundant folds. With the evaporative form, abundant tears may be present as well as foam at the eyelid margin. Very rarely, severe, advanced, chronic drying leads to significant vision loss from keratinization of the ocular surface or loss of corneal epithelium, leading to scarring, vascularization, infections, ulceration, and perforation.

Diagnosis

Diagnosis is based on characteristic symptoms and clinical appearance. The Schirmer test and tear breakup test may differentiate type.

The Schirmer test determines whether tear production is normal. A strip of filter paper is placed, without topical anesthesia, at the junction of the middle and lateral third of the lower eyelid. A person with < 5.5 mm of wetting after 5 min on 2 successive occasions has aqueous tear-deficient keratoconjunctivitis sicca.

With evaporative keratoconjunctivitis sicca, the Schirmer test is usually normal. Instillation of a small volume of highly concentrated fluorescein can make the tear film visible under cobalt blue light at the slit lamp. A blink reapplies a complete tear film. The patient then stares, and the length of time until the first dry spot develops is determined (tear breakup test). An accelerated rate of intact tear film loss (< 10 sec) is characteristic of evaporative keratoconjunctivitis sicca.

Once aqueous tear-deficient keratoconjunctivitis sicca is diagnosed, Sjögren's syndrome (see p. 264) should be suspected, especially if xerostomia is also present. Serologic tests and labial salivary gland biopsy are used for diagnosis. Patients with primary or secondary Sjögren's syndrome are at increased risk for several serious diseases, (eg, biliary cirrhosis, non-Hodgkin's lymphoma). Therefore, proper evaluation and monitoring are essential.

Treatment

Frequent use of artificial tears can be effective for both forms. More viscous artificial tears coat the ocular surface longer and are particularly useful in evaporative keratoconjunctivitis sicca. Artificial tear ointments applied before sleep are particularly useful when patients have nocturnal lagophthalmos or irritation on waking. Most cases are treated adequately throughout the patient's life with such supplementation. Using humidifiers and avoiding dry, drafty environments can often help. Not smoking and avoiding secondary smoke are important. In recalcitrant cases, occlusion of the nasolacrimal punctum may be indicated. In severe cases, a partial tarsorrhaphy can reduce tear loss through evaporation. Topical cyclosporine may be a useful adjunct in some patients.

Patients with evaporative keratoconjunctivitis sicca often benefit from treatment of concomitant blepharitis and associated rosacea with warm compresses, eyelid margin scrubs, intermittent topical eyelid antibiotic ointments (eg, bacitracin at bedtime) and/or systemic doxycycline 50 to 100 mg po once or twice/day (contraindicated in pregnant or nursing patients—see p. 886).

KERATOCONUS

Keratoconus is a bulging distortion of the cornea, leading to loss of visual acuity.

Keratoconus is a slowly progressive ectasia of the cornea (bulging due to weakness of its structural elements), usually bilateral, beginning between ages 10 and 20. Its cause is unknown. The cone shape that the cornea assumes causes major changes in the refractive characteristics of the cornea (irregular astigmatism) and necessitates frequent change of eyeglasses. Contact lenses may provide better vision correction and should be tried when eyeglasses are not satisfactory. Corneal transplant surgery may be necessary if visual acuity with contact lenses is inadequate, contact lenses are not tolerated, or a visually significant corneal scar is present.

KERATOMALACIA

(Xerotic Keratitis; Xerophthalmia)

Keratomalacia is degeneration of the cornea caused by nutritional deficiency.

Keratomalacia is typically caused by vitamin A deficiency and protein-calorie malnutrition. It is characterized by a hazy, dry cornea that becomes denuded. Corneal ulceration with secondary infection is common. The lacrimal glands and conjunctiva are also affected. Lack of tears causes extreme dryness of the eyes, and foamy spots appear on the temporal and often nasal bulbar conjunctiva (Bitot's spots). Night blindness may occur. Further details, including specific therapy, can be found under Vitamin A Deficiency on p. 34.

PERIPHERAL ULCERATIVE KERATITIS

(Marginal Keratolysis; Peripheral Rheumatoid Ulceration)

Peripheral ulcerative keratitis is inflammation and ulceration of the cornea occurring with chronic connective tissue diseases. Irritation and decreased vision result.

Peripheral ulcerative keratitis is a serious corneal ulceration that often occurs with active and/or long-standing connective tissue diseases, such as RA, Wegener's granulomatosis, and relapsing polychondritis. The high mortality rate of about 40% in 10 yr (mostly from MI) in patients with connective tissue disease and peripheral ulcerative keratitis is due to an underlying vasculitis. The mortality rate may be reduced to about 8% in 10 yr with systemic cytotoxic immunosuppression.

Patients often have decreased visual acuity, photophobia, and foreign body sensation. A crescentic area of opacification in the periphery of the cornea, due to infiltration by WBCs and ulceration, stains with fluorescein. Infectious causes, such as bacteria, fungi, and herpes simplex virus, must be ruled out by culturing the ulcer and eyelid margins.

Any patient with this type of ulcer should be promptly referred to an ophthalmologist. Treatment includes local and systemic approaches to control inflammation (eg, immunosuppression or tissue adhesive and bandage contact lenses) and repair damage (eg, patch grafts). Cyclophosphamide or other immunosuppressants treat the keratitis, life-threatening vasculitis, and underlying autoimmune disease. Additionally, helpful drugs include collagenase inhibitors, such as tetracycline or topical 20% *N*-acetylcysteine.

PHLYCTENULAR KERATOCONJUNCTIVITIS

(Phlyctenular Conjunctivitis; Phlyctenulosis)

Phlyctenular keratoconjunctivitis, a hypersensitivity reaction of the cornea and conjunctiva to bacterial antigens, is characterized by discrete nodular areas of corneal or conjunctival inflammation.

Phlyctenular keratoconjunctivitis results from a hypersensitivity reaction to bacterial antigens, primarily staphylococcal, but TB, *Chlamydia*, and other agents have been implicated. It is more common in children.

Patients have crops of small yellow-gray nodules (phlyctenules) that appear at the limbus, on the cornea, or on the bulbar conjunctiva and persist from several days to 2 wk. On the conjunctiva, these nodules ulcerate but heal without a scar. When the cornea is affected, severe lacrimation, photophobia, aching, and foreign body sensation may be prominent. Frequent recurrence, especially with secondary infection, may lead to corneal opacity and vascularization with loss of visual acuity.

Diagnosis is by characteristic clinical appearance. Testing for TB may be indicated. Treatment is with a topical corticosteroid-antibiotic combination. If phlyctenulosis is associated with seborrheic blepharitis, eyelid scrubs may reduce recurrence.

SUPERFICIAL PUNCTATE KERATITIS

Superficial punctate keratitis is corneal inflammation of diverse causes characterized by scattered, fine, punctate corneal epithelial loss or damage. Symptoms are redness, irritation, and decreased vision. Diagnosis is by slit-lamp examination. Treatment depends on cause.

Superficial punctate keratitis is a nonspecific finding often caused by viral conjunctivitis, blepharitis, keratoconjunctivitis sicca, trachoma, ultraviolet (UV) light exposure (eg, welding arcs, sunlamps, snow glare), contact lens overwear, systemic drugs (eg, adenine arabinoside), and topical drug or preservative toxicity.

Symptoms include photophobia, foreign body sensation, lacrimation, redness, and decreased vision. Slit-lamp or ophthalmoscope examination of the cornea reveals a characteristic hazy appearance with multiple punctate speckles that stain with fluorescein.

Keratitis that accompanies adenovirus conjunctivitis (the most common type of viral conjunctivitis) resolves spontaneously in about 3 wk. Blepharitis (see p. 885), keratoconjunctivitis sicca (see p. 899), and trachoma (see p. 892) require specific therapy. When caused by overwearing contact lenses, keratitis is treated with an antibiotic ointment (eg, ciprofloxacin 0.3% qid), but the eye is not patched because of the high incidence of serious infection. Patients should be examined the next day. Suspected topical drugs (active ingredient or preservative) should be stopped.

Ultraviolet keratitis: UVB light (wavelength < 300 nm) can burn the cornea, causing keratitis or keratoconjunctivitis. It can be caused by arc welding, high-voltage electric sparks, artificial sun lamps, and sunlight reflected off snow at high altitudes. UV radiation increases 4 to 6% for every 1000-ft (305-m) increase in altitude above sea level, and snow reflects 85% of UVB. Even a brief, unprotected glance at a welding arc may produce a burn.

Symptoms are usually not apparent for 8 to 12 h after exposure and last 24 to 48 h. Patients have lacrimation, pain, redness, swollen eyelids, photophobia, headache, foreign body sensation, and decreased vision. Permanent vision loss is rare. Diagnosis is by history, presence of superficial punctate keratitis, and absence of a foreign body or infection. Treatment consists of short-acting cycloplegic drugs, an antibiotic solution or ointment (eg, bacitracin or gentamicin 0.3% 2 drops q 4 h or a thin ointment strip q 8 h), and patching the more severely affected eye. Severe pain may require systemic analgesics. The corneal surface regenerates spontaneously in 24 to 48 h. The eye must be rechecked in 24 h. Dark glasses or welder's helmets that block UV light are preventive.

CORNEAL TRANSPLANTATION

(Corneal Graft; Penetrating Keratoplasty)

Corneal transplantations are performed for several reasons:

- To improve the optical qualities of the cornea and thus improve vision—eg, replacing a cornea that is scarred after a corneal ulcer; is clouded from edema (Fuchs' dystrophy or edema after cataract surgery); is opaque due to deposits of nontransparent abnormal corneal stromal proteins (eg, hereditary corneal stromal dystrophy); or has irregular astigmatism, as occurs with keratoconus
- To reconstruct the anatomic cornea to preserve the eye—eg, replacing a perforated cornea
- To preserve the eye from a disease unresponsive to medical management—eg, severe, uncontrolled fungal corneal ulcer; or to alleviate pain—eg, to relieve severe foreign body sensation due to recurrent ruptured bullae in bullous keratopathy.

The most common indications are bullous keratopathy (pseudophakic, Fuchs' endothelial dystrophy, aphakic), keratoconus, repeat graft, keratitis/postkeratitis (viral, bacterial, fungal, *Acanthamoeba*, perforation), and corneal stromal dystrophies.

Tissue matching is not routinely performed. Cadaveric donor tissue cannot be used from anyone suspected of having a communicable disease.

Corneal transplantation can be performed using general anesthesia or local anesthesia plus IV sedation.

Topical antibiotics are used for several weeks postoperatively and topical corticosteroids for several months. To protect the eye from inadvertent trauma after transplantation, the patient wears shields, glasses, or sunglasses. In some patients, corneal astigmatism can be reduced in the early postoperative period by suture adjustment or selective suture removal. Achievement of full visual potential may take up to 18 mo because of changing refraction after suture removal, wound healing, and/or corneal astigmatism. In many patients, earlier and better vision is attained with a rigid contact lens over the corneal transplant.

Complications include infection (intraocular and corneal), wound leak, glaucoma, graft rejection, graft failure, high refractive error (especially astigmatism and/or myopia), and recurrence of disease (ie, herpes simplex, hereditary corneal stromal dystrophy).

Graft rejection has been reported in up to 68%. Patients develop decreased vision, photosensitivity, ocular ache, and ocular redness. Graft rejection is treated with topical corticosteroids (eg, prednisolone 1% hourly), sometimes with a supplemental periocular injection (eg, methylprednisolone 40 mg). If graft rejection is severe or if graft function is marginal, additional corticosteroids are given orally (eg, prednisone 1 mg/kg once/day) and occasionally IV (eg, methylprednisolone 3 to 5 mg/kg once). Typically the rejection episode reverses, and graft function returns fully. The graft may fail if the rejection episode is unusually severe or long-standing or after multiple episodes of graft rejection. Regraft is possible, but the long-term prognosis is lower than for the original graft.

Prognosis

The chance of long-term transplant success is > 90% for keratoconus, corneal scars, early bullous keratopathy, or hereditary corneal stromal dystrophies; 80 to 90% for more advanced bullous keratopathy or inactive viral keratitis; 50% for active corneal infection; and 0 to 50% for chemical or radiation injury.

The generally high rate of success of corneal transplantation is attributable to many factors, including the avascularity of the cornea and the fact that the anterior chamber has venous drainage but no lymphatic drainage. These conditions promote low-zone tolerance (an immunologic tolerance that results from constant exposure to low doses of an antigen) and an active process termed anterior chamber–associated immune deviation, in which there is suppression of intraocular lymphocytes and delayed-type hypersensitivity to transplanted intraocular antigens. Another important factor is the effectiveness of the corticosteroids (topically, locally, and systemically) used to treat graft rejection.

Corneal Limbal Stem Cell Transplantation

Corneal limbal stem cell transplantation surgically replaces critical stem cells at the periphery of the cornea when the host stem cells have been too severely damaged to recover. Conditions such as severe chemical burns and severe contact lens overwear may cause persistent nonhealing corneal epithelial defects. These defects result from failure of corneal epithelial stem cells to produce sufficient epithelial cells to repopulate the cornea. Untreated, persistent nonhealing corneal epithelial defects are vulnerable to infection, which can lead to scarring and/or perforation. The stem cells of the corneal epithelium reside at the base of the epithelium at the limbus (where the conjunctiva meets the cornea). Because a corneal transplant replaces only the central cornea and not the limbus, treatment of a persistent nonhealing corneal epithelial defect requires a corneal limbal stem cell transplant. Corneal limbal stem cells can be transplanted from the patient's healthy eye or from a cadaveric donor eye. The patient's damaged corneal epithelial stem cells are removed by a partial-thickness dissection of the limbus (ie, all the epithelium and the superficial stroma of the limbus). Donor limbal tissue, which is prepared by a similar dissection, is sutured into the prepared bed. The transplanted corneal epithelial stem cells produce new cells that repopulate the cornea, healing the persistent nonhealing corneal epithelial defect.

103 GLAUCOMA

The glaucomas are a group of eye disorders characterized by progressive optic nerve damage at least partly due to increased intraocular pressure (IOP). Glaucoma is the 2nd most common cause of blindness in the US and the leading cause for black and Hispanic Americans. About 3 million Americans have glaucoma, but only ½ are aware of it. Glaucoma can occur at any age but is 6 times more common in people > 60 yr.

The glaucomas are categorized as open-angle or closed-angle (angle-closure—see TABLE 103–1). The "angle" refers to the angle formed by the junction of the iris and cornea at the periphery of the anterior chamber (see FIG. 103–1). The angle is where > 96% of the aqueous humor exits the eye via either the trabecular meshwork and Schlemm's canal (the major pathway, particularly in the elderly) or the ciliary body face and choroidal vasculature. These drainage paths are not simply a mechanical filter and drain but instead involve active physiologic processes.

Glaucomas are further subdivided into primary (cause of outflow resistance or angle closure is unknown) and secondary (outflow resistance results from another disorder), accounting for > 20 adult types.

TABLE 103–1. CLASSIFICATION OF THE GLAUCOMAS BASED ON MECHANISMS OF OUTFLOW OBSTRUCTION*

I. Open-Angle Glaucoma Mechanisms

A. Trabecular
- 1. Idiopathic
  - a. Chronic open-angle glaucoma
  - b. Juvenile glaucoma
  - c. Steroid-induced glaucoma
- 2. "Clogging" of trabecular meshwork
  - a. RBCs
    - Hemorrhagic glaucoma
    - Ghost cell glaucoma
  - b. Macrophages
    - Hemolytic glaucoma
    - Phacolytic glaucoma
    - Melanomalytic glaucoma
  - c. Neoplastic cells
    - Malignant tumors
    - Neurofibromatosis
    - Nevus of Ota
    - Juvenile xanthogranuloma
  - d. Pigment particles
    - Pigmentary glaucoma
    - Exfoliation syndrome (glaucoma capsulare)
    - Uveitis
    - Malignant melanoma
  - e. Protein
    - Uveitis
    - Lens-induced glaucoma
  - f. Viscoelastic agents
  - g. α-Chymotrypsin–induced glaucoma
  - h. Vitreous
- 3. Alterations of the trabecular meshwork
  - a. Edema
    - Iritis/uveitis (trabeculitis)
    - Scleritis and episcleritis
    - Alkali burns
  - b. Trauma (angle recession)
  - c. Intraocular foreign bodies (hemosiderosis, chalcosis)

B. Posttrabecular
- 1. Obstruction of Schlemm's canal
  - a. Collapse of canal
  - b. Clogging of canal (eg, sickled RBCs)
- 2. Elevated episcleral venous pressure
  - a. Carotid-cavernous fistula
  - b. Cavernous sinus thrombosis
  - c. Retrobulbar tumors
  - d. Thyrotropic exophthalmos
  - e. Superior vena cava obstruction
  - f. Mediastinal tumors
  - g. Sturge-Weber syndrome
  - h. Idiopathic episcleral venous pressure elevation

II. Angle-Closure Glaucoma Mechanisms

A. Anterior ("pulling" mechanism)
- 1. Contracture of membranes
  - a. Neovascular glaucoma
  - b. Iridocorneal endothelial syndrome
  - c. Posterior polymorphous dystrophy
  - d. Penetrating and nonpenetrating trauma
- 2. Contracture of inflammatory precipitates
- 3. Inflammatory membrane
  - a. Fuchs' heterochromic iridocyclitis
  - b. Luetic interstitial keratitis

B. Posterior ("pushing" mechanism)
- 1. With pupillary block
  - a. Pupillary block glaucoma
  - b. Lens-induced mechanisms
    - Intumescent lens
    - Subluxation of lens
    - Mobile lens syndrome
  - c. Posterior synechiae
    - Iris-vitreous block in aphakia
    - Pseudophakia
    - Uveitis
- 2. Without pupillary block
  - a. Plateau iris syndrome
  - b. Ciliary block (malignant) glaucoma
  - c. Lens-induced mechanisms
    - Intumescent lens
    - Subluxation of lens
    - Mobile lens syndrome
  - d. Following lens extraction (forward vitreous shift)
  - e. Uveal edema (eg, following scleral buckling, panretinal photocoagulation, central retinal vein occlusion)
  - f. Intraocular tumors
    - Malignant melanoma
    - Retinoblastoma
  - h. Cysts of the iris and ciliary body
  - i. Retrolenticular tissue contracture
    - Retinopathy of prematurity (retrolental fibroplasia)
    - Persistent hyperplastic primary vitreous

TABLE 103–1. CLASSIFICATION OF THE GLAUCOMAS BASED ON MECHANISMS OF OUTFLOW OBSTRUCTION*—Continued

III. Developmental Anomalies of the Anterior Chamber Angle

A. High insertion of peripheral iris
1. Axenfeld-Rieger syndrome
2. Peters' anomaly

B. Incomplete development of trabecular meshwork/Schlemm's canal
1. Congenital (infantile) glaucoma
2. Glaucomas associated with other developmental anomalies

C. Fine strands that contract to close angle (aniridia)

*Clinical examples cited; not an inclusive list of the glaucomas.

From Ritch R, Shields MB, Krupin T: *The Glaucomas,* ed 2. St. Louis, Mosby, 1996, p. 720; with permission.

Etiology and Pathophysiology

Axons of retinal ganglion cells travel through the optic nerve carrying images from the eye to the brain. Damage to these axons causes ganglion cell death with resultant optic nerve atrophy and patchy visual loss. Elevated IOP (normal range, 11 to 21 mm Hg) plays a role in axonal damage, either by direct nerve compression or diminution of blood flow. However, the relationship between pressure and nerve damage is variable. Many people with IOP > 21 mm Hg (ie, ocular hypertension) never develop glaucoma. Of those with elevated IOP, only about 1 to 2%/yr (roughly 10% over 5 yr) develop glaucoma. Additionally, about ⅓ of patients with glaucoma do not manifest IOPs > 21 mm Hg (low- or normal-tension glaucoma).

IOP is determined by the balance of aqueous secretion and drainage. Elevated IOP is caused by inadequate or obstructed outflow, not oversecretion. In open-angle glaucoma, IOP is elevated because outflow is inadequate despite an angle that appears unobstructed. In angle-closure glaucoma, IOP is elevated when a physical distortion of the peripheral iris mechanically blocks outflow.

Symptoms, Signs, and Diagnosis

Symptoms and signs vary with type of glaucoma, but the defining characteristic is optic nerve damage as evidenced by an abnormal optic disk and certain types of visual field deficits. Visual deficits of the optic nerve include nasal step defects (which do not cross the horizontal meridian), arcuate scotomata extending nasally from the blind spot, temporal wedge defects, and paracentral scotomata. Deficits of the more proximal visual pathways (ie, from the lateral geniculate nucleus to the occipital lobe) involve quadrants or hemispheres of the visual field. IOP may be elevated or within the average range. (For techniques of measurement, see p. 871.)

Glaucoma should be suspected in a patient with visual field defects, abnormal optic disk on funduscopy, or an elevated IOP. Such

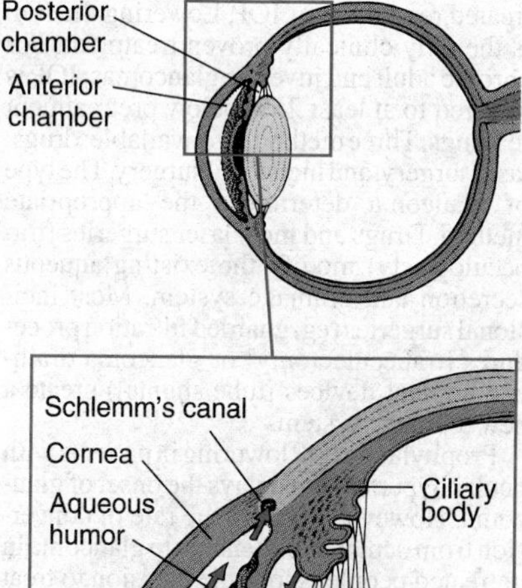

Fig. 103–1. Aqueous humor production and flow. Most of the aqueous humor, produced by the ciliary body, exits the eye at the angle formed by the junction of the iris and cornea. It exits primarily via the trabecular meshwork and Schlemm's canal.

patients (and those with any risk factors) should be referred to an ophthalmologist for a comprehensive examination that includes a thorough history, examination of the optic disks, formal visual field examination, IOP measurement, and gonioscopy (visualization of the anterior chamber angle with a special mirrored contact lens prism). Glaucoma is diagnosed when characteristic findings of optic nerve damage are present and other causes (eg, multiple sclerosis) have been excluded. Elevated IOP makes the diagnosis more likely but is not essential.

Screening can be done by primary physicians by checking visual fields with a frequency doubled perimeter and ophthalmoscopic evaluation of the optic nerve. Although IOP should be measured, screening based only on IOP has low sensitivity, low specificity, and low positive predictive value. Patients > 40 yr should receive comprehensive eye examinations q 1 to 2 yr.

Treatment

Patients with characteristic optic nerve and corresponding visual field changes are treated regardless of IOP. Lowering the IOP is the only clinically proven treatment. For chronic adult and juvenile glaucomas, IOP is lowered to at least 25% below pretreatment readings. Three methods are available: drugs, laser surgery, and incisional surgery. The type of glaucoma determines the appropriate method. Drugs and most laser surgeries (trabeculoplasty) modify the existing aqueous secretion and drainage system. Most incisional surgeries (eg, guarded filtration procedures [trabeculectomy] or glaucoma drainage implant devices [tube shunts]) create a new drainage system.

Prophylactic IOP lowering in patients with ocular hypertension delays the onset of glaucoma. However, because the rate of conversion from ocular hypertension to glaucoma in untreated people is low, the decision to treat prophylactically should be individualized by the presence of risk factors, magnitude of IOP elevation, and patient factors (ie, preference for drugs vs surgery, drug adverse effects). Generally, treatment is recommended for patients with IOP > 30 mm Hg.

PRIMARY OPEN-ANGLE GLAUCOMA

Primary open-angle glaucoma is a syndrome of optic nerve damage associated with an open anterior chamber angle and an elevated or sometimes average intraocular pressure (IOP). Symptoms occur late and involve visual field loss. Diagnosis is by funduscopy, gonioscopy, visual field examination, and measurement of IOP. Treatment includes topical β-blockers, prostaglandin analogs and other drugs, and sometimes surgical drainage.

Etiology and Pathophysiology

Although open-angle glaucoma can have numerous causes (see TABLE 103–1), 60 to 70% of cases have no identifiable cause (primary open-angle glaucoma). Both eyes usually are affected, but typically not equally.

Risk factors include older age, positive family history, black race, thinner central corneal thickness, systemic hypertension, diabetes, cardiovascular disease, and myopia. In blacks, glaucoma is more severe and develops at an earlier age, and blindness is 6 to 8 times more likely.

Elevated-pressure glaucoma: Two thirds of patients with glaucoma have elevated (>21 mm Hg) IOP. Aqueous humor drainage is inadequate, whereas production by the ciliary body is normal. Identifiable mechanisms (ie, secondary open-angle glaucomas) include developmental anomalies, scarring from trauma or infection, and plugging of channels by detached iris pigment or exfoliated anterior chamber cells.

Normal- or low-pressure glaucoma: In at least ⅓ of patients with glaucoma, IOP is within the average range, but optic nerve damage and visual field loss typical of glaucoma are present. These patients have a higher incidence of vasospastic diseases (eg, migraines, Raynaud's phenomenon) than the general population, suggesting that a primary vascular disorder compromising blood flow to the optic nerve may play a role.

Symptoms and Signs

Early symptoms are uncommon. Usually, the patient becomes aware of visual field loss only when optic nerve atrophy is quite marked; the typically asymmetric deficits contribute to delay in recognition. However, some patients have complaints, such as missing stairs if their inferior visual field has been lost, noticing portions of words missing when reading, or having difficulty with driving.

Findings on examination include an unobstructed open angle on gonioscopy and characteristic optic nerve appearance and visual field defects. IOP may be normal or high but is almost always higher in the eye with more optic nerve damage.

Optic nerve appearance: The optic nerve head (ie, disk) is normally a slightly vertically elongated circle with a centrally located depression called the cup. The neurosensory rim is the tissue between the margin of the cup and the edge of the disk and is composed of the ganglion cell axons from the retina. Characteristic optic nerve changes include increased cup:disk ratio, thinning of the neurosensory rim, pitting or notching of the rim, nerve fiber layer hemorrhage that crosses the disk margin (ie, Drance hemorrhage), vertical elongation of the cup, and quick angulations in the course of the exiting blood vessels. Thinning of the neurosensory rim over time can be solely diagnostic of glaucoma regardless of the IOP or visual field. However, most initial diagnoses of glaucoma involve some visual field change.

Visual field defects: Visual field changes caused by lesions of the optic nerve include nasal step defects (which do not cross the horizontal meridian), arcuate scotomata extending from the blind spot nasally, temporal wedge defects, and paracentral scotomata.

Diagnosis

Diagnosis is suggested by the examination, but similar findings can result from other optic neuropathies (eg, from ischemia, cytomegalovirus infection, vitamin B_{12} deficiency).

Before a diagnosis of normal-pressure glaucoma can be established, the following factors may need to be ruled out: inaccurate IOP readings, large diurnal fluctuations (producing intermittent normal readings), optic nerve damage from previous resolved glaucoma, intermittent angle-closure glaucoma, and other ocular or neurologic disorders that produce similar visual field defects.

Optic disk photography and a detailed optic disk drawing are helpful for future comparison. The frequency of follow-up examinations varies from weeks to years, depending on the patient's reliability, severity of the glaucoma, and response to treatment.

Treatment

Vision lost by glaucoma cannot be recovered. The goal is to prevent further optic nerve and visual field damage by lowering IOP. The target level is 25 to 40% below pretreatment readings. If damage progresses, the IOP goal is lowered further, and additional therapy is initiated.

Initial treatment is usually drug therapy, proceeding to laser therapy and then incisional surgery if the target IOP is not met. Surgery may be the initial treatment if IOP is extremely high.

Drug therapy: Multiple drugs are available (see TABLE 103–2). Topical agents are preferred. The most popular are the prostaglandin analogs, followed by β-blockers (particularly timolol). Other drugs include α_2-selective adrenergic agonists, cholinergic agonists, and carbonic anhydrase inhibitors. Oral carbonic anhydrase inhibitors are effective, but adverse effects limit their use.

Patients taking topical glaucoma drugs should be taught passive lid closure with punctal occlusion to help reduce systemic absorption and associated adverse effects, although the effectiveness of these maneuvers is controversial. Patients who cannot tolerate drops instilled directly onto the conjunctiva may place the drop on the nose just medial to the medial canthus, then roll the head slightly toward the eye so that the liquid flows into the eye.

Typically, to gauge effectiveness, drugs are started in only one eye (one-eye trial); once improvement in the treated eye has been confirmed at a subsequent visit (typically 1 to 4 wk later), both eyes are treated.

Surgery: Surgery for primary open-angle and normal-pressure glaucoma includes laser trabeculoplasty, a guarded filtration procedure, and possibly tube shunts or ciliodestructive procedures.

Argon laser trabeculoplasty (ALT) may be the initial treatment for patients who do not respond to or who cannot tolerate drug therapy. Laser energy is applied to either 180° or 360° of the trabecular meshwork to improve the drainage of aqueous humor. Within 2 to 5 yr, about 50% of patients require additional drug therapy or surgery because of insufficient IOP control.

Selective laser trabeculoplasty (SLT) uses a pulsed double-frequency neodymium:yttrium-aluminum-garnet laser. SLT and ALT are equally effective initially, but SLT may have greater effectiveness in subsequent treatments.

A guarded filtration procedure is the most commonly used filtration procedure. A hole is made in the limbal sclera, which is covered by a partial-thickness scleral flap that controls egress of aqueous from the eye to the subconjunctival space, forming a filtration bleb. Patients with trabeculectomies are at increased risk of endophthalmitis and should

TABLE 103–2. DRUGS USED TO TREAT GLAUCOMA

TYPE	DRUG/DOSE/ FREQUENCY	MECHANISM OF ACTION ON EYE	COMMENTS
Miotics, direct-acting (cholinergic agonists; topical)	Carbachol 1 drop bid–tid Pilocarpine 1 drop bid–qid	Cause miosis, increase aqueous outflow	Less effective as monotherapy than β-blockers; patients with darker pigmented pupils may need higher strengths; hinder dark adaptation
Miotics, indirect-acting (cholinesterase inhibitors; topical)	Demecarium 1 drop once/day–bid* Echothiophate iodide 1 drop once/day–bid* Isoflurophate 1 drop once/day–bid* Neostigmine 1 drop once/day–bid† Physostigmine 1 drop once/day–bid†	Cause miosis, increase aqueous outflow	Shorter acting, reversible inhibition Very long acting; irreversible inhibition; can cause cataracts and retinal detachment; should be avoided in angle-closure glaucoma because of the extreme miosis; hinder dark adaptation May still be excellent choices in pseudophakic patients
Carbonic anhydrase inhibitors (oral or IV)	Acetazolamide 125–250 mg po qid (or 500 mg po bid using extended-release capsules) or 500 mg IV single dose (adult) Methazolamide 25–50 mg po bid–tid	Decrease aqueous production	Used as adjunctive therapy. Cause fatigue, altered taste, anorexia, depression, paresthesias, electrolyte abnormalities, kidney stones, blood dyscrasias
Carbonic anhydrase inhibitors (topical)	Brinzolamide 1 drop bid–qid Dorzolamide 1 drop bid–tid¨		Low risk of systemic effects, but may cause bad taste in mouth
Nonselective adrenergic agonists (topical)	Dipivefrin 1 drop bid Epinephrine 1 drop bid	Cause mydriasis, increase aqueous outflow and decrease aqueous production	Often combined with a miotic (dipivefrin, a prodrug, is metabolized to epinephrine). Less reliable than selective adrenergic agents and higher incidence of allergic and toxic reactions
α_2-Selective adrenergic agonists (topical)	Apraclonidine 1 drop bid–tid Brimonidine 1 drop bid–tid‡	Decrease aqueous production; may increase uveoscleral aqueous outflow; may cause mydriasis	Apraclonidine has a high rate of allergic reaction and tachyphylaxis. Less common with brimonidine, which may cause dry mouth
β-Blockers (topical)	Timolol 1 drop once/day–bid Betaxolol 1 drop once/day–bid§ Carteolol 1 drop once/day–bid Levobunolol 1 drop once/day–bid Metipranolol 1 drop once/day–bid	Decrease aqueous production; do not affect pupil size	Systemic adverse effects include bronchospasm, depression, fatigue, confusion, erectile dysfunction, hair loss, bradycardia. May develop insidiously and be attributed by patients to aging or other processes

TABLE 103–2. DRUGS USED TO TREAT GLAUCOMA—Continued

TYPE	DRUG/DOSE/ FREQUENCY	MECHANISM OF ACTION ON EYE	COMMENTS
Prostaglandin analogs (topical)	Bimatoprost 1 drop at bedtime Latanoprost 1 drop at bedtime Travoprost 1 drop at bedtime Unoprostone 1 drop at bedtime	Increase uveoscleral outflow rather than altering conventional (trabeculocanalicular) aqueous outflow	Increased pigmentation of the iris; possible worsening of uveitis. Few systemic effects
Osmotic diuretics (oral, IV)	Glycerin 1–1.5 g/kg body weight po. May repeat 8–12 h later Mannitol 0.5–2.0 g/kg body weight IV over 30–45 min May repeat 8–12 h later	Cause increased serum osmolarity, which draws fluid from eye	Used for acute angle closure; have adverse systemic effects

*Irreversible; may be cataractogenic; increased risk of retinal detachment.
†Reversible.
‡More α_2-selective than apraclonidine.
§β_1-selective.

be instructed to report any signs or symptoms of bleb infection (blebitis) or endophthalmitis immediately.

ANGLE-CLOSURE GLAUCOMA

Angle-closure glaucoma is glaucoma associated with a closed anterior chamber angle, which may be chronic or, rarely, acute. Symptoms of acute angle closure are severe ocular pain and redness, decreased vision, colored halos, headache, nausea, and vomiting. Intraocular pressure is elevated. Immediate treatment of the acute condition with multiple topical and systemic drugs is required to prevent permanent visual loss, followed by definitive iridotomy.

Angle-closure glaucoma accounts for about 10% of all glaucomas in the US.

Etiology and Pathophysiology

Angle-closure glaucoma is caused by factors that either pull or push the iris up into the angle (ie, junction of the iris and cornea at the periphery of the anterior chamber), physically blocking the drainage of aqueous and raising intraocular pressure (IOP). Elevated IOP damages the optic nerve.

Angle closure may be primary (cause is unknown) or secondary to another condition (see TABLE 103–1) and can be acute, subacute (intermittent), or chronic.

Primary angle-closure glaucoma: Narrow angles are not present in young people. As people age, the lens of the eye continues to grow. In some but not all people, this growth pushes the iris forward, narrowing the angle. Risk factors for developing narrow angles include Asian ethnicity, hyperopia, family history, and advanced age.

In people with narrow angles, the distance between the pupillary iris and the lens is also very narrow. When the iris dilates, forces pull it centripetally and posteriorly causing iris-lens contact, which prevents aqueous from passing between the lens and iris into the anterior chamber (termed pupillary block). Pressure from the continued secretion of aqueous into the posterior chamber by the ciliary body pushes the peripheral iris anteriorly (the forward-bowing iris is called iris bombe), closing the angle. This blocks aqueous outflow, resulting in rapid (within hours) and severe elevation (> 40 mm Hg) of IOP. Because of the rapid onset, this condition is called primary acute angle-closure glaucoma and is an ophthalmic emergency requiring immediate treatment.

Intermittent angle-closure glaucoma occurs if the episode of pupillary block resolves spontaneously after several hours, usually after sleeping supine.

Chronic angle-closure glaucoma occurs if the narrowing of the angle develops slowly, allowing scarring between the peripheral iris and trabecular meshwork; IOP elevation is slow.

Pupillary dilation (mydriasis) can push the iris into the angle and precipitate acute angle-closure glaucoma in any person with narrow angles. This is of particular concern when applying topical agents (eg, homatropine, phenylephrine) to dilate the eye for examination.

Secondary angle-closure glaucoma: In these patients, the mechanical obstruction of the angle is due to a coexisting condition, such as proliferative diabetic retinopathy (PDR), ischemic central vein occlusion, uveitis, or epithelial down-growth. Contraction of a neovascular membrane (eg, in PDR) or inflammatory scarring associated with uveitis can pull the iris into the angle.

Symptoms, Signs, and Diagnosis

Acute angle-closure glaucoma: Patients have severe ocular pain and redness, decreased vision, colored halos, headache, nausea, and vomiting. The systemic complaints may be so severe that patients are misdiagnosed as having a neurologic or GI problem. Examination typically reveals conjunctival injection, a hazy cornea, a fixed mid-dilated pupil, and anterior chamber inflammation. Vision is decreased. IOP is usually 40 to 80 mm Hg. The optic nerve is difficult to visualize due to corneal edema, and visual field testing is not done because of discomfort.

Diagnosis is clinical. Gonioscopy may be difficult to perform in the involved eye because of a clouded cornea with friable epithelium. However, examination of the other eye reveals a narrow or occludable angle. If the other eye has a wide angle, then a diagnosis other than primary angle-closure glaucoma should be considered.

Chronic angle-closure glaucoma: This type of glaucoma presents similarly to open-angle glaucoma (see p. 906). Some patients have ocular redness, discomfort, blurred vision, or headache that lessens with sleep (perhaps due to sleep-induced miosis and posterior displacement of the lens by gravity). On gonioscopy, the angle is narrow, and peripheral anterior synechiae (PAS) may be seen. IOP may be normal but is usually higher in the affected eye. Diagnosis is made by the presence of PAS on gonioscopy and characteristic optic nerve and visual field changes (see under Primary Open-Angle Glaucoma on p. 907).

Treatment

Acute angle-closure glaucoma: Treatment must be initiated immediately, because vision can be lost quickly and permanently. The patient should receive several drugs at once. A suggested regimen is timolol 0.5% one drop q 30 min for 2 doses; pilocarpine 2 to 4% one drop q 15 min for the first 1 to 2 h; apraclonidine 0.5 to 1% one drop q 30 min for 2 doses; acetazolamide 500 mg po initially followed by 250 mg q 6 h; and an osmotic agent, such as oral glycerol 1 mL/kg diluted with an equal amount of cold water, mannitol 1.0 to 1.5 mg/kg IV, or isosorbide 100 g po (220 mL of a 45% solution—NOTE: *This is not isosorbide dinitrate*). Response is evaluated by measuring IOP. Miotics are generally not effective when IOP is > 40 or 50 mm Hg because of an anoxic pupillary sphincter.

Definitive treatment is with laser peripheral iridotomy, which opens another pathway for fluid to pass from the posterior to the anterior chamber. It is performed as soon as the cornea is clear and inflammation has subsided; in some cases the cornea clears within hours of lowering the IOP, whereas in other cases it can take 1 to 2 days. Because the other eye has an 80% chance of developing an acute attack, peripheral iridotomy is performed on both eyes.

The risk of complications with laser peripheral iridotomy is extremely low compared with its benefits. Diplopia, which can be bothersome, may occur if the iridotomy is not placed superiorly enough for the upper lid to cover it.

Chronic angle-closure glaucoma: Patients with chronic, subacute, or intermittent angle-closure glaucoma should also have laser peripheral iridotomy. Additionally, patients with a narrow angle on gonioscopic examination, even in the absence of symptoms, should undergo a prompt peripheral iridotomy to prevent angle-closure glaucoma.

The drug and surgical treatments are the same as with open-angle glaucoma. Laser trabeculoplasty is relatively contraindicated if the angle is so narrow that additional PAS may form after the laser procedure.

104 CATARACT

(For developmental or congenital cataracts, see p. 2446.)

A cataract is a congenital or degenerative opacity of the lens. The main symptom is gradual, painless vision blurring. Diagnosis is by ophthalmoscopy and slit-lamp examination. Treatment is surgical removal and placement of an intraocular lens.

Cataracts occur with aging. Although many people have no additional risk factors, trauma (sometimes years later), smoking, alcohol use, exposure to x-rays, heat from infrared exposure, systemic disease (eg, diabetes), uveitis, systemic drugs (eg, corticosteroids), and possibly chronic ultraviolet (UV) exposure increase risk. Some cataracts are congenital, associated with numerous syndromes and diseases.

Symptoms, Signs, and Diagnosis

Cataracts generally develop slowly over years. Early symptoms may be loss of contrast, glare, needing more light to see well, and problems distinguishing dark blue from black. Later, progressive, painless blurring of vision occurs. The degree of blurring depends on the location and extent of the opacity. When the opacity is in the central lens nucleus (nuclear cataract), myopia may develop in the early stages, changing the refractive index of the lens so that a presbyopic patient may be temporarily able to read without glasses (second sight).

Cataract beneath the posterior lens capsule (posterior subcapsular cataract) disproportionately affects vision because the opacity is located at the crossing point of incoming light rays. Such cataracts reduce visual acuity more when the pupil constricts (eg, in bright light or during reading). They are also the type most likely to produce glare, especially from bright lights or from car headlights while driving at night, and loss of contrast.

Rarely, the cataract swells, occluding the trabecular drainage meshwork and producing secondary closed-angle glaucoma and pain.

Diagnosis is best made with the pupil dilated. Well-developed cataracts appear as gray or yellow-brown opacities in the lens. Examination of the red reflex through the dilated pupil with the ophthalmoscope held about 30 cm away usually discloses subtle opacities. Small cataracts stand out as dark defects in the red reflex. A large cataract may obliterate the red reflex. Slit-lamp examination provides more details about the character, location, and extent of the opacity.

Prevention and Treatment

Many ophthalmologists recommend UV-coated eyeglasses or sunglasses as a preventive measure. Reducing risk factors such as alcohol, tobacco, and corticosteroids and controlling blood glucose in diabetes delay onset.

Frequent refractions and corrective lens prescription changes may help maintain useful vision during cataract development. Occasionally, long-term pupillary dilation (with phenylephrine 2.5% q 4 to 8 h) is helpful for small cataracts. Indirect lighting while reading minimizes pupillary constriction and may optimize vision for close tasks. Polarized lenses reduces glare.

Usual indications for surgery include maximally corrected vision < 20/40 (< 6/12) and vision that is subjectively limiting, preventing needed or desired activities (eg, driving, reading, other occupational activities). Far less common indications include cataracts that cause glaucoma or the need to examine the fundus for the management of diseases such as diabetic retinopathy and glaucoma. Early cataract removal offers no advantage.

Cataract extraction is usually performed under topical or local anesthesia and IV sedation. There are 3 extraction techniques: intracapsular cataract extraction, in which the cataract is removed in one piece (rarely performed); extracapsular cataract extraction, in which the hard central nucleus is removed in one piece and then the soft cortex is removed in multiple small pieces; and phacoemulsification, in which the hard central nucleus is dissolved by ultrasound and then the soft cortex is removed in multiple small pieces. Phacoemulsification requires the smallest incision, thus enabling the fastest healing, and is usually the preferred procedure.

A plastic or silicone lens is almost always implanted intraocularly to replace the optical focusing power and magnification lost by removal of the crystalline lens. The lens implant can be placed in front of the iris (anterior chamber lens), attached to the iris and within the pupil (iris plane lens), or placed behind the iris (posterior chamber lens). Iris plane lenses are rarely used in the US because many designs led to a high frequency of postoperative complications. Posterior chamber placement is by far the most common technique.

In most cases, a tapering schedule of topical antibiotics (eg, moxifloxacin 0.5% 1 drop qid) and topical corticosteroids (eg, prednisolone acetate 1% 1 drop qid) is used for up to 4 wk postsurgery. Patients often wear an eye shield while sleeping and should avoid the Valsalva maneuver, heavy lifting, excessive forward bending, and eye rubbing for several weeks.

Complications of cataract surgery include:

- Intraoperative: bleeding beneath the retina, causing the intraocular contents to extrude through the incision (choroidal hemorrhage), vitreous prolapsing out of the incision (vitreous loss), fragments of the cataract dislocating into the vitreous, incisional burn, and detachment of corneal endothelium and its basement membrane (Descemet's membrane)
- Within the 1st week: endophthalmitis (infection within the eye) and glaucoma
- Within the 1st month: cystoid macular edema
- Months later: bullous keratopathy, retinal detachment, and posterior capsular opacification (treatable with laser).

When preexisting disorders such as amblyopia, retinopathy, macular degeneration, and glaucoma are excluded, 95% of eyes achieve vision of 20/40 (6/12) or better. If an intraocular lens is not implanted, contact lenses or thick glasses are needed to correct the resulting hyperopia.

105 UVEITIS

Uveitis is inflammation of the uveal tract—the iris, ciliary body, and choroid. Most cases are idiopathic, but identifiable causes include various infections and systemic diseases, often autoimmune. Symptoms include decreased vision, pain, redness, photophobia, and floaters. Diagnosis is clinical, supplemented with laboratory and ancillary testing. Treatment depends on cause but typically includes topical or systemic corticosteroids with cycloplegic-mydriatic drugs and/or noncorticosteroid immunosuppressants. Infectious causes require antimicrobial therapy.

Inflammation of the uvea (uveitis) may occur with or without accompanying vitreitis, retinitis, papillitis, or optic neuritis. Uveitis is classified anatomically as anterior, intermediate, posterior, or diffuse.

Anterior uveitis is localized primarily to the anterior segment of the eye and includes iritis (inflammation in the anterior chamber alone) and iridocyclitis (inflammation in the anterior chamber and anterior vitreous). Intermediate uveitis (peripheral uveitis or chronic cyclitis) occurs in the vitreous. Posterior uveitis refers to any form of retinitis, choroiditis, or inflammation of the optic disk. Diffuse uveitis (panuveitis) implies inflammation in both the anterior and posterior chambers.

Etiology and Pathophysiology

Most cases are idiopathic and presumed to be autoimmune in origin. Identifiable causes include trauma, ocular and systemic infections, and systemic autoimmune disorders (see p. 913).

The most common cause of anterior uveitis is trauma (traumatic iridocyclitis). Other causes are spondyloarthropathies (20 to 25%), juvenile idiopathic arthritis, and herpesvirus infection; half of cases are idiopathic. Most intermediate uveitis is idiopathic; uncommon identifiable causes include multiple sclerosis, sarcoidosis, TB, syphilis, Lyme disease, and Sjögren's syndrome. The most common cause of posterior uveitis is toxoplasmosis; CMV is the most common cause in patients with AIDS. The most common cause of diffuse uveitis is sarcoidosis, but most cases are idiopathic.

Infrequently, systemic drugs cause uveitis. Examples include sulfonamides, pamidronate (an inhibitor of bone resorption), rifabutin, and cidofovir.

Systemic diseases causing uveitis and their treatment are discussed elsewhere in THE MANUAL.

Symptoms and Signs

Symptoms and signs may be subtle and vary depending on the site and severity of inflammation.

Anterior uveitis tends to be the most symptomatic, usually presenting with pain, redness, photophobia, and decreased vision. Signs include hyperemia of the conjunctiva adjacent to the cornea. Slit-lamp findings include cells and flare in the aqueous humor, keratic precipitates, and posterior synechiae.

Intermediate uveitis is typically painless and presents with floaters and decreased vision. The primary sign is cells in the vitreous humor. Aggregates and condensations of inflammatory cells often occur over the pars plana, forming "snowballs." Vision may be decreased because of floaters or cystoid macular edema, which results from fluid leakage from blood vessels in the macula. Confluent and condensed vitreous cells and snowballs in the pars plana may produce a classic "snowbank" appearance, which can be associated with neovascularization of the retinal periphery.

Posterior uveitis may give rise to diverse symptoms but most commonly causes floaters and decreased vision as occurs in intermediate uveitis. Signs include cells in the vitreous humor, white or yellow-white lesions in the retina (retinitis) and/or underlying choroid (choroiditis), exudative retinal detachments, retinal vasculitis, and optic disk edema.

Diffuse uveitis may produce any or all the above symptoms and signs.

Consequences of uveitis include profound and irreversible vision loss, especially when unrecognized and/or inadequately treated. The most frequent complications include cataract; glaucoma; retinal detachment; neovascularization of the retina, optic nerve, or iris; and cystoid macular edema, which is the most common cause of decreased vision from uveitis.

Diagnosis

Uveitis should be suspected in any patient who has pain, redness, photophobia, or decreased vision. *Patients suspected of having uveitis should be referred immediately for complete ophthalmologic evaluation.* Most findings are best appreciated with slit-lamp examination and indirect ophthalmoscopy.

Many conditions that cause intraocular inflammation can mimic uveitis and should be considered in the appropriate clinical settings. Such conditions include intraocular malignancies in the very young (typically retinoblastoma and leukemia) and in the elderly (intraocular lymphoma). Less commonly, retinitis pigmentosa (see p. 920) can manifest with mild inflammation which may be confused with uveitis.

Treatment

Treatment of active inflammation usually involves corticosteroids given topically or by periocular injection along with a cycloplegic-mydriatic drug. Antimicrobial drugs are used to treat infectious uveitis. Particularly severe or chronic cases may require systemic corticosteroids, systemic noncorticosteroid immunosuppressants, cryotherapy applied transsclerally to the retinal periphery, or surgical removal of the vitreous (vitrectomy).

Uveitis From Connective Tissue Disease

A number of connective tissue diseases produce inflammation of the uveal tract.

Spondyloarthropathies: The seronegative spondyloarthropathies (see p. 290) are a common cause of anterior uveitis. Ocular inflammation is most common with ankylosing spondylitis but also occurs with reactive arthritis; inflammatory bowel disease, which includes both ulcerative colitis and Crohn's disease; and psoriatic arthritis. Uveitis is classically unilateral, but recurrences are common and may alternate between eyes. Men are affected more commonly than women. Most patients, regardless of sex, are HLA-B27 positive. Treatment requires a topical corticosteroid and a cycloplegic-mydriatic drug. Occasionally, periocular corticosteroids are required.

Juvenile idiopathic arthritis (JIA, also known as juvenile RA): JIA characteristically causes chronic bilateral iridocyclitis in children, particularly those with the pauciarticular variety (see also p. 289). Unlike most forms of anterior uveitis, however, JIA tends not to produce pain, photophobia, and conjunctival injection, but only blurring and meiosis and is, therefore, often referred to as white iritis. JIA-associated uveitis is more common in girls than in boys. Recurrent bouts of inflammation are best treated with a topical corticosteroid and a cycloplegic-mydriatic drug. Long-term control often requires use of a noncorticosteroid immunosuppressant, such as methotrexate or mycophenolate mofetil.

Sarcoidosis: Sarcoidosis (see also p. 462) accounts for 10 to 20% of uveitis, and about 25% of patients with sarcoidosis develop uveitis. Sarcoid uveitis is more common in blacks and the elderly. Virtually any symptoms and signs of anterior, intermediate, posterior, or diffuse uveitis can occur. Suggestive findings include conjunctival granulomas, large keratic precipitates on the corneal endothelium (so-called granulomatous or mutton fat precipitates), iris granulomas, and retinal vasculitis. Biopsy of suggestive lesions provides the most secure diagnosis. Treatment usually involves topical, periocular, and systemic corticosteroids along with a topical cycloplegic-mydriatic drug. Patients with moderate to severe inflammation may require a noncorticosteroid immunosuppressant, such as methotrexate, mycophenolate mofetil, or azathioprine.

Behçet's syndrome: This condition is rare in North America but is a fairly common cause of uveitis in the Middle and Far East (see also p. 273). Typical findings include severe anterior uveitis with hypopyon (layered lymphocytes in the anterior chamber), retinal vasculitis, and optic disk inflammation. The clinical course is usually severe with multiple recurrences. Diagnosis requires the presence of associated systemic manifestations, such as oral aphthous or genital ulcers; dermatitis, including erythema nodosum; thrombophlebitis; or epididymitis. Oral aphthae may be biopsied to demonstrate an occlusive vasculitis. There are no laboratory tests for Behçet's syndrome. Treatment with local and systemic corticosteroids and a cycloplegic-mydriatic drug may alleviate acute exacerbations, but most patients eventually require systemic corticosteroids and a noncorticosteroid immunosuppressant, such as cyclosporine or chlorambucil, to control the inflammation and avoid the serious complications of long-term corticosteroid treatment.

Vogt-Koyanagi-Harada (VKH) syndrome: VKH syndrome is an uncommon systemic disorder characterized by uveitis in association with cutaneous and neurologic abnormalities. VKH syndrome is particularly common in people of Asian, Asian Indian, and American Indian descent. Women in their 20s and 30s are affected more often than men. The etiology is unknown, although an autoimmune reaction directed against melanin-containing cells in the uveal tract, skin, inner ear, and meninges is strongly suspected.

Neurologic symptoms tend to occur early and include tinnitus, dysacusis (auditory agnosia), vertigo, headache, and meningismus. Cutaneous findings frequently occur later and include patchy vitiligo (especially common on the eyelids, low back, and buttocks), poliosis (a localized patch of white hair), and alopecia, often involving the head and neck. Additional ocular complications include cataracts, glaucoma, optic disk edema, and choroiditis, commonly with exudative detachment of the overlying retina.

Early treatment includes local and systemic corticosteroids and a cycloplegic-mydriatic drug. Many patients also require a noncorticosteroid immunosuppressant such as methotrexate, azathioprine, or mycophenolate mofetil.

ENDOPHTHALMITIS

Endophthalmitis is an acute, diffuse uveitis resulting most often from bacterial infection.

Most cases of endophthalmitis are caused by gram-positive bacteria, such as *Staphylococcus epidermidis* or *S. aureus*. Gram-negative organisms can also produce endophthalmitis, tend to be more virulent, and are associated with a poorer prognosis. Fungal and protozoan causes of endophthalmitis are rare. Most cases follow penetrating ocular trauma or intraocular surgery (exogenous). Less commonly, infection reaches the eye via the bloodstream after systemic surgery or dental procedures or when IV lines or IV drugs are used (endogenous).

Endophthalmitis is a medical emergency because vision prognosis is directly related to the time from onset to treatment. Rarely, untreated intraocular infections extend beyond the confines of the eye to involve the orbit and CNS. Exogenous endophthalmitis typically causes severe pain and decreased vision. Signs include intense conjunctival hyperemia and intraocular inflammation within the anterior chamber and vitreous, occasionally with eyelid edema.

Diagnosis requires a high index of suspicion in at-risk patients, especially those with recent eye surgery or trauma. Gram stain and culture of aspirates from the anterior chamber and vitreous are standard. Patients with suspected endogenous endophthalmitis should also have blood and urine cultures.

Initial treatment includes broad-spectrum intravitreal antibiotics, most commonly vancomycin and ceftazidime. Patients with endogenous endophthalmitis should receive both intravitreal and IV antibiotics.

Vision prognosis is often poor, even with early and appropriate treatment. Therapy may need to be modified once culture and sensitivity results are obtained. Patients with count-fingers or worse vision at presentation should be considered for vitrectomy and use of intraocular corticosteroids. Corticosteroids are, however, contraindicated in fungal endophthalmitis.

Infectious Uveitis

A number of infectious diseases cause uveitis (see TABLE 105–1). The most common are herpes virus, CMV, and toxoplasmosis.

Herpes virus: Herpes simplex virus (see also p. 1606) causes anterior uveitis. Herpes zoster virus does so less commonly, although the prevalence of zoster-associated anterior uveitis increases with age. Symptoms include eye pain, photophobia, and decreased vision. Signs include redness; conjunctival injection and anterior chamber inflammation, often in association with corneal inflammation (keratitis); decreased corneal sensation; acutely elevated intraocular pressure; and patchy or sectorial iris atrophy. Treatment should include a topical corticosteroid and a cycloplegic-mydriatic drug. Acyclovir, 400 mg po 5 times/day for herpes simplex virus and 800 mg po 5 times/day for herpes zoster virus, may also be given.

Much less commonly, herpes zoster and herpes simplex viruses cause a rapidly progressing form of retinitis called acute retinal necrosis (ARN), which is classically associated with occlusive retinal vasculitis and moderate to severe vitreous inflammation. One third of ARN cases become bilateral, and ¾ result in retinal detachment. ARN may also occur in patients with HIV/AIDS, but immunocompromised patients tend to have less vitreous inflammation. Vitreous biopsy for culture and PCR analysis may be useful in diagnosing ARN. Treatment includes IV acyclovir with IV and intravitreal ganciclovir or foscarnet. Oral valganciclovir may also be used.

Toxoplasmosis: Toxoplasmosis (see also p. 1584) is the most common cause of retinitis in immunocompetent patients. Most cases are transmitted congenitally, although acquired cases occur commonly. Symptoms of floaters and decreased vision may be due to cells in the vitreous humor or to retinal lesions or scars. Concurrent anterior segment involvement can occur and may produce pain, redness, and photophobia. Laboratory testing should include serum anti-*Toxoplasma* antibody titers. Treatment is recommended in patients with posterior lesions that threaten vital visual structures, such as the optic nerve or macula, and in immunocompromised patients. Multidrug therapy is commonly prescribed, including pyrimethamine, sulfonamides, clindamycin, and, in select cases, systemic corticosteroids. Corticosteroids should not, however, be used without concurrent antimicrobial coverage.

TABLE 105–1. INFECTIOUS CAUSES OF UVEITIS

MORE COMMON	LESS COMMON	RARE
Cytomegalovirus*	Histoplasmosis	*Aspergillus*
Herpes viruses	Lyme disease	*Candida*
Pneumocystis jiroveci (formerly *P. carinii*)*	Syphilis	Coccidioidomycosis
Toxoplasmosis	Toxocariasis	*Cryptococcus*
	Tuberculosis	Cysticercosis
		Leprosy
		Leptospirosis
		Onchocerciasis
		Tropheryma whippelii

*In patients with AIDS.

Cytomegalovirus: CMV (see also p. 1605) is the most common cause of retinitis in immunocompromised patients, affecting 25 to 40% of patients with AIDS, typically as the $CD4^+$ count drops to < 50 cells/μL. CMV retinitis may also occur in neonates and in pharmacologically immunosuppressed patients but is uncommon. The diagnosis is largely clinical based on direct or indirect fundus examination; serologic tests are of limited use. Treatment in patients with HIV/AIDS is with systemic or local (implant) ganciclovir, systemic foscarnet, or valganciclovir. Therapy is typically continued indefinitely, unless immune reconstitution is achieved with combination antiretroviral therapy (typically $CD4^+$ count > 100 cells/μL for at least 3 mo).

SYMPATHETIC OPHTHALMIA

Sympathetic ophthalmia is inflammation of the uveal tract after trauma or surgery to the other eye.

Sympathetic ophthalmia is a rare granulomatous uveitis that occurs after penetrating trauma or surgery to the other eye. Sympathetic ophthalmia has been estimated to occur in up to 0.5% of nonsurgical and in < 0.1% of surgical penetrating eye wounds. The underlying mechanism is thought to be an autoimmune reaction directed against melanin-containing cells in the uvea. Uveitis appears within 2 to 12 wk after injury in about 80% of cases. Isolated cases of sympathetic ophthalmia have occurred as early as 1 wk or as late as 30 yr after the initial injury or surgery. Symptoms typically include floaters and decreased vision. Choroiditis, often with overlying exudative retinal detachment, is common. Treatment typically requires long-term corticosteroids and immunosuppressants. Prophylactic enucleation of a severely injured eye should be considered within 2 wk of vision loss to minimize the risk of sympathetic ophthalmia developing in the other eye, but only when the injured eye has no vision potential.

106 RETINAL DISORDERS

(For Retinopathy of Prematurity, see p. 2268.)

The retina is the light-sensing layer of tissue at the back of the eye containing the rods, cones, and nerve endings that transform light into neural impulses. Retinal disorders are genetic, involve vascular injury that produces nerve or choroid damage, or are idiopathic. Retinal detachment has multiple causes.

AGE-RELATED MACULAR DEGENERATION

(Senile Macular Degeneration)

Age-related macular degeneration is atrophy or degeneration of the macula. It is a common cause of worsening central vision in elderly patients. Funduscopic findings are diagnostic; fluorescein angiography assists in directing treatment. Treatment is with laser photocoagulation and low-vision devices.

Etiology and Pathophysiology

Age-related macular degeneration (AMD) is a leading cause of vision loss in the elderly. It is more common in whites than in blacks. No predisposing systemic risk factor is known, but AMD may be hereditary; an association between smoking and AMD has been shown. The role of cardiovascular disease, hypertension, and cholesterol levels remains unclear.

Two different forms occur: In atrophic AMD (dry form), often referred to as geographic atrophy, there is irregular pigmentation of the macular region but no elevated macular scar and no hemorrhage or exudation in the macular region. In exudative AMD (wet or neovascular form), which is much less common, a subretinal network of choroidal neovascularization forms. This network is often associated with hyperpigmentation of the macula and soft drusen. A localized elevation of an area of the macula or a pigment epithelial detachment may be caused by hemorrhage or fluid accumulation. Eventually, this network leaves an elevated scar at the posterior pole.

Ninety percent of the blindness caused by AMD occurs in the 10% of cases that have the exudative form.

Symptoms, Signs, and Diagnosis

Both forms of AMD are often bilateral and are preceded by development of drusen (small yellow deposits that form under the macula). In atrophic AMD, central visual acuity is lost slowly and painlessly. Rapid vision loss is more typical of exudative AMD. Although peripheral vision and color vision are generally unaffected, the patient may become legally blind (< 20/200 vision) in the affected eye(s). The first symptom of exudative AMD is visual distortion in one eye, which can be detected with an Amsler grid (see p. 871). Central blind spots (scotomas) usually develop early in atrophic AMD. Funduscopy reveals pigmentary or hemorrhagic disturbance in the macular region of the involved eye; the contralateral eye almost always shows some pigmentary disturbance and drusen in the macula. Other findings may include retinal detachment, lipid exudates, tissue atrophy, and macular scarring.

AMD is diagnosed by clinical appearance of the retina. Fluorescein angiography may reveal a neovascular membrane beneath the retina. An angiogram is obtained when findings suggestive of neovascularization are present; such findings include subretinal hemorrhage, localized retinal elevation, retinal edema, and gray discoloration of the subretinal space. Fluorescein angiography demonstrates and characterizes a subretinal choroidal neovascular membrane.

Prognosis and Treatment

Atrophic AMD produces mild to moderate reduction of vision but rarely leads to blindness. There is no recommended treatment, but patients at risk of advanced disease (eg, those with large drusen or irregular macular pigmentation) may benefit from daily supplements of zinc oxide 80 mg with copper 2 mg, vitamin C 500 mg, vitamin E 400 IU, and beta carotene 15 mg. β-carotene can cause anemia, prostatic hypertrophy, stress incontinence, and, in smokers, an increased risk of lung cancer.

If exudative AMD is untreated, vision typically deteriorates substantially, often to blindness. However, peripheral vision is usually retained. Results of treatment depend on the size, location, and type of neovascularization. Thermal laser photocoagulation of neovascularization outside the fovea may prevent severe vision loss. Photodynamic therapy, a laser treatment, provides benefit under specific circumstances. Pegaptanib is a new injectable selective vascular endothelial growth factor antagonist that can be used for the treatment of neovascular AMD. Other treatments being evaluated include transpupillary thermotherapy, subretinal surgery, and macular translocation surgery.

For patients who have lost central vision, low-vision devices, such as magnifiers, high-power reading glasses, computer monitors, and telescopic lenses, are available. Low-vision counseling is advised.

CENTRAL RETINAL ARTERY OCCLUSION

Central retinal artery occlusion is blockage of the central retinal artery, usually by an embolism. Its symptom is sudden, painless, unilateral blindness. Diagnosis is by history and characteristic retinal findings on funduscopy. Decreasing intraocular pressure is attempted within the first 24 h of occlusion.

Retinal artery occlusion may be due to embolism from atherosclerotic plaques, endocarditis, fat emboli, atrial myxoma, or thrombosis of a retinal artery. Temporal arteritis (see p. 280) is another important cause.

Symptoms, Signs, and Diagnosis

Retinal artery occlusion produces sudden painless blindness or visual field defect.

The pupil may respond poorly to direct light but constricts briskly when the other eye is illuminated. In acute cases, funduscopy discloses a pale, opaque fundus with a red fovea (cherry-red spot). Typically, the arteries are attenuated and may even appear bloodless. An embolic obstruction is sometimes visible. If a major branch is occluded rather than the entire artery, fundus abnormalities and vision loss are limited to that sector of the retina. ESR is useful for excluding temporal arteritis.

Prognosis and Treatment

Immediate treatment is indicated if occlusion occurred < 24 h earlier. Beyond 72 h, it is unlikely that increased perfusion will improve vision. Once the retina has infarcted, blindness is permanent. Reduction of intraocular pressure by ocular hypotensive drugs (eg, topical timolol 0.5% or acetazolamide 500 mg IV or po), intermittent digital massage over the closed eyelid, or anterior chamber paracentesis may dislodge an embolus and allow it to enter a smaller branch of the artery, thus reducing the area of retinal ischemia. Treatments for retinal artery occlusions rarely result in improved visual acuity. Patients with occlusion secondary to temporal arteritis should receive systemic corticosteroids.

CENTRAL RETINAL VEIN OCCLUSION

Central retinal vein occlusion is blockage of the central retinal vein by a thrombus, usually occurring in elderly patients. Its symptom is sudden, painless vision loss. Diagnosis is by funduscopy. Most treatments are ineffective or unproven.

Glaucoma, diabetes, hypertension, increased blood viscosity, and elevated Hct are predisposing factors; occlusion may also be idiopathic. The condition is uncommon in young people.

Neovascularization of the retina or iris (rubeosis iridis) with secondary (neovascular) glaucoma can occur weeks to months after occlusion. Vitreous hemorrhage may develop in the presence of retinal neovascularization.

Symptoms, Signs, and Diagnosis

Painless visual loss can be sudden or gradual over a period of days to weeks. On funduscopy, the retinal veins appear distended and tortuous, the fundus is congested and edematous, and numerous retinal hemorrhages appear. These changes are limited to one quadrant if obstruction involves only a branch of the central retinal vein.

Prognosis and Treatment

In patients in whom normal retinal perfusion is re-established, normal vision may return. The time to vision improvement varies. Those with poor perfusion are more likely to develop complications and suffer severe vision loss. Visual acuity at presentation is a good indicator of final vision. If visual acuity is at least 20/40, visual acuity will likely remain good. If visual acuity is worse than 20/200, 80% of patients will not improve or will deteriorate.

There is no generally accepted medical therapy unless neovascularization develops. In this event, panretinal photocoagulation should be initiated, which may decrease vitreous hemorrhages and prevent neovascular glaucoma.

DIABETIC RETINOPATHY

Diabetic retinopathy includes microaneurysms, hemorrhages, exudates, and macular edema occurring with diabetes of at least several years' duration. Vision rarely decreases until late in the disease. Diagnosis is by funduscopy; further details are elucidated by fluorescein angiography. Treatment includes controlling diabetes and laser coagulation of threatening lesions.

Pathophysiology

Diabetic retinopathy is a major cause of blindness and tends to be particularly severe in type 1 diabetes. The degree of retinopathy is highly correlated with both duration of diabetes and poor blood glucose control. Nonproliferative retinopathy develops first. Proliferative retinopathy is more severe and may lead to vitreous hemorrhage and retinal detachment.

Nonproliferative retinopathy (simple, or background, retinopathy) produces increased capillary permeability, microaneurysms, hemorrhages, exudates, and macular edema. Macular edema (thickening of the retina caused by fluid leakage from capillaries) causes vision loss if untreated.

Proliferative retinopathy is characterized by abnormal new vessel formation (neovascularization), which occurs on the vitreous surface of the retina and may extend into the vitreous cavity and cause vitreous hemorrhages. Fibrous tissue that forms with the vessels may contract, resulting in retinal detachment. Neovascularization may also occur in the anterior segment of the eye on the iris, which can result in neovascular membrane growth in the angle of the eye at the peripheral margin of the iris, leading to neovascular glaucoma. Vision loss with proliferative retinopathy may be severe.

Symptoms, Signs, and Diagnosis

Because early detection is important, all patients with diabetes should have annual ophthalmologic examinations. Pregnant patients with diabetes should be examined every trimester. Vision symptoms are indications for ophthalmologic referral. Diagnosis is based on clinical appearance on eye examination. Fluorescein angiography is used to determine the extent of damage, to develop a treatment plan, and to monitor the results of treatment.

Nonproliferative retinopathy: Vision symptoms are rare in the early stages; as retinopathy progresses, macular edema may cause decreased visual acuity. In late stages, cystic changes from chronic macular edema and macular ischemia from capillary occlusive disease may develop.

The first signs are often venous dilation and small red dots (capillary microaneurysms) seen on funduscopy in the posterior retinal pole. Later signs include dot and blot retinal hemorrhages, hard exudates, and cotton-wool spots (soft exudates). Cotton-wool spots are areas of microinfarction that lead to retinal opacification; they are fuzzy edged and white and obscure underlying vessels. Hard exudates are discrete, yellow, and generally deeper than retinal vessels and are manifestations of chronic edema. Macular edema can be seen on slit-lamp biomicroscopy as elevation and blurring of retinal layers.

Proliferative retinopathy: Symptoms include blurred vision and black spots or flashing lights in the field of vision. Vitreous hemorrhage or retinal detachment may occur, leading to sudden severe vision loss.

Proliferative retinopathy is diagnosed when fine preretinal capillaries are observed on the optic nerve or retinal surface. Retinal hemorrhage may develop in the vitreous cavity when these abnormal vessels are damaged. In extreme cases, retinal detachment may occur with white preretinal membranes forming over the retinal surface, especially over the major retinal vessels. Detachment and contraction of the vitreous gel contribute to retinal detachment by pulling the retina anteriorly from its attachments over the major vessels.

Prognosis and Treatment

Control of diabetes and BP is important; intensive control of blood glucose can delay onset and slow progression of retinopathy. Nonproliferative diabetic retinopathy is treated with focal laser when clinically significant macular edema develops. More extensive panretinal laser may be used when nonproliferative retinopathy becomes severe. Injection of intravitreal or periocular corticosteroids is gaining popularity as a method of managing severe macular edema and may provide better visual improvement. Prognosis with proliferative retinopathy is worse with severe retinal ischemia, extensive neovascularization, or extensive preretinal fibrous tissue formation. With the possible exceptions of vitreous hemorrhage and retinal detachment, lost vision is seldom recovered, and therapeutic interventions are designed to prevent further loss.

Panretinal laser photocoagulation may diminish or eliminate proliferative retinopathy and neovascularization and decrease the risk of neovascular glaucoma. Vitrectomy may be useful in vitreous hemorrhage. Treatment of retinal detachment is covered below.

HYPERTENSIVE RETINOPATHY

Hypertensive retinopathy is retinal vascular damage caused by high BP. Symptoms develop late. Funduscopic examination shows arteriolar constriction, arteriovenous nicking, vascular wall changes, flame-shaped hemorrhages, cotton-wool spots, yellow hard exudates, and papilledema. Treatment is directed at controlling the hypertension.

Acute BP elevation typically causes reversible vasoconstriction in retinal blood vessels. More prolonged or severe hypertension leads to exudative vascular changes, a consequence of endothelial damage and necrosis. Other changes (eg, arteriole wall thickening) typically require years of elevated BP to develop. Smoking compounds the adverse effects of hypertension on the retina. Hypertension combined with diabetes greatly increases risk of vision loss.

Symptoms, Signs, and Diagnosis

There are no symptoms until the disease is well advanced. Although early vision loss often goes unnoticed, it progresses without treatment and cannot be recovered.

In the early stages, funduscopy identifies arteriolar constriction, with a decrease in the arteriole to venule caliber ratio from the normal 2:3. If acute disease is severe, superficial flame-shaped hemorrhages and small white superficial foci of retinal ischemia (cotton-wool spots) develop. Yellow hard exudates, due to lipid deposition deep in the retina and arising from leaking retinal vessels, may appear. These exudates can form a star-shaped lesion in the macula. In severe hypertension, the optic disk becomes congested and edematous. Chronic, poorly controlled hypertension causes permanent arterial narrowing, arteriovenous crossing abnormalities called arteriovenous nicking, and arteriosclerosis with moderate vascular wall changes ("copper wiring") to more severe vascular wall hyperplasia ("silver wiring"). Sometimes, obliterative disease with total vascular occlusion occurs.

Treatment

Hypertensive retinopathy is managed primarily by controlling hypertension. Other vision-threatening conditions should also be aggressively controlled.

RETINAL DETACHMENT

Retinal detachment is separation of the neural retinal layer from the underlying retinal pigment epithelium layer. Symptoms are decreased peripheral or central vision, often described in the acute phase as a curtain coming down. Associated symptoms are painless vision disturbances, including flashing lights and numerous floaters. Diagnosis is by indirect funduscopy; ultrasonography

may determine the extent of the lesion. Immediate treatment to reattach the retina is imperative if central vision is threatened. Treatment includes systemic corticosteroids; sealing the retinal holes by laser, diathermy, or cryotherapy; scleral buckling; transconjunctival cryopexy; photocoagulation; pneumatic retinopexy; intravitreal surgery; and enucleation, depending on the cause and location of the lesion. Most reversible damage occurs early, so once the macula is detached and vision decreases, treatment is less urgent.

Rhegmatogenous detachment implies the presence of a retinal tear. It occurs more frequently in myopia, after cataract surgery, or after ocular trauma.

Nonrhegmatogenous detachment (detachment without a tear) can be produced by vitreoretinal traction (eg, as occurs in proliferative retinopathy of diabetes or sickle cell disease) or by transudation of fluid into the subretinal space (eg, severe uveitis, especially in Vogt-Koyanagi-Harada syndrome, or primary or metastatic choroidal tumors).

Symptoms, Signs, and Diagnosis

Retinal detachment is painless. Early symptoms may include dark or irregular vitreous floaters, flashes of light, and blurred vision. As detachment progresses, the patient notices a curtain or veil in the field of vision. If the macula is involved, central visual acuity fails drastically. Direct funduscopy may show retinal irregularities and a bullous retinal elevation with darkened blood vessels.

Retinal detachment is suggested by symptoms and findings on funduscopy. Indirect funduscopy with scleral depression is done to detect peripheral tears and detachment.

If vitreous hemorrhage from a retinal tear obscures the retina, retinal detachment should be suspected and B-scan ultrasonography performed.

Treatment

Although often localized, retinal detachments due to retinal tears can expand to involve the entire retina if not treated promptly. *Any patient with a suspected or established retinal detachment should be seen urgently by an ophthalmologist.*

Rhegmatogenous detachment is treated by sealing the retinal holes by laser, diathermy, or cryotherapy. The eye may be treated by scleral buckling, during which fluid may be drained from the subretinal space. Anterior retinal tears without detachment can be sealed by transconjunctival cryopexy; posterior tears can be sealed by photocoagulation. More than 90% of rhegmatogenous detachments can be reattached surgically. If tears occur in the superior ⅔ of the eye, simple detachments can be treated by pneumatic retinopexy (an office procedure).

Nonrhegmatogenous detachments due to vitreoretinal traction may be treated by surgical vitrectomy; transudative detachments due to uveitis may respond to systemic corticosteroids. Primary choroidal tumors (malignant melanomas) may require enucleation, although radiation therapy and local resection are used occasionally; choroidal hemangiomas may respond to localized photocoagulation. Metastatic choroidal tumors, most often from breast, lung, or GI tract, may respond well to radiation therapy.

RETINITIS PIGMENTOSA

Retinitis pigmentosa is a slowly progressive, bilateral degeneration of the retina and the pigmented epithelium of the choroid. The condition is of incompletely understood genetic origin. Symptoms include night blindness and altered visual fields. Diagnosis is by funduscopic findings, such as dark pigmentation in a bone-spicule configuration in the equatorial retina, narrowed retinal arteries, a waxy yellow disk, degenerative vitreous opacities, cataracts, and myopia. Electroretinography aids in the differential diagnosis. No effective treatment exists.

Abnormal gene coding for retinal proteins appears to be the cause of retinitis pigmentosa. The hereditary pattern is unclear. In most cases it appears to be autosomal recessive but may also be autosomal dominant or, infrequently, X-linked. It may occur as part of a syndrome (eg, Bassen-Kornzweig, Laurence-Moon).

Symptoms, Signs, and Diagnosis

The retinal rods are affected, producing defective night vision that may become symptomatic in early childhood. A mid-peripheral ring scotoma (detectable by visual field testing) widens gradually, so that central vision eventually is reduced.

The most conspicuous funduscopic finding is dark pigmentation in a bone-spicule configuration in the equatorial retina. The retinal arteries appear narrowed, the macula may develop cystic edema, and the disk may have a waxy yellow appearance. Other manifestations can include degenerative vitreous opacities, cataract, and myopia. Congenital hearing loss may be associated.

Diagnosis may be aided by specialized testing (eg, dark adaptation, electroretinography). Other retinopathies that can simulate retinitis pigmentosa (eg, those associated with syphilis, rubella, and phenothiazine or chloroquine toxicity) must be ruled out. Family members should be examined as necessary to establish the hereditary mode. Families with a history of a hereditary syndrome may wish to seek genetic counseling and may desire testing of family members.

Treatment

No treatment slows the course of the retinal degeneration. Vision loss is typically slow but relentless. Vision drops as the macula becomes increasingly involved and usually evolves to legal blindness.

107 OPTIC NERVE DISORDERS

The optic pathway includes the retina, the optic nerve, the optic chiasm, the optic radiations, and the occipital cortex (see FIG. 107–1). Damage along the optic pathway causes a variety of visual field changes (see TABLE 98–1 on p. 872).

HEREDITARY OPTIC NEUROPATHIES

Hereditary optic neuropathies are genetic defects that cause vision loss, occasionally with cardiac or neurologic abnormalities. There is no effective treatment.

Hereditary optic neuropathies typically present in childhood or adolescence with bilateral, symmetric central vision loss. Optic nerve damage is usually permanent and in some cases progressive. By the time optic atrophy is detected, substantial optic nerve injury has already occurred.

Dominant optic atrophy is inherited in an autosomal dominant fashion. It is believed to be the most common of the hereditary optic neuropathies, with prevalence in the range of 1:10,000 to 1:50,000. It is thought to be optic abiotrophy, premature degeneration of the optic nerve leading to progressive visual loss. Onset is in the 1st decade of life.

Leber's hereditary optic neuropathy has a mitochondrial DNA abnormality that affects cellular respiration. Although mitochondrial DNA throughout the body is affected, vision loss is the primary manifestation. Males are affected 80 to 90% of the time. The disease is inherited with a maternal inheritance pattern, meaning that all offspring of a woman carrying the trait will inherit the trait, but only females can pass on the trait, because the zygote receives mitochondria only from the mother.

Symptoms, Signs, and Diagnosis

Most patients with dominant optic atrophy have no associated neurologic abnormalities, although nystagmus and hearing loss have been reported. The only symptom is slowly progressive bilateral vision loss, usually mild until late in life. The entire optic disk or at times only the temporal part is pale without visible vessels. A blue-yellow color vision deficit is characteristic. Molecular genetic testing is available to confirm the diagnosis.

Vision loss in Leber's hereditary optic neuropathy typically begins between 15 and 35 yr (range, 1 to 80 yr). Painless central vision loss in one eye is usually followed weeks to months later by loss in the other eye. Simultaneous vision loss has been reported. Most patients lose vision to worse than 20/200 acuity. Ophthalmoscopic examination may show telangiectatic microangiopathy, swelling of the nerve fiber layer around the optic disk, and an absence of leakage on fluorescein angiography. Eventually, optic atrophy supervenes.

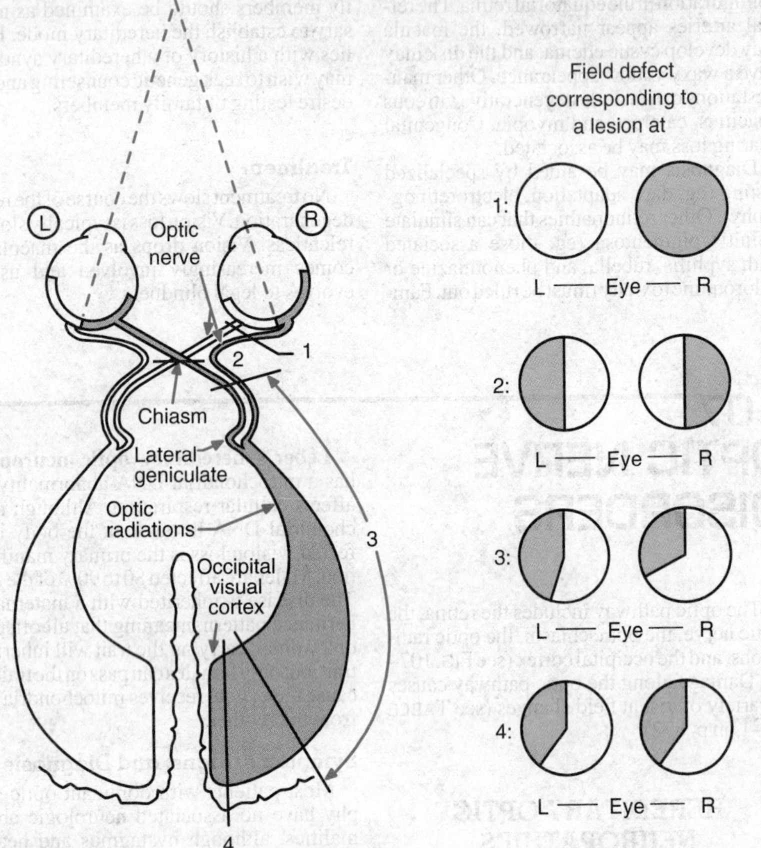

Fig. 107–1. Higher visual pathways—lesion sites and corresponding visual field defects. Note the defect typical of occipital lesions (#4).

A subgroup of patients with Leber's hereditary optic neuropathy has cardiac conduction defects, so an ECG should be obtained. Other patients may have minor neurologic abnormalities, such as a postural tremor, loss of ankle reflexes, dystonia, spasticity, or a multiple sclerosis–like illness.

Treatment

There is no effective treatment for the hereditary optic neuropathies. For Leber's hereditary optic neuropathy, corticosteroids, vitamin supplements, and antioxidants have been tried without success. A small study found benefits from quinone analogs (ubiquinone and idebenone) during the early phase. Suggestions to avoid agents like alcohol that might stress mitochondrial energy production have no proven benefit but are theoretically reasonable. Patients should avoid tobacco products and excessive alcohol intake. Cardiac and neurologic abnormalities should be referred to a specialist. Low-vision aids may be helpful. Genetic counseling is suggested.

ISCHEMIC OPTIC NEUROPATHY

(See also Retinal Artery Occlusion and other ischemic disorders in Ch. 106 on p. 916.)

Ischemic optic neuropathy is infarction of the optic disk. The only symptom is painless vision loss. Diagnosis is clinical. Treatment is ineffective.

Two varieties of optic nerve infarction exist, nonarteritic and arteritic. The nonarteritic variant occurs more frequently, typically affecting people 50 to 70 yr; vision loss tends not to be as severe as in the arteritic variant, which typically affects patients > 70.

Most ischemic optic neuropathy is unilateral. Bilateral, sequential cases occur in about 20%, but bilateral simultaneous involvement is uncommon. Atherosclerotic narrowing of the posterior ciliary arteries may predispose to nonarteritic optic nerve infarction, particularly after a hypotensive episode. Any of the inflammatory arteritides, especially temporal arteritis (see p. 280), can precipitate the arteritic form. Diagnosis of the arteritic form is important, not because anything can be done to improve the involved eye, but rather to begin preventive treatment of the other eye.

Acute ischemia causes nerve edema, which further worsens ischemia. A small optic cup to optic disk ratio is a risk for nonarteritic ischemic optic neuropathy, but cup to disk ratio does not increase risk of the arteritic variety. Usually no medical condition is apparent to cause the nonarteritic variety, although diabetes and hypertension have been detected in some patients and are thought to be risk factors. Vision loss on awakening leads investigators to suspect nocturnal hypotension as a potential cause of the nonarteritic variety.

Symptoms, Signs, and Diagnosis

Vision loss with both varieties is typically sudden and painless. Some patients notice the loss on awakening. Symptoms such as general malaise, muscle aches and pains, headaches over the temple, and jaw claudication may be present with temporal arteritis; however, such symptoms may not occur until after vision is lost. Visual acuity is reduced, and an afferent pupillary defect is present. The optic disk is swollen with surrounding hemorrhages. Visual field examination often shows a defect in the inferior and central visual fields. ESR is usually dramatically elevated in the arteritic variety and is normal in the nonarteritic variety. C-reactive protein is also a useful monitoring test. If temporal arteritis is suspected, temporal artery biopsy should be performed. For isolated cases of progressive vision loss, CT or MRI should be done to rule out compressive lesions. The most important aspect of the evaluation is to exclude the arteritic variety, because the other eye is at risk if treatment is not started quickly.

Prognosis and Treatment

There is no effective treatment, and most lost vision is not recovered; however, in the nonarteritic variety, up to 30% spontaneously recover some useful vision. The arteritic variety is treated with oral corticosteroids (prednisone 80 mg po once/day and tapered against ESR) to protect the other eye. Treatment should not be delayed while awaiting biopsy results. Treatment of the nonarteritic variety with aspirin or corticosteroids has not been helpful. Low-vision aids may be helpful.

OPTIC NEURITIS

Optic neuritis is inflammation of the optic nerve. Symptoms are usually unilateral, with eye pain and partial or complete vision loss. Diagnosis is primarily clinical. Treatment is directed at the underlying condition; most cases resolve spontaneously.

Etiology and Pathophysiology

Optic neuritis is most common in adults 20 to 40 yr. Most cases result from demyelinating disease, particularly multiple sclerosis (see p. 1888), in which case there may be recurrences. Optic neuritis is often the presenting manifestation of multiple sclerosis. Other causes include infectious disease (eg, viral encephalitis, sinusitis, meningitis, TB, syphilis, HIV); tumor metastasis to the optic nerve; chemicals and drugs (eg, lead, methanol, tobacco, quinine, arsenic, salicylates, antibiotics); and, rarely, diabetes, pernicious anemia, Graves' disease, bee stings, and trauma. Often, the cause remains obscure despite thorough evaluation.

Symptoms, Signs, and Diagnosis

The major symptom is vision loss, frequently maximal within 1 or 2 days and varying from a small central or paracentral scotoma to complete blindness. Most patients have mild eye pain.

If the optic disk is swollen, the condition is called papillitis. Otherwise, it is called retrobulbar neuritis. Testing usually reveals reduced visual acuity, a visual field deficit, an afferent pupillary defect, and disturbed color vision. Testing of color vision is a useful adjunct. About ⅔ of events are retrobulbar, producing no visible changes in the optic fundus. In the others, disk hyperemia and/or edema, edema around the disk, and vessel engorgement are present. A few exudates and hemorrhages may be present near or on the optic disk.

Optic neuritis is suspected in patients with characteristic pain and vision loss. Neuroimaging, preferably with gadolinium-enhanced MRI, may show an enlarged, enhancing, optic nerve. MRI may also help diagnose multiple sclerosis. Fluid attenuating inversion recovery (FLAIR) MRI sequences may show typical demyelinating lesions in a periventricular location if optic neuritis is related to demyelination.

Prognosis and Treatment

Prognosis and treatment depend on the underlying cause. Most events resolve spontaneously, with return of vision in 2 to 3 mo. Most patients with a typical history of optic neuritis and no underlying systemic disease, such as a connective tissue disease, recover vision, but > 25% have a recurrence in the same or the other eye. MRI is used to determine future risk of demyelinating disease. Treatment with methylprednisolone (125 to 250 mg IV qid) for 3 days followed by prednisone (1 mg/kg po once/day) for 11 days may speed recovery, but ultimate visual results are no different from observation alone. IV corticosteroids have been reported to delay onset of multiple sclerosis for at least 2 yr. Treatment with oral prednisone alone does not improve vision outcome and may increase the rate of recurrent episodes. Low-vision aids may be helpful.

PAPILLEDEMA

Papilledema is swelling of the optic disk due to increased intracranial pressure. All other causes of optic disk swelling, such as that due to malignant hypertension or thrombosis of the central retinal vein, do not involve increased intracranial pressure and therefore are not causes of papilledema. Papilledema requires an immediate search for the cause. There are no early symptoms, although transiently diminished vision lasting only seconds can occur. Diagnosis is by ophthalmoscopy with further tests, usually brain imaging, to determine cause. Treatment is directed at the underlying condition.

Papilledema is a sign of elevated intracranial pressure and is almost always bilateral. Cause can be a brain tumor or abscess, cerebral trauma or hemorrhage, meningitis, arachnoidal adhesions, cavernous or dural sinus thrombosis, or encephalitis. Papilledema also occurs with idiopathic intracranial hypertension (pseudotumor cerebri), a condition with elevated CSF pressure and no mass lesion.

Symptoms, Signs, and Diagnosis

Vision is usually not affected initially, but transient graying out of vision, flickering, or blurred or double vision may occur. Patients may have symptoms of increased intracranial pressure, such as headache or nausea and vomiting.

Evaluation begins with ophthalmoscopic examination, which reveals engorged and tortuous retinal veins, a hyperemic and swollen optic disk (optic nerve head), and retinal hemorrhages around the disk but not into the retinal periphery. Isolated disk edema (eg, from optic neuritis, ischemic optic neuropathy) without elevated CSF pressure is not considered papilledema.

In the early stages, visual acuity and pupillary response to light are usually normal and become abnormal only after the condition is well advanced. An enlarged blind spot may be detected on visual field testing. Later, nerve fiber bundle defects may be apparent.

The degree of disk swelling can be quantified by comparing the plus lens numbers needed to focus an ophthalmoscope on the most elevated portion of the disk and on the unaffected portion of the retina.

Differentiating papilledema from other causes of a swollen optic disk, such as optic neuritis, ischemic optic neuropathy, hypotony, central retinal vein occlusion, uveitis, or pseudo swollen disks (eg, optic nerve drusen) requires a thorough ophthalmologic evaluation, sometimes including CT or MRI. Lumbar puncture and measurement of CSF pressure should not be performed until intracranial mass lesions have been adequately ruled out. Lumbar puncture in the setting of intracranial mass lesions can result in brain stem herniation. If papilledema is recognized, the cause must be sought immediately by head CT or MRI. B-scan ultrasonography is the best diagnostic tool for pseudo disk edema of optic nerve drusen.

Treatment

Urgent treatment of the underlying condition is indicated. If intracranial pressure is not reduced, secondary optic nerve atrophy and vision loss eventually occur, along with other serious neurologic sequelae.

TOXIC AMBLYOPIA

(Nutritional Amblyopia)

Toxic amblyopia is reduction in visual acuity believed to be due to a toxic reaction in the orbital portion (papillomacular bundle) of the optic nerve. It is caused by multiple toxic and nutritional factors and probably other unknown factors. The symptom is painless vision loss. Diagnosis is by history and visual field examination. Treatment is avoiding suspected toxic agents and improving nutrition.

Etiology and Pathophysiology

Toxic amblyopia is usually bilateral and most often occurs in patients who use alcohol or tobacco excessively. In the former case, malnutrition may be the underlying cause. Cases of true tobacco-induced amblyopia are rare. Lead, methanol, chloramphenicol, digoxin, ethambutol, and many other chemicals can damage the optic nerve. Deficiencies of protein and antioxidants are likely risk factors. Toxic amblyopia may occur with other nutritional disorders, such as Strachan's syndrome (polyneuropathy and orogenital dermatitis).

Symptoms, Signs, and Diagnosis

Vision blurring and dimness typically develop over days to weeks. An initially small central or pericentral scotoma slowly enlarges, typically involving both the fixation and the blind spot (centrocecal scotoma) and progressively interfering with vision. Total blindness may occur in methanol ingestion, but other nutritional causes typically do not produce profound vision loss. Retinal abnormalities do not usually occur, but temporal disk pallor may develop late.

A history of malnutrition or toxic or chemical exposure combined with typical bilateral scotomata on visual field testing justifies treatment. Laboratory testing for lead, methanol, and other suspected toxins is performed.

Treatment

Vision may improve if the cause is removed quickly. Once the optic nerve has atrophied, vision usually will not recover. Chelation therapy is indicated in lead poisoning. Treatment with oral or parenteral B vitamins before vision loss becomes severe may reverse the condition in cases in which malnutrition is the presumed cause. Low-vision aids may be helpful. The role of antioxidants has not been fully characterized. Their use could be justified on a theoretic basis; however, there is no proof of efficacy, and the at-risk population who should receive such supplements has not been defined.

108 ORBITAL DISEASES

Orbital diseases may be infectious, inflammatory, or neoplastic. Cavernous sinus thrombosis causes many of the same symptoms and signs as orbital diseases. Orbital fractures are discussed on p. 2584. (See FIG. 98–1 on p. 869 for anatomy of the orbit.)

CAVERNOUS SINUS THROMBOSIS

Cavernous sinus thrombosis is septic thrombosis of the cavernous sinus, usually caused by bacterial sinusitis. Symptoms and signs include pain, exophthalmos, ophthalmoplegia, vision loss, papilledema, and fever. Diagnosis is confirmed by CT or MRI. Treatment is with IV antibiotics. Complications are common, and prognosis is poor.

Etiology and Pathophysiology

The cavernous sinuses are trabeculated sinuses located at the base of the skull that drain venous blood from facial veins. Cavernous sinus thrombosis (CST) is an extremely rare complication of common facial infections, most notably nasal furuncles (50%), sphenoidal or ethmoidal sinusitis (30%), and dental infections (10%). Most common pathogens are *Staphylococcus aureus* (70%), followed by *Streptococcus* sp; anaerobes are more common in underlying dental and sinus infections. The 3rd, 4th, and 6th cranial nerves and the ophthalmic and maxillary branches of the 5th cranial nerve are adjacent to the cavernous sinus and are commonly affected.

Complications include meningoencephalitis, brain abscess, stroke, blindness, and pituitary insufficiency.

Thrombosis of the lateral sinus (in mastoiditis) and of the superior sagittal sinus (in bacterial meningitis) occur but are rarer than CST.

Symptoms, Signs, and Diagnosis

Initial symptoms are progressively severe headache or facial pain, usually unilateral and localized to retro-orbital and frontal regions. High fever is common. Later, ophthalmoplegia (initially the 6th cranial nerve, lateral gaze), exophthalmos, and lid edema develop and often become bilateral. Facial sensation may be diminished or absent. Decreased level of consciousness, confusion, and seizures are signs of CNS spread. Patients may also demonstrate anisocoria or mydriasis (3rd cranial nerve), papilledema, and vision loss.

CST is often misdiagnosed because it is so uncommon. It may be confused with orbital cellulitis. Features that distinguish CST from orbital cellulitis include cranial nerve dysfunction, bilateral eye involvement, and mental status changes.

Diagnosis is based on CT or MRI. Useful adjunct testing may include blood cultures and lumbar puncture. Lumbar puncture demonstrates inflammatory cells (PMNs, lymphocytes, monocytes) 75% of the time; glucose is low, protein elevated, and CSF cultures positive in 25%.

Prognosis and Treatment

Mortality is 30% in all patients and 50% in those with underlying sphenoid sinusitis. An additional 30% develop serious sequelae (ophthalmoplegia, blindness, stroke, hypopituitarism) and permanent disability.

Initial treatment is high-dose IV antibiotics. Options include nafcillin or oxacillin 1 to 2 g q 4 to 6 h combined with a 3rd-generation cephalosporin (eg, ceftriaxone 1 g q 12 h). An agent for anaerobes (eg, metronidazole 500 mg q 8 h) should be added if an underlying sinusitis or dental infection is present.

In cases with underlying sphenoid sinusitis, surgical sinus drainage is indicated, especially if there is no clinical response to antibiotics within 24 h.

Secondary treatment may include corticosteroids (eg, dexamethasone 10 mg po q 6 h) for cranial nerve dysfunction; anticoagulation is controversial because most cases respond to antibiotics, and adverse effects may exceed benefits.

INFLAMMATORY ORBITAL DISEASE

Orbital inflammation (inflammatory orbital pseudotumor) can affect any or all structures within the orbit. The inflammatory response can be nonspecific, granulomatous, or vasculitic. The inflammation can be part of an underlying medical disorder or can exist in isolation. Patients of all ages can be affected. The process can be acute or chronic and can recur.

Symptoms and signs typically include a sudden onset of pain along with swelling and erythema of the eyelids. Proptosis, diplopia, and vision loss are also possible.

Similar findings occur with orbital infection (see below), but there is no history of trauma or adjacent focus of infection (ie, sinusitis). Neuroimaging with CT or MRI is required. For chronic or recurrent cases, biopsy may be used to find evidence of an underlying medical condition.

Treatment depends on the type of inflammatory response and may include oral corticosteroids, radiation therapy, and one of several immunomodulating drugs. Some initial success has occurred with monoclonal antibodies against one of the inflammatory cytokines (tumor necrosis factor-α) in difficult cases.

PRESEPTAL AND ORBITAL CELLULITIS

Preseptal cellulitis (periorbital cellulitis) is infection of the eyelid and surrounding skin anterior to the orbital septum; orbital cellulitis (postseptal cellulitis) is infection of the orbital tissues posterior to the orbital septum. Either can be caused by an external focus of infection (eg, a wound), infection that extends from the nasal sinuses or teeth, or metastatic spread from infection elsewhere. Symptoms include eyelid pain, discoloration, and swelling; orbital cellulitis also causes fever, malaise, exophthalmos, impaired eye mobility, and impaired vision. Diagnosis is based on history, examination, and neuroimaging. Treatment is with antibiotics and sometimes surgical drainage.

Preseptal and orbital cellulitis are 2 distinct diseases that share a few clinical symptoms and signs. Preseptal cellulitis usually begins superficial to the orbital septum; orbital cellulitis usually begins deep to the orbital septum.Both are more common in children; preseptal cellulitis is far more common than orbital cellulitis.

Etiology and Pathophysiology

Preseptal cellulitis is caused by contiguous spread of infection from local facial or eyelid trauma, insect bites, previous URI, conjunctivitis, or chalazion.

Orbital cellulitis is most often caused by extension of infection from adjacent sinuses, especially the ethmoid sinus (75 to 90%); it is less commonly caused by direct infection accompanying local trauma (eg, insect or animal bite, penetrating eyelid injuries) or contiguous spread of infection from the face.

Pathogens vary by etiology and age. *Streptococcus pneumoniae* is the most frequent pathogen associated with sinus infection, whereas *Staphylococcus aureus* and *Streptococcus pyogenes* predominate when infection arises from local trauma. *Haemophilus influenzae* type b, once a common cause, is now less common because of widespread vaccination. Fungi are uncommon pathogens, causing orbital cellulitis in diabetic or immunosuppressed patients. Infection in children < 9 yr is typically with a single aerobic organism; patients > 15 yr typically have polymicrobial mixed aerobic and anaerobic (*Bacteroides, Peptostreptococcus*) infections.

Because orbital cellulitis originates from large adjacent foci of fulminant infection (eg, sinusitis) separated by only a thin bone barrier, orbital infection can be extensive and severe. Subperiosteal fluid collections, some quite large, can accumulate; they are called subperiosteal abscesses, but many are sterile initially.

Complications include vision loss (3 to 11%) from ischemic retinopathy and optic neuropathy caused by increased intraorbital pressure; restricted ocular movements (ophthalmoplegia) caused by soft-tissue inflammation; and intracranial sequelae from central spread of infection, including cavernous sinus thrombosis, meningitis, and cerebral abscess.

Symptoms and Signs

Preseptal cellulitis causes tenderness, swelling, and redness or discoloration (violaceous in the case of *H. influenzae*) of the eyelid. Patients may be unable to open their eyes, but visual acuity remains normal.

Symptoms and signs of orbital cellulitis include swelling and redness of the eyelid and surrounding soft tissues, conjunctival hyperemia and chemosis, decreased ocular motility, pain with eye movements, decreased visual acuity, and exophthalmos caused by orbital swelling. Signs of the primary infection are also often present (eg, nasal discharge and bleeding with sinusitis, periodontal pain and swelling with abscess). Fever, malaise, and headache should raise suspicion of associated meningitis. Some or all of these findings may be absent early in the course of the infection.

Subperiosteal abscesses, if large enough, can cause swelling and redness of the eyelid, decreased ocular motility, exophthalmos, and decreased visual acuity.

Diagnosis

Diagnosis is suspected clinically. An ophthalmologist should be consulted when preseptal or orbital cellulitis is suspected, because visual acuity must be assessed and followed. Eyelid swelling may require the use of lid retractors for evaluation of the globe, and initial signs of complicated infection may be subtle. Preseptal and orbital cellulitis are often distinguishable clinically. Preseptal cellulitis is likely if eye findings are normal except for lid swelling, a local nidus of infection is present on the skin, and the patient has no symptoms or signs of systemic illness. If findings are equivocal, the examination is difficult (as in young children), or nasal discharge is present (suggesting sinusitis), CT should be obtained to confirm orbital cellulitis and diagnose sinusitis if present. MRI should be used if cavernous sinus thrombosis is considered.

The direction of exophthalmos may be a clue to the site of infection; eg, extension from the frontal sinus pushes the globe down and out, and extension from the ethmoid sinus pushes the globe laterally and out.

Blood cultures are often performed (ideally before beginning antibiotics) in patients with orbital cellulitis but are positive in < 33%. Lumbar puncture is performed if meningitis is suspected. Other laboratory tests are not particularly helpful.

Differential diagnosis includes noninfectious inflammation from trauma, insect bites without cellulitis, retained foreign body, allergic reaction, tumor, and other inflammatory diseases (eg, dacryocystitis, dacryoadenitis, inflammatory orbital pseudotumor). Inflammatory diseases can usually be diagnosed by location and appearance.

Treatment

Treatment of both forms of cellulitis is with antibiotics.

In patients with preseptal cellulitis, therapy should be directed against sinusitis pathogens (*S. pneumoniae*, nontypable *H. influenzae, S. aureus*, and *Moraxella catarrhalis*); in cases with dirty wounds, gram-negative infection must be considered. Amoxicillin/clavulanate 30 mg/kg po q 8 h (for children < 12 yr) or 500 mg po tid or 875 mg po bid (for adults) for 10 days is an option for outpatient treatment; ampicillin/sulbactam 50 mg/kg IV q 6 h (for children) or 1.5 to 3 g (for adults) IV q 6 h (maximum 8 g ampicillin/day) for 7 days is an option for inpatients. Outpatient treatment is an option for patients in whom orbital cellulitis has been definitively excluded and for children with no signs of systemic infection who have responsible parents or guardians.

Patients with orbital cellulitis should be hospitalized and treated with meningitis-dose antibiotics. A 2nd- or 3rd-generation cephalosporin, such as cefotaxime 50 mg/kg IV q 6 h (for children < 12 yr) or 1 to 2 g IV q 6 h (for adults) for 14 days is an option when sinusitis is present; imipenem, ceftriaxone, and piperacillin/tazobactam are other options. If cellulitis is related to trauma or foreign body, treatment should cover gram-positive (vancomycin 1 g IV q 12 h) and gram-negative (eg, ertapenem 100 mg IV once/day) pathogens and last for 7 to 10 days or until clinically improved.

Surgery to decompress the orbit and open infected sinuses is indicated if vision is compromised, suppuration or foreign body is suspected, CT demonstrates orbital or large subperiosteal abscess, or the infection does not respond to antibiotics.

TUMORS OF THE ORBIT

Orbital tumors can be benign or malignant and arise primarily within the orbit or secondarily from an adjacent source, such as the eyelid, paranasal sinus, or intracranial compartment.

An orbital mass usually causes proptosis and displacement of the globe in a direction opposite the mass. Pain, diplopia, and vision loss may also be present and depend on the type of underlying tumor. Diagnosis, in most cases, is based on the history, examination, and neuroimaging (CT and/or MRI).

Etiology and Treatment

Causes differ by age. Treatment varies by tumor type. The more common benign tumors include dermoid tumors and vascular lesions such as capillary hemangioma and lymphangioma. Treatment of dermoid tumors is excision. Capillary hemangiomas tend to spontaneously involute and therefore do not need any treatment; however, especially when located on the upper eyelid, they may affect vision and require treatment with corticosteroids or surgical debulking.

Children: The common pediatric malignant tumors include rhabdomyosarcoma or a metastatic lesion related to leukemia or neuroblastoma. If rhabdomyosarcoma is resectable, then surgery is done, followed by chemotherapy and orbital radiation therapy. Leukemic disease is usually managed by orbital radiation therapy and/or chemotherapy. Metastatic disease is typically treated with radiation therapy to the involved orbit.

Adults: The most frequent benign tumors are meningiomas, mucoceles, and cavernous hemangiomas. Sphenoid wing meningiomas are treated with debulking via craniotomy when symptomatic, sometimes followed by a course of radiation therapy. Because meningioma cells infiltrate bone of the skull base, complete resection usually is not possible. Mucoceles are treated by draining the offending lesion into the nose, because they most commonly arise from the ethmoid or frontal sinus. Cavernous hemangiomas are excised.

Frequent malignant tumors include lymphoma, squamous cell carcinoma, and metastatic disease. Lymphomas involving the orbit are usually low grade. Lymphomas can be bilateral and simultaneous and can be part of a systemic process or exist in the orbit in isolation. Radiation therapy effectively treats orbital lymphomas with few adverse effects, although the addition of monoclonal antibodies against a surface receptor on the lymphocyte is being evaluated. Most squamous cell carcinomas arise from the adjacent paranasal sinuses. Surgery and/or radiation therapy form the backbone of therapy. Metastatic disease is usually treated with radiation therapy. Metastatic disease involving the orbit is usually an unfavorable prognostic sign.

SECTION 10
DERMATOLOGIC DISORDERS

109 APPROACH TO THE DERMATOLOGIC PATIENT

History and physical examination are adequate for diagnosing many skin lesions. Some require biopsy or other testing.

History and Physical Examination

Important information includes personal or family history of atopy (suggesting atopic dermatitis); occupational exposures (contact dermatitis); long-term exposure to sunlight or other forms of radiation (benign and malignant skin tumors); systemic disease (diabetes and *Candida* or tinea, hepatitis C and cryoglobulinemia, pyoderma gangrenosum and inflammatory bowel disease); sexual history (syphilis and gonorrhea); use of medications (Stevens-Johnson syndrome, toxic epidermal necrolysis); and travel history (Lyme disease, skin infections). A negative history is as important as a positive history. The history of the particular skin lesions is also important, including time and site of initial appearance, spread, change in appearance, and triggering factors.

Visual inspection is the central evaluation tool; many skin diseases are diagnosed by the characteristic appearance or morphology of the lesions.

DESCRIPTION OF SKIN LESIONS

An extensive language has been developed to standardize description of skin lesions, including their primary morphology (lesion type), secondary morphology (configuration), texture, distribution, and color. Rash is a general term for a temporary skin eruption.

Primary Morphology

Macules are flat, nonpalpable lesions usually < 10 mm in diameter, although some apply the term to lesions of any size. Macules represent a change in color or surface texture and are not raised above the skin surface. A patch is a large macule. Examples include freckles, flat moles, tattoos, port-wine stains, and the rashes of rickettsial infections, rubella, measles, and some allergic drug eruptions.

Papules are elevated lesions usually < 10 mm in diameter that can be felt or palpated. Examples include nevi, warts, lichen planus, insect bites, seborrheic and actinic keratoses, some lesions of acne, and skin cancers. The term "maculopapular" is often loosely and improperly used to describe many red skin rashes; because it is nonspecific and easily misused, this term should be avoided.

Plaques are palpable lesions > 10 mm in diameter that are elevated above the skin surface. Plaques may resemble a mesa. Lesions of psoriasis and granuloma annulare commonly form plaques.

Nodules are firm papules or lesions that extend into the dermis or subcutaneous tissue. Examples include cysts, lipomas, and fibromas.

Vesicles are small, clear fluid-filled blisters <10 mm in diameter. Vesicles are characteristic of herpes infections, acute allergic contact dermatitis, and some autoimmune blistering disorders (eg, dermatitis herpetiformis).

Bullae are clear fluid-filled blisters >10 mm in diameter. These may be caused by burns, bites, irritant or allergic contact dermatitis, and drug reactions. Classic bullous diseases include pemphigus vulgaris and bullous pemphigoid.

Pustules are elevated lesions that contain pus. Pustules are common in bacterial infections, folliculitis, and may arise in some inflammatory diseases including pustular psoriasis.

Urticaria (wheals or hives) is characterized by elevated lesions caused by localized edema. Wheals are a common manifestation of hypersensitivity to drugs, stings or bites, autoimmunity, and less commonly, physical stimuli including temperature, pressure, and sunlight.

Scales are heaped-up accumulations of horny epithelium seen in diseases such as psoriasis, seborrheic dermatitis, and fungal infections. Pityriasis rosea and chronic dermatitis of any type may be scaly.

Crusts (scabs) consist of dried serum, blood, or pus. Crusting can occur in inflammatory or infectious skin diseases (eg, impetigo).

Erosions are open areas of skin that result from loss of part or all of the epidermis. Erosions can be traumatic or can occur with various inflammatory or infectious skin diseases. An excoriation is a linear erosion caused by scratching, rubbing, or picking.

Ulcers result from loss of the epidermis and at least part of the dermis. Causes include venous stasis dermatitis, physical trauma with or without vascular compromise (decubitus ulcers, peripheral arterial disease), infections, and vasculitis.

Petechiae are nonblanchable punctate foci of hemorrhage; causes include platelet abnormalities (thrombocytopenia, platelet dysfunction), vasculitis, and infections (eg, meningococcemia, Rocky Mountain spotted fever, other rickettsioses).

Purpura is a larger area of hemorrhage that may be palpable. Palpable purpura is considered the hallmark of leukocytoclastic vasculitis. Purpura may indicate a coagulopathy. Large areas of purpura may be called ecchymoses or bruises.

Atrophy is thinning of the skin, which may appear dry and wrinkled, resembling cigarette paper. Atrophy may be caused by chronic sun exposure, aging, and some inflammatory and/or neoplastic skin diseases including cutaneous T-cell lymphoma and lupus erythematosus. Atrophy may also result from long-term use of potent topical corticosteroids.

Scars are areas of fibrosis that replace normal skin after injury. Some scars become hypertrophic or thickened and raised. Keloids are hypertrophic scars that extend beyond the original wound margin.

Telangiectasia is small, permanently dilated blood vessels that are most often idiopathic but may occur in rosacea, systemic diseases (especially scleroderma), inherited diseases (eg, ataxia-telangiectasia, hereditary hemorrhagic telangiectasia), or following long-term therapy with topical fluorinated corticosteroids.

Secondary Morphology

Configuration is the shape of single lesions and the arrangement of clusters of lesions.

Linear lesions take on the shape of a straight line and are suggestive of some forms of contact dermatitis, linear epidermal nevi, and lichen striatus.

Annular lesions are rings with central clearing; examples include granuloma annulare, some drug eruptions, some dermatophyte infections (ringworm), and secondary syphilis.

Nummular lesions are circular or coin shaped; an example is nummular eczema.

Target (bull's-eye or iris) lesions appear as rings with central duskiness and are classic for erythema multiforme.

Serpiginous lesions have linear, branched, and curving elements; examples include some fungal and parasitic infections (eg, cutaneous larva migrans).

Reticulated lesions have a lacy or networked pattern; examples include cutis marmorata and livedo reticularis.

Herpetiform describes grouped papules or vesicles arranged like those of a herpes simplex infection. Zosteriform describes lesions clustered in a dermatomal distribution similar to herpes zoster.

Texture

Some skin lesions have visible or palpable texture that suggests a diagnosis.

Verrucous lesions have an irregular, sometimes velvety surface; warts and seborrheic keratoses are common examples.

Lichenification is thickening of the skin with accentuation of normal skin markings; it results from repeated rubbing.

Induration, or deep thickening of the skin, can result from edema, inflammation, or infiltration, including by malignancy. Indurated skin has a hard, resistant feeling. Induration is characteristic of such skin diseases as panniculitis, some skin infections, and cutaneous metastatic malignancies.

Umbilicated lesions have a central indentation and are usually viral; examples include molluscum contagiosum and herpes simplex.

Yellowish, waxy lesions such as xanthomas may occur with a lipid disorder.

Location and Distribution

It is important to note if lesions are single or multiple; if particular body parts are affected (eg, palms or soles, scalp, mucosal membranes); if the distribution is random or patterned, symmetric or asymmetric; and if lesions are on sun-exposed or protected skin.

Although few patterns are pathognomonic, some are consistent with certain diseases. Psoriasis frequently affects the scalp, extensor surfaces of the elbows and knees, umbilicus, and the gluteal cleft. Lichen planus frequently arises on the wrists, forearms, genitals, and lower legs. Vitiligo may be patchy and isolated or may group around the distal extremities and face. Lesions on sun-exposed skin of the face, especially the forehead, nose, and the conchal bowl of the ear, are characteristic of chronic cutaneous lupus erythematosus. Hidradenitis suppurativa involves skin containing a high density of apocrine glands, including the axillae and groin.

Color

Red skin can result from many different inflammatory or infectious diseases. Cutaneous tumors are often pink or red. Superficial vascular lesions such as port-wine stains may appear red.

Orange skin is most often seen in hypercarotenemia, a usually benign condition of carotene deposition following excess dietary ingestion of β-carotene.

Yellow is typical of jaundice, xanthelasmas and xanthomas, and pseudoxanthoma elasticum.

Green fingernails suggest *Pseudomonas aeruginosa* infection.

Violet skin may result from cutaneous hemorrhage or vasculitis. Vascular lesions or tumors, such as Kaposi's sarcoma and hemangiomas, can appear purple. A lilac color of the eyelids or "heliotrope" eruption is characteristic of dermatomyositis.

Shades of blue, silver, and gray can result from deposition of drugs or metals in the skin, including minocycline, amiodarone, and silver (argyria). Ischemic skin appears purple to gray in color. Deep dermal nevi appear blue.

Black skin lesions may be melanocytic, including nevi and melanoma. Black eschars can arise from vascular infarction, which may be caused by infection (eg, anthrax, angioinvasive fungi including *Rhizopus*, meningococcemia), calciphylaxis, arterial insufficiency, or vasculitis.

Other Clinical Signs

Dermatographism is the appearance after stroking the skin of an urticarial wheal in the distribution of the skin stroke. Up to 5% of normal patients may exhibit this sign, which may also be a form of physical urticaria.

Darier's sign refers to blistering of a lesion when stroked. It occurs in patients with urticaria pigmentosa or mastocytosis.

Nikolsky's sign is epidermal shearing that occurs with gentle pressure in patients with toxic epidermal necrolysis and some autoimmune bullous diseases.

Auspitz' sign is the appearance of pinpoint bleeding after removal of scale from plaques in psoriasis.

Koebner's phenomenon describes the development of lesions within areas of trauma (eg, from scratching, rubbing, injury). Psoriasis frequently exhibits this phenomenon, as may lichen planus.

DIAGNOSTIC TESTS

Diagnostic tests are indicated when the cause of a skin lesion or disease is not obvious from history and physical examination alone (for patch testing, see p. 958).

Biopsy: A skin biopsy can be performed by a primary care physician. One procedure is a punch biopsy, in which a tubular punch (diameter usually 3 mm) is inserted into deep dermal or subcutaneous tissue to obtain a specimen, which is snipped off at its base. More superficial lesions may be biopsied by scraping with a sharp curette or shaving with a scalpel. Bleeding is controlled by aluminum chloride solution or electrodesiccation; large incisions are closed by sutures. Larger or deeper biopsies can be obtained by excising a wedge of skin with a scalpel. All pigmented lesions should be excised deeply for histologic evaluation of depth; superficial biopsies are inadequate. Diagnosis and cure are achieved simultaneously for most small tumors by complete excision that includes a small border of normal skin.

Scrapings: Skin scrapings help diagnose fungal infections and scabies. For fungal infection, scales are taken from the border of the lesion, put onto a microscope slide, and a drop of 10 to 20% potassium hydroxide (KOH) is added. Hyphae and/or budding yeast confirm the diagnosis of tinea or candidiasis. For scabies, scrapings are taken from suspected burrows and placed directly under a coverslip with mineral oil; findings of mites, feces, or eggs confirm the diagnosis.

Wood's light: Wood's light (black light) can help distinguish hypopigmentation from depigmentation (depigmentation of vitiligo fluoresces ivory-white and hypopigmented lesions do not). Erythrasma fluoresces bright orange-red. Tinea capitis caused by *Microsporum canis* and *Microsporum audouinii* fluoresces a light, bright green. (NOTE: Most tinea capitis in the US is caused by *Trichophyton* species, which do not fluoresce.) The earliest clue to cutaneous *Pseudomonas* infection (eg, in burns) may be green fluorescence.

Tzanck testing: Tzanck testing can be used to diagnose viral disease, such as herpes simplex and herpes zoster, and is performed when active intact vesicles are present. Tzanck testing cannot distinguish between herpes simplex and herpes zoster infections. Cellular material is scraped with a #15 scalpel blade from the base and sides of a vesicle and stained with Wright's or Giemsa stain. Multinucleated giant cells are a sign of viral disease.

Diascopy: Diascopy is used to distinguish between hemorrhagic and inflammatory lesions. A microscope slide is pressed against a lesion to see whether it blanches. Hemorrhagic lesions (petechiae or purpura) do not blanch; inflammatory lesions do. Diascopy is sometimes used to distinguish epidermal lesions from dermal nodules; epidermal lesions disappear, while dermal nodules remain and may turn an "apple jelly" color.

PRURITUS

Pruritus (itching) can be a symptom of primary skin diseases or of systemic disease. Skin diseases notorious for causing intense pruritus include scabies, pediculosis, insect bites, urticaria, atopic and contact dermatitis, lichen planus, miliaria, and dermatitis herpetiformis.

When pruritus is prominent without any identifiable skin lesions, dry skin (especially in elderly people), systemic disease, and drugs should be considered. Systemic diseases that cause generalized pruritus include cholestatic diseases, uremia, polycythemia vera, and hematologic malignancies. Pruritus may also occur during the later months of pregnancy. Barbiturates, salicylates, morphine, and cocaine can cause pruritus. Less well-defined causes of pruritus include hyper- and hypothyroidism, diabetes, iron deficiency, and internal cancers of many types. Pruritus is rarely psychogenic.

Evaluation

History: Key elements of the history include drug exposures and an occupational/hobby history.

Physical examination: Examination should focus on identification of an underlying skin disease. Identification of lesions may be complicated by redness, papules, excoriation, fissures, lichenification, and hyperpigmentation that all may be a result of persistent scratching.

Testing: When pruritus accompanies identifiable skin lesions, biopsy is appropriate. When systemic disease is expected, testing involves CBC; measures of liver, renal, and thyroid function; and appropriate evaluation for underlying malignancy.

Treatment

Any underlying cause is treated. Supportive treatment involves proper skin care and use of topical, systemic, and/or physical agents.

Skin care involves use of cool or lukewarm (but not hot) water when bathing; limitations on use of soap, bathing duration, and bathing frequency; liberal use of emollients such as white petrolatum or other oil-based products; humidification of dry air; and avoidance of irritating or tight clothing.

Topical agents may help localized pruritus. Options include camphor/menthol lotions or creams containing 0.125 to 0.25% menthol, doxepin, phenol 0.5 to 2%, pramoxine, eutectic mixture of local anesthetics (EMLA), and corticosteroids. Topical diphenhydramine and doxepin should be avoided because they may sensitize the skin.

Systemic agents are indicated for generalized pruritus or local pruritus resistant to topical agents. Antihistamines, most notably hydroxyzine 10 to 50 mg po q 4 h prn, are effective and most commonly used. Older antihistamines must be used cautiously in elderly patients because they cause oversedation and can lead to falls; newer nonsedating antihistamines such as loratadine, fexofenadine, and cetirizine are believed to be beneficial in pruritus but have not been evaluated. Other agents include doxepin (for atopy), cholestyramine (for renal failure, cholestasis, polycythemia vera), opioid antagonists such as naltrexone and nalmefene (for biliary pruritus), cromolyn (for mastocytosis), and possibly gabapentin (for hepatic pruritus).

Physical agents that may be effective for pruritus include ultraviolet (UV) phototherapy, transcutaneous electrical nerve stimulation (TENS), and acupuncture.

URTICARIA

Urticaria (hives, wheals) are migratory, erythematous, pruritic plaques. Urticaria is classified as acute (< 6 wk) or chronic (> 6 wk). The term angioedema refers to deep dermal or subcutaneous swellings. Isolated angioedema without wheals may be due to deficiency of C1 esterase inhibitor (see p. 1350).

Etiology and Pathophysiology

There are multiple causes of urticaria, most of which involve histamine release. In acute urticaria, this generally represents a type I hypersensitivity response (see p. 1348) to any of numerous topical or systemic substances, as well as infections (typically viral or parasitic). Acute urticaria can also result from certain drugs (aspirin, NSAIDs, opioids, ACE inhibitors) and physical stimuli (cold, sunlight, exercise, rubbing), which directly trigger histamine release independently of IgE-mediated allergy.

Most cases of chronic urticaria are idiopathic, although some represent recurrent undiagnosed hypersensitivity reactions (sometimes to the barrage of substances applied to an initial dermatitis). About half of patients have a serum histamine-releasing factor (which can trigger a wheal-and-flare response if the patient's own serum is injected intradermally), and about 30 to 50% have antibodies to an IgE receptor (possibly able to functionally cross-link IgE receptors and cause mast cell degranulation), indicating an autoimmune phenomenon.

Urticarial vasculitis is an entity in which urticaria is accompanied by findings of cutaneous vasculitis; either feature may predominate. It is sometimes associated with connective tissue disorders (particularly SLE). Lesions tend to be painful (more than pruritic) and last > 24 h. They do not blanch and are often accompanied by vesicles or purpura.

Evaluation

History: Key elements include duration of the urticaria (acute vs chronic), precipitating factors (foods, drugs, physical factors), frequency of attacks, associated symptoms (mucosal swelling, wheezing), and duration of the individual lesions (> or < 24 h). Use of drugs, travel, and family history are important. Symptoms that suggest occult infection (sinus infection, tooth abscess) may be helpful.

Physical examination: A complete physical examination is appropriate, but skin lesions may be absent at the time of the visit. Evidence of any associated systemic diseases (thyroid, joint), as well as occult infections (sinus infection, tooth abscess), may be sought.

Testing: No testing is generally indicated for acute urticaria unless symptoms and signs suggest a specific disorder. Unusual or persistent cases warrant further evaluation. Although there are no specific blood tests for urticaria, an elevated eosinophil count or ESR may suggest allergic causes. Antinuclear antibodies and thyroid studies, including thyroid autoantibodies, may be obtained if clinically indicated. Testing for low serum C4 is a sensitive but nonspecific screen for C1 esterase inhibitor deficiency. Skin biopsy should be done if there is any uncertainty as to the diagnosis or if wheals persist > 24 h (to rule out urticarial vasculitis). Skin testing for allergy may be considered.

Treatment

Any identified causes are treated or remedied. Implicated drugs or foods should be stopped. Antihistamines remain the mainstay of treatment. They must be taken on a regular basis, rather than prn. Newer oral antihistamines are often preferred because of once/day dosing schedules, and some are less sedating. Appropriate choices include cetirizine 10 mg once/day, fexofenadine 180 mg once/day, and desloratadine 5 mg once/day. Older oral antihistamines (hydroxyzine 10 to 25 mg q 4 to 6 h; diphenhydramine 25 to 50 mg q 6 h) are inexpensive and quite effective; however, they can be sedating and are particularly problematic in the elderly. Systemic corticosteroids (prednisone 30 to 40 mg po once/day) may control severe outbreaks but should not be used long term. Symptomatic treatment with cool baths and avoidance of tight clothing may be helpful. Generally, topical corticosteroids are not beneficial.

SKIN MANIFESTATIONS OF INTERNAL DISEASE

The skin frequently serves as a marker for underlying internal disease. The type of lesion typically relates to a specific disease or type of disease.

Internal malignancy: Dermatomyositis is associated with breast, lung, ovarian, and GI cancers in up to 50% of affected adults. Acute onset of multiple seborrheic keratoses (Leser-Trelat sign) may indicate underlying internal malignancy, particularly adenocarcinoma. However, because of the high prevalence of seborrheic keratoses in healthy adults, this sign may be overdiagnosed. Acute febrile neutrophilic dermatosis is associated with hematologic malignancies. Acanthosis nigricans that is associated with cancer can be of rapid onset and particularly widespread. Pruritus without a clearly associated dermatitis may indicate occult malignancy, often lymphoma. Paraneoplastic pemphigus is a relatively rare autoimmune blistering disease that has been associated with various malignancies, including leukemias. The carcinoid syndrome (flushing and erythema of the neck) is associated with carcinoid tumor. Erythema gyratum repens is a rare eruption consisting of concentric erythematous lesions, resembling wood grain, which has been associated with various malignancies.

Endocrinopathies: Many skin findings associated with endocrinopathies are not specific. Patients with diabetes mellitus may have acanthosis nigricans, necrobiosis lipoidica, perforating disorders, and scleredema adultorum. Thyroid disease, both hypo- and hyperthyroidism, can affect hair, nails, and skin. Cushing's disease causes striae distensae, moon facies, and skin fragility. Addison's disease is characterized by hyperpigmentation that is accentuated in areas of trauma.

GI disease: Skin conditions commonly associated with GI diseases include pyoderma gangrenosum, which occurs in patients with inflammatory bowel disease; lichen planus and porphyria cutanea tarda, which are associated with hepatitis C infection; and diffuse hyperpigmentation, or "bronze diabetes," which occurs in hemochromatosis. Erythema nodosum may accompany inflammatory bowel disease, sarcoidosis, and various infections. Eruptive xanthomas may result from elevated serum triglycerides.

110 PRINCIPLES OF TOPICAL DERMATOLOGIC THERAPY

Topical dermatologic treatments include cleansing agents, absorbents, anti-infective agents, anti-inflammatory agents, astringents (drying agents that precipitate protein and shrink and contract the skin), emollients (skin hydrators and softeners), and keratolytics (agents that soften, loosen, and facilitate exfoliation of the squamous cells of the epidermis).

Vehicles

Topical therapies can be delivered in various vehicles, including liquids, a combination of liquid and oil, and powders. The vehicle influences a therapy's effectiveness and may itself cause adverse effects (eg, contact or irritant dermatitis). Generally, aqueous preparations are drying (because the liquid evaporates) and are used in acute inflammatory conditions. Oil-based preparations are moisturizing and are preferred for chronic inflammation.

Powders: Inert powders may be mixed with active agents (eg, antifungals) to deliver therapy. They are prescribed for lesions in moist or intertriginous areas.

Liquids: Liquid vehicles include baths and soaks, solutions, lotions, and gels.

Baths and soaks are used when therapy must be applied to large areas, such as with extensive contact dermatitis or atopic dermatitis.

Solutions are ingredients dissolved in a solvent, usually ethyl alcohol, propylene glycol, polyethylene glycol, or water. Solutions are convenient to apply (especially to the scalp for disorders such as psoriasis or seborrhea) but tend to be drying. Two common solutions are Burow's and Domeboro's.

Lotions are water-based emulsions. They are easily applied to hairy skin; they cool and dry acute inflammatory and exudative lesions, such as contact dermatitis, tinea pedis, and tinea cruris.

Gels are ingredients suspended in a solvent thickened with polymers. Gels are often more effective for controlled release of topical agents. They are often used in acne, rosacea, and psoriasis of the scalp.

Combination vehicles: Combination vehicles usually comprise oil and water but may also contain propylene or polyethylene glycol.

Creams are semi-solid emulsions of oil and water. They are used for moisturizing and cooling and when exudation is present. They vanish when rubbed into skin.

Ointments are oil based (eg, petrolatum) with little if any water. Ointments are optimal lubricants and increase drug penetration because of their occlusive nature; a given concentration of drug is generally more potent in an ointment. They are preferred for lichenified lesions and those with thick crusts or heaped-up scales, including psoriasis and lichen simplex chronicus. Ointments are less irritating than creams for erosions or ulcers.

Dressings

Dressings protect open lesions, facilitate healing, increase the absorption of drug, and protect the patient's clothing.

Nonocclusive dressings: The most common are gauze dressings. They maximally allow air to reach the wound, which is often preferred in healing, and allow the lesion to dry. Nonocclusive dressings wetted with solution, usually saline, are used to help cleanse and debride thickened or crusted lesions. The dressings are applied wet and removed after the solution has evaporated (wet to dry dressings); materials from the skin then adhere to the dressing.

Occlusive dressings: Occlusive dressings increase the absorption and effectiveness of topical therapy. Most common are transparent films such as polyethylene (plastic household wrap) or flexible, transparent, semi-permeable dressings. Hydrocolloid dressings can be applied with a gauze cover in patients with cutaneous ulceration. Zinc oxide gelatin (Unna's paste boot) is an effective occlusive dressing for patients with stasis dermatitis and ulcers. Plastic tape impregnated with flurandrenolide, a corticosteroid, can be used for isolated or recalcitrant lesions. Occlusive dressings are recommended for treating psoriasis, atopic dermatitis, skin lesions of lupus erythematosus, and chronic hand dermatitis, among other conditions. Risks include development of miliaria, skin atrophy, striae, bacterial or fungal infections, and adrenal suppression from systemic absorption of topical corticosteroids.

Other occlusive dressings are used to protect and help heal open wounds, such as burns (see p. 2592).

Categories and Indications

Major categories of topical agents include cleansing, moisturizing, drying, anti-inflammatory, antimicrobial, keratolytic, astringent, and antipruritic.

Cleansing agents: The principal cleansing agents are soaps, detergents, and solvents. Soap is the most popular cleanser, but synthetic detergents are also used. Baby shampoos are usually well tolerated around the eyes and for cleansing wounds and abrasions; they are useful for removing crusts and scales in psoriasis, eczema, and other forms of dermatitis. However, acutely irritated, weeping, or oozing lesions are most comfortably cleansed with water or isotonic saline.

Water is the principal solvent for cleansing. Organic solvents (eg, acetone, petroleum products, propylene glycol) are very drying, can be irritating, and cause irritant or less commonly allergic contact dermatitis. Removal of hardened tar and dried paint from the skin may require a petrolatum-based ointment or commercial waterless cleanser.

Moisturizing agents: Moisturizers (emollients) restore water and oils to the skin and help to maintain skin hydration. They typically contain glycerin, mineral oil, or petrolatum and are available as lotions, creams, ointments, and bath oils. Stronger moisturizers contain urea 2%, lactic acid 5 to 12%, and glycolic acid 10% (higher concentrations are used as keratinolytics, eg, for ichthyosis). They are most effective when applied to already moistened skin (eg, after a bath or shower).

Drying agents: Excessive moisture in intertriginous areas (eg, between the toes; in the intergluteal cleft, axillae, groin, and inframammary areas) can cause irritation and maceration. Powders dry macerated skin and reduce friction by absorbing moisture. However, some powders tend to clump and can be irritating if they become moist. Cornstarch and talc are most often used. Although talc is more effective, talc may cause granulomas if inhaled and is no longer used for baby powders. Cornstarch may promote fungal growth. Aluminum chloride solutions are another type of drying agent (often useful in hyperhidrosis).

Anti-inflammatory agents: Topical anti-inflammatory agents are either corticosteroids or noncorticosteroids.

Corticosteroids are the mainstay of treatment for most noninfectious inflammatory dermatoses. Lotions are useful on intertriginous areas and the face. Gels are useful on the scalp and in management of contact dermatitis. Creams are useful on the face and in intertriginous areas and for management of inflammatory dermatoses. Ointments are useful for dry scaly areas and when increased potency is required. Corticosteroid-impregnated tape is useful to protect an area from excoriation. It also increases corticosteroid absorption and therefore potency.

Topical corticosteroids range in potency from mild (Class VII) to superpotent (Class I) (see TABLE 110–1). Intrinsic differences in potency are attributable to fluorination or chlorination (halogenation) of the compound.

Topical corticosteroids are generally applied bid to tid, but high-potency formulations may require application only once/day or even less frequently. Most dermatoses are treated with mid- to high-potency formulations; mild formulations are better for mild inflammation and for use on the face or intertriginous areas, where systemic absorption is more likely. All agents can cause skin atrophy, striae, and acneiform eruptions when used > 1 mo. This effect is particularly problematic on the thinner skin of the face or genitals. Corticosteroids also promote fungal growth. Contact dermatitis in reaction to preservatives and additives is also common with prolonged use. Contact dermatitis to the corticosteroid itself may also occur. Perioral dermatitis occurs with mid- or high-potency formulations used on the face but is uncommon with mild formulations. High-potency agents may cause adrenal suppression when used in children, over extensive skin surfaces, or for long periods. Relative contraindications include conditions in which infection plays an underlying role and acneiform disorders.

Noncorticosteroid anti-inflammatory agents include tar preparations. Tar comes in the form of crude coal tar and is indicated for psoriasis. Adverse effects include irritation, folliculitis, staining of clothes and furniture, and photosensitization. Contraindications include infected skin. Several herbal products are commonly used in commercial products, although their effectiveness has not been well established. Among the most popular are chamomile and calendula.

Antimicrobials: Topical antimicrobials include antibiotics, antifungals, insecticides, and nonspecific agents.

Topical antibiotics have few indications. Topical clindamycin and erythromycin are used as primary or adjunctive treatment for acne vulgaris in patients who do not warrant or tolerate oral antibiotics. Mupirocin has excellent gram-positive (*Staphylococcus aureus*, streptococci) coverage and can be used for treatment of impetigo when deep tissues are not affected. OTC antibiotics such as bacitracin and polymyxin are often used in postoperative care of a skin biopsy site and to prevent infection in scrapes, minor burns, and excoriations. Topical neomycin causes contact dermatitis more frequently than other antibiotics. The use of topical antibiotics and washing with antiseptic soaps in healing wounds may, however, actually slow healing.

Antifungals are indicated for candidiasis, a wide variety of dermatophytoses, and other fungal infections (see TABLE 120–1 on p. 990).

Insecticides (permethrin, malathion) are used for treatment of lice infestation and scabies (see TABLE 121–1 on p. 996).

Non-antibiotic topical antiseptics include iodine solutions (povidone iodine, clioquinol), gentian violet, silver preparations (silver nitrate, silver sulfadiazine), and zinc pyrithione. Iodine is indicated for presurgical skin preparation. Gentian violet is used when an inexpensive chemically and physically stable antiseptic/antimicrobial is needed. Silver preparations (eg, silver sulfadiazine) are effective in treatment of burns and ulcers and have strong antimicrobial properties; several wound dressings are impregnated with silver. Zinc pyrithione is an antifungal and a common ingredient in shampoos for treatment of dandruff due to psoriasis or seborrheic dermatitis. Healing wounds should generally not be treated with topical antiseptics other than silver because they are irritating and tend to kill fragile granulation tissue.

TABLE 110–1. RELATIVE POTENCY OF SELECTED TOPICAL CORTICOSTEROIDS

CLASS*	DRUG	TRADE NAME
I	Betamethasone dipropionate 0.05% ointment	Diprolene
	Clobetasol propionate 0.05% cream or ointment	Temovate
	Diflorasone diacetate 0.05% ointment	Psorcon
	Halobetasol propionate 0.05% cream or ointment	Ultravate
II	Amcinonide 0.1% ointment	Cyclocort
	Betamethasone dipropionate 0.05% cream	Diprolene AF, Maxivate
	Betamethasone dipropionate 0.05% ointment	Diprosone, Maxivate
	Desoximetasone 0.25% cream, 0.05% gel, 0.25% ointment	Topicort
	Diflorasone diacetate 0.05% ointment	Florone, Maxiflor
	Fluocinonide 0.05% cream, gel, ointment, solution	Lidex
	Halcinonide 0.1% cream	Halog
	Mometasone furoate 0.1% ointment	Elocon
III	Amcinonide 0.1% cream or lotion	Cyclocort
	Betamethasone dipropionate 0.05% cream	Diprosone
	Betamethasone dipropionate 0.05% lotion	Maxivate
	Betamethasone valerate 0.1% ointment	Valisone
	Desoximetasone 0.05% cream	Topicort LP
	Diflorasone diacetate 0.05% cream	Florone, Maxiflor
	Fluocinonide cream 0.05%	Lidex E
	Fluticasone propionate 0.005% ointment	Cutivate
	Halcinonide 0.1% ointment or solution	Halog
	Triamcinolone acetonide 0.1% ointment	Aristocort A
IV	Fluocinolone acetonide 0.025% ointment	Synalar
	Flurandrenolide 0.05% ointment	Cordran
	Mometasone furoate 0.1% cream or lotion	Elocon
	Triamcinolone acetonide 0.1% ointment	Aristocort, Kenalog
	Triamcinolone acetonide 0.1% cream	Kenalog
V	Betamethasone valerate 0.1% cream	Valisone
	Desonide 0.05% ointment	Tridesilon
	Fluocinolone acetonide 0.025% cream	Synalar
	Flurandrenolide 0.05% cream	Cordran
	Fluticasone propionate 0.05% cream	Cutivate
	Hydrocortisone butyrate 0.1% cream, ointment, or solution	Locoid
	Hydrocortisone valerate 0.2% cream or ointment	Westcort
	Triamcinolone acetonide 0.1% lotion or 0.025% ointment	Kenalog
VI	Alclometasone dipropionate 0.05% cream or ointment	Aclovate
	Betamethasone valerate 0.1% lotion	Valisone
	Desonide 0.05% cream	Tridesilon
	Fluocinolone acetonide 0.01% cream or solution	Synalar

TABLE 110–1. RELATIVE POTENCY OF SELECTED TOPICAL CORTICOSTEROIDS—Continued

CLASS*	DRUG	TRADE NAME
	Flumethasone pivalate 0.03% cream	Locorten
	Triamcinolone acetonide 0.1% cream	Aristocort
	Triamcinolone acetonide 0.025% cream or lotion	Kenalog
VII	Hydrocortisone 1% or 2.5% cream, 1% or 2.5% lotion, 1% or 2.5% ointment	Hytone
	Hydrocortisone acetate (1% or 2.5% cream, 1% or 2.5% lotion, 1% or 2.5% ointment) and pramoxine hydrochloride 1%	Pramosone

*Class I is the most potent, Class VII the least potent. Potency depends on many factors, including the drug's characteristics and concentration and the base in which it is used.

Keratolytics: Keratolytics soften and facilitate exfoliation of epidermal cells. Examples include 3 to 6% salicylic acid and urea. Salicylic acid is indicated for use in psoriasis, seborrhea, acne, and warts. Adverse effects are burning and systemic toxicity if large areas are covered. It should rarely be used in children and infants. Urea is indicated for plantar keratodermas and ichthyosis. Adverse effects are irritation and intractable burning. It should not be applied to large surface areas.

Astringents: Astringents are drying agents that precipitate protein and shrink and contract the skin. The most commonly used astringents are aluminum acetate (Burow's solution) and aluminum sulfate and Ca acetate (Domeboro's solution). Usually applied with dressings or as soaks, astringents are indicated for infectious eczema, exudative skin lesions, and pressure ulcers. Witch hazel is also a popular OTC astringent.

Antipruritics: Doxepin is a topical antihistamine that is effective for itching of atopic dermatitis, lichen simplex chronic dermatitis, and nummular dermatitis. Topical benzocaine and diphenhydramine (present in certain OTC lotions) are sensitizing and not recommended. Other antipruritics include camphor 0.5 to 3%, menthol 0.1 to 0.2%, pramoxine hydrochloride, and eutectic mixtures of local anesthetics (EMLA), which contain equal parts lidocaine and prilocaine in an oil-in-water vehicle. Topical antipruritics are preferred over systemic agents (such as oral antihistamines) when smaller surface areas of skin are affected and pruritus is not intractable. Calamine lotion is soothing but not specifically antipruritic.

111 ACNE AND RELATED DISORDERS

Acne vulgaris is a common skin problem, affecting most adolescents and many adults. Perioral dermatitis and rosacea can produce similar lesions.

ACNE VULGARIS

Acne vulgaris (acne) is the formation of comedones, papules, pustules, nodules, and/or cysts as a result of obstruction and inflammation of pilosebaceous units (hair follicles and their accompanying sebaceous gland). It most often affects adolescents. Diagnosis is by examination. Treatment is a variety of topical and systemic agents intended to reduce sebum production, infection, and inflammation and normalize keratinization.

Etiology and Pathophysiology

Acne occurs when pilosebaceous units become obstructed with plugs of sebum and desquamated keratinocytes, then colonized and sometimes infected with the normal skin anaerobe *Propionibacterium acnes*. Manifestations differ depending on whether *P. acnes* stimulates inflammation in the follicle; acne can be noninflammatory or inflammatory.

Comedones, uninfected sebaceous plugs impacted within follicles, are the signature of noninflammatory acne. Comedones are termed open or closed depending on whether the follicle is dilated or closed at the skin surface. Inflammatory acne comprises papules, pustules, nodules, and cysts.

Papules appear when lipases from *P. acnes* metabolize triglycerides into free fatty acids (FFA), which irritate the follicular wall. Pustules occur when active *P. acnes* infection causes inflammation within the follicle. Nodules and cysts occur when rupture of follicles due to inflammation, physical manipulation, or harsh scrubbing releases FFAs, bacteria, and keratin into tissues, triggering soft-tissue inflammation.

The most common trigger is puberty, when surges in androgen stimulate sebum production and hyperproliferation of keratinocytes. Other triggers include hormonal changes that occur with pregnancy or throughout the menstrual cycle; occlusive cosmetics, cleansing agents, and clothing; and humidity and sweating. Associations between acne exacerbation and diet (eg, chocolate), inadequate face washing, masturbation, and sex are unfounded. Acne may improve in summer months because of sunlight's anti-inflammatory effects. Proposed associations between acne and hyperinsulinism require further investigation.

Symptoms and Signs

Cystic acne can be painful; other types cause no physical symptoms but can be a source of significant emotional distress. Lesion types frequently coexist at different stages.

Comedones appear as whiteheads or blackheads. Whiteheads (closed comedones) are flesh-colored or whitish palpable lesions 1 to 3 mm in diameter; blackheads (open comedones) are similar in appearance but with a dark center.

Papules and pustules are red lesions 2 to 5 mm in diameter. In both, the follicular epithelium becomes damaged with accumulation of neutrophils and then lymphocytes. When the epithelium ruptures, the comedone contents elicit an intense inflammatory reaction in the dermis. Relatively deep inflammation produces papules. Pustules are more superficial.

Nodules are larger, deeper, and more solid than papules. Such lesions resemble inflamed epidermoid cysts, although they lack true cystic structure.

Cysts are suppurative nodules. Occasionally, cysts become infected and form abscesses. Long-term cystic acne can cause scarring that manifests as tiny, deep pits ("icepick scars"), larger pits, shallow depressions, or areas of hypertrophic scar.

Acne conglobata is the most severe form of acne vulgaris, affecting men more than women. Patients have abscesses, draining sinuses, fistulated comedones, and keloidal and atrophic scars. The back and chest are severely involved. The arms, abdomen, buttocks, and even the scalp may be affected.

Acne fulminans is acute, febrile, ulcerative acne conglobata, characterized by sudden appearance of confluent abscesses leading to hemorrhagic necrosis. Leukocytosis and joint pain and swelling are also present.

Pyoderma faciale (also called rosacea fulminans) occurs suddenly on the midface of young women. It may be analogous to acne fulminans. The eruption consists of erythematous plaques and pustules, involving the chin, cheeks, and forehead.

Diagnosis

Diagnosis is by examination. Differential diagnosis includes rosacea (in which no comedones are seen), corticosteroid-induced acne (which lack comedones and in which pustules are usually in the same stage of development), perioral dermatitis, and acneiform drug eruptions. Acne severity is graded mild, moderate, or severe based on the number and type of lesions; a standardized system is outlined in TABLE 111–1.

Prognosis

Acne of any severity usually remits spontaneously by the early 20s, but a substantial minority of patients, usually women, may have acne into their 40s; options for treatment may be limited because of childbearing. Many adults occasionally develop mild, isolated acne lesions. Noninflammatory and mild inflammatory acne usually heals without scars. Moderate to severe inflammatory acne heals but often leaves scarring. Scarring is not only physical; acne may be a huge emotional stressor for adolescents who may withdraw, using the acne as an excuse to avoid difficult personal adjustments. Supportive counseling for patients and parents may be indicated in severe cases.

Treatment

Treatments are directed at reducing sebum production, comedone formation, inflammation, and infection (see FIG. 111–1). Selection of treatment is generally based on severity; options are summarized in TABLE 111–2. Affected areas should be cleansed daily, but extra washing, use of antibacterial soaps, and scrubbing confer no added benefit. Changes in diet are also unnecessary and ineffective. Peeling agents such as sulfur, salicylic acid, and resorcinol are minor therapeutic adjuncts.

Mild acne: Single-agent therapy is generally sufficient for comedonal acne; papulopustular generally requires dual therapy (eg, the combination of tretinoin with benzoyl peroxide or topical antibiotics). Treatment should be continued for 6 wk or until lesions respond. Maintenance treatment may be necessary to maintain control.

A mainstay of treatment for comedones is daily topical tretinoin in escalating concentrations as tolerated. Daily adapalene gel, tazarotene cream or gel, azelaic acid cream, and glycolic or salicylic acid in propylene glycol are alternatives for patients who cannot tolerate topical tretinoin. Adverse effects include erythema, burning, stinging, and peeling. Adapalene and tazarotene are retinoids; like tretinoin, they tend to be somewhat irritating and photosensitizing. Azelaic acid has comedolytic and antibacterial properties by an unrelated mechanism and may be synergistic with retinoids.

TABLE 111–1. CLASSIFICATION OF ACNE SEVERITY

SEVERITY	DEFINITION
Mild	< 20 comedones, or < 15 inflammatory lesions, or < 30 total lesions
Moderate	20 to 100 comedones, or 15 to 50 inflammatory lesions, or 30 to 125 total lesions
Severe	> 5 cysts, or total comedo count > 100, or total inflammatory count > 50, or > 125 total lesions

Mild inflammatory acne should be treated with topical benzoyl peroxide, topical antibiotics (eg, erythromycin, clindamycin), and/or glycolic acid. Combination preparations of these agents may help limit development of resistance. None have significant adverse effects other than drying and irritation (and rare allergic reactions to benzoyl peroxide).

Physical extraction of comedones using a comedone extractor is an option for patients unresponsive to topical treatment. Comedone extraction may be performed by a physician, nurse, or physician assistant. One end

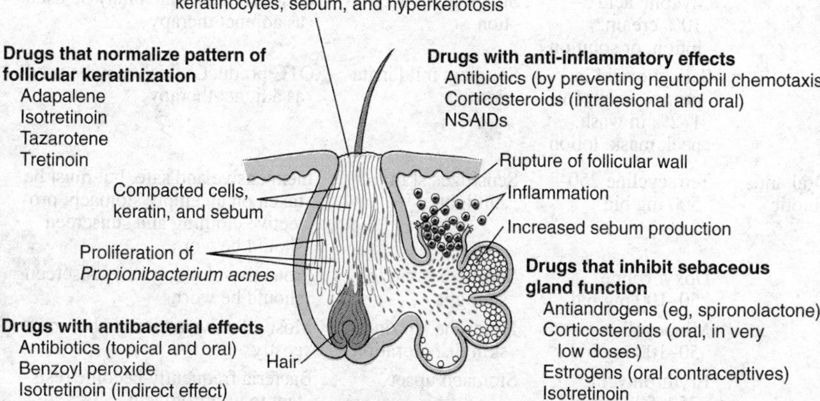

Fig. 111–1. How various drugs work in treating acne.

TABLE 111–2. DRUGS USED TO TREAT ACNE

ACTION	DRUG	ADVERSE EFFECTS	COMMENTS
Topical antibacterial	Benzoyl peroxide 2.5%, 5%, and 10% gel, lotion, or wash	Dries the skin; may bleach clothing and hair; rare allergic reactions	Should be used in all patients if tolerated. Gel product usually preferred
	Benzoyl peroxide/ erythromycin		Must be kept refrigerated
	Benzoyl peroxide/ clindamycin		—
	Clindamycin 1% gel or lotion	Diarrhea (rarely)	Avoid in patients with inflammatory bowel disease
	Erythromycin 1.5 to 2% (multiple vehicles)	—	Well tolerated
Topical comedolytic and exfoliant	Tretinoin (0.025%, 0.05%, and 0.1% cream; 0.05% liquid; 0.025% and 0.1% gel)	Irritates skin; increases sun sensitivity	If irritation occurs, reduce strength and/or frequency of use. Acne appears to worsen when tretinoin is started; may take 3 to 4 wk to notice any improvement; protective clothing and sunscreen should be worn. Avoid in pregnancy
	Tazarotene 0.05% or 0.1% cream or gel	Irritates skin; increases sun sensitivity	Acne appears to worsen when tazarotene is started; may take 3 to 4 wk to notice any improvement; protective clothing and sunscreen should be worn. Avoid in pregnancy
	Adapalene 0.1% gel	Some redness, burning, and increased sun sensitivity	As effective as tretinoin but less irritating; protective clothing and sunscreen should be worn
	Azelaic acid 20% cream	May lighten skin	Minimally irritating; may be used by itself or with tretinoin; should be used cautiously in people with darker skin because of skin-lightening effects
	Glycolic acid 5–10% cream, lotion, or solution	Stinging, mild irritation	OTC product, which may be used as adjunct therapy
	Salicylic acid in propylene glycol 1–2% in wash, peel, mask, lotion	Stinging, mild irritation	OTC product, which may be used as adjunct therapy
Oral antibiotic	Tetracycline 250–500 mg bid	Sensitizes skin to sunlight	Inexpensive and safe, but must be taken on an empty stomach; protective clothing and sunscreen should be worn
	Doxycycline 50–100 mg bid	Sensitizes skin to sunlight	Protective clothing and sunscreen should be worn
	Minocycline 50–100 mg bid	Headache, dizziness, skin discoloration	Most effective antibiotic but more costly
	Erythromycin 250–500 mg bid	Stomach upset	Bacteria frequently become resistant to erythromycin

TABLE 111–2. DRUGS USED TO TREAT ACNE—Continued

ACTION	DRUG	ADVERSE EFFECTS	COMMENTS
Oral retinoid	Isotretinoin 1–2 mg/kg once/day for 16–20 wk	Can harm a developing fetus; can affect blood cells, liver, and fat levels; dry eyes, chapped lips, drying of the mucous membranes; pain or stiffness of large joints and lower back with high dosages; has been associated with depression, suicidal thoughts, attempted suicide, and (in rare cases) completed suicide	A sexually active woman should have a pregnancy test before she starts taking isotretinoin and at monthly intervals while she is taking it; contraception or sexual abstinence should begin 1 mo before she starts taking the drug and should continue while she takes it and for 1 mo after she discontinues it. Blood tests are necessary to make sure the drug is not affecting blood cells, the liver, or fat (triglyceride and cholesterol) levels

of the comedone extractor is like a blade or bayonet that punctures the closed comedone. The other end exerts pressure to extract the comedone.

Oral antibiotics (eg, tetracycline, minocycline, doxycycline, erythromycin) can be used when wide distribution of lesions makes topical therapy impractical.

Moderate acne: Moderate acne responds best to oral systemic therapy with antibiotics. Antibiotics effective for acne include tetracycline, minocycline, erythromycin, and doxycycline. Full benefit takes ≥ 12 wk.

Tetracycline is usually a good first choice: 250 or 500 mg bid (between meals and at bedtime) for 4 wk or until lesions respond, after which it may be reduced to the lowest effective dose. Rarely, dosage must be increased to 500 mg qid. Because relapse ordinarily follows short-term treatment, therapy must be continued for months to years, although for maintenance tetracycline 250 or 500 mg once/day is often sufficient. Minocycline 50 or 100 mg bid causes fewer GI adverse effects, is easier to take, is less likely to cause photosensitization, but is the most costly option. Erythromycin and doxycycline are considered 2nd-line agents because both can cause GI adverse effects, and doxycycline is a frequent photosensitizer.

Long-term use of antibiotics may produce a gram-negative pustular folliculitis around the nose and in the center of the face. This uncommon superinfection may be difficult to clear and is best treated with oral isotretinoin after discontinuing the oral antibiotic. Ampicillin is an alternative treatment for gram-negative folliculitis. In women, prolonged antibiotic use can cause candidal vaginitis; if local and systemic therapy does not eradicate this problem, antibiotic therapy for acne must be stopped.

Severe acne: Oral isotretinoin is the best treatment for patients with moderate acne in whom antibiotics are unsuccessful and for those with severe inflammatory acne. Dosage of isotretinoin is usually 1 mg/kg once/day for 16 to 20 wk, but the dosage may be increased to 2 mg/kg once/day. If adverse effects make this dosage intolerable, it may be reduced to 0.5 mg/kg once/day. After therapy, acne may continue to improve. Most patients do not require a 2nd course of treatment; when needed, it should be resumed only after the drug has been stopped for 4 mo. Retreatment is required more often if the initial dosage is low (0.5 mg/kg). With this dosage (which is very popular in Europe), fewer adverse effects occur, but prolonged therapy is usually required.

Isotretinoin is nearly always effective, but use is limited by adverse effects, including dryness of conjunctivae and mucosae of the genitals, chapped lips, arthralgias, depression, elevated lipids, and birth defects. Petrolatum usually alleviates mucosal and cutaneous dryness. Arthralgias (mostly of large joints or the lower back) occur in about 15% of patients. Increased risk for depression and suicide is much publicized but probably rare. CBC, liver function, and fasting glucose, triglyceride, and cholesterol levels should be determined before treatment. Each should be reassessed at 4 wk and, unless abnormalities are noted, need not be repeated until the end of treatment. Triglycerides rarely increase to a level at which the drug should be stopped. Liver function is seldom affected. Because isotretinoin is teratogenic, women of childbearing age are urged to use 2 methods of contraception for 1 mo before treatment, during treatment, and at least 1 mo after stopping treatment. Pregnancy tests should be done before beginning therapy and monthly until 1 mo after therapy stops.

Intralesional injection of 0.1 mL triamcinolone acetonide suspension 2.5 mg/mL (the 10 mg/mL suspension must be diluted) is indicated for patients with firm (cystic) acne who seek quick clinical improvement and to reduce scarring. Local atrophy may occur but is usually transient. For isolated, very boggy lesions, incision and drainage are often beneficial but may result in residual scarring.

Other forms of acne: Pyoderma faciale is treated with oral corticosteroids and isotretinoin. Acne fulminans is treated with oral corticosteroids and systemic antibiotics. Acne conglobata is treated with oral isotretinoin if systemic antibiotics fail. For acne with endocrine abnormalities, antiandrogens are indicated. Spironolactone, which has some antiandrogen effects, is sometimes prescribed to treat acne at a dose of 50 to 100 mg once/day. Cyproterone acetate is used in Europe. When other measures fail, an estrogen-progesterone–containing contraceptive may be tried; therapy ≥ 6 mo is needed to evaluate effect.

Scarring: Small scars can be treated with chemical peels, laser resurfacing, or dermabrasion. Deeper, discrete scars can be excised. Wide, shallow depressions can be treated with subcision or collagen injection. Collagen implants are temporary and must be repeated every few years.

PERIORAL DERMATITIS

Perioral dermatitis is an erythematous, papulopustular facial eruption that resembles acne and/or rosacea but starts typically around the mouth.

A variety of causes have been proposed, including exposure to topical corticosteroids and/or fluoride in water and toothpaste, but etiology is unknown. Despite its name, perioral dermatitis is not a true dermatitis. It primarily affects women of childbearing age and children. Eruption classically starts at the nasolabial folds and spreads periorally, sparing a zone around the vermilion borders of the lips. But the eruption can also spread periorbitally and to the forehead.

Diagnosis is by appearance; perioral dermatitis is distinguished from acne by the absence of comedones and from rosacea by the latter's lack of lesions around the mouth and eyes. Seborrheic dermatitis and contact dermatitis must be excluded. Biopsy, which is generally not clinically necessary, shows spongiosis and a lymphohistiocytic infiltrate affecting vellus hair follicles. In the lupoid variant, granulomas may be present.

Treatment is tetracycline 250 to 500 mg po bid (between meals) for 4 wk, tapered to the lowest effective dose. Alternatives include doxycycline 50 to 100 mg bid and minocycline 50 to 100 mg bid. In contrast to acne, antibiotics can usually be stopped. Reasons for efficacy of antibiotics are unclear given the absence of evidence for infection. Topical antibiotics (eg, metronidazole 0.75% gel or cream bid) may be helpful. Isotretinoin has been successfully used to treat granulomatous perioral dermatitis.

ROSACEA

Rosacea (acne rosacea) is a chronic inflammatory disorder characterized by facial flushing, telangiectasias, erythema, papules, pustules, and in severe cases, rhinophyma. Diagnosis is based on characteristic appearance. Treatment depends on severity and includes topical metronidazole, topical and oral antibiotics, rarely isotretinoin, and, for severe rhinophyma, surgery.

Etiology and Epidemiology

The etiology of rosacea is unknown, although associations with impaired facial venous drainage, an increase in hair mites (*Demodex folliculorum*), and *Helicobacter pylori* infection have been proposed. The basic disturbance seems to be one of vasomotor control. Rosacea most commonly affects patients aged 30 to 50 with fair complexions, most notably those of Irish and Northern

European descent, but it affects and is probably under-recognized in darker-skinned patients. The age of onset helps distinguish rosacea from acne.

Symptoms and Signs

Rosacea manifests in 4 phases and is limited to the face and scalp. In the "pre-rosacea" phase, patients describe embarrassing flushing and blushing, often accompanied by uncomfortable stinging. Common reported triggers for these flares include sun exposure, emotional stress, cold or hot weather, alcohol, spicy foods, exercise, wind, cosmetics, and hot baths or hot drinks. These symptoms persist throughout other phases of the disorder.

In the vascular phase, patients develop facial erythema and edema with multiple telangiectasias, possibly as a result of persistent vasomotor instability.

An inflammatory phase often follows, in which sterile papules and pustules (leading to the designation of rosacea as "adult acne") develop. Some patients go on to develop late-stage rosacea, characterized by coarse tissue hyperplasia of the cheeks and nose (rhinophyma) caused by tissue inflammation, collagen deposition, and sebaceous gland hyperplasia.

The phases of rosacea are usually sequential. Some patients go directly into the inflammatory stage bypassing the earlier stages. Treatment may cause a patient to return to an earlier stage.

Ocular rosacea often accompanies facial rosacea and manifests as some combination of blepharoconjunctivitis, iritis, scleritis, and keratitis, causing itching, foreign body sensation, erythema, and edema of the eye.

Differential diagnosis includes acne vulgaris, SLE, sarcoidosis, photodermatitis, drug eruptions (particularly from iodides and bromides), granulomas of the skin, and perioral dermatitis.

Treatment

Primary initial treatment of rosacea involves avoidance of triggers (including use of sunscreen). Antibiotics may be used for inflammatory disease. The objective of treatment is control of symptoms, not cure.

Metronidazole cream 1%, lotion (0.75%), or gel (0.75%) and azelaic acid 20% cream, applied bid, are equally effective; 2.5% benzoyl peroxide, applied once/day or bid, can be added for improved control. Less effective alternatives include sodium sulfacetamide 10%/sulfur 5% lotion; clindamycin 1% solution, gel, or lotion; and erythromycin 2% solution, all applied bid. Many patients require indefinite treatment for chronic control.

Oral antibiotics are indicated for patients with multiple papules or pustules and those with ocular rosacea; options include tetracycline 250 to 500 mg bid, doxycycline 50 to 100 mg bid, minocycline 50 to 100 mg bid, and erythromycin 250 to 500 mg bid. Doses should be reduced to the lowest that control symptoms once a beneficial response is achieved. Recalcitrant cases may respond to oral isotretinoin.

Techniques developed for treatment of rhinophyma include dermabrasion and tissue excision; cosmetic results are good.

112 BULLOUS DISEASES

Bullae are elevated, fluid-filled blisters ≥ 5 mm across. Bullous diseases include bullous pemphigoid, dermatitis herpetiformis, epidermolysis bullosa acquisita, herpes gestationis (pemphigoid gestationis—see p. 2195), linear IgA disease, pemphigus vulgaris, and pemphigus foliaceous. Staphylococcal scalded skin syndrome (see p. 986) and toxic epidermal necrolysis (see p. 976) also cause bullae.

BULLOUS PEMPHIGOID

Bullous pemphigoid is an autoimmune skin disorder producing chronic, pruritic bullous eruptions in elderly patients. Diagnosis is by skin biopsy. Corticosteroids are used initially. Most patients require long-term maintenance therapy, for which a variety of drugs can be used.

TABLE 112–1. DISTINGUISHING PEMPHIGOID FROM PEMPHIGUS

DISORDER	APPEARANCE OF LESION	ORAL INVOLVEMENT	ITCHING	NIKOLSKY'S SIGN	PROGNOSIS
Pemphigoid	Tense bullae on normal-appearing or reddened skin	In ⅓ of patients	Common	Often negative	Usually good; occasionally fatal in the elderly
Pemphigus	Flaccid bullae of various sizes; skin or mucosa often shears off, leaving painful erosions	Typically starts in the mouth	Absent	Positive	Mortality now ≤ 10%; high without treatment

In bullous pemphigoid, antibodies are directed against the basement membrane zone of the epidermis, causing separation between the epidermis and dermis. Bullous pemphigoid must be distinguished from pemphigus (see p. 949 and TABLE 112–1), a much more serious disease.

Symptoms, Signs, and Diagnosis

Characteristic tense bullae develop on normal-appearing or reddened skin. Nikolsky's sign (see p. 950) is negative. There may be urticaria or annular, dusky-red, edematous lesions, with or without peripheral vesicles. Itching is common, usually without other symptoms. Oral lesions occur in about ⅓ of patients but heal rapidly.

Bullous pemphigoid must be differentiated from pemphigus, linear IgA disease, erythema multiforme, drug eruptions, benign mucosal pemphigoid, dermatitis herpetiformis, and epidermolysis bullosa acquisita. Patients should have a skin biopsy and serum antibody titers.

Prognosis and Treatment

Prognosis is good, and the disease usually subsides within months to years; however, the disease is potentially fatal, especially in the elderly.

Mild disease may be treated with topical corticosteroids (see p. 939). Patients with more severe disease receive prednisone 60 to 80 mg po once/day, which can be tapered to a maintenance level of ≤ 10 to 20 mg/day after several weeks. Most patients achieve remission after 2 to 10 mo. Occasional new lesions in elderly patients do not require increasing the prednisone dosage.

The disorder occasionally responds to a combination of tetracycline and nicotinamide. Other treatment options include dapsone, sulfapyridine, erythromycin, and tetracycline alone for their anti-inflammatory rather than their antibiotic properties. Most patients do not require immunosuppressants, but azathioprine, cyclophosphamide, cyclosporine, or plasmapheresis can be used.

DERMATITIS HERPETIFORMIS

Dermatitis herpetiformis is a chronic eruption characterized by clusters of intensely pruritic vesicles, papules, and urticaria-like lesions. The cause is autoimmune. Diagnosis is by skin biopsy with direct immunofluorescence testing. Treatment is usually with dapsone or sulfapyridine.

This disease usually presents in patients 30 to 40 yr old and is rare in blacks and Asians. It is an autoimmune disease. Celiac sprue is present in 75 to 90% of patients and in some of their relatives, but it is asymptomatic in most cases. The incidence of thyroid disease is also increased. Iodides may exacerbate the disease, even when symptoms are well controlled. The term "herpetiformis" refers to the clustered appearance of the lesions rather than a relationship to herpesvirus.

Symptoms, Signs, and Diagnosis

Onset is usually gradual. Vesicles, papules, and urticaria-like lesions are usually distributed symmetrically on extensor aspects (elbows, knees, sacrum, buttocks, occiput). Vesicles and papules occur in about ⅓ of patients. Itching and burning are severe, and scratching often obscures the primary lesions with eczematization of nearby skin, leading to an erroneous diagnosis of eczema.

Patients should have skin biopsy of a lesion and adjacent normal-appearing skin. IgA deposition in the dermal papillary tips is invariably present and important for diagnosis. Patients should be evaluated for celiac sprue (see p. 144).

Treatment

Strict adherence to a gluten-free diet for prolonged periods (eg, 6 to 12 mo) controls the disease in some patients, obviating or reducing the need for drug therapy. When drugs are needed, dapsone generally provides remarkable improvement. It is started at 50 mg po once/day, increased to bid or tid (or a once/day dose of 100 mg); this usually dramatically relieves symptoms, including itching, within 1 to 3 days; if so, that dose is continued. If no improvement occurs, the dose can be increased every week, up to 100 mg qid. Most patients can be maintained on 50 to 150 mg/day, and some require as little as 25 mg/wk. Although less effective, sulfapyridine may be used as an alternative for those who cannot tolerate dapsone. Initial oral dosage is 500 mg bid, increasing by 1 g/day q 1 to 2 wk until disease is controlled. Maintenance dosage varies from 500 mg twice/wk to 1000 mg once/day. Colchicine is another treatment option. Treatment continues until lesions resolve.

Patients receiving dapsone or sulfapyridine should have a baseline and weekly CBC for 4 wk, then q 2 to 3 wk for 8 wk, and q 12 to 16 wk thereafter because agranulocytosis may occur at any time. Hemolytic anemia and methemoglobinemia are the most frequently encountered adverse effects. These can be severe in people with an inherited G6PD deficiency. CNS or liver toxicity is rare. If dapsone therapy causes considerable hemolysis, significant cardiopulmonary problems, or peripheral neuropathy, sulfapyridine may be used. It usually does not induce significant hemolysis.

EPIDERMOLYSIS BULLOSA ACQUISITA

Epidermolysis bullosa acquisita is an autoimmune mucocutaneous disease causing blistering and skin fragility.

Epidermolysis bullosa acquisita usually appears in adults. Bullous lesions appear on normal-appearing skin spontaneously or caused by minor trauma. Pain and scarring are common. Because the hands and feet are often involved, disability can be significant. Occasionally, mucosa of eyes, mouth, or genitals is involved. Laryngeal and esophageal involvement also occurs. Diagnosis is by skin biopsy. Lesions respond poorly to corticosteroids. Mild disease may be treated with colchicine but more severe disease may require cyclosporine or immune globulin.

LINEAR IMMUNOGLOBULIN A DISEASE

Linear immunoglobulin A (IgA) disease is an uncommon bullous disease distinguished from bullous pemphigoid and dermatitis herpetiformis by the linear deposits of IgA in the basement membrane zone.

In linear IgA disease, vesicular or bullous skin lesions occur frequently in a clustered (herpetiform) arrangement. There is a predilection for flexural areas (eg, inguinal crease). As in dermatitis herpetiformis, severe burning and pruritus of cutaneous lesions are prominent features. It was previously considered a form of dermatitis herpetiformis, but there is no concomitant gluten-sensitive enteropathy and immunopathology. Genetic studies indicate that linear IgA disease is a separate disorder.

Diagnosis is by skin biopsy. Dapsone is the treatment of choice. Doses should be similar to those used for dermatitis herpetiformis (see above), and CBC monitoring should follow the same parameters. Other treatment options include systemic, topical, and intralesional glucocorticoids, cyclophosphamide, azathioprine, colchicine, tetracycline and nicotinamide, and cyclosporine.

PEMPHIGUS VULGARIS

Pemphigus vulgaris is an uncommon, potentially fatal, autoimmune disease characterized by intraepidermal bullae and extensive erosions on apparently healthy skin and mucous membranes. Diagnosis is by skin biopsy and serum antibody titers. Treatment is with corticosteroids and sometimes immunosuppressants. Maintenance therapy is usually required.

Autoantibodies directed against components of epidermal desmosomes cause separation of layers within the epidermis, resulting in blistering. These antibodies are present in both serum and skin during active disease. Any area of stratified squamous epithelium may be affected, including mucosal surfaces.

Pemphigus vulgaris usually occurs in middle-aged or elderly patients and is rare in children. One variant, paraneoplastic pemphigus, occurs in older patients with malignancy (primarily lymphoreticular); outcome is poor.

Symptoms and Signs

The primary lesions are flaccid bullae of various sizes, but often skin or mucosa just shears off, leaving painful erosions. Lesions typically occur first in the mouth, where they rupture and remain as chronic, often painful, erosions for variable periods before the skin is affected; dysphagia and poor oral intake are common. Lesions also may occur in the upper esophagus. Cutaneous bullae typically arise from normal-appearing skin, rupture, and leave a raw area and crusting. Itching is usually absent. Open skin lesions often become infected. If large portions of the body are affected, fluid and electrolyte loss may be significant.

Diagnosis

Pemphigus vulgaris should be suspected in any bullous disorder or chronic mucosal ulceration. It must be differentiated from other chronic oral ulcers and from other bullous dermatoses (eg, pemphigus foliaceous, bullous pemphigoid, benign mucosal [cicatricial] pemphigoid—see p. 888, drug eruptions, toxic epidermal necrolysis, erythema multiforme, dermatitis herpetiformis, bullous contact dermatitis). Two physical signs in pemphigus are helpful: lateral pressure on skin adjacent to a blister causes epidermal detachment (Nikolsky's sign) and pressure on a blister can cause the blister to extend to adjacent skin.

Patients should have biopsy of the edge of a fresh lesion and from a nearby area of normal skin; light microscopy and direct immunofluorescent staining are usually diagnostic. Serum antibodies (eg, to desmoglein-3) can be used for diagnosis and for differentiating from pemphigus foliaceous; serial titers can help follow disease activity.

Treatment

Even with treatment, pemphigus vulgaris is a serious disease with an inconsistent and unpredictable response to therapy, a prolonged course, and virtually inevitable adverse drug effects. Referral to a dermatologist with expertise in treating this disease is recommended. Hospitalization is required initially for all but the most minor cases. Cleansing and dressing of open skin lesions is similar to that done for partial-thickness burns (eg, reverse isolation, hydrocolloid or silver sulfadiazine dressings—see p. 2596).

Drug treatment aims to stop the eruption of new lesions. The mainstay is systemic corticosteroids. Some patients with few lesions may respond to oral prednisone 20 to 30 mg once/day, but most initially require IV therapy with prednisolone 1 mg/kg once/day. Some clinicians begin with much higher doses, which may slightly hasten initial response but does not appear to improve outcome. If new lesions continue to appear after 5 to 7 days, dose is increased.

Immunosuppressants such as methotrexate, cyclophosphamide, azathioprine, gold, mycophenolate mofetil, or cyclosporine can reduce the need for corticosteroids and thus minimize the undesirable effects of long-term corticosteroid use. Plasmapheresis to reduce antibody titers has also been effective.

Once no new lesions have appeared for 7 to 10 days, corticosteroid dose should be tapered monthly by about 10 mg/day (tapering slower once 20 mg/day is reached). A relapse requires return to the starting dose. If the patient has been stable after a year, a trial without treatment can be attempted but must be closely monitored.

PEMPHIGUS FOLIACEOUS

Pemphigus foliaceous is a generally benign blistering disorder. It is characterized by splitting high in the epidermis causing erosions to form on the skin.

Pemphigus foliaceous usually occurs in middle-aged patients. Foci of high incidence occur in South America, especially Brazil.

The primary lesion is a flaccid bulla. However, due to the high level of split in the epidermis, bullae are rarely seen; the blisters are so fragile that they rupture and leave shallow erosions, which may coalesce. Lesions usually begin on the trunk and may spread. Mucosal surfaces are not usually involved. In one variant, pemphigus erythematosis, lesions occur in a photo distribution and are often similar to those of cutaneous lupus erythematosus.

Diagnosis is by biopsy of a lesion and neighboring normal skin and serum antibody titers. Because the disease is much more benign than pemphigus vulgaris, treatment is generally less aggressive. Topical glucocorticosteroids may be sufficient in some cases. Others require oral prednisone and additional immunosuppressants. A combination of tetracycline 500 mg qid and nicotinamide 1.5 g/day has been effective in some patients. Plasmapheresis is an option for severe disease.

113 CORNIFICATION DISORDERS

Cornification disorders include calluses, corns, ichthyosis, and keratosis pilaris.

CALLUSES AND CORNS

(Tylomas; Helomas; Clavi)

Calluses and corns are circumscribed areas of hyperkeratosis at a site of pressure or friction. Calluses are more superficial and usually asymptomatic; corns are deeper and may be painful. Diagnosis is by appearance. Treatment is with manual abrasion and sometimes keratolytic agents. Prevention involves changing footwear.

Calluses and corns are caused by intermittent pressure or friction, usually over a bony prominence (eg, heel, metatarsal heads).

Corns consist of a sharply circumscribed keratinous plug, pea-sized or slightly larger, which extends though most of the underlying dermis. An underlying adventitial bursitis may develop. Hard corns occur over prominent bony protuberances, especially on the toes and plantar surface; soft corns occur between the toes. Most corns result from poorly fitting footwear, but small seed-sized corns on non–weight-bearing aspects of the soles and palms may represent an inherited genodermatosis (keratosis punctata).

Calluses lack a central plug and associated dermal changes and have a more even appearance. They usually occur on the hands or feet but may occur elsewhere, especially in a person whose occupation entails repeated trauma to a particular area (eg, the mandible and clavicle in a violinist).

Symptoms, Signs, and Diagnosis

Calluses are usually asymptomatic but, if friction is extreme, may become irritated, producing mild burning discomfort. At times, the discomfort may mimic that of interdigital neuralgia.

Corns may be painful or tender on pressure. A bursa or fluid-filled pocket sometimes forms beneath a corn.

A corn may be differentiated from a plantar wart or callus by trimming away the horny skin. After paring, a callus shows preserved skin markings, whereas a wart (see p. 998) appears sharply circumscribed, sometimes with soft macerated tissue or with central black dots (bleeding points) representing thrombosed capillaries. A corn, when pared, shows a sharply outlined yellowish to tan translucent core that interrupts the normal architecture of the papillary dermis. Interdigital neuralgia can be ruled out by the absence of interspace pain on palpation.

Prevention and Treatment

Although difficult to eliminate, pressure on the affected surface should be reduced and redistributed. For foot lesions, soft, well-fitting shoes are important; they should have a roomy toe box so that toes can move freely in the shoe. Stylish shoes often prevent this freedom of motion. Shoes that increase discomfort of a lesion should be eliminated from the wardrobe. Pads or rings of suitable shapes and sizes, moleskin or foam-rubber protective bandages, arch inserts (orthotics), or metatarsal plates or bars may help redistribute the pressure. For corns and calluses on the ball of the foot, an orthotic should not be full length but extend only to the ball or break of the shoe immediately behind the corn or callus. Surgical off-loading or removal of the offending bone is rarely necessary.

A nail file, emery board, or pumice stone used immediately after bathing is often a practical way to manually remove hyperkeratotic tissue. Keratolytic agents (eg, 17% salicylic acid in collodion or 40% salicylic acid plasters) can also be used, taking care to avoid applying the agent to normal skin. Normal skin may be protected by covering it with petrolatum before application of the keratolytic.

Patients with a tendency to calluses and corns may need the regular services of a podiatrist. Those with impaired peripheral circulation, especially if associated with diabetes, require expert care.

ICHTHYOSIS

Ichthyosis is scaling and flaking of skin ranging from mild but annoying dryness (xeroderma) to severe disfiguring disease (inherited ichthyosis). Ichthyosis can also be a sign of systemic disease. Diagnosis is clinical. Treatment involves emollients and sometimes oral retinoids.

Xeroderma: Xeroderma (xerosis), the mildest form of ichthyosis, is neither inherited nor associated with systemic abnormalities. It usually occurs on the lower legs of middle-aged or older patients, most often during cold weather and in those who bathe too frequently. There may be mild to moderate itching and an associated dermatitis caused by detergents or other irritants.

Inherited ichthyoses: Inherited ichthyoses, which are characterized by excessive accumulation of scale on the skin surface, are classified according to clinical and genetic criteria (see TABLE 113–1). Some occur in isolation without associated abnormalities (eg, ichthyosis vulgaris, X-linked ichthyosis, lamellar ichthyosis, epidermolytic hyperkeratosis). Other ichthyoses are part of a syndrome that involves multiple organs. For instance, Refsum's disease (see p. 2473) and Sjögren-Larsson syndrome (hereditary mental deficiency and spastic paralysis caused by a defect in fatty aldehyde dehydrogenase) are autosomal recessive conditions with skin and extracutaneous organ involvement. A dermatologist should assist in diagnosis and management, and a medical geneticist should be consulted for genetics counseling.

Acquired ichthyosis: Ichthyosis may be an early manifestation of some systemic diseases (eg, leprosy, hypothyroidism, lymphoma, AIDS). Some drugs cause ichthyosis (eg, nicotinic acid, triparanol, butyrophenones). The dry scaling may be fine and localized to the trunk and legs, or it may be thick and widespread. Biopsy of ichthyotic skin is usually not diagnostic of the systemic disease; however, there are exceptions, most notably sarcoidosis, in which a thick scaling may appear on the legs, and biopsy usually shows the typical granulomas.

Treatment

In any ichthyosis, minimizing bathing or showering is helpful. Soaps should be used only in intertriginous areas. Hexachlorophene products should not be used because of increased absorption and toxicity. An emollient—preferably plain petrolatum, mineral oil, or lotions containing urea or α-hydroxy acids (eg, lactic, glycolic, and pyruvic acids)—should be applied bid, especially after bathing while the skin is still wet. Blotting with a towel removes excess applied material. Ichthyosis caused by an underlying systemic disease may slightly improve with lubrication using propylene glycol. However, improvement is greatest if the primary disease can be corrected.

To remove the scale in inherited ichthyoses, patients can apply a preparation containing 50% propylene glycol in water under occlusion (eg, thin plastic film or bags) every night after hydration of the skin. In children, the propylene glycol preparation should be applied bid without an occlusive dressing overnight. After scaling has decreased, less frequent application is required. Other useful agents include 6% salicylic acid gel, hydrophilic petrolatum and water (in equal parts), and cold cream and the α-hydroxy acids in various bases. Topical calcipotriol cream has been used with success; however, this vitamin D derivative can result in hypercalcemia when used over broad areas, especially in small children.

Patients with epidermolytic hyperkeratosis (bullous congenital ichthyosiform erythroderma) may need long-term treatment with cloxacillin 250 mg po tid or qid or erythromycin 250 mg po tid or qid, as long as thick intertriginous scaling is present, to prevent bacterial superinfection from causing painful, foul-smelling pustules. Regular use of soaps containing chlorhexidine may also reduce the bacteria but tend to dry the skin.

Oral synthetic retinoids are effective for most ichthyoses. Acitretin (see p. 968) is effective in X-linked ichthyosis and epidermolytic hyperkeratosis. In lamellar ichthyo-

TABLE 113–1. CLINICAL AND GENETIC FEATURES OF SOME INHERITED ICHTHYOSES

DISORDER	INHERITANCE PATTERN/ PREVALENCE	ONSET	TYPE OF SCALE	DISTRIBUTION	ASSOCIATED CLINICAL FINDINGS
Ichthyosis vulgaris	Autosomal dominant 1:300	Childhood	Fine	Usually back and extensor surfaces but not flexors; usually many markings on palms and soles	Atopy; keratosis pilaris
X-linked ichthyosis	X-linked 1:6000 (males)	Birth or infancy	Large, dark (may be fine)	Prominent on neck and trunk; normal palms and soles	Corneal opacities, cryptorchidism
Lamellar ichthyosis (nonbullous congenital ichthyosiform erythroderma; collodion baby)	Autosomal recessive 1:300,000	Birth	Large, coarse	Most of body; thick palms and soles	Ectropion
Epidermolytic hyperkeratosis (bullous congenital ichthyosiform erythroderma)	Autosomal dominant 1:300,000	Birth	Thick, warty	Most of body; especially warty in flexural creases	Blisters

sis, 0.1% tretinoin cream or oral isotretinoin may be effective. The lowest effective dose should be used. Long-term (1 yr) treatment with oral isotretinoin has resulted in bony exostoses in some patients, and other long-term adverse effects may arise. (CAUTION: *Oral retinoids are contraindicated in pregnancy because of their teratogenicity, and acitretin should be avoided in women of childbearing potential because of its teratogenicity and long half-life.*)

KERATOSIS PILARIS

Keratosis pilaris is a disorder of keratinization in which horny plugs fill the openings of hair follicles.

Keratosis pilaris is common. The cause is unknown, but there is often an autosomal dominant inheritance. Multiple small, pointed keratotic follicular papules appear mainly on the lateral aspects of the upper arms, thighs, and buttocks; facial lesions may also occur, particularly in children. Lesions are most prominent in cold weather and sometimes improve in the summer. Skin may appear red. The problem is mainly cosmetic, but the disorder may cause itching or, rarely, produce follicular pustules.

Treatment is usually unnecessary and often unsatisfactory. Hydrophilic petrolatum and water (in equal parts), cold cream, or petrolatum with 3% salicylic acid may help flatten the lesions. Buffered lactic acid (ammonium lactate) lotions or creams, urea creams, 6% salicylic acid gel, or 0.1% tretinoin cream may also be effective. Acid creams should be avoided in young children because of burning and stinging. Pulse-dye laser has been used successfully to treat facial redness.

114 DERMATITIS

Dermatitis is superficial inflammation of the skin characterized by redness, edema, oozing, crusting, scaling, and sometimes vesicles. Pruritus is common. Eczema is a term often used interchangeably with dermatitis.

ATOPIC DERMATITIS

Atopic dermatitis is an immune-mediated inflammation of the skin, often with a significant genetic component. Pruritus is the primary symptom; skin lesions range from mild erythema to severe lichenification. Diagnosis is by history and examination. Treatment is moisturizers, avoidance of allergic and irritant triggers, and often topical corticosteroids.

Atopic dermatitis (AD) is IgE-mediated (extrinsic type, 70 to 80% of cases) or non-IgE-mediated (intrinsic type, 20 to 30% of cases). IgE-mediated disease is better characterized; non-IgE-mediated disease is nonfamilial and idiopathic.

Etiology and Pathophysiology

AD primarily affects children in urban areas or developed countries; at least 5% of children in the US are affected. Like asthma, it may be linked to pro-allergic/pro-inflammatory T-cell immune responses. Such responses are becoming more common in developed countries, because trends toward smaller families, cleaner indoor environments, and early use of vaccinations and antibiotics deprive children of the early exposure to infections and allergens that suppress pro-allergic T cells and induce tolerance.

AD occurs when environmental exposures trigger immunologic, usually allergic (ie, IgE-mediated), reactions in genetically susceptible people. Common environmental triggers include foods (eg, milk, eggs, soy, wheat, peanuts, fish), airborne allergens (eg, dust mites, molds, dander), and *Staphylococcus aureus* colonization on skin due to deficiencies in endogenous antimicrobial peptides. AD is common within families, suggesting a genetic component.

Eczema herpeticum (Kaposi's varicelliform eruption) is a diffuse herpes simplex infection occurring in patients with AD. Typical grouped vesicles appear in areas of active or recent dermatitis, although normal skin can be involved. High fever and adenopathy develop after several days. Skin lesions commonly become infected with staphylococci. Occasionally, viremia with internal organ infection occurs, which may be fatal. As with other herpetic infections, relapses may occur.

Fungal and nonherpetic viral skin infections, such as common warts and molluscum contagiosum, also may complicate AD.

Symptoms and Signs

AD usually appears in infancy, typically by 3 mo. In the acute phase, lasting 1 to 2 mo, red, weeping, crusted lesions appear on the face and spread to the neck, scalp, extremities, and abdomen. In the chronic phase, scratching and rubbing create skin lesions (typically erythematous macules and papules that lichenify with continued scratching). Lesions typically appear in antecubital and popliteal fossae and on the eyelids, neck, and wrists. Lesions slowly resolve to dry scaly macules (xerosis) that can fissure and facilitate exposure to irritants and allergens. In older children or adults, intense pruritus is the key feature. Patients have a reduced threshold for perceiving itch, and itch worsens with allergen exposures, dry air, sweating, local irritation, wool garments, and emotional stress.

AD may become generalized. Secondary bacterial infections and regional lymphadenitis are common. Frequent use of topical products exposes the patient to many potential allergens, and contact dermatitis may aggravate and complicate AD, as may the generally dry skin that is common in these patients.

Diagnosis

Diagnosis is clinical (see TABLE 114–1). AD is often hard to differentiate from other dermatoses (eg, seborrheic dermatitis, contact dermatitis, nummular dermatitis, psoriasis), although a family history of atopy and the distribution of lesions are helpful. Psoriasis is usually extensor rather than flexurally distributed, may involve the fingernails, and has a more shiny (micaceous) scale. Seborrheic dermatitis affects the face (eg, nasolabial folds, eyebrows, glabellar region, scalp) most commonly. Nummular dermatitis is not flexural, and lichenification is rare. Allergic precipitants of AD can be identified with skin testing and/or measurement of allergen-specific

IgE levels. Because patients can still develop other skin disorders, not all subsequent skin problems should be attributed to AD.

Prognosis and Treatment

AD in children often improves by 5 yr of age, although exacerbations are common throughout adolescence and into adulthood. Girls and patients with severe disease, early age of onset, family history, and associated rhinitis or asthma are more likely to have prolonged disease. Even in these patients, AD frequently resolves completely by age 30. AD may have long-term psychologic sequelae as children confront many challenges of living with a visible, sometimes disabling, skin disease during formative years. Patients with long-standing AD may develop cataracts in their 20s or 30s.

Treatment can usually be given at home, but patients who have exfoliative dermatitis (see p. 958), cellulitis, or eczema herpeticum may need to be hospitalized.

Supportive care: Skin care involves moisturizing. Bathing and hand washing should be infrequent and use lukewarm (not hot) water; soap use should be minimized on dermatitic areas because it may be drying and irritating. Colloidal oatmeal baths can be helpful.

Body oils or emollients such as white petrolatum, vegetable oil, or hydrophilic petrolatum (unless the patient is allergic to lanolin) applied immediately after bathing may help. Continuously wet dressings (not wet-to-dry) are an alternative for severe lesions. Coal tar cream or oil can be an effective topical antipruritic.

Antihistamines can help relieve pruritus. Options include hydroxyzine 25 mg po tid or qid (for children, 0.5 mg/kg q 6 h or 2 mg/kg in a single bedtime dose) and diphenhydramine 25 to 50 mg po at bedtime. Low-sedating H_1 blockers, such as loratadine, fexofenadine, and cetirizine, may be useful, although their efficacy has not been defined. Doxepin, a tricyclic antidepressant also with H_1 and H_2 receptor blocking activity, 25 to 50 mg po at bedtime may also help, but use is not recommended for children < 12 yr. Fingernails should be cut short to minimize excoriations and secondary infections.

Avoidance of precipitating factors: Household antigens can be controlled by using synthetic fiber pillows and impermeable mattress covers; washing bedding with hot water; removing upholstered furniture, soft toys, carpets, and pets (dust mites and animal dander); and using dehumidifiers in basements and other poorly aerated damp rooms (to reduce molds). Reduction of emotional stress is effective but often difficult. Antistaphylococcal antibiotics, both topical (mupirocin, fusidic acid) and oral (dicloxacillin, cephalexin, erythromycin, all 250 mg qid), can control *S. aureus* nasal colonization and is indicated in patients with severe disease unresponsive to specific therapies and positive nasal cultures. Extensive dietary changes intended to eliminate exposure to allergenic foods are unnecessary and probably ineffective; food hypersensitivities rarely persist beyond childhood.

Corticosteroids: Corticosteroids are the mainstay of therapy. Creams or ointments applied bid are effective for most patients with

TABLE 114–1. CLINICAL FINDINGS IN ATOPIC DERMATITIS*

Common features

Chronic or chronically relapsing
Personal or family history of atopic disease
Pruritus
Typical morphology and distribution:
  Facial and extensor eczema in infants and children
  Flexural eczema in adults

Frequent features

Cutaneous infections
Early onset
Elevated serum IgE
Nonspecific dermatitis of hands and feet
Positive type I allergy skin tests
Xerosis

Occasional features

Cataracts (anterior subcapsular)
Facial erythema
Food intolerance
Ichthyosis
Infraorbital folds
Itching with sweating
Keratoconus
Nipple eczema
Pityriasis alba
Recurrent conjunctivitis
White dermatographism
Wool intolerance

*Diagnosis requires 3 or more common features *plus* 3 or more frequent or occasional features.

mild or moderate disease. Emollients are applied between corticosteroid applications and can be mixed with them to decrease the corticosteroid amount required to cover an area. Systemic corticosteroids (prednisone 60 mg or, for children 1 mg/kg, po once/day for short courses of 7 to 14 days) are indicated for extensive or refractory disease but should be avoided whenever possible, as disease often recurs and topical therapy is safer. Prolonged, widespread use of high-potency corticosteroid creams or ointments should be avoided in infants because adrenal suppression may ensue.

Other therapies: Tacrolimus and pimecrolimus are T-cell inhibitors effective for AD. They should be used when patients do not respond to corticosteroids and tar or when corticosteroid adverse effects such as skin atrophy, stria formation, or adrenal suppression are a concern. Tacrolimus or pimecrolimus cream is applied bid. Burning or stinging after application is usually transient and abates after a few days. Flushing is less common.

Light therapy is helpful for extensive AD. Natural sun exposure ameliorates disease in many patients. Alternatively, therapy with ultraviolet A (UVA) or B (UVB) may be used. UVA therapy with psoralen (PUVA—see p. 968) is reserved for extensive, refractory AD. Adverse effects include sun damage (eg, PUVA lentigines, nonmelanoma skin cancer); for this reason, PUVA is rarely indicated for children or young adults.

Systemic immune modulators effective in at least some patients include cyclosporine, interferon-γ, mycophenolate, methotrexate, and azathioprine. All downregulate or inhibit T-cell function and have anti-inflammatory properties. These agents are indicated for widespread, recalcitrant, or disabling AD that fails to improve with topical therapy and phototherapy.

Eczema herpeticum is treated with acyclovir. Infants receive 10 to 20 mg/kg IV q 8 h; older children and adults with mild illness may receive 200 mg po 5 times/day.

CONTACT DERMATITIS

Contact dermatitis is acute inflammation of the skin caused by irritants or allergens. The primary symptom is pruritus; skin changes range from erythema to blistering and ulceration, often on or near the hands but occurring on any exposed skin surface. Diagnosis is by exposure history, examination, and sometimes skin patch testing. Treatment entails antipruritics, topical corticosteroids, and avoidance of causes.

Etiology and Pathophysiology

Irritant contact dermatitis (ICD): ICD accounts for 80% of all cases of contact dermatitis (CD). It is a nonspecific inflammatory reaction to substances contacting the skin; the immune system is not activated. Numerous substances are involved, including chemicals (eg, acids, alkalis, solvents, metal salts), soaps (eg, abrasives, detergents), plants (eg, poinsettias, peppers), and body fluids (eg, urine, saliva). Properties of the irritant (extreme pH, solubility in the lipid film on skin), environment (low humidity, high temperature, high friction), and patient (very young or old) influence the likelihood of developing ICD. ICD is more common in atopic patients, in whom ICD also may initiate immunologic sensitization and hence allergic CD.

Phototoxic dermatitis (see p. 964) is a variant in which topical (eg, perfumes, coal tar) or ingested (eg, psoralens) agents generate damaging free radicals and inflammatory mediators only after absorption of ultraviolet light.

Allergic contact dermatitis (ACD): ACD is a type IV cell-mediated hypersensitivity reaction that has 2 phases: sensitization to an antigen and response on reexposure. In the sensitization phase, allergens are captured by Langerhans' cells (dendritic epidermal cells), which migrate to regional lymph nodes where they process and present the antigen to T cells. The process may be brief (6 to 10 days for strong sensitizers such as poison ivy) or prolonged (years for weak sensitizers such as sunscreens, fragrances, and glucocorticoids). Sensitized T cells then migrate back to the epidermis and activate on re-exposure to the allergen, releasing cytokines, recruiting inflammatory cells, and leading to the characteristic symptoms and signs of ACD.

In autoeczematization, epidermal T cells activated by allergen migrate locally or through the circulation to cause dermatitis at sites remote from the initial trigger. However, contact with fluid from vesicles or blisters cannot trigger a reaction elsewhere on the patient or on another person.

Multiple allergens cause ACD (see TABLE 114–2), and cross-sensitization among agents is common (eg, between benzocaine and paraphenylene diamine).

TABLE 114–2. CAUSES OF ALLERGIC CONTACT DERMATITIS

CAUSE	EXAMPLES
Airborne substances	Ragweed pollen, insecticide spray
Chemicals used in shoe or clothing manufacturing	Particularly agents used in leather and rubber processing; tanning agents in shoes; rubber accelerators and antioxidants in gloves, shoes, underpants, and other apparel; formaldehyde in durable-press finishes
Cosmetics	Depilatories, nail polish, deodorant
Dyes	*p*-Phenylenediamine (hair and textile dyes) and others
Fragrances	Various compounds; ubiquitous in toiletries, soaps, scented household products
Industrial agents	Many compounds, including acrylic monomers, epoxy compounds, vat dyes, rubber accelerators, formaldehyde (in plastics and adhesives)
Ingredients in topical drugs:	
Antibiotics	Bacitracin, neomycin, penicillin, sulfonamides,
Antihistamines	Diphenhydramine, promethazine
Anesthetics	Benzocaine
Antiseptics	Thimerosal, hexachlorophene
Stabilizers	Ethylenediamine and derivatives
Latex	Latex gloves, condoms, catheters, balloons
Metal compounds Nickel Cobalt Chromates Mercury	Numerous occupational exposures. Also personal items, such as belt buckle, watch buckle, and jewelry
Plants	Poison ivy, oak, and sumac; ragweed; primrose; cashew shells; mango peel

ACD variants include photoallergic CD and systemically induced ACD. In photoallergic CD (see p. 964), a substance becomes sensitizing only after it undergoes structural change triggered by ultraviolet light. Typical causes include aftershave lotions, sunscreens, and topical sulfonamides. Reactions may extend to non–sun-exposed skin. In systemically induced ACD, ingestion of an allergen after topical sensitization causes diffuse dermatitis (eg, oral diphenhydramine after sensitization with topical diphenhydramine).

Symptoms and Signs

ICD is more painful than pruritic. Signs range from mild erythema to hemorrhage, crusting, erosion, pustules, bullae, and edema.

In ACD, the primary symptom is intense pruritus; pain is usually the result of excoriation or infection. Skin changes range from transient erythema through vesiculation to severe swelling with bullae and/or ulceration. Changes often occur in a pattern and/or distribution that suggest a specific exposure, such as linear streaking on an arm or leg (eg, from brushing against poison ivy) or circumferential erythema (under a wristwatch or waistband). Any surface may be involved, but hands are most common due to handling and touching potential allergens. With airborne exposure (eg, perfume aerosols), areas not covered by clothing are predominantly involved. The dermatitis is typically limited to the site of contact but may later spread due to scratching and autoeczematization. In systemically induced ACD, skin changes may be distributed over the entire body.

Diagnosis

CD can often be diagnosed by skin changes and exposure history. The patient's occupation, hobbies, household duties, vacations, clothing, topical drug use, cosmetics, and spouse's activities must be considered. The "use test," in which a suspected agent is applied far from the original area of dermatitis usually on the flexor forearm, is useful when perfumes, shampoos, or other home agents are suspected.

Patch testing is indicated when ACD is suspected and does not respond to treatment. In patch testing, standard contact allergens are applied to the upper back using adhesive-mounted patches containing minute amounts of allergen or plastic (Finn) chambers containing allergen held in place with porous tape. Thin-layer rapid use epicutaneous (T.R.U.E.) patch testing involves 2 adhesive strips that can be applied and interpreted by any provider. Skin under the patches is evaluated 48 and 96 h after application. False-positives are seen when concentrations provoke an irritant rather than allergic reaction, when reaction to one antigen triggers a nonspecific reaction to others, or with cross-reacting antigens. False-negatives are seen when patch allergens do not include the offending antigen. Definitive diagnosis requires a history of exposure to the test agent in the original area of dermatitis.

Prognosis and Treatment

Resolution may take up to 3 wk. Reactivity is usually lifelong. Patients with photoallergic CD can have flares for years when exposed to sun (persistent light reaction).

CD is treated by avoiding the trigger; patients with photosensitive CD should avoid exposure to sun. Topical treatment includes cool compresses (saline or Burow's) and corticosteroids; patients with mild to moderate ACD are given mid-potency topical corticosteroids (eg, triamcinolone 0.1% ointment or betamethasone valerate cream 0.1%). Oral corticosteroids (eg, prednisone 60 mg once/day for 7 to 14 days) can be used for severe blistering or extensive disease. Systemic antihistamines (eg, hydroxyzine, diphenhydramine) help pruritus; antihistamines with low anticholinergic potency are not as effective. Wet-to-dry dressings can soothe oozing blisters, dry the skin, and promote healing.

EXFOLIATIVE DERMATITIS

(Erythroderma)

Exfoliative dermatitis is widespread erythema and scaling of the skin caused by preexisting skin disease, drugs, malignancy, or unknown causes. Symptoms and signs are pruritus, diffuse erythema, and epidermal sloughing. Diagnosis is clinical. Treatment involves corticosteroids and correction of the cause.

Exfoliative dermatitis is a manifestation of rapid epidermal cell turnover. Its cause is unknown, but it most often occurs in the context of preexisting skin diseases (eg, atopic dermatitis, contact dermatitis, seborrheic dermatitis, psoriasis, pityriasis rubra pilaris), use of drugs (eg, penicillin, sulfonamides, isoniazid, phenytoin, barbiturates), and malignancy (eg, mycosis fungoides, leukemia, and rarely, adenocarcinomas). Up to 25% of patients have no identifiable underlying disease.

Symptoms and Signs

Symptoms include pruritus, malaise, and chills. Diffuse erythema initially occurs in patches but spreads and involves all or nearly all of the body. Extensive epidermal sloughing leads to abnormal thermoregulation, nutritional deficiencies because of extensive protein losses, increased metabolic rate with a hypercatabolic state, and hypovolemia due to transdermal fluid losses. High-output heart failure has been reported from extensive peripheral vasodilation.

Diagnosis and Treatment

Diagnosis is by history and examination. Pre-existing skin disease may underlie the extensive erythema and suggest a cause. Biopsy is often nonspecific but is indicated when mycosis fungoides is suspected. Blood tests may reveal hypoproteinemia, hypocalcemia, and iron deficiency, each a consequence of extensive protein, electrolyte, and RBC loss, but these are not diagnostic.

The disease may be life threatening; hospitalization is often necessary. Treatment is of the underlying cause if known. Because drug eruptions and contact dermatitis cannot be ruled out by history alone, all drugs should be stopped if possible or changed. Skin care is with emollients and colloidal oatmeal baths. Corticosteroids (prednisone 40 to 60 mg po once/day for 10 days, then tapered) are used for severe disease.

HAND AND FOOT DERMATITIS

Hand and foot dermatitis is not a single disease. Rather, it is a categorization of dermatitis that affects the hands and feet selectively due to one of several causes.

TABLE 114–3. DIFFERENTIAL DIAGNOSIS OF HAND DERMATITIS

LOCATION	ERYTHEMA AND SCALING	PUSTULES	VESICLES
Palm	Fingertip eczema Hyperkeratotic eczema Keratolysis exfoliativa Psoriasis Tinea	Dyshidrotic dermatitis Infection (bacterial) Psoriasis	Allergic contact dermatitis Dyshidrotic dermatitis
Dorsum	Atopic dermatitis Irritant contact dermatitis Lichen simplex chronicus Nummular eczema Psoriasis Tinea	Infection (bacterial) Psoriasis Scabies (web spaces) Tinea	Id reaction Scabies (web spaces)

Patients often present with isolated dermatitis of the hands or feet. Causes include contact dermatitis, fungal infection, psoriasis, and scabies; some cases are idiopathic. Diagnosis can sometimes be inferred from location and appearance of the skin lesions (see TABLE 114–3). Treatment of all forms of hand and feet dermatitis should be directed at the underlying cause when possible. Topical corticosteroids or antifungals may be tried empirically. Patients should also avoid prolonged contact with water.

Dyshidrotic dermatitis is characterized by pruritic vesicles or bullae on the palms, sides of the fingers, or soles. Scaling, redness, and oozing often follow vesiculation. Pompholyx is a severe form with bullae. The cause is unknown, but fungal infection, contact dermatitis, and id reactions to tinea pedis can cause a similar clinical appearance and should be ruled out. Treatment includes topical corticosteroids, tacrolimus or pimecrolimus, oral antibiotics, and ultraviolet light.

Keratolysis exfoliativa is painless patchy peeling of the palms and/or soles. The cause is unknown; treatment is unnecessary as the condition is self-resolving.

Hyperkeratotic eczema is thick yellow-brown plaques on the palms and sometimes soles. The cause is unknown. Treatment is with topical corticosteroids and keratolytics, ultraviolet A radiation with oral psoralen (PUVA), and retinoids.

Id reaction is appearance of vesicles usually on the sides of the fingers in response to active dermatitis elsewhere. The cause may be an allergic reaction.

"Housewives' eczema" affects people whose hands are frequently immersed in water. It is worsened by washing dishes, clothes, and babies because repeated exposure to even mild detergents and water or prolonged sweating under rubber gloves may irritate dermatitic skin or cause an irritant contact dermatitis.

LICHEN SIMPLEX CHRONICUS

Lichen simplex chronicus (neurodermatitis) is eczema created by repeated scratching; by several mechanisms, chronic scratching itself causes further itching, creating a vicious circle.

Lichen simplex chronicus frequently occurs in people with anxiety disorders and nonspecific emotional stress. It is characterized by pruritic, dry, scaling, hyperpigmented, lichenified plaques in irregular, oval, or angular shapes. It involves easily reached sites, most commonly the legs, arms, neck, and upper trunk.

Diagnosis is by examination. A fully developed plaque has an outer zone of discrete, brownish papules and a central zone of confluent papules covered with scales. Look-alike conditions include tinea corporis, lichen planus, and psoriasis; lichen simplex chronicus can be distinguished from these by potassium hydroxide wet mount and biopsy.

Primary treatment is patient education about the effects of scratching and rubbing. Secondary treatment is topical corticosteroids (eg, triamcinolone acetonide, fluocinonide); surgical tape impregnated with flurandrenolide (applied in the morning and replaced in the evening) may be preferred because occlusion prevents scratching. Small areas may be locally infiltrated (intralesional injections) with a long-acting corticosteroid such as triamcinolone acetonide 2.5 mg/mL (diluted with saline), 0.3 mL/cm^2 of lesion; treatment can be repeated q 3 to 4 wk. Oral H_1-blocking antihistamines may be useful.

NUMMULAR DERMATITIS

Nummular (discoid) dermatitis is inflammation of the skin characterized by coin- or disc-shaped lesions.

Nummular dermatitis is most common in middle-aged patients and is often associated with dry skin, especially during the winter. The cause is unknown. Discoid lesions often start as patches of confluent vesicles and papules that later ooze serum and form crusts. Lesions are eruptive, widespread, and pruritic. They are often more prominent on the extensor aspects of the extremities and on the buttocks but also appear on the trunk. Exacerbations and remissions may occur, and when they do, lesions tend to reappear at the sites of healed lesions.

Diagnosis is clinical based on appearance and distribution of the skin lesions.

No treatment is uniformly effective. Oral antibiotics (dicloxacillin or cephalexin 250 mg qid) may be given, along with use of tap water compresses, especially when weeping and pus are present. Less inflamed lesions may respond to tetracycline 250 mg po qid, which has a beneficial (although not necessarily antibacterial) effect. Corticosteroid cream or ointment should be rubbed in tid. An occlusive dressing with a corticosteroid cream under polyethylene film or with flurandrenolide-impregnated tape can be applied at bedtime. Intralesional corticosteroid injections may be beneficial for the few lesions that do not respond to therapy. In more widespread, resistant, and recurrent cases, ultraviolet B radiation alone or ultraviolet A radiation with oral psoralen (PUVA) may be helpful. Occasionally, oral corticosteroids are required, but long-term use should be avoided; a reasonable starting dose is prednisone 40 mg every other day.

SEBORRHEIC DERMATITIS

Seborrheic dermatitis (SD) is inflammation of skin with a high density of sebaceous glands (face, scalp, upper trunk). The cause is unknown, but *Pityrosporum ovale*, a normal skin organism, plays some role. SD occurs with increased frequency in patients with HIV and in those with certain neurologic diseases. Seborrheic dermatitis causes occasional pruritus, dandruff, and yellow, greasy scaling along the hairline and on the face. Diagnosis is clinical. Treatment is tar or other medicated shampoo and topical corticosteroids and antifungals.

Despite the name, the composition and flow of sebum are usually normal. The incidence and severity of disease seem to be affected by genetic factors, emotional or physical stress, and climate (usually worse in cold weather). SD may precede or be associated with psoriasis (seborrhiasis). Patients with neurologic disease (especially Parkinson's disease) or HIV may have severe SD. Very rarely, the dermatitis becomes generalized.

The pathogenesis of SD is unclear, but its activity has been linked to the number of *Pityrosporum* yeasts present on the skin.

Symptoms, Signs, and Diagnosis

Symptoms develop gradually, and the dermatitis is usually apparent only as dry or greasy diffuse scaling of the scalp (dandruff) with variable pruritus. In severe disease, yellow-red scaling papules appear along the hairline, behind the ears, in the external auditory canals, on the eyebrows, in the axillae, on the bridge of the nose, in the nasolabial folds, and over the sternum. Marginal blepharitis with dry yellow crusts and conjunctival irritation may develop. SD does not cause hair loss.

Newborns may develop SD with a thick, yellow, crusted scalp lesion (cradle cap); fissuring and yellow scaling behind the ears; red facial papules; and stubborn diaper rash. Older children may develop thick, tenacious, scaly plaques on the scalp that may measure 1 to 2 cm in diameter.

Diagnosis is clinical.

Treatment

In adults, zinc pyrithione, selenium sulfide, sulfur and salicylic acid, or tar shampoo should be used daily or every other day until dandruff is controlled and twice/wk thereafter. A corticosteroid lotion (eg, 0.01% fluocinolone acetonide solution, 0.025% triamcinolone acetonide lotion) can be rubbed into the scalp or other hairy areas bid until scaling and redness are controlled. For SD of the postauricular areas, nasolabial folds, eyelid margins, and bridge of the nose, 1% hydrocortisone cream is rubbed in bid or tid, decreasing to once/day when controlled; hydrocortisone cream is the safest corticosteroid for the face because fluorinated corticosteroids may produce adverse effects (eg, telangiectasia, atrophy, perioral dermatitis). In some patients, 2% ketoconazole cream or other topical imidazoles bid for 1 to 2 wk induce a remission that lasts for months. For eyelid margin seborrhea, a dilution of 1 part baby shampoo to 9 parts of water is applied with a cotton swab.

In infants, a baby shampoo is used daily, and 1% hydrocortisone cream is rubbed in bid. For thick lesions on the scalp of a young child, 2% salicylic acid in olive oil or a corticosteroid gel is applied at bedtime to affected areas and rubbed in with a toothbrush. The scalp is shampooed daily until the thick scale is gone.

STASIS DERMATITIS

Stasis dermatitis is inflammation of the skin of the lower legs caused by chronic venous insufficiency. Symptoms are itching, scaling, hyperpigmentation, and sometimes ulceration. Diagnosis is clinical. Treatment is directed at the chronic venous insufficiency.

Stasis dermatitis occurs in patients with chronic venous insufficiency (see p. 761) because blood pools in the legs, causing persistent edema.

Symptoms and Signs

Initially, hyperpigmentation and red-brown discoloration from RBC extravasation appear. Later, eczematous changes develop and manifest as erythema, scaling, weeping, and crusting, all of which can be made worse by bacterial superinfection or by contact dermatitis from the many topical treatments often applied. When chronic venous insufficiency and stasis dermatitis are both inadequately treated, stasis dermatitis progresses to frank skin ulceration, thickened fibrotic skin, or lipodermatosclerosis (a painful induration resulting from panniculitis, which if severe gives the lower leg an inverted "coke-bottle" shape with enlargement of the calf and narrowing at the ankle).

Treatment

Chronic venous insufficiency must be adequately treated with leg elevation and compression stockings (see p. 763). For acute stasis dermatitis (characterized by crusts, exudation, and superficial ulceration), continuous and then intermittent tap water compresses should be applied. For a weeping lesion, a hydrocolloid dressing may be best. For less acute dermatitis, a corticosteroid cream or ointment should be applied tid or incorporated into zinc oxide paste.

Ulcers are best treated with compresses and bland dressings (eg, zinc oxide paste); other dressings (eg, DuoDERM) are also effective (see also p. 1015). Ulcers in ambulatory patients may be healed with Unna's paste boot (zinc gelatin), the less messy zinc gelatin bandage, or a colloid dressing—all are available commercially. Colloid-type dressings used under elastic support are more effective than Unna's paste boot. It may be necessary to change the dressing q 2 or 3 days, but as edema recedes and the ulcer heals, once or twice/wk is sufficient. After the ulcer heals, an elastic support should be applied before the patient rises in the morning. Regardless of the dressing used, reduction of edema (usually with compression) is paramount for healing.

Oral antibiotics (eg, cephalosporins, dicloxacillin) are used for superimposed cellulitis. Topical antibiotics (mupirocin, silver sulfadiazine) are useful for erosions and ulcers. When edema and inflammation subside, split-thickness skin grafts may be needed for large ulcers.

Complex or multiple topical drugs or OTC remedies should not be used. The skin in stasis dermatitis is more vulnerable to direct irritants and to potentially sensitizing topical agents (eg, antibiotics; anesthetics; vehicles of topical drugs, especially lanolin or wool alcohols).

115 REACTIONS TO SUNLIGHT

The skin may respond to excessive sunlight in several ways: various chronic changes (eg, dermatoheliosis, actinic keratoses), photosensitivity, or sunburn.

Although the sun emits a wide range of ultraviolet (UV) electromagnetic radiation (ie, UVA, 320 to 400 nm; UVB, 280 to 320 nm; UVC, 10 to 280 nm), only UVA and UVB reach the earth's surface. The character and amount of such radiation vary greatly with the seasons and with changing atmospheric conditions. Exposure of skin to sunlight depends on multiple factors, eg, clothing, lifestyle, occupation, and geographic factors, such as altitude and latitude.

Sunburn-producing rays (< 320 nm) are filtered out by glass and to a great extent by smoke and smog. Sunburn-producing rays may pass through light clouds, fog, or 30 cm of clear water, causing severe burns in unsuspecting people. Snow, sand, and bright sky enhance exposure by reflecting the rays. Stratospheric ozone, which filters out shorter wavelengths of UV, is depleted by man-made chlorofluorocarbons (eg, in refrigerants and aerosols). A decreased ozone layer increases inadvertent exposure to UVA and UVB.

Sun-tanning lamps use artificial light that is more UVA than UVB, but some long-term deleterious effects should be expected. Even light sources that contain only UVA adversely affect the skin.

Pathophysiology

After exposure to sunlight, the epidermis thickens and melanocytes produce the pigment melanin at an increased rate, causing tanning, which provides some natural protection against future exposure. Exposure leads to both inactivation and loss of epidermal Langerhans' cells, which are immunologically important.

People differ greatly in their sensitivity and response to sunlight based on the amount of melanin in their skin. Skin is classified into 6 types (I to VI) in decreasing order of susceptibility to sun injury. Classification is based on skin color, UV sensitivity, and response to sun exposure. Skin type I is white to lightly pigmented, very sensitive to UV light, has no immediate pigment darkening, always burns easily, and never tans. Skin type VI is dark brown or black, least sensitive to UV light, has significant immediate pigment darkening, and tans profusely (deep black). Blacks and other dark-skinned people are not immune to the effects of the sun and can become sunburned with strong or prolonged exposure. People with blonde or red hair are especially susceptible. Uneven melanin deposition occurs in many fair-haired people and results in freckling. There is no skin pigmentation in people with albinism (see p. 1002) because of a defect in melanin metabolism, and none in areas of vitiligo (see p. 1002) because of the absence of melanocytes.

Prevention

Simple precautions help prevent sunburn and the chronic effects of sunlight and are necessary for those with photosensitivity. Initial summer exposure to bright midday sun should not be > 30 min, even in people with dark skin. In temperate zones, exposure is less hazardous before 10 am and after 3 pm because more sunburn-producing wavelengths are filtered out. Fog and clouds do not reduce risk, and risk is increased at high altitude.

Sun-exposed skin should be covered. Fabrics with a tight weave block the sun better than do those with a loose weave. Special clothing that provides high sun protection is commercially available. Broad-brimmed hats protect the face, ears, and neck. Regular use of UV-protective, wrap-around sunglasses helps shield the eyes.

Sunscreens help protect from, but do not always prevent, sunburn and chronic sun damage. In the US, the FDA rates sunscreens by sun protection factor (SPF): the higher the number, the greater the protection. Agents with SPF ≥ 15 are recommended. The SPF, however, only quantifies the protection against UVB exposure; there is no scale for UVA protection. Sunscreens are available in a wide variety of formulations, including creams, gels, foams, sprays, and sticks. Self-tanning products do not protect from UV exposure.

Most sunscreens contain several agents that function as chemical screens, absorbing light or providing a physical screen that reflects or scatters light. Common chemical sunscreen agents mostly absorb UVB rays and include the aminobenzoates, which include *p*-aminobenzoic acid (PABA), salicylates, cinnamates, benzophenones (eg, avobenzone), and the anthrilates. Of these, the benzophenones are particularly effective at screening UVA rays. Zinc oxide and titanium dioxide block both UVB and UVA rays. Micronized formulations of these products have significantly improved their cosmetic acceptability. Sunscreen failure is common and usually results from insufficient application of the product, application too late (sunscreens should optimally be applied 30 min before exposure), or failure to reapply after swimming or exercise.

Allergic or photoallergic reactions to sunscreens must be distinguished from other photosensitive skin eruptions. Patch or photopatch testing with sunscreen components may be necessary to make the diagnosis. This is usually done by dermatologists with a particular expertise in allergic contact dermatitis.

CHRONIC EFFECTS OF SUNLIGHT

Aging: Chronic exposure to sunlight ages the skin (dermatoheliosis, extrinsic aging), producing both fine and coarse wrinkles, rough leathery texture, mottled hyperpigmentation, and sometimes telangiectasia. The atrophic effects in some people may resemble those seen after x-ray therapy (chronic radiation dermatitis).

Actinic keratoses: Actinic keratoses are precancerous keratotic lesions that are a frequent, disturbing consequence of many years of sun exposure. People with blonde or red hair and skin type I or II are particularly susceptible; blacks are rarely affected.

The keratoses are usually pink, poorly marginated, and scaly or crusted on palpation, but they may be light gray or darker. They should be differentiated from warty brown seborrheic keratoses (see p. 1020), which increase in number and size with age but also occur on non–sun-exposed areas of the body and are not premalignant.

Skin cancers (see p. 1023)**:** The incidence of squamous and basal cell carcinoma in fair, light-skinned people is directly proportional to the total annual sunlight in the area. Such lesions are especially common in those who were extensively exposed to sunlight as children and teenagers and in sportsmen, farmers, ranchers, sailors, and frequent sunbathers. Sun exposure also increases the risk of malignant melanomas.

Treatment

Various combination therapies, including chemical peels, 5-fluorouracil (5-FU), topical α-hydroxy acids, and tretinoin, have been used in attempts to improve the cosmetic features of chronic sun damage. They appear to ameliorate coarse and fine wrinkling, irregular pigmentation, sallowness, roughness, and laxity but not telangiectasia. Laser resurfacing is another therapeutic option. Many chemicals are used in cosmetic products without proof that they affect the chronic effects of sunlight.

If only a few actinic keratoses are present, cryotherapy (freezing with liquid nitrogen) is the most rapid and satisfactory treatment. If there are too many lesions to freeze, topical 5-FU applied to the affected area nightly or bid for 2 to 4 wk produces dramatic results. Several strengths and formulations of 5-FU are commercially available. Many patients tolerate 0.5% 5-FU cream applied once/day for 4 wk on the face better than other concentrations. Actinic keratoses on the arms may require stronger concentrations, such as 5% cream. Topical 5-FU produces a brisk reaction, with redness, scaling, and burning, often affecting areas with no previously detected actinic keratoses. If the reaction is too brisk, application may be suspended for 2 or 3 days. Topical 5-FU has no significant adverse effects except for this unsightly and uncomfortable reaction, which can be masked by cosmetics and suppressed with topical corticosteroids. 5-FU should not be used to treat basal cell carcinomas, except those shown by biopsy to be of the superficial, multifocal type. For treatment of skin cancers, see Ch. 128 on p. 1023.

PHOTOSENSITIVITY

Photosensitivity is a poorly understood cutaneous reaction to sunlight probably involving the immune system. It may be idiopathic or occur following exposure to certain drugs or chemicals, and it is sometimes a feature of systemic diseases (eg, SLE, porphyria, pellagra, xeroderma pigmentosum). Diagnosis is clinical. Treatment varies by type.

TABLE 115–1. SOME SUBSTANCES THAT SENSITIZE THE SKIN TO SUNLIGHT

CATEGORY	SPECIFIC SUBSTANCE
Acne drugs	Isotretinoin
Antibiotics	Quinolones Sulfonamides Tetracyclines Trimethoprim
Antidepressants	Tricyclics
Antifungals	Griseofulvin
Antihyperglycemics	Sulfonylureas
Antimalarials	Chloroquine Quinine
Antipsychotics	Phenothiazines
Anxiolytics	Alprazolam Chloridazepoxide
Chemotherapy drugs	Dacarbazine Fluorouracil Methotrexate Vinblastine
Diuretics	Furosemide Thiazides
Heart drugs	Amiodarone Quinidine
Topical preparations	Antibacterials (chlorhexidine, hexachlorophene) Antifungals Coal tar Fragrances Sunscreens

In addition to the acute and chronic effects of sunlight, a variety of unusual reactions may occur soon after only a brief sun exposure. Unless the cause is obvious, patients with pronounced photosensitivity should be evaluated for systemic or cutaneous lupus erythematosus (see pp. 266 and 269) and perhaps porphyria (see p. 1221). Treatment for chemical photosensitivity is topical corticosteroids and avoidance of the causative substance.

Solar urticaria: In certain patients, urticaria develops at a site of sun exposure within a few minutes. If large areas are involved, syncope, dizziness, wheezing, and other systemic symptoms may develop. Etiology is unclear but may involve endogenous skin constituents functioning as photoallergens. Solar urticaria can be classified into 6 types based on the component of the UV spectrum that produces them. Treatment can be difficult and may include H_1 blockers, antimalarial drugs, topical sunscreens, and psoralen ultraviolet light (PUVA).

Chemical photosensitivity: Over 100 substances, ingested or applied topically, are known to predispose to cutaneous reactions following sun exposure. A limited number are responsible for most reactions (see TABLE 115–1). Reactions are divided into phototoxicity and photoallergy.

In **phototoxicity,** light-absorbing compounds directly generate free radicals and inflammatory mediators, causing tissue damage manifesting as pain and erythema (like sunburn). This reaction does not require prior exposure and can appear in any person, although reaction is highly variable. Typical causes of phototoxic reactions include topical (eg, perfumes, coal tar) or ingested (eg, tetracyclines, psoralen-containing plants) agents. Phototoxic reactions do not generalize to non–sun-exposed skin.

Photoallergy is a type IV (cell-mediated) immune response; light absorption causes structural changes in the drug or substance, allowing it to bind to tissue protein and function as a hapten. Prior exposure is required. Typical causes of photoallergic reactions include aftershave lotions, sunscreens, and sulfonamides. Reaction may extend to non–sun-exposed skin. Symptoms include erythema, pruritus, and sometimes vesicles.

Polymorphous light eruptions: These are unusual reactions to light that do not appear to be associated with systemic disease or drugs. Eruptions appear on sun-exposed areas, usually 30 min to several hours after exposure. Lesions are pruritic, erythematous, and often papular but may be papulovesicular or plaquelike. They are more common in people from northern climates when first exposed to spring or summer sun than in those exposed to sun year-round. Lesions subside within 1 wk or so. Actinic prurigo is a similar (perhaps related) phenomenon with more nodular-appearing lesions that may persist year-round, worsening with sun exposure.

Diagnosis is by exclusion, which sometimes requires reproduction of the lesions with artificial or natural sunlight when the patient is not using any medication. Treatment is by moderating sun exposure and applying topical corticosteroids. More severely affected patients may benefit from desensitization by graduated exposure to UV light with PUVA (see p. 968) or narrow band UVB (312 nm) phototherapy. Hydroxychloroquine 200 mg po bid to tid may sometimes help, especially the plaque form.

SUNBURN

Sunburn is painful erythema and sometimes blisters caused by exposure to solar UV radiation. Treatment is similar to thermal burns, including cool compresses, NSAIDs, and, for severe cases, sterile dressings and topical antimicrobials. Prevention by avoidance and use of sunscreens is crucial.

Sunburn results from overexposure of the skin to UVB rays (280 to 320 nm). Symptoms and signs appear in 1 to 24 h and, except in severe reactions, peak within 72 h. Skin changes range from mild erythema, with subsequent superficial scaling, to pain, swelling, skin tenderness, and blisters. Sunburn affecting the lower legs, particularly the pretibial surfaces, is especially uncomfortable and often slow to heal. Constitutional symptoms (fever, chills, weakness, shock), similar to a thermal burn, may develop if a large portion of the body surface is affected; these may be due to release of IL-1.

Secondary infection, blotchy pigmentation, and miliaria-like eruptions are the most common late complications. Exfoliated skin may be extremely vulnerable to sunlight for several weeks.

Treatment and Prevention

Further exposure should be avoided until sunburn has completely subsided. Cold tap-water compresses and oral NSAIDs help relieve symptoms, as may topical aloe vera. Topical corticosteroids are no more effective than cool compresses. Blistered areas should be managed similar to other partial-thickness burns (see p. 2595), with sterile dressing and topical bacitracin or silver sulfadiazine. Ointments or lotions containing local anesthetics (eg, benzocaine) should be avoided because of the risk of allergic contact dermatitis.

Early treatment of extensive, severe sunburn with a systemic corticosteroid (eg, prednisone 20 to 30 mg po bid for 4 days for adults or teenagers) may decrease the discomfort, but this use is controversial.

Simple precautions (eg, avoiding the sun especially during midday, wearing tightly woven clothing, sunscreens) prevent most cases of sunburn (see p. 962).

116 PSORIASIS AND SCALING DISEASES

Psoriasis, parapsoriasis, pityriasis rosea, pityriasis rubra pilaris, pityriasis lichenoides, lichen planus, and lichen sclerosus are dissimilar disorders grouped together because their primary lesions have similar characteristics: sharply marginated, scaling papules or plaques without wetness, crusts, fissures, and excoriations. Lesion appearance and distribution distinguish these diseases from each other.

PSORIASIS

Psoriasis is an inflammatory disease that manifests most commonly as well-circumscribed, erythematous papules and plaques covered with silvery scales. Cause is unknown, but common triggers include trauma, infection, and certain drugs. Symptoms are usually minimal with occasional mild itching, but cosmetic implications may be major. Some people develop severe disease with painful arthritis. Diagnosis is based on appearance and distribution of lesions. Treatment is with emollients, vitamin D analogues, retinoids, tar, anthralin, corticosteroids, phototherapy, and when severe, methotrexate, retinoids, biologics, or immunosuppressants.

Epidemiology and Etiology

Psoriasis is hyperproliferation of epidermal keratinocytes combined with inflammation of the epidermis and dermis. It affects about 1 to 5% of the population worldwide; light-skinned people are at greater risk. Peak onset is roughly bimodal, most often at ages 16 to 22 and at ages 57 to 60, but the condition can occur at any age. The cause is unknown, but family history is common, suggesting a genetic component in many cases. HLA antigens (CW6, B13, B17) are associated with psoriasis. An environmental trigger is thought to evoke an inflammatory response and subsequent hyperproliferation of keratinocytes. Well-identified triggers include injury (Koebner's phenomenon), sunburn, HIV, β-hemolytic streptococcal infection, drugs (especially β-blockers, chloroquine, lithium, ACE inhibitors, indomethacin, terbinafine, and interferon-α), emotional stress, and alcohol.

Symptoms and Signs

Lesions are either asymptomatic or mildly pruritic and are most often localized on the scalp, extensor surfaces of the elbows and knees, sacrum, buttocks, and penis. The nails, eyebrows, axillae, umbilicus, and/or perianal region may also be affected. The disease can be widespread, involving confluent areas of skin extending between these regions. Lesions differ in appearance depending on type. Plaque psoriasis (psoriasis vulgaris or chronic plaque psoriasis) is the most common pattern of psoriasis; lesions are discrete, oval erythematous papules or plaques covered with thick, silvery, shiny scales. Lesions appear gradually and remit and recur either spontaneously or with appearance and resolution of triggers. Subtypes exist and are described in TABLE 116–1.

Arthritis develops in 5 to 30% of patients and can be disabling (see p. 294).

Psoriasis is rarely life-threatening but can affect a patient's self-image. Besides image, the sheer amount of time required to treat extensive skin or scalp lesions and to maintain clothing and bedding may adversely affect quality of life.

Diagnosis

Diagnosis is most often by clinical appearance and distribution of lesions. Differential diagnosis includes seborrheic dermatitis, dermatophytoses, cutaneous lupus erythematosus, eczema, lichen planus, pityriasis rosea, squamous cell carcinoma in situ (Bowen's disease, especially when on the trunk), lichen simplex chronicus, and secondary syphilis. Biopsy is rarely necessary and may not be diagnostic. Disease is graded as mild, moderate, or severe largely based on the lesions' effect on the patient's ability to manage the disease.

Treatment

Treatment options are extensive and include emollients, salicylic acid, coal tar, anthralin, corticosteroids, calcipotriol, tazarotene, methotrexate, retinoids, immunosuppressants, immunotherapeutic agents, and light therapy.

Topical treatments: Emollients include emollient creams, ointments, petrolatum, paraffin, and even hydrogenated vegetable (cooking) oils. They reduce scaling and are most effective when applied bid and immediately after bathing. Lesions may appear redder as scaling decreases or becomes more transparent. Emollients are safe and should probably always be used for mild-moderate plaque psoriasis.

Salicylic acid is a keratinolytic that softens scales, facilitates their removal, and increases absorption of other topical agents. It is especially useful as a component of scalp treatments; scalp scale can be quite thick.

Coal tar ointments, solutions, or shampoos are anti-inflammatory and decrease keratinocyte hyperproliferation through an unknown effect. They are typically applied at night and washed off in the morning. They can be used in combination with topical corticosteroids or with exposure to natural or artificial ultraviolet (UV) B light (280 to 320 nm) in slowly increasing increments (Goeckerman regimen).

Anthralin is a topical antiproliferative, anti-inflammatory agent. Its mechanism is unknown. Effective dose is 0.1% cream or ointment increased to 1% as tolerated. Anthralin may be irritating and should be used with caution in intertriginous areas; it also stains. Irritation and staining can be avoided by washing off the anthralin 20 to 30 min after application. Using a liposome-encapsulated preparation may also avoid some disadvantages of anthralin.

Corticosteroids are usually used topically but may be injected into small or recalcitrant lesions. Systemic corticosteroids may precipitate exacerbations or development of pustular psoriasis and should not be used for any form of psoriasis. Topical corticosteroids are used bid, sometimes with anthralin or coal tar applied at bedtime. Corticosteroids are most effective when used overnight under occlusive polyethylene coverings or incorporated into tape; a corticosteroid cream is applied without occlusion during the day. Corticosteroid potency (see p. 939) is selected according to the extent of involvement. As lesions improve, the corticosteroid should

TABLE 116–1. SUBTYPES OF PSORIASIS

SUBTYPE	DESCRIPTION	TREATMENT AND PROGNOSIS
Guttate psoriasis	Abrupt appearance of multiple plaques 0.5 to 1.5 cm in diameter, usually on the trunk in children and young adults following streptococcal pharyngitis	*Treatment:* Antibiotics for underlying streptococcal infection *Prognosis:* Excellent, often with permanent cure
Erythrodermic psoriasis	Gradual or sudden onset of diffuse erythema, usually in patients with plaque psoriasis (though may be the first presentation); typical psoriatic plaques are less prominent or absent. Most commonly caused by inappropriate use of topical or systemic corticosteroids or light therapy	*Treatment:* Potent systemic drugs (eg methotrexate, cyclosporine) or intense inpatient topical therapy. Tars, anthralin, and phototherapy are likely to exacerbate the condition *Prognosis:* Good with elimination of triggering factors
Generalized pustular psoriasis	Explosive onset of widespread erythema and sterile pustules	*Treatment:* Systemic retinoids *Prognosis:* Can be fatal if untreated due to high-output heart failure
Pustular psoriasis of the palms and soles	Gradual onset deep pustules on palms and soles. Flare-ups may be painful and disabling. Typical psoriatic lesions may be absent	*Treatment:* Systemic retinoids *Prognosis:* Waxes and wanes
Inverse psoriasis	Psoriasis of inguinal, gluteal, axillary, inframammary, and retroauricular folds and of the glans of the uncircumcised penis. Cracks or fissures may form in the center or edge of involved areas	*Treatment:* Topical corticosteroids of minimal effective potency, with or without calcipotriol. Tar and anthralin may be irritating *Prognosis:* Waxes and wanes
Nail psoriasis	Pitting, stippling, fraying, discoloration (oil spot sign), and/or thickening of the nails, with or without separation of the nail plate (onycholysis). May resemble a fungal nail infection. Affects 30–50% of patients with other forms of psoriasis	*Treatment:* Responds best to systemic therapy; brave or stoic souls may respond to intralesional injection with corticosteroids *Prognosis:* Often unresponsive to treatment
Acrodermatitis continua of Hallopeau	Pustular psoriasis confined to distal fingers or toes, sometimes just one digit; replaced by scale and crust upon resolution	*Treatment:* Systemic retinoids; calcipotriol *Prognosis:* Waxes and wanes

be applied less frequently or at a lower potency to minimize local atrophy, striae formation, and telangiectases. Ideally, after about 3 wk, an emollient should be substituted for the corticosteroid for 1 to 2 wk (as a rest period); this limits corticosteroid dosage and prevents tachyphylaxis. Topical corticosteroid use is expensive because large quantities (about 1 oz or 30 g) are needed to cover the entire body. Topical corticosteroids applied for long duration to large areas of the body may cause systemic effects and exacerbate psoriasis. For small, thick, localized, or recalcitrant lesions, high-potency corticosteroids used with an occlusive dressing or flurandrenolide tape left on overnight and changed in the morning is effective. Relapse following discontinuation of topical corticosteroids is often faster than with other agents.

Calcipotriol is a topical vitamin D_3 analogue that induces normal keratinocyte proliferation and differentiation; it can be used in combination with topical corticosteroids (eg, calcipotriol can be applied on weekdays and corticosteroids on weekends).

Tazarotene is a topical retinoid. It is less effective than corticosteroids as monotherapy but is useful as an adjunct.

Systemic treatments: Methotrexate taken orally is the most effective treatment in severe disabling psoriasis, especially severe psoriatic arthritis or widespread erythrodermic or pustular psoriasis unresponsive to topical agents or psoralen-ultraviolet light therapy (PUVA). Methotrexate seems to interfere with the rapid proliferation of epidermal cells. Hematologic, renal, and hepatic function should be monitored. Dosage regimens vary, so only physicians experienced in its use for psoriasis should undertake methotrexate therapy.

Systemic retinoids (acitretin, isotretinoin) may be effective for severe and recalcitrant cases of psoriasis vulgaris, pustular psoriasis (in which isotretinoin may be preferred), and hyperkeratotic palmoplantar psoriasis. Because of the teratogenic potential and long-term retention of acitretin in the body, women must not be pregnant and should be warned against becoming pregnant for at least 2 yr after treatment ends. Pregnancy restrictions also apply to isotretinoin, but the agent is not retained in the body beyond 1 mo. Long-term treatment may produce diffuse idiopathic skeletal hyperostosis (DISH)—see p. 291.

Cyclosporine is an immunosuppressant that can be used for severe psoriasis. It should be limited to courses of several months (rarely, up to 1 yr) and alternated with other therapies. Its effect on the kidneys and potential long-term effects on the immune system preclude more liberal use.

Other immunosuppressants, such as hydroxyurea, 6-thioguanine, and mycophenolate mofetil, have narrow safety margins and are reserved for severe, recalcitrant psoriasis.

Immunotherapeutic agents include tumor necrosis factor (TNF)-α inhibitors (etanercept and infliximab), alefacept, and efalizumab (biologics—see p. 1328). TNF-α inhibitors lead to durable clearing of psoriasis, but their safety profile is still under study. Alefacept is a recombinant human fusion protein composed of the CD2 binding domain of leukocyte function-associated antigen (LFA) type 3 and the Fc portion of human IgG1. Alefacept reduces the number of memory T effector cells without compromising the number of naïve T cells and effectively clears plaques. Efalizumab is a monoclonal antibody that reversibly binds CD11a, a subunit of LFA-1, thereby blocking T-cell migration, binding, and activation.

Light therapy: UV light therapy (phototherapy) is typically used in patients with extensive psoriasis. The mechanism of action is unknown, although UVB light reduces DNA synthesis. In PUVA, oral methoxypsoralen, a photosensitizer, is followed by exposure to long-wave UVA light (330 to 360 nm). PUVA has an antiproliferative effect and also helps to normalize keratinocyte differentiation. Doses of light are started low and advanced as tolerated. Severe burns can result if the dose of drug or UVA is too high. Although the treatment is less messy than topical treatment and may produce remissions lasting several months, repeated treatments may increase the incidence of UV-induced skin cancer. Less UV light is required when used with oral retinoids (the so-called "re-PUVA" regimen). Narrow-band UVB light is emerging as an effective treatment and does not require psoralens. Excimer laser therapy is a type of phototherapy using extremely pure wavelengths.

Choice of therapy: Choice of specific agents and combinations requires close cooperation with the patient, always keeping in mind the untoward effects of the treatments. There is no single ideal combination or sequence of agents, but treatment should be kept as simple as possible. Monotherapy is preferred, but combination therapy is the norm. Rotational therapy refers to the substitution of one therapy for another after 1 to 2 yr to reduce the adverse effects from chronic use and to circumvent disease resistance. Sequential therapy refers to initial use of potent agents (such as cyclosporine) to quickly gain control follow by use of agents with a better safety profile.

Mild plaque psoriasis can be treated with emollients, keratolytics, tar, topical corticosteroids, calcipotriol, and/or anthralin alone or in combination. Exposure to sunlight is beneficial, but sunburn can induce exacerbations.

Moderate-severe plaque psoriasis should be treated with topical agents and either phototherapy or oral agents. Immunosuppressants are used for quick, short-term control (eg, in allowing a vacation from other modalities) and for the most severe disease. Immunotherapeutics are used for moderate to severe disease unresponsive to other agents.

Scalp plaques are notoriously difficult to treat because they resist systemic therapy, and because hair blocks application of topical agents and scale removal and shields skin from UV light. A suspension of 10% salicylic acid in mineral oil may be rubbed into the scalp at bedtime manually or with a toothbrush, covered with a shower cap (to enhance penetration and avoid messiness), and washed out the next morning with a tar (or other) shampoo. More cosmetically acceptable corticosteroid solutions can be applied to the scalp during the day. These treatments are continued until the desired clinical response is achieved. Resistant skin or scalp patches may respond to local superficial intralesional injection of triamcinolone acetonide suspension diluted with saline to 2.5 or 5 mg/mL, depending on the size and severity of the lesion. Injections may cause local atrophy, which is usually reversible.

Special treatment needs for subtypes are described in TABLE 116–1.

PARAPSORIASIS

Parapsoriasis describes a poorly understood and poorly distinguished group of diseases that share clinical features. There are 2 general forms: a small plaque type, which is usually benign, and a large plaque type, which is a precursor of cutaneous T-cell lymphoma (CTCL). Some patients with small plaque parapsoriasis eventually develop CTCL. Treatment of small plaque parapsoriasis is unnecessary but can include emollients, topical tar preparations or corticosteroids, and/or phototherapy. Treatment of large plaque parapsoriasis is phototherapy or topical corticosteroids. Course for both types is unpredictable; periodic clinical follow-up and biopsies give the best indication of risk for developing CTCL.

PITYRIASIS ROSEA

Pityriasis rosea is an inflammatory disease characterized by diffuse, scaling papules or plaques. Treatment is usually unnecessary.

Pityriasis rosea (PR) most commonly occurs between ages 10 and 35. It affects women more often and peaks in incidence in cooler months in temperate climates. The cause may be viral infection.

Symptoms and Signs

The condition classically begins with a single, primary, 2- to 10-cm "herald" patch that appears on the trunk or proximal limbs. A general centripetal eruption of 0.5- to 2-cm rose- or fawn-colored oval papules and plaques follows within 7 to 14 days. The lesions have a scaly, slightly raised border (collarette) and resemble ringworm (tinea corporis). Most patients itch, occasionally severely. Papules may dominate with little or no scaling in blacks, children, and pregnant women; the rose or fawn color is not as evident in blacks; blacks also more commonly have inverse PR (lesions in the axillae or groin that spread centrifugally). Classically, lesions orient along skin lines, giving PR a Christmas tree–like distribution when multiple lesions appear on the back. A prodrome of malaise and headache precedes the lesions in a minority of patients.

Diagnosis

Diagnosis is based on clinical appearance and distribution. Differential diagnosis includes tinea corporis, tinea versicolor, drug eruptions, psoriasis, parapsoriasis, pityriasis lichenoides chronica, lichen planus, and secondary syphilis. Serologic testing for syphilis is indicated when the palms or soles are affected, when a herald patch is not seen, or when lesions occur in an unusual sequence or distribution.

Treatment

No treatment is necessary, as the eruption usually remits within 5 wk and recurrence is rare. Artificial or natural sunlight may hasten resolution. Antipruritic therapy such as topical corticosteroids, oral antihistamines, or topical measures may be used as needed.

PITYRIASIS RUBRA PILARIS

Pityriasis rubra pilaris is a rare chronic disease that causes hyperkeratotic yellowing of the palms and soles and red follicular papules that merge to form red-orange scaling plaques and confluent areas of erythema with islands of normal skin between lesions.

The cause of pityriasis rubra pilaris is unknown. The 2 most common forms of the disease are juvenile classic, characterized by autosomal dominant inheritance and childhood onset, and adult classic, characterized by no apparent inheritance and adult onset. Atypical forms exist in both age groups. Sunlight can trigger a flare.

Diagnosis is by clinical appearance and may be supported by biopsy. Differential diagnosis includes seborrheic dermatitis (in children) and psoriasis when disease occurs on the scalp, elbows, and knees. Treatment is exceedingly difficult and empiric. Disease may be ameliorated but almost never cured; classic forms of the disease resolve slowly over 3 yr, while nonclassic forms persist. Scaling may be improved with emollients or 12% lactic acid under occlusive dressing, followed by topical corticosteroids. Oral vitamin A may be effective. Oral retinoids or methotrexate is an option when a patient is resistant to topical treatment.

PITYRIASIS LICHENOIDES

Pityriasis lichenoides is a clonal T-cell disorder that may develop in response to foreign antigens (eg, infections or drugs) and may be associated with cutaneous T-cell lymphoma.

Pityriasis lichenoides has acute and chronic forms existing in a clinical continuum. The acute form typically appears in children and young adults, with crops of asymptomatic chickenpox-like lesions that typically resolve within weeks to months. Antibiotics (tetracycline, erythromycin) or phototherapy may help.

The chronic form presents as flatter, reddish brown, scaling papules that may take months or longer to resolve. No treatment is proven effective.

LICHEN PLANUS

Lichen planus is a recurrent, pruritic, inflammatory eruption characterized by small, discrete, polygonal, flat-topped, violaceous papules that may coalesce into rough scaly patches, often accompanied by oral lesions. Diagnosis is usually clinical and supported by skin biopsy. Treatment generally requires topical or intralesional corticosteroids. Severe cases may require phototherapy or systemic immunosuppressants.

Lichen planus (LP) is thought to be caused by a T cell–mediated autoimmune reaction against basal epithelial keratinocytes in people with genetic predisposition. Drugs (especially β-blockers, NSAIDs, ACE inhibitors, sulfonylureas, gold, antimalarial agents, penicillamine, and thiazides) can cause LP; drug-induced LP (sometimes called lichenoid drug eruption) may be indistinguishable from non-drug–induced LP or may have a pattern that is more eczematous. Association with hepatitis C–induced liver insufficiency is suspected but not proven.

Symptoms and Signs

Typical lesions are pruritic, polyangular, planar papules and plaques. Lesions initially are 2 to 4 mm in diameter, with angular borders, a violaceous color, and a distinct sheen in cross-lighting. They are usually symmetrically distributed, most commonly on the flexor surfaces of the wrists, legs, trunk, glans penis, and oral and vaginal mucosae but can be widespread. The face is rarely involved. Onset may be abrupt or gradual. Children are affected infrequently. During the acute phase, new papules may appear at sites of minor skin injury (Koebner's phenomenon), such as a superficial scratch. Lesions may coalesce or change over time, becoming hyperpigmented, atrophic, hyperkeratotic (hypertrophic LP), or vesiculobullous. Although itchy, lesions are rarely excoriated or crusted. If the scalp is affected, patchy scarring alopecia (lichen planopilaris) may occur.

The oral mucosa is involved in about 50% of cases; oral lesions may occur in the absence of cutaneous lesions and usually persist for life. Reticulated, lacy, bluish-white, linear lesions (Wickham's striae) are a hallmark of oral LP, especially on the buccal mucosae. Tongue margins and gingival mucosae in edentulous areas may also be affected. An erosive form of LP may occur in which the patient develops shallow, often painful, recurrent oral ulcers, which if long-standing rarely become cancerous. Chronic exacerbations and remissions are common.

Nails are involved in up to 10% of cases. Findings vary in intensity with nail bed discoloration, longitudinal ridging and lateral thinning, and complete loss of the nail matrix and nail, with scarring of the proximal nail fold onto the nail bed (pterygium formation).

Diagnosis

Diagnosis is based on appearance and distribution of lesions and on biopsy. Biopsy shows a characteristic "lichenoid" inflammatory response of a bandlike lymphocytic infiltrate at the dermoepidermal junction, with epidermal thickening and scaling.

Differential diagnosis includes any of the papulosquamous disorders, lupus erythematosus, and secondary syphilis, among others. Oral or vaginal LP may resemble leukoplakia. Differential diagnosis of oral LP includes candidiasis, carcinoma, aphthous ulcers, pemphigus, cicatricial pemphigoid, and chronic erythema multiforme.

Prognosis and Treatment

Asymptomatic LP does not require treatment. Drugs suspected of triggering LP should be stopped. Many cases resolve without intervention, presumably because the inciting agent is no longer present. Recurrence after years may be due to reexposure to the trigger or some change in the triggering mechanism. Sometimes treatment of a previously occult infection, such as a dental abscess, results in resolution.

Few controlled studies have evaluated treatments. Options differ by location and extent of disease. Most cases of LP on the trunk or extremities can be treated with local agents. Topical corticosteroids are first-line treatment for most cases of localized disease. High-potency ointments or creams (eg, clobetasol or fluocinonide) may be used on the thicker lesions on the extremities; lower potency agents (eg triamcinolone or desonide) may be used on the face, groin, and axillae; as always, courses should be limited to reduce risk of corticosteroid atrophy). Potency may be enhanced with use of polyethylene wrapping or flurandrenolide tape. Intralesional corticosteroids (triamcinolone acetonide solution diluted with saline to 5 to 10 mg/mL) can be used q 4 wk for hyperkeratotic plaques and those resistant to other therapies.

Topical therapy is impractical for generalized LP; oral agents or phototherapy are used. Oral corticosteroids, such as prednisone 20 mg once/day for 2 to 6 wk followed by a taper, may be used for severe cases. The disease may rebound when therapy ceases; however, long-term systemic corticosteroids should not be used.

Oral retinoids (acitretin 30 mg once/day for 8 wk) is indicated for otherwise recalcitrant cases. Griseofulvin 250 mg po bid given for 3 to 6 mo may be effective. Cyclosporine can be used when corticosteroids or retinoids fail. Light therapy using psoralen plus ultraviolet A (PUVA) is an alternative to oral therapies, especially if they have failed or are contraindicated for medical reasons.

Treatment of oral LP differs slightly. Viscous lidocaine may help symptoms of erosive ulcers. Tacrolimus 0.1% ointment applied bid may induce lasting remission, although it has not been fully evaluated. Other treatment options include topical (in an adhesive base), intralesional, and systemic corticosteroids. Erosive oral LP may respond to oral dapsone or to cyclosporine rinses.

Dapsone, hydroxychloroquine, azathioprine, systemic cyclosporine, and topical tretinoin may also be useful. As with any disease with so many therapies, individual agents have not been uniformly successful.

LICHEN SCLEROSUS

Lichen sclerosus is an inflammatory dermatosis of unknown cause, possibly autoimmune, that usually affects the anogenital area.

The earliest signs are skin fragility, bruising, and sometimes blistering. Lesions typically cause mild to severe itching. When lichen sclerosus presents in children, the appearance may be confused with sexual abuse. With time, the involved tissue becomes atrophic, thinned, hypopigmented (there may be flecks of postinflammatory hyperpigmentation), fissured, and scaly. Hyperkeratotic and fibrotic forms exist. Severe and longstanding cases cause scarring and distortion of normal anogenital architecture. In women, this can even be to the point of total absorption of the labia minora and fusion over the clitoris; in men, phimosis or fusion of the foreskin to the coronal sulcus can occur.

Diagnosis can usually be based on appearance, especially in advanced cases; however, biopsy should be performed on any anogenital dermatosis that does not resolve with mild conventional therapy (eg, topical hydrocortisone or antifungal). It is especially important to biopsy any area that becomes thickened or ulcerated, as lichen sclerosus is a precursor of squamous cell carcinoma.

Treatment consists of potent topical corticosteroids (agents that otherwise should be used with extreme caution in this area). The disease is generally intractable, so long-term followup, especially to monitor for squamous cell carcinoma and sexual function and for psychologic support, is indicated.

117 HYPERSENSITIVITY AND INFLAMMATORY DISORDERS

The immune system plays a significant role in a large number of skin disorders, including dermatitis, sunlight reactions, and bullous diseases. While all of these disorders involve some level of inflammation, certain skin disorders are primarily characterized by their inflammatory component or as a hypersensitivity reaction, be it to a drug, infection, or malignancy.

ACUTE FEBRILE NEUTROPHILIC DERMATOSIS

(Sweet's Syndrome)

Acute febrile neutrophilic dermatosis is characterized by tender, indurated, dark-red papules and plaques with prominent edema in the upper dermis and dense infiltrate of neutrophils on histopathology. Cause is not known. It frequently occurs with underlying malignancy, especially hematologic malignancies.

Acute febrile neutrophilic dermatosis, when not due to malignancy, affects mostly women ages 30 to 50, with a female:male ratio of 3:1. Men who develop the condition tend to be older (60 to 90). The disease may follow an acute respiratory illness, GI infection, drug exposure, or underlying malignancy. The histopathologic pattern is that of edema in the upper dermis with a dense infiltrate of neutrophils in the dermis. Vasculitis may result but is secondary.

Patients are febrile, with an elevated neutrophil count, and have tender, dark red plaques or papules. Rarely, bullous and pustular lesions are seen. The lesions often develop in crops. Each crop is preceded by fever and persists for days to weeks.

Differential diagnosis includes erythema multiforme, erythema elevation diutinum, acute cutaneous lupus erythematosus, pyoderma gangrenosum, and erythema nodosum. An overlap between acute febrile neutrophilic dermatosis and myeloproliferative disorders exists, and acute febrile neutrophilic dermatosis may occur with chronic myelocytic leukemia, acute myelogenous leukemia, Hodgkin lymphoma, cutaneous T-cell lymphoma, multiple myeloma, hairy cell leukemia, and less commonly, nonhematologic malignancy. Treatment involves systemic corticosteroids, chiefly prednisone 60 mg po once/day tapered over 3 wk. Antipyretics are also recommended. In difficult cases, dapsone and potassium iodide can be given.

DRUG ERUPTIONS AND REACTIONS

Drugs can cause multiple skin eruptions and reactions. The most serious of these are discussed elsewhere and include Stevens-Johnson syndrome and toxic epidermal necrolysis, hypersensitivity syndrome, serum sickness, exfoliative dermatitis, angioedema and anaphylaxis, and drug-induced vasculitis. Drugs can also be implicated in hair loss, lichen planus, erythema nodosum, pigmentation changes, SLE, photosensitivity reactions, pemphigus, and pemphigoid. Other drug reactions are classified by lesion type (see TABLE 117–1).

Exanthems are the most common drug eruptions. Ampicillin is probably the most common culprit. Other drugs include sulfonamides and pantoprazole. Exanthems manifest as a morbilliform eruption that is mildly pruritic. The rash typically appears 3 to 7 days after start of the drug and is driven by T-cell–mediated immunity.

Urticaria is common (see p. 936). Mechanism is IgE-mediated. NSAIDs, including aspirin, penicillin, and sulfonamides are the drugs most often implicated. Urticaria is occasionally the first sign of impending serum sickness, with fever, joint pain, and other systemic symptoms developing within days.

Fixed drug eruptions are usually circular and recur at the same anatomic site on rechallenge with the drug. Tetracycline and phenolphthalein are common culprits.

Acneiform eruptions can be caused or exacerbated by vitamins B_2, B_6 and B_{12}. Isoniazid, phenytoin, phenobarbital, bromides, and iodides can also induce acneiform eruptions. Prednisone is also a common culprit.

TABLE 117–1. TYPES OF DRUG REACTIONS AND TYPICAL CAUSATIVE AGENTS

TYPE OF REACTION	DESCRIPTION AND COMMENTS	TYPICAL CAUSATIVE AGENTS
Acneiform eruptions	Resemble acne but lack comedones and usually begin suddenly	Corticosteroids, iodides, bromides, hydantoins, androgenic steroids, lithium
Blistering eruptions	Appear with widespread vesicles and bullae resembling autoimmune bullous disorders (see Ch. 112 on p. 947)	D-penicillamine, drugs with thiol group
Drug-induced lupus	Appears as lupus-like syndrome, although often without the rash	Hydrochlorothiazide, minocycline, hydralazine, procainamide
Erythema nodosum	Characterized by tender red nodules, predominantly in the pretibial region, but occasionally involving the arms or other areas	Sulfonamides, oral contraceptives
Exfoliative dermatitis	Characterized by redness, scaling, and thickening of the entire skin surface (see p. 958); may be fatal	Penicillin, sulfonamides, hydantoins
Fixed drug eruptions	Appear as frequently isolated, well-circumscribed, circinate or ovoid dusky red or purple lesions on the skin or mucous membranes (especially of the genitals) that reappear at the same sites each time the drug is taken	Phenolphthalein, tetracycline, sulfonamides
Lichenoid or lichen planus–like eruptions	Appear as angular papules that coalesce into scaly patches (see p. 970)	Antimalarials, gold, chlorpromazine, thiazides
Morbilliform or maculopapular eruptions	Range in appearance from a morbilliform disease to an eruption resembling pityriasis rosea	Almost any drug (especially barbiturates, analgesics, sulfonamides, ampicillin, other antibiotics)
Mucocutaneous eruptions	Vary from a few small oral vesicles or urticaria-like skin lesions to painful oral ulcers with widespread bullous skin lesions (see Erythema Multiforme on p. 974 and Stevens-Johnson Syndrome on p. 976)	Penicillin, barbiturates, sulfonamides (including derivatives used in hypertension and diabetes)
Photosensitivity eruptions	Appear as areas of dermatitis or gray-blue hyperpigmentation (phenothiazines and minocycline) on skin exposed to the sun or other ultraviolet light source	Phenothiazines, tetracyclines, sulfonamides, chlorothiazide, artificial sweeteners
Purpuric eruptions	Appear as nonblanching hemorrhagic macules that vary in size; most common on the lower extremities but may occur anywhere and may indicate a more serious purpuric vasculitis; may occur as type II cytotoxic reactions, type IV cell-mediated delayed-type allergic reactions, or type III humoral allergic immune complex vasculitis	Chlorothiazide, meprobamate, anticoagulants

Table continues on the following page.

TABLE 117–1. TYPES OF DRUG REACTIONS AND TYPICAL CAUSATIVE AGENTS—Continued

TYPE OF REACTION	DESCRIPTION AND COMMENTS	TYPICAL CAUSATIVE AGENTS
Serum sickness type drug reaction	A type III immune complex reaction; acute urticaria and angioedema occur more commonly than morbilliform or scarlatiniform eruptions; polyarthritis, myalgias, polysynovitis, fever, and neuritis may occur	Penicillin, insulin, foreign proteins
Toxic epidermal necrolysis	Characterized by large areas of loosened, easily detached epidermis that give the skin a scalded appearance (see Toxic Epidermal Necrolysis in this chapter); may be fatal in 30 to 40% of patients; staphylococcal scalded skin syndrome produces a similar condition in infants, young children, and immunosuppressed patients (see p. 986)	Barbiturates, hydantoins, penicillin, sulfonamides
Urticaria	Easily recognized by typical well-defined edematous wheals	Penicillin, aspirin, sulfonamides

Acral cyanosis can be caused by bromocriptine and bleomycin.

Skin necrosis can be caused by warfarin, heparin, barbiturates, epinephrine, norepinephrine, and vasopressin.

Diagnosis and Treatment

A detailed history is often required for diagnosis, including recent use of OTC drugs. No laboratory tests reliably aid diagnosis, although biopsy of affected skin is often suggestive. Most drug reactions resolve when drugs are stopped and require no further therapy. Whenever possible, chemically unrelated compounds should be substituted for suspect drugs. Sensitivity can be definitively established only by rechallenge with the drug, which may be hazardous and/or unethical. Pruritus can be controlled with antihistamines and topical corticosteroids.

When progression from urticaria to anaphylaxis is a concern, treatment is with aqueous epinephrine (1:1000) 0.2 mL sc or IM and with the slower-acting but more persistent soluble hydrocortisone 100 mg IV, which may be followed by an oral corticosteroid for a short period (see also p. 1360).

ERYTHEMA MULTIFORME

Erythema multiforme (EM) is an inflammatory reaction, characterized by "target" or "iris" skin lesions. Oral mucosa may be involved. Diagnosis is clinical. Lesions spontaneously resolve but frequently recur. EM can occur as reaction to a drug or an infectious agent such as herpes simplex virus (HSV) or mycoplasma. Suppressive antiviral therapy may be indicated for patients with frequent and/or symptomatic recurrence due to HSV.

EM was for years thought to represent the milder end of a spectrum of drug hypersensitivity disorders that included Stevens-Johnson syndrome and toxic epidermal necrolysis. Recent evidence suggests that EM is different from these other disorders.

Etiology

The majority of cases are caused by HSV infection (HSV-1 > HSV-2), although it is unclear if EM lesions represent a specific or nonspecific reaction to the virus. Current thinking holds that EM is caused by a T-cell–mediated cytolytic reaction to HSV DNA fragments present in keratinocytes. A genetic disposition is presumed given that EM is such a rare clinical manifestation of HSV infection. Less commonly, cases are caused by drugs, vaccines, other viral diseases (especially hepatitis C), or possibly SLE (Rowell's syndrome).

Symptoms, Signs, and Diagnosis

EM manifests as the sudden onset of asymptomatic, erythematous macules, papules, wheals, vesicles, and/or bullae on the distal extremities (including palms and soles) and face. The classic lesion is annular, with a violaceous center and pink halo separated by a pale ring (target or iris lesion). Distribution is symmetric and centripetal; spread to the trunk is common. Oral lesions include target lesions on the lips and vesicles and erosions on the palate and gingivae.

Diagnosis is by clinical appearance; biopsy is rarely necessary. Differential diagnosis includes essential urticaria, vasculitis, bullous pemphigoid, pemphigus, linear IgA dermatosis, acute febrile neutrophilic dermatosis, and dermatitis herpetiformis; oral lesions must be distinguished from aphthous stomatitis, pemphigus, herpetic stomatitis, and hand, foot, and mouth disease.

Treatment and Prognosis

EM spontaneously resolves, so treatment is usually unnecessary. Topical corticosteroids and anesthetics may ameliorate symptoms and reassure patients. Recurrences are common, and empiric oral maintenance therapy with acyclovir 400 mg q 12 h, famciclovir 250 mg q 12 h, or valacyclovir 1000 mg q 24 h can be attempted if symptoms recur more than 5 times/year, or if recurrent EM is consistently preceded by herpes flares.

ERYTHEMA NODOSUM

Erythema nodosum is a specific form of panniculitis (see p. 976) characterized by tender, red or violet, palpable subcutaneous nodules on the shins and occasionally other locations. It often occurs with an underlying systemic disease, notably streptococcal infections, sarcoidosis, and TB.

Erythema nodosum (EN) primarily affects people in their 20s and 30s but can occur at any age; women are more often affected. Etiology is unknown, but an immunologic reaction is suspected given EN's frequent association with other diseases. The most common are streptococcal infection (especially in children), sarcoidosis, and TB. Other possible triggers include other bacterial infections (*Yersinia, Salmonella*, mycoplasma, chlamydia, leprosy, lymphogranuloma venereum), fungal infections (coccidioidomycosis, blastomycosis, histoplasmosis), and viral infections (Epstein-Barr, hepatitis B); use of drugs (sulfonamides, iodides, bromides, oral contraceptives); inflammatory bowel disease; hematologic and solid malignancies; and pregnancy. Up to ⅓ of cases of EN are idiopathic.

EN manifests as erythematous, tender plaques or nodules accompanied by fever, malaise, and arthralgia. Differential diagnosis includes other forms of panniculitis and vasculitis.

Diagnosis is by clinical appearance, but EN should prompt evaluation for underlying causes, which might include biopsy, skin testing (PPD or anergy panel), antinuclear antibodies, CBC, chest x-ray, and antistreptolysin-O titer or pharyngeal culture. ESR is often high.

Erythema nodosum almost always resolves spontaneously. Treatment includes bedrest, elevation, cool compresses, and NSAIDS. Potassium iodide 300 to 500 mg po tid can be given to decrease inflammation. Systemic corticosteroids are effective but are an intervention of last resort as they can worsen an underlying occult infection. If an underlying disorder is identified, it should be treated.

GRANULOMA ANNULARE

Granuloma annulare is a benign, chronic idiopathic condition characterized by papules or nodules that spread peripherally to form a ring around normal or slightly depressed skin.

Lesions are erythematous, yellowish tan, bluish, or the color of the surrounding skin; one or more lesions may occur, most often on dorsal feet, legs, hands, or fingers. They are usually asymptomatic. Granuloma annulare is not associated with systemic diseases, except that the incidence of abnormal glucose metabolism is increased among adults with many lesions. In some cases, exposure to sunlight, insect bites, TB skin testing, trauma, and viral infections have induced disease flares.

Usually no treatment is necessary; spontaneous resolution is common. Options include the use of high-strength topical corticosteroids under occlusive dressings every night, flurandrenolide-impregnated tape, and intralesional corticosteroids. Psoralen plus ultraviolet

A (PUVA) therapy is effective and practical for patients with widespread disease.

PANNICULITIS

Panniculitis describes inflammation of the subcutaneous fat.

There are multiple causes, including infections (the most common), physical factors (eg, cold, trauma), proliferative disorders, and connective tissue disease (eg, SLE, scleroderma). Erythema nodosum is a specific form of panniculitis (see p. 975). The mechanism of action is dependent on the cause. Diagnosis is by clinical evaluation and biopsy. Treatment depends on the underlying cause.

PYODERMA GANGRENOSUM

Pyoderma gangrenosum is a chronic progressive skin necrosis of unknown etiology often associated with systemic illness.

Etiology is unknown, but pyoderma gangrenosum can be associated with vasculitis, gammopathies, RA, leukemia, lymphoma, hepatitis C, SLE, sarcoidosis, and especially inflammatory bowel disease and is thought to be due to an abnormal immune response.

Pyoderma gangrenosum begins as an inflamed erythematous papule, pustule, or nodule. The lesion, which may resemble a furuncle or an arthropod bite at this stage, then ulcerates and expands rapidly, developing a swollen necrotic base and a raised dusky to violaceous border. An undermined border is common, if not pathognomonic. Systemic symptoms such as fever, malaise, and arthralgias are common. The ulcers coalesce to form larger ulcers, often with cribriform or sieve-like scarring. A well-known feature is pathergy, wherein new lesions develop at sites of trauma. This has parallels to the Koebner phenomenon in psoriasis.

Biopsies of lesions are not often diagnostic but may be supportive; 40% of biopsies from a leading edge show vasculitis with neutrophils and fibrin in superficial vessels. Prednisone 60 to 80 mg po once/day is still the mainstay of treatment, although cyclosporine 3 mg/kg/day po is also quite effective. Dapsone, clofazimine, thalidomide, infliximab, and mycophenolate mofetil have also been used successfully.

STEVENS-JOHNSON SYNDROME AND TOXIC EPIDERMAL NECROLYSIS

Stevens-Johnson syndrome and toxic epidermal necrolysis are severe cutaneous hypersensitivity reactions. Drugs, especially sulfa drugs, antiepileptics, and antibiotics, are the most common causes. Macules rapidly spread and coalesce, leading to epidermal blistering, necrosis, and sloughing. Diagnosis is usually obvious by appearance of initial lesions and clinical syndrome. Treatment is supportive care; corticosteroids, cyclophosphamide, and other drugs may be tried. Prognosis depends on how early the syndromes are diagnosed and treated; mortality may reach 40%.

Stevens-Johnson syndrome (SJS) and toxic epidermal necrolysis (TEN) are clinically similar except for their distribution. By one commonly accepted definition, changes affect < 10% of body surface area in SJS and > 30% of body surface area in TEN; involvement of 15 to 30% of body surface area is considered SJS-TEN overlap.

The disorders affect between 1 and 5 people/million. Incidence and/or severity of both disorders may be higher in bone-marrow transplant recipients, in *Pneumocystis jiroveci* (formerly *P. carinii*)–infected HIV patients, and in patients with SLE.

Etiology and Pathophysiology

Drugs precipitate over 50% of SJS cases and up to 95% of TEN cases. Sulfa drugs (eg, co-trimoxazole, sulfasalazine), antiepileptics (eg, phenytoin, carbamazepine, phenobarbital, valproate), antibiotics (eg, aminopenicillins, quinolones, cephalosporins), and miscellaneous individual drugs (eg, piroxicam, allopurinol, chlormezanone) are most often implicated. Cases that are not due to drugs are attributed to infection (mostly with *Mycoplasma pneumoniae*), vaccination, and graft-vs-host disease. Rarely, a cause cannot be identified.

Exact mechanism is unknown; however, one theory holds that altered drug metabolism in some patients causes formation of reactive metabolites that bind to and alter cell proteins, triggering a T-cell–mediated cytotoxic reaction to drug antigens in keratinocytes. Another possible mechanism involves interactions between Fas, a cell-surface death receptor, and its ligand.

Symptoms and Signs

Within 1 to 3 wk after the start of the offending drug, patients develop a prodrome of malaise, fever, headache, cough, and conjunctivitis. Macules, often in a "target" configuration, then appear suddenly, usually on the face, neck, and upper trunk. These simultaneously appear elsewhere on the body, coalesce into large flaccid bullae, and slough over a period of 1 to 3 days. Nails and eyebrows may be lost along with epithelium.

In severe cases of TEN, large sheets of epithelium slide off the entire body at pressure points (Nikolsky's sign), exposing weepy, painful, and erythematous skin. Painful oral crusts and erosions, keratoconjunctivitis, and genital problems (such as phimosis and vaginal synechiae) accompany skin sloughing in up to 90% of cases. Bronchial epithelium may also slough, causing cough, dyspnea, pneumonia, pulmonary edema, and hypoxemia. Glomerulonephritis and hepatitis may develop.

Diagnosis

Diagnosis is often obvious from appearance of lesions and rapid progression of symptoms. Histologic examination of sloughed skin shows necrotic epithelium, a distinguishing feature. Differential diagnosis includes, in SJS and early TEN, erythema multiforme, viral exanthems, and drug rash; and, in later stages of TEN, paraneoplastic pemphigus, toxic shock/toxic strep syndrome, exfoliative erythroderma, and thermal burn. In children, TEN is less common and must be distinguished from the staphylococcal scalded skin syndrome.

Prognosis and Treatment

Severe TEN is similar to extensive burns; patients are acutely ill, may be unable to eat or open their eyes, and suffer massive fluid and electrolyte losses. They are at high risk for infection, multiorgan failure, and death. With early therapy, survival rates approach 90%.

Treatment is most successful when SJS-TEN is recognized early and treated in an inpatient dermatologic or ICU setting; burn units may be indicated for severe disease. Ophthalmology consultation is essential. Drugs should be discontinued immediately. Patients are isolated to minimize exposure to infection and are repleted aggressively with fluids, electrolytes, blood products, and nutritional supplements as needed. Skin care includes prompt treatment of secondary bacterial infections. Prophylactic antibiotics are controversial.

Treatment of STS/TEN is controversial. High-dose systemic corticosteroids (eg, 80 to 200 mg methylprednisolone IV or 80 mg prednisone po once/day for 7 to 10 days or until progression stops) or cyclophosphamide (300 mg IV q 24 h for 7 days or until significant improvement) can be given to inhibit T-cell–mediated cytolysis. However, corticosteroids are controversial and are thought by some to increase mortality. Plasmapheresis can remove reactive drug metabolites or antibodies. Early high-dose IV immune globulin (IVIG) 2.7 g/kg over 3 days blocks antibodies and Fas ligand, an apoptosis-inducing protein. Despite some remarkable results using high-dose IVIG for TEN, clinical trials involving small cohorts have reported conflicting results.

118 SWEATING DISORDERS

There are two types of sweat glands: apocrine and eccrine.

Apocrine glands are clustered in the axillae, areolae, genitals, and anus; modified apocrine glands are found in the external auditory meatus. Apocrine glands become active at puberty; their excretions are oily and viscid and are presumed to play a role in sexual olfactory messages. The most common disorders of apocrine glands are bromhidrosis and hidradenitis suppurativa (see p. 983).

Eccrine glands are sympathetically innervated, distributed over the entire body, and active from birth. Their secretions are watery and serve to cool the body in hot environments or during activity. Disorders of eccrine glands include hyperhidrosis, hypohidrosis, and miliaria.

BROMHIDROSIS

Bromhidrosis is excessive or abnormal body odor caused by decomposition by bacteria and yeasts of apocrine secretions and cellular debris.

Apocrine secretions are lipid-rich, sterile, and odorless but become odoriferous when decomposed. Eccrine bromhidrosis is not as fragrant because eccrine sweat is nearly 100% water. The cause of apocrine bromhidrosis is poor hygiene of skin and clothing.

HYPERHIDROSIS

Hyperhidrosis is excessive sweating, which can be focal or diffuse and has multiple causes. Sweating of the axillae, palms, and soles is most often due to stress; diffuse sweating is usually idiopathic but should raise suspicions for malignancies, infection, and endocrine disease. Diagnosis is obvious, but tests for underlying causes may be indicated. Treatment is topical aluminum chloride, tap water iontophoresis, botulinum toxin, and, in extreme cases, surgery.

Etiology

Hyperhidrosis can be focal or generalized.

Focal sweating: Emotional causes are common, causing sweating on the palms, soles, axillae, and forehead at times of anxiety, excitement, anger, or fear. It may be due to a generalized stress-increased sympathetic outflow. Although such sweating is a normal response, patients with hyperhidrosis sweat excessively and under conditions not causing sweating in most people.

Gustatory sweating occurs around the lips and mouth when ingesting foods and beverages that are spicy or hot in temperature. There is no known cause in most cases, but gustatory sweating can be increased in diabetic neuropathy, facial herpes zoster, cervical sympathetic ganglion invasion, CNS injury or disease, or parotid gland injury. In the latter, surgery, infection, or trauma may disrupt parotid gland innervation and lead to regrowth of parotid parasympathetic fibers into sympathetic fibers innervating local sweat glands in skin where the injury took place, usually over the parotid gland; this condition is called Frey's syndrome.

Other causes of focal sweating include pretibial myxedema (shins), hypertrophic osteoarthropathy (palms), and blue rubber bleb nevus syndrome and glomus tumor (over lesions). Compensatory sweating is intense sweating after sympathectomy.

Generalized sweating: Generalized sweating involves most of the body. Although most cases are idiopathic, numerous conditions can be involved, including endocrine disorders (especially hyperthyroidism, hypoglycemia, and hyperpituitarism induced by gonadotropin-releasing hormone agonists); pregnancy and menopause; drugs (especially antidepressants of all drug classes, aspirin, NSAIDs, hypoglycemic agents, caffeine, and theophylline); opioid withdrawal; carcinoid syndrome; autonomic neuropathy; cervical sympathetic ganglion invasion; and CNS injury or disease. Nocturnal generalized sweating (night sweats) is often benign or related to anxiety but should raise suspicions of malignancy (especially lymphoma and leukemia) and infection (especially TB, endocarditis, and systemic fungal disease).

Symptoms, Signs, and Diagnosis

Sweating is often present during examination and sometimes is extreme; clothing can be soaked, and palms or soles may become macerated and fissured. Hyperhidrosis can cause emotional distress to those who have it and may lead to social withdrawal. Palmar or plantar skin may appear pale.

Hyperhidrosis is diagnosed by history and examination but can be confirmed with the iodine and starch test (apply iodine solution to the affected area, let dry, dust on corn starch: areas of sweating appear dark). Testing is necessary only to confirm foci of sweating (as in Frey's syndrome or to locate the area needing surgical or botulinum toxin treatment) or in a semi-quantitative way when following the course of treatment.

Tests to identify a cause of hyperhidrosis are guided by a review of symptoms and might include CBC to detect leukemia, serum glucose to detect diabetes, and thyroid-stimulating hormone to screen for thyroid dysfunction.

Treatment

Initial treatment of focal and generalized sweating is similar.

Aluminum chloride hexahydrate 6 to 20% solution in absolute ethyl alcohol is indicated for topical treatment of axillary, palmar, and plantar sweating; these preparations require a prescription. The solution blocks sweat ducts and is most effective when applied nightly and covered tightly with a thin polyvinylidene or polyethylene film; it should be washed off in the morning. Sometimes an anticholinergic is taken before applying to prevent sweat from washing the aluminum chloride away. Initially, several applications weekly are needed to achieve control, then a maintenance schedule of once or twice weekly is followed. If treatment under occlusion is irritating, it should be tried without occlusion. This solution should not be applied to inflamed, broken, wet, or recently shaved skin. High-concentration, water-based aluminum chloride solutions may provide adequate relief in milder cases. Topical alternatives to aluminum chloride, including glutaraldehyde, formaldehyde, and tannic acid, are effective but can cause contact dermatitis and skin discoloration.

Tap water iontophoresis, in which salt ions are introduced into the skin using electric current, is an option for patients unresponsive to topical treatments. The affected areas (typically palms or soles) are placed in 2 tap water basins each containing an electrode across which a 15 to 25 mA current is applied for 10 to 20 min. This is performed daily for 1 wk, then repeated weekly or bimonthly. Treatments may be made more effective with topical or oral anticholinergics. Although the treatments are usually effective, the technique is time-consuming and somewhat cumbersome, and some patients tire of the routine.

Botulinum toxin A is a neurotoxin that decreases the release of acetylcholine from sympathetic nerves serving eccrine glands. Injected directly into the axillae, palms, or forehead, botulinum toxin inhibits sweating for about 5 mo depending on dosing. Complications include local muscle weakness and headache. Injections are effective but painful and expensive.

Surgery is indicated if more conservative treatments fail. Patients with axillary sweating can be treated with surgical excision of axillary sweat glands either through open dissection or by liposuction (the latter seems to have lower morbidity). Those with palmar sweating can be treated with endoscopic transthoracic sympathectomy. The potential morbidity of surgery must be considered, especially in sympathectomy. Potential complications include phantom sweating, compensatory sweating, gustatory sweating, neuralgia, and Horner syndrome.

HYPOHIDROSIS

Hypohidrosis is inadequate sweating.

Hypohidrosis due to skin abnormalities is rarely clinically significant. It is most commonly focal and caused by local skin injury (such as from trauma, radiation, infection such as leprosy, or inflammation) or by atrophy of glands from connective tissue disease (such as in scleroderma, SLE, Sjögren's syndrome). Hyphohidrosis may be due to drugs, especially those with anticholinergic properties. It is also caused by diabetic neuropathy and a variety of congenital syndromes. Heatstroke causes inadequate sweating but is a CNS rather than skin disorder (see p. 2608). A rare presentation is FUO. Diagnosis is by clinical observation of decreased sweating or by heat intolerance. Treatment is by cooling measures (eg, air-conditioning, wet garments).

MILIARIA

In miliaria, sweat flow is obstructed and trapped within the skin, causing papular lesions.

Miliaria most often occurs in warm humid weather but may occur in cool weather in an overdressed patient. Lesions vary depending on the depth of tissue at which the sweat duct is obstructed.

Miliaria crystallina is ductal obstruction in the uppermost epidermis, with retention of sweat subcorneally. It causes clear droplike vesicles that rupture with light pressure.

Miliaria rubra (prickly heat) is ductal obstruction in the mid-epidermis with retention of sweat in the epidermis and dermis. It causes irritated, pruritic papules (prickling).

Miliaria pustulosa is similar to miliaria rubra but manifests as pustules rather than papules.

Miliaria profunda is ductal obstruction at the entrance of the duct into the dermal papillae at the dermo-epidermal junction, with retention of sweat in the dermis. It causes larger, deeper-seated, frequently painful papules.

Diagnosis is by clinical appearance in the context of hot environment. Treatment is cooling and drying of the involved areas and avoidance of conditions that may induce sweating; an air-conditioned environment is ideal.

119 BACTERIAL SKIN INFECTIONS

Bacterial skin infections may be primary or a secondary infection of other skin lesions. Primary infections usually respond promptly to systemic antibiotics. Secondary infections tend to clear more slowly, requiring more complicated regimens. Recurrent skin infections should raise suspicion of colonization (eg, staphylococcal nasal carriage), malignancy, poorly controlled diabetes, or other reason for immunocompromise. Bacteria are involved in the pathophysiology of acne, but acne is not primarily considered a bacterial skin infection.

CELLULITIS

Cellulitis is acute bacterial infection of the skin and subcutaneous tissue most often caused by streptococci or staphylococci. Symptoms and signs are pain, rapidly spreading erythema, and edema; fever may occur and regional lymph nodes may enlarge. Diagnosis is by appearance; cultures are not usually necessary. Treatment is with antibiotics. Prognosis is excellent with timely treatment.

Etiology

Cellulitis is most often caused by group A β-hemolytic streptococci (eg, *S. pyogenes*) and *Staphylococcus aureus*. Streptococci cause diffuse, rapidly spreading infection because enzymes produced by the organism (streptokinase, DNAase, hyaluronidase) break down cellular components that would otherwise contain and localize the inflammation. Staphylococcal cellulitis is typically more localized and usually occurs with an open wound or cutaneous abscess.

Less common causes are group B streptococci (eg, *S. agalactiae*) in older patients with diabetes; gram-negative bacilli (eg, *Haemophilus influenzae*) in children; and *Pseudomonas aeruginosa* in patients with diabetes or neutropenia, hot tub or spa users, and hospitalized patients. Animal bites may cause cellulitis, with *Pasteurella multocida* from cats and *Capnocytophaga* sp from dogs. Immersion injuries in fresh water may result in cellulitis caused by *Aeromonas hydrophila*; in warm salt water, by *Vibrio vulnificus*.

Risk factors include skin abnormalities (eg, trauma, ulceration, fungal infection, other skin barrier compromise due to preexisting skin disease), which are common in patients with chronic venous insufficiency or lymphedema. Scars from saphenous vein removal for cardiac or vascular surgery are common sites for recurrent cellulitis, especially if tinea pedis is present. Frequently no predisposing condition or site of entry is evident.

Symptoms, Signs, and Diagnosis

Infection is most common in the lower extremities. The major findings are local erythema and tenderness, frequently with lymphangitis and regional lymphadenopathy. The skin is hot, red, and edematous, often with surface appearance resembling the skin of an orange (peau d'orange). The borders are usually indistinct, except in erysipelas (a type of cellulitis with sharply demarcated margins—see p. 982). Petechiae are common; large areas of ecchymosis, rare. Vesicles and bullae may develop and rupture, occasionally with necrosis of the involved skin. Cellulitis may mimic deep venous thrombosis but can be differentiated by one or more features (see TABLE 119–1). Fever, chills, tachycardia, headache, hypotension, and delirium may precede cutaneous findings by several hours, but many patients do not appear ill. Leukocytosis is common.

Diagnosis is by examination. Skin and (when present) wound cultures are generally not indicated because they rarely identify the infecting organism. Blood cultures are useful

TABLE 119–1. DIFFERENTIATING CELLULITIS AND DEEP VENOUS THROMBOSIS

FEATURE	CELLULITIS	DEEP VENOUS THROMBOSIS
Skin temperature	Hot	Normal or cool
Skin color	Red	Normal or cyanotic
Skin surface	Peau d'orange	Smooth
Lymphangitis and regional lymphadenopathy	Frequent	Nonexistent

in immunocompromised patients to detect or rule out bacteremia. Culture of involved tissue may be required in immunocompromised patients if they are not responding to empiric therapy or if blood cultures fail to isolate an organism.

Prognosis and Treatment

Most cellulitis resolves quickly with antibiotic therapy. Local abscesses occasionally form, requiring incision and drainage. Serious but rare complications include severe necrotizing subcutaneous infection (see p. 985) and bacteremia with metastatic foci of infection.

Recurrences in the same area are common, sometimes causing serious damage to the lymphatics, chronic lymphatic obstruction, and lymphedema.

Treatment is with antibiotics. For most patients, empiric treatment effective against both group A streptococci and *S. aureus* is used: Oral therapy is usually adequate with dicloxacillin 250 mg or cephalexin 500 mg po qid for mild infections. Levofloxacin 250 mg po once/day works as well and is easy to comply with. For more serious infections, oxacillin or nafcillin 1 g is given IV q 6 h. For penicillin-allergic patients or those with suspected methicillin-resistant *S. aureus* infection, vancomycin 1 g IV q 12 h is the drug of choice. Immobilization and elevation of the affected area help reduce edema; cool, wet dressings relieve local discomfort.

Cellulitis in a neutropenic patient requires empiric antipseudomonal antibiotics (eg, tobramycin 1.5 mg/kg IV q 8 h and piperacillin 3 g IV q 4 h) until blood culture results are available. Penicillin is the drug of choice for *P. multocida*, an aminoglycoside (eg, gentamicin) is effective against *A. hydrophila*, and tetracycline is preferred for *V. vulnificus*.

Recurrent leg cellulitis is prevented by treating concomitant tinea pedis, which often eliminates the source of bacteria residing in the inflamed, macerated tissue. If such therapy is unsuccessful or not indicated, recurrent cellulitis can sometimes be prevented by benzathine penicillin 1.2 million units IM monthly or penicillin V or erythromycin 250 mg po qid for 1 wk/mo.

CUTANEOUS ABSCESS

A cutaneous abscess is a localized collection of pus in the skin. Symptoms and signs are pain and tender, fluctuant swelling. Diagnosis is usually obvious by examination. Treatment is incision and drainage.

Bacteria causing cutaneous abscesses are typically indigenous to the skin of the involved area. For abscesses on the trunk, extremities, axillae, or head and neck, the most common organisms are *Staphylococcus aureus* and streptococci. Abscesses in the perineal (ie, inguinal, vaginal, buttock, perirectal) region contain organisms found in the stool, commonly anaerobes or a combination of aerobes and anaerobes. Carbuncles and furuncles are follicle-based cutaneous abscesses with characteristic features (see p. 983).

Cutaneous abscesses tend to form in patients with bacterial overgrowth, antecedent trauma (particularly when a foreign body is present), or immunologic or circulatory compromise.

Symptoms, Signs, and Diagnosis

Cutaneous abscesses are painful, tender, indurated, and sometimes erythematous. They vary in size, typically being 1 to 3 cm, but sometimes much larger. Initially the swelling is firm; later, as the abscess "points," the overlying skin becomes thin and feels fluctuant. The abscess may then spontaneously drain. Local cellulitis, lymphangitis, regional lymphadenopathy, fever, and leukocytosis are variable accompanying features.

Diagnosis is usually obvious by examination. Gram stain and culture are usually unnecessary except in immunocompromised patients.

Conditions resembling simple cutaneous abscesses include hidradenitis suppurativa (see p. 983) and ruptured epidermal cysts. Epidermal cysts (often incorrectly referred to as "sebaceous cysts") rarely become infected; however, rupture releases keratin into the dermis, causing an exuberant inflammatory reaction sometimes clinically resembling infection. Culture of these ruptured cysts seldom reveals any bacteria. Incision and drainage are the preferred method of treatment; antibiotics may be useful in reducing the inflammation but are not universally required if the patient has no other constitutional symptoms. Perineal abscesses may represent cutaneous emergence of a deeper perirectal abscess or drainage from Crohn's disease via a fistulous tract. These other conditions are usually recognizable by history and rectal examination.

Treatment

Some small abscesses resolve without treatment, coming to a point and draining.

Warm compresses help accelerate the process. Incision and drainage are indicated when significant pain, tenderness, and swelling are present; it is unnecessary to await fluctuance. Under sterile conditions, lidocaine injection or a freezing spray is used for local anesthesia. Patients with large, extremely painful abscesses may benefit from IV sedation and analgesia during drainage. A single puncture with the tip of a scalpel is often sufficient to open the abscess. After the pus drains, the cavity should be bluntly probed with a finger or curette to clear loculations, then irrigated with 0.9% saline solution. Some clinicians pack the cavity loosely with a gauze wick that is removed 24 to 48 h later. Local heat and elevation may hasten resolution of inflammation. Antibiotics are unnecessary unless the patient has signs of systemic infection, immunocompromise, or a facial abscess in the area drained by the cavernous sinus.

ERYSIPELAS

Erysipelas is a type of superficial cellulitis (see p. 980) with dermal lymphatic involvement.

Erysipelas should not be confused with erysipeloid, a skin infection caused by *Erysipelothrix* (see p. 1453). Erysipelas is characterized clinically by shiny, raised, indurated, and tender plaque-like lesions with distinct margins. It is most often caused by group A (or rarely group C or G) β-hemolytic streptococci and occurs most frequently on the legs and face. Erysipelas of the face must be differentiated from herpes zoster, angioneurotic edema, and contact dermatitis. It is commonly accompanied by high fever, chills, and malaise. Erysipelas may be recurrent and may result in chronic lymphedema.

Diagnosis is by characteristic appearance; blood culture is obtained in toxic-appearing patients. Diffuse inflammatory carcinoma of the breast may also be mistaken for erysipelas.

Treatment is penicillin V or erythromycin 500 mg po qid for ≥2 wk. In severe cases, penicillin G 1.2 million units IV q 6 h is indicated, which can be replaced by oral therapy after 36 to 48 h. In cases resistant to these antibiotics, cloxacillin or cephalexin can be used. Cold packs and analgesics may relieve local discomfort. Fungal foot infections may be an entry site for infection and may require antifungal treatment to prevent recurrence.

ERYTHRASMA

Erythrasma is an intertriginous infection with *Corynebacterium minutissimum* that is most common in patients with diabetes and in people living in the tropics.

Erythrasma looks like tinea or intertrigo. It is most common in the foot, where it presents as superficial scaling, fissuring, and maceration most commonly confined to the 3rd and 4th web spaces; and in the groin, where it presents as irregular but sharply marginated pink or brown patches with fine scaling. Erythrasma may also involve the axillae, submammary or abdominal folds, and perineum, particularly in obese middle-aged women and patients with diabetes.

Erythrasma fluoresces a characteristic coral-red color under Wood's light. Absence of hyphae on skin scraping also distinguishes erythrasma from tinea.

Treatment is erythromycin or tetracycline 250 mg po qid for 14 days. Topical erythromycin or clindamycin is also effective. Recurrence within 6 to 12 mo is common.

FOLLICULITIS

Folliculitis is a bacterial infection of hair follicles.

Folliculitis is usually caused by *Staphylococcus aureus* but occasionally *Pseudomonas aeruginosa* (hot-tub folliculitis) or other organisms. Hot-tub folliculitis occurs because of inadequate treatment of water with chlorine or bromine.

Signs of folliculitis are a superficial pustule or inflammatory nodule surrounding a hair follicle. Symptoms are mild pain or irritation. Infected hairs easily fall out or are removed, but new papules tend to develop. Growth of stiff hairs into the skin may cause chronic low-grade irritation or inflammation that may mimic infectious folliculitis (pseudofolliculitis barbae—see p. 1008).

Because most folliculitis is from *S. aureus*, clindamycin 1% lotion or gel may be applied topically bid for 7 to 10 days. Alternatively, benzoyl peroxide 5% wash may be used when showering for 5 to 7 days. Extensive cutaneous involvement may warrant systemic therapy (eg, cephalexin 250 to 500 mg po tid to qid for 10 days). If these measures do not result in a cure, pustules are Gram stained and cultured to rule out gram-negative etiology, and nares are cultured to rule out nasal staphylococcal carriage. Potassium hydroxide wet mount should be performed on a plucked hair to rule out fungal folliculitis.

Hot-tub folliculitis usually resolves without treatment. However, adequate chlorination of the hot tub is necessary to prevent recurrences and to protect others from infection.

FURUNCLES AND CARBUNCLES

Furuncles (boils) are tender nodules caused by staphylococcal infection. Carbuncles are clusters of furuncles connected subcutaneously, causing deeper suppuration and scarring. They are smaller and more superficial than subcutaneous abscesses (see p. 981). Diagnosis is by appearance. Treatment is warm compresses and often oral antistaphylococcal antibiotics.

Both furuncles and carbuncles may affect healthy young people but are more common in the obese, the immunocompromised (including those with neutrophil defects), the elderly, and possibly those with diabetes. Clustered cases may occur among those living in crowded quarters with relatively poor hygiene or among contacts of patients infected with virulent strains. Predisposing factors include bacterial colonization of skin or nares, hot and humid climates, and occlusion or abnormal follicular anatomy (eg, comedones in acne).

Furuncles are common on the neck, breasts, face, and buttocks. They are uncomfortable and may be painful when closely attached to underlying structures (eg, on the nose, ear, or fingers). Appearance is a nodule or pustule that discharges necrotic tissue and sanguineous pus. Carbuncles may be accompanied by fever and prostration.

Diagnosis is by examination. Material for culture should be obtained from patients with single furuncles on the nose or central face, from patients with multiple furuncles, and from immunosuppressed patients.

Treatment of a single lesion is intermittent hot compresses to allow it to point and drain spontaneously. A patient with a furuncle in the nose or central facial area or with multiple furuncles or carbuncles is given a penicillinase-resistant beta-lactam (eg, dicloxacillin or cephalexin 250 to 500 mg po qid). Systemic antibiotics are also needed for larger lesions, lesions that do not respond to topical care, evidence of expanding cellulitis, immunocompromised patients, or patients at risk for endocarditis.

Incision and drainage are occasionally necessary and are indicated to speed resolution when the furuncle or carbuncle is fluctuant.

Furuncles frequently recur and can be prevented by application of liquid soap containing either chlorhexidine gluconate with isopropyl alcohol or 2 to 3% chloroxylenol, or by maintenance antibiotics over 1 to 2 mo. Patients with recurrent furunculosis should be treated for predisposing factors such as obesity, diabetes, occupational or industrial exposure to inciting factors, and nasal carriage of *Staphylococcus aureus*.

HIDRADENITIS SUPPURATIVA

Hidradenitis suppurativa is a chronic, scarring inflammation of apocrine glands of the axillae, groin, and around the nipples and anus.

Blockage of apocrine ducts has been suggested as the cause, leading to subsequent inflammation, bacterial overgrowth, and scarring. *Staphylococcus aureus* is almost always implicated in acute cases, but gram-negative organisms such as *Proteus* may predominate in chronic cases.

Swollen, tender masses resembling cutaneous abscesses develop. Pain, fluctuance, discharge, and sinus tract formation are characteristic in chronic cases. In chronic axillary cases, coalescence of inflamed nodules causes palpable cordlike fibrotic bands. The condition may become disabling because of pain and foul odor.

Diagnosis is by examination. Bacterial cultures may be helpful if there appears to be a concomitant cellulitis or loculated abscess.

Treatment of acute cases consists of high-dose oral tetracycline (500 mg po bid) or erythromycin (250 to 500 mg po qid) until the lesions resolve. Topical clindamycin applied bid may be equally effective. Incision and drainage are necessary for an abscess or fluctuance of the affected area but alone will not resolve the problem (unlike in cutaneous abscesses). Isotretinoin 1 mg/kg po bid has also been effective in some patients, but recurrences are common. Surgical excision and repair or grafting of the affected areas are often necessary if the disease persists.

IMPETIGO AND ECTHYMA

Impetigo is a superficial skin infection with crusting or bullae caused by streptococci, staphylococci, or both. Ecthyma is an ulcerative form of impetigo.

No predisposing lesion is identified in most patients, but impetigo may follow any type of break in the skin; general risk factors seem to be moist environment, poor hygiene, and chronic nasal carriage of staphylococci. Impetigo may be bullous or nonbullous. Bullae are caused by exfoliative toxin produced by staphylococci.

Symptoms, Signs, and Diagnosis

Nonbullous impetigo typically presents as clusters of vesicles or pustules that rupture and develop a honey-colored crust (exudate from the lesion base) over the lesions. Bullous impetigo is similar except that vesicles typically enlarge rapidly to form bullae. The bullae burst and expose larger bases, which become covered with honey-colored varnish or crust. Ecthyma is characterized by small, purulent, shallow, punched-out ulcers with thick, brown-black crusts and surrounding erythema.

Impetigo and ecthyma cause mild pain or discomfort. Pruritus is common; scratching may spread infection, inoculating adjacent and nonadjacent skin.

Diagnosis is by characteristic appearance. Cultures of lesions are indicated only when the patient fails to respond to empiric therapy. Patients with recurrent impetigo should have nasal culture.

Treatment

Treatment for localized disease is mupirocin antibiotic ointment tid. Oral antibiotics (eg, dicloxacillin or cephalexin 250 to 500 mg qid, 12.5 mg/kg qid for children, for 10 days) may be needed in patients with extensive or resistant lesions.

Other therapy includes restoring a normal cutaneous barrier in patients with underlying atopic dermatitis or extensive xerosis using topical emollients and corticosteroids if warranted. Chronic staphylococcal nasal carriers are given topical antibiotics (mupirocin) for 1 wk each of 3 consecutive months.

Prompt recovery usually follows timely treatment. Delay can cause cellulitis, lymphangitis, furunculosis, and hyper- and hypopigmentation with or without scarring. Children aged 2 to 4 yr are at risk for acute glomerulonephritis if nephritogenic strains of group A streptococci are involved; nephritis seems to be more common in the southern US than in other regions.

LYMPHADENITIS

(See also Lymphangitis on p. 985.)

Lymphadenitis is an acute infection of one or more lymph nodes.

Lymphadenitis is a feature of many bacterial, viral, fungal, and protozoal infections. Focal lymphadenitis is prominent in streptococcal infection, TB or nontuberculous mycobacterial infection, tularemia, plague, cat-scratch disease, primary syphilis, lymphogranuloma venereum, chancroid, and genital herpes simplex. Multifocal lymphadenitis is common in infectious mononucleosis, cytomegalovirus infection, toxoplasmosis, brucellosis, secondary syphilis, and disseminated histoplasmosis.

Lymphadenitis typically causes pain, tenderness, and lymph node enlargement. Pain and tenderness typically distinguish lymphadenitis from lymphadenopathy. With some infections, the overlying skin is inflamed, occasionally with cellulitis. Abscesses may form, and penetration to the skin produces draining sinuses. Fever is common.

The underlying cause is usually suggested by history and examination. If not, aspiration and culture or excisional biopsy is indicated.

Treatment is directed at the cause and is usually empiric. Options include IV antibiotics, antifungals, and antiparasitics depending upon etiology or clinical suspicion. Many patients with lymphadenitis may respond to outpatient therapy with oral antibiotics. However, many also go on to form abscesses requiring surgical intervention, which, if extensive, is performed with accompanying IV antibiotics. In children, IV antibiotics are commonly needed. Hot, wet compresses may relieve some pain. Abscesses require surgical drainage. Lymphadenitis usually resolves with timely treatment, although residual, persistent nontender lymphadenopathy is common.

LYMPHANGITIS

(See also Lymphadenitis on p. 984.)

Lymphangitis is acute bacterial infection (usually streptococcal) of peripheral lymphatic channels.

Bacteria enter the lymphatic channels from an abrasion, wound, or coexisting infection (usually cellulitis). Patients with underlying lymphedema are at particular risk. Red, irregular, warm, tender streaks develop on an extremity and extend proximally from a peripheral lesion toward regional lymph nodes, which are typically enlarged and tender. Systemic manifestations (eg, fever, shaking chills, tachycardia, headache) may occur and may be more severe than cutaneous findings suggest. Leukocytosis is common. Bacteremia may occur. Rarely, cellulitis with suppuration, necrosis, and ulceration develops along the involved lymph channels as a consequence of primary lymphangitis.

Diagnosis is clinical. Isolation of the responsible organism is generally unnecessary. Most cases respond rapidly to antistreptococcal antibiotics (see Cellulitis on p. 980).

NECROTIZING SUBCUTANEOUS INFECTION

(Necrotizing Fasciitis)

Necrotizing subcutaneous infection is typically caused by a mixture of aerobic and anaerobic organisms that cause necrosis of subcutaneous tissue, usually including the fascia. This infection most commonly affects the extremities and perineum. Affected tissues become red, hot, and swollen, resembling severe cellulitis (see p. 980); in the absence of timely treatment, the area becomes gangrenous. Patients are acutely ill. Diagnosis is by history and examination and supported by evidence of overwhelming infection. Treatment involves antibiotics and surgical debridement. Prognosis is poor without early, aggressive treatment.

Etiology and Pathogenesis

Necrotizing subcutaneous infection (NSI) typically results from infection with group A streptococci (*S. pyogenes*) or a mixture of aerobic and anaerobic bacteria (*Bacteroides* sp). These organisms typically extend to subcutaneous tissue from a contiguous ulcer, infection, or after trauma. Streptococci can arrive from a remote site of infection via the bloodstream. Perineal involvement (also called Fournier's gangrene) is usually a complication of recent surgery, perirectal abscess, periurethral gland infection, or retroperitoneal infection from perforated abdominal viscera. Patients with diabetes are at particular risk for NSI.

NSI produces tissue ischemia by widespread occlusion of small subcutaneous vessels. Vessel occlusion results in skin infarction and necrosis, which facilitates the growth of obligate anaerobes (eg, *Bacteroides*) while promoting anaerobic metabolism by facultative organisms (eg, *Escherichia coli*), resulting in gangrene. Anaerobic metabolism produces hydrogen and nitrogen, relatively insoluble gases that may accumulate in subcutaneous tissues.

Symptoms and Signs

The primary symptom is intense pain. However, in areas denervated by peripheral neuropathy, pain may be minimal or absent. Affected tissue is red, hot, and swollen and rapidly becomes discolored. Bullae, crepitus (from soft-tissue gas), and gangrene may develop. Subcutaneous tissues (including adjacent fascia) necrose, with widespread undermining of surrounding tissue. Muscles are spared initially. Patients are acutely ill, with high fever, tachycardia, altered mental status ranging from confusion to obtundation, and hypotension. Patients may be bacteremic or septic and may require aggressive hemodynamic support.

Diagnosis

Diagnosis, made by history and examination, is supported by leukocytosis, soft-tissue gas on x-ray, positive blood cultures, and deteriorating metabolic and hemodynamic status.

NSI must be differentiated from clostridial soft-tissue infections, in which cellulitis, myositis, and myonecrosis often occur (see p. 1502). Such infections are anaerobic. Anaerobic cellulitis produces lots of gas but little pain, edema, or change in skin; it very seldom travels into the muscle. Anaerobic myonecrosis has pronounced skin changes, pain, and edema and usually penetrates into muscle.

Prognosis and Treatment

Mortality rate is about 30%. Old age, underlying medical problems, delayed diagnosis and therapy, and insufficient surgical debridement worsen prognosis.

Treatment of early NSI is primarily surgical. IV antibiotics are adjuncts, usually including 2 or more drugs, but regimens vary depending on Gram stain and culture (eg, penicillin G 4 million units q 4 h combined with clindamycin 600 to 900 mg q 8 h or ceftriaxone 2 g q 12 h). Evidence of bullae, ecchymosis, fluctuance, crepitus, and systemic spread of infection requires immediate surgical exploration and debridement. The initial incision should be extended until an instrument or finger can no longer separate the skin and subcutaneous tissue from the deep fascia. The most common error is insufficient surgical intervention; repeat operation q 1 to 2 days, with further incision and debridement as needed, should be carried out routinely. Amputation of an extremity may be necessary.

IV fluids may be needed in large volumes before and after surgery. Antibiotic choices should be reviewed based on Gram stain and culture of tissues obtained during surgery.

STAPHYLOCOCCAL SCALDED SKIN SYNDROME

Staphylococcal scalded skin syndrome is an acute epidermolysis caused by a staphylococcal toxin. Newborns and children are most susceptible. Symptoms are widespread bullae with epidermal sloughing. Diagnosis is by examination and sometimes biopsy. Treatment is antistaphylococcal antibiotics and local care. Prognosis is excellent with timely treatment.

Staphylococcal scalded skin syndrome (SSSS) almost always affects children < 6 yr (especially infants); it rarely occurs in older patients unless they have renal failure or are immunocompromised. Epidemics may occur in nurseries, presumably transmitted by the hands of personnel in contact with an infected infant or who are nasal carriers of *S. aureus*. Sporadic cases also occur.

SSSS is caused by group II coagulase-positive staphylococci, usually phage type 71, which elaborate exfoliatin (also called epidermolysin), a toxin that splits the upper part of the epidermis just beneath the granular cell layer (see also p. 1442). The primary infection often begins during the first few days of life in the umbilical stump or diaper area; in older children, the face is the typical site. Toxin produced in these areas enters the circulation and affects the entire skin.

Symptoms and Signs

The initial lesion is usually superficial and crusted. Within 24 h, the surrounding skin becomes painful and scarlet, changes that quickly spread to other areas. The skin may be exquisitely tender and have a wrinkled tissue paper–like consistency. Large, flaccid blisters arise on the erythematous skin and quickly break to produce erosions. Intact blisters extend laterally with gentle pressure (Nikolsky's sign). The epidermis may peel easily, often in large sheets. Widespread desquamation occurs within 36 to 72 h, and patients become very ill with systemic manifestations (eg, malaise, chills, fever). Desquamated areas appear scalded. Loss of the protective skin barrier can lead to sepsis and to fluid and electrolyte imbalance.

Diagnosis

Diagnosis is suspected clinically, but confirmation usually requires biopsy (frozen section may give earlier results). Specimens show noninflammatory superficial splitting of the epidermis. In children, skin cultures are seldom positive; in adults, they are frequently positive. Cultures should be obtained from the nose, conjunctiva, throat, and nasopharynx.

Differential diagnosis includes drug hypersensitivity, viral exanthemas, scarlet fever, thermal burns, genetic bullous diseases (eg, some types of epidermolysis bullosa), acquired bullous diseases (eg, pemphigus vulgaris, bullous pemphigoid), and toxic epidermal necrolysis (see TABLE 119–2 and p. 976). Stevens-Johnson syndrome is characterized by mucosal involvement, which is absent in SSSS.

Treatment

With prompt diagnosis and therapy, death rarely occurs; the stratum corneum is quickly replaced, and healing usually occurs within 5 to 7 days after start of treatment.

IV penicillinase-resistant antistaphylococcal antibiotics must be started immediately; nafcillin 12.5 to 25 mg/kg IV q 6 h for newborns > 2 kg and 25 to 50 mg/kg for older children is given until improvement is noted, followed by oral cloxacillin 12.5 mg/kg q 6 h (for infants and children weighing ≤ 20 kg) and 250 to 500 mg q 6 h (for older children).

TABLE 119–2. DIFFERENTIATING STAPHYLOCOCCAL SCALDED SKIN SYNDROME (SSSS) AND TOXIC EPIDERMAL NECROLYSIS (TEN)

FEATURE	SSSS	TEN
Patients affected	Infants, young children, immunocompromised adults	Older patients
Patient history	Recent staphylococcal infection, renal failure	Drug use
Level of epidermal cleavage (blister formation)*	Within the granular cell (outermost) layer of the epidermis	Between the epidermis and dermis or at the level of the basal cell

*Determined by Tzanck test or by a frozen section of a fresh specimen.

Corticosteroids are contraindicated. Topical therapy and patient handling must be minimized.

If disease is widespread and lesions are weeping, the skin should be treated as for burns (see p. 2594). Hydrolyzed polymer gel dressings may be very useful, and the number of dressing changes should be minimized.

Steps to detect carriers and prevent or treat nursery epidemics are described on p. 2329.

120 FUNGAL SKIN INFECTIONS

Fungal skin infections are caused by yeasts (*Candida* sp) or dermatophytes (*Epidermophyton, Microsporum*, and *Trichophyton* spp).

CANDIDIASIS

Candidiasis (moniliasis) is skin infection with *Candida* sp, most commonly *Candida albicans*. Infections can occur anywhere and are most common in skinfolds and web spaces, on the penis, and around fingernails. Symptoms and signs vary by site. Diagnosis is by clinical appearance and potassium hydroxide wet mount of skin scrapings. Treatment is with drying agents and antifungals.

Most candidal infections are of the skin and mucous membranes, but invasive candidiasis is common in immunosuppressed patients and can be life threatening. Systemic candidiasis is discussed in Ch. 180 (see p. 1529).

Etiology

Candida is a group of about 150 yeast species. *C. albicans* is responsible for about 70 to 80% of all candidal infections. Other significant species include *C. glabrata, C. tropicalis, C. krusei*, and *C. dubliniensis*.

Candida is a ubiquitous yeast that resides harmlessly on skin and mucous membranes until dampness, heat, and impaired local and systemic defenses provide a fertile environment for it to grow. Risk factors for candidiasis include hot weather, restrictive clothing, poor hygiene, infrequent diaper or undergarment changes in children and elderly patients, altered flora from antibiotic therapy, and immunosuppression resulting from corticosteroid and immunosuppressive drugs, pregnancy, diabetes, other endocrinopathies (eg, Cushing's disease, hypoadrenalism, hypothyroidism), blood dyscrasias, or T-cell defects.

Candidiasis occurs most commonly in intertriginous areas such as the axillae, groin, and gluteal folds (eg, diaper rash) and in digital web spaces, the glans penis, and beneath the breasts. Vulvovaginal candidiasis is common in women (see p. 2086). Candidal nail infections and paronychia may develop after improperly performed manicures and in kitchen workers and others whose hands are continually exposed to water (see p. 1010).

Oropharyngeal candidiasis is a common sign of local or systemic immunosuppression.

Chronic mucocutaneous candidiasis is a chronic infection, typically affecting the nails, skin, and oropharynx. Patients have cutaneous anergy to *Candida*, absent proliferative responses to *Candida* antigen (but normal proliferative responses to mitogens), and intact antibody response to *Candida* and other antigens. Chronic mucocutaneous candidiasis may occur as an autosomal recessive illness associated with hypoparathyroidism and Addison's disease (*Candida*-endocrinopathy syndrome).

Symptoms and Signs

Intertriginous infections manifest as pruritic, well-demarcated, erythematous patches of varying size and shape; erythema may be difficult to detect in darker-skinned patients. Primary patches may have adjacent satellite papules and pustules. Perianal candidiasis produces white maceration and pruritus ani. Vulvovaginal candidiasis causes pruritus and discharge (see p. 2086).

Candidal nail infection manifests as a full-thickness nail plate infection (onychomycosis—see p. 1010); candidal paronychia manifests as painful red periungual swelling that may develop pus (see p. 1010). Subungual infections are characterized by distal separation of one or several fingernails (onycholysis), with white or yellow discoloration of the subungual area.

Oropharyngeal candidiasis causes white plaques on oral mucus membranes that may bleed when scraped.

Chronic mucocutaneous candidiasis is characterized by red, pustular, crusted, and thickened plaques resembling psoriasis, especially on the nose and forehead and invariably associated with chronic oral candidiasis.

Diagnosis and Treatment

Diagnosis is by clinical appearance and by findings of yeast and pseudohyphae in potassium hydroxide wet mounts of scrapings from a lesion. Positive culture is usually meaningless because *Candida* is omnipresent.

Intertriginous infection is treated with drying agents as needed (eg, Burow's solution for oozing lesions, gentian violet for toe web spaces) and topical antifungals (see TABLE 120–1). Powdered formulations are ideal for dry lesions (eg, miconazole powder bid for 2 to 3 wk). Fluconazole 150 mg po once/wk for 2 to 4 wk is indicated for extensive intertriginous candidiasis; topical agents may be used at the same time.

Treatment of candidal diaper rash involves more frequent change of diapers, avoidance of disposable diapers with plastic coverings, and an imidazole cream bid. Oral nystatin is an option for infants with coexisting oropharyngeal candidiasis; 1 mL of suspension (100,000 units/mL) is placed in each buccal pouch qid.

Treatment of candidal onychomycosis and candidal paronychia is discussed on p. 1010.

Treatment of oral candidiasis is fluconazole 200 mg on the first day, then 100 mg po once/day for 2 to 3 wk thereafter.

Chronic mucocutaneous candidiasis requires long-term antifungal treatment.

DERMATOPHYTOSES

Dermatophytoses are fungal infections of keratin in the skin and nails (nail infection is called tinea unguium—see p. 1010). Symptoms and signs vary by site of infection. Diagnosis is by clinical appearance and by examination of skin scraping on potassium hydroxide wet mount. Treatment varies by site but always involves topical or oral antifungal drugs.

Dermatophytes are molds that require keratin for nutrition and must live on stratum corneum, hair, or nails to survive. All human infections are caused by *Epidermophyton, Microsporum*, and *Trichophyton* spp. These differ from candidiasis in that they are rarely if ever invasive. Transmission is person-to-person, animal-to-person, and rarely, soil-to-person. The organism may persist indefinitely. Most people do not develop clinical infection; those who do may have impaired T-cell responses from an alteration in local defenses (eg from trauma with vascular compromise) or from primary (hereditary) or secondary (eg, diabetes, HIV) immunosuppression.

Symptoms and Signs

Symptoms and signs vary by site (skin, hair, nails). Organism virulence and host susceptibility and hypersensitivity determine severity. Most often, there is little or no inflammation; asymptomatic or mildly itching lesions with a scaling, slightly raised border remit and recur intermittently. Occasionally, inflammation is more severe and manifests as sudden vesicular or bullous disease (usually of the foot) or as an inflamed boggy lesion of the scalp (kerion).

Diagnosis and Treatment

Diagnosis is based on clinical appearance and site of infection and confirmed by skin scrapings and demonstration of hyphae on potassium hydroxide (KOH) wet mount. Identification of specific organisms by culture is unnecessary except in cases of scalp infection (where an animal source may be identified and treated) and nail infection (which may be caused by a nondermatophyte). Culture may also be useful when overlying inflammation and bacterial infection are severe and/or accompanied by alopecia.

Differential diagnosis includes folliculitis decalvans, bacterial pyodermas, and entities that cause scarring alopecia, such as discoid lupus, lichen planopilaris, and pseudopelade.

Topical antifungals are generally adequate (see TABLE 120–1). In general, OTC terbinafine is best; econazole or ciclopirox may be better if candidal infection cannot be excluded. Oral agents are used for most nail and scalp infections, resistant skin infections, and patients unwilling or unable to adhere to prolonged topical regimens; doses and duration differ by site of infection.

TINEA BARBAE

Tinea barbae (barber's itch) is a dermatophyte infection of the beard area most often caused by *Trichophyton mentagrophytes* or *T. verrucosum*.

Tinea barbae presents as superficial annular lesions, but deeper infection similar to folliculitis may occur. It may also occur as an inflammatory kerion (see Tinea Capitis, below) that can result in scarring hair loss. Diagnosis is by KOH wet mount, culture, or biopsy.

Treatment is micronized griseofulvin 500 mg to 1 g po once/day until 2 to 3 wk after clinical clearance. Terbinafine 250 mg po once/day and itraconazole 200 mg po once/day have also been used. If the lesions are severely inflamed, a short course of prednisone should be added (to lessen symptoms and perhaps reduce the chance of scarring), starting with 40 mg po once/day (for adults) and tapering the dose over 2 wk.

TINEA CAPITIS

Tinea capitis is a dermatophyte infection of the scalp (scalp ringworm).

Tinea capitis mainly affects children, is contagious, and can be epidemic. *Trichophyton tonsurans* is the most common cause in the US, followed by *Microsporum canis* and *M. audouinii*; other *Trichophyton* sp (eg, *T. schoenleinii, T. violaceum*) are common elsewhere.

Tinea capitis causes the gradual appearance of round patches of dry scale and/or alopecia. *T. tonsurans* infection causes "black dot ringworm," in which hair shafts break at the scalp surface; *M. audouinii* infection causes "gray patch ringworm," in which hair shafts break above the surface, leaving short stubs. Tinea capitis less commonly manifests as diffuse scaling, like dandruff, or in a diffuse pustular pattern.

Dermatophyte infection occasionally leads to formation of a kerion, a large, boggy, inflammatory scalp mass caused by a severe inflammatory reaction to the dermatophyte. A kerion may have pustules and crusting and can be mistaken for an abscess. A kerion may result in scarring hair loss.

Diagnosis and Treatment

Tinea capitis is diagnosed by KOH wet mount of plucked hairs or of hairs and scale obtained by scraping or brushing. Spore size and appearance inside (endothrix) or outside (ectothrix) the hair shaft distinguishes organisms and can help guide treatment. Blue-green fluorescence on Wood's light examination is diagnostic for infection with *M. canis* and *M. audouinii* and can distinguish tinea from erythrasma. Differential diagnosis of tinea capitis also includes seborrheic dermatitis and psoriasis.

Treatment of children is with micronized griseofulvin suspension 10 to 20 mg/kg (doses vary by several parameters but maximum dose is generally 1 g/day), or for children > 2 y, ultramicronized griseofulvin 5 to 10 mg/kg (maximum 750 mg/day) given once/day or in 2 divided doses with meals or milk for 4 to 6 wk or until all signs of infection are gone. Some patients require up to 20 to 25 mg/kg/day. An imidazole or ciclopirox cream should be applied to the scalp to prevent spread, especially to other children, until tinea capitis is cured; selenium sulfide 2.5% shampoo should also be used at least twice/wk. Children may attend school during treatment.

Treatment of adults is with terbinafine 250 mg po once/day for 2 to 4 wk, which is more effective for endothrix infections, or

TABLE 120–1. OPTIONS FOR TREATMENT OF SUPERFICIAL FUNGAL INFECTIONS*

CLASS	AGENTS	FORMULATIONS	USES
Allylamines	Amorolfine	5% solution	Tinea unguium
	Naftifine	1% cream or gel	Dermatophytoses, skin candidiasis
	Terbinafine	1% cream or solution 250 mg tablet	Dermatophytoses
Benzylamine	Butenafine	1% cream	Dermatophytoses
Imidazoles	Butoconazole	2% cream	Vulvovaginal candidiasis
	Clotrimazole	*Topical:* 1% cream, lotion, or solution; 100, 200, and 500 mg vaginal suppository tablets *Oral:* 10 mg lozenges	Dermatophytoses, candidiasis (oropharyngeal, skin, vulvovaginal)
	Econazole	1% cream	Dermatophytoses, skin candidiasis, tinea versicolor
	Fluconazole	50 and 200 mg/5 mL solution; 50, 100, 150, 200 mg tablet	Vulvovaginal candidiasis
	Itraconazole	100 mg capsules, 10 mg/mL solution	Tinea unguium, other onychomycoses
	Ketoconazole	2% cream, 1 to 2% shampoo; 200 mg tablet	Dermatophytoses, skin candidiasis
	Miconazole	1 to 2% liquid (aerosol), 2% powder (aerosol), 1 to 2% cream and lotion, 1% solution, 2% powder or tincture; 100 to 200 mg vaginal suppositories	Dermatophytoses, candidiasis (skin, vulvovaginal)
	Oxiconazole	1% cream or lotion	Dermatophytoses, tinea versicolor
	Sulconazole	1% cream or solution	Dermatophytoses, tinea versicolor
	Terconazole	0.4% and 0.8% cream, 80 mg suppositories	Vulvovaginal candidiasis
	Tioconazole	6.5% ointment	Vulvovaginal candidiasis
Polyene	Nystatin	*Topical:* 100,000 U/g cream, ointment, powder, and vaginal tablet *Oral:* 100,000 U/mL suspension; 500,000 U tablets	Candidiasis (oropharyngeal, skin)
Miscellaneous	Carbol-fuchsin	Solution	Chronic dermatophytoses, intertrigo
	Ciclopirox	0.77% gel, 8% lacquer solution	Dermatophytoses, candidiasis, tinea versicolor, onychomycosis
	Clioquinol	3% cream	Dermatophytoses

TABLE 120–1. OPTIONS FOR TREATMENT OF SUPERFICIAL FUNGAL INFECTIONS*—Continued

CLASS	AGENTS	FORMULATIONS	USES
	Gentian violet	1 or 2% solution	Dermatophytoses, especially tinea pedis
	Griseofulvin	125, 165, 250, 330, 500 mg tablets	Dermatophytoses
	Tolnaftate	1% liquid or powder (aerosol), cream, powder, solution	Dermatophytoses, tinea versicolor
Zinc	Undecylenate/ undecylenate acid	25% solution, 10% tincture	Superficial dermatophyte infections (eg, tinea pedis)

*Advantages of one drug over another for most infections are not clear; for skin infections, allylamines have good activity against dermatophytes but weaker activity against *Candida*; imidazoles have better activity against both dermatophytes and *Candida*. Adverse effects are rare, but all topical antifungal agents can cause skin irritation, burning, allergic and contact dermatitis; oral antifungal agents can cause hepatitis and neutropenia. Oral drugs (eg, itraconazole, terbinafine) given > 1 mo require periodic laboratory monitoring of hepatic function and CBCs. Possible itraconazole drug-drug interactions include lovastatin, midazolam, pimozide, quinidine, simvastatin, and triazolam.

itraconazole 200 mg once/day for 2 to 4 wk (or 200 mg bid "pulsed" 1 wk on, 3 wk off for 2 to 3 mo). If the lesions are severely inflamed, and for kerion, a short course of prednisone should be added (to lessen symptoms and perhaps reduce the chance of scarring), starting with 40 mg once/day po (1 mg/kg for children) and tapering the dose over 2 wk.

Tinea Corporis

Tinea corporis is a dermatophyte infection of the face, trunk, and extremities (body ringworm).

Common causes are *T. mentagrophytes, T. rubrum*, and *M. canis*. Tinea corporis causes pink-to-red annular patches and plaques with raised scaly borders that expand peripherally and tend to clear centrally. A variant form appears as nummular scaling patches studded with small papules or pustules. Differential diagnosis includes pityriasis rosea, drug eruptions, nummular dermatitis, erythema multiforme, tinea versicolor, erythrasma, psoriasis, and secondary syphilis.

Treatment of mild-to-moderate lesions is an imidazole, ciclopirox, naftifine, or terbinafine in cream, lotion, or gel. The drug should be rubbed in bid continuing at least 7 to 10 days after lesions disappear, typically at about 2 to 3 wk. Extensive and resistant lesions occur in patients infected with *T. rubrum* and in people with debilitating systemic diseases. For extensive or resistant tinea corporis, the most effective therapy is oral itraconazole 200 mg once/day or terbinafine 250 mg once/day for 2 to 3 wk.

Tinea Cruris

Tinea cruris (jock itch) is a dermatophyte infection of the groin.

Common organisms include *T. rubrum* or *T. mentagrophytes*. Environmental factors associated with a moist environment (ie, warm weather, wet and restrictive clothing, obesity causing constant apposition of skin folds) are the primary risk factors. Men are affected more than women because of apposition of the scrotum and thigh. Typically, a pruritic, ringed lesion extends from the crural fold over the adjacent upper inner thigh. Infection may be bilateral. Lesions may be complicated by maceration, miliaria, secondary bacterial or candidal infection, and reactions to treatment. In addition, scratch dermatitis and lichenification can occur. Recurrence is common because fungi may repeatedly infect susceptible people. Flare-ups occur more often during summer.

Differential diagnosis includes contact dermatitis, psoriasis, erythrasma, and candidiasis. Scrotal involvement is usually absent or slight; by contrast, the scrotum is often inflamed in candidal intertrigo or lichen simplex chronicus.

Treatment is with topical antifungal cream or lotion. Choices include terbinafine, miconazole, clotrimazole, ketoconazole, econazole, naftifine, and ciclopirox applied bid for 10 to 14 days. Itraconazole 200 mg po once/day or terbinafine 250 mg po once/day for 3 to 6 wk may be needed in patients who have refractory, inflammatory, or widespread infections.

Tinea Pedis

Tinea pedis (athlete's foot) is a dermatophyte infection of the feet.

Tinea pedis is the most common dermatophytosis because moisture from foot sweating facilitates fungal growth. Tinea pedis may occur as any of 4 clinical forms or in combination: acute ulcerative, vesiculobullous, chronic hyperkeratotic, and chronic intertriginous.

Acute ulcerative tinea pedis (most often caused by *T. mentagrophytes,* var. *interdigitale*) typically begins in the 3rd and 4th interdigital spaces and extends to the lateral dorsum and/or the plantar surface of the arch. These toe web lesions are usually macerated and have scaling borders. Secondary bacterial infection, cellulitis, and lymphangitis are common complications.

Less commonly, interdigital tinea pedis flares into vesiculobullous tinea pedis, in which vesicles develop on the soles and coalesce into bullae; risk factors are occlusive shoes and environmental heat and humidity.

Chronic hyperkeratotic tinea pedis caused by *T. rubrum* causes a distinctive pattern of lesion, manifesting as scaling and thickening of the soles often extending beyond the plantar surface in a "moccasin" distribution. Differential diagnosis is sterile maceration (from hyperhidrosis and occlusive footgear), contact dermatitis (from type IV delayed hypersensitivity to various materials in shoes, particularly adhesive cement), irritant dermatitis, and/or psoriasis.

Chronic intertriginous tinea pedis is characterized by scaling, erythema, and erosion of the interdigital and subdigital skin of the feet, most commonly affecting the lateral 3 toes.

Diagnosis and Treatment

Diagnosis is usually obvious by examination and risk factors. The safest treatment is topical antifungals, but recurrence is common and treatment must often be prolonged. Alternatives that provide a more durable response include oral itraconazole 200 mg once/day for 1 mo (or pulse therapy with 200 mg bid 1 wk/mo for 1 to 2 mo) and terbinafine 250 mg po once/day for 2 to 6 wk. Concomitant topical antifungal use may reduce recurrences.

Moisture reduction on the feet and in footwear is necessary for preventing recurrence. Permeable or open-toe footwear and sock changes are important especially during warm weather. Interdigital spaces should be manually dried after bathing. Drying agents are also recommended; options include antifungal powders (eg, miconazole), gentian violet, Burow's solution soaks bid, or 20 to 25% aluminum chloride hexahydrate powder once/day.

Dermatophytid Reaction

Dermatophytid is an inflammatory reaction to dermatophytosis at a cutaneous site distant from the primary infection.

Dermatophytid (identity or "id") reactions are protean; they are not related to localized growth of the fungus but rather are an inflammatory reaction elsewhere on the body. Lesions are typically pruritic but may manifest as vesicular eruptions on the hands and feet, follicular papules, erysipelas-like plaques, erythema nodosum, erythema annulare centrifugum, or urticaria. Distribution may be extensive. Diagnosis is by KOH wet mounts that are negative at the site of the id reaction and positive at the distant site of dermatophyte infection.

Treatment of the primary infection is definitive; pending cure, topical corticosteroids and/or antipruritics (eg, hydroxyzine 25 mg qid) can be used to relieve symptoms.

INTERTRIGO

Intertrigo is skinfold changes caused by moisture and infection.

Intertrigo develops when friction and trapped moisture in intertriginous areas cause skin maceration with formation of patches or plaques; bacterial, yeast, and dermatophyte infection is common. Typical locations are the inframammary, infrapannicular, interdigital, axillary, infragluteal, and genitocrural folds. Diagnosis is by clinical appearance; potassium hydroxide wet mount and cultures can guide treatment.

If no bacteria or yeast are detected, drying agents (powders such as talc rather than cornstarch, which can support fungal growth, Burow's solution) to decrease moisture should be therapeutic. If bacteria or yeasts are present, topical antibacterial lotions or antifungal creams are given in addition to drying agents.

TINEA VERSICOLOR

Tinea versicolor is skin infection with *Malassezia furfur* that manifests as multiple asymptomatic scaly patches varying in color from white to brown. Diagnosis is based on clinical appearance and skin scrapings. Treatment is topical antifungal drugs.

Malassezia furfur is a dimorphic fungus that is normally a harmless component of normal skin flora but that in some people causes tinea versicolor. The high prevalence of tinea versicolor in young adults suggests a link to increased sebaceous secretion; other risk factors include heat and humidity and immunosuppression due to corticosteroids, pregnancy, malnutrition, diabetes, and other disorders.

Symptoms and Signs

Tinea versicolor usually causes no symptoms. Classically, it causes the appearance of multiple tan, brown, salmon, or white scaling lesions on the trunk, neck, abdomen, and occasionally face. The lesions coalesce. In whites, the condition is often diagnosed in summer months because the lesions, which do not tan, become more obvious against tanned skin.

Diagnosis and Treatment

Diagnosis is by clinical appearance and by findings of hyphae and budding cells ("spaghetti and meatballs") on potassium hydroxide wet mount. Wood's light examination reveals golden-white fluorescence.

Treatment is any topical antifungal drug. Examples include selenium sulfide shampoo 2.5% (in 10-min applications daily for 1 wk or 24-h applications weekly for 1 mo); topical azoles (eg, ketoconazole 2% daily for 2 wk); and bathing with zinc pyrithione 2% or sulfur-salicylic shampoo 2% for 1 to 2 wk.

Oral treatment is indicated for patients with extensive disease and those with frequent recurrences. Two convenient regimens are a single 400 mg dose of fluconazole and ketoconazole 200 mg once/day for 1 to 5 days.

Hypopigmentation from tinea versicolor is reversible in months to years after the yeast has cleared. Recurrence is almost universal after treatment because the causative organism is a normal skin inhabitant. Fastidious hygiene lowers the likelihood of recurrence.

121 PARASITIC SKIN INFECTIONS

Parasitic skin infections can cause severe itching and be distressing. Some systemic parasitic infections have cutaneous manifestations; these include certain nematodes (ancylostomasis, dracunculosis, strongyloidiasis, toxocariasis)—see p. 1545—and flukes (schistosomiasis—see p. 1558). Very rarely, patients have delusional parasitosis.

CUTANEOUS LARVA MIGRANS

(Creeping Eruption)

Cutaneous larva migrans is the skin manifestation of hookworm infestation.

Cutaneous larva migrans (CLM) is caused by *Ancylostoma* sp, most commonly dog or cat hookworm (*Ancylostoma braziliense*). Hookworm ova in dog or cat feces develop into infective larvae when left in warm moist ground or sand; transmission occurs when skin directly contacts contaminated soil or sand and larvae penetrate unprotected skin, usually of the feet, legs, buttocks, or back. CLM occurs worldwide but most commonly in tropical environments.

CLM causes intense pruritus; signs are erythema and papules at the site of entry, with a winding, threadlike subcutaneous trail of reddish-brown inflammation. Diagnosis is by history and clinical appearance. Topical thiabendazole 15% liquid or cream (compounded) bid to tid for 5 days is extremely effective. Oral thiabendazole is not well tolerated and not usually used. Albendazole and ivermectin can be curative and are well tolerated.

CLM may be complicated by a self-limiting pulmonary reaction called Löffler's syndrome (patchy pulmonary infiltrates and peripheral blood eosinophilia).

DELUSIONAL PARASITOSIS

Delusional parasitosis is a patient's belief that he is infested with parasites.

Patients have an unshakable belief that they are infested with insects, worms, mites, lice, or other organisms. They often provide vivid descriptions of how the organisms enter their skin and move around their bodies, and bring samples of hair, skin, and debris such as dried scabs, dust, and lint on slides or in containers (the "matchbox" sign) to prove the infestation is real. The condition is considered a "hypochondriacal psychosis," but the cause is unknown.

Diagnosis is suspected by history. Work-up requires ruling out true infestations and other physiologic disease by physical examination and judicious testing, such as skin scrapings and CBC.

Treatment is with antipsychotic drugs (see p. 1726). Typically, the patient seeks confirmation that the drug treats the infestation itself, and any suggestion that the treatment is for something else is met with resistance and/or rejection. Thus, effective treatment often requires diplomacy, and a delicate balance between offering proper treatment and respecting the patient's right-to-know.

LICE

(Pediculosis)

Lice can infect the scalp, body, pubis, and eyelashes. Head lice are transmitted by close contact; body lice in cramped, crowded conditions; and pubic lice by sexual contact. Symptoms, signs, diagnosis, and treatment differ by location of infestation.

Lice are wingless, blood-sucking insects that infest the head (*Pediculus humanus* var. *capitis*), body (*P. humanus* var. *corporis*), or pubis (*Phthirus pubis*). The 3 kinds of lice differ substantially in morphology and clinical features. Head lice and pubic lice live directly on the host; body lice, in garments. All types occur worldwide.

Head lice: Head lice are most common in girls aged 5 to 11 but can affect almost anyone; infestations are rare in blacks. Head lice are easily transmitted from person-to-person with close contact (as occurs within households and classrooms) and may be ejected from hair by static electricity or wind; transmission by these routes (or by sharing of combs, brushes, and hats) is unproven. There is no association with head lice and poor hygiene or low socioeconomic status.

Infestation typically involves the hair and scalp, but the eyebrows, eyelashes, and beard may be involved as well. Active infection usually involves ≤ 20 lice and causes severe pruritus. Examination is most often normal but may reveal scalp excoriations and posterior cervical adenopathy.

Diagnosis depends on demonstration of living lice. These are detected by a thorough combing-through of wet hair from the scalp with a fine-toothed "detection" comb; lice are usually found at the back of the head or behind the ears. Nits are ovoid, grayish white eggs fixed to the base of hair shafts. Each adult louse lays 3 to 5 eggs/day, so nits typically vastly outnumber lice and are not a measure of severity of infection.

Treatment is outlined in TABLE 121–1. Resistance is common and should be treated with oral ivermectin and by attempting to rotate pediculicides. Termination of live (viable) nits is important in preventing reinfestation; live nits fluoresce on illumination with a Wood's lamp. Most pediculicides also kill nits. Dead nits remain after successful treatment and do not signify active infection; they do not have to be removed. Nits grow away from the scalp with time; the absence of nits < $^{1}/_{4}$ inch from the scalp rules out current active infection.

Controversy surrounds the need to clean the personal items of people with lice or nits and the need to exclude children with head lice or nits from school; there are no good data supporting either approach.

Body lice: Body lice primarily live on bedding and clothing, not people, and are most frequently found in cramped, crowded conditions (eg, military barracks) and in people of low socioeconomic status. Transmission is by sharing of contaminated clothing and bedding. Body lice are important vectors of epidemic typhus, trench fever, and relapsing fever.

Body lice cause pruritus; signs are small red puncta caused by bites, usually associated with linear scratch marks, urticaria, or superficial bacterial infection. These findings are especially common on the shoulders, buttocks, and abdomen. Nits may be present on body hairs.

Diagnosis is by demonstration of lice and nits in clothing, especially at the seams. Primary treatment is thorough cleaning or replacement of clothing and bedding, which is often difficult because affected people often have few resources and little control over their environment. Secondary treatment is permethrin.

Pubic lice: Pubic lice (crabs) are sexually transmitted in adolescents and adults and may be transmitted by close parental contact in children. They may also be transmitted by fomites (towels, bedding, clothing). They most commonly infect pubic and perianal hairs but may spread to thighs, trunk, and facial hair (beard, moustache, and, in children, eyelashes).

Pubic lice cause pruritus. Physical signs are few, but some patients have excoriations and regional lymphadenopathy and/or lymphadenitis. Pale, bluish gray skin macules (maculae caeruleae) on the trunk, buttocks, and thighs are caused by anticoagulant activity of louse saliva while feeding; they are unusual but characteristic of infection. Eyelash infection manifests as eye itching, burning, and irritation.

Diagnosis is by demonstration of nits and/or living lice by close inspection (Wood's light) or microscopic analysis. A supporting sign of infection is scattering of dark brown specks (louse excreta) on skin or undergarments. Treatment is outlined in TABLE 121–1. Treatment of eyelid and eyelash infection is often difficult and involves use of petrolatum, physostigmine ointment, oral ivermectin, or physical removal of lice with forceps. Sex partners should be treated.

SCABIES

Scabies is an infestation of the skin with the mite *Sarcoptes scabiei*. Scabies causes intensely pruritic lesions with erythematous papules and burrows in web spaces, wrists, waistline, and genitals. Diagnosis is based on examination and scrapings. Treatment is with topical scabicides or rarely oral ivermectin.

Etiology

Scabies is caused by the mite *Sarcoptes scabiei* var. *hominis*, an obligate human parasite that lives in burrowed tunnels in the stratum corneum. Scabies is easily transmitted from person-to-person through physical contact; animal and fomite transmission probably also occurs. The primary risk factor is crowded conditions (as in schools, shelters, barracks, and some households); there is no clear association with poor hygiene. For unknown reasons, crusted scabies (see below) is more common in immunosuppressed patients (eg, those with HIV infection, hematologic malignancy, chronic corticosteroid or other immunosuppressant use), those with severe physical disabilities or mental retardation, and Australian Aborigines. Infestations occur worldwide. Patients in warm climates develop small erythematous papules with few burrows. Severity is related to the patient's immune status, not geography.

Symptoms, Signs, and Diagnosis

The primary symptom is intense pruritus, classically worse at night, although that timing is not specific to scabies.

Classic scabies: Erythematous papules initially appear in finger web spaces, flexor surfaces of the wrist and elbow, axillary folds, along the belt line, or on the lower buttocks. Papules can spread to any area of the body, including the breasts and penis. The face remains uninvolved in adults. Burrows are pathognomonic for disease, manifesting as fine, wavy, and slightly scaly lines several mm to 1 cm long. A tiny dark papule—the mite—is often visible at one end.

Signs of classic scabies may be atypical. In blacks and others with dark skin, scabies can manifest as granulomatous nodules. In infants, the palms, soles, face, and scalp may be involved, especially in the posterior auricular folds. In elderly patients, scabies can cause intense pruritus with subtle skin findings, making it a challenge to diagnose. In immunocompromised patients, there may be widespread nonpruritic scaling (particularly on the palms and soles in adults and on the scalp in children).

Other forms: Crusted (Norwegian) scabies is due to an impaired host immune response, allowing mites to proliferate and number in the millions. Nodular scabies is more common in infants and young children and may be due to hypersensitivity to retained

TABLE 121–1. TREATMENT OPTIONS FOR SCABIES AND LICE

DISEASE	AGENT	INSTRUCTIONS	COMMENTS
Scabies	Permethrin 5% (60 g) cream	Apply to whole body; wash off after 8–14 h	1st line treatment; re-treat in 1 wk; can cause stinging and itching
	Lindane 1% (60 mL) lotion	Apply to whole body; wash off after 8–12 h in adults, 6 h in children	Avoid in children < 2 yr, pregnant or lactating women, those with extensive dermatitis, and those with severe skin conditions with skin barrier compromise; potentially neurotoxic. Repeat in 1 wk
	Ivermectin	200 μg/kg po for 1 dose; repeat in 7–10 days	Indicated as a 2nd line to permethrin For use in institutional epidemics and immunocompromised hosts. Caution should be used when given to elderly patients with hepatic, renal, or cardiac disease May cause tachycardia Not recommended for pregnant or lactating women; safety in children < 15 kg or < 5 yr is unproven
	Crotamiton 10% cream/ lotion	Apply after bath to whole body, apply 2nd dose after 24 h, and bathe 48 h after 2nd dose	Repeat in 7 to 10 days
	Sulfur ointment 6%	Apply to whole body at bedtime for 3 nights	Very effective and safe; may be limited by its malodor
Lice			
Head	Malathion 0.5%	Apply to dry hair and scalp, wash and rinse in 8–12 h, shampoo scalp, remove nits	May re-treat in 7–9 days, if live nits are seen Unpleasant odor
	Permethrin and other pyrethroids, pyrethrins	Wash hair and apply to wet hair, behind ears and on nape, wash off in 10 min	May re-treat in 7 days, if live nits are seen Contraindicated if sensitive to chrysanthemum family of plants
	Wet combing	Should be combined with all of the therapies	
	Lindane 1% shampoo or lotion	Lather for 4–5 min, rinse, comb with fine-tooth comb or apply lotion and wash off after 12 h	Repeat in 1 wk Resistance is increasing Toxicity not typically seen with treatment of head lice but avoid in children < 2 yr and in pregnant or lactating women Do not use lindane on eyelashes
	Ivermectin	Same dose as scabies	Useful for resistant lice
Body		Topical measures not used, since body lice are found in clothing. Treat pruritus and secondary infection	

TABLE 121–1. TREATMENT OPTIONS FOR SCABIES AND LICE—Continued

DISEASE	AGENT	INSTRUCTIONS	COMMENTS
Pubic	Lindane 1% (60 ml) shampoo/lotion	Same as head lice	
	Pyrethrins with piperonyl butoxide (60 ml) shampoo	Apply to dry hair and skin, leave on for 10 min, rinse, repeat in 7–10 days	Do not apply more than twice in 24 h Pyrethrins are derivative of chrysanthemum and are combined with a piperic acid derivative (piperonyl butoxide)
	Permethrin 1% (60 ml) cream	Same as head lice	Must re-treat in 10 days
Eyelashes	Petrolatum ointment	Apply 3–4 times/day for 8–10 days	
	Fluorescein drops 10–20%	Applied to the eyelids	Provides immediate pediculocidal effect

organisms. Bullous scabies occurs more commonly in children. When it occurs in the elderly, it can mimic bullous pemphigoid, resulting in a delay in diagnosis. Scalp scabies occurs in infants and immunocompromised hosts and can mimic seborrheic dermatitis. Scabies incognito is a widespread atypical form resulting from application of topical corticosteroids.

Diagnosis is suspected by physical findings, especially burrows, and confirmed by mite, ova, or fecal pellets on microscopic examination of burrow scrapings. Scrapings should be obtained by placing glycerol, mineral oil, or immersion oil over a burrow or papule (to prevent dispersion of mites and material during scraping), which is then unroofed with the edge of a scalpel. The material is then placed on a slide and covered with a coverslip; potassium hydroxide should be avoided because it dissolves fecal pellets.

Treatment

Primary treatment is topical or oral scabicides (see TABLE 121–1). Permethrin is the 1st-line topical drug.

Older children and adults should apply permethrin or lindane to the entire body from the neck down and wash it off after 8 to 14 h. Treatments should be repeated in 7 days.

For infants and young children, permethrin should be applied to the head and neck, avoiding periorbital and perioral regions. Special attention should be given to intertriginous areas, fingernails, toenails, and umbilicus. Mittens on infants can keep permethrin out of the mouth. Lindane is not recommended in children < 2 yr and in patients with a seizure disorder because of potential neurotoxicity.

Precipitated sulfur 6 to 10% in petrolatum, applied for 24 h for 3 consecutive days, is safe and effective.

Ivermectin is indicated for patients who do not respond to topical treatment, are unable to adhere to topical regimens, or are immunocompromised with Norwegian scabies. Ivermectin has been used with success in epidemics involving close contacts, such as nursing homes. Close contacts should also be treated, and personal items (eg, towels, clothing, bedding) should be washed or isolated for at least 3 days.

Pruritus can be treated with corticosteroid ointments and/or oral antihistamines (eg, hydroxyzine 25 mg po qid). Secondary infection should be considered in patients with weeping, yellow-crusted lesions and treated with the appropriate systemic or topical antistaphylococcal and antistreptococcal antibiotic.

Symptoms and lesions take up to 3 wk to resolve despite killing of the mites, making failed treatment due to resistance, poor penetration, incompletely applied therapy, reinfection, or nodular scabies difficult to recognize. Skin scrapings can diagnose persistent scabies.

122 VIRAL SKIN DISEASES

Many systemic viral infections cause skin lesions. Molluscum contagiosum and warts are the 2 most common primary viral skin diseases without systemic manifestations. Herpes simplex virus infection is discussed in detail in Ch. 189 (see p. 1606).

MOLLUSCUM CONTAGIOSUM

Molluscum contagiosum is clusters of smooth, waxy, or pearly umbilicated papules 1 to 5 mm in diameter caused by molluscum contagiosum virus, a poxvirus.

Transmission is by direct contact; spread occurs by autoinoculation. Molluscum contagiosum can appear anywhere on the body except the palms and soles; lesions occur most commonly on the face, trunk, and extremities (children) and on the pubis, penis, or vulva (adults). Lesions may grow to 10 to 15 mm in diameter, especially in HIV and other immunocompromised patients, and yet remain asymptomatic.

Diagnosis is based on clinical appearance; hematoxylin and eosin staining of expressed fluid demonstrates inclusion bodies but is necessary only when diagnosis is uncertain. Differential diagnosis includes folliculitis, milia, and warts (for smaller lesions < 2 mm) and juvenile xanthogranuloma and Spitz nevus (for larger lesions > 2 mm).

Most lesions spontaneously regress in 6 to 9 mo, but they can remain for 2 to 3 yr. Treatment is indicated for cosmetic reasons or for prevention of sexual spread. Options include curettage, cryosurgery, laser therapy, electrocautery, trichloroacetic acid (25 to 40% solution), cantharidin, tretinoin, and imiquimod 5% cream. Especially in children, treatments producing minimal pain are used first, such as tretinoin, imiquimod, and cantharidin. Curettage or liquid nitrogen can be used after application of a topical anesthetic such as EMLA or 4% lidocaine cream. In adults, curettage is very effective but painful. Dermatologists often use combination therapy such as liquid nitrogen or cantharidin in the office and imiquimod cream at home. This form of therapy is typically successful after 1 to 2 mo in most patients.

Nondermatologists should feel comfortable using imiquimod cream. The cream is applied at night, 1 drop to each molluscum and rubbed in well, until the cream turns clear. The area is washed with soap and water. The cream can be applied 3 to 7 times/wk. Molluscum within the orbital rim should not be treated, and molluscum in the genital region can easily become irritated. Lesions should be treated until they develop a scant amount of redness; weeping and crusting should be avoided.

Cantharidin is safe and effective but can cause blistering. Cantharidin is applied in 1 small drop directly to the molluscum lesion. Areas that the patient (especially children) may rub are covered with a band-aid, because contact with the fingers should be avoided. Cantharidin should not be applied to the face or near the eyes since blistering is unpredictable. If cantharidin comes into contact with the cornea, it can scar the cornea. Cantharidin should be washed off with soap and water in 6 h. Parents should be warned about blistering. Overall, cantharidin has a very high parent and child satisfaction rate.

WARTS

Warts (verrucae vulgaris) are common, benign epidermal lesions associated with human papillomavirus infection. They can appear anywhere on the body in a variety of morphologies. Diagnosis is by examination. Warts are usually self-limited but may be treated by excision, cautery, cryotherapy, liquid nitrogen, and topical or injected agents.

Warts are almost universal in the population and affect all ages but are most frequent in children and uncommon in the elderly. Warts are caused by human papillomavirus (HPV) infection; at least 70 HPV types are linked to skin lesions. Trauma and maceration facilitate initial epidermal inoculation. Spread may then occur by autoinoculation. Local and systemic immune factors appear to influence spread; immunosuppressed patients (especially HIV and renal transplant patients) are at particular risk for developing generalized lesions that are difficult to treat.

TABLE 122–1. WART VARIANTS AND CLINICAL CORRELATIONS

CLINICAL FORM	HUMAN PAPILLOMAVIRUS	CLINICAL CORRELATIONS
Bowenoid papulosis	16, 18, 33, 39	Flat brown verrucous papules on the vulva and penis (benign); affected women and women partners should be followed closely for cervical cancer
Buschke Lowenstein tumor	6, 11	Large cauliflower-like tumors
Butcher's (meat handler's)	7	Common warts, usually benign
Cutaneous squamous cell carcinoma	38, 41, 48	Early lesions can mimic warts
Epidermodysplasia verruciformis	1–5, 7–9, 10, 12, 14, 15, 17–20, 23–25, 36, 47, 50	May develop cutaneous malignancy such as squamous cell carcinoma
Keratoacanthoma	77	Thought to be a well differentiated squamous cell carcinoma
Oral focal epithelial hyperplasia (Heck's disease)	13, 32	Benign
Warts in renal transplant patients	75–77	Often multiple and difficult to treat

Humoral immunity provides resistance to HPV infection, although cellular immunity helps established infection to regress.

Symptoms and Signs

Warts are named by their clinical appearance and location; different forms are linked to different HPV types. Unusual manifestations are listed in TABLE 122–1.

Common warts (verrucae vulgaris) are caused by HPV 1, 2, 4, 27, and 29. Generally, they are asymptomatic but sometimes cause mild pain, especially when they are located on a weight-bearing surface such as the bottom of the feet. They are sharply demarcated, rough, round or irregular, firm, and light gray, yellow, brown, or gray-black nodules 2 to 10 mm in diameter. They appear most often on sites subject to trauma (eg, fingers, elbows, knees, face) but may spread elsewhere. Variants of unusual shape (eg, pedunculated or resembling a cauliflower) are most frequent on the head and neck, especially the scalp and beard.

Filiform warts are long, narrow, frondlike growths usually on the eyelids, face, neck, or lips. They too are usually asymptomatic. This morphologically distinct variant of the common wart is benign and easy to treat.

Flat warts, caused by HPV 3, 10, 28, and 49, are smooth, flat-topped, yellow-brown papules most often on the face and along scratch marks; they are more common in children and young adults and develop by autoinoculation. They generally cause no symptoms but can be difficult to treat.

Palmar and plantar warts, caused by HPV 1, are warts on the palms and soles flattened by pressure and surrounded by cornified epithelium. They are often tender and can make walking and standing uncomfortable. They can be distinguished from corns and calluses by their tendency to pinpoint bleeding when the surface is pared away. Classically, warts hurt with "side to side" pressure, and calluses hurt with direct pressure; in reality, this is not a reliable sign.

Mosaic warts are plaques formed by the coalescence of myriad smaller, closely set plantar warts. As with other plantar warts, they are often tender.

Periungual warts appear as thickened, fissured cauliflower-like skin around the nail plate. Patients frequently lose the cuticle and are susceptible to paronychia. These warts are more common in patients who bite their nails.

Genital warts manifest as discrete flat to broad-based smooth to velvety papules on the perineal, perirectal, labial, and penile areas. Infection with high-risk HPV types (most notably types 16 and 18) are the main causes of cervical cancer. They are generally asymptomatic.

Diagnosis

Diagnosis is based on clinical appearance; biopsy is rarely needed. A cardinal sign of warts is the absence of skin lines crossing their surface and the presence of pinpoint black dots (thrombosed capillaries) or bleeding when warts are shaved. Differential diagnosis includes corns (clavi), lichen planus, seborrheic keratosis, skin tags, and squamous cell carcinomas. DNA typing is available in some medical centers but is generally not needed.

Prognosis and Treatment

Many warts regress spontaneously; others persist for years and recur at the same or different sites, even with treatment. Factors influencing recurrence appear to be related to the patient's overall immune status as well as local factors. Patients who subject themselves to local trauma (eg, athletes, mechanics, butchers) can have recalcitrant and recurrent HPV. Genital HPV infection has malignant potential, but (except in immunosuppressed patients) malignant transformation has not been generally observed in HPV-induced skin warts.

Treatment is aimed at eliciting an immune response to HPV. In most instances, this is achieved by applying an irritant (eg, salicylic acid [SCA], trichloroacetic acid, 5-fluorouracil, podophyllum resin, tretinoin, cantharidin).

These compounds can be used in combination or with a destructive method (eg, cryosurgery, electrocautery, curettage, excision, laser). Direct antiviral effects can be achieved with bleomycin and interferon-α2b, but these treatments are reserved for the most recalcitrant warts. Topical imiquimod 5% cream induces skin cells to locally produce antiviral cytokines. Topical cidofovir, HPV vaccines, and contact immunotherapy (eg, squaric acid dibutyl ester and *Candida* allergen) have been used to treat warts. Oral treatments include cimetidine, isotretinoin, and oral zinc. In most instances, modalities should be combined to increase the likelihood of success.

Common warts: In immunocompetent hosts, common warts usually spontaneously regress within 2 yr, but some linger for many years. Numerous treatments are available. Destructive methods include electrocautery, cryosurgery with liquid nitrogen, and SCA preparations. Application of these methods varies depending upon the location and severity of involvement. For example, 17% liquid SCA can be used on the fingers, and 40% plaster SCA can be used on the soles.

The most common topical agent to be used is SCA. SCA is available in a liquid, plaster, or impregnated within tape. Patients apply SCA to their warts at night and leave on for 8 to 48 h depending on the site.

Cantharidin can be used alone or in combination (1%) with SCA (3%) podophyllum (2%) in a collodion base. Cantharidin alone is removed with soap and water after 6 h; cantharidin with SCA or podophyllum is removed in 2 h. The longer these agents are left in contact with the skin, the more brisk the blistering response.

Cryosurgery is painful but extremely effective. Electrodesiccation with curettage and/or laser surgery is effective and indicated for isolated lesions but may cause scarring. Recurrent or new warts occur in about 35% of patients within 1 yr, so methods that scar should be avoided as much as possible.

Filiform warts: Treatment is removal with scalpel, scissors, curettage, or liquid nitrogen. Liquid nitrogen should be applied so that up to 2 mm of skin surrounding the wart turns white. Damage to the skin occurs when the skin thaws, which usually takes 10 to 20 sec. Blisters can occur 24 to 48 h after treatment with liquid nitrogen. Care must be taken when treating cosmetically sensitive sites, such as the face and neck, since hypopigmentation frequently occurs after treatment with liquid nitrogen. Patients with darkly pigmented skin can develop permanent depigmentation.

Flat warts: Treatment is daily tretinoin (retinoic acid 0.05% cream). If peeling is not sufficient for wart removal, another irritant (eg, 5% benzoyl peroxide) or 5% SCA cream can be applied sequentially with tretinoin. Imiquimod 5% cream can be used alone or in combination with topical drugs or destructive measures. Topical 5-fluorouracil (1% or 5% cream) can also be used. Spontaneous resolution may follow unprovoked inflammation of the lesions; however, flat warts are frequently recalcitrant to treatment.

Plantar warts: Treatment is vigorous maceration with 40% SCA plaster kept in place for several days. The wart is debrided while damp and soft, then destroyed by freezing or using caustics (eg, 30 to 70% trichloroacetic acid). Other destructive treatments (eg, CO_2 laser, pulsed-dye laser, various acids) are often effective. Duct tape is effective when applied for 6-day intervals, followed by debridement of macerated tissue.

Periungual: Combination therapy with liquid nitrogen and imiquimod 5% cream, tretinoin, or SCA is effective.

Refractory: Several methods whose long-term value and risks are not fully known are available for recalcitrant warts. Intralesional injection of small amounts of a 0.1% solution of bleomycin in saline often cures stubborn plantar and periungual warts. However, injected digits may develop Raynaud's phenomenon or vascular damage (especially when injected at the base of the digit), warranting caution. Interferon, especially interferon-α, administered intralesionally (3 times/wk for 3 to 5 wk) or IM, has also cleared recalcitrant skin and genital warts. Extensive warts sometimes improve or clear with oral isotretinoin or acitretin. Cimetidine at doses up to 800 mg po tid has been used with success but is more effective when combined with another therapy.

ZOONOTIC DISEASES

Two viral skin diseases are rarely transmitted from animals to humans.

Contagious ecthyma: Contagious ecthyma (contagious pustular dermatitis) is caused by orf virus, a poxvirus that infects ruminants (most often sheep and goats). Farmers, veterinarians, zoo caretakers, and others with direct animal contact are at risk. The cutaneous findings pass through 6 stages that last about 1 wk: (1) papular, a single red edematous papule appears on a finger (most commonly right index finder); (2) target, a larger nodule with a red center surrounded by a white ring with a red periphery; (3) acute, a rapidly growing infected-looking tumor; (4) regenerative, a nodule with black dots covered with a thin transparent crust; (5) papillomatous, a nodule with a surface studded with small projections; (6) regressive, a nodule flattened with a thick crust. Patients can develop regional adenopathy, lymphangitis, and fever.

Diagnosis is by history of contact; differential diagnosis is extensive depending upon the stage of the lesion. Acute lesions must be differentiated from milker's nodules, mycobacterium marinum, and bacterial infection; regressed lesions must be differentiated from cutaneous tumors, such as Bowen's disease or squamous cell carcinoma. Lesions spontaneously heal; no treatment is necessary.

Milker's nodules: These are caused by paravaccinia virus, a parapoxvirus that causes udder lesions in cows. Infection requires direct contact and produces macules that progress to papules, vesicles, and nodules; 6 stages have been described similar to contagious ecthyma. Fever and lymphadenopathy are uncommon. Diagnosis is by history of contact and cutaneous findings. Differential diagnosis varies depending upon morphology but includes primary inoculation TB, sporotrichosis, anthrax, and tularemia. Lesions heal spontaneously; no treatment is necessary.

123 PIGMENTATION DISORDERS

Pigmentation disorders involve hypopigmentation, depigmentation, or hyperpigmentation. Areas may be focal or diffuse.

Focal hypopigmentation is most commonly a consequence of injury, inflammatory dermatoses such as atopic dermatitis and psoriasis (postinflammatory hypopigmentation), burns, or chemical exposure. Focal hypo- or depigmentation is also a feature of vitiligo (which may involve large areas of skin), leprosy, nutritional deficiencies (kwashiorkor), and genetic conditions (tuberous sclerosis, piebaldism, Waardenburg's syndrome). Hypopigmentation can also be diffuse; the most important causes are albinism and vitiligo.

ALBINISM

Albinism (officially called oculocutaneous albinism) is an inherited defect in melanin formation that causes diffuse hypopigmentation of the skin, hair, and eyes; deficiency of melanin (and hence pigmentary dilution) may be total or partial, but all areas of the skin are involved. Ocular involvement produces strabismus, nystagmus, and decreased vision. Diagnosis is usually obvious from the skin, but ocular evaluation is necessary. No treatment for the skin involvement is available other than protection from sunlight.

Epidemiology, Symptoms, and Signs

Oculocutaneous albinism (OCA) is a group of rare inherited disorders in which melanocytes are present but melanin production is absent or greatly decreased. Cutaneous and ocular pathologies (ocular albinism) are both present. Ocular albinism is decreased retinal pigmentation with nystagmus, strabismus, reduced visual acuity, and monocular vision; these abnormalities result from abnormal optic tract CNS development manifested by foveal hypoplasia with decreased photoreceptors and misrouting of optic chiasmal fibers. Ocular albinism may occur without cutaneous abnormalities.

There are 4 main genetic forms, which have a variety of phenotypes. Almost all are autosomal recessive.

Type I OCA is caused by absent (OCA1A; 40% of all OCA) or reduced (OCA1B) tyrosinase activity; tyrosinase catalyzes several steps in melanin synthesis. OCA1A is the classic tyrosinase-negative albinism: skin and hair are milky white; eyes are blue-gray. Pigmentary dilution in OCA1B ranges from obvious to subtle.

Type II OCA (50% of all OCA) is caused by mutations in the P ("pink-eyed") gene. The function of the P protein is not yet known. Tyrosinase activity is present. There is a range of phenotypes with pigmentary dilution from minimal to moderate. Pigmented nevi and lentigines may develop with sun exposure; some lentigines may become large and dark.

Type III OCA occurs only in blacks. It is caused by mutations in a tyrosinase-related protein 1 gene whose product is important in eumelanin synthesis. Skin is brown; hair is rufous (reddish).

Type IV OCA is an extremely rare form in which the genetic defect is in a gene that codes a membrane transporter protein; the phenotype is similar to OCA2.

In a group of inherited diseases, clinical OCA occurs with bleeding disorders. In the Hermansky-Pudlak syndrome, OCA is seen in combination with platelet abnormalities and a ceroid-lipofuscin lysosomal storage disease. This syndrome is rare except in those with family origin in Puerto Rico, where its incidence is 1 in 1800. In the Chédiak-Higashi syndrome, OCA occurs (hair is silvery-gray), and a decrease in platelet dense granules results in a bleeding diathesis. Patients have severe immunodeficiency due to abnormal lymphocyte lytic granules. Progressive neurologic degeneration occurs.

Diagnosis and Treatment

Diagnosis of all types of OCA is obvious from examination of the skin, but detection of iris translucency, reduced retinal pigmentation, foveal hypoplasia, reduced visual acuity, and ocular movement disorders (strabismus and nystagmus) is necessary. Some surgical interventions may improve ocular movement disorders.

There is no treatment for albinism. Patients are at high risk for sunburn and skin cancers and should avoid sunlight, use sunglasses (with UV filtration), and use sunscreen with an SPF of ≥ 30 (see p. 962).

VITILIGO

Vitiligo is a loss of skin melanocytes that causes areas of skin depigmentation of varying sizes. Cause is unknown, but the condition may be autoimmune, as up to ⅓ of patients have evidence of other autoimmune disease. Diagnosis is often obvious on examination. Treatment often involves topical corticosteroids, psoralens plus ultraviolet A, or for severe widespread pigment loss, depigmentation ("bleaching") of residual patches of normal skin with hydroquinone.

Epidemiology and Etiology

Vitiligo affects 0.5 to 2% of the population. Etiology is unknown, but melanocytes are lacking in affected areas; some patients have antibodies to melanin. Up to 30% have other autoimmune antibodies (to thyroglobulin, adrenal cells, and parietal cells) or clinical autoimmune endocrinopathies (Addison's disease, diabetes mellitus, pernicious anemia, and thyroid dysfunction), leading to speculation that vitiligo is an autoimmune disease. However, the relationship is unclear and may be coincidental. The strongest association is with hyperthyroidism (Graves' disease) and hypothyroidism (Hashimoto's thyroiditis).

Vitiligo is both familial (autosomal dominant, with incomplete penetrance and variable expression) and acquired. Occasionally, it is the result of a direct physical injury to the involved skin (Koebner phenomenon, eg, in response to sunburn), and some patients may associate the onset with emotionally stressful life events.

Symptoms and Signs

Vitiligo is characterized by depigmented areas, usually sharply demarcated and often symmetric. Depigmentation may involve 1 or 2 spots (focal vitiligo), entire body segments (segmental vitiligo), or rarely most of the skin surface (universal vitiligo). However, vitiligo most commonly involves the face (especially around the orifices), digits, dorsal hands, flexor wrists, elbows, knees, shins, dorsal ankles, armpits, inguinal area, anogenital area, umbilicus, and nipples. Cosmetic disfigurement can be especially devastating in dark-skinned patients. Hair in vitiliginous areas is usually white.

Diagnosis and Treatment

Diagnosis is obvious on examination. Skin lesions are accentuated under Wood's light. Differential diagnosis includes postinflammatory hypopigmentation, morphea, leprosy, chemical leukoderma, and leukoderma due to melanoma. A work-up for autoimmune endocrine disease is probably unnecessary unless symptoms or signs suggest a particular disorder.

Treatment is supportive and cosmetic. Physicians must be aware of individual and ethnic sensibilities regarding uniform skin coloring; the disease can be psychologically devastating. All depigmented areas are prone to severe sunburn and must be protected with clothing or sunscreen.

Small, scattered lesions may be camouflaged with makeup. More extensive involvement requires potent topical corticosteroids, which, however, can cause hypopigmentation or atrophy in normal surrounding skin. Oral and topical psoralen plus ultraviolet A (PUVA) is often successful, although hundreds of treatments may be necessary. Khellin (in combination with PUVA) should be avoided because of hepatic toxicity. More specialized phototherapy regimens using narrowband UVB or excimer laser are under investigation. Narrowband UVB is as effective as topical PUVA and has few adverse effects.

Surgery is most reasonable for patients with stable, limited disease for whom medical therapy has failed. Therapies include autologous micrografting or suction blister grafting, as well as tattooing (the latter especially useful for difficult-to-repigment areas such as the nipples, lips, and fingertips).

Depigmentation of unaffected skin to achieve homogenous skin tone is possible with 20% monobenzyl ether of hydroquinone applied bid and is indicated when most of the skin is involved and the patient is prepared for permanent pigment loss. This treatment can be extremely irritating so a smaller test area should be treated before widespread use. Treatment for ≥ 1 yr may be required.

HYPERPIGMENTATION

Hyperpigmentation has multiple causes and may be focal or diffuse. Most but not all cases are due to an increase in melanin production and deposition. Focal hyperpigmentation is most often postinflammatory in nature, occurring after injury (eg, cuts and burns) or other causes of inflammation (eg, acne, lupus). There are also systemic and neoplastic causes.

Melasma (chloasma) consists of dark brown, sharply marginated, roughly symmetric patches of hyperpigmentation on the face (usually on the forehead, temples, and cheeks). It occurs primarily in pregnant women (melasma gravidarum, the mask of pregnancy) and in women taking oral contraceptives. Ten percent of cases occur in nonpregnant women and dark-skinned men. Melasma is more prevalent in Latinos and blacks. The mechanism is unknown, but all cases are associated with sun exposure. In women, melasma fades slowly and incompletely after childbirth or cessation of hormone use. In men, melasma rarely fades. Avoiding the sun keeps the condition from worsening. Treatment depends on whether the pigmentation is epidermal or dermal; epidermal pigmentation accentuates on Wood's light or can be diagnosed with biopsy. Only epidermal pigmentation responds to treatment. Hydroquinone 3% to 4% applied bid is often effective, but long courses are usually required; 2%

hydroquinone is useful as maintenance. Hydroquinone should be tested behind one ear or on a small patch on the forearm for 1 wk before use on the face because it may cause irritation. Bleaching agents, such as 0.1% tretinoin and azelaic acid 15 to 20% cream, can be used in place of or with hydroquinone. Chemical peeling with glycolic acid or 30 to 50% trichloroacetic acid is an option for patients with severe melasma unresponsive to topical bleaching agents.

Lentigines (singular: lentigo) are flat, tan to brown oval spots in sun-exposed areas, typically the face and back of the hands. They occur most commonly on the face and hands and are most commonly due to chronic sun exposure (solar lentigines; sometimes called "liver spots"). They are treated with cryotherapy or laser. Non-solar lentigines are sometimes associated with systemic disorders, as with Peutz-Jeghers syndrome (in which profuse lentigines of the lips occur) or multiple lentigines syndrome (Leopard syndrome); treatment is the same.

Diffuse hyperpigmentation can be caused by systemic disorders, especially Addison's disease (see p. 1207), hemochromatosis (see p. 1132), and primary biliary cirrhosis (see p. 218). Skin findings are nondiagnostic as to cause.

Drug-induced hyperpigmentation is usually diffuse but sometimes has drug-specific distribution patterns or hues (see TABLE 123–1). Mechanisms include increased melanin in the epidermis (tends to be more brown, hence "hyperpigmented"), melanin in the epidermis and high dermis (mostly brown with hints of gray or blue), increased melanin in the dermis (tends to be more grayish or blue), and dermal deposition of the drug or metabolite (usually

TABLE 123–1. HYPERPIGMENTATION EFFECTS OF SOME DRUGS AND CHEMICALS

DRUG OR CHEMICAL	EFFECT
Amiodarone	Slate-gray to violaceous discoloration of sun-exposed areas; yellowish-brown deposits in the dermis
Antimalarials	Yellow-brown to gray to bluish black discoloration of pretibial areas, face, oral cavity, and nails; drug-melanin complexes in the dermis; hemosiderin around capillaries
Bleomycin	Flagellate hyperpigmented streaks on the back, often in areas of scratching or minor trauma
Cancer chemotherapy agents, including busulfan, cyclophosphamide, dactinomycin, daunorubicin, and 5-FU	Diffuse hyperpigmentation
Desipramine and imipramine	Grayish blue discoloration on sun-exposed areas; golden-brown granules in upper dermis
Heavy metals	
Bismuth	Blue-gray discoloration of face, neck, and hands
Gold	Blue-gray deposits around the eyes (chrysiasis)
Mercury	Slate-gray discoloration of skin folds
Silver	Diffuse slate-gray discoloration (argyria), especially in sun-exposed areas
Hydroquinone	Bluish black discoloration of ear cartilage and face after long-term use (years)
Phenothiazines, including chlorpromazine	Grayish blue discoloration on sun-exposed areas; golden-brown granules in upper dermis
Tetracyclines, including minocycline	Grayish discoloration of teeth, nails, sclerae, oral mucosa, acne cysts, acne scars, and diffusely on the face

slate or bluish gray). Focal hyperpigmentation frequently follows drug-induced lichen planus (also known as lichenoid drug reactions).

In **fixed drug eruptions,** red plaques or blisters form at the same site each time a drug is taken; residual postinflammatory hyperpigmentation usually persists. Typical lesions occur on the face (especially lips), hands, feet, and genitals. Typical inciting agents include sulfonamides, tetracycline, NSAIDs (especially phenazone derivatives), barbiturates, and carbamazepine.

124 HAIR DISORDERS

Hair grows in cycles. Each cycle consists of a long growing phase (anagen) followed by a short resting phase (telogen). At the end of resting phase, the hair falls out (catagen) and a new hair starts growing in the follicle, beginning the cycle again. Eyebrows and eyelashes have a growing phase of 1 to 6 mo, and scalp hairs of 2 to 6 yr. Normally, about 100 scalp hairs reach the end of resting phase each day and fall out. When significantly more than 100 hairs/day go into resting phase (telogen effluvium), clinical hair loss may occur.

Hair growth in both men and women is regulated by androgens. Testosterone stimulates hair growth in the pubic area and underarms. Dihydrotestosterone stimulates beard hair growth.

Hair disorders include alopecia, hirsutism, and pseudofolliculitis barbae. Although most hair disorders are not serious, they are often perceived as major cosmetic issues that demand treatment. Dandruff is not a hair disorder but rather seborrheic dermatitis of the scalp (see p. 960).

ALOPECIA

(Baldness)

Alopecia has multiple causes. Diagnosis of cause can sometimes be made by gross and microscopic examination of hair. Treatment is of underlying cause.

Most alopecia is a concern for cosmetic and psychologic reasons, but it is occasionally the primary sign of an important systemic disease.

Etiology

Alopecia can be nonscarring and diffuse, nonscarring and focal, or scarring and focal.

Nonscarring diffuse loss: Causes include male-pattern baldness, female-pattern baldness, telogen effluvium, anagen effluvium, primary hair shaft abnormalities, and congenital disorders.

Male-pattern baldness (androgenetic alopecia) is common, familial, and androgenetic. Hair loss begins at the temples and/or vertex and can spread to diffuse thinning or nearly complete loss. Female-pattern baldness is hair thinning in the frontal, parietal, and crown regions. This too is androgenetic.

Telogen effluvium refers to loss of scalp hair caused by synchronicity of hair cycle so that many hairs enter the resting or telogen phase at once. At the end of this resting phase, usually several months after the inciting event, a significant increase in hair shedding is noticed. Drugs are a common cause, especially antiproliferative chemotherapeutic agents, warfarin, H_2-blockers, oral contraceptives, ACE inhibitors, β-blockers, and lithium. Other drugs that can precipitate telogen effluvium are fluorobutyrophenone, clofibrate, bezafibrate, trimethadione, valproate, captopril, penicillamine, ibuprofen, interferon, ranitidine, sulindac, tamoxifen, terfenadine, and thiamphenicol. Telogen effluvium is also common with nutritional deficiencies, after physiologic or psychologic stress (surgery, systemic illness), and with pathologic (hypothyroidism or hyperthyroidism) or physiologic (postpartum, menopause) endocrine changes.

Anagen effluvium refers to loss of scalp hair in its growth (or anagen) phase. Radiation and chemotherapeutic agents are the most common causes, but it can occur with mercury, thallium, boric acid, and vitamin A poisoning.

Primary hair shaft abnormalities (trichodystrophies) include a variety of disorders that lead to unruly or unusually wooly hair or to fractures of the hair shaft. In trichorrhexis invaginata, hairs have a ball and cup invagination (bamboo hair). This hair abnormality can occur in association with ichthyosis in the rare autosomal recessive Netherton syndrome. Bubble hair, in which bubbles are seen in the hair shaft, may occur with excessive use of hair dryers. Trichonodosis or knotting of hair occurs with excess rubbing or scratching. Monilethrix is an uncommon autosomal dominant condition that causes beaded and very brittle hair.

Other congenital disorders of the hair include wooly hair nevus (tightly coiled hair over all or portions of the scalp), the uncombable hair syndrome (scalp hair that resists all efforts to comb or brush it), trichorrhexis nodosa (hair shafts break easily and broken stumps are present over large portions of the scalp), and trichothiodystrophy (brittle hair from a defect in sulfur metabolism).

Nonscarring focal loss: Common causes include traction alopecia, tinea capitis, trichotillomania, and alopecia areata (see p. 1007). Uncommon causes include syphilis and primary hair shaft abnormalities.

Traction alopecia is hair loss primarily at the frontal and/or temporal hairline due to traction from braids, rollers, or ponytails. Tinea capitis, hair shaft infection with *Trichophyton tonsurans*, is discussed on p. 989; other less common causes of tinea capitis include *Microsporum canis, M. audouinii*, and *T. schoenleinii*. Trichotillomania—focal hair loss due to hair pulling, twisting, or teasing—is symptomatic of an obsessive-compulsive disorder (see p. 1673).

Late secondary syphilis causes hair loss ranging from localized patches to total alopecia. It may follow the distribution of the preceding exanthem. The serology is always positive. Examination reveals focal yellow-red areas with a moth-eaten appearance.

Scarring focal loss: Scarring refers to obliteration of the hair follicle with fibrosis. Scarring loss is most often due to unusual primary disorders, such as lichen planopilaris (lichen planus of the scalp), folliculitis decalvans (an idiopathic scarring alopecia associated with pustules and intact hairs clumped in a "tufted" pattern), and pseudopelade of Brocq (a particular pattern of scarring alopecia). Other causes include burns, trauma, radiation therapy, severe primary (kerion) or secondary (syphilis) infections, sarcoidosis, lupus erythematosus, and skin malignancy.

Symptoms, Signs, and Diagnosis

Symptoms, other than hair loss, are often absent and, when present (eg, itching, burning, tingling), are not specific to any cause. Except in alopecia areata (see p. 1007), some cases of infection (kerion, syphilis), lichen planus, and dissecting cellulitis of the scalp (folliculitis abscedens et suffodiens), signs of hair loss are nondiagnostic. If scarring is noted, examination should include the entire skin surface and mucous membranes to detect lesions associated with systemic disease.

Male-pattern baldness generally requires no testing. When it occurs in young males without a family history, the physician should question the patient about anabolic steroid use and other drugs. In women with significant hair loss and evidence of virilization, testosterone and dehydroepiandrosterone sulfate levels should be measured.

The "pull" test helps evaluate diffuse scalp hair loss; gentle traction is exerted on 40 to 60 hairs on at least 3 areas of the scalp, and the number of extracted hairs is counted and examined microscopically. Normally, < 6 telogen-phase hairs should come out. Extraction of > 6 hairs in telogen phase is abnormal and suggestive of telogen effluvium.

The "pluck" test is similar except that hairs are abruptly, painfully extracted. The pluck test helps diagnose a defect of telogen or anagen or an occult systemic disease.

Microscopic examination of hair from either test or from hair cuttings is almost always helpful. Anagen hairs have sheaths attached to their roots; telogen hairs have tiny bulbs without sheaths at their roots. Normally, 85 to 90% of hairs are in the anagen phase; about 10 to 15% are in telogen phase; and < 1% are in catagen phase. Telogen effluvium shows an increased percentage of telogen hairs, whereas anagen effluvium shows a decrease in telogen hairs and easy breakage. A high percentage of hairs in the catagen phase (a transitional phase between growth and rest) and trichomalacia are pathognomonic for trichotillomania. Primary hair shaft abnormalities, such as trichorrhexis invaginata and monilethrix, are usually obvious on microscopic evaluation of the hair shaft.

Scalp biopsy is indicated when alopecia persists and diagnosis is in doubt; biopsy may differentiate scarring from nonscarring forms. Specimens should be taken from an area of active inflammation, ideally at the border of a bald patch. Fungal and bacterial cultures may be useful; immunofluorescence studies may help identify lupus erythematosus, lichen planopilaris, and systemic sclerosis.

Daily hair counts can be performed by the patient to quantify hair loss when the pull test is negative. Scalp hair counts of > 100 are abnormal except after shampooing, when hair counts of up to 250 may be normal. Hairs may be brought in by the patient for microscopic examination of hair shafts and bulbs.

Treatment

Male-pattern baldness: Most treatments for hair loss have been developed for male-pattern baldness because it is so prevalent.

Minoxidil prolongs the anagen phase and may increase blood flow to the follicle; 1 mL of 2% or 5% topical drug applied bid to the scalp is most effective for vertex alopecia in male-pattern baldness affecting men or women. However, at most 30 to 40% of patients experience significant hair growth, and minoxidil is generally not effective or indicated for other causes except possibly alopecia areata. Hair growth may not be seen until 6 to 9 mo; common practice is to continue treatment as long as positive results persist.

Finasteride inhibits 5-α reductase enzyme, blocking conversion of testosterone to dihydrotestosterone, and is useful for male-pattern baldness. Finasteride 1 mg po once/day stimulates scalp hair growth. Adverse effects include decreased libido, erectile dysfunction, ejaculation disorder, and decreased ejaculate volume in about 1% of patients. The drug is not indicated for women and is contraindicated in pregnant women. Hair growth may not be seen until 6 mo; common practice is to continue treatment for 24 mo as long as positive results persist. Once treatment is discontinued, hair loss returns to previous levels.

Surgical options include follicle transplant, scalp flaps, and alopecia reduction. Few procedures have been subjected to scientific scrutiny, but patients who are self-conscious about their hair loss may consider them.

Other causes: Underlying causes are treated. Treatment for traction alopecia is elimination of physical traction or stress to the scalp. Treatment for tinea capitis is topical or oral antifungals (see p. 989). Trichotillomania is difficult to treat, but behavior modification, clomipramine 25 to 250 mg po once/day in adults or 3 mg/kg (up to 100 mg maximum) in children, and/or fluoxetine 20 to 40 mg po once/day may be of benefit.

Hair loss due to chemotherapy is temporary and is best treated with a wig. When hair regrows, it may be different in color and texture from the original hair.

Alopecia Areata

Alopecia areata is sudden patchy hair loss in people with no obvious skin disorder or systemic disease.

The scalp and beard are most frequently affected, but any hairy area may be involved. Hair loss may affect most or all of the body (alopecia universalis). Alopecia areata is thought to be an autoimmune disease affecting genetically susceptible people exposed to unclear environmental triggers, such as infection or emotional stress. It occasionally coexists with autoimmune vitiligo or thyroiditis.

Diagnosis is by inspection. Alopecia areata typically manifests as discrete circular patches of hair loss characterized by short broken hairs at the margins, which resemble exclamation points. Nails are sometimes pitted or display trachyonychia, a roughness of the nail also seen in lichen planus. Differential diagnosis includes tinea capitis, trichotillomania, discoid lupus, and secondary syphilis. Measures of TSH, vitamin B_{12}, and autoantibodies are indicated only when coexisting disease is suspected.

Treatment is with corticosteroids. Triamcinolone acetonide suspension (in doses not to exceed 0.1 mL per injection site, eg, 10 mg/mL concentration to deliver 1 mg) can be injected intradermally if the lesions are small. Potent topical corticosteroids (such as betamethasone 0.05% bid) can be used; however, they often do not penetrate to the depth of the hair bulb where the inflammatory process is located. Oral corticosteroids are effective, but hair loss recurs after cessation of therapy and adverse effects limit use. Topical anthralin (0.5 to 1% for 10 to 20 min daily, then washed off, frequency titrated as tolerated up to 30 min bid) and/or minoxidil may be used. Induction of allergic contact dermatitis using diphencyprone or squaric dibutylester leads to hair growth due to unknown mechanisms, but this intervention is best reserved for patients with diffuse involvement who are refractory to other therapies.

Alopecia areata may spontaneously regress, become chronic, or spread diffusely. Risk factors for chronicity include extensive involvement, onset before adolescence, atopy, and involvement of the peripheral scalp (ophiasis).

HIRSUTISM

(Hypertrichosis)

Hirsutism is excessive hair that occurs with or without virilization.

Hirsutism is almost exclusively a concern for women when hair takes on an appearance or distribution similar to male hair patterns. The threshold for "too much hair" is largely culturally determined. Hirsutism bothers some men when excessive hair covers the back.

Hirsutism in women may occur with virilization, in which other androgen-dependent changes such as loss of menses, voice deepening, and clitoral hypertrophy develop. Almost all cases of hirsutism with virilization are due to endocrine disorders affecting the ovaries (see p. 2078) or adrenals (see p. 1211) and are of medical, not just cosmetic, concern. Hirsutism without virilization is most often genetic or physiologic (occurring in pregnancy or after menopause) and largely of cosmetic concern. However, it may also be caused by drugs (especially phenytoin, corticosteroids, and progestins) or be a sign of endocrine (thyroid, acromegaly) or metabolic (porphyria) disease.

Diagnostic testing in men is unnecessary. In women, diagnosis is by laboratory evaluation, including serum free and total testosterone, dehydroepiandrosterone sulfate, follicle-stimulating hormone, luteinizing hormone, and prolactin; an endocrinologist may be consulted.

Mild cases can be treated without a doctor using depilatories or waxing. These treatments are temporary and tend to irritate the skin. Excess hair can be removed by diode laser or topical ornithine decarboxylase inhibitor cream and by treating any underlying endocrine abnormality.

PSEUDOFOLLICULITIS BARBAE

Pseudofolliculitis barbae is irritation of the skin due to beard hairs that penetrate the skin before leaving the hair follicle or leave the follicle and curve back into the skin, causing a foreign-body reaction.

Pseudofolliculitis barbae (PFB) predominantly affects black men. It is most noticeable around the beard and neck. It causes small papules and pustules that can be confused with bacterial folliculitis. Diagnosis is by physical examination.

Acute PFB can be treated with warm compresses and manual straightening of hairs with scissors or tweezers. Topical hydrocortisone 1% or erythromycin is used for mild inflammation, and oral tetracycline or erythromycin 500 mg bid for moderate to severe inflammation. Tretinoin (retinoic acid) 0.05% liquid or cream or 10% benzoyl peroxide cream may also be effective in mild or moderate cases but may irritate. Hairs should be allowed to grow out; grown hairs can then be cut to about 0.5 cm length. Depilatories are an alternative but may irritate. For women with hirsutism and associated PFB, an ornithine decarboxylase inhibitor can block the instigating hair growth.

125 NAIL DISORDERS

A variety of disorders can affect nails, including deformities, infections of the nail, paronychia, and ingrown toenails (see p. 345). Toenails require special attention in the elderly and in people with diabetes or peripheral vascular disease; involvement of a podiatrist is helpful to avoid local breakdown and secondary infections.

Trauma to the finger may cause changes in the nail. The nail may develop a white coloration that starts at the nail bed and grows up with the nail. Sometimes, a new nail grows below the existing nail and replaces it when fully grown in.

Most nail infections are fungal (onychomycosis—see p. 1010), but bacterial and viral infections can occur. *Pseudomonas* not infrequently causes harmless nail infection noteworthy for its striking blue-green color often associated with onycholysis; treatment is unrewarding, but patients should avoid trauma and excess moisture. Paronychia is not actually an infection of the nail but rather of periungual tissues.

Common warts (verrucae vulgaris) result from papillomavirus infection and frequently infect the proximal nail fold and sometimes the subungual area. Onychophagia (nail biting) can help to spread this infection. Warts involving these areas are especially difficult to treat. Freezing with liquid nitrogen may be effective.

DEFORMITIES

About 50% of nail deformities result from fungal infection. The remainder results from various causes, including trauma, psoriasis, lichen planus, and occasionally malignancy. Diagnosis may be obvious on examination, but sometimes fungal scrapings and culture may be performed. Once any underlying conditions are addressed, manicurists may be able to hide nail deformities with appropriate trimming and polishes.

Congenital deformities: In some congenital ectodermal dysplasias, patients have no nails (anonychia). In pachyonychia congenita, the nail beds are thickened, discolored, and hypercurved with a pincer nail deformity. Nail-patella syndrome (see p. 2383) causes triangular lunulae and partially absent thumb nails. Darier's disease is associated with red and white streaks and distal V-nicking.

Deformities associated with systemic problems: In the Plummer-Vinson syndrome, 50% of patients have koilonychia—concave, spoon-shaped nails. The yellow nail syndrome, characterized by hard, hypercurved, transversely thickened, yellow nails with loss of the cuticle, is seen in patients with lymphedema of limbs, pleural effusion, and ascites. Half-and-half nails occur with renal failure; the proximal half of the nail is white, and the distal half is pink or pigmented. White nails occur with cirrhosis, although the distal third may remain pinker.

Deformities associated with dermatologic conditions: In psoriasis, nails may demonstrate a number of changes including irregular pits, oil spots, onycholysis, and thickening and crumbling of the nail plate. Lichen planus of the nail matrix causes scarring with early nail ridging and splitting, then later leading to pterygium formation. Pterygium of the nail is characterized by scarring from the proximal nail outward in a V formation, which leads ultimately to loss of the nail. Alopecia areata is associated with regular pits that form a pattern.

Discoloration: Drugs, especially cytostatic and antimalarial drugs, can discolor nails. The drugs most commonly involved are bleomycin and cyclophosphamide and less commonly, actinomycin, doxorubicin, busulfan, 5-fluorouracil, hydroxyurea, and melphalan. Quinacrine can cause nails to appear greenish yellow or white under ultraviolet light. In argyria, the nails may be diffusely blue gray. With arsenic intoxication, the nails may turn diffusely brown. Tetracyclines, ketoconazole, phenothiazines, sulfonamides, and phenindione can all cause brownish or blue discoloration. Gold therapy can turn nails light or dark brown.

White transverse lines of the nails (Mees' lines) may occur with chemotherapy, acute arsenic intoxication, malignant tumors, MI, thallium and antimony intoxication, fluorosis, and even during etretinate therapy. They also develop with trauma to the finger, although traumatic white lines usually do not span the entire nail. The fungus *Trichophyton mentagrophytes* causes a chalky white discoloration of the nail plate.

Melanonychia striata: These are hyperpigmented longitudinal bands extending from the proximal nail fold and cuticle to the free distal end of the nail plate. In dark-skinned people, these may be a normal physiologic variant requiring no treatment. Melanonychia striata can also occur in benign melanocytic nevi and malignant melanoma. Hutchinson's sign—melanin leaching through the lunula, cuticle, and proximal nail fold—may signal a melanoma in the nail matrix. Rapid biopsy and treatment are essential.

Onychogryphosis: Onychogryphosis is a nail dystrophy in which the nail, most often on the big toe, becomes thickened and curved. It may be caused by ill-fitting shoes. It is common in the elderly. Treatment consists of trimming the deformed nails.

Onycholysis: Onycholysis is separation of the nail plate from the nail bed or complete nail plate loss. It can occur as a phototoxic reaction in patients treated with tetracyclines (photo-onycholysis), doxorubicin, 5-fluorouracil, β-blockers (particularly practolol and captopril), cloxacillin and cephaloridine (rarely), sulfamethoxazole-trimethoprim, diflunisal, etretinate, indomethacin, isoniazid, and isotretinoin. Partial onycholysis may also occur from infection with *Candida albicans*, from trauma, and in association with psoriasis or thyrotoxicosis.

Onychotillomania: In this disorder, patients pick at and self-mutilate their nails, which can lead to washboard deformity or habit-tic nails. Subungual hemorrhages can also be seen in onychotillomania. It most commonly presents in patients who habitually push back the cuticle on one finger, causing dystrophy of the nail plate as it grows.

Trachyonychia: Trachyonychia—rough, opaque nails— may occur with alopecia areata, lichen planus, atropic dermatitis, and psoriasis. It is most frequent in children.

Trauma: Damage to the nail bed, particularly crush injury, sometimes results in permanent nail deformity. Risk is reduced by primary repair at the time of injury.

Tumors: Benign and malignant tumors can affect the nail unit, causing deformity. These include benign myxoid cysts, pyogenic granulomas, glomus tumors, Bowen's disease, squamous cell carcinoma, and malignant melanoma. When malignancy is suspected, expeditious biopsy followed by referral to a surgeon is strongly advised.

ONYCHOMYCOSIS

Onychomycosis is fungal infection of the nail plate, nail bed, or both.

About 10% of the population has onychomycosis. Risk factors include tinea pedis, preexisting nail dystrophy, older age, male sex, and circulatory disease. Toenails are 10 times more commonly infected than fingernails. About 60 to 80% of cases are caused by dermatophytes (eg, *Trichophyton rubrum*); dermatophyte infection of the nails is called tinea unguium. Many of the remaining cases are caused by nondermatophyte molds (eg, *Aspergillus, Scopulariopsis, Fusarium*). Immunocompromised patients and those with chronic mucocutaneous candidiasis may have candidal onychomycosis (which is more common in the fingers).

Nails have asymptomatic patches of white or yellow discoloration and deformity. There are 3 characteristic presentations: (1) distal subungual, in which the nails thicken and yellow, keratin and debris accumulate distally and underneath, and the nail separates from the nail bed (onycholysis); (2) proximal subungual, a form that starts proximally and is a marker of immunosuppression; and (3) white superficial, in which a chalky white scale slowly spreads beneath the nail surface.

Diagnosis is by appearance and microscopic examination and culture of scrapings. Scrapings are taken from the most proximal position which can be accessed on the affected nail and examined for hyphae on potassium hydroxide wet mount and cultured. Obtaining an adequate sample of nail can be difficult because the distal subungual debris, which is easy to sample, often does not contain living fungus. Removing the distal portion of the nail with clippers before sampling or using a small curette to reach more proximally beneath the nail increases the yield. Differentiation from psoriasis or lichen planus is important, as the therapies differ.

Treatment is oral itraconazole or terbinafine. Itraconazole 200 mg bid 1 wk/mo for 3 mo, or terbinafine 250 mg once/day for 12 wk (6 wk for fingernail), achieves a high cure rate. It is not necessary to treat until all abnormal nail is gone because these drugs remain bound to the nail plate and continue to be effective after oral administration has ceased. Topical antifungal nail lacquer containing ciclopirox 8% or amorolfine 5% (not available in US) is rarely effective as primary treatment but can improve cure rate when used as an adjunct with oral drugs, particularly in resistant infections.

To limit relapse, the patient should trim nails short, dry feet after bathing, wear absorbent socks, and use antifungal foot powder. Old shoes may harbor a high density of spores and, if possible, should not be worn.

PARONYCHIA

Paronychia is infection of the periungual tissues.

Paronychia is usually acute, but chronic cases occur. In acute paronychia, the causative organisms are usually *Staphylococcus aureus* or streptococci, less commonly *Pseudomonas* or *Proteus* spp. Organisms enter through a break in the epidermis resulting from a hangnail, trauma to a nail fold, loss of the cuticle, or chronic irritation (eg, from water and detergents). Paronychia is more common in people who bite or suck their fingers. In toes, infection often begins at an ingrown toenail (see p. 345). In diabetics and those with peripheral vascular disease, toe paronychia can threaten the limb.

Symptoms and Signs

Paronychia develops along the nail margin (lateral and proximal nail folds), manifesting over hours to days with pain, warmth, redness, and swelling. Pus usually develops along the nail margin and sometimes beneath the nail. Rarely, infection penetrates deep into the finger, sometimes producing infectious flexor tenosynovitis. In diabetics and others with peripheral vascular disease, toe paronychia should be monitored for signs of cellulitis or more severe infection (eg, extension of edema or erythema, lymphadenopathy, fever).

Diagnosis and Treatment

Diagnosis is by inspection. Early treatment is warm compresses or soaks and an antistaphylococcal antibiotic (eg, dicloxacillin or cephalexin 250 mg po qid, clindamycin 300 mg po qid). Fluctuant swelling or visible pus should be drained with a Freer elevator, small hemostat, or #11 scalpel blade inserted between the nail and nail fold. Skin incision is unnecessary. A thin gauze wick should be inserted for 24 to 48 h to allow drainage.

CHRONIC PARONYCHIA

Chronic paronychia is recurrent or persistent nail fold inflammation, typically of the fingers.

Chronic paronychia occurs almost always in people whose hands are chronically wet (eg, dishwashers, bartenders, housekeepers), particularly if diabetic or immunocompromised. *Candida* is often present, but its role in etiology is unclear; fungal eradication does not always resolve the condition. The condition may be an irritant dermatitis with secondary fungal colonization.

The nail fold is painful and red as in acute paronychia, but there is almost never pus accumulation. Eventually, there is loss of the cuticle and separation of the nail fold from the nail plate. This forms a space which allows entry of irritants and microorganisms. The nail becomes distorted.

Diagnosis is clinical. Primary treatment is to keep the hands dry and to assist the cuticle in reforming to close the space between the nail fold and nail plate. Gloves or barrier creams are used if water contact is necessary. Topical corticosteroids may be helpful. Antifungal treatments are helpful only in reducing colonizing fungal organisms. Thymol 3% in ethanol applied several times a day to the space left by loss of cuticle aids in keeping this space dry and free of microorganisms.

126 PRESSURE ULCERS

(Bedsores; Decubiti; Decubitus Ulcers)

Pressure ulcers are areas of necrosis and ulceration where tissues are compressed between bony prominences and hard surfaces; they may also develop from friction and shearing forces. Risk factors include old age, impaired circulation, immobilization, malnourishment, and incontinence. Severity ranges from skin erythema to full-thickness skin loss with extensive soft-tissue necrosis. Diagnosis is clinical. Treatment includes pressure reduction, avoidance of friction and shearing forces, local care, and sometimes skin grafts or myocutaneous flaps. Prognosis is excellent for early-stage ulcers; neglected and late-stage ulcers pose risk of serious infection and nutritional stress and are difficult to heal.

Etiology and Pathophysiology

An estimated 1.3 to 3 million patients in the US have pressure ulcers (PUs); incidence is highest in older patients, especially when hospitalized or in long-term care facilities. Aging increases risk, in part because of reduced subcutaneous fat and decreased capillary blood flow. Immobility and comorbidities increase risk further.

PUs develop when soft tissues are compressed between bony prominences and contact surfaces or when friction (eg, rubbing against clothing or bedding) or shearing forces (which develop when skin clings to surfaces) cause erosion, tissue ischemia, and infarction. PUs most frequently develop over the sacrum, ischial tuberosities, trochanters, malleoli, and heels, but they can develop elsewhere, including behind the ears when nasal cannulae are used for prolonged periods. In persons wearing prosthetic devices, they often occur over bony prominences due to ill-fitting prostheses. Increased force and duration of pressure directly influence risk and severity, but PUs can develop in as little as 3 to

4 h in some settings. Ulcers are worsened when skin is overly moist and macerated (eg, from perspiration or incontinence).

Patients with cognitive impairment, immobility, or both are at higher risk. Immobility is the most important factor, either from decreased spontaneous movement (such as from stroke, sedation, severe illness) and/or inability to change position frequently because of weakness. Others include urinary and fecal incontinence; poor nutritional status, including dehydration; diabetes; and heart disease. Clinical assessment is sufficient to identify patients at risk; several scales (eg, Norton, Braden) help predict risk (see FIG. 126–1).

Other causes of skin ulcers: Chronic arterial and venous insufficiency can result in skin ulcers, particularly on the lower extremities. Although the underlying mechanism is vascular, the same forces that cause PUs can worsen these ulcers, and principles of treatment are similar.

Symptoms and Signs

Several staging systems exist; the most common classifies ulcers based on the depth of soft-tissue damage (see TABLE 126–1). Stage 1 PUs manifest hyperemia, warmth, and induration. This stage is a misnomer in the sense that an ulcer (a defect of skin into the dermis) is not present. However, ulceration will form if the course is not arrested and reversed. Stage 2 PUs involve erosion (defect of epidermis) or true ulceration; however, subcutaneous tissue is not exposed. Stage 3 and 4 PUs have deeper involvement of underlying tissue with more extensive destruction. Patients do not always progress from lower to higher stages. Sometimes the first sign is a deep, necrotic Stage 3 or 4 ulcer. When PUs develop quickly, subcutaneous tissue can become necrotic before the epidermis erodes. Any small ulcer should be thought of as an iceberg, with a potentially deep base.

PUs at any stage may be painful or pruritic but may not be noticed by patients with blunted awareness. Tenderness, erythema of surrounding skin, exudate, or foul odor suggests infection. Fever should raise suspicion of bacteremia or underlying osteomyelitis.

Nonhealing ulcers may be due to inadequate treatment but should raise suspicion of osteomyelitis or rarely squamous cell carcinoma within the ulcer (Marjolin's ulcer). Other complications of nonhealing PUs include sinus tracts, which can be superficial or connect the ulcer to deep adjacent structures (eg, to the bowel in sacral ulcers), and tissue calcification. In addition, PUs are a reservoir for hospital-acquired resistant organisms, which can slow healing and cause bacteremia and sepsis.

Diagnosis

Diagnosis is usually apparent clinically, but depth and extent can be difficult to determine. PUs are always colonized by bacteria, so wound surface cultures are uninterpretable. Underlying osteomyelitis is diagnosed with radionuclide bone scanning or gadolinium-enhanced MRI, but both have poor sensitivity and specificity. Diagnosis may require bone biopsy and culture.

Continuous assessment is mandatory for effective management. Serial photographs can also document healing.

Prognosis and Treatment

Prognosis for early-stage PUs is excellent with timely appropriate treatment, although healing typically requires weeks. Unfortunately, PUs often develop in patients with suboptimal care; if this cannot be remedied, long-term outcome is poor, even if short-term wound healing is accomplished.

Treatment requires multiple simultaneous elements.

Reducing pressure: Reducing tissue pressure is accomplished through positioning, protective devices, and modification of support surfaces. Frequent repositioning (and selection of the proper position) is most important. Bedbound patients should be turned a minimum of q 2 h, should be placed at a 30° angle to the mattress when on their side (ie, lateral decubitus) to avoid direct trochanteric pressure, and should be elevated as minimally as possible to avoid the shear forces on tissues that result from sliding down the bed. A Stryker frame facilitates turning patients with spinal cord injuries. Patients who can sit should be encouraged or stimulated to change position q 15 to 60 min.

Protective padding includes pillows or foam wedges placed between knees, ankles, and heels when a patient is on his side and pillows, foam, or sheepskin heel protectors when supine. Windows should be cut out of plaster casts at pressure sites in patients immobilized by fractures. Soft seat cushions should be provided for patients able to sit in a chair.

Patient's Name		*Evaluator's Name*		*Date of Assessment*				
SENSORY PERCEPTION Ability to respond meaningfully to pressure-related discomfort	1. *Completely limited:* Unresponsive (does not moan, flinch, or grasp) to painful stimuli, owing to diminished level of consciousness or sedation or limited ability to feel pain over most of body surface	2. *Very limited:* Responds only to painful stimuli; cannot communicate discomfort except by moaning or restlessness or has a sensory impairment that limits the ability to feel pain or discomfort over half of body	3. *Slightly limited:* Responds to verbal commands but cannot always communicate discomfort or need to be turned or has some sensory impairment that limits ability to feel pain or discomfort in 1 or 2 extremities	4. *No impairment:* Responds to verbal commands; has no sensory deficit that would limit ability to feel or voice pain or discomfort				
MOISTURE Degree to which skin is exposed to moisture	1. *Constantly moist:* Skin is kept moist almost constantly by perspiration, urine, etc: dampness is detected every time patient is moved or turned	2. *Moist:* Skin is often but not always moist; linen must be changed at least once a shift	3. *Occasionally moist:* Skin is occasionally moist, requiring extra linen change about once a day	4. *Rarely moist:* Skin is usually dry; linen changes required only at routine intervals				
ACTIVITY Degree of physical activity	1. *Bedfast:* Confined to bed	2. *Chairfast:* Ability to walk severely limited or nonexistent; cannot bear own weight or must be assisted into chair or wheelchair	3. *Walks occasionally:* Walks occasionally during day but for very short distances, with or without assistance; spends most of each shift in bed or chair	4. *Walks frequently:* Walks outside the room at least twice a day and inside room at least once every 2 h during waking hours				
MOBILITY Ability to change and control body position	1. *Completely immobile:* Does not make even slight changes in body or extremity position without assistance	2. *Very limited:* Makes occasional slight changes in body or extremity position but unable to make frequent or significant changes independently	3. *Slightly limited:* Makes frequent though slight changes in body or extremity position independently	4. *No limitations:* Makes major and frequent changes in position without assistance				
NUTRITION Usual food intake pattern	1. *Very poor:* Never eats a complete meal; rarely eats > 1/3 of any food offered; eats ≤ 2 servings of protein (meat or dairy products) per day; takes fluids poorly; does not take a liquid dietary supplement or is NPO or maintained on clear liquids or IV for > 5 days	2. *Probably inadequate:* Rarely eats a complete meal and generally eats only about half of any food offered; protein intake includes only 3 servings of meat or dairy products per day; occasionally takes a dietary supplement or receives less than optimum amount of liquid diet or tube feeding	3. *Adequate:* Eats > 1/2 of most meals; eats a total of 4 servings of protein (meat, dairy products) each day; occasionally refuses a meal, but usually takes a supplement if offered or is on a tube feeding or TPN regimen, which probably meets most of nutritional needs	4. *Excellent:* Eats most of every meal; never refuses a meal; usually eats a total of ≥ 4 servings of meat and dairy products; occasionally eats between meals; does not require supplementation				
FRICTION AND SHEAR	1. *Problem:* Requires moderate to maximum assistance in moving; complete lifting without sliding against sheets is impossible; frequently slides down in bed or chair, requiring frequent repositioning with maximum assistance; spasticity, contractures, or agitation leads to almost constant friction	2. *Potential problem:* Moves feebly or requires minimum assistance; during a move skin probably slides to some extent against sheets, chair, restraints, or other devices; maintains relatively good position in chair or bed most of the time but occasionally slides down	3. *No apparent problem:* Moves in bed and in chair independently and has sufficient muscle strength to lift up completely during move; maintains good position in bed or chair at all times					
				Total Score				

Fig. 126–1. Braden scale for predicting risk for pressure ulcers. The patient is evaluated in 6 categories: sensory perception, moisture, activity, mobility, nutrition, and friction and shear. Pressure sore risk increases as the score decreases: 15–16 = mild risk; 12–14 = moderate risk; < 12 = serious risk. Modified from Braden B, Bergstrom N: Pressure ulcers in adults: Prediction and prevention. *Clinical Practice Guideline*, no. 3, pp 14–17, May 1992. US Department of Health and Human Services.

TABLE 126–1. PRESSURE ULCER STAGING

STAGE	CHARACTERISTICS
1	Observable pressure-related changes of intact skin compared to the adjacent or opposite areas, including differences in: • Color (redness in lightly pigmented skin; red, blue, or purple hues in darkly pigmented skin) • Temperature (increased warmth or coolness) • Consistency (firm or boggy feel) • Sensation (pain, itching)
2	Partial-thickness skin loss involving the epidermis and/or dermis Ulcer is superficial and manifests as an abrasion, blister, or shallow crater
3	Full-thickness skin loss involving damage or necrosis of subcutaneous tissue, which may extend down to, but not through, underlying fascia Ulcer is a deep crater with or without undermining of adjacent tissue
4	Full-thickness skin loss with extensive tissue destruction and/or necrosis, or damage to muscle, bone, or supporting structures (such as tendons or the joint capsule)

Adapted from the National Pressure Ulcer Advisory Panel, Consensus Development Conference Statement.

Support surfaces under bedbound patients can be changed to reduce pressure. A change from standard mattress is indicated when the patient is unable to reposition himself and periodic repositioning care is unavailable. Support surfaces are static or dynamic. Static surfaces, which do not require electricity, include air, foam, gel, and water overlays and mattresses. Old-fashioned "egg crate" mattresses offer no advantage. In general, static surfaces increase surface support areas and decrease pressures and shear forces; they are indicated for high-risk patients without PUs and for patients with Stage 1 PUs. Dynamic surfaces require electricity. Alternating-air mattresses have air cells that are alternately inflated and deflated by a pump, thus shifting supportive pressure from site to site. Low-air-loss mattresses are giant air-permeable pillows that are continuously inflated with air; the air flow has a drying effect on tissues. These specialized mattresses are indicated for patients with Stage 1 ulcers who develop hyperemia on static surfaces and for patients with Stage 3 or 4 ulcers. Air-fluidized or high-air-loss mattresses contain silicone-coated beads that liquefy when air is pumped through the bed. Advantages include reduction of moisture on surfaces and cooling. They are indicated for patients with nonhealing Stage 3 and 4 ulcers or numerous truncal ulcers (see TABLE 126–2).

Ulcer care: Appropriate cleaning, debridement, and dressings are needed.

Cleaning should be performed initially and with each dressing change; ordinary soap and water is usually best. Antiseptics such as iodine and hydrogen peroxide and even antiseptic washes interfere with tissue healing and should be avoided. Cleaning involves irrigation with saline solution at pressures sufficient to remove bacteria without traumatizing tissue; this can be done with commercial syringes, squeeze bottles, or electrically pressurized systems. Alternatively, a 35-mL syringe and a 19-gauge IV catheter can be used. Irrigation should continue until no further debris can be loosened.

Debridement is necessary to remove dead tissue. There are several methods. Autolytic debridement uses synthetic occlusive dressings to facilitate digestion of dead tissues by enzymes normally present in wound fluids. Autolytic debridement may be used for small wounds with simple accumulation of tissue proteins and wounds that need to be sealed off anyway (eg, for protection from feces or urine). DuoDERM or Contreet (which is impregnated with silver and thus offers antimicrobial effects) are commonly used. Infected wounds should not be occluded.

Mechanical debridement with wet-to-dry dressings, hydrotherapy (whirlpool baths), wound irrigation, or dextranomers (small carbohydrate-based beads that help absorb exudate and liquid debris) should be used for thick exudate or loose necrotic tissue. A scalpel or scissors can be used to remove eschar (except in heel ulcers, in which eschar in the absence of edema, erythema, fluctuance, or drainage can be safely left alone) or extensive

TABLE 126–2. OPTIONS FOR SUPPORT SURFACES

	STATIC			DYNAMIC		
	Standard Hospital Mattress	**Foam**	**Static Flotation (Air or Water)**	**Alternating Air**	**Low Air Loss**	**Air Fluidized (High Air Loss)**
Support area increase	No	Yes	Yes	Yes	Yes	Yes
Pressure reduction	No	Yes	Yes	Yes	Yes	Yes
Shear reduction	No	No	Yes	Yes	Unknown	Yes
Heat reduction	No	No	No	No	Yes	Yes
Low moisture retention	No	No	No	No	Yes	Yes
Cost	Low	Low	Low	Moderate	High	High

Adapted from Bergstrom N et al: US Agency for Health Care Policy and Research. Pressure Ulcer Treatment (Quick Reference Guideline Number 15). AHCPR Publication no. 95-0653, December 1994.

areas of dead tissue. Modest eschar or tissue can be debrided at the patient's bedside, but extensive or deep areas should be debrided in the operating room. Urgent debridement is indicated in advancing cellulitis or sepsis.

Enzymatic debridement (using collagenase, papain, fibrinolysin, or streptokinase/streptodornase) is an option for patients whose caretakers are not trained to perform mechanical debridement or for patients unable to tolerate surgery. It is most effective after cross-hatching of the wound with a scalpel to improve penetration. Collagenase is especially effective as collagen comprises 75% of the dry weight of skin.

Dressings should be used for Stage 1 ulcers that are subject to friction or incontinence and for all other ulcers (see TABLE 126–3). Objectives are to keep the ulcer bed moist to retain tissue growth factors while allowing some evaporation and inflow of oxygen; to keep surrounding skin dry; to facilitate autolytic debridement; and to establish a barrier to infection. Transparent films (eg, OpSite, Tegaderm, Bioclusive) are sufficient for ulcers with limited exudate; they should not be used over cavities and must be changed q 3 to 7 days. Some experts recommend a small amount of triple antibiotic ointment under the dressing. Hydrogels (ClearSite, Vigilon, FlexiGel), which are cross-linked polymer dressings that come in sheets or gels, are indicated for very shallow wounds, such as re-epithelializing wounds with minimal exudate.

Hydrocolloids (eg, RepliCare, DuoDERM, Restore, Tegasorb), which are combinations of gelatin, pectin, and carboxymethylcellulose in the form of wafers, powders, and pastes, are indicated for light to moderate exudate; some have adhesive backings and others are typically covered with transparent films to ensure adherence to the ulcer and must be changed q 3 days. Alginates (polysaccharide seaweed derivatives containing alginic acid), which come as pads, ropes, and ribbons (AlgiSite, Sorbsan, Curasorb), are indicated for extensive exudate and for control of bleeding after surgical debridement. Foam dressings (Allevyn, LYOfoam, Hydrasorb, Mepilex, Curafoam, Contreet) are useful as they can handle a variety of levels of exudate and provide a moist environment for wound healing. Waterproof versions protect the skin from incontinence. Those with adhesive backings stay in place longer and need less frequent changing.

Pain management: Primary treatment of pain is treatment of the PU itself, but NSAIDs or acetaminophen is used for mild to moderate pain. Opioids should be avoided if possible because sedation promotes immobility (opioids may be necessary during dressing changes and debridement). In cognitively impaired patients, changes in vital signs can be used as an indication of pain.

Infection management: PUs should be continually reassessed for bacterial infection using clinical signs of erythema, warmth, increased drainage and fever; elevated WBC offers further evidence. Options for topical treatment include silver sulfadiazine, triple antibiotic, and metronidazole (the latter for anaerobic bacteria, which are often foul-smelling). Systemic antibiotics should be administered for cellulitis, bacteremia, or osteomyelitis, guided by tissue culture or clinical suspicion and not by surface culture.

Nutrition: Malnutrition is common among patients with PUs and is a risk factor for nonhealing. Markers of malnutrition include albumin < 3.5 mg/dL and/or weight < 80% of ideal. Protein intake of 1.25 to 1.5 g/kg/day is desirable for optimal healing; oral or parenteral supplementation (see p. 20) may be needed. Zinc supplementation supports wound healing, and replacement at a dose of 50 mg tid may be useful. Supplemental vitamin C 1 g/day may be provided.

Adjuncts: Multiple adjunctive treatments have been tried or are under investigation. Negative pressure therapy and the use of various topical recombinant growth factors (eg, nerve growth factor, platelet-derived growth factor-BB) and skin equivalents are showing promise in wound management; however, they do not ameliorate mechanical forces and tissue ischemia. Electrical stimulation, heat therapy, massage therapy, and hyperbaric O_2 therapy have not proven effective.

Surgery: Surgical debridement is necessary for any ulcer with devitalized tissue. Large defects, especially with exposure of musculoskeletal structures, require surgical closure. Skin grafts are useful for large, shallow defects. However, because grafts do not add to blood supply, measures must be taken to prevent pressure from developing to the point of ischemia and further breakdown. Myocutaneous flaps, because of their pressure-sharing bulk and rich vasculature, are the

TABLE 126–3. OPTIONS FOR PRESSURE ULCER DRESSINGS

ULCER TYPE*	DESCRIPTION	OBJECTIVE	USE	OPTIONS
Shallow (Stage 2)	Dry with nominal exudate	Create or retain moisture; protect from infection	Transparent films or hydrogels	*Cover with:* Transparent film, thin hydrocolloid, or thin polyurethane foam *Wrap with:* Nonadherent gauze dressing
	Wet with moderate-large exudate	Absorb exudate; facilitate autolysis; maintain moisture; protect from infection	Hydrocolloid or foam dressings	*Cover with:* Alginates, hydrocolloid with or without paste or powder, or polyurethane foam *Wrap with:* Gauze dressing or absorptive contact layer
Deep (Stages 3–4)	Dry with nominal exudate	Fill cavities, create or maintain moisture, protect from infection	Hydrocolloids, alginates, or foam dressings	*Fill with:* Copolymer starch, hydrogel, or damp gauze *Cover with:* Transparent thin film, polyurethane foam, or gauze pad
	Wet with moderate-large exudate	Fill cavities, absorb exudate, maintain moisture, protect from infection	Alginates or foam dressings	*Fill with:* Copolymer starch, dextranomer beads, calcium alginates, hydrofibers, or hydrocellular gauze or foam *Cover with:* Transparent thin film, polyurethane foam

*Dressings are not usually needed for Stage 1 ulcers.

closures of choice over large bony prominences (eg, sacrum, ischia, trochanters).

Ischemic and venous ulcers: Wound care treatments also are useful for ischemic ulcers, but the underlying pathophysiology must be addressed (eg, better control of the inflammatory process in a rheumatoid ulcer or surgical stenting or bypass surgery to improve circulation in atherosclerosis). Pentoxifylline has been tried with minimal success. Some evidence supports the use of dalteparin for diabetic foot ulcers (5000 units sc once/day until healed); however, this finding has not been corroborated. Ischemic ulcers can become infected, often with anaerobic organisms, and the infection may spread, causing septicemia or osteomyelitis.

Venous ulcers are typically sterile at first but tend to lead to cellulitis. The same local care as for PUs can be used. In addition, treatment includes measures to reduce venous hypertension, such as using compression stockings or Unna boot bandages (applied at a pressure of 35 to 40 mm Hg) and elevating the leg above the heart. Pentoxifylline 800 mg po tid for up to 24 wk may be useful.

Prevention

Prevention requires identification of high-risk patients followed by vigilant attention to skin care and hygiene. Pressure points should be checked for erythema or trauma at least once/day under adequate lighting. Patients and families must be taught a routine of daily visual inspection and palpation of sites for potential ulcer formation.

The mainstay of prevention is frequent repositioning. Pressure should not be allowed to continue over any bony surface for > 2 h. Patients who cannot move by themselves must be repositioned using pillows. Even on low pressure mattresses, the patient must be turned.

Daily attention to hygiene and dryness is necessary to prevent maceration and secondary infection. Lying on a sheepskin helps keep the skin in good condition. Protective padding, pillows, or a sheepskin can be used to separate body surfaces.

Bedding and clothing should be changed frequently; sheets should be soft, clean, and free from wrinkles and particulate matter. The skin should be sponged in hot weather and thoroughly dried afterward. For incontinent patients, ulcers should be protected from contamination; synthetic dressings are helpful for this. Skin breakdown can be prevented with careful cleansing and drying (patting and not rubbing the skin) and using anticandidal creams and moisture barrier creams or skin protective wipes (eg, Skin-Prep). Areas subject to friction may be powdered with plain talc. Cornstarch may allow fungal growth.

Oversedation should be avoided, and activity should be encouraged. Adequate nutrition is important. Adhesive tape can irritate and even tear fragile skin adjoining ulcers, and its use should be minimized.

127 BENIGN TUMORS

(See also Warts on p. 998 and Genital Warts on p. 1652.)

Most skin tumors are benign. However, because skin cancers must be treated early, proper diagnosis of unusual skin growths should always be made definitively and without undue delay.

DERMATOFIBROMA

(Fibrous Histiocytoma)

Dermatofibroma is a firm, red-to-brown, small papule or nodule composed of fibroblastic tissue usually occurring on the thighs or legs.

Dermatofibromas are common, more so in women, and typically appear in the 20s. Their cause is unknown. Lesions are usually 0.5 to 1 cm and feel like a lentil embedded in the skin. Most are asymptomatic; some itch or ulcerate following minor trauma. Diagnosis is clinical; lesions typically dimple when grasped between the fingers. They may regress spontaneously but can be excised if troublesome.

EPIDERMAL CYSTS

(Keratinous Cyst; Epidermal Inclusion Cyst; Milia; Pilar Cyst; Steatocystoma; "Sebaceous Cyst;" Wen)

Epidermal cysts are slow-growing benign cysts containing keratinous (keratinous or epidermal cysts, "sebaceous" cyst, milia),

follicular (pilar cyst, wen), or sebaceous (steatocystoma) material. They are frequently found on the scalp, ears, face, back, or scrotum.

On palpation, the cystic mass is firm, globular, movable, and nontender; it seldom causes discomfort unless it has ruptured internally, causing a rapidly enlarging, painful abscess. Keratinous cysts, the most common, often are surmounted with a punctum or pore; their contents are cheesy and often fetid (due to secondary bacterial colonization). Milia are minute superficial keratinous cysts noted on the face.

Cysts may be left or removed. A small incision may be made to evacuate the contents, then the cyst wall itself should be removed with a curet or hemostat, otherwise the lesion will recur. Surgical excision is also effective. Internally ruptured cysts should be incised and drained; a gauze drain is inserted and removed after 2 to 3 days. Antibiotics are not needed unless cellulitis is present. Milia may be evacuated with a #11 blade.

KELOIDS

Keloids are smooth overgrowths of fibroblastic tissue that arise in an area of injury (eg, surgical scars, truncal acne) or, occasionally, spontaneously.

Keloids are more frequent in blacks. They tend to appear on the upper trunk, especially the upper back and mid chest, and on deltoid areas. Unlike hyperplastic scars, keloidal scar tissue always extends beyond the area of original injury.

Keloids are shiny, firm, smooth, often dome-shaped, and slightly pink. Diagnosis is clinical. Treatment is often ineffective. Monthly corticosteroid injections (eg, triamcinolone acetonide 5 to 40 mg/mL) into the base of the lesion sometimes flatten the keloid. Surgical or laser excision may debulk lesions, but they often recur. Excision is more successful if preceded and followed by a series of intralesional corticosteroid injections. Gel sheeting (applying a soft, semiocclusive dressing made of cross-linked polymethylsiloxane polymer, or silicone) or pressure garments are other adjuncts to prevent recurrence.

KERATOACANTHOMA

Keratoacanthoma is a round, firm, usually flesh-colored nodule, with sharply sloping borders and a characteristic central crater containing keratinous material, which usually resolves spontaneously.

Etiology is unknown. Most consider these lesions to be well-differentiated squamous cell carcinomas with a tendency to involute.

Development is rapid; usually the lesion reaches its full size, which may be > 5 cm, within 1 or 2 mo. Common sites are sun-exposed areas, the face, the forearm, and the dorsum of the hand. Spontaneous involution may start within a few months. However, because this lesion cannot be relied upon to involute, biopsy or excision is recommended. Spontaneous involution may leave substantial scarring; surgery or intralesional injections with 5-fluorouracil or corticosteroids usually yield better cosmetic results, and excision allows histologic confirmation of the diagnosis. Some untreated lesions metastasize.

LIPOMAS

Lipomas are soft, movable, subcutaneous nodules of adipocytes (fat cells); overlying skin is normal.

A patient may have one or many lipomas. They occur more often in women than men and appear most commonly on the trunk, nape, and forearms. They are rarely symptomatic, but pain may occur, especially in patients with familial variants presenting with multiple lesions.

Diagnosis is usually clinical. A lipoma is usually easily moveable within the subcutis. While generally soft, some become firmer. Some superficial dimpling may occur, but frank inflammation is not normal.

A rapidly growing lesion should be biopsied, although lipomas rarely become malignant. Treatment is not usually required, but bothersome lipomas may be excised or removed by liposuction.

MOLES

(Pigmented, Melanocytic, or Nevus Cell Nevi)

Moles are pigmented macules, papules, or nodules composed of clusters of melanocytes or nevus cells. Their main significance (other than cosmetic) is their potential for being or becoming malignant. Suspect lesions (changing or highly irregular borders, color changes, becoming painful, or starting to bleed, ulcerate, or itch) are biopsied.

TABLE 127–1. CLASSIFICATION OF MOLES

TYPE	CLINICAL CHARACTERISTICS	HISTOLOGY	COMMENTS
Compound nevus	Light brown to dark brown; may be slightly or considerably elevated; 3–6 mm	Nests of melanocytes at the epidermodermal junction and within the dermis	The 2nd stage of the life cycle of melanocytic nevi
Halo nevus	Any type of melanocytic nevus surrounded by a 2- to 6-mm ring of depigmented skin	Same as for other moles but with inflammation and loss of melanocytes in halo skin	Usually resolves spontaneously but in rare cases is a sign of malignant transformation
Intradermal nevus	Flesh-colored to brown; elevated; may be smooth, hairy, or warty; 3–6 mm	Melanocytes and nevus cells confined almost entirely to the dermis	The 3rd stage of the life cycle of melanocytic nevi
Junctional nevus	Light brown to nearly black; usually flat but may be slightly elevated; 1–10 mm	Clustering of melanocytes at the epidermodermal junction	The 1st stage of the life-cycle of melanocytic nevi. Nevi on the palms, soles, and genitals are almost always junctional
Lentigo	Uniformly pigmented, brown to black; flat; sharp margins; 0.5–4 mm	An increased number of melanocytes at the epidermodermal junction	Darker, sparser, larger, and more scattered than freckles; does not darken or multiply with sun exposure. Not truly a mole

Almost everyone has a few moles, which usually appear in childhood or adolescence. They may be small or large; flesh-colored, yellow-brown, brown, or dark brown; flat or raised; smooth, hairy, or warty; broad-based or pedunculated (for classification, see TABLE 127–1). During adolescence and pregnancy, more moles often appear and existing ones may enlarge or darken.

Although an individual mole is unlikely to become malignant (the lifetime risk being about 1 in 3,000 to 10,000), the single best predictor of risk for development of melanoma is the total number of moles.

Treatment

Because moles are extremely common and melanomas are uncommon, prophylactic removal is not justifiable. However, a mole should be biopsied and examined histologically if it has characteristics of concern; the specimen must be deep enough for accurate microscopic diagnosis and should contain the entire lesion if possible, especially if the concern for malignancy is high. However, wide primary excision should not be the initial procedure, even for highly abnormal-appearing lesions, because many such lesions are not melanomas. Incisional biopsy does not increase the likelihood of metastasis if the lesion is malignant, and it avoids extensive surgery for a benign lesion.

Moles can be removed by shave or excision for cosmetic purposes, and all moles removed should be examined histologically. If hair is a concern, a hairy mole should be adequately excised rather than removed by shave. Otherwise, hair regrowth will occur.

ATYPICAL MOLES

(Dysplastic Nevi)

Atypical moles (AM) are melanocytic nevi with irregular and ill-defined borders, variegated colors usually of brown and tan tones, and macular or papular components. Management is by monitoring and biopsy of highly atypical or changed lesions. Patients should

TABLE 127–2. CHARACTERISTICS OF ATYPICAL VS TYPICAL MOLES

CRITERIA	MOLES	ATYPICAL MOLES
Age of onset	Childhood or adolescence	Continue to appear after adolescence
Color	Flesh-colored, yellow-brown, or black	Tan to dark brown with a pink background; often have a "fried egg," dark target or light target appearance; commonly have a flatter rim than center; pigment often blurs at the edges or has notching
Diameter	1–10 mm	5–12 mm
Location	Anywhere on the body	Most common on sun-exposed skin but may occur on covered areas (eg, buttocks, breast, scalp)
# of lesions	About 10	One to several dozen

reduce sun exposure and conduct regular self-examinations for new moles or changes in existing ones.

AM are nevi with a slightly different clinical and histologic appearance (disordered architecture and atypia of melanocytes). Patients with AM are at increased risk for malignant melanoma, the risk increasing with increasing number of AM as well as with increasing sun exposure. Some patients have only one or a few AM; others have many. The propensity to develop AM may be inherited (autosomal dominant) or sporadic without apparent familial association.

Familial atypical mole–melanoma syndrome refers to the presence of multiple AM and melanoma in 2 or more 1st-degree relatives. These patients are at markedly increased risk (25×) for melanoma.

Symptoms, Signs, and Diagnosis

AM are often larger than other nevi (> 6 mm diameter), primarily round (unlike many melanomas) but with indistinct borders and mild asymmetry. In contrast, melanomas have greater irregularity of color, not just tan and brown, but dark-brown, black, red, and blue or whitish areas of depigmentation. Although clinical findings suggest the diagnosis of AM (see TABLE 127–2), biopsy of the worst-appearing lesions should be performed to establish the diagnosis and to determine the degree of atypia.

If a patient with AM has a family history of melanoma (whether arising from AM or de novo) or other skin cancers, 1st-degree relatives should be examined. Patients with AM who are from melanoma-prone families (ie, 2 or more 1st-degree relatives have cutaneous melanomas) have a high lifetime risk of developing melanomas. The entire skin (including the scalp) of members of an at-risk family should be examined. A biopsy should be performed of one or more atypical-appearing lesions. Patients with multiple AM and a personal or family history of melanoma should be examined regularly (eg, yearly for family history, more often for personal history of melanoma).

Treatment

Patients with AM should avoid excessive sun exposure and use sunscreens; they should be taught self-examination to detect changes in existing moles and to recognize features of melanomas. Some experts recommend yearly photographs of the skin surface. Regular follow-up examinations may be combined with baseline and follow-up color photographs of most of the patient's body (most useful in patients with many AM).

SEBORRHEIC KERATOSES

Seborrheic keratoses are pigmented superficial epithelial lesions that are usually warty but may occur as smooth papules.

The cause is unknown. The lesions commonly occur in middle or old age and most often appear on the trunk or temples; in blacks, especially women, small keratoses often occur on the malar part of the face (dermatosis papulosa nigra).

Seborrheic keratoses vary in size and grow slowly. They may be round or oval; flesh-colored, brown, or black. They usually appear "stuck on" and may have a verrucous, velvety, waxy, scaling, or crusted surface. Diagnosis is clinical.

They are not premalignant and need no treatment unless they are irritated, itchy, or cosmetically bothersome. Lesions may be removed with little or no scarring by cryotherapy (but beware risk of hypopigmentation) or by curettage after local injection of lidocaine.

SKIN TAGS

Skin tags (acrochordons, soft fibromas) are common soft, small, flesh-colored or hyperpigmented, pedunculated lesions, usually multiple and occurring mainly on the neck, axilla, and groin.

Skin tags are usually asymptomatic but may be irritating. Irritating or unsightly skin tags can be removed by freezing with liquid nitrogen, light electrodesiccation, or excision with a scalpel or scissors. The standard of care is to submit all skin tags individually for histologic examination, especially if there is any question of the diagnosis. However, for a patient with dozens of identical lesions, the likelihood of an individual lesion being other than a skin tag is unlikely.

VASCULAR LESIONS

Vascular lesions include acquired lesions (eg, pyogenic granuloma) and those that arise at or shortly after birth (vascular birthmarks). Vascular birthmarks include vascular tumors (eg, infantile hemangioma) and vascular malformations. Vascular malformations are congenital, life-long, localized defects in vascular morphogenesis and include capillary (eg, nevus flammeus), venous, arteriovenous (eg, cirsoid aneurysm), and lymphatic malformations. Vascular birthmarks usually involve only the skin and subcutaneous tissues but rarely affect the CNS.

INFANTILE HEMANGIOMA

Infantile hemangiomas are raised, red or purplish, hyperplastic vascular lesions appearing in the 1st year of life. Most spontaneously involute; those obstructing vision, the airway, or other structures require treatment, usually with oral corticosteroids. Surgery is rarely recommended.

Infantile hemangiomas (IH) can be classified by appearance as superficial, deep, cavernous, or by descriptive terms ("strawberry hemangioma"), but all share a common pathophysiology and natural history; therefore, the inclusive term infantile hemangioma is preferred. They are the most common tumor of infancy, affecting 10 to 12% of infants by 1 yr.

IH are present at birth in 10 to 20% of those affected and almost always within the 1st several weeks of life; occasionally, deeper lesions may not be apparent until a few months after birth. Size and vascularity increase rapidly, usually peaking at about age 1 yr.

Superficial lesions have a bright red appearance; deeper lesions have a bluish color. Lesions can bleed or ulcerate from minor trauma; ulcers may be painful. IH in certain locations can interfere with function; those on the face or oropharynx may interfere with vision or obstruct the airway; those near the urethral meatus or anus may interfere with elimination. A periocular hemangioma in an infant is an emergency as even a few days of disruption of vision can result in permanent visual defects. Lumbosacral hemangiomas may be a sign of neurologic or genitourinary anomalies.

Lesions slowly involute starting at 12 to 18 mo, decreasing in size and vascularity. Generally, IH involute 10%/year of age, (eg, 50% by age 5, 60% by age 6), with maximal involution by age 10. Involuted lesions commonly have a yellowish or telangiectatic color and a wrinkled or lax fibrofatty texture; residual changes are almost always proportional to the lesion's maximal size and vascularity.

Diagnosis and Treatment

Diagnosis is clinical; the extent can be evaluated by MRI if lesions appear to encroach vital structures.

Treatment is controversial. Many physicians treat lesions early to prevent subsequent enlargement or to make them less noticeable; others do not treat unless a lesion causes (or risks) functional problems by its location. When treatment is elected, laser treatment or intralesional or systemic corticosteroids are chosen based on the location, extent, and rate of growth of the lesion. For systemic corticosteroid therapy, prednisone 1 to 3 mg/kg po bid or tid is given for ≥ 2 wk. If resolution starts, the prednisone should be decreased slowly; if not, the drug should be stopped.

Topical treatments and wound care are useful for ulcerated lesions and help prevent scarring, bleeding and pain. Compresses, topical mupirocin or metronidazole, barrier dressings (polyurethane film dressing or petrolatum-impregnated gauze), or barrier creams may be used.

Unless complications are life threatening or vital organs are compromised, surgical excision or other destructive procedures should be avoided because they frequently result in more scarring than occurs with spontaneous involution. To help parents accept nonintervention, the physician can review the natural history (photographic examples are helpful), provide serial photography of the lesion to document involution, and provide a sympathetic ear to parents' concerns.

Nevus Flammeus and Port-Wine Stain

Nevus flammeus and port-wine stains are capillary vascular malformations that are present at birth and appear as flat, pink, red, or purplish lesions.

Nevi flammei are flat pink marks that are very common on the nape, glabella, and eyelids. Lesions around the eyes disappear in a few months. Nape lesions may disappear in early childhood, only to recur in middle age.

Port-wine stains are flat, reddish to purple lesions appearing anywhere on the body. Lesions become darker and more palpable with time (often becoming quite hyperplastic by late middle age), although the lateral extent does not enlarge beyond the growth of the patient. Port-wine stains of the trigeminal area may be a component of the Sturge-Weber syndrome (in which a similar vascular lesion appears on the underlying meninges and cerebral cortex and is associated with epilepsy).

Diagnosis is clinical. Treatment with vascular lasers produces excellent results in many cases, especially if treated as early in life as possible. The lesion can also be hidden with an opaque cosmetic cream prepared to match the patient's skin color.

Nevus Araneus

(Spider Nevus; Spider Angioma; Vascular Spider)

Nevus araneus is a bright red, faintly pulsatile vascular lesion consisting of a central arteriole with slender projections resembling spider legs.

Compression of the central vessel temporarily obliterates the lesion. Lesions are acquired. One lesion or small numbers that are unrelated to internal disease may occur in children or adults. Patients with hepatic cirrhosis develop many spider angiomas that may become quite prominent. Many women develop lesions during pregnancy or while taking oral contraceptives. The lesions are asymptomatic and usually resolve spontaneously about 6 to 9 mo postpartum or after oral contraceptives are stopped. Lesions are not uncommon on the faces of children.

Diagnosis is clinical. Treatment is not usually required. If resolution is not spontaneous or treatment is desired for cosmetic purposes, the central arteriole can be destroyed with fine-needle electrodesiccation; vascular laser treatment may also be performed.

Pyogenic Granuloma

Pyogenic granuloma is a fleshy, moist or crusty, usually scarlet vascular nodule composed of proliferating capillaries in an edematous stroma.

The lesion, composed of vascular tissue, is neither of bacterial origin nor a true granuloma. It develops rapidly, often at the site of recent injury (although injury may not be recalled), and probably represents a vascular and fibrous response to injury. There is no sex or age predilection. The overlying epidermis is thin, and the lesion tends to be friable, bleeds easily, and does not blanch on pressure. The base may be pedunculated and surrounded by a collarette of epidermis. The lesions occasionally resemble and must be differentiated from melanomas or other malignant tumors. During pregnancy, pyogenic granulomas may become large and exuberant (eg, gingival pregnancy tumors, or telangiectatic epulis).

Diagnosis involves biopsy and histologic examination. Treatment consists of removal by excision or curettage and electrodesiccation, but the lesions may recur.

Lymphatic Malformations

(Lymphangioma; Lymphangioma Circumscriptum; Cystic Hygroma; Cavernous Lymphangioma)

Lymphatic vascular malformations are elevated lesions composed of dilated lymphatic vessels.

Lesions are usually yellowish tan but occasionally reddish or purple if small blood vessels are intermingled. Puncture of the lesion yields a colorless or blood-tinged fluid. Diagnosis is made clinically and by MRI. Treatment is usually not needed. If excised, recurrence is common even when there is extensive removal of dermal and subcutaneous tissues.

128 CANCERS OF THE SKIN

Skin cancers are the most common type of cancer; most arise in sun-exposed areas of skin. The incidence is highest in outdoor workers, sportsmen, and sunbathers and is inversely related to the amount of melanin skin pigmentation; light-skinned people are most susceptible. Skin cancers may also develop years after therapeutic x-ray or exposure to carcinogens (eg, arsenic ingestion).

Over one million new cases of skin cancer are diagnosed in the US yearly. About 80% are basal cell carcinoma, 16% are squamous cell carcinoma, and 4% are melanoma. Paget's disease of the nipple or extramammary Paget's (usually near the anus), Kaposi's sarcoma, tumors of adnexae, and cutaneous T-cell lymphoma (mycosis fungoides—see p. 1124) make up the remaining less common forms.

Initially, skin cancers are often symptomless. The most frequent presentation is a papule or "blind pimple" that will not go away. Any lesion that appears to be enlarging with respect to surrounding structures, with or without tenderness and mild inflammation or crusting and occasional bleeding, should be biopsied. If treated early, most skin cancers are curable.

BASAL CELL CARCINOMA

(Rodent Ulcer)

Basal cell carcinoma is a superficial slowly growing papule or nodule that derives from epidermal basal cells. Metastasis is rare, but local growth can be highly destructive. Diagnosis is by biopsy. Treatment depends on the tumor's characteristics and may involve curettage and electrodesiccation, surgical excision, cryosurgery, or, occasionally, radiation therapy.

Basal cell carcinoma is the most common type of skin cancer, with >400,000 new cases yearly in the US. It is more common in fair-skinned, sun-exposed persons and is very rare in blacks.

The clinical presentation and biologic behavior of basal cell carcinomas are highly variable. They may appear as small, shiny, firm, almost translucent nodules; ulcerated, crusted papules or nodules; flat, scarlike indurated plaques; or red, marginated, thin papules or plaques difficult to differentiate from psoriasis or localized dermatitis. Most commonly, the carcinoma begins as a shiny papule, enlarges slowly, and, after a few months or years, shows a shiny, pearly border with prominent engorged vessels (telangiectases) on the surface and a central dell or ulcer. Recurrent crusting or bleeding is not unusual, and the lesion continues to enlarge slowly. Commonly, the carcinomas may alternately crust and heal, which may unjustifiably decrease the patient's and physician's concern about the importance of the lesion. Biopsy and histologic examination are essential.

Basal cell carcinomas rarely metastasize but may invade healthy tissues. Rarely, death may ensue because the carcinoma invades or impinges on underlying vital structures or orifices (eyes, ears, mouth, bone, dura mater).

Treatment should be performed by a specialist. The clinical appearance, size, site, and histologic subtype determine choice of treatment—curettage and electrodesiccation, surgical excision, cryosurgery, or, occasionally, radiation therapy. Recurrences (about 5%), large cancers, cancers at recurrence-prone sites, and morphea-like cancers with vague borders are often treated with Mohs microscopically controlled surgery, in which tissue borders are progressively excised until specimens are tumor-free (as determined by microscopic examination during surgery).

BOWEN'S DISEASE

(Intraepidermal Squamous Cell Carcinoma)

Bowen's disease is a superficial squamous cell carcinoma in situ.

Bowen's disease is most common in sun-exposed areas but may arise at any location. The lesion can be solitary or multiple. It is red-brown and scaly or crusted, with little induration, and it frequently resembles a localized thin plaque of psoriasis, dermatitis, or a dermatophyte infection. Diagnosis is by biopsy.

Treatment depends on the tumor's characteristics and may involve curettage and electrodesiccation, surgical excision, or cryosurgery.

KAPOSI'S SARCOMA

(Multiple Idiopathic Hemorrhagic Sarcoma)

Kaposi's sarcoma is a multicentric vascular tumor caused by herpesvirus type 8. It can occur in AIDS-associated, endemic, and iatrogenic forms. Diagnosis is by biopsy. Treatment for indolent superficial lesions involves cryotherapy, electrocoagulation, or electron beam radiation therapy. Radiation therapy is used for more extensive disease. In the AIDS-associated form, antiretrovirals provide the best improvement

Kaposi's sarcoma (KS) originates from endothelial cells in response to infection by human herpesvirus 8 (HHV-8). Immunosuppression (particularly by AIDS and drugs for organ transplant recipients) markedly increases the likelihood of KS in HHV-8–infected patients. The tumor cells have a spindle shape, resembling smooth muscle cells, fibroblasts, and myofibroblasts.

Classic KS occurs most often in older (> 60 yr) men of Italian, Jewish, or Eastern European ancestry. The course is indolent, and the disease is usually confined to a small number of lesions on the skin of the lower extremities; visceral involvement occurs in < 10%. This form is usually not fatal.

AIDS-associated (epidemic) KS is the most common AIDS-associated malignancy and is more aggressive than classic KS. Multiple cutaneous lesions are typically present, often involving the face and trunk. Mucosal, lymph node, and GI involvement is common. Sometimes KS is the first manifestation of AIDS.

Endemic KS occurs in Africa independent of HIV infection. There are 2 peaks, prepubertal and adult. The prepubertal lymphadenopathic form is more aggressive and usually fatal. The adult form more resembles classic KS.

Iatrogenic (immunosuppressive) KS typically develops several years after organ transplantation. The course is more or less fulminant, depending on the degree of immunosuppression.

The lymphadenopathic type, most common in endemic KS, predominantly affects children with primary tumors involving lymph nodes (with or without skin lesions). The course is usually fulminant and fatal.

Symptoms, Signs, and Diagnosis

Cutaneous lesions are asymptomatic purple, pink, or red macules that may coalesce into blue-violet to black plaques and eventually nodules. Some edema may be present. Occasionally, nodules fungate or penetrate soft tissue and invade bone. Mucosal lesions appear as bluish to violaceous macules, plaques, and tumors. GI lesions can bleed, sometimes extensively, but usually are asymptomatic.

Diagnosis is confirmed by punch biopsy. Patients with AIDS or immunosuppression require evaluation for visceral spread by CT of the chest and abdomen. If pulmonary or GI symptoms are present, bronchoscopy or GI endoscopy should be considered if CT is negative.

Treatment

Indolent lesions often require no treatment. One or a few superficial lesions can be removed by excision, cryotherapy, or electrocoagulation. Intralesional vinblastine or interferon-α is also useful. Multiple lesions and lymph node disease are treated locally with 10 to 20 Gy of radiation therapy.

AIDS-related KS responds markedly to highly active antiretroviral therapy (HAART); this is probably a result of improvement in $CD4^+$ count and decreasing HIV viral load, but there is some evidence that protease inhibitors in this regimen may block angiogenesis. AIDS patients with indolent disease and $CD4^+$ counts > 150 /μL and HIV RNA < 500 copies/mL can be treated with IV interferon-α. Patients with more extensive or visceral disease can be given liposomal doxorubicin 20 mg/m^2 IV q 2 to 3 wk. If this regimen fails, patients may receive paclitaxel. Other agents being investigated as adjuncts include IL-12, HIV-TAT protein inhibitors, and human chorionic gonadotropin. Treatment of KS does not prolong life in most AIDS patients because infections dominate the clinical course.

Iatrogenic KS responds best to stopping immunosuppressants. In organ transplant patients, reduction of immunosuppressant dosage often results in reduction of KS lesions. If this is not possible, conventional local and systemic therapies used in other forms of KS should be instituted.

MELANOMA

(Malignant Melanoma)

Malignant melanoma arises from melanocytes in a pigmented area: skin, mucous membranes, eyes, and CNS. Metastasis is correlated with depth of dermal invasion. With spread, prognosis is poor. Diagnosis is by biopsy. Wide surgical excision is the rule for operable tumors. Metastatic disease requires chemotherapy but is difficult to cure.

About 50,000 new cases of melanoma occur yearly in the US, causing about 8000 deaths. The incidence is increasing at a faster rate than any other malignant tumor. Sun exposure is a risk, as is family history, increased numbers of melanocytic nevi, and the occurrence of lentigo maligna, large congenital melanocytic nevus, and the dysplastic nevus syndrome. Melanoma is rare in blacks.

People who have one or more 1st-degree relatives with a history of melanoma have an increased risk (up to 6 or 8 times) over those without a family history.

About 40 to 50% of melanomas develop from pigmented moles (see also p. 1018); almost all the rest arise from melanocytes in normal skin. Precancerous lesions include atypical moles (dysplastic nevi—see p. 1019). The very rare melanomas of childhood almost always arise from large pigmented moles (giant congenital nevi) present at birth. Although melanomas occur during pregnancy, pregnancy does not increase the likelihood that a mole will become a melanoma; nevi frequently change in size and darken uniformly during pregnancy. However, signs of malignant transformation should be carefully sought: change in size; irregular change in color, especially spread of red, white, and blue pigmentation to surrounding normal skin; change in surface characteristics, consistency, or shape; and especially signs of inflammation in surrounding skin, with possible bleeding, ulceration, itching, or tenderness.

Melanomas also occur on the mucosa of the oral and genital regions and conjunctiva. Mucosal melanomas (especially anorectal melanomas), which are more common in nonwhites, have an unfavorable prognosis.

Melanomas vary in size, shape, and color (usually pigmented) and in their propensity to invade and metastasize. The tumor may spread rapidly, causing death within months of its recognition, yet the 5-yr cure rate of early, very superficial lesions is nearly 100%. Thus, cure depends on early diagnosis and early treatment. Four major types of melanoma are described here.

Lentigo maligna melanoma accounts for up to 15% of melanomas. It tends to arise in older patients. It arises from lentigo maligna (Hutchinson's freckle or malignant melanoma in situ). It appears on the face or other sun-exposed areas as an asymptomatic, 2- to 6-cm, flat, tan or brown, irregularly shaped macule or patch with darker brown or black spots scattered irregularly on its surface. In lentigo maligna, both normal and malignant melanocytes are confined to the epidermis; when malignant melanocytes invade the dermis, the lesion is called lentigo maligna melanoma, and the cancer may metastasize.

Superficial spreading melanoma accounts for ⅔ of melanomas. Typically asymptomatic, it is usually diagnosed when smaller than lentigo maligna melanoma and occurs most commonly on women's legs and men's torsos. The lesion is usually a plaque with irregular raised, indurated tan or brown areas, which often show red, white, black, and blue spots or small, sometimes protuberant, blue-black nodules. Small notchlike indentations of the margins may be noted, along with enlargement or color change. Histologically, atypical melanocytes characteristically invade dermis and epidermis.

Nodular melanoma accounts for 10 to 15% of melanomas. It may occur anywhere on the body as a dark, protuberant papule or a plaque that varies from pearl to gray to black. Occasionally, a lesion contains little if any pigment or may look like a vascular tumor. Unless it ulcerates, nodular melanoma is asymptomatic, but the patient usually seeks advice because the lesion enlarges rapidly.

Acral-lentiginous melanoma, although uncommon, is the most common form of melanoma in blacks. It arises on palmar, plantar, and subungual skin and has a characteristic histologic picture similar to lentigo maligna melanoma.

Metastasis of melanoma occurs via lymphatics and blood vessels. Local metastasis results in the formation of nearby satellite papules or nodules that may or may not be pigmented. Direct metastasis to skin or internal organs may occur, and occasionally metastatic nodules or enlarged lymph nodes are discovered before the primary lesion is identified.

Diagnosis

The differential diagnosis includes basal cell and squamous cell carcinomas, seborrheic keratoses, dysplastic nevi, blue nevi, dermatofibromas, moles, hematomas (especially on the hands or feet), venous lakes, pyogenic granulomas, and warts with focal thromboses. If doubt exists, biopsy should include the full depth of the dermis and extend slightly beyond the edges of the lesion. Biopsy should be excisional for small lesions and incisional for larger lesions. By doing step sections, the pathologist can determine the maximal thickness of the melanoma. Definitive radical surgery should not precede histologic diagnosis.

Guidelines for selecting pigmented lesions for excision or biopsy include recent enlargement, darkening, bleeding, or ulceration. However, these features usually indicate that the melanoma has already invaded the skin deeply. Earlier diagnosis is possible if biopsy specimens can be obtained from lesions having variegated colors (eg, brown or black with shades of red, white, or blue), irregular elevations that are visible or palpable, and borders with angular indentations or notches. The dermatoscope, a modified ophthalmoscope used with immersion oil to examine pigmented lesions, may be useful in distinguishing melanomas from benign lesions.

The degree of lymphocytic infiltration, which represents reaction by the patient's immunologic defense system, may correlate with the level of invasion and prognosis. Chances of cure are maximal when lymphocytic infiltration is limited to the most superficial lesions and decrease with deeper levels of tumor cell invasion, ulceration, and vascular or lymphatic invasion.

The staging of melanoma is based on clinical and pathologic criteria and is categorized into local, regional, or distant disease; the stage strongly correlates with survival. A minimally invasive microstaging technique, the so-called sentinel node biopsy, is a major advance in the ability to stage patients more accurately. Staging studies are usually performed by a coordinated team that includes dermatologists, general surgeons, plastic surgeons, and dermatopathologists.

Prognosis and Treatment

For tumors of cutaneous origin (not CNS and subungual melanomas), survival rate varies depending on the thickness of the tumor at the time of diagnosis (see TABLE 128–1). Melanomas arising from mucous membranes have a poor prognosis, although they often seem quite limited when discovered. Once melanoma has metastasized, 5-yr survival is about 10%.

Treatment is by surgical excision. Although the width of margins is debated, most experts agree that a 1-cm lateral tumor-free margin is adequate for lesions < 1 mm thick. Thicker lesions may deserve more radical surgery and sentinel node biopsy.

Metastatic disease is generally inoperable. Adjuvant therapy, the active suppression of clinically inapparent micrometastasis using recombinant biological response modifiers, particularly the intensely studied interferon-α, is being evaluated. For advanced stages, studies involve infusing lymphokine-activated killer cells, or antibodies. Vaccine therapy is also being investigated. Brain metastases may

TABLE 128–1. 5-YEAR SURVIVAL FOR MALIGNANT MELANOMA, RELATIVE TO THICKNESS

TUMOR THICKNESS (mm)*	5-YR SURVIVAL (%)
< 0.76	98–100
0.76–1.5	90–94
1.51–2.25	83–84
2.26–3.0	72–77
> 3.0	46

*Tumor thickness is very difficult to assess if histologic signs of regression are present.

be treated with radiation, but the response is poor.

Lentigo maligna melanoma and lentigo maligna are usually treated with wide local excision and, if necessary, skin grafting. Intensive radiation therapy is much less effective. Early excision of lentigo maligna—before the lesion is very large—is recommended; most other treatment methods except controlled cryosurgery usually do not reach deep enough into involved follicles, which must be removed.

Spreading or nodular melanomas are usually treated by wide local excision extending down to the fascia. Lymph node dissection may be recommended when nodes are involved.

PAGET'S DISEASE OF THE NIPPLE

Paget's disease is a rare type of carcinoma that appears as a unilateral eczematous to psoriasiform plaque surrounding the nipple. It is extension to the epidermis of an underlying ductal adenocarcinoma of the breast.

Paget's disease of the nipples should not be confused with the metabolic bone disease also called Paget's disease. Often, metastatic disease is present at the time of the diagnosis. Treatment is surgical.

Paget's also occurs at other sites, most often in the groin or perianal area (extramammary Paget's disease). The bladder and rectum are the most common sites. Extramammary Paget's disease is a rare intraepithelial adenocarcinoma of apocrine gland–bearing sites. The redness, oozing, and crusting closely resemble dermatitis, but the physician should suspect carcinoma because the lesion is sharply marginated, unilateral, and unresponsive to topical therapy. Biopsy shows typical histologic changes. Treatment involves surgical removal of discovered tumors and ablation of overlying cutaneous involvement either surgically or by CO_2 laser ablation. Because of its association with underlying malignancy, systemic evaluation is required.

SQUAMOUS CELL CARCINOMA

Squamous cell carcinoma is a malignant tumor of epidermal keratinocytes that invades the dermis, usually occurring in sun-exposed areas. Local destruction may be extensive, and metastases occur in advanced stages. Diagnosis is by biopsy. Treatment depends on the tumor's characteristics and may involve curettage and electrodesiccation, surgical excision, cryosurgery, or, occasionally, radiation therapy.

Squamous cell carcinoma, the 2nd most common type of skin cancer, may develop in normal tissue, in a preexisting actinic keratosis (see p. 963) or patch of leukoplakia or in a burn scar. The incidence in the US is 80,000 to 100,000 cases annually, with 2000 deaths.

The clinical appearance is highly variable, but any nonhealing lesion on sun-exposed surfaces should be suspect. The tumor may begin as a red papule or plaque with a scaly or crusted surface and may become nodular, sometimes with a warty surface. In some, the bulk of the lesion may lie below the level of the surrounding skin. Eventually the tumor ulcerates and invades the underlying tissue. The percentage of squamous cell carcinomas on sun-exposed skin that metastasize is quite low. However, about ⅓ of lingual or mucosal cancers have metastasized before diagnosis (see p. 842). Differential diagnosis includes many types of benign and malignant lesions, such as basal cell carcinoma, keratoacanthoma, actinic keratosis, verruca vulgaris, and seborrheic keratosis. Biopsy is essential.

In general, the prognosis for small lesions removed early and adequately is excellent. Regional and distant metastases are uncommon but do occur, particularly with poorly differentiated tumors. Late-stage disease may require extensive surgery and is far more likely to metastasize, initially locoregionally to surrounding skin and lymph nodes and eventually to nearby organs. The overall 5-yr survival rate for metastatic disease is 34% despite therapy.

Treatment is the same as for basal cell carcinoma (see p. 1023), but treatment and follow-up must be monitored closely because of the greater risk of metastasis. Squamous cell carcinoma on the lip or other mucocutaneous junction should be excised; at times, cure is difficult. Recurrences should be treated aggressively with Mohs surgery, or by a team approach with surgery and radiation therapy.

Metastatic disease is responsive to radiation therapy if metastases can be identified and are isolated. Widespread metastases do not respond well to chemotherapeutic regimens.

SECTION 11 HEMATOLOGY AND ONCOLOGY

129 APPROACH TO THE PATIENT WITH ANEMIA

Red blood cell (RBC) production (erythropoiesis) takes place in the bone marrow under the control of the hormone erythropoietin (EPO). Juxtaglomerular cells in the kidney produce EPO in response to decreased O_2 delivery (as in anemia and hypoxia) and increased levels of androgens. In addition to EPO, RBC production requires adequate supplies of substrates, mainly iron, vitamin B_{12}, and folate. Vitamin B_{12} and folate are discussed in Ch. 4 (see p. 26); iron is discussed in Ch. 130 (see p. 1036).

RBCs become senescent after about 120 days. They then lose their cell membranes and are largely cleared from the circulation by the phagocytic cells of the spleen, liver, and bone marrow. Hb is broken down in these cells and in hepatocytes primarily by the heme oxygenase system with conservation (and subsequent reutilization) of iron, degradation of heme to bilirubin through a series of enzymatic steps, and reutilization of protein. Maintenance of a steady number of RBCs requires daily renewal of 1/120 of the cells; immature RBCs (reticulocytes) are continually released and constitute 0.5 to 1.5% of the peripheral RBC population.

Low levels of androgens leading to decreased EPO levels in females and in elderly patients can predispose to anemia, as does the decline in the capacity of bone marrow to produce RBCs. With aging, Hb and Hct decrease slightly, but not below normal values. In women, other factors that frequently contribute to lower concentrations of RBCs include cumulative menstrual blood loss and increased demand for iron due to multiple pregnancies.

ETIOLOGY OF ANEMIA

Anemia is a decrease in the number of RBCs, Hct, or Hb content.

The RBC mass represents the balance between production and destruction or loss of RBCs. Thus, anemia can result from one or more of 3 basic mechanisms (see TABLE 129–1): blood loss, deficient erythropoiesis, and excessive hemolysis (RBC destruction).

Blood loss can be acute or chronic. Anemia does not develop until several hours after acute blood loss, when interstitial fluid diffuses into the intravascular space and dilutes the remaining RBC mass. During the first few hours, however, concentrations of polymorphonuclear granulocytes, platelets, and, in severe hemorrhage, immature WBCs and normoblasts may rise. Chronic blood loss results in anemia if loss is more rapid than can be replaced or, more commonly, if accelerated erythropoiesis depletes body iron stores (see p. 1036).

Deficient erythropoiesis (see p. 1036) has myriad causes. Complete cessation of erythropoiesis results in a decline in RBCs of about 7 to 10%/wk (1%/day). Impaired erythropoiesis, even if not sufficient to decrease the numbers of RBCs, often causes abnormal RBC size and shape.

Excessive hemolysis (see p. 1045) can be caused by intrinsic abnormalities of RBCs or by extrinsic factors, such as the presence of

TABLE 129–1. ANEMIAS CLASSIFIED BY CAUSE

Blood loss

- Acute
- Chronic

Deficient erythropoiesis (classified by RBC indices)

- Microcytic
  - Iron deficiency
  - Iron-transport deficiency
  - Iron utilization
  - Iron reutilization
  - Thalassemias (also classified under intrinsic RBC defects)
- Normochromic-normocytic
  - Hypoproliferation
    - In kidney disease
    - In endocrine failure (thyroid, pituitary)
    - In protein depletion
  - Aplastic anemia
  - Myelophthisis
  - Myelodysplasia
- Macrocytic
  - Vitamin B_{12} deficiency
  - Folate deficiency
  - Copper deficiency
  - Vitamin C deficiency

Excessive hemolysis

- Extrinsic RBC defects
  - Reticuloendothelial hyperactivity with splenomegaly
  - Immunologic abnormalities
    - Isoimmune (isoagglutinin) hemolysis
    - Autoimmune hemolysis
      - Warm antibody hemolysis
      - Cold antibody hemolysis (paroxysmal cold hemoglobinuria)
  - Mechanical injury
    - Trauma
    - Infection
- Intrinsic RBC defects
  - Membrane alterations
    - Congenital
      - Congenital erythropoietic porphyria
      - Hereditary elliptocytosis
      - Hereditary spherocytosis
    - Acquired
      - Stomatocytosis
      - Hypophosphatemia
      - Paroxysmal nocturnal hemoglobinuria
  - Metabolic disorders (inherited enzyme deficiencies)
    - Embden-Meyerhof pathway defects
    - Glucose-6-phosphate dehydrogenase (G6PD) deficiency
  - Hemoglobinopathies
    - Sickle cell anemia (Hb S)
    - Hb C, S-C, and E diseases
    - Thalassemias (β, β-δ, and α)
    - Hb S-β-thalassemia disease

antibodies on their surface, that lead to their early destruction. An enlarged spleen sequesters and destroys RBCs more rapidly than normal. Some causes of hemolysis deform as well as destroy RBCs. Excessive hemolysis does not normally decrease reticulocyte production unless iron or other essential nutrients are depleted.

EVALUATION OF ANEMIA

Anemia is not a diagnosis; it is a manifestation of an underlying disorder. Thus, even mild, asymptomatic anemia should be investigated so that the primary problem can be diagnosed and treated. Acute or chronic blood loss is the first consideration. This diagnosis generally is based on history, examination, and a stool test for occult blood. Further testing for occult bleeding is sometimes necessary.

If blood loss is not detected, laboratory testing is usually done to determine whether anemia is due to deficient RBC production or excessive hemolysis.

History

The history should address risk factors for particular anemias, symptoms of anemia itself, and symptoms that reflect the underlying disorder.

Anemia has many risk factors. For example, a vegan diet predisposes to vitamin B_{12} deficiency anemia, whereas alcoholism increases the risk of folate deficiency anemia. A number of hemoglobinopathies are inherited, and certain drugs predispose to hemolysis. Cancer, rheumatic disorders, and chronic inflammatory disease can suppress bone marrow activity or enlarge the spleen.

The symptoms of anemia are neither sensitive nor specific and do not help differentiate between types of anemias. Symptoms reflect compensatory responses to tissue hypoxia and usually develop when Hb falls < 7 g/dL. However, they may develop at higher Hb levels in patients with limited cardiopulmonary reserve or in whom the anemia developed very rapidly. Symptoms such as weakness, seeing spots, fatigue, drowsiness, angina, syncope, and dyspnea on exertion can indicate anemia. Vertigo, headache, tinnitus, amenorrhea, loss of libido, and GI complaints may also occur. Heart failure or shock can develop with severe tissue hypoxia or hypovolemia.

Certain symptoms may suggest an underlying cause of the anemia. For example, melena, epistaxis, hematochezia, hematemesis, or menorrhagia indicates bleeding. Jaundice and dark urine suggest hemolysis. Weight loss may suggest cancer. Diffuse severe bone or chest pain may suggest sickle cell disease, and stocking-glove paresthesias may suggest vitamin B_{12} or folate deficiency.

Physical Examination

Complete physical examination is necessary. Signs of anemia itself are neither sensitive nor specific; however, pallor is common with severe anemia.

Signs of underlying disorders are often more diagnostically accurate than are signs of anemia. Heme-positive stool identifies GI bleeding. Hemorrhagic shock (eg, hypotension, tachycardia, pallor, tachypnea, diaphoresis, confusion—see p. 559) may result from acute bleeding. Jaundice may suggest hemolysis. Splenomegaly may occur with hemolysis, hemoglobinopathy, connective tissue disease, myeloproliferative disorder, infection, or cancer. Peripheral neuropathy suggests vitamin B_{12} deficiency; abdominal distention in a victim of blunt trauma suggests acute hemorrhage; petechiae develop in thrombocytopenia or platelet dysfunction; fever and heart murmurs suggest infectious endocarditis, a possible cause of hemolysis. Rarely, high-output heart failure develops as a compensatory response to anemia-induced tissue hypoxia.

Testing

Laboratory evaluation begins with a CBC, including WBC and platelet counts, RBC indices and morphology, and examination of the peripheral smear. The peripheral smear is highly accurate in determining whether anemia results from deficient RBC production or excessive RBC destruction. Subsequent tests are selected on the basis of these results and on the clinical presentation. Recognition of general diagnostic patterns can expedite the diagnosis (see TABLE 129–2).

The automated CBC directly measures Hb, RBC count, and MCV (a measure of RBC size); Hct (a measure of the percentage of blood made up of RBCs), MCH (a measure of the Hb content in individual RBCs), and MCHC (a measure of the Hb concentration in individual RBCs) are calculated values. The diagnostic criterion for anemia in men is Hb < 14 g/dL, Hct < 42%, or RBC < 4.5 million/L; for women, Hb < 12 g/dL, Hct < 37%, or RBC < 4 million/L. For infants, normal values vary with age, necessitating use of age-related tables. RBC populations are termed microcytic (small cells) if MCV is < 80 fL, and macrocytic (large cells) if MCV is > 95 fL. However, because reticulocytes are also larger than mature red cells, large numbers of reticulocytes can elevate the MCV and not represent an alteration of RBC production. Automated techniques can also determine the degree of variation in RBC size, expressed as the RBC volume distribution width (RDW). A high RDW may be the only indication of simultaneous microcytotic and macrocytotic disorders (or simultaneous microcytosis and reticulocytosis); such a pattern may result in a normal MCV, which measures only the mean value. The term hypochromia refers to RBC populations in which MCH is < 27 pg/RBC or MCHC is < 30%. RBC populations with normal MCH and MCHC values are normochromic.

The RBC indices can help indicate the mechanism of anemia and narrow the number of possible causes. Microcytic indices occur with altered heme or globin synthesis. The most common causes are iron deficiency, thalassemia, and related Hb-synthesis defects. In some patients with anemia of chronic disease, the MCV is microcytic or borderline microcytic. Macrocytic indices occur with impaired DNA synthesis (eg, due to vitamin B_{12} or folate deficiencies or chemotherapeutic drugs such as hydroxyurea and antifolate agents) and in alcoholism because of abnormalities of the cell membrane. Acute bleeding may briefly produce macrocytic indices because of the release of large young reticulocytes. Normocytic indices occur in anemias resulting from deficient EPO or inadequate response to it (hypoproliferative anemias). Hemorrhage, before iron deficiency develops, usually results in normocytic and normochromic anemia unless the number of large reticulocytes is excessive.

The peripheral blood smear is highly sensitive for excessive RBC production and hemolysis. It is more accurate than automated technologies for recognition of altered RBC structure, thrombocytopenia, nucleated RBCs,

TABLE 129–2. CHARACTERISTICS OF COMMON ANEMIAS

ETIOLOGY OR TYPE	MORPHOLOGIC CHANGES	SPECIAL FEATURES
Acute blood loss	Normochromic-normocytic, with polychromatophilia; hyperplastic marrow	If severe, possible nucleated RBCs and left shift of WBCs; leukocytosis and thrombocytosis
Chronic blood loss	Same as iron deficiency	
Iron deficiency	Microcytic, with anisocytosis and poikilocytosis; reticulocytopenia; hyperplastic marrow, with delayed hemoglobination	Possible achlorhydria, smooth tongue, and spoon nails; absent stainable marrow iron; low serum iron; increased total iron-binding capacity; low serum ferritin; low RBC ferritin
Vitamin B_{12} deficiency	Oval macrocytes; anisocytosis; reticulocytopenia; hypersegmented WBCs; megaloblastic marrow	Serum B_{12} < 180 pg/mL (< 130 pmol/L); frequent GI and CNS involvement; positive Schilling test, elevated serum bilirubin; increased LDH; antibodies to intrinsic factor in serum (common), absent gastric intrinsic factor secretion
Folate deficiency	Same as vitamin B_{12} deficiency	Serum folate < 5 ng/mL (< 11 nmol/L); RBC folate < 225 ng/mL RBCs (< 510 nmol/L); nutritional deficiency and malabsorption (sprue, pregnancy, infancy, alcoholism)
Marrow failure	Normochromic-normocytic; reticulocytopenia; failed marrow aspiration (often) or evident hypoplasia of erythroid series or of all elements	Idiopathic (> 50%) or secondary to exposure to toxic drugs or chemicals (eg, chloramphenicol, quinacrine, hydantoins, insecticides)
Sideroblastic anemia	Usually hypochromic but dimorphic with normocytes and macrocytes; hyperplastic marrow, with delayed hemoglobination; ringed sideroblasts	Inborn or acquired metabolic defect; stainable marrow iron (plentiful); response to B_6 (rare); commonly part of myelodysplastic syndrome
Acute hemolysis	Normochromic-normocytic; reticulocytosis; marrow erythroid hyperplasia	Increased serum bilirubin and LDH; increased stool and urine urobilinogen; hemoglobinuria in fulminating cases; hemosiderinuria
Chronic hemolysis	Normochromic-normocytic; reticulocytosis; marrow erythroid hyperplasia; basophilic stippling (especially in lead poisoning)	Increased serum bilirubin and LDH; shortened RBC life span; increased radio-iron turnover; hemosiderinuria
Hereditary spherocytosis	Spheroidal microcytes; normoblastic erythroid hyperplasia	Increased mean RBC Hb concentration; increased RBC fragility; shortened survival of labeled RBCs; increased radioactivity of spleen (exceeds that of liver)
Paroxysmal nocturnal hemoglobinuria	Normocytic (may be hypochromic because of iron deficiency); marrow may be hypercellular or hypocellular	Dark morning urine; hemosiderin; positive acid hemolysis (Ham's) and sugar-water tests

TABLE 129–2. CHARACTERISTICS OF COMMON ANEMIAS—Continued

ETIOLOGY OR TYPE	MORPHOLOGIC CHANGES	SPECIAL FEATURES
Paroxysmal cold hemoglobinuria	Normochromic-normocytic	Follows exposure to cold; results from a cold agglutinin or hemolysin; often associated with syphilis or other infections
Sickle cell anemia	Anisocytosis and poikilocytosis; some sickle cells in smear; all RBCs sickle in preparation with hypoxia or hyperosmolar exposure	Largely limited to blacks; urinary isosthenuria; Hb S on electrophoresis; possibly painful vaso-occlusive crises and leg ulcers; bony changes on x-ray
Thalassemia	Microcytic; thin cells; target cells; basophilic stippling; anisocytosis and poikilocytosis; nucleated RBCs in homozygotes	Decreased RBC fragility; elevated Hb A_2 and Hb F (often); Mediterranean ancestry (common); anemic homozygotes from infancy; splenomegaly; bony changes on x-ray
Infection or chronic inflammation	Normochromic-normocytic early, then microcytic; normoblastic marrow; normal iron stores	Decreased serum iron; decreased total iron-binding capacity; normal serum ferritin, RBC ferritin, and marrow iron content
Marrow replacement (myelophthisis)	Anisocytosis and poikilocytosis; nucleated RBCs; early granulocyte precursors; marrow aspiration may fail or may show leukemia, myeloma, or metastatic cells	Marrow infiltration with infectious granulomas, tumors, fibrosis, or lipid histiocytosis; possible hepatomegaly and splenomegaly; possible bony changes; radio-iron uptake greater over spleen and liver than over sacrum

or immature granulocytes and can detect other abnormalities (eg, malaria and other parasites, intracellular RBC or granulocyte inclusions) that can occur despite normal automated blood cell counts. RBC injury may be identified by finding RBC fragments, portions of disrupted cells (schistocytes), or evidence of significant membrane alterations from oval-shaped cells (ovalocytes) or spherocytic cells. Target cells (thin RBCs with a central dot of Hb) are RBCs with insufficient Hb or excess cell membrane (eg, due to hemoglobinopathies or liver disorders). The peripheral smear can also reveal variation in RBC shape (poikilocytosis) and size (anisocytosis).

The reticulocyte count is expressed as the percentage of reticulocytes (normal range, 0.5 to 1.5%) or as the absolute reticulocyte count (normal range, 50,000 to 150,000/μL). Higher values indicate excessive production, or reticulocytosis; in the presence of anemia, reticulocytosis suggests excessive RBC destruction. Low numbers in the presence of anemia indicate decreased RBC production. The reticulocyte response can usually be estimated by the number of blue cells seen in the peripheral smear stained with a supravital stain, making a reticulocyte count, which requires flow cytometry or a large amount of time, unnecessary.

Bone marrow aspiration and biopsy provide direct observation and assessment of RBC precursors. The presence of abnormal maturation (dyspoiesis) of blood cells and the amount, distribution, and cellular pattern of iron content can be assessed. Bone marrow aspiration and biopsy are performed to diagnose unexplained anemias, other cytopenias, unexplained leukocytosis, thrombocytosis, and suspected leukemia, multiple myeloma, or myelophthisis. Cytogenetic and molecular analyses can be performed on aspirate material in hematopoietic or other neoplasms or in suspected congenital lesions of RBC precursors (eg, Fanconi's anemia). Flow cytometry can be performed in suspected lymphoproliferative or myeloproliferative states to define the immunophenotype. Bone marrow aspiration and biopsy are neither technically difficult nor pose significant risk of morbidity and are safe and helpful when hematologic disease is suspected. Both usually can be performed as a single procedure. Because biopsy requires adequate bone depth, the posterior (or, less commonly, anterior) iliac crest usually is used. If only aspiration is necessary, the sternum or dorsal lumbar vertebral spine may be used.

Serum bilirubin and LDH can sometimes help differentiate between hemolysis and blood loss; both are elevated in hemolysis and normal in blood loss. Other tests are discussed under specific anemias and bleeding disorders. For tests of hemostasis (eg, bleeding time, clot retraction and observation, fibrin and fibrinogen degradation products, PTT and PT), see p. 1077.

TREATMENT OF ANEMIA

When possible, the underlying cause of anemia is treated. When the Hb falls dangerously low, eg, < 7 g/dL for those without cardiopulmonary insufficiency or higher for those with it, RBC transfusion temporarily increases O_2-carrying capacity. RBC transfusion should be reserved for patients with or at high risk of cardiopulmonary symptoms; signs of active, uncontrollable blood loss; or some form of hypoxic or ischemic end-organ failure (eg, neurologic ischemic symptoms, angina, tachycardia in patients with underlying heart failure or severe COPD). Transfusion procedures and blood components are discussed in Ch. 146 (see p. 1134).

130 ANEMIAS CAUSED BY DEFICIENT ERYTHROPOIESIS

Anemia (a decrease in the number of RBCs, Hb content, or Hct) can result from decreased RBC production (erythropoiesis), increased RBC destruction, or blood loss. Anemias due to decreased erythropoiesis are recognized by reticulocytopenia, which is usually evident on the peripheral blood smear (see p. 1033). The RBC indices, mainly the MCV, narrow the differential diagnosis of deficient erythropoiesis and determine what further testing is necessary.

Microcytic anemias result from deficient or defective heme or globin synthesis. Microcytic anemias include iron deficiency anemias, iron-transport deficiency anemias, iron-utilization anemias (including some sideroblastic anemias and lead poisoning), and thalassemias (which also cause hemolysis—see p. 1057).

Normocytic anemias result from primary bone marrow failure. They are characterized by a normal RBC distribution width (RDW) and usually normochromic indices. The mechanisms involved are hypoproliferation (deficiency of or inadequate response to erythropoietin [EPO]), hypoplasia (in aplastic anemia), myelophthisis, and myelodysplasia.

Macrocytic anemias result most often from impaired DNA synthesis, as do deficiencies of vitamin B_{12} or folate. Anemia of chronic disease may be microcytic or normocytic. Anemias due to myelodysplastic syndromes may be microcytic, normocytic, or macrocytic. Patients with microcytic anemias require testing of iron stores (see Iron Deficiency Anemia, below).

Treatment of deficient RBC production depends on the cause; however, stimulation of erythropoiesis with human recombinant EPO often is helpful. Because erythropoiesis increases the iron requirement, supplemental iron is helpful when administering any type of treatment that aims to increase erythropoiesis.

IRON DEFICIENCY ANEMIA

(Anemia of Chronic Blood Loss; Chlorosis)

Iron deficiency is the most common cause of anemia and usually results from blood loss. Symptoms are usually nonspecific. RBCs tend to be microcytic and hypochromic, and iron stores are low as shown by low serum ferritin and low serum iron with high serum transferrin. If the diagnosis is made, occult blood loss is suspected. Treatment involves

iron replacement and treatment of blood loss.

Iron is distributed in active metabolic and storage pools. Total body iron is about 3.5 g in healthy men and 2.5 g in women; the difference relates to body size, lower androgen levels, and the dearth of stored iron in women because of iron loss with menses and pregnancy. The distribution of body iron in an average man is Hb, 2100 mg; myoglobin, 200 mg; tissue (heme and nonheme) enzymes, 150 mg; and transport-iron compartment, 3 mg. Iron is stored in cells and plasma as ferritin (700 mg) and in cells as hemosiderin (300 mg).

Iron is absorbed in the duodenum and upper jejunum. Absorption of iron is determined by the type of iron molecule and by what other substances are ingested. Iron absorption is best when food contains heme iron (meat). Dietary nonheme iron must be reduced to the ferrous state and released from food binders by gastric secretions. Nonheme iron absorption is reduced by other food items (eg, vegetable fiber phytates and polyphenols; tea tannates, including phosphoproteins; bran) and certain antibiotics (eg, tetracycline). Ascorbic acid is the only common food element known to increase nonheme iron absorption.

The average American diet, which contains 6 mg of elemental iron/kcal of food, is adequate for iron homeostasis. Of about 15 mg/day of dietary iron, adults absorb only 1 mg, which is the approximate amount lost daily by cell desquamation from the skin and intestines. In iron depletion, absorption increases, although the exact signaling mechanism is not known; however, absorption rarely increases to > 6 mg/day unless supplemental iron is added. Children have a greater need for iron and appear to absorb more to meet this need.

Iron from the intestinal mucosal cell is transferred to transferrin, an iron-transport protein synthesized in the liver; transferrin can transport iron from cells (intestinal, macrophages) to specific receptors on erythroblasts, placental cells, and liver cells. For heme synthesis, transferrin transports iron to the erythroblast mitochondria, which insert the iron into protoporphyrin for it to become heme. Transferrin (plasma half-life, 8 days) is extruded for reutilization. Synthesis of transferrin increases with iron deficiency but decreases with any type of chronic disease.

Iron not used for erythropoiesis is transferred by transferrin to the storage pool, which has 2 forms. The most important is ferritin (a heterogenous group of proteins surrounding an iron core), which is a soluble and active storage fraction located in the liver (in hepatocytes), bone marrow, and spleen (in macrophages); in RBCs; and in serum. Iron stored in ferritin is readily available for any body requirement. Circulating (serum) ferritin concentration parallels the size of the body stores (1 ng/mL = 8 mg of iron in the storage pool). The 2nd storage pool of iron is in hemosiderin, which is relatively insoluble and is stored primarily in the liver (in Kupffer cells) and in the marrow (in macrophages).

Because iron absorption is so limited, the body recycles and conserves iron. Transferrin grasps and recycles available iron from aging RBCs undergoing phagocytosis by mononuclear phagocytes. This mechanism provides about 97% of the daily iron needed (about 25 mg of iron). With aging, iron stores tend to increase because iron elimination is slow.

Etiology

Because iron is poorly absorbed, most people barely meet the daily requirement. Thus, even modest losses, increased requirements, or decreased intake readily produces iron deficiency.

Blood loss is almost always the cause. In men, the most frequent cause is chronic occult bleeding, usually from the GI tract. In premenopausal women, cumulative menstrual blood loss (mean, 0.5 mg iron/day) is a common cause. Another possible cause of blood loss in men and women is chronic intravascular hemolysis (see p. 1045) if the amount of iron released during hemolysis exceeds the haptoglobin-binding capacity. Vitamin C deficiency can contribute to iron deficiency anemia by producing capillary fragility, hemolysis, and bleeding.

Increased iron requirement may contribute to iron deficiency. From birth to age 2 and during adolescence, when rapid growth requires a large iron intake, dietary iron often is inadequate. During pregnancy, the fetal iron requirement increases the maternal iron requirement (mean, 0.5 to 0.8 mg/day—see also Anemia in Pregnancy on p. 2167) despite the absence of menses. Lactation also increases the iron requirement (mean, 0.4 mg/day).

Decreased iron absorption can result from gastrectomy and upper small-bowel malabsorption syndromes. Rarely, absorption is decreased by dietary deprivation from undernutrition and certain forms of pica (eg, starch, clay, ice).

Pathophysiology, Symptoms, and Signs

Deficiency develops in stages. In the 1st stage, iron requirement exceeds intake, causing progressive depletion of bone marrow iron stores. As stores decrease, compensatory increase in absorption of dietary iron occurs. During later stages, deficiency is severe enough to impair RBC synthesis. Ultimately, anemia results in symptoms and signs.

Iron deficiency, if severe and prolonged, may cause dysfunction of iron-containing cellular enzymes. This dysfunction may contribute to fatigue and loss of stamina via mechanisms independent of the anemia itself.

In addition to the usual manifestations of anemia, some uncommon symptoms occur in severe iron deficiency; a patient may have pica, an abnormal craving to eat substances (eg, ice, dirt, paint). Other symptoms of severe deficiency include glossitis, cheilosis, concave nails (koilonychia), and, rarely, dysphagia caused by a postcricoid esophageal web.

Diagnosis

Iron deficiency anemia is suspected in patients with chronic blood loss or microcytic anemia, particularly if pica is present. In such patients, CBC, serum iron and iron-binding capacity, and serum ferritin are obtained.

Iron and iron-binding capacity (or transferrin) are usually both tested, because their relationship is important. Various tests exist; the range of normal values relates to the test used. In general, normal serum iron is 75 to 150 μg/dL (13 to 27 μmol/L) for men and 60 to 140 μg/dL (11 to 25 μmol/L) for women; total iron-binding capacity is 250 to 450 μg/dL (45 to 81 μmol/L). Serum iron concentration is low in iron deficiency and in many chronic diseases and is elevated in hemolytic disorders and in iron-overload syndromes (see p. 1131). Patients taking oral iron may have normal serum iron despite a deficiency; in such circumstances, a valid test requires cessation of iron therapy for 24 to 48 h. The iron-binding capacity increases in iron deficiency.

Serum ferritin concentrations closely correlate with total body iron stores. The range of normal in most laboratories is 30 to 300 ng/mL, and the mean is 88 in men and 49 in women. Low concentrations (< 12 ng/mL) are specific for iron deficiency. However, ferritin may also be elevated in cases of liver injury (eg, hepatitis) and in some tumors (especially acute leukemia, Hodgkin lymphoma, and GI tract tumors).

Serum transferrin receptor reflects the amount of RBC precursors available for active proliferation; levels are sensitive and specific. The range of normal is 3.0 to 8.5 μg/mL. Levels increase in early iron deficiency and when erythropoiesis increases.

The most sensitive and specific criterion for iron-deficient erythropoiesis, however, is absent marrow stores of iron, although a bone marrow examination is rarely needed.

Iron deficiency anemia must be differentiated from other microcytic anemias (see TABLE 130–1). If tests exclude iron deficiency in a patient with microcytic anemia, then anemia of chronic disease, structural Hb abnormalities (eg, hemoglobinopathies), and congenital RBC membrane abnormalities are considered. Clinical features, Hb studies (eg, Hb electrophoresis and HbA2), and genetic testing (eg, α-thalassemia) may help distinguish these entities.

Laboratory test results help stage iron deficiency anemia. Stage 1 is characterized by decreased bone marrow iron stores; Hb and serum iron remain normal, but serum ferritin concentration falls to < 20 ng/mL. The compensatory increase in iron absorption causes an increase in iron-binding capacity (transferrin level). During stage 2, erythropoiesis is impaired. Although the transferrin level is increased, the serum iron concentration decreases; transferrin saturation decreases. Erythropoiesis is impaired when serum iron falls to < 50 μg/dL (< 9 μmol/L) and transferrin saturation to < 16%. The serum ferritin receptor concentration rises (> 8.5 mg/L). During stage 3, anemia with normal-appearing RBCs and indices develops. During stage 4, microcytosis and then hypochromia develop. During stage 5, iron deficiency affects tissues, resulting in symptoms and signs.

Diagnosis of iron deficiency anemia prompts consideration of its cause, usually bleeding. Patients with obvious blood loss (eg, women with menorrhagia) may require no further testing. Men and postmenopausal women without obvious blood loss should undergo evaluation of the GI tract, because anemia may be the only indication of an occult GI cancer. Rarely, chronic epistasis or GU bleeding is underestimated by the patient and requires evaluation in patients with normal GI study results.

TABLE 130–1. DIFFERENTIAL DIAGNOSIS OF MICROCYTIC ANEMIA DUE TO DECREASED RBC PRODUCTION

DIAGNOSTIC CRITERIA	IRON DEFICIENCY	IRON-TRANSPORT DEFICIENCY	SIDEROBLASTIC IRON UTILIZATION	IRON REUTILIZATION
Peripheral blood				
Microcytosis (M) vs hypochromia (H)	M > H	M > H	M > H, may be normocytic	M > H
Polychromatophilic targeted cells	Absent	Absent	Present	Absent
Stippled RBCs	Absent	Absent	Present	Absent
RBC distribution width (RDW)	↑	↑	↑	Normal
Serum iron				
Serum iron: iron-binding capacity	↓:↑	↓:↓	↑:Normal	↓:↓
% Saturation of transferrin	< 10	0	> 50	> 10
Serum ferritin				
(normal, 30–300 ng/mL)	< 12	No data available	> 400	30–400
Bone marrow				
RBC:granulocyte ratio (normal, 1:3–1:5)	1:1–1:2	1:1–1:2	1:1–5:1	1:1–1:2
Marrow iron	Absent	Present	↑	Present
Ringed sideroblasts	Absent	Absent	Present	Absent

↑ = increased; ↓ = decreased.

Treatment

Iron therapy without pursuit of the cause is poor practice; the bleeding site should be sought even in cases of mild anemia.

Iron can be provided by various iron salts (eg, ferrous sulfate, gluconate, fumarate) or saccharated iron po 30 min before meals (food or antacids may reduce absorption). A typical initial dose is 60 mg of elemental iron (eg, as 325 mg of ferrous sulfate) given 1 or 2 times/day. Larger doses are largely unabsorbed but increase adverse effects, especially constipation. Ascorbic acid either as a pill (500 mg) or as orange juice when taken with iron enhances iron absorption without increasing gastric distress. Parenteral iron causes the same therapeutic response as oral iron but can cause adverse effects, such as anaphylactoid reactions, serum sickness, thrombophlebitis, and pain. It is reserved for patients who do not tolerate or who will not take oral iron or for patients who steadily lose large amounts of blood because of capillary or vascular disorders (eg, hereditary hemorrhagic telangiectasia). The dose of parenteral iron is determined by a hematologist. Oral or parenteral iron therapy should continue for ≥ 6 mo after correcting Hb levels to replenish tissue stores.

The response to treatment is assessed by serial Hb measurements until normal RBC values are achieved. Hb rises little for 2 wk but then rises 0.7 to 1 g/wk until near normal, at which time rate of increase tapers. Anemia should be corrected within 2 mo. A subnormal response suggests continued hemorrhage, underlying infection or malignancy, insufficient intake of iron, or, very rarely, malabsorption of oral iron.

SIDEROBLASTIC ANEMIAS

Sideroblastic anemias are iron-utilization anemias that are generally part of a myelo-

dysplastic syndrome, producing a normocytic-normochromic anemia with high RBC distribution width or a microcytic-hypochromic anemia, particularly with increased serum iron, ferritin, and transferrin saturation.

Sideroblastic anemias are among the anemias characterized by inadequate marrow utilization of iron for Hb synthesis despite the presence of adequate or increased amounts of iron (iron-utilization anemias). Other iron-utilization anemias include some hemoglobinopathies, primarily thalassemias (see p. 1057). Sideroblastic anemias are characterized by the presence of polychromatophilic, stippled, targeted RBCs (siderocytes). Sideroblastic anemias are generally part of a myelodysplastic syndrome but may be hereditary or may occur secondary to drugs (eg, chloramphenicol, cycloserine, isoniazid, pyrazinamide) or toxins (including ethanol and lead). Deficient reticulocyte production, intramedullary death of RBCs, and bone marrow erythroid hyperplasia (and dysplasia) occur. Although hypochromic RBCs are produced, other RBCs may be large, producing normochromic indices; if so, variation in RBC size (dimorphism) usually produces a high RBC distribution width (RDW).

Sideroblastic anemia is suspected in patients with microcytic anemia or a high RDW anemia, particularly with increased serum iron, serum ferritin, and transferrin saturation (see Iron Deficiency Anemia, on p. 1036). The peripheral smear shows RBC dimorphism. RBCs may appear stippled. Bone marrow examination is necessary and reveals erythroid hyperplasia; iron staining reveals the pathognomonic iron-engorged paranuclear mitochondria in developing RBCs (ringed sideroblasts). Other features of myelodysplasia are frequently evident. Serum lead is measured if sideroblastic anemia has an unknown cause.

Elimination of a toxin or drug (especially alcohol) can lead to recovery. Rarely, congenital cases respond to pyridoxine 50 mg po tid, but incompletely.

ANEMIA OF CHRONIC DISEASE

(Iron-Reutilization Anemia)

Anemia of chronic disease is a multifactorial anemia often coexistent with iron deficiency. Diagnosis generally requires the presence of chronic infection, inflammation, or cancer; microcytic or marginal normocytic anemia; and values for serum transferrin receptor and serum ferritin that are between those typical for iron deficiency and sideroblastic anemia. Treatment is to reverse the underlying disease and, if the disease is irreversible, to give erythropoietin.

Worldwide, anemia of chronic disease is the 2nd most common anemia. Early on, the RBCs are normocytic; with time they become microcytic. The major issue is that the marrow erythroid mass fails to expand appropriately in response to anemia.

Etiology and Pathophysiology

This type of anemia was thought to occur as part of a chronic disorder, most often infection, inflammatory disease (especially RA), or cancer; however, the same process appears to begin acutely during virtually any infection or inflammation. Three pathophysiologic mechanisms have been identified:

- Slightly shortened RBC survival occurs via unknown mechanisms in patients with cancer or chronic granulomatous infections.
- Erythropoiesis is impaired because of decreases in both erythropoietin (EPO) production and marrow responsiveness to EPO.
- Intracellular iron metabolism is impaired.

Reticulum cells retain iron from senescent RBCs, making iron unavailable for Hb synthesis. There is thus a failure to compensate for the anemia with increased RBC production. Macrophage-derived cytokines (eg, IL-1β, tumor necrosis factor-α, interferon-β) in patients with infections, inflammatory states, and cancer cause or contribute to the decrease in EPO production and the impaired iron metabolism.

Symptoms, Signs, and Diagnosis

Clinical findings are usually those of the underlying disease (infection, inflammation, or cancer). Anemia of chronic disease is suspected in patients with microcytic or marginal normocytic anemia with chronic infection, inflammation, or cancer. If anemia of chronic disease is suspected, serum iron, transferrin, transferrin receptor, and serum ferritin are obtained. Hb usually is > 8 μg/dL unless an additional mechanism contributes to anemia (see also TABLE 130–1). If iron deficiency is present in addition to anemia of chronic disease, serum ferritin generally remains < 100 ng/mL, and, if there is infection, inflammation, or cancer, a ferritin level of slightly < 100 ng/mL suggests that iron deficiency is superimposed on anemia of chronic disease. However, because serum ferritin may be falsely elevated as an acute-phase reactant, the serum transferrin receptor may better differentiate iron deficiency from anemia of chronic disease when serum ferritin is > 100 ng/mL.

Treatment

Treating the underlying disease is most important. Because the anemia is generally mild, transfusions usually are not required, and recombinant EPO is sufficient. Because both reduced production of and marrow resistance to EPO occur, the EPO dose may need to be 150 to 300 units/kg sc 3 times/wk. A good response is likely if after 2 wk of therapy Hb has increased > 0.5 µg/dL and serum ferritin is < 400 ng/mL. Iron supplements (see p. 1039) are required to ensure an adequate response to EPO.

HYPOPROLIFERATIVE ANEMIAS

Hypoproliferative anemias result from deficient erythropoietin (EPO) or a diminished response to it; they tend to be normocytic and normochromic. Renal, metabolic, and endocrine diseases are common causes. Treatment includes measures to correct the underlying disorder and sometimes EPO.

Hypoproliferation is a common mechanism in anemias of renal disease, hypometabolic or endocrine deficiency states (eg, hypothyroidism, hypopituitarism), and protein deprivation. The mechanism appears to be a relative or absolute decreased production of EPO. In hypometabolic states, the bone marrow may also fail to respond to EPO.

Anemia of renal disease: The deficiency in renal production of EPO and the severity of anemia correlate with the extent of renal dysfunction; anemia occurs when the creatinine clearance is < 45 mL/min. Renal glomerular lesions (eg, from amyloidosis, diabetic nephropathy), generally result in the most severe anemia for their degree of excretory failure.

The term anemia of renal disease refers only to that caused by decreased EPO, but other mechanisms may increase its severity. In uremia, mild hemolysis is common; its basis is uncertain. Less common is RBC fragmentation (traumatic hemolytic anemia), which occurs when the renovascular endothelium is injured (eg, in malignant hypertension, polyarteritis nodosa, or acute cortical necrosis). Traumatic hemolysis in children can be an acute, often fatal illness called the hemolytic-uremic syndrome (see p. 1070).

Diagnosis is based on demonstration of renal insufficiency and normocytic anemia, peripheral reticulocytopenia, and a paucity of erythroid hyperplasia for the degree of anemia. RBC fragmentation on the peripheral smear, particularly if there is thrombocytopenia, suggests simultaneous traumatic hemolysis.

Therapy is directed at improving renal function and increasing RBC production. If renal function is normalized, anemia is slowly corrected. In patients receiving long-term dialysis, erythropoiesis at typical doses may increase, but rarely to normal levels. EPO, beginning with 50 to 100 units/kg IV or sc 3 times/wk with iron supplements, is the treatment of choice. In almost all cases, maximum increases in RBCs are reached by 8 to 12 wk. Reduced doses of EPO (about ½ the induction dose) can then be given 1 to 3 times/wk. Transfusions are rarely necessary.

Other hypoproliferative anemias: Clinical and laboratory findings of other hypoproliferative normochromic-normocytic anemias are milder but otherwise mimic those of the anemia of renal disease. The mechanism of the anemia of protein depletion may be general hypometabolism. Hypometabolism may diminish the marrow response to EPO. Protein's role in hematopoiesis is unclear.

APLASTIC ANEMIA

(Hypoplastic Anemia)

Aplastic anemia is a normocytic-normochromic anemia that results from a loss of blood cell precursors, causing hypoplasia of bone marrow, RBCs, WBCs, and platelets. Symptoms result from severe anemia, thrombocytopenia (petechiae, bleeding), or leukopenia (infections). Diagnosis requires demonstration of peripheral pancytopenia and the absence of cell precursors in bone marrow. Treatment is equine antithymocyte globulin and cyclosporine. Erythropoietin, granulocyte-macrophage colony-stimulating factor, and bone marrow transplantation may also be useful.

The term aplastic anemia commonly implies a panhypoplasia of the marrow with associated leukopenia and thrombocytopenia. In contrast, pure RBC aplasia is restricted to the erythroid cell line. Although both disorders are uncommon, aplastic anemia is more common.

Etiology and Pathophysiology

True aplastic anemia (most common in adolescents and young adults) is idiopathic in about ½ of cases. Recognized causes are chemicals (eg, benzene, inorganic arsenic), radiation, and drugs (eg, antineoplastics, antibiotics, NSAIDs, anticonvulsants, acetazolamide, gold salts, penicillamine, quinacrine). The mechanism is unknown, but selective (perhaps genetic) hypersensitivity appears to be the basis.

A very rare form of aplastic anemia, Fanconi's anemia (a type of familial aplastic anemia with bone abnormalities, microcephaly, hypogonadism, and brown pigmentation of skin) occurs in children with abnormal chromosomes. Fanconi's anemia is often inapparent until some illness (especially an acute infection or inflammatory disorder) supervenes, causing peripheral cytopenias. With clearing of the supervening illness, peripheral values return to normal despite reduced marrow mass.

Pure RBC aplasia may be acute and reversible. Acute erythroblastopenia is a brief disappearance of RBC precursors from the marrow during various acute viral illnesses (particularly human parvovirus), especially in children. The anemia lasts longer than the acute infection. Chronic pure RBC aplasia has been associated with hemolytic disorders, thymomas, and autoimmune mechanisms and, less often, with drugs (eg, tranquilizers, anticonvulsants), toxins (organic phosphates), riboflavin deficiency, and chronic lymphocytic leukemia. A rare congenital form, Diamond-Blackfan anemia, usually occurs during infancy but has also been reported in adulthood. This syndrome is associated with bony abnormalities of the thumbs or digits and short stature.

Symptoms and Signs

Although onset of aplastic anemia usually is insidious, often occurring over weeks or months after exposure to a toxin, occasionally it is acute. Signs vary with the severity of the pancytopenia. Symptoms and signs of anemia (eg, pallor) usually are severe.

Severe thrombocytopenia may cause petechiae, ecchymosis, and bleeding from the gums, ocular fundi, or other tissues. Agranulocytosis commonly causes life-threatening infections. Splenomegaly is absent unless induced by transfusion hemosiderosis. Symptoms of pure RBC aplasia are generally milder and relate to the degree of the anemia or to the underlying disorder.

Diagnosis

Aplastic anemia is suspected in patients, particularly young patients, with pancytopenia (eg, WBC < 1500/μL, platelets < 50,000/μL). Pure RBC aplasia (including Diamond-Blackfan anemia) is suspected in patients with bony abnormalities and normocytic anemia. If either diagnosis is suspected, bone marrow examination is obtained.

In aplastic anemia, RBCs are normochromic-normocytic (sometimes marginally macrocytic). The WBC count reduction occurs chiefly in the granulocytes. Platelets are often far below 50,000/μL. Reticulocytes are decreased or absent. Serum iron is elevated. The bone marrow is acellular. In pure RBC aplasia, normocytic anemia, reticulocytopenia, and elevated serum iron are present, but with normal WBC and platelet counts. Bone marrow cellularity and maturation may be normal except for absence of erythroid precursors.

Treatment

In aplastic anemia, treatment of choice is equine antithymocyte globulin (ATG) 10 to 20 mg/kg diluted in 500 mL saline and infused IV over 4 to 6 h once/day for 10 consecutive days; about 60% of patients respond. Allergic reactions and serum sickness may occur; all patients require skin testing (to identify allergy to horse serum) and concomitant corticosteroids (prednisone 40 mg/m^2 po once/day beginning on day 7 for 10 days or until symptoms subside). Cyclosporine (5 to 10 mg/kg po once/day) is as effective as ATG and yields responses in about 50% of ATG failures, suggesting that its mechanism of action is different. Combined ATG and cyclosporine is also effective. If aplastic anemia is very severe or fails to respond to ATG and cyclosporine, bone marrow transplantation or treatment with cytokines (erythropoietin, granulocyte or granulocyte-macrophage colony-stimulating factor) may be effective.

Stem cell or actual bone marrow transplantation may help younger patients (particularly those < 30) but requires an identical twin or an HLA-compatible sibling. At diagnosis, siblings are evaluated for HLA compatibility.

Because transfusions pose a risk to subsequent transplantation, blood products are used only when essential.

Pure RBC aplasia has been successfully managed with immunosuppressants (prednisone, cyclosporine, or cyclophosphamide), especially when an autoimmune mechanism is suspected. Because patients with thymoma-associated pure RBC aplasia improve after thymectomy, CT is used to seek the presence of such a lesion, and surgery is considered.

MYELOPHTHISIC ANEMIA

Myelophthisic anemia is a normocytic-normochromic anemia that occurs when normal marrow space is infiltrated and replaced by nonhematopoietic or abnormal cells. Causes include tumors, granulomatous disorders, and lipid storage diseases. Marrow fibrosis often occurs. Splenomegaly may develop. Characteristic changes in peripheral blood include anisocytosis, poikilocytosis, and excessive numbers of RBC and WBC precursors. Diagnosis usually requires bone marrow biopsy. Treatment is supportive and includes measures directed at the underlying cause.

Descriptive terms used in this anemia can be confusing. Myelofibrosis, which is replacement of marrow by fibrous tissue bands, may be idiopathic (primary) or secondary. True myelofibrosis is a stem cell defect in which the fibrosis is secondary to other hematopoietic intramedullary events. Myelosclerosis is new bone formation that sometimes accompanies myelofibrosis. Myeloid metaplasia refers to extramedullary hematopoiesis in the liver, spleen, or lymph nodes that may accompany myelophthisis due to any cause. An old term, agnogenic myeloid metaplasia, indicates primary myelofibrosis with or without myeloid metaplasia.

Etiology and Pathophysiology

The most common cause is replacement of bone marrow by metastatic tumors (most often, breast or prostate; less often, kidney, lung, adrenal, or thyroid); extramedullary hematopoiesis tends to be modest. Other causes include myeloproliferative disorders (especially late-stage or spent polycythemia vera), granulomatous diseases, and (lipid) storage diseases. Myelofibrosis can occur in all of these. In children, a rare cause is Albers-Schönberg disease.

Factors that may contribute to decreased RBC production include a decreased amount of functioning hematopoietic tissue, disordered metabolism related to the underlying disease, and, in some cases, erythrophagocytosis. Extramedullary hematopoiesis or disruption of the marrow sinusoids causes release of immature cells. Abnormally shaped RBCs often result in increased RBC destruction.

Myeloid metaplasia may result in splenomegaly, particularly in patients with storage diseases. Hepatosplenomegaly is rare with myelofibrosis from malignant tumors.

Symptoms, Signs, and Diagnosis

In severe cases, symptoms of anemia and of the underlying disease may be present. Massive splenomegaly can cause abdominal pressure, early satiety, and left upper quadrant abdominal pain; hepatomegaly may be present.

Myelophthisic anemia is suspected in patients with normocytic anemia, particularly when splenomegaly or a potential underlying cause is present. If it is suspected, a peripheral smear should be obtained, because a leukoerythroblastic pattern (immature myeloid cells and nucleated RBCs, such as normoblasts in the smear) suggests myelophthisic anemia. Anemia, usually moderately severe, is characteristically normocytic but may be slightly macrocytic. RBC morphology may show extreme variation (anisocytosis and poikilocytosis) in size and shape. The WBC count may vary. The platelet count is often low, with giant bizarre-shaped platelets. Reticulocytosis often occurs; it may be caused by premature release of reticulocytes from the marrow or extramedullary sites and thus does not always indicate increased blood regeneration.

Although examination of peripheral blood can be suggestive, diagnosis usually requires bone marrow examination. Indications include a leukoerythroblastic pattern and unexplained splenomegaly. The marrow may be difficult to aspirate; marrow trephine biopsy is usually required. Findings vary according to the underlying disease. Erythropoiesis is normal or increased in some cases. However, the life span of RBCs is often reduced. Hematopoiesis may be present in the spleen and liver.

X-rays, if obtained incidentally, may disclose bony lesions (myelosclerosis) characteristic of long-standing myelofibrosis or other osseous changes (ie, osteoblastic or lytic lesions of a tumor), suggesting the cause of anemia.

Treatment

The underlying disorder is treated. In idiopathic cases, management is supportive. Erythropoietin (20,000 to 40,000 units sc once or twice/wk) and corticosteroids (eg, prednisone 10 to 30 mg po once/day) have been used, but only modest responses have been observed. Hydroxyurea (500 mg po once/day or once every other day) decreases spleen size and normalizes RBC values in many patients, but the response requires 6 to 12 mo of treatment. Thalidomide (50 to 100 mg po once/day in the evening) may provide modest responses.

MEGALOBLASTIC MACROCYTIC ANEMIAS

Megaloblastic anemias result most often from deficiencies of vitamin B_{12} and folate. Ineffective hematopoiesis affects all cell lines but particularly RBCs. Diagnosis is usually based on a CBC and peripheral smear, which may show a macrocytic anemia with anisocytosis and poikilocytosis, large oval RBCs (macro-ovalocytes), hypersegmented neutrophils, and reticulocytopenia. Treatment is directed at the underlying cause.

Macrocytes are enlarged RBCs (ie, MCV > 95 fL/cell). Macrocytic RBCs occur in a variety of clinical circumstances, many unrelated to the megaloblastosis and the resultant anemia. Macrocytosis may be due to megaloblasts or other enlarged RBCs (see sidebar 130–1). Megaloblasts are large nucleated RBC precursors with noncondensed chromatin. Megaloblastosis precedes macrocytic anemia.

Etiology

The most common cause of megaloblastic states is deficiency or defective utilization of vitamin B_{12} (see p. 37) or folate (see p. 29). Other causes include drugs (generally antineoplastics or immunosuppressants) that interfere with DNA synthesis, and rare metabolic disorders (eg, hereditary orotic aciduria); some cases are of unknown etiology.

Pathophysiology

Megaloblastic states result from defective DNA synthesis. RNA synthesis continues, resulting in a large cell with a large nucleus. All cell lines have dyspoiesis, in which cytoplasmic maturity is greater than nuclear maturity; this produces megaloblasts in the marrow before they appear in the peripheral blood. Dyspoiesis results in intramedullary cell death, making erythropoiesis ineffective and causing indirect hyperbilirubinemia and hyperuricemia. Because dyspoiesis affects all cell lines,

Sidebar 130–1. NONMEGALOBLASTIC MACROCYTOSIS

Most macrocytic (ie, MCV > 95 fL/cell) anemias are megaloblastic. Nonmegaloblastic macrocytosis occurs in various clinical states, not all of which are understood. Anemia is commonly associated but usually develops because of mechanisms independent of macrocytosis. Macrocytosis from excess RBC membrane occurs in patients with chronic liver disease in whom cholesterol esterification is defective. Macrocytosis with an MCV of about 95 to 105 fL/cell can occur with chronic alcohol use in the absence of folic acid deficiency. Mild macrocytosis can occur in aplastic anemia, especially as recovery occurs. Macrocytosis is common in myelodysplasia also. Because RBC membrane molding occurs in the spleen after cell release from the marrow, RBCs may be slightly macrocytic after splenectomy, although these changes are not associated with anemia.

Nonmegaloblastic macrocytosis is suspected in patients with macrocytic anemias in whom testing excludes vitamin B_{12} and folate deficiencies. The macro-ovalocytes on peripheral smear and the increased RDW that are typical of classic megaloblastic anemia may be absent. If nonmegaloblastic macrocytosis is unexplained clinically (eg, by the presence of aplastic anemia, chronic liver disease, or alcohol use) or if myelodysplasia is suspected, then bone marrow examination and genetic testing are performed to exclude myelodysplasia. In nonmegaloblastic macrocytosis, the marrow is not megaloblastic, but in myelodysplasia and advanced liver disease there are megaloblastoid RBC precursors with dense nuclear chromatin that differ from the usual fine fibrillar pattern in megaloblastic anemias.

reticulocytopenia and, during later stages, leukopenia and thrombocytopenia develop. Large, oval RBCs (macro-ovalocytes) enter the circulation. Hypersegmentation of polymorphonuclear neutrophils is common; the mechanism of their production is unknown.

Symptoms and Signs

Anemia develops insidiously and may not produce symptoms until it is severe. Deficiencies of vitamin B_{12} may produce neurologic manifestations, including peripheral neuropathy, dementia, and subacute combined degeneration. Folate deficiency may also produce diarrhea and glossitis; many patients with folate deficiency appear wasted, particularly with frontalis muscle mass loss.

Diagnosis and Treatment

Megaloblastic anemia is suspected in anemic patients with macrocytic indices. Diagnosis is usually based on peripheral blood smear. When fully developed, the anemia is macrocytic, with MCV > 100 fL/cell. The smear shows macro-ovalocytosis, anisocytosis, and poikilocytosis. The RBC distribution width (RDW) is high. Howell-Jolly bodies (residual fragments of the nucleus) are common. Reticulocytopenia is present. Hypersegmentation of the granulocytes develops early; neutropenia develops later. Thrombocytopenia is often present in severe cases, and platelets may be bizarre in size and shape. If the diagnosis is questionable, a bone marrow examination may be needed.

Before treatment, the cause must be identified. Deficiency of vitamin B_{12} or folate is suspected if megaloblastic anemia is recognized; these are indistinguishable on the basis of peripheral blood and bone marrow findings, so vitamin B_{12} and folate levels are required (see pp. 30 and 39).

Treatment depends on the cause. Treatment of folate and vitamin B_{12} deficiencies is discussed in Ch. 4 (see pp. 30 and 39). Drugs causing megaloblastic states may need to be eliminated or given in reduced doses.

MYELODYSPLASIA AND IRON-TRANSPORT DEFICIENCY ANEMIA

In myelodysplasia (see p. 1114), anemia is commonly prominent. The anemia can be microcytic or normochromic-normocytic, usually with a dimorphic (large and small) population of circulating cells. Bone marrow examination shows decreased erythroid activity, megaloblastoid and dysplastic changes, and, sometimes, increased numbers of ringed sideroblasts. Treatment is discussed under Sideroblastic Anemias (see p. 1040).

Iron-transport deficiency anemia (atransferrinemia) is exceedingly rare. It occurs when iron cannot move from storage sites (eg, mucosal cells, liver) to the erythropoietic precursors. The presumed mechanism is absence of transferrin or presence of a defective transferrin molecule. In addition to anemia, hemosiderosis of lymphoid tissue, especially along the GI tract, is prominent.

131 ANEMIAS CAUSED BY HEMOLYSIS

At the end of their normal life span (about 120 days), RBCs are removed from the circulation. Hemolysis involves premature destruction and hence a shortened RBC life span (< 120 days). Anemia results when bone marrow production can no longer compensate for the shortened RBC survival; this condition is termed hemolytic anemia. If the marrow can compensate, the condition is termed compensated hemolytic anemia.

Etiology

Hemolysis can result from disorders extrinsic to the RBC, or intrinsic RBC abnormalities (see TABLE 131–1).

Disorders extrinsic to the RBC include reticuloendothelial hyperactivity (hypersplenism—see p. 1091), immunologic abnormalities (eg, autoimmune hemolytic anemia, isoimmune hemolytic anemia), mechanical injury (traumatic hemolytic anemia), and infectious agents. Infectious agents may produce hemolytic anemia through the direct action of toxins (eg, from *Clostridium*

TABLE 131–1. HEMOLYTIC ANEMIAS

MECHANISM	DISORDER
Intrinsic RBC abnormalities	
Congenital RBC membrane disorders	Congenital erythropoietic porphyria Hereditary elliptocytosis Hereditary spherocytosis
Acquired RBC membrane disorders	Hypophosphatemia Paroxysmal nocturnal hemoglobinuria Stomatocytosis
Disorders of RBC metabolism	Embden-Meyerhof pathway defects G6PD deficiency
Disorders of Hb synthesis	Hb C disease Hb S-C disease Hb E disease Sickle cell diseases Thalassemias
Problems extrinsic to the RBC	
Reticuloendothelial hyperactivity	Hypersplenism
Immunologic abnormalities	Autoimmune hemolytic anemias: Warm antibody Cold antibody Paroxysmal cold hemoglobinuria
Infectious agents	*Plasmodium*, *Bartonella* spp
Mechanical trauma	Valvular heart disease, skeletal trauma, March hemoglobinuria

G6PD = Glucose-6-phosphate dehydrogenase.

perfringens, α- or β-hemolytic streptococci, or meningococci) or by invasion and destruction of the RBC by the organism (eg, *Plasmodium* and *Bartonella* spp). In hemolysis caused by defects extrinsic to the RBC, RBCs are normal; donor cells as well as autologous cells are destroyed.

Defects intrinsic to the RBC that can cause hemolysis include hereditary and acquired cell membrane disorders (hypophosphatemia, paroxysmal nocturnal hemoglobinuria, stomatocytosis), disorders of RBC metabolism (Embden-Meyerhof pathway defects; hexose monophosphate shunt defects, such as the glucose-6-phosphate dehydrogenase deficiency), and hemoglobinopathies (sickle cell disorders and the thalassemias). Quantitative and functional abnormalities of certain RBC membrane proteins (α- and β-spectrin, protein 4.1, F-actin, ankyrin) cause hemolytic anemias through unknown mechanisms.

Pathophysiology

Senescent RBCs lose membrane and are largely cleared from the circulation by the phagocytic cells of the spleen, liver, and bone marrow. Hb breakdown occurs in these cells and in hepatocytes primarily by the heme oxygenase system with conservation (and subsequent reutilization) of iron, degradation of the heme to bilirubin by a series of enzymatic steps, and reutilization of protein.

Unconjugated (indirect) hyperbilirubinemia and jaundice occur when the conversion of Hb to bilirubin exceeds the liver's capacity to form bilirubin glucuronide and excrete bilirubin into bile (see also p. 240). Bilirubin catabolism causes increased stercobilin in the stool and urobilinogen in the urine and sometimes gallstones.

Most hemolysis is extravascular and occurs in phagocytic cells of the spleen, liver, and bone marrow. The spleen usually contributes; it reduces RBC survival by destroying mildly abnormal RBCs or warm antibody coated cells. An enlarged spleen may sequester even normal RBCs. Severely abnormal RBCs or those coated with cold antibodies or complement (C3) are destroyed within the circulation or in the liver, which (because of its large blood flow) can remove damaged cells efficiently.

Intravascular hemolysis is uncommon; it results in hemoglobinuria when the Hb released into plasma exceeds the Hb-binding capacity of plasma-binding proteins (eg, haptoglobin, a globulin normally present in concentrations of about 1.0 g/L in plasma). Unbound Hb is reabsorbed into renal tubular cells, where iron is converted to hemosiderin, part of which is assimilated for reutilization and part of which reaches the urine when the tubular cells slough.

Hemolysis may be acute, chronic, or episodic. Chronic hemolysis may be complicated by aplastic crisis (temporary failure of erythropoiesis), usually caused by an infection, often parvovirus.

Symptoms and Signs

Systemic manifestations resemble those of other anemias. Hemolytic crisis (acute, severe hemolysis) is uncommon; it may be accompanied by chills, fever, pain in the back and abdomen, prostration, and shock. Severe hemolysis can cause jaundice and splenomegaly.

Diagnosis

Hemolysis is suspected in patients with anemia and reticulocytosis, particularly if splenomegaly or another possible cause is recognized. If hemolysis is suspected, peripheral blood smear is examined and serum bilirubin, LDH, and ALT obtained. If these tests are inconclusive, urinary hemosiderin and Hb as well as serum haptoglobin are obtained.

Abnormalities of RBC morphology are seldom diagnostic but are often suggestive of the presence and cause of hemolysis (see TABLE 131–2). Spherocytosis is the abnormality of RBC morphology most specific for active hemolysis. RBC fragments (schistocytes) or erythrophagocytosis on the peripheral smear suggests intravascular hemolysis. Spherocytosis increases the MCHC. Hemolysis is suggested by increased levels of serum LDH and indirect bilirubin with a normal ALT and by urinary urobilinogen. Intravascular hemolysis is suggested by decreased serum haptoglobin levels; however, haptoglobin levels can decrease because of hepatocellular dysfunction and can increase because of systemic inflammation. Intravascular hemolysis is also suggested by urinary hemosiderin or Hb. Urinary Hb, like hematuria and myoglobinuria, produces a positive benzidine reaction on dipstick testing; it can be differentiated from hematuria by the absence of RBCs on microscopic urine examination. Free Hb may make plasma reddish brown, noticeable often in centrifuged blood; myoglobin does not.

Although hemolysis can usually be identified by these simple criteria, the definitive criterion is a measure of RBC survival, preferably with a radioactive label, such as ^{51}Cr. The measured survival of radiolabeled RBCs can establish hemolysis and the sites of sequestration using body surface counting. This is rarely required, however.

Once hemolysis has been identified, the specific disorder is sought. One approach to narrowing the differential diagnosis in hemolytic anemias is to consider risk factors (eg, geographic location, genetics, underlying disease), examine the patient for splenomegaly, and obtain a direct antiglobulin (Coombs') test and peripheral smear; most hemolytic anemias produce abnormalities in one of these variables that can direct further testing. Other laboratory tests that can help discern the causes of hemolysis include quantitative Hb electrophoresis, RBC enzyme assays, flow cytometry, cold agglutinins, and the osmotic fragility, acid hemolysis, and sucrose lysis tests.

TABLE 131–2. RBC MORPHOLOGIC CHANGES IN HEMOLYTIC ANEMIAS

RBC MORPHOLOGY	CAUSES
Spherocytes	Transfused blood or warm antibody hemolytic anemia; hereditary spherocytosis
Schistocytes	Microangiopathy; intravascular prostheses
Target cells	Hemoglobinopathies (Hb S, C; thalassemias); liver dysfunction
Sickled cells	Sickle cell disorders
Agglutinated cells	Cold agglutinin disease
Heinz bodies; bite cells	Oxidant stress; unstable Hb (eg, G6PD deficiency)
Nucleated erythroblasts and basophilia	β-thalassemia major
Acanthocytes	Spur cell anemia

G6PD = Glucose-6-phosphate dehydrogenase.

Although some tests can help differentiate intravascular from extravascular hemolysis, making the distinction is sometimes difficult. During increased RBC destruction, both sites are commonly involved, although to a differing degree.

Treatment

Treatment is individualized to the specific mechanism of hemolysis. Hemoglobinuria and hemosiderinuria may necessitate iron-replacement therapy. Long-term transfusion therapy may cause excessive iron accumulation, necessitating chelation therapy. Splenectomy is beneficial in some situations, particularly when splenic sequestration is the major cause of RBC destruction. If possible, splenectomy is delayed until 2 wk after vaccination with pneumococcal, *Haemophilus influenzae*, and meningococcal vaccines.

AUTOIMMUNE HEMOLYTIC ANEMIA

Autoimmune hemolytic anemia is caused by autoantibodies that react with RBCs at temperatures ≥ 37° C (warm antibody hemolytic

anemia) or < 37° C (cold agglutinin disease). Hemolysis is usually extravascular. The direct antiglobulin (Coombs') test establishes the diagnosis and may suggest the cause. Treatment depends on the cause and may include corticosteroids, splenectomy, IV immune globulin, immunosuppressants, avoidance of blood transfusions, and withdrawal of drugs.

Etiology and Pathophysiology

Warm antibody hemolytic anemia is the most common form of autoimmune hemolytic anemia (AIHA); it is more common among women. Autoantibodies in warm antibody hemolytic anemia generally react at temperatures ≥ 37° C. They may arise spontaneously or in association with certain diseases (SLE, lymphoma, chronic lymphatic leukemia). Some drugs (eg, α-methyldopa, levodopa—see TABLE 131–3) stimulate production of autoantibodies against Rh antigens (α-methyldopa-type of AIHA). Some drugs stimulate production of autoantibodies against the antibiotic-RBC-membrane complex as part of a transient hapten mechanism; the hapten may be stable (eg, high-dose penicillin, cephalosporins) or unstable (eg, quinidine, sulfonamides). In warm antibody hemolytic anemia, hemolysis occurs primarily in the spleen. It is often severe and can be fatal. Most of the autoantibodies in warm antibody hemolytic anemia are IgG. Most are panagglutinins and have limited specificity.

Cold agglutinin disease (cold antibody disease) is caused by autoantibodies that react at temperatures < 37° C. It sometimes occurs with infections (especially mycoplasmal pneumonias or infectious mononucleosis) and lymphoproliferative states; about ½ of cases are idiopathic, which is the common form in older adults. Infections tend to cause acute disease, whereas idiopathic disease tends to be chronic. The hemolysis occurs largely in the extravascular mononuclear phagocyte system of the liver. The anemia is usually mild (Hb > 7.5 g/dL). Autoantibodies in cold agglutinin disease are usually IgM. The higher the temperature (ie, the closer to normal body temperature) at which these antibodies react with the RBC, the greater the hemolysis.

Paroxysmal cold hemoglobinuria (PCH; Donath-Landsteiner syndrome) is a rare type of cold agglutinin disease. Hemolysis results from exposure to cold, which may even be localized (eg, from drinking cold water, from washing hands in cold water). An IgG autohemolysin binds to RBCs at low temperatures and causes intravascular hemolysis after warming. It occurs most often after a nonspecific viral illness or in otherwise healthy patients, although it occurs in some

TABLE 131–3. DRUGS THAT CAN CAUSE WARM ANTIBODY HEMOLYTIC ANEMIA

AUTOANTIBODY TO RH ANTIGENS	STABLE HAPTEN	UNSTABLE HAPTEN OR UNKNOWN MECHANISM
Cephalosporins	Cephalosporins	Amphotericin B
Diclofenac	Fluorescein sodium	Antazoline
Ibuprofen	Penicillins	Cephalosporins
Interferon-α	Tetracycline	Chlorpropamide
Levodopa	Tolbutamide	Diclofenac
Mefenamic acid		Diethylstilbestrol
Methyldopa		Doxepine
Procainamide		Hydrochlorothiazide
Teniposide		Isoniazid
Thioridazine		*p*-Aminosalicylic acid
Tolmetin		Probenecid
		Quinidine
		Quinine
		Rifampin
		Sulfonamides
		Thiopental
		Tolmetin

patients with congenital or acquired syphilis. The severity and rapidity of development of the anemia varies and may be fulminant.

Symptoms and Signs

Symptoms of warm antibody hemolytic anemia tend to be due to the anemia. If the disease is severe, fever, chest pain, syncope, or heart failure may occur. Mild splenomegaly is typical.

Cold agglutinin disease presents as an acute or chronic hemolytic anemia. Other cryopathic symptoms or signs may be present (eg, acrocyanoses, Raynaud's phenomenon, cold-associated occlusive changes). Symptoms of PCH may include severe pain in the back and legs, headache, vomiting, diarrhea, and passage of dark brown urine; hepatosplenomegaly may be present.

Diagnosis

AIHA is suspected in patients with hemolytic anemia, particularly if symptoms are severe or other suggestive symptoms are present. Routine laboratory tests generally suggest extravascular hemolysis (eg, hemosiderinuria is absent; haptoglobin levels are near normal) unless anemia is sudden and severe or PCH is the cause. Spherocytosis and a high MCHC are typical.

AIHA is diagnosed by detection of autoantibodies through use of the direct antiglobulin (Coombs') test. Antiglobulin serum is added to washed RBCs from the patient; agglutination indicates the presence of immunoglobulin, generally IgG, or C3 bound to the RBCs. The test is ≤ 98% sensitive for AIHA; false-negatives can occur if antibody density is very low or if the autoantibodies are IgA or IgM. In general, the intensity of the direct antiglobulin test correlates with the number of molecules of IgG or C3 bound to the RBC and, roughly, with the rate of hemolysis. A complementary test consists of mixing the patient's plasma with normal RBCs to determine whether such antibodies are free in the plasma (the indirect antiglobulin [Coombs'] test). A positive indirect antiglobulin test and a negative direct test generally indicate an alloantibody caused by pregnancy, prior transfusions, or lectin cross-reactivity rather than immune hemolysis. Even identification of a warm antibody does not define hemolysis, because 1/10,000 normal blood donors has a positive test result.

Once AIHA has been identified by the Coombs' test, testing should differentiate between warm antibody hemolytic anemia and cold agglutinin disease as well as the mechanism responsible for warm antibody hemolytic anemia. This determination can often be made by the pattern of the direct antiglobulin reaction. Three patterns are possible: (1) The reaction is positive with anti-IgG and negative with anti-C3. This pattern is common in idiopathic AIHA and in the drug or α-methyldopa type of AIHA, usually warm antibody hemolytic anemia. (2) The reaction is positive with anti-IgG and anti-C3. This pattern is common in cases with SLE and idiopathic AIHA, usually warm antibody hemolytic anemia, and is rare in drug-associated cases. (3) The reaction is positive with anti-C3 but negative with anti-IgG. This occurs in idiopathic AIHA, usually warm antibody hemolytic anemia, when the IgG antibody is of low affinity, in some drug-associated cases, and in cold agglutinin disease and paroxysmal cold hemoglobinuria.

Other studies can suggest the cause of AIHA but are inconclusive. In cold agglutinin disease, RBCs clump on the peripheral smear, and automated cell counts often reveal an increased MCV and spuriously low Hb due to such clumping; hand warming of the tube and recounting result in values significantly closer to normal. Warm antibody hemolytic anemia can often be differentiated from cold agglutinin disease by the temperature at which the direct antiglobulin test is positive; a test that is positive at temperatures ≥ 37°C indicates warm antibody hemolytic anemia, whereas a test that is positive at lower temperatures indicates cold agglutinin disease.

If PCH is suspected, the Donath-Landsteiner test, which is specific for PCH, should be obtained. Testing for syphilis is recommended.

Treatment

In drug-induced warm antibody hemolytic anemias, drug withdrawal decreases the rate of hemolysis. With α-methyldopa-type AIHA, hemolysis usually ceases within 3 wk; however, a positive Coombs' test may persist for > 1 yr. With hapten-mediated AIHA, hemolysis ceases when the drug is cleared from the plasma. Corticosteroids have only little effect in drug-induced hemolysis; infusions of Ig appear to be more effective.

Corticosteroids (eg, prednisone 1 mg/kg po bid) are the treatment of choice in warm antibody idiopathic AIHA. In very severe hemolysis, an initial loading dose of 100 to 200 mg is recommended. Most patients have an excellent response, which in about ⅓ is sustained after 12 to 20 wk of therapy. When stable RBC values are achieved, corticosteroids are tapered slowly. In patients who relapse after corticosteroid cessation or who are not helped by corticosteroids, splenectomy is performed. About 1/3 to 1/2 of patients have a sustained response after splenectomy. In cases of fulminant hemolysis, plasma exchange has been effective. For less severe but uncontrolled hemolysis, immune globulin infusions have provided temporary control. Long-term management with immunosuppressants (including cyclosporine) has been effective after failure with corticosteroids and splenectomy.

The presence of panagglutinating antibodies in warm antibody hemolytic anemia makes cross-matching of donor blood difficult. In addition, transfusions often superimpose an alloantibody on the autoantibody, accelerating hemolysis. Thus, transfusions should be avoided whenever possible. When necessary, they should be given only in small aliquots (100 to 200 mL over 1 to 2 h, watching for hemolysis).

Therapy of cold agglutinin disease is largely supportive in acute cases, because the anemia is self-limited. In chronic cases, treatment of the underlying disease often controls the anemia. However, in idiopathic chronic cases, mild anemia (Hb, 9 to 10 g/dL) may persist for life. Avoidance of cold exposure is often helpful. Splenectomy is of no value. Immunosuppressants have only modest effectiveness. Transfusions should be given sparingly, with the blood warmed through an on-line warmer. Because the autologous RBCs have already survived the autoantibodies, autologous cell survival is better than that of transfused cells, limiting the efficacy of transfusion.

In PCH, therapy consists of strict avoidance of exposure to cold. Splenectomy is of no value. Immunosuppressants have been effective but should be restricted to progressive or idiopathic cases. Treatment of concomitant syphilis may cure PCH.

PAROXYSMAL NOCTURNAL HEMOGLOBINURIA

(Marchiafava-Micheli Syndrome)

Paroxysmal nocturnal hemoglobinuria is a rare disorder characterized by intravascular hemolysis and hemoglobinuria, the latter accentuated during sleep. Leukopenia, thrombocytopenia, and episodic crises are common. Diagnosis requires flow cytometry, although the acid hemolysis test is still valid. Treatment is supportive.

Paroxysmal nocturnal hemoglobinuria (PNH) is most common in men in their 20s, but it occurs in both sexes and at any age. It is an acquired genetic mutation resulting in a membrane defect in stem cells and their progeny, including RBCs, WBCs, and platelets. It results in unusual sensitivity to normal C3 in the plasma, leading to ongoing intravascular hemolysis of RBCs and diminished marrow production of WBCs and platelets. The defect is a missing glycosyl-phosphatidyl-inositol anchor for membrane proteins caused by an abnormality of the *PIG-A* gene, which is located on the X chromosome. Protracted urinary Hb loss may result in iron deficiency. Patients are strongly predisposed to both venous and arterial thrombi, including the Budd-Chiari syndrome. Thrombi are commonly fatal. Some patients with PNH develop aplastic anemia, and some with aplastic anemia develop PNH.

Crises may be precipitated by infection, iron use, vaccination, or menstruation. Abdominal and lumbar pain and symptoms of severe anemia may occur; gross hemoglobinuria and splenomegaly are common.

Diagnosis

PNH is suspected in patients who have typical symptoms of anemia or unexplained normocytic anemia with intravascular hemolysis, particularly if leukopenia or thrombocytopenia is present. If PNH is suspected, the sugar-water test is usually the first test performed; it relies on enhanced hemolysis of C3-dependent systems in isotonic solutions of low ionic strength, is simple to perform, and is sensitive. However, the test is nonspecific; positive results require confirmation by further testing. The most sensitive and specific test is determination of the absence of specific RBC or WBC membrane proteins by flow cytometry. An alternative is the acid hemolysis test (Ham's test). Hemolysis usually occurs if blood is acidified with HCl, incubated for 1 h, and centrifuged. If bone marrow examination is performed to exclude other disorders, hypoplasia may be present. Gross hemoglobinuria is common during crises, and the urine may contain hemosiderin.

Treatment

Treatment is symptomatic. Empiric use of corticosteroids (prednisone 20 to 40 mg po once/day) has controlled symptoms and stabilized RBC values in > 50% of patients. Generally, transfusions are reserved for crises. Transfusions containing plasma (and C3) should be avoided. Washing RBCs with saline before transfusion is no longer necessary. Heparin may be required for thromboses but can accelerate hemolysis and should be used cautiously. Oral iron supplements may be necessary. Most cases can be managed by these supportive measures for years to decades. Allogenic stem cell transplantation has been successful in a small number of cases.

TRAUMATIC HEMOLYTIC ANEMIA

(Microangiopathic Hemolytic Anemia)

Traumatic hemolytic anemia is intravascular hemolysis caused by excessive shear or turbulence in the circulation.

Trauma may originate outside the vessel, as in skeletal impact, eg, repetitive foot striking (march hemoglobinuria) or from karate or bongo playing; within the heart across a pressure gradient, as in calcific aortic stenosis or with faulty aortic valve prostheses; in arterioles, as in severe (especially malignant) hypertension, some malignant tumors, or polyarteritis nodosa; or in end arterioles, often across fibrin deposits, as in thrombotic thrombocytopenic purpura and disseminated intravascular coagulation. The trauma causes odd-shaped RBC fragments (eg, triangles, helmet shapes) called schistocytes in the peripheral blood; their appearance on the peripheral smear is diagnostic. The small schistocytes cause low MCV and high RBC distribution width (the latter reflecting the anisocytosis).

Treatment addresses the underlying process. Iron deficiency anemia occasionally is superimposed on the hemolysis as a result of chronic hemosiderinuria and, when present, responds to iron-replacement therapy.

HEREDITARY SPHEROCYTOSIS AND HEREDITARY ELLIPTOCYTOSIS

Hereditary spherocytosis and hereditary elliptocytosis are congenital RBC membrane disorders. Symptoms, generally milder in hereditary elliptocytosis, include variable degrees of anemia, jaundice, and splenomegaly. Diagnosis requires demonstration of increased RBC osmotic fragility and a negative direct antiglobulin test. Rarely, patients < 45 yr with symptomatic disease require splenectomy.

Hereditary spherocytosis (chronic familial icterus; congenital hemolytic jaundice; chronic acholuric jaundice; familial spherocytosis; spherocytic anemia) is an autosomal dominant disease with variable gene penetrance. It is characterized by hemolysis of spheroidal RBCs and anemia.

Hereditary elliptocytosis (ovalocytosis) is a rare autosomal dominant disorder in which RBCs are oval or elliptical. Hemolysis is usually absent or slight, with little or no anemia; splenomegaly is often present.

Pathophysiology

Alterations in membrane proteins cause the RBC abnormalities in both disorders. In hereditary spherocytosis, the cell membrane surface area is decreased disproportionately to the intracellular content. The decreased surface area of the cell impairs the flexibility needed for the cell to traverse the spleen's microcirculation, causing intrasplenic hemolysis.

Symptoms and Signs

Symptoms and signs of hereditary spherocytosis are usually mild, and the anemia may be so well compensated for that it is not recognized until an intercurrent viral illness transiently decreases RBC production, simulating an aplastic crisis. These episodes, however, are self-limited, with resolution of the infection. Moderate jaundice and symptoms of anemia are present in severe cases. Splenomegaly is almost invariable but only rarely causes abdominal discomfort. Hepatomegaly may be present. Cholelithiasis (pigment stones) is common and may be the presenting symptom. Congenital skeletal abnormalities (eg, tower-shaped skull, polydactylism) occasionally occur. Although usually one or more family members have had symptoms, several generations may be skipped because of variations in the degree of gene penetrance.

Clinical features of hereditary elliptocytosis are similar to those of hereditary spherocytosis but tend to be milder.

Diagnosis

These disorders are suspected in patients with unexplained hemolysis, particularly if splenomegaly, a family history of similar manifestations, or suggestive RBC indices are present. Because RBCs are spheroidal and the MCV is normal, the mean corpuscular diameter is below normal, and RBCs resemble microspherocytes. MCHC is increased. Reticulocytosis of 15 to 30% and leukocytosis are common.

If these disorders are suspected, the RBC osmotic fragility test (which mixes RBCs with varying concentrations of saline), the RBC autohemolysis test (which measures the amount of spontaneous hemolysis occurring after 48 h of sterile incubation), and, to rule out spherocytosis due to autoimmune hemolytic anemia, the direct antiglobulin (Coombs') test are obtained. RBC fragility is characteristically increased, but in mild cases it may be normal unless sterile defibrinated blood is first incubated at 37°C for 24 h. RBC autohemolysis is increased and can be corrected by the addition of glucose. The direct antiglobulin test results are negative.

Treatment

Splenectomy, after appropriate vaccination, is the only specific treatment for either disorder but is rarely needed. It is indicated in patients < 45 yr with Hb persistently < 10 g, jaundice or biliary colic, or persistent aplastic crisis. If the gallbladder has stones or other evidence of cholestasis, it should be removed during splenectomy. Although spherocytosis persists after splenectomy, the cells survive longer in the circulation. Symptoms, anemia, and reticulocytosis usually resolve. However, RBC fragility remains high.

STOMATOCYTOSIS AND ANEMIA CAUSED BY HYPOPHOSPHATEMIA

Stomatocytosis (presence of cup- or bowl-shaped RBCs) and hypophosphatemia are RBC membrane abnormalities causing hemolytic anemia.

Stomatocytosis: Stomatocytosis is a rare condition of RBCs in which a mouthlike or slitlike pattern replaces the normal central zone of pallor. These cells are associated with congenital and acquired hemolytic anemia. The symptoms result from the anemia.

The rare congenital stomatocytosis, which shows autosomal dominant inheritance, causes a severe hemolytic anemia presenting very early in life. The RBC membrane is hyperpermeable to monovalent cations (Na and K); movement of divalent cations and anions is normal. About 20 to 30% of circulating RBCs are stomatocytic; RBC fragility is increased, as is autohemolysis with inconstant correction with glucose. Splenectomy ameliorates anemia in some cases.

Acquired stomatocytosis with hemolytic anemia occurs primarily with recent excessive alcohol ingestion. Stomatocytes in the peripheral blood and hemolysis disappear within 2 wk of alcohol withdrawal.

Anemia caused by hypophosphatemia: RBC pliability varies according to intracellular ATP levels. Because the serum phosphate concentration affects RBC ATP levels, serum phosphate level < 0.5 mg/dL (< 0.16 mmol/L) depletes RBC ATP; the complex metabolic sequelae of hypophosphatemia also include 2,3-diphosphoglyceric acid depletion, a shift to the left in the O_2 dissociation curve, decreased glucose utilization, and increased lactate production. The resultant rigid, nonyielding RBCs are susceptible to injury in the capillary circulatory bed, leading to hemolysis and small, sphere-shaped RBCs (microspherocytosis).

Severe hypophosphatemia may occur in alcohol withdrawal, diabetes mellitus, refeeding after starvation, the recovery (diuretic) phase after severe burns, hyperalimentation, severe respiratory alkalosis, and in uremic patients receiving dialysis who are taking antacids. Phosphate supplements prevent or reverse the anemia and are considered for patients at risk of or who have hypophosphatemia.

EMBDEN-MEYERHOF PATHWAY DEFECTS

Embden-Meyerhof pathway defects are rare autosomal recessive RBC metabolic disorders that produce hemolytic anemia.

The most common form is pyruvate kinase deficiency. In all of these pathway defects, hemolytic anemia occurs only in homozygotes, and the exact mechanism of hemolysis is unknown. Spherocytes are absent, but small numbers of irregularly shaped spheres may be present. In general, assays of ATP and diphosphoglycerate help identify any metabolic defect and localize the defective sites for further analysis. No specific therapy exists for these hemolytic anemias, although most require no treatment other than supplemental folate (1 mg po once/day) during acute hemolysis. Hemolysis and anemia persist after splenectomy, although some improvement may occur, particularly with pyruvate kinase deficiency.

GLUCOSE-6-PHOSPHATE DEHYDROGENASE DEFICIENCY

Glucose-6-phosphate dehydrogenase (G6PD) deficiency is an X-linked enzymatic defect common in blacks that can result in hemolysis after acute illnesses or intake of oxidant drugs (including salicylates and sulfonamides). Diagnosis is based on assay for G6PD, although tests are often falsely negative during acute hemolysis. Treatment is supportive.

The only important defect in the hexose monophosphate shunt pathway is caused by glucose-6-phosphate dehydrogenase (G6PD) deficiency. Over 100 mutant forms of the enzyme have been identified. Clinically, the most common form is the drug-sensitive variety. This X-linked disorder is fully expressed in males and homozygous females and is variably expressed in heterozygous females. This defect occurs in about 10% of black males and in < 10% of black females in the US and in lower frequencies among people from the Mediterranean basin (eg, Italians, Greeks, Arabs, Sephardic Jews).

Pathophysiology

G6PD deficiency reduces energy available to maintain the integrity of the red cell membrane, which shortens RBC survival.

Hemolysis selectively affects older RBCs among affected blacks and among most affected whites. Hemolysis occurs commonly after fever, acute viral and bacterial infections, and diabetic acidosis. Less commonly, hemolysis occurs after exposure to drugs or to other substances that produce peroxide and cause oxidation of Hb and RBC membranes. These drugs and substances include primaquine, salicylates, sulfonamides, nitrofurans, phenacetin, naphthalene, some vitamin K derivatives, dapsone, phenazopyridine, nalidixic acid, methylene blue, and, in some whites, fava beans. Whether continued use of the offending drug leads to a compensated hemolytic state or lethal hemolysis depends on the degree of G6PD deficiency and the oxidant potential of the drug. Chronic congenital hemolysis (without drug use) occurs in some whites. Because older cells are selectively destroyed in blacks, hemolysis is usually self-limited, affecting < 25% of RBC mass; in whites, the deficiency is more severe, and profound hemolysis may lead to hemoglobinuria and acute renal failure.

Diagnosis and Treatment

The diagnosis is considered in any patient with acute hemolysis, particularly a black male. G6PD assay is done. Anemia, jaundice, and reticulocytosis develop during hemolysis. Heinz bodies, possibly particles of dead cytoplasm, may be visible early during the hemolytic episode but do not persist in a patient with an intact spleen because they are removed by the spleen. A specific diagnostic clue is the presence in the peripheral blood of RBCs that appear to have had one or more bites (1-μm wide) taken from the cell periphery (bite cells), possibly as a result of Heinz body removal by the spleen. Many screening tests are available. However, during and immediately after a hemolytic episode, tests may yield false-negative results because of destruction of the older, more deficient RBCs and the presence of reticulocytes rich in G6PD. Specific enzyme assays are the best diagnostic tests.

During acute hemolysis, treatment is supportive; transfusions are rarely needed. Patients are advised to avoid drugs or substances that initiate hemolysis.

SICKLE CELL ANEMIA

(Hb S Disease; Sickle Cell Disease)

Sickle cell anemia (a hemoglobinopathy—see sidebar 131–1) is chronic hemolytic anemia occurring almost exclusively in blacks, caused by homozygous inheritance of Hb S. Sickle-shaped RBCs clog capillaries, causing organ ischemia. Acute pain (crises) may develop frequently. Infection, bone marrow aplasia, or lung involvement (acute chest syndrome) can develop acutely and be fatal. Normocytic hemolytic anemia is characteristic. Diagnosis requires Hb electrophoresis and demonstration of sickling in RBCs on an unstained drop of blood. Crises are treated with analgesics and other supportive measures. Transfusions are occasionally required. Vaccines against bacterial infections,

Sidebar 131–1. HEMOGLOBINOPATHIES

Hb molecules consist of polypeptide chains whose chemical structure is genetically controlled. The normal adult Hb molecule (Hb A) consists of 2 pairs of chains designated α and β. Normal blood also contains a ≤ 2.5% concentration of Hb A_2 (composed of α and δ chains). Fetal Hb (Hb F, which has γ chains in the place of β chains) gradually decreases, particularly in the 1st months of life, until it makes up < 2% of total Hb in adults. (Hemoglobinopathies in pregnancy are discussed on p. 2168.) Hb F concentration increases in certain disorders of Hb synthesis and in aplastic and myeloproliferative states.

Some hemoglobinopathies result in anemias that are severe in homozygotes but mild in heterozygotes. Some patients are heterozygous for 2 such abnormalities and have anemia with characteristics of both traits.

Different Hbs, as distinguished by electrophoretic mobility, are alphabetically designated in order of discovery (eg, A, B, C), although the 1st abnormal Hb, sickle cell Hb, was designated Hb S. Structurally different Hbs with the same electrophoretic mobility are named for the city or location in which they were discovered (eg, Hb S Memphis, Hb C Harlem). Standard description of a patient's Hb composition places the Hb of greatest concentration first (eg, AS in sickle cell trait).

In the US, important anemias are caused by defective synthesis of Hb S or Hb C and the thalassemias; immigration of Southeast Asians has also made Hb E common.

prophylactic antibiotics, and aggressive treatment of infections prolong survival. Hydroxyurea decreases the frequency of crises.

Homozygotes (about 0.3% of blacks in the US) have sickle cell anemia; heterozygotes (8 to 13% of blacks) are not anemic.

Pathophysiology

In Hb S, valine is substituted for glutamic acid in the 6th amino acid of the β chain. Oxygenated Hb S is much less soluble than oxygenated Hb A; it forms a semisolid gel that causes RBCs to deform in a sickle shape at sites of low PO_2. Distorted, inflexible RBCs adhere to vascular endothelium and plug small arterioles and capillaries, which leads to infarction. Venous plugging predisposes to thromboses. Because sickled RBCs are fragile, the mechanical trauma of circulation produces hemolysis. Chronic compensatory marrow hyperactivity deforms the bones.

Acute exacerbations (crises) occur intermittently, often for no known reason. In some cases, fever, viral infection, or local trauma appears to be the precipitating event of a crisis. The most common type of crisis is a painful crisis, caused by ischemia and infarction, typically of the bones, but also of the spleen, lung, or kidney. Aplastic crisis occurs when marrow erythropoiesis slows during acute infection (especially viral), where an acute erythroblastopenia may occur.

Long-term consequences include impaired growth and development. Increased susceptibility to infection, particularly pneumococcal and *Salmonella* infections (including *Salmonella* osteomyelitis), also results. These infections are especially common in early childhood and can be rapidly fatal. Other consequences include avascular necrosis of the hips, renal concentrating defects, renal failure, and pulmonary fibrosis.

Symptoms and Signs

Most symptoms occur only in homozygotes and result from anemia and vaso-occlusive events resulting in tissue ischemia and infarction. Anemia is usually severe but varies highly among patients; mild jaundice and pallor are common.

Patients may be poorly developed and often have a relatively short trunk with long extremities and a tower-shaped skull. Hepatosplenomegaly is common in children, but because of repeated infarctions and subsequent fibrosis (autosplenectomy), the spleen in adults is commonly very small. Cardiomegaly and systolic ejection (flow) murmurs are common. Cholelithiasis and chronic punched-out ulcers around the ankles are common.

Painful crisis causes severe pain in long bones (eg, pretibial), the hands and feet (eg, hand-foot syndrome), and joints. Hemarthroses are common, as is avascular necrosis of the femoral head. Severe abdominal pain may develop with or without vomiting and, when due to sickling itself, is usually accompanied by back and joint pain. In children, anemia may be exacerbated by acute sequestration of sickled cells in the spleen.

Acute chest syndrome results from microvascular occlusion and is a major cause of death, with mortality rates of up to 10%. It occurs in all age groups but is most common in childhood. It is characterized by sudden onset of fever, chest pain, and pulmonary infiltrates. The infiltrates begin in the lower lobes, are bilateral in ⅓ of cases, and may be accompanied by pleural effusion. It may follow bacterial pneumonia. Hypoxemia may develop rapidly. Repeated episodes predispose to chronic pulmonary hypertension.

Priapism, a serious complication that can cause erectile dysfunction, is most common in young men. Ischemic stroke and CNS vasculitis may occur.

Heterozygotes (Hb AS) do not experience hemolysis, painful crises, or thrombotic complications except possibly during hypoxic conditions (eg, at high altitudes). Rhabdomyolysis and sudden death may occur during sustained, exhausting exercise. Impaired ability to concentrate urine (hyposthenuria) is common. Unilateral hematuria (by unknown mechanisms and usually from the left kidney) can occur but is self-limited. Typical renal papillary necrosis can occur but is more common among homozygotes.

Diagnosis

Patients with a family history but no evidence of the disease are screened with a rapid tube test that depends on the differential solubility of Hb S.

Patients with symptoms or signs suggestive of the disorder or its complications (eg, poor growth; acute, unexplained bone pain; aseptic necrosis of the femoral head), and black patients with normocytic anemia (particularly if hemolysis is present) require laboratory tests for hemolytic anemia (see p. 1047), Hb electrophoresis, and examination of RBCs for sickling. RBC count is usually between 2 and 3 million/μ L with Hb reduced proportionately; cells are normocytic (microcytosis suggests a concomitant α-thalassemia). Nucleated RBCs frequently appear in the peripheral blood, and reticulocytosis ≥10% is common. WBC count rises, often with a shift to the left during crisis or bacterial infection. Platelet count usually increases. Serum bilirubin is usually elevated (eg, 2 to 4 mg/dL [34 to 68 μmol/L]), and urine may contain urobilinogen. Dry-stained smears may show only a few sickled RBCs (crescent-shaped, often with elongated or pointed ends). The pathognomonic finding of all S-related hemoglobinopathies is sickling in an unstained drop of blood that has been prevented from drying or has been treated with a reducing drug (eg, sodium metabisulfite). Sickling may also be produced by reduced O_2 tension. Sealing a drop of blood under a coverslip with petroleum jelly provides such an environment.

Bone marrow examination, if obtained to differentiate other anemias, shows hyperplasia, with normoblasts predominating; it may become aplastic during sickling or severe infections. ESR, if obtained to exclude disorders (eg, juvenile RA causing hand and foot pain), is low. Incidental findings on skeletal x-rays may include widening of the diploic spaces of the skull and a sunray appearance of the diploic trabeculations. The long bones often show cortical thinning, irregular densities, and new bone formation within the medullary canal.

The homozygous state is differentiated from other sickle hemoglobinopathies by demonstrating only Hb S with a variable amount of Hb F on electrophoresis. The heterozygote is differentiated by the presence of more Hb A than Hb S on electrophoresis. Hb S must be distinguished from other Hb with a similar electrophoretic pattern by demonstrating the pathognomonic RBC morphology. Diagnosis is important for genetic counseling. The sensitivity of prenatal diagnosis has been greatly improved with the availability of the PCR technique.

In known sickle cell patients with acute exacerbations, including pain, fever, or other symptoms of infection, aplastic crisis is considered and Hb and reticulocyte count obtained. In patients with chest pain or difficulty breathing, acute chest syndrome and pulmonary embolism is considered; chest x-ray and assessment of arterial oxygenation is necessary. Hypoxemia or pulmonary parenchymal infiltrates on chest x-ray suggest acute chest syndrome or pneumonia. Hypoxemia without pulmonary infiltrates suggests pulmonary embolism. In patients with fever, infection and acute chest syndrome are considered; cultures and other appropriate diagnostic tests are performed. Unexplained hematuria, even among patients not suspected of having a sickle cell disorder, should prompt consideration of sickle cell trait.

Prognosis and Treatment

The life span of homozygous patients has steadily increased to > 50 yr. Common causes of death are acute chest syndrome, intercurrent infections, pulmonary emboli, infarction of a vital organ, and renal failure.

No effective in vivo anti-sickling drug is available. Splenectomy and hematinics are valueless. Complications are treated supportively. Crises are managed with liberal administration of analgesics, usually opioids. Continuous IV morphine is effective and safe; meperidine generally is avoided. Although dehydration contributes to sickling and may precipitate crises, whether vigorous hydration is helpful during crises is unclear. Nevertheless, maintaining normal intervascular volume has been a mainstay of therapy. During crises, pain and fever may persist for as long as 5 days.

Indications for hospitalization include suspected serious (including systemic) infection, aplastic crisis, acute chest syndrome, and, often, intractable pain or the need for transfusion. Patients with suspected serious bacterial infections or acute chest syndrome require broad-spectrum antibiotics immediately.

In sickle cell disease, transfusion therapy has many indications, but in most cases, efficacy has not been demonstrated. However, long-term transfusion therapy is indicated for prevention of recurrent cerebral thrombosis, especially in children < 18 yr. Transfusion is also generally indicated when Hb is < 5 g/dL. Specific indications include the need for blood volume (eg, acute splenic sequestration), aplastic crises, cardiopulmonary symptoms or signs (eg, high-output heart failure, hypoxemia with $PO_2 < 65$ mm Hg), preoperative use, priapism, and life-threatening events that would benefit from improved O_2 delivery (eg, sepsis, severe infection, acute chest syndrome, stroke, acute organ ischemia). Transfusion therapy is not helpful during an uncomplicated painful crisis; however, it may break a cycle of closely spaced painful crises. Transfusion may be needed in pregnancy.

Partial-exchange transfusion is usually preferred to simple transfusion if long-term or multiple transfusions are necessary. Partial-exchange transfusion minimizes iron accumulation and hyperviscosity. It is carried out in adults by phlebotomizing 500 mL, infusing 300 mL of normal saline, phlebotomizing another 500 mL, and then infusing 4 to 5 units of packed RBCs. Hct should be kept at < 46% and Hb S at < 60%.

In long-term management, pneumococcal, *Haemophilus influenzae*, and meningococcal vaccines; early identification and treatment of serious bacterial infection; and prophylactic antibiotics, including continuous prophylaxis with oral penicillin from age 4 mo to 6 yr, have reduced mortality, particularly during childhood.

Supplemental folate, 1 mg po once/day, is usually prescribed. Hydroxyurea, by increasing fetal Hb and thereby reducing sickling, decreases painful crises (by 50%) and decreases acute chest syndrome and transfusion requirements. The dose of hydroxyurea is variable and is adjusted to increase Hb F. Hydroxyurea may be more effective when combined with erythropoietin (eg, 40,000 to 60,000 units/wk).

Stem cell transplantation has been curative in a small number of patients but has a 5 to 10% mortality rate and so is not commonly performed. Gene therapy offers the best hope for cure.

HEMOGLOBIN C DISEASE

Hemoglobin C disease is a hemoglobinopathy (see sidebar 131–1) that causes symptoms similar to those of sickle cell disease, but milder.

Of blacks in the US, 2 to 3% have the trait, which is asymptomatic. Symptoms in homozygotes are usually similar to those of sickle cell disease, but milder. However, the abdominal crises of sickle cell anemia do not occur, and the spleen is usually enlarged. Splenic sequestration is possible.

Hemoglobin C disease is suspected in all patients with a family history and in black patients with clinical features suggesting sickle cell disease, particularly in adults with splenomegaly. The anemia is usually mild, but can be moderately severe. It is normocytic, with 30 to 100% target cells, spherocytes, and, rarely, crystal-containing RBCs seen in the smear. Nucleated RBCs may be present. The RBCs do not sickle. On electrophoresis, the Hb is type C. In heterozygotes, the only laboratory abnormality is centrally targeted RBCs.

No specific treatment is recommended. Anemia usually is not severe enough to require blood transfusion.

HEMOGLOBIN S-C DISEASE

Hemoglobin S-C disease is a hemoglobinopathy (see sidebar 131–1) that causes symptoms similar to those of sickle cell disease, but milder.

Because 10% of blacks carry the Hb S trait, the heterozygous S-C combination is more common than homozygous Hb C disease. The anemia in Hb S-C disease is like that in Hb C disease but milder; some patients even have normal Hb levels. Most symptoms are those of sickle cell anemia but usually are less frequent and less severe. However, gross hematuria, retinal hemorrhages, and aseptic necrosis of the femoral head are common. Hb S-C disease is suspected in all patients whose clinical features suggest sickle cell anemia or whose RBCs demonstrate sickling. Stained blood smears show target cells and a rare sickle cell. Sickling is identified in a sickling preparation, and Hb electrophoresis establishes the diagnosis.

HEMOGLOBIN E DISEASE

Homozygous Hb E disease (a hemoglobinopathy—see sidebar 131–1) causes a mild hemolytic anemia, usually without splenomegaly.

Hb E ($\alpha_2\beta_{22}{}^{6glu\rightarrow lys}$) is the 3rd most prevalent Hb worldwide (after Hb A and Hb S), primarily in black and Southeast Asian (> 15% incidence of homozygous disease) populations, although rarely in Chinese populations. Heterozygotes (Hb AE) are asymptomatic. Patients heterozygous for Hb E and β-thalassemia have a hemolytic disease more severe than S-thalassemia or homozygous Hb E disease and usually have splenomegaly.

In heterozygotes (Hb AE), routine laboratory test results of peripheral blood are normal. In homozygotes, a mild microcytic anemia with prominent target cells exists. Diagnosis of Hb E disorders is by Hb electrophoresis.

THALASSEMIAS

(Hereditary Leptocytosis; Mediterranean Anemia; Thalassemia Major and Minor)

Thalassemias are a group of inherited microcytic, hemolytic anemias characterized by defective Hb synthesis. They are particularly common in people of Mediterranean, African, and Southeast Asian ancestry. Symptoms and signs result from anemia, hemolysis, splenomegaly, bone marrow hyperplasia, and, if there have been multiple transfusions, iron overload. Diagnosis is based on quantitative Hb analysis. Treatment for severe forms may include transfusion, splenectomy, chelation, and stem cell transplantation.

Etiology and Pathophysiology

Thalassemia (a hemoglobinopathy—see sidebar 131–1) is among the most common inherited disorders of Hb production. It results from unbalanced Hb synthesis caused by decreased production of at least one globin polypeptide chain (β, α, γ, δ).

β-Thalassemia results from decreased production of β-polypeptide chains. Inheritance is autosomal: Heterozygotes are carriers and have asymptomatic mild to moderate microcytic anemia (thalassemia minor); homozygotes (β-thalassemia major, or Cooley's anemia) develop severe anemia and bone marrow hyperactivity. β-δ-Thalassemia is a less common form of β-thalassemia in which δ-chain as well as β-chain production are impaired and which also has heterozygous and homozygous states.

α-Thalassemia, which results from decreased production of α-polypeptide chains, has a more complex inheritance pattern, because genetic control of α-chain synthesis involves 2 pairs of genes (4 genes). Heterozygotes for a single gene defect (α-thalassemia-2 [silent]) are usually clinically normal. Heterozygotes with defects in 2 of the 4 genes (α-thalassemia-1 [trait]) tend to develop mild to moderate microcytic anemia but no symptoms. Defects in 3 of the 4 genes more severely impairs α-chain production, resulting in the formation of tetramers of excess β chains (Hb H) or, in infancy, γ chains (Bart's Hb). Defects in all 4 genes are a lethal condition in utero, because Hb that lacks α chains does not transport O_2. In blacks, the gene frequency for α-thalassemia is about 25%; only 10% have defects in more than 2 genes.

Symptoms and Signs

Clinical features of thalassemias are similar but vary in severity. β-Thalassemia major presents by age 1 to 2 yr with symptoms of severe anemia and transfusional and absorptive iron overload. Patients are jaundiced, and leg ulcers and cholelithiasis occur (as in sickle cell anemia). Splenomegaly, often massive, is common. Splenic sequestration may develop, accelerating destruction of transfused normal RBCs. Bone marrow hyperactivity causes thickening of the cranial bones and malar eminences. Long bone involvement predisposes to pathologic fractures and impairs growth, possibly delaying or preventing puberty. Iron deposits in heart muscle may cause heart failure. Hepatic siderosis is typical, leading to functional impairment and cirrhosis. Patients with Hb H disease often have symptomatic hemolytic anemia and splenomegaly.

Diagnosis

Thalassemias are suspected in patients with a family history, suggestive symptoms or signs, or microcytic hemolytic anemia. If thalassemias are suspected, laboratory tests for microcytic and hemolytic anemias and quantitative Hb studies are performed. Serum bilirubin, iron, and ferritin levels are increased.

In β-thalassemia major, anemia is severe, often with Hb ≤ 6 g/dL. RBC count is elevated relative to Hb because the cells are very microcytic. The blood smear is virtually diagnostic, with many nucleated erythroblasts; target cells; small, pale RBCs; and punctate and diffuse basophilia.

In quantitative Hb studies, elevation of Hb A_2 is diagnostic for β-thalassemia minor. In β-thalassemia major, Hb F is usually increased, sometimes to as much as 90%, and Hb A_2 is usually elevated to > 3%. The percentages of Hb F and Hb A_2 are generally normal in α-thalassemias, and the diagnosis of single or double gene defect thalassemias often is one of exclusion of other causes of microcytic anemia. Hb H disease can be diagnosed by demonstrating the fast-migrating Hb H or Bart's fractions on Hb electrophoresis. The specific molecular defect can be characterized but does not alter the clinical approach. Recombinant DNA approaches of gene mapping (particularly the PCR) have become standard for prenatal diagnosis and genetic counseling.

If bone marrow examination is performed for anemia (eg, to exclude other causes), it shows marked erythroid hyperplasia. X-rays obtained for other reasons in patients with β-thalassemia major show changes due to chronic marrow hyperactivity. The skull may show cortical thinning, widened diploic space, a sunray appearance of the trabeculae, and a granular or ground-glass appearance. The long bones may show cortical thinning, marrow space widening, and areas of osteoporosis. The vertebral bodies may have a granular or ground-glass appearance. The phalanges may appear rectangular or biconvex.

Prognosis and Treatment

Life expectancy is normal for people with β-thalassemia minor or α-thalassemia minor. The outlook for people with Hb H disease varies. Life expectancy is decreased in people with β-thalassemia major; only some live to puberty or beyond.

People with α- and β-thalassemia minor require no treatment. Splenectomy may be helpful if Hb H disease causes severe anemia or splenomegaly.

Children with β-thalassemia major should receive as few transfusions as possible to avoid iron overload. However, suppression of abnormal hematopoiesis by periodic RBC transfusion may be valuable in severely affected patients. To prevent or delay hemochromatosis, excess (transfusional) iron must be removed (eg, via chronic iron-chelation therapy). Splenectomy may help decrease transfusion requirements for patients with splenomegaly. Allogeneic stem cell transplantation has been successful, but the requirement for a histocompatible match, mortality and morbidity of the procedure, and lifelong requirement for immunosuppression have limited its usefulness.

HEMOGLOBIN S-β-THALASSEMIA DISEASE

Hemoglobin S-β-thalassemia disease is a hemoglobinopathy (see sidebar 131–1) that causes symptoms similar to those of sickle cell disease, but milder.

Because of the increased frequency of both Hb S and β-thalassemia genes in similar population groups, inheritance of both defects is relatively common. Clinically, the disorder produces symptoms of moderate anemia and signs of sickle cell anemia, which are usually less frequent and less severe. Mild to moderate microcytic anemia is usually present along with some sickled RBCs on stained blood smears. Diagnosis requires quantitative Hb studies. The Hb A_2 is > 3%. Hb S predominates on electrophoresis, and Hb A is decreased or absent. Hb F increase is variable. Treatment, if necessary, is the same as for sickle cell anemia.

132 NEUTROPENIA AND LYMPHOCYTOPENIA

Leukopenia is a reduction in the circulating WBC count to < 4000/μL. It is usually characterized by a reduced number of circulating neutrophils, although a reduced number of lymphocytes, monocytes, eosinophils, or basophils may also contribute. Thus, immune function is generally greatly decreased.

Neutropenia is a reduction in blood neutrophil count. It is more serious when accompanied by monocytopenia and lymphocytopenia. Lymphocytopenia, in which the total number of lymphocytes is < 1000/μL in adults, is not always reflected in the total WBC count, because lymphocytes account for only 20 to 40% of the count.

NEUTROPENIA

(Agranulocytosis; Granulocytopenia)

Neutropenia is a reduction in the blood neutrophil (granulocyte) count. If it is severe, the risk and severity of bacterial and fungal infections increase. Focal symptoms of infection may be muted, but fever is present during most serious infections. Diagnosis is by WBC count, but evaluation requires identification of the cause. If fever is present, infection is presumed, and immediate, empiric broad-spectrum antibiotics are necessary. Treatment with granulocyte-macrophage colony-stimulating factor or granulocyte colony-stimulating factor is sometimes helpful.

Neutrophils are the body's main defense against bacterial and fungal infections. When neutropenia is present, the inflammatory response to such infections is ineffective. Normal lower limit of the neutrophil count (total WBC × % neutrophils and bands) in whites is 1500/μL, somewhat lower in blacks (about 1200/μL).

Severity of neutropenia relates to the relative risk of infection: mild (1000 to 1500/μL), moderate (500 to 1000/μL), or severe (< 500/μL). When neutrophil counts fall to < 500/μL, endogenous microbial flora (eg, in the mouth or gut) can cause infections. If the count falls to < 200/μL, inflammatory response may be nonexistent. Acute, severe neutropenia, particularly if another factor (eg, cancer) also impairs the immune system, predisposes to rapidly fatal infections. The integrity of the skin and mucous membranes, the vascular supply to tissue, and the nutritional status of the patient also influence the risk of infections. The most frequently occurring pyogenic infections in patients with profound neutropenia are cellulitis, liver abscesses, furunculosis, pneumonia, and septicemia. Vascular catheters and other puncture sites confer extra risk of skin infections; the most common bacterial causes are coagulase-negative staphylococci and *Staphylococcus aureus*. Stomatitis, gingivitis, perirectal inflammation, colitis, sinusitis, paronychia, and otitis media often occur. Patients with prolonged neutropenia after bone marrow transplantation or chemotherapy and those receiving high doses of corticosteroids are predisposed to fungal infections.

Etiology

Acute neutropenia (occurring over hours to a few days) can develop from rapid neutrophil utilization or destruction or from impaired production. Chronic neutropenia (lasting months to years) usually arises from reduced production or excessive splenic sequestration. Neutropenia may be classified as due to an intrinsic defect in marrow myeloid cells or as secondary (due to factors extrinsic to marrow myeloid cells—see TABLE 132–1).

Neutropenia caused by intrinsic defects in myeloid cells or their precursors: This type of neutropenia is uncommon. Cyclic neutropenia is a rare congenital granulocytopoietic disorder, usually transmitted in an autosomal dominant fashion. It is characterized by regular, periodic oscillations in the number of peripheral neutrophils. The mean oscillatory period is 21 ± 3 days.

Severe congenital neutropenia (Kostmann syndrome) is a rare disorder that occurs sporadically in the US and is characterized by an arrest in myeloid maturation at the promyelocyte stage of the bone marrow, resulting in an absolute neutrophil count of < 200/μL.

Chronic idiopathic neutropenia is a group of uncommon, poorly understood disorders involving stem cells committed to the myeloid series; RBC and platelet precursors are unaffected. The spleen is not enlarged. Chronic

TABLE 132–1. CLASSIFICATION OF NEUTROPENIAS

CLASSIFICATION	ETIOLOGY
Neutropenia due to intrinsic defects in myeloid cells or their precursors*	Aplastic anemia Chronic idiopathic neutropenia, including benign neutropenia Cyclic neutropenia Myelodysplasia Neutropenia associated with dysgammaglobulinemia Paroxysmal nocturnal hemoglobinuria Severe congenital neutropenia (Kostmann syndrome) Syndrome-associated neutropenias (eg, cartilage-hair hypoplasia, dyskeratosis congenita, glycogen storage disease type IB, Schwachman-Diamond syndrome)
Secondary neutropenias†	Alcoholism Autoimmune neutropenia, including chronic secondary neutropenia in AIDS Bone marrow replacement by cancer, myelofibrosis (eg, due to granuloma), or Gaucher's cells Cytotoxic chemotherapy or radiation Drug-induced neutropenia Folate or vitamin B_{12} deficiency Hypersplenism Infection T γ-lymphoproliferative disease

*Rare disorders.
†Common disorders.

benign neutropenia is a type of chronic idiopathic neutropenia in which the rest of the immune system appears to remain intact; even with neutrophil counts < 200/μL, serious infections usually do not occur, probably because neutrophils are sometimes produced in adequate quantities in response to infection.

Neutropenia can also result from bone marrow failure due to rare syndromes (eg, cartilage-hair hypoplasia, Chédiak-Higashi syndrome, dyskeratosis congenita, glycogen storage disease type IB, Schwachman-Diamond syndrome). Neutropenia is also a prominent feature of myelodysplasia (see p. 1115—where it may be accompanied by megaloblastoid features in the bone marrow) and of aplastic anemia (see p. 1041) and can occur in dysgammaglobulinemia and paroxysmal nocturnal hemoglobinemia.

Secondary neutropenia: Secondary neutropenia can result from use of certain drugs, bone marrow infiltration or replacement, certain infections, or immune reactions.

Drug-induced neutropenia is one of the most common causes of neutropenia. It can decrease neutrophil production through toxic, idiosyncratic, or hypersensitivity mechanisms or increase peripheral neutrophil destruction through immune mechanisms. Only the toxic mechanism (eg, with phenothiazines) produces dose-related neutropenia. Idiosyncratic reactions are unpredictable and occur with a wide variety of drugs, including alternative medicine preparations or extracts, and toxins. Hypersensitivity reactions are rare and occasionally involve anticonvulsants (eg, phenytoin, phenobarbital). These reactions may last only a few days or months or years. Often, hepatitis, nephritis, pneumonitis, or aplastic anemia accompanies hypersensitivity-induced neutropenia. Immune-mediated drug-induced neutropenia, thought to arise from drugs that act as haptens to stimulate antibody formation, usually persists for about 1 wk after the drug is stopped. It may result from aminopyrine, propylthiouracil, or penicillin or other antibiotics. Severe dose-related neutropenia occurs predictably after cytotoxic cancer drugs or radiation therapy suppresses bone marrow production. Neutropenia due to ineffective marrow production can occur in megaloblastic anemias caused by vitamin B_{12} or folate deficiency. Usually, macrocytic anemia and sometimes mild thrombocytopenia develop simultaneously.

Bone marrow infiltration by leukemia, myeloma, lymphoma, or metastatic solid tumors (eg, breast, prostate) can impair neutrophil production. Tumor-induced myelofibrosis may further exacerbate neutropenia. Myelofibrosis can also occur from granulomatous infections, Gaucher's disease, and radiation therapy. Hypersplenism of any cause can lead to moderate neutropenia, thrombocytopenia, and anemia.

Infections can cause neutropenia by impairing neutrophil production or by inducing immune destruction or rapid utilization of neutrophils. Sepsis is a particularly serious cause.

Neutropenia that occurs with common childhood viral diseases develops during the first 1 to 2 days of illness and may persist for 3 to 8 days. Transient neutropenia may also result from virus- or endotoxemia-induced redistribution of neutrophils from the circulating to the marginal pool. Alcohol may contribute to neutropenia by inhibiting the neutrophilic response of the marrow during some infections (eg, pneumococcal pneumonia).

Chronic secondary neutropenia often accompanies HIV infection because of impaired production of neutrophils and accelerated destruction of neutrophils by antibodies. Autoimmune neutropenias may be acute, chronic, or episodic. They may involve antibodies directed against circulating neutrophils or neutrophil precursor cells. Most patients with autoimmune neutropenia have an underlying autoimmune disease or lymphoproliferative disorder (eg, SLE, Felty's syndrome).

Symptoms and Signs

Neutropenia is asymptomatic until infection develops. Fever is often the only indication of infection. Focal symptoms may develop but are often subtle. Patients with drug-induced neutropenia due to hypersensitivity may have a fever, rash, and lymphadenopathy from the hypersensitivity.

Some with chronic benign neutropenia and neutrophil counts < 200/μL do not experience many serious infections. Patients with cyclic neutropenia or severe congenital neutropenia tend to have oral ulcers, stomatitis, or pharyngitis and lymph node enlargement during severe chronic neutropenia. Pneumonias and septicemia often occur.

Diagnosis

Neutropenia is suspected in patients with frequent, severe, or unusual infections or in patients at risk (eg, those receiving cytotoxic or radiation therapy). Confirmation is by CBC with differential.

The first priority is to determine whether an infection is present. Because infection may be subtle, physical examination systematically assesses the most common primary sites of infection: mucosal surfaces, such as the alimentary tract (gums, pharynx, anus); lungs; abdomen; urinary tract; skin and fingernails; venipuncture sites; and vascular catheters.

If neutropenia is acute, laboratory evaluation must proceed rapidly. At least 2 sets of bacterial and fungal blood cultures are obtained from all febrile patients; if an indwelling IV catheter is present, cultures are obtained from the lumen and from a separate peripheral vein. Persistent or chronic drainage is also cultured for fungi and atypical mycobacteria. Skin lesions are aspirated or biopsied for cytology and culture. Urinalysis, urine cultures, and chest x-rays are obtained on all patients. If diarrhea is present, stool is evaluated for enteric bacterial pathogens and *Clostridium difficile* toxins.

Radiography, preferably CT scan, of the paranasal sinuses may be helpful if symptoms or signs of sinusitis (eg, positional headache, upper tooth or maxillary pain, facial swelling, nasal discharge) are present.

Next, mechanism and cause of neutropenia are determined. The history addresses all drugs, other preparations, and possible toxins ingested. Physical examination addresses the presence of splenomegaly and signs of other underlying disease (eg, arthritis, lymphadenopathy).

The presence of antineutrophil antibodies suggests immune neutropenia. In a patient at risk of deficiency, levels of folate and vitamin B_{12} are determined. The most important test is bone marrow examination, which determines whether neutropenia is due to decreased marrow production or is secondary to increased destruction or utilization of the cells (determined by normal or increased production of the cells). Bone marrow may also indicate the specific cause of the neutropenia (eg, aplastic anemia, myelofibrosis, leukemia). Additional marrow studies (eg, cytogenetic analysis; special stains and flow cytometry for detecting leukemia, other malignant disorders, and infections) are obtained. Patients who have had chronic neutropenia since infancy and a history of recurrent fevers and chronic gingivitis have WBC counts with differential obtained 3 times/wk for 6 wk, so that periodicity suggestive of cyclic neutropenia can be evaluated. Platelet and reticulocyte counts are obtained simultaneously. Eosinophils, reticulocytes, and platelets frequently cycle synchronously with the neutrophils, whereas monocytes and lymphocytes may cycle out of phase. Further testing for the cause of neutropenia may be necessary, depending on the diagnoses suspected. Differentiation between neutropenia caused by certain antibiotics and infection can sometimes be difficult. The WBC count just before the start of antibiotic treatment usually reflects the change in blood count due to the infection. If neutropenia develops during treatment with a drug known to induce low counts (eg, chloramphenicol), then switching to an alternative antibiotic may be helpful.

Treatment

Acute neutropenia: Suspected infections are always treated immediately. If fever or hypotension is present, serious infection is assumed, and empiric, high-dose, broad-spectrum antibiotics are given IV. Regimen selection is based on the most likely infecting organisms, the antimicrobial susceptibility of pathogens at that particular institution, and the regimen's potential toxicity. Because of the risk of creating resistant organisms, vancomycin is used only if gram-positive organisms resistant to other agents are suspected.

Indwelling vascular catheters can usually remain in place even if bacteremia is suspected or documented, but removal is considered in infections involving *S. aureus* or *Bacillus, Corynebacterium,* or *Candida* sp, or if blood cultures are persistently positive despite appropriate antibiotics. Infections caused by coagulase-negative staphylococci generally resolve with antimicrobial therapy alone.

If cultures are positive, antibiotic therapy is adjusted to the results of sensitivity tests. If a patient defervesces within 72 h, antibiotics are continued for at least 7 days and until the patient has no symptoms or signs of infection. When neutropenia is transient (such as that following myelosuppressive chemotherapy), antibiotic therapy is usually continued until the neutrophil count is > 500/μL; however, stopping antimicrobial coverage can be considered in selected patients with persistent neutropenia, especially those in whom symptoms and signs of inflammation have resolved, if cultures remain negative.

Fever that persists > 72 h despite antibiotic therapy suggests a nonbacterial cause, infection with a resistant species, a superinfection with a 2nd bacterial species, inadequate serum or tissue levels of the antibiotics, or localized infection, such as an abscess. Neutropenic patients with persistent fever are reassessed q 2 to 4 days with physical examination, cultures, and chest x-ray. If the patient is well except for the presence of fever, the initial antibiotic regimen can be continued. If the patient is deteriorating, alteration of the antimicrobial regimen is considered.

Fungal infections are the most likely cause of persistent fevers and deterioration. Antifungal therapy (eg, itraconazole, voriconazole, amphotericin, fluconazole) is added empirically if unexplained fever persists after 4 days of broad-spectrum antibiotic therapy. If fever persists after 3 wk of empiric therapy (including 2 wk of antifungal therapy) and the neutropenia has resolved, then stopping all antimicrobial drugs is considered and the cause of fever reevaluated.

Antibiotic prophylaxis in afebrile neutropenic patients remains controversial. Trimethoprim-sulfamethoxazole (TMP-SMX) prevents *Pneumocystis jiroveci* (formerly *P. carinii*) pneumonia in neutropenic and nonneutropenic patients with impaired cell-mediated immunity. Also, TMP-SMX may prevent bacterial infections in patients expected to be profoundly neutropenic for > 1 wk. The disadvantages of TMP-SMX prophylaxis include adverse effects, potential myelosuppression, and development of resistant bacteria and oral candidiasis. Antifungal prophylaxis is not routinely recommended for neutropenic patients, but patients at high risk of developing fungal infections (eg, after bone marrow transplantation and after receiving high doses of corticosteroids) may benefit.

Myeloid growth factors (granulocyte-macrophage colony-stimulating factor [GM-CSF] and granulocyte colony-stimulating factor [G-CSF]) are now widely used to increase the neutrophil count and to prevent infections in patients with severe neutropenia (eg, after bone marrow transplantation and intensive cancer chemotherapy). They are expensive. However, if the risk of febrile neutropenia is ≥ 30% (as assessed by neutrophil count < 500, presence of infection on a previous cycle of chemotherapy, associated comorbid disease, or age > 75), growth factors are indicated. In general, most clinical benefit occurs when the growth factor is administered beginning about 24 h after completion of chemotherapy. Patients with neutropenia caused by an idiosyncratic drug reaction may also benefit from myeloid growth factors, particularly if a delayed recovery is anticipated. The dose for G-CSF is 5 μg/kg sc once/day; for GM-CSF, 250 μg/m^2 sc once/day.

Glucocorticoids, anabolic steroids, and vitamins do not stimulate neutrophil production but can affect distribution and destruction. If acute neutropenia is suspected to be drug or toxin induced, all potentially offending agents are stopped.

Saline or hydrogen peroxide gargles every few hours, anesthetic lozenges (benzocaine 15 mg q 3 or 4 h), or chlorhexidine mouth rinses (1% solution) bid or tid may relieve the discomfort of stomatitis with oropharyngeal ulcerations. Oral or esophageal candidiasis is treated with nystatin (400,000 to 600,000 units oral rinse qid; swallowed if esophagitis) or with systemic antifungal drugs (eg, fluconazole). A semisolid or liquid diet may be necessary during acute stomatitis or esophagitis to minimize discomfort.

Chronic neutropenia: Neutrophil production in congenital, cyclic, and idiopathic neutropenia can be increased with administration of G-CSF 1 to 10 μg/kg sc once/day. Effectiveness can be maintained with daily or alternate-day G-CSF for months or years. Patients with oropharyngeal inflammation (even low grade), fever, or cellulitis or other suspected bacterial infections need appropriate antibiotics. Long-term G-CSF has also been used in other patients with chronic neutropenia, including those with myelodysplasia, HIV, and autoimmune disorders. In general, neutrophil counts increase, although clinical benefits are less clear, especially for patients who do not have severe neutropenia. For patients with autoimmune disorders or who have had an organ transplant, cyclosporine can also be beneficial.

In some patients with accelerated neutrophil destruction caused by autoimmune disorders, corticosteroids (generally, prednisone 0.5 to 1.0 mg/kg po once/day) increase blood neutrophils. This increase often can be maintained with alternate-day G-CSF therapy.

Splenectomy increases the neutrophil count in some patients with splenomegaly and splenic sequestration of neutrophils (eg, Felty's syndrome, hairy cell leukemia). However, splenectomy should be reserved for patients with severe neutropenia (ie, < 500/μL) and with serious problems with infections because it predisposes the patient to infection by encapsulated organisms.

LYMPHOCYTOPENIA

Lymphocytopenia is a total lymphocyte count of < 1000/μL in adults or < 3000/μL in children < 2 yr. Sequelae include opportunistic infections and an increased risk of malignant and autoimmune disorders. If the CBC reveals lymphocytopenia, testing for immunodeficiency and analysis of lymphocyte subpopulations should follow. Treatment is directed at the underlying cause.

The normal lymphocyte count in adults is 1000 to 4800/μL; in children < 2 yr, 3000 to 9500/μL. At age 6 yr, the lower limit of normal is 1500/μL. Both B and T cells are present in the peripheral blood; about 75% of the lymphocytes are T cells and 25% B cells. Because lymphocytes account for only 20 to 40% of the total WBC count, lymphocytopenia may go unnoticed when WBC count is checked without a differential.

Almost 65% of blood T cells are $CD4^+$ (helper) T cells. Most patients with lymphocytopenia have a reduced absolute number of T cells, particularly in the number of $CD4^+$ T cells. The average number of $CD4^+$ T cells in adult blood is 1100/μL (range, 300 to 1300/μL), and the average number of cells of the other major T-cell subgroup, $CD8^+$ (suppressor) T cells, is 600/μL (range, 100 to 900/μL).

Etiology

Inherited lymphocytopenia (see TABLE 132–2) may occur with inherited immunodeficiency diseases (see Ch. 164 on p. 1331) and disorders that involve impaired lymphocyte production. Other inherited disorders, such as Wiskott-Aldrich syndrome, adenosine deaminase deficiency, and purine nucleoside phosphorylase deficiency, may involve accelerated T-cell destruction. In many disorders, antibodies are also deficient.

Acquired lymphocytopenia can occur with a number of other disorders (see TABLE 132–2). Protein-energy malnutrition is the most common cause worldwide. AIDS is the most common infectious disease causing lymphocytopenia, which arises from destruction of $CD4^+$ T cells infected with HIV. Lymphocytopenia may also reflect impaired lymphocyte production arising from destruction of thymic or lymphoid architecture. In acute viremia due to HIV or other agents, lymphocytes may undergo accelerated destruction from active infections with the virus, may be trapped in the spleen or lymph nodes, or may migrate to the respiratory tract.

Iatrogenic lymphocytopenia is caused by cytotoxic chemotherapy, radiation therapy, or the administration of antilymphocyte globulin. Long-term treatment for psoriasis using psoralen and ultraviolet irradiation may destroy T cells. Glucocorticoids can induce lymphocyte destruction.

Lymphocytopenia may occur with autoimmune diseases such as SLE, RA, myasthenia gravis, and protein-losing enteropathy.

Symptoms, Signs, and Diagnosis

Lymphocytopenia per se generally causes no symptoms. However, findings of an associated

TABLE 132–2. CAUSES OF LYMPHOCYTOPENIA

INHERITED CAUSES	ACQUIRED CAUSES
Aplasia of lymphopoietic stem cells Ataxia-telangiectasia Cartilage-hair hypoplasia Idiopathic CD4$^+$ T lymphocytopenia Immunodeficiency with thymoma Severe combined immunodeficiency associated with defect in interleukin-2 receptor γ-chain, deficiency of ADA or PNP or unknown Wiskott-Aldrich syndrome	Infectious diseases, including AIDS, hepatitis, influenza, TB, typhoid fever, sepsis Dietary deficiency with ethanol abuse, protein-energy malnutrition, or zinc deficiency Iatrogenic after administration of cytotoxic chemotherapy, glucocorticoids, high-dose psoralen and ultraviolet A irradiation therapy, immunosuppressive therapy, radiation, or thoracic duct drainage Systemic diseases with autoimmune features; eg, aplastic anemia, Hodgkin lymphoma, myasthenia gravis, protein-losing enteropathy, RA, renal failure, sarcoidosis, SLE, thermal injury

ADA = adenosine deaminase; PNP = purine nucleoside phosphorylase.

disorder may include absent or diminished tonsils or lymph nodes, indicative of cellular immunodeficiency; skin abnormalities, such as alopecia, eczema, pyoderma, or telangiectasia; evidence of hematologic disease, such as pallor, petechiae, jaundice, or mouth ulcers; and generalized lymphadenopathy and splenomegaly, which may suggest HIV infection.

Lymphocytopenic patients experience recurrent infections or develop infections with unusual organisms. *Pneumocystis jiroveci* (formerly *P. carinii*), cytomegalovirus, rubeola, and varicella pneumonia often are fatal. Lymphocytopenia is also a risk factor for malignancy and autoimmune disorders.

Lymphocytopenia is suspected in a patient with recurrent viral, fungal, or parasitic infections but is usually detected incidentally on a CBC. *P. jiroveci*, cytomegalovirus, rubeola, or varicella pneumonia with lymphocytopenia suggests immunodeficiency. Lymphocyte subpopulations are measured in lymphocytopenic patients. Tests of antibody production with measurements of immunoglobulin levels should also be done. Patients with a history of recurrent infections undergo complete laboratory evaluation for immunodeficiency (see p. 1332), even if initial screening tests are normal.

Treatment

Lymphocytopenia usually remits with removal of the underlying factor or successful treatment of the underlying disorder. Immune globulin IV is indicated if patients have chronic IgG deficiency, lymphocytopenia, and recurrent infections. Hematopoietic stem cell transplantation can be considered for all patients with congenital immunodeficiencies and may be curative (see p. 1371).

133 THROMBOCYTOPENIA AND PLATELET DYSFUNCTION

Platelets are cell fragments that function in the clotting system. Thrombopoietin, primarily produced in the liver in response to decreased numbers of marrow megakaryocytes and circulating platelets, stimulates the bone marrow to synthesize platelets from megakaryocytes. Platelets circulate for 7 to 10 days. About 1/3 are always transiently sequestered in the spleen. The platelet count is normally 140,000 to 440,000/μL. However, the count can vary slightly according to menstrual cycle phase, decrease during near-term pregnancy (gestational thrombocytopenia), and increase in response to inflammatory cytokines (secondary, or reactive, thrombocytosis). Platelets are eventually destroyed, primarily by the spleen.

Platelet disorders include an abnormal increase in platelets (thrombocythemia, a myeloproliferative disorder; and thrombocytosis, a reactive phenomenon—see p. 1100), a decrease in platelets (thrombocytopenia), and platelet dysfunction. Any of these conditions, even conditions with increased platelets, may cause defective formation of hemostatic plugs and bleeding.

Etiology and Pathophysiology

Causes of thrombocytopenia (see TABLE 133–1) include failed platelet production, increased splenic sequestration of platelets with normal platelet survival, increased platelet destruction or consumption, dilution of platelets, and a combination of these. Increased splenic sequestration is suggested by splenomegaly.

The risk of bleeding is inversely proportional to the platelet count. When the platelet count is < 50,000/µL, minor bleeding occurs easily and the risk of major bleeding increases. Counts between 20,000 and 50,000/µL predispose to bleeding with trauma, even minor trauma; with counts < 20,000/µL, spontaneous bleeding may occur; with counts < 5000/µL, severe spontaneous bleeding is more likely. However, patients with counts < 10,000/µL may be asymptomatic for years.

Platelet dysfunction may stem from an intrinsic platelet defect or from an extrinsic factor that alters the function of normal platelets. Dysfunction may be hereditary or acquired. Hereditary disorders of platelet function consist of von Willebrand's disease, the most common hereditary hemorrhagic disease, and hereditary intrinsic platelet disorders, which are much less common. Acquired disorders of platelet function are commonly due to diseases as well as to aspirin and other drugs.

Symptoms and Signs

Platelet disorders result in a typical pattern of bleeding: multiple petechiae in the skin, typically most evident on the lower legs; scattered small ecchymoses at sites of minor trauma; mucosal bleeding (epistaxis, bleeding in the GI and GU tracts, vaginal bleeding); and excessive bleeding after surgery. Heavy GI bleeding and bleeding into the CNS may be life threatening. However, massive bleeding into tissues (eg, deep visceral hematomas or hemarthroses)

TABLE 133–1. CLASSIFICATION OF THROMBOCYTOPENIA

CAUSE	CONDITIONS
Failed platelet production	
Diminished or absent megakaryocytes in marrow	Leukemia, aplastic anemia, paroxysmal nocturnal hemoglobinuria (some patients), myelosuppressive drugs
Diminished platelet production despite the presence of megakaryocytes in marrow	Alcohol-induced thrombocytopenia, thrombocytopenia in megaloblastic anemias, HIV-associated thrombocytopenia, some myelodysplastic syndromes
Platelet sequestration in enlarged spleen	Cirrhosis with congestive splenomegaly, myelofibrosis with myeloid metaplasia, Gaucher's disease
Increased platelet destruction or use	
Immunologic destruction	Idiopathic thrombocytopenic purpura, HIV-associated thrombocytopenia, posttransfusion purpura, drug-induced thrombocytopenia, neonatal alloimmune thrombocytopenia, connective tissue disorders, lymphoproliferative disorders
Nonimmunologic destruction	Disseminated intravascular coagulation, thrombotic thrombocytopenic purpura–hemolytic-uremic syndrome, thrombocytopenia in acute respiratory distress syndrome
Dilution	Massive blood replacement or exchange transfusion (loss of platelet viability in stored blood)

TABLE 133–2. PERIPHERAL BLOOD FINDINGS IN THROMBOCYTOPENIC DISORDERS

FINDINGS	CONDITIONS
Normal RBCs and WBCs	Idiopathic thrombocytopenic purpura Gestational thrombocytopenia HIV-related thrombocytopenia Drug-induced thrombocytopenia Posttransfusion purpura
RBC fragmentation	Thrombotic thrombocytopenic purpura–hemolytic-uremic syndrome Preeclampsia with DIC Metastatic carcinoma
WBC abnormalities	Immature cells or increased mature lymphocytes in leukemia Markedly diminished granulocytes in aplastic anemia Hypersegmented polymorphonuclear leukocytes in megaloblastic anemias
Frequent giant platelets (approaching the size of RBCs)	Bernard-Soulier syndrome and other congenital thrombocytopenias
RBC abnormalities, nucleated RBCs, and immature granulocytes	Myelodysplasia

RBC = red blood cell; WBC = white blood cell; DIC = disseminated intravascular coagulation.

does not commonly occur and suggests a coagulation disorder (eg, hemophilia).

Diagnosis

Platelet disorders are suspected in patients with petechiae and mucosal bleeding. A CBC with platelet count, coagulation studies, and a peripheral blood smear are obtained. Excessive platelets and thrombocytopenia are diagnosed from the platelet count; coagulation studies are normal unless there is a simultaneous coagulopathy. If the CBC, platelet count, and INR are normal and PTT is normal or only slightly prolonged, then platelet dysfunction is suspected.

In patients with thrombocytopenia, the peripheral smear may suggest the cause (see TABLE 133–2). If the smear shows abnormalities other than thrombocytopenia, such as nucleated RBCs or abnormal or immature WBCs, then bone marrow aspiration is indicated. Bone marrow aspiration reveals the number and appearance of megakaryocytes and is the definitive test for many diseases causing marrow failure. If the bone marrow is normal but the spleen is enlarged, increased splenic sequestration is the likely cause of thrombocytopenia; if the bone marrow is normal and the spleen is not enlarged, excess platelet destruction is the likely cause. Measurement of antiplatelet antibodies is not clinically useful. HIV testing is performed in patients at risk of HIV infection.

In patients with platelet dysfunction, a hereditary cause is suspected if there is a lifelong history of easy bruising and bleeding after tooth extractions or surgery. In the case of a suspected hereditary cause, von Willebrand's antigen and factor activity studies are obtained. If a hereditary cause is not suspected, further tests are unnecessary.

Treatment

In patients with thrombocytopenia or platelet dysfunction, drugs that further impair platelet function should be avoided, particularly aspirin and other NSAIDs. Patients may require platelet transfusion, but only in limited situations (see p. 1137). Prophylactic transfusions are used sparingly because they may lose their effectiveness with repeated use due to the development of platelet alloantibodies. In platelet dysfunction or thrombocytopenia caused by decreased production, transfusions are reserved for active bleeding or severe thrombocytopenia (eg, platelet count < 10,000/μL). In thrombocytopenia caused by platelet destruction, transfusions are reserved for life-threatening or CNS bleeding.

ACQUIRED PLATELET DYSFUNCTION

Acquired platelet dysfunction may result from aspirin, other NSAIDS, or systemic disorders.

Acquired abnormalities of platelet function are very common. Aspirin is ubiquitous.

Many other drugs may also induce platelet dysfunction. Many clinical disorders (eg, myeloproliferative and myelodysplastic disorders, uremia, macroglobulinemia and multiple myeloma, cirrhosis, SLE) can impair platelet function as well. Acquired platelet dysfunction is suspected and diagnosed when an isolated prolongation of bleeding time is observed and other possible diagnoses have been eliminated. Platelet aggregation studies are unnecessary.

Aspirin and NSAIDs prevent cyclooxygenase-mediated production of thromboxane A_2. This effect can last 5 to 7 days. Aspirin modestly prolongs bleeding time in healthy people but may markedly prolong bleeding time in patients with underlying platelet dysfunction or a severe coagulation disturbance (eg, patients receiving heparin or patients with severe hemophilia). Platelets may become dysfunctional, prolonging the bleeding time as blood circulates through a pump oxygenator during cardiopulmonary bypass. The mechanism appears to be activation of fibrinolysis on the platelet surface with resultant loss of the glycoprotein Ib-IX binding site for von Willebrand's factor. Regardless of platelet count, patients who bleed excessively after cardiopulmonary bypass and who have a long bleeding time are transfused with platelets. Giving aprotinin (a protease inhibitor that neutralizes plasmin activity) during bypass may preserve platelet function, prevent prolongation of bleeding time, and reduce the need for transfusion.

Uremia may prolong bleeding via unknown mechanisms. If bleeding is observed clinically, bleeding time may be corrected transiently with vigorous dialysis, cryoprecipitate administration, or desmopressin infusion. If indicated for treatment of anemia, RBC count can be increased by transfusion or by giving erythropoietin; this process also shortens the bleeding time.

HEREDITARY INTRINSIC PLATELET DISORDERS

Hereditary intrinsic platelet disorders are rare and produce lifelong bleeding tendencies. Diagnosis is confirmed by platelet aggregation tests. Platelet transfusion is necessary to control serious bleeding.

Normal hemostasis requires platelet adhesion and activation. Adhesion requires von Willebrand's factor (VWF) and the platelet glycoprotein Ib-IX complex. Activation promotes platelet aggregation and fibrinogen binding and requires the platelet glycoprotein IIb-IIIa complex. Activation involves release of adenosine diphosphate (ADP) from platelet storage granules and conversion of arachidonic acid to thromboxane A_2 via a cyclooxygenase-mediated reaction. Hereditary intrinsic platelet disorders can involve defects in any of these steps. These disorders are suspected in patients with lifelong bleeding disorders who have normal platelet counts and coagulation studies. Diagnosis usually is based on platelet aggregation tests (see TABLE 133–3).

Disorders of amplification of platelet activation are the most common hereditary intrinsic platelet disorders and produce mild bleeding. They may result from decreased ADP in the platelet granules (storage pool deficiency),

TABLE 133–3. RESULTS OF AGGREGATION TESTS IN HEREDITARY DISORDERS OF PLATELET FUNCTION

DISORDER	COLLAGEN, EPINEPHRINE, AND LOW-DOSE ADP	HIGH-DOSE ADP	RISTOCETIN
Disorders of amplification of platelet activation	Impaired	Normal	Normal
Thrombasthenia	Absent	Absent	Normal or impaired
Bernard-Soulier syndrome	Normal	Normal	Impaired

ADP = adenosine diphosphate.

from an inability to generate thromboxane A_2 from arachidonic acid, or from an inability of platelets to aggregate in response to thromboxane A_2. Platelet aggregation tests reveal impaired aggregation after exposure to collagen, epinephrine, and low levels of ADP; and normal aggregation after exposure to high levels of ADP. The same pattern can result from use of NSAIDs or aspirin, the effect of which can persist for several days. Therefore, platelet aggregation tests should not be performed in patients who have recently taken these drugs.

Thrombasthenia (Glanzmann's disease) is a rare autosomal recessive disorder producing a defect in the platelet glycoprotein IIb-IIIa complex; platelets cannot aggregate. Patients may experience severe mucosal bleeding (eg, nosebleeds that stop only after nasal packing and transfusions of platelet concentrates). The diagnosis is suggested by a finding of single platelets without aggregates on a peripheral blood smear obtained from a finger stick. It is confirmed by the finding that platelets fail to aggregate with epinephrine, collagen, or even high levels of ADP but do aggregate transiently with ristocetin.

Bernard-Soulier syndrome is another rare autosomal recessive disorder. It impairs platelet adhesion via a defect in the glycoprotein Ib-IX complex. Bleeding may be severe. Platelets are unusually large. They do not aggregate with ristocetin but aggregate normally with ADP, collagen, and epinephrine.

Large platelets associated with functional abnormalities also occur in the May-Hegglin anomaly, a thrombocytopenic disorder with abnormal WBCs, and in the Chédiak-Higashi syndrome (see p. 1342).

IDIOPATHIC THROMBOCYTOPENIC PURPURA

Idiopathic (immunologic) thrombocytopenic purpura is a bleeding disorder caused by thrombocytopenia not associated with a systemic disease. Typically, it is chronic in adults but is usually acute and self-limited in children. Spleen size is normal. Diagnosis requires that other disorders be excluded through selective tests. Treatment includes corticosteroids, splenectomy, and, for life-threatening bleeding, platelet transfusions, and IV immune globulin.

Idiopathic thrombocytopenic purpura (ITP) usually results from development of an antibody directed against a structural platelet antigen (an autoantibody). In childhood ITP the autoantibody may be triggered by binding of viral antigen to megakaryocytes.

Symptoms, Signs, and Diagnosis

The symptoms and signs are petechiae and mucosal bleeding. The spleen is of normal size unless it is enlarged by a coexistent childhood viral infection.

ITP is suspected in patients with unexplained thrombocytopenia. Peripheral blood is normal except for reduced platelet numbers. Bone marrow is examined if blood counts or blood smear reveals abnormalities in addition to thrombocytopenia. Bone marrow examination reveals normal or possibly increased numbers of megakaryocytes in an otherwise normal marrow. Because diagnostic findings are nonspecific, diagnosis requires exclusion of other thrombocytopenic disorders suggested by clinical or laboratory test data. Because HIV-associated thrombocytopenia may be otherwise indistinguishable from ITP, HIV testing is performed if the patient has risk factors for HIV infection.

Treatment

Adults usually are given an oral corticosteroid (eg, prednisone 1 mg/kg once/day) initially. In the patient who responds, the platelet count rises to normal within 2 to 6 wk. The corticosteroid dosage is then tapered. However, most patients do not respond adequately or relapse as the corticosteroid is tapered; splenectomy can achieve a remission in about ⅔ of these patients. Because other treatments may not be effective for patients refractory to corticosteroids and splenectomy and because ITP often has a benign natural history, additional treatments may not be indicated unless platelet count is < 10,000/μL and active bleeding is present; then more intensive immunosuppressive treatment may be required with drugs such as cyclophosphamide, azathioprine, and rituximab.

Treatment of children is usually supportive, because most children spontaneously recover from severe thrombocytopenia in several days to weeks. Even after months or years of thrombocytopenia, most children have spontaneous remissions. If mucosal bleeding occurs, corticosteroids or IV immune globulin is given. Initial use of corticosteroids and IV immune globulin is controversial, because they increase platelet count but may not improve clinical outcome. Splenectomy is rarely performed in children. However, if thrombocytopenia is severe and symptomatic for > 6 mo, then splenectomy is effective.

In a child or adult with ITP and life-threatening bleeding, rapid phagocytic blockade is attempted by giving IV immune globulin 1 g/kg once/day for 1 to 2 days. This usually causes the platelet count to rise within 2 to 4 days but only for 2 to 4 wk. High-dose methylprednisolone (1 g IV once/day for 3 days) is less expensive than IV immune globulin and is easier to administer but may not be as effective. The patient with ITP and life-threatening bleeding is also given platelet transfusions. Platelet transfusions are not used prophylactically.

Oral corticosteroids or IV immune globulin may also be given when a transient increase of the platelet count is required for tooth extractions, childbirth, surgery, or other invasive procedures.

THROMBOCYTOPENIA DUE TO SPLENIC SEQUESTRATION

Increased splenic platelet sequestration can occur in various disorders that produce splenomegaly. Sequestration is expected in patients with congestive splenomegaly caused by advanced cirrhosis. The platelet count usually is > 30,000/µL unless the disorder producing the splenomegaly also impairs platelet production (eg, in myelofibrosis with myeloid metaplasia). Platelets are released from the spleen by epinephrine and therefore may be available at a time of stress. Therefore, thrombocytopenia caused only by splenic sequestration does not cause bleeding. Splenectomy corrects the thrombocytopenia but is not indicated unless severe thrombocytopenia from simultaneous marrow failure is present.

THROMBOCYTOPENIA: OTHER CAUSES

Platelet destruction can develop because of immunologic causes (HIV infection, drugs, connective tissue or lymphoproliferative disorders, blood transfusions) or nonimmunologic causes (gram-negative sepsis, acute respiratory distress syndrome). Clinical and laboratory findings are similar to those of idiopathic thrombocytopenic purpura. The history may be the only suggestion of the diagnosis. Treatment is usually correction of the underlying cause.

Acute respiratory distress syndrome: Patients with acute respiratory distress syndrome may develop nonimmunologic thrombocytopenia, possibly secondary to deposition of platelets in the pulmonary capillary bed.

Blood transfusions: Posttransfusion purpura causes immunologic platelet destruction indistinguishable from ITP, except for a history of a blood transfusion within the preceding 7 to 10 days. The patient, usually a woman, lacks a platelet antigen (PLA-1) present in most people. Transfusion with PLA-1–positive platelets stimulates formation of anti–PLA-1 antibodies, which (by an unknown mechanism) can react with the patient's PLA-1–negative platelets. Severe thrombocytopenia results, taking 2 to 6 wk to subside.

Connective tissue and lymphoproliferative disorders: Connective tissue (eg, SLE) or lymphoproliferative disorders can produce immunologic thrombocytopenia. Corticosteroids and splenectomy are often effective.

Drug-induced immunologic destruction: Quinidine, quinine, sulfa preparations, carbamazepine, methyldopa, aspirin, oral antidiabetic drugs, gold salts, and rifampin occasionally induce thrombocytopenia, typically by causing an immune reaction in which drug bound to the platelet creates a new and "foreign" antigen. This disorder is indistinguishable from idiopathic thrombocytopenic purpura (ITP) except for the history of drug ingestion. When the drug is stopped, the platelet count begins to increase within 1 to 7 days. Gold-induced thrombocytopenia is an exception, because injected gold salts may persist in the body for many weeks.

Up to 5% of patients receiving unfractionated heparin develop thrombocytopenia, which may occur even with very-low-dose heparin (eg, used in flushes to keep IV or arterial lines open). The mechanism is usually immunologic. Bleeding can occur, but more commonly platelets clump excessively, causing vessel obstruction, leading to paradoxical arterial and venous thromboses, which may be life threatening (eg, thromboembolic occlusion of limb arteries, strokes, acute MI). *Heparin should be stopped in any patient who becomes thrombocytopenic or whose platelet count decreases by more than 50%.* Because 5 days of heparin is sufficient to treat venous thrombosis and because most patients begin oral anticoagulants simultaneously with heparin, stopping heparin is usually safe. Low mol wt heparin (LMWH) may be less immunogenic than unfractionated heparin. However, LMWH is not useful if heparin-induced thrombocytopenia has already developed, because most antibodies cross-react with LMWH.

Gram-negative sepsis: Gram-negative sepsis often produces nonimmunologic thrombocytopenia that parallels the severity of the infection. The thrombocytopenia has multiple causes: disseminated intravascular coagulation, formation of immune complexes that can associate with platelets, activation of complement, and deposition of platelets on damaged endothelial surfaces.

HIV: Patients infected with HIV may develop immunologic thrombocytopenia indistinguishable from ITP except for the association with HIV. The platelet count may increase with glucocorticoids, which are often withheld unless the platelet count falls below 20,000/μL, because these drugs may further depress immune function. The platelet count also usually increases after treatment with antiviral drugs.

THROMBOTIC THROMBOCYTOPENIC PURPURA AND HEMOLYTIC-UREMIC SYNDROME

Thrombotic thrombocytopenic purpura and hemolytic-uremic syndrome are acute, fulminant disorders characterized by thrombocytopenia and microangiopathic hemolytic anemia. Other manifestations include fever, alterations in level of consciousness, and renal failure. Diagnosis requires demonstrating characteristic laboratory test abnormalities, including Coombs'-negative hemolytic anemia. Treatment is plasma exchange.

Thrombotic thrombocytopenic purpura (TTP) and hemolytic-uremic syndrome (HUS) involve nonimmunologic platelet destruction. Loose strands of fibrin are deposited in multiple small vessels, which damage passing platelets and RBCs. Platelets are also destroyed within multiple small thrombi. Multiple organs develop bland platelet-fibrin thrombi (without the vessel wall granulocytic infiltration characteristic of vasculitis) localized primarily to arteriocapillary junctions, described as thrombotic microangiopathy. TTP and HUS differ only in the relative degree of renal failure. Diagnosis and management in adults are the same. Therefore, in adults, TTP and HUS can be grouped together.

Causes and associations of TTP and HUS include congenital or acquired deficiency of the plasma enzyme ADAMTS13, which cleaves von Willebrand's factor (VWF) and thus eliminates abnormally large VWF multimers that can cause platelet thrombi; hemorrhagic colitis resulting from Shiga toxin–producing bacteria (eg, *Escherichia coli* O157:H7 and some strains of *Shigella dysenteriae*); pregnancy (often indistinguishable from severe preeclampsia or eclampsia); and drugs (such as quinine, cyclosporine, mitomycin C). Many cases are idiopathic.

Symptoms, Signs, and Diagnosis

Fever and manifestations of ischemia develop with varying severity in multiple organs. These manifestations include confusion and coma, abdominal pain, and arrhythmias caused by myocardial damage. The various clinical syndromes are indistinguishable, except that the epidemic disease of children (typically referred to as HUS) associated with enterohemorrhagic *E. coli* O157 and related Shiga toxin–producing bacteria more often localizes in the kidney and more often spontaneously remits.

TTP-HUS is suspected in patients with suggestive symptoms, thrombocytopenia, and anemia. If the disease is suspected, urinalysis, peripheral blood smear, reticulocyte count, serum LDH, renal functions, serum bilirubin (direct and indirect), and Coombs' test are obtained. The diagnosis is suggested by thrombocytopenia and anemia, with fragmented RBCs on the blood smear (helmet cells, triangular-shaped RBCs, distorted-appearing RBCs—these changes describe microangiopathic hemolysis); evidence of hemolysis (falling Hb level, polychromasia, elevated reticulocyte count, elevated serum LDH); and negative direct antiglobulin (Coombs') test. Otherwise unexplained thrombocytopenia and microangiopathic hemolytic anemia are sufficient evidence for a presumptive diagnosis. Although causes (eg, quinine sensitivity) or associations (eg, pregnancy) are clear in some patients, in most patients TTP-HUS appears suddenly and spontaneously without apparent cause. TTP-HUS is often indistinguishable, even with biopsy, from syndromes that cause identical thrombotic microangiopathies (eg, preeclampsia, scleroderma, accelerated hypertension, acute renal allograft rejection).

Prognosis and Treatment

Epidemic HUS in children associated with enterohemorrhagic infection usually spontaneously remits and is treated with supportive care and not plasma exchange. In other cases, untreated TTP-HUS is almost always fatal. With plasma exchange, however, about 85% of patients recover completely. Plasma exchange is continued daily until evidence of disease activity has subsided, which may be several days to many weeks. Corticosteroids and antiplatelet drugs (eg, aspirin) have also been used but are controversial. Most patients experience only a single episode of TTP-HUS. However, because relapses may occur years later, patients must be evaluated quickly if symptoms suggestive of a relapse develop.

VON WILLEBRAND'S DISEASE

Von Willebrand's disease is a hereditary deficiency of von Willebrand's factor (VWF), which causes platelet dysfunction. Bleeding tendency is usually mild. Screening tests show a prolonged bleeding time, normal platelet count, and, possibly, a slightly prolonged PTT. Diagnosis is based on low levels of VWF antigen and abnormal ristocetin cofactor activity. Treatment involves control of bleeding with replacement therapy (cryoprecipitate or pasteurized intermediate-purity factor VIII concentrate) or desmopressin.

Von Willebrand's factor (VWF) is synthesized and secreted by vascular endothelium to form part of the perivascular matrix. VWF promotes the platelet adhesion phase of hemostasis by binding with a receptor on the platelet surface membrane (glycoprotein Ib-IX), which connects the platelets to the vessel wall. VWF is also required to maintain normal plasma factor VIII levels. Levels of VWF can temporarily increase in response to stress, exercise, pregnancy, inflammation, or infection.

Von Willebrand's disease (VWD) involves a quantitative (type 1) or qualitative (type 2) impairment in synthesis of VWF. Type 2 VWD can result from a variety of genetic abnormalities. Inheritance of VWD is autosomal dominant. Although VWD, like hemophilia A, is a hereditary disorder that may, when severe, cause factor VIII deficiency, the deficiency is usually only moderate.

Symptoms and Signs

Bleeding manifestations are mild to moderate and include easy bruising; bleeding from small skin cuts that may stop and start over hours; sometimes, increased menstrual bleeding; and abnormal bleeding after surgical procedures (eg, tooth extraction, tonsillectomy).

Diagnosis

VWD is suspected in patients with bleeding disorders, particularly those with a family history of the disorder. Screening coagulation tests reveal a normal platelet count; normal INR; prolonged bleeding time; and, sometimes, a slightly prolonged PTT. However, stimuli that temporarily increase VWF levels can cause false-negative results in mild VWD; screening tests may need to be repeated. Definitive diagnosis requires measuring total plasma VWF antigen; VWF function, as determined by the ability of the plasma to support agglutination of normal platelets by ristocetin (ristocetin cofactor activity); and plasma factor VIII level.

In the common, type 1, form of VWD, results are concordant; ie, VWF antigen, VWF function, and plasma factor VIII level are equally depressed. The degree of depression varies from about 15 to 60% of normal and determines the severity of a patient's abnormal bleeding. Levels of VWF antigen can also be as low as 40% of normal in healthy people with type O blood.

Type 2 variants are suspected if tests are discordant, ie, VWF antigen is higher than expected for the degree of abnormality in ristocetin cofactor activity. (VWF antigen is higher than expected because the VWF defect in type 2 is qualitative, not quantitative.) Diagnosis is confirmed by demonstrating a reduced concentration of large VWF multimers on agarose gel electrophoresis. Four different type 2 variants are recognized, distinguished by different functional abnormalities of the VWF molecule.

Type 3 VWD is a rare autosomal recessive disorder in which homozygotes have no detectable VWF along with a marked deficiency of factor VIII. They have a combined defect of platelet adhesion and blood coagulation.

Treatment

Patients are treated only if they are actively bleeding or are undergoing an invasive procedure (eg, surgery, dental extraction). Treatment involves replacement of VWF by infusion of pasteurized intermediate-purity factor VIII concentrates which contain components of VWF. These concentrates are virally inactivated and therefore do not transmit HIV infection or hepatitis. Because they do not cause transfusion-transmitted infections, these concentrates are preferred to the previously common use of cryoprecipitate. High-purity factor VIII concentrates are prepared by immunoaffinity chromatography and contain no VWF.

Desmopressin is an analog of vasopressin that stimulates release of VWF into the plasma and may increase levels of factor VIII. Desmopressin can be helpful for type 1 VWD but is usually of no value in other types and may even be harmful in some. To ensure adequate response to the drug, the physician gives the patient a test dose and measures the response of VWF antigen. Desmopressin 0.3 µg/kg given in 50 mL 0.9% saline solution IV over 15 to 30 min may enable patients to undergo minor procedures (eg, tooth extraction, minor surgery) without needing replacement therapy. If a replacement product is needed, desmopressin may reduce the required dose. One dose of desmopressin is effective for about 8 to 10 h. About 48 h must elapse for new stores of VWF to accumulate, permitting a second injection of desmopressin to be as effective as the initial dose.

134 HEMOSTASIS

Hemostasis, the arrest of bleeding from an injured blood vessel, requires the combined activity of vascular, platelet, and plasma factors. Regulatory mechanisms counterbalance the tendency of clots to form. Hemostatic abnormalities can lead to excessive bleeding or thrombosis.

Vascular Factors

Vascular factors reduce blood loss from trauma through local vasoconstriction (an immediate reaction to injury) and compression of injured vessels by extravasation of blood into surrounding tissues. Vessel wall injury triggers the attachment and activation of platelets and production of fibrin; platelets and fibrin combine to form a clot.

Platelet Factors

Various mechanisms, including endothelial cell nitric oxide and prostacyclin, promote blood fluidity by preventing platelet stasis and dilating intact blood vessels. These mediators are no longer produced when the vascular endothelium is disrupted. Under these conditions, platelets adhere to the damaged intima and form aggregates. Initial platelet adhesion is to von Willebrand's factor (VWF), previously secreted by endothelial cells into the subendothelium. VWF binds to receptors on the platelet surface membrane (glycoprotein Ib/IX). Platelets anchored to the vessel wall undergo activation. During activation, platelets release mediators from storage granules, including adenosine diphosphate (ADP). Other biochemical changes resulting from activation include hydrolysis of membrane phospholipids, inhibition of adenylate cyclase, mobilization of intracellular Ca, and phosphorylation of intracellular proteins. Arachidonic acid is converted to thromboxane A_2; this reaction requires cyclooxygenase and is inhibited irreversibly by aspirin and reversibly by many NSAIDs. ADP, thromboxane A_2, and other mediators draw additional platelets to the injured endothelium (platelet aggregation) and activate them. Another receptor is assembled on the platelet surface membrane from glycoproteins IIb and IIIa. Fibrinogen binds to the glycoprotein IIa-IIIb complexes of adjacent platelets, connecting them.

Platelets provide surfaces for the assembly and activation of coagulation complexes and the generation of thrombin. Thrombin converts fibrinogen to fibrin; fibrin strands bind aggregated platelets to help secure the platelet-fibrin hemostatic plug.

Plasma Factors

Plasma coagulation factors interact to produce thrombin, which converts fibrinogen to fibrin. Radiating from and anchoring the hemostatic plug, fibrin strengthens the clot.

In the intrinsic pathway, factor XII, high mol wt kininogen, prekallikrein, and activated factor XI (factor XIa) produce factor IXa from factor IX. Factor IXa then combines with factor VIIIa and procoagulant phospholipid (present on the surface of activated platelets and tissue cells) to form a complex that activates factor X. In the extrinsic pathway, factor VIIa and tissue factor directly activate factor X (see FIG. 134–1 and TABLE 134–1).

Activation of the intrinsic or extrinsic pathway activates the common pathway, resulting in formation of the fibrin clot. Three steps are involved: (1) A prothrombin activator is produced on the surface of activated platelets and tissue cells. The activator is a complex of an enzyme, factor Xa, and 2 cofactors, factor Va and procoagulant phospholipid. (2) The prothrombin activator cleaves prothrombin into thrombin and another fragment. (3) Thrombin induces the generation of fibrin polymers from fibrinogen. Thrombin also activates factor XIII, an enzyme that catalyzes formation of stronger bonds between fibrin molecules, as well as factor VIII and factor XI.

Ca ions are needed in most thrombin-generating reactions (Ca-chelating agents [eg, citrate, ethylenediaminetetraacetic acid] are used in vitro as anticoagulants). Vitamin K–dependent clotting factors (factors II, VII, IX, and X) normally cannot bind to phospholipid surfaces through Ca bridges or function in blood coagulation when synthesized in the absence of vitamin K.

Although the coagulation pathways described above are helpful in understanding mechanisms and laboratory evaluation of coagulation disorders, in vivo coagulation is predominantly via the extrinsic pathway. People with hereditary deficiencies of factor XII, high mol wt kininogen, or prekallikrein have no bleeding abnormality. People with hereditary factor XI deficiency have a mild to moderate bleeding disorder. In vivo, factor XI

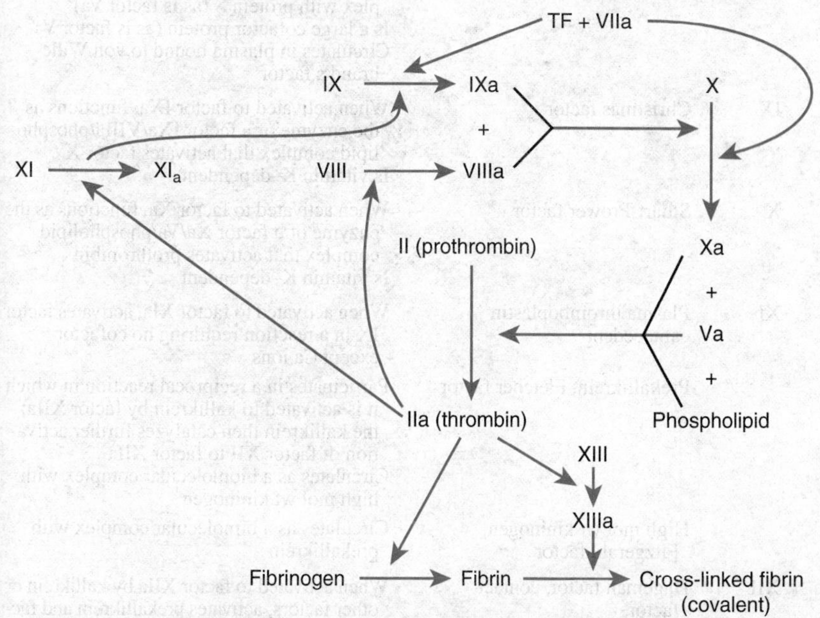

Fig. 134–1. Pathways in blood coagulation.

TABLE 134–1. COMPONENTS OF BLOOD COAGULATION REACTIONS

	COMPONENT	PURPOSE
Plasma factors		
I	Fibrinogen	A precursor of fibrin
II	Prothrombin	A precursor of thrombin, which converts fibrinogen to fibrin; thrombin activates factors V, VIII, XI, and XIII; thrombin bound to thrombomodulin activates protein C Is vitamin K–dependent
V	Proaccelerin	When activated to factor Va, serves as a cofactor for the enzyme factor Xa in a factor Xa/Va/phospholipid complex that activates prothrombin Is present in platelet α granules. Factor Va is inactivated by activated protein C in complex with protein S
VII	Proconvertin	Binds to tissue factor and is then activated to form the enzymatic component of a factor VIIa/tissue factor complex that activates factors IX and X Is vitamin K–dependent
VIII	Antihemophilic globulin	When activated to factor VIIIa, serves as a cofactor for the enzyme factor IXa in a factor IXa/VIIIa/phospholipid complex that activates factor X Is inactivated by activated protein C in complex with protein S (as is factor Va) Is a large cofactor protein (as is factor V) Circulates in plasma bound to von Willebrand's factor
IX	Christmas factor	When activated to factor IXa, functions as the enzyme of a factor IXa/VIIIa/phospholipid complex that activates factor X Is vitamin K–dependent
X	Stuart-Prower factor	When activated to factor Xa, functions as the enzyme of a factor Xa/Va/phospholipid complex that activates prothrombin Is vitamin K–dependent
XI	Plasma thromboplastin antecedent	When activated to factor XIa, activates factor IX in a reaction requiring no cofactor except Ca ions
	Prekallikrein, Fletcher factor	Participates in a reciprocal reaction in which it is activated to kallikrein by factor XIIa; the kallikrein then catalyzes further activation of factor XII to factor XIIa Circulates as a biomolecular complex with high mol wt kininogen
	High mol wt kininogen, Fitzgerald factor	Circulates as a bimolecular complex with prekallikrein
XII	Hageman factor, contact factor	When activated to factor XIIa by kallikrein or other factors, activates prekallikrein and factor XI, triggering intrinsic pathway in vitro

TABLE 134–1. COMPONENTS OF BLOOD COAGULATION REACTIONS—Continued

	COMPONENT	PURPOSE
XIII	Fibrin stabilizing factor	When activated by thrombin, catalyzes formation of peptide bonds between fibrin molecules, thus helping to stabilize the clot
	Protein C	When activated by thrombin bound to thrombomodulin, inhibits by proteolysis the cofactor activity of factors VIIIa and Va in a reaction requiring protein S and phospholipid as cofactors Is vitamin K–dependent
	Protein S	Exists in plasma as free protein S and as protein S bound to the C4b binding protein of the complement system Functions in its free form as a cofactor for activated protein C Is vitamin K–dependent
Cell surface factors		
	Tissue factor, tissue thromboplastin	Is a lipoprotein that is constitutively present on the membrane of certain tissue cells, including perivascular fibroblasts, epithelial cells at body or environmental boundaries (eg, epithelial cells of the skin, amnion, and GI and GU tracts), and glial cells of the nervous system May also develop in pathologic states on activated monocytes and macrophages, and on activated vascular endothelium Is present on some tumor cells Binds factor VIIa, which initiates the extrinsic pathway
	Procoagulant phospholipid	Acidic phospholipid (primarily phosphatidyl serine) present on the surface of activated platelets and other tissue cells Functions as a component of the factor IXa/VIIIa/phospholipid activator of factor X and of the factor Xa/Va/phospholipid activator of prothrombin Functions as the lipid moiety of tissue factor
	Thrombomodulin	Is an endothelial cell surface binding site for thrombin When bound to thrombomodulin, thrombin activates protein C

(an intrinsic pathway factor) is activated when a small amount of thrombin is generated. Factor IX (an intrinsic factor) is activated by the extrinsic pathway.

In vivo initiation of the extrinsic pathway occurs directly when injury to blood vessels brings blood into contact with the tissue factor on membranes of cells within and around the vessel walls. This contact with tissue factor generates factor VIIa/tissue factor complexes that activate factor X and factor IX (an intrinsic factor). Factor IXa, combined with its cofactor, factor VIIIa, on phospholipid membrane surfaces generates additional factor Xa. Factor X activation by both routes is required for normal hemostasis. This requirement for factors VIII and IX explains why hemophilia (deficiency of either factor VIII or

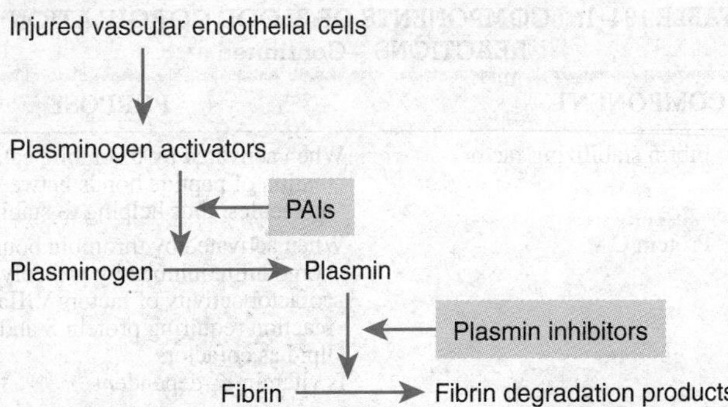

Fig. 134–2. Fibrinolytic pathway. Fibrin deposition and fibrinolysis must be balanced during repair of an injured blood vessel wall. Injured vascular endothelial cells release plasminogen activators (tissue plasminogen activator, urokinase), activating fibrinolysis. Plasminogen activators catalyze cleavage of plasminogen, creating plasmin, which dissolves clots. Fibrinolysis is controlled by plasminogen activator inhibitors (PAIs; eg, PAI-1) and plasmin inhibitors (eg, α_2-antiplasmin).

factor IX) results in bleeding despite an intact extrinsic coagulation pathway.

Regulatory Mechanisms

Several inhibitory mechanisms prevent activated coagulation reactions from amplifying uncontrollably, causing extensive local thrombosis or disseminated intravascular coagulation. These mechanisms include inactivation of procoagulant enzymes, fibrinolysis, and clearance of activated clotting factors, especially by the liver.

Inactivation of coagulation factors: Plasma protease inhibitors (antithrombin, tissue factor pathway inhibitor, α_2-macroglobulin, heparin cofactor II) inactivate coagulation enzymes. Antithrombin inhibits thrombin, factor Xa, factor XIa, and factor IXa. Heparin enhances antithrombin activity.

Two vitamin K–dependent proteins, protein C and protein S, form a complex that inactivates factors VIIIa and Va by proteolysis. Thrombin, when bound to a receptor on endothelial cells called thrombomodulin, activates protein C. Activated protein C combines with protein S and phospholipid as cofactors to proteolyze factors VIIIa and Va.

Fibrinolysis: Fibrin deposition and lysis must be balanced to maintain and remold the hemostatic seal during repair of an injured vessel wall. The fibrinolytic system dissolves fibrin by means of plasmin, a proteolytic enzyme. Fibrinolysis is activated by plasminogen activators released from vascular endothelial cells. Plasminogen activators and plasminogen from plasma bind to fibrin. Plasminogen activators catalyze cleavage of plasminogen, creating plasmin (see FIG. 134–2). Plasmin produces soluble fibrin degradation products that are swept into the circulation.

Plasminogen activators are categorized into several types. Tissue plasminogen activator (tPA), from endothelial cells, is a poor activator when free in solution but an efficient activator when bound to fibrin in proximity to plasminogen. A second type, urokinase, exists in single-chain and double-chain forms with different functional properties. Single-chain urokinase cannot activate free plasminogen but, like tPA, can readily activate plasminogen bound to fibrin. A trace concentration of plasmin cleaves single-chain to double-chain urokinase, which activates plasminogen in solution as well as plasminogen bound to fibrin. Epithelial cells that line excretory passages (eg, renal tubules, mammary ducts) secrete urokinase, which is the physiologic activator of fibrinolysis in these channels. Streptokinase, a bacterial product not normally found in the body, is another potent plasminogen activator. Streptokinase, urokinase, and recombinant tPA (alteplase) have all been used therapeutically to induce fibrinolysis in patients with acute thrombotic disorders.

Regulation of fibrinolysis: Fibrinolysis itself is regulated by plasminogen activator inhibitors (PAIs) and plasmin inhibitors that slow fibrinolysis. PAI-1, the most important PAI, inactivates tPA and urokinase and is released from vascular endothelial cells and activated platelets. The primary plasmin inhibitor is α_2-antiplasmin, which quickly inactivates free plasmin escaping from clots. Some α_2-antiplasmin is also cross-linked by factor XIIIa to fibrin during clotting; it may prevent excessive plasmin activity within clots. tPA and urokinase are rapidly cleared by the liver, which is another mechanism of preventing excessive fibrinolysis.

APPROACH TO THE PATIENT WITH A POSSIBLE BLEEDING DISORDER

A patient is evaluated for a bleeding disorder if symptoms or signs of unusual or excessive bleeding are present or if a laboratory test abnormality suggesting a bleeding disorder is found incidentally. Patients can also have disorders that produce excessive thrombosis (see p. 1080). Unusual or excessive bleeding includes unexplained nosebleeds (epistaxis), excessive or prolonged menstrual blood loss (menorrhagia), prolonged bleeding after minor cuts or trauma, easy bruising into tissues (ecchymoses) or skin (petechial or purpuric lesions), and unexplained gingival bleeding after tooth brushing or flossing.

Systemic bleeding can result from defects in blood vessels (eg, connective tissue diseases, vitamin C deficiency, hereditary hemorrhagic telangiectasia) or, more commonly, quantitative or qualitative disorders of platelets (see p. 1064) or of coagulation (see p. 1082).

Defects in platelets or blood vessels cause bleeding from superficial sites, including skin and mucous membranes; the bleeding may be spontaneous or may occur immediately after trauma. In contrast, patients with defects in coagulation (coagulopathies) bleed into tissues (eg, hemarthroses, muscle hematomas, retroperitoneal hemorrhage); after trauma, the bleeding may be delayed.

Evaluation

History: The history should address systemic diseases associated with defects in platelets or coagulation; ingestion of drugs, including aspirin, NSAIDs, or other OTC drugs that impair platelet function; excessive or unusual prior bleeding; and family history of bleeding disorders. A history of excessive or unusual prior bleeding, especially bleeding from multiple sites, suggests thrombocytopenia or a coagulopathy. Absence of a family history of excessive bleeding does not exclude an inherited coagulopathy (eg, hemophilia).

Physical examination: Signs of skin and mucous membrane bleeding include petechiae, which are pinpoint cutaneous hemorrhages that appear most conspicuously over dependent extremities (especially common in severe thrombocytopenia), ecchymoses, purpura, GI or GU tract bleeding, epistaxis, and hemoptysis. Signs of bleeding from deeper tissues may include joint tenderness and swelling, muscle bruises, and, if severe, signs of intracranial bleeding, hypovolemia, or hemorrhagic shock.

Testing: Laboratory testing of coagulation is most likely to be abnormal in patients whose history or examination reveals a bleeding risk. Abnormal results in a patient with no signs or symptoms of excessive bleeding should be repeated to exclude laboratory error. Abnormal results are not always clinically meaningful. For example, patients with deficiencies of factor XII, prekallikrein, or high mol wt kininogen in the intrinsic pathway do not bleed excessively (see TABLE 134–2).

Screening tests evaluate the components of hemostasis, including the number of circulating platelets and the plasma coagulation pathways. The most common screening tests for bleeding disorders are the platelet count, PT, and PTT. If results are abnormal, a specific test can usually pinpoint the defect. Determination of the level of fibrin degradation products measures in vivo activation of fibrinolysis.

The PT screens for abnormalities in the extrinsic and common pathways of coagulation (plasma factors VII, X, V, prothrombin, and fibrinogen). The PT is reported as the international normalized ratio (INR), which reflects the ratio of the patient's PT to the laboratory's control value; the INR controls for differences in reagents among different laboratories. Because commercial reagents and instrumentation vary widely, each laboratory should determine its own normal range for PT and PTT; a typical normal range for the PT is between 10 and 13 sec. An INR > 1.5 or a PT ≥ 3 sec longer than a laboratory's normal control value is usually abnormal and requires further evaluation. The INR is valuable in screening for abnormal coagulation in various acquired conditions (eg, vitamin K deficiency, liver disease, disseminated intravascular coagulation). It is also used to monitor

TABLE 134–2. LABORATORY TESTS OF HEMOSTASIS

PHASE OF HEMOSTASIS	TEST	PURPOSE
Formation of initial platelet plugs	Platelet count	Quantifies platelet number
	Bleeding time	Screens for overall adequacy of platelet adhesion and aggregation on injured vascular surfaces
	Platelet aggregation	Evaluates adequacy of platelet responsiveness to physiologic stimuli activating platelets (eg, collagen, adenosine diphosphate, arachidonic acid); may identify abnormal patterns in hereditary or acquired platelet functional disorders
	von Willebrand's factor antigen	Measures total concentration of plasma von Willebrand's factor protein
	von Willebrand's factor multimer composition	Evaluates distribution of VWF multimers in plasma (eg, large multimers are missing in type II variants of VWD)
	Ristocetin agglutination	Screens for presence of large multimers of VWF (often obtained as part of routine laboratory evaluation for VWD—see p. 1071)
	Ristocetin cofactor activity	Quantifies large multimers of VWF (see p. 1071)
Formation of fibrin	Prothrombin time	Screens for the factors in extrinsic and common pathways (factors VII, X, V, prothrombin, and fibrinogen)
	Partial thromboplastin time	Screens for the factors in intrinsic and common pathways (prekallikrein; high mol wt kininogen; factors XII, XI, IX, VIII, X, and V; prothrombin; and fibrinogen)
	Specific functional assays for coagulation factors	Determines activity as a percentage of normal
	Thrombin time	Screens the last step of coagulation, thrombin cleavage of fibrinogen to fibrin; is prolonged by heparin-induced antithrombin activation and with conditions resulting in qualitative abnormalities of fibrinogen or hypofibrinogenemia
	Reptilase time	Is not affected by heparin-induced antithrombin activation; if normal with a prolonged thrombin time, provides presumptive evidence that a plasma sample contains heparin (eg, residual heparin after extracorporeal bypass, or if blood sample was drawn from an IV line kept open with heparin flushes)
	Fibrinogen level	Quantifies plasma fibrinogen, which is increased in acute phase reactions and decreased in severe liver disease and severe DIC
Inhibitors of blood coagulation	Antithrombin	Quantifies plasma antithrombin, which is reduced in some patients with congenital early-onset venous thromboembolism, and during DIC or heparin therapy
	Proteins C and S	Separate tests quantify these natural anticoagulants; either may be reduced in some patients with congenital early-onset venous thromboembolism; both are reduced in DIC

TABLE 134–2. LABORATORY TESTS OF HEMOSTASIS—Continued

PHASE OF HEMOSTASIS	TEST	PURPOSE
Fibrinolysis	Clot stability on 24-h incubation in saline and in 5M urea	Causes lysis of clots in saline if fibrinolytic activity is excessive, or in 5M urea if factor XIII is deficient. Should be obtained if there is defective wound healing or frequent miscarriages
	Plasminogen activity	Quantifies plasma plasminogen, which is decreased in rare patients with congenital early-onset venous thromboembolism
	α_2-Antiplasmin	Quantifies plasma level of this fibrinolysis inhibitor, which is reduced in the rare patient with excessive bleeding as a result of increased fibrinolysis
	Serum fibrinogen/ fibrin degradation products	Screens for DIC; levels are increased when plasmin has acted on fibrinogen or fibrin in vivo (eg, in DIC); superseded by plasma D-dimer assay
	Plasma D-dimer	Is measured with either a monoclonal antibody latex agglutination test or with an ELISA; high values indicate that thrombin has been generated in vivo with resultant deposition of fibrin, activation of the cross-linking enzyme, factor XIII and secondary fibrinolysis; has the practical advantage that it can be done on citrate–plasma and, thus, unlike the test for serum fibrin degradation products, it does not require clotting blood in a special tube to prepare serum free of residual fibrinogen; is undergoing evaluation for utility in excluding in vivo thrombosis (eg, deep venous thrombosis or pulmonary embolism), especially the sensitive ELISA version

VWF = von Willebrand's factor; VWD = von Willebrand's disease; DIC = disseminated intravascular coagulation; ELISA = enzyme-linked immunosorbent assay.

therapy with the oral vitamin K antagonist, warfarin.

Partial thromboplastin time (PTT) screens plasma for abnormalities in factors of the intrinsic and common pathways (prekallikrein; high mol wt kininogen; factors XII, XI, IX, VIII, X, and V; prothrombin; fibrinogen). The PTT tests for deficiencies of all clotting factors except factor VII (measured by the PT) and factor XIII. A normal range of 28 to 34 sec is typical. A normal result indicates that at least 30% of all coagulation factors in the pathway are present in the plasma. Heparin prolongs the PTT, and the PTT is often used to monitor heparin therapy. Inhibitors that prolong the PTT include an autoantibody against factor VIII (see Hemophilia on p. 1085 and Coagulation Disorders Caused by Circulating Anticoagulants on p. 1083) and antibodies against protein-phospholipid complexes ("lupus anticoagulant"—see Coagulation Disorders Caused by Circulating Anticoagulants on p. 1083 and Thrombotic Disorders on p. 1080).

Prolongation of the INR or PTT may reflect factor deficiency or the presence of an inhibitor of a component of the coagulation system. The PT and PTT do not become prolonged until one or more of the clotting factors tested are about 70% deficient. For determining whether prolongation reflects a deficiency of one or more clotting factor or the presence of an inhibitor, the test is repeated after mixing the patient's plasma with normal plasma in a 1:1 ratio. Because this mixture provides about 50% of normal levels of all coagulation factors, failure of the mixture to correct the prolongation almost completely suggests the presence of an inhibitor in patient plasma.

Use of the bleeding time as a screening test to assess platelet–vessel wall interactions is of doubtful reliability. The test is performed with a BP cuff inflated to 40 mm Hg on the upper arm. A disposable spring-loaded device is used to make a standardized incision on the volar aspect of the forearm. Blood is absorbed onto filter paper at 30-sec intervals until bleeding stops. The bleeding time may be prolonged by thrombocytopenia, disorders of platelet function, von Willebrand's disease (VWD), and, unlike other laboratory tests, primary vessel wall abnormalities. Use of aspirin within 7 days also may prolong the bleeding time. Theoretically, the bleeding time is not prolonged by inherited or acquired coagulation disorders; in practice, however, results are unpredictable in these conditions. Because the sensitivity and reproducibility of the bleeding time are limited, its use is controversial.

Normal results on all of the screening tests exclude many bleeding disorders. Exceptions include rare, severe factor XIII deficiency, which requires a specific assay if suspected; VWD, a common entity in which the associated deficiency of factor VIII is frequently insufficient to prolong the PTT; and rare disorders of fibrinolytic control. Because prolongation of the PT or PTT requires about 70% deficiency of one or more coagulation factors, suspicion of less severe factor deficiencies (eg, patients with mild bleeding disorders) requires performance of more sensitive assays of specific factors.

In patients with bleeding disorders and symptoms suggesting occult bleeding, evaluation should be thorough. For example, CT scanning should be used for patients with severe headaches, head injuries, impairment of consciousness, or possible intraperitoneal or retroperitoneal hemorrhage.

Treatment

Treatment is directed at the underlying cause and at complications of bleeding (see p. 2554 for control of localized bleeding and p. 563 for treatment of hemorrhagic shock). For immediate treatment of bleeding due to a coagulopathy that has not yet been diagnosed, fresh frozen plasma, which contains all coagulation factors, should be infused pending definitive evaluation.

135 THROMBOTIC DISORDERS

In a healthy person, a homeostatic balance exists between procoagulant (clotting) forces and anticoagulant and fibrinolytic forces (see Ch. 134 on p. 1072). Numerous genetic, acquired, and environmental factors can tip the balance in favor of coagulation, leading to the pathologic formation of thrombi in veins (eg, deep vein thrombosis [DVT]), arteries (eg, MI, ischemic stroke), or cardiac chambers. Thrombi can obstruct blood flow at the site of formation or detach and embolize to block a distant blood vessel (eg, pulmonary embolism, stroke).

Etiology

Genetic defects that increase the propensity for venous thromboembolism include the factor V Leiden mutation, which causes resistance to activated protein C (APC); the prothrombin 20210 gene mutation; and a deficiency of protein C, protein S, protein Z, or antithrombin.

Acquired defects that predispose to venous and arterial thrombosis include heparin-induced thrombocytopenia/thrombosis, the presence of antiphospholipid antibodies, and (possibly) hyperhomocysteinemia as a result of folate, vitamin B_{12}, or vitamin B_6 deficiency.

Other disorders and environmental factors can increase the risk of thrombosis, especially if present in conjunction with one of the genetic abnormalities mentioned above.

Stasis associated with surgery or orthopedic or paralytic immobilization; heart failure; pregnancy; and obesity increase the risk of venous thrombosis. Tissue injury from trauma or surgery exposes tissue factor to blood and increases the risk of venous thrombosis.

Neoplastic cells, particularly from promyelocytic leukemia and tumors involving the lung, breast, prostate, and GI tract, predispose to venous thrombosis. They may activate coagulation by secreting a factor X–activating protease, by expressing tissue factor on exposed membrane surfaces, or both.

Sepsis and other severe infections associated with increased tissue factor exposure on monocytes and macrophages can increase the risk of venous thrombosis.

Oral contraceptives that contain estrogen increase the risk of arterial and venous thromboembolism; however, the risk with modern low-dose regimens is low. Patients who develop venous thromboembolism while taking these drugs often have a coexisting predisposing genetic abnormality.

Atherosclerosis predisposes to arterial thrombi, especially at sites of preexisting stenosis. Atherosclerotic plaques rupture and expose the contents of tissue factor–rich plaques to blood, which initiates local platelet adhesion/aggregation, coagulation factor activation, and thrombosis.

Diagnosis and Treatment

Diagnosis and treatment of thrombi are summarized elsewhere in THE MANUAL specific to their location. Predisposing factors should always be considered. In some cases, the condition is clinically obvious (eg, recent surgery or trauma, prolonged immobilization, malignancy, generalized atherosclerosis). If no predisposing factor is readily apparent, further evaluation should be conducted in patients with a family history of venous thrombosis, more than one episode of venous thrombosis, MI or ischemic stroke before age 50, or unusual sites of venous thrombosis (eg, cavernous sinus, mesenteric veins). As many as half of all patients with spontaneous DVT have a genetic predisposition.

Testing for predisposing congenital factors includes functional measurements of the activity of natural anticoagulant molecules in plasma and tests for specific gene defects. Testing begins with a group of screening tests, followed (if necessary) by specific assays.

Factor V Resistance to Activated Protein C

APC degrades factors Va and VIIIa, thus inhibiting coagulation. Any of several mutations to factor V make it resistant to inactivation by APC, increasing the tendency for thrombosis. Factor V Leiden is the most common of these mutations. Homozygous mutations increase the risk of thrombosis more than do heterozygous mutations. Its prevalence as a single gene defect in European populations is about 5%, but it rarely occurs in native Asian or African populations. It is present in 20 to 60% of patients with spontaneous venous thrombosis. Diagnosis is based on a functional plasma coagulation assay (the failure of patient plasma PTT to become prolonged in the presence of snake venom–activated patient protein C) and on molecular analysis of the factor V gene. Treatment if necessary involves anticoagulation with heparin followed by warfarin.

Protein C Deficiency

Because APC degrades factors Va and VIIIa, APC is a natural plasma anticoagulant. Decreased protein C from genetic or acquired causes promotes venous thrombosis. Heterozygous deficiency of plasma protein C has a prevalence of 0.2 to 0.5%; about 75% of people with this defect experience a venous thromboembolism (50% by age 50). Homozygous or doubly heterozygous deficiency causes neonatal purpura fulminans, ie, severe neonatal DIC. Acquired decreases occur in patients with liver disease or DIC, during cancer chemotherapy (including L-asparaginase administration), and during warfarin therapy. Diagnosis is based on antigenic and functional plasma coagulation assays (extent of prolongation of normal plasma PTT, using normal plasma depleted of protein C, as a result of the addition of patient plasma containing snake venom). Patients with symptomatic thrombosis require anticoagulation with heparin or low mol wt heparin, followed by warfarin; use of the vitamin K antagonist, warfarin, as initial therapy occasionally causes thrombotic skin infarction by lowering vitamin K–dependent protein C levels before a therapeutic decrease has occurred in most vitamin K–dependent clotting factors. Neonatal purpura fulminans is fatal without replacement of protein C (using normal plasma or purified concentrate) and anticoagulation with heparin.

Protein S Deficiency

Protein S is a cofactor for APC-mediated cleavage of factors Va and VIIIa. Heterozygous deficiency of plasma protein S predisposes to venous thrombosis and is similar to protein C deficiency in genetic transmission, prevalence, laboratory testing, treatment, and precautions. Homozygous deficiency of protein S can cause neonatal purpura fulminans that is clinically indistinguishable from that caused by homozygous deficiency of protein C. Acquired deficiencies of protein S (and protein C) occur during DIC and warfarin therapy and after L-asparaginase administration. Diagnosis is based on antigenic assays of total or free plasma protein S. (Free protein S is the form unbound to C4 binding protein.)

PROTEIN Z DEFICIENCY

Protein Z, another vitamin K–dependent protein, functions as a cofactor to down-regulate coagulation by forming a complex with the plasma protein, Z-dependent protease inhibitor. The complex inactivates factor Xa. The consequence of protein Z deficiency in the pathophysiology of thrombosis and fetal loss is unresolved.

ANTITHROMBIN DEFICIENCY

Antithrombin is a protein that inhibits thrombin and factors Xa, IXa, and XIa. Heterozygous deficiency of plasma antithrombin has a prevalence of about 0.2 to 0.4%; about half of those affected develop venous thromboses. Homozygous deficiencies are probably lethal to the fetus in utero. Acquired deficiencies occur in patients with DIC, liver disease, or nephrotic syndrome and during heparin or L-asparaginase therapy. Laboratory testing involves quantification of plasma inhibition of thrombin in the presence of heparin. Oral warfarin is used for prophylaxis against venous thromboembolism.

PROTHROMBIN 20210 GENE MUTATION

A mutation of the prothrombin gene results in increased plasma prothrombin levels and increases the risk of venous thromboembolism.

ANTIPHOSPHOLIPID ANTIBODY SYNDROME

(Anti-Cardiolipin Antibodies; Lupus Anticoagulant)

The antiphospholipid antibody syndrome consists of thrombosis and (in pregnancy) fetal demise associated with various autoimmune antibodies directed against one or more proteins (eg, β_2-glycoprotein I, prothrombin, annexin). These proteins normally bind to phospholipid membrane constituents and protect them from excessive coagulation activation. The autoantibodies displace the protective proteins and, thus, produce procoagulant endothelial cell surfaces and cause arterial or venous thromboses. In vitro clotting tests may paradoxically be prolonged because the antiprotein/phospholipid antibodies interfere with coagulation factor assembly and activation on the phospholipid components added to plasma to initiate the tests. The lupus anticoagulant is an antiphospholipid autoantibody that binds to protein-phospholipid complexes. It was initially recognized in patients with SLE, but these patients now account for a minority of those with the autoantibody. Heparin, warfarin, and aspirin have been used for prophylaxis and treatment.

HYPERHOMOCYSTEINEMIA

Hyperhomocysteinemia may predispose to arterial thrombosis and venous thromboembolism, possibly because of injury to vascular endothelial cells. Plasma homocysteine levels are elevated ≥ 10-fold in homozygous cystathionine β-synthase deficiency. Milder elevations occur in heterozygous deficiency and in other abnormalities of folate metabolism, including methyltetrahydrofolate dehydrogenase deficiency. However, by far the most common causes of hyperhomocysteinemia are acquired deficiencies of folate, vitamin B_{12}, or vitamin B_6. The diagnosis is established by measuring plasma homocysteine levels. Homocysteine levels may be normalized by dietary supplementation with folic acid, vitamin B_{12}, or vitamin B_6 (pyridoxine) alone or in combination; however, it is not clear that this therapy reduces the risk of arterial or venous thrombosis.

136 COAGULATION DISORDERS

Abnormal bleeding can result from disorders of the coagulation system (see p. 1072), of platelets, or of blood vessels. Disorders of coagulation can be acquired or hereditary. The major causes of acquired coagulation disorders are vitamin K deficiency (see p. 45), liver disease, disseminated intravascular coagulation, and development of circulating anticoagulants. Severe liver disease (eg, cirrhosis, fulminant hepatitis, acute fatty liver of pregnancy) may disturb hemostasis by impairing clotting factor synthesis. Because all coagulation factors are made in the liver, both the PT and PTT are elevated in severe liver disorders. (PT results are typically reported as INR.) Occasionally, decompensated liver disease also causes excessive fibrinolysis and bleeding due to decreased hepatic synthesis of α_2-antiplasmin.

The most common hereditary disorder of hemostasis is von Willebrand's disease (see p. 1071). The most common hereditary coagulation disorders are the hemophilias.

COAGULATION DISORDERS CAUSED BY CIRCULATING ANTICOAGULANTS

Circulating anticoagulants are usually autoantibodies that neutralize specific clotting factors in vivo (eg, an autoantibody against factor VIII or factor V) or inhibit protein-bound phospholipid in vitro. Occasionally, the latter type of autoantibody causes bleeding in vivo by binding prothrombin.

Circulating anticoagulants should be suspected in patients with excessive bleeding combined with either a prolonged PTT or PT that does not correct when the test is repeated with a 1:1 mixture of normal plasma and the patient's plasma.

Antiphospholipid antibodies (see p. 1082) typically cause thrombosis. However, in a subset of patients, the antibodies bind to prothrombin-phospholipid complexes, inducing hypoprothrombinemia; these patients may bleed excessively.

FACTOR VIII ANTICOAGULANTS

Isoantibodies to factor VIII develop in about 15 to 35% of patients with severe hemophilia A as a complication of repeated exposure to normal factor VIII molecules during replacement therapy (see Hemophilia on p. 1085). Factor VIII autoantibodies also arise occasionally in nonhemophilic patients, eg, in a postpartum woman as a manifestation of underlying systemic autoimmune disease or of transiently disordered immune regulation, or in elderly patients without overt evidence of other underlying disease. Patients with a factor VIII anticoagulant can develop life-threatening hemorrhage.

Plasma containing a factor VIII antibody has a prolonged PTT that does not correct when normal plasma or another source of factor VIII is added in a 1:1 mixture to the patient's plasma. Testing is performed immediately after mixture and again after incubation.

Therapy with cyclophosphamide and corticosteroids may suppress autoantibody production in patients without hemophilia. In postpartum women, the autoantibodies may disappear spontaneously. Management of acute hemorrhage in hemophilic patients who have factor VIII isoantibodies is discussed under Hemophilia on p. 1086.

DISSEMINATED INTRAVASCULAR COAGULATION

(Consumption Coagulopathy; Defibrination Syndrome)

Disseminated intravascular coagulation (DIC) involves abnormal, excessive generation of thrombin and fibrin in the circulating blood. During the process, increased platelet aggregation and coagulation factor consumption occur. DIC that evolves slowly (over weeks or months) causes primarily venous thrombotic and embolic manifestations; DIC that evolves rapidly (over hours or days) causes primarily bleeding. Severe, rapidly evolving DIC is diagnosed by demonstrating thrombocytopenia, an elevated PTT and PT, increased levels of serum fibrin degradation products, and a decreasing plasma fibrinogen level. Treatment includes correction of the underlying cause and replacement of platelets, coagulation factors (in fresh frozen plasma), and fibrinogen (in cryoprecipitate) to control severe bleeding. Heparin is used as therapy (or prophylaxis) in patients with slowly evolving DIC who have (or are at risk for) venous thromboembolism.

Etiology and Pathophysiology

DIC usually results from exposure of tissue factor to blood, initiating the coagulation cascade (see FIG. 134–2). DIC occurs in the following clinical circumstances:

- Complications of obstetrics—eg, abruptio placentae, saline-induced therapeutic abortion, retained dead fetus or products of conception, or amniotic fluid embolism. Placental tissue with tissue factor activity enters or is exposed to the maternal circulation.

- Infection, particularly with gram-negative organisms. Gram-negative endotoxin causes generation of tissue factor activity in phagocytic, endothelial, and tissue cells.

- Malignancy, particularly mucin-secreting adenocarcinomas of the pancreas and prostate and acute promyelocytic leukemia, in which tumor cells expose or release tissue factor activity.
- Shock from any cause that produces ischemic tissue injury and tissue factor exposure.

Less common causes of DIC include severe tissue damage from head trauma, burns, frostbite, or gunshot wounds; complications of prostate surgery that allow prostatic material with tissue factor activity (along with plasminogen activators) to enter the circulation; venomous snake bites in which enzymes enter the circulation that activate one or several coagulation factors and generate thrombin or directly convert fibrinogen to fibrin; profound intravascular hemolysis; and aortic aneurysms or cavernous hemangiomas (Kasabach-Merritt syndrome) associated with vessel wall damage and areas of blood stasis.

Slowly evolving DIC primarily causes venous thromboembolic manifestations (eg, deep venous thrombosis, pulmonary embolism), although occasionally cardiac valve vegetations occur; abnormal bleeding is uncommon. In contrast, in severe, rapidly evolving DIC, thrombocytopenia and depletion of plasma clotting factors and fibrinogen cause bleeding. Bleeding into organs, along with microvascular thromboses, may cause hemorrhagic tissue necrosis in multiple organs.

Symptoms and Signs

In slowly evolving DIC, symptoms of venous thrombosis and pulmonary embolism may be present.

In severe, rapidly evolving DIC, skin puncture sites (eg, IV or arterial punctures) bleed persistently, ecchymoses form at sites of parenteral injections, and serious GI bleeding may occur. Delayed dissolution of fibrin polymers by fibrinolysis may result in the mechanical disruption of RBCs and mild intravascular hemolysis (see Thrombotic Thrombocytopenic Purpura and Hemolytic-Uremic Syndrome on p. 1070). Occasionally, microvascular thrombosis and hemorrhagic necrosis produce dysfunction and failure in multiple organs.

Diagnosis

DIC is suspected in patients with unexplained bleeding or venous thromboembolism, especially if a predisposing condition exists. If DIC is suspected, platelet count, PT, PTT, plasma fibrinogen level, and plasma D-dimer (an indication of in vivo fibrin deposition and degradation) are obtained.

Slowly evolving DIC produces mild thrombocytopenia, a normal to minimally prolonged PT (results are typically reported as INR) and PTT, a normal or moderately reduced fibrinogen level, and an increased plasma D-dimer level. Because a variety of illnesses stimulate increased synthesis of fibrinogen as an acute-phase reactant, a declining fibrinogen level on 2 consecutive measurements can help make the diagnosis of DIC.

Severe, rapidly evolving DIC results in more severe thrombocytopenia, more prolonged PT and PTT, rapidly declining plasma fibrinogen concentrations, and a high plasma D-dimer level.

A factor VIII level can sometimes be helpful if severe, acute DIC must be differentiated from massive hepatic necrosis, which can produce similar abnormalities in coagulation studies. The factor VIII level is elevated in hepatic necrosis, because factor VIII is made in hepatocytes and released as they are destroyed; factor VIII is reduced in DIC because of the thrombin-induced generation of activated protein C, which proteolyses factor VIII.

Treatment

Immediate correction of the underlying cause is the priority (eg, broad-spectrum antibiotic treatment of suspected gram-negative sepsis, evacuation of the uterus in abruptio placentae). If treatment is effective, DIC should subside quickly. If bleeding is severe, adjunctive replacement therapy is indicated, consisting of platelet concentrates to correct thrombocytopenia; cryoprecipitate to replace fibrinogen and factor VIII; and fresh frozen plasma to increase levels of other clotting factors and natural anticoagulants (antithrombin, proteins C and S). The effects of infusion of concentrates of antithrombin or activated protein C in severe, rapidly evolving DIC are under study.

Heparin usually is not indicated in DIC. An exception is in women with a retained dead fetus and evolving DIC with a progressive decrease in platelets, fibrinogen, and coagulation factors. In this circumstance, heparin is administered for several days to control DIC, increase fibrinogen and platelets, and decrease excessive coagulation factor consumption before uterine evacuation.

HEMOPHILIA

Hemophilias are common hereditary bleeding disorders caused by deficiencies of either clotting factor VIII or IX. The extent of factor deficiency determines the probability and severity of bleeding. Bleeding into deep tissues or joints usually develops within hours of trauma. The diagnosis is suspected in a patient with an elevated PTT and normal PT and platelet count; it is confirmed by specific factor assays. Treatment includes replacement of the deficient factor if acute bleeding is suspected, confirmed, or likely to develop (eg, before surgery).

Hemophilia A (factor VIII deficiency), which affects about 80% of hemophilic patients, and hemophilia B (factor IX deficiency) have identical clinical manifestations, screening test abnormalities, and X-linked genetic transmission. Specific factor assays are required to distinguish the two.

Hemophilia is an inherited disorder that results from mutations, deletions, or inversions affecting a factor VIII or IX gene. Because these genes are located on the X chromosome, hemophilia affects males almost exclusively. Daughters of hemophilic males are obligate carriers, but sons are normal. Each son of a carrier has a 50% chance of having hemophilia, and each daughter has a 50% chance of being a carrier.

Normal hemostasis requires > 30% of normal factor VIII and IX levels. Most hemophilia patients have levels < 5%. Carriers usually have levels of about 50%; rarely, random inactivation of their normal X chromosome in early embryonic life results in a carrier having factor VIII or IX levels of < 30%.

Most hemophilia patients who were treated with plasma concentrates in the early 1980s were infected with HIV due to contaminated factor concentrates. An occasional patient develops immune thrombocytopenia secondary to HIV infection, which can exacerbate bleeding.

Symptoms and Signs

Patients with hemophilia bleed into tissues (eg, hemarthroses, muscle hematomas, retroperitoneal hemorrhage), and the bleeding may be delayed after trauma. Pain often occurs as bleeding commences, sometimes before other signs of bleeding develop. Chronic or recurrent hemarthroses can lead to synovitis and arthropathy. Even a trivial blow to the head can cause intracranial bleeding. Bleeding into the base of the tongue can cause life-threatening airway compression.

Severe hemophilia (factor VIII or IX level < 1% of normal) causes severe bleeding throughout life, usually beginning soon after birth (eg, scalp hematoma after delivery or excessive bleeding after circumcision). Moderate hemophilia (factor levels 1 to 5% of normal) usually causes bleeding after minimal trauma. In mild hemophilia (factor levels 5 to 25% of normal), excessive bleeding may occur after surgery or dental extraction.

Diagnosis

Hemophilia is suspected in patients with recurrent bleeding, unexplained hemarthroses, or a prolongation of the PTT. If hemophilia is suspected, PTT, PT, platelet count, and factor VIII and IX assays are obtained. In hemophilia, the PTT is prolonged, but the PT and platelet count are normal. Factor VIII and IX assays determine the type and severity of the hemophilia. Because factor VIII levels may also be reduced in von Willebrand's disease (VWD), von Willebrand's factor (VWF) activity, antigen, and multimer composition are measured in patients with newly diagnosed hemophilia A, particularly if the disease is mild and a family history indicates that both male and female family members are affected. Determining if a female is a true carrier of hemophilia A is sometimes possible by measuring the factor VIII level. Similarly, measuring the factor IX level often identifies a carrier of hemophilia B. PCR analysis of DNA that comprises the factor VIII gene, available at specialized centers, can be used for diagnosis of the hemophilia A carrier state and for prenatal diagnosis of hemophilia A by chorionic villus sampling at 12 wk or amniocentesis at 16 wk. These procedures carry a 0.5 to 1% risk of miscarriage.

After repeated exposure to factor VIII replacement, about 15 to 35% of patients with hemophilia A develop factor VIII isoantibodies (alloantibodies) that inhibit the coagulant activity of any additional factor VIII infused. Patients should be screened for isoantibodies (eg, by measuring the degree of PTT shortening immediately after mixing the patient's plasma with an equal volume of normal plasma, and then by repeating the measurement after incubation for 1 h), especially before an elective procedure that requires replacement therapy. If isoantibodies are present, their titers can be measured by determining the extent of factor VIII inhibition by serial dilutions of patient plasma.

Prevention and Treatment

Hemophilia patients should avoid aspirin and NSAIDs that suppress platelet function more transiently than aspirin. The newer COX-2 inhibitors have little antiplatelet activity, may produce fewer GI erosions than aspirin or other NSAIDs, and can be used with caution in hemophilia. Regular dental care is essential so that tooth extractions and other dental surgery can be avoided. Drugs should be given orally or IV; IM injections can cause hematomas. Hemophilia patients should be vaccinated against hepatitis B.

If symptoms suggest bleeding, treatment should begin immediately, even before diagnostic tests are completed. For example, treatment for headache that might indicate intracranial hemorrhage should begin before a CT scan is completed.

Replacement of the deficient factor is the primary treatment. In hemophilia A, the factor VIII level should be raised transiently to about 30% of normal to prevent bleeding after dental extraction or to abort an incipient joint hemorrhage; to 50% if major joint or IM bleeding is already evident; and to 100% before major surgery or if bleeding is intracranial, intracardiac, or otherwise life threatening. Repeated infusions at 50% of the initial calculated dose should then be given q 8 to 12 h to keep trough levels above 50% for 7 to 10 days after major surgery or life-threatening hemorrhage. Each unit/kg of factor VIII increases the factor VIII level by about 2%. Thus, to increase the level from 0% to 50%, about 25 units/kg are required.

Factor VIII can be given as purified factor VIII concentrate, which is derived from multiple donors. It undergoes viral inactivation, but this may not eliminate parvovirus or hepatitis A. Recombinant factor VIII is free of viruses but is expensive and may confer a greater risk of inducing isoantibodies. It is usually preferred unless the patient is already seropositive for HIV or for hepatitis B or C virus.

In hemophilia B, factor IX can be given as a purified or recombinant viral-inactivated product q 24 h. The target levels of factor correction are the same as in hemophilia A; however, to achieve these levels, the dose must be higher than in hemophilia A because factor IX is smaller than factor VIII and, in contrast to VIII, has an extensive extravascular distribution.

Fresh frozen plasma contains factors VIII and IX. However, unless plasma exchange is performed, sufficient whole plasma usually cannot be given to patients with severe hemophilia to raise factor VIII or IX concentrations to levels that prevent or control bleeding. Fresh frozen plasma should, therefore, be used only if rapid replacement therapy is necessary in the circumstance that factor concentrate is unavailable or the patient has a coagulopathy that is not yet defined precisely.

In hemophiliacs who develop a factor VIII inhibitor, treatment is best accomplished using recombinant factor VIIa in repeated high doses (eg, 90 μg/kg).

Adjunctive therapies may include desmopressin or an antifibrinolytic drug. As described for VWD (see p. 1072), desmopressin may temporarily raise factor VIII levels. The patient's response should be tested before desmopressin is used therapeutically. Its use after minor trauma or before elective dental surgery may obviate replacement therapy. Desmopressin should be used only for patients with mild hemophilia A (basal factor VIII levels ≥ 5%) who have demonstrated responsiveness.

An antifibrinolytic agent (ε-aminocaproic acid 2.5 to 4 g po qid for 1 wk or tranexamic acid 1.0 to 1.5 g po tid or qid for 1 wk) should be given to prevent late bleeding after dental extraction or other oropharyngeal mucosal trauma (eg, tongue laceration).

UNCOMMON HEREDITARY COAGULATION DISORDERS

Most hereditary coagulation disorders other than hemophilia are rare autosomal recessive conditions producing disease only in the homozygote (see TABLE 136–1). Factor XI deficiency is uncommon in the general population but common in descendants of European Jews (gene frequency about 5 to 9%). Bleeding typically occurs after significant injuries, including trauma or surgery, in homozygotes or compound heterozygotes.

Severe deficiency of α_2-antiplasmin (1 to 3% of normal), the major physiologic inhibitor of plasmin, can also cause bleeding.

TABLE 136–1. SCREENING LABORATORY TEST RESULTS IN INHERITED DEFECTS IN BLOOD COAGULATION

SCREENING TEST RESULTS*	DEFECT	CHARACTERISTICS
PTT long; PT normal	Factor XII, high mol wt kininogen, prekallikrein	Laboratory test abnormality without clinical bleeding; must be distinguished by specific assays from factor XI deficiency in which posttraumatic and perioperative bleeding may occur
PTT long; PT normal	Factor XI	Autosomal recessive; increased frequency in Ashkenazic Jews; posttraumatic and perioperative bleeding; diagnosis by specific assay; therapy for bleeding is to keep factor XI level > 30% with fresh frozen plasma 5–20 mL/kg/day
PTT long; PT normal	Factor VIII or IX	Factor VIII deficiency (hemophilia A); factor IX deficiency (hemophilia B); X-linked transmission; mild or severe bleeding, depending on factor VIII or IX level
PTT normal; PT long	Factor VII	Autosomal recessive; rare; severe deficiency (< 2%) results in serious bleeding; levels > 5% result in mild or no bleeding; recombinant factor VIIa is the therapy of choice
PTT long; PT long	Factor X, V, or prothrombin	Autosomal recessive; rare; bleeding may be mild to severe; diagnosed by specific assays; therapy for factor X or prothrombin deficiency is fresh frozen plasma or prothrombin complex concentrate for bleeding episodes; therapy for factor V deficiency is fresh frozen plasma with or without platelet concentrates (supply platelet factor V)
In afibrinogenemia (fibrinogen < 10 mg/dL), no clotting in PTT or PT because machine endpoint not triggered In hypofibrinogenemia (fibrinogen 70–100 mg/dL), PTT and PT often prolonged by several seconds, thrombin time long	Fibrinogen	Severe bleeding in afibrinogenemia (homozygous state); posttraumatic and perioperative bleeding in hypofibrinogenemia (heterozygous state); therapy is cryoprecipitate (5–10 bags, each containing about 250 mg fibrinogen)
PTT and PT long; thrombin time long	Dysfibrinogenemia	Manifestations vary (no, or only mild, posttraumatic and perioperative bleeding, tendency for thrombosis, wound dehiscence); fibrinogen low by clotting assay but normal by immunologic assay
PTT normal; PT normal; thrombin time normal Clot dissolves in 5M urea	Factor XIII	Autosomal recessive; rare; poor wound healing; spontaneous abortions in women; severe bleeding with < 1% of normal level; therapy is fresh frozen plasma (1–2 units q 4–6 wk is effective because half-life of factor XIII is about 10 days)
PTT and PT normal; clot lysis times in 5M urea or saline are accelerated	α_2-Antiplasmin deficiency	Severe bleeding in homozygotes; heterozygotes may have posttraumatic and perioperative bleeding; confirmation of diagnosis requires specific assay

*PT results are typically reported as INR.

Diagnosis is based on a specific α_2-antiplasmin assay. ε-Aminocaproic acid or tranexamic acid is used to control or prevent acute bleeding. Heterozygotes with α_2-antiplasmin levels of 40 to 60% of normal can occasionally experience excessive surgical bleeding if secondary fibrinolysis is extensive (eg, in patients who have had open prostatectomy).

137 BLEEDING DUE TO ABNORMAL BLOOD VESSELS

Bleeding may result from abnormalities in platelets, coagulation factors, or blood vessels. Vascular bleeding disorders are caused by defects in blood vessels, typically producing petechiae, purpura, and bruising but seldom leading to serious blood loss. Bleeding may result from deficiencies of vascular and perivascular collagen in Ehlers-Danlos syndrome and in other rare hereditary connective tissue disorders (eg, pseudoxanthoma elasticum, osteogenesis imperfecta, Marfan syndrome—see p. 2382). Hemorrhage may be a prominent feature of scurvy (see p. 40) or of Henoch-Schönlein purpura, a hypersensitivity vasculitis common during childhood (see p. 275). In vascular bleeding disorders, tests of hemostasis are usually normal. Diagnosis is clinical.

AUTOERYTHROCYTE SENSITIZATION

(Gardner-Diamond Syndrome)

Autoerythrocyte sensitization is a rare disorder affecting women. It is characterized by local pain and burning preceding painful ecchymoses that occur primarily on the extremities.

In women with autoerythrocyte sensitization, intradermal injection of 0.1 mL of autologous RBCs or RBC stroma may result in pain, swelling, and induration at the injection site. This result suggests that escape of RBCs into the tissues is involved in the pathogenesis of the lesion. However, most patients also have associated severe psychoneurotic symptoms. In addition, psychogenic factors, such as self-induced purpura, seem related to the pathogenesis of the syndrome in some patients. Diagnosis is based on examination of the site of intradermal injection of autologous RBCs and of a separate control injection site (without RBCs) 24 to 48 h after injection. Excoriation, which can complicate the test's interpretation, is prevented by making both sites difficult for the patient to reach.

DYSPROTEINEMIAS CAUSING VASCULAR PURPURA

Amyloidosis (see p. 1310) causes amyloid deposition within vessels in the skin and subcutaneous tissues, which may increase vascular fragility, producing purpura. In some patients, coagulation factor X is adsorbed by amyloid and becomes deficient, but this usually is not the cause of bleeding. Periorbital purpura or a purpuric rash that develops in a nonthrombocytopenic patient after gentle stroking of the skin suggests amyloidosis.

Cryoglobulinemia produces immunoglobulins that precipitate when plasma is cooled (ie, cryoglobulins) while flowing through the skin and subcutaneous tissues of the extremities. Monoclonal immunoglobulins formed in Waldenström's macroglobulinemia or in multiple myeloma (see p. 1129) occasionally behave as cryoglobulins, as may mixed IgM-IgG immune complexes formed in some chronic infectious diseases, most commonly hepatitis C. Cryoglobulinemia can lead to small-vessel vasculitis, which can produce purpura. Cryoglobulins can be detected by laboratory testing.

Hypergammaglobulinemic purpura is a vasculitic purpura that primarily affects women. Recurrent crops of small, palpable purpuric lesions develop on the lower legs. These lesions leave small residual brown spots. Many patients have manifestations of an underlying immunologic disorder (eg, Sjögren's syndrome, SLE). The diagnostic finding is a polyclonal increase in IgG (broad-based or diffuse hypergammaglobulinemia on serum protein electrophoresis).

Hyperviscosity syndrome (see p. 1128) resulting from a markedly elevated plasma IgM concentration may also result in purpura and other forms of abnormal bleeding (eg, profuse epistaxis) in patients with Waldenström's macroglobulinemia.

HEREDITARY HEMORRHAGIC TELANGIECTASIA

(Rendu-Osler-Weber Syndrome)

Hereditary hemorrhagic telangiectasia is a hereditary disease of vascular malformation transmitted as an autosomal dominant trait affecting men and women.

Symptoms, Signs, and Diagnosis

The most characteristic lesions are small red-to-violet telangiectatic lesions on the face, lips, oral and nasal mucosa, and tips of the fingers and toes. Similar lesions may be present throughout the mucosa of the GI tract, resulting in recurrent GI bleeding. Patients may experience recurrent, profuse nosebleeds. Some patients have pulmonary arteriovenous fistulas. These fistulas may produce significant right-to-left shunts, which can result in dyspnea, fatigue, cyanosis, or polycythemia. However, the first sign of their presence may be a brain abscess, transient ischemic attack, or stroke as a result of infected or noninfected emboli. Cerebral or spinal arteriovenous malformations occur in some families and may cause subarachnoid hemorrhage, seizures, or paraplegia.

Diagnosis is based on the finding of characteristic arteriovenous malformations on the face, mouth, nose, and digits. Endoscopy or angiography is sometimes needed, however. If a family history of pulmonary or cerebral arteriovenous malformations exists, screening at puberty and at the end of adolescence with pulmonary CT or cerebral MRI is recommended. Laboratory findings are usually normal except for iron deficiency anemia in most patients.

Treatment

Treatment for most patients is supportive, but accessible telangiectases (eg, in the nose or GI tract via endoscopy) may be treated with laser ablation. Arteriovenous fistulas may be treated by surgical resection or embolotherapy. Repeated blood transfusions may be needed; therefore, immunization with hepatitis B vaccine is important. Most patients require continuous iron therapy to replace iron lost in repeated mucosal bleeding; some patients require parenteral iron (see Iron Deficiency Anemia on p. 1036). Treatment with drugs that inhibit fibrinolysis, such as aminocaproic acid, may be beneficial.

PURPURA SIMPLEX

(Easy Bruising)

Purpura simplex is increased bruising that results from vascular fragility.

Purpura simplex is extremely common. The cause and mechanism are unknown; it may represent a heterogeneous group of disorders.

The disorder usually affects women. Bruises develop without known trauma on the thighs, buttocks, and upper arms. The history usually reveals no other abnormal bleeding, but easy bruising may be present in family members. Serious bleeding does not occur. The platelet count and tests of platelet function, blood coagulation, and fibrinolysis are normal.

No drug prevents the bruising; the patient is often advised to avoid aspirin and aspirin-containing drugs, but there is no evidence that bruising is related to or worsened by their use. The patient should be reassured that the condition is not serious.

SENILE PURPURA

Senile purpura produces ecchymoses and results from increased vessel fragility due to connective tissue damage to the dermis caused by chronic sun exposure and aging.

Senile purpura affects older patients, who develop persistent dark purple ecchymoses, which are characteristically confined to the extensor surfaces of the hands and forearms. New lesions appear without known trauma and then resolve over several days, leaving a brownish discoloration caused by deposits of hemosiderin; this discoloration may clear over weeks to months. The skin and subcutaneous tissue of the involved area often appear thinned and atrophic. No treatment hastens lesion resolution or is needed. Although cosmetically displeasing, the disorder has no serious consequences.

138 SPLEEN DISORDERS

By structure and function the spleen is like 2 organs. The white pulp, consisting of periarterial lymphatic sheaths and germinal centers, acts as an immune organ. The red pulp, consisting of macrophages and granulocytes lining vascular spaces (the cords and sinusoids), acts as a phagocytic organ.

The white pulp is a site of production and maturation of B and T cells. B cells in the spleen generate protective humoral antibodies; in certain autoimmune disorders (eg, immune thrombocytopenic purpura [ITP], Coombs'-positive immune hemolytic anemias), inappropriate autoantibodies to circulating blood elements also may be synthesized.

The red pulp removes antibody-coated bacteria, senescent or defective RBCs, and antibody-coated blood cells (as may occur in immune cytopenias such as ITP, Coombs'-positive hemolytic anemias, and some neutropenias). The red pulp also serves as a reservoir for blood elements, especially WBCs and platelets. During its culling and pitting of RBCs, the spleen removes inclusion bodies, such as Heinz bodies (precipitates of insoluble globin), Howell-Jolly bodies (nuclear fragments), and whole nuclei; thus, after splenectomy or in the functionally hyposplenic state, RBCs with these inclusions appear in the peripheral circulation. Hematopoiesis normally occurs in the red pulp only during fetal life. Beyond fetal life, hematopoiesis may occur if injury to bone marrow (eg, by fibrosis or tumors) allows hematopoietic stem cells to circulate and repopulate the adult spleen (see Myelofibrosis on p. 1101 and Myelodysplastic Syndrome on p. 1114).

SPLENOMEGALY

Splenomegaly is almost always secondary to other disorders. Its causes are myriad, as are the many possible ways of classifying them (see TABLE 138–1). Myeloproliferative diseases, lymphoproliferative diseases, storage diseases (eg, Gaucher's disease), and connective tissue diseases are the most common causes in temperate climates, whereas infectious diseases (eg, malaria, kala-azar) predominate in the tropics.

If splenomegaly is massive (spleen palpable 8 cm below the costal margin), the cause is usually chronic lymphocytic leukemia, non-Hodgkin lymphoma, chronic myelocytic leukemia, polycythemia vera, myelofibrosis with myeloid metaplasia, or hairy cell leukemia.

Splenomegaly can lead to cytopenia (see Hypersplenism on p. 1091).

Evaluation

History: Most of the presenting symptoms result from the underlying disease. However, splenomegaly itself may cause early satiety by encroachment of the enlarged spleen on the stomach. Fullness and left upper quadrant abdominal pain are also possible. Severe pain suggests splenic infarction. Recurrent infections, symptoms of anemia, or bleeding manifestations suggest cytopenia and possible hypersplenism.

Physical examination: The sensitivity for detection of ultrasound-documented splenic enlargement is 60 to 70% for palpation and 60 to 80% for percussion. Up to 3% of normal, thin, people have a palpable spleen. Also, a palpable left upper quadrant mass may indicate a problem other than an enlarged spleen.

Other helpful signs include a splenic friction rub that suggests splenic infarction and epigastric and splenic bruits that suggest congestive splenomegaly. Generalized adenopathy may suggest a myeloproliferative, lymphoproliferative, infectious, or autoimmune disorder.

Testing: If confirmation of splenomegaly is necessary because the examination is equivocal, ultrasound is the test of choice because of its accuracy and low cost. CT and MRI may provide more detail of the organ's consistency. MRI is especially useful in detecting portal or splenic vein thromboses. Nuclear scanning is accurate and can identify accessory splenic tissue but is expensive and cumbersome to perform.

Specific causes suggested clinically should be confirmed by appropriate testing (see elsewhere in THE MANUAL). If no cause is suggested, the highest priority is exclusion of occult infection, because early treatment affects the outcome of infection more than it does most other causes of splenomegaly. Testing should be thorough in areas of high geographic prevalence of infection or if the patient appears to be ill. CBC, blood cultures, and bone marrow examination and culture should be considered. If the patient is not ill, has no symptoms besides those due to splenomegaly, and has no risk factors for infection, the extent of testing is controversial but probably includes CBC, peripheral blood smear, liver function tests, and abdominal CT. Flow cytometry of peripheral blood is indicated if lymphoma is suspected.

Specific peripheral blood findings may suggest underlying causes (eg, lymphocytosis in chronic lymphocytic leukemia; leukocytosis and immature forms in other leukemias). Excessive basophils, eosinophils, or nucleated or teardrop RBCs suggest myeloproliferative disorders. Cytopenias suggest hypersplenism. Spherocytosis suggests hypersplenism or hereditary spherocytosis. Liver function test results are diffusely abnormal in congestive splenomegaly with cirrhosis; an isolated elevation of serum alkaline phosphatase suggests hepatic infiltration, as in myeloproliferative and lymphoproliferative disorders and miliary TB.

Some other tests may be useful, even in asymptomatic patients. Serum protein electrophoresis identifying a monoclonal gammopathy or decreased immunoglobulins suggest lymphoproliferative disorders or amyloidosis; diffuse hypergammaglobulinemia suggests chronic infection (eg, malaria, kala-azar, brucellosis, TB) or cirrhosis with congestive splenomegaly, sarcoidosis, or connective tissue diseases. Elevation of serum uric acid suggests a myeloproliferative or lymphoproliferative disorder. Elevation of WBC alkaline phosphatase suggests a myeloproliferative disorder, whereas decreased levels suggest chronic myelocytic leukemia.

If testing reveals no abnormalities other than splenomegaly, the patient should be reevaluated at intervals of 6 to 12 mo or when new symptoms develop.

Treatment

Treatment is directed at the underlying disorder. The enlarged spleen itself needs no treatment unless severe hypersplenism is present. Patients with palpable or very large spleens probably should avoid contact sports to decrease the risk of splenic rupture.

TABLE 138–1. COMMON CAUSES OF SPLENOMEGALY*

Congestive splenomegaly (Banti's disease)
- Cirrhosis
- External compression or thrombosis of portal or splenic veins
- Certain malformations of the portal venous vasculature

Infectious and inflammatory diseases
- Acute infections (eg, infectious mononucleosis, infectious hepatitis, subacute bacterial endocarditis, psittacosis)
- Chronic infections (eg, miliary TB, malaria, brucellosis, kala-azar, syphilis)
- Sarcoidosis
- Amyloidosis
- Connective tissue disease (eg, SLE, Felty's syndrome)

Myeloproliferative and lymphoproliferative diseases
- Myelofibrosis with myeloid metaplasia
- Lymphomas (eg, Hodgkin lymphoma)
- Leukemias, especially chronic lymphocytic and chronic myelocytic
- Polycythemia vera
- Primary thrombocythemia

Chronic, usually congenital, hemolytic anemias
- RBC shape abnormalities (eg, hereditary spherocytosis, hereditary elliptocytosis)
- Hemoglobinopathies, including thalassemias, sickle cell hemoglobin variants (eg, hemoglobin S-C disease), congenital Heinz body hemolytic anemias
- RBC enzymopathies (eg, pyruvate kinase deficiency)

Storage diseases
- Lipoid (eg, Gaucher's, Niemann-Pick, and Hand-Schüller-Christian diseases)
- Nonlipoid (eg, Letterer-Siwe disease)
- Amyloidosis

Splenic cysts
- Usually caused by resolution of previous intrasplenic hematoma

*In order of clinical frequency.

Adapted from Williams WJ et al: *Hematology*. New York, McGraw-Hill Book Company, 1976.

HYPERSPLENISM

Hypersplenism is cytopenia caused by splenomegaly.

Hypersplenism is a secondary process that can arise from splenomegaly of almost any cause (see TABLE 138–1). Splenomegaly increases the spleen's mechanical filtering and destruction of RBCs and often of WBCs and

TABLE 138–2. INDICATIONS FOR SPLENECTOMY OR RADIATION THERAPY IN HYPERSPLENISM

INDICATION	EXAMPLES
Hemolytic syndromes in which the shortened survival of intrinsically abnormal RBCs is further curtailed by splenomegaly	Hereditary spherocytosis, thalassemia
Severe pancytopenia associated with massive splenomegaly	Lipid-storage diseases (the spleen may be 30 times larger than normal)
Vascular insults involving the spleen	Recurrent infarctions, bleeding esophageal varices associated with excessive splenic venous return
Mechanical encroachment on other abdominal organs	Stomach with early satiety, left kidney with calyceal obstruction
Serious bleeding	Hypersplenic thrombocytopenia

platelets. Compensatory bone marrow hyperplasia occurs in those cell lines that are reduced in the circulation.

Symptoms, Signs, and Diagnosis

Splenomegaly is the hallmark; spleen size correlates with the degree of anemia. The spleen can be expected to extend about 2 cm beneath the costal margin for each 1-g decrease in Hb. Other clinical findings usually result from the underlying disease.

Unless other mechanisms coexist to compound their severity, anemia and other cytopenias are modest and asymptomatic (eg, platelet counts, 50,000 to 100,000/µL; WBC counts, 2500 to 4000/µL with normal WBC differential count). RBC morphology is generally normal except for occasional spherocytosis. Reticulocytosis is usual.

Hypersplenism is suspected in patients with splenomegaly and anemia or cytopenias; evaluation is similar to that of splenomegaly (see p. 1090).

Treatment

Treatment is directed at the underlying disease. However, if hypersplenism is the only serious manifestation of the disorder (eg, Gaucher's disease), then splenic ablation by splenectomy or radiation may be indicated (see TABLE 138–2). Because the intact spleen protects against serious infections with encapsulated bacteria, splenectomy should be avoided whenever possible, and patients undergoing splenectomy require vaccination against infections caused by *Streptococcus pneumoniae*, *Neisseria meningitidis*, and *Haemophilus influenzae*. Following splenectomy, patients are particularly susceptible to severe sepsis; those who develop fever should promptly consult their physician and receive empiric antibiotics.

SPLENIC RUPTURE

Splenic rupture generally results from blunt abdominal trauma.

Splenic enlargement as a result of fulminant Epstein-Barr viral disease (infectious mononucleosis or posttransplant Epstein-Barr virus-mediated pseudolymphoma) predisposes to rupture with minimal trauma or even spontaneously. Significant impact (eg, motor vehicle collision) can rupture a normal spleen.

Rupture of the splenic capsule produces marked hemorrhage into the peritoneal cavity. The manifestations, including hemorrhagic shock, abdominal pain, and distention, are usually clinically obvious. However, splenic trauma can also produce a subcapsular hematoma, which may not rupture until hours or even months after the injury.

Rupture is generally preceded by left upper quadrant abdominal pain. Splenic rupture should be suspected in patients with blunt abdominal trauma and hemorrhagic shock or left upper quadrant pain (which sometimes radiates to the shoulder); patients with unexplained left upper quadrant pain, particularly if there is evidence of hypovolemia or shock, should be asked about recent trauma. The diagnosis is confirmed by CT scan (in the stable patient), ultrasound, or peritoneal lavage (in the unstable patient).

Treatment has traditionally been splenectomy. However, splenectomy should be avoided if possible, particularly in children, to avoid the resulting permanent susceptibility to bacterial infections. In this case, treatment is transfusion as needed.

139 EOSINOPHILIC DISORDERS

Eosinophils are granulocytes derived from the same progenitor cells as monocytes-macrophages, neutrophils, and basophils. The precise functions of eosinophils are unknown. Although phagocytic, eosinophils are less efficient than neutrophils in killing intracellular bacteria. No direct evidence shows that eosinophils kill parasites in vivo, but they are toxic to helminths in vitro, and eosinophilia commonly accompanies helminthic infestations. Eosinophils may modulate immediate hypersensitivity reactions by degrading or inactivating mediators released by mast cells, such as histamine, leukotrienes (which may cause vasoconstriction and bronchoconstriction), lysophospholipids, and heparin. Prolonged eosinophilia may result in tissue damage by mechanisms that are not fully understood.

Eosinophil granules contain major basic protein and eosinophil cationic protein that are toxic to several parasites and to mammalian cells. These proteins bind heparin and neutralize its anticoagulant activity. Eosinophil-derived neurotoxin can severely damage myelinated neurons. Eosinophil peroxidase, which differs significantly from peroxidase of other granulocytes, generates oxidizing radicals in the presence of hydrogen peroxide and a halide. Charcot-Leyden crystals are primarily composed of phospholipase B and are located in sputum, tissues, and stool in diseases in which there is eosinophilia (eg, asthma, eosinophilic pneumonia).

The normal peripheral blood eosinophil count is < 350/μL, with diurnal levels that vary inversely with plasma cortisol levels; the peak occurs at night and the trough in the morning. The circulating half-life of eosinophils is 6 to 12 h, with most eosinophils residing in tissues (eg, the upper respiratory and GI tracts, skin, uterus).

Eosinophil production appears to be regulated by T cells through the secretion of the hematopoietic growth factors granulocyte-macrophage colony-stimulating factor (GM-CSF), interleukin-3 (IL-3), and interleukin-5 (IL-5). Although GM-CSF and IL-3 also increase the production of other myeloid cells, IL-5 increases eosinophil production exclusively.

EOSINOPHILIA

Eosinophilia is defined as a peripheral blood eosinophil count > 450/μL. Causes are myriad but often represent an allergic reaction or parasitic infection. Diagnosis involves selective testing directed at clinically suspected underlying causes. Treatment is directed at the underlying cause.

Eosinophilia has features of an immune response: an agent such as *Trichinella spiralis* invokes a primary response with relatively low levels of eosinophils, whereas repeated exposures result in an augmented or secondary eosinophilic response.

Factors that decrease the eosinophil count include β-blockers, corticosteroids, stress, and (sometimes) bacterial and viral infections. Several compounds released by mast cells and basophils induce IgE-mediated eosinophil production, eg, eosinophil chemotactic factor of anaphylaxis, leukotriene B4, complement complex (C5-C6-C7), and histamine (over a narrow range of concentration).

Eosinophilia may be primary (idiopathic) or secondary to numerous disorders (see TABLE 139–1). In the US, allergic or atopic diseases are the most common causes; the most common conditions are respiratory and skin diseases. Almost any parasitic invasion of tissues can elicit eosinophilia, but protozoa and noninvasive metazoa usually do not.

Of the neoplastic diseases, Hodgkin lymphoma (Hodgkin's disease) may elicit marked eosinophilia, whereas eosinophilia is less common in non-Hodgkin lymphoma, chronic myelocytic leukemia, and acute lymphoblastic leukemia. Of solid tumors, ovarian cancer is the leading cause. The pulmonary infiltrates with eosinophilia syndrome comprises a spectrum of clinical manifestations characterized by peripheral eosinophilia and eosinophilic pulmonary infiltrates (see Eosinophilic Pulmonary Diseases on p. 450 and Langerhans' Cell Histiocytosis on p. 1096) but is usually of unknown cause. Patients with eosinophilic drug reactions may be asymptomatic or have a variety of syndromes, including interstitial nephritis, serum sickness, cholestatic jaundice, hypersensitivity vasculitis, and immunoblastic lymphadenopathy. Several hundred patients were reported to have developed an eosinophilia-myalgia syndrome after taking L-tryptophan for sedation or psychotropic support. This syndrome was probably caused by a contaminant rather than by L-tryptophan.

TABLE 139–1. IMPORTANT CAUSES OF SECONDARY EOSINOPHILIA

CAUSE	EXAMPLES
Allergic or atopic diseases	Asthma, allergic rhinitis, allergic bronchopulmonary aspergillosis, occupational lung disease, urticaria, eczema, atopic dermatitis, milk-protein allergy, episodic angioedema with eosinophilia, drug reactions
Parasitic infestations (especially tissue-invasive metazoans)	Trichinosis, visceral larva migrans, trichuriasis, ascariasis, strongyloidiasis, hookworm infection, clonorchiasis, paragonimiasis, fascioliasis, cysticercosis (*Taenia solium*), echinococcosis, filariasis, schistosomiasis, *Pneumocystis jiroveci* (formerly *P. carinii*) infection
Nonparasitic infections	Aspergillosis, brucellosis, cat-scratch fever, infectious lymphocytosis, chlamydial pneumonia of infancy, acute coccidioidomycosis, infectious mononucleosis, mycobacterial disease, scarlet fever
Tumors	Carcinomas and sarcomas (lung, pancreas, colon, cervix, ovary), Hodgkin lymphoma (Hodgkin's disease), non-Hodgkin lymphomas, immunoblastic lymphadenopathy
Myeloproliferative disorders	Chronic myelocytic leukemia
Syndromes of pulmonary infiltration with eosinophilia	Simple pulmonary eosinophilia (Löffler's syndrome), chronic eosinophilic pneumonia, tropical pulmonary eosinophilia, allergic bronchopulmonary aspergillosis, Churg-Strauss syndrome
Skin disorders	Exfoliative dermatitis, dermatitis herpetiformis, psoriasis, pemphigus
Connective tissue, vasculitic, or granulomatous disorders (especially those involving the lungs)	Polyarteritis nodosa, RA, sarcoidosis, inflammatory bowel disease, SLE, scleroderma, eosinophilic fasciitis, Dressler's syndrome
Immune disorders (often with eczema)	Graft-vs-host disease, congenital immunodeficiency syndrome (eg, IgA deficiency, hyper-IgE syndrome, Wiskott-Aldrich syndrome)
Endocrine disorders	Adrenal hypofunction
Miscellaneous	Cirrhosis, radiation therapy, peritoneal dialysis, familial eosinophilia, use of L-tryptophan

The symptoms (severe muscle pain, tenosynovitis, muscle edema, skin rash) lasted weeks to months, and several deaths occurred.

Diagnosis and Treatment

When the CBC indicates eosinophilia, an absolute eosinophil count is rarely needed. A medical history, emphasizing travel, allergies, and drug use, is taken, and physical examination is performed. Specific diagnostic tests are determined by the clinical findings and may include chest x-ray, urinalysis, liver and kidney function tests, and serologic tests for parasitic and connective tissue diseases. Stool should be examined for ova and parasites, although negative findings do not rule out a parasitic cause (eg, trichinosis requires a muscle biopsy; visceral larva migrans and filarial infections require other tissue biopsies; duodenal aspirates may be needed to exclude specific parasites, eg, *Strongyloides* sp—see p. 1552). An elevated serum vitamin B_{12} or low WBC alkaline phosphatase level or abnormalities on the peripheral smear suggest an underlying myeloproliferative disorder, in which case a bone marrow aspirate and biopsy with cytogenetic studies may be helpful.

If no underlying cause is detected, the patient is followed for complications. A brief trial with low-dose corticosteroids may lower the eosinophil count if eosinophilia is secondary (eg, to allergy or parasitic infestation) rather than malignant. Such a trial is indicated if eosinophilia is persistent and progressive in the absence of a treatable cause.

IDIOPATHIC HYPEREOSINOPHILIC SYNDROME

(Disseminated Eosinophilic Collagen Disease; Eosinophilic Leukemia; Löffler's Fibroplastic Endocarditis with Eosinophilia)

Idiopathic hypereosinophilic syndrome is a condition defined by peripheral blood eosinophilia > 1500/μL persisting ≥ 6 mo with manifestations of organ system involvement or dysfunction directly related to eosinophilia in the absence of parasitic, allergic, or other causes of eosinophilia. Symptoms are myriad, depending on which organs are dysfunctional. Treatment begins with prednisone and may include hydroxyurea, interferon-α, and imatinib.

Only some patients with prolonged eosinophilia develop idiopathic hypereosinophilic syndrome. Although any organ may be involved, the heart, lungs, spleen, skin, and nervous system are typically affected. Cardiac involvement often causes morbidity and mortality. A novel fusion tyrosine kinase, FIP1L1-PDGFR, has been recognized as contributing to the pathophysiology.

Symptoms, Signs, and Diagnosis

Symptoms are diverse and depend on which organs are dysfunctional (see TABLE 139–2). The clinical syndrome follows 2 broad patterns. The first pattern involves a myeloproliferative disorder with splenomegaly, thrombocytopenia, elevated serum vitamin B_{12} levels, and hypogranular or vacuolated eosinophils. Patients with this pattern often develop endomyocardial fibrosis or (less commonly) frank leukemia. The second pattern involves a hypersensitivity-type illness with angioedema, hypergammaglobulinemia, elevated serum IgE, and circulating immune complexes. Patients with this pattern develop heart disease less often, usually require no therapy, and respond well to corticosteroids.

The diagnosis is suspected in patients with eosinophilia without an obvious cause and with symptoms suggesting organ dysfunction. Such patients should undergo testing as above to exclude any disorders causing eosinophilia secondarily. They should also undergo echocardiography to detect myocardial involvement. CBC and peripheral smear help determine which of the 2 broad patterns of disease exists. About ⅓ of patients with either of these patterns are thrombocytopenic at presentation.

TABLE 139–2. ABNORMALITIES IN PATIENTS WITH IDIOPATHIC HYPEREOSINOPHILIC SYNDROME

SYSTEM	PREVALENCE	MANIFESTATIONS
Constitutional	≅ 50%	Weakness, fatigue, anorexia, fever, weight loss, myalgias
Cardiopulmonary	> 70%	Restrictive or infiltrative cardiomyopathy or mitral or tricuspid regurgitation with cough, dyspnea, heart failure, arrhythmias, endomyocardial disease, pulmonary infiltrates, and pleural effusions, and mural thrombi with emboli
Hematologic	> 50%	Thromboembolic phenomena, anemia, thrombocytopenia, lymphadenopathy, splenomegaly
Neurologic	> 50%	Diffuse encephalopathy with altered behavior and cognitive function and spasticity, peripheral neuropathy, and cerebral emboli with focal deficits
Dermatologic	> 50%	Dermatographism, angioedema, rashes, pruritus
GI	> 40%	Diarrhea, nausea, abdominal cramps
Immunologic	≅ 40%	Elevated immunoglobulins (especially IgE), circulating immune complexes with serum sickness

Prognosis and Treatment

Hypereosinophilic syndrome used to have a poor prognosis, with death usually resulting from organ dysfunction. Current therapy has improved prognosis.

Treatment is not needed unless organ system dysfunction occurs; otherwise, the patient is evaluated q 3 to 6 mo. All therapy is designed to reduce the eosinophil count on the premise that disease manifestations result from tissue infiltration by eosinophils or the release of their contents. Focal organ system complications may need specific aggressive treatment (eg, valvular heart disease may mandate valve replacement).

Initial therapy is prednisone 1 mg/kg po once/day until clinical improvement and a normal eosinophil count are achieved; an adequate trial of prednisone should last ≥ 2 mo. If remission occurs, the dose is tapered slowly over the next 2 mo to 0.5 mg/kg once/day and then switched to 1 mg/kg once every other day. Further tapering should be done slowly to the lowest dosage that controls the disease. If ≥ 2 mo of prednisone is ineffective, if higher doses of prednisone are required, or if the dose cannot be tapered without inducing exacerbation, then hydroxyurea 0.5 to 1.5 g po once/day is added; an eosinophil count of 4,000 to 10,000/μL is the therapeutic goal.

Interferon-α is also used for patients in whom prednisone is ineffective, particularly for those with cardiac lesions. The dose is 3 to 5 million units sc 3 times/wk, depending on clinical efficacy and tolerance to adverse effects. Stopping interferon-α may exacerbate the disease.

Imatinib, an oral protein kinase inhibitor, is promising; it has been shown to normalize eosinophil counts for 3 mo in 9 of 11 patients treated.

Drug therapy and surgery may be required for cardiac manifestations (eg, infiltrative cardiomyopathy, valvular lesions, heart failure). Thrombotic complications may require the use of antiplatelet drugs (eg, aspirin, clopidogrel, ticlopidine); anticoagulation is indicated if a left ventricular mural thrombus is present or if transient ischemic attacks persist despite use of aspirin.

140 HISTIOCYTIC SYNDROMES

The histiocytic syndromes are clinically heterogeneous disorders that result from an abnormal proliferation of histiocytes—either monocyte-macrophages (antigen-processing cells) or dendritic cells (antigen-presenting cells). Classifying these disorders is difficult and has changed over time as an understanding of the biology of these cells has evolved (see TABLE 140–1 for the current classification system). Langerhans' cell histiocytosis, a dendritic cell disorder, is discussed below. Other histiocytic syndromes are described in TABLE 140–1.

LANGERHANS' CELL HISTIOCYTOSIS

(Langerhans' Cell Granulomatosis; Histiocytosis X)

(See also p. 461.)

Langerhans' cell histiocytosis is a proliferation of dendritic mononuclear cells with infiltration into organs locally or diffusely. Most cases occur in children. Manifestations may include lung infiltrates, bone lesions, skin rashes, and hepatic, hematopoietic, and endocrine dysfunction. Diagnosis is based on biopsy. Factors predicting a poor prognosis include age < 2 yr and dissemination, particularly involving the hematopoietic system, liver, and/or lungs. Treatments include supportive measures and chemotherapy or local treatment with surgery or radiation therapy as indicated by the extent of disease.

Langerhans' cell histiocytosis (LCH) is a dendritic cell disorder. It can produce distinct clinical syndromes that have been historically described as eosinophilic granuloma, Hand-Schüller-Christian disease, and Letterer-Siwe disease. Because these syndromes may be varied manifestations of the same underlying disease, and because most patients with LCH have manifestations of more than one of these syndromes, the designations of the separate syndromes are now mostly of historical significance.

The prevalence of LCH is estimated to be 1:50,000, of whom most are infants and young children, although children up to age 15 are often affected. However, the disease also affects adults, even older adults, with a male predominance.

In LCH, abnormally proliferating dendritic cells infiltrate one or more organs. Bone, skin, teeth, gingival tissue, ear, endocrine organs, lungs, liver, spleen, lymph nodes, and bone marrow may be involved. Organs may be affected by infiltration, causing dysfunction, or by compression from adjacent enlarged structures. In about half of patients, multiple organs are involved.

Symptoms and Signs

Symptoms and signs vary considerably depending on which organs are infiltrated. The syndromes are described by their historical designation, but few patients present with classic manifestations.

Eosinophilic granuloma: Solitary or multifocal eosinophilic granuloma (60 to 80% of LCH cases) occurs predominantly in older children and young adults, usually by age 30; incidence peaks between ages 5 and 10 yr. Lesions most frequently involve bone, often with pain and/or the inability to bear weight and with overlying tender (sometimes warm) swelling.

Hand-Schüller-Christian disease: This syndrome (15 to 40% of LCH cases) occurs in children aged 2 to 5 yr and in some older children and adults. It is a systemic disease that classically involves the flat bones of the skull, ribs, pelvis, and scapula. Long bones and lumbosacral vertebrae are less frequently involved; the wrists, hands, knees, feet, and cervical vertebrae are rarely involved. In classic cases, patients have exophthalmos caused by orbital tumor mass. Vision loss or strabismus caused by optic nerve or orbital muscle involvement occurs rarely. Tooth loss caused by apical and gingival infiltration is common in older patients.

Chronic otitis media and otitis externa due to involvement of the mastoid and petrous portions of the temporal bone with partial obstruction of the auditory canal are fairly common. Diabetes insipidus, the last component of the classic triad that includes flat bone involvement and exophthalmus, affects 5 to 50% of patients, with higher percentages in children who have systemic disease and involvement of the orbit and skull. Up to 40% of children with systemic disease have short stature. Hyperprolactinemia and hypogonadism may be caused by hypothalamic infiltration. Many other rare symptoms are possible.

Letterer-Siwe disease: This syndrome (10% of LCH cases), a systemic disease, is the most severe form of LCH. Typically, a child < 2 yr presents with a scaly seborrheic, eczematoid, sometimes purpuric rash involving the scalp, ear canals, abdomen, and intertriginous areas of the neck and face. Denuded skin may facilitate microbial invasion, leading to sepsis. Frequently, there is ear drainage,

TABLE 140–1. THE HISTIOCYTIC SYNDROMES

CATEGORY	DISORDERS
Disorders of varied biologic behavior	
Dendritic cell-related	Langerhans' cell histiocytosis (histiocytosis X)
	Eosinophilic granuloma
	Letterer-Siwe disease
	Hand-Schüller-Christian disease
	Other rare disorders
Macrophage-related	Hemophagocytic syndromes
	Primary hemophagocytic syndromes
	Familial
	Sporadic
	Secondary hemophagocytic syndromes
	Infection, malignancy, etc.
	Sinus histiocytosis with massive lymphadenopathy
	Other rare disorders
Malignant disorders	
	Leukemias
	Acute monocytic and myelomonocytic leukemia
	Chronic myelomonocytic leukemia (CMML)
	Adult CMML
	Childhood JMML (juvenile myelomonocytic leukemia)
	Other rare disorders

Adapted from Komp DM, Perry MC: "Introduction: The histiocytic syndromes." *Seminars in Oncology* 18:1, 1991 and Favara BE, Feller AC, Pauli M, eds.: "Contemporary classification of histiocytic disorders." *Med Pediatr Oncol* 29:157, 1997.

lymphadenopathy, hepatosplenomegaly, and, in severe cases, hepatic dysfunction with hypoproteinemia and diminished synthesis of clotting factors. Anorexia, irritability, failure to thrive, and pulmonary symptoms (eg, cough, tachypnea, pneumothorax) may also occur. Significant anemia and sometimes neutropenia occur; thrombocytopenia is of grave prognostic significance. Parents frequently report precocious eruption of teeth, when in fact the gums are receding to expose immature dentition. Patients may appear abused or neglected.

Diagnosis

LCH is suspected in patients (particularly young patients) with unexplained pulmonary infiltrates, bone lesions, or ocular or craniofacial abnormalities; and in children < 2 yr with typical rashes or severe, unexplained multiorgan disease.

Radiographs are often obtained because of presenting symptoms. Bone lesions are usually sharply marginated and round or oval, with a beveled edge giving the appearance of depth. Some lesions, however, are radiographically indistinguishable from Ewing's sarcoma, osteogenic sarcoma, other benign and malignant conditions, or osteomyelitis.

Diagnosis is based on biopsy. Langerhans' cells are usually prominent, except in older lesions. These cells are identified by a pathologist experienced in the diagnosis of LCH according to their immunohistochemical charecteristics, which include cell surface CD 1a and S-100. Once diagnosis is established, the extent of disease must be determined by appropriate imaging and laboratory studies.

Prognosis and Treatment

Disease restricted to skin, lymph nodes, or bone in patients > 2 yr has a good prognosis. Significant morbidity and mortality occur in young patients with multiorgan involvement. Disease risk is stratified in patients with multiorgan involvement. About 25% are classified as low risk. Low-risk criteria are age > 2 yr and no involvement of the hematopoietic system, liver, lungs, or spleen; at-risk criteria are age < 2 yr or involvement of these organs. The overall survival rate for multiorgan disease with treatment is about 80%. Mortality is virtually absent in low-risk patients and is most likely in at-risk patients who do not respond to initial therapy. Disease recurrence is common. A chronic remitting and exacerbating course may occur, particularly in adult patients.

Whenever possible, patients are referred to institutions experienced in the treatment of LCH. General supportive care is essential and may include scrupulous hygiene to limit ear, cutaneous, and dental lesions. Debridement and even resection of severely affected gingival tissue limit oral involvement. Seborrhea-like dermatitis of the scalp may diminish with use of a selenium-based shampoo twice/wk. If shampooing is ineffective, topical corticosteroids are used in small amounts and briefly in small areas.

Many patients require hormone replacement for diabetes insipidus or other manifestations of hypopituitarism. Patients with systemic disease are monitored for potential chronic disabilities, such as cosmetic or functional orthopedic and cutaneous disorders and neurotoxicity as well as for psychologic problems that may require psychosocial support.

Chemotherapy is indicated for patients with multiorgan involvement. Protocols sponsored by the Histiocyte Society are used; these vary according to the risk category. Almost all patients with a good response to therapy can stop treatment. Protocols for poor responders are under study.

Local surgery or radiation therapy is used for disease involving a single bone and, rarely, when multiple lesions or multiple bones are involved. Easily accessible lesions in noncritical locations undergo surgical curettage. Surgery should be avoided when it may result in significant cosmetic and/or orthopedic deformities and loss of function. Radiation therapy involving megavoltage equipment may be given to patients at risk of skeletal deformity, visual loss secondary to exophthalmos, pathologic fractures, vertebral collapse, and spinal cord injury or to patients with severe pain. Doses of radiation are considerably less than those used to treat cancer. Surgery and radiation therapy should be performed by specialists experienced in treating LCH.

Patients with multiorgan disease that progresses despite standard therapy usually respond to more aggressive chemotherapy. Patients who do not respond to salvage chemotherapy may undergo bone marrow transplantation, experimental chemotherapy, or immunosuppressive or other immunomodulatory therapy.

141 MYELOPROLIFERATIVE DISORDERS

The myeloproliferative disorders are characterized by abnormal proliferation of one or more hematopoietic cell lines or connective tissue elements. They include essential thrombocythemia, myelofibrosis, polycythemia vera, and chronic myelocytic leukemia (see p. 1113). Some hematologists also include acute leukemia, especially erythroleukemia, and paroxysmal nocturnal hemoglobinuria; however, most argue that these disorders are sufficiently different and omit them.

Each disorder is identified according to its predominant feature or site of proliferation (see TABLE 141–1). Despite overlap, each has a somewhat typical constellation of clinical features, laboratory findings, and course. Although proliferation of one cell line may dominate the clinical picture, each disorder is typically caused by clonal proliferation of a pluripotent stem cell, causing varying degrees of abnormal proliferation of RBC, WBC, and platelet precursors in the bone marrow. This abnormal clone does not, however, produce bone marrow fibroblasts. Myeloproliferative disorders, particularly chronic myelocytic leukemia, sometimes lead to acute leukemia. Recently, an abnormality of a tyrosine kinase called JAK2, involved in the marrow response to erythropoietin, has been described as contributing to the cause of polycythemia vera, essential thrombocythemia, and myelofibrosis.

TABLE 141–1. CLASSIFICATION OF MYELOPROLIFERATIVE DISORDERS

DISORDER	PREDOMINANT FEATURE
Polycythemia vera	Erythrocytosis
Myelofibrosis (or myelosclerosis) with myeloid metaplasia	Marrow fibrosis with extramedullary hematopoiesis
Essential thrombocythemia	Thrombocytosis
Chronic myelocytic leukemia	Granulocytosis

ESSENTIAL THROMBOCYTHEMIA

(Essential Thrombocytosis; Primary Thrombocythemia)

Essential thrombocythemia is characterized by an increased platelet count, megakaryocytic hyperplasia, and a hemorrhagic or thrombotic tendency. Symptoms and signs may include weakness, headaches, paresthesias, bleeding, splenomegaly, and digital ischemia. Diagnosis is based on a platelet count > 500,000/µL, normal RBC mass or normal Hct in the presence of adequate iron stores, and absence of myelofibrosis, the Philadelphia chromosome (or *ABL-BCR* rearrangement) and any other disorder that could cause thrombocytosis. Treatment is controversial but may include aspirin 81 mg/day po. Patients > 60 yr and those with multiple comorbidities require cytotoxic drugs to lower platelet counts.

Etiology and Pathophysiology

Essential thrombocythemia (ET) is a typically clonal abnormality of a multipotent hematopoietic stem cell. However, some women who fulfill diagnostic criteria for ET have polyclonal hematopoiesis. ET usually occurs between ages 50 and 70 yr.

Platelet production is increased. Platelet survival is usually normal, although it may decrease due to splenic sequestration. In elderly patients with atherosclerosis, increased platelets may lead to serious bleeding or, more commonly, thrombosis. Bleeding is more likely with extreme thrombocytosis, ie, > 1.5 million platelets/µL, due to an acquired von Willebrand's deficiency.

Symptoms, Signs, and Diagnosis

The most common symptoms are weakness, hemorrhage, nonspecific headache, and paresthesias of the hands and feet. Bleeding is usually mild and manifests as epistaxis, easy bruisability, or GI bleeding. Digital ischemia may occur, and splenomegaly (usually not extending > 3 cm below the left costal margin) occurs in 60% of patients. Hepatomegaly may also occur. In pregnant patients, thrombosis may cause recurrent spontaneous abortions.

Although symptoms are common, the course of the disease is generally benign. Serious complications are rare but can be life-threatening.

ET should be considered in patients with splenomegaly and in those who have symptoms and signs of a myeloproliferative disorder, elevated platelet counts, or abnormal platelet morphologies. If the disease is suspected, CBC, peripheral smear, bone marrow examination, and cytogenetics, including Philadelphia chromosome or *ABL-BCR* assay, should be obtained. The platelet count can be > 1,000,000/μL but may be as low as 500,000/μL. Platelet counts often decrease spontaneously during pregnancy. The peripheral smear may show platelet aggregates, giant platelets, and megakaryocyte fragments. The bone marrow shows megakaryocytic hyperplasia, with an abundance of platelets being released. Marrow iron is present. To distinguish from other myeloproliferative disorders that produce thrombocytosis, the diagnosis of ET requires a normal Hct, MCV, and iron studies; absence of the Philadelphia chromosome and *ABL-BCR* translocation (present in chronic myelocytic leukemia); and absence of teardrop-shaped RBCs and significant increase in bone marrow fibrosis (present in idiopathic myelofibrosis). Diagnosis also requires exclusion of any clinically suspected disorders that can cause secondary thrombocytosis (see TABLE 141–2).

TABLE 141–2. CAUSES OF THROMBOCYTOSIS

Chronic inflammatory disorders: RA, inflammatory bowel disease, TB, sarcoidosis, Wegener's granulomatosis
Acute infection
Hemorrhage
Iron deficiency
Hemolysis
Tumors: Cancer, Hodgkin lymphoma (Hodgkin's disease), non-Hodgkin lymphoma
Surgery: Splenectomy
Myeloproliferative and hematologic disorders: Polycythemia vera, chronic myelocytic leukemia, sideroblastic anemia, myelodysplasia (5q- syndrome), idiopathic myelodysplasia

Prognosis and Treatment

Life expectancy is near normal. Leukemic transformation occurs in < 2% of patients but may increase after exposure to cytotoxic therapy, especially alkylating agents.

Indications for therapy are controversial. For mild vasomotor symptoms (eg, headache, mild digital ischemia, erythromelalgia) and to decrease the risk of thrombosis in low-risk patients, aspirin 81 mg po once/day may be sufficient. Because the prognosis is often good, potentially toxic therapies that lower the platelet count should be used sparingly. Patients with significant bleeding need therapy to lower the platelet count. Patients > 60 yr with a previous thrombosis or with a comorbid condition that increases the risk of thrombosis should receive platelet-lowering drugs. Whether patients < 60 yr who are asymptomatic need platelet-lowering drugs needs to be studied. Most pregnant patients are given aspirin.

Myelosuppressive therapy to lower the platelet count usually consists of anagrelide, hydroxyurea, or interferon-α. The dosage and monitoring are described in the treatment of polycythemia vera (see below). The aim of therapy is a platelet count < 450,000/μL without significant clinical toxicity or suppression of other marrow elements. Because anagrelide and hydroxyurea cross the placenta, they are not used during pregnancy; interferon can be used in pregnant women.

For immediate reduction in the platelet count, plateletpheresis has been used (eg, in serious hemorrhage or thrombosis; before an emergency operation); this procedure, however, is rarely necessary. Due to the long half-life of platelets (7 days), hydroxyurea and anagrelide do not provide an immediate effect.

THROMBOCYTOSIS

(Secondary Thrombocythemia)

Thrombocytosis can develop secondary to chronic inflammatory disorders, acute infection, hemorrhage, iron deficiency, hemolysis, or tumors (see TABLE 141–2). Platelet function is usually normal. However, in myeloproliferative disorders, abnormalities of platelet aggregation occur in about 50% of patients. Unlike ET, thrombocytosis does not increase the risk of thrombotic or hemorrhagic complications unless patients have severe arterial disease or prolonged immobility. With secondary thrombocytosis, the platelet count is usually < 1,000,000/μL, and the cause may be obvious from the history, physical examination, or radiologic or blood testing. Treatment of the underlying disorder usually returns the platelet count to normal.

MYELOFIBROSIS

(Agnogenic Myeloid Metaplasia; Myelofibrosis with Myeloid Metaplasia)

Myelofibrosis is a chronic, usually idiopathic disease characterized by bone marrow fibrosis, splenomegaly, and anemia with immature and teardrop-shaped RBCs. Diagnosis requires bone marrow examination and exclusion of other conditions that can cause secondary myelofibrosis. Treatment is usually supportive.

Etiology and Pathophysiology

Myelofibrosis is excessive marrow fibrosis and loss of hematopoietic cells, with subsequent marked increase in extramedullary hematopoiesis (primarily in the liver and spleen, which enlarge significantly). It is usually a primary disorder probably resulting from neoplastic transformation of multipotent marrow stem cells; these stem cells stimulate the marrow fibroblast (which is not part of the neoplastic transformation), to secrete excessive collagen. Myelofibrosis also may occur secondary to a number of hematologic, malignant, or infectious conditions (see TABLE 141–3). Myelofibrosis may complicate chronic myelocytic leukemia and occurs in 15 to 30% of patients with polycythemia vera if they survive long enough. Large numbers of immature RBCs and granulocytes are released into the circulation (leukoerythroblastosis); they may release excess LDH into the bloodstream. Marrow failure eventually occurs, with consequent anemia and thrombocytopenia. Malignant or acute myelofibrosis, an unusual variant, has a more rapidly progressive downhill course; this may actually be a true megakaryocytic leukemia.

The peak incidence of idiopathic myelofibrosis is between 50 and 70 yr.

Symptoms, Signs, and Diagnosis

Early stages may be asymptomatic. Splenomegaly, or, in later stages, general malaise, weight loss, fever, or splenic infarction, may occur. Hepatomegaly occurs in 50% of patients. Lymphadenopathy may occur but is not typical. Rapidly progressive acute leukemia develops in about 10% of patients.

TABLE 141–3. CONDITIONS ASSOCIATED WITH MYELOFIBROSIS

CONDITION	EXAMPLES
Malignant diseases	Leukemias, polycythemia vera, multiple myeloma, Hodgkin lymphoma (Hodgkin's disease), non-Hodgkin lymphoma, cancer with marrow metastases
Infections	TB, osteomyelitis
Toxins	X- or γ-radiation, benzene, thorium dioxide
Autoimmune disorders (rarely)	SLE

Idiopathic myelofibrosis should be suspected in patients with splenomegaly, splenic infarction, anemia, or unexplained elevations in LDH. If the disease is suspected, CBC should be obtained and peripheral blood morphology and bone marrow should be examined, including cytogenetic testing. Other disorders associated with myelofibrosis (eg, chronic infections, granulomatous disorders, metastatic cancer, hairy cell leukemia, autoimmune disorders) should be excluded, usually by bone marrow examination when clinical suspicion and laboratory evaluation warrant it.

Blood cell morphology is variable. Anemia is usual and generally increases over time. RBCs are normochromic-normocytic with mild poikilocytosis, reticulocytosis, and polychromatophilia. Nucleated RBCs may be in peripheral blood. In advanced cases, RBCs are severely misshapen and teardrop-shaped; this appearance is sufficiently abnormal to suggest the diagnosis.

WBC counts are usually increased but are highly variable. Neutrophils are usually immature, and myeloblasts may be present, even in the absence of acute leukemia. Platelet counts initially may be high, normal, or decreased; however, thrombocytopenia tends to supervene as the disease progresses. Levels of progenitor cells in the peripheral blood, as measured by $CD34^+$ enumeration, may increase.

Bone marrow aspiration is usually dry. Because demonstration of marrow fibrosis is required and fibrosis may not be uniformly distributed, biopsy should be repeated at a different site if the first biopsy is nondiagnostic.

Prognosis and Treatment

The median survival is 5 yr from onset, although initial diagnosis may be delayed. Constitutional symptoms, anemia, or some cytogenetic abnormalities suggest a poor prognosis; with anemia and some cytogenetic abnormalities, median survival is as low as 2 yr. No treatment reverses or controls the underlying process. Instead, therapy is directed at symptoms and complications.

Androgens, splenectomy, chemotherapy, and splenic radiation therapy have sometimes been used for palliation. For patients with low erythropoietin (EPO) levels relative to the degree of anemia, EPO 40,000 units sc once/wk may increase Hct sufficiently; otherwise, RBC transfusion may be necessary. For younger patients with advanced disease, allogeneic marrow transplantation should be considered.

POLYCYTHEMIA VERA

(Primary Polycythemia)

Polycythemia vera is an idiopathic chronic myeloproliferative disorder characterized by an increase in RBC mass (erythrocytosis), which increases Hct and blood viscosity and may lead to thrombosis. Hepatosplenomegaly may also occur. Diagnosis may require measurement of RBC mass and exclusion of other causes of erythrocytosis. Treatment involves serial phlebotomies and sometimes myelosuppressive drugs.

Polycythemia vera (PV) is the most common of the myeloproliferative disorders; it occurs in about 5/1,000,000 people, more often in males (about 1.4:1). The mean age at diagnosis is 60 yr (range, 15 to 90 yr; rarely in childhood); 5% of patients are < 40 yr at onset.

Pathophysiology

PV involves increased production of all cell lines, including RBCs, WBCs, and platelets. Increased production confined to the RBC line is termed primary erythrocytosis. In PV, RBC production proceeds independently of erythropoietin (EPO). Extramedullary hematopoiesis occurs in the spleen, liver, and other sites with the potential for blood cell formation. Peripheral blood cell turnover increases. Eventually, about 25% of patients have reduced RBC survival and inadequate erythropoiesis. Anemia, thrombocytopenia, and myelofibrosis may develop, and RBC and WBC precursors are released into the circulation. Depending on treatment received, the incidence of transformation to acute leukemia varies between 1.5% and 10%.

In PV, blood volume expands and hyperviscosity develops, predisposing to thrombosis. Platelets function abnormally, predisposing to increased bleeding. Patients may become hypermetabolic. Increased cell turnover produces hyperuricemia.

Symptoms and Signs

PV itself is often asymptomatic. Occasionally, increased blood volume and viscosity produce weakness, headache, light-headedness, visual disturbances, fatigue, and dyspnea. Pruritus often occurs, particularly after a hot bath. The face may be red and the retinal veins engorged. The lower extremities may be red, warm, and painful, sometimes with digital ischemia (erythromelalgia). Hepatomegaly is common, and > 75% of patients have splenomegaly (which may be massive).

Thrombosis can occur in most vessels, resulting in stroke, transient ischemic attack, deep venous thrombosis, MI, retinal artery or vein occlusion, splenic infarction (often with a friction rub), or Budd-Chiari syndrome.

Bleeding (typically GI) occurs in 10 to 20% of patients.

Complications of hyperuricemia (eg, gout, renal calculi) tend to occur later in PV. Hypermetabolism can cause low-grade fevers and weight loss.

Diagnosis

PV must be considered in patients with suggestive symptoms, particularly Budd-Chiari syndrome, but is often first suspected because of an abnormal CBC (eg, Hct > 54% in men or > 49% in women). Neutrophils and platelets may be increased and morphologically abnormal. Because PV is a panmyelosis, its diagnosis is clear in patients with elevations of all 3 peripheral blood components, splenomegaly, and no cause for a secondary erythrocytosis. However, these findings are not uniformly present. With myelofibrosis, anemia and thrombocytopenia may develop, with massive splenomegaly. Additional findings include peripheral WBC and RBC precursors, marked anisocytosis and poikilocytosis, and microcytes, elliptocytes, and teardrop-shaped cells (see Table 141–4). Bone marrow examination is generally performed, showing

TABLE 141–4. CRITERIA FOR DIAGNOSIS OF POLYCYTHEMIA VERA

Erythrocytosis, absence of secondary polycythemia, and characteristic bone marrow changes (panmyelosis, enlarged megakaryocytes with clumping)

Plus

Any of the following:

- Splenomegaly
- Plasma erythropoietin level < 4 mUnits/mL
- Platelet count > 400,000 µL
- Positive endogenous colonies
- In the absence of infection, neutrophil count > 10,000/µL
- A clonal cytogenetic abnormality in the marrow

panmyelosis, large and clumped megakaryocytes, and sometimes reticulin fibers. Cytogenetic analysis of bone marrow occasionally demonstrates an abnormal clone specific for a myeloproliferative syndrome.

Because the Hct is the ratio of RBCs per unit volume of whole blood, an elevated Hct may be caused by decreased plasma volume (relative or spurious erythrocytosis, also called stress polycythemia or Gaisböck's syndrome). Measurement of RBC mass has been suggested to be an early test and helps differentiate PV from an elevated Hct due to hypovolemia. Also, in PV, plasma volume may increase, particularly if splenomegaly is present, making the Hct falsely normal despite erythrocytosis. Thus, a diagnosis of true erythrocytosis requires demonstration of an increased RBC mass. When measured with radioactive chromium (^{51}Cr)-labeled RBCs, RBC mass > 36 mL/kg in men (normal, 28.3 ± 2.8 mL/kg) and > 32 mL/kg in women (normal, 25.4 ± 2.6 mL/kg) is considered abnormal. Unfortunately, many laboratories do not perform blood volume studies.

The cause of erythrocytosis (of which there are many—see TABLE 141–5) must be sought. Secondary erythrocytosis (see p. 1105), caused by hypoxia (arterial Hb O_2 concentration < 92%); smokers' polycythemia, caused by elevated carboxyhemoglobin levels; and tumors producing erythropoietic substances are more common. Tests obtained should include arterial O_2 saturation, serum EPO levels, and P_{50} (the partial pressure of O_2 at which Hb becomes 50% saturated). P_{50} measures the affinity of Hb for O_2 and excludes a high-affinity Hb (a familial abnormality) as the cause of erythrocytosis. An alternative, but controversial, diagnostic approach is to assess causes of erythrocytosis before measuring RBC mass; if Hct is > 53% in a man or > 46% in a woman in the absence of a secondary cause for erythrocytosis, then PV is > 99% likely.

Patients with PV typically have low or low-normal serum EPO levels; those with hypoxia-induced erythrocytosis have elevated levels; and those with tumor-associated erythrocytosis have normal or elevated levels. Patients with elevated EPO levels or microscopic hematuria should undergo CT studies to seek a renal lesion or other tumor sources of EPO causing secondary erythrocytosis. Bone marrow from patients with PV, unlike that from healthy people, can form RBCs in culture without the addition of EPO (ie, positive endogenous colonies—see TABLE 141–4).

Other laboratory abnormalities may occur in PV, but most of these tests are not needed: vitamin B_{12} and B_{12}-binding capacity are frequently elevated but are not cost-effective to perform. Bone marrow biopsy is not usually necessary; if obtained, it shows hyperplasia of all cell line precursors, clumping of megakaryocytes, depletion of iron stores (best assessed in bone marrow aspirate examination), and increased reticulin. Hyperuricemia and hyperuricosuria occur in ≥ 30% of

TABLE 141–5. CAUSES OF ERYTHROCYTOSIS

TYPE	CAUSE
Primary	Polycythemia vera
Secondary	Decreased tissue oxygenation: lung disease, high altitude, intracardiac shunts, hypoventilation syndromes, abnormal Hb, smoking-induced carboxyhemoglobinemia Aberrant erythropoietin production: tumors, cysts
Relative (spurious, or Gaisböck's syndrome)	Hemoconcentration: diuretics, burns, diarrhea, stress

patients. Newer diagnostic tests recently described include increased expression of *PRV-1* gene in leukocytes and decreased expression of C-Mpl (the receptor for thrombopoietin) in megakaryocytes and platelets.

Prognosis

Without treatment, 50% of symptomatic patients die within 18 mo of diagnosis. With treatment, median survival is > 10 yr, and young patients may live many decades. Thrombosis is the most common cause of death, followed by complications of myeloid metaplasia and development of leukemia.

Treatment

Because PV is the only form of erythrocytosis for which myelosuppressive therapy may be indicated, accurate diagnosis is critical. Therapy must be individualized according to age, sex, medical status, clinical manifestations, and hematologic findings.

Phlebotomy: Phlebotomy decreases the risk of thrombosis, ameliorates symptoms, and may be the only treatment needed. It is the treatment of choice for women of childbearing age and patients < 40 yr because it is not mutagenic. Common thresholds for phlebotomy are Hct > 45% in men and > 42% in women. Initially, 300 to 500 mL of blood should be removed every other day. Less is removed (ie, 200 to 300 mL twice/wk) in elderly patients and in those with cardiac or cerebrovascular disease. Once the Hct is below the threshold value, it is rechecked monthly and maintained at this level by additional phlebotomies as needed. Elective surgery should be preceded by phlebotomy to reduce the RBC volume to normal. If necessary, intravascular volume can be maintained with crystalloid or colloid solutions.

Aspirin (81 to 100 mg po once/day) reduces the incidence of thrombotic complications. Thus, patients undergoing phlebotomy alone or phlebotomy and myelosuppression should be given aspirin unless contraindicated.

Myelosuppressive therapy: Myelosuppressive therapy may be indicated for patients with platelet counts $> 1 \times 10^6/\mu L$, with discomfort from visceral enlargement, with thrombosis despite Hct < 45, and with symptoms caused by hypermetabolism or uncontrolled pruritus as well as for patients > 60 or those with cardiovascular disease who do not tolerate phlebotomy well.

Radioactive phosphorus (^{32}P) has a success rate of 80 to 90%. Remission may last 6 mo to several years. ^{32}P is well tolerated and requires fewer follow-up visits when the disease is controlled. However, ^{32}P is associated with an increased incidence of acute leukemic transformation, and the leukemia that develops after this therapy is often resistant to induction chemotherapy. Thus, ^{32}P requires careful patient selection (eg, used only for patients who are expected to die of other disorders within 5 yr).

Hydroxyurea, which inhibits the enzyme ribonucleoside diphosphate reductase, has long been used to achieve myelosuppression; its leukemogenic potential continues to be studied. Patients are phlebotomized to an Hct < 45% and given hydroxyurea 20 to 30 mg/kg po once/day. The patient is monitored with a weekly CBC. When a steady state is achieved, the interval between CBCs is lengthened to 2 wk and then 4 wk. If the WBC count falls to < 4000/μL or the platelet count to < 100,000/μL, hydroxyurea is withheld and reinstituted at 50% of the dose when those values normalize. For poorly controlled patients who require frequent phlebotomies or who are thrombocythemic (platelet counts > 600,000/μL), the dosage can be increased monthly by 5 mg/kg. Acute toxicity is infrequent, but occasionally, patients develop a rash, GI symptoms, fever, and nail changes and skin ulcerations, which may require stopping hydroxyurea.

Interferon-α2b has been used if hydroxyurea does not control blood counts or cannot be tolerated. The typical starting dose is 3×10^6 units sc 3 times/wk.

Anagrelide is a new drug that affects megakaryocyte proliferation more specifically than do other drugs and is used to reduce platelet counts in patients with myeloproliferative disorders. Its long-term safety is under study, although it is not expected to contribute to leukemic conversion. It can cause vasodilation, producing headaches, palpitations, and fluid retention. To minimize these adverse effects, the initial dose is 0.5 mg po bid, increasing by 0.5 mg weekly, until the platelet count is < 450,000 or the dose is 5 mg po bid. The average dose required is 2 mg/day.

Most alkylating agents and, to a lesser extent, radioactive phosphate (both used previously for myelosuppression) are leukemogenic and should be avoided.

Treatment of complications: Hyperuricemia should be treated with allopurinol 300 mg po once/day if it causes symptoms or if the patient is receiving simultaneous myelosuppressive therapy. Pruritus may be managed with antihistamines but is often difficult to control; myelosuppression often is most effective. Cholestyramine 4 g po tid, cyproheptadine 4 mg po tid to qid, cimetidine 300 mg po qid, or paroxetine 20 to 40 mg po once/day may be successful. After bathing, the skin should be dried gently. Aspirin relieves symptoms of erythromelalgia. In PV, elective surgery should be postponed until the Hct is reduced to < 42% and platelets to < 600,000/μL.

SECONDARY ERYTHROCYTOSIS

(Secondary Polycythemia)

Secondary erythrocytosis is erythrocytosis that develops secondary to another factor.

Common causes of secondary erythrocytosis include smoking, chronic arterial hypoxemia, and tumor-associated erythrocytosis. Less common are high O_2-affinity hemoglobinopathies and other congenital causes.

In patients who smoke, reversible erythrocytosis may result mainly from tissue hypoxia due to elevation of blood carboxyhemoglobin concentration; levels often normalize with smoking cessation.

Patients with chronic hypoxemia (due to lung disease, right-to-left intracardiac shunts, prolonged exposure to high altitudes [see p. 2613], or hypoventilation syndromes) often develop erythrocytosis. The primary treatment is to alleviate the underlying condition, but O_2 therapy may help, and some degree of phlebotomy may decrease viscosity and alleviate symptoms.

High O_2-affinity hemoglobinopathies are very rare and are reported in certain geographic areas. This diagnosis is suggested by a family history of erythrocytosis; it is established by measuring the P_{50} (see p. 1103) and, if possible, determining the complete oxyhemoglobin dissociation curve. Standard Hb electrophoresis is usually normal and cannot reliably exclude this cause of erythrocytosis.

Tumor-associated erythrocytosis can occur when renal tumors, cysts, hepatomas, cerebellar hemangioblastomas, or uterine leiomyomas secrete EPO. Patients with erythrocytosis should have serum EPO measured and should undergo abdominal CT if serum EPO is normal or elevated. Removal of the lesion may be curative.

142 LEUKEMIAS

The leukemias are cancers of the WBCs involving bone marrow, circulating WBCs, and organs such as the spleen and lymph nodes.

Etiology and Pathophysiology

Malignant transformation usually occurs at the pluripotent stem cell level, although it sometimes involves a committed stem cell with more limited capacity for differentiation. Abnormal proliferation, clonal expansion, and diminished apoptosis (programmed cell death) lead to replacement of normal blood elements with malignant cells.

Risk of developing most leukemias increases with history of exposure to ionizing radiation (eg, post–atom bomb in Nagasaki and Hiroshima) or chemicals (eg, benzene); prior treatment with certain antineoplastic drugs, particularly procarbazine, nitrosureas (cyclophosphamide, melphalan), and epipodophyllotoxins (etoposide, teniposide); infection with viral agents (eg, human T-lymphotrophic virus 1 and 2, Epstein-Barr virus); chromosomal translocations; and preexisting conditions, including immunodeficiency disorders, chronic myeloproliferative disorders, and chromosomal disorders (eg, Fanconi's anemia, Bloom syndrome, ataxia-telangiectasia, Down syndrome, infantile X-linked agammaglobulinemia).

Manifestations of leukemia are due to suppression of normal blood cell formation and organ infiltration by leukemic cells. Inhibitory factors produced by leukemic cells and replacement of marrow space may suppress normal hematopoiesis, with ensuing anemia, thrombocytopenia, and granulocytopenia. Organ infiltration results in enlargement of the liver, spleen, and lymph nodes, with occasional kidney and gonadal involvement. Meningeal infiltration results in clinical features associated with increasing intracranial pressure (eg, cranial nerve palsies).

TABLE 142–1. FRENCH-AMERICAN-BRITISH CLASSIFICATION OF ACUTE LEUKEMIAS

LEUKEMIA AND FAB CLASSIFICATION	DESCRIPTION
Acute lymphocytic leukemia	
L1	Lymphoblasts with uniform, round nuclei and scant cytoplasm
L2	More variability of lymphoblasts; nuclei may be irregular with more cytoplasm than L1
L3	Lymphoblasts have finer nuclear chromatin and blue to deep blue cytoplasm with cytoplasmic vacuolization
Acute myelocytic leukemia	
M1	Undifferentiated myeloblastic; no cytoplasmic granulation
M2	Differentiated myeloblastic; few to many cells may have sparse granulation
M3	Promyelocytic; granulation typical of promyelocytic morphology
M4	Myelomonoblastic; mixed myeloblastic and monocytoid morphology
M5	Monoblastic; pure monoblastic morphology
M6	Erythroleukemic; predominantly immature erythroblastic morphology, sometimes megaloblastic appearance
M7	Megakaryoblastic; cells have shaggy borders that may show some budding

Classification

Leukemias were originally termed acute or chronic based on life expectancy but now are classified according to cellular maturity. Acute leukemias consist of predominantly immature, poorly differentiated cells (usually blast forms); chronic leukemias have more mature cells. Acute leukemias are divided into lymphocytic (ALL) and myelocytic (AML) types, which may be further subdivided by the French-American-British (FAB) classification (see TABLE 142–1). Chronic leukemias are described as lymphocytic (CLL) or myelocytic (CML—see TABLE 142–2).

Myelodysplastic syndromes involve progressive bone marrow failure but with an insufficient proportion of blast cells (<30%) for making a definite diagnosis of AML; 40 to 60% of cases evolve into AML.

A leukemoid reaction is marked granulocytic leukocytosis (ie, WBC > 30,000/µL) produced by normal bone marrow in response to systemic infection or cancer. Although not a neoplastic disorder, a leukemoid reaction with a very high WBC count may require testing to distinguish it from CML (see p. 1113).

ACUTE LEUKEMIA

Acute leukemia occurs when a hematopoietic stem cell undergoes malignant transformation into a primitive, undifferentiated cell with abnormal longevity. These lymphocytes (acute lymphocytic leukemia) or myeloid cells (acute myelocytic leukemia) proliferate abnormally, replacing normal marrow tissue and hematopoietic cells and inducing anemia, thrombocytopenia, and granulocytopenia. Because they are bloodborne, they can infiltrate various organs and sites, including the liver, spleen, lymph nodes, CNS, kidneys, and gonads.

Symptoms and Signs

Symptoms have usually been present for only days to weeks before diagnosis. Disrupted hematopoiesis leads to the most common presenting symptoms (anemia, infection, easy bruising and bleeding). Other presenting symptoms and signs are usually nonspecific (eg, pallor, fatigue, fever, malaise, weight loss, tachycardia, chest pain) and are attributable to anemia and a hypermetabolic state. The cause of fever often is not found, although granulocytopenia may lead to a rapidly progressing and potentially life-threatening bacterial infection. Bleeding is usually manifested by petechiae, easy bruising, epistaxis, bleeding gums, or menstrual irregularity. Hematuria and GI bleeding are uncommon. Bone marrow and periosteal infiltration may cause bone and joint pain, especially in children with ALL. Initial CNS involvement or leukemic meningitis (manifesting as headaches, vomiting, irritability, cranial nerve palsies, seizures, and papilledema) is uncommon. Extramedullary infiltration by leukemic cells may cause lymphadenopathy, splenomegaly, hepatomegaly, and leukemia cutis (a raised, nonpruritic skin rash).

Diagnosis

CBC and peripheral smear are the first tests performed; pancytopenia and peripheral blasts suggest acute leukemia. Blast cells in the blood smear may approach 90%, unless the WBC count is markedly decreased. Although the diagnosis can usually be made from the blood smear, bone marrow examination (aspiration or needle biopsy) should always be performed. Blast cells in the bone marrow are between 30 and 95%. Aplastic anemia, viral infections such as infectious mononucleosis, and vitamin B_{12} and folate deficiency should be considered in the differential diagnosis of severe pancytopenia, and leukemoid reactions to infectious disease (such as TB) can manifest as high blast counts.

Histochemical studies, cytogenetics, immunophenotyping, and molecular biology studies help distinguish the blasts of ALL from those of AML or other disease processes. Specific B-cell, T-cell, and myeloid-antigen monoclonal antibodies, together with flow cytometry, are very helpful in classifying ALL vs AML, which is critical for treatment.

Other laboratory findings may include hyperuricemia, hyperphosphatemia, hyperkalemia or hypokalemia, elevated serum hepatic transaminases or lactic dehydrogenase, hypoglycemia, and hypoxia. Lumbar puncture and head CT scan are performed in patients with CNS symptoms, B-cell ALL, high WBC count, or high LDH. Chest x-ray is performed; if a mediastinal mass is present, CT may be obtained. CT, MRI, or abdominal ultrasound may help assess splenomegaly or leukemia infiltration of other organs.

Prognosis and Treatment

Cure is a realistic goal for both ALL and AML, especially in younger patients. Prognosis is worse in infants and the elderly and in those with hepatic or renal dysfunction, CNS involvement, myelodysplasia, or a high WBC count (> 25,000/µL). Survival in untreated acute leukemia generally is 3 to 6 mo. Prognosis also varies according to karyotype.

The goal of treatment is complete remission, including resolution of abnormal clinical features, restoration of normal blood

TABLE 142–2. FINDINGS AT DIAGNOSIS IN THE MOST COMMON LEUKEMIAS

FEATURE	ACUTE LYMPHOCYTIC	ACUTE MYELOCYTIC	CHRONIC LYMPHOCYTIC	CHRONIC MYELOCYTIC
Peak age of incidence	Childhood	Any age	Middle and old age	Young adulthood
WBC concentration	H in 50% N or L in 50%	H in 60% N or L in 40%	H in 98% N or L in 2%	H in 100%
Differential WBC count	Many lymphoblasts	Many myeloblasts	Small lymphocytes	Entire myeloid series
Anemia	In > 90%, severe	In > 90%, severe	In about 50%, mild	In 80%, but mild
Platelets	L in > 80%	L in > 90%	L in 20 to 30%	H in 60% L in 10%
Lymphadenopathy	Commonly seen	Occasionally seen	Commonly seen	Infrequently seen
Splenomegaly	60%	50%	Usual and moderate	Usual and severe
Other features	CNS occurrence is common without prophylaxis	Rare CNS occurrence; Auer rods may be seen in myeloblasts	Occasional hemolytic anemia and hypogammaglobulinemia	Leukocyte alkaline phosphatase low; Philadelphia chromosome–positive in > 90%

H = high; N = normal; L = low.

counts and normal hematopoiesis with < 5% blast cells, and elimination of the leukemic clone. Although basic principles in treating ALL and AML are similar, the drug regimens differ (see pp. 1109 and 1110). The complex nature of a patient's clinical situation and the available treatment protocols necessitate an experienced team. Whenever possible, patients should be treated at specialized medical centers, particularly during critical phases (eg, remission induction).

Supportive care: Bleeding, usually the consequence of thrombocytopenia, generally responds to platelet administration. Prophylactic platelet transfusion is performed when platelets fall to < 10,000/µL; a higher threshold (20,000/µL) is used for patients with the triad of fever, disseminated intravascular coagulation, and mucositis secondary to chemotherapy. Anemia (Hb < 8 g/dL) is treated with packed RBC transfusions.

Infections are serious in the neutropenic, immunosuppressed patient and can progress quickly without the usual clinical evidence. After appropriate studies and cultures have been obtained, both febrile and afebrile patients with neutrophil counts < 500/µL should begin broad-spectrum bactericidal antibiotic treatment that includes coverage for gram-positive and gram-negative organisms (eg, ceftazidime, imipenem, and cilastatin). Fungal infections, especially pneumonias, are becoming more common and are difficult to diagnose; empiric antifungal drugs should be given if antibacterial therapy is not effective within 72 h. In patients with refractory pneumonitis, *Pneumocystis jiroveci* (formerly *P. carinii*) or a viral infection should be suspected and confirmed by bronchoscopy and bronchoalveolar lavage and treated appropriately; empiric therapy with trimethoprim-sulfamethoxazole (TMP-SMX), amphotericin, and acyclovir or other analogs, often with granulocyte transfusions, is often necessary. Granulocyte transfusions may help neutropenic patients with gram-negative or other serious sepsis but have no proven benefit as prophylaxis. In patients with drug-induced immunosuppression at risk of opportunistic infections, TMP-SMX could be given to prevent *P. jiroveci* pneumonia.

The rapid lysis of leukemic cells during initial therapy (particularly in ALL) can cause hyperuricemia, hyperphosphatemia, and hyperkalemia (tumor lysis syndrome—see p. 1170). These abnormalities can be prevented by increasing hydration (twice the daily maintenance volume), urine alkalinization (pH 7 to 8), and electrolyte monitoring. Hyperuricemia can be minimized by giving allopurinol (a xanthine oxidase inhibitor) or rasburicase (a recombinant urate-oxidase enzyme) before starting chemotherapy to reduce the conversion of xanthine to uric acid.

Psychologic support may help patients and their families weather the shock of illness and the rigors of treatment for a potentially life-threatening condition.

Acute Lymphocytic Leukemia

(Acute Lymphoblastic Leukemia)

ALL is the most common pediatric cancer; it also strikes adults of all ages. Malignant transformation and uncontrolled proliferation of an abnormally differentiated, long-lived hematopoietic progenitor cell results in a high circulating number of blasts, replacement of normal marrow by malignant cells, and the potential for leukemic infiltration of the CNS and abdominal organs. Symptoms include fatigue, pallor, infection, and easy bruising and bleeding. Examination of peripheral blood smear and bone marrow is usually diagnostic. Treatment typically includes combination chemotherapy to achieve remission, intrathecal chemotherapy for CNS prophylaxis and/or cerebral irradiation for intracerebral leukemic infiltration, consolidation chemotherapy with or without stem cell transplantation, and maintenance chemotherapy for 1 to 3 yr to avoid relapse.

Two thirds of all ALL cases occur in children, with a peak incidence at age 2 to 10 yr; ALL is the most common cancer in children and the 2nd most common cause of death in children < age 15. A 2nd rise in incidence occurs with aging after age 45.

Prognosis

Prognostic factors help determine treatment protocol and intensity. Favorable prognostic factors are age 3 to 7 yr; WBC count < 25,000/µL, FAB L1 morphology; leukemic cell karyotype with > 50 chromosomes and t(12;21); and no CNS disease at diagnosis. Unfavorable factors are a leukemic cell karyotype with chromosomes that are normal in number but abnormal in morphology (pseudodiploid) or the presence of the Philadelphia (Ph) chromosome t(9;22); increased age in adults; and a B-cell immunophenotype with surface or cytoplasmic immunoglobulin.

Regardless of risk factors, the likelihood of initial remission is ≥ 95% in children and 70 to 90% in adults. Of children, 3/4 have continuous disease-free survival for 5 yr and appear cured. Most investigatory protocols select patients with poor risk factors for more intense therapy, because the increased risk and toxicity from treatment are outweighed by the greater risk of treatment failure leading to death.

Treatment

The 4 general phases of treatment for ALL include remission induction, CNS prophylaxis, postremission consolidation or intensification, and maintenance.

Several regimens emphasize early introduction of an intensive multidrug regimen. Remission can be induced with daily oral prednisone and weekly IV vincristine with the addition of an anthracycline or asparaginase. Other drugs and combinations that may be introduced early in treatment are cytarabine and etoposide as well as cyclophosphamide. In some regimens, intermediate-dose or high-dose IV methotrexate is given with leucovorin rescue. The combinations and their dosages are modified according to the presence of risk factors. Allogeneic stem cell transplantation is recommended as consolidation of Ph chromosome–positive ALL or in 2nd or later relapses or remissions.

An important site of leukemic infiltration is the meninges; prophylaxis and treatment may include high-dose intrathecal methotrexate, cytosine arabinoside, and corticosteroids. Cranial nerve or whole-brain irradiation may be necessary and is often used for patients at high risk of CNS disease (eg, high WBC count, high serum LDH, B-cell phenotype) but has been used less often in recent years.

Most regimens include maintenance therapy with methotrexate and mercaptopurine. Therapy duration is usually 2 ½ to 3 yr but may be shorter with regimens that are more intensive in earlier phases and for B cell (L3) cases. For a patient in continuous complete remission for 2 ½ yr, the risk of relapse after therapy cessation is about 20%, usually within 1 yr. Thus, when therapy can be stopped, most patients are cured.

Relapse: Leukemic cells may reappear in the bone marrow, the CNS, or the testes. Bone marrow relapse is particularly ominous. Although a new round of chemotherapy may induce a 2nd remission in 80 to 90% of children (30 to 40% of adults), subsequent remissions tend to be brief. Only a few patients with late bone marrow relapses achieve long disease-free 2nd remissions or cure. If an HLA-matched sibling is available, stem cell transplantation offers the greatest hope of long-term remission or cure (see p. 1371).

When relapse involves the CNS, treatment includes intrathecal methotrexate (with or without cytarabine or corticosteroids) twice weekly until all signs disappear. Most regimens include systemic reinduction chemotherapy because of the likelihood of systemic spread of blast cells. The role of continued intrathecal drug use or CNS irradiation is unclear.

Testicular relapse may be evidenced clinically by painless firm swelling of the testis or may be identified on biopsy. If unilateral testicular involvement is clinically evident, the apparently uninvolved testis should undergo biopsy. Treatment is by irradiation of the involved testis and administration of systemic reinduction therapy as for isolated CNS relapse.

Acute Myelocytic Leukemia

(Acute Myelogenous Leukemia; Acute Myeloid Leukemia)

In AML, malignant transformation and uncontrolled proliferation of an abnormally differentiated, long-lived myeloid progenitor cell results in high circulating numbers of immature blood forms and replacement of normal marrow by malignant cells. Symptoms include fatigue, pallor, easy bruising and bleeding, fever, and infection; symptoms of leukemic infiltration are present in only about 5% of patients (often as skin manifestations). Examination of peripheral blood smear and bone marrow is diagnostic. Treatment includes induction chemotherapy to achieve remission and postremission chemotherapy (with or without stem cell transplantation) to avoid relapse.

The incidence of AML increases with aging; it is the more common acute leukemia in adults, with a median age of onset of 50 yr.

AML may occur as a secondary cancer after chemotherapy or irradiation for a different type of cancer.

AML has a number of subtypes that are distinguished from each other by morphology, immunophenotype, and cytochemistry. Five classes are described, based on predominant cell type, including myeloid, myeloid-monocytic, monocytic, erythroid, and megakaryocytic.

Acute promyelocytic leukemia is a particularly important subtype, representing 10 to 15% of all cases of AML, striking a younger age group (median age 31 yr) and particular ethnicity (Hispanics), in which the patient commonly presents with a coagulation disorder.

Prognosis and Treatment

Remission induction rates range from 50 to 85%. Long-term disease-free survival reportedly occurs in 20 to 40% of patients and increases to 40 to 50% in younger patients treated with stem cell transplantation.

Prognostic factors help determine treatment protocol and intensity; patients with strongly negative prognostic features are usually given more intense forms of therapy, because the potential benefits are thought to justify the increased treatment toxicity. The most important prognostic factor is the leukemia cell karyotype; unfavorable karyotypes include t(15;17), t(8;21), and inv16 (p13;q22). Other negative factors include increasing age, a preceding myelodysplastic phase, secondary leukemia, high WBC count, and absence of Auer rods. The FAB or WHO classification alone does not predict response.

Initial therapy attempts to induce remission and differs most from ALL in that AML responds to fewer drugs. The basic induction regimen includes cytarabine by continuous IV infusion or high doses for 5 to 7 days; daunorubicin or idarubicin is given IV for 3 days during this time. Some regimens include 6-thioguanine, etoposide, vincristine, and prednisone, but their contribution is unclear. Treatment usually results in significant myelosuppression, with infection or bleeding; there is significant latency before marrow recovery. During this time, meticulous preventive and supportive care is vital (see p. 1108).

In acute promyelocytic leukemia (APL) and some other cases of AML, disseminated intravascular coagulation (DIC) may be present on diagnosis and may worsen as leukemic cell lysis releases procoagulant. In APL with the translocation t(15;17), all-*trans*-retinoic acid corrects the DIC in 2 to 5 days; combined with daunorubicin or idarubicin, this regimen can induce remission in 80 to 90% of patients, and long-term survival in 65 to 70%. Arsenic trioxide is also very active in APL.

After remission, many regimens involve a phase of intensification with these or other drugs; high-dose cytarabine regimens may lengthen remission duration, particularly when given as intensification in patients < 60 yr. CNS prophylaxis usually is not given, because with better systemic disease control, CNS leukemia is a less frequent complication. Maintenance therapy has no demonstrated role in AML patients who have had intensification treatment but is somewhat useful in other situations. Extramedullary sites are infrequently involved in isolated relapse.

CHRONIC LEUKEMIA

Chronic leukemia usually presents as abnormal leukocytosis with or without cytopenia in an otherwise asymptomatic person. Findings and management differ significantly between chronic lymphocytic leukemia (CLL) and chronic myelocytic leukemia (CML).

CHRONIC LYMPHOCYTIC LEUKEMIA

(Chronic Lymphatic Leukemia)

The most common type of leukemia in the Western world, CLL involves mature-appearing defective neoplastic lymphocytes with an abnormally long life span. The peripheral blood, bone marrow, spleen, and lymph nodes undergo leukemic infiltration. Symptoms may be absent or may include lymphadenopathy, splenomegaly, hepatomegaly, and nonspecific symptoms attributable to anemia (fatigue, malaise). Diagnosis is by examination of peripheral blood smear and bone marrow aspirate. Treatment, delayed until symptoms develop, is aimed at lengthening life and decreasing symptoms and may involve chlorambucil or fludarabine, prednisone, cyclophosphamide, and/or doxorubicin. Monoclonal antibodies, such as alemtuzumab and rituximab, are increasingly being used. Palliative radiation therapy is reserved for patients whose lymphadenop-

athy or splenomegaly interferes with other organs.

Incidence of CLL increases with aging; 75% of cases are diagnosed in patients > 60 yr. CLL is twice as common in men. Although the cause is unknown, some cases are familial. CLL is rare in Japan and China and does not seem to increase among Japanese expatriates in the US, suggesting a genetic factor. CLL is more common among Jews of Eastern European descent.

Pathophysiology

In about 98% of cases, $CD5^+$ B cells undergo malignant transformation, with lymphocytes initially accumulating in the bone marrow and then spreading to lymph nodes and other lymphoid tissues, eventually inducing splenomegaly and hepatomegaly. As the disease progresses, abnormal hematopoiesis results in anemia, neutropenia, thrombocytopenia, and decreased immunoglobulin production. Many patients develop hypogammaglobulinemia and impaired antibody response, perhaps related to increased T-suppressor cell activity. Patients have increased susceptibility to autoimmune disease characterized by immunohemolytic anemias (usually Coombs' test–positive) or thrombocytopenia and a modest increase in risk of developing other cancers.

In 2 to 3% of cases, the clonal expansion is T cell in type, and even this group has a subtype (eg, large granular lymphocytes with cytopenias). In addition, other chronic leukemic patterns have been categorized under CLL: prolymphocytic leukemia, leukemic phase of cutaneous T-cell lymphoma (ie, Sézary syndrome), hairy cell leukemia, and lymphoma leukemia (ie, leukemic changes seen in advanced stages of malignant lymphoma). Differentiation of these subtypes from typical CLL is usually straightforward.

Symptoms and Signs

Onset is usually insidious; CLL is often diagnosed incidentally during routine blood tests or through evaluation of asymptomatic lymphadenopathy. The symptomatic patient usually has nonspecific complaints of fatigue, anorexia, weight loss, dyspnea on exertion, or a sense of abdominal fullness (secondary to an enlarged spleen). Initial findings include generalized lymphadenopathy and minimal-to-moderate hepatomegaly and splenomegaly. With progressive disease, there may be pallor due to anemia. Skin infiltration, either maculopapular or diffuse, may be a feature of T-cell CLL. Hypogammaglobulinemia and granulocytopenia in late CLL may predispose to bacterial, viral, and fungal infection, especially pneumonia. Herpes zoster is common and usually dermatomic.

Diagnosis

CLL is confirmed by examining the peripheral blood smear and bone marrow; the hallmark is sustained, absolute peripheral lymphocytosis (> 5000/µL) and increased lymphocytes (> 30%) in the bone marrow. Differential diagnosis is simplified by immunophenotyping. Other findings at diagnosis may include hypogammaglobulinemia (< 15% of cases) and, rarely, elevated LDH. Only 10% of cases present with moderate anemia (sometimes immunohemolytic) and/or thrombocytopenia. A monoclonal serum immunoglobulin spike of the same type may be found on the leukemic cell surface in 2 to 4% of cases.

Clinical staging is useful for prognosis and treatment. Two common approaches to staging are the Rai and the Binet, primarily based on hematologic changes and extent of disease (see TABLE 142–3).

Prognosis and Treatment

The median survival of patients with B-cell CLL or its complications is about 7 to 10 yr. A patient in stage 0 to II at diagnosis may survive for 5 to 20 yr without treatment. A patient in stage III or IV is more likely to die within 3 to 4 yr of diagnosis. Progression to bone marrow failure is usually associated with short survival. Patients with CLL are more likely to develop a secondary cancer, especially skin cancer.

Although CLL is progressive, some patients may be asymptomatic for years; therapy is not indicated until progression or symptoms occur. Cure usually is not possible, so treatment attempts to ameliorate symptoms and prolong life. Supportive care includes transfusion of packed RBCs or erythropoietin injections for anemia; platelet transfusions for bleeding associated with thrombocytopenia; and antimicrobials for bacterial, fungal, or viral infections. Because neutropenia and agammaglobulinemia limit bacterial killing, antibiotic therapy should be bactericidal. Therapeutic infusions of γ-globulin should be considered in the patient with hypogammaglobulinemia and repeated

TABLE 142–3. CLINICAL STAGING OF CHRONIC LYMPHOCYTIC LEUKEMIA

CLASSIFICATION AND STAGE	DESCRIPTION
Rai	
Stage 0	Absolute lymphocytosis of > 10,000/μL in blood and ≥ 30% lymphocytes in bone marrow (necessary for stages I–IV also)
Stage I	Plus enlarged lymph nodes
Stage II	Plus hepatomegaly or splenomegaly
Stage III	Plus anemia with Hb < 11 g/dL
Stage IV	Plus thrombocytopenia with platelet counts < 100,000/μL
Binet	
Stage A	Absolute lymphocytosis of > 10,000/μL in blood and ≥ 30% lymphocytes in bone marrow; Hb ≥ 10 g/dL, platelets > 100,000/μL, ≤ 2 involved sites*
Stage B	As for stage A, but 3–5 involved sites
Stage C	As for stage A or B, but Hb < 10 g/dL or platelets < 100,000/μL

*Sites considered: cervical, axillary, inguinal, hepatic, splenic, lymphatic.

or refractory infections or, for prophylaxis, when ≥ 2 severe infections occur within 6 mo.

Specific therapy includes chemotherapy, corticosteroids, monoclonal antibody therapy, and radiation therapy. These modalities may alleviate symptoms but have not been proven to prolong survival. *Overtreatment is more dangerous than undertreatment.*

Chemotherapy: Chemotherapy may be instituted in response to the advent of symptomatic disease, including constitutional symptoms (fever, night sweats, extreme fatigue, weight loss); significant hepatomegaly, splenomegaly, and/or lymphadenopathy; lymphocytosis exceeding 100,000/μL; and infections accompanied by anemia, neutropenia, and/or thrombocytopenia. Alkylating drugs, especially chlorambucil, alone or with corticosteroids, have long been the usual therapy for B-cell CLL. However, fludarabine is more effective. Remissions are longer than with other treatments, although survival advantage has not been demonstrated. Interferon-α, deoxycoformycin, and 2-chlorodeoxyadenosine have been highly effective for hairy cell leukemia. Patients with prolymphocytic leukemia and lymphoma leukemia usually require multidrug chemotherapy and often respond only partially.

Corticosteroid therapy: Immunohemolytic anemia and thrombocytopenia are indications for corticosteroid therapy. Prednisone 1 mg/kg po once/day may occasionally result in striking, rapid improvement in patients with advanced CLL, although response is often brief. The metabolic complications and increasing rate and severity of infections warrant caution in its prolonged use. Prednisone used with fludarabine increases the risk of *Pneumocystis jiroveci* (formerly *P. carinii*) and *Listeria* infections.

Monoclonal antibody therapy: Rituximab is the first monoclonal antibody used in the successful treatment of lymphoid cancers. The partial response rate with conventional doses in CLL is 10 to 15%. In previously untreated patients, the response rate is 75%, with 20% of patients achieving complete remission. Alemtuzumab has a 33% response rate in previously treated patients refractory to fludarabine and a 75 to 80% response rate in previously untreated patients. More problems with immunosuppression occur with alemtuzumab than with rituximab. Rituximab has been combined with fludarabine and with fludarabine and cyclophosphamide; these combinations have markedly improved the complete remission rate in both previously treated and previously untreated patients. Alemtuzumab is now being combined with rituximab and with chemotherapy to treat minimal residual disease and has effectively cleared bone marrow infiltration. Reactivation of cytomegalovirus and other opportunistic infections has occurred with alemtuzumab.

Radiation therapy: Local irradiation may be given to areas of lymphadenopathy or liver and spleen involvement for transient symptomatic palliation. Total body irradiation in small doses has been successful occasionally.

Chronic Myelocytic Leukemia

(Chronic Granulocytic Leukemia; Chronic Myelogenous Leukemia; Chronic Myeloid Leukemia)

CML occurs when a pluripotent stem cell undergoes malignant transformation and clonal myeloproliferation, leading to a striking overproduction of immature granulocytes. Initially asymptomatic, CML progression is insidious, with a nonspecific "benign" stage (malaise, anorexia, weight loss) eventually giving way to accelerated or blast phases with more ominous signs, such as splenomegaly, pallor, easy bruising and bleeding, fever, lymphadenopathy, and skin changes. Peripheral blood smear, bone marrow aspirate, and demonstration of Philadelphia chromosome are diagnostic. Treatment is with imatinib, which significantly improves response and probably survival. The curative potential of imatinib is undefined. Myelosuppressive agents (eg, hydroxyurea), stem cell transplantation, and interferon-α are also used.

CML accounts for about 15% of all adult leukemias. CML can strike at any age, although it is uncommon before age 10, and the median age at diagnosis is 45 to 55. CML may occur in either sex.

Pathophysiology

Most cases of CML appear to be induced by a translocation known as the Philadelphia (Ph) chromosome, which is demonstrable in 95% of patients. It is a reciprocal translocation t(9;22) in which a piece of chromosome 9 containing the oncogene *c-abl* is translocated to chromosome 22 and fused to the gene *BCR*. The fusion gene *ABL-BCR* is important in the pathogenesis and expression of CML and results in the production of a specific tyrosine kinase. CML ensues when an abnormal pluripotent hematopoietic progenitor cell initiates excessive production of granulocytes, primarily in the bone marrow but also in extramedullary sites (eg, spleen, liver). Although granulocyte production predominates, the neoplastic clone includes RBC, megakaryocyte, monocyte, and even some T and B cells. Normal stem cells are retained and can emerge after drug suppression of the CML clone.

CML has an initial indolent, chronic phase that may last months to years. In some cases, a secondary accelerated myeloproliferative phase develops, manifesting as treatment failure, worsening anemia, and progressive thrombocytopenia, followed by a terminal phase, in which a blast crisis ensues and blast cell tumors may develop in extramedullary sites (eg, bone, CNS, lymph nodes, skin). This development leads to fulminant complications resembling those of acute leukemia, including sepsis and bleeding. Some patients progress directly from the chronic to the blast phase.

Symptoms and Signs

Patients are often asymptomatic early on, with insidious onset of nonspecific symptoms (eg, fatigue, weakness, anorexia, weight loss, fever, night sweats, a sense of abdominal fullness), which may prompt evaluation. Initially, pallor, bleeding, easy bruising, and lymphadenopathy are unusual, but moderate or occasionally extreme splenomegaly is common (60 to 70% of cases). With disease progression, splenomegaly may increase, and pallor and bleeding occur. Fever, marked lymphadenopathy, and maculopapular skin involvement are ominous developments.

Diagnosis

CML is most frequently diagnosed by a CBC obtained incidentally or during evaluation of splenomegaly; granulocyte count is elevated, usually < 50,000/μL in the asymptomatic patient and 200,000/μL to 1,000,000/μL in the symptomatic patient; platelet count is normal or moderately increased; Hb level is usually > 10 g/dL.

Peripheral smear may help differentiate CML from leukocytosis of other etiology. In CML, peripheral blood smear shows predominantly immature granulocytes and absolute eosinophilia and basophilia, although in patients with WBC counts < 50,000/μL, immature granulocytes may be uncommon. Leukocytosis in patients with myelofibrosis is usually associated with nucleated RBCs, tear-shaped RBCs, anemia, and thrombocytopenia. Myeloid leukemoid reactions resulting from cancer or infection are not often associated with absolute eosinophilia and basophilia.

The leukocyte alkaline phosphatase score is usually low in CML and increased in leukemoid reactions. Bone marrow examination should be performed to evaluate the karyotype as well as cellularity (usually increased) and extent of myelofibrosis.

Diagnosis is confirmed by presence of the Ph chromosome on cytogenic or molecular studies, although it is absent in 5% of patients.

During the accelerated phase of disease, anemia and thrombocytopenia usually develop. Basophils may increase, and granulocyte maturation may be defective. The proportion of immature cells and the leukocyte alkaline phosphatase score may increase. In the bone marrow, myelofibrosis may develop and sideroblasts may be seen on microscopy. Evolution of the neoplastic clone may be associated with development of new abnormal karyotypes, often an extra chromosome 8 or isochromosome 17.

Further evolution may lead to a blast crisis with myeloblasts (60% of patients), lymphoblasts (30%), and megakaryocytoblasts (10%). In 80% of these patients, additional chromosomal abnormalities occur frequently.

Prognosis

Before imatinib was used, with treatment 5 to 10% of patients died within 2 yr of diagnosis; 10 to 15% died each year thereafter. Median survival was 4 to 7 yr. Most (90%) deaths follow a blast crisis or an accelerated phase of the disease. Median survival after blast crisis is about 3 to 6 mo but can be up to 12 mo with remission.

Ph chromosome–negative CML and chronic myelomonocytic leukemia have a worse prognosis than Ph chromosome–positive CML. Their clinical behaviors resemble a myelodysplastic syndrome (see below).

Treatment

Except for some cases in which stem cell transplantation can be used successfully, treatment is not curative; however, survival can be prolonged by treatment with imatinib.

Imatinib inhibits the specific tyrosine kinase that results from the *ABL-BCR* gene product. It is dramatically effective in achieving complete clinical and cytogenetic remissions of Ph chromosome–positive CML and is clearly superior to other regimens (eg, interferon ± cytosine arabinoside). Imatinib also is superior to other treatments in the accelerated and blastic phases. Combinations of chemotherapy with imatinib in blast crisis have a higher response rate than does therapy with either approach alone. Treatment tolerance is excellent. The high level of durable complete remissions associated with imatinib therapy has led to the prospect of the cure of the disease.

Older chemotherapy regimens are reserved for *ABL-BCR*–negative patients, those who relapse after receiving imatinib, and those in blast crisis. The main agents are busulfan, hydroxyurea, and interferon. Hydroxyurea is easiest to manage and has the fewest adverse effects. The starting dosage is generally 500 to 1000 mg po bid. Blood counts should be followed q 1 to 2 wk and the dosage adjusted accordingly. Busulfan often causes unexpected general myelosuppression, and interferon causes a flu-like syndrome that often is unacceptable to patients. The main benefit of these therapies is reduction in distressing splenomegaly and adenopathy and control of the tumor burden to reduce the incidence of tumor lysis and gout. None of these therapies prolongs median survival > 1 yr compared with untreated patients; thus, reduction in symptoms is the major goal, and therapy is not continued in the face of significant toxic symptoms.

Although splenic radiation is rarely used, it may be helpful in refractory cases of CML or in terminal patients with marked splenomegaly. Total dosage usually ranges from 6 to 10 Gy delivered in fractions of 0.25 to 2 Gy/day. Treatment should begin with very low doses and careful evaluation of the WBC count. Response is usually disappointing.

Splenectomy may alleviate abdominal discomfort, lessen thrombocytopenia, and relieve transfusion requirements when splenomegaly cannot be controlled with chemotherapy or irradiation. Splenectomy has not proved to play a significant role during the chronic phase of CML.

MYELODYSPLASTIC SYNDROME

Myelodysplastic syndrome involves a group of disorders typified by peripheral cytopenia, dysplastic hematopoietic progenitors, a hypercellular bone marrow, and a high risk of conversion to AML. Symptoms are referable to the specific cell line most affected and may include fatigue, weakness, pallor (secondary to anemia), increased infections and fever (secondary to neutropenia), and increased bleeding and bruising (secondary to thrombocytopenia). Diagnosis is by blood count, peripheral blood smear, and bone marrow aspiration. Treatment with 5-azacytidine may help; if AML supervenes, it is treated per the usual protocols.

Etiology and Pathophysiology

Myelodysplastic syndrome (MDS) is a group of disorders, often termed preleukemia, refractory anemias, Philadelphia chromosome–negative chronic myelocytic leukemia, chronic myelomonocytic leukemia, or agnogenic myeloid metaplasia, resulting from a somatic mutation of hematopoietic precursors. Etiology is often unknown, but risk is increased with exposure to benzene, radiation, and chemotherapeutic agents (particularly long or intense regimens and those involving alkylating agents and epipodophyllotoxins).

MDS is characterized by clonal proliferation of hematopoietic cells, including erythroid, myeloid, and megakaryocytic forms. The bone marrow is normal or hypercellular, and ineffective hematopoiesis can cause anemia (most common), neutropenia, and/or thrombocytopenia. The disordered cell production is also associated with morphologic cellular abnormalities in bone marrow and blood. Extramedullary hematopoiesis may occur, leading to hepatomegaly and splenomegaly. Myelofibrosis is occasionally present at diagnosis or may develop during the course of MDS. Classification is by blood and bone marrow findings (see TABLE 142–4). The MDS clone is unstable and tends to progress to AML.

Symptoms and Signs

Symptoms tend to reflect the most affected cell line and may include pallor, weakness, and fatigue (anemia); fever and infections (neutropenia); and increased bruising, petechiae, epistaxis, and mucosal bleeding (thrombocytopenia). Splenomegaly and hepatomegaly are common. Symptoms may also be referable to other underlying diseases; eg, in an elderly patient with preexisting cardiovascular disease, anemia from MDS may exacerbate anginal pain.

Diagnosis

MDS is suspected in patients (especially the elderly) with refractory anemia, leukopenia, or thrombocytopenia. Cytopenias secondary to congenital disorders, vitamin deficiencies, or drug adverse effects must be ruled out. Diagnosis is by examining peripheral blood and bone marrow and identifying morphologic abnormalities in 10 to 20% of cells of a particular lineage.

Anemia is the most common feature, associated usually with macrocytosis and

TABLE 142–4. MYELODYSPLASTIC SYNDROME BONE MARROW FINDINGS AND SURVIVAL

CLASSIFICATION	CRITERIA	MEDIAN SURVIVAL (YR)
Refractory anemia	Anemia with reticulocytopenia, normal or hypercellular marrow with erythroid hyperplasia and dyserythropoiesis; blasts ≤ 5%	≥ 5
Refractory anemia with sideroblasts	Same as refractory anemia with ringed sideroblasts > 15% of NMC	≥ 5
Refractory anemia with excess blasts	Some cytopenia of ≥ 2 cell lines with morphologic abnormalities of blood cells; hypercellular marrow with dyserythropoiesis and dysgranulopoiesis; blasts = 5–20% of NMC	1.5
Chronic myelomonocytic leukemia	Same as refractory anemia with excess blasts with absolute monocytosis in blood; significant increase in marrow monocyte precursors	1.5
Refractory anemia with excess blasts in transformation	Refractory anemia with excess blasts and one or more of the following: ≥ 5% blasts in blood, 20–30% blasts in marrow, Auer rods in granulocyte precursors	0.5

NMC = nucleated marrow cells.

anisocytosis. With automatic cell counters, these changes are indicated by an increased MCV and RBC distribution width. Some degree of thrombocytopenia is usual; on blood smear, the platelets vary in size, and some appear hypogranular. The WBC count may be normal, increased, or decreased. Neutrophil cytoplasmic granularity is abnormal, with anisocytosis and variable numbers of granules. Eosinophils also may have abnormal granularity. Pseudo Pelger-Huët cells (hyposegmented neutrophils) may be seen. Monocytosis is characteristic of the chronic myelomonocytic leukemia subgroup, and immature myeloid cells may occur in the less well differentiated subgroups. The cytogenetic pattern is usually abnormal, with one or more clonal cytogenetic abnormalities often involving chromosomes 5 or 7.

Prognosis and Treatment

Prognosis depends greatly on classification and on any associated disease. Patients with refractory anemia or refractory anemia with sideroblasts are less likely to progress to the more aggressive forms and may die of unrelated causes.

Azacitidine improves symptoms, decreases the rate of transformation to leukemia and the need for transfusions, and probably improves survival. Other therapy is supportive, including RBC transfusions as indicated, platelet transfusions for bleeding, and antibiotic therapy for infection. In some patients, erythropoietin to support RBC needs, granulocyte colony-stimulating factor to manage severe symptomatic granulocytopenia, and, when available, thrombopoietin for severe thrombocytopenia can serve as important hematopoietic support but have not proved to increase survival. Allogeneic stem cell transplantation is useful, and nonablative allogeneic bone marrow transplantations are now being studied for patients > 50 yr. Response of MDS to AML chemotherapy is similar to that of AML, after age and karyotype are considered.

143 LYMPHOMAS

Lymphomas are a heterogeneous group of neoplasms arising in the reticuloendothelial and lymphatic systems. The major types are Hodgkin lymphoma and non-Hodgkin lymphoma (NHL)—see TABLE 143–1.

Lymphomas were once thought to be absolutely distinct from leukemias. However, better understanding of cell markers and keen tools with which to evaluate those markers now show that the differentiation between these 2 cancers is often vague. The notion that lymphoma is relatively restricted to the lymphatic system and leukemias to the bone marrow, at least in early stages, is also not always true.

HODGKIN LYMPHOMA

(Hodgkin's Disease)

Hodgkin lymphoma is a localized or disseminated malignant proliferation of cells of the lymphoreticular system, primarily involving lymph node tissue, spleen, liver, and bone marrow. Symptoms include painless lymphadenopathy, sometimes with fever, night sweats, unintentional weight loss, pruritus, splenomegaly, and hepatomegaly. Diagnosis is based on lymph node biopsy. Treatment is curative in about 75% of cases and consists of chemotherapy and/or radiation therapy.

In the US, about 7500 new cases of Hodgkin lymphoma are diagnosed annually. The male:female ratio is 1.4:1. Hodgkin lymphoma is rare before age 10 and is most common between ages 15 and 40.

Etiology and Pathophysiology

Hodgkin lymphoma results from the clonal transformation of cells of B-cell origin, giving rise to pathognomic binucleated Reed-Sternberg cells. The cause is unknown, but genetic susceptibility and environmental associations (eg, occupation, such as woodworking; history of treatment with phenytoin, radiation therapy, or chemotherapy; infection with Epstein-Barr virus, *Mycobacterium tuberculosis*, herpesvirus type 6, HIV) play a role. Risk is slightly increased in people with certain types of immune suppression (eg, posttransplant patients taking immunosuppressants); in people with congenital immunodeficiency states (eg, ataxia-telangiectasia, Klinefelter's syndrome, Chédiak-Higashi syndrome, Wiskott-Aldrich syndrome); and in people with certain autoimmune disorders (RA, nontropical sprue, Sjögren's syndrome, SLE).

Most patients also develop a slowly progressive defect in cell-mediated immunity (T-cell function) that in advanced disease contributes to common bacterial and unusual fungal, viral, and protozoal infections. Humoral immunity (antibody production) is depressed in advanced disease. Death often results from sepsis.

Symptoms and Signs

Most patients present with painless cervical adenopathy. Although the mechanism is unclear, pain may occur in diseased areas immediately after drinking alcoholic beverages, thereby providing an early indication of the diagnosis.

Other manifestations develop as the disease spreads through the reticuloendothelial system, generally to contiguous sites. Intense pruritus may occur early. Constitutional symptoms include fever, night sweats, and unintentional weight loss (> 10% of body weight in previous 6 mo) and may signify involvement of internal nodes (mediastinal or retroperitoneal), viscera (liver), or bone marrow. Splenomegaly is often present; hepatomegaly may be present. Pel-Ebstein fever (a few days of high fever regularly alternating with a few days to several weeks of normal or below-normal temperature) occasionally occurs. Cachexia is common as disease advances.

Bone involvement is often asymptomatic but may produce vertebral osteoblastic lesions (ivory vertebrae) and, rarely, pain with osteolytic lesions and compression fracture. Intracranial, gastric, and cutaneous lesions are rare and suggest HIV-associated Hodgkin lymphoma.

Local compression by tumor masses often causes symptoms, including jaundice secondary to intrahepatic or extrahepatic bile duct obstruction; leg edema secondary to lymphatic obstruction in the pelvis or groin; severe dyspnea and wheezing secondary to tracheobronchial compression; and lung cavitation or abscess secondary to infiltration of lung parenchyma, which may simulate lobar consolidation or bronchopneumonia. Epidural invasion that compresses the spinal cord may result in paraplegia. Horner syndrome and laryngeal paralysis may result when enlarged lymph nodes compress the cervical sympathetic and recurrent laryngeal nerves. Neuralgic pain follows nerve root compression.

TABLE 143–1. COMPARISON OF HODGKIN LYMPHOMA AND NON-HODGKIN LYMPHOMA

HODGKIN LYMPHOMA	NON-HODGKIN LYMPHOMA
Localized to a specific group of nodes	Usually disseminated among more than one nodal group
Tends to spread in an orderly, contiguous fashion	Spreads noncontiguously
Does not usually affect Waldeyer's ring and the mesenteric nodes	Commonly affects the mesenteric nodes and may affect Waldeyer's ring
Infrequently involves extranodal sites	Frequently involves extranodal sites
Usually diagnosed at an early stage	Usually diagnosed at an advanced stage
In children, usually displays a favorable histologic classification	In children, usually is high grade

Diagnosis

Hodgkin lymphoma is usually suspected in patients with painless lymphadenopathy or mediastinal adenopathy detected on routine chest x-ray. Similar lymphadenopathy can result from infectious mononucleosis, toxoplasmosis, cytomegalovirus, non-Hodgkin lymphoma, or leukemia. The chest x-ray findings can resemble lung carcinoma, sarcoidosis, or TB (see also p. 488 for evaluation of a mediastinal mass).

A chest x-ray is obtained, usually followed by lymph node biopsy if findings are confirmed on torso CT or PET scan. If only mediastinal nodes are enlarged, mediastinoscopy or Chamberlain procedure (a limited left anterior thoracostomy allowing biopsy of mediastinal lymph nodes inaccessible by cervical mediastinoscopy) may be indicated. CT-guided biopsy may also be considered. CBC, ESR, alkaline phosphatase, and renal and liver function tests are generally obtained.

TABLE 143–2. HISTOPATHOLOGIC SUBTYPES OF HODGKIN LYMPHOMA (WHO CLASSIFICATION)

HISTOLOGIC TYPE	MORPHOLOGIC APPEARANCE	NEOPLASTIC CELL IMMUNOPHENOTYPE	INCIDENCE
Classic			
Nodular sclerosis	Dense fibrous tissue* surrounds nodules of Hodgkin tissue	$CD15^+$, $CD30^+$, $CD20^-$	67%
Mixed cellularity	A moderate number of Reed-Sternberg cells with a mixed background infiltrate	$CD15^+$, $CD30^+$, $CD20^-$	25%
Lymphocyte-rich	Few Reed-Sternberg cells, many B cells, fine sclerosis	$CD15^+$, $CD30^+$, $CD20^-$	3%
Lymphocyte-depleted	Numerous Reed-Sternberg cells and extensive fibrosis	$CD15^+$, $CD30^+$, $CD20^-$	Rare
Nodular lymphocyte predominant			
	Few neoplastic cells (L & H cells), many small B cells, nodular pattern	$CD15^-$, $CD30^-$, $CD20^+$, EMA^+	3%

*Shows characteristic birefringence with polarized light.

Other tests are performed depending on findings (eg, MRI for symptoms of cord compression, bone scan for evaluation of bone pain).

Biopsy reveals Reed-Sternberg cells (large binucleated cells) in a characteristically heterogeneous cellular infiltrate consisting of histiocytes, lymphocytes, monocytes, plasma cells, and eosinophils. Classic Hodgkin lymphoma has 4 histopathologic subtypes (see TABLE 143–2); there is also a lymphocyte-predominant type. Certain antigens on Reed-Sternberg cells may help differentiate Hodgkin lymphoma from NHL, and classical Hodgkin lymphoma from the lymphocyte-predominant type.

Other test results may be abnormal but nondiagnostic. CBC may show slight polymorphonuclear leukocytosis. Lymphocytopenia may occur early and become pronounced with advanced disease. Eosinophilia is present in about 20% of patients, and thrombocytosis may be present. Anemia, often microcytic, usually develops with advanced disease. In advanced anemia, defective iron reutilization is characterized by low serum iron, low iron-binding capacity, and increased bone marrow iron. Pancytopenia is occasionally caused by bone marrow invasion, usually by the lymphocyte-depleted type. Hypersplenism (see p. 1091) may appear in patients with marked splenomegaly. Elevated serum alkaline phosphatase levels may be present but do not always indicate bone marrow or liver involvement or both. Increases in leukocyte alkaline phosphatase, serum haptoglobin, ESR, and other acute-phase reactants usually reflect active disease.

Staging: After diagnosis, stage is determined to guide therapy. The commonly used Ann Arbor staging system (see TABLE 143–3) incorporates symptoms; physical examination findings; results of imaging tests, including CT of the chest, abdomen, and pelvis; and unilateral bone marrow biopsy. Laparotomy is not required for staging. Other staging tests may include PET scan and cardiac and pulmonary function tests in anticipation of therapy.

Designation of the letter A to any stage means that no systemic symptoms are being experienced. Designation of the letter B means that at least one systemic symptom is experienced. The presence of symptoms correlates with response to treatment.

Prognosis and Treatment

In Hodgkin lymphoma, disease-free survival 5 yr after therapy is considered a cure; relapse is very rare after 5 yr. Chemotherapy with or without radiation therapy achieves cure in > 75% of newly diagnosed patients. The choice of modality is complex and depends on the precise stage of disease.

TABLE 143–3. COTSWOLD MODIFICATION OF ANN ARBOR STAGING OF HODGKIN LYMPHOMA AND NON-HODGKIN LYMPHOMA

STAGE*	CRITERIA
I	In 1 lymph region only
II	In ≥ 2 lymph regions on the same side of the diaphragm
III	In the lymph nodes, spleen, or both and on both sides of the diaphragm
IV	Extranodal involvement (eg, bone marrow, lung, liver)

*Subclassification E indicates extranodal involvement adjacent to an involved lymph node (eg, disease of mediastinal nodes and hilar adenopathy with adjacent lung infiltration is classified as stage IIE). Stages can be further classified by A to indicate the absence or B to indicate the presence of constitutional symptoms (weight loss, fever, or night sweats). Constitutional symptoms generally occur with stages III and IV (20 to 30% of patients); the suffix X is used to denote bulky disease, which is > 10 cm in maximum dimension or > 1/3 the chest diameter on chest x-ray.

Stage IA, IIA, IB, or IIB disease is generally treated with chemotherapy plus radiation therapy. Such treatment cures about 80% of patients. In patients with bulky mediastinal disease, chemotherapy may be of longer duration or of a different type before radiation therapy is used.

Stage IIIA disease generally is treated with combination chemotherapy with or without radiation therapy of bulky nodal sites. Cure rates of 75 to 80% have been achieved.

Stage IIIB disease requires combination chemotherapy either alone or sometimes with radiation therapy because it is not cured by radiation therapy alone. Survival ranges from 70 to 80%.

For stage IVA and IVB disease, combination chemotherapy involving ABVD (doxorubicin [Adriamycin], bleomycin, vinblastine, dacarbazine) has become the standard regimen, producing complete remission in 70 to 80% of patients, with > 50% remaining disease-free at 10 to 15 yr. MOPP (mechlorethamine, vincristine [Oncovin], procarbazine, prednisone) is no longer used because of adverse effects, including secondary leukemia. Other effective drugs include nitrosoureas, ifosfamide, cisplatin or carboplatin, and etoposide. A promising new drug combination, Stanford V, is a 12-wk regimen. Patients who do not achieve complete remission or who relapse within 12 mo have a poor prognosis.

Autologous transplantation using peripheral cell products should be considered for all eligible patients with relapsed/refractory Hodgkin lymphoma who respond to salvage chemotherapy.

For a schedule of posttreatment surveillance, see TABLE 143–4.

Complications of treatment: Chemotherapy with MOPP-like regimens increases the risk of leukemia, which generally develops after > 3 yr. Both chemotherapy and radiation therapy increase the risk of malignant solid tumors (eg, breast, GI, lung, soft tissue). Mediastinal radiation increases the risk of coronary atherosclerosis. Breast cancer risk is increased in women beginning about 7 yr after they have received radiation treatment to adjacent nodal regions.

TABLE 143–4. HODGKIN LYMPHOMA POSTTREATMENT SURVEILLANCE

EVALUATION	SCHEDULE
History and physical examination, CBC, platelets, ESR, chemistry profile	First 2 yr, q 3 to 4 mo Yr 3 to 5, q 6 mo > 5 yr, q 12 mo
Chest x-ray at each visit if chest CT not obtained	First 2 yr, q 3 mo Yr 3 to 5, q 6 mo > 5 yr, annually
Chest CT	First 2 yr, q 6 to 8 mo Yr 3 to 5, annually > 5 yr, whenever chest x-ray abnormalities are discovered
Abdomen and pelvis CT	Stages I and II: First 5 yr, annually for 5 yr For other stages: First 2 yr, q 6 mo Yr 3 to 5, annually
Thyroid-stimulating hormone levels	q 6 mo after radiation to neck
Annual mammogram beginning at year 7	If radiation above diaphragm began at age < 30 yr
Annual mammogram beginning at age 37	If radiation above diaphragm began at age > 30 yr

NON-HODGKIN LYMPHOMAS

Non-Hodgkin lymphomas are a heterogeneous group of disorders involving malignant monoclonal proliferation of lymphoid cells in lymphoreticular sites, including lymph nodes, bone marrow, the spleen, the liver, and the GI tract. Presenting symptoms usually include peripheral lymphadenopathy. However, some forms present without adenopathy but with abnormal lymphocytes in circulation. Compared with Hodgkin lymphoma, there is a greater likelihood of disseminated disease at the time of diagnosis. Diagnosis is usually based on lymph node and/or bone marrow biopsy. Treatment includes radiation and/or chemotherapy, with stem cell transplantation usually reserved for salvage therapy after incomplete remission or relapse.

Non-Hodgkin lymphoma (NHL) is more common than Hodgkin lymphoma. It is the 6th most common cancer in the US; about 56,000 new cases are diagnosed annually in all age groups. However, NHL is not one disease but rather a category of lymphocyte malignancies. Incidence increases with age (median age, 50 yr).

Etiology and Pathophysiology

Most (80 to 85%) NHLs arise from B cells, with the remainder arising from T cells or natural killer cells. In all cases, either precursor or mature cells may be involved.

The cause of NHL is unknown, although, as with the leukemias, substantial evidence suggests a viral cause (eg, human T-cell leukemia-lymphoma virus, Epstein-Barr virus, HIV). Risk factors for NHL include immunodeficiency (secondary to posttransplant immunosuppression, AIDS, primary immune disorders, sicca syndrome, RA), *Helicobacter pylori* infection, certain chemical exposures, and previous treatment for Hodgkin lymphoma. NHL is the 2nd most common cancer in HIV-infected patients (see p. 1641), and some AIDS patients present with lymphoma. C-*myc* gene rearrangements are characteristic of some AIDS-associated lymphomas.

Overlap exists between leukemia and NHL, because both involve proliferation of lymphocytes or their precursors. A leukemia-like picture with peripheral lymphocytosis and marrow involvement may be present in up to 50% of children and in about 20% of adults with some types of NHL. Differentiation can be difficult, but generally patients with more extensive nodal involvement (especially mediastinal), fewer circulating abnormal cells, and fewer blast forms in the marrow (< 25%) are considered to have lymphoma. A leukemic phase is less common in aggressive lymphomas, except Burkitt's and lymphoblastic lymphomas.

Hypogammaglobulinemia caused by a progressive decrease in immunoglobulin production occurs in 15% of patients and may predispose to serious bacterial infection.

Classification

Pathologic classification of NHLs continues to evolve, reflecting new insights into the cells of origin and the biologic bases of these heterogeneous diseases. The WHO classification (see TABLE 143–5) is valuable because it incorporates immunophenotype, genotype, and cytogenetics; numerous other systems exist (eg, Lyon classification). Among the most important new lymphomas recognized by the WHO system are mucosa-associated lymphoid tumors (MALT—see p. 120); mantle cell lymphoma (previously diffuse small cleaved cell lymphoma); and anaplastic large cell lymphoma, a heterogeneous disorder with 75% of cases of T-cell origin, 15% of B-cell origin, and 10% unclassified. However, despite the plethora of entities, treatment is often similar except in certain T-cell lymphomas.

Lymphomas are commonly also categorized as indolent or aggressive. Indolent lymphomas are slowly progressive and responsive to therapy but are not curable. Aggressive lymphomas are rapidly progressive but responsive to therapy and often curable.

In children, NHL is almost always aggressive. Follicular and other indolent lymphomas are very rare. The treatment of these aggressive lymphomas (Burkitt's, diffuse large B cell, and lymphoblastic lymphoma) presents special concerns, including GI tract involvement (particularly in the terminal ileum); meningeal spread (requiring CSF prophylaxis or treatment); and other sanctuary sites of involvement (such as testis or brain). In addition, with these potentially curable lymphomas, treatment adverse effects as well as outcome must be considered, including late risks of secondary malignancy, cardiorespiratory sequelae, fertility preservation,

TABLE 143–5. SUBTYPES OF NON-HODGKIN LYMPHOMA (WHO CLASSIFICATION)

B-CELL ORIGIN	T-CELL AND NATURAL KILLER CELL ORIGIN
Precursor B-cell neoplasm	**Precursor T-cell neoplasm**
Precursor B-lymphoblastic leukemia/ lymphoma*	Precursor T-lymphoblastic lymphoma/ leukemia*
Mature B-cell neoplasms	**Mature T-cell neoplasms**
B-cell chronic lymphocytic leukemia/small lymphocytic lymphoma†	T-cell prolymphocytic leukemia†
B-cell prolymphocytic leukemia†	T-cell granular lymphocytic leukemia*
Lymphoplasmacytic lymphoma†	Aggressive NK cell leukemia*
Splenic marginal zone B-cell lymphoma (± villous lymphocytes)†	Adult T-cell lymphoma/leukemia* (HTLV 1-positive)
Hairy cell leukemia†	Extranodal NK/T-cell lymphoma, nasal type*
Plasma cell myeloma/plasmacytoma†	Enteropathy-type T-cell lymphoma*
Extranodal marginal zone B-cell lymphoma of the MALT type†	Hepatosplenic γ-δ T-cell lymphoma*
Nodal marginal zone B-cell lymphoma (± monocytoid B cells)†	Subcutaneous panniculitis-like T-cell lymphoma*
Follicular lymphoma†	Mycosis fungoides/Sézary syndrome†
Mantle cell lymphoma‡	Anaplastic large cell lymphoma, T/null cell, primary cutaneous type*
Diffuse large B-cell lymphomas* (includes mediastinal large B-cell lymphoma, primary effusion lymphoma)	Anaplastic large cell lymphoma, T/null cell, primary systemic type*
Burkitt's lymphoma*	Peripheral T-cell lymphoma, not otherwise characterized*
	Angioimmunoblastic T-cell lymphoma*

MALT = mucosa-associated lymphoid tissue; NK = natural killer; HTLV = human T-cell leukemia virus 1.
*Aggressive.
†Indolent.
‡Indolent but more rapidly progressive.

and developmental consequences. Current research is focused on these areas as well as on the molecular events and predictors of lymphoma in children.

Symptoms and Signs

Many patients present with asymptomatic peripheral lymphadenopathy. Enlarged lymph nodes are rubbery and discrete and later become matted. Disease is localized in some patients, but most patients have multiple areas of involvement. Mediastinal and retroperitoneal lymphadenopathy may cause pressure symptoms on various organs. Extranodal sites may dominate clinically (eg, gastric involvement can simulate GI carcinoma; intestinal lymphoma may cause a malabsorption syndrome; HIV patients who develop NHL often present with CNS involvement).

The skin and bones are initially involved in 15% of patients with aggressive lymphoma and in 7% with indolent lymphoma. Occasionally, patients with extensive abdominal or thoracic disease develop chylous ascites or pleural effusion because of lymphatic obstruction. Weight loss, fever, night sweats, and asthenia indicate disseminated disease. Patients may have hepatomegaly and splenomegaly as well.

Two problems are common in NHL but rare in Hodgkin lymphoma: Congestion and edema of the face and neck from pressure on the superior vena cava (superior vena cava or superior mediastinal syndrome) may occur. Also, ureters may be compressed by retroperitoneal and/or pelvic lymph nodes, which may interfere with urinary flow and cause secondary renal failure.

Anemia is initially present in about 33% of patients and eventually develops in most. It may be caused by bleeding from GI lymphoma, with or without low platelet levels; hemolysis from hypersplenism or Coombs'-positive hemolytic anemia; bone marrow infiltration from lymphoma; or marrow suppression from chemotherapy or radiation therapy.

The acute illness of adult T-cell leukemia-lymphoma (associated with HTLV-1) has a fulminating clinical course with skin infiltrates, lymphadenopathy, hepatosplenomegaly, and leukemia. The leukemic cells are malignant T cells, many with convoluted nuclei. Hypercalcemia often develops, related to humoral factors rather than to direct bone invasion.

Patients with anaplastic large cell lymphoma have rapidly progressive skin lesions, adenopathy, and visceral lesions. This disease may be mistaken for Hodgkin lymphoma or metastatic undifferentiated carcinoma.

Diagnosis

NHL is usually suspected in patients with painless lymphadenopathy or when mediastinal adenopathy is detected on routine chest x-ray. Painless lymphadenopathy can also result from infectious mononucleosis, toxoplasmosis, cytomegalovirus, or leukemia. The chest x-ray findings can resemble lung carcinoma, sarcoidosis, or TB. Less commonly, patients present after a finding of peripheral lymphocytosis on CBC performed for nonspecific symptoms. In such cases, the differential diagnosis includes leukemia, Epstein-Barr virus infection, and Duncan's syndrome.

Chest x-ray is obtained if not done previously, and a lymph node biopsy is performed if lymphadenopathy is confirmed on CT or PET scan. If only mediastinal nodes are enlarged, patients require CT-guided needle biopsy or mediastinoscopy. CBC, alkaline phosphatase, renal and liver function tests, LDH, and uric acid are generally obtained. Other tests are performed depending on findings (eg, MRI for symptoms of cord compression or CNS abnormalities).

Histologic criteria on biopsy include destruction of normal lymph node architecture and invasion of the capsule and adjacent fat by characteristic neoplastic cells. Immunophenotyping studies to determine the cell of origin identify specific subtypes and help define prognosis and management; these studies also can be done on peripheral cells. Demonstration of the leukocyte common antigen CD45 by immunoperoxidase rules out metastatic carcinoma, which is often in the differential diagnosis of "undifferentiated" cancers. The test for leukocyte common antigen, most surface marker studies, and gene rearrangement (to document B-cell or T-cell clonality) can be done on fixed tissues. Cytogenetics and flow cytometry require fresh tissue.

Staging: Although localized NHL does occur, the disease is typically disseminated when first recognized. Staging procedures include CT of the chest, abdomen, and pelvis; PET; and bone marrow biopsy. The final staging of NHL (see TABLE 143–3) is similar to that of Hodgkin lymphoma and is based on clinical and pathologic findings.

Prognosis

Patients with T-cell lymphomas generally have a worse prognosis than do those with B-cell types, although newer intensive treatment programs may lessen this difference.

Survival also varies with other factors. The International Prognostic Index (IPI) is frequently used in aggressive lymphomas. It considers 5 risk factors: age > 60, poor performance status (can be measured using Eastern Cooperative Oncology Group tool), elevated LDH, > 1 extranodal site, and stage III or IV. Outcome is worse with an increasing number of risk factors; actual survival varies by cell type but, eg, in large cell lymphoma, 5-yr survival for patients with 0 or 1 risk factor is 73% vs 26% for patients with 4 or 5 risk factors. Generally, patients with ≥ 2 risk factors should be considered for more aggressive or experimental treatments. A modified IPI (the FLIPI) is also being studied in indolent lymphomas.

Treatment

Treatment varies somewhat with cell type, which are too numerous to permit detailed discussion. Generalizations can be made regarding localized vs advanced disease and aggressive vs indolent forms. Burkitt's lymphoma and mycosis fungoides are discussed below.

Localized disease (stages I and II): Patients with indolent lymphomas rarely present with localized disease, but when they do, regional radiation therapy may offer long-term control. However, relapses may occur > 10 yr after radiation therapy.

About $^1/_2$ of patients with aggressive lymphomas present with localized disease, for which combination chemotherapy, with or without regional radiation, is usually curative. Patients with lymphoblastic lymphomas or Burkitt's lymphoma, even if apparently localized, must receive intensive combination chemotherapy with meningeal prophylaxis. Treatment may require maintenance chemotherapy (lymphoblastic), but cure is expected.

Advanced disease (stages III and IV): For indolent lymphomas, treatment varies considerably. A watch-and-wait approach, treatment with a single alkylating drug, or 2- or 3-drug regimens may be used. Criteria considered in selecting management options include age, general health, distribution of disease, tumor bulk, histology, and anticipated benefits of therapy. The B-cell specific anti-CD20 antibody rituximab and other biologic response modifiers may be of benefit; one of these drugs can be combined with chemotherapy or administered as single therapy. Recent reports of radiolabeled-antibody therapy also appear promising. Although survival may be prolonged in terms of years, late relapse occurs, resulting in an unfavorable long-term prognosis.

In patients with the aggressive B-cell lymphomas (eg, diffuse large B cell), the standard drug combination is R-CHOP (rituximab plus cyclophosphamide, hydroxydaunorubicin [doxorubicin], vincristine, prednisone). Complete disease regression in ≥ 70% of patients is expected, depending on the IPI category. More than 70% of complete responders are cured, and relapses after 2 yr off treatment are rare.

Autologous transplantation is being investigated as treatment at initial diagnosis. With use of the IPI, high-risk patients may be identified and selected for dose intensification. Whether this treatment provides an increased rate of cure is under study. Selected younger patients with mantle cell lymphoma may be candidates as well.

Aggressive lymphoma relapse: The first relapse after initial chemotherapy is almost always treated with autologous stem cell transplantation. Patients must be ≤ 70 yr or in equivalent health and have responsive disease, good performance status, and a source of uncontaminated and adequate number of $CD34^+$ stem cells (harvested from peripheral blood or bone marrow). Consolidation myeloablative therapy may include chemotherapy with or without irradiation. Posttreatment immunotherapy (eg, rituximab, vaccination, IL-2) is being studied.

An allogeneic transplant is the donation of stem cells from a compatible donor (brother, sister, or matched unrelated donor). The stem cells have a 2-fold effect: reconstituting normal blood counts and providing a possible graft-vs-tumor effect.

A cure may be expected in 30 to 50% of eligible patients with aggressive lymphomas undergoing myeloablative therapy. In indolent lymphomas, cure with autologous transplantation remains uncertain, although remission may be superior to that with secondary palliative therapy alone. The mortality rate of patients undergoing myeloablative transplantation has decreased dramatically to 2 to 5% for most autologous procedures and to < 15% for most allogeneic procedures.

A late sequela of standard and high-dose chemotherapy is the occurrence of second tumors, especially myelodysplasias and acute myelogenous leukemia. Chemotherapy combined with radiation therapy increases this risk, although its incidence is still only about 3%.

Burkitt's Lymphoma

Burkitt's lymphoma is a B-cell lymphoma occurring primarily in children. Endemic (African), sporadic (non-African), and immunodeficiency-related forms exist.

Burkitt's lymphoma is endemic in central Africa and constitutes 30% of childhood lymphomas in the US. The form endemic to Africa often presents as enlargement of the jaw or facial bones. In non-African Burkitt's lymphoma, abdominal disease predominates, often arising in the region of the ileocecal valve or the mesentery. The kidneys, ovaries, or breasts may be involved as well, and in adults, disease may be bulky and generalized, often with massive involvement of liver, spleen, and bone marrow. CNS involvement is often present at diagnosis or with relapsing lymphoma.

Burkitt's lymphoma is the most rapidly growing human tumor, and pathology reveals a high mitotic rate, a monoclonal proliferation of B cells, and a "starry-sky" pattern of benign macrophages that have engulfed apoptotic malignant lymphocytes. There is a distinctive genetic translocation involving the C-*myc* gene on chromosome 8 and the immunoglobulin heavy chain of chromosome 14. The disease is closely associated with Epstein-Barr virus in endemic lymphoma; however, it is uncertain whether Epstein-Barr virus plays an etiologic role. Burkitt's lymphoma occurs frequently in patients with AIDS and may be an AIDS-defining disease.

Diagnosis is based on biopsy of lymph node or tissue from another suspected disease site. Staging includes CT of the torso, bone marrow biopsy, CSF cytology, and PET scan.

Treatment must be initiated rapidly and staging studies expedited because of rapid tumor growth. An intensive alternating regimen, CODOX-M/IVAC (cyclophosphamide, vincristine, doxorubicin, methotrexate, ifosfamide, etoposide, cytarabine), has been reported to result in a cure rate of > 90% for children and adults. Meningeal prophylaxis is essential. With treatment, tumor lysis syndrome (see p. 1170) is common, and patients must receive IV hydration, allopurinol, alkalinization, and close attention to electrolytes (particularly K and Ca).

If the patient presents with bowel obstruction secondary to tumor and the tumor is completely resected at initial therapeutic/diagnostic laparotomy, then aggressive therapy is still indicated. Salvage therapy for treatment failures is generally unsuccessful, underscoring the importance of very aggressive initial therapy.

Mycosis Fungoides

Mycosis fungoides is an uncommon chronic T-cell lymphoma primarily affecting the skin and occasionally the internal organs.

Mycosis fungoides is rare compared with Hodgkin lymphoma and NHL. Unlike most other lymphomas, it is insidious in onset, sometimes appearing as a chronic, pruritic rash that is difficult to diagnose. It begins focally but may spread to involve most of the skin. Lesions are plaquelike but may become nodular or ulcerated. Eventually, systemic involvement of lymph nodes, liver, spleen, and lungs occurs, resulting in the advent of symptoms, which include fever, night sweats, and unintentional weight loss.

Diagnosis is based on skin biopsy, but histology may be equivocal early in the course because of insufficient quantities of lymphoma cells. The malignant cells are mature T cells ($T4^+$, $T11^+$, $T12^+$). Characteristic Pautrier's microabscesses are present in the epidermis. In some cases, a leukemic phase called Sézary syndrome is characterized by the appearance of malignant T cells with serpentine nuclei in the peripheral blood.

Once mycosis fungoides has been confirmed, the stage (see TABLE 143–3) is determined by CT scan of the torso and bone marrow biopsy for blood or lymph node involvement. PET scan may also be used for suspected visceral involvement.

Prognosis and Treatment

Most patients are > 50 yr at diagnosis; average life expectancy is 7 to 10 yr after diagnosis, even without treatment. Survival rates depend on stage at diagnosis. Patients who receive treatment for stage IA disease have a life expectancy analogous to that of other people without mycosis fungoides matched for age, sex, and race. Patients who receive treatment for stage IIB disease survive for about 3 yr. Patients treated for stage III disease survive an average of 4 to 6 yr. Patients treated for stage IVA or IVB disease (extracutaneous disease) survive < 1.5 yr.

Electron beam radiation therapy, in which most of the energy is absorbed in the first 5 to 10 mm of tissue, and topical nitrogen mustard have proved highly effective. Plaques may also be treated with sunlight and topical corticosteroids. Systemic treatment with alkylating drugs and folic acid antagonists produces transient tumor regression but is primarily used when other therapies have failed, after relapse, or in patients with documented extranodal and/or extracutaneous disease. Extracorporeal phototherapy with a chemosensitive drug has shown modest success. The adenosine deaminase inhibitors fludarabine and 2-chlorodeoxyadenosine also show promise.

144 PLASMA CELL DISORDERS

(Dysproteinemias; Monoclonal Gammopathies; Paraproteinemias; Plasma Cell Dyscrasias)

Plasma cell disorders are a diverse group of disorders of unknown etiology characterized by the disproportionate proliferation of one clone of B cells and the presence of a structurally and electrophoretically homogeneous (monoclonal) immunoglobulin or polypeptide subunit in serum or urine.

Pathophysiology

(For structural features and classification of the immunoglobulins, see p. 1324.)

After developing in the bone marrow, undifferentiated B cells enter peripheral lymphoid tissues, such as lymph nodes, spleen, gut, and Peyer's patches. Here, they begin to differentiate into cells, each of which can respond to a limited number of antigens. After encountering the appropriate antigen, some B cells undergo clonal proliferation into plasma cells. Each clonal plasma cell line is committed to synthesizing one specific immunoglobulin antibody that consists of one heavy chain (gamma [γ], mu [μ], alpha [α], delta [δ], or epsilon [ε]) and one light chain (kappa [κ] or lambda [λ]). A slight excess of light chains is normally produced, and urinary excretion of small amounts of free polyclonal light chains (≤ 40 mg/24 h) is normal.

Plasma cell disorders are of unknown etiology and are characterized by the disproportionate proliferation of one clone. The result is a corresponding increase in the serum level of its product, the monoclonal immunoglobulin protein (M-protein).

M-proteins may consist of both heavy and light chains or of only one type of chain. Some show antibody activity, which may produce autoimmune damage of organs, particularly the kidneys. When M-proteins are produced, production of other immunoglobulins is commonly reduced, and immunity may become impaired. M-protein may coat platelets, inactivate clotting factors, increase blood viscosity, and cause bleeding by other mechanisms. M-proteins may also produce secondary amyloidosis. The clonal cells can infiltrate bone matrix or marrow, with resultant osteoporosis, hypercalcemia, anemia, or pancytopenia.

Plasma cell disorders can vary from asymptomatic, stable conditions (in which only the protein is present) to progressive neoplasms (eg, multiple myeloma). Rarely, transient plasma cell disorders occur in patients with drug hypersensitivity (sulfonamide, phenytoin, and penicillin), presumed viral infections, and cardiac surgery. Plasma cell disorders are classified in TABLE 144–1.

Plasma cell disorders may be suspected based on clinical manifestations (often in evaluation of anemia) or because of an incidental finding of elevated serum protein or proteinuria, leading to further evaluation with serum or urine protein electrophoresis, which reveals M-protein. The M-protein is further evaluated with immunofixation electrophoresis for identification of heavy and light chain classes. Laboratory evaluation is described below.

HEAVY CHAIN DISEASES

Heavy chain diseases are neoplastic plasma cell disorders characterized by overproduction of monoclonal immunoglobulin heavy chains. Symptoms, diagnosis, and treatment vary according to the specific disorder.

Heavy chain diseases are plasma cell disorders that are generally malignant. In most plasma cell disorders, M-proteins are structurally similar to normal antibody molecules. In contrast, in heavy chain diseases, incomplete monoclonal immunoglobulins (true paraproteins) are produced. These consist of only heavy chain components (either α, γ, μ, or δ) without light chains. (ε heavy chain disease has not been described.) Most heavy chain proteins are fragments of their normal counterparts with internal deletions of variable length; these deletions appear to result from structural mutations. The clinical picture is more like lymphoma than multiple myeloma. Heavy chain diseases are considered in patients with clinical manifestations suggesting lymphoproliferative disorders.

IgA Heavy Chain (α-Chain) Disease

IgA heavy chain disease is the most common heavy chain disease and is similar to Medi-

TABLE 144–1. CLASSIFICATION OF PLASMA CELL DISORDERS

CATEGORY	SYMPTOMS	DISORDER	COMMENTS AND EXAMPLES
Monoclonal gammopathy of undetermined significance	Asymptomatic, usually nonprogressive	Associated with nonlymphoreticular tumors	Especially carcinomas of the prostate, kidney, GI tract, breast, and biliary tree
		Associated with chronic inflammatory and infectious conditions	Chronic cholecystitis, osteomyelitis, TB, pyelonephritis, RA
		Associated with various other disorders	Lichen myxedematosus, liver disease, thyrotoxicosis, pernicious anemia, myasthenia gravis, Gaucher's disease, familial hypercholesterolemia, Kaposi's sarcoma
			Occurs in apparently healthy people; age-related incidence
Malignant plasma cell disorders	Symptomatic, progressive	Macroglobulinemia	IgM
		Multiple myeloma	Most often IgG, IgA, or light chains (Bence Jones) only
		Nonhereditary primary systemic amyloidosis	Usually light chains (Bence Jones) only, but occasionally intact immunoglobulin molecules (IgG, IgA, IgM, IgD)
		Heavy chain diseases	IgG heavy chain (γ-chain) disease (sometimes benign) IgA heavy chain (α-chain) disease IgM heavy chain (μ-chain) disease IgD heavy chain (δ-chain) disease
Transient plasma cell disorders			Associated with drug hypersensitivity, viral infections, and heart surgery

terranean lymphoma or immunoproliferative small bowel disease.

IgA heavy chain disease usually appears between ages 10 and 30 and is geographically concentrated in the Middle East. The cause may be an aberrant immune response to a parasite or other microorganism. Villous atrophy and plasma cell infiltration of the jejunal mucosa is usually present and, sometimes, mesenteric lymph nodes. The peripheral lymph nodes, bone marrow, liver, and spleen usually are not involved. A respiratory tract form of the disease has been reported rarely. Osteolytic lesions do not occur.

Almost all patients present with diffuse abdominal lymphoma and malabsorption. Serum protein electrophoresis is normal in half of cases; often, there is an increased α_2 and β fraction or a decreased γ fraction. Diagnosis requires the detection of a monoclonal α chain on immunofixation electrophoresis. This chain is sometimes found in concentrated urine. If it cannot be found in serum or urine, biopsy is required. The abnormal protein can sometimes be detected in intestinal secretions. The intestinal cellular infiltrate may be pleomorphic and not overtly malignant. Bence Jones proteinuria is absent.

The course is highly variable: Some patients die in 1 to 2 yr, whereas others have remissions that last many years, particularly after treatment with corticosteroids, cytotoxic drugs, and broad-spectrum antibiotics.

IgG Heavy Chain (γ-Chain) Disease

IgG heavy chain disease is generally similar to an aggressive malignant lymphoma but is occasionally asymptomatic and benign.

IgG heavy chain disease occurs primarily in elderly men but can occur in children. Associated chronic disorders include RA, Sjögren's syndrome, SLE, TB, myasthenia gravis, hypereosinophilic syndrome, autoimmune hemolytic anemia, and thyroiditis. Reductions in normal immunoglobulin levels occur. Lytic bone lesions are uncommon. Amyloidosis sometimes develops. Common manifestations include lymphadenopathy and hepatosplenomegaly, fever, and recurring infections. Palatal edema is present in about 1/4 of patients.

The CBC may show anemia, leukopenia, thrombocytopenia, eosinophilia, and circulating atypical lymphocytes or plasma cells. Diagnosis requires demonstration by immunofixation of free monoclonal heavy chain fragments of IgG in serum and urine. Of affected patients, 1/2 have monoclonal serum components > 1 g/dL (often broad and heterogeneous), and 1/2 have proteinuria > 1 g/24 h. Although heavy chain proteins may involve any IgG subclass, the G3 subclass is especially common. Bone marrow or lymph node biopsy, performed if other tests are not diagnostic, reveals variable histopathology.

The median survival with aggressive disease is about 1 yr. Death usually results from bacterial infection or progressive malignancy. Alkylating drugs, vincristine, or corticosteroids and radiation therapy may yield transient remissions.

IgM Heavy Chain (μ-Chain) Disease

IgM heavy chain disease, which is rare, produces a clinical picture similar to chronic lymphocytic leukemia or other lymphoproliferative disorders.

IgM heavy chain disease most often affects adults > 50 yr. Visceral organ involvement (spleen, liver, abdominal lymph nodes) is common, but extensive peripheral lymphadenopathy is not. Pathologic fractures and amyloidosis may occur. Serum protein electrophoresis usually is normal or shows hypogammaglobulinemia. Bence Jones proteinuria (type κ) is present in 10 to 15% of patients. Diagnosis usually requires bone marrow examination; vacuolated plasma cells are present in 2/3 of patients and, when present, are virtually pathognomonic. Death can occur in a few months or in many years. The usual cause of death is uncontrollable proliferation of chronic lymphocytic leukemia cells. Treatment may consist of alkylating agents plus corticosteroids or may be similar to treatment of the lymphoproliferative disorder that it most closely resembles.

MACROGLOBULINEMIA

(Primary Macroglobulinemia; Waldenström's Macroglobulinemia)

Macroglobulinemia is a malignant plasma cell disorder in which B cells produce excessive amounts of IgM M-proteins. Manifestations may include hyperviscosity, bleeding, recurring infections, and generalized adenopathy. Diagnosis requires bone marrow examination and demonstration of M-protein. Treatment includes plasmapheresis as needed for hyperviscosity, and systemic therapy with alkylating agents, corticosteroids, nucleoside analogs, or rituxan.

Macroglobulinemia is clinically more similar to a lymphomatous disease than to myeloma and other plasma cell disorders. Cause is unknown. Men are affected more often than women; median age is 65.

Macroglobulinemia develops in about 12% of patients with monoclonal gammopathy. Excessive amounts of IgM M-proteins can also accumulate in other disorders, causing manifestations similar to macroglobulinemia. Small monoclonal IgM components are present in the sera of about 5% of patients with B-cell non-Hodgkin lymphoma; this circumstance is termed macroglobulinemic lymphoma. Additionally, IgM M-proteins are occasionally present in patients with chronic lymphocytic leukemia or other lymphoproliferative disorders.

Many clinical manifestations of macroglobulinemia are due to the large amount of high mol wt monoclonal IgM proteins circulating in plasma. Some of these proteins are antibodies directed toward autologous IgG (rheumatoid factors) or I antigens (cold agglutinins). About 10% are cryoglobulins. Secondary amyloidosis occurs in 5% of patients.

Symptoms and Signs

Most patients are asymptomatic, but many present with manifestations of hyperviscosity syndrome: fatigue, weakness, skin and mucosal bleeding, visual disturbances, headache, symptoms of peripheral neuropathy, and other changing neurologic manifestations. An increased plasma volume can precipitate heart failure. Cold sensitivity, Raynaud's phenomenon, or recurring bacterial infections may occur.

Examination may disclose generalized lymphadenopathy, hepatosplenomegaly, and purpura. Marked engorgement and localized narrowing of retinal veins, which resemble sausage links, suggests hyperviscosity syndrome. Retinal hemorrhages, exudates, microaneurysms, and papilledema occur in late stages.

Diagnosis

Macroglobulinemia is suspected in patients with symptoms of hyperviscosity or other typical symptoms, particularly if anemia is present. However, it is often diagnosed incidentally when protein electrophoresis reveals an M-protein that proves to be IgM by immunofixation. Laboratory evaluation includes tests used to evaluate plasma cell disorders (see Multiple Myeloma on p. 1129) as well as measurement of cryoglobulins, rheumatoid factor, cold agglutinins, coagulation studies, and direct Coombs' test.

Moderate normocytic, normochromic anemia, marked rouleau formation, and a very high ESR are typical. Leukopenia, relative lymphocytosis, and thrombocytopenia occasionally occur. Cryoglobulins, rheumatoid factor, or cold agglutinins may be present; if cold agglutinins are present, the direct Coombs' test usually is positive. Various coagulation and platelet function abnormalities may occur. Results of routine blood studies may be spurious if cryoglobulinemia or marked hyperviscosity is present. Normal immunoglobulins are decreased in ½ of patients.

Immunofixation electrophoresis of concentrated urine frequently shows a monoclonal light chain (usually κ), but gross Bence Jones proteinuria is unusual. Bone marrow studies show a variable increase in plasma cells, lymphocytes, plasmacytoid lymphocytes, and mast cells. Periodic acid-Schiff–positive material may be present in lymphoid cells. Lymph node biopsy, performed if marrow examination is normal, is frequently interpreted as diffuse well-differentiated or plasmacytic lymphocytic lymphoma. Serum viscosity is measured to confirm suspected hyperviscosity and is usually > 4.0 (normal, 1.4 to 1.8).

Prognosis and Treatment

The course is variable, with a median survival of 7 to 10 yr. Age > 60 yr, anemia, and cryoglobulinemia predict shorter survival.

Often, patients require no treatment for many years. If hyperviscosity is present, initial treatment is plasmapheresis, which rapidly reverses bleeding as well as neurologic abnormalities. Plasmapheresis often needs to be repeated.

Long-term treatment with oral alkylating drugs may be indicated for palliation, but bone marrow toxicity can occur. Nucleoside analogs (fludarabine and 2-chlorodeoxyadenosine) produce responses in large numbers of newly diagnosed patients. Rituxan can reduce tumor burden without suppressing normal hematopoiesis.

MONOCLONAL GAMMOPATHY OF UNDETERMINED SIGNIFICANCE

Monoclonal gammopathy of undetermined significance is the production of M-protein by noncancerous plasma cells in the absence of other manifestations typical of multiple myeloma.

The incidence of monoclonal gammopathy of undetermined significance (MGUS) increases with age, from 1% of people aged 25 yr to 4% of people > 70 yr. MGUS may occur in association with other diseases (see TABLE 144–1), in which case M-proteins may be antibodies produced in large amounts in response to protracted antigenic stimuli.

MGUS usually is asymptomatic, but peripheral neuropathy can occur. Although most cases are benign, up to 25% (1%/yr) progress to a B-cell malignancy, myeloma, or macroglobulinemia.

M-protein in blood or urine usually is detected incidentally during a routine examination. On laboratory evaluation, M-protein is present in low levels in serum (< 3 g/dL) or urine (< 300 mg/24 h). MGUS is differentiated from other plasma cell disorders because

M-protein levels remain stable over time, levels of other serum immunoglobulins are normal, and lytic bone lesions, anemia, and Bence Jones proteinuria are absent in most cases. Bone marrow shows only mild plasmacytosis.

No treatment is recommended. Patients should undergo evaluation q 6 to 12 mo with clinical examination and serum and urine protein electrophoresis.

MULTIPLE MYELOMA

(Myelomatosis; Plasma Cell Myeloma)

Multiple myeloma is a malignancy of plasma cells that produce monoclonal immunoglobulin and invade and destroy adjacent bone tissue. Common manifestations include bone pain, renal insufficiency, hypercalcemia, anemia, and recurrent infections. Diagnosis requires demonstration of M-protein (sometimes present in urine and not serum) and either lytic bone lesions, light-chain proteinuria, or excessive marrow plasma cells. A bone marrow biopsy is usually needed. Specific treatment includes conventional chemotherapy (usually with alkylating agents, corticosteroids, anthracyclines, or thalidomide) and high-dose melphalan followed by autologous peripheral blood stem cell transplantation.

The incidence of multiple myeloma is 2 to 4/100,000. Male:female ratio is 1.6:1, and most patients are > 40 yr. Prevalence in blacks is twice that in whites. Etiology is unknown, although chromosomal and genetic factors, radiation, and chemicals have been suggested.

Pathophysiology

Plasma cell tumors (plasmacytomas) produce IgG in about 55% of myeloma patients and IgA in about 20%; of these patients, 40% also have Bence Jones proteinuria, which is free monoclonal κ or λ light chains in the urine. In 15 to 20% of patients, plasma cells secrete only Bence Jones protein. These patients tend to have a higher incidence of lytic bone lesions, hypercalcemia, renal failure, and amyloidosis than do other myeloma patients. IgD myeloma accounts for about 1% of cases.

Diffuse osteoporosis or discrete osteolytic lesions develop, usually in the pelvis, spine, ribs, and skull. Lesions are caused by bone replacement by expanding plasmacytomas or by cytokines that are secreted by malignant plasma cells and that activate osteoclasts. The osteolytic lesions are usually multiple; occasionally, they are solitary intramedullary masses. Extraosseous plasmacytomas are unusual but may occur in any tissue, especially in the upper respiratory tract.

Hypercalcemia and anemia commonly develop. Renal failure (myeloma kidney) may occur; mechanisms include extensive cast formation in the renal tubules, atrophy of tubular epithelial cells, and interstitial fibrosis.

Susceptibility to bacterial infection results from decreased production of normal immunoglobulin and other factors. Secondary amyloidosis (see p. 1311) occurs in 10% of myeloma patients, most often in those with Bence Jones proteinuria.

Variant expressions of multiple myeloma occur (see TABLE 144–2).

TABLE 144–2. VARIANT EXPRESSIONS OF MULTIPLE MYELOMA

FORM	CHARACTERISTICS
Extramedullary plasmacytoma	Plasmacytomas that occur outside of the medullary system
Solitary plasmacytoma of bone	Single bone plasmacytomas, which usually produce no M-protein
Osteosclerotic myeloma (POEMS syndrome)	*P*olyneuropathy (chronic inflammatory polyneuropathy), *O*rganomegaly (hepatomegaly, splenomegaly, or lymphadenopathy), *E*ndocrinopathy (eg, gynecomastia, testicular atrophy), *M*-protein, and *S*kin changes (eg, hyperpigmentation, excess hair)
Nonsecretory myeloma	Absence of M-protein in serum and urine; presence of M-protein in plasma cells

Symptoms and Signs

Persistent bone pain (especially in the back or thorax), renal failure, and recurring bacterial infections are the most common presentations. Pathologic fractures are common, and vertebral collapse may lead to spinal cord compression and paraplegia. Symptoms of anemia predominate or may be the sole reason for evaluation in some patients, and a few have manifestations of hyperviscosity syndrome (see p. 1128). Peripheral neuropathy, carpal tunnel syndrome, abnormal bleeding, and symptoms of hypercalcemia (eg, polyuria, polydipsia) are common. Lymphadenopathy and hepatosplenomegaly are unusual.

Diagnosis

Multiple myeloma is suspected in patients > 40 yr with persistent unexplained bone pain, particularly at night or at rest, other typical symptoms, or unexplained laboratory abnormalities, such as elevated blood or urine protein levels, hypercalcemia, renal insufficiency, or anemia. Laboratory evaluation includes routine blood tests, protein electrophoresis, x-rays, and bone marrow examination.

Routine blood tests include CBC, ESR, and chemistry panel. Anemia is present in 80%, usually normocytic-normochromic with formation of rouleau, which are clusters of 3 to 12 RBCs that occur in stacks. WBC and platelet counts usually are normal. ESR usually is > 100 mm/h, and BUN, serum creatinine, and serum uric acid are frequently elevated. Anion gap is sometimes low. Hypercalcemia is present at diagnosis in about 10%.

Protein electrophoresis is performed on serum and, if results are inconclusive, on a urine sample concentrated from a 24-h collection. Serum electrophoresis identifies M-protein in about 80 to 90% of patients. The remaining 10 to 20% are usually those with only free monoclonal light chains (Bence Jones protein) or IgD. They almost always have M-protein detected by urine protein electrophoresis. Immunofixation electrophoresis can identify the immunoglobulin class of the M-protein and can often detect light-chain protein if the serum immunoelectrophoresis is falsely negative; immunofixation electrophoresis is obtained even if the serum test is negative if multiple myeloma is strongly suspected. Serum level of β_2-microglobulin is frequently elevated and correlates with myeloma cell mass.

X-rays include a skeletal survey. Punched-out lytic lesions or diffuse osteoporosis is present in 80% of cases. Radionuclide bone scans usually are not helpful. MRI can provide more detail and is obtained if pain or neurologic symptoms are present and plain films are nondiagnostic.

Bone marrow aspiration and biopsy are usually performed. They may reveal sheets or clusters of plasma cells diagnostic of marrow tumors. However, marrow involvement is patchy, and only increased numbers of plasma cells at various stages of maturation may be found. Still, the number of marrow plasma cells is rarely normal. Plasma cell morphology does not correlate with the class of immunoglobulin synthesized.

In the patient with serum M protein, myeloma is indicated by Bence Jones proteinuria > 300 mg/24 h, osteolytic lesions (without evidence of metastatic carcinoma or granulomatous disease), and sheets or clusters of marrow plasma cells.

Prognosis and Treatment

The disease is progressive, with median survival about 3 to 4 yr with conventional therapy and 4 to 5 yr with high-dose therapy and stem cell transplantation. Treatment improves the quality and duration of life in about 60% of patients. Unfavorable prognostic signs at diagnosis include high levels of M-protein in serum or urine, elevated serum β_2-microglobulin levels (> 6 μg/mL), diffuse bone lesions, hypercalcemia, anemia, and renal failure.

Multiple supportive measures are needed. Maintenance of ambulation helps preserve bone density. Analgesics and palliative doses of radiation therapy (18 to 24 Gy) can relieve bone pain. However, radiation therapy may impair the patient's ability to receive cytotoxic doses of systemic chemotherapy. All patients should also receive a bisphosphonate, which reduces skeletal complications, lessens bone pain, and may have an antitumor effect.

Adequate hydration prevents further renal compromise. Even patients with prolonged, massive Bence Jones proteinuria (≥ 10 to 30 g/day) may have intact renal function if they maintain urine output > 2000 mL/day. *Dehydration combined with high-osmolar IV contrast may precipitate acute oliguric renal failure in patients with Bence Jones proteinuria.*

Hydration and bisphosphonates, sometimes with prednisone 60 to 80 mg po once/day, are used to treat hypercalcemia. Although most patients do not require allopurinol, 300 mg po once/day is indicated if renal insufficiency is present or if hyperuricemia causes symptoms.

Pneumococcal and influenza vaccines are indicated to prevent infection. Antibiotics are indicated for documented bacterial infection, but prophylactic use is not routinely recommended. Prophylactic IV immune globulin may reduce the risk of infection but is generally reserved for patients with recurring infections.

Recombinant erythropoietin (40,000 units sc q wk) is used in patients whose anemia is inadequately relieved by chemotherapy. If anemia produces cardiovascular symptoms, packed RBCs are transfused. Plasmapheresis is indicated if hyperviscosity develops (see p. 1128). Chemotherapy response is indicated by decreases in serum or urine M-protein. Infection is particularly likely during chemotherapy-induced neutropenia.

Conventional chemotherapy consists of oral melphalan (0.15 mg/kg once/day) and prednisone (20 mg tid) at cycles of 6 wk with evaluation of response in 3 to 6 mo. Combination chemotherapy can be provided with a variety of IV drug regimens; it does not improve overall outcomes compared to melphalan and prednisone but may produce more rapid responses in patients with renal dysfunction. Autologous peripheral blood stem cell transplantation is considered for patients < 70 yr who have adequate cardiac, hepatic, pulmonary, and renal function, particularly those whose disease is stable or responsive after several courses of conventional chemotherapy. These patients receive initial chemotherapy with vincristine, doxorubicin, or dexamethasone or with dexamethasone and thalidomide. Adjunctive myeloid growth factor is given, and drugs that kill stem cells, such as alkylating agents and nitrosoureas, are avoided. Whether multiple courses of melphalan improves these results is under investigation. Allogeneic stem cell transplantation after nonablative therapy (eg, low-dose cyclophosphamide and fludarabine or radiation therapy) can produce myeloma-free survival of 5 to 10 yr in some patients because of decreased toxicity and the donor's allogeneic immune anti-myeloma effect. This treatment is indicated for patients < 55 yr who have good physiologic reserve. In relapsed or refractory myeloma, new therapies (eg, thalidomide, immunomodulatory drugs, proteasome inhibitors) can produce responses; these drugs are also being evaluated as 1st-line treatment for early disease.

Maintenance therapy has been tried with nonchemotherapeutic drugs, including interferon, which prolongs remission but has adverse effects. Corticosteroids are being evaluated.

145 IRON OVERLOAD

(Hemosiderosis; Hemochromatosis)

(For iron poisoning, see p. 2667.)

Iron (Fe) in excess of bodily needs is deposited in tissues as hemosiderin. Iron deposition resulting in tissue damage (or total body iron content > 5 g) is termed hemochromatosis. Focal or generalized iron deposition without associated tissue damage is hemosiderosis. Iron overload may occur as a primary (genetic) disorder of iron metabolism or secondary to other disorders that involve excessive intake or release of iron. Excess iron accumulates in nearly all tissues, but most morbidity results from deposition in the liver, thyroid, pituitary, hypothalamus, heart, pancreas, and joints. Liver involvement can lead to elevated aminotransferase (ALT and AST) levels, bridging fibrosis, or cirrhosis.

Hemosiderosis: Focal hemosiderosis can result from recurrent hemorrhage within an organ. Iron liberated from extravasated RBCs is deposited within that organ, and significant hemosiderin deposits may eventually develop. The organ usually affected is the lung, and the cause usually is recurrent pulmonary hemorrhage, either idiopathic (eg, Goodpasture's syndrome) or that occurring in conditions causing chronic pulmonary hypertension (eg, primary pulmonary hypertension, pulmonary fibrosis, severe mitral stenosis). Occasionally, iron loss from these episodes causes iron deficiency anemia, because iron in the tissue cannot be reused.

Renal hemosiderosis can result from extensive intravascular hemolysis (see p. 1045). Free Hb is filtered at the glomerulus, and iron is deposited in the kidneys. The renal parenchyma is not damaged, but severe hemosiderinuria may result in iron deficiency.

PRIMARY HEMOCHROMATOSIS

Primary hemochromatosis is an inherited disorder characterized by excessive iron accumulation causing tissue damage. Symptoms do not develop until organ damage, often irreversible, develops. Symptoms include fatigue, hepatomegaly, bronze skin pigmentation, loss of libido, arthalgias, and manifestations of cirrhosis, diabetes, or cardiomyopathy. Diagnosis is based on serum iron studies and gene assay. Treatment is with serial phlebotomies.

Etiology and Pathophysiology

Nearly all primary hemochromatosis is caused by a mutation of the *HFE* gene. Non-*HFE* primary hemochromatosis is uncommon and includes ferroportin disease, juvenile hemochromatosis, and the very rare neonatal hemochromatosis, hypotransferrinemia, and aceruloplasminemia. The clinical consequences of iron overload are the same in all types.

Over 80% of *HFE*-related hemochromatosis is caused by the homozygous C282Y or C282Y/H63D compound heterozygote mutation. The disorder is autosomal recessive, with a homozygous frequency of 1:200 and a heterozygous frequency of 1:8 in Northern Europeans. It is uncommon in blacks and rare in Asians. Of patients with clinical hemochromatosis, 83% are homozygous. The mechanism for iron overload is increased iron absorption from the GI tract, leading to chronic deposition of iron in the tissue. Hepcidin, a recently identified liver-derived peptide, is the critical control mechanism for iron absorption. Hepcidin, along with the normal *HFE* gene, prevents excessive iron absorption and storage in the normal individual.

Total body iron content can reach as high as 50 g, compared with the normal levels of about 2.5 g in women and 3.5 g in men. Iron deposition in organs catalyzes generation of reactive free hydroxyl radicals.

Symptoms and Signs

Symptoms are uncommon before middle age. Of affected men, 80 to 90% have total body iron stores > 10 g before symptoms develop. In women, symptoms are uncommon before menopause, because iron loss during menses and pregnancy provides some protection.

Because iron accumulates in multiple sites, symptoms can develop referable to many possible organs or systemically. In women, fatigue and nonspecific constitutional symptoms develop early; in men, cirrhosis or diabetes is often the initial presentation. Hypogonadism is common in both sexes as well and may predate other manifestations. Liver disease is the most common complication, and in cases that progress to cirrhosis, about 20 to 30% progress further to hepatocellular carcinoma. Ten to 15% of untreated patients develop heart failure; 90%, excessive skin pigmentation; 65%, diabetes and its potential sequelae (nephropathy, retinopathy, neuropathy); and 25 to 50%, arthropathy.

Diagnosis

Hemochromatosis is suspected in patients with typical symptoms, particularly unexplained hepatic abnormalities, and in patients with a family history. Because symptoms develop only after tissue injury, diagnosis before symptoms develop is desirable (but difficult). If hemochromatosis is suspected, testing includes serum iron, serum transferrin saturation, serum ferritin, and gene assay.

Serum iron is increased (> 300 mg/dL). Serum transferrin saturation is usually > 50% and often > 90%. Serum ferritin is increased. Gene assay establishes the diagnosis; nongenetic mechanisms of iron overload, such as congenital hemolytic states (eg, sickle cell anemia, thalassemia) must be ruled out. Hepatic iron content can be estimated with a high-intensity MRI where available. Because cirrhosis markedly affects prognosis, a liver biopsy is done if serum ferritin is unexpectedly high (eg, > 1000, but cutoffs should be adjusted for age, which can increase levels, and for elevated liver enzymes, which can decrease levels). Liver iron content can also be measured to further confirm tissue iron deposition.

First-degree relatives of people with primary hemochromatosis should be screened. Testing for C282Y and H63D identifies > 95% of cases.

Treatment

Phlebotomy is the simplest method of excess iron removal in most cases. It prolongs survival but does not prevent hepatocellular carcinoma. As soon as the diagnosis is made, about 500 mL/wk of blood (about 250 mg of iron) is removed weekly until serum iron levels are normal and transferrin saturation is < 50%. Weekly phlebotomy may be needed for several years. When iron levels are normal, further phlebotomy can be performed to maintain transferrin saturation at < 30%. Diabetes, cardiac abnormalities, erectile dysfunction, and other secondary manifestations are treated as indicated.

Ferroportin Disease

Ferroportin disease occurs largely in southern Europeans. It results from an autosomal dominant mutation in the *SLC 40 A1* gene. It manifests in the 1st decade of life as increased serum ferritin with low or normal transferrin, with progressive saturation of transferrin in the 3rd to 4th decades. Clinical manifestations are milder than in *HFE* disease, with modest liver disease and mild anemia. Tolerance to vigorous phlebotomy is poor; serial monitoring of Hb and transferrin saturation is required.

Juvenile Hemochromatosis

This is a rare autosomal recessive disease due to mutations in the *HJV* gene affecting the transcription protein hemojuvelin. It often presents in adolescents. Ferritin levels are > 1000, and transferrin saturation is > 90%. Symptoms and signs include progressive hepatomegaly and hypogonadotropic hypogonadism.

Transferrin and Ceruloplasmin Deficiency

(Hypotransferrinemia/atransferrinemia; Aceruloplasminemia)

In transferrin deficiency, absorbed iron that enters the portal system as nontransferrin-bound iron is deposited in the liver. Subsequent transfer to sites of RBC production is reduced because of the transferrin deficiency. In ceruloplasmin deficiency, lack of ferroxidase results in defective conversion of Fe^{2+} to Fe^{3+}, which is necessary for binding to transferrin; this impairs the movement of iron from intracellular stores to plasma transport, resulting in tissue iron accumulation.

These transport defects are suspected in patients with iron overload that develops at an early age or when overload is found but genetic testing results are normal. Diagnosis is based on measurement of serum transferrin (ie, iron-binding capacity) and ceruloplasmin (see Inherited Copper Toxicity on p. 51). Treatment is experimental.

An autosomal recessive form of hemochromatosis occurs with mutations in transferrin receptor 2, a protein that appears to control saturation of transferrin. Symptoms and signs are similar to *HFE* hemochromatosis.

SECONDARY IRON OVERLOAD

Secondary iron overload can result from thalassemias or sideroblastic anemias, both disorders of erythropoiesis. Secondary acquired iron overload can occur after exogenous iron administration, repeated or unusually massive transfusion, or iron-dextran treatments. Each unit of blood transfused provides 250 mg of iron. Significant tissue deposition is likely with ≥ 20 g (ie, about 80 units of blood). Overload also can occur in conditions of defective erythropoiesis, such as thalassemia, sideroblastic anemia, hemoglobinopathies, and RBC enzyme defects. With defective erythropoiesis, iron absorption increases, possibly mediated by hepcidin. These conditions of defective erythropoiesis themselves can usually be identified by clinical history. Iron overload is identified by the elevations in serum iron, transferrin saturation, and serum ferritin.

Phlebotomy may not be helpful, because these disorders sometimes cause anemia, thereby limiting the ability to remove enough blood. If anemia is present, deferoxamine (1 to 2 g once/day over 8 to 24 h in adults; 20 to 40 mg/kg/day over 8 to 12 h in children) should be given as a slow IV infusion overnight through a small portable subcutaneous pump for 5 to 7 days/wk; this process effectively reduces iron stores. Because tachyphylaxis occurs with deferoxamine therapy, continued efficacy must be evaluated (usually by urine iron measurement). Alternatively, salmon-colored urine confirms > 50 mg/day of iron in the urine. Treatment goals and monitoring (with serum iron levels and transferrin) are the same as for primary hemochromatosis (see p. 1132).

Overload of Unknown Origin

Parenchymal liver diseases, especially alcoholic liver disease, nonalcoholic steatohepatitis, and chronic hepatitis C infection, can be associated with increased iron storage. The mechanisms are unknown, although primary hemochromatosis can exist simultaneously and should be excluded. Reducing iron stores does not appear to relieve liver dysfunction if these patients do not have primary hemochromatosis.

146 TRANSFUSION MEDICINE

More than 23 million units of blood components are transfused yearly in the US. Although transfusion is probably safer than ever, risk (and the public's perception of risk) mandates informed consent whenever practical.

BLOOD COLLECTION

In the US, the collection, storage, and transport of blood and its components are standardized and regulated by the FDA, the American Association of Blood Banks, and sometimes state or local health authorities. Donor screening includes an extensive questionnaire and health interview; measurement of temperature, heart rate, and BP; and Hb determination. Some potential donors are deferred either temporarily or permanently (see TABLE 146–1). Criteria for deferral protect prospective donors from possible ill effects of donation, and recipients from disease. Donations are limited to once every 56 days. With rare exceptions, blood donors are unpaid.

TABLE 146–1. REASONS FOR BLOOD DONATION DEFERRAL OR DENIAL

DEFERRAL	DENIAL
Anemia	AIDS, participation in high-risk activity (eg, IV drug use, sexual intercourse with person with HIV), male homosexuals
Certain drugs	Bovine insulin use since 1980
Certain vaccinations	Cancer (other than mild treatable forms, eg, small skin cancers)
Malaria or exposure to malaria	Congenital bleeding disorder
Pregnancy	Hepatitis
Received transfusion within previous 12 mo	Military personnel residing on US base in UK, Germany, Belgium, Netherlands ≥ 6 mo between 1980 and 1990 or elsewhere in Europe between 1980 and 1996
Recent exposure to hepatitis	Recipient of any blood component between 1980 and present in the UK
Recent tattoo	Severe asthma
Uncontrolled hypertension	Severe heart disease
	Stay in UK (cumulative > 3 mo between 1980 and 1996), Europe (cumulative ≥ 5 yr since 1980), and France (> 5 yr since 1980)

In standard blood donation, 450 mL of whole blood is collected in a plastic bag containing an anticoagulant preservative. Whole blood or packed RBCs preserved with citrate-phosphate-dextrose-adenine may be stored for 35 days. Packed RBCs may be stored for 42 days if an adenine-dextrose-saline solution is added.

Autologous donation, which is use of the patient's own blood, is the safest method of transfusion when conditions permit. In the 2 to 3 wk preceding elective surgery, 3 or 4 units of whole blood or packed RBCs are collected, and the patient is given iron supplements. Special blood salvage procedures are also available for collecting and autotransfusing blood shed after trauma and during surgery.

Pretransfusion Testing

Donor blood testing includes ABO and Rh_0 (D) antigen typing, antibody screening, and testing for infectious disease markers (see TABLE 146–2).

Compatibility testing tests the recipient's RBCs for antigens A, B, and Rh_0(D); screens the recipient's serum for antibodies against other RBC antigens; and includes a crossmatch to ensure that the recipient's serum is compatible with antigens on donor RBCs. Compatibility testing is done before a transfusion; however, in an emergency, testing is done after releasing blood from the blood bank. It can also help in diagnosing transfusion reactions.

ABO typing of donor and recipient blood is done to prevent transfusion of incompatible RBCs (see FIG. 146–1). As a rule, blood for transfusion should be of the same ABO type as that of the recipient. In urgent situations or when the correct ABO type is in doubt or unknown, type O Rh-negative packed RBCs (not whole blood—see Acute Hemolytic Transfusion Reaction on p. 1138), which contains neither A nor B antigens, may be used for patients of any ABO type.

Rh typing determines whether the Rh factor Rh_0(D) is present (Rh-positive) or absent (Rh-negative) on the RBCs. Rh-negative patients should always receive Rh-negative blood ex-

TABLE 146–2. INFECTIOUS DISEASE TRANSMISSION TESTING

NUCLEIC ACID TESTING	ANTIGEN TESTING	ANTIBODY TESTING
Hepatitis C virus	Hepatitis B surface	Hepatitis B core
HIV	HIV-1 p24	Hepatitis C*
West Nile virus	Syphilis	HIV-1 and -2* Human T-cell lymphotropic viruses I and III

*If antibody is positive, it is confirmed by Western blot or recombinant immunoblotting assay.

cept in life-threatening emergencies when Rh-negative blood is unavailable. Rh-positive patients may receive Rh-positive or Rh-negative blood. Occasionally, RBCs from some Rh-positive people react weakly on standard Rh typing (weak D, or D^u, positive), but these people are still considered Rh-positive.

Antibody screening for unexpected anti-RBC antibodies is routinely done on blood from prospective recipients and prenatally on maternal specimens. Unexpected anti-RBC antibodies are specific for RBC blood group antigens other than A and B [eg, $Rh_0(D)$, Kell (K), Duffy (Fy)]. Early detection is important, because such antibodies can cause serious hemolytic transfusion reactions or hemolytic disease of the newborn (see p. 2272), and they may greatly complicate compatibility testing and delay procurement of compatible blood.

Indirect antiglobulin testing (the indirect Coombs' test) is used to screen for unexpected anti-RBC antibodies. This test may be positive in the presence of an unexpected blood group antibody or when free (non-RBC–attached) antibody is present in autoimmune hemolytic anemias (see p. 1047). Reagent RBCs are mixed with the patient's serum, incubated, washed, tested with antihuman globulin, and observed for agglutination. Once an antibody is detected, its specificity is determined. Knowing the specificity of the antibody is helpful for assessing its clinical significance, selecting compatible blood, and managing hemolytic disease of the newborn.

Direct antiglobulin testing (the direct Coombs' test) detects antibodies that have coated the patient's RBCs in vivo. It is used when immune-mediated hemolysis is suspected. Patients' RBCs are directly tested with antihuman globulin and observed for agglutination. A positive result, if correlated with clinical findings, suggests autoimmune hemolytic anemia, drug-induced hemolysis, a transfusion reaction, or hemolytic disease of the newborn.

Antibody titration is performed when a clinically significant, unexpected anti-RBC antibody is identified in the serum of a pregnant woman or in a patient with cold autoimmune hemolytic anemia (see p. 1047). The maternal antibody titer correlates fairly well with the severity of hemolytic disease in the incompatible fetus and is often used to guide treatment in hemolytic disease of the newborn along with ultrasonography and amniotic fluid study.

The addition of a cross-match to ABO/Rh typing and antibody screening increases detection of incompatibility by only 0.01%. If the recipient has a clinically significant anti-RBC antibody, donor blood is restricted to RBC units negative for the corresponding antigen; further testing for compatibility is performed by combining recipient serum, donor RBCs, and antihuman globulin. In recipients without clinically significant anti-RBC antibodies, an immediate spin cross-match, which omits the antiglobulin phase, confirms ABO compatibility.

Emergency transfusion is performed when not enough time (generally < 60 min) is available for thorough compatibility testing because the patient is in hemorrhagic shock.

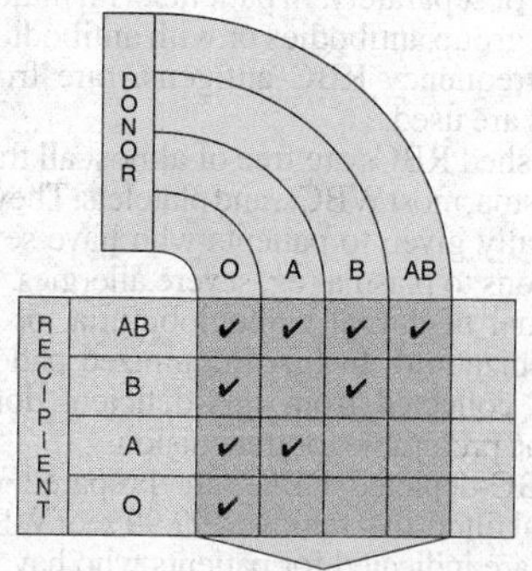

Fig. 146–1. Compatible RBC types.

When time permits (about 10 min is needed), ABO/Rh type-specific blood may be given. In more urgent circumstances, type O RBCs are transfused if the ABO type is uncertain, and Rh-negative blood is given if the Rh type is uncertain.

"Type and screen" may be requested in circumstances not likely to require transfusion, as in elective surgery. The patient's blood is typed for ABO/Rh antigens and screened for antibodies. If antibodies are absent and the patient needs blood, ABO/Rh type specific or compatible RBCs may be released without the antiglobulin phase of the cross-match. If an unexpected antibody is present, full testing is required.

BLOOD PRODUCTS

Whole blood can provide improved O_2-carrying capacity, volume expansion, and replacement of clotting factors and was previously recommended for rapid massive blood loss. However, because component therapy is equally effective and is a more efficient use of donated blood, whole blood is not generally available in the US.

RBCs are ordinarily the component of choice with which to increase Hb. Indications depend on the patient. O_2-carrying capacity may be adequate with Hb levels as low as 7 g/L in healthy patients, but transfusion may be indicated with higher Hb levels in patients with decreased cardiopulmonary reserve or ongoing bleeding. One unit of RBCs increases an average adult's Hb by about 1 g/dL and his Hct by about 3% of the pretransfusion Hct value. When only volume expansion is required, other fluids can be used concurrently or separately. In patients with multiple blood group antibodies or with antibodies to high-frequency RBC antigens, rare frozen RBCs are used.

Washed RBCs are free of almost all traces of plasma, most WBCs, and platelets. They are generally given to patients who have severe reactions to plasma (eg, severe allergies, paroxysmal nocturnal hemoglobinuria, or IgA immunization). In IgA-immunized patients, blood collected from IgA-deficient donors may be preferable for transfusion.

WBC-depleted RBCs are prepared with special filters that remove ≥99.99% of WBCs. They are indicated for patients who have experienced nonhemolytic febrile transfusion reactions, for exchange transfusions, for patients who require cytomegalovirus-negative blood that is unavailable, and possibly for the prevention of platelet alloimmunization.

Fresh frozen plasma (FFP) is an unconcentrated source of all clotting factors without platelets. Indications include correction of bleeding secondary to factor deficiencies for which specific factor replacements are unavailable, multifactor deficiency states (eg, massive transfusion, disseminated intravascular coagulation [DIC], liver failure), and urgent warfarin reversal. FFP can supplement RBCs when whole blood is unavailable for exchange transfusion. FFP should not be used simply for volume expansion.

Cryoprecipitate is a concentrate prepared from FFP. Each concentrate usually contains about 80 units each of factor VIII and von Willebrand factor and about 250 mg of fibrinogen. It also contains fibronectin and factor XIII. Although originally used for hemophilia and von Willebrand's disease, cryoprecipitate is currently used as a source of fibrinogen in acute DIC with bleeding, treatment of uremic bleeding, cardiothoracic surgery (fibrin glue), obstetric emergencies such as abruptio placentae and HELLP (*h*emolysis, *e*levated *l*iver enzymes, and *l*ow *p*latelet count) syndrome, and rare factor XIII deficiency. In general, it should not be used for other indications.

Granulocytes may be transfused when sepsis occurs in a patient with profound persistent neutropenia (WBCs < 500/μL) who is unresponsive to antibiotics. Granulocytes must be given within 24 h of harvest; however, testing for HIV, hepatitis, human T-cell lymphotrophic virus, and syphilis may not be completed before infusion. Because of improved antibiotic therapy and drugs that stimulate granulocyte production during chemotherapy, granulocytes are seldom used.

Rh immune globulin (RhIg), given IM or IV, prevents development of maternal Rh antibodies that can result from fetomaternal hemorrhage. The standard dose of intramuscular RhIg (300 μg) must be given to an Rh-negative mother immediately after abortion or delivery (live or stillborn) unless the infant is Rh_0(D) and D^u negative or the mother's serum already contains anti-Rh_0(D). If fetomaternal hemorrhage is > 30 mL, a larger dose is needed. If this is suspected, testing of the volume of fetomaternal hemorrhage begins with the screening rosette test, which, if positive, is followed by a quantitative test (eg, Kleihauer-Betke). RhIg is given IV only when IM administration is contraindicated (eg, in patients with coagulopathy).

Platelet concentrates are used to prevent bleeding in asymptomatic severe thrombocytopenia (platelet count < 10,000/μL), for bleeding patients with less severe thrombocytopenia (platelet count < 50,000/μL), for bleeding patients with platelet dysfunction due to antiplatelet drugs but with normal platelet count, for patients receiving massive transfusion that causes dilutional thrombocytopenia, and sometimes before invasive surgery, particularly with extracorporeal circulation for > 2 h (which often makes platelets dysfunctional). One platelet concentrate increases the platelet count by about 10,000/μL, and adequate hemostasis is achieved with a platelet count of about 50,000/μL. Therefore, 4 to 6 random donor platelet concentrates are commonly used in adults.

Platelet concentrates are increasingly being prepared by automated devices that harvest the platelets (or other cells) and return unneeded components (eg, RBCs, plasma) to the donor. This procedure, called cytapheresis, provides enough platelets from a single donation (equivalent to 6 random platelet units) for transfusion to an adult, which, because it minimizes infectious and immunogenic risks, is preferred to multiple donor transfusions.

Certain patients may not respond to platelet transfusions, possibly because of splenic sequestration or platelet consumption due to HLA or platelet-specific antigen alloimmunization. These patients may respond to multiple random donor platelets (because of greater likelihood that some units are HLA compatible), platelets from family members, or ABO- or HLA-matched platelets. Alloimmunization may be mitigated by transfusing WBC-depleted RBCs and WBC-depleted platelet concentrates.

Irradiated blood products are used to prevent graft-vs-host disease in patients at risk (see p. 1140).

Blood substitutes are being developed that use inert chemicals or hemoglobin solutions to carry and deliver O_2 to tissues. Perfluorocarbons are chemically and biologically inactive and are capable of dissolving O_2 and CO_2 under pressure. Because perfluorocarbons are not water miscible, they are prepared as emulsions. They are under phase II and III clinical trials. Hb-based O_2 carrier solutions are under phase III clinical trials in the US. Hb, human or bovine, is chemically modified, producing a solution capable of O_2 transport. These solutions can be stored at room temperature for up to 2 yr, making them attractive for transport to the site of trauma or to the battlefield. However, both perfluorocarbons and Hb-based O_2 carriers are cleared from plasma within 24 h.

TECHNIQUE OF TRANSFUSION

CAUTION: *Before transfusion is started, the patient's wristband, blood unit label, and compatibility test report must be checked at the bedside to ensure that the blood component is the one intended for the recipient.*

Use of an 18-gauge (or larger) needle prevents mechanical damage to and hemolysis of RBCs. A standard filter should always be used for infusion of any blood component. *Only 0.9% saline IV should be allowed into the blood bag or in the same tubing with blood.* Hypotonic solutions lyse RBCs, and the Ca in Ringer's lactate can cause clotting.

Transfusion of 1 unit of blood or blood component should be completed by 4 h; longer duration increases the risk of bacterial growth. If transfusion must be given slowly because of heart failure or hypervolemia, units may be divided into smaller aliquots in the blood bank. For children, 1 unit of blood can be provided in small sterile aliquots used over several days, thereby minimizing exposure to multiple donors.

Close observation is important, particularly during the first 15 min, and includes recording temperature, BP, pulse, and respiratory rate. Periodic observation continues throughout and after the transfusion, during which fluid status is assessed. The patient is kept covered and warm to prevent chills, which may be interpreted as a transfusion reaction. Elective transfusions at night are discouraged.

COMPLICATIONS OF TRANSFUSION

The most common complications of transfusion are febrile nonhemolytic and chill-rigor reactions. The most serious complications are acute hemolytic reaction due to ABO incompatible transfusion and transfusion-related acute lung injury, which have very high mortality rates.

Early recognition of symptoms suggestive of a transfusion reaction and prompt reporting to the blood bank are essential. The most common symptoms are chills, rigors, fever, dyspnea, light-headedness, urticaria, itching, and flank pain. If any of these symptoms (other than localized urticaria and itching) occur, the transfusion should be stopped immediately and the IV line kept open with normal saline. The remainder of the blood product and clotted and anticoagulated samples of the patient's blood should be sent to the blood bank for investigation. NOTE: *The unit in question should not be restarted, and transfusion of any previously issued unit should not be initiated.* Further transfusion should be delayed until the cause of the reaction is known, unless the need is urgent, in which case type O Rh-negative RBCs should be used.

Hemolysis of donor or recipient RBCs (usually the former) during or after transfusion can result from ABO/Rh incompatibility, plasma antibodies, or hemolyzed or fragile RBCs (eg, by overwarming stored blood or contact with hypotonic IV solutions). Hemolysis is most common and most severe when incompatible donor RBCs are hemolyzed by antibody in the recipient's plasma. Hemolytic reactions may be acute (within 24 h) or delayed (from 1 to 14 days).

Acute hemolytic transfusion reaction (AHTR): About 20 people die yearly in the US from AHTR. AHTR usually results from recipient plasma antibodies to donor RBC antigens. ABO incompatibility is the most common cause of AHTR. Antibodies against blood group antigens other than ABO can also cause AHTR. Mislabeling the recipient's pretransfusion sample at collection or failing to match the intended recipient with the blood product immediately before transfusion is the usual cause, not laboratory error.

Hemolysis is intravascular, causing hemoglobinuria with varying degrees of acute renal failure and possibly disseminated intravascular coagulation (DIC). The severity of AHTR depends on the degree of incompatibility, the amount of blood given, the rate of administration, and the integrity of the kidneys, liver, and heart. An acute phase usually develops within 1 h of initiation of transfusion, but it may occur later during the transfusion or immediately afterwards. Onset is usually abrupt. The patient may complain of discomfort and anxiety. Dyspnea, fever, chills, facial flushing, and severe pain may occur, especially in the lumbar area. Shock may develop, causing a rapid, feeble pulse; cold, clammy skin; low BP; and nausea and vomiting. Jaundice may follow acute hemolysis.

If AHTR occurs under general anesthesia, the only symptom may be hypotension, uncontrollable bleeding from incision sites and mucous membranes caused by an associated DIC, or dark urine that reflects hemoglobinuria.

If AHTR is suspected, one of the first steps is to recheck the sample and patient identifications. Diagnosis is confirmed by measuring urinary Hb, serum LDH, bilirubin, and haptoglobin. Intravascular hemolysis produces free Hb in the plasma and urine; haptoglobin levels are very low. Hyperbilirubinemia may follow.

After the acute phase, the degree of acute renal failure determines the prognosis. Diuresis and a decreasing BUN usually portend recovery. Permanent renal insufficiency is unusual. Prolonged oliguria and shock are poor prognostic signs.

If AHTR is suspected, the transfusion should be stopped and supportive treatment begun. The goal of initial therapy is to achieve and maintain adequate BP and renal blood flow with IV 0.9% saline and furosemide. IV saline is given to maintain urine output of 100 mL/h for 24 h. The initial furosemide dose is 40 to 80 mg (1 to 2 mg/kg in children), with later doses adjusted to maintain urinary flow > 100 mL/h during the first day.

Antihypertensive drugs must be administered with caution. Pressor drugs that decrease renal blood flow (eg, epinephrine, norepinephrine, high-dose dopamine) are contraindicated. If a pressor drug is necessary, dopamine 2 to 5 μg/kg/min is usually administered.

A nephrologist should be consulted as early as possible, particularly if no diuretic response occurs within about 2 to 3 h after initiating therapy, which may indicate acute tubular necrosis. Further fluid and diuretic therapy may be contraindicated, and early dialysis may be helpful.

Delayed hemolytic transfusion reaction: Occasionally, a patient who has been sensitized to an RBC antigen has very low antibody levels and negative pretransfusion tests. After transfusion with RBCs bearing this antigen, a primary or anamnestic response may result (usually in 1 to 4 wk) and cause a delayed hemolytic transfusion reaction. Delayed hemolytic transfusion reaction usually does not manifest as dramatically as AHTR. Patients may be asymptomatic or have a slight fever. Rarely, severe symptoms occur. Usually, only destruction of the transfused RBCs (with the antigen) occurs, resulting in a falling Hct and a slight rise in LDH and bilirubin. Because delayed hemolytic transfusion reaction is usually mild and self-limited, it is often unidentified, and the clinical clue may be an unexplained drop in Hb to the pretransfusion level occurring 1 to 2 wk posttransfusion. Severe reactions are treated similarly to acute reactions.

Febrile nonhemolytic transfusion reactions: Febrile reaction may occur without hemolysis. Antibodies directed against WBC HLA from otherwise compatible donor blood is one possible cause. This cause is most common in multitransfused or multiparous patients. Cytokines released from WBCs during storage, particularly in platelet concentrates, is another possible cause.

Clinically, febrile reactions consist of a temperature increase of ≥ 1° C, chills, and sometimes headache and back pain. Simultaneous symptoms of allergic reaction are common. Because fever and chills also herald a severe hemolytic transfusion reaction, all febrile reactions must be investigated as above, as with any transfusion reaction.

Most febrile reactions are treated successfully with acetaminophen and, if necessary, diphenhydramine (see below). Patients should also be treated (eg, with acetaminophen) before future transfusions. If a recipient has experienced more than one febrile reaction, special leukoreduction filters are used during future transfusions; many hospitals use prestorage leukoreduced blood components.

Allergic reactions: Allergic reactions to an unknown component in donor blood are common, usually due to allergens in donor plasma or, less often, to antibodies from an allergic donor. These reactions are usually mild, with urticaria, edema, occasional dizziness, and headache during or immediately after the transfusion. Simultaneous fever is common. Less frequently, dyspnea, wheezing, and incontinence may occur, indicating a generalized spasm of smooth muscle. Rarely, anaphylaxis occurs, particularly in IgA-deficient recipients.

In a patient with a history of allergies or an allergic transfusion reaction, an antihistamine may be given prophylactically just before or at the beginning of the transfusion (eg, diphenhydramine 50 mg po or IV). NOTE: *Drugs must never be mixed with the blood.* If an allergic reaction occurs, the transfusion is stopped. An antihistamine (eg, diphenhydramine 50 mg IV) usually controls mild urticaria and itching, and transfusion may be resumed. However, a moderate allergic reaction (generalized urticaria or mild bronchospasm) requires hydrocortisone (100 to 200 mg IV), and a severe anaphylactic reaction requires additional treatment with epinephrine 0.5 mL of 1:1000 solution sc and 0.9% saline IV (see p. 1360) along with investigation by the blood bank. Further transfusion should not occur until the investigation is completed. Patients with severe IgA deficiency require transfusion of washed RBCs, washed platelets, and plasma from IgA-deficient donor.

Volume overload: The high osmotic load of blood products, particularly whole blood, draws volume into the intravascular space over the course of hours, which can cause volume overload in susceptible patients (eg, cardiac or renal insufficiency). In such patients, whole blood is contraindicated. RBCs should be infused slowly. The patient should be observed and, if signs of heart failure (eg, dyspnea, rales) occur, the transfusion should be stopped and treatment for heart failure begun.

Typical treatment is with a diuretic such as furosemide 20 to 40 mg IV (see Pulmonary Edema on p. 664). Occasionally, patients requiring a higher volume of plasma infusion to reverse a warfarin overdose may be given a low dose of furosemide simultaneously. Patients at high risk of volume overload (eg, those with heart failure or severe renal insufficiency) are treated prophylactically with a diuretic (eg, furosemide 20 to 40 mg IV).

Acute lung injury: Transfusion-related acute lung injury is an infrequent complication caused by anti-HLA and/or anti-granulocyte antibodies in donor plasma that agglutinate and degranulate recipient granulocytes within the lung. Acute respiratory symptoms develop, and chest x-ray has a characteristic pattern of noncardiogenic pulmonary edema. After ABO incompatibility, this is the 2nd most common cause of death related to transfusion. Incidence is 1:5,000–10,000, but many cases are minor. Mild to moderate transfusion-related acute lung injury probably is commonly missed. General supportive therapy typically leads to recovery without long-lasting sequelae. Diuretics should be avoided. Cases should be reported.

Altered oxygen affinity: Blood stored for > 7 days has decreased RBC 2,3-diphosphoglycerate (DPG), which results in an increased affinity for O_2 and slower O_2 release to the tissues. There is little evidence that 2,3-DPG deficiency is clinically significant except in exchange transfusions in infants, in sickle cell patients with acute chest syndrome and stroke, and in some patients with severe heart failure. After transfusion of RBCs, 2,3-DPG regenerates within 12 to 24 h.

Graft-vs-host disease (GVHD): Transfusion-associated GVHD (see also p. 1370) is usually caused by transfusion of products containing immunocompetent lymphocytes to an immunocompromised host. The donor lymphocytes attack host tissues. GVHD can occur occasionally in immunocompetent patients if they receive blood from a donor who is homozygous for an HLA haplotype (usually a close relative) for which the patient is heterozygous. Symptoms and signs include fever, skin rash (centrifugally spreading rash becoming erythroderma with bullae), vomiting, watery and bloody diarrhea, lymphadenopathy, and pancytopenia due to bone marrow aplasia. Jaundice and elevated liver enzymes are also common. GVHD occurs 4 to 30 days after transfusion and is diagnosed based on clinical suspicion and skin and bone marrow biopsies. GVHD has > 90% mortality because no specific treatment is available.

Prevention of GVHD is with irradiation (to damage DNA of the donor lymphocytes) of all transfused blood products. This is done if the recipient is immunocompromised (congenital immune deficiency syndromes, hematologic malignancies, hematopoietic stem cell transplantation, newborns), if donor blood is obtained from a 1st-degree relative, or when HLA-matched components, excluding stem cells, are transfused. Treatment with corticosteroids and other immunosuppressants, including those used for solid organ transplantation, is not an indication for irradiation.

Complications of massive transfusion: Massive transfusion is transfusion of a volume of blood greater than or equal to one blood volume in 24 h (eg, 10 units in a 70-kg adult). When a patient receives stored blood in such large volume, the patient's own blood may be, in effect, "washed out," with only about $\frac{1}{3}$ of original blood components remaining.

In circumstances uncomplicated by prolonged hypotension or DIC, dilutional thrombocytopenia is the most likely complication. Platelets in stored blood are not fully functional. Clotting factors (except factor VIII) usually remain sufficient. Microvascular bleeding (abnormal oozing and continued bleeding from raw and cut surfaces) may result. Five to 8 (1 unit/10 kg) platelet concentrates are usually enough to correct such bleeding in an adult. Fresh frozen plasma and cryoprecipitate may be needed.

Hypothermia due to rapid transfusion of large amounts of cold blood can cause arrhythmias or cardiac arrest. Hypothermia is avoided by using an IV set with a heat-exchange device that gently warms blood. Other means of warming blood (eg, microwave ovens) are contraindicated because of potential RBC damage and hemolysis.

Citrate and K toxicities generally are not of concern even in massive transfusion; however, toxicities of both may be amplified in the presence of hypothermia. Patients with liver failure may have difficulty metabolizing citrate. Hypocalcemia can result but rarely necessitates treatment (which is 10 mL of a 10% solution of Ca gluconate IV diluted in 100 mL D_5W, given over 10 min). Patients with renal failure may have elevated K if transfused with blood stored for > 1 wk (K accumulation is usually insignificant in blood stored for < 1 wk). Mechanical hemolysis during transfusion may increase K. Hypokalemia may occur about 24 h after transfusion of older RBCs (> 3 wk), which take up K.

Infectious complications: Bacterial contamination of packed RBCs occurs rarely, possibly due to inadequate aseptic technique during collection or to transient asymptomatic donor bacteremia. Refrigeration of RBCs usually limits bacterial growth except for cryophilic organisms such as *Yersinia* sp, which may produce dangerous levels of endotoxin. All RBC units are inspected daily and before issue for bacterial growth, which is indicated by a color change. Because platelet concentrates are stored at room temperature, they have greater potential for bacterial growth and endotoxin production if contaminated. To minimize growth, storage is limited to 5 days. The risk of bacterial contamination of platelets is 1:2500. Therefore, platelets are routinely tested for bacteria.

Rarely, syphilis is transmitted in fresh blood or platelets. Storing blood for ≥ 96 h at 4 to 10° C kills the spirochete. Although federal regulations require a serologic test for syphilis on donor blood, infective donors are seronegative early in the disease. Recipients of infected units may develop the characteristic secondary rash.

Hepatitis may occur after transfusion of any blood product. The risk has been reduced by viral inactivation through heat treatment of serum albumin and plasma proteins and by the use of recombinant factor concentrates. Tests for hepatitis are required for all donor blood (see TABLE 146–2). The estimated risk of hepatitis B is 1:200,000; of hepatitis C, 1:1.5 million. Because its transient viremic phase and concomitant clinical illness likely preclude blood donation, hepatitis A (infectious hepatitis) is not a significant cause of transfusion-associated hepatitis.

HIV infection in the US is almost entirely HIV-1, although HIV-2 is also of concern. Testing for antibodies to both strains is required. Nucleic acid testing for HIV-1 antigen as well as HIV-1 p24 antigen testing is also required. Additionally, blood donors are asked about behaviors that may put them at high risk of HIV infection. HIV-0 has not been identified among blood donors. The estimated risk of HIV transmission due to transfusion is 1:2 million.

Cytomegalovirus (CMV) can be transmitted by WBCs in transfused blood. It is not transmitted through fresh frozen plasma. Because CMV does not cause disease in immunocompetent recipients, routine antibody testing of donor blood is not required. However, CMV may cause serious or fatal disease in immunocompromised patients, who should probably receive CMV-negative blood products that have been provided by CMV antibody-negative donors or by blood depleted of WBCs by filtration.

Human T-cell lymphotropic virus type I (HTLV-I), which can cause adult T-cell lymphoma/leukemia, HTLV-I–associated myelopathy, and tropical spastic paraparesis, causes posttransfusion seroconversion in some recipients. All donor blood is tested for HTLV-I and HTLV-II antibodies. The estimated risk of false-negative results on testing of donor blood is 1:641,000.

Creutzfeldt-Jakob disease has never been reported to be transfusion-transmitted, but current practice precludes donation from a person who has received human-derived growth hormone or a dura mater transplant or who has a family member with Creutzfeldt-Jakob disease. New variant Creutzfeldt-Jakob disease (mad cow disease) has not been transmitted by blood transfusion. However, donors who have spent significant time in the United Kingdom and some other parts of Europe are permanently deferred from donation (see TABLE 146–1).

Malaria is transmitted easily through infected RBCs. Many donors are unaware that they have malaria, which may be latent and transmissible for 10 to 15 yr. Storage does not render blood safe. Prospective donors must be asked about malaria or whether they have been in a region where it is prevalent. Donors who have had a diagnosis of malaria or who are immigrants, refugees, or citizens from countries in which malaria is considered endemic are deferred for 3 yr; travelers to endemic countries are deferred for 1 yr. Babesiosis has rarely been transmitted by transfusion.

THERAPEUTIC HEMAPHERESIS

Therapeutic hemapheresis includes plasmapheresis and cytapheresis, which are generally tolerated by healthy donors. However, many minor and a few major risks exist. Insertion of the large IV catheters necessary to perform hemapheresis can cause complications (eg, bleeding, infection, pneumothorax). Citrate anticoagulant may decrease serum ionized Ca. Replacement of plasma with a noncolloidal solution (eg, saline) shifts fluid from the intravascular space. Colloidal replacement solutions do not replace IgG and coagulation factors.

Most complications can be managed with close attention to the patient and manipulation of the procedure, but some severe reactions and a few deaths have occurred.

Plasmapheresis: Therapeutic plasmapheresis removes plasma components from blood. A blood cell separator extracts the patient's plasma and returns RBCs and platelets in plasma or a plasma-replacing fluid; for this purpose, 5% albumin is preferred to fresh frozen plasma (except for patients with thrombotic thrombocytopenic purpura) because it causes fewer reactions and transmits no infections. Therapeutic plasmapheresis resembles dialysis but, in addition, can remove protein-bound toxic substances. A one-volume exchange removes about 66% of such components.

To be of benefit, plasmapheresis should be used for diseases in which the plasma contains a known pathogenic substance, and plasmapheresis should remove this substance more rapidly than the body produces it. For example,

TABLE 146–3. INDICATIONS FOR PLASMAPHERESIS ACCORDING TO THE AMERICAN SOCIETY FOR APHERESIS

CATEGORY	PLASMAPHERESIS	CYTAPHERESIS
I. Standard and acceptable under certain circumstances, including primary therapy	Acute inflammatory demyelinating polyradiculoneuropathy Anti-glomerular basement membrane antibody disease Chronic inflammatory demyelinating polyradiculoneuropathy Demyelinating polyneuropathy with IgG/IgA Myasthenia gravis Phytanic acid storage disease Posttransfusion purpura Thrombotic thrombocytopenia purpura	Cutaneous T-cell lymphoma: photopheresis Erythrocytosis/polycythemia vera Familial hypercholesterolemia: *lipid adsorption* Leukocytosis syndrome: leukodepletion Sickle cell diseases: red cell exchange Thrombocytosis: platelet depletion
II. Sufficient evidence to suggest efficacy; acceptable therapy on an adjunctive basis	ABO incompatible marrow transplant (recipient) Acute CNS inflammatory demyelinating disease Coagulation factor inhibitors Cryoglobulinemia Cryoglobulinemia with polyneuropathy Familial hypercholesterolemia Lambert-Eaton syndrome Myeloma/acute renal failure Myeloma/paraproteins/hyperviscosity PANDAS (*p*ediatric *a*utoimmune *n*europsychiatric *d*isorders *a*ssociated with *s*treptococcal infections) Polyneuropathy with IgM (± Waldenström's) Rapidly progressive glomerulonephritis Sydenham's chorea	Chronic graft vs host disease: photopheresis Erythrocytosis/polycythemia vera: RBC depletion Hyperparasitemia—Malaria/babesiosis: RBC exchange Idiopathic thrombocytopenic purpura: immunoadsorption RA: immunoadsorption
III. Inconclusive evidence for efficacy or uncertain benefit-risk ratio	Acute hepatic failure Aplastic anemia/pure RBC aplasia Autoimmune hemolytic anemia Heart transplant rejection Hemolytic disease of the newborn Hemolytic uremic syndrome Inclusion-body myositis Multiple myeloma with polyneuropathy Multiple sclerosis (progressive) Multiple sclerosis (relapsing) Overdose poisoning Platelet alloimmunization and refractoriness Paraneoplastic neurologic syndromes POEMS (plasma cell dyscrasia with *p*olyneuropathy, *o*rganomegaly, *e*ndocrinopathy, *m*onoclonal protein, and *s*kin changes) syndrome Polymyositis or dermatomyositis Rasmussen's encephalitis Raynaud's phenomenon Recurrent focal glomerulosclerosis Renal transplantation (presensitization)	Cutaneous T-cell lymphoma: leukodepletion Demyelinating polyneuropathy with IgG/IgA: immunoadsorption Heart transplant rejection: photopheresis Multiple sclerosis, progressive: lymphocytapheresis Paraneoplastic neurologic syndromes: immunoadsorption Platelet alloimmunization and refractoriness: immunoadsorption Polyneuropathy with IgM (± Waldenström's): immunoadsorption

TABLE 146–3. INDICATIONS FOR PLASMAPHERESIS ACCORDING TO THE AMERICAN SOCIETY FOR APHERESIS—Continued

CATEGORY	PLASMAPHERESIS	CYTAPHERESIS
	Scleroderma/progressive systemic sclerosis SLE Stiff-man syndrome Vasculitis	
IV. Lack of efficacy in controlled trials	Renal transplantation rejection RA Systemic (AL) amyloidosis	Inclusion-body myositis: leukapheresis Polymyositis or dermatomyositis

Data from McLeod BC. *Journal of Clinical Apheresis* 15:1–5, 2000.

in rapidly progressive autoimmune disorders, plasmapheresis may be used to remove existing harmful plasma components (eg, cryoglobulins, antiglomerular basement membrane antibodies) while immunosuppressive or cytotoxic drugs suppress their future production.

There are numerous indications (see TABLE 146–3). The frequency of plasmapheresis, the volume to be removed, the replacement fluid, and other variables are individualized. Low density lipoprotein cholesterol can be removed by plasmapheresis with a recently implemented filtration method. Complications of plasmapheresis are similar to those of therapeutic cytapheresis.

Cytapheresis: Therapeutic cytapheresis removes cellular components from blood, returning plasma. It is most often used to remove defective RBCs and substitute normal ones in patients with sickle cell anemia who have the following conditions: acute chest syndrome, stroke, pregnancy, or frequent, severe sickle cell crises. Cytapheresis achieves Hb S levels of < 30% without the risk of increased viscosity that can occur because of increased Hct with simple transfusion. Therapeutic cytapheresis may also be used to reduce severe thrombocytosis or leukocytosis (cytoreduction) in acute or chronic leukemia when there is risk of hemorrhage, thrombosis, or pulmonary or cerebral complications of extreme leukocytosis (leukostasis). Cytapheresis is effective in thrombocytosis because platelets are not replaced as rapidly as WBCs. One or 2 procedures may reduce platelet counts to safe levels. Therapeutic WBC removal (leukapheresis) can remove kilograms of buffy coat in a few procedures, and it often relieves leukostasis and splenomegaly. However, the reduction in WBC count itself may be mild and only temporary.

Other uses of cytapheresis include collection of peripheral blood stem cells for autologous or allogeneic bone marrow reconstitution (an alternative to bone marrow transplantation) and collection of lymphocytes for use in immune modulation cancer therapy (adoptive immunotherapy).

147 OVERVIEW OF CANCER

Cancer is an unregulated proliferation of cells due to loss of normal controls, resulting in unregulated growth, lack of differentiation, local tissue invasion, and, often, metastasis. Cancer can develop in any tissue or organ at any age. There is often an immune response to tumors (see p. 1153). Many cancers are curable if detected at an early stage, and long-term remission is often possible in later stages. However, cure is not always possible and is not attempted in some advanced cases in which palliative care provides better quality of life than vigorous but fruitless attempts at tumor eradication.

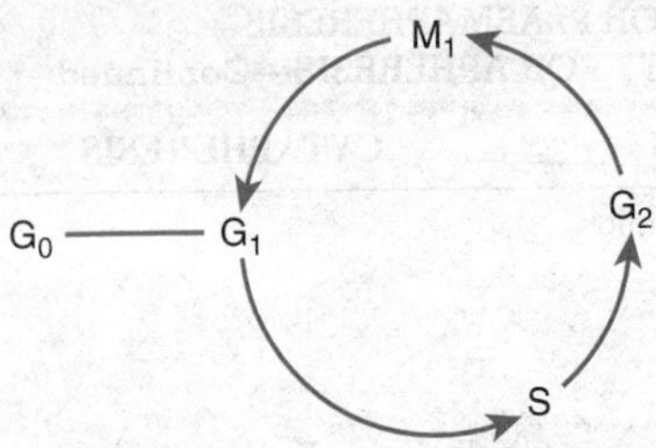

Fig. 147–1. The cell cycle. G_0 = resting phase (nonproliferation of cells); G_1 = variable pre-DNA synthetic phase (12 h to a few days); S = DNA synthesis (usually 2 to 4 h); G_2 = post-DNA synthesis (2 to 4 h)—a tetraploid quantity of DNA is found within cells; M_1 = mitosis (1 to 2 h).

CELLULAR AND MOLECULAR BASIS OF MALIGNANCY

Cellular Kinetics

Generation time is the time required for a quiescent cell to enter the cell cycle (see FIG. 147–1) and give rise to 2 daughter cells. Malignant cells usually have a shorter generation time than nonmalignant cells and a smaller percentage of cells in G_0 (resting phase), so a larger proliferation fraction exists. Initial exponential tumor growth is followed by a plateau phase when cell death equals the rate of formation of daughter cells. Compared with large tumors, small tumors have a greater percentage of actively dividing cells and thus show greater rates of proliferation.

Cellular kinetics of particular tumors are an important consideration in the design of antineoplastic drug regimens and may influence the dose schedules and timing intervals of treatment. Many antineoplastic drugs are effective only if cells are actively dividing, and some drugs work only during a specific phase of the cycle.

Tumor Growth and Metastasis

As a tumor grows, nutrients are provided by direct diffusion from the circulation. Local growth is facilitated by enzymes (eg, collagenases) and cytokines that alter or destroy adjacent tissues. As the ratio of surface area to volume becomes smaller with increased tumor growth, tumor angiogenesis factors are produced, forming the independent vascular supply required for further tumor growth.

Almost from inception, a tumor may shed cells into the circulation. From animal models, it is estimated that a 1-cm tumor sheds > 1 million cells/24 h into the venous circulation. Although most circulating tumor cells die as a result of intravascular trauma, a tiny number (much less than 1 in 1 million) adhere to the vascular endothelium and penetrate into surrounding tissues, generating independent tumors (metastases) at distant sites. Metastatic tumors grow in much the same manner as primary tumors and may subsequently give rise to other metastases.

Experiments suggest that metastasis is not a random event and that the primary tumor may regulate the growth of metastatic tumors. For example, removal of the primary tumor sometimes results in rapid growth of the metastases.

Molecular Abnormalities

Genetic mutations are largely responsible for the generation of malignant cells. These mutations alter the quantity or function of protein products that regulate cell growth and division and DNA repair. Two major categories of mutated genes are oncogenes and tumor suppressor genes.

Oncogenes are abnormal forms of normal genes (proto-oncogenes) that regulate cell growth. Mutation of these genes may result in direct and continuous stimulation of the molecular biologic pathways (eg, intracellular signal transduction pathways, transcription factors, secreted growth factors) that control cellular growth and division.

There are > 100 known oncogenes that may contribute to human neoplastic transformation. For example, the *ras* gene encodes the Ras protein, which regulates cell division. Mutations may result in the inappropriate activation of the Ras protein, leading to uncontrolled cell growth and division. In fact, the Ras protein is abnormal in about 25% of human cancers. Other oncogenes have been implicated in specific cancers. These include various protein kinases (bladder cancer, breast cancer), *bcr-abl* (chronic myelocytic leukemia, B-cell acute lymphocytic leukemia), C-*myc* (small cell lung cancer), N-*myc* (small cell lung cancer, neuroblastoma), and C-*erb* B-2 (breast cancer). Specific oncogenes may have important implications for diagnosis, therapy, and prognosis (see individual discussions under the specific cancer type).

Oncogenes typically result from acquired somatic cell mutations secondary to point mutations (eg, from chemical carcinogens), gene amplification (eg, an increase in the number of copies of a normal gene), or from insertion of viral genetic elements into host DNA. Occasionally, mutation of germ cell lines results in vertical transmission and a higher incidence of cancer development in offspring.

Tumor suppressor genes are inherent genes that play a role in cell division and DNA repair and are critical for detecting inappropriate growth signals in cells. If these genes, as a result of inherited or acquired mutations, become unable to function, genetic mutations in other genes can proceed unchecked, leading to neoplastic transformation.

As with most genes, 2 alleles are present that encode for each tumor suppressor gene. A defective copy of one gene may be inherited, leaving a person with only one functional allele for the individual tumor suppressor gene. If an acquired mutation occurs in the other allele, the normal protective mechanisms of the tumor suppressor gene are lost, and dysfunction of other protein products or DNA damage may escape unregulated, leading to cancer. For example, the retinoblastoma (*RB*) gene encodes for the protein pRB, which regulates the cell cycle by stopping DNA replication. Mutations in the *RB* gene occur in 30 to 40% of all human cancers, allowing affected cells to divide continuously.

Another mechanism that results in defective function and transcription of tumor suppressor genes is aberrant methylation of the promoter region of these genes, which inhibits gene transcription. Greater degrees of aberrant methylation and greater numbers of affected genes cause tumors to be more malignant and are associated with shortened survival in lung, bladder, and prostate cancer. In vitro alteration of the aberrant methylation has caused reversion to a nonmalignant, nonproliferative phenotype, suggesting a potential therapeutic target.

Another important regulatory protein, p53, prevents replication of damaged DNA in normal cells and promotes cell death (apoptosis) in cells with abnormal DNA. Inactive or altered p53 allows cells with abnormal DNA to survive and divide. Mutations are passed to daughter cells, conferring a high probability of neoplastic transformation. The *p53* gene is defective in many human cancers.

Gross chromosomal abnormalities (see also p. 2448) can occur through deletion, translocation, or duplication. If these alterations activate or inactivate genes that result in a proliferative advantage over normal cells, then a tumor may develop. Chromosomal abnormalities occur in certain human cancers (see TABLE 147–1). In some congenital diseases (Bloom syndrome, Fanconi

TABLE 147–1. HUMAN CANCERS CAUSED BY CHROMOSOMAL ABNORMALITIES

Lymphocytic leukemia
- Acute lymphocytic leukemia
- Chronic lymphocytic leukemia

Myeloid leukemia
- Acute monocytic leukemia
- Acute myelogenous leukemia with maturation
- Acute myelomonocytic leukemia with eosinophilia
- Acute nonlymphocytic leukemia with increased basophils
- Acute promyelocytic leukemia
- Chronic myelocytic leukemia
- Therapy-related acute myelogenous leukemia

Malignant lymphoma
- Burkitt's
- Non-Hodgkin

Myeloproliferative diseases

Solid tumors
- Benign
  - Colonic adenomas
  - Meningioma
  - Mixed tumors of salivary gland
- Adenocarcinomas
  - Bladder
  - Colon
  - Kidney
  - Ovary
  - Prostate
  - Small cell lung cancer
  - Uterus
- Sarcomas
  - Ewing's tumor
  - Extraskeletal myxoid chondrosarcoma
  - Liposarcoma, myxoid
  - Peripheral neuroepithelioma
  - Rhabdomyosarcoma (alveolar)
  - Synovial sarcoma
- Miscellaneous
  - Malignant melanoma
  - Mesothelioma
  - Neuroblastoma
  - Retinoblastoma
  - Testicular and ovarian dysgerminoma
  - Wilms' tumor

TABLE 147–2. CANCER-ASSOCIATED VIRUSES

VIRUS*	ASSOCIATED CANCER
Cytomegalovirus	Kaposi's sarcoma
Epstein-Barr virus	Burkitt's lymphoma, immunoblastic lymphoma, nasopharyngeal carcinoma
Hepatitis B virus	Hepatocellular carcinoma
Herpesvirus 8	Kaposi's sarcoma
HIV	Kaposi's sarcoma, lymphoma
Human papillomaviruses	Cervical carcinoma
Human T-cell lymphotrophic virus	T-cell lymphomas, hairy cell leukemia

*The relationship between SV40 and cancer remains uncertain and controversial.

syndrome, Down syndrome), chromosomes break easily, putting children at high risk of developing acute leukemia and other cancers.

Most cancers likely involve several of the mechanisms described above that lead to neoplastic conversion. For example, the development of tumor in familial polyposis takes place through a sequence of genetic events: epithelium hyperproliferation (loss of a suppressor gene on chromosome 5), early adenoma (change in DNA methylation), intermediate adenoma (overactivity of the *ras* oncogene), late adenoma (loss of a suppressor gene on chromosome 18), and, finally, cancer (loss of a gene on chromosome 17). Further genetic changes may be required for metastasis.

As with oncogenes, mutation of tumor suppressor genes in germ cell lines may result in vertical transmission and a higher incidence of cancer in offspring.

Telomeres are nucleoprotein complexes that cap the ends of chromosomes and maintain their integrity. Telomere shortening (with aging) results in replicative senescence, increased genetic instability, and potential tumor formation. Telomerase is an enzyme that provides for telomere synthesis and maintenance, thus telomerase may potentially allow for cellular immortality. Telomerase activity may promote tumors through multiple, complex mechanisms, especially by subverting the normal DNA synthetic checkpoints.

Environmental Factors

Viruses contribute to the pathogenesis of human malignancies (see TABLE 147–2). This may occur through the integration of viral genetic elements into the host DNA. These new genes are expressed by the host; they may affect cell growth or division, or disrupt normal host genes required for control of cell growth and division. Alternatively, viral infection may result in immune dysfunction, leading to decreased immune surveillance for early tumors.

Parasites of some types can lead to cancer. *Schistosoma haematobium* causes chronic inflammation and fibrosis of the bladder, which may lead to cancer. *Opisthorchis sinensis* has been linked to carcinoma of the pancreas and bile ducts.

Chemical carcinogens can induce gene mutations and result in uncontrolled growth and tumor formation (see TABLE 147–3). Other substances, called co-carcinogens, possess little or no inherent carcinogenic potency but enhance the carcinogenic effect of another agent when exposed simultaneously.

Ultraviolet radiation may induce skin cancer (eg, basal and squamous cell carcinoma, melanoma) by damaging DNA. This DNA damage consists of formation of thymidine dimers, which may escape repair due to inherent defects in DNA repair (eg, xeroderma pigmentosum) or through rare, random events.

Ionizing radiation is also carcinogenic. For example, survivors of the atomic bomb explosions in Hiroshima and Nagasaki have a higher-than-expected incidence of leukemia and other cancers. Similarly, the use of x-rays to treat nonmalignant disease (acne, thymic or adenoid enlargement, ankylosing spondylitis) results in higher rates of acute and chronic leukemias, Hodgkin and non-Hodgkin lymphomas, multiple myeloma, aplastic anemia terminating in acute nonlymphocytic leukemia, myelofibrosis, melanoma, and thyroid cancer. Industrial exposure (eg, to uranium by mine workers) is linked to development of lung cancer after a 15- to 20-yr latency. Long-term exposure to occupational irradiation or to internally deposited thorium dioxide predisposes people to angiosarcomas and acute nonlymphocytic leukemia.

Chronic skin irritation leads to chronic dermatitis and, in rare cases, to squamous cell carcinoma. This occurrence is presumably due to random mutations that occur more frequently because of the increased cell turnover.

Immunologic Disorders

Immune system dysfunction as a result of genetic mutation, acquired disease, aging, or immunosuppressants interferes with normal immune surveillance of early tumors and results in higher rates of cancer. Known cancer-associated immune disorders include ataxia-telangiectasia (acute lymphocytic leukemia [ALL], brain tumors, gastric cancer); Wiskott-Aldrich syndrome (lymphoma, ALL); X-linked agammaglobulinemia (lymphoma and ALL); immune deficiency secondary to immunosuppressants or HIV infection (large cell lymphoma, Kaposi's sarcoma); rheumatologic conditions, such as SLE, RA, and Sjögren's syndrome (B-type lymphoma); and general immune disorders (lymphoreticular neoplasia).

CLINICAL ASPECTS OF CANCER

Malignancy may lead to pain, wasting, neuropathy, nausea, anorexia, seizures, hypercalcemia, hyperuricemia, or obstruction. Death typically occurs as a result of sudden or progressive failure of one or multiple organ systems.

Pain in patients with metastatic cancer frequently results from bone metastases, nerve or plexus involvement, or pressure exerted by a tumor mass or effusion. Aggressive pain management is essential in the treatment of cancer and for maintenance of quality of life (see p. 1771).

Cardiac tamponade can result from malignant pericardial effusion and often occurs precipitously. The most common causes are breast cancer, lung cancer, and lymphoma. The preceding effusion may cause ill-defined chest pain or pressure that is worse when supine and better when sitting up (see p. 735). Patients with tamponade may experience signs and symptoms of decreased cardiac output (eg, dizziness or syncope). On physical examination, heart signs may be muffled and a friction rub and pulsus paradoxus may be present. X-ray may show a globular cardiac silhouette. Pericardiocentesis should be performed for diagnostic and therapeutic purposes, and a pleuropericardial window or pericardiectomy should be considered.

Pleural effusions should be drained if symptomatic and monitored for reaccumulation. If the effusion reaccumulates rapidly, thoracostomy tube drainage (see p. 380) and

TABLE 147–3. COMMON CHEMICAL CARCINOGENS

CARCINOGEN	TYPE OF CANCER
Occupational carcinogens	
Soot and mineral oil	Skin cancer
Arsenic	Lung cancer, skin cancer
Asbestos	Lung cancer, mesothelioma
Hair dyes and aromatic amines	Bladder cancer
Benzene	Leukemia
Nickel	Lung cancer, nasal sinus cancer
Formaldehyde	Nasal cancer, nasopharyngeal cancer
Vinyl chloride	Hepatic angiosarcoma
Painting materials, nonarsenic pesticides, diesel exhaust, chromates, man-made mineral fibers	Lung cancer
Lifestyle carcinogens	
Alcohol	Esophageal cancer, oropharyngeal cancer
Betel nuts	Oropharyngeal cancer
Tobacco	Head and neck cancer, lung cancer, esophageal cancer, bladder cancer
Drug carcinogens*	
Alkylating agents	Leukemia
Diethylstilbestrol	Liver cell adenoma, vaginal cancer in exposed female fetuses
Oxymetholone	Liver cancer
Thorotrast	Angiosarcoma

*Health care practitioners exposed to antineoplastic drugs are also at risk of adverse effects on reproduction.

sclerosing agents or repeated catheter drainage should be considered. Palliative surgical pleurectomy can be used for refractory effusions in advanced malignant disease.

Spinal cord compression (see p. 1913) can result from aggressive cancer spread and growth and requires immediate attention. Symptoms may include back pain, lower extremity paresthesias, and bowel and bladder dysfunction. Diagnosis is confirmed by CT or MRI. Treatment should be initiated promptly and usually consists of corticosteroids, radiation therapy, surgery, and sometimes chemotherapy.

Diagnosis

A complete history and physical examination may reveal unexpected clues to early cancer.

History: Physicians must be aware of predisposing factors and must specifically ask about familial cancer, environmental exposure (including smoking history), and prior or present illnesses (eg, autoimmune diseases, previous immunosuppressive therapy, hepatitis B and hepatitis C, HIV infection, abnormal Papanicolaou test, or human papillomavirus infection). Symptoms suggesting occult cancer can include fatigue, weight loss, fevers or night sweats, cough, hemoptysis, hematemesis or hematochezia, change in bowel habits, and persistent pain.

Physical examination: The physical examination should direct particular attention to skin, lymph nodes, lungs, breasts, abdomen, and testes. Prostate, rectal, and vaginal examinations are also important.

Testing: Tests are performed on patients with symptoms and include serum tumor markers, molecular tests, imaging tests, and biopsy.

Serum tumor markers may offer corroborating evidence in patients with findings suggestive of a specific malignancy (see p. 1155); these markers, however, are not useful for screening. α-Fetoprotein may be elevated in hepatocellular carcinoma and testicular carcinomas, carcinoembryonic antigen in colon cancer, β-human chorionic gonadotropin in choriocarcinoma and testicular carcinoma, serum immunoglobulins in multiple myeloma, DNA probes (eg, *bcr* probe to identify a chromosome 22 alteration) in chronic myelogenous leukemia, CA 125 in ovarian cancer, CA 27-29 in breast cancer, and prostate-specific antigen and prostatic acid phosphatase in prostate cancer. Restricting tumor marker testing to specific organ-related evaluations minimizes false-positive test results and does not result in missed tumors.

Molecular tests use gene-expression profiling (a genomics microassay method) and proteonomics to define tumor subtypes (eg, lymphoma, leukemias), to delineate the origin of metastatic cancers originating from an unknown primary cancer (eg, lung cancer), and to assist in recognizing inherent (or acquired) chemotherapy resistance.

Imaging tests often include plain x-rays, sonograms, CT scans, and MRIs. These tests assist in identifying abnormalities, determining qualities of a mass (solid or cystic), providing dimensions, and establishing relationship to surrounding structures, which may be important if surgery or biopsy is being considered.

Biopsy to confirm the diagnosis and tissue of origin is almost always required when cancer is suspected or detected. The choice of biopsy site is usually determined by ease of access and degree of invasiveness. If lymphadenopathy is present, fine-needle or core biopsy may yield the tumor type; if nondiagnostic, open biopsy is done. Other biopsy routes include bronchoscopy for easily accessible mediastinal or central pulmonary tumors, percutaneous liver biopsy if liver lesions are present, and CT- or ultrasound-guided biopsy. If these procedures are not suitable, open biopsy may be necessary. Consultation with an oncologist and surgeon is appropriate.

Staging

Once a histologic diagnosis is made, staging (ie, determination of the extent of disease) helps determine treatment decisions and prognosis. Clinical staging uses data from the patient's history, physical examination, and noninvasive studies. Pathologic staging requires tissue specimens. (For staging of specific neoplasms, see details in the organ-relevant chapter.)

Mediastinoscopy (see p. 377) is especially valuable in the staging of non–small cell lung cancer; if it shows mediastinal lymph node involvement, the patient would not usually benefit from a thoracotomy and lung resection but may benefit from chemoradiation and subsequent tumor resection.

Bone marrow aspiration and biopsy is especially useful in determining metastases from malignant lymphoma and small cell lung cancer, and its role in breast and prostate cancer is expanding. Marrow biopsy is positive at diagnosis in 50 to 70% of patients with malignant lymphoma (low and intermediate grade) and in 15 to 18% of patients with small cell lung cancer. Bone marrow biopsy should be performed in patients with hematologic abnormalities (ie, anemia, thrombocytopenia, pancytopenia) that cannot be explained by other mechanisms or in patients with known hematologic malignancies.

Lymph node biopsyis usually part of the evaluation of lymphoma. Regional lymph nodes are often biopsied during treatment of prostate and breast cancers.

Serum chemistries and enzymes may help staging. Elevation of liver enzymes (alkaline phosphatase, LDH, ALT) suggests the presence of liver metastases. Elevated alkaline phosphatase and serum Ca may be the first evidence of bone metastases. Elevated acid phosphatase (tartrate inhibited) suggests extracapsular extension of prostate cancer. Fasting hypoglycemia may indicate an insulinoma, hepatocellular carcinoma, or retroperitoneal sarcoma. Elevated BUN or creatinine levels may indicate an obstructive uropathy secondary to a pelvic mass, intrarenal obstruction from tubular precipitation of myeloma protein, or uric acid nephropathy from lymphoma or other cancers. Elevated uric acid levels often occur in myeloproliferative and lymphoproliferative disorders.

Imaging tests, especially CT and MRI, can detect metastases to brain, lung, spinal cord, or abdominal viscera, including the adrenal glands, retroperitoneal lymph nodes, liver, and spleen. MRI (with gadolinium contrast) is the procedure of choice for recognition and evaluation of brain tumors, both primary and metastatic. PET scanning is increasingly being used to determine the metabolic activity of the suspected cancerous mass and provides information essential for staging, treatment, and prognosis. Combined CT/PET can be valuable, especially in lung, head and neck, and breast cancer and in lymphoma. Use of imaging tests with other cancers is under study.

Ultrasonography can be used to study orbital, thyroid, cardiac, pericardial, hepatic, pancreatic, renal, and retroperitoneal areas. It may guide percutaneous biopsies and differentiate renal cell carcinoma from a benign renal cyst.

Nuclear scans can identify several types of metastases. Bone scans identify abnormal bone growth (ie, osteoblastic activity) before it is visible on plain x-ray. Thus, this technique is useless in neoplasms that are purely lytic (eg, multiple myeloma); routine bone x-rays are the study of choice in such diseases.

Grading

Grading is a histologic measure of tumor aggressiveness. It is determined from the biopsy based on the morphologic appearance of tumor cells, including the appearance of the nuclei, cytoplasm, and nucleoli; frequency of mitoses; and amount of necrosis. For many cancers, grading scales have been developed.

Screening

Screening tests are performed in asymptomatic patients at risk. The rationale is that early diagnosis may decrease cancer mortality, allow for less radical therapy, and reduce costs. Risks, however, include false-positive results, which necessitate confirmatory tests (eg, biopsy, endoscopy) that can lead to anxiety, significant morbidity, and cost, and false-negative results, which may give a mistaken sense of security, causing the patient to ignore subsequent symptoms.

Screening for cancer should be performed when a distinct high-risk group can be identified (eg, those with certain infections, exposures, or behavior); the disease has an asymptomatic period during which treatment would alter outcome; the morbidity of the disease is significant; and an intervention is available that is acceptable and effective at changing the natural history of the condition.

The screening tests themselves should satisfy the following criteria:

- Cost and convenience are reasonable
- Reliability, including accuracy, precision, and person-to-person variability, is high
- Sensitivity and specificity are adequate
- The positive predictive value is high in the population screened
- The test or procedure is acceptable to the patient.

Recommended screening schedules are constantly evolving based on ongoing studies (see TABLE 147–4).

TABLE 147–4. SCREENING PROCEDURES IN AVERAGE-RISK ASYMPTOMATIC PEOPLE AS RECOMMENDED BY THE AMERICAN CANCER SOCIETY

TYPE OF CANCER	PROCEDURE	FREQUENCY
Breast cancer	Breast self-examination	Monthly after age 20
	Breast physical examination	Every 3 yr between ages 20 and 39; then yearly
	Mammography	Yearly, starting at age 40
Cervical cancer	Papanicolaou (Pap) test	Yearly in all women who are sexually active or starting at age 18*
Cervical, uterine, and ovarian cancers	Pelvic examination	Every 1 to 3 yr between ages 18 and 40; then yearly
Prostate cancer	Rectal examination and blood test for prostate-specific antigen	Yearly after age 50 (or age 45 if in a high-risk group)
Rectal and colon cancer	Fecal occult blood or	Yearly, starting at age 50
	Flexible sigmoidoscopy or	Every 5 yr, starting at age 50
	Colonoscopy	Every 10 yr, starting at age 50

*After 3 or more consecutive normal examinations, a Pap test may be performed less often at the physician's discretion; most women > 65 yr need Pap tests less often.

Modified from the American Cancer Society guidelines published in *Cancer J Clin* 2002;52:8–22.

METASTATIC CARCINOMA OF UNKNOWN PRIMARY ORIGIN

A patient is considered to have carcinoma of unknown primary origin when a tumor is detected at one or more metastatic sites and routine evaluation fails to identify a primary tumor. Metastatic carcinoma of unknown primary origin constitutes 0.5 to 7% of all cancers and poses a therapeutic dilemma, because cancer treatment is typically directed at the specific primary tissue type.

The most common causative primary tumors are of the prostate, breast, lung, colon and rectum, and cervix; examination of these areas should be thorough. Laboratory tests should include a CBC, urinalysis, stool examination for occult blood, and serum chemistries (including prostate-specific antigen assays in males). Imaging should be limited to a chest x-ray, abdominal CT, and mammography. An upper GI series and barium enema should not be done routinely. On available cancerous tissue, a growing panel of immunocytochemical stains has begun to help determine the primary tissue site. In addition, immunoperoxidase staining for immunoglobulin, gene rearrangement studies, and electron microscopy help diagnose large cell lymphoma, whereas immunoperoxidase staining for α-fetoprotein or β-human chorionic gonadotrophin may suggest germ cell tumors. Tissue analysis for estrogen and progesterone receptors helps identify breast cancer, and immunoperoxidase staining for prostate-specific antigen helps identify prostate cancer.

Even if a precise histologic diagnosis cannot be made, one constellation of findings suggests an origin. Poorly differentiated carcinomas near or at midline regions of the mediastinum or retroperitoneum in young or middle-aged males should be considered germ cell neoplasms—even in the absence of a testicular mass. Patients with this type of carcinoma should be treated with a cisplatin-based regimen, because nearly 50% of such patients experience long disease-free intervals. For most unknown primary cancers, the responses to this regimen and to other multidrug chemotherapy programs are modest and of brief duration (eg, median survival < 1 yr).

PARANEOPLASTIC SYNDROMES

Paraneoplastic syndromes are symptoms that occur at sites distant from a tumor or its metastasis.

Although the pathogenesis remains unclear, these symptoms may be secondary to substances secreted by the tumor or may be a result of antibodies directed against tumors that cross-react with other tissue. Symptoms may occur in any organ or physiologic system. Up to 20% of cancer patients experience paraneoplastic syndromes, but often these syndromes are unrecognized.

The most common cancers associated with paraneoplastic syndromes are those that arise from the lung; others include renal carcinoma, hepatocellular carcinoma, leukemias, lymphomas, breast and ovarian tumors, neural cancers, and gastric and pancreatic tumors.

Successful treatment is best obtained by controlling the underlying malignancy, but some symptoms can be palliated with specific drugs (eg, minocycline for ectopic ADH, cyproheptadine for carcinoid syndrome, bisphosphonates and corticosteroids for hypercalcemia).

General paraneoplastic symptoms: Patients with cancer often experience fever, night sweats, anorexia, and cachexia. These may arise from release of lymphokines involved in the immune response or from mediators involved in tumor cell death, such as tumor necrosis factor-α. Alterations in liver function and steroidogenesis may also contribute.

Cutaneous paraneoplastic syndromes: Itching is the most common cutaneous symptom experienced by patients with cancer (eg, leukemia, lymphomas) and may result from hypereosinophilia. Flushing may also occur and is likely related to tumor-generated circulating vasoactive substances (eg, prostaglandins).

Various pigmented skin lesions, or keratoses, may appear, including acanthosis nigricans (GI malignancy), generalized dermic melanosis (lymphoma, melanoma, hepatocellular carcinoma), Bowen's disease (lung, GI, and GU malignancy), and large multiple seborrheic keratoses, ie, Leser-Trélat signs (lymphoma, GI malignancy). Secretion of melanin precursors from tumors may promote formation of these lesions. Ichthyosis, or desquamation of the extensor surface of the extremities, may also occur.

Hypertrichosis may manifest as sudden appearance of coarse hair on the face and ears that resolves after resection or treatment of the tumor. Alternatively, alopecia may occur with certain tumor types. The mechanism by which this occurs is not clear.

Necrotizing migrating erythema may occur with glucagonomas. Subcutaneous adipose nodular necrosis may result from release of proteolytic enzymes from various pancreatic tumors.

Herpes zoster may result from reactivation of latent virus in the context of immune system depression or dysfunction.

Endocrine paraneoplastic syndromes: Cushing's syndrome (cortisol excess, leading to hyperglycemia, hypokalemia, hypertension, central obesity, "moon facies") may result from ectopic production of ACTH or ACTH-like molecules, most often with small cell cancer of the lung.

Abnormalities in water and electrolyte balance, including hyponatremia and Ca disturbances, may result from production of ADH and parathyroid hormone–like hormones (from small cell and non–small cell lung cancer). Similarly, hypoglycemia may result from production of insulin-like growth factors or insulin production by various tumors. Hypertension may result from abnormal epinephrine and norepinephrine secretion (pheochromocytomas) or from cortisol excess (ACTH-secreting tumors). Other ectopically produced hormones include parathyroid hormone (from squamous cell lung cancer, head and neck cancer, bladder cancer), calcitonin (from breast cancer, small cell lung cancer, and medullary thyroid carcinoma), and thyroid-stimulating hormone (from gestational choriocarcinoma).

GI paraneoplastic syndromes: Watery diarrhea with subsequent dehydration and electrolyte imbalances may result from tumor-related secretion of prostaglandins or vasoactive intestinal peptide. Implicated tumors include colon cancer, some thyroid cancers, melanomas, myelomas, ovarian tumors, and CNS tumors. Protein-losing enteropathies may result from tumor mass inflammation, particularly with lymphomas.

Hematologic paraneoplastic syndromes: Patients with cancer may develop pure RBC aplasia, anemia of chronic disease, leukocytosis (leukemoid reaction), thrombocytosis, eosinophilia, basophilia, and disseminated intravascular coagulation (DIC). In addition, idiopathic thrombocytopenic purpura and a Coombs'-positive hemolytic anemia can complicate the course of lymphoid malignancies and Hodgkin lymphoma. Erythrocytosis may occur in various cancers due to ectopic production of erythropoietin or erythropoietin-like substances, and monoclonal gammopathies may sometimes be present.

Demonstrated mechanisms of hematologic abnormalities include tumor-generated substances that mimic or block normal endocrine signals for hematologic line development and generation of antibodies that cross-react with receptors or cell lines.

Neurologic paraneoplastic syndromes: Peripheral neuropathy is the most common neurologic paraneoplastic syndrome. It is usually a distal sensorimotor polyneuropathy that produces mild motor weakness, sensory loss, and absent distal reflexes. The syndrome is indistinguishable from that accompanying many chronic illnesses. It may be due to nutritional deprivation but responds poorly to nutritional therapy.

Subacute sensory neuropathy is a more specific but rare peripheral neuropathy. Dorsal root ganglia degeneration and progressive sensory loss with ataxia but little motor weakness develop; the disorder may be disabling. Anti-Hu, an autoantibody, is found in the serum of some patients with lung cancer. There is no treatment.

Guillain-Barré syndrome is more common in patients with Hodgkin lymphoma than in the general population.

The Eaton-Lambert syndrome is an immune-mediated, myasthenia-like syndrome with weakness usually affecting the limbs and sparing ocular and bulbar muscles. It is presynaptic, resulting from impaired release of acetylcholine from nerve terminals. An IgG antibody is involved. The syndrome can precede, occur with, or develop after the diagnosis of cancer. It occurs most commonly in men with intrathoracic tumors (70% have small or oat cell lung carcinoma). Symptoms and signs include fatigability, weakness, pain in proximal limb muscles, peripheral paresthesias, dry mouth, erectile dysfunction, and ptosis. Deep tendon reflexes are reduced or lost. The diagnosis is confirmed by finding an incremental response to repetitive nerve stimulation: Amplitude of the compound muscle action potential increases > 200% at rates > 10 Hz. Treatment is first directed at the underlying malignancy and sometimes induces remission. Guanidine (initially 125 mg po qid, gradually increased to a maximum of 35 mg/kg), which facilitates acetylcholine release, often lessens symptoms but may depress bone marrow and liver function. Corticosteroids and plasmapheresis benefit some patients.

Subacute cerebellar degeneration causes progressive bilateral leg and arm ataxia, dysarthria, and sometimes vertigo and diplopia. Neurologic signs may include dementia with or without brain stem signs, ophthalmoplegia, nystagmus, and extensor plantar signs, with prominent dysarthria and arm involvement. The disease usually progresses over weeks to months, often causing profound disability. Cerebellar degeneration may precede the discovery of the cancer by weeks to years. Anti-Yo, a circulating autoantibody, is found in the serum and/or CSF of some patients, especially women with breast or ovarian cancer. MRI or CT may show cerebellar atrophy, especially late in the disease. Characteristic pathologic changes include widespread loss of Purkinje cells and lymphocytic cuffing of deep blood vessels. CSF occasionally has mild lymphocytic pleocytosis. Treatment is nonspecific, but some improvement may follow successful cancer therapy.

Opsoclonus (spontaneous chaotic eye movements) is a rare cerebellar syndrome that may accompany childhood neuroblastoma. It is associated with cerebellar ataxia and myoclonus of the trunk and extremities. Anti-Ri, a circulating autoantibody, may be present. The syndrome often responds to corticosteroids and treatment of the cancer.

Subacute motor neuronopathy is a rare disorder causing painless lower motor neuron weakness of upper and lower extremities, usually in patients with Hodgkin lymphoma or other lymphomas. Anterior horn cells degenerate. Spontaneous improvement usually occurs.

Subacute necrotic myelopathy is rare. Rapid ascending sensory and motor loss occurs in gray and white matter of the spinal cord, leading to paraplegia. MRI helps rule out epidural compression from metastatic tumor—a much more common cause of rapidly progressive spinal cord dysfunction in patients with cancer. MRI may show the spinal cord necrotic lesion.

Encephalitis, or cerebritis, has been proposed, but whether it exists or is a paraneoplastic syndrome is controversial. Global encephalitis has been proposed to explain the encephalopathy that occurs most commonly in small cell lung cancer. However, the encephalopathy may be secondary to brain metastasis or extensive multidrug chemotherapy and sometimes radiation therapy. Another possible form of paraneoplastic encephalitis is limbic encephalitis, characterized by anxiety and depression, leading to memory loss, agitation, confusion, hallucinations, and behavioral abnormalities. Some patients have anti-Hu in the serum and spinal fluid.

Renal paraneoplastic syndrome: Membranous glomerulonephritis may occur in patients with colon cancer, ovarian cancer, and lymphoma as a result of circulating immune complexes.

Rheumatologic paraneoplastic syndromes: Patients with hematologic malignancies or with cancer of the colon, pancreas, or prostate may develop various arthropathies (rheumatic polyarthritis, polymyalgia) or scleroderma.

Hypertrophic osteoarthropathy is prominent with certain lung cancers and manifests as painful swelling of the joints (knees, ankles, wrists, elbows, metacarpophalangeal joints) with effusion and sometimes fingertip clubbing.

Patients with lung and gynecologic cancers may develop scleroderma or SLE.

Secondary amyloidosis may occur with myeloma, lymphomas, or renal cell carcinomas.

Dermatomyositis and, to a lesser degree, polymyositis (see p. 261) are thought to be more common in patients with cancer, especially in those > 50 yr. Typically, proximal muscle weakness is progressive with pathologically demonstrable muscle inflammation and necrosis. A dusky, erythematous butterfly rash with a heliotrope hue may develop on the cheeks with periorbital edema. Corticosteroid therapy may be helpful.

148 TUMOR IMMUNOLOGY

Tumor recognition is a complex, challenging problem for the immune system, which must distinguish proper cellular growth and organization from neoplastic transformation. This process involves recognition of tumor antigens by effector cells and induction of immunity. The development of tumors despite the presence of antigens, the significance of immune recognition in the pathogenesis of tumors, and the potential for therapeutic augmentation of immune responses remain the subject of intense investigation.

TUMOR ANTIGENS

Many neoplastic cells produce antigens, which may be released in the bloodstream or remain on the cell surface. Antigens have been identified in most of the human cancers, including Burkitt's lymphoma, neuroblastoma, malignant melanoma, osteosarcoma, renal cell carcinoma, breast carcinoma, prostate cancer, lung carcinomas, and colon cancer. A key role of the immune system is detection of these antigens to permit subsequent targeting for eradication. However, despite their foreign structure, the immune response to tumor antigens varies and is often insufficient to prevent tumor growth.

Tumor-associated antigens (TAAs) are relatively restricted to tumor cells, whereas tumor-specific antigens(TSAs) are unique to tumor cells. TSAs typically are portions of intracellular molecules expressed on the cell surface as part of the major histocompatibility complex.

Suggested mechanisms of origin for tumor antigens include (1) introduction of new genetic information from a virus (eg, human papillomavirus E6 and E7 proteins in cervical cancer); (2) alteration of oncogenes or tumor suppressor genes by carcinogens, which either generate a novel protein sequence directly or induce accumulation of proteins that are normally not expressed or are expressed at very low levels (*ras, p53*); (3) abnormally high accumulation of proteins that normally are present at substantially lower levels (eg, prostate-specific antigens, melanoma-associated antigens) or that are expressed only during embryonic development (carcinoembryonic antigens); (4) uncovering of antigens normally buried in the cell membrane because of defective membrane homestasis by neoplastic cells; and (5) release of antigens normally sequestered within the cell or its organelles when neoplastic cells die.

HOST RESPONSE TO TUMORS

The immune response to foreign antigens consists of humoral (eg, antibodies) and cellular mechanisms. Most humoral responses cannot prevent tumor growth. However, effector cells, such as T cells, macrophages, and natural killer cells, have relatively effective tumoricidal abilities. Effector cell activity is induced by antigen-presenting cells and is supported by cytokines (eg, interleukins, interferons—see p. 1326). Despite the activity of effector cells, host immunoreactivity may fail to control tumor occurrence and growth.

Cellular Immunity

The T cell is the primary cell responsible for direct recognition and killing of tumor cells. T cells carry out immunologic surveillance, then proliferate and destroy newly transformed tumor cells after recognizing tumor-associated antigens (TAAs). The T-cell response to tumors is modulated by other cells of the immune system; some require the presence of humoral antibodies directed against the tumor cells (antibody-dependent cellular cytotoxicity) to initiate the interactions that lead to the death of tumor cells. In contrast, suppressor T cells inhibit the immune response against tumors.

Cytotoxic T lymphocytes (CTLs) recognize antigens on target cells and lyse these cells. These antigens may be cell surface proteins or may be intracellular proteins (eg, TAAs) that are expressed on the surface in combination with class I major histocompatibility complex (MHC) molecules. Tumor-specific CTLs have been found with neuroblastomas, malignant melanomas, sarcomas, and carcinomas of the colon, breast, cervix, endometrium, ovary, testis, nasopharynx, and kidney.

Natural killer (NK) cells are another population of effector cells with tumoricidal activity. In contrast to CTLs, NK cells lack the receptor for antigen detection but can still recognize normal cells infected with viruses or tumor cells. Their tumoricidal activity is termed "natural" because it is not induced by a specific antigen. The mechanism by which NK cells discriminate between normal and abnormal cells is under study. Evidence suggests that class I MHC molecules on the surface of normal cells inhibit NK cells and prevent lysis. Thus, the decreased level of class I molecule expression characteristic of many tumor cells may allow activation of NK cells and subsequent tumor lysis.

Macrophages can kill specific tumor cells when activated by a combination of factors, including lymphokines (soluble factors) produced by T cells and interferon. They are less effective than T-cell–mediated cytotoxic mechanisms. Under certain circumstances, macrophages may present TAAs to T cells and stimulate tumor-specific immune response.

Dendritic cells are dedicated antigen-presenting cells present in barrier tissues (eg, skin, lymph nodes). They play a central role in initiation of tumor-specific immune response. These cells take up tumor-associated proteins, process them, and present TAAs to T cells to stimulate the CTL response against tumor. The presence of dendritic cells in tumor tissues correlates with improved prognosis.

Lymphokines produced by immune cells stimulate growth or induce activities of other immune cells. Such lymphokines include IL-2, also known as T-cell growth factor, and the interferons. IL-12 is produced by dendritic cells and specifically induces CTLs, thereby enhancing antitumor immune responses.

Humoral Immunity

In contrast to T-cell cytotoxic immunity, humoral antibodies do not appear to confer significant protection against tumor growth. Most antibodies cannot recognize TAAs. Regardless, humoral antibodies that react with tumor cells in vitro have been detected in the sera of patients with various neoplastic processes, including Burkitt's lymphoma; malignant melanoma; osteosarcoma; neuroblastoma; and lung, breast, and GI carcinomas.

Cytotoxic antibodies are directed against surface antigens of tumor cells. These antibodies can exert anti-tumor effects through complement fixation or by serving as a flag for destruction of tumor cells by T cells (antibody-dependent cell-mediated cytotoxicity). Another population of humoral antibodies, called enhancing antibodies (blocking antibodies), may actually favor rather than inhibit tumor growth. The mechanisms and relative importance of such immunologic enhancement are not well understood.

Failure of Host Defenses

Although many tumors are eliminated by the immune system (and thus are never detected), others continue to grow despite the presence of TAAs. Several mechanisms have been proposed to explain this deficient host response to the TAA, including specific immunologic tolerance to TAAs in a process that involves antigen-presenting cells and suppressor T cells, possibly secondary to prenatal exposure to the antigen; suppression of immune response by chemical, physical, or viral agents (eg, helper T-cell destruction by HIV); suppression of the immune response by cytotoxic drugs and radiation; and suppression of the immune response (decreased T, B, and antigen-presenting cell function, decreased IL-2 production, increased circulating soluble IL-2 receptors) by the tumor itself through various complex and largely uncharacterized mechanisms.

TUMOR IMMUNODIAGNOSIS

Tumor-associated antigens (TAAs) can help diagnose various tumors and sometimes determine the response to therapy or recurrence. An ideal tumor marker would be released only from tumor tissue, be specific for a given tumor type, be detectable at low levels of tumor cell burden, have a direct relationship to the tumor cell burden, and be present in all patients with the tumor. However, although most tumors release detectable antigenic macromolecules into the circulation, no tumor marker has all the requisite characteristics to provide enough specificity or sensitivity to be used in early diagnosis or mass cancer screening programs.

Carcinoembryonic antigen (CEA) is a protein-polysaccharide complex present in colon carcinomas and in normal fetal intestine, pancreas, and liver. Blood levels are elevated in patients with colon carcinoma, but the specificity is relatively low because positive results also occur in heavy cigarette smokers and in patients with cirrhosis, ulcerative colitis, and other cancers (eg, breast, pancreas, bladder, ovary, cervix). Monitoring CEA levels may be useful for detecting cancer recurrence after tumor excision if the patient initially had an elevated CEA.

α-Fetoprotein, a normal product of fetal liver cells, is also present in the sera of patients with primary hepatoma, yolk sac neoplasms, and, frequently, ovarian or testicular embryonal carcinoma.

β Subunit of human chorionic gonadotropin (β-HCG), measured by immunoassay, is the major clinical marker in women with gestational trophoblastic neoplasia (GTN)—a disease spectrum that includes hydatidiform mole, nonmetastatic GTN, and metastatic GTN (see also p. 2123)—and in about ⅔ of men with testicular embryonal carcinoma or choriocarcinoma. The β subunit is measured because it is specific for HCG.

Prostate-specific antigen (PSA), a glycoprotein located in ductal epithelial cells of the prostate gland, can be detected in low concentrations in the sera of healthy men. Using an appropriate upper limit of normal, assays with monoclonal antibodies detect elevated serum levels of PSA in about 90% of patients with advanced prostate cancer, even in the absence of defined metastatic disease. It is more sensitive than prostatic acid phosphatase. However, because PSA is elevated in benign prostatic hypertrophy, it is less specific. PSA can be used to monitor recurrence after prostatic carcinoma has been diagnosed and treated.

CA 125 is clinically useful for diagnosing and monitoring therapy for ovarian cancer, although any peritoneal inflammatory process can increase levels.

β_2-Microglobulin is often elevated in multiple myeloma and in some lymphomas. Its primary use is in prognosis.

CA 19-9 was originally developed to detect colorectal cancer but proved more sensitive for pancreatic cancer. It is primarily used to judge the response to treatment in patients with advanced pancreatic cancers. CA 19-9 can also be elevated in other GI cancers, particularly cancer of the bile ducts.

CA 15-3 is elevated in 54 to 80% of patients with metastatic breast cancer. It may also be elevated in other benign (eg, chronic hepatitis, cirrhosis, TB, sarcoidosis, SLE) and malignant (eg, lung, ovarian, endometrial, GI, and bladder carcinomas) conditions. This marker is primarily used to monitor the response to therapy.

Chromogranin A is used as a marker for carcinoid and other neuroendocrine tumors. Abnormal levels are seen in ⅓ of patients with localized disease and in ⅔ of those with metastatic cancer. Levels can be elevated in other cancers, such as lung and prostate.

Thyroglobulin is produced by the thyroid and may be elevated with various thyroid diseases. It is primarily used after complete thyroidectomy to detect recurrent thyroid cancer and to follow the response to treatment in metastatic thyroid cancer.

TA-90 is a highly immunogenic subunit of a urinary tumor–associated antigen that is present in 70% of melanomas, soft-tissue sarcomas, and carcinomas of the breast, colon, and lung. Some studies have shown that TA-90 levels can accurately predict survival and the presence of subclinical disease after surgery for melanoma.

IMMUNOTHERAPY

A number of immunologic interventions, both passive and active, can be directed against tumor cells.

Passive Cellular Immunotherapy

In passive cellular immunotherapy, specific effector cells are directly infused and are not induced or expanded within the patient.

Lymphokine-activated killer (LAK) cells are produced from the patient's endogenous T cells, which are extracted and grown in a cell culture system by exposing them to the lymphokine IL-2. The proliferated LAK cells are then returned to the patient's bloodstream. Animal studies have shown that LAK cells are more effective against cancer cells than are the original endogenous T cells, presumably because of their greater number. Clinical trials of LAK cells in humans are ongoing.

Tumor-infiltrating lymphocytes (TILs) may have greater tumoricidal activity than LAK cells. These cells are grown in culture in a manner similar to LAK cells. However, the progenitor cells consist of T cells that are isolated from resected tumor tissue. This process theoretically provides a line of T cells that has greater tumor specificity than those obtained from the bloodstream.

Concomitant use of interferon enhances the expression of major histocompatibility complex (MHC) antigens and tumor-associated antigens (TAAs) on tumor cells, thereby augmenting the killing of tumor cells by the infused effector cells. However, remissions using these agents have been infrequent. A new approach using T cells genetically modified to express receptors that recognize TAAs with high specificity to tumor cells is under study and may provide significant clinical benefit.

Passive Humoral Immunotherapy

Administration of exogenous antibodies constitutes passive humoral immunotherapy. Antilymphocyte serum has been used in the treatment of chronic lymphocytic leukemia and in T-cell and B-cell lymphomas, resulting in temporary decreases in lymphocyte counts or lymph node size.

Monoclonal antitumor antibodies may also be conjugated with toxins (eg, ricin, diphtheria) or with radioisotopes so that the antibodies deliver these toxic agents specifically to the tumor cells. Another technique involves bispecific antibodies, or linkage of one antibody that reacts with the tumor cell to a second antibody that reacts with a cytotoxic effector cell. This technique brings the effector cell in close opposition to the tumor cell, resulting in increased tumoricidal activity. However, these techniques are in the very early stages of testing; thus potential clinical benefits are uncertain.

Active Specific Immunotherapy

Approaches designed to induce cellular immunity in the tumor-bearing host are more promising than are passive immunotherapy techniques. Inducing immunity in a host that failed to spontaneously develop an effective response generally involves methods to enhance presentation of tumor antigens to host effector cells.

Autochthonous tumor cells (cells taken from the host) have been reintroduced to the host after use of ex vivo techniques (eg, irradiation, neuraminidase treatment, hapten conjugation, hybridization with other cell lines) to reduce their malignant potential and increase their antigenic activity. Genetic modulation of the tumor cells to produce immunostimulatory molecules (including cytokines such as granulocyte-macrophage colony-stimulating factor [GM-CSF] or IL-2, costimulatory molecules such as B7-1, and allogeneic class I MHC molecules) can also be performed to attract effector molecules and enhance systemic tumor targeting. Recent clinical trials with GM-CSF–modified tumor cells have produced very encouraging preliminary results.

Allogeneic tumor cells (cells taken from other patients) have been used in patients with acute lymphocytic leukemia and acute myeloblastic leukemia. Remission is induced by intensive chemotherapy and radiation therapy; irradiated allogeneic tumor cells that have been modified either genetically or chemically to increase their immunogenic potential are injected into the patient. Alternatively, allogeneic tumor cells can be injected along with bacille Calmette-Guérin (BCG) vaccine or other adjuvants (see p. 1157) to induce an enhanced immune response against the tumor. Prolonged remissions or improved reinduction rates have been reported in some series but not in most.

Defined tumor antigen–based vaccines are among the most promising approaches in cancer immunotherapy. An increasing number of tumor antigens have been unequivocally identified as the target of specific T cells grown from cancer patients.

Cellular immunity (involving cytotoxic T cells) to specific, very well defined antigens can be induced. Defined TAAs can be delivered into patients either in the form of peptides (usually co-administered with immunogenic adjuvants) or DNA that encodes specific protein (via recombinant viruses).

Recent studies have shown that the most potent responses can be achieved if TAAs are delivered using antigen-presenting cells (dendritic cells). These cells are obtained from the patient, loaded with the desired TAA, and then reintroduced intradermally to stimulate the endogenous T cell to respond to the specific antigen. Further, these cells can be genetically modified to secrete additional immune-response stimulants.

Another treatment method combines antigen-presenting cells and tumor cells in an attempt to utilize the entire spectrum of potential TAAs. Dendritic cells are either loaded with tumor cell lysates or dying tumor cells or are fused with living tumor cells. These methods are in clinical trials.

Nonspecific Immunotherapy

Interferons (IFN-α, -β, -γ) are glycoproteins that have antitumor and antiviral activity. Depending on dose, interferons may either enhance or decrease cellular and humoral immune functions. Interferons also inhibit division and certain synthetic processes in a variety of cells. Human clinical trials have indicated that interferons have antitumor activity in various neoplastic processes, including hairy cell leukemia, chronic myelocytic leukemia, AIDS-associated Kaposi's sarcoma, non-Hodgkin lymphoma, multiple myeloma, and ovarian carcinoma. However, interferons are associated with significant adverse effects, such as fever, malaise, leukopenia, alopecia, and myalgias.

Certain bacterial adjuvants (BCG and derivatives, killed suspensions of *Corynebacterium parvum*) have tumoricidal properties. They have been used with or without added tumor antigen to treat a wide variety of cancers, usually along with intensive chemotherapy or radiation therapy. For example, direct injection of BCG into neoplastic tissues has resulted in regression of melanoma and prolongation of disease-free intervals in superficial bladder carcinomas and may help prolong drug-induced remission in acute myeloblastic leukemia, ovarian carcinoma, and non-Hodgkin lymphoma.

149 PRINCIPLES OF CANCER THERAPY

Curing cancer requires eliminating all cancer cells. The major modalities of therapy are surgery and radiation therapy (for local and local-regional disease) and chemotherapy (for systemic disease). Other important methods include hormonal therapy (for selected cancers, eg, prostate, breast, endometrium), immunotherapy (monoclonal antibodies, interferons, and other biologic response modifiers and tumor vaccines—see also p. 1156), differentiating agents such as retinoids, and agents that exploit the growing knowledge of cellular and molecular biology. Overall treatment should be coordinated among a radiation oncologist, surgeon, and medical oncologist, where appropriate. Choice of modalities constantly evolves, and numerous controlled research trials continue. When available and appropriate, clinical trial participation should be considered and discussed with the patient.

Cure is defined clinically as the permanent absence of signs or symptoms of a disease; complete remission or complete response as disappearance of clinical evidence of disease; and partial response as a > 50% reduction in the size of a tumor mass or masses. Patients who appear to be cured may still have viable neoplastic cells that will eventually cause relapse. A partial response may lead to significant palliation and prolongation of life, but inevitably the tumor regrows. "Stable" disease indicates neither improvement nor worsening. The disease-free interval or disease-free survival reflects the interval between disappearance of cancer and relapse. Similarly, the duration of response refers to the time from response to the time of overt progression. Survival time refers to the time from diagnosis to death.

The disease-free interval often serves as an indicator of cure and varies with cancer type. For example, lung, colon, bladder, and testicular cancers are usually cured if a 5-yr disease-free interval occurs. Breast cancer, however, may recur even after 5 yr; thus a 10-yr disease-free interval is more indicative of cure.

Treatment decisions should weigh the likelihood of adverse effects against the likelihood of benefit; this requires frank communication and possibly the involvement of a multidisciplinary cancer team. A patient's preferences for how to live out the end of his life should be established early in the course of cancer treatment despite the difficulties of discussing death at such a sensitive time (see p. 2768).

MODALITIES OF CANCER THERAPY

Surgery

Surgery is the oldest form of effective cancer therapy. It may be used alone or in combination with other modalities.

Factors that increase operative risk in cancer patients include comorbid conditions, the debilitation associated with cancer, and, less commonly, paraneoplastic syndromes (see p. 1150). Cancer patients often have poor nutrition from anorexia and the catabolic influences of tumor growth, and these factors may inhibit or slow recovery from surgery. Patients may be neutropenic or thrombocytopenic, which increases the risk of sepsis and hemorrhage. Therefore, preoperative assessment is paramount (see p. 2742).

In the case of a primary tumor in which metastasis has not occurred, surgery may be curative. Establishing a complete margin of normal tissue around the primary tumor is critical for the success of primary tumor resection. Intraoperative examination of frozen tissue sections by a pathologist may be needed, with immediate resection of additional tissue if margins are positive for tumor cells. However, frozen tissue examination is inferior to examination of processed and stained tissue. Later review of margin tissue may prove the need for wider resection.

Surgical resection for primary tumor with local spread may also require removal of involved regional lymph nodes, resection of an involved adjacent organ, or en bloc resection. Survival rates with surgery alone are listed for selected cancers in TABLE 149–1.

In the case of metastases, in which the primary tumor has spread into adjacent normal tissues extensively, surgery may be delayed so that other modalities (eg, chemotherapy, radiation) can be used to reduce the size of the required resection. With regional lymph node metastases, nonsurgical modalities may be the best initial treatments, as in locally advanced lung cancer or head and neck cancer. Single metastases, especially those in the lung, can sometimes be resected with a reasonable rate of cure.

Patients with a limited number of metastases, particularly to the liver, brain, or lung, may benefit from surgical resection of both the primary and metastatic tumor. For example, in colon cancer with liver metastases, resection produces 5-yr survival rates of 30 to 40% if < 4 hepatic lesions exist and if adequate tumor margins can be obtained.

Cytoreduction, which is surgical resection to reduce tumor burden, is often an option when removal of all tumor tissue is impossible, as in most cases of ovarian cancer. Cytoreduction may increase the sensitivity of the remaining tissue to other treatment modalities through mechanisms that are not entirely clear. Cytoreduction has yielded favorable results in pediatric solid tumors and in ovarian cancer.

Palliative surgeryto relieve symptoms and preserve quality of life may be a reasonable alternative when cure is unlikely or when an attempt at cure produces adverse effects that are unacceptable to the patient. Tumor resection may be indicated to control pain, to reduce the risk of hemorrhage, or to relieve obstruction of a vital organ (eg, intestines, urinary tract). Nutritional supplementation with a feeding gastrostomy or jejunostomy tube may be necessary if proximal obstruction exists.

Reconstructive surgery may improve a patient's comfort or quality of life after tumor resection (eg, breast reconstruction after mastectomy).

Radiation Therapy

Radiation cannot destroy malignant cells without destroying some normal cells as well. Therefore, the risk to normal tissue must be weighed against the potential gain in treating the malignant cells. The final outcome of a dose of radiation depends on numerous factors, including nature of the delivered radiation (mode, timing, volume, dose) and properties of the tumor (cell cycle phase, molecular properties, overall sensitivity to radiation). In general, cancer cells are selectively damaged because of their high metabolic rate, and normal tissue repairs itself more effectively, resulting in greater net destruction of tumor.

The most common type of radiation therapy is external beam with a linear accelerator, which delivers photons (γ-radiation). The radiation dose to adjacent normal tissue can be limited by "conformal" technology, which reduces scatter at the field margins. Electron beam radiation therapy produces little tissue penetration and is best for skin or superficial cancers. Different energies of electrons are used based on the desired depth of penetration and type of tumor. Proton therapy, although limited in availability, can provide sharp margins and is particularly useful for base of brain and spine tumors.

Stereotactic radiation therapy is radiosurgery with precise stereotactic localization of a tumor to deliver a single high dose or multiple, fractionated doses to a small intracranial or other target. Advantages include complete tumor ablation where conventional surgery would not be possible, and minimal adverse effects. Disadvantages include limitations involving the size of the area that can be treated and the potential danger to adjacent tissues because of the high dose of radiation. In addition, it cannot be used in all areas of the body. The patient must be immobilized and the area kept completely still.

Brachytherapy involves placement of radioactive seeds through CT or ultrasonographic guidance into the tumor bed itself (eg, in the prostate or cervix). This technique achieves higher effective radiation doses over a longer period than could be accomplished by fractionated, external irradiation.

Systemic radioactive isotopes can direct radiation to cancer in organs that have specific receptors for uptake of the isotope (ie, radioactive iodine for thyroid cancer) or when using monoclonal antibodies. Isotopes can also accomplish palliation of generalized bony metastases (ie, radiostrontium for prostate cancer).

Other agents or strategies, particularly chemotherapy, can sensitize tumor tissue to the delivered radiation and increase efficacy.

Important considerations in the use of radiation include normal tissue in or adjacent to the proposed radiation field, target volume, configuration of radiation beams, dose distribution, and the modality and energy most suited to the patient's situation. Critical issues include treatment timing and dose fractionation. Treatment is tailored to take advantage of the cellular kinetics of tumor growth, with the aim of maximizing damage to the tumor while minimizing damage to normal tissues.

Radiation treatment sessions begin with the precise positioning of the patient. Foam casts or plastic masks are often constructed to ensure exact repositioning for serial treatments. Laser-guided sensors are used. Typical courses consist of large daily doses given over 3 wk for palliative treatment or smaller doses given once/day 5 days/wk for 6 to 8 wk for curative treatment.

Radiation therapy can cure many cancers (see TABLE 149–1), particularly those that are localized or that can be completely encompassed within the radiation field. Radiation therapy combined with surgery (for head and neck, laryngeal, or uterine cancer) or with chemotherapy and surgery (for sarcomas or breast, esophageal, lung, or rectal cancers) improves cure rates and allows for more limited surgery as compared with traditional surgical resection.

Radiation therapy can provide significant palliation when cure is not possible. Radiation therapy for brain tumors prolongs patient functioning; for spinal cord–compressing cancers, it can prevent progression of neurologic deficits; for superior vena caval syndromes, it can relieve venous obstruction; and for painful bone lesions, it usually relieves symptoms.

Adverse effects: Radiation can damage any intervening normal tissue. Acute adverse effects depend on the area receiving radiation and may include lethargy, fatigue, mucositis, dermatologic manifestations (erythema, pruritus, desquamation), esophagitis, pneumonitis, hepatitis, GI symptoms (nausea, vomiting, diarrhea, tenesmus), GU symptoms (frequency, urgency, dysuria), and cytopenias. Early detection and management of these adverse effects is important not only for the patient's comfort and quality of life but also to ensure continuous treatment; prolonged interruption can allow for tumor regrowth.

Late complications can include cataracts, keratitis, and retinal damage if the eye is in the treatment field; hypopituitarism; xerostomia; hypothyroidism; pneumonitis; pericarditis; esophageal stricture; hepatitis; ulcers; gastritis; nephritis; sterility; and muscular contractures. Radiation to normal tissue can lead to

TABLE 149–1. FIVE–YEAR DISEASE–FREE SURVIVAL RATES ACCORDING TO CANCER THERAPY

THERAPY	SITE	STAGE	5-YR DISEASE-FREE RATE (%)
Surgery (single modality)	Cervix	I	94
	Bladder	0 + A	81
		B_1	66
	Colon	A	81
		B	64
	Prostate	I + II	80
	Larynx	I + II	76
	Endometrium	I	74
	Ovary	I + II	72
	Oral cavity	I + II	67–76
	Kidney	I + II	67
	Testis (nonseminomatous)	I	65
	Lung (non-small cell)	I	50–70
		II	37
Radiation therapy (single modality)	Non-Hodgkin lymphoma	Pathologic stage I	60
	Hodgkin lymphoma (Hodgkin's disease)	Pathologic stage IA	80
	Testis (seminoma)	II + III	84
	Prostate	I + II	80
	Larynx	I + II	76
	Cervix	II + III	60
	Nasopharynx	I, II, III	35
	Nasal sinuses	I, II, III	35
	Esophagus		10
	Lung	III M0 (excluding Pancoast's tumor)	9
Chemotherapy	Choriocarcinoma (women)	All stages	95
	Testis (nonseminomatous)	III	88
	Hodgkin lymphoma	IIIB + IVA + B	74
	Diffuse large cell lymphoma	II, III, IV	45
	Burkitt's lymphoma	I, II, III	60
	Leukemia (childhood ALL)		85
	Leukemia (childhood, ANLL)		50
	Leukemia (< 40 yr, ANLL)		40–50
	Leukemia (> 40 yr, ANLL)		25
	Lung (small cell)	Limited	25
Surgery and radiation	Testis (seminoma)	I	94
	Endometrium	II	62
	Bladder	B_2 + C	54
	Oral cavity	III	36
	Hypopharynx	II + III	33
	Lung	III_{M0} Pancoast	32
Surgery and chemotherapy	Colon	III	70
	Ovary: carcinoma	III, IV	15

TABLE 149–1. FIVE-YEAR DISEASE-FREE SURVIVAL RATES ACCORDING TO CANCER THERAPY—Continued

THERAPY	SITE	STAGE	5-YR DISEASE-FREE RATE (%)
Radiation and chemotherapy	CNS (medulloblastoma)		70–80
	Ewing's sarcoma	All stages	70
	Anal cancer (squamous cell carcinoma)		70
	Lung (small cell cancer)	Limited	25
Surgery, radiation, and chemotherapy	Breast (with radiation therapy and +/– hormonal therapy)	I + II	70–90
	Kidney (Wilms' tumor)	All stages	80
	Embryonal rhabdomyosarcoma	All stages	80
	Oral cavity, hypopharynx	III + IV	20–40
	Rectum	II + III	50–70

ALL = acute lymphocytic leukemia; ANLL = acute nonlymphocytic leukemia.

poor healing of the tissues if further procedures or surgery is necessary. For example, radiation to the head and neck impairs recovery from dental procedures (eg, restoration, extraction) and thus should be administered only after all necessary dental work has been performed.

Radiation treatment can increase the risk of developing other malignancies, particularly leukemias and cancers of the thyroid or breast. Peak incidence occurs 5 to 10 yr after exposure and depends on the patient's age at the time of treatment. For example, chest irradiation for Hodgkin lymphoma (Hodgkin's disease) in adolescent females leads to a higher risk of breast cancer than does the same treatment for postadolescent females.

Chemotherapy

The ideal chemotherapeutic drug would target and destroy only cancer cells. Unfortunately, few such drugs exist. Common chemotherapeutic drugs and their adverse effects are described in TABLE 149–2.

The most common routes of administration are IV and oral. Frequent dosing for extended periods may necessitate subcutaneously implanted venous access devices (central or peripheral), multilumen external catheters, or peripherally inserted central catheters.

Drug resistance can occur to chemotherapy. Identified mechanisms include overexpression of target genes, drug inactivation by tumor cells, defective apoptosis in tumor cells, and loss of receptors for hormonal agents. One of the best characterized mechanisms is overexpression of the *MDR-1* gene, a cell membrane transporter that causes efflux of certain drugs (eg, vinca alkaloids, taxanes, anthracyclines). Attempts to alter *MDR-1* function and thus prevent drug resistance have been unsuccessful.

Cytotoxic drugs: Traditional cytotoxic chemotherapy, which damages cell DNA, kills many normal cells in addition to cancer cells. Antimetabolites, such as 5-fluorouracil and methotrexate, are cell cycle–specific and have no linear dose-response relationship. In contrast, other chemotherapeutic drugs (eg, DNA cross-linkers, also known as alkylating agents) have a linear dose-response relationship, producing more tumor killing as well as more toxicity at higher doses. At their highest doses, DNA cross-linkers may produce bone marrow aplasia, necessitating bone marrow transplantation to restore bone marrow function.

TABLE 149–2. COMMONLY USED ANTINEOPLASTIC DRUGS

DRUG CLASS	DRUG	MECHANISM OF ACTION	COMMONLY RESPONSIVE TUMORS	TOXICITY AND REMARKS
DNA cross-linking drugs and alkylating agents				
	Mechlorethamine (nitrogen mustard) Chlorambucil Cyclophosphamide Melphalan Ifosfamide	Form adducts with DNA, causing DNA strand breaks	Hodgkin lymphoma (Hodgkin's disease), malignant lymphoma, small cell lung cancer, breast and testicular cancer, chronic lymphocytic leukemia, multiple myeloma; malignant gliomas	Alopecia with high IV dosage; nausea and vomiting; myelosuppression; hemorrhagic cystitis (especially with cyclophosphamide and ifosfamide), which can be ameliorated with mesna; mutagenic and leukemogenic; aspermia; permanent sterility (possible)
	Procarbazine	Forms adducts with DNA, causing DNA strand breaks	Hodgkin lymphoma	Neutropenia, nausea, vomiting, secondary leukemias
	Dacarbazine	Forms adducts with DNA, causing DNA strand breaks	Melanoma	Neutropenia, nausea, vomiting, secondary leukemias
	Temozolomide	Forms adducts with DNA, causing DNA strand breaks	Malignant gliomas	Neutropenia, nausea, vomiting, secondary leukemias
Nitrosoureas	Carmustine (BiCNU)	Alkylates DNA with restricted uncoiling and replication of strands	Brain tumors, lymphoma	Myelosuppression, pulmonary toxicity (fibrosis), renal toxicity
	Lomustine	Alkylates DNA with restricted uncoiling and replication of strands	Brain tumors (astrocytoma, glioblastoma)	Myelosuppression, pulmonary toxicity (delayed), nephrotoxicity
Platinum complexes				
	Cisplatin	Establishes cross links within and between DNA strands	Lung cancer (especially small cell); testicular, breast, and gastric cancer	Anemia, ototoxicity, nausea, vomiting, peripheral neuropathy, myelosuppression
	Carboplatin	Establishes cross links within and between DNA strands	Lung, head and neck, ovarian, and breast cancer	Myelosuppression, peripheral neuropathy
	Oxaliplatin	Establishes cross links within and between DNA strands	Colon cancer	Myelosuppression, neuropathic throat pain, peripheral neuropathy

TABLE 149–2. COMMONLY USED ANTINEOPLASTIC DRUGS—Continued

DRUG CLASS	DRUG	MECHANISM OF ACTION	COMMONLY RESPONSIVE TUMORS	TOXICITY AND REMARKS
Antimetabolites				
Folate antagonist	Methotrexate	Binds to dihydrofolate reductase and interferes with thymidylate synthesis	Choriocarcinoma (female), head and neck cancer, acute lymphocytic leukemia, ovarian cancer, malignant lymphoma, osteogenic sarcoma	Mucosal ulceration; bone marrow suppression; increased toxicity with impaired renal function or ascitic fluid (with pooling of drug); leucovorin rescue can reverse toxicity at 24 h (10–20 mg q 6 h × 10 doses)
Purine antagonists	6-Mercaptopurine	Blocks de novo purine synthesis	Acute leukemia	Myelosuppression, immunosuppression
	Fludarabine	Terminates DNA synthesis	Leukemia, lymphoma	Myelosuppression, immunosuppression
	Cladribine	Inhibits ribonucleotide reductase	Leukemia, lymphoma	Myelosuppression, immunosuppression
Pyrimidine antagonists	5-Fluorouracil	Inhibits thymidylate synthase	GI tumors, breast cancer	Mucositis, alopecia, myelosuppression, diarrhea and vomiting
	Capecitabine	Inhibits thymidylate synthase	GI tumors, breast cancer	Mucositis, alopecia, myelosuppression, diarrhea and vomiting, hand/foot tenderness, ulceration
	Cytarabine	Chain termination when incorporated into DNA	Acute leukemia (especially nonlymphocytic), malignant lymphoma	Myelosuppression, nausea and vomiting, cerebellar and conjunctival toxicities at high doses, skin rash
	Gemcitabine	Chain termination when incorporated into DNA	Pancreatic, lung, and bladder cancer	Myelosuppression, hemolytic-uremic syndrome
Ribonucleotide reductase inhibitor	Hydroxyurea	Depletion of cellular deoxynucleotides	Chronic myelocytic leukemia	Myelosuppression
Spindle poison (from plants)				
Vincas	Vinblastine	Arrests mitosis by inhibiting polymerization of microtubules	Lymphomas, leukemias, breast cancer, Ewing's sarcoma, testicular cancer	Alopecia, myelosuppression, peripheral neuropathy
	Vincristine	Arrests mitosis by inhibiting polymerization of microtubules	Lymphomas and acute leukemia	Peripheral neuropathy, ileus, syndrome of inappropriate antidiuretic hormone secretion

Table continues on the following page.

TABLE 149–2. COMMONLY USED ANTINEOPLASTIC DRUGS—Continued

DRUG CLASS	DRUG	MECHANISM OF ACTION	COMMONLY RESPONSIVE TUMORS	TOXICITY AND REMARKS
	Vinorelbine	Arrests mitosis by inhibiting polymerization of microtubules	Lung and breast cancer	Myelosuppression, neuropathy
Taxanes	Paclitaxel	Promotes assembly of microtubules	Breast, lung, ovarian, head and neck, and bladder cancer	Myelosuppression, alopecia, myalgia, arthralgia, neuropathy
	Docetaxel	Promotes assembly of microtubules	Breast, lung, ovarian, and head and neck cancer	Myelosuppression, alopecia, skin rash, fluid retention
Topoisomerase inhibitors				
Podophyllotoxins	Etoposide Teniposide	Inhibit topoisomerase II and cause DNA strand breaks	Lymphoma, Hodgkin lymphoma, testicular cancer, lung cancer (especially small cell), acute leukemia	Nausea, vomiting, myelosuppression, peripheral neuropathy; cleared by liver and kidney; increased toxicity in renal failure; neutropenia
	Mitoxantrone	Inhibit topoisomerase II and cause DNA strand breaks	Acute leukemia, lymphoma	Neutropenia, nausea, vomiting
Anthracyclines	Daunorubicin Doxorubicin Epirubicin Idarubicin	Inhibit topoisomerase II and cause DNA strand breaks	Acute leukemia, lymphoma, breast and lung cancer	Doxorubicin: Nausea and vomiting, myelosuppression, alopecia; cardiac toxicity at cumulative dosage > 500 mg/m^2. Daunomycin, a related derivative, also has cardiac toxicity; its role has been limited to acute leukemia
Camptothecins	Irinotecan	Inhibits topoisomerase I and II	Colon, rectal, and lung cancer	Diarrhea, myelosuppression, alopecia
	Topotecan	Inhibits topoisomerase I and II	Ovarian and small-cell lung cancer	Myelosuppression
Tyrosine kinase inhibitors				
	Imatinib	Inhibits Bcr-Abl kinase, c-kit kinase	Chronic myelocytic leukemia, GI stromal tumors	Leukopenia, hepatocellular toxicity, edema
	Erlotinib Gefitinib	Inhibit epidermal growth factor receptor	Non–small cell lung cancer	Acne, diarrhea
Bleomycins				
	Bleomycin	Causes DNA strand breaks	Squamous cell cancer, lymphoma, testicular cancer	Anaphylaxis, chills and fever, skin rash; pulmonary fibrosis at dosage > 200 mg/m^2; requires renal excretion

TABLE 149–2. COMMONLY USED ANTINEOPLASTIC DRUGS—Continued

DRUG CLASS	DRUG	MECHANISM OF ACTION	COMMONLY RESPONSIVE TUMORS	TOXICITY AND REMARKS
Other antibiotics				
	Mitomycin	Inhibits DNA synthesis by acting as a bifunctional alkylator	Gastric adenocarcinoma; colon, breast, and lung cancer; transitional cell cancer of the bladder	Local extravasation causes tissue necrosis; myelosuppression, with leukopenia and thrombocytopenia 4 to 6 wk after treatment; alopecia; lethargy; fever; hemolytic-uremic syndrome
Biologic response modifiers				
	Interferon-α	Antiproliferative effect	Hairy cell leukemia, chronic myelocytic leukemia, lymphomas, Kaposi's sarcoma (AIDS), renal cell cancer, melanoma	Fatigue, fever, myalgias, arthralgias, myelosuppression, nephrotic syndrome (rarely)
Enzymes				
	Asparaginase	Depletion of asparagine, on which leukemic cells depend	Acute lymphocytic leukemia	Acute anaphylaxis, hyperthermia, pancreatitis, hyperglycemia, hypofibrinogenemia
Hormones				
	Tamoxifen	Binds to estrogen receptor	Breast cancer	Hot flushes, hypercalcemia, deep venous thrombosis
	Leuprolide acetate	Inhibits gonadotropin secretion	Prostate cancer	Hot flushes, decreased libido, irritation at injection site
	Megestrol acetate	Progesterone agonist	Breast and endometrial cancer	Weight gain, fluid retention
Androgen receptor blockers	Flutamide and bicalutamide	Bind to androgen receptor	Prostate cancer	Decreased libido, hot flushes, gynecomastia
Aromatase inhibitors	Anastrozole Exemestane Letrozole	Blocks conversion of androgen to estrogen	Breast cancer	Osteoporosis, hot flushes
Monoclonal antibodies				
	Gemtuzumab	Binds to CD33 on leukemic cells	Acute myelocytic leukemia	Myelosuppression
	Alemtuzumab	Binds to B and T cells	Lymphomas	Immune suppression

Table continues on the following page.

TABLE 149–2. COMMONLY USED ANTINEOPLASTIC DRUGS—Continued

DRUG CLASS	DRUG	MECHANISM OF ACTION	COMMONLY RESPONSIVE TUMORS	TOXICITY AND REMARKS
	Ibritumomab tiuxetan	Binds to CD20 on lymphoid cells	Lymphomas	Delivers radiation
	Tositumomab, iodine-131 tositumomab	Binds to CD20 on lymphoid cells	Lymphomas	Myelosuppression, fever, rash
	Rituximab	Binds to CD20 on B cells	B-cell lymphoma	Hypersensitivity
	Trastuzumab	Binds to her2/neu receptor	Breast cancer	Hypersensitivity, cardiac toxicity
	Bevacizumab	Binds to vascular endothelial growth factor	Colon cancer, renal cancer	Hypersensitivity, bleeding, hypertension

Single-drug therapy may cure selected cancers (eg, choriocarcinoma, hairy cell leukemia). More commonly, multidrug regimens incorporating drugs with different mechanisms of action and different toxicities are used to increase the tumor cell kill, reduce dose-related toxicity, and decrease the probability of drug resistance. These regimens can provide significant cure rates (eg, in acute leukemia, testicular cancer, Hodgkin lymphoma, non-Hodgkin lymphoma, and, less commonly, solid tumors such as small cell lung cancer and nasopharyngeal cancer). Multidrug regimens typically are given as repetitive cycles of a fixed combination of drugs. The interval between cycles should be the shortest one that allows for recovery of normal tissue. Continuous infusion may increase cell kill with some cell cycle-specific drugs (eg, 5-fluorouracil).

For each patient, the probability of significant toxicities should be weighed against the likelihood of benefit. End-organ function should be assessed before chemotherapeutic drugs with organ-specific toxicities are used (eg, echocardiography before doxorubicin use). Dose modification or exclusion of certain drugs may be necessary in patients with chronic lung disease (eg, bleomycin), renal failure (eg, methotrexate), or hepatic dysfunction (eg, taxanes).

Despite these precautions, adverse effects commonly result from cytotoxic chemotherapy. The normal tissues most commonly affected are those with the highest intrinsic turnover rate: bone marrow, hair follicles, and the GI epithelium.

Imaging (eg, CT, MRI, PET) is frequently performed after 2 to 3 cycles of therapy to evaluate response to treatment. Therapy continues if a clear response is seen. If the tumor progresses despite therapy, the regimen is often amended or stopped. If the disease remains stable with treatment and the patient can tolerate therapy, then a decision to continue is reasonable with the understanding that the disease will eventually progress.

Hormonal therapy: Hormonal therapy uses hormone agonists or antagonists to influence the course of cancer. It may be used alone or in combination with other treatment modalities.

Hormonal therapy is particularly useful in prostate cancer, which grows in response to testosterone. Other cancers with hormone receptors on their cells (eg, breast, endometrium) can often be palliated by hormone antagonist therapy or hormone ablation.

Use of prednisone, a glucocorticosteroid, is also considered hormonal therapy. It is frequently used to treat tumors derived from the immune system (lymphomas, lymphocytic leukemias, multiple myeloma).

Biologic response modifiers: Interferons are proteins synthesized by cells of the immune system as a physiologic immune protective response to foreign antigens (viruses, bacteria, other foreign cells). In pharmacologic amounts, they can palliate some cancers, including hairy cell leukemia, chronic myelocytic leukemia, locally advanced melanoma, metastatic renal cell cancer, and Kaposi's sarcoma. Significant toxic effects of interferon include fatigue, depression, nausea, leukopenia, chills and fever, and myalgias.

Interleukins, primarily the lymphokine IL-2 produced by activated T cells, can be used in metastatic melanomas and can provide modest palliation in renal cell cancer.

Differentiating drugs: These drugs induce differentiation in cancer cells. All-*trans*-retinoic acid has been highly effective in treating acute promyelocytic leukemia. Other drugs in this class, including phenylbutyrate, phenylacetate, arsenic compounds, vitamin D analogs, and the hypomethylating agent deoxyazacytidine, are under study. When used alone, these drugs have only transient effects, but their role in prevention and in combination with cytotoxic drugs is promising.

Antiangiogenesis drugs: Solid tumors produce growth factors that form new blood vessels necessary to support ongoing tumor growth. Several drugs that inhibit this process are available. Thalidomide is antiangiogenic, among its many effects. Avastin, a monoclonal antibody to vascular endothelial growth factor (VEGF), is effective against renal cancers and colon cancer.

Signal transduction inhibitors: Many epithelial tumors possess mutations that activate signaling pathways that contribute to their continuous proliferation and failure to differentiate. These mutated pathways include growth factors and the downstream proteins that transmit messages from growth factor receptors on the cell surface. Two such drugs, imatinib (an inhibitor of the Bcr-Abl tyrosine kinase in chronic myelocytic leukemia) and erlotinib (an inhibitor of the epidermal growth factor receptor), are now in routine clinical use. Other inhibitors of these signaling pathways are under study.

Monoclonal antibodies: Monoclonal antibodies directed against unique tumor antigens have some efficacy against neoplastic tissue (see also p. 1156). Trastuzumab, an antibody directed against a protein called Her-2 or Erb-B2, plus chemotherapy has shown benefit in metastatic breast cancer. Antibodies against CD antigens expressed on neoplastic cells, such as CD20 and CD33, are used to treat patients with non-Hodgkin lymphoma (rituximab, anti-CD20 antibody) and acute myelocytic leukemia (gemtuzumab, an antibody linked to a potent toxin).

The effectiveness of monoclonal antibodies may be increased by linking them to radioactive nuclide. One such drug, ibritumomab, is used to treat non-Hodgkin lymphoma.

Multimodality and Adjuvant Chemotherapy

In some tumors with a high likelihood of relapse despite optimal initial surgery or radiation therapy, relapse may be prevented by addition of adjuvant chemotherapy. Increasingly, combined-modality therapy (eg, radiation therapy, chemotherapy, surgery) is used. It may permit organ-sparing procedures and preserve organ function.

Adjuvant chemotherapy is systemic chemotherapy or radiation therapy given after initial surgery to eradicate residual occult tumor. Patients who have a high risk of recurrence may benefit from its use. General criteria are based on degree of local extension of the primary tumor, presence of positive lymph nodes, and certain morphologic or biologic characteristics of individual cancer cells. Adjuvant chemotherapy has increased disease-free survival and cure rate in breast and in colorectal cancer.

Neoadjuvant therapy is chemotherapy and/or radiation therapy given before surgical resection. This treatment may enhance resectability and preserve local organ function. For example, when this therapy is used in head and neck, esophageal, or rectal cancer, a smaller subsequent resection may be possible. Another advantage of neoadjuvant therapy is in assessing response to treatment; if the primary tumor does not respond, micrometastases are unlikely to be eradicated, and an alternate regimen should be considered. Neoadjuvant therapy may obscure the true pathologic stage of the cancer by altering tumor size and margins and converting histologically positive nodes to negative, complicating clinical staging. The use of neoadjuvant therapy has improved survival in inflammatory and locally advanced breast, stage IIIA lung, nasopharyngeal, and bladder cancers.

Bone Marrow Transplantation

Bone marrow or stem cell transplantation is an important component of the treatment of otherwise refractory lymphomas, leukemias, and multiple myeloma (see p. 1371 for an in-depth discussion of this topic).

Gene Therapy

Genetic modulation is under intense investigation. Strategies include the use of antisense therapy; systemic viral vector transfection; DNA injection into tumors; genetic modulation of resected tumor cells to increase their immunogenicity; and alteration of immune cells to enhance their antitumor response.

MANAGEMENT OF ADVERSE EFFECTS

Nausea and Vomiting

Nausea and vomiting are commonly experienced by the cancer patient, either from the cancer itself (eg, paraneoplastic syndromes) or from its treatment (eg, chemotherapy, radiation therapy to the brain or abdomen). However, refractory nausea and vomiting should prompt further investigation, including basic laboratory testing (electrolytes, liver function tests, amylase) and x-rays to investigate bowel obstruction or intracranial metastases.

Serotonin-receptor antagonists are the most effective drugs but are also the most expensive. Virtually no toxicity occurs with granisetron and ondansetron aside from headache and orthostatic hypotension. A 0.15-mg/kg dose of ondansetron or a 10-μg/kg dose of granisetron is given IV 30 min before chemotherapy. Doses of ondansetron can be repeated 4 and 8 h after the 1st dose. The efficacy against highly emetogenic drugs, such as the platinum analogs, can be improved with co-administration of dexamethasone (8 mg IV given 30 min before chemotherapy with repeat doses of 4 mg IV q 8 h). Aprepitant is a substance P/neurokinin-1 antagonist that can limit nausea and vomiting resulting from highly emetogenic chemotherapy. Dosage is 125 mg po 1 h before chemotherapy on day 1, then 80 mg po 1 h before chemotherapy on days 2 and 3.

Other traditional antiemetics, including phenothiazines (eg, prochlorperazine 10 mg IV q 8 h, promethazine 12.5 to 25 mg po or IV q 8 h) and metoclopramide (10 mg po or IV given 30 min before chemotherapy with repeated doses q 6 to 8 h), are alternatives restricted to patients with mild to moderate nausea and vomiting.

Dronabinol (Δ-9-tetrahydrocannabinol [THC]) is an alternative treatment for nausea and vomiting caused by chemotherapy. THC is the principal psychoactive component of marijuana. Its mechanism of antiemetic action is unknown, but cannabinoids bind to opioid receptors in the forebrain and may indirectly inhibit the vomiting center. Dronabinol is administered in doses of 5 mg/m^2 po 1 to 3 h before chemotherapy, with repeated doses q 2 to 4 h after the start of chemotherapy (maximum of 4 to 6 doses/day). However, it has variable oral bioavailability, is not effective for inhibiting the nausea and vomiting of platinum-based chemotherapy regimens, and has significant adverse effects (eg, drowsiness, orthostatic hypotension, dry mouth, mood changes, visual and time sense alterations). Smoking marijuana may be more effective. Marijuana for this purpose can be obtained legally in some states. It is used less commonly because of barriers to availability and because many patients cannot tolerate smoking.

Benzodiazepines, such as lorazepam (1 to 2 mg po or IV given 10 to 20 min before chemotherapy with repeated doses q 4 to 6 h prn), are sometimes helpful for refractory or anticipatory nausea and vomiting.

Cytopenias

Anemia, leukopenia, and thrombocytopenia may develop during chemotherapy or radiation therapy. Clinical symptoms and decreased efficacy of radiation therapy usually occur at Hct levels of < 30% or Hb levels < 10 g/mL, sooner in those with coronary artery disease or peripheral vascular disease. Recombinant erythropoietin therapy is generally started when Hct falls below 32 (a Hb < 10 mg/dL). In general, 150 to 300 units/kg sc 3 times/wk (a convenient adult dose is 10,000 units) is effective and reduces the need for transfusions. Longer-acting formulations of erythropoietin are also gaining acceptance and require less frequent dosing (darbepoietin-α 2.25 to 4.5 μg/kg sc q 1 to 2 wk). Packed RBC transfusions may be needed to relieve acute cardiorespiratory symptoms.

A platelet count < 10,000/mL, especially with bleeding, requires transfusion of platelet concentrates. Recombinant thrombopoietin and small molecules that mimic thrombopoietin are under study.

Leukocyte depletion of transfused blood products may prevent alloimmunization to platelets and should be used in patients who are expected to need platelet transfusions during multiple courses of chemotherapy or for candidates for bone marrow or stem cell transplantation. Leukocyte depletion also lowers the probability of cytomegalovirus being transferred to the patient through WBCs. Gamma irradiation of blood products to inactivate lymphocytes and prevent transfusion-induced graft-vs-host disease is also indicated in patients undergoing severely immunosuppressive chemotherapy.

Neutropenia (see also p. 1059), usually defined by an absolute neutrophil count < 500/μL, predisposes to immediate life-threatening infection. Afebrile patients with neutropenia require close outpatient follow-up for detection of fever and should be instructed to avoid contact with sick people or areas frequented by large numbers of people (eg, shopping malls, airports). Although most patients do not require antibiotics, severely immunosuppressed (ie, concomitant T-cell depletion or loss of function) leukopenic patients are sometimes given trimethoprim-sulfamethoxazole (one double-strength tablet/day) as prophylaxis for *Pneumocystis jiroveci* (formerly *P. carinii*). In transplant patients or others receiving high-dose chemotherapy, antiviral prophylaxis (acyclovir 800 mg po bid or 400 mg IV q 12 h) should be considered if serologic tests are positive for herpes simplex virus.

Fever >38° C in a neutropenic patient is an emergency. Evaluation should include immediate chest x-ray and cultures of blood, sputum, urine, stool, and any suspect skin lesions. Examination includes possible abscess sites (eg, skin, ears), skin and mucosa for presence of herpetic lesions, retina for vascular lesions suggestive of metastatic infection, and catheter sites. Rectal examination and use of a rectal thermometer are avoided if possible in neutropenic patients because of the risk of bacteremia.

Febrile neutropenic patients should receive broad-spectrum antibiotics chosen on the basis of the most likely source. Typical regimens include cefepime 2 g IV q 8 h or ceftazidime 2 g IV q 8 h immediately after cultures are obtained. If diffuse pulmonary infiltrates are present, sputum should be tested for *P. jiroveci,* and if positive, appropriate therapy should be started. If fever resolves within 72 h after starting empiric antibiotics, then antibiotics are continued until the absolute neutrophil count is > 500/μL. If fever continues for 120 h, then antifungal drugs should be added to cover possible fungal causes. Re-assessment for occult infection (often including CT of the chest and abdomen) should be undertaken at this time.

In selected patients with neutropenia related to chemotherapy, especially after high-dose chemotherapy, granulocyte colony-stimulating factor (G-CSF) or granulocyte-macrophage colony-stimulating factor (GM-CSF) may be started to shorten the leukopenic period. G-CSF 5 μg/kg sc once/day up to 14 days and longer-acting forms (eg, pegfilgrastim 6 mg sc single dose once per chemotherapy cycle) may be used to accelerate WBC recovery. These drugs should not be administered in the first 24 h after chemotherapy, and for pegfilgrastim, at least 14 days should elapse until the next planned chemotherapy dose. These drugs are begun at the onset of fever or sepsis or, in the afebrile patient, when neutrophil counts fall below 500/μL.

Many centers use outpatient treatment of selected low-risk patients with fever and neutropenia. Candidates must not have hypotension, altered mental status, respiratory distress, uncontrolled pain, or serious comorbid illnesses, such as diabetes, heart disease, or hypercalcemia. The regimen in such cases requires daily follow-up and often involves visiting nurse services and home antibiotic infusion. Some regimens involve oral antibiotics, such as ciprofloxacin 750 mg po bid plus amoxicillin-clavulanate 875 mg po bid or 500 mg po tid. If no defined institutional program for follow-up and treatment of neutropenic fever is available in an outpatient setting, then hospitalization is required.

Gastrointestinal Effects

Oral lesions, such as ulcers, infections, and inflammation, are common. Oral candidiasis can be treated with nystatin oral suspension 5 to 10 mL qid, clotrimazole troches 10 mg qid, or fluconazole 100 mg po once/day. Mucositis from radiation therapy can cause pain and preclude sufficient oral intake, leading to malnutrition and weight loss. Rinses with analgesics and topical anesthetics (2% viscous lidocaine, 5 to 10 mL q 2 h or other commercially available mixtures) before meals, a bland diet without citrus food or juices, and avoidance of temperature extremes may allow the patient to eat and maintain weight. If not, a feeding tube may be helpful if the small bowel is functional. For severe mucositis and diarrhea or an abnormally functioning intestine, parenteral alimentation may be needed.

Diarrhea from pelvic radiation therapy or from chemotherapy can be alleviated with antidiarrheal drugs as needed (kaolin/pectin suspension 60 to 120 mL regular strength, or 30 to 60 mL concentrate, po at first sign of diarrhea and after each loose stool or prn; loperamide 2 to 4 mg po; or diphenoxylate/atropine 1 to 2 tablets po). Patients receiving antibiotics should undergo stool testing for *Clostridium difficile*.

Constipation may result from opioid use. A stimulant laxative such as senna 2 to 6 tablets po at bedtime or bisocodyl 10 mg po at bedtime should be initiated when repeated opioid use is anticipated. Established constipation can be treated with a variety of drugs (eg, bisacodyl 5 to 10 mg po q 12 to 24 h, milk of magnesia 15 to 30 mL po at bedtime, lactulose 15 to 30 mL q 12 to 24 h, Mg citrate 250 to 500 mL po once). Enemas and suppositories should be avoided in neutropenic and thrombocytopenic patients.

Appetite may decrease secondary to cancer treatment or to a paraneoplastic syndrome. Corticosteroids (dexamethasone 4 mg po once/day, prednisone 5 to 10 mg po once/day) and megestrol acetate 400 to 800 mg once/day are most effective. However, the primary benefits are variably increased appetite and weight gain, not improved survival or quality of life.

Pain

Pain should be anticipated and aggressively treated (see also p. 1771). Use of multiple drug classes may provide better pain control with fewer or less severe adverse effects than single drug classes. NSAIDs should be avoided in thrombocytopenic patients. Opioids are the mainstay of treatment, given around the clock in generally efficient doses, with supplemental doses given for occasional worse pain. If the oral route is unavailable, fentanyl is given transdermally. Antiemetics and prophylactic bowel regimens are often needed with opioids. Neuropathic pain can be treated with a tricyclic antidepressant (eg, nortriptyline 25 to 75 mg po at bedtime), although most physicians prefer gabapentin. The dose required for neuropathic pain is high (≤ 3.6 g/day) but must be started low and then increased over a few weeks.

Useful nondrug treatments for pain include focal radiation therapy, nerve blockade, and surgery.

Depression

Depression is often overlooked. Patients receiving interferon can develop depression as an adverse effect. Frank discussion of a patient's fears can often relieve anxiety; depression can often be treated effectively (see p. 1704).

Tumor Lysis Syndrome

Tumor lysis syndrome may occur secondary to release of intracellular components into the bloodstream as a result of tumor cell death after chemotherapy. It occurs mainly in acute leukemias and non-Hodgkin lymphomas but can also occur in other hematologic malignancies and, uncommonly, after treatment of solid tumors. It should be suspected in patients with a large tumor burden who develop acute renal failure after initial treatment.

The diagnosis is confirmed by renal failure, hypocalcemia (< 8 mg/dL), hyperuricemia (> 15 mg/dL), and/or hyperphosphatemia (> 8 mg/dL). Allopurinol (200 to 400 mg/m^2 once/day, maximum 600 mg/day) and normal saline IV to achieve urine output > 2 L/day should be initiated with close laboratory and cardiac monitoring. Patients who have a malignancy with rapid cell turnover should receive allopurinol for at least 2 days before and during chemotherapy; for patients with high cell burden, this regimen can be continued for 10 to 14 days after therapy. All such patients should receive vigorous IV hydration to establish a diuresis of at least 100 mL/h prior to treatment. Although some physicians advocate $NaHCO_3$ IV to alkalinize the urine and increase solubilization of uric acid, alkalinization may promote Ca phosphate deposition in patients with hyperphosphatemia, and a pH of about 7 should be avoided. Alternatively, rasburicase, an enzyme that oxidizes uric acid to allantoin (a more soluble molecule), may be used to prevent tumor lysis. The dose is 0.15 to 0.2 mg/kg IV over 30 min once/day for 5 to 7 days, typically initiated 4 to 24 h before the first chemotherapy treatment. Adverse effects may include anaphylaxis, hemolysis, hemoglobinuria, and methemoglobinemia.

INCURABLE CANCER

Even in cases of incurable cancer, palliative or experimental therapy may improve quality and extent of life. But in many cases, physicians must resist the urge to administer a relatively ineffective chemotherapy drug. A better choice is to discuss the likely results of such treatments and to set realistic goals with the patient. A patient's decision to forgo cancer treatment must be respected. Another alternative is the clinical trial, the risks and benefits of which deserve discussion.

Regardless of prognosis, quality of life in cancer patients may improve with nutritional support, effective pain management, other symptomatic palliative care, and psychiatric and social support of the patient and family. Above all, the patient must know that the clinical team will remain involved and accessible for supportive care, regardless of the prognosis. Hospice or other related end-of-life care programs are important parts of cancer treatment. For more information pertaining to patients with incurable disease, see Ch. 338 on p. 2762.

CACHEXIA

Cachexia is wasting of both adipose and skeletal muscle. It occurs in many conditions and is common with many cancers when remission or control fails. Some cancers, especially pancreatic and gastric, produce profound cachexia. Such patients may lose 10 to 20% of body weight. Men tend to experience worse cachexia with cancer than do women. Neither tumor size nor the extent of metastatic disease predicts the degree of cachexia. Cachexia is associated with reduced response to chemotherapy, poor functional performance, and increased mortality.

The primary cause of cachexia is not anorexia or decreased caloric intake. Rather, this complex metabolic condition involves increased tissue catabolism. Protein synthesis is decreased and degradation increased. Cachexia is mediated by certain cytokines, especially tumor necrosis factor-α, IL-1b, and IL-6, which are produced by tumor cells and host cells in the tissue mass. The ATP-ubiquitin-protease pathway plays a role as well.

Cachexia is easy to recognize, primarily by weight loss, which is most apparent with temporalis muscle mass loss in the face. The loss of subcutaneous fat increases the risk of pressure ulcers over bony prominences.

Treatment

Treatment involves treatment of the cancer. If the cancer can be controlled or cured, regardless of modality, cachexia resolves.

Additional caloric supplementation does not relieve cachexia. Any weight gain is usually minimal and is likely to consist of adipose tissue rather than muscle. Neither function nor prognosis is improved. Thus, in most cachectic patients with cancer, high-calorie supplementation is not recommended, and parenteral nutritional support is not indicated, except in situations where oral intake of adequate nutrition is impossible.

However, other treatments can mitigate cachexia and improve function. Corticosteroids increase appetite and may improve a sense of well-being but do little to increase body weight. Likewise, cannabinoids (marijuana, dronabinol) increase appetite but not weight. Progestogens, such as megestrol, 40 mg bid or tid, may increase both appetite and body weight. Drugs to alter cytokine production and effects are being studied.

SECTION 12
ENDOCRINE AND METABOLIC DISORDERS

150 PRINCIPLES OF ENDOCRINOLOGY

The endocrine system coordinates functioning between different organs through hormones, which are released into the bloodstream from specific types of cells within endocrine (ductless) glands. Once in circulation, hormones affect function of the target tissue. Some hormones exert an effect on cells of the organ from which they were released (paracrine effect), some even on the same cell type (autocrine effect). Hormones can be peptides of various sizes, steroids (derived from cholesterol), or amino acid derivatives.

Hormones bind selectively to receptors located inside or on the surface of target cells. Receptors inside cells interact with hormones that regulate gene function (eg, corticosteroids, vitamin D, thyroid hormone). Receptors on the cell surface bind with hormones that regulate enzyme activity or affect ion channels (eg, growth hormone, thyrotropin-releasing hormone).

Hypothalamic-Pituitary Relationships

Peripheral endocrine organ functions are controlled to varying degrees by pituitary hormones (see also Ch. 151 on p. 1179). Some functions (eg, secretion of insulin by the pancreas, primarily controlled by the plasma glucose level) are controlled to a minimal extent, whereas many (eg, secretion of thyroid or gonadal hormones) are controlled to a great extent. Secretion of pituitary hormones is controlled by the hypothalamus.

The interaction between the hypothalamus and pituitary (hypothalamic-pituitary axis) is a negative feedback control system. The hypothalamus receives input from virtually all other areas of the CNS and uses it to provide input to the pituitary. In response, the pituitary releases various hormones that stimulate certain endocrine glands throughout the body. Changes in circulating levels of hormones produced by these endocrine glands are detected by the hypothalamus, which then increases or decreases its stimulation of the pituitary to maintain homeostasis.

The hypothalamus modulates the activities of the anterior and posterior lobes of the pituitary in different ways. Neurohormones synthesized in the hypothalamus reach the anterior pituitary (adenohypophysis) through a specialized portal vascular system and regulate synthesis and release of the 6 major peptide hormones of the anterior pituitary. These anterior pituitary hormones regulate peripheral endocrine glands (the thyroid, adrenals, and gonads) as well as growth and lactation. No direct neural connection exists between the hypothalamus and the anterior pituitary. In contrast, the posterior pituitary (neurohypophysis) comprises axons originating from neuronal cell bodies located in the hypothalamus. These axons serve as storage sites for 2 peptide hormones synthesized in the hypothalamus; these hormones act in the periphery to regulate water balance, milk ejection, and uterine contraction.

Virtually all hormones produced by the hypothalamus and the pituitary are released in a pulsatile fashion; periods of such release are interspersed with periods of inactivity. Some hormones (eg, adrenocorticotropic hormone, growth hormone, prolactin) have definite circadian rhythms; others (eg, luteinizing hormone and follicle-stimulating hormone during the menstrual cycle) have month-long rhythms with superimposed circadian rhythms.

Hypothalamic Controls

Thus far, 6 physiologically important hypothalamic neurohormones have been identified (see TABLE 150–1). Except for the biogenic amine dopamine, all are small peptides. Several are produced in the periphery as well as in the hypothalamus and function in local paracrine systems, especially in the GI tract. Vasoactive intestinal peptide, which also stimulates the release of prolactin, is one. Neurohormones may control the release of multiple pituitary hormones. Regulation of most anterior pituitary hormones depends on stimulatory signals from the hypothalamus; only prolactin is regulated by inhibitory stimuli. If the pituitary stalk (which connects the pituitary to the hypothalamus) is severed, prolactin release increases, whereas release of all other anterior pituitary hormones decreases.

Many hypothalamic abnormalities (including tumors and encephalitis and other inflammatory lesions) can alter the release of hypothalamic neurohormones. Because neurohormones are synthesized in different centers within the hypothalamus, some disorders affect only one neuropeptide, whereas others affect several. The result can be undersecretion or oversecretion of neurohormones. Clinical syndromes that result from the ensuing pituitary hormone dysfunction are discussed in detail in Ch. 151 on p. 1179.

Anterior Pituitary Function

The cells of the anterior lobe (which constitutes 80% of the pituitary by weight) synthesize and release several hormones necessary for normal growth and development and also stimulate the activity of several target glands.

Adrenocorticotropic hormone (ACTH): ACTH is also known as corticotropin. Corticotropin-releasing hormone (CRH) is the primary stimulator of ACTH release, but antidiuretic hormone plays a role during stress. ACTH induces the adrenal cortex to release cortisol and several weak androgens, such as dehydroepiandrosterone (DHEA). Circulating cortisol and other corticosteroids (including exogenous corticosteroids) inhibit the release of CRH and ACTH. The CRH-ACTH-cortisol axis is a central component of the response to stress. Without ACTH, the adrenal cortex atrophies and cortisol release virtually ceases.

Thyroid-stimulating hormone (TSH): TSH regulates the structure and function of the thyroid gland and stimulates synthesis and release of thyroid hormones. TSH synthesis and release are stimulated by the hypothalamic hormone thyrotropin-releasing hormone (TRH) and suppressed (by negative feedback) by circulating thyroid hormones.

Luteinizing hormone (LH) and follicle-stimulating hormone (FSH): LH and FSH control the production of the sex hormones.

TABLE 150–1. HYPOTHALAMIC NEUROHORMONES

NEUROHORMONE	HORMONES AFFECTED	EFFECT
Thyrotropin-releasing hormone	TSH Prolactin	Stimulate Stimulate
Gonadotropin-releasing hormone	LH FSH	Stimulate* Stimulate*
Dopamine	Prolactin LH FSH TSH	Inhibit Inhibit Inhibit Inhibit
Corticotropin-releasing hormone	ACTH	Stimulate
Growth hormone–releasing hormone	GH	Stimulate
Somatostatin	GH TSH Insulin	Inhibit Inhibit Inhibit

TSH = thyroid-stimulating hormone; LH = luteinizing hormone; FSH = follicle-stimulating hormone; ACTH = adrenocorticotropic hormone (corticotropin); GH = growth hormone.

*Under physiologic conditions and when administered exogenously in intermittent pulses. Continuous infusion inhibits the release of LH and FSH.

Synthesis and release of LH and FSH are stimulated by gonadotropin-releasing hormone (GnRH) and suppressed by estrogen and testosterone. In women, LH and FSH stimulate ovarian follicular development and ovulation, as discussed in Ch. 243 on p. 2069. In men, FSH acts on Sertoli cells and is essential for spermatogenesis; LH acts on Leydig cells of the testis to stimulate testosterone biosynthesis (see p. 1943).

Growth hormone (GH): GH stimulates somatic growth and regulates metabolism. Growth hormone–releasing hormone (GHRH) is the major stimulator and somatostatin is the major inhibitor of the synthesis and release of GH. GH controls synthesis of insulin-like growth factor 1 (IGF-1, also called somatomedin-C), which largely controls growth. Although IGF-1 is produced by many tissues, the liver is the major source. The metabolic effects of GH are biphasic. GH initially exerts insulin-like effects, increasing glucose uptake in muscle and fat, stimulating amino acid uptake and protein synthesis in liver and muscle, and inhibiting lipolysis in adipose tissue. Several hours later, more profound anti–insulin-like metabolic effects occur. These include inhibition of glucose uptake and use, causing plasma glucose and lipolysis to increase, which increases plasma free fatty acids. GH levels increase during fasting, maintaining plasma glucose levels and mobilizing fat as an alternative metabolic fuel. Production of GH decreases with aging. Recently ghrelin, a hormone produced in the fundus of the stomach, has been isolated. Ghrelin promotes GH release from the pituitary, increases food intake, and improves memory.

Prolactin: Prolactin is produced in cells called lactotrophs that constitute about 30% of the cells of the anterior pituitary. The pituitary doubles in size during pregnancy, largely because of hyperplasia and hypertrophy of lactotrophs. In humans, the major function of prolactin is stimulating milk production. Also, prolactin release occurs during sexual activity and stress. Prolactin may be a sensitive indicator of pituitary dysfunction; prolactin is the hormone most frequently produced in excess by pituitary tumors, and it is often the first hormone to become deficient from infiltrative disease or tumor compression of the pituitary.

Other hormones: Several other hormones are produced by the anterior pituitary. These include pro-opiomelanocortin (POMC, which gives rise to ACTH), α- and β-melanocyte-stimulating hormone (MSH), β-lipotropin (β-LPH), the enkephalins, and the endorphins. POMC and MSH can cause hyperpigmentation of the skin and are only significant clinically in disorders in which ACTH levels are markedly elevated (ie, Addison's disease, Nelson syndrome). The function of β-LPH is unknown. Enkephalins and endorphins are endogenous opioids that bind to and activate opioid receptors throughout the CNS.

Posterior Pituitary Function

The posterior pituitary releases antidiuretic hormone (also called vasopressin) and oxytocin. Both hormones are released in response to neural impulses and have half-lives of about 10 min.

Antidiuretic hormone (ADH): ADH acts primarily to promote water conservation by the kidney by increasing the permeability of the distal tubular epithelium to water. At high concentrations, ADH also causes vasoconstriction. Like aldosterone, ADH plays an important role in maintaining fluid homeostasis and vascular and cellular hydration. The main stimulus for ADH release is increased osmotic pressure of water in the body, which is sensed by osmoreceptors in the hypothalamus. The other major stimulus is volume depletion, which is sensed by baroreceptors in the left atrium, pulmonary veins, carotid sinus, and aortic arch, and then transmitted to the CNS through the vagus and glossopharyngeal nerves. Other stimulants for ADH release include pain, stress, emesis, hypoxia, exercise, hypoglycemia, cholinergic agonists, β-blockers, angiotensin, and prostaglandins. Inhibitors of ADH release include alcohol, α-blockers, and glucocorticoids.

A lack of ADH produces central diabetes insipidus (see p. 1189); an inability of the kidney to respond normally to ADH causes nephrogenic diabetes insipidus (see p. 2025). Removal of the pituitary gland usually does not result in permanent diabetes insipidus because some of the remaining hypothalamic neurons produce small amounts of ADH.

Oxytocin: Oxytocin has 2 major targets: the myoepithelial cells of the breast, which surround the alveoli of the mammary gland, and the smooth muscle cells of the uterus. Suckling stimulates the production of oxytocin, which causes the myoepithelial cells to contract. This contraction causes milk to move from the alveoli to large sinuses for ejection (ie, the milk letdown reflex of nursing mothers).

Oxytocin stimulates contraction of uterine smooth muscle cells, and uterine sensitivity to oxytocin increases throughout pregnancy. However, plasma levels do not increase sharply during parturition, and the role of oxytocin in the initiation of labor is unclear. There is no recognized stimulus for (or function of) oxytocin release in men, although men have extremely low levels.

ENDOCRINE DISORDERS

Endocrine disorders can result from dysfunction originating in the peripheral endocrine gland itself (primary disorders) or from understimulation or overstimulation by the pituitary (secondary disorders). The disorders can result in hormone overproduction (hyperfunction) or underproduction (hypofunction). Rarely, endocrine disorders (usually hypofunction) occur because of abnormal tissue responses to hormones. Clinical presentation of hypofunction disorders is often insidious and nonspecific.

Hyperfunction: Hyperfunction of endocrine glands may result from overstimulation by the pituitary but is most commonly due to hyperplasia or neoplasia of the gland itself. In some cases, cancers from other tissues can produce hormones (ectopic hormone production). Hormone excess can result from exogenous hormone administration. In some cases, patients take hormones without telling the physician (factitious disease). Tissue hypersensitivity to hormones can occur. Antibodies can stimulate peripheral endocrine glands, as occurs in hyperthyroidism of Graves' disease. Destruction of a peripheral endocrine gland can rapidly release stored hormone (eg, thyroid hormones in thyroiditis). Enzyme defects in the synthesis of a peripheral endocrine hormone can result in overproduction of hormones proximal to the block. Finally, overproduction of a hormone can occur as an appropriate response to a disease state.

Hypofunction: Hypofunction of an endocrine gland can result from understimulation by the pituitary. Hypofunction originating within the peripheral gland itself can result from congenital or acquired disorders (including autoimmune conditions, tumors, infections, vascular disorders, and toxins). Genetic disorders producing hypofunction can result from deletion of a gene or by production of an abnormal hormone. A decrease in hormone production by the peripheral endocrine gland with a resulting increase in production of pituitary regulating hormone can lead to peripheral endocrine gland hyperplasia. For example, if synthesis of thyroid hormone is defective, thyroid-stimulating hormone (TSH) is produced in excessive amounts, causing goiter.

Several hormones require conversion to an active form after secretion from the peripheral endocrine gland. Certain disorders can block this step (eg, renal disease can inhibit production of the active form of vitamin D). Antibodies to the circulating hormone or its receptor can block the ability of the hormone to bind to its receptor. Disease or drugs can cause increased rate of clearance of hormones. Circulating substances may also block the function of hormones. Abnormalities of the receptor or elsewhere in the peripheral endocrine tissue can also produce hypofunction.

Laboratory Testing

Because symptoms of endocrine disorders can begin insidiously and may be nonspecific, clinical recognition is often delayed for months or years. For this reason, biochemical diagnosis is usually essential; it typically requires measuring levels of the peripheral endocrine hormone and/or the pituitary hormone in the blood.

Free or bioavailable hormone (ie, hormone not bound to a specific binding hormone) is generally believed to be the active form. Free or bioavailable hormones are measured using equilibrium dialysis, ultrafiltration, or a solvent-extraction method to separate the free and albumin-bound hormone from the binding globulin. These methods can be expensive and time-consuming. Analog and competitive free hormone assays, although often used commercially, are not always accurate and should not be used.

Free hormone levels can also be estimated indirectly by assessing levels of the binding protein and using them to adjust levels of the total serum hormone. However, indirect methods are inaccurate if the binding capacity of the hormone-binding protein has been altered (eg, by disease).

Because most hormones have circadian rhythms, measurements need to be made at a prescribed time of day. Hormones that vary over short periods (eg, luteinizing hormone) necessitate obtaining 3 or 4 values over 1 or 2 h or using a pooled blood sample. Hormones with week-to-week variation (eg, testosterone) necessitate obtaining separate values a week apart.

In some cases, indirect estimates are used. For example, because growth hormone (GH) has a short serum half-life and is difficult to detect in serum, serum insulin-like growth factor 1 (IGF-1), which is produced in response to GH, is often measured as an index of GH activity. Sometimes, urine (eg, free cortisol when testing for Cushing's disease) or salivary hormone levels may be used. Whether measurement of circulating hormone metabolites indicates the amount of bioavailable hormone is under investigation.

In many cases, a dynamic test is necessary. Thus, in the case of hypofunctioning organs, a stimulating test can be used. In hyperfunction, a suppressive test can be used.

Treatment

Hypofunction disorders are usually treated by replacement of the peripheral endocrine hormone regardless of whether the defect is primary or secondary (an exception is GH replacement for pituitary dwarfism). If resistance to the hormone exists, drugs that reduce resistance can be used (eg, metformin or thiazolidinediones for type 2 diabetes mellitus). Occasionally, a hormone-stimulating drug is used.

Radiation therapy, surgery, and drugs that suppress hormone production are used to treat hyperfunction disorders. In some cases, a receptor antagonist is used.

Aging and Endocrinology

Hormones undergo many changes as a person ages. Most hormone levels decrease. Some remain normal, including TSH, ACTH (basal), thyroxine, cortisol (basal), 1,25-dihydroxycholecalciferol, insulin (sometimes increases), and estradiol (in men). Hormones that increase, including ACTH (response to corticotropin-releasing hormone) follicle-stimulating hormone, sex-hormone binding globulin, and activin (in men), gonadotropins (in women), epinephrine (in the oldest old), parathyroid hormone, norepinephrine, cholecystokinin, vasoactive intestinal peptide and arginine vasopressin (also loss of circadian rhythm), and atrial natriuretic factor, are associated with either receptor defects or postreceptor defects, resulting in hypofunction. Many age-related changes are similar to those in patients with hormone deficiency, leading to the hypothesis of a "hormonal fountain of youth" (ie, speculation that some changes associated with aging can be reversed by the replacement of one or more deficient hormones). Some evidence suggests that replacing certain hormones in the elderly can improve functional outcomes (eg, muscle strength, bone mineral density), but little evidence exists regarding effects on mortality. In some cases, replacing hormones may be harmful, as in estrogen replacement in most older women.

A competing theory is that the age-related decline in hormone levels represents a protective slowing down of cellular metabolism. This concept is based on the "rate of living" theory of aging (ie, the faster the metabolic rate of an organism, the quicker it dies). This concept is seemingly supported by studies on the effects of dietary restriction. Restriction decreases levels of hormones that stimulate metabolism, thereby slowing metabolic rate; this prolongs life in rodents.

Dehydroepiandrosterone (DHEA) and its sulfate levels decline dramatically with aging. Despite optimism for the role of DHEA supplementation in older people, most controlled trials failed to show any major benefits.

Pregnenolone is the precursor of all known steroid hormones. Like DHEA, its levels decline with aging. Studies in the 1940s demonstrated its safety and benefits in people with arthritis, but additional studies failed to demonstrate any beneficial effects on memory and muscle strength.

Levels of GH and its peripheral endocrine hormone (IGF-1) decline with aging. GH replacement in older people sometimes increases muscle mass but does not increase muscle strength (although it may in malnourished people). Adverse effects (eg, carpal tunnel syndrome, arthralgias, water retention) are very common. GH may have a role in the short-term treatment of some malnourished older patients, but in critically ill malnourished patients GH increases mortality. Secretagogues that stimulate GH production in a more physiologic pattern may improve benefit and decrease risk.

Levels of melatonin, a hormone produced by the pineal gland, also decline with aging. This decline may play an important role in the loss of circadian rhythms with aging. Estrogen and testosterone replacement in older patients is discussed in Ch. 245 (see p. 2082) and Ch. 227 (see p. 1947), respectively.

151 PITUITARY DISORDERS

The pituitary gland controls the functions of peripheral endocrine glands. Pituitary structure and function and relationships between the hypothalamus and the pituitary gland are discussed in Ch. 150 on p. 1174.

PITUITARY LESIONS

Patients with hypothalamic-pituitary lesions generally present with some combination of symptoms or signs of a mass lesion (eg, headaches, visual field defects—particularly bitemporal hemianopia or the hemifield slide phenomenon [images drifting apart]—altered appetite, thirst); imaging evidence of a mass lesion as an incidental finding; or hypersecretion or hyposecretion of one or more pituitary hormones.

The most common cause of hypopituitary or hyperpituitary secretion is a pituitary or hypothalamic tumor. A pituitary tumor tends to produce an enlarged sella (sella turcica). Alternatively, an enlarged sella may represent the empty sella syndrome if no endocrine or visual disorder exists.

Empty sella syndrome: In this disorder, no pituitary gland is visible by CT or MRI. The syndrome may be congenital, primary, or secondary to injury (such as ischemia after childbirth, surgery, head trauma, or radiation therapy). The typical patient is female (>80%), obese (about 75%), and hypertensive (30%) and may have idiopathic intracranial hypertension (10%) or spinal fluid rhinorrhea (10%). Pituitary functions in patients with empty sella syndrome are frequently normal (the pituitary tissue often being flattened against the sellar walls). However, hypopituitarism may occur, as may headaches and visual field defects. Occasionally, patients have small coexisting pituitary tumors that secrete growth hormone (GH), prolactin, or ACTH. Diagnosis can be confirmed by CT or MRI. No specific therapy is needed for an empty sella alone.

Anterior lobe lesions: Hypersecretion of anterior lobe hormones (hyperpituitarism) is almost always selective. The anterior pituitary hormones most commonly secreted in excess are GH (as in acromegaly, gigantism), prolactin (as in galactorrhea), and ACTH (as in the pituitary type of Cushing's syndrome). Hyposecretion of anterior lobe hormones (hypopituitarism) may be generalized, usually due to a pituitary tumor or idiopathic, or may involve the selective loss of one or a few pituitary hormones.

Posterior lobe lesions: The 2 posterior lobe hormones are oxytocin and ADH. In women, oxytocin causes myoepithelial cells of the breast and myometrial cells of the uterus to contract. Oxytocin is present in men but has no proven function. Deficiency of ADH results in central diabetes insipidus (see p. 1189). Excess ADH secretion results in the syndrome of inappropriate ADH secretion (see p. 1239).

GENERALIZED HYPOPITUITARISM

Generalized hypopituitarism refers to endocrine deficiency syndromes due to partial or complete loss of anterior lobe pituitary function. Various clinical features occur depending on the specific hormones that are deficient. Diagnosis involves imaging tests and measurement of pituitary hormone levels basally and after various provocative stimuli. Treatment depends on cause but generally includes removal of any tumor and administration of replacement hormones.

The many causes of hypopituitarism are listed in TABLE 151–1.

Symptoms and Signs

Symptoms and signs relate to the underlying cause and to the specific pituitary hormones that are deficient or absent. Onset is usually insidious and may not be recognized by the patient; occasionally, onset is sudden or dramatic.

Most commonly, gonadotropins are lost first, then growth hormone (GH), and finally thyroid-stimulating hormone (TSH) and ACTH. However, sometimes TSH and ACTH are lost first. ADH deficiency is rare in primary pituitary disease but is common with stalk and hypothalamic lesions. Function of all target glands decreases when all hormones are deficient (panhypopituitarism).

TABLE 151–1. CAUSES OF HYPOPITUITARISM

Causes primarily affecting the pituitary gland (primary hypopituitarism)

Pituitary tumors
- Adenomas
- Craniopharyngiomas

Infarction or ischemic necrosis of the pituitary
- Hemorrhagic infarction (pituitary apoplexy)
- Shock, especially postpartum (Sheehan's syndrome), or in diabetes mellitus or sickle cell anemia
- Vascular thrombosis or aneurysms, especially of the internal carotid artery

Inflammatory processes
- Meningitis (tubercular, other bacterial, fungal, malarial)
- Pituitary abscesses
- Sarcoidosis

Infiltrative disorders
- Hemochromatosis
- Langerhans' cell granulomatosis (histiocytosis—Hand-Schüller-Christian disease)

Idiopathic isolated or multiple pituitary hormone deficiencies

Iatrogenic
- Irradiation
- Surgical extirpation

Autoimmune dysfunction of the pituitary (lymphocytic hypophysitis)

Causes primarily affecting the hypothalamus (secondary hypopituitarism)

Hypothalamic tumors
- Ependymomas
- Meningiomas
- Metastatic tumors
- Pinealomas

Inflammatory processes, such as sarcoidosis

Isolated or multiple neurohormone deficiencies of the hypothalamus

Surgical transection of the pituitary stalk

Trauma (sometimes associated with basal skull fracture)

Lack of luteinizing hormone (LH) and follicle-stimulating hormone (FSH) in children leads to delayed puberty (see Hypopituitarism in Children Resulting in Short Stature on p. 1183). Premenopausal women develop amenorrhea, reduced libido, regression of secondary sexual characteristics, and infertility. Men develop erectile dysfunction, testicular atrophy, reduced libido, regression of secondary sexual characteristics, and decreased spermatogenesis with consequent infertility.

GH deficiency may contribute to decreased energy but is usually asymptomatic and clinically undetectable in adults (see p. 1184 for effects in children). Suggestions that GH deficiency accelerates atherosclerosis are unproven. TSH deficiency leads to hypothyroidism, with such symptoms as facial puffiness, hoarse voice, bradycardia, and cold intolerance. ACTH deficiency results in hypoadrenalism with attendant fatigue, hypotension, and intolerance to stress and infection. ACTH deficiency does not result in the hyperpigmentation characteristic of primary adrenal failure.

Hypothalamic lesions, which can result in hypopituitarism, can also disturb the centers that control appetite, producing a syndrome resembling anorexia nervosa.

Sheehan's syndrome, which affects postpartum women, is pituitary necrosis from hypovolemia and shock occurring in the immediate peripartum period. Lactation does not start after childbirth, and the patient may complain of fatigue and loss of pubic and axillary hair.

Pituitary apoplexy is a symptom complex caused by hemorrhagic infarction of either a normal pituitary gland or, more commonly, a pituitary tumor. Acute symptoms include severe headache, stiff neck, fever, visual field defects, and oculomotor palsies. The resulting edema may compress the hypothalamus, resulting in somnolence or coma. Varying degrees of hypopituitarism may develop suddenly, and the patient may present with vascular collapse because of deficient ACTH and cortisol. The CSF often contains blood, and MRI documents hemorrhage.

Diagnosis

Clinical features are often nonspecific, and the diagnosis must be established with certainty before committing the patient to a lifetime of hormone replacement therapy. Pituitary dysfunction must be distinguished from anorexia nervosa, chronic liver disease, myotonia dystrophica, polyglandular autoimmune disease (see TABLE 151–2), and disorders of the other endocrine glands. The clinical picture may be particularly confusing when the function of more than one gland decreases at the same time. Evidence of structural pituitary abnormalities and of hormonal deficiencies should be sought.

Imaging tests: Patients should undergo high-resolution CT or MRI, with contrast media as required (to rule out structural abnormalities, such as pituitary adenomas). PET is a research tool used in a few specialized centers and therefore is rarely done. When no modern neuroradiologic facilities are available, a simple cone-down lateral x-ray of the sella turcica can identify pituitary macroadenomas with a diameter > 10 mm. Cerebral angiography is indicated only when other imaging tests suggest perisellar vascular anomalies or aneurysms.

Laboratory testing: Initial evaluation should include testing for TSH and ACTH deficiencies, because both conditions are potentially life threatening. Testing for deficiencies of other hormones is discussed below.

Free thyroxine (T_4) and TSH should be determined. Levels of both are usually low in generalized hypopituitarism; a pattern of normal TSH level with low free T_4 may also occur. In contrast, elevated TSH levels with low free T_4 indicate a primary abnormality of the thyroid gland.

Synthetic thyrotropin-releasing hormone (TRH) 200 to 500 μg IV given over 15 to 30 sec may help identify patients with hypothalamic as opposed to pituitary dysfunction, although this test is not often performed. Plasma TSH levels are generally measured at 0, 20, and 60 min after injection. If pituitary function is intact, TSH should rise by > 5 mU/L, peaking by 30 min after injection. A delayed rise in plasma TSH levels may occur in patients with hypothalamic disease. However, some patients with primary pituitary disease also show a delayed rise.

Serum cortisol levels alone are not reliable indicators of ACTH-adrenal axis function. One of several provocative tests should be performed. One test for evaluating ACTH (as well as GH and prolactin) reserve is the insulin tolerance test. Regular insulin at a dosage of 0.1 units/kg body weight IV is given over 15 to 30 sec, and venous blood samples are obtained to determine GH, cortisol, and glucose levels at baseline (before insulin administration) and 20, 30, 45, 60, and 90 min later. If glucose drops to < 40 mg/dL (< 2.22 mmol/L) or symptoms of hypoglycemia develop, cortisol should increase by > 7 μg/dL or to > 20 μg/dL. (CAUTION: *This test is hazardous in patients with severe documented panhypopituitarism or diabetes mellitus and in the elderly and is contraindicated in those with coronary artery disease or epilepsy. A health care practitioner should be present during the test.*) Usually, only transient perspiration, tachycardia, and nervousness occur. If the patient complains of palpitations, loses consciousness, or has a seizure, the test should be stopped promptly by giving 50 mL of 50% glucose solution IV.

An insulin tolerance test alone will not differentiate between primary (Addison's disease) and secondary (hypopituitary) adrenal insufficiency. Tests to make this distinction and to evaluate the hypothalamic-pituitary-adrenal axis are described under Addison's

TABLE 151–2. DIFFERENTIATION OF GENERALIZED HYPOPITUITARISM FROM OTHER SELECTED DISORDERS

DISORDER	DIFFERENTIATING FEATURES
Anorexia nervosa	Female predominance; cachexia; abnormal ideation regarding food and body image; maintenance of secondary sexual characteristics despite amenorrhea; increased levels of basal growth hormone and cortisol
Alcoholic liver disease or hemochromatosis*	Evidence of liver disease; laboratory testing
Myotonia dystrophica	Progressive weakness; premature balding; cataracts; facial features of accelerated aging; laboratory testing
Polyglandular autoimmune disease†	Pituitary hormone levels

*May produce hypogonadism and general debility.

†If the affected glands are target glands of the pituitary.

Disease on p. 1207. An alternative provocative test that is performed much less often is the corticotropin-releasing hormone (CRH) test. CRH 1 µg/kg IV is given by rapid injection. Plasma ACTH and cortisol levels are measured 15 min before, then at baseline, and 15, 30, 60, 90, and 120 min after the injection. Adverse effects include temporary flushing, a metallic taste in the mouth, and slight and transient hypotension.

Prolactin levels are routinely measured. These levels are often elevated up to 5 times normal values when a large pituitary tumor is present, even if it does not produce prolactin. The tumor compresses the pituitary stalk, preventing dopamine, which inhibits pituitary prolactin production and release, from reaching the pituitary. Patients with such hyperprolactinemia often have hypogonadotropism and secondary hypogonadism.

Measurement of basal levels of LH and FSH is most helpful in evaluating hypopituitarism in postmenopausal women not taking exogenous estrogens in whom circulating gonadotropin concentrations are normally high (> 30 mIU/mL). Although gonadotropin levels tend to be low in other patients with panhypopituitarism, overlap exists with the normal range. Levels of both hormones should increase in response to synthetic gonadotropin-releasing hormone (GnRH) at a dose of 100 µg IV, with LH peaking about 30 min and FSH peaking 40 min after GnRH administration. However, normal, diminished, or absent responses to GnRH may occur in hypothalamic-pituitary dysfunction. Normal increases in LH and FSH in response to GnRH vary. Administration of exogenous GnRH is not helpful in distinguishing primary hypothalamic disorders from primary pituitary disorders.

Screening for GH deficiency is not recommended in adults unless GH treatment is contemplated (eg, for unexplained reduced energy and quality of life in patients with hypopituitarism otherwise fully replaced). GH deficiency is suspected if ≥ 2 other pituitary hormones are deficient. Because GH levels vary by time of day and other factors and are difficult to interpret, levels of insulin-like growth factor 1 (IGF-1), which reflect GH, are used; low levels suggest GH deficiency, but normal levels do not rule it out. A provocative test of GH release (see p. 1184) may be necessary.

Evaluation of multiple hormones is the most efficient method of evaluating pituitary function. Growth hormone–releasing hormone (1 µg/kg), CRH (1 µg/kg), TRH (200 µg), and GnRH (100 µg) are given together IV over 15 to 30 sec. Glucose, cortisol, GH, TSH, prolactin, LH, FSH, and ACTH are measured at frequent intervals for the ensuing 180 min. The usefulness of these releasing hormones in pituitary testing remains to be established. The normal responses are the same as those delineated earlier for individual testing.

Treatment

Treatment is replacement of the hormones of the hypofunctioning target glands, as discussed in the pertinent chapters in this section and elsewhere in THE MANUAL. Adults ≤ 50 yr deficient in GH are now sometimes treated with GH doses of 0.002 to 0.012 mg/kg sc once/day. Benefits of treatment include improved energy and quality of life, increased body muscle mass, and decreased body fat mass. Suggestions that GH replacement can prevent an acceleration of atherosclerosis induced by GH deficiency are unproven.

When hypopituitarism is due to a pituitary tumor, specific treatment must be directed at the tumor as well as replacing hormones. The appropriate management of such tumors is controversial. If the tumor is small and does not secrete prolactin, most endocrinologists favor transsphenoidal removal. Most endocrinologists consider dopamine agonist drugs, such as bromocriptine, pergolide, or the longer-acting cabergoline, the initial treatment of prolactinomas, regardless of size (see under Galactorrhea on p. 1187). Patients with macroadenomas > 2 cm with extremely high circulating levels of prolactin may require surgery or irradiation in addition to dopamine agonist treatment. Supervoltage irradiation of the pituitary may be added or used alone. With larger tumors and suprasellar extension, resection of the entire tumor, either transsphenoidally or transfrontally, may not be possible, and adjunctive supervoltage irradiation may be warranted.

In pituitary apoplexy, immediate surgery is warranted if visual field disturbances or oculomotor palsies develop suddenly or if somnolence progresses to coma because of hypothalamic compression. Although management with high-dose corticosteroids and general support may suffice in a few cases, transsphenoidal decompression of the tumor should generally be undertaken promptly.

Surgery and irradiation may be followed by the loss of other pituitary hormone functions.

Irradiated patients may lose endocrine function slowly over years. Therefore, posttreatment hormonal status should be evaluated frequently, preferably at 3 and 6 mo and yearly thereafter. Such evaluation should include at least assessment of thyroid and adrenal function. Patients may also develop visual difficulties related to fibrosis of the optic chiasm. Sellar imaging and visual field assessment should be performed at least q 2 yr initially for about 10 yr, particularly if residual tumor tissue is present.

SELECTIVE PITUITARY HORMONE DEFICIENCIES

Selective deficiencies of pituitary hormones may represent an early stage in the development of more generalized hypopituitarism. Patients must be observed for signs of other pituitary hormone deficiencies, and sellar imaging should be performed at intervals for signs of a pituitary tumor.

Isolated growth hormone (GH) deficiency is responsible for many cases of pituitary dwarfism (see below). Although one autosomal dominant form of complete GH deficiency is associated with a deletion of the GH structural gene, such gene defects probably account for a minority of cases. Treatment of GH deficiency in adults < 50 yr is discussed above.

Isolated gonadotropin deficiency occurs in both sexes and must be distinguished from primary hypogonadism. A eunuchoid habitus is generally present. Patients with primary hypogonadism (see p. 1944) have elevated levels of luteinizing hormone (LH) and follicle-stimulating hormone (FSH), whereas those with gonadotropin deficiency have low-normal, low, or unmeasurable levels. Although most cases of hypogonadotropic hypogonadism involve deficiencies of both LH and FSH, in rare cases the secretion of only one is impaired. Isolated gonadotropin deficiency must also be distinguished from hypogonadotropic amenorrhea secondary to exercise, diet, or mental stress (see p. 2074). Although the history may be helpful, differential diagnosis may be impossible.

In **Kallmann syndrome,** the specific lack of gonadotropin-releasing hormone (GnRH) is associated with midline facial defects, including anosmia and cleft lip or palate (see p. 2369), and with color blindness. Embryologic studies have shown that GnRH neurons originally develop in the epithelium of the olfactory placode and migrate into the septal-preoptic region of the hypothalamus early in development. In at least some cases, gene defects, localized to the X chromosome in the X-linked form of the disorder and termed the *KALIG-1* (Kallmann syndrome interval gene 1) gene, have been found in the adhesion proteins facilitating this neuronal migration. Administration of GnRH is not indicated.

Isolated ACTH deficiency is rare. Weakness, hypoglycemia, weight loss, and decreased axillary and pubic hair suggest the diagnosis. Plasma and urinary steroid levels are low and rise to normal after ACTH treatment. Clinical and laboratory evidence of other hormonal deficiencies is absent. Treatment is with cortisol replacement, as for Addison's disease (see p. 1209).

Isolated thyroid-stimulating hormone (TSH) deficiency is likely when clinical features of hypothyroidism exist, plasma TSH levels are not elevated, and no other pituitary hormone deficiencies exist. Plasma TSH levels, as measured by immunoassay, are not always lower than normal, suggesting that the TSH secreted is biologically inactive. Administration of bovine TSH increases thyroid hormone levels (see also Hypothyroidism on p. 1200).

Isolated prolactin deficiency has been noted rarely in women who fail to lactate after delivery. Basal prolactin levels are low and do not increase in response to provocative stimuli, such as thyroid-releasing hormone. Administration of prolactin is not indicated.

HYPOPITUITARISM IN CHILDREN RESULTING IN SHORT STATURE

(Pituitary Dwarfism)

Hypopituitarism in children typically results in abnormally slow growth and short stature with normal proportions. It is usually due to a pituitary tumor but may be idiopathic. Diagnosis involves measurement of growth hormone (GH) levels at baseline and in response to pharmacologic stimuli. Treatment usually involves removal of the causative tumor and GH replacement.

Hypopituitarism in children may be generalized, involving deficiency of several pituitary hormones, but is usually first expressed clinically as short stature resulting from deficiency of GH. Isolated deficiency of GH may also occur.

Hypopituitarism in children is usually due to a pituitary tumor (most commonly a craniopharyngioma) or is idiopathic. The combination of lytic lesions of the bone or skull and of diabetes insipidus suggests Langerhans' cell granulomatosis (histiocytosis—see p. 1096). Hypothalamic or pituitary hormone deficiency as well as isolated GH deficiency may occur in patients with midline defects, such as cleft palate or septo-optic dysplasia, which involves absence of the septum pellucidum, optic nerve atrophy, and hypopituitarism. GH deficiency, either alone or in patients with other abnormalities, is hereditary in about 5% of cases.

Therapeutic radiation of the CNS for various cancers causes slowing of linear growth, which can often be linked to resulting GH deficiency. Radiation of the spine, either prophylactic or therapeutic, may further impair the growth potential of the vertebrae and further jeopardize height gain.

Symptoms, Signs, and Diagnosis

In a child with hypopituitarism, height is below the 3rd percentile, and growth velocity is < 6 cm/yr before age 4 yr, < 5 cm/yr from age 4 to 8 yr, and < 4 cm/yr before puberty. Skeletal maturation, assessed by bone age determination, is > 2 yr behind chronologic age.

Although of small stature, a child with hypopituitarism retains normal proportionality between upper and lower body segments. The child fails to begin pubertal development. However, a child with isolated GH deficiency secondary to hypopituitarism may undergo delayed pubertal development.

Growth data for height and weight should be plotted on a growth chart (auxologic assessment) for all children. When growth is abnormal, bone age should be determined from an x-ray of the left hand (by convention). In GH deficiency, skeletal maturation is usually delayed to the same extent as height. Evaluating the pituitary gland and sella turcica with CT or MRI is indicated to rule out calcifications and tumors; the sella turcica is abnormally small in 10 to 20% of patients.

In mid to late childhood, insulin-like growth factor 1 (IGF-1) levels, which reflect GH activity, are measured because GH levels are highly variable and difficult to interpret. Normal IGF-1 levels help exclude GH deficiency. However, IGF-1 levels are low in conditions other than GH deficiency, such as psychosocial deprivation, malnutrition, and hypothyroidism. Because IGF-1 levels are normally low in infancy and early childhood, they do not allow reliable discrimination between normal and subnormal in this age group. For these children, IGF binding protein type 3 (IGFBP-3—the major carrier of IGF peptides) levels are measured. IGFBP-3 is less affected by malnutrition than is IGF-1.

In children with low levels of IGF-1 and IGFBP-3, GH deficiency is usually confirmed by measuring GH levels. Because basal GH levels are typically low or undetectable (except after the onset of sleep), assessment of GH levels requires provocative testing. However, provocative testing is nonphysiologic, subject to laboratory error, and poorly reproducible, and interpretation of data relies on arbitrary definitions of "normal" that vary by age and sex.

The insulin tolerance test may be the most effective provocative test for stimulating GH release. Less dangerous, but also less reliable, are tests using arginine infusion (500 mg/kg IV given over 30 min), levodopa (500 mg po to adults; 10 mg/kg to children), sleep, or 20 min of vigorous exercise. Clonidine (4 μg/kg po), another potent stimulator of GH secretion, holds promise as an alternative to insulin. Adverse effects are sleepiness and a minimal fall in BP. Generally, any GH level > 10 ng/mL or any response of > 5 ng/mL after a stimulus is sufficient to rule out GH deficiency. Increases in GH of < 5 ng/mL or to levels < 10 ng/mL are difficult to interpret.

What constitutes a normal response, however, is arbitrary, and all provocative tests of GH secretion occasionally produce misleading results. Because no single test is 100% effective in eliciting GH release, a 2nd provocative test should be performed if the first is abnormal. GH levels generally peak 30 to 90 min after administration of insulin or the onset of arginine infusion, 30 to 120 min after levodopa, 60 to 120 min after the onset of sleep or administration of clonidine, and after 20 min of vigorous exercise. Because GH responses are generally abnormal in patients with diminished thyroid or adrenal function, testing should be conducted in these patients only after adequate hormone replacement therapy.

The value of exogenous growth hormone–releasing hormone (GHRH) in evaluating GH secretion is not established. In normal people, a dose of 1 μg/kg GHRH IV administered over 15 to 30 sec results in maximal but variable release of GH, typically reaching a peak about 60 min after GHRH injection. The variability in pituitary responsiveness to GHRH is consistent with the hypothesis that intermittent secretion of somatostatin, which opposes GHRH, is responsible for modulating pituitary GH output. Presumably, absent or diminished increases in GH in response to GHRH identify patients with GH deficiency, but whether the pattern of response distinguishes primary hypothalamic disease from pituitary disease is unclear. In children with GH deficiency presumably secondary to GHRH deficiency, highly variable GH responses to GHRH occur.

Provocative testing may not detect subtle defects in the regulation of GH release. For example, in children with short stature secondary to GH secretory dysfunction, provocative testing for GH release is usually normal. However, serial measurements of GH levels over 12 to 24 h indicate abnormally low 12- or 24-h integrated GH secretion.

If diminished GH release is confirmed, secretion of other pituitary hormones and (if abnormal) hormones of their target peripheral endocrine glands also must be evaluated.

Treatment

Recombinant GH is indicated for all children with short stature who have documented GH deficiency. Dosing is usually from 0.03 to 0.05 mg/kg sc once/day. With therapy, height velocity often increases to 10 to 12 cm/yr in the first year and, although it increases more slowly thereafter, remains above pretreatment rates. Therapy is continued until an acceptable height is reached or growth rate falls below 2.5 cm/yr.

Adverse effects of GH therapy are few but include idiopathic intracranial hypertension (pseudotumor cerebri), slipped capital femoral epiphysis, and transient mild peripheral edema. Before the advent of recombinant GH, GH abstracted from pituitary glands was used. This preparation can occasionally lead to Creutzfeldt-Jakob disease 20 to 40 yr after treatment (see p. 1853). Pituitary-extracted GH was last used in the 1980s.

It is controversial whether short children with clinical features of GH deficiency but with normal GH secretion and normal IGF-1 levels should be treated with GH. Many experts recommend a trial of GH therapy for 6 to 12 mo, continuing GH only if there is a doubling of or an increase of 3 cm/yr over the pretreatment height velocity. Others object to this approach because it is expensive, is experimental, may lead to adverse effects, labels otherwise healthy children as abnormal, and raises ethical and psychosocial concerns that feed into the bias of "heightism."

Cortisol and thyroid hormone should be replaced throughout childhood, adolescence, and adulthood in patients with short stature due to pituitary dwarfism when circulating levels of these hormones are low (see pp. 1202 and 1209). When puberty fails to occur normally, treatment with gonadal sex steroids is indicated (see p. 2370).

GH therapy in children with short stature due to therapeutic radiation of the pituitary gland for cancer carries a theoretic risk of causing cancer recurrence. However, studies have not shown a greater-than-expected incidence of new cancers or a greater recurrence rate. GH replacement can probably be safely instituted at least 1 yr after the successful completion of anticancer therapy.

GIGANTISM AND ACROMEGALY

Gigantism and acromegaly are syndromes of excessive secretion of growth hormone (hypersomatotropism) that are nearly always due to a pituitary adenoma. Before closure of the epiphyses, the result is gigantism. Later, the result is acromegaly, which produces distinctive facial and other features. Diagnosis is clinical and by skull and hand x-rays and measurement of growth hormone levels. Treatment involves removal or destruction of the responsible adenoma.

Many growth hormone (GH)–secreting adenomas contain a mutant form of the G_s protein, which is a stimulatory regulator of adenylate cyclase. Cells with the mutant form of G_s protein secrete GH even in the absence of growth hormone–releasing hormone (GHRH). A few cases of ectopic GHRH-producing tumors, especially of the pancreas and lung, also have been described.

Symptoms and Signs

Pituitary gigantism: This rare condition occurs if GH hypersecretion begins in childhood, before closure of the epiphyses. Skeletal growth velocity and ultimate stature are increased but with little bony deformity.

However, soft-tissue swelling occurs, and the peripheral nerves are enlarged. Delayed puberty or hypogonadotropic hypogonadism is also frequently present, resulting in a eunuchoid habitus.

Acromegaly: In acromegaly, GH hypersecretion starts between the 20s and 40s. When GH hypersecretion begins after epiphyseal closure, the earliest clinical manifestations are coarsening of the facial features and soft-tissue swelling of the hands and feet. Appearance changes, and larger rings, gloves, and shoes are needed. Photographs of the patient are important in delineating the course of the disease.

In adults with acromegaly, coarse body hair increases and the skin thickens and frequently darkens. The size and function of sebaceous and sweat glands increase, such that patients frequently complain of excessive perspiration and offensive body odor. Overgrowth of the mandible leads to protrusion of the jaw (prognathism) and malocclusion of teeth. Cartilaginous proliferation of the larynx leads to a deep, husky voice. The tongue is frequently enlarged and furrowed. In long-standing acromegaly, costal growth leads to a barrel chest. Articular cartilaginous proliferation occurs early in response to GH excess, with the articular cartilage possibly undergoing necrosis and erosion. Joint symptoms are common, and crippling degenerative arthritis may occur.

Peripheral neuropathies occur commonly because of compression of nerves by adjacent fibrous tissue and endoneural fibrous proliferation. Headaches are common because of the pituitary tumor. Bitemporal hemianopia may develop if suprasellar extension compresses the optic chiasm. The heart, liver, kidneys, spleen, thyroid, parathyroid glands, and pancreas are larger than normal. Cardiac disease occurs in perhaps ⅓ of patients, with a doubling in the risk of death from cardiac disease. Hypertension occurs in up to ⅓ of patients. The risk of cancer, particularly of the GI tract, increases 2-fold to 3-fold. GH increases tubular reabsorption of phosphate and leads to mild hyperphosphatemia. Impaired glucose tolerance occurs in nearly ½ the cases of acromegaly and in gigantism, but clinically significant diabetes mellitus occurs in only about 10% of patients.

Galactorrhea occurs in some women with acromegaly, usually in association with hyperprolactinemia (see p.1187). However, lactation may occur with GH excess alone, because GH itself stimulates lactation. Decreased gonadotropin secretion often occurs with GH-secreting tumors. About ⅓ of men with acromegaly develop erectile dysfunction, and nearly all women develop menstrual irregularities or amenorrhea.

Diagnosis

Diagnosis can be made from the characteristic clinical findings. CT, MRI, or skull x-rays disclose cortical thickening, enlargement of the frontal sinuses, and enlargement and erosion of the sella turcica. X-rays of the hands show tufting of the terminal phalanges and soft-tissue thickening. Generally, glucose tolerance is abnormal and serum phosphate levels are elevated.

Plasma GH levels measured by radioimmunoassay are typically elevated and are the simplest way to assess GH hypersecretion. Blood should be obtained before the patient eats breakfast (basal state); in normal people, basal GH levels are < 5 ng/mL. Transient elevations of GH are normal and must be distinguished from pathologic hypersecretion. The degree of GH suppression after a glucose load remains the standard and thus should be measured in patients with elevated plasma GH; however, the results are assay-dependent, and the cut-off for normal suppression is controversial. Secretion in normal people is suppressed to < 2 ng/mL (a cutoff of < 1 ng/mL is often used) within 90 min of administration of glucose 75 g po. Most acromegalic patients have substantially higher values. Basal plasma GH levels are also important in monitoring response to therapy.

Plasma insulin-like growth factor 1 (IGF-1) should be measured in patients with suspected acromegaly; IGF-1 levels are typically substantially elevated (3-fold to 10-fold). IGF-1 levels also can be used to monitor response to therapy.

CT or MRI of the head should be performed to look for a tumor. If a tumor is not visible, excessive secretion of pituitary GH may be due to a non-CNS tumor producing excessive amounts of ectopic GHRH. Demonstration of elevated levels of plasma GHRH can confirm the diagnosis. Lungs and pancreas may be first evaluated in searching for the sites of ectopic production.

Treatment

Ablative therapy with surgery or radiation is generally indicated. Transsphenoidal resection is preferred, but choices vary at different institutions. Stereotactic supervoltage radiation, delivering about 5000 cGy to the pituitary, is used, but GH levels may not fall to normal for several years. Treatment with accelerated protons (heavy particle radiation) permits delivery of larger doses of radiation (equivalent to 10,000 cGy) to the pituitary; such therapy poses higher risk of cranial nerve and hypothalamic damage and is available only in a few centers. Development of hypopituitarism several years after irradiation is common. Because radiation damage is cumulative, proton beam therapy should *not* be used after conventional γ-irradiation. A combined surgery-radiation approach is indicated for patients with progressive extrasellar involvement by a pituitary tumor and for patients whose entire tumor cannot be resected, which is often the case.

Surgical removal of the tumor is likely to have been curative if GH levels after the glucose tolerance test and IGF-1 levels reach normal values. If one or both values are abnormal, further therapy is usually needed. If GH excess is poorly controlled, hypertension, heart failure, and a doubling in the death rate occur. If GH levels are < 5 ng/mL, however, mortality does not increase.

In general, drug therapy is indicated if surgery and radiation therapy are contraindicated, if they have not been curative, or if radiation therapy is being given time to work. In such instances, bromocriptine mesylate (1.25 to 5 mg po bid) may effectively lower GH levels in a small percentage of patients. If bromocriptine is ineffective, a somatostatin analog, octreotide, is given at 0.05 to 0.15 mg sc q 8 to 12 h; it suppresses GH secretion effectively in patients refractory to bromocriptine, surgery, or irradiation. Longer-acting somatostatin analogs, such as mannitol-modified release octreotide (octreotide LAR) given 10 to 30 mg IM q 4 to 6 wk and lanreotide given 30 mg IM q 10 to 14 days, are more convenient.

Pegvisomant, a GH receptor blocker, has been shown to reduce the effects of GH and lower IGF-1 levels in people with acromegaly, without apparent increase in pituitary tumor size. This drug may find a place in treating patients who are partially or totally unresponsive to somatostatin analogs.

GALACTORRHEA

Galactorrhea is lactation in men or in women who are not breastfeeding. It is generally due to a prolactin-secreting pituitary adenoma. Diagnosis is by measurement of prolactin levels and imaging tests. Treatment involves tumor inhibition with dopamine agonist drugs and sometimes removal or destruction of the adenoma.

Etiology

Galactorrhea is generally due to a prolactin-secreting pituitary adenoma (prolactinoma). Most tumors in women are microadenomas (< 10 mm in diameter), but a small percentage are macroadenomas (> 10 mm) when diagnosed. The frequency of microadenomas is much lower in men, perhaps because of later recognition.

Hyperprolactinemia and galactorrhea also may be caused by ingestion of certain drugs, including phenothiazines, certain antihypertensives (especially α-methyldopa), and opioids. Primary hypothyroidism can cause hyperprolactinemia and galactorrhea, because increased levels of thyroid-releasing hormone increase secretion of prolactin as well as thyroid-stimulating hormone (TSH). It is unclear why hyperprolactinemia is associated with hypogonadotropism and hypogonadism. Causes of hyperprolactinemia are listed in TABLE 151–3.

Symptoms and Signs

Abnormal lactation is not defined quantitatively; it is milk release that is inappropriate, persistent, or worrisome to the patient. Spontaneous lactation is more unusual than milk released in response to manual expression. The milk is white. Women with galactorrhea commonly also have amenorrhea or oligomenorrhea. Women with galactorrhea and amenorrhea may also have symptoms and signs of estrogen deficiency, including hot flushes and dyspareunia, due to inhibition of pulsatile luteinizing hormone and follicle-stimulating hormone release by high prolactin levels. However, estrogen production may be normal, and signs of androgen excess have been observed in some hyperprolactinemic women. Hyperprolactinemia may occur with other menstrual cycle disturbances besides amenorrhea, including infrequent ovulation and corpus luteum dysfunction.

Men with prolactin-secreting pituitary tumors typically have headaches or visual difficulties. About ⅔ of affected men have loss of libido and erectile dysfunction.

Diagnosis

Diagnosis of galactorrhea due to a prolactin-secreting pituitary adenoma is based on

TABLE 151–3. CAUSES OF HYPERPROLACTINEMIA

Physiologic

Nipple stimulation in men and women
Pregnancy
Postpartum period
Stress
Food ingestion
Sexual intercourse in some women
Sleep
Hypoglycemia
Early infancy (up to 3 mo)

Pathologic

Hypothalamic disorders
- Hypothalamic tumors
- Nontumorous hypothalamic infiltration
  - Sarcoidosis
  - TB
  - Langerhans' cell granulomatosis (histiocytosis—Hand-Schüller-Christian disease)
- Postencephalitis
- Idiopathic galactorrhea (presumed abnormality in dopamine secretion)
- Head trauma

Prolactin-secreting pituitary tumors
Tumors causing pituitary stalk compression
Surgical pituitary stalk section and other stalk lesions
Empty sella syndrome
Acromegaly
Cushing's disease
Primary hypothyroidism
Chronic renal failure
Liver disease
Ectopic production of prolactin
- Bronchogenic carcinoma (not squamous cell; mostly small cell undifferentiated)
- Hypernephroma

Chest wall lesions
- Surgical scars
- Trauma
- Chest wall tumors
- Herpes zoster

Pharmacologic

Antihypertensive drugs
- Reserpine
- α-Methyldopa
- Ca channel blockers

Oral contraceptives
Opioids
Psychoactive drugs (eg, phenothiazines, tricyclic and some other antidepressants, butyrophenones [haloperidol], benzamides [metoclopramide, sulpiride])
Thyrotropin-releasing hormone

Modified from Rebar RW: "Practical evaluation of hormonal status," in *Reproductive Endocrinology; Physiology, Pathophysiology and Clinical Management*, edited by SSC Yen and RB Jaffe. Philadelphia, WB Saunders Company, 1978, p 493; used with permission.

elevated prolactin levels. In general, prolactin levels correlate with the size of a pituitary tumor and can be used to follow patients over time. Serum gonadotropin and estradiol levels are either low or in the normal range in hyperprolactinemic women. Primary hypothyroidism is easily ruled out by absence of elevated TSH.

High-resolution CT or MRI is the method of choice in identifying microadenomas. Visual field examination is indicated in all patients with macroadenomas and in any patient who elects drug therapy or surveillance only.

Treatment

The treatment of microprolactinomas is controversial. Asymptomatic patients with prolactin levels < 100 ng/mL and with normal CT or MRI scans or those who have only microadenomas can probably be observed; serum prolactin often normalizes within years. Patients with hyperprolactinemia should be monitored with quarterly prolactin levels and undergo sellar CT or MRI annually for at least an additional 2 yr. The frequency of sellar imaging can then be reduced if prolactin levels do not increase. Indications for treatment in women include the desire for pregnancy, amenorrhea or significant oligomenorrhea (because of the risk of osteoporosis), hirsutism, low libido, and troublesome galactorrhea. Indications in men include hypogonadism (because of the risk of osteoporosis), erectile dysfunction, low libido, and troublesome infertility.

The initial treatment is usually a dopamine agonist such as bromocriptine (1.25 to 5 mg po bid), pergolide (0.05 to 0.25 mg po once/

day or bid), or the longer-acting cabergoline (0.25 to 1.0 mg po once or twice/wk). Cabergoline is the treatment of choice because it appears to be the most easily tolerated and most potent of these drugs. Women trying to become pregnant should switch to bromocriptine at least 1 mo before planned conception; long-term safety data are better established for bromocriptine than for cabergoline. Exogenous estrogen can be given to women with a microadenoma who are clinically hypoestrogenic or have low estradiol levels. Exogenous estrogen is unlikely to cause tumor expansion.

Patients with macroadenomas generally should be treated with dopamine agonists or surgically but only after thorough testing of pituitary function and evaluation for radiation therapy. Dopamine agonists are usually the initial treatment of choice and usually shrink the tumor. If prolactin levels fall and symptoms and signs of compression by the tumor abate, no other therapy may be necessary. Surgery or radiation therapy may be easier to perform or yield better results after tumor shrinkage induced by a dopamine agonist.

Radiation therapy should be used only in patients with progressive disease who do not respond to other forms of therapy. With irradiation, hypopituitarism often develops several years after therapy. Monitoring endocrine function and sellar imaging are indicated yearly for life.

CENTRAL DIABETES INSIPIDUS

(Vasopressin-Sensitive Diabetes Insipidus)

(See also syndrome of inappropriate antidiuretic hormone secretion on p. 1239 and Nephrogenic Diabetes Insipidus on p.2025.)

Diabetes insipidus (DI) results from a deficiency of vasopressin due to a hypothalamic-pituitary disorder (central DI [CDI]) or from resistance of the kidney to vasopressin (nephrogenic DI [NDI]). Polyuria and polydipsia develop. Diagnosis is by water deprivation test showing failure to maximally concentrate urine; vasopressin levels and response to exogenous vasopressin help distinguish CDI from NDI. Treatment is with intranasal DDAVP (desmopressin) or lypressin. Nonhormonal treatment includes use of diuretics (mainly thiazides) and ADH-releasing drugs, such as chlorpropamide.

Etiology and Pathophysiology

Polyuria may result from CDI, a deficiency of ADH, NDI, or compulsive or habitual water drinking (psychogenic polydipsia). The posterior lobe of the pituitary is the major site of ADH storage and release, but ADH is synthesized within the hypothalamus. Newly synthesized hormone can still be released into the circulation as long as the hypothalamic nuclei and part of the neurohypophyseal tract are intact. Only about 10% of neurosecretory neurons must remain intact to avoid CDI. The pathology of CDI thus always involves the supraoptic and paraventricular nuclei of the hypothalamus or a major portion of the pituitary stalk.

CDI may be complete (absence of vasopressin) or partial (insufficient amounts of vasopressin). CDI may be primary, in which there is a marked decrease in the hypothalamic nuclei of the neurohypophyseal system. Genetic abnormalities of the vasopressin gene on chromosome 20 are responsible for autosomal dominant forms of primary CDI, but many cases are idiopathic. CDI may also be secondary (acquired), caused by various lesions, including hypophysectomy, cranial injuries (particularly basal skull fractures), suprasellar and intrasellar tumors (primary or metastatic), Langerhans' cell granulomatosis (histiocytosis—Hand-Schüller-Christian disease), granulomas (sarcoidosis or TB), vascular lesions (aneurysm and thrombosis), and infections (encephalitis or meningitis).

Symptoms and Signs

Onset may be insidious or abrupt, occurring at any age. The only symptoms in primary CDI are polydipsia and polyuria. In secondary CDI, symptoms and signs of the associated lesions are also present. Enormous quantities of fluid may be ingested, and large volumes (3 to 30 L/day) of very dilute urine (sp gr usually < 1.005 and osmolality < 200 mOsm/L) are excreted. Nocturia almost always occurs. Dehydration and hypovolemia may develop rapidly if urinary losses are not continuously replaced.

Diagnosis

CDI must be differentiated from other causes of polyuria, particularly psychogenic polydipsia (see TABLE 151–4) and NDI. All tests for CDI (and for NDI) are based on the principle that increasing the plasma osmolality in normal people will lead to decreased excretion of urine with increased osmolality.

TABLE 151–4. COMMON CAUSES OF POLYURIA

Vasopressin-sensitive polyuria
Decreased *synthesis* of ADH
  Primary diabetes insipidus
    Hereditary (usually autosomal dominant)
    Associated with diabetes mellitus, optic atrophy, nerve deafness, and atonia of bladder and ureters
  Acquired diabetes insipidus (causes outlined in text)
Decreased *release* of ADH (psychogenic polydipsia or dipsogenic diabetes insipidus)

Vasopressin-resistant polyuria
Congenital nephrogenic diabetes insipidus (usually X-linked recessive)
Acquired nephrogenic diabetes insipidus
  Chronic renal disease
  Systemic or metabolic disease (eg, myeloma, amyloidosis, hypercalcemic or hypokalemic nephropathy, sickle cell disease)
  Drugs (lithium, demeclocycline)
Osmotic diuresis
  Glucose (diabetes mellitus)
  Poorly resorbed solutes (mannitol, sorbitol, urea)

The water deprivation test is the simplest and most reliable method for diagnosing CDI but *should be performed only while the patient is under constant supervision. Serious dehydration may result.* Additionally, those suspected of psychogenic polydipsia must be observed to prevent surreptitious drinking. The test is started in the morning by weighing the patient, obtaining venous blood to determine electrolyte concentrations and osmolality, and measuring urinary osmolality. Voided urine is collected hourly, and its sp gr or, preferably, osmolality is measured. Dehydration is continued until orthostatic hypotension and postural tachycardia appear; ≥ 5% of the initial body weight has been lost; or the urinary concentration does not increase more than 0.001 sp gr or 30 mOsm/L in sequentially voided specimens. Serum electrolytes and osmolality are again determined, and 5 units of aqueous vasopressin are injected sc. Urine for sp gr or osmolality measurement is collected one final time 60 min postinjection, and the test is terminated.

A normal response produces maximum urine osmolality after dehydration (often > 1.020 sp gr or 700 mOsm/L), exceeding the plasma osmolality; osmolality does not increase more than an additional 5% after injection of vasopressin. Patients with CDI are generally unable to concentrate urine to greater than the plasma osmolality but are able to increase their urine osmolality by > 50% after vasopressin. Patients with partial CDI are often able to concentrate urine to above the plasma osmolality but show a rise in urine osmolality of > 9% after vasopressin administration. Patients with NDI are unable to concentrate urine to greater than the plasma osmolality and show no additional response to vasopressin administration.

Measurement of circulating ADH is the most direct method of diagnosing CDI; levels at the end of the water deprivation test (before the vasopressin injection) are low in CDI and appropriately elevated in NDI. However, ADH levels are difficult to measure and the test is not routinely available. In addition, water deprivation is so accurate that direct measurement of ADH is unnecessary. Plasma vasopressin levels are diagnostic after either dehydration or infusion of hypertonic saline.

Psychogenic polydipsia: Psychogenic polydipsia may present a difficult problem in differential diagnosis. Patients may ingest and excrete up to 6 L of fluid/day and are often emotionally disturbed. Unlike patients with CDI and NDI, they usually do not have nocturia, nor does their thirst wake them at night. Continued ingestion of large volumes of water in this situation can lead to life-threatening hyponatremia (see p. 1237).

Patients with acute psychogenic water drinking are able to concentrate their urine during water deprivation. However, because chronic water intake diminishes medullary tonicity in the kidney, patients with long-standing polydipsia are not able to concentrate their urine to maximal levels during water deprivation, a response similar to that of patients with partial CDI. However, unlike CDI, patients with psychogenic polydipsia show no response to exogenous vasopressin after water deprivation. This response resembles NDI, except that basal vasopressin levels are low compared with the elevated levels present in NDI. After prolonged restriction of fluid intake to ≤ 2 L/day, normal concentrating ability returns within several weeks.

Treatment

CDI can be treated with hormone replacement and treatment of any correctable cause.

In the absence of appropriate management, permanent renal damage can result.

DDAVP (desmopressin), a synthetic analog of vasopressin with minimal vasoconstrictive properties, has prolonged antidiuretic activity lasting for 12 to 24 h in most patients and may be administered intranasally, sc, IV, or orally. DDAVP is the preparation of choice for both adults and children and is available as an intranasal solution in 2 forms. A dropper bottle with a calibrated nasal catheter has the advantage of delivering incremental doses from 5 to 20 μg but is awkward to use. A spray bottle that delivers 10 μg of DDAVP in 0.1 mL of fluid is easier to use but delivers a fixed quantity. For each patient, the duration of action of a given dose must be established, because variation among individuals is great. The duration of action can be established by following timed urine volumes and osmolality. The nightly dose is the lowest dose required to prevent nocturia. The morning and evening doses should be adjusted separately. The usual dosage range in adults is 10 to 40 μg, with most adults requiring 10 μg bid. For children age 3 mo to 12 yr, the usual dosage range is 2.5 to 10 μg bid. Overdosage can lead to fluid retention and decreased plasma osmolality, possibly resulting in seizures in small children. In such instances, furosemide can be given to induce diuresis. Headache may be a troublesome adverse effect but generally disappears if the dosage is reduced. Infrequently, DDVAP causes a slight increase in BP. Absorption from the nasal mucosa may be erratic, especially when URI or allergic rhinitis occurs. When intranasal delivery of DDAVP is inappropriate, it may be administered sc using about 1/10 the intranasal dose. DDAVP may be used IV if a rapid effect is necessary (eg, for hypovolemia). With oral DDAVP, dose equivalence with the intranasal formulation is unpredictable, so individual dose titration is needed. The initial dose is 0.1 mg po tid, and the maintenance dose is usually 0.1 to 0.2 mg tid.

Lypressin (lysine-8-vasopressin), a synthetic agent, is given by nasal spray at doses of 2 to 4 units (7.5 to 15 μg) q 3 to 8 h but, because of its short duration of action, has been largely replaced by DDAVP.

Aqueous vasopressin 5 to 10 units sc or IM can be given to provide an antidiuretic response that usually lasts ≤ 6 h. Thus, this drug has little use in long-term treatment but can be used in the initial therapy of unconscious patients and in patients with CDI who are undergoing surgery. Synthetic vasopressin can also be administered bid to qid as a nasal spray, with the dosage and interval tailored to each patient. Vasopressin tannate in oil 0.3 to 1 mL (1.5 to 5 units) IM may control symptoms for up to 96 h.

At least 3 groups of nonhormonal drugs are useful in reducing polyuria: various diuretics, primarily thiazides; ADH-releasing drugs, such as chlorpropamide, carbamazepine, and clofibrate; and prostaglandin inhibitors, which are modestly effective. These drugs have been particularly useful in partial CDI and do not cause the adverse effects of exogenous ADH.

The thiazides paradoxically reduce urine volume in partial and complete CDI (and NDI), primarily as a consequence of reducing ECF volume and increasing proximal tubular resorption. Urine volumes may fall by 25 to 50% with 15 to 25 mg/kg of chlorothiazide. Restricting salt intake may also help because it reduces urine output by reducing solute load.

Chlorpropamide, carbamazepine, and clofibrate can reduce or eliminate the need for vasopressin in some patients with partial CDI. None are effective in NDI. Chlorpropamide (3 to 5 mg/kg po once/day or bid) causes some release of ADH and also potentiates the action of ADH on the kidney. Clofibrate (500 to 1000 mg po bid) or carbamazepine (100 to 400 mg po bid) is recommended for adults only. These drugs may be used synergistically with a diuretic. However, significant hypoglycemia may result from chlorpropamide.

Prostaglandin inhibitors (such as indomethacin 0.5 to 1.0 mg/kg po tid, although most NSAIDs are effective) may reduce urine volume, but generally by no more than 10 to 25%, perhaps by decreasing renal blood flow and GFR. Together with indomethacin, restriction of Na intake and a thiazide diuretic help further reduce urine volume in NDI.

152 THYROID DISORDERS

The thyroid gland, located in the anterior neck just below the cricoid cartilage, consists of 2 lobes connected by an isthmus. Follicular cells in the gland produce the 2 main thyroid hormones, tetraiodothyronine (thyroxine, T_4), and triiodothyronine (T_3). These hormones act on cells in virtually every body tissue by combining with nuclear receptors and altering expression of a wide range of gene products. Thyroid hormone is required for normal brain and somatic tissue development in the fetus and newborn, and, in all ages, regulates protein, carbohydrate, and fat metabolism.

T_3 is the most active form; T_4 has only minimal hormonal activity. However, T_4 is much longer lasting and can be converted to T_3 (in most tissues) and thus serves as a reservoir for T_3. A 3rd form of thyroid hormone, reverse T_3 (rT_3), has no metabolic activity; levels of rT_3 increase in certain diseases.

Additionally, parafollicular cells (C cells) secrete the hormone calcitonin, which is released in response to hypercalcemia and lowers serum Ca levels (see p. 1249).

Synthesis and Release of Thyroid Hormones

Synthesis of thyroid hormones requires iodine. Iodine, ingested in food and water as iodide, is actively concentrated by the thyroid and converted to organic iodine (organification) within follicular cells by thyroid peroxidase. The follicular cells surround a space filled with colloid, which consists of thyroglobulin, a glycoprotein containing tyrosine within its matrix. Tyrosine in contact with the membrane of the follicular cells is iodinated at 1 (monoiodotyrosine) or 2 (diiodotyrosine) sites and then coupled to produce the 2 forms of thyroid hormone (diiodotyrosine + diiodotyrosine → T_4; diiodotyrosine + monoiodotyrosine → T_3).

T_3 and T_4 remain incorporated in thyroglobulin within the follicle until the follicular cells take up thyroglobulin as colloid droplets. Once inside the thyroid follicular cells, T_3 and T_4 are cleaved from thyroglobulin. Free T_3 and T_4 are then released into the bloodstream, where they are bound to serum proteins for transport, the major one being thyroxine-binding globulin (TBG), which has high affinity but low capacity for T_3 and T_4. TBG normally carries about 75% of bound thyroid hormones. The other binding proteins are thyroxine-binding prealbumin (transthyretin), which has high affinity but low capacity for T_4, and albumin, which has low affinity but high capacity for T_3 and T_4. About 0.3% of total serum T_3 and 0.03% of total serum T_4 are free and in equilibrium with bound hormones. Only free T_3 and T_4 are available to act on the peripheral tissues.

All reactions necessary for the formation and release of T_3 and T_4 are controlled by thyroid-stimulating hormone (TSH), which is secreted by pituitary thyrotropic cells. TSH secretion is controlled by a negative feedback mechanism in the pituitary: Increased levels of free T_4 and T_3 inhibit TSH synthesis and secretion, whereas decreased levels increase TSH secretion. TSH secretion is also influenced by thyrotropin-releasing hormone (TRH), which is synthesized in the hypothalamus. The precise mechanisms regulating TRH synthesis and release are unclear, although negative feedback from thyroid hormones plays a role.

Most circulating T_3 is produced outside the thyroid by monodeiodination of T_4. Only $\frac{1}{4}$ of circulating T_3 is secreted directly by the thyroid.

Laboratory Testing of Thyroid Function

TSH measurement is the best means of determining thyroid dysfunction. Normal results essentially rule out hyperthyroidism or hypothyroidism, except in rare patients with pituitary resistance to thyroid hormone or with central hypothyroidism due to disease in the hypothalamus and/or pituitary gland. Serum TSH can be falsely low in very sick people. The serum TSH level also defines the syndromes of subclinical hyperthyroidism (low serum TSH) and subclinical hypothyroidism (elevated serum TSH), both of which are characterized by normal serum T_4, free T_4, serum T_3, and free T_3 levels.

Total serum T_4 measures bound and free hormone. Changes in levels of thyroid hormone–binding serum proteins produce corresponding changes in total T_4, even though levels of physiologically active free T_4 are unchanged. Thus, a patient may be physiologically normal but have an abnormal total serum T_4 level. Free T_4 in the serum can be measured directly, avoiding the pitfalls of interpreting total T_4 levels.

Free thyroxine index (free T_4 index) is a calculated value that corrects total T_4 for the effects of varying amounts of thyroid hormone–binding serum proteins and thus gives an estimate of free T_4 when measuring total T_4. The thyroid hormone–binding ratio or T_3 resin uptake is used to estimate protein binding. Free T_4 index is readily available and compares well with direct measurement of free T_4.

Total serum T_3 and free T_3 can also be measured. Because T_3 is tightly bound to TBG (although 10 times less so than T_4), total serum T_3 levels are influenced by alterations in serum TBG level and by drugs that affect binding to TBG. Free T_3 levels in the serum are measured by the same direct and indirect methods (free T_3 index) described above for T_4 and are used mainly for evaluating thyrotoxicosis.

TBG can be measured; it is increased in pregnancy, by estrogen therapy or oral contraceptives, and in the acute phase of infectious hepatitis. TBG may also be increased by an X-linked abnormality. It is most commonly decreased by anabolic steroids and excessive corticosteroids. Large doses of certain drugs, such as phenytoin and aspirin and their derivatives, displace T_4 from its binding sites on TBG, which spuriously lowers total serum T_4 levels.

Autoantibodies to thyroid peroxidase are present in almost all patients with Hashimoto's thyroiditis (some of whom also have autoantibodies to thyroglobulin) and in most patients with Graves' disease. These autoantibodies are markers of autoimmune disease but probably do not cause disease. However, an autoantibody directed against the TSH receptor on the thyroid follicular cell is responsible for the hyperthyroidism in Graves' disease. Antibodies against T_4 and T_3 may be found in patients with autoimmune thyroid disease and may affect T_4 and T_3 measurements but are rarely clinically significant.

The thyroid is the only source of thyroglobulin, which is readily detectable in the serum of normal patients and is usually elevated in patients with nontoxic or toxic goiter. The principal use of serum thyroglobulin measurement is in evaluating patients after near-total or total thyroidectomy (with or without ^{131}I ablation) for differentiated thyroid cancer. Normal or elevated serum thyroglobulin values indicate the presence of residual normal or cancerous thyroid tissue in patients receiving TSH-suppressive doses of L-thyroxine or after withdrawal of L-thyroxine. However, thyroglobulin antibodies can interfere with thyroglobulin measurement.

Radioactive iodine uptake can be measured. A trace amount of radioiodine is administered orally or IV; a scanner then detects the amount of radioiodine taken up by the thyroid. The preferred radioiodine isotope is ^{123}I, which exposes the patient to minimal radiation (much less than ^{131}I). Thyroid ^{123}I uptake varies widely with iodine ingestion and is low in patients exposed to excess iodine. The test is valuable in the differential diagnosis of hyperthyroidism (high uptake in Graves' disease, low uptake in thyroiditis—see p. 1198). It may also help calculate the dose of ^{131}I necessary for treatment of hyperthyroidism.

Imaging by a scintillation camera can be obtained after radioisotope administration (radioiodine or technetium 99m pertechnetate) to produce a graphic representation of isotope uptake. Focal areas of increased (hot) or decreased (cold) uptake help distinguish areas of possible cancer (thyroid cancers exist in $< 1\%$ of hot nodules compared with 10 to 20% of cold nodules).

APPROACH TO THE PATIENT WITH A THYROID NODULE

Benign causes of thyroid nodules include hyperplastic colloid goiter, thyroid cysts, thyroiditis, and thyroid adenomas. Malignant causes include thyroid cancers (see p.1205).

Evaluation

Many nodules are found incidentally on thyroid imaging studies performed for other disorders. The frequency of thyroid nodules increases with age; ultrasound may reveal nodules in 10 to 67% of middle-aged and elderly patients.

History: Pain suggests thyroiditis or hemorrhage into a cyst. An asymptomatic nodule often is cancer but may be any of the benign disorders listed above. Symptoms of hyperthyroidism suggest a hyperfunctioning adenoma or thyroiditis, whereas symptoms of hypothyroidism suggest Hashimoto's thyroiditis. Risk factors for thyroid cancer include history of thyroid irradiation, especially in infancy and childhood; age < 20 yr; male sex; family history of thyroid cancer; a solitary nodule; and increasing size.

Physical examination: Signs that suggest thyroid cancer include stony hard consistency or fixation to surrounding structures, cervical lymphadenopathy, and hoarseness due to recurrent laryngeal nerve paralysis.

Testing: Initial evaluation of a thyroid nodule consists of TSH, free T_4, and antithyroid peroxidase antibody measurements. Ultrasound is useful in determining the size of the nodule but is rarely diagnostic of cancer. Thyroid cancer is suggested by ultrasound or radiographic evidence of fine, stippled psammomatous calcification (papillary carcinoma) or dense, homogeneous calcification (medullary carcinoma). Thyroid isotopic scanning is obtained if TSH is suppressed; nodules with increased radionuclide uptake (hot) are seldom malignant. Fine-needle aspiration biopsy is the best diagnostic approach for distinguishing benign from malignant nodules and is performed if initial thyroid function tests do not indicate hyperthyroidism or Hashimoto's thyroiditis. Early use of fine-needle aspiration biopsy is a more economic approach than routine use of ultrasound and radioiodine scans. Fine-needle aspiration biopsy is not routinely indicated for nodules < 1 cm on ultrasonography.

Treatment

Treatment is directed at the underlying cause. Thyroxine suppression of TSH to shrink smaller benign nodules is effective in about $\frac{1}{2}$ the cases.

EUTHYROID SICK SYNDROME

Euthyroid sick syndrome is low serum levels of thyroid hormones in clinically euthyroid patients with nonthyroidal systemic illness. Diagnosis is by excluding hypothyroidism. Treatment is of the underlying illness; thyroid hormone replacement is not indicated.

Patients with various acute or chronic nonthyroidal disorders may have abnormal thyroid function tests. Such disorders include acute and chronic illness, particularly fasting, starvation, protein-calorie malnutrition, major trauma, MI, chronic renal failure, diabetic ketoacidosis, anorexia nervosa, cirrhosis, thermal injury, and sepsis.

Decreased T_3 levels are most common. Patients with more severe or prolonged illness also have decreased T_4 levels. Serum reverse T_3 (rT_3) is increased. Patients are clinically euthyroid and do not have TSH elevations.

Pathogenesis is unknown but may include decreased peripheral conversion of T_4 to T_3, decreased clearance of rT_3 generated from T_4, and decreased binding of thyroid hormones to thyroxine-binding globulin (TBG). Pro-inflammatory cytokines (eg, tumor necrosis factor-α, IL-1) may be responsible for some changes.

Interpretation of abnormal thyroid function tests in ill patients is complicated by the effects of various drugs, including the iodine-rich contrast agents and amiodarone, which further impair the peripheral conversion of T_4 to T_3, and by drugs such as dopamine and corticosteroids, which decrease pituitary secretion of TSH, resulting in low serum TSH levels and subsequent decreased T_4 secretion.

Diagnosis and Treatment

The diagnostic dilemma is whether the patient has hypothyroidism or euthyroid sick syndrome. The best test is TSH, which in euthyroid sick syndrome is low, normal, or slightly elevated but not as high as it would be in hypothyroidism. Serum rT_3 is elevated, although this test is rarely done. Serum cortisol is often elevated in euthyroid sick syndrome and low or low-normal in hypothyroidism from pituitary-hypothalamic disease. Because tests are nonspecific, clinical judgment is required to interpret abnormal thyroid function tests in the acutely or chronically ill patient. Unless thyroid dysfunction is highly suspected, thyroid function tests should not be ordered for ICU patients.

Treatment with thyroid hormone replacement is not appropriate; when the underlying disorder is treated, thyroid tests normalize.

HASHIMOTO'S THYROIDITIS

(Autoimmune Thyroiditis; Chronic Lymphocytic Thyroiditis; Hashimoto's Struma)

Hashimoto's thyroiditis is chronic autoimmune inflammation of the thyroid with lymphocytic infiltration. Findings include painless thyroid enlargement and symptoms of hypothyroidism. Diagnosis involves demonstration of high titers of thyroid peroxidase antibodies. Lifelong thyroxine replacement is typically required.

Hashimoto's thyroiditis is believed to be the most common cause of primary hypothyroidism in North America. It is twice as prevalent in women. Incidence increases with age and in patients with chromosomal disorders, including Turner's, Down, and Klinefelter's syndromes. A family history of thyroid disorders is common.

Hashimoto's thyroiditis, like Graves' disease, is sometimes associated with other autoimmune disorders, including Addison's disease (adrenal insufficiency), type 1 diabetes, hypoparathyroidism, vitiligo, premature graying of hair, pernicious anemia, connective tissue diseases (eg, RA, SLE, Sjögren's syndrome), and Schmidt's syndrome (Addison's disease and hypothyroidism secondary to Hashimoto's thyroiditis). There may be an increased incidence of thyroid tumors, particularly thyroid lymphoma. Pathologically, there is extensive infiltration of lymphocytes with lymphoid follicles and scarring.

Symptoms, Signs, and Diagnosis

Patients complain of painless enlargement of the thyroid or fullness in the throat. Examination reveals a nontender goiter that is smooth or nodular, firm, and more rubbery than the normal thyroid. Many patients present with symptoms of hypothyroidism, but some present with hyperthyroidism.

Testing consists of T_4, TSH, and thyroid autoantibodies; early in the disease T_4 and TSH levels are normal and there are high levels of thyroid peroxidase antibodies and less commonly of antithyroglobulin antibodies. Thyroid radioactive iodine uptake may be increased, perhaps because of defective iodide organification together with a gland that continues to trap iodine. The patient later develops hypothyroidism with decreased T_4, decreased thyroid radioactive iodine uptake, and increased TSH. Testing for other autoimmune disorders is warranted only when clinical manifestations are present.

Treatment

Occasionally, the hypothyroidism is transient, but most patients require lifelong thyroid hormone replacement, typically L-thyroxine, 75 to 150 µg po once/day.

HYPERTHYROIDISM

(Thyrotoxicosis)

Hyperthyroidism is characterized by hypermetabolism and elevated serum levels of free thyroid hormones. Symptoms are many but include tachycardia, fatigue, weight loss, and tremor. Diagnosis is clinical and with thyroid function tests. Treatment depends on cause.

Hyperthyroidism can be classified on the basis of thyroid radioactive iodine uptake and the presence or absence of circulating thyroid stimulators (see TABLE 152–1).

Etiology

Hyperthyroidism may result from increased synthesis and secretion of thyroid hormones (T_4 and T_3) from the thyroid, caused by thyroid stimulators in the blood or by autonomous thyroid hyperfunction. It can also result from excessive release of thyroid hormone from the thyroid without increased synthesis. Such release is commonly caused by the destructive changes of various types of thyroiditis. Various clinical syndromes also produce hyperthyroidism.

Graves' disease (toxic diffuse goiter), the most common cause of hyperthyroidism, is characterized by hyperthyroidism and one or more of the following: goiter, exophthalmos, and pretibial myxedema. It is caused by an autoantibody against the thyroid TSH receptor; unlike most autoantibodies, which are inhibitory, this autoantibody is stimulatory, thus producing continuous synthesis and secretion of excess T_4 and T_3. Graves' disease (like Hashimoto's thyroiditis) sometimes occurs with other autoimmune disorders, including type 1 diabetes, vitiligo, premature graying of hair, pernicious anemia, connective tissue diseases, and polyglandular deficiency syndrome. The pathogenesis of infiltrative ophthalmopathy (responsible for the exophthalmos in Graves' disease) is poorly understood but may result from immunoglobulins directed to specific antigens in the extraocular muscles and orbital fibroblasts. Ophthalmopathy may also occur before the onset of hyperthyroidism or as late as 20 yr afterward and frequently worsens or improves independent of the clinical course of hyperthyroidism. Typical ophthalmopathy in the presence of normal thyroid function is called euthyroid Graves' disease.

Inappropriate TSH secretion is a rare cause. Patients with hyperthyroidism have essentially undetectable TSH except for those with a TSH-secreting anterior pituitary adenoma or pituitary resistance to thyroid hormone. TSH levels are high, and the TSH produced

TABLE 152–1. LABORATORY EVALUATION OF THYROID FUNCTION IN VARIOUS CLINICAL SITUATIONS

PHYSIOLOGIC STATE	SERUM TSH	SERUM FREE T_4	SERUM T_3	24-H RADIO-IODINE UPTAKE
Hyperthyroidism, untreated	Low	High	High	High
Hyperthyroidism, T_3 toxicosis	Low	Normal	High	Normal or high
Primary hypothyroidism, untreated	High	Low	Low or normal	Low or normal
Hypothyroidism secondary to pituitary disease	Low or normal	Low	Low or normal	Low or normal
Euthyroid, on iodine	Normal	Normal	Normal	Low
Euthyroid, on exogenous thyroid hormone	Normal	Normal on T_4, low on T_3	High on T_3, normal on T_4	Low
Euthyroid, on estrogen	Normal	Normal	High	Normal
Euthyroid sick syndrome	Normal, low, or high	Normal or low	Low	Normal

TSH = thyroid-stimulating hormone; T_4 = thyroxine; T_3 = triiodothyronine.

in both disorders is biologically more active than normal TSH. An increase in the α-subunit of TSH in the blood (helpful in differential diagnosis) occurs in patients with a TSH-secreting pituitary adenoma.

Molar pregnancy, choriocarcinoma, and hyperemesis gravidarum produce high levels of serum human chorionic gonadotropin (hCG), a weak thyroid stimulator. Levels of hCG are highest during the 1st trimester of pregnancy and result in the decrease in serum TSH and mild increase in serum free T_4 sometimes observed at that time. The increased thyroid stimulation may be caused by increased levels of partially desialated human chorionic gonadotropin (hCG), an hCG variant that appears to be a more potent thyroid stimulator than more sialated hCG. Hyperthyroidism in molar pregnancy, choriocarcinoma, and hyperemesis gravidarum is transient; normal thyroid function resumes when the molar pregnancy is evacuated, the choriocarcinoma is appropriately treated, or the hyperemesis gravidarum abates.

Nonautoimmune autosomal dominant hyperthyroidism manifests during infancy. It results from mutations in the TSH receptor gene that produce continuous thyroid stimulation.

Toxic solitary or multinodular goiter (Plummer's disease) sometimes results from TSH receptor gene mutations producing continuous thyroid stimulation. Patients with toxic nodular goiter have none of the autoimmune manifestations or circulating antibodies observed in patients with Graves' disease. Also, in contrast to Graves' disease, toxic solitary and multinodular goiters usually do not remit.

Inflammatory thyroid disease (thyroiditis) includes subacute granulomatous thyroiditis, Hashimoto's thyroiditis, and silent lymphocytic thyroiditis, a variant of Hashimoto's thyroiditis (see p. 1203). Thyrotoxicosis results from destructive changes in the gland and release of stored hormone, not from increased synthesis. Hypothyroidism may follow. High-dose radiation therapy to the neck for nonthyroid malignant disease, eg, Hodgkin lymphoma (Hodgkin's disease) or laryngeal cancer, often results in permanent hypothyroidism.

Drug-induced hyperthyroidism can result from lithium administration, producing goiter with or without hyperthyroidism or hypothyroidism. Amiodarone and interferon-α may induce thyroiditis with hyperthyroidism and other thyroid disorders. Patients receiving these drugs should be closely monitored.

Thyrotoxicosis factitia is hyperthyroidism resulting from conscious or accidental overingestion of thyroid hormone.

Excess iodine ingestion causes hyperthyroidism with a low thyroid radioactive iodine uptake. It most often occurs in patients with underlying nontoxic nodular goiter (especially elderly patients) who are given drugs that contain iodine (eg, amiodarone, iodine-containing expectorants) or who undergo radiologic studies using iodine-rich contrast agents. The etiology may be that the excess iodine provides substrate for functionally autonomous (ie, not under TSH regulation) areas of the thyroid to produce hormone. Hyperthyroidism usually persists as long as excess iodine remains in the circulation.

Metastatic thyroid cancer is a possible cause. Overproduction of thyroid hormone occurs rarely from functioning metastatic follicular carcinoma, especially in pulmonary metastases.

Struma ovarii develops when ovarian teratomas contain enough thyroid tissue to cause true hyperthyroidism. Radioactive iodine uptake occurs in the pelvis, and uptake by the thyroid is usually suppressed.

Thyroid storm, an acute form of hyperthyroidism, results from untreated or inadequately treated severe hyperthyroidism. It is rare, occurring in patients with Graves' disease or toxic multinodular goiter (a solitary toxic nodule is less common and generally less severe). It may be precipitated by infection, trauma, surgery, embolism, diabetic ketoacidosis, or toxemia of pregnancy.

Pathophysiology

In hyperthyroidism, serum T_3 usually increases more than does T_4, probably because of increased secretion of T_3 and increased conversion of T_4 to T_3 in peripheral tissues. In some patients, only T_3 is elevated (T_3 toxicosis). T_3 toxicosis may occur in any of the usual disorders that produce hyperthyroidism, including Graves' disease, multinodular goiter, and the autonomously functioning solitary thyroid nodule. If T_3 toxicosis is untreated, the patient usually also develops laboratory abnormalities typical of hyperthyroidism (ie, elevated T_4 and ^{123}I uptake). The various forms of thyroiditis commonly have a hyperthyroid phase followed by a hypothyroid phase.

Symptoms and Signs

Most symptoms and signs are the same regardless of the cause. Exceptions include infiltrative ophthalmopathy and dermopathy, which occur only in Graves' disease.

The clinical presentation may be dramatic or subtle. A goiter or nodule may be present. Many common symptoms and signs of hyperthyroidism are similar to those of adrenergic excess, such as nervousness, palpitations, hyperactivity, increased sweating, heat hypersensitivity, fatigue, increased appetite, weight loss, insomnia, weakness, and frequent bowel movements (occasionally diarrhea). Hypomenorrhea may be present. Signs may include warm, moist skin; tremor; tachycardia; widened pulse pressure; atrial fibrillation; and palpitations.

Elderly patients, particularly those with toxic nodular goiter, may present atypically (apathetic or masked hyperthyroidism) with symptoms more akin to depression or dementia. Most do not have exophthalmos or tremor. Atrial fibrillation, syncope, altered sensorium, heart failure, and weakness are more likely. Symptoms and signs may involve only a single organ system.

Eye signs include stare, eyelid lag, eyelid retraction, and mild conjunctival injection and are largely due to excessive adrenergic stimulation. They usually remit with successful treatment. Infiltrative ophthalmopathy, a more serious development, is specific to Graves' disease and can occur years before or after hyperthyroidism. It is characterized by orbital pain, lacrimation, irritation, photophobia, increased retro-orbital tissue, exophthalmos, and lymphocytic infiltration of the extraocular muscles, producing ocular muscle weakness that frequently leads to double vision.

Infiltrative dermopathy, also called pretibial myxedema (a confusing term, because myxedema suggests hypothyroidism), is characterized by nonpitting infiltration by proteinaceous ground substance, usually in the pretibial area. It rarely occurs in the absence of Graves' ophthalmopathy. The lesion is often pruritic and erythematous in its early stages and subsequently becomes brawny. Infiltrative dermopathy may appear years before or after hyperthyroidism.

Thyroid storm produces abrupt florid symptoms of hyperthyroidism with one or more of the following: fever, marked weakness and muscle wasting, extreme restlessness with wide emotional swings, confusion, psychosis, coma, nausea, vomiting, diarrhea, and hepatomegaly with mild jaundice. The patient may present with cardiovascular collapse and shock. *Thyroid storm is a life-threatening emergency requiring prompt treatment.*

Diagnosis

Diagnosis is based on history, physical examination, and thyroid function tests. Serum TSH is the best test, because TSH is suppressed in hyperthyroid patients except when the etiology is a TSH-secreting pituitary adenoma or pituitary resistance to thyroid hormone. Free T_4 is increased. However, T_4 can be falsely normal in true hyperthyroidism in patients with a severe systemic illness (similar to the falsely low levels that occur in euthyroid sick syndrome) and in T_3 toxicosis. If free T_4 is normal and TSH is low in a patient with subtle symptoms and signs of hyperthyroidism, then serum T_3 should be measured to detect T_3 toxicosis; an elevated level confirms that diagnosis.

The cause can often be diagnosed clinically (eg, exposure to a drug, the presence of signs specific to Graves' disease). If not, thyroid radioactive iodine uptake may be obtained using ^{123}I. When hyperthyroidism is due to hormone overproduction, thyroid radioactive iodine uptake is usually elevated.

TSH receptor antibodies can be measured to detect Graves' disease, but measurement is rarely necessary except during the 3rd trimester of pregnancy to assess the risk of neonatal Graves' disease; TSH receptor antibodies readily cross the placenta to stimulate the fetal thyroid. Most patients with Graves' disease have circulating antithyroid peroxidase antibodies, and fewer have antithyroglobulin antibodies.

Inappropriate TSH secretion is uncommon. The diagnosis is confirmed when hyperthyroidism occurs with elevated circulating free T_4 and T_3 concentrations and normal or elevated serum TSH.

If thyrotoxicosis factitia is suspected, serum thyroglobulin can be measured; it is usually low or low-normal—unlike in all other causes of hyperthyroidism.

In hyperthyroidism caused by excess iodine ingestion, low radioactive iodine uptake is typical because thyroid radioactive iodine uptake is inversely proportional to iodine intake.

Treatment

Treatment depends on cause.

Iodine: Iodine in pharmacologic doses inhibits the release of T_3 and T_4 within hours and inhibits the organification of iodine, a transitory effect lasting from a few days to a week, after which inhibition usually ceases. Iodine is used for emergency management of thyroid storm, for hyperthyroid patients undergoing emergency nonthyroid surgery, and (because it also decreases the vascularity of the thyroid) for preoperative preparation of hyperthyroid patients undergoing subtotal thyroidectomy. Iodine generally is not used for routine treatment of hyperthyroidism. The usual dosage is 2 to 3 drops (100 to 150 mg) of a saturated K iodide solution po tid or qid or 0.5 to 1 g Na iodide in 1 L 0.9% saline solution given IV slowly q 12 h.

Complications of iodine therapy include inflammation of the salivary glands, conjunctivitis, and rash. Na ipodate and iopanoic acid supply excess iodine and are potent inhibitors of the conversion of T_4 to T_3. The combination of one of these agents and dexamethasone, also a potent inhibitor of T_4 to T_3 conversion, can relieve symptoms of hyperthyroidism and restore serum T_3 concentration to normal within a week.

Propylthiouracil and methimazole: These antithyroid drugs block thyroid peroxidase, decreasing the organification of iodide, and impair the coupling reaction. Propylthiouracil in high doses also inhibits the peripheral conversion of T_4 to T_3. About 20 to 50% of patients with Graves' disease remain in remission after a 1- to 2-yr course of either drug. The return to normal or a marked decrease in gland size, the restoration of a normal serum TSH level, and less severe hyperthyroidism before therapy are good prognostic signs of long-term remission. The concomitant use of antithyroid drug therapy and L-thyroxine does not improve the remission rate in patients with Graves' disease. Because toxic nodular goiter rarely goes into remission, antithyroid drug therapy is given only in preparation for surgical treatment or ^{131}I therapy.

The usual starting dosage of propylthiouracil is 100 to 150 mg po q 8 h and of methimazole 5 to 20 mg tid. When T_4 and T_3 levels normalize, the dosage is decreased to the lowest effective amount, usually propylthiouracil 50 mg tid or methimazole 5 to 15 mg once/day. Usually, control is achieved in 2 to 3 mo. More rapid control can be achieved by increasing the dose of propylthiouracil to 150 to 200 mg q 8 h. Such doses or higher ones (up to 400 mg q 8 h) are generally reserved for severely ill patients, including those with thyroid storm. Maintenance doses can be continued for one or many years depending on the clinical circumstances. Carbimazole, which is used widely in Europe, is rapidly converted to methimazole. The usual starting dose is similar to that of methimazole; maintenance dosage is 5 to 20 mg once/day, 2.5 to 10 mg bid, or 1.7 to 6.7 mg tid.

Adverse effects include allergic reactions, abnormal liver function, and, in about 0.1% of patients, reversible agranulocytosis. Patients allergic to one drug can be switched to the other, but cross-sensitivity may occur. If agranulocytosis occurs, the patient cannot be switched to the other drug; other therapy (eg, radioiodine, surgery) should be used.

Each drug has advantages and disadvantages. Methimazole need only be given once/day, which improves compliance. Furthermore, when methimazole is used in dosages of < 40 mg/day, agranulocytosis is less common; with propylthiouracil, agranulocytosis may occur at any dosage. Propylthiouracil may be preferred if antithyroid drug therapy must be used during pregnancy or breastfeeding because it is less likely to cross the placenta or enter breast milk. However, methimazole has been used successfully in pregnant and nursing women without fetal or infant complications. Propylthiouracil is also preferred for the treatment of thyroid storm, because the dosages used (800 to 1200 mg/day) partially block the peripheral conversion of T_4 to T_3.

β-Blockers: Symptoms and signs of hyperthyroidism due to adrenergic stimulation may respond to β-blockers; propranolol has had the greatest use. Other manifestations typically do not respond (see TABLE 152–2).

Propranolol is indicated in thyroid storm (see TABLE 152–3). It rapidly decreases heart rate, usually within 2 to 3 h when given orally and within minutes when given IV. Propranolol is also indicated for tachycardia with hyperthyroidism, especially in elderly patients, because antithyroid drugs usually take several weeks to become fully effective. Ca channel blockers may control tachyarrhythmias in patients in whom β-blockers are contraindicated.

Radioactive sodium iodine (^{131}I, radioiodine): In the US, ^{131}I is the most common treatment for hyperthyroidism. Radioiodine is often recommended as the treatment of choice for Graves' disease and toxic nodular goiter in all patients, including children. Dosage of ^{131}I is difficult to adjust, because the response of the gland cannot be predicted; some physicians give a standard dose of 8 mCi. When sufficient ^{131}I is given to produce euthyroidism, about 25% of patients become hypothyroid 1 yr later, and the incidence continues to increase yearly. Thus, most patients eventually become hypothyroid. However, if smaller doses are used, incidence of recurrence is higher. Larger doses, such as 10 to 15 mCi, often cause hypothyroidism within 6 mo. Radioactive iodine is not used during pregnancy. There is no proof that radioiodine increases the incidence of tumors, leukemia, thyroid cancer, or birth defects in children born to women who become pregnant later in life.

TABLE 152–2. EFFECTS OF PROPRANOLOL ON HYPERTHYROIDISM

PHENOMENA IMPROVED	PHENOMENA NOT IMPROVED
Tachycardia	O_2 consumption: Although excess catecholamines (as in patients with pheochromocytoma) increase O_2 consumption, the major stimulus to O_2 consumption is thyroid hormone
Tremor	Goiter
Mental symptoms	Bruit
Heat intolerance and sweating (occasional)	Circulating thyroxine levels
Diarrhea (occasional)	Weight loss (may be stabilized, but not improved)
Proximal myopathy (occasional)	Exophthalmos
Eyelid lag	

Surgery: Surgery is indicated for patients with Graves' disease whose hyperthyroidism has recurred after courses of antithyroid drug and who refuse ^{131}I therapy, patients who cannot tolerate other drugs, patients with very large goiters, and in some younger patients with toxic adenoma and multinodular goiter. Surgery may be performed in elderly patients with giant nodular goiters.

Surgery usually restores normal function. Postoperative recurrences vary between 2 and 16%; risk of hypothyroidism is directly related to the extent of surgery and occurs in about ⅓ of patients. Vocal cord paralysis and hypoparathyroidism are uncommon complications. Saturated solution of K iodide 3 drops (about 100 to 150 mg) po tid should be

TABLE 152–3. TREATMENT OF THYROID STORM

Iodine: 5 drops saturated solution of K iodide po tid or 10 drops Lugol's solution po tid; or 1g Na iodide slowly by IV drip over 24 h or iopanoic acid 0.5 g bid

Propylthiouracil: 600 mg po given before iodine, then 400 mg q 6 h

Propranolol: 40 mg po qid; or 1 mg *slowly* IV q 4 h under close monitoring; the rate of administration should not exceed 1 mg/min; a repeat 1-mg dose may be given after 2 min

IV dextrose solutions

Correction of dehydration and electrolyte imbalance

Cooling blanket for hyperthermia

Antiarrhythmic drugs (eg, Ca channel blockers, adenosine, β-blockers) if necessary for atrial fibrillation

Treatment of underlying disease, such as infection

Corticosteroids: hydrocortisone 100 mg IV q 8 h or dexamethasone 8 mg IV once/day

Definitive therapy after control of the crisis consists of ablation of the thyroid with ^{131}I or surgical treatment

given for 10 days before surgery to reduce the vascularity of the gland. Propylthiouracil or methimazole must also be given, because the patient should be euthyroid before iodide is given. Dexamethasone and iopanoic acid can be added to rapidly restore euthyroidism. Surgical procedures are more difficult in patients who previously underwent thyroidectomy or radioiodine therapy.

Treatment of thyroid storm: A treatment regimen for thyroid storm is shown in TABLE 152–3.

Treatment of infiltrative dermopathy and ophthalmopathy: In infiltrative dermopathy (in Graves' disease), topical corticosteroids sometimes relieve the pruritus. Dermopathy usually remits spontaneously after months or years. Ophthalmopathy should be treated jointly by the endocrinologist and ophthalmologist and may require corticosteroids, orbital radiation, and surgery.

SUBCLINICAL HYPERTHYROIDISM

Subclinical hyperthyroidism is low serum TSH in patients with normal serum free T_4 and T_3 and absent or minimal symptoms of hyperthyroidism.

Subclinical hyperthyroidism is far less common than subclinical hypothyroidism (see p. 1202). Patients with serum TSH < 0.1 mU/L have an increased incidence of atrial fibrillation (particularly elderly patients), reduced bone mineral density, increased fractures, and increased mortality. Patients with serum TSH that is only slightly below normal are less likely to have these features. Many patients with subclinical hyperthyroidism are taking levothyroxine; in these patients, reduction of the dose is the most appropriate management unless therapy is aimed at maintaining a suppressed TSH in patients with thyroid cancer or nodules. The other causes of subclinical hyperthyroidism are the same as those for clinically apparent thyrotoxicosis.

Therapy is indicated for patients with endogenous subclinical hyperthyroidism (serum TSH < 0.1 mU/L), especially those with atrial fibrillation or reduced bone mineral density. The usual treatment is ^{131}I. In patients with milder symptoms (eg, nervousness), a trial of antithyroid drug therapy is worthwhile.

HYPOTHYROIDISM

(Myxedema)

Hypothyroidism is thyroid hormone deficiency. It is diagnosed by clinical features such as a typical facies, hoarse slow speech, and dry skin, and by low levels of thyroid hormones. Management includes treatment of the underlying cause and administration of thyroxine.

Hypothyroidism occurs at any age but is particularly common in the elderly. It occurs in close to 10% of women and 6% of men > 65. Although typically easy to diagnose in younger adults, it may be subtle and present atypically in the elderly.

Primary hypothyroidism: Primary hypothyroidism is due to disease in the thyroid; TSH is increased. The most common cause is probably autoimmune. It usually results from Hashimoto's thyroiditis and is often associated with a firm goiter or, later in the disease process, with a shrunken fibrotic thyroid with little or no function. The 2nd most common cause is post-therapeutic hypothyroidism, especially after radioactive iodine therapy or surgery for hyperthyroidism or goiter. Hypothyroidism during overtreatment with propylthiouracil, methimazole, and iodide abates after therapy is stopped.

Most patients with non-Hashimoto's goiters are euthyroid or have hyperthyroidism, but goitrous hypothyroidism may occur in endemic goiter. Iodine deficiency decreases thyroid hormonogenesis; in response, TSH is released, which causes the thyroid to enlarge and trap iodine avidly; thus, goiter results. If iodine deficiency is severe, the patient becomes hypothyroid, a rare occurrence in the US since the advent of iodized salt.

Iodine deficiency can cause endemic cretinism in children; endemic cretinism is the most common cause of congenital hypothyroidism in severely iodine-deficient regions and a major cause of mental deficiency worldwide.

Rare inherited enzymatic defects can alter the synthesis of thyroid hormone and cause goitrous hypothyroidism (see p. 2363).

Hypothyroidism may occur in patients taking lithium, perhaps because lithium inhibits hormone release by the thyroid. Hypothyroidism may also occur in patients taking amiodarone or other iodine-containing drugs, and in patients taking interferon-α. Hypothyroidism can result from radiation therapy for cancer of the larynx or Hodgkin lymphoma (Hodgkin's disease). The incidence of permanent hypothyroidism after radiation therapy is high, and thyroid function (through measurement of serum TSH) should be evaluated at 6- to 12-mo intervals.

Secondary hypothyroidism: Secondary hypothyroidism occurs when the hypothalamus produces insufficient thyrotropin-releasing hormone (TRH) or the pituitary produces insufficient TSH. Sometimes, deficient TSH secretion due to deficient TRH secretion is termed tertiary hypothyroidism.

Symptoms and Signs

Symptoms and signs of primary hypothyroidism are often subtle and insidious. Symptoms may include cold intolerance, constipation, forgetfulness, and personality changes. Modest weight gain is largely the result of fluid retention and decreased metabolism. Paresthesias of the hands and feet are common, often due to carpal-tarsal tunnel syndrome caused by deposition of proteinaceous ground substance in the ligaments around the wrist and ankle. Women with hypothyroidism may develop menorrhagia or secondary amenorrhea.

The facial expression is dull; the voice is hoarse and speech is slow; facial puffiness and periorbital swelling occur due to infiltration with the mucopolysaccharides hyaluronic acid and chondroitin sulfate; eyelids droop because of decreased adrenergic drive; hair is sparse, coarse, and dry; and the skin is coarse, dry, scaly, and thick. The relaxation phase of deep tendon reflexes is slowed. Hypothermia is common. Dementia or frank psychosis (myxedema madness) may occur. In the elderly, hypothyroidism may mimic dementia or parkinsonism.

Carotenemia is common, particularly notable on the palms and soles, caused by deposition of carotene in the lipid-rich epidermal layers. Deposition of proteinaceous ground substance in the tongue may produce macroglossia. A decrease in both thyroid hormone and adrenergic stimulation causes bradycardia. The heart may be enlarged, partly because of dilation but chiefly because of pericardial effusion. Pleural or abdominal effusions also may be noted. The pericardial and pleural effusions develop slowly and only rarely cause respiratory or hemodynamic distress.

Although secondary hypothyroidism is uncommon, its causes often affect other endocrine organs controlled by the hypothalamic-pituitary axis. In a woman with hypothyroidism, indications of secondary hypothyroidism are a history of amenorrhea rather than menorrhagia and some suggestive differences on physical examination. Secondary hypothyroidism is characterized by skin and hair that are dry but not very coarse, skin depigmentation, only minimal macroglossia, atrophic breasts, and low BP. Also, the heart is small, and serous pericardial effusions do not occur. Hypoglycemia is common because of concomitant adrenal insufficiency or growth hormone deficiency.

Myxedema coma is a life-threatening complication of hypothyroidism, usually occurring in patients with a long history of hypothyroidism. Its characteristics include coma with extreme hypothermia (temperature 24° to 32.2° C), areflexia, seizures, and respiratory depression with CO_2 retention. Severe hypothermia may be missed unless low-reading thermometers are used. Rapid diagnosis based on clinical judgment, history, and physical examination is imperative, because death is likely without rapid treatment. Precipitating factors include illness, infection, trauma, drugs that suppress the CNS, and exposure to cold.

Diagnosis

Serum TSH is the most sensitive test. In primary hypothyroidism, there is no feedback inhibition of the intact pituitary, and serum TSH is always elevated, whereas serum free T_4 is low. In secondary hypothyroidism, free T_4 and serum TSH are low (sometimes TSH is normal but with decreased bioactivity).

Many patients with primary hypothyroidism have normal circulating levels of T_3, probably caused by sustained TSH stimulation of the failing thyroid, resulting in preferential synthesis and secretion of the biologically active hormone T_3. Therefore, serum T_3 is not sensitive for hypothyroidism.

Anemia is often present, usually normocytic-normochromic and of unknown etiology, but it may be hypochromic because of menorrhagia and sometimes macrocytic because of associated pernicious anemia or decreased absorption of folic acid. Anemia is rarely severe (Hb > 9 g/dL). As the hypometabolic state is corrected, anemia subsides, sometimes requiring 6 to 9 mo.

Serum cholesterol is usually high in primary hypothyroidism but less so in secondary hypothyroidism.

In addition to primary and secondary hypothyroidism, other conditions may produce decreased levels of total T_4, such as serum thyroxine-binding globulin (TBG) deficiency, some drugs (see p. 1201), and euthyroid sick syndrome (see p. 1194).

Treatment

Various thyroid hormone preparations are available for replacement therapy, including synthetic preparations of T_4 (L-thyroxine), T_3 (liothyronine), combinations of the 2 synthetic hormones, and desiccated animal thyroid extract. L-Thyroxine is preferred; the average maintenance dose is 75 to 125 μg po once/day (see p. 2364 for pediatric doses). Therapy is begun with low doses, especially in the elderly, usually 25 μg once/day. The dose is adjusted q 6 wk until maintenance dose is achieved. The maintenance dose may need to be decreased in elderly patients and increased in pregnant women. Dose may also need to be increased if drugs that decrease T_4 absorption or increase its biliary excretion are administered concomitantly. The dose used should be the lowest that restores serum TSH levels to the mid-normal range (though this criterion cannot be used in patients with secondary hypothyroidism).

Liothyronine should not be used alone for long-term replacement because of its short half-life and the large peaks in serum T_3 levels it produces. The administration of standard replacement amounts (25 to 37.5 μg bid) results in rapidly increasing serum T_3 to between 300 and 1000 ng/dL (4.62 to 15.4 nmol/L) within 4 h due to its almost complete absorption; these levels return to normal by 24 h. Additionally, patients receiving liothyronine are chemically hyperthyroid for at least several hours a day, potentially increasing cardiac risks.

Similar patterns of serum T_3 occur when mixtures of T_3 and T_4 are taken po, although peak T_3 is lower because less T_3 is given. Replacement regimens with synthetic T_4 preparations reflect a different pattern in serum T_3 response. Increases in serum T_3 occur gradually, and normal levels are maintained when adequate doses of T_4 are given. Desiccated animal thyroid preparations contain variable amounts of T_3 and T_4 and should not be prescribed unless the patient has been stable on such a preparation.

In patients with secondary hypothyroidism, L-thyroxine should not be given until there is evidence of adequate cortisol secretion (or cortisol therapy is given), because L-thyroxine could precipitate adrenal crisis.

Myxedema coma is treated with a large initial dose of T_4 (300 to 500 μg IV) or T_3 (25 to 50 μg IV). The maintenance dose of T_4 is 75 to 100 μg IV once/day and of T_3, 10 to 20 μg IV bid until T_4 can be given orally. Corticosteroids are also given, because the possibility of central hypothyroidism usually cannot be initially ruled out. The patient should not be rewarmed rapidly, which may precipitate hypotension or arrhythmias. Hypoxemia is common, so PaO_2 should be monitored. If ventilation is compromised, immediate mechanical ventilatory assistance is required. The precipitating factor should be rapidly and appropriately treated and fluid replacement given carefully, because hypothyroid patients do not excrete water appropriately. Finally, all drugs should be given cautiously because they are metabolized more slowly than in healthy people.

Subclinical Hypothyroidism

Subclinical hypothyroidism is elevated serum TSH in patients with absent or minimal symp-

toms of hypothyroidism and normal serum levels of free T_4.

Subclinical thyroid dysfunction is relatively common; it occurs in nearly 15% of elderly women, particularly in those with underlying Hashimoto's thyroiditis.

In patients with serum TSH > 10 mU/L, there is a high likelihood of progression to overt hypothyroidism with low serum levels of free T_4 in the next 10 yr. These patients are also more likely to have hypercholesterolemia and atherosclerosis. They should be treated with L-thyroxine, even if they are asymptomatic. For patients with TSH levels between 4.5 and 10 mU/L, a trial of L-thyroxine is reasonable if symptoms of early hypothyroidism (eg, fatigue, depression) are present. L-Thyroxine therapy is also indicated in pregnant women and in women who plan to become pregnant to avoid deleterious effects of hypothyroidism on the pregnancy and fetal development. Patients who are not treated should have annual measurement of serum TSH and free T_4 to assess progress of the condition.

SILENT LYMPHOCYTIC THYROIDITIS

Silent lymphocytic thyroiditis is a self-limited, subacute disorder occurring most commonly in women during the postpartum period. Symptoms are initially of hyperthyroidism, then hypothyroidism, and then generally recovery to the euthyroid state. Treatment of the hyperthyroid phase is with a β-blocker. If hypothyroidism is permanent, lifelong thyroxine supplementation is needed.

The term silent refers to the absence of thyroid tenderness in contrast with subacute thyroiditis, which usually causes thyroid tenderness. Silent lymphocytic thyroiditis causes most cases of postpartum thyroid dysfunction. It occurs in about 5 to 10% of postpartum women.

Thyroid biopsy reveals lymphocytic infiltration as in Hashimoto's thyroiditis but without lymphoid follicles and scarring. Thyroid peroxidase autoantibodies and, less commonly, antithyroglobulin antibodies are almost always positive during pregnancy and the postpartum period. Thus, this disorder would appear to be a variant of Hashimoto's thyroiditis (see p. 1194).

Symptoms and Signs

The condition begins in the postpartum period, usually within 12 to 16 wk. Silent lymphocytic thyroiditis is characterized by a variable degree of painless thyroid enlargement with a hyperthyroid phase of several weeks, often followed by transient hypothyroidism due to depleted thyroid hormone stores but usually eventual recovery to the euthyroid state (as noted below for painful subacute thyroiditis). The hyperthyroid phase is self-limited and may be brief or overlooked. Many women with this disorder are diagnosed when they become hypothyroid, which occasionally is permanent.

Diagnosis

Silent lymphocytic thyroiditis is frequently undiagnosed. Suspicion of the diagnosis generally depends on clinical findings, typically once hypothyroidism has occurred. Eye signs and pretibial myxedema do not occur.

Thyroid function test results vary depending on the phase of illness. Initially, serum T_4 and T_3 are elevated and TSH is suppressed. In the hypothyroid phase, these findings are reversed. WBC count and ESR are normal. Needle biopsy provides definitive diagnosis but is usually unnecessary.

Prognosis and Treatment

Because silent lymphocytic thyroiditis lasts only a few months, treatment is conservative, usually requiring only a β-blocker (eg, propranolol) during the hyperthyroid phase (see p. 1199). Antithyroid drugs, surgery, and radioiodine therapy are contraindicated. Thyroid hormone replacement may be required during the hypothyroid phase. Most patients recover normal thyroid function, although some remain permanently hypothyroid. Therefore, thyroid function should be reevaluated after 9 to 12 mo of thyroxine therapy; replacement is stopped for 5 wk and TSH remeasured. This disorder almost always recurs after subsequent pregnancies.

SIMPLE NONTOXIC GOITER

(Euthyroid Goiter)

Simple nontoxic goiter, which may be diffuse or nodular, is noncancerous hypertrophy of the thyroid without hyperthyroidism, hypothyroidism, or inflammation. Cause is usually unknown, but it may result from chronic overstimulation by thyroid-stimulating

hormone, most commonly in response to a deficiency of iodine (endemic [colloid] goiter) or from ingestion of various foods or drugs that inhibit thyroid hormone synthesis. Except in severe iodine deficiency, thyroid function is normal and patients are asymptomatic except for an obviously enlarged, nontender thyroid. Diagnosis is clinical and with determination of normal thyroid function. Treatment is directed at the underlying cause, but partial surgical removal may be required for very large goiters.

Simple nontoxic goiter, the most common type of thyroid enlargement, is frequently noted at puberty, during pregnancy, and at menopause. The cause at these times is usually unclear. Known causes include intrinsic thyroid hormone production defects and, in iodine-deficient countries, ingestion of foods that contain substances that inhibit thyroid hormone synthesis (goitrogens, eg, broccoli, cauliflower, cabbage, cassava). Other causes include the use of drugs that can decrease the synthesis of thyroid hormone (eg, amiodarone or other iodine-containing compounds, lithium).

Iodine deficiency is rare in North America but remains the most common cause of goiter worldwide (termed endemic goiter). Compensatory small TSH elevations occur, preventing hypothyroidism, but the TSH stimulation results in goiter formation. Recurrent cycles of stimulation and involution may result in nontoxic nodular goiters. However, the true etiology of most nontoxic goiters in iodine-sufficient areas is unknown.

Symptoms, Signs, and Diagnosis

The patient may have a history of low iodine intake or overingestion of food goitrogens, but these phenomena are rare in North America. In the early stages, the goiter is typically soft, symmetric, and smooth. Later, multiple nodules and cysts may develop.

Thyroidal radioactive iodine uptake, thyroid scan, and thyroid function tests (measurements of T_4, T_3, and TSH) are performed. In the early stages, thyroidal radioactive iodine uptake may be normal or high with normal thyroid scans. Thyroid function tests are usually normal. Thyroid antibodies are measured to rule out Hashimoto's thyroiditis.

In endemic goiter, serum TSH may be slightly elevated, and serum T_4 may be low-normal or slightly low, but serum T_3 is usually normal or slightly elevated.

Treatment

In iodine-deficient areas, iodine supplementation of salt; oral or IM administration of iodized oil yearly; and iodination of water, crops, or animal fodder eliminates iodine-deficiency goiter. Goitrogens being ingested should be stopped.

In other instances, suppression of the hypothalamic-pituitary axis with thyroid hormone blocks TSH production (and hence stimulation of the thyroid). Full TSH-suppressive doses of L-thyroxine (100 to 150 μg/day po depending on the serum TSH) are useful in younger patients. L-Thyroxine is contraindicated in older patients with nontoxic nodular goiter, because these goiters rarely shrink and may harbor areas of autonomy so that L-thyroxine therapy can result in hyperthyroidism. Large goiters occasionally require surgery or ^{131}I to shrink the gland enough to prevent interference with respiration or swallowing or to correct cosmetic problems.

SUBACUTE THYROIDITIS

(de Quervain's, Giant Cell, or Granulomatous Thyroiditis)

Subacute thyroiditis is an acute inflammatory disease of the thyroid probably caused by a virus. Symptoms include fever and thyroid tenderness; initial hyperthyroidism is common. Diagnosis is clinical and with thyroid function tests. Treatment is with high doses of NSAIDs or with corticosteroids. The disease usually resolves spontaneously within months.

History of an antecedent viral URI is common. Histologic studies demonstrate less lymphocytic infiltration of the thyroid than in Hashimoto's thyroiditis or silent thyroiditis, but there is characteristic giant cell infiltration, PMNs, and follicular disruption.

Symptoms, Signs, and Diagnosis

There is pain in the anterior neck and fever of 37.8° to 38.3° C. Neck pain characteristically shifts from side to side and may settle in one area, frequently radiating to the jaw and ears. It is often confused with dental pain, pharyngitis, or otitis and is aggravated by swallowing or turning of the head. Symptoms of hyperthyroidism are common early in the disease because of hormone release from the disrupted follicles. There is more lassitude and prostration than in other thyroid disorders. On physical examination, the thyroid is asymmetrically enlarged, firm, and tender.

Laboratory findings early in the disease include an increase in free T_4 and T_3, a decrease in TSH and thyroid radioactive iodine uptake (often 0), and a high ESR. After several weeks, the thyroid is depleted of T_4 and T_3 stores, and transient hypothyroidism develops accompanied by a decrease in free T_4 and T_3, a rise in TSH, and recovery of thyroid radioactive iodine uptake. Weakly positive thyroid antibodies may be present.

Prognosis and Treatment

Subacute thyroiditis is self-limited, generally subsiding in a few months; occasionally, it recurs and may result in permanent hypothyroidism when follicular destruction is extensive.

Treatment is with high doses of aspirin or NSAIDs. In severe and protracted cases, corticosteroids (eg, prednisone 30 to 40 mg po once/day, gradually decreasing the dose over 3 to 4 wk) eradicate all symptoms within 48 h. If hypothyroidism persists, thyroid hormone replacement therapy may be required.

THYROID CANCERS

The 4 general types of thyroid cancer are papillary, follicular, medullary, and anaplastic. Papillary and follicular carcinoma together are called differentiated thyroid cancer because of their histologic resemblance to normal thyroid tissue and because differentiated function (eg, thyroglobulin secretion) is preserved. Most thyroid cancers present as asymptomatic nodules. Rarely, lymph node, lung, or bone metastases cause the presenting symptoms of small thyroid cancers. Diagnosis is often by fine-needle aspiration biopsy but may involve other tests. Except for the anaplastic form, most thyroid cancers are not highly malignant and are rarely fatal. Treatment is surgical removal, usually followed by ablation of residual tissue with radioactive iodine.

Papillary Carcinoma

Papillary carcinoma accounts for 70 to 80% of all thyroid cancers. The female-to-male ratio is 3:1. It may be familial in up to 5% of patients. Most patients present between ages 30 and 60. The tumor is often more aggressive in elderly patients. Many papillary carcinomas contain follicular elements.

The tumor spreads via lymphatics to regional lymph nodes in $\frac{1}{3}$ of patients and may metastasize to the lungs. Patients < 45 yr with small tumors confined to the thyroid have an excellent prognosis.

Treatment

Treatment for encapsulated tumors < 1.5 cm localized to one lobe is usually lobectomy and isthmectomy, although some experts recommend more extensive thyroid surgery; surgery is almost always curative. Thyroid hormone in TSH-suppressive doses is given to minimize chances of regrowth and cause regression of any microscopic remnants of papillary carcinoma. Tumors > 4 cm or that are diffusely spreading often require total or near-total thyroidectomy with postoperative radioiodine ablation of residual thyroid tissue with appropriately large doses of ^{131}I administered when the patient is hypothyroid. Treatment may be repeated q 6 to 12 mo to ablate any remaining thyroid tissue. TSH suppressive doses of L-thyroxine are given after treatment, and serum thyroglobulin levels help detect recurrent or persistent disease. About 10 to 20% of patients, mainly the elderly, have recurrent or persistent disease.

Follicular Carcinoma

Follicular carcinoma accounts for about 10% of thyroid cancers. It is more common among elderly patients and in regions of iodine deficiency. It is more malignant than papillary carcinoma, spreading hematogenously with distant metastases.

Treatment requires near-total thyroidectomy with postoperative radioiodine ablation of residual thyroid tissue as in treatment for papillary carcinoma. Metastases are more responsive to radioiodine therapy than are those of papillary carcinoma. TSH-suppressive doses of L-thyroxine are given after treatment. Serum thyroglobulin should be monitored to detect recurrent or persistent disease.

Medullary Carcinoma

Medullary (solid) carcinoma constitutes about 3% of thyroid cancers and is composed of parafollicular cells (C cells) that produce calcitonin. It may be sporadic (usually unilateral); however, it is often familial, caused by a mutation of the *ret* proto-oncogene. The familial form may occur in isolation or as a component of multiple endocrine neoplasia (MEN) syndromes types IIA and IIB (see pp. 1317 and 1318). Although calcitonin can lower serum Ca and phosphate, serum Ca is normal because the high level of calcitonin ultimately down-regulates its receptors. Characteristic amyloid deposits that stain with Congo red are also present.

Symptoms, Signs, and Diagnosis

Patients typically present with an asymptomatic thyroid nodule, although many cases are now diagnosed during routine screening of affected kindreds with MEN-IIA or IIB before a palpable tumor develops.

Medullary carcinoma may have a dramatic biochemical presentation when associated with ectopic production of other hormones or peptides (eg, ACTH, vasoactive intestinal polypeptide, prostaglandins, kallikreins, serotonin).

Metastases spread via the lymphatic system to cervical and mediastinal nodes and sometimes to liver, lungs, and bone.

The best test is serum calcitonin, which is greatly elevated. A challenge with Ca (15 mg/kg IV over 4 h) provokes excessive secretion of calcitonin. X-rays may show a dense, homogenous, conglomerate calcification.

All patients with medullary carcinoma should have genetic testing; relatives of those with mutations should have genetic testing and measurement of basal and stimulated calcitonin levels.

Treatment

Total thyroidectomy is indicated even if bilateral involvement is not obvious. Lymph nodes are also dissected. If hyperparathyroidism is present, removal of hyperplastic or adenomatous parathyroids is required. Pheochromocytoma, if present, is usually bilateral. Pheochromocytomas should be identified and removed before thyroidectomy because of the danger of provoking hypertensive crisis during the operation. Long-term survival is common in patients with medullary carcinoma and MEN-IIA; > ⅔ of affected patients are alive at 10 yr. Medullary carcinoma of the sporadic type has a worse prognosis.

Relatives with an elevated calcitonin level without a palpable thyroid abnormality should undergo thyroidectomy, because there is a greater chance of cure at this stage. Some experts recommend surgery in relatives who have normal basal and stimulated serum calcitonin but who have the *ret* proto-oncogene mutation.

Anaplastic Carcinoma

Anaplastic carcinoma is an undifferentiated cancer that accounts for about 2% of thyroid cancers. It occurs mostly in elderly patients and slightly more often in women. The tumor is characterized by rapid, painful enlargement. Rapid enlargement of the thyroid may also suggest thyroid lymphoma, particularly if found in association with Hashimoto's thyroiditis.

No effective therapy exists, and the disease is generally fatal. About 80% of patients die within 1 yr of diagnosis. In a few patients with smaller tumors, thyroidectomy followed by external radiation has been curative. Chemotherapy is mainly experimental.

Radiation-Induced Thyroid Cancer

Thyroid tumors develop in people exposed to large amounts of environmental thyroid radiation, as occurs from atomic bomb blasts, nuclear reactor accidents, or incidental thyroid irradiation due to radiation therapy. Tumors may be detected 10 yr after exposure, but risk remains increased for 30 to 40 yr. Such tumors are usually benign; however, about 7% are papillary thyroid carcinoma. The tumors are frequently multicentric or diffuse.

Patients who had thyroid irradiation should undergo yearly thyroid palpation, ultrasound, and measurement of thyroid autoantibodies (to exclude Hashimoto's thyroiditis). A thyroid scan does not always reflect areas of involvement.

If a nodule is found by ultrasound, fine-needle aspiration biopsy should be performed. In the absence of suspicious or cancerous lesions, many physicians recommend lifelong TSH-lowering doses of thyroid hormone to suppress thyroid function and thyrotropin secretion and possibly decrease the chance of developing a thyroid tumor.

Surgery is required if fine-needle aspiration biopsy suggests cancer. Near-total or total thyroidectomy is the treatment of choice, to be followed by radioiodine ablation of any residual thyroid tissue if a cancer is found (depending on the size, histology, and invasiveness).

153 ADRENAL DISORDERS

The adrenal glands, located on the cephalad portion of each kidney, consist of a cortex and medulla, each with separate endocrine functions.

The adrenal cortex produces glucocorticoids (primarily cortisol), mineralocorticoids (primarily aldosterone), and androgens (primarily dehydroepiandrosterone and androstenedione). Glucocorticoids promote and inhibit gene transcription in many cells and organ systems. Prominent effects include anti-inflammatory actions and increased hepatic gluconeogenesis. Mineralocorticoids regulate electrolyte transport across epithelial surfaces, particularly renal conservation of Na in exchange for K. Adrenal androgens' chief physiologic activity occurs after conversion to testosterone and dihydrotestosterone. Physiology of the pituitary-corticoadrenal system is further described in Chs. 150 and 151.

The adrenal medulla is composed of chromaffin cells, which synthesize and secrete catecholamines (mainly epinephrine and lesser amounts of norepinephrine). Chromaffin cells also produce bioactive amines and peptides (eg, histamine, serotonin, chromogranins, neuropeptide hormones). Epinephrine and norepinephrine, the major effector amines of the sympathetic nervous system, are responsible for the "flight or fight" response (ie, chronotropic and inotropic effects on the heart; bronchodilation; peripheral and splanchnic vasoconstriction with skeletal muscular vasodilation; metabolic effects including glycogenolysis, lipolysis, and renin release).

Most deficiency syndromes affect output of all adrenocortical hormones. Hypofunction may be primary (malfunction of the adrenal gland itself, as in Addison's disease) or secondary (due to lack of adrenal stimulation by the pituitary or hypothalamus, although some experts refer to hypothalamic malfunction as tertiary).

Hyperfunction produces distinct clinical syndromes. Hypersecretion of androgens results in adrenal virilism; of glucocorticoids, Cushing's syndrome; and of aldosterone, hyperaldosteronism (aldosteronism). These syndromes frequently have overlapping features. Hyperfunction may be compensatory, as in congenital adrenal hyperplasia, or due to acquired hyperplasia, adenomas, or adenocarcinomas. (See also Congenital Adrenal Hyperplasia on p. 2365.) Excess quantities of epinephrine and norepinephrine are produced in pheochromocytoma (see p. 1216).

ADDISON'S DISEASE

(Primary or Chronic Adrenocortical Insufficiency)

Addison's disease is an insidious, usually progressive hypofunctioning of the adrenal cortex. It produces various symptoms, including hypotension and hyperpigmentation, and can lead to adrenal crisis with cardiovascular collapse. Diagnosis is clinical and by finding elevated plasma ACTH with low plasma cortisol. Treatment depends on the cause but generally includes hydrocortisone and sometimes other hormones.

Addison's disease develops in about 4/100,000 annually. It occurs in all age groups, about equally in each sex, and tends to become clinically apparent during metabolic stress or trauma. Onset of severe symptoms (adrenal crisis) may be precipitated by acute infection (a common cause, especially with septicemia). Other causes include trauma, surgery, and Na loss from excessive sweating.

Etiology

About 70% of cases in the US are due to idiopathic atrophy of the adrenal cortex, probably caused by autoimmune processes. The remainder result from destruction of the adrenal gland by granuloma (eg, TB), tumor, amyloidosis, hemorrhage, or inflammatory necrosis. Hypoadrenocorticism can also result from administration of drugs that block corticosteroid synthesis (eg, ketoconazole, the anesthetic etomidate). Addison's disease may coexist with diabetes mellitus or hypothyroidism in polyglandular deficiency syndrome (see p. 1219).

Pathophysiology

Both mineralocorticoids and glucocorticoids are deficient.

Mineralocorticoid deficiency results in increased excretion of Na and decreased excretion of K, chiefly in urine but also in sweat, saliva, and the GI tract. A low serum concentration of Na and a high concentration of K result. Inability to concentrate the urine, combined with changes in electrolyte balance, produce severe dehydration, plasma hypertonicity, acidosis, decreased circulatory volume, hypotension, and, eventually, circulatory collapse. However, when adrenal insufficiency is caused by inadequate ACTH production (secondary adrenal insufficiency—see p. 1210), electrolyte levels are often normal or only mildly deranged.

Glucocorticoid deficiency contributes to hypotension and produces severe insulin sensitivity and disturbances in carbohydrate, fat, and protein metabolism. In the absence of cortisol, insufficient carbohydrate is formed from protein; hypoglycemia and diminished liver glycogen result. Weakness follows, due in part to deficient neuromuscular function. Resistance to infection, trauma, and other stress is diminished. Myocardial weakness and dehydration reduce cardiac output, and circulatory failure can occur. Decreased blood cortisol results in increased pituitary ACTH production and increased blood β-lipotropin, which has melanocyte-stimulating activity and, together with ACTH, produces

TABLE 153–1. TEST RESULTS SUGGESTING ADDISON'S DISEASE

Blood chemistry	Low serum Na (< 135 mEq/L)
	High serum K (> 5 mEq/L)
	Ratio of serum Na:K: < 30:1
	Low fasting blood glucose (< 50 mg/dL [< 2.78 mmol/L])
	Decreased plasma HCO_3 (< 20 mEq/L)
	Elevated BUN (> 20 mg/dL [> 7.1 mmol/L])
Hematology	Elevated Hct
	Low WBC count
	Relative lymphocytosis
	Increased eosinophils
Imaging tests	Evidence of:
	Calcification in the adrenal areas
	Renal TB
	Pulmonary TB

the hyperpigmentation of skin and mucous membranes characteristic of Addison's disease. Thus, adrenal insufficiency secondary to pituitary failure (see p. 1210) does not cause hyperpigmentation.

Symptoms and Signs

Weakness, fatigue, and orthostatic hypotension are early symptoms and signs. Hyperpigmentation is characterized by diffuse tanning of exposed and, to a lesser extent, unexposed portions of the body, especially on pressure points (bony prominences), skin folds, scars, and extensor surfaces. Black freckles are common on the forehead, face, neck, and shoulders. Areas of vitiligo develop, and bluish black discolorations of the areolae and mucous membranes of the lips, mouth, rectum, and vagina occur. Anorexia, nausea, vomiting, and diarrhea often occur. Decreased tolerance to cold, with hypometabolism, may be noted. Dizziness and syncope may occur. The gradual onset and nonspecific nature of early symptoms often lead to an incorrect initial diagnosis of neurosis. Weight loss, dehydration, and hypotension are characteristic of the later stages of Addison's disease.

Adrenal crisis is characterized by profound asthenia; severe pain in the abdomen, lower back, or legs; peripheral vascular collapse; and, finally, renal shutdown with azotemia. Body temperature may be low, although severe fever often occurs, particularly when crisis is precipitated by acute infection. A significant number of patients with partial loss of adrenal function (limited adrenocortical reserve) appear well but experience adrenal crisis when under physiologic stress (eg, surgery, infection, burns, critical illness). Shock and fever may be the only signs.

Diagnosis

Clinical symptoms and signs suggest adrenal insufficiency. Sometimes the diagnosis is considered only on discovery of characteristic abnormalities of serum electrolytes, including low Na (< 135 mEq/L), high K (> 5 mEq/L), low HCO_3 (15 to 20 mEq/L), and high BUN (see TABLE 153–1).

Differential diagnosis: Hyperpigmentation can result from bronchogenic carcinoma, ingestion of heavy metals (eg, iron, silver), chronic skin conditions, or hemochromatosis. Peutz-Jeghers syndrome is characterized by pigmentation of the buccal and rectal mucosa. Frequently, hyperpigmentation occurs with vitiligo, which may indicate Addison's disease, although other diseases can cause this association.

Weakness resulting from Addison's disease subsides with rest, unlike neuropsychiatric weakness, which is often worse in the morning than after activity. Most myopathies that cause weakness can be differentiated by their distribution, lack of abnormal pigmentation, and characteristic laboratory findings.

Patients with adrenal insufficiency develop hypoglycemia after fasting because of decreased gluconeogenesis. In contrast, patients with hypoglycemia due to oversecretion of insulin can have attacks at any time, usually have increased appetite with weight gain, and have normal adrenal function. Low serum Na due to Addison's disease must be differentiated from that of edematous patients with cardiac or liver disease (particularly those taking diuretics), the dilutional hyponatremia of the syndrome of inappropriate ADH secretion, and salt-losing nephritis. These patients are not likely to have hyperpigmentation, hyperkalemia, and increased BUN.

Testing: Laboratory tests, beginning with plasma cortisol and ACTH levels, confirm adrenal insufficiency. Elevated ACTH (≥ 50 pg/mL) with low cortisol (< 5 μg/dL [< 138 nmol/L]) is diagnostic, particularly in patients who are severely stressed or in shock. Low ACTH (< 5 pg/mL) and cortisol suggest secondary adrenal insufficiency (see p. 1210); it is important to note that ACTH levels within the normal range are inappropriate for very low cortisol levels.

If ACTH and cortisol levels are borderline and adrenal insufficiency is clinically suspected—particularly in a patient who is about to undergo major surgery—provocative testing must be performed. If time is too short (eg, emergency surgery), the patient is given hydrocortisone empirically (eg, 100 mg IV or IM), and provocative testing is performed subsequently.

Addison's disease is diagnosed by demonstrating failure of exogenous ACTH to increase plasma cortisol. Secondary adrenal insufficiency is diagnosed by a prolonged ACTH stimulation test, insulin tolerance test, or glucagon test.

ACTH stimulation testing is performed by injecting cosyntropin (synthetic ACTH) 250 μg IV or IM. (Some authorities believe that in suspected secondary adrenal insufficiency a low-dose ACTH stimulation test using 1 μg IV instead of the standard 250 μg should be performed, because such patients may react normally to the higher dose.) Patients taking glucocorticoid supplements or spironolactone should not take them on the day of the test. Normal preinjection plasma cortisol ranges from 5 to 25 μg/dL (138 to 690 nmol/L) and doubles in 30 to 90 min, reaching at least 20 μg/dL (552 nmol/L). Patients with Addison's disease have low or low-normal values that do not rise above 20 μg/dL at 30 min. A normal response to cosyntropin may occur in secondary adrenal insufficiency. However, because pituitary failure may cause adrenal atrophy (and hence failure to respond to ACTH), the patient may need to be primed with long-acting ACTH 1 mg IM once/day for 3 days before the cosyntropin test if pituitary disease is suspected.

A prolonged ACTH stimulation test (sampling for 24 h) may be used to diagnose secondary (or tertiary—hypothalamic) adrenal insufficiency. Cosyntropin 1 mg IM is given and cortisol measured at intervals for 24 h. Results for the 1st hour are similar for both the short (sampling stopped after 1 h) and prolonged tests, but in Addison's disease there is no further rise beyond 60 min. In secondary and tertiary adrenal insufficiency, cortisol levels continue to rise for ≥ 24 h. Only in cases of prolonged adrenal atrophy is adrenal priming (with long-acting ACTH, see above) necessary. The simple short test is usually done initially, because a normal response obviates the need for further investigation.

Treatment

Normally, cortisol is secreted maximally in the early morning and minimally at night. Thus, hydrocortisone (similar to cortisol) 10 mg po is usually given in the morning, with ½ as much at lunchtime and again in the early evening. The total daily dose is usually 15 to 30 mg. Night doses should generally be avoided, because they may produce insomnia. Additionally, fludrocortisone 0.1 to 0.2 mg po once/day is recommended to replace aldosterone. The easiest way to adjust the dose is to ensure that the renin level is within the normal range. Normal hydration and absence of orthostatic hypotension are evidence of adequate replacement therapy. In some patients, fludrocortisone produces hypertension, which is treated by reducing the dosage or starting a nondiuretic antihypertensive. Some clinicians tend to give too little fludrocortisone in an effort to avoid use of antihypertensives.

Intercurrent illnesses (eg, infections) are potentially serious and should be vigorously treated; the patient's hydrocortisone dosage should be doubled during the illness. If nausea and vomiting preclude oral therapy, parenteral therapy is necessary. Patients should be instructed when to take supplemental prednisone and taught to self-administer parenteral hydrocortisone for urgent situations. A pre-loaded syringe with 100 mg hydrocortisone should be available to the patient. A bracelet or wallet card giving the diagnosis and corticosteroid dose may help in case of adrenal crisis that renders the patient unable to communicate. When salt loss is severe, as in very hot climates, the dose of fludrocortisone may need to be increased.

In coexisting diabetes mellitus and Addison's disease, the hydrocortisone dose usually should not be > 30 mg/day; otherwise, insulin requirements are increased.

Adrenal crisis: Therapy should be instituted immediately upon suspicion. (CAUTION: *In adrenal crisis, a delay in instituting corticosteroid therapy, particularly if there is hypoglycemia and hypotension, may be fatal.*) If the patient is acutely ill, confirmation by an ACTH stimulation test should be postponed until the patient has recovered.

Hydrocortisone 100 mg is injected IV over 30 sec, followed by an infusion of 1 L of a 5% dextrose in 0.9% saline solution containing hydrocortisone 100 mg given over 2 h. Additional 0.9% saline is given IV until hypotension, dehydration, and hyponatremia have been corrected. Serum K may fall during rehydration, requiring replacement. Hydrocortisone therapy is given continuously at 10 mg/h for 24 h. Mineralocorticoids are not required when high-dose hydrocortisone is given. When illness is less acute, hydrocortisone 50 or 100 mg can be given IM q 6 h. Restoration of BP and general improvement should occur within 1 h after the initial dose of hydrocortisone. Inotropic agents may be needed until the effects of hydrocortisone are achieved.

A total dose of 150 mg hydrocortisone is usually given over the 2nd 24-h period if the patient has improved markedly, and 75 mg is given on the 3rd day. Maintenance oral doses of hydrocortisone (15 to 30 mg) and fludrocortisone (0.1 mg) are given daily thereafter, as described above. Recovery depends on treatment of the underlying cause (eg, infection, trauma, metabolic stress) and adequate hydrocortisone therapy.

For patients with some adrenal function who develop adrenal crisis under stress, hydrocortisone treatment is the same, but fluid requirements may be much lower.

Treatment of complications: Fever > 40.6° C occasionally accompanies the rehydration process. Except in the presence of falling BP, antipyretics (eg, aspirin 650 mg) may be given po with caution. Complications of corticosteroid therapy may include psychotic reactions. If psychotic reactions occur after the 1st 12 h of therapy, the hydrocortisone dosage should be reduced to the lowest level consistent with maintaining BP and good cardiovascular function. Antipsychotic drugs may be temporarily required but should not be prolonged.

With treatment, Addison's disease does not typically reduce life expectancy.

SECONDARY ADRENAL INSUFFICIENCY

Secondary adrenal insufficiency is adrenal hypofunction due to a lack of ACTH. Symptoms are the same as for Addison's disease (see p. 1208). Diagnosis is clinical and by laboratory findings, including low plasma ACTH with low plasma cortisol. Treatment depends on the cause but generally includes hydrocortisone.

Secondary adrenal insufficiency may occur in panhypopituitarism, in isolated failure of ACTH production, in patients receiving corticosteroids, or after corticosteroids are stopped. Inadequate ACTH can also result from failure of the hypothalamus to stimulate pituitary ACTH production, which is sometimes called tertiary adrenal insufficiency.

Panhypopituitarism (see p. 1179) may occur secondary to pituitary tumors; craniopharyngioma in younger people; and various tumors, granulomas, and, rarely, infection or trauma that destroys pituitary tissue. Patients receiving corticosteroids for > 4 wk may have insufficient ACTH secretion during metabolic stress to stimulate the adrenals to produce adequate quantities of corticosteroids, or they may have atrophic adrenals that are unresponsive to ACTH. These problems may persist for up to 1 yr after corticosteroid treatment is stopped.

Symptoms, Signs, and Diagnosis

Symptoms and signs are similar to those of Addison's disease (see p. 1208). Differentiating clinical or general laboratory features include the absence of hyperpigmentation and relatively normal electrolyte and BUN levels; hyponatremia, if it occurs, is usually dilutional.

Patients with panhypopituitarism have depressed thyroid and gonadal function and hypoglycemia, and coma may supervene when symptomatic secondary adrenal insufficiency occurs. Adrenal crisis is especially likely if a patient is treated for a single endocrine gland problem, particularly with thyroxine, without hydrocortisone replacement.

Tests to differentiate primary and secondary adrenal insufficiency are discussed under Addison's disease (see p. 1209). Patients with confirmed secondary adrenal insufficiency should have CT or MRI of the brain to rule out pituitary tumor or atrophy. Adequacy of the hypothalamic-pituitary-adrenal axis during long-term corticosteroid treatment can be determined by injecting cosyntropin 250 μg IV. After 30 min, plasma cortisol should be > 20 μg/dL (> 552 nmol/L). An insulin stress test to induce hypoglycemia and a rise in cortisol is the gold standard for testing integrity of the hypothalamic-pituitary-adrenal axis.

The corticotropin-releasing hormone (CRH) test can be used to distinguish between hypothalamic and pituitary causes but is rarely used in clinical practice. After administration of CRH 100 μg (or 1 μg/kg) IV, the normal response is a rise of plasma ACTH of 30 to 40 pg/mL; patients with pituitary failure do not respond, whereas those with hypothalamic disease usually do.

Treatment

Glucocorticoid replacement is similar to that described for Addison's disease. Each case varies regarding the type and degree of specific hormone deficiencies. Fludrocortisone is not required because the intact adrenals produce aldosterone. During acute febrile illness or after trauma, patients receiving corticosteroids for nonendocrine disorders may require supplemental doses to augment their endogenous hydrocortisone production. In panhypopituitarism, other pituitary deficiencies should be treated appropriately (see p. 1183).

ADRENAL VIRILISM

(Adrenogenital Syndrome)

Adrenal virilism is a syndrome in which excessive adrenal androgens cause virilization. Diagnosis is clinical and confirmed by elevated androgen levels with and without dexamethasone suppression; determining the underlying cause may involve adrenal imaging, with needle biopsy if a mass lesion is found. Treatment depends on the cause.

Adrenal virilism is caused by an androgen-secreting adrenal tumor or by adrenal hyperplasia. Sometimes, the tumor secretes both excess androgens and cortisol, resulting in Cushing's syndrome (see p. 1212) with suppression of ACTH secretion and atrophy of the contralateral adrenal. Adrenal hyperplasia is usually congenital; delayed virilizing adrenal hyperplasia is a variant of congenital adrenal hyperplasia. Both are caused by a defect in hydroxylation of cortisol precursors; cortisol precursors accumulate and are shunted into the production of androgens. The defect is only partial in delayed virilizing adrenal hyperplasia, so clinical disease may not develop until adulthood.

Symptoms and Signs

Effects depend on the patient's sex and age at onset and are more noticeable in women than in men. Symptoms and signs include hirsutism (sometimes the only sign in mild cases), baldness, acne, and deepening of the voice. Libido may increase. In prepubertal children, growth may accelerate. If untreated, premature epiphyseal closure and short stature occur. Affected prepubertal males may experience premature sexual maturation. Females may have amenorrhea, atrophy of the uterus, clitoral hypertrophy, decreased breast size, and increased muscularity. In adult men, the excess adrenal androgens may suppress gonadal function and cause infertility. Ectopic adrenal tissue in the testes may enlarge and simulate tumors.

Diagnosis

Adrenal virilism is suspected clinically, although mild hirsutism and virilization with hypomenorrhea and elevated plasma testosterone may also occur in polycystic ovary (Stein-Leventhal) syndrome (see p. 2078). Adrenal virilism is confirmed by demonstrating elevated levels of adrenal androgens. In adrenal hyperplasia, urinary dehydroepiandrosterone (DHEA) and its sulfate (DHEAS) are elevated, pregnanetriol excretion is often increased, and urinary free cortisol is diminished. Plasma DHEA, DHEAS, 17-hydroxyprogesterone, testosterone, and androstenedione may be elevated. A level of > 30 nmol/L of 17-hydroxyprogesterone 30 min after administration of cosyntropin 0.25 mg IM strongly suggests the most common form of adrenal hyperplasia.

Virilizing tumors are excluded if dexamethasone 0.5 mg po q 6 h for 48 h suppresses production of excess androgens. If excessive androgen excretion is not suppressed, CT or MRI of the adrenals and ultrasound of the ovaries are performed to search for a tumor.

Treatment

Recommended treatment for adrenal hyperplasia is dexamethasone 0.5 to 1 mg po at bedtime, but even these small doses may produce signs of Cushing's syndrome. Cortisol (25 mg once/day) or prednisone (5 to 10 mg once/day) can be used instead. Although most symptoms and signs of virilism disappear, hirsutism and baldness disappear slowly, the voice may remain deep, and fertility may be impaired.

Tumors require adrenalectomy. For those with cortisol-secreting tumors, hydrocortisone should be given preoperatively and postoperatively because their nontumerous adrenal cortex will be atrophic and suppressed.

CUSHING'S SYNDROME

Cushing's syndrome is a constellation of clinical abnormalities caused by chronic high blood levels of cortisol or related corticosteroids. Cushing's disease is Cushing's syndrome that results from excess pituitary production of ACTH, usually secondary to a pituitary adenoma. Typical symptoms include moon facies and truncal obesity with thin arms and legs. Diagnosis is by history of receiving corticosteroids or by elevated serum cortisol. Treatment depends on the cause.

Etiology

Hyperfunction of the adrenal cortex can be ACTH-dependent or ACTH-independent. ACTH-dependent hyperfunction may result from hypersecretion of ACTH by the pituitary gland; secretion of ACTH by a nonpituitary tumor, such as small cell carcinoma of the lung or a carcinoid tumor (ectopic ACTH syndrome); or administration of exogenous ACTH. ACTH-independent hyperfunction usually results from therapeutic administration of corticosteroids or from adrenal adenomas or carcinomas; rare causes include primary pigmented nodular adrenal dysplasia (usually in adolescents) and macronodular dysplasia (in older patients).

Whereas the term Cushing's syndrome denotes the clinical picture resulting from cortisol excess from any cause, Cushing's disease refers to hyperfunction of the adrenal cortex from pituitary ACTH excess. Patients with Cushing's disease usually have a small adenoma of the pituitary gland.

Symptoms and Signs

Clinical manifestations include moon facies with a plethoric appearance, truncal obesity with prominent supraclavicular and dorsal cervical fat pads ("buffalo hump"), and, usually, very slender distal extremities and fingers. Muscle wasting and weakness are present. The skin is thin and atrophic, with poor wound healing and easy bruising. Purple striae may appear on the abdomen. Hypertension, renal calculi, osteoporosis, glucose intolerance, reduced resistance to infection, and mental disturbances are common. Cessation of linear growth is characteristic in children. Females usually have menstrual irregularities. In adrenal tumors, increased production of androgens may lead to hypertrichosis, temporal balding, and other signs of virilism in females.

Diagnosis

Diagnosis is usually suspected based on the characteristic symptoms and signs. Confirmation, and investigation of the underlying cause, generally requires hormonal and imaging tests.

Testing begins with measurement of urinary free cortisol (UFC), the best assay for urinary excretion (normal, 20 to 100 μg/24 h [55.2 to 276 nmol/24 h]). UFC is elevated > 120 μg/24 h (> 331 nmol/24 h) in all patients with Cushing's syndrome. However, many patients with UFC elevations between 100 and 150 μg/24 h (276 and 414 nmol/24 h) have obesity, depression, or polycystic ovaries but not Cushing's syndrome. A patient with suspected Cushing's syndrome with grossly elevated UFC (> 4 times the upper limit of normal) almost certainly has Cushing's syndrome. Two to 3 normal collections virtually exclude the diagnosis. Slightly elevated levels generally necessitate further investigation.

Traditionally, further investigation is accomplished with the dexamethasone test, in which 1, 1.5, or 2 mg of dexamethasone is administered po at 11 to 12 PM and plasma cortisol is measured at 8 to 9 AM the next morning. In most normal patients, this drug suppresses morning plasma cortisol to ≤ 1.8 μg/mL (≤ 50 nmol/L), whereas patients with Cushing's syndrome virtually always have a higher level. A more specific but equally sensitive test is to give dexamethasone 0.5 mg po q 6 h for 2 days (low dose). In general, a clear failure to suppress levels in response to low-dose dexamethasone establishes the diagnosis.

If these tests are indeterminate, the patient is hospitalized for measurement of serum cortisol at midnight, which is more likely to be conclusive. Cortisol normally ranges from 5 to 25 μg/dL (138 to 690 nmol/L) in the early morning (6 to 8 AM) and declines gradually to < 1.8 μg/dL (< 50 nmol/L) at midnight. Patients with Cushing's syndrome occasionally have a normal morning cortisol but lack normal diurnal decline in cortisol production, such that the midnight plasma cortisol levels are above normal and the total 24-h cortisol production is elevated. Alternatively, salivary cortisol samples may be collected and stored in the refrigerator at home. Plasma cortisol may be spuriously elevated in patients with congenital increases of corticosteroid-binding globulin or with estrogen therapy, but diurnal variation is normal in these patients.

ACTH levels are measured to determine the cause of Cushing's syndrome. Undetectable levels, both basally and particularly in response to corticotropin-releasing hormone (CRH), suggest a primary adrenal cause. High levels suggest a pituitary cause. If ACTH is detectable (ACTH-dependent Cushing's syndrome), provocative tests help differentiate Cushing's disease from ectopic ACTH syndrome, which is rarer. In response to high-dose dexamethasone (2 mg po q 6 h for 48 h), the 9 AM serum cortisol falls by > 50% in most patients with Cushing's disease but rarely in those with ectopic ACTH syndrome. Conversely, ACTH and cortisol rise by > 50% and 20%, respectively, in response to human or ovine-sequence CRH (100 μg IV or 1 μg/kg IV) in most patients with Cushing's disease but very rarely in those with ectopic ACTH syndrome (see TABLE 153–2). An alternative approach to localization is to catheterize both petrosal veins (which drain the pituitary) and measure ACTH from these veins 5 min after a bolus of CRH 100 μg or 1 μg/kg. A central-to-peripheral ACTH ratio > 3 virtually excludes ectopic ACTH syndrome, whereas a ratio < 3 suggests a need to seek such a source.

Pituitary imaging is obtained if ACTH levels and provocative tests suggest a pituitary cause; gadolinium-enhanced MRI is most accurate, but some microadenomas are visible on CT. If testing suggests a nonpituitary cause, imaging includes high-resolution CT of the chest, pancreas, and adrenals; scintiscanning with radiolabeled octreotide; and PET scanning.

In children with Cushing's disease, pituitary tumors are very small and usually cannot be detected with MRI. Petrosal sinus sampling is particularly useful in this situation. MRI is preferred to CT in pregnant women to avoid fetal exposure to radiation.

TABLE 153–2. DIAGNOSTIC TESTS IN CUSHING'S SYNDROME

DIAGNOSIS	SERUM CORTISOL, 9 AM	SALIVARY OR SERUM CORTISOL, MIDNIGHT	URINARY FREE CORTISOL	LOW-DOSE OR OVERNIGHT DEXAMETHASONE	HIGH-DOSE DEXAMETHASONE	CORTICOTROPIN-RELEASING HORMONE
Normal	N	N	N*	S	S	N
Cushing's disease	N or ↑	↑	↑	NS	S	N or ↑
Ectopic ACTH	N or ↑	↑	↑	NS	NS	Flat
Adrenal tumor	N or ↑	↑	↑	NS	NS	Flat

*May be elevated in non-Cushing's conditions.

N = normal; S = suppression; NS = nonsuppression; flat = no significant rise in ACTH or cortisol.

Treatment

Initially, the patient's general condition should be supported by high protein intake and appropriate administration of K. If clinical manifestations are severe, it may be reasonable to block corticosteroid secretion with metyrapone 250 mg to 1 g po tid or ketoconazole 400 mg po once/day, increasing to a maximum of 400 mg tid. Ketoconazole is more readily available but slower in onset and sometimes hepatotoxic.

Pituitary tumors that produce excessive ACTH are removed surgically or extirpated with radiation. If no tumor is demonstrated on imaging but a pituitary source is likely, total hypophysectomy may be attempted, particularly in elderly patients. Younger patients usually receive supervoltage irradiation of the pituitary, delivering 45 Gy. Improvement usually occurs in < 1 yr. However, in children, irradiation may reduce secretion of growth hormone and occasionally cause precocious puberty. In special centers, heavy particle beam irradiation, providing about 100 Gy, is often successful, as is a single focused beam of radiation therapy given as a single dose—radiosurgery. Response to irradiation occasionally requires several years.

Bilateral adrenalectomy is reserved for patients with pituitary hyperadrenocorticism who do not respond to both pituitary exploration (with possible adenomectomy) and irradiation. Adrenalectomy requires life-long corticosteroid replacement.

Nelson syndrome occurs when after adrenalectomy the pituitary gland continues to expand, causing a marked increase in the secretion of ACTH and its precursors, resulting in severe hyperpigmentation. It occurs in ≤ 50% of patients who undergo adrenalectomy. The risk is probably reduced if the patient undergoes pituitary radiation. Although irradiation may arrest continued pituitary growth, many patients also require hypophysectomy. The indications for hypophysectomy are the same as for any pituitary tumor—an increase in size such that the tumor encroaches on surrounding structures, producing visual field defects, pressure on the hypothalamus, or other complications. Routine irradiation is often performed after hypophysectomy if not previously carried out. Radiosurgery, or focused radiation therapy, can be given in a single fraction when standard external beam radiation therapy has already been performed, as long as the lesion is at a reasonable distance from the optic nerve and chiasm.

Adrenocortical tumors are removed surgically. Patients must receive cortisol during the surgical and postoperative periods because their nontumorous adrenal cortex will be atrophic and suppressed. Benign adenomas can be removed laparoscopically. With multinodular adrenal hyperplasia, bilateral adrenalectomy may be necessary. Even after a presumed total adrenalectomy, functional regrowth occurs in a few patients.

Ectopic ACTH syndrome is treated by removing the nonpituitary tumor that is producing the ACTH. However, in some cases, the tumor is disseminated and cannot be excised. Adrenal inhibitors, such as metyrapone 500 mg po tid (and up to total 6 g/day) or mitotane 0.5 g po once/day, increasing to a maximum of 3 to 4 g/day, usually control severe metabolic disturbances (eg, hypokalemia). When mitotane is used, a small dose of hydrocortisone or a large dose of dexamethasone may be needed. Measures of cortisol production may be unreliable, and severe hypercholesterolemia may develop. Ketoconazole (400 to 1200 mg po once/day) also blocks corticosteroid synthesis, though it may cause liver toxicity and can cause addisonian symptoms. Alternatively, the corticosteroid receptors can be blocked with mifepristone (RU 486). Mifepristone increases plasma cortisol but blocks effects of the corticosteroid. Sometimes ACTH-secreting tumors respond to long-acting somatostatin analogs, although administration for > 2 yr requires close follow-up, because mild gastritis, gallstones, cholangitis, jaundice, and vitamin B_{12} malabsorption may develop.

PRIMARY ALDOSTERONISM

(Conn's Syndrome)

Primary aldosteronism is aldosteronism caused by autonomous production of aldosterone by the adrenal cortex (due to hyperplasia, adenoma, or carcinoma). Symptoms and signs include episodic weakness, elevated BP, and hypokalemia. Diagnosis includes measurement of plasma aldosterone levels and plasma renin activity. Treatment depends on cause. A tumor is removed if possible; in hyperplasia, spironolactone or related drugs may normalize BP and eliminate other clinical features.

Aldosterone is the most potent mineralocorticoid produced by the adrenals. It causes Na retention and K loss. In the kidney, aldosterone causes transfer of Na from the lumen of the distal tubule into the tubular cells in exchange for K and hydrogen. The same effect occurs in salivary glands, sweat glands, cells of the intestinal mucosa, and in exchanges between ICFs and ECFs.

Aldosterone secretion is regulated by the renin-angiotensin system and, to a lesser extent, by ACTH. Renin, a proteolytic enzyme, is stored in the juxtaglomerular cells of the kidney. Reduction in blood volume and flow in the afferent renal arterioles induces secretion of renin. Renin transforms angiotensinogen from the liver to angiotensin I, which is transformed by ACE to angiotensin II. Angiotensin II causes secretion of aldosterone and, to a much lesser extent, secretion of cortisol and deoxycorticosterone; it also has pressor activity. Na and water retention resulting from increased aldosterone secretion increases the blood volume and reduces renin secretion.

Primary aldosteronism is caused by an adenoma, usually unilateral, of the glomerulosa cells of the adrenal cortex or, more rarely, by adrenal carcinoma or hyperplasia. Adenomas are extremely rare in children, but the syndrome sometimes occurs in childhood adrenal carcinoma or hyperplasia. In adrenal hyperplasia, which is more common in elderly men, both adrenals are overactive, and no adenoma is present. The clinical picture can also occur with congenital adrenal hyperplasia from deficiency of 11 β-hydroxylase and the dominantly inherited dexamethasone-suppressible hyperaldosteronism.

Symptoms, Signs, and Diagnosis

Hypernatremia, hypervolemia, and a hypokalemic alkalosis may occur, producing episodic weakness, paresthesias, transient paralysis, and tetany. Diastolic hypertension and hypokalemic nephropathy with polyuria and polydipsia are common. In many cases, the only manifestation is mild to moderate hypertension. Edema is uncommon.

Diagnosis is suspected in patients with hypertension and hypokalemia. Initial laboratory testing consists of plasma aldosterone levels and plasma renin activity (PRA). Ideally, tests are performed with the patient off of drugs that affect the renin-angiotensin system (eg, thiazide diuretics, ACE inhibitors, angiotensin antagonists, β-blockers) for 4 to 6 wk. PRA is usually measured in the morning with the patient recumbent. Patients with primary aldosteronism typically have plasma aldosterone > 15 ng/dL (> 0.42 nmol/L) and low levels of PRA, with a ratio of plasma aldosterone (in nanograms/dL) to PRA (in nanograms/mL/h) > 20.

Low levels of both PRA and aldosterone suggest nonaldosterone mineralocorticoid excess (eg, due to licorice ingestion, Cushing's syndrome, or Liddle syndrome). High levels of both PRA and aldosterone suggest secondary hyperaldosteronism (see p. 1216). The principal differences between primary and secondary aldosteronism are shown in TABLE 153–3. In children, Bartter syndrome (see p. 2024) is distinguished from primary

TABLE 153–3. DIFFERENTIAL DIAGNOSIS OF ALDOSTERONISM

CLINICAL FINDING	PRIMARY ALDOSTERONISM		SECONDARY ALDOSTERONISM	
	Adenoma	Hyperplasia	Hypertension	Edema
BP	↑↑	↑	↑↑↑↑	N, ↑
Edema	Absent	Absent	Absent	Present
Serum Na	N, ↑	N, ↑	N, ↓	N, ↓
Serum K	↓	N, ↓	↓	N, ↓
Plasma renin activity*	↓↓	↓↓	↑↑	↑
Aldosterone	↑	↑	↑↑	↑

*When corrected for age. Elderly patients have lower mean renin activities.

↑↑↑↑ = very greatly increased; ↑↑ = greatly increased; ↑ = increased; ↓↓ = greatly decreased; ↓ = decreased; N = normal.

hyperaldosteronism by the absence of hypertension and marked elevation of renin.

Patients with findings suggesting primary hyperaldosteronism should undergo CT or MRI to determine whether the cause is a tumor or hyperplasia. Aldosterone levels measured on awakening and 2 to 4 h later while standing also may help make this distinction; in adenoma, levels decline and in hyperplasia, levels increase. In equivocal cases, bilateral catheterization of the adrenal veins to measure cortisol and aldosterone should confirm whether the aldosterone excess is unilateral (tumor) or bilateral (hyperplasia).

Treatment

Tumors should be removed laparoscopically. After removal of an adenoma, BP decreases in all patients; complete remission occurs in 50 to 70%. With adrenal hyperplasia, 70% remain hypertensive after bilateral adrenalectomy; thus surgery is not recommended. Hyperaldosteronism in these patients can usually be controlled by spironolactone, starting with 300 mg po once/day and decreasing to a maintenance dose, usually around 100 mg once/day over 1 mo; or by amiloride (5 to 10 mg) or another K-sparing diuretic. About $\frac{1}{2}$ of such patients need additional antihypertensive treatment (see p. 608).

SECONDARY ALDOSTERONISM

Secondary aldosteronism is increased adrenal production of aldosterone in response to nonpituitary, extra-adrenal stimuli, including renal artery stenosis and hypovolemia. Symptoms are those of primary aldosteronism. Treatment involves correcting the underlying cause.

Secondary aldosteronism is caused by reduced renal blood flow, which stimulates the renin-angiotensin mechanism with resultant hypersecretion of aldosterone. Causes of reduced renal blood flow include obstructive renal artery disease (eg, atheroma, stenosis), renal vasoconstriction (as occurs in accelerated hypertension), and edematous disorders (eg, heart failure, cirrhosis with ascites, nephrotic syndrome). Secretion may be normal in heart failure, but hepatic blood flow and aldosterone metabolism are reduced, so circulating levels of the hormone are high.

PHEOCHROMOCYTOMA

A pheochromocytoma is a catecholamine-secreting tumor of chromaffin cells typically located in the adrenals. It causes persistent or paroxysmal hypertension. Diagnosis is by measuring catecholamine products in blood or urine. Imaging tests, especially CT or MRI, help localize tumors. Treatment involves removal of the tumor when possible. Drug therapy for control of BP includes α-blockade, possibly combined with β-blockade.

The catecholamines secreted include norepinephrine, epinephrine, dopamine, and dopa in varying proportions. About 90% of pheochromocytomas are in the adrenal medulla, but they may also be located in other tissues derived from neural crest cells; possible sites include the paraganglia of the sympathetic chain, retroperitoneally along the course of the aorta, in the carotid body, in the organ of Zuckerkandl (at the aortic bifurcation), in the GU system, in the brain, in the pericardial sac, and in dermoid cysts.

Pheochromocytomas in the adrenal medulla occur equally in both sexes, are bilateral in 10% of cases (20% in children), and are malignant in < 10%. Of extra-adrenal tumors, 30% are malignant. Although pheochromocytomas occur at any age, peak incidence is between the 20s and 40s.

Pheochromocytomas vary in size but average 5 to 6 cm in diameter. They weigh 50 to 200 g, but tumors weighing several kg have been reported. Rarely, they are large enough to be palpated or cause symptoms due to pressure or obstruction. Regardless of the histologic appearance, the tumor is considered benign if it has not invaded the capsule and no metastases are found, although exceptions occur.

Pheochromocytomas may be part of the syndrome of familial multiple endocrine neoplasia (MEN), types IIA and IIB, in which other endocrine tumors (parathyroid or medullary carcinoma of the thyroid) coexist or develop subsequently (see p. 1314). Pheochromocytoma develops in 1% of patients with neurofibromatosis (von Recklinghausen's disease) and may occur with hemangiomas and renal cell carcinoma, as in von Hippel-Lindau disease. Familial pheochromocytomas and carotid body tumors may be due to mutations of the enzyme succinate dehydrogenase.

Symptoms and Signs

Hypertension, which is paroxysmal in 45% of patients, is prominent. About 1/1000 hypertensive patients has a pheochromocytoma. Common symptoms and signs are tachycardia, diaphoresis, postural hypotension, tachypnea, cold and clammy skin, severe headache, angina, palpitations, nausea, vomiting, epigastric pain, visual disturbances, dyspnea, paresthesias, constipation, and a sense of impending doom. Paroxysmal attacks may be provoked by palpation of the tumor, postural changes, abdominal compression or massage, induction of anesthesia, emotional trauma, unopposed β-blockade (which paradoxically increases BP by blocking β-mediated vasodilation), or micturition (if the tumor is in the bladder). In elderly patients, severe weight loss with persistent hypertension is suggestive of pheochromocytoma.

Physical examination, except for presence of hypertension, is usually normal unless performed during a paroxysmal attack. Retinopathy and cardiomegaly are often less severe than might be expected for the degree of hypertension, but a specific catecholamine cardiomyopathy can occur.

Diagnosis

Pheochromocytoma is suspected in patients with typical symptoms or particularly sudden, severe, or intermittent unexplained hypertension. Diagnosis involves demonstrating high levels of catecholamine products in the serum or urine.

Blood tests: Plasma free metanephrine is up to 99% sensitive. This test has superior sensitivity to measurement of circulating epinephrine and norepinephrine because plasma metanephrines are elevated continuously, unlike epinephrine and norepinephrine, which are secreted intermittently; however, grossly elevated plasma norepinephrine renders the diagnosis highly probable.

Urine tests: Urinary metanephrine is less specific than plasma free metanephrine, but sensitivity is about 95%. Two or 3 normal results render the diagnosis extremely unlikely. Measurement of urinary norepinephrine and epinephrine is nearly as accurate. The principal urinary metabolic products of epinephrine and norepinephrine are the metanephrines vanillylmandelic acid (VMA) and homovanillic acid (HVA). Healthy people excrete only very small amounts of these substances. Normal values for 24 h are as follows: free epinephrine and norepinephrine < 100 μg (< 582 nmol), total metanephrine < 1.3 mg (< 7.1 μmol), VMA < 10 mg (< 50 μmol), HVA < 15 mg (< 82.4 μmol). In pheochromocytoma and neuroblastoma, urinary excretion of epinephrine and norepinephrine and their metabolic products increases intermittently. However, elevated excretion of these compounds may also occur in other disorders (eg, coma, dehydration, sleep apnea) or extreme stress; in patients being treated with rauwolfia alkaloids, methyldopa, or catecholamines; or after ingestion of foods containing large quantities of vanilla (especially if renal insufficiency is present).

Other tests: Blood volume is constricted and may falsely elevate Hb and Hct levels. Hyperglycemia, glycosuria, or overt diabetes mellitus may be present, with elevated fasting levels of plasma free fatty acid and glycerol. Plasma insulin level is inappropriately low for the plasma glucose. After removal of the pheochromocytoma, hypoglycemia may occur, especially in patients treated with oral antihyperglycemics.

Provocative tests with histamine or tyramine *are hazardous and should not be used.* Glucagon (0.5 to 1 mg injected rapidly IV) provokes a rise in BP > 35/25 mm Hg within 2 min in normotensive patients with pheochromocytoma but is now generally unnecessary. *Phentolamine mesylate must be available to terminate any hypertensive crisis.*

The general approach is to use 24-h urinary catecholamines as a screening test and to avoid provocative tests. In patients with elevated plasma catecholamines, a suppression test using oral clonidine or IV pentolinium can be used but is rarely necessary.

Imaging tests to localize tumors are usually performed for patients with abnormal screening results. Tests should include CT and MRI of the chest and abdomen with and without contrast. With isotonic contrast media, no adrenoceptor blockade is necessary. PET has also been used successfully. Repeated sampling of plasma catecholamine concentrations during catheterization of the vena cava with sampling at different locations, including the adrenal veins, can help localize the tumor: there will be a step up in norepinephrine level in a vein draining the tumor. Adrenal vein norepinephrine-to-epinephrine ratios may help in the hunt for a small adrenal source. Radiopharmaceuticals with nuclear imaging techniques can also help localize pheochromocytomas. ^{123}I-metaiodobenzylguanidine

(MIBG) is the most used compound outside the US; 0.5 mCi is injected IV and the patient is scanned on days 1, 2, and 3. Normal adrenal tissue rarely picks up this isotope, but 90% of pheochromocytomas do. The imaging is usually positive only when the lesion is large enough to be obvious on CT or MRI, but it can help confirm that a mass is likely to be the source of the catecholamines. ^{131}I-MIBG is a less sensitive alternative.

Signs of an associated genetic disorder (eg, café-au-lait patches in neurofibromatosis) should be sought. Patients should be screened for MEN with a serum Ca (and possibly calcitonin) and any other tests as directed by clinical findings.

Treatment

Surgical removal is the treatment of choice. The operation is usually delayed until hypertension is controlled by a combination of α- and β-blockers (usually phenoxybenzamine 20 to 40 mg po tid and propranolol 20 to 40 mg po tid). β-Blockers should not be used until adequate α-blockade has been achieved. Some α-blockers, such as doxazosin, may be equally effective but better tolerated.

The most effective and safest preoperative α-blockade is phenoxybenzamine 0.5 mg/kg IV in 0.9% saline over 2 h on each of the 3 days before the operation. Na nitroprusside can be infused for hypertensive crises preoperatively or intraoperatively. When bilateral tumors are documented or suspected (as in a patient with MEN), sufficient hydrocortisone (100 mg IV bid) given before and during surgery avoids acute glucocorticoid insufficiency from bilateral adrenalectomy.

Most pheochromocytomas can be removed laparoscopically. BP must be continuously monitored via an intra-arterial catheter, and volume status is closely monitored. Anesthesia should be induced with a nonarrhythmogenic drug (eg, a thiobarbiturate) and continued with enflurane. During surgery, paroxysms of hypertension should be controlled with injections of phentolamine 1 to 5 mg IV or nitroprusside infusion (2 to 4 μg/kg/min) and tachyarrhythmias with propranolol 0.5 to 2 mg IV. If a muscle relaxant is needed, drugs that do not release histamine are preferred. The use of atropine preoperatively should be *avoided.* Preoperative blood transfusion (1 to 2 units) should be given before the tumor is removed in anticipation of blood loss. If BP has been well controlled before surgery, a diet high in salt is recommended to increase blood volume. An infusion of norepinephrine 4 to 12 mg/L of a dextrose-containing solution should be started if hypotension develops. Some patients whose hypotension responds poorly to levarterenol may benefit from hydrocortisone 100 mg IV.

Malignant metastatic pheochromocytoma should be treated with α- and β-blockers. The tumor may be indolent and survival long-lasting. However, even with rapid tumor growth, BP can be controlled. ^{131}I-MIBG prolongs life when used to treat residual disease. Radiation therapy may reduce bone pain; chemotherapy is rarely effective but can be attempted if all else fails.

NONFUNCTIONAL ADRENAL MASSES

Nonfunctional adrenal masses are space-occupying lesions of the adrenal glands that have no hormonal activity. Symptoms, signs, and treatment depend on the nature and size of the mass.

The most common nonfunctioning adrenal mass in adults is an adenoma (50%), followed by carcinomas (30%) and metastatic tumors (10%). Cysts and lipomas make up most of the remainder. However, the precise proportions depend on the clinical presentation; when discovered on incidental screening, most are adenomas. Less commonly, in newborns, spontaneous adrenal hemorrhage may produce large adrenal masses, simulating neuroblastoma or Wilms' tumor. In adults, bilateral massive adrenal hemorrhage may result from thromboembolic disease or coagulopathy. Benign cysts are observed in elderly patients and may be due to cystic degeneration, vascular accidents, bacterial infections, or parasitic infestations (*Echinococcus*). Hematogenous spread of TB organisms may cause adrenal masses. A nonfunctional adrenal carcinoma produces a diffuse and infiltrating retroperitoneal process. Hemorrhage can occur, producing adrenal hematomas.

Symptoms, Signs, and Diagnosis

Nonfunctional adrenal masses are usually found incidentally during tests such as CT or MRI conducted for other reasons. Nonfunctionality is established clinically and confirmed by adrenal hormonal measurements as described above. With any adrenal mass, adrenal insufficiency is rare unless both glands are involved.

The major signs of bilateral massive adrenal hemorrhage are abdominal pain, falling Hct, signs of acute adrenal failure, and suprarenal masses on CT or MRI. TB of the adrenals may cause calcification and Addison's disease. Nonfunctional adrenal carcinoma usually manifests as metastatic disease and may therefore not be amenable to surgery, though mitotane may afford chemotherapeutic control when used with supportive exogenous corticosteroids.

Small adrenal adenomas (< 2 cm) usually are nonfunctional, produce no symptoms, and require no special treatment but should be observed for growth or development of secretory function (such as looking for clinical signs and periodically measuring electrolytes). If metastatic disease is possible, fine-needle biopsy can be diagnostic.

Treatment

If the tumor is solid, of adrenal origin, and > 4 cm, it should be excised, because biopsy cannot always distinguish benign from malignant tumors.

Tumors 2 to 4 cm in diameter are a particularly difficult clinical problem. If scanning does not suggest cancer and hormonal function does not seem altered (eg, normal electrolytes and catecholamines, no evidence of Cushing's syndrome), it is reasonable to reevaluate periodically. However, many of these tumors secrete cortisol in quantities too small to produce symptoms, and whether they would eventually produce symptoms and morbidity if untreated is unclear. Most clinicians merely observe these patients.

154 POLYGLANDULAR DEFICIENCY SYNDROMES

(Autoimmune Polyglandular Syndromes; Polyendocrine Deficiency Syndromes)

Polyglandular deficiency syndromes are characterized by concurrent subnormal function of several endocrine glands. Etiology is most often autoimmune. Symptoms depend on the combination of deficiencies, which fall within one of 3 types. Diagnosis requires measurement of hormone levels and autoantibodies against affected endocrine glands. Treatment includes replacement of missing or deficient hormones.

Etiology and Pathophysiology

Endocrine deficiency can be caused by infections, infarctions, or tumors that produce partial or complete gland destruction. However, polyglandular endocrine deficiency is usually caused by an autoimmune reaction that produces inflammation, lymphocytic infiltration, and partial or complete gland destruction. Impairment of one gland by autoimmune disease is frequently followed by impairment of other glands, resulting in multiple endocrine failure. Three patterns of autoimmune failure have been described (see TABLE 154–1).

Type I: Onset usually occurs in childhood (particularly between ages 3 and 5) or in adulthood before age 35. Hypoparathyroidism is the most frequent endocrine deficiency (79%), followed by adrenocortical failure (72%). Gonadal failure occurs after puberty in 60% of women and in about 15% of men. Chronic mucocutaneous candidiasis is common. Malabsorption associated with cholecystokinin deficiency can occur; causative factors include intestinal lymphangiectasia, IgA deficiency, hypoparathyroidism, and bacterial overgrowth. Although ⅔ of patients have antibodies to pancreatic glutamic acid decarboxylase, type 1 diabetes mellitus occurs infrequently. Ectodermal diseases (eg, dental enamel hypoplasia, tympanic membrane sclerosis, tubulointerstitial disease, keratoconjunctivitis) also occur. Type I may be inherited, usually in an autosomal recessive pattern.

Type II (Schmidt's syndrome): Multiple glandular failure generally occurs in adults, with peak incidence at age 30. It occurs twice as often in women. It always involves the adrenal cortex and frequently the thyroid gland and the pancreatic islets, producing type 1 diabetes. Autoantibodies against the target

TABLE 154–1. CHARACTERISTICS OF TYPES I, II, AND III POLYGLANDULAR DEFICIENCY SYNDROMES

CHARACTERISTIC	TYPE I	TYPE II	TYPE III
Age at onset	Childhood (3–5 yr)	Adult (peak 30 yr)	Adult (before age 35)
HLA types	A28, A3	Primarily B8, DW3, DR3, DR4; others in specific diseases	DR3, DR4
Female/male	1.4/1.0	1.8/1.0	N/A
Clinical manifestations			
Addison's disease	67%	100%	Not seen
Thyroid disease*	10–11%	69%	100%
Pernicious anemia	13–15%	< 1%	†
Diabetes mellitus (insulin-dependent)	2–4%	52%	†
Gonadal failure	45%	3.5%	†
Hypoparathyroidism	82%	Not seen	Not seen
Vitiligo	4%	5–50%	N/A
Chronic mucocutaneous candidiasis	73–78%	Not seen	N/A
Chronic active hepatitis	11–13%	Not seen	N/A
Alopecia	26–32%	Not seen	†
Malabsorption	22–24%	Not seen	N/A
Celiac disease and myasthenia gravis	Not seen	Incidence uncertain	†
Sarcoidosis	Not seen	Not seen	†

N/A = Data not available.
*Usually chronic lymphocytic thyroiditis, but also includes Graves' disease.
†Associated; incidence uncertain.

Adapted from Trence DL, Morley JE, Handwerger BS: Polyglandular autoimmune syndromes. *American Journal of Medicine* 77(1):107–116, 1984; and from Leshin M: Polyglandular autoimmune syndromes. *American Journal of Medical Sciences* 290(2):77–88, 1985; used with permission.

glands are frequently present, especially against P-450 cytochrome adrenocortical enzymes. Both mineralocorticoid and glucocorticoid deficiency can occur. Glandular destruction results mostly from cell-mediated autoimmunity, either from depressed suppressor T-cell function or some other type of T-cell–mediated injury. Reduced systemic T-cell–mediated immunity is common, manifested by a poor response on skin testing to standard antigens. Reactivity is also reduced in about 30% of 1st-degree relatives with normal endocrine function.

Some patients have thyroid-stimulating antibodies and initially present with symptoms and signs of hyperthyroidism.

Theoretically, specific HLA types may have increased susceptibility to certain viruses that might induce the destructive reaction. Inheritance usually follows an autosomal dominant pattern with variable expressivity.

Type III: Type III is characterized by glandular failure in adults, particularly middle-aged women. It does not involve the adrenal cortex but includes at least 2 of the following: thyroid deficiency, type 1 diabetes, pernicious anemia, vitiligo, and alopecia. Inheritance may follow an autosomal dominant pattern with incomplete penetrance.

Symptoms, Signs, and Diagnosis

The clinical appearance of patients with polyglandular deficiency syndromes is the sum of the individual endocrine deficiencies. There is no specific sequence in which individual endocrine deficiencies occur. Thus, patients with one endocrine deficiency should be observed over a period of years for development of additional endocrine deficiencies through repeated clinical assessment and measurements of hormone levels. Relatives should be made aware of the diagnosis and screened when appropriate. Measurement of glutamic acid decarboxylase antibodies may be useful in determining risk.

Diagnosis is suggested clinically and confirmed by detecting deficient hormone levels. Measuring autoantibodies to the affected glandular tissue can help differentiate autoimmune polyglandular endocrine dysfunction from that of other causes (eg, tuberculous hypoadrenalism, nonautoimmune hypothyroidism).

Multiple endocrine deficiencies may suggest hypothalamic-pituitary failure. In almost all cases, elevated plasma levels of pituitary tropic hormones demonstrate the peripheral nature of the defect; however, hypothalamic-pituitary insufficiency occasionally occurs as part of type II syndrome.

Asymptomatic patients at risk need not be tested with autoantibodies because such antibodies may persist for years without causing endocrine deficiencies.

Treatment

Treatment of the various individual glandular deficiencies is discussed elsewhere in THE MANUAL. The interaction of multiple deficiencies may complicate treatment.

Chronic mucocutaneous candidiasis usually requires lifelong antifungal therapy. If given early (within the 1st few weeks to months) in the course of endocrine failure, immunosuppressive doses of cyclosporine may benefit some patients.

IPEX Syndrome

IPEX (immune dysregulation, polyendocrinopathy, enteropathy, X-linked) is a recessive syndrome involving aggressive autoimmunity.

Untreated, IPEX syndrome is usually fatal in the 1st year of life. The enteropathy leads to diarrhea. Immunosuppressants and bone marrow transplantation can prolong life but are rarely curative.

POEMS Syndrome

(Crow-Fukase Syndrome)

POEMS (polyneuropathy, organomegaly, endocrinopathy, monoclonal gammopathy, skin changes) is a nonautoimmune polyglandular deficiency syndrome.

POEMS syndrome is probably caused by circulating immunoglobulins produced by a plasma cell dyscrasia (see also p. 1125). Patients may have hepatomegaly, lymphadenopathy, hypogonadism, type 2 diabetes mellitus, primary hypothyroidism, hyperparathyroidism, adrenal insufficiency, and excess production of monoclonal IgA and IgG from plasmacytomas and skin abnormalities (eg, hyperpigmentation, dermal thickening, hirsutism, angiomas, hypertrichosis). Patients may have edema, ascites, pleural effusion, papilledema, and fever. Patients with the syndrome also have increased circulating cytokines (IL-1-β, IL-6), vascular endothelial growth factor, and tumor necrosis factor-α.

Treatment consists of chemotherapy and radiation therapy followed by autologous hematopoietic or stem cell transplantation. Five-year survival is about 60%.

155 PORPHYRIAS

Porphyrias result from genetic deficiencies of enzymes of the heme biosynthetic pathway. These deficiencies allow heme precursors to accumulate, causing toxicity. Porphyrias are defined by the specific enzyme deficiency. Two major clinical manifestations occur: neurovisceral abnormalities (generally the acute porphyrias) and cutaneous photosensitivity (generally the cutaneous porphyrias).

Heme, an iron-containing pigment, is synthesized mostly in the bone marrow (by erythroblasts and reticulocytes) and is incorporated into hemoglobin. Heme is also synthesized in the liver and incorporated into certain enzymes (eg, cytochromes). Heme synthesis requires 8 enzymes (see TABLE 155–1). These

TABLE 155–1. SUBSTRATES AND ENZYMES OF THE HEME BIOSYNTHETIC PATHWAY AND THE DISEASES ASSOCIATED WITH THEIR DEFICIENCY

SUBSTRATE AND ENZYME*	PORPHYRIA	NEUROVISCERAL SYMPTOMS	CUTANEOUS SYMPTOMS	INHERITANCE
Glycine + succinyl CoA				
δ-Aminolevulinic acid synthase	None (deficiency causes sideroblastic anemia)	No (not a porphyria)	No (not a porphyria)	X-linked recessive
δ-Aminolevulinic acid				
δ-Aminolevulinic acid dehydratase (ALAD)	ALAD-deficient porphyria	Yes	No	Autosomal recessive
Porphobilinogen				
Porphobilinogen deaminase	Acute intermittent porphyria	Yes	No	Autosomal dominant
Hydroxymethylbilane				
Uroporphyrinogen III cosynthase	Congenital erythropoietic porphyria	No	Severe, mutilating disease	Autosomal recessive
Uroporphyrinogen III				
Uroporphyrinogen decarboxylase	Porphyria cutanea tarda and hepatopatoerythropoietic porphyria	No No	Fragile skin, blisters Severe blistering	Autosomal dominant
Coproporphyrinogen III				
Coproporphyrinogen oxidase	Hereditary coproporphyria	Yes	Fragile skin, blisters	Autosomal dominant
Protoporphyrinogen IX				
Protoporphyrinogen oxidase	Variegate porphyria	Yes	Fragile skin, blisters	Autosomal dominant
Protoporphyrin IX				
Ferrochelatase	Erythropoietic protoporphyria	No	Skin pain, no lesions	Autosomal dominant
Heme				

ALAD = δ-Aminolevulinic acid dehydratase.

*Successive intermediates in the heme biosynthetic pathway, beginning with glycine and succinyl CoA and ending with heme. Deficiency of an enzyme causes buildup of precursor compounds.

enzymes produce and transform molecular species called porphyrins, which are toxic if they accumulate.

Etiology and Pathophysiology

Porphyrias result from a deficiency of any of the last 7 enzymes of the heme biosynthetic pathway (deficiency of the 1st enzyme in the pathway, δ-aminolevulinic acid [ALA] synthase, causes sideroblastic anemia). Single genes encode each enzyme; any of numerous possible mutations can incapacitate the enzyme encoded by that gene. When an enzyme of heme synthesis is deficient or defective, its substrate and any other heme precursors normally modified by that enzyme may accumulate in bone marrow, liver, skin, or other tissues and produce toxicities. These precursors may appear in excess in the blood and be excreted in urine, bile, or stool.

Most porphyrias are autosomal dominant. Homozygous states are often incompatible with life, generally causing fetal death; the exceptions are ALA dehydratase (ALAD) deficiency porphyria and uroporphyrinogen III cosynthase deficiency, in which only homozygous or double heterozygous conditions (ie, 2 separate heterozygous mutations in the same gene in the same patient) cause disease. Disease penetrance in heterozygotes varies.

Although porphyrias are most precisely defined according to the deficient enzyme, classification by major clinical features (phenotype) is often useful. Thus, porphyrias are generally divided into 2 classes: acute and cutaneous. Acute porphyrias present as intermittent attacks of abdominal, mental, and neurologic symptoms. They are typically triggered by drugs and other exogenous factors. Cutaneous porphyrias tend to produce continuous or undulating symptoms involving cutaneous photosensitivity. Some acute porphyrias also have cutaneous manifestations.

In terms of genetic prevalence, the 2 most common porphyrias are acute intermittent porphyria (AIP) and porphyria cutanea tarda (PCT). The prevalence of each is about 1/10,000; TABLE 155–2 contrasts their major features. Because of variable penetrance in heterozygous porphyrias, clinically expressed disease is less common than genetic prevalence.

Urine discoloration (red or reddish brown) may occur in the symptomatic phase of all porphyrias except erythropoietic protoporphyria (EPP) and ALAD-deficiency porphyria. Discoloration results from oxidized porphyrins and/or the porphyrin precursor porphobilinogen (PBG). Sometimes the color develops after the urine has stood in light for about 30 min, allowing time for oxidation. In the acute porphyrias, except in ALAD-deficiency porphyria, about 1 in 3 heterozygotes (more frequently in females than males) also have increased urinary excretion of PBG (and urine discoloration) in the latent phase.

Diagnosis

Patients with symptoms suggesting porphyria are screened by blood or urine tests for porphyrins or the porphyrin precursors PBG and ALA (see TABLE 155–3). Abnormal results on screening are confirmed by further testing.

Asymptomatic patients, including suspected carriers and people who are between

TABLE 155–2. MAJOR FEATURES OF THE TWO MOST COMMON PORPHYRIAS

PORPHYRIA	PRESENTING SYMPTOMS	EXACERBATING FACTORS	MOST IMPORTANT SCREENING TESTS*	TREATMENT
Acute intermittent porphyria	Neurovisceral (intermittent, acute)	Drugs (mostly P-450 inducers); fasting; alcohol ingestion; infections; stress	Urinary porphobilinogen	Glucose; heme
Porphyria cutanea tarda	Blistering skin lesions (chronic)	Iron; alcohol; estrogens; hepatitis C virus; halogenated hydrocarbons	Plasma (or urine) porphyrins	Phlebotomy; low-dose chloroquine

*In symptomatic phase.

TABLE 155–3. SCREENING FOR PORPHYRIAS

TESTING	SYMPTOMS SUGGESTING PORPHYRIA: Acute Neurovisceral Symptoms	SYMPTOMS SUGGESTING PORPHYRIA: Photosensitivity
Screening	Urinary PBG (semiquantitative, random urine sample)	Plasma porphyrins*
Confirmation (when screening tests are significantly abnormal)	Urinary ALA and PBG† (quantitative‡) Fecal porphyrins RBC PBG deaminase Plasma porphyrins*	RBC porphyrins Urinary ALA PBG and porphyrins (quantitative) Fecal porphyrins† Plasma porphyrins

PBG = porphobilinogen; ALA = δ-aminolevulinic acid.

*The preferred method is by direct fluorescent spectrophotometry.

†Urinary and fecal porphyrins are fractionated only if the total is increased.

‡Correct results according to urine creatinine concentration.

attacks, are evaluated similarly. However, the above tests are less sensitive in these circumstances; measurement of RBC or WBC enzyme activity is considerably more sensitive. Genetic analysis is highly accurate and preferentially used within families when the mutation is known; prenatal testing (involving amniocentesis or chorionic villus sampling) is possible but rarely indicated.

ACUTE PORPHYRIAS

Acute porphyrias produce intermittent attacks of abdominal pain and neurologic symptoms. Attacks are precipitated by certain drugs and other factors. Patients with variegate porphyria and hereditary coproporphyria may develop bullous eruptions from sunlight exposure. Diagnosis is based on elevated levels of δ-aminolevulinic acid and porphyrin precursor porphobilinogen in the urine during attacks. Attacks are treated with glucose or, if more severe, IV heme. Symptomatic treatment, including analgesia, is given as necessary.

Acute porphyrias include, in order of prevalence, acute intermittent porphyria (AIP), variegate porphyria (VP), hereditary coproporphyria (HCP), and the exceedingly rare ALAD-deficiency porphyria.

Among heterozygotes, acute porphyrias are rarely expressed clinically before puberty and, after puberty, in only about 20 to 30%. Among homozygotes, onset is in childhood, and symptoms are severe.

Precipitating Factors

Many precipitating factors exist, typically accelerating heme synthesis above the catalytic capacity of the defective enzyme. Accumulation of porphyrin precursor porphobilinogen (PBG) and δ-aminolevulinic acid (ALA) (or in the case of ALA dehydratase [ALAD] deficiency porphyria, ALA alone) results.

Hormonal factors are important. Women are more prone to attacks than men, particularly during periods of hormonal change (eg, just before menstruation, use of oral contraceptives, during the early weeks of gestation, just after delivery). Nevertheless, pregnancy is not contraindicated.

Other factors include drugs (including barbiturates, other antiseizure drugs, and sulfonamide antibiotics—see TABLE 155–4) and reproductive hormones (progesterone and related steroids), particularly those that induce hepatic ALA synthase and cytochrome P-450 enzymes. Attacks usually occur within 24 h after exposure to a precipitating drug. Low-calorie and low-carbohydrate diets and alcohol can also precipitate symptoms. Stress resulting from infection or other illness, surgery, and mental problems is sometimes implicated. Attacks usually result from multiple, sometimes unidentifiable, factors.

Sunlight precipitates cutaneous symptoms in VP and HCP.

Symptoms and Signs

Symptoms and signs involve the nervous system, abdomen, or both (neurovisceral). Attacks develop over hours or days and can

TABLE 155–4. DRUGS AND PORPHYRIA*

CATEGORY	UNSAFE	SAFE	PROBABLY SAFE
Analgesic	Dextropropoxyphene, diclofenac, meprobamate, propoxyphene	Aspirin, buprenorphine, caffeine, codeine, morphine, propofol	Atropine, dexibuprofen, fentanyl, hydromorphone, ketobemidone, ketoprofen, naproxen
Anesthetic (local)	Lidocaine	Bupivacaine	Articaine
Anesthetic (premedication/ induction/ maintenance)	Barbiturates	Atropine, morphine, propofol	Alfentanil, desflurane, droperidol, enflurane, fentanyl, isoflurane, remifentanil, scopolamine, sufentanil
Antidepressant		Lithium	Fluoxetine
Antidiarrheal		Active carbon, loperamide	
Antiemetic		Chlorpromazine	Granisetron, ondansetron, scopolamine, tropisetron
Antiepileptic	Barbiturates, carbamazepine, diones (paramethadione, trimethadione), felbamate, mephenytoin, phenytoin, primidone, succinimides (ethosuximide, methsuximide), valproate		Clonazepam, diazepam (active seizure), gabapentin, levetiracetam
Antihyperglycemic		Acarbose, insulin, metformin	
Anti-infective	Chloramphenicol, clindamycin, erythromycin, indinavir, ketoconazole, mecillinam, nitrofurantoin, pivampicillin, pivmecillinam, rifampin, ritonavir, sulfonamides, trimethoprim	Acyclovir, amikacin, amoxicillin, amoxicillin with β-lactamase inhibitor, ampicillin, cloxacillin, dicloxacillin, fusidic acid, ganciclovir, gentamicin, immune sera, immunoglobulins, methenamine hippurate, netilmicin, oseltamivir, penicillin G, penicillin V, piperacillin, teicoplanin, tobramycin, vaccines, valacyclovir, vancomycin, zanamivir	Amphotericin B, azithromycin, bacampicillin, cephalosporins, ciprofloxacin, didanosine, ethambutol, ertapenem, famciclovir, flucytosine, foscarnet with cilastatin, imipenem, levofloxacin, meropenem, moxifloxacin, norfloxacin, ofloxacin, piperacillin with tazobactam, phosphomycin, ribavirin

Table continues on the following page.

TABLE 155–4. DRUGS AND PORPHYRIA*—Continued

CATEGORY	UNSAFE	SAFE	PROBABLY SAFE
Anti-inflammatory/antirheumatic		Hyaluronic acid, penicillamine, salicylates	Abacavir, dexibuprofen, tenofovir disoproxil fumarate, ibuprofen, ketoprofen, lamivudine, lornoxicam, naproxen, piroxicam, tenoxicam, zalcitabine
Anti-migraine	Ergots		
Anti-peptic ulcer		Alginic acid, calcium-containing antacids, cimetidine, magnesium-containing antacids, sucralfate	Famotidine, misoprostol, nizatidine, ranitidine
Anti-osteoporosis		Bisphosphonates, calcium	
Anxiolytic, sedative-hypnotic, antipsychotic	Ethchlorvynol, glutethimide, hydroxyzine, meprobamate	Chlorpromazine, droperidol, fluoxetine, fluphenazine, haloperidol, levomepromazine, prochlorperazine, propiomazine	Alprazolam, clozapine, dixyrazine, lorazepam, olanzapine, oxazepam, perphenazine, triazolam, zopiclone
Heart, circulation	Dihydralazine, ergoloid mesylate, hydralazine, lidocaine, methyldopa, spironolactone	Amiloride, β-blockers, cholestyramine, colestipol, digitalis glycosides, enalapril, epinephrine, heparins, lisinopril, nicotinic acid, organic nitrates	ACE inhibitors, adenosine, amrinone, angiotensin II-antagonists, bendroflumethiazide, bezafibrate, bumetanide, digoxin, dobutamine, dopamine, dopexamine, doxazosin, ethacrynic acid, etilefrine, fenofibrate, furosemide, hydrochlorothiazide, milrinone, phenylephrine, prostaglandins, quinidine, spironolactone
Hormones	Danazol, progesterone and synthetic progestins	Nonreproductive hormones including glucocorticoids	Natural estrogens
Laxative		Bisacodyl, dietary fiber, lactitol, lactulose, lauryl sulfate, psyllium seed, sagrada, senna glycosides, sodium docusate, sodium picosulfate, sorbitol	

TABLE 155–4. DRUGS AND PORPHYRIA*—Continued

CATEGORY	UNSAFE	SAFE	PROBABLY SAFE
Muscle relaxants	Carisoprodol, orphenadrine	Atracurium, cisatracurium, mivacurium, pancuronium, rocuronium, suxethonium, vecuronium	Baclofen
Respiratory system	Clemastine, dimenhydrinate	Alimemazine, dornase alfa, codeine, corticosteroids, dipalmitoyl phosphatidyl choline, ephedrine, ethylmorphine, ipratropium, phenylpropanolamine, phospholipid surfactant, salbutamol	Bambuterol, cromoglycic acid, cromolyn, declorahidine, desloratadine, fexofenadine, formoterol, levocabastine, lidocaine (solution for gargling), loratadine, mizolastine, oxymetazoline, phenoterol, salmeterol, terbutaline, tiotropium

*The classifications of the drugs in the list are based on a combination of clinical observations, case reports in the literature, and theoretical considerations derived from the structure and metabolism of the substances. Clinical observations, however, may in many cases be unreliable. Also, the biochemical and molecular-biologic models for the activation of the disease are incomplete. This list is meant as guidance only and is neither complete nor applicable to all patients. Drugs must be used cautiously in patients with porphyria.

last up to several weeks. Some gene carriers experience few attacks in their lifetime. Others experience recurrent symptoms. In women, attacks often coincide with phases of the menstrual cycle.

The acute porphyric attack: Constipation, fatigue, irritability, and insomnia typically precede an acute attack. The most common symptoms with the attack are abdominal pain and vomiting. The pain may be excruciating and is disproportionate to abdominal tenderness. Abdominal manifestations may result from effects on visceral nerves or from local vasoconstrictive ischemia. Because there is no inflammation, the abdomen is nontender, without peritoneal signs. Temperature and WBC count are normal or slightly increased. Bowel distention may develop as a result of paralytic ileus. The urine is red or reddish brown and positive for PBG during an attack.

All components of the peripheral and central nervous systems may be involved. Motor neuropathy is common with severe and prolonged attacks. Muscle weakness usually begins in the extremities but can involve any motor neuron or cranial nerve and proceed to tetraplegia. Bulbar involvement can produce ventilatory failure.

CNS involvement may produce seizures or mental disturbances (eg, apathy, depression, agitation, frank psychosis, hallucinations). Seizures, psychotic behavior, and hallucinations may be due to hyponatremia or hypomagnesemia, which can also contribute to arrhythmias.

Excess catecholamines generally produce restlessness and tachycardia. Rarely, catecholamine-induced arrhythmias cause sudden death. Labile hypertension with transiently high BP may cause vascular changes progressing to irreversible hypertension if untreated. Renal failure in acute porphyria is multifactorial; acute hypertension (possibly leading to chronic hypertension) is likely a main precipitating factor.

Subacute/subchronic symptoms: Some patients experience prolonged symptoms of lesser intensity (eg, obstipation, fatigue, headache, back or thigh pain, paresthesia, tachycardia, dyspnea, insomnia, mental disturbance, seizures).

Skin symptoms in VP and HCP: Fragile skin and bullous eruptions may develop on sun-exposed areas, even in the absence of neurovisceral symptoms. Often the patient is not aware of the connection to sun exposure. Cutaneous manifestations are identical to those of PCT.

Late manifestations: Motor involvement during acute attacks may produce persistent weakness between attacks. Hepatocellular cancer, hypertension, and renal impairment become more common after middle age in AIP, and possibly also in VP and HCP, especially in patients with previous porphyric attacks.

Diagnosis

Acute attack: Misdiagnosis is common because the acute attack is confused with other causes of acute abdomen (sometimes leading to unnecessary surgery) or with a primary neurologic or mental disorder. However, in a patient previously diagnosed as a gene carrier or who has a positive family history, porphyria should be suspected. Still, even in known gene carriers, other causes must be considered.

Red or reddish brown urine, not present before onset of symptoms, is a cardinal sign and is present during full-blown attacks. A urine specimen should be examined in patients with abdominal pain of unknown cause, especially if severe constipation, vomiting, tachycardia, muscle weakness, bulbar involvement, or mental symptoms occur.

If porphyria is suspected, the urine is analyzed for PBG using a rapid qualitative or semiquantitative determination. A positive result or high clinical suspicion necessitates quantitative ALA and PBG measurements preferentially obtained from the same specimen. PBG and ALA levels > 5 times normal indicate an acute porphyric attack unless the patient is a gene carrier with increased porphyrin precursor excretion even during the latent phase of the disorder.

If urinary PBG and ALA are normal, an alternative diagnosis must be considered. Elevated ALA with normal or slightly increased PBG suggests lead poisoning or ALAD-deficiency porphyria. Analysis of a 24-h urine specimen is not useful. Instead, a random urine specimen is used, PBG and ALA concentrations being corrected for dilution by relating to the creatinine concentration of the sample. Electrolytes and Mg should be measured. Hyponatremia may be present from excessive vomiting or diarrhea with hypotonic fluid replacement or from the syndrome of inappropriate ADH secretion (SIADH).

Determination of type: Because treatment does not depend on the type of acute porphyria, identification of the specific type is valuable mainly for finding gene carriers in relatives. The different forms of acute porphyria are distinguished by characteristic patterns of porphyrin (and precursor) accumulation and excretion in plasma, urine, and stool. When urine analysis reveals increased levels of ALA and PBG, fecal porphyrins should be measured. Fecal porphyrins are usually normal or minimally increased in AIP but elevated in HCP and VP. Often, these markers are not present in the quiescent phase of the disorder. In the cutaneous acute porphyrias, plasma porphyrins with characteristic fluorescence often are found. Erythrocyte PBG deaminase levels about 50% of normal suggest AIP. Diminished WBC protoporphyrinogen oxidase and coproporphyrinogen oxidase levels suggest VP and HCP, respectively.

Family studies: Children of a gene carrier have a 50% risk of inheriting the condition. Because early diagnosis and counseling reduce the risk of morbidity, children in affected families should be tested as early as possible. Genetic testing is used if the causing mutation has been identified in the index case. If not, pertinent RBC or WBC enzyme levels are measured. Gene analysis can be used for in utero diagnosis (using amniocentesis or chorionic villus sampling) but is seldom indicated because of the favorable outlook for most gene carriers.

Prognosis and Treatment

Advances in medical care and self-care have improved the prognosis for symptomatic patients. Still, some patients develop recurrent crises or progressive disease with permanent paralysis or renal failure. Also, frequent demands for potent analgesics may give rise to drug addiction.

Treatment of all acute porphyrias is essentially identical. Possible triggers (eg, drugs) are identified and withdrawn or corrected. Unless the attack is mild, the patient is hospitalized in a darkened, quiet, private room. Heart rate, BP, and fluid and electrolyte balance are monitored. Neurologic status, bladder function, muscle and tendon function, respiratory function, and pulse oximetry are continuously monitored. Symptoms (eg, pain, vomiting) are treated with nonporphyrinogenic drugs as needed (see TABLE 155–4).

Dextrose (300 to 500 g daily) inhibits ALA synthase and decreases symptoms. It can be given by mouth if the patient is not vomiting; otherwise, it is given IV. To avoid overhydration with consequent hyponatremia, 1 L of a 50% dextrose solution can be given by central venous catheter over 24 h.

IV heme should be given immediately for severe attacks or muscle weakness. Heme usually resolves symptoms in 3 to 4 days. If heme therapy is delayed, nerve damage is more advanced and recovery is slower and possibly incomplete. Heme is available in the US as lyophilized hematin to be reconstituted with sterile water. The dose is 3 mg/kg IV once/day for 4 days. In this form, heme degradation products form rapidly and may cause phlebitis at the infusion site; they also have a transient anticoagulant effect. Adverse effects can be reduced by reconstitution with human albumin. Heme arginate is a more stable, generally toxicity-free alternative.

Prevention

People at risk should avoid potentially harmful drugs (see TABLE 155–4), alcohol, emotional stress, exposure to organic solvents (eg, in painting or dry cleaning), crash diets, or periods of starvation. Diets for obesity should provide gradual weight loss and be adopted only during periods of remission. Carriers of VP or HCP should minimize sun exposure; sunscreen that blocks only ultraviolet light is ineffective, but opaque titanium dioxide agents are beneficial. Associations for porphyria patients can provide written information and direct counseling.

Patients should be identified prominently in the medical record as carriers and should carry a card verifying the carrier state and precautions to be observed.

A high-carbohydrate diet may decrease the risk of acute attacks. A high-carbohydrate diet or a lump of sugar every hour may help relieve symptoms of an acute attack. Prolonged use should be avoided in order to decrease risk of obesity and dental caries.

Patients who experience recurrent and predictable attacks (typically women with attacks related to the menstrual cycle) may benefit from p-pills or prophylactic heme therapy given shortly before the expected onset. There is no standardized regimen; a specialist should be consulted. Frequent premenstrual attacks in some women are aborted by administration of a gonadotropin-releasing hormone analog plus low-dose estrogen. Oral contraceptives are sometimes used successfully, but the progestin component is likely to exacerbate the porphyria.

CUTANEOUS PORPHYRIAS

Cutaneous porphyrias tend to present as undulating or unremitting disease with a relatively steady production of phototoxic porphyrins in the liver or bone marrow. These porphyrins accumulate in the skin and, on sunlight exposure (visible light, including near-ultraviolet [UV], but not UV), generate cytotoxic radicals that produce cutaneous manifestations.

Cutaneous porphyrias include porphyria cutanea tarda, erythropoietic protoporphyria (EPP), and the extremely rare hepatoerythropoietic porphyria and congenital erythropoietic porphyria (see TABLE 155–5). The acute porphyrias variegate porphyria and hereditary coproporphyria also have cutaneous manifestations.

In all cutaneous porphyrias except EPP, cutaneous photosensitivity presents as fragile skin and bullous eruptions. Skin changes generally occur on sun-exposed areas (eg, face, neck, dorsal sides of fingers and hands) or traumatized skin. The cutaneous reaction is insidious, and often patients are unaware of the connection to sun exposure. In contrast, the photosensitivity in EPP occurs within minutes or hours after sun exposure, presenting as a burning pain that persists for hours, often without any objective signs on the skin.

PORPHYRIA CUTANEA TARDA

Porphyria cutanea tarda is a relatively common porphyria affecting mainly the skin. Iron plays a key role in pathogenesis. Symptoms include fragile skin and blisters on sun-exposed skin or as bruised area. Patients have an increased incidence of liver disease. Triggers include excessive sun exposure, alcohol, estrogens, hepatitis C infection, and possibly HIV infection; however, drugs, with the exceptions of iron and estrogens, are not triggers. Diagnosis is by plasma fluorescence or by porphyrin analysis in urine and stool. Treatment includes iron depletion by phlebotomy, chloroquine, and forced porphyrin excretion by treatment

TABLE 155–5. SOME LESS COMMON PORPHYRIAS

TYPE AND DESCRIPTION	SYMPTOMS AND SIGNS	DIAGNOSIS	TREATMENT
Congenital erythropoietic porphyria (Günther disease)—*deficiency of uroporphyrinogen III cosynthase*	In utero or shortly after birth: Severe cases present as nonimmune hydrops Soon after birth: skin blistering, anemia, red urine In adulthood: corneal scarring (possibly severe), hemolytic anemia, splenomegaly, erythrodontia, deposition of porphyrins in bone, bone demineralization (possibly substantial)	Porphyrins in plasma, urine, and stool usually elevated to levels higher than in other porphyrias Urinary ALA and PBG normal Low RBC uroporphyrinogen cosynthase activity confirms diagnosis For in utero diagnosis, confirm increased amniotic porphyrins	Avoid sunlight (including lights for treating neonatal hyperbilirubinemia) and/or wear sun-protective clothing Avoid skin trauma Prompt treatment of secondary bacterial infections helps prevent scarring Splenectomy may improve hemolytic anemia RBC transfusions can decrease porphyrin production Bone marrow transplantation
Hepatoerythropoietic porphyria—*deficiency of uroporphyrinogen decarboxylase*	Skin blistering Red urine Anemia	Elevated isocoproporphyrin in urine or stool Elevated zinc protoporphyrin in RBCs (to differentiate from PCT)	Phlebotomy may benefit milder cases Severe case treatment similar to that of congenital erythropoietic porphyria
Dual porphyria—*disorders resulting from deficiencies of more than 1 enzyme of the heme biosynthetic pathway*	In people with deficiencies of PBG deaminase and protoporphyrinogen oxidase or uroporphyrinogen decarboxylase: Symptoms are those of acute porphyria, cutaneous porphyria, or both	Elevated isocoproporphyrins in urine and stool, sometimes increased ALA and PBG in urine	Avoid agents that may precipitate symptoms of PCT or acute porphyria Treat acute neurovisceral symptoms (see text)

ALA = δ-aminolevulinic acid; PBG = porphobilinogen; PCT = porphyria cutanea tarda.

with hydroxychloroquine. Prevention is by avoidance of sunlight, alcohol, and iron-containing drugs.

Etiology and Pathophysiology

Porphyria cutanea tarda (PCT) results from a genetic deficiency of uroporphyrinogen decarboxylase (UPGD; see TABLE 155–1). Porphyrins accumulate in the liver and are transported to the skin, where they cause photosensitivity. The 50% decrease in UPGD activity in heterozygous patients is insufficient to cause clinical PCT. Other factors must further impair enzyme activity. Iron plays a central role, probably by generating oxygen radicals that inhibit UPGD by oxidizing its substrate; thus, hemochromatosis is a significant risk factor. Alcohol, estrogens, and chronic viral infection probably contribute in different ways by increasing iron activity in hepatic tissue. The drugs that commonly trigger acute porphyria (see TABLE 155–4) do not trigger PCT.

Liver disease is common in PCT and may be due partly to porphyrin accumulation, chronic hepatitis C infection, concomitant hemosiderosis, or excess alcohol. Cirrhosis occurs in ≤35% of patients and hepatocellular carcinoma in 7 to 24% (more common in middle-aged men).

The 2 major forms of the disease, types 1 and 2, have similar incidence, precipitants, symptoms, and treatment. Other less common forms also occur. Overall prevalence is about 1/10,000.

In type 1 PCT (sporadic), decarboxylase deficiency is restricted to the liver. It usually presents in middle age or later.

In type 2 PCT (familial), decarboxylase deficiency is inherited in an autosomal dominant fashion with limited penetrance. Deficiency occurs in all cells, including RBCs. It presents earlier than type 1, sometimes in childhood.

Secondary PCT-like conditions (pseudoporphyria) may occur with certain photosensitizing drugs (eg, furosemide, tetracyclines, validiric acid, sulfonamides, some NSAIDs). Because porphyrins are poorly dialyzed, some patients receiving long-term hemodialysis develop a skin condition that resembles PCT (pseudoporphyria of end-stage renal disease).

Symptoms and Signs

The patient presents with fragile skin, mainly on sun-exposed areas. Phototoxicity is delayed: the patient does not always connect sun exposure with symptoms.

Spontaneously or after minor trauma, tense bullae develop. Accompanying erosions and ulcers may develop secondary infection; they heal slowly, leaving atrophic scars. Sun exposure occasionally leads to erythema, edema, or itching. Hyperemic conjunctivitis may develop, but other mucosal sites are not affected. Areas of hypopigmentation or hyperpigmentation may develop, as may facial hypertrichosis and pseudosclerodermoid changes.

Diagnosis

In an otherwise healthy patient, fragile skin and blister formation suggest PCT. Differentiation from acute porphyrias with cutaneous symptoms (variegate porphyria [VP] and hereditary coproporphyria [HCP]) is important, because in patients with VP and HCP, porphyrinogenic drugs may cause neurovisceral symptoms. Previous neurologic, mental, or unexplained abdominal symptoms may suggest an acute porphyria. A history of exposure to chemicals that can cause pseudoporphyria should be sought.

Although all porphyrias that cause skin lesions produce elevated plasma porphyrins, elevated urinary uroporphyrin and heptacarboxyl porphyrin, and fecal isocoproporphyrin indicate PCT. Urinary concentration of porphyrin precursor porphobilinogen (PBG) and, usually, δ-aminolevulinic acid (ALA) is normal in PCT. RBC activity of UPGD is normal in type 1 PCT but decreased in type 2.

Because concurrent hepatitis C infection is common and may be asymptomatic, serum markers for hepatitis C (see p. 226) should be obtained.

Treatment and Prevention

Two different therapeutic strategies are available: reduction of body iron stores and increase in porphyrin excretion. These strategies can be combined.

Iron removal by phlebotomy is usually effective. A pint of blood is removed q 1 to 2 wk. When serum ferritin falls slightly below normal, phlebotomy is stopped. Usually, only 5 to 6 sessions are needed. Urine and plasma porphyrins fall gradually with treatment, lagging behind but paralleling the fall in ferritin. The skin eventually becomes normal. After remission, further phlebotomy is needed only if there is a recurrence.

Low-dose chloroquine or hydroxychloroquine (100 to 125 mg po twice/wk) removes excess porphyrins from the liver by increasing the excretion rate. Higher doses can cause transient liver damage and worsening of porphyria. When remission is achieved, the regimen is stopped.

Chloroquine and hydroxychloroquine are not effective in advanced renal disease. Phlebotomy is usually contraindicated because of underlying anemia. However, recombinant erythropoietin mobilizes excess iron and resolves the anemia enough to permit phlebotomy.

Patients should avoid sun exposure; hats and clothing protect best, as do zinc or titanium oxide sunscreens. Typical sunscreens that block UV light are ineffective, but UVA-absorbing sunscreens, such as those containing dibenzylmethanes, may help somewhat. Alcohol ingestion should be avoided permanently, but estrogen therapy can usually be resumed safely after a disease remission.

Erythropoietic Protoporphyria

EPP typically presents in infancy with burning skin pain after even short exposure to sunlight. Gallstones are common later in

life, and acute liver failure occurs in about 10%. Diagnosis is based on symptoms and increased levels of protoporphyrin in RBCs and plasma. Treatment is with β-carotene and avoidance of sunlight.

Etiology and Pathophysiology

EPP results from deficiency of the enzyme ferrochelatase in erythroid tissue. Phototoxic protoporphyrins accumulate in bone marrow and erythrocytes, enter the plasma, and are deposited in the skin or excreted by the liver into bile and stool. Heavy biliary protoporphyrin excretion can produce gallstones. These cytotoxic molecules sometimes damage the hepatobiliary tract, resulting in hepatic protoporphyrin accumulation that leads to acute liver failure; liver failure may become clinically acute within days.

Inheritance is autosomal dominant, but clinical manifestations occur only in people who possess both the defective EPP gene and an unusual low-output (but otherwise normal) allele from the healthy parent. Clinical prevalence is about 5/million.

Symptoms and Signs

Severity varies greatly, even among patients within a single family. Usually, an infant or young child with EPP cries for hours after short exposure to sun. However, because cutaneous signs are usually absent and the child cannot describe his symptoms, EPP often goes undiagnosed.

If unrecognized, EPP causes psychosocial problems because the child inexplicably refuses to go outdoors. The pain may be so distressing that it produces nervousness, tenseness, aggressiveness, or even feelings of detachment from the surroundings or suicidal thoughts.

In childhood, crusting may develop around the lips and on the back of the hands after prolonged sun exposure. Blistering and scarring do not occur. If skin protection is neglected chronically, rough, thickened, and leathery skin may develop, especially over the knuckles. Linear perioral furrows (carp mouth) may develop.

Biliary excretion of large amounts of protoporphyrin can produce cholestasis that progresses to nodular cirrhosis and acute liver failure in ≤ 10% of patients; symptoms include jaundice, malaise, upper abdominal pain, and tender hepatic enlargement.

Diagnosis

EPP should be suspected in children and adults with painful cutaneous photosensitivity who experience no blisters or scarring. Family history is usually negative. The diagnosis is confirmed by finding increased RBC and plasma protoporphyrin concentrations. A genetic marker for susceptibility to cholestatic complications has been identified.

Screening of potential carriers among relatives is by demonstrating increased RBC protoporphyrin contents and decreased ferrochelatase activity (assayed in lymphocytes) or by genetic testing if the mutation has been identified in the index case. Susceptibility for cutaneous disease in carriers is indicated by finding the low-output ferrochelatase allele.

Treatment and Prevention

Acute symptoms are alleviated by cold baths or wet towels and analgesics. Regular physician-patient consultations that provide information, discussion, and opportunities for genetic counseling together with physical checkups are important.

Patients should avoid sun exposure; opaque titanium dioxide or zinc oxide sunscreens are beneficial, and UVA-absorbing sunscreens, such as those containing dibenzylmethanes, may help somewhat. The patient should avoid alcohol and fasting, both of which increase the rate of RBC production and thus the protoporphyrin load. Drugs that trigger acute porphyrias (see TABLE 155–4) need not be avoided.

β-Carotene 120 to 180 mg po once/day in children or 300 mg once/day in adults produces a slightly yellow protective coloration of the skin and neutralizes the toxic radicals in the skin that cause symptoms. Another antioxidant, cysteine, may also lessen photosensitivity. The brown protective skin color obtained with topically applied dihydroxyacetone-3 is generally cosmetically preferable to the yellowish tint produced by β-carotene.

If the above measures are ineffective (eg, increasing photosensitivity, rising porphyrin concentrations, progressive jaundice), erythrocyte hypertransfusion (ie, to above-normal Hb levels) can reduce the production rate of porphyrin-loaded RBCs. Administration of bile acids facilitates biliary excretion of protoporphyrin. Oral cholestyramine or charcoal can interrupt the enterohepatic circulation, which increases fecal excretion. Liver failure may require immediate liver transplant.

156 FLUID AND ELECTROLYTE METABOLISM

Body fluid volume and electrolyte concentration are normally maintained within very narrow limits despite wide variations in dietary intake, metabolic activity, and environmental stresses. Homeostasis of body fluids is preserved primarily by the kidneys.

WATER AND SODIUM BALANCE

Water and Na balance are closely interdependent. Total body water (TBW) is about 60% of body weight (ranging from about 50% in obese people to 70% in lean people). Almost $\frac{2}{3}$ of TBW is in the intracellular compartment (intracellular fluid, or ICF); the other $\frac{1}{3}$ is extracellular (extracellular fluid, or ECF). Normally, about 25% of the ECF is in the intravascular compartment; the other 75% is interstitial fluid. FIG. 156–1 depicts the distribution of TBW.

The major intracellular cation is K, with an average concentration of 140 mEq/L. The extracellular K concentration is 3.5 to 5 mEq/L. The major extracellular cation is Na, with an average concentration of 140 mEq/L and an intracellular Na concentration of 12 mEq/L.

The concentration of combined solutes in water is osmolarity, which, in body fluids, is similar to osmolality. Serum osmolality can be measured in the laboratory or estimated according to the formula

$$\text{Plasma osmolality (mOsm/kg)} = 2[\text{serum Na}] + \frac{[\text{Glucose}]}{18} + \frac{[\text{BUN}]}{2.8}$$

where serum Na is expressed in mEq/L and glucose and BUN are expressed in mg/dL. Osmolality of body fluids is normally between 275 and 290 mOsm/kg. Na is the major determinant of serum osmolality. Apparent changes in osmolality may result from errors in the measurement of Na with electrodes that are not ion-sensitive (see Diagnosis under Hyponatremia on p. 1240). If measured osmolality exceeds estimated osmolality by ≥ 10 mOsm/L, then unmeasured osmotically active substances are probably present in the plasma (osmolar gap). The most common are alcohols (ethanol, methanol, isopropanol, ethylene glycol), mannitol, and glycine.

Water crosses cell membranes freely from areas of low solute concentration to areas of high solute concentration. Thus, osmolality tends to equalize across the various body fluid compartments, resulting primarily from movement of water, not solutes. Solutes such as urea that freely diffuse across cell membranes have little or no effect on water shifts (little or no osmotic activity), whereas solutes that are restricted to one fluid compartment, such as Na and K, have the greatest osmotic activity. Tonicity, or effective osmolality, reflects osmotic activity and determines the force drawing water across fluid compartments (the osmotic force). Osmotic force can be opposed by other forces. For example, plasma proteins have a small osmotic effect that tends to draw water into the plasma; this is normally counteracted by vascular hydrostatic forces that drive water out of the plasma.

The average daily fluid intake is about 2.5 L. The amount needed to replace losses from the urine and other sources is about 1 to 1.5 L/day in healthy adults. However, an average young adult with normal kidney function may ingest as little as 200 mL of water each day to excrete the nitrogenous and other wastes generated by cellular metabolism on a short-term basis. More is needed in people with any loss of renal concentrating ability (ie, the elderly; those with diabetes insipidus, certain renal diseases, hypercalcemia, severe salt restriction, chronic overhydration or hyperkalemia; and those ingesting ethanol, phenytoin, lithium, demeclocycline, or amphotericin B) and those with osmotic diuresis (eg, due to high protein diets or hyperglycemia).

Other obligatory water losses are mostly insensible losses from the lungs and skin, averaging about 0.4 to 0.5 mL/kg/h body weight or about 650 to 850 mL/day in a 70-kg adult. With fever, another 50 to 75 mL/day may be lost for each degree C of temperature elevation above normal. GI losses are usually negligible, except with marked vomiting, diarrhea, or both. Sweat losses can be significant with environmental heat.

Water intake is regulated by thirst. Thirst is triggered by receptors in the anterolateral

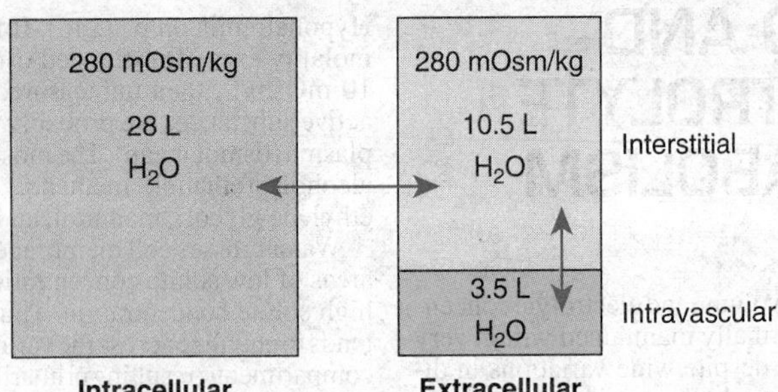

Fig. 156–1. Fluid compartments in an average 70-kg man. Total body water = 70 kg × 0.60 = 42 L.

hypothalamus that respond to increased plasma osmolality (as little as 2%) or decreased body fluid volume. Hypothalamic dysfunction decreases the capacity for thirst.

Water excretion is regulated primarily by arginine vasopressin, also known as ADH. ADH is released by the posterior pituitary and results in increased water reabsorption in the distal nephron. ADH release is stimulated by increased plasma osmolality, decreased blood volume, decreased BP, or stress. ADH release may be impaired by certain drugs (eg, ethanol, phenytoin) and diabetes insipidus (see p. 1189).

Maximum daily fluid intake can be as much as 25 L. Greater amounts exceed the diluting capacity of the kidneys and quickly lower plasma osmolality.

DISORDERS OF FLUID VOLUME

Because Na is the major osmotically active ion in the ECF, total body Na content determines ECF volume. Deficiency or excess of total body Na content causes ECF volume depletion or overload. Serum Na concentration does not necessarily reflect total body Na.

Dietary intake and renal excretion regulate total body Na content. When total Na content and ECF volume are low, the kidneys increase Na conservation. When total Na content and ECF volume are high, Na excretion (natriuresis) increases so that volume decreases.

Renal Na excretion can be adjusted widely to match Na intake. Renal Na excretion requires delivery of Na to the kidney and so depends on renal blood flow and GFR. Thus, inadequate Na excretion may be secondary to decreased renal blood flow, as in renal disease or heart failure.

The renin-angiotensin-aldosterone axis is the main regulatory mechanism of renal Na excretion. In volume-depleted states, GFR and Na delivery to the distal nephron decrease, causing release of renin. Renin cleaves angiotensinogen (renin substrate) to form angiotensin I. ACE then cleaves angiotensin I to angiotensin II. Angiotensin II increases Na retention by decreasing the filtered load of Na and enhancing proximal tubular Na reabsorption. Angiotensin II also stimulates the adrenal cortex to secrete aldosterone, which increases Na reabsorption via multiple renal mechanisms. Angiotensin I can also be transformed to angiotensin III, which stimulates aldosterone release as much as angiotensin II but has much less pressor activity. Aldosterone release is also stimulated by hyperkalemia. Several natriuretic factors have been identified, including atrial natriuretic peptide (ANP), brain natriuretic peptide (BNP), and a C-type natriuretic peptide (CNP).

ANP, in cardiac atrial tissue, increases in response to ECF volume overload (eg, heart failure, renal disease, cirrhosis with ascites) and primary aldosteronism and in some patients with essential hypertension. Decreases have occurred in some patients with nephrotic syndrome and presumed ECF volume contraction. High levels increase Na excretion and increase GFR even if BP is low.

BNP is synthesized mainly in the atria and left ventricle and has similar triggers and effects to ANP. BNP assays are available, and high BNP level is used to diagnose volume overload. CNP, in contrast to ANP and BNP, is primarily vasodilatory.

Na depletion requires inadequate Na intake plus abnormal losses from the skin, GI tract, or kidney (defective renal Na conservation). Defective renal Na conservation may be caused by primary renal disease, adrenal insufficiency, or diuretic therapy. Na overload requires higher Na intake than excretion; however, because normal kidneys can excrete large amounts of Na, Na overload generally reflects defective renal Na excretion.

Extracellular Fluid Volume Contraction

ECF volume contraction is a decrease in ECF volume caused by loss of water and total body Na content. Causes include vomiting, sweating, diarrhea, burns, diuretic use, and renal failure. Clinical features include diminished skin turgor, dry mucous membranes, tachycardia, and orthostatic hypotension. Diagnosis is clinical. Treatment involves administration of Na and water.

A decrease in ECF (ECF volume contraction [hypovolemia]) is not the same as a decrease in effective plasma volume. Decreased effective plasma volume may occur with decreased ECF, but it may also occur with an increased ECF (eg, in heart failure, hypoalbuminemia, capillary leak syndrome).

ECF volume contraction usually involves loss of Na; Na loss always causes water loss. Depending on many factors, plasma Na concentration can be high, low, or normal despite the decreased total body Na content. Common causes of ECF volume depletion are listed in TABLE 156–1.

TABLE 156–1. COMMON CAUSES OF EXTRACELLULAR FLUID VOLUME DEPLETION

Extrarenal

Bleeding

Dialysis: Hemodialysis, peritoneal dialysis

GI: Vomiting, diarrhea, nasogastric suction

Skin: Excessive sweating, burns, exfoliation

Third-space losses: Intestinal lumen, intraperitoneal, retroperitoneal

Renal/adrenal

Acute renal failure: Diuretic phase of recovery

Adrenal disease: Addison's disease (glucocorticoid deficiency), hypoaldosteronism

Bartter syndrome

Diabetes mellitus with ketoacidosis or extreme glucosuria

Diuretics

Salt-wasting renal disease (medullary cystic disease, interstitial nephritis, some cases of pyelonephritis and myeloma)

Symptoms and Signs

ECF volume depletion is suspected in patients with a history of inadequate fluid intake (especially in comatose or disoriented patients); increased fluid losses; diuretic therapy; and renal or adrenal disease.

In mild (5%) ECF volume depletion, the only sign may be diminished skin turgor. The patient may complain of thirst. Dry mucous membranes do not always correlate with volume depletion, especially in the elderly or in mouth-breathers. Oliguria is typical. When ECF volume has diminished by 5 to 10%, orthostatic tachycardia, hypotension, or both are generally present, although orthostatic changes can occur in patients without ECF volume depletion, particularly those deconditioned or bedridden. Skin turgor (best assessed at the upper torso) may be decreased. If dehydration exceeds 10%, signs of shock can occur (eg, tachypnea, tachycardia, hypotension, confusion, poor capillary refill).

Diagnosis

Diagnosis is usually clinical. If the cause is obvious and easily correctible (eg, acute gastroenteritis in an otherwise healthy patient), laboratory testing is unnecessary; otherwise, serum electrolytes, BUN, and creatinine are measured. Plasma osmolality and urine Na, creatinine, and osmolality are measured if there is suspicion of clinically meaningful electrolyte abnormality that is not clear from serum tests and for patients with cardiac or renal disease. Invasive monitoring is necessary for patients with previously unstable heart failure or arrhythmias.

Central venous pressure and pulmonary artery occlusion pressure are decreased in ECF volume depletion, but measurement is rarely required.

During ECF volume depletion, normally functioning kidneys conserve Na. Thus, the urine Na concentration is usually < 15 mEq/L; the fractional excretion of Na (urine Na/serum Na divided by urine creatinine/serum creatinine) is usually < 1%; also, urine osmo-

TABLE 156–2. PRINCIPAL CAUSES OF EXTRACELLULAR FLUID VOLUME OVERLOAD

Renal Na retention
Cirrhosis
Drugs: Minoxidil, NSAIDs, estrogens, fludrocortisone
Heart failure, including cor pulmonale
Pregnancy and premenstrual edema
Renal disease, especially nephrotic syndrome
Decreased plasma oncotic pressure
Nephrotic syndrome
Protein-losing enteropathy
Reduced albumin synthesis (liver disease, malnutrition)
Increased capillary permeability
Acute respiratory distress syndrome
Angioedema
Burns, trauma
Idiopathic edema
IL-2 therapy
Sepsis syndrome
Iatrogenic
Administration of excess Na (eg, 0.9% normal saline IV)

lality is often > 450 mOsm/kg. If metabolic alkalosis is combined with ECF volume depletion, urine Na concentration may be high; in this instance, a urine Cl concentration of < 10 mEq/L more reliably indicates ECF volume depletion. Misleadingly high urinary Na (generally > 20 mEq/L) or low urine osmolality can also occur due to renal Na losses resulting from renal disease, diuretics, or adrenal insufficiency. ECF volume depletion frequently increases the BUN and plasma creatinine levels with the ratio of BUN to creatinine often > 20:1. Values such as Hct often increase in volume depletion but are difficult to interpret unless baseline values are known.

Treatment

The cause of volume depletion is corrected and fluids are given to replace existing volume deficits as well as any ongoing fluid losses and to provide daily fluid requirements. Mild-to-moderate volume deficits may be replaced by increased oral intake of Na and water if the patient is conscious and is not vomiting severely. When volume deficits are severe or when oral hydration is impractical, IV 0.9% saline is given. Typical IV regimens are presented on p. 564; oral regimens, on p. 2293.

Extracellular Fluid Volume Expansion

ECF volume expansion is caused by an increase in total body Na content. It typically occurs in heart failure, nephrotic syndrome, and cirrhosis. Clinical features include weight gain, edema, and orthopnea. Diagnosis is clinical. Treatment aims to correct volume expansion and its cause.

An increase in total body Na is the key pathophysiologic event. It increases osmolality, which triggers compensatory mechanisms that produce water retention.

Movement of fluid between interstitial and intravascular spaces depends on Starling's forces at the capillaries. Increased capillary hydrostatic pressure, as occurs in heart failure; decreased plasma oncotic pressure, as occurs in nephrotic syndrome; or a combination, as occurs in severe cirrhosis, shifts fluid into the interstitial space, producing edema. In these conditions, subsequent intravascular volume depletion increases renal Na retention, which maintains fluid overload. Common causes of volume overload are listed in TABLE 156–2.

Symptoms and Signs

Weight gain and weakness may occur before edema formation. Dyspnea on exertion, decreased exercise tolerance, tachypnea, orthopnea, and paroxysmal nocturnal dyspnea can also occur early when volume overload is caused by left ventricular dysfunction. Elevated jugular venous pressure may produce jugular venous distention.

Early symptoms of edema may include puffy eyes on rising in the morning and tight shoes at the end of the day. Edema is often dependent in heart failure. In ambulatory patients, edema is in the feet and lower legs; patients at bed rest develop edema on the buttocks, genitals, and posterior thighs; women who lie on only one side may develop edema in the dependent breast. Edema can be accompanied by myriad findings, including pulmonary rales, elevated central venous pressure, an S_3 gallop, and an enlarged heart with pulmonary edema and/or pleural effusions on chest x-ray. In cirrhosis, edema is frequently confined to the lower extremities and accompanied by ascites. Other signs of cirrhosis include spider angiomas, gynecomastia, palmar erythema, and testicular atrophy. In nephrotic syndrome, edema is often diffuse, occasionally with generalized anasarca, pleural effusions, and ascites; periorbital edema occurs frequently, but not invariably.

Diagnosis

Symptoms and signs, including dependent edema, are usually diagnostic. Physical findings may suggest a cause. For instance, edema plus ascites suggests cirrhosis. Rales and S_3 suggest heart failure. Generally, diagnostic testing includes serum electrolytes, BUN, creatinine, and any other tests directed at the cause (eg, chest x-ray for suspected heart failure). Causes of isolated lower extremity swelling (eg, lymphedema, venous stasis, venous obstruction, local trauma) should be excluded.

Treatment

In patients with heart failure, maximizing left ventricular function (eg, by using inotropic agents or afterload reduction) can increase Na delivery to the kidneys and Na excretion. Treatment of the causes of nephrotic syndrome depends on the specific renal histopathology.

Loop diuretics, such as furosemide, inhibit Na reabsorption in the ascending limb of the loop of Henle. Thiazide diuretics inhibit Na reabsorption in the distal tubule. Both loop diuretics and thiazide diuretics increase excretion of Na and thus water. K wasting can be problematic in some patients; K-sparing diuretics, such as amiloride, triamterene, and spironolactone, inhibit Na reabsorption in the distal nephron and collecting duct. When used alone, they increase Na excretion, but only modestly. Both triamterene and amiloride have been combined with a thiazide to prevent K wasting.

Many patients respond insufficiently to diuretics; common contributing factors include inadequate treatment of the cause of volume overload, noncompliance with dietary Na restriction, hypovolemia, and renal disease. Diuresis can frequently be achieved by increasing the dose of a loop diuretic or combining it with a thiazide.

After correction of volume overload, maintenance of euvolemia may require restriction of dietary Na unless the underlying condition can be eliminated. Diets containing 3 to 4 g/day Na are generally adequate, are fairly well tolerated, and work reasonably well in mild-to-moderate volume overload diets for heart failure. Advanced cirrhosis and nephrotic syndrome often require more severe Na restriction (≤ 1 g/day). K salts are often substituted for Na salts to make Na restriction tolerable; however, care should be taken, especially in patients receiving K-sparing diuretics or ACE inhibitors and in those with renal disease, because potentially fatal hyperkalemia can result.

HYPONATREMIA

Hyponatremia is decrease in plasma Na concentration < 136 mEq/L caused by an excess of water relative to solute. Common causes include diuretic use, diarrhea, heart failure, and renal disease. Clinical manifestations are primarily neurologic (due to an osmotic shift of water into cells), especially in acute hyponatremia, and include headache, confusion, and stupor; seizures and coma may occur. Diagnosis is by measuring plasma Na; plasma and urine electrolytes and osmolality help determine the cause. Treatment involves restricting water intake and promoting its loss, replacing any Na deficit, and treating the cause.

Etiology and Pathophysiology

Hyponatremia reflects an excess of total body water (TBW) relative to total body Na content. Because total body Na content is reflected by ECF volume status, hyponatremia must be considered along with fluid status: hypovolemia, euvolemia, and hypervolemia (see TABLE 156–3).

Hypovolemic hyponatremia: Deficiencies in both TBW and total body Na exist, although proportionally more Na than water has been lost; the Na deficit produces hypovolemia. Hyponatremia can occur when fluid losses, such as those that occur with the losses of Na-containing fluids as in protracted vomiting, severe diarrhea, or sequestration of fluids in a 3rd space (see TABLE 156–4), are replaced with ingestion of free water or treated with hypotonic IV fluid. Significant ECF fluid losses also cause release of ADH, causing water retention by the kidneys, which can maintain or worsen hyponatremia. In extrarenal causes of hypovolemia, because the normal renal response to volume loss is Na conservation, urine Na concentration is typically < 10 mEq/L.

TABLE 156–3. PRINCIPAL CAUSES OF HYPONATREMIA

Hyponatremia with hypovolemia
(decreased TBW and Na; relatively greater decrease in Na)

Extrarenal losses
- GI: Vomiting, diarrhea
- Third-space losses: Pancreatitis, peritonitis, small-bowel obstruction, rhabdomyolysis, burns

Renal losses
- Diuretics
- Mineralocorticoid deficiency
- Osmotic diuresis (glucose, urea, mannitol)
- Salt-losing nephropathies

Hyponatremia with euvolemia (increased TBW; near-normal total body Na)

Diuretics
Glucocorticoid deficiency
Hypothyroidism
Primary polydipsia
States that increase release of ADH (postoperative opioids, pain, emotional stress)
Syndrome of inappropriate ADH secretion

Hyponatremia with hypervolemia
(increased total body Na; relatively greater increase in TBW)

Extrarenal disorders
- Cirrhosis
- Heart failure

Renal disorders
- Acute renal failure
- Chronic renal failure
- Nephrotic syndrome

TBW = total body water.

Renal fluid losses resulting in hypovolemic hyponatremia may occur with mineralocorticoid deficiency, diuretic therapy, osmotic diuresis, or salt-losing nephropathy. Salt-losing nephropathy encompasses a loosely defined group of intrinsic renal diseases with primarily renal tubular dysfunction. This group includes interstitial nephritis, medullary cystic disease, partial urinary tract obstruction, and, occasionally, polycystic kidney disease. Renal causes of hypovolemic hyponatremia can usually be differentiated from extrarenal causes by the history. Patients with ongoing renal fluid losses can also be distinguished from those with extrarenal fluid losses by inappropriately high urine Na concentration (> 20 mEq/L). An exception occurs with metabolic alkalosis (as occurs with protracted vomiting) where large amounts of HCO_3 are spilled in the urine, obligating the excretion of Na to maintain electrical neutrality. In metabolic alkalosis, urine Cl concentration frequently differentiates renal from extrarenal sources of volume depletion (see p. 1270).

Diuretics may also produce hypovolemic hyponatremia. Thiazide diuretics, in particular, affect the kidneys' diluting ability while increasing Na excretion. Once volume depletion occurs, the nonosmotic release of ADH causes water retention and worsens hyponatremia. Concomitant hypokalemia shifts Na intracellularly and enhances ADH release, thereby worsening hyponatremia. This effect of thiazides may last for up to 2 wk after cessation of therapy; however, hyponatremia usually responds to replacement of K and volume deficits along with judicious restriction of water intake until the drug effect dissipates. Elderly patients are especially susceptible to thiazide-induced hyponatremia, particularly if a preexisting defect in renal water excretion exists. Rarely, such patients develop severe, life-threatening hyponatremia within a few weeks after the initiation of a thiazide diuretic resulting from an exaggerated natriuresis and underlying impaired urinary diluting capacity. Loop diuretics much less commonly cause hyponatremia.

Euvolemic hyponatremia: In euvolemic hyponatremia, total body Na and thus ECF volume are normal; however, TBW is increased. Primary polydipsia can cause hy-

TABLE 156–4. COMPOSITION OF FLUIDS LOST

Fluid	(mEq/L) Na	K	Cl
Gastric	20–80	5–20	100–150
Pancreatic	120–140	5–15	90–120
Small bowel	100–140	5–15	90–130
Bile	120–140	5–15	80–120
Ileostomy	45–135	3–15	20–115
Diarrheal	10–90	10–80	10–110
Sweat	10–30	3–10	10–35
Burns	140	5	110

From: http://www.vnh.org/PediatricEmergencyManual/Electrolyte.html

TABLE 156–5. DISORDERS ASSOCIATED WITH SYNDROME OF INAPPROPRIATE ANTIDIURETIC HORMONE SECRETION

Malignancy	Brain abscess
CNS	Encephalitis
Duodenum	Guillain-Barré syndrome
Lung	Head trauma
Lymphoma	Meningitis
Pancreas	Stroke
Pulmonary disorders	Subdural or subarachnoid hemorrhage
Aspergillosis	**Endocrine disorders**
Lung abscess	Addison's disease
Pneumonia	Hypopituitarism
Positive-pressure breathing	Hypothyroidism
TB	**Miscellaneous causes**
CNS disorders	Protein-energy malnutrition
Acute intermittent porphyria	Surgery
Acute psychosis	

ponatremia only when water intake overwhelms the kidneys' ability to excrete water. Because normal kidneys can excrete up to 25 L urine/day, hyponatremia due solely to polydipsia results only from the ingestion of large amounts of water or from defects in renal diluting ability. Patients affected include those with psychosis or more modest degrees of polydipsia plus renal insufficiency. Dilutional hyponatremia may also result from excessive water intake without Na retention in the presence of Addison's disease, myxedema, or nonosmotic ADH secretion (eg, stress; postoperative states; use of drugs such as chlorpropamide or tolbutamide, opioids, barbiturates, vincristine, clofibrate, carbamazepine). Postoperative hyponatremia occurs because of a combination of nonosmotic ADH release and excessive administration of hypotonic fluids after surgery. Certain drugs (eg, cyclophosphamide, NSAIDs, chlorpropamide) potentiate the renal effect of endogenous ADH, whereas others (eg, oxytocin) have a direct ADH-like effect on the kidney. A deficiency in water excretion is common in all these conditions.

Syndrome of inappropriate ADH secretion (SIADH) is attributed to excessive ADH release. It is defined as less than maximally dilute urine in the presence of plasma hypoosmolality (hyponatremia) without volume depletion or overload, emotional stress, pain, diuretics or other drugs that stimulate ADH secretion, and with normal cardiac, hepatic, renal, adrenal, and thyroid function. SIADH is associated with myriad disorders (see TABLE 156–5).

Hypervolemic hyponatremia: Hypervolemic hyponatremia is characterized by an increase in both total body Na (and thus ECF volume) and TBW with a relatively greater increase in TBW. Various edematous disorders, including heart failure and cirrhosis, cause hypervolemic hyponatremia. Rarely, hyponatremia occurs in nephrotic syndrome, although pseudohyponatremia may be due to interference with Na measurement by elevated lipids. In each of these disorders, a decrease in effective circulating volume results in the release of ADH and angiotensin II. Hyponatremia results from the antidiuretic effect of ADH on the kidney as well as the direct impairment of renal water excretion by angiotensin II. Decreased GFR and stimulation of thirst by angiotensin II also potentiate the development of hyponatremia. Urine Na excretion is usually < 10 mEq/L and urine osmolality is high relative to plasma osmolality.

Hyponatremia in AIDS: Hyponatremia has been reported in > 50% of hospitalized patients with AIDS. Among the many potential contributing factors are administration of hypotonic fluids, impaired renal function, nonosmotic ADH release due to intravascular volume depletion, and administration of drugs that impair renal water excretion. In addition, adrenal insufficiency has become increasingly common in AIDS patients as the result of cytomegalovirus adrenalitis, mycobacterial infection, or interference with adrenal glucocorticoid and mineralocorticoid synthesis by ketoconazole. SIADH may be present because of coexistent pulmonary or CNS infections.

Symptoms and Signs

Symptoms mainly involve CNS dysfunction. However, when hyponatremia is accompanied by disturbances in total body Na content, signs of volume depletion or overload also occur (see p. 1236). The degree of hyponatremia, the rapidity with which it develops, its cause, and the patient's age and overall condition determine symptom severity. In general, older chronically ill patients with hyponatremia develop more symptoms than younger otherwise healthy patients. Symptoms are also more severe with faster-onset hyponatremia. Symptoms generally occur when the effective plasma osmolality falls to < 240 mOsm/kg. Symptoms can be subtle and consist mainly of changes in mental status, including altered personality, lethargy, and confusion. As the plasma Na falls below 115 mEq/L, stupor, neuromuscular hyperexcitability, seizures, coma, and death can result. Severe cerebral edema may occur in premenopausal women with acute hyponatremia, perhaps because estrogen and progesterone inhibit brain Na^+,K^+-ATPase and decrease solute extrusion from brain cells. Sequelae include hypothalamic and posterior pituitary infarction and occasionally brain stem herniation.

Diagnosis

Hyponatremia is diagnosed by measuring serum electrolytes. However, serum Na may be artifactually low when severe hyperglycemia increases osmolality. Water moves out of cells into the ECF. Serum Na concentration falls about 1.6 mEq/L for every 100-mg/dL (5.55-mmol/L) rise in the plasma glucose level above normal. This condition is called translational hyponatremia because no net change in the amount of TBW or Na has occurred. Pseudohyponatremia with normal plasma osmolality may occur in hyperlipidemia or extreme hyperproteinemia, because the lipid or protein occupies space in the volume of plasma taken for analysis. Newer methods of measuring plasma electrolytes with ion-selective electrodes circumvent this problem.

Determining the cause of hyponatremia can be complex. The history sometimes suggests a cause (eg, significant fluid loss from vomiting or diarrhea, renal disease, compulsive fluid ingestion, intake of drugs that stimulate ADH release or enhance ADH action).

The patient's volume status, particularly the presence of obvious volume depletion or overload, suggests certain causes (see TABLES 156–1 and 156–2). Overtly hypovolemic patients usually have an obvious source of fluid loss (typically followed by hypotonic fluid replacement). Overtly hypervolemic patients usually have a readily recognizable condition, such as heart failure or hepatic or renal disease. Euvolemic patients and those with equivocal volume status require more laboratory testing to identify a cause.

Acuity of onset helps determine permissible speed of treatment. Sudden onset of CNS dysfunction suggests acute onset of hyponatremia.

Laboratory tests should include blood and urine osmolality and electrolytes. Euvolemic patients should also have thyroid and adrenal function tested. Hypo-osmolality in an euvolemic patient should cause excretion of a large volume of dilute urine (eg, osmolality < 100 mOsm/kg and specific gravity < 1.003). Serum Na level and serum osmolality that are low and urine osmolality that is inappropriately high (120 to 150 mmol/L) with respect to the low serum osmolality suggest volume overload, volume contraction, or SIADH. Volume overload and volume contraction are differentiated clinically (see pp. 1235 and 1236). If neither appears likely, SIADH is considered. Patients with SIADH are usually normovolemic or slightly hypervolemic. BUN and creatinine values are normal, and serum uric acid is generally low. Urine Na level is usually > 30 mmol/L, and fractional excretion of Na is > 1%.

In a patient with volume contraction, if renal function is normal, Na reabsorption results in a urine Na of < 20 mmol/L. Urine Na > 20 mmol/L in a hypovolemic patient suggests mineralocorticoid deficiency or salt-losing nephropathy. Hyperkalemia suggests adrenal insufficiency.

Treatment

Rapid correction of hyponatremia, even mild hyponatremia, risks neurologic complications (see p. 1241). Generally, Na should be corrected no faster than 0.5 mEq/L/h. Increase should not exceed 10 mEq/L over the first 24 h. Any identified cause of hyponatremia is treated concurrently.

Mild hyponatremia: Mild, asymptomatic hyponatremia (ie, plasma Na > 120 mEq/L) requires restraint. In diuretic-induced hyponatremia, elimination of the diuretic may be enough; some patients need some Na or K replacement. Similarly, if mild hyponatremia results from inappropriate parenteral fluid administration in a patient with impaired water excretion, merely stopping hypotonic fluid therapy may suffice.

With hypovolemia, if adrenal function is normal, administration of 0.9% saline usually corrects both hyponatremia and hypovolemia. If the plasma Na is < 120 mEq/L, it may not completely correct upon restoration of intravascular volume; restriction of free water ingestion to ≤ 500 to 1000 mL/24 h may be needed.

In hypervolemic patients, in whom dilutional hyponatremia is due to renal Na retention (eg, heart failure, cirrhosis, nephrotic syndrome), water restriction combined with treatment of the underlying disorder is often successful. An ACE inhibitor, in conjunction with a loop diuretic, can correct refractory hyponatremia in patients with heart failure. If hyponatremia does not respond to simple fluid restriction, a loop diuretic in escalating doses can be used, sometimes in conjunction with IV 0.9% normal saline. K and other electrolytes lost in the urine must be replaced. If hyponatremia is severe and unresponsive to diuretics, intermittent or continuous hemofiltration may be needed to control ECF volume while hyponatremia is corrected with IV 0.9% normal saline.

In euvolemia, treatment is directed at the cause (eg, hypothyroidism, adrenal insufficiency, diuretic use). If SIADH is present, severe water restriction (eg, 250 to 500 mL/24 h) is required. Additionally, a loop diuretic may be combined with IV 0.9% saline as in hypervolemic hyponatremia. Lasting correction depends on successful treatment of the underlying disease. When the underlying disease is not treatable, as in metastatic lung cancer, and severe water restriction is unacceptable to the patient, demeclocycline (300 to 600 mg q 12 h) may be helpful; however, demeclocycline may cause acute renal failure; renal failure is usually reversible when the drug is stopped. Investigational selective vasopressin receptor antagonists effectively produce water diuresis without significant loss of electrolytes in the urine and may provide useful future treatment for resistant hyponatremia.

Severe hyponatremia: Severe hyponatremia (plasma Na < 109 mEq/L; effective osmolality < 238 mOsm/kg) in asymptomatic patients can be treated safely with stringent restriction of water intake. Treatment is more controversial when neurologic symptoms (eg, confusion, lethargy, seizures, coma) are present. The debate primarily concerns the pace and degree of hyponatremia correction. Many experts recommend that plasma Na be raised no faster than 1 mEq/L/h, but replacement rates of up to 2 mEq/L/h for the first 2 to 3 h have been suggested for patients with seizures. Regardless, the rise should be ≤ 10 mEq/L over the first 24 h. More vigorous correction risks precipitation of osmotic demyelination syndrome (see below).

Hypertonic (3%) saline (containing 513 mEq Na/L) may be used, but only with frequent (q 2 to 4 h) electrolyte determinations. For patients with seizures or coma, ≤ 100 mL/h may be administered over 4 to 6 h in amounts sufficient to raise the serum Na 4 to 6 mEq/L. This amount (in mEq) may be calculated using the Na deficit formula as

$$\text{(Desired change in Na)} \times \text{TBW}$$

where TBW is 0.6 × body weight in kg in men and 0.5 × body weight in kg in women.

For example, the amount of Na needed to raise the Na from 106 to 112 in a 70-kg man can be calculated as follows:

$$(112 \text{ mEq/L} - 106 \text{ mEq/L}) \times (0.6 \text{ L/kg} \times 70 \text{ kg}) = 252 \text{ mEq.}$$

Because there is 513 mEq Na/L in hypertonic saline, roughly 0.5 L of hypertonic saline is needed to raise the Na from 106 to 112 mEq/L. Adjustments may be needed, so plasma Na must be monitored closely, beginning within the first 2 to 3 h after initiation of treatment. Patients with seizures, coma, or altered mental status need supportive treatment, which may involve airway intubation and benzodiazepines (eg, lorazepam 1 to 2 mg IV q 5 to 10 min prn) for seizures.

Osmotic demyelination syndrome: Osmotic demyelination syndrome (previously called central pontine myelinolysis) may follow too-rapid correction of hyponatremia. Demyelination may affect the pons and other areas of the brain. Lesions are more common in patients with alcoholism, malnutrition, or other chronic debilitating illness. Flaccid paralysis, dysarthria, and dysphagia can evolve over a few days or weeks. The lesion may extend dorsally to involve sensory tracts and leave the patient with a locked-in syndrome (an awake and sentient state in which the patient, because of generalized motor paralysis, cannot communicate, except possibly by coded eye movements). Damage often is permanent. If Na is replaced too rapidly (eg, > 14 mEq/L/8 h) and neurologic symptoms start to develop, it is critical to prevent further plasma Na increases by stopping hypertonic fluids. In such cases, inducing hyponatremia with hypotonic fluid may mitigate the development of permanent neurologic damage.

TABLE 156–6. PRINCIPAL CAUSES OF HYPERNATREMIA

Hypernatremia with hypovolemia (decreased TBW and Na; relatively greater decrease in TBW)

- Extrarenal losses
  - GI: Vomiting, diarrhea
  - Skin: Burns, excessive sweating
- Renal losses
  - Intrinsic renal disease
  - Loop diuretics
  - Osmotic diuresis (glucose, urea, mannitol)

Hypernatremia with euvolemia (decreased TBW; near-normal total body Na)

- Extrarenal losses
  - Respiratory: Tachypnea
  - Skin: Fever, excessive sweating
- Renal losses
  - Central diabetes insipidus
  - Nephrogenic diabetes insipidus
- Other
  - Inability to access water
  - Primary hypodipsia
  - Reset osmostat

Hypernatremia with hypervolemia (increased Na; normal or increased TBW)

- Hypertonic fluid administration (hypertonic saline, $NaHCO_3$, total parenteral nutrition)
- Mineralocorticoid excess
  - Adrenal tumors secreting deoxycorticosterone
  - Congenital adrenal hyperplasia (caused by 11-hydroxylase defect)
  - Iatrogenic

TBW = total body water.

HYPERNATREMIA

(For hypernatremia in neonates, see p. 2282.)

Hypernatremia is plasma Na concentration >145 mEq/L caused by a deficit of water relative to solute. A major symptom is thirst; other clinical manifestations are primarily neurologic (due to an osmotic shift of water out of cells), including confusion, neuromuscular excitability, seizures, and coma. Diagnosis is by measuring serum Na. Treatment is usually controlled water replacement. If the response is poor, further testing (eg, monitored water deprivation or administration of ADH) is directed at detecting the underlying cause.

Etiology and Pathophysiology

Hypernatremia in adults has a mortality of 40 to 60%. Hypernatremia usually implies either an impaired thirst mechanism or limited access to water. The severity of the underlying diseases that usually result in an inability to drink and the effects of brain hyperosmolality are thought to be responsible for the high mortality. The elderly are particularly susceptible, especially in warm weather, due to a reduced thirst response and underlying diseases. Common causes of hypernatremia are listed in TABLE 156–6.

Hypernatremia associated with volume depletion occurs with Na loss accompanied by a relatively greater loss of water from the body. Common extrarenal causes include most of those that cause hyponatremia and volume depletion (see p. 1237). Either hypernatremia or hyponatremia can occur with severe volume loss, depending on the relative amounts of Na and water lost and the amount of water ingested before presentation.

Renal causes of hypernatremia and volume depletion include therapy with diuretics. Loop diuretics inhibit Na reabsorption in the concentrating portion of the nephron and can increase water clearance. Osmotic diuresis can also impair renal concentrating ability because of a hypertonic substance present in the tubular lumen of the distal nephron. Glycerol, mannitol, and occasionally urea can cause osmotic diuresis resulting in hypernatremia. Perhaps the most common cause of hypernatremia due to osmotic diuresis is hyperglycemia in diabetic patients. Because glucose does not penetrate cells in the absence of insulin, hyperglycemia further dehydrates the ICF. The degree of hyperosmolality may be obscured by artificial lowering of plasma Na resulting from movement of water out of cells into the ECF (translational hyponatremia—see Hyponatremia on p. 1237). Patients with renal disease can also be predisposed to hypernatremia if their kidneys are unable to maximally concentrate urine.

Hypernatremia with euvolemia is usually a decrease in total body water (TBW) with near-normal total body Na (pure water deficit). Extrarenal causes of water loss, such as excessive sweating, result in some Na loss, but because sweat is hypotonic, hypernatremia can result before significant hypovolemia. A deficit of almost purely water also occurs in central or nephrogenic diabetes insipidus.

Essential hypernatremia (primary hypodipsia) occasionally occurs in children with brain damage and in chronically ill elderly adults. It is characterized by an impaired thirst mechanism, altered osmotic trigger for ADH release, or both. The nonosmotic release of ADH appears intact, and these patients are generally euvolemic.

Hypernatremia in rare cases is associated with volume overload. In this case, hypernatremia results from a grossly elevated Na intake associated with limited access to water. One example is the excessive administration of hypertonic $NaHCO_3$ during CPR or during treatment of lactic acidosis. Hypernatremia can also be caused by the administration of hypertonic saline or hyperalimentation.

Hypernatremia is particularly common in the elderly. Reasons include difficulty obtaining water, impaired thirst mechanism, impaired renal concentrating ability (due to diuretics or nephron loss accompanying aging or other renal disease), and increased insensible losses. In the elderly, ADH release is enhanced in response to osmotic stimuli but is decreased in response to changes in volume and pressure. Furthermore, some elderly patients have impaired angiotensin II production, which may contribute directly to the impaired thirst mechanism, ADH release, and renal concentrating ability. Hypernatremia in the elderly is particularly common in postoperative patients and in those receiving tube feedings, parenteral nutrition, or hypertonic solutions.

Symptoms and Signs

The major symptom of hypernatremia is thirst. The absence of thirst in conscious patients with hypernatremia suggests an impaired thirst mechanism. Patients with difficulty communicating may be unable to express thirst or obtain access to water. The major signs of hypernatremia result from CNS dysfunction due to brain cell shrinkage. Confusion, neuromuscular excitability, seizures, or coma may result; cerebrovascular damage with subcortical or subarachnoid hemorrhage and venous thromboses are frequent in patients dying from severe hypernatremia.

In chronic hypernatremia, osmotically active substances occur in CNS cells (idiogenic osmoles) and increase intracellular osmolality. Therefore, the degree of brain cell dehydration and resultant CNS symptoms are less severe in chronic than in acute hypernatremia.

When hypernatremia occurs with abnormal total body Na, the typical symptoms of volume depletion or overload are present (see Extracellular Fluid Volume Contraction on p. 1235 and Extracellular Fluid Volume Expansion on p. 1236). A large volume of hypotonic urine is characteristically excreted in patients with renal concentrating defects. When losses are extrarenal, the route of water loss is often evident (eg, vomiting, diarrhea, excessive sweating), and the urinary Na concentration is low.

Diagnosis

The diagnosis is clinical and by measuring serum Na. If the patient does not respond to simple rehydration or if hypernatremia recurs despite adequate access to water, further diagnostic testing is warranted. Determination of the underlying cause requires assessment of urine volume and osmolality, particularly after water deprivation.

A water deprivation test (see p. 1190) is occasionally used to differentiate among several polyuric states, such as central and nephrogenic diabetes insipidus.

Treatment

Replacement of free water is the other main goal of treatment. Oral hydration is effective in conscious patients without significant GI dysfunction. In severe hypernatremia or in patients unable to drink because of continued vomiting or mental status changes, IV hydration is preferred. If hypernatremia lasts < 24 h, it should be corrected within 24 h. However, if hypernatremia is chronic or of unknown duration, it should be corrected over 48 h, and the plasma osmolality should be lowered at a rate of no more than 2 mOsm/L/h to avoid cerebral edema caused by excess brain solute. The amount of water necessary to replace existing deficits may be estimated by the following formula:

$$\text{Free water deficit} = \text{TBW} \times [(\text{plasma Na}/140) - 1]$$

where TBW is in liters and is estimated by multiplying weight in kilograms by 0.6; plasma Na is in mEq/L. This formula assumes constant total body Na content. In patients with hypernatremia and depletion of total body Na content (ie, who have volume depletion), the free water deficit is greater than that estimated by the formula.

In patients with hypernatremia and ECF volume overload (excess total body Na content), the free water deficit can be replaced with 5% D/W, which can be supplemented with a loop diuretic. However, too-rapid infusion of 5% D/W may produce glycosuria, thereby increasing salt-free water excretion and hypertonicity, especially in diabetes mellitus. KCl should be replaced according to the plasma K concentration.

In patients with hypernatremia and euvolemia, free water can be replaced using either 5% D/W or 0.45% saline.

Treatment of patients with central diabetes insipidus and acquired nephrogenic diabetes insipidus is discussed on pp. 1190 and 2025.

In patients with hypernatremia and hypovolemia, particularly in diabetics with nonketotic hyperglycemic coma, 0.45% saline can be administered as an alternative to a combination of 0.9% normal saline and 5% D/W to replenish Na and free water. When severe acidosis (pH < 7.10) is present, $NaHCO_3$ solution can be added to 5% D/W or 0.45% saline, as long as the final solution remains hypotonic.

DISORDERS OF POTASSIUM CONCENTRATION

K is the most abundant intracellular cation, but only about 2% of total body K is extracellular. Because most intracellular K is contained within muscle cells, total body K is roughly proportional to lean body mass. An average 70-kg adult has about 3500 mEq of K.

K is a major determinant of intracellular osmolality. The ratio between ICF and ECF K concentrations strongly influences cell membrane polarization, which in turn influences important cell processes, such as the conduction of nerve impulses and muscle (including myocardial) cell contraction. Thus, relatively small alterations in plasma K concentration can have major clinical manifestations.

In the absence of factors that shift K in or out of cells (see p. 1245), the plasma K level correlates closely with total body K content. Assuming a constant plasma pH, a decrease in plasma K concentration from 4 to 3 mEq/L indicates a total K deficit of 100 to 200 mEq. A fall in plasma K to < 3 mEq/L indicates a total K deficit of about 200 to 400 mEq.

Insulin moves K into cells; high levels of insulin thus lower plasma K concentration. Low insulin levels, as in diabetic ketoacidosis, cause K to move out of cells, thus raising plasma K, sometimes even in the presence of total body K deficiency. β-Adrenergic agonists, especially selective β_2-agonists, move K into cells, whereas β-blockade and α-agonists probably move K out of cells. Acute metabolic acidosis causes K to move out of cells, whereas acute metabolic alkalosis causes K to move into cells. However, changes in plasma HCO_3 concentration may be more important than changes in pH; acidosis caused by accumulation of mineral acids (nonanion gap, hyperchloremic acidosis) is more likely to elevate plasma K. In contrast, metabolic acidosis due to accumulation of organic acids (increased anion gap acidosis) does not cause hyperkalemia. Thus, the hyperkalemia common in diabetic ketoacidosis results more from insulin deficiency than from acidosis. Acute respiratory acidosis and alkalosis affect plasma K concentration less than metabolic acidosis and alkalosis. Nonetheless, plasma K concentration should be interpreted in the context of the plasma pH (and HCO_3 concentration).

Dietary K intake normally varies between 40 and 150 mEq/day. In the steady state, fecal losses are usually close to 10% of intake. Urinary excretion contributes to K balance. When K intake increases (> 150 mEq of K is ingested daily), about 50% of the excess K appears in the urine over the next several hours. Most of the remainder is transferred into the intracellular compartment to minimize the rise in plasma K. If elevated K intake continues, renal K excretion rises because of K-stimulated aldosterone secretion; aldosterone promotes K excretion. In addition, K absorption from stool appears to be under some regulation and may fall by 50% in chronic K excess.

When K intake falls, intracellular K again serves as a reserve against wide swings in plasma K concentration. Renal K conservation develops relatively slowly in response to decreases in dietary K and is far less efficient than the kidneys' ability to conserve Na. Thus, K depletion is a frequent clinical problem. Urinary K excretion of 10 mEq/day represents near-maximal renal K conservation and implies significant K depletion.

Acute acidosis impairs K excretion, whereas chronic acidosis and acute alkalosis can promote K excretion. Increased delivery of Na to the distal nephron, as occurs with high Na intake or loop diuretic therapy, promotes K excretion.

Pseudohypokalemia, or falsely low serum K, occasionally occurs in patients with chronic myelocytic leukemia with a WBC count > 10^5/μL if the specimen remains at room temperature before being processed because of uptake of plasma K by abnormal leukocytes in the sample. It is prevented by prompt separation of plasma or serum in blood samples.

Pseudohyperkalemia, or falsely elevated serum K, is more common, typically occurring from hemolysis and release of intracellular K. To prevent this, phlebotomy personnel should not rapidly aspirate blood through a narrow-gauge needle or excessively agitate blood samples. Pseudohyperkalemia can also result from platelet count > 10^6/μL due to release of K from platelets during clotting. In cases of pseudohyperkalemia, the plasma K (unclotted blood), as opposed to serum K, is normal.

HYPOKALEMIA

Hypokalemia is serum K concentration < 3.5 mEq/L caused by a deficit in total body K stores or abnormal movement of K into cells. The most common causes are excess losses from the kidneys or GI tract. Clinical features include muscle weakness and polyuria; cardiac hyperexcitability may occur with severe hypokalemia. Diagnosis is by serum measurement. Treatment is administration of K and addressing the cause.

Etiology and Pathophysiology

Hypokalemia can be caused by decreased intake of K but is usually caused by excessive losses of K in the urine or from the GI tract.

GI tract losses: Abnormal GI K losses occur in chronic diarrhea and include losses due to chronic laxative abuse or bowel diversion. Other causes include clay pica, vomiting, and gastric suction (which removes HCl, causing the kidneys to excrete K). Rarely, villous adenoma of the colon causes massive K loss from the GI tract. GI K losses may be compounded by concomitant renal K losses due to metabolic alkalosis and stimulation of aldosterone due to volume depletion.

Intracellular shift: The transcellular shift of K into cells may also cause hypokalemia. This can occur in glycogenesis during TPN or enteral hyperalimentation or after administration of insulin. Stimulation of the sympathetic nervous system, particularly with β_2-agonists (eg, albuterol, terbutaline) may increase cellular K uptake. Similarly, severe hypokalemia occasionally occurs in thyrotoxic patients from excessive β-sympathetic stimulation (hypokalemic thyrotoxic periodic paralysis). Familial periodic paralysis (see p. 2457) is a rare autosomal dominant disease characterized by transient episodes of profound hypokalemia thought to be due to sudden abnormal shifts of K into cells. Episodes frequently involve varying degrees of paralysis. They are typically precipitated by a large carbohydrate meal or strenuous exercise, but variants have been described without these features.

Renal losses: Various disorders can increase renal K excretion. Excretion can increase in adrenal steroid excess due to direct mineralocorticoid effects on K secretion by the distal nephron. Cushing's syndrome, primary hyperaldosteronism, rare renin-secreting tumors, glucocorticoid-remediable aldosteronism (a rare inherited disorder involving abnormal aldosterone metabolism), and congenital adrenal hyperplasia can cause hypokalemia from excess mineralocorticoid formation. Inhibition of the enzyme 11β-hydroxysteroid dehydrogenase (11β-HSDH) prevents the conversion of cortisol, which has some mineralocorticoid activity, to cortisone, which does not. Substances such as glycyrrhizin (found in natural licorice and used in the manufacture of chewing tobacco) inhibit 11β-HSDH, resulting in high circulating levels of cortisol and renal K wasting.

Liddle syndrome (see also p. 2024) is a rare autosomal dominant disorder characterized by severe hypertension and hypokalemia. Liddle syndrome is caused by unrestrained Na reabsorption in the distal nephron due to one of several mutations found in genes encoding for epithelial Na channel subunits.

Inappropriately high reabsorption of Na results in both hypertension and renal K wasting.

Bartter and Gitelman's syndromes are uncommon genetic disorders characterized by renal K and Na wasting, excessive production of renin and aldosterone, and normotension. Bartter syndrome (see also p. 2024) is caused by mutations in a loop diuretic–sensitive ion transport mechanism in the loop of Henle. Gitelman's syndrome is caused by loss of function mutations in a thiazide-sensitive ion transport mechanism in the distal nephron.

Renal K wasting can also be caused by numerous congenital and acquired renal tubular diseases, such as the renal tubular acidoses and Fanconi syndrome, an unusual syndrome resulting in renal wasting of K, glucose, phosphate, uric acid, and amino acids.

Drugs: Diuretics are by far the most commonly used drugs that cause hypokalemia. K-wasting diuretics that block Na reabsorption proximal to the distal nephron include thiazides, loop diuretics, and osmotic diuretics. By inducing diarrhea, laxatives, especially when abused, can cause hypokalemia. Surreptitious diuretic and/or laxative abuse is a frequent cause of persistent hypokalemia, particularly among patients preoccupied with weight loss and among health care practitioners with access to prescription drugs.

Other drugs that can cause hypokalemia include amphotericin B, antipseudomonal penicillins (eg, carbenicillin), and high-dose penicillin. Finally, hypokalemia occurs in both acute and chronic theophylline intoxication.

Symptoms and Signs

Mild hypokalemia (plasma K 3 to 3.5 mEq/L) rarely causes symptoms. Plasma K < 3 mEq/L generally produces muscle weakness and may lead to paralysis and respiratory failure. Other muscular dysfunction includes cramping, fasciculations, paralytic ileus, hypoventilation, hypotension, tetany, and rhabdomyolysis. Persistent hypokalemia can impair renal concentrating ability, producing polyuria with secondary polydipsia.

Cardiac effects of hypokalemia are usually minimal until plasma K levels are < 3 mEq/L. Hypokalemia produces sagging of the ST segment, depression of the T wave, and elevation of the U wave. With marked hypokalemia, the T wave becomes progressively smaller and the U wave becomes increasingly larger. Sometimes, a flat or positive T wave merges with a positive U wave, which may be confused with QT prolongation (see FIG. 156–2). Hypokalemia may produce premature ventricular and atrial contractions, ventricular and atrial tachyarrhythmias, and

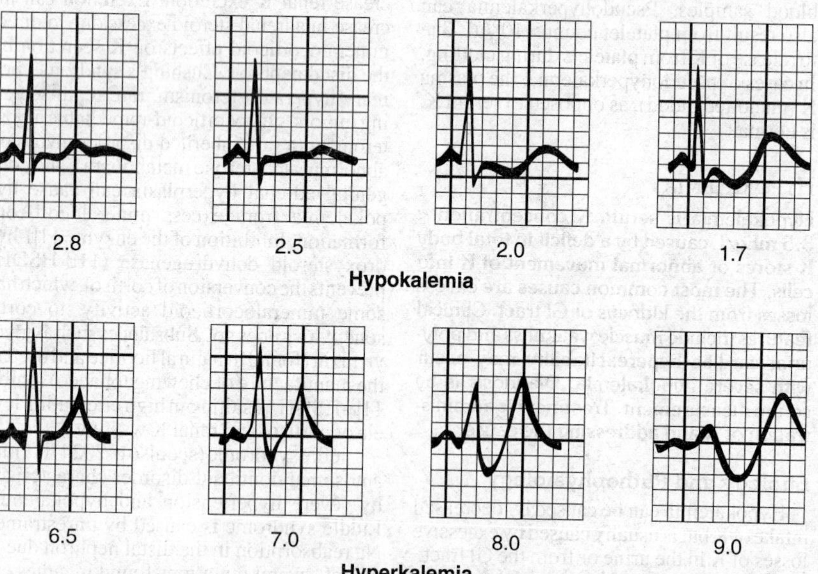

Fig. 156–2. ECG patterns in hypokalemia and hyperkalemia. (Serum K is in mEq/L.)

2nd- or 3rd-degree atrioventricular block. Such arrhythmias become more severe with increasingly severe hypokalemia; eventually, ventricular fibrillation may occur. Patients with significant preexisting heart disease and/or those receiving digoxin are at risk of cardiac conduction abnormalities even from mild hypokalemia.

Diagnosis

Hypokalemia is diagnosed on the basis of a plasma or serum K level < 3.5 mEq/L. If the cause is not apparent by history (in particular, the drug history), further investigation is warranted. After acidosis and other causes of intracellular K shift have been eliminated, 24-h urinary K is measured. In hypokalemia, K secretion is normally < 15 mEq/L. Extrarenal (GI) K loss or decreased K ingestion is suspected in chronic unexplained hypokalemia when renal K secretion is < 15 mEq/L. Secretion of ≥ 15 mEq/L suggests a renal cause for K loss. Unexplained hypokalemia with increased renal K secretion and hypertension suggests an aldosterone-secreting tumor or Liddle syndrome. Hypokalemia with increased renal K loss and normal BP suggests Bartter syndrome, but hypomagnesemia, surreptitious vomiting, and diuretic abuse are more common and should also be considered.

Treatment and Prevention

Many oral K supplements are available. Because they cause GI irritation and occasional bleeding, they are usually given in divided doses. Liquid KCl given orally elevates levels within 1 to 2 h, but it is poorly tolerated in doses > 25 to 50 mEq due to bitter taste. Wax-impregnated KCl preparations are safe and better tolerated. GI bleeding may be even less common with microencapsulated KCl preparations. Several preparations containing 8 or 10 mEq/capsule are available.

When hypokalemia is severe, is unresponsive to oral therapy, or occurs in hospitalized patients with active disease, K must be replaced parenterally. Because K solutions can irritate peripheral veins, the concentration should not exceed 40 mEq/L. The rate of correction of hypokalemia is limited because of the lag in K movement into cells. *Routine infusion rates should not exceed 10 mEq/h.* In hypokalemic-induced arrhythmia, IV KCl must be given more rapidly, usually through a central vein or using multiple peripheral veins simultaneously. Infusion of 40 mEq KCl/h can be undertaken but only with continuous cardiac monitoring and hourly plasma K determinations. Glucose solutions are avoided because elevation in the plasma insulin levels could result in transient worsening of hypokalemia.

In K deficit with high plasma K concentration, as in diabetic ketoacidosis, IV K is deferred until the plasma K starts to fall. Even when K deficits are severe, it is rarely necessary to give > 100 to 120 mEq of K in a 24-h period unless K loss continues. When hypokalemia occurs with hypomagnesemia, both the K and Mg deficiencies must be corrected to stop ongoing renal K wasting (see Hypomagnesemia on p. 1261).

Routine K replacement is not necessary in most patients receiving diuretics. However, plasma K should be monitored when diuretics are used, particularly in patients with decreased left ventricular function, receiving digoxin, with diabetes, and with asthma who are receiving β_2-agonists. Triamterene 100 mg po once/day or spironolactone 25 mg po qid do not increase K excretion and may be useful in patients who become hypokalemic but must use diuretics. If hypokalemia develops, K supplementation is indicated. When plasma K is < 3 mEq/L, oral KCl supplementation is often necessary. Because a decrease in plasma K of 1 mEq/L correlates with a 200- to 400-mEq deficit in total body K stores, usually 20 to 80 mEq/day in excess of any ongoing K losses should be given over several days to correct K deficits. The need for K supplementation may continue for several weeks during refeeding after prolonged starvation.

HYPERKALEMIA

Hyperkalemia is serum K concentration > 5.5 mEq/L resulting from excess total body K stores or abnormal movement of K out of cells. The usual cause is impairment of renal excretion; it can also occur in metabolic acidosis as in uncontrolled diabetes. Clinical manifestations are generally neuromuscular, resulting in muscle weakness and cardiac toxicity that, if severe, can degenerate to ventricular fibrillation or asystole. Diagnosis is by measuring serum or plasma K. Treatment involves giving a cation exchange resin and, in emergencies, Ca gluconate, insulin, and dialysis.

Etiology and Pathophysiology

Normal kidneys eventually excrete K loads, so sustained hyperkalemia usually implies diminished renal K excretion. Hyperkalemia also may be caused by transcellular movement of K out of cells in metabolic acidosis; hyperglycemia in the presence of insulin deficiency; moderately heavy exercise, particularly in the presence of β-blockade; digoxin intoxication; acute tumor lysis; acute intravascular hemolysis; or rhabdomyolysis. Much more unusual is hyperkalemic familial periodic paralysis, a rare inherited disorder characterized by episodic hyperkalemia due to sudden movement of K out of cells, usually precipitated by exercise (see p. 2457).

Hyperkalemia from total body K excess is particularly common in oliguric states (especially acute renal failure) and with rhabdomyolysis, burns, bleeding into soft tissue or the GI tract, and adrenal insufficiency. In chronic renal failure, hyperkalemia is uncommon until the GFR falls to < 10 to 15 mL/min unless dietary K intake is excessive or another source of excess K load is present, such as oral or parenteral K therapy, GI bleeding, tissue injury, or hemolysis. Other potential causes of hyperkalemia in chronic renal failure are hyporeninemic hypoaldosteronism (type 4 renal tubular acidosis), ACE inhibitors, K-sparing diuretics, fasting (suppression of insulin secretion), β-blockers, and NSAIDs. If sufficient KCl is ingested or given parenterally, severe hyperkalemia may result even with normal renal function. Causes are usually iatrogenic, such as giving K supplements to patients taking ACE inhibitors. Other drugs that may limit renal K output, thereby producing hyperkalemia, include cyclosporine, lithium, heparin, and trimethoprim.

Symptoms and Signs

Although flaccid paralysis occasionally occurs, hyperkalemia is usually asymptomatic until cardiac toxicity develops (see FIG. 156–2). Initial ECG changes occur with K > 5.5 mEq/L, characterized by shortening of the QT interval and tall, symmetric, peaked T waves. K > 6.5 mEq/L produces nodal and ventricular arrhythmias, widening of the QRS complex, PR interval prolongation, and disappearance of the P wave. Finally, the QRS complex degenerates into a sine wave pattern, and ventricular fibrillation or asystole ensues.

In the rare disorder hyperkalemic familial periodic paralysis, weakness frequently develops during attacks and can progress to frank paralysis.

Diagnosis

The diagnosis is made by plasma K level > 5.5 mEq/L. Because severe hyperkalemia requires prompt treatment, it should be considered in patients at high risk, such as those with renal failure, advanced heart failure treated with ACE inhibitors and K-sparing diuretics, or symptoms of urinary obstruction, particularly if arrhythmias or other electrocardiographic signs of hyperkalemia are present.

Diagnosis of the cause of hyperkalemia includes review of drugs and measurement of electrolytes, BUN, and creatinine. In cases in which renal failure is present, additional tests, including a renal ultrasound to exclude obstruction, are needed (see p. 1982).

Treatment

Mild hyperkalemia: Patients with plasma K < 6 mEq/L and no ECG abnormalities may respond to diminished K intake or stopping K-elevating drugs. The addition of a loop diuretic enhances renal K excretion. Na polystyrene sulfonate in sorbitol can be given (15 to 30 g in 30 to 70 mL of 70% sorbitol po q 4 to 6 h). It acts as a cation exchange resin and removes K through the GI mucosa. Sorbitol is administered with the resin to ensure passage through the GI tract. Patients unable to take drugs orally because of ileus or other reasons may be given similar doses by enema. About 1 mEq of K is removed per gram of resin given. Resin therapy is slow and often fails to lower plasma K significantly in hypercatabolic states. Because Na is exchanged for K when Na polystyrene sulfonate is used, Na overload may occur, particularly in oliguric patients with preexisting volume overload.

Moderate to severe hyperkalemia: Plasma K > 6 mEq/L, especially with electrocardiographic changes, requires aggressive therapy to shift K into cells. The first 2 of the following measures are performed immediately:

1. Administration of 10 to 20 mL 10% Ca gluconate (or 5 to 10 mL 22% Ca gluceptate) IV over 5 to 10 min. Ca antagonizes the effect of hyperkalemia on cardiac muscle excitability. *Caution should be used when giving Ca to patients taking digoxin because of the risk of precipitating hypokalemia-related arrhythmias.* If the ECG has deteriorated to a sine wave or asystole, Ca gluconate may be given more rapidly (5 to 10 mL IV over 2 min). CaCl can also be used but can be irritating and should be given through a central venous catheter. The effect occurs within

minutes but lasts only 20 to 30 min. Ca infusion is a temporizing measure while awaiting the effects of other treatments and may need to be repeated.

2. Administration of regular insulin 5 to 10 units IV followed immediately by or administered simultaneously with rapid infusion of 50 mL 50% glucose. Infusion of 10% D/W should follow at 50 mL/h to prevent hypoglycemia. The effect on plasma K peaks in 1 h and lasts for several hours.

3. A high-dose β-agonist, such as albuterol 10 to 20 mg inhaled over 10 min (5 mg/mL concentration) can safely lower plasma K by 0.5 to 1.5 mEq/L and may be a helpful adjunct. The peak effect occurs in 90 min.

4. Administration of IV $NaHCO_3$ is controversial. It may lower serum K over several hours. Reduction may result from alkalinization or the hypertonicity due to the concentrated Na in the preparation. The hypertonic Na that it contains may be harmful for dialysis patients who also may have volume overload. If given, the usual dose is 45 mEq (1 ampule of 7.5% $NaHCO_3$) infused over 5 min and repeated in 30 min. HCO_3 therapy has little effect when used by itself in patients with advanced renal insufficiency unless acidemia is also present.

In addition to the above strategies for lowering K by shifting it into cells, maneuvers to remove K from the body should also be performed early in the treatment of severe or symptomatic hyperkalemia. K can be removed via the GI tract by administration of Na polystyrene sulfonate (see p. 1248) or by hemodialysis. Hemodialysis should be instituted promptly after emergency measures in patients with renal failure or if emergency treatment is ineffective. Peritoneal dialysis is relatively inefficient at removing K.

DISORDERS OF CALCIUM CONCENTRATION

Ca is required for the proper functioning of muscle contraction, nerve conduction, hormone release, and blood coagulation. In addition, Ca helps regulate many enzymes.

Maintenance of the body Ca stores depends on dietary Ca intake, absorption of Ca from the GI tract, and renal Ca excretion. In a balanced diet, roughly 1000 mg of Ca is ingested each day. About 200 mg/day is lost in the bile and other GI secretions. Depending on the concentration of circulating vitamin D, particularly $1,25(OH)_2D$ (1,25-dihydroxycholecalciferol, calcitriol, or active vitamin D hormone, which is converted in the kidney from 25(OH)D, the inactive form), roughly 200 to 400 mg of Ca is absorbed from the intestine each day. The remaining 800 to 1000 mg appears in the stool. Ca balance is maintained through renal Ca excretion averaging 200 mg/day.

Both extracellular and intracellular Ca concentrations are tightly regulated by bidirectional Ca transport across the plasma membrane of cells and intracellular organelles, such as the endoplasmic reticulum, the sarcoplasmic reticulum of muscle cells, and the mitochondria. Cytosolic ionized Ca is maintained within the micromolar range (less than 1/1000 of the plasma concentration). Ionized Ca acts as an intracellular 2nd messenger; it is involved in skeletal muscle contraction, excitation-contraction coupling in cardiac and smooth muscle, and activation of protein kinases and enzyme phosphorylation. Ca is also involved in the action of other intracellular messengers, such as cyclic adenosine monophosphate (cAMP) and inositol 1,4,5-triphosphate, and thus mediates the cellular response to numerous hormones, including epinephrine, glucagon, ADH (vasopressin), secretin, and cholecystokinin.

Despite its important intracellular roles, roughly 99% of body Ca is in bone, mainly as hydroxyapatite crystals. Roughly 1% of bone Ca is freely exchangeable with the ECF and, therefore, is available for buffering changes in Ca balance. Normal total plasma Ca levels range from 8.8 to 10.4 mg/dL (2.20 to 2.60 mmol/L). About 40% of the total blood Ca is bound to plasma proteins, primarily albumin. The remaining 60% includes ionized Ca plus Ca complexed with phosphate (PO_4) and citrate. Total Ca (ie, protein-bound, complexed, and ionized Ca) is usually what is determined by clinical laboratory measurement. Ideally, the ionized or free Ca should be determined, because this is the physiologically active form of Ca in plasma; this determination, because of its technical difficulty, is usually restricted to patients in whom significant alteration of protein binding of plasma Ca is suspected. Ionized Ca is generally assumed to be roughly 50% of the total plasma Ca.

Regulation of Calcium Metabolism

The metabolism of Ca and of PO_4 (see p. 1259) are intimately related. The regulation of both Ca and PO_4 balance is greatly influenced by circulating levels of parathyroid hormone (PTH), vitamin D, and, to a lesser extent, calcitonin. Ca and inorganic PO_4 concentrations are also linked by their ability to chemically react to form $CaPO_4$. The product of concentrations of Ca and PO_4 (in mEq/L) is estimated to be 60 normally; when the product exceeds 70, precipitation of $CaPO_4$ crystals in soft tissue is much more likely. Precipitation in vascular tissue accelerates arteriosclerotic vascular disease.

PTH is secreted by the parathyroid glands. It has several actions, but perhaps the most important is to defend against hypocalcemia. Parathyroid cells sense decreases in plasma Ca and, in response, release preformed PTH into the circulation. PTH increases plasma Ca within minutes by increasing renal and intestinal absorption of Ca and by rapidly mobilizing Ca and PO_4 from bone (bone resorption). Renal Ca excretion generally parallels Na excretion and is influenced by many of the same factors that govern Na transport in the proximal tubule. However, PTH enhances distal tubular Ca reabsorption independently of Na. PTH also decreases renal PO_4 reabsorption and thus increases renal PO_4 losses. Renal PO_4 loss prevents the solubility product of Ca and PO_4 from being exceeded in plasma as Ca levels rise in response to PTH.

PTH also increases plasma Ca by stimulating conversion of vitamin D (see p. 41) to its most active form, $1,25(OH)_2D$. This form of vitamin D increases the percentage of dietary Ca absorbed by the intestine. Despite increased Ca absorption, long-term increases in PTH secretion generally result in further bone resorption by inhibiting osteoblastic function and promoting osteoclastic activity. PTH and vitamin D both function as important regulators of bone growth and bone remodeling (see Vitamin D Deficiency and Dependency on p. 41).

Testing parathyroid function includes measuring circulating PTH levels by radioimmunoassay and measuring total or nephrogenous cAMP excretion in urine. Urinary cAMP is seldom measured now that accurate assays for PTH are widely available. Assays for the intact PTH molecule are best.

Calcitonin is secreted by the thyroid parafollicular cells (C cells). Calcitonin tends to lower plasma Ca concentration by enhancing cellular uptake, renal excretion, and bone formation. The effects of calcitonin on bone metabolism are much weaker than those of either PTH or vitamin D.

HYPOCALCEMIA

(For hypocalcemia in neonates, see p. 2279.)

Hypocalcemia is total plasma Ca concentration < 8.8 mg/dL (< 2.20 mmol/L) in the presence of normal plasma protein concentrations, or a plasma ionized Ca concentration < 4.7 mg/dL (< 1.17 mmol/L). Causes include hypoparathyroidism, vitamin D deficiency, and renal disease. Manifestations include paraesthesias, tetany, and, if severe, seizures, encephalopathy, and heart failure. Diagnosis involves measurement of plasma Ca. Treatment is administration of Ca, sometimes with vitamin D.

Etiology and Pathophysiology

Hypocalcemia has a number of causes. Several are listed below.

Hypoparathyroidism: Hypoparathyroidism is characterized by hypocalcemia and hyperphosphatemia and often produces chronic tetany. Hypoparathyroidism results from deficient parathyroid hormone (PTH) often because of the accidental removal of or damage to several parathyroid glands during thyroidectomy. Transient hypoparathyroidism is common after subtotal thyroidectomy. Permanent hypoparathyroidism occurs after < 3% of thyroidectomies performed by experienced surgeons. Manifestations of hypocalcemia usually begin about 24 to 48 h postoperatively but may occur after months or years. PTH deficiency is more common after radical thyroidectomy for cancer or as the result of surgery on the parathyroid itself (subtotal or total parathyroidectomy). Risk factors for severe hypocalcemia after subtotal parathyroidectomy include severe preoperative hypercalcemia, removal of a large adenoma, and elevated alkaline phosphatase.

Idiopathic hypoparathyroidism is an uncommon sporadic or inherited condition in which the parathyroid glands are absent or atrophied. It manifests in childhood. The parathyroid glands are occasionally absent with thymic aplasia and abnormalities of the arteries arising from the brachial arches (DiGeorge syndrome). Other inherited forms include the X-linked genetic syndrome of hypoparathyroidism, Addison's disease, and mucocutaneous candidiasis.

Pseudohypoparathyroidism: Pseudohypoparathyroidism is an uncommon group of disorders characterized not by hormone deficiency but by target organ resistance to

PTH. Complex genetic transmission of these disorders occurs.

Patients with type Ia pseudohypoparathyroidism (Albright's hereditary osteodystrophy) have a mutation in the stimulatory Gs-α_1 protein of the adenylyl cyclase complex (GNAS1). The result is failure of normal renal phosphaturic response or increase in urinary cyclic adenosine monophosphate (cAMP) to PTH. Patients are usually hypocalcemic as a result of hyperphosphatemia. Secondary hyperparathyroidism and hyperparathyroid bone disease can occur. Associated abnormalities include short stature, round facies, mental retardation with calcification of the basal ganglia, shortened metacarpal and metatarsal bones, mild hypothyroidism, and other subtle endocrine abnormalities. Because only the maternal allele for GNAS1 is expressed in the kidneys, patients whose abnormal gene is paternal, although they have many of the somatic features of the disease, do not have hypocalcemia, hyperphosphatemia, or secondary hyperparathyroidism; this condition is sometimes described as pseudopseudohypoparathyroidism.

Less is known about type Ib pseudohypoparathyroidism. These patients have hypocalcemia, hyperphosphatemia, and secondary hyperparathyroidism but do not have the other associated abnormalities.

Type II pseudohypoparathyroidism is even less common than type I. In affected patients, exogenous PTH raises the urinary cAMP normally but does not raise plasma Ca or urinary phosphate (PO_4). An intracellular resistance to cAMP has been proposed.

Vitamin D deficiency: Vitamin D deficiency may result from inadequate dietary intake or decreased absorption due to hepatobiliary disease or intestinal malabsorption. It can also result from alterations in vitamin D metabolism as occur with certain drugs (eg, phenytoin, phenobarbital, rifampin) or lack of skin exposure to sunlight. The latter is an important cause of acquired vitamin D deficiency in the institutionalized elderly and in northern climates among people wearing clothing that covers them completely (eg, Muslim women in England). Type I vitamin D–dependent rickets (pseudovitamin D deficiency rickets) is an autosomal recessive disorder involving a mutation in the gene encoding the 1-α-hydroxylase enzyme. Normally expressed in the kidney, 1-α-hydroxylase is needed to convert 25(OH)D to the active form of vitamin D, $1,25(OH)_2D$. In type II vitamin D–dependent rickets, target organs cannot respond to $1,25(OH)_2D$. Vitamin D deficiency, hypocalcemia, and severe hypophosphatemia occur. Muscle weakness, pain, and typical bone deformities can occur (see p. 42).

Renal disease: Renal tubular disease, including acquired proximal renal tubular acidosis due to nephrotoxins (eg, heavy metals) and distal renal tubular acidosis, can cause severe hypocalcemia due to abnormal renal loss of Ca and decreased renal conversion to $1,25(OH)_2D$. Cadmium, in particular, causes hypocalcemia by injuring proximal tubular cells and interfering with vitamin D conversion.

Renal failure can result in hypocalcemia from diminished formation of $1,25(OH)_2D$ from direct renal cell damage as well as suppression of 1-α-hydroxylase by hyperphosphatemia.

Other causes: Mg depletion, which occurs with intestinal malabsorption or dietary deficiency, can cause hypocalcemia. Relative PTH deficiency and end-organ resistance to PTH action occur, resulting in plasma Mg concentrations of < 1.0 mg/dL (< 0.5 mmol/L); repletion improves PTH levels and renal Ca conservation.

Acute pancreatitis causes hypocalcemia when lipolytic products released from the inflamed pancreas chelate Ca.

Hypoproteinemia can reduce the protein-bound fraction of plasma Ca. Hypocalcemia due to diminished protein binding is asymptomatic. Because ionized Ca is unchanged, this entity has been termed factitious hypocalcemia.

Enhanced bone formation with inadequate Ca intake occurs particularly after surgical correction of hyperparathyroidism in patients with severe osteitis fibrosa cystica and has been termed hungry bone syndrome.

Septic shock can cause hypocalcemia due to suppression of PTH release and decreased conversion of 25(OH)D to $1,25(OH)_2D$.

Hyperphosphatemia causes hypocalcemia by poorly understood mechanisms. Patients with renal failure and subsequent PO_4 retention are particularly prone.

Drugs that produce hypocalcemia include those generally used to treat hypercalcemia (see p. 1257); anticonvulsants (phenytoin, phenobarbital) and rifampin, which alter vitamin D metabolism; transfusion of > 10 units of citrate-anticoagulated blood; and radiocontrast agents containing the divalent ion-chelating agent ethylenediaminetetraacetate.

Although excessive secretion of calcitonin might be expected to cause hypocalcemia, low plasma Ca levels rarely occur in patients with large amounts of circulating calcitonin from medullary carcinoma of the thyroid.

Symptoms and Signs

Hypocalcemia is frequently asymptomatic. The presence of hypoparathyroidism is often suggested by the clinical manifestations of the underlying condition (eg, cataracts, basal ganglia calcification, chronic candidiasis in idiopathic hypoparathyroidism).

Clinical manifestations of hypocalcemia are due to disturbances in cellular membrane potential, resulting in neuromuscular irritability. Muscle cramps involving the back and legs are common. Insidious hypocalcemia may produce mild, diffuse encephalopathy and should be suspected in a patient with unexplained dementia, depression, or psychosis. Papilledema occasionally occurs, and cataracts may develop after prolonged hypocalcemia. Severe hypocalcemia with plasma Ca < 7 mg/dL (< 1.75 mmol/L) may cause tetany, laryngospasm, or generalized seizures.

Tetany characteristically results from severe hypocalcemia but can result from reduction in the ionized fraction of plasma Ca without marked hypocalcemia, as occurs in severe alkalosis. Tetany is characterized by sensory symptoms consisting of paresthesias of the lips, tongue, fingers, and feet; carpopedal spasm, which may be prolonged and painful; generalized muscle aching; and spasm of facial musculature. Tetany may be overt with spontaneous symptoms or latent and requiring provocative tests to elicit. Latent tetany generally occurs at less severely decreased plasma Ca concentrations: 7 to 8 mg/dL (1.75 to 2.20 mmol/L).

Chvostek's and Trousseau's signs are easily elicited at the bedside to identify latent tetany. Chvostek's sign is an involuntary twitching of the facial muscles elicited by a light tapping of the facial nerve just anterior to the exterior auditory meatus. It is present in ≤ 10% of healthy people and in most people with acute hypocalcemia but is often absent in chronic hypocalcemia. Trousseau's sign is the precipitation of carpopedal spasm by reduction of the blood supply to the hand with a tourniquet or BP cuff inflated to 20 mm Hg above systolic BP applied to the forearm for 3 min. Trousseau's sign also occurs in alkalosis, hypomagnesemia, hypokalemia, and hyperkalemia and in about 6% of people with no identifiable electrolyte disturbance.

Arrhythmia or heart block occasionally develops in patients with severe hypocalcemia. In hypocalcemia, the ECG typically shows prolongation of the QT_C and ST intervals. Changes in repolarization, such as T-wave peaking or inversion, also occur.

Many other abnormalities may occur with chronic hypocalcemia, such as dry and scaly skin, brittle nails, and coarse hair. *Candida* infections occasionally occur in hypocalcemia but most commonly occur in patients with idiopathic hypoparathyroidism. Cataracts occasionally occur with long-standing hypocalcemia and are not reversible by correction of plasma Ca.

Sidebar 156–1. ESTIMATION OF IONIZED CALCIUM LEVELS

Ionized Ca levels can be estimated from routine laboratory tests, usually with reasonable accuracy. Acidosis increases ionized Ca by decreasing protein binding, whereas alkalosis decreases ionized Ca. In hypoalbuminemia, measured plasma Ca is often low, mainly reflecting low levels of protein-bound Ca, while ionized Ca can be normal. Measured total plasma Ca decreases or increases by about 0.8 mg/dL (0.20 mmol/L) for every 1-g/dL decrease or increase in albumin. Thus, an albumin level of 2.0 g/dL (normal, 4.0 g/dL) should itself reduce measured plasma Ca by 1.6 mg/dL. Similarly, increases in plasma proteins, as occur in multiple myeloma, can raise total plasma Ca.

Diagnosis

Hypocalcemia is diagnosed by a total plasma Ca level < 8.8 mg/dL (< 2.20 mmol/L). However, because low plasma protein can lower total, but not ionized, plasma Ca, ionized Ca should be estimated based on albumin level (see sidebar 156–1). Suspicion of low ionized Ca mandates its direct measurement, despite normal total plasma Ca. Hypocalcemic patients should undergo measurement of renal function (eg, BUN, creatinine), serum PO_4, Mg, and alkaline phosphatase.

If hypocalcemia has no obvious etiology (eg, alkalosis, renal failure, or massive blood transfusion), further testing is needed. Intact PTH levels should be measured. Because hypocalcemia is the major stimulus for PTH secretion, PTH should be elevated in hypocalcemia. Thus, low or even low-normal PTH levels are inappropriate and suggest hypoparathyroidism. An undetectable PTH level suggests idiopathic hypoparathyroidism. Hypoparathyroidism is characterized by low plasma Ca, high plasma PO_4, and normal alkaline phosphatase. Hypocalcemia with high plasma PO_4 suggests renal failure.

Type I pseudohypoparathyroidism can be distinguished by the presence of hypocalcemia despite normal to elevated levels of circulating PTH. Despite the presence of high levels of circulating PTH, urinary cAMP and urinary PO_4 are absent. Provocative testing by injection of parathyroid extract or recombinant human PTH fails to raise plasma or urinary cAMP. Patients with type Ia pseudohypoparathyroidism frequently also have skeletal abnormalities, including short stature and shortened 1st, 4th, and 5th metacarpals. Those with type Ib disease have renal manifestations without skeletal abnormalities.

In type II pseudohypoparathyroidism, exogenous PTH raises urinary cAMP but does not induce phosphaturia or raise plasma Ca concentration. Vitamin D deficiency must be excluded before type II pseudohypoparathyroidism is diagnosed.

In osteomalacia or rickets, typical skeletal abnormalities may be present on x-ray (see p. 43). The plasma PO_4 level is often mildly reduced, and alkaline phosphatase is elevated, reflecting increased mobilization of Ca from bone. Measurement of plasma 25(OH)D and $1,25(OH)_2D$ may help distinguish vitamin D deficiency from vitamin D–dependent states. Familial hypophosphatemic rickets is recognized by the associated renal PO_4 wasting.

Treatment

For tetany, Ca gluconate 10 mL of 10% solution IV over 10 min is given. Response can be dramatic but may last for only a few hours. Repeated infusions or the addition of a continuous infusion may be needed with 20 to 30 mL of 10% Ca gluconate in 1 L of 5% D/W over the next 12 to 24 h. Infusions of Ca are hazardous in patients receiving digoxin and should be given slowly and with continuous ECG monitoring. When tetany is associated with hypomagnesemia, it may respond transiently to Ca or K administration but is permanently relieved only by repletion of Mg (see p. 1262).

In transient hypoparathyroidism after thyroidectomy or partial parathyroidectomy, supplemental oral Ca may be sufficient. However, hypocalcemia may be particularly severe and prolonged after subtotal parathyroidectomy in patients with chronic renal failure or end-stage renal disease. Prolonged parenteral administration of Ca may be necessary postoperatively; supplementation with as much as 1 g/day of elemental Ca may be required for 5 to 10 days before oral Ca and vitamin D are sufficient. Elevated plasma alkaline phosphatase in such settings may be a sign of rapid uptake of Ca into bone. The need for large amounts of parenteral Ca usually does not fall until the alkaline phosphatase levels begin to decrease.

In chronic hypocalcemia, oral Ca and occasionally vitamin D supplements are usually sufficient. Ca may be given as Ca gluconate (90 mg elemental Ca/1 g) or Ca carbonate (400 mg elemental Ca/1 g) to provide 1 to 2 g of elemental Ca/day. Although any vitamin D preparation suffices, 1-hydroxylated compounds, such as synthetic calcitriol [$1,25(OH)_2D$], and pseudo 1-hydroxylated analogs, such as dihydrotachysterol, offer more rapid onset of action and more rapid clearance from the body. Calcitriol is particularly useful in renal failure because it requires no renal metabolic alteration. Patients with hypoparathyroidism usually respond to calcitriol in dosages of 0.5 to 2 μg/day po. Pseudohypoparathyroidism can occasionally be managed with oral Ca supplementation alone. Benefit from calcitriol requires 1 to 3 μg/day.

Vitamin D therapy is not effective unless adequate dietary or supplemental Ca (1 to 2 g elemental Ca/day) and PO_4 (see p. 1260) are supplied. Vitamin D toxicity with severe symptomatic hypercalcemia can be a serious complication of treatment with vitamin D analogs. Plasma Ca concentration should be monitored weekly at first and then at 1- to 3-mo intervals after Ca levels have stabilized. The maintenance dose of calcitriol or dihydrotachysterol usually decreases with time.

Rickets due to vitamin D deficiency responds to as little as 10 μg (400 IU/day) of vitamin D (as vitamin D_2 or D_3); if osteomalacia is present, 125 μg/day (5000 IU/day) of

TABLE 156–7. PRINCIPAL CAUSES OF HYPERCALCEMIA

Excessive bone resorption

Cancer with bone metastases: Particularly carcinoma, leukemia, lymphoma, multiple myeloma
Hyperthyroidism
Humoral hypercalcemia of malignancy, ie, hypercalcemia of cancer in the absence of bone metastases
Immobilization: Particularly in young, growing people, in those undergoing orthopedic casting and/or traction, and in those with Paget's disease of bone; also in elderly with osteoporosis, paraplegics, and quadriplegics
Parathyroid hormone excess: Primary hyperparathyroidism, parathyroid carcinoma, familial hypocalciuric hypercalcemia, advanced secondary hyperparathyroidism
Vitamin D toxicity; vitamin A toxicity

Excessive GI Ca absorption and/or intake

Milk-alkali syndrome
Sarcoidosis and other granulomatous diseases
Vitamin D toxicity

Elevated plasma protein concentration

Uncertain mechanism

Aluminum-induced osteomalacia
Infantile hypercalcemia
Lithium intoxication, theophylline intoxication
Myxedema, Addison's disease, postoperative Cushing's disease
Neuroleptic malignant syndrome
Thiazide diuretic treatment

Artifactual

Exposure of blood to contaminated glassware
Prolonged venous stasis while obtaining blood samples

vitamin D is given for 6 to 12 wk and then reduced to 10 μg/day (400 IU/day). An additional 2 g Ca/day is desirable during the early stages of treatment. In patients with rickets or osteomalacia due to lack of exposure to sunlight, treatment with increased exposure to sunlight or ultraviolet lamp treatment may be all that is required.

Type I vitamin D–dependent rickets responds to calcitriol 0.25 to 1.0 μg/day po. Patients with type II vitamin D–dependent rickets do not respond to any form of vitamin D (the more easily understood term—hereditary resistance to 1,25$(OH)_2$D—has been suggested). Treatment depends on the severity of bone lesions and hypocalcemia. Up to 6 μg/kg body weight or a total of 30 to 60 μg/day of calcitriol with up to 3 g of elemental Ca/day is needed in severe cases. Treatment with vitamin D requires monitoring of plasma Ca levels; although hypercalcemia may result, it generally responds quickly to dose adjustment of vitamin D.

HYPERCALCEMIA

Hypercalcemia is total plasma Ca concentration > 10.4 mg/dL (> 2.60 mmol/L) or ionized plasma Ca > 5.2 mg/dL (> 1.30 mmol/L). Principal causes include hyperparathyroidism, vitamin D toxicity, and cancer. Clinical features include polyuria, constipation, muscle weakness, confusion, and coma. Diagnosis is by plasma ionized Ca and parathyroid hormone levels. Treatment to increase Ca excretion and reduce bone resorption of Ca involves saline, Na diuresis, and drugs such as pamidronate.

Etiology and Pathophysiology

Hypercalcemia usually results from excessive bone resorption. The principal causes of hypercalcemia are listed here and in TABLE 156–7.

Primary hyperparathyroidism is a generalized disorder resulting from excessive secretion of parathyroid hormone (PTH) by one or more parathyroid glands. It probably is the most common cause of hypercalcemia. Incidence increases with age and is higher in postmenopausal women. It also occurs in high frequency ≥ 3 decades after neck irradiation. Familial and sporadic forms exist. Familial forms due to parathyroid adenoma occur in patients with other endocrine tumors (see p. 1314). Primary hyperparathyroidism causes hypophosphatemia and excessive bone resorption. Although asymptomatic hypercalcemia is the most frequent presentation, nephrolithiasis is also common, particularly when hypercalciuria occurs due to long-standing hypercalcemia. Histologic examination shows a parathyroid adenoma in about 90% of patients with primary hyperparathyroidism, although it is sometimes difficult to distinguish an adenoma from a normal gland. About 7% of cases are due to hyperplasia of ≥ 2 glands. Parathyroid cancer occurs in 3% of cases.

The syndrome of familial hypocalciuric hypercalcemia (FHH) is transmitted as an autosomal dominant trait. Most cases involve an inactivating mutation of the Ca-sensing receptor gene, resulting in higher levels of plasma Ca being needed to inhibit PTH secretion. Subsequent PTH secretion induces phosphate (PO_4) excretion. There is persistent hypercalcemia (usually asymptomatic), often from an early age; normal to slightly elevated levels of PTH; hypocalciuria; and hypermagnesemia. Renal function is normal, and nephrolithiasis is unusual. However, severe pancreatitis occasionally occurs. This syndrome, which is associated with parathyroid hyperplasia, is not relieved by subtotal parathyroidectomy.

Secondary hyperparathyroidism occurs when long-term hypocalcemia, which is caused by conditions such as renal insufficiency or intestinal malabsorption syndromes, stimulates increased secretion of PTH. Hypercalcemia or, less often, normocalcemia may occur. The sensitivity of the parathyroid to Ca may be diminished because of pronounced glandular hyperplasia and elevation of the Ca set point (ie, the amount of Ca necessary to reduce secretion of PTH).

Tertiary hyperparathyroidism results in autonomous hypersecretion of PTH regardless of plasma Ca concentration. Tertiary hyperparathyroidism generally occurs in patients with long-standing secondary hyperparathyroidism, as in patients with end-stage renal disease of several years' duration.

Cancer is a common cause of hypercalcemia in hospitalized patients. Although there are several mechanisms, elevated plasma Ca ultimately occurs as a result of bone resorption. Humoral hypercalcemia of cancer (ie, hypercalcemia with no or minimal bone metastases) occurs most commonly with squamous cell carcinoma, renal cell carcinoma, breast cancer, prostate cancer, and ovarian cancer. Many cases of humoral hypercalcemia of cancer were formerly attributed to ectopic production of PTH. However, some of these tumors secrete a PTH-related peptide that binds to PTH receptors in both bone and kidney and mimics many of the effects of the hormone, including osteoclastic bone resorption. Hematologic cancers, most often myeloma, but also certain lymphomas and lymphosarcomas, cause hypercalcemia through elaboration of a group of cytokines that stimulate osteoclasts to resorb bone, resulting in osteolytic lesions and/or diffuse osteopenia. Hypercalcemia may result from local elaboration of osteoclast-activating cytokines or prostaglandins and/or direct bone resorption by the metastatic tumor cells.

High levels of endogenous vitamin D [$1,25(OH)_2D$] are another possible cause. Although plasma concentrations are low in most patients with solid tumors, patients with lymphoma sometimes have elevated levels. Exogenous vitamin D in pharmacologic doses produces excessive bone resorption as well as increased intestinal Ca absorption, resulting in hypercalcemia and hypercalciuria (see Vitamin D Toxicity on p. 44).

Granulomatous disease, such as sarcoidosis, TB, leprosy, berylliosis, histoplasmosis, and coccidioidomycosis, leads to hypercalcemia and hypercalciuria. In sarcoidosis, hypercalcemia and hypercalciuria appear to be due to unregulated conversion of 25(OH)D to $1,25(OH)_2D$, presumably due to expression of the 1-α-hydroxylase enzyme in mononuclear cells within sarcoid granulomas. Similarly, elevated plasma levels of $1,25(OH)_2D$ have been reported in hypercalcemic patients with TB and silicosis. Other mechanisms must account for hypercalcemia in some instances, because depressed $1,25(OH)_2D$ levels occur in some patients with hypercalcemia and leprosy.

Immobilization, particularly complete prolonged bed rest in patients at risk (see TABLE 156–7), can result in hypercalcemia due to accelerated bone resorption. Hypercalcemia develops within days to weeks of onset of bed rest. Reversal of hypercalcemia occurs promptly on resumption of weight bearing. People with Paget's disease are particularly prone to hypercalcemia when at bed rest.

Idiopathic hypercalcemia of infancy (see Williams syndrome, in TABLE 294–1 on p. 2452) is an extremely rare sporadic disorder with dysmorphic facial features, cardiovascular abnormalities, renovascular hypertension, and hypercalcemia. PTH and vitamin D metabolism are normal, but the response of calcitonin to Ca infusion may be abnormal.

In milk-alkali syndrome, excessive amounts of Ca and absorbable alkali are ingested, usually during self-treatment with Ca carbonate antacids for dyspepsia or to prevent osteoporosis, resulting in hypercalcemia, metabolic alkalosis, and renal insufficiency. The availability of effective drugs for peptic ulcer disease and osteoporosis has greatly reduced the incidence of this syndrome.

Symptoms and Signs

In mild hypercalcemia, many patients are asymptomatic. The condition is frequently discovered during routine laboratory screening.

Clinical manifestations of hypercalcemia include constipation, anorexia, nausea and vomiting, abdominal pain, and ileus. Impairment of the renal concentrating mechanism leads to polyuria, nocturia, and polydipsia. Elevation of plasma Ca > 12 mg/dL (> 3.00 mmol/L) causes emotional lability, confusion, delirium, psychosis, stupor, and coma. Neuromuscular symptoms include skeletal muscle weakness. Hypercalciuria with nephrolithiasis is common. Less often, prolonged or severe hypercalcemia produces reversible acute renal failure or irreversible renal damage due to nephrocalcinosis (precipitation of Ca salts within the kidney parenchyma). Peptic ulcers and pancreatitis may occur in patients with hyperparathyroidism for reasons that are not related to hypercalcemia.

Severe hypercalcemia causes a shortened QT_c interval on ECG, and arrhythmias may occur, particularly in patients taking digoxin. Hypercalcemia > 18 mg/dL (> 4.50 mmol/L) may cause shock, renal failure, and death.

Diagnosis

Hypercalcemia is diagnosed by a total plasma Ca level > 10.4 mg/dL (> 2.60 mmol/L) or ionized plasma Ca > 5.2 mg/dL (> 1.30 mmol/L). Plasma Ca can be artifactually elevated (see TABLE 156–7). Hypercalcemia can also be masked by low serum protein; if protein and albumin are abnormal or if ionized hypercalcemia is clinically suspected (eg, because of symptoms of hypercalcemia), ionized plasma Ca should be measured.

The cause is apparent from the history and clinical findings in ≥ 95% of patients. Initial evaluation should include a review of the history, particularly of past plasma Ca levels; physical examination; a chest x-ray; and laboratory studies, including electrolytes, BUN, creatinine, ionized Ca, PO_4, alkaline phosphatase, and serum protein immunoelectrophoresis. Patients without an obvious cause of hypercalcemia after this evaluation should undergo measurement of intact PTH and 24-h urinary Ca.

Asymptomatic hypercalcemia that has been present for years or is present in multiple family members raises the possibility of FHH. Primary hyperparathyroidism generally presents later in life but can be present for several years before symptoms occur. If there are no obvious causes, levels of plasma Ca < 11 mg/dL (< 2.75 mmol/L) suggest hyperparathyroidism or other nonmalignant causes, whereas levels > 13 mg/dL (> 3.25 mmol/L) suggest cancer.

The chest x-ray is particularly helpful, revealing most granulomatous diseases, such as TB, sarcoidosis, and silicosis, as well as primary lung cancer and lytic and Paget's lesions in bones of the shoulder, ribs, and thoracic spine.

X-rays can also demonstrate the bony effects of secondary hyperparathyroidism, most commonly in long-term dialysis patients. In osteitis fibrosa cystica (often due to primary hyperparathyroidism), increased osteoclastic activity from overstimulation by PTH causes rarefaction of bone with fibrous degeneration and cyst and fibrous nodule formation. Because characteristic bone lesions occur only with relatively advanced disease, x-rays are not recommended in asymptomatic patients. X-rays typically show bone cysts, a heterogeneous appearance of the skull, and subperiosteal resorption of bone in the phalanges and distal clavicles.

Diagnosis of the cause of hypercalcemia often relies on laboratory studies.

In hyperparathyroidism, the plasma Ca is rarely > 12 mg/dL (> 3.00 mmol/L), but the ionized plasma Ca is almost always elevated. Low plasma PO_4 level suggests hyperparathyroidism, especially when coupled with elevated PO_4 renal excretion. When hyperparathyroidism results in increased bone turnover, plasma alkaline phosphatase is frequently increased. Increased intact PTH, particularly inappropriate elevations (ie, in the absence of hypocalcemia), is diagnostic. Primary hyperparathyroidism is suggested by an absence of a family history of endocrine neoplasia, childhood neck irradiation, or other obvious cause. Chronic renal disease suggests the presence of secondary hyperparathyroidism, but primary hyperparathyroidism can also be present. In patients with chronic renal disease, high plasma Ca and normal plasma PO_4 suggest primary hyperparathyroidism, whereas elevated PO_4 suggests secondary hyperparathyroidism.

The need for localization of parathyroid tissue before surgery on the parathyroid(s) is controversial. High-resolution CT scanning with or without CT-guided biopsy and immunoassay of thyroid venous drainage, MRI, high-resolution ultrasonography, digital subtraction angiography, and thallium 201-technetium 99 scanning all have been used and are highly accurate, but they have not improved the usually high cure rate of parathyroidectomy performed by experienced surgeons. Technetium-99 sestamibi, a radionuclide agent for parathyroid imaging, is more sensitive and specific than earlier agents and may be useful for identifying solitary adenomas.

For residual or recurrent hyperparathyroidism after initial parathyroid surgery, imaging is necessary and may reveal abnormally functioning parathyroid glands in unusual locations throughout the neck and mediastinum. Technetium-99 sestamibi is probably the most sensitive imaging test. Use of multiple imaging studies (MRI, CT, or high-resolution ultrasound in addition to technetium-99 sestamibi) before repeat parathyroidectomy is sometimes necessary.

A plasma Ca > 12 mg/dL (> 3.00 mmol/L) suggests tumors or some other cause of hypercalcemia rather than hyperparathyroidism. In humoral hypercalcemia of cancer, PTH is often decreased or undetectable; PO_4 is often decreased; and metabolic alkalosis, hypochloremia, and hypoalbuminemia are often present. Suppressed PTH differentiates this from primary hyperparathyroidism. Humoral hypercalcemia of cancer can also be diagnosed by detection of PTH-related peptide in plasma.

Simultaneous anemia, azotemia, and hypercalcemia suggest myeloma. Myeloma is confirmed by bone marrow examination or by the presence of a monoclonal gammopathy.

If Paget's disease is suspected, testing begins with plain x-rays (see p. 308).

FHH, thiazide therapy, renal failure, and milk-alkali syndrome can produce hypercalcemia without hypercalciuria. FHH is distinguished from primary hyperparathyroidism by the early age of onset, frequent occurrence of hypermagnesemia, and presence of hypercalcemia without hypercalciuria in other family members. The fractional excretion of Ca (ratio of Ca clearance to creatinine clearance) is low (< 1%) in FHH; it is almost always elevated (1 to 4%) in primary hyperparathyroidism. Intact PTH can be elevated or normal, perhaps reflecting altered feedback regulation of the parathyroid glands.

In addition to a history of increased intake of Ca antacids, milk-alkali syndrome is recognized by the combination of hypercalcemia, metabolic alkalosis, and occasionally, azotemia with hypocalciuria. The diagnosis can be confirmed if the plasma Ca level rapidly returns to normal when Ca and alkali ingestion stops, although renal insufficiency can persist if nephrocalcinosis is present. Circulating PTH usually is suppressed.

In hypercalcemia from sarcoidosis, other granulomatous disorders, and some lymphomas, plasma levels of $1,25(OH)_2D$ may be elevated. Vitamin D toxicity is also characterized by elevated $1,25(OH)_2D$ levels. In other endocrine causes of hypercalcemia, such as thyrotoxicosis and Addison's disease, typical laboratory findings of the underlying disorder help establish the diagnosis.

Treatment

There are 4 main strategies for lowering plasma Ca: decrease intestinal Ca absorption, increase urinary Ca excretion, decrease bone resorption, and remove excess Ca through dialysis. The treatment used depends on both the degree and the cause of hypercalcemia.

In mild hypercalcemia (plasma Ca < 11.5 mg/dL [< 2.88 mmol/L]), in which symptoms are mild, treatment is deferred pending definitive diagnosis. After diagnosis, the underlying cause is treated. If symptoms are significant, treatment aimed at lowering plasma Ca is necessary. Oral PO_4 can be used. When taken with meals, it binds some Ca, preventing its absorption. A starting dose is 250 mg of elemental PO_4 (as Na or K salt) qid. The dose can be increased to 500 mg qid as needed unless diarrhea develops. Another treatment is increasing urinary Ca excretion by giving isotonic saline plus a loop diuretic. Initially, 1 to 2 L of saline is given over 2 to 4 h unless significant heart failure is present, because nearly all patients with significant hypercalcemia are hypovolemic. Furosemide 20 to 40 mg IV q 2 to 4 h is given as needed to maintain a urine output of roughly 250 mL/h (monitored hourly). Care must be taken to avoid volume depletion. To avoid hypokalemia and hypomagnesemia, K and Mg are monitored as often as q 4 h during treatment and replaced intravenously as needed. Plasma Ca begins to decrease in 2 to 4 h and falls to near-normal levels within 24 h.

Moderate hypercalcemia (plasma Ca > 11.5 mg/dL [< 2.88 mmol/L] and < 18 mg/dL [< 4.51 mmol/L]) can be treated with isotonic saline and a loop diuretic as previously mentioned or, depending on its cause, agents that decrease bone resorption (usually calcitonin, bisphosphonates, or infrequently plicamycin or gallium nitrate), corticosteroids, or chloroquine.

Calcitonin (thyrocalcitonin) is a rapidly acting peptide hormone normally secreted in response to hypercalcemia by the C cells of the thyroid. Calcitonin appears to lower plasma Ca by inhibiting osteoclastic activity.

A dose of 4 to 8 IU/kg sc q 12 h of salmon calcitonin is safe. Its usefulness in the treatment of cancer-associated hypercalcemia is limited by its short duration of action, the development of tachyphylaxis, and the lack of response in ≥ 40% of patients. However, the combination of salmon calcitonin and prednisone may control plasma Ca for several months in some patients with cancer. If calcitonin stops working, it can be stopped for 2 days (while prednisone is continued) and then resumed.

Bisphosphonates inhibit osteoclasts. They are usually the drugs of choice for cancer-associated hypercalcemia. Etidronate 7.5 mg/kg IV once/day for 3 to 5 days is used to treat Paget's disease and cancer-associated hypercalcemia. Maintenance with 20 mg/kg po once/day can also be used. Pamidronate can be given for cancer-associated hypercalcemia as a one-time dose of 30 to 90 mg IV, repeated only after 7 days. It lowers plasma Ca for ≤ 2 wk. Zoledronate can also be given in doses of 4 to 8 mg IV and lowers plasma Ca for an average of > 40 days. Oral bisphosphonates (alendronate or risedronate) can be given to maintain Ca in the normal range.

Plicamycin 25 μg/kg IV once/day in 50 mL of 5% D/W over 4 to 6 h is effective in patients with hypercalcemia due to cancer but is used infrequently because other treatments are safer. Gallium nitrate is also effective in hypercalcemia due to cancer but is used infrequently because of renal toxicity and limited clinical experience.

The addition of corticosteroids (eg, prednisone 20 to 40 mg po once/day) effectively controls hypercalcemia by decreasing calcitriol production and thus intestinal Ca absorption in most patients with vitamin D toxicity, idiopathic hypercalcemia of infancy, and sarcoidosis. Some patients with myeloma, lymphoma, leukemia, or metastatic cancer require 40 to 60 mg of prednisone once/day. However, > 50% of such patients fail to respond to corticosteroids, and response, when it occurs, takes several days; thus, other treatment usually is necessary.

Chloroquine PO_4 500 mg po once/day inhibits $1,25(OH)_2D$ synthesis and reduces plasma Ca levels in patients with sarcoidosis. Routine ophthalmologic surveillance (eg, retinal examinations q 6 to 12 mo) is mandatory to detect dose-related retinal damage.

In severe hypercalcemia (plasma Ca > 18 mg/dL [> 4.50 mmol/L] or with severe symptoms), hemodialysis with low-Ca dialysate may be needed in addition to other treatments above. Although there is no completely satisfactory way to correct severe hypercalcemia in patients with renal failure, hemodialysis is probably the safest and most reliable short-term treatment.

IV PO_4 (disodium PO_4 or monopotassium PO_4) should be used only when hypercalcemia is life threatening and unresponsive to other methods and when short-term hemodialysis is not possible. No more than 1 g should be given IV in 24 h; usually 1 or 2 doses over 2 days lower plasma Ca for 10 to 15 days. Soft-tissue calcification and acute renal failure may result. NOTE: *IV infusion of Na sulfate is even more hazardous and less effective than PO_4 infusion and should not be used.*

Treatment of hyperparathyroidism in patients with renal failure is combined with dietary PO_4 restriction and PO_4-binding agents, such as Ca carbonate or sevelamer, to prevent hyperphosphatemia and metastatic calcification. Aluminum-containing compounds should be avoided in renal failure, especially in patients receiving long-term dialysis, to prevent accumulation in bone resulting in severe osteomalacia. Despite the use of PO_4 binders, dietary restriction of PO_4 is needed. Vitamin D administration is potentially hazardous in renal failure and requires frequent monitoring of Ca and PO_4. Treatment should be limited to patients with symptomatic osteomalacia (unrelated to aluminum), secondary hyperparathyroidism, or postparathyroidectomy hypocalcemia. Although oral calcitriol is often given along with oral Ca to suppress secondary hyperparathyroidism, the results are variable in patients with end-stage renal disease. The parenteral form of calcitriol, or vitamin D analogs such as paricalcitol, may better prevent secondary hyperparathyroidism in such patients, because the higher attained plasma levels of $1,25(OH)_2D$ directly suppress PTH release. Elevation of serum Ca frequently complicates vitamin D therapy in dialysis patients. Simple osteomalacia may respond to 0.25 to 0.5 μg/day of oral calcitriol, whereas correction of postparathyroidectomy hypocalcemia may require prolonged administration of as much as 2 μg of calcitriol/day and ≥ 2 g of elemental Ca/day. The calcimimetic, cinacalcet, represents a new class of drugs that decrease PTH levels in dialysis patients without increasing serum Ca. Osteomalacia caused by aluminum usually occurs in dialysis patients who have taken large amounts of aluminum-containing PO_4 binders. In these patients, removal of aluminum with deferoxamine is necessary before improvement in bone lesions occurs with calcitriol.

Symptomatic or progressive hyperparathyroidism is treated surgically. Adenomatous glands are removed. The remaining parathyroid tissue is also generally removed, because parathyroid glands are typically difficult to locate during subsequent surgical exploration. To prevent subsequent hypoparathyroidism, a small portion of a normal-appearing parathyroid gland is usually reimplanted in the belly of the sternocleidomastoid muscle or subcutaneously in the forearm. Cryopreservation of parathyroid tissue is also occasionally performed to allow for later autologous transplantation if persistent hypoparathyroidism develops.

The indications for surgery in patients with mild, primary hyperparathyroidism are controversial. A summary statement from the 2002 NIH Workshop on Asymptomatic Primary Hyperparathyroidism lists as indications for surgery the following: plasma Ca 1 mg/dL (0.25 mmol/L) > upper limits of normal; calciuria > 400 mg/day (10 mmol/day); creatinine clearance 30% < that of age-matched controls; peak bone density at the hip, lumbar spine, or radius 2.5 standard deviations below controls (T score = −2.5); age < 50 yr; and the possibility of poor compliance with followup. If surgery is not performed, patients should remain active (ie, avoid immobilization that could exacerbate hypercalcemia), follow a low-Ca diet, drink plenty of fluids to minimize the chance of nephrolithiasis, and avoid drugs that can raise plasma Ca, such as thiazide diuretics. Plasma Ca and renal function are monitored q 6 mo. Bone density is monitored q 12 mo.

Although patients with asymptomatic primary hyperparathyroidism with no indications for surgery may be treated conservatively, concerns regarding subclinical bone disease, hypertension, and longevity remain. Although FHH results from histologically abnormal parathyroid tissue, the response to subtotal parathyroidectomy is unsatisfactory. Because overt clinical manifestations are rare, occasional drug therapy is usually sufficient.

When hyperparathyroidism is mild, the plasma Ca level drops to just below normal within 24 to 48 h after surgery; plasma Ca must be monitored. In patients with severe osteitis fibrosa cystica, prolonged, symptomatic hypocalcemia may occur postoperatively unless 10 to 20 g elemental Ca is given in the days before surgery. Even with preoperative Ca administration, large doses of Ca and vitamin D may be required (see p. 1253) while bone Ca is repleted.

DISORDERS OF PHOSPHATE CONCENTRATION

Phosphorus is one of the most abundant elements in the human body. Most phosphorus in the body is complexed with oxygen as phosphate (PO_4). About 85% of the roughly 500 to 700 g of PO_4 in the body is contained in bone, where it is an important constituent of hydroxyapatite. In soft tissues, PO_4 is mainly found in the intracellular compartment as an integral component of several organic compounds, including nucleic acids and cell membrane phospholipids. PO_4 is also involved in aerobic and anaerobic energy metabolism. RBC 2,3-diphosphoglycerate (2,3-DPG) plays a crucial role in O_2 delivery to tissue. Adenosine diphosphate (ADP) and ATP contain PO_4 and use chemical bonds between PO_4 groups to store energy. Inorganic PO_4 is a major intracellular anion but is also present in plasma. The normal plasma inorganic PO_4 concentration in adults ranges from 2.5 to 4.5 mg/dL (0.81 to 1.45 mmol/L). PO_4 is ≤ 50% higher in infants and 30% higher in children, possibly because additional PO_4 is required for growth.

The typical American diet contains about 800 to 1500 mg of PO_4. This amount appears in the stool in varying amounts depending on the amount of PO_4 binding compounds (mainly Ca) in the diet. Like Ca, GI PO_4 absorption is enhanced by vitamin D. Renal PO_4 excretion roughly equals GI absorption to maintain PO_4 balance. PO_4 depletion can occur in various diseases and normally results in conservation of PO_4 by the kidneys. Bone PO_4 serves as a reservoir, which can buffer changes in plasma and intracellular PO_4.

HYPOPHOSPHATEMIA

Hypophosphatemia is plasma phosphate (PO_4) concentration < 2.5 mg/dL (0.81 mmol/L). Causes include alcoholism, burns, starvation, and diuretic use. Clinical features include muscle weakness, respiratory failure, and heart failure; seizures and

coma can occur. Diagnosis is by serum PO_4 levels. Treatment consists of PO_4 supplementation.

Etiology and Pathophysiology

Hypophosphatemia occurs in 2% of hospitalized patients but is more prevalent in certain populations (eg, it occurs in up to 10% of hospitalized patients with alcoholism). Hypophosphatemia has numerous causes, but clinically significant hypophosphatemia occurs in relatively few clinical settings, such as the recovery phase of diabetic ketoacidosis, acute alcoholism, and severe burns. Hypophosphatemia may also occur in patients receiving TPN, during refeeding after prolonged malnutrition, and in severe chronic respiratory alkalosis.

Acute hypophosphatemia with plasma PO_4 < 1 mg/dL (< 0.32 mmol/L) is most often caused by transcellular shifts of PO_4, often superimposed on chronic PO_4 depletion.

Chronic hypophosphatemia most often results from decreased renal PO_4 reabsorption. Causes include hyperparathyroidism; other hormonal disturbances, such as Cushing's syndrome and hypothyroidism; electrolyte disorders, such as hypomagnesemia and hypokalemia; theophylline intoxication; and long-term diuretic administration. Severe chronic hypophosphatemia usually results from a prolonged negative PO_4 balance. Causes include chronic starvation or malabsorption, especially if combined with vomiting or copious diarrhea, or long-term ingestion of large amounts of PO_4-binding aluminum, usually in the form of antacids. Ingestion of aluminum is particularly prone to produce PO_4 depletion when combined with decreased dietary intake and dialysis losses of PO_4 in patients with end-stage renal disease.

Symptoms, Signs, and Diagnosis

Although hypophosphatemia usually is asymptomatic, anorexia, muscle weakness, and osteomalacia can occur in severe chronic depletion. Serious neuromuscular disturbances may occur, including progressive encephalopathy, coma, and death. The muscle weakness of profound hypophosphatemia may be accompanied by rhabdomyolysis, especially in acute alcoholism. Hematologic disturbances of profound hypophosphatemia include hemolytic anemia, decreased release of O_2 from hemoglobin, and impaired leukocyte and platelet function.

Hypophosphatemia is diagnosed by a plasma PO_4 level < 2.5 mg/dL (< 0.81 mmol/L). A search for the cause (such as liver function tests or signs of cirrhosis in a patient suspected of alcoholism) is appropriate. However, most causes of hypophosphatemia (eg, diabetic ketoacidosis, burns, refeeding) are readily apparent.

Treatment

Oral PO_4 replacement is usually adequate in asymptomatic patients, even when the plasma concentration is very low. PO_4 can be given in doses ≤ 3 g/day po in tablets containing Na or K PO_4. Oral Na or K PO_4 is usually poorly tolerated because of diarrhea. Ingestion of 1 L of low-fat or skim milk provides 1 g of PO_4 and may be more acceptable. Removal of the cause of hypophosphatemia, such as stopping PO_4-binding antacids or diuretics or correcting hypomagnesemia, is preferable when possible.

Parenteral PO_4 should be administered when plasma PO_4 is < 0.5 mEq/L (< 0.16 mmol/L); rhabdomyolysis, hemolysis, or CNS symptoms are present; or oral replacement is not feasible due to underlying illness. IV administration of KPO_4 (as buffered mix of K_2HPO_4 and KH_2PO_4) is relatively safe if renal function is well preserved. The usual parenteral dose is 2 mg (8 mmol)/kg IV over 6 h. Alcoholics may require ≥ 1 g/day during TPN; supplemental PO_4 is stopped when oral intake is resumed. Plasma Ca and PO_4 levels should be monitored during therapy, particularly when PO_4 is given IV or to patients with impaired renal function. In most cases, no more than 7 mg/kg (about 500 mg for a 70-kg adult) of PO_4 should be given over 6 h. Hypocalcemia, hyperphosphatemia, metastatic calcification, and hyperkalemia may be avoided by close monitoring and avoidance of more rapid rates of PO_4 administration. $NaPO_4$ (rather than KPO_4) preparations generally should be used in patients with impaired renal function.

HYPERPHOSPHATEMIA

Hyperphosphatemia is serum phosphate (PO_4) concentration > 4.5 mg/dL (> 1.46 mmol/L). Causes include chronic renal failure, hypoparathyroidism, and metabolic or respiratory acidosis. Clinical features may be due to accompanying hypocalcemia and include tetany. Diagnosis is by serum PO_4. Treatment includes restriction of PO_4 intake

and administration of PO_4-binding antacids, such as Ca carbonate.

Hyperphosphatemia generally results from a decrease in renal excretion of PO_4. Advanced renal insufficiency (GFR < 20 mL/min) reduces excretion sufficiently to increase plasma PO_4. Defects in renal excretion of PO_4 in the absence of renal failure also occur in pseudohypoparathyroidism and hypoparathyroidism. Hyperphosphatemia can also occur with excessive oral PO_4 administration and occasionally with overzealous use of enemas containing PO_4.

Hyperphosphatemia occasionally results from a transcellular shift of PO_4 into the extracellular space that is so large that the renal excretory capacity is overwhelmed. This occurs most frequently in diabetic ketoacidosis (despite total body PO_4 depletion), crush injuries, and nontraumatic rhabdomyolysis as well as in overwhelming systemic infections and tumor lysis syndrome. Hyperphosphatemia also plays a critical role in the development of secondary hyperparathyroidism and renal osteodystrophy in patients on dialysis. Lastly, hyperphosphatemia can be spurious in cases of hyperproteinemia (multiple myeloma or Waldenström's macroglobulinemia), hyperlipidemia, hemolysis, or hyperbilirubinemia.

Symptoms, Signs, and Diagnosis

Most patients with hyperphosphatemia are asymptomatic, although symptoms of hypocalcemia, including tetany, can occur if concomitant hypocalcemia is present. Soft-tissue calcifications are common in patients with chronic renal failure, especially if the plasma Ca × PO_4 product is chronically > 70.

Hyperphosphatemia is diagnosed by PO_4 level > 4.5 mg/dL (> 1.46 mmol/L). If the etiology is not obvious (eg, rhabdomyolysis, tumor lysis syndrome, renal failure, overingestion of PO_4 laxatives), additional evaluation is warranted to exclude hypoparathyroidism or pseudohypoparathyroidism, which is end-organ resistance to PTH (see p. 1250). False elevation of serum PO_4 also should be excluded by measuring serum protein, lipid, and bilirubin levels.

Treatment

The mainstay of treatment in patients with renal failure is reduction of intake of PO_4. This is usually accomplished with avoidance of foods containing high amounts of PO_4 and with use of PO_4-binding drugs taken with meals. Because of the possibility of aluminum-related osteomalacia, Ca carbonate and Ca acetate replace aluminum-containing antacids in patients with end-stage renal disease. Recently, the possibility of excessive Ca × PO_4 products causing vascular calcification in dialysis patients taking Ca-containing binders has been recognized. For this reason, a PO_4-binding resin, sevelamer, is now widely used in dialysis patients in doses of 800 to 2400 mg tid with meals.

DISORDERS OF MAGNESIUM CONCENTRATION

Mg is the 4th most plentiful cation in the body. A 70-kg adult has about 2000 mEq of Mg. About 50% is sequestered in bone and is not readily exchangeable with other compartments. The ECF contains only about 1% of total body Mg. The remainder resides in the intracellular compartment. Normal plasma Mg concentration ranges from 1.4 to 2.1 mEq/L (0.70 to 1.05 mmol/L).

The maintenance of plasma Mg concentration is largely a function of dietary intake and effective renal and intestinal conservation. Within 7 days of initiation of a Mg-deficient diet, renal and stool Mg excretion each fall to about 1 mEq/day (0.5 mmol/day).

About 70% of plasma Mg is ultrafiltered by the kidney; the remainder is bound to protein. Protein binding of Mg is pH dependent. Plasma Mg concentration and either total body Mg or intracellular Mg content are not closely related. However, severe plasma hypomagnesemia may reflect diminished body stores of Mg.

Many enzymes are Mg activated or dependent. Mg is required by all enzymatic processes involving ATP and by many of the enzymes involved in nucleic acid metabolism. Mg is required for thiamine pyrophosphate cofactor activity and appears to stabilize the structure of macromolecules such as DNA and RNA. Mg is also related to Ca and K metabolism in an intimate but poorly understood way.

HYPOMAGNESEMIA

Hypomagnesemia is plasma Mg concentration < 1.4 mEq/L (< 0.70 mmol/L). Causes include inadequate Mg intake and absorption or increased excretion due to hypercalcemia

or drugs such as furosemide. Clinical features are often due to accompanying hypokalemia and hypocalcemia and include lethargy, tremor, tetany, seizures, and arrhythmias. Treatment is with Mg replacement.

Plasma Mg concentration, even if free Mg is measured, may be normal even with decreased intracellular or bone Mg stores. Mg depletion usually results from inadequate intake plus impairment of renal conservation or GI absorption. There are numerous causes of clinically significant Mg deficiency (see TABLE 156–8).

Symptoms, Signs, and Diagnosis

Clinical manifestations are anorexia, nausea, vomiting, lethargy, weakness, personality change, tetany (eg, positive Trousseau's or Chvostek's sign or spontaneous carpopedal spasm), and tremor and muscle fasciculations. The neurologic signs, particularly tetany, correlate with development of concomitant hypocalcemia and/or hypokalemia. Myopathic potentials are found on electromyography but are also compatible with hypocalcemia or hypokalemia. Severe hypomagnesemia may produce generalized tonic-clonic seizures, especially in children.

Hypomagnesemia is diagnosed by a serum Mg level < 1.4 mEq/L (< 0.70 mmol/L). Severe hypomagnesemia usually results in levels of < 1.0 mEq/L (< 0.50 mmol/L). Associated hypocalcemia and hypocalciuria are common in patients with steatorrhea, alcoholism, or other causes of Mg deficiency. Hypokalemia with increased urinary K excretion and metabolic alkalosis may be present. Thus, unexplained hypocalcemia and hypokalemia suggest the possibility of Mg depletion.

TABLE 156–8. CAUSES OF HYPOMAGNESEMIA

CAUSE	COMMENT
Alcoholism	Due to both inadequate intake and excessive renal excretion
GI losses	Chronic diabetes Steatorrhea
Pregnancy-related	Pre-eclampsia/eclampsia (see p. 2197) Lactation (increased Mg requirements)
Primary renal losses	Rare disorder(s). Inappropriately high urinary Mg excretion without apparent cause (eg, Gitelman's syndrome)
Secondary renal losses	Loop and thiazide diuretics Hypercalcemia After removal of parathyroid tumor Diabetic ketoacidosis Hypersecretion of aldosterone, thyroid hormones, or ADH Nephrotoxins (amphotericin B, cisplastin, cyclosporine, aminoglycosides)

Treatment

Treatment with Mg salts (sulfate or chloride) is indicated when Mg deficiency is symptomatic or persistent by < 1 mEq/L (< 0.50 mmol/L). Alcoholics are treated empirically. In such cases, deficits approaching 12 to 24 mg/kg are possible. About twice the amount of the estimated deficit should be given in patients with intact renal function, because about 50% of the administered Mg is excreted in urine. Mg gluconate 500 to 1000 mg po tid is given for 3 to 4 days. Parenteral administration is reserved for patients with severe, symptomatic hypomagnesemia or who cannot tolerate oral drugs. When Mg must be replaced parenterally, a 10% Mg sulfate ($MgSO_4$) solution (1 g/10 mL) is available for IV use and a 50% solution (1 g/2 mL) is available for IM use. The plasma Mg level should be monitored frequently during Mg therapy, particularly when Mg is given parenterally or to patients with renal insufficiency. Treatment is continued until a normal plasma Mg level is achieved.

In severe, symptomatic hypomagnesemia (eg, generalized seizures, Mg < 1 mEq/L [< 0.5 mmol/L]), 2 to 4 g of $MgSO_4$ IV is given over 5 to 10 min. If seizures persist, the dose may be repeated up to a total of 10 g over the next 6 h. If seizures stop, 10 g in 1 L of 5% D/W can be infused over 24 h, followed by up to 2.5 g q 12 h to replace the deficit in total Mg stores and prevent further drops in plasma Mg. When plasma Mg is 1 mEq/L (< 0.5 mmol/L) but symptoms are less severe, $MgSO_4$ may be given IV in 5% D/W at a rate of 1 g/h as slow infusion for up to 10 h. In less severe cases of hypomagnesemia, gradual repletion may be achieved by administration of smaller parenteral doses over 3 to 5 days until the plasma Mg level is normal.

Hypermagnesemia

Hypermagnesemia is a plasma Mg concentration > 2.1 mEq/L (> 1.05 mmol/L). The major cause is renal failure. Symptoms include hypotension, respiratory depression, and cardiac arrest. Diagnosis is by serum Mg levels. Treatment includes IV administration of Ca gluconate and possibly furosemide; hemodialysis can be helpful in severe cases.

Symptomatic hypermagnesemia is fairly uncommon. It occurs most commonly in patients with renal failure after ingestion of Mg-containing drugs, such as antacids or purgatives.

Symptoms, Signs, and Diagnosis

At plasma Mg concentrations of 5 to 10 mEq/L (2.5 to 5 mmol/L), the ECG shows prolongation of the PR interval, widening of the QRS complex, and increased T-wave amplitude. Deep tendon reflexes disappear as the plasma Mg level approaches 10 mEq/L (5.0 mmol/L); hypotension, respiratory depression, and narcosis develop with increasing hypermagnesemia. Cardiac arrest may occur when blood Mg levels exceed 12 to 15 mEq/L (6.0 to 7.5 mmol/L).

Hypermagnesemia is diagnosed when serum Mg levels are > 2.1 mEq/L (> 1.05 mmol/L).

Treatment

Treatment of severe Mg toxicity consists of circulatory and respiratory support with administration of 10% Ca gluconate 10 to 20 mL IV. Ca gluconate may reverse many of the Mg-induced changes, including respiratory depression. Administration of IV furosemide can increase Mg excretion if renal function is adequate and volume status is maintained. Hemodialysis may be valuable in severe hypermagnesemia, because a relatively large fraction (about 70%) of blood Mg is not protein bound and thus ultrafilterable. If hemodynamic compromise occurs and hemodialysis is impractical, peritoneal dialysis is an option.

157 ACID-BASE REGULATION AND DISORDERS

Metabolic processes continually produce acid and, to a lesser degree, base. H^+ is especially reactive; it can attach to negatively charged proteins and, in high concentrations, alter their overall charge, configuration, and function. To maintain cellular function, the body has elaborate mechanisms that maintain blood H^+ concentration within a narrow range—typically 37 to 43 nmol/L (pH 7.37 to 7.43, where $pH = -\log [H^+]$) and ideally 40 nmol/L (pH = 7.4). Disturbances of these mechanisms can have serious clinical consequences.

Acid-base equilibrium is closely tied to fluid and electrolyte balance, and disturbances in one of these systems often affect another. Fluid and electrolytes are discussed on p. 1233.

Acid-Base Physiology

Most acid comes from carbohydrate and fat metabolism, which generates 15,000 to 20,000 mmol of CO_2 daily. CO_2 is not an acid itself but combines with water (H_2O) in the blood to create carbonic acid (H_2CO_3), which in the presence of the enzyme carbonic anhydrase dissociates into H^+ and HCO_3^-. The H^+ binds with Hb in the blood and is released with oxygenation in the alveoli, at which time the above reaction is reversed, creating H_2O and CO_2, which is exhaled in each breath.

Lesser amounts of organic acid derive from incomplete metabolism of glucose and fatty acids into lactic acid and ketoacids; from metabolism of sulfur-containing amino acids (cysteine, methionine) into sulfuric acid; from metabolism of cationic amino acids (arginine, lysine); and from hydrolysis of dietary phosphate. This "fixed" or "metabolic" acid load cannot be exhaled and therefore must be neutralized or excreted.

Most base comes from metabolism of anionic amino acids (glutamate and aspartate) and from oxidation and consumption of organic anions such as lactate and citrate, which produce HCO_3^-.

Acid-Base Balance

Acid-base balance is maintained by chemical buffering and by pulmonary and renal elimination.

Chemical buffering: Chemical buffers provide an immediate response to acid-base disturbances. Buffers may be extracellular or intracellular; bone also plays an important buffering role. A buffer is the conjugate base of a weak acid; it accepts and relinquishes H^+, thereby minimizing changes in free H^+ concentration.

The most important physiologic buffer is the extracellular HCO_3^-/CO_2 system, described by the equation:

$$H^+ + HCO_3^- \Leftrightarrow H_2CO_3 \Leftrightarrow CO_2 + H_2O$$

An increase in H^+ drives the equation to the right and generates CO_2. This buffer system is most important and efficient because CO_2 concentrations can be finely controlled by alveolar ventilation, whereas H^+ and HCO_3^- concentrations can be finely regulated by renal excretion.

The relationship between HCO_3^- and CO_2 in the system is quantified by the Kassirer-Bleich equation, derived from the Henderson-Hasselbalch equation:

$$H^+ = 24 \times P_{CO_2}/HCO_3^-$$

This equation illustrates that acid-base balance depends on the ratio of P_{CO_2} and HCO_3^-, not on the absolute value of either one alone. Any 2 measures (usually H^+ and P_{CO_2}) can be used to calculate the other (usually HCO_3^-).

Other important physiologic buffers include intracellular organic and inorganic phosphates and proteins, including Hb in RBCs. Less important are extracellular phosphate and plasma proteins. Bone becomes an important buffer after consumption of extracellular HCO_3^-. Bone initially releases sodium carbonate ($NaHCO_3$) and potassium carbonate ($KHCO_3$) in exchange for H^+; with prolonged acid loads, bone releases calcium carbonate ($CaCO_3$) and calcium phosphate ($CaPO_4$). Long-standing acidemia therefore contributes to bone demineralization and osteoporosis.

Pulmonary regulation: CO_2 concentration is finely regulated by changes in tidal volume and respiratory rate (minute ventilation). A decrease in pH is sensed by arterial chemoreceptors and leads to increases in tidal volume or respiratory rate; CO_2 is exhaled and blood pH increases. In contrast to chemical buffering, which is immediate, pulmonary regulation occurs over minutes to hours. It is about 50 to 75% effective; it does not completely normalize pH.

Renal regulation: The kidneys control pH by adjusting the amount of HCO_3^- that is reabsorbed and the amount of H^+ that is excreted; increase in HCO_3^- is equivalent to removing free H^+. Changes in renal acid-base handling occur hours to days after changes in acid-base status.

HCO_3^- reabsorption occurs mostly in the proximal tubule and, to a lesser degree, in the collecting tubule. H_2O within the tubular cell dissociates into H^+ and OH^-; in the presence of carbonic anhydrase, the OH^- combines with CO_2 to form HCO_3^-, which is transported back into the peritubular capillary, while the H^+ is secreted into the tubular lumen and joins with freely filtered HCO_3^- to form CO_2 and H_2O, which are also reabsorbed. Thus reabsorbed HCO_3^- ions are newly generated and not the same as those that were filtered. Decreases in effective circulating volume (such as occur with diuretic therapy) increase HCO_3^- reabsorption, while increases in parathyroid hormone in response to an acid load decrease HCO_3^- reabsorption. Also, increased P_{CO_2} leads to increased HCO_3^- reabsorption, while Cl^- depletion (typically from volume depletion) leads to increased Na^+ reabsorption and HCO_3^- generation by the proximal tubule.

Acid is actively excreted into the proximal and distal tubules where it combines with urinary buffers—primarily freely filtered HPO_4^{-2}, creatinine, uric acid, and ammonia—to be transported outside the body. The ammonia buffering system is especially important because other buffers are filtered in fixed concentrations and can be depleted by high acid loads; by contrast, tubular cells actively regulate ammonia production in response to changes in acid load. Arterial pH is the main determinant of acid secretion, but excretion is also influenced by K^+, Cl^-, and aldosterone levels. Intracellular K^+ concentration and H^+ secretion are reciprocally related; K^+ depletion causes increased H^+ secretion and hence metabolic alkalosis.

ACID-BASE DISORDERS

Acid-base disorders are changes in arterial PCO_2, serum HCO_3^-, and serum pH.

Acidemia is serum pH < 7.35.

Alkalemia is serum pH > 7.45.

Acidosis refers to physiologic processes that cause acid accumulation or alkali loss.

Alkalosis refers to physiologic processes that cause alkali accumulation or acid loss.

Actual changes in pH depend on the degree of physiologic compensation and whether multiple processes are present.

Classification

Acidoses and alkaloses are defined as metabolic or respiratory based on clinical context and primary changes in serum HCO_3^- or PCO_2.

Metabolic acidosis is serum $HCO_3^- < 24$ mEq/L. Causes are increased acid production or acid ingestion, decreased renal acid excretion, and GI or renal HCO_3^- loss.

Metabolic alkalosis is serum $HCO_3^- > 24$ mEq/L. Cause is acid loss or HCO_3^- retention.

Respiratory acidosis is $PCO_2 > 40$ mm Hg (hypercapnia). Cause is a decrease in respiratory rate or volume or both (hypoventilation).

Respiratory alkalosis is $PCO_2 < 40$ mm Hg (hypocapnia). Cause is an increase in respiratory rate or volume or both (hyperventilation).

Simple acid-base disorders, discussed below, are one disorder. Mixed acid-base disorders comprise 2 or more disorders. Simple and mixed disorders may occur with or without respiratory or renal compensation (see TABLE 157–1). Compensation cannot return

TABLE 157–1. PRIMARY CHANGES AND COMPENSATIONS IN SIMPLE ACID-BASE DISORDERS

DISORDER	pH	HCO_3	PCO_2	COMPENSATION
Metabolic acidosis	< 7.35	Primary decrease	Compensatory decrease	1.2-mm Hg decrease in PCO_2 for every 1-mmol/L decrease in HCO_3 **or** $PCO_2 = (1.5 \times HCO_3) + 8\ (\pm 2)$ **or** $PCO_2 = HCO_3 + 15$ **or** PCO_2 = last 2 digits of pH × 100
Metabolic alkalosis	> 7.45	Primary increase	Compensatory increase	0.6–0.75 mm Hg increase in PCO_2 for every 1-mmol/L increase in HCO_3. PCO_2 should not rise above 60 mm Hg in compensation
Respiratory acidosis	< 7.35	Compensatory increase	Primary increase	*Acute:* 1–2 mmol increase in HCO_3 for every 10-mm Hg increase in PCO_2 *Chronic:* 3–4 mmol increase in HCO_3 for every 10-mm Hg increase in PCO_2
Respiratory alkalosis	> 7.45	Compensatory increase	Primary increase	*Acute:* 1–2 mmol decrease in HCO_3 for every 10-mm Hg decrease in PCO_2 *Chronic:* 4–5 mmol decrease in HCO_3 for every 10-mm Hg decrease in PCO_2

TABLE 157–2. CLINICAL CONSEQUENCES OF ACID-BASE DISORDERS

SYSTEM	ACIDEMIA	ALKALEMIA
Cardiovascular	Impaired cardiac contractility; arteriolar dilation; venoconstriction; centralization of blood volume; increased pulmonary vascular resistance; decreased cardiac output, systemic blood pressure, hepatorenal blood flow; decreased threshold for cardiac arrhythmias; attenuation of responsiveness to catecholamines	Arteriolar constriction; reduced coronary blood flow; reduced anginal threshold; decreased threshold for cardiac arrhythmias
Metabolic	Insulin resistance; inhibition of anaerobic glycolysis; reduction in ATP synthesis; hyperkalemia; protein degradation; bone demineralization (chronic)	Stimulation of anaerobic glycolysis; formation of organic acids; decreased oxyhemoglobin dissociation; decreased ionized Ca; hypokalemia; hypomagnesemia; hypophosphatemia
Neurologic	Inhibition of metabolism and cell-volume regulation; obtundation and coma	Tetany; seizures; lethargy; delirium; stupor
Respiratory	Compensatory hyperventilation with possible respiratory muscle fatigue	Compensatory hypoventilation with possible hypercapnia and hypoxemia

pH completely to normal and never overshoots.

Symptoms and Signs

Compensated or mild acid-base disorders cause few symptoms or signs. Severe, uncompensated disorders have multiple cardiovascular, respiratory, neurologic, and metabolic consequences described below and in TABLE 157–2 (see also FIG. 46–4 on p. 371).

Diagnosis

Evaluation is with ABG and serum electrolytes. The ABG directly measures arterial pH and PCO_2. HCO_3^- levels on ABG are calculated using the Henderson-Hasselbalch equation; levels on serum chemistry panels are directly measured and are more accurate.

The pH establishes the primary process (acidosis or alkalosis) but may normalize with compensation. Changes in PCO_2 reflect the respiratory component, and changes in HCO_3^- reflect the metabolic component. However, several calculations may be required to determine if changes in PCO_2 and HCO_3^- are primary or compensatory and whether a mixed disorder is present; in mixed disorders, values may be deceptively normal. Interpretation must also consider clinical conditions (eg, chronic lung disease, renal failure, drug overdose).

The anion gap (see sidebar 157–1) should always be calculated; elevation almost always indicates a metabolic acidosis. A normal anion gap with a low HCO_3^- (eg, < 24 mEq/L) and high serum Cl indicates a non-anion gap (hyperchloremic) metabolic acidosis. If metabolic acidosis is present, a delta-gap is calculated (see sidebar 157–1) to identify concomitant metabolic alkalosis, and Winter's formula is applied to see whether respiratory compensation is appropriate or reflects a 2nd acid-base disorder (predicted $PCO_2 = 1.5\,[HCO_3^-] + 8 \pm 2$; if PCO_2 is higher, there is also a primary respiratory acidosis—if lower, respiratory alkalosis).

Respiratory acidosis is suggested by PCO_2 > 40 mm Hg; HCO_3^- should compensate acutely by increasing 3 to 4 mEq/L for each 10-mm Hg rise in PCO_2 sustained for 4 to 12 h (there may be no increase or only 1 to 2 mEq/L, which slowly increases to 3 to 4 mEq/L over days). Greater increase in HCO_3^- implies a primary metabolic alkalosis; lesser increase suggests no time for compensation or coexisting primary metabolic acidosis.

Metabolic alkalosis is suggested by HCO_3^- > 28 mEq/L. The PCO_2 should compensate by increasing about 0.6 to 0.75 mm Hg for each 1 mEq/L increase in HCO_3^- (up to about 55 mm Hg). Greater increase implies concomitant respiratory acidosis; lesser increase, respiratory alkalosis.

Respiratory alkalosis is suggested by P_{CO_2} <38 mm Hg. The HCO_3^- should compensate over 4 to 12 h by decreasing 5 mEq/L for every 10-mm Hg decrease in P_{CO_2}. Lesser decrease means there has been no time for compensation or existence of a primary metabolic alkalosis. Greater decrease implies a primary metabolic acidosis.

Nomograms are an alternative way to diagnose mixed disorders, allowing for simultaneous plotting of pH, HCO_3^-, and P_{CO_2}.

Sidebar 157–1. THE ANION GAP

The anion gap is defined as plasma Na concentration minus the sum of Cl and HCO_3^- concentrations; $Na^+ - (Cl^- + HCO_3^-)$. The term "gap" is misleading, because the law of electroneutrality requires the same number of positive and negative charges in an open system; the gap appears on laboratory testing because certain cations (+) and anions (–) are not measured on routine laboratory chemistry panels. Thus:

Na^+ + unmeasured cations (UC) = Cl^- + HCO_3^- + unmeasured anions (UA)
and
the anion gap, $Na^+ - (Cl^- + HCO_3^-)$ = UA – UC.

The predominant unmeasured anions are PO_4^{3-}, SO_4^-, various negatively charged proteins, and some organic acids, accounting for 20 to 24 mEq/L. The predominant unmeasured extracellular cations are K^+, Ca^{++}, and Mg^{++} and account for about 11 mEq/L. Thus the typical anion gap is 23 – 11 = 12 mEq/L. The anion gap can be affected by increases or decreases in the UC or UA.

Increased anion gap is most commonly caused by metabolic acidosis in which negatively charged acids—mostly ketones, lactate, sulfates, or metabolites of methanol, ethylene glycol, and salicylate—consume (are buffered by) HCO_3^-. Other causes of increased anion gap include hyperalbuminemia and uremia (increased anions) and hypocalcemia or hypomagnesemia (decreased cations).

Decreased anion gap is unrelated to metabolic acidosis but is caused by hypoalbuminemia (decreased anions); hypercalcemia, hypermagnesemia, lithium intoxication, and hypergammaglobulinemia (increased cations); or hyperviscosity or halide (bromide or iodide) intoxication. The effect of low albumin can be accounted for by adjusting the anion gap 2.5 mEq/L upward for every 1-g/dL fall in albumin.

Negative anion gap occurs rarely as a laboratory artifact in severe cases of hypernatremia, hyperlipidemia, and bromide intoxication.

The delta gap: The difference between the patient's anion gap and the normal anion gap is termed the delta gap. This amount is considered an HCO_3^- equivalent, because for every unit rise in the anion gap, the HCO_3^- should lower by 1 (by buffering). Thus, if the delta gap is added to the measured HCO_3^-, the result should be in the normal range for HCO_3^-; elevation indicates the additional presence of a metabolic alkalosis.

Example: A vomiting, ill-appearing alcoholic patient has laboratory results showing

Na, 137; K, 3.8; Cl, 90; HCO_3^-, 22; pH, 7.40; P_{CO_2}, 41; P_{O_2}, 85

At first glance, results appear unremarkable. However, calculations show elevation of the anion gap

137 – (90 + 22) = 25 (normal, 10),

indicating a metabolic acidosis. Respiratory compensation is evaluated by Winter's formula:

Predicted P_{CO_2} = 1.5 (22) + 8 ± 2
= 39 ± 2

Predicted = measured, so respiratory compensation is appropriate.

Because there is metabolic acidosis, the delta gap is calculated, and the result is added to measured HCO_3^-:

25 – 10 = 15
15 + 22 = 37

The HCO_3^- equivalent indicates a metabolic alkalosis. Thus, the patient has a mixed disorder, with metabolic acidosis from alcoholic ketoacidosis and metabolic alkalosis from recurrent vomiting with loss of Cl and volume.

TABLE 157–3. CAUSES OF METABOLIC ACIDOSIS

High anion gap

Ketoacidosis (diabetes, chronic alcoholism, malnutrition, fasting)

Lactic acidosis

Renal failure

Toxins metabolized to acids
- Methanol (formate)
- Ethylene glycol (oxalate)
- Paraldehyde (acetate, chloracetate)
- Salicylates

Toxins causing lactic acidosis
- CO_2
- Cyanide
- Iron
- Isoniazid
- Toluene (initially high gap, subsequent excretion of metabolites normalizes gap)

Rhabdomyolysis (rare)

Normal anion gap (hyperchloremic acidosis)

GI HCO_3^- loss (diarrhea, ileostomy, colostomy, enteric fistulas, use of ion-exchange resins)

Ureterosigmoidostomy, ureteroileal conduit

Renal HCO_3^- loss
- Tubulointerstitial renal disease
- Renal tubular acidosis, types 1, 2, 4
- Hyperparathyroidism

Ingestions (acetazolamide, $CaCl_2$, $MgSO_4$)

Others
- Hypoaldosteronism
- Hyperkalemia
- Parenteral infusion of arginine, lysine, NH_4Cl
- Rapid NaCl infusion
- Toluene (late)

METABOLIC ACIDOSIS

Metabolic acidosis is primary reduction in HCO_3^-, typically with compensatory reduction in PCO_2; pH may be markedly low or slightly subnormal. Metabolic acidoses are categorized as high or normal anion gap based on the presence or absence of unmeasured anions in serum. Causes include accumulation of ketones and lactic acid, renal failure, and drug or toxin ingestion (high anion gap) and GI or renal HCO_3^- loss (normal anion gap). Symptoms and signs in severe cases include nausea and vomiting, lethargy, and hyperpnea. Diagnosis is clinical and with ABG and serum electrolytes. The underlying cause is treated; IV $NaHCO_3$ may be indicated when pH is very low.

Etiology and Pathophysiology

Metabolic acidosis is acid accumulation from increased acid production or acid ingestion; decreased acid excretion; or GI or renal HCO_3^- loss. Acidemia (arterial pH < 7.35) results when acid load overwhelms respiratory compensation. Causes are classified by their effect on the anion gap (see sidebar 157–1 and TABLE 157–3).

High anion gap acidosis: The most common causes of a high anion gap metabolic acidosis are ketoacidosis, lactic acidosis (see p. 1270), renal failure, and toxic ingestions.

Ketoacidosis is a common complication of type 1 diabetes mellitus, but it also occurs with chronic alcoholism, malnutrition, and, to a lesser degree, fasting. In these conditions, the body converts from glucose to free fatty acid (FFA) metabolism; FFAs are converted by the liver into ketoacids, acetoacetic acid, and β-hydroxybutyrate (all unmeasured anions). Ketoacidosis is also a rare manifestation of congenital isovaleric and methylmalonic acidemia.

Renal failure causes anion gap acidosis by decreased acid excretion and decreased HCO_3^- reabsorption. Accumulation of sulfates, phosphates, urate, and hippurate accounts for the high anion gap.

Toxins may have acidic metabolites or trigger lactic acidosis. Rhabdomyolysis is a rare cause of metabolic acidosis thought to be due to release of protons and anions directly from muscle.

Normal anion gap acidosis: The most common causes of normal anion gap acidosis are GI or renal HCO_3^- loss and impaired renal acid excretion. Normal anion gap metabolic acidosis is also called hyperchloremic acidosis, because instead of reabsorbing HCO_3^- with Na, the kidney reabsorbs Cl^-.

Many GI secretions are rich in HCO_3^- (eg, biliary, pancreatic, and intestinal fluids); loss from diarrhea, tube drainage, or fistulas can cause acidosis. In ureterosigmoidostomy (insertion of ureters into the sigmoid colon after obstruction or cystectomy), the colon secretes and loses HCO_3^- in exchange for urinary Cl^- and absorbs urinary ammonium, which dissociates into NH_3^+ and H^+. Ion-exchange resin uncommonly causes HCO_3^- loss by binding HCO_3^-.

The renal tubular acidoses (see p. 2026) either impair H^+ secretion (types 1 and 4) or

HCO_3^- absorption (type 2). Impaired acid excretion and a normal anion gap also occur in early renal failure, tubulointerstitial renal disease, and when carbonic anhydrase inhibitors (eg, acetazolamide) are taken.

Symptoms and Signs

Symptoms and signs (see TABLE 157–2) are primarily those of the cause. Mild acidemia is itself asymptomatic. More severe acidemia (pH < 7.10) may cause nausea, vomiting, and malaise. Symptoms may appear at higher pH if acidosis develops rapidly. The most characteristic sign is hyperpnea (long, deep breaths at a normal rate), reflecting a compensatory increase in alveolar ventilation.

Severe, acute acidemia predisposes to cardiac dysfunction with hypotension and shock; ventricular arrhythmias; and coma. Chronic acidemia causes bone demineralization disorders (rickets, osteomalacia, osteopenia).

Diagnosis

Recognition of metabolic acidosis and appropriate respiratory compensation are discussed on p. 1266. Determining the cause of metabolic acidosis begins with the anion gap.

The cause of an elevated anion gap may be clinically obvious (eg, hypovolemic shock, missed hemodialysis), but if not, blood testing should include glucose, BUN, creatinine, lactate, and tests for possible toxins. Salicylate levels can be measured in most laboratories, but methanol and ethylene glycol usually cannot; their presence may be suggested by presence of an osmolar gap. Calculated serum osmolarity (2 [Na] + [glucose]/18 + BUN/2.8 + blood alcohol/5) is subtracted from measured osmolarity. A difference > 10 implies the presence of an osmotically active substance, which in the case of a high anion gap acidosis is methanol or ethylene glycol. Although ingestion of ethanol may cause an osmolar gap and a mild acidosis, it should never be considered the cause of a significant metabolic acidosis.

If the anion gap is normal and no cause is obvious (eg, marked diarrhea), urinary electrolytes are measured and the urinary anion gap is calculated as [Na] + [K] – [Cl]. Normal (including patients with GI losses) is 30 to 50 mEq/L; an elevation suggests renal HCO_3^- loss (for evaluation of renal tubular acidosis, see p. 2027).

Treatment

Treatment is directed at the underlying cause. Hemodialysis is required for renal failure and sometimes for ethylene glycol, methanol, and salicylate poisoning.

Treatment of acidemia with $NaHCO_3$ is clearly indicated only in certain circumstances and is probably deleterious in others. When metabolic acidosis results from loss of HCO_3^- or accumulation of inorganic acids (ie, normal anion gap acidosis), HCO_3^- therapy is generally safe and appropriate. However, when acidosis results from organic acid accumulation (ie, high anion gap acidosis), HCO_3^- is controversial; it does not clearly improve mortality in these conditions, and there are several possible risks. With treatment of the underlying condition, lactate and ketoacids are metabolized back to HCO_3^-; exogenous HCO_3^- loading may therefore cause an "overshoot" metabolic alkalosis. In any condition, HCO_3^- may also cause Na and volume overload, hypokalemia, and, by inhibiting respiratory drive, hypercapnia. Furthermore, because HCO_3^- does not diffuse across cell membranes, intracellular acidosis is not corrected and may paradoxically worsen because some of the added HCO_3^- is converted to CO_2, which does cross into the cell and is hydrolyzed to H^+ and HCO_3^-.

Despite these and other controversies, most experts still recommend HCO_3^- IV for severe metabolic acidosis (pH < 7.00), with a target pH of 7.20.

Treatment requires 2 calculations. The 1st is the level to which HCO_3^- must be raised, calculated by the Kassirer-Bleich equation, using a value for $[H^+]$ of 63 nmol/L at a pH of 7.2:

$$63 = 24 \times P_{CO_2}/HCO_3^-$$

or

$$\text{desired } HCO_3^- = 0.38 \times P_{CO_2}$$

The amount of HCO_3^- needed to achieve that level is:

$$NaHCO_3 \text{ required (mEq)} = (\text{desired } [HCO_3^-] - \text{observed } [HCO_3^-]) \times 0.4 \times \text{body weight (kg)}$$

This amount of $NaHCO_3$ is given over several hours. Serum pH and HCO_3^- levels can be checked 30 min to 1 h after administration, which allows for equilibration with extravascular HCO_3^-.

Alternatives to $NaHCO_3$ include tromethamine, an amino alcohol that buffers both metabolic (H^+) and respiratory (H_2CO_3) acid; carbicarb, an equimolar mixture of $NaHCO_3$ and carbonate (the latter consumes CO_2 and generates HCO_3^-); and dichloroacetate, which enhances oxidation of lactate. These are all of unproven benefit and cause complications of their own.

K^+ depletion, common in metabolic acidosis, should also be treated as needed with oral or parenteral KCl.

LACTIC ACIDOSIS

Lactic acidosis results from overproduction, decreased metabolism, or both, of lactate.

Lactate is a normal byproduct of glucose and amino acid metabolism. The most serious form of lactic acidosis, type A, occurs when lactic acid is overproduced in ischemic tissue to generate ATP during O_2 deficit. Overproduction typically occurs during tissue hypoperfusion in hypovolemic, cardiac, or septic shock and is worsened by decreased lactate metabolism in the poorly perfused liver. It may also occur with primary hypoxia from lung disease and with various hemoglobinopathies.

Type B lactic acidosis occurs in states of normal tissue perfusion (and hence ATP production) and is less ominous. Lactate production may be increased from vigorous muscle use (eg, exertion, seizures, hypothermic shivering), alcohol ingestion, cancer, drugs such as biguanides (eg, phenformin and, less so, metformin) and nucleoside reverse transcriptase inhibitors or by various toxins (see TABLE 157–3). Metabolism may be decreased from hepatic insufficiency or thiamine deficiency.

D-Lactic acidosis is an unusual form of lactic acidosis in which D-lactic acid, the product of bacterial carbohydrate metabolism in the colon of patients with jejunoileal bypass or intestinal resection, is systemically absorbed. It persists in circulation because lactate dehydrogenase can metabolize only L-lactate.

Findings and treatment are as for other metabolic acidoses except for D-lactic acidosis. In D-lactic acidosis, the anion gap is lower than expected for the decrease in HCO_3^-, and there may be a urinary osmolar gap (difference between calculated and measured urine osmolarity). Treatment is IV fluids, restriction of carbohydrates, and sometimes antibiotics (eg, metronidazole).

METABOLIC ALKALOSIS

Metabolic alkalosis is primary increase in HCO_3^- with or without compensatory increase in PCO_2; pH may be high or nearly normal. Common causes include prolonged vomiting, hypovolemia, diuretic use, and hypokalemia. Renal impairment of HCO_3^- excretion must be present to sustain alkalosis. Symptoms and signs in severe cases include headache, lethargy, and tetany. Diagnosis is clinical and with ABG and serum electrolytes. The underlying cause is treated; oral or IV acetazolamide or HCl is sometimes indicated.

Etiology and Pathophysiology

Metabolic alkalosis is HCO_3^- accumulation from acid loss, alkali administration, intracellular shift of H^+ (as occurs in hypokalemia), or HCO_3^- retention. Regardless of initial cause, persistence of metabolic alkalosis indicates that the kidneys have increased their HCO_3^- reabsorption, because HCO_3^- is normally freely filtered by the kidney and hence excreted. Volume depletion and hypokalemia are the most common stimuli for increased HCO_3^- reabsorption, but any condition that elevates aldosterone or mineralocorticoids (which enhance Na reabsorption and K and H^+ excretion) can elevate HCO_3^-. Thus, hypokalemia is both a cause and a frequent consequence of metabolic alkalosis. Causes are listed in TABLE 157–4; the most common are volume depletion (particularly when involving loss of gastric acid and Cl from recurrent vomiting or nasogastric suction) and diuretic use.

Metabolic alkalosis involving loss or excess secretion of Cl is termed Cl-responsive, because it typically corrects with IV administration of NaCl-containing fluid. Cl-unresponsive metabolic alkalosis does not and typically involves severe Mg or K deficiency or mineralocorticoid excess. The 2 forms can coexist, eg, in patients with volume overload made hypokalemic from high-dose diuretics.

Symptoms, Signs, and Diagnosis

Symptoms and signs of mild alkalemia are usually related to the underlying etiology. More severe alkalemia increases protein binding of ionized Ca^{++}, leading to hypocalcemia and subsequent headache, lethargy, and neuromuscular excitability, sometimes with delirium, tetany, and seizures. Alkalemia also lowers threshold for anginal symptoms and

TABLE 157–4. CAUSES OF METABOLIC ALKALOSIS

CAUSE	COMMENTS
GI acid loss*	
Gastric acid loss from vomiting or nasogastric suction	Loss of HCl and acid coupled with contraction alkalosis from release of aldosterone and subsequent resorption of HCO_3
Congenital chloridorrhea	Fecal Cl loss and HCO_3 retention
Villous adenoma	Probably secondary to K depletion
Renal acid loss	
Primary hyperaldosteronism†	Including congenital adrenal hyperplasia
Secondary hyperaldosteronism†	Occurs with volume depletion, heart failure, cirrhosis with ascites, nephrotic syndrome, Cushing's syndrome or disease, renal artery stenosis, renin-secreting tumor
Use of glycyrrhizin-containing compounds† (eg, licorice, chewing tobacco, carbenoxoione, Lydia Pinkham's vegetable compound)	Glycyrrhizin inhibits enzymatic conversion of cortisol to less active metabolites
Bartter syndrome†	A rare congenital disease causing hyperaldosteronism and hypokalemic metabolic alkalosis that presents in early childhood with renal salt wasting and volume depletion
Gitelman's syndrome†	A disease like Bartter syndrome characterized in addition by hypomagnesemia and hypocalciuria and presenting in young adults
Diuretics (thiazide and loop)‡	Multiple mechanisms: secondary hyperaldosteronism from volume depletion, Cl depletion, and/or contraction alkalosis; may be Cl-unresponsive because of concomitant K depletion
Hypokalemia and hypomagnesemia†	Stimulate K and Mg reabsorption and H excretion; alkalosis unresponsive to NaCl and volume replacement until the deficiencies are corrected. Low K also causes H to shift into cells, raising extracellular pH
HCO_3 excess	
Posthypercapnic*	Persistent elevation of compensatory HCO_3 levels, often with volume, K, and Cl depletion
Postorganic acidosis	Conversion of lactic acid or ketoacid to HCO_3 worsened by HCO_3 therapy for acidosis
$NaHCO_3$ loading	Occurs with overzealous loading or loading in the setting of hypokalemia; as H shifts back into cells, the serum becomes more alkalotic
Milk-alkali syndrome	Chronic ingestion of Ca carbonate antacids provides Ca and HCO_3 load; hypercalcemia decreases and GFR prevents elimination of the excess HCO_3 load
Contraction alkalosis*	
Diuretics (all types) Sweat loss in cystic fibrosis	NaCl loss concentrates a fixed amount of HCO_3 in a smaller total body volume
Other	
Carbohydrate refeeding after starvation	Resolution of starvation ketosis/acidosis with improved cellular function
Laxative abuse*	Unclear mechanism
Some antibiotics (carbenicillin, penicillin, ticarcillin)	Contain nonreabsorbable anion, which increases K and H excretion

*Cl-responsive.
†Cl-unresponsive.
‡May be either Cl-responsive or Cl-unresponsive.

arrhythmias. Concomitant hypokalemia may cause weakness.

Recognition of metabolic alkalosis and appropriate respiratory compensation is discussed on p. 1266 and requires ABG and serum electrolytes (including Ca and Mg).

Common causes can often be determined by history and physical examination. If history is unrevealing and renal function is normal, urinary Cl^- and K^+ concentrations are measured (values are not diagnostic in renal insufficiency). Urinary Cl < 20 mEq/L indicates significant renal Cl^- reabsorption and hence a Cl-responsive cause (see TABLE 157–4). Urinary Cl > 20 mEq/L suggests a Cl-unresponsive form.

Urinary K and presence or absence of hypertension help differentiate Cl-unresponsive alkaloses. Urinary K < 30 mEq/day signifies hypokalemia or laxative misuse. Urinary K > 30 mEq/day without hypertension suggests diuretic abuse or Bartter or Gitelman's syndrome. Urinary K > 30 mEq/day with hypertension requires evaluation for hyperaldosteronism, mineralocorticoid excess, and renovascular disease; tests typically include plasma renin activity and aldosterone and cortisol levels (see pp. 1212 and 1215).

Treatment

Underlying conditions are treated, with particular attention paid to correction of hypovolemia and hypokalemia.

Patients with Cl-responsive metabolic alkalosis are given 0.9% saline solution IV; infusion rate is typically 50 to 100 mL/h greater than urinary and other sensible and insensible fluid losses until urinary Cl rises to > 25 mEq/L and urinary pH normalizes after an initial rise from bicarbonaturia. Patients with Cl-unresponsive metabolic alkalosis rarely benefit from rehydration.

Patients with severe metabolic alkalosis (eg, pH > 7.6) sometimes require more urgent correction of serum pH. Hemofiltration or hemodialysis is an option, particularly if volume overload is present. Acetazolamide 250 to 375 mg po or IV once/day or bid increases HCO_3^- excretion but may also accelerate urinary losses of K^+ and PO_4^-; volume-overloaded patients with diuretic-induced metabolic alkalosis and those with posthypercapnic metabolic alkalosis may especially benefit.

Hydrochloric acid in a 0.1 to 0.2 normal solution IV is safe and effective but must be given through a central catheter because it is hyperosmotic and scleroses peripheral veins. Dose is 0.1 to 0.2 mmol/kg/h, with frequent monitoring of ABG and electrolytes.

RESPIRATORY ACIDOSIS

Respiratory acidosis is primary increase in P_{CO_2} with or without compensatory increase in HCO_3^-; pH is usually low but may be near normal. Cause is a decrease in respiratory rate and/or volume (hypoventilation) from CNS, pulmonary, or iatrogenic conditions. Respiratory acidosis can be acute or chronic; the chronic form is asymptomatic, but the acute, or worsening, form causes headache, confusion, and drowsiness. Signs include tremor, myoclonic jerks, and asterixis. Diagnosis is clinical and with ABG and serum electrolytes. The underlying cause is treated; O_2 and mechanical ventilation are often required.

Respiratory acidosis is CO_2 accumulation (hypercapnia) from a decrease in respiratory rate and/or volume (hypoventilation). Causes of hypoventilation are discussed under Ventilatory Failure on p. 551 and include conditions impairing CNS respiratory drive; impaired neuromuscular transmission and other causes of muscular weakness; and obstructive, restrictive, and parenchymal pulmonary disorders. Hypoxia typically accompanies hypoventilation.

Respiratory acidosis may be acute or chronic. Distinction is based on the degree of metabolic compensation; CO_2 is initially buffered inefficiently, but over 3 to 5 days the kidneys increase HCO_3^- reabsorption significantly.

Symptoms and Signs

Symptoms and signs depend on the rate and degree of P_{CO_2} increase. CO_2 rapidly diffuses across the blood-brain barrier; symptoms and signs are a result of high CNS CO_2 concentrations (low CNS pH) and any accompanying hypoxemia.

Acute (or acutely worsening chronic) respiratory acidosis causes headache, confusion, anxiety, drowsiness, and stupor (CO_2 narcosis). Slowly developing, stable respiratory acidosis (as in COPD) may be well tolerated, but patients may have memory loss, sleep disturbances, excessive daytime sleepiness, and personality changes. Signs include gait disturbance, tremor, blunted deep tendon reflexes, myoclonic jerks, asterixis, and papilledema.

Diagnosis and Treatment

Recognition of respiratory acidosis and appropriate renal compensation is discussed on p. 1266 and requires ABG and measurement of serum electrolytes. Causes are usually obvious from history and examination. Calculation of the alveolar-arterial (A-a) O_2 gradient (inspired PO_2 − [arterial PO_2 + 5/4 arterial PCO_2]) can help distinguish pulmonary from extrapulmonary disease; a normal gradient essentially excludes pulmonary disorders.

Treatment is provision of adequate ventilation by either endotracheal intubation or noninvasive positive pressure ventilation (for specific indications and procedures, see Ch. 65 on p. 544). Adequate ventilation is all that is needed to correct respiratory acidosis, although chronic hypercapnia generally must be corrected slowly (eg, over several hours or more), because too-rapid PCO_2 lowering can cause a posthypercapnic "overshoot" alkalosis when the underlying compensatory hyperbicarbonatemia becomes unmasked; the abrupt rise in CNS pH that results can lead to seizures and death. Any K^+ and Cl^- deficits are corrected.

$NaHCO_3$ is generally contraindicated, because HCO_3^- can be converted to PCO_2 in serum but crosses the blood-brain barrier slowly, increasing serum pH without affecting CNS pH. One exception may be in cases of severe bronchospasm, in which HCO_3^- may improve responsiveness of bronchial smooth muscle to β-agonists.

RESPIRATORY ALKALOSIS

(See also Hyperventilation Syndrome on p. 358.)

Respiratory alkalosis is a primary decrease in PCO_2 with or without compensatory decrease in HCO_3^-; pH may be high or near normal. Cause is an increase in respiratory rate and/or volume (hyperventilation). Respiratory alkalosis can be acute or chronic. The chronic form is asymptomatic, but the acute form causes light-headedness, confusion, paresthesias, cramps, and syncope. Signs include hyperpnea or tachypnea and carpopedal spasms. Diagnosis is clinical and with ABG and serum electrolytes. Treatment is directed at the cause.

Etiology and Pathophysiology

Respiratory alkalosis is a primary decrease in PCO_2 (hypocapnia) from an increase in respiratory rate and/or volume (hyperventilation). Ventilation increase occurs most often as a physiologic response to hypoxia, metabolic acidosis, and increased metabolic demands (eg, fever), and as such is present in many serious conditions. In addition, pain and anxiety and some CNS disorders can increase respirations without a physiologic need.

Respiratory alkalosis can be acute or chronic. Distinction is based on the degree of metabolic compensation; excess HCO_3^- is buffered by extracellular H^+ within minutes, but more significant compensation occurs over 2 to 3 days as the kidneys decrease H^+ excretion.

Pseudorespiratory alkalosis is low arterial PCO_2 and high pH in patients with severe metabolic acidosis from poor systemic perfusion (eg, cardiogenic shock, during cardiopulmonary resuscitation). Pseudorespiratory alkalosis occurs when mechanical ventilation (often hyperventilation) eliminates larger-than-normal amounts of alveolar CO_2. Large amounts of alveolar CO_2 cause apparent respiratory alkalosis on the ABG, but poor systemic perfusion and cellular ischemia cause cellular acidosis, leading to acidosis of venous blood. Diagnosis is by demonstration of marked arteriovenous differences in PCO_2 and pH and by elevated lactate levels; treatment is improvement of systemic hemodynamics.

Symptoms and Signs

Symptoms and signs depend on the rate and degree of fall in PCO_2. Acute respiratory alkalosis causes light-headedness, confusion, peripheral and circumoral paresthesias, cramps, and syncope; mechanism is thought to be change in cerebral blood flow and pH. Tachypnea or hyperpnea is often the only sign; carpopedal spasm may occur in severe cases. Chronic respiratory alkalosis is usually asymptomatic and has no distinctive signs.

Diagnosis and Treatment

Recognition of respiratory alkalosis and appropriate renal compensation is discussed on p. 1266 and requires ABG and serum electrolytes. Minor hypophosphatemia and hypokalemia from intracellular shifts and decreased ionized Ca^{++} from an increase in protein binding may be present.

Presence of hypoxia or an increased alveolar-arterial (A-a) O_2 gradient (inspired PO_2 − [arterial PO_2 + 5/4 arterial PCO_2]) requires search for a cause. Other causes are often apparent on history and examination. However, because pulmonary embolism often presents without hypoxia (see p. 412), embolism must be strongly considered in a hyperventilating patient before ascribing the cause to anxiety.

Treatment is directed at the underlying disorder; respiratory alkalosis is not life threatening, so no interventions to raise pH are necessary. Increasing inspired CO_2 through rebreathing (such as from a paper bag) is common practice but may be dangerous in at least some patients with CNS disorders in whom CSF pH may already be below normal.

158 DIABETES MELLITUS AND DISORDERS OF CARBOHYDRATE METABOLISM

Diabetes mellitus and its complications (diabetic ketoacidosis, nonketotic hyperosmolar syndrome) are the most common disorders of carbohydrate metabolism, but alcoholic ketoacidosis and hypoglycemia are also important.

DIABETES MELLITUS

Diabetes mellitus is impaired insulin secretion and variable degrees of peripheral insulin resistance leading to hyperglycemia. Early symptoms are related to hyperglycemia and include polydipsia, polyphagia, and polyuria. Later complications include vascular disease, peripheral neuropathy, and predisposition to infection. Diagnosis is by measuring plasma glucose. Treatment is diet, exercise, and drugs that reduce glucose levels, including insulin and oral antihyperglycemic drugs. Prognosis varies with degree of glucose control.

There are 2 main categories of diabetes mellitus (DM)—type 1 and type 2, which can be distinguished by a combination of features (see TABLE 158–1). Terms that describe the age of onset (juvenile or adult) or type of treatment (insulin- or non-insulin–dependent) are no longer accurate because of overlap in age groups and treatments between disease types.

Impaired glucose regulation (impaired glucose tolerance, or impaired fasting glucose—see TABLE 158–2) is an intermediate, possibly transitional, state between normal glucose metabolism and DM that becomes common with age. It is a significant risk factor for DM and may be present for many years before onset of DM. It is associated with an increased risk of cardiovascular disease, but typical diabetic microvascular complications generally do not develop.

Type 1: In Type 1 DM (previously called juvenile-onset or insulin-dependent), insulin production is absent because of autoimmune pancreatic β-cell destruction possibly triggered by an environmental exposure in genetically susceptible people. Destruction progresses subclinically over months or years until β-cell mass decreases to the point that insulin concentrations are no longer adequate to control plasma glucose levels. Type 1 DM generally develops in childhood or adolescence and until recently was the most common form diagnosed before age 30; however, it can also develop in adults (latent autoimmune diabetes of adulthood). Type 1 accounts for < 10% of all cases of diabetes.

The pathogenesis of the autoimmune β-cell destruction involves incompletely understood interactions between susceptibility genes, autoantigens, and environmental factors. Susceptibility genes include those within the major histocompatibility complex (MHC)—especially HLA-DR3,DQB1*0201 and HLA-DR4,DQB1*0302, which are present in > 90% of patients with type 1 DM—and those outside the MHC, which seem to regulate insulin production and processing and confer risk for DM in concert with MHC genes. Susceptibility genes are more common in some populations than in others and explain the higher prevalence of type 1 DM

TABLE 158–1. GENERAL CHARACTERISTICS OF TYPES 1 AND 2 DIABETES MELLITUS

CHARACTERISTIC	TYPE 1	TYPE 2
Age at onset	Most commonly < 30 yr	Most commonly > 30 yr
Associated obesity	No	Very common
Propensity to ketoacidosis requiring insulin treatment for control	Yes	No
Plasma levels of endogenous insulin	Extremely low to undetectable	Variable; may be low, normal, or elevated depending on degree of insulin resistance and insulin secretory defect
Twin concordance	≤ 50%	> 90%
Associated with specific HLA-D antigens	Yes	No
Islet cell antibodies at diagnosis	Yes	No
Islet pathology	Insulitis, selective loss of most β cells	Smaller, normal-appearing islets; amyloid (amylin) deposition is common
Prone to develop diabetic complications (retinopathy, nephropathy, neuropathy, atherosclerotic cardiovascular disease)	Yes	Yes
Hyperglycemia responds to oral antihyperglycemic drugs	No	Yes, initially in many patients

in some ethnic groups (Scandinavians, Sardinians).

Autoantigens include glutamic acid decarboxylase, insulin, insulinoma-associated protein, and other proteins in β cells. It is thought that these proteins are exposed or released during normal β-cell turnover or β-cell injury (eg, from infection), activating a cell-mediated immune response resulting in β-cell destruction (insulitis). Glucagon-secreting α cells remain unharmed. Antibodies to autoantigens, which can be detected in serum, seem to be a response to (not a cause of) β-cell destruction.

Several viruses (including coxsackie, rubella, cytomegalovirus, Epstein-Barr, and retroviruses) have been linked to the onset of type 1 DM. Viruses may directly infect and destroy β cells, or they may cause β-cell destruction indirectly by exposing autoantigens,

TABLE 158–2. DIAGNOSTIC CRITERIA FOR DIABETES MELLITUS AND IMPAIRED GLUCOSE REGULATION

TEST	NORMAL	IMPAIRED GLUCOSE REGULATION	DIABETES
FPG	< 100 (< 5.6)	100–125 (5.6–6.9)	≥ 126 (≥ 7.0)
OGTT	< 140 (< 7.7)	140–199 (7.7–11.0)	≥ 200 (≥ 11.1)

FPG = fasting plasma glucose; OGTT = oral glucose tolerance test, 2 h glucose level.

NOTE: All values refer to glucose levels in mg/dL [mmol/L].

activating autoreactive lymphocytes, mimicking molecular sequences of autoantigens that stimulate an immune response (molecular mimicry), or other mechanisms.

Diet may also be a factor. Exposure of infants to dairy products (especially cow's milk and the milk protein β casein), high nitrates in drinking water, and low vitamin D consumption have been linked to increased risk of type 1 DM. Early (< 4 mo) or late (> 7 mo) exposure to gluten and cereals increases islet cell autoantibody production. Mechanisms for these associations are unclear.

Type 2: In Type 2 DM (previously called adult-onset or non-insulin–dependent), insulin secretion is inadequate. Often insulin levels are very high, especially early in the disease, but peripheral insulin resistance and increased hepatic production of glucose make insulin levels inadequate to normalize plasma glucose levels. Insulin production then falls, further exacerbating hyperglycemia. The disease generally develops in adults and becomes more common with age. Plasma glucose levels reach higher levels after eating in older than in younger adults, especially after high carbohydrate loads, and take longer to return to normal, in part because of increased accumulation of visceral/abdominal fat and decreased muscle mass.

Type 2 DM is becoming increasingly common in children as childhood obesity has become epidemic: 40 to 50% of new-onset DM in children is now type 2. Over 90% of adults with DM have type 2 disease. There are clear genetic determinants, as evidenced by the high prevalence of the disease within ethnic groups (especially American Indians, Hispanics, and Asians) and in relatives of people with the disease. No genes responsible for the most common forms of type 2 DM have been identified.

Pathogenesis is complex and incompletely understood. Hyperglycemia develops when insulin secretion can no longer compensate for insulin resistance. Although insulin resistance is characteristic in people with type 2 DM and those at risk for it, evidence also exists for β-cell dysfunction and impaired insulin secretion, including impaired 1st-phase insulin secretion in response to IV glucose infusion, a loss of normally pulsatile insulin secretion, an increase in proinsulin secretion signaling impaired insulin processing, and an accumulation of islet amyloid polypeptide (a protein normally secreted with insulin). Hyperglycemia itself may impair insulin secretion, because high glucose levels desensitize β cells and/or cause β-cell dysfunction (glucose toxicity). These changes typically take years to develop in the presence of insulin resistance.

Obesity and weight gain are important determinants of insulin resistance in type 2 DM. They have some genetic determinants but also reflect diet, exercise, and lifestyle. Adipose tissue increases plasma levels of free fatty acids that may impair insulin-stimulated glucose transport and muscle glycogen synthase activity. Adipose also appears to function as an endocrine organ, releasing multiple factors (adipocytokines) that favorably (adiponectin) and adversely, (tumor necrosis factor-α, IL-6, leptin, resistin) influence glucose metabolism. Intrauterine growth restriction and low birth weight have also been associated with insulin resistance in later life and may reflect prenatal environmental influences on glucose metabolism.

Miscellaneous types: Miscellaneous causes of DM that account for a small proportion of cases include genetic defects affecting β-cell function, insulin action, and mitochondrial DNA (eg, maturity-onset diabetes of youth); pancreatic diseases (eg, cystic fibrosis, pancreatitis, hemochromatosis); endocrinopathies (eg, Cushing's syndrome, acromegaly); toxins (eg, the rodenticide vacor); and drug-induced diabetes, most notably from glucocorticoids, β-blockers, protease inhibitors, and therapeutic doses of niacin. Pregnancy causes some insulin resistance in all women, but only a few develop gestational DM (see p. 2170).

Symptoms and Signs

The most common symptoms of DM are those of hyperglycemia: an osmotic diuresis caused by glycosuria leading to urinary frequency, polyuria, and polydipsia that may progress to orthostatic hypotension and dehydration. Severe dehydration causes weakness, fatigue, and mental status changes. Symptoms may come and go as plasma glucose levels fluctuate. Polyphagia may accompany symptoms of hyperglycemia but is not typically a primary patient concern. Hyperglycemia can also cause weight loss, nausea and vomiting, and blurred vision, and it may predispose to bacterial or fungal infections.

Patients with type 1 DM typically present with symptomatic hyperglycemia and sometimes with diabetic ketoacidosis (DKA—see p. 1290). Some patients experience a long but transient phase of near-normal glucose levels following acute onset of the disease (honeymoon phase) due to partial recovery of insulin secretion.

Patients with type 2 DM may present with symptomatic hyperglycemia but are often asymptomatic, and their condition is detected only on routine testing. In some patients, initial symptoms are those of diabetic complications (see below), suggesting that the disease has been present for some time. In some patients, hyperosmotic coma occurs initially, especially during a period of stress or when glucose metabolism is further impaired by drugs, such as corticosteroids.

Complications

Years of poorly controlled hyperglycemia lead to multiple, primarily vascular complications that affect small (microvascular) and/or large (macrovascular) vessels. The mechanisms by which vascular disease develops include glycosylation of serum and tissue proteins with formation of advanced glycation end products; superoxide production; activation of protein kinase C, a signaling molecule that increases vascular permeability and causes endothelial dysfunction; accelerated hexosamine biosynthetic and polyol pathways leading to sorbitol accumulation within tissues; hypertension and dyslipidemias that commonly accompany DM; arterial microthromboses; and pro-inflammatory and prothrombotic effects of hyperglycemia and hyperinsulinemia that impair vascular autoregulation. Immune dysfunction is another major complication and develops from the direct effects of hyperglycemia on cellular immunity.

Microvascular disease underlies the 3 most common and devastating manifestations of DM: retinopathy, nephropathy, and neuropathy. Microvascular disease also dramatically impairs skin healing, so that even minor breaks in skin integrity can develop into deeper ulcers and easily become infected. Intensive control of plasma glucose can prevent many of these complications but may not reverse them once established.

Diabetic retinopathy: Diabetic retinopathy is the most common cause of adult blindness in the US (see also p. 918). It is characterized initially by retinal capillary microaneurysms and later by macular edema and neovascularization. There are no early symptoms or signs, but focal blurring, vitreous or retinal detachment, and partial or total visual loss eventually develop; rate of progression is highly variable. Diagnosis is by retinal examination; treatment is argon laser photocoagulation or vitrectomy. Tight glycemic control, early detection, and treatment are critical to preventing vision loss.

Diabetic nephropathy: Diabetic nephropathy (see also p. 2007) is a leading cause of chronic renal failure in the US. It is characterized by thickening of the glomerular basement membrane, mesangial expansion, and glomerular sclerosis. These changes cause glomerular hypertension and progressive decline in GFR. Systemic hypertension may accelerate progression. The disease is usually asymptomatic until nephrotic syndrome or renal failure develops. Diagnosis is by detection of urinary albumin. A urine dipstick positive for protein signifies albumin excretion > 300 mg/day and advanced diabetic nephropathy (or an improperly collected or stored specimen). If the dipstick is negative for protein, the albumin:creatinine ratio on a spot urine specimen or urinary albumin in a 24-h collection should be measured. A ratio > 30 mg/g or an albumin concentration 30 to 300 mg/24 h signifies microalbuminuria and early diabetic nephropathy. Treatment is rigorous glycemic control combined with BP control. An ACE inhibitor and/or angiotensin II receptor blocker should be used to treat hypertension at the earliest sign of microalbuminuria or even before, because these drugs lower intraglomerular BP and thus have renoprotective effects.

Diabetic neuropathy: Diabetic neuropathy is the result of nerve ischemia from microvascular disease, direct effects of hyperglycemia on neurons, and intracellular metabolic changes that impair nerve function. There are multiple types, including symmetric polyneuropathy (with small- and large-fiber variants) and autonomic neuropathy. Symmetric polyneuropathy is most common and affects the distal feet and hands (stocking-glove distribution); it manifests as paresthesias, dysesthesias, or a painless loss of sense of touch, vibration, proprioception, or temperature. In the lower extremities, these symptoms can lead to blunted perception of foot trauma from ill-fitting shoes and abnormal weight bearing, which can in turn lead to foot ulceration and infection or to fractures, subluxation, and dislocation or destruction of normal foot architecture (Charcot's joint). Small-fiber neuropathy is characterized by pain, numbness, and loss of temperature sensation with preserved

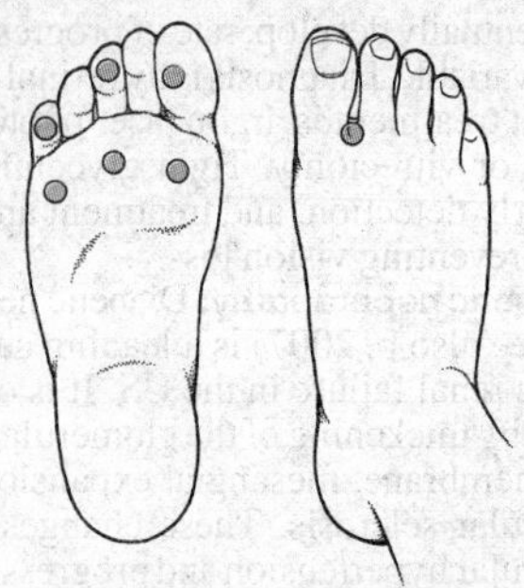

Fig. 158–1. Diabetic foot screening. A monofilament esthesiometer is touched to specific sites on each foot and is pushed until it bends. This test provides a constant, reproducible light-touch stimulus, which can be used to monitor change in sensation over time. Both feet are tested, and presence (+) or absence (–) of sensation at each site is recorded.

vibration and position sense. Patients are prone to foot ulceration and neuropathic joint degeneration and have a high incidence of autonomic neuropathy. Predominant large-fiber neuropathy is characterized by muscle weakness, loss of vibration and position sense, and lack of deep tendon reflexes. Atrophy of intrinsic muscles of the feet and foot drop are common.

Autonomic neuropathy can produce orthostatic hypotension, exercise intolerance, resting tachycardia, dysphagia, nausea and vomiting (due to gastroparesis), constipation and diarrhea (including dumping syndrome), fecal incontinence, urinary retention and incontinence, erectile dysfunction and retrograde ejaculation, and decreased vaginal lubrication.

Other forms of diabetic neuropathy include radiculopathies, cranial neuropathies, and mononeuropathies. Radiculopathies most often affect the proximal L2 through L4 nerve roots, causing pain, weakness, and atrophy of the lower extremities (diabetic amyotrophy), or the proximal T4 through T12 nerve roots, causing abdominal pain (thoracic polyradiculopathy). Cranial neuropathies cause diplopia, ptosis, and anisocoria when they affect the 3rd cranial nerve or motor palsies when they affect the 4th or 6th cranial nerves. Mononeuropathies cause finger weakness and numbness (median nerve) or foot drop (peroneal nerve). Diabetics are also prone to nerve compression disorders, such as carpal tunnel syndrome. Mononeuropathies can occur in several places simultaneously (mononeuritis multiplex). All tend to affect older people predominantly and abate spontaneously over months.

Diagnosis of symmetric polyneuropathy is by detection of sensory deficits and diminished ankle reflexes; loss of ability to detect the light touch of a nylon monofilament identifies patients at highest risk of foot ulceration (see FIG. 158–1). Electromyography and nerve conduction studies may be needed for all forms of neuropathy and are sometimes used to exclude other causes of neuropathic symptoms, such as nondiabetic radiculopathy and carpal tunnel syndrome. Strict glycemic control may lessen neuropathy. Treatments for relief of symptoms include topical capsaicin cream, tricyclic antidepressants (eg, imipramine), SSRIs (eg, duloxetine), anticonvulsants (eg, gabapentin, carbamazepine), and mexiletine. Patients with sensory loss should examine their feet daily to detect minor foot trauma and prevent it from progressing to limb-threatening infection.

Macrovascular disease: Large-vessel atherosclerosis is a result of the hyperinsulinemia, dyslipidemias, and hyperglycemia characteristic of DM. Manifestations are angina pectoris and MI, transient ischemic attacks and strokes, and peripheral arterial disease.

Diabetic cardiomyopathy is thought to result from many factors, including epicardial atherosclerosis, hypertension and left ventricular hypertrophy, microvascular disease, endothelial and autonomic dysfunction, obesity, and metabolic disturbances. Patients develop heart failure due to impairment in left ventricular systolic and diastolic function and are more likely to develop heart failure after MI. Diagnosis is by history and examination; the role of screening tests is evolving. Treatment is rigorous control of atherosclerotic risk factors, including normalization of plasma glucose, lipids, and BP, combined with smoking cessation and daily intake of aspirin and ACE inhibitors. In contrast with microvascular disease, intensive control of plasma glucose alone is not an effective preventive measure.

Infection: Diabetics are prone to bacterial and fungal infections because of adverse effects of hyperglycemia on granulocyte and T-cell function. Most common are mucocutaneous fungal infections (eg, oral and vaginal candidiasis) and bacterial foot infections (including osteomyelitis), which are typically exacerbated by lower extremity vascular insufficiency and diabetic neuropathy.

Other complications: Diabetic foot complications (skin changes, ulceration, infection, gangrene) are common and are attributable to vascular disease, neuropathy, and relative immunosuppression.

Diabetics have an increased risk of developing some rheumatologic diseases, including muscle infarction, carpal tunnel syndrome, Dupuytren's contracture, adhesive capsulitis, and sclerodactyly. They may also develop ophthalmologic disease unrelated to diabetic retinopathy (eg, cataracts, glaucoma, corneal abrasions, optic neuropathy); hepatobiliary diseases (eg, nonalcoholic fatty liver disease [steatosis and steatohepatitis], cirrhosis, gallstones); and dermatologic disease (eg, tinea infections, lower extremity ulcers, diabetic dermopathy, necrobiosis lipoidica diabeticorum, diabetic scleroderma, vitiligo, granuloma annulare, acanthosis nigricans [a sign of insulin resistance]). Depression and dementia are also more common.

Diagnosis

DM is indicated by typical symptoms and signs and confirmed by measurement of plasma glucose. Measurement after an 8- to 12-h fast (fasting plasma glucose [FPG]) or 2 h after ingestion of a concentrated glucose solution (oral glucose tolerance testing [OGTT]) is best (see TABLE 158–2). OGTT is more sensitive for diagnosing DM and impaired tolerance but is more expensive and less convenient and reproducible than FPG. It is therefore rarely used routinely, except for diagnosing gestational DM (see p. 2170) and for research purposes.

In practice, DM or impaired fasting glucose regulation is often diagnosed using random measures of plasma glucose or of glycosylated hemoglobin (HbA_{1c}). A random glucose value > 200 mg/dL (> 11.1 mmol/L) may be diagnostic, but values can be affected by recent meals and must be confirmed by repeat testing; testing twice may not be necessary in the presence of diabetic symptoms. HbA_{1c} measurements reflect glucose levels over the preceding 2 to 3 mo. Values > 6.5 mg/dL indicate abnormally high plasma glucose levels. However, assays and reference ranges are not yet standardized, and values may be falsely high or low (see Monitoring on p. 1281). For these reasons, HbA_{1c} is not yet considered as reliable as FPG or OGTT testing for diagnosing DM and should be used mainly for monitoring DM control.

Urine glucose measurement, once commonly used, is no longer used for diagnosis or monitoring because it is neither sensitive nor specific.

Those at high risk of type 1 DM (eg, siblings and children of people with type 1 DM) can be tested for the presence of islet cell or anti-glutamic acid decarboxylase antibodies, which precede onset of clinical disease. However, there are no proven preventive strategies for people at high risk, so such screening is usually reserved for research settings.

Risk factors for type 2 DM include age > 45; obesity; sedentary lifestyle; family history of DM; history of impaired glucose regulation; gestational DM or delivery of a baby > 4.1 kg; history of hypertension or dyslipidemia; polycystic ovary syndrome; and black, Hispanic, or American Indian ethnicity. Risk of insulin resistance among overweight patients (body mass index ≥ 25 kg/m^2) is increased with serum triglycerides ≥ 130 mg/dL (≥ 1.47 mmol/L); triglyceride/high density lipoprotein (HDL) ratio ≥ 3.0 (≥ 1.8); and insulin ≥ 108 pmol/L. These patients should be screened for DM with a fasting plasma glucose level at least once q 3 yr as long as plasma glucose measurements are normal and at least annually if results reveal impaired fasting glucose levels (see TABLE 158–2).

All patients with type 1 DM should begin screening for diabetic complications 5 yr after diagnosis; screening begins at diagnosis for patients with type 2 DM. Patients should have their feet examined at least annually for impaired sense of pressure, vibration, pain, or temperature, which is characteristic of peripheral neuropathy. Pressure sense is best tested with a monofilament esthesiometer (see FIG. 158–1). The entire foot, and especially skin beneath the metatarsal heads, should be examined for skin cracking and signs of ischemia, such as ulcerations, gangrene, fungal nail infections, deceased pulses, and hair loss. Funduscopic examination should be performed by an ophthalmologist; the screening interval is controversial but ranges from annually for patients with established retinopathy to q 3 yr for those without retinopathy on at least one examination. Spot or 24-h urine testing is indicated annually to detect proteinuria or microalbuminuria, and serum creatinine should be measured to assess renal function. Many people consider baseline electrocardiography important given the risk of heart disease.

Lipid profile should be checked at least annually and more often when abnormalities are present.

Treatment

Treatment involves control of hyperglycemia to improve symptoms and prevent complications while minimizing hypoglycemic episodes. Goals for treatment are maintenance of plasma glucose between 80 and 120 mg/dL (4.4 and 6.7 mmol/L) during the day and between 100 and 140 mg/dL (5.6 and 7.8 mmol/L) at bedtime (as determined by home monitoring—see Monitoring on p. 1281) and maintenance of HbA_{1c} levels < 7%. These goals may be adjusted for patients in whom strict glucose control may be inadvisable, such as the elderly; patients with a short life expectancy; patients who experience repeated bouts of hypoglycemia, especially with hypoglycemic unawareness; and patients who cannot communicate the presence of hypoglycemia symptoms (eg, young children).

Key elements for all patients are patient education, dietary and exercise counseling, and monitoring of glucose control. All type 1 diabetics require insulin. Type 2 diabetics with mildly elevated plasma glucose should be prescribed a trial of diet and exercise followed by a single oral antihyperglycemic drug if lifestyle changes are insufficient, additional oral drugs as needed (combination therapy), and insulin when ≥ 2 drugs are ineffective for meeting recommended goals. Type 2 diabetics with more significant glucose elevations at diagnosis are typically prescribed lifestyle changes and oral antihyperglycemic drugs simultaneously. Insulin is indicated as initial therapy for type 2 diabetics who are pregnant and for those who present with acute metabolic decompensation, such as nonketotic hyperosmolar syndrome (NKHS) or DKA. Patients with impaired glucose regulation should receive counseling addressing their risk of developing DM and the importance of lifestyle changes for preventing DM. They should be monitored closely for development of DM symptoms or elevated plasma glucose; ideal follow-up intervals have not been determined, but annual or biannual checks are probably appropriate.

Patient education about causes of DM; diet; exercise; drugs; self-monitoring with finger-stick testing; and the symptoms and signs of hypoglycemia, hyperglycemia, and diabetic complications is crucial to optimizing care. Most type 1 diabetics can also be taught how to titrate their insulin doses. Education should be reinforced at every physician visit and hospitalization. Formal diabetes education programs, generally conducted by diabetes nurses and nutrition specialists, are often very effective.

Diet adjusted to individual circumstances can help patients control fluctuations in their glucose level and, for type 2 patients, lose weight. In general, all diabetics need to be educated about a diet that is low in saturated fat and cholesterol and contains moderate amounts of carbohydrate, preferably from whole grain sources with higher fiber content. Although dietary protein and fat contribute to caloric intake (and thus, weight gain or loss), only carbohydrates have a direct effect on blood glucose levels. A low-carbohydrate, high-fat diet improves glucose control for some patients, but its long-term safety is uncertain. Patients with type 1 DM should use carbohydrate counting or the carbohydrate exchange system to match insulin dose to carbohydrate intake and facilitate physiologic insulin replacement. "Counting" the amount of carbohydrate in the meal is used to calculate the pre-meal insulin dose. In general, patients require 1 unit of rapid-acting insulin for each 15 g of carbohydrate in a meal. This approach requires detailed patient education and is most successful when guided by an experienced diabetes dietician. Some experts advise use of the glycemic index to delineate between rapid and slowly metabolized carbohydrates, although others believe the index adds little. Type 2 diabetics should restrict calories, eat regularly, increase fiber intake, and limit intake of refined carbohydrates and saturated fats. Some experts also recommend dietary protein restriction to ≤ 0.8 g/kg/day to prevent progression of early nephropathy (see p. 2007). Dietitian consultation should complement physician counseling; the patient and the person who prepares the patient's meals should both be present.

Exercise should involve an incremental increase in physical activity to whatever level a patient can tolerate. Some experts believe that aerobic exercise is better than isometric exercise for weight loss and protection from vascular disease, but resistance training can also improve glucose control, and all forms of exercise are beneficial. Patients who experience hypoglycemic symptoms during exercise should be advised to test their blood glucose and ingest carbohydrates or lower their insulin dose as needed to get their glucose slightly above normal just before exercise. Hypoglycemia during vigorous exercise may require carbohydrate ingestion during the workout period, typically 5 to 15 g of sucrose or another simple sugar. Patients with known or suspected cardiovascular disease may benefit from exercise stress testing before beginning an exercise program, while activity goals may need to be lowered for patients with diabetic complications such as neuropathy and retinopathy.

Monitoring: DM control can be monitored using plasma glucose, HbA_{1C}, or fructosamine levels. Self-monitoring of whole blood glucose using fingertip blood, test strips, and a glucose meter is most important. It should be used to help patients adjust dietary intake and insulin and to help physicians recommend adjustments in the timing and doses of drugs. Many different monitoring devices are available. Nearly all require test strips and a means for pricking the skin and obtaining a sample; most come with control solutions, which should be used periodically to verify proper meter calibration. Choice among devices is usually based on patient preferences for features such as time to results (usually 5 to 30 sec), size of display panel (large screens may benefit patients with poor eyesight), and need for calibration. Meters that allow for testing at sites less painful than fingertips (palm, forearm, upper arm, abdomen, thigh) are also available. Newer devices measure glucose transcutaneously, but their use has been limited by skin irritation and erratic readings; better technology may soon make near-continuous readings with such devices feasible.

Patients with poor glucose control and those given a new drug or a new dose of an existing drug may be asked to self-monitor once (usually morning fasting) to ≥ 5 times/day, depending on the patient's needs and abilities and the complexity of the treatment regimen. Most type 1 diabetics benefit from testing at least 4 times/day.

HbA_{1C} levels reflect glucose control over the preceding 2 to 3 mo and hence assess control between physician visits. HbA_{1C} should be assessed quarterly in type 1 patients and at least annually in type 2 patients whose plasma glucose appears stable (more frequently when control is uncertain). Home testing kits are useful for patients who are able to follow the testing instructions rigorously. Control suggested by HbA_{1c} values sometimes appears to differ from that suggested by daily glucose readings because of falsely elevated or normal values. False elevations may occur with renal insufficiency (urea interferes with the assay), low RBC turnover (as occurs with iron, folate, or vitamin B_{12} deficiency anemia), high-dose aspirin, and high blood alcohol concentrations. Falsely normal values occur with increased RBC turnover, as occurs with hemolytic anemias and hemoglobinopathies (eg, HbS, HbC) or during treatment of deficiency anemias.

Fructosamine, which is mostly glycosylated albumin but also comprises other glycosylated proteins, reflects glucose control in the previous 1 to 2 wk. Fructosamine monitoring may be used during intensive treatment of DM and for patients with Hb variants or high RBC turnover (which cause false HbA_{1C} results), but it is mainly used in research settings.

Urine glucose monitoring provides a crude indication of hyperglycemia and can be recommended only when blood glucose monitoring is impossible. By contrast, self-measurement of urine ketones is recommended for type 1 diabetics who experience symptoms, signs, or triggers of ketoacidosis, such as nausea or vomiting, abdominal pain, fever, cold or flu-like symptoms or unusual sustained hyperglycemia (> 250 to 300 mg/dL) on glucose self-monitoring.

Insulin: Insulin is required for all patients with type 1 DM who become ketoacidotic without it; it is also helpful for management of many type 2 patients. Insulin replacement should ideally mimic β-cell function using 2 insulin types to provide basal and prandial requirements (physiologic replacement); this requires close attention to diet and exercise as well as to insulin timing and dose. Most insulin preparations are now recombinant human, practically eliminating the once-common allergic reactions to the drug when it was extracted from animal sources. Except for rare use of regular insulin IV, insulin is administered subcutaneously; a number of analogs, created by modifications of the human insulin molecule that alter subcutaneous absorption rates, are available.

Insulin types are commonly categorized by their time to onset and duration of action (see TABLE 158–3). However, these parameters vary within and between patients depending on many factors (eg, site and technique of injection, amount of subcutaneous fat, blood flow at the injection site).

TABLE 158–3. ONSET, PEAK, AND DURATION OF ACTION OF HUMAN INSULIN PREPARATIONS*

INSULIN PREPARATION	ONSET OF ACTION	PEAK ACTION	DURATION OF ACTION
Rapid-acting			
Lispro, aspart, glulisine†	5–15 min	45–75 min	3–5 h
Short-acting			
Regular (R)†	30–60 min	2–4 h	6–8 h
Intermediate-acting			
NPH‡	2–4 h	6–10 h	12–18 h
Lente	3–4 h	8–12 h	12–18 h
Long-acting			
Ultralente	4–8 h	10–16 h	16–20 h
Glargine	1–2 h	No peak	24 h
Premixed			
70% NPH/30% R	30–60 min	Dual (NPH & R)	10–16 h
50% NPH/50% R	30–60 min	Dual (NPH & R)	10–16 h
75% NPL/25% lispro	5–15 min	Dual (NPL & lispro)	10–16 h
70% NPA/30% aspart	5–15 min	Dual (NPA & aspart)	10–16 h

R = regular; NPH = neutral protamine Hagedorn; NPL = neutral protamine lispro; NPA = neutral protamine.

*Times are approximate, assume subcutaneous administration, and may vary with injection technique and factors influencing absorption.

†Lispro and aspart are also available in premixed forms with intermediate-acting insulins.

‡Also exists in premixed form (NPH/R).

Rapid-acting insulins, including lispro and aspart, are rapidly absorbed because reversal of an amino acid pair prevents the insulin molecule from associating into dimers and polymers. They begin to reduce plasma glucose often within 15 min but have short duration of action (<4 h). These insulins are best used at mealtime to control postprandial spikes in plasma glucose.

Regular insulin is slightly slower in onset (30 to 60 min) than lispro and aspart but lasts longer (6 to 8 h). It is the only form approved for IV use.

Neutral protamine Hagedorn (NPH, or insulin isophane) and lente (insulin zinc) are intermediate-acting; they do not have significant effects on plasma glucose for up to several hours but remain active for 12 to 18 h. Ultralente (extended insulin human zinc) is the slowest onset insulin (up to 8 h) and has a duration of action of 18 to 24 h. Unlike ultralente, insulin glargine has no discernible peak of action and provides a steady basal effect over 24 h. Combinations of NPH and regular insulin and of insulin lispro and lispro protamine (a form of lispro modified to act like NPH) are commercially available in premixed preparations (see TABLE 158–3).

Different insulin types can be drawn into the same syringe for injection but should not be premixed in bottles except by a manufacturer. On occasion, mixing insulins may affect rates of insulin absorption, producing variability of effect and making glycemic control less predictable, especially if mixed >1 h before use. Insulin glargine should never be mixed with any other insulin.

Many prefilled insulin pen devices are available as an alternative to the conventional vial and syringe method. Insulin pens may be more convenient for use away from home and may be preferable for patients with limited vision or manual dexterity. Spring-loaded self-injection devices (for use with a syringe) may be useful for the occasional patient who is fearful of injection, and syringe magnifiers are available for patients with low vision.

Lispro, aspart, or regular insulin can also be given continuously using an insulin pump. Continuous subcutaneous insulin infusion pumps can eliminate the need for multiple daily injections, provide maximal flexibility in the timing of meals, and substantially reduce variability in glucose levels. Disadvantages include cost, mechanical failures leading to interruptions in insulin supply, and the inconvenience of wearing an external device. Frequent and meticulous self-monitoring and close attention to pump function are necessary for safe and effective use of the insulin pump.

Inhaled insulin has rapid onset and short duration of action like insulin lispro and may become available soon. Oligomeric or liposomal oral forms and transmucosal (eg, intranasal, oral spray) or transdermal delivery systems show promise but require further study.

Hypoglycemia is the most common complication of insulin treatment, occurring more often as patients try to achieve strict glucose control and approach near-normoglycemia. Symptoms of mild or moderate hypoglycemia include headache, diaphoresis, palpitations, light-headedness, blurred vision, agitation, and confusion. Symptoms of more severe hypoglycemia include seizures and loss of consciousness. In elderly patients, hypoglycemia may produce strokelike symptoms of aphasia or hemiparesis and is more likely to precipitate stroke, MI, and sudden death. Type 1 diabetics with long duration of disease may be unaware of hypoglycemic episodes because they no longer experience autonomic symptoms (hypoglycemia unawareness).

Patients should be taught to recognize symptoms of hypoglycemia, which usually respond rapidly to the ingestion of sugar, including candy, juice, and glucose tablets. Typically, 10 to 15 g of glucose or sucrose should be ingested. For patients who are unconscious or unable to swallow, hypoglycemia can be treated immediately with glucagon 1 mg sc or IM or a 50% dextrose solution 50 mL IV (25 g), followed, if necessary, by IV infusion of a 5 or 10% dextrose solution to maintain adequate plasma glucose levels.

Hyperglycemia may follow hypoglycemia either because too much sugar was ingested or because hypoglycemia caused a surge in counter-regulatory hormones (glucagon, epinephrine, cortisol, growth hormone). Too high a bedtime insulin dose can drive glucose down and stimulate a counter-regulatory response, leading to morning hyperglycemia (Somogyi phenomenon). A more common cause of unexplained morning hyperglycemia, however, is a rise in early morning growth hormone (dawn phenomenon). In this case, the evening insulin dose should be increased, changed to a longer-acting preparation, or injected later.

Hypokalemia may be caused by intracellular shifts of K from insulin-induced stimulation of the Na-K pump, but it is uncommon. Hypokalemia more commonly occurs in acute care settings where IV insulin is used.

Local allergic reactions at the site of insulin injections are rare, especially with the use of human insulins, but they may still occur in patients with latex allergy because of the natural rubber latex contained in vial stoppers. They can produce immediate pain or burning followed by erythema, pruritus, and induration—the latter sometimes persisting for days. Most reactions spontaneously disappear after weeks of continued injection and require no specific treatment, although antihistamines may provide symptomatic relief.

Generalized allergic reaction is extremely rare with human insulins but can occur when insulin is restarted after a lapse in treatment. Symptoms develop 30 min to 2 h after injection and include urticaria, angioedema, pruritus, bronchospasm, and anaphylaxis. Treatment with antihistamines often suffices, but epinephrine and IV glucocorticoids may be needed. If insulin treatment is needed after a generalized allergic reaction, skin testing with a panel of purified insulin preparations and desensitization should be performed.

Local fat atrophy or hypertrophy at injection sites is relatively rare and is thought to result from an immune reaction to a component of the insulin preparation. Either may resolve by rotation of injection sites.

Insulin resistance occurs mostly in type 2 diabetics. The cause is usually obesity. Circulating anti-insulin antibodies are a rare cause; it can sometimes be treated by changing insulin preparations (eg, from animal to human insulin) and by administering corticosteroids if necessary.

Insulin regimens for type 1 DM: Regimens for type 1 DM range from twice/day "split-mixed" (eg, split doses of rapid- and intermediate-acting insulins) to more physiologic "basal-bolus" regimens using multiple daily injections (eg, single fixed [basal] dose of long-acting and variable prandial [bolus] doses of rapid-acting insulin) or an insulin pump. Intensive treatment, defined as glucose monitoring ≥ 4 times/day and ≥ 3 insulin injections/day or continuous insulin infusion, is more effective than conventional treatment (1 to 2 insulin injections daily with or without monitoring) for preventing diabetic retinopathy, nephropathy, and neuropathy. However, intensive therapy may result in more frequent episodes of hypoglycemia and weight gain and is generally effective only in patients who are able and willing to take an active role in their self-care.

In general, most type 1 diabetics can start with a total dose of 0.2 to 0.8 units of insulin/kg/day; obese patients may require higher doses. Physiologic replacement involves giving 40 to 60% of the daily insulin dose as an intermediate- or long-acting preparation to cover basal needs, with the remainder given as a rapid- or short-acting preparation to cover postprandial increases. This approach is most effective when the dose of rapid- or short-acting insulin is determined by a sliding scale that takes into account preprandial blood glucose, anticipated meal content, and results of plasma glucose monitoring; dose can be adjusted 1 to 2 units for each 50 mg/dL (2.7 mmol/L) above or below target glucose level. This physiologic regimen allows greater freedom of lifestyle because patients can skip or time-shift meals and maintain euglycemia. However, no specific insulin regimen is proven more effective than others, and these recommendations are for initiation of therapy; thereafter, choice of regimens generally rests on physiologic response and patient and physician preferences.

Insulin regimens for type 2 DM: Regimens for type 2 DM also vary. Many patients are adequately controlled with lifestyle changes or oral drugs, but insulin should be added when glucose remains inadequately controlled by ≥ 2 oral drugs; insulin should replace oral drugs in women who become pregnant. The rationale for combination therapy is strongest for use of insulin with oral biguanides and insulin sensitizers. Regimens vary from a single daily injection of long- or intermediate-acting insulin (usually at bedtime) to the multiple injection regimen used by patients with type 1 DM. In general, the simplest effective regimen is preferred. Because of insulin resistance, some patients with type 2 DM require very large doses (> 2 units/kg/day). A common complication is weight gain, which is mostly attributable to reduction in loss of glucose in urine and improved metabolic efficiency.

Oral antihyperglycemic drugs: Oral antihyperglycemic drugs (see TABLE 158–4) are the primary treatment for type 2 DM, although insulin is often added when ≥ 2 oral drugs fail to provide adequate glycemic control. Oral antihyperglycemic drugs may enhance pancreatic insulin secretion (secretagogues), sensitize peripheral tissues to insulin (sensitizers), or impair GI absorption of glucose. Drugs with different mechanisms of action may be synergistic.

Sulfonylureas (SUs) are insulin secretagogues; they lower plasma glucose by stimulating pancreatic β-cell insulin secretion and may secondarily improve peripheral and hepatic insulin sensitivity by reducing glucose toxicity. First-generation drugs (see TABLE 158–4) are more likely to cause adverse effects and are used infrequently. All SUs promote hyperinsulinemia and weight gain of 2 to 5 kg, which over time may potentiate insulin resistance and limit their usefulness. All also can cause hypoglycemia; risk factors include age > 65, use of long-acting drugs (especially chlorpropamide, glyburide, glipizide), erratic eating and exercise, and renal or hepatic insufficiency. Hypoglycemia caused by long-acting drugs may last for days after treatment cessation, occasionally causes permanent neurologic disability, and can be fatal; for these reasons some practitioners hospitalize hypoglycemic patients, especially the elderly. Chlorpropamide also causes the syndrome of inappropriate antidiuretic hormone secretion. Most patients taking SUs alone eventually require additional drugs to achieve normoglycemia, suggesting that SUs may exhaust β-cell function. However, worsening of insulin secretion and insulin resistance is probably more a feature of DM itself than of drugs used to treat it.

Short-acting insulin secretagogues (repaglinide, nateglinide) stimulate insulin secretion in a manner similar to SUs. They are faster acting, however, and may stimulate insulin secretion more during meals than at other times. Thus, they may be especially effective for reducing postprandial hyperglycemia and appear to have lower risk of hypoglycemia. Like SUs, they can cause weight gain. Repaglinide appears to be as effective as SUs or metformin in lowering glucose levels; nateglinide may be somewhat less effective and therefore more appropriate for patients with mild hyperglycemia. Patients who have not responded to other oral drug classes (eg, SUs, metformin) are not likely to respond to these drugs.

Biguanides lower plasma glucose by decreasing hepatic glucose production (gluconeogenesis and glycogenolysis). They are considered peripheral insulin sensitizers, but their stimulation of peripheral glucose uptake may simply be a result of reductions in glucose from their hepatic effects. Biguanides also lower lipids and may also decrease GI nutrient absorption, increase β-cell sensitivity to circulating glucose, and decrease levels of plasminogen activating inhibitor 1, thereby exerting an antithrombotic effect. Metformin is the only biguanide commercially available in the US. It is at least as effective as SUs in reducing plasma glucose, rarely causes hypoglycemia, and can be safely used with other drugs and insulin. In addition, metformin does not cause weight gain and may even promote weight loss by suppressing appetite. However, the drug commonly causes GI adverse effects (eg, dyspepsia, diarrhea), which for most people recede with time. Less commonly, metformin causes vitamin B_{12} malabsorption, but clinically significant anemia is rare. Contribution of metformin to life-threatening lactic acidosis is controversial, but the drug is thought to be contraindicated in patients at risk of acidemia (including those with renal insufficiency [creatinine ≥ 1.4 mg/dL], heart failure, hypoxia or severe respiratory disease, alcoholism, other forms of metabolic acidosis, or dehydration). The drug should be withheld during surgery, administration of IV contrast, and any serious illness. Many people receiving metformin monotherapy eventually require an additional drug.

Thiazolidinediones (TZDs) decrease peripheral insulin resistance (insulin sensitizers), but their specific mechanisms of action are not well understood. The drugs bind a nuclear receptor primarily present in fat cells (peroxisome-proliferator-activated receptor-γ [PPARγ]) that is involved in the transcription of genes that regulate glucose and lipid metabolism. TZDs also increase HDL levels, lower triglycerides, and may have anti-inflammatory and anti-atherosclerotic effects. TZDs are as effective as SUs and metformin in reducing HbA_{1c}. Because the drug class is relatively new, data on long-term safety and effectiveness are not available. Though one TZD (troglitazone) caused acute liver failure, currently available drugs have not proven hepatotoxic; nevertheless, periodic monitoring of liver function is recommended. TZDs may cause peripheral edema, especially in patients taking insulin, and may worsen heart failure in susceptible patients. Weight gain, due to increased adipose tissue mass, is common and may be substantial (> 10 kg) in some patients.

α-Glucosidase inhibitors (AGIs) competitively inhibit intestinal enzymes that hydrolyze dietary carbohydrates; carbohydrates are digested and absorbed more slowly, thereby lowering postprandial plasma glucose. AGIs are less effective than other oral drugs in reducing plasma glucose, and patients often stop the drugs because they may cause dyspepsia, flatulence, and diarrhea. But the drugs are otherwise safe and can be used in combination with all other oral drugs and with insulin.

Glucagon-like peptide-1 (GLP-1) agonists (eg, exenatide [an incretin hormone]) enhance glucose-dependent insulin secretion and slow gastric emptying. Exenatide may also reduce appetite and promote weight loss. It is given by injection bid before meals and may be used in combination with oral antihyperglycemics. Other drugs that increase the availability of endogenous GLP-1 are being developed.

Other antihyperglycemic treatments: Transplantation of pancreatic or islet cells is an alternative means of insulin delivery; both techniques effectively transplant insulin-producing β cells into insulin-deficient (type 1) patients. Indications, tissue sources, procedures, and limitations of both procedures are discussed on pp. 1378 and 1379.

Pramlintide, a synthetic analog of the hormone amylin, is used in combination with insulin in the treatment of type 1 and type 2 diabetes. It slows gastric emptying, suppresses post-meal glucagon secretion, and promotes satiety. It is given by injection before each meal.

Other antihyperglycemic oral drugs are under investigation, including adrenoreceptor antagonists and phosphodiesterase inhibitors to augment pancreatic insulin secretion. Non-TZD insulin sensitizers, including recombinant human insulin like growth factor-1 (IGF-1), are also under development.

Adjunctive treatments: Adjunctive treatments to prevent or treat diabetic complications are critical. ACE inhibitors and/or angiotensin II receptor blockers are indicated for patients with evidence of early nephropathy (microalbuminuria or proteinuria), even in the absence of hypertension, and are a good choice for treating hypertension in diabetics who have not yet demonstrated renal impairment. ACE inhibitors also help prevent cardiovascular events in diabetic patients. Aspirin 325 mg once/day provides cardiovascular

TABLE 158–4. CHARACTERISTICS OF ORAL ANTIHYPERGLYCEMICS

GENERIC NAME	DAILY DOSAGE	DURATION OF ACTION (h)	COMMENTS
Insulin secretagogues			Augment pancreatic β-cell insulin secretion
Sulfonylureas			Can be used alone or in combination with other oral drugs and insulin. Major adverse effects are hypoglycemia and possibly weight gain
1st-Generation			
Acetohexamide	250 mg once/day–750 mg bid	12–24	
Chlorpropamide	100 mg once/day–750 mg once/day	24–36	Chlorpropamide may cause hyponatremia and flushing after alcohol ingestion
Tolbutamide	250 mg once/day–1500 mg bid	12	
Tolazamide	100 mg once/day–500 mg bid	14–16	
2nd-Generation			
Glyburide, regular-release	1.25 mg once/day–10 mg bid	12–24	No evidence of increased effectiveness of doses above 10 mg/day for glipizide and glyburide
Glyburide, micronized	0.75 mg once/day–6 mg bid	12–24	
Glipizide, regular-release	2.5 mg once/day–20 mg bid	12–24	
Glipizide, extended-release	2.5–20 mg once/day	24	
Glimepiride	1–8 mg once/day	24	
Short-acting insulin secretagogues			
Nateglinide	60–120 mg tid with meals	3–4	
Repaglinide	0.5–4 mg tid with meals	3–4	
Insulin sensitizers			
Biguanides			
Metformin, regular-release	500 mg once/day–1250 mg bid	6–10	Augments suppression of hepatic glucose production by insulin Can be used alone or in combination with other oral drugs and insulin
Metformin, extended-release	500 mg–2 g once/day	24	Major adverse effects: lactic acidosis (rare); contraindicated in at-risk patients, including those with renal insufficiency, heart failure, metabolic acidosis, hypoxia, alcoholism, and dehydration Does not cause hypoglycemia Other adverse effects: GI distress (diarrhea, nausea, pain); vitamin B_{12} malabsorption Potentiates weight loss

TABLE 158–4. CHARACTERISTICS OF ORAL ANTIHYPERGLYCEMICS—Continued

GENERIC NAME	DAILY DOSAGE	DURATION OF ACTION (h)	COMMENTS
Thiazolidinediones			Major adverse effects: weight gain, fluid retention, anemia (mild) Rosiglitazone may increase low-density lipoprotein cholesterol Hepatotoxicity is rare, but liver function monitoring is required
Pioglitazone	15–45 mg once/day	24	
Rosiglitazone	2–8 mg once/day	24	
Intestinal enzyme inhibitors			
α-Glucosidase inhibitors			Applied as monotherapy or combination therapy with other oral drugs or insulin to decrease postprandial plasma glucose levels Must be taken with the first bite of meal GI adverse effects (flatulence, diarrhea, bloating) common but may decrease over time Start with small dose (25 mg/day) and gradually titrate over several weeks
Acarbose	25–100 mg tid with meals	6–10	
Miglitol	25–100 mg tid with meals	6–10	

protection and should be used by most adults with DM in the absence of a specific contraindication. Patients with type 2 DM tend to have high levels of triglycerides and small, dense low-density lipoproteins (LDLs) and low levels of HDLs; they should receive aggressive treatment with the same treatment goals as those of patients with known coronary artery disease (LDL < 100 mg/dL [< 2.6 mmol/L], HDL > 40 mg/dL [> 1.1 mmol/L], and triglycerides < 150 mg/dL [< 1.7 mmol/L]—see TABLE 159–4 on p. 1303).

Orlistat, an intestinal lipase inhibitor, reduces dietary fat absorption; it reduces serum lipids and helps promote weight loss. It may be useful in selected patients as part of a comprehensive weight loss program. Surgical treatment for obesity, such as gastric resection or bypass, also leads to weight loss and improved glucose control in diabetic patients unable to lose weight through other means.

Regular professional podiatric care, including trimming of toenails and calluses, is important for patients with sensory loss or circulatory impairment. Such patients should be advised to inspect their feet daily for cracks, fissures, calluses, corns, and ulcers. Feet should be washed daily in lukewarm water, using mild soap, and dried gently and thoroughly. A lubricant (eg, lanolin) should be applied to dry, scaly skin; nonmedicated foot powders should be applied to moist feet. Toenails should be cut, preferably by a podiatrist, straight across and not too close to the skin. Adhesive plasters and tape, harsh chemicals, corn cures, water bottles, and electric pads should not be used on skin. Patients should change stockings daily and not wear constricting clothing (eg, garters, socks or stockings with tight elastic tops). Shoes should fit well, be wide-toed without open heels or toes, and be changed frequently. Special shoes should be prescribed to reduce trauma if the foot is deformed (eg, previous toe amputation, hammer toe, bunion). Walking barefoot should be avoided. Patients with neuropathic foot ulcers should avoid weight bearing until ulcers heal. If they cannot, they should wear appropriate orthotic protection. Because most patients with these ulcers have little or no macrovascular occlusive disease, debridement and antibiotics frequently result in good healing and may prevent major surgery (see p. 961). After the ulcer has healed, appropriate inserts or special shoes should be prescribed. In refractory cases, especially if osteomyelitis is present, surgical removal of the metatarsal head (the source of pressure) or amputation of the involved toe or transmetatarsal amputation may be required. A neuropathic joint can often be satisfactorily managed with orthopedic devices (eg, short leg braces, molded shoes, sponge-rubber arch supports, crutches, prostheses).

Finally, all diabetics should be vaccinated against *Streptococcus pneumoniae* (once) and influenza virus (annually).

Special Populations and Settings

Brittle diabetes: The term brittle diabetes refers to patients who have dramatic, recurrent swings in glucose levels that often occur for no apparent reason. Patients experience disabling episodes of hyperglycemia or hypoglycemia that typically lead to recurrent emergency department visits and hospitalizations. Labile plasma glucose levels are more likely to occur in type 1 DM patients because of complete absence of endogenous insulin production but can occur in any diabetic. Known causes include occult infection (eg, osteomyelitis, soft tissue abscess), gastroparesis (which leads to erratic absorption of dietary carbohydrates), and endocrinopathies (eg, Addison's disease, hypothyroidism). In most cases cause is unknown, and brittle diabetes is attributed to an inappropriate insulin regimen and inadequate patient education or understanding leading to errors in insulin administration and diet choices or to psychologic distress (eg, anger, depression, anxiety) that expresses itself in erratic patterns of food intake and physical activity, nonadherence to medical recommendations, and inappropriate self-titration of drugs.

The initial approach to such patients is to thoroughly review diabetes self-care techniques, including insulin preparation and injection and glucose testing. Increased frequency of self-testing may reveal previously unrecognized patterns and provides the patient with helpful feedback. A thorough dietary history, including timing of meals, should be taken to identify potential contributions to poor control. Underlying causes should be ruled out by physical examination and appropriate laboratory tests. For some insulin-treated patients, changing to a more intensive regimen that allows for frequent dose adjustments (based on glucose testing) is helpful. In some cases, the frequency of hypoglycemic and hyperglycemic episodes diminishes over time even without specific treatment, suggesting life circumstances may contribute to causation.

Adolescents: Glucose control typically deteriorates as diabetic children enter adolescence. Multiple factors contribute, including pubertal and insulin-induced weight gain; hormonal changes that decrease insulin sensitivity; psychosocial factors that lead to insulin nonadherence (eg, mood and anxiety disorders); family conflict, rebellion, and peer pressure; eating disorders that lead to insulin omission as a means of controlling weight; and experimentation with cigarettes, alcohol, and substance use. For these reasons, some adolescents experience recurrent episodes of hyperglycemia and DKA requiring emergency department visits and hospitalization.

Treatment often involves intensive medical supervision combined with psychosocial interventions (eg, mentoring or support groups), individual or family therapy, and psychopharmacology when indicated. Patient education is important so that adolescents can safely enjoy the freedoms of early adulthood. Rather than judging personal choices and behaviors, providers must continually reinforce the need for careful glycemic control, especially frequent blood sugar monitoring and use of frequent, low-dose, fast-acting insulins as needed.

Hospitalization: Diabetes can be a primary reason for hospitalization or can accompany other illnesses that require inpatient care. All diabetics with DKA, NKHS, and prolonged or severe hypoglycemia should be hospitalized. Others with SU-induced hypoglycemia, poorly controlled hyperglycemia, and acute worsening of diabetic complications may benefit from brief hospitalization, as do children and adolescents with new-onset disease. Control may worsen on discharge when insulin regimens developed in controlled inpatient settings prove inadequate to the uncontrolled conditions outside the hospital.

When other illnesses mandate hospitalization, glucose control may prove difficult, and it is often neglected when other diseases are more acute. Many patients do well without any change in drugs. Restricted physical activity and acute illness worsen hyperglycemia in some patients, whereas dietary restrictions and symptoms that accompany illness (eg, nausea, vomiting, diarrhea, anorexia) precipitate hypoglycemia in others—especially when antihyperglycemic drug doses remain unchanged. In addition, it may be difficult to control glucose adequately in hospitalized patients because usual hospital routines (eg, timing of meals, drugs, and procedures) are inflexibly timed relative to diabetes treatment regimens. Inpatients who are able to eat may continue usual outpatient regimens; others may be appropriately treated with basal insulin without or with supplemental short-acting insulin. Sliding-scale insulin should not be the only intervention to correct hyperglycemia; it is reactive rather than proactive, and no data suggest it leads to outcomes equivalent to or better than other approaches. Longer-acting insulins should be adjusted to prevent hyperglycemia rather than just using short-acting insulins to correct it.

Inpatient hyperglycemia worsens short-term prognosis for many acute conditions, most notably stroke and acute MI, and often prolongs hospital stay. Critical illness causes insulin resistance and hyperglycemia even in patients without known DM. Insulin infusion to maintain plasma glucose between 100 and 150 mg/dL (4.4 and 6.1 mmol/L) prevents adverse outcomes such as organ failure, may enhance recovery from stroke, and leads to improved survival in patients requiring prolonged (> 5 days) critical care. Severely ill patients, especially those receiving glucocorticoids or pressors, may need very high doses of insulin (> 5 to 10 units/h) because of insulin resistance. Insulin infusion should also be considered for patients receiving TPN and for type 1 patients who cannot ingest anything orally.

Surgery: The physiologic stress of surgery can increase plasma glucose in diabetics and induce DKA in type 1 DM patients. For type 1 patients, ½ to ⅔ of the usual morning dose of intermediate- or long-acting insulin can be given the morning before surgery with an IV infusion of a 5% dextrose solution at a rate of 100 to 150 mL/h. During and after surgery, plasma glucose (and ketones if hyperglycemia suggests the need) should be checked at least q 2 h. Glucose infusion is continued and monitoring continued at 2- to 4-h intervals, and regular insulin is given sc q 4 to 6 h as needed to maintain the plasma glucose level between 100 and 200 mg/dL (5.55 and 11.01 mmol/L) until the patient can be switched to oral feedings and resume the usual insulin regimen. Additional doses of intermediate- or long-acting insulin should be given if there is a substantial delay (> 24 h) in resuming the usual regimen. This approach may also be used for insulin-treated type 2 patients, but frequent measurement of ketones may be omitted.

Some physicians prefer to withhold sc insulin on the day of surgery and to administer insulin by IV infusion. One approach is to add 6 to 10 units of regular insulin to 1 L of 5% dextrose in 0.9% saline solution or water infused initially at 100 to 150 mL/h on the morning of surgery based on the plasma glucose level. Alternatively, separate insulin (1 to 2 units/h) and dextrose (75 to 125 mL/h of 5% dextrose) infusions may be used and allow for easier titration. Insulin adsorption onto IV tubing can lead to inconsistent effects, which can be minimized by preflushing the IV tubing with insulin solution. Insulin infusion is continued through recovery, with insulin adjusted based on the plasma glucose levels obtained in the recovery room and at 1- to 2-h intervals thereafter.

Most patients with type 2 DM who are treated with oral antihyperglycemic drugs maintain acceptable glucose levels when fasting and may not require insulin in the perioperative period. Most oral drugs, including SUs and metformin, should be withheld on the day of surgery, and plasma glucose levels should be measured preoperatively and postoperatively and q 6 h while patients receive IV fluids. Oral drugs may be resumed when patients are able to eat, but metformin should be withheld until normal renal function is confirmed 48 h after surgery.

Prevention

No treatments definitely prevent the onset or progression of type 1 DM. Azathioprine, corticosteroids, and cyclosporine induce remission of early type 1 DM in some patients, presumably through suppression of autoimmune β-cell destruction; however, toxicity and the need for lifelong treatment limit their use. In a few patients, short-term treatment with anti-CD3 monoclonal antibodies reduces insulin requirements for at least the 1st year of recent-onset disease by suppressing autoimmune T-cell response.

Type 2 DM usually can be prevented with lifestyle modification. Weight loss of as little as 7% of baseline body weight, combined with moderate-intensity physical activity (eg, walking 30 min/day), may reduce the incidence of DM in high-risk individuals by > 50%. Metformin has also been shown to reduce the risk of DM in patients with impaired glucose regulation. Moderate alcohol consumption (5 to 6 drinks/wk) and treatment with ACE inhibitors, angiotensin II receptor blockers, statins, and metformin, TZDs, and acarbose may also be protective, perhaps by inducing PPARγ activity, but require further study before they can be recommended for routine preventive use.

Risk of DM complications can be decreased by strict control of plasma glucose, defined as $HbA_{1c} < 7.0\%$, and by control of hypertension and lipid levels (see pp. 608 and 1302). Specific measures for prevention of progression of complications once detected are described under Complications (see p. 1277) and Treatment (see p. 1280).

DIABETIC KETOACIDOSIS

Diabetic ketoacidosis (DKA) is an acute metabolic complication of diabetes characterized by hyperglycemia, hyperketonemia, and metabolic acidosis. DKA occurs mostly in type 1 diabetes. It causes nausea, vomiting, and abdominal pain and can progress to cerebral edema, coma, and death. DKA is diagnosed by detection of hyperketonemia and anion gap metabolic acidosis in the presence of hyperglycemia. Treatment involves volume expansion, insulin replacement, and prevention of hypokalemia.

DKA is most common in type 1 diabetics and develops when insulin levels are insufficient to meet the body's basic metabolic requirements. DKA is the 1st manifestation of type 1 diabetes mellitus (DM) in a minority of patients. Insulin deficiency can be absolute (such as during lapses in the administration of exogenous insulin) or relative (such as when usual insulin doses do not meet metabolic needs during acute infection, trauma, or other physiologic stress). DKA is less common in type 2 DM, but it may occur in situations of unusual physiologic stress, such as MI.

Insulin deficiency causes the body to metabolize triglycerides and muscle instead of glucose for energy. Serum levels of glycerol and free fatty acids (FFAs) rise because of unrestrained lipolysis, as does alanine from muscle catabolism. Glycerol and alanine provide substrate for hepatic gluconeogenesis, which is stimulated by the excess of glucagon that accompanies insulin deficiency. Glucagon also stimulates mitochondrial conversion of FFAs into ketones. Insulin normally blocks ketogenesis by inhibiting the transport of FFA derivatives into the mitochondrial matrix, but ketogenesis proceeds in the absence of insulin. The major ketoacids produced, acetoacetic acid and β-hydroxybutyric acid, are strong organic acids that create metabolic acidosis. Acetone derived from the metabolism of acetoacetic acid accumulates in serum and is slowly disposed of by respiration.

Hyperglycemia caused by insulin deficiency produces an osmotic diuresis that leads to marked urinary losses of water and electrolytes. Urinary excretion of ketones obligates additional losses of Na and K. Serum Na may fall from natriuresis or rise due to excretion of large volumes of free water. K is also lost in large quantities, sometimes > 300 mEq/24 h.

K levels generally fall further during treatment as insulin therapy drives K into cells. If serum K is not monitored and replaced as needed, life-threatening hypokalemia may develop.

Symptoms and Signs

Symptoms and signs of DKA include those of hyperglycemia (see p. 1276) with the addition of nausea, vomiting, and—particularly in children—abdominal pain. Lethargy and somnolence are symptoms of more severe decompensation. Patients may be hypotensive and tachycardic from dehydration and acidosis; they may breathe rapidly and deeply to compensate for acidemia (Kussmaul's respirations). They may also have fruity breath due to exhaled acetone. Fever is not a sign of DKA itself and, if present, signifies underlying infection. In the absence of timely treatment, DKA progresses to coma and death.

Acute cerebral edema, a complication in about 1% of DKA patients, occurs primarily in children and less often in adolescents and young adults. Headache and fluctuating level of consciousness herald this complication in some patients, but respiratory arrest is the initial manifestation in others. The cause is not well understood but may be related to too-rapid reductions in serum osmolality or to brain ischemia. It is most likely to occur in children < 5 yr when DKA is the initial presentation of DM. Children with the highest BUN and lowest $Paco_2$ at presentation appear to be at greatest risk. Delays in correction of hyponatremia and use of HCO_3 during DKA treatment are additional risk factors.

Diagnosis

DKA is diagnosed by the detection of an arterial pH < 7.30 with an anion gap > 12 (see sidebar 157–1 on p. 1267) and serum ketones in the presence of hyperglycemia. A presumptive diagnosis can be made when urine glucose and ketones are strongly positive. Urine test strips and some assays for serum ketones may underestimate the degree of ketosis because they detect acetoacetic and not β-hydroxybutyric acid, which is usually the predominant ketoacid.

Other laboratory abnormalities include hyponatremia, elevated serum creatinine, and elevated serum osmolarity. Despite a significant total body deficit of K, initial serum K is typically elevated because of the extracellular migration of K in response to acidosis. As acidosis is corrected, serum K drops. An initial K level < 4.5 mEq/L indicates marked K depletion and requires immediate K supplementation. Electrocardiography can help determine the physiologic significance of high, low, and changing K levels. Serum amylase and lipase are often elevated, even in the absence of pancreatitis (which may be present in alcoholic DKA patients and in those with coexisting hypertriglyceridemia).

Prognosis and Treatment

Mortality rates for DKA are between 1 and 10%; shock or coma on admission indicates a worse prognosis. Major causes of death are circulatory collapse, hypokalemia, and infection. Among children with cerebral edema, 57% recover completely, 21% survive with neurologic sequelae, and 21% die.

The most urgent goals of treatment are rapid volume repletion, correction of hyperglycemia and acidosis, and prevention of hypokalemia. Identification of underlying precipitating factors is also important. Treatment should occur in intensive care settings because clinical and laboratory assessments are initially needed every hour or every other hour with appropriate adjustments in treatment.

Volume repletion in adults is typically achieved with rapid IV infusion of 1 to 3 L of 0.9% saline solution followed by saline infusions at 1 L/h or faster as need to raise BP, correct hyperglycemia, and keep urine flow adequate. Adults with DKA typically need a minimum of 3 L of saline over the first 5 h. When BP is stable and urine flow adequate, normal saline is replaced by 0.45% saline. When plasma glucose falls to < 250 mg/dL, IV fluid should be changed to 5% dextrose in 0.45% saline.

For children, fluid deficits are estimated at 60 to 100 mL/kg body weight; maintenance fluids (for ongoing losses) must also be provided (see p. 2291). The fluid deficit should be replaced over 36 h. Initial fluid therapy should be 0.9% saline (20 mL/kg) over 1 to 2 h, followed by 0.45% saline once BP is stable and urine output adequate. Remaining fluids should be given at 5 to 10 mL/kg/h, depending on the degree of dehydration.

Hyperglycemia is corrected by administration of regular insulin 0.15 unit/kg IV bolus initially, followed by continuous IV infusion of 0.1 unit/kg/h in 0.9% saline solution. Insulin should be withheld until serum K is ≥ 3.3 mEq/L (see p. 1292). Insulin adsorption onto IV tubing can lead to inconsistent effects, which can be minimized by pre-flushing the IV tubing with insulin solution. If plasma glucose does not fall by 50 to 75 mg/dL in the 1st hour, insulin doses should be doubled. Children should be given a continuous IV insulin infusion of 0.1 unit/kg/h or higher with or without a bolus.

Ketones should begin to clear within hours if insulin is given in sufficient doses. However, clearance of ketones may appear to lag because of conversion of β-hydroxybutyrate to acetoacetate (which is the "ketone" measured in most hospital laboratories) as acidosis resolves. Serum pH and HCO_3 levels should also quickly improve, but restoration of a normal serum HCO_3 level may take 24 h. Rapid correction of pH by HCO_3 administration may be considered if pH falls below 7, but HCO_3 is associated with development of acute cerebral edema (primarily in children) and should not be used routinely.

When plasma glucose becomes 250 to 300 mg/dL (13.88 to 16.65 mmol/L) in adults, 5% dextrose should be added to IV fluids to reduce the risk of hypoglycemia. Insulin dosage can then be reduced (minimum 1 to 2 units/h), but the continuous IV infusion of regular insulin should be maintained until the anion gap has narrowed and blood and urine are consistently negative for ketones. Insulin replacement may then be switched to regular insulin 5 to 10 units sc q 4 to 6 h. When the patient is stable and able to eat, a typical split-mixed or basal-bolus insulin regimen is begun. IV insulin should be continued for 1 to 4 h after the initial dose of sc insulin is given. Children should continue to receive 0.05 unit/kg/h insulin infusion until sc insulin is initiated and pH is > 7.3.

Hypokalemia prevention requires replacement of 20 to 30 mEq K in each liter of IV fluid to keep serum K between 4 and 5 mEq/L. If serum K is < 3.3 mEq/L, insulin should be withheld and K given at 40 mEq/h until serum K is ≥ 3.3 mEq/L; if serum K is > 5 mEq/L, K supplementation can be withheld. Initially normal or elevated serum K measurements may reflect shifts from intracellular stores in response to acidemia and belie the true K deficits that almost all DKA patients have. Insulin replacement rapidly shifts K into cells, so levels should be checked hourly or every other hour in the initial stages of treatment.

Treatment of suspected cerebral edema is hyperventilation, corticosteroids, and mannitol, but these are often ineffective after the onset of respiratory arrest.

NONKETOTIC HYPEROSMOLAR SYNDROME

Nonketotic hyperosmolar syndrome (NKHS) is a metabolic complication of diabetes mellitus (DM) characterized by hyperglycemia, extreme dehydration, hyperosmolar plasma, and altered consciousness. It most often occurs in type 2 DM, often in the setting of physiologic stress. NKHS is diagnosed by severe hyperglycemia and serum hyperosmolarity and absence of significant ketosis. Treatment is IV saline solution and insulin. Complications include coma, seizures, and death.

NKHS, also called hyperosmolar hyperglycemic state, is a complication of type 2 DM and has a mortality rate of up to 40%. It usually develops after a period of symptomatic hyperglycemia in which fluid intake is inadequate to prevent extreme dehydration from the hyperglycemia-induced osmotic diuresis. The precipitating factor may be a coexisting acute infection, drugs that impair glucose tolerance (glucocorticoids) or increase fluid loss (diuretics), medical nonadherence, or other medical conditions. Serum ketones are not present, and plasma glucose and osmolarity are typically much higher than in diabetic ketoacidosis (DKA): > 600 mg/dL (> 33 mmol/L) and > 320 mOsm/L, respectively.

Symptoms, Signs, and Diagnosis

The primary symptom of NKHS is altered consciousness varying from confusion or disorientation to coma, usually as a result of extreme dehydration with or without prerenal azotemia, hyperglycemia, and hyperosmolarity. In contrast to DKA, focal or generalized seizures and transient hemiplegia may occur. Serum K levels are usually normal, but Na may be low or high depending on volume deficits. BUN and serum creatinine levels are markedly increased. Arterial pH is usually > 7.3, but occasionally mild metabolic acidosis develops due to lactate accumulation.

The average fluid deficit is 10 L, and acute circulatory collapse is a common cause of death. Widespread thrombosis is a frequent finding on autopsy, and in some cases bleeding may occur as a consequence of disseminated intravascular coagulation. Other complications include aspiration pneumonia, acute renal failure, and acute respiratory distress syndrome.

Treatment

Treatment is 0.9% saline solution 1 L IV over 30 min, then at 1 L/h to raise BP and improve circulation and urine output. It can be replaced by 0.45% saline when BP becomes normal and plasma glucose reaches 300 mg/dL. The rate of infusion of IV fluids should be adjusted depending on BP, cardiac status, and the balance between fluid input and output.

Insulin is given at 0.15 unit/kg IV bolus followed by a 0.1 unit/kg/h infusion after the 1st liter of saline has been infused. Hydration alone can sometimes precipitously decrease plasma glucose, so insulin dose may need to be reduced; a too-quick reduction in osmolality can lead to cerebral edema. Occasional insulin-resistant type 2 DM patients with NKHS require larger insulin doses. Once plasma glucose reaches 200 to 250 mg/dL, insulin infusion should be reduced to basal levels (1 to 2 units/h) until rehydration is complete and the patient is able to eat. Addition of 5% dextrose infusion may occasionally be needed to avoid hypoglycemia. After recovery from the acute episode, patients are usually switched to adjusted doses of subcutaneous insulin. Most patients can resume using oral antihyperglycemic drugs once their condition is stable.

K replacement is similar to DKA: 40 mEq/h for serum K < 3.3 mEq/L; 20 to 30 mEq/h for serum K between 3.3 and 4.9 mEq/L; and none for serum K ≥ 5 mEq/L.

ALCOHOLIC KETOACIDOSIS

Alcoholic ketoacidosis is a metabolic complication of alcohol use and starvation char-

acterized by hyperketonemia and anion gap metabolic acidosis without significant hyperglycemia. Alcoholic ketoacidosis causes nausea, vomiting, and abdominal pain. Diagnosis is by history and findings of ketoacidosis without hyperglycemia. Treatment is IV saline solution and dextrose infusion.

Alcoholic ketoacidosis is attributed to the combined effects of alcohol and starvation on glucose metabolism. Alcohol diminishes hepatic gluconeogenesis and leads to decreased insulin secretion, increased lipolysis, impaired fatty acid oxidation, and subsequent ketogenesis. Counter-regulatory hormones are increased and may further inhibit insulin secretion. Plasma glucose levels are usually low or normal, but mild hyperglycemia sometimes occurs.

Typically, an alcohol binge leads to vomiting and the cessation of alcohol or food intake for ≥ 24 h. During this period of starvation, vomiting continues and abdominal pain develops, leading the patient to seek medical attention. Pancreatitis may occur.

Diagnosis requires a high index of suspicion; the absence of hyperglycemia makes diabetic ketoacidosis (DKA) improbable. Typical laboratory findings include a high anion gap metabolic acidosis, ketonemia, and low levels of K, Mg, and P. Detection of acidosis may be complicated by concurrent metabolic alkalosis due to vomiting. Lactic acid levels are often elevated because of the altered balance of reduction and oxidation reactions in the liver.

Treatment begins with an IV infusion of 5% dextrose in 0.9% saline solution, with added thiamin and other water-soluble vitamins and with K replacement as required. Ketoacidosis and GI symptoms usually respond rapidly. Use of insulin is appropriate only if there is any question of atypical DKA or if hyperglycemia > 300 mg/dL develops.

HYPOGLYCEMIA

Hypoglycemia unrelated to exogenous insulin therapy is an uncommon clinical syndrome characterized by low plasma glucose level, symptomatic sympathetic nervous system stimulation, and CNS dysfunction. Many drugs and disorders cause it. Diagnosis requires blood tests performed at the time of symptoms or during a 72-h fast. Treatment is provision of glucose combined with treatment of the underlying cause.

Symptomatic hypoglycemia unrelated to treatment of diabetes mellitus (DM) is relatively rare, in part because the body has extensive counter-regulatory mechanisms to compensate for low blood glucose levels. Glucagon and epinephrine levels surge in response to acute hypoglycemia and appear to be the 1st line of defense. Cortisol and growth hormone levels also increase acutely and are important in the recovery from prolonged hypoglycemia. The threshold for release of these hormones is usually above that for hypoglycemic symptoms.

Causes of physiologic hypoglycemia can be classified as reactive (postprandial) or fasting, insulin mediated or non-insulin mediated, and drug induced or nondrug induced. Insulin-mediated causes include exogenous administration of insulin or an insulin secretagogue and insulin-secreting tumors (insulinomas). A helpful practical classification is based on clinical status: whether hypoglycemia occurs in patients who appear healthy or ill. Within these categories, causes of hypoglycemia can be divided into drug-induced and other causes. Pseudohypoglycemia occurs when processing of blood specimens in untreated test tubes is delayed and cells, such as RBCs and leukocytes (especially if increased, as in leukemia or polycythemia), consume glucose. Factitious hypoglycemia is true hypoglycemia induced by nontherapeutic administration of sulfonylureas or insulin.

Symptoms and Signs

The surge in autonomic activity in response to low plasma glucose causes sweating, nausea, warmth, anxiety, tremulousness, palpitations, and possibly hunger and paresthesias. Insufficient glucose supply to the brain causes headache, blurred or double vision, confusion, difficulty speaking, seizures, and coma. In controlled settings, autonomic symptoms begin at or beneath a plasma glucose level of about 60 mg/dL (3.33 mmol/L), whereas CNS symptoms occur at or below a glucose level of about 50 mg/dL (2.78 mmol/L). However, symptoms suggestive of hypoglycemia are far more common than the condition itself. Most people with glucose levels at these thresholds have no symptoms, and most people with symptoms suggestive of hypoglycemia have normal glucose concentrations.

Diagnosis

In principle, diagnosis requires verification that a low plasma glucose level (< 50 mg/dL

[< 2.78 mmol/L]) exists at the time hypoglycemic symptoms occur and that the symptoms are responsive to glucose administration. If a practitioner is present when symptoms occur, blood should be sent for glucose testing. If glucose is normal, hypoglycemia is ruled out and no further testing is needed. If glucose is abnormally low, serum insulin, C-peptide, and proinsulin measured from the same tube can distinguish insulin-mediated from non–insulin-mediated and factitious from physiologic hypoglycemia and can obviate the need for further testing. Insulin growth factor 2 (IGF-2) levels may help identify non-islet-cell (IGF-2 secreting) tumors, which are an unusual cause of hypoglycemia.

In practice, however, it is unusual that practitioners are present when patients experience symptoms suggestive of hypoglycemia. Home glucose meters are unreliable for quantifying hypoglycemia, and there are no clear HbA_{1c} thresholds that distinguish long-term hypoglycemia from normoglycemia. So the need for more extensive diagnostic testing is based on the probability that an underlying disorder that could cause hypoglycemia exists given a patient's clinical appearance and coexisting illnesses.

A 72-h fast performed in a controlled setting is the standard for diagnosis. Patients drink only noncaloric, noncaffeinated beverages, and plasma glucose is measured at baseline whenever symptoms occur and q 4 to 6 h or q 1 to 2 h if glucose falls below 60 mg/dL (3.3 mmol/L). Serum insulin, C-peptide, and proinsulin should be measured at times of hypoglycemia to distinguish endogenous from exogenous (factitious) hypoglycemia. The fast is terminated at 72 h if the patient has experienced no symptoms and glucose remains normal; sooner if glucose decreases to ≤ 45 mg/dL (2.5 mmol/L) in the presence of hypoglycemic symptoms. End-of-fast measurements include β-hydroxybutyrate (which should be low in insulinoma), serum sulfonylurea to detect drug-induced hypoglycemia, and plasma glucose after IV glucagon injection to detect an increase characteristic of insulinoma. Sensitivity, specificity, and predictive values for detecting hypoglycemia by this protocol have not been reported. There is no definitive lower limit of glucose that unequivocally defines pathologic hypoglycemia during a 72-h fast; normal women tend to have lower fasting glucose levels than men and may have glucose levels as low as 30 mg/dL without symptoms. If symptomatic hypoglycemia has not occurred by 72 h, the patient should exercise vigorously for about 30 min. If hypoglycemia still does not occur, insulinoma is essentially excluded and further testing is generally not indicated.

Treatment

Immediate treatment of hypoglycemia involves provision of glucose. Patients able to eat or drink can drink juices, sucrose water, or glucose solutions; eat candy or other foods; or chew on glucose tablets when symptoms occur. Infants and younger children may be given 10% dextrose solution 2 to 5 mL/kg IV bolus. Adults and older children unable to eat or drink can be given glucagon 0.5 (< 20 kg) or 1 mg (≥ 20 kg) sc or IM or 50% dextrose 50 to 100 mL IV bolus, with or without a continuous infusion of 5 to 10% dextrose solution sufficient to resolve symptoms. The efficacy of glucagon depends on the size of hepatic glycogen stores; glucagon has little effect on plasma glucose in patients who have been fasting or who are hypoglycemic for long periods.

Underlying causes of hypoglycemia must also be treated. Islet cell and non-islet cell tumors must first be localized, then removed by enucleation or partial pancreatectomy; about 6% recur within 10 yr. Diazoxide and octreotide can be used to control symptoms while the patient is awaiting surgery or when a patient refuses or is not a candidate for a procedure. Islet cell hypertrophy is most often a diagnosis of exclusion after an islet cell tumor is sought but not identified. Drugs that cause hypoglycemia, including alcohol, must be stopped. Treatment of hereditary and endocrine disorders; hepatic, renal, and heart failure; and sepsis and shock are described elsewhere.

159 LIPID DISORDERS

Lipids are fats that are either absorbed from food or synthesized by the liver. Triglycerides (TGs) and cholesterol contribute most to disease, although all lipids are physiologically important. The primary function of TGs is to store energy in adipocytes and muscle cells; cholesterol is an ubiquitous constituent of cell membranes, steroids, bile acids, and signaling molecules. All lipids are hydrophobic and mostly insoluble in blood, so they require transport within hydrophilic, spherical structures called lipoproteins, which possess surface proteins (apoproteins) that are cofactors and ligands for lipid-processing enzymes. Lipoproteins are classified by size and density (defined as the ratio of lipid to protein) and are important because high levels of low-density lipoproteins (LDLs) and low levels of high-density lipoproteins (HDLs) are major risk factors for atherosclerotic heart disease (see p. 620).

Physiology

Lipids and lipoproteins are metabolized in 2 separate but closely related pathways (see also TABLE 159–1). The pathways are clinically important because pathway defects in lipoprotein synthesis, processing, and clearance can lead to accumulation of atherogenic lipids in plasma and endothelium.

Exogenous (dietary) lipid metabolism: Over 95% of dietary lipids are TGs; the rest are phospholipids, free fatty acids (FFAs), cholesterol (present in foods as esterified cholesterol), and fat-soluble vitamins. Dietary TGs are digested in the stomach and duodenum into monoglycerides (MGs) and FFAs by gastric lipase, emulsification from vigorous stomach peristalsis, and pancreatic lipase. Dietary cholesterol esters are de-esterified into free cholesterol by these same mechanisms. MGs, FFAs, and free cholesterol are then solubilized in the intestine by bile acid micelles, which shuttle them to intestinal villi for absorption. Once absorbed into the enterocyte, they are reassembled into TGs and packaged with cholesterol into chylomicrons, the largest lipoproteins.

TABLE 159–1. MAJOR APOPROTEINS AND ENZYMES IMPORTANT TO LIPID METABOLISM

COMPONENT	LOCATION	FUNCTION
Apoproteins		
Apo A-I	HDL	Major component of HDL particle
Apo A-II	HDL	Not known
Apo B-100	VLDL, IDL, LDL, Lp(a)	LDL receptor ligand
Apo C-II	Chylomicrons, VLDL, HDL	LPL cofactor
Apo E	Chylomicrons, remnants, VLDL, HDL	LDL receptor ligand
Apo(a)	Lp(a)	Not known
Enzymes		
ABCA1	Within cells	Contributes to intracellular cholesterol transport to membrane
CETP	HDL	Mediates transfer of cholesteryl esters from HDL to VLDL
LCAT	HDL	Esterifies free cholesterol for transport within HDL

Apo = apoprotein; HDL = high-density lipoprotein; VLDL = very-low-density lipoprotein; IDL = intermediate-density lipoprotein; LDL = low-density lipoprotein; LPL = lipoprotein lipase; Lp(a) = lipoprotein (a); CETP = cholesteryl ester transfer protein; LCAT = lecithin cholesterol: acyl transferase; ABCA1 = ATP-binding cassette transporter A1.

Chylomicrons transport dietary TGs and cholesterol from within enterocytes through lymphatics into the circulation. In the capillaries of adipose and muscle tissue, apoprotein C-II (apo C-II) on the chylomicron activates endothelial lipoprotein lipase (LPL) to convert 90% of chylomicron TG to fatty acids and glycerol, which are taken up by adipocytes and muscle cells for energy use or storage. Cholesterol-rich chylomicron remnants then circulate back to the liver, where they are cleared in a process mediated by apoprotein E (apo E).

Endogenous lipid metabolism: Lipoproteins synthesized by the liver transport endogenous TGs and cholesterol. Lipoproteins circulate through the blood continuously until the TGs they contain are taken up by peripheral tissues or the lipoproteins themselves are cleared by the liver. They become more cholesterol rich as they lose TGs, so factors that stimulate hepatic lipoprotein synthesis generally lead to elevated plasma cholesterol.

Very-low-density lipoproteins (VLDLs) contain apoprotein B-100 (apo B), are synthesized in the liver, and transport TGs and cholesterol to peripheral tissues. VLDL is the way the liver exports excess TGs derived from plasma FFA and chylomicron remnants; VLDL synthesis increases with increases in intrahepatic FFA, such as occurs with high-fat diets and when excess adipose tissue releases FFAs directly into the circulation (eg, in obesity, uncontrolled diabetes mellitus). Apo C-II on the VLDL surface activates endothelial LPL to break down TGs into FFAs and glycerol, which are taken up by cells.

Intermediate-density lipoproteins (IDLs) are the product of LPL processing of VLDLs and chylomicrons. IDLs are cholesterol-rich VLDL and chylomicron remnants that are either cleared by the liver or metabolized by hepatic lipase into LDL, which retains apo B.

Low-density lipoproteins (LDLs), the products of VLDL and IDL metabolism, are the most cholesterol-rich of all lipoproteins. About 40 to 60% of all LDLs are cleared by the liver in a process mediated by apo B and hepatic LDL receptors. The rest are taken up by either hepatic LDL or nonhepatic non-LDL (scavenger) receptors. Hepatic LDL receptors are down-regulated by delivery of cholesterol to the liver by chylomicrons and by increased dietary saturated fat; they can be up-regulated by decreased dietary fat and cholesterol. Nonhepatic scavenger receptors, most notably on macrophages, take up excess oxidized circulating LDLs not processed by hepatic receptors. Oxidized-LDL–rich macrophages can then migrate into endothelium in response to endothelial inflammation or other stimuli and form foam cells within atherosclerotic plaques (see p. 621). There are 2 forms of LDL: large buoyant and small dense LDL. Small, dense LDL is especially rich in cholesterol esters, associated with metabolic disturbances such as hypertriglyceridemia and insulin resistance, and especially atherogenic. The increased atherogenicity of small, dense LDL derives from less efficient hepatic LDL receptor binding, leading to prolonged circulation and exposure to endothelium and increased oxidation.

High-density lipoproteins (HDLs) are initially cholesterol-free lipoproteins that are synthesized in both enterocytes and the liver. HDL metabolism is complex, but HDL's overall role is to obtain cholesterol from peripheral tissues and other lipoproteins and transport it to where it is needed most—other cells, other lipoproteins (using cholesteryl ester transfer protein [CETP]), and the liver (for clearance). Its overall effect is anti-atherogenic. Efflux of free cholesterol from cells is mediated by ATP-binding cassette transporter A1 (ABCA1), which combines with apo A-I to produce nascent HDL. Free cholesterol in nascent HDL is then esterified by the enzyme lecithin-cholesterol acyl transferase (LCAT), producing mature HDL. Blood HDL levels may not completely represent reverse cholesterol transport.

Lipoprotein(a) [Lp(a)] is LDL that contains apolipoprotein(a), characterized by 5 cysteine-rich regions called kringles. One of these regions is homologous with plasminogen and is thought to competitively inhibit fibrinolysis and thus predispose to thrombus. The Lp(a) may also directly promote atherosclerosis. The metabolic pathways of Lp(a) production and clearance are not well characterized, but levels increase in patients with diabetic nephropathy.

DYSLIPIDEMIA

(Hyperlipidemia)

Dyslipidemia is elevation of plasma cholesterol and/or TGs or a low HDL level that contributes to the development of atherosclerosis. Causes may be primary (genetic)

or secondary. Diagnosis is by measuring plasma levels of total cholesterol, TGs, and individual lipoproteins. Treatment is dietary changes, exercise, and lipid-lowering drugs.

There is no natural cutoff between normal and abnormal lipid levels because lipid measurements are continuous. A linear relation probably exists between lipid levels and cardiovascular risk, so many people with "normal" cholesterol levels benefit from achieving still lower levels. Consequently, there are no numeric definitions of dyslipidemia; the term is applied to lipid levels for which treatment has proven beneficial. Proof of benefit is strongest for lowering elevated LDL levels; it is less strong for lowering elevated TG and increasing low HDL levels, in part because elevated TG and low HDL levels are more predictive of cardiovascular risk in women than in men.

Classification and Etiology

Dyslipidemias were traditionally classified by patterns of elevation in lipids and lipoproteins (Fredrickson phenotype—see TABLE 159–2). A more practical system categorizes dyslipidemias as primary or secondary and characterizes them by increases in cholesterol only (pure or isolated hypercholesterolemia), increases in TGs only (pure or isolated hypertriglyceridemia), or increases in both cholesterol and TGs (mixed or combined hyperlipidemias). This system does not take into account specific lipoprotein abnormalities (eg, low HDL or high LDL) that may contribute to disease despite normal cholesterol and TG levels.

Primary causes are single or multiple genetic mutations that result in either overproduction or defective clearance of TG and LDL cholesterol, or in underproduction or excessive clearance of HDL (see TABLE 159–3). Primary lipid disorders are suspected when a patient has physical signs of dyslipidemia (see p. 1301), onset of premature atherosclerotic disease (< 60 yr), a family history of atherosclerotic disease, or serum cholesterol > 240 mg/dL (> 6.2 mmol/L). Primary disorders, the most common cause of dyslipidemia in children, do not cause a large percentage of cases in adults. The names of many reflect an old nomenclature in which lipoproteins were detected and distinguished by how they separated into α (HDL) and β (LDL) bands on electrophoretic gels.

TABLE 159–2. LIPOPROTEIN PATTERNS (FREDRICKSON PHENOTYPES)

PHENOTYPE	ELEVATED LIPOPROTEIN(S)	ELEVATED LIPIDS
I	Chylomicrons	TGs
IIa	LDL	Cholesterol
IIb	LDL and VLDL	TGs and cholesterol
III	VLDL and chylomicron remnants	TGs and cholesterol
IV	VLDL	TGs
V	Chylomicrons and VLDL	TGs and cholesterol

TGs = triglycerides; LDL = low-density lipoprotein; VLDL = very-low-density lipoprotein.

Secondary causes contribute to most cases of dyslipidemia in adults. The most important secondary cause in developed countries is a sedentary lifestyle with excessive dietary intake of saturated fat, cholesterol, and trans fatty acids (TFAs). TFAs are polyunsaturated fatty acids to which hydrogen atoms have been added; they are commonly used in many processed foods and are as atherogenic as saturated fat. Other common secondary causes include diabetes mellitus, alcohol overuse, chronic renal insufficiency and/or failure, hypothyroidism, primary biliary cirrhosis and other cholestatic liver diseases, and drugs, such as thiazides, β-blockers, retinoids, highly active antiretroviral agents, estrogen and progestins, and glucocorticoids.

Diabetes is an especially significant secondary cause because patients tend to have an atherogenic combination of high TGs; high small, dense LDL fractions; and low HDLs (diabetic dyslipidemia, hypertriglyceridemic hyperapo B). Patients with type 2 diabetes are especially at risk. The combination may be a consequence of obesity and/or poor control of diabetes, which may increase circulating FFAs, leading to increased hepatic VLDL production. TG-rich VLDL then transfers TG and cholesterol to LDL and HDL, promoting formation of TG-rich, small, dense LDL and clearance of TG-rich HDL. Diabetic dyslipidemia is often exacerbated by the increased

TABLE 159–3. GENETIC (PRIMARY) DISORDERS OF LIPID METABOLISM

DISORDER	GENETIC DEFECT	INHERITANCE	PREVALENCE	CLINICAL FEATURES	TREATMENT
Familial hypercholesterolemia	LDL receptor; diminished LDL clearance	Codominant	Heterozygotes: 1/500; 5% of MIs < 60 yr Homozygotes: 1/1 million Common in French Canadians, Christian Lebanese, Afrikaners	Heterozygotes: xanthomas, arcus corneae, and premature CAD (ages 30–50); TC: 250–500 mg/dL (7–13 mmol/L) Homozygotes: xanthomas and premature CAD (before age 18); TC > 500 mg/dL (13 mmol/L)	Diet Lipid-lowering drugs, LDL apheresis (homozygotes) Liver transplantation (homozygotes) Gene therapy
Familial defective apo B-100	Apo B (LDL receptor-binding region); diminished LDL clearance	Dominant	1/700	Xanthomas, arcus senilis, and premature CAD; TC: 250–500 mg/dl (7–13 mmol/L)	Diet Lipid-lowering drugs
Polygenic hypercholesterolemia	Unknown; multiple defects and mechanisms	Variable	Common	Premature CAD; TC: 250–350 mg/dL (6.5–9.0 mmol/L)	Diet Lipid-lowering drugs
LPL deficiency	Endothelial LPL; diminished chylomicron clearance	Recessive	Rare; found worldwide	Failure to thrive (infants); xanthomas, hepatosplenomegaly, and pancreatitis; TG: > 750 mg/dL (8.5 mmol/L)	Diet: total fat restriction with fat-soluble vitamin supplementation; medium-chain TG supplementation
Apo C-II deficiency	Apo C-II (causing functional LPL deficiency)	Recessive	< 1/1 million	Adults may develop pancreatitis; often associated with metabolic syndrome TG: > 750 mg/dL (8.5 mmol/L)	Diet: total fat restriction with fat-soluble vitamin supplementation; medium-chain TG supplementation
Familial hypertriglyceridemia	Unknown, possibly multiple defects and mechanisms	Dominant	1/100	Usually no symptoms or findings; occasional hyperuricemia; TG: 200–500 mg/dL (2.3–5.7 mmol/L), can go higher with dietary factors and alcohol	Diet Weight loss Lipid-lowering drugs

Familial combined	Unknown	Dominant	1/50 to 1/100; 15% of MIs < 60 yr	Premature CAD; apo B disproportionately elevated TC: 250–500 mg/dL (6.5–13.0 mmol/L) TG: 250–750 mg/dL (2.8–8.5 mmol/L)	Diet Weight loss Lipid-lowering drugs
Familial dysbetalipoproteinemia	Apo E (usually e2/e2 homozygotes); diminished chylomicron and VLDL clearance	Recessive (more common) or dominant (less common)	1/5000; found worldwide	Xanthomas (especially palmar), yellow palmar creases, premature CAD; TC: 250–500 mg/dL (6.5–13.0 mmol/L) TG: 250–500 mg/dL (2.8–5.6 mmol/L)	Diet Lipid-lowering drugs
Primary hypoalphalipoproteinemia (familial or nonfamilial)	Unknown, possibly apo A-I, C-III, or A-IV	Dominant	About 5%	Premature CAD; HDL: 15–35 mg/dL	Exercise HDL-elevating drugs
Familial apo A/apo C-III deficiency/mutations	Apo A or apo C-III; increased HDL catabolism	Unknown	Rare	Corneal opacities, xanthomas, some premature CAD; HDL: 15–30 mg/dL	Nonspecific
Familial LCAT deficiency	LCAT gene	Recessive	Extremely rare	Corneal opacities, anemia, renal failure; HDL < 10 mg/dL	Fat restriction Renal transplantation
Fisheye disease (partial LCAT deficiency)	LCAT gene	Recessive	Extremely rare	Corneal opacities; HDL < 10 mg/dL	Nonspecific
Tangier disease	ABCA1 gene	Codominant	Rare	Some with premature CAD, peripheral neuropathy, hemolytic anemia, corneal opacities, hepatosplenomegaly, orange tonsils; HDL: < 5 mg/dL	Low-fat diet
Familial HDL deficiency	ABCA1 gene	Dominant	Rare	Premature CAD	Low-fat diet

Table continues on the following page.

TABLE 159–3. GENETIC (PRIMARY) DISORDERS OF LIPID METABOLISM—Continued

DISORDER	GENETIC DEFECT	INHERITANCE	PREVALENCE	CLINICAL FEATURES	TREATMENT
Hepatic lipase deficiency	Hepatic lipase	Recessive	Extremely rare	Premature CAD TC: 250–1500 mg/dL TG: 395–8200 mg/dL HDL: Variable	Empiric: diet, lipid-lowering drugs
Cerebrotendinous xanthomatosis	Hepatic mitochondrial 27-hydroxylase; bile acid synthesis blocked, cholesterol converted to cholestanol, which accumulates	Recessive	Rare	Cataracts, premature CAD, neuropathy, ataxia	Chenodeoxycholic acid
Sitosterolemia	ABCG5 and ABCG8 genes	Recessive	Rare	Tendon xanthomas, premature CAD	Fat restriction Bile acid sequestrants Ezetimibe
Cholesteryl ester storage and Wolman's disease	Lysosomal esterase deficiency	Recessive	Rare	Premature CAD; accumulation of cholesteryl esters and TG in lysosomes in the liver, spleen, and lymph nodes	Possibly statins Bone marrow transplantation (experimental)

LDL = low-density lipoprotein; TC = total cholesterol; CAD = coronary artery disease; TG = triglyceride; LPL = lipoprotein lipase; LCAT = lecithin cholesterol:acyl transferase; Apo = apoprotein; VLDL = very-low-density lipoprotein; HDL = high-density lipoprotein; ABCA1 = ATP-binding cassette transporter A1; ABCG5 and 8 = ATP-binding cassette subfamily G members 5 and 8.

caloric intake and physical inactivity that characterize the lifestyles of some patients with type 2 diabetes. Women with diabetes may be at special risk for cardiac disease from this form.

Symptoms and Signs

Dyslipidemia itself causes no symptoms but can lead to symptomatic vascular disease, including coronary artery disease and peripheral arterial disease. High TGs (> 1000 mg/dL [> 11.3 mmol/L]) can cause acute pancreatitis. High levels of LDL can cause eyelid xanthelasmas; arcus corneae; and tendinous xanthomas found at the Achilles, elbow, and knee tendons and over metacarpophalangeal joints. Patients with the homozygous form of familial hypercholesterolemia may have the above findings plus planar or cutaneous xanthomas. Patients with severe elevations of TGs can have eruptive xanthomas over the trunk, back, elbows, buttocks, knees, hands, and feet. Patients with the rare dysbetalipoproteinemia can have palmar and tuberous xanthomas.

Severe hypertriglyceridemia (> 2000 mg/dL [> 22.6 mmol/L]) can give retinal arteries and veins a creamy white appearance (lipemia retinalis). Extremely high lipid levels also give a lactescent (milky) appearance to blood plasma.

Diagnosis and Screening

Dyslipidemia is diagnosed by measuring serum lipids, though it may be suspected in patients with characteristic physical findings. Routine measurements (lipid profile) include total cholesterol (TC), TGs, HDL, and LDL.

TC, TGs, and HDL are measured directly; TC and TG values reflect cholesterol and TGs in all circulating lipoproteins, including chylomicrons, VLDL, IDL, LDL, and HDL. TC values vary by 10% and TGs by up to 25% day-to-day even in the absence of disease. TC and HDL can be measured in the nonfasting state, but most patients should have all lipids measured while fasting for maximum accuracy and consistency.

Testing should be postponed until after resolution of acute illness, because TGs increase and cholesterol levels decrease in inflammatory states. Lipid profiles are generally reliable within the first 24 h after an acute MI but then change.

LDL values are most often calculated as the amount of cholesterol not contained in HDL and VLDL, where VLDL is estimated by TG ÷ 5; ie, LDL = TC − [HDL + (TGs ÷ 5)] (Friedewald formula). VLDL cholesterol is estimated by TG ÷ 5 because the cholesterol concentration in VLDL particles is usually $^1/_5$ of the total lipid in the particle. This calculation is valid only when TGs are < 400 mg/dL and patients are fasting, because eating increases TGs. The calculated LDL value incorporates measures of all non-HDL, nonchylomicron cholesterol, including that in IDL and Lp(a). LDL can also be measured directly using plasma ultracentrifugation, which separates chylomicrons and VLDL fractions from HDL and LDL, and by an immunoassay method. Direct measurement may be useful in some patients with elevated TGs to determine if LDL levels are also high, but these direct measurements are not routinely necessary. The role of apo B testing is under study because values reflect all non-HDL cholesterol (in VLDL, VLDL remnants, IDL, and LDL) and may be more predictive of coronary artery disease (CAD) risk than LDL alone.

A fasting lipid profile (TC, TGs, HDL, and calculated LDL) should be obtained in all adults ≥ 20 yr and should be repeated q 5 yr. Lipid measurement should be accompanied by assessment of other cardiovascular risk factors, defined as diabetes mellitus, cigarette use, hypertension, and family history of CAD in a male 1st-degree relative before age 55 or a female 1st-degree relative before age 65.

A definite age after which patients no longer require screening has not been established, but evidence supports screening of patients into their 80s, especially in the presence of atherosclerotic cardiovascular disease.

Indications for screening patients < 20 yr are atherosclerotic risk factors, such as diabetes, hypertension, cigarette smoking, and obesity; premature CAD in a parent, grandparent, or sibling; or a cholesterol level > 240 mg/dL (> 6.2 mmol/L) or known dyslipidemia in a parent. If information on relatives is unavailable, as in the case of adopted children, screening is at the discretion of the health care practitioner.

Patients with premature atherosclerotic cardiovascular disease, cardiovascular disease with normal or near-normal lipid levels, an extensive family history of heart disease, or high LDL refractory to drug therapy should probably have Lp(a) levels measured. Lp(a) levels may also be directly measured in patients with borderline high LDL to determine if drug therapy is warranted. C-reactive protein and homocysteine measurement may be considered in the same populations.

Tests for secondary causes of dyslipidemia—including measurements of fasting glucose, liver enzymes, creatinine, thyroid stimulating hormone (TSH), and urinary protein—should be performed in most patients with newly diagnosed dyslipidemia, and when a component of the lipid profile has inexplicably changed for the worse.

Prognosis and Treatment

Prognosis varies with lipid levels and other cardiovascular risk factors.

General principles: Treatment is indicated for all patients with cardiovascular disease (secondary prevention) and for some without (primary prevention). The National Institutes of Health's National Cholesterol Education Program (NCEP) Adult Treatment Panel III (ATPIII) guidelines are the most common reference for deciding which adults should be treated (see TABLES 159–4 and 159–5). The guidelines focus primarily on reducing elevated LDL levels and secondarily on treating high TGs, low HDL, and metabolic syndrome (see p. 61). An alternate treatment guide (the Sheffield table) uses TC:HDL ratios combined with presence of CAD risk factors to predict cardiovascular risk, but this approach probably leads to undertreatment.

Treatment of children is controversial; dietary changes may be difficult to implement, and no data suggest that lowering lipid levels in childhood effectively prevents heart disease in adulthood. Moreover, the safety and effectiveness of long-term lipid-lowering treatment are questionable. Nevertheless, the American Academy of Pediatrics (AAP) recommends treatment for some children who have elevated LDL levels.

Treatment options depend on the specific lipid abnormality, although different lipid abnormalities often coexist. In some patients, a single abnormality may require several therapies; in others, a single treatment may be adequate for several abnormalities. Treatment should always include treatment of hypertension and diabetes, smoking cessation, and in those with a 10-yr risk of MI or death from CAD of ≥ 10% (as determined from the Framingham tables—see TABLES 159–6 and 159–7), low-dose daily aspirin. In general, treatment options for men and women are the same.

Elevated LDLs: ATPIII guidelines recommend treatment for adults with elevated LDL levels and a history of CAD; conditions that confer a risk for future cardiac events similar to that of CAD itself (CAD equivalents, defined as diabetes mellitus, abdominal aortic aneurysm, peripheral arterial disease, and symptomatic carotid artery disease); or ≥ 2 CAD risk factors. ATPIII guidelines recommend that these patients have LDL levels lowered to < 100 mg/dL, but accumulating evidence suggests that this target may be too high and a target LDL < 70 mg/dL is an option for patients at very high risk (eg, those with known CAD and diabetes, other poorly controlled risk factors, metabolic syndrome, or acute coronary syndrome). When drugs are used, a dose providing at least a 30 to 40% decrease in LDL is desirable (see TABLE 159–8).

The AAP recommends dietary treatment for children with LDL > 110 mg/dL. Drug therapy is recommended for children > 10 yr who are poorly responsive to dietary therapy and who have LDLs ≥ 190 mg/dL without a family history of premature cardiovascular disease. Drug therapy is also recommended for children > 10 yr with LDLs ≥ 160 mg/dL and a family history of premature cardiovascular disease or ≥ 2 risk factors for premature cardiovascular disease. Childhood risk factors besides family history and diabetes include cigarette smoking, hypertension, low HDLs (< 35 mg/dL), obesity, and physical inactivity.

Treatment options include lifestyle changes (diet and exercise), drugs, dietary supplements, procedural interventions, and experimental therapies. Many of these are also effective for treating other lipid abnormalities. Exercise directly lowers LDL in some people; it is also essential to maintain ideal body weight. Dietary changes and exercise should be the initial approach whenever feasible.

Dietary changes include decreasing intake of saturated fats and cholesterol; increasing intake of monounsaturated fats, dietary fiber, and complex carbohydrates; and maintaining ideal body weight. Referral to a dietitian is often useful, especially for older people.

The length of time for which lifestyle changes should be attempted before beginning lipid-lowering drugs is controversial. In patients at average or low cardiovascular risk, 3 to 6 mo is reasonable. Generally, 2 to 3 visits with a patient over 2 to 3 mo are sufficient to assess motivation and adherence.

Drugs are the next step when lifestyle changes are not effective. However, for patients with extremely elevated LDLs (> 200

TABLE 159–4. NATIONAL CHOLESTEROL EDUCATION PROGRAM ADULT TREATMENT PANEL III APPROACH TO DYSLIPIDEMIAS

1. Measure fasting lipoproteins (in mg/dL):

TC (mmol/L)	
< 200 (5.17)	Desirable
200–239 (5.17–6.18)	Borderline high
≥ 240 (6.20)	High
LDL	
< 100 (2.58)	Optimal
100–129 (2.58–3.33)	Near optimal/above optimal
130–159 (3.36–4.11)	Borderline high
160–189 (4.13–4.88)	High
≥ 190 (4.91)	Very high
HDL	
< 40 (1.03)	Low
≥ 60 (1.55)	High
TG	
< 150	Desirable
150–199 (1.695–2.249)	Borderline high
200–499 (2.26–5.639)	High
≥ 500 (5.65)	Very high

2. Identify CAD or CAD equivalents (if present, see TABLE 159–5)
   - CAD equivalents
     - Other atherosclerotic disease:
       - Peripheral arterial disease
       - Abdominal aortic aneurysm
       - Symptomatic carotid artery disease
     - Diabetes mellitus
     - Additional risk factors that confer 10-yr risk of MI or CAD death > 20% (see TABLES 159–6 and 159–7)
3. Identify major CAD risk factors
   - Cigarette smoking
   - Hypertension (BP ≥ 140/90 *or* on antihypertensive drug)
   - Low HDL (≤ 40 mg/dL [1.03 mmol/L])
   - Family history of premature CAD (CAD in male 1st-degree relative < 55 or in female 1st-degree relative < 65)
   - Age (men ≥ 45, women ≥ 55)
4. If ≥ 2 major risk factors are present without CAD or CAD equivalent, assess 10-yr risk of MI or CAD death using Framingham risk tables (see TABLES 159–6 and 159–7).

TC = total cholesterol; LDL = low-density lipoprotein; HDL = high-density lipoprotein; TG = triglyceride; CAD = coronary artery disease.

Data from the Third Report of the Expert Panel on Detection, Evaluation, and Treatment of High Blood Cholesterol in Adults. National Institutes of Health, National Heart, Lung, and Blood Institute, 2001.

TABLE 159–5. NATIONAL CHOLESTEROL EDUCATION PROGRAM ADULT TREATMENT PANEL III GUIDELINES FOR TREATMENT OF HYPERLIPIDEMIA

RISK CATEGORY	BEGIN LIFESTYLE CHANGES IF:	CONSIDER DRUG THERAPY IF:	LDL GOAL
High: CAD or CAD equivalents (10-yr risk > 20%)	LDL ≥ 100 mg/dL (2.58 mmol/L)	LDL ≥ 100 mg/dL (2.58 mmol/L)(drug optional if < 100 mg/dL [< 2.58 mmol/L])	< 100 mg/dL; < 70 mg/dL optional
Moderate high: ≥ 2 risk factors with 10-yr risk 10 to 20%*	LDL ≥ 130 mg/dL (3.36 mmol/L)	LDL ≥ 130 mg/dL (3.36 mmol/L)	< 130 mg/dL; < 100 mg/dL optional
Moderate: ≥ 2 risk factors with 10-yr risk < 10%*	LDL ≥ 130 mg/dL (3.36 mmol/L)	LDL ≥ 160 mg/dL (4.13 mmol/L)	< 130 mg/dL; < 100 mg/dL optional
Lower: 0–1 risk factor	LDL ≥ 160 mg/dL (4.13 mmol/L)	LDL ≥ 190 mg/dL (4.91 mmol/L) (drug optional if 160–189 mg/dL [4.13–4.88 mmol/L])	< 160 mg/dL

*For 10-yr risk, see Framingham risk tables (TABLES 159–6 and 159–7).

CAD = coronary artery disease; LDL = low-density lipoprotein.

Data from the Third Report of the Expert Panel on Detection, Evaluation, and Treatment of High Blood Cholesterol in Adults. National Institutes of Health, National Heart, Lung, and Blood Institute, 2001 and from Grundy SM, Cleeman JI, Merz CNB, et al. Implications of recent clinical trials for the National Cholesterol Education Program Adult Treatment Panel III guidelines. *Circulation* 2004;110:227–239.

mg/dL [> 5.2 mmol/L]) and those at high cardiovascular risk, drug therapy should accompany diet and exercise from the start.

Statins are the drugs and possibly treatment of choice for LDL reduction and demonstrably reduce cardiovascular mortality. Statins inhibit hydroxymethylglutaryl CoA reductase, a key enzyme in cholesterol synthesis, leading to up-regulation of LDL receptors and increased LDL clearance. They reduce LDL by up to 60% and produce small increases in HDL and modest decreases in TGs. Statins also appear to decrease intra-arterial and/or systemic inflammation by stimulating production of endothelial nitric oxide; they may also decrease LDL deposition in endothelial macrophages and decrease cholesterol in inflammatory cell membranes. This anti-inflammatory effect is antiatherogenic even in the absence of elevated lipid levels. Adverse effects are uncommon but include liver enzyme elevations and myositis or rhabdomyolysis. Muscle toxicity without enzyme elevation has also been reported. Adverse effects are more common in older patients, those with multiple diseases, and those on multiple drugs. In some people, changing from one statin to another or lowering the dose relieves the problem. Muscle toxicity seems to be most common when some of the statins are used with drugs that inhibit cytochrome P3A4 (eg, macrolide antibiotics, azole antifungals, cyclosporine) and with fibrates, especially gemfibrozil. Properties of statins differ slightly by agent, and the choice of agent should be based on patient characteristics, LDL level, and provider discretion (see TABLE 159–8).

Bile acid sequestrants block intestinal bile acid reabsorption, forcing up-regulation of hepatic LDL receptors to recruit circulating cholesterol for bile synthesis. They are proven to reduce cardiovascular mortality. Bile acid sequestrants are usually used with statins or with nicotinic acid (see p. 1308) to augment LDL reduction and are the drugs of choice for children and women who are or are planning to become pregnant. Bile acid sequestrants are safe, but their use is limited by adverse effects of bloating, nausea, cramping, and constipation. They may also increase TGs, so their use is contraindicated in patients with hypertriglyceridemia. Cholestyramine and colestipol, but not colesevelam, interfere with absorption of other drugs—notably thiazides, β-blockers, warfarin, digoxin, and thyroxine—an effect that can be minimized by administration 4 h before or 1 h after other drugs.

Ezetimibe inhibits intestinal absorption of cholesterol and phytosterol. It usually lowers LDL by 15 to 20% and causes small increases in HDL and a mild decrease in TGs. Ezetimibe can be used as monotherapy in patients intolerant to statins or added to statins for patients on maximum doses with persistent LDL elevation. Adverse effects are infrequent.

Dietary supplements that lower LDL levels include fiber supplements and commercially available margarines containing plant sterols (sitosterol and campesterol) or stanols. The latter reduce LDL by up to 10% without affecting HDL or TGs by competitively displacing cholesterol from intestinal micelles. Garlic supplements and walnuts have been advocated for LDL reduction with only minimal evidence to support their use.

Procedural approaches are reserved for patients with severe hyperlipidemia (LDL > 300 mg/dL) that is refractory to conventional therapy, such as occurs with familial hypercholesterolemia. Options include LDL apheresis (in which LDL is removed by extracorporeal plasma exchange), ileal bypass (to block reabsorption of bile acids), liver transplantation (which transplants LDL receptors), and portocaval shunting (which decreases LDL production by unknown mechanisms).

TABLE 159–6. FRAMINGHAM RISK TABLES FOR MEN

	POINT SCORE									
AGE	**20–34**	**35–39**	**40–44**	**45–49**	**50–54**	**55–59**	**60–64**	**65–69**	**70–74**	**75–79**
Age points	–9	–4	0	3	6	8	10	11	12	13
TC<160	0	0	0	0	0	0	0	0	0	0
160–199	4	4	3	3	2	2	1	1	0	0
200–239	7	7	5	5	3	3	1	1	0	0
240–279	9	9	6	6	4	4	2	2	1	1
≥280	11	11	8	8	5	5	3	3	1	1
Nonsmoker	0	0	0	0	0	0	0	0	0	0
Smoker	8	8	5	5	3	3	1	1	1	1
HDL ≥ 60	–1									
50–59	0									
40–49	1									
< 40	2									
Systolic BP < 120	Untreated 0; treated 0									
120–129	Untreated 0; treated 1									
130–139	Untreated 1; treated 2									
140–159	Untreated 1; treated 2									
≥160	Untreated 2; treated 3									

POINTS (10-yr risk of MI or CAD death %): < 0 points = < 1%; 0–4 points = 1%; 5–6 points = 2%; 7 points = 3%; 8 points = 4%; 9 points = 5%; 10 points = 6%; 11 points = 8%; 12 points = 10%; 13 points = 12%; 14 points = 16%; 15 points = 20%; 16 points = 25%; >17 points = ≥ 30%.

TC = total cholesterol; HDL = high-density lipoprotein; CAD = coronary artery disease.

Data from the Third Report of the Expert Panel on Detection, Evaluation, and Treatment of High Blood Cholesterol in Adults. National Institutes of Health, National Heart, Lung, and Blood Institute, 2001.

TABLE 159–7. FRAMINGHAM RISK TABLES FOR WOMEN

	POINT SCORE									
AGE	**20–34**	**35–39**	**40–44**	**45–49**	**50–54**	**55–59**	**60–64**	**65–69**	**70–74**	**75–79**
Age points	−7	−3	0	3	6	8	10	12	14	16
TC < 60	0	0	0	0	0	0	0	0	0	0
160–199	4	4	3	3	2	2	1	1	1	1
200–239	8	8	6	6	4	4	2	2	1	1
240–279	11	11	8	8	5	5	3	3	2	2
≥280	13	13	10	10	7	7	4	4	2	2
Nonsmoker	0	0	0	0	0	0	0	0	0	0
Smoker	9	9	7	7	4	4	2	2	1	1
HDL ≥ 60	−1									
50–59	0									
40–49	1									
< 40	2									
Systolic BP < 120	Untreated 0; treated 0									
120–129	Untreated 1; treated 3									
130–139	Untreated 2; treated 4									
140–159	Untreated 3; treated 5									
≥160	Untreated 4; treated 6									

POINTS (10 yr risk of MI or CAD death %): < 9 points = < 1%; 9–12 points = 1%; 13–14 points = 2%; 15 points = 3%; 16 points = 4%; 17 points = 5%; 18 points = 6%; 19 points = 8%; 20 points = 11%; 21 points = 14%; 22 points = 17%; 23 points = 22%; 24 points = 27%; ≥25 points = ≥ 30%.

TC = total cholesterol; HDL = high-density lipoprotein; CAD = coronary artery disease.

Data from the Third Report of the Expert Panel on Detection, Evaluation, and Treatment of High Blood Cholesterol in Adults. National Institutes of Health, National Heart, Lung, and Blood Institute, 2001.

LDL apheresis is the procedure of choice in most instances when maximally tolerated therapy fails to lower LDL adequately. Apheresis is also the usual therapy in patients with the homozygous form of familial hypercholesterolemia who have limited or no response to drug therapy.

Future therapies to reduce LDL include peroxisome proliferator–activated receptor agonists that have thiazolidinedione-like and fibrate-like properties, LDL-receptor activators, LPL activators, and recombinant apo E. Cholesterol vaccination (to induce anti-LDL antibodies and hasten LDL clearance from serum) and gene transfer are conceptually appealing therapies that are under study but years away from being available for use.

Elevated TGs: Though it is unclear if elevated TGs independently contribute to cardiovascular disease, they are associated with multiple metabolic abnormalities that contribute to CAD (eg, diabetes, metabolic syndrome). Consensus is emerging that lowering elevated TGs is beneficial (see TABLE 159–4). No target goals exist, but levels < 150 mg/dL (1.7 mmol/L) are generally considered desirable. No guidelines specifically address treatment of elevated TGs in children.

Treatment first involves lifestyle changes, including exercise, weight loss, and avoidance of concentrated dietary sugar and alcohol. Intake of 2 to 4 servings/wk of fish high in ω-3 fatty acids may be effective, but the amount of ω-3 fatty acids is often lower than

TABLE 159–8. LIPID–LOWERING DRUGS

DRUG CLASS AND AGENTS	EFFECTS	ADULT DOSES AND COMMENTS
Statins Fluvastatin Lovastatin Simvastatin Pravastatin Atorvastatin Rosuvastatin	Reduce LDL (primary); increase HDL, decrease TGs (secondary)	Fluvastatin (20–80 mg po once/day at bedtime): Least potent, no renal excretion. Dose necessary to achieve recommended 30–40% reduction of LDL: 40–80 mg Lovastatin: Immediate release (20–80 mg po once/day at dinner); extended release (20–60 mg po once/day). Dose necessary to achieve recommended 30–40% reduction of LDL: 40 mg Simvastatin (5–80 mg po once/day in the evening). Dose necessary to achieve recommended 30–40% reduction of LDL: 20–40 mg Pravastatin (10–80 mg po once/day). Dose necessary to achieve recommended 30–40% reduction of LDL: 40 mg Atorvastatin (10–80 mg po once/day): No renal excretion, long half-life. Dose necessary to achieve recommended 30–40% reduction of LDL: 10 mg Rosuvastatin (5–40 mg po once/day): Most potent, long half-life. Dose necessary to achieve recommended 30–40% reduction of LDL: 5–10 mg
Nicotinic acid (niacin)	Increases HDL, lowers TGs (low doses); lowers LDL (higher doses), lower Lp(a) (secondary)	Immediate-release: 500 mg bid–1000 mg po tid Extended-release: 500–2000 mg po once/day at bedtime Frequent adverse effects: Flushing, impaired glucose tolerance, increased uric acid. Use aspirin and give with food to minimize flushing
Bile acid sequestrants Cholestyramine Colestipol Colesevelam	Reduce LDL (primary); slightly increase HDL (secondary); may increase TGs	Cholestyramine (4 g po 1–6 times/day with meals) Colestipol (5–30 g po once/day with a meal) Colesevelam (2.4–4.5 g po once/day with a meal)
Fibrates Gemfibrozil Ciprofibrate Clofibrate Fenofibrate Bezafibrate	Reduce TGs, increase HDL, may increase LDL (in patients with high TGs)	Gemfibrozil (600 mg po bid): Decrease dose in renal insufficiency Clofibrate (1g po bid) Ciprofibrate (100–200 mg po once/day): not available in US Fenofibrate (67–201 mg po once/day): Decrease dose in renal insufficiency; may be safest fibrate for use with statins Bezafibrate (200 mg po tid or 400 mg po once/day): Requires dose reduction in renal failure; not available in US
Cholesterol absorption inhibitors Ezetimibe	Lower LDL (primary), decrease TGs, increases HDLs	Dose: 10 mg po once/day Adverse effect profile not well established
Combination agents Niacin extended release + lovastatin	Combined effects of niacin and statins	Dose: 500 mg niacin /20 mg lovastatin po once/day or 2000 mg/40 mg po once/day Not recommended as initial therapy

LDL = low density lipoprotein; HDL = high density lipoprotein; TG = triglyceride; Lp(a) = lipoprotein a.

needed; supplements may be helpful. In patients with diabetes, glucose levels should be tightly controlled. If these measures are ineffective, lipid-lowering drugs should be considered. Patients with very high TGs should begin drug therapy at diagnosis to more quickly reduce the risk of acute pancreatitis.

Fibrates reduce TGs by about 50%. They appear to stimulate endothelial LPL, leading to increased fatty acid oxidation in the liver and muscle and decreased hepatic VLDL synthesis. They also increase HDLs by up to 20%. Fibrates can cause GI adverse effects, including dyspepsia and abdominal pain. They uncommonly cause cholelithiasis. Fibrates potentiate muscle toxicity when used with statins and potentiate the effects of warfarin.

Nicotinic acid may also be useful (see Low HDLs, below).

Statins can be used in patients with TGs < 500 mg/dL if LDL elevations are also present; statins may reduce both LDLs and TGs through reduction of VLDLs. If only TGs are elevated, fibrates are the drug of choice.

Omega-3 fatty acids in high doses (1 to 6 g/day of eicosapentaenoic acid [EPA] and docosahexaenoic acid [DHA]) can be effective in reducing TGs. The ω-3 fatty acids EPA and DHA are the active ingredients in fish oil or ω-3 capsules. Adverse effects include eructation and diarrhea. These may be decreased by giving the fish oil capsules with meals in divided doses (eg, bid or tid). Omega-3 fatty acids can be a useful adjunct to other therapies.

Low HDLs: Treatment to increase HDL levels may decrease risk of death, but data are limited. ATPIII guidelines define low HDL as < 40 mg/dL [< 1.04 mmol/L]; the guidelines do not specify an HDL target level and recommend interventions to raise HDL only after LDL targets have been reached. Treatments for LDL and TG reduction often increase HDL, and the 3 objectives can sometimes be achieved simultaneously. No guidelines specifically address treatment of low HDL in children.

Treatment includes an increase in exercise and monounsaturated fat intake. Alcohol raises HDL but is not routinely recommended as a therapy because of its many other adverse effects. Drugs are useful when lifestyle changes alone are insufficient.

Nicotinic acid (niacin) is the most effective drug for increasing HDLs. Its mechanism of action is unknown, but it appears to both increase HDL production and inhibit HDL clearance; it may also mobilize cholesterol from macrophages. Niacin also decreases TGs and, in doses of 1500 to 2000 mg/day, reduces LDLs. Niacin produces flushing, pruritus, and nausea; premedication with low-dose aspirin may prevent these adverse effects; slow-release preparations cause them less often. Niacin can cause liver enzyme elevations and occasionally liver failure, insulin resistance, and hyperuricemia and gout. It may also increase homocysteine levels. In patients with average LDL and below-average HDL levels, niacin combined with statin treatment may be effective in preventing cardiovascular disease.

Fibrates increase HDLs (see above). Infusion of recombinant HDL (eg, apolipoprotein A-1 Milano, an HDL variant in which a cysteine is substituted for an arginine at position 173 allowing for dimer formation) appears promising as a treatment for atherosclerosis but requires further study. Torcetrapib, a CETP inhibitor, markedly increases HDL and decreases LDL levels, but effect on atherosclerosis is unproven and this drug also requires further study.

Elevated Lp(a): The upper limit of normal for Lp(a) is about 30 mg/dL (0.8 mmol/L), but values in African-Americans run higher. Few data exist to guide the treatment of elevated Lp(a) or to establish treatment efficacy. Niacin is the only drug that directly decreases Lp(a); it can lower Lp(a) by ≤ 20% at higher doses. The usual approach to patients with elevated Lp(a) is to lower LDL aggressively.

Secondary causes: Treatment of diabetic dyslipidemia should always involve lifestyle changes, with statins to reduce LDLs and/or fibrates to decrease TGs. Metformin lowers TGs, which may be a reason to choose it over other oral antihyperglycemic drugs when treating diabetes. Some thiazolidinediones (TZDs) increase both HDLs and LDLs (probably the less atherogenic large, buoyant type of LDLs). Some TZDs also decrease TGs. These agents should not be chosen over lipid-lowering drugs to treat lipid abnormalities in diabetic patients but may be useful adjuncts. Patients with very high TG levels and less than optimally controlled diabetes may have better response to insulin than to oral antihyperglycemic drugs.

Treatment of dyslipidemia in patients with hypothyroidism, renal disease, and/or obstructive liver disease involves treating the underlying causes primarily and lipid abnormalities secondarily. Abnormal lipid levels in patients with low-normal thyroid function (high-normal TSH levels) improve with hormone replacement. Reducing the dosage of or stopping drugs that cause lipid abnormalities should be considered.

Monitoring treatment: Lipid levels should be monitored periodically after starting treatment. No data support specific monitoring intervals, but measuring lipid levels 2 to 3 mo after starting or changing therapies and once or twice yearly after lipid levels are stabilized is common practice.

Despite the low incidence of liver and muscle toxicity with statin use (0.5 to 2% of all users), current recommendations are for baseline measurements of liver and muscle enzyme levels at the beginning of treatment. Many practitioners obtain at least one additional set of liver enzymes 4 to 12 wk after beginning treatment and annually thereafter. Statin therapy can be continued unless liver enzymes increase to > 3 times the upper limit of normal. Muscle enzyme levels need not be checked regularly unless patients develop myalgias or other muscle symptoms.

Elevated High-Density Lipoprotein Levels

Elevated HDL level is HDL > 80 mg/dL (> 2.1 mmol/L).

Elevated HDL levels decrease cardiovascular risk; high HDL levels caused by some primary genetic disorders may not protect against cardiovascular disease because of accompanying lipid and metabolic abnormalities.

Primary causes are single or multiple genetic mutations that result in overproduction or decreased clearance of HDLs. Secondary causes of high HDLs include chronic precirrhotic alcoholism, primary biliary cirrhosis, hyperthyroidism, and drugs (eg, corticosteroids, insulin, phenytoin). The unexpected finding of high HDL in a patient not taking a lipid-lowering drug should prompt a diagnostic evaluation for a secondary cause with measurements of AST, ALT, and TSH; a negative evaluation suggests a possible primary cause.

Cholesteryl ester transfer protein (CETP) deficiency is a rare autosomal recessive disorder caused by a CETP gene mutation. CETP facilitates transfer of cholesterol esters from HDL to other lipoproteins, and CETP deficiency leads to low-cholesterol LDL and slower HDL clearance. Affected patients display no symptoms or signs but have HDLs > 150 mg/dL. Protection from cardiovascular disease has not been proven. No treatment is necessary.

Familial hyperalphalipoproteinemia is an autosomal dominant condition caused by various unidentified and known genetic mutations, including those that cause apolipoprotein A-I overproduction and apolipoprotein C-III variants. The disorder is usually diagnosed incidentally when plasma HDL levels are > 80 mg/dL. Affected patients have no other symptoms or signs. No treatment is necessary.

HYPOLIPIDEMIA

Hypolipidemia is a decrease in plasma lipoprotein caused by primary (genetic) or secondary factors. It is usually asymptomatic and diagnosed incidentally on routine lipid screening. Treatment of secondary hypolipidemia involves treating underlying causes. Treatment of primary hypolipidemia is often unnecessary, but patients with some genetic disorders require high-dose vitamin E.

Classification and Etiology

Hypolipidemia is defined as a total cholesterol (TC) < 120 mg/dL (< 3.1 mmol/L) or LDL < 50 mg/dL (< 0.13 mmol/L). Secondary causes are far more common than primary causes and include hyperthyroidism, chronic infections and other inflammatory states, hematologic and other malignancies, malnutrition (including that accompanying chronic alcohol use), and malabsorption. The unexpected finding of low cholesterol or low LDLs in a patient not taking a lipid-lowering drug should prompt a diagnostic evaluation, including measurements of AST, ALT, and thyroid stimulating hormone; a negative evaluation suggests a possible primary cause.

There are 3 primary disorders in which single or multiple genetic mutations result in underproduction or increased clearance of LDLs.

Abetalipoproteinemia (Bassen-Kornzweig syndrome) is an autosomal recessive condition caused by mutations in the gene for microsomal TG transfer protein, a protein critical to chylomicron and VLDL formation. Dietary fat cannot be absorbed, and lipoproteins in both metabolic pathways are virtually absent from serum; TC is typically < 45 mg/dL (1.16 mmol/L), TGs are < 20 mg/dL (< 0.23 mmol/L), and LDLs are undetectable. The condition is often first noticed in infants with fat malabsorption, steatorrhea, and failure to thrive. Mental retardation may result. Because vitamin E is distributed to peripheral tissues via

VLDLs and LDLs, most affected individuals eventually develop severe vitamin E deficiency. Symptoms and signs include visual changes from slow retinal degeneration, sensory neuropathy, posterior column signs, and cerebellar signs of dysmetria, ataxia, and spasticity, which can eventually lead to death. RBC acanthocytosis is a distinguishing feature on blood smear. Diagnosis is made by the absence of apo B in plasma; intestinal biopsies show lack of microsomal transfer protein. Treatment is with high doses (100 to 300 mg/kg once/day) of vitamin E with supplementation of dietary fat and other fat-soluble vitamins.

Hypobetalipoproteinemia is an autosomal dominant or codominant condition caused by mutations in the gene coding for apo B. Heterozygous patients have truncated apo B, leading to rapid LDL clearance. Heterozygotes manifest no signs or symptoms except for TC < 120 mg/dL and LDLs < 80 mg/dL. TGs are normal. Homozygous patients have either shorter truncations, leading to lower lipid levels (TC < 80 mg/dL, LDLs < 20 mg/dL), or absent apo B synthesis, leading to symptoms and signs of abetalipoproteinemia. Diagnosis is by finding low levels of LDL and apo B; hypobetalipoproteinemia and abetalipoproteinemia are distinguished from one another by family history. Heterozygotes and homozygotes with low but detectable LDLs require no treatment. Treatment of homozygotes with no LDLs is the same as for abetalipoproteinemia.

Chylomicron retention disease is an autosomal recessive condition caused by an unknown mutation leading to deficient apo B secretion from enterocytes. Chylomicron synthesis is absent, but VLDL synthesis remains intact. Affected infants have fat malabsorption, steatorrhea, and failure to thrive and may develop neurologic disease similar to that in abetalipoproteinemia. Diagnosis is by intestinal biopsy of patients with low cholesterol levels and absence of postprandial chylomicrons. Treatment is supplementation of fat and fat-soluble vitamins.

160 AMYLOIDOSIS

Amyloidosis is any of a group of disparate conditions characterized by extracellular deposition of various insoluble proteins. These proteins may accumulate locally, causing relatively few symptoms, or widely, involving multiple organs and producing severe multiorgan failure. Amyloidosis can be primary or be secondary to various infectious, inflammatory, or malignant conditions. Rarely, it results from any of several inherited metabolic defects. Diagnosis is by biopsy of affected tissue. Treatment varies with the type of amyloidosis.

Etiology, Pathophysiology, and Classification

Amyloid deposits may be formed from at least 18 different proteins, including immunoglobulin fragments. Amyloid deposits are metabolically inert but interfere physically with organ structure and function. All stain positive with Congo red dye, stain pink with hematoxylin and eosin, and have apple-green birefringence under polarized light after Congo red staining. Amyloid deposits have a fibrillar, usually rigid, and nonbranching ultrastructure. They form a β-pleated sheet that can be seen by x-ray diffraction. In addition to the fibrillar amyloid protein, the deposits also contain serum amyloid P component and glycosaminoglycans. On gross inspection, affected organs appear waxy and translucent.

There are 3 major systemic forms of amyloidosis: primary, secondary, and familial. Also, there are 2 major localized forms, A β and AIAPP (which occurs in the pancreas of type 2 diabetes patients), as well as several miscellaneous forms (eg, A β_2-microglobulin associated with chronic hemodialysis).

Primary amyloidosis (AL): AL is a monoclonal plasma cell disorder in which the abnormal protein is an immunoglobulin, usually a light chain fragment (Bence Jones protein) but occasionally a heavy chain fragment (AH amyloidosis). These chains either have an aberrant structure or are processed abnormally so that some form insoluble deposits. Common sites for deposition include the skin, nerves, heart, GI tract (including tongue), kidney, liver, spleen, and blood vessels. A mild plasmacytosis occurs in the bone marrow, which is suggestive of multiple myeloma, but most patients do not have true multiple myeloma (with lytic bone lesions, renal tubular casts, and anemia). However, about 10 to 20% of patients with multiple myeloma also develop amyloidosis.

Secondary amyloidosis (AA): This form can occur secondary to several infectious, inflammatory, and malignant (eg, myeloma) conditions and is caused by the degradation of the acute-phase reactant serum amyloid A (SAA). Common causative infections include TB, bronchiectasis, osteomyelitis, and leprosy. Inflammatory conditions include RA, juvenile RA, Crohn's disease, and familial Mediterranean fever. Inflammatory cytokines (eg, IL-1, tumor necrosis factor, IL-6) that are produced in these disorders cause increased hepatic production of the precursor protein SAA, which circulates in the serum.

AA amyloidosis shows a predilection for the spleen, liver, kidneys, adrenals, and lymph nodes. The liver, spleen, and kidneys are often enlarged, firm, and rubbery. Involvement of the heart and peripheral or autonomic nerves is rare. However, no organ system is spared, and vascular involvement may be widespread.

Familial amyloidosis: The familial form results from accumulation of a mutated version of a plasma protein (most commonly transthyretin [TTR], hence ATTR). Nearly all of the abnormal protein is produced by the liver. Over 80 mutations of the gene for TTR have been identified, all inherited in an autosomal dominant pattern.

Age at onset of symptoms is highly variable, ranging from the teens to the 70s. ATTR amyloidosis produces peripheral sensory and motor neuropathy, often with an autonomic neuropathy. Carpal tunnel syndrome is common. Later in the illness, cardiovascular and renal involvement occurs. Vitreous abnormalities may also develop.

Other very rare hereditary amyloidoses result from mutations of other physiologic proteins, including apolipoprotein A-1, lysozyme, fibrinogen, gelsolin, A β protein, and cystatin C. These amyloidoses have various systemic and localized effects.

A β_2-microglobulin (dialysis-related) amyloidosis: This form occurs in patients with chronic renal failure who have been on hemodialysis or peritoneal dialysis for long periods, usually > 8 yr. The amyloid deposits consist of β_2-microglobulin, a component of the class I major histocompatibility complex, which is normally cleared by the kidneys but cannot be removed by dialysis membranes. Deposits preferentially occur in and around bones and joints and in the carpal tunnel and have been found in the GI tract and in other organs.

A β-protein amyloidosis: This occurs in patients with Alzheimer's disease. Although the exact role of amyloid deposits is unclear, the neuritic plaques characteristic of Alzheimer's disease contain amyloid deposits consisting of a β-protein fragment of β-amyloid precursor protein (a transmembrane glycoprotein). The β-protein fragment is sometimes complexed with apolipoprotein E. Within the plaques, nonfibrillar forms of the β protein are intermixed with fibrillar amyloid forms.

β-Protein amyloid deposition may also occur around cerebral blood vessels, which is thought to be a cause of nonhypertensive cerebral hemorrhage (cerebral amyloid angiopathy). The angiopathy may occur sporadically or as a hereditary syndrome (Dutch hereditary cerebral hemorrhage).

Symptoms and Signs

Symptoms and signs are nonspecific and relate to the organ or system affected. Symptoms in AA amyloidosis are often obscured by the underlying disease.

When the kidneys are affected, nephrotic syndrome is the most striking early manifestation. Initially, only slight proteinuria may occur; later, the distinctive symptom complex develops with anasarca, hypoproteinemia, and massive proteinuria.

Hepatic involvement produces painless hepatomegaly, which may be massive (liver weight > 7 kg). Except for occasional elevation of alkaline phosphatase, liver function tests remain normal. Jaundice is rare. Occasionally, portal hypertension develops, with resulting esophageal varices and ascites.

Cardiac involvement produces a restrictive cardiomyopathy, eventually leading to heart failure. Cardiomegaly and various degrees of heart block or arrhythmia may occur.

Peripheral neuropathy, with paresthesias of the fingers and toes, is a common presenting manifestation in AL and ATTR amyloidoses. Autonomic neuropathy may produce orthostatic hypotension, erectile dysfunction, sweating abnormalities, and GI motility disturbances.

Rheumatologic symptoms in patients with A β_2-microglobulin amyloidosis include carpal tunnel syndrome and chronic pain in the shoulder, wrist, and fingers. Pathologic fractures, particularly of the humerus and femur, may occur.

GI amyloid may cause motility abnormalities of the esophagus and small and large intestines. Gastric atony, malabsorption, bleeding, or pseudo-obstruction may also occur. Macroglossia is common in AL amyloidoses.

A firm, symmetric, nontender goiter resembling that found in Hashimoto's thyroiditis may result from amyloidosis of the thyroid gland. Lung involvement (mostly in AL amyloidosis) can be characterized by focal pulmonary nodules, tracheobronchial lesions, or diffuse alveolar deposits. In several hereditary amyloidoses, amyloid vitreous opacities and bilateral scalloped pupillary margins develop.

Diagnosis

Amyloidosis is suspected clinically but can be diagnosed only by biopsy. Subcutaneous abdominal fat pad aspiration and biopsy of rectal mucosa are the best approaches. Other useful biopsy sites are the gingiva, skin, nerve, kidney, and liver. Tissue sections are stained with Congo red dye and examined with a polarizing microscope for characteristic birefringence. Isotopically labeled serum AP (in which AP represents the pentagonal component of amyloid) can be used in a scintigraphic test to confirm the diagnosis.

Prognosis

Prognosis depends on the type of amyloidosis and the organ system involved. AL amyloidosis with multiple myeloma has the poorest prognosis: death within 1 yr is common. Untreated ATTR amyloidoses are fatal within 10 to 15 yr. Prognosis in other familial amyloidoses varies. In general, renal or cardiac involvement in patients with any type of amyloidosis is of particular concern.

Prognosis in AA amyloidosis depends on successful treatment of the underlying disease, although rare patients undergo spontaneous regression of the amyloid deposits without such treatment.

Treatment

Management is generally symptomatic, although treatment of the underlying cause can sometimes arrest amyloidosis. In patients with renal amyloid, kidney transplantation provides long-term survival comparable to that in other renal diseases, although mortality is higher in the early years. Amyloid ultimately recurs in a donor kidney, but several recipients have done very well and have survived up to 10 yr. Heart transplantation has been successful in carefully selected AL patients with severe cardiac involvement.

Patients with AL amyloidosis are treated with chemotherapy. A common protocol uses melphalan 0.075 mg/kg po bid and prednisone 0.2 mg/kg po qid. High-dose melphalan with bone marrow or stem cell transplantation achieves good short-term success and apparent cures in some cases.

In patients with ATTR amyloidosis, liver transplantation—which removes the site of synthesis of the mutant protein—is very effective.

For AA amyloidosis with familial Mediterranean fever, colchicine 0.6 mg once/day or bid is effective. Underlying infections in patients with AA amyloidosis of infectious origin must be treated aggressively. Treatment of amyloid resulting from cancer (eg, renal cell carcinoma) is directed at the cancer.

161 CARCINOID TUMORS

Carcinoid tumors develop from neuroendocrine cells in the GI tract (90%—see also p. 172), pancreas, and pulmonary bronchi (see also p. 510). More than 95% of all GI carcinoids originate in only 3 sites: the appendix, ileum, and rectum. Although carcinoids are often benign or only locally invasive, those affecting the ileum and bronchus are frequently malignant.

Carcinoids can be endocrinologically inert or produce a variety of hormones. The most common endocrinologic syndrome is carcinoid syndrome; however, most patients with carcinoids do not develop carcinoid syndrome. The likelihood that a tumor will be endocrinologically active varies with its site of origin, being highest for tumors originating in the ileum and proximal colon (40 to 50%). The likelihood is lower with bronchial carcinoids, lower still with appendiceal carcinoids, and essentially zero with rectal carcinoids.

Endocrinologically inert carcinoids are suspected because of their symptoms and signs (eg, pain, luminal bleeding, GI obstruction). They can be detected by angiography, CT, or MRI. Small-bowel carcinoids may exhibit filling defects or other abnormalities on barium x-rays. Definitive diagnosis is made histologically after biopsy or resection.

Endocrinologically active carcinoids are diagnosed and treated as described below.

CARCINOID SYNDROME

Carcinoid syndrome develops in some people with carcinoid tumors and is characterized by cutaneous flushing, abdominal cramps, and diarrhea. Right-sided valvular heart disease may develop after several years. The syndrome results from vasoactive substances (including serotonin, bradykinin, histamine, prostaglandins, polypeptide hormones) secreted by the tumor, which is typically a metastatic intestinal carcinoid. Diagnosis is clinical and by demonstrating increased urinary 5-hydroxyindoleacetic acid. Tumor localization may require a radionuclide scan or laparotomy. Treatment of symptoms is with somatostatin or octreotide, but surgical removal is performed where possible; chemotherapy may be used for malignant tumors.

Etiology and Pathophysiology

Endocrinologically active tumors of the diffuse peripheral endocrine or paracrine system produce various amines and polypeptides with corresponding signs and symptoms, including carcinoid syndrome. Carcinoid syndrome is usually due to endocrinologically active malignant tumors that develop from neuroendocrine cells (mostly in the ileum) and produce serotonin. It can, however, occur from tumors elsewhere in the GI tract (particularly the appendix and rectum), pancreas, bronchi, or, rarely, the gonads. Rarely, certain highly malignant tumors (eg, oat cell carcinoma of the lung, pancreatic islet cell carcinoma, medullary thyroid carcinoma) are responsible.

An intestinal carcinoid does not usually produce the syndrome unless hepatic metastases have occurred, because metabolic products released by the tumor are rapidly destroyed by blood and liver enzymes in the portal circulation (eg, serotonin by hepatic monoamine oxidase). Hepatic metastases, however, release metabolic products via the hepatic veins directly into the systemic circulation. Metabolic products released by primary pulmonary and ovarian carcinoids bypass the portal route and may similarly induce symptoms. Rare intestinal carcinoids with only intra-abdominal spread can drain directly into the systemic circulation or the lymphatics and produce symptoms.

Serotonin acts on smooth muscle to produce diarrhea, colic, and malabsorption. Histamine and bradykinin, through their vasodilator effects, cause flushing. The role of prostaglandins and various polypeptide hormones, which may be produced by paracrine cells, awaits further investigation; elevated human chorionic gonadotropin and pancreatic polypeptide levels are occasionally present with carcinoids.

Many patients develop right-sided endocardial fibrosis, leading to pulmonary stenosis and tricuspid regurgitation. Left heart lesions, which have been reported with bronchial carcinoids, are rare because serotonin is destroyed during passage through the lungs.

Symptoms and Signs

The most common (and often earliest) sign is an uncomfortable flushing, typically of the head and neck, often precipitated by emotional stress or the ingestion of food, hot beverages, or alcohol. Striking skin color changes may occur, ranging from pallor or erythema to a violaceous hue. Abdominal cramps with recurrent diarrhea occur and are often the patient's major complaint. Malabsorption syndrome may occur. Patients with valvular lesions may have a heart murmur. A few patients have asthmatic wheezing, and some have decreased libido and erectile dysfunction; pellagra develops rarely.

Diagnosis

Serotonin-secreting carcinoids are suspected on the basis of their symptoms and signs. Diagnosis is confirmed by demonstrating increased urinary excretion of the serotonin metabolite 5-hydroxyindoleacetic acid (5-HIAA). To avoid false-positive results, measurement is performed after the patient has abstained from serotonin-containing foods (eg, bananas, tomatoes, plums, avocados, pineapples, eggplant, walnuts) for 3 days. Certain drugs, including guaifenesin, methocarbamol, and phenothiazines, also interfere with the test and should be stopped temporarily before testing. On the 3rd day, a 24-h urine sample is collected for assay. Normal excretion of 5-HIAA is < 10 mg/day (< 52 μmol/day); in patients with carcinoid syndrome, excretion is usually > 50 mg/day (> 260 μmol/day).

Provocative tests with Ca gluconate, catecholamines, pentagastrin, or alcohol have been used to induce flushing. These tests may be helpful when the diagnosis is in doubt, but they must be performed with care. Localization of the tumor involves the same techniques used to localize a nonfunctioning carcinoid (see p. 1313) but may require extensive evaluation, sometimes including laparotomy. A scan with radionuclide-labeled somatostatin receptor ligand ^{111}In-pentetreotide or with ^{123}I-metaiodobenzylguanidine may demonstrate metastases.

Other conditions that present with flushing and that could, therefore, be confused with carcinoid syndrome should be excluded. In patients in whom 5-HIAA excretion is not increased, disorders that involve systemic activation of mastocytes (eg, systemic mastocytosis with increased urinary levels of histamine metabolites and increased serum tryptase level) and idiopathic anaphylaxis may be responsible. Additional causes of flushing include menopause, ethanol ingestion, drugs such as niacin, and certain tumors (eg, vipomas, renal cell carcinoma, medullary thyroid carcinoma).

Prognosis and Treatment

Despite metastatic disease, these tumors are slow growing, and survival of 10 to 15 yr is not unusual.

Resection of primary lung carcinoids is often curative. For patients with hepatic metastases, surgery is only diagnostic or palliative, and radiation therapy is unsuccessful, in part because of the poor tolerance of normal hepatic tissue to radiation. No effective chemotherapeutic regimen has been established, but streptozocin with 5-fluorouracil is most widely used, sometimes with doxorubicin.

Certain symptoms, including flushing, have been relieved by somatostatin (which inhibits release of most hormones) without lowering urinary 5-HIAA or gastrin. Numerous studies have suggested good results with octreotide, a long-acting analog of somatostatin. Octreotide is the drug of choice for controlling diarrhea and flushing. Case reports indicate that tamoxifen has been effective infrequently; leukocyte interferon (IFN-α) has temporarily relieved symptoms.

Flushing also can be treated with phenothiazines (eg, prochlorperazine 5 to 10 mg or chlorpromazine 25 to 50 mg po q 6 h). Histamine$_2$ blockers may also be used. Phentolamine (an α-blocker) 5 to 15 mg IV has prevented experimentally induced flushes. Corticosteroids (eg, prednisone 5 mg po q 6 h) may be useful for severe flushing caused by bronchial carcinoids.

Diarrhea may be controlled by codeine phosphate 15 mg po q 4 to 6 h, tincture of opium 0.6 mL po q 6 h, loperamide 4 mg po as a loading dose and 2 mg after each loose bowel to a maximum of 16 mg/day, diphenoxylate 5 mg po qid, or peripheral serotonin antagonists such as cyproheptadine 4 to 8 mg po q 6 h or methysergide 1 to 2 mg po qid.

Niacin and adequate protein intake are needed to prevent pellagra, because dietary tryptophan is diverted to serotonin by the tumor. Enzyme inhibitors that prevent the conversion of 5-hydroxytryptophan to serotonin include methyldopa 250 to 500 mg po q 6 h and phenoxybenzamine 10 mg/day.

162 MULTIPLE ENDOCRINE NEOPLASIA SYNDROMES

(Familial Endocrine Adenomatosis; Multiple Endocrine Adenomatosis)

The multiple endocrine neoplasia (MEN) syndromes comprise 3 genetically distinct familial diseases involving adenomatous hyperplasia and malignant tumors in several endocrine glands. Clinical features depend on the glandular elements present.

Each syndrome is inherited as an autosomal dominant trait with a high degree of penetrance, variable expressivity, and production of seemingly unrelated effects by a single mutant gene. The specific genetic abnormalities are not always known.

Symptoms and signs develop at any age. Proper management includes early identification of affected individuals within a kindred and surgical removal of the tumors when possible. Although these syndromes are gen-

TABLE 162–1. CONDITIONS ASSOCIATED WITH MEN SYNDROMES

CONDITION	MEN-I	MEN-IIA	MEN-IIB
Parathyroid adenomas	≥ 90%	25%	Rare
Pancreatic islet cell tumors	30–75%	—	—
Pituitary adenomas	50–65%	—	—
Medullary carcinoma of the thyroid	—	> 90%	> 90%
Pheochromocytomas	—	50%	60%
Mucosal neuromas	—	—	≅100%
Marfanoid habitus	—	—	≅100%

MEN = Multiple endocrine neoplasia.

erally considered clinically distinct, significant overlap exists (see TABLE 162–1).

MULTIPLE ENDOCRINE NEOPLASIA, TYPE I

(Multiple Endocrine Adenomatosis, Type I; Wermer's Syndrome)

Multiple endocrine neoplasia, type I (MEN-I) is a hereditary syndrome characterized by tumors of the parathyroid glands, pancreatic islet cells, and pituitary gland. Clinical features most commonly include hyperparathyroidism and asymptomatic hypercalcemia. Genetic screening is used to detect carriers. Diagnosis is by hormonal and imaging tests. Tumors are surgically removed when possible.

MEN-I is probably caused by an inactivating mutation of the tumor suppressor gene that encodes the transcription factor menin; many mutations of this gene may be responsible.

About 40% of MEN-I cases involve tumors of all 3 affected glands—the parathyroids, pancreas, and pituitary. Almost any combination of the tumors and symptom complexes outlined below is possible. A patient with a MEN-I gene mutation and one of the MEN-I tumors is at risk of developing any of the other tumors later on. Age at onset ranges from 4 to 81 yr, but peak incidence occurs in the 20s in women and 30s in men. Women are affected twice as often as men.

Symptoms and Signs

The clinical features depend on the glandular elements present (see TABLE 162–1).

Parathyroid: Hyperparathyroidism is present in ≥ 90% of patients. Asymptomatic hypercalcemia is the most common manifestation: about 25% of patients have evidence of nephrolithiasis or nephrocalcinosis. In contrast to sporadic cases of hyperparathyroidism, diffuse hyperplasia or multiple adenomas are more common than solitary adenomas.

Pancreas: Pancreatic islet cell tumors occur in 30 to 75% of patients. Tumors are usually multicentric, and multiple adenomas or diffuse islet cell hyperplasia commonly occurs. About 30% of tumors are malignant and have local or distant metastases. Malignant islet cell tumors due to MEN-I syndrome often have a more benign course than do sporadically occurring malignant islet cell tumors.

About 40% of islet cell tumors originate from a β cell, secrete insulin (insulinoma), and can cause fasting hypoglycemia. β-Cell tumors are more common in patients < 40. About 60% of islet cell tumors originate from non-β-cell elements and tend to occur in patients > 40. Non-β-cell tumors are somewhat more likely to be malignant.

Most islet cell tumors secrete pancreatic polypeptide, the clinical significance of which is unknown. Gastrin is secreted by many non-β-cell tumors (increased gastrin secretion in MEN-I also often originates from the duodenum). Increased gastrin secretion increases gastric acid, which may inactivate pancreatic lipase, leading to diarrhea and steatorrhea. Increased gastrin secretion also leads to peptic ulcers in > 50% of MEN-I patients. Usually the ulcers are multiple or atypical in location, and often bleed, perforate, or become obstructed. Peptic ulcer disease may be intractable and complicated (Zollinger-Ellison syndrome—see p. 181). Among patients presenting with Zollinger-Ellison syndrome, 20 to 60% have MEN-I.

A severe secretory diarrhea can develop and cause fluid and electrolyte depletion with non-β-cell tumors. This complex, referred to as the watery diarrhea, hypokalemia, and achlorhydria syndrome (WDHA; pancreatic cholera—see p.182), has been ascribed to vasoactive intestinal polypeptide, although other intestinal hormones or secretagogues (including prostaglandins) may contribute. Hypersecretion of glucagon, somatostatin, chromogranin, and calcitonin; ectopic secretion of ACTH (causing Cushing's syndrome); and hypersecretion of growth hormone–releasing hormone (causing acromegaly) sometimes occur in non-β-cell tumors.

Pituitary: Pituitary tumors occur in 50 to 65% of MEN-I patients. From 25 to 90% are prolactinomas. About 25% of pituitary tumors secrete growth hormone or growth hormone and prolactin. Affected patients have acromegaly clinically indistinguishable from sporadically occurring acromegaly. About 3% of tumors secrete ACTH, producing Cushing's disease. Most of the remainder are nonfunctional. Local tumor expansion may cause visual disturbance, headache, and hypopituitarism.

Other manifestations: Adenomas and adenomatous hyperplasia of the thyroid and adrenal glands occurs occasionally in MEN-I patients. Hormone secretion is rarely altered as a result, and the significance of these abnormalities is uncertain. Carcinoid tumors, particularly those derived from the embryologic foregut, occur in isolated cases. Multiple subcutaneous and visceral lipomas may also occur.

Diagnosis

Patients with tumors of the parathyroids, pancreas, or pituitary, particularly those with a family history of endocrinopathy, should undergo clinical screening for other tumors of MEN-I. Such screening includes querying for symptoms of peptic ulcer disease, diarrhea, nephrolithiasis, hypoglycemia, and hypopituitarism; examination for visual field defects, galactorrhea in women, and features of acromegaly and subcutaneous lipomas; and measurement of serum Ca, intact parathyroid hormone, gastrin, and prolactin.

Additional laboratory or radiologic tests should be performed if these screening tests suggest a MEN-I–related endocrine abnormality. An insulin-secreting β-cell tumor of the pancreas is diagnosed by fasting hypoglycemia with an elevated plasma insulin level.

A gastrin-secreting non-β-cell tumor of the pancreas or duodenum is diagnosed by elevated basal plasma gastrin levels, an exaggerated gastrin response to infused Ca, and a paradoxical rise in gastrin level after infusion of secretin. An elevated basal level of pancreatic polypeptide or gastrin or an exaggerated response of these hormones to a standard meal may be the earliest sign of pancreatic involvement. CT or MRI can help localize tumors. Because these tumors are often small and difficult to localize, other imaging tests (eg, somatostatin receptor scintigraphy, endoscopic ultrasound, intraoperative ultrasound) may be necessary.

Acromegaly is diagnosed by elevated growth hormone levels that are not suppressed by glucose administration and by elevated levels of plasma insulin-like growth factor 1.

In patients with 2 or more MEN-I–related endocrine abnormalities who are not from a known MEN-I kindred (index case), direct DNA sequencing of the MEN-I gene identifies a specific mutation in 80 to 90%. If an index case is identified, 1st-degree relatives should undergo genetic testing or clinical screening. Annual clinical screening is necessary for 1st-degree relatives whose genetic screening is positive and who have minimal symptoms, who have not undergone genetic testing, or for whom testing of the index case did not identify a specific mutation.

Treatment

Treatment of parathyroid and pituitary lesions is primarily surgical. Islet cell tumors are more difficult to manage because the lesions are often small and difficult to find and multiple lesions are common. If a single tumor cannot be found, total pancreatectomy may be required for adequate control of hyperinsulinism. Diazoxide may be a useful adjunct in treating hypoglycemia; streptozocin and other cytotoxic drugs may ameliorate symptoms by reducing tumor burden.

The treatment of gastrin-secreting non-β-cell tumors is complex. Localization and removal of the tumor should be attempted. If localization is impossible, a proton pump inhibitor frequently produces symptomatic relief from peptic ulcer disease. With the availability of these drugs, gastrectomy is rarely required.

Octreotide, a somatostatin analog, can block hormone secretion from nongastrin-secreting pancreatic tumors and is well tolerated, particularly if given as a long-acting preparation administered q 4 wk. Palliative treatments for metastatic pancreatic tumors include hepatic artery embolization and interferon-α (in combination with octreotide).

MULTIPLE ENDOCRINE NEOPLASIA, TYPE IIA

(MEN-II; Multiple Endocrine Adenomatosis, Type II; Sipple's Syndrome)

Multiple endocrine neoplasia, type IIA (MEN-IIA) is a hereditary syndrome characterized by medullary carcinoma of the thyroid, pheochromocytoma, and hyperparathyroidism. Clinical features depend on the glandular elements present. Diagnosis involves genetic testing. Hormonal and imaging tests help locate the tumors, which are removed surgically when possible.

Mutations in a specific tyrosine kinase gene, *ret*, suggest that this dominant oncogene is responsible for MEN-IIA.

Symptoms and Signs

Clinical features depend on the type of tumor present (see TABLE 162–1).

Thyroid: Almost all patients have medullary carcinoma of the thyroid (see p. 1205). The tumor usually develops during childhood and begins with thyroid hyperplasia. Tumors are frequently multicentric.

Adrenal: Pheochromocytoma usually originates in the adrenal glands. Pheochromocytoma occurs in about 50% of patients within a MEN-IIA kindred, and in some kindreds pheochromocytoma accounts for 30% of deaths. In contrast to sporadic pheochromocytoma (see p. 1216), the familial variety within MEN-IIA begins with adrenal medullary hyperplasia and is multicentric and bilateral in > 50% of cases; extra-adrenal pheochromocytomas are rare. Pheochromocytomas are almost always benign, but some tend to recur locally.

Pheochromocytomas that occur with MEN usually produce epinephrine disproportionately to norepinephrine, in contrast to sporadic cases.

Hypertensive crisis secondary to pheochromocytoma is a common presentation. Hypertension in MEN-IIA patients with pheochromocytoma is more often paroxysmal than sustained, in contrast to the usual sporadic case. Patients with pheochromocytomas may have paroxysmal palpitations, anxiety, headaches, or sweating; many are asymptomatic.

Parathyroid: About 25% of patients have evidence of hyperparathyroidism (which may be long-standing), with hypercalcemia, nephrolithiasis, nephrocalcinosis, or renal failure. In another 25% with no clinical or biochemical evidence of hyperparathyroidism, parathyroid hyperplasia is noted incidentally during surgery for medullary carcinoma of the thyroid. Hyperparathyroidism frequently involves multiple glands as either diffuse hyperplasia or multiple adenomas.

Other manifestations: Increased incidence of Hirschsprung's disease has been reported in children in at least one MEN-IIA kindred. Zollinger-Ellison syndrome occurs rarely in MEN-IIA.

Diagnosis

MEN-IIA is suspected in patients with bilateral pheochromocytoma, a familial history of MEN, or at least 2 of its characteristic endocrine manifestations. The diagnosis is confirmed with genetic testing. Many of the reported kindreds come to medical attention after bilateral pheochromocytomas are diagnosed in the index case.

Medullary carcinoma of the thyroid is diagnosed by measuring plasma calcitonin after provocative infusion of pentagastrin and Ca. In most patients with palpable thyroid lesions, basal calcitonin levels are elevated; in early disease, the basal levels may be normal, and the medullary carcinoma can be diagnosed only by an exaggerated response to Ca and pentagastrin. Early diagnosis of medullary carcinoma of the thyroid is important so that the tumor can be removed while still localized.

Because pheochromocytoma may be asymptomatic, its exclusion may be difficult (see p. 1217). The most sensitive tests are plasma free metanephrines and fractionated urinary catecholamines (particularly epinephrine). CT or MRI is useful in localizing the pheochromocytoma or establishing the presence of bilateral lesions.

Hyperparathyroidism is diagnosed by hypercalcemia, hypophosphatemia, and increased parathyroid hormone level.

Genetic testing, used to confirm the diagnosis, is highly accurate. First-degree relatives and any symptomatic relatives of the index patient should also undergo genetic testing.

Annual screening for hyperparathyroidism and pheochromocytoma should begin in early childhood and continue indefinitely. Screening for hyperparathyroidism is with measurement of serum Ca. Screening for pheochromocytoma includes questions about symptoms, measurement of BP, and laboratory testing.

Treatment

In a patient presenting with pheochromocytoma and either medullary carcinoma of the thyroid or hyperparathyroidism, the pheochromocytoma should be removed first; even if asymptomatic, it greatly increases risk of other surgeries. Chemotherapy is ineffective in treating residual or metastatic medullary carcinoma of the thyroid, but radiation therapy may lengthen survival.

In gene carriers, prophylactic thyroidectomy is recommended in infancy or early childhood, because untreated medullary carcinoma of the thyroid is fatal.

MULTIPLE ENDOCRINE NEOPLASIA, TYPE IIB

(MEN-III; Mucosal Neuroma Syndrome; Multiple Endocrine Adenomatosis, Type IIB)

Multiple endocrine neoplasia, type IIB (MEN-IIB) is a syndrome characterized by multiple mucosal neuromas, medullary carcinoma of the thyroid, and pheochromocytoma, and often a marfanoid habitus. The syndrome is sometimes hereditary. Symptoms depend on the glandular elements present. Diagnosis and treatment are the same as for MEN-IIA.

About 50% of cases have been sporadic rather than familial, although the true incidence of sporadic MEN-IIB syndrome is unknown. Men are affected twice as often as women. Hyperparathyroidism occurs rarely in MEN-IIB. Genetic studies have identified mutations in the *ret* oncogene.

Symptoms and Signs

Symptoms and signs reflect the glandular abnormalities (see TABLE 162–1). About 50% of patients have the complete syndrome with mucosal neuromas, pheochromocytomas, and medullary carcinoma of the thyroid. Fewer than 10% have neuromas and pheochromocytomas alone, whereas the remaining patients have neuromas and medullary carcinoma of the thyroid without pheochromocytoma.

Often, mucosal neuromas are the earliest sign, and they occur in most or all patients. Neuromas appear as small glistening bumps on the lips, tongue, and buccal mucosa. The eyelids, conjunctivae, and corneas also commonly develop neuromas. Thickened eyelids and diffusely hypertrophied lips are characteristic. GI abnormalities related to altered motility (constipation, diarrhea, and, occasionally, megacolon) are common and thought to result from diffuse intestinal ganglioneuromatosis. Patients may have a marfanoid habitus; skeletal abnormalities of the spine (lordosis, kyphosis, scoliosis), pes cavus, and talipes equinovarus are common.

Medullary carcinoma of the thyroid and pheochromocytoma resemble the corresponding disorders in MEN-IIA syndrome; both tend to be bilateral and multicentric. Medullary carcinoma of the thyroid, however, tends to be particularly aggressive in MEN-IIB and may be present in very young children.

Although the neuromas, facial characteristics, and GI disorders are present at an early age, the syndrome may not be recognized until medullary carcinoma of the thyroid or pheochromocytoma presents in later life.

Diagnosis and Treatment

MEN-IIB is suspected in patients with a family history of MEN-IIB, pheochromocytoma, multiple mucosal neuromas, or medullary carcinoma of the thyroid. Genetic testing is highly accurate and is done in 1st-degree relatives and any symptomatic relatives of MEN-IIB patients.

Pheochromocytoma may be suspected clinically and is confirmed by measuring plasma-free metanephrines or urinary catecholamines (see p. 1217). Laboratory testing for medullary carcinoma of the thyroid may be done (see p. 1206). MRI or CT is used to search for pheochromocytomas and medullary carcinoma of the thyroid.

Affected patients should have total thyroidectomy as soon as the diagnosis is established. Pheochromocytoma, if present, should be removed before thyroidectomy is performed. Gene carriers should undergo prophylactic thyroidectomy in infancy or early childhood.

SECTION 13
IMMUNOLOGY; ALLERGIC DISORDERS

163 BIOLOGY OF THE IMMUNE SYSTEM

The immune system distinguishes self from nonself and eliminates potentially harmful nonself molecules and cells from the body. The immune system also has the capacity to recognize and destroy abnormal cells that derive from host tissues (see p. 1153). Any molecule capable of being recognized by the immune system is considered an antigen (Ag).

Anatomic barriers, part of the body's external defenses, must be overcome before the immune system is activated to destroy foreign antigens. These barriers include the outer, keratinized epidermis; mucus of the respiratory, GI, and urogenital tracts; and cilia on respiratory epithelial cells, which help expel particles and organisms trapped by mucus. Each has specialized immune functions. For example, in the skin, keratinocytes secrete antimicrobial peptides (defensins), and sebaceous and sweat glands secrete microbe-inhibiting substances (eg, lactic acid, fatty acids). Also, many immune cells (eg, mast cells, intraepithelial lymphocytes, Ag-sampling Langerhans' cells) reside in the skin. Mucus in respiratory, GI, and GU tracts contains antimicrobial substances, such as lysozyme, lactoferrin, and secretory IgA antibody (SIgA). Breaching of anatomic barriers can trigger 2 types of immune response: innate and acquired.

Innate (natural or nonspecific) immunity does not require prior exposure to an Ag (ie, memory) to be effective. Components include phagocytic cells (neutrophils and monocytes in the blood, macrophages and dendritic cells in tissues) that ingest and destroy invading Ags; Ag-presenting cells (macrophages, dendritic cells) that present fragments of ingested Ags to T cells, which are part of acquired immunity; natural killer cells that kill virus-infected cells and some tumor cells; and certain polymorphonuclear leukocytes (eosinophils, basophils, mast cells) that release inflammatory mediators.

Acquired (adaptive or specific) immunity remembers past exposures and is Ag-specific. Components include antibody (Ab) and T and B cells (lymphocytes). Acquired immunity derived from certain T-cell responses is called cellular immunity; immunity derived from B-cell responses is called humoral immunity because B cells secrete soluble Ag-specific Ab.

Innate and acquired immune responses interact; eg, IgE (acquired immunity) binds to mast cells or basophils (innate immunity) to produce an allergic response. Many molecular components participate in innate and acquired immunity; they include complement, cytokines, and acute phase reactants.

Successful immune defense requires activation, regulation, and resolution of the immune response.

Activation: The immune system is activated when a foreign Ag is recognized by circulating Abs or cell surface receptors. These receptors may be highly specific (eg, Ig expressed on B cells or bound to phagocytes) or broadly specific (eg, pattern-recognition receptors on dendritic cells, including mannose, scavenger, and Toll-like receptors, which recognize common microbial pathogen-associated molecular patterns in ligands such as gram-negative lipopolysaccharide, unmethylated cytosine-guanosine dinucleotides [CpG motifs], and peptidoglycans). Ab-Ag and complement-microorganism complexes can also bind to surface receptors for the crystallizable fragment (Fc) region of IgG (FcγR) and for C3b and iC3b.

Once recognized, an Ag, Ag-Ab complex, or complement-microorganism complex is phagocytosed. Some microorganisms are killed after they are phagocytosed; others (eg, mycobacteria) inhibit the phagocyte's ability to kill them once they are engulfed. In such cases, T cell–derived cytokines, particularly interferon-γ(IFN-γ), stimulate the phagocyte to produce lytic enzymes and other microbicidal macrophage products, which kill the microorganism.

Unless Ag is rapidly phagocytosed and entirely degraded (an uncommon event), the acquired immune response is recruited. This response begins in the spleen for circulating Ag, in regional lymph nodes for tissue Ag, and in mucosa-associated lymphoid tissues (eg, tonsils, adenoids, Peyer's patches) for mucosal Ag. For example, Langerhans' dendritic cells in the skin phagocytose Ag and migrate to local lymph nodes; there, peptides derived from the Ag are expressed on the cell surface within class II major histocompatibility complex (MHC) molecules, which present the peptide to CD4 helper T (T_H) cells. When the T_H cell engages the complex, the cell expresses receptors for the cytokine IL-2 and secretes several cytokines. A subset of T_H cells (T_H1) secretes IFN-γ, IL-2, and lymphotoxin, which facilitate macrophage and cytotoxic T-cell responses; another subset, T_H2 cells, secretes IL-4, IL-5, IL-6, IL-10, and IL-13, which stimulate antibody production by B-cells.

In contrast to class II MHC molecules, which present extracellular Ag to CD4 T_H cells, class I MHC molecules present intracellular Ag (eg, viruses) to CD8 cytotoxic T cells. The activated cytotoxic T cell then kills the infected cell.

Regulation: The immune response must be regulated to prevent overwhelming damage to the host (eg, anaphylaxis, widespread tissue destruction). Regulatory T cells help control the immune response via secretion of immunosuppressive cytokines, such as IL-10 and transforming growth factor-β (TGF-β), or via a poorly defined cell contact mechanism. These regulatory cells help prevent autoimmune responses and probably help resolve ongoing responses to nonself Ag.

Resolution: The immune response resolves when Ag is sequestered and eliminated from the body. Without stimulation by Ag, cytokine secretion ceases, and activated cytotoxic T cells undergo apoptosis. Apoptosis tags a cell for immediate phagocytosis, which prevents spillage of the cellular contents and development of subsequent inflammation. T and B cells that have differentiated into memory cells are spared this fate.

COMPONENTS OF THE IMMUNE SYSTEM

The immune system consists of cellular and molecular components that work together to destroy antigens (Ags).

Antigen-Presenting Cells

Although some Ags can stimulate the immune response directly, T cell–dependent acquired immune responses typically require antigen-presenting cells (APCs) to present Ag-derived peptides within major histocompatibility complex (MHC) molecules. Intracellular Ag (eg, viruses) can be processed and presented to CD8 cytotoxic T cells by any nucleated cell because all nucleated cells express class I MHC molecules. However, extracellular Ag must be processed into peptides and complexed with surface class II MHC molecules on APCs to be recognized by CD4 helper T (T_H) cells. B cells, monocytes, macrophages, and dendritic cells constitutively express class II MHC molecules and therefore act as APCs for CD4 T-cell responses.

Monocytes in the circulation are precursors to tissue macrophages. Monocytes migrate into tissues, where over about 8 h, they develop into macrophages under the influence of macrophage colony-stimulating factor (M-CSF), secreted by various cell types (eg, endothelial cells, fibroblasts). At infection sites, activated T cells secrete cytokines (eg, interferon-γ[IFN-γ]) that induce production of macrophage migration inhibitory factor, preventing macrophages from leaving.

IFN-γ and granulocyte-macrophage colony-stimulating factor (GM-CSF) act as macrophage-activating factors. Activated macrophages kill intracellular organisms and secrete IL-1 and tumor necrosis factor-α (TNF-α). These cytokines potentiate the secretion of IFN-γ and GM-CSF and increase the expression of adhesion molecules on endothelial cells, facilitating leukocyte influx and destruction of pathogens.

Dendritic cells are present in the skin (as Langerhans' cells), lymph nodes, and tissues throughout the body. Dendritic cells in the skin act as sentinel APCs, taking up Ag, then travel to local lymph nodes where they can activate T cells. Follicular dendritic cells are a distinct lineage, do not express class II MHC molecules, and therefore do not present Ag to T_H cells. However, they have receptors for IgG Fc and for complement, which enable them to bind with immune complexes and present the complex to B cells in germinal centers of secondary lymphoid organs.

Polymorphonuclear Leukocytes

Polymorphonuclear (PMN) leukocytes, also called granulocytes because their cytoplasm contains granules, include neutrophils, eosinophils, basophils, and mast cells. All occur in the circulation and have multilobed nuclei except for mast cells, which are tissue-based and functionally similar to circulating blood basophils.

Neutrophils constitute 40 to 70% of total WBCs; they are a 1st line of defense against infection. Mature neutrophils have a half-life of about 2 to 3 days. During acute inflammatory responses (eg, to infection), neutrophils, drawn by chemotactic factors, leave the circulation and enter tissues. Their purpose is to phagocytose and digest pathogens. Microorganisms are killed when phagocytosis generates lytic enzymes and reactive O_2 compounds (eg, superoxide, hypochlorous acid) or triggers release of granule contents (eg, defensins, proteases, bactericidal permeability-increasing protein, lactoferrin, and lysozymes). DNA and histones are also released, and they, with granule contents such as elastase, generate fibers in the surrounding tissues that may facilitate killing by trapping bacteria and focusing enzyme activity.

Eosinophils constitute up to 5% of WBCs. They target organisms too large to be engulfed; they kill by secreting toxic substances (eg, reactive O_2 compounds similar to those produced in neutrophils), major basic protein (which is toxic to parasites), eosinophil cationic protein, and several enzymes. Eosinophils are also a major source of inflammatory mediators (eg, prostaglandins, leukotrienes, platelet-activating factor, many cytokines).

Basophils constitute < 5% of WBCs and share several characteristics with mast cells, although the 2 cell types are distinct lineages. Both have high-affinity receptors for IgE called FcεRI. When these cells encounter certain Ags, the bivalent IgE molecules bound to the receptors become cross-linked, triggering cell degranulation with release of preformed inflammatory mediators (eg, histamine, platelet-activating factor) and generation of newly synthesized mediators (eg, leukotrienes, prostaglandins, thromboxanes). Mucosal mast cell granules contain tryptase and chondroitin sulfate; connective tissue mast cell granules contain tryptase, chymase, and heparin. By releasing these mediators, mast cells play a key role in generating protective acute inflammatory responses; basophils and mast cells are the source of type I hypersensitivity reactions associated with atopic allergy (see p. 1353). Degranulation can also be triggered by the anaphylatoxin complement fragments C3a and C5a.

Lymphocytes

Lymphocytes include B cells, which mature in bone marrow, and T cells, which mature in the thymus. The 2 cell types are morphologically indistinguishable but have different immune functions. They can be distinguished by Ag-specific surface receptors and molecules called clusters of differentiation (CDs), whose presence and absence define some subsets. More than 300 CDs have been identified (for further information on CD Ags, see the CD index at http://mpr.nci.nih.gov/prow). Each lymphocyte recognizes a specific Ag via surface receptors.

B cells: About 5 to 15% of lymphocytes in the blood are B cells; they are also present in the spleen, lymph nodes, and tonsils. Their primary function is to manufacture and secrete antibodies (Abs—see p. 1324). They are identifiable by membrane expression of Ig (mIg) and by B cell–specific CD surface molecules; they also express class II MHC molecules and various other non-B cell–specific CD molecules. mIg isotype varies depending on the B cell's stage of development (mIgM on immature B cells; mIgM and mIgD on mature naive B cells; and mIgG, mIgA, or mIgE on B cells that have switched Ig isotype after encounter with Ag and with T_H cells). mIg can bind Ag, but subsequent B-cell activation depends on signaling through 2 invariable molecules (Igα and Igβ).

After random rearrangement of the genes that encode Ig, B cells have the potential to recognize an almost limitless number of unique Ags. Gene rearrangement occurs in programmed steps in the bone marrow during B-cell development. The process starts with a committed stem cell, continues through pro-B and pre-B cell stages, and results in an immature B cell. If this immature B cell interacts with Ag, it may become inactivated (tolerant) or be eliminated (by apoptosis). Immature B cells that are not inactivated or eliminated may continue to develop into mature naive B cells, leave the marrow, and enter peripheral lymphoid organs. When mature naive B cells first encounter Ag, these cells become lymphoblasts, undergo clonal proliferation, and differentiate into memory cells, which can respond to the same Ag in the future, or into mature Ab-secreting plasma cells. This response, called the primary immune response, is characterized by a latent period of days before Ab is produced. Initially, only IgM is produced. With the help of T cells, B cells can further rearrange their Ig genes and switch to production of IgG, IgA, or IgE. Thus, on first exposure, the response is slow and provides limited protective immunity.

The secondary (anamnestic or booster) immune response occurs when memory B and T_H cells are reexposed to the Ag. The memory B-cells rapidly proliferate, differentiate into mature plasma cells, and promptly produce and release large amounts of Ab (chiefly IgG because of a T cell–induced isotype switch) into the blood and other tissues where Ab can react with Ag. Thus, after reexposure, the immune response is faster and more effective.

T cells: T cells develop from bone marrow stem cells that travel to the thymus, where they go through rigorous selection. In selection, T-cells that can recognize nonself Ag complexed to self MHC molecules survive; they leave the thymus for peripheral blood and lymphoid tissues. T cells that react to self Ag presented by self MHC molecules or to self MHC molecules without Ag are eliminated by apoptosis.

Most mature T cells express either CD4 or CD8 and have Ag-binding, Ig-like surface receptors called T-cell receptors (TCRs) that are associated with invariable CD3 and ζ chains in a unit called the TCR-CD3 complex. CD3 chains (CD3γ, CD3δ, 2 CD3εs) and 2 ζ chains, analogous to Igα and Igβ molecules on the surface of B cells, transduce the activation signal through the cell membrane. Genes that encode the TCR, like Ig genes, are rearranged, resulting in defined specificity and affinity for the Ag peptide displayed in the MHC molecule of an APC. The number of T-cell specificities is almost limitless.

Most T-cells express a TCR consisting of an α chain and a β chain; αβ T cells recognize linear peptide Ag presented by MHC molecules. However, some T cells express a TCR consisting of a γ chain and a δ chain; γδ T cells recognize lipid or glycolipid Ag presented by the MHC-like molecule CD1, or sometimes they recognize Ag directly. The CD4 subset of αβ T cells recognizes only Ag peptide within class II MHC molecules, and the CD8 subset recognizes only Ag peptide within class I MHC molecules. For T cells to be activated, the TCR must engage with Ag-MHC and accessory molecules (eg, CD28 with CD80 or CD86 must interact); otherwise, the T cell becomes anergic or dies by apoptosis. Some accessory molecules inhibit previously activated T cells and thus dampen the immune response.

The 3 main types of T cells are helper, regulatory, and cytotoxic T cells.

Helper T (T_H) cells are usually CD4 but may be CD8. They differentiate from T_H0 cells, which can secrete several cytokines (eg, IFN-γ, IL-2, IL-3, IL-4, IL-5, GM-CSF), into T_H1 cells (under the influence of IFN-γ and IL-12) or into T_H2 cells (under the influence of IL-4 and IL-10). In general, T_H1 cells promote cell-mediated immunity via cytotoxic T cells and macrophages and secrete IFN-γ, IL-2, and lymphotoxin (TNF-β). T_H2 cells promote Ab production by B cells (humoral immunity) and secrete IL-4, IL-5, IL-6, IL-10, and IL-13. Both cell types secrete several other cytokines. Different patterns of cytokine production identify other T_H-cell functional phenotypes.

The distinction between T_H1 and T_H2 cells is clinically relevant. For example, a T_H1 response dominates in tuberculoid leprosy, and a T_H2 response dominates in lepromatous leprosy. A T_H1 response is characteristic of certain autoimmune disorders (eg, RA, multiple sclerosis), and a T_H2 response promotes IgE production and development of allergic disorders.

Regulatory T cells mediate suppression of immune responses. The process involves functional subsets of CD4 T cells, including Foxp3 CD25 T cells, which either secrete cytokines with immunosuppressive properties (eg, transforming growth factor-β [TGF-β], IL-10) or suppress the immune response by poorly defined mechanisms that require cell-to-cell contact. Some regulatory T cells express the CD8 T-cell phenotype.

Cytotoxic T (T_C) cells are usually CD8 but may be CD4; they are vital for eliminating intracellular pathogens, especially viruses. T_C cells play a role in organ transplant rejection.

T_C-cell development involves 3 phases: a precursor cell that can differentiate into a T_C cell when appropriately stimulated; an effector cell that has differentiated and can kill its appropriate target; and a memory cell that is quiescent (no longer stimulated) but is ready to become an effector when restimulated by the original Ag-MHC combination. Fully activated T_C cells can kill an infected target cell by inducing apoptosis.

T_C cells may be syngeneic—generated in response to self (autologous) cells modified by viral infection or other foreign proteins. Or, they may be allogeneic—generated in response to cells that express foreign MHC products (eg, in organ transplantation when the donor's MHC molecules differ from the recipient's). Some T_C cells can directly recognize foreign MHC (direct pathway); others may recognize fragments of the foreign MHC presented by self MHC molecules of the transplant recipient (indirect pathway).

Natural killer (NK) cells: Conventional NK cells are lymphocytes that do not belong to T- or B-cell lineages and do not express surface Ig or the TCR/CD3 complex on their surfaces. Normally, they constitute 5 to 15% of peripheral blood lymphocytes. NK cells have killing mechanisms similar to those of T_C cells but lack immunologic memory. The surface markers that best characterize NK cells are $CD2^+$, $CD3^-$, $CD4^-$, $CD8^+$, $CD16^+$ (a receptor for IgG-Fc), and $CD56^+$. A distinct subset of cells called NK-T cells expresses the usual NK markers with the TCR/CD3 complex; activated NK-T cells secrete IL-4 and IFN-γ and may help regulate the immune response.

Typical NK cells are thought to be important for tumor surveillance because they kill certain autologous, allogeneic, and even xenogeneic tumor cells regardless of whether the tumor cells express MHC molecules. They preferentially target cells that express few or no class I MHC molecules and can kill cells infected with certain viruses that inhibit MHC expression.

Poorly defined but ubiquitously expressed ligands on target cells activate receptors on NK cells, triggering killing. The killing mechanism of NK cells may resemble that of T_C cells or be Ab-dependent. In Ab-dependent cell-mediated cytotoxicity, Abs recognize and bind a target cell; the Fc region of the Ab can then bind its receptor (CD16) on the NK cell, forming a bridge. Once the bridge is formed, a lytic signal is delivered to the target cell, resulting in its death.

NK cells can also secrete several cytokines (eg, IFN-γ, IL-1, TNF-α); they are a major source of IFN-γ. By secreting IFN-γ, NK cells can influence the acquired immune system by promoting differentiation of T_H1 cells and inhibiting that of T_H2 cells.

Lymphokine-activated killers: Some lymphocytes develop into potent lymphokine-activated killers (LAK) capable of killing a wide spectrum of tumor target cells and abnormal lymphocytes (eg, infected with certain viruses). These cells are a phenomenon rather than a unique lymphocyte subset. LAK precursors are heterogeneous but can be classified primarily as NK-like or T-like. Typical NK cells are the main precursors.

Antibodies

Abs, produced by B cells in response to Ags, consist of 4 polypeptide chains (2 identical heavy chains and 2 identical light chains) joined by disulfide bonds to produce a Y configuration (see FIG. 163–1). Abs are Y-shaped molecules whose heavy and light chains are divided into a variable (V) and a constant (C) region.

The V regions are located at the amino-terminal ends of the Y arms; they are called variable because they contain many different amino acids, which determine the specificity of the Ig. Hypervariable regions within the V regions contain idiotypic determinants, to which certain natural (anti-idiotype) Abs can bind; this binding may help regulate B-cell responses. A B cell can switch the Ig heavy chain isotype it produces, but it retains its heavy chain V region and the entire light-chain, thereby retaining antigenic specificity. The C region contains a relatively constant sequence of amino acids that is distinctive for each Ig isotype.

The amino-terminal (variable) end of the Ab binds to Ag to form an Ab-Ag complex. The Ag-binding (Fab) portion of Ig consists of a light chain and a fragment of a heavy chain and contains the V region of the Ig molecule (ie, the combining sites). The crystallizable fragment (Fc) contains most of the C region; Fc is responsible for complement activation and binds to Fc receptors on cells. Fragmentation with pepsin produces $F(ab')_2$, consisting of the 2 Fab fragments and a part of the heavy chains still linked by disulfide bonds.

Abs recognize specific configurations (epitopes, or antigenic determinants) on the surfaces of Ags (eg, proteins, polysaccharides, nucleic acids). Abs and Ags fit tightly together because the matching areas on the surface of each molecule are relatively large. The same Ab molecule can cross-react with related Ags if their epitopes are similar enough to those of the original Ag.

Five types of heavy chains define 5 Ig classes (μ for IgM, γ for IgG, α for IgA, ε for IgE, and δ for IgD); there are also 2 types of light chains (κ and λ). Each of the 5 Ig classes can bear either κ or λ light chains.

IgM is the first Ab formed after exposure to new Ag. It has 5 Y-shaped molecules (10 heavy chains and 10 light chains), linked by a single joining (J) chain. IgM circulates primarily in the intravascular space; it complexes with and agglutinates Ag and can activate complement, thereby facilitating phagocytosis. Isohemagglutinins and many Abs to gram-negative organisms are IgM. Monomeric IgM acts as a surface Ag receptor on B cells.

IgG is the most prevalent Ig isotype in serum; it is present in intravascular and extravascular spaces. IgG is the primary circulating Ig produced after re-immunization (secondary immune response) and is the predominant isotype contained in commercial γ-globulin products. IgG protects against bacteria, viruses, and toxins and is the only Ig isotype that crosses the placenta. There are 4 subclasses of IgG: IgG1, IgG2, IgG3, and IgG4, numbered in descending order of serum concentration. IgG subclasses differ functionally mainly in their ability to activate complement; IgG1 and IgG3 are most efficient, IgG2 is less efficient, and IgG4 is inefficient. IgG1 and IgG3 are efficient mediators of Ab-dependent cellular cytotoxicity; IgG4 and IgG2 are less so.

IgA occurs at mucosal surfaces, in serum, and in secretions (saliva; tears; respiratory, GU, and GI tract secretions; colostrum), where it provides an early antibacterial and antiviral defense. J chain links IgA into a dimer to form secretory IgA. Secretory IgA is synthesized by plasma cells in the subepithelial regions of the GI and respiratory tracts.

IgD is expressed primarily on the surface of naive B cells, where it influences B-cell maturation. When an immature B cell that initially expresses surface IgM begins to coexpress IgM and IgD, the B cell transitions from being at risk of elimination when it encounters Ag into being an Ag-responsive mature B cell. Serum IgD levels are very low, and the function of circulating IgD is unknown.

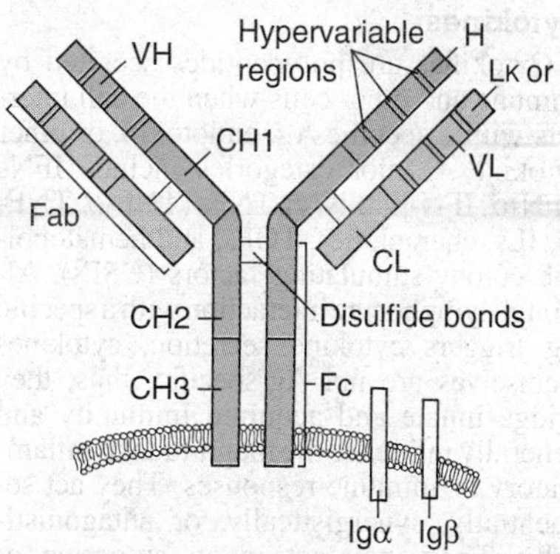

Fig. 163–1. B-cell receptor. The B-cell receptor consists of an Ig molecule anchored to the cell's surface. CH = heavy chain constant region; CL = light chain constant region; Fab = antigen-binding fragment; Fc = crystallizable fragment; VH = heavy chain variable region; VL = light chain variable region.

IgE is present in low levels in serum and respiratory and GI mucous secretions. IgE binds with high affinity to FcεRI receptors expressed at high levels on mast cells and basophils and at low levels on several other hematopoietic cells, including dendritic cells. If allergen bridges 2 IgE molecules bound to the mast cell or basophil surface, the cells degranulate, releasing chemical mediators that cause an allergic response. IgE levels are elevated in atopic disorders (eg, allergic or extrinsic asthma, hay fever, atopic dermatitis) and parasitic infections.

Acute Phase Reactants

Acute phase reactants are plasma proteins whose levels dramatically increase if infection or tissue damage occurs. Most dramatically increased are C-reactive protein and mannose-binding lectin (which fix complement and act as opsonins), the transport protein α_1-acid glycoprotein, and serum amyloid P component. Many acute phase reactants are made in the liver. Collectively, they may help limit tissue injury, enhance host resistance to infection, and promote tissue repair and resolution of inflammation.

Cytokines

Cytokines are polypeptides secreted by immune and other cells when the cell interacts with a specific Ag, endotoxin, or other cytokines. Major categories include IFNs (IFN-α, IFN-β, IFN-γ), TNFs (TNF-α, TNF-β), ILs, chemokines, TGFs, and hematopoietic colony-stimulating factors (CSFs). Although lymphocyte interaction with a specific Ag triggers cytokine secretion, cytokines themselves are not Ag-specific; thus, they bridge innate and acquired immunity and generally influence the magnitude of inflammatory or immune responses. They act sequentially, synergistically, or antagonistically. They may act in an autocrine or paracrine manner.

Cytokines deliver their signals via cell surface receptors. For example, the IL-2 receptor consists of 3 chains: α, β, and γ. The receptor's affinity for IL-2 is high if all 3 chains are expressed, intermediate if only the β and γ chains are expressed, or low if only the α chain is expressed. Mutations or deletion of the γ chain is the basis for X-linked severe combined immunodeficiency (see p. 1345).

Chemokines induce chemotaxis and migration of leukocytes. There are 4 subsets, defined by the number of intervening amino acids between the first 2 cysteine residues in the molecule. Chemokine receptors (CCR5 on memory T cells, monocytes/macrophages, and dendritic cells; CXCR4 on resting T cells) act as coreceptors for entry of HIV into cells.

HUMAN LEUKOCYTE ANTIGEN SYSTEM

The human leukocyte antigen (HLA) system, the major histocompatibility complex (MHC) in humans, is located on chromosome 6. It encodes cell surface molecules specialized to present antigenic peptides to the T-cell receptor (TCR) on T cells. MHC molecules which present antigen (Ag) are divided into 2 major classes.

Class I MHC molecules are present on the surface of all nucleated cells and platelets. These polypeptides consist of a heavy chain bound to a β_2-microglobulin molecule. The heavy chain consists of 2 peptide-binding domains, an Ig-like domain, and a transmembrane region with a cytoplasmic tail. The heavy chain of the class I molecule is encoded by genes at the HLA-A, -B, or -C loci. Lymphocytes reactive to class I molecules express CD8 molecules often associated with effector cytotoxic function.

Class II MHC molecules are present on Ag-presenting cells (B cells, macrophages, dendritic cells, Langerhans' cells), thymic epithelium, and activated (but not resting) T cells; most nucleated cells can be induced to express class II MHC molecules by interferon (IFN)-γ. Class II MHC molecules consist of 2 polypeptide (α and β) chains; each chain has a peptide-binding domain, an Ig-like domain, and a transmembrane region with a cytoplasmic tail. Both polypeptide chains are encoded by genes in the HLA-DP, -DQ, or -DR region of chromosome 6. Lymphocytes reactive to class II molecules express CD4 and are often helper T cells.

A group of important inflammatory molecules, called class III MHC molecules, include complement components (eg, C2, C4, factor B), tumor necrosis factor (TNF)-α, and heat shock proteins.

Individual alleles of each locus of the HLA system are given standard designations (eg, HLA-A1, -B5, -Cw1, -DR1). Alleles defined by DNA sequencing are named to identify the gene and to give each allele a unique number composed of the HLA locus, an asterisk, 2 numbers representing the serologic equivalent of the Ag, and 2 numbers representing the specific allele (eg, A*0201, DRB1*0103, DQA1*0102). Sometimes another number is added to identify a different subtype.

Some disorders are linked to specific HLA Ags (eg, psoriasis to HLA-Cw6, ankylosing spondylitis and reactive arthritis to HLA-B27, narcolepsy to HLA-DR2 and HLA-DQB1*0602, type I diabetes mellitus to HLA-DQ2 and HLA-DQ8, multiple sclerosis to HLA-DR2, RA to HLA-DRB1).

COMPLEMENT SYSTEM

The complement system is an enzyme cascade that helps defend against infection. This system bridges innate and acquired immunity by augmenting antibody (Ab) responses and immunologic memory, lysing foreign cells, and clearing immune complexes and apoptotic cells. Complement components have many biologic functions (eg, stimulation of chemotaxis, triggering of mast cell degranulation independent of IgE). Many complement proteins are enzymes that exist in serum as inactive precursors (zymogens); others reside on cell surfaces. There are 3 pathways of complement

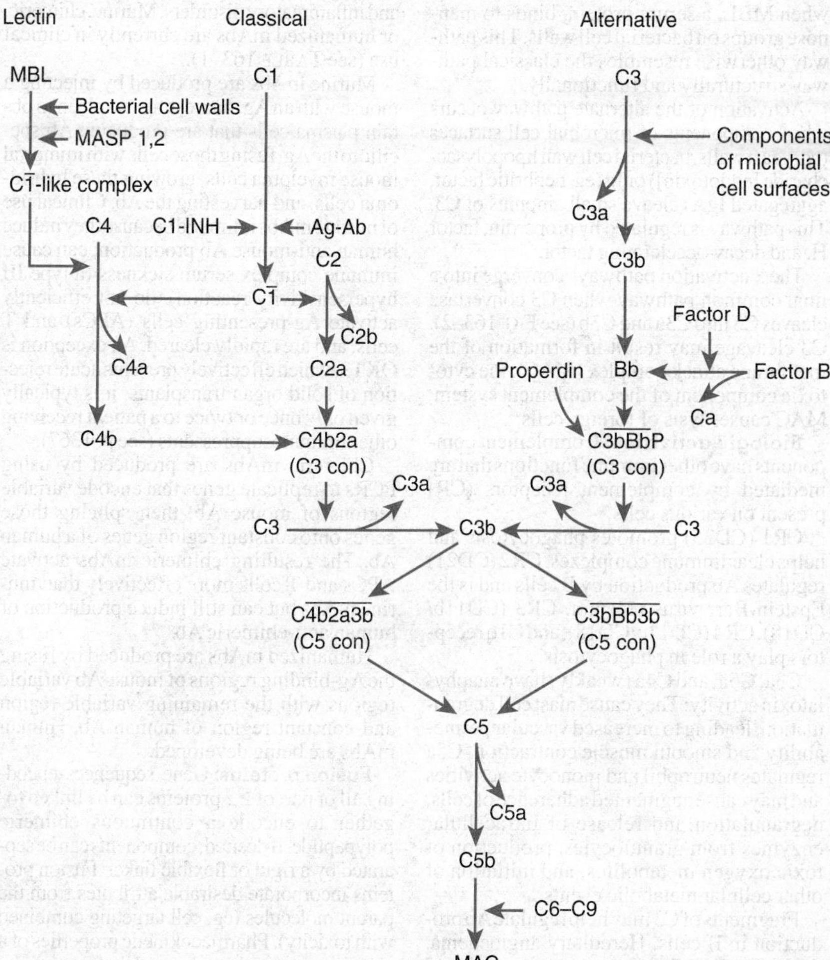

Fig. 163–2. Complement activation pathways. The classical, mannose-binding lectin (MBL), and alternative pathways converge into a final common pathway when C3 convertase (C3 con) cleaves C3 into C3a and C3b. C1-INH = C1 inhibitor; MASP = mannose-binding lectin-associated serine protease; Ag = antigen; Ab = antibody; P = properdin; MAC = membrane attack complex. Overbar indicates activation.

activation: classical, mannose-binding lectin, and alternative (see FIG. 163–2).

Classical pathway components are labeled with a C and a number (eg, C1, C3), based on the order in which they were identified. Alternative pathway components are often lettered (eg, factor B, factor D) or named (eg, properdin).

Activation of the classical pathway is Ab-dependent, occurring when C1 interacts with Ag-IgM or aggregated Ag-IgG complexes, or Ab-independent, occurring when polyanions (eg, heparin, protamine, DNA and RNA from apoptotic cells), gram-negative bacteria, or bound C-reactive protein reacts directly with C1. This pathway is regulated by C1 inhibitor (C1-INH).

Activation of the mannose-binding lectin (MBL) pathway is Ab-independent; it occurs when MBL, a serum protein, binds to mannose groups on bacterial cell walls. This pathway otherwise resembles the classical pathway structurally and functionally.

Activation of the alternate pathway occurs when components of microbial cell surfaces (eg, yeast walls, bacterial cell wall lipopolysaccharide [endotoxin]) or Ig (eg, nephritic factor, aggregated IgA) cleave small amounts of C3. This pathway is regulated by properdin, factor H, and decay-accelerating factor.

The 3 activation pathways converge into a final common pathway when C3 convertase cleaves C3 into C3a and C3b (see FIG. 163–2). C3 cleavage may result in formation of the membrane attack complex (MAC), the cytotoxic component of the complement system. MAC causes lysis of foreign cells.

Biologic activities: Complement components have other immune functions that are mediated by complement receptors (CR) present on various cells.

CR1 (CD35) promotes phagocytosis and helps clear immune complexes. CR2 (CD21) regulates Ab production by B cells and is the Epstein-Barr virus receptor. CR3 (CD11b/CD18), CR4 (CD11c/CD18), and C1q receptors play a role in phagocytosis.

C3a, C5a, and C4a (weakly) have anaphylatoxin activity: They cause mast cell degranulation, leading to increased vascular permeability and smooth muscle contraction. C5a regulates neutrophil and monocyte activities and may cause augmented adherence of cells, degranulation and release of intracellular enzymes from granulocytes, production of toxic oxygen metabolites, and initiation of other cellular metabolic events.

Fragments of C3 may help regulate Ab production in B cells. Hereditary angioedema, due to C1-INH deficiency, may be mediated by a kinin-like substance. The Bb fragment of factor B increases the spreading and adherence of macrophages.

IMMUNOTHERAPEUTICS

Therapeutic agents that use or modify immune mechanisms have been and are being developed. Use of these agents is rapidly evolving; new classes, new agents, and new uses of current agents are certain to be developed.

Monoclonal antibodies: Monoclonal antibodies (mAbs) are manufactured in vitro to recognize specific targeted Ags; they are used to treat solid and hematopoietic tumors and inflammatory disorders. Murine, chimeric, or humanized mAbs are currently in clinical use (see TABLE 163–1).

Murine mAbs are produced by injecting a mouse with an Ag, harvesting its spleen to obtain plasma cells that are producing Ab specific to the Ag, fusing those cells with immortal mouse myeloma cells, growing these hybridoma cells, and harvesting the Ab. Clinical use of murine mAbs is limited because they induce human anti-mouse Ab production, can cause immune complex serum sickness (a type III hypersensitivity reaction), do not efficiently activate Ag-presenting cells (APCs) and T cells, and are rapidly cleared. An exception is OKT3, which effectively prevents acute rejection of solid organ transplants; it is typically given only once or twice to a patient receiving other immunosuppressants (see p. 1367).

Chimeric mAbs are produced by using PCRs to replicate genes that encode variable regions of mouse Ab, then splicing those genes onto constant region genes of a human Ab. The resulting chimeric mAbs activate APCs and T cells more effectively than murine mAbs but can still induce production of human anti-chimeric Ab.

Humanized mAbs are produced by fusing the Ag-binding regions of mouse Ab variable regions with the remaining variable region and constant region of human Ab. Human mAbs are being developed.

Fusion proteins: Gene sequences encoding all or part of ≥ 2 proteins can be linked together to encode a continuous chimeric polypeptide. If desired, components can be separated by a rigid or flexible linker. Fusion proteins incorporate desirable attributes from the parent molecules (eg, cell targeting combined with toxicity). Pharmacokinetic properties of a protein can often be enhanced by fusion to another polypeptide with a long serum half-life.

Soluble cytokine receptors: Soluble versions of cytokine receptors are used as therapeutic reagents to block the action of cytokines. Etanercept, a fusion protein, consists of 2 identical chains from the CD120b tumor necrosis factor (TNF)-α receptor monomer joined together to increase affinity for TNF and linked to the Fc region of IgG to improve half-life. This agent is used to treat RA refractory to other treatments, ankylosing spondylitis, and psoriatic arthritis. Soluble IL receptors (eg, those for IL-1, IL-2, IL-4, IL-5, and IL-6) are being developed for treatment of inflammatory and allergic disorders and cancer. Anakinra, used to treat RA, is a recombi-

TABLE 163–1. SOME IMMUNOTHERAPEUTIC AGENTS IN CLINICAL USE*

AGENT	EFFECTS	INDICATIONS
Monoclonal antibodies†		
Abciximab	Anti-GP IIb/IIIa platelet fibrinogen receptor	Prevention of restenosis in patients undergoing percutaneous coronary interventions (with antiplatelet drugs and heparin)
Adalimumab	Anti-TNF-α	Moderate to severe RA refractory to standard treatments
Alemtuzumab	Anti-B cell (CD52)	B-cell chronic lymphocytic leukemia refractory to standard treatments
Basiliximab	Anti-IL-2 receptor	Prevention of acute organ rejection in kidney transplant patients
Bevacizumab	Anti-vascular endothelial growth factor	Solid tumors (eg, kidney, lung, colon, glioma) refractory to standard treatment
Cetuximab	Anti-epidermal growth factor receptor	Solid organ tumors (eg, lung, pancreas, colon) refractory to standard treatments
Daclizumab	Anti-IL-2 receptor	Prevention of acute organ rejection in renal transplant patients
Efalizumab	Anti-T cell (CD11a)	Psoriasis
Gemtuzumab	Antimyeloblast (CD33; linked to the cytotoxin calicheamicin)	Relapses of acute myeloid leukemia
Ibritumomab	Anti-B cell (CD20; linked to the radioactive agent yttrium 90)	Relapsed or refractory low-grade follicular or transformed B-cell non-Hodgkin lymphoma
Infliximab	Anti-TNF-α	Moderate to severe Crohn's disease with or without fistulization; moderate to severe RA inadequately responsive to methotrexate
Mepolizumab	Anti-IL-5	Eosinophilic dermatitis in hypereosinophilic syndrome
OKT3	Anti-T cell (CD3)	Acute treatment and prevention of kidney transplant rejection
Omalizumab	Anti-IgE	Moderate to severe asthma in patients < 12 yr with documented allergic disease inadequately controlled by inhaled corticosteroids
Palivizumab	Anti-RSV	RSV in children at high risk of severe infections
Pexelizumab	Anti-complement component C5	Coronary artery bypass graft surgery requiring cardiopulmonary bypass
Rituximab	Anti-B cell (CD20)	Relapsed or refractory low-grade or follicular B-cell non-Hodgkin lymphoma
Tositumomab	Anti-B cell (CD20; linked to the radioactive agent iodine-131)	Refractory and relapsed CD20+ follicular non-Hodgkin lymphoma

Table continues on the following page.

TABLE 163–1. SOME IMMUNOTHERAPEUTIC AGENTS IN CLINICAL USE*—Continued

AGENT	EFFECTS	INDICATIONS
Trastuzumab	Anti-epidermal growth factor receptor (anti-HER-2/*neu*)	HER-2/*neu*–positive breast cancer
Fusion proteins		
Alefacept (fusion of CD2 binding portions of CD58 to Fc region of IgG1)	Inhibition of T-cell activation; induction of T-cell apoptosis	Moderate to severe chronic plaque psoriasis
Denileukin diftitox (fusion of IL-2 to diphtheria toxin)	Delivery of toxin to CD25 component of IL-2 receptor	Cutaneous T-cell lymphoma
Etanercept (fusion of 2 CD120b TNF-α receptors to Fc region of IgG1)	Decrease in TNF levels	Moderate to severe RA, polyarticular juvenile RA
Soluble cytokine receptor		
Anakinra (soluble IL-1 receptor, sometimes pegylated for longer half-life)	Competitively inhibits IL-1α and IL-1β activities	Moderate to severe RA
Cytokines		
IFN-α	Antiproliferative and antiviral	Chronic hepatitis C infection, AIDS-related Kaposi's sarcoma, and hairy cell leukemia
IFN-β	Antiproliferative and antiviral	Reduction of number of flare-ups in relapsing multiple sclerosis
IFN-γ	Immunostimulatory and antiviral	Control of infection in chronic granulomatous disease
IL-2	Immunostimulatory	Renal cell carcinoma and metastatic melanoma
IL-11	Thrombopoietic growth factor	Prevention of thrombocytopenia after myelosuppressive chemotherapy
Erythropoietin	Stimulates erythropoiesis	Anemia associated with chronic renal failure
G-CSF	Stimulates granulocyte production	Reversal of neutropenia after chemotherapy, radiation therapy, or both
GM-CSF	Stimulates granulocyte and monocyte/macrophage production	Reversal of neutropenia after chemotherapy, radiation therapy, or both

*Does not include mAbs used for diagnostic testing and radiologic imaging.

†In mAb nomenclature, the 1st syllables vary; the next syllables represent the targeted disorder (bacteria = bac; viral = vir; immune = lim; infectious = les; cardiovascular = cir; for cancer, breast = mar, colon = col, ovarian = gov, prostate = pro, testicular = got, melanoma = mel, miscellaneous = tum), followed by a syllable representing the source (eg, o = mouse, xi = chimeric, u = human, zu = humanized); the last syllable is always "mab."

GP = glycoprotein; TNF = tumor necrosis factor; CD = cluster of differentiation; RSV = respiratory syncytial virus; Fc = crystallizable fragment; IFN = interferon; G-CSF = granulocyte colony-stimulating factor; GM-CSF = granulocyte-macrophage colony-stimulating factor.

nant nonglycosylated form of the IL-1R antagonist; this drug attaches to the IL-1 receptor and thus prevents binding of IL-1.

Recombinant cytokines: Colony-stimulating factors (CSF), such as erythropoietin, granulocyte CSF (G-CSF), and granulocyte-macrophage CSF (GM-CSF), are used in patients undergoing chemotherapy or transplantation for hematologic disorders and cancers (see TABLE 163–1). Interferon-α (IFN-α) and IFN-γ are used to treat cancer, immunodeficiency disorders, and viral infections; IFN-β is used to treat relapsing multiple sclerosis. Many other cytokines are being studied. Cells expressing cytokine receptors can be targeted by modified versions of the relevant cytokine (eg, denileukin diftitox, a fusion protein containing sequences from IL-2 and from the A and B chains of diphtheria toxin). Denileukin is used in cutaneous T-cell lymphoma to target cells expressing the CD25 component of the IL-2 receptor.

Small-molecule mimetics: Small linear peptides, cyclicized peptides, and small organic molecules have been developed as agonists or antagonists for various applications. Screening libraries of peptides or organic compounds can identify potential mimetics (eg, agonists for receptors for erythropoietin, thrombopoietin, and G-CSF).

164 IMMUNODEFICIENCY DISORDERS

Immunodeficiency disorders increase susceptibility to infection. They may be secondary or primary; secondary is more common.

Secondary immunodeficiencies: Causes include nonimmune systemic disorders (eg, diabetes, undernutrition, HIV infection) and immunosuppressive treatments (eg, chemotherapy, radiation therapy—see TABLE 164–1). Secondary immunodeficiency also occurs among critically ill, older, or hospitalized patients. Prolonged serious illness may impair immune responses; impairment is often reversible if the underlying illness resolves. Some decrease in immunity occurs with aging.

Immunodeficiency can result from loss of serum proteins (particularly IgG and albumin) through the kidneys in the nephrotic syndrome, through skin in severe burns or dermatitis, or through the GI tract in enteropathy. Enteropathy may also lead to lymphocyte loss, resulting in lymphopenia. These disorders can mimic B- and T-cell defects. Treatment focuses on the underlying disorder; a diet high in medium-chain triglycerides may decrease loss of Igs and lymphocytes from the GI tract and be remarkably beneficial.

Primary immunodeficiencies: These disorders are genetically determined; they may occur alone or as part of a syndrome. More than 100 have been described, and heterogeneity within each disorder may be considerable. The molecular basis for more than half is known. Primary immunodeficiencies typically manifest in infancy and childhood as abnormally frequent (recurrent) or unusual infections. About 80% of patients are < 20 yr at onset; because transmission is often X-linked, 70% are male. Overall incidence of symptomatic disease is about 1/10,000 people.

Primary immunodeficiencies are classified by the main component of the immune system that is deficient, absent, or defective: B cells (or Ig), T cells, natural killer (NK) cells, phagocytic cells, or complement proteins (see TABLE 164–2). As more information becomes available, classifying immunodeficiencies by their molecular defects may be more useful.

B-cell defects causing Ig and antibody deficiencies account for 50 to 60% of primary immunodeficiencies. Serum Ig and antibody titers decrease, predisposing to infections with encapsulated gram-positive bacteria. The most common B-cell disorder is selective IgA deficiency. Others include common variable immunodeficiency, hyper-IgM syndrome, transient hypogammaglobulinemia of infancy, and X-linked agammaglobulinemia.

T-cell disorders account for about 5 to 10% of primary immunodeficiencies and predispose to infection by viruses, fungi, other opportunistic organisms, and many common pathogens. T-cell disorders also cause Ig deficiencies because the B and T cell immune systems are interdependent. Examples are DiGeorge syndrome, ZAP-70 deficiency, X-linked lymphoproliferative syndrome, and chronic mucocutaneous candidiasis (see p. 988).

TABLE 164–1. SECONDARY IMMUNODEFICIENCY DISORDERS

CATEGORY	EXAMPLES
Endocrine	Diabetes mellitus
GI	Hepatic insufficiency, hepatitis, intestinal lymphangiectasia, protein-losing enteropathy
Hematologic	Aplastic anemia, cancer, graft-vs-host disease, sickle cell disease
Iatrogenic	Anticonvulsants (causing IgA deficiency), general anesthesia, immunosuppressants (eg, antithymocyte globulin, chemotherapeutic drugs, corticosteroids), radiation therapy, splenectomy
Infectious	Cytomegalovirus, Epstein-Barr virus, or HIV infection, measles, varicella
Nutritional	Alcoholism, undernutrition
Physiologic	Physiologic immunodeficiency in infants due to immaturity of immune system, pregnancy
Renal	Nephrotic syndrome, renal insufficiency, uremia
Rheumatologic	RA, SLE
Other	Burns, chromosomal abnormalities (eg, Down syndrome), congenital asplenia, critical and chronic illness, histiocytosis, sarcoidosis

Combined B- and T-cell defects account for about 20% of primary immunodeficiencies. The most important form is severe combined immunodeficiency (SCID). Others include ataxia-telangiectasia, cartilage-hair hypoplasia, cytokine deficiencies, hyper-IgE syndrome, major histocompatibility complex (MHC) deficiencies (absence of class I or II MHC molecules on immune cells), and Wiskott-Aldrich syndrome. In some forms of combined immunodeficiency (eg, purine nucleoside phosphorylase deficiency), Ig levels are normal or elevated, but because of inadequate T-cell function there is impaired antibody formation.

Natural killer cell defects are very rare and may predispose to viral infections and tumors.

Phagocytic cell defects account for 10 to 15% of primary immunodeficiencies and impair the ability of phagocytic cells (eg, monocytes, macrophages, granulocytes such as neutrophils and eosinophils) to kill pathogens. Examples are chronic granulomatous disease, leukocyte adhesion deficiency, and Chédiak-Higashi syndrome. Cutaneous staphylococcal and gram-negative infections are characteristic.

Complement deficiencies are rare (≤ 2%); they include isolated deficiencies of complement components or inhibitors and may be hereditary or acquired. Hereditary deficiencies are autosomal recessive except for deficiencies of C1 inhibitor, which is autosomal dominant, and properdin, which is X-linked. The deficiencies result in defective opsonization, phagocytosis, and lysis of pathogens and in defective clearance of antigen-antibody complexes. Recurrent infection—due to defective opsonization—and autoimmune disorders (eg, SLE, glomerulonephritis)—due to defective clearance of antigen-antibody complexes (see TABLE 164–2)—are the most serious consequences. One of these deficiencies causes hereditary angioedema.

Primary immunodeficiency syndromes are genetically determined immunodeficiencies with immune and nonimmune defects. Nonimmune manifestations are often more easily recognized than those of the immunodeficiency. Examples are DiGeorge syndrome, cartilage-hair hypoplasia, Wiskott-Aldrich syndrome, and ataxia-telangiectasia.

APPROACH TO THE PATIENT WITH SUSPECTED IMMUNODEFICIENCY

Immunodeficiency typically manifests as recurrent infections. However, more likely causes of recurrent infections in children are repeated exposures to infection at day care or school (infants and children may normally have up to 10 respiratory infections/yr), and more likely causes in children and adults are inadequate duration of antibiotic treatment, resistant organisms, and other disorders that predispose to infection (eg, congenital heart defects, allergic rhinitis, ureteral or urethral stenosis, immotile cilia syndrome, asthma, cystic fibrosis, severe dermatitis).

Immunodeficiency should be suspected when recurrent infections are severe, complicated, resistant to treatment, or caused by

TABLE 164–2. PRIMARY IMMUNODEFICIENCY DISORDERS

DISORDER	INHERITANCE	CLINICAL FINDINGS
Ig (B-cell) deficiencies		
Common variable immunodeficiency	Autosomal dominant	Similar to X-linked agammaglobulinemia but manifests later and B cells are present; also autoimmune disorders, malabsorption, nodular lymphoid hyperplasia of GI tract, bronchiectasis; lymphoma (10%)
Hyper-IgM syndrome with AID or UNG deficiencies	Autosomal recessive	Similar to X-linked hyper-IgM syndrome but with lymphoid hyperplasia; no leukopenia
Hyper-IgM syndrome with CD40 deficiency	Autosomal recessive	Similar to X-linked hyper-IgM syndrome, lymphoid hypoplasia, neutropenia
Hyper-IgM syndrome with CD40 ligand deficiency	X-linked	Similar to X-linked agammaglobulinemia but greater frequency of *Pneumocystis jiroveci* (formerly *P. carinii*) pneumonia, cryptosporidiosis, severe neutropenia, and lymphoid hypoplasia
IgA deficiency	Autosomal dominant	Sometimes asymptomatic; recurrent sinopulmonary infections, diarrhea, allergies (including anaphylactic transfusion reactions), autoimmune disorders (eg, celiac disease, inflammatory bowel disease, SLE, chronic active hepatitis)
Transient hypogammaglobulinemia of infancy	—	Low Ig but normal antibody levels
X-linked agammaglobulinemia	X-linked	Recurrent sinopulmonary and skin infections in infancy; neutropenia, lymphoid hypoplasia
T-cell disorders		
Chronic mucocutaneous candidiasis	Autosomal dominant or recessive	Persistent or recurrent candidal infection, nail dystrophy, endocrine disorders (hypoparathyroidism, Addison's disease) in recessive form
DiGeorge syndrome	Autosomal	Unusual facies with low-set ears, a congenital heart disorder (eg, aortic arch abnormalities), thymic hypoplasia or aplasia, hypoparathyroidism with hypocalcemic tetany, recurrent infections
X-linked lymphoproliferative syndrome	X-linked	Asymptomatic until onset of Epstein-Barr virus infection; then fulminant or fatal infectious mononucleosis with liver failure and, in survivors, B-cell lymphomas, aplastic anemia, hypogammaglobulinemia, or a combination
ζ-Associated protein 70 (ZAP-70) deficiency	Autosomal recessive	Common and opportunistic infections; no CD8 cells
Combined B- and T-cell defects		
Ataxia-telangiectasia	Autosomal recessive	Ataxia, telangiectasias, recurrent sinopulmonary infections, endocrine abnormalities (eg, gonadal dysgenesis, testicular atrophy, diabetes mellitus), increased risk of cancer
Cartilage-hair hypoplasia	Autosomal recessive	Short-limbed dwarfism, common and opportunistic infections

Table continues on the following page.

TABLE 164–2. PRIMARY IMMUNODEFICIENCY DISORDERS—Continued

DISORDER	INHERITANCE	CLINICAL FINDINGS
Combined immunodeficiency with low but not absent T-cell function and normal or elevated Igs	Autosomal recessive or X-linked	Common and opportunistic infections, lymphopenia, lymphadenopathy, hepatosplenomegaly, and skin lesions resembling those of Langerhans cell histiocytosis in some patients
Hyper-IgE syndrome	Autosomal dominant	Staphylococcal abscesses of skin, lungs, joints, and viscera; pulmonary pneumatoceles; pruritic dermatitis; coarse facial features; delayed shedding of baby teeth; osteopenia; recurrent fractures; tissue and blood eosinophilia
MHC deficiencies	Autosomal recessive	Common and opportunistic infections
Severe combined immunodeficiency	Autosomal recessive and X-linked	Oral candidiasis, pneumonia, diarrhea before 6 mo, failure to thrive, graft vs host disease, absent thymic shadow, lymphopenia, bony abnormalities (in ADA deficiency), exfoliative dermatitis as part of Omenn's syndrome
Wiskott-Aldrich syndrome	X-linked recessive	GI bleeding (eg, bloody diarrhea), recurrent respiratory infections, opportunistic infections, eczema, thrombocytopenia, cancer (in 10% of patients > 10 yr), varicella-zoster virus infection, herpes infection
Phagocytic cell defects		
Chédiak-Higashi syndrome	Autosomal recessive	Recurrent infections, albinism, fever, jaundice, hepatosplenomegaly, lymphadenopathy, neurologic changes, pancytopenia, bleeding diathesis
Chronic granulomatous disease	X-linked or autosomal recessive	Granulomatous lesions in the lungs, liver, lymph nodes, and GI and GU tract (causing obstruction); lymphadenitis; hepatosplenomegaly; skin, lymph node, lung, liver, and perianal abscesses; osteomyelitis; pneumonia
Leukocyte adhesion deficiency	Autosomal recessive	Soft-tissue infections, periodontitis, poor wound healing, delayed umbilical cord detachment, leukocytosis
IFN-γ receptor defects	Autosomal dominant or recessive	Mycobacterial infections
IL-12 deficiency and IL-12 receptor β1 defect	Autosomal recessive	*Salmonella* and mycobacterial infections
Complement deficiencies in the classical pathway		
C1	Autosomal recessive	SLE
C2	Autosomal recessive	SLE, recurrent pyogenic infections with encapsulated bacteria (especially pneumococcal) that start in early childhood, other autoimmune disorders (eg, glomerulonephritis, polymyositis, vasculitis, Schönlein-Henoch purpura, Hodgkin lymphoma)

TABLE 164–2. PRIMARY IMMUNODEFICIENCY DISORDERS—Continued

DISORDER	INHERITANCE	CLINICAL FINDINGS
C3	Autosomal recessive	Recurrent pyogenic infections with encapsulated bacteria that start at birth, glomerulonephritis, other antigen-antibody complex disorders, sepsis
C4	Autosomal recessive	SLE, other autoimmune disorders (eg, IgA nephropathy, progressive systemic sclerosis, Schönlein-Henoch purpura, type I diabetes mellitus, autoimmune hepatitis)
C5, C6, C7, C8, C9 (membrane attack complex)	Autosomal recessive	Recurrent *N. meningitidis* and disseminated *N. gonorrhoeae* infections
Complement deficiencies in the MBL pathway		
MBL	Autosomal recessive	Recurrent pyogenic infections with encapsulated bacteria that start at birth; unexplained sepsis; increased severity of infection in secondary immunodeficiencies due to corticosteroids, cystic fibrosis, or chronic lung disorders
MASP-2	Unknown	Autoimmune disorders (eg, inflammatory bowel disease, erythema multiforme), recurrent pyogenic infections with encapsulated bacteria (eg, *Streptococcus pneumoniae*)
Complement deficiencies in the alternative pathway		
Factor B	Autosomal recessive	
Factor D	Autosomal	Pyogenic infections
Properdin	X-linked	
Complement regulatory protein deficiencies		
C1 inhibitor	Autosomal dominant	Angioedema
Factor I	Autosomal codominant	Same as C3 deficiency
Factor H	Autosomal codominant	Same as C3 deficiency; hemolytic-uremic syndrome
Decay accelerating factor	Autosomal recessive	Paroxysmal nocturnal hemoglobinuria
Complement receptor (CR) deficiencies		
CR1	Acquired	Secondary finding in immune (antigen-antibody) complex–mediated disease
CR3	Autosomal recessive	Leukocyte adhesion deficiency syndrome (recurrent *Staphylococcus aureus* and *Pseudomonas aeruginosa* infections)

CD = clusters of differentiation; AID = activation-dependent (induced) cytidine deaminase; ADA = adenosine deaminase; MHC = major histocompatibility complex; C = complement; MBL = mannose-binding lectin; MASP = mannose-binding lectin-associated serine protease; UNG = uracil DNA glycosylase.

unusual organisms. Initially, infections due to immunodeficiency are typically upper and lower respiratory tract infections (eg, sinusitis, bronchitis, pneumonia) and gastroenteritis, but they may be serious bacterial infections (eg, meningitis, sepsis).

Immunodeficiency should also be suspected in infants or young children with chronic diarrhea and failure to thrive, especially when the diarrhea is caused by unusual viruses (eg, adenovirus) or fungi (eg, *Cryptosporidium* sp). Other signs include skin lesions (eg, eczema, warts, abscesses, pyoderma, alopecia), oral or esophageal thrush, oral ulcers, and periodontitis.

Less common manifestations include severe viral infection with herpes simplex or varicella zoster virus and CNS problems (eg, chronic encephalitis, delayed development, seizure disorder). Frequent use of antibiotics may mask many of the common symptoms and signs.

Diagnosis

History and physical examination are helpful but must be supplemented by immune function testing.

History: Whether patients have a history of risk factors for infection, as well as symptoms and risk factors for secondary immunodeficiency disorders, is determined. Onset of infections before age 12 mo suggests combined B- and T-cell defects or a B-cell defect, which becomes evident when maternal antibodies are disappearing (at about age 6 mo). In general, the earlier the age at onset in children, the more severe the immunodeficiency. Certain other primary immunodeficiencies (eg, common variable immunodeficiency [CVID]) may not manifest until adulthood. Certain infections suggest certain immunodeficiency disorders (see TABLE 164–3); however, no infection is specific to any one disorder, and

TABLE 164–3. SOME HISTORICAL FINDINGS SUGGESTING TYPE OF IMMUNODEFICIENCY

FINDING	IMMUNODEFICIENCY
Recurrent *Streptococcus pneumoniae* and *Haemophilus influenzae* infections	Ig or C2 deficiency
Recurrent *Giardia lamblia* infection	Antibody deficiency syndromes
Familial clustering of autoimmune disorders (eg, SLE, RA, pernicious anemia)	Common variable immunodeficiency or IgA deficiency
Pneumocystis infections, cryptosporidiosis, or toxoplasmosis	T-cell disorders or occasionally Ig deficiency
Viral, fungal, or mycobacterial (opportunistic) infections	T-cell disorders
Clinical infection due to attenuated live vaccines (eg, varicella, polio, BCG)	T-cell disorders
Graft-vs-host disease due to blood transfusions	T-cell disorders
Staphylococcal infections, infections with gram-negative organisms (eg, *Serratia* or *Klebsiella* sp), or fungal infections (eg, aspergillosis)	Phagocytic cell defects
Skin infections	Neutrophil defect or Ig deficiency
Recurrent gingivitis	Neutrophil defect
Recurrent neisserial infections	Certain complement deficiencies
Recurrent sepsis	Certain complement deficiencies or IgG deficiency
Family history of childhood death or of infections in a maternal uncle that are similar to those of the patient	X-linked disorders (eg, severe combined immunodeficiency, X-linked agammaglobulinemia, Wiskott-Aldrich syndrome, hyper-IgM syndrome)

certain common infections (eg, respiratory viral or bacterial infections) occur in many.

Physical examination: Patients with immunodeficiency may or may not appear chronically ill. Macular rashes, vesicles, pyoderma, eczema, petechiae, alopecia, or telangiectasia may be evident. Cervical lymph nodes and adenoid and tonsillar tissue are typically very small or absent in X-linked agammaglobulinemia, X-linked hyper-IgM syndrome, SCID, and other T-cell immunodeficiencies despite a history of recurrent infections. In certain immunodeficiencies (eg, chronic granulomatous disease), lymph nodes of the head and neck may be enlarged and suppurative. Tympanic membranes may be scarred or perforated. The nostrils may be crusted, indicating purulent nasal discharge. Chronic cough is common, as are lung crackles, especially in adults with CVID. The liver and spleen are often enlarged in patients with CVID or chronic granulomatous disease. Muscle mass and fat deposits of the buttocks are decreased. In infants, skin around the anus may break down because of chronic diarrhea. Neurologic examination may detect delayed developmental milestones or ataxia. Other characteristic findings may suggest a tentative clinical diagnosis (see TABLE 164–4).

Initial testing: If a specific secondary immunodeficiency disorder is suspected clinically, testing should focus on that disorder (eg, diabetes, HIV infection, cystic fibrosis, primary ciliary dyskinesia—see p. 442). Tests are needed to confirm a diagnosis of immunodeficiency (see TABLE 164–5). Initial screening tests should include CBC with manual differential, quantitative Ig measurements, antibody titer measurements, and skin testing for delayed hypersensitivity. If results are normal, immunodeficiency (especially Ig deficiency) can be excluded. If results are abnormal, further tests in specialized laboratories are needed to identify specific deficiencies. If chronic infections are objectively documented, initial and specific tests may be done simultaneously. Prenatal testing is available for many disorders and is indicated if there is a family history of immunodeficiency and the mutation has been identified in family members.

CBC can detect abnormalities in one or more cell types (eg WBCs, platelets) characteristic of specific disorders. However, many abnormalities are transient manifestations of infection, drug use, or other factors; thus, abnormalities should be confirmed and followed.

Neutropenia (absolute neutrophil count < 1200 cells/ μL) may be congenital or cyclic or may occur in aplastic anemia. Lymphopenia (lymphocytes < 2000/μL at birth, < 4500/μL at age 9 mo, or < 1000/μL in older children or adults) suggests a T-cell disorder because 75% of circulating lymphocytes are T cells. Leukocytosis that persists between infections may occur in leukocyte adhesion deficiency. Thrombocytopenia in male infants suggests Wiskott-Aldrich syndrome. Anemia may suggest anemia of chronic disease or autoimmune hemolytic anemia, which may occur in CVID and other immunodeficiencies.

Peripheral blood smear should be examined for Howell-Jolly bodies and other unusual RBC forms suggesting primary asplenia or impaired splenic function. Granulocytes may have morphologic abnormalities (eg, giant granules in Chédiak-Higashi syndrome).

Low serum levels of IgG, IgM, or IgA suggest antibody deficiency, but results must be compared with those of age-matched controls. An IgG level < 200 mg/dL usually indicates significant antibody deficiency, although such levels may occur in protein-losing enteropathies or nephrotic syndrome.

IgM antibodies can be assessed by measuring isohemagglutinin titers (anti-A, anti-B). All patients except infants < 6 mo and people with blood type AB have natural antibodies at a titer of ≥ 1:8 (anti-A) or ≥ 1:4 (anti-B); antibodies to A, B, and some bacterial polysaccharides are selectively deficient in certain disorders (eg, Wiskott-Aldrich syndrome, complete IgG2 deficiency). IgG antibody titers can be assessed in immunized patients by measuring antibody titers before and after administration of vaccine antigens (*Haemophilus influenzae* type B, tetanus, diphtheria, conjugated or nonconjugated pneumococcal, and meningococcal antigens); a less-than-twofold increase in titer at 2 to 3 wk suggests antibody deficiency regardless of Ig levels. Natural antibodies (eg, antistreptolysin O, heterophile antibodies) may also be measured.

Most immunocompetent adults, infants, and children react to 0.1 mL of *Candida albicans* extract (1:100 for infants and 1:1000 for older children and adults) injected intradermally. Positive reactivity, defined as erythema and induration > 5 mm at 24, 48, and 72 h, excludes a T-cell disorder. Lack of response does not confirm immunodeficiency in patients with no previous exposure to *Candida*.

Chest x-ray may be useful in some infants; an absent thymic shadow suggests a T-cell

TABLE 164–4. CHARACTERISTIC CLINICAL FINDINGS IN SOME PRIMARY IMMUNODEFICIENCY DISORDERS

AGE GROUP	FINDINGS*	DISORDER
< 6 mo	Diarrhea, failure to thrive	Severe combined immunodeficiency
	Maculopapular rash, splenomegaly	Severe combined immunodeficiency with graft-vs-host disease
	Hypocalcemic tetany, a congenital heart disorder, unusual facies with low-set ears	DiGeorge syndrome
	Recurrent pyogenic infections, sepsis	C3 deficiency
	Oculocutaneous albinism, neurologic changes, lymphadenopathy	Chédiak-Higashi syndrome
	Cyanosis, a congenital heart disorder, midline liver	Congenital asplenia
	Delayed umbilical cord detachment, leukocytosis, periodontitis, poor wound healing	Leukocyte adhesion deficiency
	Abscesses, lymphadenopathy, antral obstruction, pneumonia, osteomyelitis	Chronic granulomatous disease
	Recurrent staphylococcal abscesses of the skin, lungs, joints, and viscera, pneumatoceles, coarse facial features, pruritic dermatitis	Hyper-IgE syndrome
	Chronic gingivitis, recurrent aphthous ulcers and skin infections, severe neutropenia	Severe congenital neutropenia
	GI bleeding (eg, bloody diarrhea), eczema	Wiskott-Aldrich syndrome
6 mo to 5 yr	Paralysis after oral polio immunization	X-linked agammaglobulinemia
	Severe progressive infectious mononucleosis	X-linked lymphoproliferative syndrome
	Persistent oral candidiasis, nail dystrophy, endocrine disorders (hypoparathyroidism, Addison's disease)	Chronic mucocutaneous candidiasis
> 5 yr (including adults)	Ataxia, recurrent sinopulmonary infections, neurologic deterioration, telangiectasias	Ataxia-telangiectasia
	Recurrent *Neisseria* meningitis	C5, C6, C7, or C8 deficiency
	Recurrent sinopulmonary infections, malabsorption, splenomegaly, autoimmune disorders, nodular lymphoid hyperplasia of the GI tract, bronchiectasis	Common variable immunodeficiency
	Progressive dermatomyositis with chronic echovirus encephalitis	X-linked agammaglobulinemia

*In addition to infection.

Adapted from Stiehm, ER, Conley ME: "Immunodeficiency Diseases: General Considerations," in *Immunodeficiency Disease in Infants and Children, ed 4,* edited by ER Stiehm. Philadelphia, WB Saunders Company, 1996, p. 212.

disorder, especially if the x-ray is obtained before onset of infection or other stress that may shrink the thymus. Lateral pharyngeal x-ray may show absence of adenoidal tissue.

Additional testing: If clinical findings or initial tests suggest a specific disorder of immune cell or complement function, other tests are indicated.

If patients have recurrent infections and lymphopenia, lymphocyte phenotyping using flow cytometry and monoclonal antibodies to T, B and NK cells is indicated to check for lymphocyte deficiency. If T cells are low or absent, in vitro mitogen stimulation studies are done to assess T-cell function. If MHC deficiency is suspected, serologic (not molecular) HLA typing is indicated.

If phagocytic cell defects are suspected, a flow cytometric respiratory burst assay can detect whether O_2 radicals are produced during phagocytosis; no production is characteristic of chronic granulomatous disease.

If the type or pattern of infections suggests complement deficiency, the serum dilution required to lyse 50% of antibody-coated RBCs (CH50) is measured. This test detects complement component deficiencies in the classical or alternative complement activation pathway.

If examination or screening tests detect abnormalities suggesting lymphocyte or phagocytic cell defects, other tests can more precisely characterize specific disorders (see TABLE 164–6).

Prenatal diagnosis: An increasing number of primary immunodeficiency disorders can be diagnosed prenatally using chorionic villus sampling, cultured amniotic cells, or fetal blood sampling, but these tests are used only when a mutation in family members has already been identified (see p. 2144). X-linked agammaglobulinemia, Wiskott-Aldrich syndrome, ataxia-telangiectasia, X-linked lymphoproliferative syndrome, all forms of SCID, and all forms of chronic granulomatous disease can be detected. Sex determination by ultrasonography can be used to exclude X-linked disorders.

Prognosis

Prognosis depends on the primary immunodeficiency disorder. Most patients with an Ig or complement deficiency have a good prognosis with a near-normal life expectancy if they are diagnosed early, are treated appropriately, and have no coexisting chronic disorders (eg, a pulmonary disorder such as bronchiectasis). Other immunodeficient patients (eg, those with phagocytic cell defect or combined immunodeficiencies, such as Wiskott-Aldrich syndrome or ataxia-telangiectasia) have a

TABLE 164–5. INITIAL AND ADDITIONAL LABORATORY TESTS FOR IMMUNODEFICIENCY

TYPE	INITIAL TESTS	ADDITIONAL TESTS
B-cell deficiency	IgG, IgM, IgA, IgE levels Isohemagglutinin titers Antibody response to vaccine antigens (eg, *Haemophilus influenzae* type b, tetanus, diphtheria, conjugated and nonconjugated pneumococcal, and meningococcal antigens)	B-cell phenotyping using flow cytometry and monoclonal antibodies to B cells
T-cell deficiency	Lymphocyte count Delayed hypersensitivity skin tests (eg, using *Candida*) Chest x-ray for size of thymus in infants only T-cell count and subset analysis	T-cell phenotyping using flow cytometry and monoclonal antibodies to T cells T-cell proliferative response to mitogens
Phagocytic cell defects	Phagocytic cell count and morphology	Flow cytometric respiratory burst assay
Complement deficiency	C3 level C4 level CH50 activity	Specific component assays

CH = hemolytic complement; C = complement.

TABLE 164–6. ADVANCED LABORATORY TESTS FOR IMMUNODEFICIENCY

TYPE	TEST	INDICATIONS	INTERPRETATION
B-cell deficiency*	IgE level measurement	Abscesses, ataxia	Levels are high in patients with abscesses and pneumatoceles (hyper-IgE syndrome), partial T-cell deficiencies, allergic disorders, or parasitic infections. Levels may be high or low in patients with incomplete B-cell defects or deficiencies. Isolated deficiency is not clinically significant
	B-cell quantification via flow cytometry	Low Ig levels	No B cells suggests Omenn's syndrome; < 1% suggests X-linked agammaglobulinemia
	Lymph node biopsy	For some patients with lymphadenopathy to determine whether germinal centers are normal and to exclude cancer and infection	Interpretation varies by histology
	Mutation analysis	B cells < 1% by flow cytometry	The test can detect X-linked agammaglobulinemia
T-cell deficiency	T cell enumeration using flow cytometry and monoclonal antibodies†	Lymphopenia, suspected SCID or complete DiGeorge syndrome	Interpretation varies by molecular type of SCID
	T-cell proliferation assays to mitogens, antigens, or irradiated allogeneic WBCs	Low percentage of T cells, lymphopenia, suspected SCID or complete DiGeorge syndrome	Low or absent uptake of radioactive thymidine during cell division indicates a T-cell defect
	Detection of antigens (eg, class II MHC molecules) using monoclonal antibodies or serologic HLA typing	Suspected MHC deficiency, absence of MHC stimulation by cells	Absence of class I or class II HLA antigens by serologic HLA typing is diagnostic for MHC antigen deficiency
	RBC adenosine deaminase assay	Severe lymphopenia	Levels are low in a specific form of SCID
	Purine nucleoside phosphorylase assay	Severe persistent lymphopenia	Levels are low in combined immunodeficiency with normal or elevated Ig levels
	T-cell receptor and signal transduction assays	Phenotypically normal T cells that do not proliferate normally in response to mitogen antigen	Interpretation varies by test

TABLE 164–6. ADVANCED LABORATORY TESTS FOR IMMUNODEFICIENCY—Continued

TYPE	TEST	INDICATIONS	INTERPRETATION
Phagocytic cell defects	Assays for oxidant products (hydrogen peroxide, superoxide), proteins (CR3 [CD11] adhesive glycoproteins, NADPH oxidase components)	For patients who have a history of staphylococcal abscesses or certain gram-negative infections (eg, *Serratia marcescens*)	Abnormalities confirm phagocytic cell defects or deficiencies
Complement deficiency	Measurement of levels of specific complement components	CH50 level < 11%	Interpretation varies by test

*Measuring IgG subclass levels is rarely helpful.

†Test uses anti-CD3 for all T cells, anti-CD4 for helper T cells, anti-CD8 for cytotoxic T cells, anti-CD45RO/RA and anti-CD25 for activated T cells, and anti-CD16 and anti-CD56 for natural killer cells.

SCID = severe combined immunodeficiency; MHC = major histocompatibility complex; NADPH = nicotinamide adenine dinucleotide phosphate.

guarded prognosis; most require intensive and frequent treatment. Some immunodeficient patients (eg, those with SCID) will die during infancy unless immunity is restored through transplantation. All forms of SCID could be diagnosed at birth if a WBC count and manual differential on cord or peripheral blood were routinely done in newborns. Suspicion for SCID, a true pediatric emergency, must be high because prompt diagnosis is essential for survival. If done before patients reach age 3 mo, transplantation of bone marrow or stem cells from a matched or half-matched (haploidentical) relative is lifesaving in 95%.

Treatment

Treatment generally involves preventing infection, managing acute infection, and replacing missing immune components when possible.

Infection can be prevented by avoiding environmental exposures and live-virus vaccines (varicella, polio, measles, mumps, rubella). Patients at risk of serious infections (eg, those with SCID, chronic granulomatous disease, Wiskott-Aldrich syndrome, or asplenia) or a specific infection (eg, *Pneumocystis jiroveci* [formerly *P. carinii*] in patients with T-cell disorders) can be given prophylactic antibiotics (eg, 5 mg/kg trimethoprim-sulfamethoxazole po bid).

Management of acute infection involves timely use of antibiotics and sometimes surgery (eg, for abscesses) after attempts to obtain cultures. Antibiotics are chosen as usual. Self-limited viral infections can cause severe disease in immunocompromised patients. Antivirals (eg, amantadine, rimantadine, oseltamivir, zanamivir for influenza; acyclovir for herpes infection, including varicella-zoster; ribavirin for respiratory syncytial or parainfluenza viral infections) may be lifesaving.

When transfusions are necessary, blood products should come from cytomegalovirus-negative donors, be filtered to remove WBCs, and be irradiated (15 to 30 Gy) to prevent graft-vs-host disease.

Replacing missing immune components helps prevent infection; replacement therapies used in more than one primary immunodeficiency disorder include IV immune globulin and hematopoietic stem cell transplantation.

IV immune globulin (IVIG) is effective replacement therapy in most forms of antibody deficiency. The usual dose is 400 mg/kg at monthly intervals; treatment is begun at a low rate. Some patients need higher or more frequent doses. IVIG 800 mg/kg/mo helps some antibody-deficient patients who do not respond well to conventional doses, particularly those with a chronic lung disorder. High-dose IVIG aims to keep IgG trough levels in the normal range (> 500 mg/dL). IVIG may also be given by slow sc infusions at weekly intervals.

Hematopoietic stem cell transplantation using bone marrow, cord blood, or adult peripheral blood stem cells is effective for lethal T-cell and other immunodeficiencies. Pretransplantation chemotherapy is unnecessary in patients without T cells (eg, those with SCID). However, patients with intact T-cell function or partial T-cell deficiencies (eg, Wiskott-Aldrich syndrome, combined immunodeficiency with low but not absent T-cell function) require pretransplantation chemotherapy to ensure graft acceptance. When a matched sibling donor is unavailable, haploidentical bone marrow from a parent can be used. In such cases, mature T cells that cause graft-vs-host disease must be rigorously depleted from parental marrow before it is given. Umbilical cord blood from an HLA-matched sibling can also be used as a source of stem cells. In some cases, bone marrow or umbilical cord blood from a matched unrelated donor can be used, but immunosuppressants are required to prevent graft-vs-host disease, and their use delays restoration of immunity.

Retroviral vector gene therapy has been successful in a few patients with X-linked and ADA-deficient SCID, but this treatment is on hold because some patients developed leukemia.

ATAXIA-TELANGIECTASIA

Ataxia-telangiectasia results from a T-cell defect and causes progressive cerebellar ataxia, oculocutaneous telangiectasias, and recurrent sinopulmonary infections.

Inheritance is autosomal-recessive. Ataxia-telangiectasia is caused by mutations in the gene that encodes ataxia-telangiectasia–mutated (ATM) protein. ATM protein may be important in mitogenic signal transduction, meiotic recombination, and cell cycle control.

Onset of neurologic symptoms and evidence of immunodeficiency varies. Ataxia usually develops when children begin to walk. Progression of neurologic symptoms leads to severe disability. Speech becomes slurred, choreoathetoid movements and nystagmus develop, and muscle weakness usually progresses to muscle atrophy. Telangiectasias may not appear until age 4 to 6 yr; they are most prominent on the bulbar conjunctivae, ears, antecubital and popliteal fossae, and sides of the neck. Recurrent sinopulmonary infections lead to recurrent pneumonia, bronchiectasis, and chronic restrictive pulmonary disease. Patients often lack IgA and IgE and have a progressive T-cell defect. Endocrine abnormalities that may occur include gonadal dysgenesis, testicular atrophy, and diabetes mellitus.

Frequency of cancer (especially leukemia, brain tumors, and gastric cancer) is high, and frequency of chromosome breaks, consistent with a defect in DNA repair, is increased. Serum α_1-fetoprotein is usually elevated.

Treatment with antibiotics or IV immune globulin is of some value, but no treatment is effective for the CNS abnormalities. Thus, neurologic deterioration progresses, causing death, usually by age 30.

CHÉDIAK-HIGASHI SYNDROME

Chédiak-Higashi syndrome is characterized by impaired lysis of phagocytized bacteria, resulting in recurrent bacterial respiratory and other infections and oculocutaneous albinism.

Chédiak-Higashi syndrome is rare. Inheritance is autosomal recessive. The syndrome is caused by a mutation in a gene that regulates intracellular protein trafficking. Giant lysosomal granules develop in neutrophils and other cells (eg, melanocytes, neural Schwann cells). The abnormal lysosomes cannot fuse with phagosomes, so ingested bacteria cannot be lysed normally.

Clinical findings include oculocutaneous albinism and susceptibility to recurrent respiratory and other infections. In about 85% of patients, an accelerated phase occurs, causing fever, jaundice, hepatosplenomegaly, lymphadenopathy, pancytopenia, bleeding diathesis, and neurologic changes. Once the accelerated phase occurs, Chédiak-Higashi syndrome is usually fatal within 30 mo. Transplantation of unfractionated HLA-identical bone marrow after pretransplantation cytoreductive chemotherapy may be curative.

CHRONIC GRANULOMATOUS DISEASE

Chronic granulomatous disease is characterized by WBCs that cannot produce activated O_2 compounds and by defects in phagocytic cell microbicidal function. Manifestations include recurrent infections; multiple granulomatous lesions of the

lungs, liver, lymph nodes, and GI and GU tract; abscesses; lymphadenitis; hypergammaglobulinemia; elevated ESR; and anemia. Diagnosis is by assessing O_2 radical production in WBCs by a flow cytometric respiratory burst assay. Treatment is with antibiotics, antifungal drugs, and interferon-γ; granulocyte transfusions may be needed.

More than 50% of cases of chronic granulomatous disease (CDG) are inherited as an X-linked recessive trait and thus occur only in males; in the rest, inheritance is autosomal recessive. In CGD, WBCs do not produce hydrogen peroxide, superoxide, and other activated O_2 compounds because nicotinamide adenine dinucleotide phosphate oxidase activity is deficient. Phagocytic cell microbicidal function is defective, so that bacteria and fungi are not killed despite normal phagocytosis.

Symptoms and Signs

CGD usually begins with recurrent abscesses during early childhood, but in a few patients, onset is delayed until the early teens. Typical pathogens are catalase-producing organisms (eg, *Staphylococcus aureus*; *Escherichia coli*; *Serratia, Klebsiella,* and *Pseudomonas* sp; fungi). *Aspergillus* infections are the leading cause of death.

Multiple granulomatous lesions occur in the lungs, liver, lymph nodes, and GI and GU tract (causing obstruction). Suppurative lymphadenitis, hepatosplenomegaly, pneumonia, and hematologic evidence of chronic infection are common. Skin, lymph node, lung, liver, and perianal abscesses; stomatitis; and osteomyelitis also occur. Growth may be delayed. Hypergammaglobulinemia and anemia can occur; ESR is elevated.

Diagnosis and Treatment

Diagnosis is by a flow cytometric respiratory burst assay to detect O_2 radical production. The test can also identify female carriers of the X-linked form.

Treatment is continuous antibiotics, particularly trimethoprim-sulfamethoxazole 160/800 mg po bid alone or with cephalexin 500 mg po q 8 h. Oral antifungals are given as primary prophylaxis or are added if fungal infections occur even once; most useful are itraconazole po q 12 h (100 mg for patients < 13 yr; 200 mg for those ≥ 13 yr or weighing > 50 kg) or voriconazole po q 12 h (100 mg for those weighing < 40 kg; 200 mg for those weighing ≥ 40 kg). Interferon (IFN)-γ may reduce severity and frequency of infections, probably by increasing nonoxidative antimicrobial activity. Usual dose is 50 μg/m^2 sc 3 times/wk. Granulocyte transfusions are lifesaving when infections are severe. HLA-identical sibling bone marrow transplantation has been successful after pretransplantation chemotherapy, as has gene therapy.

COMMON VARIABLE IMMUNODEFICIENCY

Common variable immunodeficiency (acquired or adult-onset hypogammaglobulinemia) is characterized by low Ig levels with phenotypically normal B cells that can proliferate but do not develop into Ig-producing cells.

Common variable immunodeficiency (CVID) includes several different molecular defects, but in most patients, the molecular defect is unknown. CVID is clinically similar to X-linked agammaglobulinemia in the types of infections that develop, but onset tends to be later, even in adulthood. T-cell immunity may be impaired in some patients. Autoimmune disorders (eg, SLE, Addison's disease, thyroiditis, RA, alopecia areata, autoimmune hemolytic or pernicious anemia) can occur, as can malabsorption, nodular lymphoid hyperplasia of the GI tract, lymphoid interstitial pneumonia, splenomegaly, and bronchiectasis. Gastric carcinoma and lymphoma occur in 10% of patients.

Diagnosis is suggested by familial clustering of autoimmune disorders and is confirmed by measuring serum Ig and antibody titers to protein and polysaccharide vaccine antigens. If either measurement is low, B-cell quantification by flow cytometry is indicated to distinguish CVID from X-linked agammaglobulinemia and from multiple myeloma or chronic lymphocytic leukemia. Serum protein electrophoresis is indicated to screen for monoclonal gammopathies (eg, myeloma), which may be associated with reduced levels of other Ig isotypes. Treatment consists of IV immune globulin 400 mg/kg/mo and antibiotics as needed to treat infection.

DiGEORGE SYNDROME

DiGeorge syndrome is thymic and parathyroid hypoplasia or aplasia leading to T-cell immunodeficiency and hypoparathyroidism.

DiGeorge syndrome results from gene deletions in the DiGeorge chromosomal region at 22q11, mutations in genes at chromosome 10p13, and mutations in other unknown genes, which cause dysembryogenesis of structures that develop from pharyngeal pouches during the 8th wk of gestation. Most cases are sporadic; boys and girls are equally affected. DiGeorge syndrome may be partial, in which some T-cell function exists, or complete, in which T-cell function is absent.

Infants have low-set ears, midline facial clefts, a small receding mandible, hypertelorism, a shortened philtrum, and a congenital heart disorder. They also have thymic and parathyroid hypoplasia or aplasia, causing T-cell deficiency and hypoparathyroidism. Recurrent infections begin soon after birth, but the degree of immunodeficiency varies considerably, and T-cell function may improve spontaneously. Hypocalcemic tetany appears within 24 to 48 h of birth.

Prognosis often depends on severity of the heart disorder. For partial DiGeorge syndrome, hypoparathyroidism is treated with Ca and vitamin D supplementation; long-term survival is not affected. Complete DiGeorge syndrome is fatal without treatment, which is transplantation of cultured thymus tissue.

HYPER-IgE SYNDROME

Hyper-IgE syndrome is a combined B- and T-cell immunodeficiency characterized by recurrent staphylococcal abscesses of the skin, lungs, joints, and viscera starting in infancy.

Inheritance is autosomal dominant with incomplete penetrance; the genetic basis is unknown. Hyper-IgE syndrome typically causes recurrent staphylococcal abscesses of the skin, lungs, joints, and viscera with pulmonary pneumatoceles and a pruritic eosinophilic dermatitis. Patients have coarse facial features, delayed shedding of baby teeth, osteopenia, and recurrent fractures. All have tissue and blood eosinophilia and very high IgE levels (> 1000 IU/mL [> 2400 μg/L]). Treatment consists of lifelong continuous staphylococcal antibiotics (eg, dicloxacillin, cephalexin).

HYPER-IgM SYNDROME

Hyper-IgM syndrome is an Ig deficiency characterized by normal or elevated serum IgM levels and decreased or absent amounts of other serum Igs, resulting in susceptibility to bacterial infections.

Hyper-IgM syndrome may be X-linked or autosomal. Most cases are caused by mutation in a gene that is located on the X chromosome and that encodes a protein (CD154, or CD40 ligand) on the surfaces of activated helper T cells. In the presence of cytokines, normal CD40 ligand interacts with B cells and thus signals them to switch from producing IgM to producing IgA, IgG, or IgE. In X-linked hyper-IgM syndrome, T cells lack a functional CD154 and cannot signal B cells to switch. Thus, B cells produce only IgM; IgM levels may be normal or elevated. Patients with this form may have severe neutropenia and often present during infancy with *Pneumocystis jiroveci* (formerly *P. carinii*) pneumonia. Otherwise, clinical presentation is similar to that of X-linked agammaglobulinemia and includes recurrent pyogenic bacterial sinopulmonary infections during the 1st 2 yr of life. Susceptibility to *Cryptosporidium* sp may be increased. Lymphoid tissue is very small because germinal centers are missing. Many patients die before puberty, and those who live longer often develop cirrhosis or B-cell lymphomas.

At least 4 autosomal recessive forms of hyper-IgM syndrome involve a B-cell defect. In 2 of these forms (activation-induced cytidine deaminase and uracil DNA glycosylase or UNG deficiencies), serum IgM levels are much higher than in the X-linked form; lymphoid hyperplasia (including lymphadenopathy, splenomegaly, and tonsillar hypertrophy) is present and autoimmune disorders may be present.

Diagnosis is clinical and by demonstrating normal or elevated serum IgM levels and low or absent levels of other Igs. Treatment is IV immune globulin 400 mg/kg/mo. For the X-linked form, granulocyte colony-stimulating factor is also given as needed for neutropenia, and because prognosis is poor, bone marrow transplantation is preferred if an HLA-identical sibling donor is available.

IgA DEFICIENCY

IgA deficiency is an IgA level < 10 mg/dL with normal IgG and IgM levels. It is the most common primary immunodeficiency. Many patients are asymptomatic, but some develop recurrent infections and autoimmune disorders. Diagnosis is by measuring

serum Ig. Some patients develop common variable immunodeficiency, and some remit spontaneously. Treatment is avoidance of blood products that contain IgA; antibiotics are given as needed.

IgA deficiency affects up to 1/333 people. Transmission is autosomal dominant with incomplete penetrance. IgA deficiency is commonly associated with certain HLA haplotypes, and rare alleles or deletions of genes in the major histocompatibility complex (MHC) class III (see p. 1326) region are common. IgA deficiency also occurs in siblings of children with common variable immunodeficiency (CVID) and evolves into CVID in some patients. Drugs such as phenytoin, sulfasalazine, colloidal gold and D-penicillamine may lead to IgA deficiency in genetically susceptible patients.

Symptoms, Signs, and Diagnosis

Many patients are asymptomatic; others have recurrent sinopulmonary infections, diarrhea, allergies, or autoimmune disorders (eg, celiac or inflammatory bowel disease, SLE, chronic active hepatitis). Anti-IgA antibodies may develop after exposure to IgA in plasma or to immune globulin; anaphylactic reactions to IV immune globulin (IVIG) and other blood products that contain IgA may occur.

Diagnosis is suspected in patients who have recurrent infections (including giardiasis); anaphylactic transfusion reactions; or a family history of CVID, IgA deficiency, or autoimmune disorders or who are taking drugs that lead to IgA deficiency. Diagnosis is confirmed by a serum IgA level < 10 mg/dL with normal IgG and IgM levels and normal antibody titers in response to vaccine antigens.

Prognosis and Treatment

A few IgA-deficient patients develop CVID over time; others improve spontaneously. Prognosis is worse if an autoimmune disorder develops.

Treatment is avoidance of blood products that contain IgA because even trace amounts can elicit an anti-IgA–mediated anaphylactic reaction. If RBC transfusion is needed, only washed RBCs or frozen blood can be used. Antibiotics are given as needed for bacterial infections of the ears, sinuses, lungs, or GI or GU tract. IVIG is contraindicated because many patients have antibodies to IgA and because IVIG is > 99% IgG, which patients do not need. Patients are advised to wear an identification bracelet to prevent inadvertent plasma or IVIG administration, which could lead to anaphylaxis.

LEUKOCYTE ADHESION DEFICIENCY

Leukocyte adhesion deficiency results from an adhesion molecule defect that causes granulocyte and lymphocyte dysfunction and recurrent soft-tissue infections.

Inheritance is autosomal recessive. Leukocyte adhesion deficiency is caused by deficiency of adhesive glycoproteins on the surfaces of WBCs that facilitate cellular interactions, cell attachment to blood vessel walls, cell movement, and interaction with complement fragments. Deficiencies impair the ability of granulocytes (and lymphocytes) to migrate out of the intravascular compartment, to engage in cytotoxic reactions, and to phagocytose bacteria. Severity of disease correlates with degree of deficiency.

Severely affected infants have recurrent or progressive necrotic soft-tissue infections with staphylococcal and gram-negative organisms, periodontitis, poor wound healing, leukocytosis, and delayed (> 3 wk) umbilical cord detachment. WBC counts remain high even between infections. Infections become increasingly difficult to control.

Diagnosis is by demonstrating absence or severe deficiency of adhesive glycoproteins on the surface of WBCs using monoclonal antibodies (eg, anti-CD11 or anti-CD18) and flow cytometry. Leukocytosis on CBC testing is common but nonspecific. Most patients die by age 5 unless treated successfully by bone marrow transplantation, but moderately affected patients survive into young adulthood. Treatment is with antibiotics, often given continuously. Granulocyte transfusions can also help. Bone marrow transplantation is the only effective treatment and can be curative.

SEVERE COMBINED IMMUNODEFICIENCY

Severe combined immunodeficiency is characterized by absent T cells and a low, high, or normal number of B cells and natural killer cells. Most infants develop opportunistic infections within the 1st 3 mo of life.

Diagnosis is by demonstrating lymphopenia, an absence or very low number of T cells, and impaired lymphocyte proliferative responses to mitogens. Patients must be kept in protected environments; definitive treatment is bone marrow stem cell transplantation.

Severe combined immunodeficiency (SCID) is caused by mutations in at least 10 different genes that produce 4 phenotypes. In all forms, T cells are absent (T-); the number of B cells and natural killer (NK) cells may be low or none (B-; NK-) or high or normal (B+; NK+), depending on the form of SCID. However, B cells, even when normal in number, cannot function because T cells are absent. The most common form is X-linked. It affects the IL-2 receptor γ chain (a component of at least 6 cytokine receptors) and thus causes severe disease; phenotype is T- B+ NK-. For other forms, inheritance is autosomal recessive. The 2nd most common form results from adenosine deaminase (ADA) deficiency, which leads to apoptosis of precursors for B, T, and NK cells; phenotype is T- B- NK-. The next most common form results from IL-7 receptor α-chain deficiency; phenotype is T- B+ NK+.

By age 6 mo, most infants with SCID develop candidiasis, pneumonia, and diarrhea, leading to failure to thrive. Some have graft-vs-host disease due to maternal lymphocytes or blood transfusions. Other infants present at age 6 to 12 mo. Exfoliative dermatitis may develop as part of Omenn's syndrome. ADA deficiency may cause bony abnormalities.

Diagnosis, Prognosis, and Treatment

Diagnosis is by demonstrating lymphopenia, a low number of or no T cells, absent lymphocyte proliferative responses to mitogens, an absent thymic shadow on x-ray, and decreased lymphoid tissue.

All forms of SCID are fatal in infancy without early diagnosis and treatment. Treatment with IV immune globulin (IVIG) and antibiotics, including *Pneumocystis jiroveci* (formerly *P. carinii*) prophylaxis, is helpful but not curative. In 90 to 100% of infants with SCID or its variants, bone marrow stem cell transplantation from an HLA-identical, mixed leukocyte culture–matched sibling restores immunity. When an HLA-identical sibling is not available, haploidentical bone marrow from a parent that is rigorously depleted of T cells can be used. If SCID is diagnosed by age 3 mo, the survival rate after transplantation with either type of bone marrow is 95%. Pretransplantation chemotherapy is unnecessary because patients do not have T cells and therefore cannot reject a graft. Patients with ADA deficiency who do not receive a bone marrow graft may be treated with injections of polyethylene glycol–modified bovine ADA once or twice/wk. Gene therapy has been successful in X-linked SCID but has caused T-cell leukemias, precluding its current use.

TRANSIENT HYPOGAMMAGLOBULINEMIA OF INFANCY

Transient hypogammaglobulinemia of infancy is a temporary decrease in serum IgG and sometimes IgA and other Ig isotypes to levels below age-appropriate normal values.

In transient hypogammaglobulinemia of infancy, IgG levels continue to be low after the physiologic fall in maternal IgG at around age 3 to 6 mo. The condition rarely leads to significant infections and is not thought to be a true immunodeficiency. Diagnosis is by serum Ig measurements and demonstration that antibody production in response to vaccine antigens (eg, tetanus, diphtheria) is normal. Thus, this condition can be distinguished from permanent forms of hypogammaglobulinemia, in which specific antibodies to vaccine antigens are not produced. IVIG replacement therapy is unnecessary; this condition may persist for months to a few years but usually resolves.

WISKOTT-ALDRICH SYNDROME

Wiskott-Aldrich syndrome results from a combined B- and T-cell defect and is characterized by recurrent infection, atopic dermatitis, and thrombocytopenia.

Inheritance is X-linked recessive. Wiskott-Aldrich syndrome is caused by mutations in the gene that encodes the Wiskott-Aldrich syndrome protein (WASP), a cytoplasmic protein necessary for normal B- and T-cell signaling. Because B- and T-cell functions are impaired, infections with pyogenic bacteria and opportunistic organisms, particularly viruses and *Pneumocystis jiroveci* (formerly *P. carinii*), develop. The 1st manifestations often are hemorrhagic (usually bloody diarrhea), followed by recurrent respiratory infections, eczema, and thrombocytopenia. Cancers, especially Epstein-Barr virus lymphomas and acute lymphoblastic leukemia, develop in about 10% of patients > 10 yr.

Diagnosis is by demonstrating impaired antibody responses to polysaccharide antigens, cutaneous anergy, partial T-cell immunodeficiency, elevated IgE and IgA levels, low IgM levels, and low or normal IgG levels. Antibodies to polysaccharide antigens (eg, blood group antigens A and B) may be selectively deficient. Platelets are small and defective, and splenic destruction of platelets is increased, causing thrombocytopenia. Mutation analysis may be used.

Treatment is splenectomy, continuous antibiotics, IVIG, and HLA-identical bone marrow transplantation. Without transplantation, most patients die by age 15; however, some patients may survive into adulthood.

X-LINKED AGAMMAGLOBULINEMIA

(Bruton's Disease)

X-linked agammaglobulinemia is characterized by low or absent levels of Igs and antibodies and absent B cells, leading to recurrent infections with encapsulated bacteria.

X-linked agammaglobulinemia results from mutations in a gene on the X chromosome that encodes the Bruton tyrosine kinase (Btk). Btk is essential for B-cell development and maturation; without it, there are no B cells and no antibodies. As a result, male infants have very small tonsils and do not develop lymph nodes; they have recurrent pyogenic lung, sinus, and skin infections with encapsulated bacteria (eg, *Streptococcus pneumoniae, Haemophilus influenzae*). Patients are also susceptible to persistent CNS infections from live oral polio vaccine and with echoviruses and coxsackieviruses; these infections can also present as progressive dermatomyositis with or without encephalitis.

Diagnosis is by demonstrating low IgG levels (< 100 mg/dL) and absent B cells (< 1% CD19+ cells by flow cytometry). They may also have transient neutropenia. If the mutation has been identified in family members, mutational analysis of chorionic villus, amniocentesis, or percutaneous umbilical cord blood samples can provide prenatal diagnosis.

Treatment is IV immune globulin 400 mg/kg/mo. Prompt use of adequate antibiotics for each infection is crucial; bronchiectasis requires continuous rotation of antibiotics. With early diagnosis and appropriate treatment, prognosis is good unless CNS viral infections develop.

X-LINKED LYMPHOPROLIFERATIVE SYNDROME

(Duncan's Syndrome)

X-linked lymphoproliferative syndrome results from a T-cell and natural killer cell defect and is characterized by an abnormal response to Epstein-Barr virus infection, leading to liver failure, immunodeficiency, lymphoma, fatal lymphoproliferative disease, or bone marrow aplasia.

X-linked lymphoproliferative syndrome is caused by mutations in a gene on the X chromosome that encodes a T and natural killer (NK) cell–specific protein called SAP. Without SAP, lymphocytes proliferate unchecked in response to Epstein-Barr virus (EBV) infection, and NK cells do not function.

The syndrome is usually asymptomatic until EBV infection develops. Then most patients develop fulminating or fatal infectious mononucleosis with liver failure (caused by cytotoxic T cells that react to EBV-infected B or other tissue cells); survivors of initial infection develop B-cell lymphomas, aplastic anemia, hypogammaglobulinemia (resembling that in common variable immunodeficiency), or a combination.

Diagnostic findings in patients that survive initial EBV infection include hypogammaglobulinemia, decreased antibody responses to antigens (particularly to EBV nuclear antigen), impaired T-cell proliferative responses to mitogens, decreased NK-cell function, and an inverted CD4:CD8 ratio. Genetic diagnosis by mutation analysis is possible before EBV infection and symptoms develop.

About 75% of patients die by age 10, and all die by age 40 unless bone marrow transplantation is done. It is curative if done before EBV infection becomes fatal.

ZAP-70 DEFICIENCY

ZAP-70 (zeta-associated protein 70) deficiency is impaired T-cell activation caused by a signaling defect.

ZAP-70 is important in T-cell signaling and in T-cell selection in the thymus. ZAP-70 deficiency causes T-cell activation defects.

Patients who have ZAP-70 deficiency present in infancy or early childhood with recurrent infections similar to those in severe combined immunodeficiency (SCID); however, they live longer, and the deficiency may not be diagnosed until they are several years old. Patients have normal, low, or elevated serum Ig levels and normal or elevated numbers of circulating CD4 T cells but essentially no CD8 T cells. Their CD4 T cells do not respond to mitogens or allogeneic cells in vitro and do not generate cytotoxic T cells. In contrast, natural killer cell activity is normal. The disorder is fatal unless treated by bone marrow transplantation.

165 ALLERGIC AND OTHER HYPERSENSITIVITY DISORDERS

Allergic and other hypersensitivity disorders are caused by exaggerated immune reactions unrelated to injury or infection.

The Gell and Coombs classification delineates 4 types of hypersensitivity reaction. Hypersensitivity disorders often involve more than one type.

Type I reactions (immediate hypersensitivity) are IgE-mediated. Antigen binds to IgE (which is bound to tissue mast cells and blood basophils), triggering release of preformed mediators (eg, histamine, proteases, chemotactic factors) and synthesis of other mediators (eg, prostaglandins, leukotrienes, platelet-activating factor, ILs). These mediators cause vasodilation; increased capillary permeability; mucus hypersecretion; smooth muscle spasm; and tissue infiltration with eosinophils, helper type 2 T cells (T_H2), and other inflammatory cells. Type I reactions underlie atopic disorders (including allergic asthma, rhinitis, and conjunctivitis) and latex and some food allergies.

Type II reactions result when antibody binds to cellular or tissue antigens or to a hapten coupled to a cell or tissue. The antigen-antibody complex activates cytotoxic T cells or macrophages and complement, leading to cell and tissue damage (antibody-dependent cell-mediated cytotoxicity). Disorders involving type II reactions include hyperacute graft rejection of an organ transplant, Coombs'-positive hemolytic anemias, Hashimoto's thyroiditis, and Goodpasture's syndrome (see TABLE 165–1).

Type III reactions cause acute inflammation in response to circulating antigen-antibody immune complexes deposited in vessels or tissue. These complexes can activate the complement system or bind to and activate certain immune cells, resulting in release of inflammatory mediators. The consequences of immune complex formation depend in part on the relative proportions of antigen and antibody in the immune complex. Early, there is excess antigen with small antigen-antibody complexes, which do not activate complement. Later, when antigen and antibody are more balanced, immune complexes are larger and tend to be deposited in various tissues (glomeruli, blood vessels), causing systemic reactions. Type III disorders include serum sickness, SLE, RA, leukocytoclastic vasculitis, cryoglobulinemia, hypersensitivity pneumonitis, bronchopulmonary aspergillosis, and several types of glomerulonephritis.

Type IV reactions (delayed hypersensitivity) are T cell–mediated. There are 4 subtypes based on the T-cell subpopulation involved: helper type 1 T cells (IVa), helper type 2 T cells (IVb), cytotoxic T cells (IVc), and IL-8-secreting T cells (IVd). These cells, sensitized

TABLE 165–1. PUTATIVE AUTOIMMUNE DISORDERS

LIKELIHOOD	DISORDER	MECHANISM OR EVIDENCE
Highly probable	Autoimmune hemolytic anemia	Phagocytosis of antibody-sensitized RBCs
	Autoimmune thrombocytopenic purpura	Phagocytosis of antibody-sensitized platelets
	Goodpasture's syndrome	Anti-basement membrane antibody
	Graves' disease	TSH receptor antibody (stimulatory)
	Hashimoto's thyroiditis	Cell- and antibody-mediated thyroid cytotoxicity
	Insulin resistance	Insulin-receptor antibody
	Myasthenia gravis	Acetylcholine receptor antibody
	Pemphigus	Epidermal acantholytic antibody
	SLE	Circulating and locally generalized immune complexes
Probable	Adrenergic drug resistance (in some patients with asthma or cystic fibrosis)	β-adrenergic receptor antibody
	Bullous pemphigoid	IgG and complement in basement membrane
	Diabetes mellitus (some cases)	Cell- and antibody-mediated islet cell antibodies
	Glomerulonephritis	Glomerular basement membrane antibody or immune complexes
	Idiopathic Addison's disease	Antibody and possibly cell-mediated adrenal cytotoxicity
	Infertility (some cases)	Antispermatozoal antibodies
	Mixed connective tissue disease	Antibody to extractable nuclear antigen (ribonucleoprotein)
	Pernicious anemia	Antiparietal cell, microsomes, and intrinsic factor antibodies
	Polymyositis	Nonhistone ANA
	RA	Immune complexes in joints
	Systemic sclerosis with anti-collagen antibodies	Nucleolar and other nuclear antibodies
	Sjögren's syndrome	Multiple tissue antibodies, a specific nonhistone anti–SS-B antibody
Possible	Chronic active hepatitis	Smooth muscle antibody
	Endocrine gland failure	Specific tissue antibodies (in some cases)
	Post-MI, cardiotomy syndrome	Myocardial antibody
	Primary biliary cirrhosis	Mitochondrial antibody
	Urticaria, atopic dermatitis, asthma (some cases)	IgG and IgM antibodies to IgE
	Vasculitis	Ig and complement in vessel walls, low serum component, (in some cases)
	Vitiligo	Melanocyte antibody
	Many other inflammatory, granulomatous, degenerative, and atrophic disorders	No reasonable alternative explanation

ANA = antinuclear antibody; TSH = thyroid-stimulating hormone.

after contact with a specific antigen, are activated by reexposure to the antigen; they damage tissue by direct toxic effects or through release of cytokines, which activate eosinophils, monocytes and macrophages, neutrophils, or killer cells depending on type. Disorders involving type IV reactions include contact dermatitis (eg, poison ivy), hypersensitivity pneumonitis, allograft rejection, tuberculosis, and many forms of drug hypersensitivity.

ANGIOEDEMA

Angioedema is edema of the deep dermis and subcutaneous tissues. It is caused by exposure to drug, venom, dietary, or extracted allergens. The main symptom is diffuse, painful swelling, sometimes marked. Diagnosis is by examination. Treatment is elimination or avoidance of the allergen and H_1 blockers.

Acute angioedema is essentially anaphylaxis of the subcutaneous tissues. It is sometimes accompanied by urticaria (local wheals and erythema in the skin—see p. 936); the two have similar causes (eg, drug, venom, dietary, or extracted allergens). Also, angioedema is pathogenetically related to urticaria, which occurs at the epidermal-dermal junction.

Chronic (> 6 wk) angioedema is rarely IgE-mediated and is more difficult to explain. Cause is usually unknown (idiopathic), but chronic ingestion of an unsuspected drug or chemical (eg, penicillin in milk, a nonprescription drug, preservatives, other food additives) is sometimes the cause. A few cases are hereditary (see below).

Symptoms and Signs

Angioedema may be slightly pruritic or nonpruritic. It is characterized by locally diffuse and painful soft tissue swelling that may be asymmetric, especially on the eyelids, lips, face, and tongue but also on the back of hands or feet and on genitals. Edema of the upper airways may cause respiratory distress, and the stridor may be mistaken for asthma. Complete airway obstruction may occur.

Diagnosis and Treatment

The cause is often obvious, and diagnostic tests are seldom required because reactions are self-limited and nonrecurrent. No test is particularly useful. Erythropoietic protoporphyria may mimic allergic forms of angioedema and can be distinguished by measuring blood and fecal porphyrins (see p. 1231).

For acute angioedema, treatment is removing or avoiding the allergen and relieving symptoms (eg, with H_1 blockers—see p. 1355 and TABLE 165–2). Prednisone 30 to 40 mg po once/day is indicated for more severe reactions. Topical corticosteroids are useless. If a cause is not obvious, all nonessential drugs should be stopped. Pharyngeal or laryngeal angioedema requires epinephrine 0.3 mL of a 1:1000 solution sc. It may be supplemented with an IV antihistamine (eg, diphenhydramine 50 to 100 mg). Long-term treatment may involve H_1 and H_2 blockers and occasionally corticosteroids.

HEREDITARY ANGIOEDEMA

Hereditary angioedema is caused by deficiency (type 1; in 85%) or dysfunction (type 2; in 15%) of C1 inhibitor, a protein that regulates the classical complement activation pathway (see p. 1327).

Inheritance is autosomal dominant. C1 inhibitor deficiency may also develop when complement is consumed in neoplastic disorders or when C1 inhibitor autoantibody is produced in monoclonal gammopathy (acquired deficiency). Attacks are precipitated by trauma or viral illness and aggravated by emotional stress.

Symptoms and signs are similar to those of angioedema except that edema progresses until complement components have been consumed; the GI tract is often involved, causing nausea, vomiting, colic, and signs of intestinal obstruction.

Diagnosis is by detection of low levels of C2 and C4 (substrates of C1 inhibitor), normal levels of C1q (a fragment of C1), and low C1 inhibitor function. C1 inhibitor protein levels are low in type 1; levels are normal or increased in type 2. In acquired C1 inhibitor deficiency, C1q levels are low.

Treatment is attenuated androgens (eg, stanozolol 2 mg po tid or danazol 200 mg po tid) to stimulate hepatic C1 inhibitor synthesis. Some experts advocate administering fresh frozen plasma immediately before dental or medical procedures to prevent attacks, but this approach is not standard practice and could theoretically provoke an attack by providing substrate for angioedema. Purified C1

TABLE 165–2. ORAL H1 BLOCKERS

DRUG	USUAL ADULT DOSAGE	USUAL PEDIATRIC DOSAGE	AVAILABLE PREPARATIONS
Sedating*			
Azatadine maleate	1–2 mg bid	≤ 12 yr: not recommended > 12 yr: adult dose	1-mg tablets†
Brompheniramine maleate	4 mg q 4–6 h or 8 mg q 8–12 h	< 6 yr: 0.125 mg/kg q 6 h (maximum dose 6–8 mg/day) 6–12 yr: 2–4 mg q 6–8 h (maximum dose 12–16 mg/day) > 12 yr: adult dose	4-, 8-, and 12-mg tablets 2 mg/5 mL elixir 8- and 12-mg tablets (sustained-release)
Chlorpheniramine maleate	2–4 mg q 4–6 h	< 6 yr: not recommended 6–11 yr: 2 mg q 4–6 h (maximum dose 12 mg/day) ≥ 12 yr: adult dose	2-mg chewable tablets 4-, 8-, and 12-mg tablets 2 mg/5 mL syrup 8- and 12-mg tablets or capsules (timed-release)
Clemastine fumarate	1.34 mg bid to 2.68 mg tid	6–12 yr: 0.5 mg q 12 h (maximum dose 3 mg/day)‡	1.34- and 2.68-mg tablets 0.67 mg/5 mL syrup
Cyproheptadine HCl	4 mg tid or qid (maximum 0.5 mg/kg/day)	2–6 yr: 2 mg bid to tid (maximum 12 mg/day) 7–14 yr: 4 mg bid to tid (maximum 16 mg/day)	4-mg tablets† 2 mg/5 mL syrup
Dexchlorpheniramine maleate	2 mg q 4–6 h	2–5 yr: 0.5 mg q 4–6 h (maximum dose 3 mg/day) 6–11 yr: 1 mg q 4–6 h (maximum dose 6 mg/day)	2-mg tablets 2 mg/5 mL syrup 4- and 6-mg tablets (extended-release)
Diphenhydramine HCl	25–50 mg q 4–6 h	1.25 mg/kg q 6 h (maximum dose 300 mg/day)	25- and 50-mg capsules or tablets 12.5 mg/mL syrup 12.5 mg/5 mL elixir
Diphenylpyraline HCl	5 mg q 12 h	No data	5-mg capsules (sustained action)
Hydroxyzine HCl	25–50 mg tid or qid	0.7 mg/kg tid	25-, 50-, and 100-mg capsules 10-, 25-, 50-, and 100-mg tablets 10 mg/5 mL syrup 25 mg/5 mL oral suspension
Methdilazine HCl	8 mg q 6–12 h	> 3 yr: 4 mg q 6–12 h	8-mg tablets 4-mg chewable tablets 4 mg/5 mL syrup
Promethazine HCl	12.5–25 mg bid	< 2 yr: contraindicated ≥ 2 yr: 6.25–12.5 mg bid or tid	12.5-, 25-, and 50-mg tablets† 6.25 and 25 mg/5 mL syrup

Table continues on the following page.

TABLE 165–2. ORAL H_1 BLOCKERS—Continued

DRUG	USUAL ADULT DOSAGE	USUAL PEDIATRIC DOSAGE	AVAILABLE PREPARATIONS
Trimeprazine tartrate	2.5 mg qid	6 mo–3 yr, 1.25 mg at bedtime or tid > 3 yr: 2.5 mg at bedtime or tid	2.5-mg tablets 2.5 mg/5 mL syrup† 5-mg capsules (timed-release)
Tripelennamine citrate	25–50 mg q 4–6 h	1.9 mg/kg qid (maximum dose 450 mg/day)	37.5 mg/5 mL elixir (1 mL citrate = 5 mg HCl salt)
Tripelennamine HCl	25–50 mg q 4–6 h	1.25 mg/kg qid (maximum dose 300 mg/day)	25- and 50-mg tablets 100-mg tablets (timed-release)
Triprolidine HCl	2.5 mg q 4–6 h (maximum 10 mg/day)	4 mo–2 yr: 0.313 mg q 4–6 h (maximum 1.25 mg/day) 2–4 yr: 0.625 mg q 4–6 h (maximum dose 2.5 mg/day) 4–6 yr: 0.938 mg q 4–6 h (maximum dose 3.744 mg/day) 6–12 yr: 1.25 mg q 4–6 h (maximum dose 5 mg/day)§	2.5-mg tablets 1.25 mg/5 mL syrup
Nonsedating			
Acrivastine	8 mg bid or tid	< 12 yr: not recommended ≥ 12 yr: adult dose	8-mg capsules
Cetirizine	5–10 mg once/day	> 12 yr: adult dose	5- and 10-mg tablets
Desloratadine	5 mg once/day	> 12 yr: adult dose	5-mg tablets
Ebastine	10–20 mg once/day	6–12 yr: 5 mg 12–17 yr: 5–20 mg once/day	10-mg tablets
Fexofenadine	60 mg bid or 180 mg once/day	6–11 yr: 30 mg bid ≥ 12 yr: adult dose	60- and 180-mg tablets
Levocetirizine	5 mg once/day	No data	5-mg tablets
Loratadine	10 mg once/day	2–5 yr: 5 mg once/day ≥ 6 yr: adult dose	10-mg tablets, 1 mg/mL syrup
Mizolastine	10 mg once/day	No data	10-mg tablets

NA = not applicable.

*All sedating antihistamines have strong anticholinergic properties. They should generally not be used in the elderly and in patients with glaucoma, benign prostatic hyperplasia, delirium, dementia, and orthostatic hypotension. These drugs commonly cause dry mouth, blurred vision, urinary retention, constipation, and orthostatic hypotension.

†Do not increase frequency in children.

‡Not approved for children < 6 yr, but a dose of 0.05 mg/kg/day (maximum dose 1 mg/day) has been safely used in this age group.

§Higher maximum doses are used outside the US: < 1 yr: 1 mg q 8 h; 1–6 yr: 2 mg q 8 h; 6–12 yr: 3 mg q 8 h.

inhibitor and recombinant C1 inhibitor are being developed for acute treatment.

ATOPIC AND ALLERGIC DISORDERS

Type I hypersensitivity reactions underlie all atopic and many allergic disorders. The terms atopy and allergy are often used interchangeably but are different. Atopy is an exaggerated IgE-mediated immune response; all atopic disorders are type I hypersensitivity disorders. Allergy is any exaggerated immune response to a foreign antigen regardless of mechanism. Thus, all atopic disorders are considered allergic, but many allergic disorders (eg, hypersensitivity pneumonitis) are not atopic. Allergic disorders are the most common disorders among people.

Atopic disorders most commonly affect the nose, eyes, skin, and lungs. These disorders include atopic dermatitis, contact dermatitis, urticaria (see p. 936) and angioedema (which may be primary skin disorders or symptoms of systemic disorders), latex allergy (see sidebar 165–1), allergic lung disorders (eg, asthma, allergic bronchopulmonary aspergillosis, hypersensitivity pneumonitis), and allergic reactions to venomous stings.

Etiology

Complex genetic, environmental, and site-specific factors contribute to development of allergies. A role for genetic factors is suggested by familial inheritance of disease, association between atopy and specific HLA loci, and polymorphisms of genes for the high-affinity IgE receptor β chain, IL-4, and CD14.

Environmental factors interact with genetic factors to maintain helper type 2 T (T_H2) cell immune responses, which activate eosinophils and IgE production and are proallergic. Normally, early childhood exposure to bacterial and viral infections and endotoxins (eg, lipopolysaccharide) shifts native T_H2-cell responses to helper type 1 T (T_H1)-cell responses, which suppress T_H2 cells and induce tolerance to foreign antigens; the mechanism may be mediated by Toll-like receptor-4 and occur through development of a population of regulatory T (CD4+CD25+) cells that suppress T_H2-cell responses. But trends in developed countries toward smaller families with fewer children, cleaner indoor environments, and early use of vaccinations and antibiotics may deprive children of these exposures and inhibit T_H2-cell suppression; such behavioral changes may explain the increased prevalence of some allergic disorders. Other factors thought to contribute to allergy development include chronic allergen exposure and sensitization, diet, and physical activity.

Site-specific factors include adhesion molecules in bronchial epithelium and in skin and molecules in the GI tract that direct T_H2 cells to target tissues.

By definition, an allergen induces IgE-mediated and T_H2-cell immune responses. Allergic triggers are almost always low molecular weight proteins, many of which can be constituted as airborne particles. Allergens most commonly responsible for acute and chronic allergic reactions include house dust, mite feces, animal dander, pollens (tree, grass, and weed), and molds.

Pathophysiology

When allergen binds to IgE, histamine is released from intracellular granules of mast cells, which are widely distributed but most concentrated in skin, lungs, and GI mucosa; histamine reinforces immune cell activation and is the primary mediator of clinical atopy. Physical disruption of tissue and various chemicals (eg, tissue irritants, opioids, surface-active agents) can trigger histamine release directly, independent of IgE.

Sidebar 165–1. LATEX SENSITIVITY

Latex sensitivity is an exaggerated immune response to water-soluble proteins in latex products (eg, rubber gloves, dental dams, condoms, tubing for respiratory equipment, catheters, enema tips with inflatable latex cuffs), causing urticaria, angioedema, and anaphylaxis.

Reactions to latex may be acute (IgE-mediated) or delayed (cell-mediated). Acute reactions cause urticaria and anaphylaxis; delayed reactions cause dermatitis. Diagnosis is by history. Assays for detecting IgE anti-latex antibodies and patch tests for detecting anti-latex cellular immunity are being developed, but none is well-validated yet. Treatment is avoidance of latex.

Histamine causes local vasodilation (producing erythema), increased capillary permeability and edema (producing a wheal), surrounding arteriolar vasodilation mediated by neuronal reflex mechanisms (producing flare), and stimulation of sensory nerves (producing itching). Histamine causes smooth muscle contraction in the airways (bronchoconstriction) and in the GI tract (increased GI motility) and increases salivary and bronchial gland secretions. When released systemically, it is a potent arteriolar dilator and can cause extensive peripheral pooling of blood and hypotension; cerebral vasodilation may be a factor in vascular headache. Histamine increases capillary permeability; the resulting loss of plasma and plasma proteins from the vascular space can worsen circulatory shock. It triggers a compensatory catecholamine surge from adrenal chromaffin cells.

Symptoms and Signs

Common symptoms include rhinorrhea, sneezing, and nasal congestion (upper respiratory tract); wheezing and dyspnea (lower respiratory tract); and itching (eyes, skin). Signs may include nasal turbinate edema, sinus pain on palpation, wheezing, conjunctival hyperemia and edema, and skin lichenification. Stridor, wheezing, and sometimes hypotension are life-threatening signs of anaphylaxis (see p. 1360). In some children, a narrow and high-arched palate, narrow chin, and elongated maxilla with overbite (allergic facies) are thought to be associated with chronic allergy.

Diagnosis

A thorough history is generally more reliable than testing or screening. History should include questions about frequency and duration of attacks and changes over time, triggering factors if identifiable, relation to seasonal or situational settings (eg, predictably occurring during pollen seasons; after exposure to animals, hay, or dust; during exercise; or in particular places), family history of similar symptoms or of atopic disorders, and responses to attempted treatments. Age at onset may be important in asthma because childhood asthma is likely to be atopic and asthma beginning after age 30 is not.

Nonspecific tests: Certain tests can suggest but not confirm an allergic origin of symptoms.

CBC should be ordered to detect eosinophilia in all patients except those taking corticosteroids, which reduce the eosinophil count. An eosinophil differential of 5 to 15% of total WBCs suggests atopy but is nonspecific; 16 to 40% may reflect atopy or other conditions (eg, drug hypersensitivity, cancer, autoimmune disorders, parasitic infection); a differential of 50 to 90% almost never occurs in atopic disorders and is more characteristic of hypereosinophilic syndrome or visceral larva migrans. Total WBC is usually normal.

Conjunctival or nasal secretions or sputum can be examined for leukocytes; finding any eosinophils indicates that T_H2-mediated allergic inflammation is likely.

Serum IgE levels are elevated in atopic disorders but are of little help in diagnosis because they are also elevated in parasitic infections, infectious mononucleosis, autoimmune disorders, drug reactions, immunodeficiency disorders (hyper-IgE syndrome—see p. 1344—and Wiskott-Aldrich syndrome—see p. 1346), and in some forms of multiple myeloma. IgE levels are probably most helpful for following response to therapy in allergic bronchopulmonary aspergillosis (see p. 398).

Specific tests: Skin testing uses standardized concentrations of antigen introduced directly into skin and is indicated when a detailed history and physical examination do not identify the cause and triggers for symptoms. Skin testing has higher positive predictive values for diagnosing allergic rhinosinusitis and conjunctivitis than for diagnosing allergic asthma or food allergy; negative predictive value for food allergy is high. The most commonly used antigens are pollens (tree, grass, and weed), molds, house dust mites, animal danders and sera, insect venom, foods, and β-lactam antibiotics. Choice of antigens to include is based on patient history and geographic prevalence. Two techniques can be used, percutaneous (prick) and intradermal. The prick test can detect most allergies. The intradermal test is more sensitive but less specific; it can be used to evaluate sensitivity to allergens with negative or equivocal prick test results.

For the prick technique, a drop of antigen extract is placed on the skin, which is then pricked or punctured through the extract by tenting up the skin with the tip of a 27-gauge needle held at a 20° angle or with a commercially available prick device. For the intradermal technique, just enough extract to produce a 1- or 2-mm bleb (typically 0.02 mL) is injected intradermally with a 0.5- or 1-mL syringe and a 27-gauge short-bevel needle.

Prick and intradermal skin testing should include the diluent alone as a negative control and histamine (10 mg/mL for prick tests, 0.01 mL of a 1:1000 solution for intradermal tests) as a positive control. For patients who have had a recent (< 1 yr) generalized reaction to the test antigen, testing begins with the standard reagent diluted 100-fold, then 10-fold, and then the standard concentration. A test is considered positive if a wheal and flare reaction occurs and wheal diameter is 3 to 5 mm greater than that of the negative control after 15 to 20 min. False positives occur in dermatographism (a wheal and flare reaction provoked by stroking or scraping the skin). False negatives occur when allergen extracts are improperly stored or outdated or when drugs (eg, antihistamines) suppress reactivity.

Radioallergosorbent testing (RAST) detects the presence of allergen-specific serum IgE and is indicated when skin testing is contraindicated because of generalized dermatitis, dermatographism, history of anaphylaxis to the allergen, or need to continue antihistamines. A known allergen in the form of an insoluble polymer-allergen conjugate is mixed with the serum to be tested and with ^{125}I-labeled anti-IgE antibody. Any allergen-specific IgE in the serum binds the conjugate and can be quantified by measuring the ^{125}I-labeled antibody.

Provocative testing involves direct exposure of the mucosae to allergen and is indicated for patients who must document their reaction (eg, for occupational or disability claims) and sometimes for diagnosis of food allergy. Ophthalmic testing has no advantage over skin testing and is rarely used. Nasal and bronchial challenge are primarily research tools, but bronchial challenge is sometimes used when the clinical significance of a positive skin test is unclear or when no antigen extracts are available (eg, for occupation-related asthma).

Treatment

Environmental control: Removal or avoidance of allergic triggers is the primary treatment of allergy. Strategies include use of synthetic fiber pillows and impermeable mattress covers; frequent washing of bed sheets, pillowcases, and blankets in hot water; removal of upholstered furniture, soft toys, carpets, and pets; house cleaning and extermination (to eliminate cockroach exposure); and use of dehumidifiers in basements and other poorly aerated, damp rooms. Other measures may include treating homes with heat-steam, using high-efficiency particulate air (HEPA) vacuums and filters, avoiding food triggers, limiting pets to certain rooms, and frequently cleaning cloth furniture and carpets. Adjunctive nonallergenic triggers (eg, cigarette smoke, strong odors, irritating fumes, air pollution, cold temperatures, high humidity) should also be avoided or controlled when possible.

Antihistamines: Antihistamines do not affect histamine production or metabolism but block receptors. H_1 blockers are a mainstay of treatment for allergic disorders. H_2 blockers are used primarily for gastric acid suppression and have limited usefulness for allergic reactions; they may be indicated for certain atopic disorders, especially chronic urticaria.

Oral H_1 blockers provide symptomatic relief in various atopic and allergic disorders (eg, seasonal hay fever, allergic rhinitis, conjunctivitis, urticaria, other dermatoses, minor reactions to blood transfusion incompatibilities and to x-ray radiopaque dyes); they are less effective for allergic bronchoconstriction and vasodilation. Onset of action is usually 15 to 30 min, with peak effects in 1 h; duration of action is usually 3 to 6 h.

Oral H_1 blockers are classified as sedating or nonsedating (better thought of as less sedating). Sedating antihistamines are widely available without prescription. All have significant sedative and anticholinergic properties; they pose particular problems for the elderly and patients with glaucoma, benign prostatic hyperplasia, constipation, and dementia. Nonsedating (non-anticholinergic) antihistamines are preferred except when sedative effects may be therapeutic (eg, for nighttime relief of allergy or short-term treatment of insomnia in adults or nausea in younger patients). Anticholinergic effects may also partially justify use of sedating antihistamines for symptomatic relief of rhinorrhea in URIs.

Antihistamine solutions may be intranasal (azelastine to treat rhinitis) or ocular (azelastine, emedastine, ketotifen, levocabastine, and olopatadine to treat conjunctivitis—see p. 893). Topical diphenhydramine is available but should not be used; its efficacy is unproved, drug sensitization (ie, allergy) may occur, and anticholinergic toxicity can develop in young children who are simultaneously taking oral H_1 blockers.

TABLE 165–3. INHALED NASAL CORTICOSTEROIDS AND MAST CELL STABILIZERS

DRUG	DOSE PER SPRAY	INITIAL DOSE (IN SPRAYS PER NOSTRIL)	SPRAYS OR ACTUATIONS PER CANISTER
Inhaled nasal corticosteroids			
Beclomethasone dipropionate	42 µg	> 12 yr: 1 spray bid to qid 6 to 12 yr: 1 spray bid	200
Budesonide	32 µg	≥ 6 yr: 2 sprays bid or 4 daily	200
Flunisolide	50 µg	6–14 yr: 1 spray in each nostril tid or 2 sprays in each nostril bid Adult: 1–2 sprays in each nostril bid or tid	125
Fluticasone*	50 µg	4–12 yr: 1 spray in each nostril once/day > 12 yr: 2 sprays each nostril once/day	120
Triamcinolone acetonide*	55 µg	> 6 yr: 2 sprays once/day	100
Corticosteroids with systemic effects			
Dexamethasone	84 µg	> 12 yr: 2 sprays bid or tid 6–12 yr: 1–2 sprays bid	170
Mast cell stabilizers			
Cromolyn	5.2 mg	≥ 6 yr: 1 spray tid or qid	200
Nedocromil†	1.3 mg	≥ 6 yr: 1 spray in each nostril bid	200

*Not approved for use in children < 12 yr.
†Nasal form of nedocromil is not yet available in the US.

Mast cell stabilizers: Cromolyn and nedocromil are examples. These drugs block the release of mediators from mast cells; they are used when other drugs (eg, antihistamines, topical corticosteroids) are ineffective or not well tolerated. Ocular forms (eg, lodoxamide, olopatadine, pemirolast) are also available.

Anti-inflammatory drugs: NSAIDs are not useful. Corticosteroids can be given intranasally (see TABLE 165–3) or orally. Oral corticosteroids are indicated for systemic allergic disorders that are severe but self-limited (eg, seasonal asthma flares, severe widespread contact dermatitis) and for disorders refractory to other measures.

Leukotriene modifiers are indicated for treatment of mild persistent asthma (see p. 392) and seasonal allergic rhinitis.

Anti-IgE antibody (omalizumab) is indicated for moderately persistent or severe asthma refractory to standard treatment (see p. 393); it may also be useful for treatment of refractory allergic rhinitis.

Immunotherapy: Exposure to allergen in gradually increasing doses (hyposensitization or desensitization) via injection or in high doses sublingually can induce tolerance and is indicated when allergen exposure cannot be avoided and drug treatment is inadequate. Mechanism is unknown but may involve induction of IgG antibodies, which compete with IgE for allergen or block IgE from binding with mast cell IgE receptors; induction of interferon γ, IL-12, and cytokines secreted by T_H1 cells; or induction of regulatory T cells.

For full effect, injections must be given monthly. Dose typically starts at 0.1 to 1.0 biologically active units (BAU), depending on initial sensitivity, and is increased weekly or biweekly by ≤ 2 times with each injection until a maximum tolerated concentration is reached; patients should be observed for about 30 min during dose escalation because anaphylaxis may occur after injection. Maximum dose should be given q 4 to 6 wk year-round; year-round treatment is better than preseasonal or coseasonal treatment even for seasonal allergies. Allergens used are those that typically cannot be avoided: pollens, house dust mites, molds, and venom of stinging insects. Insect venoms are standardized by weight; a typical starting dose is 0.01 μg, and usual maintenance dose is 100 to 200 μg. Animal dander desensitization is ordinarily limited to patients who cannot avoid exposure (eg, veterinarians, laboratory workers), but there is little evidence that it is useful. Food desensitization is not indicated. Desensitization for penicillin and foreign (xenogeneic) serum can be done (see p. 1363).

Adverse effects are most commonly related to overdose, occasionally via an inadvertent IM or IV injection, and range from mild cough or sneezing to generalized urticaria, severe asthma, anaphylactic shock, and, rarely, death. They can be prevented by increasing the dose in small increments, repeating or decreasing the dose if local reaction to the previous injection is large (≥ 2.5 cm in diameter), and reducing the dose when a fresh extract is used. Reducing the dose of pollen extract during pollen season is recommended.

ALLERGIC RHINITIS

Allergic rhinitis is seasonal or perennial itching, sneezing, rhinorrhea, nasal congestion, and sometimes conjunctivitis, caused by exposure to pollens or other allergens. Diagnosis is by history and skin testing. Treatment is with a combination of antihistamines, decongestants, nasal corticosteroids, and, for severe, refractory cases, desensitization.

Allergic rhinitis may occur seasonally (hay fever) or throughout the year (perennial rhinitis). At least 25% of perennial rhinitis is nonallergic. Seasonal rhinitis is caused by tree pollens (eg, oak, elm, maple, alder, birch, juniper, olive) in the spring; grass pollens (eg, Bermuda, timothy, sweet vernal, orchard, Johnson) and weed pollens (eg, Russian thistle, English plantain) in the summer; and other weed pollens (eg, ragweed) in the fall. Causes differ by region, and seasonal rhinitis is occasionally caused by airborne fungal spores. Perennial rhinitis is caused by year-round exposure to indoor inhaled allergens (eg, dust mite, cockroach, animal dander, mold) or by strong reactivity to plant pollens in sequential seasons.

Allergic rhinitis and asthma frequently coexist; whether rhinitis and asthma result from the same allergic process (one airway hypothesis) or rhinitis is a discrete asthma trigger is unclear.

Nonallergic forms of perennial rhinitis include infectious, vasomotor, atrophic, hormonal, drug-induced, and gustatory rhinitis (see p. 829).

Symptoms and Signs

Patients have itching of the nose, eyes, or mouth; sneezing; rhinorrhea; and nasal and sinus obstruction. Sinus obstruction may cause frontal headaches; sinusitis is a frequent complication. Coughing and wheezing may also occur, especially if asthma is also present. The most prominent feature of perennial rhinitis is chronic nasal obstruction, which, in children, can lead to chronic otitis media; symptoms vary in severity throughout the year. Itching is less prominent.

Signs include edematous, bluish-red nasal turbinates, and, in some cases of seasonal rhinitis, conjunctival injection and eyelid edema.

Diagnosis

Allergic rhinitis can almost always be diagnosed by history alone. Diagnostic testing is not routinely needed unless patients do not improve with empiric treatment; then, skin tests showing a reaction to pollens (seasonal) or to dust mite, cockroach, animal dander, mold, or other antigens (perennial) can be used to guide additional treatment. Eosinophilia detected on nasal smear with negative skin tests suggests aspirin sensitivity or nonallergic rhinitis with eosinophilia (NARES).

For infectious, vasomotor, atrophic, hormonal, drug-induced, or gustatory rhinitis, diagnosis is usually by history or therapeutic trials.

Treatment

Treatment of seasonal and perennial allergic rhinitis is generally the same, although attempts at environmental control (eg, eliminating dust mites and cockroaches) are recommended for perennial rhinitis. The most effective 1st-line drug treatments are oral antihistamines plus oral decongestants or nasal corticosteroids with or without oral antihistamines (see TABLE 165–3). Less effective alternatives include nasal mast cell stabilizers (cromolyn and nedocromil) given bid to qid, the nasal H_1 blocker azelastine 2 puffs once/day, and nasal ipratropium 0.03% 2 puffs q 4 to 6 h, which relieves rhinorrhea. Intranasal saline, often forgotten, helps mobilize thick nasal secretions and hydrate nasal mucous membranes.

Immunotherapy may be more effective for seasonal than for allergic perennial rhinitis; it is indicated when symptoms are severe, allergen cannot be avoided, and drug treatment is inadequate. First attempts at desensitization should begin soon after the pollen season ends to prepare for the next season; adverse reactions increase when desensitization is started during the pollen season because the person's allergic immunity is already maximally stimulated.

Montelukast relieves allergic rhinitis symptoms, but its role relative to other treatments is uncertain. Anti-IgE antibody is under study for treatment of allergic rhinitis but will probably have a limited role because less expensive, effective alternatives are available.

Treatment of NARES is nasal corticosteroids. Treatment of aspirin sensitivity is aspirin avoidance, with desensitization and leukotriene blockers as needed; nasal polyps may respond to nasal corticosteroids.

FOOD ALLERGY

Food allergy is an exaggerated immune response to dietary proteins.

Food allergy should be distinguished from nonimmune reactions to food (eg, lactase intolerance, irritable bowel syndrome, infectious gastroenteritis) and reactions to additives (eg, monosodium glutamate, metabisulfite, tartrazine), which cause most food reactions. Prevalence ranges from < 1 to 3% and varies by geography and method of ascertainment; patients tend to confuse intolerance with allergy. Digestion prevents food allergy symptoms in most adults. Almost any food or food additive can be implicated, but the most common triggers in infants and young children are milk, soy, eggs, peanuts, and wheat, and the most common in older children and adults are nuts and seafood. Cross-reactivity between food and nonfood allergens exists, and sensitization may occur nonenterally. For example, patients with oral allergies (typically, pruritus, erythema, and edema of the mouth when fruits and vegetables are eaten) may have been sensitized by pollen exposure; children with peanut allergy may have been sensitized by topical creams containing peanut oil used to treat rashes. Patients allergic to latex are also often allergic to bananas, kiwis, avocadoes, or a combination. Latex dust in food handled by workers wearing latex gloves is easily confused with true food allergy.

In general, food allergy is mediated by IgE, T cells, or both. IgE-mediated allergy (eg, urticaria, asthma, anaphylaxis) is acute in onset, usually develops during infancy, and occurs most often in people with a strong family history of atopy. T cell–mediated allergy (eg, dietary protein gastroenteropathies, celiac disease) manifests gradually and is chronic. Allergies mediated by IgE and T cells (eg, atopic dermatitis, eosinophilic gastroenteropathy) tend to be delayed in onset or chronic. Eosinophilic gastroenteropathy is an unusual disorder causing pain, cramps, and diarrhea with blood eosinophilia, eosinophilic infiltrates in the gut, protein-losing enteropathy, and a history of atopic disorders. Rarely, IgG-mediated allergy to cow's milk causes pulmonary hemorrhage (pulmonary hemosiderosis) in infants.

Symptoms and Signs

Symptoms and signs vary by allergen, mechanism, and patient age. The most common manifestation in infants is atopic dermatitis alone or with GI symptoms (nausea, vomiting, diarrhea). Children usually outgrow these manifestations and react increasingly to inhaled allergens, with symptoms of asthma and rhinitis (atopic march). By age 10 yr, patients rarely have respiratory symptoms after the allergenic food is eaten, even though skin tests remain positive. If atopic dermatitis persists or appears in older children or adults, its activity seems largely independent of IgE-mediated allergy, even though atopic patients with extensive dermatitis have much higher serum IgE levels than those who are free of dermatitis.

Older children and adults who remain food allergic tend to have more severe reactions (eg, explosive urticaria, angioedema, even anaphylaxis). In a few patients, food (especially wheat and celery) triggers anaphylaxis only if they exercise soon afterward; mechanism is unknown. A few patients have food-induced or aggravated migraine, confirmed by blinded oral challenge. Occasionally, cheilitis, aphthae, pylorospasm, spastic constipation, pruritus ani, and perianal eczema are attributed to food allergy.

Diagnosis and Treatment

Severe food allergy is usually obvious in adults. When it is not and in most children, diagnosis may be difficult, and the disorder must be differentiated from functional GI problems.

If a food reaction is suspected, the relationship of symptoms to foods is assessed by skin testing or IgE-specific radioallergosorbent testing. A positive test does not prove clinically relevant allergy, but a negative test excludes it. If a skin test is positive, that food is eliminated from the diet; if symptoms are relieved, the patient is reexposed to the food (preferably in a double-blind test) to determine if symptoms recur.

Alternatives to skin testing include eliminating foods the patient suspects of causing symptoms and prescribing a diet that consists of relatively nonallergenic foods and that eliminates common food allergens (see TABLE 165–4). No foods or fluids may be consumed other than those specified. Pure products must always be used. Many commercially prepared products and meals contain an undesired food in large amounts (eg, commercial rye bread contains wheat flour) or in traces as flavoring or thickeners, and determining whether an undesired food is present may be difficult.

If no improvement occurs after 1 wk, another diet should be tried. If symptoms are relieved, one new food is added and eaten in large amounts for > 24 h or until symptoms recur. Alternatively, small amounts of the food to be tested are eaten in the physician's presence, and the patient's reactions observed. Aggravation or recrudescence of symptoms after addition of a new food is the best evidence of allergy.

When assessing an elimination diet's effect, clinicians must consider that food sensitivities may disappear spontaneously. Oral desensitization (by first eliminating the allergenic food for a time, then giving small, daily increased amounts) has not been proved effective nor has use of sublingual drops of food extracts. Antihistamines are of

TABLE 165–4. ALLOWABLE FOODS IN ELIMINATION DIETS*

FOOD	DIET NO. 1 (No beef, pork, fowl, milk, rye, corn)	DIET NO. 2 (No beef, lamb, milk, rice)	DIET NO. 3 (No lamb, fowl, rye, rice, corn, milk)
Cereal	Rice products	Corn products	None
Vegetables	Artichokes, beets, carrots, lettuce, spinach	Asparagus, corn, peas, squash, string beans, tomatoes	Beets, lima beans, potatoes (white and sweet), string beans, tomatoes
Meats	Lamb	Bacon, chicken	Bacon, beef
Flour (bread or biscuits)	Rice	Corn, 100% rye (ordinary rye bread contains wheat)	Lima beans, potatoes, soybeans
Fruits	Grapefruit, lemons, pears	Apricots, peaches, pineapple, prunes	Apricots, grapefruit, lemons, peaches
Fat	Cottonseed oil, olive oil	Corn oil, cottonseed oil	Cottonseed oil, olive oil
Beverages	Coffee (black), lemonade, tea	Coffee (black), lemonade, tea	Coffee (black), lemonade, juice from approved fruit, tea
Miscellaneous	Cane sugar, gelatin, maple sugar, olives, salt, tapioca pudding	Cane sugar, corn syrup, gelatin, salt	Cane sugar, gelatin, maple sugar, olives, salt, tapioca pudding

*Diet No. 4: If symptoms persist when patients were following any of the above 3 elimination diets and diet is still suspected, daily diet may be restricted to an elemental diet.

little value except in acute general reactions with urticaria and angioedema. Oral cromolyn has been used with apparent success. Prolonged corticosteroid treatment is helpful for symptomatic eosinophilic enteropathy. A humanized IgG1 monoclonal antibody directed against the CH3 region of IgE shows early promise as treatment of peanut allergy.

Anaphylaxis

Anaphylaxis is an acute, life-threatening, IgE-mediated allergic reaction that occurs in previously sensitized people when they are reexposed to the sensitizing antigen. Symptoms include stridor, dyspnea, wheezing, and hypotension. Diagnosis is clinical. Bronchospasm and upper airway edema are treated with inhaled or injected β-agonists and sometimes endotracheal intubation. Hypotension requires IV fluids and vasopressors.

Etiology and Pathophysiology

Anaphylaxis is typically triggered by drugs (eg, β-lactam antibiotics, insulin, streptokinase, allergen extracts), foods (eg, nuts, eggs, seafood), proteins (eg, tetanus antitoxin, blood transfusions), animal venoms, and latex. Peanut and latex allergens may be airborne. History of atopy does not increase risk of anaphylaxis but increases risk of death when anaphylaxis occurs.

Interaction of antigen with IgE on basophils and mast cells triggers release of histamine, leukotrienes, and other mediators that cause diffuse smooth muscle contraction (bronchoconstriction, vomiting, diarrhea) and vasodilation with plasma leakage.

Anaphylactoid reactions are clinically indistinguishable from anaphylaxis but do not involve IgE and do not require prior sensitization. They occur via direct stimulation of mast cells or via immune complexes that activate complement. The most common triggers are iodinated radiographic radiopaque dye, aspirin, other NSAIDs, opioids, blood transfusion, Ig, and exercise.

Symptoms, Signs, and Diagnosis

Symptoms typically involve the skin, upper or lower airways, cardiovascular system, or the GI tract. One or more areas may be affected, and symptoms do not necessarily progress, although each patient typically manifests the same reaction to subsequent exposure.

Symptoms range from mild to severe and include flushing, pruritus, sneezing, rhinorrhea, nausea, abdominal cramps, diarrhea, sense of choking or dyspnea, palpitations, and dizziness. Signs include hypotension, tachycardia, urticaria, angioedema, wheezing, cyanosis, and syncope. Shock can develop within minutes, and patients may experience seizures, become unresponsive, and die. Cardiovascular collapse can occur without respiratory or other symptoms.

Diagnosis is clinical. Risk of rapid progression to shock leaves no time for testing, although mild equivocal cases can be confirmed by 24-h urinary levels of *N*-methylhistamine or serum levels of tryptase.

Treatment

Epinephrine is the cornerstone of treatment and should be given immediately. It can be given sc or IM (usual dose 0.3 to 0.5 mL of a 1:1000 solution in adults or 0.01 mL/kg in children, repeated every 10 to 30 min); maximal absorption occurs when the drug is given IM in the lateral thigh. Patients with cardiovascular collapse or severe airway obstruction may be given epinephrine IV in a single dose (3 to 5 mL of a 1:10,000 solution over 5 min) or by continuous drip (1 mg in 250 mL 5% D/W for a concentration of 4 μg/mL, starting at 1 μg/min up to 4 μg/min [15 to 60 mL/h]). Epinephrine may also be given by sublingual injection (0.5 mL of 1:1000 solution) or through an endotracheal tube (3 to 5 mL of a 1:10,000 solution diluted to 10 mL with saline). A 2nd injection of epinephrine sc may be needed. Glucagon 1-mg bolus followed by 1-mg/h infusion should be used in patients taking oral β-blockers, which attenuate the effect of epinephrine.

Patients who have stridor and wheezing unresponsive to epinephrine should be given O_2 and be intubated. Early intubation is recommended because waiting for a response to epinephrine may allow upper airway edema to progress sufficiently to prevent endotracheal intubation, requiring cricothyrotomy.

Hypotension can usually be treated with 1 to 2 L (20 to 40 mL/kg in children) of isotonic IV fluids (eg, 0.9% saline). Hypotension refractory to fluids and IV epinephrine may require vasopressors (eg, dopamine 5 μg/kg/min).

Antihistamines—both H_1 blockers (eg, diphenhydramine 50 to 100 mg IV) and H_2 blockers (eg, cimetidine 300 mg IV)—should be given q 6 h until symptoms resolve. Inhaled β-agonists are useful for managing bronchoconstriction; albuterol 5 to 10 mg by continuous nebulization can be given. Corticosteroids have no proven role but may help prevent late-phase reaction in 4 to 8 h; methylprednisolone 125 mg IV initially is adequate.

Prevention

Primary prevention is avoidance of known triggers. Desensitization is used for allergen triggers that cannot reliably be avoided (eg, insect stings). Patients with past reactions to radiopaque dye should avoid re-exposure; when exposure is absolutely necessary, prednisone 50 mg po q 6 h is given for 3 doses starting 18 h before the procedure and diphenhydramine 50 mg po 1 h before the procedure; however, no evidence supports the efficacy of this approach (see also p. 2718).

Patients with an anaphylactic reaction to insect stings, foods, or other known substances should wear an alert bracelet and carry a prefilled epinephrine syringe (containing 0.3 mg for adults and 0.15 mg for children) for prompt self-treatment after exposure.

AUTOIMMUNE DISORDERS

In autoimmune disorders, the immune system produces antibodies to an endogenous antigen. Antibody-coated cells, like any similarly coated foreign particle, activate the complement system (see p. 1326), resulting in tissue injury. Sometimes the mechanism of injury involves deposition of antibody-antigen complexes (type III hypersensitivity reaction). Specific autoimmune disorders are discussed elsewhere in THE MANUAL (see also TABLE 165–1).

Etiology

Several mechanisms may account for the body's attack on itself.

Autoantigens may become immunogenic because they are altered chemically, physically, or biologically. Certain chemicals couple with body proteins, making them immunogenic (as in contact dermatitis). Drugs can produce several autoimmune reactions by binding covalently to serum or tissue proteins (see below). Photosensitivity exemplifies physically induced autoallergy: Ultraviolet light alters skin protein, to which the patient becomes allergic. In animal models, persistent infection with an RNA virus that combines with host tissues alters autoantigens biologically, resulting in an autoallergic disorder resembling SLE.

Antibodies produced in response to a foreign antigen may cross-react with normal autoantigens (eg, cross-reaction between streptococcal M protein and human heart muscle).

Normally, autoimmune reactions are probably restrained by specific regulatory T cells. A regulatory T-cell defect could accompany or result from any of the above mechanisms. Anti-idiotype antibodies (antibodies to the antigen-combining site of other antibodies) may interfere with regulation of antibody activity.

Genetic factors play a role. Relatives of patients with autoimmune disorders often have the same type of autoantibodies, and incidence of autoimmune disorders is higher in identical than fraternal twins. Women are affected more often than men. The genetic role appears to be one of predisposition. In predisposed people, environmental factors may provoke disease (eg, certain drugs can trigger hemolytic anemia in patients with G6PD deficiency).

DRUG HYPERSENSITIVITY

Drug hypersensitivity is an immune-mediated reaction to a drug. Symptoms range from mild to severe and include skin rash, anaphylaxis, and serum sickness. Diagnosis is clinical; skin testing is occasionally useful. Treatment is drug discontinuation, antihistamines (for symptoms), and sometimes desensitization.

Drug hypersensitivity must be distinguished from toxic and adverse effects that may be expected from the drug and from problems due to drug interactions (see p. 2515).

Pathophysiology

Some protein and large polypeptide drugs (eg, insulin, therapeutic antibodies) can directly stimulate antibody production. However, most drugs act as haptens, binding covalently to serum or cell-bound proteins, including proteins embedded in major histocompatibility complex (MHC) molecules. The binding makes the protein immunogenic, stimulating antidrug antibody production, T-cell responses against the drug, or both. Haptens may also bind directly to the MHC II molecule, directly activating T cells. Prohaptens become haptens with metabolism; for example, penicillin itself is not antigenic, but its major degradation product, benzylpenicilloic acid, can combine with tissue proteins to form benzylpenicilloyl (BPO), a major antigenic determinant. Some drugs bind and stimulate T-cell receptors (TCR) directly; the clinical significance of this nonhapten TCR binding is being determined.

How primary sensitization occurs and how the innate immune system is initially involved is unclear, but once a drug stimulates an immune response, cross-reactions within and between drug classes can occur. For example, penicillin-sensitive patients are highly likely to react to semisynthetic penicillins (eg, amoxicillin, carbenicillin, ticarcillin), and about 10% react to cephalosporins, which have a similar β-lactam structure. However, some apparent cross-reactions (eg, between sulfonamide antibiotics and nonantibiotics) are due to a predisposition to allergic reactions rather than to specific immune cross-reactivity. Also, not every apparent reaction is allergic; for example, amoxicillin causes a rash that is not immune-mediated and does not preclude future use of the drug.

Symptoms and Signs

Symptoms and signs vary by patient and drug, and a single drug may cause different reactions in different patients. The most serious is anaphylaxis; exanthema, urticaria, and fever are common. Fixed drug reactions are uncommon.

Other distinct clinical syndromes exist. Serum sickness typically occurs 7 to 10 days after exposure and causes fever, arthralgias, and rash. Mechanism involves drug-antibody complexes and complement activation. Some patients have frank arthritis, edema, or GI symptoms. Symptoms are self-limited, lasting 1 to 2 wk. β-Lactam and sulfonamide antibiotics, iron-dextran, and carbamazepine are most commonly implicated.

Hemolytic anemia may develop when an antibody-drug-RBC interaction occurs or when a drug (eg, methyldopa) alters the RBC membrane, uncovering an antigen that induces autoantibody production. Some drugs induce lung disease (see p. 450). Tubulointerstitial nephritis is the most common allergic renal reaction (see p. 2017); methicillin, antimicrobials, and cimetidine are commonly implicated. Hydralazine and procainamide can cause an SLE-like syndrome. The syndrome is relatively benign, sparing the kidneys and CNS; the antinuclear antibody test is positive. Penicillamine can cause SLE and other autoimmune disorders (eg, myasthenia gravis).

Diagnosis

Diagnosis is suggested when a reaction occurs within minutes to hours after drug administration. However, many patients report a past reaction of uncertain nature. In such cases, if an equivalent substitute (eg, penicillin to treat syphilis) cannot be found, testing should be considered.

Skin testing: Tests for immediate-type (IgE-mediated) hypersensitivity help diagnose reactions to β-lactam antibiotics, foreign (xenogeneic) serum, and some vaccines and polypeptide hormones. However, typically, only 10 to 20% of patients who report a penicillin allergy have a positive reaction on skin tests. Also, for most drugs (including cephalosporins), skin tests are unreliable and, because they detect only IgE-mediated reactions, do not predict the occurrence of morbilliform eruptions, hemolytic anemia, or nephritis.

Penicillin skin testing is needed for patients with a history of an immediate hypersensitivity reaction in whom a penicillin must be used. BPO-polylysine conjugate and penicillin G are used with histamine and saline as controls. The prick technique (see p. 1354) is used first. If the patient has a history of a severe explosive reaction, reagents should be diluted 100-fold for initial testing. If prick tests are negative, intradermal testing may follow. If skin tests are positive, treating patients with penicillin may induce an anaphylactic reaction. If tests are negative, a serious reaction is less likely but not excluded. Although the penicillin skin test has not induced de novo sensitivity in patients, patients should usually be tested only immediately before essential penicillin therapy is begun.

For xenogeneic serum skin testing, patients who are not atopic and who have not received horse serum previously should first be given a prick test with a 1:10 dilution; if this test is negative, 0.02 mL of a 1:1000 dilution is injected intradermally. A wheal > 0.5 cm in diameter develops within 15 min in sensitive patients. All patients who may have received serum previously—whether or not they reacted—and those with a suspected allergic history should be tested first with a 1:1000 dilution. A negative result rules out the possibility of anaphylaxis but does not predict incidence of subsequent serum sickness.

Other testing: For drug provocation testing, a drug suspected of causing a hypersensitivity reaction is given in escalating doses to precipitate the reaction. This test is probably safe and effective if done in a controlled setting. Tests for hematologic drug reactions include direct and indirect antiglobulin tests (see p. 1049). Tests for other specific drug hypersensitivity (eg, RAST, histamine release, basophil or mast cell degranulation, lymphocyte transformation) are unreliable or experimental.

Prognosis and Treatment

Hypersensitivity decreases with time. IgE antibodies are present in 90% of patients 1 yr after an allergic reaction but in only about 20 to 30% after 10 yr. Patients who have anaphylactic reactions are more likely to retain antibodies to the offending drug longer. People with drug allergies should be educated about avoiding the drug and carry identification or an alert bracelet; charts should always be appropriately marked.

Treatment is stopping the implicated drug; most symptoms and signs clear within a few days after the drug is stopped. Supportive treatment of acute reactions may include antihistamines for pruritus, NSAIDs for arthralgias, corticosteroids for severe reactions (eg, exfoliative dermatitis, bronchospasm), and epinephrine for anaphylaxis. Conditions such as drug fever, a nonpruritic skin rash, or mild organ system reactions require no treatment (for treatment of specific clinical reactions, see elsewhere in THE MANUAL).

Desensitization: Rapid desensitization may be necessary if sensitivity has been established and if treatment is essential and no alternative exists. If possible, desensitization should be done in collaboration with an allergist. The procedure should not be attempted in patients who have had Stevens-Johnson syndrome. Whenever desensitization is used, O_2, epinephrine, and resuscitation equipment must be available for prompt treatment of anaphylaxis.

Desensitization is based on incremental dosing of the antigen q 30 min, beginning with a minute dose to induce subclinical anaphylaxis before exposure to therapeutic doses. This procedure depends on constant presence of drug in the serum and so must not be interrupted; desensitization is immediately followed by full therapeutic doses. Hypersensitivity typically returns 24 to 48 h after discontinuation. Minor reactions (eg, itching, rash) are common during desensitization.

For penicillin, oral or IV regimens can be used; sc or IM regimens are not recommended. If only the intradermal skin test is positive, 100 units (or μg)/mL IV in a 50-mL bag (5000 units total) should be given very slowly at first. If no symptoms appear, flow rate can be increased gradually until the bag is empty, after 20 to 30 min. The procedure is then repeated with concentrations of 1,000 and 10,000 units/mL, followed by the full therapeutic dose. If any allergic symptoms develop, flow rate should be slowed, and the patient given appropriate drug treatment (see above). If the prick test for penicillin was positive or the patient has had a severe anaphylactic reaction, the starting dose should be lower.

Oral penicillin desensitization begins with 100 units (or μg); doses are doubled q 15 min up to 400,000 units (dose 13). Then, the drug is given parenterally, and if symptoms occur, they are relieved with appropriate anti-anaphylactic drugs.

For trimethoprim-sulfamethoxazole and vancomycin, regimens similar to those for penicillin can be used.

For xenogeneic serum: If a skin test to xenogeneic serum is positive, risk of anaphylaxis is high. If serum treatment is essential, desensitization must precede it. Skin tests, using weak concentrations prepared by serial dilution, are used to determine the appropriate starting dose for desensitization (ie, the concentration that produces a negative or only a weak reaction). 0.1 mL of this solution is injected sc or slowly IV; the IV route, although not standard, gives the physician control over concentration and rate of delivery. If no reaction occurs in 15 min, the dose is doubled q 15 min until 1 mL of undiluted serum is given. This dose is repeated IM, and if no reaction occurs in another 15 min, the full dose can be given. If a reaction occurs, treatment may still be possible; the dose is reduced, an antihistamine is given as for acute urticaria, and the dose is then increased by smaller increments.

MASTOCYTOSIS

Mastocytosis is mast cell infiltration of skin or other tissues and organs. Symptoms result mainly from mediator release and include pruritus, flushing, and dyspepsia due to gastric hypersecretion. Diagnosis is by skin or bone marrow biopsy or both. Treatment is with antihistamines and control of any underlying disorder.

Mastocytosis is a group of disorders characterized by proliferation of mast cells and infiltration of the skin, other organs, or both. Pathology results mainly from release of mast cell mediators, including histamine, heparin, leukotrienes, and various inflammatory cytokines. Histamine causes many symptoms, including gastric symptoms, but other mediators contribute. Significant organ infiltration may cause organ dysfunction. Mediator release may be triggered by physical touch, exercise, alcohol, NSAIDs, opioids, insect stings, or foods.

Etiology is unknown but may involve mutations in the gene coding for the mast cell tyrosine kinase receptor (c-kit) in some patients. Stem cell factor, which is the ligand for the receptor, may also be overproduced.

Classification

Mastocytosis may be cutaneous or systemic.

Cutaneous mastocytosis typically occurs in children. Most patients present with urticaria pigmentosa, a local or diffusely distributed salmon or brown maculopapular skin rash caused by multiple small mast cell collections. Less common are diffuse cutaneous mastocytosis, which is skin infiltration without discrete lesions, and mastocytoma, which is a large (1 to 5 cm) solitary collection of mast cells.

Systemic mastocytosis most commonly occurs in adults and is characterized by multifocal bone marrow lesions; it often involves other organs, most commonly skin, lymph nodes, liver, spleen, or GI tract. Systemic mastocytosis is classified as indolent mastocytosis, with no organ dysfunction and a good prognosis; mastocytosis associated with other hematologic disorders (eg, myeloproliferative disorders, myelodysplasia, lymphoma); aggressive mastocytosis, characterized by impaired organ function; or mast cell leukemia, with > 20% mast cells in bone marrow, no skin lesions, multiorgan failure, and a poor prognosis.

Symptoms and Signs

Skin involvement is often pruritic. Stroking or rubbing skin lesions causes urticaria and erythema around the lesion (Darier's sign); this reaction differs from dermatographism, which involves normal skin.

Systemic symptoms can occur with any form. The most common is flushing; the most dramatic is anaphylactoid reaction with syncope and shock. Other symptoms include epigastric pain due to peptic ulcer disease, nausea, vomiting, chronic diarrhea, arthralgias, bone pain, and neuropsychiatric changes (eg, irritability, depression, mood lability). Hepatic and splenic infiltration may cause portal hypertension with resultant ascites.

Diagnosis

Diagnosis is suggested by clinical presentation. Similar symptoms may result from anaphylaxis, pheochromocytoma, carcinoid syndrome, and Zollinger-Ellison syndrome. Diagnosis is confirmed by biopsy of skin lesions and sometimes of bone marrow. Serum gastrin level is useful to rule out Zollinger-Ellison syndrome in patients with ulcer symptoms; urinary excretion of 5-hydroxyindoleacetic acid (5-HIAA) is measured to rule out carcinoid in those with flushing. Mast cell mediators and their metabolites may be elevated in plasma and urine, but these findings are not helpful in confirming diagnosis.

Treatment

Cutaneous mastocytosis: H_1 blockers are effective for symptoms. Children with cutaneous forms require no additional treatment, because most cases resolve spontaneously. Adults with cutaneous forms may be treated with psoralen plus ultraviolet light or with topical corticosteroids once/day or bid. Mastocytoma usually involutes spontaneously and requires no treatment. Cutaneous forms rarely progress to systemic disease in children but may do so in adults.

Systemic mastocytosis: All patients should be treated with H_1 and H_2 blockers. Aspirin controls flushing but may enhance leukotriene production, thereby contributing to mast cell–related symptoms; it should not be given to children because of the risk of Reye's syndrome. Cromolyn 200 mg po qid (100 mg qid for children 2 to 12 yr; not to exceed 40 mg/kg/day) may help by preventing mast cell degranulation. No treatment can reduce the number of tissue mast cells. Ketotifen 2 to 4 mg po bid is inconsistently effective.

Interferon-α2b 4 million units sc once/wk to a maximum of 3 million units/day induces regression of bone lesions in patients with aggressive forms. Corticosteroids (eg, prednisone 40 to 60 mg po once/day for 2 to 3 wk) may be required. Splenectomy may improve survival in aggressive forms.

Cytotoxic drugs (eg, daunomycin, etoposide, 6-mercaptopurine) may be indicated for treatment of mast cell leukemia, but efficacy is unproved. Use of imatinib (a tyrosine kinase receptor inhibitor) to treat patients with c-kit mutations is under study.

166 TRANSPLANTATION

Transplants may be the patient's own tissue (autografts; eg, bone and skin grafts), genetically identical (syngeneic) donor tissue (isografts), genetically dissimilar donor tissue (allografts or homografts), or, rarely, grafts from a different species (xenografts or heterografts). Transplanted tissue may be cells (as for hematopoietic stem cell [HSC], lymphocyte, and pancreatic islet cell transplants), parts or segments of an organ (as for hepatic or pulmonary lobar transplants and skin grafts), or entire organs (as for heart transplants).

Tissues may be grafted to an anatomically normal site (orthotopic; eg, heart transplants) or abnormal site (heterotopic; eg, a kidney transplanted into the iliac fossa). Almost always, transplantation is done to improve patient survival. However, some procedures (eg, hand, larynx, tongue, and facial transplantation) attempt to improve quality of life but jeopardize quantity of life and thus are controversial.

With rare exceptions, clinical transplantation uses allografts from living related, living unrelated, or deceased donors. Living donors are often used for kidney and HSC transplants and increasingly for segmental liver, pancreas, and lung transplants. Use of deceased-donor organs (from heart-beating or non–heart-beating donors) has helped reduce the disparity between organ demand and supply; however, demand still far exceeds supply, and the number of patients waiting for organ transplants continues to grow.

Organ distribution: Allocation depends on disease severity for some organs (liver, heart) and on disease severity, time on the waiting list, or both for others (kidney, lung, bowel). In the US and Puerto Rico, organs are allocated first among 12 geographical regions, then among local Organ Procurement Organizations. If no recipient in the 1st region is suitable, organs are reallocated to recipients in other regions.

GENERAL PRINCIPLES OF TRANSPLANTATION

All allograft recipients are at risk of graft rejection; the recipient's immune system recognizes the graft as foreign and seeks to destroy it. Recipients of grafts containing immune cells are at risk of graft-vs-host disease. Risk of these complications is minimized by pretransplantation screening and immunosuppressive therapy during and after transplantation.

Pretransplantation Screening

In pretransplantation screening, recipients and donors are tested for human leukocyte antigen (HLA) and ABO antigens, and recipients are tested for presensitization to donor antigens. HLA tissue typing is most important for kidney and the most common types of hematopoietic stem cell (HSC) transplantation. Heart, liver, pancreas, and lung transplantation typically occurs quickly, often before HLA tissue typing can be completed, so the role of matching for these organs is less well established.

HLA tissue typing of peripheral blood or lymph node lymphocytes is used to match the most important known determinants of histocompatibility in the donor and recipient. More than 1250 alleles determine 6 HLA antigens (HLA-A, -B, -C, -DP, -DQ, -DR), so matching is a challenge; eg, in the US, only 2 of 6 antigens on average are matched in kidney donors and recipients. Matching of as many HLA antigens as possible significantly improves functional survival of grafts from living related kidney and HSC donors; HLA matching of grafts from unrelated donors also improves survival, although much less so because of multiple undetected histocompatibility differences. Better immunosuppressive therapy has expanded eligibility for transplantation; HLA mismatches no longer automatically disqualify patients for transplantation.

ABO compatibility and HLA compatibility are important for graft survival. ABO mismatches can underlie hyperacute rejection of highly vascular grafts (eg, kidney, heart), which have ABO antigens on the surfaces. Presensitization to HLA and ABO antigens results from prior blood transfusions, transplantations, or pregnancies and can be detected with serology tests or, more commonly, with a lymphocytotoxic test using the recipient's serum and donor's lymphocytes in the presence of complement. A positive cross-match indicates that the recipient's serum contains antibodies directed against ABO or class I HLA antigens in the donor; it is an absolute contraindication to transplantation, except possibly in infants (up to age 14 mo) who have not yet produced isohemagglutinins. High-dose IV immune globulin has been used to suppress HLA antibodies and facilitate transplantation, but long-term outcomes are unknown. A negative cross-match does not guarantee safety; when ABO antigens are compatible but not identical (eg, donor O and recipient A, B, or AB), hemolysis is a potential complication due to antibody production by transplanted (passenger) donor lymphocytes.

Matching for HLA and ABO antigens improves graft survival, but nonwhite patients are at a disadvantage because they may have different HLA polymorphisms from white donors, a higher rate of presensitization to HLA antigens, and blood types (O and B).

Exposure to common infectious pathogens and active infections must be detected before transplantation to minimize risk of infection. This screening usually includes the history; serologic tests for cytomegalovirus (CMV), Epstein-Barr virus (EBV), herpes simplex virus (HSV), varicella-zoster virus (VZV), hepatitis B and C viruses, and HIV; and tuberculin skin testing. Positive findings may require posttransplantation antiviral treatment (eg, for CMV infection or hepatitis B) or contraindicate transplantation (eg, if HIV is detected).

Immunosuppression

Immunosuppressants control graft rejection and are primarily responsible for the success of transplantation. However, they suppress all immune responses and contribute to many posttransplantation complications, including death due to overwhelming infection. Except when HLA-identical transplants are used, immunosuppressants must usually be continued long after transplantation, but initially high doses can be reduced a few weeks after the procedure, and low doses can be continued indefinitely unless rejection occurs.

Corticosteroids: A high dose is usually given at the time of transplantation, then is reduced gradually to a maintenance dose, which is given indefinitely. Several months after transplantation, corticosteroids can be given on alternate days; this regimen helps prevent growth restriction in children. If rejection occurs, high doses are reinstituted.

Calcineurin inhibitors: These drugs (cyclosporine, tacrolimus) block T-cell transcription processes required for production of cytokines, thereby selectively inhibiting T-cell proliferation and activation.

Cyclosporine is the most commonly used drug in heart and lung transplantation. It can be given alone but is usually given with other drugs (eg, azathioprine, prednisone), so that lower, less toxic doses can be used. The initial dose is reduced to a maintenance dose soon after transplantation. The drug is metabolized by the cytochrome P-450 3A enzyme, and blood levels are affected by many other drugs. The most serious adverse effect is nephrotoxicity; cyclosporine causes vasoconstriction of afferent (preglomerular) arterioles, leading to glomerular apparatus damage, refractory glomerular hypoperfusion, and, eventually, chronic renal failure. Also, B-cell lymphomas and polyclonal B-cell lymphoproliferation occur more often in patients receiving high doses of cyclosporine or combinations of cyclosporine and other immunosuppressants directed at T cells, possibly because of an association with EBV. Other adverse effects include hepatotoxicity, refractory hypertension, increased incidence of other tumors, and less serious effects (eg, gum hypertrophy, hirsutism). Serum cyclosporine levels do not correlate with effectiveness or toxicity.

Tacrolimus is the most commonly used drug in kidney, liver, pancreas, and intestinal transplantation. Tacrolimus may be started at the time of transplantation or days after the procedure. Dosing should be guided by blood levels, which are influenced by the same drug interactions as for cyclosporine. Tacrolimus may be useful when cyclosporine is ineffective or causes intolerable adverse effects. Adverse effects of tacrolimus are similar to those of cyclosporine except tacrolimus is more prone to induce diabetes; gum hypertrophy and hirsutism are less common. Lymphoproliferative disorders seem to occur more often in patients taking tacrolimus, even weeks after transplantation. If they occur and a calcineurin inhibitor is required, tacrolimus should be stopped, and cyclosporine substituted.

Purine metabolism inhibitors: Examples are azathioprine and mycophenolate mofetil. Azathioprine, an antimetabolite, is usually started at the time of transplantation. Most patients tolerate it indefinitely. The most serious adverse effects are bone marrow depression and, rarely, hepatitis. Azathioprine is often used with low doses of cyclosporine.

Mycophenolate mofetil (MMF), a prodrug metabolized to mycophenolic acid, reversibly inhibits inosine monophosphate dehydrogenase, an enzyme in the guanine nucleotide pathway that is rate-limiting in lymphocyte proliferation. MMF is given with cyclosporine and corticosteroids to patients with a kidney, heart, or liver transplant. The most common adverse effects are leukopenia, nausea, vomiting, and diarrhea.

Rapamycins: These drugs (sirolimus, everolimus) block a key regulatory kinase in lymphocytes, resulting in arrest of the cell cycle and in inhibition of lymphocyte response to cytokine stimulation.

Sirolimus is typically given with cyclosporine and corticosteroids and may be most useful for patients with renal insufficiency. Adverse effects include hyperlipidemia, impaired wound healing, and bone marrow depression with leukopenia, thrombocytopenia, and anemia.

Everolimus is typically used to prevent heart transplant rejection; adverse effects are similar to sirolimus.

Immunosuppressive Igs: Examples are antilymphocyte globulin (ALG) and antithymocyte globulin (ATG), which are fractions of animal antisera directed against human lymphocytes or thymus cells, respectively. ALG and ATG suppress cellular immunity while preserving humoral immunity. They are used with other immunosuppressants to allow those drugs to be used in lower, less toxic doses. Use of ALG or ATG to control acute episodes of rejection improves graft survival rates; use at the time of transplantation may decrease rejection incidence and allow cyclosporine to be started later, thereby reducing its toxicity. Use of highly purified serum fractions has greatly reduced incidence of adverse effects (eg, anaphylaxis, serum sickness, antigen-antibody–induced glomerulonephritis).

Monoclonal antibodies (mAbs): mAbs directed against T cells provide a higher concentration of anti-T-cell antibodies and fewer irrelevant serum proteins than do ALG and ATG. The murine mAb OKT3 is the only mAb currently available for clinical use. OKT3 inhibits T-cell receptor (TCR)–antigen binding, resulting in immunosuppression. OKT3 is used primarily to control episodes of acute rejection; it may also be used at the time of transplantation to reduce incidence or delay onset of rejection episodes. However, benefits of prophylactic use must be weighed against adverse effects, which include severe CMV infection and development of neutralizing antibodies; these effects preclude using OKT3 for an actual rejection episode. With 1st use, OKT3 binds to the TCR-CD3 complex, activating the cell and triggering release of cytokines, which cause a syndrome of fevers, rigors, myalgias, arthralgias, nausea, vomiting, and diarrhea. Pretreatment with corticosteroids, antipyretics, and antihistamines can ameliorate these symptoms. The 1st-dose reaction less commonly includes chest pain, dyspnea, and wheezing, possibly due to complement activation. Repeated use is associated with increased incidence of EBV-induced B-cell lymphoproliferative disorders. Rarely, aseptic meningitis and hemolytic uremic syndrome occur.

Anti-IL-2 receptor monoclonal antibodies inhibit T-cell proliferation by blocking the effect of IL-2, secreted by activated T cells. Basiliximab and daclizumab, two humanized anti-T_{aT} (HAT) antibodies, are increasingly being used to treat acute rejection of kidney, liver, and intestinal transplants; they are also used as adjunct immunosuppressive therapy at the time of transplantation. The only adverse effect reported is anaphylaxis, but a single trial suggests that daclizumab, when used with cyclosporine, MMF, and corticosteroids, may increase mortality rates. Also, experience with IL-2 receptor antibodies is limited, and an increased risk of lymphoproliferative disorders cannot be excluded.

Irradiation: Irradiation of a graft, local recipient tissues, or both can be used to treat kidney transplant rejection episodes when other treatment (eg, corticosteroids and ATG) is ineffective. Total lymphatic irradiation is experimental but appears to safely suppress cellular immunity, at first by stimulation of suppressor T cells and later possibly by clonal deletion of specific antigen-reactive cells.

Future therapies: Protocols and agents to induce graft antigen-specific tolerance without suppressing other immune responses are being sought. Two strategies are promising: blockade of T-cell costimulatory pathways using a cytotoxic T lymphocyte–associated antigen 4 (CTLA-4)-IgG1 fusion protein; and induction of chimerism (coexistence of donor and recipient immune cells in which graft tissue is recognized as self) using nonmyeloablative pretransplantation treatment (eg, with cyclophosphamide, thymic irradiation, ATG, and cyclosporine) to induce transient T-cell depletion, engraftment of donor HSCs, and subsequent tolerance of solid organ transplants from the same donor.

TABLE 166–1. SIGNS OF TRANSPLANT REJECTION

REJECTION TYPE	KIDNEY	LIVER	HEART	LUNG	PANCREAS	INTESTINE
Hyperacute	Fever, anuria	Fever, coagulopathy	Cardiogenic shock	Poor oxygenation, fever, cough	Pancreatic necrosis, fever	Fever, elevated lactic acid
Accelerated	Fever, oliguria, graft swelling and tenderness	Fever, coagulopathy, ascites	Arrhythmia, cardiogenic shock	Decreased FEV_1	Pancreatitis, hyperglycemia, elevated amylase and lipase	Fever, diarrhea, intestinal necrosis
Acute	Fever; increased serum creatinine; hypertension; weight gain; graft swelling and tenderness; appearance of protein, lymphocytes, and renal tubular cells in urine sediment	Anorexia, pain, fever, jaundice, light-colored bile (seen in T-tube drainage) or stools, elevated liver enzymes, dark urine	Weakness, arrhythmia	Infiltrate (seen on x-ray), interstitial perivascular infiltrate (detected by transbronchial biopsy), decreased FEV_1	Same as accelerated	Fever, diarrhea, malabsorption
Chronic	Proteinuria with or without hypertension, nephrotic syndrome	Jaundice due to intrahepatic cholestasis with preserved hepatocellular function (vanishing bile duct syndrome), ascites	Fatigue, low stress tolerance	Obliterative bronchiolitis, cough, dyspnea	Hyperglycemia, mildly elevated amylase and lipase	Diarrhea, malabsorption

FEV_1 = forced expiratory volume in 1 sec.

Posttransplantation Complications

Rejection: Rejection of solid organs may be hyperacute, accelerated, acute, or chronic (late). These categories overlap somewhat in timing but can be distinguished histopathologically. Symptoms vary by organ (see TABLE 166–1).

Hyperacute rejection occurs within 48 h of transplantation and is caused by preexisting complement-fixing antibodies to graft antigens (presensitization). It has become rare (1%) as pretransplantation screening has improved. Hyperacute rejection is characterized by small-vessel thrombosis and graft infarction. No treatment is effective except graft removal.

Accelerated rejection occurs 3 to 5 days after transplantation and is caused by preexisting noncomplement-fixing antibodies to graft antigens. Accelerated rejection is also rare. It is characterized histopathologically by cellular infiltrate with or without vascular changes. Treatment is with high-dose pulse corticosteroids or, if vascular changes occur, antilymphocyte preparations. Plasmapheresis, which may clear circulatory antibodies more rapidly, has been used.

Acute rejection is graft destruction 6 days to 3 mo after transplantation and is caused by a T cell–mediated delayed hypersensitivity reaction to allograft histocompatibility antigens. It accounts for about 1/2 of all rejection episodes that occur within 10 yr. Acute rejection is characterized by mononuclear cellular infiltration, with varying degrees of hemorrhage, edema, and necrosis. Vascular integrity is usually maintained, although vascular endothelium appears to be a primary target. Acute rejection is often reversed by intensifying immunosuppressive therapy (eg, with pulse corticosteroids and ALG). After rejection reversal, severely damaged parts of the graft heal by fibrosis, the remainder of the graft functions normally, immunosuppressant doses can be reduced to very low levels, and the allograft can survive for long periods.

Chronic rejection is graft dysfunction, often without fever, typically occurring months to years after transplantation but sometimes within weeks. Causes are multiple and include early antibody-mediated rejection, periprocedural ischemia and reperfusion injury, drug toxicity, infection, and vascular factors (eg, hypertension, hyperlipidemia). Chronic rejection accounts for most of the other 1/2 of all rejection episodes. Proliferation of neointima consisting of smooth muscle cells and extracellular matrix (transplantation atherosclerosis) gradually and eventually occludes vessel lumina, resulting in patchy ischemia and fibrosis of the graft. Chronic rejection progresses insidiously despite immunosuppressive therapy; no established treatments exist.

Infection: Immunosuppressants, secondary immunodeficiencies that accompany organ failure, and surgery make transplant patients more vulnerable to infections. Rarely, a transplanted organ is the source of infection (eg, CMV).

The most common sign is fever, often without localizing signs. Fever can also be a symptom of acute rejection but is usually accompanied by signs of graft dysfunction. If these signs are absent, the approach is similar to that for other FUO (see p. 1390); timing of symptoms and signs after transplantation helps narrow the differential diagnosis.

In the 1st month after transplantation, most infections are caused by the same hospital-acquired bacteria and fungi that infect other surgical patients (eg, *Pseudomonas* sp causing pneumonia, gram-positive bacteria causing wound infections). The greatest concern with early infection is that organisms can infect a graft or its vascular supply at suture sites, causing mycotic aneurysms or dehiscence.

Opportunistic infections occur 1 to 6 mo after transplantation (for treatment, see elsewhere in THE MANUAL). Infections may be bacterial (eg, listeriosis, nocardiosis), viral (eg, due to CMV, EBV, VZV, or hepatitis B or C virus), fungal (eg, aspergillosis, cryptococcosis, *Pneumocystis jiroveci* infection), or parasitic (eg, strongyloidiasis, toxoplasmosis, trypanosomiasis, leishmaniasis).

Risk of infection returns to baseline for about 80% of patients after 6 mo. About 10% develop complications of early infections, such as viral infection of the graft, metastatic infection (eg, CMV retinitis, colitis), or virus-induced cancers (eg, hepatitis and hepatocellular carcinoma, human papillomavirus and basal cell carcinoma). Others develop chronic rejection, require high doses of immunosuppressants (5 to 10%), and remain at high risk of opportunistic infections indefinitely.

After transplantation, most patients are given antimicrobials to reduce risk of infection. Choice of drug depends on individual risk and type of transplantation; regimens include trimethoprim/sulfamethoxazole 80/400 mg po once/day for 4 to 12 mo to prevent *P. jiroveci* infection or to prevent UTIs in kidney transplant patients. Neutropenic patients are sometimes given quinolone antibiotics (eg, levofloxacin 500 mg po or IV once/day) to prevent gram-negative infection. Inactivated vaccines can be safely given posttransplantation; risks due to live-attenuated vaccines must be balanced against their potential benefits, especially for patients taking low doses of immunosuppressants.

Renal disorders: GFR decreases 30 to 50% during the 1st 6 mo after solid organ transplantation in 15 to 20% of patients. They usually also develop hypertension. Incidence is greatest for recipients of intestinal transplants (21%) and least for recipients of heart-lung transplants (7%). Nephrotoxic and diabetogenic effects of calcineurin inhibitors are the most important contributor, but periprocedural renal insults, pretransplantation renal insufficiency or hepatitis C infection, and use of other nephrotoxic drugs also contribute. After the initial decrease, GFR typically stabilizes or decreases more slowly; nonetheless, mortality risk quadruples unless subsequent kidney transplantation is done. Renal insufficiency after transplantation may be prevented by early weaning of calcineurin inhibitors, but a safe minimum dose has not been determined.

Cancer: Long-term immunosuppression increases incidence of virus-induced cancer, especially squamous and basal cell carcinoma, lymphoproliferative disease (mainly B-cell non-Hodgkin lymphoma), anogenital (including cervical) cancer, and Kaposi's sarcoma. Treatment is similar to that of cancer in nonimmunosuppressed patients; reduction or interruption of immunosuppression is not usually required for low-grade tumors but is recommended for more aggressive tumors and lymphomas. Transfusion of partially HLA-matched cytotoxic T cells is under study as a possible treatment for some forms of lymphoproliferative disease. Surveillance with bone marrow biopsies in affected patients is recommended.

Other complications: Immunosuppressants (especially corticosteroids and calcineurin inhibitors) increase bone resorption and risk of osteoporosis for patients who are at risk before transplantation (eg, because of reduced physical activity, tobacco and alcohol use, or a preexisting renal disorder). Although not routine, use of vitamin D, bisphosphonates, or other antiresorptive drugs after transplantation may play a role in prevention.

Failure to grow, primarily as a consequence of chronic corticosteroid use, is a concern in children. Growth failure can be mitigated by tapering corticosteroids to the minimum dose that does not lead to graft rejection.

Systemic atherosclerosis can result from hyperlipidemia due to use of calcineurin inhibitors and corticosteroids; it typically occurs in kidney transplant recipients > 15 yr posttransplantation.

Graft vs host disease (GVHD) occurs when donor T cells react against recipient's self-antigens. GVHD primarily affects hematopoietic stem cell recipients but may also affect liver and small-bowel transplant recipients (see p. 1372).

Contraindications

Absolute contraindications to transplantation include active infection, cancer (except hepatocellular carcinoma confined to the liver), and pregnancy. Relative contraindications include age > 65, poor functional or nutritional status (including severe obesity), HIV infection, multiorgan insufficiency, substance abuse disorders, and high likelihood of nonadherence. Eligibility decisions for patients with relative contraindications differ by medical center; immunosuppressants are safe and effective for HIV-positive transplant recipients.

HEART TRANSPLANTATION

Heart transplantation is an option for patients who have end-stage heart failure, coronary artery disease (CAD), arrhythmias, hypertrophic cardiomyopathy, or congenital heart disease and who remain at risk of death and have intolerable symptoms despite optimal use of drugs and medical devices. Transplantation may also be indicated for patients who cannot be weaned from temporary cardiac-assist devices after MI or nontransplant cardiac surgery and for patients with cardiac sequelae of a lung disorder requiring lung transplantation. The only absolute contraindication is pulmonary hypertension; relative contraindications include organ insufficiency (eg, pulmonary, renal, hepatic) and local or systemic infiltrative disorders (eg, cardiac sarcoma, amyloidosis).

All donated hearts come from brain-dead donors, who must be < 60 and have normal cardiac and pulmonary function and no history of CAD or other heart disorders. Donor and recipient must have compatible ABO blood type and heart size. About 25% of eligible recipients die before a donor organ becomes available. LV assist devices and artificial hearts provide interim hemodynamic support for patients waiting for a transplant. However, if left in place too long, these devices put the recipient at high risk of sepsis, device failure, and thromboembolism.

Procedure

Donor hearts are preserved by hypothermic storage. They must be transplanted within 4 to 6 h. The recipient is placed on a bypass pump, and the recipient heart is removed, preserving the posterior right atrial wall in situ. The donor heart is then transplanted orthotopically with aortic, pulmonary artery, and pulmonary vein anastomoses; a single anastomosis joins the retained posterior atrial wall to that of the donor organ.

Immunosuppressive regimens vary but are similar to those for kidney or liver transplantation (eg, anti-IL-2 receptor monoclonal antibodies, a calcineurin inhibitor, corticosteroids). About 50 to 80% of patients have at least 1 episode of rejection (average 2 to 3); most patients are asymptomatic, but about 5% develop LV dysfunction or atrial arrhythmias. Incidence of acute rejection peaks at 1 mo, decreases over the next 5 mo, and levels off by 1 yr. Risk factors for rejection include younger age, female recipient, female or black donor, and HLA mismatching. Cytomegalovirus (CMV) infection may also influence risk.

Because graft damage can be irreversible and catastrophic, surveillance endomyocardial biopsy is usually done once/yr; degree and distribution of mononuclear cell infiltrate and presence of myocyte injury in specimens is determined. Differential diagnosis includes perioperative ischemia, CMV infection, and idiopathic B-cell infiltration (Quilty lesions). Mild rejection (grade 1) without detectable clinical sequelae requires no treatment; moderate or severe rejection (grades 2 to 4) or mild rejection with clinical sequelae is treated with corticosteroids and antithymocyte globulin or OKT3 as needed.

The main complication is cardiac allograft vasculopathy, a form of atherosclerosis that diffusely narrows or obliterates vessel lumina (in 25% of patients). Its cause is probably multifactorial and relates to donor age, cold and reperfusion ischemia, dyslipidemia, immunosuppressants, chronic rejection, and viral infection (adenovirus in children, CMV in adults). For early detection, surveillance stress testing or coronary angiography with or without intravascular ultrasonography is often done at the time of endomyocardial biopsy. Treatment is aggressive lipid lowering (see p. 1302) and diltiazem; everolimus 1.5 mg po bid may be preventive.

Prognosis

Survival rates at 1 yr are 85%, and annual mortality thereafter is about 4%. Pretransplantation predictors of 1-yr mortality include need for preoperative ventilation or LV assist devices, cachexia, female recipient or donor, and diagnoses other than heart failure or CAD. Posttransplantation predictors include elevated C-reactive protein and troponin levels. Cause of death within 1 yr is most often acute rejection and infection; cause after 1 yr is most often cardiac allograft vasculopathy or a lymphoproliferative disorder. Prognosis of recipients alive at > 1 yr is excellent; exercise capacity remains below normal but is sufficient for daily activities and may increase over time with sympathetic reinnervation. More than 95% of patients reach New York Heart Association class I cardiac status, and > 70% return to full-time employment.

HEMATOPOIETIC STEM CELL TRANSPLANTATION

Hematopoietic stem cell transplantation (HSCT) is a rapidly evolving technique that offers a potential cure for hematologic cancers (leukemias, lymphomas, myeloma) and other hematologic disorders (eg, primary immunodeficiency, aplastic anemia, myelodysplasia). HSCT may be autologous or allogeneic; bone marrow, peripheral blood, or umbilical cord stem cells may be used. Peripheral blood has largely replaced bone marrow as a source of stem cells, especially in autologous HSCT, because stem cell harvest is easier and neutrophil and platelet counts recover faster. Umbilical cord HSCT has been mainly restricted to children because the number of stem cells is low.

There are no contraindications to autologous HSCT. Contraindications to allogeneic HSCT are relative and include age > 50, previous HSCT, and significant comorbidities. Allogeneic HSCT is limited mainly by lack of histocompatible donors. An HLA-identical sibling donor is ideal, followed by an HLA-matched sibling donor. Because only $\frac{1}{4}$ of patients have such a sibling donor, mismatched related or matched unrelated donors (identified through international registries) are often used. However, long-term disease-free survival rates may be lower than those with HLA-identical sibling donors. The technique for umbilical cord HSCT is still being defined, but HLA-matching is probably unimportant.

Procedure

For bone marrow stem cell harvest, 700 to 1500 mL (maximum 15 mL/kg) of marrow is aspirated from the donor's posterior iliac crests; local or general anesthesia is used. For peripheral blood harvest, the donor is treated with recombinant growth factors (granulocyte colony-stimulating factor or granulocyte-macrophage colony-stimulating factor) to stimulate proliferation and mobilization of stem cells, with standard phlebotomy 4 to 6 days afterward. Fluorescence-activated cell sorting is used to identify and separate stem from other cells.

Stem cells are then infused over 1 to 2 h through a large-bore central venous catheter. In HSCT for cancer, the recipient first is given a conditioning regimen (eg, cyclophosphamide 60 mg/kg/day IV for 2 days with total body irradiation, busulfan 1 mg/kg po qid for 4 days plus cyclophosphamide without total body irradiation) to induce remission and suppress the immune system so that the graft can be accepted. Similar regimens are used for allogeneic HSCT, even when cancer is not the indication, to reduce incidence of rejection and relapse, but not for autologous HSCT. Nonmyeloablative conditioning regimens may reduce morbidity and mortality risks and may be useful for elderly patients, patients with comorbidities, and those susceptible to a graft-vs-tumor effect (eg, those with multiple myeloma).

After transplantation, recipients are given colony-stimulating factors to shorten duration of posttransplantation leukopenia, prophylactic anti-infective drugs (see p. 1369), and, in allogeneic HSCT, up to 6 mo of prophylactic immunosuppressants (typically methotrexate and cyclosporine) to prevent donor T cells from reacting against recipient major histocompatibility complex molecules (graft-vs-host disease [GVHD]). Broad-spectrum antibiotics are usually withheld unless fever develops. Engraftment typically occurs 10 to 20 days after HSCT (earlier with peripheral blood stem cells) and is defined by an absolute neutrophil count > 500×10^6/L.

Major early (< 100 days) complications include failure to engraft, rejection, and acute GVHD. Failure to engraft and rejection affect < 5% of patients and manifest as persistent pancytopenia or irreversible decline in blood counts. Treatment is corticosteroids for several weeks.

Acute GVHD occurs in recipients of allogeneic HSCTs, 40% of HLA-matched sibling graft recipients, and 80% of unrelated donor graft recipients. It causes fever, rash, hepatitis with hyperbilirubinemia, vomiting, diarrhea, abdominal pain (which may progress to ileus), and weight loss. Risk factors include HLA and sex mismatching; unrelated donor; older age of recipient, donor, or both; donor presensitization; and inadequate GVHD prophylaxis. Diagnosis is obvious by history and physical examination; treatment is methylprednisolone 2 mg/kg IV once/day, increased to 10 mg/kg if there is no response within 5 days.

Major later complications include chronic GVHD and disease relapse. Chronic GVHD may occur by itself, develop from acute GVHD, or occur after resolution of acute GVHD. It typically occurs 4 to 7 mo after HSCT (range 2 mo to 2 yr). Chronic GVHD occurs in recipients of allogeneic HSCTs, about 35 to 50% of HLA-matched sibling graft recipients, and 60 to 70% of unrelated donor graft recipients. It affects primarily the skin (eg, lichenoid rash, scleroderma) and mucous membranes (eg, keratoconjunctivitis sicca, periodontitis, orogenital lichenoid reactions) but also affects the GI tract and liver. Immunodeficiency is a primary feature; bronchiolitis obliterans similar to that after lung transplantation can also develop. Ultimately, 20 to 40% die of GVHD; mortality rate is higher with more severe reactions. Treatment may not be necessary for skin and mucous membrane disease; treatment of more extensive disease is similar to that of acute GVHD. T-cell depletion of allogeneic donor grafts using monoclonal antibodies or mechanical separation reduces incidence and severity of GVHD but also eliminates a graft-vs-tumor effect that may enhance stem cell proliferation and engraftment and reduce disease relapse rates. Relapse rates with autologous HSCT are higher for this reason and because circulating tumor cells may be transplanted. Ex vivo tumor cell purging before autologous transplantation is under study.

In patients without chronic GVHD, all immunosuppression can be stopped 6 mo after HSCT; thus, late complications are rare in these patients.

Prognosis

Prognosis varies by indication and procedure. Overall, disease relapse occurs in 40 to 75% of recipients of autologous HSCTs and in 10 to 40% of recipients of allogeneic HSCTs. Success (cancer-free bone marrow) rates are 30 to 40% for patients with relapsed, chemotherapy-sensitive lymphoma and 20 to 50% for patients with acute leukemia in remission; compared with chemotherapy alone, HSCT improves survival of patients with multiple myeloma. Success rates are low for patients with more advanced disease or with responsive solid cancers (eg, breast cancer, or germ cell tumors). Relapse rates are reduced in patients with GVHD, but overall mortality rates are increased if GVHD is severe. Intensive preparative regimens, effective GVHD prophylaxis, cyclosporine-based regimens, and improved supportive care (eg, antibiotics, herpesvirus and cytomegalovirus prophylaxis) have increased long-term disease-free survival after HSCT.

KIDNEY TRANSPLANTATION

Kidney transplantation is the most common type of solid organ transplantation; the primary indication is end-stage renal failure. Absolute contraindications include comorbidities that could compromise graft survival (eg, severe heart disorders, cancer), which can be detected via thorough screening. Relative contraindications include poorly controlled diabetes, which can lead to renal failure. Patients in their 60s may be transplant candidates if they are otherwise healthy and functionally independent with good social support, if they have a reasonably long life expectancy, and if transplantation is likely to substantially improve function and quality of life beyond simply freeing them from dialysis. Patients with type 1 diabetes may be candidates for simultaneous pancreas-kidney or pancreas-after-kidney transplantation.

More than $\frac{1}{2}$ of donated kidneys come from previously healthy, brain-dead people. About $\frac{1}{3}$ of these kidneys are marginal, with physiologic or procedure-related damage, but are used because demand is so great. The remaining donated kidneys come from living donors; because of limited supply, allografts from carefully selected living unrelated donors are being increasingly used. Living donors relinquish reserve renal capacity, may put themselves at risk of procedural and long-term morbidity, and may have psychologic conflicts about donation; therefore, they are evaluated for normal bilateral renal function, absence of systemic disease, histocompatibility, emotional stability, and ability to give informed consent. Hypertension, diabetes, and cancer (except possibly CNS tumors) usually preclude kidney donation from living donors.

Procedure

The donor kidney is removed during an open or laparoscopic procedure, perfused with cooling solutions containing relatively large concentrations of poorly permeating substances (eg, mannitol, hetastarch) and electrolyte concentrations approximating intracellular levels, then stored in an iced solution. Kidneys preserved this way usually function well if transplanted within 48 h. Although not commonly used, continuous pulsatile hypothermic perfusion with an oxygenated, plasma-based perfusate can extend ex vivo viability up to 72 h.

Dialysis may be required before transplantation to ensure a relatively normal metabolic state, but living donor allografts appear to survive better in recipients who have not begun long-term dialysis before transplantation. Nephrectomy is usually not required unless native kidneys are infected. Whether transfusions are useful for anemic patients anticipating an allograft is unclear; transfusions can sensitize patients to alloantigens, but allografts may survive better in recipients who receive transfusions but do not become sensitized, possibly because transfusions induce some form of tolerance.

The transplanted kidney is usually placed in the iliac fossa. Renal vessels are anastomosed to the iliac vessels, and the donor ureter is implanted into the bladder or anastomosed to the recipient ureter. Vesicoureteral reflux occurs in about 30% of recipients but is usually harmless.

Immunosuppressive regimens vary. Commonly, cyclosporine is given IV during or immediately after transplantation and orally thereafter in doses titrated to minimize toxicity and rejection while maintaining trough blood levels > 200 ng/mL. On the day of transplantation, IV or oral corticosteroids are also given; dose is tapered over the following 12 wk.

Despite use of immunosuppressants, most recipients have one or more rejection episodes. Most episodes are probably insignificant, subclinical, and therefore never detected;

however, they contribute to long-term insufficiency, graft failure, or both. Signs of rejection vary by type (see TABLE 166–1).

Rejection can be diagnosed by percutaneous needle biopsy if the diagnosis is unclear clinically. Biopsy may also help distinguish antibody-mediated from T-cell–mediated rejection and identify other common causes of graft insufficiency or failure (eg, calcineurin inhibitor toxicity, diabetic or hypertensive nephropathy, polyomavirus type 1 infection). Advanced tests that may improve accuracy of rejection diagnosis include measurement of urinary mRNA-encoding mediators of rejection and gene expression profiling of biopsy samples using DNA microarrays.

Chronic allograft nephropathy refers to graft insufficiency or failure ≥ 3 mo after transplantation. Most cases are attributable to one or more of the above causes. Some experts believe the term should be reserved to describe graft insufficiency or failure when biopsy shows chronic interstitial fibrosis and tubular atrophy not attributable to any other cause.

Intensified immunosuppressive therapy (eg, with high-dose pulse corticosteroids or antilymphocyte globulin) usually reverses accelerated or acute rejection. If immunosuppressants are ineffective, dose is tapered and hemodialysis is resumed until a subsequent transplant is available. Nephrectomy of the transplanted kidney is necessary if hematuria, graft tenderness, or fever develops after immunosuppressants are stopped.

Prognosis

Most rejection episodes and other complications occur within 3 to 4 mo after transplantation; most patients then return to more normal health and activity but must take maintenance doses of immunosuppressants indefinitely.

At 1 yr, survival rates with living-donor grafts are 98% for patients and 94% for grafts; rates with deceased-donor grafts are 94% and 88%, respectively. Subsequent annual graft loss rates are 3 to 5% with a living-donor graft and 5 to 8% with a deceased-donor graft.

Among patients whose graft survives the 1st year, ½ die of other causes with the graft functioning normally; ½ develop chronic allograft nephropathy with the graft malfunctioning in 1 to 5 yr. Rates of late failure are higher for blacks than for whites.

Doppler ultrasonographic measurement of peak systolic and minimal end-diastolic flow in renal segmental arteries ≥ 3 mo after transplantation may help assess prognosis, but the gold standard remains serial determination of serum creatinine.

LIVER TRANSPLANTATION

Liver transplantation is the 2nd most common type of solid organ transplantation. Indications include cirrhosis (70% of US transplants, 60 to 70% of which are attributed to hepatitis C); fulminant hepatic necrosis (about 8%); hepatocellular carcinoma (about 7%); biliary atresia and metabolic disorders, primarily in children (about 3% each); and other cholestatic (eg, primary sclerosing cholangitis) and noncholestatic (eg, autoimmune hepatitis) disorders (about 8%). For patients with hepatocellular carcinoma, transplantation is indicated for 1 tumor < 5 cm or up to 3 tumors < 3 cm (Milan criteria) and for some fibrolamellar types. For patients with liver metastases, transplantation is indicated only for neuroendocrine tumors without extrahepatic growth after removal of the primary tumor.

Absolute contraindications are elevated intracranial pressure (> 40 mm Hg) or low cerebral perfusion pressure (< 60 mm Hg) in patients with fulminant hepatic necrosis, severe pulmonary hypertension (mean pulmonary artery pressure > 50 mm Hg), sepsis, and advanced or metastatic hepatocellular carcinoma; all of these conditions lead to poor outcomes during or after transplantation.

Nearly all donated livers come from size- and ABO-matched deceased, heart-beating donors. Annually, about 500 come from living donors, who can live without their right lobe (in adult-to-adult transplantation) or the lateral segment of their left lobe (in adult-to-child transplantation). Advantages of living donation for the recipient include shorter waiting times, shorter cold ischemic times for explanted organs, and the ability to schedule transplantation to optimize the patient's condition. Disadvantages to the donor include mortality risk of 1/300 to 400 (compared with 1/3300 in living-donor kidney transplantation) and complications (especially bile leakage) in up to ¼, usually when resection is lobar (not segmental). Living donors are also at risk of psychologic coercion. A few livers come from deceased, non–heart-beating donors.

Donor (deceased or living) risk factors for graft failure in the recipient include age > 50; hepatic steatosis; elevated liver enzymes, bilirubin, or both; prolonged stay in ICU; hypotension requiring vasopressors; and hypernatremia. Transplants from female donors to male recipients may also increase risk. But because imbalance between supply and demand is greatest for liver transplants (and is growing because prevalence of hepatitis-induced cirrhosis is increasing), livers from donors > 50 and with short cold ischemia times, those with fatty infiltration, and those with viral hepatitis (for transplantation into recipients with viral hepatitis-induced cirrhosis) are increasingly being used. Additional techniques to increase supply include split liver transplantation, in which deceased-donor livers are divided into right and left lobes or right lobe and left lateral segment (done in or ex situ) and given to 2 recipients, and domino transplantation, rarely indicated, in which a deceased-donor liver is given to a recipient with an infiltrative disease (eg, amyloidosis), and the explanted diseased liver is given to an elderly recipient who can benefit from the diseased liver but is not expected to live long enough to experience adverse effects of transplant dysfunction.

Despite these innovations, many patients die waiting for transplants. Liver-assist devices (extracorporeal perfusion of cultured hepatocyte suspensions or immortalized hepatoma cell lines) are used in some centers to keep patients alive until a liver is available or acute dysfunction resolves. For distribution of available organs, patients on the national waitlist are given a prognostic score derived from creatinine, bilirubin, and INR measurements (for adults) or from age and serum albumin, bilirubin, INR, and growth failure measurements (for children). For patients with hepatocellular carcinoma, the score incorporates tumor size and waiting time (increasing with each). Patients with higher scores are more likely to die and are given higher priority for organs from ABO- and weight-matched donors.

Procedure

Deceased-donor livers are removed after exploratory laparotomy confirms absence of intra-abdominal disease that would preclude transplantation. Living donors undergo lobar or segmental resection. Explanted livers are perfused and stored in a cold preservation solution for up to 24 h before transplantation; incidence of graft nonfunction and ischemic-type biliary injury increases with prolonged storage.

Recipient hepatectomy is the most demanding part of the procedure because it is often done in patients with portal hypertension and coagulation defects. Intraoperative blood loss can total > 100 units, but use of a cell saver machine and autotransfusion devices can reduce allogeneic transfusion requirements to < 10 to 15 units. After hepatectomy, the suprahepatic vena cava of the donor graft is anastomosed to the recipient's vena cava in an end-to-side fashion ("piggy-back" technique). Donor and recipient portal veins, hepatic arteries, and bile ducts are then anastomosed. With this technique, a bypass pump is not needed to carry portal venous blood to the systemic venous circuit. Heterotopic placement of the liver provides an auxiliary liver and obviates several technical difficulties, but outcomes have been discouraging, and this technique is still experimental.

Immunosuppressive regimens vary. Commonly, anti-IL-2 receptor monoclonal antibodies are given on the day of transplantation, with a calcineurin inhibitor (cyclosporine or tacrolimus), mycophenolate mofetil, and corticosteroids. Except in patients with autoimmune hepatitis, corticosteroids can be tapered within weeks and often stopped after 3 to 4 mo. Compared with other solid organ transplantation, liver transplantation requires the lowest doses of immunosuppressants.

Liver allografts are less aggressively rejected than other organ allografts for unknown reasons; hyperacute rejection occurs less frequently than expected in patients presensitized to HLA or ABO antigens, and immunosuppressants can often be tapered relatively quickly and eventually stopped. Most episodes of acute rejection are mild and self-limited, occur in the 1st 3 to 6 mo, and do not affect graft survival. Risk factors include younger recipient age, older donor age, greater HLA mismatching, longer cold ischemia times, and autoimmune disorders; worse nutritional status (eg, in alcoholism) appears protective.

Symptoms and signs of rejection depend on the type of rejection (see TABLE 166–1). Symptoms of acute rejection occur in about 50% of patients; symptoms of chronic rejection occur in < 2%.

Differential diagnosis of acute rejection includes viral hepatitis (eg, cytomegalovirus or Epstein-Barr virus infection; recurrent hepatitis B, C, or both), calcineurin inhibitor toxicity, and cholestasis. Rejection can be diagnosed by percutaneous needle biopsy if the diagnosis is unclear clinically. Suspected rejection is treated with IV corticosteroids;

antithymocyte globulin and OKT3 are options when corticosteroids are ineffective (in 10 to 20%). Retransplantation is tried when rejection is refractory to immunosuppressants.

Immunosuppression contributes to recurrence of viral hepatitis in patients who had viral hepatitis-induced cirrhosis before transplantation. Hepatitis C recurs in nearly all patients; usually, viremia and infection are clinically silent but may cause active hepatitis and cirrhosis. Risk factors for clinically significant reinfection may be related to the recipient (older age, HLA type, hepatocellular carcinoma), donor (older age, fatty infiltration, prolonged ischemic time, and living donor), virus (high viral load, genotype 1B, failure to respond to interferon), or postprocedural events (immunosuppressant doses, acute rejection treated with corticosteroids or OKT3, and cytomegalovirus infection). Standard treatment (see p. 230) is only marginally effective. Hepatitis B recurs in all but has been successfully managed with hepatitis B immune globulin and lamivudine; coinfection with hepatitis D appears protective against recurrence.

Early (within 2 mo) complications of liver transplantation include primary nonfunction in 5 to 15%, biliary dysfunction (eg, ischemic anastomotic strictures, bile leakage, ductal obstructions, leakage around T-tube site) in 15 to 20%, portal vein thrombosis in 8 to 10%, hepatic artery thrombosis in 3 to 5% (especially in patients taking sirolimus), hepatic artery mycotic or pseudoaneurysm, and hepatic artery rupture. Typical symptoms include fever, hypotension, and elevated liver function enzymes.

The most common late complications are intrahepatic or anastomotic bile duct strictures, which produce symptoms of cholestasis and cholangitis. Strictures can sometimes be treated endoscopically or through percutaneous transhepatic cholangiographic dilation, stenting, or both, but they often ultimately require retransplantation.

Prognosis

At 1 yr, survival rates with living-donor grafts are 85% for patients and 76% for grafts; rates with deceased-donor grafts are 86% and 80%, respectively. Overall rates for patients and grafts, respectively, are 78% and 71% at 3 yr and 72% and 64% at 5 yr. Survival is better for chronic than for acute liver failure. Death after 1 yr is rare and attributable to a recurrent disorder (eg, cancer, hepatitis) rather than to posttransplantation complications.

Recurrent hepatitis C infection leads to cirrhosis in 15 to 30% of patients by 5 yr. Hepatic disorders with an autoimmune component (eg, primary biliary cirrhosis, primary sclerosing cholangitis, autoimmune hepatitis) recur in 20 to 30% by 5 yr.

LUNG TRANSPLANTATION

Lung transplantation is an option for patients who have respiratory insufficiency or failure and who remain at risk of death despite optimal medical treatment. The most common indications are COPD, idiopathic pulmonary fibrosis, cystic fibrosis, α_1-antitrypsin deficiency, and primary pulmonary hypertension. Less common indications include interstitial lung disorders (eg, sarcoidosis), bronchiectasis, and congenital heart disease. Single and double lung procedures are equally appropriate for most lung disorders without cardiac involvement; the exception is chronic diffuse infection (eg, bronchiectasis), for which double lung transplantation is best. Heart-lung transplantation is indicated for Eisenmenger's syndrome and for any lung disorder with severe ventricular dysfunction likely to be irreversible; cor pulmonale is not an indication because it often reverses after lung transplantation. Single and double lung procedures are about equally common and are at least 8 times more common than heart-lung transplantation.

Relative contraindications include age (single lung recipients must be < 65; double lung recipients, < 60; and heart and lung recipients, < 55), active cigarette smoking, previous thoracic surgery, and, for some cystic fibrosis patients and at some medical centers, lung infection with resistant strains of *Burkholderia cepacia*, which greatly increases mortality risk.

Nearly all donated lungs are from brain-dead, heart-beating donors. Rarely, living adult (usually parent-to-child) lobar transplantation is done when deceased-donor organs are unavailable. Donors must be < 65 and never-smokers and have no active lung disorder as evidenced by oxygenation ($PaO_2/FIO_2 > 250$ to 300 mm Hg), lung compliance (peak inspiratory pressure < 30 cm H_2O at V_T 15 mL/kg and positive end expiratory pressure = 5 cm H_2O), and gross appearance by bronchoscopy. Donor and recipients must be size-matched anatomically (by chest x-ray), physiologically (by total lung capacity), or both.

Timing of referral for transplantation should be determined by factors such as degree of obstructive defect (FEV_1 < 25 to 30% predicted in patients with COPD, α_1-antitrypsin deficiency, or cystic fibrosis); PaO_2 < 55 mm Hg; $PaCO_2$ > 50 mm Hg; right atrial pressure > 10 mm Hg and peak systolic pressure > 50 mm Hg for patients with primary pulmonary hypertension; and progression rate of clinical, radiographic, or physiologic disease.

Procedure

The donor is anticoagulated, and a cold crystalloid preservation solution containing prostaglandins is flushed through the pulmonary arteries into the lungs. Donor organs are cooled with iced saline slush in situ or via cardiopulmonary bypass, then removed. Prophylactic antibiotics are often given.

Single lung transplantation requires posterolateral thoracotomy. The native lung is removed, and the bronchus, pulmonary artery, and pulmonary veins of the donor lung are anastomosed to their respective cuffs. The bronchial anastomosis requires intussusception or wrapping with omentum or pericardium to facilitate adequate healing. Advantages include a simpler operation, avoidance of cardiopulmonary bypass and systemic anticoagulation (usually), more flexibility concerning size matching, and availability of the contralateral lung from the same donor for another recipient. Disadvantages include the possibility of ventilation/perfusion mismatch between the native and transplant lungs and the possibility of poor healing of the single bronchial anastomosis.

Double lung transplantation requires sternotomy or anterior transverse thoracotomy; the procedure is similar to 2 sequential single transplants. The primary advantage is definitive removal of all diseased tissue. The disadvantage is poor healing of the tracheal anastomosis.

Heart-lung transplantation requires median sternotomy with cardiopulmonary bypass. Aortic, right atrial, and tracheal anastomoses are required; the trachea is anastomosed immediately above the bifurcation. The primary advantages are improved graft function and more dependable healing of the tracheal anastomosis because of coronary-bronchial collaterals within the heart-lung block. Disadvantages include long operative time with the need for cardiopulmonary bypass, the need for close size matching, and use of 3 donor organs by one recipient.

Methylprednisolone IV is often given to recipients before reperfusion of the transplanted lung. A common immunosuppressive regimen is a calcineurin inhibitor (cyclosporine or tacrolimus), a purine metabolism inhibitor (azathioprine or mycophenolate mofetil), and methylprednisolone. Prophylactic antithymocyte globulin (ATG) or OKT3 may also be given during the 1st 2 wk after transplantation. Corticosteroids may be omitted to facilitate healing of the bronchial anastomosis; higher doses of other drugs (eg, cyclosporine, azathioprine) are substituted. Immunosuppressants are continued indefinitely.

Rejection develops in most patients despite immunosuppressive therapy. Symptoms and signs are similar in hyperacute, acute, and chronic forms and include fever, dyspnea, cough, decreased SaO_2, interstitial infiltrate on x-ray, and a decrease in FEV_1 by > 10 to 15%. Hyperacute rejection must be distinguished from early graft dysfunction caused by ischemic injury during the transplantation procedure. Diagnosis is confirmed if bronchoscopic transbronchial biopsy shows perivascular lymphocytic infiltration in small vessels. IV corticosteroids are usually effective. Treatment of recurrent or resistant cases varies and includes higher corticosteroid doses, aerosolized cyclosporine, ATG, and OKT3.

Chronic rejection (after > 1 yr) occurs in up to 50% of patients; it takes the form of obliterative bronchiolitis or, less commonly, atherosclerosis. Acute rejection may increase risk of chronic rejection. Patients with obliterative bronchiolitis present with cough, dyspnea, and decreased FEV_1 with or without physical and radiographic evidence of an airway process. Differential diagnosis includes pneumonia. Diagnosis is by bronchoscopy with biopsy. No treatment has proved effective, but options include corticosteroids, ATG or OKT3, inhaled cyclosporine, and retransplantation.

The most common surgical complication is poor healing of the bronchial or tracheal anastomosis. Up to 20% of single lung recipients develop bronchial stenosis that causes wheezing and airway obstruction; it can be treated with dilation or stent placement. Other surgical complications include hoarseness and diaphragmatic paralysis, caused by damage to the recurrent laryngeal or phrenic nerves; GI dysmotility, caused by damage to the thoracic vagus nerve; and pneumothorax. Supraventricular arrhythmias develop in some patients, probably due to conduction changes caused by pulmonary vein-atrial suturing.

Prognosis

At 1 yr, survival rates with living-donor grafts are 70% and with deceased-donor grafts 77%. Overall 5-yr patient survival rate is 45%. Mortality rate is higher for patients with primary pulmonary hypertension, idiopathic pulmonary fibrosis, or sarcoidosis and lower for those with COPD or α_1-antitrypsin deficiency. Mortality rate is higher for single lung transplantation than for double. Most common causes of death within 1 mo are primary graft failure, ischemia and reperfusion injury, and infection (eg, pneumonia) excluding cytomegalovirus; the most common cause between 1 mo and 1 yr is infection, and after 1 yr, it is obliterative bronchiolitis. Mortality risk factors include cytomegalovirus mismatching (donor positive, recipient negative), human leukocyte antigen (HLA-DR) mismatching, diabetes, and prior need for mechanical ventilation or inotropic support. Uncommonly, the disorder recurs, particularly in some patients with an interstitial lung disorder. Exercise capacity is slightly limited because of a hyperventilatory response. Overall survival rate 1 yr after heart-lung transplantation is 60% for patients and grafts.

PANCREAS TRANSPLANTATION

Pancreas transplantation is a form of pancreatic β-cell replacement that can restore normoglycemia in diabetic patients. Because the recipient exchanges risks of insulin injection for risks of immunosuppression, eligibility is limited mostly to patients who have type 1 diabetes with renal failure and who are thus candidates for kidney transplantation; > 90% of pancreas transplantations include transplantation of a kidney. At many centers, failure of standard treatment and episodes of hypoglycemic unawareness are also eligibility criteria. Relative contraindications include age > 55 and significant atherosclerotic cardiovascular disease, defined as history of MI, coronary artery bypass graft surgery, percutaneous coronary intervention, or a positive stress test; these factors dramatically increase perioperative risk.

Options include simultaneous pancreas-kidney (SPK) transplantation; pancreas-after-kidney (PAK) transplantation; and pancreas-alone transplantation. The advantages of SPK are one-time exposure to induction immunosuppression, potential protection of the newly transplanted kidney from adverse effects of hyperglycemia, and the ability to monitor rejection in the kidney; the kidney is more prone to rejection than the pancreas, where rejection is difficult to detect. The advantage of PAK is the ability to optimize HLA matching and timing of kidney transplantation using a living donor. Pancreas-alone transplantation offers an advantage to patients who do not have end-stage renal disease but have other severe diabetes complications, including labile glucose control.

Donors are usually recently deceased patients who are aged 10 to 55 and have no history of glucose intolerance or alcohol abuse. For SPK, the pancreas and kidney come from the same donor, and the same restrictions for kidney donation apply (see p. 1373). A few (< 1%) segmental transplantations from living donors have been done, but this procedure has substantial risks for the donor (eg, splenic infarction, abscess, pancreatitis, pancreatic leak and pseudocyst, secondary diabetes), which limit its widespread use.

Procedure

The donor is anticoagulated, and a cold preservation solution is flushed into the celiac artery. The pancreas is cooled in situ with iced saline slush, then removed en bloc with the liver (for transplantation into a different recipient) and the 2nd portion of the duodenum containing the ampulla of Vater.

The donor pancreas is positioned intraperitoneally and laterally in the lower abdomen. In SPK, the pancreas is placed into the right lower quadrant of the recipient's abdomen and the kidney into the left lower quadrant. The native pancreas is left in place. Anastomoses are made between the donor splenic or superior mesenteric artery and recipient iliac artery and between the donor portal vein and recipient iliac vein. Thus, endocrine secretions drain systemically, causing hyperinsulinemia; sometimes the pancreatic venous system is anastomosed to a portal vein tributary to recreate physiologic conditions, although this procedure is more demanding and its benefits are unclear. The duodenum is sewn to the bladder dome or to the jejunum for drainage of exocrine secretions.

Immunosuppression regimens vary but typically include immunosuppressive Igs, a calcineurin inhibitor, a purine synthesis inhibitor, and corticosteroids, which can be slowly tapered over 12 mo. Despite adequate immunosuppression, rejection develops in 60 to 80% of patients, primarily affecting exocrine, not endocrine, components. Compared with kidney transplantation alone, SPK has a greater risk of rejection, and rejection episodes tend to occur later, to recur more often, and to be corticosteroid-resistant. Symptoms and signs are nonspecific (see TABLE 166–1).

After SPK and PAK, pancreas rejection, detected by an increase in serum creatinine, almost always accompanies kidney rejection. After pancreas-alone transplantation, a stable urinary amylase concentration in patients with urinary drainage excludes rejection; a decrease suggests some form of graft dysfunction but is not specific to rejection. Early detection is therefore difficult. Diagnosis is confirmed by ultrasound-guided percutaneous or cystoscopic transduodenal biopsy. Treatment is with antithymocyte globulin.

Early complications affect 10 to 15% of patients and include wound infection and dehiscence, gross hematuria, intra-abdominal urinary leak, reflux pancreatitis, recurrent UTI, small-bowel obstruction, abdominal abscess, and graft thrombosis. Late complications relate to urinary loss of pancreatic $NaHCO_3^-$, causing volume depletion and non-anion gap metabolic acidosis. Hyperinsulinemia does not appear to adversely affect glucose or lipid metabolism.

Prognosis

At 1 yr, 78% of grafts survive, but > 90% of patients survive. Whether survival is higher than that of patients without transplantation is unclear; however, the primary benefits of the procedure are freedom from insulin therapy and stabilization or improvement of many diabetic complications (eg, nephropathy, neuropathy). Graft survival is 95% for SPK, 74% for PAK, and 76% for pancreas-alone transplantation; survival after PAK and pancreas-alone transplantation is presumed to be worse than SPK because they lack a reliable marker of rejection.

Pancreatic Islet Cell Transplantation

Islet cell transplantation has theoretical advantages over pancreas transplantation: The procedure is less invasive, and islets can be cryopreserved to optimize timing of transplantation. Nevertheless, the procedure is too new for these advantages to have proven benefit, but steady improvement appears to be occurring. Its disadvantages are that transplanted glucagon-secreting α cells are nonfunctional (possibly complicating hypoglycemia) and several pancreata are usually required for a single islet cell recipient (exacerbating disparities between graft supply and demand and limiting use of the procedure). Also, islet cell transplantation appears to help maintain normoglycemia in patients who require total pancreatectomy for pain due to chronic pancreatitis. Indications are the same as those for pancreas transplantation. Simultaneous islet cell–kidney transplantation may be desirable after the technique is improved.

Procedure

A pancreas is removed from a brain-dead donor; collagenase is infused into the pancreatic duct to separate islets from pancreatic tissue. A purified islet cell fraction is infused percutaneously into the portal vein. Islet cells travel into hepatic sinusoids, where they lodge and secrete insulin.

Results are best when 2 or 3 infusions of islet cells from 2 cadavers each are used, followed by an immunosuppressive regimen consisting of an anti-IL-2 receptor, monoclonal antibodies (daclizumab), tacrolimus, and sirolimus; corticosteroids are not used. Immunosuppression must be continued life long or until islet cell function ceases. Rejection is poorly defined but can be detected by deterioration in blood glucose control; treatment of rejection is not established. Procedural complications include percutaneous hepatic puncture with bleeding, portal vein thrombosis, and portal hypertension.

Successful islet cell transplantation maintains short-term normoglycemia, but long-term outcomes are unknown; additional injections of islet preparations are necessary to obtain longer-lasting insulin independence.

SMALL-BOWEL TRANSPLANTATION

Small-bowel transplantation is indicated for patients who have malabsorption because of intestinal disorders (eg, gastroschisis, Hirschsprung's disease, autoimmune enteritis) or intestinal resection (eg, for mesenteric thromboembolism or extensive Crohn's disease) and who are at high risk of death (usually due to congenital enteropathies such as microvillus inclusion disease) or who develop complications of TPN (eg, liver failure, recurrent sepsis, total loss of venous access). Patients with locally invasive tumors that cause obstruction, abscesses, fistulas, ischemia, or hemorrhage (usually desmoid tumors associated with familial polyposis) are also candidates.

Procurement from the brain-dead, beating-heart donor is complex, partly because the small bowel can be transplanted alone, with a liver, or with a stomach, liver, duodenum, and pancreas. The role of living-related donation for small-bowel allografts has yet to be defined. Procedures vary by medical center; immunosuppressive regimens also vary, but a typical regimen includes antilymphocyte globulin for induction, followed by high-dose tacrolimus and mycophenolate mofetil for maintenance.

Weekly endoscopy is indicated to monitor rejection. Symptoms and signs of rejection include diarrhea, fever, and abdominal cramping. Endoscopic findings include mucosal erythema, friability, ulceration, and exfoliation; changes are distributed unevenly, may be difficult to detect, and can be differentiated from cytomegalovirus enteritis by viral inclusion bodies. Biopsy findings include blunted villi and inflammatory infiltrates in the lamina propria. Treatment of acute rejection is high-dose corticosteroids, antithymocyte globulin, or both.

Surgical complications affect 50% of patients and include anastomotic leaks, biliary leaks and strictures, hepatic artery thrombosis, and chylous ascites. Nonsurgical complications include graft ischemia and graft-vs-host disease caused by transplantation of gut-associated lymphoid tissue.

At 3 yr, > 50% of grafts with small-bowel transplantation alone survive, but patient survival is around 65%. With liver and small-bowel transplantation, survival rate is lower because the procedure is more extensive and the recipient's condition is more serious.

TISSUE TRANSPLANTATION

Skin allografts are used for patients with extensive burns or other conditions causing massive skin loss. Allografts are used to cover broad denuded areas and thus reduce fluid and protein losses and discourage invasive infection. The allografts are ultimately rejected, but the resulting denuded areas develop well-vascularized granulations onto which autografts from the patient's healed sites take readily. Skin cells may be grown in culture, then returned to a burned patient to help cover extensive burns; artificial skin, composed of cultured cells on a synthetic underlayer, may also be used. Split-thickness skin grafts are used to accelerate healing of small wounds. A small piece of skin just a few millimeters thick is harvested, and the donor skin is then laid onto the graft site.

Cartilage transplantation is used for children with congenital nasal or ear defects and adults with severe injuries or joint destruction (eg, severe osteoarthritis). Chondrocytes are more resistant to rejection, possibly because the sparse population of cells in hyaline cartilage is protected from cellular attack by the cartilaginous matrix around them.

Bone transplantation is used for reconstruction of large bony defects (eg, after massive resection of bone cancer). No viable donor bone cells survive in the recipient, but dead matrix from allografts can stimulate recipient osteoblasts to recolonize the matrix and lay down new bone. This matrix acts as scaffolding for bridging and stabilizing defects until new bone is formed. Cadaveric allografts are preserved by freezing to decrease immunogenicity of the bone (which is dead at the time of implantation) and by glycerolization to maintain chondrocyte viability. No postimplantation immunosuppressive therapy is used. Although patients develop anti-HLA antibodies, early follow-up detects no evidence of cartilage degradation.

Corneal transplantation is discussed on p. 902.

Adrenal autografting by stereotactically placing medullary tissue within the CNS has been reported to alleviate symptoms in patients with Parkinson's disease. Allografts of adrenal tissue, especially from fetal donors, have also been proposed. Fetal ventral mesencephalic tissue stereotactically implanted in the putamen of patients with Parkinson's disease has been reported to reduce rigidity and bradykinesia. However, with the ethical and political debates about the propriety of using human fetal tissue, a controlled trial large enough to adequately assess fetal neural transplantation appears unlikely. Xenografts of endocrinologically active cells from porcine donors are being tested.

Fetal thymus implants obtained from stillborn infants may restore immunologic responsiveness in children with thymic aplasia and resulting abnormal development of the lymphoid system. Because the recipient is immunologically unresponsive, immunosuppression is not required; however, severe graft-vs-host disease may occur.

SECTION 14 INFECTIOUS DISEASES

167 BIOLOGY OF INFECTIOUS DISEASE

A healthy person lives in harmony with the microbial flora that helps protect its host from invasion by pathogens, usually defined as microorganisms that have the capacity to cause disease. The microbial flora is mostly bacteria and fungi and includes normal resident flora, which is present consistently and promptly reestablishes itself if disturbed, and transient flora, which may colonize the host for hours to weeks but does not permanently establish itself. Organisms that are normal flora can occasionally cause disease, especially when defenses are disrupted.

Tropisms, or attractions to certain tissues, determine which body sites microorganisms colonize. Normal flora is influenced by tropisms and many other factors (eg, diet, hygiene, sanitary conditions, air pollution). For example, lactobacilli are common in the intestines of people with a high intake of dairy products; *Haemophilus influenzae* colonizes the tracheobronchial tree in patients with COPD.

HOST DEFENSE MECHANISMS

Host defenses that protect against infection include natural barriers (eg, skin and mucous membranes), nonspecific immune responses (eg, phagocytic cells [neutrophils, macrophages] and their products), and specific immune responses (eg, antibodies and lymphocytes).

Natural Barriers

The skin usually bars invading microorganisms unless it is physically disrupted (eg, by injury, IV catheter, or surgical incision).

Exceptions include human papillomavirus, which can invade normal skin, causing warts, and some parasites (eg, *Schistosoma mansoni, Strongyloides stercoralis*).

Many mucous membranes are bathed in secretions that have antimicrobial properties (eg, cervical mucus, prostatic fluid, and tears containing lysozyme, which splits the muramic acid linkage in bacterial cell walls, especially in gram-positive organisms). Local secretions also contain immunoglobulins, principally IgG and secretory IgA, which prevent microorganisms from attaching to host cells.

The respiratory tract has upper airway filters. If invading organisms reach the tracheobronchial tree, the mucociliary epithelium transports them away from the lung. Coughing also helps remove organisms. If the organisms reach the alveoli, alveolar macrophages and tissue histiocytes engulf them. However, these defenses can be overcome by large numbers of organisms or by compromised effectiveness resulting from air pollutants (eg, cigarette smoke) or interference with protective mechanisms (eg, endotracheal intubation or tracheostomy).

GI tract barriers include the acid pH of the stomach and the antibacterial activity of pancreatic enzymes, bile, and intestinal secretions. Peristalsis and the normal loss of epithelial cells remove microorganisms. If peristalsis is slowed, eg, due to drugs such as belladonna or opium alkaloids, this removal is delayed and prolongs some infections, such as symptomatic shigellosis. Compromised defense mechanisms may predispose patients to particular infections (eg, achlorhydria predisposes to salmonellosis). Normal bowel flora can inhibit pathogens; alteration of this flora with antibiotics can allow overgrowth of inherently pathogenic microorganisms (eg, *Salmonella typhimurium*) or superinfection with ordinarily commensal organisms (eg, *Candida albicans*).

GU tract barriers include the length of the urethra (20 cm) in men, the acid pH of the vagina in women, and the hypertonic state of the kidney medulla. The kidney also produces and excretes large amounts of Tamm-Horsfall mucoprotein, which binds certain bacteria, facilitating their harmless excretion.

Nonspecific Immune Responses

Cytokines (including IL-1, IL-6, tumor necrosis factor, interferon-γ) are produced principally by macrophages and activated lymphocytes and mediate an acute-phase response that develops regardless of the inciting microorganism (see also p. 1326). The response involves fever and increased production of neutrophils by the bone marrow. Endothelial cells also produce large amounts of IL-8, which attracts neutrophils.

The inflammatory response directs immune system components to injury or infection sites and is manifested by increased blood supply and vascular permeability, which allows chemotactic peptides, neutrophils, and mononuclear cells to leave the intravascular compartment. Microbial spread is limited by engulfment of microorganisms by phagocytes (eg, neutrophils and macrophages). Phagocytes are drawn to microbes via chemotaxis and engulf them, releasing phagocytic lysosomal contents that help destroy microbes. Oxidative products such as hydrogen peroxide are generated by the phagocytes and kill ingested microbes. When quantitative or qualitative defects in neutrophils result in infection, the infection usually is prolonged and recurrent and responds slowly to antimicrobial agents. Staphylococci, gram-negative organisms, and fungi are the usual pathogens responsible.

Specific Immune Responses

After infection, the host can produce a variety of antibodies, complex glycoproteins known as immunoglobulins that bind to specific microbial antigenic targets. Antibodies can help eradicate the infecting organism by attracting the host's WBCs and activating the complement system. The complement system (see p. 1326) destroys cell walls, usually through the classic pathway. Complement can also be activated on the surface of some microorganisms via the alternative pathway. Antibodies can also promote the deposition of substances known as opsonins (eg, the complement protein C3b) on the surface of microorganisms, which helps to promote phagocytosis. Opsonization is important for eradication of encapsulated organisms such as pneumococci and meningococci.

FACTORS FACILITATING MICROBIAL INVASION

Microbial invasion can be facilitated by virulence factors, microbial adherence, and resistance to antimicrobials.

Virulence factors: Virulence factors assist pathogens in invasion and resistance of host defenses. For example, encapsulated pneumococci are more virulent than nonencapsulated strains and type B encapsulated *Haemophilus influenzae* is more virulent than other *H. influenzae* capsular types. Bacterial proteins with enzymatic activity (eg, protease, hyaluronidase, neuraminidase, elastase, collagenase) facilitate local tissue spread. Invasive organisms (eg, *Shigella flexneri, Yersinia enterocolitica*) can penetrate and traverse intact eukaryotic cells, facilitating entry from mucosal surfaces.

Organisms may release toxins (called exotoxins), which are protein molecules that may cause the disease (eg, diphtheria, cholera, tetanus, botulism) or increase the severity of the disease. Most toxins bind to specific target cell receptors. With the exception of preformed toxins responsible for food-borne illnesses, toxins are produced by organisms during the course of infection. Endotoxin is a lipopolysaccharide produced by gram-negative bacteria and is part of the cell wall. Endotoxin triggers humoral enzymatic mechanisms involving the complement, clotting, fibrinolytic, and kinin pathways and causes much of the morbidity in gram-negative sepsis.

Many microorganisms have mechanisms that impair antibody production by inducing suppressor cells, blocking antigen processing, and inhibiting lymphocyte mitogenesis. Some bacteria (eg, *Neisseria gonorrhoeae, H. influenzae, Proteus mirabilis,* clostridial species, *Streptococcus pneumoniae*) produce IgA-specific proteases that cleave and inactivate secretory IgA on mucosal surfaces. Others (eg, pneumococci, meningococci) have capsules that prevent opsonic antibodies from binding.

Resistance to the lytic effects of serum complement confers virulence. Among species of *N. gonorrhoeae*, resistance predisposes to disseminated rather than localized infection.

Some organisms resist the oxidative steps in phagocytosis. For example, *Legionella* and *Listeria* either do not elicit or actively suppress the oxidative step, whereas other organisms produce enzymes (eg, catalase, glutathione reductase, or superoxide dismutase) that mitigate the oxidative products.

Microbial adherence: Adherence to surfaces helps microorganisms establish a base from which to penetrate tissues. Among the factors that determine adherence are adhesins (microbial molecules that mediate attachment to a cell) and host receptors to which the adhesins bind. Host receptors include cell surface sugar residues and cell surface proteins, such as fibronectin, that enhance binding of certain gram-positive organisms (eg, staphylococci). Other determinants of adherence include fine structures on certain bacterial cells (eg, streptococci) called fibrillae, by which some bacteria bind to human epithelial cells. Other bacteria, such as Enterobacteriaceae (eg, *Escherichia coli*), have specific adhesive organelles called fimbriae or pili. Fimbriae enable the organism to attach to almost all human cells, including neutrophils and epithelial cells in the GU tract, mouth, and intestine.

Biofilm is a slime layer that can form around certain bacteria and confer resistance to phagocytosis and antibiotics. It develops around *Pseudomonas aeruginosa* in the lungs of patients with cystic fibrosis and around coagulase-negative staphylococci in synthetic medical devices, such as IV catheters, prosthetic vascular grafts, and suture material. Factors that affect the likelihood of biofilm developing on such medical devices include the material's roughness, chemical composition, and hydrophobicity.

Antimicrobial resistance: Genetic variability among microbes is inevitable. Use of antimicrobial agents eventually selects for survival of those strains that are capable of resisting them. Minimizing inappropriate use of antibiotics is important for public health. Resistance among bacteria is discussed on p. 1423.

MANIFESTATIONS OF INFECTION

Manifestations may be local (eg, cellulitis, abscess) or systemic, most often fever. Manifestations may develop in multiple organ systems. Severe, generalized infections may produce life-threatening manifestations (eg, sepsis, septic shock—see p. 566). Most manifestations improve with successful treatment of the underlying infection. Infectious diseases commonly increase the numbers of mature and immature circulating neutrophils. Mechanisms include demargination and release of immature granulocytes from bone marrow, IL-1– and IL-6–mediated release of neutrophils from bone marrow, and colony-stimulating factors elaborated by macrophages, lymphocytes, and other tissues. Exaggeration of these phenomena (eg, in trauma, inflammation, and similar stresses) can result in release of excessive numbers of immature leukocytes into the circulation (leukemoid reaction, with leukocyte counts up to 25 to 30×10^9/L).

Conversely, some infections (eg, typhoid fever, brucellosis) commonly produce neutropenia. In overwhelming, severe infections, profound neutropenia is often a poor prognostic sign. Characteristic morphologic changes in the neutrophils of septic patients include Döhle bodies, toxic granulations, and vacuolization.

Anemia can develop despite adequate tissue iron stores. If chronic, plasma iron and total iron-binding capacity may be decreased. Serious infection, particularly with gram-negative organisms, may cause disseminated intravascular coagulation (DIC—see p. 1083).

Although most infections increase the pulse rate, others, such as typhoid fever, tularemia, brucellosis, and dengue, may not elevate the pulse rate commensurate with the degree of fever. Hypotension can result from hypovolemia or septic shock.

Hyperventilation and respiratory alkalosis are common. Subsequently, pulmonary compliance may decrease, progressing to acute respiratory distress syndrome (ARDS) and respiratory muscle failure.

Renal manifestations range from minimal proteinuria to acute renal failure, which can occur due to shock and acute tubular necrosis, glomerulonephritis, or tubulointerstitial disease.

Hepatic dysfunction, including cholestatic jaundice (often a poor prognostic sign) or hepatocellular dysfunction, occurs with many infections, even though the infection does not localize to the liver. Upper GI bleeding due to stress ulceration may occur during sepsis.

Alterations in sensorium (encephalopathy) may occur in severe infection regardless of whether there is CNS infection. Encephalopathy is most common and serious in the elderly and may produce anxiety, confusion, delirium, stupor, seizures, and coma.

Endocrinologic dysfunctions include increased production of thyroid-stimulating hormone, vasopressin, insulin, and glucagon; breakdown of skeletal muscle proteins and muscle wasting secondary to increased metabolic demands; and bone demineralization. Hypoglycemia occurs infrequently in sepsis and may be an early sign of infection in diabetics.

FEVER

Fever is elevated body temperature (eg, > 37.8 ° C orally or 38.2 ° C rectally, or an elevation of body temperature above the normal daily variation). During a 24-h period, temperature varies from lowest levels in the early morning to highest in late afternoon. The maximum variation is about 0.6 ° C. Body temperature is determined by the balance between heat production from tissues, particularly the liver and muscles, and heat loss from the periphery. In health, the hypothalamic thermoregulatory center maintains body temperature of the internal organs from 37 to 38° C. Fever raises the hypothalamic set point, triggering the vasomotor center to begin vasoconstriction, shunting blood from the periphery to decrease heat loss, and sometimes inducing shivering, which increases heat production until the temperature of the blood bathing the hypothalamus reaches the new set point. Resetting the hypothalamic set point downward (eg, with antipyretic drugs) initiates heat loss through sweating and vasodilation. The capacity to generate a fever is diminished in certain patients (eg, alcoholics, the very old, the very young).

Etiology

The cause of fever may be infectious or noninfectious (eg, inflammatory, neoplastic, environmental, and drug-mediated and immunologically mediated causes). Fever may be intermittent, characterized by daily spikes followed by a return to normal temperature, or remittent, in which the temperature does not return to normal until the cause resolves.

Pyrogens are substances that cause fever. Exogenous pyrogens are usually microbes or their products. The best studied are the lipopolysaccharides of gram-negative bacteria (commonly called endotoxins) and the *Staphylococcus aureus* toxin that produces toxic shock syndrome.

Exogenous pyrogens usually cause fever by inducing release of endogenous pyrogens (IL-1, tumor necrosis factor, interferon-γ, and IL-6). These are polypeptides produced by host cells, particularly monocyte-macrophages, that elevate the hypothalamic set point. Prostaglandin E_2 synthesis appears to play a critical role.

Symptoms and Signs

Fever can be very uncomfortable. A minority of children are at risk for febrile seizures. Fever can increase O_2 demands by 13% for every 1 °C increase over 37 °C, which is particularly problematic in adults with preexisting cardiac or pulmonary insufficiency. Fever can also worsen mental status in patients with dementia.

Diagnosis

Fever is most accurately diagnosed by measuring rectal temperature. Oral temperatures are normally about 0.6°C lower. Oral measurement produces falsely low temperatures in many situations (eg, recent cold drink, mouth-breathing, hyperventilation, inadequate time of measurement [up to several minutes are occasionally required]). Measurement by tympanic membrane is inaccurate compared with rectal temperature.

Fever suggests infection. However, it can have other causes, and patients incapable of generating fever may have normal or low temperatures during severe infections. The degree of elevation in temperature usually does not predict the likelihood or cause of infection.

Treatment

Whether to treat fever due to infection is controversial. Experimental evidence, but not clinical studies, suggests that fever enhances host defenses. Patients at particular risk for whom treatment of fever is indicated include children with previous febrile seizures, adults with cardiac or pulmonary insufficiency, and those with dementia. Drugs that inhibit brain cyclooxygenase are effective in reducing fever; those used most often are acetaminophen, aspirin, and other NSAIDs. Treatment of fever in children is discussed on p. 2240.

FEVER OF UNKNOWN ORIGIN

Fever of unknown origin (FUO) was previously defined as a body temperature ≥38.3°C rectally for ≥ 3 wk without discovering the cause despite extensive investigation for at least 1 wk. This classic definition of FUO was formulated to compare retrospective and prospective clinical studies and should be interpreted liberally. Because modern imaging studies are so useful in locating sites of infection or tumors, it has been suggested that the definition of classic FUO be modified to 2 wk of fever and either 3 days of hospital investigation or 3 outpatient visits without discovering the cause.

Etiology

Among the myriad possible causes, the most common are infections, occult tumors, drugs (especially drugs recently started), and connective tissue disorders. The most common causes vary with patient age. For example, patients < 6 yr often have infection, whereas patients between 6 and 16 yr often have connective tissue disorders or inflammatory bowel disease.

Some of the connective tissue disorders associated with FUO are SLE, RA, temporal arteritis, vasculitis, and juvenile RA of adults. The most common tumors associated with FUO are lymphoma, leukemia, renal cell carcinoma, GI tumors, and metastatic ovarian carcinoma. Other causes include pulmonary embolism, sarcoidosis, and factitious fever. No cause of FUO is identified in about 10% of adults.

Diagnosis

History: Patients most often report feeling warm; they may have chills, night sweats, or a fever detected with a home thermometer. History may suggest the cause. Information on travel and exposure to certain agents or animals should be sought. For example, coccidioidomycosis and histoplasmosis should be considered in patients recently in endemic areas. Typhoid fever is suggested by a history of drinking contaminated water, and brucellosis is suggested by employment in meatpacking plants. In older adults, headache and sometimes visual changes suggest temporal arteritis; morning stiffness suggests polymyalgia rheumatica. Fever patterns usually have little or no significance in diagnosis of FUO, although there are some exceptions. A fever that occurs every other day (tertian) or every 3rd day (quartan) may suggest malaria. In cyclic neutropenia, peripheral neutrophils become depleted every 21 days; it should be considered in patients who present with fever at corresponding intervals.

The history addresses risk factors and coexisting symptoms of connective tissue disorders and cancers, including arthralgias, weight loss, and symptoms of anemia. A complete drug history is recorded.

Examination: Complete and repeated physical examinations, especially of the skin, eyes, nail beds, lymph nodes, heart, and abdomen may reveal clues of otherwise inapparent febrile disorders.

Diagnostic testing: Laboratory evaluation generally focuses on detecting infection and connective tissue and neoplastic disorders. Evaluation for infection includes bacterial, fungal, viral, and mycobacterial cultures of blood, urine, and other accessible body fluids of organs that may be infected; CBCs; and serially measured appropriate antibody titers (eg, for suspected rickettsial infections, brucellosis, and certain viral diseases). Blood may need to be sampled for culture 2 or 3 times daily to diagnose certain diseases (eg, infective endocarditis). Microscopic examination of peripheral blood is necessary to confirm certain suspected protozoal diseases (eg, malaria). Newer and more specific immunologic and molecular biologic techniques (eg, PCR) are being developed and may help in specific infections (see p. 1394). To detect connective tissue disorders, serologic tests, such as antinuclear antibody (ANA) and rheumatoid factor, are first obtained as screening tests. ESR is sensitive but not specific for temporal arteritis and polymyalgia rheumatica. To detect occult hematologic cancers, CBC is obtained. Abnormal results may indicate the need for bone marrow examination and other tests.

Imaging studies reduce the need for biopsies and other invasive procedures. The choice of study is guided by symptoms and signs. For example, fever and back pain should suggest MRI of the spine looking for infection or tumor. If blood cultures are positive or there are new heart murmurs or peripheral signs suggesting endocarditis, echocardiography is performed. Echocardiography (especially transesophageal echocardiography) is useful in demonstrating cardiac vegetations. CT is useful in delineating abnormalities in the abdomen and chest and should be performed to localize abnormalities before more definitive (invasive) testing. MRI is more sensitive than CT for detecting most causes of FUO involving the CNS and should be performed if a CNS cause is being considered. Radionuclide scanning, especially with indium-111–labeled granulocytes, helps localize many infectious or inflammatory processes but is rarely needed anymore because MRI is highly sensitive.

Biopsy is required if an undiagnosed abnormality is suspected in tissue that is accessible for biopsy, such as liver, bone marrow, skin, pleura, lymph nodes, intestine, or muscle. Biopsy specimens should be evaluated by histopathologic examination and cultured for bacteria, fungi, viruses, and mycobacteria. Muscle biopsy or skin biopsy of rashes may diagnose vasculitis. Bilateral temporal artery biopsy may diagnose temporal arteritis in the elderly patient with an unexplained ESR elevation.

ABSCESSES

Abscesses are collections of pus in confined tissue spaces, usually caused by bacterial infection. Symptoms include local pain, tenderness, warmth, and swelling (if near the skin layer) or constitutional symptoms (if deep). Imaging may be necessary for diagnosis of deep abscesses. Treatment is surgical drainage and often antibiotics.

Etiology and Pathophysiology

Numerous organisms can cause abscesses, but *Staphylococcus aureus* is most common. Organisms may enter the tissue by direct implantation (eg, penetrating trauma with a contaminated object); spread from an established, contiguous infection; dissemination via lymphatic or hematogenous routes from a distant site; or migration from a location where there are resident flora into an adjacent, normally sterile area because of disruption of natural barriers (eg, perforation of an abdominal viscus causing an intra-abdominal abscess).

Abscesses may begin in an area of cellulitis (see p. 980) or in compromised tissue where leukocytes accumulate. Progressive dissection by pus or necrosis of surrounding cells expands the abscess. Highly vascularized connective tissue may then surround the necrotic tissue, leukocytes, and debris to wall off the abscess and limit further spread.

Predisposing factors to abscess formation include impaired host defense mechanisms (eg, impaired leukocyte defenses), the presence of foreign bodies, obstruction to normal drainage (eg, in the urinary, biliary, or respiratory tracts), tissue ischemia or necrosis, hematoma or excessive fluid accumulation in tissue, and trauma.

Symptoms, Signs, and Diagnosis

The symptoms and signs of cutaneous and subcutaneous abscesses are pain, heat, swelling, tenderness, and redness. Superficial abscesses may have a punctum. Fever may occur, especially with surrounding cellulitis. For deep abscesses, local pain and tenderness and systemic symptoms, especially fever, as well as anorexia, weight loss, and fatigue are typical. The predominant manifestation of some abscesses is abnormal organ function (eg, hemiplegia with a brain abscess).

Complications of abscesses include bacteremic spread, rupture into adjacent tissue, bleeding from vessels eroded by inflammation, impaired function of a vital organ, and inanition due to anorexia and increased metabolic needs.

Diagnosis of cutaneous and subcutaneous abscesses is by physical examination. Diagnosis of deep abscesses may require imaging. Ultrasound is noninvasive and detects many soft-tissue abscesses; CT scan is accurate for most, although MRI is usually more sensitive.

Treatment

Superficial abscesses may resolve with heat and oral antibiotics. However, healing usually requires drainage. Minor abscesses may require only incision and drainage. All pus, necrotic tissue, and debris should be removed. To prevent reformation of the abscess, elimination of open (dead) space by packing with gauze or by placing drains may be necessary. Predisposing conditions, such as obstruction of natural drainage or the presence of a foreign body, require correction.

Spontaneous rupture and drainage may occur, sometimes leading to the formation of chronic draining sinuses. Without drainage, an abscess occasionally resolves slowly after proteolytic digestion of the pus produces a thin, sterile fluid that is resorbed into the bloodstream. Incomplete resorption may leave a cystic loculation within a fibrous wall that may become calcified.

If the abscess is deep or if there is surrounding cellulitis, systemic antimicrobial drugs are indicated as adjunctive therapy; they are usually ineffective without drainage. Gram stain, culture, and sensitivity results can help guide antimicrobial therapy.

BACTEREMIA

(See also Neonatal Sepsis on p. 2333 and Occult Bacteremia on p. 2353.)

Bacteremia is the presence of bacteria in the bloodstream. It can occur spontaneously, from indwelling GU or IV catheters, or after dental, GI, GU, wound care, or other procedures. Bacteremia may cause metastatic infections, including endocarditis, especially in those with valvular heart abnormalities. Transient bacteremia is often asymptomatic but may cause fever. Development of other symptoms usually suggests more serious infection, such as sepsis or septic shock (see p. 566). Patients with certain underlying heart conditions should receive prophylactic antibiotics before procedures that can cause significant bacteremia.

Bacteremia may be transient and cause no sequelae, or it may cause metastatic or systemic consequences.

Etiology and Pathophysiology

Bacteremia has many possible causes, including dental procedures or even vigorous toothbrushing; catheterization of an infected lower urinary tract; surgical treatment of an abscess or infected wound; and colonization of indwelling devices, especially IV and intracardiac catheters, urethral catheters, and ostomy devices and tubes. Gram-negative bacteremia secondary to infection usually originates in the GU or GI tract, or the skin in patients with decubitus ulcers. Chronically ill and immunocompromised patients have an increased risk of gram-negative bacteremia. They may also develop bacteremia with gram-positive cocci, anaerobes, and fungi. Staphylococcal bacteremia is common in injection drug users. *Bacteroides* bacteremia may develop in patients with infections of the abdomen and the pelvis, particularly the female genital tract. If an infection in the abdomen causes bacteremia, the organism is most likely a gram-negative bacillus. If an infection above the diaphragm causes bacteremia, the organism is most likely gram positive.

Metastatic infection of the meninges or serous cavities, such as the pericardium or larger joints, can result from transient or sustained bacteremia. Metastatic abscesses may occur almost anywhere. Multiple abscess formation is especially common with staphylococcal bacteremia. Bacteremia may cause endocarditis (see p. 724), most commonly if the pathogen is an enterococcus, streptococcus, or staphylococcus, and less commonly with gram-negative bacteremia and fungemia. Patients with valvular heart disease, prosthetic heart valves, or other intravascular prostheses are predisposed to endocarditis, which may occur after certain dental procedures. Staphylococci can cause gram-positive bacterial endocarditis, particularly in injection drug users, and may involve the tricuspid valve.

Symptoms, Signs, and Diagnosis

Development of symptoms such as tachypnea, shaking chills, persistent fever, altered sensorium, hypotension, and GI symptoms (abdominal pain, nausea, vomiting, and diarrhea) suggests sepsis or septic shock. Septic shock develops in 25 to 40% of patients with significant bacteremia.

If bacteremia, sepsis, or septic shock is suspected, cultures are obtained of blood (see p. 726) and any other appropriate specimens as described elsewhere in THE MANUAL.

Prognosis and Treatment

In patients at risk for endocarditis or who are immunocompromised, prophylactic antibiotics are indicated before procedures likely to cause significant bacteremia (see TABLES 77–3, 77–4, and 77–5). In patients with suspected bacteremia, empiric antibiotics are given after appropriate cultures are obtained. Continuing therapy involves adjusting antibiotics according to the results of culture and sensitivity testing and usually removing any internal devices that are the suspected source of bacteria.

BIOLOGICAL WARFARE AND TERRORISM

Biological warfare is the use of microbiological agents for hostile purposes. Such use is contrary to international law and in fact has rarely taken place during formal warfare in modern history, despite the extensive preparations and stockpiling of biological agents carried out in the 20th century by most major powers. For a variety of reasons—including uncertain military efficacy and the threat of massive retaliation—experts consider the use of biological agents in formal warfare unlikely. The area of most concern is the use of such agents by terrorist groups. Biological agents are thought by some people to be an ideal weapon for terrorists. These agents may be delivered clandestinely, and they have delayed effects, allowing the user to remain undetected.

Potential biological agents include anthrax, botulinum toxin, brucellosis, encephalitis viruses, hemorrhagic fever viruses (Ebola and Marburg), plague, tularemia, and smallpox. Each of these is potentially fatal and, except for anthrax and botulinum toxin, can be passed from person to person. Of these agents, anthrax is of most concern. Anthrax spores are relatively easy to prepare and, unlike most of the other agents, can be spread through the air, creating the potential for distribution by airplane. Theoretically, 1 kg of anthrax could kill 10,000 people, although technical difficulties with preparing the spores in a sufficiently fine powder would probably limit actual deaths to a fraction of this.

Despite these theoretical concerns, the only successful terrorist use of anthrax—multiple pieces of contaminated mail delivered to a variety of locations in the US in 2001—resulted in only a handful of deaths and serious infections. A larger number of people were contaminated with anthrax spores without developing illness. However, there was extreme public anxiety related to these incidents, which may have been a major goal of the terror group responsible.

In addition to the actual infections, an even greater number of false threats of anthrax have been reported. In 1999, the FBI received an average of 1 false report/day of alleged anthrax use. False reports, both hoaxes and alarmed citizens misperceiving harmless material for anthrax, increased even more following the 2001 anthrax attack in the US.

The only other successful use of a biological agent by a terror group in the US occurred in 1984. In this event, 751 people were stricken with diarrhea resulting from the intentional contamination with *Salmonella* of a salad bar in Oregon. The bacteria were introduced by a religious cult trying to influence the results of a local election. No one died.

Defense against bioterrorism involves several factors: intelligence to disrupt the terrorists before they can use the weapons, early detection, availability of protective antibiotics, and vaccination of selected populations (eg, the military).

168 LABORATORY DIAGNOSIS OF INFECTIOUS DISEASE

Laboratory tests may identify organisms directly (eg, visually, using a microscope, growing the organism in culture) or indirectly (eg, identifying antibodies to the organism). General types of tests include microscopy, culture, immunologic tests (agglutination tests such as latex agglutination, enzyme immunoassays, Western blot, precipitation tests, and complement fixation tests), and nucleic and nonnucleic acid–based identification methods. Culture is normally the gold standard for identification of organisms, but results may not be available for days or weeks, and not all pathogens can be cultured, making alternative tests useful. When a pathogen is identified, the laboratory can also assess its susceptibility to antimicrobial agents.

Some tests (eg, Gram stain, routine aerobic culture) can detect a large variety of pathogens and are obtained routinely in many suspected infectious illnesses. However, because some pathogens are missed on these tests, clinicians must know when to suspect the pathogens those tests may miss so that they can request tests specific for those organisms (eg, special stains or culture media) or advise the laboratory to select more specific tests.

MICROSCOPY

Microscopy can be performed quickly, but accuracy depends on the experience of the microscopist and quality of equipment. Regulations often limit physicians' use of microscopy for diagnostic purposes outside a certified laboratory.

Most specimens are treated with stains that color pathogens, causing them to stand out from the background, although wet mounts of unstained samples are used to detect fungi, parasites (including helminth eggs and larvae), vaginal clue cells, and motile organisms (eg, *Trichomonas*). To increase visibility of fungi, 10% potassium hydroxide (KOH), can be applied to dissolve surrounding tissues and organisms. Darkfield microscopy for the diagnosis of syphilis also uses unstained samples.

The clinician orders a stain based on the likely pathogens, although no stain is 100% specific. Most samples are treated with the Gram stain and, if mycobacteria are suspected, an acid-fast stain. However, some pathogens are not easily visible using these stains; if these organisms are suspected, different stains or other identification methods are required. Because microscopic detection usually requires a microbe concentration of about 1×10^5/mL, most body fluid specimens (eg, CSF, urine) are concentrated (eg, by centrifugation) before examination.

Gram stain: The Gram stain classifies bacteria according to whether they retain crystal violet stain (Gram positive—blue color) or not (Gram negative—red color) and highlights cell morphology (eg, bacilli or cocci) and cell arrangement (eg, clumps, chains, diploids). Such characteristics can direct antibiotic therapy pending definitive identification. To perform a Gram stain, specimen material is heat-fixed to a slide and stained by sequential exposure to Gram's crystal violet, iodine, decolorizer, and counterstain (typically safranin).

Acid-fast and moderate (modified) acid-fast stains: These stains are used to identify "acid-fast" organisms (*Mycobacterium* sp) and "moderately acid-fast" organisms (primarily *Nocardia* sp). They are also useful for staining *Rhodococcus* and related genera, as well as oocysts of some parasites (eg, *Cryptosporidium*).

Although detection of mycobacteria in sputum requires only about 5,000 to 10,000 organisms/mL, mycobacteria are often present in lower levels, so sensitivity is limited. Specificity is better, although some moderately acid-fast organisms are hard to distinguish from mycobacteria.

Fluorescent stains: These allow detection at lower concentrations (1×10^4 cells/mL). Examples include acridine orange (bacteria and fungi), auramine-rhodamine and auramine O (mycobacteria), and calcofluor white (fungi, especially dermatophytes).

Coupling a fluorescent dye to an antibody to a pathogen (direct or indirect immunofluorescence) theoretically should increase sensitivity and specificity. However, these tests are difficult to read and interpret, and few are commercially available and commonly used (eg, *Pneumocystis* and *Legionella* direct fluorescent antibody tests).

India ink (colloidal carbon) stain: This is used to detect mainly *Cryptococcus neoformans* and other encapsulated fungi in a cell suspension (eg, CSF sediment). The background field, rather than the organism itself, is stained, which makes any capsule around the organism visible as a halo. In CSF, the test is not as sensitive as cryptococcal antigen. Specificity is also limited; leukocytes may appear encapsulated.

Wright's stain and Giemsa stain: These are used for detection of parasites in blood, *Histoplasma capsulatum* in phagocytes and tissue cells, intracellular inclusions formed by viruses and chlamydia, trophozoites of *Pneumocystis jiroveci* (formerly *P. carinii*), and some intracellular bacteria.

Trichrome stain (Gomori-Wheatley stain) and iron hematoxylin stain: These are used to detect intestinal protozoa. The Gomori-Wheatley stain is used to detect microsporidia. The iron hematoxylin stain differentially stains cells, cell inclusions, and nuclei. Gomori-Wheatley stain may miss helminth eggs and larvae and does not reliably identify *Cryptosporidium*. Fungi and human cells take up the stain. With iron hematoxylin stain, helminth eggs may stain too dark to permit identification.

CULTURE

Culture is microbial growth on or in a nutritional solid or liquid medium; increased numbers of organisms simplify identification. Culture also facilitates testing of antimicrobial susceptibility.

Communication with the laboratory is essential. Although most specimens are placed on general purpose media (eg, blood or chocolate agar), some pathogens require inclusion of specific nutrients and inhibitors or other special conditions (see TABLE 168–1); if one of these pathogens is suspected or if the patient has been taking antimicrobials, the laboratory should be advised. The specimen's source is reported so that the laboratory can differentiate pathogens from site-specific normal flora.

Specimen collection is important. The wrong type of swab can produce false-negative results. Wooden-shafted swabs are toxic to some viruses. Cotton-tipped swabs are toxic for some bacteria and chlamydia. Blood cultures require decontamination and disinfection of the skin (eg, povidone iodine swab, allowed to dry, removed with 70% alcohol); multiple samples from each different site are generally used, taken nearly simultaneously with fever spikes if possible. Normal flora of skin and mucous membranes that grow in only a single blood sample are usually interpreted as contamination. If a blood specimen is obtained from a central line, a peripheral blood specimen should also be obtained to help differentiate systemic bacteremia from catheter infection. Cultures from infected catheters generally turn positive more quickly and contain more organisms than simultaneously drawn peripheral blood cultures. Some fungi, particularly molds (eg, *Aspergillus* sp), usually cannot be cultured from blood.

The specimen must be transported rapidly, in the correct medium, in conditions that limit growth of any potentially contaminating normal flora. To accurately quantify the pathogen, additional pathogen growth must be prevented; specimens should be transported to the laboratory immediately or, if transport is delayed, refrigerated.

Certain cultures have special considerations.

Anaerobic bacteria should not be cultured from sites where they are normal flora because differentiation of pathogens from normal flora may be impossible. Specimens must be shielded from air, which can be difficult. For swab specimens, anaerobic transport media are available. Specimens collected with a syringe (eg, abscess contents) should be transported in the syringe.

Mycobacteria are difficult to culture. Specimens containing normal flora must first be decontaminated and concentrated. *Mycobacterium tuberculosis* and some other mycobacteria grow slowly. In addition, few organisms may be present in a specimen. Multiple specimens from the same site may help maximize yield. Specimens should be allowed to grow for 8 wk before being discarded. If an atypical mycobacterium is suspected, the laboratory should be notified.

Viruses are generally cultured from swabs and tissue specimens usually transported in media that contain antibacterial and antifungal agents. Specimens are inoculated onto tissue cultures that support the suspected virus and inhibit all other microbes. Viruses that are highly labile (eg, varicella zoster) should be inoculated onto tissue cultures within 1 h of collection. Standard tissue cultures are most sensitive. Rapid tissue cultures (shell vials)

TABLE 168–1. COMMON BACTERIA THAT REQUIRE SPECIAL CULTURE MEDIA

ORGANISM	PREFERRED MEDIUM
Bacteroides species	Kanamycin-vancomycin laked blood agar
Bacteroides fragilis	*Bacteroides* bile-esculin (with gentamicin and bile)
Bordetella pertussis	Bordet-Gengou agar plus methicillin or cephalexin Regan-Lowe cephalexin agar Horse blood–charcoal agar
Burkholderia cepacia	*Pseudomonas cepacia* agar
Campylobacter jejuni or *C. coli*	*Campylobacter*-selective agars (eg, cefoperazone-vancomycin agar)
Corynebacterium diphtheriae	Tinsdale agar, Cystine-tellurite blood agar, Loeffler coagulated serum medium
Escherichia coli, entero-hemorrhagic (Shiga toxin producers, including O157-H7)	MacConkey-sorbitol agar; used with specific antisera
Francisella tularensis	Blood- or chocolate-cystine agar
Legionella	Buffered charcoal yeast extract agar
Leptospira	Fletcher's or Stuart's medium with rabbit serum or *Leptospira* medium with bovine serum albumin-Tween 80
Neisseria gonorrhoeae, N. meningitidis	Modified Thayer-Martin agar, New York City agar
Salmonella and *Shigella*	May grow on standard MacConkey or eosin-methylene blue. Alternative: Hektoen or xylose-lysine-desoxycholate, *Salmonella-Shigella* agar, Gram-negative or selenite enrichment broth
Vibrio	Thiosulfate-citrate-bile salts sucrose agar
Yersinia	Cefsulodin-Irgasan-novobiocin agar

may provide more rapid results. Some common viruses cannot be detected using routine culture methods and require alternative methods for diagnosis (eg, enzyme immunoassay for Epstein-Barr virus, hepatitis B and E viruses, HIV, human T-lymphotrophic virus; serologic tests for hepatitis A and D viruses; nucleic acid–based methods for HIV).

Fungi specimens must be inoculated onto media containing antibacterial agents. Specimens should be allowed to grow for 4 wk before being discarded.

SUSCEPTIBILITY TESTING

Susceptibility tests determine a microbe's vulnerability to antimicrobial drugs by exposing a standardized concentration of organism to specific concentrations of antimicrobial drugs. Susceptibility testing can be performed on bacteria, fungi, and viruses. For some organisms, results obtained with one drug predict results with similar drugs. Thus, not all potential drugs are tested.

Susceptibility testing occurs in vitro and may not account for many in vivo factors (eg, pharmacodynamics and pharmacokinetics, site-specific drug concentrations, host immune status, site-specific host defenses) that influence treatment success. Thus, susceptibility test results do not always predict treatment outcome.

Susceptibility testing can be done qualitatively, semi-quantitatively, or using nucleic acid–based methods. Testing can also determine the effect of combining different antimicrobials (synergy testing).

Qualitative methods: Qualitative methods are less precise than quantitative. Results are usually reported as susceptible (S), intermediate (I), or resistant (R). The commonly used disk diffusion method (also known as the Kirby-Bauer test) is appropriate for rapidly growing organisms. It places antibiotic-impregnated disks on agar plates inoculated with the test organism. After incubation (typically 16 to 18 h), the diameter of the zone of inhibition around each disk is measured. Each organism-antibiotic combination has different diameters signifying S, I, or R.

Other methods that require less rigid adherence to test methods can be used to rapidly screen for resistance of a single organism to a single drug or drug class or to specific antimicrobial combinations (eg, oxacillin resistance of methicillin-resistant *Staphylococcus aureus*, β-lactamase production).

Semiquantitative methods: Semiquantitative methods determine the minimal concentration of a drug that inhibits growth of a particular organism in vitro. This minimum inhibitory concentration (MIC) is reported as a numerical value that may then be translated to 1 of 3 groupings: S (sensitive), I (intermediate), or R (resistant). MIC determination is used primarily for bacteria, including mycobacteria and anaerobes but is sometimes used for fungi. Minimal killing (bactericidal) concentration (MBC) can also be determined but is technically difficult, and standards for interpretation have not been agreed upon.

The antibiotic can be diluted in agar or broth, which is then inoculated with the organism. Broth dilution is the gold standard but is labor intensive because only one drug concentration can be tested per tube. A more efficient method uses a strip of polyester film impregnated with antibiotic in a concentration gradient along its length. The strip is laid on an agar plate containing the inoculum and the MIC determined by the location on the strip at which inhibition begins; multiple antibiotics can be tested on one plate.

The MIC allows correlation between drug susceptibility of the organism and the achievable tissue concentration of the drug. If the tissue concentration is higher than the MIC, successful treatment is likely. Similarly, reports of S, I, and R are correlated with MIC but generally are not tissue concentration specific. That is, they are usually based on achievable serum or plasma concentration of drugs.

Nucleic acid–based methods: These tests incorporate nucleic acid techniques similar to those used for organism identification (see p. 1398) but modified to detect known resistance genes or mutations. An example is *mecA*, a gene for oxacillin resistance in *S. aureus*; if this gene is present, the organism is considered resistant to all β-lactam drugs regardless of apparent susceptibility results. However, although a number of such genes are known, their presence does not uniformly confer in vivo resistance. And, because new mutations or other resistance genes may be present, their absence does not guarantee drug sensitivity. For these reasons and because the tests are limited in number, expensive, and not widely available, they have not replaced standard culture and sensitivity testing.

IMMUNOLOGIC TESTS

Immunologic tests generally detect antibodies to pathogens. Handling varies, but if testing is to be delayed, the specimen should typically be refrigerated or frozen to prevent overgrowth of bacterial contaminants.

Agglutination tests: In agglutination tests (eg, latex agglutination, coaggregation), a particle (latex bead or bacterium) is coupled to a reagent antigen or antibody. The resulting particle complex is mixed with the specimen (eg, CSF, serum); if the target antibody or antigen is present in the specimen, it cross-links the particles, producing measurable agglutination.

If results are positive, the body fluid is serially diluted and tested. Agglutination with more dilute solutions indicates higher concentrations of the target antigen or antibody. The titer is correctly reported as the reciprocal of the most dilute solution yielding agglutination; eg, 32 indicates that agglutination occurred in a solution diluted to 1/32 the starting concentration.

Agglutination tests generally are rapid but less sensitive than many other methods. They can also determine serotypes of some bacteria.

Complement fixation: The complement fixation test measures complement-consuming (complement-fixing) antibody in serum or CSF. The test is used for diagnosis of some viral and fungal infections, particularly coccidioidomycosis. The specimen is incubated with known quantities of complement and the antigen that is the target of the antibody being measured. The degree of complement fixation indicates the quantity of this antibody in the specimen. The test can measure IgM and IgG antibody titers or can be modified to detect certain antigens. It is accurate but has limited applications, is labor intensive, and requires numerous controls.

Enzyme immunoassays: Enzyme immunoassays are tests that use antibodies linked to enzymes. The tests include the enzyme immunoassay (EIA) and enzyme-linked immunosorbent assay (ELISA). These tests detect antigens and detect and quantify antibodies. Because sensitivities of most enzyme immunoassays are high, they are usually used for screening. Titers can be determined by serially diluting the specimen as with agglutination tests.

Test sensitivities, although generally high, can vary, sometimes according to patient age, microbial serotype, or stage of clinical disease.

Precipitation tests: Precipitation tests are tests that measure an antigen or antibody in body fluids by the degree of visible precipitation of antigen-antibody complexes within a gel (agarose) or in solution. There are many types of precipitation tests (eg, Ouchterlony double diffusion, counter immunoelectrophoresis), but their applications are limited. Usually, a blood specimen is mixed with test antigen to detect patient antibodies, most often in suspected fungal infection or pyogenic meningitis. Because a positive result requires a large amount of antibody or antigen, sensitivity is low.

Western blot test: The Western blot detects viral or other antibodies in the patient's sample (eg, serum or other body fluid) by their reaction with target antigens (eg, viral components) that have been immobilized onto a membrane by blotting.

The Western blot typically has good sensitivity, although often less than screening tests such as ELISA, but generally is highly specific. Thus, it is usually used to confirm a positive result obtained with a screening test.

Technical modifications of the Western blot are the line immunoassay (LIA) and the recombinant immunoblot assay (RIBA), which use synthetic or recombinant-produced antigens.

NON-NUCLEIC ACID–BASED IDENTIFICATION METHODS

Once an organism has been isolated by culture, it must be identified. Non-nucleic acid–based identification methods use phenotypic (functional or morphologic) characteristics of organisms rather than genetic identification.

Characteristics of an organism's growth on culture media, such as colony size, color, and shape, provide clues to species identification and, combined with Gram stain, direct further testing. Numerous biochemical tests are available, each restricted to organisms of a certain type (eg, aerobic or anaerobic bacteria). Some assess an organism's ability to use different substrates for growth. Others assess presence or activity of key enzymes (eg, coagulase, catalase). Tests are performed sequentially, with previous results determining the next test to be used. The sequences of tests are myriad and differ somewhat among laboratories.

Non-nucleic acid–based identification tests may involve manual methods, automated systems, or chromatographic methods. Some commercially available kits contain a battery of individual tests that may be performed simultaneously using a single specimen and may be useful for a wider range of organisms. Multiple test systems can be highly accurate but may require several days to yield results.

Chromatographic methods: Microbial components or products are separated and identified using high-performance liquid chromatography (HPLC) or gas chromatography. Usually, identification is by comparison of an organism's fatty acids to a database. Chromatographic methods can be used to identify aerobic and anaerobic bacteria, mycobacteria, and fungi. Test accuracy depends on the conditions used to culture the specimen and the quality of the database, which may be inaccurate or incomplete.

NUCLEIC ACID–BASED IDENTIFICATION METHODS

Nucleic acid–based methods detect organism-specific DNA or RNA sequences extracted from the microorganism. Sequences may or may not be amplified in vitro. Nucleic acid–based methods are generally specific and highly sensitive and can be used for all categories of microbes. Results can be provided rapidly. Because each test typically is specific to a single organism, the clinician must know the diagnostic possibilities and request tests accordingly.

Nucleic acid–based tests are qualitative, but quantification methods exist for a limited number of infections (eg, HIV, cytomegalovirus, human T-cell lymphotrophic virus);

these can be useful in diagnosis and for monitoring response to treatment.

Techniques that do not involve nucleic acid amplification are used if the organism has been first cultured or is present in high concentration in the specimen (eg, in pharyngitis caused by group A *Streptococcus*, genital infections caused by *Chlamydia trachomatis* and *Neisseria gonorrhoeae*).

Amplification: Nucleic acid amplification techniques take tiny amounts of DNA or RNA and replicate them many times, which can detect minute traces of an organism in a specimen, avoiding the need for culture. These techniques are particularly useful for organisms that are difficult to culture or identify using other methods (eg, viruses, obligate intracellular pathogens, fungi, mycobacteria, some other bacteria), or are present in low numbers. These tests may involve target amplification (eg, polymerase chain reaction [PCR], reverse transcriptase–PCR [RT-PCR], strand displacement amplification, transcription amplification), signal amplification (eg, branched DNA assays, hybrid capture), probe amplification (eg, ligase chain reaction, cleavase-invader, cycling probes), or post-amplification analysis (eg, sequencing the amplified product, microarray analysis, and melting curve analysis as is done in real-time PCR).

Because amplification methods are so sensitive, false positives from trace contamination of the specimen or equipment can easily occur. Despite high sensitivity, false negatives sometimes occur even when a patient is symptomatic (eg, West Nile virus infection). False-negative results can be minimized by avoiding use of swabs with wooden shafts or cotton tips and not freezing specimens being analyzed for labile viruses when testing is delayed more than 2 h.

169 IMMUNIZATION

Immunity can be achieved actively by using antigens (eg, vaccines, toxoids) or passively by using antibodies (eg, immune globulins, antitoxins). A toxoid is a bacterial toxin modified to be nontoxic but that can still stimulate antibody formation. A vaccine is a suspension of whole (live or inactivated) or fractionated bacteria or viruses rendered nonpathogenic. TABLE 169–1 lists vaccines available in the US.

Vaccines should be given exactly as recommended on the package insert; however, the interval between a series of doses may be lengthened without losing efficacy. Injection vaccines are usually given IM into the midlateral thigh (in infants and toddlers) or into the deltoid muscle (in school-aged children and adults). Parents should keep a written history of each child's vaccinations.

ROUTINE VACCINATIONS

The schedule of vaccinations for infants and children is listed in FIG. 266–3 on p. 2235. Vaccinations to be considered for all adults are listed in TABLE 169–2. Uses of nonroutine active immunization (eg, for rabies, typhoid, yellow fever, meningococcal and mycobacterial infections) and some of the routine vaccinations are discussed under specific disorders elsewhere in THE MANUAL.

Diphtheria-tetanus-pertussis: Diphtheria (D) and tetanus (T) vaccines are toxoids prepared from *Corynebacterium diphtheriae* and *Clostridium tetani*, respectively. The whole-cell (w) pertussis (P) vaccine contains *Bordetella pertussis* cell wall fragments combined with D and T (DTwP). Acellular (a) pertussis vaccines containing semipurified or purified components of *B. pertussis* (eg, pertussis toxin; filamentous hemagglutinin; fimbriae; and pertactin, a protein) and D and T (DTaP) are usually preferred because they less often cause fever and local reactions. Vaccination is given in childhood and involves primary and booster injections. A single-shot booster of Tdap is available for adolescents aged 10 to 18 to provide added protection against pertussis.

Adverse events are rare and are mostly attributable to the pertussis component. They include encephalopathy within 7 days; a seizure, with or without fever, within 3 days; persistent, severe, inconsolable screaming or crying for ≥ 3 h; collapse or shock within 48 h; temperature of ≥ 40.5 ° C, unexplained by another cause, within 48 h; and immediate se-

TABLE 169–1. VACCINES AVAILABLE IN THE US

VACCINE	TYPE	ROUTE
Anthrax	Inactivated bacteria	sc
BCG (for mycobacteria)	Live bacteria	Intradermal or sc
Diphtheria, tetanus, acellular pertussis (DTaP or Tdap)	Toxoids and inactivated bacterial components	IM
DTaP plus *Haemophilus influenzae* b conjugate (DTaP-HbCV)	Toxoids, inactivated whole bacteria, and bacterial polysaccharide conjugated to protein	IM
DTaP-HB-IPV	Toxoids, recombinant viral antigen, and inactivated poliovirus	IM
Hepatitis A virus (HAV)	Inactivated virus	IM
Hepatitis B virus (HBV)	Recombinant viral antigen	IM
Hepatitis A virus and hepatitis B virus	Inactivated virus plus recombinant	IM
Haemophilus influenzae b (Hib) conjugate (HbCV)	Bacterial polysaccharide conjugated to protein	IM
HbCV plus HBV vaccine	Bacterial polysaccharide conjugate plus inactivated viral antigen	IM
Influenza, types A and B	Inactivated virus or viral components	IM
Influenza	Live virus	Intranasal
Japanese encephalitis	Inactivated virus	sc
Measles	Live virus	sc
Measles and rubella	Live viruses	sc
Measles and mumps	Live viruses	sc
Measles-mumps-rubella	Live viruses	sc
Measles-mumps-rubella-varicella	Live viruses	sc
Meningococcal	Bacterial polysaccharides of serotypes A/C/Y/W-135	sc
Meningococcal conjugate	Bacterial polysaccharides of serotypes A/C/Y/W-135 conjugated to diphtheria toxoid protein	IM
Mumps	Live virus	sc
Pneumococcal (polysaccharide)	Bacterial polysaccharides of 23 pneumococcal types	IM or sc
Pneumococcal (conjugate)	Polysaccharides of 7 types, conjugated to diphtheria toxin	IM
Poliovirus (IPV)	Inactivated viruses of all 3 serotypes	IM
Rabies	Inactivated virus	Intradermal* or sc
Rubella	Live virus	sc
Smallpox	Live virus	Multiple puncture intradermal
Tetanus	Inactivated toxin (toxoid)	IM†
Tetanus and diphtheria toxoids adsorbed (Td)‡ or diphtheria-tetanus (DT)	Inactivated toxins (toxoids)	IM†

TABLE 169–1. VACCINES AVAILABLE IN THE US—Continued

VACCINE	TYPE	ROUTE
Typhoid	Capsular polysaccharide	IM
Typhoid	Live attenuated vaccine	po
Varicella	Live virus	sc
Yellow fever	Live virus	sc

*Intradermal dose is lower and used only for preexposure vaccination.
†Preparations with adjuvants should be given IM.
‡Td contains the same amount of tetanus toxoid as DTP or DT but a reduced dose of diphtheria toxoid.

Modified from "General Recommendations on Immunization. Recommendations of the Advisory Committee on Immunization Practices (ACIP)." *Morbidity and Mortality Weekly Report* 43:1, January 28,1994. Updated through Center for Biologics Evaluation and Research of U.S. Food and Drug Administration, May 2004.

vere or anaphylactic reaction to the vaccine. These reactions contraindicate further use of pertussis vaccine; combined diphtheria and tetanus vaccine is available without the pertussis component.

Tetanus toxoid is combined with diphtheria toxoid in tetanus and diphtheria toxoids adsorbed (Td). Although tetanus is rare in the US, it has a high mortality rate. Because ⅓ of cases occur unpredictably (after minor or inapparent injuries), universal tetanus vaccination remains necessary. Td boosters, 0.5 mL IM, should be given routinely q 10 yr after age 6 yr to maintain immunity. Boosters given after intervals > 10 yr establish immunity but more slowly. Some authorities recommend a single booster at age 50 as an alternative to boosters q 10 yr. Adults who missed the primary series of vaccinations in childhood should receive it as adults. Children < 7 yr receive one of the other tetanus toxoid preparations, such as DT, which contains a larger dose of diphtheria toxoid than Td.

***Haemophilus influenzae* type b conjugate:** Vaccines prepared from the purified capsule of *Haemophilus influenzae* type b (Hib)—polyribosylribitol phosphate (PRP)—prevent Hib disease in children. All Hib vaccines (HbCVs) use PRP as the polysaccharide, but 4 different protein carriers produce 4 different Hib conjugate vaccines: diphtheria toxoid (PRP-D), *Neisseria meningitidis* outer membrane protein (PRP-OMP), tetanus toxoid (PRP-T), and diphtheria mutant carrier protein CRM_{197} (HbOC).

Hepatitis: Hepatitis A vaccine is prepared using inactivated virus. Hepatitis B vaccine uses recombinant DNA technology; universal vaccination is recommended. Use of the 2 vaccines is discussed in Ch. 27 (see p. 226).

Influenza: This virus undergoes antigenic drift each year, necessitating annual revaccination with new strains. Because outbreaks usually begin in early winter or midwinter, vaccine is given in the fall, usually October and November in the Northern Hemisphere. It is recommended for those at high risk for serious sequelae, including anyone > 65 yr; residents of extended-care facilities; and patients with chronic cardiovascular or pulmonary disease, metabolic disorders (especially diabetes), renal failure, hemoglobinopathies, immunosuppression, or HIV infection; and children aged 6 to 23 mo. Health care practitioners and people desiring to avoid symptoms are also vaccinated.

Measles, mumps, and rubella: This vaccine combines live attenuated viruses into one vaccine that produces protective antibodies and probably lifelong immunity to each virus in 95% of recipients. The vaccine should be given to all children in their 2nd yr of life. Adults at risk include those who have never received the vaccine and have never become naturally infected. Generally, people born before 1956 are considered immune because infection during their childhood was ubiquitous. Those born after 1956 should receive the combined vaccine if immune status is uncertain and if they are likely to become exposed (eg, college students, health care practitioners). Although the components of the vaccine can be given separately, the combined form is preferred because a person who needs one vaccine probably needs all 3, and revaccination poses no particular risk.

Measles (rubeola) vaccination should be delayed until after passively acquired maternal antibody disappears, because replication of the vaccine virus may be inhibited by preexisting maternal antibody. A mild, noncommunicable

TABLE 169–2. ROUTINE VACCINATIONS FOR ADULTS

VACCINE	DOSE	INDICATIONS	CONTRAINDICATIONS
Measles-mumps-rubella	0.5 mL sc initially and at entry to college, military	Anyone born after 1956 and never infected or who is likely to be exposed (eg, college students)	Pregnancy, immunocompromised state, history of anaphylactic reactions to either egg protein or neomycin
Tetanus and diphtheria toxoids adsorbed	0.5 mL IM initially, at 1 mo, after 6 mo (primary series); booster vaccinations are given q 10 yr	Anyone who has never been vaccinated should have primary series; all people should have booster vaccinations q 10 yr	History of severe allergic reaction to the vaccine
Hepatitis A	1 mL IM initially and at 6–12 mo	Anyone requesting vaccination or at increased risk, due to eg, travel to endemic areas, military employment, chronic liver disease, high-risk sexual behavior, illicit drug use, or a coagulopathy	Known hypersensitivity
Hepatitis B	1.0 mL IM initially, at 1–2 mo and at 4–6 mo	All adults, particularly anyone likely to have repeated exposure (eg, health care personnel, sex partner of a known carrier) or who has had an exposure (eg, needlestick injury to a hospital worker)—see p. 227	History of anaphylactic reaction to common baker's yeast
Influenza	0.5 mL IM yearly	Anyone at high risk for complications, medical personnel, and people requesting vaccination	High fever, history of anaphylactic reactions to egg protein
Meningococcal (polysaccharide or conjugate)	0.5 mL sc for polysaccharide and IM for conjugate	Asplenia; travelers to endemic areas; college students who request vaccination	Sensitivity to thimerosal for polysaccharide and sensitivity to latex for conjugate
Pneumococcal pneumonia	0.5 mL IM or sc	Anyone at high risk for pneumococcal disease	Pregnancy (relative contraindication)
Varicella	0.5 mL sc initially and at 1–2 mo	Anyone never infected, especially health care and child care workers	Pregnancy, immunocompromised state, having received an immune globulin or a blood transfusion within 5 mo, history of anaphylactic reactions to neomycin or gelatin, active TB (untreated), febrile infection

infection is produced in 15% of vaccine recipients. Symptoms occur 7 to 11 days after immunization and include fever, malaise, and a measles-like exanthem. Subacute sclerosing panencephalitis (SSPE) is a slow virus infection of the CNS that develops in 6 to 22 cases per million people infected with wild measles viruses. It has occurred in children with no history of natural measles who received measles vaccination but has almost disappeared in the postvaccine era.

Mumps vaccine produces adverse effects only rarely, including encephalitis (which occurs only with a Japanese mumps vaccine strain), seizures, nerve deafness, parotitis, purpura, rash, and pruritus.

Rubella vaccine causes joint pain, usually in the small peripheral joints 2 to 8 wk after immunization in < 1% of infants but in ≤ 26% of women. A rash or lymphadenopathy occasionally occurs. Vaccine is not recommended for pregnant women because of the theoretic risk to the fetus. However, inadvertent administration during pregnancy does not necessarily mean a therapeutic abortion is recommended, because the actual fetal risk may be nil.

A vaccine combining measles, mumps, rubella, and varicella is also available.

Pneumococcal vaccines: Pneumococcal conjugate vaccine includes 7 purified capsular polysaccharides of *Streptococcus pneumoniae*, each coupled to a variant of diphtheria toxin. It is indicated for all children < 5 yr and immunocompromised patients but should generally be deferred during pregnancy. Unlike the older 23-valent vaccine, the conjugate vaccine can stimulate antibody responses in infants. This vaccine also seems to confer greater protection against invasive pneumococcal disease than the older vaccine. Adverse effects in children are usually mild and include fever, irritability, drowsiness, anorexia, vomiting, and local erythema. Adverse effects in immunocompromised adults are unknown.

Pneumococcal polysaccharide vaccine contains antigens from the 23 most virulent of the 83 subtypes of pneumococcus. It reduces bacteremia by 56 to 81% in adults overall but less frequently among debilitated elderly people. It reduces pneumonia incidence only minimally. It should be given to anyone at high risk for pneumococcal pneumonia or its complications, including patients with HIV infection or chronic lung or cardiac disease and those with functional asplenia (eg, sickle cell disease, post-splenectomy), alcoholism, hematologic malignancy, CSF leak, and cochlear implant. It may be given simultaneously with influenza vaccine but at a different site (eg, the opposite deltoid muscle). One immunization is recommended for lifetime protection, although revaccination q 6 yr should be considered for patients at particularly high risk.

Poliomyelitis: A primary series of trivalent inactivated poliovirus vaccine (IPV), consisting of a mixture of formalin-inactivated poliovirus types 1, 2, and 3, should be given during childhood and produces immunity in > 99% of recipients. Oral poliovirus vaccine (OPV) is no longer available in the US. Serious adverse effects have not been associated with IPV.

Varicella: Varicella vaccine, a live attenuated virus vaccine, should be given to all children and to young adults not previously infected, especially health care practitioners and close contacts of immunocompromised patients, who should have levels of protective antibodies measured to determine the need for vaccination. The vaccine produces protective varicella antibodies in 97% of recipients and reduces the likelihood of clinical illness by 70% after exposure. Waning immunity in vaccine recipients has not been demonstrated but is undergoing evaluation. No immune globulins, including varicella-zoster immune globulin, should be given within 5 mo before or 2 mo after vaccination, because immune globulins may prevent development of protective antibodies. The vaccine's adverse effects are minimal; within 1 mo of vaccination, a mild maculopapular or varicella-like rash occasionally develops. A patient who develops this rash should avoid contact with immunocompromised people until it resolves. Transient injection-site pain, tenderness, or redness sometimes develops. Recipients < 16 yr should avoid salicylates for 6 wk because of the possibility of Reye's syndrome. Spread of vaccine virus from vaccine recipients to susceptible people has been documented but occurs in < 1% of vaccinees and only if the vaccinee develops a rash.

Simultaneous administration of different vaccines: Simultaneous administration may be convenient and is particularly recommended if a child may be unavailable for future vaccination. Besides measles-mumps-rubella, measles-mumps-rubella-varicella, and DPT, approved vaccine combinations include DTwP-Hib conjugate vaccine (HbCV), DTaP-HbCV, and hepatitis B vaccine-HbCV (HB-HbCV). In addition, more than one vaccine product may be given at the same time using separate injection sites and syringes. Products that can be combined include DTwP-HbCV or DTaP-HbCV with IPV or OPV and with HB vaccine and varicella with measles-mumps-rubella. If varicella and measles-mumps-rubella are not given simultaneously, they are given > 1 mo apart.

Immunizations for travelers: Immunizations may be required for travel where infectious diseases are endemic. The Centers for Disease Control and Prevention can provide information; a telephone service (404-332-4559) and web site (www.cdc.gov/travel/vaccinat.htm) are available 24 h/day.

Risks, Restrictions, and High-Risk Groups

Live-microbial vaccines should not be given simultaneously with blood, plasma, or immune globulin, which can interfere with development of desired antibodies; ideally, such vaccines should be given 2 wk before or 6 to 12 wk after the immune globulins.

Immunocompromised patients should not receive live-virus vaccines, which could provoke severe or fatal infections. In patients receiving short-term (ie, duration of < 14 days) immunosuppressive therapy (eg, corticosteroids, antimetabolites, alkylating compounds, radiation), live-virus vaccines should be withheld until after treatment. Patients receiving longer-term immunosuppressive therapy may still receive inactivated vaccines such as DTaP or DTwP; ≥ 3 mo after immunosuppressive therapy is stopped, they should be given an additional dose of inactivated vaccine and may receive live-virus vaccines.

Asplenic patients are predisposed to overwhelming bacteremic infection, usually due to *S. pneumoniae, N. meningitidis,* or *H. influenzae* type b. They should be given HbCV vaccine, meningococcal polysaccharide vaccine, annual influenza vaccination, and pneumococcal conjugate (if age < 5 yr) or polysaccharide (if age > 5 yr) vaccine. Before undergoing solid organ transplantation, patients should receive all appropriate vaccinations. Patients who have undergone hematopoietic cell transplantation should be considered unimmunized and should receive repeat doses of all appropriate vaccines.

Patients with AIDS generally should receive inactivated vaccines (eg, DTP, IPV, HbCV) but should usually not receive live-virus and bacterial vaccines (eg, measles-mumps-rubella, OPV, BCG). However, an exception can be made for measles-mumps-rubella if immunosuppression is not severe. Naturally occurring measles can cause severe, often fatal, infection in AIDS patients, and measles-mumps-rubella rarely causes serious complications. Patients with AIDS should be vaccinated according to routine recommendations.

Risks of vaccines should be discussed with patients. Parents should give written consent for vaccination of their children. In the US, selected events that occur after routine vaccination must be reported to the manufacturer, the US Department of Health and Human Services, and the Centers for Disease Control and Prevention's Vaccine Adverse Event Reporting System (VAERS). Forms and instructions can be obtained by calling 800-822-7967 (Health and Human Services) or from the web site (www.vaers.org).

A temperature of > 39 °C necessitates delaying vaccination, but minor infections, such as the common cold (even with low-grade fever), do not. Some vaccines produced in cell culture systems contain trace amounts of egg antigens. Although egg allergies are often considered contraindications to these vaccines, the vaccines do not appear to cause significant adverse reactions in patients who can eat foods that contain eggs, such as bread or cookies. A history of other allergic reactions may contraindicate use of certain vaccines (see TABLE 169–2). Pregnancy is a relative contraindication to vaccination with measles-mumps-rubella, pneumococcal pneumonia, varicella, and other live-virus vaccines. Although concern has been raised about the safety in infants of thimerosal, a mercury-based preservative present in some vaccines, there is no evidence of harm. Nevertheless, most manufacturers are developing thimerosal-free vaccines for use in infants.

Patients with fluctuating or progressive neurologic disease, such as Guillain-Barré syndrome, should not be vaccinated until their condition has stabilized for at least 1 yr because of the risk of cerebral irritation. If a neurologic disorder is stable, vaccinations should proceed normally. The risk in multiple sclerosis is unknown.

PASSIVE IMMUNIZATION

Passive immunization provides temporary immunity when vaccines for active immunization are unavailable or have not been given before exposure. Immune globulins and antitoxins available in the US are listed in TABLE 169–3.

Human immune globulin (IG): IG is a concentrated antibody solution prepared from plasma obtained from normal donors. It

TABLE 169–3. IMMUNE GLOBULINS AND ANTITOXINS* AVAILABLE IN THE US

IMMUNOBIO-LOGIC AGENT	TYPE	INDICATION(S)
Botulinum antitoxin	Specific equine antibodies	Treatment of botulism
Botulinum antitoxin (BIG)	Specific human antibodies	Treatment of botulism in infants
Cytomegalovirus immune globulin, intravenous (CMV-IGIV)	Specific human antibodies	Prophylaxis for hematopoietic stem cell and kidney transplant recipients
Diphtheria antitoxin	Specific equine antibodies	Treatment of respiratory diphtheria
Immune globulin (IG)	Pooled human antibodies	Prophylaxis for hepatitis A pre- and postexposure; measles postexposure; immunoglobulin deficiency; rubella during the 1st trimester of pregnancy; varicella (if varicella zoster immune globulin unavailable)
Immune globulin, intravenous (IVIG)	Pooled human antibodies	Replacement therapy for antibody deficiency disorders; immune thrombocytopenic purpura; hypogammaglobulinemia in chronic lymphocytic leukemia; Kawasaki disease; neurologic disorders (eg, myasthenia gravis, Guillain-Barré syndrome); prophylaxis and treatment of severe pediatric bacterial and viral infections
Hepatitis B immune globulin (HBIG)	Specific human antibodies	Prophylaxis for hepatitis B postexposure
Rabies immune globulin (HRIG)†	Specific human antibodies	Management of rabies postexposure in people not previously immunized with rabies vaccine
Respiratory syncytial virus immune globulin (RSV-IGIV)	Specific human antibodies	Prevention of RSV in infants < 35 wk gestation or children with chronic lung disease (eg, bronchopulmonary dysplasia)
Respiratory syncytial virus murine monoclonal antibody (RSV-mAb)	Murine monoclonal antibody (palivizumab)	Prevention of RSV in infants < 35 wk gestation or children with chronic lung diseases (eg, bronchopulmonary dysplasia)
Tetanus immune globulin (TIG)	Specific human antibodies	Treatment of tetanus; postexposure prophylaxis of people not adequately immunized with tetanus toxoid
Vaccinia immune globulin (VIG)	Specific human antibodies	Treatment of eczema vaccinatum, vaccinia necrosum, and ocular vaccinia
Varicella-zoster immune globulin (VZIG)	Specific human antibodies	Postexposure prophylaxis of susceptible immunocompromised people, certain susceptible pregnant women, and perinatally exposed newborns

*Immune globulin preparations and antitoxins are administered intramuscularly unless otherwise indicated.

†HRIG is administered around the wounds as well as intramuscularly.

From "General Recommendations on Immunization. Recommendations of the Advisory Committee on Immunization Practices (ACIP)." *Morbidity and Mortality Weekly Report* 43:1, January 28, 1994. Updated 2004.

consists primarily of IgG, although trace amounts of IgA, IgM, and other serum proteins may be present. IG very rarely contains transmissible viruses (eg, hepatitis B or C or HIV) and is stable for many months if stored at 4°C. IG is given IM. Because maximal serum antibody levels may not occur until about 48 h after IM injection, IG must be given as soon after exposure as possible. Half-life of IG in the circulation is about 3 wk.

IG may be used for prophylaxis in hepatitis A, measles, immunoglobulin deficiency, varicella (in immunocompromised patients when varicella-zoster IG is unavailable), and rubella exposure in the 1st trimester of pregnancy.

IG provides only temporary protection, the antibody content against specific agents varies by as much as 10-fold among preparations, administration is painful, and anaphylaxis can occur.

Hyperimmune globulin: Hyperimmune globulin is prepared from the plasma of people with high titers of antibody against a specific organism or antigen. It is derived from people convalescing from natural infections or donors artificially immunized. Hyperimmune globulins are available for hepatitis B, respiratory syncytial virus (RSV), rabies, tetanus, cytomegalovirus, vaccinia, and varicella-zoster. Administration is painful, and anaphylaxis may occur.

IV immune globulin (IVIG): IVIG was developed to provide larger and repeated doses of human immune globulin. IVIG is the product of choice for treatment and prevention of severe pediatric bacterial and viral infections, such as septicemia in preterm and low-birth-weight infants, bacterial meningitis, and Kawasaki disease. Either IVIG or a specific monoclonal antibody against RSV is available for prevention of RSV in children < 24 mo with bronchopulmonary dysplasia or with a history of premature birth (< 35 wk gestation). IVIG is used in adults for certain autoimmune and neurologic disorders (eg, myasthenia gravis, Guillain-Barré syndrome, idiopathic thrombocytopenic purpura) and as replacement therapy (eg, antibody deficiency disorders or hypogammaglobulinemia due to chronic lymphocytic leukemia). Adverse effects are uncommon, although fever, chills, headache, faintness, nausea, vomiting, hypersensitivity, anaphylactic reactions, coughing, and volume overload have occurred.

170 BACTERIA AND ANTIBACTERIAL DRUGS

Bacteria are microorganisms that have circular double-stranded DNA and (except for *Mycoplasma* sp) cell walls.Only a small number are human pathogens.Bacteria are classified by several criteria, including morphology (see TABLE 170–1). They may be cylindric (bacilli), spherical (cocci), or spiral (spirochetes). A few coccal, many bacillary, and most spirochetal species are motile. Gram-positive bacteria retain crystal violet dye after iodine fixation and alcohol decolorization, whereas gram-negative bacteria do not. Gram-negative bacteria have an additional outer membrane containing lipopolysaccharide (endotoxin). Bacteria may be additionally enclosed in capsules, which may (eg, with *Streptococcus pneumoniae* and *Haemophilus influenzae*) impair their ingestion by phagocytes. Other factors may enhance bacterial pathogenicity (see Factors Facilitating Microbial Invasion on p. 1387).

Aerobic bacteria grow in culture in the presence of air. Anaerobic bacteria do not; facultative bacteria can grow either aerobically or anaerobically. Some bacteria (eg, *Salmonella typhi, Legionella* sp, *Mycobacteria* sp, and *Chlamydia* and *Chlamydophila* spp) preferentially reside and replicate intracellularly. Most others do so extracellularly.

Antibacterial drugs are derived from bacteria or molds or from de novo synthesis. "Antibiotic," which is often used synonymously with "antibacterial drug," technically refers only to antimicrobials derived from bacteria or molds. Antibacterials have many mechanisms of action, including inhibiting cell wall synthesis, activating enzymes that destroy the cell wall, increasing cell membrane permeability, and interfering with protein synthesis and nucleic acid metabolism.

TABLE 170–1. CLASSIFICATION OF COMMON PATHOGENIC BACTERIA

AEROBIC VS ANAEROBIC	TYPE	ORGANISM
Aerobic	Gram-positive cocci, catalase-positive	*Staphylococcus aureus* (coagulase-positive), *S. epidermidis* (coagulase-negative), other coagulase-negative staphylococci
Aerobic	Gram-positive cocci, catalase-negative	*Enterococcus faecalis, E. faecium, Streptococcus agalactiae* (Group B streptococcus), *S. bovis, S. pneumoniae, S. pyogenes* (Group A streptococcus), Viridans group streptococci, *S. anginosus, S. mutans*
Aerobic	Gram-negative cocci	*Moraxella catarrhalis, Neisseria gonorrhoeae, N. meningitidis*
Aerobic	Gram-positive bacilli	*Bacillus anthracis, Corynebacterium diphtheriae, C. jeikeium, Erysipelothrix rhusiopathiae, Gardnerella vaginalis* (gram-variable)
Aerobic	Acid-fast bacilli	*Mycobacterium avium* complex, *Mycobacterium kansasii, M. leprae, M. tuberculosis, Nocardia* sp
Aerobic	Gram-negative bacilli	Enterobacteriaceae (*Citrobacter* sp, *Enterobacter aerogenes, Escherichia coli, Klebsiella* sp, *Morganella morganii, Proteus* sp, *Providencia rettgeri, Salmonella typhi,* other *Salmonella* sp, *Serratia marcescens, Shigella* sp, *Yersinia enterocolitica, Y. pestis)*
Aerobic	Fermentative, non-Enterobacteriaceae	*Aeromonas hydrophila, Chromobacterium violaceum, Plesiomonas shigelloides, Pasturella multocida, Vibrio cholerae, V. vulnificus*
Aerobic	Non-fermentative, non-Enterobacteriaceae	*Acinetobacter calcoaceticus, Flavobacterium* meningosepticum, *Pseudomonas aeruginosa, Pseudomonas alcaligenes*, other *Pseudomonas* sp, *Stenotrophomonas maltophilia*
Aerobic	Fastidious gram-negative coccobacilli and bacilli	*Actinobacillus actinomycetemcomitans, Bartonella bacilliformis, B. henselae, B. quintana, Brucella* sp, *Bordetella* sp, *Eikenella corrodens, Haemophilus influenzae*, other *Haemophilus* sp, *Legionella* sp
Aerobic	Curved bacilli	*Campylobacter jejuni, Helicobacter pylori*
Aerobic	Chlamydiaceae	*Chlamydia trachomatis, Chlamydophila pneumoniae, C. psittaci*
Aerobic	Rickettsiae	*Rickettsia prowazekii, R. rickettsii*
Aerobic	Mycoplasma	*Mycoplasma pneumoniae*
Aerobic	Treponemataceae (spiral organisms)	*Borrelia burgdorferi, Leptospira* sp, *Treponema pallidum*
Anaerobic	Gram-negative bacilli	*Bacteroides fragilis*, other *Bacteroides* sp, *Fusobacterium* sp, *Prevotella* sp
Anaerobic	Gram-negative cocci	*Veillonella* sp
Anaerobic	Non–spore-forming gram-positive bacilli	*Actinomyces* sp, *Bifidobacterium* sp, *Eubacterium* sp, *Propionibacterium* sp
Anaerobic	Endospore-forming gram-positive bacilli	*Clostridium botulinum, C. perfringens, C. tetani*, other *Clostridium* sp
Anaerobic	Gram-positive cocci	*Gemella morbillorum, Peptococcus niger, Peptostreptococcus* sp

TABLE 170–2. COMMON ANTIBIOTIC INTERACTIONS

DRUG	TOXICITY ENHANCED BY	NO CHANGE WITH
Warfarin	Azole antifungals Cefoperozone* Cefotetan* Chloramphenicol Clarithromycin Doxycycline Erythromycin Fluoroquinolones (ciprofloxacin, levofloxacin, ofloxacin) Metronidazole Rifampin (decreased PT) Sulfonamides	Aminoglycosides (IV) Cephalosporins (some) Penicillins Tetracycline Trimethoprim
Theophylline	Clarithromycin Ciprofloxacin Erythromycin Rifampin *decreases* theophylline levels	Aminoglycosides Azithromycin Cephalosporins Metronidazole Penicillins Sulfonamides Tetracycline Trimethoprim
Phenytoin	Azole antifungals Chloramphenicol Ciprofloxacin Isoniazid Macrolides (erythromycin, clarithromycin, dirithromycin) Trimethoprim-sulfamethoxazole Rifampin *decreases* phenytoin levels	Aminoglycosides Cephalosporins Penicillins Other fluoroquinolones
Digoxin	Azithromycin Clarithromycin Erythromycin Tetracycline Trimethoprim	Aminoglycosides Cephalosporins Ketoconazole Metronidazole Fluoroquinolones Penicillins Sulfonamides

*These interfere with vitamin K–dependent clotting factors and may also increase bleeding with antiplatelet drugs and thrombolytics.

Antibacterials sometimes interact with other drugs, raising or lowering serum levels of other drugs by increasing or decreasing their metabolism or various other mechanisms. The most clinically important interactions involve drugs with a low therapeutic ratio (ie, toxic levels are close to therapeutic levels); common agents are listed in TABLE 170–2.

Many antibacterials are chemically related and are thus grouped into classes. Although drugs within each class share structural and functional similarities, they often have different pharmacology and spectra of activity.

Selection and Use of Antibacterial Drugs

Antibacterials should be used only if clinical or laboratory evidence suggests *bacterial* infection. Use for viral illness or undifferentiated fever is inappropriate, subjects the patient to drug complications without any benefit, and contributes to bacterial resistance. Certain bacterial infections (eg, abscesses, infections with foreign bodies) require surgical intervention and do not respond to antibiotics alone.

Cultures and antibiotic sensitivities are essential for selecting a drug for serious infections. However, treatment often must begin before culture results are available, necessitating selection according to the most likely infecting organisms (empiric antibiotic selection). Whether chosen according to culture results or empirically, drugs used should possess the narrowest spectrum of activity that will control the infection. For empiric treatment of serious infections that may involve any one of several pathogens (eg, fever in a neutropenic patient) or that may be due to multiple pathogens (eg, polymicrobial anaerobic infection), a broad spectrum of activity is desirable. The most likely organisms and the organisms' susceptibility to antibacterials vary according to geography (within cities or even within a hospital) and can change from month to month.

Bactericidal drugs kill bacteria in vitro. Bacteriostatic drugs slow or stop in vitro bacterial growth but depend on body defenses to kill bacteria.

Quantitative methods identify the minimum in vitro concentration at which an antibiotic can inhibit growth (minimum inhibitory concentration, or MIC) or kill (minimum bactericidal concentration, or MBC). However, in vivo antibacterial effectiveness involves other factors, including pharmacology (eg, absorption, distribution, concentration in fluids and tissues, protein binding, and rate of excretion or metabolism), the presence of drug interactions or inhibiting substances, and host defense mechanisms. Usually, greater in vitro killing power is important only if local or systemic host defenses are weak (eg, in endocarditis, meningitis, serious infections in neutropenic or other immunocompromised patients).

The predominant determinant of bacteriologic response to antibiotics is either the duration that blood levels of the antibiotic exceed the MIC (time-dependence) or the peak blood level relative to MIC (concentration-dependence). The β-lactams and vancomycin exhibit time-dependent bactericidal activity. Increasing their concentrations above the MIC does not increase their rate of bactericidal activity, and their in vivo killing is generally slow. In addition, because there is either no or very brief residual inhibition of bacterial growth after concentrations fall below the MIC (postantibiotic effect, or PAE), β-lactams and vancomycin are most often effective when serum levels of free drug (ie, drug not bound to serum protein) exceed the MIC for ≥ 50% of the time. The long serum half-life of ceftriaxone allows free serum levels to exceed the MIC of very susceptible pathogens for the entire 24-h dosing interval. However, frequent dosing or continuous infusion is required for other β-lactams that have serum half-lives of ≤2 h. For vancomycin, trough levels should be maintained at 10 to 15 μg/mL.

Aminoglycosides, fluoroquinolones, and daptomycin exhibit concentration-dependent bactericidal activity. Increasing their concentrations from levels slightly above the MIC to levels far above the MIC increases their rate of bactericidal activity and decreases the bacterial load. In addition, after brief exposure to concentrations above the MIC, aminoglycosides and fluoroquinolones exhibit a PAE on residual bacteria, the duration of which is also concentration-dependent. If PAEs are long, drug levels can be below the MIC for extended periods without loss of efficacy, allowing less frequent dosing. Consequently, aminoglycosides and fluoroquinolones are usually most effective as intermittent boluses that achieve peak free serum levels ≥ 10 times the MIC of the infecting organism.

Combinations of antibiotics are often necessary in serious infections, either because they provide treatment for multiple possible species of infecting bacteria or because they act synergistically against a single species of bacteria. Synergism is usually defined as more rapid and complete bactericidal action from a combination of antibiotics (usually a cell wall–active agent, ie, a β-lactam or vancomycin, plus an aminoglycoside) than could be achieved by either antibiotic alone.

Oral administration provides excellent blood levels of many antibiotics and does so nearly as rapidly as IV administration. IV administration is preferred if oral antibiotics cannot be tolerated (eg, due to vomiting) or absorbed (eg, due to malabsorption after intestinal surgery); intestinal motility is impaired (eg, due to opioids); no oral preparation is available (eg, aminoglycosides); or a patient is critically ill, in which case GI tract perfusion may be impaired or even the brief delay with oral administration may be detrimental. Antibiotics should be continued until objective evidence of systemic infection (eg, absence of fever, symptoms, and abnormal laboratory findings) is absent for several days. Courses of therapy for some infections (eg, endocarditis, TB, osteomyelitis) are weeks or months long to prevent relapse.

Doses and scheduling of antibacterials may need to be adjusted in infants, the elderly, and patients with renal failure (see TABLE 170–3).

Text continues on page 1423.

TABLE 170–3. USUAL DOSES OF COMMONLY PRESCRIBED ANTIBIOTICS

DRUG	ADULT DOSE			CHILDREN (AGE > 1 MO) DOSE		DOSE IN RENAL FAILURE* (CrCl < 10 mL/min)
	Oral	Parenteral	Serious Infections	Oral	Parenteral	
Aminoglycosides						
Amikacin	N/A	15 mg/kg once/ day or 7.5 mg/kg q 12 h	15 mg/kg IV once/day or 7.5 mg/kg q 12 h	N/A	5–7.5 mg/kg q 12 h	1.5–2.5 mg/kg q 24–48 h
Gentamicin	N/A	5–7 mg/kg once/day or 1.7 mg/kg q 8 h	5–7 mg/kg IV once/day	N/A	1–2.5 mg/kg q 8 h	0.34–0.51 mg/kg q 24–48 h
For synergy with a cell wall–active antibiotic in enterococcal endocarditis		1 mg/kg q 8 h				
For streptococcal and *S. saureus* endocarditis		1 mg/kg q 8 h or 3 mg/kg once/ day				
Neomycin						
For preoperative gut antisepsis (po with erythromycin and mechanical cleansing)	1 g for 3 doses	N/A	N/A	15 mg/kg q 4 h × 2 days or 25 mg/kg at 1, 2, and 11 pm on the day before surgery	N/A	N/A
For hepatic coma	1–3 g qid	N/A	N/A	0.6–1.75 g/m^2 q 6 h or 0.4–1.2 g/m^2 q 4 h	N/A	N/A

Streptomycin						
For TB	N/A	15 mg/kg IM q 24 h (1.0 g/day maximum dose) initially, then 1.0 g 2–3 times/wk	N/A	N/A	20–40 mg/kg once/ day	7.5 mg/kg (maximum 1 g) q 72–96 h
For synergy with a cell wall–active antibiotic in enterococcal endocarditis	N/A	7.5 mg/kg q 12 h	N/A	N/A	N/A	N/A
Tobramycin	N/A	5–7 mg/kg once/day or 1.7 mg/kg q 8 h	5–7 mg/kg once/day or 1.7 mg/kg q 8 h	N/A	1–2.5 mg/kg q 8 h	0.34–0.51 mg/kg q 24–48 h
β-Lactams: Cephalosporins (1st Generation)						
Cefadroxil	0.5–1 g q 12 h	N/A	N/A	15 mg/kg q 12 h	N/A	0.5 g q 36 h
Cefazolin	N/A	1–2 g q 8 h	2 g IV q 8 h	N/A	16.6–33.3 mg/kg q 8 h	1–2 g q 24–48 h
Cephalexin	0.25–0.5 g q 6 h	N/A	N/A	6.25–12.5 mg/kg q 6 h or 8.0–16 mg/ kg q 8 h	N/A	0.25–0.5 g q 24–48 h
β-Lactams: Cephalosporins (2nd Generation)						
Cefaclor†	0.25–0.5 g q 8 h	N/A	N/A	10–20 mg/kg q 12 h or 6.6–13.3 mg/ kg q 8 h	N/A	0.5 g q 12 h
Cefotetan	N/A	1–3 g q 12 h	2–3 g IV q 12 h	N/A	20–40 mg/kg q 12 h	1–3 g q 48 h
Cefoxitin	N/A	1 g IVq 8 h to 2 g IV q 4 h	2 g IV q 4 h or 3 g IV q 6 h	N/A	27–33 mg/kg q 8 h or, for severe infections, 25–40 mg/kg q 6 h	0.5–1.0 g IV q 24–48 h

Table continues on the following page.

TABLE 170–3. USUAL DOSES OF COMMONLY PRESCRIBED ANTIBIOTICS—Continued

DRUG	ADULT DOSE			CHILDREN (AGE > 1 MO) DOSE		DOSE IN RENAL FAILURE* (CrCl < 10 mL/min)
	Oral	Parenteral	Serious Infections	Oral	Parenteral	
Cefprozil	0.25 g q 12 h or 0.5 g q 12–24 h	N/A	N/A	15 mg/kg q 12 h (for otitis media)	N/A	0.25 g q 12–24 h
Cefuroxime	0.125–0.5 g q 12 h	0.75–1.5 g q 6–8 h	1.5 g q 6 h	10–15 mg/kg suspension q 12 h; for older children, 125–250 mg tablets q 12 h	25–50 mg/kg q 8 h	0.25–0.5 g po q 24 h or 0.75 g IV q 24 h
For meningitis			3 g q 8 h		50–60 mg/kg q 6 h	
β-Lactams: Cephalosporins (3rd Generation)						
Cefoperazone	N/A	1 g q 12 h to 2 g q 4 h	2 g IV q 4 h	N/A	25–100 mg/kg q 12 h	1 g q 12 h to 2 g q 4 h
Cefotaxime	N/A	1 g q 12 h to 2 g q 4 h	2 g IV q 4 h	N/A	8.3–33.3 mg/kg q 4 h or 16.6–66.6 mg/kg q 6 h	1–2 g q 24 h
Cefpodoxime‡	0.1–0.4 g q 12 h	N/A	N/A	5 mg/kg q 12 h	N/A	0.1–0.4 g q 24 h
Ceftazidime	N/A	1 g q 12 h to 2 g q 8 h	2 g IV q 8 h	N/A	25–50 mg/kg q 8 h	0.5 g q 24–48 h
Ceftibuten†	0.4 g q 24 h	N/A	N/A	9 mg/kg once/day	N/A	0.1 g q 24 h
Ceftizoxime	N/A	0.5 g q 12 h to 4 g q 8 h	4 g IV q 8 h	N/A	50 mg/kg q 6–8 h	0.5 g q 24 h to 0.5–1 g q 48 h

Ceftriaxone	N/A	1–2 g q 24 h	2 g q 24 h	N/A	50–75 mg/kg q 24 h or 25–37.5 mg/kg q 12 h	1–2 g q 24 h
For meningitis	N/A	2 g q 12 h	2 g IV q 12 h	N/A	50 mg/kg q 12 h or 100 mg/kg q 24 h (not to exceed 4 g/day); a loading dose of 100 mg/kg (not to exceed 4 g) may be administered at the start of therapy	2 g q 12 h
β-Lactams: Cephalosporins (4th Generation)						
Cefepime	N/A	1–2 g q 8–12 h	2 g IV q 8 h	N/A	50 mg/kg q 8–12 h	0.25–1 g q 24 h
β-Lactams: Penicillins						
Amoxicillin	0.25–0.5 g q 8 h or 0.875 g q 12 h	N/A	N/A	12.5–25 mg/kg q 12 h or 7–13 mg/kg q 8 h	N/A	0.25–0.5 mg q 24 h
For endocarditis prophylaxis	2 g × 1 dose	N/A	N/A	50 mg/kg 1 h before procedure	N/A	2 g × 1 dose
Amoxicillin-clavulanate	0.25–0.5 g q 8 h or 0.875 g q 12 h	N/A	N/A	If > 40 kg, dose as adult	N/A	0.25–0.5 mg q 24 h
Amoxicillin-clavulanate ES-600	N/A	N/A	N/A	45 mg/kg q 12 h	N/A	N/A
Amoxicillin-clavulanate extended-release	2 g q 12 h	N/A	N/A	N/A	N/A	N/A

Table continues on the following page.

TABLE 170–3. USUAL DOSES OF COMMONLY PRESCRIBED ANTIBIOTICS—Continued

DRUG	ADULT DOSE			CHILDREN (AGE > 1 MO) DOSE		DOSE IN RENAL FAILURE* (CrCl < 10 mL/min)
	Oral	Parenteral	Serious Infections	Oral	Parenteral	
Ampicillin	N/A	0.5–2.0 g q 4–6 h	2 g IV q 4 h	N/A	25–50 mg/kg q 6 h	0.5–2.0 g q 12–24 h
For meningitis	N/A	2 g q 4 h	2 g q 4 h	N/A	50–100 mg/kg q 6 h	2 g q 12 h
Ampicillin-sulbactam (3 g = 2 g ampicillin + 1 g sulbactam)	N/A	1.5–3.0 g q 6 h	3 g IV q 6 h	N/A	25–50 mg/kg q 6 h	1.5–3.0 g q 24 h
Dicloxacillin†	0.125–0.5 g q 6 h	N/A	N/A	3.125–6.25 mg/kg q 6 h	N/A	0.125–0.5 g q 6 h
Nafcillin	Rarely used	1–2 g q 4 h	2 g IV q 4 h	N/A	12.5–25 mg/kg q 6 h or 8.3–33.3 mg/kg q 4 h	1–2 g q 4 h
Oxacillin	Rarely used	1–2 g q 4 h	2 g IV q 4 h	N/A	12.5–25 mg/kg q 6 h or 8.3–33.3 mg/kg q 4 h	1–2 g q 4 h
Penicillin G†	0.25–0.5 g q 6–12 h (penicillin V)	1–4 million units q 4–6 h	4 million units IV q 4 h	Penicillin VK 6.25–12.5 mg/kg q 8 h	6,250–100,000 units/kg q 6 h or 4,166.6–66,666 units/kg q 4 h	0.5–2 million units q 4–6 h maximum total daily dose is 6 million units/day

Drug						
Penicillin G benzathine (Bicillin L-A)						
For streptococcal pharyngitis	N/A	1.2 million units IM × 1 dose	N/A	N/A	25,000–50,000 units/kg IM as a single dose or if < 27 kg: 300,000–600,000 units as a single dose. If ≥ 27 kg: 0.9 million units as a single dose	1.2 million units IM × 1 dose
Prophylaxis for rheumatic fever	N/A	1.2 million units IM q 3–4 wk	N/A	N/A	25,000–50,000 units/kg IM q 3–4 wk	1.2 million units IM q 3–4 wk
For early syphilis	N/A	2.4 million units IM × 1 dose	N/A	N/A	50,000 units/kg IM in a single dose	2.4 million units IM × 1 dose
For late syphilis (excluding neurosyphilis)	N/A	2.4 million units IM/wk × 3 wk	N/A	N/A	50,000 units/kg IM in 3 doses 1 wk apart	2.4 million units IM × 1 dose
Penicillin G procaine (IM only)	N/A	0.3–0.6 million units q 12 h	N/A	N/A	25,000–50,000 units/kg q 24 h or 12,500–25,000 units/kg q 12 h	0.6 million units q 12 h
Piperacillin (1.9 mEq Na/g)	N/A	3 g q 4–6 h	3 g IV q 4 h	N/A	50–75 mg/kg q 6 h or 33.3–50 mg/kg q 4 h	3–4 g q 12 h
Piperacillin-tazobactam (2.25 g = 2.0 g piperacillin + 0.25 g tazobactam)	N/A	3.375 g q 4–6 h	3.375 g q 4 h	N/A	80 mg/kg q 8 h	2.25 g q 8 h to 4.5 g q 12 h

Table continues on the following page.

TABLE 170–3. USUAL DOSES OF COMMONLY PRESCRIBED ANTIBIOTICS—Continued

DRUG	ADULT DOSE			CHILDREN (AGE > 1 MO) DOSE		DOSE IN RENAL FAILURE* (CrCl < 10 mL/min)
	Oral	Parenteral	Serious Infections	Oral	Parenteral	
Ticarcillin (5.2 mEq Na/g)	N/A	3 g q 4–6 h	3 g IV q 4 h	N/A	If < 60 kg: 50 mg/kg q 4–6 h	1–2 g q 12 h
Ticarcillin-clavulanate (3.1 g = 3 g ticarcillin + 0.1 g clavulanic acid)	N/A	3.1 g q 4–6 h	3.1 g IV q 4 h	N/A	If < 60 kg: 50 mg/kg (based on ticarcillin component) q 4–6 h	2 g q 12 h
Other β-Lactams						
Aztreonam	N/A	1–2 g q 6–12 h	2 g IV q 6 h	N/A	30–40 mg/kg q 6–8 h	0.5 g q 8 h
Ertapenem	N/A	1 g q 24 h	1 g IV q 24 h	N/A	N/A	0.5 g q 24 h
Imipenem	N/A	0.5–1.0 g q 6 h	1 g IV q 6 h	N/A	Infants 4 wk to 3 mo: 25 mg/kg q 6 h; children > 3 mo: 15–25 mg/kg q 6 h	0.125–0.25 g q 12 h (may increase risk of seizures)
Meropenem	N/A	1.0 g q 8 h	1.0 g q 8 h	N/A	20–40 mg/kg q 8 h	0.5 g q 24 h
For meningitis		40 mg/kg q 8 h	40 mg/kg q 8 h	N/A		20 mg/kg q 24 h
Fluoroquinolones§						
Ciprofloxacin	0.5–0.75 g q 12 h	0.2–0.4 g q 8–12 h	0.4 g IV q 8 h	10–15 mg/kg q 12 h (in select circumstances)	10–15 mg/kg q 12 h (in select circumstances)	0.5–0.75 g po q 24 h or 0.2–0.4 g IV q 24 h
Extended release for uncomplicated cystitis	0.5 g q 24 h × 3 days	N/A	N/A	N/A	N/A	N/A

Gatifloxacin	0.2–0.4 g q 24 h	0.4 g q 24 h	0.4 g IV q 24 h	N/A	N/A	0.2 g q 24 h
Gemifloxacin	320 mg q 24 h	N/A	N/A	N/A	N/A	160 mg q 24 h
Levofloxacin	0.25–0.75 g q 24 h	0.25–0.75 g q 24 h	0.75 g IV q 24 h	N/A	N/A	0.25–0.5 g q 48 h
Moxifloxacin	0.4 g q 24 h	0.4 g q 24 h	0.4 g IV q 24 h	N/A	N/A	0.4 g q 24 h
Norfloxacin†	0.4 g q 12 h	N/A	N/A	N/A	N/A	0.4 g q 24 h
Ofloxacin†	0.2–0.4 g q 12 h	0.4 g q 12 h	0.2–0.4 g IV q 12 h	N/A	N/A	0.1–0.2 g q 24 h
Trovafloxacin	0.2 g q 24 h	0.2–0.3 g q 24 h	0.3 g q 24 h	N/A	N/A	Not recommended
Macrolides						
Azithromycin	0.5 g on day 1, then 0.25 g q 24 h × 4 days	0.5 g q 24 h	0.5 g IV q 24 h		N/A	0.5 g on day 1, then 0.25 g q 24 h po × 4 days or 0.5 g IV q 24 h
For nongonococcal cervicitis and urethritis	1 g × 1dose	N/A	N/A	N/A	N/A	N/A
For traveler's diarrhea	1 g × 1dose	N/A	N/A	5–10 mg/kg × 1 dose	N/A	N/A
For tonsillitis/pharyngitis	N/A	N/A	N/A	12 mg/kg/day × 5 days	N/A	N/A
For otitis media and community-acquired pneumonia	N/A	N/A	N/A	10 mg/kg on day 1, then 5 mg/kg once/day on days 2–5	N/A	N/A

Table continues on the following page.

TABLE 170–3. USUAL DOSES OF COMMONLY PRESCRIBED ANTIBIOTICS—Continued

DRUG	ADULT DOSE			CHILDREN (AGE > 1 MO) DOSE		DOSE IN RENAL FAILURE* (CrCl < 10 mL/min)
	Oral	Parenteral	Serious Infections	Oral	Parenteral	
Clarithromycin	0.25–0.5 g q 12 h; extended-release 1 g q 24 h	N/A	N/A	7.5 mg/kg q 12 h	N/A	0.25–0.5 g q 24 h
Dirithromycin	0.5 g q 24 h	N/A	N/A	N/A	N/A	0.5 g q 24 h
Erythromycin†						
Base	0.25–0.5 g q 6 h	N/A	N/A	10–16.6 mg/kg q 8 h or 7.5–12.5 mg/kg q 6 h	N/A	0.25 g q 6 h
Lactobionate	N/A	0.5–1 g q 6 h	1 g q 6 h	N/A	3.75–5.0 mg/kg q 6 h	0.5 g q 6 h
Gluceptate	N/A	0.5–1 g q 6 h	1 g q 6 h	N/A	3.75–5.0 mg/kg q 6 h	0.5 g q 6 h
For GI preoperative bowel preparation	1 g × 3 doses	N/A	N/A	20 mg/kg × 3 doses	N/A	N/A
Telithromycin	800 mg q 24 h	N/A	N/A	N/A	N/A	800 mg q 24 h
Sulfonamides and Trimethoprim						
Sulfisoxazole†	1.0 g q 6 h	25 mg/kg q 6 h (not available in US)	N/A	30–37.5 mg/kg q 6 h or 20–25 mg/kg q 4 h	N/A	1 g q 12–24 h
Sulfamethizole†	0.5–1 g q 6–8 h	N/A	N/A	7.5–11.25 mg/kg q 6 h	N/A	N/A

Sulfamethoxazole	1 g q 8–12 h	N/A	N/A	25–30 mg/kg q 12 h	N/A	1 g q 24 h
Trimethoprim	0.1 g q 12 h; 0.2 g q 24 h	N/A	N/A	*For urinary tract infection*: 2 mg/kg q 12 h for 10 days	N/A	0.1 g q 24 h
Trimethoprim-sulfamethoxazole†	0.16/0.8 g q 12 h	3–5 mg/kg q 6–8 h (based on TMP)	5 mg/kg q 6 h	3–6 mg TMP/kg q 12 h	3–6 mg TMP/kg q 12 h	(Not recommended if other alternatives)
For *Pneumocystis* pneumonia	0.32/1.6 g q 8 h × 21 days	5 mg/kg q 8 h (based on TMP) × 21 days	5 mg/kg q 6–8 h	5–6.6 mg TMP/kg q 8 h or 3.75–5 mg/kg q 6 h	5–6.6 mg TMP/kg q 8 h or 3.75–5 mg/kg q 6 h	If essential, 5 mg/kg q 24 h or 1.25 mg/kg q 6 h
Tetracyclines						
Doxycycline	0.1 g q 12 h	0.1 g q 12 h	0.1 mg q 12 h	Age > 8 yr: 2–4 mg/kg q 24 h or 1–2 mg/kg q 12 h	Age > 8 yr: 2–4 mg/kg q 24 h or 1–2 mg/kg q 12 h	0.1 g q 12 h
Minocycline	0.1 g q 12 h	0.1 g q 12 h	0.1 g q 12 h	N/A	N/A	0.1 g q 12 h
Tetracycline†	0.25–0.5 g q 6 h	N/A	N/A	Age > 8 yr: 6.25–12.5 mg/kg q 6 h	N/A	Use doxycycline
Others						
Clindamycin	0.15–0.45 g q 6 h	0.6 g q 6 h to 0.9 g q 8 h	0.9 g q 8 h	2.6–6.6 mg/kg q 8 h or 2–5 mg/kg q 6 h	6.6–13.2 mg/kg q 8 h or 5–10 mg/kg q 6 h	0.15–0.45 g po q 6 h or 0.6–0.9 g IV q 6–8 h
Chloramphenicol	0.25–1 g q 6 h	0.25–1.0 g q 6 h	1 g q 6 h	N/A	12.5–18.75 mg/kg q 6 h	0.25–1.0 g IV q 6 h
For meningitis	N/A	12.5 mg/kg q 6 h (maximum 4 g/day)	12.5 mg/kg q 6 h (maximum 4 g/day)	N/A	18.75–25 mg/kg q 6 h	12.5 mg/kg q 6 h (maximum 4 g/day)

Table continues on the following page.

TABLE 170–3. USUAL DOSES OF COMMONLY PRESCRIBED ANTIBIOTICS—Continued

DRUG	ADULT DOSE			CHILDREN (AGE > 1 MO) DOSE		DOSE IN RENAL FAILURE* (CrCl < 10 mL/min)
	Oral	Parenteral	Serious Infections	Oral	Parenteral	
Daptomycin	N/A	4 mg/kg IV q 24 h	4 mg/kg IV q 24 h	N/A	N/A	4 mg/kg IV q 48 h
Linezolid	0.6 g q 12 h	0.6 g q 12 h	0.6 g IV q 12 h	10 mg/kg q 8 h	10 mg/kg q 8 h	0.6 g q 12 h
Metronidazole						
For anaerobic infection	7.5 mg/kg q 6 h (not to exceed 4 g/day)	7.5 mg/kg q 6 h (not to exceed 4 g/day)	7.5 mg/kg IV q 6 h (not to exceed 4 g/day)	7.5 mg/kg q 6 h	7.5 mg/kg q 6 h	3.75 mg/kg q 6 h (not to exceed 2 g/day)
For trichomoniasis	2 g × 1 dose or 0.5 g q 12 h × 7 days	N/A	N/A	N/A	N/A	N/A
For *Clostridium difficile* colitis	0.5 g q 8 h × 10–14 days	500 mg q 6 h	500 mg q 8 h	7.5 mg/kg q 8 h	7.5 mg/kg q 6 h	250 mg q 8 h
For amebiasis	0.5–0.75 g q 8 h × 10 days followed by paromomycin po 0.5 g q 8 h × 7 days	0.75 g q 8 h × 10 days followed by paromomycin po 0.5 g q 8 h × 7 days	0.75 g q 8 h × 10 days followed by paromomycin po 0.5 g q 8 h × 7 days	11.6–16.6 mg/kg q 8 h for 7–10 days	11.6–16.6 mg/kg q 8 h × 7–10 days	N/A

For giardiasis	0.25 g q 8 h × 5–7 days	N/A	N/A	5 mg/kg q 8 h × 5 days	N/A	N/A
Nitrofurantoin macrocrystals	50–100 mg q 6 h	N/A	N/A	1.25–1.75 mg/kg q 6 h	N/A	Not recommended
Macrocrystals/ monohydrate	100 mg q 12 h	N/A	N/A	N/A	N/A	N/A
Quinupristin/ dalfopristin	N/A	7.5 mg/kg q 8–12 h	7.5 mg/kg IV q 8 h	N/A	7.5 mg/kg q 12 h for complicated skin or skin structure infection or 7.5 mg/kg q 8 h for serious infections.	7.5 mg/kg q 8–12 h
Rifampin†						
For TB	0.6 g q 24 h	0.6 g q 24 h	N/A	5–10 mg/kg q 12 h or 10–20 mg/kg q 24 h	10–20 mg/kg q 24 h	0.3–0.6 g q 24 h
For meningococcal exposure	0.6 g q 12 h × 4 doses	N/A	N/A	Age ≥ 1 mo: 10 mg/kg q 12 h × 2 days Age < 1 mo: 5 mg/kg q 12 h × 2 days	N/A	0.6 g q 12 h × 4 doses
For *Haemophilus influenzae* exposure	20 mg/kg q 24 h × 4 days (not to exceed 600 mg q 24 h)	N/A	N/A	20 mg/kg q 24 h × 4 days	N/A	20 mg/kg q 24 h × 4 days (not to exceed 500 mg q 24 h)
For staphylococcal infections (in combination with a penicillin, cephalosporin, or vancomycin)	0.3 g q 8 h or 0.6–0.9 g q 24 h	0.3 g q 8 h or 0.6–0.9 g q 24 h	0.3 g q 8 h or 0.6–0.9 g q 24 h			0.3 g q 8 h or 0.6–0.9 g q 24 h

Table continues on the following page.

TABLE 170–3. USUAL DOSES OF COMMONLY PRESCRIBED ANTIBIOTICS—Continued

DRUG	ADULT DOSE			CHILDREN (AGE > 1 MO) DOSE		DOSE IN RENAL FAILURE* (CrCl < 10 mL/min)
	Oral	Parenteral	Serious Infections	Oral	Parenteral	
Spectinomycin	N/A	2 g IM single dose	N/A	N/A	N/A	2 g IM single dose
Vancomycin	125 mg q 6 h (only effective for *C. difficile* colitis)	15 mg/kg q 12 h (often 1 g q 12)	15 mg/kg q 12 h	N/A	13 mg/kg q 8 h or 10 mg/kg q 6 h	0.5–1.0 g IV q wk
For meningitis	N/A	1 g q 8 h or 1.5 g q 12 h¶	1 g q 8 h or 1.5 g q 12 h	N/A	15 mg/kg q 6 h	15 mg/kg IV q wk

N/A = Not applicable; TMP = trimethoprim.

*Initial loading dose should be equivalent to the usual dose for a patient with normal renal function, followed by a dose adjusted for renal failure. Dosing adjustments of aminoglycosides should be assisted by measurement of peak (drawn 1 h after start of a ⅓ h IV infusion) and trough (drawn just before next dose) serum levels.

†Decreased rate or extent of absorption when taken with food.

‡Should not exceed adult dosage.

§Generally avoided in children.

¶In addition, intrathecal or intraventricular vancomycin 10 to 20 mg daily may be necessary and dose adjusted to achieve trough CSF levels of 10 to 20 µg/mL.

Commonly used antibacterials that need dose adjustment in hepatic insufficiency include cefoperazone, ceftriaxone, chloramphenicol, clindamycin, metronidazole, nafcillin, and rifampin. Penicillins, cephalosporins, and erythromycin are among the safest antibacterials during pregnancy; tetracyclines are contraindicated. Most antibiotics reach sufficient concentrations in breast milk to affect a breastfed baby, sometimes contraindicating their use in nursing women.

Complications of antibiotic therapy include superinfection by nonsusceptible bacteria or fungi and, commonly, cutaneous, renal, hematologic, and GI adverse effects. Adverse effects frequently require stopping the offending drug and substituting another antibiotic to which the pathogen is susceptible; sometimes, no alternatives exist.

Antibiotic Resistance

Resistance to an antibiotic may be inherent in a particular bacterial species or may be acquired as a result of mutations or acquisition of genes from another organism that encode for antibiotic resistance. Mechanisms for resistance that are encoded by these genes are briefly described in TABLE 170–4. Resistance genes can be transmitted between 2 bacterial cells by transformation (uptake of naked DNA from another organism), transduction (infection by a bacteriophage), or conjugation (exchange of genetic material in the form of either plasmids, which are pieces of independently replicating extrachromosomal DNA, or transposons, which are movable pieces of chromosomal DNA). Plasmids and transposons can rapidly disseminate resistance genes.

Antibiotic use preferentially eliminates nonresistant bacteria, increasing the proportion of resistant bacteria that remain. This is true not only for pathogenic bacteria but also for normal flora; resistant normal flora serves as a reservoir for resistance genes that can spread to future pathogens.

TABLE 170–4. COMMON MECHANISMS OF ANTIBACTERIAL RESISTANCE

MECHANISM	EXAMPLE
Decreased cell wall permeability	Loss of outer cell wall D2 Porin in imipenem-resistant *Pseudomonas aeruginosa*
Enzymatic inactivation	Production of β-lactamases that inactivate penicillins in penicillin-resistant *Staphylococcus aureus, Haemophilus influenzae, Escherichia coli*
	Production of aminoglycoside-inactivating enzymes in gentamicin-resistant enterococci
Changes in target	Decreased affinity of penicillin-binding proteins for β-lactam antibiotics (eg, in *S. pneumoniae* with reduced penicillin sensitivity)
	Decreased affinity of methylated ribosomal RNA target for macrolides, clindamycin, and quinupristin in MLSB-resistant *S. aureus*
	Decreased affinity of altered cell wall precursor for vancomycin (eg, *E. faecium*)
	Decreased affinity of DNA gyrase for fluoroquinolones in fluoroquinolone-resistant *S. aureus*
Increased antibiotic efflux pump	Increased efflux of tetracycline, macrolides, clindamycin, or fluoroquinolones (eg, *S. aureus*)
Bypass of antibiotic inhibition	Development of bacterial mutants that can subsist on products (eg, thymidine) present in the environment, not just products synthesized within the bacteria (eg, trimethoprim-sulfamethoxazole)

MLSB = Macrolide, lincoside, streptogramin B.

TABLE 170–5. AMINOGLYCOSIDES

Amikacin
Gentamicin
Neomycin*
Streptomycin
Tobramycin

*Should be used topically or orally only.

AMINOGLYCOSIDES

Aminoglycosides (see TABLE 170–5) are bactericidal. They bind to the 30S ribosome, thereby inhibiting bacterial protein synthesis.

Pharmacology: Aminoglycosides are poorly absorbed orally but are well absorbed from the peritoneum, pleural cavity, joints (and should never be instilled in these body cavities), and denuded skin. Aminoglycosides are distributed well into the ECF except for vitreous humor, CSF, respiratory secretions, and bile (particularly with biliary obstruction).

Aminoglycosides are excreted by glomerular filtration and have a serum half-life of 2 to 3 h; the half-life rises exponentially as the GFR falls (eg, in renal insufficiency or in the elderly). Peak serum levels of at least 10 times the minimum inhibitory concentration (MIC) are desirable.

When β-lactams, such as piperacillin or ticarcillin, are used in high doses, the high serum levels of the β-lactam may inactivate the aminoglycoside in vitro in serum specimens obtained for drug level determination from patients receiving both drugs, if the serum is not assayed immediately or frozen. If patients with renal failure are concurrently receiving both an aminoglycoside and a high-dose β-lactam, the serum aminoglycoside concentration may be lower because of prolonged interaction in vivo.

Indications: Aminoglycosides are used for serious gram-negative infections, especially *Pseudomonas aeruginosa*. They are active against most gram-negative aerobic bacilli but lack activity against anaerobes and most gram-positive bacteria, except for most staphylococci; however, some gram-negative bacilli and methicillin-resistant staphylococci are resistant. Gentamicin, tobramycin, and amikacin are active against *P. aeruginosa*, whereas streptomycin, neomycin, and kanamycin are not. Gentamicin and tobramycin have similar antimicrobial spectra against gram-negative bacilli, but tobramycin is more active against *P. aeruginosa,* and gentamicin is more active against *Serratia marcescens*. Amikacin is frequently active against gentamicin- and tobramycin-resistant pathogens.

Aminoglycosides are used alone infrequently, typically for plague and tularemia. They are used with a broad-spectrum β-lactam for severe infection due to a suspected gram-negative bacillus. However, because of increasing aminoglycoside resistance, a fluoroquinolone can be substituted for the aminoglycoside in initial empiric regimens, or the aminoglycoside can be stopped after 2 to 3 days unless an aminoglycoside-sensitive *P. aeruginosa* is identified.

Gentamicin or, less commonly, streptomycin may be used with other antimicrobials to treat endocarditis due to streptococci or enterococci. Enterococcal resistance to aminoglycosides has become a common problem. Because therapy of enterococcal endocarditis requires prolonged use of a potentially nephrotoxic and ototoxic aminoglycoside combined with a bacterial cell wall–active drug (eg, penicillin or vancomycin) to achieve bactericidal synergy, the choice of aminoglycoside must be based on special in vitro susceptibility testing. High-level aminoglycoside susceptibility in vitro will predict synergy when low-dose aminoglycoside therapy is combined with a cell wall–active drug. If the strain is susceptible to high-level gentamicin and streptomycin, gentamicin is preferred because serum levels can be readily determined. High-level resistance to gentamicin in vitro does not rule out susceptibility of these enterococcal strains to high levels of streptomycin, in which case streptomycin should be used. There are few therapeutic options available for endocarditis due to enterococci resistant to high levels of both gentamicin and streptomycin, for which no synergistic cell wall–active drug/aminoglycoside combination exists. Endocarditis due to such strains has been treated with limited success with prolonged courses of a cell wall–active drug alone or linezolid.

Streptomycin has limited uses because of resistance. It is used with other antimicrobials for TB.

Because of toxicity, neomycin and kanamycin are limited to topical use in small amounts. Neomycin is available for eye, ear, oral, and rectal use and as a bladder irrigant. Oral use as a topical agent against intestinal flora includes bowel preparation before surgery and treatment of hepatic coma.

Toxicity: All aminoglycosides produce renal toxicity (often reversible) and vestibular and auditory toxicity (often irreversible). Symptoms and signs of vestibular damage are vertigo, nausea, vomiting, nystagmus, and ataxia. Risk factors for renal, vestibular, and auditory toxicity are large doses, very high blood levels, frequent doses, longer duration of therapy (particularly > 3 days), older age, and preexisting renal disease. Other risk factors include coadministration of vancomycin, cyclosporine, amphotericin B, or radiocontrast material (for renal toxicity) and preexisting hearing problems or coadministration of loop diuretics (for auditory toxicity). Patients receiving aminoglycosides for > 2 wk or those at risk of vestibular and auditory toxicity should be monitored with serial audiograms. At the 1st sign of toxicity, the drug is stopped (if possible) or dosing adjusted.

Aminoglycosides can prolong the effect of neuromuscular blockers (eg, succinylcholine or curare-like drugs) and worsen weakness in diseases affecting neuromuscular transmission (eg, myasthenia gravis). This particularly occurs with too-rapid administration or excessively high serum levels. It sometimes resolves more rapidly with neostigmine or IV Ca. Other neurologic effects include paresthesias and peripheral neuropathy.

TABLE 170–6. DOSING FOR AMINOGLYCOSIDES IN ADULTS

1. Choose loading dose in mg/kg (ideal weight) for peak serum levels in range from below for desired aminoglycosides. Dose is based on lean body weight plus 50% of adipose mass in obese patients and total body weight in edematous patients.

AMINOGLYCOSIDE	USUAL LOADING DOSES	EXPECTED PEAK SERUM LEVELS	TARGET SERUM TROUGH LEVELS
Tobramycin, gentamicin	1.5–2.0 mg/kg	4–10 μg/mL	< 2 μg/mL
Amikacin	5.0–7.5 mg/kg	15–30 μg/mL	< 5 μg/mL

2. Choose maintenance dose (as percentage of chosen loading dose) to continue peak serum levels indicated above according to desired interval and the patient's corrected creatinine clearance. Calculate corrected creatinine clearance C(c)cr as follows:

PERCENTAGE OF LOADING DOSE REQUIRED FOR DOSAGE INTERVAL SELECTED

C(C)CR (ML/MIN)	8 H (%)	12 H (%)	24 H (%)
90	84	—	—
70	76	88	—
50	65	79	—
30	48	63	86
20	37	50	75
15	31	42	67
10	24	34	56
5	16	23	41
0	8	11	21

C(c)cr male = (140 − age)wt in kg/70 × serum creatinine.
C(c)cr female = 0.85 × C(c)cr male.
Dosing for patients with C(c)cr ≤ 90 mL/min should be assisted by measured serum levels.

Modified from Sarubbi FA Jr, Hull JH: Amikacin serum concentrations: Prediction of levels and dosage guidelines. *Annals of Internal Medicine* 89:612–618, 1978.

Hypersensitivity reactions are uncommon. Large oral doses of neomycin can produce malabsorption.

Administration: Aminoglycosides are usually given IV. Intravitreous injection is required to treat endophthalmitis. Intraventricular injection is often required to achieve adequate intraventricular levels for treatment of meningitis. Because toxicity depends more on the duration of therapeutic levels than peak levels and because drug efficacy is concentration-dependent rather than time-dependent, frequent doses are avoided. Once/day IV dosing is preferred for most indications except enterococcal endocarditis. IV aminoglycosides are given slowly (30 min for divided daily dosing or 30 to 45 min for once/day dosing). Once-daily dosing of gentamicin or tobramycin is 5 to 7 mg/kg q 24 h; the higher dose is used initially in critically ill patients, who are likely to have expanded volumes of distribution, to achieve targeted peak serum levels of 16 to 24 μg/mL and thereby facilitate concentration-dependent bactericidal activity. Peak serum levels should be determined after the 1st dose in critically ill patients. Peak and trough levels are measured after the 2nd or 3rd dose when the daily aminoglycoside dose is divided and the duration of therapy is > 3 days. Dosing is adjusted to ensure a therapeutic peak serum level and nontoxic trough level (see TABLE 170–6). Trough levels should be undetectable at 18 to 24 h after the 1st dose with once-daily dosing and between 1 and 2 mg/mL with multiple daily dosing of gentamicin or tobramycin. The peak concentration is the level 60 min after an IM injection or 30 min after the end of a 30-min IV infusion. Assuming clinical response and continued normal renal function, the once-daily dose can be reduced after the 1st few days of therapy to 5 mg/kg. Troughs are measured within 30 min before the next dose. Serum creatinine is measured q 2 to 3 days, and if stable, serum aminoglycoside levels need not be repeated.

In patients with renal insufficiency, the loading dose is the usual dose based on body weight in patients with normal renal function; usually the dosing interval is increased rather than the dose amount decreased. Nomograms calculate maintenance doses based on serum creatinine or creatinine clearance values (see TABLE 170–6), but they are not precise, and measurement of blood levels is preferred.

SPECTINOMYCIN

Spectinomycin is a bacteriostatic antibiotic chemically related to the aminoglycosides. Spectinomycin binds to the 30S subunit of the ribosome, thus inhibiting bacterial protein synthesis. Its activity is restricted to gonococci. Spectinomycin is excreted by glomerular filtration.

Spectinomycin is given for gonococcal urethritis, cervicitis, and proctitis but is not effective in gonococcal pharyngitis. It is reserved for patients who cannot be treated with ceftriaxone, cefpodoxime, cefixime, or a fluoroquinolone.

Adverse effects, including hypersensitivity reactions and fever, are rare.

β-LACTAMS

β-Lactams are antibiotics that have a β-lactam ring nucleus. Subclasses include the cephalosporins and cephamycins (cephems), carbacephems (loracarbef), penicillins, clavams, carbapenems, and monobactams. All β-lactams bind to and inactivate enzymes required for bacterial cell wall synthesis.

CEPHALOSPORINS

The cephalosporins are bactericidal with both gram-positive and gram-negative activity. Cephalosporins are classified in generations (see TABLE170–7). Higher generations

TABLE 170–7. CEPHALOSPORINS*

1st generation	3rd generation
Cefadroxil†	Cefdinir†
Cefazolin‡	Cefditoren†
Cephalexin†	Cefixime†
Cephradine†	Cefoperazone‡
	Cefotaxime‡
2nd generation	Cefpodoxime†
Cefaclor†	Ceftazidime‡
Cefotetan‡	Ceftibuten†
Cefoxitin‡	Ceftizoxime‡
Cefprozil†	Ceftriaxone‡
Cefuroxime†‡	**4th generation**
Loracarbef†	Cefepime‡

*Loracarbef is technically a carbacephem, and cefoxitin and cefotetan are technically cephamycins, but they are grouped with cephalosporins because of similar antimicrobial spectra and pharmacology.

†Oral.

‡Parenteral.

generally have expanded spectra against aerobic gram-negative bacilli. Some 3rd-generation cephalosporins have relatively poor activity against gram-positive cocci, especially methicillin-sensitive *Staphylococcus aureus*. The 4th-generation cephalosporin, cefepime, maintains activity against gram-positive cocci and has enhanced activity against gram-negative bacilli, including *Pseudomonas aeruginosa*, extended-spectrum β-lactamase (ESBL)–producing *Klebsiella pneumoniae* and *Escherichia coli*, and ampC β-lactamase–producing Enterobacteriaceae, such as *Enterobacter* sp. Cephalosporins are not active against enterococci, methicillin-resistant staphylococci, and, except for cefotetan and cefoxitin, anaerobic gram-negative bacilli.

Pharmacology: Cephalosporins penetrate well into most body fluids and the ECF of most tissues, especially in the presence of inflammation (which enhances diffusion). However, only ceftriaxone, cefotaxime, ceftazidime, and cefepime achieve CSF levels sufficient to treat meningitis. All cephalosporins penetrate poorly into ICF and the vitreous humor.

Most cephalosporins are excreted primarily in urine. Dose adjustment is needed for these drugs in renal insufficiency. Cefoperazone and ceftriaxone, which have significant biliary excretion, do not require dose adjustment in renal insufficiency.

Indications: First-generation cephalosporins have excellent activity against gram-positive cocci. Among them, oral drugs are commonly used for uncomplicated skin and soft-tissue infections, which are usually due to staphylococci and streptococci. Parenteral cefazolin is frequently used for endocarditis due to methicillin-sensitive *Staphylococcus aureus* and for prophylaxis for cardiothoracic, orthopedic, abdominal, and pelvic surgery.

Second-generation cephalosporins and cephamycins (cefoxitin and cefotetan) are often used for polymicrobial infections involving gram-negative bacilli and gram-positive cocci. Because cephamycins are active against *Bacteroides fragilis* and other *Bacteroides* sp, they can be used when anaerobes are suspected (eg, intra-abdominal sepsis, decubitus ulcers, diabetic foot infections).

Third-generation cephalosporins are active against *Haemophilus influenzae* and some Enterobacteriaceae (eg, *E. coli, K. pneumoniae, Proteus mirabilis*) that do not express ampC β-lactamase or produce ESBL. Ceftazidime and cefoperazone are active against *P. aeruginosa*. Oral cefpodoxime is used for uncomplicated skin and soft-tissue infections due to staphylococci and streptococci, but oral cefixime and ceftibuten have little activity against *S. aureus* and should be restricted to uncomplicated infections due to streptococci.

The 4th-generation drug cefepime has good activity against gram-positive cocci (similar to cefotaxime) and *Pseudomonas* (similar to ceftazidime) and enhanced activity against many Enterobacteriaceae. Third- and 4th-generation cephalosporins are often used in polymicrobial infections involving gram-negative bacilli and gram-positive cocci (eg, intra-abdominal sepsis, decubitus ulcers, diabetic foot infections), when necessary combined with other drugs to cover anaerobes or enterococci. Ceftriaxone and some other 3rd-generation drugs are often used with a macrolide (the macrolide is used to cover "atypical" pathogens—*Mycoplasma, Chlamydophila, Legionella*) in community-acquired pneumonia. Ceftriaxone and cefotaxime are used empirically for acute meningitis due to suspected *Streptococcus pneumoniae, H. influenzae,* or *Neisseria meningitides* in combination with ampicillin to cover *Listeria monocytogenes*. Pneumococcal strains that are resistant to ceftriaxone and cefotaxime have been reported, and guidelines suggest that strains cultured in meningitis that have MICs of ≥ 0.5 μg/mL should be considered resistant to 3rd-generation cephalosporins. Thus, in acute meningitis, ceftriaxone or cefotaxime is empirically combined with vancomycin to cover *Streptococcus pneumoniae* with reduced penicillin sensitivity. Ceftazidime is part of empiric therapy for postneurosurgical meningitis to cover *P. aeruginosa* and combined with vancomycin to cover methicillin-resistant *S. aureus*, which are common pathogens in this setting.

Ceftriaxone is recommended for endocarditis caused by HACEK organisms (*Haemophilus, Actinobacillus, Cardiobacterium, Eikenella,* and *Kingella* spp) and for penicillin-sensitive streptococcal endocarditis. Ceftriaxone is used for neurologic complications of Lyme disease (except isolated Bell's palsy), carditis, and arthritis. A single IM dose of ceftriaxone is used for uncomplicated gonococcal infection and for chancroid.

Toxicity: Hypersensitivity reactions are the most common systemic adverse effects;

immediate, IgE-mediated urticaria and anaphylaxis are rare. Cross-sensitivity between cephalosporins and penicillins is uncommon; cephalosporins can be given cautiously to patients with a history of delayed hypersensitivity to penicillin if necessary. However, cephalosporins should not be used in patients who have had an anaphylactic reaction to penicillin. Pain at the IM injection site and thrombophlebitis after IV use are possible.

All cephalosporins can produce *Clostridium difficile* (pseudomembranous) colitis, leukopenia, thrombocytopenia, or a positive Coombs' test (although hemolytic anemia is very uncommon).

Cefamandole, cefoperazone, and cefotetan may have a disulfiram-like effect and cause nausea and vomiting with ethanol ingestion. Cefamandole, cefoperazone, and cefotetan may elevate the PT/INR and PTT, an effect that is reversible with vitamin K.

PENICILLINS

Penicillins (see TABLE 170–8) are bactericidal by unknown mechanisms, perhaps by activating autolytic enzymes that destroy the bacterial cell wall in some organisms. Some organisms produce β-lactamase, which inactivates the drug; this effect can be blocked by adding a β-lactamase inhibitor (clavulanic acid, sulbactam, or tazobactam). However, available β-lactamase inhibitors do not inhibit ampC β-lactamases commonly produced by *Enterobacter, Serratia, P. aeruginosa, Citrobacter, Providencia,* and *Morganella* and may only partially inhibit extended-spectrum β-lactamases produced by some *K. pneumoniae, E. coli*, and other Enterobacteriaceae.

Pharmacology: Food does not interfere with absorption of amoxicillin, but penicillin G should be given 1 h before or 2 h after a meal. Amoxicillin has generally replaced ampicillin for oral use because amoxicillin is absorbed better, causes fewer GI effects, and can be given less frequently.

Penicillins are distributed rapidly in ECF of most tissues, particularly with inflammation.

Urinary excretion of all penicillins except nafcillin is high, necessitating dose reduction in patients with severe renal insufficiency. Probenecid inhibits renal tubular secretion of many penicillins, increasing blood levels. Parenteral penicillin G is rapidly excreted (serum half-life 0.5 h) except for repository forms (the benzathine or procaine salt of penicillin G), which are intended for deep IM injection only and provide a tissue depot from which absorption takes place over several hours to several days. Benzathine penicillin reaches its peak more slowly and is generally longer acting than procaine penicillin. Three benzathine penicillin G–containing products are available: Bicillin L-A (benzathine penicillin alone), Bicillin C-R (a mixture of equal amounts of benzathine and procaine penicillin G), and Bicillin® C-R 900/300 (a mixture of 0.9 MU benzathine and 0.3 MU procaine penicillin G). *Only Bicillin L-A is recommended for treating syphilis and preventing rheumatic fever.* Both Bicillin L-A and Bicillin C-R are indicated for treatment of URIs and skin and soft-tissue infections caused by susceptible streptococci. The efficacy of Bicillin C-R to treat syphilis is unknown.

Indications: Penicillin G–like drugs (including penicillin V) are primarily used for gram-positive organisms and some gram-negative cocci (eg, meningococcus); a minority of gram-negative bacilli also are susceptible to large parenteral doses of penicillin G. Most staphylococci, most *Neisseria gonorrhoeae*, many anaerobic gram-negative bacilli, and about 30% of *H. influenzae* are

TABLE 170–8. PENICILLINS

Penicillin G–like drugs
Penicillin G*†
Penicillin G benzathine†
Penicillin G procaine†
Penicillin V*
Ampicillin-like drugs
Ampicillin*†
Ampicillin plus sulbactam†
Amoxicillin*
Amoxicillin plus clavulanate*
Penicillinase-resistant penicillins
Dicloxacillin*
Nafcillin*†
Oxacillin*†
Broad-spectrum (antipseudomonal) penicillins
Carbenicillin*
Piperacillin†
Piperacillin plus tazobactam†
Ticarcillin†
Ticarcillin plus clavulanate†

*Oral.

†Parenteral.

resistant. Penicillin G is the drug of choice for syphilis and, in combination with gentamicin, for endocarditis due to susceptible enterococci.

Amoxicillin and ampicillin are more active against enterococci and certain gram-negative bacilli, such as non-β-lactamase–producing *H. influenzae, E. coli,* and *P. mirabilis*; *Salmonella*; and *Shigella*. The addition of a β-lactamase inhibitor allows use against methicillin-sensitive staphylococci, *H. influenzae, N. gonorrhoeae, Moraxella catarrhalis, Bacteroides, E. coli,* and *K. pneumoniae*. Ampicillin is indicated primarily for infections typically caused by sensitive gram-negative organisms (eg, UTI, meningococcal meningitis, biliary sepsis, respiratory infections, *Listeria* meningitis, enterococcal infections, some typhoid fever and typhoid carriers).

The penicillinase-resistant penicillins are used primarily for penicillinase-producing *S. aureus*. These drugs also treat some *S. pneumoniae*, group A streptococci, and coagulase-negative staphylococcal infections.

The broad-spectrum (antipseudomonal) penicillins have activity similar to ampicillin but are also active against some strains of *Enterobacter* and *Serratia* and many strains of *P. aeruginosa*. Ticarcillin is less active against enterococci than piperacillin. The addition of a β-lactamase inhibitor enhances activity against β-lactamase–producing methicillin-sensitive *S. aureus, E. coli, K. pneumoniae, H. influenzae*, and gram-negative anaerobic bacilli, but not against gram-negative bacilli that produce ampC β-lactamase. The broad-spectrum penicillins exhibit synergy with aminoglycosides, with which they are usually combined for *P. aeruginosa* infections.

Toxicity: Most adverse effects are hypersensitivity reactions. Immediate reactions, including anaphylaxis (which can cause death within minutes), urticaria, and angioneurotic edema, occur in 1 to 5/10,000 injections, and fatalities occur in about 0.3/10,000 injections. Delayed reactions (occurring in up to 8% of patients) include serum sickness, rashes (eg, macular, papular, morbilliform), and exfoliative dermatitis, which usually appears after 7 to 10 days of therapy. Most patients who report an allergic reaction to penicillin do not react to subsequent exposure to penicillin. Although small, the risk of an allergic reaction is about 10-fold higher for those who have had a previous allergic reaction. Many patients report adverse reactions to penicillin that are not truly allergic (eg, GI adverse effects, nonspecific symptoms). Patients with mild or vague reactions may undergo skin tests (see p. 1362). However, patients with serious reactions *should not be given any β-lactam again* (including skin testing), except with special precautions and desensitization regimens in rare circumstances when no substitute can be found.

Rashes occur more often with ampicillin and amoxicillin than with other penicillins. Patients with infectious mononucleosis often develop a nonallergic rash, typically maculopapular, usually beginning between days 4 and 7 of treatment.

CNS toxicity (eg, seizures) may occur with high penicillin doses, especially with renal insufficiency. All penicillins can cause nephritis, *C. difficile* colitis (pseudomembranous), Coombs'-positive hemolytic anemia, leukopenia, and thrombocytopenia. Leukopenia seems to occur most often with nafcillin. Although any penicillin used in very high IV doses can interfere with platelet function and cause bleeding, ticarcillin is the most common cause, especially in patients with renal insufficiency.

Other reactions include pain at the IM injection site, thrombophlebitis when the same site is used repeatedly for IV injection, and GI disturbances with oral preparations. Black tongue, due to irritation of the glossal surface and keratinization of the superficial layers, may occur more often with oral preparations. Ticarcillin may cause Na overload when used in large doses, owing to ticarcillin being a disodium salt. Ticarcillin also can cause hypokalemic metabolic alkalosis, owing to the large amount of nonabsorbable anion presented to the distal tubules, which alter H^+ ion excretion and secondarily results in K^+ loss.

OTHER β-LACTAMS

The carbapenems (imipenem, meropenem, ertapenem) are parenteral bactericidal drugs that have an extremely broad spectrum. *H. influenzae*, anaerobes, and most Enterobacteriaceae (including those that produce ampC β-lactamase and ESBL) are susceptible, although *P. mirabilis* tends to have higher imipenem MICs. *Enterococcus faecalis* and many *P. aeruginosa* strains, including those resistant to broad-spectrum penicillins and cephalosporins, are susceptible to imipenem and meropenem but are resistant to ertapenem. Carbapenems are active against methicillin-sensitive staphylococci and streptococci, including *S. pneumoniae* (except possibly strains with reduced penicillin sensitivity). Carbapenems are active synergistically with aminoglycosides against *P. aeruginosa.* Penicillin-resistant *Enterococcus faecium* and methicillin-resistant staphylococci are resistant.

Many multidrug-resistant hospital-acquired pathogens are sensitive only to carbapenems. However, expanded use of carbapenems has resulted in some carbapenem resistance.

Imipenem and meropenem penetrate into CSF with inflamed meninges. Meropenem is used for gram-negative bacillary meningitis; imipenem is not used in meningitis because it may cause seizures. Most seizures occur in patients with CNS pathology or renal insufficiency who have received inappropriately high doses.

Aztreonam is a parenteral bactericidal antibiotic as active as ceftazidime against Enterobacteriaceae that do not express ampC β-lactamase or produce an ESBL, and against *P. aeruginosa.* Aztreonam is not active against anaerobes. Unlike cephalosporins, gram-positive organisms are resistant. Aztreonam acts synergistically with aminoglycosides. Because the metabolic products of aztreonam differ from those of other β-lactams, cross-hypersensitivity is unlikely. Thus the main use of aztreonam is severe aerobic gram-negative bacillary infections, including meningitis, in patients with serious β-lactam allergy who nevertheless require β-lactam therapy. Additional antibiotics are added to cover any suspected gram-positive cocci and anaerobes. The dose is reduced in renal failure.

CHLORAMPHENICOL

Chloramphenicol is primarily bacteriostatic. It binds to the 50S subunit of the ribosome, thereby inhibiting bacterial protein synthesis.

Pharmacology: Chloramphenicol is well absorbed orally. Parenteral therapy should be IV. It is distributed widely in body fluids, including CSF, and is excreted in urine. Because of hepatic metabolism, active chloramphenicol does not accumulate with renal insufficiency.

Indications: Chloramphenicol has a wide spectrum of activity against gram-positive and gram-negative cocci and bacilli (including anaerobes), *Rickettsia, Mycoplasma,* and *Chlamydia* and *Chlamydophila.* Because of bone marrow toxicity, the availability of alternative antibiotics, and the emergence of resistance, chloramphenicol is no longer a drug of choice for any infection, except serious infections due to a few multidrug-resistant pathogens that retain susceptibility to this antibiotic. However, outcomes of chloramphenicol treatment of meningitis caused by relatively penicillin-resistant pneumococci have been discouraging.

Toxicity: Chloramphenicol can cause 2 types of bone marrow depression: a reversible dose-related interference with iron metabolism and an irreversible idiosyncratic form of aplastic anemia. The reversible form is most likely with high doses or prolonged treatment and in patients with severe liver disease. Serum iron and saturation of serum iron-binding capacity increase; reticulocytes decrease; and vacuolization of RBC precursors, anemia, leukopenia, and thrombocytopenia develop. Irreversible idiosyncratic aplastic anemia occurs in < 1/25,000 patients. Onset may be delayed until after therapy is stopped. Chloramphenicol should not be used topically because small amounts may be absorbed and, rarely, can cause aplastic anemia.

Hypersensitivity reactions are uncommon. Optic and peripheral neuritis may occur with prolonged use. Nausea, vomiting, and diarrhea may occur.

The neonatal gray baby syndrome, which involves circulatory collapse, is often fatal. The cause is high blood levels resulting from inability of the immature liver to metabolize chloramphenicol. To avoid the syndrome, infants ≤1 mo are not given > 25 mg/kg/day initially and doses are adjusted to serum levels.

DAPTOMYCIN

Daptomycin is a cyclic lipopeptide antibiotic that has a unique mechanism of action. It binds to the bacterial cell membranes, which causes rapid depolarization of the membrane due to K efflux and associated disruption of DNA, RNA, and protein synthesis resulting in rapid concentration-dependent bacterial death. Daptomycin has broad-spectrum activity against gram-positive bacteria. Cross-resistance with other classes of antimicrobials does not occur; thus, daptomycin retains activity against multidrug-resistant pathogens, such as vancomycin- and methicillin-resistant *Staphylococcus aureus,* vancomycin-resistant enterococci, and pneumococci with reduced penicillin sensitivity.

Daptomycin is inferior to ceftriaxone for pneumonia. Daptomycin is parenterally administered once/day. Over 90% is bound to serum protein. Dosing is altered for renal failure. Because daptomycin can cause reversible skeletal myopathy (although unusual with once/day dosing), patients should be monitored for muscle pain or weakness, and serum creatine phosphokinase levels should be checked weekly.

FLUOROQUINOLONES

The fluoroquinolones (see TABLE 170–9) exhibit concentration-dependent bactericidal activity by inhibiting the activity of DNA gyrase and topoisomerase, enzymes essential for bacterial DNA replication. The fluoroquinolones are divided into 2 groups, based on antimicrobial spectrum and pharmacology: the older group includes ciprofloxacin, norfloxacin, and ofloxacin, and the newer group, gatifloxacin, gemifloxacin, levofloxacin, moxifloxacin, and trovafloxacin.

Pharmacology: Ciprofloxacin, gatifloxacin, levofloxacin, moxifloxacin, ofloxacin, and trovafloxacin can be administered orally and parenterally; gemifloxacin and norfloxacin are available only orally. Several fluoroquinolones are also available as otic and ophthalmic preparations. Oral absorption is diminished by coadministration of cations (aluminum, Mg, Ca, zinc, and iron preparations). After oral and parenteral administration, fluoroquinolones are widely distributed in most extracellular and intracellular fluids and are concentrated in prostate, lung, and bile. Most are metabolized in the liver and excreted in urine, reaching high levels in urine. Moxifloxacin is primarily eliminated in bile. Dosing reduction is required in renal insufficiency, except for moxifloxacin. Older fluoroquinolones are normally given twice/day; newer ones and an extended-release form of ciprofloxacin are given once/day.

Indications: The fluoroquinolones are active against *Neisseria, Haemophilus influenzae, Moraxella catarrhalis, Mycoplasma, Chlamydia* and *Chlamydophila, Legionella,* Enterobacteriaceae, and, particularly ciprofloxacin, *Pseudomonas aeruginosa.* The fluoroquinolones are also active against *Mycobacterium tuberculosis,* some atypical mycobacteria, and methicillin-sensitive staphylococci, but nosocomial methicillin-resistant staphylococci are usually resistant.

TABLE 170–9. FLUOROQUINOLONES

Ciprofloxacin	Moxifloxacin
Gatifloxacin	Norfloxacin
Gemifloxacin	Ofloxacin
Levofloxacin	Trovafloxacin

The older fluoroquinolones have poor activity against streptococci and anaerobes. Newer fluoroquinolones have reliable activity against streptococci (including *Streptococcus pneumoniae* with reduced penicillin-sensitivity) and some anaerobes. As use has increased, resistance is developing among Enterobacteriaceae, *P. aeruginosa, S. pneumoniae,* and *Neisseria,* particularly among older fluoroquinolones.

Fluoroquinolones (except moxifloxacin) are the empiric drugs of choice for UTIs where *Escherichia coli* resistance to trimethoprim-sulfamethoxazole is > 15%. They are effective in bacterial prostatitis, *Salmonella* bacteremia, and usually typhoid fever. Fluoroquinolones have excellent activity against most bacterial causes of infectious diarrhea (*Salmonella* sp, *Campylobacter* sp, *Shigella* sp, *Vibrio* sp, and *Yersinia enterocolitica*), except that caused by *Clostridium difficile.* A 3-day course of ofloxacin is effective for chancroid, and a 7-day course of ofloxacin is recommended for infections caused by *Chlamydia trachomatis*. The newer fluoroquinolones are used often for community-acquired pneumonia; however, another regimen should be used for patients with recent fluoroquinolone use. The newer fluoroquinolones (and azithromycin) are drugs of choice for *Legionella* pneumonia. Ciprofloxacin, because of its superior activity against *P. aeruginosa*, is used empirically for hospital-acquired pneumonia, usually with another antipseudomonal drug. Ciprofloxacin is used for long-term oral treatment of gram-negative bacillary or *Staphylococcus aureus* osteomyelitis and for meningococcal prophylaxis and was used extensively for anthrax prophylaxis in the 2001 bioterrorism event in the US.

Toxicity: Serious adverse reactions are uncommon. About 5% of patients experience upper GI adverse effects due to direct GI irritation and CNS effects. Diarrhea, leukopenia, anemia, and photosensitivity are uncommon. Rash is uncommon except if gemifloxacin is used for > 1 wk, especially in women < 40 yr of age. Fluoroquinolones predispose to tendinopathy, including rupture of the Achilles tendon, even after short-term use. Nephrotoxicity is rare. CNS effects occur in < 5%, including mild headache, drowsiness, insomnia, dizziness, and mood alteration. Trovafloxacin has the highest rate of CNS adverse events, most often dizziness, lightheadness, or vertigo. Seizures are rare, but these drugs should be avoided in patients with CNS disorders. NSAIDs may enhance the CNS stimulatory effects of the fluoroquinolones. Fluoroquinolones are contraindicated in children and may cause cartilage lesions if growth plates are open. The safety of fluoroquinolones in pregnancy has not been established. Ciprofloxacin raises theophylline levels, which may result in theophylline-related adverse effects. Fluoroquinolones can prolong the QT interval, potentially leading to ventricular arrhythmias and sudden cardiac death. The risk of arrhythmias may be reduced by avoiding their use in patients with known QT interval prolongation; in those with uncorrected hypokalemia, hypomagnesemia, or significant bradycardia; and in those receiving concomitant therapy with agents known to increase the QT interval or to cause bradycardia (metoclopramide, cisapride, erythromycin, clarithromycin, classes Ia and III antiarrhythmics, and tricyclic antidepressants). In rare cases, trovafloxacin causes severe hepatotoxicity, especially if it is used for > 2 wk; thus, trovafloxacin is rarely used.

LINCOSAMIDES, OXAZOLIDINONES, AND STREPTOGRAMINS

Lincosamides (clindamycin), oxazolidinones (linezolid), streptogramins (dalfopristin, or streptogramin a, and quinupristin, or streptogramin b) are grouped together because of a similar mode of antibacterial action and similar antibacterial spectra. The macrolides (see p. 1433) and the ketolide telithromycin (see p. 1434) may be included with this group for similar reasons. All inhibit protein synthesis by binding to the 50S ribosomal subunit. Cross-resistance occurs among the macrolides, clindamycin, quinupristin, and telithromycin (to some extent) because these drugs bind to the same target. However, cross-resistance does not occur between these antibiotics and dalfopristin and linezolid, which bind to different targets.

Lincosamides

Clindamycin is primarily bacteriostatic by binding to the 50S subunit of the ribosome, thus inhibiting bacterial protein synthesis.

Pharmacology: Clindamycin is absorbed well orally and can be given parenterally. Clindamycin diffuses well into body fluids except CSF; it is concentrated in phagocytes. Most of the drug is metabolized; metabolites are excreted in bile and urine. Dose adjustments are not required for renal failure. Clindamycin is administered q 6 to 8 h.

Indications: The spectrum of activity for clindamycin is similar to that of erythromycin except that clindamycin is effective for anaerobic infections (particularly *Bacteroides* sp, including *Bacteroides fragilis*) and macrolide-resistant, clindamycin-susceptible *Streptococcus pneumoniae* and is not reliably active against *Mycoplasma, Chlamydia* and *Chlamydophila*, and *Legionella*. Aerobic gram-negative bacilli and enterococci are resistant.

Clindamycin usually is used for anaerobes. Because anaerobic infections often also involve aerobic gram-negative bacilli, additional antibiotics are also used. Clindamycin is part of combination therapy for infections caused by toxigenic streptococci because it decreases the organism's toxin production, cerebral toxoplasmosis, babesiosis, falciparum malaria, and *Pneumocystis jiroveci* (formerly *P. carinii*) pneumonia. Clindamycin cannot be used for CNS infection (other than cerebral toxoplasmosis) because penetration into the brain and CSF is poor. Topical clindamycin is used for acne.

Toxicity: Clindamycin causes *Clostridium difficile* (pseudomembranous) colitis in up to 10% of patients regardless of route, including topical. Hypersensitivity reactions may occur. Clindamycin may cause esophagitis if not swallowed with water.

Oxazolidinones

Linezolid, in addition to activity against streptococci, enterococci (both *Enterococcus faecalis* and *E. faecium*), and staphylococci, including those strains resistant to other classes of antibiotics, is active against mycobacteria and anaerobes, such as *Fusobacterium* sp, *Prevotella* sp, *Porphyromonas* sp, *Bacteroides* sp, and peptostreptococci. Adverse effects are minimal, although reversible myelosuppression, including thrombocytopenia, leukopenia, and anemia, occurs in about 3% of patients, generally when therapy is > 2 wk. Consequently, CBCs are monitored weekly, especially when the duration of therapy is > 2 wk. Peripheral neuropathy may occur with prolonged use. Linezolid also may interact with serotonergic drugs, such as SSRIs, to produce serotonin syndrome (fever, flushing, sweating, tremors, and delirium).

Streptogramins

Quinupristin/dalfopristin (Q/D) is a fixed 30/70 combination of 2 semisynthetic derivatives of pristinamycin, a naturally occurring streptogramin. Q/D is synergistically bactericidal for streptococci and staphylococci, including strains resistant to other antibiotic classes. Q/D inhibits *E. faecium*, including vancomycin-resistant strains. *E. faecalis* is resistant. Q/D is active against some gram-negative anaerobic bacilli, *Clostridium perfringens, Peptostreptococcus* sp, and atypical respiratory pathogens (*Mycoplasma pneumoniae, Chlamydophila pneumoniae,* and *Legionella pneumophila*).

Q/D is given via a central IV catheter because phlebitis frequently occurs when administered via a peripheral vein. Up to 30% of patients develop significant myalgias. Dosage reduction is not required for renal insufficiency. The dose is reduced in patients with severe hepatic insufficiency. Q/D may inhibit drugs that are metabolized by the cytochrome P450 CYP 3A4 isoenzyme system.

MACROLIDES

The macrolides (see TABLE 170–10) are primarily bacteriostatic; by binding to the 50S subunit of the ribosome, they inhibit bacterial protein synthesis.

Pharmacology: Azithromycin, clarithromycin, dirithromycin, and erythromycin are relatively poorly absorbed orally. Azithromycin and erythromycin can also be given parenterally. Dirithromycin is a pro-drug that is converted during intestinal absorption. Food increases absorption of dirithromycin and the extended-release formulation of clarithromycin, does not affect that of clarithromycin, and decreases that of azithromycin capsules and erythromycin (including the base and stearate) preparations. All macrolides diffuse well into body fluids except CSF and are concentrated in phagocytes. Excretion is mainly in bile. No dosage adjustment is required for azithromycin and dirithromycin in patients with renal insufficiency.

TABLE 170–10. MACROLIDES

Azithromycin
Clarithromycin
Dirithromycin
Erythromycin
Telithromycin

Indications: These drugs are active against aerobic and anaerobic gram-positive cocci; however, most enterococci, many *Staphylococcus aureus* strains (especially methicillin-resistant), and some *Streptococcus pneumoniae* and *S. pyogenes* strains are resistant. Macrolides also are active against *Mycoplasma pneumoniae, Chlamydia trachomatis, Chlamydophila pneumoniae, Legionella* sp, *Corynebacterium diphtheriae, Campylobacter, Treponema pallidum, Propionibacterium acnes*, and *Borrelia burgdorferi. Bacteroides fragilis* are resistant. Clarithromycin and azithromycin have enhanced activity against *Haemophilus influenzae* and activity against *Mycobacterium avium* complex.

Macrolides have been considered the drug of choice in group A streptococcal and pneumococcal infections when penicillin cannot be used. However, pneumococci with reduced penicillin sensitivity are often resistant to macrolides. Erythromycin is used for uncomplicated skin infections. Macrolides are the drugs of choice in infection due to *M. pneumoniae, Legionella*, or *Bordetella pertussis* and in *C. diphtheriae* carriers. Because of their activity against atypical respiratory pathogens, they are often used empirically for lower respiratory tract infections, but another drug is often necessary to cover macrolide-resistant pneumococci. Macrolides are used for symptomatic cat-scratch disease (*Bartonella henselae*) and bacillary angiomatosis and peliosis hepatis in patients with AIDS (*B. henselae* and *B. quintana*). Azithromycin also is used with other drugs for cerebral toxoplasmosis and babesiosis. Oral erythromycin has been used with an oral aminoglycoside for bowel preparation before GI tract surgery. Clarithromycin and azithromycin are essential in multidrug regimens for *M. avium* complex. Azithromycin is also used for *C. trachomatis* urethritis and cervicitis. Topical erythromycin is used for acne. Macrolides are not used for meningitis.

Toxicity: Erythromycin commonly causes dose-related GI disturbances, including nausea, vomiting, abdominal cramps, and diarrhea; disturbances are less common with clarithromycin and azithromycin. Erythromycin may cause dose-related tinnitus, dizziness, and reversible hearing loss. Cholestatic jaundice occurs most commonly with erythromycin estolate. Jaundice usually appears after 10 days of administration, primarily in adults, but can occur earlier if the drug has been given previously. Erythromycin is not given IM because of severe pain; it may cause phlebitis or pain when used IV. Hypersensitivity reactions are rare.

Erythromycin has numerous drug interactions because it inhibits hepatic metabolism through the cytochrome P-450 system. Erythromycin causes QT interval prolongation and predisposes to ventricular tachyarrhythmia, especially in women and in patients with known prolongation of QT interval or electrolyte abnormalities or those taking an additional drug that may lengthen the QT interval. Erythromycin and clarithromycin can further elevate the PT/INR when taken with warfarin; they can cause rhabdomyolysis with lovastatin and simvastatin; somnolence with midazolam and triazolam; nausea, vomiting, and seizures with theophylline; and elevated serum levels of tacrolimus, cyclosporine, and ergot alkaloids. Azithromycin has the least tendency to cause drug interactions.

Telithromycin

Telithromycin is a ketolide antibiotic. Ketolides are chemically related to macrolides and inhibit bacterial ribosomal protein synthesis without inducing macrolide, clindamycin, or streptogramin resistance. Telithromycin is active against erythromycin-susceptible staphylococci and streptococci and multidrug-resistant *S. pneumoniae*. Telithromycin is also active against erythromycin-susceptible enterococci, *B. pertussis, H. influenzae, Helicobacter pylori, Moraxella catarrhalis, M. pneumoniae, C. pneumoniae, Legionella* sp, *Prevotella* sp, and *Peptostreptococcus* sp. Telithromycin is rapidly absorbed orally with or without food and most is metabolized in the liver. Telithromycin is used in adults to treat community-acquired pneumonia, acute bacterial sinusitis, and acute bacterial exacerbation of COPD.

Diarrhea, nausea, vomiting, and dizziness are the most common adverse effects. Prolongation of the QT interval, exacerbation of myasthenia gravis, hyperbilirubinemia, elevation of liver enzymes, and visual disturbances are less common. Cross-sensitivity with macrolides can occur. Telithromycin inhibits cytochrome P3A4, increasing levels of digoxin, ergot alkaloids, benzodiazepines, metoprolol, statins, cisapride, pimozide, sirolimus, and tacrolimus. Cytochrome P3A4 inducers such as rifampin, phenytoin, carbamazepine, and phenobarbital decrease levels of telithromycin; the P3A4 inhibitors itraconazole and ketoconazole increase levels of telithromycin. Telithromycin decreases absorption of sotalol.

METRONIDAZOLE

Metronidazole is bactericidal and is used primarily against anaerobes and certain protozoans.

Pharmacology: Oral metronidazole is absorbed well. IV use is generally needed only for patients who cannot be treated orally. It is distributed widely in body fluids and penetrates into CSF in high concentrations. Metronidazole is metabolized presumably in the liver and excreted mainly in urine, but elimination is not decreased in patients with renal insufficiency. Doses are usually decreased 50% in patients with significant liver disease.

Indications: Metronidazole is active against all obligate anaerobic bacteria and certain protozoan parasites (eg, *Trichomonas vaginalis, Entamoeba histolytica, Giardia lamblia*).

Metronidazole is used primarily for infections caused by obligate anaerobes (eg, intra-abdominal, pelvic, soft-tissue, periodontal, and odontogenic infections, and lung abscess), often with other antimicrobials. Metronidazole is the drug of choice for bacterial vaginosis. It has been used in Crohn's disease. It is effective in meningitis, brain abscess, endocarditis, and septicemia. Metronidazole has also been used for prophylaxis after intestinal surgery. It is effective for *Clostridium difficile* colitis when given orally or, in patients unable to take oral medication, IV. Metronidazole, in combination with other drugs, is effective for peptic ulcers due to *Helicobacter pylori* and prevents relapses. Metronidazole has been used topically and orally to treat acne rosacea.

Toxicity: Nausea, vomiting, headache, seizures, syncope, other CNS reactions, and peripheral neuropathy can occur; rash, fever, and reversible neutropenia have been reported. It can cause a metallic taste and dark urine. A disulfiram-like reaction may occur if alcohol is ingested within 7 days of use. Metronidazole inhibits metabolism of warfarin and may increase its anticoagulant effect. Although metronidazole is in the FDA category B (meaning the drug is unlikely to be harmful to the fetus), metronidazole should be avoided during the 1st trimester of pregnancy because of concerns about its mutagenicity.

MUPIROCIN

Mupirocin inhibits bacterial RNA and protein synthesis. It is available only as a 2% topical preparation, which is bactericidal against staphylococci and β-hemolytic streptococci. Systemic absorption of topical mupirocin is negligible.

Mupirocin is used for impetigo and for superficial minor secondarily infected skin lesions. Mupirocin can also eradicate *Staphylococcus aureus* nasal carriage, although relapse rates may be high. Chronic therapy leads to mupirocin-resistant staphylococci.

Mupirocin is nontoxic but may cause itching and burning when applied to denuded skin or mucous membranes.

NITROFURANTOIN

Nitrofurantoin is bactericidal; the exact mechanism is unknown.

Pharmacology: Nitrofurantoin is available only as an oral preparation. It is absorbed well and excreted in urine. Adverse effects limit doses so therapeutic levels are achieved only in the urine.

Indications: It is used only for the treatment or prophylaxis of uncomplicated UTI. In women with recurrent UTIs, it may decrease the number of episodes. It is active against common uropathogens, such as *Escherichia coli, Staphylococcus saprophyticus,* and *Enterococcus faecalis*. *E. faecium*, including vancomycin-resistant strains, *Klebsiella*, and *Enterobacter* sp are less susceptible. Most strains of *Proteus, Providencia, Morganella, Serratia, Acinetobacter,* and *Pseudomonas* are resistant. There is no cross-resistance with other antibiotic classes.

Toxicity: Nitrofurantoin is contraindicated in renal insufficiency. Common adverse reactions are nausea and vomiting, which are less likely with the macrocrystalline form. Fever, rash, hypersensitivity pneumonitis, and progressive pulmonary interstitial fibrosis may occur. Paresthesias may result and may be followed by a severe ascending motor and sensory polyneuropathy if the drug is continued, especially in patients with renal failure. Leukopenia and hepatotoxicity have been reported, and hemolytic anemia can occur in patients with G6PD deficiency.

POLYPEPTIDES

Bacitracin is a polypeptide antibiotic that inhibits cell wall synthesis and is active against gram-positive organisms.

Colistin (polymyxin E) and polymyxin B are cationic polypeptide antibiotics that disrupt bacterial cell membranes and are bactericidal against gram-negative aerobic bacilli, including *Pseudomonas aeruginosa* and *Acinetobacter* (see TABLE 170–11). They are not active against gram-positive organisms or *Proteus* sp.

Indications: Polypeptides are generally used topically; systemic absorption is negligible. An ointment containing bacitracin with neomycin or polymyxin B, or both, is available, but clinical efficacy is not confirmed. Topical bacitracin is less efficacious than other treatments for eradication of *Staphylococcus aureus* nasal carriage and impetigo. Bacitracin has been used orally for *Clostridium difficile* colitis but is less effective and less palatable than oral vancomycin or metronidazole. Colistin is available as an otic suspension for otitis externa, which is commonly due to *P. aeruginosa*, and polymyxin B is available in ophthalmic ointments and solutions with other antimicrobials (eg, bacitracin, neomycin, trimethoprim-sulfamethoxazole) and corticosteroids, and as a GU irrigant. Aerosolized colistin is sometimes used in patients with cystic fibrosis and occasionally for hospital-acquired

TABLE 170–11. POLYPEPTIDES

Bacitracin
Colistin
Polymyxin B

pneumonia caused by multidrug-resistant gram-negative bacilli.

Colistin methane sulfonate (colistimethate sodium) is used IM or IV (dose reduced in renal insufficiency) for patients with severe infections due to multidrug-resistant gram-negative bacilli such as *P. aeruginosa* or *Acinetobacter*.

Toxicity: The polymyxins are nephrotoxic. Circumoral and extremity paresthesias, generalized pruritus, vertigo, slurred speech, and muscle weakness and respiratory difficulty due to neuromuscular blockade have been reported with parenteral colistin, especially in patients with renal insufficiency. Concomitant use of other drugs that block neuromuscular transmission or are nephrotoxic (eg, aminoglycosides or curare-like drugs) should be avoided.

RIFAMYCINS

Rifampin and rifabutin are bactericidal and inhibit bacterial DNA-dependent RNA polymerase, suppressing RNA synthesis. Rifampin and rifabutin have similar pharmacology, antimicrobial spectra, and adverse events.

Pharmacology: Oral absorption is good, producing wide distribution in body tissues and fluids, including CSF. Rifampin is concentrated in polymorphonuclear granulocytes and macrophages, facilitating superior clearance of bacteria from abscesses. It is metabolized in the liver and eliminated in bile and, to a much lesser extent, in urine; dose adjustments are unnecessary with renal insufficiency.

Indications: Rifampin is active against most gram-positive and some gram-negative organisms and *Mycobacterium* sp. Resistance develops rapidly, so rifampin is rarely used alone. Rifampin is used with other antimicrobials for TB (see p. 1512), atypical mycobacterial infection, leprosy, staphylococcal prosthetic valve endocarditis, staphylococcal infections involving foreign bodies (eg, prosthetic joint), staphylococcal osteomyelitis, *Legionella* infections, and pneumococcal meningitis. Rifampin can be used alone for prophylaxis of close contacts of patients with meningococcal or *Haemophilus influenzae* type b meningitis.

Rifabutin is more active than rifampin against *Mycobacterium avium* complex and is used preferentially in multidrug regimens for these infections.

Toxicity: The most serious adverse effect is hepatitis, which occurs much more often when isoniazid or pyrazinamide is used with rifampin. Rifampin may cause a transient rise during the 1st week of therapy in unconjugated serum bilirubin, which results from competition between rifampin and bilirubin for excretion. Rifampin may also increase risk of hepatotoxicity from concurrently administered isoniazide or pyrazinamide. Patients with liver disease should be given rifampin cautiously and should have liver function tests monitored prior to rifampin therapy and q 2 to 4 wk during therapy, or should be given an alternate drug.

Less serious adverse effects are common, including heartburn, nausea, vomiting, and diarrhea. CNS effects, such as headache, drowsiness, ataxia, and confusion, have been reported. Rash, fever, thrombocytopenia, leukopenia, hemolytic anemia, and renal insufficiency have occurred, probably involving a hypersensitivity mechanism. Rifampin colors urine, saliva, sweat, sputum, and tears red-orange.

Rifampin has many drug interactions because it is a potent inducer of hepatic P-450 microsomal enzymes. Rifampin is known to accelerate elimination and thereby may decrease the effectiveness of the following drugs: phenytoin, barbiturates, quinidine, tocainide, warfarin, itraconazole, fluconazole, ketoconozole, voriconazole, β-blockers, Ca channel blockers, ACE inhibitors, atovaquone, chloramphenicol, clarithromycin, dapsone, doxycycline, tricyclic antidepressants, corticosteroids, cyclosporine, tacrolimus, oral and systemic hormone contraceptives, haloperidol, sulfonylureas, theophylline, thyroxine, digoxin, opioid analgesics, protease inhibitors, and zidovudine. To maintain optimum therapeutic effect, adjustment of dosage of these drugs may be necessary when starting or stopping concomitantly administered rifampin.

RIFAXIMIN

Rifaximin is a derivative of rifamycin that is poorly absorbed after oral administration, 97% being recovered primarily unchanged in the feces. Rifaximin can be used for the empiric treatment of traveler's diarrhea, which is primarily caused by enterotoxigenic and enteraggregative *E. coli.* Rifaximin is not known to be effective for diarrhea due to enteric pathogens other than *E. coli*. The dose is 200 mg q 8 h for 3 days in adults and children older than 12 yr. Adverse reactions include nausea, vomiting, abdominal pain, and flatulence. Like rifampin, rifaximin has the propensity to lead to emergence of rifampin-resistant mutants.

SULFONAMIDES

The sulfonamides (see TABLE 170–12) are synthetic bacteriostatic antimicrobials that competitively inhibit conversion of *p*-aminobenzoic acid to dihydropteroate, which bacteria need for folic acid synthesis and ultimately purine and DNA synthesis. Humans do not synthesize folic acid but acquire it in their diet, so their DNA synthesis is less affected. Two sulfonamides, sulfisoxazole and sulfamethizole, are available as single agents for oral administration. Sulfamethoxazole in combination with trimethoprim (TMP-SMX) is discussed below. Sulfadoxine plus pyrimethamine is available (but not in the US) as an oral, fixed combination for malaria due to chloroquine-resistant *Plasmodium falciparum*. Sulfacetamide is available as ophthalmic preparations. Silver sulfadiazine and mafenide acetate are available as topical preparations. Sulfanilamide is available as a vaginal preparation.

Pharmacology: The sulfonamides are readily absorbed orally and after topical application to burns. Sulfonamides are distributed throughout the body. They are metabolized mainly by the liver and excreted by the kidneys. Use in pregnancy results in high fetal levels.

Indications: Sulfonamides have a wide spectrum against gram-positive and many gram-negative bacteria and *Plasmodium* and *Toxoplasma*. However, resistance is widespread, and resistance to one sulfonamide indicates resistance to all.

Sulfasalazine can be used orally for inflammatory bowel disease. Sulfonamides are most commonly used with other drugs, eg, in nocardiosis, UTI, and chloroquine-resistant *P. falciparum* malaria.

Several sulfonamides are available for topical use: silver sulfadiazine and mafenide acetate for burns, vaginal cream and suppositories with sulfanilamide for vaginitis, and ophthalmic sulfacetamide for superficial ocular infections.

Toxicity: Adverse effects can result from oral and sometimes topical sulfonamides; effects include hypersensitivity reactions, such as rashes, Stevens-Johnson syndrome (see p. 976), vasculitis, serum sickness, drug fever, anaphylaxis, and angioedema; crystalluria, oliguria, and anuria; gastroenteritis; hematologic reactions, such as agranulocytosis, thrombocytopenia, kernicterus in the neonate (they compete for bilirubin-binding sites on albumin, increasing fetal blood levels of unconjugated bilirubin and increasing risk for kernicterus), and hemolytic anemia in patients with G6PD deficiency; photosensitivity; and neurologic effects, such as peripheral neuritis, insomnia, and headache. Pregnant women near term and neonates should not be given sulfonamides.

TABLE 170–12. SULFONAMIDES

Sulfacetamide	Sulfamethoxazole
Sulfadiazine	Sulfanilamide
Sulfadoxine	Sulfasalazine
Sulfamethizole	Sulfisoxazole

To avoid crystalluria, patients are well hydrated (eg, to produce a urinary output of 1200 to 1500 mL/day). Sulfonamides can be used in renal insufficiency, but peak plasma levels should be measured (< 120 μg/mL). Patients with inflammatory bowel disease who use sulfasalazine may develop folic acid deficiency, which may be due in part to drug-induced decreased intestinal absorption of this nutrient, to the disease itself, and to poor dietary intake.

Other effects include hypothyroidism, hepatitis, potentiation of sulfonylureas with consequent hypoglycemia, potentiation of phenytoin adverse effects, and potentiation of coumarin anticoagulants. Activation of quiescent SLE has been reported. The incidence of adverse effects is different for the various sulfonamides, but cross-sensitivity is common. Mafenide may cause metabolic acidosis due to carbonic anhydrase inhibition.

TRIMETHOPRIM AND SULFAMETHOXAZOLE

Trimethoprim is available as a single agent or combined with sulfamethoxazole; trimethoprim-sulfamethoxazole (TMP-SMX) is a fixed combination of the 2 drugs consisting of a 1:5 ratio (80 mg TMP plus 400 mg SMX or a double-strength tablet of 160 mg TMP plus 800 mg SMX). The drugs act synergistically to block sequential steps in bacterial folic acid metabolism. TMP prevents reduction of dihydrofolate to tetrahydrofolate, and SMX inhibits conversion of *p*-aminobenzoic acid to dihydropteroate. This synergy gives maximal antibacterial activity, which is often bactericidal.

Pharmacology: Both drugs are well absorbed orally and are excreted in the urine. They have a serum half-life of about 11 h in plasma and penetrate well into tissues and body fluids, including the CSF. TMP is concentrated in prostatic tissue.

Indications: TMP and TMP-SMX are active against a broad spectrum of gram-positive organisms (including some methicillin-resistant *Staphylococcus aureus*) and gram-negative organisms but are inactive against anaerobes, *Treponema pallidum, Mycobacterium tuberculosis, Mycoplasma,* and *Pseudomonas aeruginosa*. Enterococci and many Enterobacteriaceae and *Streptococcus pneumoniae* are resistant. TMP/SMX is not clinically effective for group A streptococcal pharyngitis.

TMP or TMP-SMX may be one of the few drugs efficacious for chronic bacterial prostatitis; however, cures occur only in a minority of patients even when given for 12 wk. TMP-SMX is as effective as fluoroquinolones in empiric short-course (3-day) therapy of uncomplicated cystitis in women if the frequency of TMP-SMX resistance is < 15%. TMP-SMX is effective in prophylaxis of recurrent UTI in women and children in low doses ($^1/_2$ to 1 double-strength tablet every night or every other night), or postcoital for women with a history of recurrences after sexual intercourse; TMP-SMX is the drug of choice for treatment of *Pneumocystis jiroveci* (formerly *P. carinii*) pneumonia and in prophylaxis of this infection in patients with AIDS or cancer. TMP-SMX is effective in intestinal infections due to various pathogens (eg, *Shigella* sp, *Vibrio* sp, *Escherichia coli*), but increasing prevalence of resistance limits usefulness. TMP-SMX is also used for *Nocardia* and *Listeria monocytogenes* infections, acute exacerbations of chronic bronchitis, and, in patients intolerant of vancomycin, methicillin-resistant *S. aureus* infections.

TMP alone is especially useful for chronic bacterial prostatitis and in prophylaxis and treatment of UTI in patients allergic to sulfonamides.

Toxicity: Most adverse reactions are the same as for sulfonamides. TMP causes identical adverse reactions to SMX but less commonly. When it does, nausea, vomiting, and rash occur most often. Folate deficiency (resulting in macrocytic anemia) can also occur. AIDS patients have a high incidence of adverse effects, especially fever, rash, and neutropenia. Use of folinic acid can prevent or treat macrocytic anemia, leukopenia, or thrombocytopenia that sometimes occurs with prolonged TMP-SMX use. TMP-SMX may cause hyperkalemia and a rise in serum creatinine in patients with pre-existing renal disease, and especially in diabetes mellitus. The drug may also produce an aseptic meningitis–like picture.

TMP-SMX may increase warfarin activity and levels of phenytoin, methotrexate, and rifampin in patients on concomitant therapy. SMX can increase the hypoglycemic effects sulfonylureas.

TETRACYCLINES

The tetracyclines (see TABLE 170–13) are bacteriostatic antibiotics that bind to the 30S subunit of the ribosome, thus inhibiting bacterial protein synthesis.

Pharmacology: About 60 to 80% of tetracycline and ≥ 90% of doxycycline and minocycline are absorbed after oral administration. Because absorption is decreased by metallic cations (eg, aluminum, Ca, Mg, and iron), tetracyclines cannot be taken with preparations containing these substances (eg, antacids, many vitamin and mineral supplements). Food decreases absorption of tetracycline but not of doxycycline or minocycline.

Tetracyclines penetrate into most body tissues and fluids. All are concentrated in unobstructed bile. However, CSF levels are not reliably therapeutic. Minocycline is the only tetracycline that penetrates into tears and saliva in levels sufficient to eradicate the meningococcal carrier state. Tetracycline and minocycline are excreted primarily in the urine, may exacerbate azotemia, and should be avoided in patients with renal insufficiency.

TABLE 170–13. TETRACYCLINES

Doxycycline
Minocycline
Tetracycline

In renal failure, doxycycline is primarily excreted in the intestinal tract and requires no dose reduction. Tetracyclines cross the placenta to accumulate in fetal bones and teeth and are excreted in milk.

Indications: Tetracyclines are effective in infections caused by rickettsiae, spirochetes (*Treponema pallidum, Borrelia burgdorferi*), *Helicobacter pylori, Vibrio* sp, *Yersinia pestis, Francisella tularensis, Brucella* sp, *Bacillus anthracis, Plasmodium vivax, Plasmodium falciparum, Mycoplasma*, and *Chlamydia* and *Chlamydophila*. About 5 to 10% of pneumococcal strains and substantial numbers of group A β-hemolytic streptococci, many gram-negative bacillary uropathogens, and penicillinase-producing gonococci are resistant.

Tetracyclines are interchangeable for most indications, although minocycline has been most studied for methicillin-resistant *Staphylococcus aureus* infections. Doxycycline is usually preferred because of its better tolerability and twice-daily administration for infections caused by rickettsiae, *Chlamydia* and *Chlamydophila, Mycoplasma*, and *Vibrio* sp; acute exacerbations of chronic bronchitis; Lyme disease; brucellosis; anthrax; plague; tularemia; granuloma inguinale; and syphilis. Doxycycline is used for prophylaxis of malaria caused by chloroquine-resistant *P. falciparum*. Minocycline is an alternate to rifampin for eradicating the meningococcal carrier state.

Toxicity: All orally administered tetracyclines produce nausea, vomiting, and diarrhea and can cause *Clostridium difficile* colitis and *Candida* superinfections. They can cause esophageal erosions if not swallowed with water. Tetracyclines can cause photosensitivity. They can cause staining of teeth, hypoplasia of dental enamel, and abnormal bone growth in children ≤ 8 yr and in fetuses. *Therefore, tetracyclines should be avoided after the 1st trimester of pregnancy, in mothers who are breastfeeding, and in children < 8 yr.* In infants, idiopathic intracranial hypertension and bulging fontanelles may occur.

Excessive blood levels from large doses or renal insufficiency may lead to fatal acute fatty degeneration of the liver, especially during pregnancy. Minocycline commonly causes vestibular dysfunction, particularly in women, limiting its use. Tetracyclines may decrease the efficacy of oral contraceptives and potentiate the effects of oral anticoagulants.

Older formulations of expired tetracycline pills can degenerate, causing Fanconi syndrome if ingested.

VANCOMYCIN

Vancomycin is a bactericidal antibiotic that inhibits cell wall synthesis.

Pharmacology: Vancomycin is not appreciably absorbed orally. Given parenterally, it penetrates into bile and pleural, pericardial, synovial, and ascitic fluids. However, penetration into even inflamed CSF is low and erratic, and doses used for meningitis must be higher than usual. Vancomycin is excreted unchanged by glomerular filtration, and dose reduction is required for renal insufficiency. In critically ill patients, serum levels should be measured after the 2nd or 3rd dose and kept between 10 μg/mL (trough levels) and 30 to 45 μg/mL (peak levels).

Indications: Vancomycin is active against most gram-positive cocci and bacilli, including almost all *S. aureus* and coagulase-negative staphylococcal strains that are resistant to penicillins and cephalosporins. Vancomycin is bacteriostatic against enterococci, but many strains of enterococcus and some strains of *S. aureus* are resistant.

Vancomycin is the drug of choice for serious infection and endocarditis caused by *S. aureus*, coagulase-negative staphylococci, *Streptococcus pneumoniae*, β-hemolytic streptococci, *Corynebacterium* group JK, viridans streptococci, or enterococci when β-lactams cannot be used because of drug allergy or resistance. However, vancomycin is less effective than antistaphylococcal β-lactams for *S. aureus* endocarditis. Vancomycin is combined with other antimicrobials when treating methicillin-resistant coagulase-negative staphylococcal prosthetic valve endocarditis, and enterococcal endocarditis. Vancomycin has also been used as an alternative agent for pneumococcal meningitis caused by strains with reduced penicillin sensitivity, although the erratic penetration of vancomycin into the CSF (especially during concomitant administration of dexamethasone) and reports of clinical failures make this a less than optimal agent when used alone for the treatment of pneumococcal meningitis.

Oral vancomycin for treatment of *Clostridium difficile* colitis is reserved for patients who fail to respond to metronidazole. Vancomycin is also used for prophylaxis of endocarditis in penicillin-allergic high-risk patients undergoing GU or GI procedures likely to result in bacteremia.

Toxicity: Hypersensitivity reactions (rash, fever, and reversible neutropenia and thrombocytopenia) may occur, especially when therapy lasts for > 2 wk. Nephrotoxicity is rare unless given with an aminoglycoside. Phlebitis occurs uncommonly during IV infusion. Infusion should be given over at least 60 min to avoid the red-person syndrome, a histamine-mediated reaction that can produce pruritus and flushing on the neck and shoulder area.

171 GRAM-POSITIVE COCCI

Many gram-positive cocci are commensal organisms that cause infection only when they find their way into normally sterile areas. They are the most common cause of skin infections and a frequent cause of pneumonia and septicemia. Although generally susceptible to a broad range of antibiotics, certain strains have developed resistance to every available antimicrobial agent.

PNEUMOCOCCAL INFECTIONS

Streptococcus pneumoniae **(pneumococcus) is a gram-positive, aerobic, encapsulated diplococcus. In the US, pneumococcal infection annually causes about 7 million cases of otitis media, 500,000 cases of pneumonia, 50,000 cases of sepsis, 3,000 cases of meningitis, and 40,000 deaths. Diagnosis is by Gram stain and culture. Treatment depends on the resistance profile and includes a β-lactam, macrolide, and fluoroquinolone.**

The pneumococcus capsule consists of a complex polysaccharide that determines serologic type and contributes to virulence and pathogenicity. There are > 85 serologic types, but most serious infections are caused by types 4, 6, 9, 14, 18, 19, and 23; these account for about 90% of invasive infections in children and 60% in adults, but these patterns are slowly changing, in part because of the wide use of polyvalent vaccine.

Pneumococci commonly colonize the human respiratory tract, particularly in winter and early spring. Spread is via airborne droplets. True epidemics of pneumococcal infections are rare.

Patients most susceptible to serious and invasive pneumococcal infections are those with chronic illness (eg, chronic cardiorespiratory disease, diabetes, liver disease, alcoholism), immune suppression, functional or anatomic asplenia or sickle cell disease, residents of long-term care facilities, smokers, and Alaskan natives and certain American Indian populations. The elderly, even those without other disease, tend to have poor prognosis with infections. Damage to the respiratory epithelium by chronic bronchitis or common respiratory viruses, notably influenza, may predispose to pneumococcal invasion.

Pneumococcal Diseases

Primary infection is frequently pulmonary. It may also cause otitis media, sinusitis, meningitis, endocarditis, septic arthritis and, rarely, peritonitis. Pneumococcal bacteremia may be a primary infection in susceptible patients or it may accompany the acute phase of any pneumococcal infection. Despite treatment, it has an overall mortality rate of 15 to 20% in children and adults and 30 to 40% in the elderly. The diseases listed below are further discussed elsewhere in THE MANUAL.

Pneumonia (see p. 423), the most frequent serious infection caused by pneumococci, may present as lobar pneumonia or less commonly as bronchopneumonia. Pleural effusion is found in about 10% of cases and may resolve spontaneously during treatment. In < 3%, it becomes loculated, thick, and fibrinopurulent, forming an empyema. Lung abscess is rare.

Acute otitis media in infants (after the newborn period) and children is caused by pneumococci in about 30 to 40% of cases (see p. 797). More than 1/3 of children in most populations have an attack of acute pneumococcal otitis media in the first 2 yr of life, and recurrent pneumococcal otitis is common. Mastoiditis and lateral sinus thrombosis, fairly common complications of otitis media in the pre-antibiotic era, are now rare.

Paranasal sinusitis may be caused by pneumococci and may become chronic and polymicrobic. Most commonly the maxillary and ethmoid sinuses are affected. Infection of the frontal or sphenoidal sinus may extend into the meninges, producing bacterial meningitis.

Acute purulent meningitis is frequently caused by pneumococcus and may be secondary to bacteremia from other foci (notably pneumonia); direct extension from infection of the ear, mastoid process, or paranasal sinuses; or basilar fracture of the skull involving one of these sites or the cribriform plate.

Endocarditis may rarely result from bacteremia even in patients without valvular heart disease. Pneumococcal endocarditis may produce a corrosive valvular lesion, with sudden rupture or fenestration, leading to rapidly progressive heart failure.

Septic arthritis, similar to septic arthritis caused by other gram-positive cocci, is usually a complication of pneumococcal bacteremia from another site (see Acute Infectious Arthritis on p. 312).

Spontaneous pneumococcal peritonitis occurs most often in patients with cirrhosis and ascites, with no features to distinguish it from spontaneous bacterial peritonitis of other causes.

Diagnosis

Pneumococci are readily identified by their typical encapsulated appearance on Gram stain. The characteristic capsule is also visible in smears stained with methylene blue. Culture and serotyping (if indicated) confirm identification. Serotyping of isolates can be helpful for epidemiologic reasons to correlate the spread of specific clones and follow antimicrobial resistance patterns. Antimicrobial susceptibility testing should be done on isolated strains. Pneumococci in joints can usually be demonstrated by direct smear and culture of the aspirated purulent synovial fluid.

Treatment

If pneumococcal infection is suspected, initial therapy pending susceptibility studies should be determined by local resistance patterns. Although the preferred treatment for pneumococcal infections is β-lactam or macrolide antibiotics, treatment has become more challenging because of the emergence of resistant strains. Strains highly resistant to penicillin, ampicillin, and other β-lactams are common worldwide. The most common predisposing factor to β-lactam resistance is use of these drugs within the past several months. Intermediately resistant organisms may be treated with ordinary or high doses of penicillin G or other β-lactams. Seriously ill patients with nonmeningeal infections caused by organisms that are highly resistant to penicillin can often be treated with ceftriaxone or cefotaxime. Very high doses of parenteral penicillin G (20 to 40 million units/day IV for adults) also work, unless the minimum inhibitory concentration of the isolate is very high. All penicillin-resistant isolates have been susceptible to vancomycin so far, but parenteral vancomycin does not always yield concentrations in CSF adequate for treatment of meningitis (especially if corticosteroids are also being used). Therefore, ceftriaxone or cefotaxime and/or rifampin are commonly used with vancomycin in patients with meningitis. Newer fluoroquinolones, such as gatifloxacin, gemifloxacin, levofloxacin, and moxifloxacin, are effective for treating respiratory infections with highly penicillin-resistant pneumococci in adults.

Prevention

Infection produces type-specific immunity but does not generalize to other serotypes.

Two pneumococcal vaccines are available: a polyvalent polysaccharide vaccine directed against the 23 serotypes that account for > 80% of serious pneumococcal infections and a conjugated vaccine against 7 serotypes.

Conjugated vaccine is recommended for all children from 6 wk through 59 mo. The schedule varies depending on age and underlying medical conditions (see Fig. 266–3 on p. 2235). If begun at ≤ 6 mo, children should receive a 3-dose primary series at approximately 2-mo intervals, followed by a 4th dose at 12 to 15 mo. The customary age for the 1st dose is 2 mo. If begun between 7 and 11 mo, a 2-dose primary series and a booster are given. Between 12 and 23 mo, 2 doses and no booster are given. From 24 mo to 9 yr, children receive 1 dose.

Polysaccharide vaccine is ineffective in children < 2 yr but reduces pneumococcal bacteremia by 50% in adults. There is no documented reduction in pneumonia. Protection generally lasts many years, but revaccination after ≥ 5 yr may be desirable in highly susceptible people. The polysaccharide vaccine is indicated for adults ≥ 65 yr and people 2 to 64 yr with increased susceptibility (see p. 1440), and before splenectomy. It is not recommended for children < 2 yr or anyone hypersensitive to the vaccine's components.

For functional or anatomic asplenic children < 5 yr, penicillin V 125 mg po bid is recommended. The duration for chemoprophylaxis is empiric, but some experts continue prophylaxis throughout childhood and into adulthood for high-risk patients with asplenia. Penicillin (250 mg po bid) is also recommended for older children or adolescents for at least 1 yr after splenectomy.

STAPHYLOCOCCAL INFECTIONS

Staphylococci are gram-positive, aerobic organisms. *Staphylococcus aureus* is the most pathogenic; it typically causes skin infections and sometimes pneumonia, endocarditis, and osteomyelitis. It commonly leads to abscess formation. Some strains elaborate toxins that cause gastroenteritis, scalded skin syndrome, and toxic shock syndrome. Diagnosis is by Gram stain and culture. Treatment is usually with penicillinase-resistant β-lactams, but because antibiotic resistance is common, vancomycin may be required. Some strains are resistant to all but the newest ribosome-targeted antibiotics (eg, linezolid, quinupristin plus dalfopristin) or daptomycin (a lipopeptide antibiotic).

The ability to clot blood by producing coagulase determines the virulence of the several species of staphylococci. Coagulase-positive *Staphylococcus aureus* is among the most ubiquitous and dangerous human pathogens, both for its virulence and its ability to develop antibiotic resistance. Coagulase-negative species like *S. epidermidis* are increasingly associated with hospital-acquired infections, whereas *S. saprophyticus* causes urinary infections.

Pathogenic staphylococci are ubiquitous. They are carried, usually transiently, in the anterior nares of about 30% of healthy adults and on the skin of about 20%. Hospital patients and personnel have higher rates.

Newborns and nursing mothers are predisposed to staphylococcal infections, as are patients with influenza, chronic bronchopulmonary disorders (eg, cystic fibrosis, emphysema), leukemia, tumors, transplants, implanted prostheses or other foreign bodies, burns, chronic skin disorders, surgical incisions, diabetes mellitus, and indwelling intravascular plastic catheters. Patients receiving adrenal steroids, irradiation, immunosuppressants, or antitumor chemotherapy are also at increased risk. Predisposed patients may acquire antibiotic-resistant staphylococci from hospital personnel. Transmission via the hands of personnel is the most common means of spread, but airborne spread also can occur.

Staphylococcal Diseases

Staphylococci cause disease by direct tissue invasion and sometimes by exotoxin production. *S. aureus* bacteremia, which frequently causes metastatic foci of infection, may occur with any localized staphylococcal infection but is particularly common with infection related to intravascular catheters or other foreign bodies. It also may occur without any obvious primary site. *S. epidermidis* and other coagulase-negative staphylococci increasingly cause hospital-acquired bacteremia associated with catheters and other foreign bodies. They are important causes of morbidity (especially prolongation of hospitalization) and mortality in debilitated patients. The diseases listed below are further discussed elsewhere in THE MANUAL.

Direct invasion: Skin infections are the most common form of staphylococcal disease. Superficial infections may be diffuse, with vesicular pustules and crusting (impetigo) or sometimes cellulitis, or focal and nodular (furuncles and carbuncles). Deeper cutaneous abscesses are common. Staphylococci are commonly implicated in wound and burn infections, postoperative incision infections, and mastitis or breast abscess in nursing mothers.

Neonatal infections usually appear within 6 wk after birth and include skin lesions with or without exfoliation, bacteremia, meningitis, and pneumonia.

Pneumonia that occurs in the community setting is not common but may develop with influenza, in patients receiving corticosteroids or immunosuppressants, and in those with chronic bronchopulmonary or other high-risk diseases. However, *S. aureus* is a common cause of hospital-acquired pneumonia. Staphylococcal pneumonia is occasionally characterized by formation of lung abscesses followed by rapid development of pneumatoceles and empyema.

Endocarditis develops, particularly in IV drug abusers and patients with prosthetic heart valves. It is an acute febrile illness often accompanied by abscesses, embolic phenomena, pericarditis, subungual petechiae, subconjunctival hemorrhage, purpuric lesions, heart murmurs, and valvular heart failure.

Osteomyelitis occurs more commonly in children, causing chills, fever, and pain over the involved bone. Redness and swelling subsequently appear. Periarticular infection frequently results in effusion, suggesting septic arthritis rather than osteomyelitis.

Toxin-mediated disease: Staphylococci may produce multiple toxins. Some have local effects; others trigger cytokine release from certain T cells, causing serious systemic effects, including skin lesions, shock, organ failure, and death.

Toxic shock syndrome (see p. 1448) may occur from use of vaginal tampons or as a complication of a seemingly minor postoperative infection.

Staphylococcal scalded skin syndrome (see p. 986), which is caused by several toxins termed exfoliatins, is an exfoliative dermatitis of childhood characterized by large bullae and peeling of the upper layer of the skin. Eventually, exfoliation occurs.

Staphylococcal food poisoning is caused by ingesting a preformed heat-stable staphylococcal enterotoxin. Food can be contaminated by staphylococcal carriers or people with active skin infections. In food that is incompletely cooked or left at room temperature, staphylococci reproduce and elaborate enterotoxin. Many foods can serve as growth media, and despite contamination, they have a normal taste and odor. Severe nausea and vomiting begin 2 to 8 h after ingestion, typically followed by abdominal cramps and diarrhea. The attack is brief, often lasting < 12 h.

Diagnosis

Diagnosis is by Gram stain and culture of infected material. Susceptibility studies should be done because methicillin-resistant organisms are now common and require alternative therapy.

Staphylococcal food poisoning is usually suspected because of case clustering (eg, within a family, attendees of a social gathering, or customers of a restaurant). Confirmation (typically by the health department) entails isolating staphylococci from suspected food and sometimes testing for enterotoxins.

X-ray changes of osteomyelitis may not be apparent for 10 to 14 days, and bone rarefaction and periosteal reaction may not be detected for even longer. Abnormalities in MRIs, CT scans, or radionuclide bone scans often are apparent earlier.

Treatment

Management includes abscess drainage, debridement of necrotic tissue, removal of foreign bodies (including vascular catheters), and administration of antibiotics. Initial choice and dosage of antibiotics depend on infection site, illness severity, and probability that resistant strains are involved. Thus, it is essential to know local resistance patterns for initial therapy (and ultimately, actual drug sensitivity).

Treatment of staphylococcal intoxications, the most serious of which is toxic shock syndrome, involves decontamination of the producing area (exploration of surgical wounds, irrigation, debridement), intensive support (including vasopressors and respiratory assistance), electrolyte balancing, and antimicrobials. In vitro evidence supports a preference for protein synthesis inhibitors (eg, clindamycin 900 mg IV q 8 h) over other classes of antibiotics. IV immune globulin has benefited severe cases.

Antibiotic resistance is common in staphylococci. Staphylococci often produce penicillinase, an enzyme that inactivates several β-lactam antibiotics. Most staphylococci are resistant to penicillin G, ampicillin, and antipseudomonal penicillins. Most community-acquired strains are susceptible to penicillinase-resistant penicillins (methicillin, oxacillin, nafcillin, cloxacillin, dicloxacillin), cephalosporins, carbapenems (imipenem, meropenem, ertapenem), macrolides, gentamicin, vancomycin, and teicoplanin.

Methicillin-resistant *S. aureus* (MRSA) isolates have become common, especially in hospitals. In addition, community-acquired methicillin-resistant *S. aureus* (CA-MRSA) has emerged over the past several years. CA-MRSA tends to be less resistant to multiple drugs than hospital-acquired isolates. These strains are usually susceptible to trimethoprim-sulfamethoxazole (TMP-SMX), doxycycline, or minocycline and are often susceptible to clindamycin, but there is the potential for emergence of resistance by strains inducibly resistant to erythromycin. Vancomycin is

TABLE 171–1. ANTIBIOTIC TREATMENT OF STAPHYLOCOCCAL INFECTIONS IN ADULTS

INFECTION	DRUGS
Community-acquired cutaneous infections (non-MRSA)	Dicloxacillin or cephalexin 250–500 mg po q 6 h for 7–10 days
Penicillin-allergic patients	Erythromycin 250–500 mg po q 6 h; clarithromycin 500 mg po q 12 h; azithromycin 500 mg po on the 1st day then 250 mg po q 24 h or clindamycin 300 mg po q 8 h
Serious infections that are unlikely to be MRSA	Nafcillin or oxacillin 1–2 g IV q 4–6 h or cefazolin 1 g IV q 8 h
Penicillin-allergic patients	Clindamycin 600 mg IV q 8 h or vancomycin 15 mg/kg q 12 h
Serious infection with high likelihood of being MRSA	Vancomycin 15 mg/kg IV q 12 h or linezolid 600 mg IV q 12 h
Documented MRSA	By reported sensitivities
Vancomycin-resistant staphylococci*	Linezolid 600 mg IV q 12 h; quinupristin plus dalfopristin 7.5 mg/kg q 8 h; daptomycin 4 mg/kg q 24 h

MRSA = methicillin-resistant *Staphylococcus aureus.*

*No clinical data, but listed drugs appear to be active in vitro (doses not established).

effective for most hospital-acquired MRSA, sometimes with the addition of rifampin and an aminoglycoside for serious infections. However, vancomycin-resistant strains have appeared in the US. TABLE 171–1 summarizes treatment options.

Prevention

Aseptic precautions (eg, thoroughly washing hands between patient examinations and sterilizing shared equipment) help decrease spread in institutions. Strict isolation procedures should be used for patients harboring resistant microbes until their infections have been cured. An asymptomatic nasal carrier need not be isolated unless the strain is MRSA or is the suspected source of an outbreak. Cloxacillin, dicloxacillin, TMP-SMX, ciprofloxacin (each of these often combined with rifampin), and topical mupirocin have been useful in treating MRSA in carriers, but the organism recurs in up to 50% and frequently becomes resistant.

Staphylococcal food poisoning can be prevented by proper food preparation. Patients with staphylococcal skin infections should not handle food, and food should be consumed immediately or refrigerated and not kept at room temperature.

STREPTOCOCCAL AND ENTEROCOCCAL INFECTIONS

(See also Pneumococcal Infections on p. 1440, Rheumatic Fever on p. 2358, and Tonsillopharyngitis on p. 825.)

Streptococci are gram-positive aerobic organisms that cause many disorders, including pharyngitis, pneumonia, wound and skin infections, sepsis, and endocarditis. Symptoms vary with the organ infected. Sequelae include rheumatic fever and glomerulonephritis. Clinical diagnoses are confirmed by Gram stain and culture. Most strains are sensitive to penicillin, with the exception of enterococci, which can be resistant to multiple drugs. Recently, erythromycin-resistant strains have emerged.

Three different types of streptococci are initially differentiated by their appearance when grown on sheep blood agar. β-Hemolytic streptococci produce zones of clear hemolysis around each colony, α-hemolytic streptococci (including viridans group streptococci) are surrounded by green discoloration resulting from incomplete hemolysis, and γ-hemolytic streptococci are nonhemolytic. Subsequent classification, based on carbohydrates present in the cell wall, divides streptococci into the Lancefield groups A through H and K through T (see TABLE 171–2). Viridans streptococci form a separate group that is difficult to classify. In the Lancefield classification, enterococci were initially included among the group D streptococci. More recently,

TABLE 171–2. CLASSIFICATION OF STREPTOCOCCI

LANCEFIELD GROUP	SPECIES	HEMOLYSIS	ASSOCIATED DISEASES	TREATMENT
A	*S. pyogenes*	β	Pharyngitis, tonsillitis, wound and skin infections, septicemia, scarlet fever, pneumonia, rheumatic fever, glomerulonephritis	Penicillin, erythromycin, clindamycin
			Necrotizing fasciitis	Expeditious surgical management. β-Lactam (usually broad spectrum until etiology is identified; if GABHS is confirmed, can use penicillin or cefazolin) plus clindamycin
B	*S. agalactiae*	β	Sepsis, postpartum or neonatal sepsis, skin infections, endocarditis, septic arthritis	Penicillin or ampicillin; cephalosporin; vancomycin
C and G	*S. equi*, *S. canis*	β	Pharyngitis, pneumonia, cellulitis, pyoderma, erysipelas, impetigo, wound infections, puerperal sepsis, neonatal sepsis, endocarditis, septic arthritis	Penicillin, vancomycin, cephalosporins, macrolides (variable susceptibility)
D	Enterococcal: *E. faecalis*, *E. durans*, and *E. faecium*	α or γ	Endocarditis, UTI, intra-abdominal infection, cellulitis, and wound infection as well as concurrent bacteremia	Enterococci: penicillin, ampicillin, or vancomycin (plus an aminoglycoside if serious infection)
	Nonenterococcal: *S. bovis* and *S. equinus*			Vancomycin-resistant enterococci: Streptogramins, oxazolidinones
Viridans*	*S. mutans*, *S. sanguis*, *S. salivarius*, *S. mitior*, *A. milleri*	α or γ	Endocarditis, localized infection or abscesses	Penicillin, other based on in vitro susceptibility
	S. iniae		Cellulitis and invasive infections from fish	Penicillin

*Do not conform to specific serogroups.
GABHS = Group A β-hemolytic streptococci.

enterococci have been classified as a separate genus.

Many streptococci elaborate virulence factors, including streptolysins, DNAases, and hyaluronidase, which contribute to tissue destruction and spread of infection. A few strains release exotoxins that activate certain T cells, triggering release of cytokines, including tumor necrosis factor-α, interleukins, and other immunomodulators, which activate the complement, coagulation, and fibrinolytic systems, in turn leading to shock, organ failure, and death.

Streptococcal Diseases

The most significant streptococcal pathogen is *S. pyogenes,* which is β-hemolytic and in Lancefield Group A, thus denoted as group A β-hemolytic streptococci (GABHS). The 2 most common acute diseases due to GABHS are pharyngitis and skin infections; in addition, delayed, nonsuppurative complications (rheumatic fever and acute glomerulonephritis) sometimes occur ≥ 2 wk after infection. Disease caused by other streptococcal species is less prevalent, and usually involves soft-tissue infection or endocarditis (see Table 171–2). Some non-GABHS infections occur predominantly in certain populations (eg, group B streptococci in newborns and postpartum women, enterococci in hospitalized patients).

Infections can spread through the affected tissues and along lymphatic channels to regional lymph nodes. They also can produce local suppurative complications, such as peritonsillar abscess, otitis media, sinusitis, and bacteremia. Suppuration depends on the severity of infection and the susceptibility of tissue.

Streptococcal pharyngitis is usually caused by GABHS. About 20% of patients present with sore throat, fever, a beefy red pharynx, and a purulent tonsillar exudate. The remainder have less prominent symptoms, and the examination resembles that of viral pharyngitis. The cervical and submaxillary nodes may enlarge and become tender. Streptococcal pharyngitis can lead to peritonsillar abscess (see p. 822). Cough, laryngitis, and stuffy nose are uncharacteristic of streptococcal pharyngeal infection; their presence suggests another cause (usually viral or allergic). An asymptomatic carrier state may exist in as many as 20%.

Scarlet fever is uncommon today. Scarlet fever is caused by group A streptococcal (and occasionally other) strains that produce an erythrogenic toxin, leading to a diffuse pink-red cutaneous flush that blanches on pressure. The rash is seen best on the abdomen or the lateral chest, as dark red lines in skin folds (Pastia's lines), or as circumoral pallor. A strawberry tongue (inflamed papillae protruding through a bright red coating) also occurs and must be differentiated from that seen in toxic shock syndrome (see p. 1448) and Kawasaki disease (see p. 2399). The upper layer of the previously reddened skin often desquamates after fever subsides. Other symptoms are similar to those in streptococcal pharyngitis, and the course and management of scarlet fever are the same as for other group A infections.

Skin infections include impetigo (see p. 984) and cellulitis (see p. 980). Cellulitis may spread rapidly due to the numerous lytic enzymes and toxins produced mainly by group A streptococcus. Erysipelas (see p. 982) is a particular form of streptococcal cellulitis.

Necrotizing fasciitis due to *S. pyogenes* is a severe dermal (or rarely muscular) infection that spreads along fascial planes (see p. 985). The inoculation originates through the skin or bowel, and the defect may be surgical, trivial, distant from the disease site, or occult, as with colonic diverticula or an appendiceal abscess. It is prevalent among IV drug abusers. Formerly known as streptococcal gangrene and popularized as the "flesh-eating bacteria," the same syndrome also may be polymicrobial, involving a host of aerobic and anaerobic flora, including *Clostridium perfringens.* When it occurs in the perineum it is called Fournier's gangrene. Comorbid conditions, such as impaired immunity, diabetes, and alcoholism, are common. Symptoms begin with fever and exquisite localized pain. Thrombosis of the microvasculature causes ischemic necrosis, leading to rapid spread and disproportionally severe toxicity. In 20 to 40% of cases, adjacent muscles are invaded. Shock and renal dysfunction are common. Mortality is high, even with treatment.

Septicemia, puerperal sepsis, endocarditis, and pneumonias due to streptococci remain serious complications, especially if the organism is a multiresistant enterococcus.

Streptococcal toxic shock syndrome (see p. 1448), similar to that caused by *S. aureus,* may result from toxin-producing strains of GABHS. Patients are usually otherwise healthy children or adults with skin and soft-tissue infections.

Delayed complications: The mechanism by which certain strains of GABHS cause delayed complications is unclear but may involve cross-reactivity of streptococcal antibodies against host tissue.

Rheumatic fever (see p. 2358), an inflammatory disorder, occurs in < 3% of patients in the weeks after untreated GABHS upper respiratory tract infection. It is much less common today than in the pre-antibiotic era. Diagnosis depends on a combination of arthritis, carditis, chorea, specific cutaneous manifestations, and laboratory tests. The most important reason for treating strep throat is to prevent rheumatic fever.

Poststreptococcal acute glomerulonephritis (see p. 2001) is an acute nephritic syndrome following pharyngitis or skin infection from certain nephritogenic strains of GABHS. This sequela follows infection with a limited number of group A streptococcal serotypes. The overall attack rate after a throat or skin infection with it is about 10 to 15%. It is most common in children, occurring 1 to 3 wk after infection. Nearly all children, but somewhat fewer adults, recover without permanent renal damage. Antibiotic treatment of GABHS infection has little effect on development of glomerulonephritis.

Diagnosis

Streptococci are readily identified by culture on a sheep blood agar plate. Rapid antigen-detection tests are available that allow detection of GABHS directly from throat swabs. Many tests are based on enzyme immunoassay methodology; but more recently, tests using optical immunoassay have become available. They have high specificity (> 95%) but vary considerably in sensitivity (55% to 80 to 90% for the newer optical immunoassay test). Negative results should be confirmed by culture (particularly if a macrolide is being considered because of potential resistance).

During convalescence, evidence of infection can be obtained indirectly by demonstrating antistreptococcal antibodies in serum. Antibodies are most useful in diagnosis of post-streptococcal diseases, such as rheumatic fever and glomerulonephritis. Confirmation requires that sequential specimens show a rise in titer, because a single value may be high from a long antecedent infection. Serum specimens need not be taken more often than q 2 wk and may be taken q 2 mo. A significant rise (or fall) in titer should span at least 2 serial dilutions. The antistreptolysin O (ASO) titer rises in only 75 to 80% of infections. For completeness in difficult cases, any one of the other tests (antihyaluronidase, antideoxyribonuclease B, antinicotinamide adenine dinucleotidase, or antistreptokinase) also can be used. Penicillin given within the first 5 days for symptomatic streptococcal pharyngitis may delay the appearance and decrease the magnitude of the ASO response. Patients with streptococcal pyoderma usually do not have a significant ASO response but may have a response to other antigens (ie, anti-DNAase or antihyluronidase).

Treatment

Pharyngitis: Pharyngeal GABHS infections, including scarlet fever, ordinarily are self-limited. Antibiotics shorten the course in young children, especially those with scarlet fever, but have only modest effect on symptoms in adolescents and adults. However, they help prevent local suppurative complications and rheumatic fever.

Penicillin is the drug of choice. A single injection of benzathine penicillin G, 600,000 units IM for small children (< 27.3 kg) or 1.2 million units IM for adolescents and adults usually suffices. Oral penicillin V may be used if the patient can be trusted to maintain the regimen for the required 10 days; 500 mg of penicillin V bid or tid (250 mg for children < 27 kg) is given. Oral cephalosporins are effective. Cefdinir, cefpodoxime, and azithromycin can be used for a 5-day course of therapy. Delaying treatment 1 to 2 days until laboratory confirmation increases neither the duration of disease nor the incidence of complications.

When penicillin or a β-lactam is contraindicated, erythromycin 250 mg po qid or clindamycin 300 mg po tid may be given for 10 days, although resistance of GABHS to macrolides has been detected (some authorities recommend confirmation of in vitro susceptibility if a macrolide is to be used and there is the possibility of macrolide resistance in the community). TMP-SMX, some of the fluoroquinolones, and the tetracyclines are unreliable. Clindamycin (5 mg/kg po qid) is preferred in children who have relapses of chronic tonsillitis, possibly because of its good activity against penicillinase-producing staphylococci or anaerobes coinfecting the tonsillar crypts and inactivating penicillin G. Clindamycin also appears to halt exotoxin production more rapidly than other agents.

Sore throat, headache, fever can be treated with analgesics or antipyretics. Bed rest and isolation are unnecessary. Close contacts who are symptomatic or have a history of post-streptococcal complications should be examined for streptococci.

Skin infection: Cellulitis is often treated without performing a culture because isolating organisms can be difficult. Thus regimens effective against both streptococci and staphylococci are used (see p. 981). Necrotizing fasciitis should be treated in an ICU. Extensive (perhaps repeated) surgical debridement is required. A recommended initial antibiotic regimen is a β-lactam (often a broad-spectrum agent until the etiology is confirmed by culture) plus clindamycin. Although streptococci remain susceptible to β-lactam antibiotics, animal studies have shown that penicillin is not always effective with a large bacterial inoculum because the streptococci are not rapidly growing.

Other streptococcal infections: Drugs of choice for treating group B, C, and G infections are penicillin, ampicillin, or vancomycin. Cephalosporins or macrolides are generally effective, but susceptibility tests must guide therapy, especially in very ill, immunocompromised, or debilitated hosts and in people with foreign bodies at the infection site. Surgical wound drainage and debridement as adjuncts to antimicrobial therapy may be lifesaving.

S. bovis is relatively susceptible to antibiotics. Although vancomycin-resistant *S. bovis* isolates recently have been reported, the organism remains susceptible to penicillin and aminoglycosides.

Most viridans streptococci are often susceptible to penicillin G and other β-lactams. Resistance is growing, and therapy for such strains should be dictated by results of in vitro susceptibility tests.

Enterococcal Infections

Enterococcus faecalis and *E. faecium* cause endocarditis, UTI, intra-abdominal infection, cellulitis, and wound infection as well as concurrent bacteremia. Enterococci associated with serious infections are difficult to eradicate unless a combination of a cell wall–active drug, such as penicillin, ampicillin, or vancomycin, plus an aminoglycoside, such as gentamicin or streptomycin, is used.

Vancomycin-resistant enterococci (VRE) also may be resistant to aminoglycosides, cell wall–active β-lactams (such as penicillin G and ampicillin), and other glycopeptides (such as teicoplanin). When identified, strict isolation techniques should be used. Recommended treatment includes streptogramins (quinupristin plus dalfopristin) and oxazolidinones (linezolid).

TOXIC SHOCK SYNDROME

Toxic shock syndrome is caused by staphylococcal or streptococcal exotoxins. Symptoms include high fever, hypotension, diffuse erythematous rash, and multiple organ involvement that may rapidly progress to severe and intractable shock. Diagnosis is made clinically and by isolating the organism. Treatment includes antibiotics, intensive support, and immunoglobulin.

Etiology and Pathophysiology

Toxic shock syndrome (TSS) is caused by exotoxin-producing cocci. Strains of phage-group 1 *Staphylococcus aureus* elaborate the TSS toxin-1 (TSST-1) or related exotoxins, and certain strains of *Streptococcus pyogenes* produce at least 2 exotoxins.

Women with preexisting staphylococcal colonization of the vagina who use tampons are at highest risk. Mechanical or chemical factors related to tampon use likely enhance production of the exotoxin or facilitate its entry into the bloodstream through a mucosal break or via the uterus. Estimates made from small series suggest about 3 cases/100,000 menstruating women still occur, and cases are still reported in women who do not use tampons and in postoperative and postpartum women. About 15% of cases occur postpartum or as postoperative staphylococcal wound infections, which frequently appear insignificant. Cases also have been reported in association with influenza, osteomyelitis, and cellulitis.

Mortality from staphylococcal TSS is < 3%. Recurrences are common in women who continue to use tampons during the first 4 mo after an episode.

Streptococcal toxic shock syndrome is similar to that caused by *S. aureus* but carries a higher mortality (20 to 60%). In addition, about 50% of cases have *S. pyogenes* bacteremia, and 50% have necrotizing fasciitis (neither of which is common for staphylococcal TSS). Patients are usually otherwise healthy children or adults. Primary infections in skin and soft tissue are more common than in other sites. In contrast to staphylococcal TSS, streptococcal TSS is more likely to cause respiratory distress syndrome and less likely to cause a typical cutaneous reaction.

Symptoms and Signs

Onset is sudden, with fever (39° to 40.5°C, which remains elevated), hypotension, a diffuse macular erythroderma, and involvement of at least 2 other organ systems. Staphylococcal TSS is likely to cause vomiting and diarrhea, myalgia and elevated CPK, mucositis, hepatic damage, thrombocytopenia, and confusion. The staphylococcal TSS rash is more likely to desquamate, particularly on the palms and soles, between 3 and 7 days after onset. Streptococcal TSS commonly causes respiratory distress syndrome, coagulopathy, and hepatic damage and is more likely to cause fever, malaise, and severe pain at the site of a soft-tissue infection. Renal impairment is frequent and common to both. The syndrome may progress within 48 h to syncope, shock, and death. Less severe cases of staphylococcal TSS are fairly common.

Diagnosis

Diagnosis is made clinically and by isolating the organism from blood cultures (for *Streptococcus*) or from the local site. TSS resembles Kawasaki disease, but Kawasaki disease generally occurs in children < 5 yr of age; it does not cause shock, azotemia, or thrombocytopenia; and the skin rash is maculopapular. Other disorders to be considered are scarlet fever, Reye's syndrome, staphylococcal scalded skin syndrome, meningococcemia, Rocky Mountain spotted fever, leptospirosis, and viral exanthematous diseases. These disorders are ruled out by specific clinical differences, cultures, and serologic studies.

Specimens for culture should be taken from any lesions, the nose (for staphylococci), throat (for streptococci), vagina (for both), and blood. Continuous monitoring of renal, hepatic, bone marrow, and cardiopulmonary function is necessary.

Treatment

Patients suspected of having TSS should be hospitalized immediately and treated intensively. Tampons, diaphragms, and other foreign bodies should be removed at once. Suspected primary sites should be decontaminated thoroughly. MRI or CT scan of soft tissue is helpful in localizing sites of infection. Decontamination includes reinspection and irrigation of surgical wounds, even if they appear healthy; repeated debridement of devitalized tissues; and irrigation of potential naturally colonized sites (sinuses, vagina). Fluid and electrolyte replacement is given to prevent or treat hypovolemia, hypotension, or shock. Because fluid loss into tissues can occur throughout the body, shock may be profound and resistant. Aggressive fluid resuscitation and circulatory support are sometimes required.

Obvious infections should be treated. If *S. pyogenes* is isolated, a β-lactam (eg, penicillin) plus clindamycin (900 mg IV q 8 h) continued for 14 days is emerging as the most effective antibiotic treatment. The rationale for the use clindamycin is explained above (see under Pharyngitis on p. 1447). Antibiotics during the acute illness also may eradicate pathogen foci and prevent recurrences. Passive immunization to TSS toxins with IV immune globulin (400 mg/kg) has been helpful in severe cases of both types of TSS and lasts for weeks, but the disease itself may not induce active immunity, so recurrences are possible.

If a test for seroconversion to TSST-1 is negative, women who have had staphylococcal TSS should probably refrain from using tampons and cervical caps, plugs, and diaphragms. It seems prudent to advise all women, regardless of TSST-1 status, to change tampons frequently or use napkins instead.

172 GRAM-POSITIVE BACILLI

Gram-positive bacilli cause anthrax, diphtheria, erysipelothricosis, listeriosis, and nocardiosis. Serious symptoms from anthrax and diphtheria are due to powerful toxins produced by the organisms.

ANTHRAX

Anthrax is caused by *Bacillus anthracis*, a toxin-producing, encapsulated, facultative anaerobe. Anthrax, an often fatal disease of animals, is transmitted to humans by contact with infected animals or their products. In humans, infection typically is through the skin. Inhalation infection is less common; oropharyngeal, meningeal, and GI infections are rare. For inhalation and GI infections,

nonspecific local symptoms are typically followed in several days by severe systemic illness, shock, and often death. Empiric treatment is with ciprofloxacin or doxycycline. Vaccination is available.

The incidence of natural infection has decreased, particularly in the developed world. However, the use of anthrax as a potential biological weapon has increased fear of this pathogen.

Pathophysiology

Bacillus anthracis readily forms spores upon drying. Spores resist destruction and can remain viable in soil, wool, and animal hair for decades. Spores germinate and begin multiplying rapidly when they enter an environment rich in amino acids and glucose. Human infection is usually through the skin but has occurred after ingestion of contaminated meat when a break in the pharyngeal or intestinal mucosa facilitates invasion. Inhaling spores, particularly when an acute respiratory infection is present, may result in inhalation anthrax (woolsorter's disease), which is often fatal. Bacteremia may occur in any form of anthrax and occurs in nearly all fatal cases.

After entering the body, spores germinate inside macrophages, which migrate to regional lymph nodes where the bacteria multiply. In inhalation anthrax, spores are deposited in alveolar spaces, where they are ingested by macrophages, usually causing a hemorrhagic mediastinitis. GI infections usually result from eating inadequately cooked contaminated meat. Meningeal anthrax is hematogenous. Only the cutaneous form is contagious (mildly) by direct contact, flies, and fomites.

The bacteria produce several toxins that account for their virulence. The predominant toxins are edema toxin and lethal toxin. Protective antigen binds to target cells and facilitates cellular entry of edema toxin and lethal toxin. Edema toxin causes massive local edema. Lethal toxin triggers a massive release of cytokines from macrophages, which is responsible for the sudden death common in anthrax infections.

Anthrax is an important animal disease, occurring in goats, cattle, sheep, and horses. Anthrax also occurs in wildlife, such as hippos, elephants, and Cape buffalo. It is rare in humans and mainly occurs in countries that do not prevent industrial or agricultural exposure to infected animals or their products. Spores have been prepared in very finely powdered form (weaponized) to be used as agents of warfare and bioterrorism (see p. 1393).

Symptoms and Signs

Most cases present within 1 to 6 days of exposure, but for inhalation anthrax the incubation period can be > 6 wk.

The cutaneous form begins as a painless, pruritic, red-brown papule. It enlarges with a surrounding zone of brawny erythema and marked edema. Vesiculation and induration are present. Central ulceration follows, with serosanguineous exudation and formation of a black eschar (the malignant pustule). Local lymphadenopathy is common, occasionally with malaise, myalgia, headache, fever, nausea, and vomiting.

Initial symptoms of inhalation anthrax are insidious and resemble influenza. Within a few days, fever worsens and chest pain and severe respiratory distress develop, followed by cyanosis, shock, and coma. Severe hemorrhagic necrotizing lymphadenitis develops and spreads to adjacent mediastinal structures. Serosanguineous transudation, pulmonary edema, and pleural effusion occur. Typical bronchopneumonia does not occur. Hemorrhagic meningoencephalitis or GI anthrax may develop.

GI anthrax ranges from asymptomatic to fatal. When swallowed, anthrax spores can cause lesions from the oral cavity to the cecum. Released toxin induces hemorrhagic necrosis extending to the mesenteric lymph nodes. Fever, nausea, vomiting, abdominal pain, and bloody diarrhea are common. Intestinal necrosis and septicemia with potentially lethal toxicity ensue.

Oropharyngeal anthrax presents as a mucocutaneous lesion in the oral cavity with sore throat, fever, adenopathy, and dysphagia. Airway obstruction may occur.

Diagnosis

Occupational and exposure history is important. Patients should have cultures and Gram stains from clinically identified sites, including cutaneous lesions, pleural fluid, CSF, or stool. Sputum examination and Gram stain are unlikely to diagnose inhalation anthrax, given the frequent lack of airspace disease. A PCR test and immunohistochemical methods can help. Nasal swab testing for spores in people potentially exposed to inhalation anthrax is not recommended because the predictive value is unknown.

Chest x-ray (or CT) should be obtained if pulmonary symptoms are present. It typically shows widening of the mediastinum (because of enlarged hemorrhagic lymph nodes) and pleural effusion. Pneumonic infiltrates are uncommon. Lumbar puncture should be performed for meningeal signs or change in mental status. An enzyme-linked immunosorbent assay (ELISA) is available, but confirmation requires a 4-fold change in antibody titer from acute to convalescent specimens.

Prognosis and Treatment

In untreated inhalation and meningeal anthrax, mortality is 100%; in cutaneous anthrax, 10 to 20%; in GI anthrax, about 50%; and between 12.4 and 50% in the oral form.

People exposed to inhaled anthrax require treatment with oral ciprofloxacin 500 mg bid (10 to 15 mg/kg for children) or doxycycline 100 mg bid (2.5 mg/kg for children) for 60 days. Amoxicillin 500 mg tid (25 to 30 mg/kg for children) is an option when ciprofloxacin and doxycycline are contraindicated. Treatment for 60 days after exposure provides optimal protection. Vaccination should be given, even after exposure.

Cutaneous anthrax is treated with ciprofloxacin 500 mg po bid (10 to 15 mg/kg for children) or doxycycline 100 mg po bid (2.5 mg/kg for children) for 7 to 10 days. Treatment is extended to 60 days if concomitant inhalation exposure was possible. Mortality is rare with treatment, but the lesion will progress through the eschar phase.

Inhalation and other forms of anthrax, including cutaneous anthrax with significant edema or systemic symptoms, require therapy with 2 or 3 drugs: ciprofloxacin 400 mg IV (10 to 15 mg/kg for children) q 12 h or doxycycline 100 mg IV (2.5 mg/kg for children) q 12 h, along with penicillin, ampicillin, imipenem-cilastatin, meropenem, rifampin, vancomycin, clindamycin, or clarithromycin. Corticosteroids may be useful but have not been evaluated adequately. With early diagnosis and intensive support, including mechanical ventilation, fluids, and vasopressors, mortality may be reduced to 50%. If treatment is delayed (usually because the diagnosis is missed), death is likely.

Drug resistance is a theoretic concern. Although nominally sensitive to penicillin, *B. anthracis* manifests inducible β-lactamases, so single-drug therapy with penicillin or a cephalosporin is not recommended. Biological warfare researchers may have created strains of anthrax resistant to multiple antibiotics, but these have not yet been encountered in a clinical situation.

Prevention

An anthrax vaccine, composed of a cell-free culture filtrate, is available for people at high risk (military personnel, veterinarians, laboratory technicians, employees of textile mills processing imported goat hair). (A separate veterinary vaccine is also available.) Repeated vaccination is required to ensure protection. Local reactions from vaccine can occur. The CDC recommends that the anthrax vaccine be administered in conjunction with antibiotic prophylaxis to patients exposed to anthrax spores. Limited data suggest that cutaneous anthrax does not result in acquired immunity, particularly if there was early effective antimicrobial therapy. Inhalation anthrax may provide some immunity in those who survive, but data are very limited.

DIPHTHERIA

Diphtheria is an acute pharyngeal or cutaneous infection by *Corynebacterium diphtheriae*, some strains of which produce an exotoxin. Symptoms are either nonspecific skin infections or pseudomembranous pharyngitis followed by myocardial and neural tissue damage secondary to the exotoxin. Diagnosis is clinical and confirmed by culture. Treatment is with antitoxin and penicillin or erythromycin. Childhood vaccination should be routine.

Corynebacterium diphtheriae usually infects the nasopharynx (respiratory diphtheria) or skin. Diphtheria strains infected by a β-phage, which carries a toxin-encoding gene, produce a potent toxin. This toxin first causes inflammation and necrosis of local tissues then damages the heart, nerves, and kidneys.

Humans are the only known reservoir for *C. diphtheriae*. The organism is spread by respiratory droplets, direct contact with oropharyngeal secretions or skin lesions, or rarely by fomites. Most patients become asymptomatic nasopharyngeal carriers. Poor personal and community hygiene contributes to the spread of cutaneous diphtheria. In the US, indigent adults living in endemic areas are particularly at risk.

Symptoms and Signs

Symptoms vary depending on infection site and whether toxin is produced. Most respiratory infections are caused by toxin-producing strains. Most cutaneous infections are caused by non–toxin-producing strains. Toxin is poorly absorbed from the skin; thus toxin complications are rare in cutaneous diphtheria.

Following an incubation period, which averages 2 to 4 days, and a prodromal period between 12 and 24 h, the patient develops mild sore throat, dysphagia, low-grade fever, and tachycardia. Nausea, emesis, chills, headache, and fever are more common in children. If a toxigenic strain is involved, the characteristic membrane appears in the tonsillar area. It may initially appear as a white, glossy exudate, but typically becomes dirty gray, tough, fibrinous, and adherent so that removal causes bleeding. Local edema may produce a visibly swollen neck (bull neck), hoarseness, stridor, and dyspnea. The membrane may extend to the larynx, trachea, and bronchi and may partially obstruct the airway or suddenly detach, causing complete obstruction.

Skin lesions generally occur on the extremities and are varied in appearance, often indistinguishable from chronic skin conditions (eg, eczema, psoriasis, impetigo). In a few cases, it produces punched-out ulcers, occasionally with a grayish membrane. Pain, tenderness, erythema, and exudate are typical. If exotoxin is produced, lesions may be numb. Concomitant nasopharyngeal infection occurs in 20 to 40%.

Myocarditis is usually evident by the 10th to 14th day but can appear any time during the 1st to 6th wk. Insignificant ECG changes occur in 20 to 30% of patients, but atrioventricular dissociation, complete heart block, and ventricular arrhythmias may occur and are associated with a high mortality rate. Heart failure may develop.

Nervous system involvement usually begins in the 1st wk of illness with bulbar palsy, causing dysphagia and nasal regurgitation. Peripheral neuropathy appears from the 3rd to 6th wk. It is both motor and sensory, although motor symptoms predominate. Resolution occurs over many weeks.

Diagnosis

The appearance of the membrane suggests the diagnosis. Gram stain of the membrane may reveal gram-positive bacilli with metachromatic (beaded) staining in typical Chinese-character configuration. Material for culture should be obtained from below the membrane, or a portion of membrane itself should be submitted. The laboratory should be notified that *C. diphtheriae* is suspected.

Cutaneous diphtheria should be considered when a patient develops skin lesions during an outbreak of respiratory diphtheria. Swab or biopsy specimens should be cultured.

Treatment

Symptomatic patients should be hospitalized in ICUs to monitor for respiratory and cardiac complications. Isolation with respiratory and contact precautions is required and must continue until 2 cultures, taken 24 and 48 h after antibiotics are stopped, are negative.

Diphtheria antitoxin must be given without waiting for culture confirmation, because the antitoxin neutralizes only toxin not yet bound to cells. The use of antitoxin for cutaneous disease, without evidence of respiratory disease, is of questionable value because toxic sequelae have rarely been reported, but some experts recommend it. In the US, antitoxin must be obtained from the CDC. CAUTION: *Diphtheria antitoxin is derived from horses; hence, a skin (or conjunctival) test to rule out sensitivity should always precede administration* (see under skin testing on p. 1362). The dose, ranging from 20,000 to 100,000 units IM or IV, is determined by the severity of symptoms and complications. If allergic reaction occurs, 0.3 to 1 mL epinephrine 1:1000 (0.01 mL/kg) should immediately be injected sc, IM, or slowly IV. In the highly sensitive patient, IV administration of antitoxin is contraindicated.

Antibiotics are required to eradicate the organism and prevent spread; they are not substitutes for antitoxin. Adults may be given either procaine penicillin G 600,000 units IM q 12 h or erythromycin 250 to 500 mg po q 6 h for 14 days. Children should receive procaine penicillin G 12,500 to 25,000 units/kg q 12 h IM or erythromycin 10 to 15 mg/kg (maximum, 2 g/day) q 6 h po or IV. Organism elimination should be documented by 2 consecutive negative throat and/or nasopharyngeal cultures after completion of antibiotics.

Recovery from severe diphtheria is slow, and patients must be advised against resuming activities too soon. Even normal physical exertion may harm the patient recovering from myocarditis.

For cutaneous diphtheria, thorough cleansing of the lesion with soap and water and administration of systemic antibiotics for 10 days are recommended.

Prevention

Everyone should be vaccinated at prescribed intervals using diphtheria-tetanus-acellular pertussis (DTaP) vaccine for children and tetanus-diphtheria (Td) vaccine for adults (see p. 1399). Infection does not guarantee immunity; therefore, patients should be vaccinated after recovery. In addition, diphtheria immunization should be updated in all contacts, including hospital personnel. Protective immunity cannot be relied on > 5 yr after a booster dose. If immunization status is unknown, the vaccine should be given.

All close contacts should be examined; nasopharyngeal and/or throat cultures for *C. diphtheriae* should be obtained regardless of immunization status. Asymptomatic contacts should be treated with erythromycin 250 to 500 mg po q 6 h for adults (10 to 15 mg/kg qid for children) for 7 days or a single dose of penicillin G benzathine (600,000 units IM for those < 30 kg and 1.2 million units IM for those > 30 kg). If cultures are positive, an additional 10-day course of erythromycin should be given. Patients should be closely monitored during the treatment period. Carriers should *not* receive antitoxin. After 3 days of treatment, it is safe to resume work while taking antibiotics. Cultures should be repeated ≥ 2 wk after completion of antibiotics. Carriers who cannot be kept under surveillance should receive penicillin G benzathine, not erythromycin, for reasons of compliance.

ERYSIPELOTHRICOSIS

Erysipelothricosis is infection caused by *Erysipelothrix rhusiopathiae*. The most common symptom is erysipeloid, an acute but slowly evolving localized cellulitis. Diagnosis is by culture of a biopsy specimen or occasionally PCR testing. Treatment is with antibiotics.

Erysipelothrix rhusiopathiae (formerly *E. insidiosa*), a capsulated, nonsporulating, nonmotile, microaerophilic bacillus with worldwide distribution, is primarily a saprophyte. It may infect a variety of animals, including insects, shellfish, fish, birds, and mammals (especially swine). In humans, infection is chiefly occupational and typically follows a penetrating wound in people who handle animal matter, either edible or nonedible (infected carcasses, rendered products [grease, fertilizer], bones, and shells). Most commonly, patients handle fish or work in slaughterhouses. Nondermal infection is rare, usually occurring as arthritis or endocarditis.

Symptoms, Signs, and Diagnosis

Within 1 wk of injury, a characteristic raised, purplish red, nonvesiculated, indurated, maculopapular rash appears, accompanied by itching and burning. Local swelling, although sharply demarcated, may inhibit use of the hand, the usual site of infection. The lesion's border may slowly extend outward, causing discomfort and disability that may persist for 3 wk. The disease usually is self-limited. Regional lymphadenopathy occurs in about ⅓ of cases. It rarely becomes generalized cutaneous disease. Bacteremia is rare but may result in septic arthritis or infective endocarditis, even in people without known valvular heart disease.

Culture of a full-thickness biopsy specimen is superior to needle aspiration of the advancing edge of a lesion because organisms are located only in deeper parts of the skin. Culture of exudate obtained by abrading a florid papule may be diagnostic. Isolation from synovial fluid or blood is necessary for diagnosis of erysipelothrical arthritis or endocarditis. PCR amplification may aid rapid diagnosis.

Treatment

For localized cutaneous disease, usual treatment is penicillin V, ampicillin, or erythromycin 500 mg po qid for 7 days. Fluoroquinolones, tetracyclines, and cephalosporins are also effective. Endocarditis is treated for 4 wk with penicillin G 25,000 to 30,000 units/kg IV q 4 h. Cephalosporins and fluoroquinolones are alternatives. Although the same drugs and doses are appropriate for arthritis (given for at least 1 wk after defervescence or cessation of effusion), repeated needle aspiration drainage of the infected joint is necessary.

LISTERIOSIS

(See also Neonatal Listeriosis on p. 2330.)

Listeriosis is bacteremia, meningitis, cerebritis, dermatitis, an oculoglandular syndrome, intrauterine and neonatal infections, or rarely endocarditis caused by *Listeria* sp. Symptoms vary with the organ system affected and include intrauterine death in perinatal infection. Diagnosis is by laboratory isolation. Treatment includes penicillin, ampicillin (often with aminoglycosides), and trimethoprim-sulfamethoxazole.

Listeria are small, non–acid-fast, noncapsulated, nonsporulating, motile, facultative anaerobes that are found worldwide in the environment and in the gut of nonhuman mammals, birds, arachnids, and crustaceans. There are several species of *Listeria*, but *L. monocytogenes* is the predominant pathogen in humans. Incidence in the US is ≥ 7 cases/1,000,000 people/yr, peaking in the summer; attack rates are highest in newborns and in adults ≥ 60 yr. Immunocompromised patients are at high risk.

Infection usually occurs via ingestion of contaminated dairy products, raw vegetables, or meats and is favored by the ability of *L. monocytogenes* to survive and grow at refrigerator temperatures. Infection also may occur by direct contact and during slaughter of infected animals. Listerial infection can spread antepartum and intrapartum from mother to child and can cause abortion.

Symptoms, Signs, and Diagnosis

Primary listeremia is rare and produces high fever without localizing symptoms and signs. Endocarditis, peritonitis, osteomyelitis, cholecystitis, and pleuropneumonia may occur. Listeremia can cause intrauterine infection, chorioamnionitis, premature labor, fetal death, or newborn infection.

Meningitis is due to listeria in about 20% of cases in newborns and in patients > 60 yr. Twenty percent of cases progress to cerebritis, either diffuse encephalitis or, rarely, rhombencephalitis and abscesses; rhombencephalitis presents as altered consciousness, cranial nerve palsies, cerebellar signs, and motor or sensory loss.

Oculoglandular listeriosis can cause ophthalmitis and regional lymph node enlargement. It may follow conjunctival inoculation and, if untreated, may progress to bacteremia and meningitis.

Listerial infections are diagnosed by culture of blood or CSF. The laboratory must be informed when *L. monocytogenes* is suspected, because the organism is easily confused with diphtheroids. In all listerial infections, IgG agglutinin titers peak 2 to 4 wk after onset.

Treatment

Listerial meningitis is best treated with ampicillin 2 g IV q 4 h. Most authorities recommend adding an aminoglycoside based on synergy in vitro. Children receive ampicillin 50 to 100 mg/kg IV q 6 h. Cephalosporins are not effective.

Endocarditis and primary listeremia are treated with ampicillin 2 g IV q 4 h plus gentamicin (for synergy) given for 6 wk and 2 wk beyond defervescence, respectively. Oculoglandular listeriosis and listerial dermatitis should respond to erythromycin 10 mg/kg po q 6 h, continued until 1 wk after defervescence. Trimethoprim-sulfamethoxazole 5/25 mg/kg IV q 8 h is an alternative.

NOCARDIOSIS

Nocardiosis is an acute or chronic, often disseminated, suppurative or granulomatous infection caused by various aerobic soil saprophytes of the genus *Nocardia*. Pneumonia is typical, but skin and CNS infections are common. Diagnosis is by culture and special stains. Treatment is usually with sulfonamides.

Several *Nocardia* sp, in the family Actinomycetaceae, cause human disease. The most common human pathogen is *N. asteroides*, which usually causes pulmonary and disseminated infection. *N. brasiliensis* most commonly causes skin infection, particularly in tropical climates. Infection is via inhalation or by direct inoculation of the skin. Nocardiosis occurs worldwide in all age groups, but incidence is greater among older adults, especially men. Person-to-person spread is rare. Lymphoreticular malignancies, organ transplantation, high-dose corticosteroid or other immunosuppressive therapy, and underlying pulmonary disease are predisposing factors, but about ½ the patients have no preexisting disease. Nocardiosis is also an opportunistic infection in patients with advanced HIV infection. Other *Nocardia* sp sometimes cause localized or, occasionally, systemic infections.

Symptoms and Signs

Nocardiosis usually begins as a subacute pulmonary infection that resembles actinomycosis, but *Nocardia* is more likely to disseminate locally or hematogenously. Dissemination with abscess formation may involve any organ but most commonly affects the brain, skin, kidney, bone, or muscle.

The most common symptoms of pulmonary involvement—cough, fever, chills, chest pain, weakness, anorexia, and weight loss—are nonspecific and may resemble those of TB or suppurative pneumonia. Pleural effusion also may occur. Metastatic brain abscesses, occurring in 30 to 50% of cases, usually produce severe headaches and focal neurologic abnormalities. Infection may be acute, subacute, or chronic.

Skin or subcutaneous abscesses occur frequently, sometimes as a primary local inoculation. They may appear as a firm cellulitis, a lymphocutaneous syndrome, or an actinomycetoma. The lymphocutaneous syndrome consists of a primary pyoderma lesion and lymphatic nodules resembling sporotrichosis. An actinomycetoma begins as a nodule, suppurates, spreads along fascial planes, and drains through chronic fistulas.

Diagnosis

Diagnosis is by identification of *Nocardia* sp in tissue or culture from localized lesions identified by physical examination, x-ray, or other imaging studies. Clumps of beaded, branching filaments of gram-positive bacteria (which may be weakly acid-fast) are often seen. *Nocardia* do not develop a clubbed appearance, as does *Actinomyces israelii*.

Prognosis and Treatment

Without treatment, pulmonary and disseminated nocardiosis are usually fatal. Among patients who are treated with appropriate antibiotics, the mortality rate is highest (> 50%) in immunocompromised patients with disseminated infections and lowest (about 10%) in immunocompetent patients with lesions restricted to the lungs. Cure rates for patients with skin infection are usually > 95%.

Trimethoprim-sulfamethoxazole or high doses of a sulfonamide alone (sulfamethoxazole or sulfisoxazole) are used. Because most cases respond slowly, a dose that maintains a sulfonamide blood concentration of 12 to 15 mg/dL (eg, with sulfadiazine 4 to 6 g/day po) must be continued for several months. When sulfonamide hypersensitivity or refractory infection is present, amikacin, a tetracycline (particularly minocycline), imipenem-cilastatin, ceftriaxone, cefotaxime, or cycloserine can be used. In vitro susceptibility data should guide the choice of alternative drugs.

173 GRAM-NEGATIVE BACILLI

Gram-negative bacilli are responsible for numerous diseases. Some are commensal organisms found among normal intestinal flora. These commensal organisms plus others, from animal or environmental reservoirs, may cause disease. UTIs, diarrhea, peritonitis, and bloodstream infections are commonly caused by gram-negative bacilli. Plague, cholera, and typhoid fever are rare but serious gram-negative infections.

BARTONELLA INFECTIONS

Bartonella sp are gram-negative bacteria previously classified as Rickettsiae. They cause several uncommon diseases: cat-scratch disease, an acute febrile anemia, a chronic cutaneous eruption, and disseminated disease in immunocompromised hosts (see TABLE 173–1).

CAT-SCRATCH DISEASE

(Cat-Scratch Fever)

Cat-scratch disease is infection caused by *Bartonella henselae*. Symptoms are a local papule and regional lymphadenitis. Diagnosis is clinical and confirmed by biopsy. Treatment is with local heat application and analgesics.

The domestic cat is a major reservoir for *B. henselae*. The prevalence of *B. henselae* antibodies in US cats is 14 to 50%. About 99% of patients report contact with cats, most of which are healthy. The cat flea may be an additional vector. Children are most often affected.

Symptoms and Signs

Within 3 to 10 days after a scratch, most patients develop an erythematous, crusted papule (rarely, a pustule) at the scratch site. Regional lymphadenopathy develops within 2 wk. The

TABLE 173–1. SOME *BARTONELLA* INFECTIONS

DISEASE	SPECIES	MANIFESTATIONS*	AT RISK	INSECT VECTOR	TREATMENT
Bacillary angiomatosis	*B. henselae, B. quintana*	Protuberant berrylike skin lesions	Immunocompromised patients	Lice, ticks, ?fleas	Doxycycline,† erythromycin
Trench fever	*B. quintana, B. henselae*	Prolonged or recurrent fever	People living in conditions of crowding or with poor hygiene, immunocompromised patients at risk for disseminated infection	Body louse, tick	Doxycycline,† erythromycin, rifampin‡
Cat-scratch disease	*B. henselae*	Lymphadenopathy, fever	Owners of cats, immunocompromised patients at risk for disseminated infection	?Fleas	Doxycycline,† erythromycin, rifampin‡
Oroya fever, verruga peruana, carrion's disease	*B. bacilliformis*	Acute febrile hemolytic anemia, skin lesions, secondary infections	Residents of Andes Mountains at elevations 600–2400 m	*Phlebotomus* sandfly	Doxycycline,† chloramphenicol, penicillin, streptomycin

*In normal host.
†Doxycycline is generally the preferred drug.
‡Treatment not usually required in patients with normal immune systems.

nodes are initially firm and tender, later becoming fluctuant, and may drain with fistula formation. Fever, malaise, headache, and anorexia may accompany lymphadenopathy.

Unusual manifestations occur in 5 to 14% of patients: Parinaud's oculoglandular syndrome (conjunctivitis associated with palpable preauricular nodes) occurs in 6%; neurologic manifestations (encephalopathy, seizures, neuroretinitis, myelitis, paraplegia, cerebral arteritis) in 2%; and hepatosplenic granulomatous disease in < 1%. Severe disseminated illness may occur in patients with AIDS.

The skin lesion and lymphadenopathy subside spontaneously within 2 to 5 mo. Complete recovery is usual, except in severe neurologic or hepatosplenic disease, which may be fatal or followed by residual effects.

Diagnosis and Treatment

Diagnosis is confirmed by culture or positive antibody titers for *B. henselae*, PCR testing, or culture from lymph node aspirate.

Treatment is local heat application and analgesics. If a lymph node is fluctuant, needle aspiration usually relieves the pain. Antibiotic treatment is not clearly beneficial and generally should not be given for localized infection. Ciprofloxacin, gentamicin, doxycycline, and trimethoprim-sulfamethoxazole (TMP-SMX) have been used for bacteremia in AIDS patients. Prolonged therapy is usually necessary (eg, weeks to months) for bacteremia to clear. In vitro antibiotic susceptibilities often do not correlate with clinical results.

Oroya Fever and Verruga Peruana

Oroya fever and verruga peruana are infections caused by *Bartonella bacilliformis*. Oroya fever occurs on initial exposure; verruga peruana occurs after recovery from the primary infection.

Endemic only to the Andes Mountains in Colombia, Ecuador, and Peru, both diseases are passed from human to human by the *Phlebotomus* sandfly.

Symptoms of Oroya fever include fever and profound anemia, which may be sudden or indolent in onset. The anemia is primarily hemolytic, but myelosuppression also occurs. Muscle and joint pain, severe headache, and often delirium and coma may occur. Superimposed bacteremia caused by *Salmonella* or other coliform organisms may occur. Verruga peruana manifests as multiple skin lesions that strongly resemble bacillary angiomatosis, usually occurring on the limbs and face. These may persist for months to years and may be accompanied by pain and fever.

Diagnosis of Oroya fever is confirmed by blood cultures. Mortality rates may exceed 50% in untreated patients. Because Oroya fever is often complicated by *Salmonella* bacteremia, chloramphenicol 500 to 1000 mg po q 6 h for 7 days is the treatment of choice. Verruga peruana is diagnosed by its appearance and sometimes by biopsy showing dermal angiogenesis. Treatment of verruga peruana with most antibiotics produces remission, but relapse is common and requires prolonged therapy.

Bacillary Angiomatosis

(Epithelioid Angiomatosis)

Bacillary angiomatosis is skin infection caused by *Bartonella henselae* or *B. quintana*.

Bacillary angiomatosis almost always occurs in immunocompromised people and is characterized by protuberant, reddish, berry-like lesions on the skin, often surrounded by a collar of scale. Lesions bleed profusely if traumatized. They may resemble Kaposi's sarcoma or pyogenic granulomas. Infection is spread by lice and ticks and probably by fleas from household cats. Disease may spread throughout the reticuloendothelial system, particularly in AIDS patients. Diagnosis relies on the histopathology of the skin lesions, cultures, and PCR analysis. The laboratory should be notified that *Bartonella* is suspected, because special stains and prolonged culture growth are necessary. Treatment is with erythromycin 500 mg po q 6 h or doxycycline 100 mg po q 12 h, continued for at least 3 mo.

Trench Fever

(Wolhynia, Shin Bone, or Quintan Fever)

Trench fever is a louse- and tick-borne disease caused by *Bartonella quintana* or *B. henselae* and observed originally in military populations during World Wars I and II. Symptoms are an acute, recurring febrile illness, occasionally with a rash. Diagnosis is by blood culture. Treatment is with a macrolide or doxycycline.

Humans are the only reservoir. *B. quintana* is transmitted to humans when feces from infected lice are rubbed into abraded skin or the conjunctiva. *B. henselae* is transmitted by tick bites. The disease is endemic in Mexico, Tunisia, Eritrea, Poland, and the former Soviet Union and is reappearing in the homeless population in the US.

After a 14- to 30-day incubation period, onset is sudden, with fever, weakness, dizziness, headache, and severe back and leg pains. Fever may reach 40.5° C and persist for 5 to 6 days. In about ½ the cases, fever recurs 1 to 8 times at 5- to 6-day intervals. A transient macular or papular rash and, occasionally, hepatomegaly and splenomegaly occur. Relapses are common and have occurred up to 10 yr after the initial attack.

Trench fever should be suspected in people living where louse infestation is heavy. Leptospirosis, typhus, relapsing fever, and malaria must be considered.

The organism is identified by blood culture, although it may take 1 to 4 wk to grow. The disease is marked by persistent bacteremia during the initial attack, during relapses, and throughout the asymptomatic periods between relapses. Although recovery is usually complete in 1 to 2 mo and mortality is negligible, bacteremia may persist for months after clinical recovery, and prolonged (>1 mo) macrolide or doxycycline treatment may be needed. Body lice must be controlled (see p. 994).

BRUCELLOSIS

(Undulant, Malta, Mediterranean, or Gibraltar Fever)

Brucellosis is caused by *Brucella* sp. Symptoms begin as an acute febrile illness with few or no localized signs and progress to a chronic stage with relapses of fever, weakness, sweats, and vague aches and pains. Diagnosis is by culture, usually from the blood. Optimal treatment usually requires 2 antibiotics—doxycycline or trimethoprim-sulfamethoxazole plus streptomycin or rifampin.

Epidemiology

The causative organisms of human brucellosis are *Brucella abortus* (from cattle), *B. melitensis* (from sheep and goats), and *B. suis* (from hogs). *B. canis* (from dogs) has caused sporadic infections. The most common sources of infection are farm animals and raw dairy products. *Brucella* infections of deer, bison, horses, moose, caribou, hares, chickens, and desert rats have also occurred.

Brucellosis is acquired by direct contact with secretions and excretions of infected animals and by ingesting raw milk or milk products containing viable organisms. It is rarely transmitted from person to person. Most prevalent in rural areas, brucellosis is an occupational disease of meatpackers, veterinarians, hunters, farmers, and livestock producers. Brucellosis is rare in the US, Europe, and Canada, but cases occur in the Middle East, Mediterranean regions, Mexico, and Central America.

Symptoms and Signs

The incubation period varies from 5 days to several months and averages 2 wk. Onset may be sudden, with chills and fever, severe headache, joint and low back pain, malaise, and occasionally diarrhea. Onset may also be insidious, with mild prodromal malaise, muscular pain, headache, and pain in the back of the neck, followed by a rise in evening temperature. As the disease progresses, the temperature increases to 40 to 41° C, then subsides gradually to normal or near-normal with profuse sweating in the morning.

Typically, intermittent fever persists for 1 to 5 wk, followed by a 2- to 14-day remission when symptoms are greatly diminished or absent. In some patients, fever may be transient. In others, the febrile phase recurs once or repeatedly in waves (undulations) and remissions over months or years.

After the initial febrile phase, anorexia, weight loss, abdominal and joint pain, headache, backache, weakness, irritability, insomnia, depression, and emotional instability may occur. Constipation is usually pronounced. Splenomegaly appears, and lymph nodes may be slightly or moderately enlarged. Up to 50% of patients have hepatomegaly.

Patients with acute, uncomplicated brucellosis usually recover in 2 to 3 wk, even without treatment. Some go on to subacute, intermittent, or chronic disease. Complications are rare but include subacute bacterial endocarditis, meningitis, encephalitis, neuritis, orchitis, cholecystitis, hepatic suppuration, and osteomyelitis.

Diagnosis

Blood cultures should be obtained; growth may take > 7 days, so the laboratory should be notified of the suspicion of brucellosis. Acute and convalescent sera should be obtained 3 wk apart. A 4-fold increase or an acute titer of 1:160 or higher is considered diagnostic, particularly if a history of exposure and characteristic clinical findings are present. The WBC count is normal or reduced with relative or absolute lymphocytosis during the acute phase.

Treatment

Activity should be restricted in acute cases, with bed rest recommended during febrile episodes.

If antibiotics are given, combination therapy is preferred. Doxycycline 100 mg po bid for 3 to 6 wk plus streptomycin 1 g IM q 12 to 24 h for 14 days lowers the rate of relapses. In children < 8 yr, trimethoprim-sulfamethoxazole (TMP-SMX) and either IM streptomycin or oral rifampin for 4 to 6 wk have been used. Severe musculoskeletal pains, especially over the spine, may require analgesia.

Pasteurization of milk helps prevent brucellosis. Cheese made from unpasteurized milk that is aged < 3 mo may be contaminated. People handling animals or carcasses likely to be infected should wear goggles and rubber gloves and protect skin breaks from exposure. Programs to detect infection in animals, eliminate infected animals, and vaccinate young seronegative cattle and swine are required in the US and in several other countries. Immunity after human infection is short-lived, on the order of 2 yr.

CAMPYLOBACTER AND RELATED INFECTIONS

Campylobacter infections commonly cause diarrhea and occasionally bacteremia, with consequent endocarditis, osteomyelitis, or septic arthritis.

Epidemiology

Campylobacter sp are motile, curved, microaerophilic, gram-negative bacilli that normally inhabit the GI tract of many domestic animals and fowl. Several species are human pathogens. Most cause diarrhea in all age groups, although peak incidence appears to be from age 1 to 5 yr. *Campylobacter* accounts for more cases of diarrhea in the US than *Salmonella* and *Shigella* combined. *C. fetus* and several others typically cause bacteremia in adults, more often when underlying predisposing diseases, such as diabetes, cirrhosis, or malignancy, are present. In patients with immunoglobulin deficiencies, these organisms may cause difficult-to-treat, relapsing infections. *C. jejuni* can cause meningitis in infants.

Contact with infected animals and ingestion of contaminated food (especially undercooked poultry) or water have been implicated in outbreaks. However, for sporadic cases, the source of the infecting organism frequently is obscure. There is an association between summer outbreaks of *C. jejuni* diarrheal illness and subsequent development (up to 30% of cases) of Guillain-Barré syndrome.

Symptoms, Signs, and Diagnosis

The most common presentation is watery and sometimes bloody diarrhea. Fever (38 to 40° C), which follows a relapsing or intermittent course, is the only constant feature of systemic *Campylobacter* infection, although abdominal pain and hepatosplenomegaly are frequent. Infection can also present as subacute bacterial endocarditis, septic arthritis, meningitis, or an indolent FUO.

Diagnosis, particularly to differentiate *Campylobacter* infection from ulcerative colitis (see p. 155), requires microbiologic evaluation. Stool culture should be obtained and also blood cultures for patients with signs of focal infection or serious systemic illness. WBCs are present in stained smears of stool.

Treatment

Most enteric infections resolve spontaneously, although erythromycin 500 mg po q 6 h for 5 days may be helpful. For patients with extraintestinal infections, antibiotic treatment should be 2 to 4 wk to prevent relapses.

CHOLERA

Cholera is an acute infection of the small bowel by _Vibrio cholerae_, which secretes a toxin that produces copious watery diarrhea, leading to dehydration, oliguria, and collapse. Infection is typically through contaminated water or seafood. Diagnosis is by culture or serology. Treatment is vigorous rehydration and electrolyte replacement along with doxycycline.

Epidemiology and Pathophysiology

The causative organism, *V. cholerae*, serogroups 01 and 0139, is a short, curved, motile, aerobic bacillus that produces enterotoxin, a protein that induces hypersecretion of an isotonic electrolyte solution by the small-bowel mucosa. Both the El Tor and classic biotypes of *V. cholerae* can cause severe disease. However, mild or asymptomatic infection is much more common with the El Tor biotype.

Cholera is spread by ingestion of water, seafood, and other foods contaminated by the excrement of people with symptomatic or asymptomatic infection. Cholera is endemic in portions of Asia, the Middle East, Africa, South and Central America, and the Gulf Coast of the US. Cases transported into Europe, Japan, and Australia have caused localized outbreaks. In endemic areas, outbreaks usually occur during warm months. The incidence is highest in children. In newly affected areas, epidemics may occur during any season and all ages are equally susceptible. A milder form of gastroenteritis is caused by noncholera vibrios (see p. 1460).

Susceptibility to infection varies and is greater for people with blood type O. Because the vibrio is sensitive to gastric acid, hypochlorhydria and achlorhydria are predisposing factors. People living in endemic areas gradually acquire a natural immunity.

Symptoms, Signs, and Diagnosis

The incubation period is 1 to 3 days. Cholera can be subclinical, a mild, uncomplicated episode of diarrhea, or a fulminant, potentially lethal disease. Abrupt, painless, watery diarrhea and vomiting are usually the initial symptoms. Significant nausea is typically absent. Stool loss in adults may exceed 1 L/h but is usually much less. The resultant severe water and electrolyte depletion leads to intense thirst, oliguria, muscle cramps, weakness, and marked loss of tissue turgor, with sunken eyes and wrinkling of skin on the fingers. Hypovolemia, hemoconcentration, oliguria and anuria, and severe metabolic acidosis with K^+ depletion (but normal serum Na^+ concentration) occur. If untreated, circulatory collapse with cyanosis and stupor may follow. Prolonged hypovolemia can cause renal tubular necrosis.

Diagnosis is confirmed by stool culture and subsequent serotyping. Cholera can be distinguished from clinically similar disease caused by enterotoxin-producing strains of *Escherichia coli* and occasionally by *Salmonella* and *Shigella*. Serum electrolytes, BUN, and creatinine should be measured.

Treatment

Replacement of fluid loss is essential. Mild cases can be treated with standard oral replacement formulas (see p. 2293). Rapid correction of severe hypovolemia is lifesaving. Prevention or correction of metabolic acidosis and hypokalemia is important. For hypovolemic and severely dehydrated patients, IV replacement with isotonic fluids should be used (for details on fluid resuscitation, see pp. 564 and 2289). Water should also be given freely by mouth. To replace K^+ losses, KCl 10 to 15 mEq/L can be added to the IV solution, or $KHCO_3$ 1 mL/kg po of a 100-g/L solution can be given qid. K^+ replacement is especially important for children, who tolerate hypokalemia poorly.

Once intravascular volume is restored, amounts for replacement of continuing losses should equal measured stool volume. Adequacy of hydration is confirmed by frequent clinical evaluation (pulse rate and strength, skin turgor, urine output). Plasma, plasma volume expanders, and vasopressors should *not* be used in place of water and electrolytes.

Oral glucose-electrolyte solution is effective in replacing stool losses and may be used after initial IV rehydration, and it may be the only means of rehydration in epidemic areas where supplies of parenteral fluids are limited. Patients with mild or moderate dehydration who can drink may be rehydrated with the oral solution exclusively (about 75 mL/kg in 4 h). Those with more severe dehydration need more and may need to receive the fluid by nasogastric tube. The oral solution recommended by the WHO contains 20 g glucose; 3.5 g NaCl; 2.9 g trisodium citrate and dihydrate (or 2.5 g $NaHCO_3$); and 1.5 g KCl per liter of drinking water. This should be continued ad libitum after rehydration in amounts at least equal to continuing stool and vomitus losses. Solid food should be given only after vomiting stops and appetite returns.

Early treatment with an effective oral antimicrobial eradicates vibrios, reduces stool volume by 50%, and stops diarrhea within 48 h. The choice of antimicrobial should be based on the susceptibility of *V. cholerae* isolated from the community. Drugs effective for susceptible strains include doxycycline (in adults, a single dose of 300 mg po); furazolidone (adults, 100 mg po qid for 72 h; children, 1.5 mg/kg qid for 72 h); trimethoprim-sulfamethoxazole (TMP-SMX; adults, one double-strength tablet bid; children, 5 mg/kg bid [TMP] for 72 h).

Most patients are free of *V. cholerae* within 2 wk after cessation of diarrhea, but a few become chronic biliary tract carriers.

Prevention

To control cholera, human excrement must be properly disposed of and water supplies purified. Drinking water should be boiled or chlorinated and vegetables and fish cooked thoroughly.

A killed oral whole cell–B subunit vaccine (not available in the US) provides 85% protection against the 01 serogroup for 4 to 6 mo. Protection lasts up to 3 yr in adults but wanes rapidly in children and is greater for the classic than the El Tor biotype. There is no cross-protection between 01 and 0139 serogroups. Vaccines proven effective against both serogroups are a future goal. Parenteral cholera vaccine gives only short-term, partial protection and is not recommended. Prompt prophylaxis with doxycycline 100 mg po q 12 h in adults (TMP-SMX can be used for prophylaxis in children < 9 yr) can decrease secondary cases among household contacts of cholera patients, but mass prophylaxis is inappropriate and some strains are not sensitive.

NONCHOLERA *VIBRIO* INFECTIONS

Noncholera vibrios do not produce enterotoxin or invade the bloodstream, but they can cause dysentery, cellulitis, and septicemia. Symptoms are weakness, low-grade fever, cramping abdominal pain, watery or bloody diarrhea with tenesmus, or manifes-

tations of localized wound infection or generalized sepsis. Diagnosis is by routine cultures of stool, wounds, or blood. Treatment is with ciprofloxacin or doxycycline and fluids and electrolytes; local lesions may require surgical debridement.

Epidemiology

The noncholera vibrios are *Vibrio parahaemolyticus, V. mimicus, V. alginolyticus, V. hollisae, V. vulnificus*, and the so-called nonagglutinable vibrios. *V. parahaemolyticus* is a halophilic organism incriminated in foodborne (inadequately cooked seafood, usually shrimp) outbreaks of diarrhea in Japan and in coastal areas of the US. The organism neither produces enterotoxin nor invades the bloodstream but damages the intestinal mucosa. Severe infections with nonagglutinable vibrios have usually been reported in patients with liver disease and other immunodeficiencies, although otherwise healthy people can develop severe infections. Neither *V. alginolyticus* nor *V. vulnificus* causes enteritis, but both can cause marine wound infection.

Symptoms, Signs, and Diagnosis

After a 15- to 24-h incubation period, enteric illness begins acutely with cramping abdominal pain, large amounts of watery diarrhea (stools may be bloody and contain PMNs), tenesmus, weakness, and sometimes low-grade fever. Symptoms subside spontaneously in 24 to 48 h. Nonagglutinable vibrios may cause a cholera-like illness, and they have been isolated from wounds and blood.

Wounds infected through warm seawater can progress rapidly to cellulitis, in some cases resulting in necrotizing fasciitis with typical hemorrhagic, bullous lesions.

V. vulnificus, when ingested by a compromised host (often someone with chronic liver disease or immunodeficiency), crosses the intestinal mucosa without causing enteritis and produces septicemia with a high mortality rate.

Wound and bloodstream infections are readily diagnosed with routine cultures. When enteric infection is suspected, *Vibrio* organisms can be cultured from stool on thiosulfate citrate bile salts sucrose medium. Contaminated seafood also yields positive cultures.

Treatment

Noncholera *Vibrio* infections can be treated with a single dose of ciprofloxacin 1 g po or doxycycline 300 mg po. With diarrhea, close attention to volume repletion and replacing electrolyte losses is needed. For patients with necrotizing fasciitis, surgical debridement is also required.

ESCHERICHIA COLI INFECTIONS

***Escherichia coli* are the most numerous aerobic commensal inhabitants of the large intestine. Certain strains produce toxins that cause diarrhea, and all strains produce infection when they invade sterile tissues. Diagnosis is by standard culture techniques. Toxin assays may be helpful for diarrhea. Treatment with antibiotics is guided by sensitivity studies.**

E. coli normally inhabits the GI tract. Enterotoxigenic and enteropathogenic strains are major causes of diarrhea in infants and traveler's diarrhea in adults (see p. 137). Enterohemorrhagic strains of *E. coli*, such as type O157:H7 (see p. 1462), produce several cytotoxins, neurotoxins, and enterotoxins, including Shiga toxin, and cause bloody diarrhea, which, in 2 to 7% of cases, may lead to hemolytic-uremic syndrome (see p. 1070). Such strains have most often been acquired from undercooked ground beef. Other strains of enteroaggregative *E. coli* are emerging as potentially important causes of persistent diarrhea in patients with AIDS and in children in tropical areas.

If normal intestinal anatomic barriers are disrupted (eg, by ischemia, inflammatory bowel disease, trauma), the organism may spread to adjacent structures or invade the bloodstream.

The extraintestinal site most often infected by *E. coli* is the urinary tract, which is generally colonized by ascending infection from the perineum. Hepatobiliary, peritoneal, cutaneous, and pulmonary infections also occur. *E. coli* bacteremia may also occur without an evident portal of entry. *E. coli* bacteremia and meningitis are common in newborns, particularly preterm infants (see Neonatal Meningitis on p. 2330 and Neonatal Sepsis on p. 2333).

Samples of blood, stool, or other clinical material are sent for culture. If an enterohemorrhagic strain is suspected, the laboratory must be notified because special culture media are required.

Treatment must be started empirically and then modified on the basis of antibiotic sensitivity studies. Many strains are resistant to ampicillin and tetracyclines, so that other drugs should be used, including ticarcillin, piperacillin, the cephalosporins, aminoglycosides, trimethoprim-sulfamethoxazole (TMP-SMX), and fluoroquinolones. Surgery may be required to drain pus, debride necrotic lesions, or remove foreign bodies.

E. coli O157:H7 Infection

E. coli O157:H7 typically causes acute bloody diarrhea, which may lead to hemolytic-uremic syndrome. Symptoms are abdominal cramps and diarrhea that may be grossly bloody. Fever is not prominent. Diagnosis is by stool culture and toxin assay. Treatment is supportive; antibiotic use is controversial.

Epidemiology

Although over 100 serotypes of *E. coli* produce Shiga and Shiga-like toxins, *E. coli* O157:H7 is the most common in North America. In some parts of the US and Canada, *E. coli* O157:H7 infection may be a more common cause of bloody diarrhea than shigellosis or salmonellosis. It can occur in people of all ages, although severe infection is most common in children and the elderly. *E. coli* O157:H7 has a bovine reservoir, so outbreaks and sporadic cases occur after ingestion of undercooked beef (especially ground beef) or unpasteurized milk. Food or water contaminated with cow manure or raw ground beef can also transmit infection. The organism can also be transmitted (especially among infants in diapers) by the fecal-oral route.

After ingestion, *E. coli* O157:H7 and similar strains of *E. coli* (termed enterohemorrhagic *E. coli*) produce high levels of various toxins in the large intestine that are closely related to the potent cytotoxins produced by *Shigella dysenteriae* type 1, cholera, and other enteropathogens. These toxins appear to directly damage mucosal cells and vascular endothelial cells in the gut wall. If absorbed, they exert toxic effects on other vascular endothelia (eg, renal).

Symptoms and Signs

E. coli O157:H7 infection typically begins acutely with severe abdominal cramps and watery diarrhea that may become grossly bloody within 24 h. Some patients report diarrhea as being "all blood and no stool," which has given rise to the term hemorrhagic colitis. Fever, usually absent or low grade, may occasionally reach 39° C. Diarrhea may last 1 to 8 days in uncomplicated infections.

About 5% of cases (mostly children < 5 yr and adults > 60 yr) are complicated by the hemolytic-uremic syndrome (see p. 1070), which typically develops in the 2nd wk of illness. Death may occur, especially in the elderly, with or without this complication.

Diagnosis

E. coli O157:H7 infection should be distinguished from other infectious diarrheas by isolating the organism from stool cultures. Often, the clinician must specifically ask the laboratory to test for the organism. Because bloody diarrhea and severe abdominal pain without fever suggest various noninfectious etiologies, *E. coli* O157:H7 infection should be considered in suspected cases of ischemic colitis, intussusception, and inflammatory bowel disease. A rapid stool assay for Shiga toxin may help. Patients at risk of noninfectious diarrheas may need sigmoidoscopy. If performed, sigmoidoscopy may reveal erythema and edema; barium enema typically shows evidence of edema with thumbprinting.

Treatment and Prevention

The mainstay of treatment is supportive. Although *E. coli* is sensitive to most commonly used antimicrobials, antibiotics have not been shown to alleviate symptoms, reduce carriage of the organism, or prevent hemolytic-uremic syndrome. Fluoroquinolones are suspected of increasing release of enterotoxins.

In the week after infection, patients at high risk for developing hemolytic-uremic syndrome (eg, children < 5 yr, the elderly) should be observed for early signs, such as proteinuria, hematuria, red cell casts, and rising serum creatinine. Edema and hypertension develop later. Patients who develop complications are likely to require intensive care, including dialysis and other specific therapies, at a tertiary medical center.

Proper disposal of the stool of infected people, good hygiene, and careful hand washing with soap limit spread of infection. Preventive measures that may be effective in the day care setting include grouping children known to be infected with *E. coli* O157:H7 or requiring 2 negative stool cultures before allowing infected children to attend. Pasteurization of milk and thorough cooking of beef prevent food-borne transmission. Reporting outbreaks of bloody diarrhea to public health authorities is important, because intervention can prevent additional infections.

HAEMOPHILUS INFECTIONS

***Haemophilus* sp cause numerous mild and serious infections, including bacteremia, meningitis, pneumonia, otitis media, cellulitis, and epiglottitis. Diagnosis is by culture and serotyping. Treatment is with antibiotics.**

There are several pathogenic species of *Haemophilus*, the most common of which is *H. influenzae*, which has 6 distinct encapsulated strains, a through f, and numerous nonencapsulated, nontypeable strains. Before the use of *H. influenzae* type b (Hib) conjugate vaccine, most cases of serious, invasive disease were caused by type b. *H. influenzae* causes many childhood infections, including meningitis, bacteremia, septic arthritis, pneumonia, tracheobronchitis, otitis media, conjunctivitis, sinusitis, and acute epiglottitis. These infections, as well as endocarditis, may occur in adults, although far less commonly. These illnesses are discussed elsewhere in THE MANUAL. Occasionally, nonencapsulated strains cause invasive infections.

H. influenzae serotype *aegyptius* may cause mucopurulent conjunctivitis and bacteremic Brazilian purpuric fever. *H. ducreyi* causes chancroid (see p. 1650). *H. parainfluenzae* and *H. aphrophilus* are rare causes of bacteremia, endocarditis, and brain abscess.

Many *Haemophilus* sp are normal flora in the upper respiratory tract and rarely cause illness. Pathogenic strains enter the upper respiratory tract through droplet inhalation or direct contact. Spread is rapid in nonimmune populations. Children are at highest risk of serious infection, particularly males, blacks, and Native Americans. Overcrowded living conditions and day care center attendance predispose to infection, as do immunodeficiency states, asplenia, and sickle cell disease.

Diagnosis and Treatment

Diagnosis is by culture of blood and body fluids. Strains involved with invasive illness should be serotyped.

Treatment depends on nature and location of the infection, but doxycycline, fluoroquinolones, 2nd- and 3rd-generation cephalosporins, and carbapenems are used for invasive disease. The Hib vaccine has markedly reduced the rate of bacteremia. Children with serious illness are hospitalized with contact and respiratory isolation for 24 h after starting antibiotics. Antibiotic choices depend strongly on the site of infection and require sensitivity testing; many isolates in the US produce β-lactamase. For invasive illness, including meningitis, cefotaxime or ceftriaxone is recommended. For less serious infections, oral cephalosporins, macrolides, and amoxicillin-clavulanate are generally effective. (See individual disease entries for specific recommendations.)

Prevention

Hib conjugate vaccines are available for children ≥ 2 mo of age and have reduced invasive infections such as meningitis, epiglottitis, and bacteremia by 99%. A primary series is given at 2, 4, and 6 mo or 2 and 4 mo, depending on the vaccine product. A booster at 12 to 15 mo is indicated.

Contacts within the household may have asymptomatic *H. influenzae* carriage. Unimmunized or incompletely immunized household contacts < 4 yr are at risk for illness and should receive a dose of vaccine. In addition, all household members (except pregnant women) should receive prophylaxis with rifampin 600 mg (20 mg/kg for children) po once/day for 4 days. Nursery or day care contacts should receive prophylaxis if ≥ 2 cases of invasive disease occurred in 60 days. The benefit of prophylaxis if only one case occurred has not been established.

HACEK INFECTIONS

The HACEK group includes weakly virulent, gram-negative organisms that primarily cause endocarditis.

The HACEK group of nonmotile, gram-negative bacilli or coccobacilli contains a number of minimally pathogenic, slow-growing, fastidious genera including *Haemophilus* sp. Also included in the group are *Actinobacillus actinomycetemcomitans, Cardiobacterium hominis, Eikenella corrodens*, and *Kingella kingae*. Their primary pathology is endocarditis in susceptible people, of which about 1% is due to this group. *A. actinomycetemcomitans* is usually found along with *A. israelii* (see Actinomycosis on p. 1496). *E. corrodens* is usually found in human bite wounds, endocarditis, brain and visceral abscesses, osteomyelitis, respiratory infections, uterine infections from intrauterine devices, and mixed soft-tissue infections. *Haemophilus* strains may cause respiratory infections or, less commonly, endocarditis.

Antibiotic sensitivities differ among species, so treatment should be directed by sensitivity studies.

KLEBSIELLA, ENTEROBACTER, AND *SERRATIA* INFECTIONS

***Klebsiella, Enterobacter*, and *Serratia* are closely related normal intestinal flora that rarely cause disease in normal hosts.**

Infections with *Klebsiella, Enterobacter*, and *Serratia* are usually hospital-acquired and occur mainly in patients with diminished resistance. Usually, *Klebsiella, Enterobacter*, and *Serratia* cause infections in the respiratory or urinary tract that present as pneumonia, cystitis, or pyelitis and may progress to lung abscess, empyema, and septicemia. *Klebsiella* pneumonia, a rare and severe disease with dark brown or red currant–jelly sputum, lung abscess formation, and empyema, is most common in diabetics and alcoholics. *Serratia,* particularly *S. marcescens*, has greater affinity for the urinary tract. *Enterobacter* can cause otitis media, cellulitis, and neonatal sepsis.

Treatment is with 3rd-generation cephalosporins, cefepime, carbapenems, fluoroquinolones, piperacillin-tazobactam, or aminoglycosides. However, because some isolates are resistant to multiple antibiotics, sensitivity studies are essential. *Enterobacter* strains are prone to develop resistance to cephalosporins during treatment.

LEGIONELLA INFECTIONS

***Legionella pneumophila* most often causes pneumonia, with extrapulmonary features. Diagnosis requires specific growth media, serologic testing, or PCR analysis. Treatment is with doxycycline, macrolides, or fluoroquinolones.**

The 1st appearance of this organism was in 1976 at a convention of the American Legion, thus the name Legionnaires' disease. Nonpneumonic infection is called Pontiac fever. The organisms can be found in soil and freshwater. Manufactured water-storage containers, including water-cooled air-conditioning units, enhance its growth. Spread is most likely by aerosols of potable water.

Extrapulmonary foci of infection occur most frequently in hospitalized patients and most commonly involve the heart. Other sites include the CNS, liver, and intestines. Immunocompromised patients, cigarette smokers, the elderly, and those with chronic lung disease are principally affected.

Symptoms, Signs, and Diagnosis

Legionnaires' disease is a flu-like syndrome with acute fever, chills, malaise, myalgias, headache, or confusion. Frequently nausea, loose stools/watery diarrhea, abdominal pain, cough, and arthralgias also occur. Pneumonic manifestations may include dyspnea, pleuritic pain, and hemoptysis.

Diagnosis is by examination of sputum or bronchoalveolar lavage fluid; blood cultures are unreliable. Slow growth on laboratory media may delay identification for 3 to 5 days. Direct fluorescent antibody staining of sputum or lavage fluid is frequently used. In addition, PCR with DNA probing is available. A urinary antigen test is 70% sensitive and 100% specific 3 days after symptom onset but detects only *L. pneumophila* (serogroup 1) and not non-*pneumophila Legionella*. Paired acute and convalescent antibody assays may yield a delayed diagnosis. A 4-fold increase, or an acute titer of ≥ 1:128, is considered diagnostic. Chest x-rays usually show nonspecific changes such as infiltrates and pleural effusions.

Treatment

Doxycycline, macrolides, and fluoroquinolones are highly effective for Legionnaires' disease. Any respiratory quinolone (given IV or po) for 7 to 14 days is the recommended regimen. Rifampin may be added for severe infections. Mortality is low in otherwise healthy people but can reach 50% in hospital-acquired outbreaks.

MELIOIDOSIS

Melioidosis is infection caused by *Burkholderia* (formerly *Pseudomonas*) *pseudomallei*. Presentations include pneumonia, septicemia, and localized infection in various

organs. Diagnosis is by culture or serology. Treatment with antibiotics, such as ceftazidime, is prolonged.

The organism can be isolated from soil and water and is endemic in Southeast Asia; Australia; Central, West, and East Africa; India; and China. Humans may contract melioidosis by contamination of skin abrasions or burns, ingestion, or inhalation but not directly from infected animals or other humans. In endemic areas, melioidosis is likely to occur in patients with AIDS.

Symptoms, Signs, and Diagnosis

Infection may be asymptomatic, or remain latent for years. Mortality is < 10%, except in acute septicemic melioidosis, which is frequently fatal.

Acute pulmonary infection is the most common form. It varies from mild to overwhelming necrotizing pneumonia. Onset may be abrupt or gradual, with headache, anorexia, pleuritic or dull aching chest pain, and generalized myalgia. Fever is usually > 39° C. Cough, tachypnea, and rales are characteristic. Sputum may be blood-tinged. Chest x-rays usually show upper lobe consolidation, frequently cavitating and resembling TB. Nodular lesions, thin-walled cysts, and pleural effusion may also occur. The WBC count ranges from normal to 20,000/μL.

Disseminated septicemic infection begins abruptly, with septic shock and multiple organ involvement manifested by disorientation, extreme dyspnea, severe headache, pharyngitis, upper abdominal colic, diarrhea, and pustular skin lesions. High fever, hypotension, tachypnea, a bright erythematous flush, and cyanosis are present. Muscle tenderness may be striking. Signs of arthritis or meningitis sometimes occur. Pulmonary signs may be absent or may include rales, rhonchi, and pleural rubs.

Nondisseminated septicemic infection occurs when bacteremia involves only a single organ. It does not usually lead to shock.

Localized (chronic suppurative) infection causes secondary abscesses, most often in the skin, lymph nodes, or bone. Patients may be afebrile. An acute suppurative form is uncommon.

B. pseudomallei can be identified in exudates by methylene blue or Gram stain and by culture. Chest x-rays usually show irregular, nodular (4 to 10 mm) densities. The liver and spleen may be palpable. Liver function tests, AST, and bilirubin often are abnormal. The WBC count is normal or slightly increased.

Treatment

Asymptomatic infection needs no treatment. Mildly ill patients are given trimethoprim-sulfamethoxazole (TMP-SMX), one double-strength tablet po bid for a minimum of 30 days. Moderately or seriously ill patients are given ceftazidime 30 mg/kg IV q 6 h for 2 to 4 wk (imipenem, meropenem, and piperacillin are acceptable substitutes), then oral TMP-SMX, or amoxicillin-clavulanate for 30 to 120 days.

PERTUSSIS

(Whooping Cough)

Pertussis is a highly communicable disease occurring mostly in children and teenagers that is caused by *Bordetella pertussis*. Symptoms are initially those of nonspecific URI followed by paroxysmal or spasmodic coughing that usually ends in a prolonged, high-pitched, crowing inspiration (the whoop). Diagnosis is by nasopharyngeal culture, PCR, and serologic assays. Treatment is with macrolide antibiotics.

Etiology and Pathophysiology

Pertussis is endemic throughout the world. Its incidence in the US cycles q 3 to 4 yr. In a given unimmunized locality, it becomes epidemic q 2 to 4 yr. It occurs at all ages, but 71% occurs in children < 5 yr, and 38% of the cases, including nearly all deaths, occur in infants < 6 mo. It is also serious in the elderly. Mortality is about 1 to 2% in children aged < 1 yr and is highest in the 1st month of life. Most deaths are caused by bronchopneumonia and cerebral complications. One attack does not confer life-long natural immunity, but secondary attacks are usually mild and often unrecognized.

Transmission by aerosols of *B. pertussis* (a small, nonmotile, gram-negative coccobacillus) from infected patients, particularly in the catarrhal and early paroxysmal stages, causes disease in 90 to 100% of close contacts. Transmission by contact with contaminated articles is rare. Patients usually are not infectious after the 3rd wk of the paroxysmal phase.

Respiratory complications are most common, including asphyxia in infants. Otitis media occurs frequently. Bronchopneumonia (also common in the elderly) may be fatal at any age. Seizures are common in infants but rare in older children. Hemorrhage into the brain, eyes, skin, and mucous membranes can result from severe paroxysms and consequent anoxia. Cerebral hemorrhage, cerebral edema, and toxic encephalitis may result in spastic paralysis, mental retardation, or other neurologic disorders. Umbilical herniation and rectal prolapse occasionally occur.

Parapertussis, caused by *Bordetella parapertussis*, may be clinically indistinguishable from pertussis but is usually milder and less often fatal.

Symptoms and Signs

The incubation period averages 7 to 14 days (maximum 3 wk). *B. pertussis* invades respiratory mucosa, increasing the secretion of mucus, which is initially thin and later viscid and tenacious. Uncomplicated disease lasts about 6 to 10 wk and consists of 3 stages: catarrhal, paroxysmal, and convalescent.

The catarrhal stage begins insidiously, generally with sneezing, lacrimation, or other signs of coryza; anorexia; listlessness; and a troublesome, hacking nocturnal cough that gradually becomes diurnal. Fever is rare.

After 10 to 14 days, the paroxysmal stage begins with an increase in the severity and frequency of the cough. Repeated bouts of ≥ 5 rapidly consecutive forceful coughs occur during a single expiration and are followed by the whoop—a hurried, deep inspiration. Copious viscid mucus may be expelled or bubble from the nares during or after the paroxysms. Vomiting is characteristic. In infants, choking spells (with or without cyanosis) may be more common than whoops.

Symptoms diminish as the convalescent stage begins, usually within 4 wk of onset. The average duration of illness is about 7 wk (range 3 wk to 3 mo). Paroxysmal coughing may recur for months, usually induced in the still-sensitive respiratory tract by irritation from a URI.

Diagnosis

The catarrhal stage is often difficult to distinguish from bronchitis or influenza. Adenovirus infections and TB should also be considered.

Cultures of nasopharyngeal specimens are positive for *B. pertussis* in 80 to 90% of cases in the catarrhal and early paroxysmal stages. Because special media and prolonged incubation are required, the laboratory should be notified that pertussis is suspected. Specific fluorescent antibody testing of nasopharyngeal smears accurately diagnoses pertussis but is not as sensitive as culture. PCR can also be used. The WBC count is usually between 15,000 and 20,000/μL but may be normal or as high as 60,000/μL, usually with 60 to 80% small lymphocytes.

Parapertussis is differentiated by culture or the fluorescent antibody technique.

Treatment

Hospitalization with respiratory isolation is recommended for seriously ill infants. Isolation is continued until antibiotics have been given for 5 days.

In infants, suction to remove excess mucus from the throat may be lifesaving. O_2 and tracheostomy or nasotracheal intubation is occasionally needed. Theophylline, albuterol, and corticosteroids may ameliorate symptoms. Expectorants, cough suppressants, and mild sedation are of little value. Because any disturbance can precipitate serious paroxysmal coughing with anoxia, seriously ill infants should be kept in a darkened, quiet room and disturbed as little as possible. Patients treated at home should be quarantined, particularly from susceptible infants, for at least 4 wk from disease onset and until symptoms have subsided.

Antibiotics given in the catarrhal stage may ameliorate the disease. After paroxysms are established, antibiotics usually have no clinical effect but are recommended to limit spread. Preferred drugs are erythromycin 10 to 12.5 mg/kg po q 6 h (max 2 g/day) for 14 days or azithromycin 10 to 12 mg/kg po once/day for 5 days. Antibiotics should also be used for bacterial complications, eg, bronchopneumonia and otitis media.

Prevention

Active immunization is part of standard childhood vaccination. Five doses of vaccine are given (usually combined with diphtheria and tetanus [DTP or DTaP]) at 2, 4, and 6 mo of age; boosters are given at 15 to 18 mo and 4 to 6 yr. Significant adverse effects from the pertussis component of the vaccine include encephalopathy within 7 days; seizure, with or without fever, within 3 days; persistent, severe, inconsolable screaming or crying for ≥ 3 h; collapse or shock within 48 h; fever ≥ 40.5° C within 48 h; and immediate severe or anaphylactic reaction. These reactions contraindicate further use of pertussis vaccine; combined diphtheria and tetanus vaccine is available without the pertussis component. The acellular vaccine (DTaP) is better tolerated.

Immunity after natural infection lasts about 20 yr. Passive immunization is unreliable and is not recommended.

Close contacts < 7 yr who have had < 4 doses of vaccine should be vaccinated. Contacts of all ages, whether vaccinated or not, should receive a 10-day course of erythromycin 500 mg po qid or 10 to 12.5 mg/kg po qid.

PLAGUE AND OTHER *YERSINIA* INFECTIONS

(Bubonic Plague; Pestis; Black Death)

Plague is caused by *Yersinia pestis*. Symptoms are either severe pneumonia or massive lymphadenopathy with high fever, often progressing to septicemia. Diagnosis is epidemiologic and clinical, confirmed by culture and serology. Treatment is with a fluoroquinolone or doxycycline.

Yersinia (formerly *Pasteurella*) *pestis* is a short bacillus that often shows bipolar staining (especially with Giemsa stain) and may resemble a safety pin.

Plague occurs primarily in wild rodents (eg, rats, mice, squirrels, prairie dogs) and is transmitted from rodent to human by the bite of an infected flea vector. Human-to-human transmission occurs by inhaling droplet nuclei from patients with pulmonary infection (primary pneumonic plague), which is highly contagious. In endemic areas in the US, several cases may have been caused by household pets, especially cats. Transmission from cats can be by bite, or if the cat has pneumonic plague, by inhalation of infected droplets.

Massive human epidemics have occurred (eg, the Black Death of the Middle Ages). More recently, plague has occurred sporadically or in limited outbreaks. In the US, > 90% of human plague occurs in the Southwest, especially New Mexico, Arizona, California, and Colorado. *Yersinia* is considered a possible agent of bioterrorism.

Symptoms and Signs

In bubonic plague, the most common form, the incubation period is usually 2 to 5 days but varies from a few hours to 12 days. Onset of fever of 39.5 to 41° C is abrupt, often with chills. The pulse may be rapid and thready; hypotension may occur. Enlarged lymph nodes (buboes) appear with or shortly before the fever. The femoral or inguinal lymph nodes are most commonly involved, followed by axillary, cervical, or multiple nodes. Typically, the nodes are extremely tender and firm, surrounded by considerable edema. They may suppurate in the 2nd wk. The overlying skin is smooth and reddened but often not warm. A primary cutaneous lesion, varying from a small vesicle with slight local lymphangitis to an eschar, occasionally appears at the bite. The patient may be restless, delirious, confused, and uncoordinated. The liver and spleen may be enlarged.

Primary pneumonic plague has a 2- to 3-day incubation period, followed by abrupt onset of high fever, chills, tachycardia, and headache, often severe. Cough, not prominent initially, develops within 24 h. Sputum is mucoid at first, rapidly develops blood specks, and then becomes uniformly pink or bright red (resembling raspberry syrup) and foamy. Tachypnea and dyspnea are present, but pleurisy is not. Signs of consolidation are rare, and rales may be absent.

Septicemic plague usually occurs with the bubonic form as an acute, fulminant illness. Abdominal pain, presumably due to mesenteric lymphadenopathy, occurs in 40% of patients. Pharyngeal plague and plague meningitis are less common forms.

Pestis minor, a more benign form of bubonic plague, usually occurs only in endemic areas. Lymphadenitis, fever, headache, and prostration subside within a week.

The mortality rate for untreated patients with bubonic plague is about 60%, with most deaths occurring from sepsis in 3 to 5 days. Most untreated patients with pneumonic plague die within 48 h of symptom onset. Septicemic plague may be fatal before bubonic or pulmonary manifestations predominate.

Diagnosis

Diagnosis is made by stain and culture of the organism, typically by needle aspiration of a bubo (surgical drainage may disseminate the organism); blood and sputum cultures should also be obtained. Other tests include immunofluorescent staining and serology; a titer of > 1:16 or a 4-fold rise between acute and convalescent titers is positive. PCR testing, if available, is diagnostic. Prior vaccination does not exclude plague; clinical illness may occur in vaccinated people.

Patients with pulmonary symptoms or signs should have a chest x-ray, which shows a rapidly progressing pneumonia in pneumonic plague. The WBC count is usually 10,000 to 20,000/μL with numerous immature neutrophils.

Treatment

Immediate treatment reduces mortality to < 5%. In septicemic or pneumonic plague, treatment must begin within 24 h with streptomycin 7.5 mg/kg IM q 6 h for 7 to 10 days. Many physicians give higher initial dosages, up to 0.5 g IM q 3 h for 48 h. Doxycycline 100 mg IV or po q 12 h is an alternative. Gentamicin is probably also effective. For plague meningitis, chloramphenicol should be given in a loading dose of 25 mg/kg IV, followed by 12.5 mg/kg IV or po q 6 h.

Routine isolation precautions are adequate for patients with bubonic plague. Those with primary or secondary pneumonic plague require strict respiratory isolation. All pneumonic plague contacts should be under medical surveillance. Temperature should be taken q 4 h for 6 days. If this is not possible, tetracycline 1 g once/day po for 6 days can be given, but this can produce drug-resistant strains.

Rodents should be controlled and repellents used to minimize flea bites. Travelers should consider prophylaxis with doxycycline 100 mg po q 12 h during exposure periods.

OTHER *YERSINIA* INFECTIONS

Yersinia enterocolitica and *Y. pseudotuberculosis* occur worldwide and cause human infection.

Y. enterocolitica is a common cause of diarrheal disease and mesenteric adenitis. *Y. pseudotuberculosis* more commonly causes mesenteric adenitis and has been suspected in cases of interstitial nephritis, hemolytic-uremic syndrome, and a scarlet fever–like illness. Both species can cause pharyngitis, septicemia, focal infections in multiple organs, and reactive arthritis. Mortality from septicemia may be as high as 50%, even with treatment.

The organisms can be identified in standard cultures from normally sterile sites. Selective culture methods are required for nonsterile specimens. Serologic assays are available but difficult and not standardized. Diagnosis, particularly of the reactive arthritis, requires a high index of suspicion and close communication with the clinical laboratory.

Treatment of diarrhea is supportive because the disease is self-limited. Septic complications require β-lactamase–resistant antibiotics guided by sensitivity testing. Prevention focuses on food-handling and preparation, household pets, and epidemiology of suspected outbreaks.

PROTEEAE INFECTIONS

The Proteeae are normal fecal flora that often cause infection in patients whose normal flora have been disturbed by antibiotic therapy.

The Proteeae constitute at least 3 genera of gram-negative organisms: *Proteus* (*P. mirabilis, P. vulgaris*, and *P. myxofaciens*), *Morganella* (*M. morganii*), and *Providencia* (*P. rettgeri, P. alcalifaciens*, and *P. stuartii*). However, *P. mirabilis* causes most human infections. These organisms are normal fecal flora and can also be found in soil and water. They are often present in superficial wounds, draining ears, and sputum, particularly in patients whose normal flora has been eradicated by antibiotic therapy. They may cause bacteremia and deep-seated infections, particularly in the ears and mastoid sinuses, peritoneal cavity, and urinary tracts of patients with chronic UTIs or with renal or bladder stones.

P. mirabilis is often sensitive to ampicillin, carbenicillin, ticarcillin, piperacillin, the cephalosporins, and the aminoglycosides. The other species tend to be more resistant but generally are sensitive to the fluoroquinolones, carbapenems, piperacillin-tazobactam, 3rd-generation cephalosporins, and cefixime.

PSEUDOMONAS AND RELATED INFECTIONS

***Pseudomonas aeruginosa* and other members of this group of gram-negative bacilli are opportunistic pathogens that frequently cause hospital-acquired infections, particularly in ventilator patients, burn patients, and those with chronic debility. Many sites can be infected, and infection is usually severe. Diagnosis is by culture. Antibiotic choice varies with the pathogen and must be guided by sensitivity studies because resistance is common.**

Epidemiology

Pseudomonas is ubiquitous and favors moist environments. In humans, *P. aeruginosa* is the most common pathogen, but infection may result from *P. paucimobilis, P. putida, P. fluorescens*, and *P. acidovorans*. Other important hospital-acquired pathogens formerly classified as *Pseudomonas* include *Burkholderia cepacia* and *Stenotrophomonas maltophilia*. *Burkholderia pseudomallei* causes a distinct disease known as melioidosis that is mostly limited to the Asian tropics (see p. 1464).

P. aeruginosa can be found occasionally in the axilla and anogenital areas of normal skin but rarely in stool unless antibiotics are being given. In hospitals, the organism is frequently found in sinks, antiseptic solutions, and urine receptacles. Transmission to patients by health care practitioners may occur, especially in burn and neonatal ICUs.

Diseases Caused by *Pseudomonas*

Most *P. aeruginosa* infections occur in hospitalized patients, particularly those who are debilitated or immunocompromised. *P. aeruginosa* is the 2nd most common cause of infections in ICUs. HIV-infected patients, particularly those in advanced stages, are at risk for community-acquired *P. aeruginosa* infections.

Pseudomonas infections can develop in many anatomic sites, including skin, subcutaneous tissue, bone, ears, eyes, urinary tract, and heart valves. The site varies with the portal of entry and the patient's vulnerability. In hospitalized patients, the 1st sign may be overwhelming gram-negative sepsis.

Skin and soft-tissue infections: In burns, the region below the eschar can become heavily infiltrated with organisms, serving as a focus for subsequent bacteremia—an often lethal complication. Deep puncture wounds of the foot are often infected by *P. aeruginosa*. Draining sinuses, cellulitis, and osteomyelitis may result. Drainage from puncture wounds often has a sweet, fruity smell.

External otitis with purulent drainage, common in tropical climates, is the most common form of *Pseudomonas* infection involving the ear. A more severe form, referred to as malignant external otitis (see p. 804), can develop in diabetic patients. It is manifested by severe ear pain, often with unilateral cranial nerve palsies, and requires parenteral therapy.

Ecthyma gangrenosum in neutropenic patients is a skin lesion pathognomonic for *P. aeruginosa*. It is characterized by erythematous, centrally ulcerated, purple-black areas about 1 cm in diameter found most often in the axillary or anogenital areas.

Respiratory tract infections: *P. aeruginosa* is a frequent cause of ventilator-associated pneumonia. In HIV-infected patients, *Pseudomonas* most commonly causes pneumonia or sinusitis. *Pseudomonas* bronchitis is common late in the course of cystic fibrosis. These isolates have a characteristic mucoid colonial morphology.

Other infections: *Pseudomonas* is a common cause of UTI, especially in patients who have had urologic manipulation or obstructive uropathy or received broad-spectrum antibiotics. Ocular involvement generally presents as corneal ulceration, most often after trauma, but contamination of contact lenses or lens fluid has been implicated in some cases.

Rarely, *Pseudomonas* causes acute bacterial endocarditis, usually on prosthetic valves in patients who have had open-heart surgery or on natural valves in IV drug abusers.

Bacteremia: Many *Pseudomonas* infections can produce bacteremia. In nonintubated patients without a detectable urinary focus, especially if due to a species other than *P. aeruginosa*, bacteremia suggests contaminated IV fluids, drugs, or antiseptics used in placing the IV catheter.

Diagnosis and Treatment

Diagnosis depends on culturing the organism from the site of infection—blood, skin lesions, drainage fluid, urine, CSF, or eye. Localized infection may produce a fruity smell, and pus may be greenish.

Localized infection: External otitis is treated with 1% acetic acid irrigations or topical agents such as polymyxin B or colistin. More severe infection is treated with fluoroquinolones. Focal soft-tissue infection may require early surgical debridement of necrotic tissue and drainage of abscesses in addition to antibiotics. Small corneal ulcers are treated with ciprofloxacin 0.3% or levofloxacin 0.5%. Fortified (higher than stock concentration) antibiotic drops, such as tobramycin 15 mg/mL and cefazolin 50 mg/mL, are used for more significant ulcers. Frequent dosing (eg, q 1 h around the clock) is necessary initially. Patching is contraindicated because it produces a dark warm environment that favors bacterial growth and prevents administration of topical drugs. Patients with UTIs without systemic signs or symptoms can often be treated with levofloxacin 500 mg po once/day or ciprofloxacin 400 mg po bid.

Systemic infection: Parenteral therapy is required, generally with an aminoglycoside plus an antipseudomonal β-lactam, antipseudomonal cephalosporin (eg, cefepime, cefoperazone), or meropenem.

Right-sided endocarditis can be treated with antibiotics, but usually the infected valve must be removed to cure an infection involving the mitral, aortic, or prosthetic valve.

In neutropenic patients with marginal renal function, nonaminoglycoside combinations, such as double β-lactams or a β-lactam plus a fluoroquinolone, are also satisfactory.

P. aeruginosa resistance may occur among patients treated with ceftazidime, ciprofloxacin, gentamicin, or imipenem.

SALMONELLA INFECTIONS

The 2200 known serotypes of *Salmonella* may be grouped into:

- Those highly adapted to human hosts, including *S. typhi* and *S. paratyphi* types A, B (*S. schottmülleri*), and C (*S. hirschfeldii*), which are pathogenic only in humans and commonly cause enteric (typhoid) fever
- Those adapted to nonhuman hosts or causing disease almost exclusively in animals, although 2 strains within this group, *S. dublin* and *S. choleraesuis*, also cause disease in humans
- Those unadapted to specific hosts. This group, designated *S. enteritidis*, includes > 2000 serotypes that cause gastroenteritis and accounts for 85% of all *Salmonella* infections in the US.

TYPHOID FEVER

Typhoid fever is a systemic disease caused by *Salmonella typhi*. Symptoms are high fever, prostration, abdominal pain, and a rose-colored rash. Diagnosis is clinical and confirmed by culture. Treatment is with ceftriaxone or ciprofloxacin.

Etiology and Pathophysiology

About 400 to 500 cases of typhoid fever are reported annually in the US. Typhoid bacilli are shed in stool of asymptomatic carriers or in the stool or urine of those with active disease. Inadequate hygiene after defecation may spread *S. typhi* to community food or water supplies. In endemic areas where sanitary measures are generally inadequate, *S. typhi* is transmitted more frequently by water than by food. In developed countries, transmission is chiefly by food that has been contaminated during preparation by healthy carriers. Flies may spread the organism from feces to food. Occasional transmission by direct contact (fecal-oral route) may occur in children during play and in adults during sexual practices. Rarely, hospital personnel who have not taken adequate enteric precautions have acquired the disease when changing soiled bedclothes.

The organism enters the body via the GI tract and gains access to the bloodstream via the lymphatic channels. Ulceration, hemorrhage, and intestinal perforation may occur in severe cases.

About 3% of untreated patients, referred to as chronic enteric carriers, harbor organisms in their gallbladder and shed them in stool for > 1 yr. Some carriers have no history of clinical illness. Most of the estimated 2000 carriers in the US are elderly women with chronic biliary disease. Obstructive uropathy related to schistosomiasis may predispose certain typhoid patients to developing a urinary carrier state. Epidemiologic data indicate that typhoid carriers are more likely than the general population to acquire hepatobiliary cancer.

Symptoms and Signs

The incubation period (usually 8 to 14 days) is inversely related to the number of organisms ingested. Onset is usually gradual, with fever, headache, arthralgia, pharyngitis, constipation, anorexia, and abdominal pain and tenderness. Less common symptoms include dysuria, nonproductive cough, and epistaxis.

Untreated, the temperature rises in steps over 2 to 3 days, remains elevated (usually 39.4 to 40° C) for another 10 to 14 days, begins to fall gradually at the end of the 3rd wk, and reaches normal levels during the 4th wk. Prolonged fever is often accompanied by relative bradycardia and prostration. CNS symptoms such as delirium, stupor, or coma occur in severe cases. In about 10% of patients, discrete pink, blanching lesions (rose spots) appear in crops on the chest and abdomen during the 2nd wk and resolve in 2 to 5 days. Splenomegaly, leukopenia, anemia, liver function abnormalities, proteinuria, and a mild consumption coagulopathy are common. Acute cholecystitis and hepatitis may occur.

Late in the disease, when intestinal lesions are most prominent, florid diarrhea may occur, and the stool may contain blood (20% occult, 10% gross). In about 2% of patients, severe bleeding occurs during the 3rd wk, with a mortality rate of about 25%. An acute abdomen and leukocytosis during the 3rd wk may suggest intestinal perforation, usually involving the distal ileum, which occurs in 1 to 2% of patients. Pneumonia may develop during the 2nd or 3rd wk and is usually due to secondary pneumococcal infection, although *S. typhi* can also cause pulmonary infiltrates. Bacteremia occasionally leads to focal infections such as osteomyelitis, endocarditis, meningitis, soft-tissue abscesses, glomerulitis, or GU tract involvement. Atypical presentations such as pneumonitis, fever only, or symptoms consistent with UTI may delay diagnosis. Convalescence may last several months.

In 8 to 10% of untreated patients, symptoms and signs similar to the initial clinical syndrome recur about 2 wk after defervescence. For unclear reasons, antibiotic therapy during the initial illness increases the incidence of febrile relapse to 15 to 20%. If antibiotics are restarted at the time of relapse, the fever abates rapidly, unlike the slow defervescence that occurs during the primary illness. Occasionally, a 2nd relapse occurs.

Diagnosis

Other infections causing similar presentation include other *Salmonella* infections, the major rickettsioses, leptospirosis, disseminated TB, malaria, brucellosis, tularemia, infectious hepatitis, psittacosis, *Yersinia enterocolitica* infection, and lymphoma. Early in its clinical course, typhoid fever may resemble influenza, viral URI, or UTI.

Cultures of blood, stool, and urine should be obtained. Blood cultures are usually positive only during the first 2 wk of illness, but stool cultures are usually positive during the 3rd to 5th wk. If these cultures are negative and typhoid fever is strongly suspected, culture from a bone marrow biopsy specimen may reveal the organism.

Typhoid bacilli contain antigens (O and H) that stimulate the host to form corresponding antibodies. A 4-fold rise in O and H antibody titers in paired specimens obtained 2 wk apart suggests *S. typhi* infection. However, this test is only moderately (70%) sensitive and lacks specificity; many nontyphoidal *Salmonella* strains cross-react, and liver cirrhosis causes false positives.

Prognosis and Treatment

Without antibiotics, the mortality rate is about 12%. With prompt therapy, the mortality rate is < 1%. Most deaths occur in malnourished people, infants, and the elderly. Stupor, coma, or shock reflects severe disease and a poor prognosis. Complications occur mainly in patients who are untreated or in whom treatment is delayed.

Preferred antibiotics include ceftriaxone 1 g/kg IM or IV bid (25 to 37.5 mg/kg in children) for 7 to 10 days and various fluoroquinolones (eg, ciprofloxacin 500 mg po bid for 10 to 14 days, levofloxacin 500 mg po or IV once/day for 14 days, gatifloxacin 400 mg po or IV once/day for 14 days, moxifloxacin 400 mg po or IV once/day for 14 days). Chloramphenicol 500 mg po or IV q 6 h is still widely used, but resistance is increasing. Fluoroquinolones may be used in children. Alternative therapies, depending on in vitro sensitivity, include amoxicillin 25 mg/kg po qid, trimethoprim-sulfamethoxazole (TMP-SMX) 320/1600 bid or 10 mg/kg bid (of the TMP component), and azithromycin 1 g po on day one, then 500 mg once/day for 6 days.

Corticosteroids may be added to antibiotics to treat severe toxicity. Defervescence and clinical improvement usually follow. Prednisone 20 to 40 mg once/day po (or equivalent) for the first 3 days of treatment usually suffices. Higher doses of corticosteroids (dexamethasone 3 mg/kg IV initially, followed by 1 mg/kg q 6 h for 48 h total) are used in patients with marked delirium, coma, or shock.

Nutrition should be maintained with frequent feedings. Patients are generally kept on bed rest while febrile. Salicylates, which may cause hypothermia and hypotension, as well as laxatives and enemas, should be avoided. Diarrhea may be minimized with a clear liquid diet; parenteral nutrition may be needed temporarily. Fluid and electrolyte therapy and blood replacement may be needed.

Intestinal perforation and associated peritonitis call for surgical intervention and broader gram-negative and anti–*Bacteroides fragilis* coverage.

Relapses are treated the same as the initial illness, although duration of antibiotic therapy seldom needs to be > 5 days.

Patients must be reported to the local health department and prohibited from handling food until proven free of the organism.

Typhoid bacilli may be isolated for as long as 3 to 6 mo after the acute illness in people who do not become carriers. Thereafter, 3 stool cultures at weekly intervals must be negative to exclude a carrier state.

Carriers with normal biliary tracts should be given antibiotics. The cure rate is about 60% with amoxicillin 2 g po tid for 4 wk. In some carriers with gallbladder disease, eradication has been achieved with TMP-SMX and rifampin. In other cases, cholecystectomy with 1 to 2 days of preoperative and 2 to 3 days of postoperative antibiotics is effective.

Prevention

Drinking water should be purified, sewage should be disposed of effectively, milk should be pasteurized, chronic carriers should avoid handling food, and adequate patient isolation precautions should be implemented. Special attention to enteric precautions is important. Travelers in endemic areas should avoid ingesting raw leafy vegetables, other foods stored or served at room temperature, and untreated water. Unless water is known to be safe, it should be boiled or chlorinated before drinking.

A live attenuated oral typhoid vaccine is available (Ty21a strain) and is about 70% effective. It is administered every other day for a total of 4 doses. Because the vaccine contains living *S. typhi* organisms, it is contraindicated in patients who are immunosuppressed. In the US, the Ty21a vaccine is not used in children < 6 yr. An alternative is the single-dose, IM Vi polysaccharide vaccine, which is 64 to 72% effective and is well tolerated.

NONTYPHOIDAL *SALMONELLA* INFECTIONS

Nontyphoidal salmonellae, mainly *Salmonella enteritidis*, primarily produce gastroenteritis, bacteremia, and focal infection. Symptoms may be diarrhea, high fever with prostration, or those of focal infection. Diagnosis is by cultures of blood, stool, or site specimens. Treatment, when indicated, is with trimethoprim-sulfamethoxazole or ciprofloxacin, with surgery for abscesses, vascular lesions, and bone and joint infections.

Most nontyphoidal *Salmonella* infections are caused by *S. enteritidis*. These infections are common and remain a significant public health problem in the US. Many serotypes of *S. enteritidis* have been given names and are referred to informally as if they were separate species even though they are not. The most common *Salmonella* serotypes in the US include *S. typhimurium, S. heidelberg, S. newport, S. infantis, S. agona, S. montevideo*, and *S. saint-paul*.

Human disease occurs by direct and indirect contact with numerous species of infected animals, the foodstuffs derived from them, and their excreta. Infected meat, poultry, raw milk, eggs, and egg products are common sources of *Salmonella*. Other reported sources include infected pet turtles and reptiles, carmine red dye, and contaminated marijuana.

Subtotal gastrectomy, achlorhydria (or ingestion of antacids), sickle cell anemia, splenectomy, louse-borne relapsing fever, malaria, bartonellosis, cirrhosis, leukemia, lymphoma, and HIV infection are all risk factors for *Salmonella* infection.

Each *Salmonella* serotype can produce any or all of the clinical syndromes described below, although given serotypes tend to produce specific syndromes. Enteric fever, for instance, is caused by *S. paratyphi* types A, B, and C.

An asymptomatic carrier state may also occur. However, carriers do not appear to play a major role in large outbreaks of nontyphoidal gastroenteritis. Persistent shedding of organisms in the stool for ≥ 1 yr occurs in only 0.2 to 0.6% of patients with nontyphoidal *Salmonella* infections.

Symptoms and Signs

Salmonella infection may present as gastroenteritis, enteric fever, a bacteremic syndrome, or focal disease.

Gastroenteritis usually starts 12 to 48 h after ingestion of organisms, with nausea and cramping abdominal pain followed by diarrhea, fever, and sometimes vomiting. Usually the stool is watery but may be a pastelike semisolid. Rarely, mucus or blood is present. The disease is usually mild, lasting 1 to 4 days. Occasionally, a more severe, protracted illness occurs.

Enteric fever in a less severe form than typhoid is characterized by fever, prostration, and septicemia.

Bacteremia is relatively uncommon in patients with gastroenteritis. However, *S. choleraesuis, S. typhimurium*, and *S. heidelberg*, among others, can cause a sustained and frequently lethal bacteremic syndrome lasting ≥ 1 wk, with prolonged fever, headache, malaise, and chills but rarely diarrhea. Patients may have recurrent episodes of bacteremia or other invasive infections (eg, septic arthritis) due to *Salmonella*. Multiple *Salmonella* infections in a patient without other risk factors should prompt HIV testing.

Focal *Salmonella* infection can occur with or without sustained bacteremia, producing pain in or referred from the involved organ—the GI tract (liver, gallbladder, and appendix), endothelial surfaces (atherosclerotic plaques, ileofemoral or aortic aneurysms, heart valves), pericardium, meninges, lungs, joints, bones, GU tract, or soft tissues. Preexisting solid tumors will occasionally be seeded and develop abscesses that may, in turn, become a source of *Salmonella* bacteremia. *S. choleraesuis* and *S. typhimurium* are the most common causes of focal infection.

Diagnosis, Treatment, and Prevention

Diagnosis is by isolating the organism from stool or another infected site. In bacteremic and focal forms, blood cultures are positive, but stool cultures are generally negative. In stool specimens stained with methylene blue, WBCs are often seen, indicating inflammatory colitis.

Gastroenteritis is treated symptomatically with oral or IV fluids (see p. 136). Antibiotics do not hasten resolution, may prolong excretion of the organism, and are unwarranted in uncomplicated cases. However, in elderly nursing home residents, infants, and patients with HIV infection, increased mortality dictates treatment with antibiotics. Antibiotic resistance is more common with nontyphoidal *Salmonella* than with *S. typhi*. Trimethoprim-sulfamethoxazole (TMP-SMX) 5 mg/kg (of the TMP component) po q 12 h for children and ciprofloxacin 500 mg po q 12 h for adults are acceptable regimens. Nonimmunocompromised patients should be treated for 3 to 5 days; patients with AIDS may require prolonged suppression to prevent relapses. Systemic or focal disease should be treated with antibiotic doses as outlined above for typhoid fever. Sustained bacteremia is generally treated for 4 to 6 wk. Abscesses should be drained surgically. At least 4 wk of antibiotic therapy should follow surgery. Infected aneurysms and heart valves and bone or joint infections usually require surgical intervention and prolonged courses of antibiotics. The prognosis is usually good, unless severe underlying disease is present.

Asymptomatic carriage is usually self-limited, and antibiotic treatment is rarely required. In unusual cases (eg, in food handlers or health care workers), eradication may be attempted with ciprofloxacin 500 mg po q 12 h for 1 mo. Follow-up stool cultures should be obtained in the weeks after drug administration to document elimination of *Salmonella*.

Preventing contamination of foodstuffs by infected animals and humans is paramount. Preventive measures for travelers discussed under Typhoid Fever on p. 1472 also apply to most other enteric infections. Case reporting is essential.

SHIGELLOSIS

(Bacillary Dysentery)

Shigellosis is an acute infection of the intestine caused by *Shigella* sp. Symptoms include fever, nausea, vomiting, and diarrhea that is usually bloody. Diagnosis is clinical and confirmed by stool culture. Treatment is supportive, mostly with rehydration; antibiotics (eg, ampicillin or trimethoprim-sulfamethoxazole) are optional.

Etiology and Pathophysiology

The genus *Shigella* is distributed worldwide and is the typical cause of inflammatory dysentery, responsible for 5 to 10% of diarrheal illness in many areas. *Shigella* is divided into 4 major subgroups: A, B, C, and D, which are subdivided into serologically determined types. *S. flexneri* and *S. sonnei* are found more widely than *S. boydii* and the particularly virulent *S. dysenteriae*. *S. sonnei* is the most common isolate in the US.

The source of infection is the feces of infected people or convalescent carriers. Direct spread is by the fecal-oral route. Indirect spread is by contaminated food and fomites. Flies serve as vectors. Epidemics occur most frequently in overcrowded populations with inadequate sanitation. Shigellosis is particularly common in younger children living in endemic areas. Adults usually have less severe disease.

Convalescents and subclinical carriers may be significant sources of infection, but true long-term carriers are rare. Infection imparts little or no immunity.

Shigella organisms penetrate the mucosa of the lower intestine, causing mucus secretion, hyperemia, leukocytic infiltration, edema, and often superficial mucosal ulcerations. *Shigella dysenteriae* type 1 (not present in the US) produces Shiga toxin, which causes marked watery diarrhea and sometimes hemolytic-uremic syndrome.

Symptoms and Signs

The incubation period is 1 to 4 days. The most common presentation, watery diarrhea, is indistinguishable from other bacterial, viral, and protozoan infections that induce secretory activity of intestinal epithelial cells.

In adults, initial symptoms may be episodes of gripping abdominal pain, urgency to defecate, and passage of formed feces that temporarily relieves the pain. These episodes recur with increasing severity and frequency. Diarrhea becomes marked, with soft or liquid stools containing mucus, pus, and often blood. Rectal prolapse and consequent fecal incontinence may result from severe tenesmus. However, adults may present without fever, with nonbloody and nonmucoid diarrhea, and with little or no tenesmus. The disease usually resolves spontaneously in adults—mild cases in 4 to 8 days, severe cases in 3 to 6 wk. Significant dehydration and electrolyte loss with circulatory collapse and death occur mainly in debilitated adults and infants < 2 yr.

Rarely, shigellosis starts suddenly with rice-water or serous (occasionally bloody) stools. The patient may vomit and rapidly become dehydrated. Infection may present with delirium, seizures, and coma, but little or no diarrhea. Death may occur in 12 to 24 h.

In young children, onset is sudden, with fever, irritability or drowsiness, anorexia, nausea or vomiting, diarrhea, abdominal pain and distention, and tenesmus. Within 3 days, blood, pus, and mucus appear in the stools. The number of stools may increase to ≥ 20/day, and weight loss and dehydration become severe. If untreated, a child may die in the first 12 days. If the child survives, acute symptoms subside by the 2nd wk.

Secondary bacterial infections may occur, especially in debilitated and dehydrated patients. Severe mucosal ulcerations may cause significant acute blood loss. Other complications are uncommon but include toxic neuritis, arthritis, myocarditis, and, rarely, intestinal perforation. The hemolytic-uremic syndrome may complicate shigellosis in children. Infection does not become chronic and is not an etiologic factor in ulcerative colitis. However, patients with the HLA-B27 genotype more commonly develop reactive arthritis after shigellosis (and other enteritides).

Diagnosis

Diagnosis is facilitated by a high index of suspicion during outbreaks and in endemic areas and by the presence of fecal leukocytes on smears stained with methylene blue or Wright's stain. Stool cultures are diagnostic and should be obtained. In patients with symptoms of dysentery (bloody and mucoid stools), the differential diagnosis should include invasive *Escherichia coli, Salmonella, Yersinia, Campylobacter*, amebiasis, and viral diarrheas.

The mucosal surface, as seen through a proctoscope, is diffusely erythematous with numerous small ulcers. Although the WBC count is often reduced at onset, it averages 13,000/μL. Hemoconcentration is common, as is diarrhea-induced metabolic acidosis.

Treatment and Prevention

Fluid loss is treated symptomatically with oral or IV fluids (see p. 564). Antibiotics can reduce the symptoms and shedding of *Shigella* but are not necessary for mild illness in healthy adults. However, children, the elderly, debilitated patients, and those with severe disease generally should be treated. For adults, a fluoroquinolone, such as ciprofloxacin 500 mg po for 3 to 5 days, or trimethoprim-sulfamethoxazole (TMP-SMX) one double-strength tablet q 12 h is the treatment of choice. For children, the treatment is TMP-SMX at a dosage of 4 mg/kg po q 12 h of the TMP component. Many *Shigella* isolates are likely to be resistant to ampicillin and tetracycline.

Hands should be washed thoroughly before handling food, and soiled garments and bedclothes should be immersed in covered buckets of soap and water until they can be boiled. Proper isolation techniques (especially stool isolation) should be used with patients and carriers. A live oral vaccine is being developed, and field trials in endemic areas hold promise. Immunity is, however, generally type specific.

TULAREMIA

(Rabbit or Deer Fly Fever)

Tularemia is a febrile disease caused by *Francisella tularensis* that resembles typhoid fever. Symptoms are a primary local ulcerative lesion, regional lymphadenopathy, profound systemic symptoms, and occa-

TABLE 173–2. TYPES OF TULAREMIA*

TYPE	% OF CASES	COMMENT
Ulceroglandular	87	Primary lesions on the hands or fingers
Typhoidal	8	Systemic illness with abdominal pain and fever
Oculoglandular	3	Inflammation of ipsilateral lymph nodes, probably caused by inoculation of the eye from an infected finger or hand
Glandular	2	Regional lymphadenitis but no primary lesion and often cervical adenopathy, suggesting oral ingestion of bacteria

*Tularemic pneumonia may be primary or may occur as the ulceroglandular type of infection.

sionally, atypical pneumonia. Diagnosis is primarily epidemiologic and clinical. Treatment is with streptomycin, gentamicin, chloramphenicol, or doxycycline.

Epidemiology and Pathophysiology

The 4 types of tularemia are listed in TABLE 173–2. The causative organism, *F. tularensis*, is a small, pleomorphic, nonmotile, nonsporulating, aerobic bacillus that enters the body by ingestion, inoculation, inhalation, or contamination. It can penetrate apparently unbroken skin but may actually enter through microlesions. Type A, a more virulent serotype for humans, is found in rabbits and rodents. Type B usually produces a mild ulceroglandular infection and is found in water and aquatic animals. Transmission among animals is by blood-sucking arthropods and cannibalism.

Hunters, butchers, farmers, and fur handlers are most commonly infected. In winter months, most cases result from contact (especially during skinning) with infected wild rabbits. In summer months, infection usually follows handling of other infected animals or birds or contact with infected ticks or other arthropods. Rarely, cases result from eating undercooked infected meat, drinking contaminated water, or mowing fields in endemic areas. In the Western states, ticks, deer flies, horse flies, and direct contact with animals are other sources of infection. Human-to-human transmission has not been reported. Laboratory workers are at particular risk because infection is readily acquired during normal handling of infected specimens. Tularemia is considered a possible agent of bioterrorism.

In disseminated cases, characteristic focal necrotic lesions in various stages of evolution are scattered throughout the body. They are 1 mm to 8 cm; whitish yellow; seen externally as the primary lesions on the fingers, eyes, or mouth; and commonly found in lymph nodes, spleen, liver, kidneys, and lungs. In pneumonia, necrotic foci occur in the lungs. Although severe systemic toxicity may occur, no toxins have been demonstrated.

Symptoms and Signs

Onset occurs suddenly, 1 to 10 (usually 2 to 4) days after contact, with headache, chills, nausea, vomiting, fever of 39.5° or 40° C, and severe prostration. Extreme weakness, recurring chills, and drenching sweats develop. Within 24 to 48 h, an inflamed papule appears at the infection site (finger, arm, eye, or roof of the mouth), except in glandular or typhoidal tularemia. The papule rapidly becomes pustular and ulcerates, producing a clean ulcer crater with a scanty, thin, colorless exudate. Ulcers are usually single on the extremities but multiple in the mouth or eyes. Usually, only one eye is affected. Regional lymph nodes enlarge and may suppurate and drain profusely. A typhoid-like state frequently develops by the 5th day, and the patient may develop atypical pneumonia, sometimes accompanied by delirium. Although signs of consolidation are frequently present, reduced breath sounds and occasional rales may be the only physical findings in tularemic pneumonia. A dry, nonproductive cough is associated with a retrosternal burning sensation. A nonspecific roseola-like rash may appear at any stage of the disease. Splenomegaly and perisplenitis may occur. In untreated cases, temperature remains elevated for 3 to 4 wk and resolves gradually. Mediastinitis, lung abscess, and meningitis are rare complications.

Mortality is almost nil in treated cases and about 6% in untreated cases. Death usually results from overwhelming infection, pneumonia, meningitis, or peritonitis. Relapses can occur in inadequately treated cases. One attack confers immunity.

Diagnosis

Diagnosis is suspected by a history of contact with rabbits or wild rodents or exposure to arthropod vectors; the sudden onset of symptoms; and the characteristic primary lesion. Patients should have cultures of blood and relevant clinical material (eg, sputum, lesions) and acute and convalescent antibody titers 2 wk apart. A 4-fold rise or a single titer >1:128 is diagnostic. The serum of brucellosis patients may also cross-react to *F. tularensis* antigens but usually in much lower titers. Fluorescent antibody staining is used by some laboratories. Leukocytosis is common, but the WBC count may be normal with an increase only in the proportion of PMNs.

Because this organism is highly infectious, samples and culture media suspected of tularemia should be handled with extreme caution, and if possible, processed by a laboratory with a class B or C rating.

Treatment

The preferred drug is streptomycin 0.5 g IM q 12 h (if in a bioterrorism setting, 1 g q 12 h) until the temperature is normal, then 0.5 g once/day for 5 days. In children, the dose is 10 to 15 mg/kg IM q 12 h for 10 days. Gentamicin 1 to 2 mg/kg IM or IV tid is also effective. Chloramphenicol (oral form not available in US) or doxycycline 100 mg po q 12 h may be given until the temperature is normal, but relapses occasionally occur with these drugs, and they may not prevent node suppuration.

Continuous wet saline dressings are beneficial for primary skin lesions and may diminish the severity of lymphangitis and lymphadenitis. Surgical drainage of large abscesses is rarely necessary unless therapy is delayed. In ocular tularemia, applying warm saline compresses and using dark glasses give some relief. In severe cases, 2% homatropine 1 to 2 drops q 4 h may relieve symptoms. Intense headache usually responds to oral opioids (eg, oxycodone or hydrocodone with acetaminophen).

Prevention

When entering endemic areas, tick-proof clothing and repellents should be used. A thorough search for ticks should be done after leaving. Ticks should be removed at once (see sidebar 177–1 on p. 1491). When handling rabbits and rodents, especially in endemic areas, protective clothing, including rubber gloves and face masks, should be worn because organisms may be present in the animal and in tick feces on the animal's fur. Wild birds and game must be thoroughly cooked before eating. Water that may be contaminated must be disinfected before use.

174 SPIROCHETES

(See also Syphilis on p. 1657.)

The family Spirochaetales is distinguished by the helical shape of the bacteria. They are too thin to be visualized on routine microscopy but can be viewed using darkfield microscopy. There are 3 genera: *Treponema, Leptospira,* and *Borrelia.*

BEJEL, PINTA, AND YAWS

Bejel, pinta, and yaws (endemic treponematoses) are chronic, tropical, nonvenereal, spirochetal infections spread by body contact. Symptoms of bejel are mucous membrane and mucocutaneous lesions, followed by bone and skin gummas. Yaws causes periostitis and dermal lesions. Pinta lesions are confined to the dermis. Diagnosis is clinical and epidemiologic. Treatment is with penicillin.

The causative agents, *Treponema pallidum* subsp *endemicum* (bejel), *T. pallidum* subsp *pertenue* (yaws), and *T. carateum* (pinta), are morphologically and serologically indistinguishable from the agent of syphilis, *T. pallidum* subsp *pallidum*. Like syphilis, the typical course is an initial mucocutaneous lesion followed by diffuse secondary lesions, a latent period, and late destructive disease.

Transmission is by close skin contact—sexual or not—primarily between children living in conditions of poor hygiene. Bejel (endemic syphilis) occurs mainly in arid countries of the eastern Mediterranean and West Africa (Sahel). Transmission results from mouth-to-mouth contact or sharing eating and drinking utensils. Yaws (frambesia) is found in humid equatorial countries, where transmission is favored by scanty clothing and skin trauma. Pinta occurs among the natives of Mexico, Central America, and South America and is not very contagious. Transmission probably requires contact with broken skin.

Symptoms and Signs

Bejel begins in childhood as a mucous patch, usually on the buccal mucosa, followed by papulosquamous and erosive papular lesions of the trunk and extremities. Periostitis of the leg bones is common. Later, gummatous lesions of the nose and soft palate develop.

Yaws, after an incubation period of several weeks, begins as a granulomatous or macular lesion at the inoculation site, usually on the legs. The lesion heals but is followed by a generalized eruption of soft granulomas on the face, extremities, and buttocks, often at mucocutaneous junctions. Granulomas heal slowly and may recur. Keratotic lesions may develop on the soles, causing painful ulcerations (crab yaws). Later, destructive lesions may develop, including periostitis (particularly of the tibia), proliferative exostoses of the nasal portion of the maxillary bone (goundou), juxta-articular nodules, gummatous skin lesions, and, ultimately, mutilating facial ulcers, particularly around the nose (gangosa).

Pinta lesions are confined to the dermis. They begin at the inoculation site as small papules and progress over several months to erythematous squamous plaques, mainly on the extremities, face, and neck. Later, symmetric slate-blue patches develop, usually on the face and extremities and over bony prominences. Still later, lesions become depigmented, resembling vitiligo. Hyperkeratosis may occur on the soles and palms. Destructive lesions leave a scar.

Diagnosis and Treatment

Diagnosis is by the typical appearance of lesions in people from endemic areas. Serologic tests for syphilis (the Venereal Disease Research Laboratory [VDRL] and fluorescent treponemal antibody absorption tests) are positive; thus, differentiation from venereal syphilis is clinical. Early lesions are often darkfield-positive for spirochetes and are indistinguishable from *T. pallidum* subsp *pallidum.*

Active disease is treated with 1 dose of penicillin benzathine 1.2 million units IM. Children < 45 kg should receive 600,000 units IM. Public health control includes active case finding and treatment of family and close contacts with penicillin benzathine.

LEPTOSPIROSIS

Leptospirosis includes all infections caused by the genus *Leptospira*, regardless of serotype, including infectious (spirochetal) jaundice and canicola fever. Symptoms are biphasic. Both phases involve acute febrile episodes; the 2nd phase sometimes includes hepatic, renal, and meningeal involvement. Diagnosis is by darkfield microscopy, culture, and serology. Treatment is with doxycycline or penicillin.

Leptospirosis, a zoonosis occurring in many domestic and wild animals, may cause inapparent illness or serious, even fatal, disease. A carrier state exists in which animals shed leptospires in their urine for months. Human infections are acquired by direct contact with infected urine or tissue, or indirectly by contact with contaminated water or soil. Abraded skin and exposed mucous membranes (conjunctival, nasal, oral) are the usual entry portals. Leptospirosis can be an occupational disease (eg, of farmers or sewer and abattoir workers), but in the US, most patients are exposed incidentally during recreational activities (eg, swimming in contaminated water). Dogs and rats are other common probable sources. The 40 to 100 annual US cases occur mainly in late summer and early fall. Because distinctive clinical features are lacking, probably many more cases are not diagnosed and reported.

Symptoms and Signs

The incubation period ranges from 2 to 20 (usually 7 to 13) days. The disease is characteristically biphasic. The septicemic phase starts abruptly, with headache, severe muscular aches, chills, and fever. Conjunctival suffusion usually appears on the 3rd or 4th day. Splenomegaly and hepatomegaly are uncommon. This phase lasts 4 to 9 days, with recurrent chills and fever that often spikes to > 39° C. Defervescence follows. The 2nd, or immune, phase occurs between the 6th and 12th day of illness, correlating with appearance of antibodies in serum. Fever and earlier symptoms recur, and meningitis may develop. Iridocyclitis, optic neuritis, and peripheral neuropathy occur infrequently. If acquired during pregnancy, leptospirosis, even during the convalescent period, may cause abortion.

Weil's syndrome (icteric leptospirosis) is a severe form with jaundice from intravascular hemolysis, and usually azotemia, anemia, diminished consciousness, and continued fever. Onset is similar to that of less severe forms. However, hemorrhagic manifestations, which are due to capillary injury and include epistaxis, petechiae, purpura, and ecchymoses, then develop and rarely progress to subarachnoid, adrenal, or GI hemorrhage. Thrombocytopenia may occur. Signs of hepatocellular and renal dysfunction appear from the 3rd to 6th day. Renal abnormalities include proteinuria, pyuria, hematuria, and azotemia. Hepatic damage is minimal, and healing is complete.

Mortality is nil in anicteric patients. With jaundice, the mortality rate is 5 to 10%; it is higher in patients > 60 yr.

Diagnosis

Similar symptoms can result from viral meningoencephalitis, other spirochetal infections, influenza, and hepatitis. The history of biphasic illness may help differentiate leptospirosis. Leptospirosis should be considered in any patient with FUO who might have been exposed to leptospires.

Patients with suspected leptospirosis should have blood cultures, acute and convalescent (3 to 4 wk) antibody titers, CBC, serum chemistries, and liver function tests. Meningeal findings mandate lumbar puncture; the CSF cell count is between 10 and 1000/μL (usually < 500/μL), with predominantly mononuclear cells. CSF glucose is normal; protein is < 100 mg/dL.

The peripheral blood WBC count is normal or slightly elevated in most but may reach 50,000/μL in severely ill patients with jaundice. The presence of > 70% neutrophils helps differentiate leptospirosis from viral illnesses. In jaundiced patients, bilirubin levels are usually < 20 mg/dL (< 342 μmol/L) but may reach 40 mg/dL (684 μmol/L) in severe infection; marked intravascular hemolysis in such patients may cause significant anemia.

Treatment

Antibiotic therapy is effective even when begun relatively late. In severe illness, penicillin G 5 to 6 million units IV q 6 h or ampicillin 500 to 1000 mg IV q 6 h is recommended. In less severe cases, doxycycline 100 mg po q 12 h, ampicillin 500 to 750 mg po q 6 h, or amoxicillin 500 mg po q 6 h may be given for 5 to 7 days. In severe cases, supportive care, including fluid and electrolyte therapy, is also important. Patient isolation is not required, but urine must be handled and disposed of carefully.

Doxycycline 200 mg po given once/wk during a period of known geographic exposure prevents disease.

LYME DISEASE

Lyme disease is a tick-transmitted infection caused by *Borrelia burgdorferi*. Symptoms include an erythema migrans rash, which may be followed weeks to months later by neurologic, cardiac, or joint abnormalities. Diagnosis is primarily clinical, but acute and convalescent antibody titers may be helpful. Treatment is with antibiotics such as doxycycline or, for serious infections, ceftriaxone.

Epidemiology and Pathophysiology

Lyme disease was recognized in 1975 because of close clustering of cases in Lyme, Connecticut and is now the most commonly reported tick-borne illness in the US. It has been reported in 49 states, but > 90% of cases occur from Massachusetts to Maryland, in Wisconsin and Minnesota, and in California and Oregon. Lyme disease also occurs in Europe, across the former Soviet Union, and in China and Japan. Onset is usually in the summer and early fall. Most patients are children and young adults living in heavily wooded areas.

Lyme disease is transmitted primarily by *Ixodes scapularis*, the deer tick. In the US, the white-footed mouse is the primary animal reservoir for *Borrelia burgdorferi* and the preferred host for nymphal and larval forms of the deer tick. Deer are hosts for adult ticks but do not carry *Borrelia*. Other mammals (eg, dogs) can be incidental hosts and can develop Lyme disease. In Europe, sheep host the organism but do not develop the disease.

B. burgdorferi enters the skin at the site of the tick bite. After 3 to 32 days, the organisms migrate locally in the skin around the bite, spread in lymph to produce regional adenopathy, or disseminate in blood to organs or other skin sites. The relative paucity of organisms in involved tissue suggests that most manifestations are due to host immune response rather than to the destructive properties of the organism.

Symptoms and Signs

Lyme disease has 3 stages: early localized, early disseminated, and late. The early and late stages are usually separated by an asymptomatic interval.

Erythema migrans (EM), the hallmark and best clinical indicator of Lyme disease, is the 1st sign of the disease. It occurs in at least 75% of patients, beginning as a red macule or papule, usually on the proximal portion of an extremity or the trunk (especially the thigh, buttock, or axilla), between 3 and 32 days after a tick bite. The area expands, often with central clearing, to a diameter ≤ 50 cm. Soon after onset, nearly ½ of untreated patients develop multiple, usually smaller, lesions without indurated centers. Cultures of biopsy samples of these secondary lesions have been positive, indicating dissemination of infection. EM generally lasts a few weeks (average, 3 to 4 wk). Evanescent lesions may appear during resolution. Mucosal lesions do not occur.

Symptoms of early-disseminated disease begin days or weeks after the appearance of the primary lesion when the bacteria spread through the body. This musculoskeletal, flulike syndrome, consisting of malaise, fatigue, chills, fever, headache, stiff neck, myalgias, and arthralgias, may last for weeks. Because symptoms are often nonspecific, the diagnosis is frequently missed; a high index of suspicion is required. Frank arthritis is rare at this stage. Less common are backache, nausea and vomiting, sore throat, lymphadenopathy, and splenomegaly. Symptoms are characteristically intermittent and changing, but malaise and fatigue may linger for weeks. Some patients develop symptoms of fibromyalgia. Resolved skin lesions may reappear faintly, sometimes before recurrent attacks of arthritis, in late-stage disease.

Neurologic abnormalities develop in about 15% of patients within weeks to months of EM (generally before arthritis occurs), commonly last months, and usually resolve completely. Most common are lymphocytic meningitis (CSF pleocytosis of about 100 cells/μL) or meningoencephalitis, cranial neuritis (especially Bell's palsy, which may be bilateral), and sensory or motor radiculoneuropathies, alone or in combination.

Myocardial abnormalities occur in about 8% of patients within weeks of EM. They include fluctuating degrees of atrioventricular block (1st-degree, Wenckebach, or 3rd-degree) and, rarely, myopericarditis with chest pain, reduced ejection fractions, and cardiomegaly.

In untreated Lyme disease, the late stage begins months to years after initial infection. Arthritis develops in about 60% of patients within several months (occasionally up to 2 yr) of disease onset (as defined by EM). Intermittent swelling and pain in a few large joints, especially the knees, typically recur for several years. Affected knees commonly are much more swollen than painful; they are often hot, but rarely red. Baker cysts may form and rupture. Malaise, fatigue, and low-grade fever may precede or accompany arthritis attacks. About 10% of patients develop chronic (unremittent for ≥ 6 mo) knee involvement. Other late findings (occurring years after onset) include an antibiotic-sensitive skin lesion (acrodermatitis chronica atrophicans) and chronic CNS abnormalities, either polyneuropathy or a subtle encephalopathy with mood, memory, and sleep disorders.

Diagnosis

Cultures of blood and relevant body fluids (eg, CSF, joint fluid) may be obtained—primarily to diagnose other pathogens. Acute and convalescent antibody titers may be helpful; positive enzyme-linked immunosorbent assay (ELISA) titers should be confirmed by Western blot. However, seroconversion may be late (eg, > 4 wk) or occasionally absent, and positive IgG titers may represent previous infection. PCR testing of CSF or synovial fluid is often positive when those sites are involved. Consequently, diagnosis depends on both test results and the presence of typical findings. A classic EM rash strongly suggests Lyme disease, particularly when supported by other elements (eg, recent tick bite, exposure to endemic area, typical systemic symptoms).

In the absence of rash, diagnosis is more difficult because of the protean and often subtle symptoms. Early-disseminated disease may mimic juvenile RA in children and reactive arthritis and atypical RA in adults. Important negative findings include usually absent morning stiffness, subcutaneous nodules, iridocyclitis, mucosal lesions, rheumatoid factor, and antinuclear antibodies. Lyme disease presenting with a musculoskeletal, flulike syndrome in summer may resemble ehrlichiosis, a rickettsial infection transmitted by the same tick (see p. 1494). The lack of leukopenia, thrombocytopenia, elevated transaminases, and inclusion bodies in neutrophils helps distinguish Lyme disease. Acute rheumatic fever is considered in the occasional patient with migratory polyarthralgias and either an increased PR interval or chorea (as a manifestation of meningoencephalitis). However, patients with Lyme disease rarely have heart murmurs or evidence of a preceding streptococcal infection.

Late-stage disease lacks axial involvement, which distinguishes it from spondyloarthropathies with peripheral joint involvement. Lyme disease may cause Bell's palsy, fibromyalgia, and chronic fatigue syndrome and can mimic lymphocytic meningitis, peripheral neuropathies, and similar CNS syndromes.

In areas where Lyme disease is endemic, many patients with arthralgias, chronic fatigue, difficulty concentrating, or other troublesome but nonspecific symptoms attribute these to late-stage Lyme disease. Without a history of EM rash or other symptoms of early-localized or early-disseminated Lyme disease, few of these patients actually have Lyme disease. In such patients, elevated IgG

TABLE 174–1. GUIDELINES FOR ANTIBIOTIC TREATMENT OF ADULT LYME DISEASE*

Early Lyme disease†

Amoxicillin, 500 mg tid po for 10–21 days or 1 g po q 8 h (some advise adding probenecid 500 mg po tid; probenecid is not needed if 1 g po q 8 h is used)
Doxycycline, 100 mg po bid for 10–21 days
Cefuroxime axetil, 500 mg po bid for 10–21 days
Azithromycin, 500 mg po once/day for 7 days (less effective than other regimens)

Neurologic manifestations

Bell's palsy (no other neurologic abnormalities)
 Doxycycline as for early disease
Meningitis (with or without radiculoneuropathy or encephalitis)‡
 Ceftriaxone, 2 g IV once/day for 14–28 days
 Penicillin G, 5 million units IV q 6 h for 14–28 days
 Doxycycline, 100 mg po bid for 14–28 days
 Chloramphenicol, 500 mg po or IV qid for 14–28 days

Cardiac manifestations

Ceftriaxone, 2 g IV once/day for 14–28 days
Penicillin G, 20 million units IV once/day for 14–28 days
Doxycycline, 100 mg po bid for 21 days (for mild carditis with 1st-degree heart block, PR interval ≤ 30 sec, normal ventricular function)
Amoxicillin, 500 mg po tid or 1 g po q 8 h for 21 days (for mild carditis with 1st-degree heart block, PR interval ≤ 30 sec, normal ventricular function)

Arthritis

Amoxicillin, 500 mg po qid or 1 g po q 8 h and probenecid, 500 mg po qid for 30 days (if no neurologic involvement)
Doxycycline, 100 mg po bid for 30 days (if no neurologic involvement)
Ceftriaxone, 2 g IV once/day for 14–28 days
Penicillin G, 20 million units IV once/day for 14–28 days

Acrodermatitis chronica atrophicans

Amoxicillin, 1 g po tid for 30 days
Doxycycline, 100 mg po bid for 30 days

*Pregnant women may receive amoxicillin 500 mg tid for 21 days. No treatment is necessary for pregnant women who are seropositive but asymptomatic.

†Without neurologic, cardiac, or joint involvement. For early Lyme disease limited to a single erythema migrans lesion, 10 days is sufficient.

‡Optimal duration of therapy has not been established. There are no controlled trials of therapy > 4 wk for any neurologic manifestation of Lyme disease.

Adapted from Rahn DW, Malawista SE: "Treatment of Lyme disease (special article)." In *1994 Year Book of Medicine*, edited by GL Mandell, RC Bone, MJ Cline, et al. St. Louis, Mosby–Year Book, 1994, pp. xxi–xxxvi.

titers indicating past exposure, not persistent infection, often lead to long and fruitless courses of antibiotic therapy.

Treatment

Most features of Lyme disease respond to antibiotics, but treatment of early disease is most successful. In late-stage disease, antibiotics eradicate the bacteria, relieving the arthritis in most people. However, a few people have persistent arthritis even after all the bacteria are gone because of continued inflammation. TABLE 174–1 shows adult treatment regimens for various presentations of Lyme disease. Treatment in children is similar except that doxycycline is avoided in children < 8 yr and doses are adjusted based on weight (see TABLE 170–3 on p. 1410). Duration of treatment has not been established by controlled trials, and recommendations vary in the literature.

For symptomatic relief, NSAIDs may be used. Complete heart block may require a temporary pacemaker. Tense knee joints due to effusions require aspiration and crutches. Patients with arthritis of the knee that persists despite antibiotic therapy may respond to arthroscopic synovectomy.

Prevention

Precautions against tick bite (see sidebar 177–1 on p. 1491) should be taken by people in endemic areas. Deer tick nymphs, which attack humans, are small and difficult to see. Once attached to the skin, they gorge on blood for days. Transmission of *B. burgdorferi* does not usually occur until the infected tick has been in place for > 36 h. Thus, searching for ticks after potential exposure and removing them can help prevent infection.

A single dose of doxycycline 200 mg po has been shown to reduce the likelihood of Lyme disease after deer tick bite, but many clinicians do not recommend this treatment or limit it to patients with obviously engorged ticks. Patients with known tick bite can easily be instructed to monitor the bite site and seek care if rash or other symptoms occur; the diagnostic dilemma of Lyme is most prominent when there is no history of tick bite.

A vaccine, which was only moderately effective, has been removed from the market.

RAT-BITE FEVER

Rat-bite fever is caused by either *Streptobacillus moniliformis* or *Spirillum minus*. Symptoms of the streptobacillary form include fever, rash, and arthralgias. The spirillary form causes relapsing fever, rash, and regional lymphadenitis. Diagnosis is clinical and confirmed by culture and sometimes rising antibody titers. Treatment is with oxacillin-clavulanate or doxycycline.

Rat-bite fever is transmitted to humans in up to 10% of rat bites. However, there may be no history of rat bite. Both the streptobacillary and spirillary forms affect mainly urban dwellers living in crowded conditions and biomedical laboratory personnel. The streptobacillary form is more common.

Streptobacillary rat-bite fever: This form is caused by the pleomorphic gram-negative bacillus *Streptobacillus moniliformis*, an organism present in the oropharynx of healthy rats. Epidemics have been associated with ingestion of unpasteurized *S. moniliformis*–contaminated milk (Haverhill fever), but infection is usually a consequence of a bite by a wild rat or mouse. Other rodents and weasels have also been implicated.

The primary wound usually heals promptly, but after an incubation period of 1 to 22 (usually < 10) days, a viral-like syndrome develops abruptly, causing chills, fever, vomiting, headache, and back and joint pains. Most patients develop a morbilliform, petechial rash on the hands and feet about 3 days later. Polyarthralgia or arthritis, usually affecting the large joints asymmetrically, develops in many patients within 1 wk and may persist for several days or months if untreated. Bacterial endocarditis and abscesses in the brain or other tissues are rare but serious. Some patients have infected pericardial effusion and infected amniotic fluid.

Diagnosis is confirmed by culturing the organism from blood or joint fluid. Measurable agglutinins develop during the 2nd or 3rd wk and are diagnostically important if the titer increases. The WBC count ranges between 6,000 and 30,000/μL. The streptobacillary form usually can be differentiated clinically from the spirillary form.

Treatment includes amoxicillin-clavulanate 875/125 mg po bid, procaine penicillin G 600,000 units IM bid, or penicillin V 500 mg po qid for 7 to 10 days. Erythromycin 500 mg po qid may be used for patients allergic to penicillin. Doxycycline 100 mg bid for 14 days is an alternative.

Spirillary rat-bite fever (sodoku): *Spirillum minus* infection is acquired through a rat or, occasionally a mouse, bite. The wound usually heals promptly, but inflammation recurs at the site after 4 to 28 (usually > 10) days, accompanied by a relapsing fever and regional lymphadenitis. A roseolar-urticarial rash sometimes develops but is less prominent than the streptobacillary rash. Systemic symptoms commonly accompany fever, but arthritis is rare. In untreated patients, 2- to 4-day cycles of fever usually recur for 4 to 8 wk, but febrile episodes rarely recur for > 1 yr.

Diagnosis is by direct visualization or culture of *Spirillum* from blood smears or tissue from lesions or lymph nodes, or by Giemsa stain or darkfield examination of blood from inoculated mice. The WBC count ranges between 5,000 and 30,000/μL. The Venereal Disease Research Laboratory (VDRL) results are false-positive in ½ the patients. The disease may easily be confused with malaria, meningococcemia, or *Borrelia recurrentis* infection, all of which are characterized by relapsing fever.

Treatment is the same as for the streptobacillary form.

RELAPSING FEVER

(Tick, Recurrent, or Famine Fever)

Relapsing fever is a recurring febrile disease caused by several species of *Borrelia* and transmitted by lice or ticks. Symptoms are recurrent febrile episodes with headache, myalgia, and vomiting lasting 3 to 5 days, separated by intervals of apparent recovery. Diagnosis is clinical, confirmed by staining of peripheral blood smears. Treatment is with a tetracycline or erythromycin.

Epidemiology and Pathophysiology

The insect vector may be soft ticks of the genus *Ornithodoros* or the body louse, depending on geographic location. Louse-borne relapsing fevers are rare in the US and endemic only in parts of Africa and South America; the tick-borne, in the Americas, Africa, Asia, and Europe. In the US, the disease is generally confined to the western states, where occurrence is highest between May and September.

The louse is infected by feeding on a febrile patient. If the louse is crushed on a new host, *Borrelia* are released and can enter abraded skin or bites. Intact lice do not transmit disease. Ticks acquire the spirochetes from rodent reservoirs. Humans are infected when spirochetes in the tick's saliva or excreta enter the skin as the tick bites. Congenital borreliosis has also been reported.

The mortality rate is generally < 5% but may be considerably higher in very young, pregnant, old, malnourished, or debilitated people or during epidemics of louse-borne fever.

Symptoms and Signs

Because the tick feeds transiently and painlessly at night, most patients do not give a history of tick bite but may report an overnight exposure to caves or rustic dwellings. When present, louse infestation is usually obvious.

The incubation period ranges from 3 to 11 days (median, 6 days). Sudden chills mark the onset, followed by high fever, tachycardia, severe headache, vomiting, muscle and joint pain, and often delirium. An erythematous macular or purpuric rash may appear early over the trunk and extremities. Conjunctival, subcutaneous, or submucous hemorrhages may be present. Fever remains high for 3 to 5 days, then clears abruptly, indicating a turning point in the disease. The duration of illness ranges from 1 to 54 days (median, 18 days). Later in the several weeks' course of the disease, jaundice, hepatomegaly, splenomegaly, myocarditis, and heart failure may occur, especially in louse-borne disease. Other symptoms may include ophthalmitis, iridocyclitis, exacerbation of asthma, and erythema multiforme. Meningismus is rare. Spontaneous abortion can occur.

The patient is usually asymptomatic for several days to ≥ 1 wk between the initial episode and the 1st relapse. Relapses, related to the cyclic development of the parasites, occur with a sudden return of fever and, often, arthralgia and all the former symptoms and signs. Jaundice is more common during relapse. The illness clears as before, but 2 to 10 similar episodes may follow at intervals of 1 to 2 wk. The episodes become progressively less severe, and recovery eventually occurs as the patient develops immunity.

Diagnosis

The diagnosis is suggested by the recurrent fever and confirmed by visualization of spirochetes in the blood during a febrile episode. The spirochetes may be seen on darkfield examination or Wright's- or Giemsa-stained thick and thin blood smears. (Acridine orange stain for examining blood or tissue is more sensitive than Wright's or Giemsa stain for peripheral blood smears.) Serologic tests are unreliable. Mild polymorphonuclear leukocytosis may occur.

Differential diagnosis includes Lyme arthritis, malaria, dengue, yellow fever, leptospirosis, typhus, influenza, and the enteric fevers.

Treatment

In fever transmitted by ticks, tetracycline or erythromycin 500 mg po q 6 h is given for 5 to 10 days. A single 500-mg oral dose of either drug cures louse-transmitted fever. Doxycycline 100 mg po bid for 5 to 10 days is also effective. Children < 8 yr are given erythromycin estolate 10 mg/kg po tid. When vomiting or severe disease precludes oral administration, tetracycline 10 mg/kg in 100 or 500 mL of saline may be given IV bid or tid to children > 8 yr. Children < 8 yr are given penicillin G 25,000 units/kg IV q 6 h.

Therapy should be started early during fever or during the afebrile stage but should be avoided near the end of the episode because of the danger of Jarisch-Herxheimer reaction (see p. 1663), which can be fatal. The severity of the Jarisch-Herxheimer reaction may be lessened by giving acetaminophen 650 mg po 2 h before and 2 h after the 1st dose of doxycycline or erythromycin.

Dehydration and electrolyte imbalance should be corrected with parenteral fluids. Acetaminophen with oxycodone or hydrocodone may be used for severe headache. Nausea and vomiting should be treated with prochlorperazine 5 to 10 mg po or IM once/day to qid. If heart failure occurs, specific therapy is indicated.

175 NEISSERIACEAE

All pathogenic aerobic gram-negative cocci belong to the Neisseriaceae family, which is composed of 5 genera: *Acinetobacter, Kingella, Moraxella* (including 2 subgenera *Moraxella* and *Branhamella), Neisseria,* and *Oligella*. Of these, *Neisseria* includes the most important human pathogens, *N. meningitidis* and *N. gonorrhoeae*. Numerous saprophytic Neisseriaceae commonly inhabit the oropharynx, vagina, or colon but rarely cause human disease. *Moraxella catarrhalis* causes otitis media in children and sinusitis. Over half a dozen other *Moraxella* sp and the related *Kingella kingae* cause infections in the CNS, respiratory tract, urinary tract, endocardium, bones, and joints.

Humans are the only reservoir of *Neisseria*, and person-to-person spread is the prime mode of transmission. Both *N. meningitidis* (meningococcus) and *N. gonorrhoeae* can exist in an asymptomatic carrier state. Carrier states are particularly important with meningococcus because of its association with epidemics. Gonorrhea is discussed on p. 1653.

ACINETOBACTER INFECTIONS

Acinetobacter sp can cause suppurative infections in any organ system and are often opportunists in hospitalized patients.

Acinetobacter is ubiquitous and can survive on dry surfaces for days. Risk factors for hospital-acquired infection include length of stay, surgery, wounds, previous infection, fecal colonization with *Acinetobacter*, treatment with broad-spectrum antibiotics, parenteral nutrition, indwelling devices, ICU stay, and mechanical ventilation. Risk factors for community-acquired infection include alcoholism, cigarette smoking, chronic lung disease, diabetes mellitus, and residence in a tropical developing community.

Acinetobacter sp can cause suppurative infections in any organ system. It is often an opportunist in hospitalized patients. The significance of isolates from clinical specimens is difficult to determine because they often represent colonization.

The respiratory system is the most common site for infection. *Acinetobacter* easily colonizes tracheostomy sites. *Acinetobacter* causes community-acquired bronchiolitis and tracheobronchitis in healthy children and tracheobronchitis in immunocompromised adults. Spread in ICUs has been attributed to colonized health care practitioners, contaminated common equipment, and contaminated parenteral nutrition solutions. Hospital-acquired *Acinetobacter* pneumonias are frequently multilobar and complicated. Secondary bacteremia and septic shock are associated with a poor prognosis.

Rarely, *Acinetobacter* causes meningitis (primarily after neurosurgical procedures), cellulitis or phlebitis with an indwelling venous catheter, ocular infections, native and prosthetic valve endocarditis, osteomyelitis, septic arthritis, and pancreatic and liver abscesses.

In patients with localized cellulitis or phlebitis associated with a foreign body (eg, IV catheter or suture), removal of the foreign body with local care is generally sufficient. Tracheobronchitis after endotracheal intubation may resolve with pulmonary toilet alone. Patients with more extensive infections should be treated with antibiotics and debridement if necessary.

Acinetobacter tends to be resistant to many antimicrobials. Typically, imipenem can be used. However, outbreaks of imipenem-resistant *Acinetobacter* have occurred. Sulbactam has intrinsic bactericidal activity against many multidrug-resistant *Acinetobacter* strains. Although mild to moderate infections may respond to monotherapy, serious infections are treated with combination therapy. Bactericidal synergy occurs when several antimicrobials (eg, carbenicillin, imipenem, β-lactam/β-lactamase inhibitor) are combined with an aminoglycoside.

A hospital outbreak involving multidrug-resistant *Acinetobacter* strains with similar antibiograms should prompt an infection control investigation of compliance with hand washing, barrier precautions, ventilator care, and housekeeping.

KINGELLA INFECTIONS

***Kingella* organisms colonize the human respiratory tract. They cause skeletal infections, endocarditis, and bacteremia, and rarely pneumonia, epiglottitis, meningitis, abscesses, and ocular infections.**

Kingella are short, nonmotile, gram-negative coccobacilli that occur in pairs or short chains. The organisms are slow-growing and fastidious. *Kingella* are recovered from the human respiratory tract and are a rare cause of human disease.

Among *Kingella* species, *K. kingae* is the most frequent human pathogen. *K. kingae* frequently colonizes the respiratory mucous membranes. Children between 6 mo and 4 yr have the highest rates of colonization and invasive disease from this and other respiratory tract pathogens such as *Moraxella catarrhalis* and *Streptococcus pneumoniae*. Infection shows a seasonal distribution, with more cases in fall and winter.

The most common manifestations of *K. kingae* disease are skeletal infections, endocarditis, and bacteremia. Other rare infections include pneumonia, epiglottitis, meningitis, abscesses, and ocular infections.

The most common skeletal infection is septic arthritis, which most frequently affects large, weight-bearing joints, especially the knee and ankle. Osteomyelitis most frequently involves the bones of the lower extremity. Onset is insidious, and diagnosis is often delayed. Hematogenous invasion of the intervertebral disk can occur and has been most commonly reported in the lumbar intervertebral spaces.

Kingella endocarditis has been reported in all age groups. Endocarditis may involve both native and prosthetic valves. *Kingella* is a component of the so-called HACEK group (*Haemophilus aphrophilus* and *Haemophilus parainfluenzae, Actinobacillus, Cardiobacterium, Eikenella, Kingella*—see p. 1463), which includes fastidious bacteria capable of causing endocarditis.

Diagnosis requires laboratory isolation from suspected fluids or tissues.

Kingella organisms are generally susceptible to various penicillins and cephalosporins. However, antimicrobial susceptibility testing is needed to guide therapy. Other useful drugs include aminoglycosides, trimethoprim-sulfamethoxazole, tetracyclines, erythromycin, and ciprofloxacin.

MENINGOCOCCAL DISEASES

Meningococcus (*Neisseria meningitidis*) causes meningitis and septicemia. Symptoms, usually severe, include headache, nausea, vomiting, photophobia, lethargy, rash, multiple organ failure, shock, and disseminated intravascular coagulation. Diagnosis is clinical, confirmed by culture. Treatment is penicillin or a 3rd-generation cephalosporin.

Meningitis and septicemia account for > 90% of meningococcal infections. Infections of lungs, joints, respiratory passageways, GU organs, eyes, endocardium, and pericardium are less common.

Worldwide, the incidence of endemic disease is 0.5 to 5/100,000, with an increased number of cases in winter and spring in temperate climates. Local outbreaks occur, most frequently in sub-Saharan Africa between Senegal and Ethiopia, an area known as the meningitis belt. In major African epidemics, attack rates range from 100 to 800/100,000 population.

Meningococci can colonize the oropharynx/nasopharynx of asymptomatic carriers. A combination of factors is probably responsible for transition from carrier to invasive disease. Despite documented high rates of colonization, transition to invasive disease is rare and occurs primarily in previously uninfected patients. Transmission generally occurs via direct contact with respiratory secretions from a nasopharyngeal carrier. Carrier rates rise dramatically during epidemics.

After invading the body, *N. meningitidis* causes meningitis and severe bacteremia in both children and adults, resulting in profound vascular effects. Infection can rapidly become fulminant and is associated with a mortality rate of 10 to 15%. Of patients who recover, 10 to 15% have serious sequelae, such as permanent hearing loss, mental retardation, or loss of phalanges or limbs.

Children between 6 mo and 3 yr are the most frequently infected. Other high-risk groups include adolescents, military recruits, college freshmen living in dormitories, people with complement deficiencies, and microbiologists working with *N. meningitidis* isolates. Infection or vaccination confers type-specific immunity.

Symptoms and Signs

Patients with meningitis frequently report fever, headache, and stiff neck (see also Acute Bacterial Meningitis on p. 1858). Other symptoms include nausea, vomiting, photophobia, and lethargy. A maculopapular or hemorrhagic peticial rash often appears soon after disease onset. Meningeal signs are often apparent on physical examination. Fulminant meningococcemia syndromes include Waterhouse-Friderichsen syndrome (septicemia, profound shock, cutaneous purpura, and adrenal hemorrhage), sepsis with multiple organ failure, shock, and disseminated intravascular coagulation. A rare, chronic meningococcemia causes recurrent mild symptoms.

Diagnosis

Neisseria are small, gram-negative cocci readily identified on Gram stain and by other standard bacteriologic identification methods. Serologic methods, such as latex agglutination and coagglutination tests, permit rapid presumptive diagnosis of *N. meningitides* in blood, CSF, synovial fluid, and urine. However, both positive and negative results should be confirmed by culture. PCR for *N. meningitidis* has been developed but is not commercially available.

Treatment and Prevention

While awaiting definitive identification of the causal organism, immunocompetent adults suspected of having meningococcal infection are given a 3rd-generation cephalosporin (eg, cefotaxime 2 g IV q 6 h or ceftriaxone 2 g IV q 12 h plus vancomycin 500 mg IV q 6 h or 1 g IV q 12 h). Coverage for *Listeria monocytogenes* should be considered in immunocompromised patients by adding ampicillin 2 g IV q 4 h. Once *N. meningitidis* has been definitively identified, the preferred treatment is penicillin 4 million units IV q 4 h.

Corticosteroids decrease the incidence of neurologic complications in children. When corticosteroids are used, they should be administered with or before the 1st dose of antibiotics. Dexamethasone 0.15 mg/kg IV q 6 h in children (10 mg q 6 h in adults) is given for 4 days.

Close contacts of people with meningococcal disease are at increased risk for acquiring disease and should receive a prophylactic antibiotic. Options include rifampin 600 mg po q 12 h for 4 doses (children > 1 mo, 10 mg/kg po q 12 h for 4 doses; children < 1 mo, 5 mg/kg po q 12 h for 4 doses) or ceftriaxone 250 mg IM for 1 dose (children < 15 yr, 125 mg IM for 1 dose) or a single dose of a fluoroquinolone in adults (ciprofloxacin or levofloxacin 500 mg or ofloxacin 400 mg).

A meningococcal conjugate vaccine is available in the US. The vaccine includes 4 of the 5 serogroups of meningococcus (all but B). People who are at increased risk for developing meningococcal infection should be vaccinated. Vaccination is recommended for military recruits, travelers to endemic areas, people with laboratory or industrial exposure to *N. meningitidis* aerosols, and patients with functional or actual asplenia. Vaccination should be considered for college freshmen, especially those who live in dormitories, household or institutional contacts of people with meningococcal disease, medical and laboratory personnel at risk of exposure to meningococcal disease, and patients with immune deficiencies.

MORAXELLA CATARRHALIS INFECTION

***Moraxella catarrhalis* causes ear and upper and lower respiratory infections.**

Previously classified as *Micrococcus*, then *Neisseria,* and also known as *Branhamella catarrhalis,* this organism is a frequent cause of otitis media in children, acute and chronic sinusitis at all ages, and lower respiratory infection in adults with chronic lung disease. It is the 2nd most common bacterial cause of COPD exacerbations after nontypeable *Haemophilus influenzae*. *M. catarrhalis* pneumonia resembles pneumococcal pneumonia. Although bacteremia is rare, ½ of patients die within 3 mo due to intercurrent diseases.

The prevalence of *M. catarrhalis* colonization depends on age. About 1 to 5% of healthy adults have upper respiratory tract colonization. Nasopharyngeal colonization with *M. catarrhalis* is common throughout infancy, may be higher during winter months, and is a risk factor for acute otitis media; early colonization is a risk factor for recurrent otitis media. Substantial regional differences in colonization rates occur. Living conditions, hygiene, environmental factors (eg, household smoking), genetic characteristics of the populations, host factors, and other factors may contribute to these differences.

The organism appears to spread contiguously from its colonizing position in the respiratory tract to the infection site.

There is no pathognomic feature of *M. catarrhalis* otitis media, acute or chronic sinusitis, or pneumonia. In lower respiratory disease, patients experience increased cough, purulent sputum production, and increased dyspnea.

These gram-negative cocci resemble *Neisseria* sp but can be readily distinguished by routine biochemical tests after culture isolation from infected fluids or tissues.

All strains are now β-lactamase producers. The organism is generally susceptible to β-lactam/β-lactamase inhibitors, sulfamethoxazole, tetracyclines, extended-spectrum oral cephalosporins, aminoglycosides, macrolides, and fluoroquinolones.

OLIGELLA INFECTIONS

***Oligella* sp cause infection primarily of the GU tract.**

The genus *Oligella* contains 2 species, *Oligella urethralis* and *O. ureolytica*. *O. urethralis* is a commensal of the GU tract, and most clinical isolates are from the urine, predominantly from men. Although symptomatic infections are rare, bacteremia, septic arthritis that mimics gonococcal arthritis, and peritonitis have been reported.

O. ureolytica is also found primarily in the urine, usually from patients with long-term urinary catheters or other urinary drainage systems. These patients have a propensity to develop urinary stones, possibly because the organism hydrolyzes urea and alkalinizes the urine, leading to precipitation of phosphates. Bacteremia has occurred in a patient with obstructive uropathy.

Diagnosis is by culture. As these organisms are rarely isolated, antimicrobial susceptibility data are limited; most are sensitive to β-lactam antibiotics. However, a β-lactam–producing strain and strains resistant to ciprofloxacin have been identified.

176 CHLAMYDIA AND MYCOPLASMAS

CHLAMYDIA

Three species of *Chlamydia* cause human disease, including sexually transmitted diseases and pneumonias. Most are susceptible to azithromycin, doxycycline, and some fluoroquinolones.

Chlamydiae are nonmotile, obligate intracellular organisms. Although originally considered viruses because they require a cellular host, they are now known to be bacteria.

Three species cause human disease: *Chlamydia trachomatis, Chlamydophila* (formerly *Chlamydia*) pneumoniae, and *Chlamydophila* (formerly *Chlamydia*) *psittaci*.

C. trachomatis has 18 immunologically defined serovars. Serotypes A, B, Ba, and C cause trachoma and inclusion conjunctivitis; D through K cause sexually transmitted diseases (STDs) localized to mucosal surfaces; L1, L2, and L3 cause STDs leading to invasive lymph node disease (lymphogranuloma venereum). *C. trachomatis* is the most common bacterial cause of STDs in the US, including nongonococcal urethritis (see p. 1651) and epididymitis in men; cervicitis, urethritis, and pelvic inflammatory disease in women; and proctitis, lymphogranuloma venereum, and reactive arthritis (Reiter's syndrome) in both sexes. Maternal transmission of *C. trachomatis* causes neonatal conjunctivitis and pneumonia. The organism occasionally is isolated from the throat in adults but rarely causes symptomatic pharyngitis.

C. pneumoniae can cause pneumonia (especially in children and young adults) that may be clinically indistinguishable from pneumonia caused by *Mycoplasma pneumoniae*. From 6 to 19% of community-acquired pneumonia is due to *C. pneumoniae*, but chlamydial pneumonia is uncommon in children < 5 yr. No seasonal variations in occurrence have been observed. The organism has been found in atheromatous lesions, and infection may be associated with increased risk of coronary artery disease, although proof of a connection has not yet been established.

C. psittaci causes psittacosis. Strains causing human disease are usually transmitted from psittacine birds (eg, parrots), causing a disseminated disease characterized by pneumonitis.

Diagnosis

Diagnosis is usually presumptive because testing is difficult. Routine testing for genital infection has been recommended and is increasingly common. In cases of urethritis, diagnosis is often made by excluding gonorrhea as a cause or by presuming that both chlamydia and gonorrhea are present. *C. trachomatis* can be isolated by diagnostic cell culture, available only in larger medical centers. *C. trachomatis* can best be identified in genital samples using nucleic acid amplification tests (NAATs) such as PCR, since these tests are more sensitive than cell culture and have less stringent sample handling requirements. Antigen detection by enzyme-linked immunosorbent assay (ELISA) or direct immunofluorescent slide test is also available for genital and ocular infections, but both methods are less sensitive than culture or NAATs. Serologic tests are useful in diagnosing pneumonia in infants and lymphogranuloma venereum.

Chlamydial genital infection is so common in women that all sexually active women ≤ 25 yr are urged to undergo testing once or twice/year. Testing should also be a routine part of prenatal care.

A primary clue to diagnosis of *C. psittaci* infection is close contact with birds, typically parrots or parakeets.

Treatment

Treatment of uncomplicated lower genital tract infection is typically with a single dose of azithromycin (1 g po) or with 7-day regimens of doxycycline (100 mg po bid) or some fluoroquinolones (eg, levofloxacin 500 mg po once/day). Treatment of presumed infection is routine when gonorrhea is present (see also p. 1653). Treatment of pelvic inflammatory disease, lymphogranuloma venereum, or epididymitis is usually 2 wk.

Specific infections are discussed elsewhere in THE MANUAL. Psittacosis and *C. pneumoniae* pneumonia are discussed in Ch. 52; lymphogranuloma venereum and urethritis, in Ch. 194; epididymitis, in Ch. 239; reactive arthritis, in Ch. 34; neonatal conjunctivitis and neonatal pneumonia, in Ch. 279; and trachoma and inclusion conjunctivitis, in Ch. 101.

MYCOPLASMAS

Mycoplasmas are ubiquitous prokaryotes lacking a cell wall. They are distinct from bacteria and viruses.

Mycoplasma pneumoniae is a common cause of pneumonia, particularly community-acquired, *M. genitalium* and *Ureaplasma urealyticum* are suspected causes of nongonococcal urethritis. They (and *M. hominis*) are often present in patients with other urogenital infections (eg, vaginitis, cervicitis, pyelonephritis, pelvic inflammatory disease) and some non-urogenital infections, but whether they cause these infections is not clear.

Mycoplasmas are not visible on light microscopy. Culture is technically difficult and often unavailable, but laboratory diagnosis is sometimes possible with DNA probes or by detection of antibodies or antigens; frequently, diagnosis must be clinical. Macrolides are usually the antimicrobials of choice. Most species are also sensitive to fluoroquinolones and tetracyclines.

177 RICKETTSIAE AND RELATED ORGANISMS

Rickettsial diseases (rickettsioses) and related diseases (ehrlichiosis, Q fever) are caused by a group of gram-negative, obligately intracellular coccobacilli. Most have an arthropod vector. Symptoms generally include sudden-onset fever with severe headache, malaise, prostration, and, in most cases, a characteristic rash. Diagnosis is clinical, confirmed by immunofluorescence or PCR. Treatment is with tetracyclines or chloramphenicol.

Although rickettsiae require living cells for growth, they are true bacteria because they have metabolic enzymes and cell walls, use O_2, and are susceptible to antibiotics. Rickettsiae (except *Coxiella burnetii*, the causative agent of Q fever, which is no longer classified with the Rickettsieae) have an animal reservoir and an insect vector (usually an arthropod) that infects humans (see TABLE 177–1).

Rickettsiae multiply at the site of arthropod attachment and often produce a local lesion (eschar). They penetrate the skin or mucous membranes and multiply in the endothelial cells of small blood vessels (*Rickettsia rickettsii*), causing a vasculitis, or replicate in WBCs (*Ehrlichia*). The endovasculitis of *R. rickettsii* produces the rash, encephalitic signs, and gangrene of skin and tissues. Patients seriously ill with a rickettsial disease of the typhus or spotted fever group or with ehrlichiosis may have ecchymotic skin necrosis, digital gangrene, circulatory collapse, shock, oliguria, anuria, azotemia, anemia, hyponatremia, hypochloremia, edema, delirium, and coma.

Diagnosis

Rickettsial and related diseases must be differentiated from other acute infections, primarily meningococcemia, rubeola, and rubella. A history of louse or flea contact, tick bite, or presence in a known endemic area is helpful, but such history is often absent. Clinical features may help distinguish diseases.

In meningococcemia, the rash may be pink, macular, maculopapular, or petechial in the subacute form and petechially confluent or ecchymotic in the fulminant form. It develops rapidly in acute meningococcal disease and, when ecchymotic, usually is tender on palpation.

In rubeola, the rash begins on the face, spreads to the trunk and arms, and soon becomes confluent. The rash of rubella usually remains discrete. Postauricular lymph node enlargement and lack of toxicity favor rubella.

Rickettsial and related diseases must also be differentiated from each other. Because many rickettsiae are localized to certain geographic areas, knowledge of residence and recent travel often helps in diagnosis. However, testing is usually required. The most useful tests for *R. rickettsii* are indirect immunofluorescence assay (IFA) and PCR of a biopsy specimen of the rash. Culture is difficult and not clinically useful. For *Ehrlichia*, PCR of blood is the best test. Serologic tests are not useful for acute diagnosis as they usually become positive only on convalescence.

Clinical presentation allows some differentiation of rickettsial diseases, but overlap is considerable.

The rash of Rocky Mountain spotted fever (RMSF) usually appears on about the 4th febrile day as blanching macules on the extremities and gradually becomes petechial as it spreads to the trunk, palms, and soles over several days. Some patients with RMSF never develop a rash.

The rash of epidemic typhus usually appears initially over the axillary folds and trunk. Later it spreads peripherally, rarely involving the palms, soles, and face. Profound physiologic and pathologic abnormalities similar to those of RMSF occur.

In murine typhus, the rash is nonpurpuric, nonconfluent, and less extensive, and renal and vascular complications are uncommon.

Scrub typhus presents similarly to RMSF and epidemic typhus. However, it occurs in different geographic areas, and frequently, an eschar develops with satellite adenopathy.

Rickettsialpox is mild, and the rash, in the form of vesicles with surrounding erythema, is sparse, and may resemble varicella. African tick bite fever (*R. africae*) has symptoms similar to other rickettsial diseases with a rash characterized by multiple black eschars on the distal extremities with regional adenopathy.

TABLE 177–1. DISEASES CAUSED BY *RICKETTSIA, EHRLICHIA,* AND *COXIELLA*

GROUP/ DISEASE	ORGANISM	RASH/ ESCHAR	VECTOR	ENDEMIC REGION
Typhus				
Epidemic typhus; Brill-Zinsser disease	*Rickettsia prowazekii*	Trunk to extremities; may be absent in Brill-Zinsser disease; no eschar	Body lice	Worldwide
Murine (endemic) typhus	*R. typhi* (formerly *R. mooseri*)	Trunk to extremities; no eschar	Rat flea, cat flea	Worldwide
Scrub typhus				
Tsutsugamushi disease	*R. tsutsugamushi*	Trunk to extremities; eschar occurs	Trombiculid mite larvae (chiggers)	Asiatic-Pacific area bounded by Japan, India, and Australia
Spotted fever				
Rocky Mountain spotted fever	*R. rickettsii*	Extremities to trunk; no eschar	Ixodid ticks (*Dermacentor andersoni* [wood tick] principally in western US and *D. variabilis* [dog tick] principally in eastern and southern US)	Western Hemisphere; most of the US (except Maine, Hawaii, Alaska); Central and South America
North Asian tick-borne rickettsiosis	*R. sibirica*	Trunk, extremities, face; eschar occurs	Ixodid ticks	Armenia, Central Asia, Siberia, Mongolia
Queensland tick typhus	*R. australis*	Trunk, extremities, face; eschar occurs	Ixodid ticks	Australia
African tick bite fever	*R. africae*	Eschar on extremities (tache noir) at site of tick bite	Ixodid ticks	South Africa, Zimbabwe
Mediterranean spotted fever (fièvre boutonneuse)*	*R. conorii*	Trunk, extremities, face; eschar occurs	*Rhipicephalus sanguineus* (brown dog tick)	Africa, India, Europe and the Middle East adjacent to the Mediterranean, Black, and Caspian Seas
Rickettsialpox	*R. akari*	Vascular; trunk, extremities, face; eschar occurs	Mites	US, Russia, Korea, Africa
Ehrlichioses				
Monocytic ehrlichiosis	*Ehrlichia chaffeensis*	None; no eschar	Ticks	Southeastern and south-central US

Table continues on the following page.

TABLE 177–1. DISEASES CAUSED BY *RICKETTSIA, EHRLICHIA,* AND *COXIELLA*—Continued

GROUP/ DISEASE	ORGANISM	RASH/ ESCHAR	VECTOR	ENDEMIC REGION
Granulocytic ehrlichiosis	*Anaplasma phagocytophila* and *E. ewingii*	None; no eschar	Ticks	Southeastern and south-central US
Q fever	*Coxiella burnetii*	None; no eschar	No vector needed	Worldwide

*Often known by the area in which it occurs (eg, Indian tick typhus, Mediterranean spotted fever, Marseilles fever).

Treatment

Because diagnostic tests can take time and may be insensitive, antibiotics are generally begun presumptively to prevent significant deterioration, death, and prolonged recovery. The tetracyclines are 1st-line treatment: doxycycline 200 mg po once followed by 100 mg bid until the patient improves and has been afebrile for 24 to 48 h, but continued for at least 7 days. IV preparations are used in patients too ill to take oral drugs. Chloramphenicol 500 mg po or IV qid for 7 days is 2nd-line treatment. Both agents are rickettsiostatic, not rickettsicidal. Ciprofloxacin and other fluoroquinolones are effective against certain rickettsiae, but extensive clinical experience is lacking.

Because severely ill patients with RMSF or epidemic typhus may have a marked increase in capillary permeability in later stages, IV fluids should be given cautiously to maintain BP while avoiding worsening pulmonary and cerebral edema. Heparin is not recommended in patients who develop disseminated intravascular coagulation.

EASTERN TICK-BORNE RICKETTSIOSES

Eastern tick-borne rickettsioses are caused by various rickettsia transmitted by ixodid ticks. Symptoms are an initial skin lesion, satellite adenopathy, and an erythematous maculopapular rash.

Eastern tick-borne rickettsioses (ETBR) include North Asian tick-borne rickettsiosis, Queensland tick typhus, African tick typhus, and Mediterranean spotted fever (fièvre boutonneuse). The causative agents belong to the spotted fever group of rickettsiae.

The epidemiology of these tick-borne rickettsioses resembles that of spotted fever in the Western Hemisphere. Ixodid ticks and wild animals maintain the rickettsiae in nature. If humans intrude accidentally into the cycle, they become infected. In certain areas, the cycle of fièvre boutonneuse involves domiciliary environments, with the brown dog tick, *Rhipicephalus sanguineus*, as the dominant vector.

The symptoms and signs are similar for all ETBR and generally milder than with spotted fever. After an incubation period of 5 to 7 days, fever, malaise, headache, and conjunctival injection develop. With the onset of fever, a small buttonlike ulcer 2 to 5 mm in diameter with a black center appears (an eschar, or, in fièvre boutonneuse, tache noire). Usually the regional or satellite lymph nodes are enlarged. On about the 4th day of fever, a red maculopapular rash appears on the forearms and extends to most of the body, including the palms and soles. Fever lasts into the 2nd wk. Complications and death are rare except among elderly or debilitated patients. However, the disease should not be ignored; a fulminant form of vasculitis can occur.

For diagnosis, see p. 1488. Treatment is doxycycline 100 mg po bid for 5 days or ciprofloxacin 500 to 750 mg po bid for 5 days. Measures can be taken to prevent tick bites (see sidebar 177–1).

EPIDEMIC TYPHUS

(European, Classic, or Louse-Borne Typhus; Jail Fever)

Epidemic typhus is caused by *Rickettsia prowazekii*. Symptoms are prolonged high fever, intractable headache, and a maculopapular rash.

Sidebar 177–1. TICK BITE PREVENTION

Preventing tick access to skin includes staying on paths and trails, tucking trousers into boots or socks, wearing long-sleeved shirts, and applying repellents with diethyltoluamide (DEET) to skin surfaces. DEET should be cautiously applied to very young children because of reports of toxic reactions. Permethrin on clothing effectively kills ticks. Good personal hygiene should be practiced, with frequent searches for ticks, particularly of hairy areas and in children. Engorged ticks should be removed with care and not crushed between the fingers because of the danger of disease transmission. The tick's body should not be grasped or squeezed. Gradual traction on the head with a small forceps dislodges the tick. The point of attachment should be swabbed with alcohol. Petroleum jelly, alcohol, lit matches, and any other irritants are not effective and should not be used.

No practical means are available to rid entire areas of ticks, but tick populations may be reduced in endemic areas by controlling small-animal populations.

Humans are the natural reservoir for *R. prowazekii*, which is prevalent worldwide and transmitted by body lice when louse feces are scratched or rubbed into bite or other wounds (and sometimes the mucous membranes of the eyes or mouth). In the US, humans may occasionally contract epidemic typhus after contact with flying squirrels.

Fatalities are rare in children < 10 yr, but mortality increases with age and may reach 60% in untreated patients > 50 yr.

Symptoms and Signs

After an incubation period of 7 to 14 days, fever, headache, and prostration suddenly occur. Temperature reaches 40° C in several days and remains high, with slight morning remission, for about 2 wk. Headache is generalized and intense. Small, pink macules, which appear on the 4th to 6th day, rapidly cover the body, usually in the axillae and on the upper trunk and generally excluding the palms, soles, and face. Later the rash becomes dark and maculopapular. In severe cases, the rash becomes petechial and hemorrhagic. Splenomegaly sometimes occurs. Hypotension occurs in most seriously ill patients. Vascular collapse, renal insufficiency, encephalitic signs, ecchymosis with gangrene, and pneumonia are poor prognostic signs.

Diagnosis, Prevention, and Treatment

For details of diagnosis, see p. 1488. Primary treatment is doxycycline 200 mg po once followed by 100 mg bid until the patient improves and has been afebrile for 24 to 48 h, but continued for at least 7 days. Chloramphenicol 500 mg po or IV qid for 7 days is 2nd-line treatment.

Louse infestation is usually obvious and strongly suggests typhus in the proper setting. Immunization and louse control are highly effective for prevention. However, vaccines are not available in the US. Lice may be eliminated by dusting infested people with malathion or lindane.

Brill-Zinsser Disease

Brill-Zinsser disease is a recrudescence of epidemic typhus, occurring years after an initial attack.

Patients with Brill-Zinsser disease either had acquired epidemic typhus earlier or lived in an endemic area. Apparently, when host defenses falter, viable organisms retained in the body are activated, causing recurrent typhus; thus, disease is sporadic, occurring at any season and in the absence of infected lice. However, lice that feed on patients may acquire infection and transmit the agent.

Symptoms and signs are almost always mild and resemble epidemic typhus with similar circulatory disturbances and hepatic, renal, and CNS changes. The remittent febrile course lasts about 7 to 10 days. The rash is often evanescent or absent. Mortality is nil. For diagnosis and treatment, see p. 1491.

MURINE (ENDEMIC) TYPHUS

(Rat-Flea Typhus; Urban Typhus of Malaya)

Murine typhus is caused by *Rickettsia typhi*, which is transmitted to humans by rat fleas; it is clinically similar to, but milder than, epidemic typhus, causing chills, headache, fever, and rash.

Animal reservoirs include wild rats, mice, and other rodents. Rat fleas and probably cat fleas transmit the agent to humans. Distribution is sporadic, but worldwide; the incidence is low, but higher in rat-infested areas.

After an incubation of 6 to 18 days (mean 10 days), a shaking chill accompanies headache and fever. The fever lasts about 12 days; then temperature gradually returns to normal. The rash and other manifestations are similar to those of epidemic typhus but are much less severe. The early rash is sparse and discrete. Mortality is low, but higher in elderly patients.

Murine typhus is identified by immunofluorescence assay (IFA), immunohistology of a skin biopsy, PCR, and enzyme-linked immunosorbent assay (ELISA). Incidence has been decreased by reducing rat and rat-flea populations. No effective vaccine exists. Primary treatment is doxycycline 200 mg po once followed by 100 mg bid until the patient improves and has been afebrile for 24 to 48 h, but continued for at least 7 days. Chloramphenicol 500 mg po or IV qid for 7 days is 2nd-line treatment (for details of treatment, see p. 1490.)

RICKETTSIALPOX

(Vesicular Rickettsiosis)

Rickettsialpox is caused by *Rickettsia akari*. Symptoms are an initial local lesion and a generalized papulovesicular rash.

Rickettsialpox occurs in many areas of the US and in Russia, Korea, and Africa. The vector, a small, colorless mite, is widely distributed. It infects the house mouse and some species of wild mice. Humans may be infected by either chigger or adult mite bites.

An eschar, which appears initially about 1 wk before onset of fever as a small papule 1 to 1.5 cm in diameter, develops into a small ulcer with a dark crust that leaves a scar when it heals. Regional lymphadenopathy is present. An intermittent fever lasts about 1 wk, with chills, profuse sweating, headache, photophobia, and muscle pains. Early in the febrile course, a generalized maculopapular rash with intraepidermal vesicles appears, sparing the palms and soles. The disease is mild; no deaths have been reported.

Treatment is doxycycline 100 mg po bid for 5 days or ciprofloxacin 750 mg po bid for 5 days. For prophylaxis, mouse harborages must be destroyed and the vector controlled by residual insecticides.

ROCKY MOUNTAIN SPOTTED FEVER

(Spotted Fever; Tick Fever; Tick Typhus)

Rocky Mountain spotted fever is caused by *Rickettsia rickettsii* and transmitted by ixodid ticks. Symptoms are high fever, cough, and rash.

Epidemiology and Pathophysiology

Rocky Mountain spotted fever (RMSF) is limited to the Western Hemisphere. Initially recognized in the Rocky Mountain states, it occurs in practically all of the US, especially the Atlantic states, and throughout Central and South America. In humans, infection occurs mainly from May to September, when adult ticks are active and people are most likely to be in tick-infested areas. In southern states, sporadic cases occur throughout the year. The incidence is highest in children < 15 yr and in others who frequent tick-infested areas for work or recreation.

Hard-shelled ticks (family Ixodidae) harbor *R. rickettsii*, and infected females transmit the agent to their progeny. These ticks are the natural reservoirs. *Dermacentor andersoni* (wood tick) is the principal vector in the western US. *D. variabilis* (dog tick) is the vector in the eastern and southern US. RMSF is probably not transmitted directly from person to person.

Small blood vessels are the sites of the characteristic pathologic lesions. Rickettsiae propagate within damaged endothelial cells, and vessels may become blocked by thrombi, producing vasculitis in the skin, subcutaneous tissues, CNS, lungs, heart, kidneys, liver, and spleen. Disseminated intravascular coagulation often occurs in severely ill patients (see p. 1083).

Symptoms and Signs

A history of tick bite is elicited in about 70% of patients. The incubation period averages 7 days but varies from 3 to 12 days; the shorter the incubation period, the more severe the infection. Onset is abrupt, with severe headache, chills, prostration, and muscular pains. Fever reaches 39.5 to 40° C within several days and remains high (for 15 to 20 days in severe cases), although morning remissions may occur. Between the 1st and 6th day of fever, most patients develop a rash on the wrists, ankles, palms, soles, and forearms that rapidly extends to the neck, face, axillae, buttocks, and trunk. Initially macular and pink, it becomes maculopapular and darker. In about 4 days, the lesions become petechial and may coalesce to form large hemorrhagic areas that later ulcerate. Neurologic symptoms include headache, restlessness, insomnia, delirium, and coma, all indicative of encephalitis. Hypotension develops in severe cases. Hepatomegaly may be present, but jaundice is infrequent. Nausea and vomiting are common. Localized pneumonitis may occur. Untreated patients may develop pneumonia, tissue necrosis, and circulatory failure, sometimes with brain and heart damage. Cardiac arrest with sudden death occasionally occurs in fulminant cases.

Diagnosis and Treatment

Any seriously ill patient who lives in or near a wooded area anywhere in the Western Hemisphere and has unexplained fever, headache, and prostration, with or without a history of tick contact, should be suspected of having RMSF.

For diagnosis and treatment, see p. 1488. Starting antibiotics early significantly reduces mortality, from about 20 to 7%, and prevents most complications. When a tick bite occurs in a known endemic area but clinical signs are absent, antibiotics should not be given immediately. If fever, headache, and malaise occur with or without a rash, antibiotics should be started promptly. No effective vaccine is available. Measures can be taken to prevent tick bites (see sidebar 177–1).

SCRUB TYPHUS

(Tsutsugamushi Disease; Mite-Borne Typhus; Tropical Typhus)

Scrub typhus is a mite-borne disease caused by *Rickettsia tsutsugamushi*. Symptoms are fever, a primary lesion, a macular rash, and lymphadenopathy.

R. tsutsugamushi is transmitted by trombiculid mites, which feed on forest and rural rodents, including rats, voles, and field mice. Human infection follows a chigger (mite larva) bite.

After an incubation period of 6 to 21 days (mean 10 to 12 days), fever, chills, headache, and generalized lymphadenopathy start suddenly. At onset of fever, an eschar often develops at the site of the chigger bite. The lesion, common in whites but rare in Asians, begins as a red, indurated lesion about 1 cm in diameter that eventually vesiculates, ruptures, and becomes covered with a black scab. Regional lymph nodes enlarge. Fever rises during the 1st wk, often to 40 to 40.5° C. Headache is severe and common, as is conjunctival injection. A macular rash develops on the trunk during the 5th to 8th day of fever, often extending to the arms and legs. It may disappear rapidly or become maculopapular and intensely colored. Cough is present during the 1st wk of fever, and pneumonitis may develop during the 2nd wk. In severe cases, pulse rate increases; BP drops; and delirium, stupor, and muscular twitching develop. Splenomegaly may be present, and interstitial myocarditis is more common than in other rickettsial diseases. In untreated patients, high fever may persist ≥ 2 wk, then falls gradually over several days. With therapy, defervescence usually begins within 36 h. Recovery is prompt and uneventful.

Clearing brush and spraying infested areas with residual insecticides eliminate or decrease mite populations. Insect repellents (eg, diethyltoluamide [DEET]) should be used when exposure is likely. For details of diagnosis and treatment, see p. 1488; primary treatment is doxycycline 200 mg po once followed by 100 mg bid until the patient improves and has been afebrile for 24 to 48 h, continued for at least 7 days. Chloramphenicol 500 mg po or IV qid for 7 days is 2nd-line treatment.

EHRLICHIOSIS

Ehrlichiosis is caused by rickettsial-like bacteria of the genus *Ehrlichia* transmitted to humans by ticks. Symptoms resemble Rocky Mountain spotted fever except that a rash is present in only a minority of patients. Patients have an abrupt onset of illness with fever, chills, headache, and malaise.

Etiology and Epidemiology

Ehrlichia are obligate, intracellular bacteria that appear as small cytoplasmic inclusions in lymphocytes and neutrophils. Infections are transmitted to humans via tick bites, sometimes via contact with animals that carry the brown dog tick or deer tick. Most cases have been identified in the southeastern and south-central parts of the US. Three species of *Ehrlichia* are human pathogens in the US: *E. chaffeensis* causes human monocytic ehrlichiosis; *Anaplasma phagocytophila* (formerly *E. phagocytophila*) and *E. ewingii* cause human granulocytic ehrlichiosis. The difference in the primary target cell results in only minor differences in clinical manifestations.

Symptoms and Signs

Although some infections are asymptomatic, most cause an abrupt onset of illness with fever, chills, headache, and malaise, usually beginning about 12 days after the tick bite. Some patients develop a maculopapular or petechial rash involving the trunk and extremities, although rash is rare with *E. ewingii*. Abdominal pain, vomiting and diarrhea, disseminated intravascular coagulation, seizures, and coma may occur.

Diagnosis and Treatment

Diagnostic serologic tests are available, but PCR from blood is more sensitive and specific and can render an early diagnosis. Cytoplasmic ehrlichial inclusions in monocytes or neutrophils may occur. Hematologic and hepatic abnormalities include leukopenia, thrombocytopenia, and abnormal liver function tests, especially elevated levels of transaminases.

Treatment is best started before laboratory results return. When treatment is started early, patients generally respond rapidly and well. When treatment is delayed, serious complications may follow, including viral and fungal superinfections and death in 2 to 5%. For details on treatment, see p. 1490. Measures can be taken to prevent tick bites (see sidebar 177–1).

Q FEVER

Q fever is an acute or chronic disease caused by the rickettsial-like, *Coxiella burnetii*. Symptoms of acute disease are sudden onset of fever, headache, malaise, and interstitial pneumonitis. Chronic disease manifestations reflect the organ system affected. Diagnosis is confirmed by several serologic techniques, isolation of the organism, or PCR. Treatment is with doxycycline or chloramphenicol.

Coxiella burnetii is a small, intracellular, pleomorphic bacillus that is no longer classified with the *Rickettsia*. Molecular studies have reclassified it as a Proteobacteria in the same group as *Legionella*.

Etiology and Epidemiology

Worldwide in its distribution, Q fever is maintained as an inapparent infection in domestic or farm animals. Sheep, cattle, and goats are the principal reservoirs for human infection. *C. burnetii* persists in stool, urine, milk, and tissues (especially the placenta), so that fomites and infective aerosols form easily. *C. burnetii* is also maintained in nature through an animal-tick cycle.

Cases occur among workers whose occupations bring them in close contact with farm animals or their products. Transmission is usually by inhalation of infected aerosols, but the disease can also be contracted by ingesting infective raw milk. *C. burnetii* is very virulent, resists inactivation, and remains viable in dust and stool for months; even a single organism can cause infection.

Q fever can be acute or chronic. Acute disease produces a febrile illness that often affects the respiratory system, although sometimes the liver is involved. Chronic Q fever is usually manifested by endocarditis or hepatitis; however, osteomyelitis may occur.

Symptoms and Signs

The incubation period averages 18 to 21 days (range 9 to 28 days). Some infections are minimally symptomatic; usually, however, patients have influenza-like symptoms. Onset is abrupt, with fever, severe headache, chills, severe malaise, myalgia, anorexia, and sweats. Fever may rise to 40° C and persist 1 to > 3 wk. Respiratory symptoms, a dry nonproductive cough and pleuritic chest pain, appear 4 to 5 days after onset of illness. Lung symptoms may be particularly severe in elderly or debilitated patients. On examination, lung crackles are common, and findings suggestive of consolidation may be present. Unlike the rickettsial diseases, acute Q fever does not produce a rash.

Acute hepatic involvement, occurring in some patients, resembles viral hepatitis, with fever, malaise, hepatomegaly with right upper abdominal pain, and possibly jaundice. Headache and respiratory signs are frequently absent. Chronic Q fever hepatitis may present as FUO and must be differentiated from other causes of liver granulomas (eg, TB, sarcoidosis, histoplasmosis, brucellosis, tularemia, syphilis) by laboratory testing.

Endocarditis resembles viridans group subacute bacterial endocarditis (see p. 724); aortic valve involvement is more common, but vegetations may occur on any valve. Marked finger clubbing, arterial emboli, hepatomegaly and splenomegaly, and a purpuric rash may occur.

Q fever is fatal in only 1% of untreated patients. However, some patients with neurologic involvement have residual impairment.

Diagnosis

Early on, Q fever resembles many infections (eg, influenza, other viral infections, salmonellosis, malaria, hepatitis, brucellosis). Later, it resembles many forms of bacterial, viral, and mycoplasmal pneumonias. Contact with animals or animal products is an important clue.

Immunofluorescence assay (IFA) is the diagnostic method of choice; enzyme-linked immunosorbent assay (ELISA) is also available. Acute and convalescent serology (typically complement fixation) may be used. PCR can identify the organism in biopsy specimens. *C. burnetii* may be isolated from clinical specimens, but only by special research laboratories; routine blood and sputum cultures are negative.

Patients with respiratory signs or symptoms require chest x-ray; findings may include atelectasis, pleural-based opacities, pleural effusion, and lobar consolidation. The gross appearance of the lungs may resemble bacterial pneumonia, but histologically more resembles psittacosis and some viral pneumonias.

In acute Q fever, CBC may be normal, but about 30% of patients have an elevated WBC count. Alkaline phosphatase, AST, and ALT levels are mildly elevated to 2 to 3 times the normal level in typical cases. If obtained, liver biopsy specimens show diffuse granulomatous changes.

Treatment and Prevention

Primary treatment is doxycycline 200 mg po once followed by 100 mg po bid until the patient improves and has been afebrile for about 5 days, but continued for at least 7 days. Chloramphenicol 500 mg po or IV qid for 7 days is 2nd-line treatment. Fluoroquinolones and macrolides are also effective. For details of treatment, see p. 1490.

In endocarditis, treatment needs to be prolonged ≥ 4 wk; tetracycline is preferred. When antibiotic treatment is only partially effective, damaged valves must be replaced surgically, although some cures without surgery have occurred. Clear-cut regimens for chronic hepatitis have not been determined.

The patient is isolated. Vaccines are effective and should be used to protect slaughterhouse and dairy workers, rendering plant workers, herders, woolsorters, farmers, and others at risk. These vaccines are not available commercially but may be obtained from special laboratories, eg, the U.S. Army Medical Research Institute of Infectious Diseases in Fort Detrick, Maryland.

178 ANAEROBIC BACTERIA

Anaerobic bacteria are intolerant of O_2, replicating at low oxidation-reduction potential sites, such as necrotic, devascularized tissue. Microaerophilic organisms are tolerant of low O_2 concentrations but grow better anaerobically or with > 10% CO_2 in the air. Anaerobic organisms can be classified as strict or moderate (eg, intolerant of 0.5% O_2 vs tolerant of 2 to 8% O_2). Facultative anaerobes tolerate O_2 but grow in its absence as well. In humans, anaerobic organisms are among the normal flora (especially of the GI tract, mouth, and vagina), but when they enter sterile spaces, they can cause serious infections.

Anaerobic infections are typically suppurative, causing abscess formation and tissue necrosis, often the result of thrombophlebitis and/or gas formation. Many anaerobes produce enzymes that devitalize tissue as well as some of the most potent paralytic toxins known. Clues to the presence of anaerobic infection include gas formation in tissue, foul feculent odors, and abscess formation or tissue necrosis.

Specimens for anaerobic culture should be obtained as aspirates or biopsy material from normally sterile sites. Delivery to the laboratory should be prompt, and transport devices should provide an O_2-free atmosphere of carbon dioxide, hydrogen, and nitrogen. Swabs are best transported in an anaerobically sterilized, semisolid medium such as Cary-Blair transport medium.

Clostridia: The most notorious of the anaerobic pathogens are the clostridia—spore-forming, gram-positive bacilli found widely in dust, soil, and vegetation and as normal flora in mammalian GI tracts. Although nearly 100 *Clostridium* sp have been identified, only 25 to 30 commonly induce human or animal disease. The pathogenic species produce tissue-destructive and neural exotoxins that are responsible for disease manifestations. Clostridia may become pathogenic when tissue O_2 tension and pH are low. Such an anaerobic environment may develop in ischemic or devitalized tissue, as occurs with primary arterial insufficiency, or after severe penetrating or crushing injuries. The deeper and more severe the wound, the more prone the patient is to clostridial infection, especially if there is even minimal contamination by foreign matter. Clostridial disease can also occur after injection of street drugs. Serious noninfectious disease can occur after ingestion of home-canned foods in which clostridia have produced toxins.

The most frequent clostridial infection is minor, self-limited gastroenteritis typically from *C. perfringens* type A. Serious clostridial diseases are relatively rare but can be fatal. Enteritis necroticans is caused by *C. perfringens* type C, antibiotic-associated colitis by *C. difficile*, and neutropenic enterocolitis by *C. septicum*. Abdominal disorders, such as cholecystitis, peritonitis, ruptured appendix, and bowel perforation can involve *C. perfringens, C. ramosum*, and many others. Muscle necrosis and soft-tissue infection, which is characterized by crepitant cellulitis, myositis, and clostridial myonecrosis, can be caused by *C. perfringens*. Tissue necrosis can be caused by *C. septicum*. Tetanus is caused by *C. tetani*, botulism by *C. botulinum*. Clostridia also appear as components of mixed flora in common mild wound infections; their role in such infections is unclear.

Hospital-acquired clostridial infection is increasing, particularly in postoperative and immunocompromised patients. Severe clostridial sepsis may complicate intestinal perforation and obstruction.

Other anaerobes: Organisms of concern include *Actinomyces israelii*, a cause of chronic localized or hematogenous infection, and a host of nonsporulating anaerobes, both cocci and bacilli, most of which are commensals until they invade normally sterile spaces.

ACTINOMYCOSIS

Actinomycosis is a chronic localized or hematogenous infection caused by *Actinomyces israelii*. Symptoms are a local abscess with multiple draining sinuses, a TB-like pneumonitis, and low-grade septicemia. Diagnosis is by the typical appearance combined with laboratory identification. Treatment is with prolonged antibiotics and surgery.

The causative organisms, *Actinomyces* sp and *Propionibacterium* sp (most commonly

A. israelii), are often present commensally on the gums, tonsils, and teeth. However, many, if not most, infections are polymicrobial, with other bacteria (oral anaerobes, staphylococci, streptococci, or Enterobacteriaceae) frequently cultured from lesions.

Actinomycosis most often occurs in adult males and takes several forms. In the cervicofacial (lumpy jaw) form, the most common portal of entry is decayed teeth. In the thoracic form, pulmonary disease results from aspiration of oral secretions. In the abdominal form, disease presumably results from a break in the mucosa of a diverticulum or the appendix or during trauma. There is also a localized pelvic form of actinomycosis, a complication of certain types of intrauterine device (IUD) contraceptives. Spread from primary sites occurs rarely, presumably by hematogenous seeding.

Symptoms and Signs

The characteristic lesion is an indurated area of multiple, small, communicating abscesses surrounded by granulation tissue. Lesions tend to form sinus tracts that communicate to the skin and drain a purulent discharge containing "sulfur" granules (rounded or spherical, usually yellowish, and ≤ 1 mm in diameter). Infection spreads to contiguous tissues, but only rarely hematogenously.

The cervicofacial form usually begins as a small, flat, hard swelling, with or without pain, under the oral mucosa or the skin of the neck, or as a subperiosteal swelling of the jaw. Subsequently, areas of softening appear and develop into sinuses and fistulas that discharge the characteristic sulfur granules. The cheek, tongue, pharynx, salivary glands, cranial bones, meninges, or brain may be affected, usually by direct extension.

In the abdominal form, the intestines (usually the cecum and appendix) and the peritoneum are infected. Pain, fever, vomiting, diarrhea or constipation, and emaciation are characteristic. One or more abdominal masses that cause signs of partial intestinal obstruction occur. Draining sinuses and intestinal fistulas may develop and extend to the external abdominal wall.

In the thoracic form, lung involvement resembles TB. Extensive invasion may occur before chest pain, fever, and productive cough appear. Perforation of the chest wall, with chronic draining sinuses, may result.

In the generalized form, infection spreads hematogenously to the skin, vertebral bodies, brain, liver, kidneys, ureters, and (in women) pelvic organs. Diverse symptoms, such as back pain, headache, and abdominal pain, related to these sites may occur. A local pelvic form may occur. Symptoms include vaginal discharge along with pelvic or lower abdominal pain.

Diagnosis

Diagnosis is suspected clinically and confirmed by x-rays and identification of *A. israelii* in sputum, pus, or biopsy specimen. In pus or tissue, the microorganism appears as the distinctive sulfur granules or as tangled masses of branched and unbranched wavy bacterial filaments, pus cells, and debris, surrounded by an outer zone of radiating, club-shaped, hyaline, and refractive filaments that take hematoxylin-eosin stain in tissue but are positive on Gram stain.

Nodules in any location may simulate malignant growths. Lung lesions must be distinguished from those of TB and cancer. Most abdominal lesions occur in the ileocecal region and are difficult to diagnose, except during laparotomy or when draining sinuses appear in the abdominal wall. Aspiration liver biopsy should be avoided because it can produce a persistent sinus.

Prognosis and Treatment

The disease is slowly progressive. Prognosis relates directly to early diagnosis. It is most favorable in the cervicofacial form and progressively worse in the thoracic, abdominal, and generalized forms, especially if the CNS is involved.

Most patients respond to antibiotics, although response is usually slow because of extensive tissue induration and the relatively avascular nature of the lesions. Therefore, treatment must be continued for at least 8 wk and occasionally for ≥ 1 yr, until signs and symptoms have resolved. High doses of penicillin G (eg, 3 to 5 million units IV q 6 h) are usually effective. Penicillin V (1 g po qid) may be substituted after about 2 to 6 wk. Tetracycline 500 mg po q 6 h may be given instead of penicillin. Minocycline, clindamycin, and erythromycin also have been successful. Antibiotic regimens may be broadened to cover other pathogens cultured from lesions. Anecdotal reports suggest that hyperbaric O_2 therapy is helpful.

Extensive and repeated surgical procedures may be required. Sometimes, small abscesses can be aspirated; large ones are drained, and fistulas are excised surgically.

BOTULISM

Botulism is neuromuscular poisoning from *Clostridium botulinum* toxin. Infection is not necessary if toxin is ingested. Symptoms are weakness and paralysis. Diagnosis is clinical and with laboratory identification of toxin. Treatment is with support and antitoxin.

Etiology and Pathophysiology

C. botulinum elaborates 7 types of antigenically distinct neurotoxins, 4 of which affect humans—types A, B, E, and rarely F. Types A and B are highly poisonous proteins resistant to digestion by GI enzymes. About 50% of food-borne outbreaks in the US are caused by type A toxin, followed by types B and E. Type A toxin occurs predominantly west of the Mississippi River, type B in the eastern states, and type E in Alaska and the Great Lakes area.

Botulism occurs in 3 forms: food-borne, wound, and infant. In food-borne botulism, toxin produced in contaminated food is eaten; in wound and infant botulism, neurotoxin is elaborated in vivo by *C. botulinum* in infected tissue and in the large intestine, respectively. After absorption, toxin interferes with release of acetylcholine at peripheral nerve endings.

C. botulinum spores are highly heat-resistant and may survive boiling for several hours at 100° C. However, exposure to moist heat at 120° C for 30 min kills the spores. Toxins, on the other hand, are readily destroyed by heat, and cooking food at 80° C for 30 min safeguards against botulism. Toxin production (especially type E) can occur at temperatures as low as 3° C—ie, inside a refrigerator—and does not require strict anaerobic conditions.

Home-canned foods are the most common sources, but commercially prepared foods have been implicated in about 10% of outbreaks. Vegetables, fish, fruits, and condiments are the most common vehicles, but beef, milk products, pork, poultry, and other foods have been involved. Of outbreaks caused by seafood, type E accounts for about 50%; types A and B cause the rest. In recent years, noncanned foods (eg, foil-wrapped baked potatoes, chopped garlic in oil, patty melt sandwiches) have caused restaurant-associated outbreaks.

C. botulinum spores are common in the environment, and many cases may be caused by the ingestion or inhalation of dust, or by absorption through the eyes or a break in the skin. Infant botulism occurs most often in infants < 6 mo. The youngest reported patient was 2 wk and the oldest, 12 mo. Infant botulism results from ingestion of *C. botulinum* spores, their colonization of the large intestine, and toxin production in vivo. Unlike food-borne botulism, infant botulism is not caused by ingestion of a preformed toxin. Most cases are idiopathic, although some have been traced to ingestion of honey.

Symptoms and Signs

Food-borne botulism begins abruptly, usually 18 to 36 h after toxin ingestion, although the incubation period may vary from 4 h to 8 days. Nausea, vomiting, abdominal cramps, and diarrhea frequently precede neurologic symptoms. Neurologic symptoms are characteristically bilateral and symmetric, beginning with the cranial nerves and followed by descending weakness or paralysis. Common initial symptoms and signs include dry mouth, diplopia, ptosis, loss of accommodation, and diminished or total loss of pupillary light reflex. Symptoms of bulbar paresis (eg, dysarthria, dysphagia, dysphonia, a flaccid facial expression) develop. Dysphagia can lead to aspiration pneumonia. Muscles of respiration and of the extremities and trunk progressively weaken in a descending pattern. There are no sensory disturbances, and the sensorium usually remains clear. Fever is absent, and the pulse remains normal or slow unless intercurrent infection develops. Constipation is common after neurologic impairment appears. Major complications include respiratory failure caused by diaphragmatic paralysis and pulmonary infections.

Wound botulism is manifested by neurologic symptoms, as in food-borne botulism, but there are no GI symptoms or evidence implicating food as a cause. A history of a traumatic injury or a deep puncture wound in the preceding 2 wk may suggest the diagnosis. Careful search should be made for breaks in the skin and for skin abscesses caused by self-injection of illegal drugs.

In infant botulism, constipation is present initially in 90% of cases and is followed by neuromuscular paralysis, beginning with the cranial nerves and proceeding to peripheral and respiratory musculature. Cranial nerve deficits typically include ptosis, extraocular muscle palsies, weak cry, poor suck, decreased gag reflex, pooling of oral secretions, and an expressionless face. Severity varies from mild lethargy and slowed feeding to severe hypotonia and respiratory insufficiency.

Diagnosis

Botulism may be confused with Guillain-Barré syndrome, poliomyelitis, stroke, myasthenia gravis, tick paralysis, and poisoning caused by curare or belladonna alkaloids. Electromyography shows characteristic augmented response to rapid repetitive stimulation in most cases.

In food-borne botulism, the pattern of neuromuscular disturbances and ingestion of a likely food source are important diagnostic clues. The simultaneous presentation of at least 2 patients who ate the same food simplifies diagnosis, which is confirmed by demonstrating *C. botulinum* toxin in serum or stool or isolating the organism from stool. Finding *C. botulinum* toxin in suspect food identifies the source.

In wound botulism, finding toxin in serum or isolating *C. botulinum* organism on anaerobic culture of the wound confirms the diagnosis.

Infant botulism may be confused with sepsis, congenital muscular dystrophy, spinal muscular atrophy, hypothyroidism, and benign congenital hypotonia. Finding *C. botulinum* toxin or organisms in the stool establishes the diagnosis.

Treatment and Prevention

Anyone known or thought to have been exposed to contaminated food must be carefully observed. Administration of activated charcoal may be helpful. Patients with significant symptoms often have impaired airway reflexes, so if charcoal is used, it should be administered via gastric tube, and the airway should be protected by a cuffed endotracheal tube. Toxoids are available for active immunization of people working with *C. botulinum* or its toxins.

The greatest threat to life is respiratory impairment and its complications. Patients should be hospitalized and closely monitored with serial measurements of vital capacity. Progressive paralysis prevents patients from showing signs of respiratory distress as their vital capacity decreases. Respiratory impairment requires management in an ICU, where intubation and mechanical ventilation are readily available. Improvements in such supportive care have reduced the mortality rate to < 10%.

Nasogastric intubation is the preferred method of alimentation because it simplifies management of calories and fluids; stimulates intestinal peristalsis, which eliminates *C. botulinum* from the gut; and allows the use of breast milk in infants. In addition, it avoids the potential infectious and vascular complications inherent in IV alimentation.

Trivalent antitoxin (A, B, E) is available from the Centers for Disease Control and Prevention (CDC) through state health departments. Antitoxin does not inactivate toxin that is already bound at the neuromuscular junction; therefore, preexisting neurologic impairment cannot be reversed rapidly. (Ultimate recovery depends on regeneration of nerve endings, which may take weeks or months.) However, antitoxin may slow or halt further progression. Antitoxin should be given as soon as possible after clinical diagnosis and not delayed to await culture results. Antitoxin is less likely to be of benefit if given > 72 h after symptom onset. In the US, botulism equine trivalent antitoxin is given as a single 10-mL dose containing 7500 IU of antitoxin A, 5500 IU of antitoxin B, and 8500 IU of antitoxin E. All patients for whom the antitoxin is required must be reported to state health authorities or the CDC. Antitoxin is only available through the CDC, the telephone number is 404-639-2206 weekdays and 404-639-2888 for all other times. Because antitoxin derives from horse serum, there is a risk of anaphylaxis or serum sickness. (For precautions, see Drug Hypersensitivity on p. 1361, and for treatment, see Anaphylaxis on p. 1360.) Horse serum antitoxin is not recommended in infants. A botulism immune globulin (derived from the plasma of people immunized with *C. botulinum* toxoid) is under study for the treatment of infant botulism.

Because even minute amounts of *C. botulinum* toxin can cause serious illness, all materials suspected of containing toxin require special handling. Details regarding specimen collection and handling can be obtained from state health departments or the CDC.

Proper canning and adequate heating of home-canned food before serving are essential. Canned foods showing evidence of spoilage and swollen or leaking cans should be discarded. Infants < 12 mo should not be fed honey, which may contain *C. botulinum* spores.

CLOSTRIDIUM DIFFICILE–INDUCED DIARRHEA

(Pseudomembranous Colitis)

Toxins produced by *Clostridium difficile* strains in the GI tract cause pseudomembranous colitis, typically after antibiotic use. Symptoms are diarrhea, sometimes bloody, rarely progressing to sepsis and acute abdomen. Diagnosis is by identifying *C. difficile* toxin in stool. Treatment is oral metronidazole or vancomycin.

C. difficile is the most common cause of antibiotic-associated colitis and is typically hospital-acquired. *C. difficile*–induced diarrhea occurs in up to 8% of hospitalized patients and is responsible for 20 to 30% of cases of hospital-acquired diarrhea. Extremes of age, severe underlying disease, prolonged hospital stay, and living in a nursing home are risk factors.

C. difficile is carried asymptomatically by 15 to 70% of newborns and 3 to 8% of healthy adults and is common in the environment (soil, water, household pets). Disease may result from overgrowth of intrinsic organisms or infection from an external source. Health care workers are frequently the source of transmission.

Antibiotic-induced changes in GI flora are the dominant predisposing factor. Although most antibiotics have been implicated, cephalosporins (particularly 3rd-generation), penicillins (particularly ampicillin, amoxicillin), and clindamycin pose the highest risk. *C. difficile* colitis also may follow use of certain antineoplastic agents.

The organism secretes both a cytotoxin and an enterotoxin. The main effect is on the colon, which secretes fluid and develops characteristic pseudomembranes—discrete yellow-white plaques that are easily dislodged. Plaques may coalesce in severe cases. Toxic megacolon, which rarely develops, is somewhat more likely after use of antimotility agents.

Symptoms and Signs

Symptoms typically begin 5 to 10 days after starting antibiotics but may occur on the 1st day or up to 2 mo later. Diarrhea may be mild and semiformed or frequent and watery. Cramping or pain is common, but nausea and vomiting are rare. Limited tissue dissemination occurs very rarely, as do sepsis and acute abdomen. Reactive arthritis has occurred after *C. difficile*–induced diarrhea.

Diagnosis and Treatment

Diagnosis should be suspected in any patient developing diarrhea within 2 mo of antibiotic use or 72 h of hospital admission. Diagnosis is confirmed by stool (sample, not swab) assay for *C. difficile* toxin. A single sample is usually adequate, but repeat samples should be submitted when suspicion is high and the 1st sample is negative. Fecal leukocytes are often present but not specific.

Metronidazole 250 mg po q 6 h or 500 mg po q 8 h for 10 days is the therapy of choice. If the patient does not respond or relapses, metronidazole as above can be repeated for 21 days, or vancomycin 125 to 500 mg po q 6 h for 10 days may be given. Some patients require bacitracin 500 mg po q 6 h for 10 days, cholestyramine resin, or *Saccharomyces boullardii* yeast. Relapses occur in 15 to 20% of patients. A few patients have required total colectomy for cure.

Infection control measures are vital to reduce the spread of *C. difficile* among patients and health care workers.

CLOSTRIDIAL INTRA-ABDOMINAL INFECTIONS

Clostridia, primarily *Clostridium perfringens*, are common in mixed intra-abdominal infections due to a ruptured viscus or pelvic inflammatory disease.

Clostridium sp are common residents of the GI tract and are present in many abdominal infections, generally mixed with other enteric organisms. Clostridia are often the primary agents in emphysematous cholecystitis, gas gangrene of the uterus (previously common with septic abortion), certain other female genital tract infections (tubo-ovarian, pelvic, and uterine abscesses), and infection after perforation of colon carcinoma.

The primary organisms are *C. perfringens* and, in the case of colon carcinoma, *C. septicum*. The organism produces exotoxins (lecithinases, hemolysins, collagenases, proteases, lipases) that can cause suppuration. Gas formation is common. Clostridial septicemia may cause hemolytic anemia from the effect of lecithinase on RBC membranes. With severe hemolysis and coexisting toxicity, acute renal failure can occur.

Symptoms are similar to other abdominal infections, with pain, fever, abdominal tenderness, and a toxic appearance. In uterine infection, gas sometimes escapes through the cervix. Rarely, acute tubular necrosis develops.

Early diagnosis requires a high index of suspicion. Early and repeated Gram stains and cultures of the site, pus, lochia, and blood are indicated. Because *C. perfringens* occasionally can be isolated from the healthy vagina and lochia, cultures are not specific. X-rays may show local gas production (eg, in the biliary tree or gallbladder wall, uterus, or other sites).

Treatment is surgical debridement and penicillin G 5 million units IV q 6 h for at least 1 wk. Organ removal (eg, hysterectomy) may be necessary and can be lifesaving if debridement is insufficient. If acute tubular necrosis develops, dialysis is needed. The usefulness of hyperbaric O_2 has not been established.

CLOSTRIDIAL NECROTIZING ENTERITIS

(Enteritis Necroticans; Pigbel)

Clostridial necrotizing enteritis is necrotizing inflammation of the jejunum and ileum caused by *Clostridium perfringens*.

C. perfringens occasionally causes severe, inflammatory disease in the small bowel (primarily the jejunum). Inflammation is segmental, involving small or large patches with varying degrees of hemorrhage and necrosis. Perforation may occur.

Disease is caused by clostridial β-toxin, which is very sensitive to proteolytic enzymes and is inactivated by normal cooking. Disease occurs primarily in populations with multiple risk factors, including protein deprivation (causing inadequate synthesis of protease enzymes), poor food hygiene, episodic meat feasting, staple diets containing trypsin inhibitors (sweet potatoes), and *Ascaris* infestation (these parasites secrete a trypsin inhibitor). These factors are typically present collectively only in the hinterlands of New Guinea and parts of Africa, Central and South America, and Asia. In New Guinea, the disease is known as pigbel and is usually spread through contaminated pork, other meats, and perhaps peanuts.

Severity varies from mild diarrhea to a fulminant course of severe abdominal pain, vomiting, bloody stool, and sometimes death within 24 h. Treatment is with antibiotics (penicillin G, metronidazole). Perhaps 50% of seriously ill patients require surgery for perforation, persistent intestinal obstruction, or failure to respond to antibiotics. An experimental toxoid vaccine has been used successfully in endemic areas but is not available commercially.

Neutropenic enterocolitis is a similar syndrome that occurs in the cecum of neutropenic patients (eg, those with leukemia or receiving cancer chemotherapy). *Clostridium septicum* is the usual agent. Symptoms are fever, abdominal pain, and diarrhea. Treatment is with antibiotics, but surgery may be necessary.

Neonatal necrotizing enterocolitis (see p. 2286), which occurs in neonatal ICUs, may be caused by *C. perfringens, C. butyricum*, and *C. difficile*, although the role of these organisms needs further study.

CLOSTRIDIUM PERFRINGENS FOOD POISONING

***Clostridium perfringens* food poisoning is acute gastroenteritis caused by ingestion of contaminated food.**

C. perfringens is widely distributed in feces, soil, air, and water. Contaminated meat has caused many outbreaks. When meat contaminated with *C. perfringens* is left at room temperature, the organism multiplies and produces toxin. Outbreaks typically occur in commercial establishments and rarely at home. Once inside the GI tract, *C. perfringens* produces an enterotoxin that acts on the small bowel. Only *C. perfringens* type A has been definitively linked to this food poisoning syndrome. The enterotoxin produced is sensitive to heat (> 75° C).

Mild gastroenteritis is most common, with onset of symptoms 6 to 24 h after ingestion of contaminated food. The most common symptoms are watery diarrhea and abdominal cramps. Vomiting is unusual. Symptoms typically resolve within 24 h; severe or fatal cases rarely occur. Diagnosis is based on epidemiologic evidence and isolation of organisms in high quantity from contaminated food or from stools of affected people, or direct identification of enterotoxin in stool samples.

To prevent disease, leftover cooked meat should be refrigerated promptly and reheated thoroughly (internal temperature, 75° C) before serving. Treatment is supportive (see p. 136); antibiotics are not given.

CLOSTRIDIAL SOFT-TISSUE INFECTIONS

Clostridial soft-tissue infections include cellulitis, myositis, and clostridial myonecrosis. They usually occur after trauma. Symptoms may include edema, pain, gas with crepitation, foul-smelling exudates, intense coloration of the site, and progression to shock and renal failure. Diagnosis is by inspection and smell, confirmed by culture. Treatment is with penicillin and surgical debridement. Hyperbaric O_2 is sometimes beneficial.

Clostridium perfringens is the most common strain involved. Infection develops hours or days after injury, usually in an extremity after severe crushing or penetrating trauma devitalizes tissue, creating anaerobic conditions. The presence of foreign material (even sterile) markedly increases the risk of clostridial infection. Infection also may occur in operative wounds, particularly in patients with underlying occlusive vascular disease. Spontaneous cases occur rarely, usually involving *C. septicum* originating from occult colon perforation in patients with colon cancer, diverticulitis, or bowel ischemia. Infection typically, but not always, results in soft-tissue gas collection.

In proper conditions (low oxidation-reduction potential, low pH), as occur in devitalized tissue, infection progresses rapidly, from initial injury through shock, toxic delirium, and death within as little as 1 day.

Symptoms and Signs

Clostridial cellulitis occurs as a localized infection in a superficial wound, usually ≥ 3 days after injury. Infection may spread extensively along fascial planes, often with evident crepitation and abundant gas bubbling, but toxicity is much less severe than with extensive myonecrosis, and pain is minimal. Bullae frequently are evident, with foul-smelling, serous, brown exudate. Discoloration and gross edema of the extremity are rare. Clostridial skin infections associated with primary vascular occlusion of an extremity rarely progress to severe toxic myonecrosis or extend beyond the line of demarcation.

Clostridial myositis, suppurative infection of muscle without necrosis, is most common in parenteral drug users. It resembles staphylococcal pyomyositis and lacks the systemic symptoms of clostridial myonecrosis. Edema, pain, and frequently gas in the tissues occur. It spreads rapidly and may progress to myonecrosis.

In clostridial myonecrosis (gas gangrene), initial severe pain is common, sometimes even before other findings. The wound site may be pale initially, but it becomes red or bronze, often with blebs or bullae, and finally turns blackish green. The area is tensely edematous and tender to palpation. Crepitation is less obvious early than it is in clostridial cellulitis but is ultimately palpable in about 80%. Wounds and drainage have a particularly foul odor.

With progression, the patient appears toxic, with tachycardia, pallor, and hypotension. Shock and renal failure occur, although the patient often remains alert until the terminal stage. Unlike clostridial uterine infection, overt hemolysis is rare in gas gangrene of the extremities, even in terminally ill patients. Whenever massive hemolysis occurs, mortality of 70 to 100% can be expected due to acute renal failure and septicemia.

Diagnosis

Early suspicion and intervention are essential. Clostridial cellulitis responds well to treatment, but myonecrosis has a mortality rate of ≥ 40% with treatment and 100% without.

Although localized cellulitis, myositis, and spreading myonecrosis may be clinically distinct, differentiation often requires surgical exploration. In myonecrosis, muscle tissue is visibly necrotic; the affected muscle is a lusterless pink, then deep red, and finally gray-green or mottled purple and does not contract on stimulation. X-rays may show local gas production, and CT and MRI delineate the extent of gas and necrosis.

Wound exudate should be cultured for anaerobic and aerobic organisms. Because of their short generation time, anaerobic cultures of *Clostridia* may be positive in as little as 6 h. However, other anaerobic and aerobic bacteria, including members of the Enterobacteriaceae family and *Bacteroides, Streptococcus*, and *Staphylococcus* spp, alone or mixed, can cause clostridia-like severe cellulitis, extensive fasciitis, or clostridial myonecrosis (see Necrotizing Subcutaneous Infection on p. 985). Also, many wounds, particularly if open, are contaminated with both pathogenic and nonpathogenic clostridia that are not responsible for the infection. The presence of clostridia is significant when Gram stain shows them in large numbers, few PMNs are found in the exudates, and free fat globules are demonstrated with Sudan stain. However, if PMNs are abundant and the smear shows many chains of cocci, an anaerobic streptococcal or staphylococcal infection should be suspected. Abundant gram-negative bacilli may indicate infection with one of the Enterobacteriaceae or a *Bacteroides* sp (see also Mixed Anaerobic Infections on p. 1506). Detection of clostridial toxins in the wound or blood is useful only in the rare case of wound botulism (see p. 1498).

Treatment

When clinical signs of clostridial infection are present, such as gas or myonecrosis, rapid, aggressive intervention is mandatory. Thorough drainage and debridement are as important as antibiotics; both should be instituted rapidly. Penicillin G is the drug of choice; 1 to 2 million units IV q 2 to 3 h should be given immediately for severe cellulitis and myonecrosis. Addition of clindamycin 600 mg IV q 6 h is beneficial. If gram-negative organisms are seen or suspected, a broad-spectrum antibiotic (eg, ticarcillin combined with clavulanate, ampicillin combined with sulbactam, or piperacillin combined with tazobactam) should be added.

Hyperbaric O_2 therapy may be helpful in extensive myonecrosis, particularly in extremities, as a supplement to antibiotics and surgery. Hyperbaric O_2 therapy may have potential to salvage tissue and lessen mortality and morbidity if started early *but should not delay surgical debridement*.

TETANUS

(Lockjaw)

Tetanus is an acute poisoning from a neurotoxin produced by *Clostridium tetani*. Symptoms are intermittent tonic spasms of voluntary muscles. Spasm of the masseters accounts for the name lockjaw. Diagnosis is clinical. Treatment is immune globulin and intensive support.

Etiology and Pathophysiology

Tetanus bacilli form durable spores that can be found in soil and animal feces and remain viable for years. Worldwide, tetanus is estimated to cause over half a million deaths annually, mostly in newborns and young children, but the disease is so rarely reported that all figures are only rough estimates. However, in the US, only 37 cases were reported in 2001. Disease incidence is directly related to the immunization level in a population, attesting to the effectiveness of preventive efforts. In the US, well over $\frac{1}{2}$ of elderly patients have inadequate antibody levels and account for $\frac{1}{3}$ to $\frac{1}{2}$ of cases. Most of the rest occur in inadequately immunized patients between the ages of 20 and 59. Those < 20 yr account for < 10%. Patients with burns, surgical wounds, or a history of injection drug abuse are especially prone to developing tetanus. However, tetanus may follow trivial or even inapparent wounds. Infection may also develop postpartum in the uterus (maternal tetanus) and in a newborn's umbilicus (tetanus neonatorum).

Manifestations of tetanus are caused by an exotoxin (tetanospasmin). The toxin may enter the CNS along the peripheral motor nerves or may be bloodborne to nervous tissue. Tetanospasmin binds irreversibly to the ganglioside membranes of nerve synapses, blocking release of inhibitory transmitter from nerve terminals and thereby causing a generalized tonic spasticity, usually with superimposed intermittent tonic seizures. Once bound, the toxin cannot be neutralized.

Symptoms and Signs

The incubation period ranges from 2 to 50 days (average, 5 to 10 days). The most frequent symptom is jaw stiffness. Other symptoms include difficulty swallowing; restlessness; irritability; stiff neck, arms, or legs; headache; fever; sore throat; chills; and tonic spasms. Later, the patient has difficulty opening his jaw (trismus). Facial muscle spasm produces a characteristic expression with a fixed smile and elevated eyebrows (risus sardonicus). Rigidity or spasm of abdominal, neck, and back muscles—even opisthotonos—may occur. Sphincter spasm causes urinary retention or constipation. Dysphagia may interfere with nutrition. Characteristic painful, generalized tonic spasms with profuse sweating are precipitated by minor disturbances such as a draft, noise, or movement. Mental status is usually clear, but coma may follow repeated spasms. During generalized spasms, the patient is unable to speak or cry out because of chest wall rigidity or glottal spasm. Spasms also interfere with respiration, causing cyanosis or fatal asphyxia. The immediate cause of death may not be apparent.

The patient's temperature is only moderately elevated unless a complicating infection, such as pneumonia, is present. Respiratory and pulse rates are increased. Reflexes are often exaggerated. Moderate leukocytosis is usual. Patients with protracted tetanus may manifest a very labile and overactive sympathetic nervous system, including periods of hypertension, tachycardia, and myocardial irritability.

In generalized tetanus, skeletal muscles throughout the body are affected. Localized tetanus can occur, with spasticity of a muscle group near the wound but without trismus. Spasticity may persist for weeks.

Cephalic tetanus, tetanus infection of the brain and cranial nerves, is a form of localized tetanus. It is more common in children, in whom it may occur with chronic otitis media. Its incidence is greatest in Africa and India. All cranial nerves can be involved, especially the 7th. Cephalic tetanus may become generalized.

Tetanus in a newborn is usually generalized and frequently fatal. It often begins in improperly cleansed umbilical stumps in children born of inadequately immunized mothers. Its onset during the first 2 wk of life is characterized by rigidity, spasms, and poor feeding. Bilateral deafness has occurred in surviving newborns.

Respiratory failure is the most common cause of death. Laryngeal spasm and abdominal wall, diaphragm, and chest wall muscle rigidity and spasms cause asphyxiation. Hypoxemia can also induce cardiac arrest, and pharyngeal spasm leads to aspiration of oral secretions with subsequent pneumonia, contributing to a hypoxemic death.

Diagnosis

A history of a recent wound in a patient with muscle stiffness or spasms is a clue. Tetanus can be confused with meningoencephalitis of bacterial or viral origin, but the combination of an intact sensorium, normal CSF, and muscle spasms suggests tetanus. Trismus must be distinguished from peritonsillar or retropharyngeal abscess or another local cause. Phenothiazines can induce tetanus-like rigidity.

C. tetani can sometimes be cultured from the wound, but culture is not sensitive.

Prognosis and Treatment

Tetanus has a worldwide mortality rate of 50%, 15 to 60% in untreated adults, and 80 to 90% in newborns even if treated. Mortality is highest at the extremes of age and in drug abusers. The prognosis is poorer if the incubation period is short and symptoms progress rapidly or if treatment is delayed. The course tends to be milder when there is no demonstrable focus of infection.

Therapy requires maintaining adequate ventilation. Additional interventions include early and adequate use of human immune globulin to neutralize nonfixed toxin; prevention of further toxin production; sedation; control of muscle spasm, hypertonicity, fluid balance, and intercurrent infection; and continuous nursing care.

General principles: The patient should be kept in a quiet room. Three principles should guide all therapeutic interventions: prevent further toxin release by debriding the wound and giving metronidazole 500 mg IV q 6 to 8 h; neutralize toxin outside the CNS with human tetanus immune globulin and tetanus toxoid, taking care to inject into different body sites to avoid neutralizing the antitoxin; and minimize the effect of toxin already in the CNS.

Wound care: Because dirt and dead tissue promote *C. tetani* growth, prompt, thorough debridement, especially of deep puncture wounds, is essential. Antibiotics are not substitutes for adequate debridement and immunization.

Antitoxin: The benefit of human-derived antitoxin depends on how much tetanospasmin is already bound to the synaptic membranes—only free toxin is neutralized. For adults, human tetanus immune globulin 3000 units IM is given once (this large volume may be split and given at separate sites). Dose can range from 1,500 to 10,000 units, depending on wound severity. Antitoxin of animal origin is far less preferable because the patient's serum antitoxin level is not well maintained and a considerable risk of serum sickness exists. If horse serum must be used, however, the usual dose is 50,000 units IM or IV (CAUTION: see Drug Hypersensitivity on p. 1361). If necessary, immune globulin or antitoxin can be injected directly into the wound, but this injection is not as important as proper wound care.

Management of muscle spasm: To control rigidity and spasms, benzodiazepines are the standard of care. They block reuptake of an endogenous inhibiting neurotransmitter, γ-aminobutyric acid (GABA), at the $GABA_A$ receptor. Diazepam can help control seizures, counter muscle rigidity, and induce sedation. Dosage varies and requires meticulous titration and close observation. The most severe cases may require 10 to 20 mg IV q 3 h (do not exceed 5 mg/kg). Less severe cases can be controlled with 5 to 10 mg po q 2 to 4 h. Dosage in infants > 30 days is 1 to 2 mg slowly IV, repeated q 3 to 4 h as necessary. Young children receive 0.1 to 0.8 mg/kg/day up to 0.1 to 0.3 mg/kg q 4 to 8 h. In children > 5 yr, 5 to 10 mg IV is given q 3 to 4 h. Adults receive 5 to 10 mg po q 4 to 6 h or up to 40 mg/h IV drip. Although diazepam has been used most extensively, midazolam (adults, 0.1 to 0.3 mg/kg/h IV infusion; children, 0.06 to 0.15 mg/kg/h IV infusion) is water-soluble and preferred for prolonged therapy. Midazolam reduces the risk of lactic acidosis from propylene glycol solvent required for diazepam and lorazepam and reduces the risk of long-acting metabolites accumulating and causing coma.

Benzodiazepines may not prevent reflex spasms, and effective respiration may require neuromuscular blockade with vecuronium 0.1 mg/kg IV or other paralytic agents and mechanical ventilation. Pancuronium has been used but may worsen autonomic instability. Vecuronium is free from adverse cardiovascular effects but is short acting. Longer acting agents (eg, pipecuronium and rocuronium) also work, but no randomized clinical comparative trials have been performed.

Intrathecal baclofen (a $GABA_A$ agonist) is effective but has no clear advantage over benzodiazepines. It is given by continuous infusion; effective doses range between 20 and 2000 μg/day. A test dose of 50 μg is given first; if response is inadequate, 75 μg may be given 24 h later, and 100 μg 24 h after that. Those who do not respond to 100 μg are not candidates for chronic infusion. Coma and respiratory depression requiring ventilatory support are potential adverse effects.

Dantrolene (loading dose 1.0 to 1.5 mg/kg IV followed by infusion 0.5 to 1.0 mg/kg q 4 to 6 h for ≤ 25 days) relieves muscle spasticity. Dantrolene given orally can be used in place of infusion therapy for up to 60 days. Hepatotoxicity and expense limit its use.

Morphine may be given q 4 to 6 h to control autonomic dysfunction, especially cardiovascular; total daily dose is 20 to 180 mg. β-Blockade with long-acting agents such as propranolol is not recommended. Sudden cardiac death is a feature of tetanus, and β-blockade can increase risk; however, esmolol, a short-acting β-blocker, has been used successfully. Atropine at high doses has been used; blockade of the parasympathetic nervous system markedly reduces excessive sweating and secretions. Lower mortality has been reported in clonidine-treated patients compared with those treated with conventional therapy.

Mg sulfate at doses that maintain serum levels between 4 to 8 mEq/L (eg, 4 g bolus followed by 2 to 3 g/h) has a stabilizing effect, eliminating catecholamine stimulation. Patellar tendon reflex is used to assess overdosage. Tidal volume may be impaired, so ventilatory support must be available.

Pyridoxine (100 mg once/day) lowers mortality in newborns. Newer agents that may prove useful include Na valproate, which blocks GABA–aminotransferase, inhibiting GABA catabolism; ACE inhibitors, which inhibit angiotensin II and reduce norepinephrine release from nerve endings; dexmedetomidine, a potent α-2 adrenergic agonist; and adenosine, which reduces presynaptic norepinephrine release and antagonizes the inotropic effect of catecholamines. Corticosteroids are of unproven benefit; their use is not recommended.

Antibiotics: The role of antibiotic therapy is minor compared with wound debridement and general support. Typical antibiotics include penicillin G 6 million units IV q 6 h, doxycycline 100 mg po bid, and metronidazole 500 mg po q 8 h.

Supportive care: In moderate or severe cases, the patient should be intubated. Mechanical ventilation is essential when neuromuscular blockade is required to control muscle spasms that impair respirations. IV hyperalimentation avoids the hazard of aspiration secondary to gastric tube feeding. Because constipation is usual, stools should be kept soft. A rectal tube may control distention. Bladder catheterization is required if urinary retention occurs. Chest physiotherapy, frequent turning, and forced coughing are essential to prevent pneumonia. Analgesia with opioids is often needed.

Prevention

A series of 4 primary immunizations against tetanus, followed by boosters q 10 yr, with the adsorbed (for primary immunization) or fluid (for boosters) toxoid is superior

TABLE 178–1. GUIDELINES FOR TETANUS IMMUNIZATION

TETANUS PROPHYLAXIS IN ROUTINE WOUND MANAGEMENT

HISTORY OF ADSORBED TETANUS TOXOID	CLEAN, MINOR WOUNDS		ALL OTHER WOUNDS*	
	TD	TIG†	TD	TIG
Unknown or < 3 doses	Yes	No	Yes	Yes
≥ 3 doses	Yes if >10 yr since last dose	No	Yes if > 5 yr since last dose	No

*Such as, but not limited to, wounds contaminated with dirt, feces, soil, or saliva; puncture wounds, crush injuries, avulsions, and wounds resulting from missiles, burns, and frostbite.

†Tetanus immune globulin (human) 250–500 units IM.

to giving antitoxin at the time of injury. Tetanus toxoid comes by itself, mixed with diphtheria in both adult (Td) and child strengths (DT), and combined with both diphtheria and pertussis (DTP). Routine diphtheria, tetanus, and pertussis immunization and booster recommendations are discussed in Ch. 169 on p. 1399. Adults need to maintain immunity with regular boosters q 10 yr. Immunization in an unimmunized or inadequately immunized pregnant woman produces both active and passive immunity in the fetus and should be given at a gestational age of 5 to 6 mo with a booster at 8 mo. Passive immunity develops with maternal toxoid given before a gestational age of 6 mo.

Following injury, tetanus vaccination is given depending on wound type and vaccination history; tetanus immune globulin may also be indicated (see TABLE 178–1). Patients not previously vaccinated are given a 2nd and 3rd dose of toxoid at monthly intervals.

MIXED ANAEROBIC INFECTIONS

Anaerobes can infect normal hosts and those with compromised resistance or damaged tissues. Symptoms depend on site of infection. Anaerobes are often accompanied by aerobic organisms. Diagnosis is clinical combined with Gram stain and anaerobic cultures. Treatment is with antibiotics and surgical drainage and debridement.

Hundreds of species of nonsporulating anaerobes are part of the normal flora of the skin, mouth, GI tract, and vagina. If this commensal relationship is disrupted (eg, by surgery or other trauma, poor blood supply, tissue necrosis), a few of these species can cause infections with high morbidity and mortality. After becoming established in a primary site, organisms can spread hematogenously to distant sites. Because aerobic and anaerobic bacteria frequently are found in the same infected site, appropriate procedures for isolation and culture are necessary to keep from overlooking the anaerobes. Anaerobes can be the major cause of infection in the pleural spaces and lungs; in intra-abdominal, gynecologic, CNS, upper respiratory tract, and cutaneous diseases; and in bacteremia.

Etiology and Pathophysiology

The principal anaerobic gram-positive cocci that produce disease are the peptococci and the peptostreptococci, which are part of the normal flora of the mouth, upper respiratory tract, and large intestine. The principal anaerobic gram-negative bacilli include *Bacteroides fragilis, Prevotella melaninogenica*, and *Fusobacterium* sp. The *B. fragilis* group is part of the normal bowel flora and includes the anaerobic pathogens most frequently isolated from intra-abdominal infections. Organisms in the *Prevotella* group and *Fusobacterium* sp are part of the indigenous oral flora.

Anaerobic infections can usually be characterized by the following features:

- They tend to occur as localized collections of pus or abscesses
- The reduced O_2 tension and low oxidation-reduction potential that prevail in

avascular and necrotic tissues are critical for their survival

- When bacteremia occurs, it usually does not lead to disseminated intravascular coagulation (DIC) and purpura.

Some anaerobic bacteria possess distinct virulence factors. Those of *B. fragilis* probably account for its frequent isolation from clinical specimens despite its relative rarity in normal flora. This organism has a polysaccharide capsule that apparently stimulates abscess formation. An experimental model of intra-abdominal sepsis has shown that *B. fragilis* alone can cause abscesses, whereas other *Bacteroides* sp require the synergistic effect of another organism. Another virulence factor, a potent endotoxin, is implicated in septic shock associated with severe *Fusobacterium* pharyngitis.

Morbidity and mortality are as great from anaerobic and mixed bacterial sepsis as from sepsis caused by a single aerobic organism. Anaerobic infections are often complicated by deep-seated tissue necrosis. The overall mortality rate for severe intra-abdominal sepsis and mixed anaerobic pneumonias tends to be high. *B. fragilis* bacteremia has high mortality, especially in the elderly and in patients with cancer.

Symptoms and Signs

Patients usually have fever, rigors, and critical illness; shock may develop. DIC may occur in *Fusobacterium* sepsis.

Clinical clues to the presence of anaerobic organisms include infection adjacent to mucosal surfaces bearing anaerobic flora; ischemia, tumor, penetrating trauma, foreign body, or perforated viscus; spreading gangrene involving skin, subcutaneous tissue, fascia, and muscle; feculent odor in pus or infected tissues; abscess formation; gas in tissues; septic thrombophlebitis; and failure to respond to antibiotics that do not have significant anaerobic activity.

Specific infections caused by mixed anaerobic organisms are discussed elsewhere in THE MANUAL. A listing of these conditions appears in TABLE 178–2. Anaerobes are rare in UTI, septic arthritis, and infective endocarditis.

Diagnosis

Anaerobic infection should be suspected in any foul-smelling wound or when a Gram stain of pus from an infected site shows mixed pleomorphic bacteria. Only specimens from normally sterile sites should be cultured, because commensal contaminants may easily be mistaken for pathogens.

Gram stains and aerobic cultures should be obtained for all specimens. Gram stain, particularly in *Bacteroides* infection, and cultures, for all anaerobes, may be falsely negative. Antibiotic sensitivity testing of anaerobes is exacting, and data may not be available for ≥ 1 wk after initial culture. However, if the species is known, sensitivity patterns usually can be predicted. Therefore, many laboratories do not routinely test anaerobic organisms for sensitivity.

Treatment and Prevention

In established infection, pus is drained and devitalized tissue, foreign bodies, and necrotic

TABLE 178–2. CONDITIONS OFTEN CAUSED BY MIXED* ANAEROBIC ORGANISMS

- Anaerobic cellulitis
- Aspiration pneumonia
- Bartholin's gland infections
- Brain abscesses
- Chronic otitis media
- Chronic sinusitis
- Decubitus or ischemic ulcer infections
- Dental abscesses
- Endometritis
- Epidural and subdural empyema
- Human bite infections
- Intra-abdominal abscess
- Liver abscess
- Ludwig's angina
- Lung abscess
- Mandibular osteomyelitis
- Necrotizing gingivitis
- Necrotizing ulcerative mucositis (cancrum oris)
- Nongonococcal tubo-ovarian abscess
- Parametrial abscess
- Pelvic peritonitis
- Periodontitis
- Peritonitis
- Septic thrombophlebitis
- Skene's glands infection
- Vincent's angina

*With aerobes or other anaerobes.

tissue removed. Organ perforations must be closed or drained. Whenever possible, blood supply should be reestablished. Septic thrombophlebitis may require vein ligation as well as antimicrobial therapy.

Because anaerobic culture results may not be available for 3 to 5 days, antibiotics are started. Antibiotics sometimes work even when some of the bacterial species in a mixed infection are resistant to the antibiotic, especially if surgical debridement and drainage are adequate.

Oropharyngeal anaerobic infections should be treated with penicillin G. Infrequently, oral anaerobic infections fail to respond and require a drug effective against penicillin-resistant anaerobes (see below). Lung abscesses should be treated with clindamycin or a β-lactam/β-lactamase combination. In patients allergic to penicillin, clindamycin or metronidazole (plus an agent active against aerobes) is useful.

GI or female pelvic anaerobic infections, which likely contain *B. fragilis*, may be penicillin resistant. Resistance to 2nd-generation cephalosporins and clindamycin also occurs. No single regimen has been shown to be superior. The following drugs have excellent in vitro activity and are effective: metronidazole, imipenem-cilastatin, piperacillin-tazobactam, ampicillin-sulbactam, meropenem, and ticarcillin-clavulanic acid. All except metronidazole can be used as monotherapy because these drugs also have good activity against aerobes. Drugs that are somewhat less active in vitro but are usually effective include clindamycin, cefoxitin, and cefotetan. Metronidazole 500 to 750 mg IV q 8 h (for children, 10 mg/kg q 8 h) given with an aminoglycoside (eg, gentamicin 5 mg/kg once/day or 2 mg/kg q 8 h; to cover enteric gram-negative flora) can be used for intra-abdominal infection or any infection arising from a colonic source. Clindamycin 900 mg IV q 8 h (for children, 10 mg/kg q 8 h) is an alternative. Metronidazole is active against clindamycin-resistant *B. fragilis*, has unique anaerobic bactericidal activity, and usually avoids the pseudomembranous colitis sometimes associated with clindamycin. Concerns about its potential mutagenicity have not been of clinical consequence.

Patients undergoing elective colonic surgery should undergo bowel preparation (eg, cathartics, enemas, and oral neomycin and erythromycin). Preoperative parenteral antibiotics control bacteremia, reduce secondary or metastatic suppurative complications, and prevent local spread of infection around the surgical site. Cefoxitin or a combination of either metronidazole or clindamycin with gentamicin or tobramycin may be used.

179 MYCOBACTERIA

Mycobacteria are small, slow-growing, aerobic bacilli distinguished by a complex, lipid-rich cell envelope responsible for their characterization as "acid-fast" (ie, resistant to decolorization by acid after staining with carbolfuchsin). The most common mycobacterial infection is tuberculosis; others include leprosy and various diseases caused by *Mycobacterium avium* complex.

TUBERCULOSIS

(See also Perinatal Tuberculosis on p. 2338.)

Tuberculosis is a chronic, progressive infection with a period of latency following initial infection. It occurs most commonly in the lungs. Pulmonary symptoms include productive cough, chest pain, and dyspnea. Diagnosis is by sputum culture and smear. Treatment is with multiple antimicrobial agents.

Tuberculosis (TB) is the leading infectious cause of morbidity and mortality in adults worldwide, killing about 2 million people every year.

Etiology

TB properly refers only to disease caused by *Mycobacterium tuberculosis*. Similar disease occasionally results from *M. bovis, M. africanum*, and *M. microti*.

TB occurs almost exclusively from inhalation of droplet nuclei containing *M. tuberculosis*. They disperse primarily through coughing, singing, and other forced respiratory maneuvers by a person with active pulmonary TB whose sputum contains a significant number of organisms (typically enough to render the smear positive). People with pulmonary cavitary lesions are especially infectious. Droplet nuclei containing tubercle bacilli may float on room-air currents for several hours, increasing the chance of spread. About ¼ of household contacts acquire infection. Health care practitioners in the US who have close contact with active cases have increased risk. Transmission is enhanced by overcrowding; thus, people living in poverty or in institutions are at particular risk. Once effective treatment begins, however, cough rapidly decreases, and within weeks, TB is no longer contagious.

Less commonly, spread occurs from aerosolization of organisms after irrigation of infected wounds, in mycobacteriology laboratories, and in autopsy rooms. TB of the tonsils, lymph nodes, abdominal organs, bones, and joints was once commonly caused by ingestion of milk infected with *M. bovis*, but such infection has been largely eradicated in developed countries by slaughtering cows that test positive on a tuberculin skin test. Fomites do not appear to facilitate spread.

Epidemiology

About 1.6 billion are infected worldwide. Of these, perhaps only 15 million have active disease at any given time. Case rates vary widely by country, age, race, sex, and socioeconomic status. In the US, the case rate has declined 10-fold since 1953. There are now about 15,000 cases/yr; > 50% occur in patients born outside the US in high-prevalence areas (eg, Asia, Africa, Latin America). In the southeastern US and inner cities throughout the US, poor US-born blacks, the homeless, those in jails and prisons, and other disenfranchised minorities contribute disproportionately to the case rate.

HIV infection is the greatest single medical risk factor because cell-mediated immunity, which is impaired by HIV, is essential for defense against TB; other immunosuppressive illnesses (eg, diabetes) or therapies (eg, corticosteroids) are risks but less so than HIV. Age has traditionally been considered an independent risk factor because the elderly have more years of potential exposure and are more likely to have impaired immunity. However, in the US, the difference in prevalence is no longer as large, probably because the incidence of infectious cases (and hence lifetime risk of significant exposure) has declined.

A resurgence of TB occurred in parts of the US and other developed countries between 1985 and 1992, associated with several factors, including HIV, homelessness, a deteriorated public health infrastructure, and the appearance of multidrug-resistant–TB (MDR-TB—see p. 1514). Although substantially controlled in the US by public health and institutional infection control measures, the problem of MDR-TB appears to be growing around the world, fueled by poor treatment supervision, weak retreatment regimens, HIV coinfection, institutional transmission, and inadequate resources. Control efforts, including prolonged (eg, > 18 mo) use of 2nd-line antibiotics, treatment of drug adverse effects, community-based supervision, and social and emotional support, are raising hopes for better global control of MDR-TB.

Pathophysiology

Tubercle bacilli initially produce a primary infection, followed by a latent (dormant) phase and, in some cases, by active disease. Infection is not transmissible in the primary and latent phases.

Primary infection: Airborne droplet nuclei lodge in subpleural terminal airspaces, predominantly in the lower lung, usually in only one site. Tubercle bacilli replicate inside macrophages, ultimately killing them; inflammatory cells are attracted to the area, causing a tubercle and sometimes pneumonitis. In the early weeks of infection, some infected macrophages are borne to regional lymph nodes (eg, hilar, mediastinal). Hematogenous spread to any part of the body, particularly the apical-posterior portion of the lungs, epiphyses of the long bones, kidneys, vertebral bodies, and meninges, may occur. In 95% of cases, after about 3 wk of uninhibited growth, the immune system suppresses bacillary replication before symptoms or signs develop. Foci of infection in the lung or other sites resolve into epithelioid cell granulomas, which may have caseous and necrotic centers; tubercle bacilli can survive in this material for years, the host's resistance determining whether the infection ultimately resolves without treatment, remains dormant, or becomes active. Foci may leave nodular scars in the apices of one or both lungs (Simon foci), calcified scars from the primary infection (Ghon foci), or calcified hilar lymph nodes. The tuberculin skin test (see p. 1511) is positive.

Rarely, the primary focus immediately progresses, causing acute illness with pneumonia (sometimes cavitary), pleural effusion, and marked mediastinal or hilar lymph node enlargement (which in children may compress bronchi). Small pleural effusions are predominantly lymphocytic, typically contain few organisms, and clear within a few weeks. Primary extrapulmonary TB at any site can sometimes present without evidence of lung involvement. TB lymphadenopathy is the most common extrapulmonary presentation; however, meningitis is the most feared because of its high mortality in the very young and very old.

Active disease: In about 10% of patients overall, latent infection develops into active disease, although the percentage varies significantly by age and other risk factors. In 50 to 80% of those who develop active disease, TB reactivates within the 1st 2 yr, but it can occur decades later. Any organ initially seeded may be a site of reactivation, but reactivation occurs most often in the lung apices, where O_2 tension is highest. Ghon foci and affected hilar lymph nodes are much less likely to be sites of reactivation. Extrapulmonary TB is discussed on p. 1517.

Conditions that facilitate activation include impaired immunity (particularly HIV infection), certain immunosuppressant drugs (eg, corticosteroids, infliximab and other tumor necrosis factor blockers), gastrectomy, jejunoileal bypass surgery, silicosis, renal insufficiency, stress, diabetes, head or neck cancer, adolescence, and advanced (particularly > 70 yr) age.

TB damages tissues through delayed hypersensitivity (see p. 1348), typically producing granulomatous necrosis with a caseous histologic appearance. Lung lesions are cavitary. Pleural effusion is less common than in progressive primary TB but may occur from direct extension or hematogenous spread. Rupture of a large tuberculous lesion into the pleural space may produce empyema with or without bronchopleural fistula; it sometimes causes pneumothorax. In the prechemotherapy era, TB empyema sometimes complicated medically induced pneumothorax therapy and was usually rapidly fatal.

The course varies greatly, depending on the virulence of the organism and the state of host defenses. The course may be rapid among blacks and American Indians who have not had as many centuries of selective pressure to develop innate or natural immunity.

Acute respiratory distress syndrome, which appears to be due to hypersensitivity to TB antigens, develops rarely after diffuse hematogenous spread or rupture of a large cavity with spillage into the lungs.

Symptoms and Signs

In active pulmonary TB, even moderate or severe disease, the patient may have no symptoms except "not feeling well" or may have more specific symptoms. Cough is most common. At first, it may be minimally productive of yellow or green sputum, usually on rising, but cough may become more productive as the disease progresses. Drenching night sweats are a classic symptom but are neither common in nor specific for TB. Dyspnea may result from lung parenchymal involvement, spontaneous pneumothorax, or pleural TB with effusion. Hemoptysis occurs only with cavitary TB.

Diagnosis

Pulmonary TB is often suspected on the basis of chest x-rays taken while evaluating respiratory symptoms (cough > 3 wk, hemoptysis, chest pain, dyspnea), an unexplained illness, FUO, or a positive tuberculin skin test (see p.1511). In adults, a multinodular infiltrate above or behind the clavicle (the most characteristic location, most visible in an apical lordotic view) suggests reactivation of TB. Middle and lower lung infiltrates are nonspecific but should prompt suspicion of primary TB in patients (usually young) whose symptoms or exposure history suggests recent infection, particularly if there is pleural effusion.

Initial tests are chest x-ray, sputum examination (stain and culture), and tuberculin skin testing. If the chest x-ray is highly characteristic (upper lobe lung cavitation) in a person with TB risk factors, sputum examination is still required, but skin testing is often not done. The finding of acid-fast bacilli in a sputum smear is strong presumptive evidence of TB, but definitive diagnosis requires a positive sputum culture or a positive rapid molecular test. Culture results may take ≥ 3 wk, but examination by molecular methods usually takes only days. Rapid molecular tests can also detect a genetic mutation associated with resistance to rifampin, a key feature of MDR-TB. Positive cultures are routinely tested for resistance to isoniazid, rifampin, and ethambutol, but results take up to 8 wk by conventional bacteriologic methods.

Patients who cannot produce sputum spontaneously can have it induced by aerosolized hypertonic saline. If not, bronchial washings, which are particularly sensitive, can be obtained by fiberoptic bronchoscopy. Transbronchial biopsies should be performed on infiltrative lesions and submitted for culture, histologic evaluation, and molecular testing. Gastric washings are often positive but are no longer commonly used except in small children, who usually cannot produce a good sputum specimen. Tubercle bacilli are nominally Gram positive but take up Gram stain inconsistently; samples are best prepared with Ziehl-Neelsen or Kinyoun stains for conventional light microscopy or fluorochrome stains for fluorescent microscopy.

Skin testing: The tuberculin skin test (TST; Mantoux or PPD—purified protein derivative) is usually performed, although it is a test of infection, latent or active, and is not diagnostic of active disease. The standard dose of 5 units of PPD in 0.1 mL of solution is injected on the volar forearm. It is critical to give the injection intradermally, not subcutaneously. A well-demarcated bleb or wheal should result. The diameter of induration (not erythema) is measured 48 to 72 h after injection. Induration of ≥ 10 mm generally indicates infection with *M. tuberculosis* but does not indicate activity of the infection. Different cutoffs, intended to improve sensitivity and specificity, are sometimes appropriate; induration ≥ 5 mm is considered positive in patients with HIV infection or chest x-ray evidence of past TB and close contacts of patients with TB, whereas for patients with no known risk factors, the test is not considered positive unless induration is > 15 mm. Results can be falsely negative, most often in the febrile, elderly, HIV-infected (especially if $CD4^+$ cell count is < 200 cells/μL), and the very ill, many of whom show no reaction to any skin test (anergy). Anergy probably occurs because of inhibiting antibodies or because so many T cells have been mobilized to the disease site that too few remain to produce a significant skin reaction. Multiple-puncture devices (the tine test) are no longer recommended for general use.

Blood tests based on the production of gamma interferon by lymphocytes exposed in vitro to TB-specific antigens are now available and will likely soon replace the tuberculin skin test for routine testing for TB infection.

Prognosis and Treatment

In immunocompetent patients with drug-susceptible pulmonary TB, even severe disease and large cavities usually heal if appropriate therapy is instituted and completed. Still, TB causes or contributes to death in about 10% of cases, often in those who are debilitated for other reasons. Disseminated TB and TB meningitis may be fatal in up to 25% of cases despite optimal treatment. TB is much more aggressive in immunocompromised patients and, if not properly and aggressively treated, may be fatal in as little as 2 mo from its initial symptom. This is especially true of MDR-TB, in which mortality can approach 90%.

Most patients with uncomplicated TB and all with complicating illness (eg, AIDS, hepatitis, diabetes), adverse drug reactions, and drug resistance should be referred to a TB specialist. However, most can be treated at home with instructions on how to avoid spreading disease; these measures include staying at home, avoiding visitors (previously exposed family members may stay), and covering coughs with a tissue or hand. Surgical face masks for TB patients are stigmatizing and are generally not recommended for cooperative patients. Precautions must be continued for several weeks in or outside the hospital. The main indications for hospitalization are serious concomitant illness, need for diagnostic procedures, social issues (eg, homelessness), and need for respiratory isolation, such as people living in congregate settings where previously unexposed people would be regularly encountered.

All hospitalized patients initially should be in respiratory isolation, ideally in a negative-pressure room with 6 to 12 air changes/h. Anyone entering the room should wear a respirator that has been appropriately fitted and that meets The National Institute for Occupational Safety and Health guidelines to filter 1-micron particles.

Public health considerations: To limit transmission and development of drug-resistant strains, treatment is monitored by public health programs to ensure adherence, even if the patient is being treated by a private physician. In most states, TB care (including skin testing, chest x-rays, and drugs) is available free through public health clinics to reduce barriers to treatment.

Frequently, case management includes supervision of the ingestion of every dose of medication by public health personnel, a strategy known as directly observed therapy (DOT). DOT increases the likelihood that the full treatment course will be completed from 61% to 86% (91% with enhanced DOT, in which incentives and enablers such as transportation vouchers, child care, outreach workers, and meals are provided). DOT is particularly important for children and adolescents; for those with HIV infection, psychiatric illness, or substance abuse; and after treatment failure, relapse, or development of drug resistance.

Public health departments usually perform a home visit to evaluate potential barriers to treatment (eg, extreme poverty, unstable housing, alcoholism, or mental illness) and seek other active cases and close contacts. Close contacts are people who share the same breathing space for prolonged periods, typically household residents, but often includes people at work, school, and places of recreation. The precise duration and degree of contact that constitutes risk varies because TB patients vary greatly in infectiousness. For a patient who is highly infectious, as evidenced by multiple family members with disease or positive skin tests, even relatively casual contacts (eg, passengers on the bus he rides) should be referred for skin testing and evaluation for latent infection (see p. 1515), whereas a patient who does not infect any household contacts is less likely to infect casual contacts.

First-line drugs: The 1st-line drugs isoniazid (INH), rifampin (RIF), pyrazinamide (PZA), and ethambutol (EMB) are used together in initial treatment (for regimens and doses, see p. 1514 and TABLE 179–1).

INH is given orally once/day, has good tissue penetration, including CSF, and is highly bactericidal. It remains the single most useful and least expensive drug for TB treatment. However, decades of uncontrolled use (often as a single agent) in many countries (especially in East Asia) have greatly increased the percentage of resistant strains. In the US, about 10% of isolates are INH-resistant. INH is safe during pregnancy. Adverse reactions include rash, fever, and, rarely, anemia and agranulocytosis. INH causes harmless, transient aminotransferase elevations in up to 20% and symptomatic (usually reversible) hepatitis in about 1/1000 (more often in people > 35 yr, alcoholics, and patients with chronic liver disease). Monthly liver function testing is not recommended, but patients with unexplained fatigue, anorexia, nausea, vomiting, or jaundice may have hepatic toxicity; treatment is suspended and liver function tests obtained. Those with symptoms and any significant aminotransferase elevation (or asymptomatic elevation > 5 times normal) probably have hepatic toxicity, and INH is stopped. After recovery from mild aminotransferase elevations and symptoms, the patient can be safely challenged with a half-dose for 2 to 3 days. If this dose is tolerated (typically in about ½ of patients), the full dose may be restarted with close monitoring for symptoms and liver function deterioration. If the patient is receiving both INH and RIF, both drugs must be stopped, and the challenge performed with each drug separately. INH, rather than RIF, is more likely the cause of hepatotoxicity. Peripheral neuropathy can occur due to INH-induced pyridoxine (vitamin B_6) deficiency, most likely in pregnant or undernourished patients, alcoholics, patients with cancer or uremia, and the elderly. A daily dose of 25 to 50 mg of pyridoxine can prevent this complication, although it is usually not needed in children and healthy young adults. INH delays hepatic metabolism of phenytoin, requiring dose reduction. INH can also cause a violent reaction to disulfiram, a drug occasionally used for alcoholism.

RIF, given orally, is bactericidal, is well absorbed, penetrates well into cells and CSF, and acts rapidly. It also eliminates dormant organisms in macrophages or caseous lesions that can cause late relapse. Thus, RIF should be used throughout the course of therapy. Adverse effects include cholestatic jaundice (rare), fever, thrombocytopenia, and renal failure. RIF adds only slightly to the hepatotoxicity of INH. RIF has many significant drug interactions. It accelerates metabolism of anticoagulants, oral contraceptives, corticosteroids, digitoxin, oral antihyperglycemic drugs, methadone, and many other drugs. RIF is safe during pregnancy. Newer rifamycins, rifabutin and rifapentine, are available for special situations. Rifabutin is used for patients taking drugs (particularly antiretroviral agents) that have unacceptable interactions with RIF. Its action is similar to RIF, but it has been associated with uveitis when used with clarithromycin or fluconazole. Rifapentine is used in certain once/wk regimens (see

TABLE 179–1. DOSING OF FIRST-LINE ANTITUBERCULOSIS DRUGS*

DRUG	ADULTS/ CHILDREN	DAILY†	ONCE/ WK	2/WK	3/WK
Isoniazid	Adults (maximum)	5 mg/kg (300 mg)	15 mg/kg (900 mg)	15 mg/kg (900 mg)	15 mg/kg (900 mg)
	Children (maximum)	10–15 mg/kg (300 mg)	N/A	20–30 mg/kg (900 mg)	N/A
Rifampin	Adults (maximum)	10 mg/kg (600 mg)	N/A	10 mg/kg (600 mg)	10 mg/kg (600 mg)
	Children (maximum)	10–20 mg/kg (600 mg)	N/A	10–20 mg/kg (600 mg)	N/A
Rifabutin	Adults (maximum)	5 mg/kg (300 mg)	N/A	5 mg/kg (300 mg)	5 mg/kg (300 mg)
	Children	Dosing unknown	N/A	N/A	N/A
Rifapentine‡	Adults	N/A	10 mg/kg (600 mg)	N/A	N/A
	Children	N/A	N/A	N/A	N/A
Pyrazinamide	Adults (whole tablets)		N/A		
	40–55 kg	1 g		2 g	1.5 g
	56–75 kg	1.5 g		3 g	2.5 g
	≥ 76 kg§	2 g		4 g	3 g
	Children (maximum)	20–40 mg/kg (2 g)	N/A	15–50 mg/kg (2 g)	N/A
Ethambutol	Adults (whole tablets)		N/A		
	40–55 kg	800 mg		2000 mg	1200 mg
	56–75 kg	1200 mg		2800 mg	2000 mg
	≥ 76 kg§	1600 mg		4000 mg	2400 mg
	Children (maximum)	15–25 mg/kg (1 g)	N/A	50 mg/kg (2.5 g)	N/A

All dosing < 7 days/wk must be given as directly observed therapy.

*Specific regimens are discussed in text.
†Considered either 5 or 7 days/wk.
‡Continuation phase only.
§Maximum dose.

TABLE 179–1) but is not used in children or patients with HIV or extrapulmonary TB.

PZA, an oral bactericidal drug, when used during the intensive initial 2 mo of treatment, prevents development of resistance to RIF and shortens therapy to 6 mo. Its major adverse effects are GI upset and hepatitis. It often causes hyperuricemia, which is generally mild and only rarely induces gout. It is contraindicated in pregnancy.

EMB is given orally and is the best tolerated of the 1st-line drugs. Its main toxicity is optic neuritis, which is more common at higher doses (eg, 25 mg/kg) and in patients with impaired renal function. Patients present initially with an inability to distinguish blue from green, followed by impairment of visual acuity. Because both are reversible if detected early, patients should have a baseline test of visual acuity and color vision and should be questioned monthly regarding their vision. EMB is generally avoided in young children who cannot read eye charts but can be used if needed because of drug resistance or drug intolerance. Another drug is substituted for EMB if optic neuritis occurs. It can be used safely in pregnancy. Resistance to EMB is uncommon.

Second-line drugs: Other antibiotics are active against TB and are used primarily for MDR-TB. The 2 most important classes are the aminoglycosides and fluoroquinolones.

Streptomycin, the most commonly used aminoglycoside, is very effective and bactericidal. Resistance is still relatively uncommon in the US but is more common globally. CSF penetration is poor, and intrathecal administration should not be used if other effective drugs are available. Dose-related adverse effects include renal tubular damage, vestibular damage, and ototoxicity. The dose is about 15 mg/kg IM (usually 1 g for adults, reduced to 0.5 g for those > 60 yr, < 45 kg, or who have any degree of renal insufficiency). In patients > 60 yr with renal insufficiency, the dose is 0.25 g. To limit dose-related adverse effects, one dose is given only 5 days/wk for > 2 mo. Then it may be given twice/wk for another 2 mo if necessary. Patients should be monitored with appropriate testing of balance, hearing, and serum creatinine levels. Allergic reactions include rash, fever, agranulocytosis, and serum sickness. Flushing and tingling around the mouth commonly accompany injection but subside quickly. Streptomycin is contraindicated in pregnancy because it may damage the 8th cranial nerve in the fetus.

Kanamycin and amikacin may remain effective even if streptomycin resistance has developed. Their renal and neural toxicities are similar to those of streptomycin. Capreomycin, a related parenteral bactericidal drug, has dosage, effectiveness, and adverse effects similar to those of streptomycin. It is an important drug for MDR-TB because isolates resistant to streptomycin are often susceptible to capreomycin, and it seems somewhat better tolerated than the aminoglycosides when prolonged administration is required.

Some of the fluoroquinolones—levofloxacin, moxifloxacin, and gatifloxacin—are the most active and safe TB drugs after INH and RIF. The newer fluoroquinolones, moxifloxacin and gatifloxacin, appear almost as active with RIF as INH. Unfortunately, resistance to one fluoroquinolone usually means resistance to the others.

Other 2nd-line drugs include ethionamide, cycloserine, and para-aminosalicylic acid (PAS). These are less effective and more toxic than the 1st-line drugs but useful in treatment of MDR-TB.

Drug resistance: Treatment with any single antibiotic always results in survival of a few resistant mutant organisms. For most infections, survival of a few organisms is not a problem because immune defenses eliminate these remaining bacteria. However, resistance is a significant problem with TB because very few organisms (< 100) are required to perpetuate disease as susceptible organisms are suppressed. Thus, multiple drugs are used simultaneously; because drug resistance mutations occur separately, the possibility is remote that a given bacterium would have spontaneous mutations causing resistance to several drugs. However, once a resistant strain has developed and proliferated, it may acquire resistance to additional drugs through the same process; thus MDR-TB can occur.

Treatment regimens: All patients with new, previously untreated TB should receive a 2-mo initial phase of treatment followed by a 4- or 7-mo continuation phase.

Initial-phase therapy is with 4 antibiotics for the first 2 mo: INH, RIF, PZA, and EMB (see TABLE 179–1 for dosing). These can be given daily throughout (for all regimens, 5 days/wk is considered equivalent to daily), or daily for 2 wk followed by doses 2 or 3 times/wk for 6 wk. Intermittent dosing is possible without diminished effectiveness because of the growth characteristics of tubercle bacilli. However, regimens involving less than daily dosing must be carried out as DOT.

At 2 mo, PZA is stopped, and cultures and smears are obtained; continuation-phase treatment depends on their results and presence or absence of a cavitary lesion on the initial chest x-ray. If both culture and smear are negative, regardless of the chest x-ray, or the culture or smear is positive but x-ray showed no cavitation, INH and RIF are continued for 4 more mo (6 mo total). If the x-ray showed cavitation *and* the culture or smear is positive, INH and RIF are continued for 7 more mo (9 mo total). In either regimen, EMB is stopped if culture shows no resistance to any drug. Continuation-phase drugs can be given daily, twice weekly, or 3 times weekly. Patients with negative culture and smears and no cavitation on chest x-ray who are HIV-negative may receive once-weekly INH plus rifapentine.

For both initial and continuation phases, the total number of doses (calculated by doses/week times number of weeks) must be administered; thus if any doses are missed, treatment is extended and not stopped at the end of the time period.

Management of resistant TB varies by the pattern of drug resistance. Generally, MDR-TB requires prolonged (eg, 18 to 24 mo) treatment with the remaining active 1st-line drugs (including PZA, if susceptible) with addition of one or more 2nd-line drugs (typically a fluoroquinolone and an aminoglycoside or capreomycin). MDR-TB should always be treated by a TB specialist.

Other treatment: Surgical resection of a persistent TB cavity may occasionally be necessary. The main indication for resection is persistent, culture-positive MDR-TB in a patient with a destroyed lung region into which antibiotics cannot penetrate.

Corticosteroids are indicated in patients with acute respiratory distress syndrome, meningitis, or pericarditis. Dexamethasone 12 mg po or IV q 6 h is given to adults and children > 25 kg; children < 25 kg receive 8 mg. Treatment is continued for 2 to 3 wk. Corticosteroids that are needed for other indications pose no danger in a patient with active TB who is receiving an effective TB regimen.

Screening and Prevention

Screening is with TST. Indications for TST include close contact with people who have active pulmonary TB; chest x-ray evidence of past TB infection; risk factors for exposure to TB (eg, immigration within 5 yr from high-risk areas, indigent patients, IV drug users, selected US health care practitioners, such as respiratory therapists); and risk factors for development of active TB, particularly those with HIV infection but also others with impaired immunity, and patients with gastrectomy, jejunoileal bypass surgery, silicosis, renal insufficiency, diabetes, or head or neck cancer, and advanced age (eg, > 70 yr). In the US, most children and others without specific TB risk factors should not be skin tested to avoid false-positive reactions.

A positive result (see p. 1511 for criteria) suggests latent TB infection (LTBI). Patients with positive skin test are evaluated for other risk factors and have a chest x-ray. Those with x-ray abnormalities suggesting TB require evaluation for active TB as above, including sputum examination and culture. Updated guidelines for testing and treatment of LTBI are on the Centers for Disease Control and Prevention (CDC) web site (www.cdc.gov).

Some patients with remote TB exposure have a negative TST; however, the test itself may serve as an immune booster so that a subsequent test as little as 1 wk or as much as several years later will be positive (booster reaction). Thus, in a person who is tested regularly (eg, health care workers), the 2nd routine test will be positive, giving the false appearance of recent infection (and hence mandating further testing and treatment). In circumstances in which recurrent TST is indicated, a 2nd TST should be done 1 to 4 wk after the 1st to identify a booster reaction (because it is highly unlikely that a person would convert in that brief interval). Subsequent TST is performed and interpreted normally.

Treatment of LTBI is indicated principally in people whose TST converted from negative to positive within the previous 2 yr and in those with x-ray changes consistent with old TB and no evidence of active TB. Another indication for preventive treatment is people who, if infected, are at high risk for developing active TB (eg, HIV-infected people). Treatment is also strongly indicated for any child < 4 yr who is a close contact of a person with smear-positive TB, regardless of whether there was TST conversion.

Treatment generally consists of INH unless resistance is suspected (eg, in exposure to a known case). The dose is 300 mg once/day for 6 to 9 mo for most adults and 10 mg/kg for 9 mo for children. HIV-infected patients and people with abnormal chest x-rays consistent with old TB also require 9 mo of therapy. An alternative for patients resistant to or intolerant of INH is RIF, 600 mg once/day for 4 mo. The main limitations of treatment of LTBI are poor adherence and hepatotoxicity. Used for LTBI, INH causes clinical hepatitis in 1/1000 cases; hepatitis usually reverses if INH is stopped promptly. Patients being treated for LTBI should stop the drug if they experience any new symptoms, especially unexplained fatigue, loss of appetite, or nausea. Hepatitis due to RIF is less common than with INH, but drug interactions are frequent.

The BCG vaccine, made from an attenuated strain of *M. bovis*, is administered to > 80% of the world's children, primarily in high-burden countries. Overall average efficacy is probably only 50%. However, although BCG is not believed to prevent TB infection, it reduces the rate of extrathoracic TB in children, especially TB meningitis, and therefore is considered worthwhile. BCG has few indications in the US, except possibly unavoidable exposure to an infectious TB case that cannot be effectively treated, that is, highly resistant MDR-TB. Although BCG vaccination often converts the TST, the reaction is usually smaller than the response to natural TB infection, and it usually wanes more quickly. The TST reaction due to BCG should rarely be > 15 mm and rarely > 10 mm 15 yr after BCG administration. CDC recommends that all TST reactions in children who have had BCG be attributed to TB infection (and treated accordingly) because of the risk of serious complications of untreated latent infection. The new in vitro blood tests for TB infection based on gamma interferon production are not influenced by BCG vaccination.

Special Populations

Children: Primary TB in children often spreads to the vertebrae (Pott's disease) or the highly vascular epiphyses of long bones. Children ≤ 4 yr may also develop serious TB rapidly, possibly miliary TB, TB meningitis, or cavitary disease, before the TST becomes positive. However, in most children, there are few symptoms other than a brassy cough. The most common sign is hilar lymphadenopathy, but segmental atelectasis is possible. Adenopathy may progress, even after chemotherapy is started, and may produce lobar atelectasis, which usually clears during treatment. If hilar adenopathy is present, treatment with INH, RIF, and PZA is recommended for 6 mo (see TABLE 179–1).

The elderly: Reactivated disease can involve any organ, but particularly lungs, brain, kidneys, long bones, vertebrae, or lymph nodes. Reactivation may produce few symptoms and can be overlooked for weeks or months, delaying appropriate evaluation. Outbreaks in nursing homes may produce apical, middle, or lower lobe pneumonia as well as pleural effusion in previously tuberculin-negative residents. The pneumonia may not be recognized as TB and may persist and spread to others despite broad-spectrum antibiotic treatment. In the US, miliary TB and TB meningitis, commonly thought to afflict mainly young children, are more common in the elderly.

Patients > 60 yr with reactivated infection and no previous therapy usually respond well to RIF plus INH because they acquired the infection decades earlier, long before availability of modern drugs, and INH resistance is rare. INH, however, is hepatotoxic in up to 4 to 5% of patients > 65 yr (compared with 1 to 2% of patients < 65 yr). In the elderly, chemoprophylaxis is indicated only if the TST increases ≥ 15 mm from a previously negative reaction. In these converters, INH decreases active TB by 98.5%.

TST sensitivity can be poor in the elderly. Close contacts of an active case and others at high risk with negative TST should receive preventive treatment unless contraindicated.

HIV-infected patients: TST sensitivity is generally poor in immunocompromised patients (who may be anergic). In HIV-infected patients with LTBI, active TB develops in about 5 to 10%/yr, whereas it develops in about the same percentage over a lifetime in people who are not immunocompromised. A decade ago, ½ of HIV-infected TB patients who were untreated or infected with a resistant strain died, with median survival of only 60 days. Outcomes are somewhat better now due to earlier TB diagnosis and antiretroviral therapy, but TB in HIV patients remains a serious concern. Dissemination of bacilli during primary infection is usually much more extensive in patients with HIV infection. Consequently, a larger proportion of TB is extrapulmonary. Tuberculomas are more common and more destructive. HIV reduces both inflammatory reaction and cavitation of pulmonary lesions. As a result, a patient's chest x-ray may show a nonspecific pneumonia, or even be normal, even though acid-fast bacilli are present in sufficient numbers to appear on a sputum smear.

TB may develop early in AIDS and may be its presenting manifestation. Hematogenous dissemination of TB in people with HIV infection produces a serious, often baffling illness with symptoms of both infections. A mycobacterial illness in an AIDS patient that develops while the $CD4^+$ T cell count is ≥ 200/μL is almost always TB. By contrast, depending on the probability of TB exposure, a mycobacterial infection that develops while the $CD4^+$ count is < 50/μL is usually due to *M. avium* complex (see p. 1518), which is not contagious.

TB in HIV-infected people generally responds well to usual regimens when in vitro study shows sensitivity. For multidrug-resistant strains, however, outcomes are not as favorable because the drugs are more toxic and less effective. Therapy for susceptible TB should be continued for 6 to 9 mo after conversion of sputum cultures to negative but may be shortened to 6 mo if 3 separate pretreatment sputum smears are negative, suggesting that there are few infecting organisms. Current recommendations suggest that if the sputum culture is positive after 2 mo of therapy, treatment is prolonged to 9 mo. HIV-infected patients whose tuberculin reactions are ≥ 5 mm should receive chemoprophylaxis.

Extrapulmonary Tuberculosis

TB outside the lung usually results from hematogenous dissemination. Sometimes infection directly extends from an adjacent organ. Symptoms vary by site but generally include fever, malaise, and weight loss.

Miliary TB: Also known as generalized hematogenous TB, miliary TB occurs when a tuberculous lesion erodes into a blood vessel, disseminating millions of tubercle bacilli into the bloodstream and throughout the body. The lungs and bone marrow are most often affected, but any site may be involved. Miliary TB is most common in children < 4 yr, immunocompromised people, and the elderly.

Symptoms include fever, chills, weakness, malaise, and often progressive dyspnea. Intermittent dissemination of tubercle bacilli may lead to a prolonged FUO. Bone marrow involvement may produce anemia, thrombocytopenia, or a leukemoid reaction.

Genitourinary TB: Infection of the kidney may present as pyelonephritis (eg, fever, back pain, pyuria) without the usual urinary pathogens on routine culture ("sterile pyuria"). Infection commonly spreads to the bladder and, in men, to the prostate, seminal vesicles, or epididymis, causing an enlarging scrotal mass. Infection may spread to the perinephric space and down the psoas muscle, sometimes causing an abscess on the anterior thigh.

Salpingo-oophoritis can occur after menarche, when the fallopian tubes become vascular. Symptoms include chronic pelvic pain and sterility or ectopic pregnancy from tubal scarring.

TB meningitis: Meningitis often occurs in the absence of infection at other extrapulmonary sites. In the US, it is most common among the elderly and immunocompromised, but in areas where TB is common among children, TB meningitis usually occurs between birth and 5 yr. At any age, meningitis is the most serious form of TB and has high morbidity and mortality. It is the one form of TB believed to be prevented in childhood by vaccination with BCG.

Symptoms are low-grade fever, unremitting headache, nausea, and drowsiness, which may progress to stupor and coma. Kernig's and Brudzinski's signs may be positive. Stages are (1) clear sensorium with abnormal CSF, (2) drowsiness or stupor with focal neurologic signs, and (3) coma. Stroke may develop due to thrombosis of a major cerebral vessel. Focal neurologic symptoms suggest a tuberculous mass intracranial lesion (tuberculoma).

TB peritonitis: Peritoneal infection represents seeding from abdominal lymph nodes or from salpingo-oophoritis. Peritonitis is particularly common in alcoholics with cirrhosis.

Symptoms may be mild, with fatigue, abdominal pain, and tenderness, or severe enough to mimic acute abdomen. The "doughy abdomen" referred to in old textbooks is rarely present.

TB pericarditis: Pericardial infection may develop from foci in mediastinal lymph nodes or from pleural TB. In some high incidence parts of the world, TB pericarditis is a common cause of heart failure.

Symptoms may begin with a pericardial friction rub, pleuritic and positional chest pain, or fever. Pericardial tamponade may occur, producing dyspnea, neck vein distention, paradoxical pulse, muffled heart sounds, and possibly hypotension.

TB lymphadenitis: Usually the hilar lymph nodes are involved. Other nodes generally are not involved unless the inoculum is large or poorly contained, allowing organisms to reach the thoracic duct, where they disseminate into the bloodstream. Most infected nodes heal, but reactivation commonly occurs. Infection in supraclavicular nodes may inoculate anterior cervical nodes, eventually resulting in scrofula—TB lymphadenitis in the neck.

Affected nodes are swollen and may be mildly tender or drain. Adjacent nodes sometimes coalesce into an irregular mass.

TB of bones and joints: Weight-bearing joints are most commonly involved, but bones of the wrist, hand, and elbow also may be affected, especially after injury.

Pott's disease is spinal infection, which begins in a vertebral body and often spreads to adjacent vertebrae, with narrowing of the disk space between them. Untreated, the vertebrae may collapse, possibly impinging on the spinal cord.

Symptoms include progressive or constant pain in involved bones and chronic or subacute arthritis (usually monoarticular). In Pott's disease, spinal cord compression produces neurologic deficits, including paraplegia; paravertebral swelling may result from an abscess.

Gastrointestinal TB: Because the entire GI mucosa resists TB invasion, infection requires prolonged exposure and enormous inocula. It is very unusual in developed countries where bovine TB is rare.Ulcers of the mouth and oropharynx may develop from eating contaminated dairy products; primary lesions also may occur in the small bowel. Intestinal invasion generally produces hyperplasia and an inflammatory bowel syndrome with pain, diarrhea, obstruction, and hematochezia. It may also mimic appendicitis. Ulceration and fistulae are possible.

TB of the liver: Liver infection is common with advanced pulmonary TB and widely disseminated or miliary TB. However, the liver generally heals without sequelae when the principal infection is treated. TB in the liver occasionally spreads to the gallbladder, leading to obstructive jaundice.

Other sites: Rarely, TB may develop on abraded skin in a patient with cavitary pulmonary TB. TB may infect the wall of a blood vessel and has even ruptured the aorta. Adrenal involvement, leading to Addison's disease, formerly was common but now is rare. Trauma to a tendon sheath may cause tuberculous tenosynovitis in a patient with tuberculous involvement of any organ.

Diagnosis and Treatment

Testing is as discussed on p. 1510, including chest x-ray, TST, and microscopic analysis (with appropriate staining) and cultures of affected body fluids (CSF, urine, or pleural, pericardial, or joint fluid) and tissue for mycobacteria. However, cultures and smears are often negative because few organisms may be present; in this case, nucleic acid amplification techniques may be helpful. If all tests are negative and miliary TB is still a concern, biopsies of the bone marrow and the liver are done. Blood culture is rarely diagnostic. If TB is highly suspected by other features, (eg, granuloma on biopsy, positive TST plus unexplained lymphocytosis in pleural fluid or CSF), treatment should proceed despite inability to demonstrate TB organisms.

Chest x-ray may show signs of primary or active TB; in miliary TB, it shows thousands of 2- to 3-mm interstitial nodules evenly distributed through both lungs. TST may initially be negative, but a repeat test in a few weeks will likely be positive. If it is not, the diagnosis of TB should be questioned or causes of anergy sought.

Other imaging studies are obtained based on clinical findings. Abdominal or genitourinary involvement usually requires CT or ultrasound; renal lesions are often visible. Bone and joint involvement requires CT or MRI; MRI is preferable for spinal disease.

Body fluids typically show lymphocytosis. The most suggestive CSF constellation also includes a glucose level < 50% that in the serum and an elevated protein level.

Drug treatment is the most important modality and follows standard regimens and principles discussed on p. 1514. Six to 9 mo of therapy is probably adequate for most sites except the meninges, which require treatment for 9 to 12 mo. Corticosteroids may help in pericarditis and meningitis (for dosing, see p. 1515).

Surgery is required to drain empyema, cardiac tamponade, and CNS abscess; close bronchopleural fistulas; resect infected bowel; and decompress spinal cord encroachment. Surgical debridement is sometimes needed in Pott's disease if swelling does not subside or pain persists; fixation of the vertebral column by bone graft is required in only the most advanced cases. Adenitis should not be treated with incision and drainage, which usually produces a chronic, draining lesion. However, total resection of the involved nodes is sometimes needed (avoiding wound contamination).

OTHER MYCOBACTERIAL INFECTIONS RESEMBLING TUBERCULOSIS

Mycobacteria other than the tubercle bacillus sometimes infect humans. They are commonly present in soil and water and are less virulent than *M. tuberculosis*. Most exposures do not produce disease, which usually requires a defect in local or systemic host defenses; frail elderly are sometimes infected. *M. avium* complex (MAC)—the closely related species of *M. avium* and *M. intracellulare*—accounts for most diseases. Other causative species are *M. kansasii, M. xenopi, M. marinum, M. ulcerans*, and the *M. fortuitum* complex (*M. fortuitum* and *M. chelonei*). Person-to-person transmission is rare but can occur in compromised hosts.

The lungs are the most common site; most involve MAC, but a few are due to *M. kansasii*, *M. xenopi*, and *M. fortuitum* complex. Occasional cases involve lymph nodes, bones and joints, the skin, and wounds. However, disseminated MAC disease is increasing in HIV-infected patients, and resistance to antituberculous drugs is the rule (except in *M. kansasii* and *M. xenopi*).

Pulmonary disease: The typical patient is a middle-aged or older white man with previous lung problems such as chronic bronchitis, emphysema, healed TB, bronchiectasis, or silicosis. MAC also commonly causes pulmonary disease in middle-aged women without underlying lung abnormalities. Cough and expectoration are common, but systemic symptoms are infrequent. The course may be slowly progressive or stable for long periods. Respiratory insufficiency and persistent hemoptysis may develop. X-ray features resemble those of pulmonary TB, but cavitation tends to be thin-walled, and pleural effusion is rare.

Because the organisms are usually resistant to any single drug, susceptibility testing is of limited value. Determination of susceptibility to drug combinations can be helpful but can be obtained only in highly specialized laboratories.

In moderately symptomatic disease with positive sputum smears and cultures, clarithromycin 500 mg po bid, rifampin (RIF) 600 mg po once/day, and ethambutol (EMB) 15 to 25 mg/kg po once/day should be used for 12 to 18 mo or until cultures are negative for 12 mo. In progressive cases unresponsive to standard drugs, combinations of 4 to 6 drugs that include rifabutin 300 mg po once/day, ciprofloxacin 250 to 500 mg po or IV bid, clofazimine 100 to 200 mg po once/day, and amikacin 10 to 15 mg/kg IV once/day may be tried. Resection surgery is recommended in exceptional cases involving well-localized disease in young, otherwise healthy patients. *M. kansasii* and *M. xenopi* infections respond to standard TB regimens if RIF and clarithromycin are included.

Lymphadenitis: In children 1 to 5 yr, chronic submaxillary and submandibular cervical lymphadenitis is commonly due to MAC or *M. kansasii*. It is presumably acquired by oral ingestion. Diagnosis is usually by biopsy. Treatment with clarithromycin, RIF, and EMB is given to avoid fistulas and disfiguring scars.

Cutaneous disease: Swimming pool granuloma is a protracted but self-limited superficial granulomatous ulcerating disease usually caused by *M. marinum* contracted from contaminated swimming pools or from cleaning a home aquarium. *M. ulcerans* and *M. kansasii* are occasionally involved. Lesions, reddish bumps enlarging and turning purple, most frequently occur on the upper extremities or knees. Healing may occur spontaneously, but tetracycline (250 to 500 mg po qid) and combinations of clarithromycin, RIF, and EMB for 3 to 6 mo have been effective against *M. marinum*.

Wounds and foreign body infections: *M. fortuitum* complex has caused serious infections of penetrating wounds of the eyes and skin (especially feet) and in patients receiving contaminated materials (porcine heart valves, breast implants, bone wax). Treatment usually requires extensive debridement and removal of the foreign material. Useful drugs include clarithromycin 500 mg po bid, sulfamethoxazole 20 mg/kg po bid, doxycycline 100 to 200 mg po bid, cefoxitin 1 g IV q 6 to 8 h, and amikacin 10 to 15 mg/kg IV once/day, for 3 to 6 mo duration. Infections caused by *M. abscessus* and *M. chelonae* are resistant to most antibiotics and have proven extremely difficult or impossible to cure and should be referred to an experienced specialist.

Disseminated disease: MAC causes disseminated disease commonly in patients with advanced AIDS and occasionally in those with other immunocompromised states, including organ transplantation and hairy cell leukemia. In AIDS, disseminated MAC usually develops late (unlike TB, which develops early), occurring simultaneously with other opportunistic infections.

Disseminated MAC disease causes fever, anemia, thrombocytopenia, diarrhea, and abdominal pain—features similar to Whipple's disease. Diagnosis can be confirmed by cultures of blood, bone marrow, or small-bowel biopsy specimens. Organisms may be identified in stool and respiratory specimens, but organisms from these specimens may represent colonization rather than true disease. Combinations of antimycobacterial drugs (see under TB Treatment on p. 1514) have reduced bacteremia and temporarily lessened symptoms but are not curative; the prognosis is poor.

LEPROSY

(Hansen's Disease)

Leprosy is a chronic infection by the acid-fast bacillus *Mycobacterium leprae*, which

has a unique tropism for peripheral nerves, skin, and mucous membranes. Symptoms are myriad, including anesthetic polymorphic skin lesions and peripheral neuropathy. Diagnosis is clinical and confirmed by biopsy. Treatment is with dapsone plus other antimycobacterial drugs.

M. leprae is an obligate intracellular parasite that causes leprosy worldwide in > 1 million people. Although most cases occur in Asia, the highest prevalence is in Africa. Endemic foci also exist in Mexico, South and Central America, and the Pacific islands. Almost all of the estimated 5000 cases in the US involve immigrants from developing countries who have settled in California, Hawaii, and Texas. There are several forms; the most severe, lepromatous form, is more common in men. Leprosy may occur at any age, although the highest incidence is among those in their teens and 20s.

Until recently, humans were the only recognized natural reservoir for *M. leprae*, but 15% of wild armadillos in Louisiana and Texas are infected, and subhuman primates occasionally harbor the organism. However, except possibly for some insect vectors (eg, bedbugs, mosquitoes), zoonotic transmission is not a factor in human disease. *M. leprae* is also in soil.

The organism is thought to be transmitted by nasal droplets and secretions. Untreated lepromatous patients harbor large numbers of organisms in their nasal mucosa and its secretions, even before signs and symptoms appear, and about 50% of patients have had intimate contact with an infected person, commonly a household member. Brief contact conveys little risk of transmission. The milder tuberculoid form is probably noncontagious. Most (95%) immunocompetent people do not develop infection even after exposure. Those who do, probably have a genetic predisposition.

M. leprae grow slowly (doubling time, 2 wk). The usual incubation period ranges from 6 mo to 10 yr. Once infection develops, hematogenous dissemination can occur.

Symptoms and Signs

About 3/4 of those infected develop a single skin lesion (indeterminate leprosy) that clears spontaneously; the remainder develop clinical leprosy. Symptoms, signs, and severity of clinical disease vary, depending on the degree of cell-mediated immune response to *M. leprae*.

Tuberculoid leprosy (paucibacillary Hansen's disease) is the mildest form. Affected patients have a strong cell-mediated response, which limits disease to a few skin patches or individual nerves; lesions contain few or no bacteria. Skin lesions consist of one or a few hypoesthetic, centrally hypopigmented macules with sharp, raised borders. The rash, as in all forms of leprosy, is nonpruritic. Lesions are dry because autonomic nerve involvement impairs sweating. Peripheral nerves may be damaged and palpably enlarged, generally asymmetrically, and frequently are contiguous to skin lesions.

Lepromatous leprosy (multibacillary Hansen's disease) is the most severe form. Affected patients lack cell-mediated immunity to *M. leprae* and have systemic infection with widespread bacterial infiltration of skin, nerves, and other organs (nose, testes, kidneys). They have skin macules, papules, nodules, or plaques, often symmetric, loaded with *M. leprae*. Gynecomastia, loss of digits, and often severe peripheral neuropathy may occur. Patients may lose eyelashes and eyebrows. Disease in western Mexico and elsewhere in Latin America may produce diffuse dermal infiltration with loss of body hair and other skin appendages but no focal skin lesions, a condition termed diffuse lepromatosis or lepra bonita. Lepromatous patients may develop erythema nodosum, and those with diffuse lepromatosis may develop Lucio's phenomenon, with ulcers (especially of the legs) that often become secondarily infected, resulting in bacteremia and death.

Borderline leprosy (also termed multibacillary), of intermediate severity, is the most common form. Skin lesions resemble tuberculoid leprosy but are more numerous and irregular; large patches may affect a whole limb, and peripheral nerve involvement with weakness and loss of sensation is common. This type is unstable and may become more like lepromatous leprosy or may undergo a reversal reaction, becoming more like the tuberculoid form.

Leprosy reactions: A number of patients undergo intermittent, acute, immunologically mediated inflammatory events. There are 2 types.

Type 1 reactions result from a spontaneous increase in cell-mediated immunity. They occur in about 1/3 of patients with borderline leprosy, usually after starting therapy. The clinical consequences are a marked increase in inflammation within preexisting lesions, with skin edema, erythema, and tenderness, and neuritis with pain, tenderness, and loss of function. New lesions may also develop. These reactions contribute significantly to nerve damage, particularly if not treated early. Because the immune response is increased, these are termed reversal reactions, despite the apparent clinical worsening.

Type 2 reactions are a systemic inflammatory reaction to immune complex deposition. This is also called erythema nodosum leprosum (ENL). It previously occurred in about ½ of patients with borderline lepromatous and lepromatous leprosy within the 1st yr of treatment; it is less common since the addition of clofazimine to the drug regimen. It may also occur spontaneously before therapy. It appears to be a polymorphonuclear vasculitis or panniculitis and probably involves circulating immune complexes or increased T-helper cell function. Levels of circulating tumor necrosis factor increase. ENL involves erythematous and painful papules or nodules that may pustulate and ulcerate and produce fever, neuritis, lymphadenitis, orchitis, arthritis (particularly in large joints, usually knees), and glomerulonephritis. Hemolysis or bone marrow suppression may produce anemia, and hepatic inflammation may produce mild abnormalities in liver function tests.

Complications: Most complications are due to peripheral neuritis resulting from the infection or a leprosy reaction; distal hypoesthesia and weakness are the result. Nerve trunks and microscopic dermal nerves may be affected, particularly the ulnar nerve at the elbow, leading to clawing of the 4th and 5th digits in severe cases. The perineal, median, zygomatic branch of the facial nerve and the posterior auricular nerves may also be affected. Small nerve fibers that respond to pain and temperature or fine touch are particularly affected, while larger nerve fibers responsible for position and vibration sensation are generally spared. Tendon transfers may correct lagophthalmos and functional disabilities of the extremities but should not be performed until 6 mo after initiation of therapy.

Plantar ulcers with secondary infection are a major cause of morbidity and should be treated with debridement and appropriate antibiotics. The patient should avoid weight bearing or wear a total-contact cast (Unna boot) that allows ambulation. To prevent recurrence, calluses should be filed, and patients should wear custom-molded shoes or extra-depth shoes that do not rub the feet.

The eyes may be severely affected. With lepromatous leprosy or ENL, iritis may lead to glaucoma. Corneal insensitivity and involvement of the facial nerve's zygomatic branch (causing lagophthalmos) may lead to corneal trauma, scarring, and blindness. Patients with corneal involvement should routinely use lubricating eye drops.

The nasal mucosa and cartilage are affected in lepromatous patients, leading to chronic nasal congestion and, at times, epistaxis. Although uncommon, nasal cartilage perforation and collapse may result if leprosy goes untreated.

Hypogonadism may occur in lepromatous males from decreased serum testosterone levels and increased follicle-stimulating and luteinizing hormone levels, with erectile dysfunction, infertility, and gynecomastia. Supplemental testosterone (see p. 1947) may relieve symptoms.

Amyloidosis and consequent renal failure occasionally occur in lepromatous leprosy associated with severe, recurrent ENL.

Diagnosis

Diagnosis is suggested by the clinical picture of skin lesions and peripheral neuropathy and confirmed by microscopic examination of biopsy specimens; the organism does not grow on artificial culture media. Biopsy specimens should be taken from the advancing edge of tuberculoid lesions. In lepromatous patients, specimens should be taken from nodules or plaques, although pathologic changes may be visible even in normal-appearing skin.

Serum IgM antibodies to *M. leprae* are specific but insensitive. Lepromatous patients almost always have antibodies, but only ⅔ of patients with tuberculous leprosy have them. Because such antibodies may indicate asymptomatic infection in endemic areas, their diagnostic usefulness is limited. However, they may be useful in monitoring disease activity because antibody levels fall with effective chemotherapy and may rise with relapse.

Lepromin (heat-killed *M. leprae*) is available for skin testing but is neither sensitive nor specific and is not recommended.

Treatment and Prevention

With treatment, the medical sequelae are often minor, but cosmetic deformities may lead to ostracizing of patients and their families.

Drugs: Dapsone 50 to 100 mg po once/day is the mainstay of therapy (1 to 2 mg/kg for children). Adverse effects include hemolysis and anemia (generally mild); allergic dermatoses that can be severe; and, rarely, a syndrome including exfoliative dermatitis, high fever, and mononucleosis-like WBC differential (dapsone syndrome). Although dapsone-resistant leprosy has been reported, resistance is usually only partial, and patients respond to usual dapsone doses.

Rifampin (RIF) is primarily bactericidal for *M. leprae*. However, it is too expensive for many developing countries if given at the recommended dosage of 600 mg po once/day. Adverse effects include hepatotoxicity, flu-like syndromes, and, rarely, thrombocytopenia and renal failure when given intermittently.

Clofazimine, a phenazine dye that is similar to dapsone in activity against *M. leprae*, is given at oral dosages of 50 mg once/day to 100 mg 3 times/wk; 300 mg once/mo is moderately helpful in preventing type 2 leprosy reactions and possibly type 1 reactions. Adverse effects include GI intolerance and an uneven reddish black skin discoloration.

Ethionamide 250 to 500 mg po once/day is also effective. However, because it often causes GI irritability and may cause liver dysfunction, especially when given with RIF, it is not recommended unless liver function can be monitored regularly.

Recently, 3 antimicrobials, minocycline (100 mg po once/day), clarithromycin (500 mg po bid), and ofloxacin (400 mg po once/day), have been found to kill *M. leprae* rapidly and reduce dermal infiltration. Their combined bactericidal activity for *M. leprae* is greater than that of dapsone, clofazimine, and ethionamide, but not RIF. Only minocycline has proven safe for the long-term administration required in leprosy.

Recommended regimens: Although antimicrobial therapy is effective, optimal regimens remain uncertain. Drug sensitivity testing in mice is often recommended for lepromatous and borderline patients, particularly in the US.

The WHO recommends multidrug regimens for all forms of leprosy. Treatment for lepromatous leprosy requires more intensive regimens and a greater duration than that for tuberculoid leprosy. For affected adults, the WHO advocates dapsone 100 mg once/day, clofazimine 50 mg once/day plus 300 mg once/mo, and RIF 600 mg once/mo for at least 2 yr or until results of skin biopsies are negative (usually in about 5 yr). For tuberculoid leprosy patients without demonstrable acid-fast bacilli, the WHO recommends dapsone 100 mg once/day and RIF 600 mg once/mo for 6 mo. Many authorities in India recommend that the duration be extended to 1 yr.

In the US, lepromatous leprosy is usually treated with RIF 600 mg once/day for 2 to 3 yr plus dapsone 100 mg once/day for life. Tuberculoid leprosy is treated with dapsone 100 mg once/day for 5 yr. Advice on diagnosis and treatment is available from the National Hansen's Disease Program in Baton Rouge, LA (1-800-642-2477).

Leprosy reactions: Patients with type 1 reactions (except minor skin inflammation) are given prednisone 40 to 60 mg po once/day initially followed by low maintenance doses (often as low as 10 to 15 mg once/day) for a few months. Minor skin inflammation should not be treated.

First and 2nd episodes of ENL may be treated, if mild, with aspirin or, if significant, with 1 wk of prednisone 40 to 60 mg po once/day plus antimicrobials. For recurrent cases, thalidomide 100 to 300 mg po once/day is the drug of choice (in the US, available through the National Hansen's Disease Program). However, because of its teratogenicity, thalidomide should not be given to women who may become pregnant. Adverse effects are mild constipation, mild leukopenia, and sedation.

Prevention: BCG vaccine or dapsone has been only marginally effective and is not recommended. Because the disease is minimally contagious, historical shunning has no scientific basis. Reasonable precautions include the avoidance of direct contact with secretions and tissues of infected people.

180 FUNGI

(See also Ch. 120 on p. 987.)

Many fungi are opportunists and are not usually pathogenic except in a compromised host. Causes of compromised immunity include AIDS, azotemia, diabetes mellitus, bronchiectasis, emphysema, TB, lymphoma, leukemia, other hematologic malignancies, burns, and therapy with corticosteroids, immunosuppressants, or antimetabolites. Candidiasis, aspergillosis, mucormycosis (zygomycosis), and nocardiosis are typical opportunistic systemic fungal infections (mycoses). Systemic mycoses affecting severely immunocompromised patients often have acute presentations with rapidly progressive pneumonia, fungemia, or manifestations of extrapulmonary dissemination. Local fungal infections of the skin (see p. 987), mouth (see p. 816), and vagina (see p. 2086) occur in normal hosts.

In immunocompetent patients, systemic mycoses typically have a chronic course; disseminated mycoses with pneumonia and septicemia are rare and, if lung lesions develop, usually progress slowly. Months or years may elapse before medical attention is sought or a diagnosis is made. Symptoms are rarely intense in such chronic mycoses, but fever, chills, night sweats, anorexia, weight loss, malaise, and depression may occur.

Primary fungal infections may have a characteristic geographic distribution. For example, coccidioidomycosis is primarily confined to the southwestern US and northern Mexico; histoplasmosis occurs primarily in the eastern and midwestern US; blastomycosis is restricted to North America and Africa; and paracoccidioidomycosis, sometimes called South American blastomycosis, is confined to that continent. However, travelers can manifest disease any time after returning from endemic areas.

When a fungus disseminates from a primary focus in the lung, the manifestations may be characteristic. For example, cryptococcosis usually presents as a chronic meningitis, progressive disseminated histoplasmosis as generalized involvement of the reticuloendothelial system (liver, spleen, bone marrow), and blastomycosis as single or multiple skin lesions.

Diagnosis

Pulmonary fungal infections must be distinguished from TB, tumors, and chronic pneumonias caused by nonfungal organisms. Specimens are obtained for fungal and acid-fast bacilli culture and histopathology. Sputum samples may be adequate, but occasionally bronchoalveolar lavage, transthoracic needle biopsy, or even surgery may be required to obtain an acceptable specimen.

Infections are readily recognized as fungal by their histopathologic appearance. However, identification of the specific organism may be difficult and usually requires fungal culture. The clinical significance of positive sputum cultures may be unclear if they show commensal organisms (eg, *Candida albicans*) or those prevalent in the environment (eg, *Aspergillus* sp). Therefore, an etiologic role for these organisms typically requires confirmation of tissue invasion.

If histopathology and culture are unavailable or unrevealing, serologic tests may be used for many systemic mycoses, although few provide definitive diagnoses. Among the most useful assays are those that measure specific antigenic products of organisms, most notably *Cryptococcus neoformans, Histoplasma capsulatum,* and *Aspergillus*. Complement fixation assays for anticoccidioidal antibodies are satisfactorily specific and do not require proof of rising levels; high titers confirm the diagnosis and indicate high risk of extrapulmonary dissemination. In chronic meningitis, a positive complement fixation for anticoccidioidal antibodies in CSF often provides the only indication for aggressive antifungal therapy. Most other tests for antifungal antibodies have low sensitivity and/or specificity, and because measurement of acute and convalescent titers is required, are unhelpful in guiding initial therapy.

ANTIFUNGAL DRUGS

Drugs for systemic antifungal treatment include primarily amphotericin B (and its lipid formulations), various azole derivatives, echinocandins, and flucytosine (see TABLE 180–1).

Amphotericin B

Despite its high toxicity, amphotericin B remains standard therapy for most life-threatening systemic mycoses.

For chronic mycoses, treatment usually is started with ≥ 0.3 mg/kg IV once/day, increased as tolerated to the desired dose (0.4 mg/kg to 1.0 mg/kg, generally not > 50 mg daily); many patients tolerate the desired

TABLE 180–1. DRUGS FOR SYSTEMIC FUNGAL INFECTIONS

DRUG	USES	DOSE	ADVERSE EFFECTS
Amphotericin B	Most fungal infections	0.5–1.5 mg/kg IV once/day	Acute infusion reactions, cardiac arrest, encephalopathy, neuropathy, GI upset, renal damage, liver failure, marrow injury, thrombophlebitis, hearing loss, visual impairment, rash
Caspofungin	Aspergillosis	70 mg on day 1, then 50 mg IV once/day	Phlebitis, headache, GI upset, rash, marrow injury, myalgia, edema, fever
Fluconazole	Mucosal and systemic candidiasis, cryptococcal meningitis	3–12 mg/kg po or IV once/day	GI upset, dizziness, angioedema, anaphylaxis, seizures, exfoliative dermatitis, marrow and hepatic injury
Flucytosine	Candidiasis (systemic), cryptococcosis	12.5–37.5 mg/kg po qid	Myocardial toxicity; psychosis; neuropathy; nausea; vomiting; hepatic, renal, and marrow injury; colitis; respiratory arrest
Itraconazole	Dermatomycosis, multiple systemic mycoses	100 mg po once/day to 200 mg po bid *or* 200 mg IV bid	Liver damage, GI upset, rash, headache, dizziness, marrow suppression, hemolysis, respiratory irritation, erectile dysfunction, hypokalemia, hypertension, edema, hepatitis, hallucinations
Ketoconazole	Multiple systemic mycoses; severe, recalcitrant dermatomycosis	200 mg po once/day *or* 3.3–6.6 mg/kg po once/day (> 2 yr old)	Liver damage, GI upset, depression, itching, headache, dizziness, marrow suppression, hemolysis
Nystatin	Nonesophageal membrane GI candidiasis	500,000–1,000,000 units po tid	Rash, GI upset, tachycardia, bronchospasm, facial swelling, myalgia
Voriconazole	Invasive aspergillosis	200 mg po bid *or* 3 to 6 mg/kg IV q 12 h	Transient visual disturbances, edema, GI upset, rash, sepsis, respiratory disorder, elevated hepatic enzymes

dose on the 1st day. If patients tolerate the target dose, twice that dose can be given on a more convenient alternate-day schedule. Extended treatment courses may be even less frequent (eg, 3 times/wk).

For acute, life-threatening mycoses, amphotericin B is started at 0.6 to 1.0 mg/kg/day. For certain rapidly progressive opportunistic mycoses (eg, invasive aspergillosis), daily doses as high as 1.5 mg/kg have been used, usually divided into 2 or 3 infusions.

The standard formulation, colloidal amphotericin B deoxycholate, must always be administered in 5% D/W, because salts can precipitate the drug. It is usually administered over 2 to 3 h, although more rapid infusions over 20 to 60 min are safe in selected patients. Reactions are usually mild, but some experience chills, fever, nausea, vomiting, anorexia, headache, and, occasionally, hypotension. Amphotericin B may also cause chemical thrombophlebitis. Premedication with acetaminophen or NSAIDs is often used; if these are ineffective, hydrocortisone 25 to 50 mg IV or diphenhydramine 25 mg IV is sometimes added. Often, hydrocortisone can be tapered and omitted during extended therapy. Severe chills and rigors can be relieved or prevented by meperidine, 50 to 75 mg IV.

Intrathecal amphotericin B injections are used in chronic meningitis but are rarely needed; administration is usually via direct intracisternal injection or with a subcutaneous Ommaya-type reservoir connected to an intraventricular catheter. Headache, nausea, and vomiting may occur but may be reduced by adding dexamethasone to each intrathecal injection. Lumbar intrathecal injections are seldom used because of erratic distribution and potentially severe local inflammatory effects, which may lead to adhesive arachnoiditis. At the time of injection, 10 mL or more of CSF is withdrawn into a syringe containing amphotericin B diluted in 5% D/W to 0.2 mg/mL. Doses of 0.05 to 0.5 mg are then injected over 2 min or more. Doses are gradually increased as tolerated, peaking with a regimen of 0.5 mg 3 times/wk.

Renal impairment is the major toxic risk of amphotericin B therapy. Serum creatinine and BUN should be monitored before and at regular intervals during treatment. Amphotericin B is unique among nephrotoxic antimicrobial drugs in that it is not eliminated appreciably via the kidneys and does not accumulate as renal failure worsens. Nevertheless, dosages should be lowered if serum creatinine rises to > 3.0 to 3.5 mg/dL (> 265 to 309 μmol/L) or BUN to > 50 mg/dL (> 18 mmol urea/L). Acute nephrotoxicity can be reduced by IV hydration with saline before amphotericin B infusion. Mild to moderate renal function abnormalities induced by amphotericin B generally resolve gradually after completion of therapy. Permanent damage occurs primarily after prolonged treatment; following > 4 g total dose, about 75% have persistent renal insufficiency. Besides renal toxicity, amphotericin B frequently suppresses bone marrow function, manifested primarily by anemia. Hepatotoxicity or other untoward effects are unusual.

Several lipid vehicles reduce the toxicity of amphotericin B (particularly nephrotoxicity and infusion-related symptoms). Three preparations are available: amphotericin B lipid complex, liposomal amphotericin B, and amphotericin B cholesteryl sulfate. These drugs are expensive and generally reserved for patients with renal insufficiency (serum creatinine > 2.5 mg/dL), those with persistent infusion-related adverse effects unrelieved by pretreatment, and those in whom disease progresses after > 500 mg total dose of standard amphotericin B.

Antifungal Azoles

These drugs are not nephrotoxic and can be administered orally. They have simplified treatment of chronic mycoses in outpatient settings. The first such oral drug, ketoconazole, has largely been supplanted by more effective, less toxic triazole derivatives, such as fluconazole and itraconazole. Drug interactions are a significant problem with the azoles.

Echinocandins: Echinocandins are water-soluble lipopeptides that inhibit glucan synthase. Their mechanism of action is unique within the antifungal class of drugs, making them attractive from the standpoint of cross-resistance. Although there are several echinocandins in development, caspofungin is the only commercially available agent at this time. Caspofungin is used for salvage therapy for serious *Aspergillus* infections and as 1st-line therapy for serious candidal infections, including candidal esophagitis, candidal peritonitis, and candidemia. Caspofungin has a broad spectrum of activity against the species of *Candida* encountered most frequently in clinical settings. Therefore, it is used frequently in patients with candidal infections until the precise species of the organism is determined. The agent has minimal toxicities, and drug-drug interactions are relatively few. It is necessary to reduce doses of tacrolimus when it is used in combination with caspofungin.

Fluconazole: This drug is water-soluble and is absorbed almost completely after an oral dose. It is excreted largely unchanged in urine and has a half-life > 24 h, allowing single daily doses. It has high penetration into CSF (≥ 70% of serum levels) and has been especially useful for cryptococcal and coccidioidal meningitis. It also provides an effective, less toxic alternative to amphotericin B for candidemia in non-neutropenic patients. Doses range from 200- to 400-mg daily doses, to as high as 800 mg/day in some seriously ill patients; daily doses of ≥ 1000 mg have been given in limited trials with acceptable toxicity.

Candida krusei is typically fluconazole-resistant, and *Candida* (*Torulopsis) glabrata* is generally less sensitive than *C. albicans*. Other fluconazole-resistant *Candida* sp have been increasing recently due to widespread use, often for mucocutaneous candidiasis, which has other effective therapy (see p. 988). So far, most resistant *Candida* appear sensitive to itraconazole. Of special concern are recent reports of fluconazole-resistant *Candida* in patients without AIDS who were never previously treated with azoles.

GI discomfort and skin rash are the most common adverse effects. More severe toxicity is unusual, but fluconazole use has been associated with hepatic necrosis, Stevens-Johnson syndrome, anaphylaxis, alopecia, and congenital anomalies when used beyond the 1st trimester of pregnancy. Interactions with other drugs occur less often with fluconazole than with ketoconazole or itraconazole. However, fluconazole sometimes causes elevated serum levels of cyclosporine, rifabutin, phenytoin, tacrolimus, warfarin-type oral anticoagulants, sulfonylurea drugs such as tolbutamide, or zidovudine. Rifampin may lower fluconazole blood levels.

Itraconazole: This drug has become the standard treatment for lymphocutaneous sporotrichosis as well as mild or moderately severe histoplasmosis, blastomycosis, or paracoccidioidomycosis. It is also effective in mild cases of invasive aspergillosis, some cases of coccidioidomycosis, and certain types of chromomycosis. Itraconazole has been used successfully to clear some types of fungal meningitis, although it is not the drug of choice. Because of its high lipid solubility and protein binding, itraconazole blood levels tend to be low, but tissue levels are generally high. Drug levels are negligible in urine or CSF.

Acidic drinks (eg, cola, acidic fruit juices) or food may improve absorption. However, absorption may be lowered if itraconazole is taken with prescription or OTC drugs used to lower gastric acidity. Several drugs may decrease serum itraconazole concentrations, including rifampin, rifabutin, didanosine, phenytoin, and carbamazepine. Itraconazole also inhibits metabolic degradation of other drugs, causing blood level elevations with potentially serious consequences. Serious, even fatal, cardiac arrhythmias may occur if itraconazole is used with cisapride (not available in the US) or some antihistamines, such as terfenadine, astemizole, and perhaps loratadine. Rhabdomyolysis has been associated with itraconazole-induced elevations in blood levels of cyclosporine or statins. Blood level elevations of digoxin, tacrolimus, oral anticoagulants, or sulfonylureas also may occur when these drugs are used with itraconazole.

In doses of up to 400 mg/day, the main adverse effects are GI, but a few men have reported erectile dysfunction, and higher doses may cause hypokalemia, hypertension, and edema. Other reported adverse effects include allergic rash, hepatitis, and hallucinations.

Voriconazole: Voriconazole is a 2nd-generation azole. Voriconazole can be used for 1st-line therapy for serious *Aspergillus* infections and is now considered by most clinical mycologists to be the treatment of choice for *Aspergillus* infections in both immunocompetent and immunocompromised hosts. Voriconazole can also be used for salvage therapy of *Scedosporium apiospermum* and *Fusarium* infections. Additionally, the drug is effective in candidal esophagitis and is used as salvage therapy for candidal infections and has activity against a broader spectrum of species of *Candida* than does fluconazole. Patients taking voriconazole must be monitored for liver toxicity, visual disturbances, and dermatologic reactions. Additionally, there are numerous drug-drug interactions; the interaction of voriconazole and certain immunosuppressants used after organ transplantation is particularly important.

Flucytosine

Flucytosine, a nucleic acid analog, is water-soluble and well absorbed after oral administration. Preexisting or emerging resistance is common, so it is almost always used with another antifungal, usually amphotericin B. Flucytosine combined with amphotericin B is primarily used to treat cryptococcosis but has also proven valuable for some cases of disseminated candidiasis, other yeast infections, and severe invasive aspergillosis. Use in combination with antifungal azoles may be beneficial in cryptococcosis and some other mycoses.

The usual dose (12.5 to 37.5 mg/kg po qid) leads to high drug levels in serum, urine, and CSF. Major adverse effects are bone marrow suppression (thrombocytopenia and leukopenia), hepatotoxicity, and enterocolitis; only myelosuppression is proportional to serum levels. Because flucytosine is primarily cleared by the kidneys, blood levels rise if nephrotoxicity develops during concomitant use with amphotericin B, particularly when the latter is used in doses > 0.4 mg/kg/day. Flucytosine serum concentrations should be monitored and the dosage adjusted to keep levels between 40 and 90 μg/mL. CBC and renal and liver function tests should be obtained twice/wk. If blood levels are unavailable, therapy is begun at 25 mg/kg qid and decreased if renal function declines.

ASPERGILLOSIS

Aspergillosis is an opportunistic infection caused by inhaled spores of the mold

Aspergillus, which invade blood vessels, causing hemorrhagic necrosis and infarction. Symptoms may be those of asthma, pneumonia, sinusitis, or rapidly progressing systemic illness. Diagnosis is primarily clinical but may be aided by imaging studies, histopathology, and specimen staining and culture. Treatment is with voriconazole, amphotericin B (or its lipid formulations), caspofungin, itraconazole, or flucytosine. Fungus balls may require surgical resection. Recurrence is common.

Aspergillus sp are among the most common environmental molds, frequently present in decaying vegetation (compost heaps), on insulating materials, in air conditioning or heating vents, in operating pavilions and patient rooms, on hospital implements, and in airborne dust. Invasive infections are usually acquired by inhalation of spores or, occasionally, by direct invasion through damaged skin. Major risk factors include neutropenia, long-term high-dose corticosteroid therapy, organ transplantation (especially bone marrow transplantation), hereditary disorders of neutrophil function, such as chronic granulomatous disease, and, occasionally, AIDS. Allergic bronchopulmonary aspergillosis results in lung inflammation unrelated to fungal invasion of tissues (see p. 398).

Aspergillus tends to infect open spaces, such as pulmonary cavities from previous lung disease (eg, bronchiectasis, tumor, TB), the sinuses, or ear canals (otomycosis). Such infections tend to be locally invasive and destructive, although systemic spread sometimes occurs, particularly in immunocompromised patients. *A. fumigatus* is the most common cause of invasive pulmonary disease; *A. flavus* most often causes invasive extrapulmonary disease.

Focal infections sometimes form a fungus ball (aspergilloma), a characteristic growth of tangled masses of hyphae, with fibrin exudate and few inflammatory cells, typically encapsulated by fibrous tissue.

A chronic form of invasive aspergillosis occasionally occurs, notably in patients with the hereditary phagocytic cell defect, chronic granulomatous disease. *Aspergillus* sp can also cause endophthalmitis after trauma or surgery to the eye (or by hematogenous seeding) and infections of intravascular and intracardiac prostheses.

Primary superficial aspergillosis is uncommon but may occur in burns; beneath occlusive dressings; after corneal trauma (keratitis); or in the sinuses, mouth, nose, or ear canal.

Symptoms and Signs

Chronic pulmonary aspergillosis causes cough, often with hemoptysis and shortness of breath. Invasive pulmonary aspergillosis usually causes rapidly progressive, ultimately fatal respiratory failure if untreated.

Extrapulmonary invasive aspergillosis begins with skin lesions, sinusitis, or pneumonia; may involve the liver, kidneys, brain, and other tissues; and is often rapidly fatal.

Aspergillosis in the sinuses can form an aspergilloma, an allergic fungal sinusitis, or a chronic, slowly invasive granulomatous inflammation with fever, rhinitis, and headache. Necrosing cutaneous lesions may overlie the nose or sinuses, palatal or gingival ulcerations may be present, signs of cavernous sinus thrombosis may develop, and pulmonary or disseminated lesions may occur.

Diagnosis

Because *Aspergillus* sp are common in the environment, positive sputum cultures may be due to environmental contamination or to noninvasive colonization in patients with chronic lung disease; positive cultures are significant mainly when obtained from patients with increased susceptibility due to immunosuppression or with high suspicion due to typical imaging findings. Conversely, sputum cultures from patients with aspergillomas or invasive pulmonary aspergillosis are often negative; cavities are often walled off from airways, and invasive disease progresses mainly by vascular invasion and tissue infarction.

Chest x-ray is obtained, and CT of sinuses is done if sinus infection is suspected. A movable fungus ball within a cavitary lesion is characteristic on both, although most lesions are focal and solid. Sometimes imaging detects a halo sign, a thin air shadow surrounding a nodule representing cavitation within a necrotic lesion. Diffuse, generalized pulmonary infiltrates occur in some patients.

Tissue sample for culture and histopathology is usually necessary for confirmation, typically obtained from the lungs via bronchoscopy and the sinuses by anterior rhinoscopy. Because cultures require significant time and false-negative histopathology may occur, most decisions to treat are based on strong presumptive clinical evidence. Large vegetations often release sizable emboli that may occlude blood vessels and provide specimens for diagnosis.

Various serologic assays exist but are of limited value for rapid diagnosis of acute, life-threatening invasive aspergillosis. Detection of antigens such as galactomannans can be specific but is not sufficiently sensitive to identify most cases in their early stages. Blood cultures are almost always negative, even with rare cases of endocarditis.

Treatment

Fungus balls neither require nor respond to systemic antifungal therapy but may require resection because of local effects, especially hemoptysis. Invasive infections generally require aggressive treatment with IV amphotericin B or voriconazole (which most now consider the 1st choice). Oral itraconazole (but *not* fluconazole) can be effective in some cases. Caspofungin may be used as salvage therapy. Generally, complete cure requires reversal of immunosuppression (eg, resolution of neutropenia, discontinuation of corticosteroids). Recrudescence is common if neutropenia reoccurs. The role of combinations of antifungals as either primary or salvage therapy needs more evaluation.

BLASTOMYCOSIS

(Gilchrist's Disease; North American Blastomycosis)

Blastomycosis is a pulmonary and occasionally hematogenous disease caused by inhaling spores of the mold *Blastomyces dermatitidis*. Symptoms are from either pneumonia or dissemination to multiple organs, most commonly the skin. Diagnosis is clinical and/or with chest x-ray and confirmed by laboratory identification of the organism. Treatment is with itraconazole, fluconazole, or amphotericin B.

In North America, the endemic area for blastomycosis includes the Ohio–Mississippi River valleys, extending into the middle Atlantic and Southeastern states, the northern Midwest, upstate New York, and southern Canada. Infection also occurs in the Middle East and Africa. The incidence and severity of blastomycosis may be increased in immunocompromised patients, but it is a less common opportunistic infection than histoplasmosis or coccidioidomycosis.

Blastomyces dermatitidis grows as a mold at room temperature in soil enriched with animal excreta and in moist, decaying, acidic organic material. Inhaled spores convert in the lungs into large invasive yeasts, which form broad-based buds. Infection may remain localized to the lungs or disseminate hematogenously to cause focal infection in numerous organs, including skin, prostate, epididymis, testes, kidneys, vertebrae, ends of long bones, subcutaneous tissues, brain, oral or nasal mucosa, thyroid, lymph nodes, bone marrow, and other tissues.

Symptoms and Signs

Pulmonary blastomycosis may be an acute, self-limited disease that often goes unrecognized. Or, it can present with insidious onset that progresses to a chronic, progressive infection. Symptoms include a productive or dry hacking cough, chest pain, dyspnea, fever, chills, and drenching sweats. Pleural effusion occurs occasionally. Some patients have rapidly progressive infections, and acute respiratory distress syndrome may develop.

In extrapulmonary disseminated blastomycosis, symptoms depend on the organ involved. Skin lesions are by far the most common, may be single or multiple, and may occur with or without clinically apparent pulmonary involvement. Papules or papulopustules usually appear on exposed surfaces and spread slowly. Painless miliary abscesses, varying from pinpoint to 1 mm in diameter, develop on the advancing borders. Irregular, wartlike papillae may form on surfaces. As lesions enlarge, the centers heal, forming atrophic scars. A fully developed individual lesion appears as an elevated verrucous patch, usually ≥ 2 cm wide with an abruptly sloping, purplish red, abscess-studded border. Ulceration may occur if bacterial superinfection is present. Sometimes areas overlying bone lesions are swollen, warm, and tender. Genital lesions present as painful epididymal swelling, deep perineal discomfort, or prostatic tenderness on rectal examination.

Diagnosis

Patients should have chest x-ray. Focal or diffuse infiltrates may be present, sometimes as a patchy bronchopneumonia fanning out from the hilum. These findings must be distinguished from other mycoses, TB, and tumors. Skin lesions can be mistaken for sporotrichosis, TB, iodism, or basal cell carcinoma. Genital involvement may mimic TB.

Cultures of infected material are obtained; they are definitive when positive. The organism's characteristic appearance on microscopic examination is also frequently diagnostic. Serology is not sensitive but is useful if positive.

Treatment

Untreated blastomycosis is usually slowly progressive and ultimately fatal. Itraconazole 200 to 400 mg po once/day is used for mild to moderate disease. Fluconazole appears less effective, but 400 to 800 mg po once/day may be tried in itraconazole-intolerant patients with mild disease. IV amphotericin B is used for severe, life-threatening infections and is usually effective.

CANDIDIASIS (INVASIVE)

(Candidosis; Moniliasis)

(See also pp. 987 and 2086.)

Candidiasis is infection by *Candida* sp, most often *C. albicans,* manifested by mucocutaneous lesions, fungemia, and sometimes focal infection of multiple sites. Symptoms depend on the site of infection and include dysphagia; skin and mucosal lesions; blindness; vaginal itching, burning, and discharge; fever; shock; oliguria; renal shutdown; and disseminated intravascular coagulation. Diagnosis is confirmed by histopathology and cultures from normally sterile sites. Treatment, when necessary, is with amphotericin B, fluconazole, caspofungin, voriconazole, or flucytosine.

Etiology and Epidemiology

Candida sp are commensal organisms that inhabit the GI tract and sometimes the skin (see p. 987). Unlike other systemic mycoses, candidiasis results from endogenous organisms. Most infections are caused by *C. albicans* or *C. tropicalis*; however, *C. glabrata* (formerly *Torulopsis glabrata*) is increasingly involved in fungemia, UTIs, and, occasionally, pneumonia or other focal disease.

Candida sp account for about 80% of major systemic fungal infections. *Candida* is the most common cause of fungal infections in immunocompromised patients and one of the most common hospital-acquired infections.

Candidiasis involving the mouth and esophagus is a defining opportunistic infection in AIDS. Although mucocutaneous candidiasis is frequently present in HIV-infected patients, hematogenous dissemination is unusual until immunosuppression becomes profound. Neutropenic patients (eg, those receiving cancer chemotherapy) are at high risk for developing life-threatening disseminated candidiasis.

Candidemia may occur in non-neutropenic patients who have prolonged hospitalizations. This bloodstream infection is often related to multiple trauma or surgical procedures, multiple courses of broad-spectrum antibacterial therapy, and/or IV hyperalimentation. IV lines and the GI tract are the usual portals of entry. Candidemia often prolongs hospitalization and increases mortality from concurrent diseases. Prolonged or untreated candidemia may lead to endocarditis or meningitis as well as to focal involvement of skin, subcutaneous tissues, bones, joints, liver, spleen, kidneys, eyes, and other tissues. Endocarditis is commonly related to IV drug abuse, valve replacement, or intravascular trauma induced by indwelling intravenous catheters.

All forms of disseminated candidiasis should be considered serious, progressive, and potentially fatal.

Symptoms, Signs, and Diagnosis

Esophagitis is most often manifested by dysphagia. Symptoms of respiratory tract infections are nonspecific, such as cough. Candidemia usually causes fever, but no symptoms are specific. Sometimes, a syndrome develops resembling bacterial sepsis, with a fulminating course that may include shock, oliguria, renal shutdown, and disseminated intravascular coagulation. Candidal endophthalmitis starts as white retinal lesions that are initially asymptomatic but can progress, opacifying the vitreous and causing potentially irreversible scarring and blindness. In neutropenic patients, eye involvement is occasionally accompanied by retinal hemorrhages. Papulonodular skin lesions may also develop, especially in neutropenic patients, in whom they indicate a high prevalence of widespread hematogenous dissemination to other organs. Symptoms of other focal infection depend on the organ involved.

Because *Candida* sp are commensals, their culture from sputum, the mouth, the vagina, urine, stool, or skin does not necessarily signify an invasive, progressive infection. A characteristic clinical lesion must also be present, histopathologic evidence of tissue invasion (eg, yeasts, pseudohyphae, and/or hyphae in tissue specimens) must be documented, and other etiologies excluded. Positive cultures of blood, CSF, pericardium or pericardial fluid, or tissue biopsy specimens provide definitive evidence that systemic therapy is needed. Serologic assays do not have sufficient specificity or sensitivity to be useful.

Treatment

Predisposing conditions such as neutropenia, immunosuppression, the use of broad-spectrum antibacterial antibiotics, hyperalimentation, and indwelling lines should be reversed or controlled if possible. IV amphotericin B is recommended for most severely ill patients, especially those who are immunosuppressed. Caspofungin is an alternative to amphotericin B in adults with or without neutropenia. Fluconazole, 400 to 800 mg po once/day, is also considered a 1st-line drug (unless *C. krusei* or *C. glabrata* is involved) for non-neutropenic patients and may be effective in patients with neutropenia at the same dose.

Esophageal candidiasis is treated with fluconazole, 100 to 200 mg po or IV once/day, or itraconazole, 200 mg po once/day. Patients in whom this fails (or with severe infection) may receive voriconazole, 4 mg/kg po or IV bid, or caspofungin. Voriconazole is also effective for bloodstream and other hematogenously disseminated infections.

COCCIDIOIDOMYCOSIS

(San Joaquin Fever; Valley Fever)

Coccidioidomycosis is a pulmonary or hematogenous disease caused by the fungus *Coccidioides immitis*, usually occurring as an acute benign asymptomatic or self-limited respiratory infection. The organism occasionally disseminates to cause focal lesions in other tissues. Symptoms, if present, are those of lower respiratory infection or low-grade nonspecific disseminated disease. Diagnosis is suspected by clinical and epidemiologic characteristics and confirmed by chest x-ray, culture, and serology. Treatment, if needed, is usually with fluconazole, itraconazole, or amphotericin B.

Coccidioidomycosis is endemic in the southwestern US, including Arizona, the central valley of California, parts of New Mexico, and Texas west of El Paso. The area extends into northern Mexico, and foci occur in parts of Central America and Argentina. Infections are acquired by inhalation of spore-laden dust. Because of travel and delayed onset of clinical manifestations, infections sometimes become evident outside endemic areas.

Once inhaled, *C. immitis* spores convert to large tissue-invasive spherules. As spherules enlarge and then rupture, each releases multiple small endospores that may form new spherules. Pulmonary pathology is characterized by an acute, subacute, or chronic granulomatous reaction with varying degrees of fibrosis. Lesions may cavitate or form coin lesions.

Sometimes, progressive disease occurs, with widespread lung involvement and/or dissemination to cause focal lesions in almost any other tissue, most commonly in skin and subcutaneous tissues, bones, and meninges. Progressive disease is more common in men and is more likely to occur with HIV infection, immunosuppressive therapy, and advanced age and in the 2nd half of pregnancy or postpartum, and in certain ethnic backgrounds (Filipino, African American, Native American, Hispanic, and Asian, in decreasing order of relative risk).

Symptoms and Signs

Primary coccidioidomycosis: Most patients are asymptomatic, but nonspecific respiratory symptoms resembling influenza or acute bronchitis or, less often, acute pneumonia or pleural effusion, sometimes occur. Symptoms, in decreasing order of frequency, include fever, cough, chest pain, chills, sputum production, sore throat, and hemoptysis. Physical signs may be absent or limited to scattered rales with or without areas of dullness to percussion over lung fields. Some patients develop hypersensitivity to the localized respiratory infection, manifested by arthritis, conjunctivitis, erythema nodosum, or erythema multiforme.

Primary pulmonary lesions sometimes leave nodular coin lesions that must be distinguished from tumors and TB or other granulomatous infections. Sometimes, residual cavitary lesions develop that may vary in size over time and often appear thin-walled. A small percentage of these cavities fails to close spontaneously. Hemoptysis or the threat of rupture into the pleural space may occasionally necessitate surgery.

Progressive coccidioidomycosis: Nonspecific symptoms develop a few weeks, months, or occasionally years after primary infection, including low-grade fever, anorexia, weight loss, and weakness. Extensive pulmonary involvement may cause progressive cyanosis, dyspnea, and mucopurulent or bloody sputum. Symptoms of extrapulmonary lesions depend on the site. Draining sinus tracts sometimes connect deeper lesions to the skin. Localized extrapulmonary lesions often become chronic and recur frequently, sometimes long after completion of seemingly successful antifungal therapy.

Diagnosis

Eosinophilia may be an important clue in patients in endemic areas. Diagnosis can be established by fungal culture or by visualizing *C. immitis* spherules in sputum, pleural fluid, CSF, exudate from draining lesions, or biopsy specimens. Intact spherules are usually 20 to 80 μm in diameter, thick-walled, and filled with small (2 to 4 μm) endospores. Endospores released into tissues from ruptured spherules may be mistaken for nonbudding yeasts.

Complement fixation for IgG anticoccidioidal antibodies remains the most useful test. Titers ≥ 1:4 in serum are consistent with current or recent infection, and higher titers (≥ 1:32) signify an increased likelihood of extrapulmonary dissemination. However, immunocompromised patients may have low titers. Titers should decline during successful therapy. The presence of complement-fixing antibodies in CSF is diagnostic of coccidioidal meningitis and is important because CSF cultures are rarely positive.

Delayed cutaneous hypersensitivity to coccidioidin or spherulin usually develops within 10 to 21 days after acute infections in immunocompetent patients but is characteristically absent in progressive disease. Because this test is positive in most people in endemic areas, it is of primary value for epidemiologic studies rather than for diagnosis.

Treatment

Untreated disseminated coccidioidomycosis is usually fatal, uniformly if meningitis is present. Mortality in HIV-infected patients exceeds 70% within 1 mo of diagnosis; it is unclear whether treatment can alter mortality.

Treatment for primary coccidioidomycosis is controversial in low-risk patients. Some experts give fluconazole, since its toxicity is low and there is a small chance of hematogenous seeding, especially to bone or brain. Others feel that the immune response may be blunted by the use of fluconazole and that risks of hematogenous seeding are very low in primary infection. High complement fixation titers indicate spread and the need for treatment.

Mild to moderate nonmeningeal extrapulmonary involvement should be treated with fluconazole ≥ 400 mg po once/day or itraconazole, 200 mg po or IV bid. For severe illness, amphotericin B 0.5 to 1.0 mg/kg IV over 2 to 6 h once/day is given for 4 to 12 wk until total dose reaches 1 to 3 g, depending on the degree of infection. Patients with AIDS-associated coccidioidomycosis require maintenance therapy to prevent relapse; fluconazole 200 mg po once/day or itraconazole 200 mg bid usually is sufficient, and weekly IV amphotericin B may suffice for azole-intolerant patients. Lipid formulations of amphotericin B are used in patients refractory to or intolerant of standard amphotericin B.

For meningitis, fluconazole is used. The optimal dose is unclear; doses of 800 to 1200 mg/day may be more effective than 400 mg/day. If amphotericin B is used, intrathecal injections are needed, either intraventricularly via a subcutaneous reservoir or intracisternally. Treatment for meningeal coccidioidomycosis must be continued for many months, probably lifelong. Surgical removal of involved bone may be necessary to cure osteomyelitis.

CRYPTOCOCCOSIS

(European Blastomycosis; Torulosis)

Cryptococcosis is a pulmonary or disseminated infection acquired by inhalation of soil contaminated with the encapsulated yeast *Cryptococcus neoformans*. Symptoms are those of pneumonia, meningitis, or involvement of skin, bones, or viscera. Diagnosis is clinical and microscopic, confirmed by culture. Treatment is with azoles, amphotericin B, or flucytosine.

Distribution is worldwide. Cryptococcosis is a defining opportunistic infection for AIDS, although patients with Hodgkin lymphoma, other lymphomas, or sarcoidosis and those receiving long-term corticosteroid therapy are also at increased risk. Infections in immunocompetent patients have a self-limited, subacute, or chronic course. Progressive dissemination very rarely occurs in those who are not obviously immunosuppressed, more frequently men > 40 yr.

Symptoms and Signs

Cryptococcosis typically affects the meninges or the lungs. Meningeal inflammation typically presents with microscopic multifocal intracerebral lesions. Meningeal granulomas and larger focal brain lesions may be evident. Inflammation is not extensive; fever is usually low-grade and may be absent. Cryptococcal meningitis in patients with AIDS may produce minimal or no symptoms and normal CSF parameters except for the presence of many yeasts. Most symptoms of cryptococcal meningitis are attributable to cerebral edema and are usually nonspecific, including headache, blurred vision, confusion, depression, agitation, or other behavioral changes. Except for ocular or facial palsies, focal signs are rare until relatively late in the course. Blindness may develop due to cerebral edema or direct involvement of the optic tracts.

Pulmonary cryptococcosis often presents with asymptomatic and self-limited primary lung lesions. In immunocompetent people, these isolated pulmonary lesions sometimes heal spontaneously without disseminating, even without antifungal therapy. Pneumonia usually causes cough and other nonspecific respiratory symptoms. AIDS-associated cryptococcal pulmonary infection, however, may present with severe, progressive pneumonia with acute dyspnea and an x-ray pattern suggestive of *Pneumocystis* infection.

Disseminated involvement may occur in any infected person. Dermatologic spread is most common, presenting as pustular, papular, nodular, or ulcerated lesions, sometimes resembling acne, molluscum contagiosum, or basal cell carcinoma. Focal sites of dissemination may also occur in subcutaneous nodules, the ends of long bones, joints, liver, spleen, kidneys, prostate, and other tissues. These lesions usually cause few or no symptoms. Involved tissues typically contain cystic masses of yeasts that appear gelatinous because of accumulated cryptococcal capsular polysaccharide but have minimal or no acute inflammatory changes, especially in the brain. Rarely, pyelonephritis occurs with renal papillary necrosis.

Diagnosis

Culture is definitive. CSF, sputum, and urine yield organisms most often, and blood cultures may be positive in heavy infections, particularly in those with AIDS. In disseminated cryptococcosis with meningitis, *C. neoformans* is frequently cultured from urine, and prostatic foci of infection sometimes persist despite successful clearance of organisms from the CNS. Diagnosis is strongly suggested by identification by experienced observers of encapsulated budding yeasts in smears of body fluids, secretions, exudates, or other specimens. In fixed tissue specimens, encapsulated yeasts may also be identified and confirmed as *C. neoformans* by positive mucicarmine or Masson-Fontana staining.

Elevated CSF protein and a mononuclear cell pleocytosis are usual in cryptococcal meningitis, although neutrophilia occasionally predominates. Glucose is frequently low, and encapsulated yeasts forming narrow-based buds can be seen on India ink smears in most cases. The latex test for cryptococcal capsular antigen is positive in CSF and/or blood specimens from > 90% of patients with meningitis and is generally specific, although false-positive results may occur, usually with titers ≤ 1:8, especially in the presence of rheumatoid factor.

Treatment

Patients without AIDS: Patients may need no treatment for localized pulmonary involvement, confirmed by normal CSF parameters, negative CSF and urine cultures, and no suggestion of cutaneous, bone, or other extrapulmonary lesions; some experts give a course of fluconazole to avoid hematogenous dissemination, since its toxicity is so low.

In the absence of meningitis, localized lesions in skin, bone, or other sites require systemic antifungal therapy, typically fluconazole 400 mg po once/day for 3 to 6 mo. For more severe disease, amphotericin B 0.5 to 1.0 mg/kg once/day is used for 6 to 10 wk.

For meningitis, the standard regimen is amphotericin B 0.7 to 1.0 mg/kg IV once/day plus flucytosine 25 mg/kg po q 6 h for 6 to 10 wk; alternatively, this regimen can be used for 2 wk followed by fluconazole 400 mg po once/day for 10 wk. Following these regimens, fluconazole is given at 200 mg once/day for 10 mo. There is not universal agreement regarding the need for the addition of flucytosine.

Antigen titers should steadily decline during successful therapy. In general, cultures should become and remain negative for at least 2 wk before treatment is ended.

Patients with AIDS: All patients require treatment. In isolated pulmonary or urinary tract disease, fluconazole 400 mg po once/day is given. For more severe disease, fluconazole 400 mg po once/day plus flucytosine 25 to 37.5 mg/kg qid is used for 10 wk. For meningitis, the standard regimen is amphotericin B 0.7 to 1.0 mg/kg IV once/day plus flucytosine 25 mg po q 6 h for 6 to 10 wk; alternatively, this regimen can be used for 2 wk followed by fluconazole 400 mg po once/day for 10 wk total.

Nearly all AIDS patients need maintenance therapy for life. Fluconazole 200 mg po once/day is preferred, but itraconazole at the same dose is acceptable. Weekly doses of IV amphotericin B also can be used.

HISTOPLASMOSIS

Histoplasmosis is a pulmonary and hematogenous disease caused by *Histoplasma capsulatum*, often chronic and usually following an asymptomatic primary infection. Symptoms are either those of pneumonia or nonspecific chronic illness. Diagnosis is by chest x-ray and/or identification of the organism in sputum or tissue. Treatment is with amphotericin B or itraconazole.

Histoplasmosis occurs worldwide. The endemic areas in the US are in the Ohio–Mississippi River valleys extending into parts of northern Maryland, southern Pennsylvania, central New York, and Texas, but microfoci have been noted in other states, such as Florida. *H. capsulatum* grows as a mold in nature or when cultured at room temperature but converts to a small (1 to 5 μm in diameter) yeast cell at 37° C and when invading host cells. Infection follows inhalation of mold spores in soil or dust contaminated with bird or bat droppings. Severe disease is more common after heavy, prolonged exposure and in men, infants, or those with compromised T-cell–mediated immunity.

Initial infection is in the lungs and usually remains there but may spread hematogenously to other organs if it is not controlled by normal cell-mediated host defenses. Progressive disseminated histoplasmosis is one of the defining opportunistic infections for AIDS.

Symptoms and Signs

Most histoplasmosis infections are asymptomatic or so mild that the patient does not seek medical attention. The disease has 3 main forms.

Acute primary histoplasmosis is a syndrome with fever, cough, myalgias, chest pain, and malaise of varying severity. Acute pneumonia sometimes is evident on physical examination and chest x-ray.

Progressive disseminated histoplasmosis characteristically includes generalized involvement of the reticuloendothelial system, with hepatosplenomegaly, lymphadenopathy, bone marrow involvement, and sometimes oral or GI ulcerations. The course is usually subacute or chronic, with only nonspecific often subtle symptoms, such as fever, fatigue, weight loss, weakness, and malaise; HIV-positive patients may experience unexplained worsening in condition. CNS involvement may develop, presenting as meningitis or focal brain lesions. Adrenal infection is rare but may result in Addison's disease. Patients with AIDS may develop severe acute pneumonia with hypoxia suggestive of *Pneumocystis jiroveci* (formerly *P. carinii*) infection as well as hypotension, mental status changes, coagulopathy, or rhabdomyolysis.

Chronic cavitary histoplasmosis is characterized by pulmonary lesions that are often apical and resemble cavitary TB. Manifestations are worsening cough and dyspnea, progressing eventually to disabling respiratory dysfunction. Dissemination does not occur.

Fibrosing mediastinitis is a chronic but rare form of histoplasmosis, ultimately causing circulatory compromise. Patients with histoplasmosis may lose vision, but organisms are not present in lesions, antifungal chemotherapy is not helpful, and the link to *H. capsulatum* infection is unclear.

Diagnosis

The index of suspicion must be high because symptoms are nonspecific. Microscopic histopathology can strongly suggest the diagnosis, particularly in patients with AIDS with extensive infections in whom intracellular yeasts may be seen in Wright's- or Giemsa-stained peripheral blood or buffy coat specimens. Fungal culture confirms the diagnosis. Lysis-centrifugation or culture of buffy coat improves the yield from blood specimens. A test for *H. capsulatum* antigen is sensitive and specific, particularly when simultaneous serum and urine specimens are tested; however, cross-reactivity with other fungi has been noted (*Coccidioides immitis, Blastomyces dermatitidis, Paracoccidioides brasiliensis, Penicillium marneffei*).

Prognosis and Treatment

The acute primary form is almost always self-limited, although very rare deaths after massive infections have been reported. Chronic cavitary histoplasmosis can cause death from severe respiratory insufficiency. Untreated progressive disseminated histoplasmosis has a mortality rate > 90%.

Acute primary histoplasmosis requires no antifungal therapy unless there is no spontaneous improvement after 1 mo; itraconazole 200 mg po once/day for 6 to 12 wk is then used. Rare cases of severe pneumonia require more aggressive therapy with amphotericin B.

In the chronic form, itraconazole 200 mg po once/day or bid is given for 12 to 24 mo. Amphotericin B is used if the patient is seriously ill or does not respond to or tolerate itraconazole.

For severe disseminated histoplasmosis, amphotericin B 0.5 to 1.0 mg/kg IV once/day for 4 to 12 wk is the treatment of choice. Patients without AIDS can be switched to itraconazole 200 mg po once/day after they become afebrile and require no ventilatory or BP support. For mild disseminated disease, itraconazole 200 mg po once/day or bid for 9 mo can be used. In patients with AIDS, indefinite chronic therapy with itraconazole is used to prevent relapse. Fluconazole appears to be less effective. Intermittent doses of IV amphotericin B can be used for chronic suppression in azole-intolerant patients with AIDS.

MUCORMYCOSIS

(Phycomycosis; Zygomycosis)

Mucormycosis is infection by diverse fungal species, including *Rhizopus, Rhizomucor, Absidia*, and *Basidiobolus*. Symptoms most frequently result from invasive necrotic lesions in the nose and palate with pain, fever, orbital cellulitis, proptosis, and purulent nasal discharge. CNS symptoms may follow. Pulmonary symptoms are severe and include productive cough, high fever, and toxicity. Diagnosis is primarily clinical, requires a high index of suspicion, and may be confirmed by histopathology. Treatment is with IV amphotericin B.

Infection is most common in immunocompromised people, in patients with poorly controlled diabetes, and in patients receiving the iron-chelating drug deferoxamine.

Rhinocerebral mucormycosis is the most common form, but primary cutaneous, pulmonary, or GI lesions sometimes develop, and hematogenous dissemination to other sites can occur.

Symptoms, Signs, and Diagnosis

Rhinocerebral infections are usually severe and frequently fatal. Necrotic lesions appear on the nasal mucosa or sometimes the palate. Vascular invasion by hyphae leads to progressive tissue necrosis that may involve the nasal septum, palate, and bones surrounding the orbit or sinuses. Manifestations may include pain, fever, orbital cellulitis, proptosis, purulent nasal discharge, and mucosal necrosis. Progressive extension of necrosis to involve the brain can cause signs of cavernous sinus thrombosis, seizures, aphasia, or hemiplegia. Pulmonary infections resemble invasive aspergillosis. Cutaneous *Rhizopus* infections have developed under occlusive dressings.

Diagnosis requires a high index of suspicion and painstaking examination of tissue samples for large nonseptate hyphae with irregular diameters and branching patterns, because much of the necrotic debris contains no organisms. For unclear reasons, cultures usually are negative, even when hyphae are clearly visible in tissues. CT scans and x-rays often underestimate or miss significant bone destruction.

Treatment

Effective therapy requires that diabetes be controlled or, if at all possible, immunosuppression reversed or deferoxamine stopped. IV amphotericin B must be used because azoles are ineffective. Surgical debridement of necrotic tissue is usually needed. Most experts use high doses of lipid formulations of amphotericin B (up to 10 mg/kg/day). An experimental azole antifungal, posaconazole, has shown promising results for pulmonary mucormycosis in immunocompromised hosts, in conjunction with appropriate surgery.

MYCETOMA

(Maduromycosis; Madura Foot)

Mycetoma is a chronic, progressive, local infection caused by fungi or bacteria, involving the feet, upper extremities, or back. Symptoms include tumefaction and formation of sinus tracts. Diagnosis is clinical, confirmed by microscopy and culture. Treatment includes antimicrobials and surgical debridement.

Bacteria, primarily *Nocardia* sp and other actinomycetes, cause > ½ the cases. The remainder are caused by about 20 different fungal species. When caused by fungi, the lesions are sometimes called eumycetoma. Mycetoma occurs mainly in tropical or subtropical areas, including the southern US, and is acquired by entry of organisms through sites of local trauma on bare skin of the feet as well as on the extremities or backs of workers carrying contaminated vegetation or other objects. Men aged 20 to 40 are most often affected, presumably because of trauma incurred while working outdoors. Infections spread through contiguous subcutaneous areas, resulting in tumefaction and formation of multiple draining sinuses that exude characteristic "grains" of clumped organisms. Microscopic tissue reactions may be primarily suppurative or granulomatous depending on the specific causative agent.

Symptoms, Signs, and Diagnosis

The initial lesion may be a papule, a fixed subcutaneous nodule, a vesicle with an indurated base, or a subcutaneous abscess that ruptures to form a fistula to the skin surface. Fibrosis is common in and around early lesions. There is little or no tenderness in the absence of acute suppurative bacterial superinfection. Infection progresses slowly over the course of months or years, with gradual, progressive extension to and destruction of contiguous muscles, tendons, fascia, and bones. Neither systemic dissemination nor signs and symptoms suggesting generalized infection occur. Eventually, muscle wasting, deformity, and tissue destruction prevent use of affected limbs. In advanced infections, involved extremities appear grotesquely swollen, forming a club-shaped mass of cystic areas with multiple draining and intercommunicating sinus tracts and fistulas that discharge thick or serosanguineous exudates containing characteristic grains.

Causative agents can be identified presumptively by gross and microscopic examination of grains from exudates, which are irregularly shaped, variably colored, 0.5- to 2-mm granules. Crushing and culture of these granules provides definitive identification. Specimens may yield multiple bacteria and fungi, some of which are potential causes of superinfections.

Treatment

Treatment may be required for > 10 yr. Death may occur in neglected cases due to bacterial superinfection and sepsis. Sulfonamides and certain other antibacterial drugs, sometimes in combination, are used to treat *Nocardia* (see p. 1454). Among those infections caused by fungi, certain of the potential causative organisms may respond at least partially to amphotericin B or to itraconazole or ketoconazole, but many are resistant to all antifungal drugs. Relapses occur after antifungal therapy in most cases, and many cases do not improve or worsen during treatment. Surgical debridement is necessary, and limb amputation may be needed to prevent potentially fatal severe secondary bacterial infections.

PARACOCCIDIOIDOMYCOSIS

(South American Blastomycosis)

Paracoccidioidomycosis is a progressive mycosis of skin, mucous membranes, lymph nodes, and internal organs caused by *Paracoccidioides brasiliensis*. Symptoms are skin ulcers, adenitis, and pain from abdominal organ involvement. Diagnosis is clinical and microscopic, confirmed by culture. Treatment is with itraconazole, amphotericin B, or sulfonamides.

Infections occur only in discrete foci in South and Central America, most often in men aged 20 to 50, especially coffee growers of Colombia, Venezuela, and Brazil. Although a relatively unusual opportunistic infection, paracoccidioidomycosis sometimes occurs in immunocompromised patients, including those with AIDS. Although specific natural sites for *P. brasiliensis* remain undefined, it is presumed to exist in soil as a mold, with infection due to inhalation of spores. Spores convert to invasive yeasts within the lungs and are assumed to spread to other sites via blood and lymphatics.

Symptoms, Signs, and Diagnosis

Clinically apparent infections are generally chronic and progressive but not usually fatal. Mucocutaneous infections most often involve the face, especially at the nasal and oral mucocutaneous borders. Yeasts are usually abundantly present within pinpoint lesions throughout granular bases of slowly expanding ulcers. Regional lymph nodes enlarge, become necrotic, and discharge necrotic material through the skin. Lymphatic infections mainly involve painless enlargement of cervical, supraclavicular, or axillary nodes. Visceral infections are characterized by focal lesions causing enlargement mainly of the liver, spleen, and abdominal lymph nodes, sometimes with accompanying abdominal pain. Mixed infections involve combinations of all 3 patterns.

Culture is diagnostic, although the presence in specimens of large (often > 15 μm) yeasts forming characteristic multiple buds provides strong presumptive evidence.

Treatment

Azoles are highly effective. Oral itraconazole is generally considered the drug of choice. IV amphotericin B also can eliminate the infection and is often used in very severe cases. Sulfonamides, which are widely used in some countries because they are inexpensive, can suppress growth and improve lesions but are not curative.

PIGMENTED FUNGI

(Chromoblastomycosis; Chromomycosis; Hematomycosis; Phaeohyphomycosis; Verrucous Dermatitis)

Chromomycosis and phaeohyphomycosis are infections of subcutaneous tissues, sinuses, brain, and other tissues caused by pigmented fungi. Symptoms are ulcerating nodules on exposed body parts. Diagnosis is by appearance, histopathology, and culture. Treatment is with itraconazole or flucytosine and surgical excision.

Chromomycosis is a cutaneous infection affecting normal, immunocompetent people mostly in tropical or subtropical areas, characterized by formation of papillomatous nodules that tend to ulcerate. Pigmented fungi have been increasingly recognized as opportunists affecting immunosuppressed patients. The causative agents of these infections are many kinds of dark, melanin-pigmented dematiaceous fungi including species of *Bipolaris, Cladophialophora, Cladosporium, Drechslera, Exophiala, Fonsecaea, Phialophora, Xylohypha, Ochroconis, Rhinocladiella, Scolecobasidium,* and *Wangiella*.

Symptoms, Signs, and Diagnosis

Most infections begin on the foot or leg, but other exposed body parts may be infected, especially where the skin is broken. Early small, itchy, enlarging papules may resemble dermatophytosis (ringworm). These extend to form dull red or violaceous, sharply demarcated patches with indurated bases. Several weeks or months later, new lesions, projecting 1 to 2 mm above the skin, may appear along paths of lymphatic drainage. Hard, dull red or grayish cauliflower-shaped nodular projections may develop in the center of patches, gradually extending to cover extremities over periods as long as 4 to 15 yr. Lymphatic obstruction may occur, itching may persist, and secondary bacterial superinfections may cause ulcerations and, occasionally, septicemia.

Extracutaneous infections (termed phaeohyphomycosis) may occur. These include invasive sinusitis, sometimes with bony necrosis, as well as subcutaneous nodules or abscesses, keratitis, lung masses, osteomyelitis, mycotic arthritis, intramuscular abscess, endocarditis, brain abscess, and chronic meningitis.

Dematiaceous fungi only rarely cause fatal infections in those who have normally intact host defense mechanisms. Life-threatening illnesses occur more often in immunocompromised patients.

Late chromomycosis lesions have a characteristic appearance, but early involvement may be mistaken for dermatophytoses. Phaeohyphomycosis must be distinguished by histopathology and culture from myriad other infectious and noninfectious conditions. Dematiaceous fungi are frequently discernible in tissue specimens stained with conventional hematoxylin and eosin, appearing as septate, brownish bodies, reflecting their natural melanin content. Fontana-Masson staining for melanin confirms their presence. Culture is needed to identify the causative species.

Treatment

Itraconazole is the most effective drug, although not all patients respond. Flucytosine is sometimes added to prevent relapse. Fluconazole seldom causes lesions to regress, and amphotericin B is ineffective. Many cases require surgical excision for cure.

SPOROTRICHOSIS

Sporotrichosis is a cutaneous infection caused by the saprophytic mold *Sporothrix schenckii*. Pulmonary and hematogenous involvement is uncommon. Symptoms are cutaneous nodules that spread via lymphatics and break down into abscesses and ulcers. Diagnosis is by culture. Treatment is with itraconazole or amphotericin B.

S. schenckii is found on rose or barberry bushes, sphagnum moss, and other mulches. Horticulturists, gardeners, farm laborers, and timber workers are most often infected, typically following minor trauma involving contaminated material.

Symptoms, Signs, and Diagnosis

Lymphocutaneous infections are most common. They can occur on any body site but characteristically involve one hand and arm, although primary lesions may occur on exposed surfaces of the feet or face. A primary lesion may appear as a small, nontender papule or, occasionally, as a slowly expanding subcutaneous nodule that eventually becomes necrotic and sometimes ulcerates. Typically, a few days or weeks later, a chain of draining lymph nodes begins to enlarge slowly but progressively, forming movable subcutaneous nodules. If untreated, overlying skin reddens and may later necrose, sometimes causing an abscess, ulceration, and bacterial superinfection. Systemic signs and symptoms of infection are notably absent.

Rarely, without primary lymphocutaneous lesions, hematogenous spread leads to indolent infections of multiple peripheral joints, sometimes bones, and, less often, genitals, liver, spleen, kidneys, or meninges. Equally rare is chronic pneumonia caused by inhalation of spores and manifested by localized infiltrates or cavities, most often in patients with preexisting chronic lung disease.

The illness must be differentiated from local infections caused by *Mycobacterium tuberculosis*, atypical mycobacteria, *Nocardia*, or other organisms. During the early, nondisseminated stage, the primary lesion is sometimes misdiagnosed as a spider bite. Culture from the active infection site provides the definitive diagnosis. *S. schenckii* yeasts can be seen only rarely in fixed tissue specimens, even with special staining. Serologic tests are not widely available.

Treatment

Lymphocutaneous sporotrichosis is chronic and indolent, and potentially fatal only if bacterial superinfections cause sepsis. Oral itraconazole, given for 3 to 6 mo, is the treatment of choice. Severe infection and infection in AIDS patients require IV amphotericin B. AIDS patients may require lifelong maintenance on itraconazole.

MISCELLANEOUS OPPORTUNISTIC FUNGI

Many yeasts and molds can cause opportunistic, even life-threatening, infections in immunocompromised patients. They only rarely affect immunocompetent people. Yeasts tend to cause fungemia as well as focal involvement of skin and other sites. *Trichosporon beigelii* and *Blastoschizomyces capitatus* particularly affect neutropenic patients. Infants and debilitated adults receiving lipid-containing IV hyperalimentation infusions are susceptible to *Malassezia furfur* fungemia. *Penicillium marneffei* was recognized as an opportunistic invader in Southeast Asian patients with AIDS, and cases have been recognized in the US. *P. marneffei* skin lesions may resemble molluscum contagiosum. Especially in neutropenic patients, various environmental molds can cause focal vasculitic lesions mimicking invasive aspergillosis, including species of *Fusarium* and *Scedosporium,* both of which are becoming more frequent.

Specific diagnosis requires culture and speciation and is crucial because not all of these organisms respond to any single antifungal drug. For example, *Scedosporium* sp are typically resistant to amphotericin B. Optimal regimens of antifungal therapy for each member of this group of fungal opportunists must be defined.

181 APPROACH TO PARASITIC INFECTIONS

Parasitic infections are responsible for substantial morbidity and mortality worldwide. They are prevalent in Central and South America, Africa, and Asia. They are much less common in Australia, Canada, Europe, Japan, New Zealand, and the US. By far the greatest impact is on residents of developing areas, but parasitic infections are encountered in industrialized countries in immigrants and travelers returning from endemic regions and, on occasion, even in residents who have not traveled, particularly those with AIDS or other causes of immunodeficiency.

Many parasitic infections are spread through fecal contamination of food or water. They are most frequent in impoverished areas where sanitation and hygiene are poor. Some parasites, like the hookworm, can enter the skin during contact with infected dirt or, in the case of schistosomes, with freshwater. Others, like malaria, are transmitted by arthropod vectors. On rare occasions, parasites may be transmitted via blood transfusions or shared needles or congenitally from mother to fetus.

Some parasites are endemic in the US and other industrialized countries. Examples include the pinworm, *Enterobius vermicularis, Trichomonas vaginalis,* toxoplasmosis, and enteric parasites such as *Giardia lamblia* and *Cryptosporidium* spp.

Taxonomically, parasites can be divided into 2 major groups: protozoa, which are single-celled organisms that multiply by simple binary division (see Chs. 185 and 186), and helminths, or worms, that are multicellular and have complex organ systems. The helminths can be further divided into the roundworms (nematodes—see Ch. 182) and the flatworms (platyhelminthes), which include tapeworms (cestodes—see Ch. 184) and flukes (trematodes—see Ch. 183). Some parasites have adapted to living in the lumen of the intestine where conditions are anaerobic; others reside in the blood or tissues.

The characteristics of protozoan and helminthic infections vary in important ways. Protozoa can multiply in their human hosts, increasing in number to produce overwhelming infection. With rare exceptions, protozoan infections do not cause eosinophilia.

In contrast, helminths do not multiply in humans but can elicit eosinophilic responses when they migrate through tissue. Most helminths have complex life cycles that involve substantial time outside their human hosts. Exceptions are *Strongyloides stercoralis, Capillaria philippinensis*, and *Hymenolepis nana*, which can increase in number due to autoinfection. In strongyloidiasis, autoinfection can result in life-threatening, disseminated hyperinfections in immunosuppressed people, particularly those taking corticosteroids.

The severity of helminthic infections usually correlates with the worm burden, but exceptions exist such as when a single migrating *Ascaris* produces life-threatening pancreatitis by occluding the pancreatic duct. The worm burden depends on the degree of environmental exposure, parasite factors, and the host's genetically determined immune responses. If a person moves from an endemic area, the number of adult worms diminishes over time. Although a few parasites (eg, *Clonorchis sinensis*) can survive for decades, many species have life spans of only a few years or less.

Diagnosis

Parasitic infections should be considered in the differential diagnosis of clinical syndromes arising in residents of or travelers to areas where sanitation and hygiene are poor or where vector-borne diseases are endemic. For example, fever in the returning traveler may suggest the possibility of malaria. Recent experience indicates that immigrants from developing areas to industrialized countries who return home to visit friends and relatives are at particular risk. They frequently do not seek or cannot afford pretravel advice on disease prevention and are more likely to enter high-risk settings than tourists who stay at resort facilities. Although less frequent, the possibility of an endemic or imported parasitic infection must also be considered in residents of industrialized countries who present with suggestive clinical syndromes, even if they have not traveled.

Physicians with expertise in parasitic infections and tropical medicine are available for consultation at many major medical centers, travel clinics, and public health facilities. Historical information, physical findings, and laboratory data may also suggest specific parasitic infections. For example, eosinophilia is common when helminths migrate through tissue and suggests a parasitic infection in an immigrant or returning traveler.

Methods for the diagnosis of specific parasitic infections are discussed in the chapters to follow and are summarized in TABLE 181–1. "Laboratory Identification of Parasites of Public Health Concern" provides detailed descriptions of diagnostic methods and is available from the Centers for Disease Control and Prevention (CDC) (www.dpd.cdc.gov/dpdx). Ova or parasites of protozoa and helminths that infect the GI tract typically are shed in the stool. Routine detection requires examination of stool specimens, preferably 3 collected every other day or on 3 consecutive days, because shedding can be sporadic.

Freshly passed stools uncontaminated with urine, water, dirt, or disinfectants should be sent to the laboratory within 1 h; unformed or watery stools are most likely to contain motile trophozoites. Stools should be refrigerated, but not frozen, if not examined immediately. Portions of fresh stools should also be emulsified in fixative to preserve GI pro-

Text continues on page 1544.

TABLE 181–1. COLLECTING AND HANDLING SPECIMENS FOR MICROSCOPIC DIAGNOSIS OF PARASITIC INFECTIONS

SPECIMEN	PARASITE	OPTIMAL SPECIMEN	COLLECTION DETAILS	COMMENTS
Blood	*Plasmodium* sp	Thick and thin smears of capillary blood (ie, finger or earlobe, using disposable lancet) or 5–10 mL of fresh anticoagulated blood See accompanying text	Collect multiple samples during acute illness Be certain all alcohol disinfectant has evaporated before collecting specimen Prepare smears from capillary or anticoagulated blood within 3 h after collection Dry slowly in covered dish	Use Wright's or Giemsa stain Ensure that glass slides are very clean If any doubt exists about ability to prepare good slides, collect anticoagulated blood in a tube and send to laboratory for preparation of slides and staining
	Babesia sp	Tick and thin smears as per malaria	As per malaria	Use Wright's or Giemsa stain. Morphology similar to *Plasmodium* sp ring forms but without pigment and gametocytes. Tetrads are diagnostic of *Babesia* sp
	Trypanosoma sp	Thin smears of capillary blood or 5–6 mL of anticoagulated blood	Smear on glass slides	Use Wright's or Giemsa stain. Various concentration techniques are used to enhance the sensitivity for African trypanosomiasis
	Filarial worms	1 mL of anticoagulated blood; if 1st specimen is negative, collect 5–10 mL and concentrate by centrifugation or filtration	*Wuchereria bancrofti* and *Brugia malayi:* draw blood between 10 PM and 2 AM *Loa loa, Dipetalonema perstans,* and *Mansonella ozzardi:* draw blood between 10 AM and 6 PM	Use Wright's or Giemsa stain either directly or, for greater sensitivity, after concentration
Bone marrow or other reticuloendothelial tissue				
	Leishmania sp	Aspirates of bone marrow, spleen, liver, or lymph nodes or buffy coat smears	Smear on glass slides	Use Wright's or Giemsa stain
CNS				
	Naegleria *Acanthamoeba* *Balamuthia*	Fresh spinal fluid	Use aseptic collection technique Examine specimen as soon as possible	Examination by light or phase-contrast microscopy; parasites may be detected by their movements; can be cultured or fixed and stained with Giemsa

Table continues on the following page.

TABLE 181–1. COLLECTING AND HANDLING SPECIMENS FOR MICROSCOPIC DIAGNOSIS OF PARASITIC INFECTIONS—Continued

SPECIMEN	PARASITE	OPTIMAL SPECIMEN	COLLECTION DETAILS	COMMENTS
	Trypanosoma brucei subsp	Fresh spinal fluid	Use aseptic collection technique	Wet mount and Giemsa stained, direct or concentrated by centrifugation
Intestinal tract				
Duodenal aspirate or jejunal biopsy	*Giardia* *Cryptosporidium* sp *Isospora* *Cyclospora* Microsporida *Strongyloides*	Specimen placed in sterile jar or tube with a little saline or on glass slide with coverslip	Examine immediately or fix for histopathologic examination	Multiple stains may be required for optimal diagnosis; see below and text for details
Rectal biopsy	*Schistosoma mansoni* *Schistosoma japonicum*	For schistosomes: biopsy specimen from level of dorsal fold (Houston valve), about 9 cm from anus	Fix for histopathologic examination and crush a segment between slides for increased sensitivity	Speciation is based on the morphology of ova
Feces	*Entamoeba histolytica* *Entamoeba dispar* Other amebas	3 freshly passed stools collected in AM every other day	Examine unformed or diarrheal specimens within 15 min Keep formed stools refrigerated until examination (see also accompanying text)	Wet mounts and permanent stained slides (eg, trichomes); concentration techniques for cysts Stool should be assayed for the *E. histolytica* adherence lectin antigen to differentiate it from the nonpathologic *E. dispar*
	Giardia	3 freshly passed stools collected in AM every other day	If initial series of 3 specimens is negative, examine 3 more, 1 wk later Obtain duodenal aspirates if necessary (see accompanying text)	If immediate examination is not possible, preserve specimen in polyvinyl alcohol. Examine direct mounts and concentrated specimen for cysts and trophozoites. Assays for fecal antigens are more sensitive

Cryptosporidium sp	Multiple freshly passed stools collected daily or every other day	Refrigerate and examine fresh samples or preserve in 10% buffered formalin, acetate-acetic acid-formalin, or suspended in 2.5% aqueous K dichromate Handle with care; fresh and dichromate-preserved stools are infectious Obtain duodenal aspirate or jejunal biopsy if stool specimens are negative	Examine wet mounts by conventional light, differential interference contrast, and immunofluorescence microscopy Stain specimens with modified acid-fast or modified safranin. Assays for fecal antigens are more sensitive
Isospora	Multiple freshly passed stools collected daily or every other day	Concentration techniques enhance sensitivity	Oocysts can be visualized in wet mounts by bright-field differential interference contrast or epifluorescence microscopy. Stain fixed specimens with modified acid-fast
Cyclospora	Multiple freshly passed stools collected daily or every other day	Specimens should be refrigerated or preserved in 10% formalin or 2.5% K dichromate. Concentration techniques increase sensitivity	Examine wet mounts by conventional light, bright-field differential interference contrast, and UV fluorescence microscopy. Oocysts are autofluorescent under UV light. Fixed specimens can be stained with modified acid-fast or modified safranin
Microsporida	Multiple stools collected daily or every other day	Small-bowel biopsies may be necessary if stools are negative	Specimens stained by chromotropic methods are most widely used. Chemofluorescent agents such as Calcofluor white can also be used for quick identification. Electron microscopy is the standard and used for speciation
Trichuris *Ascaris* Hookworms *Strongyloides* Tapeworms Flukes	Up to 3 stools collected daily	Refrigerate specimen if necessary Immediate examination is not critical, but larvae from hatched hookworm eggs in old stools may be confused with those of *Strongyloides*	Active larvae are seen with *Strongyloides*, ova with the rest. The agar plate assay is more sensitive than ova and parasite examination for *Strongyloides*

Table continues on the following page.

TABLE 181–1. COLLECTING AND HANDLING SPECIMENS FOR MICROSCOPIC DIAGNOSIS OF PARASITIC INFECTIONS—Continued

SPECIMEN	PARASITE	OPTIMAL SPECIMEN	COLLECTION DETAILS	COMMENTS
	Enterobius *Taenia* sp	Ova on cellophane tape	Collect from area around anus in AM before bowel movement or bath	Ova occasionally seen in stool specimen or by Papanicolaou test of vaginal contents
Sigmoidoscopy (proctoscopy)	*Entamoeba histolytica* *Entamoeba dispar*	Fresh scrapings collected with a curet or Volkmann's spoon, a piece of mucosa snipped off with a surgical instrument, or aspirate from lesion obtained via a 1-mL serologic pipette with a rubber bulb Cotton-tipped swabs are not satisfactory	Examine specimen immediately or preserve it for later examination	Stool should be assayed for the *E. histolytica* antigen to differentiate *E. histolytica* from *E. dispar,* a nonpathogen
Respiratory tract				
Sputum, tracheal, bronchial aspirates	*Paragonimus* sp	Fresh sputum	Examine specimen as soon as possible or preserve for later examination	Concentration techniques may be necessary
	Strongyloides (hyperinfection)	Sputum; any aspirated material; also drainage material	Examine specimen as soon as possible or preserve it for later examination	Active larvae may be seen in wet mounts or can be fixed and stained with Giemsa
Lung biopsy	*Paragonimus* sp	Open lung biopsy Percutaneous biopsy under fluoroscopy or CT	Collect and place in sterile container in sterile saline	Biopsy may allow species identification if a fluke is recovered

Skin				
	Onchocerca	For patients infected in Africa, use skin snips from thigh, buttocks, iliac crest For patients infected in Latin America, use skin snips from head, scapula, buttocks	For skin snips, disinfect skin with alcohol, insert 25-gauge needle just under epidermis, raise it, and slice off small piece of tissue with a scalpel or razor blade, or use sclerocorneal punch biopsy tool	Bleeding should not occur Examine specimen suspended in saline
	Leishmania sp	Ulcer rim biopsy or slip smear scrapings	Leishmaniasis, look for amastigotes in touch preparations of lesion/ulcer wall	Use Wright's or Giemsa stained touch preparations, histopathology, and culture
Urogenital system				
Vaginal, urethral, or prostatic secretions	*Trichomonas* sp	1 sterile swab in a tube with small amount of sterile saline	Tell female patients not to douche for 3–4 days before collecting specimen Send specimen to laboratory as soon as possible	Identification of motile organisms by wet mount is the most rapid; DFA for parasites is more sensitive; culture is most sensitive but takes 3–7 days
Urine or bladder biopsy	*Schistosoma haematobium*, occasionally *S. japonicum*	Fresh urine or biopsy from area around the trigone	Recommended time for urine collection: between noon and 3 PM	Wet mount, concentrated by centrifugation

UV = ultraviolet; DFA = direct fluorescent antibody.
Based on the CDC's "Laboratory Identification of Parasites of Public Health Concern" (www.dpd.cdc.gov/dpdx).

TABLE 181–2. SEROLOGIC AND MOLECULAR TESTS FOR PARASITIC INFECTIONS

PARASITE, INFECTION	ANTIBODY	ANTIGEN OR DNA/ RNA
Protozoans		
African sleeping sickness	CATT	
Amebiasis	EIA	EIA, PCR
Babesiosis	IFA	PCR
Chagas' disease	IFA, EIA	
Cryptosporidiosis		IFA, EIA, DFA, PCR
Cyclosporiasis		PCR
Giardiasis		EIA, DFA, PCR
Leishmaniasis	IFA, EIA	
Malaria (all species)	IFA	PCR
Microsporidiosis		PCR, IIF
Toxoplasmosis	IFA, EIA (IgG and IgM)	
Roundworms		
Filariasis		EIA, PCR
Strongyloidiasis	EIA	
Trichinellosis	EIA	
Toxocariasis	EIA	
Flukes		
Paragonimiasis	IB, EIA	
Schistosomiasis	EIA, IB	
Tapeworms		
Cysticercosis	IB, EIA	
Echinococcosis	IB, EIA, IHA	

CATT = card agglutination trypanosomiasis test for *T. b. gambiense*; DFA = direct fluorescent antibody; EIA = enzyme immunoassay; IB = immunoblot; IFA = indirect fluorescent antibody test; IHA = indirect hemagglutination assay; IIF = immunofluorescence assay; PCR = polymerase chain reaction.

Note: Some antigen and parasite detection kits are available commercially. Others are available at the CDC or other reference laboratories.

Based on CDC's "Laboratory Identification of Parasites of Public Health Concern" (www.dpd.cdc.gov/dpdx).

tozoa. Concentration techniques can be used to improve sensitivity. Anal cellophane tape or swabs may demonstrate pinworm or tapeworm eggs. If strongyloidiasis is suspected, fresh stool should be smeared on an agar plate to identify larvae. Antibiotics, x-ray contrast material, purgatives, and antacids can hinder detection of ova and parasites for several weeks. Serologic assays, antigen detection tests (eg, *Giardia lamblia* or *Cryptosporidium*), or PCR testing may aid diagnosis (see TABLE 181–2). Nonetheless, laboratory testing has sensitivity that is low enough that, when clinical suspicion is strong, empirical treatment may be given.

Sigmoidoscopy or colonoscopy should be considered when routine stool examinations are negative in patients with persistent GI symptoms who are suspected of having amebiasis. Sigmoidoscopic specimens should be collected with a curet or spoon (cotton swabs are not suitable) and processed immediately for microscopy. Duodenal aspirates or small-bowel biopsies may be necessary for the diagnosis of such infections as cryptosporidiosis and microsporidiosis.

Treatment

Advice for treating parasitic infections is available from experts at major medical and public health centers and travel clinics, in textbooks of infectious diseases and tropical medicine, and in summary form from *The Medical Letter on Drugs and Therapeutics* (www.medletter.org, August 2004 issue). Drugs for unusual parasitic infections can be obtained from the manufacturer or from the CDC Drug Service.

Prevention

Despite substantial investment and research, no vaccines are yet available for prevention of human parasitic infections. Prevention is based on avoidance strategies.

Sanitary disposal of feces and provision of purified water can prevent transmission of most intestinal parasites. For the international traveler the best advice is "cook it, boil it, peel it, or forget it." When followed, these measures substantially reduce the risk of intestinal parasitic infections as well as bacterial and viral gastroenteritis. Meat, particularly pork, and fish, particularly freshwater varieties, should be thoroughly cooked before ingestion. Other safety measures include removing litter boxes from areas where food is prepared to prevent toxoplasmosis. People should not swim in freshwater lakes, streams, or rivers in areas where schistosomiasis is endemic or walk barefoot in areas where hookworms are found.

The risk of malaria and many other vector-borne diseases can be decreased by wearing long-sleeved shirts and pants and applying N, N-diethylmetatoluamide (DEET)–containing insect repellants to exposed skin and permethrin to clothing. Window screens, air conditioning, and mosquito nets impregnated with permethrin or other insecticides provide further protection. In addition, prophylactic antimalarial drugs should be taken by those traveling in endemic regions.

Travelers to rural Latin America should not sleep in adobe dwellings where reduviid bugs can transmit Chagas' disease. In Africa, travelers should avoid bright colors and wear long-sleeved shirts and pants to avoid tsetse flies in regions where African sleeping sickness is found.

Specific recommendations for travel are provided by the CDC, in hardcopy and on the web (www.cdc.gov/travel).

182 NEMATODES (ROUNDWORMS)

Nematodes are nonsegmented cylindric worms ranging from 1 mm to 1 m in length. Nematodes have a body cavity, distinguishing them from tapeworms and flukes. Depending on the species, different stages in the life cycle are infectious to humans. Hundreds of millions of humans are infected with nematodes, the most common of which are *Ascaris*, the hookworms, and *Trichuris*.

ANGIOSTRONGYLIASIS

Angiostrongyliasis is infection with larvae of worms of the genus *Angiostrongylus*; intestinal symptoms or eosinophilic meningitis occurs depending on the infecting species.

Angiostrongylus is a parasite of rats. Excreted larvae are taken up by intermediate (snails and slugs) and transport (certain crabs and freshwater shrimp) hosts. Human infection is acquired by ingestion of raw or undercooked snails or slugs or transport hosts; it is unclear if larval contamination of vegetables can cause infection.

A. cantonensis infection occurs predominantly in Southeast Asia and the Pacific Basin, although infection has been reported elsewhere. The larvae migrate from the GI tract to the meninges, where they cause eosinophilic meningitis, with fever, headache, and meningismus.

A. costaricensis infection occurs in the Americas. Adult worms reside in arterioles of the ileocecal area, and eggs can be released into the intestinal tissues resulting in local inflammation with abdominal pain, vomiting, and fever; a painful right lower quadrant mass may develop.

Diagnosis is suspected by history of ingesting potentially contaminated material. Patients with meningeal findings require lumbar puncture; CSF shows eosinophilia, but parasites are rarely visible. Diagnosis of GI infection is difficult as larvae and eggs are not present in stool.

Treatment of *A. cantonensis* meningitis is with analgesics, corticosteroids, and removal of CSF. Most patients have a self-limited course and recover completely. Anthelmintics do not appear to be effective for either *A. cantonensis* or *A. costaricensis*.

ANISAKIASIS

Anisakiasis is infection with larvae of worms of the genus *Anisakis* and related genera such as *Pseudoterranova*. Infection is acquired by eating raw or poorly cooked saltwater fish; larvae burrow into the mucosa of the GI tract, causing discomfort.

Anisakis is a parasite of the GI tract of marine mammals. Excreted eggs hatch into free-swimming larvae, which are ingested by fish and squid; human infection is acquired by ingestion of these intermediate hosts in a raw or poorly cooked state. Larvae burrow into the stomach and small bowel. Symptoms typically include abdominal pain, nausea, and vomiting; intestinal infection may create an inflammatory mass causing symptoms resembling Crohn's disease.

Diagnosis is usually made by upper endoscopy; stool examination is unhelpful, but a serologic test is available in some countries. Infection typically resolves spontaneously after several weeks but rarely persists for months. Endoscopic removal of the larvae is curative. Cooking to > 50° C (> 122° F) and freezing > 24 h destroy larvae; they may resist pickling, salting, and smoking.

ASCARIASIS

Ascariasis is infection with *Ascaris lumbricoides*. Light infections may be asymptomatic. Early symptoms are pulmonary (cough, wheezing); later symptoms are GI, with cramps or abdominal pain from obstruction of GI lumina (intestines or biliary or pancreatic ducts) by adult worms. Chronically infected children may develop malnutrition. Diagnosis is by identifying eggs or adult worms in stool, adult worms that migrate from the nose or mouth, or larvae in sputum during the pulmonary migration phase. Treatment is with albendazole, mebendazole, or pyrantel pamoate.

Etiology and Pathophysiology

Ingested eggs hatch in the duodenum, and the resulting larvae penetrate the wall of the small bowel and migrate via the portal circulation through the liver to the heart and lungs. Larvae lodge in the alveolar capillaries, penetrate alveolar walls, and ascend the bronchial tree into the oropharynx. They are swallowed and return to the small bowel, where they develop into adult worms, which mate and release eggs into the stool. The life cycle is completed in about 2 to 3 mo; adult worms live 1 to 2 yr.

A tangled mass of worms from heavy infection can produce bowel obstruction, particularly in children. Aberrantly migrating individual adult worms occasionally obstruct the biliary or pancreatic ducts, causing cholecystitis or pancreatitis; cholangitis, liver abscess, and peritonitis are less common. Fever from other illnesses or certain drugs (eg, albendazole, mebendazole, tetrachloroethylene) may provoke aberrant migration.

Ascariasis occurs worldwide. It is concentrated in tropical and subtropical areas with poor sanitation, but transmission occurs in rural areas of the southeastern US. Ascariasis is the most prevalent intestinal helminth infection in the world. Current estimates suggest that > 1.3 billion people are infected, of whom about 20,000 (mostly children) die each year from bowel or biliary obstruction. An estimated 4 million people in the US are infected.

Symptoms, Signs, and Diagnosis

Larvae migrating through the lungs may produce cough, wheezing, and occasionally hemoptysis or other respiratory symptoms. Adult worms in small numbers usually do not produce GI symptoms, although passage of an adult worm by mouth or rectum may bring an otherwise asymptomatic patient to medical attention. Bowel or biliary obstruction causes cramping abdominal pain, nausea, and vomiting. Jaundice is uncommon. Even moderate infections can lead to malnutrition in children. The pathophysiology is unclear and may include competition for nutrients, impairment of absorption, and depression of appetite.

Diagnosis is by microscopic detection of eggs in stools. Occasionally, larvae can be found in the sputum during the pulmonary phase. Eosinophilia can be marked while larvae migrate though the lungs but usually subsides later in infection when adult worms reside in the intestine. Chest x-ray during the pulmonary phase may show infiltrates (Löffler's pneumonia).

Treatment and Prevention

All infections should be treated. Albendazole (400 mg po once), mebendazole (100 mg po bid for 3 days), or ivermectin (150 μg/kg once) are effective. Mebendazole and albendazole should not be used in pregnancy. Recent data suggest that nitazoxanide is also effective at a dose of 500 mg bid for 3 days in adults; 100 mg q 12 h for 3 days in children 1 to 3 yr; and 200 mg q 12 h for 3 days in children 4 to 11 yr. Obstructive complications may respond to anthelmintic therapy or require surgical or endoscopic extraction of adult worms.

Prevention requires adequate sanitation. Uncooked or unwashed vegetables should be avoided in areas where human feces are used as fertilizer.

FILARIAL NEMATODE INFECTIONS

Threadlike adult filarial worms reside in tissues. Gravid females produce live offspring (microfilariae) that circulate in blood or migrate through tissues. When ingested by a suitable bloodsucking insect (mosquitoes or flies), microfilariae develop into infective larvae that are inoculated or deposited in the skin of the next host during the insect bite. Only a few filarial species infect humans.

DIROFILARIASIS

(Dog Heartworm Infection)

***Dirofilaria immitis* is the dog heartworm, which is transmitted to humans by infected mosquitoes.**

Symptomatic human infection is very rare, but larvae may become encapsulated in infarcted lung tissue and produce well-defined pulmonary nodules. The patient may have chest pain, cough, and occasionally hemoptysis. Many patients remain asymptomatic, and a pulmonary nodule is discovered on routine chest x-ray, which may be suggestive of a tumor. Diagnosis is by histologic examination of a surgical specimen. No treatment is indicated in humans; infection is self-limited.

DRACUNCULIASIS

(Guinea Worm Disease; Fiery Serpent)

Dracunculiasis is infection with *Dracunculus medinensis*. Symptoms are a painful, inflamed skin lesion containing an adult worm and debilitating arthritis. Diagnosis is by inspection. Treatment is slow removal of the adult worm.

Twenty years ago dracunculiasis was endemic in much of tropical Africa, Yemen, India, and Pakistan. Today, infection occurs mainly within a narrow belt of African countries and Yemen.

Humans become infected by drinking water containing infected microcrustaceans (copepods). The larvae are released, penetrate the bowel wall, and mature into adult worms in about 1 yr. The gravid female migrates through subcutaneous tissues, usually to the distal lower extremities. The cephalic end of the worm produces an indurated papule that vesiculates and eventually ulcerates. On contact with water, a loop of the uterus prolapses through the skin and discharges motile larvae. Worms that fail to reach the skin die and disintegrate or become calcified. In most endemic areas, transmission is seasonal and each infectious episode lasts about 1 yr.

Symptoms and Signs

Infection is initially asymptomatic; symptoms usually develop with eruption of the worm. Local symptoms include intense itching and a burning pain at the site of the skin lesion. Urticaria, erythema, dyspnea, vomiting, and pruritus are thought to reflect allergic reactions to worm antigens. If the worm is broken during expulsion or extraction, a severe inflammatory reaction ensues with disabling pain. Symptoms subside and the ulcer heals once the adult worm is expelled. In about 50% of cases, secondary bacterial infections occur along the track of the emerging worm. Chronic sequelae include fibrous ankylosis of joints and contraction of tendons.

Diagnosis, Treatment, and Prevention

Diagnosis is obvious once the white, filamentous adult worm appears at the cutaneous ulcer. Calcified worms can be localized with x-ray examination (they have been found in Egyptian mummies). Serodiagnostic tests are not specific.

Treatment consists of slow removal of the adult worm over days to weeks by rolling it on a stick. Surgical removal under local anesthesia is an option but is seldom available in endemic areas. The beneficial effect of metronidazole (250 mg tid for 10 days) has been ascribed to the drug's anti-inflammatory and antibacterial properties rather than to anthelmintic effects.

Filtering drinking water through a piece of cheesecloth, chlorination, or boiling effectively protects against dracunculiasis.

LOIASIS

Loiasis is infection with *Loa loa*. Symptoms include localized angioedema (Calabar swellings) and subconjunctival migration of adult worms. Diagnosis is by detecting microfilariae in peripheral blood or seeing worms migrating across the eye. Treatment is with diethylcarbamazine.

Loiasis is confined to the rain forest belt of western and central Africa. *Loa loa* are transmitted by tabanid flies (*Chrysops*, the deerfly, or horsefly). Adults migrate in subcutaneous tissues and the eye, and microfilariae circulate in blood. Occasionally, infection causes cardiomyopathy, nephropathy, or encephalitis.

Symptoms, Signs, and Diagnosis

Infection produces areas of angioedema (Calabar swellings) that develop anywhere on the body but predominantly on the extremities; they are presumed to reflect hypersensitivity reactions to allergens released by migrating adult worms. In native residents, swellings usually last 1 to 3 days but are more frequent and severe in visitors. Worms may also migrate subconjunctivally across the eyes. This may be unsettling, but residual eye damage is uncommon.

Nephropathy generally presents as proteinuria with or without mild hematuria and is believed to be due to immune complex deposition. Encephalopathy is usually mild, with vague CNS symptoms.

Microscopic detection of microfilariae in peripheral blood establishes the diagnosis. Blood samples should be drawn around noontime, when microfilaremia levels are the highest. Serodiagnostic tests do not differentiate *Loa loa* from other filarial nematode infections.

Treatment and Prevention

Diethylcarbamazine (DEC) is the only drug that kills microfilariae and adult worms. DEC is given as 50 mg po on day 1, 50 mg po tid on day 2, 100 mg tid on day 3, then 3 mg/kg tid on days 4 through 14. A single dose of 6 mg/kg once has been used in mass treatment programs and is recommended by some. Multiple courses may be necessary before there is complete resolution. DEC transiently exacerbates proteinuria and, in heavily infected patients, may trigger encephalopathy, leading to coma and death. Lower doses of DEC (0.5 to 1.0 mg/kg once/day) and simultaneous corticosteroids may be used in heavily infected people. Such patients may benefit from apheresis or initial treatment with albendazole. Ivermectin administration in heavily infected patients may also cause encephalopathy and death.

DEC (300 mg po once/wk) can be used to prevent infection. Insect repellents may reduce exposure to infected flies.

Bancroftian and Brugian Lymphatic Filariasis

Lymphatic filariasis is infection with any of 3 species of *Filarioidea*. Acute symptoms include fever, lymphadenitis, lymphangitis, funiculitis, and epididymitis. Chronic symptoms include abscesses, hyperkeratosis, polyarthritis, hydroceles, lymphedema, and elephantiasis. Tropical pulmonary eosinophilia with bronchospasm, fever, and pulmonary infiltrates is another manifestation of infection. Diagnosis is by detection of microfilariae in blood, ultrasound visualization of adult worms, or serology. Treatment is with diethylcarbamazine; antibiotics are used for complicating bacterial cellulitis.

Etiology and Pathophysiology

Lymphatic filariasis is caused by *Wuchereria bancrofti, Brugia malayi*, and *B. timori*, which are spread by mosquitoes. Infective larvae from the mosquito migrate to the lymphatics, where they develop into threadlike adult worms within 6 to 12 mo. Gravid adult females produce microfilariae that circulate in blood.

Bancroftian filariasis is present in tropical and subtropical areas of Africa, Asia, the Pacific, and the Americas, including Haiti. Brugian filariasis is endemic in South and Southeast Asia. Current estimates suggest that about 129 million people are infected.

Symptoms and Signs

Infection often leads to microfilaremia without overt clinical manifestations. However, acute inflammatory filariasis consists of 4- to 7-day episodes (often recurrent) of fever and inflammation of lymph nodes with lymphangitis, termed acute adenolymphangitis (ADL), or acute epididymitis and spermatic cord inflammation. Localized involvement of an affected limb may result in an abscess that drains externally and leaves a scar. ADL is often associated with secondary bacterial infections.

Extralymphatic signs include chronic microscopic hematuria and proteinuria and mild polyarthritis, all presumed to result from immune complex deposition.

Chronic filarial disease develops insidiously after many years. In most patients, asymptomatic lymphatic dilatation occurs, but chronic inflammatory responses to adult worms and secondary bacterial infections may result in chronic lymphedema of the affected body area or to scrotal hydroceles. Chronic pitting lymphedema of the lower extremity can progress to elephantiasis. Increased local susceptibility to bacterial and fungal infections contributes to the development of elephantiasis. Other forms of chronic filarial disease are caused by disruption of lymphatic vessels or aberrant drainage of lymph fluid, leading to chyluria and chyloceles.

ADL episodes usually precede onset of chronic disease by ≥ 2 decades. Acute filariasis is more severe in previously unexposed immigrants to endemic areas than in native residents. Microfilaremia gradually disappears after leaving the endemic area.

Tropical pulmonary eosinophilia (TPE) is an uncommon manifestation with recurrent bronchospasm, transitory lung infiltrates, low-grade fever, and marked eosinophilia. It is most likely due to hypersensitivity reactions to microfilariae. Chronic TPE can lead to pulmonary fibrosis.

Diagnosis

Microscopic detection of microfilariae in blood establishes the diagnosis. Filtered or centrifuged concentrates of blood are more sensitive than thick blood films. Blood samples must be obtained when peak microfilaremia occurs—at night, where *W. bancrofti* is endemic, but during the day in many Pacific islands where *B. malayi* and *B. timori* occur. Viable adult worms can be visualized in dilated lymphatics by ultrasonography; their movement has been called the filarial dance.

A sensitive and specific rapid antigen test is available for *W. bancrofti* but not for other filariae. Measurement of antifilarial IgG is available from the National Institutes of Health and is very sensitive as an initial screen, but it cannot differentiate past exposure from current active infection; thus, it is most helpful in visitors to endemic areas. PCR-based assays for DNA of *W. bancrofti* and *B. malayi* are available in research settings.

Treatment and Prevention

Diethylcarbamazine (DEC) kills microfilariae and a variable proportion of adult worms. A recommended dose is 50 mg po on day 1, 50 mg po tid on day 2, 100 mg po tid on day 3, then 2 mg/kg tid on days 4 to 14. A single dose of albendazole (400 mg po) with either ivermectin (200 μg/kg po) or DEC (6 mg/kg) rapidly reduces microfilaremia levels, but ivermectin alone does not kill adult worms. Acute attacks of ADL generally resolve spontaneously, although antibiotics may be required to control secondary bacterial infections. Whether DEC therapy prevents or lessens chronic lymphedema remains controversial.

Chronic lymphedema requires meticulous skin care, including use of systemic antibiotics to treat secondary bacterial infections, which may slow or prevent progression to elephantiasis. Conservative measures such as elastic bandaging of the affected limb reduce swelling. Surgical decompression using nodal-venous shunts to improve lymphatic drainage offers some long-term benefit in extreme cases of elephantiasis. Massive hydroceles can also be managed surgically.

TPE responds to DEC (2 mg/kg tid for 12 to 21 days), but relapses may occur in up to 25% of cases, requiring additional courses of therapy.

Avoiding mosquito bites in endemic areas is the best protection. Chemoprophylaxis with DEC or combinations of antifilarial drugs (ivermectin/albendazole or ivermectin/DEC) can suppress microfilaremia. DEC has even been used as an additive to table salt in some endemic areas.

Onchocerciasis

(River Blindness)

Onchocerciasis is infection with the filarial nematode *Onchocerca volvulus*. Symptoms are subcutaneous nodules, pruritus, adenopathy and lymphatic obstruction, chronic skin disease, and eye lesions that may lead to blindness. Diagnosis is by finding microfilariae in skin snips, the cornea, or anterior chamber of the eye; identifying adult worms in subcutaneous nodules; or using PCR or DNA probes. Treatment is with ivermectin.

Etiology and Pathophysiology

Onchocerciasis is spread by blackflies (*Simulium* sp) that breed in swiftly flowing streams (hence the term river blindness). Infective larvae inoculated into the skin during the bite of a blackfly develop into adult worms in 12 to 18 mo. Adult female worms may live up to 15 yr in subcutaneous nodules. Mature female worms produce microfilariae that migrate mainly through the skin and invade the eyes.

About 18 million people are infected, of whom about 270,000 are blind and an additional 500,000 are visually impaired. Onchocerciasis is the 2nd leading cause of blindness worldwide (after trachoma). Onchocerciasis is most common in tropical and sub-Saharan regions of Africa. Small foci exist in Yemen, southern Mexico, Guatemala, Ecuador, Colombia, Venezuela, and the Brazilian Amazon. Blindness is fairly rare in the Americas.

Symptoms and Signs

The subcutaneous (or deeper) nodules (onchocercoma) that contain adult worms may be visible or palpable but otherwise asymptomatic. They are composed of inflammatory cells and fibrotic tissue in various proportions. Old nodules may caseate or calcify.

Onchocercal dermatitis is caused by the microfilarial stage of the parasite. Intense pruritus may be the only symptom in lightly infected people. Skin lesions usually consist of a nondescript maculopapular rash with secondary excoriations, scaling ulcerations and lichenification, and mild to moderate lymphadenopathy. Premature wrinkling, skin atrophy, enlargement of inguinal or femoral nodes, lymphatic obstruction, patchy hypopigmentation, and transitory localized areas of edema and erythema can occur. Onchocercal dermatitis is generalized in most patients, but a localized and sharply delineated form of eczematous dermatitis with hyperkeratosis, scaling, and pigment changes (Sowdah) is common in Yemen and Saudi Arabia.

Eye disease ranges from mild visual impairment to complete blindness. Lesions of the anterior eye include punctate (snowflake) keratitis, an acute inflammatory infiltrate surrounding dying microfilariae that resolves without causing permanent damage; sclerosing keratitis, an ingrowth of fibrovascular scar tissue that may cause subluxation of the lens and blindness; and anterior uveitis or iridocyclitis that may deform the pupil. Chorioretinitis, optic neuritis, and optic atrophy may also occur.

Diagnosis

Demonstration of microfilariae in skin snips is the traditional diagnostic method (see TABLE 181–1 on p. 1539). Microfilariae may also be visible in the cornea and anterior chamber of the eye by slit-lamp examination. PCR-based methods to detect parasite DNA in skin snips may be more sensitive than standard techniques but are available only in research settings. Serodiagnostic tests are also available in specialty laboratories, but the specificity depends on the antigen, and substantial cross-reactivity exists between *Onchocerca* and other helminths. Serology cannot differentiate past from current infection.

Palpable nodules (or deep nodules detected by ultrasonography or MRI in industrialized countries) can be excised and examined for adult worms.

Treatment and Prevention

Ivermectin is given as a single oral dose of 150 μg/kg, repeated q 6 to 12 mo until asymptomatic. Ivermectin reduces microfilariae in the skin and eyes and decreases production of microfilariae for several months. It does not appear to kill adult worms in standard regimens but inhibits microfilarial release from female worms. Adverse effects are qualitatively similar to those of diethylcarbamazine (DEC) but are much less common and less severe. DEC is no longer used for onchocerciasis because it can cause a severe hypersensitivity (Mazzotti) reaction, which can further damage skin and eyes and lead to cardiovascular collapse. Doxycycline, which targets an endosymbiont of the adult filaria, is still being studied.

No drug has been shown to protect against infection with *O. volvulus*. However, annual or semiannual administration of ivermectin effectively controls disease and may decrease transmission. Surgical removal of accessible onchocercomas can reduce skin microfilaria counts, but it has been replaced by ivermectin therapy.

In theory it is possible to minimize *Simulium* bites by avoiding fly-infested areas, wearing protective clothing, and liberally using insect repellents.

HOOKWORM INFECTION

(Ancylostomiasis)

Ancylostomiasis is infection with *Ancylostoma duodenale* or *Necator americanus*. Symptoms include rash at the site of larval entry and sometimes abdominal pain or other GI symptoms during early infection. Later, iron deficiency may develop. Hookworms are a major cause of iron deficiency anemia in endemic regions. Diagnosis is by finding eggs in stool. Treatment is albendazole, mebendazole, or pyrantel pamoate.

Etiology and Pathophysiology

Both hookworm species have similar life cycles. Eggs passed in the stool hatch in 1 to 2 days (if they are deposited in a warm, moist place on loose soil) and release rhabditiform larvae, which molt once to become slender filariform larvae in 5 to 10 days. Filariform larvae penetrate human skin, reach the lungs via blood vessels, penetrate into pulmonary alveoli, ascend the respiratory tree to the epiglottis, and are swallowed. The larvae develop into adults that attach to the wall of the small bowel, feeding on blood. Chronic blood loss leads to iron deficiency anemia. The development of anemia depends on worm burden and the amount of absorbable iron in the diet. Adult worms may live ≥ 2 yr.

The estimated prevalence of hookworm infection is about 1 billion, mostly in tropical latitudes. Both *A. duodenale* and *N. americanus* are found in Africa, Asia, and the Americas. Only *A. duodenale* is found in the Middle East, North Africa, and southern Europe. *N. americanus* predominates in the Americas and Australia. It was once widely distributed in the southern US. It is still endemic on islands of the Caribbean and in Central and South America.

Infection with *A. caninum*, which ordinarily infects dogs, is a common cause of eosinophilic enteritis in Queensland, Australia. Several cases have been diagnosed in the US. Eggs of *A. caninum* are not usually found in human stool. Infection may be asymptomatic or cause acute abdominal pain and eosinophilia.

Symptoms and Signs

Hookworm infection is often asymptomatic. However, a pruritic papulovesicular rash (ground itch, cutaneous larva migrans—see p. 993) may develop at the site of larval penetration. Migration of large numbers of larvae though the lungs occasionally causes Löffler's pneumonia, with cough, wheezing, and sometimes hemoptysis. During the acute phase, adult worms in the intestine may cause colicky epigastric pain, anorexia, flatulence, diarrhea, and weight loss. Chronic infection can lead to iron deficiency anemia and hypoproteinemia, causing pallor, dyspnea, weakness, tachycardia, lassitude, and peripheral edema. A low-grade eosinophilia is often present. Chronic blood loss may lead to severe anemia, growth retardation, heart failure, and anasarca.

Diagnosis, Treatment, and Prevention

A. duodenale and *N. americanus* produce thin-shelled oval eggs that are readily detected in fresh stool. If the stool is not kept cold and examined within several hours, the eggs may hatch and release larvae that may be confused with those of *Strongyloides stercoralis*. Nutritional status, anemia, and iron stores should be evaluated.

Albendazole (a single dose of 400 mg po) or mebendazole (100 mg po bid for 3 days) is given. Cure rates are > 99%. Pyrantel pamoate (11 mg/kg po once/day [1 g maximum] for 3 days) is also effective. These drugs should not be used in pregnancy. General support and correction of iron deficiency anemia are needed if infection is heavy.

Preventing unhygienic defecation and avoiding direct skin contact with the soil are effective in preventing infection but difficult to implement in many endemic areas. Periodic mass treatment of susceptible populations at 3- to 4-mo intervals has been used in high-risk areas.

PINWORM INFESTATION

(Enterobiasis; Oxyuriasis)

Enterobiasis is an intestinal infestation by *Enterobius vermicularis*, usually in children. Its major symptom is perianal itching. Diagnosis is by visual inspection for thread-like worms in the perianal area or the cellophane tape test for ova. Treatment is with pyrantel pamoate, mebendazole, or albendazole.

Pathophysiology

Infestation usually results from transfer of ova from the perianal area to fomites (clothing, bedding, furniture, rugs, toys), from which the ova are picked up by the new host, transmitted to the mouth, and swallowed. Thumb sucking is a risk factor. Reinfestation (autoinfestation) easily occurs through finger transfer of ova from the perianal area to the mouth.

Pinworms reach maturity in the lower GI tract within 2 to 6 wk. The female worm migrates to the perianal region (usually at night) to deposit ova. The sticky, gelatinous substance in which the ova are deposited and the movements of the female worm cause perianal pruritus. The ova can survive on fomites as long as 3 wk at normal room temperature. Pinworm infestation is the most common helminthic infection in the US, with an estimated 40 million people infected.

Symptoms, Signs, and Diagnosis

Most of those infected have no symptoms or signs, but some experience perianal pruritus and develop perianal excoriations from scratching. Rarely, migrating female worms ascend the human female genital tract, causing vaginitis and, on rare occasion, peritoneal lesions. Many other conditions have been attributed to pinworm infestation (eg, abdominal pain, insomnia, seizures), but a causal relationship is unlikely. Pinworms have been found obstructing the appendiceal lumen in cases of appendicitis, but the presence of the parasites may be coincidental.

Pinworm infestation can be diagnosed by finding the female worm, which is about 10 mm long (males average 3 mm), in the perianal region 1 or 2 h after a child goes to bed at night or in the morning, or by low-power microscopic identification of ova on cellophane tape. The ova are obtained in the early morning before the child arises by patting the perianal skinfolds with a strip of cellophane tape, which is then placed sticky side down on a glass slide and viewed microscopically. The 50 × 30 μm ova are oval with thin shells that contain a curled-up larva. A drop of toluene placed between tape and slide dissolves the adhesive and eliminates air bubbles under the tape that can hamper identification of the ova. This procedure should be repeated on 5 successive mornings if necessary. Eggs may also be encountered, but less frequently, in stool, urine, or vaginal smears.

Treatment

Because pinworm infestation is seldom harmful, prevalence is high, and reinfestation is common, treatment is indicated only for symptomatic infections. However, most parents actively seek treatment when their children have pinworms. A single dose of mebendazole 100 mg po (regardless of age) or albendazole 400 mg, repeated in 2 wk, is effective in eradicating pinworms (but not ova) in >90% of cases. A single dose of pyrantel pamoate 11 mg/kg po (maximum 1 g) initially and repeated after 2 wk is also effective. Reinfestation is common, because viable ova may be excreted for 1 wk after therapy, and ova deposited in the environment before therapy can survive 3 wk. Because multiple infestations within the household are the rule, treatment of the entire family may be necessary. Clothing, bedding, and other articles should be washed frequently and the environment vacuumed.

Carbolated petrolatum or other antipruritic creams or ointments used in the perianal region bid to tid may relieve itching.

STRONGYLOIDIASIS

(Threadworm Infection)

Strongyloidiasis is infection with *Strongyloides stercoralis*. Findings include rash and pulmonary symptoms (including cough and wheezing), eosinophilia, and abdominal pain with diarrhea. Diagnosis is by finding larvae in stool or small-bowel contents or by the detection of antibodies in blood. Treatment is with ivermectin, thiabendazole, or albendazole.

Etiology and Pathophysiology

Strongyloidiasis is endemic throughout the tropics and subtropics, including rural areas of the southern US, at sites where there is exposure of bare skin to contaminated soil and unsanitary conditions.

Adult worms live in the mucosa and submucosa of the duodenum and jejunum. Released eggs hatch in the bowel lumen, liberating rhabditiform larvae. Most of these larvae are excreted in the stool. After a few days in soil, they develop into infectious filariform larvae. Like hookworms, *Strongyloides* larvae penetrate the skin of humans, migrate via the bloodstream to the lungs, break through pulmonary capillaries, ascend the respiratory tract, are swallowed, and reach the intestine, where they mature in about 2 wk. In the soil, larvae that do not contact humans may develop to free-living adult worms that can reproduce for several generations before their larvae reenter a human host.

Some rhabditiform larvae convert within the intestine to infectious filariform larvae that immediately reenter the bowel wall, short-circuiting the life cycle (internal autoinfection). Sometimes filariform larvae are passed in stool and reenter through the skin of the buttocks and thighs. Autoinfection can result in extremely high worm burdens (hyperinfection syndrome) and explains why strongyloidiasis persists for many decades. Hyperinfection usually occurs in patients taking corticosteroids or with impaired cell-mediated immunity, particularly those infected with the human T-lymphotropic virus 1 (HTLV-1). Hyperinfection may represent activation of a previously asymptomatic or newly acquired *Strongyloides* infection. However, disseminated strongyloidiasis is less common than might be predicted among patients with AIDS, even those living in areas where *Strongyloides* is highly endemic.

Symptoms and Signs

Infection may be asymptomatic. Cutaneous symptoms sometimes result from an allergic reaction to migrating larvae; larva currens, a serpiginous, migratory, urticarial lesion, is pathognomonic, but nonspecific maculopapular or urticarial eruptions may occur. Pulmonary symptoms are uncommon, although heavy infections may produce Löffler's pneumonia, with cough, wheezing, and eosinophilia. GI symptoms include anorexia, epigastric pain and tenderness, diarrhea, nausea, and vomiting. In heavy infections, malabsorption and protein-losing enteropathy may result in weight loss and cachexia.

The hyperinfection syndrome can result in disseminated disease involving the CNS, lungs, skin, liver, and heart. Immunosuppression increases risk. GI and pulmonary symptoms are often prominent. Ileus, obstruction, massive GI bleeding, severe malabsorption, and peritonitis may occur. Pulmonary symptoms include dyspnea, hemoptysis, and respiratory failure. Infiltrates may be seen on chest x-ray. Other symptoms depend on the organ involved. CNS involvement includes parasitic meningitis, brain abscess, and diffuse invasion of the brain. Secondary gram-negative meningitis and bacteremia, which occurs with high frequency, probably reflects disruption of bowel mucosa and/or carriage of bacteria on migrating larvae. Liver infection may result in cholestatic and granulomatous hepatitis. Infection may be fatal in immunocompromised patients, even with treatment.

Diagnosis

Microscopic visualization of larvae in a single stool sample is successful about 25% of the time in uncomplicated infections. Repeated examination of concentrated stool or the agar-plate method raises the sensitivity to ≥ 85%. If the specimen stands at room temperature for several hours, rhabditiform larvae may transform into longer filariform larvae, leading to erroneous diagnosis of hyperinfection. Sampling of proximal small bowel by aspiration may be positive in low-level infections. The latter should be done endoscopically to permit biopsy of suspicious duodenal and jejunal lesions. In the hyperinfection syndrome, filariform larvae may be found in stool, duodenal contents, sputum, and bronchial washings, and uncommonly in CSF, urine, or pleural or ascitic fluid. Chest x-rays may show diffuse interstitial infiltrates, consolidation, or abscess.

Enzyme-linked immunosorbent assay (ELISA) for serum anti–*S. stercoralis* antibodies is > 90% sensitive but may be falsely positive in patients infected with other intestinal nematodes or filariasis. Specificity varies with the assay used.

Eosinophilia is often present but can be suppressed by drugs such as corticosteroids or cytotoxic chemotherapeutic agents.

Treatment and Prevention

Ivermectin (200 μg/kg po once/day for 1 or 2 days or single doses given at an interval of 2 wk) is effective for uncomplicated infection and is generally well tolerated. Doses of 200 μg/kg once/wk for 4 wk have been used for hyperinfection. Albendazole (400 mg bid for 2 days) is an alternative, but failures occur. Albendazole and ivermectin can be used together in hyperinfections. Cure should be documented by repeated stool examinations.

Thiabendazole was the drug of choice for strongyloidiasis, but it is more toxic than ivermectin and is no longer commercially available in the US. When thiabendazole is used, uncomplicated infection is treated with 25 mg/kg po bid for 2 days (maximum 3 g/day) and results in 80 to 90% cure. Repeated courses may be required. In hyperinfection syndrome, 25 mg/kg po bid should be given for a minimum of 5 to 7 days, but therapy should be continued for at least several days after parasites have disappeared from all sites. Adverse effects of thiabendazole, which are frequent and occasionally disabling, are nausea, vomiting, abdominal pain, dizziness, headache, paresthesia, malaise, pruritus, and flushing. Cure should be documented by repeated stool examination.

Prevention of primary infections is the same as for hookworms. To prevent potentially fatal hyperinfection syndrome, patients with possible exposure to *Strongyloides* (even in the distant past), patients with unexplained eosinophilia, and patients with symptoms suggestive of strongyloidiasis should undergo several stool examinations and serologic testing before receiving corticosteroids or other immunosuppressants. If infected, treatment for strongyloidiasis should be instituted and parasitologic cure documented before immunosuppression. Immunosuppressed people who have recurrent strongyloidiasis require additional courses of treatment until cured.

TOXOCARIASIS

(Visceral or Ocular Larva Migrans)

Toxocariasis is human infection with nematode ascarid larvae that ordinarily infect animals. Symptoms are fever, anorexia,

hepatosplenomegaly, rash, pneumonitis, asthma, or visual impairment. Diagnosis is by serologic assay. Treatment is with albendazole or mebendazole. Corticosteroids may be added for severe symptoms or eye involvement.

Etiology and Pathophysiology

The eggs of *Toxocara canis, T. cati*, and other animal ascarid helminths mature in soil and infect dogs, cats, and other animals. Eggs in their stools may be ingested by humans and hatch in the human intestine. Larvae penetrate the bowel wall and may migrate through liver, lungs, CNS, eyes, or other tissues. The larvae usually do not complete their development in the human body but can remain alive for many months.

Symptoms and Signs

Visceral larva migrans (VLM) consists of fever, anorexia, hepatosplenomegaly, rash, pneumonitis, and asthmatic symptoms, depending on the affected organs. Hyperglobulinemia, leukocytosis, and marked eosinophilia are common. Tissue damage is caused by focal eosinophilic granulomatous reactions to the migrating larvae. VLM occurs mostly in 2- to 5-yr-old children with a history of geophagia. The syndrome is self-limiting in 6 to 18 mo if egg intake ceases. Deaths due to invasion of the brain or heart occur rarely. Fatal infections have been reported in people infected with the raccoon ascarid, *Baylisascaris procyonis*, which may cause CNS infection in humans.

Ocular larva migrans (OLM), also called ocular toxocariasis, usually presents with no or very mild systemic manifestations. OLM lesions consist mostly of granulomatous reactions to a larva in the retina that may cause visual impairment. OLM occurs in older children and less commonly in young adults. The lesion may be confused with retinoblastoma or other intraocular tumor.

Diagnosis

Diagnosis is based on clinical, epidemiologic, and serologic findings. There is a highly specific enzyme-linked immunosorbent assay (ELISA) for antibodies to *T. canis*. Biopsies of the liver or other affected organs may show eosinophilic granulomatous reactions, but larvae are difficult to find in tissue sections and biopsies are low yield. Stool examinations are worthless. OLM should be distinguished from retinoblastoma to prevent unnecessary surgical enucleation of the eye.

Treatment and Prevention

No proven treatment for VLM is available, but mebendazole 100 to 200 mg po bid for 5 days or albendazole 400 mg po bid for 5 days is often used. Antihistamines may suffice for mild symptoms. Corticosteroids (prednisone 20 to 40 mg po once/day) are indicated in those with severe symptoms. Corticosteroids, both local and oral, are also indicated for acute OLM. Laser photocoagulation has been used to kill larvae in the retina.

Infection in puppies with *T. canis* is common in the US. Infection with *T. cati* in cats is less common, but both should be dewormed regularly. Contact with dirt or sand contaminated with animal feces should be minimized.

TRICHINOSIS

(Trichiniasis)

Trichinosis is infection with *Trichinella spiralis* or related *Trichinella* species. Symptoms include initial GI irritation followed by periorbital edema, muscle pain, fever, and eosinophilia. Diagnosis is clinical and with serologic tests. Muscle biopsy may be diagnostic but is seldom necessary. Treatment is with mebendazole or albendazole plus prednisone if symptoms are severe.

Etiology and Pathophysiology

Trichinosis occurs worldwide. In addition to the classic agent *T. spiralis*, trichinosis can be caused by *T. pseudospiralis, T. nativa, T. nelsoni*, and *T. britovi*. The life cycle is maintained by animals that are fed (eg, pigs, horses) or eat (eg, bears, foxes, boars) other animals whose striated muscles contain encysted infective larvae (eg, rodents). Humans become infected by eating raw, undercooked, or processed meat from infected animals, most commonly pigs, wild boar, or bear. Larvae undergo excystation in the small bowel, penetrate the mucosa, and become adults in 6 to 8 days. Mature females release living larvae for 4 to 6 wk and then die or are expelled. Newborn larvae migrate through the bloodstream and body but ultimately survive only within striated skeletal muscle cells. Larvae fully encyst in 1 to 2 mo and remain viable for several years as intracellular parasites. Dead larvae eventually are resorbed or calcify. The cycle continues only if encysted larvae are ingested by another carnivore.

Symptoms and Signs

Many infections are asymptomatic or mild. During the 1st wk, nausea, abdominal cramps, and diarrhea may occur. One to 2 wk after infection, systemic symptoms and signs begin: facial or periorbital edema, myalgia, persistent fever, headache, and subconjunctival hemorrhages and petechiae. Eye pain and photophobia often precede myalgia.

Symptoms from muscle invasion may mimic polymyositis. The muscles of respiration, speech, mastication, and swallowing may be painful. Severe dyspnea may occur in heavy infections.

Fever is generally remittent, rising to 39° C or higher, remaining elevated for several days, and then falling gradually. Eosinophilia usually begins when newborn larvae invade tissues, peaks 2 to 4 wk after infection, and gradually declines as the larvae encyst.

In heavy infections, the inflammation may cause cardiac (myocarditis, heart failure, arrhythmia), neurologic (encephalitis, meningitis, visual or auditory disorders, seizures), or pulmonary (pneumonitis, pleurisy) complications. Death may result from myocarditis or encephalitis.

Signs and symptoms gradually improve, and most disappear by about the 3rd mo, when the larvae have become fully encysted in muscle cells and eliminated from other organs and tissues. Vague muscular pains and fatigue may persist for months. Recurrent infections with *T. nativa* can cause chronic diarrhea.

Diagnosis

No specific tests to diagnose the intestinal stage are available. After the 2nd wk of infection, a muscle biopsy may disclose larvae and cysts but is seldom necessary. Diffuse inflammation in muscle tissue indicates recent infection.

Serologic tests are performed for those with suspected infection. Because results may be falsely negative, especially if done within the first 2 to 3 wk of infection, tests should be repeated after 1 mo. Because antibodies may persist for years, serologic tests are of most value if they are initially negative and then turn positive. Serology and muscle biopsy are complementary tests: either one can be negative in a given patient. Skin testing with larval antigens is unreliable.

Muscle enzymes (creatine phosphokinase and LDH) are elevated in 50% of patients and correlate with abnormal electromyograms.

Trichinosis must be differentiated from acute rheumatic fever, acute arthritis, angioedema, and myositis; febrile illnesses such as TB, typhoid fever, sepsis, and undulant fever; pneumonitis; the neurologic manifestations of meningitis, encephalitis, and poliomyelitis; and eosinophilia from Hodgkin lymphoma, eosinophilic leukemia, polyarteritis nodosa, and disease caused by other migrating nematodes.

Treatment and Prevention

Anthelmintics, mebendazole (200 to 400 mg po tid for 3 days, then 400 to 500 mg tid for 10 days) or albendazole (400 mg bid for 8 to 14 days), eliminate adult worms from the GI tract, but probably have little effect on encysted larvae.

Analgesics (eg, NSAIDs or opioids) may be required for muscle pains. For severe allergic manifestations or myocardial or CNS involvement, prednisone 20 to 60 mg po once/day is given for 3 or 4 days then tapered over 10 to 14 days.

Trichinosis is prevented by cooking meat thoroughly until brown (71° C [160° F] throughout). Larvae can usually be killed by freezing the meat at −17° C (5° F) for 3 wk or −30° C (−20° F) for 6 days, but *T. nativa* is relatively resistant. Smoking or salting meat does not reliably kill larvae. Domestic swine should not be fed uncooked meat products.

TRICHURIASIS

(Whipworm Infection; Trichocephaliasis)

Trichuriasis is infection with *Trichuris trichiura*. Symptoms may include abdominal pain, diarrhea, and in heavy infections, anemia and malnutrition. Diagnosis is by finding eggs in stool. Treatment is with mebendazole or albendazole.

Infection is spread via the fecal-oral route. Ingested eggs hatch in the duodenum, where the larvae invade and mature in the mucosa before migrating to the large bowel. Adult whiplike worms embed their heads into the superficial mucosa of the colon and cecum, where they may live 7 to 10 yr.

The parasite occurs principally in the tropics and subtropics. Mild asymptomatic infections occur in rural parts of the southern US.

Light infections are often asymptomatic. Heavy infections cause abdominal pain, anorexia, and diarrhea and may result in anemia or retarded growth. Very heavy infections may cause weight loss, anemia, and rectal prolapse, particularly in children.

The characteristic lemon-shaped eggs with clear opercula at both ends are readily found in feces.

Mebendazole 100 mg po bid for 3 days and albendazole 400 mg po once are recommended. When albendazole is used for heavy infections, most experts recommend 400 mg once/day for 3 days. Ivermectin and nitazoxanide are alternatives. These drugs should not be used during pregnancy. Prevention requires adequate sanitation and good personal hygiene.

183 TREMATODES (FLUKES)

Flukes are parasitic flat worms that infect the blood vessels, GI tract, lungs, or liver. They are often categorized according to the organ system they invade. *Schistosoma* sp infect the vasculature of the GI or GU systems; *Fasciolopsis buski, Heterophyes heterophyes*, and related organisms, the lumen of the GI tract; *Clonorchis sinensis, Fasciola hepatica*, and *Opisthorchis* sp, the liver; and *Paragonimus westermani* and related sp, the lungs and other organs such as the CNS.

CLONORCHIASIS

(Oriental Liver Fluke Infection)

Clonorchiasis is infection with the liver fluke *Clonorchis sinensis*. Infection is through undercooked freshwater fish. Symptoms include fever, chills, epigastric pain, tender hepatomegaly, diarrhea, and mild jaundice. Diagnosis is by identifying eggs in the feces or duodenal contents or occasionally by percutaneous transhepatic cholangiography. Treatment is with praziquantel or albendazole.

Adult *C. sinensis* worms live in the bile ducts. Eggs are passed in the stool and ingested by snails. Cercariae released from infected snails subsequently infect a variety of freshwater fish. Humans become infected by eating raw, dried, salted, or pickled fish containing encysted metacercariae. The latter are released in the duodenum, enter the common bile duct, and migrate to smaller intrahepatic ducts (or occasionally the gallbladder and pancreatic ducts), where they mature into adult worms in about 1 mo. The adults may live ≥ 20 yr.

Clonorchis is endemic in the Far East, especially in Korea, Japan, Taiwan, and southern China, and infection occurs elsewhere among immigrants and those eating fish imported from endemic areas.

Light infections are usually asymptomatic. Heavier infections can cause fever, chills, epigastric pain, tender hepatomegaly, mild jaundice, and eosinophilia. Later, diarrhea may occur. Chronic cholangitis in heavy infections may progress to atrophy of liver parenchyma, portal fibrosis, and cirrhosis. Jaundice may occur if a mass of flukes obstructs the biliary tree. Other complications include suppurative cholangitis, chronic pancreatitis, and, late in the course, cholangiocarcinoma.

Diagnosis is by finding eggs in the feces or duodenal contents. The eggs are difficult to distinguish from those of *Metagonimus, Heterophyes*, and *Opisthorchis*. Other tests are nondiagnostic but may be abnormal; alkaline phosphatase, bilirubin, and eosinophil counts may be elevated. A plain abdominal x-ray occasionally shows intrahepatic calcification. Hepatic ultrasound may show ductal irregularities and evidence of scarring.

Treatment is with praziquantel 25 mg/kg po tid for 1 day or albendazole 10 mg/kg po once/day for 7 days. Biliary obstruction may require surgery. Freshwater fish from endemic waters should be thoroughly cooked and not eaten raw, pickled, or wine-soaked.

FASCIOLIASIS

Fascioliasis is infection with the liver fluke *Fasciola hepatica*, which is acquired by eating contaminated watercress.

F. hepatica is the sheep and cattle liver fluke. Incidental human fascioliasis, acquired by eating watercress contaminated by sheep or cattle dung, occurs in Europe, Africa, China, and South America but is rare in the US.

In acute infection, larvae migrate through the intestinal wall, the peritoneal cavity, the liver capsule, and the parenchyma of the liver before maturing to adulthood. Acute infection causes abdominal pain, intermittent fever, eosinophilia, malaise, and weight loss due to liver damage. Chronic infection may be asymptomatic or lead to intermittent biliary tract obstruction.

CT scans frequently reveal hypodense lesions in the liver. Antibody detection assays are useful in the early stages of disease. Eggs may be recovered in the stool or in duodenal or biliary materials during chronic infection.

Treatment is with triclabendazole, where it is available, or bithionol 30 to 50 mg/kg po every other day for 10 to 15 doses. Treatment failures are common with praziquantel.

FASCIOLOPSIASIS

Fasciolopsiasis is infection with the intestinal fluke *Fasciolopsis buski*, which is acquired by eating aquatic plants.

F. buski is present in the intestine of pigs in many parts of Asia. Human infection is acquired by eating aquatic plants, such as water chestnuts, bearing infectious metacercariae. Adult worms attach to and ulcerate the mucosa of the proximal small bowel, thereby causing diarrhea, abdominal pain, and signs of malabsorption. Treatment is with praziquantel 25 mg/kg po tid for 1 day.

HETEROPHYIASIS AND RELATED TREMATODE INFECTIONS

Heterophyiasis is infection with the intestinal fluke *Heterophyes heterophyes*, which is acquired by eating infected, raw or undercooked freshwater fish.

Heterophyes heterophyes and several related trematodes are endemic in the Far East, Southeast Asia, Nile Delta, and other areas of the world. Infection is acquired by eating infected, raw or undercooked fish from freshwater or brackish water. Salmon live part of their lives in freshwater and can be infected with *Nanophyetus salmincola*. Adult flukes can cause abdominal pain and diarrhea. Treatment with praziquantel is the same as for fasciolopsiasis.

OPISTHORCHIASIS

Opisthorchiasis is infection with 1 of 2 species of the liver fluke *Opisthorchis*, which is acquired by eating infected, raw or undercooked fish.

Opisthorchiasis occurs in cats and dogs in eastern and central Europe, Siberia, and parts of Asia, such as Thailand and Cambodia. The life cycle of *Opisthorchis* requires both snails and fish. Human disease resembles clonorchiasis and is acquired by eating raw or undercooked freshwater fish that contains infectious metacercariae. Infection may lead to cholangiocarcinoma. Praziquantel 25 mg/kg po tid for 1 day is the treatment of choice.

PARAGONIMIASIS

(Oriental Lung Fluke Infection; Endemic Hemoptysis)

Paragonimiasis is infection with the lung fluke *Paragonimus westermani* and related sp. Human infection is through raw, pickled, or poorly cooked freshwater crustaceans. Symptoms include dyspnea, chronic cough, chest pain, and hemoptysis. Allergic skin reactions and CNS abnormalities, including seizures, aphasia, paresis, and visual disturbances, can also occur. Diagnosis is by identifying eggs in sputum, stool, or pleural or peritoneal fluid. Serologic tests are also available. Praziquantel is the treatment of choice; bithionol is an alternative.

Although > 30 species of *Paragonimus* can infect humans, *P. westermani* is the most frequent cause of disease. The most important endemic areas are in the Far East, principally Korea, Japan, Taiwan, the highlands of China, and the Philippines. Endemic foci also exist in West Africa and in parts of South and Central America.

Eggs passed in sputum or feces develop for 2 to 3 wk in freshwater before miracidia hatch. The miracidia invade snails; larvae develop and multiply and eventually emerge as cercariae. Cercariae penetrate freshwater crabs or crayfish and encyst to form metacercariae. Humans become infected by eating raw, pickled, or poorly cooked crustaceans. Metacercariae excyst in the human GI tract, penetrate the intestinal wall into the peritoneum, migrate to and through the diaphragm into the pleural cavity, enter lung tissue, encyst, and develop into hermaphroditic adult worms. Worms may also develop in the brain, liver, lymph nodes, skin, and spinal cord. Adult flukes may persist for 20 to 25 yr.

Symptoms, Signs, and Diagnosis

Most damage is to the lungs, but other organs may be involved. About 25 to 45% of all extrapulmonary infections affect the CNS. Manifestations of pulmonary infection develop slowly and include chronic cough, chest pain, hemoptysis, and dyspnea. The clinical picture resembles, and is often confused with, TB. Cerebral infections present as space-occupying lesions, often within a year after the onset of pulmonary disease. Seizures, aphasia, paresis, and visual disturbances are common. Migratory allergic skin lesions similar to those of cutaneous larva migrans are common in infections with *P. skriabini* but also occur with other species.

Diagnosis is by identifying the characteristic large operculated eggs in sputum or stool. Occasionally, eggs may be found in pleural or peritoneal fluid. Eggs may be difficult to find because they are released intermittently and in small numbers. Concentration techniques increase sensitivity. X-rays provide ancillary information but are not diagnostic; chest x-rays may show a diffuse infiltrate, nodules and annular opacities, cavitations, lung abscesses, pleural effusion, and pneumothorax. Serologic tests may assist in diagnosis of light or extrapulmonary infections.

Treatment and Prevention

Praziquantel 25 mg/kg po tid for 2 days cures 80 to 100% of pulmonary infections and is the drug of choice. Bithionol 30 to 50 mg/kg po every other day for 10 to 15 doses is an alternative but has more adverse effects. Praziquantel is used to treat extrapulmonary infections, but multiple courses may be required. Surgery may be needed to excise skin lesions or, rarely, brain cysts.

The best prevention is to avoid eating raw or undercooked freshwater crabs and crayfish from endemic waters.

SCHISTOSOMIASIS

(Bilharziasis)

Schistosomiasis is infection with blood flukes of the genus *Schistosoma*, which are acquired transcutaneously by swimming or wading in contaminated waters. The organisms infect the vasculature of the GI or GU system. Acute symptoms are dermatitis, followed several weeks later by fever, chills, nausea, abdominal pain, diarrhea, malaise, and myalgia. Chronic symptoms vary with species but include bloody diarrhea and hematuria. Diagnosis is by identifying eggs in stool, urine, or biopsy specimens. Serologic tests are sensitive and specific. Treatment is with praziquantel.

Etiology and Pathophysiology

Schistosomiasis is by far the most important trematode infection. *Schistosoma* is the only trematode that invades through the skin; all other trematodes infect only via ingestion. About 200 million people are infected worldwide. The risk of infection is spreading as new dams are built in endemic areas.

There are 5 species of schistosomes, all with similar life cycles involving freshwater snails. *S. haematobium*, which causes urinary tract disease, is widely distributed over the African continent with smaller foci in the Middle East and India. The other *Schistosoma* sp cause intestinal disease. *S. mansoni* is widespread in Africa and is the only species in the Western Hemisphere, endemic in Brazil, Surinam, Venezuela, and on some Caribbean islands. *S. japonicum* is present only in Asia, mainly in China and the Philippines. *S. mekongi* is in Laos and Cambodia; *S. intercalatum* is in Central Africa. The disease may be imported in travelers and immigrants from endemic areas, but transmission does not occur within the US and Canada.

Adult worms live and copulate within the veins of the mesentery or bladder, depending on the species. Some eggs penetrate the intestinal or bladder mucosa and are passed in stool or urine; other eggs remain within the host organ or are transported through the portal system to the liver, and occasionally to other sites (eg, lungs, CNS, spinal cord). Excreted eggs hatch in freshwater, liberating miracidia that enter snails. After multiplication, thousands of free-swimming cercariae are released. These penetrate human skin within a few minutes after exposure and transform into schistosomulae, which travel through the bloodstream to the lungs, where they mature in about 6 wk. Subsequently they migrate to their ultimate home in the intestinal veins or the venous plexus of the GU tract. Eggs appear in stool or urine 1 to 3 mo after cercarial penetration. Estimates of the adult worm life span range from 3 to 37 yr.

Symptoms and Signs

Schistosome dermatitis is a pruritic papular rash where the cercariae penetrate the skin (see also Dermatitis Caused by Avian and Animal Schistosomes, below) in previously sensitized people.

Acute schistosomiasis (Katayama fever) occurs with onset of egg laying, typically 2 to 4 wk after heavy exposure. Symptoms include fever, chills, nausea, abdominal pain, malaise, myalgia, urticarial rashes, and marked eosinophilia, resembling serum sickness. Manifestations are more common and usually more severe in visitors than in residents of endemic areas and typically last for several weeks.

Chronic schistosomiasis results mostly from host responses to eggs retained in tissues. Early on, intestinal mucosal ulcerations caused by *S. mansoni* or *S. japonicum* may bleed and produce bloody diarrhea. As lesions progress, focal fibrosis, strictures, fistulas, and papillomatous growths may develop. With *S. haematobium*, ulcerations in the bladder wall may cause dysuria, hematuria, and urinary frequency. Over time, chronic cystitis develops. Strictures may lead to hydroureter and hydronephrosis. Papillomatous masses in the bladder are common, and squamous cell carcinoma may develop. Blood loss from both GI and GU tracts frequently results in anemia.

Secondary bacterial infection of the GU tract and persistent *Salmonella* septicemia associated with *S. mansoni* are also common. Several species, notably *S. haematobium*, can cause genital disease in both men and women, resulting in numerous symptoms including infertility.

Granulomatous reactions to eggs of *S. mansoni* and *S. japonicum* in the liver usually do not compromise liver function but may produce fibrosis and cirrhosis, which can lead to portal hypertension and subsequent hematemesis from esophageal varices. Eggs in the lungs may produce granulomas and focal obliterative arteritis, which may cause pulmonary hypertension and cor pulmonale. Eggs lodged in the spinal cord can cause transverse myelitis, and those in the CNS can cause seizures.

Diagnosis

Eggs are sought in the stool (*S. japonicum, S. mansoni, S. mekongi, S. intercalatum*) or urine (*S. haematobium* and occasionally *S. japonicum*). Repeated examinations using concentration techniques may be necessary. Geography is a primary determinant of species, so a history of exposure should be communicated to the laboratory. If the clinical picture suggests schistosomiasis but no eggs are found on repeated examination of urine or feces, intestinal or bladder mucosa can be biopsied for eggs.

Serologic tests are highly sensitive and specific for infection but do not provide information on worm burdens, clinical status, or prognosis.

Treatment and Prevention

Single-day oral treatment with praziquantel (20 mg/kg bid for *S. haematobium, S. mansoni*, and *S. intercalatum*; 20 mg/kg tid for *S. japonicum* and *S. mekongi*) is recommended. However, treatment does not affect developing schistosomulae and thus may not abort an early infection. Adverse effects are generally mild and include abdominal pain, diarrhea, headache, and dizziness. Therapeutic failures have been reported, but it is difficult to determine whether they are due to reinfection or drug-resistant strains. Oxamniquine (not available in the US) is effective only against *S. mansoni*. African strains are more resistant to this drug than South American strains and require larger doses (30 mg/kg po once/day for 1 or 2 days vs 15 mg/kg once). Oxamniquine-resistant cases have been observed.

Patients should be examined for living eggs 3 and 6 mo after treatment. Retreatment is indicated if egg excretion has not decreased markedly. In the future, antigen detection tests may supplant quantitative egg counts as tools to monitor response to chemotherapy.

Scrupulously avoiding contact with contaminated water prevents infection. The sanitary disposal of urine and feces reduces the likelihood of infection. Adult residents of endemic areas are more resistant to reinfection than children, suggesting the possibility of acquired immunity. Vaccine development is under way.

DERMATITIS CAUSED BY AVIAN AND ANIMAL SCHISTOSOMES

(Cercarial Dermatitis; Swimmers' Itch; Clam Diggers' Itch)

Cercarial dermatitis is a skin condition that develops when *Schistosoma* sp that cannot develop in humans penetrate the skin.

Cercariae of *Schistosoma* sp that infect birds and mammals other than humans can penetrate the skin. Although the organisms do not develop in humans, humans may become sensitized and develop pruritic maculopapular skin lesions at the site of penetration. Skin lesions may be accompanied by a systemic febrile response that runs for 5 to 7 days and resolves spontaneously.

Saltwater schistosome dermatitis (clam diggers' itch) occurs on all Atlantic, Gulf, Pacific, and Hawaiian coasts. It is very common in muddy flats off Cape Cod. Freshwater schistosome dermatitis (swimmers' itch) is common in lakes of northern Michigan, Wisconsin, and Minnesota. Diagnosis is based on clinical findings. Most cases do not require medical attention. Treatment is symptomatic with cool compresses, baking soda, or antipruritic lotions. Topical corticosteroids can also be used.

184 CESTODES (TAPEWORMS)

All tapeworms (cestodes) cycle through 3 stages—eggs, larvae, and adults. Adults inhabit the intestines of definitive hosts, mammalian carnivores. Several of the adult tapeworms that infect humans are named after their intermediate host: the fish tapeworm (*Diphyllobothrium latum*), the beef tapeworm (*Taenia saginata*), and the pork tapeworm (*Taenia solium*). Eggs are excreted with feces into the environment and ingested by an intermediate host (typically another species) in which larvae develop, enter the circulation, and encyst in the musculature or other organs. When the intermediate host is eaten, cysts develop into adult tapeworms in the intestines of the definitive host, restarting the cycle. With some cestode species (eg, *T. solium*), the definitive host can also serve as an intermediate host and develop tissue cysts instead of intestinal worms if eggs are ingested.

Adult cestodes are typically long, multisegmented flat worms that lack a digestive tract and absorb nutrients directly from the host's small bowel. The longest parasite in the world is the 40-m whale tapeworm, *Polygonoporus sp.* Tapeworms have 3 recognizable portions. The scolex (head) functions as an anchoring organ that attaches to intestinal mucosa. The neck is an unsegmented region of high regenerative capacity. If treatment fails to eliminate the neck and scolex, the entire worm may regenerate. The rest of the worm consists of numerous proglottids (segments). Proglottids closest to the neck are undifferentiated. As proglottids move caudally, each develops hermaphroditic sex organs. Distal proglottids are gravid and contain eggs in a uterus.

In contrast to adult tapeworms, larvae can cause severe and even lethal disease, most importantly in the brain, but also in the liver, lungs, eyes, muscles, and subcutaneous tissues. In humans, *T. solium* causes cysticercosis, and *Echinococcus granulosus* and *E. multilocularis cause* hydatid disease. *Sparganum mansoni* and *T. multiceps* larvae also can infect humans.

Symptoms, Signs, and Diagnosis

Adult tapeworms are so well adapted to their hosts that they cause minimal symptoms. Larvae, however, may elicit intense immunologic reactions as they travel through tissues (hence inducing immunity) and cause severe disease when they settle in extraintestinal sites.

Adult tapeworm infections are diagnosed by identifying eggs or gravid proglottid segments in stool. Larval disease is best identified by imaging studies, such as brain CT or MRI, and for some species, serologic tests.

Treatment and Prevention

The anthelmintic agents, praziquantel and niclosamide, are effective for most intestinal tapeworm infections. Some extraintestinal infections respond to anthelmintic treatment, whereas others require surgical intervention.

Prevention and control are by thorough cooking (to temperature > 57° C [> 135° F]) of pork, beef, lamb, game meat, and fish; regular worming of dogs and cats; preventing recycling through hosts, such as dogs eating dead game or livestock; reduction and avoidance of intermediate hosts such as rodents, fleas, and grain beetles; meat inspection; and sanitary treatment of human waste. Prolonged freezing of meat is effective, pickling is variably effective, and smoking and drying are ineffective.

DIPHYLLOBOTHRIASIS

(Fish Tapeworm Infection)

Diphyllobothriasis is infection with the freshwater fish intestinal tapeworm, *Diphyllobothrium latum*. Treatment is with praziquantel.

D. latum is the largest parasite of humans (up to 10 m in length). It and *Sparganum mansoni* are the only human tapeworms with aquatic life cycles. In freshwater, eggs of *D. latum* from human feces hatch free-swimming larvae, which are ingested by microcrustaceans that are themselves ingested by fish, in which the larvae become infective. Diphyllobothriasis occurs worldwide, especially where cool lakes are contaminated by sewage. Infections in the US and northern Europe occur in people who eat raw freshwater fish. Infection is less common with current sewage treatment.

Infection is usually asymptomatic, but mild GI symptoms may be noted. Fish tapeworms take up dietary vitamin B_{12}, which occasionally results in B_{12} deficiency and megaloblastic anemia. Diagnosis is by identification of characteristic operculated eggs or broad proglottids in the stool.

Treatment is with a single oral dose of praziquantel, 5 to 10 mg/kg. Vitamin B_{12} may be needed to correct the anemia. Thorough cooking of freshwater fish or freezing at −10° C (14° F) for 48 h prevents infection.

DIPYLIDIUM CANINUM INFECTION

***Dipylidium caninum* can cause intestinal infection, which is typically asymptomatic.**

D. caninum, the double-pored tapeworm, is present in dogs and cats. Fleas are the intermediate host. Ingestion of an infected flea, usually by a young child, produces an asymptomatic, self-limited infection, but proglottids may be seen in the stool.

ECHINOCOCCOSIS

(Hydatid Disease)

Echinococcosis is infection with larvae of *Echinococcus granulosus* or *E. multilocularis* (alveolar hydatid disease). Symptoms, such as jaundice, abdominal discomfort, cough, chest pain, and hemoptysis, arise from cysts in vital organs. Cyst rupture can cause fever, urticaria, and serious anaphylactic reactions. Diagnosis is with imaging tests, examination of cyst fluid, or serologic tests. Treatment is with albendazole and/or surgery or cyst aspiration and instillation of a scolicidal agent.

Echinococcus granulosus is common in sheep-raising areas of the Mediterranean, Middle East, Australia, New Zealand, South Africa, and South America. It requires canines as definitive hosts and herbivores (eg, sheep, horses, deer) or humans as intermediate hosts. Foci also exist in regions of Canada, Alaska, and California.

E. multilocularis worms are present in foxes, and the hydatid larvae are found in small wild rodents. Infected dogs and other canines are the main link to occasional human infection. *E. multilocularis* occurs mainly in Central Europe, Alaska, Canada, and Siberia. Its range of natural infection in the continental US extends from Wyoming and the Dakotas to the upper Midwest. On rare occasion, *E. vogelii* or *E. oliganthus* cause polycystic hydatid disease in humans, primarily in the liver.

Etiology and Pathophysiology

Ingested eggs from animal feces (which may be present in the fur of dogs or other animals) hatch in the gut; penetrate the intestinal wall; migrate via the circulation; and lodge in the liver or lungs, or, less frequently, in the brain, bone, or other organs. *E. granulosus* larvae develop slowly (usually over many years) into large unilocular, fluid-filled lesions—hydatid cysts. Brood capsules containing numerous small infective protoscolices form within these cysts. Large cysts may contain > 1 L of highly antigenic hydatid fluid as well as millions of protoscolices. Daughter cysts sometimes form within or outside primary cysts. If the cyst leaks or ruptures, infection can spread to the peritoneum. *E. multilocularis* produces spongy masses that are locally invasive and difficult or impossible to treat surgically. Cysts are found primarily in the liver but can metastasize to the lungs, lymph nodes, and other tissues.

Symptoms and Signs

Although many infections are acquired in childhood, clinical signs may not appear for years, except when cysts are in vital organs. Symptoms and signs may resemble those of a space-occupying tumor. In the liver, they eventually produce abdominal pain or a palpable mass. Jaundice may occur if the bile duct is obstructed. Rupture into the bile duct, abdominal or peritoneal cavity, or lung may produce fever, urticaria, or a serious anaphylactic reaction. Pulmonary cysts are usually discovered on routine chest x-ray as round, often irregular, pulmonary masses. Pulmonary cysts can rupture, causing cough, chest pain, and hemoptysis.

Diagnosis

CT, MRI, and ultrasound scans may be pathognomonic if daughter cysts and hydatid sand (protoscolices and debris) are present, but simple hydatid cysts may be difficult to differentiate from simple benign cysts, abscesses, or benign or malignant tumors. The presence of hydatid sand in aspirated cyst fluid is diagnostic. Serologic tests (enzyme immunoassay, immunofluorescent assay) are variably sensitive but are useful if positive and should be obtained. Eosinophilia on CBC may be present.

Treatment

For *E. granulosis*, albendazole 400 mg po bid for 1 to 6 mo (7.5 mg/kg bid in children) is curative in 30 to 40% of patients and can be used to suppress growth in inoperable cases. Surgery, sometimes via laparoscopy, can be curative. Albendazole is often given before surgery to prevent metastatic infections if there is spillage of cyst contents. Some centers perform percutaneous aspiration under CT guidance followed by instillation of a scolecocidal agent (eg, hypertonic saline) and reaspiration (the PAIR technique—percutaneous aspiration-injection-reaspiration).

Prognosis for *E. multilocularis* infection is poor unless the entire larval mass can be removed. Surgery is indicated if it is feasible, which depends on the size, location, and manifestations of the lesion. Albendazole in the above doses can suppress the growth of inoperable lesions. Liver transplantation has been lifesaving in a few patients.

HYMENOLEPIS NANA INFECTION

(Dwarf Tapeworm Infection)

***Hymenolepis nana*, a small intestinal tapeworm, is the most common human cestode; it is treated with praziquantel.**

H. nana is only 15 to 40 mm long. It requires only one host but can also cycle through two. Its larvae migrate only within the gut wall, and its life span is relatively short (4 to 6 wk). *H. nana* is more frequent in populations living under conditions of poverty and poor hygiene, particularly when fleas are present.

H. nana has 3 modes of infection: (1) an indirect 2-host cycle involving rodents as primary definitive hosts and grain beetles, fleas, or other insects that feed on contaminated rodent droppings as intermediate hosts; (2) an oral-anal cycle in which eggs are passed from one human to another or recycle externally in a single host; and (3) internal autoinfection, whereby eggs hatch within the gut and initiate a 2nd generation without ever exiting the host. Autoinfection can result in massive numbers of worms, which can produce nausea, vomiting, diarrhea, abdominal pain, weight loss, and nonspecific systemic symptoms. The pronounced cellular and humoral response to the tissue phase of *H. nana* infection probably provides some protection for adults living in endemic areas.

Diagnosis is made by finding eggs in stool samples. Praziquantel 25 mg/kg po once is the treatment of choice.

HYMENOLEPIS DIMINUTA INFECTION

***Hymenolepis diminuta* can cause intestinal infection.**

H. diminuta, the rat tapeworm, has a life cycle similar to the indirect cycle of *Hymenolepis nana*, involving grain insects (see above). It rarely infects humans but can cause mild diarrhea. Diagnosis is by finding characteristic eggs in stool. Infection is effectively treated with praziquantel.

MULTICEPS INFECTION

***Multiceps* sp, a rare cause of human infection, is acquired by accidental ingestion of dog feces.**

Canines are the definitive hosts for adult *Multiceps* tapeworms; sheep and other herbivorous animals are intermediate hosts. Unwitting ingestion of dog feces causes human disease. The larva, termed a coenurus, forms a cyst in human tissues.

Symptoms require several years to develop and depend on the organ infected. Involvement of the brain causes increased intracranial pressure, seizures, loss of consciousness, and focal neurologic deficits. Diagnosis usually comes after surgical resection of a space-occupying lesion.

SPARGANOSIS

Sparganosis is infection with larvae of the tapeworm *Sparganum mansoni*.

S. mansoni affects dogs, cats, and other carnivores. Eggs are passed into freshwater where they are ingested by copepods (eg, *Cyclops*). Frogs, reptiles, and various small mammals ingest them and serve as intermediate hosts. Humans can become infected by accidental ingestion of copepods from water contaminated by cat or dog feces, ingestion of inadequately cooked flesh from another intermediate host, or contact with poultices containing flesh from these sources. In humans, larvae typically migrate to subcutaneous tissue or muscle and form slowly growing masses. Other sites, including the CNS, may be involved but are much less common. Symptoms are caused by mass effect, and disease may be discovered through imaging studies.

Diagnosis is typically made after surgical removal. Praziquantel has been used to treat cerebral sparganosis, although its efficacy is undocumented.

TAENIASIS SAGINATA

(Beef Tapeworm Infection)

Infection with the beef tapeworm, *Taenia saginata*, may produce mild GI upset or passage of a motile segment in the stool. It is treated with praziquantel.

Cattle are intermediate hosts for *T. saginata*. Humans are infected by eating cysticerci in raw or undercooked beef. The larvae mature in about 2 mo to adult worms (usually only 1 to 2 are present) that can live for several years.

Infection occurs worldwide but especially in cattle-raising regions of the tropics and subtropics in Africa, the Middle East, Eastern Europe, Mexico, and South America. Infection is uncommon in US cattle and is monitored by federal inspection.

Passage of a motile segment often brings an otherwise asymptomatic patient to medical attention. Other patients may have mild digestive symptoms. The stool should be examined for proglottids and eggs; eggs may also be present on anal swabs. The ova of *T. saginata* are indistinguishable from those of *T. solium* (pork tapeworm), as are the clinical features and management of intestinal infections.

Treatment is with a single oral dose of praziquantel, 5 or 10 mg/kg. Alternatively, a single 2-g dose of niclosamide is given as 4 tablets (500 mg each) that are chewed one at a time and swallowed with a small amount of water (40 to 50 mg/kg once for children). Both drugs have cure rates of about 90%. Treatment can be considered successful when no proglottids are passed for 4 mo.

TAENIASIS SOLIUM AND CYSTICERCOSIS

(Pork Tapeworm Infection)

Taeniasis solium is infection with adult worms that follows ingestion of contaminated pork. Cysticercosis is infection with larvae of *Taenia solium* from ova in human feces. Adult worms may produce mild GI symptoms or passage of a motile segment in the stool. Symptoms with cysticercosis are usually absent unless larvae invade the CNS, which can cause seizures and various other neurologic signs. Neurocysticercosis may be recognized on brain imaging studies. Less than half of patients with neurocysticercosis have adult *T. solium* in their intestines and thus eggs or proglottids in their stool. Adult worms can be eradicated with praziquantel. Treatment of symptomatic neurocysticercosis is with corticosteroids, anticonvulsants, and, in some situations, albendazole or praziquantel. Surgery may be required.

Etiology and Pathophysiology

Humans infected with adult *T. solium* worms are asymptomatic or have mild GI complaints. The presentation, diagnosis, and management are similar to beef tapeworm infection (see above). However, humans may also act as intermediate hosts for *T. solium* larvae if they ingest *T. solium* eggs from human excreta. It has also been postulated that if an adult tapeworm is present in the intestine, gravid proglottids may be passed retrograde from the intestine to the stomach, where oncospheres (immature form of the parasite) may hatch and migrate to subcutaneous tissue, muscle, viscera, and CNS.

Cysticercosis is prevalent, and neurocysticercosis is a major cause of epilepsy in Latin America, Africa, Southeast Asia, and Eastern Europe. Infection in the US is most common in immigrants from those areas but has occurred in North Americans who have not traveled abroad; they have apparently been infected through exposure to immigrants harboring adult *T. solium*.

Symptoms, Signs, and Diagnosis

Viable cysticerci in most organs cause minimal or no tissue reaction, but death of the cysts in the CNS can elicit an intense tissue response. Thus, symptoms often do not appear for years after infection. Infection in the brain may result in severe symptoms, resulting from mass effect and inflammation after degeneration of the cysticercus.

Patients may present with seizures, signs of increased intracranial pressure, hydrocephalus, focal neurologic signs, altered mental status, or aseptic meningitis. Cysticerci may also infect the spinal cord, muscles, subcutaneous tissues, and the eye. Substantial secondary immunity develops after larval infection.

Eggs are present in ≤ 50% of stool samples from patients with cysticercosis. Diagnosis is usually made when CT or MRI is performed to evaluate neurologic symptoms. Scans may show solid nodules, cysts, calcified cysts, ring-enhancing lesions, or hydrocephalus. Enzyme-linked immunosorbent assay (ELISA) and other serologic assays can be performed to identify antibodies, but many infected people are negative. Infection with adult *T. solium* worms can usually be diagnosed from stool samples.

Treatment

Corticosteroids (prednisone 60 mg po once/day or dexamethasone 6 mg once/day) and anticonvulsants should be administered to patients with symptomatic neurocysticercosis to reduce inflammation and symptoms. The treatment of choice for cerebral cysticercosis is controversial. Not all patients respond to treatment, and not all patients must be treated (cysts may already be dead and calcified, or the inflammatory response to treatment may be worse than the disease). Albendazole 400 mg po bid for 8 to 14 days is the drug of choice; praziquantel 20 to 35 mg/kg po tid for 30 days can also be used. Neither albendazole nor praziquantel should be used in patients with ocular or spinal cord involvement.

Surgery may be necessary for obstructive hydrocephalus (due to intraventricular cysticerci), infection of the 4th ventricle, and spinal and ocular cysticercosis.

Intestinal infection is treated with praziquantel 5 to 10 mg/kg as a single dose to eliminate adult worms.

185 INTESTINAL PROTOZOA

The most important intestinal protozoan pathogens are *Entamoeba histolytica, Cryptosporidium* sp, *Giardia lamblia, Isospora belli, Cyclospora cayetanensis,* and members of the phylum Microsporidia. Multiple pathogenic parasites and nonpathogenic commensal organisms may be present in the intestine. Nonintestinal protozoan infections are covered in other chapters: extraintestinal protozoal diseases (malaria, babesiosis, leishmaniasis, toxoplasmosis, trypanosomiasis) in Ch. 186, nematodes in Ch. 182, flukes in Ch. 183, and tapeworms in Ch. 184.

Intestinal protozoa are passed by the fecal-oral route, so infections are widespread in areas with inadequate sanitation. They are also common within the US in settings where fecal incontinence and poor hygiene prevail, such as in mental institutions and day care centers. Some GI protozoa are spread sexually, especially with practices involving oral-anal contact, and several protozoan species cause severe opportunistic infections in patients with AIDS.

Clinical diagnosis is often difficult; microscopic examination of suitable stool specimens is usually necessary. Diagnosis may require several samples, concentration methods, special stains, or semi-invasive diagnostic techniques such as endoscopic biopsy (see Table 181–1 on p. 1539). Sensitive and specific fecal antigen tests are available for *G. lamblia, Cryptosporidium* sp, and *E. histolytica.*

AMEBIASIS

(Entamebiasis)

Amebiasis is infection with *Entamoeba histolytica*. It is commonly asymptomatic, but mild diarrhea to severe dysentery may occur. Extraintestinal infections include liver abscesses. Diagnosis is by identifying *E. histolytica* in stool specimens or by serologic tests. Treatment for symptomatic disease is with metronidazole or tinidazole followed by paromomycin or other drugs active against cysts in the lumen.

Two species of *Entamoeba* are morphologically indistinguishable: *E. histolytica* is pathogenic, but *E. dispar* harmlessly colonizes the colon. They exist in 2 forms: the trophozoite and the cyst. The motile trophozoite feeds on bacteria and tissue, reproduces, colonizes the lumen and the mucosa of the large intestine, and sometimes invades tissues and organs. Trophozoites predominate in liquid stools but rapidly die outside the body. Some trophozoites in the colonic lumen become cysts that are excreted with stool. Cysts predominate in formed stools and are resistant to the external environment. They may spread either directly from person to person or indirectly via food or water. Amebiasis can be sexually transmitted by oral-anal contact.

E. histolytica trophozoites adhere to and kill colonic epithelial cells and PMNs and can cause dysentery with blood and mucus. They also secrete proteases that degrade the extracellular matrix and permit invasion into the intestine wall and beyond. Trophozoites can spread via the portal circulation and cause necrotic liver abscesses. Infection may spread by direct extension from the liver or through the bloodstream to the lungs, brain, and other organs.

Symptoms and Signs

Most infected people are asymptomatic but chronically pass cysts in stools. Symptoms that occur with tissue invasion include intermittent diarrhea and constipation, flatulence, and cramping abdominal pain. Tenderness over the liver or ascending colon may occur, and stools may contain mucus and blood.

Amebic dysentery, common in the tropics, presents with episodes of frequent semiliquid stools that often contain blood, mucus, and live trophozoites. Abdominal findings range from mild tenderness to frank abdominal pain, with high fevers and toxic systemic symptoms. Abdominal tenderness frequently accompanies amebic colitis. Between relapses, symptoms diminish to recurrent cramps and loose or very soft stools, but emaciation and anemia may develop. Symptoms suggestive of appendicitis may occur. Surgery in such cases may result in peritoneal spread of amebas.

Chronic amebic infection can mimic inflammatory bowel disease and presents as intermittent nondysenteric diarrhea with abdominal pain, mucus, flatulence, and weight loss. Chronic infection may also present as tender, palpable masses or annular lesions (amebomas) in the cecum and ascending colon that resemble carcinomas.

Extraintestinal disease originates from infection in the colon and can involve any organ, but a liver abscess, usually single and in the right lobe, is the most common. It can present in patients without prior symptoms, is more common in men than in women (7:1 to 9:1), and may develop insidiously. Symptoms include pain or discomfort over the liver, which is occasionally referred to the right shoulder; intermittent fever; sweats; chills; nausea; vomiting; weakness; and weight loss. Jaundice is unusual and low grade when present. The abscess may perforate into the subphrenic space, right pleural cavity, right lung, or other adjacent organs. Skin lesions are occasionally observed, especially around the perineum and buttocks in chronic infection, and may also occur in traumatic or operative wounds.

Diagnosis

Nondysenteric amebiasis may be misdiagnosed as irritable bowel syndrome, regional enteritis, or diverticulitis. Amebic dysentery may be confused with shigellosis, salmonellosis, schistosomiasis, or ulcerative colitis. In amebic dysentery, stools are usually less frequent and watery than those in bacillary dysentery. They characteristically contain tenacious mucus and flecks of blood. Unlike stools in shigellosis, salmonellosis, and ulcerative colitis, amebic stools do not contain large numbers of WBCs. Hepatic amebiasis and amebic abscess must be differentiated from other hepatic infections and tumors.

Diagnosis of amebiasis is supported by finding amebic trophozoites and/or cysts in the stool or tissues; however, pathogenic *E. histolytica* are morphologically indistinguishable from nonpathogenic *E. dispar*. Identification of intestinal amebas may require examination of 3 to 6 stool specimens and concentration methods (see TABLE 181–1on

p. 1539). Antibiotics, antacids, antidiarrheals, enemas, and intestinal radiocontrast agents interfere with recovery of the parasite and should not be given until the stool has been examined. *E. histolytica* also has to be distinguished from nonpathogenic amebas such as *Entamoeba coli, Endolimax nana*, and others.

In symptomatic patients, proctoscopy often shows characteristic flask-shaped mucosal lesions, which should be aspirated and the material examined for trophozoites. Biopsy specimens from rectosigmoid lesions may also show trophozoites.

Extraintestinal amebiasis is more difficult to diagnose. Stool examination is usually negative, and recovery of trophozoites from aspirated pus is uncommon. If a liver abscess is suspected, ultrasound, CT, or MRI should be performed. They are of similar sensitivity; however, no technique can differentiate amebic from pyogenic abscess with certainty. Needle aspiration is usually reserved for lesions of uncertain etiology, those in which rupture seems imminent, or those that respond poorly to drug therapy. Abscesses contain thick, semifluid material ranging from yellow to chocolate-brown. A needle biopsy may show necrotic tissue, but motile amebas are difficult to find in abscess material, and amebic cysts are not present. A therapeutic trial of an amebicide is often the most helpful diagnostic tool for an amebic liver abscess.

Serologic tests are positive in about 95% of patients with amebic liver abscess, > 70% of those with active intestinal infection, and 10% of asymptomatic carriers. The indirect hemagglutination and enzyme-linked immunosorbent assays are most sensitive. Antibody titers can confirm *E. histolytica* infection but may persist for months or years, making it impossible to differentiate acute from past infection in residents from areas with a high prevalence of infection. *E. histolytica* and *E. dispar* are morphologically indistinguishable, so microscopic examination cannot be used to differentiate them. A sensitive and specific antigen detection assay for the *E. histolytica* adherence lectin has been developed. PCR-based assays are available in research settings.

Treatment

For mild to moderate GI symptoms, 7 to 10 days of oral metronidazole is recommended (500 to 750 mg tid for adults, 12 to 17 mg/kg tid for children). Metronidazole should not be given to pregnant women. Alcohol must be avoided because of the drug's disulfiram-like effect. Alternatively, tinidazole can be used (2 g po once/day can be given for 3 days in adults or 50 mg/kg [maximum 2 g] once/day for 3 days in children). Tinidazole is generally better tolerated than metronidazole.

For severe intestinal and extraintestinal amebiasis, metronidazole 750 mg tid for 7 to 10 days is used in adults or 12 to 17 mg/kg tid for 7 to 10 days in children. Alternatively, tinidazole 2 g once/day for 5 days can be used in adults and 50 mg/kg once/day (maximum 2 g) for 5 days in children.

A course of metronidazole or tinidazole should be followed by a 2nd oral drug to eradicate residual cysts in the lumen. The options are iodoquinol (650 mg po tid for 20 days for adults or 10 to 13 mg/kg tid for 20 days for children [maximum of 2 g/day]); paromomycin (8 to 11 mg/kg tid for 7 days); and diloxanide furoate (500 mg tid for 10 days for adults or 7 mg/kg tid for 10 days for children).

Therapy should include rehydration with fluid and electrolytes and other supportive measures.

Asymptomatic people who pass *E. histolytica* cysts should be treated with paromomycin, iodoquinol, or diloxanide furoate (see above for doses). Metronidazole and tinidazole are not sufficiently active against *E. histolytica* cysts to be used alone.

Treatment is not necessary for *E. dispar* infections.

Prevention

Contamination of food and water with human feces must be prevented, a problem complicated by the high incidence of asymptomatic carriers. Uncooked foods, including salads and vegetables, and potentially contaminated water and ice should be avoided in developing areas. Boiling water kills *E. histolytica* cysts. The effectiveness of chemical disinfection with iodine- or chlorine-containing compounds depends on the temperature of the water and amount of organic debris in it. Portable filters provide various degrees of protection. Work has begun on the development of a vaccine, but none is available now.

CRYPTOSPORIDIOSIS

Cryptosporidiosis is infection with *Cryptosporidium*. The primary symptom is watery diarrhea, often with other signs of GI distress. Illness is typically self-limited in immu-

nocompetent patients but can be persistent and severe in those with AIDS. Diagnosis is by identification of the organism or antigen in stool. Treatment, when necessary, is with nitazoxanide.

Cryptosporidia are coccidian protozoa that replicate in small-bowel epithelial cells. Infective oocysts are shed into the lumen and passed in stool. After ingestion by another vertebrate, the oocyst releases sporozoites that transform into trophozoites in epithelial cells, replicate, and then produce oocysts that are released into the lumen of the intestine to complete the cycle. Thin-walled oocysts are involved in autoinfection.

C. parvum and *C. hominis* are responsible for most human cases. Infections result from fecally contaminated food or water, direct person-to-person contact, or zoonotic spread. The disease occurs worldwide. More than 400,000 people were affected in a waterborne outbreak in Milwaukee, Wisconsin in 1993. Children, travelers to foreign countries, immunocompromised patients, and medical personnel caring for patients with cryptosporidiosis are at increased risk. Cryptosporidiosis is responsible for up to 0.6 to 7.3% of diarrheal illness in industrialized countries and an even higher percentage in areas with poor sanitation. Outbreaks have occurred in day care centers. Severe, chronic diarrhea due to cryptosporidiosis is a problem in patients with AIDS.

Symptoms and Signs

The incubation period is about 1 wk, and clinical illness occurs in > 80% of infected people. Onset is acute, with profuse watery diarrhea, abdominal cramping, and, less commonly, nausea, anorexia, fever, and malaise. Symptoms generally persist 1 to 2 wk, rarely ≥ 1 mo, and then abate. Fecal excretion of oocysts may continue for several weeks after symptoms have subsided. Asymptomatic shedding of oocysts is common among older children in developing countries.

In the immunocompromised host, onset may be more gradual, but diarrhea can be more severe. Unless the underlying immune defect is corrected, infection can persist, causing profuse intractable diarrhea for life. Fluid losses of > 5 to 10 L/day have been reported in some AIDS patients. The intestine is the most common site of infection in immunocompromised hosts; however, other organs may be involved.

Diagnosis

Identifying the acid-fast oocysts in stool confirms the diagnosis, but conventional methods of stool examination are unreliable. Oocyst excretion is intermittent, and multiple stool samples may be needed. Several concentration techniques increase the yield. *Cryptosporidium* oocysts can be identified by phase-contrast microscopy or by staining with modified Ziehl-Neelsen or Kinyoun techniques. Immunofluorescence microscopy with fluorescein-labeled monoclonal antibodies allows for greater sensitivity and specificity. Intestinal biopsy can demonstrate *Cryptosporidium* within epithelial cells. Enzyme-linked immunosorbent assay for fecal *Cryptosporidium* antigen is more sensitive than microscopic examinations for oocysts.

Treatment and Prevention

In immunocompetent people, cryptosporidiosis is self-limited. Nitazoxanide is used in children. The recommended dose for children 12 to 47 mo is 100 mg q 12 h for 3 days. For ages 4 to 11 yr, it is 200 mg q 12 h for 3 days. Use in adults is currently being investigated, but a dose of 500 mg bid for 3 days has been used. Treatment failures are common with nitazoxanide in patients with AIDS. Symptoms of cryptosporidiosis have abated after effective highly active antiretroviral therapy in some AIDS patients. Supportive measures, oral and parenteral rehydration, and hyperalimentation are indicated in immunocompromised patients.

Stools of patients with cryptosporidiosis are highly infectious; strict stool precautions should be observed. Special biosafety guidelines have been developed for handling clinical specimens. Boiling water is the most reliable decontamination method; only filters with pore sizes ≤ 1 μm (specified as "absolute 1 micron" or certified by NSF Standard No. 53) remove *Cryptosporidium* cysts.

GIARDIASIS

Giardiasis is infection with the flagellated protozoan *Giardia lamblia*. Infection can be asymptomatic or cause symptoms ranging from intermittent flatulence to chronic malabsorption. Diagnosis is by identifying the organism in fresh stool or duodenal contents or by assays of *Giardia* antigen in stool. Treatment is with metronidazole, tinidazole, or nitazoxanide; alternatives include furazolidone and paromomycin.

Giardia trophozoites firmly attach to the duodenal and proximal jejunal mucosa and multiply by binary fission. Some organisms transform into environmentally resistant cysts that are spread by the fecal-oral route. Waterborne transmission is the major source of giardiasis. Transmission can also occur by direct person-to-person contact, especially in mental institutions and day care centers or between sex partners. *Giardia* cysts remain viable in surface water and are resistant to routine levels of chlorination. Wild animals may also serve as reservoirs. Thus, mountain streams as well as chlorinated but poorly filtered municipal water supply systems have been implicated in waterborne epidemics.

Symptoms, Signs, and Diagnosis

Many cases are asymptomatic. However, asymptomatic people can pass infective cysts. Symptoms of acute giardiasis generally appear 1 to 2 wk after infection. They are usually mild and include watery malodorous diarrhea, abdominal cramps and distention, flatulence and eructation, intermittent nausea, epigastric discomfort, and sometimes low-grade malaise and anorexia. Acute giardiasis usually lasts 1 to 3 wk. Malabsorption of fat and sugars can lead to significant weight loss in severe cases. Neither blood nor WBCs are found in the stool.

A subset of infected patients develops chronic diarrhea with foul stools, abdominal distention, and malodorous flatus. Substantial weight loss may occur. Chronic giardiasis occasionally causes failure to thrive in children.

Characteristic trophozoites or cysts in stool are diagnostic, but parasite excretion is intermittent and at low levels in chronic infections. Thus, diagnosis may require repeated stool examinations. Enzyme-linked immunosorbent assay to detect parasite antigen in stool is more sensitive. Sampling of the upper intestinal contents can also yield trophozoites but is seldom necessary. Specific DNA probes are under evaluation.

Treatment and Prevention

For symptomatic infections, metronidazole (250 mg po tid for 5 days in adults; 5 mg/kg po tid for 5 days in children) can be used. Adverse effects include nausea, headaches, and a disulfiram-like effect if alcohol is consumed concurrently. Tinidazole (2 g once in adults or 50 mg/kg [maximum 2 g] in children) is as effective as, and less toxic than, metronidazole. Neither of these drugs should be administered with alcohol. Nitazoxanide is available in liquid form for children (see under Cryptosporidiosis on p. 1567 for doses) and as tablets for adults (500 mg bid for 3 days). Furazolidone (100 mg po qid for 7 to 10 days in adults; 1.5 mg/kg po qid for 7 to 10 days in children) is also available but is less effective and has more adverse effects.

Metronidazole and tinidazole should not be given to pregnant women. If therapy cannot be delayed because of severe symptoms, the nonabsorbable aminoglycoside paromomycin (8 to 11 mg/kg po tid for 7 days) is an option.

Treatment of asymptomatic cyst passers can theoretically reduce the spread of infection, but whether it is cost effective remains unclear. Water can be decontaminated by boiling. *Giardia* cysts resist routine levels of chlorination. Disinfection with iodine-containing compounds is variably effective and depends on the turbidity and temperature of the water and duration of treatment. Some hand-held filtration devices can remove *Giardia* cysts from contaminated water, but the efficacy of various filter systems has not been fully assessed.

ISOSPORIASIS AND CYCLOSPORIASIS

Isosporiasis and cyclosporiasis are infections with the coccidian protozoa *Isospora belli* and *Cyclospora cayetanensis*, respectively. Symptoms include watery diarrhea with accompanying GI and systemic complaints. Diagnosis is by detection of characteristic oocysts in stool or intestinal biopsy specimens. Treatment is usually with trimethoprim-sulfamethoxazole.

The life cycles of *I. belli* and *C. cayetanensis* are similar to that of *Cryptosporidium*, except that oocysts must sporulate before becoming infective. Human isosporiasis and cyclosporiasis are most common in tropical and subtropical climates. Transmission is by the fecal-oral route via contaminated food or drink. In North America, outbreaks of *C. cayetanensis* have been caused by ingestion of imported raspberries from Guatemala.

Symptoms, Signs, and Diagnosis

The primary complaint is acute, nonbloody, watery diarrhea, with fever, abdominal cramps, nausea, anorexia, malaise, and weight loss. In immunocompetent people, the illness usually resolves spontaneously but can last weeks.

In hosts with depressed cell-mediated immunity as in AIDS, isosporiasis and cyclosporiasis may cause severe, intractable, voluminous diarrhea resembling cryptosporidiosis. Extraintestinal disease in patients with AIDS may include cholecystitis and disseminated infection.

Diagnosis is by detection of oocysts by microscopic examination of the stool. Detection is facilitated by staining stool samples with modified acid-fast stain. Multiple stool specimens may be needed. Diagnosis is sometimes made only when intracellular parasite stages are detected in biopsies of intestinal tissue. In isosporiasis, the stool may contain Charcot-Leyden crystals (hexagonal, double-pointed, and often needlelike crystals) derived from eosinophils. Unlike other protozoan infections, peripheral blood eosinophilia may also occur with *I. belli*.

Treatment

Treatment of choice for both isosporiasis and cyclosporiasis is double-strength trimethoprim-sulfamethoxazole (TMP-SMX) 160 mg TMP and 800 mg SMX po bid for 10 days. Children are given 5 mg/kg TMP and 25 mg/kg SMX bid. In patients with AIDS, higher doses and longer duration may be needed. Treatment of acute infection is usually followed by long-term suppressive therapy in those with AIDS. Ciprofloxacin 500 mg po bid for 7 days has also been used in isosporiasis and cyclosporiasis but appears to be less effective then TMP-SMX.

Prevention is as for cryptosporidiosis.

MICROSPORIDIOSIS

Microsporidiosis is infection with microsporidia. Symptomatic disease develops predominantly in patients with AIDS and includes chronic diarrhea, disseminated infection, and corneal disease. Diagnosis is by demonstrating organisms in biopsy specimens, stool, urine, other secretions, or corneal scrapings. Treatment is with albendazole, depending on the infecting species and clinical syndrome, with topical fumagillin added in eye disease.

Microsporidia are obligate intracellular spore-forming protozoan parasites. At least 14 of the > 1200 species are associated with human disease. Organisms are acquired by ingestion, inhalation, direct contact with the conjunctiva, animal contact, or person-to-person transmission. Inside the host, they uncoil, harpoon a host cell, and inoculate it with an infective sporoplasm. Intracellular division then produces sporoblasts that mature into spores, which can disseminate throughout the body or pass into the environment via respiratory aerosols, stool, or urine. An inflammatory response develops when spores are liberated from host cells.

Little is known about routes of transmission to humans or possible animal reservoirs. Microsporidia probably are a common cause of subclinical or mild self-limited illness in otherwise healthy people, but only a few cases of human infection were reported in the pre-AIDS era.

Microsporidia have emerged as opportunistic pathogens in patients with AIDS. *Encephalitozoon bieneusi* and *E.* (formerly *Septata*) *intestinalis* can cause chronic diarrhea in patients with AIDS and $CD4^+$ cell counts < 100/µL. Microsporidian species can also infect the biliary tract, cornea, muscles, respiratory tract, genitourinary system, and, occasionally, the CNS.

Symptoms, Signs, and Diagnosis

Clinical illness caused by microsporidia varies with the parasite species and the immune status of the host. In patients with AIDS, various species cause chronic diarrhea, cholangitis, punctate keratoconjunctivitis, peritonitis, hepatitis, myositis, or sinusitis. Infections of kidneys, gallbladder, and sinuses have occurred. *Vittaforma (Nosema) corneum* and several other species can cause ocular infections ranging from punctuate keratopathy with redness and irritation to severe, vision-threatening stromal keratitis.

Infecting organisms can be demonstrated in specimens of affected tissue obtained by biopsy; in stool, urine, CSF, bile, or sputum; or in corneal scrapings. Microsporidia are best seen with special staining techniques and may require electron microscopy. Fluorescence brighteners (fluorochromes) have been used for quick detection of spores in tissues and smears. Immunoassay and PCR-based tests hold promise for the future.

Treatment

Microsporidia infections are usually self-limited in immunocompetent patients, and therapy is seldom necessary. In immunocompromised patients, albendazole (400 mg po bid for 21 days in adults) may be effective in controlling intestinal infection with *E. intestinalis*. The drug reduces the number of organisms in small-bowel biopsies but does not eliminate infection. Fumagillin 20 mg po tid for 14 days has been used for *E. bieneusi*, but it has adverse effects. Ocular lesions caused by *E. hellem* and *E. cuniculi* have been treated with albendazole 400 mg bid plus fumagillin eyedrops. These drugs are also used for *V. corneum*, but they frequently fail and keratoplasty may be required. Albendazole 400 mg bid has been used for patients with disseminated disease caused by numerous microsporidian species. There is no established treatment for *Pleistophora* infections. Treatment of AIDS with highly active antiretroviral therapy is important and can lead to improvement in symptoms.

186 EXTRAINTESTINAL PROTOZOA

Protozoa are motile, single-celled organisms that are found worldwide. Many of those that cause extraintestinal infections are transmitted by arthropod vectors. They include African trypanosomiasis, Chagas' disease, leishmaniasis, and malaria. Toxoplasmosis is acquired through contaminated food. Free-living amebas are acquired through contact with water or soil.

AFRICAN TRYPANOSOMIASIS

(African Sleeping Sickness)

African trypanosomiasis is infection with protozoa of the genus *Trypanosoma* transmitted by the bite of a tsetse fly. Symptoms include characteristic skin lesions, intermittent fever, headache, rigors, transient edema, generalized lymphadenopathy, and often-fatal meningoencephalitis. Diagnosis is by identifying the organism in blood, lymph node aspirate, or CSF, or sometimes serologic tests. Treatment is with suramin, pentamidine, melarsoprol, or eflornithine, depending on the subspecies and clinical stage.

Etiology and Pathophysiology

African trypanosomiasis is caused by *T. brucei gambiense* in West and Central Africa and by *T. brucei rhodesiense* in East Africa, which are transmitted by tsetse flies. Both species are endemic in Uganda. Metacyclic trypomastigotes inoculated by flies transform into bloodstream trypomastigotes that multiply by binary fission and spread through the lymphatics and bloodstream after inoculation. Bloodstream trypomastigotes multiply until specific antibodies produced by the host sharply reduce parasite levels. However, a subset of parasites escapes immune destruction by a change in their variant surface glycoprotein and starts a new multiplication cycle. The cycle of multiplication and lysis repeats. Late in the course of infection, trypanosomes appear in the interstitial fluid of many organs, including the myocardium and eventually the CNS. African trypanosomiasis can also be transmitted by blood transfusion.

Symptoms and Signs

A papule may develop at the site of the tsetse fly bite within a few days to 2 wk. It evolves into a dusky red, painful, indurated nodule (trypanosomal chancre). A chancre is seen in about half of Caucasians with *T.b. rhodesiense* but is seldom evident in Africans with *T.b. gambiense.* Over several months in *T.b. gambiense* infection, but a period of weeks with *T.b. rhodesiense*, intermittent fever, headaches, rigors, and transient swellings occur. An evanescent, circinate erythematous rash may develop. It is most readily visible in light-skinned patients. Generalized lymphadenopathy often occurs. Winterbottom's sign (enlarged lymph nodes in the posterior cervical triangle) is characteristic with *T.b. gambiense* sleeping sickness.

In the Gambian form, CNS involvement occurs months to several years after onset of acute disease. In the Rhodesian form, disease is more fulminant, and CNS invasion occurs within a few weeks to several months. CNS involvement causes persistent headache, inability to concentrate, personality changes (eg, progressive lassitude and indifference), daytime somnolence, hyperphagia, tremor, ataxia, and terminal coma. If untreated, death usually occurs within months of disease onset with *T.b. rhodesiense* and during the 2nd or 3rd yr with *T.b. gambiense*. Untreated patients die in coma from malnutrition or secondary infections.

Diagnosis

Early in the disease, diagnosis is made by finding trypanosomes in wet mounts or in Giemsa-stained thin or thick smears of peripheral blood (more useful in the Rhodesian type) or in fluid aspirated from an enlarged lymph node (more useful in the Gambian type). Centrifugation of blood or fluid samples may be useful in concentrating trypanosomes. In advanced stages, trypanosomes may be found only in centrifuged CSF. Serologic tests (immunofluorescent assay, enzyme-linked immunosorbent assay, card agglutination) are useful for *T.b. gambiense*.

When the CNS is involved, CSF pressure is increased, and CSF levels of lymphocytes (≥ 5 cells/μL), total protein, and IgM are elevated. In addition to trypanosomes, characteristic Mott cells (morula-like plasma cells filled with immunoglobulin) may be present. Laboratory findings include anemia, monocytosis, and markedly elevated serum levels of polyclonal IgM.

Treatment

Suramin and pentamidine are each effective against bloodstream stages of both *T. brucei* subspecies but do not cure CNS infection. Pentamidine is preferred for *T.b. gambiense*, and suramin for *T.b. rhodesiense*. The dosage of pentamidine isethionate is 4 mg/kg IM once/day for 10 days. An initial test dose of suramin 100 mg IV (to exclude hypersensitivity) is followed by 20 mg/kg IV up to 1 g on days 1, 3, 7, 14, and 21 for adults. For children, 20 mg/kg IV is given after the 100-mg test on days 1, 3, 7, 14, and 21. Eflornithine (availability limited) is effective against both early and late stages of *T.b. gambiense* (not *T.b. rhodesiense*) trypanosomiasis. It is given 100 mg/kg IV qid for 14 days. It is the drug of choice for *T.b. gambiense* when available.

Melarsoprol is used in most African countries for CNS disease. It is usually given as 3-day courses of 2 to 3.6 mg/kg IV once/day. After 7 days, 3.6 mg/kg once/day is given for 3 days. Seven days later, the 3-day course of therapy is repeated. Alternative regimens have been proposed for debilitated patients with severe CNS involvement. Serious adverse effects include reactive encephalopathy and exfoliative dermatitis in addition to the usual toxicity of arsenicals on the GI and renal systems. Corticosteroids decrease the risk of reactive encephalopathy.

Prevention

Prevention includes avoiding endemic areas and protecting against tsetse flies. Visitors to game parks should wear substantial wrist- and ankle-length clothing (tsetse flies bite through thin clothes) and use insect repellents with DEET appropriately.

Pentamidine confers some protection against *T.b. gambiense*, but because pentamidine may cause renal failure and hypoglycemia and lead to diabetes, it is not warranted for prophylaxis.

BABESIOSIS

Babesiosis is infection with *Babesia* sp. Infections can be asymptomatic or produce a malaria-like illness with fever and hemolytic anemia. Disease is most severe in asplenic patients, the elderly, and those with AIDS. Diagnosis is by identifying *Babesia* in a peripheral blood smear, serology, or PCR. Treatment, when needed, is with azithromycin plus atovaquone or with quinine plus clindamycin.

Etiology and Pathophysiology

In the US, *Babesia microti* is the most common cause of babesiosis. Rodents are the principal natural reservoir, and deer ticks of the family Ixodidae are the usual vectors. Larval ticks become infected while feeding on an infected rodent, then transform into nymphs that transmit the parasite to another animal or to a human. Adult ticks ordinarily feed on deer but also may transmit the parasite to humans. *Babesia* enter RBCs, mature, and then divide asexually. Infected erythrocytes eventually rupture and release organisms that invade other RBCs.

Endemic areas in the US include the islands and the mainland bordering Nantucket Sound in Massachusetts, eastern Long Island and Shelter Island in New York, coastal Connecticut, and New Jersey as well as foci in Wisconsin, Georgia, and California. Other *Babesia* sp transmitted by different ticks infect humans in areas of Europe. Babesiosis can also be transmitted by blood transfusion.

Symptoms, Signs, and Diagnosis

Asymptomatic infection may persist for months to years and remain subclinical throughout its course in otherwise healthy people, especially those < 40 yr. When symptomatic, the illness usually starts after a 1- to 2-wk incubation period with malaise, fatigue, chills, fever, headache, myalgia, and arthralgia that may last for weeks. Hepatosplenomegaly with jaundice, mild to moderately severe hemolytic anemia, mild neutropenia, and thrombocytopenia may occur.

Infection is sometimes fatal, particularly in the elderly, asplenic patients, and those with AIDS. In such patients, babesiosis may resemble falciparum malaria, with high fever, hemolytic anemia, hemoglobinuria, jaundice, and renal failure. Splenectomy may cause previously acquired asymptomatic parasitemia to become symptomatic.

Most patients do not remember a tick bite. Diagnosis is usually made by finding *Babesia* in blood smears. Tetrad forms, although not common, are helpful diagnostic clues. Serologic and PCR tests are available.

Treatment and Prevention

Asymptomatic patients require no treatment, but therapy is indicated for cases with persistent high fever, rapidly increasing parasitemia, and falling Hct. The combination of atovaquone 750 mg po q 12 h and azithromycin 500 mg po on day 1 and 250 to 500 mg once/day thereafter for 7 to 10 days is as effective as traditional therapy with quinine plus clindamycin and has fewer adverse effects. Pediatric dosage is atovaquone 20 mg/kg bid and azithromycin 12 mg/kg once/day for 7 to 10 days. Alternatively, quinine 650 mg po tid for 7 days plus clindamycin 600 mg po tid or 1.2 g IV bid for 7 to 10 days can be used. Pediatric dosage is quinine 8 mg/kg po tid plus clindamycin 7 to 14 mg/kg po tid. Exchange transfusion has been lifesaving in hypotensive patients with high parasitemia.

Standard tick precautions (see sidebar 177–1 on p. 1491) should be taken by all in endemic areas. Asplenic people should be particularly cautious.

CHAGAS' DISEASE

(American Trypanosomiasis)

Chagas' disease is infection with *Trypanosoma cruzi*, transmitted by Triatominae bug bites. Symptoms begin with a skin lesion or unilateral periorbital edema; progress to fever, malaise, generalized lymphadenopathy, and hepatosplenomegaly; in some, chronic cardiomyopathy, megaesophagus, or megacolon occurs. Diagnosis is by detecting trypanosomes in peripheral blood or aspirates from infected organs. PCR, serologic tests, and xenodiagnosis may be helpful. Treatment is with nifurtimox or benznidazole.

Etiology and Pathophysiology

T. cruzi is transmitted by Triatominae (reduviid, kissing, or assassin) bugs. While biting, infected bugs deposit feces containing metacyclic trypomastigotes on the skin. These infective forms enter through the bite wound or penetrate mucous membranes. The parasites then invade macrophages at the site of entry, transform into amastigotes that multiply by binary fission, and are released as trypomastigotes into the blood and tissue spaces, whence they infect other cells. Cells of the reticuloendothelial system, myocardium, muscles, and nervous system are most commonly involved. Reservoirs include dogs, cats, opossums, rats, and other animals. Infection can also be transmitted by blood transfusion, organ transplantation, or transplacentally.

Infected Triatominae are found in North, Central, and South America. More than 20 million people in the Americas are infected with *T. cruzi*, but the prevalence has been decreasing due to control measures. In some rural parts of South America, Chagas' disease has been a leading cause of death. Vector-borne disease is rare in the US, but some Latin American immigrants living in the US are chronically infected. These people are potential sources of transmission by blood transfusion or organ donation.

Symptoms and Signs

Acute infection is followed by a latent (indeterminate) period, which may remain asymptomatic or progress to chronic disease. Immunosuppression may reactivate latent infection, with high parasitemia and a 2nd acute stage, skin lesions, or brain abscesses. Congenital transmission occurs in 1 to 5% of pregnancies and results in abortion, stillbirth, or chronic neonatal disease with high mortality.

Acute infection in endemic areas usually occurs in childhood and can be asymptomatic. When present, symptoms start 1 to 2 wk after exposure. An indurated, erythematous skin lesion (a chagoma) appears at the site of parasite entry. When the inoculation site is the conjunctiva, unilateral periocular and palpebral edema with conjunctivitis and preauricular lymphadenopathy are collectively called Romaña's sign. Acute Chagas' disease is fatal in a small percentage of patients due to acute myocarditis with heart failure or acute meningoencephalitis. In the remainder, symptoms subside without treatment. Primary acute Chagas' disease in immunocompromised patients, such as those with AIDS, may be severe and atypical, with skin lesions and brain abscesses, although the latter are rare.

Chronic disease develops in 20 to 40%, after a latent phase that may last years or decades. Chronic cardiomyopathy leads to flaccid enlargement of all chambers, apical aneurysms, and localized degenerative lesions in the conduction system, producing heart failure, syncope, sudden death due to heart block or ventricular arrhythmia, and thromboembolism. ECG may show right bundle branch or complete heart block. GI disease produces symptoms resembling achalasia or Hirschsprung's disease. Chagas' megaesophagus presents as dysphagia and may lead to pulmonary infections from aspiration or to severe malnutrition. Megacolon may result in prolonged periods of obstipation and intestinal volvulus.

Diagnosis

The number of trypanosomes in peripheral blood is high during the acute phase and readily detected by examination of thin or thick smears. In contrast, few parasites are present in blood during latent infection or chronic disease. Definitive diagnosis may be made by examination of aspirates from organs such as lymph nodes. Serologic tests are sensitive but may yield false-positive results in patients with visceral or mucocutaneous leishmaniasis or other diseases. Other diagnostic approaches include xenodiagnosis (by examining the rectal contents of laboratory-raised bugs after they take a blood meal from a suspected patient) and detecting PCR-amplified parasite DNA in blood or tissue fluids.

Treatment and Prevention

Treatment in the acute stage rapidly reduces parasitemia, shortens the clinical illness, and reduces risk of mortality but often does not eradicate the infection. Treatment of children and young adults with indeterminate infections has been recommended, but many are not cured. Treatment in the chronic stage is symptomatic. Chronic organ damage, which may be caused in part by host inflammatory responses, appears to be largely irreversible. Supportive measures include drugs for heart failure, pacemakers, antiarrhythmic drugs, cardiac transplantation, esophageal dilation, and GI tract surgery.

The only effective drugs are nifurtimox (2 to 2.5 mg/kg po qid for 3 to 4 mo in adults; 4 to 5 mg/kg qid for 3 mo in 1- to 10-yr-old children; 3 to 3.75 mg/kg qid for 3 mo in 11- to 16-yr-old children) or benznidazole (2.5 to 3.5 mg/kg po bid for 1 to 3 mo for adults; 5.0 mg/kg bid for children ≤ 12 yr). These long treatment courses are often associated with severe GI adverse effects, peripheral neuropathy, poor tolerance, and low compliance.

Plastering walls and replacing thatched roofs or repeated spraying of houses with residual insecticides can control Triatominae bugs. Infection in travelers is rare and can be avoided by not sleeping in such dwellings or by using bed nets if forced to do so.

Transfusion-induced Chagas' disease is a major health problem in endemic areas. A small number of cases have been reported in the US. Although screening for antibodies has been proposed, US blood banks currently rely on historical information to exclude potentially infected donors. Transfusion-induced Chagas' disease can also be prevented by adding gentian violet to blood in endemic areas if blood screening with serologic tests is not possible.

FREE-LIVING AMEBAS

Free-living amebas are protozoa that live independently in soil or water and do not require a human or an animal host. They rarely cause disease, unlike the parasitic ameba *Entamoeba histolytica*, which is a common cause of intestinal infection (see p. 1565). Pathogenic free-living amebas are of the genera *Naegleria, Acanthamoeba*, and *Balamuthia*.

Three major syndromes occur, primary amebic meningoencephalitis, granulomatous amebic encephalitis, and amebic keratitis. *Acanthamoeba* can also cause skin lesions.

PRIMARY AMEBIC MENINGOENCEPHALITIS

Primary amebic meningoencephalitis is a generally fatal, acute CNS infection caused by *Naegleria fowleri*.

N. fowleri inhabits fresh water worldwide. Swimming in contaminated water exposes nasal mucosa to the organism, which can enter the CNS via olfactory neuroepithelium and the cribriform plate. Most patients are healthy children or young adults.

Symptoms begin within 1 to 2 wk of exposure, sometimes with alteration of smell and taste. Fulminant meningoencephalitis ensues with headache, meningismus, and mental status change, progressing to death within 10 days, usually from cerebral herniation.

Diagnosis is suspected by history of swimming in fresh water, but confirmation is difficult because CT and routine CSF tests, although necessary to exclude other causes, are nonspecific. Wet mount of CSF should be performed, which may demonstrate motile amebic trophozoites (which are destroyed by Gram stain techniques).

Only a few patients have survived, so optimal treatment is unclear. A reasonable regimen uses amphotericin B intravenously and intrathecally; effective doses are unclear. Some have added oral rifampin, oral and intrathecal miconazole, and oral sulfisoxazole. Experimental evidence suggests azithromycin might be of benefit.

Granulomatous Amebic Encephalitis

Granulomatous amebic encephalitis is a generally fatal subacute CNS infection in immunocompromised or debilitated hosts caused by *Acanthamoeba* sp or *Balamuthia mandrillaris*.

Acanthamoeba sp and *Balamuthia mandrillaris* are present worldwide in water, soil, and dust. Human exposure is common, but infection is rare. *Acanthamoeba* infection occurs almost entirely in immunocompromised or otherwise debilitated patients, but *B. mandrillaris* may also infect healthy hosts; manifestations are otherwise similar. The entry portal is thought to be the skin or lower respiratory tract, with subsequent hematogenous dissemination to the CNS.

Onset is insidious, often with focal neurologic manifestations. Mental status change, seizures, and headache are common. Survival is highly unlikely (and only in immunocompetent patients), death occurring between 7 and 120 days after onset (average, 39 days).

Diagnosis is often postmortem. CT and routine CSF tests are obtained but are nonspecific. CT may show multiple nonenhancing lucent areas, and CSF shows elevated WBC count (predominantly lymphocytes), but trophozoites are rarely demonstrated in the CSF. Visible skin lesions often show amebas and should be biopsied; if detected, amebas may be cultured and tested for drug sensitivity. Brain biopsy is often positive.

Against *Acanthamoeba*, the diamidine derivatives (propamidine, pentamidine, dibromopropamidine) appear to have the greatest activity in vitro. Other agents include trimethoprim-sulfamethoxazole, ketoconazole, itraconazole, miconazole, paromomycin, neomycin, 5-fluorocytosine, and, to a lesser extent, amphotericin B. Recent studies suggest that *B. mandrillaris* is sensitive to pentamidine in vitro, and this drug may be beneficial in treatment of CNS infections.

Amebic Keratitis

Amebic keratitis is corneal infection by *Acanthamoeba* sp, typically occurring in contact lens wearers.

Acanthamoeba sp can cause chronic and progressively destructive keratitis. The main risk factor (85% of cases) is contact lens use, particularly if lenses are worn while swimming or if unsterile lens cleaning solution is used. Some infections follow corneal abrasion.

Lesions are typically very painful with foreign body sensation. Initially, lesions have a dendriform appearance resembling herpes simplex keratitis. Later there are patchy stromal infiltrates, and sometimes a characteristic ring-shaped lesion. Most have an associated anterior uveitis. Vision is diminished.

Diagnosis is confirmed by examining Giemsa- or trichrome-stained corneal scrapings and by culture on special media. Viral culture is obtained if herpes is considered.

Early, superficial infection responds better to treatment. The encysted stage of the life cycle appears to cause most problems. Epithelial lesions are debrided, and intensive drug therapy is applied. Combination therapy with ≥ 2 antimicrobials works best. Polyhexamethylene biguanide 0.02% and propamidine isethionate 0.1% have been applied hourly for the first 3 days. Other topical agents, such as clotrimazole 1%, chlorhexidine, fluconazole, natamycin, or neomycin-polymyxin B-gramicidin, are sometimes added. Systemic treatment with fluconazole or itraconazole has also been used, particularly in patients with anterior uveitis or involvement of the sclera. Early recognition and treatment have eliminated the need for therapeutic keratoplasty in most instances, but it remains an option in cases in which pharmacologic therapy fails. Intensive treatment is required for the 1st month, being tapered per clinical response, but often continuing for 6 to 12 mo. Recurrence is common if treatment is stopped prematurely.

LEISHMANIASIS

Leishmaniasis is a group of diseases caused by species of *Leishmania*. Manifestations include visceral, cutaneous, and mucocutaneous syndromes. Visceral leishmaniasis causes irregular fever, hepatosplenomegaly, pancytopenia, and polyclonal hypergammaglobulinemia with high untreated mortality. Cutaneous leishmaniasis produces painless nodular skin lesions that enlarge, ulcerate centrally, and persist for months to years but eventually heal. Mucocutaneous disease affects nasopharyngeal tissues and can cause gross mutilation of the nose and palate. Diagnosis is by demonstrating parasites in smears or cultures of splenic or bone marrow aspirates in visceral leishmaniasis or of lesions in cutaneous leishmaniasis. Treatment is with pentavalent antimony compounds, liposomal amphotericin B, amphotericin B deoxycholate, or miltefosine, depending on the causative species and clinical syndrome.

Etiology and Pathophysiology

Leishmaniasis is present worldwide in tropical and some temperate areas. *Leishmania* are transmitted by tiny sand flies (*Phlebotomus* sp and *Lutzomyia* sp) and survive in the vertebrate host as intracellular amastigotes. Vector flies are infected by biting humans or animals. Animal reservoirs vary with the *Leishmania* species and location and include canines, rodents, humans, and other animals. Infection is spread rarely by blood transfusion, shared needles, congenitally, or sexually.

Visceral leishmaniasis (kala-azar; Dumdum fever) is typically caused by *L. donovani* or *L. infantum/L. chagasi* and occurs in India, Africa (particularly the Sudan), Central Asia, the Mediterranean basin, South and Central America, and infrequently China. Parasites disseminate from the skin to the lymph nodes, spleen, liver, and bone marrow and cause symptoms. Subclinical infections are common; only a minority of infected persons develop progressive visceral disease.

Cutaneous leishmaniasis is also known as oriental or tropical sore, Delhi or Aleppo boil, uta or chiclero ulcer, or forest yaws. The causative agents are *L. major* and *L. tropica* in southern Europe, Asia, and Africa; *L. mexicana* and related species in Mexico and Central and South America; and *L. braziliensis* and related species in Central and South America. Outbreaks have occurred among US military personnel training in Panama or serving in Iraq and Afghanistan. Isolated cases have been reported in travelers to endemic areas in Central and South America, Israel, and elsewhere.

Mucocutaneous leishmaniasis (espundia) is caused mainly by *L. braziliensis*, but it occasionally occurs with other *Leishmania* species.

Symptoms and Signs

For visceral leishmaniasis, the clinical manifestations usually develop gradually over weeks to months after inoculation of the parasite. Irregular fever, hepatosplenomegaly, pancytopenia, and polyclonal hypergammaglobulinemia with reversed albumin:globulin ratio occur. In some patients, there are twice-daily temperature spikes. Emaciation and death occur within 1 to 2 yr in 80 to 90% of untreated symptomatic patients. Those with asymptomatic, self-resolving infections and survivors (after successful treatment) are resistant to further attacks unless cell-mediated immunity is impaired (eg, AIDS). After treatment for visceral leishmaniasis, patients in the Sudan and India may develop post kala-azar dermal leishmaniasis with flat or nodular cutaneous lesions full of parasites. These lesions develop at the end of or within 6 mo of therapy in patients in the Sudan and 1 to 2 yr later in India. The lesions persist for a few months to a year in most patients in the Sudan but can last for years in India.

Cutaneous leishmaniasis produces a well-demarcated skin lesion at the site of a sand fly bite after several weeks to months. Multiple lesions may occur after multiple infective bites or with metastatic spread. The initial lesion is often a papule that slowly enlarges, ulcerates centrally, and develops a raised, erythematous border where intracellular parasites are concentrated. Ulcers are painless and cause no systemic symptoms unless secondarily infected. Leishmanial lesions generally heal spontaneously after months but may persist for years. They leave a depressed, burn-like scar. The course depends on the species and the host's immune status. In the Americas, skin lesions can be followed by metastatic mucocutaneous lesions if they are caused by *L. braziliensis* or related species (see mucocutaneous leishmaniasis, below). Diffuse cutaneous leishmaniasis is an uncommon form characterized by widespread nodular skin lesions resembling those of lepromatous leprosy. It is presumed to result from cell-mediated anergy to the organism.

Mucocutaneous leishmaniasis starts with a primary cutaneous ulcer. This skin lesion heals spontaneously, but parasites can metastasize to nasopharyngeal tissues. Months to years later, mucosal lesions develop, sometimes resulting in gross mutilations of the nose, palate, and face.

Diagnosis

A definite diagnosis is made by demonstrating organisms in Giemsa-stained smears or cultures of aspirates from the spleen, bone marrow, liver, or lymph nodes in visceral leishmaniasis or biopsy, aspirates, or touch preparations from the border of a cutaneous lesion. Parasites are usually difficult to isolate from mucosal lesions. Organisms causing simple cutaneous leishmaniasis can be differentiated from those capable of causing mucocutaneous leishmaniasis with specific DNA probes or monoclonal antibodies, or by analysis of isoenzyme patterns of cultured parasites.

Serologic tests are available. A recombinant antigen (rk39) is positive in patients with visceral leishmaniasis, but not in subclinical cases or persons with cutaneous leishmaniasis. Skin tests may be available outside the US.

Treatment and Prevention

The drugs of choice depend on the infecting species and the geographic locations. Pentavalent antimony compounds have been used for visceral and cutaneous disease. Drugs include Na stibogluconate (Na antimony gluconate) or meglumine antimonate 20 mg/kg slowly injected IV or IM once/day for 20 to 28 days. Adverse effects include nausea, vomiting, malaise, and elevated amylase and liver enzymes. If cardiotoxicity develops, administration should be stopped. In industrialized countries, liposomal amphotericin B 3 mg/kg once/day for 5 days, then 3 mg/kg once/day on days 14 and 21, is the drug of choice for immunocompetent patients. Higher doses and longer regimens are used in those with AIDS. Alternatives are amphotericin B deoxycholate 0.5 to 1 mg/kg by slow infusion every day or every other day for up to 8 wk or pentamidine isethionate 2 to 4 mg/kg IV once/day or every other day for up to 15 doses.

Drug resistance has become a problem with antimonials, particularly in India in persons with visceral leishmaniasis. Miltefosine, given 100 mg once/day (2.5 mg/kg for children 2 to 11 yr) for 28 days, is effective. Adverse effects include nausea and vomiting, transient transaminase elevations, and dizziness. It is not available in the US.

Treatment of cutaneous disease depends on several factors, including the causative *Leishmania* sp, extent of lesion, and whether dissemination to the mucosa is a concern. Parenteral pentavalent antimonials are often used, particularly for *Leishmania* sp that can disseminate to cause mucosal leishmaniasis. Fluconazole or itraconazole is effective in some cases. Topical paromomycin has been used for *L. major* infections. Mucosal disease frequently relapses, as does visceral disease in patients with AIDS. Diffuse cutaneous leishmaniasis is relatively resistant to treatment.

Supportive measures may be needed for patients with visceral leishmaniasis, including adequate nutrition, transfusions, and antibiotics for secondary bacterial infection. Reconstructive surgery may be required for mucocutaneous disease with gross distortion of the nose or palate, but surgery should be delayed for 6 to 12 mo after therapy to avoid loss of grafts to relapses.

For prevention, treatment of cases in a geographic area, reduction of the vector population, and elimination of nonhuman reservoirs where appropriate may help. Insect repellents containing DEET provide protection. Insect screens, bed nets, and clothing are more effective if treated with permethrin or pyrethrum, because the tiny flies can penetrate mechanical barriers. Vaccines are not currently available.

MALARIA

Malaria is infection with any of 4 species of *Plasmodium*. Symptoms are fever, which may be periodic, chills, sweating, hemolytic anemia, and splenomegaly. Diagnosis is by seeing *Plasmodium* in a peripheral blood smear. Treatment and prophylaxis depend on the species and drug sensitivity and include chloroquine, quinine, atovaquone and proguanil, mefloquine, doxycycline, and artemisinin derivatives. Patients infected

with *P. vivax* and *P. ovale* also receive primaquine.

Malaria is endemic in Africa, much of South and Southeast Asia, Central America, and northern South America. There are between 300 and 500 million infected people worldwide, with between 1 and 2 million deaths yearly, most in children < 5 yr. Malaria once was endemic in the US but has been virtually eliminated from North America. About 1000 cases/yr occur in the US, nearly all acquired abroad; a small number result from blood transfusions or rare autochthonous transmission by local mosquitoes that feed on infected immigrants.

Etiology and Pathophysiology

The 4 *Plasmodium* species that infect humans are *P. falciparum, P. vivax, P. ovale*, and *P. malariae*. The basic elements of the life cycle are the same for all. Transmission begins when a female *Anopheles* mosquito feeds on a person with malaria and ingests blood containing gametocytes. During the following 1 to 2 wk, gametocytes inside the mosquito reproduce sexually and produce infective sporozoites. When the mosquito feeds again on a human, it transmits sporozoites, which quickly infect hepatocytes. The parasites mature into tissue schizonts within hepatocytes. Each schizont produces 10,000 to 30,000 merozoites, which are released into the bloodstream 1 to 3 wk later when the hepatocyte ruptures. Each merozoite can invade an RBC and there transform into a trophozoite. Trophozoites grow and develop into erythrocyte schizonts, which produce further merozoites, which 48 to 72 h later rupture the RBC and are released in plasma. These merozoites then rapidly invade new RBCs, repeating the cycle.

Tissue schizonts in the liver may persist as hypnozoites for up to 3 yr with *P. vivax* and *P. ovale* but not with *P. falciparum* or *P. malariae*. These dormant forms serve as "time-release capsules," which cause relapses and complicate chemotherapy because they are not killed by most drugs.

The pre-erythrocytic (hepatic) stage of the malarial life cycle is bypassed when infection is transmitted by blood transfusions, sharing of contaminated needles, or congenitally. Therefore, these modes of transmission do not produce latent disease and delayed recurrences.

Rupture of RBCs during release of merozoites is responsible for the clinical symptoms. If severe, hemolysis produces anemia and jaundice, which are worsened by phagocytosis of infected RBCs in the spleen.

Unlike other forms of malaria, *P. falciparum* causes microvascular obstruction because infected RBCs adhere to vascular endothelial cells. Ischemia develops with resultant tissue hypoxia, particularly in the brain, kidneys, lungs, and GI tract; hypoglycemia; and lactic acidosis.

Resistance: Most West Africans have complete resistance to *P. vivax* because their RBCs lack the Duffy blood group, which is required for *P. vivax* invasion of RBCs; many African Americans are resistant. The development of *Plasmodium* in RBCs is also retarded in patients with hemoglobin S, hemoglobin C, thalassemia, G6PD deficiency, or Melanesian elliptocytosis.

Previous infections provide partial immunity. Once residents of hyperendemic areas leave, acquired immunity lasts only for a period of months, and symptomatic malaria may develop if they return home and become infected.

Symptoms and Signs

The incubation period is usually 12 to 17 days for *P. vivax*, 9 to 14 days for *P. falciparum*, 16 to 18 days or longer for *P. ovale*, and about 1 mo (18 to 40 days) or longer (years) for *P. malariae*. However, some strains of *P. vivax* in temperate climates may not cause clinical illness for months to more than a year after infection.

Manifestations common to all forms of malaria include fever, anemia, jaundice, splenomegaly, hepatomegaly, and the malarial paroxysm (rigor) that coincides with release of merozoites from ruptured RBCs. The classic paroxysm starts with malaise, abrupt chills and fever rising to 39 to 41° C, rapid and thready pulse, polyuria, and increasing headache and nausea. After 2 to 6 h, fever falls and profuse sweating occurs for 2 to 3 h, followed by extreme fatigue. Fever is often hectic at the start of infection. In established infections, malarial paroxysms typically occur about every 2 to 3 days depending on species; intervals are not rigid.

Anemia may be severe in *P. falciparum* infection or chronic *P. vivax* and tends to be mild in *P. malariae*. Splenomegaly usually becomes palpable by the end of the 1st week of clinical disease but may not occur with *P. falciparum*. The enlarged spleen is soft and prone to traumatic rupture. Splenomegaly may decrease with recurrent attacks of malaria as functional immunity develops. After many bouts, the spleen may become fibrotic and firm and occasionally becomes massively enlarged (tropical splenomegaly). Hepatomegaly usually accompanies splenomegaly.

P. falciparum causes the most severe disease because of its microvascular effects. It is the only species likely to cause fatal disease if untreated; nonimmune patients may die within days of their initial symptoms. Patients with cerebral malaria may develop symptoms ranging from irritability to seizures and coma. Respiratory distress syndrome, diarrhea, icterus, epigastric tenderness, retinal hemorrhages, algid malaria (a shocklike syndrome), and severe thrombocytopenia may also occur. Renal insufficiency may result from volume depletion, vascular obstruction by parasitized erythrocytes, or immune complex deposition. Hemoglobinemia and hemoglobinuria resulting from intravascular hemolysis may progress to blackwater fever (so named from the dark color of the urine), either spontaneously or after treatment with quinine. Hypoglycemia is common and may be aggravated by quinine treatment and associated hyperinsulinemia. Placental involvement may lead to spontaneous abortion, stillbirth, or, rarely, congenital infection.

P. vivax*, *P. ovale, and ***P. malariae*** typically do not compromise vital organs. Mortality is rare and is mostly due to splenic rupture or uncontrolled hyperparasitemia in asplenic patients. The clinical course with *P. ovale* is similar to that of *P. vivax*. In established infections, temperature spikes occur at 48-h intervals. *P. malariae* infections often cause no acute symptoms, but low-level parasitemia may persist for decades and lead to immune complex–mediated nephritis or nephrosis or tropical splenomegaly; when symptomatic, fever tends to occur at 72-h intervals.

In a person who has been taking chemoprophylaxis (see p. 1584), malaria may be atypical. The incubation period may extend weeks after the drug is stopped. Those infected may develop headache, backache, and irregular fever. Parasites may initially be difficult to find in blood samples.

Diagnosis

Fever and chills (particularly recurrent attacks) in a traveler returning from an endemic region should prompt immediate assessment for malaria, even as much as 1 to 2 yr after return. Malaria is typically diagnosed by finding parasites on microscopic examination of thick or thin blood smears. The infecting species is identified by characteristic features on smears (see TABLE 186–1). The species

TABLE 186–1. DIAGNOSTIC FEATURES OF *PLASMODIUM* SPECIES IN BLOOD FILMS

CHARACTERISTIC	***PLASMODIUM* SPECIES***		
	Vivax	*Falciparum*	*Malariae*
Infected RBCs enlarged	Yes	No	No
Schüffner's dots	Yes†	No	No
Maurer's dots or clefts	No	Yes†	No
Multiple infections in RBCs	Rare	Yes	No
Rings with 2 chromatin dots	Rare	Frequent	No
Crescentic gametocytes	No	Yes	No
Bayonet or band trophozoites	No	No	Yes†
Schizonts present in peripheral blood	Yes	Rare	Yes
Number of merozoites per schizont (mean [range])	16 (12–24)	12 (8–24)‡	8 (6–12)

*RBCs infected with *P. ovale* are fimbriated, oval, and slightly enlarged; the parasites otherwise resemble *P. malariae*.

†Not always visible.

‡Schizonts are trapped in viscera and usually are not present in peripheral blood.

determines therapy and prognosis. Blood smears should be repeated at 4- to 6-h intervals if the initial smear is negative.

Thick films are prepared by spreading a large drop of blood circularly over a 15-mm area of a glass slide so that blood cells are layered on top of each other. The slide is allowed to dry thoroughly. Thick films are stained with Giemsa or Wright's-Giemsa solutions. After staining, slides can be rinsed in buffered water and then air-dried (not blotted). Since RBCs are hemolyzed by water in unfixed thick smears, parasites appear as extracellular organisms against a uniform background of red cell stroma. Thin films, which are fixed in methanol before staining, are less sensitive than thick films but require less diagnostic expertise to interpret.

Bedside dipstick tests using monoclonal antibodies for histidine-rich protein-2 appear to be of comparable accuracy to blood smears in diagnosis of *P. falciparum* and require less training than microscopy. PCR and species-specific DNA probes may be used but are not widely available. Serologic tests may reflect prior exposure and are not appropriate to diagnose acute malaria.

Treatment

Malaria is particularly dangerous in children < 5 yr, pregnant women, and previously unexposed visitors to endemic areas. In case of a febrile illness during travel in an endemic region, prompt professional medical evaluation is essential; when this is not possible, self-medication with atovaquone-proguanil can be used pending evaluation.

If *P. falciparum* is suspected, therapy should be initiated immediately, even if the initial smear is negative. *P. falciparum* and, more recently, *P. vivax* have become increasingly resistant to antimalarial drugs. Recommended dosages of antimalarial drugs are listed in TABLES 186–2 and 186–3. Common adverse effects and contraindications are listed in TABLE 186–4.

Treatment of the acute attack: Chloroquine is the drug of choice against *P. malariae, P. ovale*, and chloroquine-sensitive *P. falciparum* and *P. vivax*. Chloroquine resistance is common among *P. falciparum* strains throughout endemic areas, with the exception of Central America west of the Panama Canal, Haiti, and the Dominican Republic. Chloroquine resistance is not always complete, but chloroquine should be used only for malaria acquired in areas where *Plasmodium* sp are known to be sensitive.

Uncomplicated chloroquine-resistant *P. falciparum* can be treated with atovaquone-proguanil or quinine plus doxycycline. If the patient is pregnant, quinine plus clindamycin can be used. Mefloquine at treatment doses is an option, but adverse effects are common. IV quinidine or quinine dihydrochloride is used in patients unable to take oral drugs. These drugs should be used with hemodynamic and ECG monitoring; the infusion is slowed or temporarily suspended if the QT interval is > 0.6 sec or the QRS widens > 25% beyond baseline. Parenteral therapy should be continued until oral medication is tolerated. It is customary to supplement quinine and quinidine with doxycycline or clindamycin to prevent late recrudescences. These antibiotics act too slowly to be used alone for the treatment of acute malaria. Halofantrine (not available in the US) may prolong the QT interval and has been associated with sudden death. Artesunate and several other artemisinin derivatives are available overseas but not in the US; they are usually combined with a 2nd drug (eg, lumefantrine) to prevent recrudescence.

The patient must be monitored closely for hypoglycemia and proper hydration. Exchange transfusions have been used in some patients with high parasitemia to remove infected RBCs, but there is not uniform agreement on this approach. After successful treatment, the patient usually shows improvement in 24 to 48 h, but symptoms can persist for 5 days with *P. falciparum*.

Chloroquine-resistant *P. vivax* is common in Papua New Guinea and Indonesia. It is treated with quinine plus doxycycline or with mefloquine.

Curative therapy for hypnozoites: To prevent relapses of *P. vivax* or *P. ovale* malaria, the hypnozoite stage must be eliminated from the liver with primaquine. Primaquine may be given simultaneously with chloroquine or afterward. Some *P. vivax* strains are less sensitive and require repeated treatment with higher doses. Primaquine therapy is not necessary for *P. falciparum* or *P. malariae,* because these *Plasmodium* sp do not have a persistent hepatic phase.

Prevention

Prophylactic antimalarial drugs and insect repellants reduce but do not eliminate risk of malaria. No vaccine is currently available.

TABLE 186–2. TREATMENT OF MALARIA

INFECTION	DRUG*	ADULT DOSAGE	PEDIATRIC DOSAGE
Chloroquine-resistant *P. falciparum*			
Oral drugs of choice	Atovaquone-proguanil[a]	4 adult tablets daily × 3 days	< 5 kg: not indicated 5–8 kg: 2 pediatric tablets once/day × 3 days 9–10 kg: 3 pediatric tablets once/day × 3 days 11–20 kg: 1 adult tablet once/day for 3 days 21–30 kg: 2 adult tablets once/day × 3 days 31–40 kg: 3 adult tablets once/day × 3 days > 40 kg: 4 adult tablets once/day × 3 days
	or		
	Quinine sulfate **plus**	650 mg q 8 h × 3–7 days[b]	10 mg/kg q 8 h × 3–7 days[b]
	Doxycycline	100 mg bid × 7 days[c]	2 mg/kg bid × 7 days[c]
	or plus		
	Tetracycline	250 mg qid × 7 days[c]	6.25 mg/kg qid × 7 days[c]
	or plus		
	Pyrimethamine-sulfadoxine[d]	3 tablets once on the last day of quinine	< 5 kg: 1/4 tablet once on last day of quinine 5–10 kg: 1/2 tablet once on last day of quinine 11–20 kg: 1 tablet once on last day of quinine 21–30 kg: 1 1/2 tablets once on last day of quinine 31–40 kg: 2 tablets once on last day of quinine > 40 kg: 3 tablets once on last day of quinine
	or plus		
	Clindamycin	7 mg/kg tid × 7 days	7 mg/kg tid × 7 days
Alternatives	Mefloquine[e]	750 mg followed 12 h later by 500 mg	15 mg/kg followed 12 h later by 10 mg/kg
	or		
	Artesunate **plus**	4 mg/kg once/day × 3 days	4 mg/kg once/day × 3 days
	Mefloquine[e]	750 mg followed 12 h later by 500 mg	15 mg/kg followed 12 h later by 10 mg/kg
Chloroquine-resistant *P. vivax*			
Oral drugs of choice	Quinine sulfate **plus**	650 mg q 8 h × 3–7 days[b]	10 mg/kg q 8 h × 3–7 days[b]
	Doxcycline	100 mg bid × 7 days[c]	2 mg/kg bid × 7 days[c]
	or		
	Mefloquine[e]	750 mg followed 12 h later by 500 mg	15 mg/kg followed 12 h later by 10 mg/kg

TABLE 186–2. TREATMENT OF MALARIA—Continued

INFECTION	DRUG*	ADULT DOSAGE	PEDIATRIC DOSAGE
Alternatives	Chloroquine **plus**	8.3 mg base/kg q 16 h for 3 doses	8.3 mg base/kg q 16 h for 3 doses
	Primaquine	30 mg base once/day × 14 days	0.6 mg/kg once/day × 14 days
All *Plasmodium* except chloroquine-resistant *P. falciparum* and chloroquine-resistant *P. vivax*			
Oral drug of choice	Chloroquine phosphate[f]	1 g (600 mg base), then 500 mg (300 mg base) 6 h later, then 500 mg (300 mg base) at 24 and 48 h	10 mg base/kg (maximum 600 mg base), then 5 mg base/kg 6 h later, then 5 mg/kg at 24 and 48 h
All *Plasmodium*			
Parenteral drug of choice	Quinidine gluconate[g]	10 mg/kg loading dose (maximum 600 mg) in normal saline over 1–2 h, followed by continuous infusion of 0.02 mg/kg/min until oral therapy can be started	10 mg/kg loading dose (maximum 600 mg) in normal saline over 1–2 h, followed by continuous infusion of 0.02 mg/kg/min until oral therapy can be started
	or		
	Quinine dihydrochloride[g]	20 mg/kg loading dose in 5% dextrose over 4 h, followed by 10 mg/kg over 2–4 h q 8 h (maximum 1800 mg/day) until oral therapy can be started	20 mg/kg loading dose in 5% dextrose over 4 h, followed by 10 mg/kg over 2–4 h q 8 h (maximum 1800 mg/day) until oral therapy can be started
Alternative	Artemether	3.2 mg/kg IM, then 1.6 mg/kg once/day × 5–7 days	3.2 mg/kg IM, then 1.6 mg/kg once/day × 5–7 days
Prevention of relapses: *P. vivax* and *P. ovale* only			
Drug of choice	Primaquine phosphate	30 mg base once/day × 14 days	0.6 mg base/kg once/day × 14 days

*See TABLE 186–4 for adverse reactions and contraindications.

a. Atovaquone plus proguanil is available as a fixed-dose combination tablet: adult tablets (250 mg atovaquone/100 mg proguanil) and pediatric tablets (62.5 mg atovaquone/25 mg proguanil). To enhance absorption, it should be taken with food or a milky drink.

b. In Southeast Asia, relative resistance to quinine has increased, and treatment should be continued for 7 days.

c. Use of tetracyclines is contraindicated in pregnancy and in children ≤ 8 yr old.

d. Combination tablets contain 25 mg of pyrimethamine and 500 mg of sulfadoxine. Resistance to pyrimethamine-sulfadoxine has been reported from Southeast Asia, the Amazon basin, sub-Saharan Africa, Bangladesh, and Oceania.

e. Resistance to mefloquine has been reported in some areas, eg, the Thailand-Myanmar and Thailand-Cambodia borders and the Amazon basin, where 25 mg/kg should be used. In the US, a 250-mg tablet of mefloquine contains 228 mg mefloquine base. Outside the US, each 275-mg tablet contains 250 mg base.

f. If chloroquine phosphate is not available, hydroxychloroquine sulfate is as effective; 400 mg of hydroxychloroquine sulfate is equivalent to 500 mg of chloroquine phosphate.

g. For problems with quinidine availability, call the manufacturer or the Centers for Disease Control and Prevention Malaria Hotline (770-488-7788). Quinidine may have greater antimalarial activity than quinine. The loading dose should be decreased or omitted in patients who have received quinine or mefloquine. If > 48 h of parenteral treatment is required, the quinine or quinidine dose should be reduced by 30 to 50%.

Used with permission from *The Medical Letter on Drugs and Therapeutics*, The Medical Letter, Inc., August 2004.

Prophylaxis against mosquitoes includes using permethrin- or pyrethrum-containing residual insecticide sprays on clothing or in homes and outbuildings, placing screens on doors and windows, using mosquito netting (preferably impregnated with permethrin or pyrethrum) around beds, using mosquito repellents such as DEET, and wearing protective

TABLE 186–3. PREVENTION OF MALARIA

INFECTION	DRUG*	ADULT DOSAGE	PEDIATRIC DOSAGE
Chloroquine-sensitive areas			
Drug of choice	Chloroquine phosphate **or**	500 mg (300 mg base) once/wk[a]	5 mg/kg base once/wk, up to adult dose of 300 mg base[a]
	Atovaquone-proguanil[b]	1 adult tablet/day[c]	11–20 kg: 1 pediatric tablet/day[c] 21–30 kg: 2 pediatric tablets/day[c] 31–40 kg: 3 pediatric tablets/day[c] > 40 kg: 1 adult tablet/day[c]
	Plus[d]		
	Primaquine	30 mg base once/day for last 2 wk of prophylaxis	0.6 mg/kg base once/day for last 2 wk of prophylaxis
Chloroquine-resistant areas			
Drug of choice	Atovaquone-proguanil[b]	1 adult tablet/day[c]	11–20 kg: 1 pediatric tablet/day[c] 21–30 kg: 2 pediatric tablets/day[c] 31–40 kg: 3 pediatric tablets/day[c] > 40 kg: 1 adult tablet/day[c]
	Doxycycline	100 mg once/day[e]	2 mg/kg once/day, up to 100 mg/day[e]
	Mefloquine[f]	250 mg once/wk[a]	5–10 kg: 1/8 tablet once/wk[a] 11–20 kg: 1/4 tablet once/wk[a] 21–30 kg: 1/2 tablet once/wk[a] 31–45 kg: 3/4 tablet once/wk[a] > 45 kg: 1 tablet once/wk[a]
	Plus[d]		
	Primaquine	30 mg base once/day for last 2 wk of prophylaxis	0.6 mg/kg base once/day for last 2 wk of prophylaxis
Alternatives	Primaquine **or**	30 mg base once/day[g]	0.6 mg/kg base once/day[g]
	Chloroquine phosphate	500 mg (300 mg base) once/wk[a]	5 mg/kg base once/wk, up to 300 mg base[a]
	Plus		
	Proguanil	200 mg once/day[h]	< 2 yr: 50 mg once/day[h] 2–6 yr: 100 mg once/day[h] 7–10 yr: 150 mg once/day[h] > 10 yr: 200 mg once/day[h]

*See TABLE 186–4 for adverse reactions and contraindications.

a. Beginning 1 to 2 wk before travel and continuing weekly for the duration of stay and for 4 wk after leaving.

b. Atovaquone plus proguanil is available as a fixed-dose combination tablet: adult tablets (250 mg atovaquone/100 mg proguanil) and pediatric tablets (62.5 mg atovaquone/25 mg proguanil). To enhance absorption, it should be taken with food or a milky drink.

c. Beginning 1 to 2 days before travel and continuing for the duration of stay and for 1 wk after leaving.

d. Recommended by some experts for prevention of attack after departure from areas where *P. vivax* and *P. ovale* are endemic, which includes almost all areas where malaria is found (except Haiti). Others prefer to avoid the toxicity of primaquine and rely on surveillance to detect cases when they occur, particularly when exposure was limited or doubtful.

e. Beginning 1 to 2 days before travel and continuing for the duration of stay and for 4 wk after leaving. Use of tetracyclines is contraindicated in pregnancy and in children ≤ 8 yr.

f. Resistance to mefloquine has been reported in some areas, such as the Thailand-Myanmar and Thailand-Cambodia borders; in these areas, atovaquone-proguanil or doxycycline should be used for prophylaxis. Many experts no longer recommend mefloquine because of its potential for serious neuropsychiatric effects.

g. Beginning 1 day before travel and continued until 3 to 7 days after leaving may provide effective prophylaxis against chloroquine-resistant *P. falciparum*. Some studies have shown less efficacy against *P. vivax*. Nausea and abdominal pain can be diminished by taking with food.

h. Prophylaxis is recommended during exposure and for 4 wk after.

Adapted with permission from *The Medical Letter on Drugs and Therapeutics*. The Medical Letter, Inc., August 2004.

TABLE 186–4. ADVERSE REACTIONS AND CONTRAINDICATIONS OF ANTIMALARIAL DRUGS

DRUG	ADVERSE REACTIONS	CONTRAINDICATIONS
Atovaquone-proguanil	GI disturbances, headache, dizziness, pruritus	Hypersensitivity, pregnancy, breastfeeding, severe renal impairment (creatinine clearance < 30 mL/min)
Chloroquine phosphate Chloroquine HCl Hydroxychloroquine sulfate	GI disturbances, headaches, dizziness, blurred vision, rashes or pruritus, exacerbation of psoriasis, blood dyscrasias, alopecia, ECG changes, retinopathy, psychosis (rare)	Hypersensitivity, retinal or visual field changes
Clindamycin	Hypotension, bone marrow toxicity, renal dysfunction, rashes, jaundice, tinnitus, pseudomembranous colitis	Hypersensitivity
Doxycycline	GI upset, photosensitivity, vaginal candidiasis, pseudomembranous colitis, erosive esophagitis	Pregnancy, children ≤ 8 yr
Halofantrine	Prolongation of PR and QT intervals, cardiac arrhythmia, hypotension, GI disturbances, dizziness, mental changes, seizures, sudden death	Cardiac conduction defects, familial QT prolongation, drugs that affect QT interval, hypersensitivity, pregnancy
Mefloquine	Bad dreams, neuropsychiatric symptoms, dizziness, vertigo, confusion, psychosis, seizures, sinus bradycardia, GI disturbances	Hypersensitivity, history of seizures or psychiatric disorders, drugs that may prolong cardiac conduction (eg, β-blockers, Ca channel blockers, quinine, quinidine, halofantrine) in patients with heart disease, occupations requiring fine coordination and spatial discrimination, pregnancy
Quinine sulfate Quinine dihydrochloride	GI disturbances, tinnitus, visual disturbances, allergic reactions, mental changes, arrhythmias, cardiotoxicity	Hypersensitivity, G6PD deficiency, optic neuritis, tinnitus, pregnancy (relative contraindication), past adverse quinine reaction (continuous ECG, BP [when given IV], and glucose monitoring recommended)
Quinidine gluconate	Arrhythmias, prolonged Q-Tc interval, hypotension	Hypersensitivity, thrombocytopenia (continuous ECG, BP, and glucose monitoring recommended)
Primaquine phosphate	Severe intravascular hemolysis in people with G6PD deficiency, GI disturbances, leukopenia, methemoglobinuria	Concomitant quinacrine, potentially hemolytic or bone marrow suppressing agents, G6PD deficiency, pregnancy
Pyrimethamine-sulfadoxine	Erythema multiforme, Stevens-Johnson syndrome, toxic epidermal neurolysis, urticaria, exfoliative dermatitis, serum sickness, hepatitis, seizures, mental changes, GI disturbances, stomatitis, pancreatitis, bone marrow toxicity, hemolysis, fever, nephrosis	Hypersensitivity, folate deficiency anemia, infants ≤ 2 mo, pregnancy, breastfeeding

clothing, especially between dusk and dawn, when *Anopheles* mosquitoes are active.

Chemoprophylaxis: Regimens and dosing vary by geographic location and patient characteristics (see TABLE 186–3). If exposure to *P. vivax* or *P. ovale* was intense or prolonged or the traveler was splenectomized, a 14-day prophylactic course of primaquine phosphate on return helps reduce the risk of recurrence. The major adverse effect is hemolysis in people with G6PD deficiency.

Malaria during pregnancy poses a serious threat to both the mother and fetus. If travel to an endemic area is unavoidable, chemoprophylaxis with at least chloroquine should be given. The safety of mefloquine during pregnancy has not been documented, but limited experience suggests that it may be used when the benefits are judged to outweigh the risks. Doxycycline, atovaquone-proguanil, and primaquine should not be used during pregnancy.

TOXOPLASMOSIS

Toxoplasmosis is infection with *Toxoplasma gondii*. Symptoms range from none, to benign lymphadenopathy, a mononucleosis-like illness, or life-threatening CNS disease in immunocompromised people. Retinochoroiditis, seizures, and mental retardation occur in congenital infection. Diagnosis is by serologic tests, histology, or PCR. Treatment is most often with pyrimethamine plus sulfadiazine or clindamycin. Corticosteroids are administered concurrently for retinochoroiditis.

Human exposure to toxoplasmosis is common wherever cats are found; 20 to 40% of healthy adults in the US are seropositive. The risk of developing disease is very low except for a fetus infected in utero and those who are immunocompromised.

Etiology and Pathophysiology

T. gondii is ubiquitous in birds and mammals. This obligate intracellular parasite invades and multiplies asexually as tachyzoites within the cytoplasm of any nucleated cell. When host immunity develops, multiplication of tachyzoites ceases and tissue cysts form, which persist for years, especially in brain and muscle. Sexual reproduction of *T. gondii* occurs only in the intestinal tract of cats; the resultant oocysts passed in the feces remain infectious in moist soil for months.

Ingestion of oocysts from cat feces is the most common mode of oral infection in the US. Infection can also occur by eating raw or undercooked meat containing tissue cysts, most commonly lamb, pork, or rarely beef. Toxoplasmosis can be transmitted transplacentally if the mother becomes infected or if immunosuppression reactivates a prior infection during pregnancy. Transmission may also occur via transfusion of whole blood or WBCs or via transplantation of an organ from a seropositive donor. Reactivation occurs primarily in immunocompromised patients. In otherwise healthy people, congenital or acquired infection can reactivate in the retina. Past infection confers resistance to reinfection.

Symptoms and Signs

Infection is usually asymptomatic but may cause mild, self-resolving cervical or axillary lymphadenopathy. Symptomatic infections may present in several ways.

Acute toxoplasmosis may mimic infectious mononucleosis with lymphadenopathy, fever, malaise, myalgia, hepatosplenomegaly, and less commonly, pharyngitis. Atypical lymphocytosis, mild anemia, leukopenia, and slightly elevated liver enzymes are common. The syndrome may persist for weeks to months but is almost always self-limited.

Severe disseminated toxoplasmosis is rare in immunocompetent people. Latent toxoplasmosis reactivates in 30 to 40% of AIDS patients who are not taking antibiotic prophylaxis, but the widespread use of trimethoprim-sulfamethoxazole for *Pneumocystis* prophylaxis has dramatically reduced the incidence. Most patients with AIDS who develop toxoplasmosis present with life-threatening encephalitis or meningoencephalitis; myocarditis, pneumonitis, orchitis, involvement of other organs, and disseminated disease are much less common. CNS toxoplasmosis can cause focal neurologic deficits, such as motor or sensory loss, cranial nerve palsies, visual abnormalities, focal seizures, and generalized CNS abnormalities, such as headache, altered mental status, seizures, coma, and fever.

Disseminated disease, which occurs primarily in severely immunocompromised patients, is characterized by pneumonitis, myocarditis, meningoencephalitis, polymyositis, diffuse maculopapular rash, high fevers, chills, and prostration. In toxoplasmic pneumonitis, diffuse interstitial infiltrates may progress rapidly to consolidation and cause respiratory failure, whereas endarteritis may lead to infarction of small lung segments. Myocarditis, wherein conduction defects are common but often asymptomatic, may rapidly lead to heart failure. Untreated disseminated infections are usually fatal.

Congenital toxoplasmosis results from a primary (and often asymptomatic) acute infection acquired by the mother during pregnancy. Women infected before conception ordinarily do not transmit toxoplasmosis to the fetus unless the infection is reactivated during pregnancy by immunosuppression. Spontaneous abortion and stillbirth may occur. The percentage of surviving fetuses born with toxoplasmosis increases from 15% to 30% to 60% for maternal infections acquired in the 1st, 2nd, or 3rd trimester of pregnancy, respectively. Disease in the newborn may be severe, particularly if acquired early in pregnancy, with jaundice, rash, hepatosplenomegaly, and the characteristic tetrad of abnormalities: bilateral retinochoroiditis, cerebral calcifications, hydrocephalus or microcephaly, and psychomotor retardation. Prognosis is poor. Many children with less severe infections and most infants born to mothers infected during the 3rd trimester appear healthy at birth but are at high risk of seizures, mental retardation, retinochoroiditis, or other symptoms developing months or even years later.

Ocular toxoplasmosis usually results from congenital infection that is reactivated, often in the teens and 20s, but it can occur with acquired infections. Focal necrotizing retinitis and a secondary granulomatous inflammation of the choroid occur. Relapses of retinochoroiditis are common and may lead to ocular pain, blurred vision, and sometimes blindness.

Diagnosis

The diagnosis is usually made serologically. Specific IgM antibodies appear during the first 2 wk of acute illness, peak within 4 to 8 wk, and eventually become undetectable, but they may be present for as long as 18 mo after acute infection. IgG antibodies arise more slowly, peak in 1 to 2 mo, and may remain high and stable for months to years. Specific IgM antibodies with low IgG are consistent with recent infection in immunocompetent patients. Acute infection should also be suspected if the IgG is positive in the presence of encephalitis in an immunocompromised host. *Toxoplasma*-specific IgG antibody levels in AIDS patients are usually low to moderate but may occasionally be absent. Past infection in a healthy person typically produces a negative IgM test, and a positive IgG indicates resistance to reinfection. Low titers of IgG antibodies are usually present, but specific IgM antibody is not detected in patients with retinochoroiditis.

Detection of specific IgM antibody in newborns suggests congenital infection (maternal IgG crosses the placenta but IgM does not). Detection of *Toxoplasma*-specific IgA antibodies is more sensitive than IgM in congenitally infected infants, but it is available only at special reference facilities.

Serologic testing is not useful for confirming the diagnosis of toxoplasmic encephalitis in patients with AIDS. IgM antibodies are not present during reactivation, and IgG antibodies to *T. gondii* do not distinguish between latent and reactivated infection.

The parasite, on occasion, can be demonstrated histologically. Tachyzoites, which are present during acute infection, take up Giemsa or Wright's stain but may be difficult to find in routine tissue sections. Tissue cysts do not distinguish acute from chronic infection. *Toxoplasma* must be distinguished from other intracellular organisms, such as *Histoplasma, Trypanosoma cruzi,* and *Leishmania.* PCR tests for parasite DNA in blood, CSF, or amniotic fluid are available at several reference laboratories. PCR-based analysis of amniotic fluid is the preferred method to diagnose toxoplasmosis during pregnancy.

If CNS toxoplasmosis is suspected, patients should have head CT with contrast agent and/or MRI and a lumbar puncture if there are no signs of increased intracranial pressure. MRI is more sensitive than CT. CSF may show lymphocytic pleocytosis and elevated protein levels. CT typically shows single or multiple dense, rounded, ring-enhancing lesions. Although these lesions are not pathognomonic, their presence in patients with AIDS and CNS symptoms warrants a trial of chemotherapy for *T. gondii*. If the suspected diagnosis of toxoplasmosis is correct, clinical or radiographic improvement should become evident within 7 to 14 days. If symptoms persist, a brain biopsy should be considered.

Treatment

Most immunocompetent patients do not require therapy unless visceral disease is present or severe symptoms persist. However, specific treatment is indicated for acute toxoplasmosis of newborns, pregnant women, and immunocompromised patients.

The most effective regimen is pyrimethamine 50 to 100 mg po bid for 1 day, then 50 to 100 mg once/day for 3 to 4 wk in adults (1 mg/kg q 12 h for 3 days, then 1 mg/kg once/day for 4 wk in children) plus sulfadiazine 1 to 1.5 g po qid for adults for 4 wk (25 to 50 mg/kg qid for 4 wk for children). Pyrimethamine bone marrow suppression can be minimized with leucovorin (not folate, which blocks the therapeutic effect) 10 to 25 mg once/day (for adults). Patients with ocular toxoplasmosis should also receive corticosteroids.

Congenitally infected infants should be given pyrimethamine 1 mg/kg bid for 2 or 3 days then 1 mg/kg once/day plus sulfadiazine 50 mg/kg bid for 6 mo; after 6 mo, pyrimethamine is given 3 times/wk and sulfadiazine is continued daily to complete a year of total therapy. Infants also receive leucovorin 5 to 10 mg po 3 times/wk while receiving pyrimethamine and for 1 wk after pyrimethamine is stopped.

Treatment of acutely infected pregnant women can decrease the incidence of fetal infection. However, pyrimethamine should not be used until after the 1st trimester of pregnancy. Spiramycin 1 g po tid has been used safely to reduce the risk of transmission in pregnant women during the 1st trimester but is less active than pyrimethamine-sulfonamide combinations and does not cross the placenta. It is continued until fetal infection is documented or excluded at the end of the 1st trimester. If no transmission has occurred, spiramycin can be continued to term. If the fetus is infected, therapy with pyrimethamine and sulfadiazine is begun.

Relapses are common in patients with AIDS, and suppressive treatment should continue indefinitely. In patients with acute toxoplasmosis who are unable to tolerate sulfonamides, pyrimethamine plus clindamycin 600 mg po or IV qid can be used. Atovaquone and azithromycin are other alternatives for sulfa-intolerant patients.

Prevention

Washing hands thoroughly after handling raw meat, soil, or cat litter is essential. Food possibly contaminated with cat feces should be avoided. Meat should be cooked to 165 to 170° F.

Chemoprophylaxis is recommended for patients with HIV and positive IgG *T. gondii* serology once $CD4^+$ cell counts are < 100/μL. The combination of trimethoprim-sulfamethoxazole in the same doses used for prophylaxis against *Pneumocystis jiroveci* (eg, 1 double-strength tablet once/day) is one effective regimen. Two other regimens are pyrimethamine with dapsone and atovaquone with or without pyrimethamine.

187 VIRUSES

Viruses are the smallest parasites, ranging from 0.02 to 0.3 μm. They depend completely on cells (bacterial, plant, or animal) to reproduce. Viruses have an outer cover of protein, and sometimes lipid, and an RNA or DNA core. For infection to occur, the virus first attaches to the host cell. The viral DNA or RNA then separates from the outer cover (uncoating) and replicates inside the host cell in a process that requires specific enzymes. Most RNA viruses replicate their nucleic acid in the cytoplasm, whereas most DNA viruses do so in the nucleus. The host cell typically dies, releasing new viruses that infect other host cells.

Some infections are asymptomatic or latent. In latent infection, viral RNA or DNA remains in host cells but does not cause disease unless some trigger causes symptom recurrence. Latency may facilitate person-to-person spread. Herpesviruses exhibit latency.

Several hundred different viruses infect humans (see TABLE 187–1). Viruses that primarily infect humans often spread via respiratory and enteric excretions. Some are transmitted sexually and through transfer of blood. Viruses exist worldwide, but their spread is limited by inborn resistance, prior immunizing infections or vaccines, sanitary and other public health control measures, and prophylactic antiviral drugs.

Zoonotic viruses pursue their biologic cycles chiefly in animals; humans are secondary or accidental hosts. These viruses are limited to areas and environments able to support

Text continues on page 1592.

TABLE 187–1. SELECTED VIRUSES THAT INFECT HUMANS*

VIRUS GROUPS AND CATEGORIES	PRINCIPAL SYNDROMES	PREVALENCE AND DISTRIBUTION	THERAPY	PREVENTION
Respiratory				
Influenza viruses A, B, and C	Influenza; AFRD; acute bronchitis and pneumonia; croup	Epidemic, occasionally pandemic (A, B); endemic (C)	Amantadine, rimantadine (A), oseltamivir, zanamivir (A and B)	Vaccine (A and B); oseltamivir, zanamivir (A and B); amantadine and rimantadine (A)
Parainfluenza viruses 1–4	AFRD (children); acute bronchitis and pneumonia; croup	Local epidemics (1); widespread in children (1, 2, 3)	None	Vaccines under investigation
Adenoviruses	AFRD (children); ARD (adults); acute pharyngoconjunctival fever; epidemic keratoconjunctivitis; viral pneumonia; acute follicular conjunctivitis; diarrhea; hemorrhagic cystitis	Global, mostly children	None	Vaccine (4, 7) for military epidemics
Epstein-Barr virus	Infectious mononucleosis	Widespread; infection apparent chiefly in young adults	None	None
Respiratory syncytial virus	Lower respiratory illness (infants); mild upper respiratory illness (adults)	Widespread in children	Ribavirin for high-risk infants	None
Rhinoviruses	Common cold; acute coryza with or without fever	Universal, especially in cold months	None	None
Gastroenteritis				
Epidemic gastroenteritis viruses	Epidemic nausea and vomiting; diarrhea	Local epidemics (children); increased in colder months Rotavirus (children); adenovirus 40, 41 (infants); coronavirus-like agents (infants)	None	Rotavirus vaccines under investigation
Exanthematous				
Rubeola virus	Measles; encephalomyelitis	Global; incidence decreasing due to vaccine; CNS involvement rare	None	Vaccines

Table continues on the following page.

TABLE 187–1. SELECTED VIRUSES THAT INFECT HUMANS*—Continued

VIRUS GROUPS AND CATEGORIES	PRINCIPAL SYNDROMES	PREVALENCE AND DISTRIBUTION	THERAPY	PREVENTION
Rubella virus	German measles	Universal; birth defects from infection during pregnancy	None	Vaccines
Human parvovirus B19	Erythema infectiosum (fifth disease); rash; malaise; arthritis; hydrops fetalis (infection during pregnancy); anemia (infection in immunocompromised hosts or those with hemoglobinopathies)	Sporadic outbreaks	IV immune globulin (severe anemia)	None
Human herpesvirus type 6	Roseola infantum (exanthem subitum)	Widespread; young children	None	None
Varicella-zoster virus	Chickenpox; zoster	Almost universal (children), occasionally in adults (chickenpox); common in adults; reactivation of latent virus (zoster)	Acyclovir (chickenpox); acyclovir; famciclovir; valacyclovir (zoster)	Immune globulins, vaccine (chickenpox)
Variola	Smallpox	Natural disease eradicated	None	Vaccine
Alphaviruses (some)	Chikungunya disease	Africa, Southeast Asia, India	Possibly ribavirin	None
	Mayaro disease	South America, Trinidad	Possibly ribavirin	None
Molluscum contagiosum virus	Molluscum contagiosum papules	Genital (adults); exposed skin (children); more severe (AIDS)	Cryotherapy; curettage	None
Hepatitis				
Type A	Hepatitis A (acute)	Widespread; often epidemic	None	γ-Globulin; vaccine
Type B	Hepatitis B (acute and chronic)	Widespread	Interferon, antivirals	Strict aseptic precautions; screening for hepatitis B surface antigen; vaccine; γ- or hyperimmune globulin
Type C	Hepatitis C (acute and chronic)	Widespread	Interferon, ribavirin	Aseptic precautions; screening for hepatitis C

TABLE 187–1. SELECTED VIRUSES THAT INFECT HUMANS*—Continued

VIRUS GROUPS AND CATEGORIES	PRINCIPAL SYNDROMES	PREVALENCE AND DISTRIBUTION	THERAPY	PREVENTION
Type D	Hepatitis D (delta); severe hepatitis	Associated with IV drug abuse; can infect only in the presence of hepatitis B infection	None	None
Type E	Hepatitis E	Outbreaks; developing world; severe in pregnancy	None	Avoid contaminated water, food
Neurologic				
Polioviruses	Poliomyelitis (paralytic); aseptic meningitis	Global; incidence now low due to vaccine	None	Vaccines; live (oral), killed (injected)
Alphaviruses (some)	Western equine encephalitis	North and South America	Possibly ribavirin	None
	Eastern equine encephalitis	North and South America	Possibly ribavirin	Vaccine available to protect equines only
	Venezuelan equine encephalitis	Gulf states to South America	Possibly ribavirin	Vaccine available for equines; investigation vaccine has been used to vaccinate lab workers at risk
Flaviviruses (some)	Japanese encephalitis	Southeast Asia, Japan, Korea, China, India, Philippines, eastern former Soviet Union	Possibly ribavirin	Vaccine
	Murray Valley encephalitis	Australia, New Guinea	Possibly ribavirin	None
	St. Louis encephalitis	North and South America	Possibly ribavirin	None
	Russian spring-summer encephalitis	Former Soviet Union, eastern and central Europe, Malaysia	Possibly ribavirin	None
	Powassan encephalitis	North America	Possibly ribavirin	None
	West Nile virus encephalitis	Africa, Middle East, southern France, former Soviet Union, India, Indonesia, US	Possibly ribavirin	None

Table continues on the following page.

TABLE 187–1. SELECTED VIRUSES THAT INFECT HUMANS*—Continued

VIRUS GROUPS AND CATEGORIES	PRINCIPAL SYNDROMES	PREVALENCE AND DISTRIBUTION	THERAPY	PREVENTION
Flaviviruses (*continued*)	Tick-borne encephalitis	Europe, Balkans, former Soviet Union	Possibly ribavirin	Vaccine is available in Europe and Russia
Bunyaviruses (some)	California encephalitis and related types	Probably worldwide; common in midwestern US	None	None
Arenaviruses (some)	Lymphocytic choriomeningitis	Worldwide; chief reservoir, rodents	None	None
Rabies virus	Rabies	Worldwide	None	Vaccine; postexposure rabies immune globulin
Hemorrhagic fever				
Flaviviruses (some)	Omsk hemorrhagic fever	Former Soviet Union	Possibly ribavirin	None
	Kyasanur Forest disease	India	Possibly ribavirin	None
	Yellow fever	Africa, Central and South America	Possibly ribavirin	Vaccine
	Dengue fever	Tropics and subtropics, worldwide	Possibly ribavirin	None
Bunyaviruses (some)	Hantaan virus	Northern Asia, Europe, southwestern US		None
Filoviruses (some)	Marburg virus	Africa	None	None
	Ebola virus	Africa	None	None
Arenaviruses (some)	Lassa fever	Africa	Ribavirin	None
	Machupo (Bolivian hemorrhagic fever)	South America	Convalescent plasma; ribavirin	None
	Junin (Argentinian hemorrhagic fever)	South America	Convalescent plasma; ribavirin	Vaccine under investigation
Nairovirus	Crimean-Congo hemorrhagic fever	Former Soviet Union, central Africa, western Pakistan	None	None

TABLE 187–1. SELECTED VIRUSES THAT INFECT HUMANS*—Continued

VIRUS GROUPS AND CATEGORIES	PRINCIPAL SYNDROMES	PREVALENCE AND DISTRIBUTION	THERAPY	PREVENTION
Recurrent or chronic skin/mucous membrane lesions				
Herpes simplex virus	Herpes labialis; herpetic gingivostomatitis; dermatitis; keratoconjunctivitis; encephalitis; vulvovaginitis; neonatal disseminated disease	Recurrent labial, almost universal; gingivostomatitis frequent in infants and children	Acyclovir; famciclovir; valacyclovir; penciclovir	None
Human papillomavirus	Warts (verrucae); genital warts; cervical cancer	Universal; common; often recurrent	Cryotherapy; interferon (possibly for genital); podophyllin (genital); imiquimod	None
Multisystem				
Coxsackieviruses	Herpangina; epidemic pleurodynia; aseptic meningitis; meningoencephalitis; neonatal sepsis; myocarditis; pericarditis; AFRD (children); paralytic disease; fever and exanthem	Varies with types; most persons infected; increased in warm months and in children	None	None
Echoviruses† and "high-numbered" enteroviruses	Aseptic meningitis; fever and exanthem; meningoencephalitis; aseptic meningitis; neonatal sepsis; paralytic disease; myocarditis; pericarditis; ARD	As for coxsackieviruses	None	None
Cytomegalovirus	Congenital defects (cytomegalic inclusion disease); hepatitis (cytomegalovirus mononucleosis); immunocompromised host (including AIDS): retinitis, GI disease, CNS disease; pneumonia	Widespread; congenital; immunosuppressed	Ganciclovir; foscarnet; cidofovir; CMV I6 in specialized circumstances (eg, organ transplant recipient with CMV pneumonitis)	Ganciclovir
Nonspecific acute febrile illness				
Orbivirus	Colorado tick fever	Western US	None	None
Phleboviruses (some)	Phlebotomus (sandfly) fever	Mediterranean basin, Balkans, Middle East, Pakistan, India, China, eastern Africa, Panama, Brazil	None	None

Table continues on the following page.

TABLE 187–1. SELECTED VIRUSES THAT INFECT HUMANS*—Continued

VIRUS GROUPS AND CATEGORIES	PRINCIPAL SYNDROMES	PREVALENCE AND DISTRIBUTION	THERAPY	PREVENTION
Phleboviruses (*continued*)	Rift Valley fever	Eastern Africa, Egypt	None	Vaccine available for livestock; human vaccine under investigation
Other				
Mumps virus	Parotitis; orchitis; meningoencephalitis	Global; mostly children; some adults	None	Vaccine
Hantavirus	Hantavirus pulmonary syndrome	US (west of Mississippi River), Canada, Brazil, Bolivia, Paraguay, Argentina	None	
Reoviruses	Often asymptomatic	Widespread in children	None	None

AFRD = acute febrile respiratory disease; ARD = acute respiratory disease.

*Developments are so rapid that no summary can be fully up-to-date. In many cases, therapy and preventive measures are unknown.

†Echovirus types 9, 10, and 28 have been reclassified; these numbers are no longer used; more recently described enteroviruses have been designated as types 68 to 72.

their nonhuman natural cycles of infection (vertebrates, arthropods, or both). Most are discussed in Ch. 191 on p. 1617.

Some viruses are oncogenic. Human T-lymphotropic virus 1 predisposes to human leukemia and lymphoma. Epstein-Barr virus predisposes to malignancies such as nasopharyngeal carcinoma, Burkitt's lymphoma, Hodgkin lymphoma, and lymphomas in immunosuppressed organ transplant recipients. Hepatitis B and C viruses predispose to hepatocellular carcinoma. Human herpesvirus 8 predisposes to Kaposi's sarcoma, primary effusion lymphomas, and Castleman disease (a lymphoproliferative disorder).

Slow viral diseases have lengthy incubations (months or years) and are often due to reactivation of a virus that caused an earlier infection. They cause some chronic degenerative diseases, including subacute sclerosing panencephalitis (measles virus), progressive rubella panencephalitis, and progressive multifocal leukoencephalopathy (JC virus). Creutzfeldt-Jakob disease and bovine spongiform encephalopathy have characteristics similar to slow viral diseases, but they are caused by prions (see p. 1853).

Diagnosis

Some viral diseases can be diagnosed clinically or epidemiologically (eg, by well-known viral syndromes such as measles, rubella, roseola infantum, erythema infectiosum, and chickenpox, or during epidemic outbreaks such as influenza). For others, definitive diagnosis is necessary mainly when specific treatment may be helpful or when the agent may be a public health threat (eg, severe acute respiratory syndrome [SARS]). Such cases require testing.

Serologic examination during acute and convalescent stages is sensitive and specific but slow; more rapid diagnosis can sometimes be made using culture, PCR, or viral antigen tests. Histopathology with electron (not light) microscopy can sometimes help. Specific diagnostic procedures are described in Ch. 168 on p. 1394. For many less common diseases (eg, rabies, smallpox, Eastern equine encephalitis), state health laboratories and the Centers for Disease Control and Prevention can analyze specimens.

Treatment and Prevention

Antiviral drugs: Progress in the use of antiviral drugs is occurring rapidly. Antiviral chemotherapy can be directed at various phases of viral replication. It can interfere with viral particle attachment to host cell membranes or uncoating of viral nucleic acids, inhibit a cellular receptor or factor required for viral replication, or block specific virus-coded enzymes and proteins produced in the host cells that are essential for viral replication but not for normal host cell metabolism. Antiviral drugs are most often used therapeutically or prophylactically against herpesviruses (including cytomegalovirus—see Ch. 189), respiratory viruses (see Ch. 188), and HIV (see Ch. 192). However, some drugs are effective against many different kinds of viruses. Some drugs against HIV are being evaluated for other viral infections such as hepatitis B virus (HBV).

Interferons: Interferons are compounds released from infected host cells in response to viral or other foreign antigens. There are many different interferons, which have numerous effects that include blocking translation and transcription of viral RNA and stopping viral replication without disturbing normal host cell function. Interferons are sometimes given attached to polyethylene glycol (pegylated formulations), which allow a slow, sustained release of the interferon.

Interferon therapy for viral infection is used for hepatitis B and C and human papillomavirus. Interferon is indicated for patients with chronic infection with HBV or hepatitis C virus (HCV) plus abnormal liver function tests and either detectable viral loads or biopsy-documented active disease. Interferon-α2b can be used as a treatment for HBV at doses of 5 million units sc once/day or 10 million units sc 3 times/wk for 16 wk; treatment may induce clearance of HBV DNA and the hepatitis B e antigen (HBeAg) from serum and improve liver function tests and liver histology. Higher doses are required if there is coexistent delta hepatitis. HCV is treated with ribavirin plus either pegylated interferon-α2b 1.5 μg/kg sc once/wk or pegylated interferon-α2a 180 μg sc once/wk; treatment may decrease HCV RNA level and improve liver function and liver histology. Interferon-α-n3, intralesionally or IM, has also cleared intractable condyloma acuminata of skin and genitals, but its optimal administration and long-term effects are unclear. A recombinant form of endogenous interferon-α is being studied in hairy cell leukemia, Kaposi's sarcoma, human papillomavirus, and respiratory viruses.

Adverse effects include fever, chills, weakness, and myalgia, typically starting 7 to 12 h after the 1st injection and lasting up to 12 h. Depression, hepatitis, and, when used at high doses, bone marrow suppression are also possible.

Vaccines and immune globulins: Vaccines work by stimulating native immunity. Viral vaccines in general use include influenza, measles, mumps, poliomyelitis, rabies, rubella, hepatitis A, hepatitis B, varicella, and yellow fever. Adenovirus and smallpox vaccines are available but used only in high-risk groups (eg, military recruits).

Immune globulins are available for passive immune prophylaxis in limited situations. Some are used postexposure (eg, rabies, hepatitis immune globulins). Others may help in treating disease.

188 RESPIRATORY VIRUSES

(See also Bronchiolitis on p. 2305 and Croup on p. 2307.)

Viral infections commonly affect the upper or lower respiratory tract. Although these infections can be classified by the causative virus (eg, influenza), they are generally classified clinically according to syndrome (eg, the common cold, bronchiolitis, croup). Although specific pathogens commonly produce characteristic clinical manifestations (eg, rhinovirus and the common cold or respiratory syncytial virus [RSV] and bronchiolitis), each is capable of causing any of the viral respiratory syndromes.

The severity of viral respiratory illness varies widely, with severe disease more likely in the elderly and infants. Morbidity may result directly from viral infection or may be indirect, due to exacerbation of underlying cardiopulmonary conditions or bacterial superinfection of the lung, paranasal sinuses, or middle ear.

Detection of viral pathogens by PCR, culture, or serology is generally too slow to be useful for patient care but is useful for epidemiologic surveillance. More rapid diagnostic tests are available for influenza and RSV, but the utility of these tests for routine care is not clear. Management decisions are generally based on clinical data and epidemiology.

Treatment

Treatment of viral respiratory infections is usually supportive. Antibacterial drugs are ineffective against viral pathogens, and prophylaxis against secondary bacterial infections is not recommended. Antibiotics should be given only when secondary bacterial infections develop. In patients with chronic lung disease, antibiotics may be given with less restriction. Aspirin should not be used in children with respiratory infections because of the risk of Reye's syndrome. Some patients continue to have cough for weeks after resolution of an URI. Symptoms may improve with an inhaled bronchodilator or corticosteroids.

In some cases, antiviral drugs play a role. Amantadine, rimantadine, oseltamivir, and zanamivir are effective for influenza. Ribavirin, a guanosine analog that inhibits replication of many RNA and DNA viruses, may be considered in severely immunocompromised patients with lower respiratory tract infection due to RSV.

ADENOVIRUS INFECTIONS

Infection with one of the many adenoviruses may be asymptomatic or result in specific syndromes, including mild respiratory infections, keratoconjunctivitis, gastroenteritis, and primary pneumonia. Diagnosis is clinical. Treatment is supportive.

Adenoviruses are DNA viruses classified according to 3 major capsid antigens (hexon, penton, and fiber). Adenoviruses are commonly acquired by contact with secretions (including finger transmission) from an infected person or by contact with a contaminated object (eg, towel, instrument). Infection may be airborne or waterborne (eg, acquired by swimming). Respiratory or GI viral shedding may continue for months, even if infection is asymptomatic.

Symptoms, Signs, and Diagnosis

In immunocompetent hosts, most adenovirus infections are asymptomatic; when symptomatic, a broad spectrum of clinical manifestations is possible. The most common syndrome, especially in children, involves fever that tends to be > 39° C and to last > 5 days. Sore throat, cough, rhinorrhea, or other respiratory symptoms may occur. A separate syndrome involves conjunctivitis, pharyngitis, and fever (pharyngoconjunctival fever). Rare adenoviral syndromes in infants include severe bronchiolitis (see p. 2305) and pneumonia. In closed populations of young adults (eg, military recruits), outbreaks of respiratory illness may occur; symptoms include fever and lower respiratory tract symptoms, usually tracheobronchitis but occasionally pneumonia. Epidemic keratoconjunctivitis (see p. 890) is sometimes severe and occurs both sporadically and in epidemics. Conjunctivitis is frequently bilateral. Preauricular adenopathy may develop. Chemosis, pain, and punctate corneal lesions that are visible with fluorescein staining may be present. Systemic symptoms and signs are mild or absent. Epidemic keratoconjunctivitis usually resolves within 3 or 4 wk, although corneal lesions may persist much longer. Nonrespiratory adenoviral syndromes include hemorrhagic cystitis, diarrhea in infants, and meningoencephalitis.

Laboratory diagnosis of adenovirus infection rarely affects management. During the acute illness, virus can be isolated from respiratory and ocular secretions and frequently from stool and urine. A 4-fold rise in the serum antibody titer indicates recent adenoviral infection.

Prognosis, Treatment, and Prevention

Most patients recover fully. Even severe primary adenoviral pneumonia is not fatal except for rare fulminant cases, predominantly in infants, military recruits, and immunocompromised patients.

Treatment is symptomatic and supportive.

To minimize transmission, heath care practitioners should change gloves and wash hands after examining infected patients, properly sterilize instruments, and avoid using ophthalmologic instruments in multiple patients.

Vaccines containing live adenovirus types 4 and 7, given orally in an enteric-coated capsule, have previously reduced lower respiratory disease in military populations; however, these vaccines are no longer available.

COMMON COLD

(Upper Respiratory Infection)

The common cold is an acute, usually afebrile, self-limited viral infection involving upper respiratory symptoms, such as rhinorrhea, cough, and sore throat. Diagnosis is clinical. Hand washing helps prevent its spread. Treatment is supportive.

About 50% of all colds are caused by one of the > 100 serotypes of rhinoviruses. Coronaviruses cause some outbreaks, and infections caused by influenza, parainfluenza, and respiratory syncytial viruses may also manifest as the common cold, particularly in patients who are experiencing reinfection.

Rhinovirus infections are most common during fall and spring and are less common during winter months. Rhinoviruses are most efficiently spread by direct person-to-person contact, although spread may also occur via large-particle aerosols.

The most potent deterrent to infection is the presence of specific neutralizing antibodies in the serum and secretions, induced by previous exposure to the same or a closely related virus. Susceptibility to colds is not affected by exposure to cold temperature, host health and nutrition, or upper respiratory tract abnormalities (eg, enlarged tonsils or adenoids).

Symptoms, Signs, and Diagnosis

After an incubation period of 24 to 72 h, symptoms begin with a "scratchy" or sore throat, followed by sneezing, rhinorrhea, nasal obstruction, and malaise. Temperature is usually normal, particularly when the pathogen is a rhinovirus or coronavirus. Nasal secretions are watery and profuse during the first days but then become more mucoid and purulent. Mucopurulent secretions do not indicate a bacterial superinfection. Cough is usually mild but often lasts into the 2nd wk. Most symptoms due to uncomplicated colds resolve within 10 days. In patients with asthma and chronic bronchitis, colds may exacerbate the illness. Purulent sputum or significant lower respiratory tract symptoms are unusual with rhinovirus infection. Purulent sinusitis and otitis media may result from the viral infection itself or secondary bacterial infection.

Diagnosis is generally made clinically and presumptively, without diagnostic tests. Allergic rhinitis is the most important consideration in differential diagnosis.

Treatment and Prevention

No specific treatment exists. Antipyretics and analgesics may relieve fever or sore throat. Nasal obstruction may improve with nasal decongestants. Topical nasal decongestants are more effective than oral decongestants, but the use of topical drugs for > 3 to 5 days may result in rebound congestion. Rhinorrhea may improve with 1st-generation antihistamines (eg, chlorpheniramine) or intranasal ipratropium bromide (2 sprays of a 0.03% solution bid or tid); these, however, should be avoided in the elderly and people with benign prostatic hypertrophy or glaucoma. First-generation antihistamines frequently produce sedation, but 2nd-generation (nonsedating) antihistamines are ineffective for treating the common cold.

Zinc, echinacea, and vitamin C have all been evaluated as common cold therapies but none have been clearly demonstrated to be beneficial.

There are no vaccines. Polyvalent bacterial vaccines, citrus fruits, vitamins, ultraviolet light, glycol aerosols, and other folk remedies do not prevent the common cold. Hand washing and use of surface disinfectant in a contaminated environment may reduce spread of infection.

Antibiotics should not be given unless there is evidence of secondary bacterial infection. In patients with chronic lung disease, antibiotics may be given with less restriction.

INFLUENZA

(Flu; Grippe; Grip)

Influenza is a viral respiratory infection causing fever, coryza, cough, headache, and malaise. Mortality is possible during epidemics, particularly among high-risk patients (eg, those who are institutionalized, at the extremes of age, have cardiopulmonary insufficiency, or are in late pregnancy). Diagnosis is usually clinical and depends on local epidemiologic patterns. High-risk patients, their caregivers and household contacts, health care practitioners, and all

children aged 6 to 24 mo should receive annual influenza vaccination. Antiviral treatments include the neuraminidase inhibitors zanamivir and oseltamivir, which are effective for both influenza A and B, and amantadine and rimantadine, which are effective only against influenza A.

Influenza refers to illness caused by the influenza viruses, but the term is commonly and incorrectly used to refer to similar illnesses caused by other viral respiratory pathogens. Influenza viruses are classified as types A, B, or C by their nucleoproteins and matrix proteins. Influenza C virus infection does not cause typical influenza illness and is not discussed here.

Hemagglutinin (HA) is a glycoprotein on the influenza surface that allows the virus to bind to cellular sialic acid and fuse with the host membrane. Neuraminidase (NA), another surface glycoprotein, enzymatically removes sialic acid, promoting viral dispersion from the infected cell. Relatively minor mutations in HA and NA of influenza A and B result in the frequent emergence of new viral strains (antigenic drift). The result is decreased protection by antibody generated to the previous strain. In contrast to antigenic drift, a major change in NA or HA occurs in influenza A (antigenic shift) at infrequent intervals (10 to 40 yr during the last century); as a result, the population has no immunity to the new virus, and pandemic influenza may occur.

Epidemiology

Influenza produces widespread sporadic illness yearly during fall and winter in temperate climates. Epidemics in the US occur about every 2 to 3 yr, most often caused by influenza A viruses. Pandemics caused by new influenza A serotypes may cause particularly severe disease. Influenza B viruses typically produce mild disease but can cause epidemics with moderate or severe disease, usually occurring in 3- to 5-yr cycles. Although most influenza epidemics result from a single serotype, different influenza viruses may appear sequentially in one location or may appear simultaneously, with one virus predominating in one location and another virus predominating elsewhere.

Seasonal epidemics often occur in 2 waves—the 1st in schoolchildren and their household contacts (generally younger people) and the 2nd mostly in housebound or institutionalized people, particularly the elderly.

Influenza viruses may be spread by airborne droplets, person-to-person contact, or contact with contaminated items. Airborne spread appears to be the most important mechanism.

Patients with underlying cardiopulmonary disease, metabolic disease (especially diabetes mellitus) that requires regular medical attention, renal insufficiency, hemoglobinopathies, or immunodeficiency are at increased risk for severe disease. Women in the 2nd or 3rd trimester of pregnancy, children < 24 mo, and adults > 65 yr are also at increased risk. Morbidity and mortality in these patients may be due to exacerbation of underlying illness, primary influenza pneumonia, or secondary bacterial pneumonia.

Symptoms and Signs

The incubation period ranges from 1 to 4 days with an average of about 48 h. In mild cases, many symptoms are like those of a common cold (eg, sore throat, rhinorrhea); mild conjunctivitis may also occur. Typical influenza in adults is characterized by the sudden onset of chills, fever, prostration, cough, and generalized aches and pains (especially in the back and legs). Headache is prominent, often with photophobia and retrobulbar aching. Respiratory symptoms may be mild at first, with scratchy sore throat, substernal burning, nonproductive cough, and sometimes coryza. Later, lower respiratory tract illness becomes dominant; cough can be persistent, raspy, and productive. Children may have prominent nausea, vomiting, or abdominal pain, and infants may present with a sepsis-like syndrome. After 2 to 3 days, acute symptoms rapidly subside, although fever may last up to 5 days. Cough, weakness, sweating, and fatigue may persist for several days or occasionally for weeks.

Pneumonia is suggested by a worsening cough, purulent or bloody sputum, dyspnea, and rales. Secondary bacterial pneumonia is suggested by persistence or recurrence of fever, cough, and other respiratory symptoms in the 2nd wk.

Encephalitis, myocarditis, and myoglobinuria develop infrequently, usually during convalescence. The cause is unclear, but they occur more frequently after influenza A pandemics. Reye's syndrome (see p. 2401), characterized by encephalopathy, fatty liver, hypoglycemia, and lipidemia, is strongly associated with epidemics of influenza B, particularly in children who have ingested aspirin.

Diagnosis

The diagnosis is generally made clinically in patients with a typical syndrome when influenza is known to be present in the community. Although many rapid diagnostic tests are available, their sensitivities and specificities vary widely among different studies. The use of rapid tests to select patients who might benefit from antiviral therapy remains controversial. Definitive diagnosis requires cell culture of nasopharyngeal swabs or aspirate or acute and convalescent antibody titers. This testing takes several days or more and is useful primarily for establishing the presence of influenza in the community and detecting antigenic changes.

Patients with lower respiratory tract signs and symptoms, such as dyspnea, hypoxia, or rales on lung examination, should have a chest x-ray to detect pneumonia. Primary influenza pneumonia typically appears as diffuse interstitial infiltrates or as acute respiratory distress syndrome. Secondary bacterial pneumonia is more likely to be lobar or segmental.

Prognosis and Treatment

Most patients recover fully, although full recovery often takes 1 or 2 wk. However, influenza and influenza-related pneumonia are important causes of death in high-risk patients, young children, the elderly, and those with chronic disease. The efficacy of antiviral treatment in these cases is unknown. Appropriate antibacterial therapy decreases the mortality rate from secondary bacterial pneumonia.

Treatment for most patients is symptomatic, including rest, hydration, and antipyretics as needed, but aspirin is avoided in children. Complicating bacterial infections require appropriate antibiotics.

Antiviral drugs given within 1 to 2 days of symptom onset decrease symptom duration slightly. Treatment with antiviral drugs is generally recommended in high-risk patients who develop influenza-like symptoms, but proof of benefit in such patients is lacking.

Resistance to amantadine and rimantadine develops frequently during treatment, and resistance to either drug makes both ineffective. Resistance that develops during treatment does not affect the efficacy of treatment for the index patient but may result in transmission of resistant virus to contacts. Resistance to oseltamivir and zanamivir occurs but is not clinically relevant. In children, oseltamivir may decrease the incidence of otitis media; however, no other data indicate that treatment of influenza prevents complications.

Amantadine and rimantadine inhibit virus penetration or uncoating. They are effective against influenza A viruses but not against influenza B. Treatment is stopped after 3 to 5 days or 1 to 2 days after symptoms resolve. For both drugs, 100 mg po bid can be used. To avoid adverse effects due to drug accumulation, the dose is reduced for children (2.5 mg/kg bid to a maximum of 150 mg/day for children < 10 yr or 200 mg/day for children ≥ 10 yr). In patients with impaired renal function, dose is adjusted according to the creatinine clearance. The dose of rimantadine should not exceed 100 mg/day if hepatic dysfunction exists. Dose-related nervousness, insomnia, or other CNS effects occur in about 10% of people receiving amantadine and in about 2% of people receiving rimantadine. These effects usually occur within 48 h after starting the drug, are more prominent in the elderly and in those with CNS diseases or impaired renal function, and often resolve during continued use. Anorexia, nausea, and constipation may also occur.

The NA inhibitors zanamivir and oseltamivir are effective against both influenza A and B. The dose of zanamivir is 2 puffs (10 mg) bid. Oseltamivir is given at 75 mg po bid for patients > 12 yr. The dose is decreased in younger patients. These drugs have relatively few adverse effects. Zanamivir should not be given to patients with underlying reactive airway disease because of possible bronchospasm due to the inhalation route. Oseltamivir may produce occasional nausea and vomiting.

Prevention

Influenza infections can be prevented by annual vaccination. Chemoprophylaxis with antiviral agents is also useful in certain situations. Prevention is indicated for all patients, but is especially important for high-risk patients and health care practitioners.

Vaccination: Vaccines are modified annually to include the most prevalent strains (usually 2 strains of influenza A and 1 of influenza B). When the vaccine contains the same HA and NA as the strains in the community, vaccination decreases infections by 70 to 90% in healthy adults. In the institutionalized elderly, vaccines are less effective for prevention but decrease pneumonia and death by 60 to 80%. Vaccine-induced immunity is decreased by antigenic drift and is absent if there is antigenic shift.

Vaccination is indicated for patients > 65 yr; patients with cardiopulmonary disorders; residents of chronic care facilities; patients who are under routine medical care for chronic metabolic diseases (eg, diabetes mellitus), renal failure, hemoglobinopathies, or immunosuppression; children on long-term aspirin therapy; and women who will reach the 2nd or 3rd trimester of pregnancy during influenza season (between November and March in the US). Household contacts and people who care for these high-risk patients should also be immunized. Vaccination of all children 6 to 24 mo of age and their household contacts is also recommended. Influenza vaccine is given annually to maintain antibody titers and allow vaccine modification to compensate for antigenic drift. Vaccine is best given in the fall, so that antibody titers will be high during the winter influenza season.

Inactivated influenza vaccines are given by IM injection. Adults receive a single 0.5-mL dose. Because children have had fewer opportunities for exposure to influenza virus, both a primary and a booster dose (0.5 mL each for children 3 to 10 yr, 0.25 mL each for children 6 to 35 mo) 1 mo apart are recommended unless vaccination has been administered in prior years. Adverse effects associated with the vaccine are usually limited to mild pain at the injection site that lasts no more than a few days. Fever, myalgia, and other systemic effects are uncommon. The vaccine is contraindicated in patients who have a history of anaphylactic reactions to chicken or to egg protein.

A live attenuated influenza vaccine has recently become available in the US for healthy people between age 5 and 50 yr. The vaccine should not be given to patients in high-risk groups, pregnant women, household contacts of patients with immunodeficiency, or children who are receiving chronic aspirin therapy. The vaccine is given intranasally at a dose of 0.25 mL in each nostril. Children between 5 and 8 yr who have not been previously vaccinated with the live attenuated vaccine should receive a 2nd dose at least 6 wk after the 1st dose. Adverse effects associated with the vaccine are mild, most often rhinorrhea.

Antiviral drugs: Vaccination is the preferred method of prevention, but antiviral drugs are also effective. Antiviral drugs are indicated for patients who have been vaccinated only within the previous 2 wk, patients for whom vaccination is contraindicated, and patients who are immunocompromised and thus may not respond to vaccination. Drugs do not impair development of immunity from the vaccine. Antiviral drugs can be stopped 2 wk after vaccination. If vaccine cannot be given, antiviral drugs are continued for the duration of the epidemic.

Amantadine and rimantadine prevent influenza A, which accounts for most influenza illness. The NA inhibitors zanamivir and oseltamivir prevent both influenza A and B. Prophylactic doses of these antivirals are the same as treatment doses except for oseltamivir, for which the prophylactic dose is 75 mg once/day.

AVIAN INFLUENZA

Avian influenza (bird flu) is caused by strains of influenza A that normally infect only wild birds (and sometimes pigs). Infections due to these strains have recently been detected in humans.

Most human infections are caused by strains of avian influenza type H5N1, but H7N7, H7N3, and H9N2 have caused some human infections. Infections with these strains are asymptomatic in wild birds but can cause highly lethal illness in domestic birds.

The 1st human cases were discovered in Hong Kong in 1997. Spread to humans was contained by culling domestic bird populations. In 2003 and 2004, however, humans were infected with avian influenza strains in several Asian nations (H9N2 and, continuing into 2005, H5N1), Canada (H7N3), and the Netherlands (H7N7). Although most cases occurred through exposure to infected birds, some human-to-human transmission probably occurred in the Netherlands and may have occurred in Asia.

All influenza viruses are capable of rapid mutation, raising the possibility that avian strains could acquire the ability to spread more easily from person-to-person. This could occur by direct mutation or by recombination with human strains in a human or porcine host. Many experts are concerned that, should these strains acquire the ability for efficient human-to-human spread, an influenza pandemic could result.

Human infection with avian influenza H5N1 strains can cause severe respiratory symptoms. Mortality was 33% in the 1997 outbreak and almost 80% in the 2004 outbreak. Infection with the H7 strains most commonly causes conjunctivitis, although in the Netherlands outbreak a few patients had flu-like symptoms and one patient (of 83) died.

An appropriate clinical syndrome in the setting of exposure to a known infected individual or exposure to birds in an area with an ongoing avian influenza outbreak should prompt consideration of this infection. History of recent travel to Asia with exposure to birds or infected individuals should prompt testing for influenza A by reverse transcription–PCR. Culture of the organism should not be attempted. Suspected and confirmed cases are reported to the Centers for Disease Control and Prevention.

Treatment with oseltamivir or zanamivir at usual doses is indicated. The strain of H5N1 in the 2004 outbreak is resistant to amantadine and rimantadine. Containment is achieved by culling infected flocks.

PARAINFLUENZA VIRUS INFECTIONS

Parainfluenza viruses include several closely related viruses causing many respiratory illnesses varying from the common cold to an influenza-like syndrome or pneumonia, with croup as the most common severe manifestation. Diagnosis is usually clinical. Treatment is supportive.

The parainfluenza viruses are paramyxoviruses types 1, 2, 3, and 4. They share antigenic cross-reactivity but tend to cause diseases of different severity. Type 4 has antigenic cross-reactivity with mumps and appears to be an uncommon cause of respiratory disease.

Childhood outbreaks of parainfluenza virus infections can occur in nurseries, pediatric wards, and schools. Types 1 and 2 tend to cause epidemics in the autumn, with each serotype occurring in alternate years. Type 3 disease is endemic and infects most children < 1 yr. Parainfluenza viruses can cause repeated infections, but reinfection generally produces milder illness. Thus, in immunocompetent adults, most infections are asymptomatic or mild.

The most common illness in children is an upper respiratory illness with no or low-grade fever.

Parainfluenza type 1 probably causes croup (laryngotracheobronchitis—see p. 2307), primarily in infants aged 6 to 36 mo. Croup begins with common cold symptoms. Later, there is fever and a "barking" cough, hoarseness, and stridor. Respiratory failure due to upper airway obstruction is a rare but potentially fatal complication.

Parainfluenza virus type 3 may produce pneumonia and bronchiolitis in young infants (see p. 2305). These illnesses are generally indistinguishable from disease caused by respiratory syncytial virus (see below) but are often less severe.

A specific viral diagnosis is unnecessary. Treatment is symptomatic.

RESPIRATORY SYNCYTIAL VIRUS AND HUMAN METAPNEUMOVIRUS INFECTIONS

Respiratory syncytial virus (RSV) and human metapneumovirus infections cause seasonal lower respiratory tract disease, particularly in infants and young children. Disease may be asymptomatic, mild, or severe, including bronchiolitis and pneumonia. Although diagnosis is usually clinical, laboratory diagnosis is readily available. Treatment is supportive.

RSV is an RNA virus, classified as a pneumovirus. Subgroups A and B have been identified. Human metapneumovirus (hMPV), a similar but separate virus, was recently discovered. RSV is ubiquitous; almost all children are infected by age 4 yr. Outbreaks occur annually in winter or early spring. Because the immune response to RSV does not protect against reinfection, the attack rate is about 40% for all exposed people. However, antibody to RSV decreases illness severity. The seasonal epidemiology of hMPV appears to be similar to that of RSV, but the incidence of infection and illness appears to be substantially lower. RSV is the most common cause of lower respiratory tract illness in young infants.

Symptoms, Signs, and Diagnosis

The most recognizable clinical syndromes are bronchiolitis and pneumonia. These illnesses typically begin with upper respiratory symptoms and fever and then progress over several days to dyspnea, cough, and wheezing. Apnea may be the initial symptom of RSV in infants < 6 mo. In healthy adults and older children, illness is usually mild and may be inapparent or manifested only as an afebrile common cold. However, patients who are elderly or immunocompromised or have underlying cardiopulmonary disorders may develop severe disease. RSV and hMPV illness appear to be similar.

RSV (and possibly hMPV) infection is suspected in infants and young children with bronchiolitis or pneumonia during RSV season. Because antiviral treatment is not generally recommended, a specific laboratory diagnosis is unnecessary for patient management. However, a laboratory diagnosis may facilitate hospital infection control by allowing segregation of children infected with the same virus. Rapid antigen tests with high sensitivities for RSV are available for use in children; these methods are insensitive in adults.

Treatment and Prevention

Treatment of RSV and hMPV infections is supportive, including supplemental O_2 and hydration as needed (see Bronchiolitis on p. 2305). Corticosteroids and bronchodilators are not generally helpful. Antibiotics are reserved for patients with fever and evidence of pneumonia on chest x-ray. Palivizumab is not effective for treatment. Ribavirin, an antiviral drug with activity against RSV, has little or no efficacy, is potentially toxic to health care practitioners, and is no longer recommended except for infection in the severely immunocompromised host.

Passive prophylaxis with monoclonal antibody to RSV (palivizumab) decreases the frequency of hospitalization in high-risk infants. It is cost effective only for infants at high risk for hospitalization (ie, those age < 2 yr with hemodynamically significant congenital heart disease or chronic lung disease requiring medical treatment in the preceding 6 mo, those born at < 29 wk gestation who are < 1 yr old at the start of RSV season, and those born at 29 to 32 wk gestation who are < 6 mo old at the start of the season). The dose is 15 mg/kg IM. The 1st dose is given just before the usual onset of the RSV season (early November in North America). Subsequent doses are given at 1-mo intervals for the duration of the RSV season (usually a total of 5 doses).

SEVERE ACUTE RESPIRATORY SYNDROME

Severe acute respiratory syndrome (SARS) is caused by a coronavirus, is probably spread by respiratory droplets, and has an incubation of 2 to 10 days. It produces an influenza-like illness that occasionally leads to progressively severe respiratory insufficiency. The mortality rate is 10%. Diagnosis is clinical. To prevent spread, patients are isolated. Treatment is supportive.

Coronaviruses are enveloped RNA viruses. Coronaviruses 229E and OC43 have long been known to produce the common cold. In late 2002, an outbreak of a viral respiratory illness labeled SARS occurred. SARS is caused by a coronavirus (SARS-CoV) that is genetically dissimilar from known human or animal coronaviruses.

SARS-CoV appears to be a new human pathogen that was first detected in the Guangdong province of China in November 2002. Evidence of SARS-CoV infection has also been found in masked palm civets, raccoon dogs, and the Chinese ferret badger. SARS has spread to > 30 countries. As of mid-July 2003, over 8000 cases had been reported worldwide, with over 800 deaths (about 10% case mortality rate); since late 2003, naturally occurring cases appear to be contained to China.

Transmission of SARS-CoV is probably mainly by respiratory droplets and generally requires close personal contact. However, transmission can occur after very casual contact and possibly by aerosol spread. Infection primarily involves people between the ages of 15 and 70 yr.

Symptoms, Signs, and Diagnosis

The incubation period is 2 to 10 days (median 5 days). Initial symptoms resemble influenza, with fever, cough, chills, rigor, and myalgia. Upper respiratory symptoms (runny nose, sore throat) are uncommon. Most patients have a mild illness and recover within 1 to 2 wk. Other patients develop respiratory distress, usually > 1 wk after symptom onset, with marked dyspnea, hypoxemia, and occasionally acute respiratory distress syndrome (ARDS). Death is due to respiratory failure.

Because initial symptoms are nonspecific, SARS is suspected in patients with likely exposure (based on epidemiologic factors) as well as fever and suggestive clinical symptoms. Suspected cases are reported to the state health department and evaluated by standard procedures for severe community-acquired pneumonia. Chest x-ray is frequently normal early in the illness. As respiratory symptoms worsen, focal interstitial infiltrates are common, which occasionally become generalized and sometimes progress to ARDS.

Typical laboratory tests are nonspecific, but WBC counts are usually normal or decreased, sometimes with a decrease in absolute lymphocyte count. Transaminases, CPK, or LDH may be elevated, but renal function remains normal. If chest CT is obtained, it may show peripheral, subpleural ground-glass opacifications.

Viral cultures for known respiratory pathogens (eg, influenza, respiratory syncytial virus) are obtained using swabs from the oropharynx and nasopharynx, and the laboratory is notified that SARS is suspected. Although serologic and PCR tests have been developed for detection of SARS-CoV, they are not useful for clinical management. For epidemiologic surveillance, acute and convalescent (3-wk) serum specimens are sent to state or local health departments to be forwarded to the Centers for Disease Control and Prevention for testing.

Prognosis, Treatment, and Prevention

Predictors of death appear to be age > 60 yr, comorbidity, increased LDH levels, and increased absolute neutrophil count. Treatment of SARS is supportive, with mechanical ventilation as needed. Oseltamivir, ribavirin, and corticosteroids have been used, but there is no current evidence of benefit.

Patients suspected of having SARS should be placed in isolation in a negative-pressure room. Contact and respiratory precautions should be taken. Staff should use N-95 masks, eye protection, gloves, and gowns.

People exposed to patients suspected of having SARS (eg, family members, airline personnel, health care practitioners) should be alert for symptoms of illness. In the absence of symptoms, such people may attend work, school, and other activities as usual. If fever or respiratory symptoms develop, they should limit their public activities and seek medical evaluation. If symptoms do not progress to meet suspect SARS criteria within 72 h, they may return to normal activity as tolerated.

189 HERPESVIRUSES

Eight types of herpesviruses infect humans (see TABLE 189–1). After initial infection, all herpesviruses remain latent within specific host cells and may subsequently reactivate or be shed. Herpesviruses do not survive long outside a host; thus transmission usually requires intimate contact, although varicella-zoster virus (VZV) may spread by aerosol. Because the virus remains latent, transmission sometimes occurs from asymptomatic infected people. Epstein-Barr virus (EBV) and human herpesvirus type 8 (HHV-8), also known as Kaposi's sarcoma–associated herpesvirus (KSHV), are tightly linked with malignancy.

Drug Treatment

Drugs that have activity against herpesviruses include acyclovir, cidofovir, famciclovir, fomivirsen, foscarnet, ganciclovir, idoxuridine, penciclovir, trifluridine, valacyclovir, valganciclovir, and vidarabine.

Acyclovir: Acyclovir is a purine nucleoside analog with activity against herpesviruses (in order of potency): herpes simplex virus type 1 (HSV-1), herpes simplex virus type 2 (HSV-2), VZV, and EBV. It has minimal activity against cytomegalovirus (CMV). It terminates viral DNA synthesis in a process that requires viral thymidine kinase; immunocompromised patients who require prolonged treatment may develop resistance via a mutation in viral thymidine kinase. Adverse effects are infrequent with oral administration but may include nausea, vomiting,

TABLE 189–1. HERPESVIRUSES THAT INFECT HUMANS

COMMON NAME	OTHER NAME	TYPICAL MANIFESTATIONS
Herpes simplex virus type 1	Human herpesvirus 1	Gingivostomatitis; keratoconjunctivitis; cutaneous herpes; genital herpes; encephalitis; herpes labialis; esophagitis*; pneumonia*; hepatitis*†
Herpes simplex virus type 2	Human herpesvirus 2	Genital herpes; cutaneous herpes; gingivostomatitis; neonatal herpes; aseptic meningitis; disseminated infection*; hepatitis*†
Varicella-zoster virus	Human herpesvirus 3	Chickenpox; herpes zoster; disseminated herpes zoster*
Epstein-Barr virus	Human herpesvirus 4	Infectious mononucleosis; hepatitis; encephalitis; nasopharyngeal carcinoma; lymphoproliferative syndromes*; oral hairy leukoplakia*
Cytomegalovirus	Human herpesvirus 5	Infectious mononucleosis; hepatitis; congenital cytomegalic inclusion disease; hepatitis*; retinitis*; pneumonia*; colitis*
Human herpesvirus 6		Roseola infantum; otitis media with fever; encephalitis
Human herpesvirus 7		Roseola infantum
Human herpesvirus 8	Kaposi's sarcoma–associated herpesvirus	Not a known cause of acute illness but has a causative role in Kaposi's sarcoma (see p. 1024)* and AIDS-related non-Hodgkin lymphomas that grow primarily in the pleural, pericardial, or abdominal cavities as lymphomatous effusions

*In immunocompromised hosts.
†Uncommonly causes fulminant hepatitis in the absence of cutaneous lesions in immunocompetent hosts.

diarrhea, headache, and rashes. IV acyclovir is indicated when a higher serum drug level is required, as in herpes encephalitis. Adverse effects include renal failure, phlebitis, rash, and neurotoxicity (lethargy, confusion, seizures, coma). Thrombotic thrombocytopenic purpura/hemolytic uremic syndrome (TTP/HUS) has been reported in immunocompromised patients receiving acyclovir.

Cidofovir: Cidofovir is a nucleotide analog that has a long duration of action and in vitro inhibition of a broad spectrum of viruses, including HSV-1, HSV-2, VZV, CMV, EBV, KSHV, adenovirus, human papillomavirus (HPV), and human polyomavirus. Topical cidofovir is used for mucocutaneous HSV unresponsive to oral or IV acyclovir.

Famciclovir: Famciclovir is a prodrug of the active antiviral penciclovir and has an antiviral spectrum similar to acyclovir. It inhibits viral DNA polymerase in a thymidine kinase–dependent process. Famciclovir is as effective as acyclovir for genital herpes and herpes zoster and is more bioavailable. Strains resistant to acyclovir are also resistant to famciclovir. Adverse effects of famciclovir are similar to those of oral acyclovir.

Fomivirsen: Fomivirsen is a phosphorothioate oligonucleotide. Oligonucleotides bind to viral RNA, blocking its expression (antisense mechanism). Fomivirsen has potent activity against CMV; it inhibits CMV protein synthesis. It is given by intravitreal injection for patients with HIV infection and CMV retinitis that is resistant to other therapies. Adverse effects include increased intraocular pressure and corticosteroid-responsive uveitis.

Foscarnet: Foscarnet is an organic analog of inorganic pyrophosphate. It selectively inhibits virus-specific DNA polymerase and reverse transcriptase. Its mechanism does not involve viral thymidine kinase; it is active against EBV, KSHV, human herpesvirus 6, acyclovir-resistant (and acyclovir-susceptible) HSV and VZV, and ganciclovir-resistant (and ganciclovir-susceptible) CMV. Foscarnet's efficacy is similar to that of ganciclovir for treating and delaying progression of CMV retinitis, and it has some anti-HIV activity.

Ganciclovir and valganciclovir: Ganciclovir is a nucleoside analog of 2′-deoxyguanosine that differs only slightly from acyclovir chemically. It has in vitro activity against all herpesviruses, including CMV, but HSV strains resistant to acyclovir are cross-resistant to ganciclovir. Ganciclovir is primarily used in patients with both HIV and CMV retinitis. It inhibits viral DNA synthesis by competitive inhibition of viral DNA polymerase in a viral thymidine kinase–dependent process. Its primary adverse effect is bone marrow suppression, particularly neutropenia. Severe neutropenia (< 500 neutrophils/μL) requires bone marrow stimulation with granulocyte colony-stimulating factor or granulocyte-macrophage colony-stimulating factor or drug discontinuation. Less common adverse effects include rash, fever, azotemia, liver function abnormalities, nausea, and vomiting. Oral ganciclovir is only 6 to 9% bioavailable. The formulation, which requires 12 capsules/day for a standard dose (1 g tid), limits its usefulness. A more bioavailable formulation is valganciclovir, which is taken as two 450-mg tablets once/day or bid.

Idoxuridine: Idoxuridine (IDU) irreversibly replaces thymidine in newly synthesized DNA, rendering DNA essentially nonfunctional in viral as well as host cells. Because of its high systemic toxicity, IDU has been limited to topical therapy of herpes simplex keratoconjunctivitis. IDU may cause irritation, pain, photophobia, pruritus, and inflammation or edema of the eyelids; allergic reactions occur rarely.

Penciclovir: Penciclovir is a phosphorylated guanosine analog that competitively inhibits viral DNA polymerase. Penciclovir cream is used for recurrent herpes labialis in adults.

Trifluridine: Trifluridine (trifluorothymidine), a thymidine analog, impairs DNA synthesis and is effective in treating primary keratoconjunctivitis and recurrent keratitis or ulceration caused by HSV-1 and HSV-2. Trifluridine is as effective as vidarabine and may be effective in patients who have not responded to IDU or vidarabine. The marrow-suppressive effect of trifluridine precludes systemic use. Adverse effects include ocular stinging, palpebral edema, and, less frequently, punctate keratitis and allergic reactions.

Valacyclovir: Valacyclovir is converted to acyclovir by 1st-pass metabolism, which makes it 3 to 5 times more bioavailable than acyclovir. Its antiviral spectrum and adverse effects are similar to acyclovir. Because patients with advanced HIV and transplant recipients who have received high-dose valacyclovir have had TTP/HUS, it should be used with caution in these patients.

Vidarabine: Vidarabine (adenine arabinoside, ara-A) impairs viral DNA synthesis and is effective against HSV infections. Vidarabine appears less susceptible to the development of drug resistance than IDU, and IDU-resistant infections often respond to vidarabine. Ophthalmic preparations of vidarabine are effective for acute keratoconjunctivitis and recurrent superficial keratitis caused by HSV-1 and HSV-2. Possible adverse effects include superficial punctate keratitis with tearing, irritation, pain, and photophobia.

CHICKENPOX

(Varicella)

Chickenpox is an acute, systemic, usually childhood infection caused by the varicella-zoster virus (human herpesvirus type 3). It usually begins with mild constitutional symptoms that are followed shortly by skin lesions appearing in crops and characterized by macules, papules, vesicles, and crusting. Patients at risk of severe neurologic or other systemic complications (eg, pneumonia) include adults, newborns, and patients who are immunocompromised or have certain underlying medical conditions. Diagnosis is clinical. Those at risk of severe complications receive postexposure prophylaxis with immune globulins, and, if disease develops, treatment with antiviral drugs (eg, valacyclovir, famciclovir, acyclovir). Vaccination provides effective prevention.

Chickenpox is caused by the varicella-zoster virus (human herpesvirus type 3), chickenpox being the acute invasive phase of the virus and herpes zoster (shingles) representing reactivation of the latent phase (see p. 1609). Chickenpox, which is extremely contagious, is spread by infected droplets and is most communicable during the prodrome and early stages of the eruption. It is communicable from 48 h before the 1st skin lesions appear until the final lesions have crusted. Indirect transmission (by immune carriers) does not occur.

Epidemics occur in winter and early spring in 3- to 4-yr cycles. Some infants may have partial immunity, probably acquired transplacentally, until age 6 mo.

Symptoms, Signs, and Diagnosis

In immunocompetent children, chickenpox is rarely severe. In adults and immunocompromised children, infection can be serious. Mild headache, moderate fever, and malaise may occur 11 to 15 days after exposure, about 24 to 36 h before lesions appear. This prodrome is more likely in patients > 10 yr and is usually more severe in adults.

The initial rash, a macular eruption, may be accompanied by an evanescent flush. Within a few hours, lesions progress to papules and then characteristic, sometimes pathognomonic, teardrop vesicles, often intensely itchy, on red bases. Lesions initially develop on the face and trunk and erupt in successive crops; some macules appear just as earlier crops begin to crust. The eruption may be generalized (in severe cases) or more limited but almost always involves the upper trunk. Ulcerated lesions may develop on the mucous membranes, including the oropharynx and upper respiratory tract, palpebral conjunctiva, and rectal and vaginal mucosa. In the mouth, vesicles rupture immediately, are indistinguishable from those of herpetic gingivostomatitis, and often cause pain on swallowing. Scalp lesions may produce tender, enlarged suboccipital and posterior cervical lymph nodes. New lesions usually cease to appear by the 5th day, and the majority are crusted by the 6th day; most crusts disappear < 20 days after onset.

Secondary bacterial infection (typically streptococcal or staphylococcal) of the vesicles may occur, causing cellulitis or rarely streptococcal toxic shock. Pneumonia may complicate severe chickenpox in adults, newborns, and immunocompromised patients of all ages but usually not in immunocompetent young children. Myocarditis, transient arthritis or hepatitis, and hemorrhagic complications may also occur.

Encephalopathy occurs in < 1/1000 cases, usually as the disease resolves or within the next 2 wk. Complete neurologic recovery is likely, although rarely persistent deficits or death occurs. One of the most common neurologic complications is acute postinfectious cerebellar ataxia. Transverse myelitis, cranial nerve palsies, and multiple sclerosis–like clinical manifestations have also occurred. Reye's syndrome (see p. 2401), a rare but severe childhood complication, may begin 3 to 8 days after onset of the rash; aspirin increases the risk. In adults, encephalitis, which can be life threatening, occurs in 1 to 2/1000 cases of chickenpox.

Chickenpox is suspected in patients with the characteristic rash, which is usually the basis for diagnosis. The rash may be confused with that of other viral skin infections. If the diagnosis is in doubt, laboratory confirmation can be performed; it requires immunofluorescent detection of viral antigen in lesions or culture or serologic findings. Samples are generally obtained with scraping and transported to the laboratory in viral media.

Prognosis and Treatment

Chickenpox in childhood is rarely severe. Severe or fatal disease is more likely in adults, patients with depressed T-cell immunity (eg, lymphoreticular malignancy), and those receiving corticosteroids or chemotherapy.

Mild cases require only symptomatic treatment. Relief of itching and prevention of scratching, which predisposes to secondary bacterial infection, may be difficult. Wet compresses, or, for severe itching, systemic antihistamines and colloidal oatmeal baths may help. Simultaneous use of large doses of systemic and topical antihistamines can produce encephalopathy and should be avoided.

To prevent secondary bacterial infection, patients should bathe regularly and keep their underclothing and hands clean and their nails clipped. Antiseptics should not be applied unless lesions become infected; infection is treated with antibiotics.

Oral antivirals, when given to immunocompetent hosts within 24 h of the onset of rash, slightly decrease symptom duration and severity. However, because the disease is generally benign in children, antiviral treatment is not routinely recommended. Oral valacyclovir, famciclovir, or acyclovir should be strongly considered for immunocompromised patients and for healthy people at risk for moderate to severe disease, including all patients ≥ 12 yr, those with skin disorders (particularly eczema) or chronic lung disease, and those receiving salicylate or corticosteroid therapy. The dose of famciclovir is 500 mg tid and of valacyclovir is 1 g tid. Acyclovir is a less desirable choice because of its poorer oral bioavailability but can be given at 20 mg/kg qid with a maximum daily dose of 3200 mg. Immunocompromised children > 1 yr should be given 500 mg/m^2 q 8 h.

Patients should not return to school or work until the final lesions have crusted.

Prevention

Infection provides lifelong protection. All healthy children and susceptible adults should receive doses of live attenuated varicella vaccine (see FIG. 266–3 on p. 2235). Vaccination is particularly important in women of child-bearing age and adults with underlying chronic medical conditions. Serologic testing to determine immune status before vaccination in adults is usually not required. Vaccination is contraindicated in patients with moderate to severe concurrent illness, immunocompromised patients, pregnant women, patients on high doses of systemic corticosteroids, and children using salicylates. Although the vaccine may cause chickenpox in immunocompetent patients, disease is usually mild (< 10 papules or vesicles) and brief and produces few systemic symptoms.

Following exposure, chickenpox can be prevented or attenuated by IM administration of varicella-zoster immune globulin (VZIG), prepared from pooled plasma containing high titers of specific antibody. Candidates for postexposure prophylaxis include people with leukemia, immunodeficiencies, or other severe debilitating illness; susceptible pregnant women; and newborns whose mothers developed chickenpox within 5 days before or 2 days after delivery. VZIG 12.5 units/kg IM (100 units/mL) up to 625 units must be given within 4 days of exposure. Postexposure vaccination may modify or prevent varicella if administered within 3 days (and possibly up to 5 days) after exposure. Vaccination should be given as soon as possible in susceptible patients eligible for vaccination. Potentially susceptible individuals should take strict precautions to avoid people capable of transmitting the infection.

CYTOMEGALOVIRUS INFECTION

(Cytomegalic Inclusion Disease)

(See also Congenital and Perinatal Cytomegalovirus Infection on p. 2320.)

Cytomegalovirus (CMV, human herpesvirus type 5) can cause infections that have a wide range of severity. A syndrome that is similar to infectious mononucleosis but lacks severe pharyngitis is common. Severe focal disease, including retinitis, can develop in HIV-infected patients and rarely in organ transplant recipients and other immunocompromised patients. Severe systemic disease can develop in newborns and immunocompromised patients. Laboratory diagnosis, helpful for severe disease, may involve culture, serology, biopsy, or antigen or nucleic acid detection. Ganciclovir and other antiviral drugs are used to treat severe disease, particularly retinitis.

CMV is transmitted through blood, body fluids, or transplanted organs. Infection may be acquired transplacentally or during birth. Prevalence increases with age; 60 to 90% of adults have had CMV infection. Lower socioeconomic groups tend to have a higher prevalence.

Congenital infection may cause infection ranging from asymptomatic to abortion, stillbirth, or postnatal death (see p. 2320). Complications include extensive hepatic or CNS damage.

Acquired infections are often asymptomatic. An acute febrile illness, termed CMV mononucleosis or CMV hepatitis, may cause hepatitis with elevated aminotransferases, atypical lymphocytosis similar to infectious mononucleosis, and splenomegaly.

Postperfusion/posttransfusion syndrome can develop 2 to 4 wk after transfusion with blood products containing CMV. It produces fever lasting 2 to 3 wk and manifestations similar to CMV hepatitis.

In immunocompromised patients, CMV is a major cause of morbidity and mortality. Disease often results from reactivation of latent virus. Patients may have pulmonary, GI, or CNS involvement. In the terminal phase of AIDS, CMV infection causes retinitis in up to 40% of patients and causes funduscopically visible retinal abnormalities. Ulcerative disease of the colon, with abdominal pain and GI bleeding, or of the esophagus, with odynophagia, may occur.

Diagnosis

CMV infection is suspected in healthy people with mononucleosis-like syndromes; immunocompromised patients with GI, CNS, or retinal symptoms; and newborns with systemic disease. CMV mononucleosis can sometimes be differentiated from infectious (Epstein-Barr virus) mononucleosis by the absence of pharyngitis, a negative heterophil antibody test, and serology. CMV infection can be differentiated from viral hepatitis by hepatitis serology. Laboratory confirmation of primary CMV infection is necessary only to differentiate it from other, particularly treatable, conditions or for serious disease. Especially in the immunocompromised host, CMV may be isolated from urine, other body fluids, or tissues. However, CMV can be excreted for months or years after infection, so its identification does not necessarily indicate active disease. Seroconversion can be demonstrated by development of CMV antibodies. In immunocompromised patients, biopsy showing CMV-induced pathology is often necessary to demonstrate invasive disease; also, PCR or antigen detection from peripheral blood can quantitatively measure CMV loads, which can be helpful. Diagnosis in infants can be made by urine culture.

Treatment and Prevention

CMV retinitis (see p. 915), which occurs mostly in AIDS patients, is treated with antivirals. Most patients receive induction therapy with either ganciclovir, 5 mg/kg IV bid for 2 to 3 wk, or valganciclovir, 900 mg po bid for 21 days. If induction fails more than once, another drug should be used. After induction, patients receive maintenance or suppressive therapy with valganciclovir 900 mg po once/day to delay progression. Maintenance therapy with ganciclovir 5 mg/kg IV once/day can also be used to prevent recurrence. Alternatively, foscarnet can be given with or without ganciclovir. Foscarnet dose is 90 mg/kg IV q 12 h for 2 to 3 wk for induction followed by 90 to 120 mg/kg IV once/day for maintenance therapy. Adverse effects of IV foscarnet are significant and include nephrotoxicity, symptomatic hypocalcemia, hypomagnesemia, hyperphosphatemia, hypokalemia, and CNS effects. Combination therapy with ganciclovir and foscarnet increases efficacy as well as adverse effects. Cidofovir therapy consists of 5 mg/kg IV once/wk (induction) for 2 wk followed by similar maintenance doses every other week. Efficacy is similar to ganciclovir or foscarnet. Significant adverse effects, including renal failure, limit its use. To reduce potential nephrotoxicity, probenecid and pre-hydration should be given with each dose. However, the adverse effects of probenecid, including rash, headache, and fever, may be significant enough to prevent its use.

Ganciclovir ocular implants can also be used for prolonged treatment in some patients. Intraocular injections into the vitreous are given sometimes, primarily if other measures have failed or are contraindicated (salvage therapy). Such treatments include injection of ganciclovir or foscarnet. Potential adverse effects of ocular injection therapy include direct retinal toxicity, vitreous hemorrhage, endophthalmitis, retinal detachment, cystoid macular edema, and cataract formation. Cidofovir may cause iritis or ocular hypotony. Even patients receiving ocular injections or those with implants need systemic therapy to prevent CMV in the contralateral eye and extraocular tissues. Ultimately, improvement of $CD4^+$ count to > 200 cells/μL with systemic retroviral therapy should prevent the need for ocular implants and chemoprophylaxis.

Anti-CMV drugs are used to treat severe disease other than retinitis but are less consistently effective than in retinitis. Ganciclovir plus immune globulin has been used to treat CMV pneumonia in bone marrow transplant recipients.

Prophylaxis of CMV disease is necessary for solid organ or hematopoietic cell transplant recipients at risk for CMV disease. Drugs used include ganciclovir, valganciclovir, and valacyclovir.

HERPES SIMPLEX VIRUS INFECTIONS

Herpes simplex viruses (human herpesviruses 1 and 2) commonly cause recurrent infection affecting the skin, mouth, lips, eyes, and genitals. Common severe infections include encephalitis, meningitis, neonatal herpes, and, in immunocompromised patients, disseminated infection. Mucocutaneous infections cause clusters of small painful vesicles on an erythematous base. Diagnosis is clinical; laboratory confirmation by culture, PCR, direct immunofluorescence, or serology can be performed.

Treatment is symptomatic; antiviral therapy with acyclovir, valacyclovir, or famciclovir is helpful for severe infections and, if begun early, in recurrent or primary infections.

Both types of herpes simplex virus (HSV), HSV-1 and HSV-2, can cause oral or genital infection. Most often, HSV-1 causes gingivostomatitis, herpes labialis, and herpes keratitis. HSV-2 usually causes genital lesions. Transmission of HSV occurs from close contact with an individual who is actively shedding virus. Viral shedding generally occurs from lesions but can occur even when lesions are not apparent.

After the initial infection, HSV remains dormant in nerve ganglia from which it can periodically emerge, causing symptoms. Recurrent herpetic eruptions are precipitated by overexposure to sunlight, febrile illnesses, physical or emotional stress, immunosuppression, or unknown stimuli. Recurrent eruptions are generally less severe, and generally occur less frequently over time.

Diseases Caused by Herpes Simplex

Mucocutaneous infection is most common. Ocular infection (herpes keratitis), CNS infection, and neonatal herpes are unusual but more serious manifestations. HSV rarely causes fulminant hepatitis in the absence of cutaneous lesions. In patients with HIV infection, herpetic infections can be particularly severe. Progressive and persistent esophagitis, colitis, perianal ulcers, pneumonia, encephalitis, and meningitis may occur.

HSV outbreaks may be followed by erythema multiforme (see p. 974) possibly from an immune reaction to the virus. Eczema herpeticum is a complication of HSV infection in which patients have severe disease in skin regions with eczema.

Mucocutaneous infection: Lesions may appear anywhere on the skin or mucosa but are most frequent around or in the mouth or on the lips, conjunctiva and cornea, and genitals. Generally, after a prodromal period (typically < 6 h in recurrent HSV-1) of tingling discomfort or itching, clusters of small, tense vesicles appear on an erythematous base. Clusters vary in size from 0.5 to 1.5 cm but may coalesce. Lesions on the nose, ears, eyes, fingers, or genitals may be particularly painful. Vesicles typically persist for a few days, then dry, forming a thin, yellowish crust. Healing generally occurs 8 to 12 days after onset. Lesions usually heal completely, but recurrent lesions at the same site may cause atrophy and scarring. Skin lesions can develop secondary bacterial infection. In patients with depressed cell-mediated immunity from HIV infection or other causes, prolonged or progressive lesions may persist for weeks or longer. Localized infections can disseminate, particularly—and often dramatically—in immunocompromised patients.

Acute herpetic gingivostomatitis usually results from primary infection with HSV-1, typically in children. Occasionally, through oral-genital contact, the cause is HSV-2. Intraoral and gingival vesicles rupture, usually within several hours to 1 or 2 days, to form ulcers. Fever and pain often occur. Difficulty in eating and drinking may lead to dehydration. After resolution, the virus resides dormant in the semilunar ganglion.

Herpes labialis is usually a secondary outbreak of HSV. It develops as ulcers (cold sores) on the vermilion border of the lip or, much less commonly, as ulcerations of the mucosa of the hard palate.

Herpetic whitlow, a swollen, painful, erythematous lesion of the distal phalanx, results from inoculation of HSV through the skin and is most common in health care practitioners (see p. 334).

Genital herpes is the most common ulcerative sexually transmitted disease in developed countries. It is usually caused by HSV-2, although 10 to 30% involve HSV-1. Primary lesions develop 4 to 7 days after contact. The vesicles usually erode to form ulcers that may coalesce. Lesions may occur on the prepuce, glans penis, and penile shaft in men and on the labia, clitoris, perineum, vagina, and cervix in women. They may occur around the anus and in the rectum in men or women who engage in receptive rectal intercourse. Genital HSV infection may cause urinary hesitancy, dysuria, urinary retention, or constipation. Severe sacral neuralgia may occur. Scarring may follow healing, and recurrences occur in 80% with HSV-2 and 50% with HSV-1. Primary genital lesions are usually more painful, prolonged, and widespread and are more likely to be bilateral and involve regional adenopathy and constitutional symptoms than recurrent genital lesions. Recurrent lesions may have severe prodromal symptoms and may involve the buttock, groin, or thigh.

Herpes simplex keratitis: HSV infection of the corneal epithelium produces pain, tearing, photophobia, and corneal ulcers that often have a branching pattern (see p. 897).

Neonatal herpes simplex: Infection develops in newborns, including in those whose mothers have no suggestion of current or past herpes infection. It is often transmitted during birth and usually involves HSV-2. It usually develops between the 1st and 4th wk of life, often causing mucocutaneous vesicles or CNS involvement. It causes major morbidity and mortality (see p. 2328).

CNS infection: Herpes encephalitis (see also p. 1851) occurs sporadically and may be severe. Multiple early seizures are characteristic. Aseptic meningitis (see p. 1864) may result from HSV-2. It is usually self-limited and may involve lumbosacral myeloradiculitis, which may produce urinary retention or obstipation.

Diagnosis

Diagnosis is often clinical based on characteristic lesions. Laboratory confirmation can be helpful, especially if infection is severe, the patient is immunocompromised or pregnant, or lesions are atypical. A Tzanck test (a superficial scraping from the base of a freshly ruptured vesicle stained with Wright's-Giemsa stain) often reveals multinucleate giant cells in HSV or varicella-zoster virus infection. Definitive diagnosis is with culture, seroconversion involving the appropriate serotype (in primary infections), and biopsy. Material for culture should be obtained from a vesicle or the base of a freshly ulcerated lesion. HSV can sometimes be identified using direct immunofluorescence assay of scrapings of lesions. PCR of CSF and MRI are used to diagnose HSV encephalitis.

HSV should be distinguished from herpes zoster, which rarely recurs and usually causes more severe pain and larger groups of lesions that are distributed along a dermatome. Clusters of vesicles or ulcers on an erythematous base are unusual in genital ulcers other than herpes.

Patients with herpes infections that recur frequently, fail to heal, or fail to respond to antiviral drugs as expected should be suspected of being immunocompromised, possibly from HIV infection.

Treatment

Mucocutaneous infection: Isolated infections often go untreated without consequence. Acyclovir, valacyclovir, or famciclovir can be used for treatment of infection, especially when it is primary. Infection with acyclovir-resistant HSV is rare and occurs almost exclusively in immunocompromised patients. Foscarnet may be effective for acyclovir-resistant infections. Secondary bacterial infections are treated with topical antibiotics (eg, mupirocin or neomycin-bacitracin) or, if severe, with systemic antibiotics (eg, penicillinase-resistant β-lactams). All mucocutaneous herpes infections are treated symptomatically. Systemic analgesics may help.

Gingivostomatitis typically requires only symptom relief with topical anesthetics applied directly with a swab (eg, dyclonine 0.5% liquid or benzocaine 2 to 20% ointment q 2 h as needed). When many large areas are affected, 5% lidocaine viscous may be used as a mouth rinse 5 min before mealtime. (NOTE: *Lidocaine must not be swallowed because it anesthetizes the oropharynx, hypopharynx, and possibly the epiglottis. Children must be watched for signs of aspiration.*) Severe cases can be treated with acyclovir, valacyclovir, or famciclovir.

Herpes labialis responds to oral and topical acyclovir. The duration of a recurrent eruption may be decreased by about a day by applying penciclovir 1% cream q 2 h while awake for 4 days, beginning during the prodrome or when the 1st lesion appears. Toxicity appears to be minimal. Acyclovir-resistant strains are resistant to penciclovir. Docosanol 10% cream may be effective when used 5 times/day.

Genital herpes is treated with antiviral drugs. Acyclovir 200 mg po 5 times/day for 10 days, valacyclovir 1 g po bid for 10 days, or famciclovir 250 mg po tid for 7 to 10 days can be used for primary eruptions. These drugs reduce viral shedding and symptoms in severe primary infections. However, even early treatment of primary infections does not prevent recurrences.

In recurrent eruptions, symptom duration and severity can be reduced marginally by antiviral treatment, particularly during the prodromal phase. Acyclovir 200 mg po q 4 h for 5 days, valacyclovir 500 mg po bid for 3 days, or famciclovir 125 mg po bid for 5 days can be used. Beginning at the 1st symptom or sign of recurrence, patients with frequent eruptions (eg, > 6 eruptions/yr) may receive suppressive antiviral therapy with acyclovir 400 mg po bid, valacyclovir 500 to 1000 mg po once/day, or famciclovir 250 mg po bid. Doses should be adjusted for renal insufficiency. Adverse effects are infrequent with oral administration but may include nausea, vomiting, diarrhea, headache, and rash.

Herpes simplex keratitis: Treatment involves topical antivirals, such as idoxuridine or trifluridine, and should be supervised by an ophthalmologist (see p. 897).

Neonatal herpes simplex: Acyclovir 20 mg/kg IV q 8 h for 14 to 21 days should be used. A dose of 20 mg/kg IV q 8 h for 21 days is indicated for CNS and disseminated HSV disease.

CNS infection: Encephalitis is treated with acyclovir 10 mg/kg IV q 8 h for 14 to 21 days. Aseptic meningitis is usually treated with IV acyclovir. Adverse effects include phlebitis, rash, and neurotoxicity (lethargy, confusion, seizures, coma).

HERPES ZOSTER

(Shingles; Acute Posterior Ganglionitis)

Herpes zoster is infection that results when varicella-zoster virus reactivates from its latent state in a posterior dorsal root ganglion. Symptoms usually begin with pain along the affected dermatome, followed in 2 to 3 days by a vesicular eruption that is usually diagnostic. Treatment is antiviral drugs and possibly corticosteroids given within 72 h after skin lesions appear.

Chickenpox and herpes zoster are caused by the varicella-zoster virus (human herpesvirus type 3), chickenpox being the acute invasive phase of the virus (see p. 1603) and herpes zoster (shingles) representing reactivation of the latent phase. Herpes zoster inflames the sensory root ganglia; the skin of the associated dermatome; and sometimes the posterior and anterior horns of the gray matter, meninges, and dorsal and ventral roots. Herpes zoster frequently occurs in elderly and HIV-infected patients and is more severe in immunocompromised patients. There are no clear-cut precipitants.

Symptoms and Signs

Lancinating, dysesthetic, or other pain develops in the involved site, followed in 2 to 3 days by a rash, usually crops of vesicles on an erythematous base. The site is usually ≥ 1 adjacent dermatomes in the thoracic or lumbar region. Lesions are typically unilateral. The site is usually hyperesthetic, and pain may be severe. Lesions usually continue to form for about 3 to 5 days. Herpes zoster may disseminate to other regions of the skin and to visceral organs, especially in immunocompromised patients.

Fewer than 4% of patients with herpes zoster experience another outbreak. However, many, particularly the elderly, have persistent or recurrent pain in the involved distribution (postherpetic neuralgia), which may persist for months, years, or permanently. Infection in the trigeminal nerve is particularly likely to lead to severe, persistent pain. The pain of postherpetic neuralgia may be sharp and intermittent or constant and may be debilitating.

Geniculate zoster (Ramsay Hunt syndrome) results from involvement of the geniculate ganglion. Ear pain, facial paralysis, and sometimes vertigo occur. Vesicles erupt in the external auditory canal, and taste may be lost in the anterior ⅔ of the tongue (see also Herpes Zoster Oticus on p. 793).

Ophthalmic herpes zoster (see also p. 897) results from involvement of the gasserian ganglion, with pain and vesicular eruption in and around the eye, in the distribution of the ophthalmic division of the 5th cranial nerve. Vesicles on the tip of the nose (Hutchinson's sign) indicate involvement of the nasociliary branch and often severe ocular disease. However, eye involvement may occur in the absence of lesions on the tip of the nose.

Intraoral zoster is uncommon but may produce a sharp unilateral distribution of lesions. No intraoral prodromal symptoms occur.

Diagnosis

Herpes zoster is suspected in patients with the characteristic rash and sometimes in patients with typical pain in a dermatomal distribution. Diagnosis is usually based on the virtually pathognomonic rash. If the diagnosis is equivocal, demonstrating multinucleate giant cells with a Tzanck test can confirm infection with a herpes virus. Herpes simplex virus (HSV) may produce nearly identical lesions, but unlike herpes zoster, HSV tends to recur and is not dermatomal. Viruses can be differentiated by culture. Antigen detection from a biopsy sample can be useful.

Treatment and Prevention

Wet compresses are soothing, but systemic analgesics are often necessary. Treatment with oral antivirals decreases the severity and duration of the acute eruption, the incidence of postherpetic neuralgia, and the rate of serious complications in immunocompromised patients and pregnant women. Treatment should start as soon as possible, ideally during the prodrome, and is likely ineffective if given > 72 h after skin lesions appear. Famciclovir 500 mg po tid for 7 days and valacyclovir 1 g po tid for 7 days have better bioavailability with oral dosing than acyclovir and therefore are generally preferred to oral acyclovir 800 mg 5 times/day for 7 to 10 days for herpes zoster. Corticosteroids increase the rate of healing and resolution of acute pain moderately but do not decrease the incidence of postherpetic neuralgia.

For immunocompromised patients, acyclovir is recommended at a dosage of 10 mg/kg IV q 8 h for 7 days for adults and 500 mg/m^2 IV q 8 h for 7 to 10 days for children ≥ 1 yr.

Prevention involves preventing primary infection (chickenpox) by use of the varicella vaccine (see p. 1605) in children and susceptible adults. In a large study, use of a more potent vaccine to boost the immune response in elderly patients who previously had chickenpox was recently shown to decrease the incidence of zoster.

Management of postherpetic neuralgia can be particularly difficult. Treatments include gabapentin, cyclic antidepressants, and topical capsaicin or lidocaine ointment. Opioid analgesics may be necessary. Intrathecal methylprednisolone may be of benefit.

For treatment of ophthalmic herpes zoster, an ophthalmologist should be consulted (see p. 898). For treatment of otic herpes zoster, an otolaryngologist should be consulted (see p. 793).

INFECTIOUS MONONUCLEOSIS

Infectious mononucleosis is caused by Epstein-Barr virus (EBV, human herpesvirus type 4), characterized by fatigue, fever, pharyngitis, and lymphadenopathy. Fatigue may persist weeks or months. Severe complications, including splenic rupture and neurologic syndromes, occasionally occur. Diagnosis is clinical or with heterophil antibody testing. Treatment is supportive.

Etiology and Pathophysiology

EBV is a herpesvirus that infects 50% of children before age 5. Its host is humans. After initial replication in the nasopharynx, the virus infects B cells, which are induced to secrete immunoglobulins, including heterophil antibodies. Morphologically abnormal (atypical) lymphocytes develop, mainly from CD8$^+$ T cells.

After primary infection, EBV remains within the host, primarily in B cells, for life and undergoes intermittent asymptomatic shedding from the oropharynx. It is detectable in oropharyngeal secretions of 15 to 25% of healthy EBV-seropositive adults. Shedding increases in frequency and titer in immunocompromised patients (eg, organ allograft recipients, HIV-infected people).

EBV has not been recovered from environmental sources and is not very contagious. Transmission may occur by transfusion of blood products but much more frequently occurs by kissing between an uninfected and an EBV-seropositive person who is shedding the virus asymptomatically. Only about 5% of patients acquire EBV from someone who has acute infection. Early childhood transmission occurs more frequently among lower socioeconomic groups and in crowded conditions.

EBV is statistically associated with and likely has a causal role in Burkitt's lymphoma, certain B-cell tumors in immunocompromised patients, and nasopharyngeal carcinoma. EBV does not cause chronic fatigue syndrome. However, it may occasionally cause a syndrome of fever, interstitial pneumonitis, pancytopenia, and uveitis (ie, chronic active EBV).

Symptoms and Signs

In most young children, primary EBV infection is asymptomatic. Symptoms of infectious mononucleosis develop most often in older children and adults.

The incubation period is about 30 to 50 days. Usually, fatigue develops initially, lasting several days to a week or longer, followed by fever, pharyngitis, and adenopathy. However, some of these symptoms may not develop. Fatigue can last months, but is usually maximal in the first 2 to 3 wk. Fever usually peaks in the afternoon or early evening, with a temperature around 39.5° C, although it may reach 40.5° C. When fatigue and fever predominate (the so-called typhoidal form), onset and resolution may be much slower. Pharyngitis may be severe, painful, and exudative and may resemble streptococcal pharyngitis. Adenopathy is usually symmetric and may involve any group of nodes, particularly the anterior and posterior cervical chains. Adenopathy may be the only manifestation.

Splenomegaly, which occurs in about 50% of cases, is maximal during the 2nd and 3rd wk and usually produces only a barely palpable splenic tip. Mild hepatomegaly and hepatic percussion tenderness may occur. Less frequent findings include maculopapular eruptions, jaundice, periorbital edema, and palatal enanthema.

Complications: Although recovery is usually complete, complications may be dramatic.

Neurologic complications include encephalitis, seizures, Guillain-Barré syndrome, peripheral neuropathy, aseptic meningitis, myelitis, cranial nerve palsies, and psychosis. Encephalitis may present with cerebellar dysfunction or it may be global and rapidly progressive, similar to herpes simplex encephalitis, but usually is self-limited.

Hematologic complications are usually self-limited. They include granulocytopenia, thrombocytopenia, and hemolytic anemia. Transient mild granulocytopenia or thrombocytopenia occurs in about 50% of patients; severe cases, associated with bacterial infection or bleeding, occur less frequently. Hemolytic anemia is often due to anti-i–specific antibodies.

Splenic rupture can cause severe consequences. It can result from splenic enlargement and capsular swelling, which are maximal 10 to 21 days after presentation. A history of trauma is present only about half of the time. Rupture is usually painful but occasionally causes painless hypotension. Treatment is discussed on p. 1092.

Respiratory complications include, rarely, upper airway obstruction due to pharyngeal or paratracheal lymphadenopathy; respiratory complications may respond to corticosteroids. Clinically silent interstitial pulmonary infiltrates occur mostly in children and are usually visible on x-rays.

Hepatic complications include elevated aminotransferase levels (about 2 to 3 times normal, returning to baseline over 3 to 4 wk), which occur in about 95% of cases. If jaundice or more severe enzyme elevations occur, other causes of hepatitis should be investigated.

Overwhelming infection with EBV occurs sporadically but may cluster in families, particularly those with X-linked lymphoproliferative syndrome (see also p. 1347). These survivors of primary EBV infection are at risk for developing agammaglobulinemia or lymphoma.

Diagnosis

Infectious mononucleosis should be suspected in patients with typical symptoms and signs. Exudative pharyngitis, anterior cervical lymphadenopathy, and fever may be clinically indistinguishable from those caused by group A β-hemolytic streptococci; however, posterior cervical or generalized adenopathy or hepatosplenomegaly suggest infectious mononucleosis. Moreover, detection of streptococci in the oropharynx does not exclude infectious mononucleosis. Cytomegalovirus (CMV) may produce a syndrome similar to infectious mononucleosis, with atypical lymphocytosis as well as hepatosplenomegaly and hepatitis but usually not with severe pharyngitis. Toxoplasmosis, hepatitis B, rubella, primary HIV infection, or atypical lymphocytes associated with adverse drug reactions can also produce infectious mononucleosis–like syndromes, but these can usually be distinguished by other clinical features.

Laboratory diagnosis usually involves a CBC and a heterophil antibody test. Lymphocytes that are morphologically atypical account for up to 80% of the WBCs. Although individual lymphocytes may resemble leukemic lymphocytes, lymphocytes are heterogeneous, which is unlikely with leukemia.

Heterophil antibodies are measured using various card-agglutination (monospot) tests. The antibodies are present in only 50% of patients < 5 yr but are present in 90% of adolescents and adults with primary EBV infection. The titer and prevalence of heterophil antibodies rise during the 2nd and 3rd wk of illness. Thus, if the diagnosis is strongly suspected but the heterophil antibody test is negative, repeating the test after 7 to 10 days of symptoms is reasonable. If the test remains negative, then antibodies to EBV should be measured. If EBV antibody titers do not reveal acute EBV infection, then a heterophil antibody-negative infectious mononucleosis–like syndrome such as CMV should be considered. Heterophil antibodies may persist 6 to 12 mo after recovery.

In children ≤ 4 yr, in whom heterophil antibodies may never be detectable, IgM antibodies to the EBV viral capsid antigen (VCA) indicate primary EBV infection. These antibodies disappear within 3 mo after infection. Only some laboratories have the capability to measure them. IgG EBV-VCA antibodies persist for life in high titers and do not discriminate between acute and past infection.

Prognosis and Treatment

Infectious mononucleosis is usually self-limited. Duration of illness varies; the acute phase lasts about 2 wk. Generally, 20% of patients can return to school or work within 1 wk and 50% within 2 wk. Fatigue may persist for several more weeks, or, in 1 to 2% of cases, for months. Death occurs in < 1%, mostly due to complications (eg, encephalitis, splenic rupture, airway obstruction).

Treatment is supportive. Patients are encouraged to rest during the acute phase but should quickly resume activity when fever, pharyngitis, and malaise abate. To prevent splenic rupture, heavy lifting and contact sports should be avoided for 1 mo after presentation and until splenomegaly (which can be monitored by ultrasound) resolves.

Although corticosteroids hasten defervescence and relieve pharyngitis, they should not generally be used in uncomplicated disease. Corticosteroids can be helpful for complications such as impending airway obstruction, severe thrombocytopenia, and hemolytic anemia. Although oral or IV acyclovir decreases oropharyngeal shedding of EBV, there is no convincing evidence to warrant its clinical use.

ROSEOLA INFANTUM

(Exanthem Subitum; Pseudorubella)

Roseola infantum is an infection of infants or very young children caused by human herpesvirus 6 (HHV-6) or, less commonly, HHV-7. It causes high fever and a rubelliform eruption that occurs during or after defervescence, but localizing symptoms or signs are absent. Diagnosis is clinical, and treatment is symptomatic.

Roseola infantum is the most well-described illness to result from HHV-6. HHV-6 may also produce visceral disease in immunocompromised patients, eg, organ transplant recipients. Roseola infantum occurs most often in the spring and fall. Minor local epidemics have been reported.

Symptoms and Signs

The incubation period is about 5 to 15 days. Fever of 39.5 to 40.5° C begins abruptly and persists 3 to 5 days without any localizing symptoms or signs. Despite the high fever, the child is usually alert and active, although febrile seizures may occur. Cervical and posterior auricular lymphadenopathy often develops. Encephalitis or hepatitis occurs rarely.

The fever usually falls rapidly on the 4th day, and if it occurs, a macular or maculopapular eruption generally appears prominently on the chest and abdomen and, to a lesser extent, on the face and extremities; it lasts for a few hours to 2 days and may be unnoticed in mild cases. In 70% of HHV-6 infections, the classic exanthem does not occur.

Diagnosis and Treatment

If roseola is known to be in the community, it may be suspected when a child aged 6 mo to 3 yr develops typical symptoms and signs. Testing is rarely needed, but diagnosis can be confirmed by culture, PCR, or serologic tests.

Treatment is generally symptomatic. Foscarnet or ganciclovir have been used to treat some immunosuppressed patients with severe disease, although controlled trials are lacking. Foscarnet is more consistently active than ganciclovir against HHV-6.

190 ENTEROVIRUSES

Enteroviruses, along with rhinoviruses (see Common Cold on p. 1595), are picornaviruses (*pico,* or small, RNA viruses). Enteroviruses include the polioviruses types 1 to 3, coxsackieviruses A1 to A22 and A24 and B1 to 6, echoviruses 2 to 9, 11 to 21, 24 to 27, and 29 to 33, and enteroviruses 68 to 71 and 73. Coxsackieviruses and echoviruses (*e*nteric *c*ytopathic *h*uman *o*rphan viruses) are antigenically heterogeneous. They are shed in oral secretions, stool, blood, and CSF and have wide geographic distribution.

Enteroviruses cause various syndromes (see TABLE 190–1). Enteroviral diseases/

TABLE 190–1. SYNDROMES CAUSED BY ENTEROVIRUSES

SYNDROME	SEROTYPES MOST OFTEN IMPLICATED	COMMENTS
Aseptic meningitis	Coxsackieviruses A2, 4, 7, 9, and others and B2–5; polioviruses 1–3; echoviruses 4, 6, 7, 9, 11 and, less commonly, others	Most common in infants and children; course usually benign; may involve rash or encephalitis; virus can often be isolated from the throat, stool, or CSF
Conjunctivitis (hemorrhagic)	Enterovirus 70 (conjunctivitis is rarely accompanied by transient radiculomyelopathy or poliomyelitis-like paralysis); echovirus 7; coxsackievirus A24 (conjunctivitis with less subconjunctival hemorrhage)	May produce subconjunctival hemorrhage and keratitis; outbreaks are rare in the US; recovery usually in 1–2 wk
Epidemic pleurodynia (Bornholm disease)	Coxsackieviruses B1–6	May affect any age group. Chest and upper abdominal pain
Hand-foot-and-mouth disease	Coxsackievirus A16; enterovirus 71	Most common in young children; vesicular exanthem usually brief and benign
Herpangina	Coxsackieviruses A2, 4–6, 8, 10; probably coxsackievirus 3 and others	Most common in infants and children; characteristic palatal and pharyngeal lesions
Myopericarditis	Coxsackieviruses B1–5; coxsackieviruses A4 and 16; echoviruses 9 and 22	May occur at any age; disease at birth (myocarditis neonatorum) produces fever and heart failure and has high mortality; in other forms there is often complete recovery; diagnosis may require PCR of myocardial tissue
Paralysis	Polioviruses 1–3; coxsackieviruses A7 and others; echoviruses 4, 6, and others; enterovirus 71	Transient mild paresis with aseptic meningitis may occur at any age; younger children generally have milder disease; severe paralysis is possible with poliovirus
Rash	Coxsackieviruses A9 and B1, 3, 4, and 5; coxsackieviruses A4–6, and 16 also implicated; echovirus 9 and 16; echoviruses 2, 4, 11, 14, 19, and 25 also implicated; rash with aseptic meningitis may result from coxsackieviruses A9 and B4, echoviruses 4 and 16, and enterovirus 71	Fever is common; rash is usually nonpruritic, does not desquamate, and occurs on the face, neck, chest, and extremities; may be maculopapular, morbilliform, or occasionally hemorrhagic, petechial, or vesicular; course usually benign
Respiratory disease	Echoviruses 4, 8, 9, 11, 20, and others; coxsackieviruses A21 and 24 and B1 and 3–5	Sore throat, coryza, cough and fever most common; course usually mild; may produce GI symptoms in children

epidemics in the US occur in summer-fall. Epidemic pleurodynia, hand-foot-and-mouth disease, herpangina, and poliomyelitis are caused almost exclusively by enteroviruses. Other disorders caused by enteroviruses may also have other causes.

Aseptic meningitis is frequently caused by a group A or B coxsackievirus or an echovirus in infants and young children. In older children and adults, other enteroviruses as well as other viruses may cause aseptic meningitis. A rash may accompany enteroviral aseptic meningitis. Rarely, encephalitis, possibly severe, also occurs.

Hemorrhagic conjunctivitis occurs rarely in epidemics in the US. Importation of the virus from Africa, Asia, Mexico, and the Caribbean may make outbreaks more common. The eyelids rapidly swell. Often, unlike uncomplicated conjunctivitis, subconjunctival hemorrhages or keratitis develops, causing pain, tearing, and photophobia. Systemic illness is unusual, although a few cases of transient lumbosacral radiculomyelopathy or poliomyelitis-like illness have occurred when hemorrhagic conjunctivitis was due to enterovirus 70. Recovery is usually complete within 1 to 2 wk of onset. Coxsackievirus A24 also causes hemorrhagic conjunctivitis, but subconjunctival hemorrhage is less frequent.

Myopericarditis caused by group B coxsackieviruses and some echoviruses occurs in newborns infected after birth (myocarditis neonatorum) or rarely in utero. Usually, several days after birth, the newborn suddenly develops a picture resembling sepsis with fever, lethargy, disseminated intravascular coagulation, bleeding, and multiple organ (including cardiac) failure. CNS, hepatic, pancreatic, or adrenal lesions may occur simultaneously. Recovery may occur within a few weeks, but death may occur from circulatory collapse or, if the liver is involved, hepatic failure. In older children or adults, myocarditis may result from a group B coxsackievirus, or less likely a group A coxsackievirus or an echovirus. There may be complete recovery.

Rashes may result from certain coxsackieviruses and echoviruses, often during epidemics. They are usually nonpruritic, do not desquamate, and occur on the face, neck, chest, and extremities. They are sometimes maculopapular or morbilliform but occasionally hemorrhagic, petechial, or vesicular. Fever is common. Aseptic meningitis may develop simultaneously.

Respiratory infections may result from enteroviruses. Symptoms include fever, coryza, pharyngitis, and, in some infants and children, vomiting and diarrhea. Bronchitis and interstitial pneumonia have occasionally occurred in adults and children.

Diagnosis and Treatment

Diagnosis of enteroviral diseases is clinical. Laboratory diagnosis is usually unnecessary but can often be accomplished by culturing the virus, demonstrating seroconversion, or sometimes demonstrating viral RNA by reverse transcriptase–PCR. Enteroviruses that cause aseptic meningitis can be cultured from the throat, stool, blood, or CSF. Treatment of enteroviral disease is supportive, although antiviral drugs are under development.

EPIDEMIC PLEURODYNIA

(Bornholm Disease)

Epidemic pleurodynia is a febrile disorder caused by a group B coxsackievirus. Infection produces severe pleuritic chest or abdominal pain.

Epidemic pleurodynia may occur at any age but is most common in children. There is sudden onset of severe, frequently intermittent, often pleuritic pain in the epigastrium or lower anterior chest, with fever and often headache, sore throat, and malaise. The involved truncal muscles may become swollen and tender. Symptoms usually subside in 2 to 4 days but may recur within a few days and persist or recur for several weeks. Up to 5% of cases are complicated by aseptic meningitis, orchitis, and, less commonly, myopericarditis. After recovery, subsequent infection with another group B coxsackievirus is possible.

Diagnosis may be obvious in a child who has unexplained severe pleuritic pain during an epidemic. However, symptoms may be hard to distinguish from other causes of pain. Laboratory diagnosis is not routinely necessary; it consists of demonstrating seroconversion or isolating the virus on a throat or stool culture.

Treatment includes NSAIDs and other symptomatic measures.

HAND-FOOT-AND-MOUTH DISEASE

Hand-foot-and-mouth disease is a febrile disorder usually caused by coxsackievirus A16. Infection produces a vesicular eruption of skin and mucosa.

The disease is most common among young children. The course is similar to that of herpangina, but vesicles are distributed over the buccal mucosa and tongue, the hands and feet, and occasionally the buttocks or genitals. Treatment is symptomatic.

HERPANGINA

Herpangina is a febrile disorder caused by numerous group A coxsackieviruses and occasionally other enteroviruses. Infection produces oropharyngeal mucosal vesicular and ulcerative lesions.

Herpangina tends to occur in epidemics, most commonly in infants and children. It is characterized by sudden onset of fever with sore throat, headache, anorexia, and frequently, neck pain. Infants may vomit. Within 2 days after onset, up to 20 (mean, 4 to 5 per patient) 1- to 2-mm diameter grayish papules develop and become vesicles with erythematous areolae. They occur most frequently on the tonsillar pillars but also on the soft palate, tonsils, uvula, or tongue. During the next 24 h, the lesions become shallow ulcers, seldom > 5 mm in diameter, that heal in 1 to 7 days. Complications are unusual. Lasting immunity to the infecting strain follows, but repeated episodes caused by other group A coxsackieviruses or other enteroviruses are possible.

Diagnosis is based on symptoms and characteristic oral lesions. It is best confirmed by isolating the virus from the lesions or by demonstrating a rise in specific antibody titer, but such testing is not generally recommended. Recurrent aphthous ulcers may appear similar. Bednar's aphthous ulcers rarely occur in the pharynx but generally are not associated with systemic symptoms. Herpetic stomatitis occurs sporadically and produces larger, more persistent and more numerous ulcers throughout the oropharynx than herpangina. Coxsackievirus A10 causes lymphonodular pharyngitis, which is similar except that the papules become 2- to 3-mm whitish to yellowish nodules instead of vesicles and ulcers.

Treatment of herpangina is symptomatic.

POLIOMYELITIS

(Infantile Paralysis; Acute Anterior Poliomyelitis)

Poliomyelitis is an acute infection caused by a poliovirus. Manifestations include a nonspecific minor illness, sometimes aseptic meningitis without paralysis (nonparalytic poliomyelitis), and less often flaccid weakness of various muscle groups (paralytic poliomyelitis). Diagnosis is clinical, although laboratory diagnosis is possible. Treatment is supportive.

Polioviruses have 3 serotypes. Type 1 is the most paralytogenic and the most common cause of epidemics. Humans are the only natural host. Infection is highly transmittable via direct contact. Asymptomatic or minor infections exceed paralytic infections by ≥ 60:1 and are the main source of spread. Extensive vaccination has almost eradicated the disease in developed countries. However, cases still occur in regions with incomplete immunization, such as sub-Saharan Africa and southern Asia.

Virus enters the mouth via the fecal-oral route, multiplies in lymphoid tissues resulting in primary viremia and later, several days of secondary viremia, culminating in development of antibodies and development of symptoms. Virus reaches the CNS via secondary viremia or migration up peripheral nerves. Virus is present in the throat and feces during incubation and, after symptom onset, persists 1 to 2 wk in the throat and ≥ 3 to 6 wk in feces.

Significant damage occurs in only the spinal cord and brain. Inflammation compounds damage produced by primary viral invasion. Factors predisposing to serious neurologic damage include increasing age (throughout life), recent tonsillectomy or intramuscular injection, pregnancy, impairment of B-lymphocyte function, and physical exertion concurrent with onset of the CNS phase.

Symptoms and Signs

Symptomatic disease may be major (paralytic or nonparalytic) or minor. Most symptomatic infections, particularly in young children, are minor, with 1 to 3 days of slight fever, malaise, headache, sore throat, and vomiting, which develop 3 to 5 days after exposure. There are no neurologic symptoms.

Major poliomyelitis usually develops without a preceding minor illness, particularly in older children and adults. Incubation is usually 7 to 14 days. Common manifestations may include aseptic meningitis, deep muscle pain, hyperesthesias, paresthesias, and, during active myelitis, urinary retention and muscle spasms. Asymmetric flaccid paralysis may develop. Dysphagia, nasal regurgitation, and nasal voice are early signs of bulbar involvement. Encephalitic signs occasionally predominate. Infrequently, respiratory failure develops.

Some patients develop postpoliomyelitis syndrome (see below).

Diagnosis

Nonparalytic poliomyelitis may resemble other viral meningitides, with CSF usually revealing normal glucose, mildly elevated protein, and a cell count of 10 to 500/μL (predominantly lymphocytes). Isolation of the virus from the throat or feces or demonstration of a rise in specific antibody titer confirms poliomyelitis.

Asymmetric flaccid limb paralysis or bulbar palsies without sensory loss during an acute febrile illness in a nonimmunized child or young adult almost always indicates paralytic poliomyelitis. Rarely, certain group A and B coxsackieviruses (especially A7), several echoviruses, and enterovirus type 71 may produce similar findings. West Nile virus infection can also cause an acute flaccid paralysis that is clinically indistinguishable from paralytic poliomyelitis due to polio viruses. Epidemiologic clues as well as specific serologic testing for West Nile virus can differentiate these disorders. Guillain-Barré syndrome (see p. 1894) produces flaccid paralysis, but usually it produces no fever, muscle weakness is symmetric, sensory deficits occur in 70% of cases, and CSF protein is usually elevated with a normal cell count.

Prognosis

In nonparalytic forms, recovery is complete. In paralytic forms, about ⅔ of patients have residual permanent weakness. Bulbar paralysis is more likely to resolve than peripheral paralysis. Mortality is 4 to 6% but increases to 10 to 20% in adults and in those with bulbar disease.

Postpoliomyelitis syndrome—muscle fatigue and decreased endurance, often accompanied by weakness, fasciculations, and atrophy—may develop years or decades after paralytic poliomyelitis, particularly in older patients and in those more severely affected initially. Damage usually occurs in previously affected muscle groups. The cause may be related to further loss of anterior horn cells due to aging in a population of neurons already depleted by earlier poliovirus infection. It rarely produces severe increases in disability.

Treatment

Standard treatment is supportive, including rest, analgesics, and antipyretics as needed. Specific antiviral therapy is still investigational.

During active myelitis, precautions to avoid complications of bed rest (eg, deep venous thrombosis, atelectasis, UTI) and prolonged immobility (eg, contractures) may be necessary. Respiratory failure may require mechanical ventilation. Mechanical ventilation or bulbar paralysis requires intensive pulmonary toilet measures.

Treatment of postpoliomyelitis syndrome is supportive.

Prevention

All infants and children should be immunized. The American Academy of Pediatrics recommends vaccination at 2 mo, 4 mo, and 6 to 18 mo and a booster dose at 4 to 6 yr (see also p. 1403 and Fig. 266–3 on p. 2235). Childhood vaccination produces immunity in > 95% of recipients. Salk inactivated poliovirus vaccine (IPV) is preferred to Sabin live attenuated oral polio vaccine (OPV), which causes paralytic poliomyelitis in about 1 case per 2,400,000 doses and is thus no longer available in the US. Serious adverse effects have not been associated with IPV. Adults are not routinely vaccinated. Nonimmunized adults traveling to endemic or epidemic areas should receive primary vaccination with IPV, including 2 doses given 4 to 8 wk apart and a 3rd given 6 to 12 mo later. At least 1 dose is given before travel. Immunized adults traveling to endemic or epidemic areas should receive 1 dose of IPV. Immunocompromised hosts and their household contacts should not receive OPV.

191 ARBOVIRIDAE, ARENAVIRIDAE, BUNYAVIRIDAE, AND FILOVIRIDAE

Arbovirus (*ar*thropod-*bo*rne *virus*) is a term applied to a group of viruses that are transmitted to vertebrates by certain types of blood-eating insects, chiefly mosquitoes and ticks (arthropods). Arbovirus is not part of the current viral classification system. Families in the current classification system that have some arbovirus members include the Bunyaviridae, Flaviviridae, Reoviridae, and Togaviridae. Bunyaviridae includes bunyaviruses, phleboviruses, nairoviruses, and hantaviruses. Arenaviridae and Filoviridae, including Marburg and Ebola viruses, are not arboviruses.

Arboviruses number > 250 and are distributed worldwide; at least 80 cause human disease. Birds are often reservoirs for arboviruses, which are transmitted by mosquitoes to horses, other domestic animals, and humans. Most arboviral diseases are not transmissible by humans. Reservoirs for the Bunyaviridae include insects and vertebrates, often rodents. They spread to humans directly from their reservoirs, but human-to-human transmission may occur. Arenaviruses are usually transmitted by rodents and their excreta; in the case of Lassa fever, human-to-human transmission is possible. Reservoirs for the Marburg and Ebola viruses are unknown, and human-to-human transmission occurs readily.

Many infections are asymptomatic. When symptomatic, they generally begin with a minor nonspecific flu-like illness that may evolve to one of a few syndromes (see TABLE 191–1). These include lymphadenopathy, rashes, aseptic meningitis, encephalitis, arthralgias, arthritis, and noncardiogenic pulmonary edema. Many produce fever and bleeding tendencies (hemorrhagic fever); decreased synthesis of vitamin K–dependent coagulation factors, disseminated intravascular coagulation, and altered platelet function contribute to bleeding. Laboratory diagnosis often involves viral cultures, PCR, electron microscopy, and antigen and antibody detection where available.

Diseases transmitted by mosquitoes or ticks can often be prevented by wearing clothing that covers as much of the body as possible, using insect repellants, and minimizing the likelihood of exposure to the insect (eg, for mosquitoes, limiting time outdoors in wet areas; for ticks, see sidebar177–1 on p. 1491). Diseases transmitted by rodent excreta can be prevented by sealing sites of potential rodent entry into homes and nearby buildings, preventing rodent access to food, and eliminating potential nesting sites around the home. Guidelines for cleaning and working in areas with potential rodent excreta are available through the Centers for Disease Control and Prevention (CDC).

Treatment for most of these infections is supportive. In hemorrhagic fevers, bleeding may require phytonadione (see under Vitamin K Deficiency on p. 46). Transfusion of packed RBCs or fresh frozen plasma may also be necessary. Aspirin and NSAIDs are contraindicated because of antiplatelet activity.

Ribavirin (30 mg/kg IV loading dose followed by 16 mg/kg IV q 6 h for 4 days, then 8 mg/kg q 8 h for 6 days) is effective in Lassa fever, Rift Valley fever, and Crimean-Congo hemorrhagic fever. For dosage in hemorrhagic fever with renal syndrome, see p. 1621. Antiviral treatment for other syndromes has not been adequately studied.

DENGUE

(Breakbone Fever; Dandy Fever)

Dengue is a mosquito-borne disease caused by a flavivirus. Dengue fever usually results in the abrupt onset of high fever, headache, myalgias, arthralgias, lymphadenopathy, and a rash that appears with a 2nd temperature rise after an afebrile period. Respiratory symptoms, such as cough, sore throat, and rhinorrhea, can occur. Dengue can also cause potentially fatal hemorrhagic fever with bleeding tendency and shock. Diagnosis involves PCR and serologic testing. Treatment is symptomatic, including meticulously adjusted intravascular volume replacement.

TABLE 191–1. ARBOVIRUS, ARENAVIRUS, AND FILOVIRUS DISEASES

MAJOR CLINICAL SYNDROME	VIRAL AGENT/ DISEASE	FAMILY	VECTOR	MAJOR DISTRIBUTION
Fever, malaise, headaches, myalgia	Colorado tick fever	Reoviridae (Orbivirus)	Tick	Western US, western Canada
	Phlebotomus fever	Bunyaviridae (Phlebovirus)	Sandfly	Mediterranean basin, Balkans, Middle East, Pakistan, India, China, eastern Africa, Panama, Brazil
	Venezuelan equine encephalitis	Togaviridae (Alphavirus)	Mosquito	Argentina, Brazil, northern South America, Panama, Mexico, Florida
	Rift Valley fever	Bunyaviridae (Phlebovirus)	Mosquito	South Africa, eastern Africa, Egypt
Fever, malaise, headaches, myalgia, lymphadenopathy, rash	Dengue fever	Flaviviridae	Mosquito	Southeast Asia, Africa, Oceania, Australia, South America, Mexico, Caribbean
	West Nile fever	Flaviviridae	Mosquito	Africa, Middle East, southern France, former Soviet Union, India, Indonesia
Fever, malaise, headaches, myalgia, arthralgia, rash	Chikungunya disease	Togaviridae (Alphavirus)	Mosquito	Africa, India, Guam, Southeast Asia, New Guinea
	Mayaro virus	Togaviridae (Alphavirus)	Mosquito	Brazil, Bolivia
	Ross River virus	Togaviridae (Alphavirus)	Mosquito	Australia, New Guinea, Solomon Islands, Samoa, Cook Islands
	Barmah Forest virus	Togaviridae (Alphavirus)	Mosquito	Australia
	Sindbis virus disease (Ockelbo disease, Karelian fever)	Togaviridae (Alphavirus)	Mosquito	Africa, Australia, former Soviet Union, Finland, Sweden
Fever with CNS involvement	Eastern equine encephalitis	Togaviridae (Alphavirus)	Mosquito	Atlantic and Gulf coasts of US, Caribbean, upper New York, western Michigan
	Western equine encephalitis	Togaviridae (Alphavirus)	Mosquito	US, Canada, Central and South America
	West Nile virus	Flaviviridae	Mosquito	Africa, Middle East, southern France, former Soviet Union, India, Indonesia, US
	St. Louis encephalitis	Flaviviridae	Mosquito	US, Caribbean
	Venezuelan equine encephalitis	Togaviridae (Alphavirus)	Mosquito	Argentina, Brazil, northern South America, Panama, Mexico, Florida
	La Crosse encephalitis	Bunyaviridae	Mosquito	North Central States, New York

TABLE 191–1. ARBOVIRUS, ARENAVIRUS, AND FILOVIRUS DISEASES—Continued

MAJOR CLINICAL SYNDROME	VIRAL AGENT/ DISEASE	FAMILY	VECTOR	MAJOR DISTRIBUTION
	Japanese encephalitis	Flaviviridae	Mosquito	Japan, Korea, China, India, Philippines, Southeast Asia, former Soviet Union (eastern)
	Powassan virus	Flaviviridae	Tick	Eastern Canada, New York
	Murray Valley encephalitis	Flaviviridae	Mosquito	Australia, New Guinea
	Kyasanur Forest disease	Flaviviridae	Tick	India
	Tick-borne encephalitis	Flaviviridae	Tick	Europe, Balkans, former Soviet Union
	Lymphocytic choriomeningitis	Arenaviridae	Rodent	US, Argentina, Germany, Balkans
Fever, malaise, headaches, myalgia, hemorrhagic signs	Yellow fever	Flaviviridae	Mosquito	Central and South America, Africa
	Dengue hemorrhagic fever	Flaviviridae	Mosquito	Southeast Asia, Oceania, Caribbean
	Kyasanur Forest disease	Flaviviridae	Tick	India
	Omsk hemorrhagic fever	Flaviviridae	Tick	Former Soviet Union
	Crimean-Congo hemorrhagic fever	Bunyaviridae (Nairovirus)	Tick	Africa, eastern Europe, Middle East, former Soviet Union
	Hantaan virus	Bunyaviridae (Hantavirus)	Rodent	Korea, Japan, China, Southeast Asia, Europe
	Seoul virus	Bunyaviridae (Hantavirus)	Rodent	Korea, Japan
	Puumala virus (Nephropathia epidemica)	Bunyaviridae (Hantavirus)	Rodent	Scandinavia, former Soviet Union
	Machupo virus	Arenaviridae	Rodent	Bolivia
	Junin virus	Arenaviridae	Rodent	Argentina
	Guanaritovirus	Arenaviridae	Rodent	Venezuela
	Lassa fever	Arenaviridae	Rodent, human to human	West Africa
	Marburg virus	Filoviridae	Unknown, human to human	Zimbabwe, Kenya, Uganda
	Ebola virus	Filoviridae	Unknown, human to human	Zaire, Sudan
Fever, malaise, headaches, myalgia, noncardiogenic pulmonary edema	Hantavirus: Sin Nombre, Black Creek Canal, Bayou, New York-1, Rio Mamore	Bunyaviridae (Hantavirus)	Rodent	US (west of Mississippi River), Canada, Brazil, Bolivia, Paraguay, Argentina

Dengue is endemic to the tropical regions of the world in latitudes from about 35° north to 35° south. Outbreaks are most prevalent in Southeast Asia but also occur in the Caribbean, including Puerto Rico and the US Virgin Islands, Oceania, and the Indian subcontinent; more recently, dengue incidence has increased in Central and South America. Each year about 100 to 200 cases are imported to the US by returning tourists. The causative agent, a flavivirus with 4 serogroups, is transmitted by the bite of *Aedes* mosquitoes.

Symptoms and Signs

After an incubation period of 3 to 15 days, chills, headache, retro-orbital pain with eye movement, lumbar backache, and severe prostration begin abruptly. Extreme aching in the legs and joints occurs during the first hours, which accounts for the traditional name of breakbone fever. The temperature rises rapidly to up to 40° C, with hypotension and relative bradycardia. Bulbar and palpebral conjunctival injection, a transient flushing or pale pink macular rash, particularly of the face, and a palpable spleen are common. Cervical, epitrochlear, and inguinal lymph nodes are usually enlarged.

Fever and other symptoms persist 48 to 96 h, followed by rapid defervescence with profuse sweating. Patients then feel well for about 24 h, after which fever usually occurs again, typically with a lower peak temperature than the first. Simultaneously, a blanching maculopapular rash spreads from the extremities to cover the body diffusely except the face or to cover the trunk and extremities in a patchy distribution. The palms and soles may be bright red, swollen, and itchy.

Mild cases of dengue, usually lacking lymphadenopathy, remit in < 72 h. In more severe disease, asthenia may last several weeks. Death is rare. Immunity to the infecting strain is long-lasting, whereas broader immunity to other strains lasts only 2 to 12 mo.

Diagnosis

Dengue fever is suspected in patients in endemic areas who develop sudden fever, headache, myalgias, and adenopathy, particularly with the characteristic rash or recurrent fever. Evaluation should rule out alternative diagnoses, especially malaria and leptospirosis. Diagnostic studies include PCR of blood and serology. Serology involves hemagglutination inhibiting or complement fixation tests using paired sera, but cross-reactions with other flavivirus antibodies are possible. Although rarely performed, cultures can be done using mosquitoes or specialized cell lines. CBC may show leukopenia by the 2nd day of fever; by the 4th or 5th day, the WBC count may be 2000 to 4000/μL with only 20 to 40% granulocytes. Urinalysis may show moderate albuminuria and a few casts.

Treatment and Prevention

Treatment is symptomatic. People in endemic areas should try to prevent mosquito bites. To prevent further transmission by mosquitoes, patients with dengue should be kept under mosquito netting until the 2nd bout of fever has resolved. Vaccines are being evaluated.

Dengue Hemorrhagic Fever

(Philippine, Thai, or Southeast Asian Hemorrhagic Fever; Dengue Shock Syndrome)

Dengue hemorrhagic fever (DHF) is a variant presentation that occurs primarily in children < 10 yr living where dengue is endemic. DHF requires prior exposure to the dengue virus. It is an immunopathologic disease.

DHF is suspected in children with World Health Organization (WHO)–defined clinical criteria for the diagnosis: sudden fever that stays high for 2 to 7 days; hemorrhagic manifestations, including at least a positive tourniquet test and petechiae, purpura, ecchymoses, bleeding gums, hematemesis, or melena; and hepatomegaly. The tourniquet test is performed by inflating a BP cuff to midway between the systolic and the diastolic BP for 15 min. The number of petechiae that form within a 2.5-cm diameter circle are counted; > 20 petechiae suggests capillary fragility. Shock may ensue. CBC, coagulation tests, urinalysis, liver function tests, and dengue serologic tests should be obtained. Thrombocytopenia (< 100,000 platelets/μL) and a prolonged PT characterize the coagulation abnormalities. There may be mild proteinuria and increases in AST levels. Complement fixation antibody titers against flaviviruses are usually high. Patients with WHO-defined clinical criteria plus thrombocytopenia (≤100,000/μL) or hemoconcentration (Hct increased by ≥20%) are presumed to have the disease.

In adults, DHF begins with abrupt fever and headache and is initially indistinguishable from classic dengue. Shock and increasing illness may develop rapidly 2 to 6 days after onset. Bleeding tendencies occur, usually as purpura, petechiae, or ecchymoses at injection sites; sometimes as hematemesis, melena, or epistaxis; and occasionally as subarachnoid hemorrhage. Hepatomegaly is common, as is bronchopneumonia with or without bilateral pleural effusions. Myocarditis can occur.

Mortality ranges from 6 to 30%; most deaths occur in infants. Patients require intensive treatment to maintain euvolemia. Both hypovolemia (which can produce shock) and overhydration (which can produce acute respiratory distress syndrome) should be avoided. Urine output and the degree of hemoconcentration can be used to monitor intravascular volume. No antivirals have been shown to improve outcome.

HANTAVIRUS INFECTION

The genus Hantavirus consists of at least 4 serogroups with 9 viruses causing 2 major, sometimes overlapping, clinical syndromes: hemorrhagic fever with renal syndrome (HFRS) and hantavirus pulmonary syndrome (HPS). Viruses causing HFRS are Hantaan, Seoul, Dobrava (Belgrade), and Puumala. Those causing HPS are Sin Nombre, Black Creek Canal, Bayou, and New York-1. Hantaviruses occur in wild rodents throughout the world, who shed it throughout life in urine and feces. Transmission occurs between rodents. Transmission to humans is through inhalation of aerosols of rodent excreta. Recent evidence suggests human-to-human transmission may occur on rare occasions. Naturally and laboratory-acquired infections are becoming more common.

Laboratory diagnosis of Hantavirus infection is established by serologic tests and reverse transcriptase–PCR (rt-PCR). Serologic tests include enzyme-linked immunosorbent assay (ELISA) and Western and strip immunoblot assays. Growth of the virus is technically difficult and requires a biosafety level 3 laboratory.

Hemorrhagic Fever With Renal Syndrome

(Epidemic Nephrosonephritis; Korean Hemorrhagic Fever; Nephropathia Epidemica)

Hemorrhagic fever with renal syndrome begins as a flu-like illness and may progress to shock, bleeding, and renal failure. Diagnosis is with serologic tests and PCR. Mortality is 6 to 15%. Treatment includes IV ribavirin.

Some forms of hemorrhagic fever with renal syndrome (HFRS) are mild (eg, nephropathia epidemica, caused by Puumala virus, occurring in Scandinavia, the western part of the former Soviet Union, and Europe), while others are severe (eg, those caused by Hantaan, Seoul, and Dobrava viruses as occur in Korea or the Balkans).

Symptoms, Signs, and Diagnosis

Incubation is about 2 wk. In mild forms, infection is often asymptomatic. When symptoms occur, onset is sudden, with high fever, headache, backache, and abdominal pain. On the 3rd or 4th day, subconjunctival hemorrhages, palatal petechiae, and a truncal petechial rash may appear. Diffuse reddening of the face that resembles sunburn, with dermatographism, occurs in > 90%. Relative bradycardia is present, and transient mild hypotension occurs in about ½ with shock in a minority. After the 4th day, renal failure develops. About 20% of patients become mentally obtunded. Seizures or severe focal neurologic symptoms occur in 1%. The rash subsides; the patient develops polyuria and recovers over several weeks. Proteinuria, hematuria, and pyuria may develop.

HFRS is suspected in patients with possible exposure who have fever, a bleeding tendency, and renal failure. If suspected, CBC, electrolytes, renal function tests, coagulation tests, and urinalysis are obtained. During the hypotensive phase, the Hct increases and leukocytosis and thrombocytopenia develop. Albuminuria, hematuria, RBC and WBC casts may develop, usually between the 2nd and 5th day. During the diuretic phase, electrolyte abnormalities are common. Diagnosis of HFRS is ultimately based on serology or PCR.

Prognosis and Treatment

Death can occur during the diuretic phase secondary to volume depletion, electrolyte disturbances, and secondary infections. Recovery usually takes 3 to 6 wk but may take up to 6 mo. Overall mortality is 6 to 15%, almost all of which occurs in the more severe forms. Residual renal dysfunction is uncommon except with severe disease that occurs in the Balkans.

Treatment is with IV ribavirin (loading dose 30 mg/kg, then 16 mg/kg q 6 h for 4 days, then 8 mg/kg q 8 h for 3 days). Supportive care, which may include renal dialysis, is critical, particularly during the diuretic phase.

Hantavirus Pulmonary Syndrome

Hantavirus pulmonary syndrome occurs primarily in the southwestern US. It begins as a flu-like illness and within days produces noncardiogenic pulmonary edema. Diagnosis is with serologic tests and reverse transcriptase–PCR. Mortality is 50 to 75%. Treatment is supportive.

Most cases of hantavirus pulmonary syndrome (HPS) are caused by the Sin Nombre hantavirus (Four Corners virus, Muerto Canyon virus); others occur in patients with Black Creek Canal virus, Andes virus, or Laguna Negra virus. Infection is transmitted to humans via inhalation of excreta of sigmodontine rodents (especially the deer mouse). Most cases occur west of the Mississippi River in spring or summer, typically after heavy rains.

Symptoms, Signs, and Diagnosis

HPS begins as a nonspecific flu-like illness, with acute fever, myalgia, headache, and GI symptoms. Two to 15 days later (median 4 days), the patient rapidly develops noncardiogenic pulmonary edema and hypotension. Several patients have had a combination of HFRS and HPS. Mild cases of HPS have also been recognized.

HPS is suspected in patients with possible exposure who have unexplained clinical or radiographic pulmonary edema. The chest x-ray may show increased vascular markings, Kerley B lines, bilateral infiltrates, or pleural effusions. If suspected, echocardiogram should be obtained to exclude cardiogenic pulmonary edema. CBC, liver function tests, and urinalysis are also usually obtained. There is mild neutrophilic leukocytosis, hemoconcentration, and thrombocytopenia. Modest elevation of LDH, AST, and ALT, with decreased serum albumin, is typical. Urinalysis shows minimal abnormalities. Diagnosis is with serologic testing or reverse transcriptase–PCR.

Prognosis and Treatment

Patients who survive the first few days improve rapidly and recover completely over 2 to 3 wk, often without sequelae. Mortality is 50 to 75%.

Treatment is supportive. Mechanical ventilation, meticulous volume control, and vasopressors may be required. For severe cardiopulmonary insufficiency, extracorporal mechanical oxygenation may be life-saving. IV ribavirin is ineffective.

LASSA FEVER

Lassa fever is an often fatal arenavirus infection that occurs mostly in Africa. It may involve multiple organ systems but spares the CNS. Diagnosis is with serologic tests and PCR. Treatment includes IV ribavirin.

Lassa fever outbreaks have occurred in Nigeria, Liberia, and Sierra Leone. Cases have been imported to the US and the United Kingdom. The reservoir is *Mastomys natalensis*, a rat that commonly inhabits houses in Africa. Most human cases probably result from contamination of food with rodent urine, but human-to-human transmission can occur via urine, feces, saliva, vomitus, or blood.

Symptoms and Signs

The incubation period is 5 to 16 days. Symptoms begin with gradually progressive fever, weakness, malaise, and GI symptoms (eg, nausea, vomiting, diarrhea, dysphagia, stomach ache); symptoms and signs of hepatitis may occur. Over the subsequent 4 to 5 days, symptoms progress to prostration with sore throat, cough, chest pain, and vomiting. The sore throat becomes more severe during the 1st wk; patches of white or yellow exudate may appear on the tonsils, often coalescing into a pseudomembrane. Sixty to 80% of patients have systolic BPs of < 90 mm Hg with pulse pressures of < 20 mm Hg, and relative bradycardia is possible. Facial and neck swelling and conjunctival edema occur in 10 to 30%. Occasionally, patients have tinnitus, epistaxis, bleeding from the gums and venipuncture sites, maculopapular rash, cough, and dizziness. Twenty percent of patients develop sensorineural hearing loss, often permanent. In patients who will recover, defervescence occurs; fatally ill patients often develop shock, delirium, rales, pleural effusion, and, occasionally, generalized seizures. Pericarditis occasionally occurs. The degree of fever and the aminotransferase levels correlate with disease severity. Late sequelae include alopecia, iridocyclitis, and transient blindness.

Diagnosis

Lassa fever is suspected in patients with possible exposure who have a viral prodrome followed by unexplained disease of any organ system except the CNS. If suspected, liver function tests, urinalysis, serologic tests, and possibly CBC should be obtained. Proteinuria is common and may be massive. AST and ALT levels rise (10×normal), as do LDH levels. The most rapid diagnostic test is PCR, although demonstrating either Lassa IgM antibodies or a 4-fold rise in IgG antibody titer using an indirect fluorescent antibody technique is also diagnostic. Although the virus can be grown in cell culture, cultures are not routine. Due to the risk of infection, particularly in patients with hemorrhagic fever, cultures must be handled only in a biosafety level 4 laboratory. Chest x-rays, obtained if lung involvement is suspected, may show basilar pneumonitis and pleural effusions.

Prognosis, Treatment, and Prevention

Recovery or death generally occurs 7 to 31 days (average 12 to 15 days) after symptoms begin. Mortality occurs in 16 to 45%. Disease is severe during pregnancy. Mortality is 50 to 92% in women who are pregnant or who have delivered within 1 mo. Most pregnant women lose the fetus.

Ribavirin may reduce mortality up to 10-fold if begun within the first 6 days. All patients with AST levels ≥ 150 U/mL should be treated with IV ribavirin 30 mg/kg once followed by 16 mg/kg qid for 4 days followed by 8 mg/kg tid for an additional 7 days. Anti–Lassa fever plasma may be used as adjunctive therapy in very ill patients. Supportive treatment, including correction of fluid and electrolyte imbalances, is imperative. For infected pregnant women, particularly during the 3rd trimester, uterine evacuation appears to reduce maternal mortality.

Universal precautions, airborne isolation (including use of goggles, high-efficiency masks, a negative-pressure room, and positive-pressure filtered air respirators), and surveillance of contacts are recommended.

LYMPHOCYTIC CHORIOMENINGITIS

Lymphocytic choriomeningitis is caused by an arenavirus. It usually produces a flu-like illness or aseptic meningitis, sometimes with rash, arthritis, orchitis, parotitis, or encephalitis. Diagnosis is by viral isolation or indirect immunofluorescence. Treatment is supportive.

Lymphocytic choriomeningitis is endemic in rodents. Human infection results most commonly from exposure to dust or food contaminated by the gray house mouse or hamsters, which harbor the virus and excrete it in urine, feces, semen, and nasal secretions. When transmitted by mice, the disease occurs primarily in adults during autumn and winter.

Symptoms and Signs

The incubation period is 1 to 2 wk. Most patients have no or minimal symptoms. Some develop a flu-like illness. Fever, usually 38.5 to 40° C, with rigors is accompanied by malaise, weakness, myalgia (especially lumbar), retro-orbital headache, photophobia, anorexia, nausea, and lightheadedness. Sore throat and dysesthesia occur less often. After 5 days to 3 wk, patients may improve for 1 or 2 days. Many relapse with recurrent fever, headache, skin rashes, swelling of metacarpophalangeal and proximal interphalangeal joints, meningeal signs, orchitis, parotitis, or alopecia of the scalp. Aseptic meningitis occurs in the minority of patients. Rarely, frank encephalitis, ascending paralysis, bulbar paralysis, transverse myelitis, or acute Parkinson's disease can occur. Neurologic sequelae are rare in meningitis but occur in up to 33% of patients with encephalitis. Infection may cause fetal abnormalities, including hydrocephalus and chorioretinitis.

Diagnosis and Treatment

Lymphocytic choriomeningitis is suspected in patients with murine exposure and an acute illness, particularly aseptic meningitis or encephalitis. Aseptic meningitis may lower CSF glucose mildly but occasionally to as low as 15 mg/dL. CSF WBCs range from a few hundred to a few thousand cells, usually with > 80% lymphocytes. WBC counts of 2000 to 3000/μL and platelet counts of 50,000 to 100,000/μL typically occur during the 1st wk of illness. Diagnosis can be made by isolating the virus from the blood or CSF or by indirect immunofluorescence assays of inoculated cell cultures.

Treatment is supportive.

MARBURG AND EBOLA VIRUS INFECTIONS

Marburg and Ebola are filoviruses that cause hemorrhage, multiple organ failure, and high mortality rates. Diagnosis is with enzyme-linked immunosorbent assay, PCR, or electron microscopy. Treatment is supportive. Strict isolation and quarantine measures are necessary to contain outbreaks.

Epidemics have occurred rarely and sporadically. Most index cases involve exposure to nonhuman primates from sub-Saharan Africa or the Philippines; however, the vector and reservoir are unknown.

Human-to-human transmission occurs via skin and mucous membrane contact with an infected person or other primate. Aerosol transmission has been postulated.

Symptoms, Signs, and Diagnosis

After an incubation period of 5 to 10 days, fever, myalgia, and headache occur, often with abdominal (nausea, vomiting, pain, diarrhea) and upper respiratory (cough, chest pain, pharyngitis) symptoms. Photophobia, conjunctival injection, jaundice, and lymphadenopathy also occur. Delirium, stupor, and coma may occur, indicating CNS involvement. Hemorrhagic symptoms begin within the 1st few days and include petechiae, ecchymoses, and frank bleeding around puncture sites and mucous membranes. A maculopapular rash, primarily on the trunk, begins around day 5. During the 2nd wk of symptoms, either defervescence occurs and patients begin recovery or patients develop fatal multiple organ failure. Recovery is prolonged and may be complicated by recurrent hepatitis, uveitis, transverse myelitis, and orchitis. Mortality ranges from 25 to 90% (higher with Ebola).

Marburg or Ebola virus infection is suspected in patients with bleeding tendencies, fever, and travel to endemic areas or exposure to primates from these areas. If suspected, CBC, routine blood chemistries, liver function and coagulation tests, and urinalysis are obtained. Diagnostic tests include the enzyme-linked immunosorbent blood assay and PCR. The gold standard is detection of characteristic virions on electron microscopy, performed on infected tissue (especially liver) or blood.

Treatment and Prevention

No vaccine or effective antiviral therapy exists, although a vaccine is currently in development. Treatment is supportive and includes minimizing invasive procedures and replacing depleted coagulation factors.

Mask-gown-glove precautions, thorough equipment sterilization, hospital closures, and community education have shortened epidemics. All suspected cases and their cadavers require strict isolation and special handling. The US has strict quarantine procedures to prevent importation of infected monkeys. Case reporting is required.

YELLOW FEVER

Yellow fever is a mosquito-borne flavivirus infection endemic in tropical South America and sub-Saharan Africa. Symptoms may include sudden onset of fever, relative bradycardia, headache, and, if severe, jaundice, hemorrhage, and multiple organ failure. Diagnosis is with viral culture and serologic tests. Prevention involves vaccination and mosquito control. Treatment is supportive.

In urban yellow fever, virus is transmitted by the bite of an *Aedes aegypti* mosquito infected about 2 wk previously by feeding on a viremic person. In jungle (sylvatic) yellow fever, the virus is transmitted by *Haemagogus* and other forest canopy mosquitoes that acquire the virus from wild primates. Incidence is highest during months of peak rainfall, humidity, and temperature in South America and during the late rainy and early dry seasons in Africa.

Symptoms and Signs

Infection ranges from asymptomatic (in 5 to 50% of cases) to a hemorrhagic fever with 50% mortality. Incubation lasts 3 to 6 days. Onset is sudden, with fever of 39 to 40° C, chills, headache, dizziness, and myalgias. The pulse, usually rapid initially, by the 2nd day becomes slow for the degree of fever (Faget's sign). The face is flushed and the eyes are injected. Nausea, vomiting, constipation, severe prostration, restlessness, and irritability are common. Mild disease may resolve after 1 to 3 days. In moderate or severe cases, however, the fever falls suddenly 2 to 5 days after onset, and a remission of several hours or days ensues. The fever recurs, but the pulse remains slow. Jaundice, extreme albuminuria, and epigastric tenderness with hematemesis often occur together after 5 days of illness. There may be oliguria, petechiae, mucosal hemorrhages, confusion, and apathy.

Disease may last > 1 wk with rapid recovery and no sequelae. In the most severe (malignant) cases, delirium, intractable hiccups, seizures, coma, and multiple organ failure may occur terminally. During recovery, bacterial superinfections, particularly pneumonia, can occur.

Diagnosis

Yellow fever is suspected in patients in endemic areas who develop sudden fever with relative bradycardia and jaundice; mild disease often escapes diagnosis. CBC, urinalysis, liver function tests, coagulation tests, viral blood culture, and serologic tests should be obtained. Leukopenia with a relative neutropenia is common, as are thrombocytopenia, prolonged clotting, and increased PT. Bilirubin and aminotransferase levels may be elevated acutely and for several months. Albuminuria, which occurs in 90% of patients, may reach 20 g/L; it helps differentiate yellow fever from hepatitis. In the most severe form, called malignant yellow fever, hypoglycemia and hyperkalemia may occur terminally.

Diagnosis is confirmed by culture, serologic tests, PCR, or by finding characteristic midzonal hepatocyte necrosis at autopsy. Suspected or confirmed cases must be quarantined. Needle biopsy of the liver during illness is contraindicated by the risk of hemorrhage.

Prognosis and Treatment

Up to 10% of patients with disease severe enough to be diagnosed die.

Treatment is mainly supportive. Bleeding may be treated with Ca gluconate 1 g IV once or twice/day or with phytonadione. Prophylaxis against GI bleeding with a proton pump inhibitor or an H_2 blocker should be used in all patients ill enough to require hospitalization.

Prevention

The most effective way to prevent outbreaks is to reduce the number of mosquitoes and limit mosquito bites by using diethyltoluamide (DEET), mosquito netting, and protective attire. During jungle outbreaks, people should evacuate the area until they are immunized and mosquitoes are controlled. For people traveling to endemic areas, active immunization with the 17D strain of live, attenuated yellow fever vaccine (0.5 mL sc q 10 yr) is indicated and is effective in 95%. In the US, the vaccine is given only at US Public Health Service–authorized Yellow Fever Vaccination Centers. The vaccine is contraindicated in pregnant women and in those with compromised immunity.

To prevent further mosquito transmission, infected patients should be isolated in rooms that are well screened and sprayed with insecticides.

192 HUMAN IMMUNODEFICIENCY VIRUS

(See also Human Immunodeficiency Virus Infection in Children on p. 2341.)

Human immunodeficiency virus (HIV) infection results from 1 of 2 similar retroviruses (HIV-1 and HIV-2) that destroy $CD4^+$ lymphocytes and impair cell-mediated immunity, increasing risk of certain infections and cancers. Initial infection may produce nonspecific febrile illness. The risk of subsequent manifestations—related to immunodeficiency—is proportional to the level of $CD4^+$ lymphocytes. Manifestations range from asymptomatic carriage to the acquired immune deficiency syndrome (AIDS), which is defined by serious opportunistic infections or cancers. HIV infection is diagnosable by antibody or antigen testing. Treatment aims to suppress HIV replication by combinations of drugs that inhibit HIV enzymes.

Retroviruses are enveloped RNA viruses, several of which produce human diseases. Retroviruses are defined by their mechanism of replication via reverse transcription to produce DNA copies that integrate in the host cell genome. Other retroviruses include human T-lymphotropic virus (see sidebar 192–1).

Sidebar 192–1.
HTLV INFECTIONS

Infection with human T-lymphotropic virus (HTLV) 1 and 2 can cause T-cell leukemias and lymphomas, lymphadenopathy, hepatosplenomegaly, skin lesions, and occasionally immunocompromise. Some immunocompromised patients develop infections similar to those that occur in AIDS. HTLV-1 can also cause a myelopathy (see Tropical Spastic Paraparesis on p. 1916). HTLV-1 can be transmitted sexually and through blood. Most cases are transmitted from mother to child by breastfeeding.

AIDS is defined as HIV infection that leads to any of the disorders listed in category B or C of TABLE 192–1 or a CD4$^+$ T lymphocyte (helper cell [see p. 1323]) count of < 200/μL. The disorders listed in categories B and C of TABLE 192–1 are serious opportunistic infections; certain cancers, such as Kaposi's sarcoma and non-Hodgkin lymphoma, to which defective cell-mediated immunity predisposes; and neurologic dysfunction.

HIV-1 causes most cases in the Western Hemisphere, Europe, Asia, and Central, South, and East Africa. HIV-2 causes most cases in parts of West Africa and appears less virulent than HIV-1. In certain areas of West Africa, both organisms are prevalent and may coinfect patients.

TABLE 192–1. CLINICAL CATEGORIES OF HIV INFECTION*

Category A
Asymptomatic
Symptoms of acute primary HIV infection
Persistent generalized adenopathy

Category B
Bacillary angiomatosis
Candidiasis, oropharyngeal (thrush)
Candidiasis, vulvovaginal; persistent, frequent, or poorly responsive to therapy
Cervical dysplasia (moderate or severe)/cervical carcinoma in situ
Constitutional symptoms, such as fever ≥ 38.5° C) or diarrhea lasting > 1 mo
Hairy leukoplakia, oral
Herpes zoster (shingles), involving at least 2 distinct episodes or > 1 dermatome
Immune thrombocytopenic purpura
Listeriosis
Pelvic inflammatory disease, particularly if complicated by tubo-ovarian abscess
Peripheral neuropathy

Category C
Candidiasis of bronchi, trachea, or lungs
Candidiasis, esophageal
Cervical cancer, invasive†
Coccidioidomycosis, disseminated or extrapulmonary
Cryptococcosis, extrapulmonary
Cryptosporidiosis, chronic intestinal (> 1 mo duration)
Cytomegalovirus disease (other than liver, spleen, or lymph nodes)
Cytomegalovirus retinitis (with loss of vision)
Encephalopathy, HIV-related
Herpes simplex: chronic ulcer(s) (> 1 mo duration); or bronchitis, pneumonitis, or esophagitis
Histoplasmosis, disseminated or extrapulmonary
Isosporiasis, chronic intestinal (> 1 mo duration)
Kaposi's sarcoma
Lymphoma, Burkitt's (or equivalent term)
Lymphoma, immunoblastic (or equivalent term)
Lymphoma, primary, of brain
Mycobacterium avium complex or *M. kansasii*, disseminated or extrapulmonary
M. tuberculosis, any site (pulmonary† or extrapulmonary)
Mycobacterium, other species or unidentified species, disseminated or extrapulmonary
Pneumocystis jiroveci (formerly *P. carinii*) pneumonia
Pneumonia, recurrent†
Progressive multifocal leukoencephalopathy
Salmonella septicemia, recurrent
Toxoplasmosis of brain
Wasting syndrome due to HIV

*1993 CDC clinical categories by increasing severity based on opportunistic infections and tumors. Categories B and C represent AIDS-defining illnesses. Although categories correspond roughly with disease progression, they are less predictive of prognosis in patients receiving current treatment regimens.

†Added in the 1993 expansion of the AIDS surveillance case definition.

HIV-1 originated in rural central Africa in the 1st half of the 20th century, when a closely related chimpanzee virus first infected humans. Epidemic global spread began in the late 1970s, and AIDS was recognized in 1981. More than 40 million people are infected worldwide. Of the 3 million annual deaths and 14,000 new daily infections, 95% occur in the developing world, $\frac{1}{2}$ are in women, and $\frac{1}{7}$ are in children < 15 yr.

Transmission and Epidemiology

Transmission of HIV requires contact with body fluids—specifically blood, semen, vaginal secretions, breast milk, saliva, or exudates from wounds or skin and mucosal lesions—that contain free virions or infected cells. Transmission is more likely with higher concentrations of virions, which can be very high during primary infection, even if asymptomatic. Transmission by saliva or droplets produced by coughing or sneezing, although conceivable, is extremely unlikely. HIV is not transmitted by casual contact or even by the close nonsexual contact that occurs at work, school, or home. Transmission is generally by direct transfer of bodily fluids through sexual relations, sharing of blood-contaminated needles, childbirth, breastfeeding, or medical procedures (eg, transfusions or exposure to contaminated instruments).

Sexual practices such as fellatio and cunnilingus appear to be relatively low risk but not absolutely safe (see TABLE 192–2). Risk does not increase significantly if semen or vaginal secretions are swallowed. However, open sores in the mouth may increase risk. The sexual practices with the highest risks are those that produce mucosal trauma, typically intercourse. Anal-receptive intercourse poses the highest risk. Mucous membrane inflammation facilitates HIV transmission; sexually transmitted infections such as gonorrhea, chlamydia, trichomoniasis, and those that produce ulceration (eg, chancroid, herpes, syphilis) increase risk.

HIV is transmitted from mother to offspring transplacentally or perinatally in 30 to 50% of cases. HIV is excreted in breast milk, and breastfeeding can transmit HIV to about 75% of at-risk infants who had previously escaped infection. Infection of large numbers of women of childbearing age has increased the incidence of AIDS in children (see p. 2341).

The risk of transmission after skin penetration with a medical instrument contaminated with infected blood is about 1/300 on average without treatment; immediate antiretroviral treatment probably reduces that risk to 1/1500. Risk appears to be higher if the wound is deep or if blood is inoculated (eg, with a contaminated hollow-bore needle). The risk of transmission from infected medical personnel who take appropriate precautions to uninfected patients is unclear but appears minimal. In the 1980s, one dentist transmitted HIV to ≥ 6 of his patients by unknown means. However, extensive investigations of patients cared for by other HIV-infected physicians, including surgeons, have uncovered few other cases.

Although screening of blood donors has minimized the risk of transmission via transfusion, a small risk still exists because screening tests may miss early infections (see Prevention on p. 1639).

HIV has spread in 2 epidemiologically distinct patterns. The 1st pattern primarily

TABLE 192–2. HIV TRANSMISSION RISK OF SEVERAL SEXUAL ACTIVITIES

No risk (unless sores are present)

- Dry kissing
- Body-to-body rubbing and massage
- Using unshared inserted sexual devices
- Being masturbated by a partner, without semen or vaginal fluids
- Bathing and showering together
- Contact of intact skin with feces or urine

Theoretical risk (extremely low risk unless sores are present)

- Wet kissing
- Oral sex performed on male (with or without ejaculation, with or without ingestion of semen)
- Oral sex performed on female (with or without barrier)
- Oral-anal contact
- Digital vaginal or anal penetration, with or without a glove
- Using shared but disinfected inserted sexual devices

Low risk

- Vaginal or anal intercourse (with proper use of a condom)
- Using shared but not disinfected inserted sexual devices

High risk

- Vaginal or anal intercourse (with or without ejaculation, condom not used or used improperly) involves male homosexual intercourse or contact with infected blood (eg, IV drug abusers who share needles and, before effective screening of donors, transfusion recipients); this pattern predominates in the US and Europe. In the 2nd pattern, heterosexual intercourse is the major mode of transmission (thus affecting men and women nearly equally); this pattern predominates in Africa, South America, and southern Asia. In some countries (eg, Brazil, Thailand), there is no predominant mode. In areas where heterosexual transmission is dominant, HIV infection follows routes of trade, transportation, and economic migration to cities and spreads secondarily to rural areas. In Africa, particularly southern Africa, the HIV epidemic has killed tens of millions of young adults, creating millions of orphans. Factors that perpetuate spread include poverty and poor education, a deficient system of medical care, and lack of effective drugs.

Many opportunistic infections are reactivations of latent infections; thus, epidemiologic factors, which determine the likelihood of latent pathogens, also influence the risk of specific opportunistic infections. Toxoplasmosis and TB have a high prevalence in the general population in many developing countries. Similarly, coccidioidomycosis is common in the American Southwest and histoplasmosis in the American Midwest. In the US and Europe, human herpesvirus 8 infection, which causes Kaposi's sarcoma, is common in homosexual and bisexual men but uncommon in other HIV patients. Thus, > 90% of US AIDS patients who develop Kaposi's sarcoma are in this risk group.

Pathophysiology

HIV attaches to and penetrates host T cells via $CD4^+$ molecules and chemokine receptors. After attachment, HIV RNA and enzymes are released into the host cell. Viral replication requires that reverse transcriptase, an RNA-dependent DNA polymerase, copy HIV RNA, producing proviral DNA; this copying is prone to errors, resulting in frequent mutations. Proviral DNA enters the host cell's nucleus and is integrated into host DNA in a process that involves HIV integrase. With each cell division, the integrated proviral DNA is duplicated along with host DNA. Proviral HIV DNA is transcribed to viral RNA and translated to HIV proteins, including the envelope glycoproteins 40 and 120. The HIV proteins are assembled into HIV virions at the inner cell membrane and budded from the cell surface; each host cell may produce thousands of virions. Protease, another HIV enzyme, cleaves viral proteins after budding, converting the virion into an infectious form.

Infected $CD4^+$ lymphocytes produce > 98% of plasma HIV virions. A subset of infected $CD4^+$ lymphocytes constitutes a reservoir of HIV that can reactivate (eg, if antiviral treatment is stopped). Virions have a plasma half-life of about 6 h. In moderate to heavy HIV infection, about 10^8 to 10^9 virions are created and destroyed daily. With this much viral replication, the high frequency of transcription errors by HIV reverse transcriptase results in many mutations, increasing the chance of developing strains resistant to host immunity and drugs.

The main consequence of HIV infection is damage to the immune system, specifically loss of $CD4^+$ T lymphocytes, which are involved in cell-mediated and, to a lesser extent, humoral immunity. $CD4^+$ lymphocyte depletion may result from direct cytotoxic effects of HIV replication, cell-mediated immune cytotoxicity, and thymic damage that impairs lymphocyte production. Infected $CD4^+$ lymphocytes have a half-life of about 2 days. Rates of $CD4^+$ lymphocyte destruction correlate with plasma HIV level. Typically, during the initial or primary infection, HIV levels are highest (> 10^6 copies/mL), and circulating $CD4^+$ lymphocyte counts drop rapidly. Normal $CD4^+$ counts are about 750/μL, and immunity is minimally affected if counts are > 500/μL.

HIV virion concentrations in plasma stabilize at values (set points) that vary widely among patients but average about 4 to 5 $\log_{10}$/mL). They are measured by nucleic acid amplification assays and expressed as HIV RNA copies/mL of plasma. The higher the set point, the sooner $CD4^+$ counts fall to levels that seriously impair immunity (< 200/μL) and result in AIDS. For every 3-fold (0.5 $\log_{10}$) increase in plasma HIV RNA in untreated patients, the risk of progression to AIDS or death over the next 2 to 3 yr without treatment increases about 50%.

Humoral immunity is also affected. Hyperplasia of B (antibody-producing) cells in lymph nodes causes lymphadenopathy and increased secretion of antibodies to previously encountered antigens, often leading to hyperglobulinemia. Total antibody levels (especially IgG and IgA) and titers against previous antigens (eg, cytomegalovirus [CMV]) may be unusually high. However, response to new antigens is defective or absent. Response to immunizations declines as $CD4^+$ counts decline.

Antibodies to HIV are measurable usually within a few weeks after primary infection; however, antibodies cannot eliminate infection because mutated forms of HIV are generated that are not controlled by the patient's current antibodies.

The risk and severity of opportunistic infections, AIDS, and AIDS-related cancers are determined by 2 factors: $CD4^+$ lymphocyte count and the patient's exposure to potentially opportunistic pathogens. For example, the risk of *Pneumocystis* pneumonia, *Toxoplasma* encephalitis, and cryptococcal meningitis begins when the $CD4^+$ count is around 200/μL, and the risk of CMV and *Mycobacterium avium* complex (MAC) infections begins when the $CD4^+$ count is around 50/μL. Without treatment, the risk of progression from HIV infection to AIDS is about 1 to 2%/yr in the first 2 to 3 yr of infection and about 5 to 6%/yr thereafter; eventually, AIDS almost invariably develops.

HIV also infects nonlymphoid cells, such as dendritic skin cells; macrophages; brain microglia; and cardiac, renal, and other cells, causing disease in the corresponding organ systems. The HIV strains in several compartments such as the nervous system (brain and CSF) and genital tract (semen) are genetically distinct from those in plasma. Thus, in those tissues, HIV levels and resistance patterns may differ from those in plasma.

Symptoms and Signs

Initially, primary HIV infection may be asymptomatic or cause transient nonspecific symptoms (acute retroviral syndrome). Acute retroviral syndrome usually begins within 1 to 4 wk of infection and lasts 3 to 14 days, with fever, malaise, rash, arthralgia, generalized lymphadenopathy, and sometimes aseptic meningitis. Symptoms are often mistaken for infectious mononucleosis or benign nonspecific viral syndromes.

Most patients have a period of months to years during which other symptoms are few, mild, intermittent, and nonspecific. Symptoms reflect either direct effects of HIV or opportunistic infections. Asymptomatic, diffuse lymphadenopathy; oral candidiasis; herpes zoster; diarrhea; fatigue; and fever are most common. Some patients have progressive wasting. Asymptomatic, mild-to-moderate cytopenias (eg, leukopenia, anemia, thrombocytopenia) are common.

Eventually, when $CD4^+$ counts drop < 200/μL, symptoms worsen and AIDS-defining illnesses (those in category B or C of TABLE 192–1), often many, develop. Evaluation may reveal infection by *Mycobacterium* sp, *Pneumocystis jiroveci* (formerly *P. carinii*), *Cryptococcus neoformans*, or other fungi. Other infections that are common but suggest AIDS by their unusual severity or recurrence include herpes zoster, herpes simplex, vaginal candidiasis, and recurrent *Salmonella* sepsis. TABLE 192–3 lists common syndromes and aspects of diagnosis and treatment as well as comments that pertain specifically to HIV infection. Some patients present with cancers (eg, Kaposi's sarcoma, B-cell lymphomas) that occur with increased frequency or severity or have unique features in patients with HIV infection (see p. 1641). In others, neurologic dysfunction may occur.

Diagnosis

Screening (antibody) tests should be offered periodically to those at risk. For those at highest risk, especially sexually active people with multiple partners who do not practice safe sex, testing should be repeated q 6 mo. Such testing is confidential and available, often free of charge, in many public and private facilities throughout the world.

HIV infection is suspected in patients with persistent, unexplained, generalized adenopathy or any of the conditions listed in category B or C in TABLE 192–1. It may also be suspected in high-risk patients with nonspecific symptoms that could represent acute primary HIV infection. When HIV is diagnosed, staging with plasma HIV level and $CD4^+$ counts should be pursued. The $CD4^+$ count is calculated as the product of the WBC count, the percentage of lymphocytes among the WBCs, and the percentage of lymphocytes that bear the $CD4^+$ marker. Normal $CD4^+$ counts in adults are about 750 ± 250/μL.

Detection of antibodies to HIV is sensitive and specific except during the first few weeks after infection. The enzyme-linked immunosorbent assay (ELISA) test for HIV antibodies is highly sensitive, but results can rarely be falsely positive. Positive ELISA tests are therefore confirmed with a more specific test such as the Western blot. Newer rapid tests for

Text continues on page 1634.

TABLE 192–3. COMMON MANIFESTATIONS OF HIV INFECTION BY ORGAN SYSTEM

SYNDROME	CAUSE	DIAGNOSTIC EVALUATION	TREATMENT	SYMPTOMS/ COMMENTS
Neurologic				
Mild to severe dementia Cognitive impairment with or without motor deficits	Direct virus-induced brain damage	HIV RNA in CSF; CT or MRI (showing brain atrophy) is nonspecific	Antiretroviral drugs may reverse damage and improve function	Does not always progress to AIDS dementia
Ascending paralysis	Guillain-Barré syndrome or CMV polyradiculopathy	Spinal cord MRI, CSF testing	Treat CMV polyradiculopathy or provide support for Guillain-Barré syndrome	CMV polyradiculopathy causes neutrophilic pleocytosis
Acute or subacute focal encephalitis (see p. 1851)	*Toxoplasma gondii*	Ring-enhancing lesions on CT or MRI, especially near basal ganglia; antibodies are sensitive but not specific; response to empiric antiviral treatment; brain biopsy (rarely indicated)	Pyrimethamine, folinic acid, and sulfadiazine (clindamycin if allergic to sulfa—see p.1586)	Prophylaxis with clindamycin and pyrimethamine or trimethoprim-sulfamethizole (as for *Pneumocystis* pneumonia) indicated for patients with $CD4^+$ count < 200/µL and previous toxoplasmosis or positive antibodies
Subacute encephalitis	CMV (see p. 1605); less often herpes simplex virus or varicella-zoster virus	CSF PCR; response to treatment	Treat cause	CMV often presents with delirium, cranial nerve palsies, myoclonus, seizures, and progressively impaired consciousness and often responds rapidly to treatment
Myelitis or polyradiculopathy (see p. 1910)	CMV	Spinal cord MRI, CSF PCR	Antiviral drugs (see p. 1593)	Simulates Guillain-Barré syndrome
Progressive encephalitis of white matter only	Progressive multifocal leukoencephalopathy (see p. 1855) or HIV	Brain MRI, CSF tests	Antiretroviral drugs	Usually fatal within a few months; may respond to antiretrovirals

TABLE 192–3. COMMON MANIFESTATIONS OF HIV INFECTION BY ORGAN SYSTEM—Continued

SYNDROME	CAUSE	DIAGNOSTIC EVALUATION	TREATMENT	SYMPTOMS/ COMMENTS
Subacute meningitis	Cryptococcal, *Histoplasma*, or TB meningitis	CT or MRI, CSF stains and cultures	Treat cause	Good outcomes for patients treated early
Peripheral neuropathy (see p. 1903)	Direct effects of HIV, or CMV, antiviral toxicity	History, sensory and motor testing	Treat causative agent or remove toxic drugs	Very common; not quickly reversible
Ophthalmologic				
Retinitis	CMV	Direct retinoscopy	Specific anti-CMV drugs (see p. 1606)	Requires specialist examination
Cardiac				
Cardiomyopathy	Direct viral damage to cardiac myocytes	Echocardiography	Antiretroviral drugs	Symptoms of heart failure
Renal				
Nephrotic syndrome or renal insufficiency	Direct viral damage, resulting in focal glomerulosclerosis	Renal biopsy	May respond to antiretroviral drugs or ACE inhibitors	Increased incidence in African Americans and patients with lower $CD4^+$ counts
Oral				
Oral candidiasis (see p. 1529)	Immunosuppression by HIV	Examination	Systemic antifungals (see p. 1523)	May be painless in early stages
Intraoral ulcers	Herpes simplex virus; aphthous ulcers	See p. 817	See p. 817	May be severe and result in undernutrition
Periodontal disease	Mixed oral bacterial flora	Examination	Improve hygiene and nutrition; antibiotics	May be severe, with bleeding, swelling, and tooth loss
Painless intraoral mass	Kaposi's sarcoma; lymphoma	Biopsy	Treat cause	
Painless white filiform patches on the sides of the tongue (oral hairy leukoplakia)	Epstein-Barr virus	Examination	Acyclovir	Usually asymptomatic
GI				
Esophagitis	Candidiasis; CMV; herpes simplex virus	Esophagoscopy with biopsy of ulcers	Treat cause	Dysphagia, anorexia

Table continues on the following page.

TABLE 192–3. COMMON MANIFESTATIONS OF HIV INFECTION BY ORGAN SYSTEM—Continued

SYNDROME	CAUSE	DIAGNOSTIC EVALUATION	TREATMENT	SYMPTOMS/ COMMENTS
Gastroenteritis or colitis	Intestinal *Salmonella*, MAC, *Cryptosporidium*, CMV, *Microsporidia, Isospora belli*, or *Clostridium difficile*	Cultures and stains of stools, or biopsy, but determination of the cause may be difficult	Treat cause and symptoms supportively	Diarrhea, weight loss, abdominal cramping
Cholecystitis or cholangitis	CMV or *Cryptosporidium*	Ultrasound or endoscopy	Treat cause (CMV) or provide antiretrovirals (*Cryptosporidium*)	May cause pain or obstruction
Anal, rectal, and perirectal lesions	Herpes simplex virus, human papillomavirus, anal cancer; causes may be multiple	Examination; microbiologic methods; biopsy	Treat cause(s)	High incidence in homosexual men
Hepatocellular damage from hepatitis viruses, opportunistic infections, or antiviral toxicity	TB, MAC, CMV, or peliosis (bartonellosis). HIV may also worsen chronic hepatitis B or C	Need to differentiate from hepatitis due to antiretroviral or other drugs. Liver biopsy sometimes necessary	Treat cause	Symptoms of hepatitis such as anorexia, nausea, vomiting, or jaundice
Skin				
Herpes zoster	Varicella-zoster virus	Usually clinical (see p. 1609)	Acyclovir or related drugs	Common, prodrome of mild to severe pain or tingling may precede skin lesions
Herpes simplex ulcers	Herpes simplex virus	Usually clinical (see p. 1608)	Antivirals if severe, extensive, persistent, or disseminated	Atypical lesions of herpes simplex: extensive, severe, persistent
Scabies	*Sarcoptes scabiei*	See p. 995	See p. 997	May produce severe hyperkeratotic lesions
Violaceous or red papules or nodules	Kaposi's sarcoma; bartonellosis	Biopsy	Treat cause	
Centrally umbilicated skin lesions	Cryptococcosis or molluscum contagiosum	See pp. 998 and 1532	See pp. 998 and 1532	May be presenting sign of cryptococcemia

TABLE 192–3. COMMON MANIFESTATIONS OF HIV INFECTION BY ORGAN SYSTEM—Continued

SYNDROME	CAUSE	DIAGNOSTIC EVALUATION	TREATMENT	SYMPTOMS/ COMMENTS
Pulmonary				
Subacute (occasionally acute) pneumonia	Mycobacteria, fungi such as *Pneumocystis jiroveci* (formerly *P. carinii*), *Cryptococcus neoformans, Histoplasma capsulatum, Coccidioides immitis, Aspergillus*	Mild hypoxia or increased alveolar-arterial O_2 gradient may occur before evidence of pneumonia on x-ray. Skin tests may be falsely negative due to anergy; bronchoscopy may be necessary	Treat cause	May present with cough, tachypnea, chest discomfort
Acute (occasionally subacute) pneumonia	Typical pathogens or *Haemophilus, Pseudomonas, Nocardia,* or *Rhodococcus*	See Ch. 52 on p. 423. In patients with known or suspected HIV and pneumonia, opportunistic or unusual pathogens are excluded	Treat cause	May present with cough, tachypnea, chest discomfort
Tracheobronchitis	*Candida*, herpes simplex virus		Treat cause	May present with cough, tachypnea, chest discomfort
Subacute or chronic pneumonia or mediastinal adenopathy	Kaposi's sarcoma, B-cell lymphoma	Chest CT scan, bronchoscopy	Treat cause	May present with cough, tachypnea, chest discomfort
Systemic septicemia from disseminated opportunistic infections	*Mycobacterium tuberculosis, Mycobacterium avium, Histoplasma capsulatum*	Blood cultures, bone marrow examination	Treat cause	
Gynecologic				
Vaginal candidiasis	*Candida*	See p. 2086	See p. 2086	May be increased in severity or recurrent
Pelvic inflammatory disease	Usual pathogens (see p. 2087)	See p. 2088	See p. 2089	May be increased in severity, atypical, and difficult to treat

Table continues on the following page.

TABLE 192–3. COMMON MANIFESTATIONS OF HIV INFECTION BY ORGAN SYSTEM—Continued

SYNDROME	CAUSE	DIAGNOSTIC EVALUATION	TREATMENT	SYMPTOMS/ COMMENTS
Hematologic				
Anemia	Multifactorial: HIV-induced marrow suppression; immune-mediated peripheral destruction; anemia of chronic disease; infections, particularly human parvovirus B-19 and disseminated MAC or histoplasmosis; cancer	See p. 1032; parvovirus diagnosed by bone marrow showing multinucleated erythroblasts or by serum PCR	Treat cause; transfusion as needed; erythropoietin for anemia due to antineoplastic drugs or due to zidovudine if severity is sufficient to warrant transfusion and erythropoietin level is < 500 mU/L; IVIG for parvovirus	Parvovirus may produce acute severe anemia
Thrombocytopenia	Immune thrombocytopenia, (see p. 1068); drug toxicity; HIV-induced marrow suppression; immune-mediated peripheral destruction; infections; cancer	CBC, clotting, PTT, peripheral smear, bone marrow biopsy or von Willebrand's factor	Antiretroviral drugs; IVIG for bleeding or preoperatively; possibly anti-Rho (D) IgG, vincristine, danazol, or interferon; splenectomy if severe and intractable	Often asymptomatic and may occur in otherwise asymptomatic HIV infection
Neutropenia	HIV-induced marrow suppression, immune-mediated peripheral destruction, infections, cancer, drug toxicity	See p. 1061	For severe neutropenia (< 200–500/μL) plus fever, immediate broad-spectrum antibiotics (see p. 1062). If drug-induced, granulocyte or granulocyte-macrophage colony-stimulating factors	

MAC = *Mycobacterium avium* complex; CMV = cytomegalovirus; IVIG = intravenous immune globulin.

blood and saliva can be done quickly without technically complex procedures or equipment, allowing testing in a variety of settings and immediate reporting to patients. Positive results should be confirmed by standard blood tests.

If HIV infection is suspected despite negative antibody test results (eg, during the first few weeks), plasma may be tested for HIV RNA. The nucleic acid amplification assays used are sensitive and specific. Measurement of p24 HIV antigen by ELISA is a less sensitive and specific alternative for directly detecting HIV in blood. HIV RNA (virion) concentration assays require advanced technology, such as reverse transcription–PCR (RT-PCR) or branched DNA (bDNA) measurement, which are sensitive to extremely low HIV RNA levels. Quantitative plasma HIV RNA assays are used for determining prognosis and monitoring treatment. Plasma level or viral load reflects HIV replication rates. Higher set point levels (the relatively stable virus levels that occur after primary infection) predict increased risk of $CD4^+$ count decline and opportunistic infection, even in patients without symptoms or evidence of current immunocompromise (ie, patients with > 500/μL).

HIV infection can be staged according to clinical manifestations (in order of increasing severity, category A, B, or C, see TABLE 192–1) and $CD4^+$ count (≥ 500, 200 to 499, or < 200/μL). The clinical category is determined by the most severe manifestation the patient has had, past or present, so the patient is never restaged to a less severe category.

Diagnosis of the various opportunistic infections, tumors, and other syndromes that occur in HIV-infected patients is discussed elsewhere in THE MANUAL. Many aspects unique to HIV are included in TABLE 192–1 and the section on cancers (see p. 1641).

Hematologic abnormalities are common, and bone marrow aspiration and biopsy may be useful to evaluate some syndromes (eg, cytopenias, lymphomas, cancers). It can also aid in diagnosis of disseminated infections with MAC, *Mycobacterium tuberculosis, Cryptococcus, Histoplasma*, human parvovirus B19, *Pneumocystis jiroveci* (formerly *P. carinii*), and *Leishmania*. Most patients have normocellular or hypercellular marrow despite peripheral cytopenia, reflecting peripheral destruction. Iron stores are usually normal or increased, reflecting anemia of chronic disease (an iron-reutilization defect). Mild to moderate plasmacytosis, lymphoid aggregates, increased numbers of histiocytes, and dysplastic changes in hematopoietic cells are common.

Differentiation of HIV-associated neurologic syndromes often requires contrast-enhanced CT or MRI. These syndromes are listed in TABLE 192–4 and discussed elsewhere in THE MANUAL.

Prognosis

As discussed above, the risk of AIDS and/or death is predicted by $CD4^+$ count in the short term and by plasma viral RNA level in the longer term. For every 3-fold (0.5 $\log_{10}$) increase in viral load, mortality over the next 2 to 3 yr increases about 50%. However, $CD4^+$ counts rise and HIV RNA levels fall dramatically with effective treatment. HIV-associated morbidity and mortality are uncommon when $CD4^+$ count is ≥ 500/μL; low with counts of 200 to 499/μL; moderate with counts of 50 to 200/μL; and high if counts fall < 50/μL.

Because adequate antiviral therapy can cause significant long-term morbidity, it is not recommended for everyone. Current indications include $CD4^+$ count of < 350/μL and HIV RNA level of > 55,000 copies/mL. Use of potent combinations of antiretroviral drugs for HIV therapy (highly active antiretroviral therapy [HAART]) aims to reduce plasma HIV RNA levels and increase $CD4^+$ lymphocyte counts (immune restoration or reconstitution). The lower the pretreatment $CD4^+$ count and the higher the HIV RNA level, the less likely treatment is to succeed; however, some improvement is likely even in those with advanced immunosuppression. The increase in $CD4^+$ count indicates a corresponding decrease in the risk of opportunistic infections, other complications, and death. With immune restoration, even complications for which no specific treatment exists (eg, HIV-induced cognitive dysfunction) or that were previously considered untreatable (eg, progressive multifocal leukoencephalopathy) may improve. Cancers (eg, lymphoma and Kaposi's sarcoma) and opportunistic infections have improved outcomes as well. Vaccines that may enhance immunity to HIV among infected patients have been under investigation for many years but are not yet available.

Treatment

HAART aims to suppress viral replication nearly totally. Total suppression to undetectable levels is usually possible if patients take their drugs > 95% of the time. However, maintaining this degree of adherence is difficult. Partial suppression (failure to lower plasma levels to undetectable levels) selects for resistant HIV and makes subsequent treatment more likely to fail. Patients beginning HAART sometimes experience clinical deterioration, despite rising $CD4^+$ counts, as an immune reaction to subclinical opportunistic infections or to residual microbial antigens after successful treatment of opportunistic infections. These sometimes serious

TABLE 192–4. MOST COMMON NEUROLOGIC SYNDROMES OF HIV

- AIDS dementia
- Cryptococcal meningitis
- Cytomegalovirus encephalitis
- Primary CNS lymphoma
- Progressive multifocal leukoencephalopathy
- TB meningitis or focal encephalitis
- Toxoplasma encephalitis

TABLE 192–5. ANTIRETROVIRAL DRUGS

GENERIC NAME	ABBREVIATION	USUAL ADULT DOSE (ORAL)	ADVERSE EFFECTS*
Nucleoside Reverse Transcriptase Inhibitors			
Abacavir	ABC	300 mg bid	Severe hypersensitivity reactions (especially on rechallenge), anorexia, nausea, vomiting
Didanosine	ddI	400 mg once/day if > 60 kg; 250 mg once/day if < 60 kg	Peripheral neuropathy,† pancreatitis,‡ lactic acidosis, diarrhea
Emtricitabine	FTC	200 mg once/day	Minimal
Lamivudine	3TC	150 mg bid or 300 mg once/day	Peripheral neuropathy,† rarely pancreatitis
Stavudine	d4T	40 mg bid if > 60 kg; 30 mg bid if < 60 kg	Peripheral neuropathy,† rarely pancreatitis, lactic acidosis, fat redistribution with lipoatrophy of face and extremities
Zalcitabine	ddC	0.75 mg tid	Peripheral neuropathy,† pancreatitis,‡ oral ulcers
Zidovudine	ZDV, AZT	300 mg bid	Anemia and leukopenia,§ rarely pancreatitis, myositis
Nucleotide Reverse Transcriptase Inhibitor			
Tenofovir	TDF	300 mg once/day	Increases levels of ddI, otherwise minimal
Non-Nucleoside Reverse Transcriptase Inhibitors			
Delavirdine	DLV	400 mg q 8 h	Rashes, inhibits cytochrome P-450 metabolism of indinavir, serious effects may occur if given together with certain nonsedating antihistamines, sedative hypnotics, antiarrhythmics, Ca channel blockers, ergot alkaloid preparations, amphetamines, or cisapride
Efavirenz	EFV	600 mg at bedtime	Rash and CNS symptoms, falsely positive cannabinoid test, excessive blood levels if taken after fatty meals
Nevirapine	NVP	200 mg once/day for 2 wk, then 200 mg bid	Rashes, increases cytochrome P-450, so decreases levels of PIs
Protease Inhibitors‖			
Amprenavir	APV	1200 mg bid with food	Diarrhea, nausea, rashes
Atazanavir	ATV	400 mg once/day	Hyperbilirubinemia
Fosamprenovir	None	1400 mg bid	Diarrhea, vomiting, rash
Indinavir	IND	800 mg tid on empty stomach (600 mg for patients taking DLV; should not be given with ddI)	Kidney stones, occasionally obstructive (patients should ingest 1300 mL of fluid daily); cross-resistance with other protease inhibitors, especially ritonavir
Lopinavir	LPV	400 mg q 12 h (in fixed combination with 100 mg ritonavir) with food	Diarrhea

TABLE 192–5. ANTIRETROVIRAL DRUGS—Continued

GENERIC NAME	ABBREVIATION	USUAL ADULT DOSE (ORAL)	ADVERSE EFFECTS*
Nelfinavir	NLF	1250 mg bid with food	Diarrhea
Ritonavir	RIT	600 mg bid with food	Diarrhea, nausea, abdominal pain, altered taste, circumoral paresthesias; dose reduction may decrease incidence and severity of adverse effects
Saquinavir	SQV	1200 mg tid, within 2 h of a meal; combination with RIT may increase SQV trough levels and efficacy	Nausea, vomiting, diarrhea
Tipronavir	TPV	500 mg with ritonavir 100 mg bid	Hepatitis
Fusion Inhibitor			
Enfuviritide	T-20	90 mg sc bid	Hypersensitivity, local injection site reactions

*All classes of antiretroviral drugs may contribute to chronic metabolic adverse effects, which include elevated cholesterol and triglycerides, insulin resistance, and centripetal redistribution of body fat (see text).

†Peripheral neuropathy may be reversible when the drug is stopped and can be treated symptomatically with partial relief.

‡Symptoms of pancreatitis, such as nausea and vomiting or back and abdominal pain, require that ddI or ddC be immediately stopped until pancreatitis is confirmed or excluded.

§Can be treated with transfusions or other drugs such as erythropoietin for anemia or colony-stimulating factor (granulocyte colony-stimulating factor or granulocyte-macrophage colony-stimulating factor) for leukopenia.

||Class effects include bleeding tendency. All are metabolized by cytochrome P-450 system, creating potential for many drug interactions.

reactions are termed immune reconstitution inflammatory syndromes (IRIS).

The success of HAART is assessed by measuring plasma viral (RNA) levels q 4 to 8 wk for the first months and q 3 to 4 mo thereafter. With successful therapy, HIV RNA becomes undetectable (ie, < 50 copies/mL) within 3 to 6 mo. Increasing levels are the earliest evidence of treatment failure. If treatment fails, drug susceptibility (resistance) assays can determine the susceptibility of the dominant HIV strain to all available drugs as a guide for revising therapy. Maintaining patients on failing drug regimens contributes to development of HIV mutants that are more drug-resistant but, compared to wild-type HIV, appear to have less capacity to reduce $CD4^+$ counts.

The antivirals used in HAART are listed by class in TABLE 192–5. Three of the 5 classes inhibit reverse transcriptase, blocking its RNA-dependent and DNA-dependent DNA polymerase activity. Nucleoside reverse transcriptase inhibitors (NRTIs) are phosphorylated to active metabolites that compete for incorporation into viral DNA. They inhibit the HIV reverse transcriptase enzyme competitively and terminate synthesis of DNA chains. Nucleotide reverse transcriptase inhibitors (nRTIs) inhibit HIV reverse transcriptase enzyme like NRTIs but do not require initial phosphorylation. Non-nucleoside reverse transcriptase inhibitors (NNRTIs) bind directly to the reverse transcriptase enzyme. Protease inhibitors (PIs) inhibit the viral protease enzyme that is crucial to maturation of HIV variants following budding from host cells. Fusion inhibitors (FIs) block binding of HIV to $CD4^+$ lymphocyte receptors that is required for HIV to enter cells.

To fully suppress replication of naturally occurring HIV, combinations of 3 or 4 drugs from different classes are usually necessary.

The specific drugs are chosen on the basis of factors such as concomitant diseases (eg, hepatic dysfunction) and other drugs being taken (to avoid drug interactions). Compliance is maximized by making the regimen affordable and tolerable and using once/day (preferable) or bid dosing. Guidelines from expert panels for initiating, selecting, switching, and interrupting therapy and special issues in treating women and children change regularly and are updated at www.aidsinfo.nih.gov/guidelines.

Interactions between antiretrovirals may synergistically increase efficacy. For example, a subtherapeutic dose of ritonavir (100 mg) can be combined with another PI (eg, lopinavir, amprenavir, indinavir, atazonavir, tipronavir). Ritonavir inhibits the hepatic enzyme that metabolizes the other PI, increasing the other drug's levels and efficacy. Another example is the combination of lamivudine (3TC) with zidovudine (ZDV). Use of either drug as monotherapy quickly results in resistance, but the mutation producing resistance in response to 3TC increases the susceptibility of HIV to ZDV. Thus, they are synergistic.

Conversely, interactions between antiretrovirals may decrease the efficacy of each drug. One drug may increase elimination of another drug (eg, by inducing hepatic cytochrome P-450 enzymes responsible for elimination). A 2nd, poorly understood effect of some NRTI combinations (eg, ZDV and stavudine [d4T]) results in decreased antiviral activity without increasing drug elimination.

Combining drugs often increases the risk that either individual drug will result in an adverse effect. One possible mechanism is hepatic metabolism of PIs by cytochrome P-450, which decreases metabolism (and increases levels) of other drugs. A 2nd mechanism is additive toxicities; eg, combining NRTIs such as d4T and didanosine (ddI) increases the chance of adverse metabolic effects and peripheral neuropathy. Since many drugs may interfere with antiretrovirals, interactions should always be checked before any new drug is started. In addition to drug interactions, grapefruit juice and St. John's wort can decrease activity of some antiretroviral drugs and should be avoided.

Adverse effects: The serious adverse effects of antiretrovirals are listed in TABLE 192–5. Some of them, notably anemia, pancreatitis, hepatitis, and glucose intolerance, can be detected by blood tests before they cause symptoms. Patients should be screened regularly, both clinically and with appropriate laboratory testing (CBC and chemistry panels), especially when starting new drugs or developing unexplained symptoms.

Metabolic effects consist of interrelated syndromes of fat redistribution, hyperlipidemia, and insulin resistance. A common development is redistribution of subcutaneous fat from the face and distal extremities to the trunk and abdomen. The cosmetic effect can stigmatize and distress patients. Facial treatments with injected collagen or polylactic acid can be beneficial. Hyperlipidemia and hyperglycemia due to insulin resistance and nonalcoholic steatohepatitis may occur with lipodystrophy. Drugs from all classes appear to contribute to these metabolic effects: some, such as ritonavir or d4T, do so commonly, others, such as atazanavir, appear to have minimal effects on lipid levels.

Mechanisms accounting for metabolic effects appear to be multiple; one is mitochondrial toxicity. The risk of mitochondrial toxicity and metabolic effects varies by drug class (highest with NRTIs and PIs) and within drug classes: eg, among NRTIs, highest with d4T. Effects are dose dependent and often begin in the first 1 to 2 yr of treatment. The long-term effects and optimal management of metabolic effects are unclear. Lipid-lowering (statins) and insulin-sensitizing drugs (glitazones) may be helpful.

Bone complications of HAART include asymptomatic osteopenia and osteoporosis, which are common among patients with metabolic effects. Uncommonly, avascular necrosis of large joints such as the hip and shoulder produces severe joint pain and dysfunction. Mechanisms of bone complications are poorly understood.

Interruption of HAART is generally safe if all drugs are stopped simultaneously. Interruption may be necessary for treatment of intervening illnesses or if drug toxicity is intolerable or needs to be evaluated. After interruption, to determine which drug is responsible for toxicity, restarting drugs as monotherapy for up to a few days is safe for most drugs. The most important exception is abacavir; *patients who had fever or rash during previous exposure to abacavir may develop severe and potentially fatal hypersensitivity reactions with re-exposure.*

End-of-life care: Although life expectancy for those with AIDS has increased dramatically due to new therapies, many patients deteriorate and die. Death is rarely sudden; thus, patients usually have time to make plans. Nonetheless, plans should be recorded early in a durable power of attorney for health care (see p. 2771), with clear instructions for end-of-life care. Other legal documents, including powers of attorney and wills, should be in place. These documents are particularly important for homosexual patients because of the lack of protection of assets and rights (including visitation and decision-making) for partners.

As patients near the end of life, physicians may need to prescribe drugs to relieve pain, anorexia, agitation, and other distressing symptoms. The profound weight loss of many people in the last stages of living with AIDS makes good skin care of paramount importance. The comprehensive support of hospice programs is a very good match for many patients facing death with AIDS, since hospice providers are usually supportive of individual decision-making and of caregiving by whoever is willing and able, and since their support is at home.

Prevention

Vaccines against HIV have been difficult to develop because of the extreme mutability of HIV surface proteins that results in an enormous diversity of antigenic types. Nonetheless, many candidates are at various stages of investigation for their ability to prevent or ameliorate infection.

Prevention of transmission: Public education is effective and appears to have decreased rates of infection in some countries, notably Thailand and Uganda. Because sexual contact accounts for most cases, education to avoid unsafe sex practices is the most relevant measure. Unless both partners are known to be free of HIV and remain monogamous, safe sex practices are essential (see TABLE 192–2). Condoms offer the best protection, but oil-based lubricants may dissolve latex, increasing the risk of latex condom failure. Antiretroviral therapy of HIV-infected people reduces their risk of sexual transmission, but the extent of reduction is unclear.

Safe sex practices remain advisable to protect HIV-positive patients as well as their partners. For example, unprotected sex between HIV-infected people may expose an individual to resistant or more virulent strains of HIV and to other viruses (eg, cytomegalovirus, Epstein-Barr virus, herpes simplex virus, hepatitis B) that cause severe disease in AIDS patients.

Parenteral drug users should be counseled about the risk of sharing needles. Counseling is probably more effective if combined with provision of sterile needles and with treatment of drug dependence and rehabilitation.

Confidential testing for HIV infection, which also mandates the availability of pretest and post-test counseling, should be offered to anyone requesting it. Pregnant women who test positive are advised of the risk of maternal-fetal transmission; risk is decreased by ⅔ using monotherapy with ZDV or nevirapine, and probably even more using combinations of 2 or 3 drugs. Therapy can be toxic to the fetus or mother and cannot be guaranteed to prevent transmission. Some women choose to terminate their pregnancy for this or other reasons.

In parts of the world where donated blood and organs are screened universally using current methods (eg, ELISA), the risk of transmitting HIV by blood transfusion is probably between 1/10,000 and 1/100,000 per unit transfused. Transmission is still possible, because antibody results may be falsely negative during early infection. Currently, screening of blood for both antibody and p24 antigen is mandated in the US and probably further reduces the risk of transmission. To reduce risk further, people with risk factors for HIV infection, even those with recent negative HIV antibody test results, are asked not to donate blood or organs for transplantation.

To prevent HIV transmission from patients, medical and dental professionals should wear gloves in situations that may involve contact with any patient's mucous membranes or body fluids and be taught how to avoid needle-stick accidents. Home caregivers should wear gloves if their hands may be exposed to body fluids. Surfaces or instruments contaminated by blood or other body fluids should be cleaned and disinfected. Effective disinfectants include heat, peroxide, alcohols, phenolics, and hypochlorite (bleach). Isolation of HIV-infected patients is unnecessary unless indicated because of an opportunistic infection (eg, TB). Consensus regarding measures to prevent transmission from infected professionals to patients has not been reached.

Postexposure prophylaxis: Preventive treatment is indicated after penetrating injuries involving HIV-infected blood (usually needle sticks) or heavy mucous membrane (eye or mouth) exposure. Risk of infection after percutaneous exposure is overall about

TABLE 192–6. POSTEXPOSURE PROPHYLAXIS

EXPOSURE TYPE	INFECTION STATUS OF SOURCE: HIV-Positive Class 1*	HIV-Positive Class 2*	HIV Status of Source Unknown†	Unknown Source‡	HIV-Negative
Less severe (eg, solid needle and superficial injury)	Recommend basic 2-drug PEP	Recommend expanded 3-drug PEP	Generally, no PEP warranted; however, consider basic 2-drug PEP§ for source with HIV risk factors‖	Generally, no PEP warranted; however, consider basic 2-drug PEP§ in settings where exposure to HIV-infected persons is likely	No PEP warranted
More severe (eg, large-bore hollow needle, deep puncture, visible blood on device, or needle used in patient's artery or vein)	Recommend expanded 3-drug PEP	Recommend expanded 3-drug PEP	Generally, no PEP warranted; however, consider basic 2-drug PEP§ for source with HIV risk factors‖	Generally, no PEP warranted; however, consider basic 2-drug PEP§ in settings where exposure to HIV-infected persons is likely	No PEP warranted

PEP = Postexposure prophylaxis.

*HIV-positive, Class 1: asymptomatic HIV infection or known low viral load (eg, < 1500 RNA copies/mL). HIV-positive, Class 2: symptomatic HIV infection, AIDS, acute seroconversion, or known high viral load. If drug resistance is a concern, obtain expert consultation. Initiation of PEP should not be delayed pending expert consultation, and, because expert consultation alone cannot substitute for face-to-face counseling, resources should be available to provide immediate evaluation and follow-up care for all exposures.

†Source of unknown HIV status (eg, deceased source person with no samples available for HIV testing).

‡Unknown source (eg, a needle from a sharps disposal container).

§PEP is optional and should be based on an individualized decision between the exposed person and the treating clinician.

‖If PEP is offered and taken and the source is later determined to be HIV-negative, PEP should be discontinued.

From *MMWR* June 29, 2001/50 (RR11); 1-42.

0.3% and about 0.09% after mucous membrane exposure. Risk appears proportional to the amount of inoculum (eg, greater with visibly contaminated needles, hollow-bore needles), depth of injury, and viral load of the source blood.

Combinations of 2 NRTIs (eg, ZDV and 3TC) or 3 drugs (2 NRTIs plus a PI or NNRTI; nevirapine is avoided because of rare but severe hepatitis) for 1 mo is currently recommended to reduce risk of infection, depending on the degree of risk conferred by the exposure (see TABLE 192–6). Although evidence is not conclusive, ZDV alone probably reduces risk of transmission after needlestick injuries by about 80%. For detailed recommendations, see www.cdc.gov/mmwr/PDF/rr/rr5011.pdf or www.ucsf.edu/hivcntr/PEPline.

Prevention of opportunistic infections: Effective chemoprophylaxis is available for many opportunistic infections and reduces rates of disease from *P. jiroveci, Candida, Cryptococcus,* and MAC. In patients who experience immune reconstitution from therapy, restoration of $CD4^+$ counts to above threshold values for > 3 mo allows prophylaxis to be stopped.

Patients with $CD4^+$ counts < 200/μL should receive primary prophylaxis against *P. jiroveci* pneumonia and *Toxoplasma* encephalitis. Double-strength trimethoprim-sulfamethoxazole (TMP-SMX) tablets are effective for both when given once/day or 3 times/wk. Some adverse effects can be minimized with the 3 times/wk dose or by gradual dose escalation. Some patients who cannot tolerate TMP-SMX can tolerate dapsone (100 mg once/day). For the minority of patients treated with either drug in whom a troublesome adverse effect occurs (eg, fever, neutropenia, rash), aerosolized pentamidine (300 mg once/day) or atovaquone 1500 mg once/day can be used.

Patients with $CD4^+$ counts < 75 should receive primary prophylaxis against disseminated MAC with azithromycin, clarithromycin, or rifabutin. Azithromycin is preferred because it can be given weekly as two 600-mg tablets, provides protection (70%) similar to daily clarithromycin, and does not interact with other drugs. Patients with suspected latent TB (at any $CD4^+$ count) should receive treatment to prevent reactivation with daily rifampicin or rifabutin plus pyrazinamide for 2 mo or isoniazid for 9 mo.

For primary prophylaxis against some fungal infections (eg, esophageal candidiasis, cryptococcal meningitis or pneumonia), oral fluconazole taken daily (100 to 200 mg once/day) or weekly (400 mg) is successful, but infrequently used because the cost per infection prevented is high and diagnosis and treatment of these diseases are usually successful.

Patients receive secondary prophylaxis with fluconazole if they have had recurrent oral, vaginal, or esophageal candidiasis or cryptococcal infections. Previous histoplasmosis is an indication for prophylactic itraconazole (see p. 1533). Patients with latent toxoplasmosis, as indicated by serum antibodies (IgG) to *Toxoplasma gondii*, receive TMP-SMX (in doses used to prevent *Pneumocystis* pneumonia) to prevent reactivation and consequent *Toxoplasma* encephalitis. Latent infection is uncommon (about 15% of adults) in the US compared with Europe and most developing countries. Secondary prophylaxis is also indicated for patients with previous *Pneumocystis* pneumonia, herpes simplex infection (see p. 1606), and possibly aspergillosis (see p. 1526).

Detailed guidelines for prophylaxis of fungal (including *Pneumocystis*), viral, mycobacterial, and *Toxoplasma* infections are at www.aidsinfo.nih.gov/guidelines.

CANCERS COMMON IN HIV-INFECTED PATIENTS

Kaposi's sarcoma, non-Hodgkin lymphoma, and cervical cancer are AIDS-defining neoplasms in HIV-infected patients. Other cancers that appear to be increased in incidence or severity include Hodgkin lymphoma (especially the mixed cellularity and lymphocyte-depleted subtypes), primary CNS lymphoma, anal cancer, testicular cancer, melanoma and other skin cancers, and lung cancer. Leiomyosarcoma is a rare complication of HIV infection in children. For full discussion of Kaposi's sarcoma, see p. 1024.

Non-Hodgkin lymphoma: Non-Hodgkin lymphoma (see also p. 1120) incidence increases 50- to 200-fold in HIV-infected patients. Most are B-cell, aggressive, high-grade histologic subtype lymphomas. At diagnosis, extranodal sites are usually involved, such as bone marrow, GI tract, and other sites that are unusual in non–HIV-associated non-Hodgkin lymphoma, eg, the CNS and body cavities (eg, pleural, pericardial, peritoneal).

Common presentations include rapidly enlarging lymph nodes or extranodal masses or systemic symptoms such as weight loss, night sweats, or fevers. Diagnosis is by biopsy with histopathologic and immunochemical analysis of tumor cells. Abnormal circulating lymphocytes or unexpected cytopenias suggest involvement of the bone marrow, mandating marrow biopsy. Tumor staging may require CSF examination and CT or MRI of the chest, abdomen, and other areas where tumor is suspected. Poor prognosis is predicted by $CD4^+$ count < 100, age > 35 yr, poor functional status, bone marrow involvement, a history of opportunistic infections, and a high-grade histologic subtype.

Non-Hodgkin lymphoma is treated with systemic, multidrug chemotherapy (eg, with cyclophosphamide, doxorubicin, vincristine, and prednisone), usually combined with antiretrovirals, prophylactic antibiotics and antifungals, and hematologic growth factors. Therapy may be limited by profound myelosuppression, particularly when using combinations of myelosuppressive antitumor or antiretroviral drugs. Another possible treatment is IV anti-CD20 monoclonal antibody (rituximab), which is effective for non-Hodgkin lymphoma in patients without HIV. Radiation therapy may debulk large tumors and control pain or bleeding.

Primary central nervous system lymphoma: Primary CNS lymphomas (PCNSLs) occur with increased frequency in HIV-infected patients (see also p. 1923). PCNSLs consist of intermediate- or high-grade malignant B-cells, originating in CNS tissue. Presenting symptoms include headache, seizures, neurologic deficits (eg, cranial nerve palsies), and mental status change.

Acute treatment requires control of cerebral edema and whole-brain radiation therapy. Radiographic response is common, but median survival is < 6 mo. The role of antitumor chemotherapy is unclear, but survival is improved by highly active antiretroviral therapy (HAART).

Cervical cancer: Cervical cancer (see also p. 2125) is difficult to cure in HIV-infected patients. HIV-infected women have increased human papillomavirus (HPV) infection rates, persistence of oncogenic subtypes (types 16, 18, 31, 33, 35, and 39), and cervical intraepithelial dysplasia (CIN, incidence of up to 60%), but no proven increase in cervical cancer rates. However, cervical cancers are more extensive, are more difficult to cure, and have higher recurrence rates after treatment. Confirmed risk factors in HIV-infected women include infection with HPV subtype 16 or 18, $CD4^+$ counts < 200/μL, and age > 34 yr. HIV infection does not affect management of CIN or cervical cancer. Frequent Papanicolaou smears are important to monitor for progression. HAART may produce resolution of HPV infection and regression of CIN but has no clear effects on cancer.

Squamous cell cancer of the anus and vulva: Squamous cell cancers of the anus (see also p. 177) and vulva (see also p. 2129) are caused by HPV and occur more commonly in HIV-infected patients. The reason for the increased incidence in HIV appears to be the increased rate of high-risk behaviors, eg, anal-receptive intercourse, rather than HIV itself. Anal dysplasia is common, and squamous cell cancers can be very aggressive. Treatments include surgical extirpation, radiation therapy, and combined modality chemotherapy with mitomycin or cisplatin and 5-fluorouracil.

193 OTHER VIRUSES

The number of viral diseases affecting humans is large. Most of these are discussed elsewhere in THE MANUAL, including Chs. 187, 188, 189, 190, 191, and 192. A few are not easily categorized and are separated here for discussion. Most of these tend to present in children but can occur in adults.

MEASLES

(Rubeola; Morbilli; 9-Day Measles)

Measles is a highly contagious, viral infection that is most common in children. It is characterized by fever, cough, coryza, conjunctivitis, enanthem (Koplik's spots) on the buccal or labial mucosa, and a maculopapular rash that spreads cephalocaudally. Diagnosis is usually clinical. Treatment is supportive. Vaccination is highly effective.

Worldwide, measles infects about 30 to 40 million annually, causing about 800,000 deaths, primarily in children. It is less common in the US because of routine childhood vaccination; about 100 to 300 cases occur annually.

Etiology and Epidemiology

Measles is caused by a paramyxovirus. It is extremely communicable and is spread mainly by secretions from the nose, throat, and mouth during the prodromal or early eruptive stage or by airborne droplets. Communicability continues from several days before until several days after the rash appears. Measles is not communicable once desquamation begins.

An infant whose mother has had measles receives antibodies transplacentally that are protective for most of the 1st year of life. Lifelong immunity is conferred by infection. In the US, many measles cases are imported by travelers or immigrants.

Symptoms and Signs

Measles begins, after a 7- to 14-day incubation period, with a prodrome of fever, coryza, hacking cough, and tarsal conjunctivitis. The pathognomonic Koplik's spots appear 2 to 4 days later, usually on the buccal mucosa opposite the 1st and 2nd upper molars. They resemble grains of white sand surrounded by red areolae. They may be extensive, producing diffuse mottled erythema of the buccal mucosa. Sore throat develops.

The rash appears 3 to 5 days after symptom onset, usually 1 to 2 days after Koplik's spots appear. It begins on the face in front of and below the ears and on the side of the neck as irregular macules, soon mixed with papules. Within 24 to 48 h, lesions spread to the trunk and extremities, including the palms and soles, as they begin to fade on the face. Petechiae or ecchymoses may occur with severe rashes.

During peak disease severity, the temperature may exceed 40° C, with periorbital edema, conjunctivitis, photophobia, a hacking cough, extensive rash, prostration, and mild itching. Constitutional symptoms and signs parallel the severity of the eruption and the epidemic. In 3 to 5 days, the fever falls, the patient feels more comfortable, and the rash fades rapidly, leaving a coppery brown discoloration followed by desquamation.

Immunocompromised patients may not have a rash and can develop severe, progressive giant cell pneumonia.

Atypical measles syndrome usually occurs in people previously immunized with the original killed virus measles vaccines, which have been unavailable since 1968. The older vaccines can alter disease expression. Atypical measles syndrome may begin abruptly, with high fever, prostration, headache, abdominal pain, and cough. The rash may appear 1 to 2 days later, often beginning on the extremities, and may be maculopapular, vesicular, urticarial, or purpuric. Edema of the hands and feet may occur. Pneumonia and hilar adenopathy are common, and may be prolonged; chest x-ray abnormalities may persist for weeks to months. Symptomatic hypoxemia may occur.

Bacterial superinfections include pneumonia, otitis media, and others. Measles transiently suppresses delayed hypersensitivity, which can worsen active TB and temporarily prevent reaction to tuberculin and histoplasmin antigens on skin tests. Bacterial superinfection is suggested by pertinent focal signs or a relapse of fever, leukocytosis, or prostration.

Acute thrombocytopenic purpura may occur after infection resolves and produce a mild, self-limited bleeding tendency, although occasionally bleeding is severe.

Encephalitis occurs in 1/1000 to 2000 cases, usually 2 days to 1 wk after onset of the rash, often beginning with high fever, headache, seizures, and coma. CSF usually has a lymphocyte count of 50 to 500/μL and a mildly elevated protein level but may be normal initially. Encephalitis may resolve in about 1 wk or may persist longer, causing morbidity or death.

Subacute sclerosing panencephalitis (SSPE) is a late complication (see p. 1649).

Diagnosis

Typical measles may be suspected in an exposed patient who has coryza, conjunctivitis, photophobia, and cough but usually is suspected only after the rash appears. Diagnosis is usually clinical, by identifying Koplik's spots or the rash. CBC is unnecessary but, if obtained, may show leukopenia with a relative lymphocytosis. Laboratory identification is necessary only for public health and outbreak control purposes and is rarely performed to make the diagnosis. It is most easily done by demonstrating the presence of measles IgM in an acute serum specimen or, alternatively, by rapid immunofluorescent staining of pharyngeal or urinary epithelial cells, by reverse transcription–PCR of throat swabs or urine samples, or by viral growth in tissue culture. A rise in IgG antibody levels between acute and convalescent sera is highly accurate but delays diagnosis.

Differential diagnosis includes rubella, scarlet fever, drug rashes (eg, from phenobarbital or sulfonamides), serum sickness, roseola infantum, infectious mononucleosis, erythema infectiosum (see p. 2340), and echovirus and coxsackievirus infections (see also TABLE 187–1). Atypical measles, because of its greater variability, can simulate even more conditions than typical measles. Features that distinguish rubella from typical measles can include the absence of a recognizable prodrome, absence or milder severity of fever and other constitutional symptoms, enlarged (and usually tender) postauricular and suboccipital lymph nodes, and short duration. Drug rashes often resemble the measles rash but can usually be distinguished by the absence of a prodrome, cephalocaudal progression, or cough and the history. Roseola infantum can produce a skin rash similar to that of measles, but it seldom occurs in children > 3 yr. It can usually be differentiated by the high initial temperature, absence of Koplik's spots and malaise, and the simultaneity of defervescence and appearance of the rash.

Prognosis and Treatment

Mortality is about 2/1000 in the US but much higher in the developing world. Undernutrition and vitamin A deficiency may predispose to mortality. Vitamin A supplementation is recommended in populations at risk.

Cases of suspected measles should be reported immediately to local or state health departments without waiting for laboratory confirmation. Treatment is supportive, including for encephalitis. Vitamin A reduces morbidity and mortality in malnourished children but is not needed in others. For children > 1 yr with ophthalmologic evidence of vitamin A deficiency, 200,000 international units (IU) po is given daily for 2 days and repeated in 4 wk. Children living in regions where vitamin A deficiency is common receive a single dose of 200,000 IU. Children 6 mo to 1 yr receive a single dose of 100,000 IU.

Prevention

A live attenuated virus vaccine is routinely given to children in most developed countries (see also p. 1401 and FIG. 266–3 on p. 2235). The 1st dose is recommended at age 12 to 15 mo but can be given as young as 6 mo during a measles outbreak. Two doses are recommended. Infants immunized at < 1 yr of age still require 2 further doses given after the first birthday. Vaccine provides long-lasting immunity and has decreased measles incidence in the US by 99%. The vaccine produces mild, or inapparent, noncommunicable infection. Fever > 38° C occurs 5 to 12 days after inoculation in < 5% of vaccinees and can be followed by a rash. CNS reactions are exceedingly rare; the vaccine does not cause autism.

Contraindications to the vaccine include generalized malignancies (eg, leukemia, lymphoma), immunodeficiency, and therapy with immunosuppressants, such as corticosteroids, irradiation, alkylating agents, or antimetabolites. HIV infection is a contraindication only if there is severe immunosuppression(CDC immunologic category 3 with $CD4^+$ < 15%); if not, the risks of wild measles outweigh the risk of acquiring measles from the live vaccine. Reasons to defer vaccination include pregnancy, serious febrile illness, active untreated TB, or administration of antibody (as whole blood, plasma, or any immune globulin). The duration of deferral depends on the type and dose of immune globulin preparation given but may be as long as 11 mo.

Prevention in susceptible contacts is possible by giving the vaccine within 3 days of exposure. If vaccine should be deferred, immune serum globulin 0.25 mL/kg IM (maximum dose 15 mL) is given immediately, with vaccination given 5 to 6 mo later if medically appropriate (eg, patient no longer pregnant). An exposed immunodeficient patient with a contraindication to vaccination is given immune serum globulin 0.5 mL/kg IM (maximum, 15 mL). Immune serum globulin should not be given simultaneously with vaccine.

MONKEYPOX

Monkeypox virus is structurally related to the smallpox virus and causes similar, but milder, illness.

Monkeypox, like smallpox, is a member of the Orthopoxvirus group. Although the reservoir is unknown, monkeypox is endemic among rodents and monkeys in the rain forests of Africa, mostly in western and central Africa. Human disease occurs in Africa sporadically and in occasional epidemics. It is probably transmitted from animals via wounds or mucous membranes. Person-to-person transmission occurs inefficiently, with an attack rate of 8 to 9%. Most patients are children. People who have received smallpox vaccine may be at reduced risk. In Africa, mortality ranges from 4 to 22%.

Clinically, monkeypox is similar to smallpox; however, skin lesions occur more often in crops and lymphadenopathy may be more common. Clinical differentiation of monkeypox from smallpox and chickenpox may be impossible. Diagnosis is by culture, PCR, immunohistochemistry, or electron microscopy, depending on which tests are available. Treatment is supportive. Cases are reported to public health authorities.

MUMPS

(Epidemic Parotitis)

Mumps is an acute, contagious, systemic viral disease, usually causing painful enlargement of the salivary glands, most commonly the parotids. Complications may include orchitis, meningoencephalitis, and pancreatitis. Diagnosis is usually clinical. Treatment is supportive. Vaccination is highly effective.

The causative agent, a paramyxovirus, is spread by droplets or saliva. The virus probably enters through the nose or mouth. It is in saliva up to 6 days before salivary gland swelling appears. It is also in blood and urine and in CSF if there is CNS involvement. One attack usually confers permanent immunity.

Mumps is less communicable than measles. It is endemic in certain heavily populated areas but may occur in epidemics when people are crowded. It occurs mainly in unimmunized populations, with peak incidence during late winter and early spring. Disease occurs at any age, but usually between 5 and 10 yr; it is unusual in children < 2 yr, particularly those < 1 yr. About 25 to 30% of cases are clinically inapparent.

Symptoms and Signs

After a 14- to 24-day incubation period, most people develop headache, anorexia, malaise, and a low- to moderate-grade fever. Involvement of salivary glands occurs 12 to 24 h later, accompanied by fever up to 39.5 or 40° C. Fever persists 24 to 72 h. Glandular swelling peaks about the 2nd day and lasts 5 to 7 days. Involved glands are extremely tender during the febrile period.

Parotitis is usually bilateral. Pain on chewing or swallowing, especially on swallowing acidic liquids such as vinegar or citrus juice, is its earliest symptom. It later produces swelling beyond the parotid in front of and below the ear. Occasionally, the submandibular and sublingual glands also swell; more rarely, these are the only glands affected. Submandibular gland involvement produces neck swelling beneath the jaw, and suprasternal edema may develop, perhaps due to lymphatic obstruction by enlarged salivary glands. With sublingual gland involvement, the tongue may swell. The oral duct openings of the affected glands are edematous and slightly inflamed. The skin over the glands may become tense and shiny.

Mumps may involve organs other than the salivary glands, particularly in postpubertal patients. About 20% of postpubertal male patients develop testicular inflammation (orchitis), usually unilateral, pain, tenderness, edema, erythema, and warmth of the scrotum. Some testicular atrophy may ensue, but testosterone production and fertility are usually preserved. In females, gonadal involvement (oophoritis) is less commonly recognized, far less painful, and does not impair fertility.

Meningitis, typically with headache, vomiting, stiff neck, and CSF pleocytosis, occurs in 1 to 10%. Encephalitis, with drowsiness, seizures, or coma, occurs in about 1/1000 to 5000 cases. About 50% of CNS mumps infections occur without parotitis.

Pancreatitis, typically with sudden severe nausea, vomiting, and epigastric pain, may occur toward the end of the 1st wk. These symptoms disappear in about 1 wk, leading to complete recovery.

Prostatitis, nephritis, myocarditis, mastitis, polyarthritis, and lacrimal gland involvement occur extremely rarely. Inflammation of the thyroid and thymus glands may cause edema and swelling over the sternum, but sternal swelling more often results from submandibular gland involvement.

Diagnosis

Mumps is suspected in patients with salivary gland inflammation and typical systemic symptoms, particularly if there is parotitis or a known mumps outbreak. Laboratory testing is not needed. Other conditions that can cause similar glandular involvement are listed in TABLE 193–1. Mumps is also suspected in unexplained aseptic meningitis or encephalitis during mumps outbreaks. Lumbar puncture is necessary for patients with meningeal signs.

Laboratory diagnosis is necessary if disease is unilateral, recurrent, occurs in previously immunized patients, or produces prominent involvement of tissues other than the salivary glands. Acute and convalescent sera are tested by complement fixation, hemagglutination inhibition, or enzyme-linked immunosorbent assays (ELISA). If the laboratory is capable, the virus can usually be cultured from the throat, CSF, and occasionally the urine. Other laboratory tests are generally unnecessary, although serum amylase level can also be measured; elevation suggests mumps. WBC count is nonspecific; it may be normal but usually shows slight leukopenia and neutropenia. In meningitis, CSF glucose is usually normal but is occasionally between 20 and 40 mg/dL (1.1 and 2.2 mmol/L), as in bacterial meningitis.

Prognosis, Treatment, and Prevention

Uncomplicated mumps generally resolves, although a relapse occurs rarely after about 2 wk. Prognosis of meningitis is usually good, although permanent sequelae, such as unilateral (rarely bilateral) nerve deafness or facial paralysis, may result. Postinfectious encephalitis, acute cerebellar ataxia, transverse myelitis, and polyneuritis occur rarely.

TABLE 193–1. CAUSES OF PAROTID AND OTHER SALIVARY GLAND ENLARGEMENT

Suppurative bacterial parotitis
HIV parotitis
Other viral parotitis
Metabolic disorders (uremia, diabetes mellitus)
Mikulicz's syndrome (a chronic, usually painless parotid and lacrimal gland swelling of unknown etiology that occurs with TB, sarcoidosis, SLE, leukemia, and lymphosarcoma)
Malignant and benign salivary gland tumors
Drug-related parotid enlargement (eg, from iodides, phenylbutazone, or propylthiouracil)

Treatment of mumps and its complications is supportive. The patient is isolated until glandular swelling subsides. A soft diet reduces pain caused by chewing. Acidic substances (eg, citrus fruit juices) that cause discomfort should be avoided.

Repeated vomiting due to pancreatitis may necessitate IV hydration. For orchitis, bed rest and supporting the scrotum in cotton on an adhesive-tape bridge between the thighs to minimize tension, or applying ice packs, often relieves pain. Corticosteroids have not been shown to hasten resolution of the orchitis.

Mumps immune globulin and serum immune globulin are not helpful. Vaccination with live mumps virus vaccine (see p. 1401 and FIG. 266–3 on p. 2235) provides effective prevention, produces no significant local or systemic reactions, and requires only one injection. Postexposure vaccination does not protect against mumps from that exposure.

RUBELLA

(German Measles; 3-Day Measles)

(See also Congenital Rubella on p. 2321.)

Rubella is a contagious viral infection that may produce adenopathy, rash, and sometimes constitutional symptoms that are usually mild and brief. Infection during early pregnancy can cause spontaneous abortion, stillbirth, or congenital defects. Diagnosis is usually clinical. Treatment is usually unnecessary. Vaccination is effective.

Rubella is caused by an RNA virus, rubella virus, which is spread by respiratory droplets through close contact or through the air. A patient can transmit rubella from asymptomatic infection or from 10 days before until 15 days after the onset of the rash. Congenitally infected infants may transmit rubella for many months after birth. Rubella is less contagious than measles. Immunity appears to be life long after natural infection. However, 10 to 15% of young adults have not had childhood infection and are susceptible. The incidence in the US at present is at a historic low.

Symptoms and Signs

Many cases are mild. After a 14- to 21-day incubation period, a 1- to 5-day prodrome, usually consisting of fever, malaise, and lymphadenopathy, occurs in adults but may be minimal or absent in children. Tender swelling of the suboccipital, postauricular, and posterior cervical glands is characteristic. There is pharyngeal injection at the onset.

The rash is similar to that of measles but less extensive and more evanescent. It begins on the face and neck and quickly spreads to the trunk and extremities. At onset, a blanching, macular erythema may appear, particularly on the face. On the 2nd day, it often becomes more scarlatiniform (pinpoint) with a reddish flush. Petechiae form on the soft palate (Forschheimer's spots), later coalescing into a red blush. The rash lasts 3 to 5 days.

Constitutional symptoms in children are absent or mild and may include malaise and occasional arthralgias. Adults usually have few or no constitutional symptoms but occasionally have fever, malaise, headache, stiff joints, transient arthritis, and mild rhinitis. Fever generally resolves by the 2nd day of the rash.

Encephalitis has occurred rarely during large military outbreaks. Complete resolution is typical, but it is occasionally fatal. Thrombocytopenic purpura and otitis media occur rarely.

Diagnosis

Rubella is suspected in patients with characteristic adenopathy and rash. Laboratory diagnosis is necessary only for pregnant women, patients with encephalitis, and newborns. A ≥ 4-fold rise between acute and convalescent (4 to 8 wk) antibody titers is confirmatory.

Differential diagnosis includes measles, scarlet fever, secondary syphilis, drug rashes, erythema infectiosum (see p. 2340), and infectious mononucleosis as well as echo- and coxsackievirus infections (see also TABLE 187–1). Infections with enteroviruses and parvovirus B19 (erythema infectiosum) may be clinically indistinguishable. Rubella is differentiated from measles by the milder, more evanescent rash; milder and briefer constitutional symptoms; and absence of Koplik's spots, photophobia, and cough. Within a day of onset, scarlet fever usually produces more severe constitutional symptoms and pharyngitis than rubella. In secondary syphilis, adenopathy is not tender and the rash is usually prominent on the palms and soles. Laboratory diagnosis of syphilis is also usually readily available. Infectious mononucleosis can be differentiated by its more severe pharyngitis, more prolonged malaise, and atypical lymphocytosis and by antibody testing (see p. 1610).

Treatment and Prevention

Treatment is symptomatic. No specific therapy for encephalitis is available.

Live-virus vaccine is given routinely (see FIG. 266–3 on p. 2235). It produces immunity for ≥ 15 yr in > 95% of recipients and does not appear to cause viral transmission. Because certain other infections are clinically indistinguishable from rubella, a history of rubella does not guarantee immunity.

Vaccination is given to children and all susceptible postpubertal persons, especially college students, military recruits, health care practitioners, recent immigrants, and those working with young children. *Vaccine should not be given to any immunosuppressed person.* Routine vaccination is recommended for all susceptible mothers immediately after delivery. Screening women of childbearing age for rubella antibodies and immunizing those susceptible is also suggested. However, women receiving the vaccine should prevent conception for at least 28 days afterward. The vaccine virus may be capable of infecting a fetus during early pregnancy. Although it does not cause the congenital rubella syndrome, the risk of fetal damage is estimated at ≤ 3%; *use of vaccine is contraindicated throughout pregnancy.*

Fever, rash, lymphadenopathy, polyneuropathy, arthralgia, and arthritis occur rarely with vaccination in children; painful joint swelling occasionally follows vaccination in adults, usually women.

PROGRESSIVE RUBELLA PANENCEPHALITIS

Progressive rubella panencephalitis is a neurologic disorder occurring in a child with congenital rubella. It is presumably due to persistence or reactivation of rubella virus infection.

Some children with congenital rubella syndrome (eg, with deafness, cataracts, microcephaly, and mental retardation) develop neurologic deficits in the early teens.

The diagnosis is considered when a child with congenital rubella develops progressive spasticity, ataxia, mental deterioration, and seizures. Testing involves at least CSF examination and serology. Elevated CSF total protein and globulin and elevated rubella antibody titers in CSF and serum occur. CT may show ventricular enlargement due to cerebellar atrophy and white matter disease. Brain biopsy may be necessary to exclude other causes of encephalitis or encephalopathy. Rubella virus usually cannot be recovered by viral culture or immunohistologic testing. No specific treatment exists.

SMALLPOX

(Variola)

Smallpox is a highly contagious disease caused by the smallpox virus, an orthopoxvirus. It causes death in up to 30%. Indigenous infection has been eradicated. The main concern for outbreaks is from bioterrorism. Severe constitutional symptoms and a characteristic pustular rash develop. Treatment is supportive. Prevention involves vaccination, which, because of its risks, is performed selectively.

No cases of smallpox have occurred in the world since 1977, due to worldwide vaccination. In 1980, the World Health Organization (WHO) recommended discontinuation of routine smallpox vaccination. Routine vaccination in the US ended in 1972. Because humans are the only natural host of the smallpox virus and because the virus cannot survive > 2 days in the environment, WHO has declared natural infection eradicated. Recent concerns about terrorist access to existing stockpiles of smallpox virus raise the possibility of a recurrence (see p. 1393).

Because immunity declines over time, nearly all people—even those previously vaccinated—are now susceptible to smallpox.

Etiology and Pathophysiology

There are at least 2 strains of smallpox virus. The more virulent strain causes variola major (classic smallpox); the less virulent strain causes variola minor (alastrim).

Smallpox is transmitted person-to-person by direct contact or inhalation of droplet nuclei. Contaminated clothing or bed linens can also transmit infection. The infection is most communicable for the first 7 to 10 days after the rash appears. Once crusts form on the skin lesions, infectivity declines.

The attack rate is as high as 85% in unvaccinated people, and infection may lead to as many as 10 to 20 secondary cases from each primary case.

The virus invades the oropharyngeal or respiratory mucosa and multiplies in regional lymph nodes. It eventually localizes in small blood vessels of the dermis and the oropharyngeal mucosa. Other organs are seldom clinically involved, except for occasionally the CNS, with encephalitis. Skin lesions may develop secondary bacterial infection.

Symptoms and Signs

Variola major has a 10- to 12-day incubation period (range 7 to 17 days), followed by a 2- to 3-day prodrome of fever, headache, backache, and extreme malaise. Sometimes severe abdominal pain and vomiting occur. Following the prodrome, a maculopapular rash develops on the oropharyngeal mucosa, face, and arms, spreading shortly thereafter to the trunk and legs. The oropharyngeal lesions quickly ulcerate. After 1 or 2 days, the cutaneous lesions become vesicular, then pustular. Pustules are denser on the face and extremities than on the trunk, and they may appear on the palms. The pustules are round, tense, and appear deeply embedded. The skin lesions of smallpox, unlike those of chickenpox, are all at the same stage of development on a given body part. After 8 or 9 days, the pustules become crusted. Severe residual scarring is typical. Mortality is about 30%, due to a massive inflammatory response causing shock and multiple organ failure, and usually occurs in the 2nd wk of illness.

Variola minor results in symptoms that are similar but much less severe, with a less extensive rash. Mortality is < 1%.

About 10% of people with smallpox develop either a hemorrhagic or malignant variant. The hemorrhagic form is rarer and has a shorter, more intense prodrome followed by generalized erythema and cutaneous and mucosal hemorrhage. It is uniformly fatal within 5 or 6 days. The malignant form has a similar, severe prodrome, followed by development of confluent, flat, nonpustular skin lesions. In the rare survivors, the epidermis frequently peels.

Diagnosis

Diagnosis is confirmed by electron microscopy or viral culture of material scraped from skin lesions. PCR testing of vesicular or pustular samples identifies viral strains. Suspected smallpox must be reported immediately to local public health agencies or the Centers for Disease Control and Prevention (CDC) at 770-488-7100. These agencies will arrange for testing in a laboratory with high-level containment capability (biosafety level 4).

Treatment and Prevention

Treatment is generally supportive, with antibiotics for the occasional secondary bacterial infection. Antivirals have never been used clinically, but cidofovir may be considered for use under an investigational new drug protocol sponsored by the CDC.

Smallpox vaccine consists of live vaccinia virus, which is related to smallpox and provides cross-immunity. Vaccine is administered with a bifurcated needle dipped in reconstituted vaccine. The needle is rapidly jabbed 15 times in an area about 5 mm in diameter with sufficient force to draw a trace of blood. The vaccine site is covered with a dressing to prevent spread of the vaccine virus to other body sites. Fever, malaise, and myalgias are common the week after vaccination. Successful vaccination is indicated by development of a pustule by about the 7th day. Revaccination may produce only a papule surrounded by erythema, which peaks between 3 and 7 days. People without such signs of successful vaccination should receive another dose of vaccine.

Until an outbreak demonstrates release of smallpox in the population, pre-exposure vaccination remains recommended only for people at high risk for exposure to the virus (eg, laboratory technicians, health care practitioners, and mortuary attendants). Risk factors for complications include extensive skin disorders (particularly eczema), immunosuppressive diseases or therapies, ocular inflammation, and pregnancy. Widespread vaccination is not recommended because of risk. Serious complications occur in about 100 per million primary vaccines. Postvaccinial encephalitis occurs in about 1 of 300,000 recipients of primary vaccination, typically 8 to 15 days post vaccination. Progressive vaccinia results in a nonhealing vaccinial (vesicular) skin lesion that spreads to adjacent skin and ultimately other skin areas, bones, and viscera. Progressive vaccinia may occur with both primary vaccination and revaccination but almost exclusively in patients with an underlying defect in cell-mediated immunity; it can be fatal. Eczema vaccinatum results in vaccinial skin lesions appearing on areas of active or even healed eczema. Generalized vaccinia results from hematogenous dissemination of the vaccinia virus and produces vaccinia lesions at multiple body locations; it is usually benign. If there is inadvertent ocular viral implantation, vaccinia keratitis occurs rarely.

Some serious vaccine complications are treated with vaccinia immune globulin (VIG). In the past, high-risk patients who required vaccination because of viral exposure were simultaneously given VIG to try to prevent complications. The efficacy of this practice is unknown, and it is not recommended by the CDC. VIG is available only from the CDC.

Postexposure vaccination can prevent or significantly limit the severity of illness and is indicated for family and close personal contacts of smallpox patients. Early administration is most effective, but some benefit is realized up to 4 days postexposure.

Isolation of people with smallpox is essential. In limited outbreaks, patients may be isolated in a hospital in negative-pressure rooms equipped with high-efficiency particulate (HEPA) filters. In mass outbreaks, home isolation may be required. Contacts should be placed under surveillance, typically with daily temperature measurement, and isolated at home for temperature > 38° C or other sign of illness.

SUBACUTE SCLEROSING PANENCEPHALITIS

Subacute sclerosing panencephalitis is a progressive, usually fatal, brain disorder occurring months to usually years after an attack of measles. It produces mental deterioration, myoclonic jerks, and seizures. Diagnosis involves EEG, CT, CSF examination, and measles serology. Treatment is supportive.

Subacute sclerosing panencephalitis (SSPE) is probably a persistent measles virus infection (see p. 1642). Affected patients have measles virus in brain tissue.

SSPE occurs in about 6 to 22 cases per million people who had wild measles and in about 1 case per million people receiving measles vaccine; some cases may be due to unrecognized measles before vaccination. Males are more often affected. Onset is usually before age 20. SSPE is exceedingly rare in the US and Western Europe.

Symptoms and Signs

Often, the first signs are subtle—diminished performance in schoolwork, forgetfulness, temper tantrums, distractibility, and sleeplessness. However, hallucinations and myoclonic jerks may then occur, followed by generalized seizures. There is further intellectual decline and speech deterioration. Dystonic movements and transient opisthotonos occur. Later, muscular rigidity, dysphagia, cortical blindness, and optic atrophy may occur. Focal chorioretinitis and other funduscopic abnormalities are common. In the final phases, hypothalamic involvement may produce intermittent hyperthermia, diaphoresis, and pulse and BP disturbances.

Diagnosis

SSPE is suspected in young patients with dementia and neuromuscular irritability. EEG, CT or MRI scan, CSF examination, and measles serology are obtained. EEG shows periodic complexes with high-voltage diphasic waves occurring synchronously throughout the recording. CT or MRI may show cortical atrophy or white matter lesions. CSF examination usually reveals normal pressure, cell count, and total protein content; however, CSF globulin is almost always elevated, constituting up to 20 to 60% of the CSF protein. Serum and CSF contain elevated levels of measles virus antibodies. Anti-measles IgG appears to increase as the disease progresses. If test results are inconclusive, brain biopsy may be needed.

Prognosis and Treatment

The disease is almost invariably fatal within 1 to 3 yr (often pneumonia is the terminal event), although some have a more protracted course. A few patients have remissions and exacerbations.

Antiepileptics and other supportive measures are the only accepted treatments. Isoprinosine, interferon-α, and lamivudine are controversial, and antiviral drugs have generally not proved helpful.

194 SEXUALLY TRANSMITTED DISEASES

Sexually transmitted microorganisms vary widely in size, life cycle, symptoms, and susceptibility to available treatments. Bacterial sexually transmitted diseases (STDs) include syphilis, gonorrhea, chancroid, lymphogranuloma venereum, granuloma inguinale, and syndromes caused by chlamydia, mycoplasma, and ureaplasma infections. Viral STDs include genital and anorectal warts, genital herpes (see p. 1607), molluscum contagiosum (see p. 998), and HIV infection (see p. 1625). Parasitic infestations that can be sexually transmitted include trichomoniasis (caused by a protozoan), scabies (caused by a mite—see p. 995), pediculosis pubis (caused by a louse—see p. 995), amebiasis (see p. 1565), and giardiasis (see p. 1567). Many other infections not considered primarily to be STDs, including candidiasis, salmonellosis, shigellosis, campylobacteriosis, hepatitis A, B, and C, and cytomegalovirus infection, can be transmitted sexually.

Because sexual activity can include close contact of skin and mucous membranes of the genitals, mouth, and rectum, organisms spread among people efficiently. Inflammation or ulceration caused by some STDs (eg, herpes and chancroid) predisposes to transmission of others (eg, HIV). STD prevalence rates remain high in most of the world, despite diagnostic and therapeutic advances that can rapidly render patients with many STDs noninfectious. Factors impeding control of STDs include increased multipartnered and unprotected sexual activity, the difficulty that both physicians and patients have communicating about sexual issues, inadequate funding, susceptibility to reinfection with the same organism if both partners are not treated simultaneously, development of drug-resistant organisms, and increased international travel.

STDs are diagnosed and treated in various settings, in some of which diagnostic tests are limited or patient follow-up is not assured. Initial treatment is often syndromic, ie, directed at organisms most likely to cause the presenting syndrome (eg, urethritis, cervicitis, genital ulcers, pelvic inflammatory disease). Identification of the causative organism is pursued if tests are available and the diagnosis is unclear, disease is severe, initial treatment has failed, or for other reasons such as public health surveillance and psychosocial factors.

STD control depends on good facilities for diagnosis and treatment; public health programs for locating and treating patients' sexual contacts; following those who received treatment to ensure that they have been cured; educating health care practitioners and the public; and patients avoiding high-risk behaviors. Condoms and vaginal dams greatly decrease risk if used correctly. Vaccines are generally unavailable, except for hepatitis A and B.

CHANCROID

Chancroid is an infection of the genital skin or mucous membranes caused by *Haemophilus ducreyi* and characterized by painful ulcers and suppuration of the inguinal lymph nodes. Diagnosis is usually clinical because of difficulty culturing the organism. Treatment is with a macrolide, ceftriaxone, or ciprofloxacin.

H. ducreyi is a short, slender, gram-negative bacillus with rounded ends. Chancroid is rare in the US but is common throughout much of the developing world. As for other STDs causing genital ulceration, it appears to increase the risk of HIV transmission. Chancroid may coexist with other causes of genital ulcers.

Symptoms, Signs, and Diagnosis

After an incubation period of 3 to 7 days, small, painful papules appear and rapidly break down into shallow, soft, painful ulcers with ragged, undermined edges (ie, with overhanging tissue) and a red border. Ulcers vary in size and often coalesce. Deeper erosion occasionally leads to marked tissue destruction. The inguinal lymph nodes become tender, enlarged, and matted together, forming a fluctuant abscess (bubo). The skin over the abscess may become red and shiny and may break down to form a sinus. Autoinoculation may result in new lesions. Phimosis, urethral stricture, and urethral fistula may result from chancroid.

Chancroid is suspected in patients with unexplained genital ulcers or buboes, which may be mistaken for abscesses. Diagnosis is based on clinical findings; culture of the organism is difficult (it requires media containing hemin and albumin and growth is slow), and microscopic identification is confounded by mixed flora in ulcers. However, a sample of pus from a bubo or exudate from the edge of an ulcer should be sent to a laboratory that has the capability to identify *H. ducreyi*. If a bubo is aspirated to obtain material for diagnosis, antimicrobial treatment should be given promptly. Other causes of genital ulcers should be excluded as should HIV; serologic test for syphilis and culture for herpes should be routinely performed. If laboratory testing for chancroid is impractical, patients treated for other causes of genital ulcers can be treated with antibiotic regimens that also cover chancroid.

Treatment

Single-dose regimens include azithromycin 1 g po or ceftriaxone 250 mg IM. Erythromycin 500 mg po q 6 h for 7 days or ciprofloxacin 500 mg po bid for 3 days is also recommended. It is safe for buboes to be either aspirated for diagnosis or incised for symptomatic relief if patients also receive effective antimicrobial therapy. Sexual contacts should be examined and the patient followed for 3 mo. Treatment of patients with HIV, particularly with single-dose regimens, may be ineffective.

CHLAMYDIAL, MYCOPLASMAL, AND UREAPLASMAL INFECTIONS

Sexually transmitted urethritis, cervicitis, proctitis, and pharyngitis not due to gonorrhea are caused predominantly by chlamydia and infrequently by mycoplasma or ureaplasma. Chlamydia may also cause salpingitis, epididymitis, perihepatitis, neonatal conjunctivitis, and infant pneumonia. Untreated chlamydial salpingitis can become chronic, causing minimal symptoms but leading to serious consequences. Diagnosis is by culture, immunoassay for antigens, or genetic methods. Treatment is with single-dose azithromycin or a week of ofloxacin, levofloxacin, erythromycin, or a tetracycline.

Because the organisms causing most cases of nongonococcal sexually transmitted cervicitis in women and of urethritis, proctitis, and pharyngitis in both sexes have been identified, the previously used terms nonspecific urethritis and nongonococcal urethritis are imprecise. Causal agents include *Chlamydia trachomatis* (responsible for about 50% of such cases of urethritis and most such cases of mucopurulent cervicitis), *Mycoplasma genitalium, Ureaplasma urealyticum,* and *Trichomonas vaginalis* (see p. 1663). Chlamydia may also cause lymphogranuloma venereum (see p. 1656).

Symptoms and Signs

Men develop symptomatic urethritis after a 7- to 28-day incubation period, usually beginning with mild dysuria, discomfort in the urethra, and a clear to mucopurulent discharge. Although discharge may be slight and symptoms mild, they are frequently more marked early in the morning, when the urethral meatus is often red and the opening is blocked with dried secretions, which may also stain underclothes. Occasionally, onset is more acute, with dysuria, frequency, and copious, purulent discharge that simulates gonococcal urethritis. Epididymitis, or after rectal or orogenital contact, proctitis or pharyngitis may develop.

Women are generally asymptomatic, although vaginal discharge, dysuria, frequency, pelvic pain, and dyspareunia as well as symptoms of proctitis and pharyngitis may occur. Cervicitis with yellow, mucopurulent exudate and cervical ectopy (expansion of the red endocervical epithelium onto the vaginal surfaces of the cervix) are characteristic. Salpingitis may occur, producing lower abdominal discomfort, typically bilateral, and marked tenderness on palpation of the abdomen, adnexa, and cervix. Fitz-Hugh-Curtis syndrome, (perihepatitis) may produce right upper quadrant pain, fever, and vomiting.

Reactive arthritis (previously called Reiter's syndrome—see p. 292) caused by immunologic reactions to both genital and GI pathogens is an infrequent complication of adult chlamydial infections. It sometimes produces skin and eye lesions and noninfectious recurrent urethritis.

Infants born to women with chlamydial cervicitis may develop chlamydial ophthalmia neonatorum and pneumonia (see Neonatal Conjunctivitis on p. 2325).

Diagnosis

Diagnosis is suspected in patients with urethritis, salpingitis, cervicitis, or unexplained proctitis, pharyngitis, or lower UTIs; similar symptoms can result from gonococcal infection. If clinical evidence for urethritis is equivocal, urine samples with ≥ 5 WBCs/high-power field confirm the diagnosis. First-voided, morning samples are most sensitive. Samples of cervical or male urethral exudates are obtained to detect chlamydia by cell culture assays, immunoassay for antigens, or genetic methods. Nonculture methods, such as immunofluorescent staining, enzyme-linked immunosorbent assay (ELISA), or detection by specific nucleic acid probes with or without amplification, enable most laboratories to detect *C. trachomatis* in genital secretions. Nucleic acid amplification techniques are highly sensitive and specific and can be used on urine specimens, enabling simultaneous testing for gonococci on the same genital or urine specimen. Their use should be routine. Urine testing is especially useful for screening large numbers of asymptomatic people because genital examination is not necessary. Detection of mycoplasma and ureaplasma is currently impractical in routine practice.

Treatment

Uncomplicated documented or suspected chlamydial infections are treated with azithromycin 1 g po once or 7 days of ofloxacin 300 mg po bid, levofloxacin 500 mg po once/day, or doxycycline 100 mg po bid. The fluoroquinolones, but not the tetracyclines, are sufficient to treat simultaneous gonorrhea in many regions. In pregnant women, azithromycin 1 g po once should be used.

Patients who relapse (about 10%) are coinfected with microbes that do not respond to antichlamydial therapy or have been reinfected since treatment. They require further diagnostic evaluation, treatment of sex partners, and repeated or longer courses (21 to 28 days). If chlamydial genital infections are untreated, symptoms and signs subside within 4 wk in about 60 to 70% of patients. However, in women, asymptomatic cervical infection may persist, resulting in chronic endometritis, salpingitis, or pelvic peritonitis and their sequelae—pelvic pain, infertility, and increased risk of ectopic pregnancy.

Patients should abstain from sexual intercourse until they and their partners complete treatment. Because infection is often asymptomatic, treatment of sex partners is particularly important in eradication of infection and its damaging sequelae in women.

GENITAL WARTS

(Condylomata Acuminata; Venereal Warts; Anogenital Warts)

Genital warts are hyperplastic, sometimes pedunculated lesions of the skin or mucous membranes of the genitals caused by human papillomaviruses (HPVs). Some HPV types cause flat endocervical or anal lesions that are precancerous. Diagnosis is clinical. Multiple treatments exist, but few are highly effective. Genital warts may resolve without treatment in immunocompetent patients but may persist and spread in patients with decreased cell-mediated immunity (eg, HIV infection).

Certain HPV types are transmitted sexually and can cause anogenital warts after an incubation period of 1 to 6 mo. Some types (eg, 16 and 18) usually cause flat endocervical or anal warts that are difficult to see and diagnose clinically but increase the risk of cervical, anorectal, and bladder cancers and bowenoid papulosis of the skin. Other types cause easily visible warts.

Symptoms, Signs, and Diagnosis

Visible anogenital warts are usually soft, moist, minute pink or gray polyps that enlarge, may become pedunculated, and usually cluster. The surfaces resemble the surface of a cauliflower. In men, they occur most commonly under the foreskin, on the coronal sulcus, within the urethral meatus, and on the penile shaft. They may occur around the anus and in the rectum, especially in homosexual men. In women, they occur most commonly on the vulva, vaginal wall, cervix, and perineum. They may be more severe and difficult to treat in immunocompromised patients. Growth rates vary, but pregnancy, immunosuppression, or maceration of the skin may accelerate both the growth of lesions and their spread.

Genital warts are usually diagnosed clinically. Their appearance generally differentiates them from condyloma lata of secondary syphilis, which are flat-topped. However, serologic tests for syphilis should be performed initially and after 3 mo. Biopsies of atypical or persistent warts may be necessary to exclude carcinoma. Endocervical and anal warts can be visualized only by colposcopy. Staining to enhance visualization increases the yield. Nucleic acid amplification (PCR) assays allow typing of HPV, but their role in HPV management is not yet clear.

Treatment

No treatment is completely satisfactory; relapse is frequent and requires retreatment. However, in immunocompetent people, genital warts may resolve without treatment. Before topical treatments, surrounding tissue should be protected with petroleum jelly. Patients should be warned that after treatment the area may be painful. Treatment of rectal warts may require application of lidocaine ointment or jelly before bowel movements. Genital warts may be removed by cryotherapy, electrocauterization, laser, or surgical excision using a local or general anesthetic. Removal with a resectoscope using a general anesthetic may be the most effective treatment. Topical antimitotics (eg, podophyllotoxin, podophyllin, 5-fluorouracil), caustics (eg, trichloroacetic acid), and interferon inducers (eg, imiquimod) are widely used but usually require multiple applications over weeks to months and frequently fail. Interferon-α, intralesionally or IM, has cleared intractable lesions of skin and genitals, but its optimal administration and long-term effects are unclear. Also, in some patients with bowenoid papulosis of the genitals (caused by type 16 HPV), lesions initially disappeared after treatment with interferon-β but reappeared as invasive cancers.

For urethral lesions, thiotepa has been effective. In men, 5-fluorouracil applied bid to tid is highly effective for urethral lesions but produces acute urethral obstruction on rare occasions. Endocervical lesions should not be treated until Papanicolaou test results have ruled out other cervical abnormalities (eg, dysplasia or cancer) that may dictate treatment.

Sexual contacts should be examined. Circumcision may prevent recurrences in men. Women with endocervical warts, who are at risk for cervical dysplasia or carcinoma (see p. 2125), require regular follow-up (eg, cervical cytologic or colposcopic examination semiannually). Sex partners of these women and of patients with bowenoid papulosis also should be counseled and followed for HPV-related lesions.

GONORRHEA

Gonorrhea is caused by the bacterium *Neisseria gonorrhoeae*. It typically infects epithelia of the urethra, cervix, rectum, pharynx, or eyes, causing irritation and purulent discharge. Dissemination to skin and joints occurs infrequently. Diagnosis is by culture or genetic methods. Several antibiotic regimens—oral or parenteral—can be used.

N. gonorrhoeae is an aerobic, gram-negative diplococcus, transmission of which is almost always by sexual contact. Urethral and endocervical infections are most common, but infection also occurs in the pharynx or rectum after oral or anal intercourse. Transmission per episode of vaginal intercourse is about 20% from women to men but may be more efficient from men to women. Newborns can acquire conjunctival infection from the birth canal (see p. 2325). Children may develop gonorrhea through sexual abuse.

In 10 to 20% of women, the infection ascends via the endometrium to the salpinges and pelvic peritoneum (pelvic inflammatory disease—see p. 2087). Chlamydia or enteric organisms may be causative as well. Endocervical gonorrhea is commonly accompanied by infection of the urethra, Skene's ducts, and Bartholin's glands, which may be symptomatic. In a small fraction of men, ascending urethritis progresses to unilateral epididymitis. Disseminated gonococcal infection (DGI) from hematogenous spread occurs in < 1% of cases, predominantly in women. DGI typically affects the skin, tendon sheaths, and joints. Pericarditis, endocarditis, meningitis, and perihepatitis occur rarely.

Concomitant infection with *Chlamydia trachomatis* occurs in 15 to 25% of heterosexual men and 35 to 50% of women.

Symptoms and Signs

About 10 to 20% of infected women and very few infected men are asymptomatic. About 25% of men have minimal symptoms.

Male urethritis has an incubation period from 2 to 14 days. Onset is usually marked by mild discomfort in the urethra, followed a few hours later by dysuria and a purulent discharge. Urinary frequency and urgency may develop as the disease spreads to the posterior urethra. Examination reveals a purulent, yellow-green urethral discharge, and the meatus may be inflamed.

Epididymitis usually causes unilateral scrotal pain, tenderness, and swelling. A secondary hydrocele may follow. Rarely, men develop abscesses of Tyson's and Littre's glands; periurethral abscesses; or infection of Cowper's glands, the prostate, and the seminal vesicles.

Cervicitis usually has an incubation period of < 10 days. Urethritis may occur concurrently. Symptoms range from mild to severe and include dysuria, frequency, and vaginal discharge. The cervix may be reddened and friable, with a mucopurulent or purulent discharge. Pus may be expressed from the urethra on pressure against the symphysis pubis or from Skene's ducts or Bartholin's glands. Rarely, infections in sexually abused prepubertal girls cause dysuria, purulent vaginal discharge, and vulvar irritation, erythema, and edema.

Pelvic inflammatory disease (PID) occurs in 10 to 20% of infected women. It may include salpingitis, pelvic peritonitis, and pelvic abscesses and may produce lower abdominal discomfort, typically bilateral, dyspareunia, and marked tenderness on palpation of the abdomen, adnexa, and cervix.

Fitz-Hugh-Curtis syndrome is gonococcal (or chlamydial) perihepatitis that occurs predominately in women and produces right upper quadrant abdominal pain, fever, nausea, and vomiting, often mimicking biliary or hepatic disease.

Rectal gonorrhea is usually asymptomatic. It occurs predominately in homosexual men but also can occur in women who participate in anal sex, producing itching, purulent discharge, bleeding, tenesmus, and constipation, all of varying severity. Proctoscopy may show erythema or mucopurulent exudate on the rectal wall.

Gonococcal pharyngitis is uncommonly symptomatic but may cause sore throat. Since *Neisseria meningitidis* is often carried in the throat without causing symptoms or harm, the 2 organisms must be distinguished.

Disseminated gonococcal infection (DGI, or arthritis-dermatitis syndrome) reflects bacteremia and typically presents with fever, malaise, migratory polyarthralgia, and skin lesions. Many patients develop tenosynovitis, typically in the flexor tendons of the wrist or the Achilles tendon. Skin lesions are small and slightly painful, with a red base; may be papular, pustular, or vesicular; and typically occur on the distal extremities. Genital gonorrhea, the usual source of disseminated infection, may be asymptomatic. DGI can mimic other disorders that cause fever, skin lesions, and polyarthritis (eg, the prodrome of hepatitis B infection or meningococcemia), some of which may produce genital symptoms (eg, reactive arthritis—see p. 292).

Gonococcal arthritis is a more focal form of DGI that results in a frank septic arthritis with effusion. Some patients have previous or coincident symptoms of DGI. Usually only 1 or 2 joints are involved, primarily the knees, ankles, wrists, and elbows. Onset is often acute, with fever, severe pain, and limitation of movement but may occur without constitutional symptoms. Infected joints are swollen, and the overlying skin may be warm and red.

Diagnosis

Diagnosis is by Gram stain, culture, or a number of commercially available genetic techniques. Confirmed cases should be reported to the public health system. Reporting is mandatory throughout the US. A serologic test for syphilis (STS) and a screen for chlamydia infection should be obtained.

Urethral samples are obtained by inserting a small swab about 2 to 4 cm into the urethra. Rectal and pharyngeal swabs for culture can be obtained with any sterile cotton-tipped swab. Endocervical or rectal swabs should be inserted at least 2 cm and rotated for 10 sec. Gram stain is sensitive and specific for samples from men with urethral discharge but not for samples from other sites or from women. Rectal and pharyngeal infections cannot be accurately evaluated by Gram stain. Culture requires an atmosphere with added CO_2 and an enriched medium, such as the modified Thayer-Martin agar, containing antibiotics that selectively suppress normal flora.

For urethral and cervical infections, assays based on nucleic acid probes can detect gonococcal (and chlamydial) infections rapidly and reliably. If preceded by amplification (eg, PCR or ligase chain reaction), they can be used to detect infections using urine. This approach facilitates screening asymptomatic patients at high risk without invasive procedures to collect samples from genital sites.

In 30 to 40% of patients with DGI, blood cultures are positive in the 1st wk of illness. With septic arthritis, blood cultures are less often positive, but joint fluids are more often positive. Isolated, frank, acute arthritis in a sexually active patient requires joint aspiration to diagnose gonococcal infection. Fluid is usually purulent (WBCs > 20,000/μL). Cultures of joint fluid are positive in 40 to 50%, but organisms are rarely visible on Gram stain. PCR testing may be more sensitive but has not been evaluated.

Treatment

Uncomplicated gonococcal infection of the urethra, cervix, rectum, and pharynx can be treated with a single dose of ceftriaxone 125 mg IM or a fluoroquinolone, such as ciprofloxacin 500 mg, ofloxacin 400 mg, or levofloxacin 250 mg once only. In some regions, such as the west coast of the US, fluoroquinolone-resistant gonococci are sufficiently common that these drugs are not recommended. Alternatively, spectinomycin 2 g IM is given. Patients are also empirically treated for chlamydia infection (see p. 1652), which is often asymptomatic or masked by symptoms of gonorrhea. A single 2-g oral dose of azithromycin is effective against both gonococci and chlamydia but frequently causes GI adverse effects and is not recommended.

DGI with gonococcal arthritis is initially treated parenterally with ceftriaxone 1 g IM or IV q 24 h, ceftizoxime 1 g IV q 8 h, cefotaxime 1 g IV q 8 h, ciprofloxacin 400 mg IV q 12 h, ofloxacin 400 mg IV q 12 h, or spectinomycin 2 g IM q 12 h. Parenteral therapy is continued for 24 to 48 h after clinical improvement and followed by 4 to 7 days of oral therapy with either ciprofloxacin 500 mg bid, cefixime 400 mg bid, or ofloxacin 400 mg bid. Concomitant chlamydia therapy is also given.

For gonococcal arthritis, therapeutic joint drainage is usually not required. Initially the joint may be immobilized in a functional position. Passive range-of-motion exercises should be started as soon as possible. Once pain subsides, more active exercises, with stretching, active range of motion, and muscle strengthening, should begin. Over 95% of patients treated for gonococcal arthritis recover complete joint function. Because sterile joint effusions may persist for prolonged periods, an anti-inflammatory drug may be beneficial.

Posttreatment cultures are unnecessary if symptomatic response is adequate. However, for patients with symptoms for > 7 days, cultures are repeated with antimicrobial sensitivity testing. All patients with gonorrhea should abstain from sexual activity until treatment is completed. The patient's sexual contacts should be tested for gonorrhea and other STDs as appropriate, and if exposed within 2 wk, treated for gonorrhea presumptively (epidemiologic treatment).

GRANULOMA INGUINALE

(Donovanosis)

Granuloma inguinale is a progressive infection of genital skin caused by *Calymmatobacterium granulomatis.* Skin lesions are beefy red, raised, and often ulcerated. Diagnosis is with clinical criteria and microscopy. Treatment is with antibiotics, usually tetracyclines, macrolides, or trimethoprim-sulfamethoxazole.

Granuloma inguinale is caused is *C.* (formerly *Donovania*) *granulomatis*, a gram-negative bacillus. It is very rare in most of the world. Current epidemiologic data are unavailable, but historical foci have been in Papua New Guinea, northern Australia, southern Africa, and parts of Brazil and India.

Symptoms, Signs, and Diagnosis

After an incubation period of about 1 to 12 wk, a painless, beefy red nodule slowly enlarges, becoming an elevated, velvety, malodorous, granulating, ulcerated plaque. Sites of infection are the penis, scrotum, groin, and thighs in men; the vulva, vagina, and perineum in women; the anus and buttocks in patients who have anal-receptive intercourse; and the face in both sexes. Lymphadenopathy is absent, and the disease spreads by contiguity and autoinoculation. Lesions progress slowly but eventually may cover the genitals. Healing is slow with scarring. Secondary infection is common and can cause gross tissue destruction. Hematogenous dissemination to bones, joints, or liver occurs occasionally, and anemia, cachexia, and death may occur without treatment.

Granuloma inguinale is suspected in patients from endemic areas with bright, beefy red, moist, smooth, raised lesions. Diagnosis is confirmed microscopically by presence of Donovan bodies (numerous bacilli in the cytoplasm of macrophage demonstrated by Giemsa or Wright's stain) in smears of fluid from scrapings of the edge of lesions. Tissue smears contain many plasma cells. Biopsy specimens are taken if the diagnosis is unclear or if adequate tissue fluid is unobtainable because lesions are dry, sclerotic, or necrotic. The organism does not grow on ordinary culture media.

Treatment

Tetracyclines, macrolides, and trimethoprim-sulfamethoxazole (TMP-SMX) are most effective, followed by ceftriaxone, aminoglycosides, fluoroquinolones, and chloramphenicol. Recommended oral regimens include doxycycline 100 bid, TMP-SMX one double-strength tablet bid, erythromycin 500 mg bid, or azithromycin 1 g/wk for 3 wk. Ceftriaxone 1 g IM or IV once/day for 14 days is an alternative.

Response to treatment should begin within 7 days, but healing of extensive disease may be slow and lesions may recur, requiring more prolonged therapy. HIV-infected patients may also require prolonged or intensive treatment. Follow-up should continue for 6 mo after apparently successful treatment. Sexual contacts should be examined.

LYMPHOGRANULOMA VENEREUM

Lymphogranuloma venereum is a chlamydial disease characterized by a transitory primary skin lesion followed by suppurative lymphadenitis and lymphangitis. Lymphatic obstruction, fistula formation, and proctitis are also possible. Diagnosis is often clinical, but laboratory confirmation with serologic or immunofluorescent testing is usually possible. Treatment is with 21 days of a tetracycline or erythromycin.

Lymphogranuloma venereum (LGV) is caused by serotypes (L1-L3) of *Chlamydia trachomatis* other than those that cause trachoma, inclusion conjunctivitis, urethritis, and cervicitis. These LGV strains invade and reproduce in regional lymph nodes but can also cause mucosal infections.

LGV occurs sporadically in the US but is endemic in parts of Africa, India, Southeast Asia, South America, and the Caribbean. It is diagnosed much more commonly in men than women.

Symptoms and Signs

After an incubation period of ≥ 3 days, a nonindurated vesicle forms, ulcerates, and heals so quickly that it may pass unnoticed. Usually about 2 to 4 wk later, the inguinal lymph nodes enlarge, become tender, and coalesce, forming a large, tender, fluctuant mass (bubo) that adheres to the deep tissues and inflames the overlying skin. Fever, malaise, headache, joint pains, anorexia, and vomiting are possible. Backache is common in women, in whom the initial lesions may be on the cervix or upper vagina, resulting in enlargement and suppuration of perirectal and pelvic lymphatics.

Multiple sinuses may develop and discharge pus or blood. Healing eventually occurs with scar formation, but sinuses can persist or recur. Chronic inflammation obstructs the lymphatic vessels, producing edema, ulcers, fistulas, and possibly eventual genital elephantiasis. The genital or rectal areas may develop large polypoid lymphedematous masses. Involvement of the rectal wall in women or homosexual men may result in ulcerative proctitis with bloody purulent rectal discharges and, if chronic, strictures. Systemic spread occurs rarely.

Diagnosis

LGV is suspected in patients with genital ulcers, inguinal adenitis, or proctitis who are from or have sexual contacts with people from areas where infection is endemic. It is also suspected in patients with buboes, which may be mistaken for abscesses caused by other bacteria. Diagnosis by cell culture, the standard, is available in only a few laboratories. Complement fixing antibodies to chlamydia at titers of ≥ 1:64 usually occur at presentation or shortly thereafter. Immunoassays (eg, enzyme-linked immunosorbent assay [ELISA]) for chlamydia antigens, immunofluorescence using monoclonal antibodies for staining of pus, and nucleic acid amplification methods used to diagnose other chlamydial infections may prove helpful for diagnosis of LGV but have not been evaluated.

Treatment

Doxycycline 100 mg po bid, erythromycin 500 mg po qid, or tetracycline 500 mg po qid, each for 21 days, rapidly heals early disease. Azithromycin 1 g po weekly for 1 to 3 wk is probably effective but has not been fully evaluated; neither has clarithromycin.

Lymphedema in later stages may not resolve despite elimination of the organism. Fluctuant buboes may be aspirated or incised if necessary for symptomatic relief, but most patients respond quickly to antibiotics. Buboes and fistulas may require surgery, but rectal strictures can usually be dilated. Elephantiasis is treated by plastic surgery. Sexual contacts should be examined and tested, and the patient should be followed for 6 mo after apparently successful treatment.

SEXUALLY TRANSMITTED ENTERIC INFECTIONS

Various bacterial (*Shigella, Campylobacter*, or *Salmonella*), viral (hepatitis A, B, and C), and parasitic (*Giardia* or amebiasis) pathogens are transmitted by sexual practices, especially those that facilitate fecal-oral contamination (in order of decreasing frequency, ororectal, anogenital, orogenital, genital intercourse). Although bacterial pathogens may coexist with or cause proctitis, they usually produce symptoms (diarrhea, fever, bloating, nausea, abdominal pain) that suggest disease more proximal in the GI tract. Multiple coinfections are frequent, especially in people with many sex partners. Asymptomatic infections also occur with all these pathogens and are the rule with *Entamoeba dispar*, which is common in homosexual men in Western countries and was previously known as nonpathogenic *Entamoeba histolytica*. Diagnosis and treatment of these conditions are discussed in other sections of THE MANUAL.

SYPHILIS

(See also Congenital Syphilis on p. 2322.)

Syphilis is a systemic disease caused by *Treponema pallidum*, characterized by 3 sequential clinical stages and by years of latency. Common symptoms include genital ulcers, skin lesions, meningitis, aortic disease, and neurologic syndromes. Diagnosis is by serologic tests and adjunctive studies selected on the basis of the stage of disease. Penicillin is the drug of choice.

Syphilis is caused by *T. pallidum*, a spirochete that cannot survive for long outside the human body. In sexually acquired syphilis, *T. pallidum* enters through the mucous membranes or skin, reaches the regional lymph nodes within hours, and rapidly disseminates throughout the body.

Syphilis occurs in primary, secondary, and tertiary stages (see TABLE 194–1), with latent periods between them. A person with syphilis remains infective through the 1st 2 stages. Perivascular infiltration of lymphocytes, plasma cells, and later, fibroblasts causes swelling and proliferation of the endothelium of smaller blood vessels, leading to endarteritis obliterans.

Infection is usually transmitted by sexual contact, including orogenital and anorectal contact, and by contact with the skin lesions of primary or secondary syphilis. Risk of transmission is about 30% from a single sexual encounter with a person with primary syphilis. Prior infection does not confer immunity against reinfection.

Symptoms and Signs

Syphilis may be diagnosed at any stage and may affect multiple or single organs, mimicking many other diseases. Syphilis may be accelerated by coexisting HIV infection; in these cases, eye involvement, meningitis, and other neurologic complications are more common and more severe.

Primary syphilis: After an incubation period of 3 to 4 wk (range 1 to 13 wk), a primary lesion (chancre) develops at the site of inoculation. The initial red papule quickly erodes to form an ulcer that is at most minimally painful, has an indurated base, and when abraded, exudes a clear serum containing numerous spirochetes. Regional lymph nodes are firm, discrete, and nontender. Chancres can occur anywhere but are most common on the penis, anus, and rectum in men; on the vulva, cervix, rectum, and perineum in women; and on the lips or in the oropharynx in either sex.

Secondary syphilis: In secondary syphilis, bacteremia with widespread dissemination, generalized mucocutaneous lesions, adenopathy, and protean organ manifestations

TABLE 194–1. CLASSIFICATION OF SYPHILIS

TYPE	STAGE	DESCRIPTION
Acquired	Primary	Chancre; regional lymphadenopathy
	Secondary (immediately follows primary stage)	Varied dermatologic lesions that mimic several disorders—eg, rashes, erosion of mucous membranes, alopecia, and multiple other manifestations
	Latent (asymptomatic; may persist indefinitely or be followed by late stage)	Early latent syphilis (infection < 2 yr duration†), infectious lesions may recur; late latent syphilis (infection > 2 yr duration†), recurrences are rare
	Late or tertiary (symptomatic; not contagious)	Includes benign tertiary syphilis, cardiovascular syphilis, and neurosyphilis (asymptomatic neurosyphilis, meningovascular neurosyphilis, parenchymatous neurosyphilis, tabes dorsalis)
Congenital*	Early	Symptomatic, the overt disease seen in infants up to age 2 yr
	Late	Symptomatic; stigmas occur later in life—eg, Hutchinson's teeth, scars of interstitial keratitis, bony abnormalities

*Can also exist in permanently latent, or asymptomatic, state.
†For reporting purposes, the division is sometimes made on a 4-yr rather than a 2-yr basis.

may occur, typically beginning 4 to 10 wk after the chancre appears. About 25% have a residual chancre. Systemic symptoms of fever, malaise, anorexia, nausea, and fatigability as well as headache and bone pain are common.

Over 80% of patients have mucocutaneous lesions; a wide variety of rashes and lesions occur, and any body surface can be affected. Lesions may be transitory, persistent for months, or recurrent, but all eventually heal, usually without scarring.

Syphilitic dermatitis is usually symmetric; is more marked on the flexor and volar surfaces, especially the palms and soles; generally occurs as macules, papules, and pustules; and is rarely vesicular or bullous. The individual lesions are pigmented or barely visible in heavily pigmented skin and are pink, pale red, or brown in less pigmented skin. They are round, often scale, and may become confluent and indurated, but generally do not itch or hurt. After lesions resolve, hyperpigmentation or depigmentation can occur. If the scalp is involved, patchy hair loss often occurs (alopecia areata).

Condyloma lata are hypertrophic, flattened, dull pink or gray papules at mucocutaneous junctions and in moist areas of the skin (eg, perianal area, under breasts) that are extremely infectious. The mucous membranes frequently erode, forming mucous patches that are circular, raised, and often gray to white with a red areola. These occur mostly on the oral mucosa, palate, pharynx, or larynx; on the glans penis or vulva; or in the anal canal and rectum.

Virtually any organ system can be affected. About 50% of patients have lymphadenopathy, usually generalized, with nontender, firm, discrete nodes, and often with hepatosplenomegaly. About 10% of patients have lesions of the eyes (uveitis), bones (periostitis), joints, meninges, kidneys (glomerulitis), liver (hepatitis), or spleen. About 10 to 30% of patients have mild CSF pleocytosis, but < 1% have symptoms of meningitis, which can include headache, neck stiffness, cranial nerve lesions, deafness, and papilledema.

Latent period: The latent period is characterized by absence of signs and symptoms, normal CSF, and positive serologic test results. Because symptoms of primary and secondary syphilis are occasionally minimal or overlooked, patients frequently are diagnosed in the latent stage by serologic tests for syphilis. Syphilis may remain latent permanently. However, relapses with contagious mucocutaneous lesions may occur but almost always in the early latent period (< 2 yr after infection). In patients given antibiotics for other diseases, latent syphilis may be cured, which could account for the rarity of late-stage disease in developed countries.

Late or tertiary syphilis: About 1/3 of untreated people develop late syphilis, though sometimes not until many years after the initial infection. Lesions may be clinically described as benign tertiary syphilis, cardiovascular syphilis, or neurosyphilis. All are now rare in developed countries.

Benign tertiary gummatous syphilis usually develops within 3 to 10 yr of infection and may involve the skin, bones, and viscera. Gummas are granulomatous masses that are sometimes necrotic and surrounded by vasculitis. They are frequently localized but may diffusely infiltrate an organ or tissue, grow and heal slowly, and leave scars. In the skin, they often result in nodular, ulcerative, or scaling eruptions. When subcutaneous, they result in punched-out ulcers with bases resembling washed leather. Healed ulcers typically leave atrophic scars. Though most common on the leg, upper trunk, face, and scalp, gummas may occur almost anywhere, including submucosal tissues (especially of the palate, nasal septum, pharynx, and larynx) and lead to perforation of the palate or septum.

Benign tertiary syphilis of bone results in either periostitis with bone formation or osteitis with destructive lesions causing a deep, boring pain, characteristically worse at night. A lump or swelling may be palpable. The GI and respiratory tracts may also be involved.

Cardiovascular syphilis usually presents as a dilated, fusiform aneurysm of the ascending aorta, narrowing of the coronary ostia, or aortic valvular insufficiency, typically 10 to 25 yr after the initial infection. Syphilitic aneurysms may produce symptoms by compressing or eroding adjacent structures in the mediastinum and chest wall. Such symptoms include brassy cough and stridor from pressure on the trachea, bronchial stenosis and subsequent infection from esophageal compression, hoarseness from compression of the recurrent laryngeal nerve, and painful erosion of the sternum and ribs or spine from repeated pulsations of the dilated aorta.

Neurosyphilis, if it develops during the 1st 5 to 10 yr after infection, involves principally the meninges and blood vessels, causing asymptomatic, acute, or meningovascular neurosyphilis. Parenchymatous neurosyphilis and tabes dorsalis usually occur 2 to 3 decades later.

Asymptomatic neurosyphilis produces abnormal CSF (eg, lymphocytic pleocytosis and increased protein) in about 15% of those originally diagnosed as having latent syphilis, in 25 to 40% of those with secondary syphilis, in 12% of those with cardiovascular syphilis, and in 5% of those with benign tertiary syphilis. It evolves to symptomatic neurosyphilis in 5% without treatment. A person whose CSF is normal > 2 yr after the initial infection is unlikely to develop neurosyphilis.

Various symptomatic forms of neurosyphilis, but hardly any other disorder, can produce an Argyll Robertson pupil, a small irregular pupil that accommodates normally with convergence but does not react to light.

Acute syphilitic meningitis produces fever and meningismus as well as abnormal CSF. It usually develops within 1 yr after the initial infection, sometimes with other signs of secondary syphilis. Cranial nerve dysfunction may be clinically indistinguishable from meningovascular neurosyphilis.

Meningovascular neurosyphilis is vasculitis of large- to medium-sized arteries of the brain or spinal cord that causes brain infarction, often multifocal and accompanied by CSF pleocytosis. Symptoms may begin with headache, neck stiffness, dizziness, bizarre behavior, poor concentration, memory loss, lassitude, insomnia, and blurred vision. Hemiparesis, confusion, seizures, papilledema, aphasia, and cranial nerve palsies usually indicate basilar vasculitis.

Spinal cord involvement may produce weakness and wasting of shoulder girdle and arm muscles, slowly progressive spastic paraplegia with urinary and/or fecal incontinence, and, in rare cases, transverse myelitis with sudden flaccid paraplegia and loss of sphincter control.

Parenchymatous neurosyphilis (general paresis or dementia paralytica) results from chronic meningoencephalitis that causes destruction of cortical parenchyma. It usually develops 15 to 20 yr after initial infection, generally not affecting patients before their 40s or 50s. It produces progressive behavioral deterioration and may mimic a mental illness or dementia. Irritability, difficulty concentrating, deterioration of memory, defective judgment, headaches, insomnia, fatigue, and lethargy are common, and seizures, aphasia, and transient hemiparesis are possible. The patient's hygiene and grooming deteriorate. Emotional instability, wasting, depression, and delusions of grandeur with lack of insight may occur.

TABLE 194–2. FEATURES THAT MAY HELP DIFFERENTIATE COMMON SEXUALLY TRANSMITTED GENITAL ULCERS OR PAPULES

FEATURES	CAUSE
Solitary ulcer; indurated; rubbery; painless, and only slightly tender; relatively nontender adenopathy	Syphilitic chancre
Clusters of small, superficial ulcers on an erythematous base; painful; sometimes with vesicles; inguinal adenopathy	Herpes simplex virus
Shallow ulcer; nonindurated; painful; ragged, undermined edges; red border; ulcers vary in size and often coalesce; buboes	Chancroid
Small papule or ulcer, often asymptomatic or unnoticed; severely tender and painful buboes, sometimes with distal lymphedema or drainage to the skin; fever possible	Lymphogranuloma venereum
Multiple, shallow lesions; other systemic symptoms (eg, fever, rash, and adenopathy)	Primary HIV infection
Multiple, shallow lesions; in scabies, presence of characteristic extragenital lesions and burrows; in pediculosis pubis, presence of lice	Excoriated scabies or pediculosis pubis
Elevated; velvety; malodorous; granulating lesions; no inguinal adenopathy	Granuloma inguinale

Signs include tremors of the mouth, tongue, outstretched hands, and whole body; pupillary abnormalities (see p. 1659); dysarthria; hyperreflexia; and, in some cases, extensor plantar responses. Handwriting usually is shaky and illegible.

Tabes dorsalis (locomotor ataxia) involves slow, progressive degeneration of the posterior columns and nerve roots. It typically develops 20 to 30 yr after initial infection by an unknown mechanism. The earliest and most characteristic symptom usually is an intense, stabbing (lightning) pain in the back and legs that recurs irregularly. Gait ataxia, hyperesthesia, and paresthesia may produce a sensation of walking on foam rubber. Loss of bladder sensation leads to urine retention, incontinence, and recurrent infections. Erectile dysfunction is common.

Most patients with tabes dorsalis are thin and have characteristic sad facies and Argyll Robertson pupils (pupils that accommodate but do not respond to light). Optic atrophy may occur. Examination of the legs discloses hypotonia, hyporeflexia, impaired vibratory and joint position sense, ataxia in the heel-shin test, absence of deep pain sensation, and Romberg's sign. Tabes dorsalis tends to be intractable even with treatment.

Visceral crises are usually considered a variant of tabes dorsalis. They cause paroxysms of pain in various organs, the most common being gastric crises with vomiting. Rectal, bladder, and laryngeal crises also occur.

Other lesions: Trophic lesions, secondary to hypoesthesia of the skin or periarticular tissues, may develop in the later stages. Trophic ulcers may develop on the soles of the feet and penetrate as deeply as the underlying bone. Charcot's arthropathy, a painless joint degeneration with bony swelling and an abnormal range of movement, is common (see also p. 297).

Diagnosis

Syphilis is suspected in patients with typical mucocutaneous lesions or unexplained neurologic disorders, particularly in areas of high disease prevalence. In such areas, it should also be considered in patients with a broad range of unexplained findings. Because it has such diverse clinical manifestations and advanced stages are now relatively rare in most developed countries, it may escape recognition. Patients with HIV and syphilis may have atypical or accelerated disease. Diagnostic tests performed depend on what stage of syphilis is suspected. Diagnostic tests for syphilis include reaginic tests, treponemal tests, and darkfield microscopy.

Diagnostic tests for syphilis: These include serologic tests for syphilis (STS) and darkfield examination of fluids from lesions. STS consist of screening (reaginic) and confirmatory (treponemal) tests. The organism cannot be grown in the laboratory.

Reaginic tests use lipid antigens (cardiolipin, ie, bovine heart lipids) to detect reagin (ie, human antibodies that bind to lipids). The Venereal Disease Research Laboratory (VDRL) and the rapid plasma reagin (RPR) tests are sensitive, simple, and inexpensive reaginic tests that are used for screening but are not specific for syphilis. Results may be presented qualitatively (eg, reactive, weakly reactive, borderline, or nonreactive) and quantitatively as titers (eg, positive at 1:16 dilution). Multiple conditions other than treponemal infections (eg, SLE, antiphospholipid antibody syndromes) can produce a positive reagin test (biologically false positive). CSF testing with reaginic tests is reasonably sensitive for early disease but less so in late neurosyphilis. CSF reagin tests can be used to diagnose neurosyphilis or to monitor response to treatment by measuring titers.

Treponemal tests detect antitreponemal antibodies. These qualitative tests include the fluorescent treponemal antibody absorption (FTA-ABS) test, the microhemagglutination assay for antibodies to *T. pallidum* (MHA-TP), and the *T. pallidum* hemagglutination assay (TPHA). Treponemal tests are very specific for syphilis, and their failure to confirm treponemal infection identifies a biologically false-positive reaction. Although application of treponemal tests to CSF is controversial, some authorities believe FTA-ABS test is sensitive.

Neither reaginic nor treponemal tests become positive until 3 to 6 wk after the initial infection. Thus, an STS in early primary syphilis may be negative, and a negative result does not exclude syphilis until after 6 wk. Reaginic titers decline after effective treatment, becoming negative by 1 yr in primary and by 2 yr in secondary syphilis. Treponemal tests usually remain positive for many decades, despite effective treatment.

Darkfield microscopy directs light obliquely through a slide of exudate from a chancre or lymph node aspirate. Although infrequently available, darkfield microscopy is the most sensitive and specific test for early primary syphilis. The spirochetes appear against a dark background as bright, motile, narrow coils that are about 0.25 μm wide and from 5 to 20 μm long. They must be distinguished morphologically from nonpathogenic spirochetes, which may be part of the normal flora, especially of the mouth.

Primary syphilis: Primary syphilis is usually suspected based on genital, but occasionally extragenital, relatively painless ulcers. Differentiating characteristics of some causes of sexually transmitted genital ulcers are described in TABLE 194–2. Causes of ulcers that are not listed in the table include mucous patches of secondary syphilis, erosive balanitis, gummatous ulceration of tertiary syphilis, Behçet's syndrome, epithelioma, and trauma. Coinfections with 2 pathogens (eg, herpes simplex virus and *T. pallidum*) are not rare.

Darkfield microscopy (if available) of exudate from a chancre or lymph node aspirate is diagnostic. If results are negative or the test is unavailable, STS is done. If STS is negative or cannot be immediately performed, but a skin lesion has been present for < 3 wk (before STS become positive) and clinical suspicion for an alternate diagnosis is low, treatment may be instituted and STS repeated in 2 to 4 wk. Patients with syphilis should be encouraged to undergo testing for other STDs including HIV at diagnosis and 6 mo later.

Secondary syphilis: Because it can mimic many diseases, syphilis should be considered in any undiagnosed cutaneous eruption or mucosal lesion, particularly if there is generalized lymphadenopathy, lesions on the palms or soles, or condylomalata, or if the patient has risk factors (eg, HIV, multiple sex partners). Secondary syphilis may be clinically mistaken for a drug eruption, rubella, infectious mononucleosis, erythema multiforme, pityriasis rubra pilaris, fungal infection, or, particularly, pityriasis rosea. Condyloma lata may be mistaken for warts, hemorrhoids, or pemphigus vegetans, and scalp lesions for ringworm or idiopathic alopecia areata.

Secondary syphilis is excluded by a negative reaginic STS, which is virtually always reactive in this stage, often with a high titer. A compatible syndrome with a positive STS (either reagin or treponemal) is grounds for treatment. Uncommonly, this combination will represent latent syphilis coexisting with another skin disease. Secondary syphilis patients should be tested for other STDs and for asymptomatic neurosyphilis.

Latent syphilis: Asymptomatic, latent syphilis is diagnosed when reaginic and treponemal STS are positive in the absence of symptoms or signs of active syphilis. Such patients should have thorough examination to exclude secondary and tertiary syphilis, particularly genital, skin, neurologic, and cardiovascular examinations. Treatment and serologic follow-up for up to several years may be needed to ensure the success of therapy because reaginic STS titers fall slowly. Latent acquired syphilis must be differentiated from latent congenital syphilis (see p. 2322), latent yaws, and other treponemal diseases.

Late or tertiary syphilis: Patients with symptoms or signs of tertiary syphilis (particularly unexplained neurologic abnormalities) should have STS. If it is reactive, lumbar puncture for CSF examination (including STS), imaging of the brain and aorta, and screening of any other organ systems in which involvement is clinically suspected should follow. Reaginic STS is nearly always positive, except in a few cases of tabes dorsalis.

In benign tertiary syphilis, differentiation from other inflammatory mass lesions or ulcers may be difficult without biopsy. In cardiovascular syphilis, symptoms of aneurysmal compression of adjacent structures, particularly stridor or hoarseness, may be suggestive and clinical evaluation may be nearly pathognomonic. Syphilitic aortitis is suggested by aortic insufficiency without aortic stenosis, and, on chest x-ray, widening of the aortic root, and linear calcification on the walls of the ascending aorta. Diagnosis of aneurysm is confirmed with aortic imaging (transesophageal echocardiogram, CT, or MRI).

Except for the Argyll Robertson pupil, most symptoms and signs of neurosyphilis are nonspecific, so that diagnosis relies heavily on a high index of suspicion. Asymptomatic neurosyphilis is diagnosed based on abnormal CSF (typically lymphocytic pleocytosis and elevated protein) and reactive CSF reaginic test. In parenchymatous neurosyphilis, the CSF reaginic and serum treponemal tests are reactive and the CSF typically has lymphocytic pleocytosis and elevated protein. Because HIV produces mild pleocytosis and a variety of other neurologic symptoms, it may confound the diagnosis. In tabes dorsalis, serum reaginic tests may be negative if a patient has been previously treated, but serum treponemal tests are usually positive. Although the CSF usually shows a lymphocytic pleocytosis, elevated protein, and sometimes a positive reaginic or treponemal result, in many treated cases CSF is normal.

Treatment

The treatment of choice in all stages of syphilis, including during pregnancy, is sustained-release penicillin. Case reporting to public health agencies is required. All sexual contacts within the past 3 mo (in primary syphilis) and within 1 yr (in secondary syphilis) should be evaluated and treated if infected.

Primary, secondary, and latent syphilis: Benzathine penicillin G 2.4 million units IM once produces blood levels that are sufficiently high for 2 wk to cure primary, secondary, and early (< 1 yr) latent syphilis. Doses of 1.2 million units are usually given in each buttock to reduce local reactions. Additional injections of 2.4 million units should be given 7 and 14 days later for latent syphilis that is late (≥ 1 yr) or of unknown duration because of occasional treponemal persistence in the CSF after single-dose regimens.

For penicillin-allergic patients, ceftriaxone 125 mg IM once/day for 10 days, azithromycin 1 g po once, or doxycycline 100 mg po bid for 14 days may be used, but efficacy of these drugs is not well defined, particularly for late latent syphilis, and the 14-day regimen requires good compliance.

Late or tertiary syphilis: Benign or cardiovascular tertiary syphilis can be treated in the same way as late latent syphilis.

For ocular or neurosyphilis, either aqueous penicillin 3 to 4 million units IV q 4 h for 10 days (best penetrates the CNS but may be impractical) or procaine penicillin G 2.4 million units IM once/day plus 500 mg probenecid po qid, both for 10 to 14 days, followed by benzathine penicillin 2.4 million units weekly for 3 doses, is recommended. Ceftriaxone 2 g IM or IV daily for 14 days has been successful in patients with serous penicillin allergies who cannot be desensitized. Treatment of asymptomatic neurosyphilis appears to prevent the development of new neurologic deficits. Symptomatic treatment of neurosyphilis may include oral or IM antipsychotics, which may help control paresis. Patients with tabes dorsalis and lightning pains should receive analgesics as needed, and carbamazepine 200 mg po tid or qid is sometimes helpful.

Jarisch-Herxheimer reaction (JHR): Over 50% of patients with primary or secondary syphilis, especially those with secondary syphilis, have a JHR within 6 to 12 h of initial treatment. The mechanism is not understood. It typically presents as malaise, fever, headache, sweating, rigors, anxiety, or a temporary exacerbation of the syphilitic lesions. It may be misdiagnosed as an allergic reaction. JHR usually subsides within 24 h and poses no danger. However, patients with general paresis or a high CSF cell count may manifest a more serious reaction, including seizure or stroke, and should be warned and observed accordingly. Unanticipated JHR may occur in patients with undiagnosed syphilis who are given antitreponemal antibiotics for other conditions.

Posttreatment Surveillance

The importance of repeated tests to confirm cure should be explained to the patient before treatment. Examinations and reaginic titers should be performed 3, 6, and 12 mo after treatment and annually thereafter until nonreactive. Failure to decline by 4-fold at 6 mo suggests treatment failure and indicates need for retreatment. After successful treatment, primary lesions heal rapidly, and reaginic titers fall and usually become qualitatively negative within 9 to 12 mo. Treponemal tests usually remain positive for decades or permanently and need not be measured serially.

Patients with neurosyphilis should undergo CSF testing at 3 and 6 mo and q 6 mo thereafter until CSF has been normal for 2 yr. Normal CSF, serologic tests, and examination for 2 yr indicates probable cure. Serologic or clinical relapse occasionally occurs after the 6th to 9th mo, usually affecting the nervous system; reinfection should also be considered. Indications for retreatment with a more intensive regimen of antibiotics include a reaginic test that remains positive for > 1 yr, an increasing titer, and clinical relapse. If CSF remains abnormal after 6 to 12 mo of maximal treatment, the need for continuing maximal treatment is unclear.

TRICHOMONIASIS

Trichomoniasis is infection of the vagina or male genital tract with *Trichomonas vaginalis*. It can be asymptomatic or produce urethritis, vaginitis, or occasionally cystitis, epididymitis, or prostatitis. Diagnosis is by microscopic examination of vaginal or prostatic secretions or by urethral culture. Patients and sexual contacts are treated with metronidazole.

T. vaginalis is a flagellated, sexually transmitted protozoan that infects men less commonly than women (about 20% of women of reproductive age). Infection may be asymptomatic in either sex, particularly in men; the organism may persist for long periods in the GU tract, resulting in unsuspected transmission to a sex partner. It may account for 5 to 15% of male urethritis in some areas. Coinfection with gonorrhea and other STDs is common.

Symptoms and Signs

Women may have symptoms ranging from none to copious, yellow-green, frothy vaginal discharge with soreness of the vulva and perineum with dyspareunia and dysuria. Previously asymptomatic infection may become symptomatic at any time with inflammation of the vulva and perineum and edema of the labia. The vaginal walls and surface of the cervix may have punctate, red "strawberry" spots. Urethritis and possibly cystitis may also occur.

Men are usually asymptomatic; however, sometimes urethritis results in a discharge that may be transient, frothy, or purulent or causes dysuria and frequency, usually early in the morning. Often urethral discharge is milder and causes only minimal urethral irritation, occasional moisture at the urethral meatus; minimal discharge may be noticeable under the foreskin. Epididymitis and prostatitis are rare complications.

Diagnosis

Trichomoniasis is suspected in women with vaginitis, in men with urethritis, and in their partners. Suspicion is high if symptoms persist after evaluation and treatment for other infections such as gonorrhea, chlamydia, mycoplasma, and ureaplasma.

In women, bedside diagnosis is attempted by microscopic examination immediately after mixing vaginal secretion from the posterior fornix with a drop of saline. The exudate contains numerous neutrophils, while the causative organism is pear-shaped with flagella, often motile, and averages 7 to 10 μm (about the size of WBCs), but occasionally reaches 25 μm. Cultures are more sensitive than microscopy. Trichomoniasis is also commonly diagnosed on a Papanicolaou test. As with diagnosis of any STD, patients with trichomoniasis should undergo testing to exclude other common STDs such as gonorrhea and chlamydia.

In men, microscopy of urine is insensitive, although occasionally organisms are visible in a 1st-voided morning specimen or a centrifuged specimen. Cultures of urine and urethral swabs are most sensitive. If poor compliance with follow-up is likely, treatment can be initiated in sex partners of patients with documented trichomoniasis without confirming the diagnosis in the partner.

Treatment

Metronidazole 2 g po in a single dose cures up to 95% of women if sex partners are treated simultaneously. Effectiveness of single-dose regimens in men is not as clear, so treatment is typically with 500 mg bid for 5 to 7 days. IV metronidazole has cured some women resistant to repeated oral doses.

Metronidazole may cause leukopenia, disulfiram-like reactions to alcohol, or candidal superinfections. It is relatively contraindicated in early pregnancy, although it may not be dangerous to the fetus after the 1st trimester. Sex partners should be screened and treated for other STDs.

SECTION 15
PSYCHIATRIC DISORDERS

195 APPROACH TO THE PATIENT WITH MENTAL COMPLAINTS

Patients with mental complaints or concerns present in a variety of clinical settings, including primary care and emergency treatment centers. Complaints or concerns may be new or a continuation of a history of mental problems. Many complaints are related to coping with physical conditions. The method of assessment depends on whether the complaints constitute an emergency or occur in a scheduled clinical setting. In an emergency, the physician may have to focus on more immediate history, symptoms, and behavior to be able to make a management decision. In a scheduled visit, a more thorough assessment is appropriate.

ROUTINE PSYCHIATRIC ASSESSMENT

Assessment includes a general medical and psychiatric history and a mental status examination.

History

The physician must determine whether the patient can provide a history, ie, whether the patient readily and coherently responds to initial questions. If not, information is sought from family and caregivers. Close family members may provide information that the patient has omitted. Receiving information that is not solicited by the physician does not violate patient confidentially. Previous psychiatric assessments and treatments are reviewed and records from such care obtained as soon as possible.

Conducting an interview hastily and indifferently with closed-ended queries (following a rigid system review) often prevents the patient from revealing relevant information. Tracing the history of the presenting illness with open-ended questions, so that the patient can tell his story in his own words, takes the same amount of time and enables the patient to describe associated social circumstances and reveal emotional reactions.

The interview should include psychiatric history, including previous treatment courses; medical history; social background, including educational level and marital, employment, and legal histories; family health history; and the patient's response to important life events and changes. Developmental history, including the family atmosphere during childhood, behavior during schooling, handling of different family and social roles, stability and effectiveness at work, sexual adaptation, pattern of social life, and quality and stability of marriage, helps in appraising personality. The physician should tactfully ask about use or abuse of alcohol, drugs, and tobacco; behavior while driving; and other aspects of everyday conduct. Responses to the usual vicissitudes of life—failures, setbacks, losses, previous illnesses—may help determine coping mechanisms (see TABLE 201–1 on p. 1718). When appropriate, the physician must ask about suicidal thoughts and plans.

The personality profile that emerges may suggest traits that are adaptive (eg, resilience, conscientiousness) or maladaptive (eg, self-centeredness, dependency, poor tolerance of frustration). The interview may reveal obsessions (unwanted and distressing thoughts or impulses), compulsions (urges to perform irrational or apparently useless acts), and delusions (fixed false beliefs) and may determine whether distress is expressed in physical symptoms (eg, headache, abdominal pain), mental symptoms (eg, phobic behavior, depression), or social behavior (eg, withdrawal, rebelliousness). The patient should also be asked about attitudes regarding psychiatric treatments, including drugs and psychotherapy, so that this information can be incorporated into the treatment plan.

The interviewer should establish whether a physical condition is causing or worsening a mental condition. Many physical conditions cause enormous stress and require coping mechanisms to withstand the stress-related pressures. Most people with severe physical conditions experience some kind of adjustment disorder, and those with underlying mental disorders may become unstable.

Observation during an interview may provide evidence of mental or physical disorders. Body language may reveal evidence of attitudes and feelings denied by the patient. For example, does the patient fidget or pace back and forth despite denying anxiety? Does the patient seem sad despite denying feelings of depression? General appearance may provide clues as well. For example, is the patient clean and well-kempt? Is a tremor or facial droop present?

Mental Status Examination

A mental status examination uses observation and questions to evaluate several domains of mental function, including speech, emotional expression, thinking and perception, and cognitive functions. Brief standardized screening questionnaires are available for assessing certain components of the mental status examination, including those specifically designed to assess orientation and memory. Screening questionnaires cannot take the place of a broader, more detailed mental status examination, however (see sidebar 206–1 on p. 1749).

Speech can be assessed by noting spontaneity, syntax, and rate and volume. A patient with depression might speak slowly and softly, whereas a patient with mania might speak rapidly and loudly. Abnormalities such as dysarthrias and aphasias may indicate an underlying physical cause of mental status changes, such as head injury, stroke, brain tumor, or multiple sclerosis.

Emotional expression can be assessed by asking patients to describe their feelings. The patient's tone of voice, posture, hand gestures, and facial expressions are all considered. If there is evidence of feelings of depression or anxiety, suicide risk should be assessed (see p. 1743).

Thinking and perception can be assessed by noticing not only what is communicated but also how it is communicated. Abnormal content might take the form of delusions, ideas of reference (notions that everyday occurrences have special meaning or significance personally meant for or directed to the patient), or obsessions. The physician can assess whether ideas seem to be linked and goal-directed and whether transitions from one thought to the next are logical. Psychotic or manic patients may have disorganized thoughts or an abrupt flight of ideas.

Cognitive functions include the patient's level of alertness; attentiveness or concentration; orientation to person, place, and time; memory; abstract reasoning; insight; and judgment. Abnormalities of cognition most often occur with delirium or dementia and with substance abuse or withdrawal but can also occur with depression.

TABLE 195–1. SELECTED PHYSICAL DISORDERS CAUSING MENTAL SYMPTOMS

DISORDER	SYMPTOMS
Neurologic	
Cerebral arteritis	Confusion, delirium
Epilepsy	Hallucination, personality change, inattention
Limbic encephalitis	Memory impairment, confusion, hallucination
Mass lesion	Variable, depending on location: hallucination, personality change, impaired motor or visual function
Migraine	Hallucination
Multiple sclerosis	Mood symptoms, euphoria, irritability, delusions
Subdural hematoma	Dementia
Vascular infarct	Delirium, dementia
Endocrine	
Cushing's syndrome	Depression, mania if exogenous steroid use
Diabetes mellitus	Anxiety, depression
Hyperthyroidism	Anxiety, insomnia, emotional lability, inattention
Hypothyroidism	Depression, memory loss, poor concentration, slow speech
Infectious	
Herpes encephalitis	Confusion, agitation, hallucination, disorientation
HIV/AIDS	Delirium, dementia, mood symptoms
Lyme disease	Dementia, fatigue
Neurosyphilis	Dementia

MEDICAL ASSESSMENT OF THE PATIENT WITH MENTAL SYMPTOMS

Numerous physical disorders produce symptoms mimicking specific mental disorders (see TABLE 195–1). Other physical disorders may not mimic specific mental syndromes but, rather, cause change in mood and energy. New-onset mental symptoms, qualitatively different symptoms in a patient with a known or stable mental disorder, and atypical symptoms or those that begin at an atypical age necessitate a medical assessment. The medical assessment looks at new or changed drug dosages and use of illicit drugs; use of intoxicants, including alcohol; signs and symptoms (eg, fever, dyspnea, morning headache, diarrhea); and family and personal history of comorbid medical conditions.

Vital signs as well as cardiovascular, pulmonary, and neurologic function are assessed. A physical disorder as the cause of mental symptoms is most likely indicated by confusion and inattention (reduced clarity of awareness of the environment—see p. 1808); lateralizing findings on neurologic examination; incontinence; and meningeal signs.

Testing

Generally, testing in the acute or emergency setting is based on routine orders. In some situations, blood alcohol and drug levels and urine toxicology screens are obtained to rule out substance abuse or withdrawal. A head CT scan is done if mental symptoms are new or if delirium, headache, recent trauma, or focal neurologic findings (eg, weakness of an extremity) are present. Lumbar puncture is performed in patients with meningeal signs or a normal head CT with fever, headache, or delirium. If indicated, testing for SLE, syphilis, and HIV are performed. In the nonacute setting, testing is guided by symptoms.

PSYCHIATRIC EMERGENCIES

Patients who present with severe changes in mood, thoughts, or behavior and those experiencing severe, potentially life-threatening drug adverse effects need urgent psychiatric assessment and treatment. Nonspecialists are often the first care providers, but whenever possible, such cases should be evaluated by a psychiatrist.

When a patient's mood, thoughts, or behavior is highly unusual or disorganized, assessment must first determine if the patient's or other people's safety is threatened. The threat to the patient can include inability to perform self-care (leading to self-neglect) or suicidal behavior (see p.1741). The threat to others can include aggression and violence.

Aggressive, violent patients are often psychotic and have diagnoses such as schizophrenia, delusional disorder, delirium, acute mania, and dementia. Such behavior can also result from intoxication with alcohol or other substances, particularly phencyclidine (PCP), amphetamines, or cocaine. Aggressive, potentially violent behavior is usually managed with some combination of seclusion, physical restraints, close monitoring that may involve constant observation by a trained sitter, and drug therapy. The decrease in noise and activity afforded by seclusion may be enough to reduce agitation and aggressiveness. Restraints may still be needed, however, to hold the patient long enough to undergo a complete assessment (see sidebar 195-1). Drug therapy, if used, should target control of specific symptoms. Rapid calming or tranquilizing of a patient is usually achieved with a benzodiazepine or an antipsychotic (typically a conventional antipsychotic, but a 2nd-generation drug may also be used) administered IM or IV (see TABLE 195–2). Benzodiazepines act more quickly (within a few minutes) but may cause confusion and often have erratic IM absorption. Sometimes a combination of both drugs is most effective.

Nonaggressive, nonviolent patients may have highly unusual or disorganized mood, thoughts, or behavior and may not be able to explain their complaints or concerns coherently. In such instances, other sources of information must be found and consulted immediately so that a more complete assessment can be undertaken. Information from available family members or loved ones may be invaluable. Some nonaggressive, nonviolent, incoherent patients are psychotic, but others have panic disorder, delirium, or complex-partial seizures. Self-neglect is a particular concern for patients with psychotic disorders, dementia, or substance abuse because of impaired ability to obtain food, clothing, and appropriate protection from the elements.

Moving the patient to a calm, quiet environment and responding in a supportive, reassuring manner may improve the likelihood of obtaining a useful history directly from the patient. In some cases, drug therapy may also be used, especially if it is targeted to address specific symptoms that have not responded to other measures.

Adverse effects of antipsychotic drugs: Antipsychotics, particularly dopamine-receptor antagonists, at therapeutic as well as toxic doses, can cause acute extrapyramidal

Sidebar 195–1. USE OF PHYSICAL RESTRAINTS IN AGGRESSIVE, VIOLENT PATIENTS

Restraints are used to prevent clear, imminent harm to the patient or others; to prevent the patient's treatment from being significantly disrupted; to prevent damage to physical surroundings; and to decrease sensory overstimulation. Contraindications include use in patients with extremely unstable physical and mental conditions unless absolutely indicated and accompanied by direct supervision; in delirious or demented patients unable to tolerate an environment of reduced stimulation; in overtly suicidal patients who could use the restraint as a suicide device; and for punishment or the convenience of staff. In preparation for applying restraints, one person should be positioned at each extremity and another at the patient's head. Restraints should be applied only by staff members adequately trained in protecting patient rights and safety. Hospital accreditation standards now require that patients in restraints be continuously observed by a trained sitter. Immediately after restraints have been applied, the patient must be monitored for signs of injury; circulation and range of motion; nutrition and hydration; vital signs, hygiene, and elimination; physical and mental comfort; and readiness for discontinuation of restraints as appropriate. These assessments should be performed every 15 min.

Recently, the Joint Commission on Accreditation of Healthcare Organizations issued revised guidelines for use of restraints in the psychiatric setting. Restraints must be applied under the direction of a licensed independent practitioner (LIP). The LIP must provide an assessment within the 1st hour of restraint placement. The order for continued restraint may be written for up to 4 h at a time. The patient must be evaluated by an LIP or registered nurse during the interval and before further continuation of the restraint order. At 8 h, the LIP must re-evaluate the patient in person before continuing the restraint order.

The use of physical restraints should be considered a last resort, when other steps have not sufficiently controlled aggressive, potentially violent behavior. However, when restraints are needed for such a situation, they are legal in all states if their use is properly documented in the patient's medical record. Restraints have the advantage of being immediately removable, whereas drugs may alter symptoms enough or in such a way as to delay an assessment.

adverse effects (see TABLE 195–3), including acute dystonia. These adverse effects may be dose dependent and may resolve once the drug is stopped. Several antipsychotics, including thioridazine, haloperidol, olanzapine, risperidone, and ziprasidone can cause long QT interval syndrome and ultimately increase the risk of fatal arrhythmias.

TABLE 195–2. DRUG THERAPY FOR AGITATED PSYCHIATRIC PATIENTS

DRUG	DOSAGE	COMMENTS
Lorazepam	0.5–2 mg q 1 h IM (deltoid), or IV prn	IV preferred. Absorption from IM injection may be erratic. Respiratory depression
Haloperidol	1–10 mg po, IM (deltoid), or IV q 1 h prn (1–2.5 mg for mild agitation and for frail or older patients; 2.5–5 mg for moderate; 5–10 mg for severe)	Usually required only if psychosis is clear. Can make some substance intoxications (eg, phencyclidine) worse and may cause dystonia. Liquid concentrate may be used for rapid absorption if the patient can take the drug po. No respiratory depression
Ziprasidone	10–20 mg, may repeat 10-mg dose q 2 h or 20-mg dose q 4 h; maximum, 40 mg/day	ECG monitoring may be needed. Avoid concomitant use with carbamazepine and ketoconazole

TABLE 195–3. TREATMENT OF ACUTE ADVERSE EFFECTS OF ANTIPSYCHOTICS

SYMPTOMS	TREATMENT	COMMENTS
Acute dystonic reactions (eg, oculogyric crisis, torticollis)	Benztropine 2 mg IV or IM, may be repeated once in 20 min Diphenhydramine 50 mg IV or IM q 20 min × 2	Benztropine 2 mg po may prevent dystonia when given with an antipsychotic
Laryngeal dystonia	Lorazepam 4 mg IV over 10 min, then 1–2 mg IV slowly	Intubation may be needed
Akinesia, severe parkinsonian tremors, bradykinesia	Benztropine 1–2 mg po bid Diphenhydramine 25–50 mg po tid	With akinesia, the antipsychotic may have to be stopped and one with a lower potency used
Akathisia (with other extrapyramidal symptoms)	Amantadine 100–150 mg po bid Benztropine 1–2 mg po bid Biperiden 1–4 mg po bid Procyclidine 2.5–10 mg po bid Propranolol 10–30 mg tid po Trihexyphenidyl 2–7 mg po bid (1–5 mg po tid or can use sustained-release form 2–7 mg bid)	The causative drug should be stopped or a lower dose used
Akathisia associated with extreme anxiety	Lorazepam 1 mg tid po Clonazepam 0.5 mg bid po	

Neuroleptic malignant syndrome is a hypermetabolic reaction to antipsychotics, particularly dopamine-receptor antagonists (see p. 1727), although any antipsychotic can be involved. This syndrome usually occurs early in treatment or after an increase in dosage and rarely during maintenance treatment unless other physical conditions such as dehydration occur. It develops in up to 3% of patients started on antipsychotics. Risk is increased in agitated males who have received large and rapidly increased doses. No genetic component is apparent. Its pathophysiologic basis is believed to be blockade of dopamine D_2 receptors.

Characteristic signs are "lead pipe" muscle rigidity, hyperpyrexia, tachycardia, hypertension, tachypnea, change in mental status, confusion, and diaphoresis. Common complications include MI, aspiration pneumonia, respiratory failure, acidosis, and rhabdomyolysis. Less common complications include thromboembolism and renal failure. Mortality approaches 30%.

Diagnosis is based on clinical findings. Similar presentation occurs with bacterial meningitis, sepsis, environmental or malignant hyperthermia, and pheochromocytoma. Patients should undergo CBC, electrolyte, BUN and creatinine, and liver function tests. PT and PTT are done to check for disseminated intravascular coagulation. Serum CK should be done to detect rhabdomyolysis. A head CT and lumbar puncture are done if a CNS cause is suspected. Diagnosis is confirmed by muscle biopsy, with demonstration of abnormal augmentation of in vitro muscle contraction after pretreatment with halothane. Laboratory abnormalities include respiratory and metabolic acidosis, myoglobinuria, elevated CK, and leukocytosis.

Treatment is usually administered in an ICU. Treatment includes immediate discontinuation of the presumed causative drug, supportive care, and aggressive treatment of myoglobinuria, fever, and acidosis. Evaporative cooling is the treatment of choice to reduce the core body temperature to 39.5° C. The dopamine agonist bromocriptine 2.5 to 7.5 mg po tid or dantrolene 1 to 3 mg/kg IV q 4 to 6 h may be used as a muscle relaxant.

Legal Considerations

Patients with severe changes in mood, thoughts, or behavior are usually hospitalized when their condition is likely to deteriorate without psychiatric intervention and when appropriate alternatives are not available.

If a patient refuses hospitalization, the physician must decide whether to hold him against his will. Doing so may be necessary to ensure the immediate safety of the patient or of others or to allow completion of an assessment and implementation of treatment. Criteria and procedures for involuntary hospitalization vary by jurisdiction. Usually, temporary restraint requires a physician or psychologist and one additional clinician or family member to certify that the patient has a mental disorder, is a danger to himself or to others, and refuses voluntary treatment. Danger to self includes, but is not limited to, suicidal ideation or attempts and failure to obtain basic needs, including nutrition, shelter, and needed drugs. In most jurisdictions, knowledge of intent to commit suicide requires a medical practitioner to act immediately to prevent the suicide, such as notifying the police or other responsible agency. Danger to others includes homicidal intent, placing others in peril, or failing to provide for the needs or safety of dependents because of the mental disorder.

In most states, when a patient expresses the intention to harm a particular person, the evaluating physician is required to warn the intended victim and notify a specified law enforcement agency. Specific requirements vary by state. Typically, state regulations also require reporting suspected abuse of children, the elderly, and spouses.

196 ANXIETY DISORDERS

Everyone periodically experiences fear and anxiety. Fear is an emotional, physical, and behavioral response to an immediately recognizable external threat (eg, an intruder, a runaway car). Anxiety is a distressing, unpleasant emotional state of nervousness and uneasiness; its causes are less clear. Anxiety is less tied to the exact timing of a threat; it can be anticipatory before a threat, or it can persist after a threat has passed or occur without an identifiable threat. Anxiety is often accompanied by physical changes and behaviors similar to those caused by fear.

Some degree of anxiety is adaptive; it can help people prepare, practice, and rehearse so that their functioning is improved and help them be appropriately cautious in potentially dangerous situations. However, beyond a certain level, anxiety causes dysfunction and undue distress. At this point, it is maladaptive and considered a disorder.

Anxiety occurs in a wide range of physical and mental disorders, but it is the predominant symptom of several. Anxiety disorders are more common than any other class of psychiatric disorder. However, they often are not recognized and consequently not treated. Left untreated, chronic, maladaptive anxiety can contribute to or interfere with treatment of some physical disorders.

Etiology

The causes of anxiety disorders are not fully known, but both mental and physical factors are involved. Many people develop anxiety disorders without any identifiable antecedent triggers. Anxiety can be a response to environmental stressors, such as the ending of a significant relationship or exposure to a life-threatening disaster. Some physical disorders can directly produce anxiety, including hyperthyroidism, pheochromocytoma, hyperadrenocorticism, heart failure, arrhythmias, asthma, and COPD. Other physical causes include use of drugs; effects of corticosteroids, cocaine, amphetamines, and even caffeine may mimic anxiety disorders. Withdrawal from alcohol, sedatives, and some illicit drugs may also cause anxiety.

Symptoms, Signs, and Diagnosis

Anxiety can arise suddenly, as in panic, or gradually over many minutes, hours, or even days. Anxiety may last from a few seconds to years; longer duration is more characteristic of anxiety disorders. Anxiety ranges from barely noticeable qualms to complete panic. The ability to tolerate a given level of anxiety varies from person to person.

Anxiety disorders can be so distressing and disruptive that depression may result. Alternatively, an anxiety disorder and depressive disorder may coexist, or depression may develop first, with symptoms and signs of an anxiety disorder occurring later.

Deciding when anxiety is so dominant or severe that it constitutes a disorder depends on several variables, and physicians differ at what point they make the diagnosis. Physicians must first determine, by history, physical examination, and appropriate lab tests, if anxiety is due to a physical disorder or drug. They must also determine if anxiety is better accounted for by another mental disorder. If other causes are not found and if anxiety is very distressing, interferes with functioning, and does not stop spontaneously within a few days, then an anxiety disorder is present and merits treatment.

Diagnosis of a specific anxiety disorder is based on its characteristic symptoms and signs. A family history of anxiety disorders (except acute and posttraumatic stress disorders) helps in making the diagnosis, because some patients appear to inherit a predisposition to the same anxiety disorders that their relatives have as well as a general susceptibility to other anxiety disorders. However, some patients may appear to acquire the same disorders as their relatives through learned behavior.

GENERALIZED ANXIETY DISORDER

Generalized anxiety disorder is characterized by excessive, almost daily, anxiety and worry for ≥ 6 mo about many activities or events. The cause is unknown, although it commonly coexists in people who have alcohol abuse, major depression, or panic disorder. Diagnosis is based on history and physical examination. Treatment is psychotherapy, drug therapy, or both.

Generalized anxiety disorder (GAD) is common, affecting about 3% of the population within a 1-yr period. Women are twice as likely to be affected as men. The disorder often begins in childhood or adolescence but may begin at any age.

Symptoms and Signs

The focus of the worry is not restricted as it is in other mental disorders (eg, to having a panic attack, being embarrassed in public, or being contaminated); the patient has multiple worries, which often shift over time. Common worries include work responsibilities, money, health, safety, car repairs, and chores. To meet the criteria of the *Diagnostic and Statistical Manual of Mental Disorders,* Fourth Edition (DSM-IV), a person must also experience ≥ 3 of the following: restlessness, unusual fatigability, difficulty concentrating, irritability, muscle tension, or disturbed sleep. The course is usually fluctuating and chronic, with worsening during stress. Most people with GAD have one or more other comorbid psychiatric disorders, including major depression, specific phobia, social phobia, and panic disorder.

Treatment

Antidepressants, including SSRIs (eg, paroxetine, starting dose of 20 mg once/day), serotonin-norepinephrine reuptake inhibitors (eg, venlafaxine extended-release, starting dose 37.5 mg once/day), and tricyclics (eg, imipramine, starting dose 10 mg once/day), are effective but typically only after being taken for at least a few weeks. Benzodiazepines (anxiolytics—see TABLE 196–1) in small to moderate doses are also often effective, although sustained use usually causes physical dependence. One strategy involves starting with concomitant use of a benzodiazepine with an antidepressant. Once the antidepressant becomes effective, the benzodiazepine is tapered.

Buspirone is also effective at a starting dose of 5 mg bid or tid. However, buspirone can take at least 2 wk before it begins to help.

Psychotherapy, usually cognitive-behavioral therapy, can be both supportive and problem-focused. Relaxation and biofeedback may be of some help, although few studies have documented their efficacy.

OBSESSIVE-COMPULSIVE DISORDER

Obsessive-compulsive disorder is characterized by anxiety-provoking ideas, images, or impulses (obsessions) and by urges (compulsions) to do something that will lessen that anxiety. The cause is unknown. Diagnosis is based on history. Treatment consists of psychotherapy, drug therapy, or, in severe cases, both.

Obsessive-compulsive disorder occurs about equally in men and women and affects about 2% of the population.

TABLE 196–1. BENZODIAZEPINES

DRUG	STARTING ORAL DOSE	MAINTENANCE ORAL DOSE	ONSET/ DURATION
Alprazolam	0.25 mg bid; XR form, 0.5 mg once/day	1 mg tid; XR form, 3 mg once/day	Intermediate/intermediate
Chlordiazepoxide*	5 mg tid	25 mg tid	Intermediate/long
Clonazepam	0.25 mg once/day	1 mg tid	Intermediate†/long
Clorazepate*	7.5 mg bid	7.5 mg tid or 15 mg bid; SD form, 22.5 mg once/day after stabilized on 7.5 mg tid	Rapid/long
Diazepam*	2 mg tid	5 mg tid	Rapid/long
Lorazepam	0.5 mg tid	1 mg tid	Intermediate/short
Oxazepam	10 mg tid	15 mg qid	Slow/short

XR = extended release; SD = single dose (sustained release).
*Generally not recommended in the elderly because of substantial increase in half-life.
†A rapid-onset oral disintegrating tablet (wafer) is available.

Symptoms and Signs

The dominant theme of the obsessive thoughts may be harm, risk, or danger or contamination, doubt, loss, or aggression. Typically, affected people feel compelled to perform repetitive, purposeful rituals to balance their obsessions: eg, washing balances contamination; checking, doubt; and hoarding, loss. They may avoid people whom they fear behaving aggressively against. Most rituals, such as hand washing or checking locks, are observable, but some, such as repetitive counting or statements under one's breath, are not.

At some point, people with obsessive-compulsive disorder recognize that their obsessions do not reflect real risks and that the behaviors they perform to relieve their concern are unrealistic and excessive. Preservation of insight, although sometimes slight, differentiates obsessive-compulsive disorder from psychotic disorders, in which contact with reality is lost.

Because people with this disorder fear embarrassment or stigmatization, they often conceal their obsessions and rituals, on which they may spend several hours each day. Relationships often deteriorate, and performance in school or at work may decline. Depression is a common secondary feature.

Diagnosis and Treatment

Diagnosis is clinical based on criteria in the *Diagnostic and Statistical Manual of Mental Disorders,* Fourth Edition (DSM-IV).

Exposure and ritual prevention therapy is effective; its essential element is exposure to situations or people that trigger the anxiety-provoking obsessions and rituals. After exposure, the patient forgoes rituals, allowing the anxiety triggered by exposure to diminish through habituation. Improvement often continues for years, especially in patients who master the approach and use it even after formal treatment has ended. However, a few people have incomplete responses.

Many experts believe that combining psychotherapy and drug therapy is best, especially for severe cases. SSRIs (see p. 1708) and clomipramine (a tricyclic antidepressant with potent serotonergic effects) are effective. For most SSRIs, lower doses (eg, fluoxetine 20 mg once/day, fluvoxamine 100 mg once/day, sertraline 50 mg once/day, paroxetine 40 mg once/day) are often as effective as large ones.

PANIC ATTACKS AND PANIC DISORDER

A panic attack is the sudden onset of a discrete, brief period of intense discomfort or

fear accompanied by somatic or cognitive symptoms. Panic disorder is occurrence of repeated panic attacks typically accompanied by fears about future attacks or changes in behavior to avoid situations that might predispose to attacks. Diagnosis is clinical. Isolated panic attacks may not require treatment. Panic disorder is treated with drug therapy, psychotherapy (eg, exposure therapy, cognitive-behavioral therapy), or both.

Panic attacks are common, affecting as many as 10% of the population in a single year. Most people recover without treatment; a few develop panic disorder. Panic disorder is uncommon, affecting 2 to 3% of the population in a 12-mo period. Panic disorder usually begins in late adolescence or early adulthood and affects women 2 to 3 times more often than men.

Symptoms, Signs, and Diagnosis

A panic attack involves the sudden onset of at least 4 of the 13 symptoms listed in TABLE 196–2. Symptoms usually peak within 10 min and dissipate within minutes thereafter, leaving little for a physician to observe. Although uncomfortable—at times extremely so—panic attacks are not medically dangerous.

Panic attacks may occur in any anxiety disorder, usually in situations tied to the core features of the disorder (eg, a person with a phobia of snakes may panic upon seeing a snake). In pure panic disorder, however, some of the attacks occur spontaneously.

Most people who have a panic disorder anticipate and worry about another attack (anticipatory anxiety) and avoid places or situations where they have previously panicked. People with panic disorder often worry that they have a dangerous heart, lung, or brain disorder and repeatedly visit their family physician or an emergency department seeking help. Unfortunately, in these settings, attention is focused on physical symptoms, and the correct diagnosis often is not made. Many people with panic disorder also have symptoms of major depression.

Panic disorder is diagnosed after physical disorders that can mimic anxiety are eliminated and symptoms meet diagnostic criteria stipulated in the *Diagnostic and Statistical Manual of Mental Disorders*, Fourth Edition (DSM-IV).

Treatment

Some people recover without treatment, particularly if they continue to confront situations in which attacks have occurred. For others, especially without treatment, panic disorder follows a chronic waxing and waning course.

Patients should be told that treatment usually helps control symptoms. If avoidance behaviors have not developed, reassurance, education about anxiety, and encouragement to continue to return to and remain in places where panic attacks have occurred may be all that is needed. However, with a long-standing disorder that involves frequent attacks and avoidance behaviors, treatment is likely to require drug therapy combined with more intensive psychotherapy.

Many drugs can prevent or greatly reduce anticipatory anxiety, phobic avoidance, and the number and intensity of panic attacks. The different classes of antidepressants—SSRIs, serotonin-norepinephrine reuptake inhibitors (SNRIs), serotonin modulators, tricyclics (TCAs), and monoamine oxidase inhibitors (MAOIs)—are similarly effective. However, SSRIs and SNRIs offer a potential advantage of fewer adverse effects in comparison with other antidepressants. Benzodiazepines (anxiolytics—see TABLE 196–1) work more rapidly than antidepressants but are more likely to cause physical dependence and such adverse effects as somnolence, ataxia, and memory problems. Antidepressants and benzodiazepines are sometimes used in combination initially, with a slow taper from the benzodiazepine after the antidepressant

TABLE 196–2. SYMPTOMS OF A PANIC ATTACK

Cognitive

Fear of dying
Fear of going crazy or of losing control
Feelings of unreality, strangeness, or detachment from the environment

Somatic

Chest pain or discomfort
Dizziness, unsteady feelings, or faintness
Feeling of choking
Flushes or chills
Nausea or abdominal distress
Numbness or tingling sensations
Palpitations or accelerated heart rate
Sensations of shortness of breath or smothering
Sweating
Trembling or shaking

becomes effective. Panic attacks often recur when drugs are stopped.

Different forms of psychotherapy are effective. Exposure therapy, in which the patient confronts what he fears, helps diminish the fear and complications caused by fearful avoidance. For example, patients who fear fainting are asked to spin in a chair or to hyperventilate until they feel faint, thereby learning that they will not faint when experiencing that symptom. Cognitive-behavioral therapy involves teaching patients to recognize and control their distorted thinking and false beliefs and to modify their behavior so that it is more adaptive. For example, patients who describe acceleration of their heart rate or shortness of breath in certain situations or places and fear that they are having a heart attack are taught that their worries are unfounded and to respond instead with slow, controlled breathing or other methods that promote relaxation.

PHOBIC DISORDERS

Phobic disorders consist of persistent, unreasonable, intense fears (phobias) of situations, circumstances, or objects. The fears provoke anxiety and avoidance. Phobic disorders are classified as general (agoraphobia and social phobia) or specific. The causes of phobias are unknown. Phobic disorders are diagnosed based on history. Treatment for agoraphobia and social phobia is drug therapy, psychotherapy (eg, exposure therapy, cognitive-behavioral therapy), or both. Some phobias are treated mainly with exposure therapy.

Categories

Agoraphobia: Agoraphobia is fear of and anticipatory anxiety about being trapped in situations or places without a way to escape easily and without help if intense anxiety develops. The situations are avoided or they may be endured but with substantial anxiety. Agoraphobia can occur alone or as part of panic disorder.

Agoraphobia without panic disorder affects about 4% of women and 2% of men during any 12-mo period. Peak age at onset is the early 20s; first appearance after age 40 is unusual. Common examples of situations or places that create fear and anxiety include standing in line at a bank or at a supermarket checkout, sitting in the middle of a long row in a theater or classroom, and using public transportation, such as a bus or an airplane. Some people develop agoraphobia after a panic attack in a typical agoraphobic situation. Others simply feel uncomfortable in such a situation and may never, or only later, have panic attacks there. Agoraphobia often interferes with function and, if severe enough, can cause a person to become housebound.

Social phobia (social anxiety disorder): Social phobia is fear of and anxiety about being exposed to certain social or performance situations. These situations are avoided or endured with substantial anxiety. People with social phobia recognize that their fear is unreasonable and excessive.

Social phobia affects about 9% of women and 7% of men during any 12-mo period, but the lifetime prevalence may be at least 13%. Men are more likely than women to have the most severe form of social anxiety, avoidant personality disorder (see p. 1720).

Fear and anxiety in people with social phobia often centers on being embarrassed or humiliated if they fail to meet expectations. Often the concern is that anxiety will be apparent through sweating, blushing, vomiting, or trembling (sometimes as a quavering voice) or that the ability to keep a train of thought or find words to express oneself will be lost. Usually, the same activity performed alone produces no anxiety. Situations in which social phobia is common include public speaking, acting in a theatrical performance, and playing a musical instrument. Other potential situations include eating with others, signing one's name before witnesses, or using public bathrooms. A more generalized type of social phobia produces anxiety in a broad array of social situations.

Specific phobias: A specific phobia is fear of and anxiety about a particular situation or object. The situation or object is usually avoided when possible, but if exposure occurs, anxiety quickly develops. The anxiety may intensify to the level of a panic attack. People with specific phobias typically recognize that their fear is unreasonable and excessive.

Specific phobias are the most common anxiety disorders. Among the most frequent are fear of animals (zoophobia), heights (acrophobia), and thunderstorms (astraphobia, brontophobia). Specific phobias affect about 13% of women and 4% of men during any 12-mo period. Some cause little inconvenience—eg, fear of snakes (ophidiophobia) in a city dweller, unless he is asked to hike in an area where snakes are found. However, others interfere severely with functioning—eg, fear of closed places (claustrophobia), such as elevators, in a person who must work on an upper floor of a skyscraper. Phobia of blood (hemophobia), injections and pins (trypanophobia, belonephobia), or injury (traumatophobia) occurs to some degree in at least 5% of the population. People with a phobia of blood, needles, or injury, unlike those with other phobias or anxiety disorders, can actually faint because an excessive vasovagal reflex produces bradycardia and orthostatic hypotension.

Diagnosis

Diagnosis is clinical based on criteria in the *Diagnostic and Statistical Manual of Mental Disorders*, Fourth Edition (DSM-IV).

Prognosis and Treatment

If untreated, agoraphobia usually waxes and wanes in severity. Agoraphobia may disappear without formal treatment, possibly because some affected people conduct their own form of exposure therapy. But if agoraphobia interferes with functioning, treatment is needed. Social phobia is almost always chronic, and treatment is needed. The prognosis for specific phobias is more variable when untreated, because it may be easy to avoid the situation or object that causes fear and anxiety.

Because many phobic disorders involve avoidance, exposure therapy, a form of psychotherapy, is the treatment of choice. With structure and support from a clinician, patients seek out, confront, and remain in contact with what they fear and avoid until their anxiety is gradually relieved through a process called habituation. Exposure therapy helps > 90% of those who carry it out faithfully and is almost always the only treatment needed for specific phobias. Cognitive-behavioral therapy is effective for agoraphobia and social phobia. Cognitive-behavioral therapy involves teaching patients to recognize and control their distorted thinking and false beliefs as well as instructing them on exposure therapy. For example, patients who describe acceleration of their heart rate or shortness of breath in certain situations or places learn that their worries about having a heart attack are unfounded and are taught to respond with slow, controlled breathing or other methods that promote relaxation when in those situations.

Very short-term therapy with a benzodiazepine (eg, lorazepam 0.5 to 1.0 mg po) or a β-blocker (propranolol is generally preferred—10 to 40 mg po), ideally about 1 to 2 h before the exposure, is occasionally useful when exposure to an object or situation cannot be avoided (eg, when a person who has a phobia of flying must fly on short notice) or when cognitive-behavioral therapy is either unwanted or has not been successful.

Many people with agoraphobia also have panic disorder, and many of them benefit from drug therapy with an SSRI. SSRIs and benzodiazepines are effective for social phobia, but SSRIs are probably preferable in most cases, because unlike benzodiazepines, they are unlikely to interfere with cognitive-behavioral therapy. β-Blockers are useful for performance phobia.

STRESS DISORDERS

Stress disorders can take the form of acute stress disorder or posttraumatic stress disorder.

Acute Stress Disorder

Acute stress disorder is a brief period of intrusive recollections occurring very soon after a witnessed or experienced overwhelming traumatic event.

In acute stress disorder, the person has been through a traumatic event, has recurring recollections of the trauma, avoids stimuli that remind him of the trauma, and has increased arousal. Symptoms begin within 4 wk of the traumatic event and last a minimum of 2 days but, unlike posttraumatic stress disorder, last no more than 4 wk. A person with this disorder experiences 3 or more dissociative symptoms: a sense of numbing, detachment, or absence of emotional responsiveness; reduced awareness of surroundings (eg, being dazed); a feeling that things are not real; a feeling that he is not real; or amnesia for an important part of the trauma.

Many people recover once they are removed from the traumatic situation and shown understanding, empathy, and an opportunity to describe what happened and their reaction to it. Some experts recommend systematic debriefing to assist those who were involved in or witness to the traumatic event as they process what has happened and reflect on its effect. In one approach to debriefing, the event is referred to as the critical incident and the debriefing is referred to as critical incident stress debriefing (CISD). Other experts have expressed concern that CISD may be not be as helpful as supportive, empathic interviewing and may be quite distressful for some patients.

Drugs to assist sleep may help, but other drugs are generally not indicated.

Posttraumatic Stress Disorder

Posttraumatic stress disorder is recurring, intrusive recollections of an overwhelming traumatic event. The pathophysiology of the disorder is incompletely understood. Symptoms also include avoidance of stimuli associated with the traumatic event, nightmares, and flashbacks. Diagnosis is based on history. Treatment consists of exposure therapy and drug therapy.

When terrible things happen, many people are lastingly affected; in some, the effects are so persistent and severe that they are debilitating and constitute a disorder. Generally, events likely to evoke posttraumatic stress disorder (PTSD) are those that invoke feelings of fear, helplessness, or horror. These events might include experiencing serious injury or the threat of death or witnessing others being seriously injured, threatened with death, or actually dying.

Lifetime prevalence approaches 8%, with a 12-mo prevalence of about 5%.

Symptoms, Signs, and Diagnosis

Most commonly, patients have frequent, unwanted memories replaying the triggering event. Nightmares of the event are common. Much rarer are transient waking dissociative states in which events are relived as if happening (flashback), sometimes causing the patient to react as if in the original situation (eg, loud noises such as fireworks might trigger a flashback of being in combat, which in turn might cause a person to seek shelter or prostrate himself on the ground for protection).

The person avoids stimuli associated with the trauma and often feels emotionally numb and disinterested in daily activities. Sometimes the onset of symptoms is delayed, occurring many months or even years after the traumatic event. PTSD is considered chronic if present > 3 mo. Depression, other anxiety disorders, and substance abuse are common in people with chronic PTSD.

In addition to trauma-specific anxiety, patients may experience guilt because of their actions during the event or because they survived when others did not.

Diagnosis is clinical based on criteria in the *Diagnostic and Statistical Manual of Mental Disorders*, Fourth Edition (DSM-IV).

Treatment

If untreated, chronic PTSD often diminishes in severity without disappearing, but some people remain severely handicapped. The primary form of psychotherapy used, exposure therapy, involves exposure to situations that the person avoids because they may trigger recollections of the trauma. Repeated exposure in fantasy to the traumatic experience itself usually lessens distress after some initial increase in discomfort. Stopping certain ritual behaviors, such as excessive washing to feel clean after a sexual assault, also helps.

Drug therapy is effective, particularly with SSRIs (see p. 1708). Drugs with mood-stabilizing effects, such as valproate, carbamazepine, and topirimate, can help reduce arousal, nightmares, and flashbacks.

Because the anxiety is often intense, supportive psychotherapy plays an important role. Therapists must be openly empathic and sympathetic, recognizing and acknowledging patients' mental pain and the reality of the traumatic events. Therapists must also encourage patients to face the memories through behavioral desensitization and learning techniques to control anxiety. For survivor guilt, psychotherapy aimed at helping patients understand and modify their self-critical and punitive attitudes may be helpful.

197 DISSOCIATIVE DISORDERS

Everyone occasionally experiences a failure in the normal automatic integration of memories, perceptions, identity, and consciousness. For example, a person may drive somewhere and then realize that he does not remember many aspects of the drive because of preoccupation with personal concerns, a program on the radio, or conversation with a passenger. Typically, such a failure, referred to as dissociation, does not disrupt everyday activities.

People with a dissociative disorder may totally forget a series of normal behaviors occupying minutes or hours and may sense missing a period of time in their experience. Dissociation thus disrupts the continuity of self and the recollection of life events; when memory is poorly integrated, dissociative amnesia is present. When identity is fragmented along with memory, dissociative fugue or dissociative identity disorder is present. When the experience and perception of self are disrupted, depersonalization disorder is present.

Dissociative disorders are usually attributed to overwhelming stress. Such stress may be generated by traumatic events or by intolerable inner conflict.

DEPERSONALIZATION DISORDER

Depersonalization disorder consists of persistent or recurrent feelings of being detached from one's body or mental processes, usually with a feeling of being an outside observer of one's life. It is often triggered by severe stress. Diagnosis is by history. Treatment consists of psychotherapy.

The experience of depersonalization is common, frequently occurring in connection with life-threatening danger, such as accidents, assaults, and serious illnesses and injuries; it can occur as a symptom in many mental disorders and seizure disorders. When depersonalization occurs independently of any other mental or physical disorder and is persistent or recurrent, depersonalization disorder is present. It is estimated to occur in about 2% of the general population.

Symptoms, Signs, and Diagnosis

Patients have a distorted perception of themselves, their bodies, and their lives, which can make them profoundly uncomfortable. A person may feel unreal, as if he is an automaton or is dreaming. Often the symptoms are transient and accompanied by anxiety, panic, or phobic symptoms. However, symptoms can be chronic.

Patients often have great difficulty describing their symptoms and may fear or believe they are going crazy. They always retain the knowledge that their "unreal" experiences are not real but, rather, are just the way that they feel.

Diagnosis is based on the symptoms, after ruling out physical disorders, substance abuse, and other general mental disorders (especially anxiety and depression) and other dissociative disorders. Psychologic tests and special interviews are helpful.

Prognosis and Treatment

The feeling of depersonalization is often transient and resolves spontaneously. Even when it persists or is recurrent, some patients are minimally impaired if they can suppress the feeling of depersonalization by keeping their mind busy and focusing on other thoughts. Other patients become disabled by the chronic sense of estrangement or by the accompanying anxiety or depression.

Complete recovery is possible for many patients, especially those whose symptoms occur in connection with stresses that can be dealt with in treatment and those whose symptoms have not been protracted. Some patients gradually improve without intervention. Some may progress to more chronic and refractory depersonalization.

Treatment must address all stresses associated with the onset of the disorder as well as earlier stresses, such as childhood emotional abuse or neglect, which may have predisposed patients to later mental insults that trigger the onset of depersonalization. Various psychotherapies (eg, psychodynamic psychotherapy, cognitive behavior therapy, hypnosis) are successful for some patients. Cognitive techniques can help block obsessive thinking about the unreal state of being. Behavioral techniques can help patients engage in tasks that distract them from the depersonalization. Grounding techniques may help patients feel more well-grounded and real in the moment.

Other mental disorders, which are often associated with or precipitated by depersonalization, must be treated. Anxiolytics and antidepressants help some patients, mainly those in whom coexisting anxiety or depression accentuates the depersonalization.

DISSOCIATIVE AMNESIA

Dissociative amnesia is an inability to recall important personal information that is too extensive to be explained by normal forgetfulness. The cause is usually trauma or severe stress. Diagnosis is based on history after ruling out other causes. Treatment is psychotherapy, sometimes combined with hypnosis or drug-facilitated interviews.

The information lost would normally be part of conscious awareness that could be described as autobiographic memory—eg, who one is; what one did; where one went; to whom one spoke; what was said, thought, experienced, and felt. The forgotten information sometimes continues to influence behavior.

The incidence is unknown, but dissociative amnesia is most commonly diagnosed in young adults. The amnesia appears to be caused by traumatic or stressful experiences endured or witnessed (eg, physical or sexual abuse, rape, combat, abandonment during natural disasters, death of a loved one, financial troubles) or tremendous internal conflict (eg, turmoil over guilt-ridden impulses, apparently unresolvable interpersonal difficulties, criminal behaviors).

Symptoms, Signs, and Diagnosis

The main symptom is memory loss. Characteristically, one or more episodes are experienced, in which some patients forget some, but not all, events that occurred during a period of time; others cannot recall any information. These periods, or gaps in memory, may represent only a few hours or can encompass years or even an entire lifetime. Usually the forgotten period of time is clearly demarcated. Patients seen shortly after they become amnestic may appear confused and depressed. Some are very distressed, whereas others are indifferent.

Diagnosis requires a medical and psychiatric examination, including blood and urine tests to rule out toxic causes, such as illicit drug use. An EEG can help rule out a seizure disorder as the cause. Psychologic tests can help characterize the nature of the dissociative experiences.

Prognosis and Treatment

Most patients recover their missing memories and resolve their amnesia. However, some are never able to reconstruct their missing past. The prognosis is determined mainly by the patient's life circumstances, particularly stresses and conflicts associated with the amnesia, and by the patient's overall mental adjustment.

If the loss of memory is of a very short time period, treatment other than supportive intervention may not be warranted, especially if the necessity or benefit of recovering the memory of some painful event is not apparent. Treatment for more severe memory loss begins with creation of a safe and supportive environment. This measure alone frequently leads to gradual recovery of missing memories. When it does not or when the need to recover memories is urgent, questioning the patient while he is under hypnosis or, rarely, in a drug-induced (methohexital) semihypnotic state is often successful. These strategies are performed gently, because the circumstances that stimulated memory loss are likely to be recalled and to be very upsetting. The questioner must be careful to phrase questions so as not to suggest existence of an event and risk creating a false memory. The accuracy of memories recovered with such strategies can only be determined by external corroboration. However, regardless of the degree of historical accuracy, filling in the gap as much as possible is often therapeutically useful in restoring continuity to the patient's identity and sense of self and creating a cohesive narrative. Once the amnesia is lifted, treatment helps to give meaning to the underlying trauma or conflict and to resolve problems associated with the amnestic episode.

DISSOCIATIVE FUGUE

Dissociative fugue is one or more episodes of amnesia in which the inability to recall some or all of one's past is combined with either the loss of one's identity or the formation of a new identity. The episodes, called fugues, result from trauma or stress. Dissociative fugue often manifests as sudden, unexpected, purposeful travel away from home. Diagnosis is based on the history after ruling out other causes of amnesia. Treatment consists of psychotherapy, sometimes combined with hypnosis or drug-facilitated interviews, but response rates are low.

The incidence of dissociative fugue has been estimated at 0.2%, but the rate increases in connection with wars, accidents, and natural disasters.

Etiology

Causes are similar to those of dissociative amnesia (see p. 1679), with some additional factors. Fugues are often mistaken for malingering, because fugues may remove the person from accountability for his actions, absolve him of certain responsibilities, or reduce his exposure to hazardous situations. However, fugues are spontaneous, not planned, and not faked. Many fugues appear to represent disguised wish fulfillment. For example, a financially distressed executive leaves his hectic life and lives as a farm hand in the country. A fugue may remove the patient from an embarrassing situation or intolerable stress or may be related to issues of rejection or separation. For example, the fugue may say, in effect, "I am not the man who found his wife to be unfaithful." Some fugues may protect the person from suicidal or homicidal impulses.

Symptoms, Signs, and Diagnosis

The length of a fugue may range from hours to months, occasionally longer. During the fugue, the person may appear and act normal or is only mildly confused. The person may assume a new name and identity and engage in complex social interactions. However, at some point, confusion about the new identity or a return of the original identity may make the person aware of amnesia or cause distress. When the fugue ends, shame, discomfort, grief, depression, intense conflict, and suicidal or aggressive impulses may appear—the person must deal with what he left behind. Failure to remember events that occurred during the fugue may cause confusion, distress, or even terror.

A fugue in progress is rarely recognized. It is suspected when a person seems confused over his identity, puzzled about his past, or confrontational when his new identity is challenged. Often the fugue is not diagnosed until the person abruptly returns to his prefugue identity and is distressed to find himself in unfamiliar circumstances. The diagnosis is usually made retrospectively based on documentation of the circumstances before travel, the travel itself, and the establishment of an alternate life. When there is suspicion that a fugue is faked, cross-checking information from multiple sources may reveal inconsistencies that preclude the diagnosis.

Prognosis and Treatment

Most fugues are brief and self-limited. Impairment after the fugue ends is usually mild and short-lived. However, if the fugue was prolonged and complications due to behavior before or during the fugue are significant, the person may have considerable difficulties trying to return to his prefugue identity—eg, a soldier who returns after a fugue may be charged with desertion, or a person who marries during a fugue may have inadvertently become a bigamist.

In the rare case in which the person is identified while still in a fugue, recovering information (possibly with help from law enforcement and social services personnel) about his true identity, figuring out why it was abandoned, and facilitating its restoration are important.

Treatment after the fugue ends involves psychotherapy, sometimes combined with hypnosis or drug-facilitated (methohexital) interviews. However, efforts to restore memory of the fugue period are often unsuccessful. A psychiatrist may help the person explore his handling of the types of situations, conflicts, and moods that precipitated the fugue to help prevent recurrences.

DISSOCIATIVE IDENTITY DISORDER

Dissociative identity disorder, formerly called multiple personality disorder, is characterized by 2 or more identities or personalities that alternate and by an inability to recall important personal information relating to some of the identities. The cause is typically overwhelming childhood trauma. Diagnosis is based on history, sometimes supplemented by hypnosis or drug-facilitated interviewing. Treatment is psychotherapy, sometimes combined with drug therapy.

What is not known by one identity may be known by another. Some identities may appear to know and interact with others in an elaborate inner world.

Etiology

Dissociative identity disorder is attributed to the interaction of overwhelming stress (typically extreme mistreatment), insufficient nurturing and compassion in response to overwhelmingly hurtful experiences during childhood, and dissociative capacity (ability to uncouple one's memories, perceptions, or identity from conscious awareness).

Children are not born with a sense of a unified identity—it develops from many sources and experiences. In overwhelmed children, many parts of what should have blended together remain separate. Chronic and severe abuse (physical, sexual, or emotional) during childhood is frequently reported by and documented in patients with dissociative identity disorder. Some patients have not been abused but have experienced an important early loss (such as death of a parent), serious medical illness, or other overwhelmingly stressful events.

In contrast to most children who achieve cohesive, complex appreciation of themselves and others, severely mistreated children may go through phases in which different perceptions and emotions are kept segregated. Such children may develop an ability to escape the mistreatment by "going away" or "retreating" into their own mind. Each developmental phase may be used to generate different selves.

Symptoms and Signs

Several symptoms are characteristic: fluctuating symptom pictures; fluctuating levels of function, from highly effective to disabled; severe headaches or other bodily pain; time distortions, time lapses, and amnesia; and depersonalization and derealization. Depersonalization refers to feeling unreal, removed from one's self, and detached from one's physical and mental processes. The patient feels like an observer of his life, as if he were watching himself in a movie. Patients may even feel as if transiently they do not inhabit their bodies. Derealization refers to experiencing familiar people and surroundings as if they were unfamiliar, strange, or unreal.

Patients may discover objects, productions, or samples of handwriting that they cannot account for or recognize. They may refer to themselves in the first person plural (we) or in the third person (he, she, they).

The switching of identities and the amnestic barriers between them frequently result in chaotic lives. Because the identities often interact with each other, patients typically report hearing inner conversations between other personalities, which comment on or address the patient. Thus, a patient may be misdiagnosed with psychosis. Although these voices are experienced as hallucinations, they have a distinctly different quality from the typical hallucinations of psychotic disorders like schizophrenia.

Patients often have a remarkable array of symptoms that can resemble those of anxiety disorders, mood disorders, posttraumatic stress disorder, personality disorders, eating disorders, schizophrenia, and seizure disorders. Suicidal ideation and attempts are common, as are episodes of self-mutilation. Many affected patients abuse substances.

Diagnosis

Patients typically give histories of having had 3 or more different mental disorders and of prior treatment failures. The skepticism of some physicians regarding the validity of dissociative identity disorder can also contribute to misdiagnosis.

The diagnosis requires specific questions about dissociative phenomena. Prolonged interviews, hypnosis, or drug-facilitated (methohexital) interviews are sometimes used, and the patient may be asked to keep a journal between visits. All of these measures encourage a shift of personality states during the evaluation. Specially designed questionnaires can help.

The psychiatrist may also attempt to directly contact other identities by asking to speak to the part of the mind involved in behaviors for which the patient had amnesia or that were experienced in a depersonalized or derealized fashion.

Prognosis

Symptoms wax and wane spontaneously, but dissociative identity disorder does not resolve spontaneously. Patients can be divided into 3 groups. Those in the 1st group have mainly dissociative symptoms and posttraumatic features and generally function well and recover completely with treatment. Those in a 2nd group have dissociative symptoms combined with symptoms of other disorders, such as personality disorders, mood disorders, eating disorders, and substance abuse disorders. They improve more slowly, and treatment may be less successful or longer and more crisis-ridden. Patients in the 3rd group not only have severe symptoms from coexisting mental disorders but also may remain emotionally attached to their alleged abusers. These patients often require long-term treatment, which typically aims to help control symptoms more than to achieve integration.

Treatment

Integration of the identity states is the most desirable outcome. Medications help manage symptoms of depression, anxiety, impulsivity, and substance abuse, but treatment to achieve integration centers on psychotherapy. For patients who cannot or will not strive for integration, treatment aims to facilitate cooperation and collaboration among the identities and to reduce symptoms.

The first priority of psychotherapy is to stabilize the patient and ensure safety, before evaluating traumatic experiences and exploring problematic identities. Some patients benefit from hospitalization, in which continuous support and monitoring are provided as painful memories are addressed. Hypnosis is often used to explore traumatic memories and diffuse their effect. Hypnosis may also help with accessing the identities, facilitating communication between them, and stabilizing and interpreting them. As the reasons for the dissociations are addressed, therapy can move to the point at which the patient's selves and relationships and social functioning can be reconnected, integrated, and rehabilitated. Some integration occurs spontaneously. Integration can be encouraged by negotiating with and arranging the unification of the identities or facilitated with imagery and hypnotic suggestion.

198 DRUG USE AND DEPENDENCE

Among people who use drugs, some do so in large enough amounts often enough and long enough to become dependent. A single definition for drug dependence is elusive. Concepts that aid in defining drug dependence are tolerance and psychologic and physical dependence.

Tolerance describes the need to progressively increase the drug dose to produce the effect originally achieved with smaller doses.

Psychologic dependence includes feelings of satisfaction and a desire to repeat the drug experience or to avoid the discontent of not having it. This anticipation of effect is a powerful factor in the chronic use of psychoactive drugs and, with some drugs, may be the only obvious factor associated with intense craving and apparent compulsive use. Craving and compulsion to use a drug leads to its use in larger amounts or over a longer period than was intended when use began. Psychologic dependence involves giving up social, occupational, or recreational activities because of drug use and persistent use despite knowledge of having a physical or mental problem that is likely caused or exacerbated by using the drug. Drugs that cause psychologic dependence often have one or more of the following effects: reduced anxiety and tension; elation, euphoria, or other mood changes pleasurable to the user; feelings of increased mental and physical ability; altered sensory perception; and changes in behavior. Drugs that cause chiefly psychologic dependence include marijuana, amphetamine, 3,4-methylenedioxymethamphetamine (MDMA), and hallucinogens, such as lysergic acid diethylamide (LSD), mescaline, and psilocybin.

Physical dependence is manifested by a withdrawal (abstinence) syndrome, in which untoward physical changes occur when the drug is stopped or when its effect is counteracted by a specific antagonist that displaces the agonist from its binding site on cell receptors. Drugs that cause strong physical dependence include heroin, alcohol, and cocaine.

Addiction, a concept without a consistent, universally accepted definition, is used in this chapter to refer to compulsive use and overwhelming involvement with a drug, including spending an increasing amount of time obtaining the drug, using the drug, or recovering from its effects; it may occur without physical dependence. Addiction implies the risk of harm and the need to stop drug use, regardless of whether the addict understands and agrees.

Drug abuse is definable only in terms of societal disapproval. It may involve experimental and recreational use of drugs, which is usually illegal; unsanctioned or illegal use of psychoactive drugs to relieve problems or symptoms; or use of drugs first for the previous 2 reasons but later because of dependence and the need to continue at least partially to prevent withdrawal. Illicit drug use, although considered abuse simply because it involves illegality, does not always involve dependence. Conversely, use of legal substances, such as alcohol, may involve dependence and abuse. Abuse of prescription and illegal drugs cuts across socioeconomic groups and includes people with advanced education and professional status.

Recreational drug use has increasingly become a part of Western culture, although in general, it is not sanctioned by society. Some users apparently are unharmed; they tend to use drugs episodically in relatively small doses, precluding clinical toxicity and development of tolerance and physical dependence. Many recreational drugs (eg, crude opium, alcohol, marijuana, caffeine, hallucinogenic mushrooms, coca leaf) are "natural," ie, close to plant origin; they contain a mixture of relatively low concentrations of psychoactive compounds and are not isolated psychoactive chemicals. Recreational drugs are most often taken orally or inhaled. Taking these drugs by injection makes it harder to predict and control desired and unwanted effects. Recreational use is often accompanied by ritualization, with a set of observed rules, and is seldom practiced alone. Most drugs used this way are psychostimulants or hallucinogens designed to induce a "high" or altered consciousness rather than to relieve mental distress; depressant drugs are difficult to use in this controlled way.

Intoxication refers to development of a reversible substance-specific syndrome of mental and behavioral changes that may involve cognitive impairment, impaired judgment, impaired physical and social functioning, mood lability, and belligerence.

In the US, the Comprehensive Drug Abuse Prevention and Control Act of 1970 and subsequent modifications require the pharmaceutical industry to maintain physical security and strict record keeping for certain of these classes. Controlled substances are divided into 5 schedules (or classes) on the basis of their potential for abuse, accepted medical use, and accepted safety under medical supervision. Schedule I substances have a high potential for abuse, no accredited medical use, and a lack of accepted safety. Schedule V substances are least likely to be abused. The schedule classification determines how a substance must be controlled. Schedule I drugs can be used only under government-approved research conditions. Prescriptions for Schedule II to IV drugs must bear the physician's federal Drug Enforcement Administration (DEA) license number. Some drugs in Schedule V do not require a prescription. State schedules may vary from federal schedules.

Etiology of Drug Dependence

Commonly used psychoactive drugs vary in their potential for creating dependence. Drug dependence develops in a manner both complex and unclear. The process is influenced by the properties of the psychoactive drugs; the user's predisposing physical characteristics (probably including genetic predisposition), personality, and socioeconomic class; and the cultural and social setting. The psychology of the user and the availability of the drug determine the choice of psychoactive drug and, at least initially, the pattern and frequency of use.

Progression from experimentation to occasional use and then to dependence is only partially understood. Factors leading to increased use and dependence or addiction may include peer or group pressure, emotional distress that is symptomatically relieved by specific drug effects, sadness, social alienation, and environmental stress (particularly if accompanied by feelings of impotence to effect change or to accomplish goals). Physicians may inadvertently contribute to harmful use of psychoactive drugs by overzealously prescribing them to patients under stress and may fall victim to manipulative patients. Many social factors and the mass media may contribute to the expectation that drugs can safely relieve distress or gratify needs. Stated simply, the outcome of drug use depends on interaction between the drug, the user, and the setting.

Few differences exist between the biochemical, drug dispositional, and physical responsiveness of people who become addicted or dependent and those who do not, although such differences have been vigorously sought. Exceptions exist, however; nonalcoholic relatives of alcoholics have a diminished physical response to alcohol. Because of their higher tolerance, they need to drink more to get the desired effect.

A neural substrate for reinforcement (the tendency to seek more drugs and other stimuli) has been identified in animal models. In these studies, self-administration of such drugs as opioids, cocaine, amphetamine, nicotine, and benzodiazepines (anxiolytics) is associated with enhanced dopaminergic transmission in specific midbrain and cortical circuits. This finding suggests the existence of a brain reward pathway involving dopamine in the mammalian brain. However, evidence that hallucinogens and cannabinoids activate this system is insufficient, and not everyone who experiences these "rewards" becomes dependent or addicted.

An addictive personality has been described variously by behavioral scientists, but little scientific evidence backs this claim. Some experts describe addicts as escapists, ie, people who cannot face reality and who run away. Others describe addicts as people with schizoid traits, such as fearfulness, withdrawal from others, feelings of depression, and a history of frequent suicide attempts and numerous self-inflicted injuries. Addicts have also been described as dependent and grasping in their relationships, frequently exhibiting overt, unconscious rage and immature sexuality. However, before people develop drug dependence, they generally do not exhibit the deviant, pleasure-oriented, irresponsible behavior usually attributed to addicts. Clinicians, patients, and the culture often perceive drug abuse within the context of a dysfunctional life or life episode yet blame the drug exclusively rather than place any blame on the addict's psychologic characteristics. Sometimes addicts justify drug use as a way to alleviate temporary anxiety or depression resulting from a crisis, job pressure, or a family catastrophe. Most addicts abuse alcohol along with other drugs, and they may have repeated hospital admissions for overdose, adverse reactions, or withdrawal problems.

ALCOHOL

Excessive alcohol use can result in serious physical and mental problems. Chronic excessive use that involves a compulsion to drink, increased tolerance, and withdrawal symptoms is called alcohol dependence or, alternatively, alcoholism.

Alcohol abuse generally refers to a maladaptive pattern of episodic drinking resulting in failure to fulfill obligations, exposure to physically hazardous situations, legal problems, or social and interpersonal problems without evidence of dependence.

Alcohol dependence refers to frequent consumption of large amounts of alcohol over time, resulting in tolerance, psychologic dependence, and physical dependence and a dangerous withdrawal syndrome. Alcoholism is often used as an equivalent term for alcohol dependence, especially when drinking results in significant clinical toxicity and tissue damage.

About ⅔ of American adults drink alcohol. The male:female ratio is about 4:1. Lifetime prevalence of alcohol abuse and dependence combined is about 15%.

People who abuse or who are dependent on alcohol usually experience serious social consequences from their drinking. Frequent intoxication is obvious and destructive; it interferes with the ability to socialize and work. Eventually, drunkenness may lead to failed relationships as well as job loss due to absenteeism. People may be arrested for drunkenness or be apprehended for driving while intoxicated, adding to the social consequences they incur from their drinking. In the US, the legal blood alcohol concentration (BAC) while driving is ≤ 80 mg/dL (0.08%) in most states.

Female alcoholics are, in general, more likely to drink alone and are less likely to experience some of the social stigma. Alcoholics may seek medical treatment for their drinking. Eventually, they may be hospitalized for delirium tremens (DT) or cirrhosis. Injuries are common. The earlier in life these behaviors are evident, the more crippling the disorder.

Etiology of Disorders

Drinking to the point of becoming intoxicated or forming a maladaptive pattern of drinking that constitutes alcohol abuse begins with a desire to reach a state of feeling high. Some drinkers who find the feeling rewarding then focus on repeatedly reaching that state.

Certain personality traits are more common in those who abuse alcohol chronically or become dependent on alcohol: isolation, loneliness, shyness, depression, dependency, hostile and self-destructive impulsivity, and sexual immaturity. Alcoholics frequently come from a broken home and have a disturbed relationship with their parents. Societal factors—attitudes transmitted through the culture or child rearing—affect patterns of drinking and consequent behavior.

The incidence of alcoholism is higher in biologic children of alcoholics than in adoptive children, and the percentage of children of alcoholics who are problem drinkers is greater than that of the general population. Thus, in some populations and countries, prevalence is high. There is evidence of genetic or biochemical predisposition, including data that suggests some people who become alcoholics are less easily intoxicated, ie, they have a higher threshold for CNS effects.

Symptoms and Signs

Acute use: Alcohol is absorbed into the blood, principally from the small bowel. It accumulates in blood because absorption is more rapid than oxidation and elimination. About 5 to 10% of ingested alcohol is excreted unchanged in urine, sweat, and expired air; the remainder is oxidized to CO_2 and water at a rate of 5 to 10 mL/h (of absolute alcohol); each milliliter furnishes about 7 kcal. Alcohol chiefly depresses the CNS.

A BAC of 50 mg/dL produces sedation or tranquility; 50 to 150 mg/dL, lack of coordination; 150 to 200 mg/dL, delirium; and 300 to 400 mg/dL, unconsciousness. BAC > 400 mg/dL may be fatal. Sudden death from either respiratory depression or arrhythmias may occur when large quantities are drunk rapidly. This problem is emerging in US colleges but has been known in other countries in which the syndrome is more common.

Chronic use: People who drink large amounts of alcohol repetitively over time become tolerant to its effects, such that eventually, similar amounts have less of an intoxicating effect. Tolerance is caused by adaptational changes of CNS cells (cellular, or pharmacodynamic, tolerance). People who develop tolerance may reach an incredibly high BAC. However, ethanol tolerance is incomplete, and some degree of intoxication and impairment occurs with a high-enough dose. Even tolerant drinkers may die of respiratory depression secondary to alcohol overdose. Alcohol-tolerant people are susceptible to alcoholic ketoacidosis (see p. 1292), especially during binge drinking. Alcohol-tolerant people are cross-tolerant to many other CNS depressants (eg, barbiturates, nonbarbiturate sedatives, benzodiazepines).

The physical dependence accompanying tolerance is profound, and withdrawal produces potentially fatal adverse effects. Alcoholism eventually leads to organ damage, most commonly hepatitis and cirrhosis (see p. 211); gastritis; pancreatitis; cardiomyopathy, often accompanied by arrhythmias; peripheral neuropathy (see p. 1903); and brain damage (including Wernicke's encephalopathy [see p. 1688], Korsakoff's psychosis [see p. 1689], Marchiafava-Bignami disease [see p. 1689] and alcoholic dementia).

A continuum of symptoms and signs accompanies alcohol withdrawal, usually beginning 12 to 48 h after cessation of intake. The mild withdrawal syndrome includes tremor, weakness, sweating, hyperreflexia, and GI symptoms. Some patients have generalized tonic-clonic seizures, but usually not more than 2 in short succession (alcoholic epilepsy, or rum fits).

Alcoholic hallucinosis follows abrupt abstinence from prolonged, excessive alcohol use. Symptoms include auditory illusions and hallucinations that frequently are accusatory and threatening; the patient is usually apprehensive and may be terrified by the hallucinations and by vivid, frightening dreams. The syndrome may resemble schizophrenia, although thought usually is not disordered and the history is not typical of schizophrenia. Symptoms do not resemble the delirious state of an acute organic brain syndrome as much as does DT or other pathologic reactions associated with withdrawal. Consciousness remains clear, and the signs of autonomic lability seen in DT are usually absent. When hallucinosis occurs, it generally precedes DT and is transient. Recovery usually occurs in 1 to 3 wk; recurrence is likely if the patient resumes drinking.

DT usually begins 48 to 72 h after alcohol withdrawal along with anxiety attacks, increasing confusion, poor sleep (accompanied by frightening dreams or nocturnal illusions), marked sweating, and profound depression. Fleeting hallucinations that arouse restlessness, fear, and even terror are common. Typical of the initial delirious, confused, and disoriented state is a return to a habitual activity; eg, the patient frequently imagines that he is back at work and attempts to perform some related activity. Autonomic lability, evidenced by diaphoresis and increased pulse rate and temperature, accompanies the delirium and progresses with it. Mild delirium is usually accompanied by marked diaphoresis, a pulse rate of 100 to 120 beats/min, and a temperature of 37.2 to 37.8° C. Marked delirium, with gross disorientation and cognitive disruption, is associated with significant restlessness, a pulse of > 120 beats/min, and a temperature of > 37.8° C.

During DT, the patient is suggestible to many sensory stimuli, particularly to objects seen in dim light. Vestibular disturbances may cause the patient to believe that the floor is moving, the walls are falling, or the room is rotating. As the delirium progresses, resting tremor of the hand develops, sometimes extending to the head and trunk. Ataxia is marked; care must be taken to prevent self-injury. Symptoms vary among patients but are usually the same for a particular patient with each recurrence.

Treatment

Acute use: When people drink to the point of intoxication, the 1st priority of treatment is to stop them from drinking any additional alcohol, which could lead to unconsciousness and death. The 2nd priority is to ensure their safety and the safety of others by preventing drinkers from operating a motor vehicle or any other mode of transportation or from engaging in any other activity that would create a high risk of death or injury while impaired by alcohol. Somnolent patients may become alert and combative as their BAC decreases.

Chronic use: Medical evaluation is needed initially to detect intercurrent illness that might complicate withdrawal and to rule out CNS injury that might mimic or be masked by the withdrawal syndrome. Withdrawal symptoms must be identified and treated. Steps must be taken to prevent Wernicke-Korsakoff syndrome (see p. 1689).

Some drugs commonly used to treat withdrawal resemble alcohol in their pharmacologic effects. All patients entering withdrawal are candidates for CNS depressants, but not all need them. Many patients can be detoxified without drugs if proper attention is paid to psychologic support and reassurance and if the approach and environment are nonthreatening. However, these methods may not be possible in general hospitals or emergency departments.

Benzodiazepines are the mainstay of therapy. Dosage depends on vital signs and mental status. In most situations, chlordiazepoxide, initially 50 to 100 mg po, is recommended; doses may need to be repeated q 2 to 4 h. Diazepam, given 5 to 10 mg IV or po hourly until sedation occurs, is a useful alternative. Compared with short-acting benzodiazepines (lorazepam, oxazepam), long-acting benzodiazepines (eg, chlordiazepoxide, diazepam) provide less frequent dosing and, when the dose is tapered, a smoother decrease in serum levels. For significant liver disease, a short-acting benzodiazepine (lorazepam) or one metabolized by glucuronidation (oxazepam) is preferred. (NOTE: Benzodiazepines may cause intoxication, physical dependence, and withdrawal in alcoholics and therefore should not be continued after the detoxification period. Carbamazepine 200 mg po qid may be used as an alternative and then tapered.)

Isolated seizures need no specific therapy; repeated seizures respond to diazepam 1 to 3 mg IV. Routine administration of phenytoin is unnecessary. Outpatient therapy with phenytoin is almost always a waste of time and drug, because seizures occur only under the stress of alcohol withdrawal, and patients who are withdrawing or heavily drinking do not take their anticonvulsants.

Although DT may begin to resolve within 24 h, it may be fatal and thus must be treated promptly. Patients with DT are extremely suggestible and respond well to reassurance. They generally should not be restrained. Fluid balance must be maintained, and large doses of B and C vitamins, particularly thiamin, must be given promptly. Appreciably elevated temperature with DT is a poor prognostic sign. If improvement is not marked within 24 h, other disorders, such as subdural hematoma, a hepatic or renal disorder, or other mental disturbances, should be suspected.

Maintenance: Maintaining sobriety is difficult. The patient should be warned that after a few weeks, when he has recovered from his last bout, he is likely to find an excuse to drink. He should also be told that he may be able to practice controlled drinking for a few days or, rarely, a few weeks, but he will most likely lose control eventually.

A rehabilitation program is often the best approach. Most inpatient rehabilitation programs last 3 to 4 wk and are conducted in a center that does not permit leaving for the duration of the course of treatment. Rehabilitation programs combine medical supervision and psychotherapy, including one-on-one and group therapy. Psychotherapy involves techniques that enhance motivation and teach patients to avoid circumstances that precipitate drinking. Social support of abstinence is important, including the support of family and friends.

Alcoholics Anonymous (AA) has benefited alcoholics more than any other approach. The patient must find an AA group in which he is comfortable. AA provides the patient with nondrinking friends who are always available and a nondrinking environment in which to socialize. The patient also hears others confess before the group every rationalization he has ever used for his own drinking. The help he gives other alcoholics may give him the self-regard and confidence formerly found only in alcohol. In the US, unlike in other countries, AA groups include a high proportion of nonvoluntary enrollees whose attendance is mandated by court or probation officer order. Many alcoholics are reluctant to go to AA and find individual counseling or group or family treatment more acceptable. Alternative organizations, such as LifeRing Recovery (Secular Organizations for Sobriety), exist for those seeking a more secular approach.

Drug therapy should be used in combination with psychotherapy. Disulfiram interferes with the metabolism of acetaldehyde (an intermediary product in the oxidation of alcohol) so that acetaldehyde accumulates. Drinking alcohol within 12 h of taking disulfiram produces facial flushing in 5 to 15 min, then intense vasodilation of the face and neck with suffusion of the conjunctivae, throbbing headache, tachycardia, hyperpnea, and sweating. With high doses of alcohol, nausea and vomiting may follow in 30 to 60 min and may lead to hypotension, dizziness, and sometimes fainting and collapse. The reaction can last up to 3 h. Few patients risk ingesting alcohol while taking disulfiram because of the intense discomfort. Drugs that contain alcohol (eg, tinctures; elixirs; some OTC liquid cough/cold preparations, which contain as much as 40% alcohol) must also be avoided. Disulfiram is contraindicated during pregnancy and in patients with cardiac decompensation. It may be given on an outpatient basis after 4 or 5 days of abstinence. The initial dosage is 0.5 g po once/day for 1 to 3 wk, followed by a maintenance dosage of 0.25 g once/day. Effects may persist for 3 to 7 days after the last dose. Periodic physician visits are needed to encourage continuation of disulfiram as part of an abstinence program. Disulfiram's general usefulness has not been established, and many patients are noncompliant. Compliance usually requires adequate social support, such as observation of ingestion.

Naltrexone, an opioid antagonist (see p. 1699), decreases the relapse rate in most patients who take it consistently. Naltrexone is given as 50 mg po once/day. It is unlikely to be useful without supportive counseling. Acamprosate, a synthetic analogue of gamma-aminobutyric acid, is given as 2 g po once/day. Acamprosate decreases the relapse rate and drinking days in patients who relapse; like naltrexone, it works best when combined with counseling. Nalmefene and topiramate are under investigation for their ability to decrease alcohol craving.

WERNICKE'S ENCEPHALOPATHY

Wernicke's encephalopathy is a disorder characterized by acute onset of confusion, nystagmus, partial ophthalmoplegia, and ataxia due to thiamin deficiency. Diagnosis is primarily clinical. The disorder may remit with treatment, persist, or degenerate into Korsakoff's psychosis. Treatment consists of thiamin and supportive measures.

Wernicke's encephalopathy results from inadequate intake or absorption of thiamin plus continued carbohydrate ingestion. Severe alcoholism is a common underlying condition. Excessive alcohol intake interferes with thiamin absorption from the GI tract and hepatic storage of thiamin; the poor nutrition associated with alcoholism often precludes adequate thiamin intake. Wernicke's encephalopathy may also result from other conditions that cause prolonged undernutrition or vitamin deficiency (eg, recurrent dialysis, hyperemesis, starvation, gastric plication, cancer, AIDS). Loading carbohydrates in patients with thiamin deficiency (ie, refeeding after starvation or giving IV dextrose-containing solutions to high-risk patients) can trigger Wernicke's encephalopathy.

Not all thiamin-deficient alcohol abusers develop Wernicke's encephalopathy, suggesting that other factors may be involved. Genetic abnormalities that result in a defective form of transketolase, an enzyme that processes thiamin, may be involved.

Characteristically, lesions are symmetrically distributed around the 3rd ventricle, aqueduct, and 4th ventricle. Changes in the mamillary bodies, dorsomedial thalamus, locus ceruleus, periaqueductal gray matter, ocular motor nuclei, and vestibular nuclei are common.

Symptoms and Signs

Clinical changes occur acutely. Oculomotor abnormalities, including horizontal and vertical nystagmus and partial ophthalmoplegias (eg, lateral rectus palsy, conjugate gaze palsies), are common. Pupils may be abnormal; they are usually sluggish or unequal.

Vestibular dysfunction without hearing loss is common, and the oculovestibular reflex may be impaired. Gait ataxia may result from vestibular disturbances and cerebellar dysfunction, gait is wide-based and slow, with short-spaced steps.

Global confusion is often present, characterized by profound disorientation, indifference, inattention, drowsiness, or stupor. Peripheral nerve pain thresholds are often elevated, and many patients develop severe autonomic dysfunction characterized by sympathetic hyperactivity (eg, tremor, agitation) or hypoactivity (eg, hypothermia, postural hypotension, syncope). In untreated patients, stupor may progress to coma, then to death.

Diagnosis, Prognosis, and Treatment

Diagnosis is clinical and depends on recognition of underlying undernutrition or vitamin deficiency. There are no characteristic abnormalities in CSF, evoked potentials, brain imaging, or EEG. However, these tests, as well as laboratory tests (eg, blood tests, glucose, CBC, liver function tests, arterial blood gas measurements, toxicology screening), should be done to rule out other etiologies.

Prognosis depends on timely diagnosis. If begun in time, treatment may correct all abnormalities. Ocular symptoms usually begin to abate within 24 h after early thiamin administration. Ataxia and confusion may persist days to months. Untreated, the disorder progresses; mortality is 10 to 20%. Of surviving patients, 80% develop Korsakoff psychosis (the combination is called Wernicke-Korsakoff syndrome).

Treatment consists of immediate administration of thiamin 100 mg IV or IM, continued daily for at least 3 to 5 days. Mg is a necessary cofactor in thiamin-dependent metabolism, and hypomagnesemia should be corrected using Mg sulfate 1 to 2 g IM or IV q 6 to 8 h or Mg oxide 400 to 800 mg po once/day. Supportive treatment includes rehydration, correction of electrolyte abnormalities, and general nutritional therapy, including multivitamins. Patients with advanced disease require hospitalization. Alcoholism cessation is mandatory.

Because Wernicke's encephalopathy is preventable, all malnourished patients should be treated with parenteral thiamin (typically 100 mg IM followed by 50 mg po daily) plus vitamin B_{12} and folate (both 1 mg/day po), particularly if IV dextrose is necessary. Thiamin is also prudent before any treatment is begun in patients who present with a reduced level of consciousness. Patients who are malnourished should continue to receive thiamin as outpatients.

KORSAKOFF'S PSYCHOSIS

Korsakoff's psychosis is a late complication of persistent Wernicke's encephalopathy that results in memory deficits, confusion, and behavioral changes.

Korsakoff's psychosis (Korsakoff's amnestic syndrome) occurs in 80% of untreated patients with Wernicke's encephalopathy. A severe or repeated attack of postalcoholic delirium tremens can trigger Korsakoff's psychosis whether or not a typical attack of Wernicke's encephalopathy has occurred first. Other triggers include subarachnoid hemorrhage, thalamic hemorrhage, thalamic ischemic stroke, and, infrequently, tumors affecting the paramedian posterior thalamic region. Why Korsakoff's psychosis develops in only some patients with Wernicke's encephalopathy is unclear.

Symptoms and Signs

Immediate memory is severely affected; retrograde and anterograde amnesia occurs in varying degrees. Patients tend to draw on memory of remote events, which appears to be less affected than memory of recent events. Disorientation to time is common. Emotional changes are common; they include apathy, blandness, or mild euphoria with little or no response to events, even frightening ones. Spontaneity and initiative may be decreased.

Confabulation is often a striking early feature; bewildered patients unconsciously fabricate imaginary or confused accounts of events they cannot recall; these fabrications may be so convincing that the underlying disorder is not detected.

Prognosis and Treatment

Prognosis is fairly good for patients with head injury, subarachnoid hemorrhage, or both; the amnesia is transient. Prognosis is poor when the cause is thiamin deficiency or infarct; prolonged institutional care is required for about 25% of patients, and only about 20% recover completely. However, they may improve up to 12 to 24 mo after onset, and patients should not be prematurely institutionalized. Treatment consists of thiamin and adequate hydration.

MARCHIAFAVA-BIGNAMI DISEASE

Marchiafava-Bignami disease is a rare demyelination of the corpus callosum that occurs in chronic alcoholics, predominantly men.

The pathology and circumstances link this disorder to osmotic demyelination syndrome (previously called central pontine myelinolysis), of which it may be a variant (see p. 1241). In Marchiafava-Bignami disease, agitation and confusion occur with progressive dementia and frontal release signs. Some patients recover over several months; others experience seizures and coma, which may precede death.

AMPHETAMINES

Amphetamines can be taken as pills, injected, snorted, or smoked. Amphetamines can cause elevated mood; increased wakefulness, alertness, concentration, and intensified physical performance; and a feeling of well-being. Prolonged use can cause dependence.

Among the drugs classified as amphetamines are amphetamine and methamphetamine (commonly known as ice, crystal, crystal meth, speed, crank, or glass).

Methamphetamine, sometimes used medically (for attention-deficit hyperactivity disorder, obesity, and narcolepsy), is easily manufactured illicitly, and its use has become widespread in Holland, Great Britain, and North America. Illicit use of methamphetamine is the chief type of amphetamine abuse in North America.

Symptoms and Signs

Acute use: The psychologic effects of using amphetamines are similar to those produced by cocaine and include alertness, euphoria, and feelings of competence and power. Amphetamines typically cause erectile dysfunction in men but enhance sexual desire. Use is associated with unsafe sex practices, and users are at higher risk of sexually transmitted infections, including HIV infection.

Chronic use: Repeated use of amphetamines has been shown to cause death of large numbers of brain cells. Repeated use also induces dependence. Tolerance develops slowly, but amounts several hundred-fold greater than the amount originally used may eventually be ingested or injected. Tolerance to various effects develops unequally, so that tachycardia and enhanced alertness diminish, but hallucinations and delusions may occur. However, even massive doses are rarely fatal. Long-term users have reportedly injected as much as 15,000 mg of amphetamine in 24 h without observable acute illness.

Amphetamine abusers are prone to accidents, because the drug produces excitation and grandiosity followed by excess fatigue and sleeplessness. Taken IV, amphetamine may lead to serious antisocial behavior and can precipitate a schizophrenic episode.

A paranoid psychosis may result from long-term use of high IV or oral doses. Rarely, the psychosis is precipitated by a single high dose or by repeated moderate doses. Typical features include delusions of persecution, ideas of reference, and feelings of omnipotence. People who use high IV doses usually accept that they will eventually experience paranoia and often do not act on it. Nevertheless, with very intense drug use or near the end of weeks of use, awareness may fail and the user may respond to the delusions. Recovery from even prolonged amphetamine psychosis is usual. Thoroughly disorganized and paranoid users recover slowly but completely. The more florid symptoms fade within a few days or weeks, but some confusion, memory loss, and delusional ideas commonly persist for months.

An exhaustion syndrome occurs with repeated use of methamphetamine, involving intense fatigue and need for sleep after the stimulation phase. Methamphetamine can also produce a psychosis in which the person misinterprets others' actions, hallucinates, and becomes unrealistically suspicious. Some users experience a prolonged depression, during which suicide is possible. Methamphetamine use has also led to deaths attributed to severe dehydration, disseminated intravascular coagulation, and renal failure. Users have a high rate of severe tooth decay affecting multiple teeth; causes involve decreased salivation, acidic combustion products, and poor oral hygiene.

Although no stereotypical withdrawal syndrome occurs upon stopping methamphetamine or other amphetamines, EEG changes occur, considered by some to fulfill the physical criteria for dependence. Abruptly stopping use may uncover underlying depression or precipitate a serious depressive reaction. Withdrawal is often followed by 2 or 3 days of intense fatigue or sleepiness and depression.

Treatment

Acute use: People in the acute agitated psychotic state, with paranoid delusions and auditory and visual hallucinations, respond well to phenothiazines; chlorpromazine 25 to 50 mg IM rapidly reverses this state but may produce severe postural hypotension. Haloperidol 2.5 to 5 mg IM is effective; it rarely produces hypotension but may produce an alarming acute extrapyramidal motor reaction. Usually, reassurance and a quiet, nonthreatening environment are conducive to recovery and are often all that is needed. Ammonium chloride 1 g po q 2 to 4 h to acidify the urine hastens amphetamine excretion.

Chronic use: Cognitive-behavioral therapy (a form of psychotherapy) is effective in some patients. Depression sometimes occurs when amphetamines are stopped and may respond to antidepressants if depressive symptoms persist for weeks.

ANABOLIC STEROIDS

Anabolic steroids are used to enhance physical performance and muscle growth. When used chronically at high doses and without medical supervision, they can cause erratic and irrational behavior and a wide range of physical adverse effects.

Anabolic steroids include testosterone and any drugs chemically and pharmacologically related to testosterone that promote muscle growth. Anabolic steroids have androgenic effects (eg, changes in hair or in libido, aggressiveness) and anabolic effects (eg, increased protein utilization, muscle mass changes). The androgenic effects cannot be separated from the anabolic, but some anabolic steroids have been synthesized to minimize the androgenic effects.

Testosterone is rapidly degraded by the liver; oral testosterone is inactivated too rapidly to be effective, and injectable testosterone must be modified (eg, by esterification) to retard absorption or delay breakdown. Analogs modified by 17-α-alkylation are often effective orally but may have increased adverse effects. Transdermal preparations also are available.

Adverse effects vary significantly by dose and drug. There are few adverse effects at physiologic replacement doses (eg, methyltestosterone 10 to 50 mg/day or its equivalent). Athletes may use doses of 10 to 50 times this range. At high doses, some effects are clear, whereas others are equivocal (see TABLE 198–1). Uncertainties exist because most studies involve abusers who may not report doses accurately and who also use black market drugs, many of which are counterfeit and contain (despite labeling) varying doses and substances.

Anabolic steroids are used clinically to treat low testosterone levels (see Male Hypogonadism on p. 1944). Additionally, because anabolic steroids are anticatabolic and improve protein utilization, they are sometimes given to burn, bedridden, or other debilitated patients to prevent muscle wasting. Some physicians prescribe them to patients with AIDS-related wasting and to those with cancer. There are few data, however, to recommend such therapy and little guidance on how supplemental androgens may affect underlying diseases. Testosterone has been reputed to benefit wound healing and muscle injury, although there are no data to support these claims.

Anabolic steroids are abused to increase lean muscle mass and strength; these effects are enhanced when combined with resistance training and proper diet. There is no direct evidence that anabolic steroids increase endurance or speed, but substantial anecdotal evidence suggests that athletes taking them can perform more frequent high-intensity workouts. Muscle hypertrophy is unequivocal.

Estimates of lifetime incidence of anabolic steroid abuse range from 0.5 to 5% of the population, but subpopulations vary significantly (eg, higher rates in bodybuilders and competitive athletes). In the US, the reported rate of use is 6 to 11% among high school–aged males, including an unexpected number of nonathletes, and about 2.5% among high school–aged females.

TABLE 198–1. ADVERSE EFFECTS OF ANABOLIC STEROIDS

Clearly demonstrated
- Erythrocytosis
- Abnormal lipid profile (decreased HDL, increased LDL)
- Liver abnormalities: peliosis hepatitis, adenoma
- Mood disorders (with high dose)
- Androgenic effects: acne, baldness, virilization and hirsutism in females
- Gonadal suppression (decreased sperm count, testicular atrophy)
- Gynecomastia
- Premature closure of epiphyses

Equivocal
- Hypertension/LVH
- Worsening of prostatic hypertrophy or preexisting carcinoma
- Hepatic carcinoma

Poorly shown
- Increased risk of sudden death in athletes
- Significant mood disorder with low dose
- Predominantly with 17α-alkylated agents

HDL = high-density lipoprotein; LDL = low-density lipoprotein; LVH = left ventricular hypertrophy.

Athletes may take steroids for a certain period, stop, then start again (cycling) several times a year. Intermittent discontinuation of the drugs is believed to allow endogenous testosterone levels, sperm count, and the hypothalamic-pituitary-gonadal axis to return to normal. Anecdotal evidence suggests that cycling may decrease harmful effects and the need for increasing drug doses to attain the desired effect.

Athletes frequently use many drugs simultaneously (a practice called stacking) and alternate routes of administration (oral, IM, or transdermal). Increasing the dose through a cycle (pyramiding) may result in doses 5 to 100 times the physiologic dose. Stacking and pyramiding are intended to increase receptor binding and minimize adverse effects, but these benefits have not been proved.

Symptoms and Signs

The most characteristic sign is a rapid increase in muscle bulk. The rate and extent of increase is directly related to the doses taken. Patients taking physiologic doses will have slow and often unnoticeable growth; those taking mega-doses may increase lean body weight at several pounds/mo. Increases in energy level and libido (in men) occur but are more difficult to identify.

Psychologic effects (generally only with very high doses) are often noticed by the family: wide and erratic mood swings, irrational behavior, increased aggressiveness ("roid rage"), irritability, increased libido, and depression.

Increased acne and gynecomastia are common complaints, as are virilizing effects in females. Some of these effects (eg, alopecia, enlarged clitoris, hirsutism, deepened voice) may be irreversible. Additionally, breast size may decrease; vaginal mucosa may atrophy; menstruation may change or stop; libido may increase or, less commonly, decrease; and aggressiveness and appetite may increase.

Diagnosis, Prevention, and Treatment

A urine screen usually detects users of anabolic steroids. Metabolites of anabolic steroids can be detected in urine up to 6 mo (even longer for some types of anabolic steroids) after the drugs are stopped.

Physicians caring for adolescents and young adults should be alert to the signs of steroid abuse and educate patients about its risks. Education about anabolic steroids should start by the beginning of middle school.

ANXIOLYTICS AND SEDATIVES

Use of anxiolytics and sedatives (hypnotics) for medical purposes is common. Intoxication, with physical and mental impairment, can occur with acute use. Repetitive use can lead to abuse or dependence.

Tolerance and tachyphylaxis develop irregularly and incompletely, so considerable behavioral, mood, and cognitive disturbances persist, even in a regular user, depending on the dosage and the drug's pharmacodynamic effects. Some cross-tolerance exists between alcohol and barbiturates and nonbarbiturate anxiolytics and sedatives, including benzodiazepines. (Barbiturates and alcohol are strikingly similar in the dependence, withdrawal symptoms, and chronic intoxication they produce.) When intake of anxiolytics and sedatives is reduced below a critical level, a self-limited withdrawal syndrome ensues.

Symptoms and Signs

Acute use: The signs of progressive anxiolytic and sedative intoxication are depression of superficial reflexes, fine lateral-gaze nystagmus, slightly decreased alertness with coarse or rapid nystagmus, ataxia, slurred speech, and postural unsteadiness. Further progression results in nystagmus on forward gaze, somnolence, marked ataxia with falling, confusion, deep sleep, constricted pupils, respiratory depression, and, ultimately, death. Patients taking large doses of sedatives frequently have difficulty thinking, slow speech and comprehension (with some dysarthria), poor memory, faulty judgment, narrowed attention span, and emotional lability.

Chronic use: In susceptible patients, psychologic dependence on the drug may develop rapidly, and after only a few weeks, attempts to stop using the drug exacerbate insomnia and result in restlessness, disturbing dreams, frequent awakening, and feelings of tension in the early morning. The extent of physical dependence is related to dose and duration of use; eg, pentobarbital 200 mg/day taken for many months may not induce significant tolerance, but 300 mg/day for > 3 mo or 500 to 600 mg/day for 1 mo may induce a withdrawal syndrome when the drug is stopped.

Withdrawal from barbiturates taken in large doses produces an abrupt withdrawal syndrome in the form of a severe, frightening, and potentially life-threatening illness similar to delirium tremens. Occasionally, even after properly managed withdrawal over 1 to 2 wk, a seizure occurs. Within the first 12 to 20 h after withdrawal of a short-acting barbiturate, the untreated patient becomes increasingly restless, tremulous, and weak. By the 2nd day, the tremulousness becomes more prominent, deep tendon reflexes may be increased, and the patient becomes weaker. During the 2nd and 3rd days, seizures occur in 75% of patients who were taking ≥ 800 mg/day. Seizures may progress to status epilepticus and death. From the 2nd to the 5th day, the untreated withdrawal syndrome includes delirium, insomnia, confusion, and frightening visual and auditory hallucinations. Hyperpyrexia and dehydration often occur.

Withdrawal from benzodiazepines produces a similar withdrawal syndrome, although it is rarely as severe or life threatening. Onset may be slow because the drugs remain in the body a long time. A withdrawal syndrome of varying severity has been reported in people who have taken therapeutic doses, although the prevalence of this unusual phenomenon is unknown. Withdrawal may be most severe in those who used drugs with rapid absorption and quick decline in serum levels (eg, alprazolam, lorazepam, triazolam). Many people who misuse benzodiazepines have been or are heavy users of alcohol, and a delayed benzodiazepine withdrawal syndrome may complicate alcohol withdrawal.

Treatment

Acute intoxication generally requires nothing more than observation. On occasion, intoxication is severe enough to require respiratory support. The benzodiazepine receptor antagonist flumazenil can be used for treatment of severe sedation secondary to benzodiazepine overdose. Its clinical usefulness is not well defined, because most people who overdose on benzodiazepines recover without intervention. Occasionally, when used to reverse sedation, flumazenil precipitates seizures.

The procedure for managing dependence on sedatives, particularly barbiturates, is to withdraw the drug on a strict schedule, monitoring signs of withdrawal. Often it is best to switch to a long-acting compound, which is easier to taper. Before withdrawal is begun, sedative tolerance can be evaluated with a test dose of pentobarbital 200 mg po given to a nonintoxicated, fasting patient; if the patient is not tolerant, the dose produces drowsiness or shallow sleep 1 to 2 h later. A patient with intermediate levels of tolerance may show some sedation; a patient tolerant of ≥ 900 mg shows no signs of intoxication. If the 200-mg dose has no effect, the tolerance level can be determined by repeating the test q 3 to 4 h with a larger dose. Severe anxiety or agitation may increase the patient's tolerance. Once the 24-h dose still tempered by tolerance is determined, that dose is usually given qid for 2 or 3 days to stabilize the patient and is then decreased by 10%/day. Withdrawal should be undertaken in the hospital. Once the withdrawal syndrome has begun, reversing it is difficult, but with close monitoring, symptoms can be minimized. The reestablishment of CNS stability requires about 30 days.

Alternatively, phenobarbital can be used. It does not produce the high of more rapidly acting drugs. Rapid-onset barbiturates, other sedatives, or minor anxiolytics can be replaced by a dose of phenobarbital equivalent to ⅓ the average daily dose of the drug on which the patient is dependent; eg, for secobarbital 1000 mg/day, the stabilizing dose of phenobarbital is 300 mg/day, typically given as 75 mg q 6 h. Phenobarbital is given orally qid, and the initial phenobarbital dose is reduced by 30 mg/day until the patient is drug-free. Because the initial daily dose must be estimated from the patient's history, a potential for error exists, and the patient must be observed closely for the first 72 h. If he remains agitated or anxious, the dose should be increased; if he is drowsy or dysarthric or has nystagmus, the dose should be decreased. While the patient is being detoxified, other sedatives and psychoactive drugs should be avoided. However, if the patient is also taking antidepressants, especially tricyclics, the antidepressant should not be abruptly stopped; the dose should be reduced over 3 to 4 days.

COCAINE

High doses of cocaine can cause euphoric excitement or schizophrenic-like symptoms. Psychologic and physical dependence can lead to profound addiction.

Most cocaine users are episodic recreational users who voluntarily curtail their use. However, cocaine use and the development of addictive behavior in some users has increased in North America, although recent declines are recorded. Availability of highly biologically active forms, such as crack cocaine, has worsened the problem of cocaine dependence.

Although most cocaine in the US is snorted, smoking crack cocaine has become widely publicized. The hydrochloride salt is converted to a more volatile form, usually by adding $NaHCO_3$, water, and heat. The converted material is combusted and the resultant smoke inhaled. Onset of effect is quicker, and intensity of the high is magnified. Crack use has not expanded to the suburbs or to the urban middle class: Low-income Americans continue to be the primary users.

Tolerance to cocaine occurs, and withdrawal from heavy use is characterized by somnolence, increased appetite, and depression.

The tendency to continue taking the drug is strong after a period of withdrawal.

Symptoms and Signs

Acute use: Effects differ with different modes of use. When injected or smoked, cocaine produces hyperstimulation, alertness, euphoria, and feelings of competence and power. The excitation and high are similar to those produced by injecting amphetamine. These feelings are less intense and disruptive in users who snort cocaine powder.

An overdose may produce tremors, seizures, and delirium. Death may result from MI, arrhythmias, and heart failure. Patients with extreme clinical toxicity may, on a genetic basis, have decreased (atypical) serum cholinesterase, an enzyme needed for clearance of cocaine. The concurrent use of cocaine and alcohol produces a condensation product, cocaethylene, which has stimulant properties and may contribute to toxicity.

Chronic use: Because cocaine is a very short-acting drug, heavy users may inject it or smoke it q 10 to 15 min. This repetition produces toxic effects, such as tachycardia, hypertension, mydriasis, muscle twitching, sleeplessness, and extreme nervousness. Hallucinations, paranoid delusions, and aggressive behavior may develop, which can make the person dangerous. Pupils are maximally dilated, and the drug's sympathomimetic effect increases heart and respiration rates and BP.

Severe toxic effects occur in the compulsive heavy user. Rarely, repeated snorting causes nasal septal perforation due to local ischemia. Repeatedly smoking volatile crack cocaine in high doses can have serious toxic cardiovascular and behavioral consequences.

Treatment

Treatment of acute cocaine intoxication is generally unnecessary because the drug is extremely short-acting. If an overdose requires intervention, IV barbiturates or diazepam may be used, but close observation and supportive care is the appropriate approach. Anticonvulsants do not prevent seizures due to cocaine overdose. Hyperthermia or significantly elevated BP, which rarely results, must be treated.

Stopping sustained use requires considerable assistance, and the depression that may result requires close supervision and treatment. Many nonspecific therapies, including support and self-help groups and cocaine hotlines, exist. Extremely expensive inpatient therapy is available.

Treatment of infants born to cocaine-addicted mothers is discussed under Prenatal Drug Exposure on p. 2283.

GAMMA HYDROXYBUTYRATE

Gamma hydroxybutyrate causes intoxication resembling alcohol or ketamine intoxication and can lead to respiratory depression and death, especially when combined with alcohol.

Gamma hydroxybutyrate (GHB, also called "G") is taken by mouth. It is similar to ketamine in its effects but lasts longer and is far more dangerous.

GHB produces feelings of relaxation and tranquility. It may also cause fatigue and disinhibition. At higher doses, GHB may produce dizziness and loss of coordination, nausea, and vomiting. Seizures and coma may also occur and can lead to respiratory failure and death. Combining GHB and any other sedative, especially alcohol, is extremely dangerous. Most deaths have occurred when GHB was taken with alcohol.

Withdrawal symptoms occur if GHB is not taken for several days after previous frequent use.

Treatment is needed only for overdose. Use of a ventilator may be needed if breathing is affected. Most people recover rapidly, although effects may not fade for 1 to 2 h.

HALLUCINOGENS

Hallucinogens can cause intoxication, with altered perception and impaired judgment. Chronic use can further impair judgment and lead to depression, anxiety, or psychosis.

Hallucinogens include lysergic acid diethylamide (LSD), psilocybin, and mescaline. Some other drugs, including marijuana, also have hallucinogenic properties. The term hallucinogen persists, although use of these drugs may not produce hallucinations. Alternative terms, such as psychedelic and psychotomimetic, are even less appropriate.

Symptoms and Signs

Acute use: Hallucinogens induce intoxication in the form of CNS excitation and central autonomic hyperactivity manifested as changes in perception and mood (usually euphoric, sometimes depressive). True hallucinations are rare.

Responses to the hallucinogens depend on several factors, including the user's expectations, his ability to cope with perceptual distortions, and the setting. Untoward reactions (anxiety attacks, extreme apprehensiveness, or panic states) to LSD are rare. Most often, these reactions quickly subside with appropriate treatment in a secure setting. However, some people (especially after using LSD) remain disturbed and may show a persistent psychotic state. Whether drug use has precipitated or uncovered a preexisting psychotic potential or can produce this state in a previously stable person is unresolved.

Chronic use: The main features of chronic use are the psychologic effects and impaired judgment, which can lead to dangerous decision making or accidents. A high degree of tolerance for LSD develops and disappears rapidly. Users tolerant of any of these drugs are cross-tolerant of the others. Psychologic dependence varies greatly but usually is not intense, and no evidence of physical dependence is detected when the drugs are abruptly withdrawn.

Some people, especially those who are long-term or repeat users (particularly of LSD), experience apparent drug effects long after they have stopped drug use. These episodes (flashbacks) most commonly consist of visual illusions but can include distortions of virtually any sensation (including self-image or perceptions of time or space) and hallucinations. Flashbacks can be precipitated by use of marijuana, alcohol, or barbiturates or by stress or fatigue or can occur without apparent reason. The mechanisms of flashbacks are not known. Flashbacks tend to subside within 6 to 12 mo.

Treatment

Acute use: Reassurance that the bizarre thoughts, visions, and sounds are due to the drug and not to a nervous breakdown usually suffices. Phenothiazine antipsychotics must be used with extreme caution because of the danger of hypotension. Anxiolytics, such as chlordiazepoxide and diazepam, may help reduce frightening anxiety.

Chronic use: Withdrawal is usually easily accomplished; some people may need psychiatric treatment for associated problems. A helpful relationship with a physician, with frequent contact, can be beneficial.

Persistent psychotic states or other mental disorders require appropriate psychiatric care. Flashbacks that are transient or not unduly distressing to the patient require no special treatment. However, flashbacks associated with anxiety and depression may require therapy similar to that for acute adverse reactions.

KETAMINE

Ketamine (also called "K" or Special K) can cause intoxication, sometimes with confusion or a catatonic state. Overdose can cause collapse.

Ketamine is an anesthetic. When used illicitly, it is generally snorted.

A giddy euphoria occurs with lower doses, often followed by bursts of anxiety or mood lability. Higher doses produce a withdrawn state (disassociation); when doses are higher still, disassociation can become severe (known as a "K-hole") with ataxia, dysarthria, muscular hypertonicity, and myoclonic jerks. Cardiovascular status is usually unaffected. With very high doses, coma and severe hypertension may occur; deaths are unusual. Acute effects generally fade after 30 min.

The patient should be kept in a nonstimulatory environment and closely observed. Further treatment is rarely needed.

MARIJUANA (CANNABIS)

Marijuana is the most commonly used illicit drug. Psychologic dependence can develop with chronic marijuana use, but there is very little clinically apparent physical dependence.

Any drug that causes euphoria and diminishes anxiety can cause dependence, and marijuana is no exception. However, heavy use and reports of inability to stop are unusual. Marijuana is most commonly used episodically without evidence of social or psychologic dysfunction. A mild withdrawal syndrome may occur similar to that of benzodiazepine withdrawal when the drug is stopped, but some heavy users report disrupted sleep and nervousness when they stop.

In the US, marijuana is commonly smoked in cigarettes made from the flowering tops and leaves of the dried plant or as hashish, the pressed resin of the plant. Dronabinol, a synthetic form of Δ-9-tetrahydrocannabinol (the principal active constituent of marijuana), is used to treat nausea and vomiting associated with cancer chemotherapy and to enhance appetite in AIDS patients. This form is not sold on the street.

Symptoms and Signs

Smoked marijuana produces a dreamy state of consciousness in which ideas seem disconnected, unanticipated, and free-flowing. Time, color, and spatial perceptions may be altered. In general, a feeling of well-being and relaxation (a high) results. These effects last 2 to 3 h after inhalation. There is no persuasive evidence of a prolonged or hangover effect. Tachycardia, conjunctival injection, and dry mouth occur regularly. Many of the psychologic effects seem to be related to the setting in which the drug is taken. Panic reactions and paranoia have occurred, particularly in naive users, but have become unusual as the culture has become more familiar with the drug. Communicative and motor abilities are decreased, depth perception and tracking are impaired, and the sense of timing is altered—all hazardous in certain situations (eg, driving, operating heavy equipment). Appetite often increases. Psychotic symptoms may be exacerbated or even precipitated in schizophrenics by marijuana, even in patients being treated with antipsychotics.

Critics of marijuana cite much scientific data regarding adverse effects, but most of the claims regarding severe biologic impact are unsubstantiated. Findings are sparse even among relatively heavy users and in areas intensively investigated, such as immunologic and reproductive function. However, high-dose smokers develop pulmonary symptoms (episodes of acute bronchitis, wheezing, coughing, and increased phlegm), and pulmonary function may be altered. Such alteration is manifested by large airway changes of unknown significance. Even daily smokers do not develop obstructive airway disease. Lung cancer has not been reported in people who smoke only marijuana, possibly because less smoke is inhaled than during cigarette smoking, and the smoke contains fewer carcinogenic substances. However, biopsies of bronchial tissue sometimes show precancerous changes, so cancer may occur. In a few case-control studies, diminished cognitive function was found in small samples of long-term high-dose users; this finding awaits confirmation.

The effect of prenatal marijuana use on newborns is not clearly known. Decreased fetal weight has been reported, but when all factors (eg, maternal alcohol and tobacco use) are accounted for, the effect on fetal weight decreases. Δ-9-Tetrahydrocannabinol is secreted in breast milk. Although harm to breastfed babies has not been shown, breastfeeding mothers, as with pregnant women, should avoid using marijuana.

Because cannabinoid metabolites persist, urine tests after each use can remain positive for days or weeks after stopping use. Tests that identify an inactive metabolite identify use only, not dysfunction; the smoker may be free of drug effect by the time his urine is tested. The test can detect extremely small amounts and so is of little value in identifying the pattern of use.

METHYLENEDIOXYMETH-AMPHETAMINE

(Ecstasy)

3,4-Methylenedioxymethamphetamine (MDMA—commonly known as ecstasy or Adam or "E") is an amphetamine analog. MDMA is usually taken as a pill. It has both stimulant and hallucinogenic effects. Prolonged use can cause dependence.

MDMA is often used at dance clubs, concerts, and "rave" parties. Ecstasy produces a state of excitement and disinhibition and accentuates physical sensation. Like amphetamines, ecstasy energizes but to a far lesser extent. Unlike amphetamines, its use has not been associated with unsafe sexual practices and the spread of sexually transmitted diseases. Although the toxic effects of this drug remain controversial, the brain death caused by typical amphetamines has not been shown. The effects of intermittent, occasional use are uncertain. Fulminant hepatic failure may occur rarely. Chronic, repeated use may produce problems similar to that of amphetamines. Some users develop paranoid psychosis. Cognitive decline may also occur with repeated, frequent use. Treatment for dependency is similar to that for amphetamines, although treatment for acute overdose is rarely needed.

OPIOIDS

Use of opioids for medical purposes but without the supervision of health care practitioners and all use for nonmedical purposes can lead to consequences such as

delirium and injury. Chronic use can lead to dependence. Dependence is marked by an overpowering compulsion to continue taking opioids, the development of tolerance so that the dosage must be increased to obtain the initial effect, and physical dependence that increases in intensity with increased dosage and duration of use.

Dependence on opioids is increasing. Heroin is the most commonly used recreational opioid, whereas opium use is uncommon. Dependence on prescription analgesic opioids, such as morphine and oxycodone, is increasing, with some of the increase accounted for by people who are taking them for legitimate medical purposes. Additionally, many people find that opioid use allows them to bear what they once considered the unbearable stresses of life.

Physical dependence necessitates continued use of the same opioid or a related one to prevent withdrawal. Withdrawal of the drug or administration of an antagonist precipitates a characteristic, self-limited withdrawal syndrome.

Therapeutic doses taken regularly over 2 to 3 days can lead to some tolerance and dependence, and when the drug is stopped, the user may have mild withdrawal symptoms which are scarcely noticed or are flu-like.

Patients with chronic pain requiring long-term use should not be labeled addicts, although they may have some problems with tolerance and physical dependence. Opioids induce cross-tolerance so that abusers can substitute one for another. People who have developed tolerance may show few signs of drug use and may function normally in their usual activities, but obtaining the drug is an ever-present problem. Tolerance to the various effects of these drugs frequently develops unevenly. Heroin users, for example, may become largely tolerant to the drug's euphoric and lethal effects but continue to have constricted pupils and constipation.

Symptoms and Signs

Acute intoxication (overdose) is characterized by euphoria, flushing, itching (particularly with morphine), miosis, drowsiness, decreased respiratory rate and depth, hypotension, bradycardia, and decreased body temperature.

Physical dependence is suggested by a history of ≥ 3 opioid injections/day, fresh needle marks, withdrawal symptoms and signs, or morphine glucuronide in a urine specimen (heroin is biotransformed to morphine, conjugated with glucuronide, and excreted). Because heroin is often snorted, the nasal septum may be perforated.

The withdrawal syndrome generally includes symptoms and signs of CNS hyperactivity. Severity of the syndrome increases with the size of the opioid dose and the duration of dependence. Symptoms appear as early as 4 h after withdrawal and, for heroin, peak within 72 h. Anxiety and a craving for the drug are followed by increased resting respiratory rate (> 16 breaths/min), usually with yawning, perspiration, lacrimation, and rhinorrhea. Other symptoms include mydriasis, piloerection (gooseflesh), tremors, muscle twitching, hot and cold flashes, aching muscles, and anorexia. The withdrawal syndrome in people who were taking methadone (which has a long half-life) develops more slowly and is overtly less severe than heroin withdrawal, although users may describe it as worse.

Complications: Complications of heroin addiction may be related to the unsanitary administration of the drug or to the drug's inherent properties, overdose, or intoxicated behavior accompanying drug use. Common complications are pulmonary, bone, and neurologic disorders; hepatitis; and immunologic changes.

Aspiration pneumonitis, pneumonia, lung abscess, septic pulmonary emboli, and atelectasis may occur. Pulmonary fibrosis from talc granulomatosis may develop when opioid analgesic tablets are injected. Chronic heroin addiction results in a decreased vital capacity and a mild to moderate decrease in diffusion capacity. These effects are distinct from the pulmonary edema that may occur acutely with heroin injection. Many opioid addicts smoke ≥ 1 pack of cigarettes/day, making them particularly susceptible to a variety of pulmonary infections.

Viral hepatitis types A, B, and C may develop. The combination of viral hepatitis and the frequently high alcohol intake may account for the high incidence of liver dysfunction.

Osteomyelitis (particularly lumbar vertebral) is the most common musculoskeletal complication, probably due to hematogenous spread of organisms from unsterile injections. Infectious spondylitis and sacroiliitis may occur. In myositis ossificans (drug abuser's elbow), the brachialis muscle is damaged by inept needle manipulation, followed by replacement of the muscle bundle with a calcific mass (extraosseous metaplasia).

Hypergammaglobulinemia of both IgG and IgM occurs in ≤ 90% of addicts. The reason is unknown but may reflect repeated antigenic stimulation from infections or from daily parenteral injection of foreign substances. Hypergammaglobulinemia diminishes with methadone maintenance. Heroin addicts and other IV drug users are at extremely high risk of HIV infection and AIDS. In communities in which sharing of needles and syringes is common, the spread of AIDS is devastating.

Neurologic disorders in heroin addicts are usually noninfectious complications of coma and cerebral anoxia. Toxic amblyopia (apparently due to adulteration of heroin by quinine), transverse myelitis, various mononeuropathies and polyneuropathies, and Guillain-Barré syndrome may occur. Cerebral complications include those secondary to bacterial endocarditis (bacterial meningitis, mycotic aneurysm, brain abscess, and subdural and epidural abscesses), those due to viral hepatitis or tetanus, and acute cerebral falciparum malaria. Some neurologic complications may be due to allergic responses to the heroin-adulterant mixture.

Superficial cutaneous abscesses, cellulitis, lymphangitis, lymphadenitis, and phlebitis from contaminated needles may occur. Many heroin addicts begin with subcutaneous injections (skin popping) and may return to this mode when extensive scarring makes their veins inaccessible. As addicts become more desperate, cutaneous ulcers in unlikely sites may be found. Contaminated needles and inoculum may lead to bacterial endocarditis, hepatitis, and HIV infection. These complications follow frequent injection. Because heroin potency has recently increased, more users are snorting and smoking, which may diminish problems with infectious contamination.

Some problems of the heroin-addicted mother are transferred to the fetus. Because heroin and methadone freely cross the placental barrier, the fetus readily becomes physically dependent. A mother infected with HIV or hepatitis B virus may transmit the virus to her newborn. Pregnant addicts seen early enough should be encouraged to enter a methadone maintenance program. Abstinence is better for the fetus, but abstinent mothers often revert to heroin use and withdraw from prenatal care. Withdrawal of heroin or methadone from pregnant women late in the 3rd trimester may precipitate early labor; thus, pregnant women seen at or near term may best be stabilized with methadone rather than disturbed by attempts to withdraw opioids. The methadone-maintained mother may nurse her newborn without causing any apparent clinical problems in the child, because concentration of the drug in breast milk is minimal.

Infants of opioid-dependent mothers may present with tremors, a high-pitched cry, jitters, seizures (rarely), and tachypnea. Problems of the newborn, including drug withdrawal and fetal alcohol syndrome, are discussed under Prenatal Drug Exposure on p. 2283.

Treatment

Acute use: Overdose is usually managed with the opioid antagonist naloxone (0.4 to 2 mg IV) because it has no respiratory depressant properties (see also TABLE 326–8 on p. 2688). It rapidly reverses unconsciousness due to an opioid. Because some patients become agitated, delirious, and combative as they recover from a comatose state, physical restraints may be required and should be applied before the antagonist is given. All patients treated for overdose should be hospitalized and observed for at least 24 h because the action of naloxone is relatively short. Also, respiratory depression may recur within several hours, especially with methadone, at which time methadone should be re-administered at an appropriate dose. Severe pulmonary edema, which may cause death from hypoxia, is usually not responsive to naloxone and has an unclear relationship to overdose.

Chronic use: The clinical management of opioid addicts is extremely difficult. The AIDS epidemic has provoked a harm-reduction movement, seeking to offer services that reduce the harm of drug use without requiring cessation. For example, providing clean needles and syringes for injection users reduces the spread of HIV. Despite this evidence of harm reduction, US federal funding cannot be used to establish needle or syringe provision to IV users. Other harm-reduction approaches, including easy access to methadone or buprenorphine maintenance, alternative maintenance strategies, and eased restrictions on the prescribing of psychoactive drugs, are more prevalent in some European countries than in the US, where programs viewed as abetting drug consumption behavior are resisted.

Physicians must be fully aware of federal, state, and local regulations. Treatment is complicated by the need to deal with the societal attitudes toward the treatment of addicts (including the attitudes of law enforcement officers and other physicians and health care practitioners). In most cases, the physician should refer addicts to specialized treatment centers rather than attempt to care for them alone.

To legally use an opioid drug in treating an addict, a physician must establish the existence of physical opioid dependence. However, many addicts who seek treatment use low-grade heroin, which may not cause physical dependence. Low-grade opioid dependence (as may occur in people who have used opioid analgesics for a long time) can be treated by reducing the opioid dose slowly, by substituting a weak opioid (eg, propoxyphene), or by using benzodiazepines (which are not cross-tolerant to opioids) in decreasing doses.

The withdrawal syndrome is self-limited and, although severely uncomfortable, is not life threatening. Minor metabolic and physical withdrawal effects may persist up to 6 mo. Whether this protracted withdrawal syndrome contributes to relapse is unclear. The patient's drug-seeking behavior usually begins with the first symptoms of withdrawal, and hospital personnel must be aware that he will try to obtain drugs. Visitors may have to be restricted. Many patients with withdrawal symptoms have other medical problems that must be diagnosed and treated.

Methadone substitution is the preferred method of opioid withdrawal for more seriously addicted patients because of its long half-life and less profound sedation and euphoria. Methadone is given orally in the smallest amount (generally, 15 to 40 mg once/day) that will prevent severe but not necessarily all symptoms of withdrawal. Higher doses should be given when evidence of withdrawal is observed. Doses of ≥ 25 mg can produce unconsciousness if the person has not developed tolerance. After the appropriate dose has been established, it should be reduced progressively by not more than 20%/day. Patients commonly become angry and request additional medication. The withdrawal syndrome induced by methadone resembles that of heroin, but onset is more gradual and delayed, beginning 36 to 72 h after stopping the drug. Acute manifestations of withdrawal usually subside within 10 days, but patients often report deep muscle aches. Weakness, insomnia, and severe pervasive anxiety are common for several months. Methadone withdrawal for addicts coming from a methadone maintenance program may be particularly difficult because their dose of methadone may be as high as 100 mg once/day. In general, detoxification should be started by reducing the dose to 60 mg once/day over several weeks before attempting complete detoxification.

The central adrenergic drug clonidine can halt almost all signs of opioid withdrawal. It probably decreases central adrenergic outflow secondary to stimulation of central receptors (the same mechanism by which clonidine lowers BP). However, clonidine can cause hypotension and drowsiness, and its withdrawal may precipitate restlessness, insomnia, irritability, tachycardia, and headache. Clonidine may help people withdraw from heroin or methadone before they begin oral naltrexone treatment. The mixed opioid agonist-antagonist buprenorphine also has been successfully used in withdrawal.

Maintenance: No consensus exists regarding long-term treatment of opioid-dependent users. In the US, thousands of opioid addicts are in methadone maintenance programs, which are intended to meet the supply problems of addicts by providing large doses of oral methadone, thus enabling addicts to be socially productive. Methadone blocks the effects of injected heroin and alleviates the user's drug hunger. For many, the program has worked. However, the widespread use of methadone has provoked societal and political anger, and many people distrust its usefulness as treatment.

Buprenorphine, an agonist-antagonist, is available as maintenance treatment for opioid addicts and is becoming preferred over methadone. It blocks receptors, thereby interfering with illicit use of heroin or of other opioid analgesics. Buprenorphine can be prescribed by specially trained physicians certified by the federal government. Typical dose is an 8- or 16-mg tablet once/day. For many opioid addicts, this option is preferable to methadone maintenance because it eliminates the need for attending a methadone maintenance clinic.

Levomethadyl acetate (LAAM) is a longer-acting opioid related to methadone. QT interval abnormalities have been found in some patients taking LAAM. Its use is therefore discouraged, and patients receiving it are best transferred to methadone therapy. LAAM is used 3 times/wk, thereby diminishing the expense and the problems of daily client visits or take-home drugs. A dose of 100 mg 3 times/wk is comparable to methadone 80 mg once/day.

Naltrexone, an orally bioavailable opioid antagonist, blocks the effects of heroin. It has little agonist effect, and many opioid addicts will not voluntarily consume it. The usual dose is 50 mg once/day or 350 mg/wk in 2 or 3 divided doses.

The therapeutic community concept, pioneered by Daytop Village and Phoenix House, involves nondrug treatment in communal residential centers, where drug users receive training, education, and redirection to help them build new lives. Residency is usually 15 mo. These communities have helped, even transformed, some users. However, initial dropout rates are extremely high. How well these communities work, how many will be opened, and how much funding society will give remain unanswered.

VOLATILE NITRITES

Nitrites (poppers, as amyl, butyl, or isobutyl, sold as Locker Room and Rush) may be inhaled to enhance sexual pleasure. Use is particularly prominent among urban male homosexuals. There is little evidence of significant hazard, although nitrites and nitrates produce vasodilation, with brief hypotension, dizziness, and flushing, followed by reflex tachycardia (see also TABLE 326–8 on p. 2687). They are, however, dangerous when combined with drugs used for erectile enhancement; the combination can lead to severe hypotension and death.

VOLATILE SOLVENTS

Inhalation of volatile industrial solvents and solvents from aerosol sprays can produce a state of intoxication. Chronic use can result in neuropathies and hepatoxocity.

Use of volatile solvents continues to be an endemic problem among adolescents. About 10% of adolescents in the US have reportedly inhaled volatile solvents. Volatile solvents (eg, aliphatic and aromatic hydrocarbons, chlorinated hydrocarbons, ketones, acetates, ether, chloroform, alcohol) produce temporary stimulation before depressing the CNS. Partial tolerance and psychologic dependence develop with frequent use, but a withdrawal syndrome does not occur.

Acute symptoms of dizziness, drowsiness, slurred speech, and unsteady gait occur early. Impulsiveness, excitement, and irritability may occur. As effects on the CNS increase, illusions, hallucinations, and delusions develop. The user experiences a euphoric, dreamy high, culminating in a short period of sleep. Delirium with confusion, psychomotor clumsiness, emotional lability, and impaired thinking develops. The intoxicated state may last from minutes to > 1 h.

Complications of chronic use may result from the effect of the solvent or from other toxic ingredients, such as lead in gasoline. Carbon tetrachloride may cause a syndrome of hepatic and renal failure. Injuries to brain, liver, kidneys, and bone marrow may result from heavy exposure or hypersensitivity. Death most often results from respiratory arrest, arrhythmias, or asphyxia due to airway occlusion.

Treatment of solvent-dependent adolescents is difficult, and relapse is frequent. However, most users stop solvent use by the end of adolescence. Intensive attempts to broadly improve the patients' social skills and status in family, school, and society may help. For symptoms and treatment of poisoning with specific solvents, see throughout TABLE 326–8 on p. 2671.

SUBSTANCE USE IN CHILDREN AND ADOLESCENTS

Substance use disorders are common among children, especially in adolescents. Regardless of economic or ethnic background, alcohol, tobacco, and marijuana are consistently the most commonly used substances. Use of other substances, including amphetamines and methamphetamine, inhalants, hallucinogens, cocaine, anabolic steroids, opioids, and so-called date rape drugs and club drugs (eg, MDMA, ketamine, gamma hydroxybutyrate), is less common, and the prevalence of use of each is more variable over time. Of growing concern is a reported increase in random mixing of date rape and club drugs at parties.

Children and adolescents use drugs for a variety of reasons. Some may do so as a means of escaping from perceived pressures (eg, parental pressure, societal pressure), or of challenging authority. Influence of peers and portrayal of substances such as alcohol in the media are other commonly cited reasons. Parental attitudes and the examples that parents set in their own use of alcohol, tobacco, prescription drugs, and other substances are a powerful influence.

Primary care physicians should be prepared to provide their adolescent patients with adequate screening, counseling, and, when necessary, referral to other treatment services and resources.

199 EATING DISORDERS

Eating disorders are grouped into 3 categories: anorexia nervosa, bulimia nervosa, and binge eating disorder.

ANOREXIA NERVOSA

Anorexia nervosa is characterized by a relentless pursuit of thinness, a morbid fear of obesity, a refusal to maintain a minimally normal body weight, and, in women, amenorrhea. Diagnosis is clinical. Treatment is with cognitive-behavioral therapy; olanzapine may help with weight gain, and SSRIs, especially fluoxetine, may help prevent relapse.

Severe anorexia nervosa is uncommon, affecting < 0.5% of the general population. However, most mild cases are probably undiagnosed. About 95% of people with anorexia nervosa are female. Onset is usually during adolescence.

The exact etiology is unknown. Other than being female, few risk factors have been identified. In Western society, obesity is considered unattractive and unhealthy, and the desire to be thin is pervasive, even among children. More than 50% of prepubertal girls diet or take other measures to control their weight. Excessive concern about weight or a history of dieting appears to predict increased risk, potentially in people genetically predisposed to anorexia nervosa. Studies of identical twins have shown a concordance of >50%. Family and social factors probably play a role. Many patients belong to middle or upper socioeconomic classes; are meticulous, compulsive, and intelligent; and have very high standards for achievement and success.

Symptoms and Signs

Anorexia nervosa may be mild and transient or severe and long-standing. Most patients are lean yet are concerned about body weight and restrict food intake. Preoccupation and anxiety about weight increase, even as emaciation develops.

Anorexia is a misnomer, because appetite remains until the patient becomes cachectic. Patients are preoccupied with food: They study diets and calories; hoard, conceal, and waste food; collect recipes; and prepare elaborate meals for others. Patients are often manipulative, lying about food intake and concealing behavior, such as induced vomiting. Binge eating followed by induced vomiting and the use of laxatives and diuretics (binge-purge behavior—see Bulimia Nervosa on p. 1702) occurs in 50%. The others simply restrict their food intake. Most anorectics exercise excessively to control weight.

Reports of bloating, abdominal distress, and constipation are common. Patients usually lose interest in sex. Depression occurs frequently. Common physical findings include bradycardia, low BP, hypothermia, lanugo hair or slight hirsutism, and edema. Even patients who appear cachectic tend to remain very active (including pursuing vigorous exercise programs), are free of symptoms of nutritional deficiencies, and have no unusual susceptibility to infections.

Endocrine changes include prepubertal or early pubertal patterns of luteinizing hormone secretion, low levels of thyroxine and triiodothyronine, and increased cortisol secretion. In a severely malnourished patient, virtually every major organ system may malfunction. Menses usually cease. Dehydration and metabolic alkalosis may occur, and serum K may be low; all are aggravated by induced vomiting and laxative or diuretic use. Cardiac muscle mass, chamber size, and output decrease. Some patients have prolonged QT intervals (even when corrected for heart rate), which, with the risks imposed by electrolyte disturbances, may predispose to tachyarrhythmias. Sudden death, most likely due to ventricular tachyarrhythmias, may occur.

Diagnosis

Denial is a prominent feature, and patients resist evaluation and treatment. They are usually brought to the physician's attention by their families or by intercurrent illness. Anorexia nervosa is usually apparent based on the characteristic symptoms and signs, particularly the loss of ≥ 15% of body weight in a young person who fears obesity, becomes amenorrheic, denies illness, and otherwise appears well. Body fat is usually very low. The key to diagnosis is eliciting the central "fear of fatness," which is not diminished by weight loss. In females, amenorrhea is required for the diagnosis. In severe cases, marked depression or symptoms suggesting another disorder, such as schizophrenia, may require differentiation. Rarely, a severe physical disorder, such as regional enteritis or a CNS tumor, is misdiagnosed as anorexia nervosa. Amphetamine abuse may produce similar symptoms.

Prognosis and Treatment

Without treatment, mortality rates approach 10%, although unrecognized mild disease probably rarely leads to death. With treatment, ½ of patients regain most or all lost weight and reverse any endocrine and other complications. About ¼ have intermediate outcomes and may relapse. The remaining ¼ have poor outcomes, including relapses and persistent physical and mental complications.

Treatment may require life-saving short-term intervention to restore body weight. All patients need long-term therapy to improve mental functioning and prevent relapse.

When weight loss has been severe or rapid or when weight has fallen below about 75% of ideal, prompt restoration of weight becomes critical, and hospitalization should be considered. Nutritional therapy, which begins by providing about 30 to 40 kcal/kg/day, can produce weight gains of up to 1.5 kg/wk during inpatient care and 0.5 kg/wk during outpatient care. If any doubt exists, the patient should be hospitalized. Removing the patient from her home sometimes reverses a downhill course, although ongoing psychiatric treatment is also required.

Loss of bone mass must be treated with elemental Ca 1200 to 1500 mg/day, vitamin D 600 to 800 IU/day, and, if severe, a bisphosphonate.

Once nutritional, fluid, and electrolyte status has been stabilized, long-term treatment begins. Treatment is complicated by the patient's abhorrence of weight gain, denial of illness, and manipulative behavior. The physician should attempt to provide a calm, concerned, stable relationship while encouraging a reasonable caloric intake. Individual psychotherapy—particularly cognitive–behavioral therapy—may be helpful, as is family therapy for younger patients. Second-generation antipsychotics (eg, olanzapine 10 mg once/day) may help produce weight gain and relieve the morbid fear of obesity. Fluoxetine may help prevent relapse after weight has been restored, beginning with 20 mg once/day.

BULIMIA NERVOSA

Bulimia nervosa is recurrent episodes of binge eating followed by self-induced vomiting, laxative or diuretic abuse, vigorous exercise, or fasting. Diagnosis is based on history and examination. Treatment is with psychotherapy and SSRIs, especially fluoxetine.

Bulimia nervosa afflicts 1 to 3% of adolescent and young women. Those affected are persistently and overly concerned about body shape and weight. Unlike patients with anorexia nervosa, however, those with bulimia nervosa are usually of normal weight.

Symptoms and Signs

Patients typically describe binge-purge behavior. Binges involve rapid consumption of food, especially high-calorie foods, such as ice cream and cake. Binges vary in amount of food consumed, sometimes involving thousands of calories. They tend to be episodic, are often triggered by psychosocial stress, may occur as often as several times a day, and are carried out in secret.

Most symptoms and physical complications result from purging. Self-induced vomiting leads to erosion of dental enamel of the front teeth and to painless salivary gland enlargement. Serious fluid and electrolyte disturbances, especially hypokalemia, occur occasionally. Very rarely, the stomach ruptures or the esophagus is torn during a binge, leading to life-threatening complications. Cardiomyopathy may result from long-term abuse of syrup of ipecac to induce vomiting.

Patients with bulimia nervosa tend to be more aware of and remorseful or guilty about their behavior than those with anorexia nervosa and are more likely to acknowledge their concerns when questioned by a sympathetic physician. They also appear less introverted and more prone to impulsive behavior, drug and alcohol abuse, and overt depression.

Diagnosis

The diagnosis is suspected when patients express marked concern about weight gain and have wide fluctuations in weight, especially with excessive laxative use or unexplained hypokalemia. Although bulimic patients express concern about becoming obese and may be obese, most tend to fluctuate around a normal body weight. Swollen parotid glands, scars on the knuckles (from induced vomiting), and dental erosion are danger signs. However, the diagnosis depends on the patient's description of binge-purge behavior.

Two binge-eating episodes a week for at least 3 mo are required for the diagnosis according to the *Diagnostic and Statistical Manual of Mental Disorders,* Fourth Edition (DSM-IV). However, a sensible physician is not constrained by these criteria.

Treatment

Treatment is with psychotherapy and drug therapy. Psychotherapy, usually cognitive-behavioral therapy, has both short- and long-term benefits. SSRIs alone are somewhat effective in reducing binge eating and vomiting, but they enhance the effectiveness of cognitive-behavioral therapy, and this combination is the treatment of choice.

BINGE EATING DISORDER

Binge eating disorder is characterized by binge eating that is not followed by inappropriate compensatory behavior, such as self-induced vomiting or laxative abuse. Diagnosis is clinical. There is increasing evidence that the most effective treatment is a standard behavioral weight-loss program.

Binge eating disorder affects 2 to 4% of the general population and becomes more prevalent with increasing body weight, reaching 30% among obese people in some weight-reduction programs.

Unlike bulimia nervosa, binge eating disorder occurs most commonly in obese people and contributes to excessive caloric intake. People with binge eating disorder tend to be older than those with anorexia nervosa or bulimia nervosa, and more (nearly 50%) are men.

People with binge eating disorder are generally distressed by it, especially if they are trying to lose weight. About 50% of obese binge eaters are depressed compared with < 5% of obese non–binge eaters.

Treatment

Most people are treated in conventional weight-loss programs, which pay little attention to binge eating. Patients tend to accept this intervention because they are usually more concerned about their weight than about their binge eating. The presence of binge eating apparently does not limit weight loss in these programs.

Evaluation of treatment is compromised by the lability of binge eating disorder. Untreated people may improve, and placebo response rates are very high. Cognitive-behavioral therapy is effective in controlling binge eating but has little effect on body weight, presumably because of compensatory (nonbinge) eating. Drug therapy with SSRIs controls both binge eating and weight, but discontinuation is frequently followed by relapse. Paradoxically, the most effective treatment of binge eating disorder is a standard behavioral weight-loss program, which not only produces weight loss but also controls binge eating.

Self-help groups that follow the principles of Alcoholics Anonymous, such as Overeaters Anonymous and Food Addicts Anonymous, have helped some people with binge eating disorder.

The presence of binge eating disorder does not preclude the use of surgical approaches for severely obese patients.

200 MOOD DISORDERS

(For mood disorders in children, see p. 2502.)

Mood disorders are emotional disturbances consisting of prolonged periods of excessive sadness, excessive joyousness, or both. Mood disorders are categorized as depressive or bipolar. Anxiety and related disorders (see p. 1672) also affect mood.

Sadness and joy (elation) are part of everyday life. Sadness is a universal response to defeat, disappointment, and other discouraging situations. Joy is a universal response to success, achievement, and other encouraging situations. Grief, a form of sadness, is considered a normal emotional response to a loss. Bereavement refers specifically to the emotional response to death of a loved one.

A mood disorder is diagnosed when sadness or elation is overly intense, continues longer than expected for a causative event, or occurs without cause; function must also be impaired. In such cases, intense sadness is termed depression, and intense elation is termed mania. Depressive disorders are characterized by depression; bipolar disorders are characterized by varying combinations of depression and mania. However, certain features of depressive and bipolar disorders can overlap, especially when they first occur.

Lifetime risk of suicide (see p. 1741) for people with a depressive disorder is 2 to 15%, depending on severity of the disorder. Risk is highest initially after hospital discharge, when treatment has been initiated and psychomotor activity is returning to normal but mood is still dark; risk remains high for 1 yr after discharge. Risk is also increased during mixed bipolar states, the premenstrual state, and personally significant anniversaries. Alcohol and substance use increases risk.

Other complications include disability ranging from mild to complete inability to function, maintain social interaction, and participate in routine activities; impaired food intake; and alcoholism and other drug dependencies.

DEPRESSIVE DISORDERS

Depressive disorders are characterized by sadness severe enough or persistent enough to interfere with function and sometimes by decreased interest or pleasure in activities. Exact cause is unknown but probably involves heredity, changes in neurotransmitter levels, altered neuroendocrine function, and psychosocial factors. Diagnosis is based on history. Treatment usually consists of drugs, psychotherapy, or both, and sometimes electroconvulsive therapy.

The term depression is often used to refer to any of several depressive disorders. Three are classified in the *Diagnostic and Statistical Manual of Mental Disorders*, Fourth Edition (DSM-IV) by specific symptoms: major depressive disorder (often called major depression), dysthymia, and depressive disorder not otherwise specified. Two others are classified by etiology: depressive disorder due to a general physical condition and substance-induced depressive disorder.

Depressive disorders occur at any age but typically develop during the mid teens, 20s, or 30s. In primary care settings, as many as 30% of patients report depressive symptoms, but < 10% have major depression.

The term depression is often used to describe the low or discouraged mood that results from disappointments or losses. However, a better term for such a mood is demoralization. The negative feelings of demoralization, unlike those of depression, resolve when circumstances or events improve; the low mood usually lasts days rather than weeks or months, and suicidal thoughts and prolonged loss of function are much less likely.

Etiology

Exact cause is unknown. Heredity has an uncertain role; depression is more common among 1st-degree relatives of depressed patients, and concordance between identical twins is high. Hereditary genetic polymorphisms for the serotonin transporter active in the brain may be triggered by stress. People who have a history of child abuse or other major life stresses and have the short allele for this transporter are about twice as likely to develop depression as those who have the long allele.

Other theories focus on changes in neurotransmitter levels, including abnormal regulation of cholinergic, catecholaminergic (noradrenergic or dopaminergic), and serotonergic (5-hydroxytryptamine) neurotransmission. Neuroendocrine deregulation may be a factor, with particular emphasis on 3 axes: hypothalamic-pituitary-adrenal, hypothalamic-pituitary-thyroid, and growth hormone.

Psychosocial factors also seem involved. Major life stresses, especially separations and losses, commonly precede episodes of major depression; however, such events do not usually cause lasting, severe depression except in people predisposed to a mood disorder.

People who have had an episode of major depression are at higher risk of subsequent episodes. People who are introverted and who have anxious tendencies may be more likely to develop a depressive disorder. Such people often lack the social skills to adjust to life pressures. Depression may also develop in people with other mental disorders.

Women are at higher risk, but no theory explains why. Possible factors include greater exposure to or heightened response to daily stresses, higher levels of monoamine oxidase (the enzyme that degrades neurotransmitters considered important for mood), and endocrine changes that occur with menstruation and at menopause. In postpartum depression (see p. 2210), symptoms develop within 4 wk after delivery; endocrine changes have been implicated, but the specific cause is unknown. Also, thyroid function is more commonly dysregulated in women.

In seasonal affective disorder, symptoms develop in a seasonal pattern, typically during autumn or winter; the disorder tends to occur in climates with long or severe winters. Depressive symptoms or disorders may occur with various physical disorders, including thyroid and adrenal gland disorders, benign and malignant brain tumors, stroke, AIDS, Parkinson's disease, and multiple sclerosis (see TABLE 200–1). Certain drugs, such as corticosteroids, some β-blockers, antipsychotics (especially in the elderly), and reserpine, can also result in depressive disorders. Abuse of some recreational drugs (eg, alcohol, amphetamines) can lead to or accompany depression. Toxic effects or withdrawal of drugs may cause transient depressive symptoms.

Symptoms and Signs

Depression causes cognitive, psychomotor, and other types of dysfunction (eg, poor concentration, fatigue, loss of sexual desire, menstrual abnormalities) as well as a depressed mood. Other mental symptoms or disorders (eg, anxiety and panic attacks) commonly coexist, sometimes complicating diagnosis and treatment. Patients with all forms of depression are more likely to abuse alcohol or other recreational drugs in an attempt to self-treat sleep disturbances or anxiety symptoms; however, depression is a less common cause of alcoholism and drug abuse than was once thought. Patients are also more likely to become heavy smokers and to neglect their health, increasing their risk of development or progression of other disorders (eg, COPD). Depression may reduce protective immune responses. Depression increases risk of MIs and stroke because cytokines and factors that increase blood clotting are released during depression.

Major depression (unipolar disorder): Periods (episodes) that include ≥ 5 mental or physical symptoms and last ≥ 2 wk are classified as major depression. Symptoms must include sadness deep enough to be described as despondency or despair (often called depressed mood) or loss of interest or pleasure in usual activities (anhedonia). Other mental symptoms include feelings of worthlessness or guilt, recurrent thoughts of death or suicide, reduced ability to concentrate, and occasionally agitation. Physical symptoms include changes in weight or appetite, loss of energy, fatigue, psychomotor retardation or agitation, and sleep disorders (insomnia, hypersomnia, early morning awakening). Patients may appear miserable, with tearful eyes, furrowed brows, down-turned corners of the mouth, slumped posture, poor eye contact, lack of facial expression, little body movement, and speech changes (eg, soft voice, lack of prosody, use of monosyllabic words). The appearance may be confused with Parkinson's disease. In some patients, depressed mood is so deep that tears dry up; they report that they are unable to experience usual emotions and feel that the world has become colorless and lifeless. Nutrition may be severely impaired, requiring immediate intervention. Some depressed patients neglect personal hygiene or even their children, other loved ones, or pets.

Major depression is often divided into subgroups. The psychotic subgroup is characterized by delusions, often of having committed unpardonable sins or crimes, harboring incurable or shameful disorders, or of being persecuted. Patients may have auditory or visual hallucinations (eg, accusatory or condemning voices). The catatonic subgroup is characterized by severe psychomotor retardation or excessive purposeless activity, withdrawal, and, in some patients, grimacing and mimicry of speech (echolalia) or movement (echopraxia). The melancholic subgroup is characterized by loss of pleasure in nearly all activities, inability to respond to pleasurable stimuli, unchanging emotional expression, excessive or inappropriate guilt, early morning awakening, marked psychomotor retardation or agitation, and significant anorexia or weight loss. The atypical subgroup is characterized by a brightened mood in response to positive events and rejection sensitivity, resulting in depressed overreaction to perceived criticism or rejection, feelings of leaden paralysis or anergy, weight gain or increased appetite, and hypersomnia.

Dysthymia: Low-level or subthreshold depressive symptoms are classified as dysthymia. Symptoms typically begin insidiously during adolescence and follow a low-grade course over many years or decades (diagnosis requires a course of ≥ 2 yr); dysthymia may intermittently be complicated by episodes of major depression. Affected patients are habitually gloomy, pessimistic, humorless, passive, lethargic, introverted, hypercritical of self and others, and complaining.

TABLE 200–1. SOME CAUSES OF SYMPTOMS OF DEPRESSION AND MANIA

TYPE OF DISORDER	DEPRESSION	MANIA
Connective tissue	SLE	Rheumatic fever SLE
Endocrine	Addison's disease Cushing's disease Diabetes mellitus Hyperparathyroidism Hyperthyroidism and hypothyroidism Hypopituitarism	Hyperthyroidism
Infectious	AIDS General paresis (parenchymatous neurosyphilis) Influenza Infectious mononucleosis TB Viral hepatitis Viral pneumonia	AIDS General paresis Influenza St. Louis encephalitis
Neoplastic	Cancer of the head of the pancreas Disseminated carcinomatosis	
Neurologic	Cerebral tumors Complex partial seizures (temporal lobe) Head trauma Multiple sclerosis Parkinson's disease Sleep apnea Stroke (left frontal)	Complex partial seizures (temporal lobe) Diencephalic tumors Head trauma Huntington's disease Multiple sclerosis Stroke
Nutritional	Pellagra Pernicious anemia	
Other*	Coronary artery disease Fibromyalgia Renal or hepatic failure	
Pharmacologic	Amphetamine withdrawal Amphotericin B Anticholinesterase insecticides Barbiturates Cimetidine Corticosteroids Cycloserine Indomethacin Mercury Metoclopramide Phenothiazines Reserpine Thallium Vinblastine Vincristine	Amphetamines Certain antidepressants Bromocriptine Cocaine Corticosteroids Levodopa Methylphenidate Sympathomimetic drugs
Mental	Alcoholism and other substance use disorders Antisocial personality Dementing disorders in the early phase Schizophrenic disorders	

*Depression is highly associated with these disorders, but no causal relationship has been established.

Depression not otherwise specified (NOS): Clusters of symptoms that do not meet criteria for other depressive disorders are classified as depression NOS. For example, minor depressive disorder may involve ≥ 2 wk of any of the symptoms of major depression but fewer than the 5 required for diagnosing major depression. Brief depressive disorder involves the same symptoms required for diagnosing major depression but lasts only 2 days to 2 wk. Premenstrual dysphoric syndrome involves a depressed mood, anxiety, and decreased interest in activities but only during most menstrual cycles, beginning in the luteal phase and ending within a few days after onset of menses.

Mixed anxiety-depression: Although not considered a type of depression in DSM-IV, this condition, also called anxious depression, refers to concurrent mild symptoms common to anxiety and depression. The course is usually chronically intermittent. Because depressive disorders are more serious, patients with mixed anxiety-depression should be treated for depression. Obsessions, panic, and social phobias with hypersomniac depression suggest bipolar II disorder.

Diagnosis

Diagnosis is based on identifying the symptoms and signs described above. Several brief questionnaires are available for screening. They help elicit some depressive symptoms but cannot be used alone for diagnosis. Specific close-ended questions help determine whether patients have symptoms required by DSM-IV criteria for diagnosis of major depression.

Severity is assigned by the degree of pain and disability (physical, social, and occupational); duration of symptoms also helps determine severity. The presence of suicidal risk (manifested as suicidal ideas, plans, or attempts—see p. 1741) indicates that the disorder is severe. A physician should gently but directly ask patients about any thoughts and plans to harm themselves or others. Psychosis and catatonia indicate severe depression. Melancholic features indicate severe or moderate depression. Coexisting physical conditions, substance abuse disorders, and anxiety disorders may add to severity.

No laboratory findings are pathognomonic for depressive disorders. Tests for limbic-diencephalic dysfunction are rarely indicated or helpful. They include the thyrotropin-releasing hormone stimulation test, dexamethasone suppression test, and sleep EEG for rapid eye movement latency, which is sometimes abnormal in depressive disorders. Sensitivity of these tests is low; specificity is better. PET scanning may show a decrease in brain metabolism of glucose in the dorsal frontal lobes and an increase in metabolism in the amygdala, cingulate, and subgenual cortex (all moderators of anxiety); these changes normalize with successful treatment.

Laboratory testing is necessary to exclude physical conditions that can cause depression. Tests include CBC, thyroid-stimulating hormone levels, and routine electrolyte, vitamin B_{12}, and folate levels. Testing for illicit drug use is sometimes appropriate.

Depressive disorders must be distinguished from demoralization. Other mental disorders (eg, anxiety disorders) can mimic or obscure the diagnosis of depression. Sometimes more than one disorder is present. Major depression (unipolar disorder) must be distinguished from bipolar disorder (see p. 1713).

In elderly patients, depression can manifest as dementia of depression (formerly called pseudodementia), which causes many of the symptoms and signs of dementia—psychomotor retardation and decreased concentration (see p. 1811). However, early dementia may cause depression. In general, when the diagnosis is uncertain, treatment of a depressive disorder should be tried.

Differentiating chronic depressive disorders, such as dysthymia, from substance abuse disorders may be difficult, particularly because they can coexist and may contribute to each other.

Physical disorders must also be excluded as a cause of depressive symptoms. Hypothyroidism often causes symptoms of depression and is common, particularly among the elderly. Parkinson's disease, in particular, may manifest with symptoms that mimic depression (eg, loss of energy, lack of expression, paucity of movement). A thorough neurologic examination is needed to exclude this disorder.

Prognosis and Treatment

With treatment, symptoms often remit. Mild depression may be treated with general support and psychotherapy. Moderate to severe depression is treated with drugs, psychotherapy, or both, and sometimes electroconvulsive therapy. Some patients require > 1 drug or a combination of drugs. Improvement may require 1 to 4 wk of taking drugs as prescribed. Depression, especially in patients who have had > 1 episode, is likely to recur; therefore, severe cases often warrant long-term maintenance drug therapy.

Most people with depression are treated as outpatients. Patients with significant suicidal ideation, particularly when family support is lacking, require hospitalization, as do those with psychotic symptoms or physical debilitation.

Depressive symptoms in patients with substance abuse disorders often resolve within a few months of cessation of substance use. If a physical disorder or drug toxicity could be the cause, treatment is directed first at the disorder. If the diagnosis is in doubt or if symptoms are disabling or include suicidal ideation or hopelessness, a therapeutic trial with an antidepressant or a mood-stabilizing drug may help.

Initial support: A physician should see patients weekly or biweekly to provide support and education and to monitor progress. Telephone calls may supplement office visits. Patients and loved ones may be worried or embarrassed about the idea of having a mental disorder. The physician can help by explaining that depression is a serious medical disorder caused by biologic disturbances and requiring specific treatment and that depression is most often self-limiting and the prognosis with treatment is good. Patients and loved ones should be reassured that depression does not reflect a character flaw (eg, laziness). Telling patients that the path to recovery often fluctuates helps them put feelings of hopelessness in perspective and improves compliance.

Encouraging patients to gradually increase simple activities (eg, taking walks, exercising regularly) and social interactions must be balanced with acknowledging their desire to avoid activities. The physician can suggest that patients avoid self-blame and explain that dark thoughts are part of the disorder and will go away.

Psychotherapy: Individual psychotherapy, often as cognitive-behavioral therapy (individual or group) alone is often effective for milder forms of depression. Cognitive-behavioral therapy is increasingly used to combat the inertia and self-defeating mental set of depressed patients. However, cognitive-behavioral therapy is most useful when used with antidepressants to treat moderate to severe depression. Cognitive-behavioral therapy may improve coping skills and enhance gains by providing support and guidance, by removing cognitive distortions that prevent adaptive action, and by encouraging the patient to gradually resume social and occupational roles. Couple therapy may help reduce conjugal tensions and disharmony. Long-term psychotherapy is unnecessary except for patients who have long-term interpersonal conflicts or who are unresponsive to brief therapy.

Selective serotonin reuptake inhibitors (SSRIs): These drugs prevent reuptake of serotonin (5-hydroxytryptamine [5-HT]). SSRIs include citalopram, escitalopram, fluoxetine, fluvoxamine, paroxetine, and sertraline. Although these drugs have the same mechanism of action, differences in their clinical properties make selection important. SSRIs have a wide therapeutic margin; they are relatively easy to administer, with little need for dose adjustment (except for fluvoxamine).

By preventing reuptake of 5-HT presynaptically, SSRIs result in more 5-HT to stimulate postsynaptic 5-HT receptors. SSRIs are selective to the 5-HT system but not specific for the different 5-HT receptors. Thus, they stimulate 5-HT_1 receptors, with antidepressant and anxiolytic effects, but they also stimulate 5-HT_2, commonly causing anxiety, insomnia, and sexual dysfunction, and 5-HT_3 receptors, commonly resulting in nausea and headache. Thus, SSRIs can paradoxically relieve and cause anxiety.

A few patients may seem more agitated, depressed, and anxious within a week of starting SSRIs or increasing the dose. Patients and their loved ones should be warned of this possibility and instructed to call the physician if symptoms worsen with treatment. This situation should be closely monitored because some patients, especially younger children and adolescents, become increasingly suicidal if agitation, increased depression, and anxiety are not detected and rapidly treated. Recent studies have determined that children and adolescents have an increased rate of suicidal ideation, suicide gestures, and suicide attempts during the first few months of taking SSRIs (the same concern may apply to serotonin modulators, serotonin-norepinephrine reuptake inhibitors, and dopamine-norepinephrine reuptake inhibitors); physicians must balance this risk with clinical need.

Sexual dysfunction (especially difficulty achieving orgasm but also decreased libido and erectile dysfunction) occurs in ≥ ⅓ of patients. Some SSRIs cause weight gain. Others, especially fluoxetine, cause anorexia in the first few months. SSRIs have few anticholinergic, adrenolytic, and cardiac conduction effects. Sedation is minimal or nonexistent, but in the early weeks of treatment, some patients tend to be sleepy during the day. Loose stools or diarrhea occurs in some patients.

Drug interactions are relatively uncommon; however, fluoxetine, paroxetine, and fluvoxamine can inhibit CYP450 isoenzymes, which can lead to serious drug interactions. For example, fluoxetine and fluvoxamine can inhibit the metabolism of certain β-blockers, including propranolol and metoprolol, potentially resulting in hypotension and bradycardia.

Serotonin modulators (5-HT_2 blockers): These drugs block primarily the 5-HT_2 receptor and inhibit reuptake of 5-HT and norepinephrine. Serotonin modulators include nefazodone, trazodone, and mirtazapine. Serotonin modulators have antidepressant and anxiolytic effects but do not cause sexual dysfunction. Unlike most antidepressants, nefazodone does not suppress REM sleep and produces restful sleep. Nefazodone can significantly interfere with drug-metabolizing liver enzymes and has been associated with liver failure.

Trazodone is related to nefazodone but does not inhibit 5-HT reuptake presynaptically. Unlike nefazodone, trazodone has caused priapism (in 1/1000) and, as an α_1-noradrenergic blocker, may cause orthostatic (postural) hypotension. It is very sedating, so its use in antidepressant doses (> 200 mg/day) is limited. It is most often given in 50- to 100-mg doses at bedtime to depressed patients with insomnia.

Mirtazapine inhibits 5-HT reuptake and blocks α_2-adrenergic autoreceptors as well as 5-HT_2 and 5-HT_3 receptors. The result is more efficient serotonergic function and increased noradrenergic function without sexual dysfunction or nausea. It has no cardiac adverse effects, has minimal interaction with drug-metabolizing liver enzymes, and is generally well tolerated, except for sedation and weight gain mediated by H_1 (histamine) blockade.

Serotonin-norepinephrine reuptake inhibitors: These drugs (eg, venlafaxine, duloxetine) have a dual 5-HT and norepinephrine mechanism of action, as do tricyclic antidepressants. However, their toxicity approximates that of SSRIs; nausea is the most common problem during the first 2 wk. Venlafaxine has some potential advantages over SSRIs: It may work better in some patients with severe or refractory depression, and because it is not highly protein bound and has virtually no interaction with drug-metabolizing liver enzymes, it poses little risk when given with other drugs. However, withdrawal symptoms (irritability, anxiety, nausea) often occur if the drug is stopped suddenly. Duloxetine resembles venlafaxine in effectiveness and adverse effects.

Dopamine-norepinephrine reuptake inhibitors: By mechanisms not clearly understood, they favorably influence catecholaminergic, dopaminergic, and noradrenergic function. These drugs do not affect the 5-HT system.

Bupropion is currently the only drug in this class. It can help depressed patients with concurrent attention-deficit hyperactivity disorder or cocaine dependence and those trying to stop smoking. Bupropion causes hypertension in a very few patients but has no other effects on the cardiovascular system. Bupropion can cause seizures in 0.4% of patients taking doses > 150 mg tid (or > 200 mg sustained-release [SR] bid or > 450 mg extended-release [XR] once/day); risk is increased in patients with bulimia. Bupropion does not have sexual adverse effects and interacts little with coadministered drugs, although it does inhibit the CYP2D6 hepatic enzyme. Agitation, which is common, is considerably attenuated by using the sustained-release or extended-release form. Bupropion may result in dose-related recent memory loss that is reversible with dose reduction.

Heterocyclic antidepressants: This group of drugs, once the mainstay of treatment, includes tricyclic (tertiary amines amitriptyline and imipramine and their secondary amine metabolites nortriptyline and desipramine), modified tricyclic, and tetracyclic antidepressants. Acutely, these drugs increase the availability of primarily norepinephrine and, to some extent, 5-HT by blocking reuptake in the synaptic cleft. Long-term use downregulates α_1-adrenergic receptors on the postsynaptic membrane—a possible final common pathway of their antidepressant activity. Although effective, these drugs are now rarely used because overdose causes toxicity and they have more adverse effects. The more common adverse effects of heterocyclics are due to their muscarinic-blocking, histamine-blocking, and α_1-adrenolytic actions. Many heterocyclics have strong anticholinergic properties and are thus unsuitable for the elderly and for patients with benign prostatic hypertrophy, glaucoma, or chronic constipation. All heterocyclics, particularly maprotiline and clomipramine, lower the threshold for seizures.

Monoamine oxidase inhibitors (MAOIs): These drugs inhibit the oxidative deamination of the 3 classes of biogenic amines (norepinephrine, dopamine, and 5-HT) and other phenylethylamines. MAOIs have little or no effect on normal mood. Their primary value is their effectiveness when other antidepressants are ineffective (eg, for atypical depression when SSRIs are ineffective).

MAOIs marketed as antidepressants in the US (eg, phenelzine, tranylcypromine, isocarboxazid) are irreversible and nonselective (inhibiting MAO-A and MAO-B). They can cause hypertensive crises if a sympathomimetic drug or food containing tyramine or dopamine is ingested concurrently. This effect is called the cheese reaction because mature cheese has a high tyramine content. MAOIs are underused because of concern about this reaction. More selective and reversible MAOIs (eg, moclobemide, befloxatone), which inhibit MAO-A, are not yet available in the US; they are relatively free of these interactions. To prevent hypertension and febrile crises, patients taking MAOIs should avoid sympathomimetic drugs (eg, pseudoephedrine), dextromethorphan, reserpine, and meperidine as well as malted beers, Chianti wines, sherry, liqueurs, and overripe, aged foods that contain tyramine or dopamine (eg, bananas, fava or broad beans, yeast extracts, canned figs, raisins, yogurt, cheese, sour cream, soy sauce, pickled herring, caviar, liver, extensively tenderized meats). Patients can carry 25-mg tablets of chlorpromazine and, as soon as signs of such a hypertensive reaction occur, take 1 or 2 tablets as they head for the nearest emergency department.

Common adverse effects include erectile dysfunction (least common with tranylcypromine), anxiety, nausea, dizziness, insomnia, pedal edema, and weight gain. MAOIs should not be used with other classes of antidepressants, and at least 2 wk (5 wk with fluoxetine, which has a long half-life) should elapse between use of the 2 classes of drugs. MAOIs used with antidepressants that affect the 5-HT system (eg, SSRIs, nefazodone) could cause a neuroleptic malignant syndrome (malignant hyperthermia, muscle breakdown, renal failure, seizures, and eventual death—see p. 1671). Patients who are taking MAOIs and who also need antiasthmatic, antiallergic, local anesthetic, or general anesthetics should be treated by a psychiatrist and an internist, a dentist, or an anesthesiologist with expertise in neuropsychopharmacology.

Drug choice and administration: Choice of drug may be guided by past response to a specific antidepressant. Otherwise, SSRIs are the starting drugs of choice. Although the different SSRIs are equally effective for typical cases, certain properties of the drugs make them more or less appropriate for certain patients (see TABLE 200–2).

If one SSRI is ineffective, another SSRI can be substituted, but an antidepressant from a different class is more likely to help. Tranylcypromine in high doses (20 to 30 mg po bid) is often effective for depression refractory to sequential trials of other antidepressants; it should be given by a physician experienced in use of MAOIs. Psychologic support of patients and loved ones is particularly important in refractory cases.

Insomnia, a common adverse effect of SSRIs, is treated by reducing the dose or adding a low dose of trazodone or another sedating antidepressant. Initial nausea and loose stools usually resolve, but throbbing headaches do not always go away, necessitating a change in drug class. An SSRI should be stopped if it causes agitation (most common with fluoxetine). When decreased libido, impotence, or anorgasmia occur during SSRI therapy, dose reduction may help, or a change can be made to another drug class.

SSRIs, which tend to stimulate many depressed patients, should be given in the morning. Giving the entire heterocyclic antidepressant dose at bedtime usually makes sedatives unnecessary, minimizes adverse effects during the day, and improves compliance. MAOIs are usually given in the morning and early afternoon to avoid excessive stimulation.

Therapeutic response with most classes of antidepressants usually occurs in about 2 to 3 wk (sometimes as early as 4 days or as late as 8 wk). For a first episode of mild or moderate depression, the antidepressant should be given for 6 mo, then tapered gradually over 2 mo. If the episode is severe or a recurrence or if there is suicidal risk, the dose that produces full remission should be continued during maintenance. For psychotic depression, maximal doses of a venlafaxine or a heterocyclic antidepressant (eg, nortriptyline) can be given for 3 to 6 wk; if necessary, an antipsychotic (eg, risperidone starting at 0.5 to 1 mg po bid and titrated to 4 to 8 mg once/day, olanzapine starting at 5 mg po once/day and titrated to 10 to 20 mg once/day, quetiapine starting at 25 mg po bid and titrated to 200 to 375 mg po bid) can be added. To reduce risk

TABLE 200–2. ANTIDEPRESSANTS

DRUG	STARTING DOSE	MAINTENANCE DOSE	PRECAUTIONS
Heterocyclics			Contraindicated in patients with coronary artery disease, certain arrhythmias, angle-closure glaucoma, benign prostatic hypertrophy, or esophageal hiatus hernia; can cause orthostatic hypotension leading to falls and fractures; potentiates effect of alcohol; raises blood level of antipsychotics
Amitriptyline	25 mg once/day	50 mg bid	Causes weight gain
Amoxapine	25 mg bid	200 mg bid	Can have extrapyramidal adverse effects
Clomipramine	25 mg once/day	75 mg tid	Lowers seizure threshold at doses of > 250 mg/day
Desipramine	25 mg once/day	300 mg once/day	Not to be used in patients < 12 yr
Doxepin	25 mg once/day	150 mg bid	Causes weight gain
Imipramine	25 mg once/day	200 mg once/day	May cause excessive sweating and nightmares
Maprotiline	75 mg once/day	225 mg once/day	—
Nortriptyline	25 mg once/day	150 mg once/day	Effective within therapeutic window
Protriptyline	5 mg tid	20 mg tid	Difficult to dose because of complex pharmacokinetics
Trimipramine	50 mg once/day	300 mg once/day	Causes weight gain
MAOIs			Serotonergic syndrome possible when taken with an SSRI or nefazodone; hypertensive crisis possible when taken with other antidepressants, sympathomimetic or other selective drugs, or certain foods and beverages
Isocarboxazid	10 mg bid	20 mg tid	Causes orthostatic hypotension
Phenelzine	15 mg tid	30 mg tid	Causes orthostatic hypotension
Tranylcypromine	10 mg bid	30 mg bid	Causes orthostatic hypotension; has amphetamine-type stimulant effects and modest abuse potential
SSRIs			
Citalopram	20 mg once/day	40 mg once/day	Lower potential for drug interactions due to less effect on CYP450 isoenzymes
Escitalopram	10 mg once/day	20 mg once/day	—
Fluoxetine	10 mg once/day	60 mg once/day	Has very long half-life. The only antidepressant proven effective in children
Fluvoxamine	50 mg once/day	150 mg bid	Can cause clinically significant elevation of theophylline, warfarin, and clozapine blood levels

Table continues on the following page.

TABLE 200–2. ANTIDEPRESSANTS—Continued

DRUG	STARTING DOSE	MAINTENANCE DOSE	PRECAUTIONS
Paroxetine	20 mg once/day 25 mg CR once/day	50 mg once/day 62.5 mg CR once/day	Has greater potential for interactions between its active metabolites and HCAs, carbamazepine, antipsychotics, or type IC antiarrhythmics than other SSRIs; may cause the most ejaculatory inhibition
Sertraline	50 mg once/day	200 mg once/day	Of SSRIs, has highest incidence of loose stools
Serotonin-norepinephrine reuptake inhibitors			
Duloxetine	20 mg bid	30 mg bid	Modest dose-dependent increase in systolic and diastolic BP; may cause mild urinary hesitancy in males
Venlafaxine	25 mg tid 37.5 mg XR once/day	125 mg tid 225 mg XR once/day	Modest dose-dependent increase in diastolic BP Rare increase in systolic BP (not dose-dependent) Causes discontinuation symptoms if stopped abruptly
Serotonin modulators (5-HT$_2$ blockers)			
Mirtazapine	15 mg once/day	45 mg once/day	Causes weight gain and sedation
Nefazodone	100 mg once/day	300 mg bid	May cause liver failure
Trazodone	50 mg tid	100–200 mg tid	May cause priapism May cause orthostatic hypotension
Dopamine-norepinephrine reuptake inhibitor			
Bupropion	100 mg bid 150 mg SR once/day 150 mg XL once/day	150 mg SR tid 450 mg XL once/day	Contraindicated in patients who have bulimia or who are seizure-prone; may interact with HCAs, increasing the risk of seizures; may cause dose-dependent recent memory loss

MAOIs = monoamine oxidase inhibitors; HCAs = heterocyclic antidepressants; CR = continuous release; XR = extended release; 5-HT = 5-hydroxytryptamine (serotonin); SR = sustained release; XL = extended release.

of tardive dyskinesia, the physician should give the antipsychotic in the lowest effective dose and stop it as soon as possible.

Continued therapy with an antidepressant for 6 to 12 mo (up to 2 yr in patients > 50 yr) is usually needed to prevent relapse. Most antidepressants, especially SSRIs, should be tapered off (by decreasing the dose by about 25%/wk) rather than discontinued abruptly; stopping SSRIs abruptly may result in serotonergic syndrome (nausea, chills, muscles aches, dizziness, anxiety, irritability, insomnia, and fatigue).

Medicinal herbs are used by some patients. St. John's wort (see p. 2732) may be effective for mild depression, although data are contradictory. St. John's wort may interact with other antidepressants.

Electroconvulsive therapy (ECT): Severe suicidal depression, depression with agitation or psychomotor retardation, or depression during pregnancy is often treated with ECT if drugs are ineffective. Patients who have stopped eating may need ECT to prevent death. ECT is also effective for psychotic depression. Response to 6 to 10 ECT treatments is usually dramatic and may be lifesaving. Relapse after ECT is common, and drug therapy is often maintained after ECT is stopped.

Phototherapy: Phototherapy may be used in patients with seasonal depression. Treatment can be provided at home with 2,500 to 10,000 lux at a distance of 30 to 60 cm for 30 to 60 min/day (longer with a less intense light source). In patients who go to sleep late at night and rise late in the morning, phototherapy is most effective in the morning, sometimes supplemented with 5 to 10 min of exposure between 3 and 7 PM. For patients who go to sleep and rise early, phototherapy is most effective between 3 PM and 7 PM.

BIPOLAR DISORDERS

Bipolar disorders are characterized by mania and depression, which usually alternate. Exact cause is unknown, but heredity, changes in the level of brain neurotransmitters, and psychosocial factors may be involved. Diagnosis is based on history. Treatment consists of drugs, sometimes with psychotherapy.

Bipolar disorders usually begin in the teens, 20s, or 30s. Lifetime prevalence is about 1%. Rates are about equal for men and women.

Bipolar disorders are classified partly based on long-term patterns of episodes of more intense symptoms as bipolar I disorder, bipolar II disorder, or bipolar disorder not otherwise specified (NOS). Forms associated with a disorder or drug use are classified as bipolar disorder due to their general physical condition or substance-induced bipolar disorder.

Etiology

Exact cause is unknown. Heredity plays some role. There is also evidence of dysregulation of serotonin and norepinephrine. Psychosocial factors may also be involved. Stressful life events are often associated with initial development of symptoms and later exacerbations, although cause and effect have not been established.

Bipolar disorders or symptoms of bipolar disorders can occur with several physical disorders, as adverse effects of many drugs, or as part of several other mental disorders (see TABLE 200–1).

Symptoms and Signs

Bipolar disorder begins with an acute phase of symptoms and is followed by a repeating course of relapse and remission. Relapses are episodes marked by more intense symptoms, lasting about 3 to 6 mo. Episodes are manic, depressive, hypomanic, or a mixture (of depressive and manic features). Cycles—time from onset of one episode to that of the next—vary in length. Cyclicity is particularly accentuated in rapid-cycling forms of bipolar disorder (usually defined as ≥ 4 episodes/yr). Disruption of developmental and social functioning is common, especially when onset occurs between ages 13 and 18.

Psychotic symptoms may be present. In full-blown manic psychosis, the mood is usually elation, but irritability and frank hostility with cantankerousness are not uncommon.

Bipolar I disorder is defined by alternation of full-fledged manic and major depressive episodes. It commonly begins with depression. Depression can occur immediately before or after mania, or depression and mania can be separated by months or years.

Bipolar II disorder is defined by a history of at least one major depressive episode and at least one hypomanic episode. Depressive episodes alternate with hypomania. During the hypomanic period, mood brightens, the need for sleep decreases, and psychomotor activity accelerates. Often, the switch follows circadian factors (eg, going to bed depressed and waking early in the morning in a hypomanic state). Hypersomnia and overeating are characteristic and may recur seasonally (eg, in autumn or winter); insomnia and poor appetite occur during the depressive phase. For some patients, hypomanic periods are adaptive because they produce high energy, confidence, and supernormal social functioning.

Bipolar disorder NOS refers to disorders with clear bipolar features that do not meet the specific criteria for other bipolar disorders.

Mania: A manic episode is defined as ≥ 1 wk of a persistently elevated, expansive, or irritable mood, accompanied by ≥ 3 additional symptoms: inflated self-esteem or grandiosity, decreased need for sleep, greater talkativeness than usual, persistent elevation of mood, flight of ideas or racing of thoughts, distractibility, increased goal-directed activity, and excessive involvement in pleasurable activities with a higher risk of undesirable consequences (eg, injury, loss of money). Symptoms impair functioning.

Typically, patients in a manic episode are exuberant and flamboyantly or colorfully dressed; they have an authoritative manner with a rapid, unstoppable flow of speech.

Patients make clang associations: New thoughts are triggered by word sounds rather than meaning. Easily distracted, patients may constantly shift from one theme or endeavor to another. However, they tend to believe they are in their best mental state. Lack of insight and an increased capacity for activity often lead to intrusive behavior and can be a dangerous combination. Interpersonal friction results and may lead to paranoid delusions that they are being unjustly treated or persecuted. Accelerated mental activity is experienced as racing thoughts by patients, is observed as flights of ideas by the physician, and, in its extreme form, is difficult to distinguish from the loose associations of schizophrenia. Psychotic symptoms develop in some patients with bipolar I disorder. Need for sleep is decreased. Manic patients are inexhaustibly, excessively, and impulsively involved in various activities without recognizing the inherent social dangers.

Hypomania: A hypomanic episode is a distinct episode of ≥ 4 days that is distinctly different from the patient's usual nondepressed mood. The episode is marked by ≥ 4 symptoms that occur during a manic episode, but the symptoms are relatively less intense, so that functioning is not markedly impaired.

Mixed state: A mixed episode blends depressive and manic or hypomanic features. The most typical examples are momentary switches to tearfulness during the height of mania or racing thoughts during a depressive period. In at least ⅓ of people with bipolar disorder, the entire episode is mixed. A common presentation consists of a dysphorically excited mood, crying, curtailed sleep, racing thoughts, grandiosity, psychomotor restlessness, suicidal ideation, persecutory delusions, auditory hallucinations, indecisiveness, and confusion. This presentation is called dysphoric mania (ie, prominent depressive symptoms superimposed on manic psychosis).

Diagnosis

Some patients who experience hypomania or mania do not report it unless they are specifically questioned. Skillful questioning may reveal morbid signs (eg, excesses in spending, impulsive sexual escapades, stimulant drug abuse). Such information is more likely to be provided by relatives. Diagnosis is based on the symptoms and signs described above. All patients must be asked gently but directly about suicidal ideation, plans, or activity.

A review of substance (especially amphetamines, particularly methamphetamine—see p. 1689) and prescription drug use and of body systems is needed to exclude drugs and physical disorders. Although no laboratory findings are pathognomonic for bipolar disorders, routine blood tests should be done to screen for physical disorders; thyroid-stimulating hormone (TSH) excludes hyperthyroidism. Other physical disorders (eg, pheochromocytoma) occasionally confuse the diagnosis. Anxiety disorders (eg, social phobia, panic attacks, obsessive-compulsive disorders) may also confuse the diagnosis.

Prognosis and Treatment

Most patients with hypomania can be treated as outpatients. Acute mania usually requires inpatient management. Typically, mood stabilizers are used to induce remission in patients with acute mania or hypomania. Lithium and certain anticonvulsants, especially valproate, carbamazepine, oxcarbazepine, and lamotrigine, act as mood stabilizers and are similarly effective. Choice of a mood stabilizer depends on the patient's medical history and adverse effects of the specific mood stabilizer.

Two thirds of patients with uncomplicated bipolar disorder respond to lithium. Several therapeutic mechanisms have been proposed but are unproved. Predictors of a good response include a euphoric mania as part of a primary mood disorder, < 2 episodes/yr, and a personal and family history of response to lithium. Lithium is less effective in patients with a mixed state, rapid-cycling forms of bipolar disorder, comorbid anxiety, substance abuse, or a neurologic disorder.

Lithium carbonate is started at 300 mg po bid or tid and increased over 7 to 10 days until a blood level of 0.8 to 1.2 mEq/L is reached. Lithium levels should be maintained between 0.8 and 1.0 mEq/L, usually by giving 450 to 900 mg sustained-release po bid. Adolescents, whose glomerular function is excellent, need higher doses of lithium; elderly patients need lower doses. During a manic episode, patients retain lithium and excrete Na; oral dosage and lithium blood level need to be higher during acute treatment than during maintenance prophylaxis.

Because lithium's onset of action has a 4- to 10-day latency period, an antipsychotic may be necessary initially; it is given as needed until the manic stage is controlled. Acute manic psychosis is being increasingly managed with 2nd-generation antipsychotics, such as risperidone (usually 4 to 6 mg po once/day), olanzapine (usually 10 to 20 mg po once/day), quetiapine (200 to 400 mg po bid), ziprasidone (40 to 80 mg po bid), and aripiprazole (10 to 30 mg once/day) because risk of extrapyramidal adverse effects is minimal. For extremely hyperactive psychotic patients with poor food and fluid intake, giving an antipsychotic IM with supportive care for 1 wk before initiating lithium is preferable. Noncompliant, cantankerous manic patients are customarily given a depot phenothiazine (eg, fluphenazine 12.5 to 25 mg IM q 3 to 4 wk) instead of an oral antipsychotic. Many patients with bipolar disorder and mood-incongruent psychotic features beyond the usual boundaries of pure mood disorder require intermittent courses of depot antipsychotics. Lorazepam or clonazepam 2 to 4 mg IM or po tid given early in acute management can reduce the doses need of the antipsychotic.

Although lithium attenuates bipolar mood swings, it has no effect on normal mood. It also appears to have an antiaggressive action, but whether this action occurs in people without a bipolar disorder is unclear. Lithium can cause sedation and cognitive impairment directly or indirectly by causing hypothyroidism. The most common acute, mild adverse effects are fine tremor, fasciculation, nausea, diarrhea, polyuria, thirst, polydipsia, and weight gain (partly attributed to drinking high-calorie beverages). These effects are usually transient and often respond to decreasing the dose slightly, dividing the dose (eg, tid), or using slow-release forms. Once dosage is established, the entire dose should be given after the evening meal. This dosing may improve compliance, and the troughs in blood levels are believed to protect the kidneys. A β-blocker (eg, atenolol 25 to 50 mg po once/day) can control severe tremor. Some β-blockers may worsen depression.

Lithium toxicity is manifested initially by gross tremor, increased deep tendon reflexes, persistent headache, vomiting, and confusion and may progress to stupor, seizures, and arrhythmias. Toxicity is more likely to occur in elderly patients and in patients with decreased creatinine clearance or with Na loss, which may result from fever, vomiting, diarrhea, or use of diuretics. NSAIDs other than aspirin may contribute to hyperlithemia. Lithium blood levels should be measured, including each time the dose is changed and at least q 6 mo. Lithium may precipitate hypothyroidism, particularly when there is a family history of hypothyroidism. Therefore, TSH levels should be monitored when lithium is started and at least annually if there is a family history or if symptoms suggest thyroid dysfunction or at least biannually for all other patients.

Lithium commonly and chronically exacerbates acne and psoriasis and can cause nephrogenic diabetes insipidus, which may respond to dose reduction or temporary interruption of lithium. Patients with a history of parenchymal renal disease may be at risk of structural damage to the distal tubule. Renal function should be assessed at baseline, and serum creatinine levels should be monitored over time.

Anticonvulsants that act as mood stabilizers, especially valproate, carbamazepine, and oxcarbazepine, are often used for acute mania and for mixed states (mania and depression). Their precise therapeutic action in bipolar disorder is unknown but may involve γ-aminobutyric acid mechanisms and ultimately G-protein signaling systems. Their main advantages over lithium include a wider therapeutic margin and lack of renal toxicity. The loading dose is 20 mg/kg, then 250 to 500 mg po tid for valproate. Carbamazepine should not be loaded; the dose should be increased gradually to reduce risk of toxicity. Oxcarbazepine has fewer adverse effects and is moderately effective.

Combining mood stabilizers is often necessary for optimal results, especially when episodes of mania or mixed states are severe. Electroconvulsive therapy is sometimes used for cases refractory to mood stabilizers.

Treatment of an initial manic or hypomanic episode with a mood stabilizer should continue for at least 6 mo, then tapered and stopped. The mood stabilizer is restarted for recurrent episodes and maintained if episodes are < 3 yr apart. Maintenance therapy with lithium should be initiated after 2 classic manic episodes < 3 yr apart.

In patients with recurrences, depressive episodes should be treated with antidepressants and mood stabilizers (the anticonvulsant lamotrigine may be particularly effective) because antidepressants (especially heterocyclics), given alone, may trigger hypomania.

Prevention of rapid cycling: Antidepressants, even when given with a mood stabilizer, can induce rapid cycling in some patients (eg, patients with bipolar II disorder). Antidepressants should not be used prophylactically unless previous depressive episodes have been severe and, if used, should be given for only 4 to 12 wk. When disruptive psychomotor acceleration or mixed states supervene, adding 2nd-generation antipsychotics (eg, risperidone, olanzapine, quetiapine) to the regimen can stabilize the patient.

For an established case of rapid cycling, antidepressants, stimulants, caffeine, benzodiazepines, and alcohol must be gradually stopped. Hospitalization may be required. Lithium (or divalproex) may be given with bupropion. Carbamazepine may also be useful. Some experts combine an anticonvulsant with lithium, trying to keep both drugs at ½ to ⅔ their usual dose and blood levels in an appropriate and safe range. Because borderline hypothyroidism also predisposes to rapid cycling (especially in women), TSH should be checked. Thyroid replacement should be given if TSH is high.

Phototherapy: Phototherapy is a relatively new approach to seasonal bipolar or bipolar II disorder (with autumn-winter depression and spring-summer hypomania). It is probably most useful as augmentation (see p. 1713).

Precautions during pregnancy: Most drugs used to treat bipolar disorder must be tapered and stopped before pregnancy or during early pregnancy. Women who wish to have a baby should have at least 2 yr of maintenance therapy with no episodes before lithium is stopped. Lithium is stopped during the 1st trimester to avoid risk of Epstein's anomaly, a heart defect. Carbamazepine and divalproex should also be stopped during the 1st trimester because they may cause neural tube defects. Other mood stabilizers (eg, lamotrigine, oxcarbazepine), if absolutely necessary, can be used during the 2nd and 3rd trimesters but should be stopped 1 to 2 wk before delivery and resumed a few days postpartum. For a severe relapse during the 1st trimester, electroconvulsive therapy is safer. For early manic recurrence, potent antipsychotics are relatively safe. Women taking mood stabilizers should not breastfeed because these drugs pass into the milk.

Education and psychotherapy: Enlisting the support of loved ones is crucial to preventing major episodes. Group therapy is often recommended for patients and their partner; there, they learn about bipolar disorder, its social sequelae, and the central role of mood stabilizers in treatment. Individual psychotherapy may help patients better cope with problems of daily living and adjust to a new way of identifying themselves.

Patients, particularly those with bipolar II disorder, may not comply with mood-stabilizer regimens because they believe that these drugs make them less alert and creative. The physician can explain that decreased creativity is relatively uncommon because mood stabilizers usually provide opportunity for a more even performance in interpersonal, scholastic, professional, and artistic pursuits.

Patients should be counseled to avoid stimulant drugs and alcohol, to minimize sleep deprivation, and to recognize early signs of relapse. If patients tend to be financially extravagant, finances should be turned over to a trusted family member. Patients with a tendency to sexual excesses should be given information about conjugal consequences (eg, divorce) and infectious risks of promiscuity, particularly AIDS.

CYCLOTHYMIC DISORDER

Cyclothymic disorder is characterized by hypomanic and mini-depressive periods that last a few days, follow an irregular course, and are less severe than in bipolar disorder. Diagnosis is clinical and based on history. Management consists primarily of education, although some patients with functional impairment require drug therapy.

Cyclothymic disorder is commonly a precursor of bipolar II disorder. However, it can also occur as extreme moodiness without becoming a major mood disorder. In chronic hypomania, a form rarely seen clinically, elated periods predominate, with habitual reduction of sleep to < 6 h. People with this form are constantly overcheerful, self-assured, overenergetic, full of plans, improvident, overinvolved, and meddlesome; they rush off with restless impulses and accost people.

For some people, cyclothymic and chronic hypomanic dispositions contribute to success in business, leadership, achievement, and artistic creativity; however, they more often have serious detrimental interpersonal and social results. Results often include instability with an uneven work and schooling history, impulsive and frequent changes of residence, repeated romantic or marital breakups, and an episodic abuse of alcohol and drugs.

Treatment

Patients should be taught how to live with the extremes of their temperamental inclinations; however, living with cyclothymic disorder is not easy because interpersonal relationships are often stormy. Jobs with flexible hours are advised. Patients with artistic inclinations should be encouraged to pursue careers in the arts because the excesses and fragility of cyclothymia may be better tolerated there.

The decision to use a mood stabilizer depends on the balance between functional impairment and the social benefits or creative spurts that patients may experience. Divalproex 500 to 1000 mg/day is often better tolerated than equivalent doses of lithium. Antidepressants should be avoided unless depressive symptoms are severe and prolonged because switching and rapid cycling are risks.

201 PERSONALITY DISORDERS

(See also Dissociative Identity Disorder on p. 1681.)

Personality disorders are pervasive, inflexible, and stable patterns of behavior that cause significant distress or functional impairment. Ten distinct personality disorders have been identified and grouped into 3 clusters. All are believed to be caused by a combination of genetic and environmental factors. Diagnosis is clinical. Treatment is with psychotherapy and sometimes drug therapy.

Personality traits are patterns of thinking, perceiving, reacting, and relating that are relatively stable over time and in various situations. Personality traits are usually evident from late adolescence or early adulthood, and although many traits persist throughout much of life, some fade with aging and some can be modified. Personality disorders exist when these traits become so rigid and maladaptive that they impair functioning. Mental coping mechanisms (defenses) that are used unconsciously at times by everyone tend to be immature and maladaptive in people with personality disorders (see TABLE 201–1).

People with personality disorders are often frustrating and even infuriating to those around them (including physicians). Most are distressed about their lives and experience impaired work or social relationships. Personality disorders often coexist with mood, anxiety, substance abuse, and eating disorders. People with severe personality disorders are at high risk of hypochondriasis and violent or self-destructive behaviors. They may have inconsistent, detached, overemotional, abusive, or irresponsible styles of parenting, leading to physical and mental problems in their children.

About 13% of the general population is affected. Antisocial personality disorder occurs in about 2% of the population, with men outnumbering women 6:1. Borderline personality disorder occurs in about 2% of the population, with women outnumbering men 3:1.

Diagnosis and Classification

Patients' emotional reactions and their perspectives on what causes their problems and how others treat them can provide information about their disorder. Diagnosis is based on observing repetitive patterns of behavior or perceptions that cause distress and impair social functioning. The patient often lacks insight into these patterns; thus evaluation may be sought initially by others who interact with the patient. Often, suspicion of a personality disorder arises from the physician's discomfort, typically if the physician begins to feel angry or defensive.

The general criteria in the *Diagnostic and Statistical Manual of Mental Disorders*, Fourth Edition (DSM-IV) emphasize the need to consider whether other mental or physical disorders (eg, depression, substance abuse, hyperthyroidism) can account for the patient's patterns of behavior. The DSM-IV recognizes 10 distinct personality disorders and divides them into 3 clusters: (A) odd/eccentric, (B) dramatic/erratic, and (C) anxious/fearful.

Cluster A: Patients in cluster A tend to be detached and distrustful.

Paranoid personality involves coldness and distancing in relationships, with a need for control and a tendency toward jealousy if attachments are formed. Affected people are often secretive and untrusting. They tend to be suspicious of changes and frequently find hostile and malevolent motives behind other people's acts. Often these hostile motives represent projections (see TABLE 201–1) of their own hostilities onto others. Their reactions

TABLE 201–1. COPING MECHANISMS

MECHANISM	DEFINITION	RESULT	PERSONALITY DISORDERS INVOLVED
Projection	Attribution of one's unacknowledged feelings to others	Leads to prejudice, rejection of intimacy through paranoid suspicion, overvigilance for external danger, and injustice collecting	Typical of paranoid and schizotypal personalities; used by people with borderline, antisocial, or narcissistic personality when under acute stress
Splitting	Black-or-white, all-or-nothing perceptions or thinking, in which people are divided into all-good idealized saviors or all-bad evildoers	Avoids the discomfort of feeling ambivalent (ie, having loving and angry feelings for the same person), uncertain, and helpless	Typical of borderline personality
Acting out	A direct behavioral expression of an unconscious wish or impulse that enables a person to avoid being conscious of the accompanying painful or pleasurable affect	Leads to many delinquent, reckless, promiscuous, and substance-abusing acts, which can become so habitual that the actor remains unaware and dismissive of the feelings that initiated the acts	Very common in people with antisocial, cyclothymic, or borderline personality
Turning aggression against self	Turning angry feelings directed toward others toward the self; when indirect, called passive aggression, when direct, called self-mutilation	Internalizes feelings about other people's failures; engages in silly, provocative clowning	Underlies passive-aggressive and depressive personality; dramatic in people with borderline personality, who express anger toward others in self-mutilation
Fantasy	A tendency to use imaginary relationships and private belief systems to resolve conflict and relieve loneliness	Leads to eccentricity and avoidance of intimacy	Used by people with avoidant or schizoid personality, who in contrast to psychotic people, do not believe in and thus do not act on their fantasies
Hypochondriasis	Uses physiologic complaints to gain attention	May gain nurturant attention from others; may express anger toward others without their knowing it	Used by people with dependent, histrionic, or borderline personality (see p. 1738)

sometimes surprise or scare others. They then use the resulting anger of or rejection by others (ie, projective identification) to justify their original feelings. Paranoid people tend to feel a sense of righteous indignation and often take legal action against others. These people may be highly efficient and conscientious, although they usually need to work in relative isolation. This disorder must be differentiated from paranoid schizophrenia.

Schizoid personality is characterized by introversion, social withdrawal, isolation, and emotional coldness and distancing. Affected people are often absorbed in their own thoughts and feelings and fear closeness and intimacy with others. They are reticent, are given to daydreaming, and prefer theoretical speculation to practical action.

Schizotypal personality, like schizoid personality, involves social withdrawal and emotional coldness but also oddities of thinking, perception, and communication, such as magical thinking, clairvoyance, ideas of reference, or paranoid ideation. These oddities suggest schizophrenia (see p. 1722) but are never severe enough to meet its criteria. People with schizotypal personality are believed to have a muted expression of the genes that cause schizophrenia.

Cluster B: These patients tend to be emotionally unstable, impulsive, and intense.

Borderline personality is marked by unstable self-image, mood, behavior, and relationships. Affected people tend to believe they were deprived of adequate care during childhood and consequently feel empty, angry, and entitled to nurturance. As a result, they relentlessly seek care and are sensitive to its perceived absence. Their relationships tend to be intense and dramatic. When feeling cared for, they appear like lonely waifs who seek help for depression, substance abuse, eating disorders, and past mistreatments. When they fear the loss of the caring person, they frequently express inappropriate and intense anger. These mood shifts are typically accompanied by extreme changes in their view of the world, themselves, and others—eg, from bad to good, from hated to loved. When they feel abandoned, they dissociate or become desperately impulsive. Their concept of reality is sometimes so poor that they have brief episodes of psychotic thinking, such as paranoid delusions and hallucinations. They often become self-destructive and may self-mutilate or attempt suicide. They initially tend to evoke intense, nurturing responses in caretakers, but after repeated crises, vague unfounded complaints, and failures to comply with therapeutic recommendations, are viewed as help-rejecting complainers. Borderline personality tends to become milder or to stabilize with age.

Antisocial personality is marked by the callous disregard for the rights and feelings of others. Affected people exploit others for materialistic gain or personal gratification. They become frustrated easily and tolerate frustration poorly. Characteristically, they act out (see TABLE 201–1) their conflicts impulsively and irresponsibly, sometimes with hostility and violence. They usually fail to anticipate the consequences of their behaviors and typically do not feel remorse or guilt afterward. Many of them have a well-developed capacity for glibly rationalizing their behavior or blaming it on others. Dishonesty and deceit permeate their relationships. Punishment rarely modifies their behavior or improves their judgment. Antisocial personality often leads to alcoholism, drug addiction, promiscuity, failure to fulfill responsibilities, frequent relocation, and difficulty abiding by laws. Life expectancy is decreased, but the disorder tends to diminish or stabilize with age.

Narcissistic personality involves grandiosity. Affected people have an exaggerated sense of superiority and expect to be treated with deference. Their relationships are characterized by a need to be admired, and they are extremely sensitive to criticism, failure, or defeat. When confronted with a failure to fulfill their high opinion of themselves, they can become enraged or seriously depressed and suicidal. They often believe others envy them. They may exploit others because they think their superiority justifies it.

Histrionic personality involves conspicuous attention seeking. Affected people are also overly conscious of appearance and are dramatic. Their expression of emotions often seems exaggerated, childish, and superficial. Still, they frequently evoke sympathetic or erotic attention from others. Relationships are often easily established and overly sexualized but tend to be superficial and transient. Behind their seductive behaviors and their tendency to exaggerate somatic problems (ie, hypochondriasis [see TABLE 201–1]) often lie more basic wishes for dependency and protection.

Cluster C: These patients tend to be nervous and passive or rigid and preoccupied.

Dependent personality is characterized by the surrender of responsibility to others. Affected people may submit to others to gain and maintain support. For example, they often allow the needs of those people they depend on to supersede their own. They lack self-confidence and feel intensely inadequate about taking care of themselves. They believe that others are more capable, and they are reluctant to express their views for fear that their aggressiveness will offend the people whom they need. Dependency in other personality disorders may be hidden by obvious behavioral problems; eg, histrionic or borderline behaviors mask underlying dependency.

Avoidant personality is marked by hypersensitivity to rejection and fear of starting relationships or anything new because of the risk of failure or disappointment. Because of their strong conscious desire for affection and acceptance, affected people are openly distressed by their isolation and inability to relate comfortably to others. They respond to even small hints of rejection by withdrawing.

Obsessive-compulsive personality is characterized by conscientiousness, orderliness, and reliability, but inflexibility often makes affected people unable to adapt to change. They take responsibilities seriously, but because they hate mistakes and incompleteness, they can become entangled with details and forget their purpose. As a result, they have difficulty making decisions and completing tasks. Such problems make responsibilities a source of anxiety, and they rarely enjoy much satisfaction from their achievements. Most obsessive-compulsive traits are adaptive, and as long as they are not too marked, people who have them often achieve much, especially in the sciences and other academic fields in which order, perfectionism, and perseverance are desirable. However, they can feel uncomfortable with feelings, interpersonal relationships, and situations in which they lack control or must rely on others or in which events are unpredictable.

Other personality types: Several other personality types have been described but are not classified as disorders in the DSM-IV.

Passive-aggressive (negativistic) personality typically produces the appearance of ineptness or passivity, but these behaviors are covertly designed to avoid responsibility or to control or punish others. Passive-aggressive behavior is often evidenced by procrastination, inefficiency, or unrealistic protests of disability. Frequently, affected people agree to perform tasks they do not want to perform and then subtly undermine completion of the tasks. Such behavior usually serves to deny or conceal hostility or disagreements.

Cyclothymic personality (see also p. 1716) alternates between high-spirited buoyancy and gloom and pessimism; each mood lasts weeks or longer. Characteristically, the rhythmic mood changes are regular and occur without justifiable external cause. When these features do not interfere with social adaptation, cyclothymia is considered a temperament and is present in many gifted and creative people.

Depressive personality is characterized by chronic moroseness, worry, and self-consciousness. Affected people have a pessimistic outlook, which impairs their initiative and disheartens others. Self-satisfaction seems undeserved and sinful. They unconsciously believe their suffering is a badge of merit needed to earn the love or admiration of others.

Treatment

Although treatment differs according to the type of personality disorder, some general principles apply. Family and friends can act in ways that either reinforce or diminish the patient's problematic behavior or thoughts, so their involvement is helpful and often essential. An early effort should be made to get the patient to see that the problem is really based on who he is. Another principle is that treating a personality disorder takes a long time. Repetitious confrontation in prolonged psychotherapy or by peer encounters is usually required to make such people aware of their defenses, beliefs, and maladaptive behavior patterns.

Because personality disorders are particularly difficult to treat, therapists with experience, enthusiasm, and an understanding of the patient's expected areas of emotional sensitivity and usual ways of coping are important. Kindness and direction alone do not change personality disorders. Treatment of personality disorders may involve a combination of psychotherapy and drug therapy. However, symptoms typically are not very responsive to drugs.

Relief of anxiety or depression is the first goal, and drug therapy can be helpful. Reducing environmental stress can also quickly relieve such symptoms. Maladaptive behaviors, such as recklessness, social isolation, lack of assertiveness, or temper outbursts, can be changed in months. Group therapy and behavior modification, sometimes within day hospital or residential settings, are effective. Participation in self-help groups or family therapy can also help change socially undesirable behaviors. Behavioral change is most important for patients with borderline, antisocial, or avoidant personality disorder. Dialectical behavioral therapy (DBT) has proved effective for borderline personality disorder. DBT, which involves weekly individual psychotherapy and group therapy as well as telephone contact with therapists between scheduled sessions, seeks to help patients understand their behaviors and teach them problem solving and adaptive behaviors. Psychodynamic therapy is also highly effective for patients with borderline and avoidant personality disorders. An important component of such therapies is to help patients with personality disorders reorganize feeling states in themselves and to think about the effect their behaviors have on others.

Interpersonal problems, such as dependency, distrust, arrogance, and manipulativeness, usually take > 1 yr to change. The cornerstone for effecting interpersonal changes is individual psychotherapy that helps the patient understand the sources of his interpersonal problems. A therapist must repeatedly point out the undesirable consequences of the patient's thought and behavior patterns and must sometimes set limits on the patient's behavior. Such therapy is essential for patients with histrionic, dependent, or passive-aggressive personality disorder. For some patients with personality disorders that involve how attitudes, expectations, and beliefs are mentally organized (eg, narcissistic or obsessive-compulsive types), psychoanalysis is recommended, usually for ≥ 3 yr.

202 SCHIZOPHRENIA AND RELATED DISORDERS

Schizophrenia and related disorders—brief psychotic disorder, delusional disorder, schizoaffective disorder, and schizophreniform disorder—are characterized by psychotic symptoms. Psychotic symptoms include delusions, hallucinations, disorganized thinking and speech, and bizarre and inappropriate behavior.

BRIEF PSYCHOTIC DISORDER

Brief psychotic disorder consists of delusions, hallucinations, or other psychotic symptoms for at least 1 day but < 1 mo, with eventual return to normal premorbid functioning. It is typically caused by severe stress in susceptible people.

Brief psychotic disorder is uncommon. Preexisting personality disorders (eg, paranoid, histrionic, narcissistic, schizotypal, borderline) predispose to its development. A major stressor, such as loss of a loved one, may precipitate the disorder. The disorder causes at least one psychotic symptom: delusions, hallucinations, disorganized speech, or grossly disorganized or catatonic behavior. This disorder is not diagnosed if a psychotic mood disorder, a schizoaffective disorder, schizophrenia, a physical disorder, or adverse drug effect (prescribed or illicit) better accounts for the symptoms. Differentiating between brief psychotic disorder and schizophrenia in a patient without any prior psychotic symptoms is based on duration of symptoms; if the duration exceeds 1 mo, the patient no longer meets required diagnostic criteria for brief psychotic disorder.

Treatment is similar to that of an acute exacerbation of schizophrenia; supervision and short-term treatment with antipsychotics may be required.

DELUSIONAL DISORDER

Delusional disorder is characterized by nonbizarre delusions (false beliefs) that persist for at least 1 mo, without other symptoms of schizophrenia.

Delusional disorder is distinguished from schizophrenia by the presence of delusions without other symptoms of schizophrenia. The delusions tend to be nonbizarre and involve situations that could occur, such as being followed, poisoned, infected, loved at a distance, or deceived by one's spouse or lover.

In contrast to schizophrenia, delusional disorder is relatively uncommon. Onset generally occurs in middle or late adult life. Psychosocial functioning is not as impaired as it is in schizophrenia, and impairments usually arise directly from the delusional belief.

When delusional disorder occurs in older patients, it is sometimes called paraphrenia. It may coexist with mild dementia. The physician must be careful to distinguish delusions from elder abuse being reported by a mildly demented elderly patient.

Symptoms and Diagnosis

Delusional disorder may arise in the context of a preexisting paranoid personality disorder (see p. 1717). In such people, a pervasive distrust and suspiciousness of others and their motives begins in early adulthood and extends throughout life. Early symptoms may include the feeling of being exploited, preoccupation with the loyalty or trustworthiness of friends, a tendency to read threatening meanings into benign remarks or events, persistent bearing of grudges, and a readiness to respond to perceived slights.

Several subtypes of delusional disorder are recognized. In the erotomanic subtype, the patient believes that another person is in love with him. Efforts to contact the object of the delusion through telephone calls, letters, surveillance, or stalking are common. People with this subtype may have conflicts with the law related to this behavior. In the grandiose subtype, the patient believes he has a great talent or has made an important discovery. In the jealous subtype, the patient believes that his spouse or lover is unfaithful. This belief is based on incorrect inferences supported by dubious evidence. Physical assault may be a significant danger. In the persecutory subtype, the patient believes that he is being plotted against, spied on, maligned, or harassed. He may repeatedly attempt to obtain justice through appeals to courts and other government agencies and may resort to violence in retaliation for the imagined persecution. In the somatic subtype, the delusion relates to a bodily function; eg, the patient believes he has a physical deformity, odor, or parasite.

Diagnosis largely depends on making a clinical assessment, obtaining a thorough history, and ruling out other specific conditions associated with delusions. Assessment of dangerousness, especially the extent to which the patient is willing to act on his delusion, is very important.

Prognosis and Treatment

Delusional disorder does not generally lead to severe impairment or change in personality, but delusional concerns may gradually progress. Most patients can remain employed.

Treatment aims to establish an effective physician-patient relationship and to manage complications. If the patient is assessed to be dangerous, hospitalization may be required. Insufficient data are available to support the use of any particular drug, although antipsychotics sometimes suppress symptoms. A long-term treatment goal of shifting the patient's major area of concern away from the delusional locus to a more constructive and gratifying area is difficult but reasonable.

SCHIZOAFFECTIVE DISORDER

Schizoaffective disorder is characterized by significant mood symptoms, psychosis, and other symptoms of schizophrenia. It is differentiated from schizophrenia by occurrence of one or more episodes of depressive or manic symptoms.

Schizoaffective disorder is considered when a psychotic patient also demonstrates mood symptoms. The diagnosis requires that significant mood symptoms (depressive or manic) be present for a substantial portion of the total duration of illness, concurrent with symptoms of schizophrenia. Differentiating schizoaffective disorder from schizophrenia and mood disorders may require longitudinal assessment of symptoms and symptom progression. The prognosis is somewhat better than that for schizophrenia but worse than that for mood disorders.

Because schizoaffective disorder often leads to long-term disability, comprehensive treatment (including drugs, psychotherapy, and community support) is often required. For treatment of the manic type, antipsychotics combined with lithium, carbamazepine, or valproate may be more effective than antipsychotics alone. For treatment of the depressive type, antipsychotics are commonly combined with antidepressants. Antidepressants should generally be introduced once positive psychotic symptoms are stabilized. SSRIs are preferred because of their safety profile. Second-generation antipsychotics may be more effective than conventional antipsychotics in alleviating depression associated with psychosis.

SCHIZOPHRENIA

Schizophrenia is characterized by psychosis (loss of contact with reality), hallucinations (false perceptions), delusions (false beliefs), disorganized speech and behavior, flattened affect (restricted range of emotions), cognitive

deficits (impaired reasoning and problem solving), and occupational and social dysfunction. The cause is unknown, but evidence for a genetic component is strong. Symptoms usually begin in adolescence or early adulthood. One or more episodes of symptoms must last ≥ 6 mo before the diagnosis is made. Treatment consists of drug therapy, psychotherapy, and rehabilitation.

Worldwide, the prevalence of schizophrenia is about 1%. The rate is comparable among men and women and relatively constant cross-culturally. The rate is higher among lower socioeconomic classes in urban areas, perhaps because its disabling effects lead to unemployment and poverty. Similarly, a higher prevalence among single people may reflect the effect of illness or illness precursors on social functioning. The average age at onset is 18 yr in men and 25 yr in women. Onset is rare in childhood, but early adolescent or late-life onset (when it is sometimes called paraphrenia) may occur.

Etiology

Although its specific cause is unknown, schizophrenia has a biologic basis, as evidenced by alterations in brain structure, such as enlarged cerebral ventricles and decreased size of the anterior hippocampus and other brain regions, and on changes in neurotransmitters, especially involving altered activity of dopamine and glutamate. Some experts suggest that schizophrenia occurs in people with neurodevelopmental vulnerabilities and that the onset, remission, and recurrence of symptoms are the result of interactions between these enduring vulnerabilities and environmental stressors.

Neurodevelopmental vulnerability to schizophrenia may result from genetic predisposition; intrauterine, birth, or postnatal complications; or viral CNS infections. Maternal exposure to famine and influenza in the 2nd trimester of pregnancy, birth weight below 2500 g, Rh incompatibility in a 2nd pregnancy, and hypoxia increase risk. Although most people with schizophrenia do not have a family history, genetic factors have been implicated. People who have a 1st-degree relative with schizophrenia have about a 10% risk of developing the disorder, compared with a 1% risk among the general population. Monozygotic twins have a concordance of about 50%. Sensitive neurologic and neuropsychiatric tests suggest that aberrant smooth-pursuit eye tracking, impaired cognition and attention, and deficient sensory gating occur more commonly among patients with schizophrenia than among the general population. These markers (endophenotypes) also occur among 1st-degree relatives of people with schizophrenia and may represent the inherited component of vulnerability.

Environmental stressors can trigger the emergence or recurrence of symptoms in vulnerable people. Stressors may be primarily biochemical (eg, substance abuse, especially marijuana) or social (eg, becoming unemployed or impoverished, leaving home for college, breaking off a romantic relationship, joining the Armed Forces); these stressors are not, however, causative. There is no evidence that schizophrenia is caused by poor parenting. Protective factors that may mitigate the effect of stress on symptom formation or exacerbation include good social support, coping skills, and antipsychotics (see Treatment on p. 1726).

Symptoms and Signs

Schizophrenia is a chronic illness that may progress through several phases, although the duration and patterns of phases can vary. Patients with schizophrenia tend to develop psychotic symptoms an average of 12 to 24 mo before presenting for medical care. In the premorbid phase, patients may show no symptoms or may have impaired social competence, mild cognitive disorganization or perceptual distortion, a diminished capacity to experience pleasure (anhedonia), and other general coping deficiencies. Such traits may be mild and recognized only in retrospect or may be more noticeable, with impairment of social, academic, and vocational functioning. In the prodromal phase, subclinical symptoms may emerge, including withdrawal or isolation, irritability, suspiciousness, unusual thoughts, perceptual distortions, and disorganization. Onset of overt schizophrenia (delusions and hallucinations) may be sudden (over days or weeks) or slow and insidious (over years). In the middle phase, symptomatic periods may be episodic (with identifiable exacerbations and remissions) or continuous; functional deficits tend to worsen. In the late illness phase, the illness pattern may be established, and disability may stabilize or even diminish.

Generally, symptoms are categorized as positive, disorganized, negative, and cognitive. Positive symptoms are characterized by an excess or distortion of normal functions;

negative symptoms, by diminution or loss of normal functions. Disorganized symptoms include thought disorder and bizarre behavior. Cognitive symptoms are deficits in information processing and problem solving. A person may have symptoms from one or all categories.

Positive symptoms can be further categorized as delusions and hallucinations or thought disorder and bizarre behavior. Delusions are erroneous beliefs. In persecutory delusions, the patient believes he is being tormented, followed, tricked, or spied on. In delusions of reference, the patient believes that passages from books, newspapers, song lyrics, or other environmental cues are directed at him. In delusions of thought withdrawal or thought insertion, the patient believes that others can read his mind, that his thoughts are being transmitted to others, or that thoughts and impulses are being imposed on him by outside forces. Hallucinations may be auditory, visual, olfactory, gustatory, or tactile, but auditory hallucinations are by far the most common. The patient may hear voices commenting on his behavior, conversing with one another, or making critical and abusive comments. Delusions and hallucinations may be extremely vexing to the patient.

Thought disorder involves disorganized thinking, with rambling, non–goal-directed speech that shifts from one topic to another. Speech can range from mildly disorganized to incoherent and incomprehensible. Bizarre behavior may include childlike silliness, agitation, and inappropriate appearance, hygiene, or conduct. Catatonia is an extreme behavior that can include maintaining a rigid posture and resisting efforts to be moved or engaging in purposeless and unstimulated motor activity.

Negative (deficit) symptoms include blunted affect, poverty of speech, anhedonia, and asociality. With blunted affect, the patient's face appears immobile, with poor eye contact and lack of expressiveness. Poverty of speech refers to decreased speech and terse replies to questions, creating the impression of inner emptiness. Anhedonia may be reflected by a lack of interest in activities and increased purposeless activity. Asociality is demonstrated by a lack of interest in relationships. Negative symptoms often lead to poor motivation and a diminished sense of purpose and goals.

Cognitive deficits include impairment in attention, processing speed, working memory, abstract thinking, problem solving, and understanding social interactions. The patient's thinking may be inflexible, and the ability to problem solve, understand the viewpoints of other people, and learn from experience may be diminished. Symptoms of schizophrenia typically impair the ability to function and often markedly interfere with work, social relations, and self-care. Unemployment, isolation, deteriorated relationships, and diminished quality of life are common outcomes. Severity of cognitive impairment is a major determinant of overall disability.

Subtypes: Five subtypes of schizophrenia have been described: paranoid, disorganized, catatonic, residual, and undifferentiated. Paranoid schizophrenia is characterized by delusions or auditory hallucinations, with preservation of cognition and affect. Disorganized schizophrenia is characterized by disorganized speech, disorganized behavior, and flat or inappropriate affect. In catatonic schizophrenia, physical symptoms, including either immobility or excessive motor activity and the assumption of bizarre postures, predominate. In undifferentiated schizophrenia, symptoms are mixed. In residual schizophrenia, there is a clear history of schizophrenia with more prominent symptoms followed by a prolonged period of mild negative symptoms.

Alternatively, some experts classify schizophrenia into deficit and nondeficit subtypes based on the presence and severity of negative symptoms, such as blunted affect, lack of motivation, and diminished sense of purpose. Patients with the deficit subtype have prominent negative symptoms unaccounted for by other factors (eg, depression, anxiety, an understimulating environment, drug adverse effects). Those with the nondeficit subtype may have delusions, hallucinations, and thought disorders but are relatively free of negative symptoms.

Suicide: About 10% of patients with schizophrenia commit suicide. Suicide is the major cause of premature death among people with schizophrenia and explains, in part, why on average the disorder reduces the life span of those affected by 10 yr. Patients who have paranoid subtypes with late onset and good premorbid functioning—the very patients with the best prognosis for recovery—are also at the greatest risk of suicide. Because these patients retain the capacity for grief and anguish, they may be more prone to act in despair based on a realistic recognition of the effect of their disorder (see also p. 1741).

Violence: Schizophrenia is a relatively modest risk factor for violent behavior. Threats of violence and minor aggressive outbursts are far more common than seriously dangerous behavior. Patients more likely to engage in significant violence include those with substance abuse, persecutory delusions, or command hallucinations and those who do not take their prescribed drugs. Very rarely, a severely depressed, isolated, paranoid person attacks or murders someone whom he perceives as the single source of his difficulties (eg, an authority, a celebrity, his spouse). Patients with schizophrenia may present in an emergency setting with threats of violence to obtain food, shelter, or needed care.

Diagnosis

No definitive test for schizophrenia exists. Diagnosis is based on a comprehensive assessment of history, symptoms, and signs. Information from collateral sources, such as family, friends, teachers, and coworkers, is often important. According to the *Diagnostic and Statistical Manual of Mental Disorders*, Fourth Edition (DSM-IV), 2 or more characteristic symptoms (delusions, hallucinations, disorganized speech, disorganized behavior, negative symptoms) for a significant portion of a 1-mo period are required for the diagnosis, and prodromal or attenuated signs of illness with social, occupational, or self-care impairments must be evident for a 6-mo period that includes 1 mo of active symptoms.

Psychosis due to other medical disorders or substance abuse must be ruled out by history and examination that includes laboratory tests and neuroimaging studies (see p. 1668). Although some patients with schizophrenia have structural brain abnormalities on imaging, these are insufficiently specific to have diagnostic value.

Other mental disorders with similar symptoms include several that are related to schizophrenia: brief psychotic disorder, schizophreniform disorder, schizoaffective disorder, and delusional disorder. In addition, mood disorders can produce psychosis in some people. Certain personality disorders (especially schizotypal) manifest symptoms similar to those of schizophrenia, although they are usually milder and do not involve psychosis.

Prognosis

During the first 5 yr after onset of symptoms, functioning may deteriorate and social and work skills may decline, with progressive neglect of self-care. Negative symptoms may increase in severity, and cognitive functioning may decline. Thereafter, the level of disability tends to plateau. Some evidence suggests that severity of illness may lessen in later life, particularly among women. Spontaneous movement disorders may develop in patients who have severe negative symptoms and cognitive dysfunction, even when antipsychotics are not used.

Prognosis varies depending on the subtype. Patients with paranoid schizophrenia tend to be less severely disabled and more responsive to available treatments. Patients with the deficit subtype are typically more disabled, have a poorer prognosis, and are more resistant to treatment.

Schizophrenia can occur with other mental disorders. When associated with significant obsessive-compulsive symptoms (see p. 1674), it has a particularly poor prognosis; with symptoms of borderline personality disorder (see p. 1719), a better prognosis. About 80% of people with schizophrenia will experience one or more episodes of major depression at some time in their life.

For the 1st year after diagnosis, prognosis is closely related to adherence to prescribed psychoactive drugs. Overall, ⅓ of patients achieve significant and lasting improvement; ⅓ improve somewhat but have intermittent relapses and residual disability; and ⅓ are severely and permanently incapacitated. Only about 15% of all patients fully return to their pre-illness level of functioning. Factors associated with a good prognosis include good premorbid functioning (eg, good student, strong work history), late and/or sudden onset of illness, a family history of mood disorders other than schizophrenia, minimal cognitive impairment, few negative symptoms, and paranoid or nondeficit subtype. Factors associated with a poor prognosis include early age at onset, poor premorbid functioning, a family history of schizophrenia, and disorganized or deficit subtype with many negative symptoms. Men have poorer outcomes than women; women respond better to treatment with antipsychotics.

Substance abuse is a significant problem in up to 50% of patients with schizophrenia. Anecdotal evidence suggests that use of marijuana and other hallucinogens is highly disruptive for patients with schizophrenia and should be strongly discouraged. Comorbid substance abuse is a significant predictor of poor outcome and may lead to drug noncompliance, repeated relapse, frequent rehospitalization, declining function, and loss of social support, including homelessness.

TABLE 202–1. CONVENTIONAL ANTIPSYCHOTICS

CLASS	DRUG	DAILY DOSE (RANGE)*	USUAL ADULT DOSE	COMMENTS
Phenothiazines				
Aliphatic	Chlorpromazine†‡	30–800	400 mg po at bedtime	Prototypic low-potency drug. Also available as a rectal suppository
Piperidines	Thioridazine‡	150–800	400 mg po at bedtime	Only drug with an absolute maximum (800 mg/day)—it causes pigmentary retinopathy at higher doses and has a significant anticholinergic effect. Warning added to label due to QTc prolongation
Piperazines	Trifluoperazine†‡	2–40	10 mg po at bedtime	
	Fluphenazine†‡	0.5–40	7.5 mg po at bedtime	Also available as fluphenazine decanoate and fluphenazine enanthate, which are IM depot forms (dose equivalents are not available)
	Perphenazine†‡	12–64	16 mg po at bedtime	
Dibenzoxazepines	Loxapine	20–250	60 mg po at bedtime	Has affinity for dopamine-2 and 5-hydroxytryptamine (serotonin)-2 receptors
Dihydroindolones	Molindone	15–225	60 mg po at bedtime	Possibly associated with weight reduction
Thioxanthenes	Thiothixene†‡	8–60	10 mg po at bedtime	Has high incidence of akathisia
Butyrophenones	Haloperidol†‡	1–15	4 mg po at bedtime	Prototypic high-potency drug; haloperidol decanoate (IM depot) form is available. Akathisia common
Diphenylbutylpiperidines	Pimozide	1–10	3 mg po at bedtime	Approved only for Tourette's syndrome

QTc = QT interval corrected for heart rate.

*Current recommended dosing for conventional antipsychotic agents is to initiate at low range of displayed values and titrate upwards gradually to a single dose; dosing at bedtime is recommended. No evidence that rapid dose escalation is more effective.

†Available in an IM form for acute treatment.

‡Available as an oral concentrate.

Treatment

The time between onset of psychotic symptoms and first treatment correlates with the rapidity of initial treatment response, quality of treatment response, and severity of negative symptoms. When treated early, patients tend to respond more quickly and fully. Without ongoing use of antipsychotics after an initial episode, 70 to 80% of patients have a subsequent episode within 12 mo. Continuous use of antipsychotics can reduce the 1-yr relapse rate to about 30%.

General goals are to reduce severity of psychotic symptoms, prevent recurrences of symptomatic episodes and associated deterioration of functioning, and help patients function at the highest level possible. Antipsychotics, rehabilitation with community support services, and psychotherapy are the major components of treatment. Because schizophrenia is a long-term and recurrent illness, teaching patients illness self-management skills is a significant overall goal.

Drugs are divided into conventional antipsychotics and 2nd-generation antipsychotics (SGAs) based on their specific neurotransmitter receptor affinity and activity. SGAs may offer some advantages both in terms of modestly greater efficacy (although for some of the SGAs the modest advantage is questionable) and reduced likelihood of involuntary movement disorder and related adverse effects.

Conventional antipsychotics: These drugs (see TABLE 202–1) act primarily by blocking the dopamine-2 receptor (dopamine-2 blockers). Conventional antipsychotics can be classified as high, intermediate, or low potency. High-potency antipsychotics have a higher affinity for dopamine receptors and less for α-adrenergic and muscarinic receptors. Low-potency antipsychotics, which are rarely used, have less affinity for dopamine receptors and relatively more affinity for α-adrenergic, muscarinic, and histaminic receptors. Different drugs are available in tablet, liquid, and short- and long-acting IM preparations. A specific drug is selected primarily based on adverse effect profile, required route of administration, and the patient's previous response to the drug.

Two conventional antipsychotics and one SGA are available as long-acting depot preparations (see TABLE 202–2). These preparations are useful for ruling out drug noncompliance. They may also help patients who because of disorganization, indifference, or denial of illness cannot reliably take daily oral drugs.

Conventional antipsychotics produce several adverse effects, such as sedation, cognitive blunting, dystonia and muscle stiffness, tremors, elevated prolactin levels, and weight gain (for treatment of adverse effects, see TABLE 195–3 on p. 1671). Akathisia (motor restlessness) is particularly unpleasant and may

TABLE 202–2. DEPOT ANTIPSYCHOTIC DRUGS

DRUG*	DOSAGE	PEAK LEVEL†
Fluphenazine decanoate	12.5–50 mg q 2–4 wk	1 day
Fluphenazine enanthate	12.5–50 mg q 1–2 wk	2 days
Haloperidol decanoate	25–150 mg q 28 days (3–5 wk range is acceptable)	7 days
Risperidone microspheres‡	25–50 mg q 2 wk	35 days

*Given IM with Z-track technique.
†Time until peak level after a single dose.
‡Because of 3-wk lag time between 1st injection and achievement of adequate blood levels, patients should continue on oral antipsychotics for 3 wk after 1st injection. Assessment of tolerability with oral risperidone recommended prior to initiating therapy.

lead to noncompliance. These drugs may also cause tardive dyskinesia, an involuntary movement disorder most often characterized by puckering of the lips and tongue and/or writhing of the arms or legs. The incidence of tardive dyskinesia is about 5%/yr of drug exposure among patients taking conventional antipsychotics. In about 2%, tardive dyskinesia is severely disfiguring. In some patients, tardive dyskinesia persists indefinitely, even after the drug is stopped. Because of this risk, patients receiving long-term maintenance therapy should be evaluated at least q 6 mo. Rating instruments, such as the Abnormal Involuntary Movement Scale, may be used (see TABLE 202–3). Neuroleptic malignant syndrome, a rare but potentially fatal adverse effect, is characterized by rigidity, fever, autonomic instability, and elevated creatinine phosphokinase (see also p. 1671).

About 30% of patients with schizophrenia do not respond to conventional antipsychotics. They may respond to clozapine, a 2nd-generation antipsychotic.

Second-generation antipsychotics: SGAs act by blocking both dopamine and serotonin receptors (serotonin-dopamine receptor antagonists). SGAs tend to alleviate positive symptoms; may lessen negative

TABLE 202–3. ABNORMAL INVOLUNTARY MOVEMENT SCALE

1. Observe gait on the way into the room.
2. Have patient remove gum or dentures, if ill-fitting.
3. Determine if patient is aware of any movements.
4. Have patient sit on a firm, armless chair with hands on knees, legs slightly apart, and feet flat on the floor. Now and throughout the examination, look at the entire body for movements.
5. Have patient sit with hands unsupported, dangling over the knees.
6. Ask patient to open mouth twice. Look for tongue movements.
7. Ask patient to protrude tongue twice.
8. Ask patient to tap thumb against each finger for 15 sec with each hand. Observe face and legs.
9. Have patient stand with arms extended forward.

Rate each item on a 0 to 4 scale for the greatest severity observed. 0 = none; 1 = minimal, may be extreme normal; 2 = mild; 3 = moderate; 4 = severe. Movements that occur only on activation merit 1 point less than those that occur spontaneously.

Facial and oral movements	Muscles of facial expression	0 1 2 3 4
	Lips and perioral area	0 1 2 3 4
	Jaw	0 1 2 3 4
	Tongue	0 1 2 3 4
Extremity movements	Arms	0 1 2 3 4
	Legs	0 1 2 3 4
Trunk movements	Neck, shoulders, hips	0 1 2 3 4
Global judgments	Severity of abnormal movements	0 1 2 3 4
	Incapacitation due to abnormal movements	0 1 2 3 4
	Patient's awareness of abnormal movements (0 = unaware; 4 = severe distress)	0 1 2 3 4

Modified from *ECDEU Assessment Manual for Psychopharmacology* by W. Guy. Copyright 1976 by US Department of Health, Education and Welfare.

symptoms to a greater extent than do conventional antipsychotics (although such differences have been questioned); may cause less cognitive blunting; are less likely to cause extrapyramidal (motor) adverse effects; have a lower risk of causing tardive dyskinesia; and for some SGAs produce little or no elevation of prolactin.

Clozapine is the only SGA demonstrated to be effective in up to 50% of patients resistant to conventional antipsychotics. Clozapine reduces negative symptoms, produces few or no motor adverse effects, and has minimal risk of causing tardive dyskinesia, but it produces other adverse effects, including sedation, hypotension, tachycardia, weight gain, type 2 diabetes, and increased salivation. It also may cause seizures in a dose-dependent fashion. The most serious adverse effect is agranulocytosis, which can occur in about 1% of patients. Consequently, frequent monitoring of WBCs is required, and clozapine is generally reserved for patients who have responded inadequately to other drugs.

Newer SGAs (see TABLE 202–4) provide many of the benefits of clozapine without the risk of agranulocytosis and are generally preferable to conventional antipsychotics for treatment of an acute episode and for prevention of recurrence. Newer SGAs are very similar to each other in efficacy but differ in adverse effects, so drug choice is based on individual response and on other drug characteristics. For example, olanzapine, which has a relatively high rate of sedation, may be prescribed for patients with prominent agitation or insomnia; less sedating drugs might be preferred in patients with lethargy. A 4- to 8-wk trial is usually required to assess efficacy. After acute symptoms have stabilized, maintenance treatment is initiated, in which the lowest dose that prevents symptom recurrence is used.

TABLE 202–4. SECOND-GENERATION ANTIPSYCHOTICS*

CLASS	DRUG	DOSE RANGE	USUAL ADULT DOSE	COMMENT†
Dibenzodiazepine	Clozapine	150–450 mg po bid	400 mg po at bedtime	First SGA, demonstrated efficacy in patients resistant to treatment. Frequent WBC counts required because of risk of agranulocytosis; increased risk of seizures, weight gain
Benzisoxazole	Risperidone	4–10 mg po at bedtime	4 mg po at bedtime	May cause extrapyramidal symptoms at doses > 6 mg; dose-dependent prolactin elevation; only SGA with a long-acting injectable form available
Thienobenzodiazepine	Olanzapine	10–20 mg po at bedtime	15 mg po at bedtime	Somnolence, weight gain, and dizziness are most common adverse effects
Dibenzothiazepine	Quetiapine	150–375 mg po bid	200 mg po bid	Low potency allowing wide dosing; no anticholinergic effect. Dose titration required because of blocking of α_2 receptors, requires twice-daily dosing
Benzisothiazolylpiperazine	Ziprasidone	40–80 mg po bid	80 mg po bid	Inhibition of serotonin and norepinephrine reuptake may convey antidepressant properties. Shortest half-life of new drugs; requires twice-daily dosing with food. IM form available for acute treatment. Low tendency for weight gain
Dihydrocarostyril	Aripiprazole	10–30 mg po at bedtime	15 mg po at bedtime	Dopamine-2 partial agonist, low tendency for weight gain

SGA = Second-generation antipsychotic.

*Monitoring for weight gain and type 2 diabetes recommended for this class of antipsychotics.

†All 2nd-generation antipsychotics have been associated with an increase in mortality in elderly patients with dementia.

Risperidone is the only SGA available in a long-acting injectable formulation.

Weight gain, hyperlipidemia, and elevated risk of type 2 diabetes are the major adverse effects of SGAs. Thus, before treatment with SGAs is begun, all patients should be screened for risk factors, including personal/family history of diabetes, weight, waist circumference, BP, and fasting plasma glucose and lipid profile. Patient and family education regarding signs and symptoms of diabetes (polyuria, polydipsia, weight loss), including diabetic ketoacidosis (nausea, vomiting, dehydration, rapid respiration, clouding of sensorium), should be provided. In addition, nutritional and physical activity counseling should be provided to all patients beginning an SGA. All patients undergoing ongoing treatment with an SGA require periodic monitoring of weight, BMI, and fasting blood glucose and referral for specialty evaluation of patients who develop hyperlipidemia or type 2 diabetes.

Rehabilitation and community support services: Psychosocial skill training and vocational rehabilitation programs help many patients work, shop, and care for themselves; manage a household; get along with others; and work with mental health professionals. Supported employment, in which patients are placed in a competitive work setting and provided with an on-site job coach to promote adaptation to work, may be particularly valuable. In time, the job coach acts only as a backup for problem solving or for communication with employers.

Support services enable many patients with schizophrenia to reside in the community. Although most can live independently, some require supervised apartments where a staff member is present to ensure drug compliance. Programs provide a graded level of supervision in different residential settings, ranging from 24-h support to periodic home visits. These programs help promote patient autonomy while providing sufficient care to minimize the likelihood of relapse and need for inpatient hospitalization. Assertive community treatment programs provide services in the patient's home or other residence and are based on high staff-to-patient ratios; treatment teams directly provide all or nearly all required treatment services.

Hospitalization or crisis care in a hospital alternative may be required during severe relapses, and involuntary hospitalization may be necessary if the patient poses a danger to himself or others. Despite the best rehabilitation and community support services, a small percentage of patients, particularly those with severe cognitive deficits and those resistant to drug therapy, require long-term institutional or other supportive care.

Psychotherapy: The goal of psychotherapy is to develop a collaborative relationship between the patient, family, and physician so that the patient can learn to understand and manage his illness, take drugs as prescribed, and handle stress more effectively. Although individual psychotherapy in combination with drug therapy is a common approach, few empirical guidelines are available. Psychotherapy that begins by addressing the patient's basic social service needs, provides support and education regarding the nature of the illness, promotes adaptive activities, and is based on empathy and a sound dynamic understanding of schizophrenia is likely to be most effective. Many patients need empathic psychologic support to adapt to what is often a lifelong illness that can substantially limit functioning.

For patients who live with their families, psychoeducational family interventions can reduce the rate of relapse. Support and advocacy groups, such as the National Alliance for the Mentally Ill, are often helpful to families.

SCHIZOPHRENIFORM DISORDER

Schizophreniform disorder is characterized by symptoms identical to those of schizophrenia but that last ≥ 1 mo but < 6 mo.

At presentation, schizophrenia is likely to be suspected. Psychosis secondary to substance abuse or to a physical disorder must also be ruled out. Differentiating between schizophreniform disorder and schizophrenia in a patient without any prior psychotic symptoms is based on duration of symptoms; if the duration exceeds 6 mo, the patient no longer meets required diagnostic criteria for schizophreniform disorder. Persistence of symptoms or disability beyond 6 mo suggests schizophrenia, but the acute psychosis may also evolve into a psychotic mood disorder, such as bipolar or schizoaffective disorder. Longitudinal observation is often required to establish the diagnosis and appropriate treatment.

Treatment with antipsychotics and supportive psychosocial care is indicated. After symptoms resolve, drug treatment is continued for 12 mo and then gradually tapered accompanied by close monitoring for the return of psychotic symptoms.

SUBSTANCE-INDUCED PSYCHOTIC DISORDER

Psychotic symptoms, particularly delusions and hallucinations, can result from a wide variety of substances, including alcohol, amphetamines, marijuana, cocaine, hallucinogens, inhalants, opioids, phencyclidine, and certain sedatives and anxiolytics. The diagnosis is made when symptoms begin during or less than 1 mo after intoxication with or withdrawal from the implicated substance and after other psychotic disorders are ruled out. Because symptoms may overlap with brief psychotic disorder, schizophreniform disorder, and acute episodes of psychotic mania or schizophrenia, differentiating these conditions may be difficult. Diagnosis may require several days of observation. Treatment may vary depending on the drug involved. Hallucinogen and phencyclidine psychosis may not respond well to antipsychotics. A supportive approach is preferred, with reassuring, structured, and protective surroundings. Agitation may respond best to short-acting benzodiazepines, such as lorazepam given po or IM.

203 SEXUALITY AND SEXUAL DISORDERS

(For sexual dysfunction in men, see p. 1947; for sexual dysfunction in women, see p. 2099.)

Accepted norms of sexual behavior and attitudes vary greatly within and among different cultures. Health professionals should never be judgmental of sexual behaviors, even when societal influences pressure them to do so. Generally, what is normal and abnormal cannot be defined by health professionals. When sexual behavior or difficulties bother a patient or the patient's partner or cause harm, then treatment is warranted.

Masturbation, once widely regarded as a perversion and a cause of mental disorders, is now recognized as normal sexual activity throughout life; it is considered abnormal only when it inhibits partner-oriented behavior, is performed in public, or is sufficiently compulsive to cause distress. About 97% of males and 80% of females masturbate. Although masturbation is harmless, guilt created by the disapproval and punitive attitudes of others may cause considerable distress and impair sexual performance.

Homosexuality has not been considered a disorder by the American Psychiatric Association for > 3 decades. About 4 to 5% of the population identify themselves as exclusively homosexual for their entire lives. Like heterosexuality, homosexuality results from complex biologic and environmental factors leading to an ability to become sexually aroused by people of the same sex. Like heterosexuality, homosexuality is not a matter of choice.

Frequent sexual activity with many partners, often involving anonymous or one-time-only encounters, may indicate a diminished capacity for intimacy. However, promiscuity is not in itself evidence of a psychosexual disorder. Casual sex is common, although the fear of AIDS has resulted in a decrease. Most cultures discourage extramarital sexuality but accept premarital or nonmarital sexual activity as normal. In the US, most people engage in sexual activity before marriage or without marriage as part of the trend toward more sexual freedom in developed countries. Extramarital sex occurs frequently among married people despite social taboos.

Accepted norms of sexual behavior and attitudes are influenced greatly by parents. A forbidding, puritanical rejection of physical sexuality, including touching, by a parent engenders guilt and shame in a child and inhibits his capacity for enjoying sex and developing healthy intimate relationships as an adult. Relations with parents may be damaged by excessive emotional distance, by punitive behaviors, or by overt seductiveness and sexual exploitation. Children exposed to verbal and physical hostility, rejection, and cruelty are likely to develop problems with sexual and emotional intimacy.

For example, love and sexual arousal may become dissociated, so that emotional bonds can be formed with people from the same social class or intellectual circle, but sexual relationships can be formed only with those considered inferior, such as prostitutes, with whom there is no emotional intimacy.

Well-informed physicians can offer sensitive, disciplined advice on sexuality and should not miss opportunities for helpful intervention. Behaviors that place patients at risk of sexually transmitted diseases must be addressed. Physicians have an opportunity to recognize and address psychosexual issues, including sexual dysfunction (see pp. 1947 and 2099), gender identity problems, and paraphilias.

GENDER IDENTITY DISORDER AND TRANSSEXUALISM

Gender identity disorder is a strong, persistent cross-gender identification condition in which people believe they are victims of a biologic accident and are cruelly imprisoned in a body incompatible with their subjective gender identity. Those with the most extreme form of gender identity disorder are called transsexuals.

Core gender identity is a subjective sense of knowing to which gender one belongs, ie, the awareness that "I am a male" or "I am a female." Gender identity is the inner sense of masculinity or femininity. Gender role is the objective, public expression of being male, female, or androgynous (blended). It is everything that one says and does to indicate to others or to oneself the degree to which one is male or female. For most people, gender identity and role are congruous. Those with gender identity disorder, however, experience some degree of incongruity between their anatomic sex and their gender identity. The incongruity experienced by transsexuals is usually complete, severe, disturbing, and long-standing. Labeling the condition as a "disorder" can add to the distress that frequently occurs, and the term should not be construed as being judgmental. Treatment is aimed at helping patients adapt rather than trying to dissuade them from their identity.

Etiology and Pathophysiology

Although biologic factors, such as genetic complement and the prenatal hormonal milieu, largely determine gender identity, the formation of a secure, unconflicted gender identity and gender role is influenced by social factors, such as the character of the parents' emotional bond and the relationship that each of them has with the child.

When sex labeling and rearing are confusing (eg, in cases of ambiguous genitals or genetic syndromes altering genital appearance, such as androgen insensitivity), children may become uncertain about their gender identity or role, although the level of importance of environmental factors remains controversial. However, when sex labeling and rearing are unambiguous, even the presence of ambiguous genitals often does not affect a child's gender identity. Transsexuals usually have had gender identity problems in early childhood. However, most children with gender identity conflicts do not develop into adults with transsexualism.

Childhood gender identity problems are usually present by age 2. For some people, however, gender identity disorder does not manifest until adulthood. Children experiencing difficulty with gender identity commonly prefer cross-dressing, insist that they are of the other sex, intensely and persistently desire to participate in the stereotypical games and activities of the other sex, and have negative feelings toward their genitals. For example, a young girl may insist she will grow a penis and become a boy; she may stand to urinate. A boy may sit to urinate and wish to be rid of his penis and testes. Most children with these disorders are not evaluated until they are age 6 to 9, at a point when the disorder is already chronic.

Diagnosis

Diagnosis in children requires the presence of both cross-gender identification (the desire to be or insistence that one is the other sex) and a sense of discomfort about one's sex or of substantial inappropriateness in one's gender role. Cross-gender identification must not be merely a desire for perceived cultural advantages of being the other sex. For example, a boy who says he wants to be a girl so that he will receive the same special treatment his younger sister receives is not likely to have gender identity disorder. Gender role behaviors fall on a continuum of traditional masculinity or femininity, with a growing cultural recognition of the presence of people who do not fit into the traditional male-female dichotomy. Western cultures are more tolerant of tomboyish behaviors in young girls (generally not considered a gender identity disorder) than effeminate or "sissy" behaviors in boys. Many boys role-play as girls or mothers, including trying on their sister's or mother's clothes. Usually, this behavior is part of normative development. Only in extreme cases does this behavior and an associated expressed wish to be the other sex persist. Most boys with gender identity disorder of childhood do not have the disorder as adults, but many are homosexual or bisexual.

Assessment of adults focuses on determining whether there is significant distress or obvious impairment in social, occupational, or other important areas of functioning. Cross-gender behavior, such as cross-dressing, may not require any treatment if it occurs without concurrent psychologic distress or functional impairment or if a person has a physical intersex condition (eg, congenital adrenal hyperplasia, ambiguous genitals, androgen insensitivity syndrome).

Rarely, transsexualism is associated with genital ambiguity or genetic abnormality (eg, Turner's syndrome, Klinefelter's syndrome). Most transsexuals who request treatment are natal males who claim a feminine gender identity and regard their genitals and masculine features with repugnance. Their primary objective in seeking help is not to obtain psychologic treatment but to obtain hormones and genital surgery that will make their physical appearance approximate their gender identity. The combination of psychotherapy, hormonal reassignment, and sex reassignment surgery is often curative.

Male-to-female transsexualism often first manifests in early childhood with participation in girls' games, fantasies of being female, avoidance of rough-and-tumble play and competitive games, and distress at the physical changes of puberty, often followed by a request during adolescence for feminizing somatic treatments. Many transsexuals adopt a convincing public feminine gender role. Some are satisfied with mastering a more feminine appearance and obtaining an identity card in the female role (eg, driver's license) that helps allow them to work and live in society as women. Others experience problems, which may include depression and suicidal behavior. The likelihood of a more stable adjustment may be increased by taking moderate doses of a feminizing hormone (eg, ethinyl estradiol 0.1 mg once/day) and with electrolysis and other feminizing treatments. Many transsexuals request sex reassignment surgery. The decision for surgery often raises important social problems for the patient. In follow-up studies, genital surgery has helped selected transsexuals live happier and more productive lives and so is justified in highly motivated, properly assessed and treated transsexuals who have completed a 1- to 2-yr real-life experience in the opposite gender role. Before surgery, patients often need assistance with "passing" in public, including gestures and voice modulation. Participation in gender support groups, available in most large cities, is usually helpful.

Female-to-male transsexualism is increasingly seen in medical and psychiatric practice as treatments improve. Patients ask for mastectomy early, then hysterectomy and oophorectomy. Androgenic hormones (eg, IM testosterone ester preparations 300 to 400 mg q 3 wk or equivalent doses of androgen transdermal patches or gels) are given to permanently alter the voice, induce a more masculine muscle and fat distribution, and enable growth of facial and body hair. Patients may opt for an artificial phallus (neophallus) to be fashioned from skin transplanted from the inner forearm (phalloplasty) or for a micropenis to be created from fat tissue removed from the testosterone-hypertrophied clitoris (metoidioplasty). Surgery may help certain patients achieve greater adaptation and life satisfaction. As with male-to-female transsexuals, such patients should meet the criteria established by the Harry Benjamin International Gender Dysphoria Association and have lived in the male gender role for at least 1 yr. Anatomic results of neophallus surgical procedures are often less satisfactory than neovaginal procedures for male-to-female transsexuals. Complications are common, especially in procedures that involve extending the urethra into the neophallus.

PARAPHILIAS

Paraphilias are recurrent, intense, sexually arousing fantasies, urges, or behaviors that are distressing or disabling and that involve inanimate objects, children or other nonconsenting adults, or suffering or humiliation of oneself or one's partner.

Sexual preferences that seem unusual to another person or health practitioner do not constitute paraphilia simply because they are unusual. The arousal patterns are considered pathologic only when they become obligatory for sexual functioning (ie, erection or orgasm cannot occur without the stimulus), involve inappropriate partners (eg, children, nonconsenting adults), and cause significant distress or impairment in social, occupational, or other important areas of functioning. People with a paraphilia may have an impaired or nonexistent capacity for affectionate, reciprocal emotional and sexual intimacy with a partner. Other aspects of personal and emotional adjustment may be impaired as well.

The pattern of erotic arousal is usually fairly well developed before puberty. At least 3 processes are involved: Anxiety or early emotional trauma interferes with normal psychosexual development; the standard pattern of arousal is replaced by another, sometimes through early exposure to highly charged sexual experiences that reinforce the person's experience of sexual pleasure; and the pattern of sexual arousal often acquires symbolic and conditioning elements (eg, a fetish symbolizes the object of arousal but may have been chosen because the fetish was accidentally associated with sexual curiosity, desire, and excitement). Whether all paraphilic development results from these psychodynamic processes is controversial, and some evidence for altered brain functioning is present in some paraphilias (eg, pedophilia).

In most cultures, paraphilias are far more common among males. Biologic reasons for the unequal distribution may exist but are poorly defined.

Many of the paraphilias are rare. The most common are pedophilia, voyeurism, and exhibitionism. Only a small subset of people with paraphilias break the law and become sex offenders. Some of these offenders have significant personality disorders (eg, antisocial or narcissistic), which makes treatment difficult.

FETISHISM

Fetishism is use of an inanimate object (the fetish) as the preferred method of producing sexual excitement. However, in common parlance, the word is often used to describe particular sexual interests, such as sexual role-playing, preference for certain physical characteristics, and preferred sexual activities.

Common fetishes include aprons, shoes, leather or latex items, and women's underclothing. The fetish may replace typical sexual activity with a partner or may be integrated into sexual behavior with a willing partner. Minor fetishistic behavior as an adjunct to consensual sexual behavior is not considered a disorder because distress, disability, and significant dysfunction are absent. More intense, obligatory fetishistic arousal patterns may cause problems in a relationship.

Transvestic fetishism: Heterosexual males who dress in women's clothing generally begin such behavior in late childhood (see also Gender Identity Disorder and Transsexualism, on p. 1732). This behavior is associated, at least initially, with sexual arousal.

Cross-dressing per se is not a disorder. Personality profiles of cross-dressing men are generally similar to age- and race-matched norms. When their partners are cooperative, these men have intercourse in partial or full feminine attire. When their partners are not cooperative, they may feel anxiety, depression, guilt, and shame associated with the desire to cross-dress.

Most transvestites do not present for treatment. Those who do are brought in by unhappy spouses, are referred by courts, or are self-referred out of concern about experiencing negative social and employment consequences. Some cross-dressers present for treatment of comorbid gender dysphoria, substance abuse, or depression. Social and support groups for cross-dressers are generally helpful.

EXHIBITIONISM

Exhibitionism is characterized by achievement of sexual excitement through genital exposure, usually to an unsuspecting stranger. It may also refer to a strong desire to be observed by others during sexual activity.

The exhibitionist (usually male) may masturbate while exposing himself or while fantasizing about exposing himself. He may be aware of his need to surprise, shock, or impress the unwilling observer. The victim is almost always a female adult or a child of either sex. Actual sexual contact is almost never sought. Age at onset is usually the mid 20s; occasionally, the first act occurs during preadolescence or middle age. About 30% of apprehended male sex offenders are exhibitionists. They have the highest recidivism rate of all sex offenders; about 20 to 50% are rearrested. Most exhibitionists are married, but the marriage is often troubled by poor social and sexual adjustment, including frequent sexual dysfunction. Very few females are diagnosed as exhibitionists, although society sanctions some exhibitionistic behaviors in females (through media and entertainment venues).

For some people, exhibitionism is expressed as a strong desire to have others watch their sexual acts. It is not the act of surprising an audience but, rather, of being seen by a consenting audience that appeals to such people. People with a compulsion for this form of exhibitionism may make pornographic films or become adult entertainers. They are rarely troubled by this sexual need.

When laws are broken and sex offender status is conferred, treatment generally begins with psychotherapy, support groups, and SSRIs (see p. 1736). If these drugs are ineffective, antiandrogens should be considered, with full informed consent and appropriate monitoring of liver function and serum testosterone levels.

Voyeurism

Voyeurism is achievement of sexual arousal by observing people who are naked, disrobing, or engaging in sexual activity. When observation is of unsuspecting people, this sexual behavior often leads to problems.

Desire to watch others in sexual situations is common and not in itself abnormal. Voyeurism usually begins in adolescence or early adulthood. Adolescent voyeurism is generally viewed more leniently; few teenagers are arrested. When pathologic, voyeurs spend considerable time seeking out viewing opportunities. Orgasm is usually achieved by masturbating during or after the voyeuristic activity. The voyeur does not seek sexual contact with those being observed.

Voyeurs have ample legal opportunities to watch sexual activity in many cultures. When laws are broken and sex offender status is conferred, treatment generally begins with therapy, support groups, and SSRIs (see p. 1736). If these drugs are ineffective, antiandrogens should be considered, with full informed consent and appropriate monitoring of liver function and serum testosterone levels.

Sexual Masochism

Sexual masochism is intentional participation in an activity in which one is humiliated, beaten, bound, or otherwise abused to experience sexual excitement.

Sadomasochistic fantasies and sexual behavior between consenting adults is very common. Masochistic activity tends to be ritualized and chronic. For most practitioners, the humiliation and beating are simply acted out in fantasy, with participants knowing that it is a game and carefully avoiding actual humiliation or injury. However, some masochists increase the severity of their activity with time, potentially leading to serious injury or death.

Masochistic activities may be the preferred or exclusive mode of producing sexual excitement. People may act on their masochistic fantasies themselves (eg, binding themselves, piercing their skin, applying electrical shocks, burning themselves) or seek out a partner who may be a sexual sadist. Activities with a partner include bondage, blindfolding, spanking, flagellation, humiliation by means of urination or defecation on the person, forced cross-dressing, or simulated rape.

Sexual Sadism

Sexual sadism is infliction of physical or mental suffering (humiliation, terror) on the sex partner to stimulate sexual excitement and orgasm.

Generally, the person has insistent, persistent fantasies in which sexual excitement results from suffering inflicted on the partner, consenting or not. Mild sadism is a common sexual practice; when it become pathologic is a matter of degree. Sexual sadism is not rape, a complex amalgam of sex and power over the victim. Sexual sadism is diagnosed in < 10% of rapists.

Most sadistic sexual behavior occurs between consenting adults. As is the case with masochism, sadism is generally limited in scope and not harmful. In some people, the behaviors escalate to the point of harm. When practiced with nonconsenting partners, sexual sadism constitutes criminal activity and is likely to continue until the sadist is apprehended. Sexual sadism is particularly dangerous when associated with antisocial personality disorder (see p. 1719).

Pedophilia

(See also p. 2508.)

Pedophilia is a preference for sexual activity with prepubertal children. Pedophilia often leads to imprisonment; medical management should include pharmacotherapy and psychotherapy.

Sexual offenses against children constitute a significant proportion of reported criminal sexual acts. Arbitrarily, the age of a person with pedophilia is set at ≥ 16 yr, with the age difference between the offender and the child victim set at ≥ 5 yr. The age of the child is generally ≤ 13 yr. For older adolescents with pedophilia, no precise age difference is specified; clinical and legal judgment is relied on.

Most pedophiles are male. Pedophiles prefer opposite-sex to same-sex children 2:1. In most cases, the adult is known to the child and may be a family member, stepparent, or a person with authority. Looking or touching seems more prevalent than genital contact. Homosexual males typically have less close acquaintanceship with the child. Exclusive pedophiles are attracted only to children; nonexclusive types may also be attracted to adults.

Some pedophiles limit their sexual activities to their own children or to close relatives (incest). Predatory pedophiles, many of whom have antisocial personality disorder, may use force and threaten to physically harm the child or the child's pets if the abuse is disclosed. The course of pedophilia is chronic, and perpetrators often develop substance abuse or dependence, depression, and marital conflict. Many cases of sexual abuse of children occur in the context of substance abuse and pervasive family dysfunction.

Identifying a pedophile often poses an ethical crisis for a physician. The physician can try to protect the privacy of the patient but must protect the community of children. Physicians should know the reporting requirements in their state.

Long-term individual or group psychotherapy is usually necessary and may be especially helpful when part of multimodal treatment that includes social skills training, treatment of comorbid physical and mental disorders (eg, seizure disorders, attention deficit disorder, depression), and drug treatment. Treatment is less effective when court ordered, although many adjudicated sex offenders have benefited from treatments, such as group psychotherapy and antiandrogens.

In the US, IM medroxyprogesterone is the treatment of choice; cyproterone is used in Europe. Typical doses are medroxyprogesterone 200 mg IM 2 to 3 times/wk for 2 wk, followed by 200 mg 1 to 2 times/wk for 4 wk, then 200 mg q 2 to 4 wk. Serum testosterone should be monitored and maintained in the normal female range (< 62 ng/dL). Treatment is usually long-term, because deviant fantasies usually recur weeks to months after discontinuation of treatment. Gonadotropin-releasing hormone agents (eg, leuprolide, gosarelin) have also been used IM. The usefulness of antiandrogens in female pedophiles is less well established. In addition to antiandrogens, SSRIs (eg, high-dose fluoxetine 60 to 80 mg once/day or fluvoxamine 200 to 300 mg once/day) may be useful. Drugs are most effective when used as part of a multimodal treatment program.

204 SOMATOFORM AND FACTITIOUS DISORDERS

Somatization is the expression of mental phenomena as physical (somatic) symptoms. Typically, the symptoms cannot be explained by a physical disorder. Disorders characterized by somatization extend in a continuum from those in which symptoms develop unconsciously and nonvolitionally to those in which symptoms develop consciously and volitionally. This continuum includes somatoform disorders, factitious disorders, and malingering. Somatization typically leads to seeking medical evaluation and treatment.

Somatoform disorders are characterized by physical symptoms or by perceived defects in appearance. Development of the symptoms or perceived defects is unconscious and nonvolitional. Symptoms or perceived defects cannot be explained by an underlying physical disorder. Somatoform disorders are distressing and often interfere with social, occupational, or other functioning. These disorders include body dysmorphic disorder, conversion disorder, hypochondriasis, pain disorder, somatization disorder, undifferentiated somatoform disorder, and somatoform disorder not otherwise specified.

Factitious disorders involve the conscious and volitional feigning of symptoms in the absence of any external incentive (eg, time off work) and is thus distinguished from malingering. The patient gains gratification from assuming the sick role through the simulation, exaggeration, or aggravation of signs and symptoms. Signs and symptoms may be mental, physical, or both. The most severe form is Munchausen syndrome.

Malingering is recurrent intentional feigning of physical and mental symptoms motivated by an external incentive (eg, feigning illness to avoid work or military duty, evade criminal prosecution, or obtain financial compensation or drugs for abuse). Malingering is suspected when a patient reports severe symptoms, yet little is revealed through unannounced observation, a physical examination, or laboratory testing. Malingering may also be suspected when a patient does not cooperate with efforts to diagnose or treat potential underlying causes of symptoms.

BODY DYSMORPHIC DISORDER

Body dysmorphic disorder is preoccupation with an imagined or slight defect in appearance that causes significant distress or interference with social, occupational, or other functioning. Diagnosis is based on history. Treatment consists of drug therapy and psychotherapy.

Body dysmorphic disorder usually begins in adolescence and appears to occur in men and women equally.

Symptoms and Signs

Symptoms may develop gradually or abruptly. Although intensity may vary, typically there are few symptom-free intervals. Symptoms commonly involve the face or head but may involve any body part or several parts and may change from one part to another. A patient may be concerned about thinning hair, acne, wrinkles, scars, vascular markings, color of complexion, or excessive facial hair or may focus on the shape or size of the nose, eyes, ears, mouth, breasts, buttocks, or other body part. Men may have a form of the disorder called muscle dysmorphia, which involves a preoccupation with the idea that their body is not sufficiently lean and muscular.

Patients usually spend many hours a day thinking about their perceived defect. Most check themselves often in mirrors, others avoid mirrors, and still others alternate between the 2 behaviors. Most try to camouflage their imagined defect—eg, by growing a beard to hide perceived scars or by wearing a hat to cover slightly thinning hair. Many undergo medical, dental, or surgical treatment to correct their perceived defect, but such treatment is usually unsuccessful and may intensify their preoccupation. Men with muscle dysmorphia may use androgen supplements.

Many patients avoid appearing in public. Some leave their homes only at night; others, not at all. Social isolation, repeated hospitalization, and suicidal behavior may result.

Diagnosis and Treatment

Because patients with the disorder are reluctant to reveal their symptoms, the disorder may go undiagnosed for years. It is distinguished from normal concerns about appearance because it is time-consuming, causes significant distress, and impairs functioning.

Diagnosis is based on history. If the only concern is body shape and weight, anorexia nervosa may be the more accurate diagnosis (see p. 1701); if the only concern is sex characteristics, gender identity disorder may be considered (see p. 1732).

SSRIs are often effective, although relatively high doses are often required. Cognitive-behavioral therapy may also help.

CONVERSION DISORDER

Conversion disorder consists of symptoms or deficits that develop unconsciously and nonvolitionally and usually involve motor or sensory function. Manifestations resemble a neurologic or other general medical condition but rarely conform to known pathophysiologic mechanisms or anatomic pathways. Onset and maintenance of conversion symptoms are typically attributed to mental factors, such as stress. Diagnosis is based on history after excluding physical disorders. Treatment begins by establishing a consistent, supportive physician-patient relationship; psychotherapy can help, as may hypnosis or drug-facilitated interviews.

Conversion disorder tends to develop during adolescence or early adulthood but may occur at any age. It is somewhat more common among women. Isolated conversion symptoms may not fully meet the criteria of conversion disorder or somatization disorder.

Symptoms, Signs, and Diagnosis

Symptoms often develop abruptly, and onset can usually be linked to a stressful event. Symptoms are limited to those that affect voluntary motor or sensory function and suggest a neurologic or general medical condition (eg, impaired coordination or balance, weakness, or paralysis of an arm or a leg or loss of sensation in a body part). Other symptoms can include seizures, blindness, double vision, deafness, aphonia, difficulty in swallowing, sensation of a lump in the throat, and urinary retention.

The symptoms are severe enough to cause distress or disrupt social, occupational, or other important areas of functioning. A patient may have a single episode or sporadic repeated ones; symptoms may become chronic. Typically, episodes are brief.

The diagnosis is considered only after an examination and tests rule out physical disorders that can fully account for the symptoms and their effects.

Treatment

A consistently trusting and supportive physician-patient relationship is essential. After the physician has excluded a physical disorder and reassured the patient that the symptoms do not indicate a serious underlying disorder, the patient usually begins to feel better and symptoms fade. When a mentally distressing situation has preceded symptom onset, psychotherapy can be effective.

Other treatments are not widely effective. Hypnotherapy, drug-facilitated interviewing, and behavior modification therapy, including relaxation training, may help.

HYPOCHONDRIASIS

Hypochondriasis is a fear of having a serious disease based on misinterpretation of physical symptoms or normal bodily functions. Hypochondriasis is nonvolitional; the exact cause is unknown. Diagnosis is confirmed when fears and symptoms persist for ≥ 6 mo despite reassurance after thorough medical evaluation. Treatment includes establishing a consistent, supportive physician-patient relationship; psychotherapy and drug therapy may help.

Hypochondriasis usually begins in early adulthood and appears to occur equally among men and women.

Symptoms, Signs, and Diagnosis

A wide array of fears derive from misinterpretation of nonpathologic physical symptoms or normal bodily functions (eg, borborygmi, abdominal bloating and crampy discomfort, cardiac awareness, sweating). The location, quality, and duration of symptoms are often described in minute detail, but symptoms are generally not associated with abnormal physical findings. Symptoms adversely affect social and occupational functioning or cause significant distress.

The diagnosis is suggested by the history and confirmed when symptoms persist ≥ 6 mo after examination and reassurance by a physician fail to relieve the concerns. The symptoms are not better accounted for by depression or another mental disorder.

Prognosis and Treatment

The course is often chronic—fluctuating in some, steady in others; some patients recover. Treatment is difficult because the patient believes that something is seriously wrong and that the physician has failed to find the real cause. A trusting relationship with a caring, reassuring physician can still prove beneficial. If symptoms are not adequately relieved, the patient may benefit from a psychiatric referral while continuing under the care of the primary physician. Treatment with SSRIs may be helpful, as may cognitive-behavioral therapy.

MUNCHAUSEN SYNDROME

Munchausen syndrome, a severe and chronic form of factitious disorder, consists of repeated production of feigned physical symptoms without an external incentive; the motivation for this behavior is to assume the sick role. Symptoms are usually acute, dramatic, and convincing and are accompanied by a tendency to wander from one physician or hospital to another for treatment. The exact cause is unknown, although stress and borderline personality disorder are often implicated.

Munchausen patients may simulate many physical symptoms or conditions (eg, MI, hematemesis, hemoptysis, diarrhea, FUO). A patient's abdominal wall may be crisscrossed by scars, or a digit or a limb may have been amputated. Fevers are often due to self-inflicted injection with bacteria; *Escherichia coli* is often the infecting organism. Munchausen patients initially and sometimes interminably become the responsibility of medical or surgical clinics. Nevertheless, the disorder is a mental problem, is more complex than simple dishonest simulation of symptoms, and is associated with severe emotional difficulties. Patients may have prominent histrionic or borderline personality features but are usually intelligent and resourceful. They know how to simulate disease and are sophisticated regarding medical practices. They differ from malingerers because, although their deceits and simulations are conscious and volitional, it is unclear what they gain beyond medical attention for their suffering, and their motivations and quest for attention are largely unconscious and obscure.

There may be an early history of emotional and physical abuse. Patients may also have experienced a severe illness during childhood or had a seriously ill relative. Patients appear to have problems with their identity, inadequate impulse control, a deficient sense of reality, and unstable relationships. Feigning illness may be a way to increase or protect self-esteem by means of blaming failures on their illness, being associated with prestigious physicians and medical centers, and appearing unique, heroic, or medically knowledgeable and sophisticated.

Diagnosis is based on history and examination, including any tests necessary to exclude physical disorders. Less severe and chronic forms of factitious disorder may also involve the production of physical symptoms. Other forms of factitious disorder may involve feigning of mental (rather than physical) signs and symptoms, eg, depression, hallucinations, and delusions or symptoms of posttraumatic stress disorder. In these cases, too, the patient's apparent goal is to assume the sick role. In other cases, patients may produce both mental and physical symptoms.

Treatment

Treatment is rarely successful. Patients get initial relief by having their treatment demands met, but their provocations typically escalate, ultimately surpassing what physicians are willing or able to do. Confrontation or refusal to meet treatment demands often results in angry reactions, and patients generally move on to another physician or hospital. Psychiatric treatment is usually refused or circumvented, but consultation and follow-up care may be accepted, at least to help resolve a crisis. However, management is generally limited to recognizing the disorder early and avoiding risky procedures and excessive or unwarranted use of drugs.

Munchausen patients or those with a more limited factitious disorder can be nonaggressively and nonpunitively confronted with the diagnosis without suggesting guilt or reproach by redefining it as a cry for help. Alternatively, some experts recommend a nonconfrontational approach that offers patients a way to recover from their illness without admitting their role in its cause. In either case, it is helpful to convey that the physician and patient can cooperatively resolve the problem.

MUNCHAUSEN SYNDROME BY PROXY

Munchausen syndrome by proxy is a variant in which adults (usually parents) intentionally produce or feign symptoms in a person who is under their care (usually a child).

The adult falsifies history and may injure the child with drugs or other agents or add blood or bacterial contaminants to urine specimens to simulate disease. The parent seeks medical care for the child and appears to be deeply concerned and protective. The child typically has a history of frequent hospitalizations, usually for a variety of nonspecific symptoms, but no firm diagnosis. Victimized children may be seriously ill and sometimes die.

PAIN DISORDER

(Somatoform Pain Disorder)

Pain disorder consists of pain in one or more anatomic sites severe enough to cause distress or impairment of social, occupational, or other functioning. Mental factors seem to have a dominant role in the onset, severity, exacerbation, or maintenance of symptoms, but the pain is not intentionally produced or feigned. Some patients may recall an initial stimulus that produced acute pain. Diagnosis is based on history. Treatment begins by establishing a consistent, supportive physician-patient relationship; psychotherapy can also help.

The proportion of people whose chronic pain is dominated by mental factors is unknown. However, pain is rarely, if ever, "all in a patient's head"; apperception of pain involves sensory and emotional components (see p. 1769).

Symptoms, Signs, and Diagnosis

Pain dominated by mental factors is common in mood and anxiety disorders, but in pain disorder, pain is the predominant complaint. Any body part may be affected, but the back, head, abdomen, and chest are most common. The pain may be acute or chronic (> 6 mo). An underlying physical disorder or injury may explain the pain but not its severity and duration or the degree of disability.

Diagnosis is based on history after excluding a physical disorder that would adequately explain the pain and its severity, duration, and degree of disability. Detection of mental or social stressors may help explain the disorder.

Treatment

A thorough medical evaluation, followed by strong reassurance, may be sufficient. Sometimes, empathetically pointing out a relationship with an obvious mental or social stressor is effective. However, many patients develop chronic problems and are very difficult to treat. Patients are often reluctant to associate their problem with the psychosocial stressors and typically reject psychotherapy. They may visit many physicians with an expressed wish to find a cure and are at risk of developing dependence on opioids or benzodiazepines. Thorough regular reevaluations by a caring, empathetic physician, who remains alert to the possibility of a new significant physical disorder while protecting the patient from unnecessary and potentially costly or dangerous tests or procedures, offers the best hope for long-term palliation.

SOMATIZATION DISORDER

Somatization disorder is characterized by multiple physical complaints (which include pain and GI, sexual, and neurologic symptoms) over several years that cannot be explained fully by a physical disorder. Symptoms usually begin before age 30 and are not intentionally produced or feigned. Diagnosis is based on history after excluding physical disorders. Treatment focuses on establishing a consistent, supportive physician-patient relationship that avoids exposing the patient to unnecessary and potentially unsafe diagnostic testing and therapies.

Somatization disorder is often familial, yet the etiology is unknown. The disorder occurs more often in women. Male relatives of affected women have an increased risk of antisocial personality and substance-related disorders.

Symptoms and Signs

Recurring and multiple physical complaints usually begin before age 30. Severity fluctuates, but symptoms persist. Complete symptom relief for any extended period is rare. Some people become more overtly depressed, and their references to suicide become more ominous.

Any body part may be affected, and specific symptoms and their frequency vary among cultures. In the US, typical symptoms include headache, nausea and vomiting, bloating, abdominal pain, diarrhea or constipation, dysuria, dysmenorrhea, dyspareunia, and loss of sexual desire. Men frequently complain of erectile or ejaculatory dysfunction. Neurologic symptoms are common. Anxiety and depression may also occur. Typically, patients are dramatic and emotional when recounting their symptoms, often referring to them as "unbearable," "beyond description," or "the worst imaginable."

Patients may become extremely dependent. They increasingly demand help and emotional support and may become enraged when they feel their needs are not met. They are sometimes considered exhibitionistic and seductive. They may also threaten or attempt suicide. Often dissatisfied with their medical care, they typically go from one physician to another or seek treatment from several physicians concurrently.

The intensity and persistence of symptoms reflect the patient's strong desire to be cared for. Symptoms may help the patient avoid responsibilities, but they may also prevent pleasure and act as punishment, suggesting underlying feelings of unworthiness and guilt.

Diagnosis and Treatment

Patients are unaware of their underlying mental problem and believe that they have physical ailments, so they pressure physicians for tests and treatments. Physicians usually conduct many examinations and tests to eliminate a physical disorder as the cause. Because such patients may develop concurrent physical disorders, appropriate examinations and tests should also be performed when symptoms change significantly or when objective signs develop. Patients are commonly referred to a psychiatrist, even those patients who have a satisfactory relationship with a primary physician.

Specific diagnostic criteria include onset of many physical symptoms before age 30, treatment-seeking or impaired functioning, and a history of pain affecting at least 4 body parts, 2 or more GI symptoms, at least 1 sexual or reproductive symptom, and at least 1 neurologic symptom (excluding pain). The diagnosis is supported by the dramatic nature of the complaints and the patient's sometimes exhibitionistic, dependent, and suicidal behavior.

Somatization disorder is distinguished from generalized anxiety disorder, conversion disorder, and major depression by the predominance, multiplicity, and persistence of physical symptoms. Patients with about 6 mo of at least 1 physical symptom unexplained by a physical disorder who do not fully meet the specific diagnostic criteria for somatization disorder are said to have undifferentiated somatoform disorder.

Treatment is difficult. Patients tend to be frustrated and angered by suggestions that their symptoms are mental. Drug treatment may help concurrent mental disorders (eg, depression). Psychotherapy, particularly cognitive-behavioral therapy, emphasizes self-management of the disorder. It is important for the patient to have a supportive relationship with a physician who offers symptomatic relief, sees the patient regularly, and protects the patient from unnecessary tests and procedures.

205 SUICIDAL BEHAVIOR

Suicidal behavior includes 3 types of self-destructive acts: completed suicide, attempted suicide, and suicide gestures. Thoughts and plans about suicide are referred to as suicide ideation.

Completed suicide is a suicidal act that results in death. Attempted suicide is an act intended to be self-lethal, but one that does not result in death. Frequently, suicide attempts involve at least some ambivalence about wishing to die and may be a cry for help. Suicide gestures are attempts that involve an action with a very low lethal potential (eg, inflicting superficial scratches on the wrist, overdosing on vitamins). Suicide gestures and suicide ideation are most often pleas for help from people who still wish to live. They are predominantly ways of communicating feelings of desperation and hopelessness. However, they should not be dismissed lightly.

Epidemiology

Statistics on suicidal behavior are based mainly on death certificates and inquest reports and underestimate the true incidence. Suicide ranks 11th among causes of death in the US, with 30,622 completed suicides in 2001. It is the 3rd leading cause of death among people 15 to 24 yr. Men ≥ 75 yr have the highest rate of death by suicide. Among all age groups, male deaths by suicide outnumber female deaths by 4:1.

Each year, it is estimated that > 700,000 people attempt suicide. About 25 attempts are made for every death that occurs by suicide. However, 10% of people who make an attempt will eventually die by suicide, because many people make repeated attempts. About 20 to 30% of people who attempt suicide try again within 1 yr. About 3 females attempt suicide for every male that makes an attempt. The rate of attempts is disproportionately high among adolescent girls. Suicide runs in families.

People in a secure relationship have a significantly lower suicide rate than single people. Attempted and completed suicide rates are higher among those who live alone. Suicide is less common among practicing members of most religious groups (particularly Roman Catholics).

Group suicides, whether of many people or only 2 (such as lovers or spouses), represent an extreme form of personal identification with others.

Suicide notes are left by about 1 in 6 people who complete suicide. The content may indicate the mental disorder that led to the suicidal act.

Etiology

The primary remediable risk factor in suicide is depression. Other factors include social factors (disappointment and loss) and personality abnormalities (impulsivity and aggression). Traumatic childhood experiences, particularly the distresses of a broken home, parental deprivation, and abuse, are significantly more common among people who commit suicidal acts. Suicide is sometimes the final act in a course of self-destructive behavior, such as alcoholism, reckless driving, and violent antisocial acts. Often, one factor (commonly disruption of an important relationship) is the last straw. Serious physical disorders, especially those that are chronic and painful, play an important role in about 20% of suicides among the elderly.

Alcohol and drugs of abuse may increase disinhibition and impulsivity as well as worsen mood, a potentially lethal combination. About 30% of people who attempt suicide have consumed alcohol before the attempt, and about ½ of them were intoxicated at the time. Alcoholics are suicide-prone even when sober.

Some patients with schizophrenia commit suicide, sometimes from depression, to which these patients are prone. The suicide method may be bizarre and violent. Attempted suicide is uncommon, although it may be the first sign of psychiatric disturbance, occurring early in schizophrenia.

People with personality disorders are prone to attempted suicide—especially emotionally immature people with a borderline or an antisocial personality disorder, because they tolerate frustration poorly and react to stress impetuously with violence and aggression.

Aggression toward others is sometimes evident in suicidal behavior. In rare instances, former lovers or estranged spouses are involved in murder-suicides, in which one person murders another, then commits suicide.

Methods

The choice of methods is determined by cultural factors and availability as well as the seriousness of intent. Some methods (eg, jumping from heights) make survival virtually impossible, whereas others (eg, drug ingestion) make rescue possible. However, using a method that proves not to be fatal does not necessarily imply that the intent was less serious. A bizarre method suggests an underlying psychosis. Drug ingestion is the most frequent method used in suicide attempts. Violent methods, such as shooting and hanging, are uncommon among attempted suicides. Some methods, such as driving over cliffs, can endanger others. Suicide by police is a bizarre form of suicide in which a person commits an act (eg, brandishing a weapon) that forces law enforcement agents to kill him.

For completed suicides, firearms are most commonly used by both men (74%) and women (31%), followed by hanging in men and drug ingestion in women.

Management of Suicidal Acts

A health professional who becomes aware that a patient is contemplating suicide is, in most jurisdictions, required to inform an empowered agency to intervene. Failure to do so can result in criminal and civil actions. Such patients should not be left alone until they are in a secure environment. Transportation to the psychiatric facility should be accompanied by trained professionals (eg, ambulance, police), never by family members or friends.

Any suicidal act, regardless of whether it is a gesture or an attempt, must be taken seriously. Every person with a serious self-injury should be evaluated and treated for the physical injury. If an overdose of a potentially lethal drug is confirmed, immediate steps are taken to prevent absorption and expedite excretion, administer any available antidote, and provide supportive treatment (see Ch. 326 on p. 2651).

Initial assessment can be performed by any medical personnel trained in the assessment and management of suicidal behavior. However, psychiatric assessment should be performed as soon as possible for all patients. A decision must be made as to whether the person needs to be admitted and whether involuntary commitment or restraint is necessary. Patients with a psychotic disorder, delirium, or epilepsy and some with severe depression and an unresolved crisis should be admitted to a psychiatric unit.

After a suicide attempt, the patient may deny any problems, because the severe depression that led to the suicidal act may be followed by a short-lived mood elevation. Nonetheless, the risk of later, completed suicide is high unless the patient's problems are resolved.

The psychiatric assessment identifies some of the problems that contributed to the attempt and helps the physician plan appropriate treatment. It consists of establishing rapport; understanding the suicide attempt, its background, the events preceding it, and the circumstances in which it occurred; appreciating the current difficulties and problems; thoroughly understanding personal and family relationships, which are often pertinent to the suicide attempt; fully assessing the patient's mental state, with particular emphasis on recognizing depression, anxiety, agitation, panic attacks, severe insomnia, or other mental disorders and alcohol or drug abuse, which require specific treatment in addition to crisis intervention; interviewing close family members and friends; and contacting the family physician.

Prevention

Prevention requires identifying at-risk people and initiating appropriate interventions (see TABLE 205–1).

Although some attempted or completed suicides are a surprise and shock, even to close relatives and associates, clear warnings may have been given to family members, friends, or medical personnel. Warnings are often explicit, such as actually discussing plans or suddenly writing or changing a will. However, warnings can be more subtle, such as making comments about having nothing to live for or being better off if dead.

On average, primary care physicians encounter ≥6 potentially suicidal people in their practice each year. About 77% of people who commit suicide were seen by a physician within one year before killing themselves, and about 32% had been under psychiatric care during the preceding year. Because severe, painful physical disorders; substance abuse; and mental disorders, particularly depression, are so often a factor in suicide, recognition of these possible factors and initiating appropriate treatment are important contributions a physician can make to suicide prevention.

Each depressed patient should be questioned about thoughts of suicide. The fear that such inquiry may implant the idea of self-destruction is baseless. Inquiry helps the physician obtain a clearer picture of the depth of the depression, encourages constructive discussion, and conveys the physician's awareness of the patient's deep despair and hopelessness.

The risk of suicide is increased early in the treatment of depression, when psychomotor retardation and indecisiveness may be ameliorated but a depressed mood is only partially lifted. Psychoactive drugs must therefore be chosen carefully and dispensed in sublethal amounts so that ingestion of the entire contents of a prescription bottle would not be fatal. There is some evidence that certain antidepressants increase risk of suicidal behavior, especially in teenagers. Patients should be warned when starting antidepressants that their condition can worsen initially, possibly due to the drug itself, and they should be instructed to call their physician should they begin to feel worse.

Even in people threatening imminent suicide (eg, a patient who calls and declares that he is going to take a lethal dose of a drug or a person who threatens to jump from a high height), there may be some desire to live. The physician or another person to whom the person appeals for help must support the desire to live. Emergency psychiatric aid includes

TABLE 205–1. RISK FACTORS AND WARNING SIGNS FOR SUICIDE

Personal and Social Factors

Male sex

Age > 65 yr

Previous suicide attempt

Making detailed suicide plans, taking steps to implement plan (obtaining gun, pills), taking precautions against being discovered

Personally significant anniversaries

Family history of suicide or of affective disorder

Unemployment or financial difficulties, particularly if causing a drastic fall in economic status

Recent separation, divorce, or widowhood

Social isolation with real or imagined unsympathetic attitude of relatives or friends

Clinical Features

Depressive illness, especially at onset or near end of illness

Marked motor agitation, restlessness, and anxiety with severe insomnia

Marked feelings of guilt, inadequacy, and hopelessness; self-denigration or nihilistic delusion

Delusion or near-delusional conviction of a physical disorder (eg, cancer, heart disease, sexually transmitted disease)

Command hallucinations

Impulsive, hostile personality

Alcohol or drug abuse, especially of recent onset

A chronic, painful, or disabling physical disorder, especially in formerly healthy patients

Use of drugs that may contribute to suicidal behavior (eg, abruptly stopping paroxetine and certain other antidepressants can result in increased depression and anxiety, which in turn increases the risk of suicidal behavior)

establishing a relationship and open communication with the person; reminding him of his identity (ie, using his name repeatedly); helping sort out the problem that has caused the crisis; offering constructive help with the problem; encouraging the person to take positive action; and reminding him that family and friends care for him and want to help.

Effect of Suicide

Any suicidal act has a marked emotional effect on all involved. The physician, family, and friends may feel guilt, shame, and remorse at not having prevented it as well as anger toward the deceased or others. The physician can provide valuable assistance to the deceased's family and friends in dealing with their feelings of guilt and sorrow.

Assisted Suicide

Assisted suicide refers to the assistance given by physicians or other professionals to a person who wishes to end his life. Assistance may be requested as to drugs that can be saved up to take a lethal dose, instructions on a painless way to commit suicide, or administration of a lethal dose of drug. Assisted suicide is controversial and is illegal in most states in the US. Nonetheless, patients with painful, debilitating, and untreatable conditions may initiate a discussion about it with a physician. Assisted suicide may pose difficult ethical issues for physicians.

SECTION 16
NEUROLOGIC DISORDERS

206 APPROACH TO THE NEUROLOGIC PATIENT

Neurologic symptoms are common. History and neurologic examination can usually identify disorders requiring emergency action. Substituting CT, MRI, and laboratory tests for thorough clinical evaluation can lead to error and unnecessary cost. The neurologic evaluation aims to identify the pathophysiology of the problem and to determine where the abnormality originates: muscle, neuromuscular junction, peripheral nerve, plexus, nerve root, spinal cord, brain stem, or cerebrum.

History

The history is the most important part of the neurologic evaluation. Patients should be put at ease and allowed to tell their story in their own words. Usually, a clinician can quickly determine whether a reliable history is forthcoming or whether a family member should be interviewed instead. Specific questions clarify the quality, intensity, distribution, duration, and frequency of each symptom. What aggravates and attenuates the symptom and whether past treatment was effective or not should be determined. Specific disabilities should be described quantitatively (eg, walks at most 25 ft before stopping to rest), and their effect on the patient's daily routine noted. Past medical history and a complete review of systems are essential because neurologic complications are common in other disorders, especially alcoholism, diabetes, cancer, vascular disorders, and HIV infection. Family history is important because migraine and many metabolic, muscle, nerve, and neurodegenerative disorders are inherited. Social, occupational, and travel history provides information about unusual infections and exposure to toxins and parasites.

Sometimes neurologic symptoms and signs are functional or hysterical, reflecting a psychiatric disorder. Typically, such symptoms and signs do not conform to the rules of anatomy and physiology, and the patient is often depressed or unusually frightened. However, functional and physical disorders sometimes coexist and distinguishing them can be challenging.

Neurologic Examination

The neurologic examination begins with careful observation of the patient entering the examination area and during history taking. The patient's speed, symmetry, and coordination while moving to the examining table are noted, as are posture and gait. The patient's demeanor, dress, and responses provide information about mood and social adaptation. Abnormalities in language, speech, or praxis; neglect of space; unusual posturing; and other disorders of movement may be apparent before formal testing.

As information is obtained, a skilled examiner may include certain components of the examination and exclude others based on a preliminary hypothesis about anatomy and pathophysiology of the problem. If the examiner is less skilled, a complete neurologic screening is done.

Sidebar 206-1. EXAMINATION OF MENTAL STATUS

The mental status examination is an assessment of current mental capacity through evaluation of general appearance, behavior, any unusual or bizarre beliefs and perceptions (eg, delusions, hallucinations), mood, and all aspects of cognition (eg, attention, orientation, memory).

Examination of mental status is done as part of the routine physical examination in older patients and in those who have experienced head trauma or any new bout of confusion. Many screening tools are available: The Mini-Mental State is one of the most commonly used, but many others exist. Baseline results are recorded, and the examination is repeated yearly and whenever a change in mental status is suspected. Patients should be told that recording of mental status is routine.

The examination is performed in a quiet room, and the examiner should make sure that the patient can hear the questions clearly. Patients who do not speak English as their primary language should be questioned in the language they speak fluently.

Mental status examination evaluates the different parameters of cognitive function. The examiner must first establish that the patient is attentive—eg, by asking the patient to immediately repeat 3 words. It is not useful to test an inattentive patient further.

The parameters of cognitive function to be tested include the following:

Orientation	Test the 3 parameters of orientation: (1) person (What is your name?), (2) time (What is today's date?), and (3) place (What is the name of this place?)
Short-term memory	Ask the patient to repeat 3 objects after a 1-min delay.
Long-term memory	Ask the patient a question about the past, such as "What color suit did you wear at your wedding?" or "What was the make of your first car?"
Math	Use any simple mathematical test. Serial 7s are common: The patient is asked to start with 100 and to subtract 7, then 7 from that, etc.
Word finding	Ask the patient to name as many objects in a single category, such as articles of clothing or animals, as possible in 1 min.
Spelling	Ask the patient to spell a 5-letter word forward and backward.
Object identification	Hold up an object, such as a pen, book, or ruler, and ask the patient to name it.
Following commands	Start with a 1-step command, such as "Touch your nose with your right hand." Then test a 3-step command, such as "Take this piece of paper in your right hand. Fold it in half. Put the paper on the desk."
Writing	Ask the patient to write a sentence. The sentence should contain a subject and an object and should make sense. Spelling errors should be ignored.
Spacial orientation	Ask the patient to draw a clock and mark it with a specific time. Or ask the patient to copy a simple and then a more complex geometric shape.
Reasoning	Ask the patient to explain similarities between 3 or 4 objects or to explain a proverb.
Judgment	Have the patient explains what he would do in a hypothetical situation: "What would you do if you found a fire in your kitchen?"

Mental status (see also Ch. 195 on p. 1667): The patient's attention span is assessed first; an inattentive patient cannot cooperate fully and hinders testing. Any hint of cognitive decline requires examination of mental status (see sidebar 206–1), which involves testing of multiple aspects of cognitive function (eg, orientation to time, place, and person; memory; verbal and mathematical abilities; judgment; reasoning). Loss of orientation to person occurs only when obtundation, delirium, or dementia is severe; as an isolated symptom, it suggests malingering. Insight into illness and fund of knowledge in relation to educational level are assessed, as are affect and mood (see p. 1703).

The patient is asked to perform a complex command that involves 3 body parts and discriminates between right and left (eg, "Put your right thumb in your left ear, and stick out your tongue"). The patient is asked to name simple objects and body parts and to read, write, and repeat simple phrases; if deficits are noted, other tests of aphasia are needed (see p. 1788). Spatial perception can be assessed by asking the patient to imitate simple and complex finger constructions and to draw a clock, cube, house, or interlocking pentagons; the effort expended is often as informative as the final product. This test may identify impersistence, perseveration, micrographia, and hemispatial neglect. Praxis can be assessed by asking the patient to use a toothbrush or comb or to snap the fingers.

Cranial nerves (see also Ch. 219 on p. 1867): Smell, a function of the 1st (olfactory) cranial nerve, is usually evaluated only after head trauma or when lesions of the anterior fossa are suspected or patients report abnormal smell or taste. The patient is asked to identify odors (eg, soap, coffee, cloves) presented to each nostril. Alcohol, ammonia, and other irritants, which test the nociceptive receptors of the 5th (trigeminal) cranial nerve, are used only when malingering is suspected.

Evaluation of the 2nd (optic), 3rd (oculomotor), 4th (trochlear), and 6th (abducens) cranial nerves involves the visual system. For the 2nd cranial nerve, visual acuity is tested using a Snellen chart for distance vision and a hand-held chart for near vision; each eye is assessed individually, with the other eye covered. Color perception is tested using standard pseudoisochromatic Ishihara or Hardy-Rand-Ritter plates that have numbers or figures embedded in a field of specifically colored dots. Visual fields are tested by directed confrontation in all 4 visual quadrants. Direct and consensual pupillary response are tested (see also p. 1868). For the 3rd, 4th, and 6th cranial nerves, eyes are observed for symmetry of movement, globe position, asymmetry or droop of the eyelids (ptosis), and twitches or flutters of globes or lids. Extraocular movements controlled by these nerves are tested by asking the patient to follow a moving target (eg, examiner's finger, penlight) to all 4 quadrants (including across the midline); this test can detect nystagmus and palsies of ocular muscles. The pupillary light response is tested for symmetry and briskness. Funduscopic examination is also done.

To evaluate the 5th (trigeminal) nerve's 3 sensory divisions (ophthalmic, maxillary, and mandibular), an examiner uses a pin to test facial sensation and brushes a wisp of cotton against the lower or lateral cornea to evaluate the corneal reflex. If facial sensation is lost, the angle of the jaw should be examined; sparing of this area (innervated by spinal root C2) suggests a trigeminal deficit. A weak blink due to facial weakness (eg, 7th cranial nerve paralysis) should be distinguished from a depressed or absent corneal response, which is common in contact lens wearers. A patient with facial weakness feels the cotton wisp normally on both sides, even though blink is decreased. Trigeminal motor function is tested by palpating the masseter muscles while the patient clenches the teeth and by asking the patient to open the jaw against resistance. If a pterygoid muscle is weak, the jaw deviates to that side.

The 7th (facial) cranial nerve is evaluated by checking for hemifacial weakness. Asymmetry of facial movements is often more obvious during spontaneous conversation, especially when the patient smiles or, if obtunded, grimaces at a noxious stimulus; on the weakened side, the nasolabial fold is depressed and the palpebral fissure is widened. If the patient has only lower facial weakness (ie, furrowing of the forehead and eye closure are preserved), 7th nerve weakness is central rather than peripheral. Taste in the anterior ⅔ of the tongue can be tested with sweet, sour, salty, and bitter solutions placed on both sides of the tongue. Hyperacusis may be detected with a vibrating tuning fork held next to the ear.

Because the 8th (vestibulocochlear, acoustic, auditory) cranial nerve carries auditory and vestibular input, evaluation involves testing hearing (see p. 784) and balance (see p. 780).

The 9th (glossopharyngeal) and 10th (vagus) cranial nerves are usually evaluated together. Whether the palate elevates symmetrically is noted, and each side of the posterior pharynx is touched with a tongue blade to check for the gag reflex; bilateral absence of the gag reflex is common among healthy people and may not be significant. In an unresponsive, intubated patient, suctioning the endotracheal tube normally triggers coughing. If hoarseness is noted, the vocal cords are inspected. Isolated hoarseness (with normal gag and palatal elevation) should prompt a search for lesions (eg, mediastinal lymphoma, aortic aneurysm) compressing the recurrent laryngeal nerve.

The 11th (spinal accessory) cranial nerve is evaluated by testing the muscles it supplies. For the sternocleidomastoid, the patient is asked to turn the head against resistance supplied by the examiner's hand while the examiner palpates the active muscle (opposite the turned head). For the upper trapezius, the patient is asked to elevate the shoulders against resistance supplied by the examiner.

The 12th (hypoglossal) cranial nerve is evaluated by asking the patient to extend the tongue and inspecting it for atrophy, fasciculations, and weakness (deviation is toward the side of a lesion).

Motor system: The limbs and shoulder girdle should be fully exposed, then inspected and palpated for atrophy, hypertrophy, asymmetric development, fasciculations, myotonia, tremor, and other involuntary movements, including chorea (brief, jerky movements), athetosis (continuous, writhing movements), and myoclonus (shocklike contractions of a muscle). Passive flexion and extension of the limbs in a relaxed patient provide information about muscle tone. Decreased muscle bulk indicates atrophy, but bilateral atrophy or atrophy in large or concealed muscles, unless advanced, may not be obvious. In the elderly, loss of some muscle mass is common. Hypertrophy occurs when one muscle must work harder to compensate for weakness in another; pseudohypertrophy occurs when muscle tissue is replaced by excessive connective tissue or storage material.

Fasciculations (brief, fine, irregular twitches of the muscle visible under the skin) are relatively common. Although they can occur in normal muscle, particularly in calf muscles of the elderly, fasciculations usually indicate lesions of the lower motor neuron (eg, nerve degeneration or injury and regeneration). Myotonia (slowed relaxation of muscle after a sustained contraction or direct percussion of the muscle) indicates myotonic dystrophy and may be demonstrated by inability to quickly open a clenched hand. Increased resistance followed by relaxation (clasp-knife phenomenon) and spasticity indicates upper motor neuron lesions. Lead-pipe rigidity, often with cogwheeling, suggests a basal ganglia disorder.

Muscle strength: Patients who report weakness may mean fatigue, clumsiness, or true muscle weakness. Thus, the examiner must define the precise character of symptoms, including exact location, time of occurrence, precipitating and ameliorating factors, and associated symptoms and signs. Limbs are inspected for weakness (an extended weak limb drifts downward), tremor, and other involuntary movements. The strength of specific muscle groups is tested against resistance, comparing one side of the body against the other. However, pain may preclude a full effort during strength testing. With hysterical weakness, resistance to movement may be initially normal, followed by a sudden giving way.

Subtle weakness may be indicated by decreased arm swing while walking, pronator drift in an outstretched arm, decreased spontaneous use of a limb, an externally rotated leg, slowing of rapid alternating movements, or impairment of fine dexterity (eg, ability to fasten a button, open a safety pin, or remove a match from its box).

Strength should be graded. One useful scale assigns 0 to no visible muscle contraction, 1 to trace movement, 2 to limb movement when gravity is eliminated, 3 to movement against gravity but not resistance, 4 to movement against resistance supplied by the examiner, and 5 to normal strength. The difficulty with this and similar scales is the large range in strength possible between grades 4 and 5. Distal strength can be semiquantitatively measured with a handgrip ergometer or with an inflated BP cuff squeezed by the patient.

Functional testing often provides a better picture of the relationship between strength and disability. As the patient performs various maneuvers, deficiencies are noted and quantified as much as possible (eg, number of squats done or steps climbed). Rising from a squatting position or stepping onto a chair tests proximal leg strength; walking on the heels and on tiptoe tests distal strength. Pushing with the arms to get out of a chair indicates quadriceps weakness. Swinging the body to move the arms indicates shoulder girdle weakness. Rising from the supine position by turning prone, kneeling, and using the hands to climb up the thighs to slowly push erect (Gowers' sign) suggests pelvic girdle weakness.

Gait, stance, and coordination: Normal gait, stance, and coordination require integrity of the motor, vestibular, and proprioceptive pathways (see also Ch. 221 on p. 1879). A lesion in any of the pathways produces characteristic deficits: Cerebellar ataxia requires a wide gait for stability; dropfoot causes a steppage gait (lifting the leg higher than normal to avoid catching the foot on surface irregularities); pelvic muscle weakness causes waddling; and spastic leg causes scissoring and circumduction. Patients with impaired proprioception must constantly observe placement of their feet to avoid tripping or falling. Coordination can be tested with finger-to-nose or knee-to-shin maneuvers, which help detect ataxic movements.

Sensation: The best screening test for sensory loss uses a safety pin to lightly prick the face, torso, and 4 limbs; the patient is asked whether the pinprick feels the same on both sides and whether the sensation is dull or sharp. The pin is discarded after use to avoid transmission of HIV and hepatitis. Cortical sensory function is evaluated by asking the patient to identify a familiar object (eg, coin, key) placed in the palm of the hand (stereognosis) and numbers written on the palm (graphesthesia) and to distinguish between feeling 2 points and 1 point on the palm and on the fingers. Temperature sense can be tested with a cold tuning fork that has one prong rubbed warm by the palm or with test tubes containing warm and cold water. Joint position is tested by moving the terminal phalanges of the patient's fingers, then the toes, up or down. If the patient cannot identify these movements with eyes closed, the next most proximal joints are tested (eg, ankles if toe movement is not perceived). Pseudoathetosis refers to involuntary writhing, snakelike movements of a limb (athetosis) that result from loss of position sense; motor pathways, including those of the basal ganglia, are preserved. The brain cannot sense where the limb is in space so the limb moves on its own and the patient must use vision to control the limb's movements. Typically, when the eyes are closed, the patient cannot locate the limb in space. Inability to stand with feet together and eyes closed (Romberg test) indicates impaired postural sense. To test vibration sense, the examiner places a finger under the patient's distal interphalangeal joint and presses a lightly tapped 128-cycle tuning fork on top of the joint. The patient should note the end of vibration about the same time as the examiner, who feels it through the patient's joint. A cotton wisp can be used to test light touch.

If sensation is impaired, the anatomic pattern suggests location of the lesion: Stocking-glove distribution suggests peripheral nerves; dermatomal distribution, isolated nerves (mononeuritis multiplex) or nerve roots (radiculopathy); sensation reduced below a certain level, the spinal cord; crossed face-body pattern, the brain stem; and hemisensory loss, the brain (see FIGS. 206–1, 206–2, and 206–3). Location of the lesion is confirmed by determining whether motor weakness and reflex changes follow a similar pattern. Patchy sensory, motor, and reflex deficits in a limb suggest lesions of the brachial or pelvic plexus.

Reflexes: Deep tendon (muscle stretch) reflex testing evaluates the afferent nerve, synaptic connections within the spinal cord, motor nerves, and descending motor pathways. Lower motor neuron lesions (eg, affecting the anterior horn cell, spinal root, or peripheral nerve) depress reflexes; upper motor neuron lesions (ie, non–basal ganglia disorders anywhere above the anterior horn cell) increase reflexes (see p. 1897).

Reflexes tested include the biceps (innervated by C5 and C6), radial brachialis (by C6), triceps (by C7), quadriceps knee jerk (by L4), and ankle jerk (by S1). Any asymmetric increase or depression is noted. Jendrassik's maneuver can be used to augment hypoactive reflexes: The patient locks the hands together and pulls vigorously apart as a tendon in the lower extremity is tapped.

Lightly stroking the 4 quadrants of the abdomen should elicit a superficial abdominal reflex. Depression of this reflex may be due to a central lesion, obesity, or lax skeletal muscles (eg, after pregnancy); its absence may indicate spinal cord injury.

Pathologic reflexes (eg, Babinski's, Chaddock's, Oppenheim, snout, root, grasp) are reversions to primitive responses and indicate loss of cortical inhibition. Babinski's, Chaddock's, and Oppenheim reflexes all evaluate the plantar response. The normal reflex response is flexion of the great toe. An abnormal response is slower and consists of extension of the great toe with fanning of the other toes and often knee and hip flexion. This reaction is of spinal reflex origin and indicates spinal disinhibition due to an upper motor neuron lesion. For Babinski's reflex, the lateral sole of the foot is firmly stroked; stroking should not be too medial or it may inadvertently induce a primitive grasp reflex. In sensitive patients, the reflex response may be masked by quick voluntary withdrawal of the foot, which is not a problem in Chaddock's or Oppenheim reflex testing. For Chaddock's reflex, the lateral foot, from lateral malleolus to small toe, is stroked with a blunt instrument. For the Oppenheim reflex, the anterior tibia, from just below the patella to the foot, is firmly stroked with a knuckle.

The snout reflex is present if tapping a tongue blade across the lips causes pursing of the lips. The rooting reflex is present if stroking

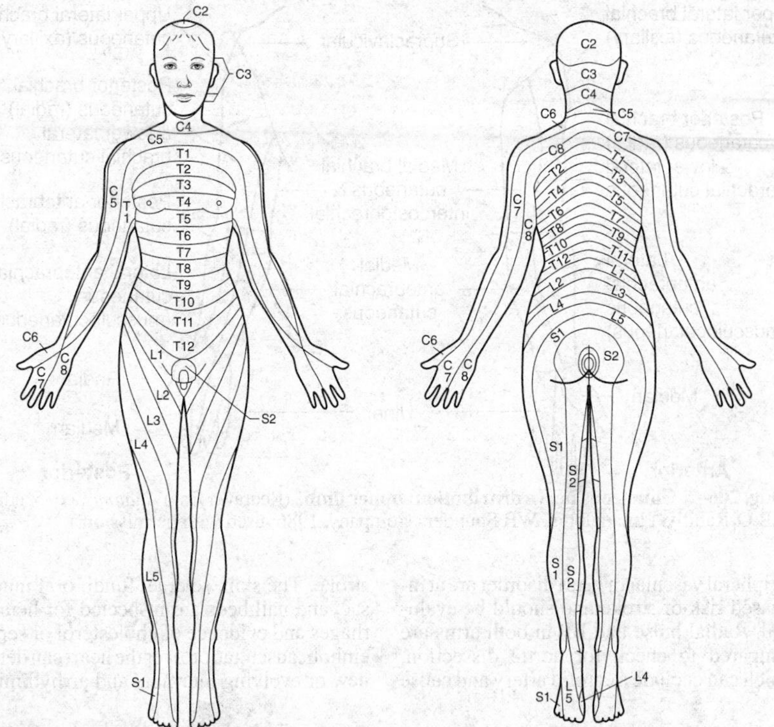

Fig. 206–1. Sensory dermatomes. (Redrawn from Keegan JJ, Garrett FD, *Anatomical Record* 102:409–437, 1948; used with permission of The Wistar Institute, Philadelphia, Pennsylvania.)

the lateral upper lip causes movement of the mouth toward the stimulus. The palmomental reflex is present if stroking the palm of the hand causes contraction of the ipsilateral mentalis muscle of the lower lip. Hoffman's sign is present if tapping the nail on the 3rd or 4th finger elicits involuntary flexion of the distal phalanx of the thumb and index finger.

For the glabellar sign, the forehead is tapped to induce blinking; normally, each of the 1st 5 taps induces a single blink, then the reflex fatigues. Blinking persists in patients with diffuse cerebral dysfunction.

Testing for clonus (rhythmic, rapid alternation of muscle contraction and relaxation caused by sudden, passive tendon stretching) is done by rapid dorsiflexion of the foot at the ankle. Sustained clonus suggests damage to an upper motor neuron.

Sphincteric reflexes may be tested during the rectal examination. When the perianal region is touched lightly (to test S4 to S5 nerve root levels), normal response is contraction of the external anal sphincter (anal wink); however, absence is not always pathologic. For the bulbospongiosus reflex, which tests S2 to S4 levels, the dorsum of the penis is tapped; normal response is contraction of the bulbospongiosus muscle. For the cremasteric reflex, which tests the L2 level, the area just below the inguinal crease is stroked; normal response is elevation of the ipsilateral testicle.

Autonomic nervous system (see also p. 1766): Assessment involves checking for postural hypotension, heart rate changes in response to the Valsalva maneuver, decreased or absent sweating, and evidence of Horner's syndrome (unilateral ptosis, pupillary constriction, and facial anhidrosis). Disturbances of bowel, bladder, sexual, and hypothalamic function should be noted.

Cerebrovascular examination: Patients, particularly the elderly, and those with hypertension, diabetes, hypercholesterolemia, or a

Upper lateral brachial cutaneous (axillary)
Supraclavicular
Posterior brachial cutaneous (radial) & lower lateral brachial cutaneous
Medial brachial cutaneous & intercostobrachial
Posterior antebrachial cutaneous (radial)
Lateral antebrachial cutaneous (musculocutaneous)
Medial antebrachial cutaneous
Radial
Median
Ulnar
Anterior
Posterior

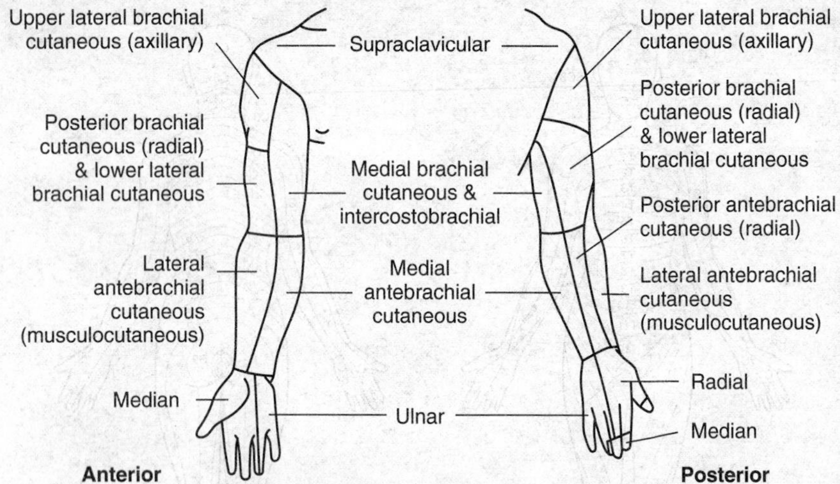

Fig. 206–2. Cutaneous nerve distribution: upper limb. (Redrawn from *Anatomy,* ed. 5, edited by R O'Rahilly. Philadelphia, WB Saunders Company, 1986; used with permission.)

peripheral vascular or heart disorder are at increased risk of stroke and should be evaluated. Radial pulse and BP in both arms are compared to check for aortic dissection, which can occlude a carotid artery and cause stroke. The skin, sclerae, fundi, oral mucosae, and nail beds are inspected for hemorrhages and evidence of cholesterol or septic emboli; auscultation over the heart can detect new or evolving murmurs and arrhythmias.

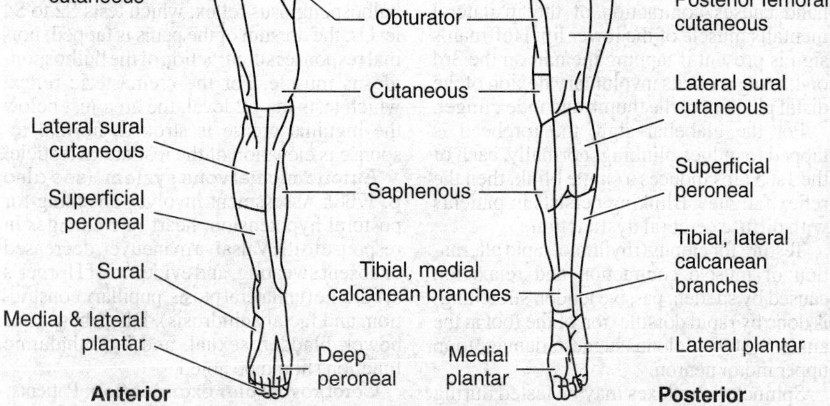

Ventral rami, spinal
Iliohypogastric
Genitofemoral
Lateral femoral cutaneous
Ilioinguinal
Lateral femoral cutaneous
Posterior femoral cutaneous
Obturator
Cutaneous
Lateral sural cutaneous
Lateral sural cutaneous
Saphenous
Superficial peroneal
Superficial peroneal
Sural
Tibial, medial calcanean branches
Tibial, lateral calcanean branches
Medial & lateral plantar
Lateral plantar
Deep peroneal
Medial plantar
Anterior
Posterior

Fig. 206–3. Cutaneous nerve distribution: lower limb. (Redrawn from *Anatomy,* ed. 5, edited by R O'Rahilly. Philadelphia, WB Saunders Company, 1986; used with permission.)

Bruits over the cranium may indicate an arteriovenous malformation or fistula or, occasionally, redirected blood flow across the circle of Willis after carotid occlusion. Auscultation over the carotid arteries can detect bruits near the bifurcation; vigorous palpation should be avoided. By running the bell of the stethoscope down the neck toward the heart, the examiner may identify a change in character that can distinguish a bruit from a systolic heart murmur. Decreased vigor of the carotid upstroke suggests a stenotic lesion. Peripheral pulses are palpated to check for peripheral vascular disease. The temporal arteries are palpated; enlargement or tenderness may suggest temporal arteritis.

NEUROLOGIC DIAGNOSTIC PROCEDURES

Diagnostic procedures should not be used for preliminary screening, except perhaps in emergencies when a complete neurologic evaluation is impossible. Evidence uncovered during the history and physical examination should guide testing.

Lumbar puncture (spinal tap): Lumbar puncture is used to evaluate intracranial pressure and CSF composition (see TABLE 206–1) and to administer intrathecal drugs or radiopaque agent for myelography. Relative contraindications include infection at the puncture site, bleeding diathesis, increased intracranial pressure, and Chiari I type malformation obstructing CSF flow. If papilledema or focal neurologic deficits are present, CT or MRI should be used before lumbar puncture to rule out presence of a mass that could precipitate transtentorial or cerebellar herniation.

For the procedure, the patient is typically in the left lateral decubitus position. A cooperative patient is asked to hug the knees and curl up as tightly as possible. Assistants may have to hold patients who cannot maintain this position, or the spine may be flexed better by having patients, particularly obese patients, sit on the side of the bed and lean over a bedside tray table. An area 20 cm in diameter is washed with iodine, then wiped with alcohol to remove the iodine and prevent its introduction into the subarachnoid space. An LP needle with stylet is inserted into the L4 to L5 interspace (the L4 spinous process is typically on a line between the posterior-superior iliac crests); the needle is aimed rostrally toward the patient's umbilicus and always kept parallel to the floor. Entrance into the subarachnoid space is usually accompanied by a discernible pop; the stylet is withdrawn to allow CSF to flow out. Opening pressure is measured with a manometer; 4 tubes are each filled with about 5 to 10 mL of CSF for testing. The puncture site is then covered with a sterile adhesive strip. A postlumbar puncture headache (see p. 1849) occurs in about 10% of patients.

Normal CSF is clear and colorless; ≥ 300 cells/μL produces cloudiness or turbidity. Bloody fluid may indicate a traumatic puncture (pushing the needle in too far, into the venous plexus along the anterior spinal canal) or subarachnoid hemorrhage. A traumatic puncture is distinguished by gradual clearing of the CSF between the 1st and 4th tubes (confirmed by decreasing RBC count), absence of xanthochromia (yellowish CSF due to lysed RBCs) in a centrifuged sample, and fresh, uncrenated RBCs. With intrinsic subarachnoid hemorrhage, the CSF remains uniformly bloody throughout collection; xanthochromia is often present if several hours have passed after ictus; and RBCs are usually older and crenated. Faintly yellow fluid may also be due to senile chromogens, severe jaundice, or increased protein (> 100 mg/dL).

Cell count and differential glucose and protein counts aid in the diagnosis of many neurologic disorders (see TABLE 206–1). If infection is suspected, the centrifuged CSF sediment is stained for bacteria (Gram stain), for TB (acid-fast stain or immunofluorescence), and for *Cryptococcus* sp (India ink). Larger amounts of fluid (10 mL) improve the chances of detecting the pathogen, particularly acid-fast bacilli and certain fungi, in stains and cultures. In early meningococcal meningitis or severe leukopenia, CSF protein may be too low for bacterial adherence to the glass slide during Gram staining, producing a false-negative result. Mixing a drop of aseptic serum with CSF sediment prevents this problem. When hemorrhagic meningoencephalitis is suspected, a wet mount is used to search for amebas. Latex particle agglutination and coagglutination tests may allow rapid bacterial identification, especially when stains and cultures are negative (eg, in partially treated meningitis). CSF should be cultured aerobically and anaerobically and for acid-fast bacilli and fungi. Except for enteroviruses, viruses are seldom isolated from the CSF. Viral antibody panels are available.

TABLE 206–1. CEREBROSPINAL FLUID ABNORMALITIES IN VARIOUS DISORDERS

CONDITION	PRESSURE	WBC/μL	PREDOMINANT CELL TYPE	GLUCOSE	PROTEIN
Normal	100–200 mm H_2O	0–3	L	50–100 mg/dL (2.78–5.55 mmol/L)	20–45 mg/dL
Acute bacterial meningitis	↑	100–10,000	PMN	↓	> 100 mg/dL*
Subacute meningitis (TB, *Cryptococcus* infection, sarcoidosis, leukemia, carcinoma)	N or ↑	100–700	L	↓	↑
Acute syphilitic meningitis	N or ↑	25–2000	L	N	↑
Paretic neurosyphilis	N or ↑	15–2000	L	N	↑
Lyme disease of CNS	N or ↑	0–500	L	N	N or ↑
Brain abscess or tumor	N or ↑	0–1000	L	N	N or ↑
Viral infections	N or ↑	100–2000	L	N	N or ↑
Pseudotumor cerebri	↑	N	L	N	N or ↓
Cerebral hemorrhage	↑	Bloody	RBCs	N	↑
Cerebral thrombosis	N or ↑	0–100	L	N	N or ↑
Spinal cord tumor	N	0–50	L	N	N or ↑
Guillain-Barré syndrome	N	0–100	L	N	> 100 mg/dL
Lead encephalopathy	↑	0–500	L	N	↑

L = lymphocyte; N = normal; PMN = polymorphonuclear leukocyte; ↑ = increased; ↓ = decreased.
*Up to 14% of patients may have a CSF protein level < 100 mg/dL on the initial lumbar puncture.

NOTE: Figures given for pressure, cell count, and protein are approximations; exceptions are common. Similarly, PMNs may predominate in disorders usually characterized by lymphocyte response, especially early in the course of viral infections or tuberculous meningitis. Alterations in glucose are less variable and more reliable.

Venereal Disease Research Laboratories (VDRL) testing and cryptococcal antigen testing are often routinely done. PCR tests for herpes simplex virus and other CNS pathogens are available.

Normally, CSF:blood glucose ratio is about 0.6, and except in severe hypoglycemia, CSF glucose is typically > 50 mg/dL (2.78 mmol/L). Increased CSF protein (> 50 mg/dL) is a sensitive but nonspecific index of disease; protein increases to > 500 mg/dL in purulent meningitis, advanced TB meningitis, complete block by spinal cord tumor, or a bloody puncture. Special examinations for globulin (normally < 15%), oligoclonal banding, and myelin basic protein aid in diagnosis of a demyelinating disorder.

CT: CT provides rapid, noninvasive imaging of the brain and skull. A radiopaque agent helps detect brain tumors and abscesses. Noncontrast CT is used to rapidly detect acute hemorrhage and various gross structural changes without concern about contrast allergy or renal failure. With an intrathecal agent, CT can outline abnormalities encroaching on the brain stem, spinal cord, or spinal nerve roots (eg, meningeal carcinoma, herniated disk) and may detect a syrinx in the spinal cord. CT angiography can show the cerebral blood vessels, obviating the need for MRI or angiography.

MRI: MRI provides better resolution of neural structures than CT. This difference is most significant clinically for visualizing brain stem lesions and other abnormalities of the posterior fossa; CT images of this region are often marred by bony streak artifacts. Also, MRI is better for detecting demyelinating plaques, early infarction, subclinical brain edema, cerebral contusions, incipient transtentorial herniation, abnormalities of the craniocervical junction, and syringomyelia. It is especially valuable for identifying spinal abnormalities (eg, tumor, abscess) compressing the spinal cord and requiring emergency intervention. Visualization of inflammatory, demyelinated, and neoplastic lesions may require enhancement with IV paramagnetic contrast agents (eg, gadolinium). Use of diffusion-weighted MRI allows rapid, early detection of ischemic stroke. MRI is contraindicated in patients who have had a pacemaker, cardiac or carotid stents for < 6 wk or who have ferromagnetic aneurysm clips or other metallic objects that may overheat or be displaced within the body by the intense magnetic field.

Magnetic resonance angiography (MRA) uses MRI with or without a contrast agent to show cerebral vessels and major arteries and their branches in the head and neck. Although MRA has not replaced cerebral angiography, it is used when cerebral angiography cannot be done (eg, because the patient refuses or has increased risk). As a check for stroke, MRA tends to exaggerate severity of arterial narrowing and thus does not usually miss occlusive disease of large arteries.

Magnetic resonance venography (MRV) uses MRI to show the major veins and dural sinuses of the cranium. MRV obviates the need for cerebral angiography in diagnosing cerebral venous thrombosis and is useful for monitoring thrombus resolution and guiding the duration of anticoagulation. Magnetic resonance spectroscopy can measure metabolites in the brain regionally to distinguish tumors from abscess or stroke.

Echoencephalography: Ultrasonography can be used at the bedside (usually in the neonatal ICU) to detect hemorrhage and hydrocephalus in children < 2 yr. CT has replaced echoencephalography in older children and adults.

Cerebral angiography: X-rays taken after a radiopaque agent is injected show arterial and venous circulation in the brain. With digital data processing (digital subtraction angiography), small amounts of agent can produce high-resolution images. Cerebral angiography supplements CT and MRI in delineating the site and vascularity of intracranial lesions; it is the gold standard for diagnosing stenotic or occluded arteries, congenitally absent vessels, aneurysms, and arteriovenous malformations. Vessels as small as 0.1 mm can be visualized. Angiographic interventions (eg, angioplasty, stent placement, intra-arterial thrombolysis, aneurysm obliteration) can be done.

Duplex Doppler ultrasonography: This noninvasive procedure can assess dissection, stenosis, occlusion, and ulceration of the carotid bifurcation. It is safe and rapid, but it does not provide the detail of angiography. It is preferable to periorbital Doppler ultrasonography and oculoplethysmography for evaluating patients with carotid artery transient ischemic attacks and is useful for following an abnormality over time. Transcranial Doppler ultrasonography helps evaluate residual blood flow after brain death, vasospasm of the middle cerebral artery after subarachnoid hemorrhage, and vertebrobasilar stroke.

Myelography: X-rays are taken after a radiopaque agent is injected into the subarachnoid space via lumbar puncture. MRI has replaced myelography for evaluation of intraspinal abnormalities, but CT myelography is still done when MRI is unavailable. Contraindications are the same as those for lumbar puncture. Myelography may exacerbate the effects of spinal cord compression, especially if too much fluid is removed too rapidly.

EEG: Electrodes are distributed over the brain to detect electrical changes associated with seizure disorders, sleep disorders, and metabolic or structural encephalopathies. Twenty electrodes are distributed symmetrically over the scalp. The normal awake EEG shows 8- to 12-Hz, 50-μV sinusoidal alpha waves that wax and wane over the occipital and parietal lobes and > 12-Hz, 10- to 20-μV beta waves frontally, interspersed with 4- to 7-Hz theta waves. The EEG is examined for asymmetries between the 2 hemispheres (suggesting a structural disorder), for excessive slowing (appearance of 1- to 4-Hz, 50- to 350-μV delta waves, as occurs in depressed consciousness, encephalopathy, and dementia), and for abnormal wave patterns.

Abnormal wave patterns may be nonspecific (eg, epileptiform sharp waves) or diagnostic (eg, 3-Hz spike and wave for absence seizures, 1-Hz periodic sharp waves for Creutzfeldt-Jakob disease). The EEG is particularly useful for appraising episodic altered consciousness of uncertain etiology. If a seizure disorder is suspected and the routine EEG is normal, maneuvers that electrically activate the cortex (eg, hyperventilation, photic stimulation, sleep, sleep deprivation) can sometimes elicit evidence of a seizure disorder. Nasopharyngeal leads can sometimes detect a temporal lobe seizure focus when the EEG is otherwise uninformative. Continuous ambulatory monitoring of the EEG (with or without video monitoring) over 24 h can often determine whether fleeting memory lapses, subjective auras, or unusual episodic motor behavior is due to seizure activity.

Measurement of evoked responses (potentials): Visual, auditory, or tactile stimuli are used to activate corresponding areas of the cerebral cortex, resulting in focal cortical electrical activity. Ordinarily, these small potentials are lost in EEG background noise, but computer processing cancels out the noise to reveal a waveform. Latency, duration, and amplitude of the evoked responses indicate whether the tested sensory pathway is intact.

Evoked responses are particularly useful for detecting clinically inapparent deficits in a demyelinating disorder, appraising sensory systems in uncooperative infants, substantiating deficits suspected to be histrionic, and following the subclinical course of disease. For example, visual evoked responses may detect unsuspected optic nerve damage by multiple sclerosis. When integrity of the brain stem is in question, brain stem auditory evoked responses is an objective test. Somatosensory evoked responses may pinpoint the physiologic disturbance when a structural disorder (eg, metastatic carcinoma that invades the plexus and spinal cord) affects multiple levels of the neuraxis.

Electromyography and nerve conduction velocity studies: When determining whether weakness is due to nerve, muscle, or neuromuscular junction disorder is clinically difficult, these studies can identify the affected nerves and muscles.

In electromyography, a needle is inserted in a muscle, and electrical activity is recorded while the muscle is contracting and resting. Normally, resting muscle is electrically silent; with minimal contraction, action potentials of single motor units appear. As contraction increases, the number of potentials increases, forming an interference pattern. Denervated muscle fibers are recognized by increased activity with needle insertion and abnormal spontaneous activity (fibrillations and fasciculations); fewer motor units are recruited during contraction, producing a reduced interference pattern. Surviving axons branch to innervate adjacent muscle fibers, enlarging the motor unit and producing giant action potentials. In muscle disorders, individual fibers are affected without regard to their motor units; thus, amplitude of their potentials is diminished, but the interference pattern remains full.

In nerve conduction velocity studies, a peripheral nerve is stimulated with electrical shocks at several points along its course to a muscle, and the time to initiation of contraction is recorded. The time an impulse takes to traverse a measured length of nerve determines conduction velocity. The time required to traverse the segment nearest the muscle is called distal latency. Similar measurements can be made for sensory nerves. When weakness is due to a muscle disorder, nerve conduction is normal. In neuropathy, conduction is often slowed, and the response pattern may show a dispersion of potentials due to unequal involvement of myelinated and unmyelinated axons. A nerve can be repeatedly stimulated to evaluate the neuromuscular junction for fatigability; eg, a progressive decremental response occurs in myasthenia gravis.

207 NEUROTRANSMISSION

A neuron generates and propagates an action potential along its axon, then transmits this signal across a synapse by releasing neurotransmitters, which trigger a reaction in another neuron or an effector cell (eg, muscle cells; most exocrine and endocrine cells). The signal may stimulate or inhibit the receiving cell, depending on the neurotransmitter and receptor involved.

In the CNS, interconnections are complex. An impulse from one neuron to another may pass from axon to cell body, axon to dendrite (a neuron's receiving branches), cell body to cell body, or dendrite to dendrite. A neuron simultaneously receives many impulses—excitatory and inhibitory—from other neurons and integrates them into various patterns of firing.

Propagation: Action potential propagation along an axon is electrical, caused by the exchanges of Na^+ and K^+ ions across the axonal membrane. A particular neuron generates an identical action potential after each stimulus, conducting it at a fixed velocity along the axon. Velocity depends on axonal diameter and degree of myelination and ranges from 1 to 4 m/sec in small, unmyelinated fibers to 75 m/sec in large myelinated ones. Propagation speed is higher in myelinated fibers because the myelin cover has regular gaps (nodes of Ranvier) where the axon is exposed. The electrical impulse jumps from one node to the next, skipping the myelinated section of the axon. Thus, disorders that alter the myelin cover (eg, multiple sclerosis) interfere with impulse propagation, causing various neurologic symptoms.

Transmission: Impulse transmission is chemical, caused by release of specific neurotransmitters from the nerve ending (terminal). Neurotransmitters diffuse across the synaptic cleft and bind briefly to specific receptors on the adjoining neuron or effector cell. Depending on the receptor, the response may be excitatory or inhibitory.

One type of synapse, the electrical synapse, does not involve neurotransmitters; ion channels directly connect the cytoplasm of the presynaptic and postsynaptic neurons. This type of transmission is the fastest.

The nerve cell body produces enzymes that synthesize most neurotransmitters, which are stored in vesicles at the nerve terminal (see FIG. 207–1). The amount in one vesicle (usually several thousand molecules) is a quantum. An action potential arriving at the terminal opens axonal Ca channels; Ca inflow releases neurotransmitter molecules from many vesicles by fusing the vesicle membranes to the nerve terminal membrane. Membrane fusion generates an opening through which the molecules are expelled into the synaptic cleft via exocytosis.

The amount of neurotransmitters in the terminal is typically independent of nerve activity and kept relatively constant by modifying uptake of neurotransmitter precursors or the activity of enzymes involved in neurotransmitter synthesis or destruction. Stimulation

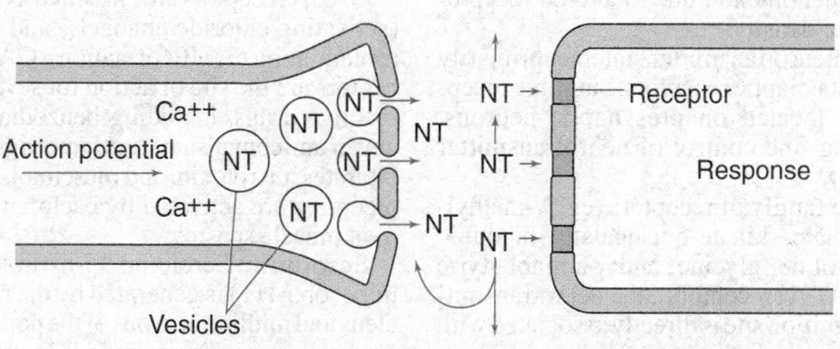

Fig. 207–1. Neurotransmission. Action potentials open the axonal Ca channels (not shown). Ca^{++} activates release of neurotransmitters (NT) from vesicles where they are stored. NT molecules fill the synaptic cleft. Some bind to postsynaptic receptors, initiating a response. The others are pumped back into the axon and stored or diffuse into the surrounding tissues.

of presynaptic receptors can decrease presynaptic neurotransmitter synthesis, and blockade can increase it.

The neurotransmitter-receptor interaction must be terminated quickly to allow rapid, repeated activation of receptors. The neurotransmitter is quickly pumped back into the presynaptic nerve terminals by active, ATP-dependent processes (reuptake), is destroyed by enzymes near the receptors, or diffuses into the surrounding area and is removed. Neurotransmitters taken up by the nerve terminals are repackaged in vesicles for reuse.

Disorders or substances that alter the production, release, reception, breakdown, or reuptake of neurotransmitters or that change the number and affinity of receptors can cause neurologic or psychiatric symptoms and disorders (see TABLE 207–1). Drugs that modify neurotransmission can alleviate many of these disorders (eg, Parkinson's disease, depression).

Receptors: Neurotransmitter receptors are protein complexes that span the cell membrane. Their nature determines whether a given neurotransmitter is excitatory or inhibitory. Receptors that are continuously stimulated by neurotransmitters or drugs become desensitized (downregulated); those that are not stimulated by their neurotransmitter or are chronically blocked by drugs become supersensitive (upregulated). Downregulation or upregulation of receptors strongly influences the development of tolerance and physical dependence. These concepts are particularly important in organ or tissue transplantation, in which denervation deprives receptors of their neurotransmitter. Withdrawal symptoms can be explained at least in part by a rebound phenomenon due to altered receptor affinity or density.

Most neurotransmitters interact primarily with postsynaptic receptors, but some receptors are located on presynaptic neurons, providing fine control of neurotransmitter release.

In one family of receptors (eg, *N*-methyl-D-glutamate, kinate-quisqualate, nicotinic acetylcholine, glycine, and γ-aminobutyric acid [GABA] receptors), the neurotransmitter recognition site is directly associated with an ion channel, thus providing a rapid response. In the other family (eg, serotonin, α- and β-adrenergic, and dopaminergic receptors), receptor activation causes another molecule (2nd messenger) to carry the message to the effector. The 2nd messenger is commonly an enzyme that catalyzes a chain of events resulting in protein phosphorylation or Ca mobilization; responses mediated by a 2nd messenger system are slower. Far more neurotransmitters activate specific receptors than 2nd messengers.

Major Neurotransmitters and Receptors

At least 100 substances can act as neurotransmitters; about 18 are of major importance. Several occur in slightly different forms.

Glutamate and aspartate: These amino acids are the major excitatory neurotransmitters in the CNS. They occur in the cortex, cerebellum, and spinal cord. In neurons, synthesis of nitric oxide (NO) increases in response to glutamate. Excess glutamate can be toxic, increasing intracellular Ca, free radicals, and proteinase activity. These neurotransmitters may contribute to tolerance to opioid therapy and mediate hyperalgesia.

Glutamate receptors are classified as NMDA (*N*-methyl-D-aspartate) receptors and non-NMDA receptors. Phencyclidine (PCP, also known as angel dust) and memantine (used to treat Alzheimer's disease) bind to NMDA receptors.

GABA: GABA is the major inhibitory neurotransmitter in the brain. It is an amino acid derived from glutamic acid, which is decarboxylated by glutamate decarboxylase. After interaction with its receptors, GABA is actively pumped back into nerve terminals and metabolized. Glycine, which resembles GABA in its action, occurs principally in interneurons (Renshaw cells) of the spinal cord and in circuits that relax antagonist muscles.

GABA receptors are classified as $GABA_A$ (activating chloride channels) and $GABA_B$ (potentiating cAMP formation). $GABA_A$ receptors are the site of action for several neuroactive drugs, including benzodiazepines, newer anticonvulsants (eg, lamotrigine), barbiturates, picrotoxin, and muscimol. $GABA_B$ receptors are activated by baclofen, used to treat muscle spasms.

Serotonin: Serotonin (5-hydroxytryptamine, or 5-HT) is generated by the raphe nucleus and midline neurons of the pons and upper brain stem. Tryptophan is hydroxylated by tryptophan hydroxylase to 5-hydroxytryptophan, then decarboxylated to serotonin. Serotonin levels are controlled by the uptake of tryptophan and intraneuronal monoamine oxidase (MAO).

TABLE 207–1. EXAMPLES OF DISORDERS ASSOCIATED WITH DEFECTS IN NEUROTRANSMISSION

DISORDER	PATHOPHYSIOLOGY	TREATMENT
Neurotransmitter imbalance		
Alzheimer's disease	Loss of brain cells in the limbic system (eg, hippocampus) and the association area of the cortex, especially neurons that synthesize and use acetylcholine	Cholinesterase inhibitors (donepezil, rivastigmine, galantamine) delay synaptic degradation of acetylcholine and thus modestly improve cognitive function and memory. Memantine, an NMDA-receptor antagonist, may slow progression of the disease and increase autonomy
Anxiety	May reflect reduced activity of GABA, perhaps due to imbalance of endogenous inhibitors, stimulators of the GABA receptor, or both	Benzodiazepines increase the probability of opening Cl^-channels modulated by GABA through $GABA_A$ receptor activation
Autism	Possible hyperserotonemia, which occurs in 30–50% of autistic people, with no evidence of central 5-HT abnormalities	No specific drug therapy exists
Brain injury	Injury (eg, trauma, hypoxia, prolonged seizures) stimulating excessive glutamate release, which leads to increased Ca and Na and neuronal death	Ca channel blockers, glycine, and older NMDA-receptor antagonists (eg, dextromethorphan, ketamine) may reduce the extent of neuronal loss in experimental ischemia but are not effective in people. Memantine, a newer NMDA-receptor antagonist, is under study
Depression	Reduced norepinephrine and 5-HT levels and an increased number of β-adrenergic $5\text{-}HT_2$ receptors; possible overactivity of α_2-adrenergic presynaptic receptors that regulate norepinephrine release, reducing the amount of norepinephrine in the synaptic cleft; possible involvement of other hormones and neuropeptides (eg, substance P, CRF, neuropeptide Y, vasopressin V1b, glutamate, acetylcholine)	Antidepressants downregulate receptors indirectly or directly by inhibiting reuptake of 5-HT (as with SSRIs) and norepinephrine or by blocking MAO. Activation of $5\text{-}HT_2$ receptors (as with nefazodone) is also involved in the antidepressant effect. Substance P (neurokinin-1 [NK1]) and CRF-1 antagonists show promise in the treatment of depression
Seizure disorders	Seizures consisting of sudden synchronous high-frequency firing by localized groups of neurons in certain brain areas, perhaps caused by reduced activity of GABA	Phenytoin stabilizes neuronal membranes and reduces excessive neurotransmitter release. Phenobarbital binds to the $GABA_A$ receptor–Cl channel complex, enhancing the opening time of the Cl^- channel modulated by activation of $GABA_4$ receptors by GABA

Table continues on the following page.

TABLE 207–1. EXAMPLES OF DISORDERS ASSOCIATED WITH DEFECTS IN NEUROTRANSMISSION—Continued

DISORDER	PATHOPHYSIOLOGY	TREATMENT
Huntington's disease (chorea)	Major neuronal damage in cortex and striatum due to polyglutamine expansion (encoded by CAG repeat), produced by an abnormal gene on chromosome 4; the abnormal gene overproduces the protein huntingtin, which may combine with molecules that induce excessive stimulation of cells by excitatory amino acid neurotransmitters (eg, glutamate), exacerbating oxidative apoptosis	No specific treatment exists, but drugs that block NMDA receptors may block the toxic effects of excess glutamate. GABA-mimetic drugs are ineffective
Mania	Increased norepinephrine levels, reduced 5-HT levels, and a decreased number of adrenergic receptors	Lithium is the drug of choice. It reduces norepinephrine release and 2nd-messenger synthesis, thereby upregulating receptors. However, its ability to decrease PIP_2 seems to be the principal mechanism of action. Valproate is beneficial
Neuroleptic malignant syndrome	Blockage of D_2 receptors by drugs (eg, antipsychotic drugs, methylphenidate) or abrupt withdrawal of a dopaminergic agonist, resulting in muscle rigidity, fever, change in mental status, and autonomic instability	Treatment with a D_2 agonist (eg, bromocriptine) reverses the disorder
Pain	Involves various initiators (eg, bradykinins, prostaglandins) and neurotransmitters in the neuronal pain pathways; the latter can be stimulatory (eg, substance P, which transmits nerve impulses) or inhibitory (eg, enkephalins and endorphins, which interfere with nerve impulses)	NSAIDs inhibit prostaglandin synthesis selectively (with COX-2 inhibitors—eg, celecoxib, parecoxib) or nonselectively (with COX-1 and -2 inhibitors—eg, ibuprofen, naproxen) and reduce pain impulse formation; opioid analgesics (eg, morphine) activate endorphin-enkephalin (μ, δ, and κ) receptors, reducing pain impulse transmission
Parkinsonism	Inhibition of dopaminergic system due to blockage of dopaminergic receptors by antipsychotic drugs	Anticholinergic drugs reduce cholinergic activity and restore balance between cholinergic and dopaminergic systems
Parkinson's disease	Loss of dopaminergic neurons of the pars compacta in the substantia nigra and other areas, with reduced levels of dopamine and metenkephalin, resulting in striatal acetylcholine overactivity	L-dopa reaches the synaptic cleft, is taken up by the axon, and is decarboxylated to dopamine, which is secreted into the cleft to activate dendritic dopamine receptors. Amantadine increases the presynaptic release of dopamine; pergolide, like dopamine, stimulates D_1 and D_2 receptors. Anticholinergic drugs reduce activity of the cholinergic system, restoring the balance of dopamine and acetylcholine. MAO-B inhibitors prevent reuptake of dopamine, increasing its levels. Selegiline, an MAO-B inhibitor, prolongs the response to levodopa and allows the dosage of carbidopa/levodopa to be reduced

TABLE 207–1. EXAMPLES OF DISORDERS ASSOCIATED WITH DEFECTS IN NEUROTRANSMISSION—Continued

DISORDER	PATHOPHYSIOLOGY	TREATMENT
Schizophrenia	Increased presynaptic release, synthesis of dopamine, sensitivity or density of postsynaptic dopamine receptors, or a combination	Antipsychotic drugs block dopamine receptors and reduce dopaminergic overactivity to normal. Haloperidol preferentially blocks D_2 and D_3 receptors (high affinity) and D_4 receptors (low affinity) in mesocortical areas. Clozapine has a high affinity for binding D_4 and 5-HT_2 receptors, suggesting 5-HT system involvement in the pathogenesis of schizophrenia and its response to treatment. Clozapine has a significant risk of leukopenia. Olanzapine and risperidone, similar to haloperidol, also have high affinity for 5-HT_2 D_2 receptors
Tardive dyskinesia	Hypersensitive dopamine receptors due to chronic blockade by antipsychotic drugs	Reducing doses of antipsychotics may reduce hypersensitivity of dopamine receptors
Normal neurotransmitters but nonfunctional receptors		
Myasthenia gravis	Reflects inactivation of acetylcholine receptors and postsynaptic histochemical changes at the neuromuscular junction due to autoimmune reactions	Anticholinesterase drugs inhibit acetylcholinesterase, increase acetylcholine levels at the junction, and stimulate remaining receptors, increasing muscle activity
Decreased neuronal uptake of neurotransmitters		
Amyotrophic lateral sclerosis	Possible destruction of motor neurons resulting from increased glutamate stimulation, which induces nitric oxide production, causing neuronal toxicity	Riluzole, which inhibits glutamate transmission, modestly extends survival
Normal neurotransmitters but ion channel defects		
Episodic ataxia/myokymia	Defective voltage-gated K channels, producing distal rippling and incoordination	Carbamazepine may be helpful for myokymia
Hyperkalemic periodic paralysis	Decreased Na channel inactivation, producing episodic weakness	Attacks may be terminated by Ca gluconate, glucose, and insulin. Acetazolamide can reduce the number of attacks
Hypokalemic periodic paralysis	Defective voltage-gated Ca channels, producing sustained membrane depolarization	Acute attacks can be terminated by K salts. Acetazolamide is effective for prevention
Lambert-Eaton syndrome	Antibodies, often generated by small cell lung carcinoma, that antagonize Ca channels of the presynaptic neuromuscular junction, reducing acetylcholine release	Corticosteroids, immunosuppression, plasmapheresis, and IV immune globulins are effective
Paramyotonia congenita	Defective voltage-gated Na channels, producing cold-induced myotonia and episodic weakness	Hydrochlorothiazide prevents attacks. Ca gluconate is beneficial during severe attacks

Table continues on the following page.

TABLE 207–1. EXAMPLES OF DISORDERS ASSOCIATED WITH DEFECTS IN NEUROTRANSMISSION—Continued

DISORDER	PATHOPHYSIOLOGY	TREATMENT
Rasmussen's encephalitis	Glutamate-gated channels; most distinctive form of epilepsia partialis continua	Corticosteroids and antiviral drugs are usually ineffective. Functional hemispherectomy can control seizures if spontaneous remission does not occur
Startle disease	Glycine-gated channels (disorder characterized by hyperreflexia and falling)	Valproate or clonazepam may induce improvement
Poisoning		
Botulism	Inhibition of acetylcholine release from motor neurons by toxin from *Clostridium botulinum*	No specific drug therapy exists; tiny amounts of poison are used to treat certain dystonias or spasticity
Mushroom poisoning	*Amanita muscaria:* Inhibition of anticholinesterase and blockade of acetylcholine receptors by isoxazole derivatives	Intensive supportive care for hepatic and renal failure is provided
	Inocybe and *Clitocybe* spp: Stimulation of muscarinic receptors by muscarine and related compounds	Atropine protects muscarinic receptors
Organophosphates	Irreversible inhibition of acetylcholinesterase and marked increase in acetylcholine levels in synaptic cleft	Pralidoxime removes toxin from acetylcholinesterase; atropine protects receptors from high acetylcholine levels
Snake venom (*Bungarus multicinctus*)	Blocks acetylcholine receptors at neuromuscular junction by α-*Bungarus* toxin	Antivenom is available

NMDA = *N*-methyl-D-aspartate; GABA = γ-aminobutyric acid; 5-HT = serotonin; CRF = corticotrophin (ACTH)-releasing factor; MAO = monoamine oxidase; PIP_2 = phosphatidylinositol 4,5-bisphosphate; D = dopaminergic; COX-2 = cyclooxygenase-2; MAO-B = MAO type B.

Serotoninergic (5-HT) receptors (with at least 15 subtypes) are classified as $5\text{-}HT_1$ (with 4 subtypes), $5\text{-}HT_2$, and $5\text{-}HT_3$. Selective serotonin receptor agonists (eg, sumatriptan) can abort migraines.

Acetylcholine: Acetylcholine is the major neurotransmitter of the bulbospinal motor neurons, autonomic preganglionic fibers, postganglionic cholinergic (parasympathetic) fibers, and many neurons in the CNS (eg, basal ganglia, motor cortex). It is synthesized from choline and acetyl coenzyme A by choline acetyltransferase, and its action is rapidly terminated via local hydrolysis to choline and acetate by acetylcholinesterase. Acetylcholine levels are regulated by choline acetyltransferase and by choline uptake. Levels of this neurotransmitter are decreased in patients with Alzheimer's disease.

Cholinergic receptors are classified as nicotinic N_1 (in the adrenal medulla and autonomic ganglia) or N_2 (in skeletal muscle) or muscarinic M_1 through M_5 (widely distributed in the CNS). M_1 occurs in the autonomic nervous system, striatum, cortex, and hippocampus; M_2 occurs in the autonomic nervous system, heart, intestinal smooth muscle, hindbrain, and cerebellum.

Dopamine: Dopamine interacts with receptors on some peripheral nerve fibers and many central neurons (eg, in the substantia nigra, midbrain, ventral tegmental area, and hypothalamus). The amino acid tyrosine is taken up by dopaminergic neurons and converted by tyrosine hydroxylase to 3,4-dihydroxyphenylalanine (dopa), which is decarboxylated by aromatic-L-amino-acid decarboxylase to dopamine. After release and interaction with receptors, dopamine is actively pumped back (reuptake) into the nerve terminal. Tyrosine hydroxylase and MAO regulate dopamine levels in nerve terminals.

Dopaminergic receptors are classified as D_1 through D_5. D_3 and D_4 receptors play a role in thought control (limiting the negative symptoms of schizophrenia); D_2 receptor activation controls the extrapyramidal system.

Norepinephrine: Norepinephrine is the neurotransmitter of most postganglionic sympathetic fibers and many central neurons (eg, in the locus caeruleus and hypothalamus). The precursor tyrosine is converted to dopamine, which is hydroxylated by dopamine β-hydroxylase to norepinephrine. After release and interaction with receptors, some norepinephrine is degraded by catechol *O*-methyltransferase (COMT), and the remainder is actively taken back into the nerve terminal, where it is degraded by MAO. Tyrosine hydroxylase and MAO regulate intraneuronal norepinephrine levels.

Adrenergic receptors are classified as α_1 (postsynaptic in the sympathetic system), α_2 (presynaptic in the sympathetic system and postsynaptic in the brain), β_1 (in the heart), or β_2 (in other sympathetically innervated structures).

Endorphins and enkephalins: Endorphins are polypeptides that activate many central neurons (eg, in the hypothalamus, amygdala, thalamus, and locus caeruleus). The cell body contains a large polypeptide called pro-opiomelanocortin, the precursor of α-, β-, and γ-endorphins. This polypeptide is transported down the axon and cleaved into fragments; one is β-endorphin, contained in neurons that project to the periaqueductal gray matter, limbic structures, and major catecholamine-containing neurons in the brain. After release and interaction with receptors, β-endorphin is hydrolyzed by peptidases.

Met-enkephalin and leu-enkephalin are small peptides present in many central neurons (eg, in the globus pallidus, thalamus, caudate, and central gray matter). Their precursor, proenkephalin, is formed in the cell body, then split by specific peptidases into the active peptides. These substances are also localized in the spinal cord, where they act as neuromodulators of pain signals. The neurotransmitters of pain signals in the posterior horn of the spinal cord are glutamate and substance P. Enkephalins decrease the amount of neurotransmitter released and hyperpolarize (make more negative) the postsynaptic membrane, reducing the generation of action potentials and pain perception at the level of the postcentral gyrus. After release and interaction with peptidergic receptors, enkephalins are hydrolyzed into smaller, inactive peptides and amino acids. Rapid inactivation prevents these substances from being clinically useful. More stable molecules (eg, morphine) are used as analgesics instead.

Endorphin-enkephalin (opioid) receptors are classified as μ_1 and μ_2 (affecting sensorimotor integration and analgesia), δ_1 and δ_2 (affecting motor integration, cognitive function, and analgesia), and κ_1, κ_2, and κ_3 (affecting water balance regulation, analgesia, and food intake). σ-Receptors, currently classified as nonopioid and mostly localized in the hippocampus, bind PCP. New data suggest the presence of many more receptor subtypes, with pharmacologic implications. Components of the molecular precursor to the receptor protein can be rearranged during receptor synthesis to produce several receptor variants (eg, 19 splice variants of the μ opioid receptor). Also, 2 receptors can combine (dimerize) to form a new receptor.

Other neurotransmitters: Dynorphins are a group of 7 peptides with similar amino acid sequences. They coexist with enkephalins.

Substance P, a peptide, occurs in central neurons (habenula, substantia nigra, basal ganglia, medulla, and hypothalamus) and is highly concentrated in the dorsal root ganglia. Its release is triggered by intense afferent painful stimuli.

Nitric oxide (NO) is a labile gas that mediates many neuronal processes. It is generated from arginine by NO synthase, an enzyme that activates soluble guanylate cyclase by binding to Ca/calmodulin complexes. Thus, neurotransmitters that increase intracellular Ca (eg, substance P, glutamate, acetylcholine) stimulate NO synthesis in neurons that express NO synthetase. NO may be an intracellular messenger; it may diffuse out of a cell into a 2nd neuron and produce physiologic responses (eg, long-term potentiation [a form of learning], neurotransmitter release and reuptake) or enhance glutamate (NMDA) receptor-mediated neurotoxicity.

Substances with less firmly established roles in neurotransmission include histamine, vasopressin, vasoactive intestinal peptide, carnosine, bradykinin, cholecystokinin, bombesin, somatostatin, corticotropin releasing factor, neurotensin, and possibly adenosine.

208 AUTONOMIC NERVOUS SYSTEM

The autonomic nervous system (ANS) regulates physiologic processes. Regulation occurs without conscious control, ie, autonomously. The 2 major divisions are the sympathetic and parasympathetic systems.

Disorders of the ANS can affect any system of the body. They can originate in the peripheral or central nervous system and may be primary or secondary to other disorders.

Anatomy

The sympathetic and parasympathetic systems each consist of 2 sets of nerve bodies: one set (called preganglionic) in the CNS, with connections to another set in ganglia outside the CNS. Efferent fibers from the ganglia (postganglionic fibers) lead to effector organs.

The preganglionic cell bodies of the sympathetic system are located in the intermediolateral horn of the spinal cord between T1 and L2 or L3. The sympathetic ganglia are adjacent to the spine and consist of the vertebral (sympathetic chain) and prevertebral ganglia, including the superior cervical, celiac, superior mesenteric, and aorticorenal ganglia. Long fibers run from these ganglia to effector organs, including the smooth muscle of blood vessels, viscera, lungs, scalp (piloerector muscles), and pupils; the heart; and glands (sweat, salivary, and digestive).

The preganglionic cell bodies of the parasympathetic system are located in the brain stem and sacral portion of the spinal cord. Preganglionic fibers exit the brain stem with the 3rd, 7th, 9th, and 10th (vagus) cranial nerves; the vagus nerve contains about 75% of all parasympathetic fibers. Parasympathetic ganglia are located within the effector organs, and postganglionic fibers are only 1 or 2 mm long. Thus, the parasympathetic system can produce specific, localized responses in effector organs, including blood vessels of the head, neck, and thoracoabdominal viscera; lacrimal and salivary glands; smooth muscle of viscera and glands (eg, liver, spleen, colon, kidneys, bladder, genitals); and ocular muscles.

The ANS receives input from parts of the CNS that process and integrate stimuli from the body and external environment. These parts include the hypothalamus, nucleus of the solitary tract, reticular formation, amygdala, hippocampus, and olfactory cortex.

Physiology

The ANS controls BP, heart rate, body temperature, weight, digestion, metabolism, fluid and electrolyte balance, sweating, urination, defecation, sexual response, and other processes. Many organs are controlled primarily by either the sympathetic or parasympathetic system, although they may receive input from both; occasionally, functions are reciprocal (eg, sympathetic input increases heart rate; parasympathetic decreases it).

The sympathetic nervous system is catabolic and activates fight-or-flight responses. Thus, sympathetic output increases heart rate and contractility, bronchodilation, hepatic glycogenolysis and glucose release, BMR, and muscular strength; it also causes sweaty palms. Less immediately life-preserving functions (eg, digestion, renal filtration) are decreased. Ejaculation is a sympathetic function.

The parasympathetic nervous system is anabolic; it conserves and restores. GI secretions and motility (including evacuation) are stimulated, heart rate is slowed, and BP decreases. Erection is a parasympathetic function.

Two major neurotransmitters in the ANS are acetylcholine and norepinephrine. Fibers that secrete acetylcholine are termed cholinergic; they include all preganglionic fibers and all postganglionic parasympathetic fibers. Fibers that secrete norepinephrine are termed adrenergic; they include most postganglionic sympathetic fibers, except for those that innervate piloerectors, sweat glands, and blood vessels, which are cholinergic. However, sweat glands on the palms and soles also respond to adrenergic stimulation to some degree. There are different subtypes of adrenergic (see p. 1765) and cholinergic (see p. 1764) receptors, varying by location.

Evaluation

History: Symptoms suggesting autonomic dysfunction include orthostatic hypotension, heat intolerance, and loss of bladder and bowel control. Erectile dysfunction is an early symptom. Other possible symptoms include dry eyes and dry mouth, but they are nonspecific.

Physical examination: In a normally hydrated patient, a sustained decrease of > 20 mm Hg in systolic BP or a decrease of > 10 mm Hg in diastolic BP with standing suggests autonomic dysfunction. Heart rate change with respiration and standing should be noted; absence of physiologic sinus arrhythmia and failure of heart rate to increase with standing indicate autonomic dysfunction.

Miosis and mild ptosis (Horner's syndrome) suggest a sympathetic lesion. A dilated, unreactive pupil (Adie's pupil) suggests a parasympathetic lesion.

Abnormal GU and rectal reflexes may indicate ANS deficits. Testing includes the cremasteric reflex (normally, stroking the thigh results in retraction of the testes), anal wink reflex (normally, stroking perianal skin results in contraction of the anal sphincter), and bulbocavernosus reflex (normally, squeezing the glans penis or clitoris results in contraction of the anal sphincter).

Laboratory testing: If patients have symptoms and signs suggesting autonomic dysfunction, sudomotor, cardiovagal, and adrenergic tests are usually done to help determine severity and distribution of the dysfunction.

The quantitative sudomotor axon-reflex test evaluates integrity of postganglionic neurons using iontophoresis; electrodes filled with acetylcholine are placed on the legs and wrist to stimulate sweat glands, and the volume of sweat is then measured. The test can detect decreased, absent, or persistent (after stimulus discontinuation) sweat production. The thermoregulatory sweat test evaluates both preganglionic and postganglionic pathways. After a dye is applied to the skin, patients enter a closed compartment that is heated to cause maximal sweating. Sweating causes the dye to change color, so that areas of anhidrosis and hypohidrosis are apparent and can be calculated as a percentage of BSA.

Cardiovagal testing evaluates heart rate response (via ECG rhythm strip) to deep breathing and to the Valsalva maneuver. If the ANS is intact, heart rate varies with these maneuvers; the ratio of longest to shortest R-R interval (Valsalva ratio) should be ≥ 1.4.

Adrenergic testing evaluates response of beat-to-beat BP to the head-up tilt and Valsalva maneuver. The head-up tilt shifts blood to dependent parts, causing reflex responses. The Valsalva maneuver increases intrathoracic pressure and reduces venous return, causing BP changes and reflex vasoconstriction. In both tests, the pattern of responses is an index of adrenergic function.

AUTONOMIC NEUROPATHIES

Autonomic neuropathies are peripheral nerve disorders with disproportionate involvement of autonomic fibers.

The best known autonomic neuropathies are those accompanying peripheral neuropathy due to diabetes, amyloidosis, or autoimmune disorders. Autoimmune autonomic neuropathy often develops after a viral infection, and onset may be subacute.

Common symptoms include orthostatic hypotension, neurogenic bladder, erectile dysfunction, gastroparesis, and obstinate constipation. When somatic fibers are involved, sensory loss in a stocking-and-glove distribution and distal weakness may occur (see also Ch. 223 on p. 1891).

Diagnosis is based on demonstration of autonomic failure and a specific cause of neuropathy (eg, diabetes, amyloidosis). Autoimmune autonomic neuropathy may be suspected after a viral infection. Ganglionic anti–acetylcholine receptor antibody A_3 is present in about ½ of patients.

Underlying disorders are treated. Autoimmune autonomic neuropathy may respond to immunotherapy; plasma exchange or IV γ-globulin can be used for more severe cases.

HORNER'S SYNDROME

Horner's syndrome is ptosis, miosis, and anhidrosis due to dysfunction of cervical sympathetic output.

Horner's syndrome results when the cervical sympathetic pathway running from the hypothalamus to the eye is disrupted. The syndrome may be central, preganglionic, or postganglionic in origin; it may be primary or secondary to another disorder. Central lesions include brain stem ischemia, syringomyelia, and brain tumor; peripheral lesions include Pancoast tumor, cervical adenopathy, neck and skull injuries, aortic or carotid dissection, and thoracic aortic aneurysm. A congenital form exists.

Symptoms include ptosis, miosis, anhidrosis, and hyperemia of the affected side. In the congenital form, the iris does not become pigmented and remains blue-gray. Liquid cocaine 10% can be applied to the affected eye; poor pupillary dilation after 30 min indicates Horner's syndrome. If results are positive, 1% hydroxyamphetamine solution or 5% n-methyl hydroxyamphetamine can be applied to the eye 48 h later to determine whether the lesion is preganglionic (if the pupil dilates) or postganglionic (if the pupil does not dilate). Patients with Horner's syndrome require MRI or CT of the brain, spinal cord, chest, or neck, depending on clinical suspicion.

Any identifiable causes are treated; there is no treatment for primary Horner's syndrome.

MULTIPLE SYSTEM ATROPHY

Multiple system atrophy is a relentlessly progressive neurodegenerative disorder causing pyramidal, cerebellar, and autonomic dysfunction. It includes 3 disorders previously thought to be distinct: olivopontocerebellar atrophy, striatonigral degeneration, and Shy-Drager syndrome. Symptoms include hypotension, urinary retention, constipation, ataxia, rigidity, and postural instability. Diagnosis is clinical. Treatment is symptomatic, with volume expansion, compression garments, and vasoconstrictor drugs.

Multiple system atrophy affects about twice as many men as women. Mean age at onset is about 53 yr; after symptoms appear, patients live about 9 to 10 yr.

Etiology is unknown, but neuronal degeneration occurs in several areas of the brain; the area and amount damaged determine initial symptoms. A characteristic finding is cytoplasmic inclusion bodies containing α-synuclein within oligodendroglial cells.

Symptoms and Signs

Initial symptoms vary but include a combination of parkinsonism unresponsive to levodopa, cerebellar abnormalities, and autonomic symptoms.

Parkinsonian symptoms (predominant in striatonigral degeneration) include rigidity, bradykinesia, postural instability, and jerky postural tremor. High-pitched, quavering dysarthria is common. In contrast to Parkinson's disease, resting tremor and dyskinesia are uncommon, and symptoms respond poorly and transiently to levodopa.

Symptoms of cerebellar dysfunction (predominant in olivopontocerebellar atrophy) include ataxia, dysmetria, dysdiadochokinesia (difficulty performing rapidly alternating movements), poor coordination, and abnormal eye movements.

Typical symptoms of autonomic failure are orthostatic hypotension (symptomatic fall in BP when a person stands, often with syncope—see p. 581), urinary retention or incontinence, constipation, and erectile dysfunction.

Other autonomic symptoms, which may occur early or late, include decreased sweating, problems with breathing and swallowing, fecal incontinence, and decreased tearing and salivation. Sleep apnea and respiratory stridor are common.

Diagnosis

Diagnosis is suspected clinically, based on the combination of autonomic failure and parkinsonism or cerebellar symptoms. Similar symptoms may result from Parkinson's disease, Lewy body dementia, pure autonomic failure, autonomic neuropathies, progressive supranuclear palsy, multiple cerebral infarcts, or drug-induced parkinsonism.

No diagnostic test is definitive, but MRI abnormalities in the striatum, pons, and cerebellum are highly suggestive. Multiple system atrophy can be diagnosed antemortem based on these findings plus symptoms of generalized autonomic failure and lack of response to levodopa.

Treatment

There is no specific treatment, but symptoms are managed.

Treatment of orthostatic hypotension includes intravascular volume expansion with salt and water supplementation; sometimes fludrocortisone 0.1 to 0.4 mg po once/day is used. Use of compression garments for the lower body (eg, abdominal binder, Jobst stockings) and α-adrenoreceptor stimulation with midodrine 10 mg po tid may help. However, midodrine also increases peripheral vascular resistance and supine BP, which may be problematic. Raising the head of the bed about 10 cm reduces nocturnal polyuria and supine hypertension and may reduce morning orthostatic hypotension.

Levodopa/carbidopa 25/100 mg po at bedtime or pergolide 0.1 mg po once/day, titrated upward to 0.25 to 1.0 mg tid, may be tried to relieve rigidity and other parkinsonian symptoms, but these drugs are usually ineffective. Urinary incontinence secondary to detrusor hyperreflexia may be treated with oxybutynin chloride 5 mg po tid or tolterodine 2 mg po bid. Many patients must self-catheterize their bladder. Constipation can be treated with a high-fiber diet and stool softeners; for refractory cases, enemas may be necessary. Erectile dysfunction can be treated with drugs such as sildenafil 50 mg po prn and with various physical means (see p. 1949).

PURE AUTONOMIC FAILURE

Pure autonomic failure results from neuronal loss in autonomic ganglia, causing orthostatic hypotension and other autonomic symptoms.

Pure autonomic failure, previously called idiopathic orthostatic hypotension or Bradbury-Eggleston syndrome, denotes generalized autonomic failure without CNS involvement. This disorder differs from multiple system atrophy because it lacks central or preganglionic involvement. Pure autonomic failure affects more women, tends to begin in a person's 40s or 50s, and does not progress to death.

Etiology is usually unknown; some cases are due to an autoimmune autonomic neuropathy.

The main symptom is orthostatic hypotension; there may be other autonomic symptoms (eg, decreased sweating, heat intolerance, urinary retention, erectile dysfunction, fecal incontinence or constipation, pupillary abnormalities). Diagnosis is by exclusion. The norepinephrine level is usually < 100 pg/mL supine and does not increase with standing.

Treatment is symptomatic: vasopressors and support hose for orthostatic hypotension, a high-fiber diet and stool softeners for constipation, bladder antispasmodics for urinary problems, and avoidance of hot conditions for sweating abnormalities.

209 PAIN

(See also entries under Pain in the Index.)

Pain is the most common reason patients seek medical care. It has sensory and emotional components and is often classified as acute (< 1 mo) or chronic. Acute pain is frequently associated with anxiety and hyperactivity of the sympathetic nervous system (eg, tachycardia, increased respiratory rate and BP, diaphoresis, dilated pupils). Chronic pain does not involve sympathetic hyperactivity but may be associated with vegetative signs (eg, fatigue, loss of libido, loss of appetite) and depressed mood. People vary considerably in their tolerance for pain.

Etiology and Pathophysiology

Acute pain, which occurs in response to tissue injury, results from activation of peripheral pain receptors (nociceptors) and their specific sensory nerve fibers (A delta fibers and C fibers). Chronic pain (see p. 1776) related to ongoing tissue injury is presumably caused by persistent activation of these fibers. Chronic pain may also result from neuropathic pain. Neuropathic pain (see p. 1779) is caused by damage or dysfunction of the peripheral or central nervous system, rather than stimulation of pain receptors.

Nociceptive pain results from ordinary injury or illness; it may be somatic or visceral. Somatic pain receptors are located in skin, subcutaneous tissues, fascia, other connective tissues, periosteum, endosteum, and joint capsules. Stimulation of these receptors produces sharp or dull localized pain. Visceral pain receptors are located in most viscera and the surrounding connective tissue. Visceral pain due to injury of a hollow organ is a poorly localized, deep aching or cramping, which may be referred to remote cutaneous sites. Visceral pain due to injury of organ capsules or other deep connective tissues may be more localized and sharp.

Although pain of purely psychologic origin, a form of somatic delusion, is rare, psychologic factors commonly contribute to chronic pain and may predominate in some patients. Pain that is understood to be caused predominantly by psychologic factors is sometimes called psychogenic pain; psychophysiologic pain is a more accurate term because the pain results from interaction of physiologic and psychologic phenomena. This type of pain can be categorized using descriptions of somatoform disorders (eg, chronic pain disorders, somatization disorders, hypochondriasis—see p. 1736) in the *Diagnostic and Statistical Manual of Mental Disorders,* Fourth Edition (DSM-IV).

Many pain syndromes are multifactorial. For example, chronic low back pain and most cancer pain syndromes have a prominent nociceptive component but may also involve neuropathic pain due to nerve damage.

Pain modulation: Pain fibers enter the spinal cord at the dorsal root ganglia, travel up the lateral columns to the thalamus and then to the cerebral cortex. All along this pathway, the pain signal is modulated by excitatory and inhibitory nerve impulses and various neurochemical mediators. These modulators interact in poorly understood ways to exaggerate or reduce the perception of and response to pain.

Repetitive stimulation (eg, from a prolonged painful condition) can sensitize neurons in the dorsal horn of the spinal cord so that a lesser peripheral stimulus causes pain (windup phenomenon). Peripheral nerves and nerves at other levels of the CNS may also be sensitized, with long-term synaptic changes in cortical receptive fields (remodeling) that maintain exaggerated pain perception.

Substances released when tissue is injured, including those involved in the inflammatory cascade, can sensitize peripheral nociceptors. These substances include vasoactive peptides (eg, calcitonin gene-related protein, substance P, neurokinin A) and other mediators (eg, prostaglandin E_2, serotonin, bradykinin, epinephrine).

Psychologic factors are important modulators. They not only affect verbal expression of pain (ie, whether patients appear stoic or sensitive) but also generate neural output that modulates neurotransmission along pain pathways. Psychologic reaction to protracted pain interacts with other CNS factors to induce long-term changes in pain perception.

The many neuromodulators (eg, serotonin, norepinephrine) involved in pain modulation pathways account for the potential benefit of nonanalgesic drugs (eg, antidepressants, anticonvulsants, membrane stabilizers) in the treatment of chronic pain.

Evaluation

Clinicians should evaluate the cause, severity, and nature of the pain and its effect on activities and psychologic well-being. Evaluation of the cause of acute pain (eg, back pain, chest pain) is discussed elsewhere in THE MANUAL; that of chronic pain is discussed below.

The history should include quality (eg, burning, cramping, aching, deep, superficial, boring, shooting), severity, location, patterns of referred pain, duration, course, timing (including frequency of remissions), pattern and degree of fluctuation, and exacerbating and relieving factors. The patient's level of function should be assessed, focusing on activities of daily living (eg, dressing, bathing), employment, avocations, and personal relationships (including sexual).

What pain means to the patient should be determined, with emphasis on psychologic issues, depression, and anxiety. Reporting pain is more socially acceptable than reporting anxiety or depression, and appropriate therapy often depends on sorting out these divergent perceptions. Pain and suffering should also be distinguished, especially in a cancer patient (see p. 1170); suffering may be due as much to loss of function and fear of impending death as to pain. Whether secondary gain (external, incidental benefits of a disorder—eg, time off, disability payments) contributes to pain or pain-related disability should be determined. The patient's perception of pain can represent more than the disorder's intrinsic pathology.

Information about the use, efficacy, and adverse effects of prescription and OTC drugs and other treatments should be elicited. Alcohol and recreational or illicit drug use should be assessed. The patient should be asked if litigation is ongoing or financial compensation for injury will be sought. A personal or family history of chronic pain can often illuminate the current problem. Possible contribution of family members to perpetuation of chronic pain should be considered.

Pain severity: Because external signs (eg, crying, wincing, rocking) and spontaneous complaints of pain vary by culture and among individuals, severity should be formally measured. Baseline measurements also help assess effectiveness of interventions.

Formal measures include verbal category scales (eg, mild, moderate, severe), numerical scales, and Visual Analogue Scale (VAS). For the numerical scale, patients are asked to rate their pain from 0 to 10 (0 = no pain; 10 = "the worst pain ever"). For the VAS, patients make a hash mark representing their degree of pain on an unmarked 10-cm line with the left side labeled "no pain" and the right side labeled "unbearable pain." The pain score is distance in mm from the left end of the line. Children and patients with limited literacy or known developmental problems may select from images of faces ranging from smiling to contorted with pain or from fruits of varying sizes to convey their perception of pain severity.

Treatment of Pain

Nonopioid and opioid analgesics are the mainstay of pain treatment. Antidepressants, anticonvulsants, and other CNS-active drugs may be used for chronic or neuropathic pain. Neuraxial infusion, nerve stimulation, injection therapies, and neural blockade can help selected patients. Cognitive interventions (eg, relaxation techniques, hypnosis, biofeedback) and behavioral therapy (eg, graduated exercise, incremental gains in function, changes in relationships in the home) may help patients modify their emotional and behavioral response to pain.

Nonopioid Analgesics

Acetaminophen and NSAIDs are often effective for mild to moderate pain (see TABLE 209–1). Of these, only ketorolac can be given parenterally. Nonopioids do not cause physical dependence or tolerance.

Acetaminophen has no anti-inflammatory or anti-platelet effects and does not cause gastric irritation.

NSAIDs include nonselective COX-1 and COX-2 inhibitors and selective COX-2 inhibitors (coxibs); all are effective analgesics. Aspirin is the least expensive but has prolonged antiplatelet effects. Coxibs have lowest risk of ulcer formation and GI upset. Some studies

TABLE 209–1. NONOPIOID ANALGESICS

CLASS	DRUG	USUAL DOSAGE RANGE* (mg)
Indoles	Etodolac	200–400 q 6–8 h
	Indomethacin	25–50 q 8–12 h
	Sulindac	150 q 12 h
	Tolmetin	200–400 q 6–8 h
Naphthylalkanone	Nabumetone	1000–2000 q 24 h
Oxicam	Piroxicam	20 q 24 h
Para-aminophenol derivative	Acetaminophen	650–1000 q 4–6 h
Propionic acids	Fenoprofen	200–600 q 6 h
	Flurbiprofen	50–150 q 12 h
	Ibuprofen	400 q 4 h to 800 q 6 h
	Ketoprofen	50–75 q 6–8 h
	Naproxen	250–500 q 12 h
	Naproxen sodium	275–550 q 12 h
	Oxaprozin	600–1200 q 24 h
Salicylates	Aspirin	650–1000 q 4–6 h
	Choline Mg trisalicylate	750–2000 q 12 h
	Diflunisal	500 q 8–12 h
Fenamates	Meclofenamate	50–100 q 6–8 h
	Mefenamic acid	250 q 6 h
Pyrazole	Phenylbutazone	100 q 6–8 h up to 7 days
Pyrrolo-pyrrolo derivative	Ketorolac	30 IV or IM q 6 h or 20 po, followed by 10 po q 4–6 h for maximum 5 days
Selective COX-2 inhibitor	Celecoxib	100–200 q 12 h

*Route is oral, except for ketorolac, which can be given parenterally.

suggest that coxibs can be prothrombotic, increasing the risk of MI, stroke, and claudication. This effect appears to be dose- and duration-related. One study suggests risk with some nonselective COX-1 and COX-2 inhibitors. All the data are limited and often conflicting.

Some clinicians continue to use coxibs first; others limit use to patients predisposed to GI toxicity (eg, the elderly, those on corticosteroids, those with a history of peptic ulcer disease or GI distress due to other NSAIDs) and those who are not doing well with or who have a history of intolerance to nonselective NSAIDs. Long-term use of any NSAID, particularly a coxib, should be approached cautiously in patients with cardiovascular risk factors. All NSAIDs should be used cautiously in patients with renal insufficiency; coxibs are not renal-sparing.

If initial recommended doses provide inadequate analgesia, a higher dose is given, up to the conventional safe maximum dose. If analgesia remains inadequate, the drug should be stopped. If pain is not severe, another NSAID may be tried because response varies from drug to drug. Long-term use of NSAIDs requires monitoring for occult blood in stool and changes in CBC, electrolytes, and hepatic and renal function.

Opioid Analgesics

"Opioid" is a generic term for natural or synthetic substances that bind to specific opioid receptors in the CNS, producing an agonist action. Opioids are also called narcotics. Some opioids used for analgesia have both agonist and antagonist actions; potential for abuse is slightly less with them than with pure agonists, but antagonist activity may induce a withdrawal syndrome in patients already physically dependent on opioids. In general, acute pain is best treated with short-acting drugs; chronic pain is best treated with longer-acting drugs (see TABLES 209–2 and 209–3).

Opioid analgesics are useful in managing severe acute or chronic pain. They are often underused, resulting in needless pain and suffering, because clinicians often underestimate the required dosage, overestimate the duration of action and risks of adverse effects, and have unreasonable concerns about addiction (see p. 1696). Physical dependence (development of withdrawal symptoms when a drug is stopped) should be assumed to exist in all patients treated with opioids for more than a few days. However, addiction (compulsive use of a substance, with craving and psychologic dependence) is very rare in patients with no history of substance abuse. Careful assessment before initiation of opioids should enable a physician to infer whether risk of abuse is relatively high. If it is, treatment may still be appropriate, but more controls (eg, small prescriptions, frequent visits, no refills for "lost" prescriptions) are then used.

Route of administration: Almost any route can be used. The oral or transdermal route is preferred for long-term use; both are effective and provide stable blood levels. Modified-release oral and transdermal forms allow less frequent dosing, which is particularly important for providing overnight relief. Fentanyl lozenges deliver the drug through the oral mucosa; they are used for sedation in children and as treatment of breakthrough pain.

The IV route provides most rapid onset and hence easiest titration, but duration of analgesia is short. A bolus effect (toxicity at peak levels early in the dosing interval or later breakthrough pain at trough levels) can be prominent. Continuous IV infusion, sometimes with patient-controlled supplemental doses, eliminates this effect but requires an expensive pump; this approach is usually used for postoperative pain.

The IM route provides analgesia longer than IV but is painful, and absorption can be erratic; it is not recommended.

Intraspinal opioids (eg, morphine 5 to 10 mg epidurally or 0.5 to 1 mg intrathecally) can provide relief up to 24 h; they are typically used postoperatively. Implanted infusion devices can provide long-term neuraxial infusion. These devices can also be used with other drugs (eg, local anesthetics, clonidine).

Dosing and titration: Initial dose is modified according to the patient's response; it is increased incrementally until analgesia and adverse effects are balanced acceptably. Sedation, respiratory rate, and BP must be monitored; they are monitored frequently when opioids are given parenterally to relatively opioid-naive patients. The elderly are more sensitive to opioids and are predisposed to adverse effects; they require lower doses than younger patients. Newborns, especially when premature, are also sensitive to opioids, because they lack adequate metabolic pathways to eliminate them.

For moderate, transient pain, an opioid may be given prn. For severe or ongoing pain, doses should be given regularly, without

TABLE 209–2. OPIOID ANALGESICS

DRUG	DOSE*	PEDIATRIC DOSE†	COMMENTS
Opioid agonists‡ for mild-to-moderate pain			
Codeine	Parenteral and oral: 30–60 mg q 4 h	0.5–1 mg/kg	
Hydrocodone	Oral: 5–10 mg q 4 h	0.135 mg/kg	Similar to codeine
Propoxyphene	Oral: Propoxyphene hydrochloride 65 mg q 4 h or propoxyphene napsylate 100 mg q 4 h		Effectiveness at these doses similar to aspirin
Opioid agonists for moderate-to-severe pain			
Fentanyl	Transdermal: 25 μg/h q 3 days	Transmucosal: 5–15 μg/kg	Short-acting (< 1 h) parenteral form used for anesthesia; transmucosal form used in hospitals for procedural sedation or analgesia and for breakthrough pain
Hydromorphone	Oral: 2–4 mg q 4–6 h Parenteral: 1–2 mg q 4–6 h Rectal: 3 mg q 6–8 h		Short half-life. Rectal form used at bedtime
Levorphanol	Oral: 4 mg q 6–8 h Parenteral: 2 mg q 6–8 h		Long half-life
Meperidine	Oral: 50–300 mg q 4 h Parenteral: 1 mg/kg q 4 h	1.1–1.75 mg/kg	Not preferred because its active metabolite (normeperidine) causes dysphoria and CNS excitation (eg, myoclonus, tremulousness, seizures) and accumulates for days after dosing is begun, particularly in patients with renal failure
Methadone	Oral: 10 mg q 6–8 h Parenteral: 5 mg q 6–8 h	Not recommended	Most often used for treatment of heroin withdrawal, long-term maintenance treatment of opioid addiction, and analgesia for chronic pain. Establishment of a safe, effective dose for analgesia complicated by its long half-life (usually much longer than duration of analgesia). Requires close monitoring for several days or more after amount or frequency of dose is increased because serious toxicity can occur as the plasma level rises to steady state

Table continues on the following page.

TABLE 209–2. OPIOID ANALGESICS—Continued

DRUG	DOSE*	PEDIATRIC DOSE†	COMMENTS
Morphine	Oral immediate-release: 10–30 mg q 4 h Oral controlled-release: 15 mg q 12 h Oral sustained-release: 30 mg q 24 h Parenteral: 5–10 mg q 4 h	0.05–0.2 mg/kg q 4 h	Standard of comparison. Triggers histamine release more often than other opioids, causing itching
Oxycodone	Oral: 5–10 mg q 4 h Oral controlled-release: 10–20 mg q 12 h		
Oxymorphone	IM or sc: 1–1.5 mg q 4 h IV: 0.5 mg Rectal: 5 mg q 4–6 h		Rapid onset
Opioid agonist/antagonists			
Buprenorphine	IV or IM: 0.3 mg q 6 h	Use only if > 13 yr (same dose)	Psychotomimetic effects less prominent than those of other agonist-antagonists, but other effects similar. Respiratory depression that may not be fully reversible with naloxone
Butorphanol	IV: 1 (0.5–2) mg q 3–4 h IM: 2 (1–4) mg q 3–4 h Nasal: 1 mg (1 spray), repeated in 1 h prn	Not recommended	2-dose nasal sequence may be repeated q 3–4 h
Nalbuphine	Parenteral: 10 mg q 3–6 h	Not recommended	Psychotomimetic effects less prominent than those of pentazocine but more prominent than those of morphine
Pentazocine	Oral: 50–100 mg q 3–4 h Parenteral: 30 mg q 3–4 h (not to exceed 360 mg/day)	Not recommended	Usefulness limited by ceiling effect on analgesia at higher doses, by potential for opioid withdrawal in patients physically dependent on opioid agonists, and by risk of psychotomimetic effects, especially for nontolerant, nonphysically dependent patients with acute pain. Available in tablets combined with naloxone, aspirin, or acetaminophen. Can cause confusion and anxiety, especially in the elderly

*Doses for opioid-naive patients; patients with opioid tolerance or severe pain may require substantially higher doses.

† Not all drugs are appropriate for analgesia in children.

‡ Often combined with acetaminophen.

waiting for severe pain; a supplemental dose should also be available prn. A common error is prescribing short-acting drugs at long intervals, allowing breakthrough pain.

For patient-controlled analgesia, a bolus dose (in a postoperative setting, typically morphine 1 mg q 6 min) is provided when patients push a button; a baseline infusion (eg, morphine 0.5 to 1 mg/h) may or may not be given. The physician controls the amount and interval of the bolus. Patients with prior opioid exposure or chronic pain require a higher baseline infusion and bolus dose, which is further adjusted based on response.

Tolerance to analgesic effects (need for increasing doses to maintain effects) may occur with opioid use, as does tolerance to adverse effects (eg, respiratory depression, nausea, sedation); tolerance to constipation is least likely to occur. Most patients identify a dose providing satisfactory analgesia and take that dose for a long time; a subsequent need for an increase to maintain pain relief usually reflects worsening of the underlying disorder. Thus, fear of tolerance should not inhibit appropriate early, aggressive use of an opioid.

Nonopioid analgesics (eg, acetaminophen, NSAIDs) are often given concomitantly. Products containing both drugs are convenient, but the nonopioid limits upward titration of the opioid dose.

Adverse effects: Common adverse effects include respiratory depression, sedation, constipation, nausea, and vomiting. Because steady-state plasma levels are not approached until 4 to 5 half-lives have passed, drugs with a long half-life (particularly levorphanol and methadone) pose a risk of delayed toxicity as plasma levels rise. Modified-release opioids typically require several days to approach steady-state levels.

In the elderly, opioids tend to have more adverse effects (commonly, constipation and confusion). Opioids frequently cause urinary retention in middle-aged men with benign prostatic hyperplasia.

Opioids should be used cautiously in patients with renal failure, COPD (because of respiratory depression), hepatic disorders, encephalopathy, or dementia.

Constipation is common among patients taking opioids for more than a few days; for prevention in predisposed patients (eg, the elderly), dietary fiber and fluids should be increased, and a stimulant laxative (eg, senna—see p. 76) should be given. Persisting constipation can be managed with Mg citrate 90 mL po q 2 to 3 days, lactulose 15 mL po bid, or propylethylene glycol powder (dose adjusted as needed).

TABLE 209–3. EQUIANALGESIC DOSES OF OPIOID ANALGESICS*

DRUG	IM (mg)	ORAL (mg)
Butorphanol	2	—
Codeine	130	200
Hydromorphone	1.5	7.5
Levorphanol	2	4
Meperidine	75	300
Methadone	10	20
Morphine	10	30
Nalbuphine	10	—
Oxycodone	15	30
Oxymorphone	1	—
Pentazocine	60	180

*Equivalences are based on single-dose studies.

Cross-tolerance between drugs is incomplete, so when one drug is substituted for another, the equianalgesic dose should be reduced by 50%; methadone should be reduced by 75–90%.

In some patients, sedation can be treated specifically with methylphenidate (initially, 5 to 10 mg po bid), dextroamphetamine (initially, 2.5 to 10 mg po bid), or modafinil (initially, 100 to 200 mg po once/day). These drugs are typically given in the morning and as needed later. Maximum dose of methylphenidate seldom exceeds 60 mg/day. For some patients, caffeine-containing beverages provide enough stimulation. Stimulants may also potentiate analgesia.

Nausea can be treated with hydroxyzine 25 to 50 mg po q 6 h, metoclopramide 10 to 20 mg po q 6 h, or an antiemetic phenothiazine (eg, prochlorperazine 10 mg po or 25 mg rectally q 6 h).

Respiratory depression is rare with conventional doses and with long-term use. If it occurs acutely, ventilatory assistance may be needed until the opioid's effect can be reversed by an opioid antagonist.

Opioid antagonists: These opioid-like substances bind to opioid receptors but produce little or no agonist activity. They are used mainly to reverse symptoms of opioid overdose, particularly respiratory depression.

Naloxone acts in < 1 min when given IV and slightly less rapidly when given IM. However, opioid-induced respiratory depression usually lasts longer than the duration of antagonism; thus, *repeated doses of naloxone and close monitoring are necessary*. The dose for acute opioid overdosage is 0.4 mg IV q 2 to 3 min prn. For patients receiving long-term opioid therapy, naloxone should be used only to reverse respiratory depression and must be given more cautiously to avoid precipitating withdrawal or recurrent pain. A reasonable regimen is 1 mL of a dilute solution (0.4 mg in 10 mL saline) IV q 1 to 2 min, titrated to adequate respirations (not alertness).

Naltrexone, an orally bioavailable opioid antagonist, is given as an adjunct in opioid and alcohol addiction. It is long-acting and generally well tolerated.

Adjuvant Drugs

Adjuvant analgesic drugs include anticonvulsants, antidepressants (eg, tricyclics, venlafaxine, bupropion), oral local anesthetics, and corticosteroids (see TABLE 209–4). These drugs have many uses, most notably to relieve pain with a neuropathic component. Gabapentin is the most widely used drug for such purposes. The dose often needs to be high, up to 1200 mg tid or sometimes higher.

Topical drugs are also widely used. Capsaicin cream, other compounded creams (eg, local anesthetic and NSAIDs), and a lidocaine 5% patch have little risk of adverse effects; they should be considered for many types of pain.

Neural Blockade

Interrupting nerve transmission in peripheral or central pain pathways by drugs or physical methods provides short-term and sometimes long-term relief. Pathway destruction (neuroablation) is used rarely, typically reserved for patients with advanced disorders and a short life expectancy.

Local anesthetic drugs (eg, lidocaine) can be given IV, intrathecally, intrapleurally, transdermally, sc, or epidurally. Epidural analgesia using local anesthetics or opioids is particularly useful for some types of postoperative pain. Long-term epidural drug administration is occasionally used for patients with localized pain and a short life expectancy. For long-term neuraxial drug administration, an intrathecal route via an implanted pump is preferred.

Neuroablation involves interrupting a nociceptive pathway surgically or with a radiofrequency lesion. The procedure is used mainly for cancer pain. Somatic pain is more responsive than visceral pain. Neuroablation of the ascending spinothalamic tract (cordotomy) is usually used; it provides relief for several years, although numbness and dysesthesias develop. Neuroablation of the dorsal roots (rhizotomy) is used when a specific dermatome can be identified.

Nerve Stimulation

Nerve stimulation (neuroaugmentation) may decrease pain, presumably by activating endogenous pain modulatory pathways. The most common method is transcutaneous electrical nerve stimulation (TENS), which applies a small current to the skin. Also, electrodes may be implanted along peripheral nerves or along the dorsal columns in the epidural space. Stimulation of brain structures (deep brain stimulation and motor cortex stimulation) has also been used, but evidence of benefit is slight.

CHRONIC PAIN

(See also Fibromyalgia on p. 321.)

Chronic pain is pain that persists or recurs for > 3 mo, persists > 1 mo after resolution of an acute tissue injury, or accompanies a nonhealing lesion. Causes include chronic disorders (eg, cancer, arthritis, diabetes) and injuries (eg, herniated disk, torn ligament). Various drugs and psychologic treatments are used.

Unresolved, long-lasting disorders (eg, cancer, RA, herniated disk) that produce ongoing nociceptive or neuropathic stimuli may account completely for chronic pain. However, chronic pain stimuli sensitize and remodel the nervous system—from peripheral receptors to the cerebral cortex. With sensitization, discomfort that is due to a nearly resolved disorder and might otherwise be perceived as mild or trivial is instead perceived as significant pain. Psychologic factors may also amplify persistent pain. Thus, chronic pain commonly appears out of proportion to identifiable physical processes. In some cases (eg, chronic back pain after injury), the original precipitant of pain is obvious; in others (eg, chronic headache, atypical facial pain, chronic abdominal pain), the precipitant is remote or occult.

In most patients, physical processes are undeniably involved in sustaining chronic pain and are sometimes (eg, in cancer pain) the main factor. However, even in these patients,

TABLE 209–4. DRUGS FOR NEUROPATHIC PAIN

CLASS/DRUG	DOSE*	COMMENTS
Anticonvulsants†		
Carbamazepine	200–400 mg bid	Monitor WBCs when starting treatment
Gabapentin	300 mg bid to 1200 mg tid	Preferred drug in this class; starting dose usually 300 mg once/day
Phenytoin	300 mg once/day	Limited data; second-line drug
Pregabalin	75–300 mg bid	Mechanism similar to gabapentin but more stable pharmacokinetics
Valproate	250–500 mg bid	Limited data, but strong support for treatment of headache
Antidepressants		
Amitriptyline	10–25 mg at bedtime	May increase dose to 75–150 mg over 1–2 wk, particularly if significant depression is present; may not need high doses; not recommended for the elderly or patients with a heart disorder because it has strong anticholinergic effects
Desipramine	10–25 mg at bedtime	Better tolerated than amitriptyline; may increase dose to 150 mg or sometimes higher
Paroxetine	20 mg once/day	Better tolerated than tricyclic antidepressants; may increase dose to 60 mg once/day
Central α-2 adrenergic agonists		
Clonidine	0.1 mg once/day	Also can be used transdermally or intrathecally
Tizanidine	2–20 mg bid	Less likely to cause hypotension than clonidine
Corticosteroids		
Dexamethasone	0.5–4 mg qid	Used only for pain with an inflammatory component
Prednisone	5–60 mg once/day	Used only for pain with an inflammatory component
NMDA-receptor antagonists		
Amantadine	100 mg bid	Limited evidence of efficacy
Dextromethorphan	30–120 mg qid	Usually considered second-line
Oral local anesthetic		
Mexiletine	150 mg once/day to 300 mg q 8 h	Consider cardiac evaluation in those with significant heart disease
Topical		
Capsaicin 0.025–0.075%	tid	Some evidence of efficacy in neuropathic pain and arthritis
EMLA®	tid, under occlusive dressing if possible	Usually considered for a trial if lidocaine patch is ineffective; expensive
Lidocaine 5%	Daily	Available as patch
Other		
Baclofen	20–60 mg bid	May act via $GABA_B$ receptor; helpful in trigeminal neuralgia; used in other types of neuropathic pain
Pamidronate	60–90 mg/mo	Evidence of efficacy in complex regional pain syndrome

*All oral unless otherwise indicated.

† Newer anticonvulsants have fewer adverse effects.

NMDA = *N*-methyl-D-aspartate; EMLA = eutectic mixture of local anesthetics; GABA = γ-aminobutyric acid.

psychologic factors usually also play a role. Patients who have to continually prove that they are sick to obtain medical care, insurance coverage, or work relief may unconsciously reinforce their pain perceptions, particularly when litigation is involved. This response differs from malingering, which is conscious exaggeration of symptoms for secondary gain (eg, time off, disability payments). Various factors in the patient's environment (eg, family members, friends) may reinforce behaviors that perpetuate chronic pain.

Chronic pain can lead to psychologic problems. Constant, unremitting pain limits activities and may cause depression and anxiety, interrupt sleep, and interfere with almost all activities. Distinguishing cause from effect is often difficult.

Symptoms and Diagnosis

Chronic pain often leads to vegetative signs (eg, lassitude, sleep disturbance, decreased appetite, loss of taste for food, weight loss, diminished libido, constipation), which develop gradually; depression may develop. Patients may become inactive, withdraw socially, and become preoccupied with physical health. Psychologic and social impairment may be severe, causing virtual lack of function.

Some patients, particularly those without a clear-cut ongoing cause, have a history of failed medical and surgical treatments, multiple (and duplicative) diagnostic tests, use of many drugs (sometimes involving abuse or addiction), and inappropriate use of health care.

An organic cause should always be sought—even if a prominent psychologic contribution to the pain is likely. Physical processes associated with the pain should be evaluated appropriately and characterized. However, once a full evaluation is done, repeating tests in the absence of new findings is not useful. The best approach is often to stop testing and focus on relieving pain and restoring function.

The effect of pain on the patient's life should be assessed; evaluation by an occupational therapist may be necessary. Formal psychiatric evaluation should be considered if a coexisting psychiatric disorder (eg, major depression) is suspected as cause or effect.

Treatment

Specific causes should be treated. Early, aggressive treatment of acute pain may limit or prevent sensitization and remodeling and hence prevent progression to chronic pain.

Drugs or physical methods may be used. Psychologic and behavioral treatments are usually helpful. Many patients who have marked functional impairment or who do not respond to a reasonable attempt at management by their physician benefit from the multidisciplinary approach available at a pain clinic.

Drugs: Analgesics include NSAIDs, opioids, and adjuvant analgesics (eg, antidepressants, anticonvulsants—see p. 1776 and Table 209–4). One or more drugs may be appropriate. Adjuvant analgesics are most commonly used for neuropathic pain. For persistent, moderate-to-severe pain that impairs function, opioids should be considered after determining the following: what conventional treatment practice is, whether other treatments are reasonable, whether an opioid is likely to be effective, and whether the patient has an unusually high risk of adverse effects from an opioid or is likely to be a responsible drug user. Prescription drug abuse is an increasing problem, and physicians should not offer long-term opioid therapy unless they can assess risk of abuse, monitor patients appropriately, and respond reasonably to problematic drug use. As pain lessens, patients usually need help reducing use of opioids. If depression coexists with pain, antidepressants should be used.

Depending on the condition, trigger point injection, joint or spinal injections, nerve blocks, spinal cord stimulation, or neuraxial infusion is appropriate.

Physical methods: Many patients benefit from physical therapy or occupational therapy. Spray-and-stretch techniques can relieve myofascial trigger points. Some patients require an orthosis.

Psychologic treatments: Behavioral treatments can improve patient function, even without reducing pain. Patients should keep a diary of daily activities to pinpoint areas amenable to change. The physician should make specific recommendations for gradually increasing physical activity and social engagement. Activities should be prescribed in gradually increasing units of time; pain should not, if at all possible, be allowed to abort the commitment to greater function. When activities are increased in this way, reports of pain often decrease.

Various cognitive techniques of pain control (eg, relaxation training, distraction techniques, hypnosis, biofeedback) may be useful. Patients may be taught to use distraction by guided imagery (organized fantasy evoking calm and comfort; eg, imagining resting on a beach or lying in a hammock). Other cognitive-behavioral techniques (eg, self-hypnosis) may require training by specialists. Behavior of family members or fellow workers that reinforces pain behavior (eg, constant inquiries about the patient's health or insistence that the patient perform no chores) should be discouraged. The physician should avoid reinforcing pain behavior, disapprove of maladaptive behaviors, applaud progress, and provide pain treatment while emphasizing return of function.

NEUROPATHIC PAIN

Neuropathic pain results from damage to or dysfunction of the peripheral or central nervous system, rather than stimulation of pain receptors. Diagnosis is suggested by pain out of proportion to tissue injury, dysesthesia (eg, burning, tingling), and signs of nerve injury detected during neurologic examination. Although neuropathic pain responds to opioids, treatment is often with adjuvant drugs (eg, antidepressants, anticonvulsants, baclofen, topical drugs).

Pain can develop after injury to any level of the nervous system, peripheral or central, and may involve the sympathetic nervous system (sympathetically maintained pain). Specific syndromes include postherpetic neuralgia (see p. 1609), root avulsions, painful traumatic mononeuropathy, painful polyneuropathy (particularly due to diabetes), central pain syndromes (potentially caused by virtually any lesion at any level of the nervous system), postsurgical pain syndromes (eg, postmastectomy syndrome, postthoracotomy syndrome, phantom pain), and complex regional pain syndrome (reflex sympathetic dystrophy and causalgia—see p. 1780).

Etiology and Pathophysiology

Peripheral nerve injury or dysfunction can result in neuropathic pain. Typical causes include nerve compression (eg, by neuroma, tumor, or herniated disc) and various metabolic neuropathies (see Table 223–1 on p. 1892). Mechanisms presumably vary and may involve an increased number of Na channels on regenerating nerves.

Central neuropathic pain syndromes appear to involve reorganization of central somatosensory processing; the main categories are deafferentation pain and sympathetically maintained pain. Both are complex and, although presumably related, differ substantially.

Deafferentation pain is due to partial or complete interruption of peripheral or central afferent neural activity. Examples are postherpetic neuralgia, central pain (pain after CNS injury), and phantom pain (pain felt in the region of an amputated body part). Mechanisms are unknown but may involve sensitization of central neurons, with lower activation thresholds and expansion of receptive fields.

Sympathetically maintained pain depends on efferent sympathetic activity. Complex regional pain syndrome sometimes involves sympathetically maintained pain. Other types of neuropathic pain may have a sympathetically maintained component. Mechanisms probably involve abnormal sympathetic-somatic nerve connections (ephapses), local inflammatory changes, and changes in the spinal cord.

Symptoms and Diagnosis

Dysesthesias (spontaneous or evoked burning pain, often with a superimposed lancinating component) are typical, but pain may also be deep and aching. Other sensations—eg, hyperesthesia, hyperalgesia, allodynia (pain from a nonnoxious stimulus), hyperpathia (particularly unpleasant, exaggerated pain response)—may also occur. Symptoms are long-lasting, typically persisting after resolution of the primary cause (if one was present), because the CNS has been sensitized and remodeled.

Neuropathic pain is suggested by its typical symptoms when nerve injury is known or suspected; the cause (eg, amputation, diabetes) may be readily apparent. If not, the diagnosis often can be assumed based on the description. Pain that is ameliorated by sympathetic nerve block is sympathetically maintained pain.

Treatment

Without concern for diagnosis, rehabilitation, and psychosocial issues, treatment has a limited chance of success. For peripheral nerve lesions, mobilization is needed to prevent trophic changes, disuse atrophy, and joint ankylosis. Surgery may be needed to alleviate compression. Psychologic factors must be constantly considered from the start of treatment. Anxiety and depression must be treated appropriately. When dysfunction is entrenched, patients may benefit from the comprehensive approach provided by a pain clinic.

Several classes of drugs are moderately effective (see TABLE 209–4), but complete or near-complete relief is unlikely. Antidepressants and anticonvulsants are most commonly used. Evidence of efficacy is strong for several tricyclic antidepressants and for the anticonvulsant gabapentin but is weaker for the newer (and better tolerated) antidepressants and for many other anticonvulsants.

Opioid analgesics can provide some relief but are less effective than for nociceptive pain; adverse effects may prevent adequate analgesia. Topical drugs and a lidocaine-containing patch may be effective for peripheral syndromes. Sympathetic blockade is usually ineffective except for some patients with complex regional pain syndrome.

COMPLEX REGIONAL PAIN SYNDROME

(Reflex Sympathetic Dystrophy and Causalgia)

Complex regional pain syndrome is chronic neuropathic pain that follows soft tissue or bone injury (type I) or nerve injury (type II) and persists out of proportion in intensity and duration to the original tissue damage. Other manifestations include autonomic changes (eg, sweating, vasomotor abnormalities), motor changes (eg, weakness, dystonia), and trophic changes (eg, skin or bone atrophy, hair loss, joint contractures). Diagnosis is clinical. Treatment includes drugs, physical therapy, and sympathetic blockade.

Complex regional pain syndrome (CRPS) type I was previously known as reflex sympathetic dystrophy, and type II as causalgia. Both types occur most often in young adults and are 2 or 3 times more common among women.

Etiology and Pathophysiology

CRPS type I typically follows an injury (usually of a hand or foot), most commonly after crush injuries, especially in a lower limb. It may follow acute MI, stroke, or cancer (eg, lung, breast, ovary, CNS); no precipitant is apparent in about 10% of patients. CRPS type II is similar to type I but involves overt damage to a peripheral nerve.

Pathophysiology is unclear, but peripheral nociceptor and central sensitization and release of neuropeptides (substance P, calcitonin gene-related peptide) help maintain pain and inflammation. The sympathetic nervous system is more involved in CRPS than in other neuropathic pain syndromes: Central sympathetic activity is increased, and peripheral nociceptors are sensitized to norepinephrine (a sympathetic neurotransmitter); these changes may lead to sweating abnormalities and poor blood flow due to vasoconstriction. Nonetheless, only some patients respond to sympathetic manipulation (ie, central or peripheral sympathetic blockade).

Symptoms and Signs

Symptoms vary greatly and do not follow a pattern; they include sensory, focal autonomic (vasomotor or sudomotor), and motor abnormalities.

Pain—burning or aching—is common. It does not follow the distribution of a single peripheral nerve; it may worsen with changes in environment or emotional stress. Allodynia and hyperalgesia may occur. Pain often causes patients to limit use of an extremity.

Cutaneous vasomotor changes (eg, red, mottled, or ashen color; increased or decreased temperature), sudomotor abnormalities (dry or hyperhidrotic skin) may be present. Edema may be considerable and locally confined. Other symptoms include trophic abnormalities (eg, shiny, atrophic skin; cracking or excess growth of nails; bone atrophy; hair loss) and motor abnormalities (weakness, tremors, spasm, dystonia with fingers fixed in flexion or equinovarus position of foot). Range of motion is often limited, sometimes leading to joint contractures. Symptoms may interfere with fitting prostheses to amputated limbs.

Psychologic distress (eg, depression, anxiety, anger) is common, fostered by the poorly understood cause, lack of effective therapy, and prolonged course.

Diagnosis

Diagnosis is clinical. Standard criteria require occurrence of pain (usually burning), allodynia or hyperalgesia; focal autonomic dysregulation (vasomotor or sudomotor abnormalities); and no evidence of another disorder that could explain the symptoms. If another disorder is present, CRPS should be considered possible or probable.

Other symptoms and findings may support the diagnosis: edema, trophic abnormalities, or a change in temperature of the affected area. Thermography may be used to document the temperature change if clinical evaluation is equivocal and if this finding would help establish the diagnosis. Bone changes (eg, demineralization on x-ray or increased uptake on a triple-phase radionuclide bone scan) also may be detected and are usually evaluated only if the diagnosis is equivocal.

Imaging tests are not specific because they may be abnormal after trauma in patients without CRPS.

Sympathetic nerve block (cervical stellate ganglion or lumbar) can be used for diagnosis and treatment. However, false-positive and false-negative results are common because not all CRPS pain is sympathetically maintained and nerve block may also affect nonsympathetic fibers. In another test of sympathetic involvement, a patient is given IV infusions of saline (placebo) or phentolamine 1 mg/kg over 10 min while pain scores are recorded; a decrease in pain after phentolamine but not placebo indicates sympathetically maintained pain.

Prognosis and Treatment

Prognosis varies and is difficult to predict. CRPS may remit or remain stable for years; in a few patients, it progresses, spreading to other areas of the body.

Treatment is complex and often unsatisfactory, particularly if begun late. It includes drugs, physical therapy, sympathetic blockade, psychologic treatments, and neuromodulation. Few controlled trials have been done.

Many of the drugs used for neuropathic pain, including tricyclic antidepressants, anticonvulsants, and corticosteroids (see TABLE 209–4), may be tried; none is known to be superior. Long-term treatment with opioid analgesics may be useful for selected patients.

In some patients with sympathetically maintained pain, regional sympathetic blockade relieves pain, so that physical therapy is possible. Oral analgesics (NSAIDs, opioids, and various adjuvant analgesics) may also relieve pain sufficiently to allow rehabilitation.

For neuromodulation, implanted spinal cord stimulators are being increasingly used. Transcutaneous electrical nerve stimulation (TENS), applied at multiple locations with different stimulation parameters, should be given a long trial. Other methods of neuromodulation include brisk rubbing of the affected part (counterirritation) and acupuncture. No one form of neuromodulation is known to be more effective than another, and a poor response to one form does not mean a poor response to another. Neuraxial infusion with opioids, anesthetics, and clonidine may help, and intrathecal baclofen has reduced dystonia in a few patients.

Physical therapy is essential. Goals include mobilization, strengthening, increased range of motion, and vocational rehabilitation.

210 FUNCTION AND DYSFUNCTION OF THE CEREBRAL LOBES

The cerebrum is divided by a longitudinal fissure into 2 hemispheres, each containing 5 discrete lobes. The frontal, temporal, parietal, and occipital lobes cover the brain's surface; the insula is hidden beneath the temporal lobe (see FIG. 210–1). Although specific functions are attributed to each lobe, most activities require coordination of multiple areas in both hemispheres. For example, although the occipital lobe is essential to visual processing, parts of the parietal, temporal, and frontal lobes on both sides also process complex visual stimuli.

Function is extensively lateralized. Visual, tactile, and motor activities of the left side of the body are directed predominately by the right hemisphere and vice versa. Certain complex functions manifest bilaterally but are directed predominantly by one hemisphere (cerebral dominance). For example, the left hemisphere is typically dominant for language, and the right is dominant for spatial attention.

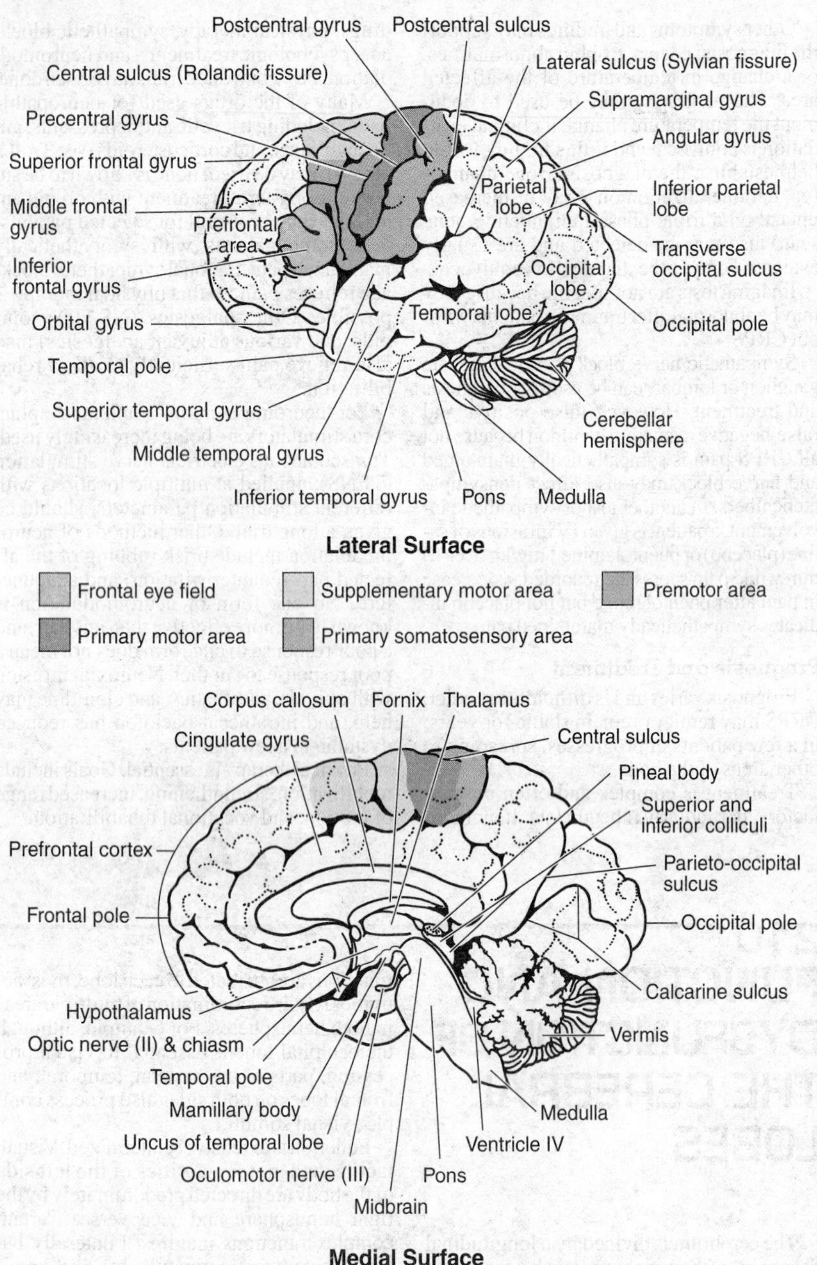

Fig. 210–1. Areas of the brain.

The cerebral cortex contains the primary sensory and motor areas as well as multiple association areas. The primary sensory areas directly receive somesthetic, auditory, visual, olfactory, and gustatory stimuli from peripheral receptors. Sensory stimuli are further processed in association areas that relate to one or more senses. The primary motor cortex generates volitional body movements; motor association areas help plan and execute complex motor activity.

Heteromodal association areas in the frontal, temporal, and parietal lobes integrate sensory data, motor feedback, and other information with instinctual and acquired memories. This integration facilitates learning and creates thought, expression, and behavior.

Frontal lobes: The frontal lobes are essential for planning and executing learned and purposeful behaviors; they are also the site of many inhibitory functions. There are at least 4 functionally distinct areas in the frontal lobes: the primary motor cortex in the precentral gyrus (the most posterior part) and the medial, orbital, and lateral frontal areas (termed the prefrontal areas).

The medial frontal area is important in arousal and motivation. The orbital frontal area helps modulate social behaviors. The inferolateral frontal area is specialized for expressive language function; the dorsolateral frontal area manipulates very recently acquired information, a function called working memory.

Patients with large medial frontal lesions extending to the most anterior frontal pole sometimes become abulic (apathetic, inattentive, and markedly slow to respond). Patients with orbital frontal lesions can become emotionally labile, indifferent to the implications of their actions, or both. They may be alternately euphoric, facetious, vulgar, and indifferent to social nuances. Bilateral acute trauma to this part of the prefrontal areas may make patients boisterously talkative, restless, and socially intrusive. With aging and especially with many types of dementia, the frontal lobe degenerates, leading to disinhibition and abnormal behaviors.

Lesions of the inferolateral frontal area (Broca's area) cause expressive aphasia (impaired comprehension or expression of words—see p. 1787). Lesions of the dorsolateral frontal area can impair the ability to retain information and process it in real time (eg, to spell words backwards, to alternate between letters and numbers sequentially).

In the primary motor cortex, all of the moving parts on one side of the body are controlled by the contralateral side (shown on a spatial map called a homunculus—see FIG. 210–2). Because 90% of motor fibers from each hemisphere cross the midline in the brain stem, damage to the motor cortex of one hemisphere causes weakness or paralysis on the opposite side of the body.

Parietal lobes: The postrolandic area (postcentral gyrus) of the parietal lobes (primary somatosensory cortex) integrates somesthetic stimuli for recognition and recall of form, texture, and weight. In the primary somatosensory cortex, located in the anterior parietal lobes, all of the somatosensory functions on one side of the body are controlled by the contralateral side (on a homunculus—see FIG. 210–2). More posterolateral areas of the parietal lobes generate visual-spatial relationships and integrate these perceptions with other sensations to create awareness of trajectories of moving objects. These areas also generate proprioception (awareness of the position of body parts). In the dominant hemisphere, Gerstmann's area, located in the midparietal lobule, is important to abilities such as calculation, writing, left-right orientation, and finger recognition. The nearby angular gyrus is important for naming and other aspects of word recognition. The nondominant parietal lobe integrates the contralateral side of the body with its environment and is important for attention to space and for abilities such as drawing.

Lesions of the anterior part of the parietal lobe can cause difficulty recognizing objects by touch (astereognosis). Lesions in more lateral areas can impair naming and other language functions or cause deficits in writing, calculating, left-right disorientation, and finger-naming (Gerstmann's syndrome). Acute injury to the nondominant parietal lobe may cause neglect of the contralateral side (usually the left), resulting in decreased awareness of that part of the body, its environment, and any associated injury to that side (anosognosia). For example, patients with large right parietal lesions may deny the existence of left-sided paralysis; they may lapse into global confusion. Patients with smaller lesions may become confused when performing learned motor tasks (eg, dressing, other well-learned activities)—a spatial-manual deficit called apraxia.

Temporal lobes: The temporal lobes are integral to auditory perception, receptive

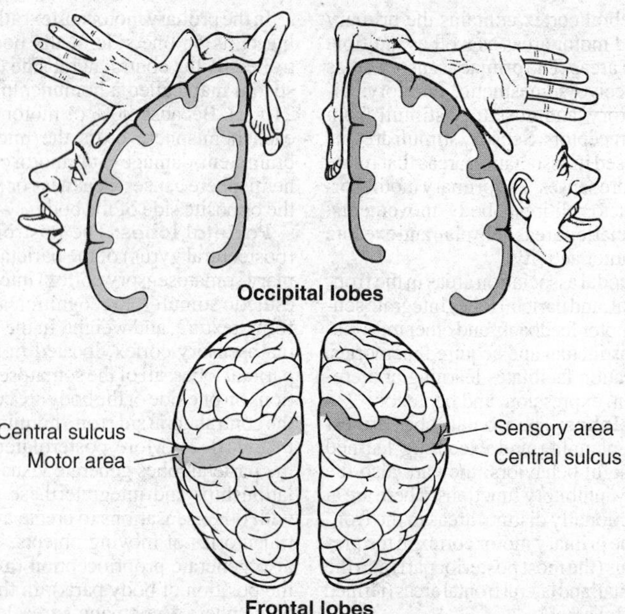

Fig. 210–2. Homunculus. Specific parts of the cortex control specific motor and sensory functions on the contralateral side of the body. The amount of cortical space given to a body part varies; eg, the area of the cortex that controls the hand is larger than the area that controls the shoulder. The map of these parts is called the homunculus ("little person").

components of language, declarative and visual memory, and emotion. Patients with right temporal lobe lesions commonly lose acuity for nonverbal auditory stimuli (eg, music). Left temporal lobe lesions interfere greatly with the recognition, memory, and formation of language. Patients with epileptogenic foci in the medial limbic-emotional parts of the temporal lobe commonly have complex partial seizures, characterized by uncontrollable feelings and autonomic, cognitive, or emotional dysfunction. Occasionally, such patients have personality changes, characterized by humorlessness, philosophic religiosity, and obsessiveness; in men, libido may be decreased.

Occipital lobe: The occipital lobe contains the primary visual cortex and visual association areas. Lesions in the primary visual cortex lead to a form of central blindness called Anton's syndrome; patients become unable to recognize objects by sight and are generally unaware of their deficits. Seizures in the occipital lobe can cause visual hallucinations, often consisting of lines or meshes of color superimposed on the contralateral visual field.

Insula: The insula integrates sensory and autonomic information from the viscera. It plays a role in certain language functions, as evidenced by aphasia in patients with some insular lesions. The insula processes aspects of pain and temperature sensation and possibly taste.

Pathophysiology

Cerebral dysfunction may be focal or global. Focal and global processes may also affect subcortical systems, altering arousal (eg, causing stupor or coma) or integration of thought (eg, causing delirium).

Focal dysfunction usually results from structural abnormalities (eg, tumors, stroke, trauma, malformations, gliosis, demyelination). Manifestations depend on the lesion's location, size, and development rate. Lesions < 2 cm in diameter and very slow developing lesions may be asymptomatic. Larger lesions, rapidly developing lesions (over weeks or months rather than years), and lesions that affect both hemispheres simultaneously are more likely to become symptomatic.

Global dysfunction is caused by toxic-metabolic disorders or sometimes by diffuse inflammation, vasculopathy, major trauma, or disseminated cancer; these disorders affect multiple dimensions of cerebral function.

Focal lesions in white matter can interrupt the connectivity between brain areas and cause the disconnection syndrome (inability to perform a task that requires coordinated activity of ≥ 2 brain regions, despite retention of basic functions of each region).

Recovery from brain injury depends in part on the degree of plasticity of the remaining cerebrum, a capacity that varies among different individuals and as a function of age and general health. Plasticity (ability of an area of the brain to alter its function) is most prominent in the developing brain. For example, if the dominant hemisphere language areas are severely damaged before age 8 yr, the opposite hemisphere can often assume near-normal language function. Although there is considerable capacity for recovery from brain injury after the 1st decade of life, severe damage more often results in permanent deficits. Gross reorganization of brain function after injury in adults is uncommon, although plasticity remains operative on the local level in many brain areas throughout life.

Cerebral dysfunction syndromes: Specific syndromes include agnosia, amnesia, aphasia, and apraxia. Psychiatric conditions (eg, depression, psychosis, anxiety disorders) sometimes include similar elements. In general, diagnosis is clinical, often assisted by neuropsychologic testing. Diagnosis of the cause usually requires laboratory tests (blood and CSF analysis, ECG, EEG) and brain imaging, either structural (CT, MRI) or functional (PET, SPECT).

AGNOSIA

Agnosia is inability to identify an object using one or more of the senses. Diagnosis is clinical, often including neuropsychologic testing, with brain imaging (CT, MRI) to identify cause. Prognosis depends on the nature and extent of damage and patient age. There is no specific treatment, but occupational therapy may help patients compensate.

Agnosias are uncommon. They result from damage (eg, by infarct, tumor, trauma) or degeneration to areas of the brain that integrate perception, memory, and identification.

Discrete brain lesions can cause different forms of agnosia, which may involve any sense. Typically, only one sense is affected; ability to identify objects with other senses is unaffected. Examples are inability to identify objects through sound such as a ringing telephone (auditory agnosia), taste (gustatory agnosia), smell (olfactory agnosia), touch (tactile agnosia), or sight (visual agnosia).

Other forms of agnosia involve very specific and complex processes within one sense. For example, prosopagnosia is inability to identify well-known faces, including close friends, or to otherwise distinguish individual objects among a class of objects, despite the ability to identify generic facial features and objects.

Anosognosia often accompanies damage to the right, nondominant parietal lobe. Patients deny their deficit, insisting that nothing is wrong even when one side of their body is completely paralyzed. When shown the paralyzed body part, patients may deny that it is theirs. In an often related phenomenon, patients ignore the paralyzed or desensitized body parts (hemi-inattention) or the space around them (hemineglect). Hemineglect most often involves the left side of the body.

Occipitotemporal lesions may cause an inability to recognize familiar places (environmental agnosia), visual disturbances (visual agnosia), or color blindness (achromatopsia). Right-sided temporal lesions may cause an inability to interpret sounds (auditory agnosia) or impaired music perception (amusia).

Diagnosis

Patients are asked to identify common objects through sight, touch, or another sense. If hemineglect is suspected, patients are asked to identify the paralyzed parts of their body or objects in their hemivisual fields. Neuropsychologic testing may help identify more subtle agnosias. Tests to detect deficits in sensation and comprehension must be done to distinguish such defects from agnosia.

Brain imaging (eg, CT or MRI with or without angiographic protocols) is required to characterize the central lesion (eg, infarct, hemorrhage, mass) and to check for atrophy suggesting a degenerative disorder. Physical examination can typically detect primary deficits in individual senses that may confound testing.

Prognosis and Treatment

There is no specific treatment. Rehabilitation with speech or occupational therapists can help patients learn to compensate for their deficits. Recovery may be influenced by size and location of lesions, degree of impairment, and patient age. Most recovery occurs within the 1st 3 mo but may continue to a variable degree up to a year.

AMNESIAS

Amnesia is partial or total inability to recall past experiences. It may result from traumatic brain injury, degeneration, metabolic disorders, seizure disorders, or psychologic disturbances. Diagnosis is clinical, often including neuropsychologic testing and brain imaging (CT, MRI). Treatment is directed at the cause.

Processing of memories involves registration (taking in new information), encoding (forming associations, time stamps, and other processes necessary for retrieval), and retrieval. Deficits in any of these steps can cause amnesia.

Amnesia can be classified as retrograde (for events before the cause), anterograde (inability to store new memories after the cause), global (for information related to all senses and past times), and sense-specific (for events processed by one sense—eg, an agnosia). Amnesia may be transient (as occurs after brain trauma), fixed (as occurs after a serious event such as encephalitis, global ischemia, or cardiac arrest), or progressive (as occurs with degenerative dementias, such as Alzheimer's disease). Memory deficits more commonly involve facts (declarative memory) and, less commonly, skills (procedural memory).

Pathophysiology and Etiology

Amnesia can result from diffuse cerebral impairment, bilateral lesions, or multifocal injuries that impair memory-storage areas in the cerebral hemispheres. Predominant pathways for declarative memory occur along the medial parahippocampal region and hippocampus as well as in the inferomedial temporal lobes, orbital surface of the frontal lobes, and diencephalon. Of these, the hippocampal gyri, hypothalamus, nuclei of the basal forebrain, and dorsomedial thalamic nuclei are critical. The amygdaloid nucleus contributes emotional amplifications to memory. The thalamic intralaminar nuclei and activated brain stem reticular formation stimulate the imprinting of memories. Bilateral damage to the medial and dorsal thalamus and to the brain stem reticular formation and adrenergic system severely impairs recent memory and the ability to form new memories; the most common causes are thiamin deficiency, hypothalamic tumors, and ischemia. Bilateral damage to the medial temporal lobes, especially the hippocampus, can cause semipermanent declarative amnesia.

Severe, irreversible memory loss is most commonly caused by degenerative dementias, severe brain trauma, brain anoxia or ischemia, alcoholic-nutritional disorders (eg, Wernicke's encephalopathy, Korsakoff's psychosis—see pp. 1688–1689), and various drug intoxications (eg, chronic solvent sniffing, amphotericin B or lithium toxicity).

Posttraumatic amnesias for the periods immediately before and after concussion or more severe head trauma seem to result from medial temporal lobe injury. More severe injuries may affect larger areas of memory storage and recall, as can many diffuse cerebral disorders that cause dementia.

Psychologic disturbances of memory result from extreme psychologic trauma or stress (see p. 1679).

With aging, many people gradually develop noticeable problems with memory, often first for names, then for events, and occasionally for spatial relationships. This widely experienced so-called benign senescent forgetfulness has no proven relationship to dementia, although some similarities are hard to overlook. People who have a subjective memory problem, who perform worse on objective memory tests, but who otherwise have intact cognition and daily function may have amnestic mild cognitive impairment (amnestic MCI). People with amnestic MCI are more likely to develop Alzheimer's disease than age-matched people without memory problems.

Diagnosis and Treatment

Simple bedside tests (eg, 3-item recall, location of objects previously hidden in the room) and formal tests (eg, word list learning tests such as the California Verbal Learning Test and the Buschke Selective Reminding Test) can help identify verbal memory loss. Assessment of nonverbal memory is more difficult but may include recall of visual designs or a series of tones. Clinical findings usually suggest causes and hence the necessary tests.

Any underlying disorder or psychologic cause (see p. 1680) must be treated. However, some patients with acute amnesia improve spontaneously. Certain disorders that cause amnesia (eg, Alzheimer's disease, Korsakoff's psychosis, herpes encephalitis) can be treated; however, treatment of the underlying disorder may or may not lessen the amnesia. If it does not, no specific measures can hasten recovery or improve the outcome.

Transient Global Amnesia

Transient global amnesia is disturbed memory caused by central vascular or ischemic lesions. Diagnosis is primarily clinical but includes laboratory tests and CT, MRI, or both to evaluate central circulation. The amnesia typically remits spontaneously but may recur. There is no specific treatment, but underlying abnormalities are corrected.

Transient global amnesia is typically caused by transient ischemia (eg, atherosclerosis, thrombosis, thromboembolic disease) affecting the posteromedial thalamus or hippocampus bilaterally, but it can be caused by seizure activity or migraines.

A distinct benign form of transient global amnesia can follow excessive alcohol ingestion, moderately large sedative doses of barbiturates, use of several illicit drugs, or sometimes relatively small doses of benzodiazepines (especially midazolam and triazolam).

Symptoms, Signs, and Diagnosis

Patients present with acute global amnesic confusion that lasts from as little as 30 to 60 min to ≥ 12 h. Patients have a retrograde memory deficit that can extend back for several years; they are often disoriented to time and place but usually not to personal identity. Smaller disturbances occur in anterograde memory. Many patients are anxious or agitated and may repeatedly ask questions about transpiring events. Language function, attention, visual-spatial skills, and social skills are retained. Impairments gradually resolve as the episode subsides. Usually, episodes do not recur, except when the cause is seizures or migraines.

The benign transient amnesia (blackout) after substance ingestion is distinct because it is selectively retrograde (ie, for events during and preceding intoxication), relates specifically to drug-accompanied events, does not cause confusion (once acute intoxication resolves), and recurs only if similar amounts of the same drug are ingested.

Diagnosis is primarily clinical. Neurologic examination typically does not detect any abnormalities other than disturbed memory.

Prognosis and Treatment

Prognosis is good. Symptoms typically last < 24 h. As the disorder resolves, the amnesia lessens, but memory for events during the attack may be lost. Lifetime recurrence rate is about 5 to 25%.

Evaluation to rule out central ischemia (eg, due to stroke, thrombosis, or thromboembolic disease) is required (see p. 1793). Laboratory tests should include CBC, coagulation tests, and evaluation for hypercoagulable states. CT, MRI, or both with or without angiographic protocols is done. EEG may show nonspecific abnormalities and hence is unnecessary unless a seizure is suspected or episodes recur.

No specific treatment is indicated. However, underlying ischemia (see p. 1794) or seizure (see p. 1826) should be treated accordingly.

APHASIA

Aphasia is language dysfunction that may involve impaired comprehension or expression of words or nonverbal equivalents of words. It results from dysfunction of the language centers in the cerebral cortex and basal ganglia or of the white matter pathways that connect them. Diagnosis is clinical, often including neuropsychologic testing, with brain imaging (CT, MRI) to identify cause. Prognosis depends on the nature and extent of damage and patient age. There is no specific treatment, but speech therapy may promote recovery.

Language function resides predominantly in the posterosuperior temporal lobe, adjacent inferior parietal lobe, inferolateral frontal lobe, and subcortical connection between those regions—usually in the left hemisphere, even in left-handed people. Damage to any part of this roughly triangular area (eg, by infarct, tumor, trauma, or degeneration) interferes with some aspect of language function. Prosody (quality of rhythm and emphasis that adds meaning to speech) is usually influenced by both hemispheres but is sometimes affected by dysfunction of the nondominant hemisphere alone.

Aphasia is distinct from developmental disorders of language and from dysfunction of the motor pathways and muscles that produce speech (dysarthria). It is broadly divided into receptive and expressive aphasia.

Receptive (sensory, or Wernicke's) aphasia is inability to comprehend words or to recognize auditory, visual, or tactile symbols. It is caused by a disorder of the posterosuperior temporal gyrus of the language-dominant hemisphere. Often, alexia (loss of the ability to read words) is also present. In expressive (motor, or Broca's) aphasia, comprehension and ability to conceptualize are relatively preserved, but the ability to create words is impaired. It is due to a disorder of the posteroinferior part of the frontal lobe. It often causes agraphia (loss of the ability to write) and impairs oral reading.

Symptoms and Signs

Patients with Wernicke's aphasia speak normal words fluently, often including meaningless phonemes, but do not know their meaning or relationships. The result is a jumble of words or "word salad." Patients with Wernicke's aphasia are typically unaware that their speech is incomprehensible to others. A right visual field cut commonly accompanies Wernicke's aphasia because the visual pathway is near the affected area.

Patients with Broca's aphasia can comprehend and conceptualize relatively well, but their ability to form words is impaired. Usually, the impairment affects speech production and writing (agraphia, dysgraphia), greatly frustrating patients' attempts to communicate. Broca's aphasia may include anomia (inability to name objects) and impaired prosody.

Diagnosis

Verbal interaction can typically identify gross aphasias. Testing to identify specific deficits should include assessment of spontaneous speech, naming, repetition, comprehension, speech production, reading, and writing. Spontaneous speech is assessed for fluency, number of words spoken, ability to initiate speech, presence of spontaneous errors, word-finding pauses, hesitations, circumlocutions, and prosody. Initially, Wernicke's aphasia may be mistaken for delirium. However, Wernicke's aphasia is a pure language disturbance without other features of delirium (eg, fluctuating level of consciousness, hallucinations, inattention).

Formal cognitive testing by a neuropsychologist or speech and language therapist may detect finer levels of dysfunction and assist in planning treatment and assessing potential for recovery. Various formal tests for diagnosing aphasia (eg, Boston Diagnostic Aphasia Examination, Western Aphasia Battery, Boston Naming Test, Token Test, Action Naming Test) are available.

Brain imaging (eg, CT or MRI with or without angiographic protocols) is required to characterize the lesion (eg, infarct, hemorrhage, mass). Further tests are done to determine the etiology of the lesion as indicated (see pp. 1793 and 1825).

Prognosis and Treatment

Effectiveness of treatment is unclear, but most clinicians think that treatment by qualified speech therapists helps and that patients treated soon after onset improve most.

Recovery is also influenced by size and location of lesions, extent of language impairment, and, to a lesser degree, the age, education, and general health of the patient. Children < 8 yr often regain language function after severe damage to either hemisphere. After that age, most recovery occurs within the 1st 3 mo, but improvement continues to a variable degree up to a year.

APRAXIA

Apraxia is inability to execute purposeful, previously learned motor tasks, despite physical ability and willingness, as a result of brain damage. Diagnosis is clinical, often including neuropsychologic testing, with brain imaging (CT, MRI) to identify cause. Prognosis depends on the nature and extent of damage and patient age. There is no specific treatment, but physical and occupational therapy may modestly improve functioning and patient safety.

Apraxia results from brain damage (eg, by infarct, tumor, or trauma) or degeneration, usually in the parietal lobes or their connections, which retain memories of learned movement patterns. Less commonly, damage to other areas of the brain (premotor cortex, corpus callosum, frontal lobe) or diffuse damage related to degenerative dementias results in apraxia.

Symptoms, Signs, and Diagnosis

Patients cannot conceptualize or perform learned complex motor tasks despite an ability to perform the individual component movements. For example, patients with constructional apraxia may be unable to copy a simple geometric shape despite being able to see and recognize the stimulus, hold and use a pen, and understand the task. Typically, patients do not recognize their deficits.

Tests include asking patients to perform or imitate common learned tasks (eg, waving good-bye; saluting; beckoning come here, stop, or go; opening a lock with a key; using a screwdriver; using scissors; taking a deep breath and holding it). Strength in all relevant muscle groups must be assessed to exclude motor weakness as the cause of symptoms. Neuropsychologic testing or assessment by a physical or occupational therapist may help identify more subtle apraxias.

Caregivers should be asked about the patient's ability to perform activities of daily living, especially those that involve household tools (eg, correct and safe use of eating utensils, toothbrush, kitchen utensils to prepare a meal, hammer, and scissors) and writing.

Brain imaging (eg, CT or MRI with or without angiographic protocols) is required to determine whether a central lesion (eg, infarct, hemorrhage, mass, focal atrophy) is present. Physical examination can typically detect underlying neuromuscular disorders or musculoskeletal injuries that may be confused with apraxia.

Prognosis and Treatment

In general, patients become dependent, requiring help with activities of daily living and at least some degree of supervision. Patients with stroke may have a stable course and even improve somewhat.

There is no specific medical treatment. Drugs that slow the symptomatic progression of dementia do not appear beneficial. Physical and occupational therapy may modestly improve functioning but is more often useful for making the environment safer and for providing devices that help patients circumvent the primary deficit.

211 STROKE

(Cerebrovascular Accident)

Strokes are a heterogeneous group of disorders involving sudden, focal interruption of cerebral blood flow, causing neurologic deficit. Strokes can be ischemic (80%), typically resulting from thrombosis or embolism; or hemorrhagic (20%), resulting from vascular rupture (eg, subarachnoid or intracerebral hemorrhage). Stroke symptoms lasting < 1 h are termed a transient ischemic attack (TIA). Strokes damage brain tissue; TIA often does not, and when damage occurs, it is less extensive than in stroke. In Western countries, stroke is the 3rd most common cause of death and the most common cause of neurologic disability.

Etiology and Pathophysiology

Strokes involve the arteries of the brain (see FIG. 211–1), either the anterior circulation, consisting of branches of the internal carotid artery; or the posterior circulation, consisting of branches of the vertebral and basilar arteries.

Neurologic deficits reflect the involved area of brain (see TABLE 211–1). Anterior circulation stroke typically produces unilateral symptoms, whereas posterior circulation stroke often causes bilateral deficits and is more likely to affect level of consciousness.

Neurologic deficits generally do not reflect the type of stroke, but other manifestations are often suggestive. Sudden, severe headache may result from subarachnoid hemorrhage. Impaired consciousness or coma, often accompanied by headache, nausea, and vomiting, suggests increased intracranial pressure (see p. 1917), which can occur 48 to 72 h after large ischemic strokes and earlier with many hemorrhagic strokes; fatal brain herniation may result (see p. 1800).

Stroke risk factors include prior stroke, older age, family history of stroke, alcoholism, male sex, hypertension, cigarette smoking, hypercholesterolemia, diabetes, and use of certain drugs (eg, cocaine, amphetamines). Certain risk factors predispose to a particular type of stroke (eg, hypercoagulability predisposes

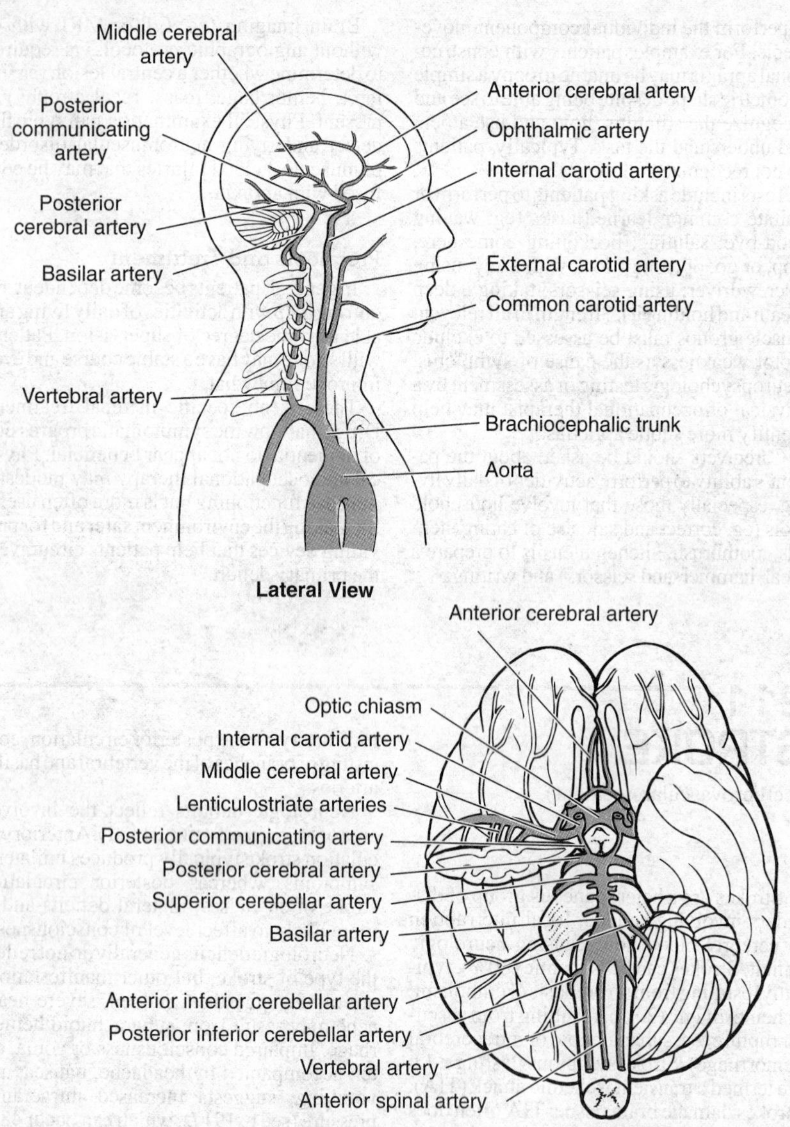

Fig. 211–1. Arteries of the brain. The anterior cerebral artery supplies the medial portions of the frontal and parietal lobes and corpus callosum. The middle cerebral artery supplies large portions of the frontal, parietal, and temporal lobe surfaces. Branches of the anterior and middle cerebral arteries (lenticulostriate arteries) supply the basal ganglia and anterior limb of the internal capsule.

The vertebral and basilar arteries supply the brain stem, cerebellum, posterior cerebral cortex, and medial temporal lobe. The posterior cerebral arteries bifurcate from the basilar artery to supply the medial temporal (including the hippocampus) and occipital lobes, thalamus, mammillary and geniculate bodies.

The anterior and posterior circulation communicate in the circle of Willis.

TABLE 211–1. SELECTED STROKE SYNDROMES

SYMPTOMS AND SIGNS	SYNDROME
Contralateral hemiparesis (maximal in the leg), urinary incontinence, apathy, confusion, poor judgment, mutism, grasp reflex, gait apraxia	Anterior cerebral artery (uncommon)
Contralateral hemiparesis (worse in arm and face than in leg), dysarthria, hemianesthesia, contralateral homonymous hemianopia, aphasia (if dominant hemisphere is affected) or apraxia and sensory neglect (if nondominant hemisphere is affected), monocular loss of vision (if internal carotid is affected)	Middle cerebral artery (common)
Contralateral homonymous hemianopia, unilateral cortical blindness, memory loss, unilateral 3rd cranial nerve palsy, hemiballismus	Posterior cerebral artery
Unilateral or bilateral cranial nerve deficits (eg, nystagmus, vertigo, dysphagia, dysarthria, diplopia, blindness), spastic paresis, crossed sensory and motor deficits*; impaired consciousness, coma, death (if basilar artery occlusion is complete)	Vertebrobasilar system
Unilateral pure sensory or motor deficits without cortical deficits	Lacunar infarcts

*Ipsilateral facial sensory loss or motor weakness with contralateral body hemianesthesia or hemiparesis indicates a lesion at the pons or lower.

to thrombotic stroke, atrial fibrillation to embolic stroke, intracranial aneurysms to subarachnoid hemorrhage).

Evaluation

Evaluation aims to establish whether stroke has occurred, whether it is ischemic or hemorrhagic, and whether immediate treatment is required.

Stroke is suspected by sudden neurologic deficits compatible with brain damage in an arterial territory; a particularly sudden, severe headache; sudden, unexplained coma; or sudden impairment of consciousness. Such patients should have immediate head CT to differentiate hemorrhagic from ischemic stroke and to detect signs of increased intracranial pressure. CT is particularly sensitive for intracranial blood but may be normal or show only subtle changes in anterior circulation ischemic stroke during the 1st hours of symptoms. CT also misses some small posterior circulation strokes and up to 3% of subarachnoid hemorrhages. If consciousness is impaired with no or equivocal lateralizing signs, further tests for non-stroke causes are obtained (see full discussion in Ch. 212 on p. 1800). If stroke is clinically suspected but not identified on CT, MRI can help in the diagnosis of ischemic stroke.

After type of stroke is determined, the most common causes for that type of stroke are sought as discussed below. Patients are also evaluated for coexisting acute general disorders (eg, infection, dehydration, hypoxia, hyperglycemia, hypertension).

Treatment

Stabilization may need to precede complete evaluation. Comatose or obtunded patients may require airway support (see p. 544). If increased intracranial pressure is suspected, intracranial pressure monitoring (see p. 516) and measures to reduce cerebral edema (see p. 2577) may be necessary. Supportive care and correction of coexisting abnormalities (eg, fever, hypoxia, dehydration, hyperglycemia, sometimes hypertension) are vital acutely and during convalescence. Specific acute treatments vary by type of stroke. During convalescence, measures to prevent aspiration, deep venous thrombosis, UTI, decubitus ulcers, and undernutrition may be necessary (eg, in bedridden patients). Passive exercises, particularly of paralyzed limbs, and breathing exercises are started early to prevent contractures, atelectasis, and pneumonia. Most patients require occupational and physical therapy (see p. 2748) to maximize functional recovery. Some need additional therapies (eg, speech therapy, feeding restrictions). Depression after stroke may require antidepressants; many patients benefit from counseling. For rehabilitation, an interdisciplinary approach is best. Life tyle modifications (eg, stopping cigarette smoking) are encouraged.

ISCHEMIC STROKE

Ischemic stroke is focal brain infarction that produces sudden neurologic deficits persisting > 1 h. Common causes are (in order of incidence) nonthrombotic occlusion of small, deep cortical arteries (lacunar infarction); embolism due to cardiac sources; arterial thrombosis with hemodynamic disturbance leading to decrease of cerebral blood flow; and artery-to-artery embolism. Diagnosis is clinical, but CT or MRI is done to confirm presence and extent of stroke. Thrombolytic therapy may be useful acutely in certain patients. Depending on the cause of stroke, carotid endarterectomy, antiplatelet drugs, or warfarin may help reduce risk of subsequent strokes.

Etiology

Ischemia usually results from thrombi or emboli. Atheromas, particularly if ulcerated, predispose to thrombi. Atheromas may affect any major cerebral artery and are common at areas of turbulent flow, particularly the carotid bifurcation and internal carotid branches. Intracranial thrombosis occurs most often at the main trunk of the middle cerebral artery and its branches but is also common in the large arteries at the base of the brain, in deep perforating arteries, and in small cortical branches. The basilar artery and the segment of the internal carotid artery between the cavernous sinus and supraclinoid process are often affected.

Less common causes of thromboses include vascular inflammation secondary to disorders such as acute or chronic meningitis, vasculitic disorders, and syphilis; dissection of intracranial arteries or the aorta; hypercoagulability disorders (eg, antiphospholipid syndrome, hyperhomocysteinemia); hyperviscosity disorders (eg, polycythemia, thrombocytosis, hemoglobinopathies, plasma cell disorders); and rare disorders (eg, moyamoya disease, Binswanger's disease) as well as use of sympathomimetic drugs (eg, cocaine, amphetamines). Older oral contraceptive formulations increased risk of thrombosis.

Emboli may lodge anywhere in the cerebral arterial tree. Embolic sources include cardiac thrombi, especially in atrial fibrillation, in rheumatic heart disease (usually mitral stenosis), after MI, from vegetations on heart valves in bacterial or marantic endocarditis, or from prosthetic heart valves; clots that form after open-heart surgery; and atheromas in neck arteries. Another source is atheromas in the aortic arch. Rarely, emboli consist of fat (from fractures of long bones), air (in decompression sickness), or venous clots that pass from the right to the left side of the heart through a patent foramen ovale with shunt (paradoxical emboli). Emboli may dislodge spontaneously or after invasive cardiovascular procedures (eg, catheterization).

Ischemic stroke can also result from lacunar infarcts. These small (≤ 1.5 cm) infarcts occur in patients with nonatherothrombotic obstruction of the small, perforating arteries that supply deep cortical structures (a process called lipohyalinosis). Whether emboli cause lacunar infarcts is controversial. Lacunar infarcts tend to occur in elderly patients with diabetes or poorly controlled hypertension.

Less commonly, ischemic stroke results from vasospasm (eg, during migraine, after subarachnoid hemorrhage) or venous infarction (eg, during intracranial infection, postoperatively, peripartum, or secondary to a hypercoagulation disorder).

Pathophysiology

Inadequate blood flow in a single brain artery can often be compensated for by an efficient collateral system, particularly between the carotid and vertebral arteries via anastomoses at the circle of Willis, and, to a lesser extent, between major arteries supplying the cerebral hemispheres. However, normal variations in the circle of Willis and in the caliber of various collateral vessels, atherosclerosis, and other acquired arterial lesions can interrupt collateral flow, increasing the chance that blockage of one artery will cause brain ischemia.

Injury becomes irreversible if blood flow is < 5% of normal for more than about 30 min or < 40% of normal for > 3 to 6 h. Injury occurs more rapidly during hyperthermia and more slowly during hypothermia. If tissues are ischemic but not yet irreversibly damaged, promptly restoring blood flow may reduce or reverse injury. Mechanisms of ischemic injury include edema, microvascular thrombosis, programmed cell death (apoptosis), and infarction with cell necrosis. Inflammatory mediators (eg, IL-1B, tumor necrosis factor-α) contribute to edema and microvascular thrombosis. Edema, if severe or extensive, can increase intracranial pressure. Many factors may contribute to necrotic cell death; they include loss of ATP stores, loss of ionic homeostasis (including intracellular Ca accumulation), lipid peroxidative damage to cell membranes by free radicals (an iron-mediated process), excitatory neurotoxins (eg, glutamate), and intracellular acidosis due to accumulation of lactate.

Symptoms and Signs

Symptoms and signs depend on the part of brain affected. Although patterns of neurologic deficits often suggest the affected artery (see TABLE 211–1), correlation is often inexact.

Deficits may become maximal within several minutes of onset, typically in embolic stroke. Less often, deficits evolve slowly, usually over 24 to 48 h (called evolving stroke or stroke in evolution), typically in thrombotic stroke. In most evolving strokes, unilateral neurologic dysfunction (often beginning in one arm, then spreading ipsilaterally) extends without producing headache, pain, or fever. Progression is usually stepwise, interrupted by periods of stability. A stroke is considered submaximal when there is residual function in the affected area (implying viable tissue at risk of damage).

Embolic strokes often occur during the day; headache may precede neurologic deficits. Thrombi tend to occur during the night and thus are first noticed on awakening. Lacunar infarcts may produce one of the classic lacunar syndromes (eg, pure motor hemiparesis, pure sensory hemianesthesia, ataxic-hemiparesis, dysarthria–clumsy hand); signs of cortical dysfunction (eg, aphasia) are absent. Multiple lacunar infarcts may result in multi-infarct dementia.

Deterioration during the 1st 48 to 72 h after onset of symptoms, particularly impaired consciousness, results more often from cerebral edema than from extension of the infarct. Unless the infarct is large or extensive, function commonly improves within the 1st few days; further improvement occurs gradually for up to 1 yr.

Diagnosis

Diagnosis is suggested by sudden neurologic deficits referable to a specific arterial territory. Ischemic stroke must be distinguished from other causes of similar focal deficits (eg, hypoglycemia, migraine, postictal [Todd's] paralysis, hemorrhagic stroke). Headache, coma or stupor, and vomiting are more likely with hemorrhage.

Although diagnosis is clinical, neuroimaging and bedside glucose testing are mandatory. CT is done first to exclude intracerebral hemorrhage, subdural or epidural hematoma, and a rapidly growing, bleeding, or suddenly symptomatic tumor. CT evidence of even large anterior circulation ischemic stroke during the 1st few hours may be subtle and may include effacement of sulci or the insular cortical ribbon, loss of the gray-white junction between cortex and white matter, and a dense middle cerebral artery sign. After 24 h of ischemia, infarcts are usually visible as hypodensities, except for small infarcts of the pons and medulla, which may be obscured by bone artifacts. Diffusion-weighted MRI (highly sensitive for early ischemia) and magnetic resonance angiography (to rule out arterial stenosis) can be done immediately after CT.

Clinical distinction between lacunar, embolic, and thrombotic stroke is not reliable, so tests to identify common or treatable causes and risk factors are routinely performed. These typically include carotid duplex ultrasonography, ECG, transesophageal echocardiography, and various blood tests (CBC, platelet count, PT/PTT, fasting blood glucose, lipid profile, homocysteine, ESR, and, for at-risk patients, syphilis serology). Many clinicians also obtain magnetic resonance or CT angiography. Other tests are done based on clinically suspected disorders, such as antiphospholipid antibodies.

Prognosis

Stroke severity and progression are often assessed using standardized measures such as the National Institutes of Health Stroke Scale (see TABLE 211–2); the score on this scale correlates with extent of functional impairment and prognosis. During the 1st days, progression and outcome can be difficult to predict. Older age, impaired consciousness, aphasia, and brain stem signs suggest a poor prognosis. Early improvement and younger age suggest a favorable prognosis.

About 50% of patients with moderate or severe hemiplegia and most with milder deficits can take care of their basic needs, have a clear sensorium, and eventually can walk

TABLE 211–2. THE NATIONAL INSTITUTES OF HEALTH STROKE SCALE*

CRITERION	FINDING	SCORE
Level of consciousness (LOC)	Alert	0
	Drowsy	1
	Stuporous	2
	Comatose	3
LOC questions†	Answers both correctly	0
	Answers one correctly	1
	Answers both incorrectly	2
LOC commands‡	Obeys both correctly	0
	Obeys one correctly	1
	Obeys both incorrectly	2
Gaze	Normal	0
	Partial gaze palsy	1
	Forced deviation	2
Visual field	No visual loss	0
	Partial hemianopia	1
	Complete hemianopia	2
	Bilateral hemianopia	3
Facial palsy	None	0
	Minor	1
	Partial	2
	Complete	3
Motor arm function (score for both left and right sides)	No drift	0
	Drift	1
	No resistance to gravity	2
Motor arm function (*continued*)	No effort against gravity	3
	No Movement	4
Motor leg function (score for both left and right sides)	No drift	0
	Drift	1
	No resistance to gravity	2
	No effort against gravity	3
	No movement	4
Limb ataxia	Absent	0
	Present in one limb	1
	Present in two limbs	2
	Untestable	—
Sensory	Normal	0
	Mild to moderate loss	1
	Severe loss	2
Best language function	No aphasia	0
	Mild to moderate dysarthria	1
	Severe aphasia	2
	Mute	3
Dysarthria	Normal articulation	0
	Mild to moderate dysarthria	1
	Severe dysarthria (unintelligible or worse)	2
	Untestable	—
Neglect	No neglect	0
	Partial neglect	1
	Complete neglect	2

*Total score is the sum of the scores for individual items.
† Patients are asked their age and the current month.
‡ Patients are asked to open and close the eyes and to make a fist.

adequately. Complete neurologic recovery occurs in about 10%. Use of the affected limb may be limited, and most deficits that remain after 12 mo are permanent. Subsequent strokes often occur, and each tends to worsen neurologic function. About 20% of patients die in the hospital; mortality rate increases with age.

Treatment

Acute: Patients with acute ischemic strokes are hospitalized unless they have expressed prior wishes otherwise. Supportive measures (see p. 1791) may be needed during initial evaluation and stabilization. Perfusion of an ischemic brain area may require a high BP because autoregulation is lost; thus, BP should not be decreased unless it exceeds 220 mm Hg systolic or 120 mm Hg diastolic on 2 successive readings > 15 min apart, there are signs of other end-organ damage (eg, aortic dissection, acute MI, pulmonary edema, hypertensive encephalopathy, retinal hemorrhages, acute renal failure), or use of recombinant tissue plasminogen activator (tPA) is likely. For hypertension, nicardipine 5 mg/h IV is given initially; dose is increased by 2.5 mg/h q 5 min to a maximum of 15 mg/h as needed to decrease systolic BP by 10% to 15%. Alternatively, IV labetalol can be used.

Antithrombotic therapy may include tPA, thrombolysis-in-situ, antiplatelet drugs, and anticoagulants. Most patients are not candidates for thrombolytic therapy; they should be given antiplatelet therapy with aspirin (81 to 325 mg po once/day) within 24 to 48 h. Contraindications to antiplatelet drugs include aspirin- or NSAID-induced asthma or urticaria, other hypersensitivity to aspirin or to tartrazine, acute GI bleeding, G6PD deficiency, and use of warfarin.

Recombinant tPA is used for patients with acute ischemic stroke of < 3 h duration and who do not have contraindications to tPA. Although tPA can cause fatal or other symptomatic brain hemorrhage, patients treated with tPA strictly following protocol have a higher likelihood of functional neurologic recovery. Only physicians experienced in stroke management should use tPA to treat patients with acute stroke; inexperienced physicians are more likely to violate protocols, resulting in more brain hemorrhages and deaths. tPA must be given within 3 h of symptom onset—a difficult requirement. The precise time of symptom onset may not be known; also, brain hemorrhage must be excluded by CT before treatment with tPA. Factors that exclude use of tPA must be ruled out (see TABLE 211–3). Dose is 0.9 mg/kg IV (maximum dose 90 mg); 10% is given by rapid IV injection, and the remainder by constant infusion over 60 min. Vital signs are closely monitored for 24 h after treatment (systolic BP < 185 mm Hg or diastolic BP < 110 mm Hg), and any bleeding complications are aggressively managed. Anticoagulants and antiplatelet drugs are not used within 24 h of treatment with tPA.

Thrombolysis-in-situ (angiographically directed intra-arterial thrombolysis) of a thrombus or embolus can sometimes be used for major strokes if symptoms have begun > 3 h but < 6 h ago, particularly for strokes due to large occlusions in the middle cerebral artery. This treatment, although standard of care in some large stroke centers, is often unavailable in other hospitals.

Anticoagulation with heparin or low mol wt heparin is used for stroke caused by cerebral venous thrombosis, emboli due to atrial fibrillation, and when stroke due to presumed progressive thrombosis continues to evolve despite use of antiplatelet drugs and cannot be treated any other way (eg, with tPA or invasive methods). Warfarin is begun simultaneously. Before anticoagulation is given, hemorrhage must be excluded by CT. Constant heparin infusion is used to increase PTT to 1.5 to 2 times baseline values until warfarin has increased

TABLE 211–3. EXCLUSION CRITERIA FOR USE OF TISSUE PLASMINOGEN ACTIVATOR IN STROKE*

Intracranial hemorrhage on CT scan

Multilobar infarct (hypodensity > ⅓ of the territory supplied by the middle cerebral artery) on CT scan

Rapidly decreasing symptoms

Presentation suggesting subarachnoid hemorrhage even if CT is negative

History of intracranial hemorrhage, AVM, aneurysm, or brain tumor

History of stroke or head trauma within the past 3 mo

Systolic BP > 185 mm Hg or diastolic BP > 110 mm Hg after antihypertensive treatment

Arterial puncture at noncompressible site or lumbar puncture in the past 7 days

Major surgery or serious trauma in the past 14 days

GI or urinary tract hemorrhage in the past 21 days

Platelet count < 100,000/μL

Use of heparin within 48 h and PTT > 40 sec

Current use of oral anticoagulants, INR > 1.7, or PT > 15

Seizure at onset of stroke

Blood glucose < 50 or > 400 mg/dL (< 2.78 or > 22.2 mmol/L)

Bacterial endocarditis or suspected pericarditis

Known or suspected pregnancy

*Initiation of treatment is required within 3 h of symptom onset. CT and, for women of childbearing age, a pregnancy test are required.

AVM = arteriovenous malformation.

the INR to 2 to 3 (3 in hypercoagulable disorders). Warfarin predisposes to bleeding, so its use should be restricted to patients likely to be compliant with dosage and monitoring requirements and not prone to falls.

Long term: Supportive care is continued during convalescence. Controlling general medical risk factors (especially hyperglycemia and fever) can limit brain damage after stroke, leading to better functional outcomes.

Carotid endarterectomy is indicated for patients with recent nondisabling stroke attributed to an ipsilateral carotid obstruction of 70% to 99% of the arterial lumen or by an ulcerated plaque. In symptomatic patients, endarterectomy, with or without antiplatelet therapy, is indicated for carotid obstruction of ≥ 60% with or without ulceration and life expectancy of at least 5 yr. The procedure should be done by surgeons who have a morbidity and mortality rate of < 3% with the procedure in the hospital where it will be done.

Oral antiplatelet drugs are used to prevent subsequent strokes (secondary prevention). Aspirin 81 to 325 mg once/day, clopidogrel 75 mg once/day, or the combination product aspirin 25 mg/extended-release dipyridamole 200 mg bid may be used. In patients taking warfarin, antiplatelet drugs additively increase risk of bleeding and are thus usually avoided; however, aspirin is occasionally used simultaneously with warfarin in certain high-risk patients.

Transient Ischemic Attack

A transient ischemic attack (TIA) is focal brain ischemia producing sudden neurologic deficits that last < 1 h. Diagnosis is clinical. Carotid endarterectomy, antiplatelet drugs, and warfarin decrease risk of stroke after certain types of TIA.

TIA is similar to ischemic stroke except that symptoms last < 1 h; most TIAs last < 5 min. Although the definition is clinical and currently being revised, infarction is very unlikely if deficits resolve within 1 h. TIAs are most common among the middle-aged and elderly. TIAs markedly increase risk of stroke, beginning in the 1st 24 h.

Etiology

Most TIAs are caused by emboli, usually from carotid or vertebral arteries, although most of the causes of ischemic stroke (see p. 1792) can also result in TIAs. Uncommonly, TIAs result from impaired perfusion due to severe hypoxemia, reduced O_2-carrying capacity of blood (eg, profound anemia, carbon monoxide poisoning), or increased blood viscosity (eg, severe polycythemia), particularly in brain arteries with preexisting stenosis. Ischemia does not result from systemic hypotension unless it is severe or arterial stenosis preexists because brain blood flow is maintained at near-normal levels over a wide range of systemic BPs (autoregulation).

In subclavian steal syndrome, a subclavian artery stenosed proximal to the origin of the vertebral artery "steals" blood from the vertebral artery (in which blood flow reverses) to supply the arm during exertion, causing signs of vertebrobasilar ischemia.

Occasionally, TIAs occur in children with a severe cardiovascular disorder that produces emboli or a very high Hct.

Symptoms and Signs

Neurologic deficits are similar to those of strokes (see TABLE 211–1). Transient monocular blindness (amaurosis fugax), which usually lasts < 5 min, may occur when the ophthalmic artery is affected. Symptoms begin suddenly, usually last 2 to 30 min, then resolve completely. Patients may have several TIAs daily or only 2 or 3 over several years. Symptoms are usually similar in successive carotid attacks but vary somewhat in successive vertebrobasilar attacks.

Diagnosis and Treatment

Diagnosis is made in retrospect when sudden neurologic deficits referable to ischemia in an arterial territory resolve within 1 h. Isolated peripheral facial nerve palsy, loss of consciousness, or impaired consciousness does not suggest TIA. TIAs must be distinguished from other causes of similar symptoms (eg, hypoglycemia, migraine aura, postictal [Todd's] paralysis). Because infarct, a small hemorrhage, and even a mass lesion cannot be excluded clinically, neuroimaging is required. CT is best for excluding hemorrhage. MRI usually detects evolving infarction within hours; CT may not identify infarcts for >24 h. Diffusion-weighted MRI is the most accurate imaging test to rule out an infarct in patients with presumed TIA but is not always available.

The cause of a TIA is sought as for that of ischemic strokes, including tests for carotid stenosis, cardiac sources of emboli, atrial fibrillation, and hematologic abnormalities and screening for stroke risk factors. Because risk of subsequent ischemic stroke is high and immediate, evaluation proceeds rapidly, usually as an inpatient.

Treatment is aimed at preventing strokes; antiplatelet drugs are used (see p. 1795). Carotid endarterectomy or arterial angioplasty and stenting can be useful for selected patients, particularly those who have no neurologic deficits but who are at high risk of stroke. Warfarin is indicated if cardiac sources of emboli are present. Control of modifiable stroke risk factors may prevent stroke.

INTRACEREBRAL HEMORRHAGE

Intracerebral hemorrhage is focal bleeding from blood vessels within the brain parenchyma. The cause is usually hypertension. Typical symptoms include focal neurologic deficits, often with abrupt onset of headache, nausea, and impairment of consciousness. Diagnosis is by CT. Treatment includes BP control, supportive measures, and, in some cases, surgical evacuation.

Intracerebral hemorrhage includes hemorrhage within basal ganglia, brain stem, midbrain, or cerebellum as well as the cerebral hemispheres. Most intracerebral hemorrhages occur in the basal ganglia, cerebral lobes, cerebellum, or pons.

Intracerebral hemorrhage usually results from rupture of an arteriosclerotic small artery that has been weakened, primarily by chronic arterial hypertension. Hypertensive intracerebral hemorrhage is usually large, single, and catastrophic. Use of cocaine or, occasionally, other sympathomimetic drugs can cause transient severe hypertension and hemorrhage. Less often, the cause is congenital aneurysm, arteriovenous or other vascular malformation (see sidebar 211–1), trauma, mycotic aneurysm, brain infarct, primary or metastatic brain tumor, excessive anticoagulation, blood dyscrasia, or a bleeding or vasculitic disorder.

Lobar intracerebral hemorrhages (hematomas in the cerebral lobes, outside the basal ganglia) usually result from angiopathy due to amyloid deposition in cerebral arteries (cerebral amyloid angiopathy), which affects primarily the elderly.

Blood from an intracerebral hemorrhage accumulates as a mass that can dissect through and compress adjacent brain tissues, causing neuronal dysfunction. Large hematomas increase intracranial pressure. Pressure from supratentorial hematomas and the accompanying edema may cause transtentorial brain herniation, compressing the brain stem and often causing secondary hemorrhages in the midbrain and pons (see Fig. 212–1). If the hemorrhage ruptures into the ventricular system (intraventricular hemorrhage), blood may cause acute hydrocephalus. Cerebellar hematomas can expand to block the ventricular system, causing acute hydrocephalus, or they can dissect into the brain stem. Brain herniation, midbrain or pontine hemorrhage, intraventricular hemorrhage, acute hydrocephalus, or dissection into the brain stem can impair consciousness and cause coma and death.

Symptoms and Signs

Symptoms typically begin with sudden headache, often during activity. Loss of consciousness is common, often within a few minutes. Nausea, vomiting, delirium, and focal or generalized seizures are also common. Neurologic deficits are usually sudden and progressive. Large hemorrhages, when located in the hemispheres, produce hemiparesis; when located in the posterior fossa, they produce cerebellar or brain stem deficits (eg, conjugate eye deviation or ophthalmoplegia, stertorous breathing, pinpoint pupils, coma). Large hemorrhages are fatal within a few days in about ½ of patients. In survivors, consciousness returns and neurologic deficits gradually diminish to various degrees as the extravasated blood is resorbed.

Small hemorrhages may cause focal deficits without impairment of consciousness and with minimal or no headache and nausea. Small hemorrhages may mimic ischemic stroke.

Diagnosis and Treatment

Diagnosis is suggested by sudden onset of headache, focal neurologic deficits, and impaired consciousness, particularly in patients with risk factors. Intracerebral hemorrhage must be distinguished from ischemic stroke, subarachnoid hemorrhage, and other causes of acute neurologic deficits (eg, seizure, hypoglycemia).

Immediate CT and bedside blood glucose measurement are necessary. If CT shows no hemorrhage and subarachnoid hemorrhage is clinically suspected, lumbar puncture is necessary.

Treatment includes supportive measures and control of general medical risk factors.

Sidebar 211-1. VASCULAR LESIONS IN THE BRAIN

Common brain vascular lesions include arteriovenous malformations and aneurysms.

Arteriovenous malformations (AVMs): AVMs are tangled, dilated blood vessels in which arteries flow directly into veins. AVMs occur most often at the junction of cerebral arteries, usually within the parenchyma of the frontal-parietal region, frontal lobe, lateral cerebellum, or overlying occipital lobe. They can bleed or directly compress brain tissue; seizures or ischemia may result. Neuroimaging may detect them incidentally; contrast or noncontrast CT can usually detect AVMs > 1 cm. Occasionally, a cranial bruit suggests an AVM. Arteriography is required for definitive diagnosis and determination of whether the lesion is operable. Superficial AVMs are usually obliterated by a combination of microsurgery, radiosurgery, and endovascular surgery. AVMs that are deep or < 3 cm in diameter are treated with stereotactic radiosurgery, endovascular therapy (eg, preresection embolization or thrombosis via an intra-arterial catheter), or coagulation with focused proton beams.

Aneurysms: Aneurysms are focal dilations within arteries. They occur in about 5% of people. Common contributing factors may include arteriosclerosis, hypertension, and hereditary connective tissue disorders (eg, Ehlers-Danlos syndrome, pseudoxanthoma elasticum, autosomal dominant polycystic kidney syndrome). Occasionally, septic emboli cause mycotic aneurysms. Brain aneurysms are most often < 2.5 cm in diameter and saccular (noncircumferential), sometimes with small, thin-walled, often multiple outpouchings (berry aneurysm). Most aneurysms occur along the middle or anterior cerebral arteries or the communicating branches of the circle of Willis, particularly at arterial bifurcations. Mycotic aneurysms usually develop distal to the 1st bifurcation of the arterial branches of the circle of Willis.

Many aneurysms are asymptomatic, but a few produce symptoms by compressing adjacent structures. Ocular palsies, diplopia, squint, and orbital pain may indicate pressure on the 3rd, 4th, 5th, or 6th cranial nerves. Visual loss and a bitemporal field defect may indicate pressure on the optic chiasm. Aneurysms may bleed into the subarachnoid space, producing subarachnoid hemorrhage. Aneurysms may not cause headache before rupture, but some experts believe that preceding warning leaks may produce headaches. Neuroimaging may detect aneurysms incidentally.

Diagnosis requires arteriography or magnetic resonance angiography. If < 7 mm, asymptomatic aneurysms in the anterior circulation rarely rupture and do not warrant the risks of treatment. If aneurysms are larger, are in the posterior circulation, or produce symptoms due to bleeding or to compression of neural structures, endovascular therapy, if feasible, is required.

Anticoagulants and antiplatelet drugs are contraindicated. If patients have used anticoagulants, the effects are reversed when possible by giving fresh frozen plasma, vitamin K, or platelet transfusions as indicated. Hypertension should be treated only if mean arterial pressure is > 130 mm Hg or systolic BP is > 185 mm Hg. Nicardipine 5 mg/h IV is given initially; dose is increased by 2.5 mg/h q 5 min to a maximum of 15 mg/h as needed to decrease systolic BP by 10% to 15%. For patients with cerebellar hemisphere hematomas that are > 3 cm in diameter and cause the brain to shift, surgical evacuation is often lifesaving. Early evacuation of large lobar cerebral hematomas may also be lifesaving, but rebleeding occurs frequently, sometimes increasing neurologic deficits. Early evacuation of deep cerebral hematomas is seldom indicated because surgical mortality is high and neurologic deficits are usually severe. Some patients have surprisingly few neurologic deficits because hemorrhage is less destructive to brain tissue than infarction.

SUBARACHNOID HEMORRHAGE

Subarachnoid hemorrhage is sudden bleeding into the subarachnoid space. The most common cause of spontaneous bleeding is a ruptured aneurysm. Symptoms include sudden, severe headache, usually with loss

or impairment of consciousness. Secondary vasospasm (causing focal brain ischemia), meningismus, and hydrocephalus (causing persistent headache and obtundation) are common. Diagnosis is by CT or, if CT is normal, CSF analysis. Patients are treated in a referral center with supportive measures and neurosurgery.

Subarachnoid hemorrhage is due to bleeding between the arachnoid and pia mater from a ruptured aneurysm. In general, head trauma is the most common cause, but traumatic subarachnoid hemorrhage is usually considered a separate disorder (see p. 2572). Spontaneous (primary) subarachnoid hemorrhage results from ruptured aneurysms, most often a congenital intracranial saccular or berry aneurysm, in about 85% of patients. Bleeding may stop spontaneously. Aneurysmal hemorrhage may occur at any age but is most common from age 40 to 65. Less common causes are mycotic aneurysms, arteriovenous malformations, and bleeding disorders.

Blood in the subarachnoid space produces a chemical meningitis that commonly increases intracranial pressure for days or a few weeks. Secondary vasospasm may produce focal brain ischemia; about 25% develop signs of a TIA or ischemic stroke. Brain edema is maximal and risk of vasospasm and subsequent infarction (called angry brain) is highest between 72 h and 10 days. Secondary acute hydrocephalus is also common. A 2nd rupture (rebleeding) sometimes occurs, most often within about 7 days.

Symptoms and Signs

Headache is usually severe, peaking within seconds. Loss of consciousness may follow, usually immediately but sometimes not for several hours. Severe neurologic deficits may develop and become irreversible within minutes or a few hours. Sensorium may be impaired, and patients may become restless. Seizures are possible. Initially, the neck is usually not stiff unless the cerebellar tonsils herniate. However, within 24 h, chemical meningitis produces moderate to marked meningismus, vomiting, and sometimes bilateral extensor plantar responses. Heart or respiratory rate is often abnormal. Fever, continued headaches, and confusion are common during the 1st 5 to 10 days. Secondary hydrocephalus may produce headache, obtundation, and motor deficits that persist for weeks. Rebleeding may cause recurrent or new symptoms.

Diagnosis

Diagnosis is suggested by characteristic symptoms. Testing should proceed as rapidly as possible, before damage becomes irreversible. Noncontrast CT is > 90% sensitive. False-negative results occur if volume of blood is small. If subarachnoid hemorrhage is suspected clinically but not identified on CT or if CT is not immediately available, lumbar puncture is done. Lumbar puncture is contraindicated if increased intracranial pressure is suspected because the sudden decrease in CSF pressure may lessen the tamponade of a clot on the ruptured aneurysm, causing further bleeding.

CSF findings suggesting subarachnoid hemorrhage include numerous RBCs, xanthochromia, and increased pressure. RBCs in CSF may also be caused by traumatic lumbar puncture. Traumatic lumbar puncture is suspected if the RBC count decreases in tubes of CSF drawn sequentially during the same lumbar puncture (see p. 1755). Also, about 6 h or more after a subarachnoid hemorrhage, RBCs become crenated and lyse, resulting in a xanthochromic CSF supernatant and visible crenated RBCs on microscopic CSF examination; these findings indicate that subarachnoid hemorrhage preceded the lumbar puncture. If there is still doubt, hemorrhage should be assumed, or the lumbar puncture should be repeated in 8 to 12 h. In patients with subarachnoid hemorrhage, cerebral arteriography is done as soon as possible after the initial bleeding episode. All 4 cerebral vessels should be evaluated, because multiple aneurysms may be present.

On ECG, subarachnoid hemorrhage may produce ST-segment elevation or depression. It can produce syncope, mimicking MI. Other possible ECG abnormalities include prolongation of the QRS or QT intervals and peaking or deep, symmetric inversion of T waves.

Prognosis and Treatment

About 35% of patients die after the 1st aneurysmal subarachnoid hemorrhage; another 15% die within a few weeks because of a subsequent rupture. After 6 mo, a 2nd rupture occurs at a rate of about 3%/yr. In general, prognosis is grave with an aneurysm, better with an arteriovenous malformation, and best when 4-vessel arteriography does not detect a lesion, presumably because the bleeding source is small and has sealed itself. Among survivors, neurologic damage is common, even when treatment is optimal.

Patients with subarachnoid hemorrhage should be treated in referral centers whenever possible. Hypertension should be treated only if mean arterial pressure is > 130 mm Hg; euvolemia is maintained, and IV nicardipine is titrated as for ischemic stroke (see p. 1795). Bed rest is mandatory. Restlessness and headache are treated symptomatically. Stool softeners are given to prevent constipation, which can lead to straining. *Anticoagulants and antiplatelet drugs are contraindicated.*

Nimodipine 60 mg po q 4 h is given for 21 days to prevent vasospasm, but BP needs to be maintained in the desirable range. Clinical signs of acute hydrocephalus should prompt consideration of ventricular drainage.

Obliteration of the aneurysm reduces risk of rebleeding. If the aneurysm is accessible, surgery to clip the aneurysm or bypass its blood flow can be done, especially for patients with an evacuable hematoma or acute hydrocephalus. If patients are arousable, most vascular neurosurgeons operate within the 1st 24 h to minimize risk of rebleeding and risks due to angry brain. If > 24 h have elapsed, some neurosurgeons delay surgery until 10 days have passed, decreasing risks due to angry brain but increasing risk of rebleeding and overall mortality. Alternatively, detachable coils can be inserted during angiography to occlude the aneurysm, especially when it is in the anterior cerebral artery complex or in the posterior circulation.

212 STUPOR AND COMA

Stupor and coma are disturbances in consciousness resulting from dysfunction of both cerebral hemispheres or the reticular activating system. Stupor is unresponsiveness from which the patient can be aroused only briefly by vigorous, repeated stimulation. Coma is unresponsiveness from which the patient generally cannot be aroused. Causes may be structural or global (often metabolic). Diagnosis is clinical; identification of cause usually requires laboratory tests and CNS imaging. Treatment is immediate stabilization and specific management of the cause. For long-term stupor or coma, adjunctive treatment includes passive range-of-motion exercises, enteral feedings, and prevention of pressure ulcers. Prognosis varies by cause.

The alert state requires intact function of the cerebral hemispheres and preservation of arousal mechanisms in the reticular activating system (RAS)—an extensive network of nuclei and interconnecting fibers in the upper pons, midbrain, and posterior diencephalon.

Etiology and Pathophysiology

Various structural and global CNS disorders cause stupor or coma (see TABLE 212–1). A decrease in consciousness results from dysfunction of the RAS or both cerebral hemispheres; unilateral cerebral hemisphere disorders may produce severe neurologic deficits but not coma. With increasing injury, stupor progresses to coma, and coma to brain death. Other forms of altered consciousness include delirium (marked by agitation rather than lethargy), syncope, and seizures; in the last two, consciousness is briefly lost.

Structural disorders may cause stupor or coma through direct, mechanical disruption of the RAS or through the indirect influence of mass effect and edema. A unilateral massive hemispheric focal lesion (eg, left middle cerebral artery stroke) rarely disturbs consciousness unless the contralateral hemisphere is already compromised or becomes edematous. Infarcts of the upper brain stem cause various degrees of stupor or coma, depending on their extent.

Global or systemic disorders that can cause stupor or coma often involve cerebral anoxia or ischemia. Psychiatric disorders (eg, psychogenic unresponsiveness) can mimic disturbed consciousness but are usually distinguished from true stupor or coma by a normal physical and neurologic examination.

Herniation syndromes: Because the skull is rigid (after infancy), intracranial masses or edema may increase intracranial pressure, which can cause brain tissue to herniate through a rigid intracranial barrier.

In transtentorial (uncal) herniation, the temporal lobe shifts across the edge of the tentorium cerebelli (a tentlike structure on which the temporal lobe normally rests). The uncus—the medial edge of the herniating lobe—crushes the diencephalon and upper brain stem, causing compression ischemia and infarction of the tissues containing the RAS (see FIG. 212–1). Herniation of both temporal lobes (central herniation), usually because of bilateral masses or diffuse edema, causes bilateral compression of the midbrain and brain stem.

Tonsillar herniation results from infratentorial masses (usually) or supratentorial masses. The cerebellar tonsils, forced through the foramen magnum, compress the brain stem and obstruct CSF flow, causing acute hydrocephalus. Transtentorial and tonsillar herniation are life threatening.

In subfalcine herniation, the cingulate gyrus herniates under the falx cerebri.

Symptoms, Signs, and Diagnosis

Repeated noxious stimuli do not arouse comatose patients; stuporous patients are aroused only briefly. In comatose patients, stimulation may trigger primitive reflex movements (eg, decerebrate or decorticate posturing).

Diagnosis and initial stabilization should occur simultaneously. Airway, breathing, and circulation must first be ensured; patients with infrequent, shallow, or strenuous respirations or low O_2 saturation (by pulse oximetry or arterial blood gas measurements) require intubation. Hypotension must be corrected (see p. 564). Finger-stick glucose testing is required. Patients with low glucose levels should be given thiamin 100 mg IM (to prevent Wernicke's encephalopathy in susceptible patients) and 50 mL of 50% dextrose. If opioid overdose is suspected, naloxone 2 mg IV is given. If trauma is involved, the neck is stabilized with a hard collar until an x-ray can be taken to check for fractures.

History: Medical identification bracelets or the contents of a wallet or purse may provide clues (eg, hospital identification card, drugs). Relatives, paramedics, and police officers should be questioned about onset of the disturbance (eg, whether seizure, headache, vomiting, head trauma, or drug was involved). They should describe the environment in which the patient was found; containers that may have held food, alcohol, drugs, or poisons should be examined and saved for chemical analysis and possible legal evidence. Relatives should be asked about recent infections, psychiatric problems, and previous illnesses. Medical records should be reviewed if available.

TABLE 212–1. COMMON CAUSES OF STUPOR AND COMA

CAUSE	EXAMPLES
Structural disorders	Aneurysm rupture and subarachnoid hemorrhage Brain abscess Brain tumor Cranial trauma (concussion, cerebral lacerations or contusions, epidural or subdural hematoma) Hydrocephalus (acute) Upper brain stem infarct or hemorrhage
Global disorders	CNS vasculitis Drugs and toxins (eg, barbiturates, carbon monoxide, ethyl alcohol, methyl alcohol, opioids) Hypothermia Infections (meningitis, encephalitis, sepsis) Metabolic disorders (eg, diabetic ketoacidosis, hepatic coma, hypoglycemia, hyponatremia, hypoxia, uremia)

Physical examination: Physical examination should be focused and efficient. Signs of head trauma include periorbital ecchymosis (raccoon eyes), ecchymosis behind the ear (Battle's sign), hemotympanum, instability of the maxilla, and CSF rhinorrhea and otorrhea. Scalp contusions and small bullet holes can be missed unless the head is carefully inspected. The fundi should be examined for papilledema, hemorrhages, and exudates. Passive neck flexion, possible in the absence of trauma, may detect stiffness, suggesting subarachnoid hemorrhage or meningitis. The cervical spine or neck should be immobilized until clinical history, physical examination, or imaging tests exclude fracture.

Fever or petechial rash suggests CNS infection. Needle marks may suggest drug overdose (eg, of opioids or insulin). A bitten tongue suggests seizure. Breath odor may indicate alcohol intoxication.

Neurologic examination: The neurologic examination determines whether the brain stem is intact and where the lesion is located within the CNS. State of consciousness, pupils, eye movements, respirations, and motor functions help determine the level of CNS dysfunction.

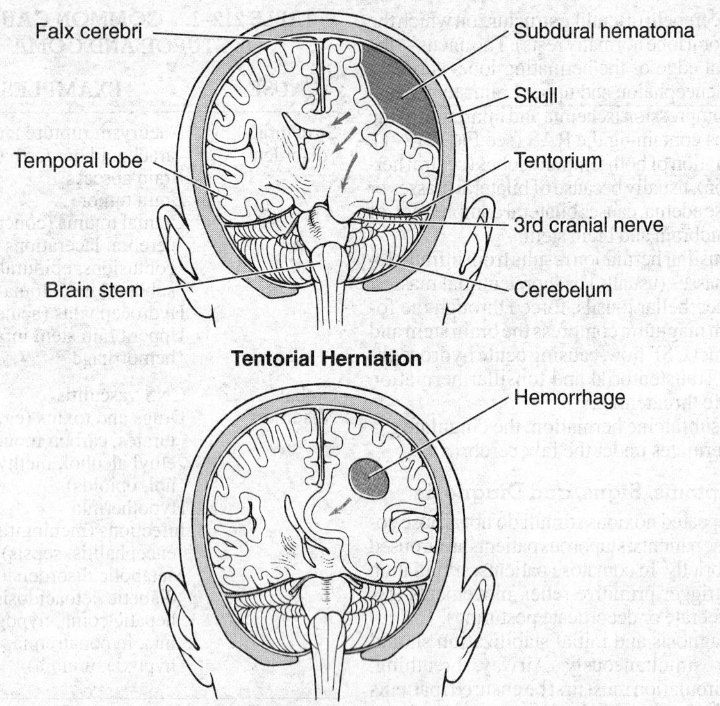

Fig. 212–1. Tentorial and subfalcine herniation. Because the skull is rigid after infancy, intracranial masses or swelling may increase intracranial pressure, which can cause protrusion (herniation) of brain tissue through a rigid intracranial barrier: falx cerebri (subfalcine herniation of the cingulate gyrus), tentorial notch (tentorial herniation), or foramen magnum (tonsillar herniation). Transtentorial and tonsillar herniation are life threatening.

In tentorial herniation, one medial temporal lobe may herniate, usually because of a unilateral mass, and cause unilateral damage. The 1st structure compressed may be the ipsilateral 3rd cranial nerve, causing a unilateral dilated fixed pupil and oculomotor paresis; the posterior cerebral artery, causing a homonymous hemianopia; or the opposite cerebral peduncle, causing ipsilateral hemiparesis. Then, the midbrain and brain stem can be compressed, causing impaired consciousness, abnormal breathing patterns, pupils fixed in midposition, loss of oculocephalic and oculovestibular reflexes (the eyes do not move in response to head rotation or to caloric stimulation, respectively), bilateral motor paresis with decerebrate rigidity or flaccidity, and Cushing's reflex (hypertension, particularly systolic, and bradycardia). Herniation of both temporal lobes (central herniation), usually because of bilateral masses, causes bilateral, symmetric damage, compressing the midbrain and brain stem and producing many of the same symptoms as tentorial herniation.

Tonsillar herniation results from infratentorial masses (usually) or supratentorial masses. The cerebellar tonsils, forced through the foramen magnum, compress the brain stem and obstruct CSF flow, causing acute hydrocephalus. Symptoms include obtundation, headache, vomiting, meningismus, dysconjugate eye movements, and abrupt respiratory and cardiac arrest.

Arousal is evaluated by attempting to wake patients first with verbal commands, then with nonnoxious stimuli, and finally with noxious stimuli (eg, pressure to the supraorbital ridge, nail bed, or sternum). The Glasgow Coma Scale (see TABLE 212–2) assigns points based on the responses to stimuli. Eye opening, facial grimacing, and purposeful withdrawal of limbs from the noxious stimulus indicates that the depth of unconsciousness is relatively light. Asymmetric motor responses to pain may indicate a focal hemispheric lesion.

As stupor deepens into coma, noxious stimuli may trigger stereotypic reflex posturing. Decorticate posturing (arm flexion and adduction with leg extension) indicates hemispheric damage to the corticospinal tract with preservation of the brain stem. Decerebrate rigidity (neck, back, and limb extension with clenched jaws) suggests upper brain stem damage and represents a deterioration in motor response. Flaccidity without movement suggests severe injury throughout the neuraxis and represents the worst possible motor response. Asterixis and multifocal myoclonus accompany metabolic disorders such as uremia, hepatic failure, anoxia, and drug toxicity. In psychogenic unresponsiveness, motor response is typically absent, but muscle tone and reflexes remain normal.

In transtentorial herniation, the herniating temporal lobe may first compress the ipsilateral 3rd cranial nerve, causing a unilateral dilated fixed pupil and oculomotor paresis; the posterior cerebral artery, causing homonymous hemianopia; or the opposite cerebral peduncle, causing ipsilateral hemiparesis. Then, the midbrain and brain stem can be compressed, causing impaired consciousness, abnormal breathing patterns, pupils fixed in midposition, loss of oculocephalic and oculovestibular reflexes, bilateral motor paresis with decerebrate rigidity or flaccidity, and Cushing's reflex (hypertension, particularly systolic, and bradycardia); these midbrain findings also occur with central herniation.

In tonsillar herniation, symptoms include obtundation, headache, vomiting, meningismus, dysconjugate eye movements, and abrupt respiratory and cardiac arrest.

Ophthalmic examination: This examination provides information about brain stem function (see TABLE 212–3). It includes pupillary responses, extraocular movements, funduscopic examination (for papilledema or hemorrhage), and assessment of other neuro-ophthalmic reflexes. Pupils usually become fixed early if a structural lesion is present, but the pupil response is preserved until very late in metabolic coma.

When eye movements are absent, the oculocephalic reflex is tested by the doll's-eye maneuver: The eyes are observed while passively rotating the patient's head from side to side. This maneuver should not be attempted after trauma unless cervical spine fracture is excluded. If consciousness is normal and visual fixation is possible, the eyes follow head movement. If consciousness is depressed and

TABLE 212–2. GLASGOW COMA SCALE*

AREA ASSESSED	RESPONSE	POINTS
Eye opening	Open spontaneously; open with blinking at baseline	4
	Open to verbal command, speech, or shout	3
	Open in response to pain applied to the limbs or sternum	2
	None	1
Verbal	Oriented	5
	Confused conversation, but able to answer questions	4
	Inappropriate responses; words discernible	3
	Incomprehensible speech	2
	None	1
Motor	Obeys commands for movement	6
	Responds to pain with purposeful movement	5
	Withdraws from pain stimuli	4
	Responds to pain with abnormal (spastic) flexion (decorticate posture)	3
	Responds to pain with abnormal (rigid) extension (decerebrate posture)	2
	None	1

*Combined scores < 8 are typically regarded as coma.

Adapted from Teasdale G, Jennett B: "Assessment of coma and impaired consciousness. A practical scale." *Lancet* 2:81–84; 1974.

TABLE 212–3. INTERPRETATION OF PUPILLARY RESPONSE AND EYE MOVEMENTS

AREA ASSESSED	FINDING	INTERPRETATION
Pupils	Sluggish light reactivity retained until all other brain stem reflexes are lost	Metabolic disorders
	Unilateral pupillary dilation, pupil unreactive to light	3rd cranial nerve compression (eg, in transtentorial herniation)
	Pupils fixed in midposition	Midbrain failure or dysfunction due to structural damage (infarction or hemorrhage) or metabolic depression by drugs or toxins
	Pupils tiny (1 mm wide)	Massive pontine hemorrhage or opioid coma
Eye movements	Abnormal pupillary and oculomotor signs from the start	Primary brain stem lesion
	Spontaneous, conjugate roving eye movements (associated with an intact brain stem)	Early metabolic coma
	Gaze preference to one side	Brain stem lesion on the opposite side or cerebral hemisphere lesion on the same side
	Absent eye movements	Further testing required

brain stem is intact, gaze appears fixed on the ceiling as the head rotates. If brain stem function is destroyed, the eyes move with head movement as if they are fixed in their sockets.

If the oculocephalic reflex is absent, oculovestibular (cold caloric) testing is done. After integrity of the tympanic membrane is confirmed, a syringe connected to a flexible catheter is used to irrigate the external auditory canal with 10 to 40 mL of ice water over a 30-sec period. In conscious patients (eg, with psychogenic coma), this test causes deviation of the eyes toward the irrigated ear with nystagmus beating away from the irrigated ear. In comatose patients with preserved brain stem function, both eyes deviate toward the irrigated ear but without nystagmus. Responses are absent or dysconjugate when the brain stem is impaired by a structural lesion or by deepening metabolic coma.

Respiratory patterns: Dysfunction of both hemispheres or the diencephalon may cause periodic cycling of breathing (Cheyne-Stokes and Biot's respirations—see p. 354); midbrain or upper pontine dysfunction may cause central neurogenic hyperventilation, with respiratory rates of > 40 breaths/min. Pontine or medullary lesions typically cause an inspiratory gasp (apneustic breathing), which often progresses to respiratory arrest.

Tests: Initially, pulse oximetry, finger-stick blood glucose measurements, and cardiac monitoring are done. Blood tests include a comprehensive metabolic panel, CBC with differential and platelets, coagulation tests, and ammonia level. Arterial blood gases are measured, and if the diagnosis remains unclear, carboxyhemoglobin, sulfhemoglobin, and methemoglobin levels are checked. Blood and urine should be obtained for Gram stain, culture, and routine toxicology screening; alcohol levels are also measured. Testing for certain drugs (eg, salicylates, acetaminophen, tricyclic antidepressants) should be done when toxic ingestion is suspected because several drugs are often coingested. ECG (12-lead) should be done.

Unless a cause is immediately apparent, noncontrast head CT should be rapidly done to check for mass lesions, hemorrhage, edema, and hydrocephalus. If this test is not diagnostic, contrast CT or MRI may detect isodense subdural hematomas, multiple metastases, sagittal sinus thrombosis, herpes encephalitis, or another cause missed by routine CT. Chest x-rays should also be taken.

If infection is suspected, lumbar puncture is done to check opening pressure. CSF analysis includes cell and differential counts, protein, glucose, Gram stain, cultures, and sometimes, depending on the clinical context, specific tests (eg, cryptococcal antigen, Venereal Disease Research Laboratory [VDRL] tests, PCR for herpes simplex). In unconscious patients, CT must be done before lumbar puncture to exclude an intracranial mass or obstructive hydrocephalus because in such cases, suddenly lowering CSF pressure by lumbar puncture could trigger fatal herniation.

EEG may be done if diagnosis remains uncertain; in the rare patient with nonconvulsive status epilepticus, EEG shows spikes, sharp waves, or spike and slow complexes. However, in most comatose patients, EEG shows slowing and reductions in wave amplitude that are nonspecific and often occur in metabolic encephalopathy.

Prognosis and Treatment

Prognosis depends on the specific cause, duration, and depth of stupor or coma. After trauma, a Glasgow Coma Scale score of 3 to 5 may indicate fatal brain damage, especially if pupils are fixed or oculovestibular reflexes are absent. If pupils are unreactive or motor response to noxious stimuli is absent or reflex 3 days after cardiac arrest, patients have virtually no chance of a good neurologic recovery. If the cause is barbiturate overdose or a reversible metabolic disorder, patients may lose all brain stem reflexes and all motor response but may recover fully.

Immediate stabilization and support are provided during diagnosis. Most patients with stupor or coma require admission to an ICU for ventilatory support and for monitoring of neurologic state. Specific treatment depends on the cause (see elsewhere in THE MANUAL).

For herniation, treatment includes mannitol 25 to 100 g infused IV, endotracheal intubation, and controlled ventilation with a target P_{CO_2} of 25 to 30 mm Hg. For herniation due to tumors, a corticosteroid (eg, dexamethasone 16 mg IV, followed by dexamethasone 4 mg po or IV q 6 h) is also required. Mass lesions should be surgically decompressed as soon as possible.

Stuporous or comatose patients require meticulous long-term care. Stimulants and opioids should be avoided. Enteral feeding is started with precautions to avoid aspiration (eg, elevation of the head of the bed); a percutaneous endoscopic jejunostomy tube is placed if necessary. Early attention to skin breakdown and pressure points is required to prevent pressure ulcers. Topical agents to prevent desiccation of the eyes are beneficial. Passive range-of-motion exercises done by physical therapists may reduce deconditioning, and taping or dynamic flexion splitting of the extremities may prevent contractures.

VEGETATIVE STATE

A vegetative state is prolonged unresponsiveness in a state of wakefulness without awareness. It is due to overwhelming dysfunction of the cerebral hemispheres, with sufficient sparing of the diencephalon and brain stem to preserve autonomic and motor reflexes and sleep-wake cycles. Patients may have complex reflexes, including eye movements, yawning, and involuntary movements to noxious stimuli but show no awareness of self or environment. Diagnosis is clinical and based on duration of condition. Prognosis is bleak, and treatment is supportive. Withdrawal of care should be discussed with family members.

Unlike patients in a coma, patients in a vegetative state can open their eyes and have sleep-wake cycles, but like those in a coma, they lack awareness of their environment. This condition occurs when the reticular activating system (RAS) remains functional but the cortex is severely damaged. Hypothalamic and brain stem autonomic function is sufficient for survival if medical and nursing care is adequate.

Symptoms, Signs, and Diagnosis

Patients show no evidence of awareness of self or environment and cannot interact with others. Sustained, purposeful responses to external stimuli are absent, as are language comprehension and expression.

Signs of an intact reticular formation (eg, eye opening, intermittent wakefulness with irregular sleep-wake cycles) and an intact brain stem (eg, reactive pupils, oculocephalic reflex) are present. More complex brain stem reflexes, including yawning, chewing, swallowing, and, uncommonly, guttural vocalizations, are also present. Arousal and startle reflexes may be preserved; eg, loud sounds or blinking with bright lights may elicit eye opening. Eyes may water and produce tears. Spontaneous roving eye movements—usually slow, of constant velocity, and without saccadic jerks—may be misinterpreted as volitional tracking and can upset family members.

The limbs may move, but only primitively purposeful motor responses (eg, grasping an object that contacts the hand) occur. Pain may elicit decorticate or decerebrate postures or only semipurposeful or no purposeful avoidance. Patients have fecal and urinary incontinence. Cranial nerve and spinal reflexes are typically preserved.

Diagnosis is based on typical symptoms and signs in the context of a CNS insult. Brain imaging, EEG, and somatosensory evoked potentials usually do not add anything to diagnosis.

Prognosis and Treatment

Recovery from a vegetative state is rare after 3 mo if brain damage is nontraumatic and after 12 mo if brain damage is traumatic. At best, recovery involves moderate to severe disability. Rarely, improvement occurs late; after 5 yr, about 3% of patients may recover the ability to communicate and comprehend, but a return to independence in daily activities is even rarer; no patients regain normal function.

Most patients in a persistent vegetative state die within 6 mo of a pulmonary infection, a UTI, generalized system failure, or sudden death of unknown cause. For the rest, life expectancy is about 2 to 5 yr, although a few patients live for decades.

Treatment aims to prevent systemic disorders (eg, pneumonia, UTI), provide good nutrition, prevent pressure ulcers, and provide physical therapy to prevent limb contractures. Patients cannot perceive pain but can react to pain with reflex motor responses. Decisions about life-sustaining care should involve social services, hospital ethics committee, and frequent meetings with family members. Maintaining patients, especially those without advanced directives to guide decisions about terminating treatment (see p. 2768), in a persistent vegetative state for > 6 mo leads to societal and ethical problems.

LOCKED-IN SYNDROME

Locked-in syndrome is a state of wakefulness and awareness with inability to show facial expression, move, speak, or communicate, except by coded eye movements.

Locked-in syndrome typically results from a pontine hemorrhage or infarct that disrupts and damages the centers that mediate horizontal gaze.

Patients have intact cognitive function and are awake, with eye opening and sleep-wake cycles. They cannot move their lower face, chew, swallow, speak, breathe, or move their limbs. Vertical eye movement is possible; patients can open and close their eyes or blink a specific number of times to answer questions.

Diagnosis is primarily clinical. Brain imaging helps identify cause and shows sequelae over time. EEG shows a normal awake pattern during arousal and normal phases of sleep.

Mortality rate is high; most patients die within a month. Recovery to independence is rare but can occur over a period of months when the cause is partly reversible (eg, severe widespread paralysis due to Guillain-Barré syndrome). Positive prognostic features include early recovery of lateral eye movements and evoked potentials produced by magnetic stimulation of the motor cortex. Patients have survived in the locked-in state up to 18 yr.

Treatment aims to prevent systemic disorders (eg, pneumonia, UTI), provide good nutrition, prevent pressure ulcers, and provide physical therapy to prevent limb contractures. Speech therapists may help establish a communication code using eye blinks or movements. Because cognitive function is intact, patients should make their own health care decisions if communication can be established.

BRAIN DEATH

Brain death involves unconsciousness, absence of sustainable spontaneous respirations, and persistent absence of brain stem reflexes; spinal reflexes, including deep tendon, plantar flexion, and withdrawal reflexes, may remain.

The concept of brain death developed because ventilators and drugs can perpetuate cardiopulmonary functions despite complete cessation of brain function. Thus, the definition of a person's death as the total cessation of integrated brain function, especially that of the brain stem, has been widely accepted legally and societally.

Diagnosis and Prognosis

For a physician to declare brain death, a structural or known metabolic cause of brain damage must be present, and use of potentially anesthetizing or paralyzing drugs, especially self-administered, must be ruled out. Hypothermia below 32° C must be corrected, and status epilepticus should not be present.

TABLE 212–4. GUIDELINES FOR DETERMINING BRAIN DEATH (IN PATIENTS > 1 YR)

All 9 items must be confirmed to declare brain death:

1. Reasonable efforts were made to notify the patient's next of kin or other close people.
2. Cause of coma is known and sufficient to account for irreversible loss of all brain function.
3. CNS depressant drugs, hypothermia (< 32° C), and hypotension (MAP < 55 mm Hg) have been excluded. No neuromuscular blockers contribute to the neurologic findings.
4. Any observed movements can be attributed entirely to spinal cord function.
5. Cough, pharyngeal reflexes, or both are absent.
6. Corneal and pupillary light responses are absent.
7. No caloric responses follow iced water siphoned against the tympanic membrane.
8. An apnea test of a minimum of 8 min shows no respiratory movements with a documented increase in $Pa{CO_2}$ of > 20 mm Hg from pretest baseline.
PROCEDURE: Apnea testing is done by disconnecting the ventilator from the endotracheal tube. Oxygen (6 L/min) can be supplied by diffusion from a cannula placed through the endotracheal tube. Despite the ventilatory stimulus of the passively rising $Pa{CO_2}$, no spontaneous respirations are seen over an 8- to 12-min period.
NOTE: The apnea test should be done with extreme caution to minimize risks of hypoxia and hypotension. If arterial BP falls significantly during the test, the test should be stopped, and an arterial blood sample drawn to determine whether $Pa{CO_2}$ has risen either > 55 mm Hg or increased by > 20 mm Hg. This finding validates the clinical diagnosis of brain death.
9. At least one of the following 4 criteria has been established:
   a. Items 2–8 have been confirmed by 2 examinations separated by at least 6 h.
   b. Items 2–8 have been confirmed. AND
      An EEG shows electrocortical silence.
      A 2nd examination at least 2 h after the 1st confirms items 2–8.
   c. Items 2–8 have been confirmed. AND
      Arteriography reveals no intracranial blood flow.
      A 2nd examination at least 2 h after the 1st confirms items 2–8.
   d. If any of items 2–8 cannot be determined because the injury or condition prohibits evaluation (eg, extensive facial injury precludes caloric testing), the following criteria apply:
      Items that are assessable are confirmed.
      No intracranial blood flow is evident.
      A 2nd examination 6 h after the 1st confirms all assessable items.

MAP = mean arterial pressure; $Pa{CO_2}$ = partial pressure of arterial CO_2.

Adapted from American Academy of Neurology Guidelines (1995).

Sequential testing over 6 to 24 h is necessary (see TABLE 212–4). Examination includes assessment of pupil reactivity, oculovestibular and oculocephalic reflexes, corneal reflexes, and apnea testing. EEG may be used to confirm absence of activity and provide additional evidence to family members but is not required.

Recovery after appropriate diagnosis of brain death has not been reported, and even with mechanical ventilation, asystole typically occurs within several days. Cessation of ventilatory support results in terminal arrhythmias. Spinal motor reflexes may occur during terminal apnea; they include arching of the back, neck turning, stiffening of the legs, and upper extremity flexion (the so-called Lazarus sign). Family members who wish to be present when the ventilator is shut off need to be warned of such reflex movements.

213 DELIRIUM AND DEMENTIA

Delirium (sometimes called acute confusional state) and dementia are the most common causes of cognitive impairment, although affective disorders (eg, depression) also can disrupt cognition. Delirium and dementia are separate disorders but are sometimes difficult to distinguish. In both, cognition is disordered, but dementia affects mainly memory and delirium affects mainly attention.

Other specific characteristics help distinguish between the 2 disorders (see TABLE 213–1). Delirium is typically caused by acute illness or drug toxicity (sometimes life threatening) and is often reversible, whereas dementia is typically caused by anatomic changes in the brain, has slower onset, and is generally irreversible. Delirium often develops in patients with dementia. Mistaking delirium for dementia in an elderly patient—a common clinical error—must be avoided, particularly when delirium is superimposed on chronic dementia. No laboratory test can definitively establish the cause of cognitive impairment; a thorough history and physical examination as well as knowledge of baseline function are essential.

DELIRIUM

Delirium is an acute, transient, usually reversible, fluctuating disturbance in attention, cognition, and consciousness level. Causes include almost any disorder, intoxication, or drug. Diagnosis is clinical, with laboratory and imaging tests to identify the cause. Treatment is correction of the cause and supportive measures.

Delirium may occur at any age but is more common among the elderly. At least 10% of elderly patients who are admitted to the hospital have delirium; 15 to 50% experience delirium at some time during hospitalization. Delirium is also common among nursing home residents. When delirium occurs in younger people, it is usually due to drug use or a life-threatening systemic disorder.

Etiology and Pathophysiology

Many conditions and drugs (particularly anticholinergics, psychoactive drugs, and opioids) can cause delirium (see TABLE 213–2). In about 10 to 20% of patients, no cause is identified.

Mechanisms are not fully understood but may involve reversible impairment of cerebral oxidative metabolism, multiple neurotransmitter abnormalities, and generation of cytokines. Stress of any kind upregulates sympathetic tone and downregulates parasympathetic tone, impairing cholinergic function and thus contributing to delirium. The elderly are particularly vulnerable to reduced cholinergic transmission, increasing their risk of delirium. Regardless of cause, the cerebral hemispheres or arousal mechanisms of the thalamus and brain stem reticular-activating system become impaired.

Predisposing factors include brain disorders (eg, dementia, stroke, Parkinson's disease), advanced age, sensory impairment, and multiple coexisting disorders. Precipitating factors include use of ≥ 3 new drugs, infection, dehydration, immobility, undernutrition, and use of bladder catheters. Recent exposure to anesthesia also increases risk, especially if exposure is prolonged and if anticholinergics are given during surgery. Decreased sensory stimuli at night may trigger delirium in at-risk patients. For elderly patients in an ICU, risk of delirium (ICU psychosis) is particularly high.

Symptoms and Signs

Delirium is characterized primarily by difficulty focusing, maintaining, or shifting attention (inattention). Consciousness level fluctuates; patients are disoriented to time, place, and sometimes person. They may have hallucinations. Confusion regarding day-to-day events and daily routines is common, as are changes in personality and affect. Thinking becomes disorganized, and speech is often disordered, with prominent slurring, rapidity, neologisms, aphasic errors, or chaotic patterns. Symptoms fluctuate over minutes to hours; they may lessen during the day and worsen at night.

Symptoms may include inappropriate behavior, fearfulness, and paranoia. Patients may become irritable, agitated, hyperactive, and hyperalert, or they may become quiet, withdrawn, and lethargic. Some patients alternate between the two. Usually, patterns of sleeping and eating are grossly distorted. Because of the many cognitive disturbances, insight is poor, and judgment impaired. Other symptoms and signs depend on the cause.

TABLE 213–1. DIFFERENCES BETWEEN DELIRIUM AND DEMENTIA*

FEATURE	DELIRIUM	DEMENTIA
Development	Sudden, with a definite beginning point	Slow and gradual, with an uncertain beginning point
Duration	Days to weeks, although it may be longer	Usually permanent
Cause	Almost always another condition (eg, infection, dehydration, use or withdrawal of certain drugs)	Usually a chronic brain disorder (eg, Alzheimer's disease, Lewy body dementia, vascular dementia)
Course	Usually reversible	Slowly progressive
Effect at night	Almost always worse	Often worse
Effect on attention	Greatly impaired	No effect until dementia has become severe
Effect on consciousness level	Varies, ranging from sluggishness to alertness	No effect until dementia has become severe
Orientation to time and place	Varies	Impaired
Use of language	Slow, often incoherent, and inappropriate	Sometimes difficulty finding the right word
Memory	Varies	Lost, especially for recent events
Need for medical attention	Immediate	Required but less urgently

*Differences are generally true and helpful diagnostically, but exceptions are not rare. For example, traumatic brain injury occurs suddenly but may result in severe, permanent dementia; hypothyroidism may produce the slowly progressive picture of dementia but be completely reversible with treatment.

Diagnosis

Diagnosis is clinical. All patients with any sign of cognitive impairment require a formal mental status examination (see sidebar 206–1 on p. 1749). Attention is assessed first. Simple tests include immediate repetition of the names of 3 objects, digit span (ability to repeat 7 digits forward and 5 backward), and naming the days of the week forward and backward. Inattention (patient does not register directions or other information) must be distinguished from poor short-term memory (patient registers information but rapidly forgets it). Further cognitive testing is futile for patients who cannot register information.

After initial assessment, standard diagnostic criteria, such as the *Diagnostic and Statistical Manual of Mental Disorders* (DSM) or Confusion Assessment Method (CAM) may be used. Features required for diagnosis are an acute change in cognition that fluctuates during the day, inattention (eg, difficulty focusing or following what is said), plus another feature: with DSM, disturbance of consciousness (ie, less clarity); with CAM, either an altered level of consciousness (eg, hyperalert, lethargic, stuporous, comatose) or disorganized thinking (eg, rambling, irrelevant conversation, illogical flow of ideas).

Interviewing family members, caregivers, and friends can determine whether the change in mental status is recent and is distinct from any baseline dementia (see TABLE 213–1). The history helps distinguish a psychiatric disorder from delirium. Psychiatric disorders, unlike delirium, almost never cause inattention or fluctuating consciousness, and onset of psychiatric disorders is nearly always subacute. History should also include use of alcohol and illicit, OTC, and prescription drugs, focusing particularly on drugs with CNS effects and on new additions, discontinuations, or changes in dose, including overdosing.

TABLE 213–2. CAUSES OF DELIRIUM

CATEGORY	EXAMPLES
Drugs	Alcohol, anticholinergics, antiemetics, antihistamines (eg, diphenhydramine), antihypertensives, antiparkinsonian drugs (levodopa), antipsychotics, antispasmodics, benzodiazepines, cimetidine, corticosteroids, digoxin, hypnotics, muscle relaxants, opioids, recreational drugs, sedatives, tricyclic antidepressants
Endocrine disorders	Hyperparathyroidism, hyperthyroidism, hypothyroidism
Infections	Encephalitis, fever, meningitis, pneumonia, sepsis, systemic infections, UTIs
Metabolic disorders	Acid-base disturbances, fluid and electrolyte abnormalities, hepatic or uremic encephalopathy, hyperthermia, hypoglycemia, hypoxia, Wernicke's encephalopathy
Neurologic disorders	Postconcussion syndrome, postictal state, transient ischemia
Structural disorders	Brain abscesses, cerebral hemorrhage, cerebral infarction, primary or metastatic brain tumors, subarachnoid hemorrhage, subdural hematomas, vascular occlusion
Vascular/circulatory disorders	Anemia, cardiac arrhythmias, heart failure, hypoperfusion states, shock
Vitamin deficiency	Thiamin, vitamin B_{12}
Withdrawal syndromes	Alcohol, barbiturates, benzodiazepines, opioids
Other causes	Change of environment, fecal impaction, long stays in ICU, postoperative states, sensory deprivation, sleep deprivation, urinary retention

The physical examination can detect signs of CNS trauma or infection (eg, fever, meningismus, Kernig and Brudzinski signs). Tremor and myoclonus suggest uremia, hepatic failure, or drug intoxication. Ophthalmoplegia and ataxia suggest Wernicke-Korsakoff syndrome (see p. 1689). Focal neurologic findings (eg, cranial nerve palsies, motor or sensory deficits) or papilledema suggests a structural CNS disorder.

Tests should include serum glucose, thyroid function tests, toxicology screening, CBC with differential, serum electrolytes, urinalysis, appropriate cultures (especially urine), and cardiac and pulmonary evaluation (eg, ECG, pulse oximetry, chest x-ray).

CT or MRI should be done if clinical findings suggest a CNS lesion or if initial testing has not identified the cause of delirium, especially in patients ≤ 65 yr, because a primary CNS disorder is more likely. Lumbar puncture may be indicated to rule out meningitis, encephalitis, or subarachnoid hemorrhage. If nonconvulsive status epilepticus, a rare cause, is suspected (based on history, subtle motor twitches, automatisms, or presence of a steadier but less intense pattern of bewilderment and drowsiness), EEG should be done.

Prognosis

Morbidity and mortality rates are higher in patients who have delirium when they are hospitalized and in those who develop delirium during hospitalization.

Certain causes of delirium (eg, hypoglycemia, intoxication, infection, iatrogenic factors, drug toxicity, electrolyte imbalance) typically resolve rapidly with treatment. However, recovery may be slow (days to even weeks or months), especially in the elderly, resulting in longer hospital stays, increased complications, increased costs, and long-term disability. Some patients never fully recover from delirium. For up to 2 yr after delirium occurs, risk of cognitive and functional decline, institutionalization, and death is increased.

Treatment

Treatment consists of correcting the cause and removing aggravating factors (eg, stopping drugs, treating infection), providing support for the patient and family members, and managing agitation to ensure patient safety. Adequate fluid and nutrition should be provided, and nutritional deficiencies (eg, of thiamin or vitamin B_{12}) should be corrected.

The environment should be stable, quiet, and well-lit and include visual cues to orient the patient (eg, calendar, clocks, family photographs). Frequent reorientation and reassurance by hospital staff or family members may also help. Patients' sensory deficits should be minimized (eg, by replacing hearing-aid batteries, by encouraging patients who need eyeglasses or hearing aids to use them).

Approach to treatment should be multidisciplinary (with a physician, physical and occupational therapists, nurses, and social workers); it should involve strategies to enhance mobility and range of motion, treat pain and discomfort, prevent skin breakdown, ameliorate incontinence, and minimize risk of aspiration.

Agitation may threaten the well-being of the patient, a caregiver, or a staff member. Simplifying drug regimens and avoiding use of IV lines, Foley catheters, and physical restraints (particularly in the long-term care setting) as much as possible can help prevent exacerbation of agitation and reduce risk of injury. However, in certain circumstances, physical restraints may be needed to prevent patients from harming themselves or others. Restraints should be applied by a staff member trained in their use; they should be released at least every 2 h to prevent injury and discontinued as soon as possible. Use of hospital-employed assistants (sitters) as constant observers may help avoid the need for restraints.

Drugs, typically low-dose haloperidol (0.5 to 1.0 mg po, IV, or IM), may lessen agitation or psychotic symptoms but do not correct the underlying cause and may prolong or exacerbate delirium. Second-generation (atypical) antipsychotics (eg, risperidone 0.5 to 3 mg po q 12 h, olanzapine 2.5 to 15 mg po once/day) may be used instead because they have fewer extrapyramidal adverse effects; however, long-term use in the elderly may increase risk of stroke. These drugs are not typically given IV or IM. Benzodiazepines (eg, lorazepam 0.5 to 1.0 mg) have a more rapid onset of action (5 min after parenteral administration) than antipsychotics but commonly worsen confusion and sedation in patients with delirium. Overall, antipsychotics and benzodiazepines are equally effective for managing agitation in delirium, but antipsychotics have fewer adverse effects. Benzodiazepines are preferred for delirium attributed to sedative withdrawal and for patients intolerant of antipsychotics (eg, those with Parkinson's disease or Lewy body dementia). Dose of these drugs should be reduced as quickly as possible.

DEMENTIA

Dementia is chronic, global, usually irreversible deterioration of cognition. Diagnosis is clinical; laboratory and imaging tests are used to identify treatable causes. Treatment is supportive. Cholinesterase inhibitors can sometimes temporarily improve cognitive function.

Dementia may occur at any age but affects primarily the elderly (about 5% of those aged 65 to 74 and 40% of those > 85). It accounts for more than ½ of nursing home admissions. At least 4 to 5 million people in the US have dementia.

Etiology and Classification

Dementias can be classified in several ways: Alzheimer's or non-Alzheimer's type, cortical or subcortical, irreversible or potentially reversible, or common or rare. Dementias may be primary neurodegenerative disorders or due to another condition (see Table 213–3).

The main types are Alzheimer's disease, vascular dementia, Lewy body dementia, frontal-temporal dementias, and HIV-associated dementia. Other disorders associated with dementia include Parkinson's disease, Huntington's disease, progressive supranuclear palsy, Creutzfeldt-Jakob disease, Gerstmann-Sträussler-Scheinker syndrome, other prion disorders, and neurosyphilis. Distinguishing type or cause of dementia is difficult; definitive diagnosis often requires postmortem pathologic examination of brain tissue. Patients can have > 1 type (mixed dementia).

Some structural brain disorders (eg, normal-pressure hydrocephalus, subdural hematoma), metabolic disorders (eg, hypothyroidism, vitamin B_{12} deficiency), and toxins (eg, lead) cause a slow deterioration of cognition that may resolve with treatment. This impairment is sometimes called reversible dementia, but some experts restrict the term dementia to irreversible cognitive deterioration. Depression may mimic dementia (and was formerly called pseudodementia); the 2 disorders often

TABLE 213–3. CLASSIFICATION OF SOME DEMENTIAS

CLASSIFICATION	EXAMPLES
Primary neurodegenerative (cortical)	Alzheimer's disease Frontotemporal dementias Mixed dementia with an Alzheimer's component
Vascular	Lacunar disease (eg, Binswanger's disease) Multi-infarct dementia
Associated with Lewy bodies	Diffuse Lewy body disease Parkinson's disease with dementia Progressive supranuclear palsy Corticobasal ganglion degeneration
Due to ingestion	Dementia due to chronic alcohol abuse Dementia due to heavy metal or other toxin exposures
Due to infections	Dementia due to fungal infections (eg, cryptococcal) Dementia due to spirochetes (eg, syphilis, Lyme disease) Dementia due to viral infections (eg, HIV, postencephalitic)
Due to prions	Creutzfeldt-Jakob disease
Due to structural brain disorders	Brain tumor Normal-pressure hydrocephalus Subdural hematomas (chronic)

coexist. Changes in cognition occur with aging, but they are not dementia.

Any disorder may exacerbate cognitive deficits in patients with dementia. Delirium often occurs in patients with dementia. Drugs, particularly benzodiazepines and anticholinergics (eg, some tricyclic antidepressants, antihistamines, antipsychotics, benztropine), may temporarily cause or worsen symptoms of dementia, as may alcohol, even in moderate amounts. New or progressive renal or hepatic failure may reduce drug clearance and cause drug toxicity after years of taking a stable drug dose (eg, of propranolol).

Symptoms and Signs

Dementia impairs cognition globally. Often, loss of short-term memory is the 1st sign. Although symptoms exist in a continuum, they can be divided into early, intermediate, and late. Personality changes and behavioral disturbances may develop early or late. Motor and other focal neurologic deficits occur at different stages, depending on the type of dementia; they occur early in vascular dementia and late in Alzheimer's disease. Incidence of seizures is somewhat increased during all stages. Psychosis—hallucinations, delusions, or paranoia—occurs in about 10% of patients with dementia, although a higher percentage may experience these symptoms temporarily.

Early: Recent memory is impaired; learning and retaining new information become difficult. Language problems (especially with word finding), mood swings, and personality changes develop. Patients may have progressive difficulty with independent activities of daily living (eg, balancing their checkbook, finding their way around, remembering where they put things). Abstract thinking, insight, or judgment may be impaired. Patients may respond to loss of independence and memory with irritability, hostility, and agitation.

Agnosia (impaired ability to identify objects despite intact sensory function—see p. 1785), apraxia (impaired ability to perform previously learned motor activities despite intact motor function—see p. 1788), or aphasia (impaired ability to comprehend or use language—see p. 1787) may further limit functional ability.

Although early dementia may not compromise sociability, family members may report strange behavior accompanied by emotional lability.

Intermediate: Patients become unable to learn and recall new information. Memory of remote events is reduced but not totally lost. Patients may require help with basic activities of daily living (eg, bathing, eating, dressing, toileting). Personality changes may progress. Patients may become irritable, anxious, self-centered, inflexible, or angry more easily, or they may become more passive, with a flat affect, depression, indecisiveness, lack of spontaneity, or general withdrawal from social situations. Behavior disorders may develop: Patients may wander or become suddenly and inappropriately agitated, hostile, uncooperative, or physically aggressive (see p. 1821).

By this stage, patients have lost all sense of time and place, because they cannot effectively use normal environmental and social cues. Patients often get lost; they may be unable to find their own bedroom or bathroom. They remain ambulatory but are at risk of falls or accidents secondary to confusion. Altered sensation or perception may culminate in psychosis with hallucinations and paranoid and persecutory delusions. Sleep patterns are often disorganized.

Late (severe): Patients cannot walk, feed themselves, or perform any other activities of daily living; they may become incontinent. Recent and remote memory is completely lost. Patients may be unable to swallow. They are at risk of undernutrition, pneumonia (especially due to aspiration), and pressure ulcers. Because they depend completely on others for care, placement in a long-term care facility often becomes necessary. Eventually, patients become mute.

Because such patients cannot relate any symptoms to a physician and because elderly patients often have no febrile or leukocytic response to infection, a physician must rely on experience and acumen whenever a patient appears ill. End-stage dementia results in coma and death, usually due to infection.

Diagnosis

Diagnosis focuses on distinguishing dementia from delirium and identifying the cerebral areas affected and potentially reversible causes. Distinguishing between dementia and delirium is crucial (because delirium is usually reversible with prompt treatment) but can be difficult. Attention is assessed first. If a patient is inattentive, the diagnosis is likely to be delirium, although advanced dementia also severely impairs attention. Other features that suggest delirium rather than dementia (eg, duration of cognitive impairment—see Table 213–1) are determined by the history, physical examination, and tests for specific causes.

Dementia must also be distinguished from age-associated memory impairment; the elderly have a relative deficiency in recall, particularly compared with recall during their youth. This change is not progressive and does not affect daily function. If such people are given enough time to learn new information, their intellectual performance is good. Mild cognitive impairment involves a subjective memory complaint; memory is impaired compared with that of age-matched controls, but other cognitive domains and daily function are not affected. Up to 50% of patients with mild cognitive impairment develop dementia within 3 yr.

Dementia should also be distinguished from the dementia of depression; this cognitive disturbance resolves with treatment of depression. Depressed older patients may experience cognitive decline, but unlike patients with dementia, they tend to exaggerate their memory loss and rarely forget important current events or personal matters. Neurologic examinations are normal except for signs of psychomotor slowing. When tested, patients with depression make little effort to respond, but those with dementia often try hard but respond incorrectly. When depression and dementia coexist, treating depression does not fully restore cognition.

The best screening test for dementia is a short-term memory test (eg, registering 3 objects and recalling them after 5 min); patients with dementia forget simple information within 3 to 5 min. Another test assesses the ability to name objects within categories (eg, lists of animals, plants, or pieces of furniture). Patients with dementia struggle to name a few; those without dementia easily name many.

In addition to loss of short-term memory, diagnosis of dementia requires at least one of the following cognitive deficits: aphasia, apraxia, agnosia, or impaired ability to plan, organize, sequence, or think abstractly (executive dysfunction). Each cognitive deficit must substantially impair function and represent a significant decline from a previous level of functioning. Also, the deficits must not occur only during delirium.

History and physical examination should focus on signs of systemic disorders that may indicate delirium or on treatable disorders that cause cognitive impairment (vitamin B_{12} deficiency, advanced syphilis, hypothyroidism, depression—see Table 213–2).

A formal mental status examination (see sidebar 206–1 on p. 1749) should be done. When delirium is absent, a score of < 24 points suggests dementia; adjustments for education improve diagnostic accuracy. If the diagnosis remains in doubt, patients should be referred for full neuropsychologic testing, which may help characterize specific deficits due to dementia.

Tests should include CBC, liver function tests, and thyroid-stimulating hormone and vitamin B_{12} levels. If clinical findings suggest a specific disorder, other tests (eg, HIV tests, syphilis serology) are indicated. Lumbar puncture is rarely needed but should be considered if a chronic infection or neurosyphilis is suspected. Other tests may be used to exclude causes of delirium.

CT or MRI should be done in the initial evaluation of dementia or after any sudden change in cognition or mental status. Brain imaging can identify potentially reversible structural disorders (eg, normal-pressure hydrocephalus, brain tumors, subdural hematoma) and metabolic disorders (eg, Hallervorden-Spatz disease, Wilson's disease). Occasionally, EEG is useful (eg, to evaluate episodic lapses in attention or bizarre behavior). Functional MRI or single-photon emission CT can provide information about cerebral perfusion patterns and help with differential diagnosis.

Prognosis and Treatment

Dementia is usually progressive. However, progression rate varies widely and depends on the cause. Dementia shortens life expectancy, but survival estimates vary.

Measures to ensure patient safety and to provide an appropriate environment are essential to treatment, as is caregiver assistance. Several drugs are available.

Patient safety: Occupational and physical therapists can evaluate the home for safety; the goals are to prevent accidents (particularly falls), to manage behavior disorders, and to plan for change as dementia progresses

How well patients function in various settings (ie, kitchen, automobile) should be evaluated using simulations. If patients have deficits and remain in the same environment, protective measures (eg, unplugging the stove, removing the car, confiscating car keys) may be required. Some states require physicians to notify the Department of Motor Vehicles of patients with dementia because at some point, such patients can no longer drive safely. If patients wander, signal monitoring systems can be installed. Ultimately, assistance (eg, housekeepers, home health aides) or a change of environment (living facilities without stairs, assisted-living facility, skilled nursing facility) may be indicated.

Environmental measures: An appropriate environment can help preserve feelings of self-control and personal dignity. Measures include frequent reinforcement of orientation; a bright, cheerful, familiar environment; minimal new stimulation; and regular, low-stress activities.

Large calendars and clocks and a routine for daily activities can help with orientation; medical staff members can wear large name tags and repeatedly introduce themselves. Changes in surroundings, routines, or people should be explained to patients precisely and simply, omitting nonessential procedures. Patients require time to adjust and become familiar with the changes. Telling patients about what is going to happen (eg, about a bath or feeding) may avert resistance or violent reactions. Frequent visits by staff members and familiar people encourage patients to remain social.

The room should be reasonably bright and contain sensory stimuli (eg, radio, television, night-light) to help patients remain oriented and focus their attention. Quiet, dark, private rooms should be avoided.

Activities can help patients function better; those related to interests before dementia began are good choices. Activities should be enjoyable, provide some stimulation, but not involve too many choices or challenges. Exercise to reduce restlessness, improve balance, and maintain cardiovascular tone should be done daily. Exercise can also help improve sleep and reduce behavior disorders. Occupational and music therapy helps maintain fine motor control and provides nonverbal stimulation. Group therapy (eg, reminiscence therapy, socialization activities) may help maintain conversational and interpersonal skills.

Drugs: Eliminating or limiting drugs with CNS activity often improves function. Sedating and anticholinergic drugs, which tend to worsen dementia, should be avoided.

The cholinesterase inhibitors donepezil, rivastigmine, and galantamine (see p. 1816) are somewhat effective in improving cognitive function in patients with Alzheimer's disease or Lewy body dementia and may be useful in other forms of dementia. These drugs inhibit acetylcholinesterase, increasing the acetylcholine level in the brain. A new drug, memantine, may help to slow progression of moderate to severe dementia and can be used with a cholinesterase inhibitor.

Other drugs (eg, antipsychotics) have been used to control behavior disorders (see p. 1822). Patients with dementia and signs of depression should be treated with nonanticholinergic antidepressants, preferably SSRIs.

Caregiver assistance: Immediate family members are largely responsible for care of a patient with dementia. Nurses and social workers can teach them and other caregivers how to best meet the patient's needs (eg, how to deal with daily care and handle financial issues); teaching should be ongoing. Other resources (eg, support groups, educational materials, Internet web sites) are available. Caregivers may experience substantial stress. Stress may be caused by worry about protecting the patient and frustration, exhaustion, anger, and resentment from having to do so much to care for someone. Health care practitioners should watch for early symptoms of caregiver stress and burnout and, when needed, suggest support services (eg, social worker, nutritionist, nurse, home health aide). If a patient with dementia has an unusual injury, the possibility of elder abuse should be investigated.

End-of-life issues: Because insight and judgment deteriorate in patients with dementia, appointment of a family member, guardian, or lawyer to oversee finances may be necessary. Early in dementia, before the patient is incapacitated, the patient's wishes about care should be clarified, and financial and legal arrangements (eg, durable power of attorney, durable power of attorney for health care) should be made. When these documents are signed, the patient's capacity should be evaluated, and evaluation results recorded (see also p. 2769).

Alzheimer's Disease

Alzheimer's disease causes progressive cognitive deterioration and is characterized by senile plaques, β-amyloid deposits, and neurofibrillary tangles in the cerebral cortex and subcortical gray matter.

Alzheimer's disease is the most common cause of dementia; it accounts for > 65% of dementias in the elderly. The disease is twice as common among women as among men, partly because women have a longer life expectancy. Alzheimer's disease affects about 4% of people aged 65 to 74 and 30% of those > 85. Prevalence in industrialized countries is expected to increase as the proportion of the elderly increases.

Etiology and Pathophysiology

Most cases are sporadic, with late onset (> 60 yr) and unclear etiology. However, about 5 to 15% are familial; ½ of these cases have an early onset (< 60 yr) and are typically related to specific genetic mutations.

Typically, extracellular β-amyloid deposits, intracellular neurofibrillary tangles (paired helical filaments), and senile plaques develop, and neurons are lost. Cerebrocortical atrophy is common, and use of cerebral glucose is reduced, as is perfusion in the parietal lobe, temporal cortices, and prefrontal cortex.

At least 5 distinct genetic loci, located on chromosomes 1, 12, 14, 19, and 21, influence initiation and progression of Alzheimer's disease. Genes for the amyloid precursor proteins presenilin I and presenilin II are involved. Mutations in these genes may alter the processing of amyloid precursor protein, leading to deposition and fibrillar aggregation of β-amyloid. β-Amyloid may lead to neuronal death and formation of the neurofibrillary tangles and senile plaques, which consist of degenerated axonal or dendritic processes, astrocytes, and glial cells around an amyloid core.

Other genetic determinants include the apolipoprotein (apo) E alleles (ε). Apo E proteins influence β-amyloid deposition, cytoskeletal integrity, and efficiency of neuronal repair. Risk of Alzheimer's disease is substantially increased in people with 2 ε4 alleles and may be decreased in those who have the ε2 allele.

Other common abnormalities include increased brain and CSF concentrations of the tau protein (a component of neurofibrillary tangles and β-amyloid) and reduced levels of choline acetyltransferase and various neurotransmitters (eg, somatostatin).

The relationship of environmental factors (eg, low hormone levels, metal exposure) and Alzheimer's disease is under study, but no link has been established.

Symptoms, Signs, and Diagnosis

Symptoms and signs of Alzheimer's disease are similar to those of other dementias, with early, intermediate, and late stages (see p. 1812). Loss of short-term memory is often the first sign. The disease progresses gradually but may plateau for periods of time. Behavior disorders (eg, wandering, agitation, yelling) are common (see p. 1821)

Generally, diagnosis is similar to that of other dementias (see p. 1813). Traditional diagnostic criteria for Alzheimer's disease include dementia established by physical examination and documented by a formal mental status examination; deficits in ≥ 2 areas of cognition; gradual onset and progressive worsening of memory and other cognitive functions; no disturbance of consciousness; onset after age 40, most often after age 65; and no systemic or brain disorders that could account for the progressive deficits in memory

TABLE 213–4. MODIFIED HACHINSKI ISCHEMIC SCORE

FEATURE	POINTS*
Abrupt onset of symptoms	2
Stepwise deterioration (eg, decline-stability-decline)	1
Fluctuating course	2
Nocturnal confusion	1
Personality relatively preserved	1
Depression	1
Somatic complaints (eg, arm tingling, arm clumsiness)	1
Emotional lability	1
History or presence of hypertension	1
History of stroke	2
Evidence of coexisting atherosclerosis (eg, PAD, MI)	1
Focal neurologic symptoms (eg, hemiparesis, homonymous hemianopia, aphasia)	2
Focal neurologic signs (eg, unilateral weakness, sensory loss, asymmetric reflexes, Babinski's sign)	2

PAD = peripheral arterial disease.

*Total score is determined: < 4 suggests primary dementia (eg, Alzheimer's disease); 4–7 = indeterminate; and > 7 suggests vascular dementia.

and cognition. However, deviations from these criteria do not exclude a diagnosis of Alzheimer's disease.

Distinguishing Alzheimer's disease from other dementias is difficult. Assessment tools (eg, Hachinski Ischemic Score—see Table 213–4) can help distinguish vascular dementia from Alzheimer's disease. Fluctuations in cognition, parkinsonian symptoms, well-formed visual hallucinations, and relative preservation of short-term memory suggest Lewy body dementia rather than Alzheimer's disease (see Table 213–5). Patients with Alzheimer's disease are often better-groomed and neater than patients with other dementias. For about 85% of patients with Alzheimer's disease, a thorough history and standard neurologic examination provide a correct diagnosis.

Prognosis and Treatment

Although progression rate varies, cognitive decline is inevitable. Average survival from time of diagnosis is 7 yr, although this figure is debated.

General treatment of Alzheimer's disease is the same as that of all dementias (see p. 1814).

Cholinesterase inhibitors modestly improve cognitive function and memory in some patients. Four are approved for use; generally, donepezil, rivastigmine, and galantamine are equally effective, but tacrine is rarely used because of its hepatotoxicity. Donepezil is a 1st-line drug because it has once/day dosing and is well-tolerated. The recommended dose is 5 mg once/day for 4 to 6 wk, then increased to 10 mg once/day. Treatment should be continued if functional improvement is apparent after several months, but otherwise it should be stopped. The most common adverse effects are GI (eg, nausea, diarrhea). Rarely, dizziness and cardiac arrhythmias occur. Adverse effects can be minimized by increasing the dose gradually (see Table 213–6).

The recently approved *N*-methyl-D-aspartate receptor antagonist memantine (5 to 10 mg po bid) appears to slow the progression of Alzheimer's disease. Efficacy of high-dose vitamin E (1000 IU po once/day or bid), selegiline, NSAIDs, *Ginkgo biloba* extracts, and statins is unclear. Estrogen therapy does not appear useful in prevention or treatment and may be harmful.

VASCULAR DEMENTIA

Vascular dementia is acute or chronic cognitive deterioration due to diffuse or focal cerebral infarction that is most often related to cerebrovascular disease.

Vascular dementia is the 2nd most common cause of dementia among the elderly. It is more common among men and usually begins after age 70. It occurs more often in people who have vascular risk factors (eg, hypertension, diabetes mellitus, hyperlipidemia, smoking) and in those who have had several strokes. Many patients have both vascular dementia and Alzheimer's disease.

Vascular dementia occurs when multiple small cerebral infarcts (or sometimes hemor-

TABLE 213–5. DIFFERENCES BETWEEN ALZHEIMER'S DISEASE AND LEWY BODY DEMENTIA

FEATURE	ALZHEIMER'S DISEASE	LEWY BODY DEMENTIA
Pathology	Senile plaques, neurofibrillary tangles, and β-amyloid deposits in the cerebral cortex and subcortical gray matter	Lewy bodies in neurons of the cortex
Epidemiology	Affects twice as many women	Affects twice as many men
Inheritance	Familial in 5–15% cases	Rarely familial
Day-to-day fluctuation	Some	Prominent
Short-term memory	Lost early in the disease	Less affected; deficits in alertness and attention more than in memory acquisition
Parkinsonian symptoms	Very rare, occurring late in the disease; normal gait	Prominent, obvious early in the disease; axial rigidity and unstable gait
Autonomic dysfunction	Rare	Common
Hallucinations	Occur in about 20% of patients, usually when disease is moderately advanced	Occur in about 80%, usually when disease is early; most commonly, visual
Adverse effects with antipsychotics	Common; may worsen symptoms of dementia	Common; acutely worsen extrapyramidal symptoms and may be severe or life threatening

rhages) cause enough neuronal or axonal loss to impair brain function. Vascular dementia results from disease of small vessels (lacunar disease) or of medium-sized vessels (multi-infarct dementia).

Binswanger's dementia (subcortical arteriosclerotic encephalopathy) is an uncommon variant of small-vessel dementia associated with severe, poorly controlled hypertension and systemic vascular disease. It involves multiple lacunar infarcts in deep hemispheric white and gray matter.

Symptoms and Signs

Symptoms and signs are similar to those of other dementias (see p. 1812). However, because infarction is the cause, vascular dementia tends to progress in discrete steps; each episode is accompanied by intellectual decline, sometimes followed by modest recovery. As the disease progresses, focal neurologic deficits often develop; they include exaggeration of deep tendon reflexes, extensor plantar response, gait abnormalities, weakness of an extremity, hemiplegias, pseudobulbar palsy with pathologic laughing and crying, and other signs of extrapyramidal dysfunction. However, with small-vessel ischemic damage, the decline is gradual. Cognitive loss may be focal. Patients with partial aphasia may be more aware of their deficits; thus, depression may be more common than in other dementias.

Diagnosis

Diagnosis is similar to that of other dementias (see p. 1813). If focal signs or evidence of cerebrovascular disease is present, a thorough evaluation for stroke should be done (see p. 1791).

CT and MRI may show bilateral multiple infarcts in the dominant hemisphere and limbic structures, multiple lacunar strokes, or periventricular white-matter lesions extending into the deep white matter. In Binswanger's dementia, imaging shows leukoencephalopathy in the cerebrum semiovale adjacent to the cortex, often with multiple lacunae affecting structures deep in the gray matter (eg, basal ganglia, thalamic nuclei).

The Hachinski Ischemic Score is sometimes used to help differentiate vascular dementia from Alzheimer's disease (see Table 213–4).

TABLE 213–6. DRUGS FOR DEMENTIA

DRUG NAME	STARTING DOSE	MAXIMUM DOSE	COMMENTS
Donepezil	5 mg once/day	10 mg once/day	Generally well-tolerated but can cause nausea or diarrhea
Galantamine	4 mg bid Extended-release: 8 mg once/day in the AM	12 mg bid Extended-release: 24 mg once/day in the AM	Possibly more beneficial for behavioral symptoms than other drugs; modulates nicotinic receptors and appears to stimulate release of acetylcholine and enhances its effect
Memantine	5 mg bid	10 mg bid	Appears to slow the progression of Alzheimer's disease
Rivastigmine	1.5 mg bid	6 mg bid	Available in liquid solution

Prognosis and Treatment

The 5-yr mortality rate is 61%, which is higher than that for most forms of dementia, presumably because other atherosclerotic disorders coexist.

Generally, treatment is the same as that of other dementias (see p. 1814). However, vascular dementia may be preventable, and its progression may be slowed by BP control, cholesterol-lowering therapy, regulation of blood sugar (90 to 150 mg/dL), and smoking cessation.

The efficacy of cognition-enhancing drugs, including cholinesterase inhibitors, is uncertain. However, because many patients also have Alzheimer's disease, these drugs may have some benefit. Adjunctive drugs for depression, psychosis, and sleep disorders are useful.

Lewy Body Dementia

Lewy body dementia is chronic cognitive deterioration characterized by cellular inclusions called Lewy bodies in the cytoplasm of cortical neurons.

Lewy body dementia is the 3rd most common dementia. Age of onset is typically > 60.

Lewy bodies are spherical, eosinophilic, neuronal cytoplasmic inclusions composed of aggregates of α-synuclein, a synaptic protein. They occur in the cortex of some patients with primary Lewy body dementia and in the substantia nigra of patients with Parkinson's disease (see p. 1882). In Lewy body dementia, neurotransmitter levels and neuronal pathways between the striatum and the neocortex are abnormal. But whether the Lewy bodies cause or result from disease is unclear.

Symptoms and Signs

Initial cognitive deterioration resembles that of other dementias (see p. 1812). But extrapyramidal symptoms differ from those of Parkinson's disease: In Lewy body dementia, tremor does not occur early, axial rigidity with gait instability occurs early, and deficits tend to be symmetric.

Fluctuating cognitive function is a relatively specific feature of Lewy body dementia. Periods of being alert, coherent, and oriented may alternate with periods of being confused and unresponsive to questions, usually over a period of days to weeks but sometimes during the same interview. Memory is impaired, but the impairment appears to result more from deficits in alertness and attention than in memory acquisition; thus, short-term recall is affected less than digit span memory (ability to repeat 7 digits forward and 5 backward). Excessive daytime drowsiness is common. Visuospatial and visuoconstructional abilities (tested by block design, clock drawing, or figure copying) are affected more than other cognitive deficits. Thus, Lewy body dementia may be difficult to distinguish from delirium, and all patients presenting with these symptoms and signs should be evaluated for delirium.

Visual hallucinations are common and often threatening, unlike the benign hallucinations of Parkinson's disease. Auditory, olfactory, and tactile hallucinations are less common. Delusions occur in 50 to 65% of patients and are often complex and bizarre, compared with the simple persecutory ideation common in Alzheimer's disease. Autonomic dysfunction is common, and unexplained syncope may result. Autonomic dysfunction may occur simultaneously with or after onset of cognitive deficits. Extreme sensitivity to antipsychotics is typical.

Diagnosis, Prognosis, and Treatment

Diagnosis is clinical, but sensitivity and specificity are generally poor. Diagnosis is considered probable if 2 of 3 features—fluctuations in cognition, visual hallucinations, and parkinsonism—are present and possible if only one is present. Supportive evidence consists of repeated falls, syncope, and antipsychotic sensitivity. Overlap in symptoms between Lewy body dementia and Parkinson's disease may complicate diagnosis. When motor deficits of Parkinson's disease precede and are more severe than cognitive impairment, Parkinson's disease is usually diagnosed. When early cognitive impairment and behavioral disturbances predominate, Lewy body dementia is usually diagnosed.

CT and MRI show no characteristic changes but are helpful initially in ruling out other causes of dementia. Positron emission tomography with fluorine-18-labeled deoxyglucose and single-photon emission CT (SPECT) with ^{123}I-FP-CIT (N-w-fluoropropyl-2b-carbomethoxy-3b-[4-iodophenyl]-tropane), a fluoroalkyl analog of cocaine, may help identify Lewy body dementia but are not routinely done. Definitive diagnosis requires autopsy samples of brain tissue.

Lewy body dementia progresses; prognosis is poor. Treatment is generally supportive (see p. 1814). Rivastigmine 1.5 mg po bid, titrated upward as needed to 6 mg bid, may improve cognition. Other cholinesterase inhibitors may also be useful. In about ½ of patients, extrapyramidal symptoms respond to antiparkinsonian drugs (see p. 1883), but psychiatric symptoms may worsen. If such drugs are needed, levodopa is preferred.

Traditional antipsychotics, even at very low doses, tend to acutely worsen extrapyramidal symptoms and are best avoided.

HIV-Associated Dementia

HIV-associated dementia is chronic cognitive deterioration due to brain infection by HIV or opportunistic organisms.

HIV-associated dementia (AIDS dementia complex) may occur in the late stages of HIV infection. Unlike almost all other forms of dementia, it tends to occur in younger people. The dementia may result from HIV infection or from secondary infection with JC virus causing progressive multifocal leukoencephalopathy. Other opportunistic infections (eg, fungal, bacterial, viral, protozoan) may also contribute.

In purely HIV-associated dementia, subcortical pathologic changes result when infected macrophages or microglial cells infiltrate into the deep gray matter (ie, basal ganglia, thalamus) and white matter.

Prevalence of HIV dementia in late-stage HIV infection ranges from 7 to 27%, but 30 to 40% may have milder forms. Incidence is inversely proportional to $CD4^+$ count.

Symptoms and Signs

Symptoms and signs may be similar to those of other dementias (see p. 1812). Early manifestations include slowed thinking and expression, difficulty concentrating, and apathy; insight is preserved, and manifestations of depression are few. Motor movements are slowed; ataxia and weakness may be evident. Abnormal neurologic signs may include paraparesis, lower-extremity spasticity, ataxia, and extensor-plantar responses. Mania or psychosis is sometimes present.

Diagnosis, Prognosis, and Treatment

Generally, diagnosis is similar to that of other dementias (see p. 1813) except for the search for a cause.

HIV patients with untreated dementia have a worse prognosis (average life expectancy of 6 mo) than HIV patients without dementia. With treatment, cognitive impairment stabilizes, and some improvement may occur.

When a patient with HIV infection presents or when cognitive function changes acutely, lumbar puncture and CT or MRI should be done to check for CNS infection. MRI is more useful than CT because it can exclude other CNS causes of dementia (eg, toxoplasmosis, progressive multifocal leukoencephalopathy, cerebral lymphoma). Late-stage findings may include diffuse nonenhancing white matter hyperintensities, cerebral atrophy, and ventricular enlargement.

The primary treatment is highly active antiretroviral therapy, which increases $CD4^+$

counts and improves cognitive function (see p. 1635). Supportive measures are similar to those for other dementias (see p. 1814).

FRONTOTEMPORAL DEMENTIA

Frontotemporal dementia refers to sporadic hereditary disorders that affect the frontal and temporal lobes, including Pick's disease.

Frontotemporal dementia (FTD) accounts for up to 10% of dementias. Age at onset is typically younger (age 55 to 65) than in Alzheimer's disease. FTDs affect men and women about equally. Pick's disease is a variant of FTD, which may be pathologically characterized by severe atrophy, neuronal loss, gliosis, and presence of abnormal neurons (Pick cells) containing inclusions (Pick bodies).

About ½ of FTDs are inherited; most gene mutations involve tau on chromosome 17q21-22 and result in abnormalities of the microtubule-binding tau protein; thus, FTDs are considered tauopathies. Some experts classify supranuclear palsy and corticobasal degeneration with FTDs because they share similar pathology and gene mutations affecting the tau protein. Symptoms do not always correspond to the gene mutation or to pathology and vice versa. For example, the same mutation causes FTD symptoms in one family member but symptoms of corticobasal degeneration in another, and Pick's cells may be absent in patients with typical symptoms of Pick's disease.

Symptoms and Signs

Generally, FTD affects personality, behavior, and usually language function (syntax and fluency) more and memory less than does Alzheimer's disease. Abstract thinking and attention (maintaining and shifting) are impaired; responses are disorganized. Orientation is preserved, but retrieval of information may be impaired. Motor skills are generally preserved. Patients have difficulty sequencing tasks, although visual-spatial and constructional tasks are less affected.

Frontal release signs (grasp, root, suck, snout, and palmomental reflexes and glabellar sign—see pp. 1752–1753) appear late in the disease but also occur in other dementias. Some patients develop motor neuron disease with generalized muscle atrophy, weakness, fasciculations, bulbar symptoms (eg, dysphagia, dysphonia, difficulty chewing), and increased risk of aspiration pneumonia and early death.

Frontal variant FTD: Social behavior and personality change because the orbitobasal frontal lobe is affected. Patients become impulsive and lose their social inhibitions (eg, they may shoplift); they neglect personal hygiene. Some have Klüver-Bucy syndrome, which involves emotional blunting, hypersexual activity, hyperorality (eg, bulimia, sucking and smacking of lips), and visual agnosias. Impersistence (impaired concentration), inertia, and mental rigidity appear. Behavior becomes repetitive and stereotyped (eg, patients may walk to the same location every day). Patients may pick up and manipulate random objects for no reason (called utilization behavior). Verbal output is reduced; echolalia, perseveration (inappropriate repetition of a response), and eventually mutism occur.

Primary progressive aphasia: Language function deteriorates because of asymmetric (worse on left) anterolateral temporal lobe atrophy; hippocampus and memory are relatively spared. Most patients present with difficulty finding words. Attention (eg, digit span) may be severely impaired. Many patients have aphasia, with decreased fluency and difficulty comprehending language; hesitancy in speech production and dysarthria are also common. In some patients, aphasia is the only symptom for ≥ 10 yr; in others, global deficits develop within a few years.

Semantic dementia is a type of primary progressive aphasia. When the left side of the brain is affected most, the ability to comprehend words is progressively lost. Speech is fluent but lacks meaning (eg, a generic or related term is used instead of the specific name of an object). When the right side is affected most, patients have progressive anomia (inability to name objects and prosopagnosia (inability to recognize familiar faces). They cannot remember topographic relationships. Some patients with semantic dementia also have Alzheimer's disease.

Diagnosis, Prognosis, and Treatment

Diagnosis is suggested by typical clinical findings. As for other dementias, cognitive deficits are evaluated (see p. 1813). CT and MRI are done to determine location and extent of brain atrophy and to exclude other possible causes (eg, brain tumors, abscesses, stroke).

FTDs are characterized by severely atrophic, sometimes paper-thin gyri in the temporal and frontal lobes. Because MRI or CT may not show the regionally prominent cortical atrophy until late in FTD, neuroimaging may be less useful for excluding Alzheimer's disease (which affects the hippocampus and parietal lobes early), but clinical differences may help distinguish them. For example, primary progressive aphasia differs from Alzheimer's disease in that memory and visuospatial function are preserved and syntax and fluency are impaired.

FTDs usually progress gradually, but progression rate varies; if symptoms are limited to speech and language, progression to general dementia may be slower. There is no specific treatment for Pick's disease. Treatment is generally supportive (see p. 1814).

BEHAVIOR DISORDERS IN DEMENTIA

Disruptive actions are common in patients with dementia and are the primary reason for up to 50% of nursing home admissions. Actions include wandering, restlessness, yelling, throwing, hitting, refusing treatment, interrupting staff members, insomnia, and crying. Behavior disorders in dementia have not been well characterized, and their treatment is poorly understood.

Deciding what actions constitute a behavior disorder is highly subjective. Tolerability (what actions caregivers can tolerate) depends partly on the patient's living arrangements, particularly safety. For example, wandering may be tolerable if a patient lives in a safe environment (with locks and alarms on all doors and gates); however, if the patient lives in a nursing home or hospital, wandering may be intolerable because it disturbs other patients or interferes with the operation of the institution. Many behaviors (eg, wandering, repeatedly questioning, being uncooperative) are better tolerated during the day. Whether sundowning (exacerbation of disruptive behaviors at sundown or early evening) is a matter of tolerability or true diurnal variation is unknown. In nursing homes, 12 to 14% of patients with dementia have more behavior disturbances during the evening than during the day.

Etiology

Behavior disorders may result from functional changes related to dementia: Reduced ability to control behavior, misinterpretation of visual and auditory cues, impaired short-term memory (eg, patients repeatedly ask for things already received), and reduced ability or inability to express needs (eg, they wander because they are lonely, frightened, or looking for something or someone).

Patients with dementia often adapt poorly to the regimentation of institutional living. For many elderly patients with dementia, behavior disorders develop or worsen after they are moved to a more restrictive environment.

Physical problems (eg, pain, shortness of breath, urinary retention, constipation, physical abuse) can exacerbate behavior disorders partly because patients may be unable to adequately communicate. Physical problems can lead to delirium, and delirium superimposed on chronic dementia may worsen the behavior disorder.

Evaluation

The best approach is to characterize and classify the behavior, rather than to label all such behaviors agitation, a term with too many meanings to be useful. Specific behaviors, precipitating events (eg, feeding, toileting, drug administration, visits), and time the behavior started and resolved should be recorded, which helps identify changes in pattern or intensity of a behavior and makes planning a management strategy easier. If behavior changes, a physical examination should be done to exclude physical disorders and physical abuse, but environmental changes (eg, a different caregiver) should also be noted, because they, rather than a patient-related factor, may be the reason.

Psychotic behavior must be identified because management differs. Presence of delusions or hallucinations indicates psychosis. Delusions and hallucinations must be distinguished from disorientation, fearfulness, and misunderstanding, which are common among patients with dementia. Delusions without paranoia may be confused with disorientation, but delusions are usually fixed (eg, a nursing home is repeatedly called a prison), and disorientation varies (eg, a nursing home is called a prison, a restaurant, and a home).

Treatment

Management of behavior disorders in dementia is controversial and has been inadequately studied. Supportive measures are preferred; however, drugs are commonly used.

Environmental measures: The environment should be safe and flexible enough to accommodate behaviors that are not dangerous. Signs to help patients find their way and doors equipped with locks or alarms can help ensure the safety of patients who wander. Flexible sleeping hours and organization of beds can help patients with sleeping problems. Measures used to treat dementia generally also help minimize behavior disorders: providing cues about time and place, explaining care before giving it, and encouraging physical activity (see p. 1814). If an institution cannot provide an appropriate environment for a particular patient, transferring the patient to one that can may be preferable to drug treatment.

Caregiver support: Learning how dementia leads to behavior disorders and how to respond to disruptive behavior can help family members and other caregivers provide care for and cope with the patient better. Learning how to manage stress, which may be considerable, is essential.

Drugs: Drugs are used only when other approaches are ineffective and when drugs are essential for safety. The need for continued treatment should be reassessed at least every month. Drugs should be selected to target the most intolerable behaviors. Antidepressants, preferably SSRIs, should be prescribed only for patients with signs of depression.

Antipsychotics are often used even though their efficacy has been shown only in psychotic patients (see p. 1726). Other patients are unlikely to benefit and likely to experience adverse effects, particularly extrapyramidal symptoms. Tardive dyskinesia or tardive dystonia may develop; they often do not resolve when the dose is reduced or the drug withdrawn.

Choice of antipsychotic depends on relative toxicity. Of conventional antipsychotics, haloperidol is relatively nonsedating and has less potent anticholinergic effects but is most likely to cause extrapyramidal symptoms; thioridazine and thiothixene are less likely to cause extrapyramidal symptoms but are more sedating and have more anticholinergic effects than haloperidol. Second-generation (atypical) antipsychotics (eg, olanzapine, risperidone) are minimally anticholinergic and produce fewer extrapyramidal symptoms than conventional antipsychotics; however, these drugs, used for an extended period, may be associated with an increased risk of hyperglycemia and all-cause mortality. Also, risk of cerebrovascular events may be increased in elderly patients with dementia-related psychosis using these drugs.

If antipsychotics are used, they should be given in a low dose (eg, olanzapine 2.5 to 15 mg po once/day; risperidone 0.5 to 3 mg po q 12 h; haloperidol 0.5 to 1.0 mg po, IV, or IM) and for a short period.

The anticonvulsants carbamazepine, valproate, gabapentin, and lamotrigine may be useful in controlling violent outbursts. Evidence suggests that β-blockers (eg, propranolol 10 mg bid initially, slowly increased, if needed, to 40 mg bid) can be useful in some patients with violent physical outbursts. Patients should be monitored for hypotension, bradycardia, and depression.

Sedatives (eg, short-acting benzodiazepines) are sometimes used in the short term to alleviate anxiety but are not recommended in the long term.

214 SEIZURE DISORDERS

(See also Febrile Seizures on p. 2374 and Neonatal Seizure Disorders on p. 2375.)

A seizure is an abnormal, unregulated electrical discharge that occurs within the brain's cortical gray matter and transiently interrupts normal brain function. A seizure typically produces altered awareness, abnormal sensations, involuntary movements, or convulsions.

An isolated seizure can be provoked in a normal brain by reversible stressors (eg, hypoxia, hypoglycemia; in children, fever). A seizure disorder (epilepsy) is diagnosed when a patient has ≥ 2 seizures not related to reversible stressors.

TABLE 214–1. CAUSES OF SEIZURES

CONDITION	EXAMPLES
Autoimmune disorders	Cerebral vasculitis, multiple sclerosis (rarely)
Cerebral edema	Eclampsia, hypertensive encephalopathy, ventricular obstruction
Cerebral ischemia	Adams-Stokes syndrome, cerebral venous thrombosis, embolic cerebral infarcts, vasculitis
Cerebral trauma	Birth injury, skull fracture, penetrating injuries
CNS infections	AIDS, brain abscess, falciparum malaria, meningitis, neurocysticercosis, neurosyphilis, rabies, toxoplasmosis, viral encephalitis
Congenital or developmental abnormalities	Genetic disorders (eg, fifth day fits*, lipid storage diseases such as Tay-Sachs disease), neuronal migration disorders (eg, heterotopias)
Drugs	Cause seizures: Cocaine, other CNS stimulants, cyclosporine, tacrolimus, pentylenetetrazol, picrotoxin, strychnine Lower seizure threshold: Aminophylline, antidepressants, sedating antihistamines, antimalarial drugs, some antipsychotics (eg, clozapine), buspirone, fluoroquinolones, theophylline
Expanding brain lesions	Intracranial hemorrhage, tumors
Hyperpyrexia	Fever, heatstroke
Metabolic disturbances	Commonly, hypocalcemia, hypoglycemia, hyponatremia; less commonly, aminoacidurias, hyperglycemia, hypomagnesemia, hypernatremia
Pressure-related	Decompression illness, hyperbaric O_2 treatments
Withdrawal syndromes	Alcohol, anesthetics, barbiturates, benzodiazepines

*Fifth day fits (benign neonatal seizures) are tonic-clonic seizures occurring between 4 and 6 days of age in otherwise healthy infants; one form is inherited.

Etiology and Classification

Seizure disorders are considered symptomatic (ie, a symptom of a known cause such as a brain tumor or stroke—see TABLE 214–1) or idiopathic (no known cause). Idiopathic seizure disorders probably have some genetic basis.

Seizures are classified as generalized or partial. In generalized seizures, the aberrant electrical discharge diffusely involves the entire cortex of both hemispheres from the onset, and consciousness is usually lost. Generalized seizures result most often from metabolic disorders and sometimes from genetic disorders. Generalized seizures include infantile spasms and absence, tonic-clonic, atonic, and myoclonic seizures.

Partial seizures (those of focal onset) are often due to structural abnormalities. The excess neuronal discharge begins in one cerebral cortex. Partial seizures may be simple (no impairment of consciousness) or complex (reduced but not complete loss of consciousness). Partial seizures may spread and activate the entire cerebrum bilaterally, manifesting as a generalized seizure. Activation may occur so rapidly that the initial partial seizure is not clinically apparent, or a generalized seizure may follow a brief partial seizure (called secondary generalization).

Idiopathic seizure disorders generally begin between ages 2 and 14. Incidence of symptomatic seizures is highest at birth and among the elderly. Seizures before age 2 are usually caused by developmental defects, birth injuries, or metabolic disorders. Many seizures that begin in adults are secondary to

TABLE 214–2. MANIFESTATIONS OF PARTIAL SEIZURES BY SITE

FOCAL MANIFESTATION	SITE OF DYSFUNCTION
Bilateral tonic posture	Frontal lobe (supplementary motor cortex)
Simple contralateral movements (eg, limb twitching, jacksonian march)	Frontal lobe
Head and eye version with posturing	Supplementary motor cortex
Abnormal taste sensation (dysgeusia)	Insula
Visceral or autonomic (eg, epigastric aura, salivation)	Insular-orbital-frontal cortex
Olfactory hallucinations	Anteromedial temporal lobe
Chewing movements, salivation, speech arrest	Amygdala, opercular region
Complex automatic behaviorisms	Temporal lobe
Visual hallucinations (formed images)	Posterior temporal lobe or amygdala-hippocampus
Localized sensory disturbances (eg, tingling or numbness of a limb or ½ the body)	Parietal lobe (sensory cortex)
Visual hallucinations (unformed images)	Occipital lobe

cerebral trauma, alcohol withdrawal, tumors, or cerebrovascular disease; for 50% of seizures, cause is unknown. Seizure disorders in the elderly are often due to tumors or strokes. Posttraumatic seizures occur after 25 to 75% of head injuries that cause skull fractures, intracranial hemorrhages, or focal neurologic deficits.

Sometimes patients with psychiatric disorders simulate seizures (called nonepileptic seizures or pseudoseizures).

Symptoms and Signs

Seizures may be preceded by an aura of sensory or psychic manifestations (eg, smell of rotting flesh, stomach butterflies). Most seizures end spontaneously in 1 to 2 min. A postictal state may follow a seizure (most commonly, generalized) and is characterized by deep sleep, headache, confusion, and muscle soreness; this state lasts from minutes to hours. Sometimes the postictal state includes Todd's paralysis, a transient neurologic deficit on the side contralateral to the seizure focus.

Most patients appear neurologically normal between seizures, although high doses of anticonvulsants can reduce alertness. Any progressive mental deterioration is usually related to the neurologic disorder that caused the seizures rather than seizures themselves. Rarely, seizures are unremitting.

Simple partial seizures: Motor, sensory, or psychomotor symptoms occur without loss of consciousness. Specific symptoms reflect the affected area of the brain (see TABLE 214–2). In jacksonian seizures, focal motor symptoms begin in one hand, then march up the arm. Other focal seizures affect the face first, then spread to an arm and sometimes a leg. Some partial motor seizures begin with an arm raising and the head turning toward the moving arm. Some proceed to generalized convulsions.

Complex partial seizures: An aura often precedes the seizure. During the seizure, patients may stare, perform automatic purposeless movements, utter unintelligible sounds without understanding what is said, and resist assistance. Consciousness is impaired, but patients have some awareness of the environment (eg, they purposefully withdraw from noxious stimuli). Motor symptoms subside after 1 to 2 min, but confusion and disorientation may continue for another 1 or 2 min.

Patients may lash out if restrained during the seizure or while recovering consciousness after a generalized seizure. However, unprovoked aggressive behavior is unusual.

Left temporal lobe seizures may cause verbal memory abnormalities; right temporal lobe seizures may cause visual spatial memory abnormalities. Incidence of psychiatric disorders is higher in patients with a temporal lobe seizure than in the general population: 33% have psychologic difficulties, and 10% have schizophreniform or depressive psychoses.

Between seizures, many patients develop new behaviors, such as religiosity, hypergraphia (compulsion to write copiously), extreme dependence on other people, and altered sexuality.

Epilepsia partialis continua: This rare form of focal motor seizures usually involves the hand or one side of the face; seizures recur every few seconds or minutes for days to years at a time. In adults, the cause is usually a structural lesion (eg, stroke). In children, it is usually a focal cerebral cortical inflammatory process (eg, Rasmussen encephalitis), possibly caused by a chronic viral infection or autoimmune processes.

Generalized seizures: Consciousness is usually lost, and motor function is abnormal from the onset.

Infantile spasms are characterized by sudden flexion of the arms, forward flexion of the trunk, and extension of the legs. Seizures last a few seconds and recur many times a day. They occur only in the 1st 5 yr of life, then are replaced by other types of seizures. Developmental defects are usually present.

Absence seizures (formerly called petit mal) consist of 10- to 30-sec loss of consciousness with eyelid fluttering; axial muscle tone may or may not be lost. Patients do not fall or convulse; they abruptly stop activity, then just as abruptly resume it, with no postictal symptoms or knowledge that a seizure has occurred. Absence seizures are genetic and occur predominantly in children. Without treatment, such seizures are likely to occur many times a day. Seizures often occur when patients are sitting quietly, can be precipitated by hyperventilation, and rarely occur during exercise. Atypical absence seizures last longer, are accompanied by more pronounced jerking or automatic movements, and cause less complete loss of awareness. Many patients have a history of damage to the nervous system, developmental delay, and other types of seizures. Atypical absence seizures usually continue into adulthood.

Atonic seizures occur in children. They are characterized by brief, complete loss of muscle tone and consciousness. Children fall or pitch to the ground, risking trauma, particularly head injury.

Generalized tonic-clonic (sometimes called primarily generalized) seizures typically begin with an outcry; they continue with loss of consciousness and falling, followed by tonic, then clonic contractions of muscles of the extremities, trunk, and head. Urinary and fecal incontinence and frothing at the mouth sometimes occur. Seizures usually last 1 to 2 min. Secondarily generalized tonic-clonic seizures begin with a simple partial or complex partial seizure.

Myoclonic seizures are brief, lightning-like jerks of a limb, several limbs, or the trunk. They may be repetitive, leading to a tonic-clonic seizure. Unlike other seizures with bilateral motor movements, consciousness is not lost unless a generalized seizure occurs.

Juvenile myoclonic epilepsy appears during childhood or adolescence. Seizures begin with a few bilateral, synchronous myoclonic jerks, followed in 90% by generalized tonic-clonic seizures. They often occur on awakening in the morning, especially after sleep deprivation or alcohol use.

Febrile seizures occur with fever and in the absence of intracranial infection; they should be considered a type of provoked seizure. They affect about 4% of children aged 3 mo to 5 yr (see p. 2374). Benign febrile seizures are brief, solitary, and generalized tonic-clonic in appearance. Complicated febrile seizures are focal, last > 15 min, or recur ≥ 2 times in < 24 h. Overall, 2% of patients with febrile seizures develop a subsequent seizure disorder. However, incidence of seizure disorders and risk of recurrent febrile seizures are much greater among children with complicated febrile seizures, preexisting neurologic abnormalities, onset before age 1 yr, or a family history of seizure disorders.

Status epilepticus: Generalized convulsive status epilepticus is tonic-clonic seizure activity lasting > 5 to 10 min or ≥ 2 seizures between which patients do not fully regain consciousness. The previous definition of > 30 min duration was revised to encourage more prompt identification and treatment. Untreated generalized seizures lasting > 60 min may result in permanent brain damage; longer-lasting seizures may be fatal. There are many causes, including rapid withdrawal of anticonvulsants. Complex partial and absence status epilepticus often manifest as prolonged confusion.

Diagnosis

Evaluation must determine whether a seizure (vs, eg, syncope, cardiac arrhythmia, or drug overdose) occurred, then identify possible causes or precipitants. Patients with new-onset seizures are evaluated in an emergency department; they can sometimes be discharged after thorough assessment. Those with a known seizure disorder may be evaluated in a physician's office.

History: Classic seizure activity, bitten tongue, incontinence, prolonged loss of consciousness followed by confusion, or presence of aura suggests a seizure. History should include information about the 1st and subsequent seizures (eg, duration, frequency, sequential evolution, longest and shortest interval between seizures, aura, postictal state, precipitating factors). Risk factors for seizures (eg, prior head trauma or CNS infection, known neurologic disorders, drug use or withdrawal, anticonvulsant noncompliance, family history of seizures or neurologic disorders) should be identified.

Physical examination: Physical examination is almost always normal when seizures are idiopathic but may provide significant findings when seizures are symptomatic. Fever and stiff neck suggest meningitis, subarachnoid hemorrhage, or encephalitis. Papilledema suggests increased intracranial pressure. Focal neurologic defects (eg, asymmetry of reflexes or muscle strength) may indicate a structural abnormality (eg, tumor). Skin lesions may indicate a neurocutaneous disorder (eg, axillary freckling or café-au-lait spots in neurofibromatosis, hypomelanotic skin macules or shagreen patches in tuberous sclerosis).

Testing: For patients with a known seizure disorder and a normal or unchanged neurologic examination, little testing is required except for blood anticonvulsant levels, unless symptoms or signs of trauma or a metabolic disorder are present.

For patients with new-onset seizures or with a newly abnormal neurologic examination, head CT is required immediately to exclude a mass or hemorrhage. Follow-up MRI is recommended when CT is negative; it provides better resolution for brain tumors and abscesses and can detect cerebral venous thrombosis and herpes encephalitis. Laboratory tests for metabolic disorders should be done, including CBC; serum glucose, BUN, creatinine, Na, Ca, Mg, and P; and liver function tests. If meningitis or CNS infection is suspected in any patient, head CT is done, and if it is normal, a lumbar puncture is required. EEG is done; it may be needed to diagnose complex partial or absence status epilepticus. Alert and oriented patients with normal imaging and laboratory tests can undergo EEG as outpatients.

In complex partial seizures of temporal lobe origin, temporal lobe foci (spikes or slow waves) occur between seizures (interictal). In generalized-at-onset tonic-clonic seizures, interictal EEG abnormalities may manifest as symmetric bursts of sharp and slow, 4- to 7-Hz activity. In secondarily generalized seizures, the EEG may show focal electrical discharges. In absence seizures, spikes and slow-wave discharges appear at a rate of 3/sec. In juvenile myoclonic epilepsy, a 4- to 6-Hz polyspike and wave abnormality is characteristic.

However, diagnosis is clinical and cannot be excluded by a normal EEG. EEG is less likely to detect abnormalities if seizures are infrequent. Of patients ultimately confirmed to have a seizure disorder, 30% have a normal 1st EEG; a 2nd EEG done after sleep deprivation detects abnormalities in $\frac{1}{2}$. Some patients never have an abnormal EEG.

Inpatient combined video-EEG monitoring for 1 to 5 days may help determine type and frequency of seizures (eg, frontal lobe seizure vs a pseudoseizure) and guide treatment.

Prognosis and Treatment

With treatment, seizures are eliminated in $\frac{1}{3}$ of patients, and frequency of seizures is reduced by > 50% in another $\frac{1}{3}$. About 60% of patients whose seizures are well-controlled by anticonvulsants can eventually stop the drugs and remain seizure-free.

Optimal treatment is to eliminate the causes whenever possible (see elsewhere in THE MANUAL). If the cause cannot be corrected or identified, anticonvulsants are often required, particularly after a 2nd seizure; usefulness of anticonvulsants after a single seizure is controversial, and risks and benefits should be discussed with the patient.

During a seizure, injury should be prevented by loosening clothing around the neck and placing a pillow under the head. Attempting to protect the tongue is futile and likely to damage the patient's teeth or the rescuer's fingers. Patients should be rolled onto their side to prevent aspiration. These measures should be taught to the patient's family members and coworkers.

Until seizures are controlled, patients should refrain from activities in which loss of consciousness could be life threatening (eg, driving, swimming, climbing, bathing in a bathtub). After seizures are completely controlled (typically for > 6 mo), many such activities can be done if appropriate safeguards (eg, lifeguards) are used, and patients should be encouraged to lead a normal life, including exercise and social activities. In a few states, physicians must report patients with seizures to the Department of Motor Vehicles. However, most states allow automobile driving after seizures have been absent for 6 mo to 1 yr.

Cocaine and some other illicit drugs (eg, phencyclidine, amphetamines) can trigger seizures and should be avoided. Alcohol intake should be minimized. Some drugs (eg, haloperidol, phenothiazines) may lower seizure threshold and should be avoided if possible.

Family members must be taught a commonsense approach toward the patient. Overprotection should be replaced with sympathetic support that lessens negative feelings (eg, of inferiority or self-consciousness); invalidism should be prevented. Institutional care is rarely advisable and should be reserved for severely retarded patients and for patients with seizures so frequent and violent despite drug treatment that they cannot be cared for elsewhere.

Acute seizures and status epilepticus: Most seizures remit spontaneously in several minutes and do not require emergency drug treatment. Status epilepticus and most seizures lasting > 5 min require drugs to terminate the seizures, with monitoring of respiratory status. Intubation is necessary if there is any indication of airway compromise. IV access should be quickly obtained, and lorazepam 0.05 to 0.1 mg/kg IV is given at a rate of 2 mg/min. Large doses are sometimes required. However, if seizures continue after about 8 mg is given, fosphenytoin 10 to 20 PE (phenytoin equivalents)/kg IV is given at a rate of 100 to 150 PE/min; phenytoin 15 to 20 mg/kg IV at a rate of 50 mg/min is a 2nd choice. Additional seizures require an additional 5 to 10 PE/kg of fosphenytoin or 5 to 10 mg/kg of phenytoin. Persistent seizures after lorazepam and phenytoin defines refractory status epilepticus. Recommendations for a 3rd anticonvulsant vary and include phenobarbital, propofol, midazolam, and valproate. Phenobarbital 15 to 20 mg/kg IV at 100 mg/min (3 mg/kg/min in children) is given; continued seizures require another 5 to 10 mg/kg. A loading dose of valproate 10 to 15 mg/kg IV is an alternative. At this point, if status epilepticus has not abated, intubation and general anesthesia are necessary. The optimal anesthetic to use is controversial, but many physicians use propofol 15 to 20 mg/kg at 100 mg/min or pentobarbital 5 to 8 mg/kg (loading dose) followed by infusion of 2 to 4 mg/kg/h until EEG manifestations of seizure activity have been suppressed. Inhalational anesthetics are rarely used. After initial treatment, the cause for status epilepticus must be identified and treated.

Posttraumatic seizures: Prophylactic anticonvulsants are given if head injury causes skull fracture, intracranial hemorrhage, or focal neurologic deficits. These drugs reduce risk of seizures during the 1st week after injury but do not prevent permanent posttraumatic epilepsy months or years later. They should be stopped after 1 wk unless seizures occur.

Long-term treatment: No single anticonvulsant controls all types of seizures, and different patients require different drugs. Patients occasionally require multiple drugs.

The drug of choice for the particular seizure disorder is started at a relatively low dose, which is gradually increased over 1 to 2 wk to the standard therapeutic dose, based on the patient's lean body mass. Dose should be tailored to the patient's tolerance of the drug. After the target dose range is reached, trough blood drug levels are measured. If seizures continue or the blood level is subtherapeutic, the daily dose is increased by small increments. If toxicity develops before seizures are controlled, the dose is reduced to the pretoxicity dose. Then, another anticonvulsant is gradually added until seizures are controlled. Patients should be closely monitored because drug interactions can interfere with either drug's rate of metabolic degradation. The initial, ineffective anticonvulsant is then slowly tapered and eventually withdrawn completely. Use of multiple anticonvulsants should be avoided because incidence of adverse effects and drug interactions increases significantly; adding a 2nd drug helps about 10% of patients, but incidence of adverse effects more than doubles. Many drugs alter the blood level of anticonvulsants and vice versa. Physicians should be aware of all potential drug-drug interactions before prescribing a new drug.

Once seizures are controlled, the drug should be continued without interruption until patients have been seizure-free for at least 1 to 2 yr. At that time, stopping the drug should be considered. Most anticonvulsants can be tapered by 10% q 2 wk. Relapse is more likely in patients who have had a seizure disorder since childhood, require more than one anticonvulsant to be seizure-free, had seizures while taking an anticonvulsant, have partial or myoclonic seizures, have an underlying static encephalopathy, or have had an abnormal EEG within the last year. Of those who relapse, about 60% do so within 1 yr, and 80% within 2 yr. Patients who have a relapse when they are not taking anticonvulsants and those who have important social reasons for avoiding seizures should be treated indefinitely.

The most effective anticonvulsants for long-term use and their initial doses for children and adults are listed in TABLE 214–3.

TABLE 214–3. DRUGS USED IN SEIZURE DISORDERS

DRUG[a]	INDICATIONS	CHILDREN	ADULTS[b]	THERAPEUTIC	TOXIC	ADVERSE EFFECTS
Acetazolamide	Refractory absence seizures	4–15 mg/kg bid (not to exceed 1 g/day)	4–15 mg/kg bid (not to exceed 1g/day)	Not determined	> 25 µg/mL	Renal calculi, dehydration
Carbamazepine[c]	Partial seizures, generalized seizures, mixed seizures (not absence or myoclonic seizures)	< 6 yr: Tablets: 5–10 mg/kg bid Suspension: 2.5–5 mg/kg qid 6–12 yr: Tablets: 100 mg bid Suspension: 2.5 mL qid >12 yr: Tablets 200 mg bid Suspension: 5 mL qid	200–600 mg bid	4–12 µg/mL (17–51 µmol/L)	> 14 µg/mL (> 59 µmol/L)	Diplopia, dizziness, nystagmus, GI upset, dysarthria, lethargy, low WBC count (3000–4000/µL) Idiosyncratic: granulocytopenia, thrombocytopenia, liver toxicity, aplastic anemia
Clonazepam	Lennox-Gastaut syndrome (absence seizure variant), akinetic and myoclonic seizures (as monotherapy or adjunctive therapy); possibly absence seizures refractory to succinimide anticonvulsants (eg, ethosuximide)	Initially, 0.01mg/kg bid to tid (maximum: 0.05 mg/kg/day); increased by 0.25–0.5 mg q 3 days until seizures are controlled or adverse effects occur For maintenance, usually 0.03–0.06 mg/kg tid	Initially, 0.5 mg tid For maintenance, up to 5–7 mg tid; (maximum: 20 mg/day)	25 to 30 ng/mL	> 80 ng/mL	Drowsiness, ataxia, behavioral abnormalities; serious reactions rare, but partial or complete tolerance to beneficial effects usual in 1–6 mo
Ethosuximide	Absence seizures	3–6 yr: 250 mg once/day (usual maximum daily dose: 20–40 mg/kg) > 6 yr: Initially, 250 mg bid; increased by 250 mg/day as needed q 4–7 days (usual maximum daily dose: 1500 mg)	250 mg bid; increased in 250-mg increments (usual maximum daily dose: 1500 mg)	40–100 µg/mL (283–708 µmol/L)	> 100 µg/mL (> 708 µmol/L)[d]	Nausea, lethargy, dizziness, headache Idiosyncratic: leukocytopenia or pancytopenia, dermatitis, SLE

Fosphenytoin	Status epilepticus, same indications as for IV phenytoin	10–20 PE/kg IV once; maximum infusion rate: 150 mg/min (heart and BP monitoring needed at maximum rate but not at slower rates)	Same as for children	10–20 μg/mL (40–80 μmol/L)	> 25 μg/mL (> 99 μmol/L)	Ataxia, dizziness, somnolence, headache, pruritus, paresthesias
Gabapentin	≥ 12 yr: Partial seizures with and without secondarily generalized tonic-clonic seizures (as adjunctive therapy) 3 to 12 yr: Partial seizures (as adjunctive therapy)	≥ 12 yr: 300 mg tid (usual maximum dose: 1200 mg tid) 3–12 yr: 12.5–20 mg/kg bid (usual maximum dose: 50 mg/kg bid)	300 mg tid (usual maximum dose: 1200 mg tid)	Not determined	Not determined	Drowsiness, dizziness, weight gain, headache 3–12 yr: Somnolence, aggressive behavior, mood lability, hyperactivity
Lamotrigine[e]	≥ 16 yr: Partial seizures (as adjunctive therapy) ≥ 2 yr (including adults): Generalized seizures in Lennox-Gastaut syndrome (as adjunctive therapy) ≥ 16 yr (including adults): Partial or generalized seizures after withdrawal of concomitantly used enzyme-inducing anticonvulsants[f]	< 16 yr: With enzyme-inducing anticonvulsants and without valproate: Initially, 1 mg/kg bid for 2 wk, followed by 2.5 mg/kg bid for 2 wk, then 5 mg/kg bid (usual maximum daily dose: 15 mg/kg or 250 mg) With enzyme-inducing anticonvulsants and valproate: Initially, 0.1 mg/kg bid for 2 wk, followed by 0.2 mg/kg bid for 2 wk, then 0.5 mg/kg bid (usual maximum daily dose: 5 mg/kg or 250 mg) With valproate and without enzyme-inducing anticonvulsants: Initially, 0.1–0.2 mg/kg bid for 2 wk, followed by 0.1–0.25 mg/kg bid for 2 wk, then 0.25–0.5 mg/kg bid (usual	With enzyme-inducing anticonvulsants: 50 mg once/day for 2 wk, followed by 50 mg bid for 2 wk, then increased by 100 mg/day q 1–2 wk to usual maintenance dose (150–250 mg bid) With valproate (with or without enzyme-inducing anticonvulsants): 25 mg once every other day for 2 wk, followed by 25 mg once/day for 2 wk, then increased by 25–50 mg/day q 1–2 wk to usual maintenance dose (100 mg once/	No significant relationship observed between blood levels and pharmacologic effect		Commonly, headache, dizziness, drowsiness, insomnia, fatigue, nausea, vomiting, diplopia, ataxia, tremor,[g] rash (in 2–3%); rash progressing to Stevens-Johnson syndrome (in 1/50–100 children and 1/1000 adults), exacerbation of severe myoclonic epilepsy

Table continues on the following page.

TABLE 214–3. DRUGS USED IN SEIZURE DISORDERS—Continued

DRUG[a]	INDICATIONS	CHILDREN	ADULTS[b]	THERAPEUTIC	TOXIC	ADVERSE EFFECTS
Lamotrigine[e] *(continued)*		maximum daily dose: 2 mg/kg or 150 mg)	day to 200 mg bid)			
Levetiracetam	≥ 6 yr: Partial seizures (as adjunctive therapy)	250 mg bid (maximum dose: 1500 mg po bid)	500 mg bid (maximum dose: 1500 mg bid)	No significant relationship observed between blood levels and pharmacologic effect		Fatigue, weakness, muscle incoordination, mood and behavioral changes, increased risk of infection
Phenobarbital	Generalized tonic-clonic and partial seizures, status epilepticus, neonatal seizures	Newborns: 3–4 mg/kg once/day, then increased[h] Infants: 5–8 mg/kg once/day 1–5 yr: 3–5 mg/kg once/day 6–12 yr: 4–6 mg/kg once/day[i] For status epilepticus: 10–20 mg/kg (maximum dose: 100 mg/min or 2 mg/kg/min)	1.5–4 mg/kg at bedtime For status epilepticus: 15–20 mg/kg (maximum: 60 mg/min or 2 mg/kg/min)	10–40 µg/mL (43–129 µmol/L)	> 40 µg/mL (> 151 µmol/L)	Drowsiness, paradoxical hyperactivity in children, nystagmus, ataxia, learning difficulties Idiosyncratic: anemia, rash
Phenytoin	Tonic-clonic seizures, complex partial seizures, prevention of seizures secondary to neurosurgery or head trauma, convulsive status epilepticus	Newborns: Initially, 2.5 mg/kg bid (usual maintenance dose: 2.5–4 mg/kg bid) For status epilepticus: 6 mo–3 yr: 8–10 mg/kg 4–6 yr: 7.5–9 mg/kg 7–9 yr: 7–8 mg/kg 10–16 yr: 6–7 mg/kg	4–7 mg/kg at bedtime For status epilepticus: 15–20 mg/kg IV	10–20 µg/mL (40–80 µmol/L)	> 25 µg/mL (> 99 µmol/L)	Megaloblastic anemia, gingival hyperplasia, osteopenia, hirsutism, adenopathy At high blood levels: nystagmus, ataxia, dysarthria, lethargy, irritability, nausea, vomiting, confusion Idiosyncratic: rash, exfoliative dermatitis, seizure exacerbation (rare)

Primidone	Partial and generalized tonic-clonic seizures	< 8 yr: Initially, 50–125 mg at bedtime, increased by 50–125 mg/day q 3–7 days (usual maintenance dose: 3–8 mg/kg tid)	Initially, 100–125 mg at bedtime, followed by 100–125 mg bid days 4–6 and 100–125 mg tid days 7–9, then 250 mg tid	5–12 µg/mL (23–55 µmol/L)	> 15 µg/mL (> 69 µmol/L)	Same as for phenobarbital
Tiagabine	≥ 12 yr (including adults): Adjunctive therapy for partial seizures	4 mg once/day	4 mg once/day increased by 4–8 mg/day every wk to max dose of 56 mg/day (28 mg bid or 14 mg qid)	No significant relationship observed between blood levels and pharmacologic effect		Dizziness, lightheadedness, cognitive difficulties, fatigue, tremor, abdominal pain
Topiramate	≥ 2 yr (including adults): Partial-onset generalized tonic-clonic seizures	2–16 yr: 0.5–1.5 mg/kg bid (not to exceed 25 mg/day)	50 mg once/day (usual maximum dose: 200 mg bid)	5–20 µg/mL (probably)		Confusion, depression even at low doses (in 5%), anorexia, weight loss, nephrolithiasis (in 1–5%), psychosis (in 1%)
Valproate	Absence, complex absence, partial, tonic-clonic, or myoclonic seizures, juvenile myoclonic epilepsy, infantile spasms, neonatal, or febrile seizures	Initially, 5 mg/kg bid or tid, increased by 5–10 mg/kg/day at weekly intervals (usual maintenance dose: 10–20 mg/kg tid)[j] Extended-release dose is about 8–20% higher than total dose of regular form	5 mg/kg tid (started low and increased slowly, especially if other drugs are being taken; maximum dose: 20 mg/kg tid)	50–100 µg/mL (before AM dose) (347–693 µmol/L)	> 150 µg/mL (> 900 µmol/L)	Nausea and vomiting, GI intolerance, weight gain, reversible alopecia (in 5%), transient drowsiness, transient neutropenia Idiosyncratic: hyperammonemic encephalopathy Rarely, fatal hepatic necrosis in young neurologically impaired children treated with multiple anticonvulsants

Table continues on the following page.

TABLE 214–3. DRUGS USED IN SEIZURE DISORDERS—Continued

DRUG[a]	INDICATIONS	CHILDREN	ADULTS[b]	THERA-PEUTIC	TOXIC	ADVERSE EFFECTS
Zonisamide	≥ 16 yr (including adults): Partial seizures (as adjunctive therapy)	1–2 mg/kg bid	100 mg once/day to 300 mg bid	15–40 µg/mL (at > 30 µg/mL, possible increase in CNS adverse effects)	> 40 µg/mL	Sedation, fatigue, dizziness, ataxia, confusion, cognitive impairment (eg, impaired word finding), weight loss, anorexia; less commonly, depression, psychosis, urinary calculi

PE = Phenytoin equivalents.

[a]Route is po unless otherwise specified.
[b]70 kg if not weight based.
[c]Same starting dose for regular and extended-release tablets.
[d]Not well established.
[e]May have special synergistic effect when used with valproate.
[f]Metabolism of the 1st anticonvulsant increased by enzyme-inducing anticonvulsants and decreased by enzyme-inhibiting anticonvulsants.
[g]Incidence of rash reduced with slower rates of dosage escalation (especially if lamotrigine is added to valproate).
[h]Increases in dose based on clinical response and blood levels.
[i]Divided doses may be used.
[j]Possibly fewer adverse effects with extended slow-release formulation, which may improve compliance.

Once drug response is known, blood levels are less useful to follow than is the clinical course. Some patients have toxic symptoms at low levels; others tolerate high levels without symptoms. Blood drug levels are only guidelines. The appropriate dose of any anticonvulsant is the lowest dose that stops all seizures with the fewest adverse effects regardless of blood drug level.

For generalized tonic-clonic seizures, phenytoin, carbamazepine, and valproate are preferred. For adults, phenytoin can be given in divided doses or in a single dose at bedtime. If seizures continue, the total daily dose can be increased cautiously to 600 mg while trough blood levels are monitored. At a higher dose, dividing the daily dose may reduce toxic symptoms.

For partial seizures, treatment begins with carbamazepine, carbamazepine derivatives (eg, oxcarbazepine), or phenytoin. Valproate is generally less effective but may be considered. Newer drugs (eg, gabapentin, lamotrigine, tiagabine, topiramate, vigabatrin, zonisamide) appear effective, but their efficacy vs that of standard anticonvulsants has not been established.

For pure absence seizures, ethosuximide is preferred. For atypical absence seizures or absence seizures associated with other seizure types, valproate is preferred. Although clonazepam is effective, tolerance to this drug often develops. Acetazolamide is reserved for refractory cases.

Infantile spasms, atonic seizures, and myoclonic seizures are difficult to treat. Valproate is preferred, followed by clonazepam. Ethosuximide is sometimes effective, as is acetazolamide (same dosages as for absence seizures). Lamotrigine may have some benefit; it is often used with other anticonvulsants, which affect the dosage of lamotrigine. Phenytoin has limited effectiveness. For infantile spasms, corticosteroids for 8 to 10 wk are often effective. The optimal regimen is controversial. ACTH 20 to 60 units IM once/day may be used. A ketogenic diet may help but is difficult to maintain. Carbamazepine may make certain patients with primary generalized epilepsies and multiple seizure types worse.

Juvenile myoclonic epilepsy responds only to certain anticonvulsants (eg, valproate) and can be exacerbated by others (eg, carbamazepine); lifetime treatment is usually recommended.

Anticonvulsants are not recommended for febrile seizures unless a child has a subsequent seizure in the absence of febrile illness. Previously, many physicians gave anticonvulsants to children with complicated febrile seizures to prevent development of nonfebrile seizures, but this treatment does not appear effective, and long-term phenobarbital use reduces learning capacity.

Adverse effects: All anticonvulsants may cause an allergic scarlatiniform or morbilliform rash, and none is completely safe during pregnancy (see TABLE 214–3).

For patients taking carbamazepine, CBC should be monitored routinely for the 1st year of therapy. If the WBC count decreases significantly, the drug should be stopped. Dose-dependent neutropenia (ie, neutrophil count < 1000/μL) is common and, if no other anticonvulsant can be readily substituted, can be managed by decreasing the dose. Patients taking valproate should have liver function tests q 3 mo for 1 yr; if serum transaminases or ammonia levels increase significantly (> 2 times the upper limit of normal), the drug should be stopped. An increase in ammonia up to 1.5 times the upper limit of normal can be tolerated safely.

Fetal antiepileptic drug syndrome (cleft lip, cleft palate, cardiac defects, microcephaly, growth retardation, developmental delay, abnormal facies, digital hypoplasia) occurs in 4% of the children of women who take anticonvulsants during pregnancy. Among commonly used anticonvulsants, carbamazepine appears to be the least teratogenic, but only slightly so; valproate may be the most teratogenic. Yet, because uncontrolled generalized seizures during pregnancy can lead to fetal injury and death, continued treatment with anticonvulsants is generally advisable (see p. 2183). The risk should be put in perspective: Ethyl alcohol is more toxic to the developing fetus than any anticonvulsant. Folate supplements help reduce risk of neural tube defects and should be used.

Surgery: About 10 to 20% of patients have seizures that are refractory to medical treatment. For most patients whose seizures originate from a local area of abnormal brain, function improves markedly when the epileptic focus is resected. Some patients remain seizure-free, but most still require anticonvulsants. Because surgery requires extensive testing and monitoring, these patients are best treated in specialized seizure disorder centers.

Vagus nerve stimulation: Intermittent electrical stimulation of the left vagus nerve with an implanted pacemaker-like device reduces the number of partial seizures by $\frac{1}{3}$. After the device is programmed, patients can activate it with a magnet when they sense a seizure is imminent. Vagus nerve stimulation is used as an adjunct to an anticonvulsant. Adverse effects include deepening of the voice during stimulation, cough, and hoarseness. Complications are minimal. Duration of effectiveness is unclear.

215 SLEEP AND WAKEFULNESS DISORDERS

(See also Sleep Apnea on p. 499; for sleep problems in children, see p. 2241.)

Almost $\frac{1}{2}$ of all people in the US report sleep-related problems. Disordered sleep can cause emotional disturbance, memory difficulty, poor motor skills, decreased work efficiency, and increased risk of traffic accidents. It can even contribute to cardiovascular disorders and mortality.

Most commonly reported are insomnia and excessive daytime sleepiness (EDS). Insomnia is difficulty falling or staying asleep or a sensation of unrefreshing sleep. EDS is the tendency to fall asleep during normal waking hours. Insomnia and EDS are not disorders themselves but are symptoms of various sleep-related disorders (see TABLE 215–1). Parasomnias are abnormal sleep-related events.

Physiology

There are 2 types of sleep: nonrapid eye movement (NREM) and rapid eye movement (REM). Both are marked by characteristic physiologic changes.

NREM sleep constitutes about 75 to 80% of total sleep time in adults. It consists of 4 stages in increasing depth of sleep. Progression through the stages occurs cyclically 4 to 5 times a night (see FIG. 215–1). The EEG slows from 4- to 8-Hz (theta) activity in stage 1 to $\frac{1}{2}$- to 2-Hz (delta) activity in stages 3 and 4. Slow, rolling eye movements, which characterize quiet wakefulness and early stage 1 sleep, disappear in deeper sleep stages. Muscle activity decreases as well. Stages 3 and 4

TABLE 215–1. DIFFERENTIAL DIAGNOSIS OF INSOMNIA AND EXCESSIVE DAYTIME SLEEPINESS

DISORDER	INSOMNIA	EXCESSIVE DAYTIME SLEEPINESS
Inadequate sleep hygiene	√	√
Adjustment sleep disorder	√	
Psychophysiologic insomnia	√	
Physical or mental sleep disorders	√	√
Insufficient sleep syndrome		√
Drug-dependent and drug-induced sleep disorders	√	√
Obstructive sleep apnea		√
Central sleep apnea	√	
Circadian rhythm sleep disorders	√	√
Narcolepsy		√
Periodic limb movement disorder	√	√
Restless legs syndrome	√	

√ = present.

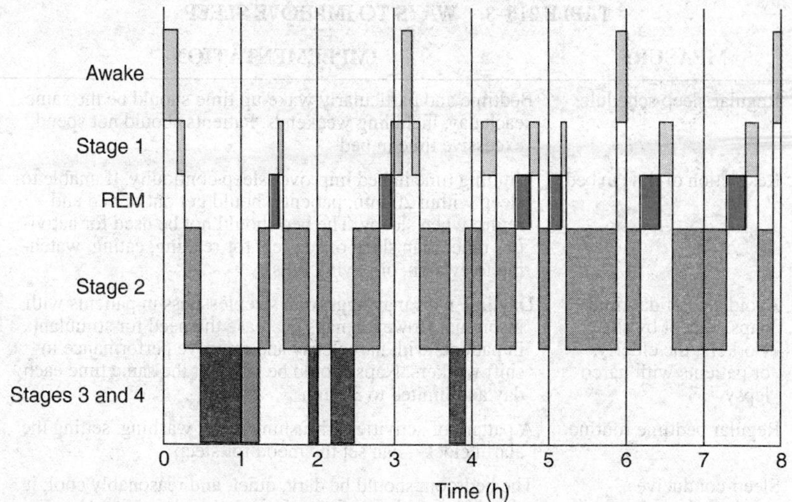

Fig. 215–1. Typical sleep pattern in young adults. Rapid eye movement (REM) sleep occurs cyclically throughout the night q 90–120 min. Stage 1 accounts for 2–5% of sleep time; stage 2, for 45–55%; stage 3, for 3–8%; stage 4, for 10–15%; and REM, for 20–25%. Brief awakenings normally occur throughout the night, especially at the end of each sleep cycle.

are referred to as deep sleep because arousal threshold is high; people perceive these stages as high-quality sleep.

REM sleep follows each cycle of NREM sleep. It is characterized by low-voltage fast activity on the EEG and postural muscle atonia. Respiration rate and depth fluctuate dramatically. Most dreams occur during REM.

Individual sleep requirements vary widely, ranging from 4 to 10 h/24 h. Infants sleep a large part of the day; with age, total sleep time and deep sleep tend to decrease, and sleep becomes more interrupted. In the elderly, stage 4 may disappear. These changes may be responsible for increasing EDS and fatigue with age, but their clinical significance is unclear.

Evaluation

History: Quality and quantity of sleep should be assessed by determining bedtime, latency of sleep (time from bedtime to falling asleep), number and time of awakenings, final morning awakening and arising times, and frequency and duration of naps. Having the patient keep a sleep log for several weeks is more accurate than questioning. Bedtime events (eg, food or alcohol consumption, physical or mental activity) should be evaluated. Intake of and withdrawal from drugs, alcohol, caffeine, and nicotine as well as level and timing of the patient's physical activity should also be included. Mental symptoms, particularly depression, anxiety, mania, and hypomania, should be recorded.

TABLE 215–2. EPWORTH SLEEPINESS SCALE

Situation
Sitting and reading
Watching TV
Sitting inactive in a public place
Riding as a car passenger for 1 h continuously
Lying down to rest in the afternoon
Sitting and talking to someone
Sitting quietly after lunch (no alcohol)
Sitting in a car stopped for a few minutes in traffic

For each situation, probability of dozing is self-rated as none (0), slight (1), moderate (2), or high (3). A score of ≥ 10 suggests abnormal daytime sleepiness.

TABLE 215–3. WAYS TO IMPROVE SLEEP

MEASURE	IMPLEMENTATION
Regular sleep schedule	Bedtime and particularly wake-up time should be the same each day, including weekends. Patients should not spend excessive time in bed
Restriction of time in bed	Limiting time in bed improves sleep continuity. If unable to sleep within 20 min, patients should get out of bed and return when sleepy. The bed should not be used for activities other than sleep or sex (eg, for reading, eating, watching television, or paying bills)
Avoidance of daytime naps, except by shift workers, the elderly, or patients with narcolepsy	Daytime naps may aggravate sleeplessness in patients with insomnia. However, naps decrease the need for stimulants in patients with narcolepsy and improve performance in shift workers. Naps should be taken at the same time each day and limited to 30 min
Regular bedtime routine	A pattern of activities—brushing teeth, washing, setting the alarm clock—can set the mood for sleep
Sleep-conducive environment	The bedroom should be dark, quiet, and reasonably cool; it should be used only for sleep and sexual activity. Heavy curtains or a sleep mask can eliminate light, and earplugs, fans, or white-noise devices can help eliminate disturbing noise
Pillows	Pillows between the knees or under the waist can increase comfort. For patients with back problems, lying supine with a large pillow under the knees can help
Regular exercise	Exercise promotes sleep and reduces stress, but if done in the late evening, it can stimulate the nervous system and interfere with falling asleep
Relaxation	Stress and worry interfere with sleep. Reading or taking a warm bath before bedtime can aid relaxation. Techniques such as visual imagery, progressive muscle relaxation, and breathing exercises can be used. Patients should not watch the clock
Avoidance of stimulants and diuretics	Drinking alcoholic or caffeinated beverages, smoking, eating caffeinated foods (eg, chocolate), taking appetite suppressants, and taking prescription diuretics—especially near bedtime—should be avoided
Bright light exposure while awake	Light exposure during the day can help rectify circadian rhythms

Difficulty falling asleep (initial insomnia) should be distinguished from difficulty maintaining sleep (sleep maintenance insomnia). The former suggests delayed sleep phase syndrome, chronic psychophysiologic insomnia, inadequate sleep hygiene, restless legs syndrome, or childhood phobias. The latter suggests advanced sleep phase syndrome, major depression, central sleep apnea syndrome, periodic limb movement disorder, or aging.

If EDS is the problem, severity should be quantified based on the propensity for falling asleep in different situations. The Epworth Sleepiness Scale (see TABLE 215–2) may be used; a cumulative score ≥ 10 represents abnormal daytime sleepiness.

Clinicians should ask about symptoms of specific sleep disorders (eg, snoring, interrupted breathing patterns, other nocturnal respiratory disturbances, restlessness in the extremities, jerking leg movements); bed partners or other family members can best identify these symptoms.

General medical history should focus on symptoms of COPD or asthma, heart failure, hyperthyroidism, gastroesophageal reflux, neurologic disorders (particularly movement and degenerative disorders), and any painful disorders (eg, RA) that may interfere with sleep.

Physical examination: The physical examination is useful mainly for identifying signs associated with obstructive sleep apnea. Signs include obesity with fat distributed around the neck or midriff; mandibular hypoplasia and retrognathia; nasal obstruction; enlarged tonsils, tongue, uvula, or soft palate; decreased pharyngeal patency; and redundant pharyngeal mucosa. The chest should be examined for expiratory wheezes and kyphoscoliosis. Signs of right ventricular failure should be noted. A thorough neurologic examination should be done.

Testing: Tests are usually done when the clinical diagnosis is in doubt or when response to initial presumptive treatment is inadequate. Patients with obvious problems (eg, poor sleep habits, transient stress, or shift work) do not require testing.

Polysomnography is particularly useful when obstructive sleep apnea, narcolepsy, or periodic limb movement disorder is suspected. This test monitors EEG, eye movements, heart rate, respirations, O_2 saturation, and muscle tone and activity during sleep. Video recording may be used to identify abnormal movements during sleep. Polysomnography is typically done in a sleep laboratory; equipment for home use has been devised but is not widely available.

The multiple sleep latency test assesses speed of sleep onset in 5 daytime nap opportunities 2 h apart. The patient lies in a darkened room and is asked to sleep. Onset and stage of sleep (including REM) are monitored by polysomnography. For the maintenance of wakefulness test, the patient is asked to stay awake in a quiet room; this test is probably a more accurate measure of sleep tendency in everyday situations. Patients with EDS typically also require laboratory tests of renal, liver, and thyroid function.

Treatment

Specific conditions are treated. Good sleep hygiene (see TABLE 215–3) is important whatever the cause and is often the only treatment patients with minor problems need.

TABLE 215–4. GUIDELINES FOR THE USE OF HYPNOTICS

Define a clear indication and treatment goal.

Prescribe the lowest effective dose.

Limit duration of use to a few weeks.

Individualize the dose for each patient.

Use lower doses when used with a CNS depressant or alcohol, in the elderly, and in patients with hepatic or renal disorders.

Avoid in patients who have sleep apnea syndrome or history of abuse and in pregnant patients.

For patients who need longer-term treatment, consider intermittent therapy.

Avoid abrupt drug discontinuation (ie, taper).

Re-evaluate drug treatment regularly; assess efficacy and adverse events.

Hypnotics: General guidelines for use of hypnotics (see TABLE 215–4) aim at minimizing abuse, misuse, and addiction.

Common hypnotics are listed in TABLE 215–5. All hypnotics act at the benzodiazepine recognition site on the γ-aminobutyric (GABA) receptor and augment the inhibitory effects of GABA. The drugs differ primarily in elimination half-life and onset of action. Drugs with a short half-life are used for sleep-onset insomnia. Drugs with a longer half-life are needed for sleep-maintenance insomnia; they have greater potential for daytime carryover effects, especially after prolonged use or in the elderly. Patients who experience daytime sedation, incoordination, or other daytime effects should avoid activities requiring alertness (eg, driving), and the dose should be reduced, the drug stopped, or, if needed, another drug used. Other adverse effects include amnesia, hallucinations, incoordination, and falls.

Hypnotics should be used cautiously in patients with pulmonary insufficiency. In the elderly, any hypnotic, even in small doses, can cause restlessness, excitement, or exacerbation of delirium and dementia.

Prolonged use is discouraged because tolerance can develop (see p. 1692) and because abrupt discontinuation can cause rebound insomnia or even anxiety, tremor, and seizures. These effects are more common with benzodiazepines (particularly triazolam). Difficulties can be minimized by using the lowest

TABLE 215–5. ORAL HYPNOTICS IN COMMON USE

DRUG	HALF LIFE* (h)	DOSE (mg)†	COMMENTS
Benzodiazepines			
Flurazepam	40–250	15–30	High risk of next-day residual sedation; not recommended for the elderly
Quazepam	40–250	7.5–15	High lipophilicity, which may mitigate residual sedation in 1st 7–10 days of continuous use
Estazolam	10–24	0.5–2	Effective for sleep induction and maintenance
Temazepam	8–22	7.5–15	Longest latency for sleep induction
Triazolam	< 6	0.125–0.5	May cause anterograde amnesia; high likelihood of tolerance and rebound after repeated use
Imidazopyridine			
Zolpidem	2.5	5–10	Effective for sleep induction and maintenance
Pyrazolopyrimadine			
Zaleplon	1	5–20	Ultrashort-acting; can be given for initial insomnia or after nocturnal awakening (minimum of 4 h from arising); when given at normal bedtime, least likely to have residual effects

*Includes parent and active metabolites.
†Dose given at bedtime.

effective dose for brief periods and by tapering the dose before stopping the drug (see also p. 1693). A new intermediate-acting hypnotic, eszopiclone (nightly dose of 1 to 3 mg), does not appear to produce tolerance with prolonged use (up to 6 mo) or withdrawal symptoms.

Other sedatives: Many drugs not specifically indicated for insomnia are used to induce and maintain sleep.

Alcohol is widely used but is a poor choice because, after prolonged use and at higher doses, it produces unrefreshing, disturbed sleep with frequent nocturnal awakenings, often increasing daytime sleepiness. Alcohol can also further impair respiration during sleep in patients with obstructive sleep apnea.

OTC antihistamines (eg, doxylamine, diphenhydramine) can often induce sleep. However, efficacy is unpredictable, and these drugs have adverse effects such as daytime sedation, confusion, and systemic anticholinergic effects, which are particularly worrisome in the elderly.

Low doses of some antidepressants at bedtime may improve sleep: eg, doxepin 25 to 50 mg, trazodone 50 mg, trimipramine 75 to 200 mg, and paroxetine 5 to 20 mg. However, they should be used mainly when standard hypnotics are not tolerated (rare) or depression is present.

Melatonin is a hormone secreted by the pineal gland. Darkness stimulates secretion, and light inhibits it. By binding with melatonin receptors in the suprachiasmatic nucleus, melatonin mediates circadian rhythm, especially in physiologic sleep onset. Oral melatonin (typically 0.5 to 5 mg at bedtime) may be effective for sleep problems due to shift work, jet lag, or blindness; delayed sleep phase syndrome; and sleep fragmentation in the elderly. It must be taken at the appropriate time (when endogenous melatonin is normally secreted); taken at the wrong time, it can aggravate sleep problems. Its efficacy is unproved, and it appears to stimulate coronary artery disease in animals. Available preparations of melatonin are unregulated, so content and purity cannot be assured, and the effects of long-term use are unknown. Its use should be supervised by a physician. Melatonin occurs naturally in some foods.

CIRCADIAN RHYTHM SLEEP DISORDERS

Circadian rhythm sleep disorders are desynchronization between internal and environmental sleep-wake rhythms. Patients typically have insomnia, excessive daytime

sleepiness, or both, which typically resolve as the body clock realigns itself. Diagnosis is clinical. Treatment depends on the cause.

Circadian rhythm disorders may result from external changes (eg, jet lag, shift work) or from an internal misalignment of the body clock with the day/night cycle (eg, delayed or advanced sleep phase syndrome).

Desynchronization of sleep due to external changes also alters other circadian body rhythms, including temperature and hormone secretion; in addition to insomnia and sleepiness, these alterations may cause nausea, malaise, irritability, and depression. Repetitive circadian shifts (eg, frequent long-distance travel, rotating shift work) are particularly difficult. Symptoms resolve over several days as rhythms readjust. Because light is the strongest determinant of circadian rhythm, exposure to bright light (sunlight or artificial light of 5,000 to 10,000 lux intensity) after desired awakening time speeds readjustment. Melatonin may be tried (see p. 1838).

Patients with circadian rhythm disorders often misuse alcohol, hypnotics, and stimulants.

Time zone change (jet lag) syndrome: This syndrome is caused by rapid travel across >2 time zones. Eastward travel (advancing the sleep cycle) causes more severe symptoms than westward travel (delaying sleep).

If possible, travelers should gradually shift their sleep-wake schedule before travel to approximate that of their destination and maximize exposure to daylight (particularly in the morning) in the new locale. Short-acting hypnotics or wake-promoting drugs (eg, modafinil) may be used for brief periods after arrival.

Shift work sleep disorder: Severity of symptoms is proportional to the frequency of shift changes, the magnitude of each change, and the frequency of counterclockwise (sleep-advancing) changes. Fixed-shift work (ie, full-time night or evening) is preferable; rotating shifts should go clockwise (ie, day to evening to night). However, even fixed-shift workers have difficulties because daytime noise and light interfere with sleep quality, and workers often shorten sleep times to participate in social or family events.

Shift workers should maximize their exposure to bright light (sunlight or, for night workers, artificial light) at times when they should be awake and ensure that the bedroom is as dark and quiet as possible during sleep. Sleep masks and white-noise devices are helpful. When symptoms persist and interfere with functioning, judicious use of hypnotics with a short half-life and wake-promoting drugs is appropriate.

Altered sleep phase syndromes: In these syndromes, patients have normal sleep quality and duration with a 24-h circadian rhythm cycle, but the cycle is out of synch with desired or necessary wake times. Less commonly, the cycle is not 24 h, and patients awaken and sleep earlier or later each day. If able to follow their natural cycle, patients have no symptoms.

Patients with delayed sleep phase syndrome consistently go to sleep and awaken late (eg, 3 AM and 10 AM). This pattern is more common during adolescence. If required to awaken earlier for work or school, EDS results; patients often present because of poor school performance or missed morning classes. They can be distinguished from people who stay up late by choice because they cannot fall asleep earlier even if they try. Mild phase delay (<3 h) is treated by progressive earlier arising plus morning bright light therapy, perhaps with melatonin at desired bedtime.

Advanced sleep phase syndrome (early to bed and early to rise) is more common among the elderly and responds to treatment with bright light in the evening.

INSOMNIA AND EXCESSIVE DAYTIME SLEEPINESS

Sleep disorders may manifest with insomnia or excessive daytime sleepiness (EDS).

Inadequate sleep hygiene: Sleep is impaired by certain behaviors. They include consumption of caffeine or sympathomimetic or other stimulant drugs (typically near bedtime, but even in the afternoon for people who are particularly sensitive), late evening exercise or excitement (eg, a thrilling TV show), and an irregular sleep-wake schedule. Patients who compensate for lost sleep by sleeping late or by napping fragment nocturnal sleep further. Insomniacs should adhere to a regular awakening time and avoid naps regardless of the amount of nocturnal sleep. Adequate sleep hygiene measures are important (see TABLE 215–3).

Adjustment sleep disorder: Acute emotional stressors (eg, job loss, hospitalization) can cause insomnia. Symptoms typically remit shortly after the stressors abate; insomnia is usually transient and brief. Nevertheless, if daytime sleepiness and fatigue develop, especially if they interfere with daytime functioning, short-term treatment with hypnotics is warranted. Persistent anxiety may require specific treatment.

Psychophysiologic insomnia: Insomnia, regardless of cause, may persist well beyond resolution of precipitating factors. The main reason is usually anticipatory anxiety about the prospect of another sleepless night followed by another day of fatigue. Patients often spend hours in bed focusing on and brooding about their sleeplessness. Patients typically have greater difficulty falling asleep in their own bedroom than falling asleep away from home.

Optimal treatment combines behavioral strategies and drugs. Although behavioral strategies are more difficult to implement and take longer, effects are longer lasting. Behavioral strategies include sleep hygiene, education, relaxation training, stimulus control, and cognitive therapy. Hypnotics are suitable for patients who need rapid relief and whose insomnia has had daytime effects such as EDS and fatigue. These drugs must not be used indefinitely.

Physical sleep disorders: Physical disorders may interfere with sleep and cause EDS. Disorders that cause pain or discomfort (eg, arthritis, cancer, herniated disks), particularly those that worsen with motion, cause transient awakenings and poor sleep quality. Treatment is directed at the underlying disorder and relief of symptoms (eg, with bedtime analgesics).

Mental sleep disorders: Most major mental disorders are associated with EDS and insomnia, which are reported by 90% of patients with major depression. Conversely, 60 to 69% of chronic insomniacs have a major mental disorder, most commonly a mood disorder.

Patients with depression may have initial sleeplessness or sleep maintenance insomnia. Sometimes in bipolar disorder and seasonal affective disorder, sleep is uninterrupted, but patients complain of unrelenting daytime sleepiness.

If depression is accompanied by sleeplessness, antidepressants that provide more sedation (eg, amitriptyline, doxepin, mirtazapine, nefazodone, trazodone) may be chosen. These drugs are used at regular, not low, doses to ensure correction of the depression.

If depression is accompanied by EDS, antidepressants with activating qualities, such as bupropion, venlafaxine, or SSRIs (eg, fluoxetine, sertraline) may be chosen.

Insufficient sleep syndrome (sleep deprivation): Patients with this syndrome do not sleep enough at night (for various social or employment reasons) to stay alert when awake. This syndrome is probably the most common cause of EDS, which disappears when sleep time is increased (eg, on weekends or vacations).

Drug-related sleep disorders: Insomnia and EDS can result from chronic use of CNS stimulants (eg, amphetamines, caffeine), hypnotics (eg, benzodiazepines), other sedatives, antimetabolite chemotherapy, anticonvulsants (eg, phenytoin), oral contraceptives, methyldopa, propranolol, alcohol, and thyroid hormone preparations. Insomnia can also develop during withdrawal of CNS depressants (eg, barbiturates, opioids, sedatives), tricyclic antidepressants, monoamine oxidase inhibitors, or illicit drugs (eg, cocaine, heroin, marijuana, phencyclidine). Commonly prescribed hypnotics can disrupt REM sleep, causing irritability and apathy and reducing mental alertness. Abrupt withdrawal of hypnotics and sedatives can cause nervousness, tremors, and seizures. Many psychoactive drugs can induce abnormal movements during sleep.

NARCOLEPSY

Narcolepsy is characterized by excessive daytime sleepiness, often with sudden loss of muscle tone (cataplexy), sleep paralysis, and hypnagogic phenomena. Diagnosis is by polysomnography and a multiple sleep latency test. Treatment is with modafinil or various stimulants.

The cause is unknown. Narcolepsy is strongly associated with specific HLA haplotypes, and children of patients with narcolepsy have a 40-fold increased risk, suggesting a genetic cause. However, concordance in twins is low (25%), suggesting a prominent role for environmental factors, which often trigger the disorder. The neuropeptide hypocretin-1 is deficient in CSF of narcoleptic animals and most human patients, suggesting that the cause may be HLA-associated autoimmune destruction of hypocretin-containing neurons in the lateral hypothalamus. Narcolepsy is equally common in both sexes.

Narcolepsy features dysregulation of the timing and control of REM sleep. Therefore, REM sleep intrudes into wakefulness and into the transition from wakefulness to sleep. Many symptoms of narcolepsy result from postural muscle paralysis and vivid dreaming, which characterize REM.

Symptoms and Signs

The main symptoms are excessive daytime sleepiness (EDS), cataplexy, hypnagogic hallucinations, and sleep paralysis; about 10% of patients have all 4. Many patients also have disturbed nocturnal sleep. Symptoms usually begin in adolescents or young adults without prior illness, although onset can be precipitated by an illness, stressor, or period of sleep deprivation. Once established, narcolepsy persists throughout life; life span is unaffected.

EDS can occur anytime. Sleep episodes vary from few to many per day, and each may last minutes or hours. Patients can resist the desire to sleep only temporarily but can be roused as readily as from normal sleep. Sleep tends to occur during monotonous conditions (eg, reading, watching television, attending meetings) but may also occur during complex tasks (eg, driving, speaking, writing, eating). Patients may also experience sleep attacks—episodes of sleep that strike without warning. Patients may feel refreshed when they awaken yet fall asleep again in a few minutes. Nighttime sleep may be unsatisfying and interrupted by vivid, frightening dreams. Consequences include low productivity, breaches in interpersonal relationships, poor concentration, low motivation, depression, a dramatic reduction in quality of life, and potential for physical injury (particularly due to motor vehicle collisions).

Cataplexy is momentary muscular weakness or paralysis without loss of consciousness evoked by sudden emotional reactions, such as mirth, anger, fear, joy, or, often, surprise. Weakness may be confined to the limbs (eg, patients may drop the rod when a fish strikes their line) or may cause a limp fall during hearty laughter (as in "weak with laughter") or sudden anger. These attacks resemble the loss of muscle tone that occurs during REM sleep. Cataplexy occurs in about ¾ of patients.

Sleep paralysis is momentary inability to move when just falling asleep or immediately after awakening. These occasional episodes may be very frightening. They resemble the motor inhibition that accompanies REM sleep. Sleep paralysis occurs in about ¼ of patients but also in some healthy children and, less commonly, in healthy adults.

Hypnagogic phenomena are particularly vivid auditory or visual illusions or hallucinations that may occur when just falling asleep or, less often, immediately after awakening. They are difficult to distinguish from intense reverie and are somewhat similar to vivid dreams, which are normal in REM sleep. Hypnagogic phenomena occur in about ⅓ of patients, are common among healthy young children, and occasionally occur in healthy adults.

Diagnosis

A delay of 10 yr from onset to diagnosis is common. A history of cataplexy strongly suggests narcolepsy in patients with EDS. Nocturnal polysomnography, followed by multiple sleep latency testing (MSLT), is diagnostic. Findings include REM episodes during at least 2 of 5 daytime nap opportunities, an average sleep latency (time to fall asleep) of ≤5 min, and no other diagnostic abnormalities on nocturnal polysomnography. The maintenance of wakefulness test does not help with diagnosis but does help monitor treatment efficacy.

Other disorders that can cause chronic hypersomnia are usually suggested by the history and physical examination; brain imaging and blood and urine tests can confirm the diagnosis. These disorders include space-occupying lesions affecting the hypothalamus or upper brain stem, increased intracranial pressure, and certain forms of encephalitis. Hypothyroidism, hyperglycemia, hypoglycemia, anemia, uremia, hypercapnia, hypercalcemia, hepatic failure, seizure disorders, and multiple sclerosis can also cause hypersomnia. Acute, relatively brief hypersomnia commonly accompanies acute systemic disorders such as influenza.

The Kleine-Levin syndrome, a very rare disorder in adolescent boys, produces episodic hypersomnia and hyperphagia. Etiology is unclear but may be an autoimmune response to an infection.

Treatment

Patients who have occasional episodes of sleep paralysis or hypnagogic phenomena and mild EDS may need no treatment. For others, stimulant drugs are used. Patients should also get enough sleep at night and take brief naps (< 30 min) at the same time every day (typically afternoon).

Patients with mild to moderate sleepiness benefit from modafinil, a long-acting wake-promoting drug. Its mechanism of action is unclear, but it is not a stimulant. Typically, modafinil 100 to 200 mg po is given in the morning. Dose is increased to 400 mg as needed, but some patients require considerably more. If effects do not last into the evening, a small 2nd dose (eg, 100 mg) at noon or 1 PM may be used, although this dose sometimes interferes with nocturnal sleep. Adverse effects include nausea and headache, which are mitigated by lower initial doses and slower titration.

Patients who do not respond to modafinil are usually given amphetamine derivatives instead of or with modafinil. Methylphenidate 5 mg po bid to 20 mg po tid may be most effective and is especially useful for immediate management because modafinil's onset is delayed. Methamphetamine 5 to 20 mg po bid or dextroamphetamine 5 mg po bid to 20 mg po tid may be used; all are available in long-acting preparations and therefore can be dosed once/day in many patients. Adverse effects include agitation, hypertension, tachycardia, and mood changes (eg, manic reactions); abuse potential is high. Pemoline, although less addictive than amphetamines, is rarely used because it may be hepatotoxic and liver enzymes must be monitored q 2 wk. The anorexiant mazindol (2 to 8 mg po once/day in the morning) can be used.

Tricyclic antidepressants (particularly imipramine, clomipramine, and protriptyline) and monoamine oxidase inhibitors are useful in treating cataplexy, sleep paralysis, and hypnagogic phenomena. Clomipramine 25 to 150 mg po once/day in the morning seems to be the most potent anticataplectic but should be taken only during the day to reduce nocturnal arousal. The newest anticataplectic, Na oxybate, is given 2.75 to 4.5 g po twice during the night. Its use is highly controlled because of the potential for illicit use.

Idiopathic Hypersomnia

Idiopathic hypersomnia is an increase in nocturnal sleep hours plus EDS; it is differentiated from narcolepsy by lack of cataplexy, hypnagogic hallucinations, and sleep paralysis.

Diagnosis is by exclusion; polysomnography shows long nocturnal sleep without evidence of other sleep pathology. MSLT shows short sleep latencies without REM periods. Treatment is similar to that of narcolepsy, except that anticataplectic drugs are unnecessary.

PARASOMNIAS

Parasomnias are behavioral disturbances that occur during sleep. They are most common among children and adolescents and sometimes disappear by adulthood. Diagnosis is clinical. Treatment may include drugs and psychotherapy.

Somnambulism is sitting, walking, or other complex behavior during sleep, usually with the eyes open but without evidence of recognition. It is most common during late childhood and adolescence and occurs just after NREM stage 3 and 4 sleep. Prior sleep deprivation and poor sleep hygiene increase the likelihood of these episodes, and risk is higher for 1st-degree relatives. Patients may mumble repetitiously, and some injure themselves on obstacles or stairs. There is no accompanying dream. Usually, patients do not remember the episode. Treatment is directed at protecting patients from injury. It includes using electronic alarms to awaken patients when they leave the bed, using a low bed, and removing obstacles from the bedroom. Benzodiazepines, particularly clonazepam 0.5 to 2 mg po, at bedtime may help.

Night terrors are fearful, screaming, flailing episodes often accompanied by sleepwalking. They are more common among children and occur during NREM stages 3 and 4 sleep; thus, they do not represent nightmares. In adults, night terrors are often associated with mental difficulties or alcoholism. Intermediate- or long-acting benzodiazepines (eg, clonazepam 1 to 2 mg po, diazepam 2 to 5 mg po) at bedtime may help.

Nightmares (frightening dreams) affect children more frequently than adults. They occur during REM sleep, more commonly when fever or excess fatigue is present or after alcohol has been ingested. Treatment is directed at any underlying mental distress.

REM sleep behavior disorder is verbalization (sometimes profane) and often violent movements (eg, waving the arms, punching, kicking) during REM sleep. These behaviors may represent acting out dreams by patients who, for unknown reasons, do not have the atonia normally present during REM sleep. This disorder is more common among the elderly, particularly those with CNS degenerative disorders (eg, Parkinson's or Alzheimer's disease, vascular dementia, olivopontocerebellar degeneration, multiple system atrophy, progressive supranuclear palsy). It can also occur in narcolepsy and with use of norepinephrine reuptake inhibitors (eg, atomoxetine, reboxetine). Polysomnography may detect excessive motor activity during REM; audiovisual monitoring may detect abnormal body movements and vocalizations. Treatment is with clonazepam 0.5 to 2 mg po at bedtime. Bed partners should be warned about the possibility of harm.

Nocturnal leg cramps of the calf or foot muscles commonly occur in otherwise healthy middle-aged and elderly patients during sleep. Diagnosis is based on the history and lack of physical signs or disability. Prevention includes stretching the affected muscles for several minutes before sleep. Stretching as soon as cramps occur relieves symptoms promptly and is preferable to drug treatment. Numerous drugs (eg, quinine, Ca and Mg supplements, diphenhydramine, benzodiazepines, mexiletine) have been used; none is likely to be effective, and adverse effects may be significant (particularly with quinine and mexiletine). Avoiding caffeine and other sympathetic stimulants may help.

PERIODIC LIMB MOVEMENT DISORDER AND RESTLESS LEGS SYNDROME

These disorders are characterized by abnormal motions of and sometimes sensations in the legs, which interfere with sleep.

Periodic limb movement disorder (PLMD) and restless legs syndrome (RLS) are more common during middle and older age. The mechanism is unclear but may involve abnormalities in dopamine neurotransmission in the CNS. The disorders can occur in isolation or during drug withdrawal, with intake of stimulants or certain antidepressants, or in chronic renal and hepatic failure, pregnancy, anemia, and other disorders.

PLMD is characterized by repetitive (usually q 20 to 40 sec) twitching or kicking of the lower extremities during sleep. Patients usually complain of interrupted nocturnal sleep or excessive daytime sleepiness. They are typically unaware of the movements and brief arousals that follow and have no abnormal sensations in the extremities.

In RLS, patients complain of a creeping or crawling sensation in the lower extremities when reclining. To relieve symptoms, patients move the affected extremity by stretching, kicking, or walking. As a result, they have difficulty falling asleep, repeated nocturnal awakenings, or both.

Diagnosis may be suggested by the patient's or bed partner's history but, if not, is usually apparent on sleep studies. Patients with either disorder should be evaluated medically (eg, with blood tests for anemia and iron deficiency—see p. 1033—and hepatic and renal function tests).

Numerous drugs are used (including dopaminergic drugs, benzodiazepines, anticonvulsants, and vitamins and minerals), although none is specific for PLMD or RLS.

Dopaminergic drugs, although often effective, may have adverse effects such as augmentation (symptoms are felt later in the day), rebound (symptoms worsen after stopping the drug), nausea, and insomnia. Two D_2 and D_3 dopamine agonists, pramipexole and ropinirole, are effective and have few adverse effects. Pramipexole 0.125 mg is given 2 h before onset of severe symptoms and increased, as needed, by 0.125 mg every 2 nights until symptoms are relieved (maximum dose 4 mg). Augmentation is less frequent with pramipexole than with levadopa. Ropinerole 0.5 mg is given 2 h before symptoms occur and is increased, as needed, by 0.25 mg nightly (maximum dose 3 mg).

Benzodiazepines may improve sleep continuity but do not reduce limb movements; they should be used cautiously to avoid tolerance and daytime sleepiness. Gabapentin beginning with 300 mg at bedtime can help when RLS is accompanied by pain; dose is increased by 300 mg weekly, maximum dose 2700 mg. Opioids may also work but are used as a last resort because of tolerance, adverse effects, and abuse potential.

216 HEADACHE

Headache is one the most common reasons patients seek medical attention. Most patients with recurrent, episodic headaches have a primary headache disorder (ie, not associated with a demonstrable structural abnormality). These disorders include migraine (with or without aura), cluster headache (episodic or chronic), tension-type headache (episodic or chronic), chronic paroxysmal hemicrania, and hemicrania continua. Patients with new-onset, persistent headache may have a secondary headache disorder, due to various intracranial, extracranial, and systemic disorders (see TABLE 216–1 and elsewhere in THE MANUAL).

TABLE 216–1. CAUSES OF SECONDARY HEADACHE

CAUSE	EXAMPLES
Extracranial disorders	Carotid or vertebral artery dissection Cervical spine disorders CSF leak with low-pressure headache Dental disorders (infection, temporomandibular joint dysfunction) Glaucoma Sinusitis
Intracranial disorders	Brain tumors and mass lesions Chiari type I malformation Hemorrhage (intracerebral, subdural, subarachnoid) Idiopathic intracranial hypertension Infections (eg, cerebritis, encephalitis, meningitis) Obstructive hydrocephalus Vascular disorders (eg, moyamoya disease, vascular malformations, vasculitis, venous sinus thrombosis)
Systemic disorders	Accelerated hypertension Bacteremia Fever Hypercapnia Hypoxia (including altitude sickness) Viremia
Drugs and toxins	Analgesic rebound Caffeine withdrawal Hormones (eg, estrogen) Nitrates Proton pump inhibitors

Evaluation

History and physical examination usually suggest a diagnosis and guide subsequent testing.

History: Headache characteristics helpful in diagnosis include age at onset; frequency, duration, location, and severity of the headache; factors associated with initiation, exacerbation, or remission; accompanying symptoms (eg, fever, stiff neck, nausea, vomiting, mental status changes, photophobia); and preceding conditions (ie, head trauma, cancer, immunosuppression).

Recurrent episodic, severe headache with onset in adolescence or early adulthood suggests a primary headache disorder. Sudden-onset, very severe (thunderclap) headache suggests possible subarachnoid hemorrhage. A subacute, progressively worsening daily headache suggests a space-occupying lesion. Headache with onset after age 50 and accompanied by scalp tenderness, jaw claudication, or visual changes suggests temporal arteritis.

Confusion, seizure, fever, or focal neurologic symptoms suggest a serious cause requiring further evaluation.

History of a coexisting disorder may suggest the cause of headache; eg, recent head trauma, hemophilia, alcoholism, or anticoagulant therapy may suggest subdural hematoma.

Physical examination: A neurologic examination (see p. 1748), including ophthalmoscopy, mental status examination, and evaluation for meningeal signs, is necessary. Recurring episodic headaches in a patient who appears well and has a normal neurologic examination rarely have an ominous cause.

Neck stiffness with flexion (but not rotation) indicates meningeal irritation due to infection or subarachnoid hemorrhage; fever suggests infection, but low-grade fever may occur with hemorrhage. Tenderness on palpation of the temporal arteries in patients > 50 suggests temporal arteritis. Papilledema indicates increased intracranial pressure, which may be due to idiopathic intracranial hypertension, accelerated hypertension, a mass lesion, or sagittal sinus thrombosis. Focal neurologic symptoms or mental status changes typically accompany structural lesions (eg, tumor, stroke, abscess, hematoma).

Testing: Imaging and laboratory tests are necessary only if history or examination findings are worrisome or abnormal.

Patients requiring very urgent CT or MRI to look for hemorrhage, increased intracranial pressure, and other structural causes of headache include those with

- Sudden-onset thunderclap headache
- Altered mental status, including seizure
- Focal neurologic deficits
- Papilledema
- Severe hypertension

Because an unremarkable CT scan does not entirely rule out subarachnoid hemorrhage, meningitis, encephalitis, or inflammatory processes, lumbar puncture is indicated when these disorders are suspected.

Patients requiring prompt but not immediate imaging include those with a change in prior headache pattern, new onset of headache after age 50, systemic symptoms (eg, weight loss), secondary risk factors (eg, cancer, HIV, head trauma), or chronic unexplained headache. For these patients, MRI (typically using gadolinium with magnetic resonance angiography or venography) is preferred; it can show many unusual but important causes of headache that can be missed on CT (eg, carotid dissection, cerebral vein thrombosis, pituitary apoplexy, vascular malformations, cerebral vasculitis, Chiari type I malformation).

Patients with unusual, persistent headaches may also require lumbar puncture to check for chronic meningitis (eg, infectious, granulomatous, neoplastic) and idiopathic intracranial hypertension (assessed by CSF pressure).

Other tests are used if specific disorders are suspected (eg, ESR for temporal arteritis, intraocular pressure measurement for glaucoma, dental x-rays for tooth abscess).

CLUSTER HEADACHE

Cluster headaches cause excruciating, unilateral periorbital or temporal pain, with ipsilateral autonomic symptoms (ptosis, lacrimation, rhinorrhea, nasal congestion). Diagnosis is clinical. Acute treatment is with O_2, triptans, ergotamine, or a combination. Prevention is with verapamil, methysergide, lithium, valproate, or a combination.

Cluster headache affects primarily men, typically beginning at age 20 to 40; prevalence in the US is 0.4%. Usually, cluster headache is episodic; for 1 to 3 mo, patients experience ≥ 1 attack/day, followed by remission for months to years. Some patients have cluster headaches without remission.

Pathophysiology is unknown, but the periodicity suggests hypothalamic dysfunction. Alcohol intake triggers cluster headache during the attack period but not during remission.

Symptoms, Signs, and Diagnosis

Symptoms are distinctive. Attacks usually occur at the same time each day, often awakening patients from sleep in the middle of the night. Pain is always unilateral in an orbitotemporal distribution. It is excruciating, peaking within minutes; it usually subsides spontaneously within 30 min to 1 h. Cluster headache patients are agitated, restlessly pacing the floor, unlike migraine patients who prefer to lie quietly in a darkened room.

Autonomic features, including nasal congestion, rhinorrhea, lacrimation, facial flushing, and Horner's syndrome, are prominent, occurring on the same side as the headache.

Diagnosis is based on the distinctive symptom pattern and exclusion of intracranial pathology.

Other unilateral primary headache syndromes with autonomic symptoms include chronic paroxysmal hemicrania, in which attacks are more frequent (> 5/day) and much briefer (usually just minutes) than in cluster headache; and hemicrania continua, characterized by moderately continuous unilateral head pain with superimposed brief episodes of more intense pain. These 2 painful disorders, unlike cluster headache and migraine, respond dramatically to indomethacin, but not to other NSAIDs.

Treatment

Acute attacks of cluster headache can be aborted with injections of a triptan or dihydroergotamine (see TABLE 216–2) or 100% O_2 inhalation. All patients require preventive drugs because cluster headache is frequent, severe, and incapacitating. Prednisone (eg, 60 mg po once/day) can provide prompt temporary prevention while preventive drugs with slower onset of action (eg, verapamil, lithium, methysergide, valproate, topiramate) are initiated.

TABLE 216–2. DRUGS FOR MIGRAINE AND CLUSTER HEADACHES

DRUG	DOSAGE	COMMENTS
Preventive		
Amitriptyline	10–100 mg po at bedtime	Has anticholinergic effects; causes weight gain; helpful for patients with insomnia; small doses often effective
β-Blockers	Atenolol 25–100 mg po once/day Metoprolol 50–200 mg po once/day Nadolol 20–160 mg po once/day Propranolol 20–160 mg po bid Timolol 5–20 mg po once/day	β-Blockers without intrinsic sympathomimetic activity are used; they should be avoided in patients with bradycardia, hypotension, or asthma
Divalproex	Regular-release: 250–500 mg po bid Extended-release: 500–1000 mg po once/day	Alopecia, GI upset, hepatic dysfunction, thrombocytopenia, tremor, weight gain
Topiramate	50–200 mg po usually once/day	Weight loss, cognitive adverse effects (eg, confusion, depression)
Verapamil*	240 mg once/day to tid	Hypotension, constipation; most useful for patients with basilar artery migraine
Migraine-specific		
Dihydroergotamine	0.5–1 mg sc or IV 4 mg/mL nasal spray	Nausea; contraindicated in patients with hypertension or coronary artery disease; cannot be used concurrently with triptans
Triptans	Almotriptan 12.5 mg po Eletriptan 20–40 mg po Frovatriptan 2.5 mg po Naratriptan 2.5 mg po Rizatriptan 10 mg po Sumatriptan 50–100 mg po, 5–20 mg nasal spray, or 6 mg sc Zolmitriptan 2.5–5 mg po or 5 mg nasal spray	Flushing, paresthesias, sense of pressure in chest or throat; can repeat doses up to 3 times/day if headache recurs; contraindicated in patients with coronary artery disease or uncontrolled hypertension

*Generally used in the regular-release formulation.

IDIOPATHIC INTRACRANIAL HYPERTENSION

(Benign Intracranial Hypertension; Pseudotumor Cerebri)

Idiopathic intracranial hypertension involves increased intracranial pressure without a mass lesion or hydrocephalus; CSF composition is normal.

Idiopathic intracranial hypertension usually occurs in women of childbearing age. Incidence is 1/100,000 in normal-weight women but 20/100,000 in obese women. Intracranial pressure is markedly elevated (> 250 mm H_2O); the cause is unknown but may involve obstruction of cerebral venous outflow.

Symptoms and Signs

Almost all patients have daily or near daily generalized headache of fluctuating intensity,

TABLE 216–3. CONDITIONS ASSOCIATED WITH PAPILLEDEMA AND IDIOPATHIC INTRACRANIAL HYPERTENSION

CONDITION	EXAMPLES
Obstruction of cerebral venous drainage	Cerebral venous sinus thrombosis Jugular vein thrombosis
Disorders	Addison's disease COPD Hypoparathyroidism Iron deficiency anemia if severe Menstrual changes (menarche, irregular menses, pregnancy) Renal failure Right ventricular heart failure with pulmonary hypertension Sleep apnea
Drugs	Anabolic steroids Corticosteroid withdrawal after prolonged use Growth hormone in deficient patients Nalidixic acid and nitrofurantoin Tetracycline and tetracycline derivatives Vitamin A in large doses

at times with nausea. They may also have transient obscuration of vision, diplopia (due to 6th cranial nerve dysfunction), and pulsatile intracranial tinnitus. Vision loss begins peripherally and may not be noticed by the patient until late in the course. Permanent vision loss is the main danger.

Bilateral papilledema is almost always present. A few patients are asymptomatic but have papilledema discovered during routine ophthalmoscopic examination. Neurologic examination may detect partial 6th cranial nerve palsy but is otherwise unremarkable.

Diagnosis and Treatment

Diagnosis is suspected clinically and established by normal brain imaging (preferably MRI with magnetic resonance venography) and lumbar puncture showing elevated opening pressure and normal CSF composition. Rarely, certain drugs and disorders can cause a clinical picture resembling idiopathic intracranial hypertension (see TABLE 216–3).

Treatment is aimed at reducing pressure and relieving symptoms with serial lumbar punctures and diuretics (eg, acetazolamide 250 mg po qid). Headache may respond to NSAIDs or drugs used for migraine. Obese patients should be encouraged to lose weight. If vision loss occurs despite serial lumbar punctures and drug treatment, optic nerve sheath fenestration or lumboperitoneal shunting may be indicated.

Frequent ophthalmologic assessment (including quantitative visual fields) is required to monitor response to treatment; merely testing visual acuity is not sensitive enough to warn of impending vision loss.

MIGRAINE

Migraine is a chronic, episodic primary headache. Symptoms typically last 4 to 72 h and may be severe. Pain is often but not always unilateral, throbbing, worse with exertion, and accompanied by autonomic symptoms (eg, nausea; sensitivity to light, sound, or odors). Fortification spectra and other transient focal neurologic deficits occur in a few patients, usually just before the headache. Diagnosis is clinical. Treatment is with serotonin 1B,1D receptor agonists, antiemetics, and analgesics. Preventive regimens include lifestyle modifications (eg, of sleeping habits or diet) and drugs (eg, β-blockers, amitriptyline, valproate, topiramate).

Epidemiology and Pathophysiology

Migraine is the most common cause of recurrent moderate to severe headache; lifetime prevalence is 18% for women and 6% for men in the US. It most commonly begins during puberty or young adulthood, waxing and waning in frequency and severity over the ensuing years and usually diminishing after age 50. Studies show familial aggregation of migraine.

Migraine is thought to be a neurovascular pain syndrome with altered central neuronal processing (activation of brain stem nuclei, cortical hyperexcitability, and spreading cortical depression) and involvement of the trigeminovascular system (triggering neuropeptide release, which produces painful inflammation in cranial vessels and the dura mater).

The triggering mechanism for specific attacks is often unclear. However, many potential migraine triggers have been identified; they include drinking red wine, skipping meals, excessive afferent stimuli (eg, flashing lights, strong odors), weather changes, sleep deprivation, stress, and hormonal factors. Head trauma, neck pain, or temporomandibular joint dysfunction sometimes triggers or exacerbates migraine.

Fluctuating estrogen levels are a potent migraine trigger. Many women have onset of migraine at menarche, severe attacks during menstruation (menstrual migraine), and worsening during menopause. For most women, migraines remit during pregnancy (but sometimes there is an exacerbation during the 1st or 2nd trimester). Oral contraceptives and other hormone therapy occasionally trigger or worsen migraine and have been associated with stroke in women who have migraine with aura.

Symptoms and Signs

In some patients, some migraine attacks are preceded or accompanied by a neurologic aura (prodrome) lasting minutes to an hour (migraine with aura). Most commonly, auras involve visual symptoms (fortification spectra—eg, binocular flashes, arcs of scintillating lights, bright zigzags, scotomata). Paresthesias and numbness (typically starting in one hand and marching to the ipsilateral arm and face), speech disturbances, and transient brain stem–thalamic dysfunction are less common than visual auras. Some patients have attacks of migraine aura with little or no headache.

Pain varies from moderate to severe, and attacks last from hours to days, typically resolving with sleep. The pain can be bilateral or unilateral, most often in a frontotemporal distribution, and is described as aching, squeezing, or sometimes throbbing.

Migraine is more than a headache. Autonomic symptoms such as nausea (and occasionally vomiting), photophobia, sonophobia, and osmophobia are prominent. Patients report difficulty concentrating during attacks. Routine physical activity usually aggravates migraine headache; this effect, plus the photophobia and sonophobia, encourages most patients to lie in a dark, quiet room during attacks. Severe attacks can be incapacitating, disrupting family and work life.

Attacks vary significantly in frequency and severity. Many patients have several types of headache, including milder attacks without nausea or photophobia; these attacks may resemble tension headache.

Rare forms of migraine include basilar artery migraine, with combinations of vertigo, ataxia, visual field loss, sensory disturbances, focal weakness, and altered level of consciousness. Abdominal migraine (periodic syndrome), which affects children with a family history of migraine, is characterized by 2-h bouts of abdominal pain, flushing or pallor, nausea, and vomiting. These children often develop typical migraines later in life.

Diagnosis

Diagnosis is based on characteristic symptoms and a normal physical (including neurologic) examination. Typical cases without worrisome findings (see p. 1845) do not require CNS imaging.

Common diagnostic errors include not realizing that migraine often causes bilateral pain and is not always described as throbbing. Autonomic and visual symptoms of migraine often lead to a misdiagnosis of sinus headache or eyestrain. A dangerous error is to assume that any headache in patients known to have migraine represents another migraine attack. A thunderclap headache or change in the previous headache pattern may indicate a new, potentially serious disorder.

In older patients, migraine with aura can be mistaken for a transient ischemic attack, especially when the aura occurs without headache. In younger patients, several unusual disorders can mimic migraine with aura: dissection of the carotid or vertebral artery, antiphospholipid antibody syndrome, cerebral vasculitis, moyamoya disease, CADASIL (cerebral autosomal dominant arteriopathy with subcortical infarcts and leukoencephalopathy), and MELAS (mitochondrial encephalopathy, lactic acidosis, and strokelike episodes) syndrome.

Prognosis and Treatment

For some patients, migraine is an infrequent, tolerable inconvenience. For others, it is a devastating malady resulting in frequent periods of incapacity, loss of productivity, and severely impaired quality of life. Consequently, treatment is stratified based on frequency, duration, and severity of attacks. A thorough explanation of the disorder helps patients understand that although migraine cannot be cured, it can be controlled, enabling them to better participate in treatment.

Patients are urged to keep a written head-
che diary to document the number and tim-
ng of attacks, possible triggers, and response
o treatment. Identified triggers are eliminated
vhen possible. Behavioral interventions (bio-
eedback, stress management, psychotherapy)
re used when stress is a major trigger or when
nalgesics are being overused.

Acute migraine headache: Mild to mod-
rate attacks are treated with NSAIDs or ace-
aminophen. Analgesics containing opioids,
affeine, or butalbital are helpful for infre-
uent, mild attacks but are prone to being over-
sed, sometimes leading to rebound headache
nd daily headache syndrome.

In patients whose mild attacks often evolve
nto incapacitating migraine or whose attacks
re severe from the onset, triptans are used.
riptans are selective serotonin 1B, 1D recep-
or agonists. They are not analgesic per se but
pecifically block the release of vasoactive
europeptides that trigger migraine pain.
riptans are most effective when taken at the
nset of attacks. They are available in oral, in-
ranasal, and sc forms (see TABLE 216–2); sc
orms are more effective but have more ad-
erse effects. Combining a triptan with an
ntiemetic at the onset of attacks is effective
vhen nausea is prominent.

IV dihydroergotamine with a dopamine
ntagonist antiemetic (eg, metoclopramide
0 mg IV, prochlorperazine 5 to 10 mg IV) is
elpful for aborting very severe, persistent at-
acks. The antiemetic alone may relieve mild
ttacks.

Triptans and dihydroergotamine can cause
oronary artery constriction and are thus con-
raindicated in patients with coronary artery
isease or uncontrolled hypertension; they
nust be used with caution in older patients
nd in patients with vascular risk factors.

A good response to dihydroergotamine or
triptan should not be interpreted as diagnos-
c for migraine because these drugs may re-
eve headache due to subarachnoid hemor-
hage and other structural abnormalities.

Opioids should be a last resort (rescue
rug) for severe headache when other mea-
ures are ineffective.

revention

Daily preventive therapy is warranted when
requent migraines interfere with activity de-
pite acute treatment. For patients who use an-
lgesics frequently, particularly those with re-
ound headache, preventive drugs (see TABLE
16–2) should be combined with a program for stopping overused analgesics. Choice of drug can be guided by coexisting disorders: eg, a small bedtime dose of amitriptyline for patients with depression or insomnia; a β-blocker for patients with hypertension or coronary artery disease; or topiramate, which can induce weight loss, for obese patients.

Periodic injections of small doses of botulinum toxin into the scalp reduces the number and severity of migraine attacks in some patients unresponsive to other preventive treatments.

POST–LUMBAR PUNCTURE AND LOW-PRESSURE HEADACHE

Headache can result from reduction in CSF volume and pressure due to lumbar puncture or spontaneous CSF leaks.

Removal of CSF by lumbar puncture (LP) reduces CSF volume and pressure, as do spontaneous CSF leaks (eg, from arachnoid cysts along the spinal canal, which may rupture with coughing or sneezing). Head elevation with sitting up or with standing stretches the pain-sensitive basal meninges, causing headache. Headaches are intense, postural, and often accompanied by neck pain, meningismus, and vomiting. Headache is alleviated only by lying completely flat.

Headache after LP is common, usually occurring hours to a day or 2 afterward, and can be debilitating. Younger patients with small body mass are at greatest risk. Using smaller, noncutting needles decreases risk. The amount of CSF removed and duration of recumbency after LP do not affect incidence.

Post-LP headache is clinically obvious and testing is rarely used; other low-pressure headaches may require imaging. If obtained, brain MRI with gadolinium often shows diffuse enhancement of the pachymeninges and, in severe cases, downward sagging of the brain. CSF pressure is typically low or unobtainable if patients have been upright for any length of time (gravity accelerates CSF loss).

The 1st line of treatment is recumbency, hydration, an elastic abdominal binder, mild analgesics, and caffeine. If post-LP headache persists after a day of such treatment, an epidural blood patch (injection of a few mL of the patient's clotted venous blood into the lumbar epidural space) is usually effective. Spontaneous CSF leaks rarely require surgical closure.

TENSION-TYPE HEADACHE

Tension-type headache produces mild generalized pain without the incapacity, nausea, or photophobia associated with migraine.

Episodic tension-type headache is common; most patients obtain relief with OTC analgesics and do not seek medical attention. Many patients with frequent tension-type headache also have migraine; in many, tension-type headache is a forme fruste of migraine. Depression, sleep disturbances, and anxiety disorders are often also present in patients with frequent tension-type headaches.

Chronic tension-type headaches cause very frequent or continuous mild pain that lasts hours to days. Sometimes described as viselike, these headaches originate in the occipital or bifrontal region and spread over the entire head. Tension-type headaches are typically absent when patients awaken and worsen as the day progresses.

Diagnosis is based on characteristics of the headache and a normal physical (including neurologic) examination. Potential triggers for chronic tension-type headache (eg, sleep disorders, stress, temporomandibular joint dysfunction, neck pain, eyestrain) should be evaluated and treated.

Drugs used to prevent migraine, particularly amitriptyline, can help prevent chronic tension-type headache. Because patients with these headaches commonly overuse analgesics, behavioral and psychologic interventions (eg, relaxation and stress management techniques) are important.

217 BRAIN INFECTIONS

Inflammation of the brain (encephalitis) is usually secondary to viral infection. Other brain infections include brain abscesses, helminthic infections, prion diseases, and subdural empyema. Meningitis (inflammation of the brain and spinal cord—see p. 1858), cytomegalovirus infection (see p. 1605), and HIV infection (see p. 1625) can also affect the brain. Slow virus infections, such as progressive multifocal leukoencephalopathy (see p. 1855), are characterized by long incubations and a prolonged course. They may be caused by the JC virus, the measles virus, or the rubella virus (see p. 1646).

BRAIN ABSCESS

A brain abscess is an intracerebral collection of pus. Symptoms may include headache, lethargy, fever, and focal neurologic deficits. Diagnosis is by contrast-enhanced CT or MRI and sometimes culture. Treatment is with antibiotics and usually surgical drainage.

A brain abscess can result from direct extension of cranial infections (eg, osteomyelitis, mastoiditis, sinusitis, subdural empyema), penetrating head wounds (including neurosurgical procedures), hematogenous spread (eg, in bacterial endocarditis, congenital heart disease with right-to-left shunt, IV drug abuse), or unknown causes.

The bacteria involved are usually anaerobic and sometimes mixed, often including anaerobic streptococci or *Bacteroides*. Staphylococci are common after cranial trauma, neurosurgery, or endocarditis. Enterobacteriaceae are common with an ear source. Fungi (eg, *Aspergillus*) and protozoa (eg, *Toxoplasma gondii*, particularly in HIV-infected patients) can cause abscesses.

An abscess forms when an area of cerebral inflammation becomes necrotic and encapsulated by glial cells and fibroblasts. Edema around the abscess may increase intracranial pressure.

Symptoms, Signs, and Diagnosis

Symptoms result from increased intracranial pressure and mass effect. Headache, nausea, vomiting, lethargy, seizures, personality changes, papilledema, and focal neurologic deficits develop over days to weeks. Fever, chills, and leukocytosis may develop before the infection is encapsulated, then subside.

When symptoms suggest an abscess, contrast-enhanced CT or MRI is done. An abscess appears as an edematous mass with ring enhancement, which may be difficult to distinguish from a tumor or occasionally infarction; culture and drainage may be necessary. Lumbar puncture is not done because it may precipitate transtentorial herniation and because CSF findings are nonspecific (see TABLE 206–1 on p. 1756).

Treatment

All patients receive antibiotics for ≥ 4 to 8 wk. Initial empiric antibiotics include cefotaxime 2 g IV q 4 h or ceftriaxone 2 g IV q 12 h; both are effective against streptococci, Enterobacteriaceae, and most anaerobes but not against *Bacteroides fragilis,* which requires metronidazole 7.5 mg/kg IV q 6 h. If *Staphylococcus aureus* is suspected, vancomycin 1 g q 12 h is used until sensitivity to nafcillin (2 g q 4 h) is determined. Response to antibiotics is best monitored by serial CT or MRI. Drainage, stereotactic or open, provides optimal therapy and is necessary for most abscesses that are solitary and surgically accessible, particularly those > 2 cm in diameter. Patients with increased intracranial pressure may benefit from a short course of high-dose corticosteroids. Anticonvulsants are sometimes recommended to prevent seizures.

ENCEPHALITIS

Encephalitis is inflammation of the parenchyma of the brain, resulting from direct viral invasion or hypersensitivity initiated by a virus or another foreign protein. Encephalomyelitis is the same process but involves the brain and spinal cord. These disorders can be caused by many viruses. Symptoms include fever, headache, and altered mental status, often accompanied by seizures or focal neurologic deficits. Diagnosis requires CSF analysis and neuroimaging. Treatment is supportive and, for certain causes, includes antiviral drugs.

Etiology and Pathophysiology

Encephalitis may be a primary manifestation or a secondary complication of viral infection. Viruses causing primary encephalitis may be epidemic (eg, arbovirus, poliovirus, echovirus, coxsackievirus) or sporadic (eg, herpes simplex, rabies, varicella-zoster, or mumps virus). Mosquito-borne arboviral encephalitides infect people during the summer and early fall when the weather is warm. Incidence in the US varies from 150 to > 4000 cases yearly, mostly in children. Most cases occur during epidemics. Among arboviruses, La Crosse virus (California virus) is identified as a cause primarily in the north central US. However, the virus is geographically widespread, and La Crosse encephalitis probably is underrecognized and accounts for most cases of arbovirus encephalitis in children. Mortality rate is probably < 1%. Until 1975, St. Louis encephalitis occurred every 10 yr, mostly in the central and eastern US; it is now rare. As of 2003, West Nile encephalitis has spread from the East Coast, where it first appeared in 1999, to all but a few western states. Mortality rate is about 9%. Small epidemics of eastern equine encephalitis occur every 10 to 20 yr in the eastern US, mainly among young children and people > 55. Mortality rate is about 50 to 70%. For unknown reasons, western equine encephalitis has largely disappeared from the US since 1988.

In the US, the most common sporadic encephalitis is caused by herpes simplex virus (HSV); hundreds to several thousand cases occur yearly. Most are due to HSV type 1, but HSV type 2 may be more common among immunocompromised patients. HSV encephalitis occurs at any time of the year, tends to affect patients < 20 or > 40 yr, and is often fatal if untreated.

Primary encephalitis can occur as a late consequence of a viral infection. The best known types are HIV encephalopathy, which causes dementia (see p. 1819), and subacute sclerosing panencephalitis (see p. 1649), which occurs years after a measles infection. The mechanism is probably reactivation of the original infection.

Encephalitis can occur as a secondary immunologic complication of certain viral infections or vaccinations. Inflammatory demyelination of the brain and spinal cord can occur 1 to 3 wk later (as acute disseminated encephalomyelitis); the immune system attacks one or more CNS antigens that resemble proteins of the infectious agent. The most common causes used to be measles, rubella, chickenpox, and mumps (all now uncommon because childhood vaccination is widespread); smallpox vaccine; and live-virus vaccines (eg, the older rabies vaccines prepared from sheep or goat brain). In the US, most cases now result from influenza A or B virus, enteroviruses, Epstein-Barr virus, hepatitis A or B virus, or HIV.

In acute encephalitis, cerebral edema and petechial hemorrhages occur throughout the hemispheres, brain stem, cerebellum, and, occasionally, spinal cord. Direct viral invasion of the brain usually damages neurons, sometimes with visible inclusion bodies. Severe infection, particularly untreated HSV encephalitis, can produce brain hemorrhagic necrosis. Acute disseminated encephalomyelitis is characterized by perivenous demyelination and absence of virus in the brain.

Symptoms and Signs

Symptoms include fever, headache, and altered mental status, often accompanied by seizures and focal neurologic deficits. A GI or respiratory prodrome may precede these symptoms. Meningeal signs are typically mild and less prominent than other manifestations. Status epilepticus, particularly convulsive status epilepticus, or coma suggests severe brain inflammation and a poor prognosis.

Diagnosis

Encephalitis is suspected in patients with unexplained alterations in mental status. Clinical presentation and differential diagnoses may suggest certain diagnostic tests, but MRI and CSF analysis (including PCR for HSV) are usually done, sometimes with other tests to identify the causative virus. MRI is sensitive for early HSV encephalitis, showing edema in the orbitofrontal and temporal areas, which HSV typically infects. MRI can also exclude lesions that mimic viral encephalitis (eg, brain abscess, sagittal sinus thrombosis). CT is much less sensitive than MRI for HSV but can help because it is rapidly available and can exclude disorders that make lumbar puncture risky (eg, mass lesions, hydrocephalus, cerebral edema). If encephalitis is present, CSF is characterized by lymphocytic pleocytosis, normal glucose, mildly elevated protein, and an absence of pathogens using Gram stain and culture (similar to CSF in aseptic meningitis). CSF abnormalities may not develop until 8 to 24 h after onset of symptoms. Hemorrhagic necrosis can introduce many RBCs and some neutrophils into CSF, elevate protein, and modestly lower glucose.

PCR for HSV in CSF is sensitive and specific. However, results may not be available rapidly. CSF viral cultures grow enteroviruses but not most other viruses. Paired acute and convalescent serologic tests of CSF and blood must be drawn several weeks apart; they can detect an increase in viral titers specific for certain viral infections. Despite extensive testing, the cause of most cases of encephalitis remains unknown. Brain biopsy may be indicated for patients who are worsening, who are responding poorly to treatment with acyclovir or another antimicrobial, or who have a lesion that is still undiagnosed.

Prognosis and Treatment

Mortality rate varies with cause, but severity of epidemics due to the same virus varies during different years. Permanent neurologic deficits are more likely to occur in infants.

If HSV encephalitis is suspected, acyclovir 10 mg/kg IV q 8 h is started promptly and continued usually for 14 days. Acyclovir is relatively nontoxic but can cause liver function abnormalities, bone marrow suppression, and transient renal failure. Giving acyclovir IV slowly over 1 h helps prevent nephrotoxicity.

Supportive therapy includes treatment of fever, dehydration, electrolyte disorders, and seizures. Euvolemia should be maintained.

HELMINTHIC INFECTIONS

Parasitic helminthic worms infect the CNS of millions of people in developing countries. Infected people who visit or immigrate to nonendemic areas, including the US, may present there. Worms may produce meningitis, encephalitis, cerebral masses, hydrocephalus, stroke, and myelopathy.

Neurocysticercosis (see also p. 1563): Among about 20 helminths that can cause neurologic disorders, the pork tapeworm *Taenia solium* causes by far the most cases in the Western Hemisphere. The resulting disorder is neurocysticercosis. After a person eats food contaminated with the worm's eggs, larvae migrate to tissues, including the brain, spinal cord, and CSF pathways, and form cysts. Cyst diameter rarely exceeds 1 cm in neural parenchyma but may exceed 5 cm in CSF spaces. Brain parenchymal cysts cause few symptoms until death of the worms triggers local inflammation, gliosis, and edema, causing seizures (most commonly), cognitive or focal neurologic deficits, or personality changes. Larger cysts in CSF pathways may cause obstructive hydrocephalus. Cysts may rupture into CSF, inducing subacute eosinophilic meningitis. Mortality rate for symptomatic neurocysticercosis is up to 50%.

Neurocysticercosis is suspected in patients who come from developing countries and who have eosinophilic meningitis or unexplained seizures, cognitive or focal deficits, or personality changes. It is suggested by multiple calcified cystic lesions seen on CT or MRI; a contrast agent may enhance the lesions. Diagnosis requires serum and CSF serologic tests and occasionally cyst biopsy.

Albendazole (7.5 mg/kg po q 12 h for 8 to 30 days; maximum daily dose, 800 mg) is the antimicrobial of choice. Alternatively, praziquantel 20 to 33 mg/kg po tid may be given for 30 days. Dexamethasone 8 mg once/day IV or po for the 1st 2 to 4 days may lessen the acute inflammatory response as the worms die. Short- or long-term anticonvulsant treatment may be required. Surgical excision of cysts and ventricular shunts may also be required.

Other infections: In schistosomiasis (see p. 1558), necrotizing eosinophilic granulomas develop in the brain, causing seizures, increased intracranial pressure, and diffuse and focal neurologic deficits. Large, solitary echinococcal cysts (see Echinococcosis on p. 1561) can cause focal deficits and, occasionally, seizures. Coenurosis, caused by tapeworm larvae, usually produces grapelike cysts that may obstruct CSF outflow in the 4th ventricle. Gnathostomiasis, a rare infection, results in necrotic tracts surrounded by inflammation along nerve roots, spinal cord, and brain or in subarachnoid hemorrhage, causing low-grade fever, stiff neck, photophobia, headache, migratory neurologic deficits (occasionally, affecting the 6th or 7th cranial nerve), and paralysis.

PRION DISEASES

(Transmissible Spongiform Encephalopathies)

Prion diseases are progressive, fatal, and untreatable degenerative brain disorders. They include Creutzfeldt-Jakob disease (CJD, the prototypic example), Gerstmann-Sträussler-Scheinker syndrome (GSS), fatal insomnia (FI), variant CJD (vCJD), and kuru. Prion diseases usually occur sporadically, with a worldwide annual incidence of about 1/1 million.

Prion diseases result from misfolding of a normal brain protein called prion protein (PrP), whose exact function is unknown. Misfolded prion proteins (or prions) induce previously normal PrP to misfold and are markedly resistant to degeneration (similar to β-amyloid, which they resemble), resulting in slow but inexorable proliferation. Gradual accumulation of prions causes gliosis and characteristic histologic vacuolar (spongiform) changes, resulting in dementia and other neurologic deficits. Symptoms and signs develop months to years after exposure.

Prion diseases can be caused by spontaneous or hereditary defects of the PrP gene, contained in the short arm of chromosome 20. Some defects cause familial CJD, some GSS, and others FI. Small abnormalities in particular codons may determine the predominant symptoms and rate of disease progression.

Prion diseases can also be transmitted by infected tissue. Cannibalism caused the spread of kuru in New Guinea, and prions can be transmitted via organ transplants. Prion diseases can be transmitted between species via the food chain (eg, in vCJD). Prion diseases occur in mink, elk, deer, domestic sheep and cattle, and other mammals. In several Western US states and Canada, chronic wasting disease of elk and deer, a prion disease, is a concern; whether this disease can be transmitted to people who hunt, butcher, or eat affected animals is unknown.

Prion diseases should be considered in all patients with dementia. Treatment of prion diseases is symptomatic. Prions resist standard disinfection techniques and pose risks to surgeons, pathologists, and technicians who handle contaminated tissues and instruments.

CREUTZFELDT-JAKOB DISEASE

Creutzfeldt-Jakob disease is a sporadic or familial prion disease. Bovine spongiform encephalopathy (mad cow disease) is a variant form. Symptoms include dementia, myoclonus, and other CNS deficits; death occurs in 1 to 2 yr. Transmission can be prevented by taking precautions when handling infected tissues and using bleach to clean contaminated instruments. Treatment is supportive.

CJD typically affects people > 40 yr (median, about 60 yr). It occurs worldwide; incidence is higher among Northern African Jews. Most cases are sporadic, but 5 to 15% are familial, with autosomal dominant transmission. In the familial form, age at onset is earlier and duration of disease is longer. CJD can be transmitted iatrogenically (eg, after cadaveric corneal or dural transplants, use of stereotactic intracerebral electrodes, or use of growth hormone prepared from human pituitary glands).

vCJD is most common in the United Kingdom (UK). In the early 1980s, because of relaxed regulations for processing animal by-products, tissue from sheep infected with scrapie, a prion disease, was introduced into cattle feed. Thousands of cattle developed bovine spongiform encephalopathy (BSE), called mad cow disease. Some people who ate meat from affected cattle developed vCJD.

Because the incubation period in BSE is long, a connection between BSE and contaminated feed was not recognized in the UK until BSE had become an epidemic, which was controlled by massive slaughter of cattle. In the UK, the annual number of cases of vCJD between 2000 and 2002 has ranged from 17 to 28. Whether incidence is decreasing is unclear. Although vCJD has been restricted to the UK and Europe thus far, BSE has been reported in North American cattle.

Symptoms, Signs, and Prognosis

About 70% of patients present with memory loss and confusion, which eventually occur in all patients; 15 to 20% present with incoordination and ataxia, which often develop early in the disease. Myoclonus provoked by noise or other sensory stimuli (startle myoclonus) often develops in the middle to late stages of disease. Although dementia, ataxia, and myoclonus are most characteristic, other neurologic abnormalities (eg, hallucinations, seizures, neuropathy, various movement disorders) can occur. Ocular disturbances (eg, visual field defects, diplopia, dimness or blurring of vision, visual agnosia) are common. Death typically occurs after 6 to 12 mo, commonly due to pneumonia. vCJD develops at a younger average age than in sporadic CJD, and life expectancy is longer (averaging 1.5 yr).

Diagnosis and Prevention

CJD should be considered in elderly patients with rapidly progressive dementia, especially if accompanied by myoclonus or ataxia; however, CNS vasculitis, hyperthyroidism, and bismuth intoxication must be excluded. vCJD is considered in younger patients who have ingested processed beef in the UK; Wilson's disease should be excluded.

Diagnosis may be difficult. MRI may show cerebral atrophy. Diffusion-weighted MRI may show basal ganglia and cortical abnormalities. CSF is typically normal, but characteristic 14-3-3 protein is often detected. EEG may show characteristic periodic sharp waves. Brain biopsy is usually unnecessary.

Workers handling fluids and tissues from patients suspected of having CJD must wear gloves and avoid mucous membrane exposure. Contaminated skin can be disinfected by 5 to 10 min of exposure to 4% Na hydroxide, followed by extensive washing with water. Steam autoclaving of materials at 132° C for 1 h or immersion in 4% Na hydroxide or 10% Na hypochlorite solution for 1 h is recommended. Standard methods of sterilization (eg, exposure to formalin) are ineffective.

Gerstmann-Sträussler-Scheinker Disease

GSS disease is an autosomal dominant prion brain disease that begins in middle age.

GSS occurs worldwide and is similar to but about 100-fold less common than CJD. It develops at an earlier age (40 vs 60 yr), and average life expectancy is longer (5 yr vs 6 mo).

Patients have cerebellar dysfunction with unsteady gait, dysarthria, and nystagmus. Gaze palsies, deafness, dementia, parkinsonism, hyporeflexia, and extensor plantar responses are also common. Myoclonus is much less common than in CJD. GSS disease should be considered in patients with characteristic symptoms and signs and a family history, particularly if they are ≤ 45 yr. Genetic testing can confirm the diagnosis.

Fatal Insomnia

Fatal insomnia is a typically hereditary prion disorder causing difficulty sleeping, motor dysfunction, and death.

FI, a very rare disease, usually results from an autosomal dominant mutation, but several sporadic cases have been identified. Average age at onset is 40 yr (ranging from the late 30s to the early 60s).

Common early symptoms include difficulty falling asleep and intermittent motor dysfunction (eg, myoclonus, spastic paresis). This stage can last for months but eventually progresses to severe insomnia, myoclonus, sympathetic hyperactivity (eg, hypertension, tachycardia, hyperthermia, sweating), and dementia. Death occurs in an average of 13 mo.

FI should be considered in patients with motor dysfunction, sleep disturbances, and a amily history. Genetic testing can confirm he diagnosis.

PROGRESSIVE MULTIFOCAL LEUKOENCEPHALOPATHY

Progressive multifocal leukoencephalopathy is a slow virus infection that usually occurs in patients with impaired cell-mediated immunity. It produces subacute and progressive CNS demyelination, multifocal neurologic deficits, and death, usually within a year. Diagnosis is with contrast-enhanced CT or MRI plus CSF PCR. Treatment is supportive.

Progressive multifocal leukoencephalopathy (PML) is probably caused by reactivation of the JC virus, a ubiquitous human papovavirus that is typically acquired during childhood and remains latent in the kidneys and possibly other sites (eg, mononuclear cells, CNS). The reactivated virus has a tropism for oligodendrocytes. Most patients have depressed cell-mediated immunity due to AIDS (the most common risk factor), reticuloendothelial system disorders (eg, leukemia, lymphoma), or other conditions (eg, Wiskott-Aldrich syndrome, organ transplantation). The risk in AIDS increases with increasing HIV viral load; prevalence of PML has decreased because of widespread use of more effective antiretrovirals.

Symptoms and Signs

Clumsiness may be the 1st symptom. Hemiparesis is the most common finding. Aphasia, dysarthria, and hemianopia are also common. Multifocal cortical damage produces cognitive impairment in ⅔ of patients. Sensory, cerebellar, and brain stem deficits may be present. Occasionally, transverse myelitis develops. Headaches and convulsive seizures are rare and occur most often in patients with AIDS. Gradual, relentless progression culminates in death, usually 1 to 9 mo after symptoms begin.

Diagnosis and Treatment

PML is suspected in patients with unexplained progressive brain dysfunction, particularly in those with depressed cell-mediated immunity. Contrast-enhanced MRI or CT is done and may strongly suggest PML, showing single or multiple white matter lesions. MRI shows hyperintense T-2–weighted images. A contrast agent enhances, usually faintly and peripherally, 5 to 15% of lesions. CT usually shows low-density, nonenhancing lesions. CSF is analyzed for JC viral antigen using PCR; a positive result with compatible neuroimaging findings is nearly pathognomonic. Routine CSF analysis is usually normal. Serologic tests are not helpful. Stereotaxic biopsy can provide a definitive diagnosis but is rarely warranted.

Treatment is supportive. Cidofovir and other antivirals are under study but do not appear to provide much benefit. Patients with AIDS may improve as antivirals reduce the HIV viral load.

RABIES

Rabies is a viral encephalitis transmitted by the saliva of infected bats and certain infected mammals. Symptoms include depression and fever, followed by agitation, excessive salivation, and hydrophobia. Diagnosis is by serologic tests or biopsy. Vaccination is indicated for people at high risk of exposure. Postexposure prophylaxis involves wound care and passive and active immunoprophylaxis. The disorder is almost universally fatal. Treatment is supportive.

Rabies causes > 50,000 human deaths worldwide annually, mostly in Latin America, Africa, and Asia, where canine rabies is endemic. In the US, vaccination of domestic animals has reduced rabies cases in people to < 6/yr, mostly transmitted by infected bats. Infected raccoons, skunks, and foxes can also transmit rabies.

Rabid animals transmit the infection through their saliva, usually by biting. Rarely, the virus can enter through a skin abrasion or across mucous membranes of the eyes, nose, or mouth. The virus travels from the site of entry via peripheral nerves to the spinal cord (or to the brain stem when the face is bitten), then to the brain. It spreads from the CNS via peripheral nerves to other parts of the body. Involvement of the salivary glands and oral mucosa is responsible for transmissibility.

Symptoms and Signs

Pain or paresthesias may develop at the site of the bite. Rapidity of progression depends on the viral inoculum and proximity of the wound to the brain. The incubation period averages 1 to 2 mo but may be > 1 yr. Initial symptoms are nonspecific: fever, headache, and malaise. Within days, encephalitis ("furious" rabies; in 80%) or paralysis ("dumb" rabies; in 20%) develops. Encephalitis causes restlessness, confusion, agitation, bizarre behavior, hallucinations, and insomnia. Salivation is excessive, and attempts to drink produce painful spasms of the laryngeal and pharyngeal muscles (hydrophobia). In the paralytic form, ascending paralysis and quadriplegia develop without delirium and hydrophobia.

Diagnosis and Treatment

Rabies is suspected in patients with encephalitis or ascending paralysis and a history of an animal bite or exposure to bats; bat bites may be superficial and overlooked. Direct fluorescence antibody testing of a biopsy specimen of skin from the nape of the neck is the diagnostic test of choice. Diagnosis can also be made by PCR of CSF, saliva, or tissue. Specimens tested for rabies antibodies include serum and CSF. CT, MRI, and EEG are normal or show nonspecific changes.

Death usually occurs 3 to 10 days after symptoms begin. Only a handful of patients have survived, all of whom received immunoprophylaxis before onset of symptoms. Treatment is only supportive and includes sedation and comfort measures.

Prevention

Rabid animals can often be recognized by their strange behavior; they may be agitated and vicious, weak, or paralyzed and may show no fear of people. Nocturnal animal (eg, bats, skunks, raccoons) may be out dur

TABLE 217–1. RABIES POSTEXPOSURE PROPHYLAXIS

ANIMAL TYPE	EVALUATION AND DISPOSITION OF ANIMAL	POSTEXPOSURE PROPHYLAXIS*
Skunks, raccoons, bats,† foxes, and most other carnivores	Regarded as rabid unless proved negative by laboratory tests‡	Consider immediate vaccination
Dogs, cats, and ferrets	Healthy and available for 10 days of observation	Do not begin immunoprophylaxis unless animal develops symptoms of rabies§
	Unknown (escaped)	Consult public health officials¶
	Rabid or suspected rabid	Vaccinate immediately
Livestock, small rodents (eg, squirrels, hamsters, guinea pigs, gerbils, chipmunks, rats, mice), lagomorphs (rabbits and hares), large rodents (woodchucks and beavers), and other mammals	Consider individually	Consult public health officials; immunoprophylaxis almost never required for bites of squirrels, hamsters, guinea pigs, gerbils, chipmunks, rats, mice, other small rodents, or lagomorphs

*Clean all bites immediately with soap and water.

†Because detecting bat bites is difficult, vaccination is indicated if a bite is reasonably likely, a when a person awakens with a bat in the room or a young child is found with a bat.

‡The animal should be euthanized and tested as soon as possible. Holding for observation is no recommended. Vaccine is discontinued if rabies immunofluorescence tests of the animal are negative

§If the animal remains healthy during the 10-day observation period, it was not infective at the tim of bite. However, treatment with rabies immune globulin (RIG) and human diploid cell vaccin (HDCV) or rabies vaccine is begun at the 1st sign of rabies in a dog, cat, or ferret that has bitte someone. A symptomatic animal should be immediately euthanized and tested.

¶If expert consultation is not available locally and rabies is possible, immediate vaccination shoul be considered.

Adapted from "Rabies prevention—United States 1999: Recommendations of the Immunizatio Practices Advisory Committee (ACIP)." *Morbidity and Mortality Weekly Report* 48(RR-1):1–21, 1999.

ing the day. Bats may make unusual noises and have difficulty flying. An animal suspected of having rabies should not be approached. Local health authorities should be contacted to remove the animal.

Exposure is considered to be a bite that breaks the skin or any contact between mucous membrane or broken skin and animal saliva. If exposure occurs, prompt, meticulously executed prophylaxis almost always prevents human rabies. The wound is cleansed immediately and thoroughly with soap and water or benzalkonium chloride. Deep puncture wounds are flushed with soapy water using moderate pressure. Wounds are usually left open.

Postexposure prophylaxis (PEP) with rabies vaccine and rabies immune globulin is given depending on the biting animal and circumstances (see TABLE 217–1). PEP is begun, and the animal's brain is tested for virus. Local or state health departments or the Centers for Disease Control and Prevention usually conduct testing and can advise on other treatment issues.

For PEP, rabies immune globulin (RIG) 20 IU/kg is infiltrated around the wound for passive immunization; if injection volume is too much for distal areas (eg, fingers, nose), some RIG may be given IM. This treatment is accompanied by human diploid cell rabies vaccine (HDCV) for active immunization. HDCV is given in a series of 5 1-mL IM injections (deltoid area is preferred), beginning on the day of exposure (day 0), in a limb other than the one used for RIG. Subsequent injections occur on days 3, 7, 14, and 28. The WHO also recommends a 6th injection on day 90. Rarely, a serious systemic or neuroparalytic reaction occurs; then, completion of vaccination is weighed against the patient's risk of developing rabies. Rabies antibody titer is measured to help assess risk of discontinuing vaccination.

PEP for a person previously vaccinated against rabies includes 1-mL IM injections of HDCV on days 0 and 3 but no RIG.

HDCV is safe and recommended for preexposure prophylaxis for people at risk, including veterinarians, animal handlers, spelunkers, workers who handle the virus, and travelers to endemic areas.

SUBDURAL EMPYEMA

Subdural empyema is a collection of pus between the dura mater and arachnoid. Symptoms include fever, lethargy, focal neurologic deficits, and seizures. Diagnosis is by contrast-enhanced CT or MRI. Treatment is with surgical drainage and antibiotics.

Subdural empyema is usually a complication of sinusitis (especially frontal and ethmoid), but it can follow ear infections, cranial trauma or surgery, or bacteremia. Pathogens are similar to those that cause brain abscess. In children < 5 yr, the usual cause is bacterial meningitis; because childhood meningitis is now uncommon, childhood subdural empyema is uncommon. Cortical venous thrombosis and brain abscess are common complications.

Symptoms, Signs, and Diagnosis

Fever, headache, lethargy, focal neurologic deficits, and seizures evolve over several days. Meningeal signs, vomiting, and papilledema are common. Without treatment, coma and death occur rapidly.

Diagnosis is by contrast-enhanced CT or MRI. Blood and surgical specimens are cultured aerobically and anaerobically. Lumbar puncture provides little useful information and may precipitate transtentorial herniation. If subdural empyema is suspected (eg, based on symptom duration of several days, focal deficits, or risk factors) in patients with meningeal signs, lumbar puncture is contraindicated until neuroimaging excludes a mass lesion. In infants, a subdural tap may be diagnostic and may relieve pressure.

Treatment

Emergency surgical drainage of the empyema and any underlying sinusitis should be done. Pending culture results, antibiotic coverage is the same as that for brain abscess except in young children, who may require antibiotics for any accompanying meningitis (see TABLES 218–2 and 218–3 on pp. 1863 and 1864). Anticonvulsants and measures to reduce intracranial pressure may be needed.

218 MENINGITIS

(For Brain Infections, see p. 1850.)

Meningitis is inflammation of the meninges of the brain or spinal cord. It is often infectious and is one of the most common CNS infections. Sometimes inflammation involves both the meninges and brain parenchyma (meningoencephalitis). Meningitis may become evident over hours or days (acute) or a longer period (subacute or chronic).

The most common types of acute meningitis are acute bacterial meningitis and aseptic meningitis. Acute bacterial meningitis is a severe illness characterized by purulent CSF. It is rapidly progressive and, without treatment, fatal. Aseptic meningitis is milder and typically self-limited; it is usually caused by viruses but sometimes by bacteria, fungi, parasites, or noninfectious inflammation.

Symptoms and Signs

Many cases of infectious meningitis begin with a vague prodrome of viral symptoms. The classic meningitis triad of fever, headache, and nuchal rigidity develops over hours or days. Passive flexion of the neck is restricted and painful, but rotation and extension are typically not as painful. In severe cases, attempts at neck flexion may induce flexion of the hip or knee (Brudzinski's sign), and there may be resistance to passive extension of the knee while the hip is flexed (Kernig's sign). Neck stiffness and Brudzinski's and Kernig's signs are termed meningeal signs or meningismus; they occur because tension on nerve roots passing through inflamed meninges causes irritation.

Although brain parenchyma is not typically involved early in meningitis, lethargy, confusion, seizures, and focal deficits may develop, particularly in untreated bacterial meningitis.

Diagnosis and Treatment

Acute meningitis is a medical emergency that requires rapid diagnosis and treatment. After IV access and blood cultures are obtained, lumbar puncture is done to obtain CSF for Gram stain, culture, cell count and differential, and glucose and protein content. These tests must be done as rapidly as possible. However, patients with signs compatible with a mass lesion (eg, focal deficits, papilledema, deterioration in consciousness, seizures) require head CT before lumbar puncture because there is a small possibility that lumbar puncture can cause cerebral herniation if a brain abscess or other mass lesion is present.

CSF findings aid in the diagnosis of meningitis (see TABLE 218–1). Presence of bacteria on Gram stain or growth of bacteria in culture is diagnostic of bacterial meningitis. Gram stain is positive about 80% of the time in bacterial meningitis and usually differentiates among the common causative pathogens. CSF lymphocytosis and absence of pathogens suggest aseptic meningitis but may represent partially treated bacterial meningitis.

If patients appear ill and have findings of meningitis, antibiotics (see p. 1862) are started as soon as blood cultures are drawn. If patients do not appear very ill and the diagnosis is less certain, antibiotics can await CSF results.

ACUTE BACTERIAL MENINGITIS

(For neonatal meningitis, see p. 2330.)

Acute bacterial meningitis is fulminant, often fatal pyogenic infection beginning in the meninges. Symptoms include headache, fever, and stiff neck. Without rapid treatment, obtundation and coma follow. Diagnosis is by CSF tests. Treatment requires antibiotics, often beginning empirically with a 3rd- or 4th-generation cephalosporin, vancomycin, and ampicillin; corticosteroids are usually given. Residual morbidity is common.

Etiology

Many bacteria can cause meningitis, but most common are group B streptococci during the 1st 2 mo of life and, thereafter, *Neisseria meningitidis* (meningococci) and *Streptococcus pneumoniae* (pneumococci). Meningococci exist in the nasopharynx of about 5% of people and spread by respiratory droplets and close contact. Only a small fraction of carriers develop meningitis; what makes them susceptible is unknown. Meningococcal meningitis occurs most often in the 1st year of life. It also tends to occur in epidemics among closed populations (eg, in military barracks, college dormitories, boarding schools).

TABLE 218–1. CEREBROSPINAL FLUID ABNORMALITIES IN VARIOUS INFECTIONS

CONDITION	PRESSURE	CELLS/μL	PREDOMINANT CELL TYPE	GLUCOSE	PROTEIN	EXAMPLES
Normal	100–200 mm H_2O	0–5	Lymphocytes	50–100 mg/dL	20–45 mg/dL	—
Bacterial or other purulent meningitis	> 300	100–10,000	PMNs	> 25	> 100*	Acute bacterial meningitis, fulminant fungal meningitis, fulminant amebic meningoencephalitis
Aseptic meningitis	N or ↑	10–1000	Lymphocytes (sometimes some PMNs)	N	N or ↑ (< 100 mg/dL)	Many infectious and noninfectious causes, partially treated bacterial meningitis, early listerial meningitis
Subacute or chronic meningitis	N or ↑	25–2000	Lymphocytes	↓	↑ or ↑↑	Meningitis due to TB, cryptococci, other fungi, sarcoidosis, Lyme disease, syphilis, cysticercosis, or tumor

PMNs = polymorphonuclear leukocytes; ↑ = increased; ↑↑ = greatly increased; ↓ = decreased; N = normal.

*Up to 14% of patients may have a CSF protein level < 100 mg/dL on the initial lumbar puncture.

NOTE: Figures given for pressure, cell count, and protein are approximations; exceptions are common. Similarly, PMNs may predominate in disorders usually characterized by lymphocyte response, especially early in the course of viral infections or tuberculous meningitis. Alterations in glucose are less variable and more reliable.

Pneumococci are the most common cause of meningitis in adults. Especially at risk are alcoholics and people with chronic otitis, sinusitis, mastoiditis, CSF leaks, recurrent meningitis, pneumococcal pneumonia, sickle cell disease, or asplenia. Incidence of pneumococcal meningitis is decreasing because of routine vaccination.

Gram-negative meningitis (most often due to *Escherichia coli, Klebsiella* sp, or *Enterobacter* sp) can occur in immunocompromised patients or after CNS surgery, CNS trauma, bacteremia (eg, due to GU manipulation), or hospital-acquired infections. *Pseudomonas* sp occasionally causes meningitis in immunocompromised or colonized patients. *Haemophilus influenzae* type b meningitis, now uncommon because of widespread vaccination, can occur in immunocompromised patients or after head trauma in unvaccinated people.

Staphylococcal meningitis can occur after penetrating head wounds or neurosurgical procedures (often as part of a mixed infection) or after bacteremia (eg, due to endocarditis). Listerial meningitis can occur at all ages and is particularly common among patients immunocompromised because of chronic renal failure, hepatic disorders, or corticosteroid or cytotoxic therapy after organ transplantation.

Bacteria typically reach the meninges by hematogenous spread from sites of colonization in the nasopharynx or other foci of infection (eg, pneumonia). Why some bacteria are more prone to colonize CSF is not clear, but binding pili and encapsulation appear to play a role. Receptors for pili and other bacterial surface components in the choroid plexus facilitate penetration into CSF.

Bacteria can also enter CSF by direct extension from nearby infections (eg, sinusitis, mastoiditis) or through exterior openings in normally closed CSF pathways (eg, due to meningomyelocele, spinal dermal sinus, penetrating injuries, neurosurgical procedures).

Pathophysiology

Bacterial surface components, complement, and inflammatory cytokines (eg, tumor necrosis factor, IL-1) draw neutrophils into the CSF space. The neutrophils release metabolites that damage cell membranes including those of the vascular endothelium. The result is vasculitis and thrombophlebitis, causing focal ischemia or infarction, and brain edema. Vasculitis also disrupts the blood-brain barrier, further increasing brain edema. The purulent exudate in the CSF blocks CSF reabsorption by the arachnoid villi, causing hydrocephalus. Brain edema and hydrocephalus increase intracranial pressure.

Systemic complications include hyponatremia due to the syndrome of inappropriate antidiuretic hormone (SIADH), disseminated intravascular coagulation (DIC), and septic shock. Occasionally, bilateral adrenal hemorrhagic infarction (Waterhouse-Friderichsen syndrome) results.

Symptoms and Signs

A respiratory illness or sore throat often precedes the more characteristic symptoms of fever, headache, stiff neck, and vomiting. Kernig's and Brudzinski's signs appear in about $\frac{1}{2}$ of patients. Adults may become desperately ill within 24 h, and children even sooner. Seizures occur in about 30%. Cranial nerve abnormalities (eg, 3rd [oculomotor] or 7th [facial] cranial nerve palsy; occasionally, deafness) and other focal deficits occur in 10 to 20%. In patients > 2 yr, changes in consciousness progress through irritability, confusion, drowsiness, stupor, and coma. Opisthotonic posturing may occur.

Dehydration is common, and vascular collapse produces shock. Infection, particularly meningococcal, may be disseminated widely, to the joints, lungs, sinuses, and elsewhere. A petechial or purpuric rash commonly occurs in meningococcal meningitis. Examination of the head, ears, spine, and skin may reveal a source or route of infection. Spinal dimples, sinuses, nevi, or tufts of hair suggest a meningomyelocele.

In children < 2 yr, meningeal signs may be absent. In those < 2 mo, symptoms and signs are often nonspecific, particularly in early disease. Fever, hypothermia, poor feeding, lethargy, vomiting, and irritability are common presenting symptoms. Seizures, a high-pitched cry, and bulging or tight fontanelles are possible but often occur late. Subdural effusions may develop after several days; typical signs are seizures, persistent fever, and enlarging head size.

The elderly may have nonspecific symptoms (eg, confusion with or occasionally without fever). Meningeal signs may be absent or mild. Arthritis may restrict neck motion, often in multiple directions, and should not be mistaken for meningismus.

Partially treated meningitis: Patients seen early in the disease, before typical findings of meningitis appear, are sometimes diagnosed with otitis media or sinusitis and given oral antibiotics. Depending on the drug, the infection may be partially (but temporarily) suppressed. Patients may not appear as ill and have milder meningeal signs and slower disease progression. This situation can significantly hamper recognition of meningitis.

Diagnosis

Acute bacterial meningitis is suspected in children < 2 yr with lethargy, progressive irritability, a high-pitched cry, a bulging fontanelle, meningeal signs, or hypothermia. It is suspected in patients > 2 yr with meningeal signs or unexplained alterations in consciousness, particularly in those with fever or risk factors.

Because acute bacterial meningitis, especially meningococcal, can be lethal within hours, it must be diagnosed and treated rapidly. Prompt lumbar puncture is required but should not delay immediate treatment with antibiotics and corticosteroids.

CSF pressure may be elevated. Gram stain shows organisms in CSF in 80% of patients. CSF neutrophil count usually exceeds 2000/µL. Glucose is usually < 40 mg/dL because of impaired CNS glucose transport and glucose consumption by neutrophils and bacteria. Protein is typically > 100 mg/dL. Cultures are positive in 90%; they may be falsely negative in patients who are partially treated. Latex agglutination tests can be used to detect antigens of meningococci, *H. influenzae* type b, pneumococci, group B streptococci, and *E. coli* K1 strains. However, these tests are not always routinely done because they probably add little to other routine CSF tests. The limulus amebocyte lysate test can detect endotoxin in gram-negative meningitis. This test and the latex agglutination tests may be helpful when patients have received prior antibiotics (partial treatment), when patients are immunocompromised, or when other CSF tests do not identify the causative organism. PCR can occasionally be useful if CSF cultures reveal no organisms.

CT may be normal or show small ventricles, effacement of the sulci, and contrast enhancement over the convexities. MRI with gadolinium is more sensitive for subarachnoid inflammation but is not commonly used. Scans should be scrutinized for evidence of brain abscess, sinusitis, mastoiditis, skull fracture, and congenital malformations. Evidence of venous infarctions or communicating hydrocephalus may appear after days or weeks.

Disorders that resemble bacterial meningitis can usually be differentiated by clinical presentation, neuroimaging, and routine CSF tests. Viral meningitis can cause fever, headache, and stiff neck, but patients do not appear as ill and CSF test results are different (see TABLE 218–1). Subarachnoid hemorrhage causes severe headache and a stiff neck, but onset is explosive and fever is usually absent; CT shows hemorrhage, or the CSF contains RBCs or is xanthochromic. Brain abscess can cause fever, headache, and impaired consciousness, but the neck is typically supple unless abscess contents have ruptured into the CSF space, producing a fulminant secondary meningitis. Severe systemic infections (eg, sepsis, infective endocarditis) can impair cognition or consciousness by producing fever and compromising tissue perfusion; CSF is normal or contains a small number of WBCs, and the neck is supple. Cerebellar tonsillar herniation can cause impaired consciousness (secondary to obstructive hydrocephalus) and neck stiffness but usually not fever, and it can be differentiated by CT or MRI. Cerebral vasculitis (eg, due to SLE) and cerebral venous thrombosis can cause mild fever, headache, altered mental status, and mild to moderate meningeal inflammation, typically producing CSF test results similar to those of viral encephalitis.

Occasionally, fungal meningitis or amebic (*Naegleria*) meningoencephalitis can cause acute, fulminant meningitis with clinical findings and routine CSF test results similar to those of bacterial meningitis. Gram stain and routine cultures show no bacteria. Microscopic examination or culture of CSF can detect fungi (see p. 1867). In amebic meningoencephalitis, ameboid movement can be detected in unspun wet mounts of CSF, and the ameba can be cultured. TB meningitis is usually subacute or chronic but is occasionally acute; CSF characteristics are usually intermediate between those of acute bacterial and aseptic meningitis and special stains (eg, acid-fast, immunofluorescent) are needed to identify TB.

Peripheral blood tests include blood cultures (positive in 50%), cell count with differential, electrolytes, glucose, renal function, and coagulation tests. Serum Na is monitored for evidence of SIADH, and coagulation results are monitored for evidence of DIC. Urine and any nasopharyngeal or respiratory secretions and skin lesions are cultured.

Waterhouse-Friderichsen syndrome should be suspected in any febrile patient who remains in shock despite adequate volume replacement and who has rapidly evolving purpura and evidence of DIC. Serum cortisol level is measured, and CT, MRI, or ultrasonography of the adrenal glands is done.

Prognosis and Treatment

Early antibiotics and supportive care have reduced the mortality rate of acute bacterial meningitis to < 10%. However, if meningitis is treated late or occurs in neonates, the elderly, or immunocompromised patients, death is common. A poor outcome is predicted by persistent leukopenia or development of Waterhouse-Friderichsen syndrome. Survivors occasionally have deafness, other cranial nerve deficits, cerebral infarction, recurrent seizures, or mental retardation.

If acute bacterial meningitis is suspected, antibiotics and corticosteroids are given as soon as blood cultures are drawn (see TABLE 218–2). If the diagnosis is unclear and the patient is not very ill, antibiotics may be withheld pending CSF test results. Giving antibiotics before lumbar puncture slightly increases the probability of false-negative cultures, particularly with pneumococci, but does not affect other test results.

Dexamethasone 0.15 mg/kg IV q 6 h in children and 10 mg IV q 6 h in adults should be given 15 min before the 1st dose of antibiotics and continued for 4 days. Dexamethasone may prevent hearing loss and other neurologic sequelae, possibly by inhibiting release of proinflammatory cytokines triggered by antibiotic-induced bacterial lysis. Dexamethasone should not be given to patients with immunodeficiency because it may impair host defenses against nonbacterial meningitis.

If no pathogen is identified in the CSF, addition of antibiotics for TB should be considered. If no bacteria grow in culture or are otherwise identified after 24 to 48 h, corticosteroids are stopped; corticosteroids continued for > 1 day without appropriate antibiotic coverage could worsen the infection. Corticosteroids impede vancomycin's penetration of CSF, so the vancomycin dose may have to be increased.

When initial CSF tests are inconclusive, a repeat lumbar puncture in 8 to 24 h (or sooner if the patient deteriorates) may help. If clinical and CSF findings continue to suggest aseptic meningitis, antibiotics are withheld. If the patient's condition is serious, especially if antibiotics have been given (possibly producing falsely sterile cultures), antibiotics should be continued.

Choice of antibiotics depends on pathogen and patient age (see TABLE 218–2; for antibiotic doses, see TABLE 218–3). Third-generation cephalosporins (eg, ceftriaxone, cefotaxime) are effective against pathogens common in patients of all ages. Cefepime, a 4th-generation cephalosporin, can be substituted for a 3rd-generation cephalosporin in children and can be useful for *Pseudomonas* infection. However, because cephalosporin-resistant pneumococci are becoming increasingly prevalent, vancomycin, with or without rifampin, is usually added. Ampicillin is added to cover *Listeria* sp. Aminoglycosides penetrate the CNS poorly but are still used empirically to cover gram-negative bacteria in neonates (see p. 2332). When CSF Gram stain and culture results become available, antibiotics are adjusted.

Lumbar puncture should be repeated 24 to 48 h after starting antibiotics to confirm CSF sterility and conversion to lymphocytic predominance. Generally, antibiotics are continued for ≥ 1 wk after fever subsides and CSF is nearly normal (complete normalization may take weeks). Drug doses are not reduced when clinical improvement occurs because drug penetration commonly decreases as meningeal inflammation decreases.

Supportive therapy includes treatment of fever, dehydration, electrolyte disorders, seizures, and shock. If Waterhouse-Friderichsen syndrome is suspected, high-dose hydrocortisone (eg, 100 to 200 mg IV q 4 to 6 h or as a continuous infusion after an initial bolus is given; treatment should not be delayed pending hormone levels.

Cerebral edema can be minimized by avoiding overhydration. If brain herniation is suspected, hyperventilation (Pa_{CO_2}, 25 to 30 mm Hg), mannitol (0.25 to 1.0 g/kg IV), and additional dexamethasone (4 mg IV q 4 h) can be used; monitoring intracranial pressure may be helpful. If ventricles are enlarged, intracranial pressure may be monitored and CSF drained, but outcome is usually poor.

For infants up to 1 yr of age with subdural effusion, daily subdural taps through the cranial sutures usually help. *No more than 20 mL/day of CSF should be removed from one side* to avoid sudden shifts in intracranial contents. If effusion persists after 3 to 4 wk of taps, surgical exploration for possible excision of a subdural membrane is indicated.

Patients with severe meningococcal meningitis may benefit from drotrecogin alfa (activated protein C), which downregulates the

TABLE 218–2. ANTIBIOTIC THERAPY FOR ACUTE BACTERIAL MENINGITIS

ORGANISM	AGE GROUP	ANTIBIOTIC*	COMMENT
Unknown	Infants < 1 mo	Ampicillin and cefotaxime and gentamicin (tobramycin or amikacin†)	See p. 2332
	Children > 1 mo	Ampicillin and cefotaxime (ceftriaxone) and vancomycin	—
	Adults	Ampicillin and ceftriaxone (cefotaxime) and vancomycin	—
Gram-positive organisms (unidentified)	Children and adults	Vancomycin and ceftriaxone (cefotaxime) and ampicillin‡	—
Gram-negative bacilli (unidentified)	Children and adults	Ceftazidime (ceftriaxone or cefotaxime) and gentamicin (tobramycin or amikacin†)	—
Haemophilus influenzae type b	Children and adults	Ceftriaxone (cefotaxime)	—
Meningococci	Children and adults	Penicillin G (ampicillin) plus ceftriaxone (cefotaxime)	Penicillin G is used for susceptible strains after sensitivities are known
Streptococci (pneumococci)	Children and adults	Vancomycin and ceftriaxone (cefotaxime) with or without rifampin	Penicillin G may be used for susceptible strains after sensitivities are known
Staphylococci	Children and adults	Vancomycin or nafcillin (oxacillin) with or without rifampin	Vancomycin is used for methicillin-resistant strains; nafcillin or oxacillin is used for susceptible strains after sensitivities are known. Rifampin is added if no improvement occurs with vancomycin or nafcillin
Listeria sp	Children and adults	Ampicillin (penicillin G) or trimethoprim-sulfamethoxazole and gentamicin (tobramycin or amikacin†)	Penicillin G is used for susceptible strains after sensitivities are known; trimethoprim-sulfamethoxazole is used in patients allergic to penicillin
Enteric gram-negative bacteria (*Escherichia coli, Klebsiella* sp, *Proteus* sp)	Children and adults	Ceftriaxone (cefotaxime) and gentamicin (tobramycin or amikacin†)	—
Pseudomonas sp	Children and adults	Ceftazidime or cefepime (usually alone, can add an aminoglycoside); alternatives: meropenem or aztreonam	—

*Alternative antibiotics are in parentheses. Among 3rd-generation cephalosporins, cefotaxime may be preferred for children; ceftriaxone, for adults.

†Amikacin is used in areas where gentamicin resistance is common. Because aminoglycosides have poor CSF penetration, they may have to be given intrathecally or via an Ommaya reservoir, especially in patients with *Pseudomonas* meningitis. When aminoglycosides are used, renal function should be monitored.

‡If the gram-positive organisms are pleomorphic, ampicillin is included to cover *Listeria* sp.

TABLE 218–3. COMMON IV ANTIBIOTIC DOSAGES FOR BACTERIAL MENINGITIS*

ANTIBIOTIC	DOSAGE	
	Children > 1 mo	Adults
Ceftriaxone	50 mg/kg q 12 h	2 g q 12 h
Cefotaxime	50 mg/kg q 6 h	2 g q 4–6 h
Ceftazidime	50 mg/kg q 8 h	2 g q 8 h
Cefepime	2 g q 12 h	2 g q 8–12 h
Ampicillin	75 mg/kg q 6 h	2–3 g q 4 h
Penicillin G	4 million units q 4 h	4 million units q 4 h
Nafcillin and oxacillin	50 mg/kg q 6 h	2 g q 4 h
Vancomycin†	15 mg/kg q 6 h	500–750 mg q 6 h
Gentamicin and tobramycin†	2.5 mg/kg q 8 h	2 mg/kg q 8 h
Amikacin†	10 mg/kg q 8 h	7.5 mg/kg q 12 h
Rifampin	6.7 mg/kg q 8 h	600 mg q 24 h
Chloramphenicol	25 mg/kg q 6 h	1 g q 6 h

*See Table 279–1 on p. 2314 for neonatal dosages.
†Renal function should be monitored.

inflammatory response. A greater frequency of intracranial bleeding occurs with or without drotrecogin alfa treatment in patients septic due to meningitis.

Prevention

A conjugated pneumococcal vaccine effective against 7 serotypes, including > 80% of organisms that cause meningitis, is recommended for all children (see p. 1403 and FIG. 266–3 on p. 2235). Routine vaccination for *H. influenzae* type b is highly effective and begins at age 2 mo. A quadrivalent meningococcal vaccine is given to children ≥ 2 yr with immunodeficiencies or functional asplenia, travelers to endemic areas, and laboratory personnel who routinely handle meningococcal specimens. Meningococcal vaccine should also be considered for students living in dormitories and for military recruits.

Spread of meningitis is prevented by keeping patients in respiratory isolation (droplet precautions) for the 1st 24 h of therapy. Gloves, masks, and gowns are used. Anyone who has face-to-face contact with the patient (eg, family and medical staff members) should receive postexposure prophylaxis. For meningococcal meningitis, it consists of meningococcal vaccine and chemoprophylaxis. Vaccination is especially important for containing epidemics. Chemoprophylaxis against meningococci is oral rifampin for 48 h (adults, 600 mg q 12 h; children, 10 mg/kg q 12 h; infants < 1 mo, 5 mg/kg q 12 h). Alternatives include a single dose of IM ceftriaxone (adults, 250 mg; children, 125 mg) or a single dose of ciprofloxacin 500 mg po (adults only). Chemoprophylaxis against *H. influenzae* type b is rifampin 20 mg/kg po once/day (maximum 600 mg) for 4 days. There is no consensus on whether children < 2 yr require prophylaxis for exposure at day care. Chemoprophylaxis is not usually needed for contacts of patients with pneumococcal meningitis.

ASEPTIC MENINGITIS

Aseptic meningitis is inflammation of the meninges with CSF lymphocytic pleocytosis and no cause apparent after routine CSF stains and cultures. Viruses are the most common cause. Other causes may be infectious or noninfectious. Symptoms include fever, headache, and meningeal signs. Viral aseptic meningitis is usually self-limited. Treatment is usually symptomatic.

Etiology

Causes may be infectious (eg, rickettsiae, spirochetes, parasites) or noninfectious (eg, intracranial tumors and cysts, drugs, systemic disorders—see TABLE 218–4).

Enteroviruses, including echovirus and coxsackievirus, cause most cases. Mumps virus is a common cause worldwide but has been minimized in the US by vaccination. Enteroviruses and the mumps virus enter via the respiratory or GI tract and spread via the bloodstream. Mollaret's meningitis is a syndrome of self-limited, recurrent aseptic meningitis characterized by large atypical monocytes (once thought to be endothelial cells) in the CSF; it presumably is caused by herpes simplex virus type 2 or other viruses. Viruses that cause encephalitis typically also produce a low-grade aseptic meningitis.

Bacteria may also cause aseptic meningitis; they include spirochetes (in syphilis, Lyme disease, or leptospirosis) and rickettsiae (in typhus, Rocky Mountain spotted fever, or ehrlichiosis). CSF abnormalities may be transient or chronic. Bacterial infections such as mastoiditis, sinusitis, brain abscess, and infective endocarditis can result in CSF with characteristics of aseptic meningitis because widespread inflammation produces vasculitis, which leads to CSF pleocytosis without bacteria in the CSF.

TABLE 218–4. CAUSES OF ASEPTIC MENINGITIS*

TYPE	EXAMPLES
Infectious	
Bacterial	Brucellosis, cat-scratch disease, cerebral Whipple's disease, leptospirosis, Lyme disease (neuroborreliosis), lymphogranuloma venereum, mycoplasmal infection, rickettsial infection, syphilis, TB
Postinfectious	Multiple viruses (eg, measles, rubella, smallpox, vaccinia, varicella)
Viral	Chickenpox (varicella-zoster); coxsackievirus, echovirus, and poliovirus infections; West Nile virus infection; eastern and western equine encephalitis; herpes simplex virus infection; HIV infection, cytomegalovirus infections; infectious hepatitis; infectious mononucleosis; lymphocytic choriomeningitis; mumps; St. Louis encephalitis
Fungi and parasites†	Ameboid infection, coccidioidomycosis, cryptococcosis, malaria, neurocysticercosis, toxoplasmosis, trichinosis
Noninfectious	
Drugs	Azathioprine, carbamazepine, ciprofloxacin, cytosine arabinoside (high-dose), immune globulin, muromonab CD3, isoniazid, NSAIDs (eg, ibuprofen, naproxen, sulindac, tolmetin), OKT3 monoclonal antibody, penicillin, phenazopyridine, ranitidine, trimethoprim-sulfamethoxazole
Meningeal disease	Behçet's syndrome with neurologic involvement, leakage of an intracranial epidermoid tumor or craniopharyngioma into the CSF, meningeal leukemia, neoplastic meningitis, sarcoidosis
Parameningeal disease	Brain tumor, chronic sinusitis or otitis, multiple sclerosis, stroke
Reaction to intrathecal injections	Air, antibiotics, chemotherapeutic drugs, spinal anesthetics, iophendylate, other dyes
Vaccine reactions	Many, especially pertussis, rabies, smallpox
Other	Lead, Mollaret's meningitis

*Aseptic refers here to conditions in which a bacterial pathogen is not readily identified with routine stains and cultures. This includes some bacteria.

†Fungi and protozoa can cause a prurulent meningitis with sepsis and CSF changes similar to bacterial meningitis, except that organisms are not seen on Gram stain; thus, they are included in this category.

Noninfectious causes of meningeal inflammation include neoplastic infiltration, leakage of the contents of an intracranial cyst, intrathecal drugs, lead poisoning, and radiopaque agents. Infrequently, inflammation results from certain systemically administered drugs, presumably as a hypersensitivity reaction. The most common causative drugs are NSAIDs (especially ibuprofen), antimicrobials (especially sulfa drugs), and immune modulators (eg, IV immune globulins, OKT3 monoclonal antibodies, cyclosporine, vaccines).

Symptoms and Signs

Aseptic meningitis often follows a flu-like syndrome and usually produces fever and headache, but coryza is not prominent. Meningeal signs are less marked and slower to develop than in acute bacterial meningitis. Patients are usually not critically ill; systemic or nonspecific symptoms may predominate. Focal neurologic symptoms are absent. Patients with noninfectious meningeal inflammation are often afebrile.

Diagnosis and Treatment

Aseptic meningitis is suspected in any patient with fever, headache, and meningeal signs. Head CT or MRI is done before lumbar puncture if a brain mass is suspected (eg, by focal neurologic signs or papilledema). CSF findings (see TABLE 218–2) include mildly or markedly elevated pressure and presence of 10 to > 1000 lymphocytes/μL. Occasionally, a few neutrophils appear during the 1st few hours of viral meningitis. CSF glucose is normal, and CSF protein is normal or moderately elevated. CSF PCR is usually done to identify viral pathogens. Diagnosis of Mollaret's meningitis is by CSF PCR for herpes simplex type 2 DNA. Drug-induced aseptic meningitis is a diagnosis of exclusion. Tests are done to diagnose causes that are suspected clinically (eg, rickettsial infection, Lyme disease, syphilis).

Differentiating bacterial meningitis, which requires specific, rapid treatment, from aseptic meningitis, which usually does not, is sometimes difficult. Even a few CSF neutrophils, which may be present in early viral meningitis, should prompt consideration of early bacterial meningitis. Bacterial meningitis that is partially treated can result in CSF with characteristics similar to those in aseptic meningitis. *Listeria* sp may be difficult to detect on Gram stain and may produce a meningitis with CSF monocytosis, which is more characteristic of aseptic than most bacterial meningitis. TB is notoriously difficult to identify microscopically and may produce CSF with characteristics similar to those in aseptic meningitis; clues to TB meningitis are clinical findings, elevated CSF protein, and mildly decreased CSF glucose (see p. 1867). Idiopathic intracranial hypertension sometimes mimics aseptic meningitis.

In most patients, the diagnosis is clear, and treatment requires only hydration, analgesics, and antipyretics. If listerial, partially treated, and early bacterial meningitis cannot be excluded, antibiotics effective against bacterial meningitis are given pending results of cultures or repeat CSF tests. Drug-induced aseptic meningitis resolves when the causative drug is withdrawn. Mollaret's meningitis may be treated with acyclovir (see p. 1601).

SUBACUTE AND CHRONIC MENINGITIS

Meningeal inflammation that lasts > 2 wk (subacute meningitis) or > 1 mo (chronic meningitis) may have infectious or noninfectious causes (eg, cancer). Diagnosis requires CSF analysis, usually after CT or MRI. Treatment is directed at the cause.

Etiology

Subacute or chronic meningitis may have infectious or noninfectious causes and may be an aseptic meningitis (see TABLE 218–4). Infectious causes include fungi (most commonly *Cryptococcus neoformans*), TB, Lyme disease, AIDS, actinomyces, and syphilis; noninfectious causes include sarcoidosis, vasculitis, Behçet's syndrome, and cancers such as lymphomas, leukemia, melanomas, certain carcinomas, and gliomas (particularly glioblastoma, ependymoma, and medulloblastoma). Other causes include chemical reactions to certain intrathecal injections.

Immunosuppressants and the AIDS epidemic have increased the incidence of fungal meningitis. *Cryptococcus* sp (see p. 1531) is the most common cause in patients with AIDS, Hodgkin lymphoma, or lymphosarcoma and in those taking high-dose, long-term corticosteroids. *Coccidioides, Candida, Actinomyces, Histoplasma*, and *Aspergillus* spp are less common causes (see Ch. 180 on p. 1523).

Symptoms and Signs

Most manifestations are similar to those of acute meningitis but evolve over weeks. Fever may be minimal. Headache, backache, and cranial nerve or spinal nerve root deficits are common. Communicating hydrocephalus may develop and produce dementia. Intracranial pressure may remain elevated and produce headache, vomiting, and decreased alertness for days or weeks. Without treatment, death can occur within a few weeks or months (eg, with TB or tumor), or symptoms can continue for years (eg, with Lyme disease).

Diagnosis and Treatment

The diagnosis is suspected if meningeal symptoms or signs develop over > 2 wk, with or without symptoms of cerebral dysfunction, particularly if a potential cause of meningitis (eg, active TB, cancer) exists. The diagnosis requires CSF analysis. CT or MRI is done to exclude mass lesions that produce slowly evolving cerebral dysfunction (eg, tumors, abscesses, subdural effusions) and to determine whether lumbar puncture can be done safely. CSF pressure is often elevated but may be normal. CSF cell count is elevated with a lymphocytic predominance; glucose is slightly reduced, and protein is high (see TABLE 218–1).

Other CSF tests (eg, special stains, fungal and acid-fast bacillus culture) are determined by the patient's risk factors. For example, TB is suspected in patients who are alcoholic, HIV-positive, or from areas where TB is endemic (see p. 1509). Identification of TB by microscopy requires acid-fast staining or immunofluorescence and an exhaustive microscopic search of at least 30 to 50 mL of CSF, which requires 3 to 5 lumbar punctures. Positive cultures are the gold standard for diagnosis but also require 30 to 50 mL of CSF, and results take 2 to 6 wk. Measurement of CSF tubulostearic acid by gas-liquid chromatography is specific but technically complex and not widely used. PCR is the most promising method for rapid TB diagnosis but may be false-positive or false-negative, partly because standards between different laboratories vary.

Fungi are detected microscopically in wet mounts or, for *Cryptococcus* sp, in India ink preparations (see also p. 1532). CSF cultures grow *Cryptococcus* and *Candida* spp in a few days or, with less common fungal infections, weeks. CSF cryptococcal antigen is highly specific and sensitive. Neurosyphilis is diagnosed using the CSF Venereal Disease Research Laboratories (VDRL) test (see p. 1661). In Lyme disease (see p. 1478), definitive diagnosis requires intrathecal antibodies against *Borrelia burgdorferi*.

Diagnosis of neoplastic meningitis requires detecting cancer cells in CSF; detection depends on adequate CSF volume, frequency of collection (malignant cells may shed periodically; multiple samples increase the yield), sampling site (cisternal CSF is more often positive), and prompt fixation to preserve cell morphology. For 95% sensitivity, 30 to 50 mL of CSF (requiring 5 lumbar punctures) is collected and delivered to the laboratory promptly. For suspected neurosarcoidosis, ACE in CSF is measured; it is elevated in up to 50% of patients. For certain tumors, CSF tumor markers (eg, soluble CD27 for lymphoid cancers, such as acute lymphoblastic leukemia and non-Hodgkin lymphoma) can help with diagnosis or monitoring disease activity. Some causes of subacute or chronic meningitis (eg, Behçet's syndrome) cannot be diagnosed by CSF analysis and must be diagnosed clinically.

Treatment depends on the cause (see elsewhere in THE MANUAL).

219 NEURO-OPHTHALMOLOGIC AND CRANIAL NERVE DISORDERS

(See also Chs. 85, 91, 107, and 206 and Horner's Syndrome on p. 1767.)

Neuro-ophthalmologic disorders involve the eye, pupil, optic nerve, extraocular muscles and their nerves, or the central pathways that control and integrate ocular movement and vision. Tumors, inflammation, trauma, systemic disorders, and degenerative or other processes can affect these structures, causing vision loss, diplopia, ptosis, pupillary abnormalities, periocular pain, and headache. Cranial nerve disorders can involve dysfunction of smell, vision, hearing, taste, balance, facial expression, phonation, chewing, or swallowing (see TABLE 219–1). One or several cranial nerves may be affected.

Evaluation includes detailed questioning about symptoms, examination of the visual system, and tests to detect nystagmus (see sidebar 84–1 on p. 776). Visual system examination includes visual acuity, visual fields, ophthalmoscopy, ocular motility (see TABLE 219–2), eyelids, pupils (see also p. 869 and TABLE 219–3), and cranial nerve examination (see also p. 1750). Neuroimaging with CT or MRI is also usually required.

Extraocular movements are checked by having the patient hold his head steady, then track the examiner's finger as it moves to the far right, left, upward, downward, diagonally to either side, and inward toward the patient's nose (to assess accommodation). However, such examination may miss mild paresis of ocular movement sufficient to cause diplopia.

Diplopia can result from a defect in bilateral coordination of extraocular movements (eg, in neural pathways) or in the 3rd (oculomotor), 4th (trochlear), or 6th (abducens) cranial nerve. Evaluation involves asking the patient to close each eye separately. If diplopia occurs when one eye is closed (monocular diplopia), the cause is probably a nonneurologic eye disorder (see p. 874). If diplopia disappears when either eye is closed (binocular diplopia), the cause is probably a disorder of ocular motility. The eye that, when closed, eliminates the more peripheral image is paretic. Placing a red glass over one eye can help identify the paretic eye. When the red glass covers the paretic eye, the more peripheral image is red (see also p. 874).

Pupils are inspected for size, equality, and regularity. Normally, the pupils constrict promptly (within 1 sec) and equally during accommodation and during exposure to direct light and to light directed at the other pupil (consensual light). If the light reflex is diminished in one eye, a swinging flashlight test may discriminate between an afferent (eg, retinal or optic nerve) and an efferent (eg, 3rd cranial nerve or pupillary muscle) defect. If a pupil constricts in response to consensual but not to direct light and paradoxically enlarges when light is quickly brought from the unaffected side, the defect is afferent (called Marcus Gunn pupil). If the pupillary response to direct and consensual light is sluggish or absent, the defect is efferent.

Treatment of neuro-ophthalmologic and cranial disorders depends on the cause.

CONJUGATE GAZE PALSIES

A conjugate gaze palsy is inability to move both eyes in a single horizontal (most commonly) or vertical direction.

Gaze palsies most commonly affect horizontal gaze; some affect upward gaze, and even fewer affect downward gaze.

Horizontal gaze palsies: Conjugate horizontal gaze is controlled by neural input from the cerebral hemispheres, cerebellum, vestibular nuclei, and neck. Neural input from these sites converges at the horizontal gaze center (parapontine reticular formation, or para-abducens nucleus) and is integrated into a final command to the adjacent 6th cranial nerve nucleus, which controls the lateral rectus on the same side and the oculomotor nucleus on the opposite side via the medial longitudinal fasciculus (MLF), which controls the medial rectus.

The most common and devastating impairment of horizontal gaze results from pontine lesions that affect the horizontal gaze center and the 6th cranial nerve nucleus. Strokes are a common cause, resulting in loss of horizontal gaze ipsilateral to the lesion. Palsies due to stroke can be unresponsive to any stimulus (eg, voluntary or vestibular). Milder palsies may cause only nystagmus or inability to maintain fixation.

The 2nd most common site of lesions is the contralateral cerebral hemisphere rostral to the frontal gyrus. These lesions can be caused by a stroke. The resulting palsy may be temporary, and horizontal conjugate gaze that occurs independent of the hemisphere (eg, in response to cold-water caloric stimulation) is preserved. Lesions in other areas may affect horizontal gaze because its anatomy is complex.

Vertical gaze palsies: Upward and downward gaze depends on input from one fiber path that ascends from the vestibular system through the MLF on both sides. A separate system descends, presumably from the cerebral hemispheres, through the midbrain pretectum to the 3rd cranial nerve nuclei. The rostral interstitial nucleus of the MLF integrates the neural input into a final command for vertical gaze. Vertical gaze diminishes with age.

Vertical gaze palsies commonly result from midbrain lesions, usually infarcts and tumors. A bilateral upward gaze palsy may result from Parinaud's syndrome, due to a tumor or, less commonly, an infarct of the midbrain pretectum.

TABLE 219–1. CRANIAL NERVES

NERVE	FUNCTION	EXAMPLES OF DISORDERS	CAUSES OF DISORDERS*
Olfactory (1st)	Provides sensory input for smell	Anosmia	Head trauma; tumors of the cranial fossa, nasal cavity, and paranasal sinuses; paranasal sinusitis
Optic (2nd)	Provides sensory input for vision	Amaurosis fugax (transient monocular blindness)	Ipsilateral internal carotid disease, embolism of retinal arteries
		Retrobulbar neuritis	Acute demyelinating disease or ischemia of the 2nd cranial nerve, postinfectious or disseminated encephalomyelitis, posterior uveitis
		Toxic-nutritional optic neuropathy (toxic amblyopia)	Severe nutritional deprivation; vitamin B_{12} deficiency; methanol ingestion; use of chloramphenicol, ethambutol, isoniazid, streptomycin, sulfonamides, digitalis, chlorpropamide, ergot, disulfiram, or organic mercury
		Bitemporal hemianopia	Suprasellar extension of pituitary adenoma, craniopharyngioma, saccular aneurysm in the cavernous sinus, meningioma of tuberculum sellae
Oculomotor (3rd)	Raises eyelids; moves eyes up, down, and medially; adjusts amount of light entering eyes; focuses lenses	Palsies	Aneurysm of posterior communicating artery; transtentorial herniation due to intracranial mass (eg, subdural hematoma, tumor, abscess); ischemia of the 3rd cranial nerve (often due to small-vessel disease as occurs in diabetes) or of the midbrain
Trochlear (4th)	Moves eye in and down via the superior oblique muscle	Palsies	Often idiopathic; head trauma, infarction often due to small-vessel disease (eg, in diabetes), tentorial meningioma, pinealoma
Trigeminal (5th)			
Ophthalmic division	Provides sensory input from eye surface, tear glands, scalp, forehead, and upper eyelids	Trigeminal neuralgia	Vascular loop compressing the nerve root, occasionally multiple sclerosis lesions of cavernous sinus or superior orbital fissure
Maxillary and mandibular divisions	Provides sensory input from teeth, gums, lip, lining of palate, and skin of face; moves masticatory muscles (chewing, grinding the teeth)	Trigeminal neuropathy	Meningiomas, schwannomas, metastatic tumors at skull base

Table continues on the following page.

TABLE 219–1. CRANIAL NERVES—Continued

NERVE	FUNCTION	EXAMPLES OF DISORDERS	CAUSES OF DISORDERS*
Abducens (6th)	Moves eye outward (abduction) via lateral rectus muscle	Palsies	Often idiopathic, increased intracranial pressure, infarction (may be mononeuritis multiplex), nasopharyngeal carcinoma, pontine or cerebellar tumors, head trauma, infections or tumors affecting the meninges, Wernicke's encephalopathy, multiple sclerosis, pontine infarction
Facial (7th)	Moves muscles of facial expression, innervates tear glands and salivary glands; provides sensory input for taste in anterior ⅔ of the tongue	Palsies	Bell's palsy, Ramsay Hunt syndrome, Lyme disease, sarcoidosis, tumors that invade the temporal bone, acoustic neuromas, infarcts and tumors of the pons, Guillain-Barré syndrome, uveoparotid fever (Heerfordt's syndrome), Melkersson-Rosenthal syndrome
		Hemifacial spasm	Artery loop compressing nerve root
Vestibulocochlear (8th)	Provides sensory input for equilibrium and hearing	Meniere's disease	Perilymphatic edema
		Benign paroxysmal positional vertigo	Otolithic aggregation in semicircular canal, labyrinthine concussion, otitis media, ear surgery, occlusion of the anterior vestibular artery
		Vestibular neuronitis	Possibly viral infection
		Hearing loss or disturbance	Cerebellopontine angle tumors, acoustic neuromas, possibly viral infection, aging, exposure to loud noises
Glossopharyngeal (9th)	Provides sensory input from pharynx, tonsils, posterior tongue, and carotid arteries; moves muscles of swallowing and salivary glands; helps regulate BP	Glossopharyngeal neuralgia	Ectatic artery or tumor (less common) compressing the nerve
		Glossopharyngeal neuropathy	Tumor or aneurysm in the posterior fossa or jugular foramen
Vagus (10th)	Moves muscles of speech and swallowing; transmits impulses to heart and smooth muscles of visceral organs	Dysphagia and dysphonia Vasovagal syncope	Infectious or carcinomatous meningitis, medullary tumors or ischemia (eg, lateral medullary syndrome), herpes zoster, motor neuron disorders (eg, amyotrophic lateral sclerosis)

TABLE 219–1. CRANIAL NERVES—Continued

NERVE	FUNCTION	EXAMPLES OF DISORDERS	CAUSES OF DISORDERS*
Accessory (11th)	Turns head; shrugs shoulders	Partial or complete paralysis of sternocleidomastoid and trapezius	Tumors at skull base or meninges, surgical trauma (eg, due to lymph node biopsy), idiopathic
Hypoglossal (12th)	Moves tongue	Atrophy and fasciculation of tongue	Intramedullary lesions (eg, motor neuron disorders, tumors, poliomyelitis), lesions of the basal meninges or occipital bones (eg, platybasia, Paget's disease of skull base), surgical trauma (eg, due to endarterectomy)

*Systemic disorders (eg, myasthenia gravis, botulism, variant Guillain-Barré syndrome, poliomyelitis with bulbar involvement, progressive supranuclear palsy) can cause diffuse cranial nerve dysfunction. Amyotrophic lateral sclerosis may cause prominent tongue fasciculations.

Pupils are dilated (about 6 mm) and respond poorly to light but better to accommodation; nystagmus occurs during attempted upward gaze. Isolated downward gaze palsies are rare because they require separate symmetric midbrain lesions that skip the area that controls upward gaze. Downward paralysis is pathognomonic for progressive supranuclear palsy (see p. 1885).

INTERNUCLEAR OPHTHALMOPLEGIA

Internuclear ophthalmoplegia is unilateral or bilateral paresis of eye adduction in lateral horizontal gaze but not in convergence.

During horizontal gaze, the medial longitudinal fasciculus (MLF) on each side of the brain stem allows abduction of one eye to be coordinated with adduction of the other. The MLF connects the 6th cranial nerve nucleus (which controls the lateral rectus, responsible for abduction) and adjacent horizontal gaze center with the contralateral 3rd cranial nerve nucleus (which controls the medial rectus, responsible for adduction). The MLF also connects the vestibular nuclei with the 3rd cranial nerve nuclei.

Internuclear ophthalmoplegia results from a lesion in the MLF. In young people, the disorder is commonly caused by multiple sclerosis and is often bilateral. In the elderly, it is typically caused by stroke and is unilateral. Occasionally, the cause is neurosyphilis, Lyme disease, tumor, or drug intoxication (eg, tricyclic antidepressants).

A lesion in the MLF blocks signals from the horizontal gaze center to the 3rd cranial nerve; the eye on the affected side cannot adduct (or adducts weakly) past the midline. The affected eye adducts normally in convergence because convergence does not require signals from the horizontal gaze center. This finding distinguishes internuclear ophthalmoplegia from 3rd cranial nerve palsy, which impairs adduction in convergence. During horizontal gaze to the side opposite the affected eye, images are horizontally displaced, causing diplopia; nystagmus often occurs in the abducting eye. Sometimes vertical bilateral nystagmus occurs during attempted upward gaze. Treatment is directed at the underlying disorder.

One-and-a-half syndrome: This uncommon syndrome occurs if a lesion affects the pontine horizontal gaze center and the MLF on the same side. The eyes cannot move horizontally to either side except the eye on the side opposite the lesion can abduct; convergence is unaffected. Causes include multiple sclerosis, infarction, hemorrhage, and tumor. Improvement may occur (eg, with radiation therapy for a tumor or treatment of multiple sclerosis) but is often limited after infarction.

TABLE 219–2. COMMON DISTURBANCES OF OCULAR MOTILITY

CLINICAL FINDING	DEFICIT	COMMON CAUSES
Pareses		
Paresis of horizontal gaze in one direction, usually bilateral	Conjugate horizontal gaze palsy	Lesions in both the pontine horizontal gaze center and 6th cranial nerve ipsilaterally or lesion in the frontal cortex contralaterally
Bilateral paresis of all horizontal gaze movements except for abduction of the eye contralateral to the lesion; convergence unaffected	One-and-a-half syndrome	Lesion in the medial longitudinal fasciculus and ipsilateral pontine lateral gaze center
Unilateral or bilateral paresis of eye adduction in horizontal lateral gaze but not in convergence	Internuclear ophthalmoplegia	Lesion in the medial longitudinal fasciculus
Bilateral paresis of upward gaze with dilated pupils and poor light reflex	Parinaud's syndrome (a type of conjugate vertical gaze palsy)	Pineal tumor or midbrain infarct
Bilateral paresis of downward gaze	Conjugate downward gaze palsy	Progressive supranuclear palsy
Unilateral paresis of eye abduction and upward and downward gaze, ptosis, and often a dilated pupil	3rd cranial nerve palsy	Aneurysms, transtentorial herniation, nerve or midbrain ischemia
Unilateral paresis of vertical gaze in adduction; may be subtle, producing symptoms but no signs	4th cranial nerve palsy	Idiopathic, head trauma
Unilateral paresis of eye abduction	6th cranial nerve palsy	Idiopathic, infarct, vasculitis, increased intracranial pressure, Wernicke's encephalopathy, multiple sclerosis
Involuntary or abnormal movements		
Rhythmic involuntary movements, usually bilateral	Nystagmus	See sidebar 84–1 on p. 776
Fast downward jerk; slow upward return to midposition	Ocular bobbing	Extensive pontine destruction or dysfunction
Gaze overshoot followed by several oscillations	Ocular dysmetria	Cerebellar pathway disorders
Rapid oscillations about a point of fixation	Ocular flutter	Cerebellar pathway disorders
Rapid, conjugate, chaotic movements, often with widespread myoclonus	Opsoclonus	Many causes: postanoxic encephalopathy, occult neuroblastoma, ataxia-telangiectasia

THIRD CRANIAL NERVE PALSY

Third cranial nerve palsy impairs ocular motility and sometimes pupillary function.

Symptoms and signs include diplopia, ptosis, paresis of eye abduction and upward gaze, and, if the pupil is affected, pupil dilation and impaired light reflexes. If the pupil is affected, CT is done as soon as possible.

Third cranial (oculomotor) nerve palsies that affect the pupil are caused commonly by aneurysm (especially of the posterior communicating artery) and transtentorial brain herniation (see p. 1800) and less commonly by meningitis affecting the brain stem (eg, TB meningitis). The most common cause of palsies that spare the pupil, particularly partial palsies, is ischemia of the 3rd cranial nerve (usually due to diabetes) or of the midbrain. Occasionally, a posterior communicating artery aneurysm causes oculomotor paralysis and spares the pupil.

Symptoms, Signs, and Diagnosis

Manifestations include diplopia and drooping of the upper eyelid (ptosis). The affected eye may deviate out and down in straight-ahead gaze; adduction is slow and cannot proceed past the midline. Upward gaze is impaired. When downward gaze is attempted, the superior oblique muscle causes the eye to adduct. The pupil may be normal or dilated; its response to direct or consensual light may be sluggish or absent (efferent defect). Pupil dilation (mydriasis) may be an early sign.

Differential diagnosis includes intraorbital structural lesions that restrict ocular motility, ocular myopathies (eg, due to hypothyroidism, mitochondrial disorders, or polymyositis), and disorders of the neuromuscular junction (eg, due to myasthenia gravis or botulism). Exophthalmos or enophthalmos, a history of severe orbital trauma, or an obviously inflamed orbit

TABLE 219–3. COMMON PUPILLARY ABNORMALITIES

FINDING	COMMON CAUSES
Asymmetry of 1–2 mm between pupils, preserved light responses, no symptoms	Physiologic anisocoria (unequal pupils)
Asymmetry, impaired light responses, preserved response to accommodation	Argyll Robertson pupil, suggesting neurosyphilis
Bilateral constriction	Opioids, organophosphate or cholinergic toxins, pontine hemorrhage, most commonly miotic eye drops for glaucoma (cause unilateral constriction if single eye is used)
Bilateral dilation, preserved light reflexes	Hyperadrenergic states (eg, withdrawal syndromes, drugs such as sympathomimetics or cocaine, thyrotoxicosis)
Bilateral dilation, impaired light response	Mydriatic eye drops (eg, sympathomimetics such as phenylephrine; cycloplegics such as cyclopentolate, tropicamide, homatropine, and atropine); brain herniation, hypoxic or ischemic encephalopathy
Unilateral dilation, afferent pupillary defect	Lesions of the eye, retina, or 2nd cranial (optic) nerve
Unilateral dilation, efferent pupillary defect	Third cranial (oculomotor) nerve palsies, often due to compression (eg, due to aneurysm of the posterior communicating artery or to transtentorial herniation); mydriatic eye drops*
Unilateral dilation with minimal or slow direct and consensual light reflexes, pupil constriction in response to accommodation	Tonic (Adie's) pupil†

*Transtentorial herniation and mydriatic eye drops can often be distinguished by instilling a drop of pilocarpine ocular solution into the dilated pupil; failure to constrict in response suggests mydriatic eye drops.

†A tonic pupil is permanent but nonprogressive abnormal dilation of the pupil due to damage of the ciliary ganglion. It usually occurs in women aged 20–40. Onset is usually sudden. The only symptoms are slight blurring of vision, impaired dark adaptation, and sometimes accompanied by absent deep tendon reflexes.

suggests an intraorbital structural disorder. Myopathy should be considered if ocular paresis is mild and the pupil is spared.

CT or MRI is required. If a patient has a dilated pupil and a sudden, severe headache (suggesting ruptured aneurysm) or is increasingly unresponsive (suggesting herniation), CT is done immediately. If ruptured aneurysm is suspected and CT does not show blood or is not available rapidly, other tests such as lumbar puncture or cerebral angiography are required.

FOURTH CRANIAL NERVE PALSY

Fourth cranial nerve palsy impairs the superior oblique muscle, causing paresis of vertical gaze, mainly in adduction.

Fourth cranial (trochlear) nerve palsy is often idiopathic. Few causes have been identified, but of those, a common one is closed head injury, particularly due to motorcycle accidents, which may cause unilateral or bilateral palsies. Rare causes include aneurysms, tumors (eg, tentorial meningioma, pinealoma), and multiple sclerosis.

Because the superior oblique muscle is paretic, the eyes do not adduct normally. Patients see double images, one above and slightly to the side of the other; thus, going down stairs, which requires looking down and inward, is difficult. However, tilting the head to the side opposite the palsied muscle can compensate and eliminate the double images. Examination may detect subtle impaired ocular motility, causing symptoms but not signs.

Oculomotor exercises may help restore concordant vision. Surgery can help by weakening the muscles responsible for the greatest deviation of gaze, usually the inferior oblique.

SIXTH CRANIAL NERVE PALSY

Sixth cranial nerve palsy affects the lateral rectus muscle, impairing eye abduction and causing eye adduction. The palsy is often idiopathic or secondary to infarction or increased intracranial pressure. Determining the cause requires MRI and often lumbar puncture and evaluation for vasculitis.

Sixth cranial (abducens) nerve palsy is often due to small-vessel occlusion, particularly in diabetics as part of a process called mononeuritis multiplex (multiple mononeuropathy). Sixth cranial nerve palsy is often idiopathic, particularly when no other cranial nerves are affected. It may result from compression of the nerve by lesions in the cavernous sinus (eg, nasopharyngeal tumors), orbit, or base of the skull. Palsy may also result from anything that causes the brain to shift, such as increased intracranial pressure and head trauma. Other causes include meningitis, meningeal carcinomatosis, meningeal tumors, Wernicke's encephalopathy, aneurysm, vasculitis, multiple sclerosis, pontine stroke, and, rarely, lumbar puncture. In children, respiratory infection may cause recurrent palsy.

Symptoms include binocular horizontal diplopia. The eye is slightly adducted in straight-ahead gaze; it abducts sluggishly, and even when abduction is maximal, the lateral sclera is exposed. With complete paralysis, the eye cannot abduct past midline. Palsy resulting from nerve compression by a clot, tumor, or aneurysm in the cavernous sinus causes severe head pain, chemosis (conjunctival edema), anesthesia in the distribution of the 1st division of the 5th cranial nerve, compression with vision loss, and paralysis of the 3rd and 4th cranial nerves. Both sides are typically affected.

Diagnosis of 6th nerve palsy is usually obvious, but the cause must be identified. If retinal venous pulsations are seen during ophthalmoscopy, increased intracranial pressure is unlikely. CT is generally done, although MRI is more sensitive for multiple sclerosis and lesions in the posterior fossa. If either study is normal but meningitis or increased intracranial pressure is suspected, lumbar puncture is done. If vasculitis is suspected clinically, evaluation begins with measurement of ESR, antinuclear antibodies, and rheumatoid factor. In children, if increased intracranial pressure is excluded, respiratory infection is considered.

In many patients, 6th cranial nerve palsies resolve once the underlying disorder is treated. Idiopathic palsy usually abates within 2 mo.

TRIGEMINAL NEURALGIA

(Tic Douloureux)

Trigeminal neuralgia is severe paroxysmal, lancinating facial pain due to a disorder of the 5th cranial nerve. Diagnosis is clinical. Treatment is usually with carbamazepine or gabapentin; sometimes surgery is required.

Trigeminal neuralgia is thought to be caused by abnormal pulsations of intracranial arterial or, less often, venous loops that compress the 5th cranial (trigeminal) nerve root where it enters the brain stem. The disorder is occasionally due to multiple sclerosis. Trigeminal neuralgia affects mainly adults, especially the elderly.

Symptoms, Signs, and Diagnosis

Pain occurs along the distribution of one or more sensory divisions of the trigeminal nerve, most often the maxillary, and lasts seconds up to 2 min. It is lancinating, excruciating, and sometimes incapacitating. Pain is often precipitated by touching a facial trigger point or by moving (eg, chewing, brushing the teeth).

Symptoms are almost pathognomonic. Postherpetic pain is differentiated by its persistence, typical antecedent rash, scarring, and predilection for the ophthalmic division; migraine, which may produce atypical facial pain, is differentiated by pain that is more prolonged and often throbbing. Neurologic examination is normal. Thus, neurologic deficits suggest an alternate cause for pain (eg, tumor, multiple sclerosis plaque, vascular malformation, other lesions that compress the nerve or its brain stem pathways, or stroke). A pontine lesion disrupts trigeminal nerve sensation, corneal reflex, and motor function. Loss of pain and temperature sensation and loss of the corneal reflex with preservation of motor function suggest a medullary lesion. Trigeminal nerve deficits may occur in Sjögren's syndrome or RA but with a sensory deficit that is often perioral and nasal.

Treatment

Carbamazepine 200 mg po tid or qid is usually effective for long periods; hepatic and hematopoietic function should be checked after 2 wk, then every 3 to 6 mo. If carbamazepine is ineffective or has adverse effects, gabapentin 300 to 900 mg po tid, phenytoin 100 to 200 mg po bid or tid, baclofen 10 to 30 mg po tid, or amitriptyline 25 to 200 mg po taken at bedtime may be tried. Peripheral nerve block provides temporary relief.

If pain is severe despite these measures, neuroablative treatments are considered; however, efficacy may be temporary, and improvement may be followed by persistent pain that is even more severe than the preceding episodes. In a posterior fossa craniectomy, a small pad can be placed to separate the pulsating vascular loop from the trigeminal root. In radiosurgery, a gamma knife can be used to cut the proximal trigeminal nerve. Electrolytic or chemical lesions or balloon compression of the trigeminal (gasserian) ganglion can be made via a percutaneous stereotaxically positioned needle. Occasionally, as a last resort to relieve intractable pain, the trigeminal nerve fibers between the gasserian ganglion and brain stem are cut.

HEMIFACIAL SPASM

Hemifacial spasm is unilateral painless, irregular contractions of the facial muscles due to impairment of the 7th cranial (facial) nerve. Pathophysiology and treatment are similar to those of trigeminal neuralgia except botulinum toxin can also be used effectively.

BELL'S PALSY

Bell's palsy is sudden, idiopathic, unilateral peripheral 7th cranial nerve palsy. Symptoms are hemifacial paresis involving the upper and lower face. There are no specific tests for diagnosis. Treatment may include corticosteroids, lubrication of the eye, and intermittent use of an eye patch.

Cause is unknown, but the mechanism is presumably swelling of the 7th cranial (facial) nerve due to an immune or viral disorder (possibly herpes simplex virus infection). The nerve is compressed, resulting in ischemia and paresis because the nerve's passageway through the temporal bone is narrow. The orbicularis oculi and frontalis muscles are paretic in peripheral but not in central 7th cranial nerve palsies because these muscles receive input from left and right 7th cranial nerve nuclei.

Symptoms and Signs

Pain behind the ear often precedes facial paresis. Paresis, often with complete paralysis, develops within hours and is usually maximal within 48 to 72 h. Patients may complain of a numb or heavy feeling in the face. The affected side becomes flat and expressionless; ability to wrinkle the forehead, blink, and grimace is limited or absent. In severe cases, the palpebral fissure widens and the eye does not close, often irritating the conjunctiva and drying the cornea. Sensory examination is normal except for the external auditory canal and a small patch behind the ear. If the nerve lesion is proximal, salivation, taste, and lacrimation are impaired, and hyperacusis is present.

Diagnosis

There are no specific diagnostic tests. Bell's palsy can be distinguished from a central 7th cranial nerve lesion (eg, due to stroke or tumor), which causes weakness only of the lower face (grimace). Many disorders cause peripheral 7th cranial nerve palsies; examples are geniculate herpes (Ramsay Hunt syndrome, due to herpes zoster), middle ear or mastoid infections, sarcoidosis (particularly in black patients), Lyme disease (particularly where it is endemic), petrous bone fractures, carcinomatous or leukemic nerve invasion, chronic meningitis, and cerebellopontine angle or glomus jugulare tumors. These disorders typically develop more slowly than Bell's palsy and may have other distinguishing symptoms or signs. If the diagnosis is in doubt, MRI with contrast agent may enhance the 7th cranial nerve in Bell's palsy; CT, usually negative in Bell's palsy, is done if a fracture is suspected or if there is the possibility of stroke. Acute and convalescent serologic tests for Lyme disease are done if patients have been in a geographic area where ticks are endemic. A chest x-ray and serum ACE are checked for sarcoidosis. Viral titers are not helpful.

Prognosis and Treatment

The extent of nerve damage determines outcome. If some function remains, full recovery usually occurs within several months. Nerve conduction studies and electromyography predict likelihood of complete recovery after total paralysis in 90% if nerve branches in the face retain normal excitability to supramaximal electrical stimulation and in only about 20% if electrical excitability is absent.

Regrowth of nerve fibers may be misdirected, innervating lower facial muscles with periocular fibers and vice versa. The result is contraction of unexpected muscles during voluntary facial movements (synkinesia) or crocodile tears during salivation. Chronic disuse of the facial muscles may lead to contractures.

No treatment has proved effective for idiopathic Bell's palsy. Corticosteroids, if begun within 48 h after onset, may slightly reduce duration and degree of residual paralysis. Prednisone 60 to 80 mg po once/day is given for 1 wk, then decreased gradually over the 2nd wk. Antiviral drugs effective against herpes simplex virus (eg, valacyclovir 1 g tid for 7 to 10 days, famciclovir 500 mg po tid for 5 to 10 days, acyclovir 400 mg po 5 times/day for 10 days) are also usually given.

Corneal drying must be prevented by frequent use of natural tears, isotonic saline, or methylcellulose drops and by intermittent use of tape or a patch to help close the eye, particularly during sleep. Tarsorrhaphy is occasionally required.

GLOSSOPHARYNGEAL NEURALGIA

Glossopharyngeal neuralgia is recurrent attacks of severe pain in the 9th cranial nerve distribution (posterior pharynx, tonsils, back of the tongue, middle ear). Diagnosis is clinical. Treatment is usually with carbamazepine or gabapentin.

Glossopharyngeal neuralgia sometimes results from nerve compression by an aberrant, pulsating artery similar to that in trigeminal neuralgia and facial hemispasm. Rarely, the cause is a tumor in the cerebellopontine angle or the neck. Often, no cause is identified. The disorder is rare, more commonly affecting men, usually after age 40.

As in trigeminal neuralgia, paroxysmal attacks of unilateral brief, excruciating pain occur spontaneously or are precipitated by certain movements (eg, chewing, swallowing, talking, sneezing). The pain, lasting seconds to a few minutes, usually begins in the tonsillar region or at the base of the tongue and may radiate to the ipsilateral ear. In 1 to 2% of patients, increased vagus nerve activity causes sinus arrest with syncope; episodes may be very infrequent.

Diagnosis and Treatment

Diagnosis is clinical. Glossopharyngeal neuralgia must be distinguished from trigeminal neuralgia: Location of the pain is different; also, in glossopharyngeal neuralgia, swallowing or touching the tonsils with an applicator tends to precipitate pain, and applying lidocaine to the throat temporarily eliminates spontaneous or evoked pain. Tonsillar, pharyngeal, and cerebellopontine angle tumors and metastatic lesions in the anterior cervical triangle must be ruled out by MRI.

Treatment is the same as that for trigeminal neuralgia (see p. 1875). If oral drugs are ineffective, topical cocaine applied to the pharynx may provide temporary relief, and surgery to decompress the nerve from a pulsating artery may be necessary. If pain is restricted to the pharynx, surgery can be restricted to the extracranial part of the nerve; if pain is widespread, surgery must involve the intracranial part of the nerve.

220 CRANIOCERVICAL JUNCTION ABNORMALITIES

Craniocervical junction abnormalities are congenital or acquired abnormalities of the occipital bone, foramen magnum, or first 2 cervical vertebrae that decrease the space for the lower brain stem and cervical cord. These abnormalities can result in neck pain; syringomyelia; cerebellar, lower cranial nerve, and spinal cord deficits; and vertebrobasilar ischemia. Diagnosis is by MRI or CT. Treatment often involves reduction, followed by stabilization with surgery or an external device.

Neural tissue is flexible and susceptible to compression. Several types of craniocervical abnormalities can cause or contribute to cervical spinal cord or brain stem compression. Fusion of the atlas (C1) and occipital bone causes spinal cord compression if the anteroposterior diameter of the foramen magnum behind the odontoid process is < 19 mm. Basilar invagination (upward bulging of the occipital condyles) results in a short neck and compression that can affect the cerebellum, brain stem, lower cranial nerves, and spinal cord. Atlantoaxial subluxation or dislocation (displacement of the atlas anteriorly in relation to the axis) causes acute or chronic spinal cord compression. The Klippel-Feil malformation (fusion of cervical vertebrae) deforms and limits motion of the neck but usually does not have neurologic consequences. Platybasia (flattening of the skull base so that the angle formed by the intersection of the clival and anterior fossa planes is > 135°), seen on lateral skull x-ray, may be asymptomatic or cause cerebellar or spinal cord deficits or normal-pressure hydrocephalus.

Etiology

Most craniocervical junction abnormalities result from congenital or acquired abnormalities.

Congenital abnormalities include os odontoideum (anomalous bone that replaces all or part of the odontoid process), atlas assimilation (congenital fusion of the atlas and occipital bone), atlas hypoplasia, and Chiari malformations (descent of the cerebellar tonsils or vermis into the cervical spinal canal—see p. 2441). In achondroplasia (impaired epiphyseal bone growth, resulting in shortened, malformed bones), the foramen magnum sometimes narrows, compressing the spinal cord or brain. Down syndrome, Morquio's syndrome (mucopolysaccharidosis IV), or osteogenesis imperfecta can cause atlantoaxial subluxation or dislocation.

Acquired abnormalities may result from injury or disease. Injuries may involve bone, ligaments, or both and are usually caused by vehicle or bicycle accidents and falls (particularly diving). Many such injuries are immediately fatal. RA (the most common disease cause), metastatic tumors, and Paget's disease of the cervical spine can cause atlantoaxial dislocation or subluxation. Slowly growing craniocervical junction tumors (eg, meningioma, chordoma) can impinge on the brain stem or spinal cord. RA and Paget's disease can cause basilar invagination, which can compress the spinal cord or brain stem, or platybasia.

Symptoms and Signs

Symptoms and signs can occur after minor neck injury or spontaneously and may vary in progression. Presentation varies by degree of compression and structures affected. Some abnormalities (eg, platybasia, basilar invagination, Klippel-Feil malformation) affect the neck. It may be short with limited motion, webbed (skinfold running approximately from the sternocleidomastoid to the shoulder), or in an abnormal position (eg, torticollis in Klippel-Feil malformation).

The most common manifestations are neck pain, often spreading to the arms, and spinal cord compression (myelopathy). An occipital headache radiating to the skull vertex is common; it is attributed to compression of the C2 root and greater occipital nerve and to local musculoskeletal dysfunction. Neck pain and headache usually worsen with head movement and can be precipitated by coughing or bending forward. If patients with Chiari malformation have hydrocephalus, being upright may aggravate the hydrocephalus and result in headaches.

Spinal cord deficits involve the upper cervical cord. They include spastic paresis in the arms, legs, or both, caused by compression of motor tracts. Joint position and vibration senses (posterior column function) are commonly impaired. Tingling down the back, often into the legs, with neck flexion (Lhermitte's sign) may occur. Uncommonly, pain and temperature senses (spinothalamic tract function) are impaired in a stocking-glove pattern.

Cerebellar, brain stem, and cranial nerve deficits may occur when the brain is compressed (eg, due to platybasia, basilar invagination, or craniocervical tumors). Brain stem and cranial nerve deficits include sleep apnea, internuclear ophthalmoplegia (ipsilateral weakness of eye adduction plus contralateral horizontal nystagmus in the abducting eye with lateral gaze), downbeat nystagmus (fast component downward), hoarseness, dysarthria, and dysphagia. Cerebellar deficits usually impair coordination (see p. 1886).

Changing head position can trigger symptoms of vertebrobasilar ischemia, including intermittent syncope, drop attacks, vertigo, confusion or altered consciousness, weakness, and visual disturbance.

Syringomyelia (cavity in the central part of the spinal cord—see p. 1915) is common in patients with Chiari malformation. It may cause segmental flaccid weakness and atrophy of the distal upper extremities; pain and temperature senses may be lost in a capelike distribution over the neck and proximal upper extremities, but light touch is preserved.

Diagnosis

A craniocervical abnormality is suspected when patients have pain in the neck or occiput plus neurologic deficits referable to the lower brain stem, upper cervical spinal cord, or cerebellum. Lower cervical spine disorders can usually be distinguished clinically (based on level of spinal cord dysfunction) and by neuroimaging.

If a craniocervical abnormality is suspected, MRI or CT of the upper spinal cord and brain, particularly the posterior fossa and craniocervical junction, is done. Acute or suddenly progressive deficits are an emergency, requiring immediate imaging. Sagittal MRI best identifies associated neural lesions (eg, hindbrain, cerebellar, spinal cord, and vascular abnormalities; syringomyelia) and soft-tissue lesions. CT shows bony structures more accurately than MRI and may be done more easily in an emergency. If MRI and CT are unavailable, plain x-rays (lateral view of the skull showing the cervical spine, anteroposterior view, and oblique views of the cervical spine) are taken. If MRI is unavailable or inconclusive and CT is inconclusive, CT myelography (CT after intrathecal injection of a radiopaque agent) is done. If MRI or CT suggests vascular abnormalities, magnetic resonance angiography or vertebral angiography is done.

Treatment

If neural structures are compressed, treatment consists of reduction (traction or changes in head position to realign the craniocervical junction and thus relieve neural compression). After reduction, the head and neck are immobilized.

Acute or suddenly progressive spinal cord compression requires emergency reduction. For most patients, reduction involves skeletal traction with a crown halo ring and weight of up to about 4 kg. Reduction with traction may take 5 to 6 days. If reduction is achieved, the neck is immobilized in a halo vest for 8 to 12 wk; then x-rays must be taken to confirm stability. If reduction does not relieve neural compression, surgical decompression, using a ventral or a dorsal approach, is necessary. If instability persists after decompression, posterior fixation (stabilization) is required. For some abnormalities (eg, due to RA) external immobilization alone is rarely successful; then posterior fixation or anterior decompression and stabilization are required.

Several different methods of instrumentation (eg, plates or rods with screws) can be used for temporary stabilization until bones fuse and stability is permanent. In general, all unstable areas must be fused.

Radiation therapy and a hard cervical collar often help patients with metastatic bone tumors. Calcitonin, mithramycin, and bisphosphonates may help patients with Paget's disease.

221 MOVEMENT AND CEREBELLAR DISORDERS

Movement disorders (dyskinesias) are characterized by decreased or slow purposeful movements (hypokinesia) or excessive voluntary or abnormal involuntary movements (hyperkinesia). Although disorders involving the cerebellum impair the rate, range, and force of movement, they, except for tremors, are not considered movement disorders (see p. 1886).

Voluntary movement requires interaction of corticospinal (pyramidal) tracts, which pass through the medullary pyramids to connect the cerebral cortex to lower motor centers of the brain stem and spinal cord; the basal ganglia (caudate nucleus, putamen, globus pallidus, and substantia nigra, forming the extrapyramidal system), which are located deep in the forebrain and whose output is directed mainly rostrally through the thalamus to the cerebral cortex; and the cerebellum, the center for motor coordination. Most neural lesions that cause movement disorders occur in the extrapyramidal system; thus, movement disorders are also called extrapyramidal disorders.

Hypokinesia: Most hypokinetic disorders are parkinsonian disorders.

Hyperkinesia: There are numerous hyperkinetic disorders; they are initially characterized as rhythmic or nonrhythmic.

Rhythmic disorders are primarily tremors—regular alternating or oscillatory movements, which can occur mainly at rest or during attempted movement (as intention tremor).

Nonrhythmic disorders are characterized as slow or sustained (eg, athetosis, dystonias) or rapid. Rapid disorders are characterized as suppressible (eg, tics) or nonsuppressible (eg, hemiballismus, chorea, myoclonus).

Athetosis is nonrhythmic, slow, writhing, sinuous movements, predominantly in distal muscles; alternating postures of the proximal limbs often blend continuously to produce a flowing stream of movement. Athetosis often occurs with chorea as choreoathetosis.

Dystonias are sustained involuntary muscle contractions, often distorting body posture.

Tics are nonrhythmic, rapid, suppressible movements that are simple or complex, idiosyncratic, repetitive, and done almost unconsciously. They can be suppressed only for brief periods and with conscious effort. Simple tics (eg, eye blinking) often begin as nervous mannerisms in childhood or later, then disappear spontaneously. Tics tend to be more complex than myoclonus and less flowing than choreic movements. Tic disorders include Tourette's syndrome (see p. 2379).

Hemiballismus is a nonrhythmic, rapid, nonsuppressible movement characterized usually by unilateral, violent, flinging movements of the proximal arm.

Chorea is a nonrhythmic, jerky, rapid, nonsuppressible movement that involves mostly distal muscles or the face; movements may merge imperceptibly into purposeful or semipurposeful acts that mask the involuntary movement. It often occurs as part of choreoathetosis. Chorea occurs in Huntington's disease (see p. 1881).

Myoclonus is nonrhythmic, rapid, nonsuppressible, shocklike twitching movements that may occur in multiple muscles simultaneously.

CHOREA, ATHETOSIS, AND HEMIBALLISMUS

Chorea is involuntary movements mostly of distal muscles or the face; movements may merge imperceptibly into purposeful or semipurposeful acts that mask the involuntary motion. Athetosis is writhing, sinuous movements predominantly in distal muscles, often alternating with postures of the proximal limbs to produce a continuous, flowing stream of movement. Chorea and athetosis often occur together (as choreoathetosis). Hemiballismus is usually a unilateral, violent, flinging movement of the proximal arm.

Chorea and athetosis are manifestations of dopaminergic overactivity in the basal ganglia. Huntington's disease (see p. 1881) is the most common degenerative disease causing chorea. Other causes include thyrotoxicosis, SLE affecting the CNS, drugs (eg, antipsychotics), and rheumatic fever (Sydenham's chorea—see p. 2360). A tumor or infarct of the caudate nucleus can cause acute unilateral chorea (hemichorea).

Chorea gravidarum occurs during pregnancy, often in patients who had rheumatic fever. Chorea usually begins during the 1st trimester and resolves spontaneously by or after delivery. Treatment is sedation with barbiturates; other sedatives may harm the fetus. Rarely, a similar disorder occurs in women taking oral contraceptives.

Hemiballismus is caused by a lesion, usually an infarct, around the contralateral subthalamic nucleus. Although disabling, hemiballismus is usually self-limited, lasting 6 to 8 wk. Treatment with antipsychotics is often effective.

DYSTONIAS

Dystonias are sustained involuntary muscle contractions, often distorting body posture. Dystonias can be primary or secondary, and they can be generalized, focal, or segmental. Diagnosis is clinical. Treatment is with an anticholinergic drug or reserpine for generalized dystonia and botulinum toxin for focal or segmental dystonias.

Dystonia may be primary (idiopathic) or secondary to degenerative or metabolic CNS disorders (eg, Wilson's disease, Hallervorden-Spatz disease, various lipidoses, cerebral palsy, stroke) or drugs (most often phenothiazines, thioxanthenes, butyrophenones, and antiemetics).

Generalized dystonia (dystonia musculorum deformans): This rare dystonia is progressive and characterized by movements that result in sustained, often bizarre postures. It is often hereditary, usually as an autosomal dominant disorder with partial penetrance; asymptomatic siblings of patients often have a forme fruste of the disorder. The causative gene may be linked to chromosome 9q, but the anatomic basis is unknown. Symptoms usually begin in childhood with inversion and plantar fixation of the foot while walking. Patients with the most severe form may become twisted into grotesque fixed postures. Mental function is usually preserved.

Focal dystonias: These dystonias affect a single body part. They typically start in a person's 30s or 40s and affect women more often. Initially, spasms may be periodic, occurring randomly or during stress; they are triggered by certain movements of the affected body part and disappear during rest. Over days, weeks, or many years, spasms may progress; they may be triggered by movements of unaffected body parts and may continue during rest. Eventually, the affected body part remains distorted, sometimes in a painful position, resulting in severe disability. Symptoms vary depending on the specific muscles involved.

Meige's disease (blepharospasm-oromandibular dystonia) consists of involuntary blinking, jaw grinding, and grimacing, usually beginning in late middle age. It may mimic buccal-lingual-facial movements of tardive dyskinesia.

Occupational dystonia consists of focal dystonic spasms initiated by performing skilled acts (eg, writer's or typist's cramp).

Spastic dystonia consists of a strained, hoarse, or creaky voice due to abnormal involuntary contraction of laryngeal muscles.

Torticollis begins with a pulling sensation followed by sustained torsion and deviation of the head and neck. In early stages, it can be voluntarily overcome.

Diagnosis and Treatment

Diagnosis is clinical. Treatment is often unsatisfactory. For generalized dystonia, a high-dose anticholinergic drug (trihexyphenidyl 2 to 10 mg po tid, benztropine 3 to 15 mg po once/day), reserpine 0.1 to 0.6 mg po once/day, or both are most often used. Reserpine depletes dopamine. Levodopa and carbamazepine benefit a few patients.

For focal or segmental dystonias or for generalized dystonia that severely affects specific body parts, local injection of purified botulinum A toxin into the affected muscles by an experienced practitioner is the treatment of choice. Botulinum toxin weakens muscular contractions but does not alter the abnormal neural stimulus. Toxin injection is particularly effective for blepharospasm and torticollis. Dosage varies greatly. Treatments must be repeated every 3 to 6 mo.

FRAGILE X–ASSOCIATED TREMOR/ATAXIA SYNDROME

Fragile X–associated tremor/ataxia syndrome is a genetic disorder affecting mostly men and causing tremor, ataxia, and dementia.

Fragile X–associated tremor/ataxia syndrome (FXTAS), a newly recognized disorder, affects about 1/3000 men. Affected men carry the gene that causes fragile X syndrome in children; most are grandfathers of such children. FXTAS develops in about 30% of carriers. Women may also carry the gene but do not appear to develop the disorder.

Symptoms usually develop in older age; they include tremor that resembles essential tremor, ataxia, and dementia. Diagnosis is by genetic testing. Tremor can often be relieved with many of the drugs used to control the tremors of Parkinson's disease.

HUNTINGTON'S DISEASE

(Huntington's Chorea; Chronic Progressive Chorea; Hereditary Chorea)

Huntington's disease is an autosomal dominant disorder characterized by chorea and progressive cognitive deterioration, usually beginning in middle age. Diagnosis is by genetic testing. Treatment is supportive. First-degree relatives are encouraged to undergo genetic testing.

Huntington's disease affects both sexes equally. The caudate nucleus atrophies, the small-cell population degenerates, and levels of the neurotransmitters γ-aminobutyric acid (GABA) and substance P decrease.

Huntington's disease results from a gene mutation that causes abnormal expansion of the repetitive DNA sequence CAG that codes for the amino acid glutamine. The gene product, a large protein called huntingtin, has an expanded stretch of polyglutamine residues, which leads to disease via unknown mechanisms. The more CAG repetitions, the earlier the disease begins and the more severe the clinical course. The number of repeats can increase with successive generations and, over time, lead to a more severe phenotype within a family tree.

Symptoms, Signs, and Diagnosis

Symptoms and signs develop insidiously, starting at about age 35 to 50. Dementia or psychiatric disturbances (eg, depression, apathy, irritability, anhedonia, antisocial behavior, full-blown bipolar or schizophreniform disorder) develop before or simultaneously with the movement disorder. Abnormal movements appear; they include flicking of the extremities, a lilting gait, inability to sustain a motor act such as tongue protrusion (motor impersistence), facial grimacing, ataxia, and dystonia.

The disorder progresses, making walking impossible, swallowing difficult, and dementia severe. Because most patients eventually require institutionalization, end-of-life care should be discussed early (see p. 2762).

Diagnosis is based on typical symptoms and signs plus a positive family history and is confirmed by genetic testing. Neuroimaging is done to exclude other disorders; in advanced Huntington's disease, MRI and CT coronal views show boxcar ventricles (ie, squared-off edges due to atrophy of the caudate head).

Treatment

Treatment is supportive. Chorea and agitation may be partially suppressed by antipsychotics (eg, chlorpromazine 25 to 300 mg po tid, haloperidol 5 to 45 mg po bid) or reserpine 0.1 mg po once/day; dose is increased until intolerable or undesirable adverse effects (eg, lethargy, parkinsonism; with reserpine, hypotension) occur. Experimental therapies aim to reduce glutamatergic neurotransmission via the *N*-methyl-D-aspartate receptor and bolster mitochondrial energy production. Treatment to supplement GABA in the brain has been ineffective.

Genetic testing and counseling (see also p. 2143) are important because the disorder is asymptomatic until after childbearing age. People who have a family history and are interested in testing are referred to centers that have expertise in dealing with the complex ethical and psychologic issues involved.

MYOCLONUS

Myoclonus is a brief, shocklike contraction of a muscle or group of muscles.

Physiologic myoclonus may occur as a person falls asleep (nocturnal myoclonus). Myoclonus occurs secondary to other disorders, including metabolic disorders (eg, uremia), degenerative disorders (eg, Alzheimer's disease, progressive myoclonic epilepsy), prion diseases (eg, Creutzfeldt-Jakob disease), slow virus infections (eg, subacute sclerosing panencephalitis), and brain damage. Myoclonus due to severe closed head trauma or hypoxic-ischemic brain damage may worsen with purposeful movements (action myoclonus) or may occur spontaneously when movement is limited because of injury.

Diagnosis and Treatment

Diagnosis is clinical. Treatment begins with correction of underlying metabolic disorders. Clonazepam 0.5 to 2 mg po tid is often effective. Valproate 250 to 500 mg po bid may be effective; rarely, other anticonvulsants help. Many forms of myoclonus respond to the serotonin precursor 5-hydroxytryptophan (initially, 25 mg po qid, increased to 150 to 250 mg po qid), which must be used with the oral decarboxylase inhibitor carbidopa (50 mg every morning and 25 mg at noon or 50 mg every evening and 25 mg at bedtime).

PARKINSON'S DISEASE

Parkinson's disease is an idiopathic, slowly progressive, degenerative CNS disorder characterized by slow and decreased movement, muscular rigidity, resting tremor, and postural instability. Diagnosis is clinical. Treatment is with levodopa plus carbidopa, other drugs, and, for refractory symptoms, surgery.

Parkinson's disease affects about 1% of people ≥ 65 yr and 0.4% of those > 40 yr. The mean age at onset is about 57 yr. Rarely, Parkinson's disease begins in childhood or adolescence (juvenile parkinsonism).

Etiology and Pathophysiology

In Parkinson's disease, pigmented neurons of the substantia nigra, locus ceruleus, and other brain stem dopaminergic cell groups are lost. Loss of substantia nigra neurons, which project into the caudate nucleus and putamen, depletes dopamine in these areas. The cause is unknown.

Secondary parkinsonism results from loss of or interference with dopamine's action in the basal ganglia due to other degenerative disorders, drugs, or exogenous toxins. The most common cause is ingestion of phenothiazine, thioxanthene, butyrophenone antipsychotic drugs, or reserpine, which block dopamine receptors. Less common causes include carbon monoxide or manganese poisoning, hydrocephalus, structural brain lesions (eg, tumors, infarcts affecting the midbrain or basal ganglia), subdural hematoma, Wilson's disease, and idiopathic degenerative disorders (eg, striatonigral degeneration, multiple system atrophy). N-MPTP (n-methyl-1,2,3,4-tetrahydropyridine), an illicit drug that was made unintentionally during unsuccessful attempts to synthesize meperidine and is used parenterally, can cause severe, sudden, irreversible parkinsonism. Encephalitis can affect basal ganglia, resulting in parkinsonism.

Symptoms and Signs

In most patients, the disease begins insidiously with a resting tremor (pill-rolling tremor) of one hand. The tremor is slow and coarse. The tremor is maximal at rest, lessens during movement, and is absent during sleep; it is enhanced by emotional tension or fatigue. Usually, the hands, arms, and legs are most affected, in that order. The jaw, tongue, forehead, and eyelids may also be affected, but not the voice. Tremor may become less prominent as the disease progresses.

Many patients develop rigidity without tremor. As rigidity progresses, movement becomes slow (bradykinesia), decreased (hypokinesia), and difficult to initiate (akinesia). Rigidity and hypokinesia may contribute to muscular aches and sensations of fatigue. The face becomes masklike, with mouth open and reduced blinking. Early on, patients may appear depressed because facial expression is lacking and movements are decreased and slowed. Speech becomes hypophonic, with characteristic monotonous, stuttering dysarthria. Hypokinesia and impaired control of distal musculature cause micrographia (writing in very small letters) and make activities of daily living increasingly difficult. When a clinician moves a rigid joint, sudden, rhythmic jerks due to variations in the intensity of the rigidity occur, producing a ratchet-like effect (cogwheel rigidity).

The posture becomes stooped. Patients have difficulty starting to walk, turning, and stopping; the gait becomes shuffling with short steps, and the arms are held flexed to the waist and do not swing with the stride. Steps may inadvertently quicken, and patients may break into a run to keep from falling (festination). A tendency to fall forward (propulsion) or backward (retropulsion) when the center of gravity is displaced results from loss of postural reflexes.

Dementia and depression are common. Patients may have orthostatic hypotension, constipation, or urinary hesitancy. Many have difficulty swallowing and thus aspirate.

Patients cannot perform rapidly alternating movements. Sensation and strength are usually normal. Reflexes are normal but may be difficult to elicit because of marked tremor or rigidity. Seborrheic dermatitis is common. Postencephalitic parkinsonism causes forced, sustained deviation of the head and eyes (oculogyric crises), other dystonias, autonomic instability, and personality changes.

Diagnosis

Diagnosis is clinical. Parkinson's disease is suspected in patients with characteristic resting tremors, decreased movement, or rigidity. Bradykinesia due to Parkinson's disease must be differentiated from decreased movement and spasticity due to lesions of the corticospinal tracts. Unlike Parkinson's disease, corticospinal tract lesions cause paresis (weakness or paralysis), preferentially in distal antigravity muscles, and cause extensor plantar responses (Babinski's sign). Spasticity due to corticospinal tract lesions increases muscle tone and deep tendon reflex responses; muscle tone increases in proportion to rate and degree of stretch placed on a muscle until resistance suddenly melts away (clasp-knife phenomenon).

Diagnosis is confirmed by the presence of other characteristic signs (eg, infrequent blinking, lack of facial expression, impaired postural reflexes, characteristic gait abnormalities). Tremor without other characteristic signs suggests early disease or another diagnosis. In the elderly, reduced spontaneous movements or a short-stepped (rheumatic) gait may result from depression or dementia; such cases may be difficult to distinguish from Parkinson's disease.

Causes can be identified primarily by the history and neuroimaging. History should include questions about head trauma, stroke, hydrocephalus, exposure to drugs and toxins, and symptoms or history of other degenerative neurologic disorders.

Treatment

Drugs: Traditionally, levodopa is the first drug used. However, some experts believe that early use of levodopa hastens development of adverse effects and failure of drug response; they prefer to withhold levodopa if possible and use anticholinergic drugs, amantadine, or dopamine agonists first.

Levodopa, the metabolic precursor of dopamine, crosses the blood-brain barrier into the basal ganglia, where it is decarboxylated to form dopamine. Coadministration of the peripheral decarboxylase inhibitor carbidopa prevents levodopa catabolism, thus lowering the levodopa dosage requirements and minimizing adverse effects. Levodopa is most effective at relieving bradykinesia and rigidity, although tremor is often substantially reduced. Mildly affected patients who take levodopa may return to nearly normal, and bedridden patients may become ambulatory.

Central adverse effects of levodopa include nightmares, orthostatic hypotension, drowsiness, dyskinesias, and, particularly in elderly and demented patients, occasional hallucinations or toxic delirium. Peripheral adverse effects include nausea, vomiting, flushing, abdominal cramping, and palpitations. The dose at which dyskinesias occur tends to decrease as treatment continues. In some patients, the lowest dose that reduces parkinsonian symptoms also produces dyskinesias.

Carbidopa/levodopa is available in fixed-ratio tablets of 10/100, 25/100, 25/250, and, in a controlled-release tablet, 50/200 mg. Treatment is begun with one 25/100-mg tablet tid. Dosage is increased q 4 to 7 days as tolerated until maximum benefit is reached. Adverse effects may be minimized by increasing the dose gradually and by giving the drug with or after meals (although high-protein meals may impair absorption of levodopa). If peripheral adverse effects predominate, increasing the amount of carbidopa may help. Most patients with Parkinson's disease require 400 to 1000 mg/day of levodopa in divided doses q 2 to 5 h. Some require up to 2000 mg/day.

Occasionally, levodopa must be used to maintain motor function despite levodopa-induced hallucinations or toxic delirium. Psychosis can sometimes be treated with oral quetiapine or clozapine; these drugs aggravate parkinsonian symptoms much less than other antipsychotics (eg, risperidone, olanzapine) or not at all. Haloperidol should be avoided. Quetiapine can be started at 25 mg once/day or bid and increased in 25-mg increments q 1 to 3 days up to 800 mg/day as tolerated. Use of clozapine is limited because agranulocytosis occurs in 1% of patients. When clozapine is used, the dose is 12.5 to 50 mg once/day to 12.5 to 25 mg bid; CBC is done weekly for 6 mo and q 2 wk thereafter.

After 2 to 5 yr of treatment, most patients experience fluctuations in their response to levodopa (on-off effect). Whether dyskinesias and the on-off effect result from levodopa therapy or the underlying disease is controversial. Eventually, the period of improvement after each dose shortens, and drug-induced dyskinesias result in swings from intense akinesia to uncontrollable hyperactivity. Traditionally, such swings are managed by keeping the levodopa dose as low as possible and using dosing intervals as short as q 1 to 2 h. Alternative methods include adjunctive use of dopamine-agonists, controlled-release levodopa/carbidopa, and selegiline.

Amantadine 100 mg po once/day to tid is useful as monotherapy for early, mild parkinsonism in 50% of patients and later can be used to augment levodopa's effects. It may augment dopaminergic activity, anticholinergic effects, or both. If used as monotherapy, amantadine often loses its effectiveness after several months. Amantadine may ameliorate Parkinson's disease secondary to use of antipsychotic drugs. Adverse effects include lower extremity edema, livedo reticularis, and confusion.

Dopamine agonists directly activate dopamine receptors in the basal ganglia. Drugs (all oral) include bromocriptine 1.25 to 50 mg bid, pergolide 0.05 mg once/day to 1.5 mg tid, ropinirole 0.25 to 8 mg tid, and pramipexole 0.125 to 1.5 mg tid. They can be used as monotherapy but, as such, are rarely sufficient for more than a few years. They may be useful at all stages of the disease. Using these drugs early in treatment, with small doses of levodopa, may delay emergence of dyskinesias and on-off effects, possibly because dopamine agonists stimulate dopamine receptors longer than levodopa does. This type of stimulation is more physiologic and better preserves the receptors. Dopamine agonists are particularly useful in later stages when response to levodopa decreases or on-off effects are prominent. Adverse effects (eg, sedation, nausea, orthostatic hypotension, confusion, delirium, psychosis) may limit use of dopamine agonists. Reducing the levodopa dose may minimize adverse effects of dopamine agonists. Rarely, pergolide causes pleural, retroperitoneal, or cardiac valvular fibrosis.

Selegiline, a selective monoamine oxidase type B (MAO-B) inhibitor, inhibits one of the 2 major enzymes that break down dopamine in the brain, thereby prolonging the action of each dose of levodopa. In some patients with mild on-off effects, selegiline helps prolong levodopa's effect. Used initially as monotherapy, selegiline can delay the initiation of levodopa by about 1 yr. Selegiline may slow progression of Parkinson's disease by potentiating residual brain dopamine in early disease or by reducing oxidative metabolism of brain dopamine. A dose of 5 mg po bid does not cause hypertensive crisis (when tyramine cheeses are eaten), common with nonselective MAO inhibitors, which block the A and B isoenzymes. Although virtually free of adverse effects, selegiline can potentiate dyskinesias, mental and psychiatric adverse effects, and nausea due to levodopa use, requiring reduction in the levodopa dose.

Rasagiline, a new MAO-B inhibitor that is not metabolized to amphetamine, appears to be effective and well-tolerated in early and late disease. Whether rasagiline's effects are purely symptomatic or also neuroprotective remains unknown.

Anticholinergic drugs can be used as monotherapy in early disease and later to supplement levodopa. Commonly used anticholinergic drugs include benztropine 0.5 mg po at night to 2 mg tid and trihexyphenidyl 2 to 5 mg po tid. Antihistamines with anticholinergic effects (eg, diphenhydramine 25 to 50 mg po bid to qid, orphenadrine 50 mg po once/day to qid) are useful for treating tremor. An anticholinergic drug (eg, benztropine) may ameliorate symptoms of Parkinson's disease secondary to use of antipsychotic drugs. Anticholinergic tricyclic antidepressants (eg, amitriptyline 10 to 150 mg po at bedtime), if used for depression, may be useful as an adjunct to levodopa. Doses of anticholinergic drugs are increased very slowly. Adverse effects include dry mouth, urinary retention, constipation, and blurred vision; confusion, delirium, and impaired thermoregulation due to decreased sweating are particularly troublesome adverse effects in the elderly.

Catechol *O*-methyltransferase (COMT) inhibitors (eg, entacapone, tolcapone) inhibit the breakdown of dopamine and therefore appear to be useful adjuncts to levodopa. A combination of levodopa, carbidopa, and entacapone can be used. For each dose of levodopa taken per day, 200 mg of entacapone is given po in a once/day dose to a maximum of 1600 mg/day (eg, for levodopa taken 5 times/day, 1 g of entacapone is given once/day). Tolcapone is rarely used because of liver toxicity.

Surgery: If drugs are ineffective and disease is advanced, surgery is considered; high-frequency electrical stimulation of the subthalamic nucleus is the treatment of choice. For patients with levodopa-induced dyskinesias, stereotactic ablation of the posteroventral globus pallidus (pallidotomy) significantly reduces off-effect bradykinesia and levodopa-induced dyskinesias for up to 4 yr. For patients with severe tremor, deep brain stimulation of the ventral intermediate nucleus in the thalamus may help. Transplantation of fetal dopamine neurons is an experimental treatment that may replete dopamine in the brain.

Physical measures: Maximizing activity is a goal. Patients should perform daily activities to the extent possible. If they cannot, a regular exercise program or physical therapy may help condition them physically and teach them adaptive strategies. Because the disease, antiparkinsonian drugs, and inactivity can lead to constipation, patients should consume a high-fiber diet. Dietary supplements (eg, psyllium) and stimulant laxatives (eg, bisacodyl 10 to 20 mg po once/day) can help.

PROGRESSIVE SUPRANUCLEAR PALSY

(Steele-Richardson-Olszewski Syndrome)

Progressive supranuclear palsy is a rare, degenerative CNS disorder causing loss of voluntary eye movements, bradykinesia, muscular rigidity with progressive axial dystonia, pseudobulbar palsy, and dementia.

The cause of progressive supranuclear palsy is unknown. Neurons in the basal ganglia and brain stem degenerate; neurofibrillary tangles containing an abnormally phosphorylated tau protein are also present. Multiple lacunar strokes may occur in the basal ganglia and deep white matter.

Symptoms usually begin in late middle age. The 1st symptom may be difficulty looking up without extending the neck or difficulty climbing up and down stairs. Voluntary eye movements, particularly vertical, are difficult, but reflexive eye movements are unaffected. Movements are slowed, muscles become rigid, and axial dystonia develops. Patients tend to fall backward. Dysphagia and dysarthria with emotional lability (pseudobulbar palsy) is common; these deficits occur in a stepwise progression as occurs with multiple strokes. Dementia eventually occurs.

Diagnosis is clinical. Treatment is unsatisfactory. Occasionally, dopamine agonists and amantadine partially relieve rigidity.

TREMOR

Tremors are rhythmic, alternating, or oscillatory movements. A tremor can be a normal exaggeration of movement, a primary disorder, or a symptom of a cerebellar disorder or Parkinson's disease. Diagnosis is usually clinical. Treatment varies by etiology.

Tremors must be differentiated from asterixis, which typically causes repetitive, nonrhythmic, nonoscillatory wrist flexion during attempted wrist extension.

Tremors include resting tremors, postural (sustention) tremors, and intention tremors. Resting tremors are maximal at rest and decrease with activity; they are usually a symptom of Parkinson's disease. Postural tremors are maximal when a limb is maintained in a fixed position against gravity; gradual onset suggests physiologic or essential tremor, and acute onset suggests a toxic or metabolic disorder. Intention tremors are maximal during movement toward a target, as in finger-to-nose testing; they suggest a cerebellar disorder but may result from multiple sclerosis or Wilson's disease. Tremors can be characterized by frequency of oscillation (usually 4 to 13 cycles/sec or Hz) and amplitude of movement (fine or coarse).

Physiologic tremor: Physiologic tremor is present normally but usually causes such small movements that it is noticeable only under certain conditions. It is predominantly a postural or intention tremor. The tremor is fine and rapid (8 to 13 Hz). It is most easily visible when hands are outstretched. Physiologic tremor may be enhanced (increased amplitude) by anxiety, stress, fatigue, metabolic disorders (eg, hyperadrenergic states such as alcohol or drug withdrawal or thyrotoxicosis), or certain drugs (eg, caffeine, other phosphodiesterase inhibitors, β-adrenergic agonists, corticosteroids). Alcohol and other sedatives usually suppress the tremor.

No treatment is necessary unless symptoms are bothersome. Physiologic tremors enhanced by alcohol withdrawal or thyrotoxicosis respond to treatment of the underlying condition. Oral benzodiazepines tid or qid (eg, diazepam 2 to 10 mg, lorazepam 1 to 2 mg, oxazepam 10 to 30 mg) may be useful for people with tremor and chronic anxiety, but continuous use should be avoided. Propranolol 20 to 80 mg po qid (and other β-blockers) is often effective for tremor enhanced by drugs or acute anxiety (eg, stage fright). Primidone 50 to 250 mg po tid may be tried if β-blockers are ineffective or poorly tolerated. For some patients, a small amount of alcohol is effective.

Essential tremor (benign hereditary tremor, senile tremor): The tremor is coarse or fine, slow (4 to 8 Hz), and usually bilateral; it can affect the hands, head, and voice. It tends to increase with age and may be incorrectly called senile tremor. In 50% of patients, inheritance is autosomal dominant. The tremor is minimal or absent at rest. It may be enhanced by any factor that enhances physiologic tremor, but it can occur without such factors, differentiating it from physiologic tremor, although the difference is not always obvious.

Propranolol 20 to 80 mg po qid (and other β-blockers) is often effective. Primidone 50 to 250 mg po tid may be tried if β-blockers are ineffective or poorly tolerated.

Tremor of cerebellar disease: This tremor is an intention tremor. No effective drug is available; physical measures (eg, weighting the affected limbs or teaching patients to brace the proximal limb during activity) sometimes help.

CEREBELLAR DISORDERS

Cerebellar disorders have numerous causes, including congenital malformations, hereditary ataxias, and acquired disorders. Symptoms vary with cause but typically involve ataxia (an abnormal, wide-based gait due to impaired muscle coordination). Diagnosis is clinical and also often by imaging and sometimes genetic testing. Treatment is usually only supportive unless the cause is acquired and reversible.

The cerebellum has 3 parts. The archicerebellum (vestibulocerebellum) includes the flocculonodular lobe, which is located in the medial zone. It helps maintain equilibrium and coordinate eye, head, and neck movements; it is closely interconnected with the vestibular nuclei. The midline vermis (paleocerebellum) helps coordinate trunk and leg movements. Vermis lesions result in abnormalities of stance and gait. The lateral hemispheres (neocerebellum) control quick and finely coordinated limb movements, predominantly of the arms.

Ataxia is the archetypal sign of cerebellar dysfunction, but many other motor abnormalities may occur (see TABLE 221–1).

Etiology, Symptoms, and Signs

Congenital malformations: Such malformations are almost always sporadic, often occurring as part of complex malformation syndromes (eg, Dandy-Walker malformation—see p. 2441) that affect other parts of the CNS. Malformations manifest early in life and are nonprogressive. Manifestations vary markedly depending on the structures involved; ataxia is usually present.

TABLE 221–1. SIGNS OF CEREBELLAR DISORDERS

DEFICIT	MANIFESTATION
Ataxia	Reeling, wide-based gait
Decomposition of movement	Inability to correctly sequence fine, coordinated acts
Dysarthria	Inability to articulate words correctly, with slurring and inappropriate phrasing
Dysdiadochokinesia	Inability to perform rapid alternating movements
Dysmetria	Inability to control range of movement
Hypotonia	Decreased muscle tone
Nystagmus	Involuntary, rapid oscillation of the eyeballs in a horizontal, vertical, or rotary direction, with the fast component maximal toward the side of the cerebellar lesion
Scanning speech	Slow enunciation with a tendency to hesitate at the beginning of a word or syllable
Tremor	Rhythmic, alternating, oscillatory movement of a limb as it approaches a target (intention tremor) or of proximal musculature when fixed posture or weight bearing is attempted (postural tremor)

Hereditary ataxias: Hereditary ataxias may be autosomal recessive or autosomal dominant. Autosomal recessive ataxias include Friedreich's ataxia (the most prevalent), ataxia-telangiectasia, abetalipoproteinemia, ataxia with isolated vitamin E deficiency, and cerebrotendinous xanthomatosis.

Friedreich's ataxia results from a gene mutation that causes abnormal expansion of the repetitive DNA sequence GAA in the gene that codes for the mitochondrial protein frataxin. Decreased frataxin levels lead to mitochondrial iron overload and impaired mitochondrial function. Gait unsteadiness begins between ages 5 and 15; it is followed by upper extremity ataxia, dysarthria, and paresis, particularly of the lower extremities. Mental function often declines. Tremor, if present, is minor. Reflexes and vibration and position senses are lost. Talipes, scoliosis, and progressive cardiomyopathy are common.

Spinocerebellar ataxias (SCAs) are the main autosomal dominant ataxias. Currently, 15 different gene loci are recognized (SCA 1 to 8, 10 to 14, 16, and 17); the 9 that have been fully characterized involve expanded DNA sequence repeats. At least 6 involve a repetition of the DNA sequence CAG that codes for the amino acid glutamine, similar to that in Huntington's disease. Manifestations vary. SCAs 1 to 3, among the most common, affect multiple areas in the central and peripheral nervous systems; neuropathy, pyramidal signs, and restless leg syndrome, as well as ataxia, are common. SCAs 5, 6, 8, 11, and 15 usually cause only cerebellar ataxia.

Acquired ataxias: Acquired ataxias may result from nonhereditary neurodegenerative disorders (eg, multiple system atrophy—see p. 1768), systemic disorders, or toxin exposure, or they may be idiopathic. Systemic disorders include alcoholism (alcoholic cerebellar degeneration), celiac sprue, hypothyroidism, and vitamin E deficiency. Toxins include carbon monoxide, heavy metals, lithium, phenytoin, and certain solvents.

In children, primary brain tumors (medulloblastoma, cystic astrocytoma) may be the cause; the midline cerebellum is the most common site of such tumors. Rarely, in children, reversible diffuse cerebellar dysfunction follows viral infections.

Diagnosis and Treatment

Diagnosis is clinical and includes a thorough family history and search for acquired systemic disorders. Neuroimaging, typically MRI, is done. Genetic testing is done if family history is suggestive.

Some systemic disorders (eg, hypothyroidism, celiac sprue) and toxin exposure can be treated; occasionally, surgery for structural lesions (tumor, hydrocephalus) is beneficial. However, treatment is usually only supportive.

222 DEMYELINATING DISORDERS

Myelin sheaths cover many nerve fibers in the central and peripheral nervous system; they accelerate axonal transmission of neural impulses. Disorders that affect myelin interrupt nerve transmission; symptoms may reflect deficits in any part of the nervous system.

Myelin formed by oligodendroglia in the CNS differs chemically and immunologically from that formed by Schwann cells peripherally. Thus, some myelin disorders (eg, Guillain-Barré syndrome, chronic inflammatory demyelinating polyneuropathy, some other peripheral neuropathies—see p. 1903) tend to affect primarily the peripheral nerves, and others affect primarily the CNS (see TABLE 222–1). The most commonly affected areas in the CNS are the brain, spinal cord, and optic nerves.

Demyelination is often secondary to an infectious, ischemic, metabolic, or hereditary disorder. In primary demyelinating disorders, cause is unknown, but an autoimmune mechanism is suspected because the disorder sometimes follows a viral infection or viral vaccination.

Demyelination tends to be segmental or patchy, affecting multiple areas simultaneously or sequentially. Remyelination often occurs, with repair, regeneration, and complete recovery of neural function. However, extensive myelin loss is usually followed by axonal degeneration and often cell body degeneration; both may be irreversible.

TABLE 222–1. DISORDERS THAT CAUSE CNS DEMYELINATION

CATEGORY	DISORDERS
Hereditary disorders	Phenylketonuria and other aminoacidurias; Tay-Sachs, Niemann-Pick, and Gaucher's diseases; Hurler's syndrome; Krabbe's disease and other leukodystrophies*; adrenoleukodystrophies*; adrenomyeloneuropathy*; Leber's hereditary optic atrophy and related mitochondrial disorders
Hypoxia and ischemia	Carbon monoxide toxicity and other syndromes of delayed hypoxic cerebral demyelination, progressive subcortical ischemic demyelination
Nutritional deficiencies	Central pontine myelinolysis (may also be caused by Na fluxes), demyelination of the corpus callosum (Marchiafava-Bignami disease), vitamin B_{12} deficiency
Direct viral invasion of CNS	Progressive multifocal leukoencephalopathy, subacute sclerosing panencephalitis, tropical spastic paraparesis/HTLV-1–associated myelopathy
Primary demyelinating disorders	Recurrent, progressive disorders (multiple sclerosis and its variants); monophasic disorders such as optic neuritis, acute transverse myelitis, and acute encephalitis (acute disseminated encephalomyelitis and acute hemorrhagic leukoencephalitis)

*Some subtypes may also cause peripheral demyelination.

HTLV-1 = human T-lymphotropic virus 1.

Demyelination should be considered in any patient with unexplained neurologic deficits. Primary demyelinating disorders are suggested by diffuse or multifocal deficits; sudden onset, particularly in young adults; onset within weeks of an infection or vaccination; deficits that wax and wane; and symptoms suggesting a specific demyelinating disorder (eg, unexplained optic neuritis or internuclear ophthalmoplegia suggesting multiple sclerosis). Specific tests and treatment depend on the specific disorder.

MULTIPLE SCLEROSIS

Multiple sclerosis is characterized by disseminated patches of demyelination in the brain and spinal cord. Common symptoms include visual and oculomotor abnormalities, paresthesias, weakness, spasticity, urinary dysfunction, and mild cognitive impairment. Typically, neurologic deficits are multiple, with remissions and exacerbations gradually producing disability. Diagnosis is by history of remissions and exacerbations plus objective demonstration of at least 2 separate neurologic abnormalities by clinical signs or test results, MRI lesions, or other criteria, depending on symptoms. Treatment includes corticosteroids for acute exacerbations, immunomodulatory drugs to prevent exacerbations, and supportive measures.

Multiple sclerosis (MS) is believed to involve an immunologic mechanism. One postulated cause is infection by a latent virus (unidentified), which, when activated, triggers a secondary immune response. An increased incidence among certain families and human leukocyte antigen (HLA) allotypes (HLA-DR2) suggests genetic susceptibility. MS is more common among people who spend their 1st 15 yr of life in temperate climates (1/2000) than in those who spend them in the tropics (1/10,000). Cigarette smoking also appears to increase risk. Age at onset ranges from 15 to 60 yr, typically 20 to 40 yr; women are affected somewhat more often.

Pathophysiology

Localized areas of demyelination (plaques) occur, with destruction of oligodendroglia, perivascular inflammation, and chemical changes in lipid and protein constituents of myelin in and around the plaques. Axonal damage is possible, but cell bodies and axons tend to be relatively preserved. Fibrous gliosis develops in plaques that are disseminated throughout the CNS, primarily in white matter, particularly in the lateral and posterior columns (especially in the cervical regions), optic nerves, and periventricular areas. Tracts in the midbrain, pons, and cerebellum are also affected. Gray matter in the cerebrum and spinal cord can be affected but to a much lesser degree.

Symptoms and Signs

MS is characterized by varied CNS deficits, with remissions and recurring exacerbations. Exacerbations average about 3/yr, but frequency varies greatly. The most common initial symptoms are paresthesias in one or more extremities, in the trunk, or on one side of the face; weakness or clumsiness of a leg or hand; and visual disturbances (eg, partial loss of vision and pain in one eye due to retrobulbar optic neuritis, diplopia due to ocular palsy, scotomas). Other common early symptoms include slight stiffness or unusual fatigability of a limb, minor gait disturbances, difficulty with bladder control, vertigo, and mild affective disturbances; all usually indicate scattered CNS involvement and may be subtle. Excess heat (eg, warm weather, a hot bath, fever) may temporarily exacerbate symptoms and signs.

Mild cognitive impairment is common. Apathy, poor judgment, or inattention may occur. Affective disturbances, including emotional lability, euphoria, or, most commonly, depression, are common. Depression may be reactive or partly due to cerebral lesions of MS. A few patients have seizures.

Cranial nerves: Unilateral or asymmetric optic neuritis and bilateral internuclear ophthalmoplegia are typical. Optic neuritis produces loss of vision (ranging from scotomas to blindness), eye pain, and sometimes abnormal visual fields, a swollen optic disk, or a partial or complete afferent pupillary defect (see p. 923). Internuclear ophthalmoplegia results from a lesion in the medial longitudinal fasciculus connecting the 3rd, 4th, and 6th nerve nuclei. During horizontal gaze, adduction of one eye is decreased, with nystagmus of the other (abducting) eye; convergence is intact. Rapid, small-amplitude eye oscillations in straight-ahead (primary) gaze (pendular nystagmus) are uncommon but characteristic of MS. Vertigo is common. Intermittent unilateral facial numbness or pain (resembling trigeminal neuralgia), palsy, or spasm may occur. Mild dysarthria may occur, caused by bulbar weakness, cerebellar damage, or disturbance of cortical control. Other cranial nerve deficits are unusual but may be secondary to brain stem injury.

Motor: Weakness is common. It usually reflects corticospinal tract damage in the spinal cord, affects the lower extremities preferentially, and is bilateral and spastic. Deep tendon reflexes (eg, knee and ankle jerks) are usually increased, and an extensor plantar response (Babinski's sign) and clonus are often present. Spastic paraparesis produces a stiff, imbalanced gait; in advanced cases, it may confine patients to a wheelchair. Painful flexor spasms in response to sensory stimuli (eg, bedclothes) may occur late. Cerebral lesions may result in hemiplegia, which sometimes is the presenting symptom.

Intention tremors, in which the limb oscillates during linear movement, may simulate cerebellar dysmetria (ataxic limb movements). Resting tremor may also occur and is especially obvious when the head is unsupported.

Cerebellar: In advanced MS, cerebellar ataxia plus spasticity may be severely disabling; other cerebellar manifestations include slurred speech, scanning speech (slow enunciation with a tendency to hesitate at the beginning of a word or syllable), and Charcot's triad (intention tremor, scanning speech, and nystagmus).

Sensory: Paresthesias and partial loss of any type of sensation are common and often localized (eg, to the hands or legs). Various painful sensory disturbances (eg, burning or electric shocklike pains) can occur spontaneously or in response to touch, especially if the spinal cord is affected. An example is Lhermitte's sign, an electric shocklike pain that radiates down the spine or into the legs when the neck is flexed. Objective sensory changes tend to be transient and difficult to demonstrate.

Spinal cord: Involvement commonly causes bladder dysfunction (eg, urinary urgency or hesitancy, partial retention of urine, mild urinary incontinence). Constipation, erectile dysfunction in men, and genital anesthesia in women may occur. Frank urinary and fecal incontinence may occur in advanced MS.

A variant of MS called optic neuromyelitis (Devic disease) causes acute optic neuritis, sometimes bilateral, plus demyelination of the cervical or thoracic spinal cord, resulting in visual loss and paraparesis. Another variant causes spinal cord motor weakness but no other deficits (progressive myelopathy).

Diagnosis

MS is suspected in patients with optic neuritis, internuclear ophthalmoplegia, or other symptoms that suggest MS, particularly if deficits are multifocal or intermittent. Most diagnostic criteria for MS require a history of exacerbations and remissions plus objective demonstration by examination or testing of ≥ 2 separate neurologic abnormalities. Brain and sometimes spinal MRI is done. If MRI plus the clinical data are inconclusive, additional testing may be necessary to objectively demonstrate separate neurologic abnormalities. Such testing usually begins with CSF analysis and, if necessary, includes evoked potentials.

MRI is the most sensitive imaging test for MS and can exclude other treatable disorders that may mimic MS, such as nondemyelinating lesions at the junction of the spinal cord and medulla (eg, subarachnoid cyst, foramen magnum tumors). Gadolinium-contrast enhancement can distinguish actively inflamed from older plaques. Alternatively, contrast-enhanced CT can be done. The sensitivity of MRI and CT is increased by giving twice the dose of contrast agent and delaying scanning (double-dose delayed scan).

CSF IgG is usually increased as a percentage of CSF protein (normally < 11%), of CSF albumin (normally < 27%), or of other CSF indexes. IgG levels correlate with disease severity. Oligoclonal bands can usually be detected by agarose electrophoresis of CSF. Myelin basic protein may be elevated during active demyelination. CSF lymphocyte count and protein content may be slightly increased.

Evoked potentials (delays in electrical responses to sensory stimulation—see p. 1758) are often more sensitive for MS than symptoms or signs. Visual evoked responses are sensitive and particularly helpful in patients with no confirmed cranial lesions (eg, those with lesions only in the spinal cord). Somatosensory evoked potentials and brain stem evoked potentials are sometimes also measured. In some cases, systemic disorders (eg, SLE) and infections (eg, Lyme disease) must be excluded by routine blood tests.

Prognosis and Treatment

The course is highly varied and unpredictable. In most patients, especially when MS begins with optic neuritis, remissions can last months to > 10 yr. However, some patients, particularly men with onset in middle age, have frequent attacks and are rapidly incapacitated. Cigarette smoking may accelerate the course. Life span is shortened only in very severe cases.

Goals include shortening acute exacerbations, decreasing frequency of exacerbations, and relieving symptoms; maintaining the patient's ability to walk is particularly important. Acute exacerbations that produce objective deficits sufficient to impair function (eg, loss of vision, strength, or coordination) are treated with brief courses of corticosteroids (prednisone 60 to 100 mg po once/day tapered over 2 to 3 wk, methylprednisolone 500 to 1000 mg IV once/day for 3 to 5 days). Although they may shorten acute attacks and perhaps slow progression, corticosteroids have not been shown to affect long-term outcome. However, methylprednisolone may delay progression from acute severe optic neuritis to MS.

Immunomodulatory therapy decreases frequency of acute exacerbations and delays eventual disability. Immunomodulatory drugs include interferons (IFNs), such as IFN-β1b 8 million IU sc every other day, IFN-β1a 6 million IU (30 μg) IM weekly, and IFN-β1a 44 μg sc 3 times weekly. Common adverse effects include flu-like symptoms and depression (which tend to decrease over time), development of neutralizing antibodies after months of therapy, and cytopenias. Glatiramer acetate 20 mg sc once/day may be used. IFN-β and glatiramer are not considered immunosuppressants. The immunosuppressant mitoxantrone, 12 mg/m^2 IV q 3 mo for 24 mo, may be helpful, particularly for steadily progressive MS. Natalizumab, an anti-α_4 integrin antibody, inhibits passage of leukocytes across the blood-brain barrier; given as a monthly infusion, it reduces number of attacks and new brain lesions, but marketing has been suspended pending evaluation of a possible association with progressive multifocal leukoencephalopathy. If immunomodulatory drugs are ineffective, monthly IV immune globulin may help. Immunosuppressants other than mitoxantrone (eg, methotrexate, azathioprine, mycophenolate, cyclophosphamide, cladribine) have been used for more severe, progressive MS but are controversial.

Spasticity is treated with escalating doses of baclofen 10 to 20 mg po tid to qid or tizanidine 4 to 8 mg po tid. Gait training and range-of-motion exercises can help weak, spastic limbs. Painful sensory neuropathy is usually treated with gabapentin 100 to 600 mg po tid; alternatives include tricyclic antidepressants (eg, amitriptyline 25 to 75 mg po at bedtime, desipramine 25 to 100 mg po at bedtime if amitriptyline has intolerable anticholinergic effects), carbamazepine 200 mg po tid, and opioids. Depression is treated with counseling and antidepressants. Bladder dysfunction is treated based on its underlying mechanism (see p. 1950).

Encouragement and reassurance help. Regular exercise (eg, stationary biking, treadmill, swimming, stretching) is recommended, even for patients with advanced MS, because it conditions the heart and muscles, reduces spasticity, prevents contractures, and has psychologic benefits. Patients should maintain as normal and active a life as possible but should avoid overwork, fatigue, and exposure to excess heat. Vaccination does not appear to increase risk of exacerbations. Debilitated patients require measures to prevent pressure ulcers and UTIs; intermittent urinary self-catheterization may be necessary.

223 PERIPHERAL NERVOUS SYSTEM DISORDERS

The peripheral nervous system refers to the cranial nerves (see Ch. 219 on p. 1867) and spinal nerves from their origin to their end. The afferent (sensory) system begins in the periphery and ends in the CNS; the efferent (motor) system begins in the CNS and ends at the target muscle.

Anatomy and Physiology

Thirty of the 31 pairs of spinal nerves consist of an anterior (ventral) motor root and a posterior (dorsal) sensory root; C1 has no sensory root. Efferent motor fibers emerge from anterior horn cells located in the gray matter of the spinal cord. A motor unit consists of an anterior horn cell, its motor axon, the muscle fibers it innervates, and the connection between them (neuromuscular junction). The cell bodies of the afferent sensory fibers lie in dorsal root ganglia, located outside the spinal cord. The ventral and dorsal roots combine to form a spinal nerve, which exits via an intervertebral foramen. Because the spinal cord is shorter than the vertebral column, the more caudal the spinal nerve, the further the foramen is from the corresponding cord segment. Thus, in the lumbosacral region, nerve roots from lower cord segments descend within the spinal column in a near-vertical sheaf, forming the cauda equina.

The cervical and lumbosacral spinal nerves anastomose peripherally into plexuses, then branch into nerve trunks that terminate up to 1 m away in peripheral structures. The intercostal nerves are segmental.

The term peripheral nerve refers to the part of a spinal nerve distal to the root and plexus. Peripheral nerves are bundles of nerve fibers ranging in diameter from 0.3 to 22 μm. Schwann cells form a thin cytoplasmic tube around each fiber and further wrap larger fibers in a multilayered insulating membrane (myelin sheath), which enhances impulse conduction. The largest and most heavily myelinated fibers conduct quickly; they convey motor, touch, and proprioceptive impulses. The less myelinated and unmyelinated fibers conduct more slowly; they convey pain, temperature, and autonomic impulses. Because nerves are metabolically active tissues, they require nutrients, supplied by blood vessels called the vasa nervorum.

Etiology and Pathophysiology

Disorders can result from damage to or dysfunction of the cell body, myelin sheath, axons, or neuromuscular junction. Disorders can be genetic or acquired (due to toxic, metabolic, traumatic, infectious, or inflammatory conditions—see TABLE 223–1). Peripheral neuropathies may affect one nerve (mononeuropathy), several discrete nerves (multiple mononeuropathy, or mononeuritis multiplex), or multiple nerves diffusely (polyneuropathy). Some conditions involve a plexus (plexopathy) or nerve root (radiculopathy). More than one site can be affected (eg, in the most common variant of Guillain-Barré syndrome).

Because sensory and motor cell bodies are in different locations, a nerve cell body disorder typically affects either the sensory or motor component but rarely both.

TABLE 223–1. CAUSES OF PERIPHERAL NERVE DISORDERS

SITE	TYPE	EXAMPLES
Motor neuron	Inherited	Spinal muscular atrophy types I–IV
	Acquired, acute	Polio, infections by coxsackievirus and other enteroviruses (rare disorders)
	Acquired, chronic	Amyotrophic lateral sclerosis, paraneoplastic syndrome, postpolio syndrome, progressive bulbar palsy
Nerve root	Acquired	Herniated disk, infections, metastatic cancer, neurofibroma, trauma
Plexus	Acquired	Acute brachial neuritis, diabetes mellitus, hematoma, local tumors (eg, schwannoma), metastatic cancer, neurofibromatosis (rare), traction during birth, severe trauma
Peripheral nerve	Hereditary	Hereditary adult-onset neuropathies, hereditary sensorimotor neuropathies, hereditary sensory and autonomic neuropathies
	Infectious	Hepatitis C, HIV infection, Lyme disease, syphilis. In undeveloped nations, diphtheria, parasites
	Inflammatory	Chronic inflammatory demyelinating polyradiculoneuropathy, Guillain-Barré syndrome and variants, vasculitis
	Metabolic	Amyloidosis, diabetes mellitus, dysproteinemic neuropathy, ethanol with undernutrition (particularly deficiency of B vitamins), ICU neuropathy, leukodystrophies (rare), renal insufficiency
Neuromuscular junction		Botulism in infants, congenital myasthenia (very rare), Eaton-Lambert syndrome, myasthenia gravis, toxic neuromuscular junction disorders (eg, due to nerve agents)
Muscle fiber	Dystrophies	Distal muscular dystrophy (late distal hereditary myopathy; rare), Duchenne's muscular dystrophy and related dystrophies, fascioscapulohumeral muscular dystrophy, limb-girdle muscular dystrophy, oculopharyngeal dystrophy (rare)
	Channelopathies (myotonic)	Familial periodic paralysis, myotonia congenita (Thomsen's disease), myotonic dystrophy (Steinert's disease)
	Congenital	Central core disease, centronuclear myopathy, nemaline myopathy (very rare)
	Endocrine	Diabetes mellitus, hypothyroidism, thyrotoxic myopathy, acromegaly, Cushing's syndrome
	Inflammatory	Infection (viral more than bacterial), polymyositis/dermatomyositis
	Metabolic	Acid maltase deficiency, carnitine deficiency, glycogen storage and lipid storage diseases (rare)

Modified from Tandan R, Bradley WA: "Amyotrophic lateral sclerosis. Part I: Clinical features, pathology and ethical issues in management." *Annals of Neurology* 18:271–280, 1985; used with permission of Little, Brown and Company.

Damage to the myelin sheath (demyelination—see p. 1887) slows nerve conduction. Demyelination affects predominantly heavily myelinated fibers, causing large-fiber sensory dysfunction (buzzing and tingling sensations), motor weakness, and diminished reflexes. Profound motor weakness with minimal atrophy is a hallmark of an acquired demyelinating polyneuropathy.

Because the vasa nervorum do not reach the center of a nerve, centrally located fascicles are most vulnerable to vascular disorders (eg, vasculitis, ischemia). These disorders result in small-fiber sensory dysfunction (sharp pain and burning sensations), motor weakness proportional to atrophy, and less severe reflex abnormalities than in other nerve disorders. The distal ⅔ of a limb is affected most. Initially, deficits tend to be asymmetric because the vasculitic or ischemic process is random. However, multiple infarcts may later coalesce, causing symmetric deficits (multiple mononeuropathy).

Toxic-metabolic or genetic disorders usually begin symmetrically. Immune-mediated processes may be symmetric or, early in rapidly evolving processes, asymmetric.

Damage to the axon transport system for cellular constituents, especially microtubules and microfilaments, causes significant axon dysfunction. First affected are the smaller fibers (because they have greater metabolic requirements) and the most distal part of the nerve. Then, axonal degeneration slowly ascends, producing the characteristic distal-to-proximal pattern of symptoms (stocking-glove sensory loss, weakness).

Recovery: Damage to the myelin sheath (eg, by injury or Guillain-Barré syndrome) can often be repaired by surviving Schwann cells in about 6 to 12 wk.

After axonal damage, the fiber regrows within the Schwann cell tube at about 1 mm/day once the pathologic process ends. However, regrowth may be misdirected, causing aberrant innervation (eg, of fibers in the wrong muscle, of a touch receptor at the wrong site, or of a temperature instead of a touch receptor). Regeneration is virtually impossible when the cell body dies and is unlikely when the axon is completely lost.

Evaluation

History and physical examination should determine whether one or more limbs are affected, whether symptoms involve one or several nerve territories, and whether deficits are pure motor, pure sensory, or mixed (sensorimotor). These determinations narrow diagnostic possibilities and guide further testing.

Onset site (eg, distal vs proximal) and tempo (eg, rapid vs slowly progressive), distribution (symmetric vs asymmetric), and presence or absence of cranial nerve, limb girdle, and autonomic function involvement are determined. Family history, toxic exposures, and past medical history are also important.

Sensation (using pinprick and light touch for small fibers and vibration for large fibers), proprioception, motor strength, and deep tendon reflexes are evaluated (see pp. 1751–1752). Proportionality of motor weakness to the degree of atrophy is noted, as are type and distribution of reflex abnormalities.

Generally, nerve conduction velocity studies and electromyography (collectively called EMG) are done (see p. 1758). These tests help identify level of involvement (nerve, plexus, root) and distinguish demyelinating disorders (very slow conduction) from axonal disorders.

CERVICAL SPONDYLOSIS

Cervical spondylosis is degenerative changes in the intervertebral disk and annulus and formation of bony osteophytes, which narrow the cervical canal or neural foramina, causing radiculopathy and sometimes myelopathy.

A congenitally narrow canal increases the risk of cervical spondylosis. If the spinal cord is compressed, progressive myelopathy and a spastic gait typically develop. Pain may predominate with radicular signs in the dermatome most affected, usually between C5 and C6 or C6 and C7. Neural foraminal root compression causes arm weakness and atrophy with segmental reflex loss; spinal cord compression causes hyperreflexia, increased muscle tone, vibratory impairment, and extensor plantar responses in the legs.

Diagnosis and Treatment

If symptoms of cervical root or cord impingement occur, MRI and electrodiagnostic tests (eg, electromyography, somatosensory evoked potentials, motor evoked potentials) are indicated. Spinal x-rays, including oblique views of the neural foramina, may show degenerative changes with osteophytes and narrowing of disk space, but these findings are neither sensitive nor specific. If the sagittal diameter of the cervical canal is < 10 mm, risk of cord compression is higher.

Occasionally, signs lessen or stabilize spontaneously. Conservative treatment includes a soft collar and NSAIDs or other mild analgesics. Decompressive laminectomy is indicated for patients with myelopathy and cord compression or, if conservative treatment is ineffective, for patients with radiculopathy and electrodiagnostic evidence of neurologic dysfunction.

DISORDERS OF NEUROMUSCULAR TRANSMISSION

Disorders of neuromuscular transmission affect the neuromuscular junction. They may involve postsynaptic receptors (eg, in myasthenia gravis—see p. 1899), presynaptic release of acetylcholine (eg, in botulism), or breakdown of acetylcholine within the synapse (eg, due to drugs or neurotoxic chemicals). Common features of these disorders include fluctuating fatigue and muscle weakness.

Eaton-Lambert syndrome (see p. 1152) is due to impaired acetylcholine release from presynaptic nerve terminals.

Botulism (see full discussion on p. 1498) is also due to impaired release of acetylcholine from presynaptic nerve terminals. Botulism develops when toxin produced by *Clostridium botulinum* spores irreversibly binds to the terminal cholinergic nerve twigs, resulting in severe weakness, sometimes with respiratory compromise. Other systemic symptoms may include mydriasis, dry mouth, constipation, urinary retention, and tachycardia due to unopposed sympathetic nervous system activity. These systemic findings are absent in myasthenia gravis. In botulism, electromyography (EMG) shows a mild decremental response to low-frequency (2- to 3-Hz) repetitive nerve stimulation but a pronounced incremental response after 10 sec of exercise or with rapid (50-Hz) repetitive nerve stimulation.

Drugs or toxic chemicals may block neuromuscular junction function. Cholinergic drugs, organophosphate insecticides, and most nerve gases block neuromuscular transmission by excessive acetylcholine action that depolarizes postsynaptic receptors. Miosis, bronchorrhea, and myasthenic-like weakness result. Aminoglycoside and polypeptide antibiotics decrease presynaptic acetylcholine release and sensitivity of the postsynaptic membrane to acetylcholine. At high serum levels, these antibiotics may increase neuromuscular block in patients with latent myasthenia gravis. Long-term penicillamine treatment may cause a reversible syndrome that clinically and electromyographically resembles myasthenia gravis. Excessive Mg po or IV (with blood levels approaching 8 to 9 mg/dL) can also induce severe weakness resembling a myasthenic syndrome. Treatment consists of eliminating the drug or toxic chemical and providing necessary respiratory support and intensive nursing care. Atropine 0.4 to 0.6 mg po tid decreases bronchial secretions in patients with cholinergic excess. Higher doses (eg, 2 to 4 mg IV q 5 min) may be necessary for organophosphate insecticide or nerve gas poisoning.

Stiff-person syndrome is characterized by insidious onset of progressive stiffness in the trunk and abdomen and, to a lesser degree, in the legs and arms. Patients are otherwise normal, and examination detects only muscle hypertrophy and stiffness. EMG shows only the electrical activity of normal contraction. The syndrome may be autoimmune and can occur as a paraneoplastic syndrome (most often with breast, lung, or colon cancer or with Hodgkin lymphoma). Autoantibodies against several proteins involved with GABA (γ-aminobutyric acid)-glycine synapses are present, affecting primarily inhibitory neurons that originate in the anterior horn of the spinal cord. Only symptomatic therapy is available. Diazepam is the only drug that consistently relieves muscle stiffness. Results of plasmapheresis are inconsistent.

Isaacs' syndrome produces predominantly limb symptoms. Cause is unknown. Abnormalities are thought to originate in a peripheral nerve because they are abolished by curare but usually persist after general anesthesia. The sine qua non is myokymia—continuous muscle twitching described as "bag of worms" movements. Other symptoms include carpopedal spasms, intermittent cramps, increased sweating, and pseudomyotonia (impaired relaxation after a strong muscle contraction but without the typical waxing-and-waning EMG abnormality of true myotonia). Carbamazepine or phenytoin may relieve these symptoms.

GUILLAIN-BARRÉ SYNDROME

(Acute Idiopathic Polyneuritis; Landry's Paralysis; Acute Inflammatory Demyelinating Polyradiculoneuropathy)

Guillain-Barré syndrome is an acute, usually rapidly progressive inflammatory polyneuropathy characterized by muscular weakness and mild distal sensory loss. Cause is thought to be autoimmune. Diagnosis is clinical. Treatment includes plasmapheresis, γ-globulin, and, for severe cases, mechanical ventilation.

Guillain-Barré syndrome is the most common acquired inflammatory neuropathy. Although the cause is not fully understood, it is thought to be autoimmune. There are several variants. In some, demyelination predominates; others affect the axon.

In about ⅔ of patients, the syndrome begins 5 days to 3 wk after a banal infectious disorder, surgery, or vaccination. Infection is the trigger in > 50% of patients; common pathogens include *Campylobacter jejuni,* enteric viruses, herpesviruses (including cytomegalovirus and those causing infectious mononucleosis), and *Mycoplasma* sp. A cluster of cases followed the swine flu vaccination program in 1975.

Symptoms and Signs

Flaccid weakness predominates in most patients; it is always more prominent than sensory abnormalities and may be most prominent proximally. Relatively symmetric weakness with paresthesias usually begins in the legs and progresses to the arms, but it occasionally begins in the arms or head. In 90% of patients, weakness is maximal at 3 wk. Deep tendon reflexes are lost. Sphincters are usually spared. Facial and oropharyngeal muscles are weak in > 50% of patients with severe disease. Respiratory paralysis severe enough to require endotracheal intubation and mechanical ventilation occurs in 5 to 10%.

A few patients (possibly with a variant form) have significant, life-threatening autonomic dysfunction causing BP fluctuations, inappropriate ADH secretion, cardiac arrhythmias, GI stasis, urinary retention, and pupillary changes. An unusual variant (Fisher variant) may cause only ophthalmoparesis, ataxia, and areflexia.

Diagnosis

Diagnosis is clinical. Similar acute weakness can result from myasthenia gravis, botulism, poliomyelitis (primarily outside the US), tick paralysis, West Nile virus infection, and metabolic neuropathies, but these disorders can be distinguished. Myasthenia gravis is intermittent and worsened by exertion. Botulism may cause fixed dilated pupils (in 50%) and prominent cranial nerve dysfunction with normal sensation. Poliomyelitis usually occurs in epidemics. Tick paralysis causes ascending paralysis but spares sensation. West Nile virus causes headache, fever, and asymmetric flaccid paralysis but spares sensation. Metabolic neuropathies occur with a chronic metabolic disorder.

If Guillain-Barré syndrome is suspected, patients should be admitted to a hospital for electromyography (EMG), CSF analysis, and measurement of forced vital capacity every 6 to 8 h. Initial EMG detects slow nerve conduction velocities and evidence of segmental demyelination in ⅔ of patients; however, a normal EMG does not exclude the diagnosis and should not delay treatment. CSF analysis may detect albuminocytologic dissociation (increased protein but normal WBC count), but it may not appear for up to 1 wk and does not develop in 10% of patients.

Prognosis

Most patients improve considerably over a period of months, but about 30% of adults and even more children have some degree of residual weakness at 3 yr. Patients with residual defects may require retraining, orthopedic appliances, or surgery. This syndrome is fatal in < 2%.

After initial improvement, 3 to 10% of patients develop chronic relapsing polyneuropathy. Pathology and laboratory findings are similar to those in the acute syndrome, but weakness may be more asymmetric and progress more slowly. Eventually, nerves may become palpable because of repeated episodes of segmental demyelination and remyelination.

Treatment

Guillain-Barré syndrome is a medical emergency, requiring constant monitoring and support of vital functions, typically in an ICU. Forced vital capacity should be measured frequently so that respiration can be assisted if necessary; if vital capacity is < 15 mL/kg, endotracheal intubation is indicated. Inability to lift the head off the pillow by flexing the neck is another danger sign; it frequently develops simultaneously with phrenic nerve (diaphragm) weakness.

Fluid intake should be sufficient to maintain a urine volume of at least 1 to 1.5 L/day. Extremities should be protected from trauma and from the pressure of bed rest. Heat helps relieve pain, making early physical therapy possible. Immobilization, which may cause ankylosis, should be avoided. Passive full-range joint movement should be started immediately, and active exercises should be initiated when acute symptoms subside. Heparin 5000 units sc bid helps prevent deep vein thrombosis in bedbound patients.

Corticosteroids do not improve the outcome and should not be used. Plasmapheresis (see p. 1141) helps when done early in the syndrome and is the treatment of choice in acutely ill patients. It is relatively safe, shortens the disease course and hospital stay, and reduces mortality risk and incidence of permanent paralysis. Immune globulin (γ-globulin) 400 mg/kg IV once/day for 5 consecutive days is equally effective when given early, with benefit demonstrated up to 1 mo from disease onset. However, because plasmapheresis removes any previously administered γ-globulin, negating its benefits, γ-globulin is typically used if plasmapheresis is ineffective or unavailable.

In chronic relapsing polyneuropathy, corticosteroids lessen weakness and may be needed for a long time. Immunosuppressants (eg, corticosteroids, azathioprine), γ-globulin, and plasmapheresis benefit some patients.

HEREDITARY NEUROPATHIES

Hereditary neuropathies are a variety of congenital degenerative neurologic disorders.

Hereditary neuropathies are classified as sensorimotor neuropathies or sensory neuropathies (for hereditary motor neuropathies, see Motor Neuron Disorders on p. 1897).

Sensorimotor neuropathies: There are 3 main types (I, II, and III); all begin in childhood. Some less common types begin at birth and result in greater disability.

Types I and II (Charcot-Marie-Tooth disease, peroneal muscular atrophy) are the most common; they are usually autosomal dominant disorders characterized by weakness and atrophy, primarily in peroneal and distal leg muscles. Patients may also have other degenerative disorders (eg, Friedreich's ataxia) or a family history of them. Patients with type I present in middle childhood with footdrop and slowly progressive distal muscle atrophy, producing "stork legs." Intrinsic muscle wasting in the hands begins later. Vibration, pain, and temperature sensation decreases in a stocking-glove pattern. Deep tendon reflexes are absent. High pedal arches or hammertoes may be the only signs in less affected family members who carry the disease. Nerve conduction velocities are slow, and distal latencies are prolonged. Segmental demyelination and remyelination occur. Enlarged peripheral nerves may be palpated. The disease progresses slowly and does not affect life span. Type II evolves more slowly; weakness usually develops later in life. Patients have relatively normal nerve conduction velocities but low amplitude sensory nerve action potentials and compound muscle action potentials. Biopsies detect axonal (wallerian) degeneration.

Type III (hypertrophic interstitial neuropathy, Dejerine-Sottas disease), a rare autosomal recessive disorder, begins in childhood with progressive weakness and sensory loss and absent deep tendon reflexes. Although initially it resembles Charcot-Marie-Tooth disease, the motor weakness progresses more quickly. Demyelination and remyelination occur, producing enlarged peripheral nerves and onion bulbs, detected by nerve biopsy.

Sensory neuropathies: In hereditary sensory neuropathies, which are rare, loss of distal pain and temperature sensation is more prominent than loss of vibratory and position sense. The main complication is pedal mutilation due to pain insensitivity, resulting in a high risk of infections and osteomyelitis.

Diagnosis and Treatment

The characteristic distribution of motor weakness, foot deformities, and family history suggests the diagnosis, which should be confirmed by electrophysiologic testing. Genetic analysis is available, but there are no specific treatments. Bracing helps correct footdrop; orthopedic surgery to stabilize the foot may help. Vocational counseling to prepare young patients for disease progression may be useful.

HEREDITARY MOTOR NEUROPATHY WITH LIABILITY TO PRESSURE PALSIES

Hereditary motor neuropathy with liability to pressure palsies is a hereditary disorder in which nerves become increasingly sensitive to pressure and stretch.

In hereditary motor neuropathy with liability to pressure palsies (HNPP), nerves lose their myelin sheath and do not conduct nerve impulses normally. The cause is loss of one copy of peripheral myelin protein-22 gene

(*PMP22*), located on the short arm of chromosome 17. A duplication (extra copy) results in Charcot-Marie-Tooth disease type I. Two copies of the gene are needed for normal function. Incidence of HNPP is estimated to be 2 to 5/100,000.

The pressure palsies can be mild or severe and last from minutes to months. Numbness and weakness occur in affected areas.

HNPP should be suspected in patients with recurrent demyelinating polyneuropathy, compression mononeuropathy, multiple mononeuropathy of unknown origin, or a family history of carpal tunnel syndrome. Electromyography, nerve biopsy, and genetic testing aid in diagnosis, but biopsy is rarely required. Treatment is symptomatic and involves avoiding or modifying activities that cause symptoms. Wrist splints and elbow pads can reduce pressure, prevent reinjury, and allow the nerve to repair the myelin over time. Surgery is rarely indicated.

MOTOR NEURON DISORDERS

Motor neuron disorders are characterized by steady, relentless, progressive degeneration of corticospinal tracts, anterior horn cells, bulbar motor nuclei, or a combination. Symptoms vary in severity and may include muscle weakness and atrophy, fasciculations, emotional lability, and respiratory muscle weakness. Diagnosis involves nerve conduction velocity studies, electromyography, and exclusion of other disorders via neuroimaging and laboratory tests. Treatment is supportive.

Several motor neuron disorders (MNDs) exist. Usually, etiology is unknown. Nomenclature and symptoms vary according to the part of the motor system most affected. Myopathies, which mimic findings of MNDs, are disorders of the muscle membrane, contractile apparatus, or organelles (see p. 2457).

Classification, Symptoms, and Signs

MNDs can be classified as upper and lower; some disorders (eg, amyotrophic lateral sclerosis) have features of both.

Upper MNDs (eg, primary lateral sclerosis) affect neurons between the motor cortex and brain stem (corticobulbar tracts) or spinal cord (corticospinal tracts). Generally, symptoms consist of stiffness, clumsiness, and awkward movements, usually affecting first the mouth, throat, or both, then spreading to the limbs.

Lower MNDs affect the anterior horn cells or their efferent axons to the skeletal muscles. In bulbar palsies, only the cranial nerve motor nuclei in the brain stem (bulbar nuclei) are affected. Patients usually present with facial weakness, dysphagia, and dysarthria. When anterior horn cells of spinal (not cranial) nerves are affected, as in spinal muscular atrophies (see p. 1907), symptoms usually include muscle weakness and atrophy, fasciculations (visible muscle twitches), and muscle cramps, initially in a hand, a foot, or the tongue. Poliomyelitis, an enteroviral infection that attacks anterior horn cells, and postpolio syndrome are also lower MNDs (see p. 1615).

Physical findings help differentiate upper and lower MND (see TABLE 223–2) and weakness from lower MND from myopathy (see TABLE 223–3).

Amyotrophic lateral sclerosis (ALS): ALS (Lou Gehrig disease, Charcot's syndrome) is the most common MND. Patients present with random, asymmetric symptoms, consisting of cramps, weakness, and muscle atrophy of the hands (most commonly) or feet. Fasciculations, spasticity, hyperactive deep tendon reflexes, extensor plantar reflexes, clumsiness, stiffness of movement, weight loss, fatigue, and difficulty controlling facial expression and tongue movements soon follow. Other symptoms include hoarseness, dysphagia, slurred speech, and a tendency to choke on liquids. Late in the disorder, inappropriate, involuntary, and uncontrollable excesses of laughter or crying (pseudobulbar

TABLE 223–2. DISTINGUISHING UPPER FROM LOWER MOTOR NEURON LESIONS

FEATURE	UPPER LESION	LOWER LESION
Reflexes	Hyperactive	Diminished or absent
Atrophy	Absent*	Present
Fasciculations	Absent	Present
Tone	Increased	Decreased or absent

*May appear with prolonged limb disuse.

TABLE 223–3. DISTINGUISHING NEUROGENIC* FROM MYOGENIC† MUSCLE WEAKNESS

FEATURE	DUE TO NEURO-PATHY	DUE TO MYO-PATHY
Distribution	Distal > proximal	Proximal > distal
Fasciculations	May be present	Absent
Reflexes	Diminished	Often preserved
Sensory signs/ symptoms	May be present	Absent

*Weakness due to neuropathy: lower motor neuron.

†Weakness due to myopathy: nerve function intact.

affect) occur. Sensory systems, consciousness, cognition, voluntary eye movements, sexual function, and urinary and anal sphincters are usually spared. Death is usually caused by failure of the respiratory muscles; 50% of patients die within 3 yr of onset, 20% live 5 yr, and 10% live 10 yr. Survival > 30 yr is rare.

Progressive bulbar palsy: The muscles innervated by cranial nerves and corticobulbar tracts are predominantly affected, causing progressive difficulty with chewing, swallowing, and talking; nasal voice; reduced gag reflex; fasciculations and weak movement of the facial muscles and tongue; and weak palatal movement. A pseudobulbar affect, with emotional lability, may occur if the corticobulbar tract is affected. Patients with dysphagia have a very poor prognosis; respiratory complications due to aspiration frequently result in death within 1 to 3 yr.

Progressive muscular atrophy: In many cases, especially those with childhood onset, inheritance is autosomal recessive. Other cases are sporadic. The disorder can develop at any age. Anterior horn cell involvement occurs alone or is more prominent than corticospinal involvement, and progression tends to be more benign than that of other MNDs. Fasciculations may be the earliest manifestation. Muscle wasting and marked weakness begin in the hands and progress to the arms, shoulders, and legs, eventually becoming generalized. Patients may survive ≥ 25 yr.

Primary lateral sclerosis and progressive pseudobulbar palsy: Muscle stiffness and signs of distal motor weakness gradually increase, affecting the limbs in primary lateral sclerosis and the lower cranial nerves in progressive pseudobulbar palsy. Fasciculations and muscle atrophy may follow many years later. These disorders usually take several years to produce total disability.

Diagnosis

Diagnosis is suggested by progressive, generalized motor weakness without significant sensory abnormalities. Other neurologic disorders that cause pure muscle weakness include disorders of neuromuscular transmission and various myopathies. Acquired causes of pure motor weakness include noninflammatory myopathies, polymyositis, dermatomyositis, thyroid and adrenal disorders, electrolyte abnormalities (hypokalemia, hypercalcemia, hypophosphatemia), and various infections (eg, syphilis, Lyme disease, hepatitis C).

When cranial nerves are affected, a secondary treatable cause is less likely. Upper and lower motor neuron signs plus weakness in facial muscles strongly suggest ALS.

Electrodiagnostic tests should be done to check for evidence of disorders of neuromuscular transmission or demyelination. Such evidence is not present in MNDs; nerve conduction velocities are usually normal until late in the disease process. Needle electromyography (EMG) is the most useful test, showing fibrillations, positive waves, fasciculations, and sometimes giant motor units, even in unaffected limbs.

Brain MRI is required. MRI of the cervical spine is indicated when there is no clinical or EMG evidence of cranial nerve motor weakness.

Laboratory tests are done to identify treatable disorders. Tests include CBC, electrolytes, creatine phosphokinase, thyroid tests, serum and urine protein electrophoresis with immunofixation for monoclonal antibodies, anti-myelin-associated glycoprotein (MAG) antibodies, and a 24-h urine collection to check for heavy metals in patients who may have been exposed to them. A lumbar puncture should be done; elevated WBCs or protein levels strongly suggest an alternative diagnosis.

Serum Venereal Disease Research Laboratories (VDRL) tests, ESR, and measurement of certain antibodies (rheumatoid factor, Lyme titer, HIV, hepatitis C virus, antinuclear [ANA], anti-Hu paraneoplastic) are indicated only if suggested by risk factors or history. Genetic testing (eg, superoxide dismutase gene mutation) and enzyme measurements (eg, hexosaminidase A) should not be done unless patients are interested in genetic counseling; disorders detected by these tests have no known treatment.

Treatment

There is no specific treatment. However, an antiglutamate drug, riluzole 50 mg po bid, prolongs life in patients with bulbar-variant ALS. A multidisciplinary team approach helps patients cope with progressive neurologic disability. Physical therapy may help maintain muscle function. Occupational therapists can recommend adaptive braces and walking devices to help with activities of daily living. Speech and language therapists may provide alternative communication devices. Patients with pharyngeal weakness should be fed with extreme care and may require percutaneous endoscopic gastrostomy. Pulmonary specialists are crucial as respiratory weakness develops; they may recommend noninvasive respiratory support (eg, bilevel positive airway pressure) or tracheostomy and full ventilatory support.

Baclofen may help reduce spasticity; quinine or phenytoin may help decrease cramps. A strong anticholinergic drug (eg, glycopyrrolate, amitriptyline, benztropine, trihexyphenidyl, transdermal hyoscine, atropine) may be used to decrease saliva production. Amitriptyline and fluvoxamine are options for managing pseudobulbar affect. Pain in late stages of these disorders may require opioids and benzodiazepines. Surgery to improve swallowing has had limited success in patients with progressive bulbar palsy.

Early in the disorder, health care practitioners must talk frankly with patients, family members, and caregivers to determine the level of intervention acceptable (see p. 2768). These decisions should be reviewed and confirmed at various stages of the disorder.

MYASTHENIA GRAVIS

Myasthenia gravis is an autoimmune disorder of episodic muscle weakness and easy fatigability caused by antibody- and cell-mediated destruction of acetylcholine receptors. It is more common among young women and older men but may occur at any age. Symptoms worsen with muscle activity and lessen with rest. Diagnosis is by IV edrophonium challenge, which briefly lessens the weakness. Treatment includes anticholinesterase drugs, immunosuppressants, corticosteroids, thymectomy, and plasmapheresis.

Myasthenia gravis results from an autoimmune attack on postsynaptic acetylcholine receptors, which disrupts neuromuscular transmission. The trigger for autoantibody production is unknown, but the disorder is associated with abnormalities of the thymus, thyrotoxicosis, and other autoimmune disorders. The role of the thymus in myasthenia is unclear, but 65% of patients have thymic hyperplasia, and 10% have a thymoma. Precipitating factors include infection, surgery, and certain drugs (eg, aminoglycosides, quinine, Mg sulfate, procainamide, Ca channel blockers).

Rare forms: Ocular myasthenia gravis involves only extraocular muscles. Congenital myasthenia is a rare autosomal recessive disorder that begins in childhood; it results from structural abnormalities in the postsynaptic receptor rather than an autoimmune disorder. Ophthalmoplegia is common.

Neonatal myasthenia affects 12% of infants born to women with myasthenia gravis. It is due to IgG antibodies that passively cross the placenta. It causes generalized muscle weakness, which resolves in days to weeks as antibody titers decline. Thus, treatment is usually supportive.

Symptoms and Signs

The most common symptoms are ptosis, diplopia, and muscle weakness after exercise. Weakness resolves when the affected muscles are rested but recurs when they are used again. Ocular muscles are affected initially in 40% of patients and eventually in 85%. If generalized myasthenia is going to develop after ocular symptoms, it usually does so within the 1st 3 yr. Proximal limb weakness is common. Some patients present with bulbar symptoms (eg, altered voice, nasal regurgitation, choking, dysphagia). Sensation and deep tendon reflexes are normal. Manifestations fluctuate in intensity over hours to days.

Myasthenic crisis, a severe generalized quadriparesis or life-threatening respiratory muscle weakness, occurs in about 10% of patients. It is often due to a supervening infection that reactivates the immune system. Once respiratory insufficiency begins, respiratory failure may occur rapidly.

Diagnosis

Diagnosis is suggested by symptoms and signs and confirmed by tests. An anticholinesterase test using the short-acting (< 5 min) drug edrophonium is positive in most patients who have myasthenia with overt weakness. A muscle with obvious weakness is tested. Patients are asked to exercise the affected muscle until fatigue occurs (eg, hold the eyes open until ptosis occurs or count aloud until slurred speech develops); then, edrophonium 2 mg IV is given. If no adverse reaction (eg, bradycardia, atrioventricular block) occurs within 30 sec, another 8 mg is given. Rapid (< 2 min) recovery of muscle function is a positive result. However, a positive result is not definitive for myasthenia gravis because such improvement may occur in other neuromuscular disorders. The test may cause weakness due to cholinergic crisis to worsen (see below). Resuscitation equipment and atropine (as an antidote) must be available during the test.

Even if the anticholinesterase test is unequivocally positive, serum acetylcholine receptor antibody levels, electromyography (EMG), or both are required to confirm the diagnosis. The antibodies are present in 90% of patients with generalized myasthenia but in only 50% with the ocular form. Antibody levels do not correlate with disease severity.

EMG using repetitive stimuli (2 to 3/sec) shows a significant decrease in amplitude of the compound muscle action potential response in 60% of patients. Single-fiber EMG can improve the yield to > 95%.

Once myasthenia is diagnosed, CT or MRI of the thorax should be done to check for a thymoma. Other tests should be done to screen for autoimmune disorders frequently associated with myasthenia gravis (eg, vitamin B_{12} deficiency, hyperthyroidism, RA, SLE). Bedside pulmonary function tests (eg, forced vital capacity) help detect impending respiratory failure. Patients in myasthenic crisis require evaluation for an infectious trigger.

Treatment

Patients with respiratory failure require intubation and mechanical ventilation. Anticholinesterase drugs and plasmapheresis relieve symptoms; corticosteroids, immunosuppressants, and thymectomy lessen the severity of the autoimmune reaction. In patients with congenital myasthenia, anticholinesterase drugs and immunomodulating treatments are not beneficial and should be avoided.

Symptomatic treatment: Anticholinesterase drugs are the mainstay of symptomatic treatment but do not alter the underlying disease process. Moreover, they rarely relieve all symptoms, and myasthenia may become refractory to these drugs. Pyridostigmine is begun at 30 to 60 mg po q 3 to 4 h and titrated up to a maximum of 180 mg/dose based on symptoms. Patients who have severe dysphagia particularly in the morning can take 180-mg long-acting capsules at night, but these capsules tend to be less effective. When parenteral therapy is necessary (eg, because of dysphagia), neostigmine (1 mg = 60 mg of pyridostigmine) may be substituted. Anticholinesterase drugs can cause abdominal cramps and diarrhea, which are treated with oral atropine 0.4 to 0.6 mg or propantheline 15 mg tid to qid.

Cholinergic crisis is muscular weakness caused by a dose of neostigmine or pyridostigmine that is too high. A mild crisis may be difficult to differentiate from worsening myasthenia. Severe cholinergic crisis usually results in excess lacrimation, salivation, tachycardia, and diarrhea, which do not result from myasthenia gravis. The approach to deterioration in patients who have been responding well to treatment is controversial. Some experts believe an edrophonium test is useful because strength improves only in myasthenic crisis. Others recommend simply initiating respiratory support and stopping anticholinesterase drugs for several days.

Immunomodulating treatment: Immunosuppressants interrupt the autoimmune reaction and slow the disease course, but they do not relieve symptoms rapidly. When given IV immune globulin 400 mg/kg once/day for 5 days, 70% of patients improve in 1 to 2 wk. Effects may last 1 to 2 mo.

Corticosteroids are necessary as maintenance therapy in many patients but have little immediate effect in myasthenic crisis. Over ½ of patients worsen acutely after starting high-dose corticosteroids. Initially, prednisone 20 mg po once/day is given; dose is increased by 5 mg q 2 to 3 days up to 60 or 70 mg, which is then given every other day. Improvement may take several months; then, the dose should be reduced to the minimum necessary.

Azathioprine 2.5 to 3.5 mg/kg po once/day may be as effective as corticosteroids, although significant benefit may not occur for many months. Cyclosporine 2 to 2.5 mg/kg po bid may allow the corticosteroid dose to be reduced. These drugs require the usual precautions. Other drugs that may be beneficial include methotrexate, cyclophosphamide, and mycophenolate mofetil.

Thymectomy is an option for most patients < 60 yr with generalized myasthenia and should be done in all patients with a thymoma. Subsequently, for 80%, remission occurs or the maintenance drug dose can be lowered.

Plasmapheresis may be useful during myasthenia crisis and before thymectomy in refractory patients.

NERVE ROOT DISORDERS

Nerve root disorders result in predictable segmental radicular symptoms (pain or paresthesias in a dermatomal distribution, weakness of muscles innervated by the root). Diagnosis may require neuroimaging, electromyography, and systemic testing for underlying disorders. Treatment depends on cause but includes symptomatic relief with NSAIDs and other analgesics.

Nerve root disorders (radiculopathies) are precipitated by chronic pressure on a root in or adjacent to the spinal column. The most common cause is a herniated intervertebral disk. Bone changes due to RA or osteoarthritis, especially in the cervical and lumbar areas, may also compress isolated nerve roots. Less commonly, carcinomatous meningitis produces patchy multiple root dysfunction. Rarely, mass spinal lesions (eg, epidural abscesses and tumors, spinal meningiomas, neurofibromas) may manifest with radicular symptoms instead of the usual spinal cord dysfunction (see p. 1909). Diabetes can cause a painful thoracic or extremity radiculopathy. Infectious disorders, such as fungal (eg, histoplasmosis) and spirochetal diseases (eg, Lyme disease, syphilis), sometimes affect nerve roots. Herpes zoster infection usually causes a painful radiculopathy with dermatomal sensory loss and characteristic rash, but it may cause a motor radiculopathy with myotomic weakness and reflex loss.

Symptoms and Signs

Nerve root disorders tend to cause characteristic radicular syndromes of pain and segmental neurologic deficits based on the affected cord level (see TABLE 223–4). Muscles innervated by the affected motor root become weak and atrophy; they also may be flaccid with fasciculations. Sensory root involvement causes sensory impairment in a dermatomal distribution. Corresponding segmental deep tendon reflexes may be diminished or absent.

TABLE 223–4. SYMPTOMS OF COMMON RADICULOPATHIES BY CORD LEVEL

LEVEL	SYMPTOMS
C6	Pain in the trapezius ridge and tip of the shoulder, often radiating to the thumb, with paresthesias and sensory impairment in the same areas; weakness of biceps; and decreased biceps brachii and brachioradialis reflexes
C7	Pain in the shoulder blade and axilla, radiating to the middle finger; weakness of triceps; and decreased triceps brachii reflex
T (any)	Bandlike dysesthesias around thorax
L5	Pain in the buttock, posterior lateral thigh, calf, and foot; footdrop with weakness of the anterior tibial, posterior tibial, and peroneal muscles; and sensory loss over the shin and dorsal foot
S1	Pain along posterior aspect of the leg and buttock, weakness of the medial gastrocnemius muscle with impaired ankle plantar flexion, loss of ankle jerk, and sensory loss over the lateral calf and foot

Pain may be exacerbated by movements that transmit pressure to the nerve root through the subarachnoid space (eg, moving the spine, coughing, sneezing, Valsalva maneuver). Lesions of the cauda equina, which affect multiple lumbar and sacral roots, cause radicular symptoms in both legs and may impair sphincter and sexual function.

Findings indicating spinal cord compression include a sensory level (an abrupt change in sensation below a horizontal line across the spine), flaccid paraparesis or quadriparesis, reflex abnormalities below the site of compression, early-onset hyporeflexia followed later by hyperreflexia, and sphincter dysfunction.

Diagnosis and Treatment

Radicular symptoms require CT or MRI of the affected area. Myelography is sometimes used if multiple levels are affected. The area imaged depends on symptoms and signs; if the level is unclear, electromyography (EMG) should be done to localize the affected root, but EMG cannot identify the cause.

If imaging does not detect an anatomic abnormality, CSF analysis is done to check for infectious or inflammatory causes, and fasting blood glucose is measured to check for diabetes.

Specific causes are treated (see elsewhere in THE MANUAL). Acute pain requires appropriate analgesics (eg, NSAIDs, sometimes opioids). Use of low-dose tricyclic antidepressants at bedtime may help. Muscle relaxants, sedatives, and topical treatments rarely provide additional benefit. Chronic pain can be difficult to manage (see p. 1778); NSAIDs are often only partly effective, and opioids have a high risk of addiction. Tricyclic antidepressants and anticonvulsants may be effective, as may physical therapy and consultation with a mental health practitioner. For a few patients, alternative medical treatments (eg, transdermal electrical nerve stimulation, spinal manipulation, acupuncture, medicinal herbs) may be helpful.

HERNIATED NUCLEUS PULPOSUS

(Herniated, Ruptured, or Prolapsed Intervertebral Disk)

Herniated nucleus pulposus is prolapse of the central area of an intervertebral disk through the surrounding annulus. Symptoms occur when the disk impinges on an adjacent nerve root, causing segmental radiculopathy with paresthesias and weakness in the distribution of the affected root. Diagnosis is by CT, MRI, or CT-myelography. Treatment of mild cases is with NSAIDs and other analgesics if needed. Bed rest is rarely indicated. Patients with progressive neurologic deficits, intractable pain, or sphincter dysfunction may require urgent surgery (eg, diskectomy, laminectomy).

Spinal vertebrae are separated by cartilaginous disks consisting of an outer annulus fibrosus and an inner nucleus pulposus. When degenerative changes (with or without trauma) result in protrusion or rupture of the nucleus through the annulus fibrosus in the lumbosacral or cervical area, the nucleus is displaced posterolaterally or posteriorly into the extradural space. Radiculopathy occurs when the herniated nucleus compresses or irritates the nerve root. Posterior protrusion may compress the cord or cauda equina, especially in a congenitally narrow spinal canal (spinal stenosis). In the lumbar area, > 80% of disk ruptures affect L5 or S1 nerve roots; in the cervical area, C6 and C7 are most commonly affected. Herniated disk is common, often causing no symptoms.

Symptoms and signs are similar to those of other nerve root disorders (see p. 1901 and TABLE 223–4), although pain is somewhat more likely to develop suddenly if the disk herniates, and the cord may be compressed. In patients with lumbosacral herniation, straight-leg raises, which stretch the roots, may cause back or leg pain (bilateral if disk herniation is central); with cervical herniation, neck flexion or tilting is painful. Cervical cord compression may cause spastic paresis of the lower limbs. Cauda equina compression often results in urine retention or incontinence due to loss of sphincter function.

Diagnosis and Treatment

CT, MRI, or CT-myelography of the affected area is done. Electromyography may help identify the involved root. Because asymptomatic herniated disk is quite common, the clinician must carefully correlate symptoms with MRI abnormalities before invasive procedures are considered.

Because up to 95% of patients with herniated disk recover without surgery within about 3 mo, treatment should be conservative, unless neurologic deficits are progressive or severe. Heavy or vigorous physical activity is restricted, but ambulation and light activity (eg, lifting objects < 5 to 10 lb) are permitted as tolerated; prolonged bed rest (including traction) is contraindicated. NSAIDs and other analgesics should be used as needed to relieve pain.

If lumbar radiculopathies result in persistent or worsening objective neurologic deficits (weakness, sensory deficits) or in severe, intractable nerve root pain, invasive procedures should be considered. Microscopic diskectomy and laminectomy with surgical removal of herniated material are usually the procedures of choice. Percutaneous approaches to remove bulging disk material are being evaluated. Dissolving herniated disk material with local injections of the enzyme chymopapain is not recommended. Lesions acutely compressing the spinal cord or cauda equina (eg, producing urine retention or incontinence) require immediate surgical evaluation.

If cervical radiculopathies result in signs of spinal cord compromise, surgical decompression is needed immediately; otherwise, it is done electively when nonsurgical treatments are ineffective.

PERIPHERAL NEUROPATHY

Peripheral neuropathy is dysfunction of a spinal nerve or nerves distal to a plexus or root. It includes numerous syndromes characterized by varying degrees of sensory disturbances, pain, muscle weakness and atrophy, diminished deep tendon reflexes, and vasomotor symptoms, alone or in any combination. Initial classification is based on history and physical examination and must be confirmed with electromyography and nerve conduction velocity studies. Treatment is aimed mainly at the cause.

Peripheral neuropathy may affect a single nerve (mononeuropathy), ≥ 2 discrete nerves in separate areas (multiple mononeuropathy), or many nerves simultaneously (polyneuropathy).

MONONEUROPATHIES

Single and multiple mononeuropathies are characterized by sensory disturbances and weakness in the distribution of the affected nerve or nerves. Diagnosis is clinical but should be confirmed with electrodiagnostic tests. Treatment is directed at the cause, sometimes with splinting, NSAIDs, corticosteroid injections, and, for severe cases of nerve entrapment, surgery.

Trauma is the most common cause of acute mononeuropathy. Violent muscular activity or forcible overextension of a joint may cause focal neuropathy, as may repeated small traumas (eg, tight gripping of small tools, excessive vibration from air hammers). Prolonged, uninterrupted pressure at bony prominences can cause pressure neuropathy, usually affecting superficial nerves (ulnar, radial, peroneal), particularly in thin people; such pressure may occur during sound sleep, intoxication, bicycle riding, or anesthesia. Compression of nerves in narrow canals causes entrapment neuropathy (eg, in carpal tunnel syndrome). Nerve compression by a tumor, bony hyperostosis, a cast, crutches, or prolonged cramped postures (eg, during gardening) may cause compression paralysis. Hemorrhage into a nerve, exposure to cold or radiation, or direct tumor invasion may cause neuropathy.

Multiple mononeuropathy (mononeuritis multiplex) is usually secondary to connective tissue disorders (eg, polyarteritis nodosa, SLE, Sjögren's syndrome, RA), sarcoidosis, metabolic disorders (eg, diabetes, amyloidosis), or infectious disorders (eg, Lyme disease, HIV infection, leprosy). Diabetes usually causes sensorimotor distal polyneuropathy (see p. 1904).

Symptoms and Signs

Single and multiple mononeuropathies are characterized by pain, weakness, and paresthesias in the distribution of the affected nerve or nerves. Pure motor nerve involvement begins with painless weakness; pure sensory nerve involvement begins with sensory disturbances without weakness. Multiple mononeuropathy is often asymmetric at its onset; nerves may be involved all at once or progressively. Extensive involvement of many nerves may simulate polyneuropathy.

Ulnar nerve palsy of the elbow is often caused by trauma to the nerve in the ulnar groove of the elbow by repeated leaning on the elbow or by asymmetric bone growth after a childhood fracture (tardy ulnar palsy). The ulnar nerve can also be compressed at the cubital tunnel. Compression at the level of the elbow can cause paresthesias and a sensory deficit in the 5th digit and medial half of the 4th digit; the thumb adductor, 5th digit abductor, and interosseous muscles are weak and may be atrophied. Severe chronic ulnar palsy causes a clawhand deformity.

Carpal tunnel syndrome (see also p. 334) may be unilateral or bilateral. It results from compression of the median nerve in the volar aspect of the wrist between the transverse superficial carpal ligament and the flexor tendons of the forearm muscles. The compression causes paresthesias in the radial-palmar aspect of the hand and pain in the wrist and palm. Pain may also occur in the forearm and shoulder. Pain may be more severe at night. A sensory deficit in the palmar aspect of the 1st 3 fingers may follow, and the muscles that control thumb abduction and opposition may become weak and atrophied. Sensory symptoms due to this syndrome should be distinguished from C6 root dysfunction due to cervical radiculopathy, by electromyography (EMG) if needed.

Peroneal nerve palsy is usually caused by compression of the nerve against the lateral aspect of the fibular neck. It is most common among emaciated bedbound patients and thin people who habitually cross their legs. It causes footdrop (weakened dorsiflexion and eversion of the foot) and, occasionally, a sensory deficit in the anterolateral aspect of the lower leg and the dorsum of the foot or in the web space between the 1st and 2nd metatarsals.

Radial nerve palsy (Saturday night palsy) is caused by compression of the nerve against the humerus, as when the arm is draped over the back of a chair for a long time (eg, during intoxication or deep sleep). Typical symptoms include wristdrop (weakness of the wrist and finger extensors) and sensory loss in the dorsal aspect of the 1st dorsal interosseous muscle.

Diagnosis and Treatment

Electrodiagnostic tests are generally obtained, either to clarify diagnosis or to assess severity and prognosis.

Underlying disorders are treated. Treatment of compression neuropathy depends on cause. Often, fixed compression (eg, by tumor) must be relieved surgically. Symptoms of transient compression usually resolve with rest, heat, NSAIDs, and avoidance or modification of causative activity. Patients with carpal tunnel syndrome sometimes benefit from corticosteroid injections. For all types, braces or splints are often used pending resolution. Surgery should be considered when progression occurs despite conservative treatment.

Polyneuropathy

A polyneuropathy is a diffuse peripheral nerve disorder not confined to the distribution of a single nerve or a single limb. Electrodiagnostic tests should always be performed to classify the nerve structures involved, distribution, and severity of the disorder in order to focus the search for the underlying cause. Treatment is directed toward attenuating or removing the underlying cause.

Some polyneuropathies (eg, due to lead toxicity, dapsone use, tick bite, porphyria, or Guillain-Barré syndrome) affect primarily motor fibers; others (eg, due to dorsal root ganglionitis of cancer, leprosy, AIDS, diabetes mellitus, or chronic pyridoxine intoxication) affect primarily sensory fibers. Some disorders (eg, Guillain-Barré syndrome, Lyme disease, diabetes, diphtheria) can also affect cranial nerves. Certain drugs and toxins can affect sensory or motor fibers or both (see TABLE 223–5).

TABLE 223–5. TOXIC CAUSES OF NEUROPATHIES

TYPE	CAUSES
Axonal motor	Gangliosides; with prolonged exposure, lead, mercury, misoprostol, tetanus, tick paralysis
Axonal sensorimotor	Acrylamide, alcohol (ethanol), allyl chloride, arsenic, cadmium, carbon disulfide, chlorphenoxy compounds, ciguatoxin, dapsone, colchicine, cyanide, DMAPN, disulfiram, ethylene oxide, lithium, methyl bromide, nitrofurantoin, organophosphates, podophyllin, polychlorinated biphenyls (PCBs), saxitoxin, Spanish toxic oil, taxol, tetrodotoxin, thallium, trichloroethylene, TOCP, vacor (PNU), vinca alkaloids
Axonal sensory	Almitrine, bortezomib, chloramphenicol, dioxin, doxorubicin, ethambutol, ethionamide, etoposide, gemcitabine, glutethimide, hydralazine, ifosfamide, interferon-α, isoniazid, lead, metronidazole, misonidazole, nitrous oxide, nucleosides (didanosine [ddI], stavudine [d4T], zalcitabine [ddC]), phenytoin, platinum analogs, propafenone, pyridoxine, statins, thalidomide
Demyelinating	Buckthorn, chloroquine, diphtheria, hexachlorophene, muzolimine, perhexiline, procainamide, tacrolimus tellurium, zimeldine
Mixed	Amiodarone, ethylene glycol, gold, hexacarbons, n-hexane, Na cyanate, suramin

DMAPN = dimethylaminopropionitrile; TOCP = triorthocresyl phosphate; PNU = N-3 pyridilmethyl-N′-nitrophenyl urea.

Symptoms and Signs

Because pathophysiology and symptoms are related, polyneuropathies are often classified by area of dysfunction: myelin, vasa nervorum, or axon. Hereditary neuropathies are discussed below.

Myelin dysfunction: Myelin dysfunction polyneuropathies most often result from a parainfectious immune response triggered by an encapsulated bacterium (eg, *Campylobacter* sp), virus (eg, enteric or influenza viruses, HIV), or vaccine (eg, influenza vaccine). Presumably, antigens in these agents cross-react with antigens in the peripheral nervous system, causing an immune response (cellular, humoral, or both) that culminates in varying degrees of myelin dysfunction. In acute cases (eg, in Guillain-Barré syndrome—see p. 1894), rapidly progressive weakness and respiratory failure may develop.

Myelin dysfunction usually results in large-fiber sensory disturbances (paresthesias), significant muscle weakness greater than expected for degree of atrophy, and significantly diminished reflexes. Trunk musculature and cranial nerves may be involved. Abnormalities typically occur along the entire length of a nerve, producing proximal and distal symptoms. There may be side-to-side asymmetries, and more rostral parts of the body may be affected before distal extremities. Muscle bulk and tone are relatively preserved.

Vasa nervorum compromise: Chronic arteriosclerotic ischemia, vasculitis, and hypercoagulable states can compromise the vascular supply to the nerves.

Usually, small-fiber sensory and motor dysfunction occurs first. Patients typically have painful, often burning sensory disturbances. Abnormalities tend to be asymmetric early in the disorder and rarely affect the proximal ⅓ of the limb or trunk muscles. Cranial nerve involvement is rare, except in diabetes, which commonly affects the 3rd cranial (oculomotor) nerve. Later, symptoms and signs may appear symmetric if nerve lesions coalesce. Dysautonomia and skin changes (eg, atrophic, shiny skin) sometimes occur. Muscle weakness tends to be proportional to atrophy, and reflexes are rarely lost completely.

Axonopathy: Axonopathies tend to be distal; they may be symmetric or asymmetric.

Symmetric axonopathies result most often from toxic-metabolic disorders. Common causes include diabetes mellitus, chronic renal insufficiency, and adverse effects of chemotherapy drugs (eg, vinca alkaloids). Axonopathy may result from nutritional deficiencies (most commonly, of vitamin B) or from excess intake of vitamin B_6 or alcohol. Less common metabolic causes include hypothyroidism, porphyria, sarcoidosis, and amyloidosis. Other causes include certain infections (eg, Lyme disease), drugs (eg, nitrous oxide), and exposure to certain chemicals (eg, to Agent Orange, n-hexane) or heavy metals (eg, lead, arsenic, mercury). In a paraneoplastic syndrome associated with small-cell lung cancer, loss of dorsal root ganglia and their sensory axons results in subacute sensory neuropathy.

Primary axon dysfunction may begin with symptoms of large- or small-fiber dysfunction or both. Usually, the resulting neuropathy has a distal symmetric, stocking-glove distribution; it evenly affects the lower extremities before the upper extremities and progresses symmetrically from distal to proximal areas.

Asymmetric axonopathy can result from parainfectious or vascular disorders.

Diagnosis

Clinical findings, particularly tempo of onset, aid in diagnosis and identification of the cause. Asymmetric neuropathies suggest a disorder affecting the myelin sheath or vasa nervorum. Symmetric, distal neuropathies suggest toxic or metabolic causes. Slowly progressive, chronic neuropathies tend to be inherited or due to long-term toxic exposure or metabolic disorders. Acute neuropathies suggest an autoimmune response, vasculitis, or a postinfectious cause. Rash, skin ulcers, and Raynaud's phenomenon in patients with an asymmetric axonal neuropathy suggest a hypercoagulable state or parainfectious or autoimmune vasculitis. Weight loss, fever, lymphadenopathy, and mass lesions may suggest a tumor or paraneoplastic syndrome.

Electrodiagnostic tests: Regardless of clinical findings, electromyography (EMG) and nerve conduction velocity studies are necessary to classify type of neuropathy. At a minimum, EMG of both lower extremities should be done to assess for asymmetry and full extent of axon loss. Because EMG and nerve conduction studies assess primarily large myelinated fibers in distal limb segments, EMG may be normal in patients with proximal myelin dysfunction (eg, early in Guillain-Barré syndrome) and in patients with primarily small-fiber dysfunction. In such cases, quantitative sensory or autonomic testing or both may be done depending on the presenting symptoms.

Laboratory tests: Baseline laboratory tests for all patients include CBC, electrolytes, renal function tests, rapid plasma reagin test, and measurement of fasting blood sugar, hemoglobin A_{1C}, vitamin B_{12}, folate, and thyroid-stimulating hormone. Some clinicians include serum protein electrophoresis. The need for other tests is determined by polyneuropathy subtype.

The approach to patients with acute myelin dysfunction neuropathies is the same as that to those with Guillain-Barré syndrome (see p. 1894); forced vital capacity is measured to check for incipient respiratory failure. In acute or chronic myelin dysfunction, tests for infectious disorders and immune dysfunction, including tests for hepatitis and HIV and serum protein electrophoresis, are done. In addition, anti-myelin-associated glycoprotein (MAG) antibodies are measured if motor dysfunction predominates; anti-sulfatide antibodies are measured if primary sensory dysfunction is present. A lumbar puncture should also be done; myelin dysfunction due to an autoimmune response often causes albuminocytologic dissociation: increased CSF protein (> 45 mg%) but normal WBC count (≤ 5/μL).

For asymmetric axonal polyneuropathies, tests for hypercoagulable states and parainfectious or autoimmune vasculitis, particularly if suggested by clinical findings, should be done; the minimum is ESR, serum protein electrophoresis, and measurement of rheumatoid factor, antinuclear antibodies, and serum CPK. CPK may be elevated when rapid onset of disease results in muscle infarction. Coagulation studies (eg, protein C, protein S, antithrombin III, anticardiolipin antibody, homocysteine levels) should be done only if suggested by personal or family history. Tests for sarcoidosis, hepatitis C, or Wegener's granulomatosis should be done only if suggested by symptoms and signs. If no cause is identified, nerve and muscle biopsy should be done. An affected sural nerve is usually biopsied. A muscle adjacent to the biopsied sural nerve or a quadriceps, biceps brachii, or deltoid muscle may be biopsied. The muscle should be one with moderate weakness that has not been tested by needle EMG. Yield is higher if the contralateral muscle has EMG abnormalities. Nerve biopsies tend to be more useful in asymmetric axonopathies than in other polyneuropathy subtypes.

If initial tests do not identify the cause of distal symmetric axonopathies, a 24-h urine collection is tested for heavy metals, and urine protein electrophoresis is done. If chronic heavy metal poisoning is suspected, testing of hairs from the pubis or axillary region may help. History and physical examination should determine whether tests for other causes are needed.

Treatment

Treatment focuses on correcting the causes when possible (see elsewhere in THE MANUAL); a causative drug or toxin can be eliminated, or a dietary deficiency corrected. Although these actions may halt progression and lessen symptoms, recovery is slow and may be incomplete. If the cause cannot be corrected, treatment focuses on minimizing disability and pain. Physical and occupational therapists can recommend useful assistive devices. Amitriptyline, gabapentin, mexiletine, and topical lidocaine may relieve neuropathic pain (eg, diabetic burning feet).

For myelin dysfunction polyneuropathies, immune system–modifying treatments are usually used: plasmapheresis or IV immune globulin for acute myelin dysfunction and corticosteroids or antimetabolite drugs for chronic myelin dysfunction.

PLEXUS DISORDERS

Disorders of the brachial or lumbosacral plexus cause a painful mixed sensorimotor disorder of the corresponding limb.

Because several nerve roots intertwine within the plexus, the symptom pattern does not fit the distribution of individual roots or nerves. Disorders of the rostral brachial plexus affect the shoulders, those of the caudal brachial plexus affect the hands, and those of the lumbosacral plexus affect the legs.

Plexus disorders (plexopathies) are usually due to physical compression or injury. In infants, traction during birth may cause plexopathy. In adults, the cause is usually trauma (typically, for the brachial plexus, a fall that forces the head away from the shoulder) or invasion by metastatic cancer (typically, breast or lung cancer for the brachial plexus and intestinal or GU tumors for the lumbosacral plexus). In patients receiving anticoagulants, a hematoma may compress the lumbosacral plexus. Neurofibromatosis (see p. 2377) occasionally involves a plexus. Other causes include postradiation fibrosis (eg, after radiation therapy for breast cancer) and diabetes.

Acute brachial neuritis (neuralgic amyotrophy) occurs primarily in men and typically in young adults, although it can occur at any age. Cause is unknown, but viral or immunologic inflammatory processes are suspected.

Symptoms and Signs

Manifestations include extremity pain and motor or sensory deficits that do not correspond to an isolated nerve root. For acute brachial neuritis, symptoms include severe supraclavicular pain, weakness, and diminished reflexes, with minor sensory abnormalities in the distribution of the brachial plexus. Weakness and decreased reflexes usually occur as pain resolves. Severe weakness develops within 3 to 10 days, then typically regresses over the next few months. The most commonly affected muscles are the serratus anterior, other muscles innervated by the upper trunk, and muscles innervated by the anterior interosseus nerve (in the forearm).

Diagnosis and Treatment

Diagnosis is suggested clinically. Electromyography and somatosensory evoked potentials should be done to clarify the anatomic distribution (including possible nerve root involvement). MRI of the appropriate plexus and adjacent spine is indicated for all nontraumatic plexopathies that are not a typical case of brachial neuritis.

Treatment is directed at the cause. Corticosteroids, although commonly prescribed, have no proven benefit. Surgery may be indicated for injuries, hematomas, and benign or metastatic tumors. Metastases should also be treated with radiation therapy, chemotherapy, or both. Glycemic control can benefit patients with a diabetic plexopathy.

SPINAL MUSCULAR ATROPHIES

Spinal muscular atrophies include several types of hereditary disorders characterized by skeletal muscle wasting due to progressive degeneration of anterior horn cells in the spinal cord and of motor nuclei in the brain stem. Manifestations may begin in infancy or childhood. They vary by the specific type and may include hypotonia; hyporeflexia; difficulty sucking, swallowing, and breathing; unmet developmental milestones; and, in more severe types, very early death. Diagnosis is by genetic testing. Treatment is supportive.

Spinal muscular atrophies usually result from autosomal recessive mutations of a single gene locus on the short arm of chromosome 5, causing a homozygous deletion. There are 4 main types.

Type I spinal muscular atrophy (Werdnig-Hoffmann disease) is present in utero or becomes symptomatic by about age 6 mo. Affected infants have hypotonia (often notable at birth), hyporeflexia, tongue fasciculations, and pronounced difficulty sucking, swallowing, and eventually breathing. Death, usually due to respiratory failure, occurs within the 1st yr in 95% and by age 4 yr in all.

In **type II (intermediate) spinal muscular atrophy,** symptoms usually manifest between age 3 and 15 mo; < 25% of affected children learn to sit, and none walk or crawl. Children have flaccid muscle weakness and fasciculations, which may be hard to see in young children. Deep tendon reflexes are absent. Dysphagia may be present. The disorder is often fatal in early life, frequently resulting from respiratory complications. However, progression can stop spontaneously, leaving children with permanent, nonprogressive weakness and a high risk of severe scoliosis and its complications.

Type III spinal muscular atrophy (Wohlfart-Kugelberg-Welander disease) usually manifests between age 15 mo and 19 yr. Findings are similar to those of type I, but progression is slower and life expectancy is longer; some patients have a normal life span. Some familial cases are secondary to specific enzyme defects (eg, hexosaminidase deficiency). Symmetric weakness and wasting progress from proximal to distal areas and are most evident in the legs, beginning in the quadriceps and hip flexors. Later, arms are affected. Life expectancy depends on whether respiratory complications develop.

Type IV spinal muscular atrophy can be recessive, dominant, or X-linked, with adult onset (age 30 to 60 yr) and slow progression of primarily proximal muscle weakness and wasting. Differentiating this disorder from amyotrophic lateral sclerosis that involves predominantly lower motor neurons may be difficult.

Diagnosis and Treatment

EMG and nerve conduction velocity studies should be done; muscles innervated by cranial nerves should be included. Conduction is normal, but affected muscles, which are often clinically unaffected, are denervated. Definitive diagnosis is by genetic testing, which detects the causative mutation in about 95% of patients. Muscle biopsy is done occasionally. Serum enzymes (eg, CK, aldolase) may be slightly increased. Amniocentesis is often diagnostic.

There is no specific treatment. Physical therapy, braces, and special appliances can benefit patients with static or slowly progressive disease by preventing scoliosis and contractures. Adaptive devices available through physical and occupational therapists may improve children's independence and self-care by enabling them to feed themselves, write, or use a computer.

THORACIC OUTLET COMPRESSION SYNDROMES

Thoracic outlet compression syndromes are a group of poorly defined disorders characterized by pain and paresthesias in the hand, neck, shoulder, or arms. They appear to involve compression of the lower trunk of the brachial plexus (and perhaps the subclavian vessels) as it traverses the thoracic outlet below the scalene muscles and over the 1st rib before entering the axilla, but this involvement is unclear. Diagnostic techniques have not been established. Treatment includes physical therapy, analgesics, and, in severe cases, surgery.

Pathogenesis is often unknown but sometimes involves compression by a cervical rib, an abnormal 1st thoracic rib, abnormal insertion or position of the scalene muscles, or a malunited clavicle fracture. These syndromes are more common among women and usually develop between age 35 and 55.

Pain and paresthesias usually begin in the neck or shoulder and extend to the medial aspect of the arm and hand and sometimes the adjacent anterior chest wall. Many patients have mild to moderate sensory impairment in the C8 to T1 distribution on the painful side; a few have prominent vascular-autonomic changes in the hand (eg, cyanosis, swelling). In even fewer, the entire affected hand is weak. Rare complications include Raynaud's phenomenon and distal gangrene.

Diagnosis and Treatment

Diagnosis is suggested by distribution of symptoms. Various maneuvers are alleged to demonstrate compression of vascular structures (eg, by extending the brachial plexus), but sensitivity and specificity are not established. Auscultating bruits at the clavicle or apex of the axilla or finding a cervical rib by x-ray can aid in diagnosis. Although angiography may detect kinking or partial obstruction of axillary arteries or veins, neither finding is incontrovertible evidence of disease. Other testing is controversial, but evaluation as for brachial plexopathy (eg, electrodiagnostic tests, MRI—see p. 1907) may be reasonable.

Most patients without objective neurologic deficits respond to physical therapy, NSAIDs, and low-dose tricyclic antidepressants. If cervical ribs or subclavian artery obstructions are identified, an experienced specialist should decide whether surgery is necessary. With few exceptions, surgery should be reserved for patients who have significant or progressive neurovascular deficits and who do not respond to conservative treatment.

224 SPINAL CORD DISORDERS

Spinal cord disorders can cause permanent severe neurologic disability. For some patients, such disability can be avoided or minimized if evaluation and treatment are rapid. Spinal cord disorders include arteriovenous malformations, infections (eg, bacterial; fungal; TB; syphilis, which can cause tabes dorsalis—see p. 1660), multiple sclerosis, spondylitic myelopathy, trauma (see p. 2579), vitamin B_{12} deficiency (which causes subacute combined degeneration—see p. 38), syrinx, transverse myelopathy (due to certain disorders), spinal cord compression, and spinal cord tumors (see p. 1924).

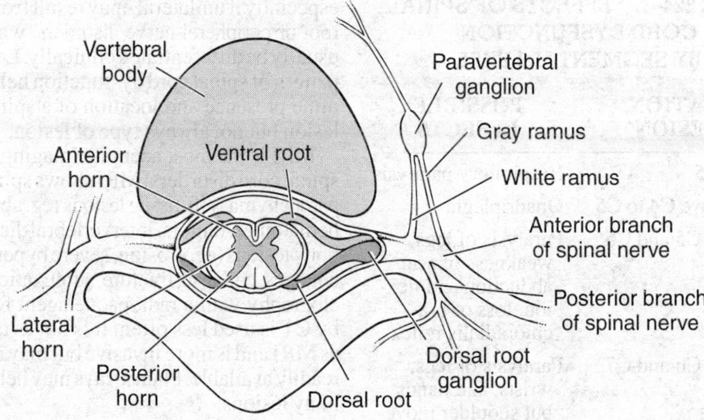

Fig. 224–1. Spinal nerve.

Anatomy

The spinal cord extends caudally from the medulla at the foramen magnum and terminates at the upper lumbar vertebrae. In the lumbosacral region, nerve roots from lower cord segments descend within the spinal column in a nearly vertical sheaf, forming the cauda equina.

The white matter at the cord's periphery contains ascending and descending tracts of myelinated sensory and motor nerve fibers. The central H-shaped gray matter is composed of cell bodies and nonmyelinated fibers (see FIG. 224–1). The anterior (ventral) horns of the "H" contain lower motor neurons, which receive impulses from the motor cortex via the descending corticospinal tracts; the axons of these cells are the efferent fibers of the spinal nerves. The posterior (dorsal) horns contain sensory fibers that originate in cell bodies in the dorsal root ganglia. The gray matter also contains many internuncial neurons that carry motor, sensory, or reflex impulses from dorsal to ventral nerve roots, from one side of the cord to the other, or from one level of the cord to another. The spinothalamic tract transmits pain and temperature sensation contralaterally in the spinal cord; most other tracts transmit information ipsilaterally. The cord is divided into functional segments (levels) corresponding approximately to the attachments of the 31 pairs of spinal nerve roots.

Pathophysiology, Symptoms, and Signs

Neurologic dysfunction due to spinal cord disorders develops at the involved spinal cord segment (see TABLE 224–1 and FIG. 206–1 on p. 1753) and at all segments below it. The exception is the central cord syndrome (see TABLE 224–2), which may spare segments below.

Spinal cord disorders produce various patterns of deficits depending on which nerve tracts within or spinal roots outside of the spinal cord are damaged. Disorders affecting spinal nerves but not directly affecting the cord cause sensory or motor abnormalities or both in the areas supplied by those spinal nerves.

Spinal cord dysfunction produces paresis, loss of sensation, reflex changes, and autonomic dysfunction (eg, bowel, bladder, and erectile dysfunction; loss of sweating). Dysfunction may be partial (incomplete). Autonomic and reflex abnormalities are generally the most conclusive signs of cord dysfunction; sensory abnormalities are the least conclusive. Corticospinal tract lesions produce upper motor neuron dysfunction. Acute injury causes flaccid paresis (decreased muscle tone, hyporeflexia, and no extensor plantar responses), which over days to weeks evolves into spastic paresis (increased muscle tone, hyperreflexia, and clonus). Extensor plantar responses and autonomic dysfunction are present. More chronic flaccid paresis suggests lower motor neuron lesions (eg, Guillain-Barré syndrome). However, spinal shock with flaccid paresis can result from sudden, severe spinal cord dysfunction (eg, due to infarction or severe trauma).

Specific cord syndromes include transverse sensorimotor myelopathy, Brown-Séquard syndrome, central cord syndrome, anterior cord syndrome, and conus medullaris syndrome (see TABLE 224–2).

TABLE 224–1. EFFECTS OF SPINAL CORD DYSFUNCTION BY SEGMENTAL LEVEL

LOCATION OF LESION*	POSSIBLE EFFECTS
Above C5	Respiratory paralysis
At or above C4 to C5	Quadriplegia
Between C5 and C6	Paralysis of legs, weakness of arm abduction and flexion, loss of brachioradialis reflex
Between C6 and C7	Paralysis of legs, wrists, and hands, but shoulder movement and elbow flexion usually possible
Between C7 and C8	Loss of biceps jerk reflex, paralysis of legs
At C8 to T1	Horner's syndrome (constricted pupil, ptosis, facial anhidrosis), paralysis of legs
Between T11 and T12 and between T12 and L1	Paralysis of leg muscles from the hips down
Conus medullaris at L1 (or 3rd, 4th, and 5th sacral nerve roots)	Complete loss of bladder and bowel control

*Abbreviations refer to vertebrae; the cord is shorter than the spine, so that moving down the spine, cord segments and vertebral levels are increasingly out of alignment.

Cauda equina syndrome, which involves damage to nerve roots at the caudal end of the cord, is not a spinal cord syndrome. However, it mimics conus medullaris syndrome, causing sensory loss in and around the perineum and anus (saddle anesthesia) and bladder, bowel, and pudendal dysfunction (eg, urinary retention, urinary frequency, urinary or fecal incontinence, erectile dysfunction, loss of rectal tone, and abnormal bulbocavernosus and anal wink reflexes).

Diagnosis

Neurologic deficits at segmental levels suggest a spinal cord disorder. Similar deficits, especially if unilateral, may result from nerve root or peripheral nerve disorders, which can usually be differentiated clinically. Level and pattern of spinal cord dysfunction help determine presence and location of a spinal cord lesion but not always type of lesion.

MRI is the most accurate imaging test for spinal cord disorders; MRI shows spinal cord parenchyma, soft-tissue lesions (eg, abscesses, hematomas, tumors, intervertebral disks), and bony lesions (eg, erosion, severe hypertrophic changes, collapse, fracture, subluxation). Myelography with a radiopaque agent followed by CT is used less often. It is not as accurate as MRI and is more invasive but may be more readily available. Plain x-rays may help detect bony lesions.

ACUTE TRANSVERSE MYELITIS

Acute transverse myelitis is acute inflammation of gray and white matter in one or more adjacent spinal cord segments, usually thoracic. Among the causes are postinfectious inflammation, multiple sclerosis, autoimmune inflammation, vasculitis, and drugs. Symptoms include bilateral motor, sensory, and sphincter deficits below the level of the lesion. Diagnosis is usually by MRI, CSF analysis, and blood tests. IV corticosteroids and plasma exchange may be helpful early. Otherwise, treatment is supportive measures and correction of any causes.

Acute transverse myelitis can occur in patients with vasculitis, multiple sclerosis, mycoplasmal infections, Lyme disease, syphilis, TB, or viral meningoencephalitis and in patients using amphetamines, IV heroin, or antiparasitic or antifungal drugs. The mechanism is often unknown, but some cases follow viral infection or vaccination, suggesting an autoimmune reaction. Inflammation tends to involve the spinal cord diffusely at one or more levels, affecting all spinal cord functions.

Symptoms and Signs

Pain in the neck, back, or head may occur. A bandlike tightness around the chest or abdomen, weakness, tingling, numbness of the feet and legs, and difficulty voiding develop over hours to a few days. Deficits may progress over several more days to a complete transverse sensorimotor myelopathy, producing paraplegia, loss of sensation below the lesion, urinary retention, and fecal incontinence. Occasionally, position and vibration sensation is spared, at least initially. The syndrome occasionally recurs in patients with multiple sclerosis, SLE, or antiphospholipid syndrome. About 10 to 20% of patients in whom the cause is unknown eventually develop multiple sclerosis.

Diagnosis, Prognosis, and Treatment

Diagnosis is suggested by transverse sensorimotor myelopathy with segmental deficits. Guillain-Barré syndrome (see p. 1894) does not localize to a specific spinal segment. Diagnosis requires MRI and CSF analysis. MRI typically shows cord swelling and helps exclude other treatable causes of spinal cord dysfunction (eg, spinal cord compression). CSF usually contains monocytes, protein content is slightly increased, and IgG index is elevated (normal, ≤ 0.85).

Tests for treatable causes should include chest x-ray; PPD; serologic tests for mycoplasma, Lyme disease, and HIV; vitamin B_{12} and folate levels; ESR; antinuclear antibodies; and CSF and blood Venereal Disease Research Laboratory (VDRL) tests. History may suggest a drug as a cause. Brain MRI is done: Multiple sclerosis develops in 50% in whom multiple periventricular T2 bright lesions are present and 5% in whom they are absent.

Generally, the more acute the progression is, the worse the prognosis. Pain suggests more intense inflammation. About $\frac{1}{3}$ of patients recover, $\frac{1}{3}$ retain some weakness and urinary urgency, and $\frac{1}{3}$ are bedridden and incontinent.

Treatment is directed at the cause or associated disorder but is otherwise supportive. In idiopathic cases, because an autoimmune cause is possible, high-dose corticosteroids are often given and sometimes followed by plasma exchange. Efficacy of such a regimen is uncertain.

TABLE 224–2. SPINAL CORD SYNDROMES

SYNDROME	CAUSE	SYMPTOMS AND SIGNS
Anterior cord syndrome	Lesions disproportionately affecting the anterior spinal cord, commonly due to occlusion of the anterior spinal artery and to infarction	Tendency for all tracts except the posterior columns to malfunction, thus sparing position and vibratory sensation
Brown-Séquard syndrome (rare)	Unilateral spinal cord lesions, typically due to penetrating trauma	Ipsilateral paresis; ipsilateral loss of touch, position, and vibratory sensation; and contralateral loss of pain and temperature sensation*
Central cord syndrome	Lesions affecting the center of the spinal cord, mainly central gray matter, and crossing spinothalamic tracts; commonly due to trauma, syrinx, and tumors in the central spinal cord	Paresis tending to be more severe in the upper than in the lower extremities and sacral regions; tendency to lose pain and temperature sensation in a capelike distribution over the upper neck, shoulders, and upper trunk, with light touch, position, and vibratory sensation relatively preserved (dissociated sensory loss)
Conus medullaris syndrome	Lesions around T12	Distal leg paresis, perianal loss of sensation, erectile dysfunction, urinary retention, hypotonic anal sphincter
Transverse myelopathy	Lesions affecting the entire spinal cord at ≥ 1 segmental levels	Deficits in all functions mediated by the spinal cord (because all tracts are affected to some degree)

*Occasionally, only part of one side of the spinal cord is dysfunctional (partial Brown-Séquard syndrome).

ARTERIOVENOUS MALFORMATIONS

Arteriovenous malformations in or around the spinal cord can cause cord compression, ischemia, parenchymal hemorrhage, subarachnoid hemorrhage, or a combination. Symptoms may include gradually progressive, ascending, or waxing and waning segmental neurologic deficits, and radicular pain; or sudden back pain with sudden segmental neurologic deficits. Diagnosis is by MRI. Treatment is with surgery or stereotactic radiosurgery and may include angiographic embolization.

Arteriovenous malformations (AVMs) are the most common spinal vascular malformations. Most are in the thoracolumbar region, posterior, and outside the cord (extramedullary). The rest are cervical or upper thoracic and often intramedullary. AVMs may be small and localized or may affect up to ½ the cord. They may compress or even replace normal spinal cord parenchyma, or they may rupture, causing focal or generalized hemorrhage.

A cutaneous angioma sometimes overlies a spinal AVM. AVMs commonly compress nerve roots, causing pain that radiates down the distribution of a nerve root (radicular pain), or compress the spinal cord, causing segmental neurologic deficits that gradually progress or wax and wane. Combined lower and upper motor neuron deficits are common. AVMs may rupture into the spinal cord parenchyma, producing sudden, severe back pain and sudden segmental neurologic deficits. High cervical AVMs rarely rupture into the subarachnoid space, producing sudden and severe headache, nuchal rigidity, and impaired consciousness (see p. 1798).

Spinal cord AVMs may be detected incidentally on imaging tests. AVMs are suspected clinically in patients with unexplained segmental neurologic deficits or subarachnoid hemorrhage, particularly those who have sudden, severe back pain or cutaneous midline angiomas. Diagnosis is by MRI, magnetic resonance angiography, selective arteriography, or, occasionally, myelography plus CT.

Surgery is indicated if spinal cord function is threatened, but expertise in specialized microtechniques is required. Stereotactic radiosurgery is helpful if the AVM is small and located in a surgically inaccessible location. Angiographic embolization occludes feeder arteries and often precedes surgical removal or stereotactic radiosurgery.

CERVICAL SPONDYLOSIS AND SPONDYLOTIC CERVICAL MYELOPATHY

Cervical spondylosis is osteoarthritis of the cervical spine causing stenosis of the canal and sometimes cervical myelopathy from encroachment of bony osteoarthritic growths (osteophytes) on the lower cervical spinal cord, sometimes with involvement of lower cervical nerve roots (radiculomyelopathy).

Cervical spondylosis due to osteoarthritis is common. Occasionally, particularly in those with a congenitally narrow (< 10 mm) spinal canal, it leads to stenosis of the canal and bony impingement on the cord, producing myelopathy. Osteophytes in the neural foramina, most commonly between C5 and C6 or C6 and C7, can produce radiculopathy (see also Nerve Root Disorders on p. 1901). Manifestations vary according to the neural structures involved.

Cord compression commonly causes gradual spastic paresis, paresthesias, or both in the hands and feet; reflexes may be increased. Neurologic deficits may be asymmetric, nonsegmental, and aggravated by cough or Valsalva maneuvers. A central cord syndrome may develop. Eventually, muscle atrophy and flaccid paresis may develop in the upper extremities at the level of the lesion, with spasticity below the level of the lesion.

Nerve root compression commonly causes early radicular pain; later there may be weakness, diminished reflexes, and muscle atrophy.

Cervical spondylosis is suspected when characteristic neurologic deficits occur in patients who are elderly, have osteoarthritis, or have radicular pain at the C5 or C6 levels. Diagnosis is by MRI or CT. For those with cord involvement, cervical laminectomy is generally needed; a posterior approach can relieve the compression but leaves anterior compressive osteophytes and may result in spinal instability and kyphosis; thus, an anterior approach with spinal fusion is being used increasingly. Those with only radiculopathy may try nonsurgical treatment with NSAIDs and a soft cervical collar; if this is ineffective, surgical decompression may be required.

HEREDITARY SPASTIC PARAPARESIS

Hereditary spastic paraparesis is a group of rare hereditary disorders characterized by progressive, spinal, nonsegmental, spastic leg paresis, sometimes with mental retardation, seizures, and other extraspinal deficits.

The genetic basis of hereditary spastic paraparesis varies and, for many forms, is unknown. In all forms, the descending corticospinal tracts and, to a lesser extent, the dorsal columns and spinocerebellar tracts degenerate, sometimes with loss of anterior horn cells.

Symptoms and signs include spastic leg paresis, with progressive gait difficulty, hyperreflexia, clonus, and extensor plantar responses. Sensation and sphincter function are usually spared. The arms may also be affected. Deficits are not localized to a spinal cord segment. Onset occurs at various ages, from the 1st year of life to old age, depending on the specific genetic form. In some forms, patients also have extraspinal neurologic deficits (eg, spinocerebellar and ocular symptoms, extrapyramidal symptoms, optic atrophy, retinal degeneration, mental retardation, dementia, polyneuropathy).

Hereditary spastic paraparesis is suggested by a family history and any signs of spastic paraparesis. Diagnosis is by exclusion of other causes and sometimes by genetic testing.

Treatment for all forms is symptomatic. Baclofen 10 mg po bid, increased as needed up to 40 mg po bid, is given for spasticity. Alternatives include diazepam, clonazepam, dantrolene, botulinum toxin, and tizanidine.

SPINAL CORD INFARCTION

(Ischemic Myelopathy)

Spinal cord infarction usually results from ischemia originating in an extravertebral artery. Symptoms include sudden and severe back pain, bilateral flaccid limb weakness, and loss of sensation, particularly pain and temperature. Diagnosis is by MRI. Treatment is generally supportive.

The primary vascular supply for the posterior $\frac{1}{3}$ of the spinal cord is the posterior spinal arteries and for the anterior $\frac{2}{3}$, the anterior spinal arteries. The anterior spinal artery has only a few feeder arteries in the upper cervical region and one large feeder, the artery of Adamkiewicz, in the lower thoracic region. The feeder arteries originate in the aorta.

Because collateral circulation for the anterior spinal artery is sparse in places, certain cord segments (eg, those around the 2nd to 4th thoracic segments) are especially vulnerable to ischemia. Injury to an extravertebral feeder artery or the aorta (eg, atherosclerosis, dissection, clamping during surgery) causes infarction more commonly than do intrinsic disorders of spinal arteries. Thrombosis is an uncommon cause, and polyarteritis nodosa is a rare cause.

Sudden pain in the back with tightness radiating circumferentially is followed by segmental bilateral flaccid weakness and sensory loss. Pain and temperature sensation are disproportionately impaired; the anterior spinal artery is typically affected, resulting in an anterior cord syndrome (see TABLE 224–2). Position and vibration sensation, conducted by the posterior columns, and often light touch are relatively spared. If the infarct is small and affects primarily tissue farthest away from an occluded artery, a central cord syndrome is also possible. Neurologic deficits may partially resolve after the 1st few days.

Infarction is suspected when severe back pain and characteristic deficits develop suddenly. Diagnosis is by MRI. Acute transverse myelitis, spinal cord compression, and demyelinating disorders may cause similar findings but are usually more gradual and are excluded by MRI and by CSF analysis. Occasionally, the cause of infarction (eg, aortic dissection, polyarteritis nodosa) can be treated, but often the only possible treatment is supportive.

SPINAL CORD COMPRESSION

Various lesions can compress the spinal cord, causing segmental sensory, motor, reflex, and sphincter deficits. Diagnosis is by MRI. Treatment is directed at relieving compression.

Compression is far more commonly caused by lesions outside the spinal cord (extramedullary) than by lesions within it (intramedullary). Compression may be acute, subacute, or chronic.

Acute compression develops within hours. It is usually due to trauma (eg, vertebral crush fracture with displacement of fracture fragments, severe bony or ligamentous injury causing hematoma, or vertebral subluxation or dislocation), or a spontaneous epidural hematoma. Acute compression may follow subacute and chronic compression, especially if the cause is abscess and tumor.

Subacute compression develops over days to weeks. It is usually caused by a metastatic extramedullary tumor, a subdural or epidural abscess or hematoma, or a cervical or, rarely, thoracic intervertebral disk rupture.

Chronic compression develops over months to years. It may be caused by bony or cartilaginous protrusions into the cervical, thoracic, or lumbar spinal canal (eg, due to osteophytes or spondylosis, especially in patients with a congenitally narrow spinal canal as in lumbar spinal stenosis—see p. 328). Other causes include arteriovenous malformations, intramedullary tumors, and slow-growing extramedullary tumors.

Atlantoaxial subluxation and other craniocervical junction abnormalities (see pp. 328 and 1877) may cause acute, subacute, or chronic spinal cord compression.

Lesions that compress the spinal cord may also compress nerve roots or, rarely, occlude the spinal cord's blood supply, causing infarction.

Symptoms and Signs

Acute or advanced spinal cord compression produces segmental deficits, paraparesis or quadriparesis, hyperreflexia, extensor plantar responses, loss of sphincter tone (with bowel and bladder dysfunction), and sensory deficits. Subacute or chronic compression may begin with local back pain, often radiating down the distribution of a nerve root (radicular pain), and sometimes hyperreflexia and loss of sensation. Sensory loss may begin in the sacral segments. Complete loss of function may follow suddenly and unpredictably, possibly resulting from secondary spinal cord infarction. Spinal percussion tenderness is prominent if the cause is metastatic carcinoma, abscess, or hematoma.

Intramedullary lesions tend to cause poorly localized burning pain rather than radicular pain and to spare sensation in sacral dermatomes. These lesions are more likely to result in spastic paresis.

Diagnosis and Treatment

Spinal cord compression is suggested by spinal or radicular pain with reflex, motor, or sensory deficits, particularly at a segmental level. MRI is always done if available. If MRI is unavailable, myelography plus CT is done. A small amount of iohexol, a nonionic, low osmolar radiopaque agent, is introduced via a lumbar puncture and allowed to run cranially to check for complete CSF block. If a block is detected, a radiopaque agent is introduced via a cervical puncture to determine the rostral extension of the block. Plain spinal x-rays are useful for rapid evaluation of bony abnormalities (eg, fracture, dislocation, subluxation) due to trauma.

Treatment is directed at relieving pressure on the cord. Incomplete or very recent complete loss of function may be reversible, but complete loss of function rarely is; thus, *for acute compression, diagnosis and treatment must occur immediately.*

If compression is due to tumor, IV dexamethasone 100 mg is given immediately, followed by 25 mg q 6 h and immediate surgery or radiation therapy. If neurologic deficits worsen despite nonsurgical treatments, surgical decompression may help. Surgery is also indicated if a biopsy is needed, if the spine is unstable, if tumors recur after radiation therapy, or if an abscess or a compressive subdural or epidural hematoma is suspected.

SPINAL SUBDURAL OR EPIDURAL ABSCESS

A spinal subdural or epidural abscess is an accumulation of pus in the subdural or epidural space that can mechanically compress the spinal cord.

Spinal subdural or epidural abscesses usually occur in the thoracic or lumbar regions. An underlying infection is often present; it may be remote (eg, endocarditis, furuncle, dental abscess) or contiguous (eg, vertebral osteomyelitis, decubitus ulcer, retroperitoneal abscess). In about ⅓ of cases, the cause cannot be determined. The most common causative organism is *Staphylococcus aureus,* followed by *Escherichia coli* and mixed anaerobes. Rarely, the cause is a tuberculous abscess of the thoracic spine (Pott's disease).

Symptoms begin with local or radicular back pain and percussion tenderness, which become severe. Fever is common. Spinal cord compression may develop; compression of lumbar spinal roots may produce lower extremity paresis (cauda equina syndrome). Deficits progress over hours to days.

The diagnosis is suggested by back pain worsened by recumbency, leg paresis, and bowel and bladder dysfunction, particularly if accompanied by fever or recent infection. Diagnosis is by MRI; myelography followed by CT can be used if MRI is not available. Samples from blood and infectious areas are cultured. Lumbar puncture is contraindicated because it may trigger cord herniation if the abscess produces complete obstruction. Plain x-rays are not routinely indicated but may show osteomyelitis in about $^1/_3$ of patients.

Antibiotics with or without parenteral needle aspiration may be sufficient; however, abscesses producing neurologic compromise are immediately drained surgically. Pus is gram-stained and cultured. Antibiotics to cover staphylococcus and anaerobes are given as for brain abscess (see p. 1851). If the abscess developed after a neurosurgical procedure, an aminoglycoside is added for gram-negative coverage.

SPINAL SUBDURAL OR EPIDURAL HEMATOMA

A spinal subdural or epidural hematoma is an accumulation of blood in the subdural or epidural space that can mechanically compress the spinal cord.

Spinal subdural or epidural hematoma (usually thoracic or lumbar) is rare but may result from back trauma, anticoagulant or thrombolytic therapy, or, in patients with bleeding diatheses, lumbar puncture. Symptoms begin with local or radicular back pain and percussion tenderness; they are often severe. Spinal cord compression may develop; compression of lumbar spinal roots may cause cauda equina syndrome and lower extremity paresis. Deficits progress over minutes to hours.

Hematoma is suspected in patients with acute, nontraumatic spinal cord compression or sudden, unexplained lower extremity paresis, particularly if a possible cause (eg, trauma, bleeding diathesis) is present. Diagnosis is by MRI or, if MRI is not immediately available, by myelography plus CT. Treatment is immediate surgical drainage. Patients taking coumarin anticoagulants are given phytonadione (vitamin K_1) 2.5 to 10 mg sc and fresh frozen plasma as needed to normalize INR. Patients with thrombocytopenia are given platelets (see p. 1066).

SYRINX

A syrinx is a fluid-filled cavity within the spinal cord (syringomyelia) or brain stem (syringobulbia). Predisposing factors include craniocervical junction abnormalities, spinal cord trauma, and spinal cord tumors. Symptoms include flaccid weakness of the hands and arms and deficits in pain and temperature sensation (but not light touch) in a capelike distribution over the back and neck. Diagnosis is by MRI. Treatment includes correction of cause and surgical procedures to drain the syrinx or otherwise open CSF flow.

Syrinxes usually result from lesions that partially obstruct CSF flow. At least $^1/_2$ of syrinxes occur in patients with congenital anomalies of the craniocervical junction (eg, herniation of cerebellar tissue into the spinal canal, called Chiari malformation) or dysraphic syndromes (eg, encephalocele, myelomeningocele—see p. 2441). For unknown reasons, these congenital anomalies often expand during the teen or young adult years. A syrinx can also develop when such congenital anomalies are absent in patients who have a spinal cord tumor, previous spinal trauma (and scarring), or no known predisposing factors. About 30% of people with a spinal cord tumor eventually develop a syrinx.

Syringomyelia is a paramedian, usually irregular and longitudinal cavity. It commonly begins in the cervical area but may extend downward along the entire length of the spinal cord. Syringobulbia, which is rare, usually occurs as a slitlike gap within the lower brain stem and may disrupt or compress the lower cranial nerves or ascending sensory or descending motor pathways.

Symptoms and Signs

Symptoms usually begin insidiously between adolescence and age 45. Syringomyelia develops in the center of the spinal cord, causing a central cord syndrome (see TABLE 224–2). Pain and temperature sensory deficits occur early but may not be recognized for years. The 1st abnormality recognized may be a painless burn or cut. Syringomyelia typically causes weakness, atrophy, and often fasciculations and hyporeflexia of the hands and arms; a deficit in pain and temperature sensation (but not light touch or position and vibration sensation) in a capelike distribution over the shoulders and back is characteristic. Later, spastic leg weakness develops. Deficits may be asymmetric.

Syringobulbia may cause vertigo, nystagmus, unilateral or bilateral loss of facial sensation, lingual atrophy and weakness, dysarthria, dysphagia, hoarseness, and sometimes peripheral sensory or motor deficits due to medullary compression.

Diagnosis and Treatment

A syrinx is suggested by an unexplained central cord syndrome or other characteristic neurologic deficits, particularly pain and temperature sensory deficits in a capelike distribution. MRI of the entire spinal cord and brain is done. Gadolinium enhancement is useful for detecting any associated tumor.

Underlying problems (eg, craniocervical junction abnormalities, postoperative scarring, spinal tumors) are corrected when possible. Commonly, the syrinx is surgically drained via a shunt, but procedures that open the CSF pathways without invading the spinal cord (eg, by going through the posterior fossa and 4th ventricle if possible) may be as or more effective. Surgery usually cannot reverse severe neurologic deterioration.

TROPICAL SPASTIC PARAPARESIS/HTLV-1–ASSOCIATED MYELOPATHY

Tropical spastic paraparesis/HTLV-1–associated myelopathy is a slowly progressive viral immune-mediated disorder of the spinal cord caused by the human T-lymphotrophic virus 1 (HTLV-1). It produces spastic weakness of both legs. Diagnosis is by serologic and PCR tests of serum and CSF. Treatment includes supportive care and possibly immunosuppressive therapies.

The human T-lymphotrophic virus 1 (HTLV-1) retrovirus is transmitted via sexual contact, IV drug use, or blood transfusion or, from mother to child, via breastfeeding. It is most common among prostitutes, IV drug users, hemodialysis patients, and patients from endemic areas such as equatorial regions, southern Japan, and parts of South America. HTLV-2 may cause a similar disorder.

The virus resides in T cells in blood and CSF. Perivascular and parenchymal infiltration with $CD4^+$ memory T cells, $CD8^+$ cytotoxic T cells, and macrophages occurs in the spinal cord, as does astrocytosis. Inflammation of spinal gray and white matter progresses for several years after onset of neurologic symptoms, causing preferential degeneration of the lateral and posterior columns. Myelin and axons in the anterior columns are also lost.

Spastic weakness develops gradually in both legs, with extensor plantar responses and bilateral symmetric loss of vibratory sensation in the feet. Achilles tendon reflexes are often absent. Urinary incontinence and urgency are common. The disorder usually progresses over several years.

Diagnosis and Treatment

The disorder is suggested by typical neurologic deficits that are unexplained, particularly in patients with risk factors. Serum and CSF serologic and PCR tests and spinal cord MRI are indicated. If CSF-to-serum ratio of HTLV-1 antibodies is > 1 or PCR detects HTLV-1 antigen in CSF, the diagnosis is very likely. Protein and Ig levels in CSF may also be elevated, often with oligoclonal bands; lymphocytic pleocytosis occurs in up to 50%. Spinal cord lesions often appear hyperintense on T2-weighted MRI.

No treatment has proved effective, but interferon-α, IV immune globulin, and oral methylprednisolone may have some benefit. Treatment of spasticity is symptomatic.

225 INTRACRANIAL AND SPINAL TUMORS

Intracranial tumors may involve the brain or other structures (eg, cranial nerves, meninges). Brain tumors are found in about 2% of routine autopsies. The tumors usually develop during early or middle adulthood but may develop at any age; they are becoming more common among the elderly. Some tumors are benign, but because the cranial vault allows no room for expansion, even these tumors can be serious.

Classification

Some primary intracranial tumors (eg, gliomas, medulloblastomas, ependymomas) originate in brain parenchyma; others (eg, meningiomas, acoustic neuromas, other schwannomas) originate in extraneural structures. Extracranial tumors may metastasize to any intracranial structure or to the skull. In the brain, metastases are about 10 times more common than primary tumors.

Type of tumor varies somewhat by site (see TABLE 225–1) and patient age. In children, common primary tumors are cerebellar astrocytomas and medulloblastomas, ependymomas, gliomas of the brain stem or optic nerve, germinomas, and congenital tumors. Congenital tumors include craniopharyngiomas, chordomas, germinomas, teratomas, dermoid cysts, angiomas, and hemangioblastomas. The most common metastatic tumors in children are neuroblastoma (usually epidural) and leukemia (meningeal).

In adults, common primary tumors include meningiomas, schwannomas, primary lymphomas, and gliomas of the cerebral hemispheres (particularly glioblastoma multiforme and anaplastic astrocytoma, which are malignant, and astrocytoma and oligodendroglioma, which are more benign). In adults, the most common sources of metastases are bronchogenic carcinoma, adenocarcinoma of the breast, malignant melanoma, and any cancer that has spread to the lungs; however, any metastatic cancer can spread to the brain.

Pathophysiology

Neurologic dysfunction may result from tumor invasion and destruction of brain tissue, from direct compression of adjacent tissue by the tumor, or, rarely, from paraneoplastic syndromes (see p. 1150). Neurologic dysfunction can also result from increased intracranial pressure (which may develop because of the space occupied by the tumor), cerebral edema, obstructed dural venous sinuses (especially by bony or extradural metastatic tumors), obstructed CSF drainage (occurring early with 3rd ventricle or posterior fossa tumors), or obstructed CSF absorption (eg, when leukemia or carcinoma involves the meninges). A malignant tumor can develop new internal blood vessels, which can bleed or become occluded, resulting in necrosis; either problem can cause neurologic dysfunction that mimics stroke.

Benign tumors grow slowly. They may become quite large before causing symptoms, partly because often there is no cerebral edema. Malignant tumors grow rapidly but rarely spread beyond the CNS. Death results from local tumor growth and thus can result from benign as well as malignant tumors. Therefore, distinguishing between benign and malignant is prognostically less important for brain tumors.

Symptoms and Signs

Many symptoms result from increased intracranial pressure. The most common is headache. Headache may be most intense when patients awake from deep non-REM sleep (usually several hours after falling asleep) because hypoventilation, which increases cerebral blood flow and thus intracranial pressure, is usually maximal during non-REM sleep. When intracranial pressure is very high, the headache may be accompanied by vomiting, which may occur with little preceding nausea. Papilledema develops in about 25% of patients with a brain tumor but may be absent even if intracranial pressure is increased. In infants and very young children, increased intracranial pressure may enlarge the head. If intracranial pressure increases sufficiently, brain herniation occurs (see p. 1800).

Deterioration in mental status is the 2nd most common symptom. Manifestations include drowsiness, lethargy, personality changes, disordered conduct, and impaired cognition, particularly with malignant brain tumors. Generalized seizures may occur, more often with primary than metastatic brain tumors. Impaired consciousness (see p. 1800) can result from herniation, brain stem dysfunction, or diffuse bilateral cortical dysfunction. Airway reflexes may be impaired.

Some symptoms may result from focal brain dysfunction. Focal neurologic deficits, endocrine dysfunction, or focal seizures (sometimes with secondary generalization) may develop depending on the tumor's location (see TABLE 225–1). Focal symptoms and signs often suggest the tumor's location. However, sometimes focal deficits do not correspond to the tumor's location. An example of these deficits, called false localizing signs, is unilateral or bilateral lateral rectus palsy; it causes paresis of eye abduction due to increased intracranial pressure compressing the 6th cranial nerve, ipsilateral hemiplegia due to compression of the contralateral cerebral peduncle against the tentorium (Kernohan's notch), and ipsilateral visual field defect due to ischemia in the contralateral occipital lobe.

Some tumors cause meningeal inflammation, resulting in subacute or chronic meningitis (see p. 1858).

TABLE 225–1. COMMON LOCALIZING MANIFESTATIONS OF BRAIN TUMORS

TUMOR SITE	FINDINGS	COMMON PRIMARY TUMOR TYPES*
Anterior corpus callosum	Cognitive impairment	Astrocytoma, oligodendroglioma
Basal ganglia	Hemiparesis (contralateral), movement disorders	Astrocytoma
Brain stem	Unilateral or bilateral motor or sensory loss, cranial nerve deficits (eg, gaze palsies, hearing loss, vertigo, palatal paresis, facial weakness), ataxia, intention tremor, nystagmus	Astrocytoma (most often juvenile pilocytic astrocytoma)
Cerebellopontine angle	Tinnitus and hearing loss (both ipsilateral), vertigo, loss of vestibular response to caloric stimulation; if tumor is large, ataxia, loss of facial sensation and facial weakness (both ipsilateral), possibly other cranial nerve or brain stem deficits	Acoustic neuroma, schwannoma, meningioma
Cerebellum	Ataxia, nystagmus, tremor, hydrocephalus with suddenly increased intracranial pressure	Astrocytoma, medulloblastoma, ependymoma
2nd cranial (optic) nerve	Loss of vision	Astrocytoma (most often juvenile pilocytic astrocytoma)
5th cranial (trigeminal) nerve	Loss of facial sensation, jaw weakness	Meningioma
Frontal lobe	Generalized or focal (contralateral) seizures; gait disorders; urinary urgency or incontinence; impaired attention and cognition and apathy, particularly if tumor is bilateral; expressive aphasia if tumor is in dominant hemisphere; hemiparesis; anosmia if tumor is at base of lobe	Astrocytoma, oligodendroglioma
Hypothalamus	Eating and drinking disorders (eg, polydipsia), precocious puberty (especially in boys), hypothermia	Astrocytoma
Occipital lobe	Generalized seizures with visual aura, visual hallucinations, hemianopia or quadrantanopia (contralateral)	Astrocytoma, oligodendroglioma
Parietal lobe	Deficits in position sensation and in 2-point discrimination (contralateral), anosognosia (no recognition of bodily defects), denial of illness, hemianopia (contralateral), generalized or focal seizures, receptive aphasia if tumor is in dominant hemisphere, inability to perceive (extinguishing) a contralateral stimulus when stimuli are applied to both sides of the body (called double simultaneous stimulation)	Astrocytoma, oligodendroglioma
Pineal region	Paresis of upward gaze, ptosis, loss of pupillary light and accommodation reflexes, sometimes hydrocephalus with suddenly increased intracranial pressure	Germ cell tumor, pineocytoma (rare)

TABLE 225–1. COMMON LOCALIZING MANIFESTATIONS OF BRAIN TUMORS—Continued

TUMOR SITE	FINDINGS	COMMON PRIMARY TUMOR TYPES*
Pituitary or suprasellar region	Endocrinopathies, monocular visual loss, headache without increased intracranial pressure, bitemporal hemianopia	Craniopharyngioma, pituitary adenoma, pituitary carcinoma (rare)
Temporal lobe	Complex partial seizures, generalized seizures with or without aura, hemianopia (contralateral), mixed expressive and receptive aphasia or anomia	Astrocytoma, oligodendroglioma
Thalamus	Sensory impairment (contralateral)	Astrocytoma

*Similar manifestations may result from brain parenchymal metastases or from tumors around the dura (eg, metastatic tumors; meningeal tumors such as meningiomas, sarcomas, or gliomas) or skull lesions (eg, granulomas, hemangiomas, osteitis deformans, osteomas, xanthomas) that compress the underlying brain.

Diagnosis

Early-stage brain tumors are often misdiagnosed. A brain tumor should be considered in patients with progressive focal or global brain neurologic deficits; new seizures; persistent, unexplained, recent-onset headaches, particularly if worsened by sleep; or evidence of increased intracranial pressure (eg, papilledema, unexplained vomiting). Similar findings can result from other intracranial masses (eg, abscess, aneurysm, arteriovenous malformation, intracerebral hemorrhage, subdural hematoma, granuloma, parasitic cysts such as neurocysticercosis) or ischemic stroke. Tumors should also be considered as causes in patients with a pituitary or hypothalamic endocrinopathy.

A complete neurologic examination, neuroimaging, and chest x-rays (for a source of metastases) should be done. T1-weighted MRI with gadolinium is the study of choice. CT with contrast agent is an alternative. MRI usually detects low-grade astrocytomas and oligodendrogliomas earlier than CT and shows brain structures near bone (eg, the posterior fossa) more clearly. If whole-brain imaging does not show sufficient detail in the target area (eg, sella turcica, cerebellopontine angle, optic nerve), closely spaced images or other special views of the area are obtained. If neuroimaging is normal but increased intracranial pressure is suspected, idiopathic intracranial hypertension (see p. 1846) should be considered and lumbar puncture performed.

Radiographic clues to the type of tumor, mainly location (see TABLE 225–1) and pattern of enhancement on MRI, may be inconclusive; brain biopsy may be required. Specialized tests (eg, molecular and genetic tumor markers in blood and CSF) can help in some cases: In patients with AIDS, Epstein-Barr virus titers in CSF typically increase as CNS lymphoma develops.

Treatment

Patients with coma or impaired airway reflexes require endotracheal intubation. Brain herniation due to tumors is treated with mannitol 25 to 100 g infused IV, a corticosteroid (eg, dexamethasone 16 mg IV, followed by 4 mg po or IV q 6 h), and endotracheal intubation. Mass lesions should be surgically decompressed as soon as possible.

Increased intracranial pressure due to tumors but without herniation is treated with corticosteroids (eg, dexamethasone as above or prednisone 30 to 40 mg po bid).

Treatment of the brain tumor depends on pathology and location (for acoustic neuroma, see p. 790). Surgical excision should be used for diagnosis and symptom relief. It may cure benign tumors. For tumors infiltrating the brain parenchyma, treatment is multimodal. Radiation therapy is required, and chemotherapy appears to benefit some patients.

Treatment of metastatic tumors includes radiation therapy and sometimes stereotactic radiosurgery. For patients with a solitary metastasis, surgical excision of the tumor before radiation therapy improves outcome.

End-of-life issues: If brain tumors are expected to soon be fatal, end-of-life issues should be considered (see p. 2762).

Radiation Therapy and Neurotoxicity

Radiation therapy may be directed diffusely to the whole head for diffuse or multicentric tumors or locally for well-demarcated tumors. Localized brain radiation therapy may be conformal, targeting the tumor with the aim of sparing normal brain tissue, or stereotactic, involving implantation of radioactive stable iodine ($^{125}I_3$) or iridium-192 ($^{192}Ir_4$), called brachytherapy, or use of a gamma knife or linear accelerator. Gliomas are treated with conformal radiation therapy; a gamma knife or linear accelerator is useful for metastases. Giving radiation daily tends to maximize efficacy and minimize damage to normal CNS tissue (neurotoxicity).

Degree of neurotoxicity depends on cumulative radiation dose, individual dose size, duration of therapy, volume of tissue irradiated, and individual susceptibility (see also p. 2601). Because susceptibility varies, prediction of radiation toxicity is imprecise. Symptoms of toxicity can develop in the 1st few days (acute) or months of treatment (early-delayed) or several months to years after treatment (late-delayed). Rarely, radiation causes gliomas, meningiomas, or peripheral nerve sheath tumors years after therapy.

Acute brain radiation toxicity in children and adults is characterized by headache, nausea, vomiting, somnolence, and sometimes worsening focal neurologic signs. It is particularly likely if intracranial pressure is high. Using corticosteroids to lower intracranial pressure can prevent or treat acute toxicity. Acute toxicity lessens with subsequent treatments.

Early-delayed brain toxicity can cause an encephalopathy in children or adults that must be distinguished from worsening or recurrent brain tumor by MRI or CT. It occurs in children who have received prophylactic whole-brain radiation therapy for leukemia; they develop somnolence, which lessens spontaneously over several days to weeks, possibly more rapidly if corticosteroids are used. After radiation therapy to the neck or upper thorax, early-delayed toxicity can result in a myelopathy, characterized by Lhermitte's sign (an electric shock–like sensation radiating down the back and into the legs when the neck is flexed). The myelopathy resolves spontaneously.

Late-delayed toxicity develops in most children and adults who receive diffuse brain radiation therapy if they survive long enough. The most common cause in children is diffuse therapy given to prevent leukemia or to treat medulloblastoma. After diffuse therapy, the main symptom is progressive dementia; many adults also develop an unsteady gait. MRI or CT shows cerebral atrophy. Toxicity after localized therapy more often involves focal neurologic deficits. MRI or CT shows a mass that may be enhanced by contrast agent and that may be difficult to distinguish from recurrence of the primary tumor. Excisional biopsy of the mass is diagnostic and often ameliorates symptoms.

After radiation therapy for extraspinal tumors (eg, due to Hodgkin lymphoma), late-delayed myelopathy can develop. It is characterized by progressive paresis and sensory loss, often as a Brown-Séquard syndrome (ipsilateral paresis and proprioceptive sensory loss, and contralateral loss of pain and temperature sensation). Most patients eventually become paraplegic.

GLIOMAS

Gliomas are primary tumors that originate in brain parenchyma. Symptoms and diagnosis are similar to those of other brain tumors. Treatment involves surgical excision, radiation therapy, and, for some tumors, chemotherapy. Excision rarely cures.

Gliomas include astrocytomas, oligodendrogliomas, medulloblastomas, and ependymomas. Many gliomas infiltrate brain tissue diffusely and irregularly.

Astrocytomas are the most common gliomas. They are classified, in ascending order of malignancy, as grade 1 or 2 (low-grade astrocytomas), grade 3 (anaplastic astrocytomas), or grade 4 (glioblastomas, including glioblastoma multiforme, the most malignant). Low-grade or anaplastic astrocytomas tend to develop in younger patients and can evolve into glioblastomas (secondary glioblastomas). Glioblastomas contain chromosomally heterogeneous cells. They can develop de novo (primary glioblastomas), usually in middle-aged or elderly people. Primary and secondary glioblastomas have distinct genetic characteristics, which can change as the tumors evolve.

Oligodendrogliomas are among the most benign gliomas. They affect mainly the cerebral cortex, particularly the frontal lobes.

Medulloblastomas develop mainly in children and young adults, usually near the 4th ventricle. Ependymomas are uncommon. They develop mainly in children, usually near the 4th ventricle. Medulloblastomas and ependymomas predispose to obstructive hydrocephalus.

Symptoms and signs vary by location (see TABLE 225–1). Diagnosis is the same as that of other brain tumors.

Treatment

Anaplastic astrocytomas and glioblastomas are treated with surgery, radiation therapy, and chemotherapy to reduce tumor mass. Excising as much tumor as possible is safe, prolongs survival, and improves neurologic function. After surgery, patients receive a full tumor dose (60 Gy) of radiation therapy; ideally, conformal radiation therapy, which targets the tumor and spares normal brain tissue, is used. Chemotherapy includes a nitrosourea (eg, carmustine, lomustine) used alone or in combination. Instead of combination chemotherapy, temozolomide can be given for 5 days/mo at 150 mg/m^2 po once/day during the 1st month, followed by 200 mg/m^2 in subsequent months. Patients receiving chemotherapy require a CBC at varying intervals but at least 24 to 48 h before each chemotherapy session. Investigational therapies (eg, chemotherapy wafers, stereotactic radiosurgery, new chemotherapeutic drugs, gene or immune therapy) should also be considered. After conventional multimodal treatment, the survival rate for patients with anaplastic astrocytomas or glioblastomas is about 50% at 1 yr, 25% at 2 yr, and 10 to 15% at 5 yr. Prognosis is better if patients are < 45 yr, if histology is anaplastic astrocytoma (rather than glioblastoma multiforme), or if initial excision improves neurologic function and leaves minimal or no residual tumor.

Low-grade astrocytomas are excised if possible, followed by radiation therapy. When radiation therapy should begin is controversial: Early treatment may maximize efficacy but may cause brain damage earlier. With treatment, 5-yr survival rate is about 40 to 50%.

Oligodendrogliomas are treated with excision and radiation therapy, similarly to low-grade astrocytomas. Chemotherapy is sometimes also used. With treatment, 5-yr survival rate is about 50 to 60%.

Medulloblastomas are treated with whole-brain radiation therapy using about 35 Gy, a posterior fossa boost using 15 Gy, and spinal cord radiation therapy using about 35 Gy. Chemotherapy may be given as adjunctive therapy and for recurrences. Several drugs—including the nitrosoureas, procarbazine, vincristine alone or in combination, intrathecal methotrexate, combination chemotherapy (eg, mechlorethamine, vincristine [Oncovin], procarbazine, and prednisone [MOPP]), cisplatin, and carboplatin—are effective for certain patients, but no regimen is consistently effective. With treatment, survival rates are at least 50% at 5 yr and about 40% at 10 yr.

Ependymomas are usually treated with surgery to excise the tumor and open CSF pathways, followed by radiation therapy. For histologically benign ependymomas, radiation therapy is directed at the tumor; for more malignant tumors with residual tumor after surgery, whole-brain radiation therapy is used. For tumors with evidence of dissemination, radiation therapy is directed at the whole brain and spinal cord. How much of the tumor is excised may predict survival best. With treatment, overall 5-yr survival rate is about 50%; however, for patients with no residual tumor, the 5-yr survival rate is > 70%.

MENINGIOMAS

Meningiomas are benign tumors of the meninges that can compress adjacent brain tissue. Symptoms depend on the tumor's location. Diagnosis is by MRI with contrast agent. Treatment may include excision, stereotactic radiosurgery, and sometimes radiation therapy.

Meningiomas, particularly those < 2 cm in diameter, are among the most common intracranial tumors. Meningiomas are the only brain tumor more common among women. They tend to occur between ages 40 and 60 yr but can occur during childhood. These benign tumors can develop wherever there is dura, most commonly over the convexities near the venous sinuses, along the base of the skull, in the posterior fossa, and rarely within ventricles. Multiple meningiomas may develop. Meningiomas compress but do not invade brain parenchyma. They can invade and

TABLE 225–2. SYMPTOMS OF MENINGIOMAS BY SITE

SITE	FINDINGS
Base of skull	Visual loss, oculomotor palsies, exophthalmos
Cerebral convexities	Focal seizures; cognitive deficits; ultimately, signs of increased intracranial pressure
Clivus and apical petrous bone	Gait disturbance; limb ataxia; deficits referable to the 5th, 7th, and 8th cranial nerves
Foramen magnum	Ipsilateral suboccipital pain and paresis that begins in the ipsilateral arm and progresses to the ipsilateral leg, then to the contralateral leg and arm; sometimes Lhermitte's sign; cranial nerve deficits (eg, dysphagia, dysarthria, nystagmus, diplopia, facial hypoesthesia)
Olfactory groove	Anosmia, sometimes papilledema and visual loss
Parasagittal or falx	Spastic paresis or sensory loss, usually beginning in the contralateral leg, but occasionally bilateral; cognitive deficits
Posterior fossa tentorial tumors that extend superiorly or inferiorly	Hydrocephalus
Sphenoid wing:	
Medial (growing into the cavernous sinus)	Oculomotor palsies, facial numbness
Middle (growing anteriorly into the orbit)	Visual loss, exophthalmos
Lateral (as a globular mass or a meningioma en plaque—ie, spread into the dura, with dural thickening and invasion of adjacent bone, sometimes growing into the temporal bone)	Seizures, headaches
Tuberculum sellae	Visual loss, bony changes sometimes visible with imaging

distort adjacent bone. There are many histologic types; all follow a similar clinical course, and some become malignant.

Symptoms depend on which part of the brain is compressed and thus on the tumor's location (see TABLE 225–2). Midline tumors in the elderly can cause dementia with few other focal neurologic findings. Diagnosis is similar to that of other brain tumors, usually by MRI with a paramagnetic contrast agent. Bony abnormalities (eg, brain atrophy, hyperostosis around the cerebral convexities, changes in the tuberculum sellae) may be seen incidentally on CT or plain x-rays.

Treatment

Asymptomatic meningiomas can be followed with serial neuroimaging. Symptomatic or enlarging meningiomas should be excised if possible. If they are large, encroach on blood vessels (usually surrounding veins), or are close to critical brain areas (eg, brain stem), surgery may cause more damage than the tumor and is thus deferred. Stereotactic radiosurgery is used for surgically inaccessible meningiomas and electively for other meningiomas. It is also used when tumor tissue remains after surgical excision or when the patient is elderly. If stereotactic radiosurgery is impossible or if a meningioma recurs, radiation therapy may be useful.

PINEAL REGION TUMORS

Pineal region tumors are usually germ cell tumors (eg, germinoma, choriocarcinoma, yolk-sac tumor, teratoma). Other primary

pineal tumors include pineocytoma and the rare malignant pineoblastoma.

Pineal region tumors tend to occur during childhood but can occur at any age. They may increase intracranial pressure by compressing the aqueduct of Sylvius. They may also cause paresis of upward gaze, ptosis, and loss of pupillary light and accommodation reflexes by compressing the pretectum rostral to the superior colliculi. These tumors may cause precocious puberty, especially in boys, probably because the hypothalamus is compressed. Germinomas are the most common pineal region tumor.

CSF β-human chorionic gonadotropin or α-fetoprotein may be elevated, depending on the tumor type. Elevated levels suggest the diagnosis; levels may be measured to monitor response to treatment. Prognosis and treatment depend on tumor histology. Radiation therapy, chemotherapy, radiosurgery, and surgery are used alone or in combination. Germinomas are very sensitive to radiation therapy and are often cured.

PITUITARY TUMORS

Most pituitary tumors are adenomas. Symptoms include headache and endocrinopathies; endocrinopathies result when the tumor produces hormones or destroys hormone-producing tissue. Diagnosis is by MRI. Treatment includes surgery or radiation therapy and correction of any endocrinopathy.

Most tumors of the pituitary and suprasellar region are pituitary adenomas. Rarely, pituitary tumors are carcinomas. Meningiomas, craniopharyngiomas, metastases, and dermoid cysts may also develop in the region of the sella turcica.

Adenomas may be secretory or nonsecretory. Secretory adenomas produce pituitary hormones; many secretory adenomas are < 10 mm in size (microadenomas). Secretory adenomas can be classified by histologic staining characteristics (eg, acidophilic, basophilic, chromophobe [nonstaining]). The hormone produced often correlates with these characteristics; eg, acidophilic adenomas overproduce growth hormone, and basophilic adenomas overproduce ACTH. The hormone most commonly overproduced is prolactin.

Any tumor that grows out of the pituitary can compress optic nerve tracts, including the chiasm. Tumors may also compress or destroy pituitary or hypothalamic tissue, impairing hormone production or secretion.

Symptoms and Signs

Headache may result from an enlarging pituitary adenoma, even when intracranial pressure is not increased. Visual manifestations such as bitemporal hemianopia, unilateral optic atrophy, and contralateral hemianopia may develop if a tumor compresses optic nerve tracts (see FIG. 107–1 on p. 922).

Many patients present with an endocrinopathy due to hormone deficiency or excess. Diabetes insipidus may develop if less vasopressin is released because the hypothalamus is compressed. Amenorrhea and galactorrhea in women and, less commonly, erectile dysfunction and gynecomastia in men may result from overproduction of prolactin. Gigantism before puberty or acromegaly after puberty may result from overproduction of growth hormone, and Cushing's syndrome from overproduction of ACTH. Rarely, hemorrhage into a pituitary tumor causes pituitary apoplexy, with sudden headache, ophthalmoplegia, and visual loss.

Diagnosis and Treatment

Pituitary tumors are suspected in patients with unexplained headaches, characteristic visual abnormalities, or endocrinopathies. Neuroimaging with 1-mm thick slices is done. MRI is usually much more sensitive than CT, particularly for microadenomas.

Endocrinopathies are treated. Pituitary tumors that secrete ACTH, growth hormone, or thyroid-stimulating hormone are surgically excised, usually using a transsphenoidal approach. Sometimes, particularly for surgically inaccessible or multifocal tumors, radiation therapy is required. Dopaminergic agonists (eg, bromocriptine, pergolide, cabergoline) are effective for adenomas that produce prolactin; surgery and radiation therapy are usually unnecessary.

PRIMARY BRAIN LYMPHOMAS

Primary brain lymphomas originate in neural tissue and are usually B-cell tumors. Diagnosis requires neuroimaging and sometimes CSF analysis, Epstein-Barr titers, or brain biopsy. Treatment includes corticosteroids, chemotherapy, and radiation therapy.

Incidence of primary brain lymphomas is increasing, particularly among immunocompromised patients and the elderly. Lymphomas tend to infiltrate the brain diffusely, often as multicentric masses adjacent to the ventricles, but may occur as solitary brain masses. Lymphomas may also occur in the meninges, uvea, or vitreous humor. Most are B-cell tumors, often immunoblastic. The Epstein-Barr virus may contribute to development of lymphomas in immunocompromised patients. Most patients do not develop subsequent systemic lymphoma.

MRI can suggest the diagnosis. Neuroimaging may be unable to distinguish cerebral toxoplasmosis, which is common among patients with AIDS, from lymphoma. If there are meningeal signs, CSF is examined; it may contain lymphoma cells. In immunocompromised patients, Epstein-Barr virus DNA may be detected in CSF. If CSF does not contain lymphoma cells or Epstein-Barr virus DNA, guided-needle or open biopsy is required. Because lymphoma is initially highly sensitive to corticosteroids, giving these drugs just before biopsy may cause the lesion to disappear, resulting in a false-negative biopsy.

Most primary brain lymphomas are difficult to cure because they infiltrate the brain diffusely. Treatment includes corticosteroids, chemotherapy, and radiation therapy. Many chemotherapy regimens, particularly those containing methotrexate (delivered as high-dose IV infusions), are effective; with methotrexate, median survival may approach 4 yr. Methotrexate can also be delivered intrathecally. It is sometimes infused into the carotid artery after general anesthesia is induced and 25% mannitol is given IV to open the blood-brain barrier. Most chemotherapy regimens are followed by radiation therapy, usually after 12 to 16 wk but sometimes delayed until the tumor recurs to reduce radiation toxicity.

SPINAL CORD TUMORS

Spinal cord tumors may develop within the spinal cord parenchyma, directly destroying tissue, or outside the cord parenchyma, often compressing the cord or nerve roots. Symptoms include progressive back pain and neurologic deficits referable to the spinal cord or spinal nerve roots. Diagnosis is by MRI. Treatment may include corticosteroids, surgical excision, and radiation therapy.

Spinal cord tumors may be intramedullary (within the cord parenchyma) or extramedullary (outside the parenchyma). The most common intramedullary tumors are gliomas (eg, ependymomas, low-grade astrocytomas). Extramedullary tumors may be intradural or extradural. Most intradural tumors are benign, usually meningiomas and neurofibromas, which are the most common primary spinal tumors. Most extradural tumors are metastatic, usually from carcinomas of the lung, breasts, prostate, kidneys, or thyroid or from lymphoma (eg, Hodgkin lymphoma, lymphosarcoma, reticulum cell sarcoma).

Intramedullary tumors infiltrate and destroy cord parenchyma and may extend over multiple spinal cord segments; an intramedullary tumor may result in a syrinx (see p. 1915). Intradural and extradural tumors cause neurologic damage by compressing the spinal cord or nerve roots. Most extradural tumors invade and destroy bone before compressing the cord.

Symptoms and Signs

Pain is an early symptom. It is progressive, unrelated to activity, and worsened by recumbency. Pain may occur in the back, radiate along the sensory distribution of a particular dermatome (radicular pain), or both. Usually, neurologic deficits referable to the spinal cord eventually develop. Common examples are spastic weakness, incontinence, and dysfunction of some or all of the sensory tracts at a particular segment of the spinal cord and below. Deficits are usually bilateral.

Many patients with extramedullary tumors present with pain, but some present with sensory deficits of the distal lower extremities or segmental neurologic deficits and spinal cord compression. Symptoms of spinal cord compression tend to worsen rapidly because most extradural tumors are metastatic. Symptoms of nerve root compression are also common; they include pain and paresthesias followed by sensory loss, muscular weakness, and, if compression is chronic, wasting, which occurs along the distribution of the affected roots.

Diagnosis and Treatment

Spinal tumors are suggested by progressive, unexplained, or nocturnal back or radicular pain; segmental neurologic deficits; or unexplained neurologic deficits referable to the spinal cord or nerve roots. They are also suggested by unexplained back pain in patients with primary tumors of the lungs, breasts, prostate, kidneys, or thyroid or with lymphoma. Diagnosis is by MRI of the affected area of the spinal cord. CT is an alternative but is less accurate. *Patients with segmental neurologic deficits or suspected spinal cord compression require emergency diagnosis and treatment.*

If MRI does not show a spinal cord tumor, other spinal masses (eg, abscesses, arteriovenous malformations—see Ch. 224 on p. 1908) and paravertebral tumors are considered. Spinal x-rays, taken for other reasons, may show bone destruction, widening of the vertebral pedicles, or distortion of paraspinal tissues, especially if the tumor is metastatic.

For patients with neurologic deficits, corticosteroids (eg, dexamethasone, 50 mg IV, then 10 mg po qid) are begun immediately to reduce spinal cord edema and preserve function. Tumors compressing the spinal cord are treated as soon as possible. Some well-localized primary spinal cord tumors can be excised surgically. Deficits resolve in about $\frac{1}{2}$ of these patients. For tumors that cannot be surgically excised, radiation therapy is used, with or without surgical decompression. Compressive metastatic extradural tumors are usually surgically excised from the vertebral body, then treated with radiation therapy. Noncompressive metastatic extradural tumors may be treated with radiation therapy alone but may require excision if radiation therapy is ineffective.

SECTION 17
GENITOURINARY DISORDERS

226 APPROACH TO THE GENITOURINARY PATIENT

Although some disorders affect both the kidneys and the lower urinary tract (eg, pyelonephritis), renal and urologic disorders usually require different approaches. Common GU symptoms include dysuria, hematospermia, hematuria, proteinuria, scrotal mass, and testicular pain. For incontinence, see p. 1951; for UTI, see p. 1968; and for priapism, see p. 2039.

APPROACH TO THE RENAL PATIENT

History

History plays a limited role because symptoms are nonspecific. Many patients who report bloody urine have highly concentrated urine; myoglobinuria, hemoglobinuria, and bilirubinuria are also often mistaken for hematuria (see p. 1939). High concentrations of urinary protein cause frothy or sudsy urine. Urinary frequency should be distinguished from polyuria in patients who report excessive urination (see p. 1941). Nocturia may be a feature of either but is often the result of excess fluid intake too close to bedtime. Family history is useful for identifying inheritance patterns and risk of polycystic kidney disease or hereditary nephropathy (Alport's syndrome).

Physical Examination

Patients with acute renal failure may be drowsy, confused, or inattentive; speech may be slurred. Those with chronic renal failure generally appear pale, wasted, or ill. Deep (Kussmaul's) respirations signify acidemia.

Inspection: Visual fullness of the upper abdomen is an unusual, nonspecific finding of polycystic kidney disease. Visibly asymmetric growth of one side of the body (hemihypertrophy) is a rare sign of Wilms' tumor. Chronic renal failure has several dermatologic manifestations, including xerosis due to sebaceous and eccrine sweat gland atrophy, pallor due to anemia, hyperpigmentation due to melanin deposition, sallow or yellow-brown skin due to urochrome deposition, and petechiae or ecchymoses due to platelet dysfunction. Cutaneous fibrosis can affect patients undergoing dialysis. Uremic frost, the deposition of white-to-tan urea crystals on the skin after sweat evaporation, is rare.

Auscultation: A soft, lateralizing abdominal bruit is occasionally heard in renal artery stenosis; presence of a diastolic component increases the probability of renovascular hypertension. Pericardial and pleuritic friction rubs can be signs of uremia.

Percussion: Pain elicited by blunt percussion of the back, flanks, and angle formed by the 12th rib and lumbar spine (costovertebral tenderness) with a fist may indicate pyelonephritis or calculi.

Palpation: Normal kidneys are not usually palpable. However, in some women, the lower pole of the right kidney can occasionally be felt with palpation upward at the rear flank during deep inspiration, and large kidneys or masses can sometimes be felt without special maneuvers. In newborns, the kidneys can be felt with the thumbs when the thumbs are placed anterior and the fingers posterior to the costovertebral angle.

Other maneuvers: Transillumination can distinguish solid from cystic renal masses in some children < 1 yr if the kidney and mass are manipulated against the abdominal wall. Asterixis (uremic flap), a manifestation of chronic renal or hepatic failure, can be detected in handwriting or by observation of outstretched hands maximally extended at the wrists; after several seconds in this position, a hand flap in the flexor direction is asterixis.

Testing

Urinalysis and measurement of serum creatinine are the 1st steps in evaluation of renal disorders. Other urine, blood, and imaging tests (eg, ultrasonography, CT, MRI) are done in specific circumstances.

Ideally, after the urethral meatus is cleaned, the urine specimen is collected midstream in the 1st void of the morning (clean-catch specimen); the urine should be examined immediately because delays can lead to changes in test results. When no alternatives exist, bladder catheterization or suprapubic aspiration can be used for collection, but the trauma may falsely increase the number of RBCs in the specimen. A specimen from a catheter collection bag is not acceptable for microscopic and bacteriologic tests.

Urinalysis: A complete urinalysis includes visual inspection for color and appearance; measurement of pH, specific gravity, protein, glucose, RBCs, nitrites, and WBC esterase by dipstick reagents; and microscopic analysis for casts, crystals, and cells (urine sediment). Bilirubin and urobilinogen, although a standard part of many dipstick tests, no longer play a significant role in evaluation of renal or hepatic disorders.

Color change to red, orange, or brown may indicate the presence of RBCs, myoglobin, bilirubin, or porphyrins; these changes may also be caused by some drugs (eg, levodopa, methyldopa, phenazopyridine, rifampin) and foods (eg, beets). Cloudy white urine may reflect infection (pyuria), lymph (chyluria) due to filariasis or to obstructed retroperitoneal lymphatics, or precipitated phosphate crystals. Green urine may indicate *Pseudomonas* infection or use of certain drugs (eg, amitriptyline, methylene blue, propofol). Rarely, urine in collection bags of catheterized bedbound patients turns purple (purple urine bag syndrome) when urinary gram-negative bacteria metabolize a tryptophan metabolite (indican) in alkaline urine into indigo; this reaction is clinically insignificant. Dark brown or black urine may result from oxidation of excessive homogentisic acid or melanogen (from melanoma) when urine is exposed to air for several hours.

Odor, often unintentionally noted during visual inspection, conveys useful information only in rare cases of inherited disorders of amino acid metabolism when urine has a distinctive smell (eg, maple syrup in maple syrup urine disease, sweaty feet in isovaleric acidemia, or tomcat urine in multiple carboxylase deficiency).

pH is normally 5.0 to 6.0 (range 4.5 to 8.0). Delay in processing a specimen may elevate pH because ammonia is released as bacteria break down urea. Measuring with a glass pH electrode is recommended when precise values are necessary for decision making, as when diagnosing renal tubular acidosis; in these cases, a layer of oil should be added to the urine specimen to prevent escape of CO_2. Infection with urease-producing pathogens can spuriously increase pH.

Specific gravity provides a rough measure of urine concentration (osmolality). Normal range is 1.001 to 1.035; values may be higher in the elderly, who are less able to dilute and concentrate urine. It is measured by hydrometer or refractometer or estimated with a dipstick. Accuracy of the dipstick is controversial, but the test may be sufficient for patients who have calculi and are advised to self-monitor urine concentration to maintain dilute urine. Specific gravity by dipstick may be spuriously elevated when urine pH is < 6 or low when pH is > 7. Hydrometer and refractometer measurements may be elevated by high levels of large molecules (eg, radiocontrast, albumin, glucose, carbenicillin) in the urine.

Protein in urine may be normal, but albumin never is. Dipsticks measure albumin, classified as negative (< 10 mg/dL), trace (15 to 30 mg/dL), or 1+ (50 to 100 mg/dL) through 4+ (> 2000 mg/dL). High pH, presence of cells, and radiocontrast cause false elevations. Dilute urine causes falsely low or negative results.

Glucose appears in urine erratically when serum glucose increases to > 180 mg/dL (10.1 mmol/L). Threshold for detection by urine dipstick is 50 mg/dL (2.8 mmol/L). Any amount is abnormal. Ascorbic acid, ketones, aspirin, and dilute urine cause falsely low or negative results.

RBCs lyse on a dipstick test strip, releasing Hb and causing a color change. Range is from negative (0) to 4+. Trace blood (3 to 5 RBCs/HPF) is normal under some circumstances (eg, exercise) in some people. Because the test strip reagent reacts with Hb, free Hb (eg, due to intravascular hemolysis) or myoglobin (eg, due to rhabdomyolysis) causes a positive result. Hemoglobinuria and myoglobinuria can be distinguished from hematuria by the absence of RBCs on microscopic examination and by the pattern of color change on the test strip. RBCs create a dotted or speckled pattern; free Hb and myoglobin create a uniform color change. Povidone iodine causes false-positive results; ascorbic acid causes false-negative results.

Nitrites are produced when bacteria reduce urinary nitrates derived from amino acid metabolism. Nitrites are not normally present and signify bacteriuria. The test is either positive or negative. False-negative results may occur with certain pathogens that cannot convert nitrate to nitrite (eg, *Enterococcus faecalis, Neisseria gonorrhoeae, Mycobacterium tuberculosis, Pseudomonas* sp) or when time is inadequate (< 4 h) for conversion of nitrate to nitrite, when urinary excretion of nitrate is low, or when bacterial enzymes reduce nitrates to nitrogen. Nitrites are used mainly with WBC esterase testing to follow patients with recurrent urine infections, particularly children with vesicoureteral reflux.

WBC esterase is released by lysed neutrophils. Its presence in urine reflects acute inflammation, most commonly due to bacterial infection. Threshold for detection is about 5 WBCs/HPF, and test results range from negative (0 WBCs/HPF) to 4+. The test is not very sensitive for detection of infection. Contamination of a urine specimen with vaginal flora is the most common cause of false-positive results. False-negative results may result from very concentrated urine; glycosuria; urobilinogen; or use of phenazopyridine, nitrofurantoin, rifampin, or large amounts of vitamin C. WBC esterase is used mainly with nitrite testing to follow patients with recurrent urine infections. If both tests are negative, the likelihood of a positive urine culture is small.

Microscopic analysis: Detection of solid elements (cells, casts, crystals) requires microscopic analysis, ideally viewed immediately after voiding and dipstick testing. The specimen is prepared by centrifuging 10 to 15 mL of urine at 1500 to 2500 rpm for 5 min. The supernatant is fully decanted; a small amount of urine remains with the residue at the bottom of the centrifuge tube. The residue can be mixed back into solution by gently agitating the tube or tapping the bottom. A single drop is pipetted onto a slide and covered with a coverslip. For routine microscopic analysis, staining is optional. The specimen is examined under reduced light with the low-power objective and under full-intensity light with the high-power objective; the latter is typically used for semiquantitative estimates (eg, 10 to 15 WBCs/HPF). Polarized light and phase-contrast microscopy are used in special circumstances. Phase-contrast microscopy enhances identification of cells and casts.

Epithelial cells (renal tubular, transitional, squamous) frequently appear in urine; most common are squamous cells lining the end of the urethra and contaminants from the vagina. Only renal tubular cells are diagnostically important; however, except when found in casts, they are difficult to distinguish from transitional cells. A few renal tubular cell casts appear in normal urine, but a large number suggests tubular injury (eg, acute tubular necrosis, tubulointerstitial nephropathy, nephrotoxins, nephrotic syndrome).

RBCs < 3/HPF may be normal, and any hematuria should be interpreted in clinical context (see p. 1939). Microscopic analysis may be useful for distinguishing glomerular from nonglomerular RBCs. Glomerular RBCs are dysmorphic, with spicules, folding, and blebs; nonglomerular RBCs retain their normal shape.

WBCs < 5/HPF may be normal; special staining can distinguish eosinophils from neutrophils (see p. 1933). Pyuria is defined as ≥ 8 WBCs/μL of uncentrifuged urine, which corresponds to 2 to 5 WBCs/HPF in spun sediment.

Lipiduria is most characteristic of the nephrotic syndrome; renal tubular cells absorb filtered lipids, which appear microscopically as oval fat bodies, and cholesterol, which produces a Maltese cross pattern under polarized light. Lipids and cholesterol can also be free floating or incorporated into casts.

Crystals in urine are common and usually clinically insignificant. Crystal formation depends on urine concentration of crystal constituents, pH, and absence of crystallization inhibitors. The 4 most common types of crystals are Ca oxalate, uric acid, cystine, and Mg ammonium phosphate. Ca oxalate crystals occur in several shapes but are most easily recognized when they form small, octahedral, envelope-like shapes. When present in large numbers, they strongly suggest ethylene glycol poisoning or, rarely, short small bowel syndrome, hereditary oxalosis and oxaluria, and high doses of vitamin C. Ca oxalate crystals are also important in evaluation of calculi. Uric acid crystals are amorphous in acidic, highly concentrated, cool urine but may be diamond- or needle-shaped or rhomboid. They may indicate mild dehydration in newborns and tumor lysis syndrome in patients with cancer or renal failure. Cystine crystals are perfect hexagons, may occur alone as flat plates or as overlapping crystals of varying sizes, and are diagnostic of cystinuria, a rare hereditary cause of calculi. Mg ammonium phosphate crystals, which may resemble coffin lids or quartz crystals, often occur in normal alkaline urine and in urine of patients with struvite calculi. Drugs (eg, acyclovir, some sulfonamides, indinavir, high-dose methotrexate) are an underrecognized cause of crystal formation. Crystals of acyclovir are birefringent and needle-shaped; they exist free or engulfed in leukocytes. Crystals of indinavir form a starburst shape or individual needle-shaped crystals and are best seen under polarized light. Sulfa and ampicillin crystals are also needle-shaped and best seen when polarized. Sulfa crystals can also appear in clusters.

Casts are made up of glycoprotein of unknown function (Tamm-Horsfall protein) secreted from the thick ascending loop of Henle. They differ in constituents and appearance (see TABLE 226–1).

Other urine tests: Other tests are useful in specific instances.

Sulfosalicylic acid (SSA) test strips can be used to detect protein other than albumin (eg,

TABLE 226–1. URINARY CASTS

TYPE	DESCRIPTION	SIGNIFICANCE
Plain casts		
Hyaline	Glycoprotein matrix secreted by tubules	Nonspecific; present in normal urine but may also appear in patients with low urine flow (eg, due to dehydration or after diuretic therapy), physiologic stress, an acute renal disorder with other abnormalities, or a chronic renal disorder (as broad casts formed in dilated tubules)
Waxy	Glycoprotein matrix with degraded protein; formed in atrophic tubules; highly refractile with waxy appearance	Present in advanced renal failure; predicts a poor prognosis
Casts with inclusions		
RBC	Glycoprotein matrix with RBCs; often appears red-orange	Virtually pathognomonic of glomerulonephritis; rarely occurs with cortical necrosis, acute tubular injury, or hematuria in runners
Epithelial cell	Protein matrix variably filled with tubular cells	Occurs in acute tubular injury, glomerulonephritis, or nephrotic syndrome
WBC	Protein matrix variably filled with WBCs	Suggests pyelonephritis but can indicate other causes of tubulointerstitial inflammation; may occur in the exudative stage of proliferative glomerulonephritis
Granular	Glycoprotein matrix with protein or cellular debris	Occasionally occurs with exercise or dehydration and normal renal function; more often indicates glomerular or tubulointerstitial disorders
Pigment	Tubular cell or granular casts with pigment stain	Usually occurs in acute renal failure due to hemolysis or rhabdomyolysis or in acute tubular necrosis when jaundice is present
Fatty	Free fat droplets or tubular cells with fat droplets in a protein matrix	May occur in various types of tubulointerstitial disorders; in large numbers, strongly suggests nephrotic syndrome or Fabry's disease
Mixed	Hyaline cast with various cells (eg, RBCs, WBCs, tubular cells)	Usually occurs in proliferative glomerulonephritis
Miscellaneous	Crystals or bacteria	With crystals, may suggest a metabolic disorder or a cause of calculi; with bacteria, pathognomonic of bacterial pyelonephritis
Pseudocasts		
	Clumped urates, WBCs, bacteria, and artifacts	Important not to confuse with true casts

Igs in multiple myeloma) when dipstick urine tests are negative; urine supernatant mixed with SSA becomes turbid if protein is present. The test is semiquantitative with a scale of 0 (no turbidity) to 4+ (flocculent precipitates). Readings are falsely elevated by radiocontrast agents.

Protein excretion can be measured in a 24-h collection or can be estimated by the protein-to-creatinine ratio, which, in a random urine sample, correlates well with values in g/1.73 m^2 BSA from a 24-h collection (eg, 400 mg/dL protein and 100 mg/dL creatinine in a random sample equal 4 g/1.73 m^2 in a 24-h collection).

Microalbuminuria is albumin excretion persistently between 30 and 300 mg/day (20 to 200 μg/min). Normally, albumin excretion is < 20 mg/day (< 15 μg/min); > 300 mg/day (> 200 μg/min) is considered overt proteinuria. Use of the urine albumin-to-urine creatinine ratio is a reliable and more convenient screening test because it avoids timed urine specimens and correlates well with 24-h values. A value > 30 mg/g (>0.03 mg/mg) suggests microalbuminuria. The reliability of the test is best when a midmorning specimen is used, vigorous exercise is avoided before the test, and unusual creatinine production (cachectic or very muscular patients) is not present. In diabetics, microalbuminuria usually indicates diabetic nephropathy and provides an early way to detect the disorder. Microalbuminuria is a risk factor for cardiovascular disorders and early cardiovascular mortality independent of diabetes or hypertension.

Ketones spill into urine with ketonemia, but use of test strips to measure urinary ketones is no longer widely recommended because they measure only acetoacetic acid and acetone, not β-hydroxybutyric acid. Thus, a false-negative result is possible even without an exogenous cause (eg, vitamin C, phenazopyridine, *N*-acetylcysteine); direct measurement of serum ketones is more accurate. Ketonuria is caused by endocrine and metabolic disorders and does not reflect renal dysfunction.

Osmolality, the total number of solute particles per unit volume (mOsm/kg [mmol/kg]), can be measured directly by osmometer. Normally, osmolality is 50 to 1200 mOsm/kg. Measurement is most useful for evaluating hypernatremia, hyponatremia, syndrome of inappropriate antidiuretic hormone secretion (SIADH), and diabetes insipidus.

Electrolyte measurements help diagnose specific disorders. Na level can help distinguish whether volume depletion (urine Na < 20 mEq/L) or acute tubular necrosis (urine Na > 40 mEq/L) is the cause of acute renal insufficiency or failure. The fractional excretion of Na (FE_{Na}), which is the ratio of excreted to filtered Na, is defined as

$$\frac{(U_{Na})(\dot{V})}{(P_{Na})(Cl_{Cr})}$$

where U_{Na} is urine Na, P_{Na} is plasma Na, $\dot{V}$ is urine flow (mL/min), P_{Cr} is plasma creatinine, U_{Cr} is urine creatinine, and Cl_{Cr} is the creatine clearance in mL/min. Because $Cl_{Cr} = (U_{Cr})(U\text{vol})/P_{Cr}$, the flow terms cancel out and the equation can be rewritten as

$$\frac{(U_{Na})(P_{Cr})}{(P_{Na})(U_{Cr})}$$

This ratio is a more reliable measure than U_{Na} alone because U_{Na} levels between 20 and 40 mEq/L are nonspecific. FE_{Na} < 1% suggests volume depletion; > 1% suggests acute tubular necrosis. Other useful measurements include fractional excretion of HCO_3 in evaluation of renal tubular acidosis (see p. 2026); Cl levels and urine anion gap for diagnosis of metabolic acidosis (see p. 1269); K levels, occasionally useful in treatment of hypokalemia; and levels of Ca, Mg, and constituents such as uric acid, oxalate, citrate, and cystine in evaluation of calculi.

Eosinophils, cells that stain bright red or pink-white with Wright's or Hansel staining, most commonly indicate acute interstitial nephritis, rapidly progressive glomerulonephritis, acute prostatitis, or renal atheroembolism.

Cytology is used to screen for cancer in high-risk populations (eg, petrochemical workers), to evaluate painless hematuria due to nonrenal disorders, and to check for recurrence after bladder tumor resection. Sensitivity is about 90% for carcinoma in situ; however, sensitivity is considerably lower for low-grade transitional cell carcinomas. Inflammatory or reactive hyperplastic lesions or cytotoxic drugs for carcinoma may produce false-positive results. Accuracy for detecting bladder tumors may be increased by vigorous bladder lavage with a small volume of 0.9% saline solution (50 mL pushed in, then aspirated by syringe through a catheter). Cells collected in the saline are concentrated and examined.

Gram stain and cultures with susceptibility testing are indicated when GU tract infections are suspected; a positive test must be interpreted in the clinical context (see p. 1968).

Amino acids are normally filtered and reabsorbed by the proximal tubules. They may appear in urine when a hereditary or acquired tubular transport defect (eg, Fanconi syndrome, cystinuria) is present. Measuring type and amount of amino acids may help in the diagnosis of certain types of calculi, renal tubular acidosis, and inherited disorders of metabolism.

Creatinine clearance: Creatinine clearance (CrCl) is a measure of GFR, the amount of blood filtered through the kidney per minute, because creatinine is produced at a constant rate by muscle metabolism and is freely filtered without reabsorption or metabolism by the kidneys. However, enough additional creatinine is secreted that CrCl overestimates GFR by about 10 mL/min/1.73 m^2 BSA, or by 10 to 20%. Using a timed urine collection, CrCl can be calculated as

$$\text{CrCL} = \frac{(\text{UCr}[\text{mg/dL}])(\text{urine volume}[\text{mL/min}])}{(\text{serum creatinine}[\text{mg/dL}])}$$

where UCr is urine creatinine concentration. Normal values (adjusted by dividing by BSA in m^2) are 70 ± 14 mL/min/m^2 for men and 60 ± 10 mL/min/m^2 for women. CrCl increases throughout childhood and progressively decreases after about age 40, so that by age 80, CrCl is normally ½ what it was in young adulthood. Up to 50% of the glomerular filtering surface may be lost before the serum creatinine begins to rise because of hypertrophy of residual glomeruli. Thus, a normal CrCl cannot exclude mild renal disease and is not useful for detecting early kidney damage.

Blood tests: Serum creatinine levels can estimate CrCl on the premise that urine volume and creatinine in the above equation are roughly constant. Levels are affected by diet, age, and muscle mass; the last 2 are reflected in the following equation:

$$\text{CrCL}_{(\text{est})} = \frac{(140 - \text{age}[\text{yr}])(\text{body wt}[\text{kg}])}{(72)(\text{serum creatinine}[\text{mg/dL}])}$$

For women, the calculated value is multiplied by 0.85. GFR (in mL/min/1.73 m^2) has been shown to be more accurately predicted by

$$186 \times (\text{SCr})^{-1.154} \times (\text{age})^{-0.203} \times 0.747 (\text{if female}) \times 1.210 (\text{if African-American})$$

but the difficulty of calculating this equation has limited its use. In general, serum creatinine values > 1.3 mg/dL (> 114 μmol/L) in men and > 1 mg/dL (> 90 μmol/L) in women are abnormal. Values may be falsely elevated by consumption of large amounts of meat and use of some drugs (cimetidine, trimethoprim, cefoxitin, flucytosine). With aging, CrCl decreases but so does creatinine production due to decreasing muscle mass and turnover; thus, serum creatinine tends to remain stable at about 1.0.

ACE inhibitors and angiotensin II receptor blockers reversibly decrease GFR and increase creatinine because they vasodilate efferent more than afferent glomerular arterioles. Creatinine levels vary inversely but nonlinearly with GFR, so that small changes just above normal in creatinine indicate a more dramatic decline in GFR than do larger changes well above normal. Thus, creatinine measurements are better used to follow changes in renal function over time rather than to detect renal disorders.

BUN/creatinine ratio is used to distinguish prerenal from renal or postrenal (obstructive) azotemia; a value > 15 is considered abnormal and may occur in prerenal and some cases of postrenal azotemia. However, BUN is affected by protein intake and by multiple nonrenal processes (eg, trauma, infection, GI bleeding, corticosteroids) and, although suggestive, is generally unreliable for evaluating renal disorders.

Serum chemistries (eg, Na, K, HCO_3) may become abnormal in acute and chronic renal failure and should be monitored periodically.

CBC may detect anemia in chronic renal disorders or, rarely, polycythemia in renal cell carcinoma or polycystic kidney disease. Anemia is often multifactorial (eg, due to erythropoietin deficiency, blood loss in dialysis circuits or the GI tract); it may be microcytic or normocytic, and may be hypochromic or normochromic.

Renin, a proteolytic enzyme, is stored in the juxtaglomerular cells of the kidneys. Renin secretion is stimulated by reduced blood volume and flow in afferent renal arterioles and is inhibited by Na and water retention. Plasma renin is assayed by measuring renin activity as the amount of angiotensin I generated per hour. Specimens should be drawn from well-hydrated, Na- and K-replete patients who have been supine for at least 15 min. Plasma renin activity should be measured in evaluation of adrenal insufficiency, hyperaldosteronism, and refractory hypertension. Renal vein renin level is still occasionally measured to determine the functional significance of renal artery obstruction (see Renovascular Hypertension on p. 616).

APPROACH TO THE UROLOGIC PATIENT

History

Pain originating in the kidneys or ureters is usually vaguely localized to the flanks or lower back and may radiate into the ipsilateral iliac fossa, upper thigh, testis, or labium. Typically, pain caused by stones is colicky and may be prostrating; it is more constant if caused by infection. Acute urinary retention distal to the bladder causes agonizing suprapubic pain; chronic urinary retention may be asymptomatic. Dysuria is a symptom of bladder or urethral irritation (see p. 1938). Prostatic pain manifests as vague discomfort or fullness in the perineal, rectal, or suprapubic regions.

Symptoms of bladder obstruction in men include urinary hesitancy, straining, decrease in force and caliber of the urinary stream, and terminal dribbling. Incontinence has various forms (see p. 1951). Enuresis after age 3 to 4 yr may be a symptom of urethral stenosis in girls, posterior urethral valves in boys, psychologic distress, or, if onset is new, infection.

Pneumaturia (air passed with urine) suggests a vesicovaginal, vesicoenteric, or ureteroenteric fistula; the last 2 may be caused by diverticulitis, abscess, or colon cancer.

Physical Examination

Inspection: Inspection of the penis can detect hypospadias or epispadias in young boys, Peyronie's disease in adults, and testicular masses in either group. Visual fullness of the upper abdomen is an extremely rare and nonspecific finding of hydronephrosis.

Percussion: Pain elicited by blunt percussion of the back, flanks, and angle formed by the 12th rib and lumbar spine (costovertebral tenderness) with a fist may indicate pyelonephritis, calculi, or urinary tract obstruction. Dullness to percussion in the lower abdomen indicates bladder distention; normally, even a full bladder cannot be percussed above the symphysis pubis. Some practitioners use percussion to detect and monitor the size of large renal masses, but accuracy and consistency are questionable.

Palpation: Fibrous plaques on the penile shaft are signs of Peyronie's disease. Rubbery fullness above the testis, often described as a bag of worms, indicates a varicocele. A firm mass in or just above the testis signifies tumor or hydrocele.

During digital rectal examination, prostatitis may be detected as a boggy, tender prostate or a focal nodule, which must be distinguished from prostate cancer.

Bladder palpation can be used to confirm distention and urinary retention. Rarely, ureteral stones can be palpated close to the bladder junction in women during gynecologic examination.

Other maneuvers: Transillumination can be used to distinguish hydroceles from solid testicular masses. Pelvic examination is performed on women.

Testing

Urinalysis (see p. 1930) is critical for evaluating urologic disorders. Imaging tests (eg, ultrasonography, CT, MRI) are frequently required. For semen testing, see p. 2138.

Bladder tumor antigen testing for transitional cell cancer of the urinary tract is more sensitive than urinary cytology in detecting low-grade cancer; it is not sensitive enough to replace endoscopic examination. Urine cytology is the best test to detect high-grade cancer.

Prostate-specific antigen (PSA) is a glycoprotein with unknown function produced by prostatic epithelial cells. Levels can be elevated in prostate cancer and in some common noncancerous disorders (eg, benign prostatic hyperplasia, infection, trauma). PSA is measured to detect recurrence of cancer after treatment; its widespread use for cancer screening is controversial (see p. 2052).

IMAGING TESTS

X-rays: Abdominal x-rays without radiocontrast are virtually useless in evaluation of renal and urologic disorders; these x-rays show only about 15% of renal calculi (Ca oxalate calculi and rarely staghorn calculi). However, x-rays taken after administration of water-soluble radiocontrast agents highlight the kidneys and urinary collecting system. Nonionic iso-osmolal agents (eg, iohexol, iopamidol) are now widely used; they have fewer adverse effects than older hyperosmolal agents but still pose a risk of acute renal insufficiency or failure (contrast nephropathy—see p. 2016 and 2718).

In urography, an x-ray is taken after IV, percutaneous antegrade or retrograde, or cystoscopic retrograde administration of radiopaque contrast. Primary contraindications for all are iodine allergy and risk factors for contrast nephropathy.

IVU (IV urography or pyelography) has been largely superseded by rapid multidimensional CT and MRI with or without a contrast agent. Abdominal compression during IVU may improve visualization of the renal pelvis and proximal ureters (with application) and distal ureters (after release). Additional x-rays at 12 and 24 h may be indicated for postrenal obstruction or hydronephrosis.

For **percutaneous anterograde urography,** radiopaque contrast is introduced through an existing nephrostomy tube or, less commonly, through percutaneous puncture of the renal pelvis guided by fluoroscopy. Occasionally, a ureterostomy or an ileal conduit can be used. This technique is used when existing percutaneous access makes it practical or when IVU, CT, or MRI is unsuccessful or unsatisfactory because of impaired renal function or proximal obstruction. Anterograde urography is indicated when retrograde urography is unsuccessful (eg, because of tumor obstruction at bladder level), when large kidney stones requiring percutaneous surgery must be evaluated, when transitional cell carcinoma of the upper collecting system is suspected, or when patients cannot tolerate general anesthesia for retrograde urography. Complications relate to placement of the nephrostomy tube and include bleeding, sepsis, and injury to adjacent organs; microscopic hematuria, pain, and urinary extravasation are less serious.

Retrograde urography uses cystoscopy and ureteral catheterization to introduce radiocontrast directly into the ureters and renal collecting system. Sedation or general anesthesia is required. This technique is used when CT or MRI is unsuccessful; when the degree, type, cause, and length of ureteral obstruction must be defined; or when patients are allergic to radiopaque contrast. It is useful for detailed examination of the pelvicaliceal collecting system, ureters (eg, to check for ureterovaginal fistulas), and bladder. However, overdistention and backflow may distort calyces and obscure detail. Risk of infection is higher than that with other types of urography; acute ureteral edema and secondary stricture formation are rare.

For **cystourethrography,** radiopaque contrast is introduced directly into the urethra and bladder. This technique is more precise than IVU for evaluation of vesicoureteral reflux, urinary incontinence, recurrent UTIs, urethral strictures, and suspected urethral or bladder trauma. Voiding cystourethrograms are taken during urination and used to identify posterior urethral valves. No patient preparation is necessary. Adverse effects include UTIs and urosepsis; severe urethral strictures are a relative contraindication.

Angiography: Angiography has been largely replaced by noninvasive vascular imaging (eg, ultrasonography, CT, MRI, radionuclide scanning). Remaining indications include renal vein renin testing and angioplasty and stenting in patients with renal artery stenosis. Arteriography is also rarely used for evaluation and treatment of renal hemorrhage and before kidney-sparing surgery. Digital subtraction angiography is no longer used when rapid-sequence multidimensional CT or helical CT is available.

Ultrasonography: Doppler ultrasonography is widely used to image the kidneys, bladder, prostate, testes, and penis. The test is safe but provides no information about renal function, and renal images may be difficult to obtain in overweight or obese patients. Also, there is no means to improve distinction between types of tissues, and test quality is operator-dependent. No patient preparation is necessary, but a full bladder facilitates its imaging. Ultrasonography can show urine volume after micturition (postvoiding residual). Doppler ultrasonography in patients with testicular pain helps distinguish torsion from other causes.

CT: CT provides a broad view of renal, urologic, and surrounding structures. Conventional or helical scanners are used for most purposes with or without IV radiocontrast agents. Helical (spiral) CT without radiocontrast is used mainly to evaluate calculi. Use of radiocontrast with either technique resembles IVU but provides additional detail of urologic and surrounding structures. CT without radiocontrast is best for evaluation of trauma and other disorders that may involve acute hemorrhage (which appears bright white and can be confused with contrast agents) or urine extravasation.

MRI: MRI is safer than CT for patients at risk of contrast nephropathy. Magnetic resonance angiography, used to enhance blood vessels, has virtually replaced angiography for evaluating renal artery stenosis and renal vein thrombosis. Other uses include distinction between hemorrhage and infection within renal cysts; determination of extent of tumor invasion within the bladder wall; and precise imaging of the pelvis and genitals using a pelvic or endorectal coil. MRI with IV lymphotropic superparamagnetic nanoparticles (eg, monocrystalline iron oxide) can identify lymph node metastases in prostate cancer but is not widely available. MRI poorly defines intrarenal calcifications because they have few mobile protons.

Radionuclide scanning: Cortical tracers that bind to proximal tubular cells (eg, technetium-99m dimercaptosuccinic acid [^{99m}Tc DMSA]) are used to image the renal parenchyma; excretory tracers that are rapidly filtered and secreted into urine (eg, ^{99m}Tc diethylenetriamine pentaacetic acid [DTPA], ^{99m}Tc mercaptoacetyltriglycine-3 [MAG3]) are used to assess and quantify excretory function. Radionuclide scanning provides more information about segmental renal emboli, renal parenchymal scarring due to vesicoureteral reflux, functional significance of renal artery stenosis, and renal transplant function than does IVU or cross-sectional imaging. ^{99m}Tc pertechnetate can be used to image blood flow to the testes and to distinguish torsion from epididymitis in patients with acute testicular pain, although Doppler ultrasonography is used more commonly because it is quicker. No patient preparation is necessary, but patients should be asked about known allergies to the tracer.

PROCEDURES

Bladder catheterization: Bladder catheterization is used to obtain urine for examination, measure residual urine volume, relieve urinary retention or incontinence, deliver radiopaque contrast or drugs directly to the bladder, and irrigate the bladder. Catheters vary by caliber, tip configuration, number of ports, balloon size, type of material, and length.

Caliber is standardized in French (F) units—also known as Charrière (Ch) units. Each unit is 0.33 mm, so a 14-F catheter is 4.6 mm in diameter. Sizes range from 14 to 24 F for adults and 8 to 12 F for children. Smaller catheters are usually sufficient for uncomplicated urinary drainage and useful for urethral strictures and bladder neck obstruction; bigger catheters are indicated for bladder irrigation and some cases of hemorrhage (eg, postoperatively or in hemorrhagic cystitis) and pyuria, because clots could obstruct smaller caliber catheters.

Straight-tipped catheters (eg, Robinson, whistle-tip) can be used for intermittent urethral catheterization (ie, catheter is removed immediately after bladder drainage). Foley catheters have a straight tip and an inflatable balloon for self-retention. Other self-retaining catheters may have an expanded tip shaped like a mushroom (de Pezzer catheter) or a 4-winged perforated mushroom (Malecot catheter); they are used in suprapubic catheterization or nephrostomy. Elbowed (coudé) catheters, which may have balloons for self-retention, have a bent tip to ease catheterization through strictures or obstructions.

All catheters have ports for urinary drainage and may have ports for balloon inflation and irrigation (eg, 3-way Foley).

Balloons on self-retaining catheters have different volumes, from 2.5 to 5 mL in children's and 10 to 30 mL in adult's catheters. Larger balloons and catheters are generally used to manage bleeding; traction on the catheter pulls the balloon against the base of the bladder and puts pressure on vessels, while the larger caliber facilitates clearance of blood clots.

Choice of catheter material depends on use: plastic, latex, or polyvinyl chloride for intermittent use; or latex with silicone, hydrogel, or polymer (to diminish bacterial colonization) for continuous use. Silicone catheters are used in patients with latex allergy.

Stylets are flexible metal guides inserted through the catheter to give it stiffness and to facilitate insertion through strictures or obstructions.

Catheterization may be urethral or suprapubic. Urethral catheters can be inserted by any health care practitioner and sometimes by patients themselves. No patient preparation is necessary. Relative contraindications are urethral strictures and current UTI. After careful cleaning of the urethral meatus with an antibacterial solution, the catheter is lubricated with sterile gel and gently advanced through the urethra into the bladder.

Complications include urethral or bladder trauma with bleeding, creation of false passages, scarring and strictures, UTI, and bladder perforation.

Suprapubic catheterization via percutaneous cystostomy is performed by a urologist or other experienced physician. No patient preparation is necessary. Indications include drainage after urethral reconstruction or bladder surgery, repair after trauma, and long-term bladder drainage. Contraindications include prior lower abdominal surgery. After the abdomen above the pubic area is numbed with a local anesthetic, a spinal needle in inserted into the bladder. A catheter is then placed through a special trocar or over a guide wire threaded through the spinal needle. Complications include UTI, intestinal injury, and bleeding.

Cystoscopy: Cystoscopy is insertion of a rigid or flexible fiberoptic instrument into the bladder. It is used to help diagnose urologic disorders (eg, bladder tumors or calculi), to manage urethral strictures, and to access the bladder for ureteral x-rays or placement of JJ stents (stents with coiled ends placed in the renal pelvis and bladder). The main contraindication is active UTI. Cystoscopy is usually performed in an outpatient setting with local anesthesia or, when necessary, conscious sedation or general anesthesia. Prophylactic antibiotics are required. Complications include UTI, bleeding, and bladder and urethral trauma.

Biopsy: Biopsy requires a trained specialist (nephrologist, urologist, or interventional radiologist).

For renal biopsy, relative contraindications include bleeding diatheses, a solitary kidney, and an uncooperative patient. Mild preoperative sedation with opioids and atropine may be needed. Complications include severe renal bleeding requiring transfusion or even surgical intervention.

For bladder biopsy, contraindications include bleeding diathesis and acute tuberculous cystitis. Preoperative antibiotics are only necessary if active UTI is present. The biopsy instrument is inserted into the bladder through a cystoscope; rigid or flexible instruments can be used. The biopsy site is cauterized to prevent bleeding, and a drainage catheter is left in place to facilitate healing and drainage of clots. Complications include excessive bleeding, UTI, and bladder perforation.

For prostate biopsy, contraindications include bleeding diathesis, acute prostatitis, and UTIs. Patient preparation includes stopping maintenance aspirin a week before biopsy, preoperative antibiotics (usually a fluoroquinolone), and an enema to clear the rectum. With the patient in a lateral position, the prostate is located by palpation or ultrasonography. Overlying structures (perineum or rectum) are anesthetized, a spring-loaded biopsy needle is inserted into the prostate, and 6 to 12 tissue cores are obtained from various sites. Complications include urosepsis, hemorrhage, urinary retention, hematuria, and hematospermia (often for 3 to 6 mo after biopsy).

Urethral dilation: Urethral dilation is used to manage urethral strictures, urethral (urgency-frequency) syndrome, and meatal stenosis. In cases of stricture, a fine filiform probe is passed through, then followers (dilators) of progressively larger diameter are attached to the distal end of the filiform probe and passed behind the probe to dilate the stricture until urine stream becomes adequate; the procedure is usually performed over several sessions.

DYSURIA

Dysuria is painful or uncomfortable urination. It is an extremely common symptom in women (most commonly due to UTIs), but it can affect men, can occur at any age, and has many noninfectious causes (see TABLE 226–2).

Evaluation

History and physical examination: Localization of symptoms is often nonspecific but may help identify the site of infection or inflammation (eg, periurethral symptoms suggest urethritis or vaginitis; suprapubic symptoms suggest cystitis). History of frequent UTIs suggests recurrence. Vaginal discharge, dyspareunia, and use of douches or other topical agents suggests vaginosis, vulvovaginitis, or vestibulitis. Fever or flank pain suggests pyelonephritis. Back or joint pain or conjunctivitis suggests spondyloarthropathy.

Penile discharge suggests urethritis; scrotal tenderness or erythema suggests epididymitis; changes in prostate consistency and prostate tenderness suggest prostatitis. Atrophy or erythema of vaginal folds and vaginal discharge suggest vulvovaginitis.

Testing: No single testing protocol is correct. Many clinicians use antibiotics without any testing to treat dysuria in young, otherwise healthy women. An evaluation always begins with urinalysis. If a dipstick test of a portion of a clean-catch specimen detects WBCs, routine urine culture is indicated, although doing both tests simultaneously is common practice. A finding of > 1000 bacteria colony-forming units/mL suggests infection. WBCs in a sterile culture suggest sexually transmitted infection, vulvovaginosis, vulvovaginitis, prostatitis, TB, tumor, calculi, or interstitial nephritis. Any vaginal discharge warrants a wet mount, and cervical (women) and urethral (men) smear should be sent for gonococcus and chlamydia culture or PCR. If there is no response to empiric antibiotics and test results are negative, imaging of the urinary tract may be indicated to check for obstruction, calculi, cancer, or other abnormalities.

Treatment

Phenazopyridine 200 mg po tid can be used to relieve acute, intolerable dysuria in the 1st 24 to 48 h. The drug turns urine red-orange; patients should be cautioned not to confuse this effect with progression of infection or hematuria. Definitive treatment is directed at the cause; a short course of antibiotics is effective in most patients (see p. 1971).

TABLE 226–2. CAUSES OF DYSURIA

TYPE	EXAMPLES
Infectious*	Cervicitis Cystitis Epididymo-orchitis Prostatitis Urethritis Vulvovaginitis
Inflammatory	Spondyloarthropathies (reactive arthritis or Behçet's syndrome) Vestibulitis
Physical	Catheterization Obstruction of bladder neck (benign prostatic hyperplasia) or urethra (strictures)
Other	Hypoestrogenism Tumors

*Common pathogens include nonsexually transmitted bacteria (mostly *Escherichia coli*) and sexually transmitted pathogens (eg, *Neisseria gonorrhoeae*, *Chlamydia trachomatis*, *Ureaplasma urealyticum*, *Trichomonas vaginalis*, herpes simplex virus).

HEMATOSPERMIA

Hematospermia is blood in semen. It is often frightening to patients but is almost always benign. Most cases are idiopathic. The most common known cause is prostate biopsy; other causes include benign prostatic hyperplasia, infections, disorders of the seminal vesicles, and tumors. The relative frequency and importance of each cause is unknown.

Urinalysis is required to check for infection. Semen inspection is necessary only when travel history suggests possible exposure to *Schistosoma haematobium* or *S. mansoni*. If patients are at risk of sexually transmitted infections, urethral cultures are indicated for *Neisseria gonorrhoeae* infection, chlamydia, and trichomoniasis. Prostate-specific antigen testing in elderly patients at risk of prostate cancer is controversial.

Treatment is directed at the cause if known. For almost all men, reassurance that hematospermia is not a sign of cancer and does not affect sexual function is the only intervention necessary.

ISOLATED HEMATURIA

Hematuria is RBCs in urine; the urine may be red (macroscopic hematuria), bloody (gross hematuria), or not discolored (microscopic hematuria). Hematuria commonly occurs with other urine abnormalities (eg, proteinuria); isolated hematuria is urinary RBCs without other symptoms or urinary abnormalities. In people < 50, hematuria may be transient, resulting from exercise or sexual intercourse. Likely causes of persistent hematuria differ by age (see TABLE 226–3).

Evaluation

History and physical examination: Isolated hematuria may be obvious based on red or bloody urine or detected only by urinalysis and microscopy. History, especially age, and physical examination occasionally give clues to the cause. However, urine and blood tests are required, and imaging tests are often needed.

Testing: Hematuria detected by urine dipstick should be confirmed by microscopic

TABLE 226–3. CAUSES OF ISOLATED HEMATURIA

AGE (yr)	COMMON	UNCOMMON
0–15	Calculi and hypercalciuria Congenital anomalies with obstruction Contamination of urine specimen with menstrual blood Glomerulopathy, such as IgA nephropathy, hereditary nephritis (Alport's syndrome), thin basement membrane disease (benign familial hematuria), and acute poststreptococcal glomerulonephritis Sexual intercourse Sickle cell disease UTIs Viral infection	Factitious Fever Hemolytic-uremic syndrome Hemophilia Henoch-Schönlein purpura *Schistosoma haematobium* infection
15–50	Calculi and hypercalciuria Contamination of urine specimen with menstrual blood Exercise Papillary necrosis Polycystic kidney disease Sexual intercourse Sickle cell disease UTIs Viral infection	Arteriovenous malformations or fistulas Disseminated intravascular coagulation Factitious Fever Goodpasture's syndrome Loin pain–hematuria syndrome Medullary sponge kidney Renal infarction Renal vein thrombosis *Schistosoma haematobium* infection
> 50	Benign prostatic hyperplasia Cancer (renal, ureteral, bladder, or prostate) Overanticoagulation Polycystic kidney disease Prostatitis	Arteriovenous malformations or fistulas Cyclic hematuria in women Endometriosis of the urethra Factitious Loin pain–hematuria syndrome Renal vein thrombosis Thrombotic thrombocytopenic purpura Toxins, such as cantharidin or djenkol bean

examination; absence of RBCs suggests myoglobinuria or hemoglobinuria. In patients < 50 (including children), a 2nd negative dipstick implies transient hematuria and is usually sufficient to exclude serious causes unless patients have risk factors for renal calculi or bladder cancer (see p. 2047). If the 2nd dipstick is positive, a urine specimen should be sent for culture; positive culture warrants treatment with antibiotics. If hematuria resolves after treatment and no other symptoms are present, no further evaluation is required for patients < 50, especially women. When hematuria is confirmed microscopically and is of unknown origin, assessment of RBC morphology can help identify possible causes. RBCs of glomerular origin (dysmorphic, with spicules, folding, and blebs; nonglomerular RBCs retain their normal shape) should prompt evaluation and follow-up for intrinsic renal disorders; RBCs of nonglomerular origin suggest renal calculi or abnormalities of the GU tract, which should be evaluated by ultrasonography or CT with contrast. All patients ≥ 50 yr require cystoscopy, as do patients who are < 50 and who have risk factors for bladder cancer. If evaluation does not suggest a cause, men require prostate examination and possibly prostate-specific antigen testing to check for prostate disorders.

Collection of urine into 3 consecutive tubes is thought by some experts to distinguish urethral (in 1st tube) from bladder (in 3rd tube) sources of RBCs, but it is not a standard evaluation.

Treatment

Treatment involves treating the cause.

POLYURIA AND FREQUENCY

Polyuria is urine output of > 3 L/day; it must be distinguished from frequency, which is the need to urinate many times during the day or night but in normal or less than normal volumes. Either problem can include nocturia.

Etiology

Polyuria implies water or solute diuresis. Causes of water diuresis include central or nephrogenic diabetes insipidus, psychogenic polydipsia, and hypotonic IV infusions. Causes of solute diuresis include diabetes mellitus, IV saline infusions, high-protein tube feedings, relief of urinary tract obstruction, and Na-wasting nephropathy.

The most common causes of frequency include UTIs, urinary incontinence, benign prostatic hyperplasia (BPH), and urinary tract calculi.

Evaluation

History and physical examination: History can sometimes distinguish polyuria from frequency and suggest a cause. Polyuria caused by diabetes insipidus is suggested by a history of malignancy or chronic granulomatous disease (via hypercalcemia), use of certain drugs (lithium, cidofovir, foscarnet), and less common conditions (eg, sickle cell disease, renal amyloidosis, sarcoidosis, Sjögren's syndrome) whose manifestations are often more prominent than and precede the polyuria.

Abrupt onset of polyuria at a precise time suggests central diabetes insipidus (see p. 1189), as does preference for extremely cold or iced water. Polyuria caused by diuresis is suggested by a history of diuretic use or diabetes mellitus, and that caused by polydipsia is suggested by a history of psychiatric illness (bipolar disorder, schizophrenia). Dysuria suggests frequency from UTI or calculi; prior pelvic surgery suggests incontinence, and weak urinary stream suggests frequency caused by BPH.

Physical examination generally plays a limited role in the evaluation of polyuria and frequency.

Testing: Measures of urinary volume in 24 h distinguish polyuria (> 3 L/day) from frequency if the difference is not obvious by history alone; output > 5 L/day suggests central diabetes insipidus, lithium toxicity, or polydipsia. Urinalysis should be performed to detect UTI or glycosuria. Serum Na measurements can distinguish polydipsia (Na < 137 mEq/L) from diabetes insipidus (Na >142 mEq/L). Diagnosis of diabetes insipidus is made by completely restricting free water intake, then measuring urine volume and osmolarity, and serum Na and osmolarity (see pp. 1190 and 2025).

Treatment

Treatment varies by cause.

PROTEINURIA

Proteinuria is protein, usually albumin, in urine. In many renal disorders, it occurs with other urinary abnormalities (eg, hematuria). Isolated proteinuria is urinary protein without other symptoms or abnormalities. Causes may be categorized as glomerular, tubular, overflow, or physiologic (see TABLE 226–4). Exercise proteinuria, sometimes with hematuria, hemoglobinuria, or myoglobinuria, is proteinuria of unknown cause that may occur in runners, boxers, and other people engaged in vigorous exercise.

Proteinuria may be transient, orthostatic (occurring only when upright and almost always between adolescence and age 30), or persistent. Most patients with physiologic causes (and many with acute tubulointerstitial disorders) have transient proteinuria; those with transient or orthostatic proteinuria usually excrete < 1 g protein/day with no deterioration of renal function, and the proteinuria resolves spontaneously.

Evaluation

History and physical examination: High concentrations of protein cause frothy or sudsy urine; patients, especially men, occasionally report this symptom. But diagnosis of proteinuria requires urinalysis; it is most often detected incidentally. History and physical examination occasionally give clues to cause.

TABLE 226–4. CAUSES OF PROTEINURIA

TYPE	EFFECT	EXAMPLES
Glomerular	Increased permeability	Glomerular disorders (primary or secondary)
Tubular	Decreased reabsorption	Fanconi syndrome Tubulointerstitial or glomerular disorders
Overflow	Increased protein production	Acute monocytic leukemia with lysozymuria Monoclonal gammopathy Multiple myeloma Myelodysplastic syndromes
Physiologic	Increased renal hemodynamics	Acute illness Emotional stress Fever Intense activity

Testing: If urine dipstick assay detects proteinuria, it should be repeated 1 to 2 times; resolution suggests an initial false-positive result or a transient cause. Persistent proteinuria should be quantified with a 24-h urine collection, although calculation of a protein:creatinine ratio (see p. 1933) in a random sample may be sufficient. Nephrotic syndrome is defined as proteinuria > 3.5 g/day.

Microscopic analysis should be performed to detect casts, lipiduria, and other signs of glomerular disorders. Orthostatic proteinuria is diagnosed with a 24-h urine collection split between a 16-h upright daytime specimen (in which protein is present) and an 8-h recumbent nighttime specimen (in which protein should be < 50 mg).

Treatment

Treatment is directed at the cause.

SCROTAL MASS

A scrotal mass should trigger suspicion for testicular cancer (see p. 2057) in young men, but it has many noncancerous causes (see p. 2041), including testicular torsion, epididymo-orchitis, hydrocele, inguinal hernia, varicocele, hematoma following vasectomy, and spermatocele. Diagnosis is often obvious from examination. Diagnostic testing should include ultrasonography if examination cannot clearly distinguish solid from cystic masses; and β-human chorionic gonadotropin (hCG), and α-fetoprotein if the mass is solid and testicular cancer is suspected. Treatment is usually surgical regardless of cause, although varicoceles are harmless and require no intervention.

SCROTAL PAIN

Medical emergencies that cause scrotal pain include testicular torsion, incarcerated hernia, appendicitis, trauma, and referred pain from ruptured abdominal aortic aneurysms or acute aortic dissection (rare). Other causes include appendiceal torsion, epididymo-orchitis, testicular tumor, hydrocele, varicocele, prostatitis, vasculitis (eg, Henoch-Schönlein purpura, polyarteritis nodosa), and referred pain from ureteral calculi.

Evaluation

History and physical examination: The focus is to distinguish emergency from other causes. Aortic catastrophes occur in older patients (> 50 yr); the other emergency conditions can occur at any age. Severe, instantaneous onset pain suggests torsion; pain with incarcerated hernia or appendicitis is more gradual. Tenderness localized to the upper testicular pole suggests appendiceal torsion. Bilateral pain suggests infection or a referred cause. An inguinal mass suggests hernia; scrotal mass is nonspecific. A normal scrotal examination suggests referred pain. Relief of pain with testicular elevation suggests epididymo-orchitis.

Testing: Urinalysis is always required. Findings of UTI suggest epididymitis. If the etiology of acute testicular pain is equivocal, color Doppler ultrasonography is generally performed to rule out testicular torsion. If Doppler ultrasonography is not available, radionuclide scanning may be useful but is less sensitive and specific.

Treatment

Analgesics are indicated for control of acute pain; morphine or other opioids may be indicated for conditions requiring surgical treatment. Definitive treatment is directed at the cause.

227 MALE REPRODUCTIVE ENDOCRINOLOGY

Male sexual development and function depend on a complex feedback circuit involving the hypothalamus, pituitary, and testes. Male sexual dysfunction can be secondary to hypogonadism or numerous other disorders.

Physiology

The hypothalamus produces gonadotropin-releasing hormone (GnRH), which is released in a pulsatile fashion q 60 to 120 min. The anterior pituitary responds to each pulse of GnRH by producing a corresponding pulse of luteinizing hormone (LH) and, to a lesser degree, follicle-stimulating hormone (FSH). Continuous stimulation by GnRH (as might occur therapeutically) suppresses pituitary release of LH and FSH.

The Leydig cells of the testes respond to LH by producing between 5 and 10 mg of testosterone daily. Testosterone levels are highest in early morning, except in older men, who may lose circadian variation.

Testosterone is synthesized from cholesterol through several intermediate compounds, including dehydroepiandrosterone (DHEA) and androstenedione. Circulating testosterone is mostly protein-bound, about 40% to sex hormone–binding globulin (SHBG) and 58% to albumin. Because testosterone is avidly bound to SHBG, only albumin-bound testosterone (which is less avidly bound) and the 1 to 2% that constitute free testosterone are bioavailable.

About 4 to 8% of testosterone is converted to a more potent metabolite, dihydrotestosterone (DHT), by the enzyme 5α-reductase in target tissues. DHT has important trophic effects in the prostate and mediates androgenic alopecia. In adults, spermatogenesis requires adequate intratesticular testosterone, but the role of DHT in spermatogenesis is controversial.

Testosterone and DHT also have metabolic effects, including increasing protein anabolism and nitrogen retention, increasing bone density and muscle mass, and modulating the immune system. Testosterone undergoes conversion to estradiol; estrogen mediates much of the effect of testosterone on organs such as bone and the brain.

Testosterone, DHT, and estradiol provide negative feedback on the hypothalamic-pituitary axis. In males, estradiol is the main inhibitor of LH production, whereas both estradiol and inhibin B, a peptide produced by Sertoli cells of the testes, inhibit production of FSH. In the presence of testosterone, FSH stimulates the Sertoli cells and induces spermatogenesis. In spermatogenesis, each germinal cell (spermatogonium), located adjacent to the Sertoli cells, undergoes differentiation into 16 primary spermatocytes, each of which generates 4 spermatids. Each spermatid matures into a spermatozoon. Spermatogenesis takes 72 to 74 days and yields about 100 million new spermatozoa each day. Upon maturation, spermatozoa are released into the rete testis, where they migrate to the epididymis and eventually to the vas deferens. Migration requires an additional 14 days. Before ejaculation, spermatozoa are mixed with secretions from the seminal vesicles, prostate, and bulbourethral glands.

Sexual Differentiation, Adrenarche, and Puberty

In the embryo, the presence of a Y chromosome triggers development and growth of the testes, which begin secreting testosterone and a müllerian-duct inhibitor by about 7 wk of gestation. Testosterone virilizes the wolffian duct (which develops into the epididymis, vas deferens, and seminal vesicles).

DHT promotes development of the remainder of the male genitals. Testosterone levels peak in the 2nd trimester and fall to almost zero by birth. Testosterone production rises briefly during the first 6 mo of life, the function of which is unclear. Thereafter, testosterone levels remain low until puberty.

LH and FSH are elevated at birth but fall to low levels within a few months, remaining low or undetectable throughout the prepubertal years. Through an unknown mechanism, blood levels of the adrenal androgens DHEA and DHEA sulfate begin to increase several years before puberty. Their conversion to testosterone in small amounts initiates pubic and axillary hair growth (adrenarche).

The mechanisms that initiate puberty are unclear, although early in puberty the hypothalamus becomes less sensitive to the inhibitory effects of sex hormones. This increases secretion of LH and FSH, stimulating testosterone production. Secretion of LH and FSH increases initially only during sleep; later, secretion increases throughout the 24-h period. LH increases more than FSH. The increased testosterone levels in boys cause pubertal changes, the first of which are growth of the testes (> 2.5 cm on the long axis, > 3 to 4 mL in volume) and thinning of scrotal skin. Later, penile length, muscle mass, and bone density increase; the voice deepens; and pubic and axillary hair becomes denser and thicker.

Effects of Aging

Both hypothalamic secretion of GnRH and the response of Leydig cells to FSH and LH diminish with aging. Beginning at about age 30, a man's serum total testosterone level declines by 1%/yr. Men aged 70 to 80 tend to have serum testosterone levels that are about $\frac{1}{2}$ to $\frac{2}{3}$ of those of men in their 20s. In addition, SHBG levels increase with aging, causing an even greater decline in serum free and bioavailable testosterone. FSH and LH levels tend to be normal or high-normal. This change is sometimes referred to as the andropause, although there is no abrupt change in hormone levels as occurs in the menopause. The decline in testosterone may contribute to age-related muscle loss, osteopenia, loss of libido, and cognitive decline. Supplementation for men with low-normal levels of testosterone is controversial. Some experts recommend a trial of testosterone supplementation in older men with symptoms or signs of hypogonadism and whose serum testosterone levels are below the lower limit of normal for men aged 20 to 40 yr. No data favor any of the testosterone preparations specifically for use in older men.

MALE HYPOGONADISM

(See also Male Hypogonadism in Children on p. 2367.)

Hypogonadism is defined as testosterone deficiency with associated symptoms or signs, deficiency of spermatozoa production, or both. It may result from a disorder of the testes (primary hypogonadism) or of the hypothalamic-pituitary axis (secondary hypogonadism). Both may be congenital or acquired as the result of aging, disease, drugs, or other factors. Additionally, a number of congenital enzyme deficiencies cause varying degrees of target organ androgen resistance. Diagnosis is confirmed by hormone levels. Treatment varies with etiology but typically includes testosterone replacement.

Etiology

Primary hypogonadism involves failure of the testes to respond to follicle-stimulating hormone (FSH) and luteinizing hormone (LH). When primary hypogonadism affects testosterone production, testosterone is insufficient to inhibit production of FSH and LH; hence, FSH and LH levels are elevated. The most common cause of primary hypogonadism is Klinefelter's syndrome. It involves seminiferous tubule dysgenesis and a 47,XXY karyotype (see p. 2454).

Secondary hypogonadism is failure of the hypothalamus (or pituitary) to produce enough FSH and LH. With secondary hypogonadism, testosterone levels are low, but levels of FSH and LH are low or inappropriately normal. Any acute systemic illness can cause temporary secondary hypogonadism. Some syndromes of hypogonadism have both primary and secondary causes (mixed hypogonadism). TABLE 227–1 lists some common causes of hypogonadism by category.

Some syndromes of hypogonadism (eg, cryptorchidism, some systemic disorders) affect spermatozoon production more than testosterone levels.

Symptoms and Signs

Age at onset of testosterone deficiency dictates the clinical presentation: congenital, childhood-onset, and adult-onset hypogonadism. Congenital hypogonadism may be of 1st-, 2nd-, or 3rd-trimester onset.

TABLE 227–1. CAUSES OF HYPOGONADISM*

TYPE	CONGENITAL CAUSES	ACQUIRED CAUSES
Primary (testicular)	Klinefelter's syndrome Anorchia (bilateral) Cryptorchidism Myotonic dystrophy Enzymatic defects in testosterone synthesis Leydig cell aplasia Noonan syndrome	Chemotherapy/radiation therapy Testicular infection (mumps, echovirus, group B arbovirus) High doses of certain drugs (eg, cimetidine, spironolactone, ketoconazole, flutamide, cyproterone)
Secondary (hypothalamic-pituitary)	Kallmann syndrome Prader-Willi syndrome Dandy-Walker malformation Isolated luteinizing hormone deficiency Idiopathic	Any acute systemic illness Hypopituitarism (tumor, infarction, infiltrative disease, infection, trauma, radiation-induced) Hyperprolactinemia Iron overload (hemochromatosis) Certain drugs (eg, estrogens, psychotropics, metoclopramide, opioids, leuprolide) Cushing's syndrome Cirrhosis Morbid obesity Idiopathic
Mixed		Aging Alcoholism Systemic disease (uremia, liver failure, AIDS, sickle cell disease) Drugs (ethanol, corticosteroids)

* In approximate order of frequency.

First-trimester onset results in inadequate male sexual differentiation. Complete absence of testosterone effect results in normal-appearing female external genitals. Partial testosterone deficiency results in abnormalities ranging from ambiguous external genitals to hypospadias. Second- or 3rd-trimester onset of testosterone deficiency results in microphallus and undescended testes.

Childhood-onset testosterone deficiency (see p. 2367) has few consequences and usually is unrecognized until puberty is delayed. Untreated hypogonadism impairs development of secondary sexual characteristics. As adults, affected patients have poor muscle development, a high-pitched voice, a small scrotum, decreased phallic and testicular growth, sparse pubic and axillary hair, and an absence of body hair. They may develop gynecomastia and eunuchoidal body proportions (span > height by 5 cm and pubic to floor length > crown to pubic length by > 5 cm) because of delayed fusion of the epiphyses and continued long bone growth.

Adult-onset testosterone deficiency has varied manifestations depending on the degree and duration of the deficiency. Decreased libido; erectile dysfunction; decline in cognitive skills, such as visual-spatial interpretation; sleep disturbances; and mood changes, such as depression and anger, are common. Decreased lean body mass, increased visceral fat, testicular atrophy, osteopenia, gynecomastia, and sparse body hair typically take months to years to develop.

Diagnosis

Congenital and childhood-onset hypogonadism are often suspected because of delayed puberty or developmental abnormalities.

Adult-onset hypogonadism should be suspected by symptoms or signs but is easily missed because these are insensitive and nonspecific. Klinefelter's syndrome should be considered in adolescent males, young men with hypogonadism, and all adult men with very small testes. Hypogonadism requires confirmatory testing.

Diagnosis of primary and secondary hypogonadism: Increases in FSH and LH are more sensitive for primary hypogonadism than are decreases in testosterone levels. Levels of FSH and LH also help determine whether hypogonadism is primary or secondary; high gonadotropin levels, even with low-normal testosterone levels, indicate primary hypogonadism, whereas gonadotropin levels that are low or lower than expected for the level of testosterone indicate secondary hypogonadism. Alternatively, in boys of short stature with delayed puberty, low testosterone plus low gonadotropin levels might result from constitutional delay. Elevation of serum FSH with normal levels of serum testosterone and LH often occurs when spermatogenesis is impaired but testosterone production is normal. Primary hypogonadism requires no further evaluation, although some clinicians perform a karyotype to definitively diagnose Klinefelter's syndrome.

Total (or calculated free and weakly bound) serum testosterone, serum FSH, and serum LH levels are measured simultaneously. The normal range for total testosterone is 300 to 1200 ng/dL (10.5 to 41.5 nmol/L). The initial screening testosterone level may be done at any time of day, but a second testosterone level should be drawn in the morning to confirm hypogonadism. Because of the increase in sex hormone–binding globulin (SHBG) with aging, total testosterone is a poor measure of hypogonadism after age 50. Although serum free testosterone more accurately reflects functional testosterone levels, its measurement requires equilibrium dialysis, which is technically difficult and not widely available. Some commercially available kits, including the analog free testosterone assay, attempt to measure serum free testosterone levels, but the results are often inaccurate, particularly in conditions such as type 2 diabetes, obesity, and hypothyroidism that alter SHBG levels. Free testosterone levels can be calculated based on SHBG, albumin, and testosterone values using a calculator available at www.issam.ch. Because of the pulsatile secretion of FSH and LH, they are sometimes measured as a pooled sample of 3 venipunctures taken at 20-min intervals. Serum FSH and LH levels are usually < 5 mIU/mL before puberty and between 5 and 15 mIU/mL in adulthood.

Sperm count can be useful and should be assessed in men who are seeking fertility treatment. In adolescents or adults, a semen sample collected by masturbation after 2 days of abstinence from ejaculation provides an excellent index of seminiferous tubular function. A normal semen sample has a volume of > 2.5 mL with > 20 million sperm/mL, of which 60% are of normal morphology and are motile (see also Sperm Disorders on p. 2138).

Evaluation of secondary hypogonadism: Because any systemic illness, which may be unrecognized, can temporarily decrease levels of testosterone, FSH, and LH, secondary hypogonadism should be confirmed by measuring these levels again after a 6-wk interval. To confirm secondary hypogonadism in adolescents, the gonadotropin-releasing hormone (GnRH) test is sometimes performed. If, in response to IV GnRH, levels of FSH and LH increase, puberty is simply delayed. If levels do not increase, true hypogonadism is likely.

To help determine the cause of confirmed secondary hypogonadism, testing should include serum prolactin level and screening tests for hemochromatosis (serum iron and transferrin—see p. 1132). If serum prolactin is elevated (suggesting a possible pituitary mass), hemochromatosis is excluded, or testosterone levels are < 200 ng/dL, CT or MRI is obtained to rule out a pituitary adenoma or other mass. Also, if there are symptoms or signs of Cushing's syndrome, 24-h urine collection for free cortisol or a dexamethasone suppression test is obtained (see p. 1212).

Treatment

Treatment of hypogonadism is directed toward providing adequate androgen replacement conveniently and safely. Although patients with primary hypogonadism will not become fertile with any endocrine therapy, patients with secondary hypogonadism often become fertile with gonadotropin therapy.

Testosterone therapy: Males who have no signs of puberty and are near age 15 may be given long-acting testosterone enanthate 50 mg IM once/mo for 4 to 8 mo. These low doses should cause some virilization and induce puberty without restricting adult height.

Older adolescents with testosterone deficiency receive long-acting testosterone enanthate or cypionate at a dose that is increased gradually over 18 to 24 mo from 50 to up to 200 mg IM q 1 to 3 wk. Transcutaneous gel may also be used, although it is more expensive and more difficult to titrate. It is reasonable to convert older adolescents to testosterone gel 1% at adult dosages when their IM dosage has been titrated up to the equivalent of 100 to 200 mg q 2 wk.

Adults with established testosterone deficiency may benefit from replacement therapy. Treatment prevents or attenuates osteopenia, muscle loss, vasomotor instability, loss of libido, and occasionally erectile dysfunction. Replacement therapy is possible with testosterone gel 1% (5 to 10 g daily to deliver 5 to 10 mg daily), IM testosterone (100 mg q 7 days or 200 mg q 10 to 14 days), or transdermal testosterone patches (5 to 6 mg daily). Testosterone gel maintains physiologic blood levels more consistently than other treatments, but IM or patch systems are sometimes used because of their lower cost.

Potential adverse effects of testosterone and its analogs include erythrocytosis (particularly in men > 50 yr receiving IM testosterone), acne, gynecomastia, and very rarely prostatic enlargement or edema. Treatment may enhance growth of an existing prostate carcinoma but probably does not cause prostate cancer. Injectable or transdermal forms of testosterone are preferable to most oral formulations, which, except for testosterone undecanoate, carry a significant risk of hepatocellular dysfunction and hepatic adenoma.

Hct should be checked q 6 to 12 mo, and digital rectal examination and serum prostate-specific antigen (PSA) testing should be offered annually in men > 50. If Hct is ≥ 54%, the testosterone dose should be reduced by $\frac{1}{4}$ or $\frac{1}{3}$. With testosterone replacement, PSA levels increase to age-adjusted normal ranges. The increase is usually only 10 to 30% but may reach 100% without evidence of prostate cancer.

Treatment of infertility due to hypogonadism: Infertility, which has many possible causes other than hypogonadism, is discussed in full on p. 2138. Infertility due to primary hypogonadism does not respond to hormonal therapy. Men with primary hypogonadism occasionally have a few intratesticular sperm that can be harvested with various microsurgical techniques and used to fertilize an egg by an assisted reproductive technique (eg, intracytoplasmic injection).

Infertility due to secondary hypogonadism usually responds to gonadotropin replacement therapy. Other symptoms of secondary hypogonadism respond well to testosterone replacement therapy alone. If secondary hypogonadism results from pituitary disease, gonadotropin replacement therapy usually is successful. Therapy begins with LH replacement. After all exogenous androgens are stopped, LH replacement is generally initiated at a low dosage (375 to 750 IU) and increased if necessary to high-dosage (1000 to 2000 IU) human chorionic gonadotropin (hCG) sc 2 to 3 times/wk. The dose is adjusted after 3 mo to achieve normal serum testosterone. Sperm counts are performed monthly, but counts are not expected to increase for at least 4 mo. FSH replacement, which is expensive, begins if 6 to 12 mo of LH replacement does not stimulate spermatogenesis. FSH replacement uses human menotropic gonadotropin or human recombinant FSH, beginning with 75 to 150 IU 3 times/wk. The dose may be doubled if conception has not occurred within 6 mo of combination therapy with hCG. Many men become fertile with treatment despite sperm counts that do not usually result in fertility (eg, < 5 million/mL).

Secondary hypogonadism due to a hypothalamic defect (eg, Kallmann syndrome) is treated initially with LH and FSH because of their ready availability; if these are ineffective, GnRH replacement therapy (q 2 h sc by a programmable minipump) might be more effective. Most (80 to 90%) of men respond successfully to these regimens.

MALE SEXUAL DYSFUNCTION

Male sexual dysfunction is a problem with 1 of the 4 main components of male sexual function (libido, erection, ejaculation, orgasm) that interferes with interest in or ability to engage in sexual relations. Many drugs and numerous physical and psychologic disorders affect sexual function.

Libido: Libido is the cognitive component of sexual function. Decreased libido manifests as a lack of sexual interest or a decrease in the frequency and intensity of sexual thoughts, either spontaneous or in response to erotic stimuli. Libido is sensitive to testosterone levels as well as to general nutrition, health, and drugs. Conditions particularly likely to decrease libido include hypogonadism (see p. 1944), uremia, and depression. Drugs that sometimes decrease libido include weak androgen receptor antagonists, such as spironolactone or cimetidine, and virtually all drugs that are active in the CNS, such as SSRIs, tricyclic antidepressants, and antipsychotics. Loss of libido due to SSRIs or tricyclic antidepressants may be partly reversible with the addition of bupropion or trazodone.

Erection: Erection occurs as the result of a complex neuropsychologic process. Higher cortical input and a sacrally mediated parasympathetic reflex arc combine to stimulate erection. Nerve output travels through the pudendal nerves, which traverse the posterolateral aspect of the prostate. Terminating in the penis, these nonadrenergic/noncholinergic nerves activate nitric oxide synthase, producing nitric oxide, which relaxes smooth muscle lining the sinusoidal spaces that connect the arterioles and venules within the corpus cavernosa. The blood flow within the sinusoids increases markedly, distending them and compressing the venules, causing veno-occlusion. The increased inflow and veno-occlusion together produce penile rigidity. Many factors affect the ability to have an erection (see below).

Ejaculation and orgasm: Ejaculation is controlled by the sympathetic nervous system. α-Adrenergic stimulation produces contractions of the epididymis, vas deferens, prostate, and muscles of the pelvic floor. In addition, the neck of the bladder closes, preventing retrograde ejaculation of semen into the bladder. SSRIs may delay or inhibit ejaculation.

Orgasm is the highly pleasurable sensation that occurs in the brain generally simultaneously with ejaculation. Anorgasmia may be a physical phenomenon due to decreased penile sensation (eg, from neuropathy).

Ejaculatory insufficiency is reduced or absent semen volume that may result from retrograde ejaculation or interruption of sympathetic stimulation. Retrograde ejaculation (prostatic fluid flowing backward into the bladder) is common in diabetics and can also be caused by surgery on the neck of the bladder or transurethral resection of the prostate. Sympathetic interruption, either from surgery or with drugs (eg, guanethidine, phentolamine, phenoxybenzamine, thioridazine), diminishes ejaculatory volume.

Premature ejaculation is ejaculation occurring sooner than desired by the man or his partner. It is usually caused by sexual inexperience, anxiety, and other psychologic factors instead of disease. It can be treated successfully with sex therapy and SSRIs.

Erectile Dysfunction

(Impotence)

Erectile dysfunction is the inability to attain or sustain an erection satisfactory for sexual intercourse. Most erectile dysfunction is related to vascular, neurologic, and hormonal disorders; drug use and sometimes psychologic disorders are also causes. Evaluation typically includes screening for underlying diseases and measuring testosterone levels. Treatment options include oral phosphodiesterase inhibitors or apomorphine, intraurethral or intracavernosal prostaglandins, mechanical pump devices, and surgical implants.

The term impotence has been replaced by the term erectile dysfunction (ED). In the US, at least 10 to 20 million men > 18 are affected. The prevalence is about 50% in men 40 to 70 and increases with aging. However, many men can be successfully treated.

Etiology

Primary ED (ie, the man has never been able to attain or sustain erections) is rare and is almost always due to psychologic factors (guilt, fear of intimacy, depression, severe anxiety) or clinically obvious anatomic abnormalities. Most often, ED is secondary (ie, a man who previously could attain and sustain erections no longer can). Over 80% of secondary ED cases have an organic etiology. However, in many men with organic disease, ED leads to secondary psychologic difficulties that compound the problem. Psychologic factors must be considered in every case.

Psychologic causes may relate to performance anxiety, stress, or mood disorder (particularly depression). ED may be situational, involving a particular place, time, or partner.

The major organic causes of ED are vascular and neurologic disorders, often stemming from atherosclerosis and diabetes. Complications of surgery, usually prostate surgery, are another common cause. Other causes include hormonal disorders, drugs, and structural disorders of the penis (eg, Peyronie's disease).

The most common vascular cause is atherosclerosis of penile arteries, often secondary to diabetes. Atherosclerosis and aging decrease the capacity for dilation of arterial blood vessels and smooth muscle relaxation, limiting the amount of blood that can enter the penis. Inadequate impedance of venous outflow (venous leaks) may cause ED or, more commonly, failure to maintain tumescence as long as desired. Venous leaks make it difficult for blood to remain in the penis during erection, so erections occur but cannot be sustained. Priapism, particularly as in sickle cell disease, may damage penile vasculature and lead to ED.

Stroke, partial complex seizures, multiple sclerosis, peripheral and autonomic neuropathies, and spinal cord injuries are among the neurologic causes. Diabetic neuropathy and surgical injury are particularly common causes.

Any endocrinopathy associated with testosterone deficiency (hypogonadism) may decrease libido and cause ED. However, erectile function only rarely improves with normalization of serum testosterone levels.

Numerous drug causes are possible (see TABLE 227–2). Alcohol can cause temporary ED.

Of men who have undergone transurethral resection of the prostate, 15 to 40% experience problems with erections because of disruption of the pudendal nerve. ED is more common after more extensive prostatic resection. Prolonged perineal pressure (as occurs during bicycle riding) can cause temporary ED.

Diagnosis

Evaluation should include history of drug and alcohol use, smoking, diabetes, hypertension, and atherosclerosis; symptoms of vascular, hormonal, neurologic, and psychologic disorders. It is vital to screen for depression, which may not always be apparent. The Beck Depression Scale or the Yesavage Geriatric Depression Scale in older men is easy to administer and may be useful. Satisfaction with sexual relationships should also be explored. Partner sexual dysfunction (eg, atrophic vaginitis, depression) must be considered and evaluated.

Examination is focused on the genitals and extragenital signs of hormonal, neurologic, and vascular disorders. Genitals are examined for anomalies, signs of hypogonadism, and fibrous bands or plaques (Peyronie's disease). Poor rectal tone, perineal sensation, or abnormal anal wink or bulbocavernosus reflexes may indicate neurologic dysfunction.

TABLE 227–2. COMMONLY USED DRUGS THAT CAN CAUSE ERECTILE DYSFUNCTION

CLASS	DRUGS
Antihypertensives	Clonidine, thiazides, probably loop diuretics, spironolactone, β-blockers
CNS drugs	Monoamine oxidase inhibitors, SSRIs, tricyclics, anxiolytics, alcohol, opioids, cocaine
Other	Anticholinergics, estrogens, cimetidine, antimetabolites, anticancer drugs, amphetamines

Diminished peripheral pulses suggest vascular dysfunction.

A psychologic cause should be suspected in young healthy men with abrupt onset of ED, particularly if onset is associated with a specific emotional event or if the dysfunction occurs only in certain settings. A history of ED with spontaneous improvement also suggests psychologic origin (psychogenic ED). Men with psychogenic ED usually have normal nocturnal erections and erections upon awakening, whereas men with organic ED often do not.

Laboratory assessment should always include measurement of testosterone level; if the level is low or low-normal, follicle-stimulating hormone (FSH) and luteinizing hormone (LH) should be measured (see p. 1946). Evaluation for occult diabetes, dyslipidemias, hyperprolactinemia, thyroid disease, and Cushing's syndrome should be performed based on clinical suspicion.

A penile pressure–brachial pressure index (systolic BP in the penis divided by systolic BP in the arm) < 0.6 indicates impaired blood flow to the penis, but this test is seldom performed in general clinical practice.

Treatment

Underlying organic disorders require appropriate treatment. Drugs that are temporally related to onset of ED should be stopped or switched. Depression may require treatment. For all patients, reassurance and education (including of the patient's partner whenever possible) are important.

For further therapy, noninvasive methods (mechanical devices and drugs) are tried first. Men who can develop but not sustain an erection may use a constriction ring. As soon as erection occurs, a metal or elastic ring or a leather band with snaps (sold by prescription in pharmacies or OTC in sex paraphernalia stores as a "cock ring") is placed around the base of the penis, preventing venous outflow. If the man cannot develop an erection, a vacuum device can draw blood into the penis, after which the band or ring is placed at the base of the penis to retain the erection. Bruising of the penis, coldness of the tip of the penis, and lack of spontaneity are some drawbacks to this modality. A constriction ring and vacuum devices might also be useful adjuncts for patients who do not respond satisfactorily to drug therapy.

Virtually all patients prefer drug therapy for ED. The primary drugs for ED are oral phosphodiesterase inhibitors, oral apomorphine (not available in the US), and intracavernosal or intraurethral prostaglandins.

Oral selective inhibitors of cyclic guanosine monophosphate (cGMP)-specific phosphodiesterase type 5 (PDE5), the predominant phosphodiesterase isoform in the penis, include sildenafil, vardenafil, and tadalafil. By increasing cGMP, these drugs enhance the nitric oxide release essential for normal erection. Vardenafil and tadalafil are more selective for the penile vasculature (and therefore may have fewer adverse effects) than sildenafil. Although there are no head-to-head comparison clinical trials, all 3 drugs appear to be equally effective (60 to 75%). Sildenafil is taken 1 to 4 h before sexual intercourse. The dose is 50 mg, although most men respond best to 100 mg. Tadalafil has a significantly longer half-life than sildenafil, which might lead to more convenient dosing. The usual dosage for tadalafil and vardenafil is 10 to 20 mg 1 h before sex, not more often than daily. The maximal dosage is usually 20 mg. All PDE5 inhibitors cause direct coronary vasodilation and potentiate the hypotensive effects of other nitrates, including those used to treat cardiovascular disease as well as recreational amyl nitrate ("poppers"). Thus, all nitrates are contraindicated for 24 h after the administration of any PDE5 inhibitor. Other adverse effects of PDE5 inhibitors include flushing, visual abnormalities, and headache. Vardenafil should not be administered with α-blockers, such as prazosin, doxazosin, and tamsulosin, because of the risk of prolonged hypotension. One study showed that sildenafil may be safely administered with doxazosin.

Apomorphine increases erectile neurogenic signals by CNS mechanisms. It appears to be only moderately effective and can cause nausea, somnolence, and hypotension.

Intraurethral insertion or intracavernosal injection of the prostaglandin alprostadil (PGE_1) can produce erections with a mean duration of about 60 min. It causes priapism in ≤ 1% (see p. 2039) and penile pain in about 10%. The intracavernosal dose is adjusted by the physician to minimize priapism; the patient can then self-inject at home. Priapism is less common with intraurethral therapy, but intraurethral therapy is much less effective than intracavernosal injection, the most effective pharmacotherapy for erectile dysfunction (80 to 90%). Combination therapy with a PDE5 inhibitor and alprostadil may be useful for some patients who fail to respond to oral PDE5 inhibitors alone.

For patients who do not respond to drug therapy, invasive treatment options include implantation of a penile prosthesis. Prostheses can be rigid plastic rods or hydraulically operated devices. Both involve the risks of general anesthesia, infection, and prosthetic malfunction.

228 VOIDING DISORDERS

Voiding disorders affect urine storage or release; both are controlled by the same neural and urinary tract mechanisms. The result is incontinence or retention.

For normal urinary function, the autonomic and voluntary nervous systems must be intact, and muscles of the urinary tract must be functional. Normally, bladder filling stimulates stretch receptors in the bladder wall to send impulses via spinal nerves S2 to S4 to the spinal cord, then to the sensory cortex, where the need to void is perceived. A threshold volume, which differs from person to person, triggers awareness of the need to void. However, the external urinary sphincter at the bladder outlet is under voluntary control and usually remains contracted until a person decides to urinate. The micturition inhibitory center in the frontal lobe also helps control urination. When the decision is made, voluntary signals in the motor cortex initiate urination. These impulses are transmitted to the pontine micturition center, which coordinates simultaneous signals to contract detrusor smooth muscle throughout the bladder (via parasympathetic cholinergic nerve fibers) and to relax the internal sphincter (via alpha sympathetic nerve fibers) and striated muscle of the external sphincter and pelvic floor. In addition to normal urinary function, continence requires normal cognitive function (including motivation), mobility, access to a toilet, and manual dexterity.

Damage to or dysfunction of any of the components involved in urinary function can cause urinary incontinence or retention.

URINARY INCONTINENCE

Urinary incontinence is involuntary loss of urine; some experts consider it present only when a patient thinks it a problem. The disorder is greatly underrecognized and underreported; the common estimate of 13 million people affected in the US is low. Incontinence can occur at any age but is more common among the elderly and among women, affecting about 30% of elderly women and 15% of elderly men.

Incontinence greatly reduces quality of life by causing embarrassment, stigmatization, isolation, and depression. Many elderly patients are institutionalized because incontinence is a burden to caregivers. In bedbound patients, urine irritates and macerates skin, contributing to sacral pressure ulcer formation. Elderly people with urgency are at increased risk of falls and fractures.

Types: Incontinence may manifest as near-constant dribbling or as intermittent voiding with or without awareness of the need to void. Some patients have extreme urgency (irrepressible need to void) with little or no warning and may be unable to inhibit voiding until reaching a bathroom. Incontinence may occur or worsen with maneuvers that increase intra-abdominal pressure. Postvoid dribbling is extremely common and probably a normal variant in men. Identifying the clinical pattern is sometimes useful, but causes often overlap and much of treatment is the same.

Urge incontinence is an urgent, irrepressible need to void that occurs just before uncontrolled urine leakage (of moderate to large volume); nocturia and nocturnal incontinence are common. Urge incontinence is the most common type of incontinence in the elderly but may affect younger people. It is often precipitated by use of a diuretic and is exacerbated by inability to quickly reach a bathroom.

Stress incontinence is urine leakage due to abrupt increases in intra-abdominal pressure (eg, with coughing, sneezing, laughing, bending, or lifting). Leakage volume is usually low to moderate. It is the 2nd most common type of incontinence in women, largely because of complications of childbirth and development of atrophic urethritis. Stress incontinence is typically more severe in obese people because of pressure from abdominal contents on the top of the bladder.

Overflow incontinence is dribbling of urine from an overly full bladder. Volume is usually small, but leaks may be constant, resulting in large total losses. Overflow incontinence is the 2nd most common type of incontinence in men.

Functional incontinence is urine loss due to cognitive or physical impairments (eg, due to dementia or stroke) or environmental barriers that interfere with control of voiding. Neural and urinary tract mechanisms that maintain continence may be normal.

Mixed incontinence is any combination of the above types. The most common combinations are urge with stress incontinence and urge or stress with functional incontinence.

Pathophysiology and Etiology

The disorder tends to differ among age groups. With age, bladder capacity decreases, ability to inhibit urination declines, involuntary bladder contractions (detrusor overactivity) occur more often, and bladder contractility is impaired. Thus, voiding becomes more difficult to postpone and tends to be incomplete. Postvoid residual volume increases, probably to ≤ 100 mL (normal < 50 mL). Endopelvic fascia weakens. In postmenopausal women, decreased estrogen levels lead to atrophic urethritis and to decreasing urethral resistance, length, and maximum closure pressure. In men, prostate size increases, partially obstructing the urethra and leading to incomplete bladder emptying and strain on the detrusor muscle. These changes occur in many normal, continent elderly people and may facilitate incontinence but do not cause it.

In younger patients, incontinence often begins suddenly, may cause little leakage, and usually resolves quickly with little or no treatment. Often, incontinence has one cause in younger patients but has several in the elderly.

Conceptually, categorization into reversible (transient) or established causes may be useful. However, causes and mechanisms often overlap and occur in combination.

Transient incontinence: A useful mnemonic for many reversible causes is DIAPPERS (with an extra P): *D*elirium, *I*nfection (commonly, symptomatic UTIs), *A*trophic urethritis and vaginitis, *P*harmaceuticals (eg, those with α-adrenergic, cholinergic, or anticholinergic properties; diuretics; sedatives), *P*sychiatric disorders (especially depression), *E*xcess urine output (polyuria), *R*estricted mobility, and *S*tool impaction (see TABLE 228–1).

Established incontinence: Established incontinence is caused by a persistent problem affecting nerves or muscles. Mechanisms usually used to describe these problems are detrusor overactivity or underactivity, bladder outlet incompetence or obstruction, detrusor-sphincter dyssynergia, or a combination (see TABLE 228–2). However, these mechanisms are also involved in some reversible causes.

Detrusor overactivity is a common cause of urge incontinence in elderly and younger patients. The detrusor muscle contracts intermittently for no apparent reason, usually when the bladder is partially or nearly full. Detrusor overactivity may be idiopathic or may result from dysfunction of the frontal micturition inhibitory center (commonly due to age-related changes or dementia) or outlet obstruction. Detrusor overactivity (hyperactivity) with impaired contractility (DHIC) is a variant of urge incontinence characterized by urgency, frequency, a weak flow rate, urinary retention, bladder trabeculation, and a postvoid residual volume of > 50 mL. This variant may mimic prostatism in men or stress incontinence in women.

Outlet obstruction is a common cause of incontinence in men, but most men with obstruction are not incontinent. Obstruction commonly results from benign prostatic hyperplasia, prostate cancer, or urethral stricture. In women, outlet obstruction is rare but can result from previous surgery for incontinence or from a prolapsed cystocele that causes the urethra to kink during straining to void. In both sexes, fecal impaction can cause obstruction. Obstruction leads to a chronically overdistended bladder, which loses its ability to contract; then the bladder does not empty completely, resulting in overflow. Obstruction also may lead to detrusor overactivity and urge incontinence; if the detrusor decompensates, overflow incontinence may follow. Some causes of outlet obstruction (eg, large bladder diverticulum; cystocele; bladder infections, calculi, and tumors) are reversible.

Detrusor-sphincter dyssynergia (loss of coordination between bladder contraction and external urinary sphincter relaxation) may cause outlet obstruction, with resultant overflow incontinence. Dyssynergia is often due to a spinal cord lesion that interrupts pathways to the pontine micturition center, which coordinates sphincter relaxation and bladder contraction. Rather than relaxing when the bladder contracts, the sphincter contracts, obstructing the bladder outlet. Dyssynergia causes severe trabeculation, diverticula, a "Christmas tree" deformation of the bladder, hydronephrosis, and renal failure.

Outlet incompetence is a common cause of stress incontinence in women. It is usually due to weakness of the pelvic floor or of endopelvic fascia. Such weakness commonly results from multiple vaginal deliveries, pelvic surgery (including hysterectomy), age-related changes (including atrophic urethritis), or a combination. As a result, the urethrovesical junction descends, the bladder neck and urethra become hypermobile, and pressure in the urethra falls below that of the bladder. In men, a common cause is damage to the sphincter or to the bladder neck and external urethra after radical prostatectomy, resulting in stress incontinence.

Detrusor underactivity causes urinary retention and overflow incontinence in about 5% of patients with incontinence. It may be caused by injury to the spinal cord (see pp. 1908 and 2579) or to nerves supplying the bladder (eg, by disk compression, tumor, or surgery), by peripheral or autonomic neuropathies, or by other neurologic disorders (see TABLE 228–2). Anticholinergics and opioids greatly decrease detrusor contractility; these drugs are common transient causes. The detrusor may become underactive in men with chronic outlet obstruction as the detrusor is replaced by fibrosis and connective tissue, preventing the bladder from emptying even when the obstruction is removed. In women, detrusor

TABLE 228–1. CAUSES OF TRANSIENT INCONTINENCE

CATEGORY	CAUSES	COMMENTS
GI disorders	Fecal impaction	Mechanism may involve mechanical disturbance of the bladder or urethra. Patients usually present with urge or overflow incontinence, typically with fecal incontinence
GU disorders	Atrophic vaginitis	Thinning of urethral epithelium and submucosa may cause local irritation and decrease urethral resistance, length, and maximum closure pressure with loss of the mucosal seal. The disorder is usually characterized by urgency and occasionally by scalding dysuria
	Urinary calculi and foreign bodies	Bladder irritation precipitates spasm
	UTIs	Only symptomatic UTIs cause incontinence; dysuria and urgency can prevent patients from reaching the toilet before voiding
	Excess urine output (due to drug or alcohol use or to various medical disorders)	Frequency, urgency, and nocturia can result
Neuropsychiatric disorders	Delirium Depression Psychosis	Awareness of the need or ability to void is impaired
Restricted mobility	Weakness, injury, use of physical restraints	Access to toilet is impaired
Drugs	Alcohol	Alcohol has a diuretic effect and can cause sedation, delirium, or immobility, which can result in functional incontinence
	α-Adrenergic antagonists (eg, alfuzosin, doxazosin, prazosin, terazosin, tamsulosin)	Bladder neck muscle in women or prostate smooth muscle in men is lax, sometimes causing stress incontinence
	α-Adrenergic agonists (eg, pseudoephedrine)	Prostate and bladder neck tone is increased, sometimes causing urinary retention and overflow incontinence
	Anticholinergics (eg, antihistamines, tricyclic antidepressants, antipsychotics, benztropine)	Bladder contractility can be impaired, sometimes causing urinary retention and overflow incontinence; these drugs also can cause delirium, constipation, and fecal impaction
	Ca channel blockers (eg, diltiazem, nifedipine, verapamil)	Detrusor contractility is decreased, sometimes causing urinary retention, overflow incontinence, nocturia due to peripheral edema, constipation, and fecal impaction
	Diuretics (eg, bumetanide [not thiazides], furosemide, theophylline, caffeine)	Urine production and output are increased, causing polyuria, frequency, urgency, and nocturia
	Misoprostol	Misoprostol relaxes the urethra and thus may cause stress incontinence
	Opioids	Opioids cause urinary retention, constipation, fecal impaction, sedation, and delirium
	Psychoactive drugs (eg, antipsychotics, benzodiazepines, sedative-hypnotics, tricyclic antidepressants)	Awareness of the need to void is blunted, and dexterity and mobility are decreased; these drugs can precipitate delirium

TABLE 228–2. CAUSES OF ESTABLISHED INCONTINENCE

URODYNAMIC DIAGNOSIS	SOME NEUROLOGIC CAUSES	SOME NONNEUROLOGIC CAUSES
Bladder outlet incompetence	Lower motor neuron lesion (rare) In men, radical prostatectomy*	In women, multiple vaginal deliveries, pelvic surgery (eg, hysterectomy), or age-related changes (eg, atrophic urethritis) In men, prostate surgery Intrinsic sphincter deficiency Urethral hypermobility
Bladder outlet obstruction	Spinal cord lesion causing detrusor-sphincter dyssynergia (rare)	Anterior urethral stricture Bladder diverticula (if large) and calculi Bladder neck suspension surgery In women, cystocele if large In men, benign prostatic hyperplasia or prostate cancer
Detrusor overactivity	Alzheimer's disease Cervical spondylosis or stenosis Multiple sclerosis Stroke	Bladder carcinoma Cystitis Idiopathic Outlet obstruction or incompetence
Detrusor underactivity	Autonomic neuropathy (eg, due to diabetes, alcoholism, or vitamin B_{12} deficiency) Disk compression Plexopathy Spinal neural tube defect (may less often cause overactivity) Surgical damage (eg, anteroposterior resection) Tumor	Chronic bladder outlet obstruction Idiopathic (common among women)

*Other prostate surgery rarely causes neurogenic incontinence.

underactivity is usually idiopathic. Less severe detrusor weakness is common among elderly women. Such weakness does not cause incontinence but can complicate treatment if other causes of incontinence coexist.

Functional impairment (eg, cognitive impairment, reduced mobility, reduced manual dexterity, coexisting disorders, lack of motivation), particularly in the elderly, may contribute to established incontinence but rarely causes it.

Evaluation

Most patients, embarrassed to mention incontinence, do not volunteer information about it, although they may mention related symptoms (eg, frequency, nocturia, hesitancy). All adults should therefore be screened with a question such as "Do you ever leak urine?"

Clinicians should not assume that incontinence is irreversible just because it is longstanding. Also, urinary retention (see p. 1960) must be excluded before treatment for detrusor overactivity is started.

History: History focuses on duration and patterns of voiding, bowel function, drug use, and obstetric and pelvic surgical history. A voiding diary can provide clues to causes; over 48 to 72 h, the patient or caregiver records volume and time of each void and each incontinent episode in relation to associated activities (especially eating, drinking, and drug use) and during sleep. The amount of urine leakage can be estimated as drops, small, medium, or soaking; or by pad tests (measuring the weight of urine absorbed by feminine pads during a 24-h period). If the volume of most nightly voids is much smaller than functional bladder capacity (defined as the largest single voided volume recorded in the diary), the cause is a sleep-related problem (patients void because they are awake anyway) or a bladder abnormality.

Of men with obstructive symptoms (hesitancy, weak urinary stream, intermittency, feeling of incomplete bladder emptying), about $\frac{1}{3}$ have detrusor overactivity without obstruction.

Urgency or an abrupt gush of urine without warning or without preceding increase in intra-abdominal pressure (often called reflex or unconscious incontinence) typically indicates detrusor overactivity.

Physical examination: Neurologic, pelvic, and rectal examinations are the focus. If functional incontinence due to impaired mobility is suspected, ambulation is tested.

Neurologic examination involves assessing mental status, gait, and lower extremity function and checking for signs of peripheral or autonomic neuropathy, including orthostatic hypotension. Neck and upper extremities should be checked for signs of cervical spondylosis or stenosis, and the spinal column for evidence of prior surgeries and for deformities, dimples, or hair tufts suggesting neural tube defects.

Innervation of the external urethral sphincter, which shares the same sacral roots as the anal sphincter, can be tested by assessing perineal sensation; volitional anal sphincter contraction (S2 to S4); the anal wink reflex (S4 to S5), which is anal sphincter contraction triggered by lightly stroking perianal skin; and the bulbocavernosus reflex (S2 to S4), which is anal sphincter contraction triggered by pressure on the glans penis or clitoris. However, the absence of these reflexes is not necessarily pathologic, and their presence does not exclude detrusor underactivity.

Pelvic examination in women can identify atrophic vaginitis and urethritis, urethral hypermobility, and pelvic floor weakness. Pale, thin vaginal mucosae with loss of rugae indicate atrophic vaginitis. Urethral hypermobility can be seen during coughing when the posterior vaginal wall is stabilized with a speculum. A cystocele, an enterocele, a rectocele, or uterine prolapse suggests pelvic floor weakness (see p. 2097). When the opposite wall is stabilized with a speculum, bulging of the anterior wall indicates a cystocele, and bulging of the posterior wall indicates a rectocele or enterocele. Pelvic floor weakness does not suggest a cause, unless a large, prolapsed cystocele is present.

Rectal examination can identify fecal impaction, rectal masses, and, in men, prostate nodules or masses. Prostate size should be noted but correlates poorly with outlet obstruction. Suprapubic palpation and percussion to detect bladder distention are usually of little value except in extreme acute cases of urinary retention.

If stress incontinence is suspected, urinary stress testing can be done on the examination table; it has a sensitivity and specificity of > 90%. The bladder must be full; a patient sits upright or close to upright with the legs spread, relaxes the perineal area, and coughs vigorously once. Immediate leakage that starts and stops with the cough confirms stress incontinence. Delayed or persistent leakage suggests detrusor overactivity triggered by the cough. If cough triggers incontinence, the maneuver can be repeated while the examiner places 1 or 2 fingers inside the vagina to elevate the urethra (Marshall-Bonney test); incontinence that is corrected by this maneuver may respond to surgery. Results can be false-positive if patients have an abrupt urge to void during the test or false-negative if patients do not relax, the bladder is not full, the cough is not strong, or a large cystocele is present (in women). In the last case, the test should be repeated with the patient supine and the cystocele reduced, if possible.

Testing: Urinalysis, urine culture, and measurement of BUN and serum creatinine are required. Other tests may include serum glucose and Ca (with albumin for estimation of protein-free Ca levels) if the voiding diary suggests polyuria, electrolytes if patients are confused, and vitamin B_{12} levels if clinical findings suggest a neuropathy.

Postvoid residual volume should be determined by catheterization or ultrasonography. Postvoid residual volume plus voided volume estimates total bladder capacity and helps assess bladder proprioception. A volume < 50 mL is normal; < 100 mL is usually acceptable in patients > 65 but abnormal in younger patients; and > 100 mL may suggest detrusor underactivity or outlet obstruction.

Urodynamic testing is indicated when examination and the above tests are not diagnostic or when abnormalities must be precisely characterized before surgery.

Cystometry may help diagnose urge incontinence, but sensitivity and specificity are unknown. Sterile water is introduced into the bladder in 50-mL increments using a 50-mL syringe and a 12- to 14-F urethral catheter until the patient experiences urgency or bladder contractions, detected by changes in fluid level in the syringe. If < 300 mL causes urgency or contractions, detrusor overactivity and urge incontinence are likely.

Peak urinary flow rate testing with a flow meter is used to confirm or exclude outlet obstruction in men. Results depend on initial bladder volume, but a peak flow rate of < 12 mL/sec with a urinary volume of 200 mL and prolonged voiding suggests outlet obstruction or detrusor underactivity; a rate of ≥ 12 mL/sec excludes obstruction and may suggest detrusor overactivity. During testing, patients are instructed to place their hand on their abdomen to check for straining during urination, especially if stress incontinence is suspected and surgery is contemplated; straining suggests detrusor weakness that may predispose patients to postoperative retention.

In cystometrography, pressure-volume curves and bladder sensation are recorded while the bladder is filled with sterile water; provocative testing (with bethanechol or ice water) is used to stimulate bladder contractions. Electromyography of perineal muscle is used to assess sphincter innervation and function. Urethral, abdominal, and rectal pressures may be measured. Pressure-flow video studies, usually done with voiding cystourethrography (see p. 1936), can correlate bladder contraction, bladder neck competency, and detrusor-sphincter synergy, but equipment is not widely available.

Other tests (eg, urine cytology, cystoscopy, bladder biopsy) may be indicated in specific instances (eg, for patients with sterile hematuria, suprapubic or perineal discomfort, or a high risk of bladder cancer).

Treatment

Specific causes are treated, and drugs that can cause or worsen incontinence are stopped or the dosing schedule is altered (eg, a diuretic dose is timed so that a bathroom is near when the drug takes effect). Other treatment is based on type of incontinence. Regardless of type and cause, some general measures are usually helpful.

General measures: Patients may benefit from bladder training (to change voiding habits) and changes in fluid intake. Bladder training usually involves timed voiding (every 2 to 3 h) while patients are awake. Prompted voiding is used for cognitively impaired patients; they are asked about every 2 h whether they need to void or whether they are wet or dry. A voiding diary helps establish how often and when voiding is indicated and whether patients can sense a full bladder. Patients are instructed to limit fluid intake at certain times (eg, before going out, 3 to 4 h before bedtime), to avoid fluids that irritate the bladder (eg, caffeine-containing fluids), and to drink 48 to 64 oz (1500 to 2000 mL) of fluid a day (because concentrated urine irritates the bladder).

Pelvic muscle exercises (eg, Kegel exercises) are often effective, especially for stress incontinence. Patients must contract the pelvic muscles (pubococcygeus and paravaginal) rather than the thigh, abdominal, or buttock muscles; the muscles are contracted for 10 sec, then relaxed for 10 sec 10 to 15 times tid. Re-instruction is often necessary, and biofeedback is often useful. In women < 75 yr, cure rate is 10 to 25%, and improvement occurs in an additional 40 to 50%, especially if patients are motivated; do the exercises as instructed; and receive written instructions, follow-up visits for encouragement, or both. Pelvic floor electrical stimulation is an automated version of Kegel exercises; it uses electrical current to inhibit detrusor overactivity and contract pelvic muscles. Advantages are improved compliance and contraction of the correct pelvic muscles, but benefits over behavioral changes alone are unclear.

Some patients, especially those with restricted mobility or cognitive impairment, benefit from a portable commode. Others use absorbent pads or specialized padded undergarments. These products can greatly improve the quality of life of patients and their caregivers. However, they should not be substituted for measures that can control or eliminate incontinence, and they must be changed often to avoid skin irritation and development of UTIs.

Drugs are often useful (see TABLE 228–3). Such drugs include anticholinergics and antimuscarinics, which relax the detrusor, and α-agonists, which increase sphincter tone. Estrogens are used to treat atrophic urethritis in women, and α-antagonists and 5 α-reductase inhibitors may be used to treat outlet obstruction in men with urge or overflow incontinence.

Urge incontinence: Treatment aims to reduce detrusor overactivity; it begins with bladder training, Kegel exercises, and relaxation techniques (eg, biofeedback). Drugs may also be needed, as may intermittent self-catheterization (eg, when postvoid residual volume is large). Infrequently, sacral nerve stimulation, intravesical therapies, and surgery are used.

Bladder training helps patients tolerate and ultimately inhibit detrusor contractions. Regular voiding intervals are gradually lengthened (eg, ½ h every 3 days that urinary control is maintained) to improve tolerance of detrusor contractions. Relaxation techniques can improve emotional and physical responses to the urge to void. Relaxing, standing in place or sitting down (rather than rushing to the toilet), and tightening pelvic floor muscles can help patients suppress the urge to void.

Drugs (see TABLE 228–3) should supplement, not replace, behavioral changes. The most commonly used are oxybutynin and tolterodine; both are anticholinergic and antimuscarinic and can be taken po once/day. Oxybutynin is available as a skin patch changed twice/wk. Drugs may be required to suppress urgency symptoms due to DHIC. Drugs with a rapid onset of action (eg, immediate-release oxybutynin) can be used prophylactically if incontinence occurs at predictable times. Combinations of drugs may increase both efficacy and adverse effects, possibly limiting this approach in the elderly.

Sacral nerve stimulation is indicated for patients with severe urge incontinence refractory to other treatments. It is thought to work by centrally inhibiting bladder sensory afferents. The procedure begins with percutaneous nerve stimulation for at least 3 days; if patients respond, a neurostimulator is permanently implanted.

Rarely, intravesical instillation of capsaicin or resiniferatoxin (a capsaicin analog) is used when urge incontinence results from spinal cord injuries and other CNS disorders. This experimental treatment desensitizes C-fiber bladder afferents responsible for reflex bladder emptying. Injecting botulinum toxin into the detrusor muscle is under study as an alternative.

Surgery is a last resort, usually used only for younger patients with severe urge incontinence refractory to other treatments. Augmentation cystoplasty, in which a section of intestine is sewn into the bladder to increase bladder capacity, is most common. Intermittent self-catheterization may be required if patients have weak bladder contractions and cannot coordinate abdominal pressure (Valsalva maneuver) with sphincter relaxation. Detrusor myomectomy and urinary diversion are alternatives. Choice of procedure is based on presence of other disorders, physical limitations, and patient preference. Neuromodulation, in which electrodes are implanted around the spinal nerve roots, is under study.

Stress incontinence: Treatment includes bladder training and Kegel exercises. Drugs, surgery, other procedures, or, in women, occlusive devices are also usually needed. Treatment is generally directed at outlet incompetence but includes treatments for urge incontinence if detrusor overactivity is present. Avoiding physical stresses that provoke incontinence can help. Losing weight may help lessen incontinence in obese patients.

Drugs (see TABLE 228–3) include pseudoephedrine, which may be useful in women with outlet incompetence; imipramine, which may be used for mixed stress and urge incontinence or for either separately; and duloxetine. If stress incontinence is due to atrophic urethritis, topical estrogen (0.3 mg conjugated or 0.5 mg estradiol once/day for 3 wk, then twice/wk after) is often effective.

Surgery and other procedures provide the best chance of cure when noninvasive treatments are ineffective. Bladder neck suspension is used to correct urethral hypermobility; suburethral slings, injection of periurethral bulking agents, or surgical insertion of an artificial sphincter is used to treat sphincter deficiency. Choice depends on the patient's ability to tolerate surgery and need for other surgeries (eg, hysterectomy, cystocele repair) and on local experience.

Occlusive devices may be used in elderly women with or without bladder or uterine prolapse if surgical risks are high or if prior surgery for stress incontinence was ineffective. Pessaries may be effective; they elevate the bladder neck, correct the vesicourethral angle, and increase urethral resistance by pressing the urethra against the pubic symphysis. Newer, possibly more acceptable alternatives include silicone suction caps over the urethral meatus, intraurethral occlusive devices inserted with an applicator, and intravaginal bladder neck support prostheses. Removable intraurethral plugs are under study.

Exercise regimens using vaginal cones—in which progressively heavier cones are inserted into the vagina and retained for 15 min bid by contracting pelvic floor muscles—are also under study.

Overflow incontinence: Treatment depends on whether the cause is outlet obstruction, detrusor underactivity, or both.

Outlet obstruction due to benign prostatic hyperplasia (see p. 2045) or cancer (see p. 2053) is treated with drugs or surgery; that due to urethral stricture is treated with dilation or stenting. Cystoceles in women are treated with surgery or can be reduced using a pessary (see p. 2098); unilateral suture

TABLE 228–3. DRUGS USED TO TREAT INCONTINENCE

DRUG	MECHANISMS	DOSE	COMMENTS
Detrusor overactivity in urge or stress incontinence			
Oxybutynin	Smooth muscle relaxant, anticholinergic, and local anesthetic	Immediate-release: 2.5–5 mg po tid to qid Extended-release: 5–30 mg po once/day Transdermal: 3.9 mg twice/wk	Oxybutynin is most effective; efficacy may increase over time. Adverse effects include anticholinergic effects (eg, dry mouth, constipation), which may worsen compliance and incontinence; adverse effects are less severe with extended-release and transdermal forms
Tolterodine	M_3 muscarinic antagonist	Immediate-release: 1–2 mg po bid Extended-release: 2–4 mg po once/day	Efficacy and adverse effects are similar to those of oxybutynin, but long-term experience is less. Because M_3 receptors are targeted, adverse effects are less severe than those of oxybutynin
Propantheline	Anticholinergic	7.5–30 mg po 3–5 times/day	Propantheline has largely been replaced by newer drugs that have fewer adverse effects. This drug must be taken on an empty stomach
Hyoscyamine	Anticholinergic	Tablet or liquid: 0.125–0.25 mg q 4 h Extended-release tablet: 0.375 mg bid	Hyoscyamine is not well studied
Imipramine	Tricyclic antidepressant, anticholinergic, and α-agonist	10–25 mg po 1 to 4 times/day	Imipramine is useful for nocturia
Flavoxate	Smooth muscle relaxant	100–200 mg po tid to qid (up to 1200 mg/day)	Flavoxate is available but is usually ineffective. Adverse effects (eg, nausea, vomiting, dry mouth, blurred vision) are tolerable with doses up to 1200 mg/day
Dicyclomine	Smooth muscle relaxant and anticholinergic	10–20 mg po tid to qid	Dicyclomine is not well studied
Outlet incompetence in stress incontinence			
Duloxetine	Centrally acting serotonin and norepinephrine reuptake inhibitor	20 mg po bid to 80 mg po once/day	Duloxetine increases urinary sphincter striated muscle tone. It appears to be effective, but experience with it is limited, and it is not yet widely available
Pseudoephedrine	α-Agonist	30–60 mg po qid	Pseudoephedrine stimulates urethral smooth muscle contraction. Adverse effects include insomnia, anxiety, and, in men, urinary retention; this drug is not recommended for people with heart disorders, hypertension, glaucoma, or diabetes

TABLE 228–3. DRUGS USED TO TREAT INCONTINENCE—Continued

DRUG	MECHANISMS	DOSE	COMMENTS
Outlet obstruction in men with urge or overflow incontinence			
Doxazosin Prazosin Tamsulosin Terazosin	α-Adrenergic blockers	1 to 8 mg po once/day 0.5 to 2 mg po bid 0.4 to 0.8 mg po once/day 1 to 10 mg po once/day	In men, these drugs relieve symptoms of outlet obstruction, may reduce postvoid residual volume and outlet resistance, and may increase urinary flow rate. Effect occurs within days to weeks. Adverse effects include hypotension, fatigue, asthenia, and dizziness
Finasteride	5 α-Reductase inhibitor	5 mg po once/day	Finasteride reduces prostate size and obstructive symptoms and makes transurethral resection of prostate glands > 50 g less likely to be needed. Adverse effects are minimal and consist of sexual dysfunction (eg, decreased libido, erectile dysfunction)
Detrusor underactivity in overflow incontinence			
Bethanechol	Cholinergic agonist	10 to 50 mg po qid	Bethanechol is usually ineffective and may cause skin flushing, tachycardia, abdominal cramps, and malaise

removal or urethral adhesiolysis may be effective if cystoceles resulted from surgery. If urethral hypermobility coexists, bladder neck suspension should be done.

Detrusor underactivity requires bladder decompression (reduction of residual volume) by intermittent self-catheterization or, rarely, temporary use of an indwelling catheter. Several weeks of decompression may be required to restore bladder function. If bladder function is not fully restored, maneuvers to augment voiding (eg, double voiding, Valsalva maneuver, application of suprapubic pressure [Credé's method] during voiding) are used. A completely acontractile detrusor requires intermittent self-catheterization or use of an indwelling catheter. Using antibiotics or methenamine mandelate to prevent UTIs in patients who require intermittent self-catheterization is controversial but probably indicated if they have frequent symptomatic UTIs or a valvular or orthopedic prosthesis. Such prophylaxis is not helpful with indwelling catheters.

Additional treatments that may induce bladder contraction and promote emptying include electrical stimulation and the cholinergic agonist bethanechol. However, bethanechol is usually ineffective and has adverse effects (see TABLE 228–3).

Refractory incontinence: Absorbent pads, special undergarments, and intermittent self-catheterization may be needed. Indwelling urethral catheters are an option for patients who cannot walk to the toilet or who have urinary retention and cannot self-catheterize; these catheters are not recommended for urge incontinence because they may exacerbate detrusor contractions. If a catheter is necessary (eg, to allow healing of a pressure ulcer in patients with refractory detrusor overactivity), a narrow catheter with a small balloon should be used to minimize irritability and consequent leakage around the catheter. For men who can comply with treatment, condom catheters may be preferable because they reduce risk of UTIs; however, these catheters may cause skin breakdown and reduce motivation to become dry. New external collection devices may be effective in women. If involuntary bladder contractions persist, oxybutynin or tolterodine can be used. If mobility is restricted, measures to prevent skin irritation and breakdown due to urine are essential (see p. 1017).

INCONTINENCE IN CHILDREN

Incontinence in children has different causes and treatment than that in adults. It may be nocturnal (enuresis [bedwetting]—see p. 2481) or diurnal. It affects boys more than girls.

Etiology

The most common cause of diurnal incontinence after age 5 yr (when >90% of children are continent during the day) is detrusor instability (bladder spasm). Some girls have giggle incontinence; bladder spasm occurs only when they laugh. Incontinence in girls may also result from infrequent voiding or incorrect position during voiding, causing urine to reflux into the vagina, then dribble out after standing (urethrovaginal reflux, or vaginal voiding). Common reversible causes include UTIs, constipation, and emotional stress. Less common, irreversible causes include detrusor-sphincter dyssynergia, epispadias, and ureteral ectopia (a congenital disorder in which the ureter inserts distal to the external sphincter). To prevent leakage, children with incontinence may cross their legs or use other postures, which increase their risk of UTIs.

Evaluation and Treatment

Diagnosis can often be based on a complete history, including documentation of voiding and bowel habits. A complete physical examination is indicated to exclude neurologic disorders. If congenital malformations are suspected, renal ultrasonography, spinal x-rays, and voiding cystourethrography are indicated.

An anticholinergic drug (eg, oxybutynin) and fluid restriction may be tried if detrusor instability is suspected. Managing constipation, gradually lengthening voiding intervals (bladder training), and changing other behaviors may be effective depending on cause. Frequent voiding or intermittent catheterization may be necessary for children with urinary retention.

URINARY RETENTION

Urinary retention is incomplete emptying of the bladder or cessation of urination; it may be acute or chronic. Causes include impaired bladder contractility, bladder outlet obstruction, detrusor-sphincter dyssynergia (lack of coordination between bladder contraction and sphincter relaxation), or a combination. Retention is most common among men, in whom prostate abnormalities or urethral strictures cause outlet obstruction. In either sex, retention may be due to drugs (particularly those with anticholinergic effects, including many OTC drugs), severe fecal impaction (which increases pressure on the bladder trigone), or neurogenic bladder in patients with diabetes, multiple sclerosis, Parkinson's disease, or prior pelvic surgery resulting in bladder denervation.

Urinary retention can cause urinary frequency and urge or overflow incontinence. It may cause abdominal distention and pain. When retention develops slowly, pain may be absent. Long-standing retention predisposes to UTI and can increase bladder pressure, causing obstructive uropathy (see p. 1963).

Diagnosis is obvious in patients who cannot void. In those who can void, diagnosis is by postvoid catheterization showing a residual urine volume > 100 mL. Other tests (eg, urinalysis, blood tests, ultrasonography, urodynamic testing, cystoscopy, cystography) are done based on clinical findings.

Relief of acute urinary retention requires urethral catheterization. Subsequent treatment depends on cause. No treatment is effective for impaired bladder contractility or a neurogenic bladder; intermittent self-catheterization or indwelling catheterization is usually required.

NEUROGENIC BLADDER

Neurogenic bladder is bladder dysfunction (flaccid or spastic) caused by neurologic damage. The primary symptom is overflow incontinence; risk of serious complications (eg, recurrent infection, vesicoureteral reflux, autonomic dysreflexia) is high. Diagnosis involves imaging and cystoscopy or urodynamic testing. Treatment involves catheterization or measures to trigger urination.

Any condition that impairs bladder and bladder outlet afferent and efferent signaling can cause neurogenic bladder. Causes may involve the CNS (eg, stroke, spinal injury, meningomyelocele, amyotrophic lateral sclerosis), peripheral nerves (eg, diabetic, alcoholic, or vitamin B_{12} deficiency neuropathies; herniated disks; damage due to pelvic surgery), or both (eg, Parkinson's disease, multiple sclerosis, syphilis). Bladder outlet obstruction often coexists and may exacerbate symptoms.

In flaccid (hypotonic) neurogenic bladder, volume is large, pressure is low, and contractions are absent. It may result from peripheral nerve damage or spinal cord damage at the S2 to S4 level. After acute cord damage, initial flaccidity may be followed by long-term flaccidity or spasticity, or bladder function may improve after days, weeks, or months.

In spastic bladder, volume is normal or small, and involuntary contractions occur. It usually results from brain damage or spinal cord damage above T12. Precise symptoms vary by site and severity of the lesion. Bladder contraction and external urinary sphincter relaxation are typically uncoordinated (sphincter dyssynergia).

Mixed patterns (flaccid and spastic bladder) may be caused by many disorders, including syphilis, diabetes mellitus, brain or spinal cord tumors, stroke, ruptured intervertebral disk, and demyelinating or degenerative disorders (eg, multiple sclerosis, amyotrophic lateral sclerosis).

Symptoms and Signs

Overflow incontinence is the primary symptom. Patients with flaccid bladder retain urine and have constant overflow dribbling; men typically also have erectile dysfunction. Patients with spastic bladder may have frequency, nocturia, and urgency or spastic paralysis with sensory deficits.

Common complications include recurrent UTIs and urinary calculi. Hydronephrosis with vesicoureteral reflux is particularly common because the large urine volume puts pressure on the vesicoureteral junction, causing dysfunction with reflux and, in severe cases, nephropathy. Patients with high thoracic or cervical spinal cord lesions are at risk of autonomic dysreflexia (a life-threatening syndrome of malignant hypertension, bradycardia or tachycardia, headache, piloerection, and sweating due to unregulated sympathetic hyperactivity). This disorder may be triggered by acute bladder distention (due to urinary retention) or bowel distention (due to constipation or fecal impaction).

Diagnosis

Diagnosis is suspected clinically. Usually, postvoid residual volume is measured, renal ultrasonography is done to detect hydronephrosis, and serum creatinine is measured to assess renal function. Further studies are often not obtained in patients who are not able to self-catheterize or ask to go to the bathroom (eg, severely debilitated elderly or post-stroke patients). Occasionally, however, cystography is used to evaluate bladder capacity and detect reflux. Cystoscopy is used to evaluate duration and severity of retention (by detecting bladder trabeculations) and to check for bladder outlet obstruction. Cystometrography can determine whether bladder volume and pressure are high or low; if done during the recovery phase of flaccid bladder after spinal cord injury, it can help evaluate detrusor functional capacity and predict rehabilitation prospects. Urodynamic testing of voiding flow rates and sphincter electromyography can show whether bladder contraction and sphincter relaxation are coordinated.

Prognosis and Treatment

Prognosis is good if the disorder is diagnosed and treated before kidneys are damaged.

Specific treatment involves catheterization or measures to trigger urination. General treatment includes renal function monitoring, control of UTIs, high fluid intake to decrease risk of UTIs and urinary calculi (although this measure may exacerbate incontinence), early ambulation, frequent changes of position, and dietary Ca restriction to inhibit calculus formation.

For flaccid bladder, especially if the cause is an acute spinal cord injury, immediate continuous or intermittent catheterization is needed. Intermittent self-catheterization is preferable to indwelling urethral catheterization, which has a high risk of recurrent UTIs and, in men, a high risk of urethritis, periurethritis, prostatic abscesses, and urethral fistulas. Suprapubic catheterization may be used if patients cannot self-catheterize.

For spastic bladder, treatment depends on the patient's ability to retain urine. Patients who can retain normal volumes can use techniques to trigger voiding (eg, applying suprapubic pressure, scratching the thighs); anticholinergics may be effective. For patients who cannot retain normal volumes, treatment is the same as that of urge incontinence (see p. 1956), including drugs (see TABLE 228–3) and sacral nerve stimulation.

Surgery is a last resort. It is usually indicated if patients have had or are at risk of severe acute or chronic sequelae or if social circumstances, spasticity, or quadriplegia prevent use of continuous or intermittent bladder drainage. Sphincterotomy (for men) converts the bladder into an open draining conduit. Sacral (S3 and S4) rhizotomy converts a spastic into a flaccid bladder. Urinary diversion may involve an ileal conduit or ureterostomy.

An artificial sphincter, surgically inserted, is an option for patients who have adequate bladder capacity and upper extremity motor skills and who can comply with instructions for use of the device; if patients do not comply, life-threatening situations (eg, renal failure, urosepsis) can result.

INTERSTITIAL CYSTITIS

Interstitial cystitis is noninfectious bladder inflammation that causes pain (suprapubic, pelvic, and abdominal), urinary frequency, and urgency with incontinence. Diagnosis is by history and exclusion of other disorders. With treatment, most patients improve, but cure is rare. Treatment varies but includes dietary changes, bladder training, pentosan, analgesics, and intravesical therapies.

Incidence of interstitial cystitis is unknown, but the disorder appears to be more common than once thought and may underlie other clinical syndromes (eg, chronic pelvic pain). Whites are more susceptible, and 90% of cases occur in women.

Cause is unknown but may involve loss of protective urothelial mucin, with penetration of urinary K and other substances into the bladder wall, activation of sensory nerves, and smooth muscle damage. Mast cells may mediate the process, but their role is unclear.

Symptoms, Signs, and Diagnosis

Interstitial cystitis is initially asymptomatic, but symptoms appear and worsen over years as the bladder wall is damaged. Suprapubic and pelvic pressure or pain occurs, usually with urinary frequency (up to 60 times/day) or urgency. These symptoms worsen as the bladder fills and diminish when patients void; in some people, symptoms worsen during ovulation, menstruation, seasonal allergies, physical or emotional stress, or sexual intercourse. Foods with high K content (eg, citrus fruits, chocolate, caffeinated drinks, tomatoes) may cause exacerbations. If the bladder wall becomes scarred, bladder compliance and capacity decrease, causing urinary urgency and frequency.

Diagnosis is suggested by symptoms after testing has excluded more common disorders that cause similar symptoms (eg, UTIs, pelvic inflammatory disease, chronic prostatitis or prostatodynia, diverticulitis). Cystoscopy sometimes reveals benign bladder (Hunner's) ulcers; biopsy is required to exclude bladder cancer. Assessment of symptoms with a standardized symptom scale or during intravesical KCl infusion (K sensitivity testing) may improve diagnostic accuracy but is not yet routine practice.

Treatment

Up to 90% of patients improve with treatment, but cure is rare. Treatment should involve avoidance of tobacco, alcohol, foods with high K content, and spicy foods as well as bladder training, drugs, intravesical therapies, and surgery as needed. Stress reduction and biofeedback may help. No treatment has been proved effective, but a combination of ≥ 2 nonsurgical treatments is recommended before surgery is considered.

The most commonly used drug is pentosan, a heparin similar to urothelial glycosaminoglycan; doses of 100 mg po tid may help restore the bladder's protective surface lining. Improvement may not be noticed for 2 to 4 mo. Intravesical instillation of 15 mL of a solution containing 100 mg of pentosan or 40,000 units of heparin plus 80 mg of lidocaine and 3 mL of Na bicarbonate may benefit patients unresponsive to oral drugs. Tricyclic antidepressants (eg, imipramine 25 to 50 mg po once/day) and NSAIDs in standard doses may relieve pain. Antihistamines (eg, hydroxyzine 10 to 50 mg once before bedtime) may help by directly inhibiting mast cells or by blocking allergic triggers.

Dimethyl sulfoxide instilled into the bladder through a catheter and retained for 15 min may deplete substance P and trigger mast cell granulation; 50 mL q 1 to 2 wk for 6 to 8 wk, repeated as needed, relieves symptoms in up to $\frac{1}{2}$ of patients. Intravesical instillation of BCG and hyaluronic acid are under study.

Bladder hydrodistention, cystoscopic resection of a Hunner's ulcer, and sacral nerve root (S3) stimulation help some patients.

Surgery (eg, partial cystectomy, bladder augmentation, neobladder, and urinary diversion) is a last resort for patients with intolerable pain refractory to all other treatments. Outcome is unpredictable; in some patients, symptoms persist.

229 OBSTRUCTIVE UROPATHY

(Urinary Tract Obstruction)

Obstructive uropathy is structural or functional hindrance of normal urine flow, sometimes leading to renal dysfunction (obstructive nephropathy). Symptoms, less likely in chronic obstruction, are pain radiating to the T11 to T12 dermatomes, anuria, nocturia, or polyuria. Diagnosis is based on bladder catheterization, ultrasonography, CT, cystourethroscopy, cystourethrography, or pyelography, depending on the level of obstruction. Treatment, depending on cause, may require prompt drainage, instrumentation, surgery (eg, endoscopy, lithotripsy), and/or hormonal therapy.

Each year about 2/1000 people in the US are hospitalized for obstructive uropathy. The condition has a bimodal distribution. In childhood, it is due mainly to congenital anomalies of the urinary tract. Incidence then declines until after age 60, when incidence rises, particularly in men because of the increased incidence of benign prostatic hyperplasia (BPH) and prostate cancer. Overall, obstructive uropathy is responsible for about 4% of end-stage renal disease. Hydronephrosis is found at postmortem examination in 2 to 4% of patients.

Etiology and Pathophysiology

Many conditions can cause obstructive uropathy, which may be acute or chronic, partial or complete, and unilateral or bilateral (see TABLE 229–1). Obstruction may occur at any level, from the renal tubules (casts, crystals) to the external urethral meatus, and may result in increased intraluminal pressure, urinary stasis, UTI, or calculus formation (which may also cause obstruction). It is much more common in males, but acquired and congenital urethral strictures and meatal stenosis occur in both males and females. In females, urethral obstruction may occur secondary to tumor, radiation therapy, surgery, or urologic instrumentation (usually repeated dilation).

Obstructive nephropathy (renal insufficiency, renal failure, or tubulointerstitial damage) may result from increased intratubular pressure, local ischemia, or, often, associated UTI. Renal damage may also result from infiltration by inflammatory T cells and macrophages, an autoimmune response to refluxed urinary Tamm-Horsfall mucoprotein (a normal secretion of epithelial cells in the loop of Henle), and vasoactive hormones.

Pathologic findings consist of dilation of the collecting ducts and distal tubules and chronic tubular atrophy with little glomerular damage. Obstructive uropathy without dilation can occur when fibrosis or a retroperitoneal tumor encases the collecting systems, when obstructive uropathy is mild and renal function is not impaired, in the presence of an intrarenal pelvis, or within 3 days after the onset of obstructive uropathy, when the collecting system is relatively noncompliant and less likely to dilate.

Symptoms and Signs

Symptoms and signs vary with the site, degree, and rapidity of onset of obstructive uropathy.

Pain is common because of distention of the bladder, collecting system, or renal capsule. Upper ureteral or renal pelvic lesions cause flank pain or tenderness, whereas lower ureteral obstruction causes pain that may radiate to the ipsilateral testicle or labia. Pain may be severe, accompanied by nausea and vomiting, with acute complete ureteral obstruction (eg, a ureteral calculus). A large fluid load (eg, from beer drinking or osmotic diuresis due to an IV radiocontrast agent) produces dilation and pain if urine production increases to a level greater than the flow rate through the area of obstruction. Pain is typically minimal or absent with partial or slowly developing obstructive uropathy (eg, ureteropelvic junction obstruction, pelvic tumor). Ureteropelvic obstruction may cause hydronephrosis, occasionally producing a palpable flank mass, particularly in massive hydronephrosis of infancy and childhood.

Urine volume does not diminish in unilateral obstruction unless it occurs in the only functioning kidney. Absolute anuria occurs with complete obstruction at the level of the bladder or urethra. Partial obstruction at that level may cause difficulty voiding or abnormalities of the urine stream. Polyuria occurs rarely with partial obstructive uropathy if the ensuing nephropathy causes impaired renal concentrating capacity and Na reabsorption.

TABLE 229–1. CAUSES OF OBSTRUCTIVE UROPATHY

Anatomic abnormalities
- Abnormal anterior or posterior valve (urethra)
- Contracture of the vesical neck
- Diverticulum (urethra)
- Polyp (ureter)
- Straddle injury (urethra)
- Stricture: phimosis, meatal stenosis, paraphimosis, pelvic fracture (urethra)

Compression from extrinsic masses or processes
- Female reproductive system: pregnancy, uterine prolapse, tumor, abscess, Gartner's duct cyst, tubo-ovarian abscess
- GI tract: Crohn's disease, diverticulitis, appendiceal abscess, tumor (including pancreatic), abscess, cyst
- GU tract: Periurethral abscess, benign prostatic hyperplasia, fibrosed chronic prostatitis, prostatic cancer
- Blood vessels: aneurysm, aberrant vessel, retrocaval ureter, puerperal ovarian vein thrombophlebitis
- Retroperitoneum: fibrosis (idiopathic, surgical, drug-induced), TB, sarcoidosis, lymphoma, metastatic tumor, lymphocele, hematoma, pelvic lipomatosis

Functional abnormalities
- Neurogenic disorders or drugs (bladder)
- Ureteropelvic or ureterovesical junction dysfunction, bladder neck dysfunction

Mechanical obstruction of the lumen of the urinary tract
- Blood clot (renal pelvis or ureter)
- Fungus ball (renal pelvis or ureter)
- Renal papillae (renal pelvis or ureter)
- Uric acid crystals (renal tubule)
- Urolithiasis (renal pelvis or ureter)

Long-standing nephropathy may also result in hypertension.

Infection may produce dysuria, pyuria, urinary urgency and frequency, pain in the referral pattern for kidneys and ureters (T11), costovertebral angle tenderness, fever, and, occasionally, septicemia.

Diagnosis

Obstructive uropathy should be considered in all patients with diminished or absent urine output or unexplained renal insufficiency. The history may suggest symptoms of BPH, prior malignancy, or urolithiasis. Most obstructions can be corrected; early diagnosis and treatment prevent irreversible renal damage.

Urinalysis and serum chemistries (serum electrolytes, BUN, creatinine) should be obtained. Other tests are performed depending on symptoms and suspected level of obstruction. Infection associated with urinary obstruction is an emergency and requires immediate evaluation and treatment.

If urine output is diminished or absent, bladder catheterization should be performed. If catheterization results in a normal flow of urine or the catheter is difficult to pass, a urethral obstruction (eg, prostatic enlargement, stricture, or valve) is suspected. Such patients should have cystourethroscopy along with voiding cystourethrography. Voiding cystourethrography diagnoses nearly all bladder neck and urethral obstructions as well as vesicoureteral reflux, adequately displaying the anatomy and postvoiding residuals.

In an asymptomatic patient with long-standing obstructive uropathy, urinalysis may be normal or reveal only a few casts, WBCs, or RBCs. However, if bilateral obstruction is complete or nearly so, acute or chronic renal failure may follow.

With unilateral obstructive uropathy and a normal contralateral kidney, the plasma creatinine concentration is usually near normal. Anuria and acute renal failure rarely occur due to autonomic-mediated vascular or ureteral spasm in the functioning kidney.

Other findings may include hyperkalemia secondary to type 1 renal tubular acidosis due to reduced distal hydrogen and K secretion, and Na wasting that predisposes to ECF volume depletion.

Imaging tests: Several diagnostic imaging techniques are available. The choice and sequencing depend on the suspected pathology, its presumed location, and the results of earlier tests.

Abdominal ultrasonography is the initial test of choice in most patients without urethral abnormalities because it avoids potential allergic and toxic complications of radiocontrast agents and allows assessment of associated renal parenchymal atrophy. However, the false-positive rate is 25% if only minimal criteria (visualization of the collecting systems) are considered in the diagnosis. The combination of ultrasonography, plain abdominal x-ray, and, if necessary, CT diagnoses obstructive uropathy in > 90% of patients, but ultrasonography and CT may not be able to differentiate hydronephrosis from multiple renal or parapelvic cysts.

Duplex Doppler ultrasonography can usually diagnose unilateral obstructive uropathy in the first few days of acute obstruction before the collecting system dilates by detecting an increased resistive index (a reflection of increased renal vascular resistance) in the affected kidney. Increased vascular resistance results from activation of the rennin-angiotensin system and increased production of thromboxane A_2 and endothelin. This modality is less useful in obesity and in bilateral obstruction, which cannot be distinguished from intrinsic renal disease.

IVU (contrast urography, intravenous pyelogram [IVP], excretory urography) has been largely superseded by CT and MR imaging (with or without contrast). However, when CT cannot identify the level of obstructive uropathy and when acute obstructive uropathy is thought to be caused by calculi, sloughed papilla, or blood clot, IVU or retrograde pyelography may be indicated.

Radionuclide scans also require some renal function but can detect obstruction without the use of contrast agents. When a kidney is assessed as nonfunctioning, a radioisotope scan can determine perfusion and identify functional renal parenchyma. Because this test cannot detect specific areas of obstruction, it is mainly used in conjunction with diuresis renography to evaluate hydronephrosis without apparent obstruction.

Antegrade or retrograde pyelography is preferred in the azotemic patient. Retrograde studies are done through a cystoscope, whereas antegrade studies require placement of a catheter percutaneously into the renal pelvis. Patients with intermittent obstruction should be studied when they are having symptoms; otherwise, the obstruction may be missed.

Diuresis renography evaluates back or flank pain in the presence of hydronephrosis without evident obstructive uropathy. A loop diuretic (eg, furosemide 0.5 mg/kg IV) is given before a radionuclide renal scan (or an IVU). If obstruction is present, the rate of washout of the radionuclide (or radiocontrast agent) during renal imaging is reduced despite increased urine flow. If the renogram is negative or equivocal but the patient is symptomatic, a perfusion pressure flow study is performed via percutaneous insertion of a catheter into the dilated renal pelvis, followed by fluid perfusion into the pelvis at 10 mL/min. If obstructive uropathy is present, in spite of the marked increase in urine flow, the rate of washout of the radioisotope during renal scanning is delayed, and there will be further dilation of the collecting system on IVU and elevation of the renal pelvic pressure to > 22 mm Hg during perfusion. A renogram or perfusion study that causes pain similar to the patient's initial complaint is interpreted as positive. If the perfusion study is negative, the pain probably has a nonrenal cause. False-positive and false-negative results are common for both tests.

Prognosis

Most obstruction can be corrected, but a delay in therapy can lead to irreversible renal damage. Outcome varies depending on the underlying pathology, the presence or absence of UTI, and the degree and duration of the obstruction. In general, acute renal failure due to a ureteral calculus is reversible, with adequate return of renal function. With chronic progressive obstructive uropathy, renal dysfunction may be partially or completely irreversible.

Treatment

Treatment consists of eliminating the obstruction by surgery, instrumentation (eg, endoscopy, lithotripsy), or drug therapy (eg, hormonal therapy for prostate cancer). Prompt drainage in hydronephrosis is indicated if renal function is compromised, UTI persists, or pain is significant. Lower obstructive uropathy may require catheter drainage or urinary diversion. Indwelling pigtail ureteral catheters can be placed for acute or long-term drainage in selected patients. Temporary drainage using a percutaneous technique may be needed in severe obstructive uropathy, UTI, or calculi. Intensive treatment for UTI and renal failure is imperative.

In the case of hydronephrosis without evident obstruction, surgery should be considered if the patient has pain and a positive diuretic renogram. However, no therapy is necessary in an asymptomatic patient with a negative diuretic renogram or with a positive diuretic renogram but normal renal function.

URINARY CALCULI

(Nephrolithiasis; Stones; Urolithiasis)

Urinary calculi are solid particles in the urinary system. They may cause pain, nausea, vomiting, hematuria, and, possibly, chills and fever from secondary infection. Diagnosis is based on urinalysis and noncontrast spiral CT. Treatment is with analgesics, antibiotics for infection, and, sometimes, instrumentation, shock wave lithotripsy, or endoscopic surgery.

About 1/1000 adults is hospitalized annually in the US because of urinary calculi, which are also found in about 1% of all autopsies. Calculi vary from microscopic crystalline foci to stones several centimeters in diameter. A large calculus, called staghorn calculus, can fill an entire renal calyceal system.

Etiology

About 80% of calculi in the US are composed of Ca, mainly Ca oxalate; 10% are uric acid; 2% are cystine; and the remainder are Mg ammonium phosphate.

General risk factors include disorders that increase urinary salt concentration, either by increased excretion of Ca or uric acid salts, or decreased urine volume.

For **Ca calculi,** the main risk factor in the US is hypercalciuria, a hereditary condition present in 50% of men and 75% of women with Ca calculi. Patients have normal serum Ca but elevated urinary Ca: > 300 mg/day (> 7.5 mmol/day) in men and > 250 mg/day (> 6.2 mmol/day) in women. About 5% of patients with Ca calculi have primary hyperparathyroidism. Rare causes are sarcoidosis, vitamin D intoxication, hyperthyroidism, renal tubular acidosis, multiple myeloma, metastatic cancer, and hyperoxaluria. Hyperoxaluria (urinary oxalate > 40 mg/day [> 440 μmol/day]) can be primary or caused by excess ingestion of oxalate-containing foods (eg, rhubarb, spinach, cocoa, nuts, pepper, tea) or by excess oxalate absorption due to various enteric diseases (eg, bacterial overgrowth syndromes, chronic pancreatic or biliary disease) or ileojejunal surgery. Hypocitruria (urinary citrate < 350 mg/day [1820 μmol/day]), present in about 40 to 50% of Ca calculi-formers, promotes Ca calculi because citrate normally binds urinary Ca and inhibits the crystallization of Ca salts.

Uric acid calculi develop with increased urine acidity (urine pH < 5.5), which crystallizes undissociated uric acid. Uric acid crystals may comprise the entire calculus or, more commonly, provide a nidus on which Ca or mixed Ca and uric acid calculi can form. Hyperuricosuria, defined as urinary uric acid > 750 mg/day (> 4 mmol/day) in women or > 800 mg/day (> 5 mmol/day) in men, is almost always caused by excess intake of purine (in meat, fish, and poultry).

Cystine calculi occur only in the presence of cystinuria (see p. 2438).

Mg ammonium phosphate calculi (struvite, infection calculi) indicate the presence of a UTI caused by urea-splitting bacteria. The calculi must be treated as infected foreign bodies. Unlike other types of calculi, Mg ammonium phosphate calculi occur 3 times more frequently in women.

Pathophysiology

Urinary calculi may remain within the renal parenchyma or pelvis or be passed into the ureter and bladder. During passage they irritate the ureter and may become lodged, obstructing urine flow and causing hydroureter and sometimes hydronephrosis. Common areas of lodgment include the ureteropelvic junction, the distal ureter (at the level of the iliac vessels), and the ureterovesical junction. Typically, a calculus must have a diameter > 5 mm to become lodged; those ≤ 5 mm are likely to pass spontaneously.

Even partial obstruction causes decreased glomerular filtration, which may persist briefly after the calculus has passed. With hydronephrosis and elevated glomerular pressure, renal blood flow declines, which further worsens renal function. Generally, however, permanent renal dysfunction occurs only after about 28 days of complete obstruction.

Secondary infection can occur with longstanding obstruction, but most patients with Ca-containing calculi do not have infected urine.

Symptoms and Signs

Even large calculi remaining in the renal parenchyma or pelvis are usually asymptomatic. However, passage of smaller stones, particularly with obstruction, can cause significant symptoms with severe pain, often accompanied by nausea and vomiting, and sometimes gross hematuria. Pain (renal colic) is typically excruciating and intermittent, usually originating in the flank or kidney area and radiating across the abdomen along the course of the ureter, frequently into the genital region. Calculi in the distal ureter or bladder may cause suprapubic pain along with urinary urgency and frequency. Urinary frequency and urgency are common, particularly as a calculus passes through the distal ureter.

On examination, patients are in obvious extreme discomfort, often ashen and diaphoretic. They are unable to lie still and may pace, writhe, or constantly shift position. The abdomen may be somewhat tender on the affected side as palpation increases pressure in the already-distended ureter, but peritoneal signs (guarding, rebound, rigidity) are lacking.

Diagnosis

The symptoms and signs suggest the diagnosis. Similar symptoms can result from appendicitis, cholecystitis, peptic ulcer, pancreatitis, ectopic pregnancy, and dissecting aortic aneurysm.

Patients suspected of having renal colic require urinalysis, an imaging study, and, if confirmed, evaluation of underlying cause, including calculus composition testing. General evaluation of acute abdominal pain is discussed on p. 97.

Urinalysis: Macroscopic or microscopic hematuria is common, but urine may be normal despite multiple calculi. Pyuria with or without bacteria may be present. A calculus and various crystalline substances may be present in the sediment, but the calculus' composition should be determined by crystallography. The only exception is the presence of the typical hexagonal crystals of cystine in a concentrated, acidified specimen, which strongly suggests cystinuria.

Imaging tests: Noncontrast spiral CT should be obtained. A noncontrast renal CT can detect the location of a calculus as well as the degree of obstruction. Moreover, spiral CT may also reveal another cause of the pain (eg, aortic aneurysm).

Although most urinary calculi are demonstrable on plain x-ray, neither their presence nor their absence obviates the need for more definitive imaging, so this study can be eschewed. Both renal ultrasonography and IVU can identify calculi and hydronephrosis, but ultrasound is less sensitive for small calculi without hydronephrosis, and IVU is time consuming and exposes the patient to the risk of IV contrast; these studies are generally used if spiral CT is unavailable.

Identifying the underlying cause: The calculus is obtained during operative removal or by straining the urine and sent to the laboratory for crystallography. Some are brought in by patients. Patients with a single Ca calculus without additional risk factors for calculi require only urinalysis and plasma Ca concentration on 2 occasions to exclude hyperparathyroidism. Predisposing factors, such as a high-protein diet or vitamin C or D supplements, should be sought. However, in patients with a strong family history of calculi, associated medical conditions that might predispose to calculi formation (eg, sarcoidosis, bone disease), or conditions that would make it difficult to treat calculi (eg, solitary kidney, urinary tract anomalies), a complete metabolic evaluation is warranted.

Treatment

Colic may be relieved by opioids, but ketorolac 30 mg IV is rapidly effective and nonsedating. Vomiting usually resolves with pain but if persistent can be treated with an antiemetic (eg, metoclopramide 10 mg IV).

Although increasing fluids (either oral or IV) has traditionally been recommended, it has not been proved to speed the passage of calculi. Calculi with a diameter of < 5 mm and larger calculi without hydronephrosis may be treated with analgesics; if the patient is comfortable and able to drink, he may go home to await calculi passage. Larger calculi and those not passed within 6 wk typically require removal. Infected calculi should always be removed immediately. Shock wave lithotripsy is the usual therapy for symptomatic calculi < 1.5 cm in diameter in the renal pelvis or proximal ureter. Percutaneous nephrolithotomy or ureteroscopy may be used to remove larger renal or ureteral calculi, respectively. Calculi impacted in the renal pelvis or ureter may require endoscopic removal, particularly when associated with infection. Calculi along the entire course of the ureter may be approached endoscopically from below (ureteroscopically) or from above (percutaneously). If the calculus is small enough to be removed intact, direct-vision basketing under ureteroscopic control may be performed. However, for most ureteral calculi, a form of intracorporeal lithotripsy with calculus fragmentation (electrohydraulic, laser, or pneumatic lithotripsy) can fragment the calculus into smaller pieces, which can then be extracted. Uric acid calculi in the upper or lower urinary tract occasionally may be dissolved by prolonged alkalinization of the urine with HCO_3 or citrate 20 mEq po bid to tid, but chemical dissolution of other calculi is not possible.

Prevention

In a patient who has passed a 1st Ca calculus, the likelihood of forming a 2nd calculus is about 15% at 1 yr, 40% at 5 yr, and 80% at 10 yr. Recovery and analysis of the calculus, measurements of calculus-forming substances in the urine, and the clinical history are needed to plan prophylaxis. In < 3% of patients, no metabolic abnormality is found. These patients seemingly cannot tolerate normal amounts of calculus-forming salts in their urine without crystallization. Thiazide diuretics, K citrate, and increased fluid intake may reduce their calculus production rate.

Hypercalciuria patients may receive thiazide diuretics (eg, chlorthalidone 25 mg po once/day or indapamide 1.25 mg po once/day), which lower urine Ca excretion and supersaturation with Ca oxalate. Patients are encouraged to increase their fluid intake to ≥ 3 L/day. K replacement with K citrate (20 mEq bid) reduces the risk of hypokalemia and supplements citrate excretion in patients with hypocitruria. A low Ca diet and Na cellulose phosphate should be used cautiously because they may produce a chronic negative Ca balance or hyperoxaluria. A "normal" Ca intake is recommended. Oral orthophosphate has not been thoroughly studied.

Hyperoxaluria prevention varies. Patients with small-bowel disease can be treated with a combination of Ca loading (usually in the form of Ca citrate 400 mg po bid), cholestyramine, and a low-oxalate, low-fat diet. Hyperoxaluria may respond to pyridoxine 5 to 500 mg po once/day, possibly by increasing transaminase activity responsible for the conversion of glyoxylate, the immediate oxalate precursor to glycine.

In **hyperuricosuria,** intake of meat, fish, and poultry should be reduced. If the diet cannot be changed, allopurinol 300 mg each morning lowers uric acid production. For uric acid calculi, the urine pH must be increased to between 6 and 6.5 with oral K alkalinizing drugs (eg, K citrate as above), along with increased fluid intake.

Urea-splitting bacteria infection requires antibiotics (eg, nitrofurantoin). If eradication of infection is impossible, long-term suppressive therapy may be necessary. In addition, acetohydroxamic acid can be used to reduce the recurrence of struvite calculi.

Urinary cystine levels must be reduced to < 250 mg cystine/L of urine to prevent recurrent cystine calculi. Any combination of increasing urine volume along with a reduction of cystine excretion (α-mecaptopropionylglycine or D-penicillamine) should reduce the urinary cystine concentration.

231 URINARY TRACT INFECTIONS

Urinary tract infections (UTIs) can be divided into upper tract infections, which involve the kidneys, and lower tract infections, which involve the bladder, urethra, or prostate. However, in practice, and particularly in children, differentiating between the sites may be difficult or impossible. Moreover, infection often moves from one area to the other.

Most UTIs are caused by enteric bacteria. The remainder are due to sexually transmitted pathogens (see Ch. 194 on p. 1650), mycobacteria (see p. 1508), fungi (see pp. 1523 and 1974), and parasites. The predominant parasitic diseases are filariasis, trichomoniasis, leishmaniasis, malaria, and schistosomiasis; these are discussed in other chapters of THE MANUAL. Of the parasites, only trichomoniasis is common in the US. Adenoviruses are implicated in hemorrhagic cystitis.

BACTERIAL URINARY TRACT INFECTIONS

(See also Ch. 173 on p. 1455; Prostatitis on p. 2045; pediatric UTI on p. 2356.)

Bacterial UTIs can involve the urethra, prostate, bladder, or kidneys. Symptoms may be absent or include urinary frequency, urgency,

and dysuria; lower abdominal pain; and flank pain. Systemic symptoms and even sepsis may occur with kidney infection. Diagnosis is based on analysis and culture of urine. Treatment is with antibiotics.

Among adults aged 20 to 50 yr, UTIs are about 50-fold more common in women. The incidence increases in patients > 50 yr, but the female:male ratio decreases because of the increasing frequency of prostate disease.

Pathophysiology

The urinary tract, from the kidneys to the urethral meatus, is normally sterile and resistant to bacterial colonization despite frequent contamination of the distal urethra with colonic bacteria. Mechanisms that maintain the tract's sterility include urine acidity, emptying of the bladder at micturition, ureterovesical and urethral sphincters, and various immunologic and mucosal barriers.

About 95% of UTIs occur when bacteria ascend the urethra to the bladder and, in the case of acute uncomplicated pyelonephritis, ascend the ureter to the kidney. The remainder of infections are hematogenous. Systemic infection can result from UTI, particularly in the elderly; about 6.5% of cases of hospital-acquired bacteremia are attributable to UTI.

Complicated UTI is considered to be present when there are underlying factors that predispose to ascending bacterial infection; these include urinary instrumentation (eg, catheterization, cystoscopy), anatomic abnormalities, and obstruction of urine flow or poor bladder emptying. A common consequence of anatomic abnormality is vesicoureteral reflux (VUR), which is present in 30 to 45% of young children with symptomatic UTI. VUR is usually caused by a congenital defect that results in incompetence of the ureterovesical valve; it is most often due to a short intramural segment (the ureter normally transits the bladder wall at an angle; the resultant lengthy segment is more readily closed by muscular contraction than the shorter segment occurring when the ureter passes straight through the wall). VUR can also be acquired in patients with a flaccid bladder due to spinal cord injury. Other anatomic abnormalities predisposing to UTI include urethral valves, delayed bladder neck maturation, and urethral duplications. Urine flow can be compromised by calculi, tumors, and prostatic enlargement. Bladder emptying can be impaired by neurogenic dysfunction (see p. 1960), pregnancy, uterine prolapse, and presence of a cystocele. UTI caused by congenital factors presents most commonly in childhood; most other factors are more common in the elderly.

Uncomplicated UTI occurs without underlying abnormality or impairment of urine flow. It is most common in young women but also can occur in younger men who have unprotected anal intercourse, an uncircumcised penis, unprotected intercourse with a woman whose vagina is colonized with uropathogens, or AIDS. Risk factors in women include sexual intercourse, diaphragm-spermicide use, antibiotic use, and a history of recurrent UTIs. Even use of spermicide-coated condoms increases risk of UTI in women. The increased risk of UTI in women using antibiotics or spermicides probably occurs from alterations in vaginal flora that allow overgrowth of *Escherichia coli*. In elderly women, soiling of the perineum from fecal incontinence increases risk. Patients of both sexes with diabetes have an increased incidence and severity of infections.

Etiology

Commensal colonic gram-negative aerobic bacteria cause most bacterial UTIs. In relatively normal tracts, strains of *E. coli* with specific attachment factors for transitional epithelium of the bladder and ureters are the most frequent. The remaining gram-negative urinary pathogens are other enterobacteria, especially *Klebsiella, Proteus mirabilis*, and *Pseudomonas aeruginosa*. Enterococci (group D streptococci) and coagulase-negative staphylococci (eg, *Staphylococcus saprophyticus*) are the most frequently implicated gram-positive organisms.

E. coli causes > 75% of community-acquired UTIs in all age groups; *S. saprophyticus* accounts for about 10%. In hospitalized patients, *E. coli* accounts for about 50% of cases; the gram-negative species *Klebsiella, Proteus, Enterobacter*, and *Serratia*, for about 40%; and the gram-positive bacterial cocci *Enterococcus faecalis* and *S. saprophyticus* and *Staphylococcus aureus* for the remainder.

Classification

Urethritis: Bacterial infection of the urethra occurs when organisms that gain access to it acutely or chronically colonize the numerous periurethral glands in the bulbous and pendulous portions of the male urethra and in the entire female urethra. The sexually transmitted pathogens *Chlamydia trachomatis* (see p. 1651), *Neisseria gonorrhoeae* (see p. 1653), and herpes simplex (see p. 1606) are common causes in both sexes.

Cystitis: In women, sexual intercourse usually precedes uncomplicated cystitis (honeymoon cystitis). In men, bacterial infection of the bladder is usually complicated and generally results from ascending infection from the urethra or prostate or is secondary to urethral instrumentation. The most common cause of recurrent cystitis in men is chronic bacterial prostatitis.

Unsterile urine (asymptomatic bacteruria): Certain patients, primarily elderly women, have persistent bacteriuria with changing flora that is both asymptomatic and refractory to treatment. WBC count in urine may be modestly elevated. Most of these patients are best left untreated, because the usual result of treatment is the establishment of highly resistant organisms.

Acute pyelonephritis: Pyelonephritis is bacterial infection of the kidney parenchyma, and the term should not be used to describe tubulointerstitial nephropathy unless infection is documented. About 20% of community-acquired bacteremias in women are from pyelonephritis. Pyelonephritis is uncommon in men with a normal urinary tract.

Although obstruction (strictures, calculi, tumors, prostatic hypertrophy, neurogenic bladder, VUR) predisposes to pyelonephritis, most women with pyelonephritis have no demonstrable functional or anatomic defects. Cystitis alone or anatomic defects may produce reflux. This tendency is greatly enhanced when ureteral peristalsis is inhibited (eg, during pregnancy, by obstruction, by endotoxins of gram-negative bacteria). Pyelonephritis or focal abscess may be due to hematogenous UTI, which is infrequent and usually results from bacteremia with virulent bacilli (eg, *Salmonella* sp, *S. aureus*). Pyelonephritis is common in young girls and in pregnant women after instrumentation or bladder catheterization.

The kidney usually is enlarged because of inflammatory PMNs and edema. Infection is focal and patchy, beginning in the pelvis and medulla and extending into the cortex as an enlarging wedge. Chronic inflammatory cells appear within a few days, and medullary and subcortical abscesses may develop. Normal parenchymal tissue between foci of infection is common. Papillary necrosis may be evident in acute pyelonephritis associated with diabetes, obstruction, sickle cell disease, or analgesic nephropathy. Although acute pyelonephritis is frequently associated with renal scarring in children, similar scarring in adults is not detectable in the absence of reflux or obstruction.

Symptoms and Signs

In the elderly, UTIs are often asymptomatic. Elderly patients, and those with a neurogenic bladder or an indwelling catheter, may present with sepsis and delirium but without symptoms referable to the urinary tract.

When symptoms are present, they may not correlate with location of the infection within the urinary tract because there is considerable overlap; however, some generalizations are useful.

In urethritis, the main symptom is dysuria, and, primarily in males, urethral discharge. Discharge tends to be purulent when due to *N. gonorrhoeae* and whitish mucoid when not.

Cystitis onset is usually sudden, typically with frequency, urgency, and burning or painful voiding of small volumes of urine. Nocturia, with suprapubic and often low back pain, is common. The urine is often turbid, and gross hematuria occurs in about 30% of patients. A low-grade fever may develop. Pneumaturia (passage of air in the urine) can occur when infection results from a vesicoenteric or vesicovaginal fistula.

In acute pyelonephritis, symptoms may be the same as those of cystitis; $\frac{1}{3}$ have frequency and dysuria. However, with pyelonephritis, symptoms typically include chills, fever, flank pain, nausea, and vomiting. If abdominal rigidity is absent or slight, a tender, enlarged kidney is sometimes palpable. Costovertebral percussion tenderness is generally present on the infected side. In children, symptoms often are meager and less characteristic (see p. 2356).

Diagnosis

Diagnosis requires demonstration by culture of significant bacteriuria in properly collected urine.

Urine collection: If a sexually transmitted disease (STD) is suspected, a urethral swab for STD testing is obtained prior to voiding. Urine collection is then by clean-catch or catheterization.

To obtain a clean-catch, midstream-voided specimen, the urethral opening is washed with a mild nonfoaming disinfectant, and the area is dried with a sterile swab. Contact of the urinary stream with the mucosa should be minimized by spreading the labia in women and by pulling back the foreskin in uncircumcised men. The first 5 mL of urine is not captured; the next 5 to 10 mL is collected in a sterile container. From men, samples are considered positive when colony counts are > 10^4/mL; from women, colony counts must be > 10^5/mL.

A catheter specimen is preferable in older women (who typically have difficulty performing a clean-catch), and women with vaginal bleeding or discharge. Many clinicians also obtain a catheterized specimen if evaluation includes a pelvic examination. Because external contamination is minimal, > 10^3 colonies/mL usually are significant. Specimens from indwelling catheters are unreliable and should not be used for diagnosing UTIs.

Urine testing: Microscopic examination of urine is useful but not definitive. Pyuria is defined as ≥ 8 WBCs/μL of uncentrifuged urine, which corresponds to 2 to 5 WBCs/high-power field in spun sediment. Most truly infected patients have > 10 WBCs/μL. The presence of bacteria in the absence of pyuria, especially when various strains are found, is usually due to contamination during sampling. Microscopic hematuria occurs in up to 50% of patients, but gross hematuria is uncommon. WBC casts, which require special stains to differentiate from renal tubular casts, indicate only an inflammatory reaction; they can be present in pyelonephritis, glomerulonephritis, and noninfective tubulointerstitial nephritis.

Dipstick tests also are commonly used. A positive nitrite test on a freshly voided specimen (bacterial replication in the container renders results unreliable if the specimen is not tested rapidly) is highly specific for UTI, but the test is not very sensitive. The leukocyte esterase test is very specific for the presence of > 10 WBCs/μL and is fairly sensitive. In uncomplicated cases with typical symptoms, most clinicians consider positive microscopic and dipstick tests sufficient; in these cases, given the likely pathogens, cultures are unlikely to change treatment but add significant expense.

Cultures are recommended when symptoms are suggestive but urinalysis is nondiagnostic; for apparent complicated UTI, including patients with diabetes, immunosuppression, recent hospitalization or urethral instrumentation, or recurrent UTI; patients > 65 yr; and perhaps those with symptoms of pyelonephritis. Urine should be cultured as soon as possible or stored at 4° C if a delay of > 10 min is expected. Samples contaminated with large numbers of epithelial cells are likely to be unhelpful; an uncontaminated specimen should be obtained for culture. Occasionally, UTI is present despite low colony counts, possibly because of prior antibiotic therapy, very dilute urine (specific gravity < 1.003), or obstruction to the flow of grossly infected urine. Repeating the culture improves the diagnostic accuracy of a positive result.

Infection localization: Clinical differentiation between upper and lower UTI is impossible in many patients, and testing is not usually advisable. When the patient has high fever, costovertebral angle tenderness, and gross pyuria with casts, pyelonephritis is highly likely. The best noninvasive technique for differentiating bladder from kidney infection appears to be the response to a short course of antibiotic therapy.

Symptoms similar to cystitis and urethritis can occur with vaginitis, which may cause dysuria from the passage of urine across inflamed labia. Vaginitis can often be distinguished by the presence of vaginal discharge, vaginal odor, and dyspareunia.

Other testing: Seriously ill patients require evaluation for sepsis, typically with CBC, electrolytes, BUN, creatinine, and blood cultures. Those with abdominal pain or tenderness are evaluated for other causes of an acute abdomen (see p. 94 for causes and diagnosis); pyuria can be present with appendicitis, inflammatory bowel disease, and other extrarenal disorders.

Most adults do not require assessment for structural abnormalities unless infections recur or are complicated; nephrolithiasis is suspected; there is painless hematuria or new renal insufficiency; or a febrile patient does not defervesce within 48 to 72 h. Imaging choices include IVU, ultrasound, and CT (see further discussion on p. 2357). Urologic investigation is not routinely needed in women with recurrent cystitis, be it symptomatic or asymptomatic, because it does not influence therapy.

Treatment

Treatment of all forms of UTI requires antibiotics. Obstructive uropathy, anatomic abnormalities, and neuropathic GU lesions usually require surgical correction. Catheter drainage of an obstructed urinary tract aids in prompt control of UTI. Occasionally, a renal cortical abscess or perinephric abscess requires surgical drainage. Instrumentation of the lower urinary tract in the presence of infected urine should be deferred if possible. Sterilization of the urine before instrumentation and antibiotic therapy for 3 to 7 days after instrumentation can prevent life-threatening urosepsis.

Urethritis: Sexually active patients with symptoms are usually treated presumptively for STDs pending test results; a typical regimen is ceftriaxone 125 mg IM plus either azithromycin 1 g po once or doxycycline 100 mg po bid for 7 days. For non-STD urethritis in men, trimethoprim-sulfamethoxazole (TMP-SMX) or a fluoroquinolone is given for 10 to 14 days; women are treated with a regimen for cystitis.

Cystitis: A 3-day oral course of TMP-SMX or a fluoroquinolone effectively treats acute cystitis and eradicates potential bacterial pathogens in vaginal and GI reservoirs. Single-dose therapy results in higher recurrence rates and is not recommended. Longer courses of therapy (7 to 14 days) are prescribed for patients with a history of recent UTI, diabetes mellitus, or symptoms lasting > 1 wk.

If pyuria but not bacteriuria is present in a sexually active woman, then *C. trachomatis* urethritis is diagnosed presumptively, and appropriate treatment is given to the patient and her sex partner. If symptoms recur with a positive urinalysis and a cultured organism sensitive to the 3-day antimicrobial therapy or if pyelonephritis is suspected, treatment is for a kidney infection with a 14-day course of TMP-SMX or a fluoroquinolone. Some patients with low colony counts develop an acute urethral syndrome due to trauma or inflammation of the urethra or occasionally caused by *N. gonorrhoeae*, TB, or fungal disease.

Asymptomatic bacteriuria: Ordinarily, asymptomatic bacteriuria in patients with diabetes, elderly patients, or those with chronic indwelling bladder catheters should not be treated. However, asymptomatic bacteriuria in pregnant women is actively sought and treated as a symptomatic UTI, although few antibiotics can be safely used. Oral β-lactams, sulfonamides, and nitrofurantoin are considered safe in early pregnancy, but sulfonamides should be avoided near parturition because of a possible role in the development of kernicterus.

Treatment may also be indicated in asymptomatic UTI in neutropenic patients, those with recent renal transplantation, patients scheduled for instrumentation of the urinary tract (after removal of a bladder catheter that has been in place for > 1 wk), young children with gross VUR, and patients with frequent UTI symptoms from a struvite calculus that cannot be removed. Therapy typically consists of an appropriate antimicrobial (based on culture results) for 3 to 14 days or long-term suppressive therapy for untreatable obstructive problems (eg, calculi, reflux).

Acute pyelonephritis: Outpatient treatment with oral antimicrobials is possible if the patient is reliable in following medical advice and has no nausea or vomiting, signs of volume depletion, or evidence of septicemia; typical regimens are 14 days of TMP-SMX 160/800 mg po bid or ciprofloxacin 500 mg po bid. Otherwise, patients should be hospitalized and given parenteral therapy selected by local sensitivity patterns of the most common strains. Common regimens include ampicillin plus gentamicin, TMP-SMX and a fluoroquinolone, and broad-spectrum cephalosporins (eg, ceftriaxone). Aztreonam, β-lactam/β-lactam inhibitor combinations (ampicillin-sulbactam, ticarcillin-clavulanate, piperacillin-tazobactam), and imipenem-cilastatin are generally reserved for patients with more complicated pyelonephritis (eg, obstruction, calculi, resistant bacteria, hospital-acquired infection) or recent urinary tract instrumentation. Parenteral therapy is continued until defervescence and other signs of clinical improvement occur. In > 80% of patients, improvement occurs within 72 h. Oral therapy can then begin, and the patient can be discharged for the remainder of the 14-day treatment course. For complicated cases, prolonged antibiotic suppression may be needed with urologic correction of anatomic defects.

When pyelonephritis is diagnosed during pregnancy, hospitalization and parenteral therapy with a β-lactam with or without an aminoglycoside is appropriate.

Prevention

In women who experience ≥ 3 UTIs/yr, voiding immediately after sexual intercourse and avoiding use of a diaphragm may be helpful. Drinking cranberry juice reduces pyuria and bacteriuria.

If these techniques are unsuccessful, low-dose oral antimicrobial prophylaxis greatly reduces the incidence of recurrent UTIs—eg, TMP-SMX 40/200 mg once/day or 3 times/wk, nitrofurantoin (macrocrystals) 50 or 100 mg once/day, or a fluoroquinolone (eg, ciprofloxacin, norfloxacin, ofloxacin, lomefloxacin, enoxacin). Postcoital TMP-SMX or a fluoroquinolone may be effective. If UTI recurs after 6 mo of this therapy, prophylaxis may be reinstituted for 2 or 3 yr.

Because of potential injury to a fetus, users of fluoroquinolones should also use effective contraception. Some antibiotics (macrolides, tetracyclines, rifampin, metronidazole, penicillins, and TMP-SMX) interfere with the effectiveness of oral contraceptives by interrupting the enterohepatic recycling of estrogen or by inducing hepatic estrogen metabolism. Women who use oral contraceptives should use barrier contraceptives while they are taking these antibiotics.

Effective prophylaxis of UTI in pregnant women is similar to that in nonpregnant women. Appropriate patients include those with acute pyelonephritis during a previous pregnancy, patients with bacteriuria during pregnancy who have had a posttreatment recurrence, and patients who required prophylaxis for recurrent UTI before pregnancy.

Antimicrobial prophylaxis for postmenopausal women is similar to that described above. Additionally, topical estrogen therapy markedly reduces the incidence of recurrent UTI in those with atrophic vaginitis/urethritis.

CHRONIC PYELONEPHRITIS

(Chronic Infective Tubulointerstitial Nephritis)

Chronic pyelonephritis is chronic pyogenic infection of the kidney that occurs only in patients with major anatomic abnormalities. Symptoms include fever, malaise, and flank discomfort. Diagnosis is with urinalysis, culture, and imaging tests. Treatment is with antibiotics and correction of any structural disorders.

Reflux of infected urine into the renal pelvis is the usual mechanism; causes include obstructive uropathy, struvite calculi, and, most commonly, VUR.

Pathologically there is atrophy and calyceal deformity with overlying parenchymal scarring. The disease may progress to renal failure; chronic pyelonephritis causes about 2 to 3% of end-stage renal disease.

Xanthogranulomatous pyelonephritis (XPN) is an unusual variant that typically occurs in middle-aged women with a history of recurrent UTIs. It is a complication of obstruction due to renal calculi and is typically associated with *Proteus* infections. The kidney is enlarged, and perirenal fibrosis and adhesions to adjacent retroperitoneal structures are common. The disease is almost always unilateral and appears to represent an abnormal inflammatory response to infection. Giant cells, lipid-laden macrophages, and cholesterol clefts account for the yellow color of the infected tissue. The disease may also occur in children.

Symptoms and Signs

Symptoms and signs are often vague and inconsistent; some have fever, flank or abdominal pain, malaise, or anorexia. In XPN, a unilateral renal mass can usually be palpated.

Diagnosis

A history of recurrent UTI and acute pyelonephritis is helpful but infrequently present except in children with VUR.

Urinalysis and culture and usually imaging tests are obtained. On urinalysis, proteinuria is absent, minimal, or intermittent even when renal scarring is far advanced. Urinary sediment is usually scant, but renal epithelial cells, granular casts, and occasionally WBC casts are found. When both kidneys are involved, defects in concentrating ability and hyperchloremic acidosis may appear before significant azotemia occurs. Urine culture may be sterile or positive for gram-negative organisms.

IVU may show irregular renal contour with partial or almost complete loss of visible parenchyma between the calyces and the renal capsule. Focal scarring is rarely absent on IVU. Ureteral dilation may be present, reflecting the changes induced by chronic severe reflux. Similar changes can occur with urinary tract TB (see Tuberculosis on p. 1508). A voiding cystourethrogram may not show reflux, which frequently ceases spontaneously (after puberty) because of the increased length of the submucosal portion of the terminal ureter. However, cystoscopy shows evidence of previous reflux at most ureteral orifices. An abnormal voiding cystourethrogram suggests the diagnosis only in a patient with otherwise unexplained proteinuria (occasionally nephrotic range) and renal insufficiency. In such cases, renal biopsy shows focal glomerulosclerosis typical of advanced reflux nephropathy.

In XPN, urinalysis and urine culture indicate the presence of infection, but diagnosis is confirmed by radiologic examination. CT can exclude renal carcinoma and other lesions and is preferred over IVU. Blood tests reveal nonspecific findings including anemia and mild liver dysfunction.

Treatment

If obstruction cannot be eliminated and recurrent UTI is common, long-term therapy with antimicrobials (eg, TMP-SMX, trimethoprim, a fluoroquinolone, nitrofurantoin) is useful and may be required indefinitely. Complications of uremia or hypertension must be treated appropriately.

For XPN, an initial course of antimicrobials should be given to control local infection, followed by en bloc nephrectomy with removal of all involved tissue and closure of any fistulas.

The course of chronic pyelonephritis is extremely variable, but the disease typically progresses very slowly; most patients have adequate renal function for ≥ 20 yr after onset. Frequent exacerbations of acute pyelonephritis, although controlled, usually further deteriorate renal structure and function. Continued obstruction predisposes to or perpetuates pyelonephritis and increases intrapelvic pressure, which damages the kidney directly.

FUNGAL URINARY TRACT INFECTIONS

Fungal infections of the urinary tract primarily affect the bladder and kidneys.

Species of *Candida*, the most common cause, are normal commensals in humans. Differentiating *Candida* colonization from infection requires evidence of tissue reaction. All invasive fungi (eg, *Cryptococcus neoformans, Aspergillus* sp, *Mucoraceae* sp, *Histoplasma capsulatum*, *Blastomyces* sp, *Coccidioides immitis*) may infect the kidneys as part of systemic or disseminated mycotic infection (see full discussion in Ch. 180 on p. 1523). Their presence alone is sufficient for diagnosis.

Lower UTI with *Candida* usually occurs with urinary catheters, typically after bacteriuria and antibiotic therapy, although candidal and bacterial infections frequently occur simultaneously. *C. albicans* prostatitis occurs infrequently in patients with diabetes, usually after instrumentation.

Renal candidiasis is usually spread hematogenously and commonly originates from the GI tract. Ascending infection also occurs from nephrostomy tubes, other permanent indwelling devices, and stents. At high risk are patients who are immunocompromised because of tumor, AIDS, chemotherapy, or immunosuppressants. A major source of candidemia in such high-risk hospitalized patients is an indwelling intravascular catheter. Renal transplantation increases the risk because of the combination of indwelling catheters, stents, antibiotics, anastomotic leaks, obstruction, and immunosuppressive therapy.

Symptoms and Signs

Most patients with candiduria are asymptomatic but have easily identifiable predisposing factors. Whether *Candida* can cause symptomatic urethritis (mild urethral itching, dysuria, watery discharge) is controversial. A fungal cause for these symptoms in men should be considered only when all other causes of urethritis have been excluded. Candidal urethritis is rare in women; however, in candidal vaginitis, dysuria may result from the urine coming into contact with inflamed periurethral tissue.

Cystitis due to *Candida* may result in frequency, urgency, dysuria, and suprapubic pain. Hematuria is common, and, in patients with poorly controlled diabetes, pneumaturia and emphysematous cystitis have occurred. One or more fungus balls or bezoars may be present in the bladder lumen from local or upper tract formation and occasionally obstruct the urethra.

Most patients with hematogenous renal candidiasis lack symptoms referable to the kidney but may have antibiotic-resistant fever, candiduria, and unexplained deteriorating renal function. Ascending infection commonly produces fungus ball elements in the ureter and renal pelvis. These masses frequently produce hematuria and urinary obstruction. Occasionally, papillary necrosis occurs, and intrarenal and perinephric abscesses may form. Clinical manifestations of dissemination to other sites (CNS, skin, eyes, liver, spleen) may be present.

Diagnosis

Diagnosis is by culture, usually from urine. The level at which candiduria reflects true *Candida* UTI and not merely colonization or contamination is unknown. Cystitis is usually diagnosed in high-risk patients with candiduria by the presence of bladder inflammation or irritation. Cystoscopy and ultrasonography of the kidney and bladder may help detect bezoars and obstruction.

Fever, candiduria, and occasionally passage of fungus balls suggest ascending renal candidiasis. Although renal function often declines, severe renal failure is rare without postrenal obstruction. Imaging of the urinary tract may help evaluate the degree of involvement. Blood cultures for *Candida* are often negative.

Unexplained candiduria should prompt evaluation of urinary tract structural abnormalities.

Treatment

Fungal colonization of catheters does not require treatment. Asymptomatic candiduria rarely requires therapy. Candiduria should be treated in symptomatic patients, neutropenic patients, and those with renal allografts or undergoing urologic manipulation. Urinary stents and Foley catheters should be removed (if possible). Treatment with fluconazole (200 mg po once/day for 7 to 14 days) and with amphotericin B (see regimens on p. 1523) has been successful. In the absence of renal insufficiency, flucytosine (25 mg/kg po qid) may help eradicate candiduria due to non-*albicans* species of *Candida*; however, resistance may emerge rapidly when this compound is used as a single agent. Bladder irrigation with amphotericin B may transiently clear candiduria but is rarely indicated. Even with apparently successful local or systemic antifungal therapy for candiduria, relapse is frequent, and this likelihood is increased by continued use of a urinary catheter.

In patients with renal candidiasis, amphotericin B and high-dose fluconazole (≥ 400 mg/day) are equally effective in the primary treatment of invasive infection with *C. albicans* and *C. tropicalis.* Even when amphotericin B is used initially, oral fluconazole should be substituted early in the course of treatment. However, some less common *Candida* species are not susceptible to fluconazole.

232 CYSTIC KIDNEY DISEASE

Cystic kidney disease may be hereditary (polycystic kidney disease, nephronophthisis, medullary cystic disease), congenital (renal cystic dysplasia, medullary sponge kidney), part of a malformation syndrome, or acquired (single or multiple cysts)—see TABLE 232–1.

ACQUIRED RENAL CYSTS

Acquired renal cysts are simple cysts that must be distinguished from more serious causes of cystic disease.

Acquired cysts are usually simple, ie, they are round and sharply demarcated with smooth walls. They may be single or multiple.

Single cysts are isolated (or few in number) and are most often detected incidentally. They are clinically insignificant but must be distinguished from other more significant cystic renal disorders and renal masses such as renal cell carcinoma, which is typically irregular or multiloculated with irregular walls, septae, and areas of unclear demarcation.

Multiple cysts are most common in patients with chronic renal failure, especially those undergoing hemodialysis. Cause is unknown, but the cysts may be due to compensatory hyperplasia of residually functioning nephrons. Criterion for diagnosis is ≥ 4 cysts in each kidney on ultrasonography or CT.

Acquired cysts are significant only because patients have a higher incidence of renal carcinoma; whether the cysts become malignant is unknown. For this reason, some physicians periodically screen patients with acquired cysts for renal carcinoma using ultrasonography or CT.

CONGENITAL RENAL CYSTIC DYSPLASIA

Congenital renal cystic dysplasia is a broad category of sporadic congenital malformations involving metanephric malformation or congenital obstructive uropathies.

TABLE 232–1. MAJOR GROUPS OF CYSTIC NEPHROPATHIES

DISORDER	CLINICAL FEATURES
Hereditary	
Medullary cystic disease	Similar to nephronophthisis but ESRD in adulthood
Nephronophthisis	Small to normal-sized kidneys, hypertension, renal tubular acidosis, ESRD in childhood
Polycystic kidney disease	
Autosomal dominant	Abdominal pain, hematuria, hypertension, large kidneys, extrarenal cysts (liver, pancreas, intestine), ESRD in adulthood
Autosomal recessive	Large kidneys, hepatic fibrosis, hypertension, ESRD in childhood
Congenital	
Renal cystic dysplasia	Associated with urinary structural obstruction or metanephric malformation; degree of dysplasia asymmetric between kidneys
Malformation syndromes	
Ehlers-Danlos	Joint hyperextensibility, increased skin elasticity
Ellis-van Creveld	Short limb dwarfism, polydactyly, heart defects frequently
Goldston	Cerebellar malformations
Ivemark's	Spleen agenesis, cyanotic heart disease, gut malrotation
Jeune's	Dwarfism involving chest, arm, legs
Laurence-Moon	Hypogonadism, mental retardation, retinopathy, polydactyly
Meckel-Gruber	Occipital encephalocele, polydactyly, craniofacial dysplasia
Melnick-Fraser	Branchial fistulae and cysts, preauricular pits or tags, hearing loss
Oral-digital-facial	Partial clefts in lip, tongue, and alveolar ridges; hypoplasia of nasal cartilage; microcysts in kidneys
Trisomy 13	Profound developmental delay, microphthalmia, cleft lip and palate, polydactyly
Trisomy 18	Profound developmental delay, malformations of head, face, hands, and feet
Trisomy 21	Mild to moderate developmental delay, low-set ears, small jaw, congenital heart defects
Tuberous sclerosis	Benign tumors of brain, kidney, and skin
Von Hippel-Lindau	Angioma proliferation in the retina, brain, spinal cord, adrenal glands
Zellweger (cerebrohepatorenal)	Brain and liver defects, developmental delay, high serum iron and copper levels, muscular hypotonia
Acquired	
Isolated simple cysts	Low risk for renal disease or hypertension
Acquired cystic disease	Associated with long-term dialysis; high risk for renal carcinoma

ESRD = end-stage renal disease.

Urologic abnormalities include ureteropelvic and ureterovesicular junction obstruction, neurogenic bladder, ureterocele, posterior urethral valves, and prune-belly syndrome (a triad of abdominal wall muscle defects, urinary tract abnormalities [eg, dilated ureters, enlarged bladder and urethra], and bilateral cryptorchidism—see p. 2437).

Symptoms and signs vary by how much renal parenchyma is preserved and whether involvement is unilateral or bilateral. Some degree of renal insufficiency or renal failure develops. Congenital renal cystic dysplasias are commonly discovered by ultrasonography prenatally or during early childhood.

Prognosis is highly unpredictable due to an inability to quantify residual functional parenchyma. Treatment is surgical correction of any associated GU abnormalities and, if renal insufficiency or renal failure is present, renal replacement therapy.

MEDULLARY SPONGE KIDNEY

Medullary sponge kidney is formation of diffuse, bilateral medullary cysts caused by abnormalities in pericalyceal terminal collecting ducts.

The cause of medullary sponge kidney is unknown, but genetic transmission occurs in < 5% of cases. The disorder is more common among patients with Ehlers-Danlos, Marfan, or Beckwith-Wiedemann syndromes; congenital hemihypertrophy; or congenital dilation of intrahepatic bile ducts (Caroli's disease).

Most patients are asymptomatic, and the disorder usually remains undiagnosed. It predisposes to calculus formation and UTI, so the most common presenting symptoms are renal colic, hematuria, and dysuria. Urinalysis typically shows evidence of incomplete distal renal tubular acidosis (overt metabolic acidosis is rare) and decreased urine-concentrating ability without symptomatic polyuria.

Diagnosis is generally by CT, but IVU can be used. Ultrasonography is not helpful because cysts are small and located deep in the medulla. Differential diagnosis includes renal cystic dysplasia, papillary necrosis, pyelonephritic cysts, TB, and other conditions that cause nephrocalcinosis.

Medullary sponge kidney is benign, and long-term prognosis is excellent. Obstruction by renal calculi may transiently reduce GFR and increase serum creatinine. Treatment is indicated only for UTIs and for recurrent calculus formation. Thiazides (eg, hydrochlorothiazide 25 mg bid) and high fluid intake inhibit calculus formation and may reduce incidence of obstructive complications.

NEPHRONOPHTHISIS AND MEDULLARY CYSTIC KIDNEY DISEASE COMPLEX

Nephronophthisis and medullary cystic kidney disease are inherited disorders that cause cysts restricted to the renal medulla or corticomedullary border and, eventually, renal failure.

Nephronophthisis and medullary cystic kidney disease are grouped together because they share many features. Pathologically, they cause cysts restricted to the renal medulla or corticomedullary border, as well as a triad of tubular atrophy, tubular basement membrane disintegration, and interstitial fibrosis. They probably share similar mechanisms, although these are not well characterized. Both disorders cause a vasopressin-resistant urine-concentrating defect that leads to polyuria and polydipsia; Na wasting severe enough to require supplementation; hypertension; and anemia. Growth retardation and bone disease are key features in affected children. However, in many patients, these problems develop slowly over years and are so well compensated for that they are not recognized as abnormal until significant uremic symptoms appear. Both disorders eventually cause renal failure.

Nephronophthisis: Inheritance is autosomal recessive. Nephronophthisis accounts for 10 to 20% of chronic renal failure in children and young adults (< 20 yr). There are 4 types: juvenile (types 1 and 4; median age at onset, 13 yr), infantile (type 2; median age at onset, 1 to 3 yr), and adolescent (type 3; median age at onset, 19 yr). Mutations in genes that code for tubular ciliary proteins (nephrocystin for types 1, 2, and 4; inversin for type 2) presumably cause ciliary dysfunction; the mechanism leading to cystic transformation may be similar to that in polycystic kidney disease but is unclear.

The mutation responsible for type 1 causes extrarenal manifestations, including oculomotor apraxia, retinitis pigmentosa (Senior-Loken syndrome), liver fibrosis, cone-shaped epiphyses (Mainzer-Saldino syndrome), and optic nerve coloboma with cerebellar vermis aplasia (Joubert's syndrome type B).

Diagnosis is by history and imaging, but cysts often occur only late in disease. Ultrasonography, CT, or MRI may show smooth renal outlines with normal-sized or small kidneys, loss of corticomedullary differentiation, and multiple cysts at the corticomedullary junction. PCR testing for the gene deletion causing type 1 disease is available.

In early disease, treatment involves management of hypertension, electrolyte and acid-base disorders, and anemia. Children with growth retardation may respond to nutritional supplements and growth hormone therapy. Ultimately, all patients develop renal failure and require dialysis or transplantation.

Medullary cystic kidney disease: Inheritance is autosomal dominant. The disease affects people in their 30s through 70s. There are 2 types, which differ by median age at onset (type 1, 62 yr; type 2, 32 yr) and by genetic mutation (type 1 is localized to chromosome 1; type 2, to chromosome 16). About 15% of patients have no family history, suggesting a sporadic new mutation. Hyperuricemia and gout are the only extrarenal manifestations. End-stage renal disease typically develops at age 30 to 50. Diagnosis and treatment are similar to those of nephronophthisis.

POLYCYSTIC KIDNEY DISEASE

Polycystic kidney disease is a hereditary disorder of renal cyst formation causing gradual enlargement of both kidneys, sometimes with progression to renal failure. Almost all forms are caused by a familial genetic mutation. Symptoms and signs include flank and abdominal pain, hematuria, and hypertension. Diagnosis is by CT or ultrasonography. Treatment is symptomatic before renal failure and with dialysis or transplantation afterward.

Etiology and Pathophysiology

Inheritance of polycystic kidney disease (PKD) is autosomal dominant or recessive; sporadic cases occur rarely. Autosomal dominant polycystic kidney disease (ADPKD) has an incidence of 1/1000 and accounts for 5 to 10% of patients with end-stage renal disease requiring replacement therapy. Clinical manifestations are rare before adulthood, but penetrance is essentially complete; all patients ≥ 80 yr have some signs. Autosomal recessive PKD is rare; incidence is 1/10,000. It frequently causes renal failure during childhood.

In 86 to 96% of cases, ADPKD is caused by mutations in the *PKD1* gene on chromosome 16, which codes for the protein polycystin 1; most other cases are caused by mutations in the *PKD2* gene on chromosome 4, which codes for polycystin 2. A few familial cases are unrelated to either locus. Polycystin 1 may regulate tubular epithelial cell adhesion and differentiation; polycystin 2 may function as an ion channel, with mutations causing fluid secretion into cysts. Mutations in these proteins may alter the function of renal cilia, which enable tubular cells to sense flow rates. A leading hypothesis proposes that tubular cell proliferation and differentiation are linked to flow rate and that ciliary dysfunction may thus lead to cystic transformation.

Early in the disease, tubules dilate and slowly fill with glomerular filtrate. Eventually, the tubules separate from the functioning nephron and fill with secreted rather than filtered fluid, forming cysts. Hemorrhage into cysts may occur, causing hematuria; patients are also at higher risk for acute pyelonephritis and urinary calculi (in 20%). Vascular sclerosis and interstitial fibrosis eventually develop via unknown mechanisms and typically affect < 10% of tubules; nonetheless, renal failure develops in about 35 to 45% of patients by age 60.

Extrarenal manifestations are common. About 1/3 of patients have hepatic cysts, which typically do not affect liver function but may cause right upper quadrant pain if they enlarge or become infected. Patients also have a higher incidence of pancreatic and intestinal cysts, colonic diverticula, and inguinal and abdominal wall hernias.

Valvular heart disorders (most often mitral valve prolapse and aortic regurgitation) can be detected by cardiac ultrasonography in 25 to 30% of patients. Aortic regurgitation results from aortic root dilation due to arterial wall changes (including aortic aneurysm); other valvular disorders may be due to collagen abnormalities. Coronary artery aneurysms also occur.

About 4% of young adults and up to 10% of elderly patients have cerebral aneurysms. Aneurysms rupture in 65 to 75% of patients, usually before age 50; risk factors include family history of aneurysm or rupture, larger aneurysms, and poorly controlled hypertension.

Symptoms and Signs

ADPKD usually causes no symptoms initially; 1/2 of patients remain asymptomatic, never develop renal insufficiency or failure, and are never diagnosed. Most patients who develop symptoms do so by the end of their 20s.

Symptoms include low-grade flank, abdominal, and lower back pain due to cystic enlargement and symptoms of infection. Acute pain, when it occurs, is usually due to hemorrhage into cysts or passage of a calculus; fever is common with acute pyelonephritis. Hepatic cysts may cause right upper quadrant pain. Valvular disorders rarely cause symptoms but occasionally require valvular replacement. Symptoms and signs of unruptured cerebral aneurysm include headache, nausea and vomiting, and cranial nerve deficits; these warrant immediate intervention (see sidebar 211–1 on p. 1798).

Signs are nonspecific and include hematuria (64%), hypertension (50%), and proteinuria (20%). Anemia is less common than in other types of chronic renal failure, presumably because erythropoietin production is preserved. In advanced disease, the kidneys may become grossly enlarged and palpable, causing fullness in the upper abdomen and flank.

Diagnosis

Diagnosis is by history, family history, physical examination, and imaging. Ultrasonography or CT is the imaging test of choice, showing extensive cystic changes throughout the kidneys and a moth-eaten appearance due to cysts that displace functional tissue. Urinalysis detects mild proteinuria and microscopic or macroscopic hematuria. Gross hematuria may be due to a dislodged calculus or to hemorrhage from a ruptured cyst. Pyuria is common even without bacterial infection. Initially, BUN and creatinine are normal or only mildly elevated, but they slowly increase, especially when hypertension is present. Rarely, CBC detects polycythemia.

Patients with symptoms of cerebral aneurysm require high-resolution CT or magnetic resonance angiography; however, there is no consensus on whether asymptomatic patients should be screened for cerebral aneurysm, at what age, and how often. A reasonable approach is to screen patients with ADPKD and a family history of hemorrhagic stroke or cerebral aneurysm.

Genetic testing for *PKD* mutations is currently reserved for patients with PKD and no known family history. Genetic counseling is recommended for 1st-degree relatives of patients with ADPKD.

Prognosis

By age 75, 50 to 75% of patients with ADPKD require renal replacement therapy (dialysis or transplantation). Predictors of more rapid progression to renal failure include earlier age at diagnosis, male sex, black race, *PKD1* genotype, larger renal volume, gross hematuria, rapid increase in kidney size, hypertension, hepatic cysts (in women), and UTIs (in men). ADPKD does not increase risk of renal cancer, but if patients with ADPKD develop renal cancer, it is more likely to be bilateral. Without dialysis or transplantation, patients usually die of uremia or complications of hypertension; about 10% die of intracranial hemorrhage from a ruptured cerebral aneurysm. With dialysis or transplantation, patients die of valvular cardiomyopathy, disseminated infection, or ruptured cerebral aneurysm.

Treatment

Strict BP control is essential, and protein intake must often be restricted to 0.6 to 0.7 g/kg/day. UTIs should be treated promptly. Percutaneous aspiration of cysts may help manage severe pain due to hemorrhage or compression but has no effect on long-term outcome. Nephrectomy is an option to relieve severe symptoms due to massive kidney enlargement or recurrent UTIs. Hemodialysis, peritoneal dialysis, or kidney transplantation is required in patients who develop chronic renal failure. ADPKD does not recur in grafts. With dialysis, patients with ADPKD maintain higher Hb levels than any other group of patients with renal failure.

RENAL CYSTIC DISEASE IN MALFORMATION SYNDROMES

Renal cysts are a prominent feature of several congenital systemic disorders.

Disorders include oral-facial-digital syndrome, von Hippel-Lindau disease, tuberous sclerosis, cerebrohepatorenal (Zellweger), Joubert's, Ivemark's, Meckel-Gruber, Laurence-Moon, Ehlers-Danlos, Ellis-van Creveld, Goldston, and Melnick-Fraser syndromes and asphyxiating thoracic dystrophy (Jeune's syndrome). Trisomies 13, 18, and 21 are also associated with renal cysts (see TABLE 232–1).

Renal cystic dysplasia is congenital renal cystic disease isolated solely to one or both kidneys. Hence, renal cystic dysplasia may be part of a syndrome (with other associated clinical features) or it may be an isolated congenital anomaly.

233 RENAL FAILURE

Renal failure is traditionally categorized as acute or chronic. The former develops rapidly, often over days, whereas the latter progresses slowly over months to years. Some causes overlap.

ACUTE RENAL FAILURE

Acute renal failure is a rapid decrease in renal function over days to weeks, causing an accumulation of nitrogenous products in the blood (azotemia). It often results from major trauma, illness, or surgery but in some cases is caused by a rapidly progressive, intrinsic renal disease. Symptoms include anorexia, nausea, and vomiting, progressing to seizures and coma if the condition is untreated. Fluid, electrolyte, and acid-base disorders develop quickly. Diagnosis is based on laboratory tests of renal function, including serum creatinine, renal failure index, and urinary sediment. Other tests are needed to determine the cause. Treatment is directed at the cause but also includes fluid and electrolyte management and sometimes dialysis.

Etiology and Pathophysiology

Causes of acute renal failure (ARF) can be classified as prerenal, renal, and postrenal (see TABLE 233–1). In all cases, creatinine and urea build up in the blood over several days, and fluid and electrolyte disorders develop. The most serious of these disorders are hyperkalemia and fluid overload (possibly causing pulmonary edema). Phosphate retention leads to hyperphosphatemia. Hypocalcemia is thought to occur from loss of calcitriol production by the injured kidney as well as by Ca phosphate precipitation in the tissues from hyperphosphatemia. Acidosis develops from inability to excrete hydrogen ions. With significant uremia, coagulation may be impaired, and pericarditis may develop. Urine output varies with the type and cause of ARF.

Prerenal azotemia is due to inadequate renal perfusion. The main causes are ECF volume depletion and cardiovascular disease. Prerenal conditions cause about 50 to 80% of ARF but do not cause permanent renal damage (and hence are potentially reversible) unless hypoperfusion is severe enough to produce tubular ischemia. Hypoperfusion of an otherwise functioning kidney leads to enhanced reabsorption of Na and water, resulting in oliguria with high urine osmolality and low urine Na.

Renal causes of ARF involve intrinsic renal disease or damage. Overall, the most common causes are prolonged renal ischemia and nephrotoxins (including IV use of iodinated radiocontrast agents—see Contrast Nephropathy on p. 2016). Disorders may involve the glomeruli, tubules, or interstitium. Glomerular disease reduces GFR and increases glomerular capillary permeability to proteins; it may be inflammatory (glomerulonephritis) or the result of vascular damage from ischemia or vasculitis. Tubules also may be damaged by ischemia and may become obstructed by cellular debris, protein or crystal deposition, and cellular or interstitial edema. Tubular damage impairs reabsorption of Na, so urinary Na tends to be elevated, which is helpful diagnostically. Interstitial inflammation (nephritis) usually involves an immunologic or allergic phenomenon. These factors are complex and interdependent, rendering the previously popular term acute tubular necrosis an inadequate description.

Postrenal azotemia (obstructive nephropathy—see also p. 1963) is due to various types of obstruction in the voiding and collecting parts of the urinary system and is responsible for about 5 to 10% of cases. Obstruction can also occur within the tubules when crystalline or proteinaceous material precipitates. This form of renal failure is often grouped with postrenal failure because the mechanism is obstructive. Obstructed ultrafiltrate flow in tubules or more distally increases pressure in the urinary space of the glomerulus, reducing GFR. Obstruction also affects renal blood flow, initially increasing the flow and pressure in the glomerular capillary by reducing afferent arteriolar resistance. However, within 3 to 4 h, the renal blood flow is reduced, and by 24 h, it has fallen to < 50% of normal because of increased resistance of renal vasculature. Renovascular resistance may take up to a week to return to normal after relief of a 24-h obstruction. To produce significant azotemia, obstruction at the level of the ureter requires involvement of both ureters unless the patient has only a single functioning kidney. Bladder outlet obstruction is probably the most common cause of sudden, and often total, cessation of urinary output in men.

TABLE 233–1. MAJOR CAUSES OF ACUTE RENAL FAILURE

TYPE AND CAUSE	EXAMPLES
Prerenal	
ECF volume depletion	Excessive diuresis, hemorrhage, GI losses, transcellular fluid accumulation (ascites, peritonitis, pancreatitis, burns)
Low cardiac output	Cardiomyopathy, MI, cardiac tamponade, pulmonary embolism
Low systemic vascular resistance	Septicemia, liver failure, antihypertensive agents
Increased renal vascular resistance	Liver failure, NSAIDs, cyclosporine, tacrolimus, anesthesia, renal artery obstruction, renal vein thrombosis, sepsis, hepatorenal syndrome
Renal	
Acute tubular injury	Ischemia (prolonged or severe prerenal state): surgery, hemorrhage, arterial or venous obstruction, NSAIDs, ACE inhibitors, cyclosporine, tacrolimus, radiocontrast, amphotericin B Toxins: aminoglycosides, amphotericin B, foscarnet, radiocontrast, ethylene glycol, hemoglobinuria, myoglobinuria, ifosfamide, heavy metals, methotrexate, streptozotocin
Acute glomerulonephritis	ANCA-associated: crescentic glomerulonephritis, polyarteritis nodosa, Wegener's granulomatosis Anti-GBM glomerulonephritis: Goodpasture's syndrome Immune-complex: lupus glomerulonephritis, postinfectious glomerulonephritis, cryoglobulinemic glomerulonephritis
Acute tubulointerstitial nephritis	Drug reaction (β-lactams, NSAIDs, sulfonamides, ciprofloxacin, thiazide diuretics, furosemide, cimetidine, phenytoin, allopurinol, and others), pyelonephritis, papillary necrosis
Acute vascular nephropathy	Vasculitis, malignant hypertension, thrombotic microangiopathies, scleroderma, atheroembolism
Infiltrative diseases	Lymphoma, sarcoid, leukemia
Postrenal	
Tubular precipitation	Uric acid (tumor lysis), sulfonamides, triamterene, acyclovir, indinavir, methotrexate, Ca oxalate (ethylene glycol ingestion), myeloma protein, myoglobin*
Ureteral obstruction	Intrinsic: calculi, clots, sloughed renal tissue, fungus ball, edema, malignancy, congenital defects Extrinsic: malignancy, retroperitoneal fibrosis, ureteral trauma during surgery or high impact injury
Bladder obstruction	Mechanical: prostatic hypertrophy or cancer, bladder cancer, urethral strictures, phimosis, urethral valves, obstructed indwelling urinary catheter Neurogenic: anticholinergics, upper or lower motor neuron lesion

ANCA = antineutrophil cytoplasmic antibody; GBM = glomerular basement membrane.

*Myoglobin also has toxic effects on the kidney.

Urine output: Prerenal causes typically present with oliguria, not anuria. Anuria usually occurs only in obstructive uropathy or, less commonly, in bilateral renal artery occlusion, acute cortical necrosis, or rapidly progressive glomerulonephritis.

A relatively preserved urine output of 1 to 2.4 L/day is initially present in most renal causes. In acute tubular injury, output may have 3 phases. The prodromal phase, with usually normal urine output, varies in duration depending on causative factors (eg, the amount of toxin ingested, the duration and severity of hypotension). The oliguric phase, with output typically between 50 and 400 mL/day, lasts an average of 10 to 14 days but varies from 1 day to 8 wk. However, many patients are never oliguric. Nonoliguric patients have a lower mortality, morbidity, and need for dialysis. In the postoliguric phase, urine output gradually returns to normal, but serum creatinine and urea levels may not fall for several more days. Tubular dysfunction may persist and is manifested by Na wasting, polyuria (possibly massive) unresponsive to vasopressin, or hyperchloremic metabolic acidosis.

Symptoms and Signs

Initially, weight gain and peripheral edema may be the only findings; often, predominant symptoms are those of the underlying illness or surgical procedure that precipitated renal deterioration. Later, as nitrogenous products accumulate, symptoms of uremia may develop, including anorexia, nausea and vomiting, weakness, myoclonic jerks, seizures, confusion, and coma; asterixis and hyperreflexia may be present on examination. Chest pain, a pericardial friction rub, and findings of pericardial tamponade may occur if uremic pericarditis is present. Fluid accumulation in the lungs may cause dyspnea and crackles on auscultation.

Other findings depend on the cause. Urine may be cola-colored in glomerulonephritis or myoglobinuria. A palpable bladder may be present with outlet obstruction.

Diagnosis

ARF is suspected when urine output falls or serum BUN and creatinine rise. Evaluation should determine the presence and type of ARF and seek an underlying cause. Blood tests generally include CBC, BUN, creatinine, electrolytes (including Ca and PO_4). Urine tests include Na and creatinine concentration and microscopic analysis of sediment. Early detection and treatment increase the chances of reversing renal failure.

A progressive daily rise in serum creatinine is diagnostic of ARF. Serum creatinine can increase by as much as 2 mg/dL/day (180 μmol/L) depending on the amount of creatinine production (which varies with lean body mass) and total body water. A rise of > 2 mg/dL/day suggests overproduction due to rhabdomyolysis.

Urea nitrogen may increase by 10 to 20 mg/dL/day (3.6 to 7.1 mmol urea/L), but BUN may be misleading because it is frequently elevated in response to increased protein catabolism resulting from surgery, trauma, corticosteroids, burns, transfusion reactions, or GI or internal bleeding.

When creatinine is rising, 24-h urine collection for creatinine clearance and the various formulas used to calculate creatinine clearance from serum creatinine are inaccurate and should not be used in estimating GFR, because the rise in serum creatinine concentration is a delayed function of GFR decline.

Other laboratory findings are progressive acidosis, hyperkalemia, hyponatremia, and anemia. Acidosis is ordinarily moderate, with a plasma HCO_3 content of 15 to 20 mmol/L. Serum K concentration increases slowly, but when catabolism is markedly accelerated, it may rise by 1 to 2 mmol/L/day. Hyponatremia usually is moderate (serum Na, 125 to 135 mmol/L) and is related to a surplus of water. The hematologic picture is that of a normochromic-normocytic anemia with an Hct of 25 to 30%.

Hypocalcemia is common and may be profound in patients with myoglobinuric ARF, apparently due to the combined effects of Ca deposition in necrotic muscle, reduced calcitriol production, and resistance of bone to parathyroid hormone (PTH). During recovery from ARF, hypercalcemia may supervene as renal calcitriol production increases, as the bone becomes responsive to PTH, and as Ca deposits are mobilized from damaged tissue.

Cause: Immediately reversible prerenal or obstructive causes must be excluded first. The drug history must be accurately reviewed and all potentially renal toxic drugs stopped.

Prerenal causes are often apparent clinically. If so, correction of an underlying hemodynamic abnormality (eg, with volume infusion) should be attempted. Abatement of ARF confirms a prerenal cause. Urinary indexes (see TABLE 233–2) are particularly helpful in distinguishing prerenal azotemia from acute

TABLE 233–2. DIAGNOSTIC INDICES IN ACUTE RENAL FAILURE

INDEX	PRERENAL	POSTRENAL	TUBULAR INJURY	AGN
U/P osmolality	> 1.5	1 to 1.5	1 to 1.5	1 to 1.5
Urine Na (mmol/L)	< 20	> 40	> 40	< 30
Fractional excretion of Na (FE_{Na})*	< 0.01	> 0.04	> 0.02	< 0.01
Renal failure index†	< 1	> 2	> 2	< 1

*U/P Na ÷ U/P creatinine.
†Urine Na ÷ U/P creatinine ratio.
AGN = acute glomerulonephritis; U/P = urine-to-plasma ratio.

Adapted from Miller TR, et al: "Urinary diagnostic indices in acute renal failure." *Annals of Internal Medicine* 89(1):47–50, 1978; used with permission of the American College of Physicians and the author.

tubular injury, which are the 2 most common causes of ARF in the hospital setting.

Postrenal azotemia should be sought in the absence of obvious prerenal factors. Immediately after the patient voids, a urethral catheter is placed or a bedside ultrasound is used to determine the residual urine in the bladder. A postvoiding residual urine volume > 200 mL suggests bladder outlet obstruction, although detrusor muscle weakness and neurogenic bladder may also cause this. The catheter may be kept in for the 1st day to monitor hourly output but is removed once oliguria is confirmed (if bladder outlet obstruction is not present) to decrease risk of infection. Renal ultrasound is then obtained to diagnose more proximal obstruction. However, ultrasound sensitivity for obstruction is only 80 to 85% because the collecting system is not always dilated, especially when the condition is acute, the ureter is encased (eg, in retroperitoneal fibrosis or neoplasm), or the patient has concomitant hypovolemia. If obstruction is strongly suspected, antegrade or retrograde contrast studies can establish the site of obstruction and guide therapy.

The urinary sediment may provide etiologic clues. Granular casts and cells occur in prerenal azotemia and sometimes in obstructive uropathy. With renal tubular injury, the sediment characteristically contains tubular cells, tubular cell casts, and many brown pigmented granular casts. Urinary eosinophils suggest allergic tubulointerstitial nephritis; RBC casts indicate glomerulonephritis or vasculitis.

Some renal causes are suggested clinically. Patients with glomerulonephritis (see Ch. 235 on p. 1996) often have edema, marked proteinuria (nephrotic syndrome), or signs of arteritis in the skin and retina, often without a history of intrinsic renal disease. Hemoptysis suggests Wegener's granulomatosis or Goodpasture's syndrome; a rash suggests polyarteritis, SLE, or Henoch-Schönlein purpura. Tubulointerstitial nephritis and drug allergy are suggested by a history of drug ingestion and a maculopapular or purpuric rash.

To further differentiate renal causes, antistreptolysin-O and complement titers, antinuclear antibodies, and antinuclear cytoplasmic antibodies are obtained. Renal biopsy may be performed if the diagnosis remains elusive.

In addition to renal ultrasound, other imaging tests are occasionally of use. If evaluating for ureteral obstruction, a noncontrast CT scan is now preferred over antegrade and retrograde urography. In addition to its ability to delineate soft-tissue structures and Ca-containing calculi, CT can detect nonradiopaque calculi. Renal arteriography or venography may be indicated if vascular causes are suggested clinically. Magnetic resonance angiography is increasingly used for diagnosing renal artery stenosis as well as thrombosis of both arteries and veins. Its advantage over radiographic angiography and spiral CT is that it uses gadolinium rather than iodinated contrast and thus is much safer for patients at risk of contrast nephropathy. Kidney size, as obtained from imaging tests, is helpful to know, because a normal or enlarged kidney favors reversibility, whereas a small kidney suggests chronic renal insufficiency.

Prognosis

Although many causes are reversible if diagnosed and treated early, the overall survival rate remains about 50% because many patients with ARF have significant underlying disorders (eg, sepsis, respiratory failure); death is usually the result of these disorders rather than the renal failure itself. Most survivors have adequate kidney function; about 10% require dialysis or transplant—½ right away and the others as renal function slowly deteriorates.

Treatment

Emergency treatment: Life-threatening complications are addressed, preferably in a critical care unit. Pulmonary edema (see p. 663) is treated with O_2, IV vasodilators (eg, nitroglycerin), and diuretics (often ineffective in ARF). Hyperkalemia (see p. 1247) is treated with IV infusion of 10% Ca gluconate, 10 mL; dextrose, 50 g; and insulin, 5 to 10 units. These drugs do not reduce total body K, so further (but slower acting) treatment with oral or rectal Na polystyrene sulfonate 30 g is begun. Although correction of an anion gap metabolic acidosis with $NaHCO_3$ is controversial, the nonanion gap portion of severe metabolic acidosis (pH < 7.20) may with less controversy be treated with IV $NaHCO_3$ in the form of a slow infusion (≤ 150 mEq $NaHCO_3$ in 1 L of 5% D/W). The non-anion gap portion is determined by calculating the increase in anion gap above normal and then subtracting this number from the decrease in HCO_3. HCO_3 is given to raise the serum HCO_3 by this difference.

Hemodialysis or hemofiltration (see also pp. 1991–1992) is initiated when severe electrolyte abnormalities cannot otherwise be controlled (for example K > 6.0) or when pulmonary edema, metabolic acidosis unresponsive to drug treatment, or uremic symptoms occur (eg, vomiting thought to be due to uremia, asterixis, encephalopathy, pericarditis, or seizures). BUN and creatinine levels are probably not the best guides for initiating dialysis in ARF. In asymptomatic patients who are not as seriously ill, particularly those in whom return of renal function is considered likely, dialysis can be deferred until symptoms occur, thus avoiding the need of placing a central venous catheter and its attendant complications.

General measures: Nephrotoxic drugs are stopped, and all drugs excreted by the kidneys (eg, digoxin, some antibiotics) are adjusted; serum levels are useful.

Daily water intake is restricted to a volume equal to the previous day's urine output plus measured extrarenal losses (eg, vomitus) plus 500 to 1000 mL/day for insensible loss. Water intake can be further restricted for hyponatremia or increased for hypernatremia. Although weight gain indicates excess fluid, water intake is not decreased if serum Na remains normal; instead, dietary Na is restricted.

Na and K intake is minimized except with prior deficiencies or GI losses. An adequate diet should be provided, including daily protein intake of about 0.8 to 1 g/kg. If oral intake is impossible, parenteral nutrition is used, but in ARF, risks of fluid overload, hyperosmolality, and infection are increased by IV nutrition. Ca salts (carbonate, acetate) or synthetic non-Ca–containing phosphate binders before meals help maintain serum PO_4 at < 5 mg/dL (< 1.78 mmol/L). To help maintain serum K at < 6 mmol/L in the absence of dialysis, a cation-exchange resin, Na polystyrene sulfonate, is given 15 g po or rectally 1 to 4 times/day as a suspension in water or in a syrup (eg, 70% sorbitol). An indwelling bladder catheter is rarely needed and should be used only when necessary because of an increased risk of UTI and urosepsis.

In many patients, a brisk and even dramatic diuresis after relief of obstruction is a physiologic response to the expansion of ECF during obstruction and does not compromise volume status. However, polyuria accompanied by the excretion of large amounts of Na, K, Mg, and other solutes may cause hypokalemia, hyponatremia, hypernatremia, hypomagnesemia, or marked contraction of ECF volume with peripheral vascular collapse. In this postoliguric phase, close attention to fluid and electrolyte balance is mandatory. Overzealous administration of salt and water after relief of obstruction can prolong diuresis. When postoliguric diuresis occurs, replacement of urine output with 0.45% saline at about 75% of urine output prevents volume depletion and the tendency for excessive free water loss while allowing the body to eliminate excessive volume if this is the cause of the polyuria.

Prevention

ARF can often be prevented by maintaining normal fluid balance, blood volume, and BP in patients with trauma, burns, or major hemorrhage and in those undergoing major surgery. Infusion of isotonic saline and blood may be helpful. If additional pressure support is required, dopamine 1 to 3 μg/kg/min IV may be used; although it can augment renal blood flow and urine output, there is no evidence that dopamine can avert ARF. In incipient ARF, furosemide 40 to 80 mg IV may reestablish normal urine flow or convert oliguric to nonoliguric ARF (mannitol may be beneficial in myoglobinuric ARF); this does not improve renal outcome, but day-to-day fluid management is easier in nonoliguric renal failure.

Use of contrast agents should be minimized, particularly in at-risk groups (eg, the elderly, those with preexisting renal insufficiency, volume depletion, diabetes, or heart failure). If contrast agents are necessary, risk can be lowered by minimizing volume of IV contrast, using non-ionic and low osmolal or iso-osmolal contrast agents, making sure patients are well hydrated before the procedure, avoiding NSAIDs, and pretreating with 0.45% saline at 1 mL/kg/h IV for 12 h before the test. N-acetylcysteine (600 mg po bid the day before and the day of IV contrast) has been used to prevent contrast nephropathy, but reports are conflicting.

Before initiating cytolytic therapy in patients with certain neoplastic diseases (eg, lymphoma, leukemia), treatment with allopurinol should be considered along with alkalinizing the urine (oral $NaHCO_3$ or acetazolamide) and increasing urine flow with increased oral or IV fluids to reduce urate crystalluria.

The renal vasculature is very sensitive to endothelin, a potent vasoconstrictor that reduces renal blood flow and GFR. Endothelin is implicated in progressive renal damage, and endothelin receptor antagonists have successfully slowed or even halted experimental renal disease. Antiendothelin antibodies or endothelin-receptor antagonists are being studied to protect the kidney against ischemic ARF.

CHRONIC RENAL FAILURE

Chronic renal failure is long-standing, progressive deterioration of renal function. Symptoms develop slowly and include anorexia, nausea, vomiting, stomatitis, dysgeusia, nocturia, lassitude, fatigue, pruritus, decreased mental acuity, muscle twitches and cramps, water retention, malnutrition, GI ulceration and bleeding, peripheral neuropathies, and seizures. Diagnosis is based on laboratory testing of renal function, sometimes followed by renal biopsy. Treatment is primarily directed at the underlying condition but includes fluid and electrolyte management and often dialysis and/or transplantation.

Etiology and Pathophysiology

Chronic renal failure (CRF) may result from any cause of renal dysfunction of sufficient magnitude (see TABLE 233–3). The most common cause in the US is diabetic nephropathy (see p. 1277), followed by hypertensive nephroangiosclerosis and various primary and secondary glomerulopathies. Metabolic syndrome (see p. 61), in which hypertension and type 2 diabetes are present, is a large and growing cause of renal damage.

CRF can be roughly categorized as diminished renal reserve, renal insufficiency, and renal failure (end-stage renal disease). Initially, as renal tissue loses function, there are few abnormalities because the remaining tissue increases its performance (renal functional adaptation); a loss of 75% of renal tissue produces a fall in GFR to only 50% of normal. Occasionally, secondary hyperparathyroidism is an early manifestation.

Decreased renal function interferes with the kidneys' ability to maintain fluid and electrolyte homeostasis. Changes proceed predictably, but considerable overlap and individual variation exist. The ability to concentrate urine declines early and is followed by decreases in ability to excrete phosphate, acid, and K. With advanced renal failure (GFR ≤ 10 mL/min/1.73 m^2), the ability to dilute urine is lost, thus urine osmolality is usually fixed close to that of plasma (300 to 320 mOsm/kg), and urinary volume does not respond readily to variations in water intake.

Plasma concentrations of creatinine and urea (which are highly dependent on glomerular filtration) begin a nonlinear rise as GFR diminishes. These changes are minimal early on. When the GFR falls below 6 mL/min/1.73 m^2 (normal = 100 mL/min/1.73 m^2), their levels increase rapidly and are usually associated with systemic manifestations (uremia). Urea and creatinine are not major contributors to the uremic symptoms; they are markers for many other substances, some not yet well defined, that cause the symptoms.

Despite a diminishing GFR, Na and water balance is well maintained by increased fractional excretion of Na and a normal response to thirst. Thus, the plasma Na concentration is typically normal, and hypervolemia is infrequent despite unmodified dietary intake of Na. However, imbalances may occur if Na

TABLE 233–3. MAJOR CAUSES OF CHRONIC RENAL FAILURE

CAUSE	EXAMPLES
Chronic tubulointerstitial nephropathies	(see TABLE 236–3 on p. 2019)
Glomerulopathies	Primary glomerular diseases Focal glomerulosclerosis Idiopathic crescentic glomerulonephritis IgA nephropathy Membranoproliferative glomerulonephritis Membranous nephropathy Glomerulopathies associated with systemic disease Amyloidosis Diabetes mellitus Hemolytic-uremic syndrome Postinfectious glomerulonephritis SLE Wegener's granulomatosis
Hereditary nephropathies	Alport's syndrome Medullary cystic disease Nail-patella syndrome Polycystic kidney disease
Hypertension	Malignant glomerulosclerosis Nephroangiosclerosis
Obstructive uropathy	Benign prostatic hyperplasia Ureteral obstruction (congenital, calculi, malignancies) Vesicoureteral reflux
Renal macrovascular disease (vasculopathy of renal arteries and veins)	

and water intakes are very restricted or excessive. Heart failure can occur from Na and water overload, particularly in patients with underlying cardiac disease.

For substances that are excreted mainly through distal nephron secretion (eg, K), adaptation usually produces a normal plasma concentration until advanced renal failure occurs unless K-sparing diuretics, ACE inhibitors, β-blockers, or angiotensin receptor blockers are used.

Abnormalities of Ca, PO_4, parathyroid hormone (PTH), vitamin D metabolism, and renal osteodystrophy can occur. Typically, hypocalcemia and hyperphosphatemia are present.

Moderate acidosis (plasma HCO_3 content, 15 to 20 mmol/L) and anemia are characteristic. The anemia of CRF is normochromic-normocytic, with an Hct of 20 to 30% (35 to 50% in patients with polycystic kidney disease). It is usually caused by deficient erythropoietin production due to a reduction of functional renal mass (see also Ch. 130 on p. 1036). Other causes include deficiencies of iron, folate, and vitamin B_{12}.

Symptoms and Signs

Patients with mildly diminished renal reserve are asymptomatic, and renal dysfunction can be detected only by laboratory testing. Even a patient with mild to moderate renal insufficiency may have no symptoms despite elevated BUN and creatinine. Nocturia is often noted, principally due to a failure to concentrate the urine. Lassitude, fatigue, anorexia, and decreased mental acuity often are the earliest manifestations of uremia.

With more significant renal insufficiency (eg, creatinine clearance < 10 mL/min for patients without diabetes and < 15 mL/min for those with diabetes), neuromuscular symptoms include coarse muscular twitches, peripheral neuropathies with sensory and motor phenomena, muscle cramps, and seizures (usually the result of hypertensive or metabolic encephalopathy). Anorexia, nausea, vomiting, stomatitis, and an unpleasant taste in the mouth are almost uniformly present. The skin may be yellow-brown. Occasionally, urea from sweat crystallizes on the skin as uremic frost. Pruritus may be especially uncomfortable. Malnutrition leading to generalized tissue wasting is a prominent feature of chronic uremia.

In advanced CRF, pericarditis and GI ulceration and bleeding are common. Hypertension is present in > 80% of patients with advanced renal insufficiency, is usually related to hypervolemia, and is occasionally the result of activation of the renin-angiotensin-aldosterone system. Cardiomyopathy (hypertensive, ischemic) and renal retention of Na and water may lead to dependent edema and heart failure.

Renal osteodystrophy (abnormal bone mineralization resulting from hyperparathyroid function, calcitriol deficiency, elevated serum PO_4, or low or normal serum Ca) usu-

TABLE 233–4. CLASSIFICATION OF ACUTE VERSUS CHRONIC RENAL FAILURE

FINDING	COMMENT
Prior known increase in serum creatinine	Most reliable evidence of CRF
Renal sonogram showing small kidneys	High association with CRF
Renal sonogram showing normal or enlarged kidneys	May be associated with ARF and some forms of CRF (diabetic nephropathy, PCKD, myeloma, malignant nephroangiosclerosis, rapidly progressive glomerulonephritis)
Oliguria, daily increases in serum creatinine and BUN	Probably ARF or ARF superimposed on CRF
Eye-band keratopathy	Probably CRF
No anemia	Probably ARF or CRF from PCKD
Severe anemia, hyperphosphatemia, hypocalcemia	Possibly CRF but seen also in ARF
Subperiosteal erosions on radiography	Probably CRF
Chronic symptoms or signs (eg, fatigue, nausea, pruritus, nocturia, hypertension)	High association with CRF

CRF = chronic renal failure; ARF = acute renal failure; PCKD = polycystic kidney disease.

ally takes the form of hyperparathyroid bone disease (osteitis fibrosa).

Diagnosis

CRF is usually first suspected when serum creatinine rises. The initial step is to determine whether the renal failure is acute, chronic, or acute superimposed on chronic (ie, an acute disease that further compromises renal function in a patient with CRF—see TABLE 233–4).

Diagnosis can often be made based on the history, physical examination, and simple laboratory tests, including urinalysis with microscopic evaluation, electrolytes, urea nitrogen, and creatinine, phosphate, Ca, and CBC. Sometimes specific serologic tests are needed. Distinguishing acute from chronic renal failure is most helped by a history of an elevated creatinine or abnormal urinalysis. An ultrasound of the kidneys is usually helpful in evaluating for obstructive uropathy and in distinguishing acute from chronic renal failure based on kidney size. Except in certain conditions (see TABLE 233–4), chronic renal failure is associated with small shrunken kidneys (usually < 10 cm in length) with thinned, hyperechoic cortex. Obtaining a precise diagnosis becomes increasingly difficult as the patient approaches end-stage renal disease. The definitive diagnostic tool is renal biopsy, but it is not recommended when ultrasonography indicates small, fibrotic kidneys.

Urinalysis findings depend on the nature of the underlying disease, but broad (> 3 WBC diameters wide) or especially waxy (highly refractile) casts often are prominent in advanced renal insufficiency of any cause.

Classification: Chronic kidney disease has been classified into 5 stages.

- Stage 1: Normal GFR (> 90 mL/min/1.73 m^2) and persistent albuminemia
- Stage 2: GFR 60 to 89 mL/min/1.73 m^2
- Stage 3: GFR 30 to 59 mL/min/1.73 m^2
- Stage 4: GFR 15 to 29 mL/min/1.73 m^2
- Stage 5: GFR < 15 mL/min/1.73 m^2

GFR (in mL/min/1.73 m^2) in chronic kidney disease can be estimated by: $186.3 \times (\text{serum creatinine})^{-1.154} \times (\text{age})^{-0.203}$. The result is multiplied by 0.742 if the patient is female and by 1.21 if African American. For female African Americans, the result is multiplied by 0.742 × 1.21.

Prognosis and Treatment

Progression of CRF is indicated in most cases by the degree of proteinuria. Patients with nephrotic-range proteinuria (> 3 g/24 h or urine protein/creatinine > 3) usually have a poorer prognosis and progress to renal failure more rapidly. Progression may occur even if the underlying disorder is not active. Patients with urine protein < 1.5 g/24 h usually progress much more slowly if at all. Hypertension is associated with more rapid progression as well.

Underlying diseases and factors must be controlled. In particular, controlling hyperglycemia in patients with diabetic nephropathy and controlling hypertension in all patients substantially slows deterioration of GFR. ACE inhibitors and angiotensin receptor blockers decrease the rate of decline in GFR in patients with diabetic nephropathy and perhaps also nondiabetic proteinuric patients.

Activity need not be restricted, although fatigue and lassitude usually limit a patient's capacity for exercise. Pruritus may respond to phosphate binders if serum phosphate is elevated. If patients do not respond, ultraviolet phototherapy may help.

Diet: Severe protein restriction in renal disease is controversial. The data are conflicting: ACE inhibitors or angiotensin receptor blocking agents may accomplish the same or a greater hemodynamic benefit than protein restriction. However, protein restricted to 0.6 g/kg/day is safe and easy for most patients to tolerate. Some experts recommend 0.6 g/kg/day for patients with diabetes and > 0.8 g/kg/day for patients without diabetes if GFR is 25 to 55 mL/min/1.73 m^2 or 0.6 g/kg/day if GFR is 13 to 24 mL/min/1.73 m^2. Many uremic symptoms markedly lessen when protein catabolism and urea generation are reduced. Daily protein may be increased if urinary protein loss is significant. Sufficient carbohydrate and fat are given to meet energy requirements and prevent ketosis.

Because dietary restrictions may reduce necessary vitamin intake, patients should take a multivitamin containing water-soluble vitamins. Administration of vitamin A or E is unnecessary. Vitamin D in the form of 1,25-dihydroxyvitamin D (calcitriol) or its analogs should be given under the guidance of PTH levels. When the intact PTH level is >65 pg/mL in stage 3 chronic renal disease or > 100 pg/mL in stage 4 disease, calcitriol 0.25 μg po once/day or 1 to 4 μg 2 times/wk (or a calcitriol analog) should be initiated as long as serum phosphate is not significantly elevated. The dose should be titrated to maintain PTH levels between 100 pg/mL and 300 pg/mL in stage 4 and end-stage renal disease. PTH levels are not corrected to normal to avoid adynamic bone disease. In some patients without secondary hyperparathyroidism, oral calcitriol may be necessary to avoid hypocalcemia despite high oral Ca intake.

Dietary modification may be helpful for hypertriglyceridemia. In the patient with hypercholesterolemia, a statin drug is effective. Fibric acid derivatives (clofibrate, gemfibrozil) may increase risk of rhabdomyolysis in renal failure, especially if taken with statin drugs, whereas ezetimibe (which reduces cholesterol absorption) appears relatively safe in CRF. Correction of hypercholesterolemia may slow progression of the underlying renal disease and reduce coronary risk.

Fluid and electrolytes: Water intake is restricted only when a serum Na concentration of 135 to 145 mmol/L is not maintained. Na restriction of 3 to 4 g/day benefits patients, especially those with edema, heart failure, or hypertension. However, restricting both water and Na intake is often ill advised. K intake is closely related to meat, vegetable, and fruit ingestion and usually does not require adjustment. However, foods (especially salt substitutes) rich in K should generally be avoided. Hyperkalemia is infrequent (except for hyporeninemic hypoaldosteronism or K-sparing diuretic therapy) until end-stage renal failure, when intake may need to be restricted to ≤ 50 mmol/day. Mild hyperkalemia (< 6 mmol/L) can be treated by reducing protein intake and correcting metabolic acidosis. More severe hyperkalemia (> 6 mmol/L) warrants urgent treatment (see pp. 1248 and 1984).

In early renal failure (GFR > 50 mL/min/1.73 m^2, serum phosphate < 5 mg/dL [< 1.6 mmol/L]), dietary PO_4 < 1 g/day is sufficient to delay secondary hyperparathyroidism. When the GFR is < 30 mL/min/1.73 m^2 (serum creatinine concentration about 3 to 5 mg/dL [260 to 440 μmol/L]) and serum phosphate is > 5 mg/dL, phosphate-binding Ca salts (acetate or carbonate but avoid citrate) or non-Ca–containing phosphate binders (sevelamer) should be started to achieve serum phosphate 4.5 to 5.5 mg/dL.

Mild acidosis (pH 7.30 to 7.35) requires no therapy. However, chronic metabolic acidosis (pH < 7.3) is usually associated with a plasma HCO_3 content < 15 mmol/L and symptoms of anorexia, lassitude, dyspnea, and exaggerated protein catabolism and renal osteodystrophy. $NaHCO_3$ 2 g po once/day is increased gradually until symptoms are relieved (HCO_3 content is about 20 mmol/L) or until evidence of Na overloading prevents further therapy.

Anemia and coagulation disorders: Anemia is treated to keep the Hb between 11 and 12 g/dL. Anemia slowly responds to recombinant human erythropoietin (eg, epoetin alfa 50 to 150 units/kg sc 1 to 3 times/wk). Because of increased iron utilization with stimulated erythropoiesis, iron stores must be replaced, usually with parenteral iron. Iron concentrations, iron-binding capacity, and ferritin concentrations should be followed closely. Transfusion should not be undertaken unless anemia is severe (Hb < 8 g/dL) or symptomatic.

The bleeding tendency in CRF rarely needs treatment. Cryoprecipitate, RBC transfusions, desmopressin (0.3 to 0.4 μg/kg [20 μg maximum] in 20 mL of isotonic saline IV over 20 to 30 min), or conjugated estrogens (2.5 to 5 mg po once/day) help when needed. The effects of these treatments last 12 to 48 h, except for conjugated estrogens, which may last for several days.

Heart failure: Symptomatic heart failure is treated with Na restriction and diuretics (see p. 660). If left ventricular function is depressed, ACE inhibitors should be used. Digoxin may be added, but the dosage must be reduced. Diuretics such as furosemide usually are effective even when renal function is markedly reduced, although large doses may be needed. Moderate or severe hypertension should be treated to avoid its deleterious effects on cardiac and renal function. Patients who do not respond to moderate reduction in Na intake (4 g/day) need further dietary Na restriction (2 g/day) and diuretic therapy (furosemide, 80 to 240 mg po bid). Hydrochlorothiazide 50 mg po bid or metolazone 5 to 10 mg po once/day may be added to high-dose furosemide therapy if hypertension or edema is not controlled; even in renal failure, the combination of a thiazide with a loop diuretic is quite potent and must be used with caution to avoid over diuresis. If reduction of the ECF volume does not control BP, conventional antihypertensives are added. Azotemia may increase with such treatment but is acceptable short-term, even if temporary dialysis is required.

Drugs: Impaired renal excretion of drugs must be considered in the care of any patient with renal failure. Common drugs that require revised dosing include penicillins, cephalosporins, aminoglycosides, fluoroquinolones, vancomycin, and digoxin. Hemodialysis reduces the serum concentrations of some drugs, which should be supplemented after hemodialysis. It is strongly recommended that physicians consult a reference on drug dosing in renal failure before prescribing drugs to these very vulnerable patients.

Certain drugs should be avoided entirely in patients undergoing dialysis. They include nitrofurantoin, metformin, and phenazopyridine.

Dialysis: Dialysis is initiated when a patient's creatinine clearance has reached ≤ 10 mL/min in a nondiabetic or ≤ 15 mL/min in a diabetic. Patients with uremic symptoms (eg, anorexia, vomiting, weight loss, fluid overload) without other explanation should be started on dialysis even if renal function has not reached these levels. (For dialysis preparation, see p. 1991.)

If a living kidney donor is available, better long-term outcomes occur when a patient receives the transplanted kidney early, even before beginning dialysis. Patients who are transplant candidates but have no living donor should receive a cadaveric renal transplant as early after initiating dialysis as possible (see p. 1373).

234 RENAL REPLACEMENT THERAPY

Renal replacement therapy (RRT) replaces nonendocrine kidney function in patients with renal failure and is occasionally used for some forms of poisoning. Techniques include intermittent hemodialysis, continuous hemofiltration and hemodialysis, and peritoneal dialysis. All modalities exchange solute and remove fluid from the blood, using dialysis and filtration across permeable membranes.

RRT does not correct the endocrine abnormalities (decreased erythropoietin and 1,25-dihydroxyvitamin D_3 production) of renal failure. In dialysis, serum solute (eg, Na, Cl, K, HCO_3, Ca, Mg, phosphate, urea, creatinine, uric acid) diffuses passively between fluid compartments down a concentration gradient (diffusive transport). In filtration, serum water passes between compartments down a hydrostatic pressure gradient, dragging solute with it (convective transport). The two processes are often used in combination (hemodiafiltration). Hemoperfusion is a rarely used technique that removes toxins by flowing blood over a bed of adsorbent material (usually a resin compound or charcoal). Kidney transplantation (see p. 1373) is considered a form of RRT.

Dialysis and filtration can be performed intermittently or continuously. Continuous therapy is used exclusively for acute renal failure; benefits over intermittent therapy are improved tolerability as a result of slower removal of solute and water. All forms of RRT except peritoneal dialysis require vascular access; continuous techniques require a direct arteriovenous or venovenous circuit.

The choice of technique depends on multiple factors, including the primary need (eg, solute and/or water removal), underlying indication (eg, acute or chronic failure, poisoning), vascular access, hemodynamic stability, availability, local expertise, and patient preference. TABLE 234–1 lists indications and contraindications for the common forms of RRT.

Care of patients requiring long-term RRT ideally involves a nephrologist, psychiatrist, social worker, renal dietitian, dialysis nurses, and the transplant surgical team. Patient assessment should begin when end-stage renal failure is anticipated but before RRT is needed, so that care can be coordinated and the patient can be educated about his options, evaluated for resources and needs, and have vascular access created. Psychosocial evaluation is important because RRT makes the patient

TABLE 234–1. INDICATIONS AND CONTRAINDICATIONS TO COMMON RENAL REPLACEMENT THERAPIES

RENAL REPLACEMENT THERAPY	INDICATIONS	CONTRAINDICATIONS
Hemodialysis	Renal insufficiency or failure (acute or chronic) with Fluid overload Hyperkalemia Hypercalcemia Metabolic acidosis Pericarditis Uremic syndrome GFR < 10 mL/min/1.73 m^2 BSA (no diabetes) GFR < 15 mL/min/1.73 m^2 BSA (diabetes) Some poisonings (see Ch. 326 on p. 2651) Pretransplantation (awaiting donor kidney)	Uncooperative or hemodynamically unstable patient
Peritoneal dialysis	Same indications as for hemodialysis (except for poisonings) in patients who Have inadequate vascular access Prefer self-therapy	Absolute: Recent abdominal wounds, surgery, fistulas; extensive abdominal adhesions Relative: Pulmonary disease, connective tissue diseases (eg, scleroderma, vasculitis), malignant hypertension, or peritoneal fibrosis
Hemoperfusion	Some poisonings (eg, barbiturate, ethchlorvynol, meprobamate, acetaminophen, paraquat, glutethimide)	Uncooperative or hemodynamically unstable patient

GFR = glomerular filtration rate (see p. 1934 for calculation); BSA = body surface area.

socially and emotionally vulnerable. It interrupts routine work, school, and leisure activities; creates anger, frustration, tension, and guilt surrounding dependency; and alters body image because of reduced physical energy, loss or change in sexual function, changed appearance due to access surgery, dialysis catheter placement, needle marks, bone disease, or other physical deterioration. Some patients express these feelings by nonadherence or by being uncooperative with the treatment team. Personality traits that improve prognosis for successful long-term adjustment include adaptability, independence, self-control, tolerance for frustration, and optimism. Emotional stability, family encouragement, consistent treatment team support, and patient and family participation in decision making are also important. Programs that encourage patient independence and maximal resumption of former life interests are more successful in decreasing psychosocial problems.

HEMODIALYSIS

(Intermittent Hemodialysis)

In hemodialysis, a patient's blood is pumped into a dialyzer containing two fluid compartments configured as bundles of hollow fiber capillary tubes or as parallel, sandwiched sheets of semipermeable membranes. In either configuration, blood in the 1st compartment is pumped along one side of a semipermeable membrane while a crystalloid solution (dialysate) is pumped along the other side, in a separate compartment, in the opposite direction. Concentration gradients of solute between blood and dialysate lead to desired changes in the patient's serum solutes, such as a reduction in urea nitrogen and creatinine; an increase in HCO_3; and equilibration of Na, Cl, K, and Mg. The dialysate compartment is under negative pressure relative to the blood compartment to prevent filtration of dialysate into the bloodstream and to remove the excess fluid from the patient. The dialyzed blood is then returned to the patient.

The patient is usually systemically anticoagulated during hemodialysis, but hemodialysis treatment may also be done with regional anticoagulation of the extracorporeal circuit with heparin or trisodium citrate or with saline flush, in which 50 to 100 mL of saline every 15 to 30 min clears the dialysis circuit of any blood clots.

The immediate objectives of hemodialysis are to correct electrolyte and fluid imbalances. Longer-term objectives are to optimize patient's functional status, comfort, and BP; prevent uremia and its complications; and improve survival. The optimal "dose" of hemodialysis is uncertain, but most patients do well with 3 to 5 h of hemodialysis 3 times/wk. Adequacy of each session is defined as a urea reduction ratio (predialysis BUN − postdialysis BUN)/predialysis BUN ≥ 65% or by KT/V ≥ 1.2 (where K is the urea clearance of the dialyzer in mL/min, T is dialysis time in minutes, and V is volume of distribution of urea [total body water] in mL). Hemodialysis dose can be increased by upward changes in dialysis time, blood flow, and increases in membrane surface area or porosity, but benefits are unproven. Short (1.5 to 2.5 h) daily hemodialysis sessions and nightly sessions (6 to 8 h, 5 to 6 days/wk) are being studied as ways to increase effectiveness and decrease complications.

Vascular access: Hemodialysis requires vascular access, achieved by temporary central vein catheterization or by surgical creation of an arteriovenous fistula. Temporary central vein catheterization is generally used only when an arteriovenous fistula has not yet been created or is not ready for use. The primary advantage is that the catheter can be placed quickly in patients who require dialysis urgently; primary disadvantages include a relatively narrow caliber that does not allow for blood flow high enough to achieve optimal clearance, and a high risk of catheter site infection and thrombosis. Catheter-based access can be best achieved by catheterization of the right internal jugular vein. Most internal jugular vein catheters remain useful for 2 to 6 wk if strict aseptic skin care is practiced and if the catheter is used only for hemodialysis. Also, catheters with a subcutaneous tunnel and fabric cuff have a longer life span (50% functional at 1 yr) and may be useful for patients in whom conventional access is impossible.

Surgically created arteriovenous fistulas are better than central venous catheters because they are more durable and less likely to become infected. But they are also prone to complications (thrombosis, infection, aneurysm and pseudoaneurysm). A newly created fistula may take 3 to 6 mo to mature and be useable, so in patients with chronic renal failure, the fistula should be created early, when GFR is between 25 and 30 mL/min. The surgical procedure anastomoses the radial, brachial, or femoral artery to an adjacent vein in an end-of-the-vein to the side-of-the-artery fashion. When the adjacent vein is not suitable for access creation, a piece of prosthetic graft is used. For patients who have poor veins, an autogenous saphenous vein graft is also an option.

Vascular access complications significantly limit the quality of hemodialysis that can be delivered, increase long-term morbidity and mortality, and are common enough that patients and practitioners should be vigilant for changes suggesting infection, thrombosis, and pseudoaneurysm or aneurysm. These changes include pain, erythema, breaks in the skin overlying the access, absence of bruit and pulse in the access, hematoma around the access, and prolonged bleeding from the dialysis cannula puncture site.

The fistula may be monitored for patency by serial ultrasonographic measurements or by measurement of the venous chamber pressure. Treatment of thrombosis, pseudoaneurysm, or aneurysm may involve angioplasty, stenting, and surgery.

Complications: Complications are listed in TABLE 234–2. Hypotension is most common and has multiple causes, including too-rapid water removal, osmotic fluid shifts, acetate in dialysate, heat-related vasodilation, and underlying conditions (eg, autonomic neuropathy, myocardial ischemia, arrhythmias). Many patients also experience cramps, pruritus, nausea and vomiting, headache, and chest and back pain. In most cases, these complications occur for unknown reasons, but some may be part of a first-use syndrome (when the patient's blood is exposed to cuprophane or cellulose membranes in the dialyzer) or dialysis disequilibrium syndrome. More severe cases of dialysis disequilibrium present as disorientation, restlessness, blurred vision, confusion, and seizures. Cause is thought to be cerebral edema. Dialysis amyloidosis affects patients who have been on hemodialysis for years and manifests as carpal tunnel syndrome, bone cysts, arthritis, and cervical spondyloarthropathy.

Prognosis: Overall annual mortality of hemodialysis-dependent patients is 25%, mostly attributable to cardiovascular disease (50%), infection (15 to 20%), and withdrawal from hemodialysis (20%). The 5-yr survival rate for hemodialysis is 35% lower for diabetics (20%) and higher for patients with glomerulonephritis. Blacks have a higher survival rate in all age groups. Nonhemodialysis contributors to mortality include comorbities (eg, hyperparathyroidism, diabetes), age, malnourishment, and late referral for dialysis.

CONTINUOUS HEMOFILTRATION AND HEMODIALYSIS

Continuous hemofiltration and hemodialysis procedures filter and dialyze blood without interruption; the principal advantage is the ability to remove large volumes of fluid while avoiding the hypotensive episodes caused by intermittent hemodialysis. These procedures are therefore indicated for managing patients with acute renal failure who are hemodynamically unstable and/or who must receive large volumes of fluid (eg, patients with multiple organ system failure or shock who require hyperalimentation and/or vasopressor drips).

In continuous hemofiltration, water and solutes up to 20,000 D in molecular weight filter from the blood by convection through a permeable membrane; the filtrate is discarded, and the patient must receive infusions of physiologically balanced water and electrolytes. A dialysis circuit can be added to the filter to improve solute clearance. Procedures may be arteriovenous or venovenous. In arteriovenous procedures, the femoral artery is cannulated, and arterial pressure pushes blood through the filter into the femoral vein. Filtration rates are typically low, especially in hypotensive patients. In continuous venovenous procedures, a pump is required to push blood from one large vein (femoral, subclavian, or internal jugular) through the dialysis circuit and back into the venous circulation. Using a double-lumen catheter, blood is drawn from and returned to the same vein. Advantages include better control of BP and filtration rate with smoother removal of fluid. Neither procedure is proven more effective than the other. All require systemic anticoagulation.

Continuous arteriovenous hemofiltration has the advantage of being usable in a hypotensive patient, but it requires cannulation of both artery and vein, whereas continuous venovenous hemofiltration requires only cannulation of one vein and provides more predictable ultrafiltration but needs a higher BP.

PERITONEAL DIALYSIS

Peritoneal dialysis uses the peritoneum as a natural permeable membrane through which water and solutes can equilibrate. Peritoneal dialysis is less physiologically stressful than hemodialysis, does not require vascular ac-

TABLE 234–2. COMPLICATIONS OF RENAL REPLACEMENT THERAPY

COMPLICATION	HEMODIALYSIS	PERITONEAL DIALYSIS
Mechanical	Thrombosis, infection, and hemorrhage of the arteriovenous fistula Stenosis or thrombosis of the subclavian vein or superior vena cava due to recurrent use of subclavian and internal jugular vein catheters	Hematoma in the pericatheter tract Intra-abdominal bleeding Perforation of a viscus (early and late), spontaneous or due to catheter insertion Dialysate leakage around the catheter Dissection of fluid into the abdominal wall Catheter obstruction by clots, fibrin, omentum, or fibrous encasement
Infectious	Vascular access cellulitis or abscess Colonization of temporary central venous catheters Bacteremia, meningitis, endocarditis, osteomyelitis	Peritonitis* Catheter exit site infection*
Cardiovascular	Hypotension due to excessive ultrafiltration* Arrhythmia Air embolism Cardiac tamponade	Hypotension Pulmonary edema Arrhythmia
Pulmonary	Dyspnea due to anaphylactic reaction to hemodialysis membrane	Atelectasis Pleural effusion Pneumonia
Metabolic	Hyponatremia and hypernatremia Hypokalemia	Hyperglycemia Hypoalbuminemia Hypertriglyceridemia Obesity
Miscellaneous	Fever due to bacteremia, pyrogens, or overheated dialysate Hemorrhage (GI, intracranial, retroperitoneal, intraocular) Pruritus Seizures Muscle cramps Restlessness Insomnia Amyloid deposits	Peritoneal sclerosis Hypothermia Seizures Abdominal and inguinal hernias

*Most common.

cess, can be performed at home, and allows patients much greater flexibility. However, it requires much more patient involvement. Of the total estimated resting splanchnic blood flow of 1200 mL/min, only about 70 mL/min comes into contact with the peritoneum, so solute equilibration occurs much more slowly than in hemodialysis. But because solute and water clearance is a function of contact time and peritoneal dialysis is performed nearly continuously, efficacy in terms of solute removal is equivalent to that obtained with hemodialysis.

In general, dialysate is instilled through a catheter into the peritoneal space, is left to dwell, and then drained. In the double-bag technique, the patient drains the fluid instilled in the abdomen in one bag and then infuses fluid from the other bag into the peritoneal cavity.

Continuous ambulatory peritoneal dialysis (CAPD) is most commonly used because of ease of performance and lack of need for a machine to perform the exchanges. A typical adult infuses 2 to 3 L (children, 30 to 40 mL/kg) of dialysate 4 to 5 times/day; dialysate is allowed to remain for 4 h during the day and 8 to 12 h at night. The solution is manually drained. Flushing the infusion set before filling reduces peritonitis rates.

Continuous cyclic peritoneal dialysis (CCPD) uses a long (12 to 15 h) daytime dwell and 3 to 6 nighttime exchanges performed with an automated cycler. Patients have more freedom during the day, but cumbersome equipment inhibits nighttime mobility. Some patients require a combination of CAPD and CCPD to achieve adequate clearances.

Intermittent peritoneal dialysis (IPD) may be manual or automated. Manual IPD is simplest, achieves the highest solute clearance, and is useful chiefly in the treatment of acute renal failure. In adults, 2 to 3 L (in children, 30 to 40 mL/kg) of dialysate, warmed to 37° C, is infused over 10 to 15 min, allowed to dwell in the peritoneal cavity for 30 to 40 min, and drained in about 10 to 15 min. Multiple exchanges may be needed over 12 to 48 h. Automated cycler IPD uses an automated system that cycles the infusion and removal of dialysate. The cycler is generally set up at bedtime, and treatment occurs while the patient sleeps.

Access: Peritoneal dialysis requires intraperitoneal access, usually via a soft silicone rubber or porous polyurethane catheter. The catheter may be implanted in the operating room under direct visualization or at the bedside by blind insertion of a trocar or under visualization through a peritoneoscope. Most catheters incorporate a polyester fabric cuff that allows tissue ingrowth from the skin or preperitoneal fascia, ideally resulting in a watertight, bacteria-impervious seal and preventing introduction of organisms along the catheter tract. Allowing 10 to 14 days between catheter implantation and use improves healing and reduces the frequency of early pericatheter leakage of dialysate. Double-cuff catheters are better than single-cuff catheters. Also, a caudally directed exit site lowers the incidence of exit site infections.

Once access is established, the patient undergoes a peritoneal equilibration test, in which dialysate drained after a 4 h dwell time is analyzed and compared with serum to determine solute clearance rates. This procedure helps determine the patient's peritoneal transport characteristics, the dose of dialysis required, and the most appropriate technique. In general, adequacy is defined as a weekly $KT/V \geq 2.0$ (where K is the urea clearance in mL/min, T is dialysis time in minutes, and V is volume of distribution of urea [total body water] in mL) and a weekly creatinine clearance of ≥ 50 L/wk/per 1.73 m^2 BSA.

Complications: (see also TABLE 234–2): The most important and common are peritonitis and catheter exit site infection. Symptoms and signs of peritonitis include abdominal pain, cloudy peritoneal fluid, fever, nausea, and tenderness to palpation. Diagnosis is made by Gram stain and culture of peritoneal fluid and WBC count with differential. Gram stain is often unrevealing, but cultures are positive in > 90%. About 90% also have > 100 WBCs/μL, usually neutrophils (lymphocytes with fungal peritonitis). Negative cultures and WBC counts < 100/μL do not exclude peritonitis; they may be due to prior antibiotic use, catheter exit site or tunnel infection, or sampling of too little fluid. Treatment is initially with a combination of a 1st-generation cephalosporin and a 3rd-generation cephalosporin (eg, ceftazidime) or an aminoglycoside (eg, gentamicin); drugs are adjusted based on the result of peritoneal dialysis fluid culture. Antibiotic therapy is usually given IV or IP (intraperitoneally) for peritonitis and orally for exit site infections.

Catheter tunnel exit site infection manifests as tenderness over the tunnel or at the exit site along with crusting, erythema, or drainage. Diagnosis is clinical. Treatment of infection without drainage is topical antiseptics (eg, povidone iodine, chlorhexidine); otherwise a 1st-generation cephalosporin or a penicillinase-resistant penicillin is used.

Prognosis: Most cases of peritonitis respond to prompt antibiotic therapy, but those caused by staphylococci or fungi also require dialysis catheter removal. Overall, 5-yr survival rate in peritoneal dialysis patients is similar to that in hemodialysis patients (about 35%).

MEDICAL ASPECTS OF LONG-TERM RENAL REPLACEMENT THERAPY

All long-term RRT patients develop accompanying metabolic and other disorders.

These require appropriate attention and adjunctive treatment. Approach varies by patient but typically includes nutritional modifications and management of multiple metabolic abnormalities (see also p. 1988).

Diet should be tightly controlled. Generally, hemodialysis patients tend to be anorexic and should be encouraged to eat a daily diet of 35 kcal/kg ideal body weight (in children, 40 to 70 kcal/kg/day depending on age and activity). Daily Na intake should be limited to 2 g (88 mEq), K to 60 mEq, and P to 800 to 1000 mg. Fluid intake is limited to 1000 to 1500 mL/day and monitored by weight gain between dialysis treatments. Patients undergoing peritoneal dialysis need a more liberal intake of protein (1.25 to 1.5 g/kg) to replace peritoneal losses (10 to 20 g/day). Survival is best among patients (both hemodialysis and peritoneal dialysis) who maintain a serum albumin > 3.5 g/dL; serum albumin is the best predictor of survival in these patients.

Anemia of renal failure should be treated with recombinant human erythropoietin and iron supplementation (see p. 1988). Because the absorption of oral iron is limited, many patients require IV iron during hemodialysis (Na ferric gluconate, iron dextran, iron sucrose). Iron stores are assessed using serum iron, total iron-binding capacity, and serum ferritin, typically before the start of erythropoietin therapy and thereafter every other month. Iron deficiency is the most common reason for erythropoietin resistance. However, some dialysis patients who have received multiple blood transfusions have iron overload (see p. 1131) and should not be given iron supplements.

Coronary artery disease risk factors must be managed aggressively because many patients who require RRT are hypertensive, dyslipidemic, or diabetic; smoke cigarettes; and ultimately die of cardiovascular disease. Continuous peritoneal dialysis is more effective in removing fluid; as a result, these patients require fewer antihypertensive drugs. Hypertension can also be controlled in about 80% of hemodialysis patients by filtration alone. Antihypertensives are required in the remaining 20%. Patients given ACE inhibitors or angiotensin receptor blockers may need closer monitoring of serum K^+ to prevent hyperkalemia. For approaches to dyslipidemia and diabetes management, see p. 1302 and p. 1274, respectively, and for smoking cessation, see p. 2733.

Hyperphosphatemia, a consequence of phosphate retention from low GFR, increases risk for soft-tissue calcification, especially in coronary arteries and heart valves, when Ca × P > 70. It also stimulates development of secondary hyperparathyroidism. Initial treatment is Ca-based antacids (Ca carbonate 1 to 6 g po tid, Ca acetate 1334 to 2668 mg po tid with meals), which function as phosphate binders and reduce P levels. Constipation and abdominal bloating are complications of chronic use. Patients should be monitored for hypercalcemia. Sevelamer hydrochloride 800 to 1600 mg or lanthanum carbonate 250 to 1000 mg with each meal is an option for patients who develop hypercalcemia while taking these antacids. Some patients require addition of aluminum-based phosphate binders, but these should be used short-term only (eg, 1 to 2 wk as needed) to prevent aluminum toxicity (see below).

Hypocalcemia and secondary hyperparathyroidism often coexist as a result of impaired renal production of vitamin D. Treatment of hypocalcemia is with calcitriol either orally (0.25 to 1.0 μg po once/day) or IV (1 to 3 μg in adults and 0.01 to 0.05 μg/kg in children per dialysis treatment). Treatment can increase serum phosphate level and should be withheld until the level is normalized to avoid soft-tissue calcification. Doses are titrated to suppress parathyroid hormone (PTH) levels to 100 to 300 pg/mL (PTH reflects bone turnover better than serum Ca). Oversuppression decreases bone turnover and leads to adynamic bone disease, which carries a high risk of fracture. The vitamin D analogs doxercalciferol and paricalcitol have less effect on Ca and P absorption from the gut but suppress PTH equally well. Early hints that these agents may reduce mortality compared with calcitriol require confirmation. Cinacalcet, a calcimimetic drug, increases sensitivity of parathyroid Ca-sensing receptors to Ca and may also be indicated for hyperparathyroidism, but its role in routine practice has yet to be defined. Its ability to decrease PTH levels by as much as 75% may decrease the need for parathyroidectomy in these patients.

Aluminum toxicity is much less common than it once was, but it remains a risk in hemodialysis patients because of exposure to aluminum-based phosphate binders. Manifestations are osteomalacia, microcytic anemia (iron-resistant), and probably dialysis dementia (a constellation of memory loss, dyspraxia, hallucinations, facial grimaces, myoclonus, seizures, and a characteristic EEG). Diagnosis is by measurement of plasma aluminum before and 2 days after IV infusion of deferoxamine 5 mg/kg. A rise in aluminum level of ≥50 μg/L suggests toxicity. Aluminum-related osteomalacia can also be diagnosed by needle biopsy of bone (requires special stains for aluminum). Treatment is avoidance of aluminum-based binders plus IV or intraperitoneal deferoxamine.

Bone disease (renal osteodystrophy) has multiple causes, including vitamin D deficiency, secondary hyperparathyroidism, chronic metabolic acidosis, and aluminum toxicity; treatment is that of the underlying cause.

Vitamin deficiencies result from dialytic loss of water-soluble vitamins (eg, B, C, folic acid) and can be replenished with daily multivitamin supplements.

Calciphylaxis is a rare disorder of systemic arterial calcification causing diffuse tissue ischemia and necrosis. Cause is unknown, though hyperparathyroidism, vitamin D supplementation, and elevated Ca and P levels are thought to contribute. It manifests as painful, violaceous, purpuric plaques and nodules that ulcerate, form eschars, and become infected. Treatment is supportive.

Constipation is a minor but troubling aspect of long-term RRT and, because of resulting bowel distention, may interfere with catheter drainage in peritoneal dialysis. Many patients require osmotic (eg, sorbitol) or bulk (eg, psyllium) laxatives. Laxatives containing Mg or phosphate should be avoided.

235 GLOMERULAR DISEASES

Glomerular diseases are classified as those that present predominantly with hematuria (nephritic syndrome), high-level proteinuria (nephrotic syndrome), or both (see TABLE 235–1). The diseases may be primary or have secondary causes (see TABLES 235–2 and 235–3). The pathophysiology of nephritic and nephrotic diseases differs substantially, but their clinical overlap is considerable—eg, several diseases may present with the same clinical picture—and the presence of hematuria or proteinuria does not itself predict response to treatment and prognosis.

The diagnosis of glomerular disease is usually made when screening or diagnostic testing reveals elevated serum creatinine and abnormal urinalysis (hematuria with or without casts, proteinuria, or both). Approach to the patient involves distinguishing predominant-nephritic from predominant-nephrotic features and identifying likely causes by patient age (see TABLE 235–1), accompanying illness (see TABLES 235–2 and 235–3), and other elements of the history (eg, time course, systemic manifestations, family history). Renal biopsy is indicated when diagnosis is unclear from history or when histology influences choice of treatment and outcomes (eg, lupus nephritis).

NEPHRITIC SYNDROME

Nephritic syndrome is defined by hematuria and RBC casts on microscopic examination of urinary sediment. Often one or more elements of mild to moderate proteinuria, edema, hypertension, elevated serum creatinine, and oliguria are also present. It has both primary and secondary causes. Diagnosis is based on history, physical examination, and sometimes renal biopsy. Treatment and prognosis vary by cause.

Nephritic syndrome is a manifestation of glomerular inflammation (glomerulonephritis [GN]) and occurs at any age. Causes differ by age (see TABLE 235–1), and mechanisms differ by cause. Acute and chronic forms exist. Postinfectious GN is the prototype of acute GN, but the condition may be caused by other glomerulopathies and by systemic diseases such as connective tissue disorders and paraproteinemias (see TABLE 235–2). Chronic GN has features similar to acute GN but develops slowly and may display mild to moderate proteinuria. Examples include IgA nephropathy and hereditary nephritis.

TABLE 235–1. GLOMERULAR DISEASES BY AGE AND PRESENTATION

AGE (yr)	NEPHRITIC SYNDROME	NEPHROTIC SYNDROME	MIXED NEPHRITIC AND NEPHROTIC SYNDROME
< 15	Mild PIGN IgA nephropathy Thin basement membrane disease Hereditary nephritis Henoch-Schönlein purpura Lupus nephritis	Minimal change disease Focal and segmental glomerulosclerosis Lupus (membranous nephropathy)	Lupus nephritis Membranoproliferative GN
15–40	IgA nephropathy Thin basement membrane disease Lupus nephritis Hereditary nephritis Mesangial proliferative GN RPGN PIGN	Focal and segmental glomerulosclerosis Minimal change disease Membranous nephropathy Diabetic nephropathy Preeclampsia Late PIGN IgA nephropathy	Membranoproliferative GN Fibrillary and immunotactoid GN* IgA nephropathy
> 40	IgA nephropathy RPGN Vasculitides PIGN	Focal and segmental glomerulosclerosis Membranous nephropathy Diabetic nephropathy Minimal change disease IgA nephropathy Amyloidosis (primary) Light chain deposition disease Benign nephrosclerosis Late PIGN	IgA nephropathy Fibrillary and immunotactoid GN*

*More commonly manifests as nephrotic syndrome.

PIGN = postinfectious glomerulonephritis; GN = glomerulonephritis, RPGN = rapidly progressive glomerulonephritis

Adapted from Rose BD. *Pathophysiology of Renal Disease* (2nd edition). New York: McGraw-Hill, 1987, p. 167.

HEREDITARY NEPHRITIS

(Alport's Syndrome)

Hereditary nephritis is a genetically heterogenous disorder characterized by hematuria, impaired renal function, sensorineural deafness, and ocular abnormalities. Cause is a gene mutation affecting type IV collagen. Symptoms and signs are those of nephritic syndrome with sensorineural deafness and, less commonly, those of ophthalmologic diseases. Diagnosis is by family history and urinalysis. Treatment is that of chronic renal failure.

Hereditary nephritis is caused by a mutation in the *COL4A5* gene that encodes the α-5 chain of type IV collagen and produces altered type IV collagen strands. The mechanism by which this causes glomerular disease is unknown, but impaired structure and function are presumed; in most families, thickening and thinning of the glomerular and tubular basement membranes occur, with multilamination of the lamina densa in a focal or local distribution. Although autosomal recessive varieties exist, the disease is most commonly inherited in X-linked fashion.

Symptoms and Signs

Because of X-linked transmission, women usually are asymptomatic and have little functional impairment. Most men eventually develop renal symptoms and signs similar to those of acute nephritic syndrome and progress to renal insufficiency between ages 20 and 30.

TABLE 235–2. CAUSES OF GLOMERULONEPHRITIS

TYPE	EXAMPLES	TYPE	EXAMPLES
Primary GN			Parasitic:
Idiopathic	Fibrillary GN Idiopathic crescentic GN IgA nephropathy Membranoproliferative GN		Malaria (*Plasmodium falciparum, P. malariae*) Schistosomiasis (*Schistosoma haematobium, S. mansoni*) Toxoplasmosis
Secondary GN			Other: Fungi (*Candida albicans, Coccidioides immitis*) Rickettsiae
Postinfectious GN	Bacterial: Group A β-streptococcal infection *Mycoplasma* *Neisseria meningitidis* Staphylococcal infections (especially bacterial endocarditis) *Streptococcus pneumoniae* Visceral abscesses (*Escherichia coli, Pseudomonas, Proteus, Klebsiella, Clostridium*)	Connective tissue diseases	Henoch-Schönlein purpura Polyarteritis nodosa SLE Wegener's granulomatosis
		Hematologic dyscrasias	Mixed IgG-IgM cryoglobulinemia Serum sickness Thrombotic thrombocytopenic purpura–hemolytic-uremic syndrome
	Viral: Coxsackievirus Cytomegalovirus Epstein-Barr virus Hepatitis B virus Hepatitis C virus Herpes zoster virus Measles Mumps Varicella	Glomerular basement membrane diseases	Goodpasture's syndrome

GN = glomerulonephritis.

Sensorineural deafness frequently is present, affecting higher frequencies. Some patients have nerve deafness alone without renal disease but can transmit the renal disease to a subsequent generation. Ophthalmologic abnormalities—cataracts (most common), anterior lenticonus, spherophakia, nystagmus, retinitis pigmentosa, blindness—also occur but less frequently than deafness. Other nonrenal manifestations include polyneuropathy and thrombocytopenia.

Diagnosis and Treatment

Diagnosis is suggested by personal and family history and by findings of microscopic hematuria on urinalysis or recurrent episodes of gross hematuria, particularly if abnormalities of hearing or vision are present. The urine may contain small amounts of protein, WBCs, and casts of various types. Nephrotic syndrome occurs rarely. No distinguishing histologic changes are seen on light or immunofluorescence microscopy. Although not widely available, immunohistochemistry for the α-5 chain in skin and, in particular, genetic analysis may become the diagnostic techniques of choice.

Treatment is indicated only when uremia occurs; its management is the same as for other causes of chronic renal failure (see p. 1987). Transplantation has also been successful. Genetic counseling is indicated.

IMMUNOGLOBULIN A NEPHROPATHY

IgA nephropathy is deposition of IgA immune complexes in glomeruli, manifesting as slowly progressive hematuria, proteinuria, and, often, renal insufficiency. Diagnosis is based on urinalysis and renal biopsy. Prognosis is generally good. Treatment options include ACE inhibitors, corticosteroids, and ω-3 polyunsaturated fatty acids.

IgA nephropathy is a form of chronic GN characterized by the deposition of IgA immune complexes in glomeruli. It is the most common form of GN worldwide. It occurs at all ages, with a peak onset in the teens and 20s; affects men 2 to 6 times more frequently than women; and is more common in whites and Asians than in blacks. Prevalence estimates are 5% in the US, 10 to 20% in southern Europe and Australia, and 30 to 40% in Asia.

Cause is unknown, but evidence suggests that IgA nephropathy may arise through multiple pathogenetic mechanisms, including increased IgA1 production, defective IgA1 glycosylation causing increased binding to mesangial cells, decreased IgA1 clearance, a defective mucosal immune system, and overproduction of cytokines stimulating mesangial cell proliferation. Familial clustering has also been observed, suggesting genetic factors at least in some cases.

Renal function is initially normal, but symptomatic renal disease may develop. A few patients present with acute or chronic renal failure, severe hypertension, or nephrotic syndrome.

Symptoms and Signs

The most common presentation is persistent or recurrent macroscopic hematuria

TABLE 235–3. CAUSES OF NEPHROTIC SYNDROME

CAUSES	EXAMPLES
Primary causes	
Idiopathic	Fibrillary and immunotactoid GN, focal segmental glomerulosclerosis, IgA nephropathy*, membranoproliferative GN, membranous nephropathy, minimal change disease, rapidly progressive GN*
Secondary causes	
Metabolic	Amyloidosis, diabetes mellitus
Immunologic	Cryoglobulinemia, erythema multiforme, Henoch-Schönlein purpura, polyarteritis nodosa, serum sickness, Sjögren's syndrome, SLE
Idiopathic	Castleman disease, sarcoidosis
Neoplastic	Carcinoma (bronchus, breast, colon, stomach, kidney), leukemia, lymphomas, melanoma, multiple myeloma
Drug-related	Gold, heroin, interferon, lithium, NSAIDs, mercury, pamidronate, penicillamine
Infectious	Bacterial (infective endocarditis, leprosy, postinfectious GN, syphilis, vascular prosthetic nephritis)
	Viral (Epstein-Barr virus, hepatitis B and C, herpes zoster virus, HIV)
	Protozoal (filariasis, helminthic, malaria, schistosomiasis)
Allergic	Antitoxins, insect stings, poison ivy or oak, snake venoms
Genetic syndromes	Alport's syndrome*, congenital nephrotic syndrome (Finnish type), corticosteroid-resistant nephrotic syndrome, Denys-Drash syndrome, Fabry's disease, familial FSGS
Physiologic	Adaptation to reduced nephrons, morbid obesity, oligomeganephronia
Miscellaneous	Chronic allograft nephropathy, malignant hypertension, preeclampsia

*More commonly manifests as nephritic syndrome.

GN = glomerulonephritis; FSGS = focal segmental glomerulonephritis.

(90% of involved children) or asymptomatic microscopic hematuria with mild proteinuria. Other symptoms are usually not prominent.

Gross hematuria in IgA nephropathy usually begins 1 or 2 days after a febrile mucosal (upper respiratory, sinus, enteral) illness, thus mimicking acute GN, except the onset of hematuria is earlier, coinciding with or immediately after the febrile illness and may be accompanied by loin pain. Hypertension is unusual at diagnosis.

Diagnosis

Diagnosis is suggested by urinalysis and confirmed by biopsy. Urinalysis demonstrates microscopic hematuria, usually with dysmorphic RBCs and RBC casts. Mild proteinuria (< 1 g/day) is typical and may occur without hematuria; nephrotic syndrome develops in ≤ 20%.

Serum creatinine and complement concentrations are usually normal. Plasma IgA concentration may be increased, and circulating IgA-fibronectin complexes are present; however, these findings are of dubious value.

Renal biopsy shows granular deposition of IgA and C3 on immunofluorescent staining in an expanded mesangium with foci of segmental proliferative or necrotizing lesions. Importantly, mesangial IgA deposits are nonspecific and also occur in many other diseases, including Henoch-Schönlein purpura (HSP), hepatic cirrhosis, inflammatory bowel disease, psoriasis, HIV infection, lung cancer, and multiple connective tissue diseases. Glomerular IgA deposition is a primary feature of HSP, and the 2 disorders may be indistinguishable on biopsy, leading to the proposal that HSP may be a systemic form of IgA nephropathy. However, HSP is clinically distinct from IgA nephropathy, usually manifesting as purpuric rash, arthralgias, and abdominal pain (see p. 275).

Prognosis

IgA nephropathy usually progresses slowly; renal insufficiency and hypertension develop within 10 yr in 15 to 20% of cases. Progression to end-stage renal disease occurs in 25% of patients after 20 yr. When IgA nephropathy is diagnosed in childhood, prognosis is usually good. However, persistent hematuria invariably leads to hypertension, proteinuria, and renal insufficiency. Older age at onset, hypertension, persistent severe proteinuria, absence of recurrent macroscopic hematuria, elevated serum creatinine, and advanced glomerular sclerosis or crescent formation and tubulointerstitial disease are risk factors for progression to renal failure.

Treatment

Normotensive patients with intact renal function (creatinine < 1.2 mg/dL) and only mild proteinuria (< 1 g/day) usually are not treated unless renal function worsens or proteinuria progresses. Patients with renal insufficiency and more severe proteinuria and hematuria are usually offered treatment, which ideally should be started before significant renal insufficiency.

ACE inhibitors are used on the premise that they reduce BP and proteinuria, but data on efficacy are contradictory. Patients with the DD genotype for the ACE gene may be at greater risk of disease progression and more likely to respond. For patients with hypertension, ACE inhibitors or angiotensin receptor blockers are the antihypertensives of choice even for relatively mild renal disease. Combination ACE inhibitor–angiotensin receptor blocker therapy should be given if monotherapy does not control hypertension or reduce proteinuria.

Corticosteroids have been used for many years, but benefit is not well documented. One protocol uses methylprednisolone 1 g IV once/day for 3 days at the beginning of months 1, 3, and 5 plus prednisone 0.5 mg/kg po every other day for 6 mo. Because of the risk of adverse effects, corticosteroids should probably be reserved for patients whose disease progresses, as shown by worsening proteinuria or renal function, or for patients who present with heavy proteinuria (> 2 g/24 h) or significant renal insufficiency (creatinine clearance < 60 mL/min). Combinations of corticosteroids, cyclophosphamide, and azathioprine are also used, but efficacy and safety compared with corticosteroids alone are uncertain. Mycophenolate is also under investigation. None of these drugs, however, prevents recurrence in transplant patients.

ω-3 Polyunsaturated fatty acids, available in fish oil supplements, have been used to treat IgA nephropathy, but data on efficacy are contradictory. Mechanism of effect may include alterations in inflammatory cytokines. Other interventions have been tried to lower IgA overproduction and to inhibit mesangial proliferation. Elimination of gluten, dairy products, eggs, and meat from the diet; tonsillectomy; and immune globulin (1 g/kg IV 2 days/mo for 3 mo followed by immune globulin

0.35 mL/kg of 16.5% solution IM q 2 wk for 6 mo) all theoretically reduce IgA production. Heparin, dipyridamole, and statins are just a few examples of in vitro mesangial cell inhibitors. Data supporting any of these interventions are limited or absent, and none can be recommended for routine treatment.

Renal transplantation is better than dialysis because of excellent long-term disease-free survival. The condition recurs in ≤ 15% of graft recipients.

POSTINFECTIOUS GLOMERULONEPHRITIS

Postinfectious GN occurs after infection, usually with a nephritogenic strain of group A β-hemolytic streptococcus. Diagnosis is suggested by history and urinalysis and confirmed by low complement. Prognosis is excellent. Treatment is supportive.

Etiology

Postinfectious GN (PIGN) is the most common cause of glomerular disease in children between 5 and 15 yr; it is rare in children < 2 yr and in adults > 40 yr.

Most cases are caused by nephritogenic strains of group A β-hemolytic streptococcus, most notably types 12 (pharyngitis) and 49 (impetigo); an estimated 5 to 10% of patients with streptococcal pharyngitis and about 25% of those with impetigo develop the condition. A latency period of 6 to 21 days between infection and GN onset is typical, but latency may extend up to 6 wk.

Less common pathogens are nonstreptococcal bacteria, viruses, parasites, rickettsiae, and fungi (see TABLE 235–2). Bacterial endocarditis and ventriculoatrial shunt infections are additional important conditions in which PIGN develops; ventriculoperitoneal shunts are more resistant to infection.

The mechanism of disease is unknown, but microbial antigens are thought to bind to the glomerular basement membrane and activate complement both directly and via interaction with circulating antibodies, causing glomerular damage, which may be focal or diffuse.

Symptoms and Signs

Symptoms and signs range from asymptomatic hematuria (in about 50%) and mild proteinuria to full-blown nephritis with microscopic or gross hematuria (cola-colored, brown, smoky, or frankly bloody), proteinuria, oliguria, edema, hypertension, and renal insufficiency. Severe, late disease is a relatively uncommon cause of nephrotic syndrome. Flank pain may be attributable to stretching of the renal capsule. Renal failure that causes fluid overload with heart failure and urgent or malignant hypertension and requires dialysis affects 1 to 2% of patients and may present as a pulmonary-renal syndrome with hematuria and hemoptysis (see p. 486). Fever is unusual and suggests persistent infection.

Clinical manifestations of nonstreptococcal PIGN may mimic other diseases (eg, polyarteritis nodosa, renal emboli, antimicrobial drug–induced acute interstitial nephritis).

Diagnosis

Streptococcal PIGN is suggested by history of pharyngitis or impetigo and urinalysis. Biopsy confirms the diagnosis but is rarely necessary; demonstration of hypocomplementemia is essentially confirmatory. Serum creatinine may rise rapidly but usually peaks below a level requiring dialysis.

Antistreptolysin O, the most common test of recent streptococcal infection, increases and remains elevated for several months in about 75% of patients with pharyngitis and in about 50% of patients with impetigo, but it is not specific. An increase in antihyaluronidase and antideoxyribonuclease titers is more specific for detecting recent streptococcal skin infection but is not widely available.

Urinalysis shows proteinuria (0.5 to 2 g/m^2/day); dysmorphic RBCs; WBCs; renal tubular cells; and RBC, WBC, and granular casts. Random urinary protein/creatinine ratio may be < 2 (normal, < 0.2).

C3 and total hemolytic complement activity (CH_{50}) levels fall during active disease and return to normal within 6 to 8 wk in 80% of PIGN cases; C1q, C2, and C4 levels are only minimally decreased or remain normal. Cryoglobulinemia may appear and persist for several months, whereas circulating immune complexes are detectable for only a few weeks.

Biopsy shows enlarged and hypercellular glomeruli, initially with neutrophilic or eosinophilic infiltration and later with mononuclear infiltration. Epithelial cell hyperplasia is a common early, transient feature. Microthrombosis may occur; if damage is severe, hemodynamic changes produce oliguria, frequently accompanied by epithelial crescents (formed within Bowman's space from epithelial cell hyperplasia). Endothelial and mesangial cells multiply, and the mesangial regions often are greatly expanded by edema and contain neutrophils, dead cells, cellular debris, and subepithelial deposits of electron-dense material. Immunofluorescence microscopy usually shows immune complex deposition with IgG and complement in a granular pattern. On electron microscopy, these deposits are semilunar or hump-shaped and are located in the subepithelial area. The presence of these deposits initiates a complement-mediated inflammatory reaction that leads to glomerular damage. Although the immune complex is presumed to contain an antigen related to streptococcal organisms, no such antigen has been found.

Prognosis and Treatment

Normal renal function is retained or regained by 85 to 95% of patients. GFR usually returns to normal over 1 to 3 mo, but proteinuria may persist for 6 to 12 mo and microscopic hematuria for several years. Transient changes in urinary sediment may recur with minor URIs. Renal cellular proliferation disappears within weeks, but residual sclerosis is common. In 10% of adults and 1% of children, PIGN evolves into rapidly progressive GN (see below).

No specific treatment exists. Treatment is supportive and may include restriction of dietary protein, Na, and fluid and treatment of edema and hypertension in more severe cases. Dialysis is occasionally necessary. Antimicrobial therapy is preventive only when given within 36 h of infection and before GN becomes established.

Rapidly Progressive Glomerulonephritis

(Crescentic Glomerulonephritis)

Rapidly progressive GN causes microscopic glomerular crescent formation with progression to renal failure within weeks to months. Diagnosis is based on history, urinalysis, serologic tests, and renal biopsy. Treatment is with corticosteroids, with or without cyclophosphamide, and sometimes plasmapheresis.

Rapidly progressive GN (RPGN) is extensive glomerular crescent formation seen on biopsy that, if untreated, progresses to end-stage renal disease over weeks to months. It is relatively uncommon, affecting 10 to 15% of patients with GN, and occurs predominantly in patients 20 to 50 yr. Types and causes are classified by findings on immunofluorescence microscopy (see TABLE 235–4).

Anti-glomerular basement membrane (GBM) antibody disease (type 1 RPGN) is autoimmune GN and accounts for 10% of RPGN cases. It may arise when respiratory exposures (eg, cigarette smoke, viral URI) expose alveolar capillary collagen, triggering formation of anticollagen antibodies. The anticollagen antibodies cross-react with GBM, fixing complement and triggering a cell-mediated inflammatory response in the kidneys and lungs. The combination of GN and alveolar hemorrhage in the presence of anti-GBM antibodies is called Goodpasture's syndrome (see p. 486). Immunofluorescent staining of renal biopsy tissue demonstrates linear IgG deposits.

Immune complex RPGN (type 2 RPGN) complicates numerous infectious and connective tissue disorders and also occurs with other primary glomerulopathies. Immunofluorescent staining demonstrates nonspecific granular immune deposits. The condition accounts for 40% of RPGN cases. Pathogenesis is usually unknown.

Pauci-immune RPGN (type 3 RPGN) is distinguished by the absence of immune complex or complement deposition on immunofluorescent staining. It constitutes 50% of all RPGN cases. Almost all patients have elevated antineutrophil cytoplasmic antibodies (ANCAs) and systemic vasculitis.

Symptoms and Signs

Presentation is usually insidious, with weakness, fatigue, fever, nausea and vomiting, anorexia, arthralgia, and abdominal pain. Some patients present similarly to those with PIGN, with abrupt-onset hematuria. About 50% of patients have edema and a history of an acute influenza-like illness within 4 wk of onset of renal failure, usually followed by severe oliguria. Nephrotic syndrome is present in 10 to 30%. Hypertension is uncommon and rarely severe. Patients with anti-GBM antibody disease may have pulmonary hemorrhage, which can present with hemoptysis or be detectable only by diffuse alveolar infiltrates on chest x-ray (pulmonary-renal or diffuse alveolar hemorrhage syndrome—see p. 485).

Diagnosis

Diagnosis is suggested by history and urinalysis and confirmed by serologic tests and renal biopsy. Serum creatinine is almost always elevated. Hematuria and RBC casts are

TABLE 235–4. SEROLOGIC CLASSIFICATION OF RAPIDLY PROGRESSIVE GLOMERULONEPHRITIS

TYPE	CAUSES
Type 1: Anti-GBM antibody–mediated (10%)	Anti-GBM GN (without lung hemorrhage) Goodpasture's syndrome (with lung hemorrhage)
Type 2: Immune complex (40%)	Postinfectious causes Antistreptococcal antibodies (eg, poststreptococcal GN) Infectious endocarditis Vascular prosthetic nephritis Viral hepatitis B infection Visceral abscess or sepsis Connective tissue diseases Anti-DNA autoantibodies (eg, lupus nephritis) IgA immune complexes (eg, Henoch-Schönlein purpura GN) Mixed IgG-IgM cryoglobulins (eg, cryoglobulinemic GN) Other glomerulopathies IgA nephropathy Membranoproliferative GN
Type 3: Pauci-immune (50%)	Pulmonary necrotizing granulomas (eg, Wegener's granulomatosis) Renal-limited disease (eg, idiopathic crescentic GN) Systemic necrotizing arteritis (eg, polyarteritis nodosa)

GBM = glomerular basement membrane; GN = glomerulonephritis.

always present, and "telescopic" sediment (ie, sediment with multiple elements, including WBCs and granular, waxy, and broad casts) is common. Anemia is always present, and leukocytosis is common.

Serologic testing should include anti-GBM antibodies (anti-GBM antibody disease); antistreptolysin O antibodies, anti-DNA antibodies, or cryoglobulins (immune complex RPGN), depending on clinical presentation; and ANCA titers (pauci-immune RPGN). Complement measurement may be of use in suspected immune complex RPGN, because hypocomplementemia is common.

Early renal biopsy is essential. The feature common to all types of RPGN is focal proliferation of glomerular epithelial cells, sometimes interspersed with numerous neutrophils, that forms a crescentic cellular mass (crescents) and that fills Bowman's space in >50% of glomeruli. The glomerular tuft usually appears hypocellular and collapses. Necrosis within the tuft or involving the crescent may occur and may be the most prominent abnormality. In such patients, histologic evidence of vasculitis should be sought.

Immunofluorescence microscopy differs for the 3 RPGN types. In anti-GBM antibody disease, linear or ribbon-like deposition of IgG along the GBM is most prominent and is often accompanied by linear and sometimes granular deposition of C3. In immune complex RPGN, immunofluorescence reveals diffuse irregular mesangial IgG and C3 deposits, commonly with proliferation of intraglomerular cells and crescent formation. In pauci-immune RPGN, immune staining and deposits are not detected. However, fibrin occurs within the crescents, regardless of the fluorescence pattern.

Prognosis

Spontaneous remission is rare, and 80 to 90% of untreated patients progress to end-stage renal disease within 6 mo. Prognosis improves with early treatment; predictors of response include early anti-GBM disease (before oliguria, creatinine < 7 mg/dL [616 μmol/L]) and

PIGN, SLE, Wegener's granulomatosis, or polyarteritis nodosa as an underlying cause. Prognosis with or without treatment is poorest in patients > 60 yr, those with oliguric renal failure or higher serum creatinine, and those in whom > 75% of glomeruli contain circumferential crescents. About 30% of patients with pauci-immune RPGN do not respond to treatment; about 40% of nonresponders require dialysis, and 33% die within 4 yr. In contrast, < 20% of those who respond to treatment require dialysis, and about 3% die. Patients who recover normal renal function demonstrate residual histologic changes principally in glomeruli, consisting chiefly of hypercellularity, with little or no sclerosis within the glomerular tuft or the epithelial cells and minimal fibrosis of the interstitium.

Death is usually due to infectious or cardiac causes, providing that a uremic death is prevented by dialysis.

Treatment

Treatment varies by disease type, although no regimens have been rigorously studied. Therapy should be instituted early, ideally when serum creatinine is < 5 mg/dL (< 440 μmol/L) and before the biopsy shows crescentic involvement of all glomeruli or organizing crescents as well as fibrotic interstitium and atrophic tubules. Treatment becomes less effective as these features become more prominent and may be harmful in some populations (eg, the elderly and patients with infection).

For anti-GBM antibody disease, plasmapheresis (daily 3- to 4-L exchanges for 14 days) is recommended; the role of plasmapheresis is less well defined for immune complex and pauci-immune RPGN. Plasmapheresis is believed to be effective because it rapidly removes free antibody, intact immune complexes, and mediators of inflammation (eg, fibrinogen, complement). Prednisone and cyclophosphamide are typically started and continued to minimize new antibody formation.

For immune complex and pauci-immune RPGN, corticosteroids (methylprednisolone 1 g IV once/day over 30 min for 3 to 5 days followed by prednisone 1 mg/kg po once/day) may reduce serum creatinine or delay dialysis for > 3 yr in 50% of patients. Cyclophosphamide 1.5 to 2 mg/kg po once/day may also benefit ANCA-positive patients; monthly pulse regimens may lessen adverse effects, but their role is not defined.

Lymphocytapheresis, a technique to remove peripheral lymphocytes from circulation, may benefit pauci-immune RPGN but requires further investigation.

Renal transplantation is effective for all types, but disease may recur in the graft; risk diminishes with time. In anti-GBM antibody disease, the anti-GBM titers should be undetectable for at least 12 mo before transplantation.

Thin Basement Membrane Disease

(Benign Familial Hematuria)

Thin basement membrane disease is diffuse thinning of the glomerular basement membrane from a width of 300 to 400 nm in normal subjects to 150 to 225 nm.

Thin basement membrane disease is hereditary and usually transmitted in autosomal dominant fashion. Not all genetic mutations have been characterized, but some families with thin basement membrane disease have been identified with mutation in the type IV collagen alpha 4 gene. Prevalence is estimated to be 5 to 9%. Most patients are asymptomatic and are incidentally noted to have microscopic hematuria on routine urinalysis, although mild proteinuria and gross hematuria are occasionally present. Renal function is typically normal, but a few patients develop progressive renal failure for unknown reasons. Recurrent flank pain, similar to that in IgA nephropathy, is a rare presentation.

Diagnosis is based on family history and findings of hematuria without other symptoms or pathology, particularly if asymptomatic family members also have hematuria. Renal biopsy is unnecessary but is often performed as part of a hematuria evaluation. Early on, thin basement membrane disease may be difficult to differentiate from hereditary nephritis because of histologic similarities. Anti-GBM antibodies are usually present in thin basement membrane disease.

Long-term prognosis is excellent, and no treatment is necessary in most cases. Patients with frequent gross hematuria or flank pain may benefit from ACE inhibitors, which may lower intraglomerular pressure.

NEPHROTIC SYNDROME

Nephrotic syndrome is urinary excretion of > 3 g of protein/day due to glomerular disease. It is more common in children and has

both primary and secondary causes. Diagnosis is by measurement of a spot urine protein/creatinine ratio or a 24-h urinary protein; underlying causes are diagnosed based on history, physical examination, and renal biopsy. Treatment and prognosis vary by cause.

Etiology and Pathophysiology

Nephrotic syndrome (NS) occurs at any age but is more prevalent in children, mostly between ages 1 ½ and 4 yr. At younger ages, boys are affected more often than girls, but both are affected equally at older ages. Causes differ by age (see TABLE 235–1). The most common primary causes are minimal change disease, focal segmental glomerulosclerosis, and membranous nephropathy. Secondary causes account for < 10% of childhood cases but > 50% of adult cases, most commonly diabetic nephropathy and preeclampsia (see TABLE 235–3). Amyloidosis is an underrecognized cause of 4% of cases.

Proteinuria occurs because of changes to capillary endothelial cells, the glomerular basement membrane (GBM), or podocytes, which normally filter serum protein selectively by size and charge. The mechanism of damage to these structures is unknown in primary glomerular disease, but evidence suggests that T cells up-regulate a circulating permeability factor or down-regulate an inhibitor of permeability factor in response to unidentified immunogens and cytokines. The result is urinary loss of macromolecular proteins, primarily albumin but also opsonins, immunoglobulins, erythropoietin, transferrin, hormone-binding proteins, and antithrombin III in conditions that cause nonselective proteinuria. As a result, patients with NS develop peripheral edema, ascites, and effusions and are at increased risk for infection (especially cellulitis and, in 2 to 6%, spontaneous bacterial peritonitis); anemia; abnormal thyroid function; and thromboembolism (especially renal vein thrombosis and pulmonary embolism in up to 5% of children and 40% of adults). Thromboembolism may develop not only because of urinary loss of antithrombin III but also because of increased hepatic synthesis of clotting factors, platelet abnormalities, and hyperviscosity from hypovolemia. Chronic complications of NS include malnutrition in children, coronary artery disease in adults, chronic renal failure, and bone disease. Malnutrition may mimic kwashiorkor, including brittle hair and nails, alopecia, and stunted growth. Coronary artery disease develops because NS causes hyperlipidemia, hypertension, and hypercoagulability. Complications of chronic renal failure are discussed on p. 1986. Bone disease develops because of vitamin D deficiency and corticosteroid use. Other chronic complications include hypothyroidism from loss of thyroid-binding globulin and proximal tubular dysfunction causing glucosuria, aminoaciduria, K depletion, phosphaturia, and renal tubular acidosis.

Renal failure is rarely a presenting finding but may occur after a prolonged illness. However, patients with NS due to a secondary cause frequently have renal insufficiency at onset or soon thereafter.

Symptoms and Signs

Primary symptoms include anorexia, malaise, and frothy urine caused by high concentrations of protein. Edema may cause dyspnea (pleural effusion or laryngeal edema), chest discomfort (pericardial effusion), arthralgia (hydrarthrosis), or abdominal pain (ascites or, in children, mesenteric edema). Edema may obscure signs of muscle wasting and cause parallel white lines in fingernail beds (Muehrcke's lines).

Other symptoms and signs are attributable to the many complications of NS (see above).

Diagnosis

Diagnosis is suspected in patients with edema and proteinuria on urinalysis and confirmed by 24-h measurement of urinary protein. The cause may be suggested by history (eg, cancer); when the cause is unclear, serologic testing and renal biopsy are indicated.

A finding of 3 g protein in a 24-h urine collection is diagnostic. The protein/creatinine ratio in a random specimen estimates grams of protein/1.73 m^2 BSA in a 24-h collection (eg, values of 40 mg/dL protein and 10 mg/dL creatinine on a random urine sample are equivalent to the finding of 4 g/1.73 m^2 in a 24-h specimen). The use of spot urine protein/creatinine ratio may be less reliable when creatinine excretion is extremely high (eg, during athletic training) or low (eg, in cachexia) and in disorders in which proteinuria may vary daily (eg, in diabetic nephropathy).

Besides proteinuria, urinalysis may demonstrate RBCs and casts (hyaline, granular, fatty, waxy, RBC, or epithelial cell). Lipiduria, the presence of free lipid or lipid within tubular cells (oval fat bodies), within casts (fatty casts), or as free globules, is primarily present with glomerular disease causing NS. Urinary cholesterol can be detected with plain microscopy and demonstrates a "Maltese cross" pattern under polarized light; Sudan staining must be used to show triglycerides. WBCs are prominent in exudative diseases and SLE.

Adjunctive testing helps characterize severity and complications. BUN and creatinine concentrations vary by degree of renal impairment. Albumin often is < 2.5 g/dL. Total cholesterol and triglyceride levels are typically increased. It is not routinely necessary to measure levels of α- and γ-globulins, immunoglobulins, hormone binding proteins, ceruloplasmin, transferrin, and complement components, but these may also be low.

The role of testing for secondary causes (see TABLE 235–3) is controversial, because yield may be low. Tests, including serum glucose or glycosylated hemoglobin (HbA_{1c}), antinuclear antibodies, and hepatitis B and C serologic tests, are indicated by clinical context and may alter management and preclude the need for biopsy. For example, demonstration of cryoglobulins suggests mixed cryoglobulinemia (eg, from chronic inflammatory disorders such as SLE, Sjögren's syndrome, or hepatitis C virus infection), whereas demonstration of a monoclonal protein on serum or urine protein electrophoresis suggests a monoclonal gammopathy (eg, multiple myeloma), especially in patients > 50 yr.

In adults, a renal biopsy is indicated to diagnose the underlying cause of idiopathic NS. Idiopathic NS in children is most likely minimal change disease and is usually presumed without biopsy unless the patient fails to improve on a trial of corticosteroids. Specific biopsy findings are discussed under individual disease entities below.

Prognosis

Prognosis varies by cause. Complete remissions may occur spontaneously or with treatment. The prognosis generally is favorable in corticosteroid-responsive disorders.

In all cases, prognosis may be worsened by infection; hypertension; significant azotemia; hematuria; or thromboses in cerebral, pulmonary, peripheral, or renal veins. The recurrence rate is high in kidney transplantation patients with focal segmental glomerulosclerosis, SLE, IgA nephropathy, and membranoproliferative glomerulonephritis (especially type II).

Treatment

Specific treatment is discussed under individual disorders below. Supportive therapy includes treatment of secondary causes when they exist and dietary restrictions, antihypertensives, and measures to prevent complications. Rarely, severe NS requires nephrectomy because of persistent hypoalbuminemia.

Treatment of underlying causes may include prompt treatment of infections (eg, staphylococcal and *Streptococcus viridans* endocarditis, vascular prosthetic nephritis, malaria, syphilis, schistosomiasis), allergic desensitization (eg, for poison oak or ivy and insect antigen exposures), and stopping drugs (eg, gold, penicillamine, NSAIDs); these measures may cure NS in specific instances.

Protein restriction is no longer recommended because of lack of demonstrated effect on disease progression. However, saturated fat and cholesterol intake should be limited, and Na restriction (< 100 mmol/day) is recommended to control symptomatic edema.

ACE inhibitors are indicated to reduce systemic and intraglomerular BP and proteinuria. They may cause or exacerbate hyperkalemia in patients with moderate to severe renal insufficiency.

Loop diuretics are usually required to control edema but may worsen preexisting renal insufficiency and hypovolemia, hyperviscosity, and hypercoagulability.

Anticoagulants are indicated for thromboembolism, but few data exist to support their use as primary prevention. Statins are indicated for hyperlipidemia. All patients should receive pneumococcal vaccination; the use of prophylactic penicillin is controversial.

CONGENITAL NEPHROTIC SYNDROMES

Congenital nephrotic syndromes include diffuse mesangial sclerosis and Finnish-type nephrotic syndrome.

Diffuse mesangial sclerosis is rare. Inheritance is unknown. A patient with severe proteinuria may require bilateral nephrectomy because of severe hypoalbuminemia; dialysis should be initiated early in the disease to ameliorate nutritional deficits and mitigate failure to thrive. The disease usually recurs in a renal graft.

Finnish-type NS, an autosomal recessive disease, affects 1/8200 Finnish newborns and is caused by a mutation in the *NPHS1* gene, which codes for a podocytic slit-diaphragm protein (nephrin). Finnish-type NS is rapidly progressive and usually necessitates dialysis within 1 yr. Most patients die within 1 yr, but a few have been supported nutritionally until renal failure occurs and then managed with dialysis or transplantation.

Other rare congenital nephrotic syndromes are now genetically characterized. These include corticosteroid-resistant nephrotic syndrome (defective *NPS2* gene coding for podocin), familial focal segmental glomerulosclerosis (defective *ACTN4* gene coding for alpha-actin 4), and Denys-Drash syndrome (defective *WT1* gene).

Diabetic Nephropathy

(See also p. 1277.)

Diabetic nephropathy is glomerular sclerosis and fibrosis caused by the metabolic and hemodynamic changes of diabetes mellitus. It manifests as slowly progressive albuminuria with worsening hypertension and renal insufficiency. Diagnosis is based on history, physical examination, urinalysis, and serum creatinine. Treatment is strict glucose control, ACE inhibitors and/or angiotensin receptor blockers, and control of BP and lipids.

Diabetic nephropathy (DN) is the most common cause of NS and of end-stage renal disease in the US, accounting for up to 80% of cases of the latter. The prevalence of renal failure among patients with type 2 diabetes mellitus is most likely underestimated at 20 to 30%; renal failure is particularly common in blacks, Asians, and Hispanics with type 2 diabetes. Prevalence increases with duration and poor control of disease; renal failure usually takes ≥ 10 yr to develop.

Pathophysiology

Pathogenesis is complex, involving glycosylation of proteins, hormonally influenced cytokine release (eg, transforming growth factor-β), deposition of mesangial matrix, and alteration of glomerular hemodynamics. Hyperfiltration, an early functional abnormality, is only a relative predictor for the development of renal failure.

Hyperglycemia causes glycosylation of glomerular proteins, which may be responsible for mesangial cell proliferation and matrix expansion and vascular endothelial damage. The GBM classically becomes thickened.

Lesions of diffuse or nodular intercapillary glomerulosclerosis are distinctive. There is marked hyalinosis of afferent and efferent arterioles as well as arteriosclerosis; interstitial fibrosis and tubular atrophy may be present. Only mesangial matrix expansion appears to correlate with progression to end-stage renal disease.

DN begins as glomerular hyperfiltration (increased GFR); GFR normalizes with early renal injury and mild hypertension, which worsens over time. Microalbuminuria, urinary excretion of albumin in a range of 30 to 300 mg albumin/day, then occurs. Urinary albumin in these concentrations is called microalbuminuria because it cannot be detected by routine urinalysis. Microalbuminuria progresses to proteinuria > 0.5 g/day, and NS usually precedes end-stage renal disease by 3 to 5 yr. Overall progression to chronic renal failure takes 10 to 20 yr. Other urinary tract abnormalities commonly occurring with DN that may accelerate the decline of renal function include papillary necrosis, type IV renal tubular acidosis, and UTIs.

Symptoms, Signs, and Diagnosis

DN is asymptomatic in early stages. Proteinuria (especially with albumin) on routine urinalysis is often the earliest warning. Hypertension and some measure of dependent edema eventually develop in most untreated patients. In later stages, patients develop symptoms and signs of uremia (eg, nausea, vomiting, anorexia) earlier (ie, with higher GFR) than do patients without DN, possibly because the combination of end-organ damage due to diabetes (eg, neuropathy) and renal failure worsens symptoms.

Diagnosis is suggested by proteinuria, diabetic retinopathy and/or hypertension, and a history of diabetes. Other renal diseases should be considered if there is heavy proteinuria with a short diabetic history, absence of diabetic retinopathy, rapid onset of heavy proteinuria, gross hematuria, RBC casts, or a rapid decline in GFR. Renal biopsy can confirm the diagnosis but is rarely necessary.

If proteinuria is evident on urinalysis, testing for microalbuminuria is unnecessary because the patient already has macroalbuminuria suggestive of diabetic renal disease. Patients with type 1 diabetes without known renal disease should be screened for microalbuminuria and proteinuria beginning 5 yr after diagnosis and at least annually thereafter. Patients with type 2 diabetes should be screened at the time of diagnosis and annually thereafter.

In patients without proteinuria on urinalysis, a microalbumin-to-creatinine ratio should be measured on a 1st morning void urine specimen. A ratio ≥ 0.03 (≥ 30 mg/g) indicates microalbuminuria if it is present on at least 2 of 3 measures within 3 to 6 mo and if it cannot be explained by infection or exercise. Some experts recommend that microalbuminuria be measured from a 24-h urine collection, but this approach is less convenient, and many patients have difficulty accurately collecting a specimen. The spot urine albumin/creatinine ratio overestimates 24-h collection of microalbuminuria in up to 30% of patients > 65 due to reduced creatinine production from reduced muscle mass.

Prognosis and Treatment

Prognosis is good for patients who are meticulously treated and monitored. Such care is often difficult in practice, however, and most patients slowly lose renal function; even prehypertension (BP 120 to 139/80 to 89 mm Hg) or stage 1 hypertension (BP 140 to 159/90 to 99 mm Hg) may accelerate injury. Systemic atherosclerotic disease (stroke, MI, peripheral arterial disease) predicts an increase in mortality.

Primary treatment is strict glucose control to maintain glycosylated hemoglobin ≤ 7.0; maintenance of euglycemia reduces microalbuminuria but may not retard disease progression once DN is well established. Glucose control must also be accompanied by strict control of BP to < 130/80 mm Hg (some experts suggest 110 to 120/< 75 mm Hg). ACE inhibitors or angiotensin receptor blockers are the antihypertensives of choice; they reduce BP and proteinuria and slow the progression of DN. The combination of both drugs may exert greater antiproteinuric and renoprotective effects than either drug alone. They should be started when microalbuminuria is detected regardless of whether hypertension is present; some experts recommend they be used even before signs of renal disease appear. Angiotensin receptor blockers can be used alone if persistent cough precludes the use of ACE inhibitors.

Nondihydropyridine Ca channel blockers (diltiazem and verapamil) are also antiproteinuric and renoprotective and are reasonable alternatives for patients with hyperkalemia or other contraindications to ACE inhibitors or angiotensin receptor blockers. In contrast, dihydropyridine Ca channel blockers (eg, nifedipine, felodipine, amlodipine) are relatively contraindicated because they may worsen proteinuria and renal function. ACE inhibitors and nondihydropyridine Ca channel blockers have greater antiproteinuric and renoprotective effects when used together, and their antiproteinuric effect is enhanced by Na restriction.

Dietary restriction of protein yields mixed results. The American Diabetic Association recommends that people with diabetes and overt nephropathy be restricted to ≤ 0.8 g protein/kg/day. Some experts recommend restriction to 0.6 g/kg when disease progression is documented. Significant protein restriction should be done only with close dietary monitoring to ensure a balanced supply of amino acids, because malnutrition may be a significant risk.

Kidney transplantation with or without simultaneous or subsequent pancreas transplantation (see p. 1373) is an option for patients with end-stage renal disease. The 5-yr survival rate for patients with type 2 diabetes receiving a kidney transplant is almost 60%, compared with 2% for dialysis-dependent patients who do not undergo transplantation (though this statistic probably represents significant selection bias). Renal allograft survival rate is > 85% at 2 yr.

Focal Segmental Glomerulosclerosis

Focal segmental glomerulosclerosis is scattered (segmental) mesangial sclerosis in some but not all (focal) glomeruli. It is most often idiopathic but may be secondary to heroin use, HIV infection, obesity, or nephron loss (eg, in reflux nephropathy or subtotal nephrectomy). Manifestations are insidious onset of proteinuria, mild hematuria, hypertension, and azotemia, mainly in adolescents but also in young and middle-aged adults. Diagnosis is indicated by history, physical examination, and urinalysis; it is confirmed by renal biopsy. Treatment is with corticosteroids and occasionally cytotoxic drugs.

Focal segmental glomerulosclerosis (FSGS) is now the most common cause of idiopathic NS among adults in the US. It is especially common in black men. Though usually idiopathic, FSGS can occur in association with injection drug use, obesity, analgesic nephropathy, and diseases causing nephron loss (eg, reflux nephropathy, subtotal nephrectomy).

Familial cases exist. HIV-associated nephropathy (HIVAN) is characterized by a lesion similar to FSGS and seems to be more common in black patients with HIV who are injection drug users. Infection of renal cells with HIV may contribute. HIVAN should be distinguished from the many other disorders that occur with higher frequency in HIV-infected patients and cause renal disease, such as thrombotic microangiopathy (hemolytic-uremic syndrome and thrombotic thrombocytopenic purpura), immune complex–mediated glomerulonephritis, and drug-induced interstitial nephritis (indinavir, ritonavir) and rhabdomyolysis (statins).

Symptoms, Signs, and Diagnosis

FSGS patients commonly present with heavy proteinuria, hypertension, and renal dysfunction, although asymptomatic non-nephrotic–range proteinuria is sometimes the only sign. Microscopic hematuria is occasionally found. Proteinuria is typically nonselective (both size and charge ultrafiltration barriers are defective). IgG levels are frequently depressed. Diagnosis is confirmed by renal biopsy, which shows focal and segmental hyalinization of the glomeruli, often with immunostaining showing IgM and C3 deposits in a nodular and coarse granular pattern. Electron microscopy reveals diffuse effacement of podocyte foot processes. Global sclerosis may occur, leading to atrophic glomeruli.

HIVAN may accompany symptoms of AIDS. At presentation, mild azotemia and signs of NS, including nephrotic-range proteinuria, are often found. The kidneys are enlarged and highly echogenic on ultrasonography. Light microscopy shows capillary collapse of varying severity (collapsing glomerulopathy) and differing degrees of increased mesangial matrix. Tubular cells show marked degenerative changes and tubular atrophy or microcytic dilation. Interstitial immune cell infiltrate, fibrosis, and edema are common. Tubular reticular inclusions, similar to those in SLE, are found within endothelial cells but are now rare with more effective HIV therapy. Normotension and persistent enlarged kidneys help to differentiate HIVAN from FSGS.

Prognosis

Prognosis is poor. Spontaneous remissions occur in < 10% of patients. Renal failure occurs in > 50% of patients within 10 yr; in 20%, end-stage renal disease occurs within 2 yr, despite treatment. The disease is more rapidly progressive in adults than in children. The presence of segmental sclerosis consistently at the glomerular pole where the tubule originates (tip lesion) may portend a more favorable response to corticosteroid therapy. Another variant, in which the capillary walls are wrinkled or collapsed (collapsing glomerulopathy), suggests more severe disease and rapid progression to renal failure. Pregnancy may exacerbate FSGS.

FSGS recurs after renal transplantation in 20 to 30% of patients; proteinuria sometimes returns within hours of transplantation. Of patients with recurrent FSGS, 30 to 50% lose their graft; risk is highest in young children, patients who develop renal failure < 3 yr after disease onset, and patients with mesangial proliferation.

Heroin addicts with NS due to FSGS can experience complete remission if they cease taking heroin early in the disease.

Most patients with HIVAN experience rapid progression to end-stage renal disease within 1 to 4 mo.

Treatment

Treatment often is not effective. Corticosteroids (eg, prednisone 1 mg/kg po once/day or 2 mg/kg every other day) are recommended for at least 2 mo, although some experts recommend up to 9 mo. Response rates of 30 to 50% have been reported with prolonged therapy. After a 2-wk remission of proteinuria, the corticosteroid is slowly tapered over ≥ 2 mo. Secondary and familial cases are more likely to be corticosteroid-resistant.

If only slight improvement or relapse occurs, cyclophosphamide (2 to 3 mg/kg po once/day for 12 wk) or cyclosporine (5 mg/kg po once/day in adults or 6 mg/kg once/day in children for 16 wk) may induce remission. Patients with corticosteroid-resistant, advanced primary FSGS should be treated with a prolonged course of ACE inhibitors. An alternative is plasmapheresis with tacrolimus immunosuppression.

Treatment of HIVAN is antiretroviral therapy. Control of the underlying HIV infection may improve the renal lesion. ACE inhibitors are probably of some benefit. The role of corticosteroids is not well defined. Dialysis is usually required.

Membranous Nephropathy

Membranous nephropathy is deposition of immune complexes on the GBM with GBM thickening. Cause is usually unknown,

although secondary causes include drugs, infections, autoimmune diseases, and cancer. Symptoms and signs include insidious onset of edema, heavy proteinuria, benign urinary sediment, normal renal function, and normal or elevated BP. Diagnosis is by renal biopsy. Treatment is usually with corticosteroids and cyclophosphamide, although many patients undergo spontaneous remission.

Membranous nephropathy (MN) mostly affects adults. It is usually idiopathic but may be caused by drugs (eg, gold, penicillamine, NSAIDs), infections (eg, hepatitis B virus), autoimmune disease (eg, SLE), thyroiditis, or cancer. Depending on the patient's age, 4 to 20% have an underlying cancer, including solid cancers of the lung, colon, stomach, breast, or kidney; Hodgkin or non-Hodgkin lymphoma; chronic lymphocytic leukemia; and melanoma.

MN is rare in children and when it occurs is usually due to hepatitis B virus infection or SLE.

Renal vein thrombosis is especially frequent in MN but is usually clinically silent unless it progresses to pulmonary embolism.

Symptoms, Signs, and Diagnosis

Patients typically present with edema and nephrotic-range proteinuria and occasionally with microscopic hematuria and hypertension. Symptoms and signs of chronic immune complex or connective tissue disease, chronic infection, or tumor may be present initially.

Diagnosis is indicated by history and urinalysis and confirmed by biopsy. Only 20% have non-nephrotic–range proteinuria. C3 and C4 levels are normal. The GFR is normal or decreased. Immune complexes are seen as dense deposits on electron microscopy (see FIG. 235–1). Subepithelial dense deposits occur with early disease, with spikes of lamina densa between the deposits. Later, deposits appear within the GBM, and marked thickening occurs. A diffuse, granular pattern of IgG deposition occurs along the GBM without cellular proliferation, exudation, or necrosis.

A search for occult cancer should be undertaken, particularly in a patient who has lost weight, has unexplained anemia or heme-positive stools, or is elderly. Drug-induced MN should also be considered.

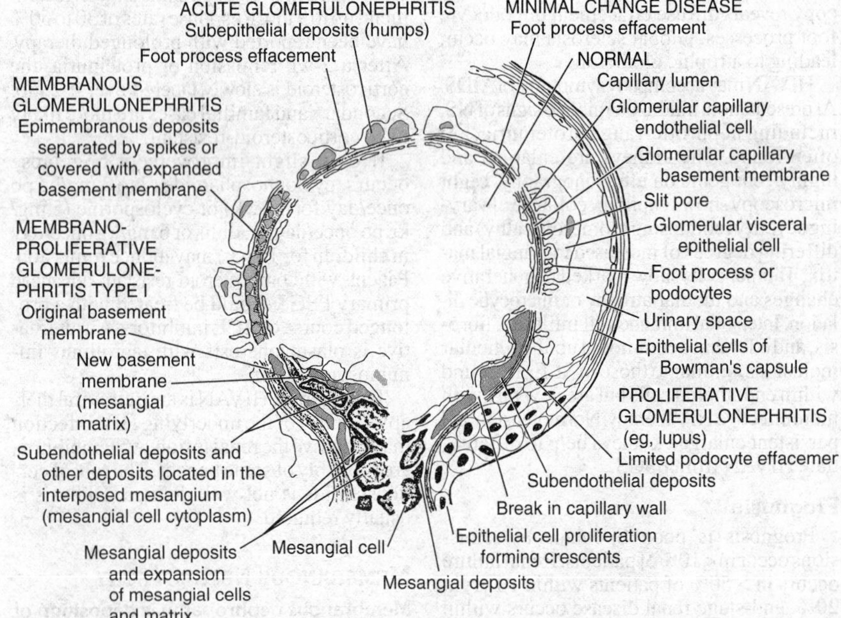

Fig. 235–1. Electron microscopic features in immunologic glomerular diseases.

Prognosis

About 25% of patients undergo spontaneous remission, 25% develop persistent non-nephrotic–range proteinuria, 25% develop persistent NS, and 25% progress to end-stage renal disease. Women, children, and young adults with non-nephrotic–range proteinuria and those with persistent normal renal function 3 yr after diagnosis tend to have little disease progression.

Men > 50 yr with proteinuria ≥ 10 g/day, patients with increased β-microglobulinuria, and patients with an initially elevated serum creatinine are at greatest risk of progression to renal failure.

Treatment

Primary treatment is that of underlying causes. Among patients with idiopathic MN, asymptomatic patients with non-nephrotic–range proteinuria do not require treatment; renal function should be monitored periodically, however. Patients with nephrotic-range proteinuria who are asymptomatic or who have edema that can be controlled with diuretics should be followed, because ≥ 50% will have a partial or complete remission within 3 to 4 yr.

Immunosuppressants should be considered only for patients with symptomatic idiopathic NS and for those most at risk of progressive disease (see Prognosis, above). No consensus protocol exists, but one approach uses methylprednisolone 1 g IV for 3 days, after which prednisone 0.5 mg/kg po once/day for the next 27 days is given. The following month, chlorambucil 0.2 mg/kg po once/day is given for 1 mo. These 2 monthly regimens are alternated for a total of 6 mo. This protocol remains controversial and should be used with caution, especially in the elderly because of the increased risk of infection.

For patients intolerant of cytotoxic drugs, cyclosporine 4 to 6 mg/kg po once/day for 4 mo may be beneficial. Patients with hypertension should be given an ACE inhibitor or angiotensin receptor blocker; these drugs may also benefit patients without hypertension by reducing proteinuria. Therapies of unproven long-term value include IV immune globulin and NSAIDs.

Minimal Change Disease

(Lipoid Nephrosis; Nil Disease)

Minimal change disease causes abrupt onset of edema and heavy proteinuria, mostly in children. Renal function is typically normal. Diagnosis is made empirically or by renal biopsy. Prognosis is excellent. Treatment is with corticosteroids or, in patients who do not respond, cyclophosphamide or cyclosporine.

Minimal change disease (MCD) is the most common cause of NS in children 4 to 8 yr (80 to 90% of childhood NS), but it also occurs in adults (20% of adult NS). The cause is almost always unknown, although rare cases may occur secondary to drug use (especially NSAIDs) and hematologic malignancies (especially Hodgkin lymphoma).

MCD causes NS without hypertension or azotemia; microscopic hematuria occurs in about 20% of patients. Azotemia can occur in nonidiopathic cases and in patients > 60 yr. Albumin is lost in the urine of patients with MCD more so than larger serum proteins, probably because MCD causes changes in the charge barrier rather than the size barrier in the glomerular capillary wall.

Diagnosis

Diagnosis in children is most often clinical, but biopsy is required in atypical cases and in adults. Electron microscopy demonstrates edema with diffuse swelling (effacement) of foot processes of the epithelial podocytes (see FIG. 235–1). Although effacement is not observed in the absence of proteinuria, heavy proteinuria may occur with normal foot processes.

Treatment

Spontaneous remissions occur in 40% of cases, but most patients are given corticosteroids. About 80 to 90% of patients respond to initial corticosteroid therapy (prednisone 60 mg/m^2 po once/day for 4 to 6 wk in children and 1 to 1.5 mg/kg po once/day for 6 to 8 wk in adults), but 40 to 60% of responders relapse. Patients who respond (ie, cessation of proteinuria or a diuresis if edema is present) should continue prednisone for another 2 wk and change to a maintenance regimen to minimize toxicity (2 to 3 mg/kg on alternate days for 4 to 6 wk in children and for 8 to 12 wk in adults, tapering during the next 4 mo). More prolonged initial therapy and slower tapering of prednisone lower relapse rates. Nonresponsiveness may be due to underlying focal sclerosis.

In corticosteroid nonresponders (< 5% of children; > 10% of adults), frequent relapsers, and corticosteroid-dependent patients, prolonged remission may be achieved with an oral cytotoxic drug (usually cyclophosphamide

2 to 3 mg/kg once/day for 12 wk or chlorambucil 0.15 mg/kg once/day for 8 wk). However, these drugs may suppress gonadal function (most serious in prepubertal adolescents), and cyclophosphamide may cause hemorrhagic cystitis and suppress bone marrow and lymphocyte function. Dosage should be monitored with frequent CBCs, and hemorrhagic cystitis should be sought by urinalysis. Adults, particularly if older or hypertensive, are prone to adverse effects from these cytotoxic drugs. Another alternative is cyclosporine 3 mg/kg po bid, adjusted to obtain a whole-blood trough concentration of 50 to 150 μg/L (40 to 125 nmol/L). Complete remission occurs in > 80% of patients, and treatment is usually continued for 1 to 2 yr. Patients responsive to cyclosporine frequently relapse when the drug is stopped.

For patients unresponsive to these interventions, most respond to alternative therapies, including ACE inhibitors, thioguanine, levamisole, azathioprine, and mycophenolate mofetil; < 5% progress to renal failure.

NEPHRITIC AND NEPHROTIC SYNDROMES

Several glomerular diseases typically present with both nephritic and nephrotic features. These include fibrillary and immunotactoid glomerulopathies, membranoproliferative glomerulonephritis (GN), and lupus nephritis.

Fibrillary and Immunotactoid Glomerulopathies

Fibrillary and immunotactoid glomerulopathies are rare conditions defined pathologically by organized deposition of nonamyloid microfibrillar or microtubular structures within the renal mesangium and basement membrane.

Fibrillary and immunotactoid glomerulopathies, found in about 0.6% of renal biopsies, occur equally in men and women and have been described in patients ≥ 10 yr. Mechanism is unknown, although deposition of immunoglobulin, particularly IgG κ and λ light chains and complement, suggests immune system dysfunction. Patients may have accompanying paraproteinemia, cryoglobulinemia, plasma cell dyscrasia, or SLE, or they may have a primary renal disease without evidence of systemic disease.

All patients have proteinuria, > 60% in the nephrotic range. Microscopic hematuria is present in about 60%; hypertension, in about 70%. Slightly > ½ have renal insufficiency at presentation.

Diagnosis is suggested by laboratory data and confirmed by renal biopsy. Urinalysis usually shows a mixed nephritic and nephrotic picture. Serum complement is occasionally decreased. Light microscopy of a biopsy specimen shows mesangial expansion by eosinophilic deposits and mild mesangial hypercellularity. Congo red staining is negative for amyloid. Immunostaining reveals IgG and complement in the area of the deposits. Electron microscopy shows glomerular deposits consisting of extracellular, elongated, nonbranching microfibrils or microtubules. The diameter of the microfibrils and microtubules varies from 9 nm to > 50 nm. Some experts distinguish immunotactoid from fibrillary glomerulopathy by the presence of microtubular (as opposed to microfibrillar) structures in the deposits; others distinguish it by the absence of a related systemic illness such as a paraproteinemia, cryoglobulinemia, or SLE.

The condition is usually slowly progressive with renal insufficiency, progressing to end-stage renal disease in 50% of patients by 2 to 4 yr. A more rapid decline is predicted by the presence of hypertension, nephrotic-range proteinuria, and renal insufficiency at presentation.

Immunosuppressants have been used without documented success except anecdotally; success may be greater with corticosteroids when serum complement is decreased.

Membranoproliferative Glomerulonephritis

(Mesangiocapillary Glomerulonephritis; Lobular Glomerulonephritis)

Membranoproliferative GN is a heterogeneous group of diseases that share mixed nephritic and nephrotic features and microscopic findings. They mostly affect children. Cause is immune complex deposition that is idiopathic or secondary to systemic disease. Diagnosis is by renal biopsy. Prognosis is generally poor. Treatment is with corticosteroids and antiplatelet drugs.

Membranoproliferative GN is a group of immune-mediated disorders characterized histologically by glomerular basement membrane (GBM) thickening and proliferative changes on light microscopy. There are 3 types, each of which may have primary (idiopathic) or secondary causes. Primary forms affect children and young adults between ages 8 and 30 and account for 10% of NS in children, while secondary causes tend to affect adults > 30. Men and women are affected equally; reported familial cases of some types suggest genetic factors play a role in at least some cases.

Type I (mesangial proliferation with immune deposits) accounts for 80 to 85% of cases. It most commonly occurs secondary to systemic immune complex disease (eg, SLE, mixed cryoglobulinemia, Sjögren's syndrome), chronic infection (eg, bacterial endocarditis, HIV, hepatitis B and C, visceral abscess, ventriculoatrial shunt), malignancy (eg, chronic lymphocytic leukemia, lymphomas, melanoma), and other disorders (eg, partial lipodystrophy, C2 or C3 deficiencies, sarcoidosis, thrombotic microangiopathies).

Type II (similar to type I with less mesangial proliferation and with GBM dense deposits) accounts for 15 to 20%. It is probably an autoimmune disease in which an IgG autoantibody (C3 nephritic factor) binds C3 convertase, rendering C3 resistant to inactivation; immunofluorescent staining identifies C3 around dense deposits and in mesangium.

Type III is thought to be a disorder similar to type I. Cause is unknown but may be related to immune complex (IgG, C3) deposition. An IgG autoantibody against the terminal component of complement is found in 70% of patients.

Symptoms and Signs

Symptoms and signs are those of nephrotic syndrome in 60 to 80% of cases. Symptoms and signs of nephritic syndrome (acute GN) are presenting features in 15 to 20% of cases of type I and III disease and in a higher percentage of type II disease. At diagnosis, 30% of patients have hypertension and 20% have renal insufficiency; hypertension often develops even before GFR declines. Patients with type II disease have a greater incidence of ocular abnormalities (basal laminar drusen, diffuse retinal pigment alterations, diskiform macular detachment, choroidal neovascularization), which ultimately impair vision.

Diagnosis

Diagnosis is by renal biopsy. Serum complement profiles are more frequently abnormal in membranoproliferative GN than in other glomerular diseases and provide supportive evidence of the diagnosis; hypocomplementemia is multifactorial in origin and is considered a marker, not a cause. In type I disease, C3 is depressed more often than C4 at diagnosis, decreases further during follow-up, but eventually normalizes. C3 is more frequently and severely reduced in type II disease. C3 is reduced but C4 is normal in type III disease. C3 nephritic factor is detectable in 80% of patients with type II and in some patients with type I disease. Terminal complement nephritic factor is detectable in 20% of type I, rare cases of type II, and 70% of cases of type III disease.

Serologic tests (eg, for SLE, hepatitis B and C, and cryoglobulinemia) are warranted to check for secondary causes of type I disease. CBC, often obtained in the course of diagnostic evaluation, demonstrates normochromic-normocytic anemia, often out of proportion to the stage of renal insufficiency (possibly because of hemolysis), and thrombocytopenia from platelet consumption.

Prognosis and Treatment

Type I membranoproliferative GN often progresses slowly; type II progresses more rapidly. In general, the long-term prognosis is poor. End-stage renal disease occurs in 50% of patients at 3 to 5 yr and in 75% at 10 yr; at 5 yr, only 25% have normal renal function. Spontaneous remission occurs in < 5%. Type I membranoproliferative GN recurs in 30% of kidney transplantation patients; type II recurs in 90%.

Specific therapy is probably not indicated in patients with non-nephrotic–range proteinuria because the disease usually progresses slowly. In nephrotic children, treatment with prednisone 2.5 mg/kg po once/day on alternate days (maximum 80 mg) for 1 yr, followed by tapering to a maintenance dose of 20 mg on alternate days for 3 to 10 yr, may stabilize renal function. However, corticosteroid treatment may retard growth and cause hypertension. In adults, dipyridamole (225 mg po once/day) with aspirin (975 mg po once/day) for 1 yr seems to stabilize renal function at 3 to 5 yr, but at 10 yr there is no difference from placebo. Prolonged therapy may be required.

Alternate therapies include α-interferon (with addition of ribavirin if creatinine clearance is > 50 mL/min) for hepatitis C virus–associated disease and plasmapheresis with corticosteroids for concomitant severe cryoglobulinemia or rapidly progressive GN. ACE inhibitors may decrease proteinuria and help control hypertension.

Lupus Nephritis

Lupus nephritis is GN caused by SLE. Clinical findings include hematuria, nephrotic-range proteinuria, and azotemia in more advanced stages. Diagnosis is based on renal biopsy. Treatment is of the underlying disorder and usually involves corticosteroids, cytotoxic drugs, and immune-modifying antimetabolites.

Lupus nephritis is diagnosed in about 50% of SLE patients (see p. 266). However, the total incidence is probably > 90%, because renal biopsy in patients with suspected SLE without clinical evidence of renal disease shows changes of GN.

Pathophysiology involves immune complex deposition with development of GN. The immune complexes consist of nuclear antigens (especially DNA), high-affinity complement-fixing IgG antinuclear antibodies, and antibodies to DNA. Subendothelial, intramembranous, or subepithelial deposits are characteristic. Wherever immune complexes are deposited, immunofluorescence staining is positive for complement and for IgG, IgA, and IgM in varying proportions.

Lupus nephritis should be distinguished from antiphospholipid syndrome nephropathy, which may occur independently or coexist in up to ⅓ of patients with lupus. In the antiphospholipid antibody syndrome, circulating lupus anticoagulant (see p. 1082) causes microthrombi, endothelial damage, and cortical ischemic atrophy. Antiphospholipid syndrome nephropathy increases a patient's risk of hypertension and renal insufficiency or failure compared with lupus nephritis alone.

Symptoms, Signs, and Diagnosis

The most prominent symptoms and signs are those of SLE; patients who present with renal disease may have edema, foaming urine, and/or hypertension.

Diagnosis is suspected by proteinuria, with or without microscopic hematuria and RBC casts, in a patient with SLE. Lupus nephritis usually develops within 1 yr of diagnosis of SLE, and a search for renal disease with urinalysis and serum creatinine is indicated whenever SLE is diagnosed or suspected.

Diagnosis is confirmed by renal biopsy. Histology is classified (WHO criteria) as normal (class I); immune complexes in the mesangium only (mesangial proliferative—class II—10 to 20% of cases); cellular proliferation and inflammation in < 50% of glomeruli usually in a segmental distribution (focal proliferative—class III—10 to 20%); cellular proliferation and inflammation in > 50% of glomeruli (diffuse proliferative—class IV—40 to 70%); and thickening of the glomerular basement membrane with subepithelial and intramembranous immune complex deposition (membranous—class V—10 to 20%). Some of these subtypes are similar to other glomerulopathies; eg, membranous and diffuse proliferative lupus nephritis are histologically similar to idiopathic membranous GN and type I membranoproliferative GN, respectively. Overlap between these categories is substantial, but the classification system is useful because clinical and prognostic features differ by category.

Renal function and SLE activity should be monitored regularly. A rising serum creatinine reflects deteriorating renal function, while a falling serum complement level or a rising anti-DNA antibody titer suggests increased disease activity.

Prognosis

Renal biopsies are scored with a semiquantitative "activity" and a "chronicity" index, which describe the degree of inflammation and scarring, respectively; the chronicity index (based on presence of glomerular sclerosis, fibrous crescents, tubular atrophy, or interstitial fibrosis) predicts progression of lupus nephritis to renal failure. Many experts believe that a mild to moderate chronicity index should provoke more aggressive therapy (eg, with cytotoxic drugs), whereas more severe chronicity scores may indicate irreversible disease, suggesting that the risk/benefit ratio of aggressive treatment might be unacceptable. The activity score (based on cellular proliferation, fibrinoid necrosis, cellular crescents, hyaline thrombi, wire loop lesions, glomerular leukocyte infiltration, or interstitial mononuclear cell infiltration) is less well correlated with disease progression, perhaps because it is based on more inflammatory disease that is more reversible with treatment.

Prognosis and indications for treatment of membranous lupus nephritis are poorly defined and controversial.

Treatment

Treatment usually combines cytotoxic drugs, antimetabolites, and corticosteroids. Induction is with cyclophosphamide, which is usually given in IV boluses (monthly for up to 6 mo) beginning with 0.75 g/m^2 and, assuming a WBC count > 3000/μL, increasing to a maximum of 1 g/m^2 in a saline solution over 30 to 60 min. Oral or IV fluid administration to create rapid urine flow minimizes the bladder toxicity of cyclophosphamide. Prednisone 60 to 80 mg po once/day is tapered according to response to 20 to 25 mg every other day over 6 to 12 mo. The amount of prednisone is determined by the extrarenal manifestations and number of relapses. Recurrences are usually treated with increasing doses of prednisone.

Many experts are replacing the more toxic cyclophosphamide maintenance regimens (after induction with 6 or 7 monthly IV cyclophosphamide doses) with protocols using mycophenolate (500 mg to 1 g po bid) or azathioprine (2 mg/kg po once/day, maximum 150 to 200 mg/day). Low-dose prednisone is continued (0.05 to 0.20 mg/kg once/day) and titrated based on disease activity. Duration of maintenance therapy is minimally 1 yr.

Anticoagulation is of theoretical benefit for patients with antiphospholipid syndrome nephropathy, but the value of such treatment has not been established.

236 TUBULOINTERSTITIAL DISEASES

Tubulointerstitial diseases are clinically heterogeneous disorders that share similar features of tubular and interstitial injury. In severe and prolonged cases, the entire kidney may become involved, with glomerular dysfunction and even renal failure. The primary categories of tubulointerstitial disease are acute tubular necrosis and acute or chronic tubulointerstitial nephritis.

Pathophysiology: The kidney has the highest blood supply of all tissues (about 3.5 mL/g/min), and unbound solutes leave the circulation via glomerular filtration at ≥ 100 mL/min; toxic agents are thus delivered at a rate 50 times that of other tissues and in much higher concentrations. When urine is concentrated, the luminal surfaces of tubular cells may be exposed to molecule concentrations 300 to 1000 times greater than that of plasma. The fine brush border of proximal tubular cells exposes an enormous surface area. A countercurrent flow mechanism increases ionic concentration of the interstitial fluid of the medulla (and thereby increases urine concentration) up to 4 times the plasma concentration.

In addition, tubular transport mechanisms separate drugs from their binding proteins, which normally protect cells from toxicity. Transcellular transport exposes the interior of the cell and its organelles to newly encountered chemicals. Binding sites of some agents (eg, sulfhydryl groups) may facilitate entry but retard exit (eg, heavy metals). General inhibition (eg, alkalinization, acidification) may alter transport in either direction. Blockade of transport receptors may alter tissue exposure (eg, diuresis from blockade of adenosine A receptor). Finally, the kidney has the highest O_2 and glucose consumption/g and is therefore vulnerable to toxins affecting cell energetics.

ACUTE TUBULAR NECROSIS

Acute tubular necrosis is characterized by acute tubular cell injury and dysfunction causing renal insufficiency or failure. Common causes are hypotension causing renal hypoperfusion and nephrotoxic drugs. The condition is asymptomatic unless it causes renal failure. The diagnosis is suspected when azotemia develops after a hypotensive event or drug exposure and is distinguished from prerenal azotemia by urine and blood chemistries. Treatment is supportive.

The most common causes of acute tubular necrosis (ATN) are hypotension and nephrotoxins. Common agents include aminoglycoside antibiotics, amphotericin, cisplatin, and radiocontrast (particularly > 100 mL). Major surgery and advanced hepatobiliary disease, poor perfusion states, and advanced age increase the risk of aminoglycoside toxicity. Less common causes include heme pigments (myoglobin and hemoglobin), poisons (ethylene glycol), and herbal and folk remedies (eg, ingestion of fish gallbladder in Southeast

TABLE 236–1. DISTINGUISHING ACUTE TUBULAR NECROSIS FROM PRERENAL AZOTEMIA

TEST*	ACUTE TUBULAR NECROSIS	PRERENAL AZOTEMIA
Rate of creatinine rise	0.3–0.5 mg/dL/day	Variable and fluctuates
BUN/creatinine ratio	10–15:1	> 20:1
Urine osmolality (mOsm/kg)	> 500	< 450
Urine Na (mEq/L)	> 40	< 20
Urine/plasma creatinine ratio	< 20	> 40
Fractional excretion of Na (%)	> 2	< 1
Urinary sediment	Muddy brown granular casts, epithelial cell casts, free epithelial cells	Normal or with hyaline casts
Response to saline expansion	Variable, typically no immediate reduction in serum creatinine	Serum creatinine normalizes in volume-depleted states

*Criteria may not apply in the setting of chronic renal failure and recent diuretic use.

Asia). Certain drug combinations (eg, aminoglycosides with amphotericin B) may be especially nephrotoxic. Toxic exposures cause patchy, segmental, tubular luminal occlusion with casts and cellular debris or segmental tubular necrosis. ATN is more likely to develop in those with a baseline creatinine clearance < 47 mL/min, diabetes mellitus, and preexisting hypovolemia or poor renal perfusion.

Symptoms, Signs, and Diagnosis

ATN is usually asymptomatic but may cause symptoms or signs of acute renal failure (see p. 1980), at which time oliguria is common. The condition is suspected when serum creatinine rises ≥ 0.5 mg/dL/day above baseline after a hypotensive event or after exposure to a nephrotoxin; the rise in creatinine may occur days after exposure to some nephrotoxins. Criteria for distinguishing ATN from prerenal azotemia, important to determining treatment, are listed in TABLE 236–1.

Prognosis, Treatment, and Prevention

Prognosis is good in otherwise healthy patients when the underlying insult is corrected; serum creatinine typically returns to normal or near-normal within 1 to 3 wk. In sick patients, even with mild acute renal failure, morbidity and mortality are increased; prognosis is better in a non-ICU (32% mortality) compared with an ICU (72% mortality) setting. Predictors of mortality include oliguria; high severity of illness; acute MI, stroke, or seizure; chronic immunosuppression; and the need for mechanical ventilation. Causes of death are usually infection or the underlying disease.

Treatment is supportive and includes discontinuation of nephrotoxins whenever possible, maintenance of euvolemia, and nutritional support. Diuretics are commonly used to maintain urine output in oliguric ATN but are of unproven benefit. Treatment of acute renal failure is discussed on p. 1984.

Prevention includes maintaining euvolemia and renal perfusion in critically ill patients, avoiding nephrotoxic drugs when possible and closely monitoring renal function when use is necessary, and taking various measures to avert contrast nephropathy (see below). Ineffective and possibly harmful agents include loop diuretics, dopamine, natriuretic peptides, and Ca channel blockers.

CONTRAST NEPHROPATHY

All iodinated radiocontrast agents are nephrotoxic. The precise mechanism of toxicity is unknown but is suspected to be some combination of renal vasoconstriction and ATN, perhaps through formation of reactive oxygen species. Risk factors for nephrotoxicity are older age, preexisting renal insufficiency (serum creatinine > 2 mg/dL), diabetes mellitus, heart failure, multiple myeloma, and high doses of hyperosmolar contrast agent (eg, during percutaneous coronary interventions). Factors that reduce renal perfusion, such as volume depletion or the concurrent use of NSAIDs or ACE inhibitors, also increase risk.

Diagnosis is based on a progressive rise in serum creatinine 24 to 48 h after a contrast study. Contrast nephropathy should be distinguished from renal atheroembolism, especially after femoral artery catheterization.

Treatment is supportive. Prevention involves mild volume expansion with $NaHCO_3$, which is preferred over isotonic NaCl. The infusion is as 3 mL/kg/h of $NaHCO_3$ at 154 mEq/L, beginning 1 h before contrast is given, followed by 1 mL/Kg/h for 6 h after the procedure. Nephrotoxic drugs are avoided before and after the procedure. Nonionic iso-osmolal contrast (eg, iodixanol) or nonionic low-osmolal contrast (eg, iohexol, iopamidol)—which has lower osmolality than ionic contrast but is still hyperosmolal relative to blood—is used. Acetylcysteine is an antioxidant that may be helpful; protocols vary, but it may be given 600 mg po bid the day before and the day of the procedure, combined with $NaHCO_3$ infusion. Acetylcysteine and volume expansion may be most helpful in patients with mild preexisting renal disease and exposure to a low dose of contrast. Periprocedural continuous venovenous hemofiltration may be more effective at preventing acute renal failure in patients with chronic renal insufficiency who require high doses of contrast.

TUBULOINTERSTITIAL NEPHRITIS

Tubulointerstitial nephritis is primary injury to renal tubules and interstitium resulting in decreased renal function. The acute form is most often due to allergic drug reactions or to infections. The chronic form is associated with a diverse array of diseases, including genetic, metabolic obstructive uropathy, and chronic environmental toxins, or to certain drugs and herbs. Diagnosis is suggested by history and urine and blood tests and confirmed by biopsy. Treatment and prognosis vary by the etiology and potential reversibility of the disorder at the time of diagnosis.

Etiology

Tubulointerstitial nephritis can be primary or can be secondary to glomerular damage (see Ch. 235 on p. 1996) and renovascular disease (see Ch. 238 on p. 2028). Primary tubulointerstitial nephritis may be acute or chronic (see TABLES 236–2 and 236–3).

Acute tubulointerstitial nephritis (ATIN) is associated with an inflammatory infiltrate and edema involving the renal interstitium that often develops over days to months. Over 95% of cases result from infection or an allergic drug reaction; a syndrome of ATIN associated with uveitis (renal-ocular syndrome) also occurs and is idiopathic. ATIN causes acute renal insufficiency or failure; severe cases, delayed therapy, or continuance of an offending drug can lead to permanent injury with chronic renal failure.

Chronic tubulointerstitial nephritis (CTIN) arises when chronic tubular insults cause gradual interstitial infiltration and fibrosis, tubular atrophy and dysfunction, and a gradual deterioration of renal function, usually over years. Glomerular involvement (glomerulosclerosis) is much more common in CTIN than in ATIN. Causes of CTIN are myriad; immunologically mediated diseases are most important, followed by infections, reflux or obstructive nephropathy, drugs, and other diseases. CTIN due to toxins, metabolic diseases, hypertension, and inherited disorders results in symmetric and bilateral disease; with other causes, renal scarring may be unequal and involve only one kidney. Some well-characterized forms of CTIN (analgesic, metabolic, heavy metal, and reflux nephropathy and myeloma kidney) are discussed in detail on pp. 2020–2022; hereditary cystic kidney diseases are discussed in Ch. 232 on p. 1975.

Symptoms and Signs

Symptoms and signs of ATIN include fever and urticarial rash, but the classically described triad of fever, rash, and eosinophilia is unreliable. Onset may be as long as several weeks after a 1st toxic exposure or as soon as 3 to 5 days after a 2nd exposure; extremes in latency range from 1 day with rifampin to 18 mo with an NSAID. Abdominal pain, weight loss, and bilateral renal masses (caused by interstitial edema) may also occur and with fever may mistakenly suggest renal malignancy or polycystic kidney disease. Many patients develop polyuria and nocturia (defect in concentration and Na reabsorption). Peripheral edema and hypertension are uncommon unless renal insufficiency or renal failure occurs.

Symptoms and signs are generally absent in CTIN. Edema usually is not present, and BP is normal or only mildly elevated in the

TABLE 236–2. CAUSES OF ACUTE TUBULOINTERSTITIAL NEPHRITIS

CAUSE	EXAMPLES
Drugs*	Antibiotics
	β-lactam agents
	Ciprofloxacin
	Ethambutol
	Isoniazid
	Macrolides
	Rifampin
	Tetracycline
	Trimethoprim-sulfamethoxazole
	Vancomycin
	Anticonvulsants
	Carbamazepine
	Phenobarbital
	Phenytoin
	Diuretics
	Furosemide
	Thiazides
	Triamterene
	NSAIDs
	Other
	Allopurinol
	Aristocholic acid
	Cimetidine
	Interferon
	Ranitidine
Idiopathic without and with uveitis	
Immunologic	Cryoglobulinemia
	IgA nephropathy
	Renal transplant rejection
	SLE (rare)
	Sjögren's syndrome
	Wegener's granulomatosis
Metabolic	Hyperoxaluria (eg, ethylene glycol poisoning)
	Hyperuricosuria (eg, tumor lysis syndrome)
Neoplastic	Lymphoma
	Myeloma
Renal parenchymal infection	Bacterial
	Legionella
	Leptospira
	Mycobacterium
	Mycoplasma
	Rickettsia
	Treponema pallidum
	Yersinia
	Fungal
	Candida
	Parasitic
	Toxoplasma gondii
	Viral
	Cytomegalovirus
	Epstein-Barr virus
	Hantavirus
	Hepatitis C
	Mumps
	Polyomavirus
Systemic infection	*Corynebacterium diphtheriae*
	Streptococcus species

* Most common listed; > 120 drugs implicated.

early stages. Symptoms of tubular dysfunction are similar to those of ATIN.

Symptoms and signs of acute or chronic renal insufficiency or failure may develop if tubulointerstitial nephritis significantly impairs renal function.

Diagnosis

Diagnosis is based on history, physical examination, and laboratory and imaging tests.

In ATIN, an active urine sediment with WBCs, RBCs, and WBC casts is typical; marked hematuria and dysmorphic RBCs are uncommon. Eosinophiluria has a positive predictive value of 50% and a negative predictive value of 90% for ATIN; thus, the presence of urinary eosinophils is not diagnostic, but their absence significantly excludes disease. Proteinuria is usually minimal but may reach nephrotic range with combined ATIN-glomerular disease induced by NSAIDs, ampicillin, rifampin, interferon, or ranitidine. Blood test findings of tubular dysfunction include hyperkalemia (defect in K excretion) and metabolic acidosis (defect in acid excretion). The kidneys may be greatly enlarged and echogenic by ultrasound examination because of interstitial inflammatory cells and edema. They may also avidly take up radioactive gallium-67 or radionuclide-labeled WBCs on radionuclide scans; positive scans strongly suggest ATIN, but a negative scan does not exclude the diagnosis.

Findings of CTIN are generally similar to those of ATIN, though urinary RBCs and WBCs are uncommon. Because CTIN is insidious in onset and is associated with interstitial fibrosis, imaging tests may show small kidneys with evidence of scarring and asymmetry.

Renal biopsy is not often performed for diagnostic purposes but has helped characterize the nature and progression of tubulointerstitial disease. In ATIN, glomeruli usually are normal. The earliest finding is interstitial edema, typically followed by interstitial infiltration with lymphocytes, plasma cells, eosinophils, and a few PMNs. In severe cases, inflammatory cells can be seen invading the space between the cells lining the tubular basement membrane (tubulitis); in other specimens, granulomatous reactions secondary to methicillin, sulfonamides, mycobacteria, and fungus may be seen. The presence of noncaseating granulomas suggests sarcoidosis. Immunofluorescence or electron microscopy seldom reveals any pathognomonic changes.

In CTIN, glomeruli vary from normal to completely destroyed. Tubules may be absent or atrophied. Tubular lumina vary in diameter but may show marked dilation, with homogeneous casts. The interstitium contains varying degrees of inflammatory cells and fibrosis. Nonscarred areas appear almost normal. Grossly, the kidneys are small and atrophic.

Prognosis

In drug-induced ATIN, renal function usually recovers within 6 to 8 wk when the offending drug is withdrawn, although some residual scarring is common. Recovery may be incomplete, with persistent azotemia above baseline. When other factors cause ATIN, histologic changes usually are reversible if the cause is recognized and removed; however, some severe cases progress to fibrosis and renal failure. Regardless of cause, diffuse rather

TABLE 236–3. CAUSES OF CHRONIC TUBULOINTERSTITIAL NEPHRITIS

CAUSE	EXAMPLES	CAUSE	EXAMPLES
Balkan nephropathy		Idiopathic	
Cystic diseases	Acquired cystic disease Medullary cystic disease Medullary sponge kidney Nephronophthisis Polycystic kidney disease	Immunologic	Amyloidosis Cryoglobulinemia Goodpasture's syndrome IgA nephropathy Renal transplant rejection Sarcoidosis Sjögren's syndrome SLE
Drugs	Analgesics Antineoplastics (cisplatin, nitrosourea) Immunosuppressives (cyclosporine, tacrolimus) Lithium	Infection	Renal parenchymal Hantavirus—Puumula type (nephropathia epidemica) Pyelonephritis Systemic
Granulomatous	Inflammatory bowel disease Sarcoidosis Tuberculosis Wegener's granulomatosis	Mechanical	Obstructive uropathy Reflux nephropathy
Heavy metals	Cadmium Lead	Metabolic	Chronic hypokalemia Cystinosis Hypercalcemia, hypercalciuria Hyperoxaluria Hyperuricemia, hyperuricosuria
Hematologic	Aplastic anemia Lymphoma Multiple myeloma Sickle cell anemia		
Hereditary nephropathy associated with hyperuricemia and gout		Radiation nephritis	
		Vascular	Atheroembolism Hypertension Renal vein thrombosis

than patchy interstitial infiltrates, delayed response to prednisone, and persistent acute renal failure (> 3 wk) suggest irreversible injury.

In CTIN, prognosis depends on the cause and on the ability to recognize and stop the process before irreversible fibrosis occurs. Many genetic (cystic kidney disease), metabolic (cystinosis), and toxic (heavy metal) causes may not be modifiable, in which case CTIN usually evolves to end-stage renal disease.

Treatment

Treatment of both ATIN and CTIN is management of the underlying causes. For immunologically induced disease in ATIN and perhaps CTIN, corticosteroids (eg, prednisone 1 mg/kg po once/day for 3 days and decreased over the next 7 to 10 days) may accelerate recovery. Also in patients with CTIN and progressive renal insufficiency, ACE inhibitors or angiotensin receptor blockers may slow disease progression.

Analgesic Abuse Nephropathy

Analgesic abuse nephropathy (AAN) is CTIN caused by cumulative lifetime use of large amounts (eg, ≥ 2 kg) of certain analgesics.

AAN was originally described in conjunction with overuse of combination analgesics containing phenacetin (typically with aspirin, acetaminophen, codeine, or caffeine). However, despite removal of phenacetin from the market, AAN continued to occur. Studies to identify the causal agent are equivocal, but acetaminophen, aspirin, and other NSAIDs have been implicated. Mechanism is unclear. Whether COX-2 inhibitors cause AAN is not known, but these drugs probably can cause ATIN and nephrotic syndrome due to minimal change disease or membranous nephropathy.

AAN predominates in women (peak incidence, 50 to 55 yr) and, in the US, is responsible for 3 to 5% of cases of end-stage renal disease (13 to 20% in Australia and South Africa).

Patients present with renal insufficiency, a bland urinary sediment, and non-nephrotic proteinuria. Hypertension and impaired urinary concentration are common. Flank pain and hematuria are signs of papillary necrosis that occur late in the course of disease. Chronic complaints of musculoskeletal pain, headache, malaise, and dyspepsia may be precipitants of long-term analgesic use rather than effects of AAN.

Diagnosis is based on history and noncontrast CT. CT signs of AAN are decreased renal size; "bumpy" contours, defined as at least 3 indentations in the normally convex outline of the kidney; and papillary calcifications, which have a sensitivity of 92% and a specificity of 100% for early diagnosis.

Renal function stabilizes when analgesics are stopped unless renal insufficiency is advanced, in which case it may progress to renal failure. Patients with AAN are at greater risk of transitional cell carcinomas of the urinary tract.

Metabolic Nephropathies

Acute urate nephropathy: This is not a true form of ATIN but rather an intraluminal obstructive uropathy caused by uric acid crystal deposition within the lumen of renal tubules; acute oliguric or anuric renal failure results. It most commonly occurs from tumor lysis syndrome (see p. 1170) after treatment of lymphoma, leukemia, or other myeloproliferative diseases, but it also occurs after seizures or treatment of solid tumors and with rare primary disorders of urate overproduction (hypoxanthine-guanine phosphoribosyltransferase deficiency) or overexcretion due to decreased proximal tubule reabsorption (Fanconi-like syndromes).

Diagnosis is suspected when acute renal failure (ARF) occurs with marked hyperuricemia (> 15 mg/dL). Typically, no symptoms are present. Urinalysis may be normal or may show urate crystals.

Prognosis for complete recovery of renal function is excellent if treatment is initiated rapidly. Treatment is supportive and may include hemodialysis to remove excess circulating urate in severe cases where diuresis cannot be induced with a loop diuretic and IV saline.

Prevention is by alkalinization of the urine to pH > 6.5 and use of allopurinol 300 mg bid to tid plus saline loading to maintain a urine output > 2.5 L/day before chemotherapy or radiation therapy. Urate oxidase (rasburicase), which catalyzes urate to a much more soluble compound, is also preventative but is not widely used because it must be given IV and can cause anaphylaxis, hemolysis, and other adverse effects.

Chronic urate nephropathy: This condition is CTIN caused by deposition of Na urate crystals in the medullary interstitium in the setting of chronic hyperuricemia. Sequelae are chronic inflammation and fibrosis, with ensuing chronic renal insufficiency and renal failure. Chronic urate nephropathy was once common in patients with tophaceous gout but is now rare because of treatment. A bland urine sediment and hyperuricemia disproportionate to the degree of renal insufficiency (eg, urate > 9 mg/dL with serum creatinine < 1.5 mg/dL, or > 10 mg/dL with serum creatinine 1.5 to 2 mg/dL, and > 12 mg/dL with more advanced renal failure) are suggestive but nonspecific; many causes of tubulointerstitial diseases may have these findings, lead nephropathy being the most common (see below). Treatment is that of hyperuricosuria (see p. 302).

Hyperoxaluria: Hyperoxaluria is a cause of both acute and chronic tubulointerstitial nephritis. ATIN and ARF may develop in susceptible patients who ingest high-oxalate foods (eg, tea, chocolate, spinach, rhubarb, star fruit) or who are exposed to exogenous substances that are metabolized into oxalate (eg, ethylene glycol ingestion, methoxyflurane anesthesia, large doses of ascorbic acid). CTIN and progressive chronic renal failure develop in patients with inherited disorders of excessive oxalate production (types I and II primary hyperoxaluria) or acquired GI diseases (eg, short bowel syndrome with increased gut absorption). Oxalate is highly insoluble when combined with Ca, and urinary excretion of greater than normal amounts leads to Ca oxalate precipitation and subsequent nephrolithiasis, ARF, or tubulointerstitial damage. Symptoms and signs differ by form of disease and include hematuria and renal colic from oxalate calculi, UTI and pyuria, hypertension, and renal tubular acidosis.

Treatment involves correcting the underlying cause if possible. High-oxalate foods should be avoided, and fluid intake should be increased to increase urinary volume. Other interventions may include Ca carbonate (1 g po once/day to qid) to bind gut oxalate; pyridoxine supplements (3 to 3.5 mg/kg po once/day) to promote conversion of glyoxalate to glycine rather than to oxalate; neutral phosphate (orthophosphate—10 to 13 mg/kg tid) to increase the urinary excretion of pyrophosphate, an inhibitor of Ca precipitation (the extra oral phosphate can also modestly reduce urinary Ca excretion by binding dietary Ca in the intestinal lumen); K citrate (10 to 20 mEq tid with meals) to increase urinary Ca oxalate solubility; or thiazide diuretics to reduce urinary Ca excretion. Treatment when end-stage renal disease occurs due to an inherited disorder is combined liver and kidney transplantation.

Hypercalcemia: Hypercalcemia (see p. 1254) causes nephropathy by 2 mechanisms. Severe (> 12 mg/dL) temporary hypercalcemia may cause reversible renal insufficiency by renal vasoconstriction and natriuresis-induced volume depletion. Long-standing hypercalcemia and hypercalciuria lead to CTIN with calcification and necrosis of tubular cells, interstitial fibrosis, and calcification (nephrocalcinosis). Diagnosis is based on presence of hypercalcemia and unexplained renal insufficiency; nephrocalcinosis can be detected by ultrasonography or noncontrast CT. Treatment is management of hypercalcemia. Nephrolithiasis, renal tubular acidosis, and nephrogenic diabetes insipidus are common associated findings.

Chronic hypokalemia: Chronic hypokalemia of a moderate to severe degree may produce nephropathy with impaired urinary concentration and vacuolation of proximal tubular cells and occasionally of distal tubular cells. Chronic interstitial inflammatory changes, fibrosis, and renal cysts have been found in renal biopsies of patients with hypokalemia of ≥ 1 mo. Treatment consists of correction of underlying causes and oral K supplements. Although the hypokalemia as well as the number and size of the cysts is reversible, the CTIN and renal insufficiency may be irreversible.

Heavy Metal Nephropathy

Lead: CTIN results as lead accumulates in proximal tubular cells. Short-term lead exposure causes proximal tubular dysfunction, including decreased urate secretion and hyperuricemia (the substrate for saturnine gout), aminoaciduria, and renal glucosuria. Chronic lead exposure (5 to 30 yr) causes progressive tubular atrophy, interstitial fibrosis, hypertension, and gout. Chronic low-level exposure may cause renal insufficiency and hypertension independent of tubulointerstitial disease. Children exposed to lead paint dust or chips, welders, battery workers, and drinkers of moonshine alcohol are most at risk. Diagnosis is usually made by whole blood lead levels. Alternatively, x-ray fluorescence may be used to detect increased bone lead concentrations, which reflect high cumulative lead exposure. Treatment with chelation therapy (see p. 2670) can stabilize renal function, but recovery may be incomplete.

Cadmium: Cadmium from contaminated water, food, and tobacco and from workplace exposures can cause nephropathy. Early manifestations are those of tubular dysfunction, including low mol wt tubular proteinuria (eg, β_2-microglobulin), aminoaciduria, and renal glucosuria. Symptoms and signs, when they occur, are attributable to chronic renal insufficiency and failure. Renal disease follows a dose-response curve. Diagnosis is suggested by a history of occupational exposure, increased levels of urinary β_2-microglobulin, and increased urinary cadmium levels (> 7 μg/g creatinine). Treatment is elimination of cadmium exposure; chelation with Na calcium edetate (EDTA) may increase cadmium nephrotoxicity. Tubular proteinuria usually is irreversible.

Other heavy metals: Those that are nephrotoxic include copper, gold, uranium, arsenic, iron, mercury, bismuth, and chromium. All cause tubular damage and dysfunction (eg, tubular proteinuria, aminoaciduria) as well as tubular necrosis, but glomerulopathies may predominate with some compounds (mercury, gold). Treatment involves removal of the patient from further exposure and chelating agents (copper, arsenic, bismuth) or dialysis (chromium, arsenic, bismuth).

Reflux Nephropathy

Reflux nephropathy is renal scarring induced by vesicoureteral reflux of infected urine into the renal parenchyma.

Chronic pyelonephritis also may play a role, but UTI without intrarenal reflux is unlikely to cause nephropathy. Vesicoureteral reflux (VUR) affects about 1% of newborns and 30 to 45% of young children with a UTI (see p. 2356); it is present in almost all children with renal scars and, for unknown reasons, is less common in black children. Children with gross reflux (up to the renal pelvis plus ureteral dilatation) are at highest risk of scarring.

Reflux requires incompetent ureterovesical valves or mechanical obstruction in the lower urinary tract. Young children with concave papillary tips are most susceptible because the papillary collecting duct orifices are normally wide open at the upper and lower poles; normal growth usually results in spontaneous cessation of intrarenal and vesicoureteral reflux by age 5. New scars in children > 5 yr are unusual but may occur after acute pyelonephritis.

Few symptoms and signs are present in young children, and the diagnosis is often overlooked until adolescence, when patients present with proteinuria, hypertension, and/or renal insufficiency.

Diagnosis

Diagnosis and staging of reflux is made by a voiding cystourethrogram (VCUG), which can demonstrate the degree of ureteral dilatation; radionuclide cystography can be used to diagnose but not to stage the condition. Renal scarring is diagnosed with 99m-technetium dimercaptosuccinic acid (DMSA) radionuclide scanning or with IVU, which is less sensitive. In older children in whom reflux is no longer active, a VCUG may not show reflux, although the DMSA scan shows scarring; cystoscopy can demonstrate evidence of previous reflux at ureteral orifices. Renal biopsy at this late stage shows CTIN and focal glomerulosclerosis, the cause of mild (1 to 1.5 g/day) to nephrotic range proteinuria.

Treatment

Many children require no treatment. Children with low-grade reflux are usually given antibiotics because they are at low risk of developing severe renal disease. However, drug therapy is associated with a higher incidence of new episodes of acute pyelonephritis; incidence of new renal scars is similar in surgical and drug treatment groups. Patients with severe reflux can be given antibiotic prophylaxis or undergo surgical interventions, including ureteral reimplantation or endoscopic injection of materials behind the ureter to prevent reflux (bladder contraction during voiding compresses the ureter between the bladder and the material).

Reflux spontaneously resolves in about 80% of young children within 5 yr. Persistent VUR may cause slowly progressive renal failure.

Myeloma-Related Kidney Disease

Patients with multiple myeloma overproduce monoclonal Ig light chains (Bence Jones proteins); these light chains are filtered by glomeruli, are nephrotoxic, and can damage virtually all areas of the kidney parenchyma.

The mechanisms of nephrotoxicity are unknown. Tubulointerstitial and glomerular damage are most common.

Tubulointerstitial disease: Light chains saturate the reabsorptive capacity of the proximal tubule, reach the distal nephron, and combine with filtered proteins and Tamm-Horsfall mucoprotein (secreted by the thick ascending limb cells) to form obstructive casts. The term myeloma kidney generally refers to renal insufficiency caused by the tubulointerstitial damage that results. Factors that predispose to cast formation include low urine flow, elevation of luminal NaCl concentration (eg, due to a loop diuretic), radiocontrast agents, and increased intratubular Ca from the hypercalcemia frequently occurring from bone lysis in multiple myeloma.

Other types of tubulointerstitial lesions associated with Bence Jones proteinuria include proximal tubular transport dysfunction producing Fanconi syndrome and light chain interstitial deposition with inflammatory infiltrates and active tubular damage.

Glomerulopathies: Myeloma glomerulopathy has 2 common mechanisms: AL amyloidosis (see also p. 1310) and glomerular light chain deposition. AL amyloidosis results in mesangial and/or subepithelial glomerular deposition of AL amyloid, randomly oriented, nonbranching fibrils composed of the variable regions of λ light chains. Light chain deposition disease (LCDD), which also can occur with lymphoma and Waldenström's macroglobulinemia, is glomerular deposition of nonpolymerized light chains, generally the constant regions of κ chains.

Less commonly, a nonproliferative, noninflammatory glomerulopathy that causes nephrotic range proteinuria can develop in advanced myeloma-related renal disease, and a proliferative glomerulonephritis occasionally develops as an early form of LCDD with progression to membranoproliferative glomerulonephritis and nodular glomerulopathy reminiscent of diabetic nephropathy.

Symptoms, Signs, and Diagnosis

Symptoms and signs are predominantly those of the myeloma (skeletal pain, pathologic fractures, diffuse osteoporosis) and a normochromic-normocytic anemia.

Diagnosis of myeloma-related kidney disease is suggested by findings of renal insufficiency, usually accompanied by bland urine sediment and a negative or trace-positive dipstick for protein (unless urine albumin is elevated in a patient with an accompanying nephrotic syndrome). Diagnosis of light chain tubulointerstitial disease is confirmed by a markedly positive urine sulfosalicylic acid test suggesting significant nonalbumin proteins and/or urine protein electrophoresis (UPEP). Diagnosis of glomerulopathy is confirmed by renal biopsy. Renal biopsy may demonstrate light chain deposition in 30 to 50% of patients despite the absence of detectable serum or urine paraproteins by immunoelectrophoresis.

Prognosis and Treatment

Prognosis is good for patients with tubulointerstitial and glomerular LCDD who receive treatment. Prognosis is worse for patients with AL amyloidosis, in whom amyloid deposition continues and progresses to renal failure in most cases. In either form without treatment, virtually all renal lesions progress to renal failure.

Treatment is management of multiple myeloma (see p. 1130) combined with prevention of volume depletion and maintenance of a high urine flow rate. Alkalinization of the urine helps change the net charge of the light chain and reduces charge interaction with Tamm-Horsfall mucoprotein, making the light chains more soluble. Colchicine decreases Tamm-Horsfall mucoprotein secretion into the lumen and decreases the interaction with light chains, thus decreasing toxicity. Avoidance of loop diuretics prevents volume depletion and high distal Na concentrations that can worsen myeloma-related kidney disease.

237 ABNORMAL RENAL TRANSPORT SYNDROMES

Many substances are secreted or reabsorbed in the renal tubule system, including electrolytes, protons, HCO_3 molecules, and free water. Dysfunction of these processes can result in clinical syndromes.

BARTTER SYNDROME

Bartter syndrome is a constellation of fluid, electrolyte, and hormonal abnormalities characterized by renal K, Na, and Cl wasting; hypokalemia; hyperaldosteronism; hyperreninemia; and normal BP. The condition affects children, producing electrolyte and growth abnormalities. Diagnosis is assisted by urine electrolyte measurements and hormone assays but is typically a diagnosis of exclusion. Treatment consists of NSAIDs, K-sparing diuretics, low-dose ACE inhibitors, and electrolyte replacement.

Bartter syndrome results from deranged NaCl transport in the ascending thick limb of the loop of Henle and the distal tubule. Subsequent K, Na, and Cl wasting leads to increased renin and aldosterone release, metabolic alkalosis, hyperuricemia, hypomagnesemia, hypercalciuria, and increased prostaglandin secretion. Further, Na wasting results in a chronically low plasma volume reflected by a normal BP despite high renin and angiotensin levels.

Bartter syndrome usually appears in childhood as a sporadic or familial disorder (usually autosomal recessive).

Symptoms and Signs

Bartter syndrome can manifest antenatally with intrauterine growth restriction and polyhydramnios. After birth, affected children have poor growth rates and appear malnourished. Most patients have low or low-normal BP and may have signs of volume depletion. Inability to retain K, Ca, or Mg can lead to muscle weakness, spasms, tetany, or palpitations. Polydipsia, polyuria, and vomiting may also be present. Mental retardation and nephrocalcinosis sometimes result.

Diagnosis

Bartter syndrome is typically a diagnosis of exclusion but should be suspected in children with an unexplained constellation of symptoms as described above. Measurement of urine electrolytes demonstrates high levels of Na, K, and Cl that are inappropriate for the euvolemic or hypovolemic state of the patient. Plasma levels of renin and aldosterone are increased, and the absence of hypertension and edema can distinguish the disorder from primary and secondary aldosteronism (see TABLE 153–3 on p. 1215).

In adult patients, bulimia nervosa, vomiting, and surreptitious laxative abuse must be excluded as causes. In these conditions, the urinary Cl is usually low (< 20 mmol/L). Diuretic abuse can also mimic this condition and can only be confirmed by a urine assay for diuretics.

Definitive diagnosis is through genetic testing, which is not commercially available and thus is rarely performed.

Prognosis and Treatment

Bartter syndrome may result in premature birth and severe electrolyte disorders and symptoms but does not typically lead to chronic renal insufficiency.

The combination of NSAIDs (indomethacin, 1 to 2 mg/kg po once/day) and a K-sparing diuretic (spironolactone, 150 mg po bid, or amiloride, 10 to 20 mg po bid) corrects most features. Further improvement in plasma electrolytes can be gained with low-dose ACE inhibitors. However, no therapy can completely eliminate K wasting, and K supplementation (KCl 20 to 40 mEq po once/day or bid) is often necessary. Mg and Ca supplements may also be needed.

Exogenous growth hormone is sometimes used to treat short stature in affected children.

LIDDLE SYNDROME

Liddle syndrome is a rare hereditary disorder in which the kidneys excrete K but retain too much Na and water, leading to hypertension. Symptoms are of hypertension, fluid

retention, and metabolic alkalosis. Diagnosis is through measurement of urinary electrolytes. K-sparing diuretics provide the best treatment.

Liddle syndrome is a rare autosomal dominant disorder of renal epithelial transport that clinically resembles primary aldosteronism (see p. 1214), with hypertension and hypokalemic metabolic alkalosis but without elevated plasma renin or aldosterone levels. The syndrome results from an inherently increased activity of the luminal membrane Na channels, which accelerates Na resorption and K secretion in the collecting tubule.

Patients with Liddle syndrome present at < 35 yr. Hypertension is present as are signs and symptoms of hypokalemia and metabolic alkalosis.

Diagnosis is suggested by the presence of hypertension, low urine Na (< 20 mEq), normal plasma renin and aldosterone levels, family history, and response to empiric treatment. Definitive diagnosis can be achieved through genetic testing but is rarely performed.

Triamterene (100 to 200 mg po bid) or amiloride (5 to 20 mg po once/day) are effective because they close Na channels. Spironolactone is ineffective.

NEPHROGENIC DIABETES INSIPIDUS

(See also Central Diabetes Insipidus on p. 1189.)

Nephrogenic diabetes insipidus is an inability to concentrate urine due to impaired renal tubule response to ADH (vasopressin), which leads to excretion of large amounts of dilute urine (in central diabetes insipidus, inadequate ADH production leads to the same sequelae). It can be inherited or secondary to conditions that impair renal concentration. Symptoms and signs include polyuria and those related to dehydration and hypernatremia. Diagnosis is based on measurement of urine osmolarity changes after water deprivation and/or administration of exogenous ADH. Treatment consists of adequate free water intake, thiazide diuretics, NSAIDs, and a low-salt, low-protein diet.

Nephrogenic diabetes insipidus (NDI) can be inherited, most commonly as an X-linked trait, but in rare cases is recessive. Homozygotes are completely unresponsive to ADH. Heterozygotes have normal or slightly impaired responsiveness to ADH.

Acquired NDI can occur when disorders disrupt the medulla or distal nephrons and impair urine concentrating ability, making the kidneys appear insensitive to ADH. These disorders include medullary and polycystic disease; sickle cell nephropathy; release of obstructing periureteral fibrosis; medullary sponge kidney; pyelonephritis; hypokalemic and hypercalcemic nephropathies; amyloidosis; Sjögren's syndrome; and myeloma. Certain nephrotoxins, especially lithium and demeclocycline, can cause NDI.

A mild form of acquired NDI can occur in any patient who is elderly or sick or who has acute or chronic renal insufficiency. An unusual form of transient ADH resistance also occurs in some women in the latter half of pregnancy (gestational diabetes insipidus).

Symptoms and Signs

Generation of large amounts of dilute urine (3 to 20 L/day) is the hallmark. Patients typically have a good thirst response, and serum Na remains near normal. However, patients who do not have good access to water or who cannot communicate their thirst (eg, infants, elderly patients with dementia) typically develop hypernatremia from extreme dehydration.

Infants with inherited NDI may develop brain damage with permanent mental retardation if treatment is not started early. Even with treatment, physical growth is often retarded in affected children presumably because of frequent dehydration.

Diagnosis

NDI is suspected in any patient producing a large amount of dilute urine. Glycosuria must be excluded. Serum Na is mildly elevated (142 to 145 mEq/L) in patients with adequate free water intake but can be dramatically elevated in patients who do not have adequate access to free water. Urine osmolality is typically < 200 despite clinical signs of hypovolemia.

The diagnosis is confirmed by a water deprivation test, which assesses the maximum urine-concentrating ability and response to exogenous ADH. After 3 to 6 h of water deprivation, the maximal osmolality of urine in NDI patients is abnormally low (< 400 mOsm/kg). NDI can be distinguished from central diabetes insipidus (lack of ADH) by administering exogenous ADH (5 units of aqueous vasopressin sc or desmopressin 10 μg intranasally). In patients with central diabetes insipidus (see p. 1189), urine osmolality increases 50 to 100% over the 2 h after administration of exogenous ADH, whereas patients with NDI have only minimal rise in urine osmolality (< 50 mOsm/kg).

Treatment

Treatment consists of ensuring adequate free water intake and correcting the underlying cause or discontinuing any likely nephrotoxin. Serious sequelae are rare if the patient can drink at will.

Some drugs can lower urine output. Thiazide diuretics (hydrochlorothiazide, 25 mg once/day or bid) can paradoxically reduce urine output by diminishing water delivery to ADH-sensitive sites in the collecting tubules. NSAIDs (indomethacin), amiloride, and a low-salt, low-protein diet can also be of benefit.

RENAL GLUCOSURIA

(Renal Glycosuria)

Renal glucosuria is glucose in the urine without hyperglycemia; it results from an inherited, isolated defect in glucose transport or occurs with other renal tubule disorders.

Renal glucosuria is the excretion of glucose in the urine in the presence of normal blood glucose levels. The condition usually involves a reduction in the glucose transport maximum (the maximum rate at which glucose can be resorbed) and subsequent escape of glucose in the urine.

The disorder is usually inherited as an autosomal dominant trait but is occasionally recessive. Renal glucosuria may occur without any other abnormalities of renal function or as part of a generalized defect in proximal tubule function (see type 2 renal tubular acidosis on p. 2027). It also may occur with various systemic disorders, including Fanconi syndrome, cystinosis, Wilson's disease, hereditary tyrosinemia, and oculocerebrorenal syndrome (Lowe syndrome).

Renal glucosuria is asymptomatic and without serious sequelae. In cases of glucosuria associated with a generalized defect in proximal tubular function, symptoms and signs may include hypophosphatemic rickets, volume depletion, short stature, muscle hypotonia, ocular changes of cataracts or glaucoma (oculocerebrorenal syndrome) or Kayser-Fleischer rings (Wilson's disease). With such findings, transport defects other than glucosuria should be sought.

The disorder is typically initially noted on routine urinalysis. Diagnosis is based on finding > 500 mg glucose in a 24-h urine collection (on a diet containing 50% carbohydrate) in the absence of hyperglycemia (serum glucose < 140 mg/dL). To confirm that the excreted sugar is glucose and to exclude pentosuria, fructosuria, sucrosuria, maltosuria, galactosuria, and lactosuria, the glucose oxidase method should be used for all laboratory measurements.

Isolated renal glucosuria is benign; no treatment is necessary.

RENAL TUBULAR ACIDOSIS

Renal tubular acidosis is acidosis and electrolyte disturbances due to impaired renal hydrogen ion excretion (type 1), impaired HCO_3 resorption (type 2), or abnormal aldosterone production or response (type 4). (Type 3 is extremely rare and is not discussed.) Patients may be asymptomatic, display symptoms and signs of electrolyte derangements, or progress to chronic renal failure. Diagnosis is based on characteristic changes in urine pH and electrolytes in response to acid or base loading. Treatment corrects pH and electrolyte imbalance using alkaline agents, electrolytes, and, rarely, drugs.

Renal tubular acidosis (RTA) defines a class of disorders in which excretion of hydrogen ions or reabsorption of filtered HCO_3 is impaired, leading to a chronic metabolic acidosis (see p. 1268) with a normal anion gap. Hyperchloremia is usually present, and secondary derangements in other electrolytes, such as K and Ca, frequently occur.

Chronic RTA is often associated with structural damage to renal tubules and may progress to chronic renal failure (see p. 1985).

Type 1 (distal) RTA is an impairment in hydrogen ion secretion in the distal tubule, resulting in a persistently high urine pH (> 5.5) and systemic acidosis. Plasma HCO_3 is usually < 15 mEq/L, and hypokalemia, hypercalciuria, and decreased citrate excretion are often present. This syndrome is rare. Sporadic cases occur most often in adults and may be primary (nearly always in women) or secondary to various diseases (eg, autoimmune disease with hypergammaglobulinemia, particularly Sjögren's syndrome or RA; kidney transplantation; nephrocalcinosis; renal medullary sponge kidney; or chronic renal obstruction) or drugs (amphotericin B, ifosfamide, lithium). Familial cases usually present in childhood and are most often autosomal dominant; they typically are associated with hypercalciuria and nephrocalcinosis.

Type 2 (proximal) RTA is an impairment in HCO_3 resorption in the proximal tubules, producing a urine pH > 7 if plasma HCO_3 concentration is normal, and a urine pH < 5.5 if plasma HCO_3 concentration is already depleted from ongoing losses. This syndrome may occur as part of a generalized dysfunction of proximal tubules and can be associated with increased urinary excretion of glucose, uric acid, phosphate, amino acids, and protein. The disorder is rare and most often occurs in the context of Fanconi syndrome, light chain nephropathy, multiple myeloma, or various drug exposures (acetazolamide, sulfonamides, ifosfamide, outdated tetracycline, streptozocin). Other etiologies include vitamin D deficiency, chronic hypocalcemia with secondary hyperparathyroidism, kidney transplantation, heavy metal exposure, and other inherited diseases (eg, fructose intolerance, Wilson's disease, oculocerebrorenal syndrome [Lowe syndrome], cystinosis).

Type 4 (generalized) RTA results from aldosterone deficiency or unresponsiveness of the distal tubule to aldosterone. Because aldosterone triggers Na resorption in exchange for K and H, there is reduced K excretion, causing hyperkalemia, reduced ammonia production, and reduced acid excretion. However, urine pH is usually normal. Plasma HCO_3 is usually in the lower range of normal. This disorder is the most common form of RTA. It typically occurs sporadically secondary to an impairment in the renin-aldosterone-renal tubule axis (hyporeninemic hypoaldosteronism). It may also occur in the context of diabetes mellitus, HIV nephropathy, or interstitial renal damage (SLE, obstructive uropathy, sickle cell disease), infection (cytomegalovirus, *Mycobacterium avium* complex), and various drugs (eg, NSAIDs, ACE inhibitors, angiotensin II receptor blockers, K-sparing diuretics, trimethoprim, pentamidine, heparin). Other causes include adrenal insufficiency, congenital adrenal hyperplasia, and genetic disorders (eg, aldosterone synthase type I or II deficiency, pseudohypoaldosteronism type I or II).

Symptoms and Signs

RTA is usually asymptomatic. However, signs of chronic electrolyte abnormalities may become apparent. Ca derangements in type 1 RTA may result in bony involvement (eg, bone pain, osteomalacia, rickets) or calculus formation (eg, nephrolithiasis, nephrocalcinosis).

Severe electrolyte disturbances are rare but can be life threatening. People with type 1 or 2 RTA may show signs and symptoms of hypokalemia, including muscle weakness, hyporeflexia, and paralysis. Type 4 RTA is usually asymptomatic with only mild acidosis, but cardiac arrhythmias or paralysis may develop if hyperkalemia is severe. Signs of ECF volume depletion may develop from urinary water loss accompanying electrolyte excretion.

Diagnosis

RTA is suspected in any patient with unexplained metabolic acidosis (low plasma HCO_3 and low blood pH) with normal anion gap.

Type 1 RTA is confirmed by a urine pH that remains > 5.5 during systemic acidosis. The acidosis may occur spontaneously or be induced by an acid load test (administration of ammonium Cl, 100 mg/kg po). Normal kidneys reduce urine pH to < 5.2 within 6 h of acidosis.

Type 2 RTA is diagnosed by measurement of the urine pH and fractional HCO_3 excretion during an HCO_3 infusion ($NaHCO_3$, 0.5 to 1.0 mEq/kg/h IV). In type 2, urine pH rises above 7.5, and the fractional excretion of HCO_3 is > 15%.

Type 4 RTA is considered in any patient with metabolic acidosis and persistent hyperkalemia without an obvious cause, such as severe renal failure, excessive intake of K supplements, or use of a K-sparing diuretic. A low transtubular K concentration gradient (< 5) indicates inappropriately low urinary K excretion and suggests hypoaldosteronism or tubular unresponsiveness to aldosterone. The gradient is calculated by

$$\text{Transtubular K gradient} = \frac{\text{Urine K/Plasma K}}{\text{Urine osmolality/Plasma osmolality}}$$

Definitive diagnosis can be obtained by measuring plasma renin and aldosterone levels after a stimulus has been applied (eg, administration of a loop diuretic, having the patient remain in the upright position for 3 h) but is usually not necessary.

Treatment

Treatment consists of correction of pH and electrolyte balance with alkali therapy. Failure to treat RTA in children slows growth.

Alkaline agents such as $NaHCO_3$ or Na citrate help achieve a relatively normal plasma HCO_3 concentration (22 to 24 mEq/L). K citrate can be substituted when persistent hypokalemia or Ca stone disease is present. Vitamin D (ergocalciferol, 400 IU po once/day) and Ca supplements (Ca carbonate, 1250 mg po tid or 500 mg elemental Ca^{2+}) may also be needed to help reduce skeletal deformities resulting from osteomalacia or rickets.

Type 1 RTA: Adults are given $NaHCO_3$ or Na citrate (0.25 to 0.5 mEq/kg po q 6 h). In children, the total daily dose may need to be as much as 2 mEq/kg q 8 h; this dose can be adjusted as the child grows.

Type 2 RTA: Plasma HCO_3 cannot be restored to the normal range, but HCO_3 replacement should exceed the acid load of the diet ($NaHCO_3$, 1 mEq/kg q 6 h in adults or 2 to 4 mEq/kg q 6 h in children). However, excess HCO_3 replacement increases $KHCO_3$ losses in the urine. Thus, citrate salts can be substituted for $NaHCO_3$ and may be better tolerated. K supplements or K citrate may be required in patients who become hypokalemic when given $NaHCO_3$ but is not recommended in patients with normal or high serum K levels. In difficult cases, treatment with low-dose hydrochlorothiazide (25 mg po bid) may stimulate proximal tubule transport functions. In cases of generalized proximal tubule disorder, hypophosphatemia and bone disorders are treated with phosphate and vitamin D supplementation to normalize the plasma phosphate concentration.

Type 4 RTA: Hyperkalemia is treated with volume expansion, dietary K restriction, and K-wasting diuretics (eg, furosemide 20 to 40 mg po once/day or bid titrated to effect). A few patients need mineralocorticoid replacement therapy (fludrocortisone, 0.1 to 0.2 mg po once/day); this should be used with caution, because it may exacerbate underlying hypertension, heart failure, or edema.

238 RENOVASCULAR DISORDERS

(See also Renovascular Hypertension on p. 616.)

Vascular disorders of the kidneys may involve partial or complete occlusion of large, medium, or small renal vessels and most commonly affect the glomeruli (see p. 1996). Systemic vasculitis (see p. 272) also may affect glomeruli.

BENIGN HYPERTENSIVE ARTERIOLAR NEPHROSCLEROSIS

Benign hypertensive arteriolar nephrosclerosis is progressive renal impairment due to chronic, poorly controlled hypertension. Symptoms and signs of chronic renal failure may develop, as may signs of end-organ damage secondary to hypertension. Diagnosis is primarily clinical, supported by laboratory tests. Treatment is strict BP control and support of renal function.

Benign hypertensive arteriolar nephrosclerosis results when chronic hypertension damages small blood vessels, glomeruli, renal tubules, and interstitial tissues. As a result, progressive renal failure develops.

Risk factors include older age, poorly controlled moderate to severe hypertension, and other renal disorders (eg, diabetic nephropathy). Blacks are at high risk; it is unclear if this is because poorly treated hypertension is common or they are genetically susceptible to hypertension-induced renal damage.

Benign nephrosclerosis progresses to end-stage renal disease in only a small percentage of patients. However, because chronic hypertension and benign nephrosclerosis are common, benign nephrosclerosis is one of the most common diagnoses in patients with end-stage renal disease.

Symptoms, Signs, and Diagnosis

Symptoms and signs of chronic renal failure may develop (see p. 1986). Signs of hypertension-related end-organ damage may occur in the vasculature of the eyes and in the skin, CNS, and periphery.

The diagnosis may be initially suspected when routine blood tests indicate deteriorating renal function. Diagnosis is primarily by history and evidence of hypertension-related end-organ damage (eg, retinal changes, left ventricular hypertrophy) on physical examination.

Laboratory tests can confirm chronic renal insufficiency or failure (eg, indicated by elevated creatinine and BUN and by hyperphosphatemia) and exclude other causes of renal failure. Typically, urinalysis shows few cells or casts in the sediment. Protein excretion is usually < 1 g/day but is occasionally in the nephrotic range.

Ultrasonography is done only if other causes of renal failure must be excluded. It may show that kidney size is reduced. Renal biopsy is done only if the diagnosis remains unclear.

Prognosis and Treatment

Prognosis usually depends on BP control and degree of renal failure. Usually, renal impairment progresses slowly; after 5 to 10 yr, only 2% of patients develop clinically significant renal dysfunction.

Treatment involves strict BP control (see p. 608). The BP goal is < 140/90 mm Hg, although < 130/80 mm Hg is more appropriate for patients with diabetes or chronic renal failure. Most experts suggest low-dose thiazide diuretic therapy with an ACE inhibitor or angiotensin II receptor blocker for proteinuric patients. Ca channel blockers and β-blockers can be added as needed. Most patients require combination therapy for BP control. Weight loss, exercise, and salt and water restriction also help control BP. Chronic renal failure should be managed (see p. 1987).

MALIGNANT HYPERTENSIVE ARTERIOLAR NEPHROSCLEROSIS

Malignant hypertensive arteriolar nephrosclerosis is abrupt deterioration of renal function secondary to a hypertensive emergency. Symptoms and signs of renal failure and symptoms associated with severe hypertension develop. Diagnosis is primarily clinical, supported by laboratory tests. With BP control, most patients recover renal function. Treatment is rapid normalization of BP and sometimes dialysis.

In malignant hypertensive arteriolar nephrosclerosis, rapidly progressive renal failure results from renal arteriolar necrosis, proliferative endarteritis, and glomerular fibrinoid necrosis. The disorder occurs in < 1% of hypertensive patients, more often in blacks. Peak incidence is during their 40s and 50s for men and about 10 yr earlier for women.

The disorder usually develops in patients with uncontrolled chronic severe hypertension. Primary hypertension is the most common cause, but nephrosclerosis may result from secondary hypertension due to acute glomerulonephritis, chronic renal failure, renal artery stenosis, renal vasculitis, and, rarely, an endocrine disorder (eg, pheochromocytoma, primary aldosteronism, Cushing's syndrome).

Symptoms and Signs

Onset of acute renal failure is abrupt and patients have severe hypertension. The hypertension can cause headache, nausea, vomiting, blurred vision, dyspnea, restlessness, confusion, and seizures. Signs of end-organ damage (eg, left ventricular hypertrophy, retinal changes) may be present but are often absent if the onset of hypertension is recent. Papilledema and hypertensive retinopathy may be detected by funduscopy.

Diagnosis

Diagnosis involves recognizing acute renal failure in the setting of severe hypertension. Imaging tests and renal biopsy are not helpful except to rule out other causes of renal failure.

Laboratory tests can confirm acute renal failure. Urinalysis usually shows proteinuria, occasionally in the nephrotic range, and microscopic hematuria. RBC casts may be present.

Prognosis and Treatment

Occasionally, renal function improves, usually within the 1st 6 to 12 mo. Survival rates after treatment are about 75 to 85% at 1 yr, 60 to 70% at 5 yr, and 45 to 50% at 10 yr. Death usually results from uremia (40%), heart failure (10%), stroke (24%), or MI (11%).

BP must be promptly controlled. Hypertensive emergencies require BP control within 1 h; in hypertensive urgencies, BP should be lowered within 24 h (see p. 618). If progressive renal insufficiency is present, dialysis may be required.

RENAL ARTERY OCCLUSION

Renal artery occlusion is acute or chronic interruption of blood flow through one or both of the main renal arteries or its branches, usually due to thromboemboli, atherosclerosis, or fibromuscular dysplasia. Symptoms of acute occlusion include steady, aching flank pain, abdominal pain, fever, nausea, vomiting, and hematuria; acute renal failure may develop. Chronic, progressive occlusion causes refractory hypertension and may lead to chronic renal failure. Diagnosis is by imaging tests (eg, CT, magnetic resonance angiography). Treatment of acute occlusion is with anticoagulation and sometimes thrombolytics, and/or surgical or catheter-based embolectomy. Treatment of chronic, progressive occlusion includes angioplasty with stenting, surgical bypass, and removal of an infarcted kidney.

Renal artery occlusion may be unilateral or bilateral. Renal hypoperfusion results in hypertension (see Renovascular Hypertension on p. 616), renal failure, or renal infarction and necrosis.

Acute occlusion: The most common cause is thromboembolism. Emboli may originate in the heart (in atrial fibrillation, after MI, or from vegetations due to bacterial endocarditis) or the aorta (as atheroemboli); less often, fat or tumor emboli are the cause. Thrombosis may occur in a renal artery spontaneously or after trauma, surgery, angiography, or angioplasty. Other causes of occlusion include dissection or rupture of a renal artery aneurysm.

Rapid, total occlusion of large renal arteries for 30 to 60 min results in infarction. The infarct is typically wedge-shaped, radiating outward from the affected vessel. Arterial occlusion for < 30 to 60 min usually causes a rapid reduction in renal function.

Chronic progressive occlusion (stenosis): The renal artery is narrowed by atherosclerosis or fibromuscular dysplasia.

Atherosclerosis develops primarily in men > 50 and usually affects the aortic orifice or proximal segment of the main renal artery. Chronic occlusion tends to become clinically evident after about 10 yr, causing renal atrophy and chronic renal failure.

Fibromuscular dysplasia is pathologic thickening of the arterial wall, most often of the distal main renal artery or the intrarenal branches. This disorder develops primarily in younger adults, particularly in women aged 20 to 50.

Symptoms and Signs

Manifestations depend on acuteness, extent, and duration of renal hypoperfusion. Partial occlusion of one renal artery is often asymptomatic for a considerable time.

Acute complete occlusion of one or both main renal arteries causes steady and aching flank pain, abdominal pain, fever, nausea, and vomiting. Gross hematuria, oliguria, or anuria may occur; hypertension is rare. After about 24 h, symptoms and signs of acute renal failure may develop (see p. 1982). If the cause was thromboembolic, other features of thromboembolism (eg, blue toes, livedo reticularis, retinal lesions with visual changes) also may be present.

Chronic progressive occlusion causes hypertension, which may begin at atypical ages (eg, < 30 yr or > 50 yr) and which may be refractory to control despite use of multiple antihypertensives. Physical examination may detect an abdominal bruit or signs of atherosclerosis. Symptoms and signs of chronic renal failure (see p. 1986) develop slowly.

Diagnosis

Diagnosis is suspected based on history, supported by laboratory tests, and confirmed by imaging tests. Which tests are done depends on the patient's renal function and other characteristics and on test availability.

For patients with adequate renal function, CT angiography (CTA) may be used because it is noninvasive, quick, and generally available. However, it requires an IV radiocontrast agent, which may be nephrotoxic; this risk is much lower with the nonionic contrast agents that are now in widespread use (see p. 2718).

For patients with impaired renal function, magnetic resonance angiography (MRA), which does not require use of a nephrotoxic contrast agent, is the diagnostic test of choice. However, because it is expensive, has limited availability, and may cause problems for patients with claustrophobia or obesity,

MRA is usually done when other tests, such as Doppler ultrasonography or radionuclide renography, are nondiagnostic.

Doppler ultrasonography is relatively inexpensive and noninvasive. With it, renal artery anatomy and function can be assessed. Although sensitivity and specificity can exceed 90%, this test is highly operator-dependent and time-consuming; lack of local expertise and patient obesity preclude its widespread use.

Radionuclide renography can provide information about renal blood flow. Use of captopril improves sensitivity and specificity for the diagnosis of chronic progressive occlusion. This technique is more useful in unilateral than in bilateral occlusion.

When other tests are inconclusive or negative but clinical suspicion is strong, arteriography is necessary for definitive diagnosis. Arteriography may also be needed before invasive interventions. However, it increases risk of atheroembolism and may exacerbate renal failure because it requires a radiocontrast agent. IV subtraction angiography uses smaller amounts of radiocontrast and obviates the need for arterial access that may produce atheroemboli. Carbon dioxide angiography avoids the need for radiocontrast entirely, but its availability is limited.

When a thromboembolic disorder is suspected, ECG (to detect atrial fibrillation), echocardiography (to detect intraventricular thrombi or valvular vegetations), and hypercoagulability studies may be needed to identify treatable embolic sources.

Blood and urine tests are nondiagnostic but are done to confirm acute or chronic renal failure, indicated by elevated creatinine and BUN and by hyperkalemia. These tests may show leukocytosis, gross or microscopic hematuria, and proteinuria.

Treatment

Treatment depends on the cause.

Acute renal artery occlusion: A renal thromboembolic disorder may be treated with a combination of anticoagulation, thrombolytics, and surgical or catheter-based embolectomy. Treatment within 3 h of symptom onset is likely to improve renal function. However, a complete recovery is unusual, and early and late mortality rates are high because of extrarenal embolization or underlying atherosclerotic heart disease.

Patients presenting within 3 h may benefit from thrombolytic therapy (eg, streptokinase, alteplase) given IV or by local intra-arterial infusion (see p. 647). However, such rapid diagnosis and treatment are rare.

All patients with a thromboembolic disorder require anticoagulation with IV heparin, unless contraindicated. Long-term anticoagulation with oral warfarin can be initiated immediately if no invasive intervention is planned. Anticoagulation should be continued for at least 6 to 12 mo—indefinitely for patients with a recurrent thromboembolic disorder or a hypercoagulability disorder.

Surgery to restore vascular patency has a higher mortality rate than thrombolytic therapy, and it has no advantage in recovery of renal function. However, surgery, particularly if done within the 1st few hours, is preferred for patients with traumatic renal artery thrombosis. If patients with severe renal failure do not recover function after 4 to 6 wk of drug therapy, surgical revascularization (embolectomy) can be considered, but it helps only a few.

If the cause is thromboemboli, the source should be identified and treated appropriately (see Deep Venous Thrombosis on p. 754).

Chronic progressive renal artery occlusion: Treatment is indicated for unilateral occlusion with renal insufficiency, bilateral occlusion, main renal artery occlusion in a solitary functioning kidney, occlusion of one or both main renal arteries with hypertension refractory to treatment with ≥ 3 drugs, and any occlusion of a main renal artery that is > 80%.

Treatment is with percutaneous transluminal angioplasty (PTA) plus stenting, or with surgical bypass of the stenotic segment. Usually, an extensively infarcted kidney must be removed if revascularization is not expected to result in functional recovery. Surgery is usually more effective than PTA for atherosclerotic occlusion; it cures or attenuates hypertension in 60 to 70% of patients. PTA is preferred for fibromuscular dysplasia; risk is minimal, success rate is high, and restenosis rate is low. If PTA is ineffective, surgical revascularization is needed.

Renovascular hypertension: Treatments are typically ineffective unless vascular patency (see p. 617) is restored. ACE inhibitors or angiotensin II receptor blockers can be used in unilateral but not in bilateral renal artery occlusion. These drugs can reduce GFR and increase serum BUN and creatinine levels. In such cases, Ca channel blockers (eg, amlodipine, felodipine) or vasodilators (eg, hydralazine, minoxidil) should be added or substituted (see p. 609).

RENAL ATHEROEMBOLISM

Renal atheroembolism is occlusion of renal arterioles by emboli, causing progressive renal impairment. It results from rupture of atheromatous plaques. Symptoms are those of renal failure; symptoms and signs of widespread arterial embolic disease may be present. Diagnosis is by renal biopsy. Long-term prognosis is usually poor. Treatment aims to prevent further embolization and preserve renal function.

Atheromatous plaques may rupture from aortic manipulation (eg, during vascular surgery, angioplasty, or arteriography) or spontaneously, usually in patients who have diffuse erosive atherosclerosis or who are being treated with anticoagulants or thrombolytic drugs.

Atheroemboli tend to produce incomplete occlusion with secondary ischemic atrophy rather than renal infarction. A foreign body immune reaction often follows embolization, leading to continued deterioration in renal function for 3 to 8 wk. Acute renal impairment may also result from massive or recurrent episodes of embolization.

Symptoms and Signs

Symptoms are usually those of insidiously developing renal failure (see p. 1982). Hypertension is rare. Abdominal pain, nausea, and vomiting can result from compromised arterial microcirculation of abdominal organs (eg, pancreas, GI tract). Sudden blindness and formation of bright yellow retinal plaques (Hollenhorst plaques) can result from emboli in retinal arterioles. Signs of widespread peripheral embolism (eg, livedo reticularis, painful muscle nodules, overt gangrene) are sometimes present.

Diagnosis

Diagnosis is suggested by signs of atheroemboli and presence of renal failure. If suspicion of atheroembolism is high in patients with renal failure, diagnosis is by percutaneous renal biopsy, which has a sensitivity of about 75%. Cholesterol crystals in the emboli dissolve during tissue fixation, leaving pathognomonic biconcave, needle-shaped clefts in the occluded vessel. Sometimes skin, muscle, or GI biopsy can provide the same information and indirectly helps establish the diagnosis.

Blood and urine tests can confirm the diagnosis of acute or chronic renal failure but do not establish cause. Urinalysis typically shows microscopic hematuria and minimal proteinuria; however, proteinuria is occasionally in the nephrotic range. Eosinophilia, eosinophiluria, and transient hypocomplementemia may be present.

If renal or systemic emboli recur and their source is unclear, transesophageal echocardiography can detect atheromatous lesions in the ascending and thoracic aorta; dual helical CT may help characterize the ascending aorta and aortic arch. However, because atherosclerosis is common among the elderly, these tests are typically positive and do not yield meaningful data.

Prognosis and Treatment

About 25% of patients with renal impairment due to atheroemboli partially recover renal function. However, long-term prognosis is usually poor; 1-yr mortality rate is 25 to 70%. Whether the poor prognosis results directly from renal impairment or the underlying atherosclerosis is unclear.

No direct treatment of the emboli is effective. Corticosteroids, antiplatelet drugs, vasodilators, and plasma exchange are not helpful. There is no convincing evidence that anticoagulation is beneficial; in some cases, anticoagulation may encourage atherosclerotic plaque embolization.

Treatment of renal failure includes control of hypertension and management of electrolytes and fluid status; sometimes dialysis is required. Modifying risk factors for atherosclerosis may slow its progression and induce regression. Strategies include management of hypertension, hyperlipidemia, and diabetes; smoking cessation; and encouragement of regular aerobic exercise and good nutrition (see p. 624).

RENAL CORTICAL NECROSIS

Renal cortical necrosis is destruction of cortical tissue resulting from renal arteriolar injury and leading to renal failure. This rare disorder typically occurs in newborns and in pregnant or postpartum women when sepsis or pregnancy complications occur.

Symptoms and signs include gross hematuria, flank pain, decreased urine output, fever, and symptoms of renal failure, but symptoms of the underlying disorder may predominate. Diagnosis is by MRI, CT, ultrasonography, isotopic renal scanning, or renal biopsy. Mortality rate at 1 yr is > 50%. Treatment is directed at the underlying disorder and at preserving renal function.

In renal cortical necrosis, bilateral renal arteriolar injury results in destruction and calcification of cortical tissues and acute renal failure. The juxtamedullary cortex, medulla, and area just under the capsule are spared. Injury usually results from reduced renal artery perfusion secondary to vascular spasm, microvascular injury, or intravascular coagulation.

Renal cortical necrosis is rare. About 10% of cases occur in infants and children. Pregnancy complications increase risk of this disorder in newborns and in women, as does bacterial sepsis. Other causes (eg, disseminated intravascular coagulation [DIC]) are less common (see TABLE 238–1).

Symptoms and Signs

Gross hematuria, flank pain, and sometimes decreased urine output or abrupt anuria occur. Fever is common, and renal failure with hypertension develops. However, these symptoms are often overshadowed by symptoms of the underlying disorder.

Diagnosis

Diagnosis is suspected when typical symptoms occur in patients with a potential cause.

Imaging tests can sometimes confirm the diagnosis. Magnetic resonance angiography is accurate and does not require a nephrotoxic contrast agent but takes a long time, which may be difficult for critically ill patients. In such cases, CT angiography may be preferred. However, it requires an IV radiocontrast agent, which may be nephrotoxic.

An alternative is isotopic renal scanning using diethylenetriamine pentaacetic acid. It shows enlarged, nonobstructed kidneys, with little or no renal blood flow. Renal biopsy is done only if the diagnosis is unclear and no contraindications exist. It provides definitive diagnosis and prognostic information.

Blood and urine tests often confirm the diagnosis of acute or chronic renal failure (eg, indicated by elevated creatinine and BUN and by hyperkalemia) and suggest a cause.

TABLE 238–1. CAUSES OF RENAL CORTICAL NECROSIS

PATIENT GROUP	CAUSES
Neonates	Abruptio placentae (> 50% of cases) Congenital heart disease (severe) Dehydration Feto-maternal transfusion Hemolytic anemia (severe) Perinatal asphyxia Renal vein thrombosis Sepsis
Children	Bacterial sepsis Dehydration Hemolytic-uremic syndrome Shock
Pregnant and postpartum women	Pregnancy complications (> 50% of cases): abruptio placentae, amniotic fluid embolism, intrauterine death, placenta previa, preeclampsia, puerperal sepsis, uterine hemorrhage Bacterial sepsis (30%)
Others	Burns Disseminated intravascular coagulation Drugs (eg, NSAIDs, nephrotoxic contrast agents) Hyperacute renal allograft rejection Incompatible blood transfusions Pancreatitis Poisoning (eg, phosphorus, arsenic) Snakebites Trauma

Severe electrolyte abnormalities may be present depending on the cause. Blood tests often detect leukocytosis (even when sepsis is not the cause) and may detect anemia and thrombocytopenia if hemolysis, DIC, or sepsis is the cause. Transaminases may be increased in relative hypovolemic states (eg, septic shock, postpartum hemorrhage). If DIC is the cause, coagulation studies may detect low fibrinogen levels, increased fibrin-degradation products, and an increasing INR. Urinalysis typically detects proteinuria, hematuria, and casts.

Prognosis and Treatment

Prognosis depends on the cause and amount of surviving cortex but is usually poor. Without dialysis, 1-yr mortality rate is > 50%. A few patients regain enough renal function to discontinue maintenance dialysis after several months; however, long-term dialysis or renal transplantation is usually necessary. There is no specific treatment except control of the underlying disorder.

RENAL VEIN THROMBOSIS

Renal vein thrombosis is occlusion of one or both main renal veins, resulting in acute or chronic renal failure. Common causes include nephrotic syndrome, primary hypercoagulability disorders, malignant renal tumors, and extrinsic compression. Symptoms of renal failure and sometimes nausea, vomiting, flank pain, gross hematuria, decreased urine output, or systemic manifestations of venous thromboembolism may occur. Diagnosis is by magnetic resonance venography or CT. With treatment, prognosis is generally good. Treatment is anticoagulation, support of renal function, and treatment of the underlying disorder. Some patients benefit from thrombectomy or nephrectomy.

Renal vein thrombosis usually results from local and systemic hypercoagulability due to nephrotic syndrome associated with membranous or membranoproliferative glomerulonephritis (see p. 2012). Other causes include SLE, sickle cell nephropathy, amyloidosis, diabetic nephropathy, renal vasculitis, allograft rejection, pregnancy, estrogen therapy, and primary hypercoagulability disorders (eg, antithrombin III deficiency, protein C or S deficiency, factor V Leiden mutations). Less common causes are related to reduced renal vein blood flow and include malignant renal tumors that extend into the renal veins (typically renal cell carcinoma), extrinsic compression of the renal vein or inferior vena cava (eg, vascular abnormalities, tumor, retroperitoneal disease, ligation of the inferior vena cava, pregnancy, aortic aneurysm), oral contraceptives, trauma, dehydration, and, rarely, thrombophlebitis migrans.

Symptoms, Signs, and Diagnosis

Usually, onset of renal failure (see p. 1980) is insidious. However, onset may be acute, causing renal infarction with nausea, vomiting, flank pain, gross hematuria, and decreased urine output.

When the cause is a hypercoagulability disorder, signs of venous thromboembolic disorders (eg, pulmonary embolism) may occur. When the cause is a renal malignancy, its signs (eg, hematuria, weight loss) predominate.

Renal venography of the inferior vena cava is diagnostic. However, magnetic resonance venography, if available, is preferred because it can also show the kidneys and associated vascular structures and does not require a nephrotoxic contrast agent. CT provides good detail with similar sensitivity and specificity and is faster and cheaper but requires a radiocontrast agent, which may be nephrotoxic. Doppler ultrasonography sometimes detects renal vein thrombosis but has high false-negative and false-positive rates.

Laboratory tests confirm deterioration of renal function. Microscopic hematuria is often present. Proteinuria may be in the nephrotic range.

If no cause is apparent, testing for hypercoagulability disorders should be initiated (see p. 1080). Renal biopsy is nonspecific but may detect a coexisting renal disorder.

Prognosis and Treatment

Death is rare and usually related to complications such as pulmonary embolism and those due to nephrotic syndrome or a malignant tumor.

The underlying disorder should be treated. Treatment of renal vein thrombosis consists of anticoagulation with IV heparin. Long-term anticoagulation with oral warfarin should be started immediately if no invasive intervention is planned. Anticoagulation minimizes risk of new thrombi, promotes recanalization of existing clots, and improves renal function. Anticoagulation should be continued for at least 6 to 12 mo or, if a hypercoagulability disorder (eg, persistent nephrotic syndrome) is present, indefinitely.

Surgical thrombectomy is rarely used but may help if anticoagulation is ineffective or contraindicated in patients with bilateral renal vein thrombosis and renal failure, if infarction is total (in certain cases), or if the underlying disorder (eg, malignant tumor) warrants it. Inferior vena cava filters may also be used in these cases.

Nephrectomy is done only if infarction is total (in certain cases) or if the underlying disorder warrants it.

SCLERODERMA RENAL DISEASE

Scleroderma renal disease results when scleroderma (systemic sclerosis) affects the kidneys, sometimes leading to renal failure. Symptoms and signs include those of scleroderma as well as those of chronic renal failure and hypertension. **Scleroderma renal crisis** is abrupt onset of symptoms of a hypertensive emergency and renal failure, usually preceded by worsening of scleroderma skin symptoms. Diagnosis is primarily clinical. Without strict BP control, prognosis is poor. Treatment focuses on scleroderma, support of renal function, and strict BP control.

Scleroderma (see p. 270), a systemic connective tissue disorder, causes thickening of the arterial wall and narrowing of the arterial lumen of various arteries. In about ½ of patients, scleroderma affects the kidneys, causing glomerular disruption and intimal proliferation, medial thinning, and increased collagen deposition in the adventitial layer of small interlobular renal arteries. Secondary changes (eg, fibrin thrombi, fibrinoid necrosis, immune reactions, increased vasomotor tone) contribute to renal dysfunction.

Scleroderma renal disease is more prevalent in patients with diffuse, rapidly progressive skin symptoms, in blacks, and in patients taking high-dose corticosteroids.

Scleroderma renal crisis occurs in 10 to 20% of patients with scleroderma renal disease; renal function deteriorates abruptly and rapidly.

Symptoms and Signs

Renal disease usually begins relatively early in scleroderma, almost invariably within the 1st 5 yr. Extrarenal symptoms and signs of scleroderma are also present. Most patients present with symptoms of insidiously developing renal failure (see p. 1982) and moderate to severe hypertension.

In scleroderma renal crisis, symptoms of a hypertensive emergency (eg, headache, nausea, vomiting, blurred vision, dyspnea, restlessness, confusion, seizures) and renal failure occur abruptly. Before renal crisis, skin symptoms often rapidly worsen.

Diagnosis

Diagnosis is primarily clinical. Urinalysis typically shows mild proteinuria with few cells or casts. Blood tests show signs of renal failure (eg, elevated creatinine and BUN, hyperkalemia). Microscopic hematuria can occur. Blood tests sometimes detect microangiopathic hemolytic anemia. Additional testing is not needed unless another cause of deteriorating renal function is suspected.

Renal biopsy is usually unnecessary and is not definitive because the vascular lesions are indistinguishable from other forms of thrombotic microangiopathy (eg, that is associated with malignant hypertensive arteriolar nephrosclerosis, thrombotic thrombocytopenic purpura, hemolytic-uremic syndrome, radiation nephritis, chronic transplant rejection, or lupus anticoagulant).

In all patients with scleroderma, renal function should be monitored; serum creatinine is measured and urinalysis for proteinuria is done every 4 mo during the 1st 5 yr after diagnosis. Weekly ambulatory BP monitoring is indicated. Patients are instructed to contact their health care practitioners if BP is high.

Prognosis and Treatment

Prognosis is usually poor. Without treatment, scleroderma renal crisis leads to advanced renal failure within 1 to 2 mo. However, aggressive BP control, if started early, can stabilize or improve renal function in up to 70% of patients.

Scleroderma renal crisis requires rapid BP reduction, usually with IV labetalol or nitroprusside. Later, BP can be maintained with oral drugs (see p. 608).

For scleroderma renal disease, aggressive BP control is key. ACE inhibitors or angiotensin II receptor blockers are the antihypertensives of choice because they have the most beneficial effects on renal function and overall morbidity and mortality. If these drugs increase serum creatinine levels, Ca channel blockers (eg, amlodipine, felodipine) or vasodilators (eg, hydralazine, minoxidil) should be added or substituted. Once azotemia develops, hypertension may become more difficult to control, and dialysis is often required within 1 to 2 yr.

Renal failure should be treated. Use of renal transplantation is often limited because of severe extrarenal manifestations, and scleroderma renal disease may recur in the renal allograft.

Extrarenal manifestations are typically treated with immunosuppressants or other drugs (see p. 272). However, these drugs usually do not alleviate renal manifestations and may precipitate renal crisis.

SICKLE CELL NEPHROPATHY

(See also Sickle Cell Anemia on p. 1053.)

Sickle cell nephropathy is progressive renal dysfunction resulting from RBC sickling in renal capillaries. Symptoms include those of renal failure, with painless gross hematuria, UTIs, and polyuria. Diagnosis is primarily clinical. Prognosis is poor. Treatment is prevention of RBC sickling and support of renal function.

Sickle cell nephropathy occurs when RBCs in the renal medullary vasa recta capillaries sickle, producing focal areas of hemorrhage or necrosis, interstitial inflammation and fibrosis, tubular atrophy, and papillary infarcts. These abnormalities lead to renal failure and may progress to end-stage renal disease. Similar abnormalities occur to a lesser extent in patients with sickle cell trait and occasionally lead to end-stage renal disease.

Conditions associated with sickle cell disease crisis (eg, dehydration, hypoxemia) and use of NSAIDs may predispose to renal papillary necrosis.

Symptoms, Signs, and Diagnosis

Patients present with symptoms of insidiously developing renal failure. Painless gross hematuria is common. Dysuria may also occur because renal papillary necrosis increases risk of repeated UTIs. Impaired ability to concentrate urine causes mild polyuria. Dehydration may precipitate sickle cell crisis.

Diagnosis is primarily clinical. Laboratory tests confirm deterioration of renal function. Hematuria is often present. Proteinuria is common and reaches nephrotic range in about 4% of patients. Urinary acidification may be abnormal, causing distal renal tubular acidosis with hyperkalemia and hyperchloremic metabolic acidosis (type 4 renal tubular acidosis).

No imaging tests are indicated, unless required to rule out other causes. Renal biopsy is nonspecific; it may be done if the cause is unclear and a treatable renal disorder is suspected to coexist. Biopsy may show membranous or membranoproliferative glomerulopathy or focal and segmental glomerular sclerosis.

Prognosis and Treatment

The course is progressive, leading to renal failure and ultimately end-stage renal disease. Median survival time for patients with sickle cell nephropathy is 4 yr; median age at death is 27 yr.

No specific therapy can reverse the process. However, early aggressive treatment of sickle cell crises (see p. 1055) may prevent or slow progression. Blood transfusions can temporarily correct impaired ability to concentrate urine in patients < 10 yr but not in older patients. ACE inhibitors may reduce degree of proteinuria, but whether they can preserve renal function in patients with sickle cell disease is unclear.

Renal failure should be treated. End-stage renal disease is usually treated with dialysis. Less often, renal transplantation is tried. Posttransplantation survival of patients with sickle cell nephropathy is similar to that of patients with other types of end-stage renal disease. Occasionally, sickle cell nephropathy recurs in the renal allograft.

239 PENILE AND SCROTAL DISORDERS

Abnormalities of the external male genitals are psychologically disturbing and sometimes serious (see pp. 2435 and 2436 for congenital defects).

BALANITIS, POSTHITIS, AND BALANOPOSTHITIS

Balanitis is inflammation of the glans penis; posthitis is inflammation of the prepuce; and balanoposthitis is inflammation of both.

Inflammation of the head of the penis may be a complication of candidiasis, gonococcal or chlamydial urethritis, chancroid, trichomoniasis, herpes simplex, scabies, or primary or secondary syphilis. Noninfectious causes include reactive arthritis (formerly, Reiter's syndrome), which can produce shallow, painless ulcers of the glans (balanitis circinata); fixed drug eruptions; contact dermatitis; psoriasis; lichen planus; seborrheic dermatitis; balanitis xerotica obliterans; and erythroplasia of Queyrat. Often, no cause can be found. Balanoposthitis often occurs in patients with a tight prepuce (phimosis), which interferes with adequate hygiene. The subpreputial secretions may become infected with anaerobic bacteria, resulting in inflammation. Diabetes mellitus predisposes to balanoposthitis. Isolated balanitis occurs mainly in circumcised patients.

Soreness, irritation, and a subpreputial discharge often occur 2 or 3 days after sexual intercourse. Phimosis, superficial ulcerations, and inguinal adenopathy may follow.

The conditions listed above, especially candidiasis, should be investigated and the urine tested for glucose. The patient's skin should be examined for lesions that suggest genital involvement with a dermatosis. History should include investigation of latex condom use. Nonspecific hygienic measures should be instituted and specific causes treated. Subpreputial irrigation to remove secretions and detritus may be necessary. Once inflammation has resolved, circumcision or preputial plasty should be considered in patients with persistent phimosis.

CUTANEOUS PENILE LESIONS

Common skin diseases that may affect the penis include psoriasis, infections, squamous cell carcinoma, papulosquamous or systemic diseases, fixed drug reactions, and allergic and irritant contact dermatitides. Sexually transmitted diseases (see also Ch. 194 on p. 1650) causing penile lesions include syphilis, chancroid, granuloma inguinale, genital warts, and genital herpes. Rare infectious penile lesions include those due to TB, fungi, and herpes zoster.

Balanitis xerotica obliterans, another name for lichen sclerosus et atrophicus in males, is an indurated, blanched area near the tip of the glans surrounding and often constricting the meatus. It results from chronic inflammation and may lead to phimosis or paraphimosis. Topical testosterone and antibacterial and anti-inflammatory drugs may be helpful, but meatotomy, laser vaporization, or meatoplasty is required in severe cases.

Erythroplasia of Queyrat and Bowen's disease of the penis are well-circumscribed, premalignant areas of reddish, velvety pigmentation in the genital area, usually on the glans or at the corona, primarily in uncircumcised men. Both conditions (and Bowenoid papulosis, which involves smaller, often multiple papules on the shaft of the penis) are considered intraepithelial neoplasia or carcinoma in situ and should be biopsied. Treatment consists of 5% fluorouracil cream, local excision, or laser therapy. Close follow-up is indicated.

Penile lichen planus occurs as small papules or annular lesions on the glans or shaft and may be mistaken for pemphigoid or erythema multiforme. A more severe form of erosive lichen planus occurs on both oral and genital mucosa and is known as penogingival syndrome in men and vulvovaginal-gingival syndrome in women. Lichen planus usually resolves spontaneously. If asymptomatic, it may not require treatment. Topical corticosteroids may help relieve symptoms.

Pearly penile papules are small, harmless angiofibromas that appear on the corona of the penis as dome-shaped or hairlike projections. They may also appear on the distal shaft. They are common, occurring in up to 10% of male patients. They are not associated with human papillomavirus, although they may be mistaken for genital warts. Treatment is not required.

Contact dermatitis (see also p. 956) of the penis has become more common with the widespread use of latex condoms. Dermatitis appears as red, pruritic lesions, sometimes with weeping or fissures. Treatment is with topical corticosteroids and use of nonlatex condoms (but not natural condoms, which do not provide adequate protection against HIV).

EPIDIDYMITIS

Epididymitis is inflammation of the epididymis, occasionally accompanied by inflammation of the testis (epididymo-orchitis). Scrotal pain and swelling usually occur unilaterally. Diagnosis is based on physical examination. Treatment is with antibiotics, analgesics, and scrotal support.

Etiology

Bacterial: Most epididymitis (and epididymo-orchitis) is caused by bacteria. When inflammation involves the vas deferens, vasitis ensues. When the entire spermatic cord structures also are involved, the diagnosis is funiculitis. Rarely, abscess, pyocele, or testicular infarction occurs.

In men < 35 yr, most cases are due to a sexually transmitted pathogen, especially *Neisseria gonorrhoeae* or *Chlamydia trachomatis*. In men > 35 yr, most cases are due to gram-negative coliform bacilli and typically occur in patients with urologic abnormalities, indwelling catheters, or recent urologic procedures. Tuberculous epididymitis, syphilitic gummas, and mycotic causes (actinomycosis, blastomycosis) are now rare in the US except in immunocompromised (eg, HIV-infected) patients.

Nonbacterial: Epididymitis and epididymo-orchitis of noninfectious etiology may be due to chemical irritation secondary to a retrograde flow of urine into the epididymis, which may occur with Valsalva maneuver (eg, with heavy lifting) or after local trauma.

Symptoms, Signs, and Diagnosis

Scrotal pain occurs in both bacterial and nonbacterial epididymitis. Pain can be severe and is sometimes referred to the abdomen. In bacterial epididymitis, the patient may also have fever, nausea, or urinary symptoms. Urethral discharge may be present if the cause is urethritis.

Physical examination reveals swelling, induration, erythema, and marked tenderness of a portion of or all of the affected epididymis and, sometimes, the adjacent testis.

Urethritis suggests a sexually transmitted pathogen, and a urethral swab is sent for gonococcus and chlamydia culture or PCR. Otherwise, the infecting organism usually can be identified by urine culture. Urinalysis and culture are normal in nonbacterial causes.

Unless findings are clearly isolated to the epididymis, testicular torsion (see p. 2042) must also be considered in patients < 30 yr; color Doppler ultrasonography is indicated. A GU evaluation is indicated if the cause is unclear or disease is recurrent.

Treatment

Treatment consists of bed rest, scrotal elevation, scrotal ice packs, anti-inflammatory analgesics, and oral antimicrobial therapy with a broad-spectrum antibiotic such as ciprofloxacin 500 mg po bid or levofloxacin 500 mg po once/day for 21 to 30 days. Alternatively, doxycycline 100 mg po bid or trimethoprim-sulfamethoxazole double-strength (160/800 mg) po bid may by used. If sepsis is suspected, an IV aminoglycoside such as tobramycin 1 mg/kg q 8 h or a 3rd-generation cephalosporin such as ceftriaxone 1 to 2 g/day may be useful until the infecting organism and its sensitivities are known. Cultures are important for establishing adequacy of treatment. Abscess and pyocele usually require surgical drainage.

Recurrent bacterial epididymitis secondary to incurable chronic urethritis or prostatitis occasionally can be prevented by vasectomy. An epididymectomy, occasionally done for chronic epididymitis, may not relieve symptoms. Patients who must continuously wear an indwelling urethral catheter are prone to develop recurrent epididymitis and epididymo-orchitis. Placement of a suprapubic cystostomy or institution of a self-catheterization regimen may be useful.

Treatment of nonbacterial epididymitis includes the above general measures, but antimicrobial therapy is not warranted. Nerve block of the spermatic cord with local anesthesia can relieve symptoms in severe, persistent cases.

ORCHITIS

Orchitis is infection of the testes, typically with mumps virus. Symptoms are testicular pain and swelling. Diagnosis is clinical. Treatment is symptomatic, with antibiotics if bacterial infection is identified.

Isolated orchitis is nearly always viral in origin, and most cases are due to mumps. Rare causes include congenital syphilis, TB, leprosy, echovirus, lymphocytic choriomeningitis, coxsackievirus, infectious mononucleosis, varicella, and group B arborviruses. Most bacterial causes also involve the epididymis (epididymo-orchitis) and are discussed under Epididymitis (see p. 2037).

Orchitis develops in 20 to 25% of males with mumps; 80% of cases occur in patients < 10 yr. Two thirds of cases are unilateral and ⅓ bilateral. Sixty percent of patients with mumps orchitis develop unilateral testicular atrophy. The incidence of tumor does not appear to be increased, but unilateral disease diminishes fertility in ¼ of men after unilateral mumps orchitis and in ⅔ of men who have had bilateral disease. Atrophy is unrelated to fertility or to the severity of the orchitis.

Symptoms and Signs

Unilateral mumps orchitis develops acutely between 4 and 7 days after parotid swelling in mumps. In 30% of cases, the disease spreads to the other testis in 1 to 9 days. Pain may be of any degree of severity. In addition to pain and swelling of the testes, systemic symptoms may develop, such as malaise, fever, nausea, headache, and myalgias. Testicular examination reveals tenderness, enlargement, and induration of the testis and edema and erythema of the scrotal skin.

Other infectious agents produce similar symptoms with a speed of onset and an intensity related to their pathogenicity.

Diagnosis and Treatment

History and physical examination usually indicate the diagnosis. Urgent differentiation of orchitis from testicular torsion and other causes of acute scrotal swelling and pain is accomplished with color Doppler ultrasonography. Mumps can be confirmed by serum immunofluorescence antibody testing. Other infectious agents may be identified by urine culture or serology.

Supportive care with analgesics and hot or cold packs is sufficient if bacterial infection has been ruled out. Bacterial causes are treated with appropriate antibiotics. Urologic follow-up is recommended.

PEYRONIE'S DISEASE

Peyronie's disease is fibrosis of the cavernous sheaths leading to contracture of the investing fascia of the corpora, resulting in a deviated and sometimes painful erection.

The disease occurs in adults. The cause is unknown but appears to be similar to that of Dupuytren's contracture. The contracture usually results in deviation of the erect penis to the involved side, occasionally causes painful erections, and may prevent intromission. Fibrosis may extend into the corpus cavernosum, compromising tumescence distally.

Resolution may occur spontaneously over many months. Mild Peyronie's disease that does not cause sexual dysfunction does not warrant treatment.

Treatment results are unpredictable. Oral vitamin E and K para-aminobenzoate have had varied success. Surgical removal of the fibrosis and replacement with a patch graft may be successful or may result in further scarring and exaggeration of the defect. A series of local injections of verapamil or high-potency corticosteroids into the plaque may be effective, but oral corticosteroids are not. To assist potency, a prosthesis may be implanted but may require a patch procedure to straighten the penis.

PHIMOSIS AND PARAPHIMOSIS

Phimosis is inability to retract the foreskin; paraphimosis is entrapment of the foreskin in the retracted position.

Phimosis: Phimosis is normal in children and typically resolves by adolescence. Treatment is not required in the absence of complications such as balanitis, urinary infections, unresponsive dermatologic disease, or suspicion of carcinoma.

Three months of betamethasone cream 0.05% bid to tid applied to the tip of the foreskin and the area touching the glans is often effective. Stretching the foreskin gently with 2 fingers or over an erect penis for 2 to 3 wk with care not to produce paraphimosis is also successful. An "I"-plasty is a foreskin-preserving procedure that is simple and effective and does not remove any tissue. Circumcision is always an option.

Paraphimosis: Paraphimosis is frequently iatrogenic, occurring during catheterization or physical examination. If the retracted foreskin is somewhat tight, it functions as a tourniquet, causing the glans to swell, both blocking the foreskin from returning to its normal position and worsening the constriction. It should be regarded as an emergency, because constriction leads quickly to vascular compromise and necrosis. Firm circumferential compression of the glans with the hand may relieve edema sufficiently to allow the foreskin to be restored to its normal position. If this is ineffective, a dorsal slit performed using a local anesthetic relieves the condition temporarily. Circumcision is then performed when edema has resolved.

PRIAPISM

Priapism is painful, persistent, abnormal erection unaccompanied by sexual desire or excitation. Diagnosis is clinical. Treatment is with injected vasoconstrictors, large-bore

needle decompression, or sometimes spinal anesthesia or surgery. Successful management depends on etiology and time between onset and treatment.

The mechanisms of priapism are poorly understood but probably involve complex vascular and neurologic abnormalities.

Ischemic: The most common type is ischemic (venoocclusive, low-flow), with a marked decrease or absence of cavernous blood flow. The corpora cavernosa contains thick, dark venous blood of motor oil consistency. The corpus spongiosum and glans penis are not affected. Severe pain from ischemia occurs after 4 h. Cavernosal ABG demonstrates metabolic acidosis. If prolonged > 4 h, priapism can lead to corporeal fibrosis and subsequent erectile dysfunction or even penile necrosis and gangrene.

Historically, pelvic vascular thrombosis was most often the cause in adults.

Drug therapy for erectile dysfunction (see p. 1949) has become the most common cause. This includes intracavernosal injection therapy and oral treatment with alprostadil, sildenafil, or vardenafil. Other less common drug causes include trazodone, lithium, chlorpromazine, methaqualone, prazosin, tolbutamide, certain antihypertensives, anticoagulants, cocaine, amphetamines, and corticosteroids. Priapism associated with total parenteral nutrition has been reported.

Rare causes include pelvic hematoma or tumor, cerebrospinal disease (eg, syphilis, tumor), and genital infection and inflammation (eg, prostatitis, urethritis, cystitis), especially if complicated by a bladder calculus. In children, blood dyscrasias such as leukemia and sickle cell disease are most common. Priapism may be idiopathic and recur.

Nonischemic: Nonischemic (arterial, high-flow) priapism can occur after penile trauma if vascular damage causes unregulated arterial inflow; this type is nonpainful and does not lead to necrosis, but subsequent erectile dysfunction is common.

Diagnosis

If the underlying cause is not obvious, screening is done for hemoglobin S, leukemia, UTI, and other causes. During the physical examination, the physician looks for penile or perineal trauma; pelvic inflammatory, neurologic, or vascular disorders; and pelvic malignancy, such as prostate cancer, that could spread to the corpora or disrupt venous outflow. Intracavernosal ABG may help differentiate between ischemic and nonischemic priapism. Angiography is diagnostic and may also be therapeutic if the cause is unregulated arterial inflow and embolization is possible.

Treatment

Treatment is often difficult and sometimes unsuccessful, even when the etiology is known. Ice packs to the penis and perineum are begun immediately. Walking up stairs may produce an "arterial steal" and result in detumescence. If ischemic priapism is suspected, terbutaline 5 mg po is given, followed by another 5 mg 15 min later. If terbutaline fails, α-agonists are injected if onset is < 4 h. Intracavernous phenylephrine can be effective, particularly if priapism is due to intracavernous injection of phentolamine, papaverine, or alprostadil. The dosage, which can be given q 5 min, is 100 to 500 μg (1 mL of 10 mg/mL phenylephrine is added to 19 mL 0.9% saline to make 500 μg/mL) until detumescence. Phenylephrine may also be administered by irrigation with a dilute solution (10 mg in 499 mL of 0.9% saline). Adverse effects include hypertension, headaches, heart palpitations, and arrhythmias.

If the time to presentation is > 4 h, the corpora should be decompressed by introducing a large-bore needle (under penile blockade with lidocaine). A 12- or 16-gauge needle is inserted transversely, avoiding the urethra on the bottom and the neurovascular bundle on top, with evacuation and irrigation. Aspiration of one side is usually sufficient, because there are adequate connections between the 2 corpora. After decompression, intracavernous injection or irrigation with phenylephrine should be performed. Repetitive aspiration and irrigation may be necessary, because priapism tends to recur. This management does not often resolve priapism if > 36 h from onset. Permanent corporeal fibrosis and erectile dysfunction are likely, and more invasive procedures are usually necessary.

Creation of a fistula between the glans and corpus cavernosum with a biopsy needle has been successful. Semipermanent diversion by means of a saphenous vein shunt from one or both corpora or a cavernosa-spongiosum shunt may result in detumescence of sufficient duration to permit reestablishment of pelvic circulation.

Complications of aspiration and irrigation include hematoma, cellulitis, corporeal abscess, urethral stricture, urethrocutaneous fistula, and even penile gangrene. Invasive surgical shunting procedures may cause temporary, and sometimes permanent, erectile dysfunction.

If priapism is nonischemic, then angiographic embolization of the aberrant artery is recommended.

Underlying causes should be treated. Sickle cell patients sometimes require oxygenation, alkalinization, erythropheresis, or exchange transfusion to reduce the hemoglobin S percentage. Leukemia patients may require chemotherapy. Neurogenic priapism may be alleviated by continuous caudal or spinal anesthesia.

SCROTAL MASSES

Scrotal masses may be due to inflammation of the scrotal wall or contents, trauma, tumors of the testis or testicular appendages (see p. 2057), or mechanical abnormalities involving the scrotal contents or adjacent structures (see also Testicular Torsion on p. 2042).

Scrotal abscesses may complicate epididymo-orchitis (see under Epididymitis on p. 2037), especially when treatment is delayed. Some abscesses drain spontaneously, but most require surgery, usually orchiectomy with drainage.

Urethral stricture and **diverticulum** may be accompanied by abscess formation with swelling of the scrotum, pain, erythema, and extravasation of urine into the scrotum and perineum. Incision and drainage as well as antibiotics are often indicated; urinary diversion by suprapubic cystostomy is needed only in severe cases with abscess. Persistent strictures can usually be treated successfully by dilation or endoscopy (internal urethrotomy). In difficult or recurrent cases, a permanent stent may be placed endoscopically. Open surgery is occasionally indicated.

Hydrocele, a common intrinsic scrotal mass, results from excessive accumulation of sterile fluid within the tunica vaginalis. A communicating hydrocele (usually congenital) fills with abdominal fluid when the patient is upright or increases intra-abdominal pressure and empties when he lies down. Noncommunicating hydroceles may fluctuate in size when an imbalance occurs between production and absorption of fluid. Overproduction occurs during inflammation of the testis or its appendages, whereas diminished resorption can be due to lymphatic or venous obstruction in the cord or retroperitoneal space. Usually, a hydrocele appears as a painless scrotal swelling that can be transilluminated. Some men have pain or discomfort from its mass effect. There are no signs of inflammation in most cases. However, inflammatory hydrocele with epididymitis may be painful. Treatment of persistent, symptomatic hydrocele is surgical (hydrocelectomy). Aspiration is a temporary measure, but aspiration with injection of sclerotic drugs may produce resolution after multiple procedures. Aspiration poses the risk of secondary infection and vascular injury.

Pyocele of the scrotum is not sterile and usually represents a complication of severe epididymitis (see p. 2037).

Hematocele (accumulation of blood within the tunica vaginalis) is usually secondary to trauma. Unlike hydrocele, it is a painful swelling and does not transilluminate. Treatment is surgical if the hematocele is large and does not absorb with conservative management, becomes infected, or is associated with laceration of the tunica albuginea.

Spermatocele (spermatic cyst) usually occurs at the upper pole of the testis adjacent to the epididymis and appears as a cystic scrotal mass. A large spermatocele may be difficult to differentiate from a hydrocele, which also is cystic and painless and transilluminates. Ultrasonography may assist diagnosis. Surgical excision is indicated if the spermatocele becomes large and bothersome.

Inguinal hernia (see p. 102) may extend into the scrotal compartment. It must be differentiated from hydrocele and hematocele. With an inguinal hernia, the cord is not palpable above the mass, whereas with a hydrocele or hematocele, normal cord structures usually are palpable above the mass. A hernia can often be reduced when the patient lies down. By definition, a congenital inguinal hernia includes a hydrocele (persistent processus vaginalis). Surgery is recommended because of the probability of progression and possibilities of incarceration and strangulation.

Varicocele (a collection of large veins, usually in the left scrotum, that feels like a bag of worms) is present in the upright position and should empty in the supine position. Incompetent venous valves result in dilation and venous stasis. Surgery may be indicated if it is symptomatic (eg, pain, a feeling of fullness) or associated with infertility (see p. 2138). Treatment may be recommended in children if there is a marked decrease in testis size on the affected side.

Lymphedema of the scrotum may result from abdominal lymphatic or venous compression, an intra-abdominal tumor, cirrhosis with ascites, filariasis, or Milroy disease (idiopathic lymphedema). It appears as a painless enlargement of the scrotal sac. Treatment is directed at the underlying cause; symptoms may lessen with scrotal suspension, although resection and scrotoplasty may be necessary in severe cases.

TESTICULAR TORSION

Testicular torsion is an emergency condition due to rotation of the testis and consequent strangulation of its blood supply. Symptoms are acute scrotal pain and swelling, nausea, and vomiting. Diagnosis is based on physical examination and confirmed by color Doppler. Treatment is immediate manual detorsion followed by surgical intervention.

Anomalous development of the tunica vaginalis and spermatic cord predisposes the testis to twisting on its cord spontaneously or after trauma. The predisposing anomaly is present in about 12% of males. Torsion is most common between the ages of 12 and 18, with a secondary peak in infancy. It is uncommon over the age of 30. It is more common in the left testis.

Symptoms, Signs, and Diagnosis

Immediate symptoms are rapid onset of severe local pain, nausea, and vomiting, followed by scrotal edema and induration. Fever and urinary frequency may be present. The testis is tender and may be elevated and horizontal. The cremasteric reflex is usually absent on the affected side.

Torsion must be rapidly identified. Similar symptoms result mainly from epididymitis; tumor pain and swelling are less acute. A clinical diagnosis usually is sufficient to proceed to treatment. An equivocal diagnosis may be resolved by color Doppler scrotal ultrasonography. Radioisotope scrotal scan is also diagnostic but takes longer and is less preferred.

Treatment

Immediate manual detorsion without radiographic delay is advised when torsion is strongly suspected on the initial examination. It is successful in 30 to 70% of cases. Because testes usually rotate inward, for detorsion the testis is rotated in an outward direction (eg, for the left testis, detorsion is clockwise when viewed from the front). More than one rotation may be needed to resolve the torsion; pain relief guides the procedure. If detorsion fails, immediate surgery is indicated, because exploration within a few hours offers the only hope of testicular salvage. Testicular salvage drops rapidly from 80 to 100% at 6 to 8 h to near zero at 12 h. Fixation of the contralateral testis is also performed to prevent torsion on that side, because the anatomic defect is usually bilateral.

240 PROSTATE DISEASE

(See also Prostate Cancer on p. 2052.)

The prostate can be affected by hyperplasia, infection, and malignancy (see p. 2052). The normal prostate is a walnut-sized organ composed of glandular tissue that makes ejaculatory fluid, its only known function. Because prostatic tissue surrounds the urethra, enlargement or other abnormalities may affect urination. The prostate may be examined by digital rectal examination to determine its size, symmetry, texture, and nodularity.

BENIGN PROSTATIC HYPERPLASIA

(Benign Prostatic Hypertrophy)

Benign prostatic hyperplasia is nonmalignant adenomatous overgrowth of the periurethral prostate gland. Symptoms are those of bladder outlet obstruction—urinary frequency, urgency, nocturia, hesitancy, incomplete emptying, terminal dribbling, overflow incontinence, or complete urinary retention. Diagnosis is based on digital rectal

examination, cystoscopy, transrectal ultrasonography, or IVU. Treatment options include 5α-reductase inhibitors, α-blockers, and surgery.

Using the criteria of a prostate volume > 30 mL and a high American Urological Association Symptom Score (see TABLE 240–1), the prevalence of benign prostatic hyperplasia (BPH) in men aged 55 to 74 without prostate cancer is 19%. But if voiding criteria of a maximal urinary flow rate < 10 mL/sec and a postvoid residual urine volume > 50 mL are included, the prevalence is only 4%. Based on autopsy studies, the prevalence of BPH increases from 8% in men aged 31 to 40 to 40

TABLE 240–1. AMERICAN UROLOGICAL ASSOCIATION SYMPTOM SCORE FOR BENIGN PROSTATIC HYPERPLASIA

OVER ABOUT THE PAST MONTH	NEVER	< 1 IN 5 TIMES	< 50% OF THE TIME	ABOUT 50% OF THE TIME	> 50% OF THE TIME	ALMOST ALWAYS
How often have you had a sensation of not emptying your bladder completely after you finish urinating?	0	1	2	3	4	5
How often have you had to urinate again < 2 h after you finished urinating?	0	1	2	3	4	5
How often have you stopped and started again several times when urinating?	0	1	2	3	4	5
How often have you found it difficult to postpone urination?	0	1	2	3	4	5
How often has your urinary stream been weak?	0	1	2	3	4	5
How often have you had to push or strain to begin urination?	0	1	2	3	4	5
How many times did you most typically get up to urinate between going to bed at night and waking in the morning?	none (0)	once (1)	twice (2)	3 times (3)	4 times (4)	≥ 5 times (5)

American Urological Association Symptom Score = total ______

Adapted from Barry MJ, Fowler FJ, O'Leary MP, et al: The American Urological Association symptom index for benign prostatic hyperplasia. *Journal of Urology* 148:1549, 1992.

to 50% in men aged 51 to 60 and to > 80% in men > 80.

Etiology and Pathophysiology

The etiology is unknown but probably involves hormonal changes associated with aging. Multiple fibroadenomatous nodules develop in the periurethral region of the prostate, probably originating within the periurethral glands rather than in the true fibromuscular prostate (surgical capsule), which is displaced peripherally by progressive growth of the nodules.

As the lumen of the prostatic urethra narrows and lengthens, urine outflow is progressively obstructed; increased pressure associated with micturition and bladder distention produces hypertrophy of the bladder detrusor, trabeculation, cellule formation, and diverticula. Incomplete bladder emptying causes stasis and predisposes to calculus formation as well as infection with secondary inflammatory changes in the bladder, prostate (chronic prostatitis—see p. 2045), and upper urinary tract. Prolonged obstruction, even if incomplete, can cause hydronephrosis and compromise renal function.

Symptoms and Signs

Symptoms include progressive urinary frequency, urgency, and nocturia due to incomplete emptying and rapid refilling of the bladder. Decreased size and force of the urinary stream produce hesitancy and intermittency. Sensations of incomplete emptying, terminal dribbling, almost continuous overflow incontinence, or complete urinary retention may ensue. Straining to void can cause congestion of superficial veins of the prostatic urethra and trigone, which may rupture and produce hematuria, and dilation of hemorrhoidal veins or inguinal hernias. Straining may also cause vasovagal syncope.

Some patients present with sudden, complete urinary retention, with marked discomfort and bladder distention. Retention may be precipitated by prolonged attempts to retain urine; immobilization; exposure to cold; use of anesthetics, anticholinergics, or sympathomimetics; or alcohol ingestion. Symptoms can be quantitated by the 7-question American Urological Association Symptom Score (see TABLE 240–1). This score allows physicians to follow the progress of obstruction and to match treatment recommendations from the literature with an individual patient's condition. Scores > 10 are usually considered abnormal.

On rectal examination, the prostate usually is enlarged, has a rubbery consistency, and in many cases has lost the median furrow. However, digital rectal examination of prostate size may be misleading; an apparently small prostate on rectal examination may cause obstruction. If distended, the urinary bladder may be palpable or percussible on abdominal examination.

Diagnosis

BPH and prostate cancer may coexist and cause similar symptoms and signs. Although carcinoma may produce a stony, hard, nodular prostate, most patients a have benign-feeling, enlarged prostate. Patients with symptoms or palpable prostatic abnormalities should undergo testing to rule out carcinoma and infection and to estimate the degree of obstruction. More severe symptoms or the presence of hematuria or UTI warrants evaluation by a urologist.

The 1st test measures levels of serum prostate-specific antigen (PSA). PSA is moderately elevated in 30 to 50% of patients with BPH, depending on prostate size and degree of obstruction. If the PSA is > 4 ng/mL or if the digital rectal examination indicates an abnormality, then a transrectal biopsy is recommended (see also Prostate Cancer on p. 2052). For young men or populations at high risk for prostate cancer, PSA > 2.5 may be considered abnormal. However, PSA is notoriously nonspecific; thus, clinical judgment must be used to evaluate the need for further testing. PSA provides prognostic information about the growth rate of the prostate, the probability of urinary retention, and the need for surgery.

Transrectal ultrasonography is often obtained to estimate gland size and guide biopsy. It also may help determine postvoid residual urine volume and differentiate vesical neck contracture, chronic prostatitis, and other obstructive phenomena. IVU or ultrasonography may disclose upward displacement of the terminal portions of the ureters (fishhooking) and a defect at the base of the bladder compatible with prostate enlargement. With prolonged obstruction, the ureters dilate and hydronephrosis occurs.

Urethral catheterization, cystoscopy, or ultrasonography after voiding measures residual urine, and catheterization permits preliminary drainage to stabilize renal function. Instrumentation should be avoided until definitive therapy has been decided, because manipulation may increase obstruction, cause trauma, or introduce infection.

Treatment

Complete obstruction requires immediate decompression. A standard urinary catheter is the 1st choice, but because it is flexible, it may not pass through a narrowed prostatic urethra. A stiffer catheter or one with a coudé tip may be effective. If this catheter cannot be passed, flexible cystoscopy or insertion of filiforms and followers (guides and dilators that progressively open the urinary passage) may be necessary (generally performed by a urologist). Suprapubic percutaneous decompression of the bladder may be used.

For partial obstruction, all anticholinergics, sympathomimetics, and opioids should be stopped, and any infection should be treated with antibiotics. For patients with mild to moderate obstructive symptoms, α-adrenergic blockers (eg, terazosin, doxazosin, tamsulosin, alfuzosin) may improve voiding. The 5α-reductase inhibitors (finasteride, dutasteride) may reduce prostate size, improving voiding over months, especially in patients with larger (> 30 mL) glands. 5α-Reductase inhibitors may be better than α-adrenergic blockers in preventing urinary retention and the need for surgery. A combination of both classes of drugs is superior to monotherapy.

Surgery is performed when patients do not respond to drug therapy or develop UTI and upper tract dilation. Transurethral resection of the prostate (TURP) is the standard. The incidence of erectile dysfunction after TURP is between 5% and 35%; of incontinence, about 1%. Sexual potency and continence are usually retained, although about 5 to 10% of patients experience some postsurgical problems, most commonly retrograde ejaculation. Larger prostates (usually > 75 g) require open surgery in rare cases; a suprapubic or retropubic approach has a much higher risk of erectile dysfunction and incontinence than after TURP. All surgical methods require postoperative catheter drainage for 1 to 5 days.

Less invasive procedures include intraurethral stents, balloon dilation, microwave thermotherapy, high-intensity focused ultrasound thermotherapy, laser ablation, electrovaporization, and radiofrequency vaporization. The circumstances under which these procedures should be used have not been firmly established, but those done in the physician's office (microwave thermotherapy, interstitial laser, and interstitial radiofrequency procedure) are being more commonly used and do not require anesthesia. Their long-term ability to alter the natural history of BPH is under study.

PROSTATITIS

(Prostatodynia)

Prostatitis refers to a disparate group of disorders that presents with a combination of irritative or obstructive urinary symptoms and perineal pain. Some result from bacterial infection of the prostate gland and others from a poorly understood combination of noninfectious inflammatory factors and/or spasm of the muscles of the urogenital diaphragm. Diagnosis is clinical, along with microscopic examination and culture of urine samples obtained before and after prostate massage. Treatment is with a fluoroquinolone if the cause is bacterial. Nonbacterial causes are treated with warm sitz baths, muscle relaxants, and anti-inflammatory drugs or anxiolytics.

Etiology

Prostatitis can be bacterial or, more commonly, nonbacterial. However, differentiating bacterial and nonbacterial causes can be difficult, particularly in chronic prostatitis.

Bacterial prostatitis can be acute or chronic and is usually caused by typical urinary pathogens (eg, *Klebsiella, Proteus, Escherichia coli*) and possibly *Chlamydia*. How they enter and infect the prostate is unknown. Chronic infections may be caused by sequestered bacteria that antibiotics have not eradicated.

Nonbacterial prostatitis can be inflammatory or noninflammatory. The mechanism is unknown but may involve incomplete relaxation of the urinary sphincter and dyssynergic voiding. The resultant elevated urinary pressure may cause urine reflux into the prostate (triggering an inflammatory response) or increased pelvic autonomic activity leading to chronic pain (see p. 1776) without inflammation.

Classification

Prostatitis is classified into 4 categories (see TABLE 240–2). These categories are differentiated by clinical findings and by the presence or absence of signs of infection and inflammation in 2 urine samples. The 1st sample is a midstream collection. The patient then undergoes digital prostate massage and voids immediately; the first 10 mL of urine constitutes the 2nd sample. Infection is defined by bacterial growth on urine culture; inflammation, by presence of WBCs on urinalysis.

TABLE 240–2. NIH CONSENSUS CLASSIFICATION SYSTEM FOR PROSTATITIS

CATEGORY	CHARACTERISTICS	URINE FINDING	PREMAS-SAGE	POSTMAS-SAGE
I Acute bacterial prostatitis	Acute symptoms of urinary infection	WBC	+/–	+
		Bacteria	+/–	+
II Chronic bacterial prostatitis	Recurrent urinary infection with same organism	WBC	+/–	+
		Bacteria	+/–	+
III Chronic prostatitis/ Chronic pelvic pain syndrome	Primarily complaints of pain, voiding, and sexual dysfunction			
IIIa Inflammatory		WBC	–	+
		Bacteria	–	–
IIIb Noninflammatory	Previously termed prostatodynia	WBC	–	–
		Bacteria	–	–
IV Asymptomatic inflammatory prostatitis	Discovered incidentally during urologic evaluation (eg, prostate biopsy, seminal fluid analysis) for other conditions	WBC	–	+

Symptoms and Signs

Symptoms vary by category but typically involve some degree of urinary irritation or obstruction and pain. Irritation is manifested by frequency and urgency; obstruction, by a sensation of incomplete bladder emptying, a need to void again shortly after urinating, or nocturia. Pain is typically in the perineum but may be perceived at the tip of the penis, lower back, or testicles. Some patients report painful ejaculation.

Acute bacterial prostatitis often produces such systemic symptoms as fever, chills, malaise, and myalgias. The prostate is exquisitely tender and focally or diffusely swollen, boggy, and/or indurated. A generalized sepsis syndrome may result, with tachycardia, tachypnea, and sometimes hypotension.

Chronic bacterial prostatitis presents with recurrent episodes of infection with or without complete resolution between bouts. Symptoms and signs tend to be milder than in acute prostatitis.

Chronic prostatitis/chronic pelvic pain syndrome typically has pain as the predominant complaint, often including pain with ejaculation. The discomfort can be significant and often markedly interferes with quality of life. Symptoms of urinary irritation or obstruction also may be present. On examination, the prostate may be tender but usually is not boggy or swollen.

Asymptomatic inflammatory prostatitis causes no symptoms and is discovered incidentally during evaluation for other prostate diseases when WBCs are present in the urine.

Diagnosis

Diagnosis is suspected clinically. Similar findings can result from urethritis, perirectal abscess, or urinary tract infection.

Febrile patients with typical symptoms and signs of acute bacterial prostatitis usually have a positive midstream urinalysis. Prostate massage to obtain a postmassage urine sample is thought to be unnecessary and possibly dangerous in these patients (although this remains unproved). Blood cultures should be obtained on toxic-appearing patients, whose symptoms include weakness, fever, confusion, and disorientation. For afebrile patients, urine samples before and after massage are adequate for diagnosis.

Other tests to consider are transrectal ultrasonography (to rule out prostatic abscess or destruction and inflammation of the seminal vesicles) and cystoscopy (to rule out other pathology).

Treatment

Treatment varies significantly with etiology.

Acute bacterial prostatitis: Nontoxic patients can be treated at home with bed rest, analgesics, stool softeners, and hydration. Therapy with a fluoroquinolone (eg, ofloxacin 300 mg po bid) is usually effective and can be given until culture and sensitivity results are known. If the clinical response is satisfactory, treatment is continued for about 30 days to prevent chronic bacterial prostatitis. Some clinicians have recommended frequent ejaculation but it is probably of no benefit.

If sepsis is suspected, the patient is hospitalized and given broad-spectrum antibiotics IV (eg, ampicillin plus gentamicin) until the bacterial sensitivity is known. If the clinical response is adequate, IV therapy is continued until the patient is afebrile for 24 to 48 h, followed by oral therapy for 4 to 6 wk.

Rarely, prostate abscess develops, requiring surgery.

Chronic bacterial prostatitis: Chronic bacterial prostatitis is treated with oral antibiotics such as fluoroquinolones for at least 6 wk. Therapy is guided by culture results; empiric antibiotic treatment of those with equivocal or negative cultures has a low success rate. Other treatments include anti-inflammatory drugs; muscle relaxants (cyclobenzaprine); α-adrenergic blockers; and other symptomatic measures, such as sitz baths.

Chronic prostatitis/chronic pelvic pain syndrome: Treatment is difficult and often unrewarding. In addition to the above treatments, anxiolytics (eg, SSRIs, benzodiazepines), sacral nerve stimulation, and microwave therapy may be considered.

Asymptomatic inflammatory prostatitis: Asymptomatic prostatitis requires no treatment.

PROSTATE ABSCESS

Prostate abscesses are focal purulent collections that develop as complications of acute prostatitis.

The usual infecting organisms are aerobic gram-negative bacilli or, less frequently, *Staphylococcus aureus*. Urinary frequency, dysuria, and urinary retention are common. Perineal pain, evidence of acute epididymitis, hematuria, and a purulent urethral discharge are less common. Fever is sometimes present. Rectal examination may show prostate tenderness and fluctuance, but prostate enlargement is often the only abnormality, and sometimes the gland feels normal.

Abscess is suspected in patients with continued or recurrent UTIs despite antimicrobial therapy and persistent perineal pain. Such patients should undergo prostate ultrasound and possibly cystoscopy. Many abscesses, however, are discovered unexpectedly during prostate surgery or endoscopy; bulging of a lateral lobe into the prostatic urethra or rupture during instrumentation reveals the abscess. Leukocytosis is common. Although pyuria and bacteriuria are frequent, urine may be normal. Blood cultures are positive in some patients. Treatment involves appropriate antibiotics plus drainage by transurethral evacuation or transperineal aspiration and drainage.

241 GENITOURINARY CANCER

(Gynecologic cancers are discussed in Ch. 254 on p. 2118.)

GU cancers (renal, renal pelvic, ureteral, bladder, prostate, urethral, penile, and testicular) account for about 42% of cancers in men (primarily as prostate cancer) and 4% in women.

BLADDER CANCER

Bladder cancer is usually transitional cell carcinoma. Symptoms include hematuria; later, urinary obstruction can cause pain. Diagnosis is by urinary imaging or cystoscopy and biopsy. Treatment is with surgery, fulguration, intravesical instillations, or chemotherapy.

In the US, > 60,000 new cases of bladder cancer and about 12,700 deaths occur each year. Bladder cancer is the 4th most common cancer among men and is less common among women; male:female incidence is about 3:1.

Bladder cancer is more common among whites than blacks, and incidence increases with age. In > 40% of patients, tumors recur at the same or another site in the bladder, particularly if tumors are large, poorly differentiated, or multiple. Expression of tumor gene p53 may be associated with progression.

Smoking is the most common risk factor and causes ≥ 50% of new cases. Risk is also increased by excess phenacetin use (analgesic abuse); long-term cyclophosphamide use; chronic irritation (eg, in schistosomiasis, by bladder calculi); and exposure to hydrocarbons, tryptophan metabolites, or industrial chemicals, notably aromatic amines (aniline dyes, such as naphthylamine used in the dye industry) and chemicals used in the rubber, electric, cable, paint, and textile industries.

More than 90% of bladder cancers are transitional cell carcinomas. Most are papillary carcinomas, which tend to be superficial and well-differentiated and to grow outward; sessile tumors are more insidious, tending to invade early and metastasize. Squamous cell carcinoma is less common and usually occurs in patients with parasitic bladder infestation or chronic mucosal irritation. Adenocarcinoma may occur as a primary tumor but may reflect metastasis from intestinal carcinoma, which should be ruled out. Bladder cancer tends to metastasize to the lymph nodes, lungs, liver, and bone. In the bladder, carcinoma in situ is high grade but noninvasive and usually multifocal; it tends to recur.

Symptoms, Signs, and Diagnosis

Most patients present with unexplained hematuria (gross or microscopic). Some present with anemia, and hematuria is detected during evaluation. Irritative voiding symptoms (dysuria, burning, frequency) and pyuria are also common at presentation. Pelvic pain occurs with advanced cancer, when a pelvic mass may be palpable.

Bladder cancer is suspected clinically. IVU (see p. 1936) and cystoscopy (see p. 1938) with biopsy of abnormal areas are usually done initially because these tests are needed even if urine cytology, which may detect cancerous cells, is negative. The role for urinary antigen and genetic marker tests is not yet established.

For obviously superficial tumors (comprising 70 to 80% of tumors), cystoscopy with biopsy is sufficient for staging. For other tumors, abdominal and pelvic CT and chest x-ray are done to determine tumor extent and to check for metastases. Bimanual examination using anesthesia and MRI may help. The standard TNM staging system is used (see TABLE 241–1).

Prognosis and Treatment

Superficial bladder cancer rarely causes death. For patients with deep invasion of the bladder musculature, the 5-yr survival rate is about 50%, but adjuvant chemotherapy may improve these results. Generally, prognosis for patients with progressive or recurrent invasive bladder cancer is poor. Prognosis for patients with squamous cell carcinoma of the bladder is also poor, because this cancer is usually highly infiltrative and detected only at an advanced stage.

Early superficial cancers, including superficial invasion of the bladder musculature, can be completely removed by transurethral resection or fulguration. Repeated bladder instillations of chemotherapeutic drugs, such as doxorubicin, mitomycin C, or thiotepa (rarely used), may reduce risk of recurrence. BCG instillation after transurethral resection is generally more effective than chemotherapy instillations for carcinoma in situ and other high-grade, superficial, transitional cell carcinomas. Even when the tumor cannot be completely resected, some patients may benefit from bladder instillations. Intravesical BCG plus interferon may successfully treat some patients who recur after BCG alone.

Tumors that penetrate deeply into or through the bladder wall usually require radical cystectomy (removal of bladder and adjacent structures) with concomitant urinary diversion; partial cystectomy is possible for < 5% of patients. Cystectomy is being performed after initial chemotherapy in patients with locally advanced disease with increasing frequency. Urinary diversion traditionally involves routing urine through an ileal conduit to an abdominal stoma and collecting it in an external bag. Alternatives such as orthotopic neobladder or continent cutaneous diversion are very common and are appropriate for many, if not most, patients. For both procedures, an internal reservoir is constructed from the intestine. For orthotopic neobladder, the reservoir is connected to the urethra. Patients empty the reservoir by relaxing the pelvic floor muscles and increasing abdominal pressure, so that urine passes through the urethra almost naturally. Most patients maintain urinary control during the day, but some incontinence may occur at night. For continent cutaneous urinary diversion, the reservoir is connected to a continent abdominal stoma. Patients empty the reservoir by self-catheterization at regular intervals throughout the day.

If surgery is contraindicated or refused, radiation therapy alone or with chemotherapy may provide 5-yr survival of 20 to 40%. Radiation therapy may cause radiation cystitis or proctitis or bladder contracture.

Patients should be monitored q 3 to 6 mo for progression or recurrence. Metastases require chemotherapy, which is frequently effective but rarely curative unless metastases are confined to lymph nodes.

Treatment of recurrent cancer depends on clinical stage and site of recurrence, and previous treatment. Recurrence after transurethral resection of superficial or locally invasive tumors is treated with a 2nd resection or fulguration. Combination chemotherapy may prolong life in patients with metastatic disease.

METASTATIC RENAL CANCER

Nonrenal cancers may metastasize to the kidneys.

The most common are melanomas and solid tumors, particularly lung, breast, stomach, gynecologic, intestinal, and pancreatic. Leukemia and lymphoma may invade the kidneys, which then appear enlarged, often asymmetrically.

Despite extensive interstitial involvement, symptoms are rare, and renal function may not change from baseline. Proteinuria is absent or insignificant, and blood urea and creatinine levels rarely increase unless a complication (eg, uric acid nephropathy, hypercalcemia, bacterial infection) occurs.

Renal metastases are usually discovered during evaluation of the primary tumor or incidentally during abdominal imaging. If there is no known primary tumor, diagnosis proceeds as for renal cell carcinoma (see p. 2055). Treatment is systemic therapy for the primary tumor, rarely surgery.

PENILE CANCER

Most penile cancers are squamous cell carcinomas and usually occur in elderly uncircumcised men, particularly those with poor local hygiene.

Human papillomavirus, particularly types 16 and 18, plays a role in etiology. Precancerous lesions include erythroplasia of Queyrat, Bowen's disease, and bowenoid papulosis. Erythroplasia of Queyrat and Bowen's disease progress to invasive squamous cell carcinoma in 5 to 10% of patients; bowenoid papulosis does not appear to do so. The 3 lesions have different clinical presentations and biologic effects but are virtually the same histologically; they may be more appropriately called intraepithelial neoplasia or carcinoma in situ.

Most squamous cell carcinomas originate on the glans, in the coronal sulcus, or under the foreskin. They usually begin as a small erythematous lesion and are confined to the skin for a long time. These carcinomas may be fungating and exophytic or ulcerative and infiltrative. The latter type metastasizes more commonly, usually to the superficial and deep inguinofemoral and pelvic nodes. Metastases to distant sites (eg, lungs, liver, bone, brain) are rare until late in the disease.

Most patients present with a sore that has not healed, subtle induration of the skin, or sometimes a pus-filled or warty growth. The sore may be shallow or deep with rolled edges. Many patients do not notice the cancer or do not report it promptly. Pain is uncommon.

Diagnosis

If cancer is suspected, biopsy is required; if possible, tissue under the lesion should be included. MRI and ultrasonography help in staging localized cancer, checking for invasion of the corpora, and evaluating lymph nodes. The standard TNM staging system is used (see TABLE 241–1).

Treatment

Untreated penile cancer progresses, typically causing death within 2 yr. Treated early, penile cancer can usually be cured.

Circumcision or laser ablation may be effective for small, superficial lesions, but total penectomy, often with ilioinguinal lymphadenectomy, is required for larger, infiltrative lesions. Partial penectomy is appropriate if the tumor can be completely excised with adequate margins, leaving a penile stump that permits urination and sexual function. If tumors are high-grade or invade the corpora cavernosa, bilateral ilioinguinal lymphadenectomy is required. The role of radiation therapy is controversial. For advanced, invasive cancer, palliation may include surgery and radiation therapy, but cure

TABLE 241–1. GENITOURINARY CANCER STAGING

AJCC/ TNM*	RENAL CELL CARCINOMA	BLADDER	PROSTATE	URETHRA	PENIS	TESTIS
T1	≤ 7 cm in greatest dimension; limited to kidney	Invades subepithelial connective tissue	Clinically inapparent by palpation or imaging	Invades subepithelial connective tissue	Invades subepithelial connective tissue	Limited to testis and epididymis without vascular or lymphatic invasion; may invade tunica albuginea but not tunica vaginalis
T1a	≤ 4 cm in greatest dimension		Incidentally found in ≤ 5% of resected tissue			
T1b	> 4 cm but ≤ 7 cm in greatest dimension		Incidentally found in > 5% of resected tissue			
T1c			Identified by needle biopsy done for elevated prostate-specific antigen level			
T2	> 7 cm in greatest dimension; limited to kidney	Invades muscle	Is palpable or reliably visible by imaging; confined to prostate	Infiltrates periurethral muscle or corpus spongiosum or prostate	Invades corpus spongiosum or cavernosum	Limited to testis and epididymis with vascular or lymphatic invasion; or extends through tunica albuginea and involves tunica vaginalis
T2a		Invades superficial muscle (inner half)	Involves $\frac{1}{2}$ of one lobe or less			
T2b		Invades deep muscle (outer half)	Involves > $\frac{1}{2}$ of one lobes but not both lobes			
T2c			Involves both lobes			

T3	Extends into major veins or invades adrenal gland or perinephric tissues but not beyond Gerota's fascia	Invades perivesical tissue	Extends through the prostatic capsule	Infiltrates beyond periurethral tissue (vagina, labia, or muscle in women; corpus cavernosum or muscle in men)	Invades urethra or prostate	Invades spermatic cord with or without vascular or lymphatic invasion
T3a	Directly invades adrenal gland or perirenal and/or renal sinus fat	Invades perivesical tissue microscopically	Extends through the prostatic capsule unilaterally or bilaterally			
T3b	Grossly extends into the renal vein, its segmental branches, or vena cava below the diaphragm	Invades perivesical tissue macroscopically (extravesical mass)	Invades seminal vesicles			
T3c	Grossly extends into vena cava above diaphragm or invades the wall of the vena cava					
T4	Invades beyond Gerota's fascia	Invades any of the following:	Is fixed or invades adjacent structures other than seminal vesicles		Invades other adjacent structures	Invades scrotum with or without vascular or lymphatic invasion
T4a		Prostate or uterus or vagina				
T4b		Pelvic or abdominal wall				

*AJCC/TNM staging also includes number of regional lymph nodes involved (not assessable = NX; N0 = no evidence of tumor; N1 up to N3, depending on primary location, nodes affected, and size of nodal metastasis) and presence of distant metastases (not assessable = MX, none = M0, present = M1). Further distinctions within a category may be indicated by a lower-case letter.

is unlikely. Chemotherapy for advanced cancer has had limited success.

PROSTATE CANCER

Prostate cancer is usually adenocarcinoma. Symptoms are rare until urethral obstruction occurs. Diagnosis is suggested by digital rectal examination or prostate-specific antigen measurement and confirmed by biopsy. Prognosis for most patients with prostate cancer, especially when it is localized or regional, is very good; more men die with prostate cancer than of it. Treatment is with prostatectomy, radiation therapy, or, for some elderly patients, watchful waiting.

Adenocarcinoma of the prostate is the most common nondermatologic cancer in men > 50 in the US. In the US, about 230,100 new cases and about 29,900 deaths (in 2004) occur each year. Incidence increases with each decade of life; autopsy studies show prostate cancer in 15 to 60% of men age 60 to 90 yr, with incidence increasing with age. Median age at diagnosis is 72, and > 75% of prostate cancers are diagnosed in men > 65. Risk is highest for black men. Sarcoma of the prostate is rare, occurring primarily in children. Undifferentiated prostate cancer, squamous cell carcinoma, and ductal transitional carcinoma also occur. Hormonal influences contribute to adenocarcinoma but almost certainly not to other types of prostate cancer.

Prostatic intraepithelial neoplasia (PIN) is precancerous histologic change. It may be low- or high-grade; high-grade is considered a precursor of invasive cancer.

Symptoms and Signs

Prostate cancer usually progresses slowly and rarely causes symptoms until advanced. In advanced disease, hematuria and symptoms of bladder outlet obstruction (eg, straining, hesitancy, weak or intermittent urine stream, a sense of incomplete emptying, terminal dribbling) may appear. Bone pain may result from osteoblastic metastases to bone (commonly pelvis, ribs, vertebral bodies).

Diagnosis

Sometimes stony hard induration or nodules are palpable on digital rectal examination (DRE), but the examination is often normal; induration and nodularity suggest cancer but must be differentiated from granulomatous prostatitis, prostatic calculi, and other prostate disorders. Extension of induration to the seminal vesicles and lateral fixation of the gland suggest locally advanced prostate cancer. Prostate cancers detected by DRE tend to be large, and > 50% extend through the capsule.

Screening: Most cases are detected by screening with DRE and serum prostate-specific antigen (PSA) levels, which is commonly performed annually in men > 50 yr. Abnormal findings require histologic confirmation, most commonly by transrectal ultrasound (TRUS)–guided transrectal needle biopsy, which can be done in a clinic without general anesthesia. Hypoechoic areas are more likely to represent cancer. Although there appears to be a drop in death rate from prostate cancer and a drop in incidence of distant disease since routine screening was initiated, the value of such screening is unproved. Occasionally, prostate cancer is diagnosed incidentally in tissue removed during surgery for benign prostatic hyperplasia (BPH).

Serum PSA is somewhat problematic as a screening test. Although it is elevated in 25 to 92% of patients with prostate cancer (depending on tumor volume), it also is moderately elevated in 30 to 50% of patients with BPH (depending on prostate size and degree of obstruction), in some smokers, and for several weeks after prostatitis. A level of ≥ 4 ng/mL has traditionally been considered an indication for biopsy in men > 50 yr (in younger patients, levels > 2.5 ng/mL probably warrant biopsy, because BPH, the most common cause of PSA elevation, is rare). Although very high levels are significant (suggesting extracapsular extension of the tumor or metastases), and it is clear that likelihood of cancer increases with increasing PSA levels, there is no cut-off below which there is no risk. In asymptomatic patients, positive predictive value for cancer is 67% for PSA > 10 ng/mL and 25% for PSA 4 to 10 ng/mL; recent evidence indicates a 15% prevalence of cancer in men ≥ 55 yr with PSA < 4 ng/mL and a 10% incidence with PSA between 0.6 and 1.0 ng/mL. Cancer present in those with lower levels tends to be smaller (often < 1 mL) and of lower grade, although high-grade cancer (Gleason score 7 to 10) can be present at any level of PSA; perhaps 15% of cancers presenting with PSA < 4 ng/mL are high grade. Although it appears that a cut-off of 4 ng/mL will miss some cancers, the clinical significance of this is unclear. There are no data yet that performing biopsy in patients > 50 yr with levels < 4 ng/mL improves disease-free outcome for patients with rapidly rising levels (> 2 ng/mL/yr); the intrinsic biology of the tumor may make those patients incurable regardless of early diagnosis.

Assays that determine the free-to-bound PSA ratio and complex PSA are more specific than standard PSA measurements and may reduce the frequency of biopsies in patients without cancer. Prostate cancer is associated with less free PSA; no standard cut-off has been established, but generally, levels < 15 to 25% warrant biopsy. Other isoforms of PSA and new markers for prostate cancer are being studied.

Staging and grading: Prostate cancer is staged to define extent of the tumor (see TABLE 241–1). TRUS may provide information for staging, particularly about capsular penetration and seminal vesicle invasion. Elevated serum acid phosphatase—especially the enzymatic assay—correlates well with the presence of metastases, particularly in lymph nodes. However, this enzyme may also be elevated in BPH (slightly after vigorous prostatic massage), multiple myeloma, Gaucher's disease, and hemolytic anemia. Radionuclide bone scanning is done to check for metastases to bone (sometimes detected by x-rays). Reverse transcriptase–PCR assays for circulating prostate cancer cells are being studied as a staging and prognostic tool.

Grading, based on the resemblance of tumor architecture to normal glandular structure, helps define the aggressiveness of the tumor. Grading takes into account histologic heterogeneity in the tumor. The Gleason score is commonly used: The most prevalent pattern and the next most prevalent pattern are each assigned a grade of 1 to 5, and the 2 grades are added (total score: 2 to 4 = well differentiated, 5 to 7 = moderately differentiated, and 8 to 10 = undifferentiated); in another scaling system ≤ 6 is considered well differentiated, 7 moderately, and 8 to 10 poorly differentiated. The lower the score, the less aggressive and invasive is the tumor and the better is the prognosis. For localized tumors, the Gleason score helps predict the likelihood of capsular penetration, seminal vesicle invasion, or spread to lymph nodes. Gleason score, clinical stage, and PSA together (using tables or nomograms) predict pathologic stage and prognosis better than any of them alone.

Both acid phosphatase and PSA levels decrease after treatment and increase with recurrence, but PSA is the most sensitive marker for monitoring cancer progression and response to treatment.

Prognosis

Prognosis for most patients with prostate cancer, especially when it is localized or regional, is very good. Prognosis for elderly men with prostate cancer differs little from age-matched men without prostate cancer. For many patients, long-term local control, even cure, is possible. Potential for cure, even when cancer is clinically localized, depends on the tumor's grade and stage. Without early treatment, patients with high-grade, poorly differentiated cancer have a poor prognosis. Undifferentiated prostate cancer, squamous cell carcinoma, and ductal transitional carcinoma respond poorly to the usual control measures. Metastatic cancer has no cure; median life expectancy is 1 to 3 yr, although some patients live for many years.

Treatment

Treatment is guided by PSA, grade and extent of tumor, patient age, coexisting disorders, and life expectancy.

Most patients, regardless of age, prefer definitive therapy. However, watchful waiting may be appropriate for asymptomatic patients > 70 with localized prostate cancer, particularly if it is well or moderately well differentiated and low volume or if life-limiting disorders coexist; in these patients, risk of death due to other causes is greater than that due to prostate cancer. This approach requires periodic DRE, PSA measurement, and monitoring of symptoms. If symptoms worsen, treatment is required. In elderly men, watchful waiting results in the same overall survival rate as prostatectomy; however, patients who had surgery had a significantly lower risk of distant metastases and disease-specific mortality.

Radical prostatectomy (removal of prostate with adnexal structures and regional lymph nodes) is probably best for patients < 70 with a tumor confined to the prostate. Prostatectomy is appropriate for some elderly patients, based on life expectancy, coexisting disorders, and ability to tolerate surgery and anesthesia. Complications include urinary incontinence (about 5 to 10%), bladder neck contracture or urethral stricture (about 7 to 20%), erectile dysfunction (about 30 to 100%—heavily dependent on age and current function), and fecal incontinence (1 to 2%). Major complications occur in > 25%, more often in elderly patients. Nerve-sparing radical prostatectomy reduces the likelihood of erectile dysfunction but cannot always be done, depending on tumor stage and location.

Cryotherapy (destruction of prostate cancer cells by freezing with cryoprobes, followed by thawing) is less well established; long-term outcomes are unknown. Adverse effects include bladder outlet obstruction, urinary incontinence, erectile dysfunction, and rectal pain or injury.

Results with radiation therapy and prostatectomy may be comparable, especially for patients with low pretreatment PSA levels. Standard external beam radiotherapy usually delivers 70 Gy in 7 wk. Conformal 3-dimensional radiation therapy or intensity modulated radiation therapy (IMRT) safely deliver doses approaching 80 Gy to the prostate; data indicate that the rate of local control is higher, especially for high-risk patients. For most patients, some decrease in erectile function occurs in at least 40%. Other adverse effects include radiation proctitis, cystitis, diarrhea, fatigue, and, possibly urethral strictures, particularly in patients with a prior history of transurethral resection of the prostate.

Whether brachytherapy (radioactive seed implants) can produce equivalent results is being studied; results appear to be comparable for patients with low PSA levels and low-grade localized tumors. Brachytherapy also decreases erectile function, although it may be delayed and patients may be more responsive to phosphodiesterase type 5 (PDE5) inhibitors than patients whose neurovascular bundles are resected or injured during surgery. Urinary frequency, urgency, and, less often, retention are common but usually subside over time. Other adverse effects include increased bowel movements; rectal urgency, bleeding, or ulceration; and prostatorectal fistulas.

For larger, less differentiated tumors, especially with a Gleason score 8 to 10 and when the PSA is > 10, pelvic lymph nodes should be assessed. Assessment can usually be done by CT or MRI, and suspicious nodes can be further evaluated by needle biopsy. If pelvic metastases are detected preoperatively, radical prostatectomy is not usually done.

For short-term palliation, one or more drugs may be used, including antiandrogens, chemotherapy drugs (eg, mitoxantrone, estramustine, taxanes), corticosteroids, and ketoconazole; docetaxel plus prednisone is a common combination. Local radiation therapy is usually palliative for patients with symptomatic bone metastases.

Patients with a locally advanced tumor or metastases may benefit from androgen deprivation by castration, either surgically with bilateral orchiectomy or medically with luteinizing hormone-releasing hormone (LHRH) agonists, such as leuprolide, goserelin, and buserelin, with or without radiation therapy. Reduction in serum testosterone with LHRH agonists equals that with bilateral orchiectomy. All of these treatments cause loss of libido and erectile dysfunction and may cause hot flashes. LHRH agonists may cause PSA levels to increase temporarily. Some patients benefit from adding antiandrogens (eg, flutamide, bicalutamide, nilutamide, cyproterone acetate [not available in US]) for total androgen blockade. Maximal androgen blockade usually refers to LHRH agonists, plus antiandrogens, but its benefits appear minimally better than those of an LHRH agonist (or orchiectomy) alone. Another approach is intermittent androgen blockade which is purported to delay emergence of androgen-independent prostate cancer. Total androgen ablation is given until PSA levels are reduced (usually to undetectable levels), then stopped; treatment is started again when PSA levels rise again. The optimal schedules for treatment and time off treatment have not been determined and vary widely among practitioners. Androgen deprivation may impair quality of life significantly (eg, patients' self-image, attitude toward the cancer and its treatment, energy levels) and cause osteoporosis, anemia, and loss of muscle mass with long-term treatment. Exogenous estrogens are rarely used because they have a risk of cardiovascular and thromboembolic complications. There is no standard therapy for hormone-refractory prostate cancer.

Cytotoxic and biologic drugs (eg, genetically designed vaccines, antisense therapy, monoclonal antibodies), angiogenesis inhibitors (eg, thalidomide, endostatin), and matrix metalloproteinase inhibitors are being studied and may provide palliation and prolong survival, but their superiority over corticosteroids alone has not been proved.

For high-grade tumors that extend beyond the prostatic capsule, several treatment protocols exist. Chemotherapy, with or without hormonal therapy, is used before surgery in some protocols and along with radiation in others. Chemotherapy regimens vary by center and trial.

RENAL CELL CARCINOMA

(Hypernephroma; Adenocarcinoma of the Kidneys)

Renal cell carcinoma is the most common renal cancer. Symptoms appear late and include hematuria, flank pain, a palpable mass, and FUO. Diagnosis is by CT or MRI and occasionally by biopsy. Treatment is with surgery for early disease and typically an experimental protocol for advanced disease.

Renal cell carcinoma (RCC), an adenocarcinoma, accounts for 90 to 95% of primary malignant renal tumors. Less common primary renal tumors include transitional cell carcinoma, Wilms' tumor, and sarcoma.

In the US, about 31,900 cases of RCC and 11,900 deaths occur each year. RCC occurs slightly more often in men. Risk factors include smoking (in 20 to 30% of patients); obesity; excess use of phenacetin; acquired cystic kidney disease in dialysis patients; adult polycystic kidney disease; and exposure to certain radiopaque dyes, asbestos, cadmium, and leather tanning and petroleum products. In some familial syndromes, particularly von Hippel-Lindau disease, incidence of RCC is high.

RCC tends to trigger thrombus formation in the renal vein which occasionally propagates into the vena cava; tumor invasion of the vein wall is uncommon. RCC metastasizes most often to the lymph nodes, lungs, adrenal glands, liver, and bone.

Symptoms and Signs

Symptoms usually do not appear until late, when the tumor may already be large and metastatic. Gross or microscopic hematuria is the most common presentation, followed by flank pain, a palpable mass, and FUO. Sometimes hypertension results from segmental ischemia or pedicle compression, and polycythemia results from increased erythropoietin activity. Hypercalcemia is common and may require treatment (see p. 1257). Paraneoplastic syndromes occur in 20% of patients.

Diagnosis

A renal mass may be detected incidentally during abdominal imaging (eg, CT, ultrasonography) done for other reasons. Otherwise, diagnosis is suggested by clinical findings and confirmed by abdominal CT with and without a radiocontrast agent or by MRI. A renal mass that is enhanced by radiocontrast strongly suggests RCC. CT and MRI also provide information about local extension and nodal and venous involvement. MRI provides further information about extension into the renal vein and vena cava and has replaced inferior vena cavography. Ultrasonography and IVU may show a mass but provide somewhat less information and do not show nonrenal causes of symptoms as accurately as CT or MRI. Often, noncancerous and cancerous masses can be distinguished radiographically, but sometimes surgery is needed for diagnosis. Needle biopsy does not have sufficient sensitivity when findings are equivocal; it is recommended only when there is an infiltrative pattern instead of a discrete mass, when the renal mass may be a metastasis from another known cancer, or sometimes to confirm a diagnosis prior to chemotherapy for metastases.

Three-dimensional CT, CT angiography, and magnetic resonance angiography are used before surgery, particularly before nephron-sparing surgery, to define the nature of RCC, to more accurately determine the number of renal arteries present, and to delineate the vascular pattern. These imaging techniques have virtually replaced aortography and selective renal artery angiography.

A chest x-ray and liver function tests are essential. If chest x-ray is abnormal, chest CT is done. If alkaline phosphatase is elevated, bone scanning may be needed. Serum electrolytes, BUN, creatinine, and Ca are measured. BUN and creatinine are unaffected unless both kidneys are diseased.

Staging: Information from the evaluation makes preliminary staging possible. Robson's system is still used in the US, but the TNM system is more precise and is being increasingly used (see TABLE 241–1). In the Robson system, stage I is tumor confined to the renal capsule. Stage II is tumor not extending beyond Gerota's fascia. Stage III is spread to the vena cava or the renal vein (IIIA) or to regional lymph nodes (IIIB). Stage IV is invasion of adjacent organs and distant metastases. At diagnosis, RCC is localized in 45%, locally invasive in about 33%, and spread to distant organs in 25%.

Prognosis and Treatment

Five-year survival rates range from 66% for stage I to 11% for stage IV. Prognosis is poor for patients with metastatic or recurrent RCC because treatments are usually ineffective, although useful for palliation.

Early RCC is treated surgically, and advanced RCC typically with an experimental protocol. Radical nephrectomy (removal of kidney, adrenal gland, perirenal fat, and Gerota's fascia) with removal of regional nodes is standard treatment for localized RCC and provides a reasonable chance for cure. Results with open or laparoscopic procedures are comparable. Nephron-sparing surgery (partial nephrectomy) is possible and appropriate for many patients, even in patients with a normal contralateral kidney if the tumor is < 4 cm. Nonsurgical destruction of renal tumors via freezing (cryosurgery) or thermal energy (radiofrequency ablation) is being done in highly selected patients, but long-term data about efficacy and indications are not yet available.

For tumors involving the renal vein and vena cava, surgery may be curative if no nodal or distant metastases exist.

If both kidneys are affected, partial nephrectomy of one or both kidneys is usually preferable to bilateral radical nephrectomy if technically feasible.

Whether external beam radiation therapy before or after nephrectomy improves survival may still be unclear, but it is virtually never used anymore. It may be palliative when surgery is contraindicated and perhaps for metastatic RCC, particularly in bone, although metastatic RCC is radioresistant.

Traditional chemotherapeutic drugs, alone or combined, and progestins are ineffective. Palliation can include nephrectomy, tumor embolization, and external beam radiation therapy. Resection of metastases, if limited in number, prolongs life in some patients, particularly those with a long interval between initial treatment (nephrectomy) and development of metastases. For some patients, immunotherapy reduces tumor size and prolongs life. About 10 to 20% of patients respond to interferon-α or IL-2, although the response is long-lasting in < 5%. Most 1st-line treatments (except IL-2) are experimental. They include stem cell transplantation, other interleukins, antiangiogenesis therapy (eg, bevacizumab, thalidomide), and vaccine therapy.

RENAL PELVIC AND URETERAL CANCERS

Cancers of the renal pelvis and ureters are usually transitional cell carcinomas and occasionally squamous cell carcinomas. Symptoms include hematuria and sometimes pain. Diagnosis is by CT, cytology, and sometimes biopsy. Treatment is surgery.

Transitional cell carcinoma (TCC) of the renal pelvis accounts for about 7% of all kidney tumors; TCC of the ureters accounts for about 4% of upper tract tumors. Risk factors are the same as those for bladder cancer. Also, inhabitants of the Balkans with endemic familial nephropathy are inexplicably predisposed to develop upper tract TCC.

Most patients present with hematuria; dysuria and frequency may occur if the bladder also is involved. Colicky pain may accompany obstruction (see p. 1963). Uncommonly, hydronephrosis results from a renal pelvic tumor.

Evaluation typically includes ultrasound or CT with contrast. Diagnosis must be confirmed by cytologic or histologic analysis. Ureteroscopy, nephroscopy, or both are done when biopsy of the upper tract is needed or when urine cytology is positive but no source of the malignant cells is obvious. Staging for obviously superficial tumors is probably unnecessary. For other tumors, abdominal and pelvic CT and chest x-ray are done to determine tumor extent and to check for metastases. The standard TNM staging system is used (see TABLE 241–1).

Prognosis

Prognosis depends on depth of penetration into or through the uroepithelial wall, which is difficult to determine. Likelihood of cure is >90% for patients with a superficial, localized tumor but is 10 to 15% for those with a deeply invasive tumor. If tumors penetrate the wall or distant metastases occur, cure is unlikely.

Treatment

Usual treatment is radical nephroureterectomy, including excision of a cuff of bladder. Partial ureterectomy is indicated in some cases (eg, in patients with a distal ureteral tumor, decreased renal function, or a solitary kidney). Laser fulguration for accurately staged and adequately visualized renal pelvic or low-grade ureteral tumors is sometimes possible. Occasionally, a chemotherapeutic drug, such as mitomycin C or BCG, is instilled. However, efficacy of laser therapy and chemotherapy has not been established.

Periodic cystoscopy is indicated because renal pelvic and ureteral cancers tend to recur in the bladder, and such recurrence, if detected at an early stage, may be treated by fulguration, transurethral resection, or intravesical instillations. Management of metastases is the same as that for metastatic bladder cancer.

TESTICULAR CANCER

Testicular cancer begins as a scrotal mass, which may be painful. Diagnosis is by ultrasonography and biopsy. Treatment is with orchiectomy and sometimes lymph node dissection, sometimes followed by radiation therapy and chemotherapy, depending on histology and stage.

Testicular cancer is the most common solid cancer in males aged 15 to 35. Incidence is 2.5 to 20 times higher in patients with cryptorchidism, even when the undescended testis has been brought down surgically. Cancer can also develop in the normally descended testis. The cause of testicular cancer is unknown.

Most testicular cancers originate in primordial germ cells. Germ cell tumors are categorized as seminomas (40%) or nonseminomas (tumors containing any nonseminomous elements). Nonseminomas include teratomas, embryonal carcinomas, endodermal sinus tumors (yolk sac tumors), and choriocarcinomas. Histologic combinations are common; eg, teratocarcinoma contains teratoma plus embryonal carcinoma. Functional interstitial cell carcinomas of the testis are rare.

Even patients with apparently localized tumors may have occult nodal or visceral metastases. Risk of metastases is highest for choriocarcinoma and lowest for teratoma.

Tumors originating in the epididymis, testicular appendages, and spermatic cord are usually benign fibromas, fibroadenomas, adenomatoid tumors, and lipomas. Sarcomas, most commonly rhabdomyosarcoma, occur occasionally, primarily in children.

Symptoms, Signs, and Diagnosis

Most present with a scrotal mass, which is painless or sometimes associated with dull, aching pain. In a few patients, hemorrhage into the tumor may cause acute local pain and tenderness. Many discover the mass themselves after minor scrotal trauma triggers self-examination.

The origin and nature of scrotal masses must be determined accurately because most testicular masses are cancerous, but most extratesticular masses are not; distinguishing between the two during physical examination may be difficult. Scrotal ultrasonography can confirm testicular origin. If a testicular mass is confirmed, serum markers α-fetoprotein and β-human chorionic gonadotropin should be measured, and a chest x-ray taken. Then, inguinal exploration is indicated; the spermatic cord is exposed and clamped before the abnormal testis is manipulated. If cancer is confirmed, abdominal and pelvic CT is needed for staging using the standard TNM system (see TABLE 241–1).

Prognosis and Treatment

Prognosis depends on histology and extent of the tumor. The 5-yr survival rate is > 95% for patients with a seminoma or nonseminoma localized to the testis or with a nonseminoma and low-volume metastases in the retroperitoneum. The 5-yr survival rate for patients with extensive retroperitoneal metastases or with pulmonary or other visceral metastases ranges from 48% (for some nonseminomas) to > 80%, depending on site, volume, and histology of the metastases, but even patients with advanced disease at presentation may be cured.

Radical inguinal orchiectomy, the cornerstone of treatment, provides important histopathologic information, particularly about the proportion of histologic types and presence of intratumoral vascular or lymphatic invasion. A few patients may be candidates for testis-sparing surgery (partial orchiectomy). Pathologic information obtained by surgery helps plan further treatment and can accurately predict risk of occult lymph node metastases. Thus, it helps identify which low-risk patients with normal x-rays and serum markers, especially those with nonseminomas, may be candidates for surveillance with frequent serum marker measurements, chest x-rays, and CT. Seminomas recur in about 15% of these patients and can usually be cured by radiation therapy when small, or chemotherapy when larger. Nonseminoma recurrences are promptly treated with chemotherapy, although delayed retroperitoneal lymph node dissection may be appropriate for some.

Standard treatment for seminoma after unilateral orchiectomy is radiation therapy, usually 20 to 40 Gy (higher dose is used for patients with a nodal mass) to the para-aortic regions up to the diaphragm, the ipsilateral ilioinguinal region is not routinely treated.

Occasionally, the mediastinum and left supraclavicular regions are also irradiated, depending on clinical stage. For nonseminomas, many consider standard treatment to be retroperitoneal lymph node dissection (RPLND); for early-stage tumors, a nerve-sparing dissection may be possible. Alternatives include surveillance for clinical stage I tumors without prognostic factors that predict relapse. At the time of orchiectomy, almost 30% of patients with nonseminomas have microscopic retroperitoneal lymph node metastases. Intermediate-sized retroperitoneal nodal masses may require retroperitoneal lymph node dissection and chemotherapy (eg, bleomycin, etoposide, cisplatin), but the optimal sequence is undecided. Laparoscopic lymph node dissection is under study. The most common adverse effect of lymph node dissection is failure to ejaculate. If tumor volume is low and a nerve-sparing procedure is used, ejaculation is usually preserved. Fertility is often impaired, but no risk to the fetus has been proved if pregnancy does occur.

A cosmetic testicular prosthesis may be placed during orchiectomy, but these prostheses are not widely available because of the problems with silicone breast implants. However, saline implants have been developed.

Nodal masses > 10 cm, lymph node metastases above the diaphragm, or visceral metastases require initial platinum-based combination chemotherapy followed by surgery for residual masses. Such treatment commonly controls the tumor long term.

URETHRAL CANCER

Urethral cancer is rare and occurs in both sexes; it may be squamous or transitional cell carcinoma or, occasionally, adenocarcinoma.

Urethral tumors invade adjacent structures early and thus tend to be advanced when diagnosed. External groin or pelvic (obturator) lymph nodes are usually the 1st sites of metastasis.

Most women present with hematuria and obstructive voiding symptoms or urinary retention. Most have a history of urinary frequency or urethral syndrome (hypersensitivity of the pelvic floor muscles). Most men present with symptoms of urethral stricture; only a few present with hematuria or a bloody discharge. Sometimes if the tumor is advanced, a mass is felt.

Diagnosis is suggested clinically and confirmed by cystourethroscopy. Biopsy may be required to differentiate urethral carcinoma, prolapse, and caruncle. CT or MRI (which is more accurate in men) is used for staging.

Prognosis depends on the precise location in the urethra and extent of the cancer, particularly depth of invasion. The 5-yr survival rates are > 60% for patients with distal tumors and 10 to 20% for those with proximal tumors; recurrence rate is > 50%.

For superficial or minimally invasive distal tumors in the anterior urethra, treatment is with radiation therapy (interstitial, or a combination of interstitial and external beam), open surgical excision, fulguration, or laser. Larger and more deeply invasive anterior tumors and proximal tumors in the posterior urethra require multimodal therapy with radical surgery and urinary diversion, usually in combination with radiation therapy. Surgery includes bilateral pelvic and sometimes inguinal lymph node dissection, often with removal of part of the symphysis pubis and inferior pubic rami. The value of chemotherapy, which is sometimes used, has not been established.

SECTION 18 GYNECOLOGY AND OBSTETRICS

242 APPROACH TO THE GYNECOLOGIC PATIENT

Gynecologic evaluation may be necessary to assess a specific problem such as pelvic pain, vaginal bleeding, or vaginal discharge (see also Ch. 246 on p. 2083). Women also need routine gynecologic evaluations, which may be provided by a gynecologist, an internist, or a family practitioner; evaluations are recommended every year for all women who are sexually active or > 18 yr. Many women expect their gynecologist to provide general as well as gynecologic health care. Obstetric evaluation focuses on issues related to pregnancy (see Ch. 259 on p. 2149).

GENERAL GYNECOLOGIC EVALUATION

Most women, particularly those seeking general preventive care, require a complete history and physical examination as well as a gynecologic evaluation.

History

Gynecologic history consists of the problem prompting the visit; menstrual, obstetric, and sexual history; and history of gynecologic symptoms, disorders, and treatments.

Menstrual history includes age at menarche, number of days of menses, length and regularity of the interval between cycles, start date of the last menstrual period (LMP), dates of the preceding period (previous menstrual period, or PMP), color and volume of flow, and any symptoms that occur with menses (eg, cramping, loose stools). Usually, menstrual fluid is medium or dark red, and flow lasts for 5 (± 2) days, with 21 to 35 days between menses; average blood loss is 30 mL (range, 13 to 80 mL), with the most bleeding on the 2nd day. A saturated pad or tampon absorbs 5 to 15 mL. Cramping is common on the day before and on the 1st day of menses. Vaginal bleeding that is painless, scant, and dark, is abnormally brief or prolonged, or occurs at irregular intervals suggests absence of ovulation (anovulation).

A complete obstetric history includes dates and outcomes of all pregnancies and previous ectopic or molar pregnancies (see p. 2149).

Sexual history includes frequency of sexual activity, number and sex of partners, use of contraception, participation in unsafe sex, and effects of sexual activity (eg, pleasure, orgasm, dyspareunia). The examiner should be professional and nonjudgmental.

The patient is asked about any symptoms present: for pelvic pain, its location, duration, character, quality, and triggering and relieving factors; for abnormal vaginal bleeding, its quantity, duration, and relation to the menstrual cycle. Patients of reproductive age are asked about symptoms of pregnancy (eg, morning sickness, breast tenderness, delayed menses).

Screening for domestic violence should be routine. Methods include self-administered questionnaires and a directed interview by a staff member or physician. In patients who do not admit to experiencing abuse, findings that suggest past abuse include inconsistent explanations for injuries, delay in seeking treatment for injuries, unusual somatic complaints, psychiatric symptoms, frequent emergency department visits, head and neck injuries, and having given birth to a low-birth-weight infant.

Physical Examination

The examiner should explain the examination, which includes breasts (see p. 2108), abdomen, and pelvis, to the patient.

For the pelvic examination, the patient lies supine on an examination table with her legs in stirrups and is usually draped. A chaperone may be required. The pubic area and hair are inspected for lesions, folliculitis, and lice. The perineum is inspected for redness, swelling, excoriations, abnormal pigmentation, and lesions (eg, ulcers, pustules, nodules, warts, tumors). Structural abnormalities due to congenital malformations or female genital mutilation are noted. A vaginal opening that is < 3 cm may indicate infibulation, a severe form of genital mutilation (see p. 2512).

Next, the introitus is palpated between the thumb and index finger for cysts or abscesses in Bartholin's glands. While spreading the labia and asking the patient to bear down, the examiner checks the vaginal opening for signs of pelvic relaxation: an anterior bulge (suggesting cystocele), a posterior bulge (suggesting rectocele), and displacement of the cervix toward the introitus (suggesting prolapsed uterus—see p. 2098).

Before speculum and bimanual examination, the patient is asked to relax her legs and hips and breathe deeply. If a Papanicolaou (Pap) test or cervical culture is planned, the speculum is rinsed with warm water; if not, it is lubricated. Then, it is inserted with the handle horizontal (blades vertical) while widening the vagina by pressing 2 fingers on the posterior vaginal wall. The speculum is fully inserted, then rotated so that the handle is down, and opened, pulling back as needed to visualize the cervix. Normally, the cervix is pink and shiny, without discharge. A specimen for the Pap test is taken from the endocervix and external cervix with a brush and plastic spatula; both are rinsed in a liquid, producing a cell suspension to be analyzed for cancerous cells and human papillomavirus. Specimens for detection of sexually transmitted diseases (STDs) are taken from the endocervix. The speculum is withdrawn, taking care not to pinch the labia with the speculum blades.

For the bimanual examination, the index and middle fingers of the dominant hand are inserted to just below the cervix. The other hand is placed just above the pubic symphysis and gently presses down to determine the size, position, and consistency of the uterus and, if possible, the ovaries. Normally, the uterus is about 6 cm by 4 cm and tilts anteriorly (anteversion), but it may tilt posteriorly (retroversion) to various degrees. The uterus also may be bent at an angle anteriorly or posteriorly (anteflexion and retroflexion, respectively). The uterus is movable and smooth; irregularity suggests uterine fibroids (leiomyomas). Normally, the ovaries are about 2 cm by 3 cm in young women and not palpable in postmenopausal women. With ovarian palpation, mild nausea and tenderness are normal. Significant pain when the cervix is gently moved from side to side (cervical motion tenderness) suggests pelvic inflammation.

After bimanual palpation, the examiner palpates the rectovaginal septum by inserting the index finger in the vagina and the middle finger in the rectum.

For children, the examination should be adjusted according to their psychosexual development and is usually limited to inspection of the external genitals. Young children can be examined on their mother's lap. Older children can be examined in the knee-chest position or on their side with one knee drawn up to their chest. Vaginal discharge can be collected, examined, and cultured. Sometimes a small catheter attached to a syringe of saline is used to obtain washings from the vagina. If cervical examination is required, a fiberoptic vaginoscope, pediatric cystoscope, or flexible hysteroscope with saline lavage should be used. In children, pelvic masses may be noted during palpation of the abdomen.

Testing

Most women who are of reproductive age and have gynecologic symptoms are tested for pregnancy (see p. 2156). Urine assays of the β subunit of human chorionic gonadotropin (β-hCG) are specific and highly sensitive; they become positive within about 1 wk of conception. Serum assays are specific and even more sensitive.

Specimens of cervical cells taken for the Pap test are examined for signs of cervical cancer; the examination may also detect uterine cancer and human papillomavirus. Pap tests are done routinely for most of a woman's life (see p. 2129).

Microscopic examination of vaginal secretions helps identify vaginal infections (eg, trichomoniasis, bacterial vaginosis, yeast infection—see Ch. 246 on p. 2083).

Culture or molecular methods (eg, PCR) are used to analyze specimens for specific STD organisms (eg, *Neisseria gonorrhoeae, Chlamydia trachomatis*) if patients have symptoms or risk factors; in some practices, such analysis is always done.

Bedside inspection of a cervical mucus specimen by a trained examiner can provide information about the menstrual cycle and hormone states; this information may help in assessment of menstrual dysfunction, infertility, suspected endocrine disorders, and time of ovulation. The specimen is placed on a slide, allowed to dry, and assessed for degree of microscopic crystallization (ferning—see p. 2073), which reflects levels of circulating estrogens. Just before ovulation, cervical mucus is clear and copious with abundant ferning because estrogen levels are high. Just after ovulation, cervical mucus is thick and ferns little. Pituitary and hypothalamic hormones (see p. 1174) and ovarian hormones (see p. 2071) may also be measured.

Imaging of suspected masses and other lesions usually involves ultrasonography, which may be done in the office; both transvaginal and transabdominal probes are used. MRI is highly specific but expensive. CT is usually less desirable because it is somewhat less accurate and involves significant radiation exposure and often radiopaque agent.

Laparoscopy detects structural abnormalities too small to be detected by imaging, as well as abnormalities on the surfaces of internal organs (eg, endometriosis, inflammation, scarring); it is also used to sample tissue.

Culdocentesis, now rarely used, is needle puncture of the posterior vaginal fornix to obtain fluid from the cul-de-sac (which is posterior to the uterus) for culture and for tests to detect blood from a ruptured ectopic pregnancy or ovarian cyst.

Endometrial aspiration is done if women > 35 have unexplained vaginal bleeding. A thin, flexible, plastic cannula is inserted through the cervix (often dilation is not required) to the level of the internal cervical os. Suction is applied to the device, which is turned and moved up and down a few times to sample different parts of the endometrial cavity. Sometimes the uterus must be stabilized with a cervical tenaculum.

PELVIC MASS

(See also Chs. 249 and 254.)

A pelvic mass may be detected during routine gynecologic examination.

Etiology

Pelvic masses may originate from gynecologic organs (cervix, uterus, or uterine adnexa) or from other pelvic organs (intestine, bladder, ureters, skeletal muscle, or bone).

Type of mass tends to vary by age group. Rarely, during the 1st few months of life, in utero maternal hormones may stimulate development of adnexal cysts. At puberty, menstrual fluid may accumulate and form a vaginal mass (hematocolpos) because outflow is obstructed; the cause is usually an imperforate hymen; other causes include congenital malformations of the uterus, cervix, or vagina.

In women of reproductive age, the most common cause of symmetric uterine enlargement is pregnancy, which may be unsuspected. Another common cause is myomas, which may extend outward. Common adnexal masses include graafian follicles (usually 5 to 8 cm) that develop normally but do not release an egg (called functional ovarian cysts). These cysts often resolve spontaneously within a few months. Adnexal masses may also result from ectopic pregnancy, ovarian or fallopian tube cancers, benign tumors (eg, benign cystic teratomas), or hydrosalpinges. Endometriosis can cause single or multiple masses anywhere in the pelvis, usually on the ovaries.

In postmenopausal women, masses are more likely to be cancerous. Many benign ovarian masses (eg, endometriomas, myomas) depend on ovarian hormone secretion and thus become less common after menopause.

Evaluation

History: General medical and complete gynecologic histories are obtained. Vaginal bleeding and pelvic pain suggest ectopic pregnancy or, rarely, gestational trophoblastic disease. Dysmenorrhea suggests endometriosis. In young girls, precocious puberty may indicate a masculinizing or feminizing ovarian tumor. In women, virilization may indicate a masculinizing ovarian tumor; menometrorrhagia or postmenopausal bleeding may indicate a feminizing ovarian tumor.

Examination: During the general examination, the examiner should look for signs of nongynecologic (eg, GI, endocrine) disorders and for ascites. A complete gynecologic examination is done. Distinguishing uterine from adnexal masses may be difficult. Endometriomas are usually nonmobile cul-de-sac masses. Adnexal cancers, benign tumors (eg, benign cystic teratomas), and adnexal masses due to ectopic pregnancy are mobile. Hydrosalpinges are usually fluctuant, tender, nonmobile, and sometimes bilateral. In young girls, pelvic organ masses may be palpable in the abdomen because the pelvis is too small to contain a large mass.

Testing: If the presence or origin (gynecologic vs nongynecologic) of a mass cannot be determined clinically, an imaging test can usually do so. Usually, pelvic ultrasonography is done first. If it does not clearly delineate size, location, and consistency of the mass, another imaging test (eg, CT, MRI) may. Ovarian masses with radiographic characteristics of cancer (eg, a solid component, surface excrescences, irregular shape) require needle aspiration or biopsy. Tumor markers may help in the diagnosis of specific tumors (see p. 1155).

Women of reproductive age are tested for pregnancy; if the test is positive, imaging is not always necessary (see p. 2150) unless ectopic pregnancy is suspected. In women of reproductive age, simple, thin-walled cystic adnexal masses 5 to 8 cm (usually follicular) do not require further investigation unless they persist for > 3 menstrual cycles.

PELVIC PAIN

Pelvic pain is extremely common and may have many causes. It may originate in gynecologic organs (cervix, uterus, or uterine adnexa) or nongynecologic organs. Sometimes the cause is unknown.

Some gynecologic disorders (eg, premenstrual syndrome, dysmenorrhea—see Ch. 244 on p. 2073) cause cyclic pain, which tends to recur at the same phase of the menstrual cycle. Dysmenorrhea (cramping or sharp pain during menses) can be a primary disorder or a symptom of another disorder. Mittelschmerz (severe but self-limited midcycle pain that occurs during ovulation) probably results from mild, brief peritoneal irritation due to a ruptured follicular cyst. Endometriosis typically causes pain before menses and during early menses but may eventually cause pain unrelated to menstrual cycles.

Some gynecologic disorders cause pain that is usually unrelated to menstrual cycles. Sudden, often severe pain can result from rupture of an ectopic pregnancy (see p. 2192), acute degeneration of a uterine fibroid (see p. 2092), adnexal torsion, or rupture or bleeding of ovarian cysts or masses (see p. 2096). Adnexal torsion usually indicates a preexisting ovarian abnormality such as enlargement (eg, due to follicular cysts or hyperstimulation with fertility drugs) or destabilization (eg, due to previous surgery). More gradual pain can result from pelvic inflammatory disease (PID—see p. 2087), pelvic tumors, or pelvic adhesions due to previous infection or surgery.

Nongynecologic disorders that can cause pelvic pain may be GI (eg, gastroenteritis, inflammatory bowel disease, appendicitis, diverticulitis, tumors, constipation, intestinal obstruction, perirectal abscess, irritable bowel syndrome), urinary (eg, cystitis, interstitial cystitis, pyelonephritis, calculi), musculoskeletal (eg, diastasis of the pubic symphysis due to previous vaginal deliveries, abdominal muscle strains), or psychogenic (eg, somatization; effects of previous physical, psychologic, or sexual abuse).

Evaluation

Diagnosis must be made expeditiously because some causes of pelvic pain (eg, ectopic pregnancy, adnexal torsion) require immediate treatment.

History and examination: A complete gynecologic history and physical examination are necessary. Acuity and severity of pain and its relationship to menstrual cycles can suggest the most likely possibilities. Quality and location of pain and associated findings also provide clues (see TABLE 242–1).

Testing: A pregnancy test is done; if it is positive, ectopic pregnancy is assumed until excluded by ultrasonography or, if ultrasonography is indeterminate, by other tests (see p. 2193). Other tests are determined by which disorders are clinically suspected. If a patient cannot be adequately examined (eg, because of pain or inability to cooperate) or if a mass is suspected, pelvic ultrasonography is done. Pelvic masses are evaluated (see p. 2065). If the cause of severe or persistent pain remains unidentified, laparoscopy is done.

Treatment

The underlying disorder is treated when possible. Pain is initially treated with oral NSAIDs. Patients who do not respond well to one NSAID may respond to another. If NSAIDs are ineffective, other analgesics or hypnosis may be tried. Musculoskeletal pain may also require rest, heat, physical therapy, or trigger point injection. For patients with intractable pain due to dysmenorrhea or some other disorders, uterosacral nerve ablation or presacral neurectomy can be tried. If all measures are ineffective, hysterectomy can be done, but it may be ineffective or even worsen the pain.

VAGINAL BLEEDING

Abnormal vaginal bleeding includes menses that are prolonged (menorrhagia), excessive (menorrhagia or hypermenorrhea), or too frequent (polymenorrhea) or that is unrelated to menses, occurring frequently and irregularly between menses (metrorrhagia) or postmenopausally. In women > 50, postmenopausal bleeding > 6 mo after the last normal menses should be evaluated. Total menstrual blood loss is usually < 80 mL. Prolonged or excessive bleeding, regardless of cause, may result in iron deficiency and anemia (see

TABLE 242–1. CLUES TO DIAGNOSIS OF PELVIC PAIN

FINDING	POSSIBLE DIAGNOSIS
Syncope or hemorrhagic shock	Ruptured ectopic pregnancy, possibly ovarian cyst
Vaginal discharge, fever, and bilateral pain and tenderness	PID
Severe, intermittent colicky pain, sometimes with nausea, which may develop and reach peak intensity within seconds or minutes	Adnexal torsion
Nausea followed by anorexia, fever, and right-sided pain	Appendicitis
Constipation, diarrhea, and relief or worsening of pain with defecation	GI disorder
Left lower quadrant pain in women > 40	Diverticulitis
Generalized abdominal tenderness or peritoneal signs	Peritonitis (eg, due to appendicitis, diverticulitis, another GI disorder, PID, adnexal torsion, or rupture of an ovarian cyst or ectopic pregnancy)
Tenderness in the anterior vaginal wall	Bladder or urethral pain due to a lower urinary tract disorder
Uterine fixation detected by bimanual examination	Adhesions, endometriosis, or late-stage cancer
Tender adnexal mass or tenderness with cervical motion	Ectopic pregnancy, PID, ovarian cyst or tumor, or adnexal torsion
Tenderness of the pubic bone in parous women, particularly if pain occurs during ambulation	Diastasis of the pubic symphysis
Painful defecation plus localized tender mass felt during internal or external examination of rectum, with or without fever	Perirectal abscess
Gross or microscopic rectal blood	GI disorder

PID = pelvic inflammatory disease.

p. 1036). For bleeding during pregnancy, see pp. 2153 and 2155.

Etiology

Most abnormal vaginal bleeding results from hormonal abnormalities in the hypothalamic-pituitary-ovarian axis, but bleeding may also result from structural gynecologic disorders. Rarely, the cause is a bleeding disorder. With hormonal causes, ovulation does not occur or occurs infrequently; as a result, estrogen, unopposed by progesterone, stimulates endometrial growth. As a result, the endometrium sloughs and bleeds irregularly, incompletely, and sometimes excessively or for a long time.

Common causes of vaginal bleeding vary by age and menstrual status (see TABLE 242–2). Among children, vaginal bleeding is very uncommon.

In women of reproductive age, bleeding can result from complications of an unsuspected pregnancy. Products of conception retained after spontaneous or therapeutic abortion may cause bleeding within hours or, occasionally, after weeks.

TABLE 242–2. COMMON CAUSES OF ABNORMAL VAGINAL BLEEDING

PATIENT CHARACTERISTICS	COMMON CAUSES
Infants	In utero endometrial stimulation by placental estrogens (causing minimal bleeding)
Children	Trauma, vaginal foreign body with vaginitis, prolapse of the urethral meatus, precocious puberty with premature menses
Women of reproductive age with syncope or hemorrhagic shock	Ruptured ectopic pregnancy
Women of reproductive age with positive pregnancy test	Spontaneous complete or incomplete abortion, ectopic pregnancy, gestational trophoblastic disease, endometritis secondary to retained products of conception
Women of reproductive age with negative pregnancy test	**Hormonally related:** Dysfunctional uterine bleeding (most common), brain lesions, drugs (eg, hormonal contraceptives), hypothyroidism, adrenal or ovarian tumors. **Structural:** Vaginal disorders (eg, cancers, adenosis, trauma, granulomas secondary to previous surgery). Cervical (eg, cancer, polyps, myomas, condylomata acuminata). Uterine (eg, cancers, adenomyosis such as benign invasion of the myometrium by the endometrium, endometrial polyps, submucous and pedunculated fibroids; occasionally, delayed endometritis secondary to retained products of conception). Ovarian (eg, tumors)
Postmenopausal women	Structural disorders of the vagina (eg, cancer; atrophic vaginitis), cervix (eg, cancer, polyps), uterus (eg, endometrial cancer, atrophy, hyperplasia [endometrium > 5 mm], polyps), or ovaries (eg, tumors)

Evaluation

History: A complete gynecologic history is obtained. For all age groups, history should include quantity and duration of bleeding, relationship of bleeding to menses, and questions about trauma. Symptoms of abnormal bleeding (eg, easy bruising, excessive gingival bleeding with toothbrushing, excessive bleeding from lacerations or venipuncture) suggest a bleeding disorder.

Pregnancy-related bleeding is considered in all women of reproductive age, particularly those with pelvic pain, irregular menses, or symptoms of pregnancy. Light-headedness, syncope, or other symptoms of hemorrhagic shock without excessive vaginal bleeding may indicate profuse internal bleeding due to an ectopic pregnancy or a ruptured ovarian cyst. Bleeding with pelvic pain, fever, and vaginal discharge, particularly in women who have had a recent spontaneous or therapeutic abortion, suggests retained products of conception, endometritis, or both. Hirsutism, particularly with obesity, suggests polycystic ovary syndrome (see p. 2078), a common cause of dysfunctional bleeding. Virilization, symptoms and signs of hypothyroidism, or galactorrhea suggests other hormonal abnormalities. In postmenopausal women, vaginal bleeding suggests a gynecologic cancer.

Examination: A general examination, including assessment for signs of hemorrhagic shock (eg, tachycardia, tachypnea, poor capillary refill, confusion, hypotension), is done. The skin is examined for signs of bleeding disorders (eg, petechiae, purpura, ecchymoses). A complete gynecologic examination is also done.

If vaginal bleeding occurs late in pregnancy (eg, during the 3rd trimester), digital pelvic examination is contraindicated until placental position is determined. Such bleeding may indicate placenta previa (see p. 2196); if placenta previa is present, examination can result in sudden, massive bleeding. In other cases, speculum examination helps determine whether bleeding originates from the vagina, cervix, or uterus. If no blood is seen, rectal examination is done to determine whether bleeding is GI in origin.

In women of reproductive age, hemorrhagic shock suggests copious external bleeding, which is usually clinically obvious, or some concealed bleeding, often due to ruptured ectopic pregnancy. Pelvic examination may reveal masses, lesions, or other signs characteristic of structural gynecologic disorders. A tender pelvic mass with bleeding suggests rupture of an ectopic pregnancy or ovarian cyst.

In children, breast development and pubic or axillary hair suggest precocious puberty and premature menses.

Testing: All women of reproductive age are tested for pregnancy. Vaginal bleeding during pregnancy involves a specific approach (see pp. 2154 and 2155). *Suspected ectopic pregnancy requires immediate pelvic ultrasonography and measurement of Hb or Hct and serum levels of the β subunit of human chorionic gonadotropin plus, if hemorrhagic shock is suspected, blood typing and cross-matching.* In women who are not pregnant, Hb or Hct is measured if bleeding is unusually heavy (eg, > 1 pad or tampon/h) or has lasted at least several days or if there are symptoms of anemia or hypovolemia. If anemia is identified and is not obviously due to iron deficiency, iron studies are done. Pelvic ultrasonography, particularly using intrauterine saline, which contrasts with uterine tissue, can help identify submucous or pedunculated fibroids, endometrial polyps, and endometrial hyperplasia.

If examination and ultrasonography do not detect any abnormalities in women > 35, endometrial sampling by aspiration or, if the cervical canal requires dilation, D & C is done. If cancer is suspected, specific tests are done. If a bleeding disorder is suspected, von Willebrand's factor, platelet count, PT, and PTT are measured.

Treatment

Hemorrhagic shock is treated (see p. 562). Iron deficiency anemia may require supplemental iron. Definitive treatment of vaginal bleeding is directed at the cause. Hormones, usually oral contraceptives, are used to treat dysfunctional uterine bleeding (see p. 2077).

243 FEMALE REPRODUCTIVE ENDOCRINOLOGY

Hormonal communication between the hypothalamus, anterior pituitary gland, and ovaries regulates the female reproductive system. The hypothalamus secretes a small peptide, gonadotropin-releasing hormone (GnRH), also known as luteinizing hormone–releasing hormone; GnRH regulates release of the gonadotropins luteinizing hormone (LH) and follicle-stimulating hormone (FSH) from specialized cells (gonadotropes) in the anterior pituitary gland (see FIG. 243–1 and p. 1175). These hormones are released in short bursts (pulses) every 1 to 4 h. LH and FSH promote ovulation and stimulate secretion of the sex hormones estradiol (an estrogen) and progesterone from the ovaries.

Estrogen and progesterone circulate in the bloodstream almost entirely bound to plasma proteins. Only unbound estrogen and progesterone appear to be biologically active. They stimulate the target organs of the reproductive system (eg, breasts, uterus, vagina). They usually inhibit but, in certain situations (eg, around the time of ovulation), may stimulate gonadotropin secretion.

Puberty

Puberty is the sequence of events in which a child acquires adult physical characteristics and capacity for reproduction. Circulating LH and FSH levels are elevated at birth but fall to low levels within a few months and remain low until puberty. Until puberty, few qualitative changes occur in reproductive target organs.

Over the last 150 yr, the age at which puberty begins has been decreasing, primarily because of improved health and nutrition, but this trend has stabilized. Puberty often occurs earlier than average in moderately obese girls and later than average in severely under-

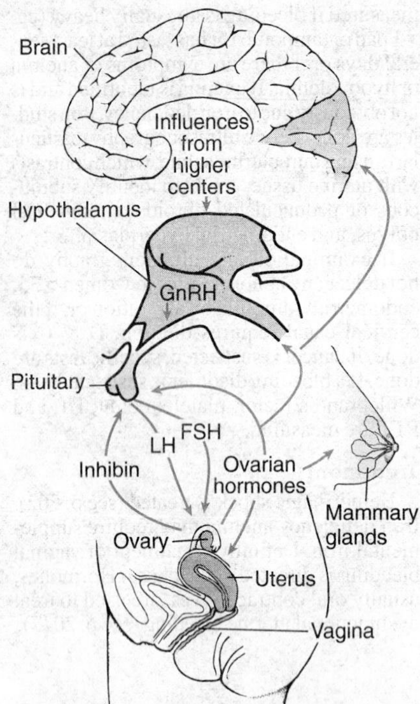

Fig. 243–1. The CNS-hypothalamic-pituitary-gonadal–target organ axis. Ovarian hormones have direct and indirect effects on other tissues (eg, bone, skin, muscle). FSH = follicle-stimulating hormone; GnRH = gonadotropin-releasing hormone; LH = luteinizing hormone.

weight and malnourished girls. Such observations suggest that a critical body weight is necessary for puberty. Puberty occurs earlier in girls whose mothers matured earlier and, for unknown reasons, in girls who live in urban areas or who are blind.

Physical changes of puberty occur sequentially during adolescence (see FIG. 243–2). Breast budding (see FIG. 243–3) and onset of the growth spurt are usually the 1st changes recognized. Then, pubic and axillary hair appears (see FIG. 243–4), and the growth spurt peaks. Menarche (the 1st menstrual period) occurs about 2 yr after breast budding. Height growth peaks early in puberty; it is limited after menarche. Body habitus changes; the pelvis and hips widen. Body fat increases and accumulates in the hips and thighs.

Mechanisms initiating puberty are unclear. Central influences may inhibit release of GnRH during childhood, then initiate its release to induce puberty in early adolescence. Early in puberty, hypothalamic GnRH release becomes less sensitive to inhibition by estrogen and progesterone. The resulting increased release of GnRH promotes LH and FSH secretion, which stimulates production of sex hormones, primarily estrogen. Estrogen stimulates development of secondary sexual characteristics. Pubic and axillary hair growth may be stimulated by the adrenal androgens dehydroepiandrosterone (DHEA) and DHEA sulfate; production of these androgens increases several years before puberty in a process called adrenarche.

Ovarian Follicular Development

A female is born with a finite number of egg precursors (germ cells). Germ cells begin as primordial oogonia that proliferate markedly by mitosis through the 4th mo of gestation. During the 3rd mo, some oogonia begin to undergo meiosis, which reduces the number of chromosomes by ½. By the 7th mo, all viable germ cells develop a surrounding layer of

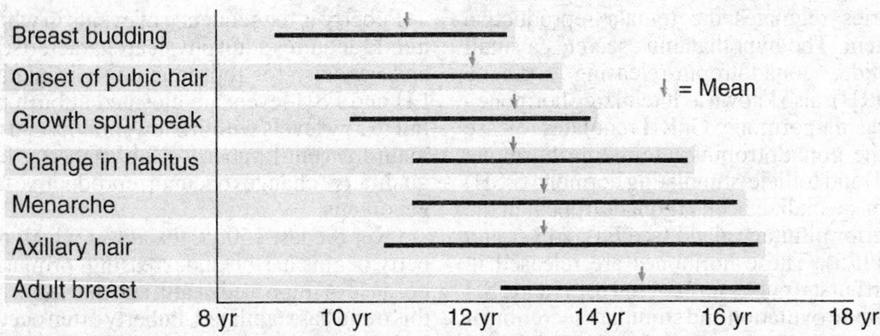

Fig. 243–2. Puberty—when female sexual characteristics develop. Bars indicate normal ranges.

granulosa cells, forming a primordial follicle, and are arrested in meiotic prophase; these cells are primary oocytes. Beginning after the 4th mo of gestation, oogonia (and later oocytes) are lost spontaneously in a process called atresia; eventually, 99.9% are lost. In older mothers, the long time that surviving oocytes spend arrested in meiotic prophase may account for the increased incidence of genetically abnormal pregnancies.

During each menstrual cycle, 3 to 30 follicles are recruited for accelerated growth. Usually in each cycle, only one follicle is selected for ovulation. This dominant follicle releases its oocyte at ovulation and promotes atresia of the other recruited follicles.

Menstrual Cycle

Menstruation is the periodic discharge of blood and sloughed endometrium (collectively called menses or menstrual flow) through the vagina; menstruation occurs throughout a woman's reproductive life in the absence of pregnancy. Menopause is the permanent cessation of menses (see p. 2081).

Average duration of menses is 5 (±2) days. Blood loss per cycle averages 30 mL (normal range, 13 to 80 mL) and is usually greatest on the 2nd day. A saturated pad or tampon absorbs 5 to 15 mL. Menstrual blood does not usually clot (unless bleeding is very heavy), probably because fibrinolysin and other factors inhibit clotting.

The median menstrual cycle length is 28 days (usual range, about 25 to 36 days). Generally, variation is maximal and intermenstrual intervals are longest in the years immediately after menarche and immediately before menopause, when ovulation occurs less regularly. The menstrual cycle begins and ends with the 1st day of menses (day 1).

The menstrual cycle can be divided into follicular (preovulatory), ovulatory, and luteal (postovulatory) phases (see FIG. 243–5).

Follicular phase: This phase varies in length more than other phases do. In the 1st half of the follicular phase (early follicular phase), the primary event is growth of recruited follicles. At this time, the gonadotropes in the anterior pituitary contain little LH and FSH, and estrogen and progesterone production is low. As a result, overall FSH secretion increases slightly, stimulating growth of recruited follicles. Also, circulating LH levels increase slowly, beginning 1 to 2 days after the increase in FSH. The recruited ovarian follicles soon increase production of estradiol; estradiol stimulates LH and FSH synthesis but inhibits their secretion.

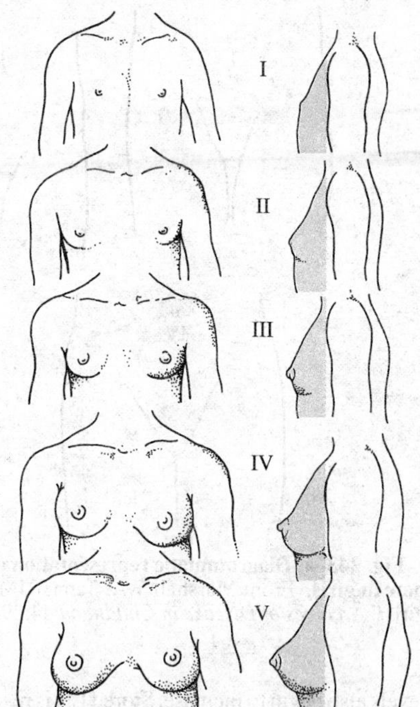

Fig. 243–3. Diagrammatic representation of Tanner stages I to V of human breast maturation. From Marshall WA, Tanner JM: "Variations in patterns of pubertal changes in girls." *Archives of Disease in Childhood* 44:291–303, 1969; used with permission.

During the 2nd half of the follicular phase (late follicular phase), the follicle selected for ovulation matures and accumulates hormone-secreting granulosa cells; its antrum enlarges with follicular fluid, reaching 18 to 20 mm before ovulation. FSH levels decrease; LH levels are affected less. FSH and LH levels diverge partly because estradiol inhibits FSH secretion more than LH secretion. Also, developing follicles produce the hormone inhibin, which inhibits FSH secretion but not LH secretion. Other contributing factors may include disparate half-lives (20 to 30 min for LH; 2 to 3 h for FSH) and unknown factors. Levels of estrogen, particularly estradiol, increase exponentially.

Ovulatory phase: Ovulation (ovum release) occurs. Estradiol levels usually peak as the ovulatory phase begins. Progesterone

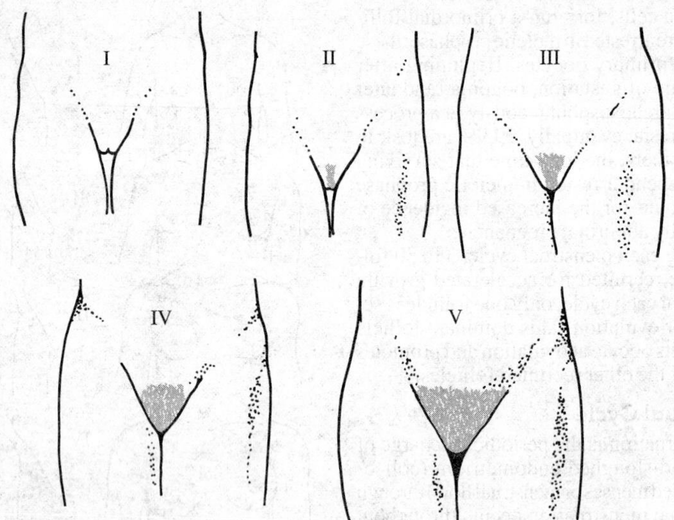

Fig. 243–4. Diagrammatic representation of Tanner stages I to V for development of pubic hair in girls. From Marshall WA, Tanner JM: "Variations in patterns of pubertal changes in girls." *Archives of Disease in Childhood* 44:291–303, 1969; used with permission.

levels also begin to increase. Stored LH is released in massive amounts (LH surge), usually over 36 to 48 h, with a smaller increase in FSH. The LH surge occurs because at this time, high levels of estradiol trigger LH secretion by gonadotropes (positive feedback). The LH surge is also stimulated by GnRH and progesterone. During the LH surge, estradiol levels decrease, but progesterone levels continue to increase. The LH surge stimulates enzymes that initiate breakdown of the follicle wall and release of the now mature ovum within about 16 to 32 h. The LH surge also triggers completion of the 1st meiotic division of the oocyte within about 36 h.

Luteal phase: The follicle is transformed into a corpus luteum. The length of this phase is the most constant, averaging 14 days, after which the corpus luteum degenerates. The corpus luteum secretes primarily progesterone in increasing quantities, peaking at about 25 mg/day 6 to 8 days after ovulation. Progesterone stimulates development of the secretory endometrium, which is necessary for embryonic implantation. Because progesterone is thermogenic, basal body temperature increases by 0.5° C for the duration of this phase. Because levels of circulating estradiol, progesterone, and inhibin are high during most of the luteal phase, LH and FSH levels decrease. Estradiol and progesterone levels decrease late in this phase.

If implantation occurs, the corpus luteum does not degenerate but remains, supported by human chorionic gonadotropin that is produced by the developing embryo.

Cyclic Changes in Other Reproductive Organs

Endometrium: The endometrium, which consists of glands and stroma, has a basal layer, an intermediate spongiosa layer, and a layer of compact epithelial cells that line the uterine cavity. The spongiosa and epithelial layers are sloughed during menses, leaving the endometrium about 2 mm thick with a dense stroma and with narrow, straight glands lined with low columnar epithelium. As estradiol levels increase, the intact basal layer regenerates the endometrium to a maximum thickness of 11 mm late in the follicular phase. The mucosa thickens and the tubular glands lengthen and coil. During the luteal phase, progesterone stimulates the tubular glands to dilate, fill with glycogen, and become secretory, while stromal vascularity increases. As estradiol and progesterone levels decrease late in the luteal phase, the stroma becomes edematous, and the endometrium and its blood vessels undergo necrosis, leading to bleeding and menstrual flow.

Because histologic changes are specific to the phase of the menstrual cycle, the cycle phase or tissue response to sex hormones can be determined accurately by endometrial biopsy. The endometrium can also be seen using transvaginal ultrasonography; late in the follicular phase, it characteristically has a trilaminar pattern, with hyperechoic basal and luminal layers and an intervening hypoechoic layer. After ovulation, the endometrium appears homogeneously echogenic.

Cervix: During the follicular phase, increasing estradiol levels increase cervical vascularity and edema and cervical mucus quantity, elasticity, and NaCl concentration. The external os opens slightly and fills with mucus at ovulation. During the luteal phase, increasing progesterone levels make the cervical mucus thicker and less elastic. Menstrual cycle phase can sometimes be identified by microscopic examination of cervical mucus dried on a glass slide; ferning (palm leaf arborization of mucus) indicates increased NaCl in cervical mucus. Ferning becomes prominent just before ovulation, when estrogen levels are high; it is minimal or absent during the luteal phase.

Vagina: Early in the follicular phase, when estradiol levels are low, the vaginal epithelium is thin and pale. Later in the follicular phase, as estradiol levels increase, squamous cells mature and become cornified, causing epithelial thickening. During the luteal phase, the number of precornified intermediate cells increases, and the number of leukocytes and amount of cellular debris increase as mature squamous cells are shed. Changes in the vaginal epithelium can be quantitated histologically and used as a qualitative index of estrogenic activity.

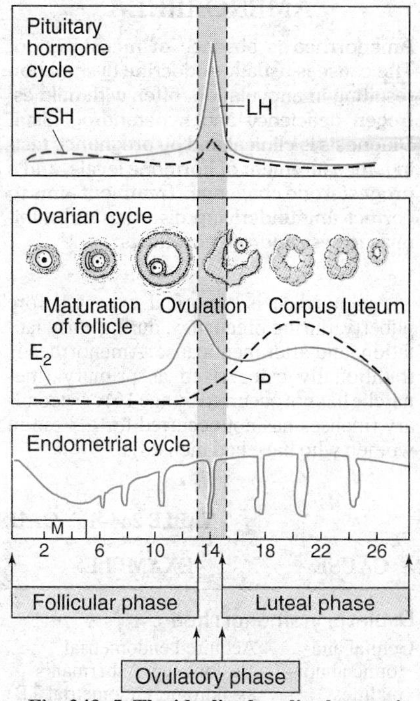

Fig. 243–5. The idealized cyclic changes in pituitary gonadotropins, estradiol (E_2), progesterone (P), and uterine endometrium during the normal menstrual cycle. Days of menstrual bleeding are indicated by M. FSH = follicle-stimulating hormone; LH = luteinizing hormone. (Adapted from Rebar RW: "Normal physiology of the reproductive system." In *Endocrinology and Metabolism Continuing Education Program, American Association of Clinical Chemistry*, November 1982. Copyright 1982 by the American Association for Clinical Chemistry; reprinted with permission.)

244 MENSTRUAL ABNORMALITIES

(For description of menstrual cycle, see p. 2071.)

Menstrual abnormalities include amenorrhea, dysfunctional uterine bleeding, dysmenorrhea (primary or secondary), and premenstrual syndrome. Irregular or absent menses and nonmenstrual vaginal bleeding have many causes, but in women of reproductive age, pregnancy should always be suspected. Abnormal vaginal bleeding in nonpregnant women (see p. 2066) is evaluated differently from vaginal bleeding in pregnant women (see pp. 2153 and 2155).

AMENORRHEA

Amenorrhea is absence of menstruation. The cause is usually endocrine dysfunction resulting in anovulation, often with mild estrogen deficiency and hyperandrogenism. Diagnosis is clinical and by pregnancy testing, measurement of hormone levels, and a progesterone challenge. Treatment aims to correct any underlying disorder and minimize excess androgenic effects.

Amenorrhea is abnormal except before puberty, during pregnancy, during early lactation, and after menopause. Amenorrhea is traditionally categorized as primary (menarche has not occurred by age 16) or secondary (menses has not occurred for ≥ 3 mo in women who have had menses).

Etiology

Amenorrhea has many causes, typically divided into anovulatory and ovulatory (see TABLE 244–1).

Anovulatory amenorrhea, in which both ovulation and menses are absent, is the most common and results from functional rather than structural causes. The hypothalamic-pituitary axis is intact and ovaries are functional, but gonadotropin secretion is decreased, resulting in mild estrogen deficiency. Causes are hypothalamic, pituitary, ovarian, or other endocrine dysfunction and some genetic disorders. Hypothalamic causes may be multifactorial and may include unknown factors. Endocrine causes may involve inappropriate hormonal feedback, which can result from altered levels of free testosterone, other androgens, or estrogen (see TABLE 244–1)

TABLE 244–1. CAUSES OF AMENORRHEA

CAUSE	EXAMPLES
Ovulatory amenorrhea	
Genital anatomic abnormalities	Acquired endometrial lesions (eg, Asherman's syndrome, endometrial TB) Cervical stenosis (rare) Imperforate hymen Male pseudohermaphroditism Transverse vaginal septum Vaginal and uterine aplasia
Anovulatory amenorrhea	
Hypothalamic dysfunction	Anorexia nervosa* Excessive exercise Hypothalamic chronic anovulation* Kallmann's syndrome Prader-Willi syndrome Psychogenic factors (eg, severe stress) Tumors (eg, hamartomas, craniopharyngiomas, gliomas) Weight loss (acute) Undernutrition (chronic)
Pituitary dysfunction	Amenorrhea-galactorrhea (hyperprolactinemia)* Benign pituitary adenoma Hypopituitarism* (eg, due to Sheehan's syndrome, head trauma, or tumor) Isolated gonadotropin deficiency* Panhypopituitarism* Pituitary tumors* (eg, Forbes-Albright syndrome) Antipsychotic drugs (eg, olanzapine)
Ovarian failure	Autoimmune disorders Chemotherapy and pelvic irradiation Congenital thymic aplasia Galactosemia Gonadal dysgenesis
Other endocrine dysfunction	Congenital or adult-onset adrenal virilism Cushing's syndrome* Drug-induced virilization (by antidepressants) Hyperthyroidism* Hypothyroidism* Liver disorders (chronic) Obesity* Polycystic ovary syndrome* Tumors producing androgens, estrogens, or human chorionic gonadotropin*
Genetic disorders	Androgen insensitivity syndrome Turner's syndrome (see p. 2453)

*These disorders cause chronic anovulation.

due to lack of sex hormone–binding globulin (eg, in chronic liver disorders), excessive extraglandular production of estrogen (eg, in obesity), ovarian or adrenal androgen excess, or polycystic ovary syndrome.

Ovulatory amenorrhea, which is less common, results from anatomic genital abnormalities in women with normal hormonal function. Many congenital anatomic abnormalities physically obstruct menstrual flow through the uterine outflow tract, causing amenorrhea. Hematocolpos (accumulation of menstrual blood in the vagina), which can cause the vagina to bulge, and hematometra (accumulation of blood in the uterus), which can cause uterine distention or a mass, may also occur. Because ovarian function is normal, the external genitals and other secondary sexual characteristics develop normally; however, some congenital disorders (eg, that cause vaginal aplasia or a vaginal septum) also cause urinary tract and skeletal abnormalities.

Diagnosis

Girls are evaluated if no signs of puberty occur by age 13 or if menarche has not occurred by age 16 or ≥ 5 yr since the onset of puberty. Women of reproductive age should have a pregnancy test after missing one menses; they are evaluated for amenorrhea if they are not pregnant and have missed menstrual cycles for ≥ 3 mo, have < 9 menses a year, or have a sudden change in menstrual pattern.

History and physical examination: The history should address the possibility of pregnancy, risk factors (eg, abnormal growth and development, family history of genetic defects, dietary deficiencies, excessive exercise, environmental stresses), and symptoms of endocrine disorders, particularly virilization (eg, increased libido).

Virilization reflects excess androgen effects, suggesting true hermaphroditism, pseudohermaphroditism, gonadal dysgenesis, polycystic ovary syndrome, a virilizing ovarian or adrenal tumor, Cushing's syndrome, adrenal virilism, or a genetic disorder. Signs of virilization include hirsutism, temporal balding, voice deepening, increased muscle mass, clitoral enlargement, and a decrease in previously normally developed secondary sexual characteristics (defeminization), such as decreased breast size and vaginal atrophy. Hypertrichosis (excessive growth of hair on the extremities, head, and back), which is common in some families, is differentiated from true hirsutism, which is characterized by excess hair on the upper lip and chin and between the breasts. Obesity in hirsute women may suggest polycystic ovary syndrome but is nonspecific. Moon facies, truncal obesity, abdominal striae, and thin extremities may indicate Cushing's syndrome.

Absence or delayed development of secondary sexual characteristics (breasts, pubic and axillary hair, genitals) suggests absent or decreased estrogen levels. Staging breast and pubic hair development using the Tanner method (see FIGS. 243–3 on p. 2071 and 243–4 on p. 2072) helps in evaluation of secondary sexual characteristics.

With the patient seated, the physician checks for breast secretion by applying pressure to all sections of the breast, beginning at the base and moving toward the nipple. Galactorrhea (breast milk secretion not temporally associated with childbirth—see p. 1187) suggests hyperprolactinemia, which usually reflects a pituitary disorder.

Pelvic examination may detect anatomic genital disorders or signs of such disorders (eg, bulging vagina, uterine mass). Ambiguous genitals may indicate virilization, true hermaphroditism, or male or female pseudohermaphroditism. Fused labia and an enlarged clitoris (clitoromegaly) usually indicate exposure to androgens during the 1st 3 mo of fetal development, suggesting congenital adrenal virilism (see Congenital Adrenal Hyperplasia on p. 2365), true hermaphroditism, or drug-induced virilization. Development of significant clitoromegaly postnatally requires marked hormonal stimulation and, if there is no history of exogenous anabolic steroid use, strongly suggests an androgen-secreting tumor, most of which originate in the ovaries. If the cervix and uterus appear absent, external genitals appear normal, and secondary sexual characteristics are not fully developed, androgen insensitivity syndrome (testicular feminization) is considered.

Testing: Routine testing includes a pregnancy test, a progesterone challenge, and measurement of hormone levels. If a genetic defect is suspected (eg, in primary amenorrhea), karyotype is determined.

The progesterone challenge helps assess contributions of estrogen deficiency, structural endometrial lesions, and uterine outflow obstruction to amenorrhea. Medroxyprogesterone 5 to 10 mg po once/day for 5 days or progesterone 5 to 10 mg IM once/day for 5 to 10 days is given. If bleeding occurs, amenorrhea is probably not caused by significant estrogen deficiency, an endometrial lesion, or uterine outflow obstruction; chronic anovulation is often the cause. If bleeding does not occur, estradiol and follicle-stimulating hormone (FSH) levels can be measured to confirm primary or secondary estrogen deficiency and distinguish between them. If results are normal, oral estrogen (usually an oral contraceptive) is given; if bleeding does not occur, amenorrhea is probably caused by an endometrial abnormality (eg, Asherman's syndrome, TB affecting the endometrium) or by uterine outflow obstruction (eg, by a congenital anatomic genital abnormality).

Serum levels of FSH, prolactin, and thyroid-stimulating hormone (TSH) are measured in all women with amenorrhea. Increased FSH (> 30 IU/L) suggests ovarian failure. Decreased FSH (< 7 IU/L) suggests a pituitary tumor. Prolactin is increased (usually > 20 ng/mL [> 888 pmol/L]) in > 30% of women with amenorrhea), often spuriously; consequently, high levels must be confirmed a few weeks later. If prolactin is persistently increased and TSH is normal (< 5 mU/L), a prolactin-secreting pituitary tumor may be the cause. Increased TSH indicates primary hypothyroidism if the prolactin level is normal and possibly even if it is elevated, because primary hypothyroidism increases prolactin secretion in some women.

If FSH level is normal and prolactin and TSH levels are normal or low, further evaluation is based on clinical presentation. If hypothyroidism is suspected, thyroid hormone levels are measured. If virilization is suspected, total serum testosterone and dehydroepiandrosterone sulfate (DHEAS) levels are measured. Testosterone levels > 200 ng/dL suggest an ovarian androgen-producing tumor. DHEAS levels that are modestly increased may suggest an adrenal tumor. If women have a serum DHEAS level of ≥ 500 μg/dL, severe hirsutism that began at puberty, a strong family history of hirsutism, or shorter stature than expected in relation to family members, adult-onset forms of adrenal virilism (see p. 1211) are considered.

Mildly elevated levels of testosterone or DHEAS suggest polycystic ovary syndrome, but levels can be elevated in women with hypothalamic or pituitary dysfunction and are sometimes normal in hirsute women with polycystic ovary syndrome. The cause of elevated levels can be determined by measuring basal serum luteinizing hormone (LH). In polycystic ovary syndrome, circulating LH levels are often increased, increasing the ratio of LH to FSH. If LH or FSH levels are < 7 IU/L, hypothalamic or pituitary dysfunction, particularly a pituitary tumor, is considered.

Treatment

Treatment is directed at the underlying disorder when possible. Therapy may also be required to induce ovulation if pregnancy is desired (see Ovulatory Dysfunction on p. 2140), to minimize hirsutism and long-term effects of hyperandrogenism (eg, cardiovascular disorders, hypertension), to treat symptoms of estrogen deficiency (see p. 2081), and to prevent osteoporosis due to estrogen deficiency.

For hirsutism with elevated testosterone levels (the most common type), physical treatments (eg, bleaching, electrolysis, plucking, waxing, depilation) are encouraged. Eflornithine cream 13.9% bid may help remove unwanted facial hair. No systemic drug is ideal or completely effective; oral contraceptives are used initially. They suppress gonadotropin and sex hormone secretion and increase production of sex hormone–binding globulin, thus reducing biologically active free testosterone. Results are delayed for several months and are rarely dramatic. All formulations appear equally effective, but oral contraceptives with minimal androgenic adverse effects are preferred (see p. 2131). If oral contraceptives are contraindicated or not desired, an oral progestin (medroxyprogesterone 5 to 20 mg once/day) can be used. Contraception is recommended because medroxyprogesterone has possible, although unproven, teratogenic effects. Progestins may cause breast pain, bloating, and depression. Gonadotropin-releasing hormone agonists and antagonists (eg, leuprolide 3.75 mg IM q mo, goserelin 3.6 mg sc q 28 days) may also help by suppressing gonadotropins and thus sex hormone secretion.

If neither testosterone nor DHEAS levels are elevated, spironolactone 100 to 200 mg po once/day can be used. It inhibits androgen synthesis and competes for androgen receptors in target tissues. It may cause diuresis, orthostatic hypotension, breast pain, and irregular uterine bleeding; contraception is recommended.

DYSFUNCTIONAL UTERINE BLEEDING

(Functional Uterine Bleeding)

Dysfunctional uterine bleeding is abnormal uterine bleeding in the absence of clinical or ultrasonographic evidence of structural abnormalities, inflammation, or pregnancy. Treatment is usually with oral contraceptives.

Dysfunctional uterine bleeding (DUB), the most common cause of abnormal uterine bleeding, occurs most often in women > 45 (> 50% of cases) and in adolescents (20% of cases). The cause is usually estrogen production unopposed by progesterone, which can lead to endometrial hyperplasia. The endometrium sloughs and bleeds incompletely, irregularly, and sometimes profusely or for a long time. Endometrial hyperplasia, particularly atypical adenomatous hyperplasia, predisposes to endometrial cancer.

Most women with DUB are anovulatory. Anovulation is usually secondary to polycystic ovary syndrome or idiopathic; the cause is sometimes hypothyroidism. Some women are anovulatory despite normal gonadotropin levels; the cause is idiopathic. About 20% of women with endometriosis (see p. 2089) have DUB due to unknown mechanisms.

Symptoms, Signs, and Diagnosis

Bleeding may occur more frequently than typical menses (< 21 days apart—polymenorrhea), last longer or involve more blood loss than menses (> 7 days or > 80 mL—menorrhagia or hypermenorrhea), or occur frequently and irregularly between menses (metrorrhagia).

Diagnosis is suspected when unexplained vaginal bleeding occurs. DUB must be distinguished from disorders that cause similar bleeding: pregnancy and pregnancy-related disorders (eg, ectopic pregnancy, spontaneous abortion), structural gynecologic lesions (eg, fibroids, cancer, polyps), gynecologic foreign bodies, gynecologic inflammation (eg, cervicitis), or bleeding disorders (see p. 2066). If bleeding is ovulatory, structural abnormalities should be excluded.

History and physical examination focus on detecting inflammation and masses. For women of reproductive age, a pregnancy test is done. If volume of bleeding is significant, Hct or Hb is measured. Thyroid-stimulating hormone is measured. Transvaginal ultrasonography is done to detect structural abnormalities. Whether bleeding is anovulatory or ovulatory can be determined by serum progesterone levels; a level ≥ 3 ng/mL (9.75 nmol/L) during the luteal phase suggests that ovulation has occurred. Biopsy is usually necessary to rule out hyperplasia or cancer in women with any of the following: age ≥ 35, obesity, polycystic ovary syndrome, ovulatory bleeding, irregular cycles that suggest chronic anovulatory bleeding, endometrial thickness > 4 mm, or inconclusive ultrasound findings. Women without these characteristics and with endometrial thickness ≤ 4 mm, including those with irregular cycles suggesting only brief periods of anovulation, do not require further testing. Women with atypical adenomatous hyperplasia require hysteroscopy and fractional D & C.

Treatment

For anovulatory DUB, oral contraceptives are usually effective (see p. 2131). For heavy bleeding, an oral contraceptive may be given qid for 3 days, tid for 3 days, bid for 3 days, and then once/day; for very heavy bleeding, conjugated estrogens 25 mg IV q 6 to 12 h may be given until bleeding abates. After acute bleeding is controlled, a combination (estrogen-progestin) oral contraceptive is given continually for about 3 mo to prevent recurrence.

If estrogen is contraindicated or if after 3 mo of oral contraceptive therapy, spontaneous cyclic menses do not resume and pregnancy is not desired, a progestin (eg, medroxyprogesterone 5 to 10 mg po once/day for 10 to 14 days/mo) can be used. If pregnancy is desired and bleeding is not heavy, ovulation induction with clomiphene (50 mg po on days 5 through 9 of the menstrual cycle) can be tried.

If bleeding persists despite hormone therapy, hysteroscopy with D & C is indicated.

Atypical adenomatous endometrial hyperplasia is treated with medroxyprogesterone acetate 20 to 40 mg po once/day for 3 to 6 mo. If repeat endometrial biopsy indicates resolution of hyperplasia, cyclic medroxyprogesterone acetate (5 to 10 mg po once/day for 10 to 14 days each month) or, if pregnancy is desired, clomiphene citrate may be used. If biopsy shows persistent or progressive atypical hyperplasia, hysterectomy is necessary. More benign cystic or adenomatous hyperplasia can usually be treated with cyclic medroxyprogesterone acetate; biopsy is repeated after about 3 mo.

DYSMENORRHEA

Dysmenorrhea is pelvic pain with menses. Primary dysmenorrhea begins during adolescence and cannot be explained by structural gynecologic disorders. Usually, secondary dysmenorrhea begins during adulthood and is due to underlying pelvic abnormalities. Diagnosis is clinical and by exclusion of structural disorders with pelvic ultrasonography and tests directed at any other clinically suspected causes. Underlying disorders are treated. Pain is treated with NSAIDs and sometimes with low-dose estrogen-progestin contraceptives.

Primary dysmenorrhea is common. It usually starts during adolescence and tends to lessen with age and after pregnancy. Pain is thought to result from uterine contractions and ischemia, probably mediated by prostaglandins produced in secretory endometrium. Contributing factors may include passage of menstrual tissue through the cervix, a narrow cervical os, a malpositioned uterus, lack of exercise, and anxiety about menses.

Common causes of secondary dysmenorrhea include endometriosis, uterine adenomyosis, fibroids, and, in a few women, an extremely tight cervical os (secondary to conization, cryocautery, or thermocautery) that becomes painful when the uterus attempts to expel tissue. Pain occasionally results from a pedunculated submucosal fibroid or an endometrial polyp extruding through the cervix.

Symptoms, Signs, and Diagnosis

Pelvic pain may occur with menses or precede menses by 1 to 3 days. Pain tends to peak 24 h after onset of menses and subside after 2 to 3 days. It is usually sharp but may be a dull, constant ache; it may radiate to the lower back or legs. Headache, nausea, constipation or diarrhea, and urinary frequency are common; vomiting occurs occasionally. Symptoms of premenstrual syndrome may occur during part or all of menses. Sometimes endometrial clots or casts are expelled.

Primary dysmenorrhea is suspected if symptoms begin soon after menarche or during adolescence. Secondary dysmenorrhea is suspected if symptoms begin after adolescence. Diagnosis requires a history of characteristic, recurrent symptoms. To differentiate primary and secondary dysmenorrhea, structural gynecologic disorders are excluded by clinical assessment, pelvic ultrasonography, and tests for other clinically suspected disorders.

Treatment

Underlying disorders are treated. Symptomatic treatment begins with adequate rest and sleep and regular exercise. Women with primary dysmenorrhea are reassured about the absence of structural gynecologic disorders. Persistent pain due to primary or secondary dysmenorrhea requires drug therapy; an NSAID is usually started 24 to 48 h before and continued until 1 or 2 days after menses begins. If these measures are ineffective, suppression of ovulation with a low-dose estrogen-progestin oral contraceptive is advisable. Hypnosis is occasionally useful. For intractable pain of unknown origin, interruption of uterine nerves by presacral neurectomy and division of the sacrouterine ligaments may help.

POLYCYSTIC OVARY SYNDROME

(Hyperandrogenic Chronic Anovulation)

Polycystic ovary syndrome is characterized by mild obesity, irregular menses or amenorrhea, and signs of androgen excess (hirsutism, acne). Typically, the ovaries contain multiple cysts. Diagnosis is by pregnancy testing, hormone level measurement, and imaging to exclude a virilizing tumor. Treatment is symptomatic.

Polycystic ovary syndrome is a common female endocrinopathy occurring in 5 to 10% of women and involving anovulation and androgen excess of unclear etiology. It is defined by symptoms, not by the presence of ovarian cysts. Ovaries may be enlarged with smooth, thickened capsules or may be normal in size. Typically, ovaries contain many 2- to 6-mm follicular cysts and sometimes larger cysts containing atretic cells. Estrogen levels are elevated, increasing risk of endometrial hyperplasia and, eventually, endometrial cancer. Androgen levels are often elevated, increasing risk of metabolic syndrome (see p. 61) and causing hirsutism.

Symptoms, Signs, and Diagnosis

Symptoms typically begin during puberty and worsen with time; a clear-cut history of regular menses for a time following menarche makes the diagnosis unlikely. Examination usually detects abundant cervical mucus, reflecting high estrogen levels. The diagnosis is suspected if women have at least 2 typical symptoms (mild obesity, hirsutism, and irregular menses or amenorrhea).

Testing includes pregnancy testing and measurement of serum estradiol, follicle-stimulating hormone, prolactin, and thyroid-stimulating hormone. Diagnosis is confirmed by ultrasonography showing > 10 follicles per ovary; follicles usually occur in the periphery and resemble a string of pearls.

If ovarian follicles or hirsutism is present, serum testosterone and dehydroepiandrosterone sulfate (DHEAS) levels are measured. Abnormal levels are evaluated as for amenorrhea (see p. 2075).

Treatment

For women who are anovulatory (ie, with a history of absent or irregular menses and no evidence of progesterone production), who are not hirsute, and who do not desire pregnancy, an intermittent progestin (eg, medroxyprogesterone 5 to 10 mg po once/day for 10 to 14 days q 1 to 2 mo) or oral contraceptives should be given to reduce risk of endometrial hyperplasia and cancer and to reduce circulating androgens.

For women who are anovulatory, who are hirsute, and who do not desire pregnancy, treatment aims to reduce hirsutism and is guided by testosterone and DHEAS levels (see p. 2076). For women who desire pregnancy, infertility treatments are used (see p. 2141).

PREMATURE OVARIAN FAILURE

(Premature Menopause)

In premature ovarian failure, ovaries do not produce enough estrogen despite high levels of circulating gonadotropins (especially follicle-stimulating hormone) in women < 40.

Premature ovarian failure has various causes (see TABLE 244–2). Genetic disorders that confer a Y chromosome increase risk of ovarian cancer, which is usually evident by age 35.

Symptoms, Signs, and Diagnosis

Typically, amenorrhea or irregular bleeding and symptoms or signs of estrogen deficiency (eg, osteoporosis, atrophic vaginitis,

TABLE 244–2. COMMON CAUSES OF PREMATURE OVARIAN FAILURE

CAUSE	EXAMPLES
Enzyme defects	Galactosemia 17α-Hydroxylase deficiency
Genetic defects	Accelerated ovarian follicle atresia (idiopathic) Gonadal dysgenesis (eg, Turner's syndrome [45,X], pure [46,XX or 46,XY] or mixed gonadal dysgenesis) Myotonic dystrophy Reduced germ cell number Trisomy X with or without chromosomal mosaicism
Immune disturbances	Autoimmune disorders (most commonly, thyroiditis, Addison's disease, hypoparathyroidism, diabetes mellitus, myasthenia gravis, vitiligo, pernicious anemia, and mucocutaneous candidiasis) Congenital thymic aplasia Isolated ovarian failure
Physical and environmental factors	Chemotherapeutic (especially alkylating) drugs Cigarette smoking Irradiation of the gonads Surgical extirpation of the gonads or adnexa Viral infections

decreased libido) occur. Diagnosis is suspected in women < 40 with these symptoms. A pregnancy test is done, and serum gonadotropin and estradiol levels are measured weekly for 2 to 4 wk; if follicle-stimulating hormone levels are high (usually > 30 mIU/mL) and estradiol levels are low (usually < 20 pg/mL), ovarian failure is confirmed. Then, further tests are done based on which cause is suspected. Karyotype is determined if women with confirmed ovarian failure are < 35.

Treatment

Women who do not desire pregnancy are given estrogen-progesterone replacement therapy (see p. 2082) until about age 51. For those who desire pregnancy, in vitro fertilization of donated oocytes plus exogenous estrogen and a progestin, which enable the endometrium to support the transferred embryo (see p. 2142), can be tried. Women with a Y chromosome require laparotomy or laparoscopy and excision of all gonadal tissue.

PREMENSTRUAL SYNDROME

(Premenstrual Tension)

Premenstrual syndrome is characterized by irritability, anxiety, emotional lability, depression, edema, breast pain, and headaches, occurring during the 7 to 10 days before and usually ending a few hours after onset of menses. Diagnosis is clinical. Treatment is symptomatic and includes diet, drugs, and counseling.

Premenstrual syndrome (PMS) appears to be caused by multiple endocrine factors (eg, hypoglycemia, other changes in carbohydrate metabolism, hyperprolactinemia, fluctuations in levels of circulating estrogen and progesterone, abnormal responses to estrogen and progesterone, excessive aldosterone or ADH). Estrogen and progesterone can cause transitory fluid retention, as can excess aldosterone or ADH.

Symptoms and Signs

Type and intensity of symptoms vary from woman to woman and from cycle to cycle. Symptoms last a few hours to ≥ 10 days, usually ending when menses begins. In perimenopausal women, symptoms may persist until after menses.

The most common symptoms are irritability, anxiety, agitation, anger, insomnia, difficulty concentrating, lethargy, depression, and severe fatigue. Fluid retention causes edema, transient weight gain, and breast fullness and pain. Pelvic heaviness or pressure and backache may occur. Some women, particularly younger ones, have dysmenorrhea when menses begins. Other nonspecific symptoms may include headache, vertigo, paresthesias of the extremities, syncope, palpitations, constipation, nausea, vomiting, and changes in appetite. Acne and neurodermatitis may also occur. Existing skin disorders may worsen, as may respiratory (eg, allergies, infection) and eye (eg, visual disturbances, conjunctivitis) problems.

Treatment

Treatment is symptomatic, beginning with adequate rest and sleep and regular exercise. Dietary changes—increasing protein, decreasing sugar, and taking vitamin B complex (especially pyridoxine) or Mg supplements—may help, as may counseling and avoiding stressful activities. Fluid retention may be relieved by reducing Na intake and taking a diuretic (eg, hydrochlorothiazide 25 to 50 mg po once/day in the morning) just before symptoms are expected. However, minimizing fluid retention does not relieve all symptoms and may have no effect. SSRIs (eg, fluoxetine 20 mg po once/day) may be used to reduce anxiety, irritability, and other emotional symptoms, particularly if stress cannot be avoided.

For some women, hormonal manipulation is effective. Options include oral contraceptives (eg, norethindrone 5 mg once/day), progesterone by vaginal suppository (200 to 400 mg once/day), an oral progestin (eg, micronized progesterone 100 mg at bedtime) for 10 to 12 days premenstrually, or a long-acting progestin (eg, medroxyprogesterone 200 mg IM q 2 to 3 mo). For severe or refractory symptoms, a gonadotropin-releasing hormone agonist (eg, leuprolide 3.75 mg IM, goserelin 3.6 mg sc q mo) with low-dose estrogen-progestin (eg, estradiol 0.5 mg once/day plus micronized progesterone 100 mg at bedtime) may minimize cyclic fluctuations. Spironolactone, bromocriptine, and monoamine oxidase inhibitors are not useful.

245 MENOPAUSE

Menopause is physiologic or iatrogenic cessation of menses (amenorrhea) due to decreasing ovarian function. Manifestations may include hot flushes, atrophic vaginitis, and osteoporosis. Diagnosis is clinical: absence of menses for 1 yr. Manifestations may be treated (eg, with hormone therapy or SSRIs).

Physiologic menopause is established when menses have been absent for 1 yr. In the US, average age of physiologic menopause is 51. Perimenopause refers to the years before (duration varies greatly) and the 1 yr after the last menses. Perimenopause is usually characterized initially by an increase in frequency of menses, followed by a decrease (oligomenorrhea), but any pattern is possible; conception is possible during perimenopause. Climacteric refers to a longer phase in which women lose reproductive capacity; it begins before perimenopause.

As ovaries age, their response to the pituitary gonadotropins follicle-stimulating hormone (FSH) and luteinizing hormone (LH) decreases, initially causing shorter follicular phases (with shorter and more irregular cycles), fewer ovulations, and thus decreased progesterone production (see FIG. 243–5 on p. 2073). Eventually, follicles do not respond, producing little estradiol. Estrogens (now mainly estrone) still circulate; they are produced by peripheral tissues (eg, fat, skin) from androgens (eg, androstenedione, testosterone). However, the total estrogen level is much lower. Around menopause, androstenedione levels decrease by half, but the decrease in testosterone levels, which begins gradually in young adulthood, does not accelerate during menopause because the stroma of the postmenopausal ovary and adrenal gland continue to secrete substantial amounts. Decreased levels of ovarian inhibin and estrogen, which inhibit pituitary release of LH and FSH, result in a substantial increase in circulating LH and FSH levels.

Premature menopause (premature ovarian failure—see p. 2079) is cessation of menses due to noniatrogenic ovarian failure before age 40. Contributory factors may include smoking, living at high altitude, and undernutrition. Iatrogenic (artificial) menopause results from medical interventions (eg, oophorectomy, chemotherapy, pelvic irradiation, any intervention that impairs ovarian blood supply).

Symptoms and Signs

Perimenopausal changes in menstruation usually begin during a woman's 40s. Menstrual flow and cycle length can vary. Menses become irregular, then are skipped. Large daily fluctuations in estrogen levels usually begin at least 1 yr before menopause and are thought to cause perimenopausal symptoms. Symptoms can last from 6 mo to about 10 yr and range from nonexistent to severe.

Hot flushes (flashes) and sweating due to vasomotor instability affect 75 to 85% of women and usually begin before menses stop. Hot flushes continue for > 1 yr in most women and for > 5 yr in 50%. Women feel warm or hot and may perspire, sometimes profusely; core temperature increases. The skin, especially of the head and neck, may become red and warm. The episodic flush, which may last from 30 sec to 5 min, may be followed by chills. Flushes may manifest during the night as night sweats. The mechanism of hot flushes is unknown, but they may be triggered by cigarette smoking, hot beverages, foods containing nitrites or sulfites, spicy food, alcohol, and possibly caffeine.

Neuropsychiatric changes (eg, poor concentration, memory loss, depression, anxiety) may accompany menopause but are not directly related to decreased estrogen. Recurrent night sweats, which can disrupt sleep, can contribute to insomnia, fatigue, irritability, and poor concentration.

Decreased estrogen leads to vaginal and vulvar dryness and thinning, which may result in inflammation of the vaginal mucosa (atrophic vaginitis). Atrophy may cause irritation, dyspareunia, and dysuria and may increase vaginal pH. The labia minora, clitoris, uterus, and ovaries decrease in size. Intermittent lightheadedness, paresthesias, and palpitations may occur. Nausea, constipation, diarrhea, arthralgia, myalgia, and cold hands and feet can occur. Weight gain with increased central adiposity and decreased muscle mass are also common but may result partly from aging.

Although menopause is normal, health problems can occur, and for some, quality of life may decrease. Risk of osteoporosis increases because estrogen is decreased, increasing bone resorption by osteoclasts (see p. 305). The most rapid loss occurs during the 1st 2 yr after estrogen begins to decrease.

Diagnosis

Diagnosis is clinical. Menopause is likely if menses have gradually decreased in frequency and have been absent for 6 mo. Women with amenorrhea are examined to exclude pregnancy if they are < 50 and are always examined to exclude ovarian tumors (for evaluation of amenorrhea, see p. 2075). Abnormal pelvic masses are evaluated (see p. 2065). If women in their 50s have a history of irregular menses followed by cessation of menses, with or without symptoms of estrogen deficiency, and no other abnormal findings, no diagnostic testing is necessary.

Measuring FSH levels may be done but is rarely necessary. Consistently elevated levels predict menopause, sometimes many months to a year in advance.

Postmenopausal women who have risk factors for osteoporosis and all women > 65 should be screened for osteoporosis (see p. 306).

Treatment

Discussing the physiologic causes of menopause and possible symptoms and signs with patients is important. Treatment is symptomatic.

For hot flushes, avoiding triggers and wearing clothing in layers that can be removed as needed may help. Black cohosh, which may have estrogenic effects, may have some efficacy, but long-term safety is unknown. Soy protein has been used, but its efficacy has not been confirmed. Other medicinal herbs, vitamin E, and acupuncture do not appear helpful. Regular exercise, stress avoidance, and relaxation techniques may improve sleep and reduce irritability; relaxation techniques can also reduce vasomotor symptoms. Nonhormonal drug treatments for hot flushes include SSRIs (eg, fluoxetine, sustained-release paroxetine, sertraline), serotonin-norepinephrine reuptake inhibitors (eg, venlafaxine), and clonidine 0.1 mg transdermally once/day. Dose requirements for SSRIs vary; starting doses can be lower than those used to treat depression and increased as needed.

OTC vaginal lubricants and moisturizers help relieve vaginal dryness. Measures to prevent and treat osteoporosis are considered (see p. 307).

Hormone therapy: Hormone therapy may be used for moderate to severe menopausal symptoms. For women who have had a hysterectomy, estrogen should be used alone, orally or as a transdermal patch, lotion, or gel. Women who have a uterus, if given any type of estrogen, are also given a progestin (as combination therapy) because unopposed estrogen increases risk of endometrial cancer. For most women, risks of oral hormone therapy outweigh benefits. Benefits include reduction in hot flushes, night sweats (and consequent sleep disturbance), and vaginal dryness. Combination therapy decreases yearly incidence (per 10,000 women treated) of osteoporosis (from 15 to 10) and colorectal cancer (from 16 to 10). For asymptomatic women, overall effects of therapy on quality of life are not very meaningful.

Risks of combination therapy are reflected in an increased yearly incidence (per 10,000 women treated) of breast cancer (from 30 to 38), ischemic stroke (from 21 to 29), pulmonary embolism (from 16 to 34), dementia (from 22 to 45), and coronary artery disease (from 30 to 37). Risk of coronary artery disease almost doubles during the 1st year of therapy and is particularly high for women with high pretreatment low density lipoprotein levels; aspirin and statins do not prevent the increase in risk. Also, the breast cancers that develop are larger and more likely to be metastatic, and false-positive mammograms are more common.

Estrogen-only therapy does not affect incidence of coronary artery disease but increases incidence (per 10,000 women treated) of ischemic stroke (from 32 to 44) and decreases incidence of hip fractures (from 17 to 11); effects on breast cancer, dementia, colorectal cancer, and pulmonary embolism are less clear.

For vaginal dryness or atrophy, topical forms of estrogen (eg, creams, vaginal tablets or rings) are as effective as oral forms. When estrogen cream is used, women with a uterus are also given a progestin. Hormone therapy is not recommended for prevention and treatment of osteoporosis because other effective measures (eg, bisphosphonates) are available.

Progestins (eg, megestrol acetate 10 to 20 mg po once/day, medroxyprogesterone acetate 10 mg po once/day or depot 150 mg IM once/mo) may relieve hot flushes but not vaginal dryness. Progestins may have adverse effects (eg, abdominal bloating, breast tenderness, increased breast density, headache, increased low density lipoprotein, decreased high density lipoprotein); micronized progesterone appears to have fewer adverse effects. There are no long-term safety data about use of progestins.

246 VAGINITIS AND PELVIC INFLAMMATORY DISEASE

The lower and upper female genital tracts are separated by the cervix. Vaginitis is inflammation of the lower tract: the vagina and vulva. Pelvic inflammatory disease is infection of the upper tract: the cervix, uterus, fallopian tubes, and, if infection is severe, ovaries (one or both).

VAGINITIS

Vaginitis is infectious or noninfectious inflammation of the vaginal mucosa and sometimes the vulva. Symptoms include vaginal discharge, irritation, pruritus, and erythema. Diagnosis is by in-office testing of vaginal secretions. Treatment is directed at the cause and at any severe symptoms.

Vaginitis is one of the most common gynecologic disorders. Some of its causes affect the vulva alone (vulvitis) or in addition (vulvovaginitis).

Etiology

The most common causes vary by patient age.

In children, vaginitis usually involves infection with GI tract flora (nonspecific vulvovaginitis). Common contributing factors in girls aged 2 to 6 yr include poor perineal hygiene (eg, wiping from back to front after bowel movements; not washing hands after bowel movements; fingering, particularly in response to pruritus). Chemicals in bubble baths or soaps may cause inflammation. Foreign bodies (eg, tissue paper) may cause nonspecific vaginitis with a bloody discharge. Sometimes childhood vulvovaginitis is due to infection with a specific pathogen (eg, streptococci, staphylococci, *Candida* sp; occasionally, pinworm).

In women of reproductive age, vaginitis is usually infectious. The most common types are trichomonal vaginitis (see p. 1663), which is sexually transmitted; bacterial vaginosis (see p. 2085); and candidal vaginitis (see p. 2086). Normally in women of reproductive age, *Lactobacillus* sp is the predominant constituent of normal vaginal flora. Colonization by these bacteria keeps vaginal pH in the normal range (3.8 to 4.2), thereby preventing overgrowth of pathogenic bacteria and fungi. Also, high estrogen levels maintain vaginal thickness, bolstering local defenses. Factors that predispose to overgrowth of bacterial and fungal vaginal pathogens may include an alkaline vaginal pH due to menstrual blood, semen, or a decrease in lactobacilli; tight, nonporous underclothing; poor hygiene; and frequent douching. Vaginitis may result from foreign bodies (eg, forgotten tampons). Inflammatory vaginitis, which is noninfectious, is uncommon.

After menopause, the marked decrease in estrogen causes vaginal thinning, increasing vulnerability to infection and inflammation. Some treatments (eg, oophorectomy, pelvic radiation, certain chemotherapy) also result in loss of estrogen. Poor hygiene (eg, in patients who are incontinent or bedridden) can lead to chronic vulvar inflammation due to chemical irritation from urine or feces, or nonspecific infection. Bacterial vaginosis, candidal vaginitis, and trichomonal vaginitis are uncommon among postmenopausal women but may occur in those with risk factors.

At any age, conditions that predispose to vaginal or vulvar infection include fistulas between the intestine and genital tract, which allow intestinal flora to seed the genital tract, and pelvic radiation or tumors, which break down tissue and thus compromise normal host defenses. Noninfectious vulvitis may occur at any age because of hypersensitivity or irritant reactions to hygiene sprays or perfumes, menstrual pads, laundry soaps, bleaches, fabric softeners, fabric dyes, synthetic fibers, bathwater additives, toilet tissue, or, occasionally, spermicides, vaginal lubricants or creams, latex condoms, vaginal contraceptive rings, or diaphragms.

Symptoms and Signs

Vaginitis produces vaginal discharge, which must be distinguished from normal discharge. Normal discharge is common when estrogen levels are high—eg, during the 1st 2 wk of life, because maternal estrogens are transferred before birth (slight bleeding often occurs when estrogen levels abruptly decrease), and during the few months before menarche, when estrogen production increases.

Normal vaginal discharge is commonly milky white or mucoid, odorless, and nonirritating; it can result in vaginal wetness that dampens underwear. Discharge due to vaginitis is accompanied by pruritus, erythema, and sometimes burning, pain, or mild bleeding. Pruritus may interfere with sleep. Dysuria or dyspareunia may occur. In atrophic vaginitis, discharge is scant, dyspareunia is common, and vaginal tissue appears thin and dry. Although symptoms vary among particular types of vaginitis, there is much overlap (see TABLE 246–1).

Vulvitis can cause erythema, pruritus, and sometimes tenderness and discharge from the vulva.

Cervical discharge due to cervicitis (eg, due to pelvic inflammatory disease [PID]) can resemble that of vaginitis; abdominal pain, cervical motion tenderness, or cervical inflammation suggests PID. Discharge that is watery, bloody, or both may result from vulvar or vaginal cancers; cancers can be differentiated from vaginitis by examination and Papanicolaou (Pap) tests. If children have vaginal discharge, a vaginal foreign body is suspected. Vaginal pruritus and discharge may result from skin disorders (eg, psoriasis, tinea versicolor), which can usually be differentiated by history and skin findings.

Diagnosis

Vaginitis is diagnosed using clinical criteria and in-office testing. First, vaginal secretions are obtained with a water-lubricated speculum, and pH paper is used to measure pH in 0.2 intervals from 4.0 to 6.0. Then, secretions are placed on 2 slides with a cotton swab and diluted with 0.9% NaCl on the 1st slide (saline wet mount) and with 10% K hydroxide on the 2nd (KOH wet mount). The KOH wet mount is checked for a fishy odor (whiff test), which results from amines produced in trichomonas vaginitis or bacterial

TABLE 246–1. COMMON TYPES OF VAGINITIS

DISORDER	SYMPTOMS AND SIGNS	CRITERIA FOR DIAGNOSIS	MICROSCOPIC FINDINGS	DIFFERENTIAL DIAGNOSIS
Inflammatory vaginitis	Purulent discharge, vaginal dryness and thinning, dyspareunia, dysuria; usually in postmenopausal women	pH > 6, negative whiff test, and characteristic microscopy findings	Increased PMNs and cocci; decreased bacilli; parabasal cells	Erosive lichen planus
Bacterial vaginosis	Gray, fishy-smelling discharge, often with pruritus and irritation; no dyspareunia	Three of the following: gray discharge, pH > 4.5, fishy odor, and clue cells	Clue cells; decreased bacilli; increased coccobacilli	Trichomonal vaginitis
Candidal vaginitis	Thick, white discharge; vaginal and sometimes vulvar pruritus with or without burning, irritation, or dyspareunia	Typical discharge, pH < 4. 5, and microscopic findings*	Budding yeast, pseudohyphae, or mycelia; best examined with 10% K hydroxide diluent	Contact irritant or allergic vulvitis, chemical irritation, vulvodynia
Trichomonal vaginitis	Often, profuse, malodorous, yellow-green discharge; dysuria; dyspareunia; erythema	Identification of causative organism by microscopy* (occasionally by culture)	Motile, flagellated protozoa; increased PMNs	Bacterial vaginosis, inflammatory vaginitis

*Culture is needed if microscopic findings are negative or symptoms persist.

vaginosis. The saline wet mount is examined microscopically as soon as possible to detect trichomonads, which can become immotile and more difficult to recognize within minutes after slide preparation. The KOH dissolves most cellular material except for yeast hyphae, making identification easier. If clinical criteria and in-office test results are inconclusive, the discharge may be cultured for fungi.

If children have trichomonal vaginitis, evaluation for sexual abuse is required; if they have unexplained vaginal discharge, cervicitis, which may be due to a sexually transmitted infection, should be considered. If women have bacterial vaginosis or trichomonal vaginitis (and thus are at increased risk of sexually transmitted diseases), cervical tests for *Neisseria gonorrhoeae* and *Chlamydia trachomatis*, common causes of sexually transmitted PID, are done.

Treatment

Measures to reduce vulvar moisture and microbial growth include keeping the vulva clean and wearing loose, absorbent cotton clothing that allows air circulation. Soaps and unnecessary topical preparations (eg, feminine hygiene sprays) should be avoided. Intermittent use of ice packs or warm sitz baths with or without baking soda may reduce soreness and pruritus.

If symptoms are moderate or severe or do not respond to other measures, drugs may be needed. For pruritus, topical corticosteroids (eg, topical 1% hydrocortisone bid prn) can be applied to the vulva but not in the vagina. Oral antihistamines decrease pruritus and cause drowsiness, helping patients sleep.

Any infection or other cause is treated. Foreign bodies are removed. Prepubertal girls are taught good perineal hygiene (eg, wiping front to back after bowel movements and voiding, washing hands, avoiding fingering the perineum). If chronic vulvar inflammation is due to being bedridden or incontinent, better vulvar hygiene may help.

Bacterial Vaginosis

Bacterial vaginosis is vaginitis due to a complex alteration of vaginal flora in which lactobacilli are decreased and anaerobic pathogens overgrow. Symptoms include a gray, thin, fishy-smelling vaginal discharge and itching. Diagnosis is clinical and by testing of vaginal secretions. Treatment is usually with oral or topical metronidazole or topical clindamycin.

Bacterial vaginosis is the most common infectious vaginitis. The cause is unknown. Anaerobic pathogens that overgrow include *Prevotella* sp, *Peptostreptococcus* sp, *Gardnerella vaginalis, Mobiluncus* sp, and *Mycoplasma hominis*, which increase in concentration 10-fold to 100-fold and replace the normally protective lactobacilli. Risk factors include those for sexually transmitted diseases (see p. 1650). However, bacterial vaginosis can occur in virgins, and treating the male sex partner does not appear to affect subsequent incidence in sexually active women. Use of an intrauterine device is also a risk factor.

Bacterial vaginosis, once considered inconsequential, appears to increase risk of PID, postabortion and postpartum endometritis, posthysterectomy vaginal cuff infection, chorioamnionitis, premature rupture of membranes, preterm labor, and preterm birth.

Symptoms, Signs, and Diagnosis

Vaginal discharge is malodorous, gray, thin, and profuse. Usually, a fishy odor is present, often becoming stronger when the discharge is more alkaline—after coitus and menses. Pruritus and irritation are common. Erythema and edema are uncommon.

For the diagnosis, 3 of 4 criteria must be present: gray discharge, vaginal secretion pH > 4.5, fishy odor, and clue cells. Clue cells (bacteria adherent to epithelial cells obscuring their cell margins) are identified by microscopic examination of a saline wet mount. Presence of WBCs on a saline wet mount suggests a concomitant infection, possibly trichomonal, gonorrheal, or chlamydial cervicitis, and the need for additional testing.

Treatment

Metronidazole 0.75% vaginal gel bid for 5 days or 2% clindamycin vaginal cream once/day for 7 days is the treatment of choice. Oral metronidazole 500 mg bid for 7 days or 2 g po once is effective but can have systemic adverse effects. Women who use clindamycin cream cannot use latex products (ie, condoms or diaphragms) for contraception because the drug weakens latex. Treatment of asymptomatic sex partners is unnecessary. For vaginitis during the 1st trimester of pregnancy, metronidazole vaginal gel should be used, although treatment during pregnancy has not been shown to lower the risk of pregnancy complications. Before an abortion, metronidazole may be given prophylactically to all patients or given only if tests of vaginal secretions are positive for bacterial vaginosis.

Candidal Vaginitis

Candidal vaginitis is vaginal infection with *Candida* sp, usually *C. albicans*.

Most fungal vaginitis is caused by *C. albicans*, which colonizes 15 to 20% of nonpregnant and 20 to 40% of pregnant women (see also p. 987). Risk factors for candidal vaginitis include diabetes, use of a broad-spectrum antibiotic or corticosteroids, pregnancy, constrictive undergarments, immunocompromise, and use of an intrauterine device. Candidal vaginitis is uncommon among postmenopausal women except among those taking systemic hormone therapy.

Typical symptoms and signs include vaginal or vulvar pruritus, burning, or irritation (which may be worse with intercourse) and a thick, white, cottage cheese–like vaginal discharge that adheres to the vaginal walls. Symptoms and signs increase the week before menses. Erythema, edema, and excoriation are common. Infected male sex partners may or may not have symptoms.

Vaginal pH is <4.5; budding yeast, pseudohyphae, or mycelia are visible on a wet mount, especially with KOH.

Treatment

Topical or oral drugs are highly effective (see TABLE 246–2). A one-dose oral regimen of fluconazole 150 mg improves compliance. Topical butoconazole, clotrimazole, miconazole, and tioconazole are available OTC. However, patients should be warned that topical creams and ointments containing mineral oil or vegetable oil weaken latex-based condoms. If symptoms persist or worsen during topical therapy, hypersensitivity to topical antifungals should be considered. Recurrences are uncommon. Frequent recurrences require long-term suppression with oral drugs (fluconazole 150 mg weekly to monthly or ketoconazole 100 mg once/day).

Inflammatory Vaginitis

Inflammatory vaginitis is vaginal inflammation in the absence of the usual infectious causes of vaginitis.

Etiology may be autoimmune. Vaginal epithelial cells slough superficially, and streptococci overgrow. The major risk factor is

TABLE 246–2. DRUGS FOR CANDIDAL VAGINITIS

TYPE	DRUG	DOSAGE
Topical or vaginal	Butoconazole	2% cream 5 g once/day for 3 days
		Sustained-release preparation of 2% cream 5 g as a single application
	Clotrimazole	1% cream 5 g once/day for 7 to 14 days
		Vaginal tablet 100 mg once/day for 7 days or 200 mg once/day for 3 days or 500 mg once
	Miconazole	2% cream 5 g once/day for 7 days
		Vaginal suppository 100 mg once/day for 7 days or 200 mg once/day for 3 days
	Nystatin	Vaginal tablet 100,000 units once/day for 14 days
	Terconazole	0.4% cream 5 g once/day for 7 days or 0.8% cream 5 g once/day for 3 days
		Vaginal suppository 80 mg once/day for 3 days
	Tioconazole	6.5% ointment 5 g once
Oral	Fluconazole	150 mg in a single dose

estrogen loss, which can result from menopause or ovarian insufficiency (eg, due to oophorectomy, pelvic radiation, or chemotherapy). Genital atrophy predisposes to inflammatory vaginitis and increases risk of recurrence.

Purulent vaginal discharge, dyspareunia, dysuria, and vaginal irritation are common. Vaginal pruritus, erythema, and sometimes burning, pain, or mild bleeding can occur. Vaginal tissue may appear thin and dry. Vaginitis may recur.

Because symptoms overlap with other forms of vaginitis, testing (eg, vaginal fluid pH measurement, microscopy, whiff test) is necessary. The diagnosis is made if vaginal fluid pH is > 6, whiff test is negative, and microscopy shows predominantly WBCs and parabasal cells.

Treatment

Treatment is with clindamycin vaginal cream 5 g every evening for 1 wk. After treatment with clindamycin, women are evaluated for genital atrophy. Genital atrophy, if present, can be treated with topical estrogens (eg, 0.01% estradiol vaginal cream 2 to 4 g once/day for 1 to 2 wk, followed by 1 to 2 g once/day for 1 to 2 wk, then 1 g 1 to 3 times weekly; estradiol hemihydrate vaginal tablets 25 μg twice/wk; estradiol rings q 3 mo). Topical therapy is usually preferred due to concerns about the safety of oral hormonal therapy (hormone replacement therapy).

PELVIC INFLAMMATORY DISEASE

Pelvic inflammatory disease is infection of the upper female genital tract: the cervix, uterus, fallopian tubes, and ovaries; abscesses may occur. Common symptoms and signs include lower abdominal pain, cervical discharge, and irregular vaginal bleeding. Long-term complications include infertility, chronic pelvic pain, and ectopic pregnancy. Diagnosis is clinical and by PCR of cervical specimens for *Neisseria gonorrhoeae* and chlamydiae; a saline wet mount; and occasionally, ultrasonography or laparoscopy. Treatment is with antibiotics.

Pelvic inflammatory disease (PID) results from microorganisms ascending from the vagina and cervix into the endometrium, fallopian tubes, and peritoneum. Infection of the cervix (cervicitis) causes mucopurulent discharge. Infection of the fallopian tubes (salpingitis), uterus (endometritis), and ovaries (oophoritis) tends to occur together.

Neisseria gonorrhoeae and *Chlamydia trachomatis* are common causes of PID; they are transmitted sexually. PID usually also involves other aerobic and anaerobic bacteria, including pathogens involved in bacterial vaginosis (see p. 2085).

PID commonly occurs in women < 35. It is rare before menarche, after menopause, and during pregnancy. Risk factors include previous PID and presence of bacterial vaginosis or any sexually transmitted infection. Other risk factors, particularly for gonorrheal or chlamydial PID, include younger age, nonwhite race, low socioeconomic status, and multiple or new sex partners.

Symptoms and Signs

Lower abdominal pain, fever, cervical discharge, and abnormal uterine bleeding are common, particularly during or after menses.

Cervicitis: The cervix appears red and bleeds easily. Mucopurulent discharge is common; usually, it is yellow-green and can be seen exuding from the endocervical canal.

Acute salpingitis: Lower abdominal pain is usually present and bilateral but may be unilateral, even if both tubes are involved. Pain can also occur in the upper abdomen. Nausea and vomiting are common when pain is severe. Irregular bleeding and fever occur in up to $^1/_3$ of patients. In the early stages, signs may be mild or absent. Later, cervical motion tenderness, guarding, and rebound tenderness are common. Occasionally, dyspareunia or dysuria occurs. Many women have minimal or no symptoms.

PID due to *N. gonorrhoeae* is usually more acute and produces more severe symptoms than that due to *C. trachomatis*, which can be indolent.

Complications: Acute gonococcal or chlamydial salpingitis may lead to the Fitz-Hugh-Curtis syndrome (perihepatitis that causes upper right quadrant pain). Infection may become chronic, characterized by intermittent exacerbations and remissions.

A tubo-ovarian abscess (collection of pus in the adnexa) develops in about 15% of women with salpingitis. It can accompany acute or chronic infection and is more likely if treatment is late or incomplete. Pain, fever, and peritoneal signs are usually present and may be severe. The abscess may rupture, causing progressively severe symptoms and possibly septic shock. Hydrosalpinx (fimbrial obstruction and tubal distention with nonpurulent fluid) is usually asymptomatic but can cause pelvic pressure, chronic pelvic pain, or dyspareunia. Tubo-ovarian abscess, pyosalpinx (pus confined to one or both fallopian tubes), and hydrosalpinx may produce a palpable adnexal mass and may lead to infertility.

Salpingitis may cause tubal scarring and adhesions. Common complications include chronic pelvic pain, menstrual irregularities, infertility, and increased risk of ectopic pregnancy.

Diagnosis

PID is suspected when women of reproductive age, particularly those with risk factors, have lower abdominal pain or cervical or

TABLE 246–3. REGIMENS FOR TREATMENT OF PELVIC INFLAMMATORY DISEASE*

TREATMENT	REGIMEN A	REGIMEN B	ALTERNATIVE REGIMENS
Inpatient	Cefotetan 2 g IV q 12 h *or* Cefoxitin 2 g IV q 6 h *plus* Doxycycline 100 mg po or IV q 12 h†	Clindamycin 900 mg IV q 8 h *plus* Gentamicin 2 mg/kg (loading dose) IV or IM, followed by 1.5 mg/kg q 8 h‡	Ofloxacin 400 mg IV q 12 h *or* Levofloxacin 500 mg IV once/day *with or without* Metronidazole 500 mg IV q 8 h *or* Ampicillin/sulbactam 3 g IV q 6 h *plus* Doxycycline 100 mg po or IV q 12 h
Outpatient	Ofloxacin 400 mg po q 12 h for 14 days *or* Levofloxacin 500 mg po once/day for 14 days *with or without* Metronidazole 500 mg po q 12 h for 14 days	Ceftriaxone 250 mg IM in a single dose *or* Cefoxitin 2 g IM and probenecid 1 g po, each in a single dose, *or* Another 3rd-generation parenteral cephalosporin (eg, ceftizoxime, cefotaxime) *plus* Doxycycline 100 mg po q 12 h for 14 days *with or without* Metronidazole 500 mg po bid for 14 days	Alternatives are under study

*Recommendations are from the Centers for Disease Control and Prevention: "Sexually transmitted diseases treatment guidelines 2002." www.cdc.gov/std/treatment

†This regimen is given for at least 24 h after patients show substantial clinical improvement; then doxycycline 100 mg po q 12 h is given for an overall total of 14 days of therapy. For tubo-ovarian abscess, clindamycin or metronidazole may be added to doxycycline after parenteral therapy is stopped.

‡Once/day dosing of gentamicin can also be used. This regimen is given for at least 24 h after patients show substantial clinical improvement; then doxycycline 100 mg po q 12 h or clindamycin 450 mg po qid is given for an overall total of 14 days of therapy. For tubo-ovarian abscess, clindamycin is preferred.

unexplained vaginal discharge. PID is considered when irregular vaginal bleeding, dyspareunia, or dysuria is unexplained. PID is more likely if lower abdominal tenderness, unilateral or bilateral adnexal tenderness, and cervical motion tenderness are present. A palpable adnexal mass suggests tubo-ovarian abscess. Because even minimally symptomatic infection may have severe sequelae, index of suspicion should be high.

If PID is suspected, PCR of cervical specimens for *N. gonorrhoeae* and *C. trachomatis* (which is nearly 100% sensitive and specific) and a pregnancy test are done. If PCR is unavailable, cultures are done. Cervical discharge may be examined using a Gram stain or saline wet mount to confirm purulence, but these tests are neither sensitive nor specific. If a patient cannot be adequately examined because of tenderness, ultrasonography is done as soon as possible. WBC count may be elevated but is not helpful diagnostically.

If the pregnancy test is positive, ectopic pregnancy, which can produce similar findings, should be considered. Other common causes of pelvic pain include endometriosis, adnexal torsion, ovarian cyst rupture, and appendicitis (for differentiating features of these disorders, see p. 2066). Fitz-Hugh-Curtis syndrome may mimic acute cholecystitis but can generally be differentiated by findings of salpingitis during pelvic examination and, if necessary, with ultrasonography.

If an adnexal or pelvic mass is suspected clinically or if patients do not respond to antibiotics within 48 to 72 h, ultrasonography is done as soon as possible to exclude tubo-ovarian abscess, pyosalpinx, and disorders unrelated to PID (eg, ectopic pregnancy, adnexal torsion). If the diagnosis is uncertain after ultrasonography, laparoscopy should be done; purulent peritoneal material obtained by laparoscopy is the diagnostic gold standard.

Treatment

Antibiotics are given empirically to cover *N. gonorrhoeae* and *C. trachomatis* and are modified based on laboratory test results. Patients with cervicitis or clinically mild to moderate PID do not require hospitalization. Outpatient treatment regimens usually also aim to eradicate bacterial vaginosis, which often coexists (see TABLE 246–3). Partners of patients with *N. gonorrhoeae* or *C. trachomatis* infection should be treated.

General indications for inpatient treatment include severe illness (eg, peritonitis, dehydration), moderate or severe vomiting, pregnancy, suspicion of a pelvic mass, and inability to exclude a surgical emergency (eg, appendicitis). In these cases, IV antibiotics (see TABLE 246–3) are started as soon as cultures are obtained and are continued until patients have been afebrile for 24 h.

Tubo-ovarian abscess may require more prolonged IV antibiotics and hospitalization. Treatment with ultrasound- or CT-guided percutaneous or transvaginal drainage is under study. Laparoscopy or laparotomy is sometimes required for drainage. Suspicion of a ruptured tubo-ovarian abscess requires immediate laparotomy. In women of reproductive age, surgery should aim to preserve the pelvic organs (with the hope of preserving fertility).

247 ENDOMETRIOSIS

Endometriosis is a noncancerous disorder in which functioning endometrial tissue is implanted outside the uterine cavity. Symptoms depend on location of the implants and may include dysmenorrhea, dyspareunia, infertility, dysuria, and pain during defecation. Diagnosis is by biopsy, usually via laparoscopy. Treatment includes anti-inflammatory drugs, drugs to suppress ovarian function and endometrial tissue growth, surgical ablation and excision of endometriotic implants, and, for severe disease if no childbearing is planned, hysterectomy plus oophorectomy.

Endometriosis is usually confined to the peritoneal or serosal surfaces of abdominal organs, commonly the ovaries, broad ligaments, posterior cul-de-sac, and uterosacral ligaments. Less common sites include the serosal surfaces of the small and large intestines, ureters, bladder, vagina, cervix, surgical scars, pleura, and pericardium. Bleeding from peritoneal implants is thought to initiate inflammation, followed by fibrin deposition, adhesion formation, and, eventually, scarring, which distorts peritoneal surfaces of organs and pelvic anatomy.

Etiology and Pathophysiology

The most widely accepted hypothesis is that endometrial cells are transported from the uterine cavity and subsequently become implanted at ectopic sites. Retrograde flow of menstrual tissue through the fallopian tubes could transport endometrial cells intra-abdominally; the lymphatic or circulatory system could transport endometrial cells to distant sites (eg, the pleural cavity). Another hypothesis is coelomic metaplasia: Coelomic epithelium is transformed into endometrium-like glands.

Microscopically, endometriotic implants consist of glands and stroma identical to intrauterine endometrium. These tissues contain estrogen and progesterone receptors and thus usually grow, differentiate, and bleed in response to changes in hormone levels during the menstrual cycle.

Incidence of endometriosis is increased in 1st-degree relatives of women with endometriosis, suggesting that heredity is a factor. Incidence is also increased in women who delay childbearing, who have shortened menstrual cycles (<27 days) with menses that are abnormally long (> 8 days), or who have müllerian duct anomalies.

Reported incidence varies but is probably about 10 to 15% in actively menstruating women aged 25 to 44. Average age at diagnosis is 27, but endometriosis also occurs among adolescents. About 25 to 50% of infertile women have endometriosis. In patients with severe endometriosis and distorted pelvic anatomy, incidence of infertility is high because mechanisms of ovum pickup and tubal transport are impaired. Some patients with minimal endometriosis and normal pelvic anatomy are also infertile. In these patients, fertility may be decreased because incidence of luteal phase dysfunction or luteinized unruptured ovarian follicle syndrome (trapped oocyte) is increased, peritoneal prostaglandin production or peritoneal macrophage activity is increased (resulting in phagocytosis), or endometrium is nonreceptive.

Potential protective factors seem to be multiple pregnancies, use of low-dose oral contraceptives (continuous or cyclic), regular exercise (especially if begun before age 15, if done for > 7 h/wk, or both).

TABLE 247–1. STAGES OF ENDOMETRIOSIS

STAGE	DISEASE	DESCRIPTION
I	Minimal	A few superficial implants
II	Mild	More, slightly deeper implants
III	Moderate	Many deep implants, small endometriomas on one or both ovaries, and some filmy adhesions
IV	Severe	Many deep implants, large endometriomas on one or both ovaries, and many dense adhesions, sometimes with the rectum adhering to the back of the uterus

Symptoms and Signs

Pelvic pain, pelvic mass, alteration of menses, and infertility are typical. Some women with extensive endometriosis are asymptomatic; some with minimal disease have incapacitating pain. Dyspareunia and midline pelvic pain before or during menses, particularly beginning after several years of pain-free menses, may develop. Such dysmenorrhea is an important diagnostic clue.

Implants on the large intestine may cause pain during defecation, abdominal bloating, or rectal bleeding during menses; those in the bladder may cause dysuria, hematuria, suprapubic pain, or a combination during urination. Implants on the ovary can form a cystic mass that is 2 to 10 cm and localized to an ovary (endometrioma); those on adnexal structures can form adnexal adhesions, resulting in a pelvic mass. Occasionally, an endometrioma ruptures or leaks, causing acute abdominal pain and peritoneal symptoms. Nonpelvic endometriosis can cause vague abdominal pain.

Pelvic examination may be normal, or rarely, lesions can be seen on the vulva or cer-

TABLE 247–2. DRUGS USED TO TREAT ENDOMETRIOSIS

CLASS	DRUG	DOSAGE	ADVERSE EFFECTS
Combination estrogen/progestin oral contraceptives	Ethinyl estradiol 30–35 μg plus a progestin	1 tablet once/day for 4–6 mo	Abdominal swelling, breast tenderness, increased appetite, edema, nausea, breakthrough bleeding, deep vein thrombosis
Progestins	Medroxyprogesterone acetate	20–30 mg po once/day for 6 mo, followed by 100 mg IM q 2 wk for 2 mo, then 200 mg IM monthly for 4 mo	Breakthrough bleeding, emotional lability, depression, atrophic vaginitis
Androgen	Danazol	100–400 mg po bid for 3–6 mo	Weight gain, acne, lowering of voice, hirsutism, hot flushes, atrophic vaginitis, edema, muscle cramps, breakthrough bleeding, decreased breast size, emotional lability, liver dysfunction, carpal tunnel syndrome, adverse effects on lipid levels
GnRH agonists	Leuprolide	1 mg sc once/day	Hot flushes, atrophic vaginitis, bone demineralization, emotional lability
	Leuprolide depot	3.75 mg IM q 28 days *or* 11.25 mg IM q 3 mo, not to exceed 6 mo	
	Nafarelin	200–400 μg intranasally bid	

GnRH = gonadotropin-releasing hormone.

vix or in the vagina, umbilicus, or surgical scars. Findings may include a retroverted and fixed uterus, enlarged ovaries, fixed ovarian masses, thickened rectovaginal septum, induration of the cul-de-sac, or nodularity of the uterosacral ligament.

Diagnosis

Diagnosis is suspected based on typical symptoms but must be confirmed by biopsy, usually via pelvic laparoscopy but sometimes via laparotomy, vaginal examination, sigmoidoscopy, or cystoscopy. Both endometrial glands and stroma must be present to diagnose endometriosis. Macroscopic appearance (eg, clear, red, brown, black) and size of implants vary during the menstrual cycle; however, typically, areas of endometriosis on the pelvic peritoneum are punctate red, blue, or purplish brown spots that are > 5 mm, often called powder burn lesions.

Other procedures (eg, ultrasonography, barium enema, IV urography, CT, MRI) sometimes show the extent of endometriosis and help monitor the disorder but are not specific or adequate for diagnosis. Investigational serum markers for endometriosis (eg, serum cancer antigen 125 [> 35 units/mL], antiendometrial antibody) may help monitor the disorder but require further refinement before being used routinely. Testing for other infertility disorders may be indicated (see p. 2138).

Staging the disorder helps physicians formulate a treatment plan and evaluate response to therapy. According to the American Society for Reproductive Medicine, endometriosis may be classified as stage I (minimal), II (mild), III (moderate), or IV (severe), based on number, location, and depth of implants and presence of filmy or dense adhesions (see TABLE 247–1). Another staging system is based primarily on pelvic pain. However, because intraobserver and interobserver variability is high in the staging systems, a more reliable method of staging is being sought.

Treatment

Symptomatic treatment begins with NSAIDs. More definitive treatment must be individualized based on the patient's age, symptoms, and desire to preserve fertility and the extent of the disorder. Options include drugs to suppress ovarian function and the growth and activity of endometriotic implants, conservative surgical resection of as much endometriotic tissue as possible, and conservative surgery plus drugs. If disease is severe or patients are approaching or past menopause, total abdominal hysterectomy with bilateral salpingo-oophorectomy may be done. Drugs and conservative surgery are symptomatic treatments; in most patients, endometriosis recurs after treatment is stopped unless ovarian function is permanently and completely ablated.

Drugs to suppress ovarian function and endometrial tissue growth include continuous oral contraceptives (commonly used), gonadotropin-releasing hormone (GnRH) agonists, and danazol (see TABLE 247–2). GnRH agonists temporarily suppress estrogen production; however, treatment is limited to ≤ 6 mo because long-term use may result in bone loss. If treatment lasts > 4 to 6 mo, add-back therapy, usually daily use of a low-dose oral contraceptive, can be given. Danazol, a synthetic androgen and an antigonadotropin, inhibits ovulation. However, its androgenic adverse effects limit its use. Cyclic or continuous oral contraceptives given after danazol or GnRH agonists may slow disease progression and are warranted for women who wish to delay childbearing. After drug treatment, fertility rates range from 40 to 60%. Whether treating minimal or mild endometriosis improves fertility rates is unclear.

Moderate to severe cases are treated most effectively by ablating or excising as many implants as possible while preserving reproductive potential. Indications for surgery include presence of endometriomas, significant pelvic adhesions, fallopian tube obstruction, incapacitating pelvic pain, and a desire to preserve fertility. Microsurgical techniques are used to prevent adhesions. Laparoscopy can sometimes be used to remove lesions; peritoneal or ovarian lesions can sometimes be electrocauterized or be vaporized or excised with a laser. After this treatment, fertility rates are 40 to 70% and are inversely proportional to severity of the endometriosis. If resection is incomplete, use of oral contraceptives or GnRH agonists may increase fertility rates. Laparoscopic resection of the uterosacral ligaments with electrocautery or a laser may reduce midline pelvic pain. Some patients require presacral neurectomy.

Hysterectomy should be reserved for patients who have intractable pelvic pain and who have completed childbearing. After removal of the uterus and both ovaries, estrogen can be started postoperatively or, if a significant amount of endometriotic tissue remains, may be delayed for 4 to 6 mo; during this interval, suppressive drugs may be necessary. Continuous progestin (eg, medroxyprogesterone acetate 2.5 mg po once/day) should be given with estrogen because if estrogen is given alone, residual tissue may grow and hyperplasia or cancers may develop.

248 UTERINE FIBROIDS

(Leiomyomas; Myomas; Fibromyomas)

Uterine fibroids are benign uterine tumors of smooth muscle origin. Fibroids frequently cause abnormal vaginal bleeding (eg, menorrhagia, menometrorrhagia), pelvic pain and pressure, urinary and intestinal symptoms, and pregnancy complications. Diagnosis is by pelvic examination and imaging. Treatment of symptomatic patients depends on the patient's desire for fertility and desire to keep her uterus and may include oral contraceptives, brief presurgical gonadotropin-releasing hormone therapy to shrink fibroids, and more definitive surgical procedures (eg, myomectomy, hysterectomy, endometrial ablation).

Uterine fibroids are the most common pelvic tumor, occurring in about 70% of women.

However, many fibroids are small and asymptomatic. About 25% of white and 50% of black women have symptomatic fibroids. Risk factors for fibroids include being a woman of color and having a high body mass index. Potentially protective factors include parturition and cigarette smoking.

Most fibroids in the uterus are mucosal, followed by intramural, then submucosal. Occasionally, fibroids occur primarily in the broad ligaments (intraligamentous), fallopian tubes, or cervix. Some fibroids are pedunculated. Fibroids are usually multiple, but all develop from a single monoclonal smooth muscle cell. Because they have estrogen receptors, fibroids tend to enlarge during the reproductive years and regress after menopause.

Degeneration is initiated by loss of blood supply and is described as hyaline, myxomatous, calcific, cystic, fatty, red (usually only during pregnancy), or necrotic. Although patients are often concerned about cancer in fibroids, sarcomatous change is extremely rare.

Symptoms and Signs

Fibroids can cause menorrhagia or menometrorrhagia. If fibroids grow, degenerate, or hemorrhage, or if pedunculated fibroids twist, severe acute or chronic pressure or pain can result. Urinary symptoms (eg, urinary frequency or urgency) can result from bladder compression, and intestinal symptoms (eg, constipation) can result from intestinal compression. Fibroids may prevent pregnancy; during pregnancy, they may cause recurrent miscarriages, premature contractions, or abnormal presentation or make cesarean section necessary.

Diagnosis and Treatment

The diagnosis is likely if bimanual pelvic examination detects an enlarged, mobile, irregular uterus that is palpable above the pelvic symphysis. Confirmation requires imaging, usually with ultrasonography, especially sonohysterography. In sonohysterography, saline is instilled into the uterus, enabling the sonographer to more specifically locate the fibroid in the uterus. If ultrasonography is inconclusive, MRI, the most accurate imaging test, is done.

Asymptomatic fibroids do not require treatment. For symptomatic fibroids, medical options, including suppression of estrogen to stop the bleeding, are suboptimal and limited. Gonadotropin-releasing hormone (GnRH) agonists may be given before surgery to shrink fibroid tissues, often stopping menses and allowing blood counts to increase. Menorrhagia or menometrorrhagia should be treated before surgery is considered.

Drugs: Exogenous progestins can partially suppress estrogen stimulation of uterine fibroid growth. Medroxyprogesterone acetate 5 to 10 mg po once/day or megestrol acetate 10 to 20 mg po once/day given 10 to 14 days each menstrual cycle can limit heavy bleeding, beginning after 1 or 2 cycles. Alternatively, oral therapy every day of the month (continuous therapy) may be given; it often reduces bleeding and provides contraception. Depot medroxyprogesterone acetate 150 mg IM q 3 mo and continuous oral therapy have similar effects. Before IM therapy, oral progestins should be tried to determine whether patients can tolerate the adverse effects (eg, weight gain, depression, irregular bleeding).

Danazol, an androgenic agonist, can suppress fibroid growth but has a high rate of adverse effects (eg, weight gain, acne, hirsutism, edema, hair loss, deepening of the voice, flushing, sweating, vaginal dryness) and is thus often less acceptable to patients.

GnRH agonists (eg, leuprolide 3.75 mg IM q mo, goserelin 3.6 mg sc q 28 days) given IM or by sc injection, subdermal pellet, or nasal spray can decrease estrogen production. Agonists are most helpful when given preoperatively to reduce fibroid and uterine volume, making surgery technically more feasible and reducing blood loss. In general, these drugs should not be used in the long term because rebound growth to pretreatment size within 6 mo is common and bone loss may occur. Generally, after GnRH therapy is stopped, women < 35 recoup bone mass, but women ≥ 35 cannot. Whether simultaneous estrogens given for symptoms prevent bone loss is being studied.

Surgery: Surgery is usually reserved for women with a rapidly enlarging pelvic mass, recurrent uterine bleeding refractory to medical therapy, persistent or intolerable pain or pressure, or urinary or intestinal symptoms. Surgical options include myomectomy and hysterectomy; both are major surgery and have similar indications. However, myomectomy is used only when women want to conceive or keep their uterus. In about 55% of women with infertility due to fibroids alone, myomectomy can restore fertility, resulting in pregnancy after about 15 mo. Multiple myomectomy can be much more difficult to perform than hysterectomy. Patient choice is important but must be based on full information about anticipated difficulties and sequelae of myomectomy vs hysterectomy. Hysterectomy may worsen quality of life.

Newer procedures may relieve symptoms, but their efficacy in restoring fertility has not been evaluated. Such procedures include laparoscopic surgery, resectoscopic surgery (using an instrument with a wide-angle telescope and electrical wire loop for excision), endometrial ablation (using heated water or a cryoprobe), high-intensity focused sonography, and MRI-directed cryoprobe of the uterine myoma. Indications include a large fibroid, abnormal bleeding, and submucous fibroids. These surgical procedures also can be used for patients who wish to keep their uterus; if the risk of surgery is too high for such patients, uterine artery embolization is an option.

249 BENIGN GYNECOLOGIC LESIONS

Benign gynecologic lesions include vulvar and vaginal cysts, cervical stenosis and polyps, uterine myomas, and benign ovarian masses, which can predispose to adnexal torsion.

VULVAR INCLUSION AND EPIDERMAL CYSTS

Vulvar inclusion cysts contain epithelial tissue; vulvar epidermal cysts develop from sebaceous glands. Both cysts eventually enlarge with cellular debris and sometimes become infected.

Inclusion cysts are the most common vulvar cysts; they may also occur in the vagina. They may result from trauma (eg, laceration, episiotomy repair) that entraps viable epithelial tissue below the surface, or they may develop spontaneously. Epidermal cysts result from obstruction of sebaceous gland ducts.

Uninfected cysts are usually asymptomatic but occasionally cause irritation; they are white or yellow and usually < 1 cm. Infected cysts may be red and tender and cause dyspareunia.

Diagnosis is clinical. Treatment, indicated only for symptomatic cysts, is excision; a local anesthetic can be used.

BARTHOLIN'S GLAND CYSTS

Bartholin's gland cysts are mucus-filled and occur on either side of the vaginal opening. They are the most common large vulvar cysts. Symptoms of large cysts include vulvar irritation, dyspareunia, pain with walking, and vulvar asymmetry. Bartholin's cysts may form abscesses, which are painful and usually red. Diagnosis is by physical examination. Large cysts and abscesses require drainage with or without excision; abscesses sometimes require antibiotics.

Bartholin's glands are round, very small, nonpalpable, and located deep in the posterolateral vaginal orifice. Obstruction of the Bartholin duct causes the gland to enlarge with mucus, resulting in a cyst. Cause of obstruction is usually unknown. Rarely, the cysts result from a sexually transmitted disease (eg, gonorrhea). A cyst may become infected, forming an abscess.

Symptoms, Signs, and Diagnosis

Most cysts are asymptomatic, but large cysts can be irritating, interfering with intercourse and walking. Most cysts are nontender, unilateral, and palpable near the vaginal orifice. Cysts distend the affected labia majora, causing vulvar asymmetry. Abscesses cause severe vulvar pain and sometimes fever; they are tender and typically erythematous.

Diagnosis is usually by physical examination. Vulvar cancers (see p. 2129), some of which develop from Bartholin's glands, may resemble cysts. Consequently, cysts are biopsied in women > 40.

Treatment

In women < 40, asymptomatic cysts do not require treatment. Symptomatic cysts may require surgery. Because cysts often recur after simple drainage, surgery aims to produce a permanent opening from the duct to the exterior. A small balloon-tipped catheter may be inserted, inflated, and left in the cyst for 4 to 6 wk; this procedure stimulates fibrosis and produces the permanent opening. Another procedure is marsupialization (suturing the everted edges of the cyst to the exterior). Recurrent cysts may require excision. In women > 40, all cysts require exploration and biopsy. Abscesses are treated with oral broad-spectrum antibiotics (eg, cephalexin 500 mg q 6 h for 7 to 10 days) and insertion of a balloon-tipped catheter.

VULVAR ENDOMETRIOMAS

Vulvar endometriomas are rare, painful cysts that result from extrauterine implantation of functioning endometrial tissue (endometriosis—see p. 2089).

Endometriosis rarely occurs in the vulva (or the vagina), sometimes producing cysts (endometriomas), often at the site of previous surgery (eg, episiotomy).

Endometriomas usually develop in the midline. They may be painful, particularly during intercourse; during menstruation, pain and endometrioma size may increase. Endometriomas are tender and may be blue.

Diagnosis is by physical examination and biopsy. Endometriomas are differentiated from other vulvar cysts by biopsy. Treatment involves excisional biopsy.

SKENE'S DUCT CYST

Skene's duct cysts develop adjacent to the distal urethra, sometimes causing perineal discharge, dyspareunia, urinary obstruction, or abscess formation.

Skene's glands are periurethral glands, located adjacent to the distal urethra. Cysts form if the duct is obstructed, usually because of infection. They occur mainly in adults. Cysts may form abscesses or cause urethral obstruction and recurrent UTIs.

Most cysts are < 1 cm and asymptomatic. Some are larger and cause dyspareunia. The 1st symptoms may be those of urinary outflow obstruction (eg, hesitancy, dribbling, retention) or UTIs. Abscesses are painful, swollen, tender, and erythematous but typically do not cause fever.

Diagnosis is usually clinical. Most symptomatic cysts and abscesses are palpable adjacent to the distal urethra; however, a diverticulum of the distal urethra may be clinically indistinguishable, requiring ultrasonography or cystoscopy for differentiation.

Symptomatic cysts are excised. Abscesses are treated initially with oral broad-spectrum antibiotics (eg, cephalexin 500 mg q 6 h for 7 to 10 days) and are excised or marsupialized.

CERVICAL STENOSIS

Cervical stenosis is stricture of the internal cervical os.

Cervical stenosis may be congenital or acquired. The most common acquired causes are menopause, surgery (eg, conization, cautery), infection, cervical or uterine cancer, and radiation therapy. Cervical stenosis may be complete or partial. It may result in a hematometra (accumulation of blood in the uterus) or, in premenopausal women, retrograde flow of menstrual blood into the pelvis, possibly causing endometriosis. A pyometra (accumulation of pus in the uterus) may also develop, particularly in women with cervical or uterine cancer.

Common symptoms in premenopausal women include amenorrhea, dysmenorrhea, abnormal bleeding, and infertility. Postmenopausal women may be asymptomatic for long periods. Hematometra or pyometra may cause uterine distention or sometimes a palpable mass.

Diagnosis and Treatment

Diagnosis may be suspected based on symptoms and signs or on inability to obtain endocervical cells or an endometrial sample for diagnostic tests (eg, for a Papanicolaou [Pap] test). Diagnosis of complete stenosis is established if a 1- to 2-mm diameter probe cannot be passed into the uterine cavity. If cervical stenosis causes symptoms or uterine abnormalities, cervical cytology and endometrial biopsy should be done to exclude the respective cancers. In postmenopausal women with no history of abnormal Pap tests, no further evaluation is needed.

Treatment is indicated only if symptoms or uterine abnormalities are present and may involve cervical dilation.

CERVICAL MYOMAS

Cervical myomas are smooth, benign tumors of the cervix.

Cervical myomas are uncommon. Uterine myomas (fibroids) usually coexist. Large cervical myomas may partially obstruct the urinary tract or may prolapse into the vagina. Prolapsed myomas sometimes ulcerate, become infected, bleed, or a combination.

Most cervical myomas are asymptomatic. The main symptom is bleeding, which may be irregular or heavy. Infection may develop. Rarely, symptoms result from prolapse, urinary outflow obstruction (eg, hesitancy, dribbling, retention), or UTIs. Cervical myomas, particularly if prolapsed, may be visible with use of a speculum. Some are palpable during bimanual examination.

Diagnosis and Treatment

Diagnosis is by physical examination. Transvaginal ultrasonography is done only to confirm an uncertain diagnosis, to exclude urinary outflow obstruction, or to identify additional myomas. CBC is done to exclude anemia. Cervical cytology is done to exclude cervical cancer.

Treatment is similar to that of fibroids (see p. 2093). Small, asymptomatic myomas are not treated. Most symptomatic cervical myomas are removed, by myomectomy if possible (if childbearing capacity is important) or by hysterectomy. Prolapsed, infected myomas are removed transvaginally if possible.

CERVICAL POLYPS

Cervical polyps are common benign growths of the cervix and endocervix.

Cervical polyps originate in the endocervical canal. They occur in about 2 to 5% of women. Endocervical polyps are probably caused by chronic inflammation.

Most cervical polyps are asymptomatic. Endocervical polyps may bleed between menses or after intercourse or become infected, causing purulent vaginal discharge (leukorrhea). Endocervical polyps are usually reddish pink, < 1 cm in all dimensions, and friable. They are rarely malignant.

Diagnosis is by speculum examination. However, if symptoms persist after treatment, cervical cytology and endometrial biopsy are done to exclude the respective cancers. Polyps are excised in the office without use of anesthetics. Bleeding after excision is rare and can be controlled with chemical cautery.

BENIGN OVARIAN MASSES

Benign ovarian masses include functional cysts and tumors; most are asymptomatic.

Functional cysts develop from Graafian follicles (follicular cysts) or the corpus luteum (corpus luteum cysts). Most functional cysts are < 1.5 cm in diameter; few exceed 8 cm, although a very few reach 15 cm. Functional cysts usually resolve spontaneously over days to weeks. Corpus luteum cysts may hemorrhage into the cyst cavity, distending the ovarian capsule or rupturing into the peritoneum.

Benign ovarian tumors usually grow slowly and rarely undergo malignant transformation. Benign cystic teratomas are the most common benign ovarian tumor. They are also called dermoid cysts because, although derived from all 3 germ cell layers, they consist mainly of ectodermal tissue. Fibromas, the most common solid benign ovarian tumors, are slow-growing and usually < 7 cm in diameter. Cystadenomas may be serous or mucinous.

Symptoms, Signs, and Diagnosis

Most functional cysts and benign tumors are asymptomatic. Hemorrhagic corpus luteum cysts may produce pain or signs of peritonitis. Occasionally, severe abdominal pain occurs because adnexal torsion of a cyst or mass, usually > 4 cm, occurs.

Masses are usually detected incidentally but may be suggested by symptoms and signs. A pregnancy test is done to exclude ectopic pregnancy. Transvaginal ultrasonography can usually confirm the diagnosis. If results are indeterminate, MRI or CT may help. Masses with radiographic characteristics of cancer (eg, cystic and solid components, surface excrescences, multilocular appearance, irregular shape) require excision. Tumor markers may help in the diagnosis of specific tumors (see p. 2119). In women of reproductive age, simple, thin-walled cystic adnexal masses 5 to 8 cm (usually follicular) without characteristics of cancer do not require further investigation unless they persist for > 3 menstrual cycles.

Treatment

Most ovarian cysts < 8 cm resolve without treatment; serial ultrasonography is done to document resolution. Cyst removal (ovarian cystectomy) via laparoscopy or laparotomy may be necessary for cysts ≥ 8 cm, cysts that persist for > 3 menstrual cycles, and hemorrhagic corpus luteum cysts with peritonitis. Cystic teratomas require removal via cystectomy if possible. Oophorectomy is done for fibromas, cystadenomas, cystic teratomas > 10 cm, and cysts that cannot be surgically removed separately from the ovary.

ADNEXAL TORSION

Adnexal torsion is twisting of the ovary and sometimes the fallopian tube, sometimes obstructing the arterial supply and causing ischemia.

Adnexal torsion is uncommon, occurring most often during reproductive years. It usually indicates an ovarian abnormality. Risk factors include pregnancy, induction of ovulation, and ovarian enlargement to >4 cm (eg, particularly by benign tumors or hyperstimulation with fertility drugs). Torsion of normal adnexa, which is rare, is more common among children than adults.

Torsion causes sudden severe pelvic pain and sometimes nausea and vomiting. For days or occasionally weeks before the sudden pain, intermittent, colicky pain may occur, presumably resulting from intermittent torsion that spontaneously resolves. Cervical motion tenderness, a unilateral tender adnexal mass, and peritoneal signs are usually present.

Adnexal torsion is suspected based on typical symptoms and unexplained peritoneal signs plus severe cervical motion tenderness or an adnexal mass without evidence of pelvic inflammatory disease. Diagnosis is usually confirmed by color Doppler transvaginal ultrasonography. Immediate laparoscopy or laparotomy is done if torsion is suspected or confirmed by ultrasonography. Treatment aims to salvage the ovary and fallopian tube by untwisting them via laparoscopy or laparotomy. Salpingo-oophorectomy is required for nonviable tissue, which may not be necrotic yet.

250 PELVIC RELAXATION SYNDROMES

Pelvic relaxation syndromes result from laxities (similar to hernias) in the ligaments, fascia, and muscles supporting the pelvic organs (pelvic floor). Common contributing factors include childbirth, obesity, aging, injury (eg, due to pelvic surgery), and chronic straining. Less common factors include congenital malformations, increased abdominal pressure (eg, due to ascites, abdominal tumors, or chronic respiratory disorders), sacral nerve disorders, and connective tissue disorders. Pelvic relaxation syndromes involve different sites of prolapse and include cystocele, urethrocele, rectocele, and uterine and vaginal prolapse. Usually, prolapse occurs in multiple sites.

CYSTOCELES, URETHROCELES, AND RECTOCELES

Cystoceles, urethroceles, and rectoceles are protrusions of the bladder, urethra, and rectum, respectively, into the vaginal canal. Symptoms include pelvic or vaginal fullness or pressure. Diagnosis is clinical. Treatment includes pessaries, pelvic muscle exercises, and surgery.

Cystocele, urethrocele, and rectocele are particularly likely to occur together. Cystocele and urethrocele commonly develop when the pubocervical vesical fascia is weakened.

Severity of cystocele can be graded based on level of protrusion: to the upper vagina (1st degree), to the introitus (2nd degree), or external to the introitus (3rd degree). Rectocele results from disruption of the levator ani muscles and is graded similarly to cystocele.

Symptoms and Signs

Pelvic or vaginal fullness, pressure, and a sensation of organs falling out are common. Organs may bulge into the vaginal canal or introitus, particularly during straining or coughing. Stress incontinence often accompanies cystocele or urethrocele. Rectocele may cause constipation and incomplete defecation; patients may have to manually press the posterior vaginal wall to defecate.

Diagnosis

Diagnosis is confirmed by examination. Cystoceles or urethroceles are detected by applying a speculum against the posterior vaginal wall while the patient is in the lithotomy position. Asking the patient to strain makes cystoceles or urethroceles visible or palpable as soft reducible masses bulging into the anterior vaginal wall. Inflamed paraurethral (Skene's) glands are differentiated by their more anterior and lateral urethral location, tenderness, and occasionally expression of pus during palpation. Enlarged Bartholin's glands can be differentiated because they develop in the medial labia majora and may be tender if infected. Rectoceles are detected by retracting the anterior vaginal wall while the patient is in the lithotomy position. Asking the patient to strain makes rectoceles visible and palpable during rectovaginal examination.

Treatment

Treatment may initially consist of a pessary and Kegel exercises. Pessaries are prostheses inserted in the vagina to maintain reduction of the prolapsed structures. Pessaries are of varying shapes and sizes, some are inflatable; they may cause vaginal ulceration if not properly sized and routinely cleansed. Kegel exercises involved isometric contractions of the pubococcygeus muscle. Isolation of the proper muscle is difficult (about 50% of patients cannot do this) but important, as a Valsalva maneuver is detrimental, and buttock or thigh contraction is unhelpful. Contraction of the proper muscle is best initiated by asking the patient to simulate attempting to hold in urine. Three sets of 8 to 10 contractions are performed daily; contractions are initially held for 1 to 2 sec and increased up to 10 sec each when possible. Exercises can be facilitated by use of weighted vaginal cones, which help patients focus on contracting the correct muscle, by biofeedback devices, or by electrical stimulation, which causes the muscle to contract.

If symptoms are severe or do not resolve with nonsurgical treatment, surgical repair of supporting structures (anterior and posterior colporrhaphy) is possible. Surgical shortening and tightening of the perineum (perineorrhaphy) may also be needed. Colporrhaphy is usually deferred, if possible, until future childbearing is no longer desired because subsequent vaginal birth may disrupt the repair. Urinary incontinence can be surgically treated at the same time as colporrhaphy. After surgery, patients should avoid heavy lifting for 2 mo. After surgery to repair a cystocele or urethrocele, a urethral catheter is used for 24 h or, rarely, for several days.

UTERINE AND VAGINAL PROLAPSE

Uterine prolapse is descent of the uterus toward or past the introitus. Vaginal prolapse is descent of the vagina or vaginal cuff after hysterectomy. Symptoms include vaginal pressure and fullness. Diagnosis is clinical. Treatment includes reduction, pessaries, and surgery.

A prolapsed uterus is graded based on level of descent: to the upper vagina (1st degree), to the introitus (2nd degree), or external to the introitus (3rd degree or total, sometimes referred to as procidentia). Vaginal prolapse may be 2nd or 3rd degree.

Symptoms, Signs, and Diagnosis

Symptoms tend to be minimal with 1st-degree uterine prolapse. In 2nd- or 3rd-degree uterine prolapse, fullness, pressure, and a sensation of organs falling out are common.

Third-degree uterine prolapse manifests as a bulge or protrusion of the cervix or cuff, although spontaneous reduction may occur before patients present. Vaginal mucosa may become dried, thickened, chronically inflamed, secondarily infected, and ulcerated. Ulcers may be painful or bleed and may resemble vaginal cancer. The cervix, if protruding, may also become ulcerated.

Symptoms of vaginal prolapse are similar. Cystocele or rectocele is usually present.

Diagnosis is confirmed by speculum or bimanual pelvic examination. Vaginal ulcers are biopsied to exclude cancer.

Treatment

Asymptomatic 1st- and 2nd-degree prolapse does not require treatment. Symptomatic or 3rd-degree prolapse can be treated nonsurgically if the perineum can structurally support a pessary. Severe or persistent symptoms require surgery, usually hysterectomy with surgical repair of the pelvic support structures (colporrhaphy) and suspension of the vagina (suturing of the upper vagina to a stable structure nearby). Surgery is delayed until all ulcers have healed. Vaginal prolapse is treated similarly to uterine prolapse.

251 SEXUAL DYSFUNCTION IN WOMEN

Many women initiate or agree to sexual activity because they seek emotional intimacy or wish to increase their sense of well-being, confirm their desirability, please or placate a partner, or a combination. Especially in established relationships, women often have little or no initial sense of sexual desire but access sexual desire (responsive desire) once sexual stimulation triggers excitement and pleasure (subjective arousal) and genital congestion (physical genital arousal). Desire for sexual satisfaction, which may or may not include one or multiple orgasms, builds as sexual activity and intimacy continue, and a physically and emotionally rewarding experience fulfills and reinforces the woman's original motivations. A woman's sexual response cycle is strongly influenced by the quality of the relationship with her partner. Initial desire typically lessens with age but increases with a new partner at any age.

Physiology of the female sexual response is incompletely understood but involves hormonal and CNS regulation of subjective and physical arousal and of orgasm. Estrogens and androgens both appear to influence arousal. Postmenopausal ovarian androgen production stays relatively constant, but adrenal androgen production begins to decrease during a woman's 40s; whether this decrease plays any role in diminishing sexual desire, interest, or arousal is unclear. Androgens probably act via both androgen receptors and estrogen receptors (after intracellular conversion of testosterone to estradiol).

Arousal involves activation of brain areas involved in cognition, emotion, motivation, and organization of genital congestion. Neurotransmitters acting on specific receptors are involved; dopamine, norepinephrine, and serotonin play a role, even though serotonin is usually sexually inhibitory, as are prolactin and γ-aminobutyric acid (GABA).

Genital congestion is a reflexive autonomic response occurring within seconds of an erotic stimulus and causing genital engorgement and lubrication. Smooth muscle cells around blood spaces in the vulva, clitoris, and vaginal arterioles dilate, increasing blood flow (engorgement) and, in the vagina, transudation of interstitial fluid across the vaginal epithelium (lubrication). Women are not always aware of congestion, and it may occur without subjective arousal. As women age, basal genital blood flow decreases, but genital congestion in response to erotic stimuli (eg, erotic videos) may not.

Orgasm is an experience of peak excitement and release characterized by contractions of pelvic muscles every 0.8 sec and slow release of genital congestion. Thoracolumbar sympathetic outflow tracts appear to be involved, but orgasm is possible even after complete spinal cord transection (eg, when a vibrator is used to stimulate the cervix). Prolactin, ADH, and oxytocin are released at orgasm and may contribute to the sense of well-being, relaxation, or fatigue that follows. However, many women experience a sense of well-being and relaxation without experiencing orgasm.

Classification

There are 5 major categories of female sexual dysfunction: sexual desire/interest disorder, sexual arousal disorders, orgasmic disorder, vaginismus, and dyspareunia. Disorder is diagnosed when symptoms cause distress. Some women may not be distressed or bothered by decreased or absent sexual desire, interest, arousal, or orgasm. Overlap is often marked, and almost all women with sexual dysfunction have features of more than one disorder. For example, chronic dyspareunia of vestibulitis often leads to sexual desire/interest and arousal disorders; impaired arousal may make sex less enjoyable or even painful, decreasing the likelihood of orgasm and subsequent spontaneous desire. However, dyspareunia due to impaired lubrication may occur as an isolated symptom in women with a high level of sexual desire, interest, and subjective arousal.

Female sexual disorders may be secondarily categorized as lifelong or acquired; situation-specific or generalized; and mild, moderate, or severe based on the degree of distress it causes the woman. These disorders probably apply equally to women in heterosexual and same-sex relationships. Little is known about the latter, but for some women, these disorders may be a manifestation of transitioning sexual identity or orientation.

Sexual desire/interest disorder is absence of or a decrease in sexual interest, desire, sexual thoughts, and fantasies and an absence of responsive desire. Motivations to become sexually aroused are scarce or absent. The decrease is greater than what might be expected based on a woman's age, life circumstances, and relationship duration.

Sexual arousal disorders can be categorized as subjective, combined, or genital. All definitions are clinically based, distinguished in part by the woman's awareness of her genital response to stimulation. In subjective sexual arousal disorder, subjective arousal in response to any type of sexual stimulation (eg, kissing, dancing, watching an erotic video, genital stimulation) is absent or low, but the woman is aware of normal genital arousal (genital congestion). In combined sexual arousal disorder, subjective arousal in response to any type of sexual stimulation is absent or low, and women report absent or impaired physical genital arousal (ie, they are unaware of it). In genital arousal disorder, subjective arousal in response to nongenital stimulation (eg, erotic video) is normal, but subjective arousal, awareness of genital congestion, and sexual sensations in response to genital stimulation (including intercourse) are absent or low. Genital arousal disorder typically affects postmenopausal women and is often described as "genital deadness". Laboratory studies confirm reduced genital congestion in response to sexual stimulation in some women; in others, the sexual sensitivity of the normally engorged tissues seems reduced.

Orgasmic disorder is orgasm that is absent, markedly diminished in intensity, or markedly delayed in response to stimulation, despite high levels of subjective arousal.

Vaginismus is reflexive tightening around the vagina when vaginal entry is attempted (eg, using a penis, finger, dildo, or any object), despite the woman's expressed desire for penetration, in the absence of structural or other physical abnormalities. The disorder is often associated with anticipation, fear, or experience of pain and phobic avoidance of attempted penetration.

Dyspareunia is pain during attempted or completed vaginal penetration or intercourse; the pain may occur at the moment of penetration (superficial/introital), with deeper entry, with penile movement, or postcoitally.

Etiology

The traditional separation of psychologic and physical etiologies is artificial; psychologic distress causes changes in physiology, and physical changes may generate major distress. There are often several causes of symptoms within and between categories of dysfunction, and the cause is often unclear.

Historical psychologic causes are experiences that affect a woman's psychosexual development. For example, past negative sexual or other experiences may lead to low self-esteem, shame, or guilt. Emotional, physical, or sexual abuse during childhood or adolescence can teach children to control and hide emotions—a useful defense mechanism—but such inhibition can make expressing sexual feelings difficult later. Early traumatic loss of a parent or another loved one may inhibit intimacy with a sex partner for fear of similar loss. Women with desire/interest disorders tend to be anxious, to have a low self-image, and to have mood instability even in the absence of a clinical mood disorder. Women with orgasmic disorder often have difficulty relinquishing control in nonsexual circumstances. A subgroup of women with dyspareunia and vulvar vestibulitis (see p. 2101) have high expectations of self and fear of negative evaluation by others.

Contextual psychologic causes are specific to a woman's current circumstances.

They include negative feelings or reduced attraction toward a sex partner (eg, due to the partner's behaviors or to a growing awareness of attraction to women), nonsexual sources of anxiety or distraction (eg, family, work, finances, cultural restrictions), concerns about privacy, and concerns about unwanted outcomes (eg, unwanted pregnancy, sexually transmitted diseases, inability to have an orgasm, erectile dysfunction in a partner).

Medical conditions that may lead to dysfunction include conditions causing fatigue or debility, hyperprolactinemia, hypothyroidism, atrophic vaginitis, bilateral oophorectomy in younger women, and psychiatric disorders (eg, anxiety disorder, depression). Drugs, most notably SSRIs, β-blockers, and hormones, may play a role. Oral estrogen and oral contraceptives increase sex hormone–binding globulin (SHBG), decreasing the amount of free androgen available for tissue receptor binding. Antiandrogens (eg, spironolactone, gonadotropin-releasing hormone agonists) may also reduce sexual desire and arousal.

Some pelvic muscle hypertonicity, manifest as voluntary guarding and high muscle tension, is a common finding in all types of chronic dyspareunia. The most common type of superficial/introital dyspareunia is vulvar vestibulitis. Vulvar vestibulitis (localized vulvar dysesthesia) is probably a form of chronic pain syndrome (see p. 1776) of the vulva, in which the nervous system, from peripheral receptors to the cerebral cortex, is sensitized and remodeled for unknown reasons. With sensitization, discomfort due to a stimulus that might otherwise be perceived as mild or trivial (eg, touch) is instead perceived as significant pain (allodynia). Some women have accompanying GU disorders (eg, vulvovaginal candidiasis, hyperoxaluria), but the etiologic role of these disorders is unproven. Some women also have other pain disorders (eg, irritable bowel syndrome—see p. 82, interstitial cystitis—see p. 1962). Pain due to vestibulitis typically occurs immediately with introital pressure, with penile movement, and with the man's ejaculation. Vestibulitis may also cause postcoital vulvar burning and dysuria. Vaginismus causes similar pain with introital pressure and penile containment and movement, but pain due to vestibulitis typically stops when penile movement stops and resumes when it starts again; pain due to vaginismus continues when penile movement stops but may progressively fade during intercourse despite continued penile movement.

Other causes of superficial/introital dyspareunia include atrophic vaginitis, vulvar lesions or disorders (eg, lichen sclerosus, vulvar dystrophies), congenital malformations, radiation fibrosis, postsurgical introital narrowing, and recurrent tearing of the posterior fourchette.

Causes of deep dyspareunia include pelvic muscle hypertonicity and uterine or ovarian disorders (eg, fibroids, endometriosis). Penile size and depth of penetration influence presence and severity of symptoms.

Damage to genital sensory or autonomic nerves and, much more commonly, use of SSRIs may lead to acquired orgasmic disorder.

Diagnosis

Diagnosis of sexual dysfunction and its causes is by history and physical examination. Ideally, history is taken from both partners, interviewed separately as well as together; it begins by asking the woman to describe the problem in her own words. Important elements of the history are listed in TABLE 251–1. Problematic areas (eg, past negative sexual experiences, negative sexual self-image) identified at the 1st visit can be investigated more fully at a follow-up visit.

Physical examination is most important for determining causes of dyspareunia; the technique may differ slightly from that used in a routine gynecologic examination. An explanation of what will occur during the examination helps the woman relax and should be repeated as the examination is done. Asking her to sit up and view her genitals in a mirror during the examination imparts a sense of control.

Evaluation of superficial/introital dyspareunia focuses on inspection of all of the vulvar skin, including the creases between the labia minora and majora (for fissures typical of chronic candidiasis), and the clitoral hood, urethral meatus, hymen, and openings of major vestibular gland ducts (for atrophy, signs of inflammation, and skin lesions typical of lichen sclerosus). Vulvar vestibulitis can be diagnosed using a cotton swab to elicit allodynia; nonpainful external areas are touched before moving to more typically painful areas (ie, outer edge of the hymenal ring, clefts adjacent to the urethral meatus). Pelvic muscle hypertonicity may be suspected if pain similar to that which occurs during intercourse can be elicited by palpating the deep levator

TABLE 251–1. COMPONENTS OF THE SEXUAL HISTORY WHEN ASSESSING FEMALE SEXUAL DYSFUNCTION

AREA	SPECIFIC ELEMENTS
Medical history (past and current)	General health (including physical energy level and mood), drugs, pregnancies, pregnancy terminations, STDs, contraception, safer practices
Relationship with partner	Emotional intimacy, trust, respect, attraction, communication, fidelity, anger, hostility, resentment, sexual orientation
Current sexual context	Sexual dysfunction in partner, what occurs in the hours before attempts at sexual activity, is there inadequate sexual stimulation, unsatisfactory sexual communication, disagreement with partner about sexual practices, lack of privacy
Effective triggers of desire and arousal	Books, videos, dates, showering together, dancing, music; physical or nonphysical, genital or nongenital stimulation
Inhibitors of arousal	Distractions; negative past sexual experiences; poor sexual self-image; fears about outcome, including loss of control, unwanted pregnancy, or confirmed infertility; stress; fatigue; depression
Orgasms	Presence or absence; whether distressed by absence or not; differences in responses with partner and with masturbation
Outcome	Emotional and physical satisfaction or dissatisfaction
Location of dyspareunia	Superficial/introital or deep vaginal tissues
Timing of dyspareunia	During partial or full entry, deep thrusting, penile movement, the man's ejaculation, or subsequent urination after intercourse
Self-image	Self-confidence, feelings about desirability, body, genitals, sexual competence
Developmental history	Relationship with caregivers and siblings; traumas; loss of loved one; emotional, physical, or sexual abuse; consequences of expressing emotions as a child; cultural or religious restrictions
Past sexual experiences	Desired, coercive, abusive, or a combination; pleasing and successful sexual practices, self-stimulation
Personality factors	Ability to trust, comfort with vulnerability, suppressed anger causing suppression of sexual emotions, need to feel in control, unreasonable expectations of self

STDs = sexually transmitted diseases.

ani muscles, particularly around the ischial spines. Palpating the urethra and bladder may identify abnormal tenderness.

Evaluation of deep dyspareunia requires a careful bimanual examination to elicit pain with cervical motion or with uterine or adnexal palpation and to check for nodules in the cul-de-sac or vaginal fornices. A rectal examination may also be indicated to check the rectovaginal septum and posterior surface of the uterus and adnexa.

Diagnosis of vaginismus requires exclusion of physical causes by physical examination after treatment makes examination possible. While sitting up, using a mirror, and in control, the woman may spread her labia and insert her or the examiner's gloved finger past the hymen as she bears down. This simple digital examination can simultaneously confirm a normal vagina and the presumed diagnosis of vaginismus.

Wet-preparation examination of vaginal discharge and Gram stain with culture or DNA probe for *Neisseria gonorrhoeae* and chlamydiae are indicated when history or examination suggests vulvitis, vaginitis, or pelvic inflammatory disease. Although low estrogen and testosterone levels may contribute to sexual dysfunction, measuring levels is rarely indicated. An exception may be measuring testosterone using well-validated assays to monitor investigational testosterone therapy.

Treatment

Treatment varies by disorder and cause; often, more than one treatment is required because disorders overlap. Sympathetic understanding of the patient and careful evaluation may themselves be therapeutic. Because SSRIs may contribute to several categories of sexual dysfunction, substitution with antidepressants that have fewer negative sexual adverse effects (eg, bupropion, meclobomide, mirtazapine, venlafaxine) may be considered. Phosphodiesterase inhibitors (eg, sildenafil, tadalafil, vardenafil) may be recommended for empiric use in some cases defined below, but efficacy is unproven.

Sexual desire/interest and subjective and combined sexual arousal disorders: If factors that limit trust, respect, attraction, and emotional intimacy between partners are the cause, the couple should be counseled that emotional intimacy is a normal requirement for female sexual response and needs to be developed with or without professional help. Education about sufficient and appropriate stimuli may help; women may need to remind their partner of their need for nonphysical, physical nongenital, and nonintercourse genital stimulation. Recommendations for more intensely erotic stimuli and fantasies may help eliminate distractions; practical suggestions to improve privacy and a sense of security can help when fear of discovery, pregnancy, or sexually transmitted diseases inhibits arousability. For patient-specific psychologic factors, psychotherapy may be required, although simple awareness of the importance of these factors may be sufficient for women to change patterns of thinking and behavior.

Hormonal abnormalities require targeted treatment: eg, topical estrogen for atrophic vulvovaginitis and bromocriptine for hyperprolactinemia. Benefits and risks of testosterone supplementation are under study. In the absence of interpersonal, contextual, and intrapersonal factors, investigational supplementation (eg, with oral methyltestosterone 1.5 mg once/day or transdermal testosterone 300 μg daily) is considered by some clinicians experienced in both women's sexual disorders and endocrinology for the following: postmenopausal women who are taking estrogen therapy and who develop sexual dysfunction in their 40s and 50s when adrenal androgens are declining, women who develop sexual dysfunction after surgical or chemotherapy-induced menopause, and women with adrenal or pituitary disorders. Careful follow-up is essential. Tibolone, a synthetic steroid used extensively in Europe, has tissue-specific estrogenic, progestogenic, and androgenic activity and appears to increase sexual desire, arousability, and vaginal congestion. In low doses, it does not stimulate endometrium, increases bone density, and does not have estrogenic effects on lipids and lipoproteins. However, its effect on risk of breast cancer is unclear, and it is currently unavailable in the US.

Drug substitutions (eg, transdermal for oral estrogen or oral contraceptives, or barrier methods for oral contraceptives) may also be indicated.

Genital arousal disorder: Initial treatment is local estrogen (or systemic estrogen if indicated for other perimenopausal symptoms) when estrogen deficiency is present. Use of a phosphodiesterase inhibitor may be tried empirically for symptoms refractory to estrogen therapy; it will benefit only those with reduced genital congestion. Other investigational therapy includes a trial of 0.2 mL topical 2% testosterone in petrolatum prepared by a pharmacist and applied to the clitoris.

Orgasmic disorder: Data support encouraging self-stimulation. A vibrator placed on the mons close to the clitoris may help, as may increasing the number and intensity of stimuli (mental, visual, tactile, auditory, written), simultaneously if necessary. Psychotherapy may help women identify and manage fear of relinquishing control, fear of vulnerability, or issues of trust with a partner. Phosphodiesterase inhibitors may be used empirically for acquired orgasmic disorder with autonomic nerve damage, although no scientific evidence supports their use.

Vaginismus: Treatment is behavioral and incremental, involving experiences of neutral self-touch remote from the introitus and moving slowly toward it, to reduce fear of subsequent pain. The woman should be encouraged to touch herself daily as close to the introitus as possible, separating the labia with her fingers. Once her fear and anxiety from introital self-touch has diminished, she can insert her finger past her hymen, pushing or bearing down as she inserts her finger to ease entry. If finger insertion causes no discomfort, vaginal cones graded in size can be prescribed for progressive insertion; they allow perivaginal muscles to become accustomed to gently increasing pressure without reflex contraction. The woman first inserts the cones into her vagina; when comfortable with them, she can allow her partner to help her insert one during a sexual encounter to confirm that it can go in comfortably when she is sexually excited. If this insertion is comfortable, the couple should be encouraged to include penile vulvar stimulation during sexual play so that the woman becomes accustomed to feeling the penis on her vulva. Ultimately, the woman can insert her partner's penis partially or fully, holding it like an insert. She may feel more confident in the woman superior position. Some men experience situational erectile dysfunction in this process and may benefit from a phosphodiesterase inhibitor.

Dyspareunia: Treatment is aimed at specific causes (eg, endometriosis, lichen sclerosus, vulvar dystrophies, vaginal infections, congenital malformations, radiation fibrosis—see elsewhere in THE MANUAL). Optimal treatment of vulvar vestibulitis is unclear; many approaches are currently used, and there are probably as yet undefined subtypes of the disorder that require different treatment. Commonly used but unproven approaches involve avoiding topical irritants and using systemic drugs (eg, tricyclic antidepressants, anticonvulsants) or topical drugs (eg, 2% cromoglycate or 2 or 5% lidocaine in glaxal base) to interrupt chronic pain circuits. Cromoglycate stabilizes WBC membranes, including those of mast cells, interrupting the neurogenic inflammation thought to underlie vestibulitis. Cromoglycate or lidocaine must be placed precisely on the area of allodynia using a 1-mL syringe without a needle. Physician supervision and use of a mirror (at least initially) are helpful. Psychotherapy and sex therapy may also help some women with vestibulitis.

Topical estrogen is helpful for atrophic vulvovaginitis (see p. 2082) and recurrent posterior fourchette tearing.

Women with pelvic muscle hypertonicity may benefit from pelvic physical therapy using pelvic floor muscle training, possibly with biofeedback to teach pelvic muscle relaxation.

While specific causes are being managed, couples should be encouraged to develop satisfying forms of nonpenetrative sex and treated for coexisting disorders of desire/interest and arousal.

252 MEDICAL EXAMINATION OF THE RAPE VICTIM

Although legal and medical definitions vary, rape is typically defined as some oral, anal, or vaginal penetration that involves threats or force against an unwilling person. Sexual assault is rape or any other sexual contact that results from coercion, including when a child is seduced by offers of affection or bribes; it includes being touched, grabbed, kissed, or shown genitals. Rape and sexual assault, including childhood sexual assault, are common; lifetime prevalence estimates for both range from 2 to 30% but tend to be about 15 to 20%.

Typically, rape is an expression of aggression, anger, or need for power; psychologically, it is more violent than sexual. Physical trauma occurs in about 50% of rapes of females.

Females are raped and sexually assaulted more often than males. Rape of males is often committed by another man and often occurs in prison. Males who are raped are more likely than females to be physically injured and to be unwilling to report the crime, and multiple assailants are more likely to be involved.

Symptoms and Signs

Rape may result in extragenital or genital injury, psychologic symptoms, sexually transmitted diseases (eg, hepatitis, syphilis, gonorrhea, chlamydial infection, trichomoniasis, rarely HIV infection), and, occasionally, pregnancy. Most physical injuries are relatively minor, but some lacerations of the upper vagina are severe. Additional injuries may result from being struck, stabbed, or shot.

Overall, psychologic symptoms of rape are potentially the most prominent. In the short term, most patients experience fear, nightmares, sleep problems, anger, embarrassment, and/or shame. Immediately after an assault, patient behavior can range from talkativeness, tenseness, crying, and trembling to shock and disbelief with dispassion, quiescence, and smiling. The latter responses rarely indicate lack of concern; rather, they reflect avoidance reactions, physical exhaustion, or coping mechanisms that require control of emotion. Anger may be displaced onto hospital staff members.

Friends, family members, and officials often react judgmentally, derisively, or in another negative way. Such reactions can impede recovery after an assault.

Eventually, most patients recover; however, long-range effects of rape may include posttraumatic stress disorder (PTSD—see p. 1678), particularly among women. PTSD is an anxiety disorder; symptoms include re-experiencing (eg, flashbacks, intrusive upsetting thoughts or images), avoidance (eg, of trauma-related situations, thoughts, and feelings), and hyperarousal (eg, sleep difficulties, irritability, concentration problems). Symptoms last for > 1 mo and significantly impair social and occupational functioning.

Evaluation

If patients seek advice before medical evaluation, they are told not to throw out or change clothing, wash, shower, douche, brush their teeth, or use mouthwash; doing so may destroy evidence.

Whenever possible, all people who are raped are referred to a local rape center, often a hospital emergency department; such centers are staffed by specially trained practitioners (eg, sexual assault nurse examiners [SANE]—see www.sane-sart.com). Benefits of a rape evaluation are explained, but a patient is free to consent to or decline the evaluation. The police are notified if the patient consents. Most patients are greatly traumatized, and their care requires sensitivity, empathy, and compassion. Females may feel more comfortable with a female physician; a female staff member should accompany all males evaluating a female. Patients are provided privacy and quiet whenever possible.

Goals of rape evaluation are medical (assessment and treatment for injuries; assessment, treatment, and prevention of pregnancy and STDs), collection of forensic evidence, and psychological evaluation and support. A form (sometimes part of a rape kit) is used to record legal evidence and medical findings (for typical elements in the form, see TABLE 252–1); it should be adapted to local requirements. Because the medical record may be used in court, results should be written legibly and in nontechnical language that can be understood by a jury.

History and examination: Before beginning, the examiner asks the patient's permission. Because recounting the events often frightens or embarrasses the patient, the examiner must be reassuring, empathetic, and nonjudgmental and should not rush the patient. Privacy should be ensured. The examiner elicits specific details, including the type of injuries sustained (particularly the mouth, breasts, vagina, and rectum); whether the patient or assailant had any bleeding or abrasions (to help assess the risks of transmission of HIV and hepatitis); orifices penetrated and whether ejaculation occurred or a condom was used; assailant's aggression, threats, weapons, and violent behavior; and a description of the assailant. Many rape forms include most or all of these questions (see TABLE 252–1). The patient should be told why questions are being asked (eg, information about contraceptive use helps determine risk of pregnancy after rape; information about previous coitus helps determine validity of sperm testing).

The examination should be explained step by step as it proceeds. Results should be reviewed with the patient. When feasible, photographs of possible injuries are taken. The mouth, breasts, genitals, and rectum are examined closely. Common sites of injury include the labia minora and posterior vagina. Examination using a Wood's lamp may reveal semen on the skin. Colposcopy is particularly sensitive for subtle genital injuries. Some colposcopes have cameras attached, making it possible to detect and photograph injuries simultaneously.

Testing and evidence collection: Routine testing includes a pregnancy test and serologic tests for syphilis, hepatitis B, and HIV; if done within a few hours of rape, these

TABLE 252–1. TYPICAL EXAMINATION FOR ALLEGED RAPE

CATEGORY	SPECIFICS
General information	Demographic data about the patient
	Name, address, and phone number of guardian, if the patient is under age
	Name of police officer, badge number, and department
	Date, time, and location of examination
History	Circumstances of attack, including date, time, location (familiar to patient?), information about assailants (number, name if known), description, weapon, type of sexual contact (vaginal, oral, rectal; condom used?), types of extragenital injuries sustained, whether bleeding (either the patient or the assailant) occurred, and occurrence and location of ejaculation by the assailant
	Activities of the patient after the attack (eg, douche, bath, urination, defecation, clothing change, use of toothpaste, mouthwash, or drugs)
	Last menstrual period
	Date of previous coitus and time, if recent
	Contraceptive history (eg, oral, intrauterine device)
Physical examination	General (extragenital) trauma to any area
	Genital trauma to the perineum, hymen, vulva, vagina, cervix, and anus
	Foreign material on the body (eg, stains, hair, dirt, twigs)
	Examination with Wood's lamp or colposcopy when available
Data collection	Condition of clothing (eg, damaged, stained, foreign material adhering)
	Small samples of clothing, including an unstained sample, given to police or laboratory
	Hair samples, including loose hairs adhering to the patient or clothing, semen-encrusted pubic hair, and clipped pubic hair of victim—at least 10 (for comparison) scalp and pubic hairs
	Semen taken from the cervix, vagina, rectum, mouth, and thighs
	Blood taken from the patient
	Dried samples of the assailant's blood taken from the patient's body and clothing
	Urine
	Saliva
	Smears of buccal mucosa
	Fingernail clippings and scrapings
	Other specimens, as indicated by the history or physical examination
Laboratory testing	Acid phosphatase to detect presence of sperm*
	Saline suspension from vagina† (for sperm motility)
	Semen analysis for sperm morphology and presence of A, B, or H blood group substances‡
	Baseline serologic test for syphilis in the patient
	Baseline testing for sexually transmitted diseases in the patient
	Blood typing (using blood from the patient and dried samples of the assailant's blood)
	Urine testing, including drug screen§ and pregnancy tests
	Other tests, as indicated by the history or physical examination
Treatment, referral, physician's clinical comments	Specify

TABLE 252–1. TYPICAL EXAMINATION FOR ALLEGED RAPE—Continued

CATEGORY	SPECIFICS
Witness to examination	Signature
Disposition of evidence	Name of the person who delivered the evidence and the person who received it Date and time of delivery and receipt

*Particularly useful if the assailant had a vasectomy, is oligospermic, or used a condom, which may cause sperm to be absent. If the test cannot be done immediately, a specimen should be placed in a freezer.
†Should be done by the examining physician if done in time to detect motile sperm.
‡In 80% of cases, blood group substances are found in semen.
§Many authorities recommend not including comments or tests regarding the presence of alcohol or drugs.

tests provide information about pregnancy or infections present before the rape but not those that develop after the rape. Vaginal discharge is examined to check for trichomonal vaginitis and bacterial vaginosis, and samples from every penetrated orifice (vaginal, oral, or rectal) are obtained for gonorrheal and chlamydial testing. If the patient has amnesia for events around the time of rape, drug screening for flunitrazepam (the "date rape drug") and gamma hydroxybutyrate should be considered. Follow-up tests are done for gonorrhea, chlamydial infection, human papillomavirus infection (initially using a cervical sample from a Papanicolaou test), syphilis, and hepatitis at 6 wk; HIV infection at 90 days; and syphilis, hepatitis, and HIV infection at 6 mo. If the vagina was penetrated and the pregnancy test was negative at the 1st visit, the test is repeated within the next 2 wk. Patients with laceration of the upper vagina, especially children, may require laparoscopy to determine depth of the injury.

Evidence that can provide proof of rape is collected; it typically includes clothing; smears of the buccal, vaginal, and rectal mucosa; combed samples of scalp and pubic hair as well as control samples (pulled from the patient); fingernail clippings and scrapings; blood and saliva samples; and, if available, semen (see TABLE 252–1). Many types of evidence collection kits are available commercially, and some states recommend specific kits. Evidence is often absent or inconclusive after showering, changing clothes, douching, and as time passes, particularly > 36 h; however, evidence may be collected up to 5 days after rape. A chain of custody, in which evidence is in the possession of an identified person at all times, must be maintained. Thus, specimens are placed in individual packages, labeled, dated, sealed, and held until delivery to another person (typically, law enforcement or laboratory personnel), who signs a receipt. In some jurisdictions, samples for DNA testing to identify the assailant are collected.

Treatment

After the evaluation, the patient is provided with facilities to wash, change clothing, use mouthwash, and urinate or defecate if needed. A local rape crisis team can provide referrals for medical, psychologic, and legal support services.

Most injuries are minor and are treated conservatively (see elsewhere in THE MANUAL). Vaginal lacerations may require surgical repair.

Sometimes examiners can use commonsense measures (eg, reassurance, general support, nonjudgmental attitude) to relieve strong emotions of guilt or anxiety. Possible psychologic and social effects are explained, and the patient is introduced to a specialist trained in rape crisis intervention. Because the full psychologic effects cannot always be ascertained at the 1st examination, follow-up visits are scheduled at 2-wk intervals. Severe psychologic effects (eg, persistent flashbacks, significant sleep disruption, fear leading to significant avoidance) or psychologic effects still present at follow-up visits warrant psychiatric or psychologic referral. Family members and friends can provide vital support, but they may need help from rape crisis specialists in handling their own negative reactions. PTSD can be effectively treated psychosocially and pharmacologically (see p. 1678).

Routine empiric prophylaxis for sexually transmitted diseases consists of ceftriaxone 250 mg IM in a single dose (for gonorrhea), metronidazole 2 g po in a single dose (for trichomoniasis and bacterial vaginosis), and either doxycycline 100 mg po bid for 7 days or azithromycin 1 g po once (for chlamydial infection). Alternatively, azithromycin 2 g po can be given (which covers gonorrhea and chlamydial infection) with metronidazole 2 g po, both in single doses.

Empiric prophylactic treatment of hepatitis B and HIV after rape is controversial. For hepatitis B, the CDC recommends hepatitis B vaccination unless the patient has been previously vaccinated and has documented immunity. The vaccine is repeated 1 and 6 mo after the first dose. Hepatitis B immune globulin (HBIG) is not given. For HIV, most authorities recommend offering prophylaxis; however, the patient should be told that the risk after rape from an unknown assailant is only about 0.2% (higher if bleeding occurred). Treatment is best begun < 4 h after penetration and should not be given at > 72 h. Usually, a fixed-dose combination of 300 mg zidovudine (ZDV) and 150 mg lamivudine (3TC) is given bid for 4 wk. If risk is higher (eg, if bleeding occurred or if the assailant is at high risk), a protease inhibitor is added (see p. 1639).

Although pregnancy caused by rape is rare (except in the few days before ovulation), emergency contraception (see p. 2136) should be offered to all women with a negative pregnancy test. Usually, oral contraceptives are used; if used > 72 h after rape, they are much less likely to be effective. An antiemetic may help if nausea develops. An intrauterine device may be effective if used up to 10 days after rape. If pregnancy results from rape, the patient's attitude toward the pregnancy and abortion should be determined, and if appropriate, the option of elective termination should be discussed.

253 BREAST DISORDERS

Breast symptoms (eg, pain, lumps, nipple discharge) are common, accounting for > 15 million physician visits/yr. Although > 90% of symptoms have benign causes, breast cancer is always a concern. Because breast cancer is common and may mimic benign disorders, the approach to all breast symptoms and findings is to conclusively exclude cancer.

History includes duration of symptoms; relation of symptoms to menses and pregnancy; presence and type of pain, discharge, and skin changes; use of drugs, including hormone therapy; personal and family history of breast cancer; and date and results of last mammogram.

Breast examination: Principles of examination are similar for physician and patient. Breasts are inspected for asymmetry in shape, nipple inversion, bulging, and dimpling (see FIG. 253–1A and B for usual positions). Although size differential is common, each breast should have a regular contour. An underlying cancer is sometimes detected by having the patient press both hands against the hips or the palms together in front of the forehead (see FIG. 253–1C and D). In these positions, the pectoral muscles are contracted, and a subtle dimpling of the skin may appear if a growing tumor has entrapped a Cooper's ligament.

The axillary and supraclavicular lymph nodes are most easily examined with the patient seated or standing (see FIG. 253–1E). Supporting the patient's arm during the axillary examination allows the arm to be fully relaxed so that nodes deep within the axilla can be palpated.

The breast is palpated with the patient seated and again with the patient supine, the ipsilateral arm above the head, and a pillow under the ipsilateral shoulder (see FIG. 253–1F). The latter position is also used for breast self-examination; the patient examines the breast with her contralateral hand. Having the patient roll to one side, so that the breast on the examined side falls medially, may help differentiate breast and chest wall tenderness because the chest wall can be palpated separately from breast tissue.

The breast should be palpated with the palmar surfaces of the 2nd, 3rd, and 4th fingers,

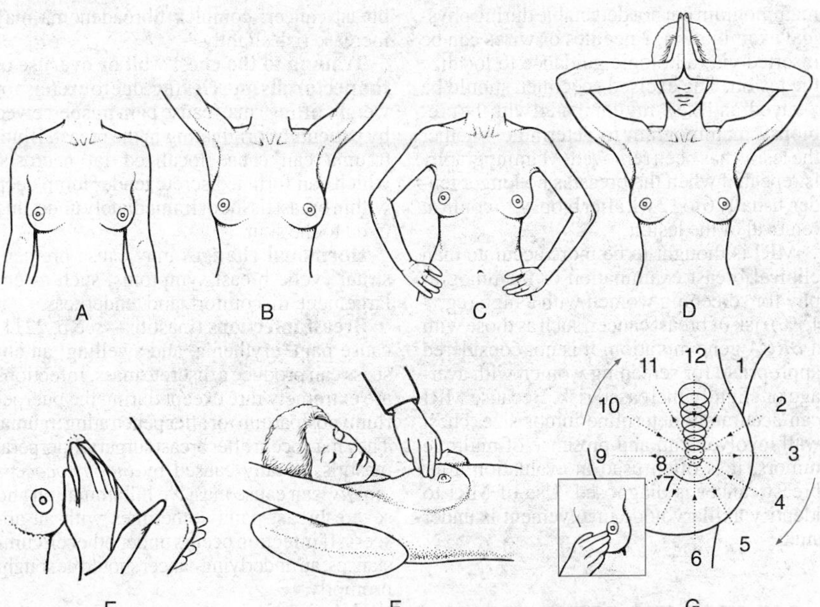

Fig. 253–1. Breast examination. Positions include patient seated or standing (A) with arms at sides; (B) with arms raised over the head, elevating the pectoral fascia and breasts; (C) with hands pressed firmly against hips; or (D) with palms pressed together in front of the forehead, contracting the pectoral muscles. (E) Palpation of axilla; arm supported as shown, relaxing the pectoral muscles. (F) Patient supine with pillow under the shoulder and with the arm raised above the head on the side being examined. (G) Palpation of breast in circular pattern from the nipple outward.

moving systematically in a small circular pattern from the nipple to the outer edges (see FIG. 253–1G). Precise location and size (measured with a caliper) of any abnormality should be noted on a drawing of the breast, which becomes part of the patient's record. A written description of the consistency of the abnormality and degree to which it can be distinguished from surrounding breast tissue should also be included. Detection of abnormalities during physical examination largely determines whether a biopsy is needed, even if a subsequent mammogram shows no abnormalities.

Testing: Imaging tests are used for screening and for evaluation of breast abnormalities. Annual screening mammography is recommended for women ≥ 50 yr and sometimes for women 40 to 50 yr (see p. 2114). Mammography is more effective in older women because with aging, fibroglandular tissue in breasts tends to be replaced with fatty tissue, which can be more easily distinguished from abnormal tissue. Low-dose x-rays of both breasts are taken in 1 (oblique) or 2 views (oblique and craniocaudal). Only about 10% of abnormalities detected result from cancer. Accuracy of mammography depends partly on the techniques used and experience of the mammographer; false-negative results may exceed 15%. Some centers use computer analysis of digitized mammography images to help in diagnosis. Such systems are not recommended for stand-alone diagnosis, but they appear to improve sensitivity for detecting small cancers by radiologists.

Mammography is also used diagnostically to evaluate lumps, pain, and nipple discharge. It can determine size and location of a lesion and provide images of surrounding tissues and lymph nodes. Diagnostic mammography requires more views than screening mammography. For biopsy of a lesion seen on a mammogram but not detectable during physical examination, 2 needles or wires can be inserted via radiologic guidance to localize the lesion. The excised specimen should be x-rayed, and the x-ray compared with the prebiopsy mammogram to determine whether the lesion has been removed. Mammography is repeated when the breast is no longer tender, usually 6 to 12 wk after biopsy, to confirm removal of the lesion.

MRI is thought to be more accurate than clinical breast examination or mammography for screening women with a high (eg, > 15%) risk of breast cancer, such as those with a *BRCA* gene mutation. It is not considered appropriate for screening women with average or slightly increased risk. Because MRI can accurately determine tumor size, chest wall involvement, and presence of multiple tumors, it is often used in evaluation after breast cancer is diagnosed. Use of MRI to identify axillary node involvement is under study.

MASTALGIA AND BREAST LUMPS

Etiology

Fibrocystic changes (previously, fibrocystic disease) is a catchall term that refers to mastalgia, breast cysts, and nondescript lumpiness, which may occur in isolation or together; breasts have a nodular and dense texture and are frequently tender when palpated. Fibrocystic changes cause the most commonly reported breast symptoms and have many causes. Most causes are not associated with increased risk of cancer; they include adenosis, ductal ectasia, simple fibroadenoma, fibrosis, mastitis, mild hyperplasia, cysts, and apocrine or squamous metaplasia. Other causes, particularly if fibrocystic changes require biopsy, may slightly increase risk of breast cancer (see p. 2111). Fibrocystic changes are more common among women who had early menarche, who had their 1st live birth at age > 30, or who are nulliparous.

Fibroadenomas are typically painless lumps that feel like small, slippery marbles. They usually develop in young women, often in teenagers, and may be mistaken for cancer although they are benign and tend to be more circumscribed and mobile. Simple fibroadenoma does not appear to increase risk of breast cancer; complex fibroadenoma may increase risk slightly.

Trauma to the chest wall or overuse of the pectoralis muscles (eg, due to exercise or weight lifting) may cause pain misperceived by patients as originating in the breast. Blunt trauma can cause localized fat necrosis, which can form a discrete tender lump deep within breast tissue or immediately under and fixed to the skin.

Hormonal changes may cause premenstrual cyclic breast symptoms, such as enlargement, discomfort, and tenderness.

Breast infections (mastitis—see p. 2211) cause pain, erythema, and swelling; an abscess can produce a discrete mass. Infections are extremely rare except during the puerperium (postpartum) or after penetrating trauma. They may occur after breast surgery. Puerperal mastitis, usually caused by *Staphylococcus aureus,* can cause massive inflammation and severe breast pain, sometimes with an abscess. If infection occurs under other circumstances, an underlying cancer should be sought promptly.

Galactocele is a round, easily movable milk-filled cyst that usually occurs up to 6 to 10 mo after lactation stops. Such cysts rarely become infected.

Cancers of various types can manifest as a lump or as pain (about 5%).

Evaluation and Treatment

Painful, tender, rubbery lumps in a younger woman with previous history of similar findings suggest fibrocystic changes. A stony hard, irregular lump with skin dimpling suggests cancer. However, because manifestations of benign and malignant lesions overlap considerably and because failing to recognize cancer has serious consequences, tests are done to conclusively exclude breast cancer.

Initially, physicians try to differentiate solid from cystic lumps because cysts are rarely cancerous. Typically, ultrasonography is done. Lesions that appear cystic are sometimes aspirated, and solid lumps are evaluated with mammography followed by imaging-guided biopsy. Some physicians evaluate all lumps with needle aspiration; if no fluid is obtained or if aspiration does not eliminate the lump, mammography followed by imaging-guided biopsy is done.

Fluid aspirated from a cyst is sent for cytology only if it is bloody, if minimal fluid is obtained, or if a mass remains after aspiration. Patients are reexamined in 4 to 8 wk. If the cyst is no longer palpable, it is considered benign; if the cyst has recurred, it is reaspirated, and any fluid is sent for cytology regardless of appearance. A 3rd recurrence or persistence of the mass after initial aspiration (even if cytology was negative) requires biopsy.

Fibroadenomas can usually be excised using a local anesthetic, but they frequently recur. After patients have had several fibroadenomas established as benign, they may decide against having subsequent ones excised. Acetaminophen, NSAIDs, vitamin E, and athletic bras to reduce trauma can be used to relieve symptoms of fibrocystic changes.

NIPPLE DISCHARGE

Nipple discharge can be serous, mucinous, milky, bloody, or purulent. It is not necessarily abnormal, even among postmenopausal women. Cancer (usually intraductal carcinoma or invasive ductal carcinoma) is the cause in < 10% of cases. The rest result from endocrine disorders or benign ductal disorders (eg, ductal ectasia, fibrocystic changes, intraductal papilloma).

Endocrine causes involve elevated prolactin levels, which lead to galactorrhea (breast milk secretion not temporally associated with childbirth—see p. 1187). Causes include pituitary tumors, hypothyroidism, chronic renal failure, and some drugs (see Table 151–3).

Evaluation and Treatment

A general examination is done; breast examination focuses on whether a lump or inflammation is present and which ducts (one, multiple, or bilateral) are involved. Although appearance is not diagnostic, bloody (and perhaps guaiac-positive) discharge suggests breast cancer; bilateral milky discharge from multiple ducts suggests galactorrhea.

Mammography is done. If a lump is palpable or apparent on mammogram, evaluation proceeds as for breast lumps (see p. 2110). If no lump is palpable and mammogram is normal, cancer is highly unlikely. If the discharge is milky, endocrine evaluation is indicated. If discharge from a single duct is persistent and the cause remains unclear, diagnosis may require ductography with or without ductoscopy. Any identified lesions are excised.

Endocrine causes are treated medically. If the discharge is persistent and annoying and the cause is benign, a nipple-flap duct resection, usually done as an outpatient procedure using a local anesthetic, can eliminate the discharge and relieve the patient's anxiety.

GYNECOMASTIA

Gynecomastia is hypertrophy of breast tissue in males.

During puberty, enlargement of the male breast is normal. It is usually transient, bilateral, smooth, firm, and symmetrically distributed under the areola; breasts may be tender. Similar changes may occur during old age but are more often unilateral. Most of the enlargement is due to proliferation of stroma, not of breast ducts.

Gynecomastia may be caused by various disorders (especially hepatic and renal failure; less commonly, endocrine disorders), drugs (eg, anabolic steroid abuse, antineoplastic drugs, Ca channel blockers, cimetidine, digitalis, estrogens, isoniazid, ketoconazole, methadone, metronidazole, reserpine, spironolactone, theophylline), and marijuana.

Gynecomastia is rarely confused with cancer, which is asymmetric, hard, and often fixed to dermis or fascia. Usually, the only imaging or other diagnostic test needed is mammography.

In most cases, no specific treatment is needed because gynecomastia usually remits spontaneously or disappears after any causative drug (except perhaps anabolic steroids) is stopped or underlying disorder is treated. If cosmetic appearance is unacceptable, surgical removal of excess breast tissue (eg, suction lipectomy alone or with cosmetic surgery) may be used.

BREAST CANCER

Breast cancer most often involves glandular breast cells in the ducts or lobules. Most patients present with an asymptomatic lump discovered during examination or screening mammography. Diagnosis is confirmed by biopsy. Treatment usually includes surgical excision, often with radiation therapy and adjuvant systemic therapy.

About 203,000 new cases were identified in 2003. It is the 2nd leading cause of cancer

TABLE 253–1. BREAST CANCER RISKS

AGE (yr)	RISK OF DEVELOPING (OR DYING OF*) BREAST CANCER (%)		
	In 10 yr	In 20 yr	In 30 yr
30	0.4 (0.1)	2.0 (0.6)	4.3 (1.2)
40	1.6 (0.5)	3.9 (1.1)	7.1 (2.0)
50	2.4 (0.7)	5.7 (1.6)	9.0 (2.6)
60	3.6 (1.0)	7.1 (2.0)	9.1 (2.6)
70	4.1 (1.2)	6.5 (1.9)	7.1 (2.0)

*Percentage for dying of breast cancer equals that for developing it divided by 3.5.

Based on Feuer EJ, Wun LM, Boring CC, et al: The lifetime risk of developing breast cancer. *Journal of the National Cancer Institute* 85(11): 892–897, 1993.

death in women (after lung cancer), with about 40,000 deaths in 2003. Male breast cancer accounts for < 1% of total cases; manifestations, diagnosis, and management are the same, although men tend to present later.

Risk Factors

In the US, cumulative risk of developing breast cancer is 12% (1 in 8) by age 95, and risk of dying of it is about 4%. Much of the risk is incurred after age 60 (see TABLE 253–1). These statistics can be misleading because cumulative risk of developing the cancer in any 20-yr period is considerably lower.

Family history of breast cancer in a 1st-degree relative (mother, sister, daughter) doubles or triples risk of developing the cancer, but history in more distant relatives increases risk only slightly. When ≥ 2 1st-degree relatives have breast cancer, risk may be 5 to 6 times higher. About 5% of women with breast cancer carry a mutation in one of the 2 known breast cancer genes, *BRCA1* or *BRCA2*. If relatives of such a woman also carry the gene, they have a 50 to 85% lifetime risk of developing breast cancer. Women with *BRCA1* mutations also have a 20 to 40% lifetime risk of developing ovarian cancer; risk among women with *BRCA2* mutations is increased less. Women without a family history of breast cancer in at least 2 1st-degree relatives are unlikely to carry this gene and thus do not require screening for *BRCA1* and *BRCA2* mutations. Men who carry a *BRCA2* mutation also have an increased risk of developing breast cancer. The genes are more common among Ashkenazi Jews.

History of in situ or invasive breast cancer increases risk: Risk of developing cancer in the contralateral breast after mastectomy is about 0.5 to 1%/yr of follow-up.

Early menarche, late menopause, or late 1st pregnancy increases risk. Women who have a 1st pregnancy after age 30 are at higher risk than those who are nulliparous.

History of fibrocystic changes requiring biopsy for diagnosis increases risk slightly. Women with multiple breast lumps but no histologic confirmation of a high-risk pattern should not be considered at high risk. Benign lesions that may slightly increase risk of developing invasive breast cancer include complex fibroadenoma, moderate or florid hyperplasia (with or without atypia), sclerosing adenosis, and papilloma. Atypical ductal or lobular hyperplasia increases risk of breast cancer 4- to 5-fold; risk increases to about 10-fold in patients who also have a family history of invasive breast cancer in a 1st-degree relative.

Oral contraceptive use increases risk very slightly (by about 5 more cases per 100,000 women). Risk increases primarily during the years of contraceptive use and tapers off during the 10 yr after stopping. Risk is highest in women who began to use contraceptives before age 20 (although absolute risk is still very low).

Postmenopausal hormone (estrogen plus a progestin) therapy appears to increase risk modestly after only 3 yr of use (see also p. 2082). With prolonged use, risk is increased by about 7 or 8 cases per 10,000 women for each year of use. Use of estrogen alone does not appear to increase risk of breast cancer. Selective estrogen-receptor modulators (eg, raloxifene) may reduce risk of developing breast cancer.

Diet may play a role in causing or promoting growth of breast cancers, but conclusive evidence about the effect of a particular diet (eg, one high in fats) is lacking. Obese postmenopausal women are at increased risk, but there is no evidence that dietary modification decreases risk. For obese women who are still menstruating, risk may be decreased.

Exposure to radiation therapy before age 30 increases risk. Mantle-field radiation therapy for Hodgkin lymphoma about quadruples risk of breast cancer over the next 20 to 30 yr.

Pathology

Most breast cancers are epithelial tumors that develop from cells lining ducts or lobules; less common are nonepithelial cancers of the supporting stroma (angiosarcoma, primary stromal sarcomas, phyllodes tumor). Cancers are divided into carcinoma in situ and invasive cancer.

Carcinoma in situ is proliferation of cancer cells within ducts or lobules and without invasion of stromal tissue. Usually, ductal carcinoma in situ (DCIS) is detected only by mammography and is localized to one area; it may become invasive. Lobular carcinoma in situ (LCIS) is a nonpalpable lesion usually discovered via biopsy; it is rarely visualized with mammography. LCIS is not malignant, but its presence indicates increased risk of subsequent invasive carcinoma in either breast; about 1 to 2% of patients with LCIS develop cancer annually.

Invasive carcinoma is primarily adenocarcinoma. About 80% is the infiltrating ductal type; most of the remainder is infiltrating lobular. Rare forms include medullary, mucinous, and tubular carcinomas.

Paget's disease of the nipple (not to be confused with the metabolic bone disease also called Paget's disease) is a form of ductal carcinoma in situ that extends into the overlying skin of the nipple and areola, manifesting with an inflammatory skin lesion (see p. 1027). Characteristic malignant cells called Paget cells are present in the epidermis. The cancer may be in situ or invasive.

Breast cancer invades locally and spreads initially through the regional lymph nodes, bloodstream, or both. Metastatic breast cancer may affect almost any organ in the body—most commonly, lungs, liver, bone, brain, and skin. Most skin metastases occur in the region of the breast surgery; scalp metastases also are common. Metastatic breast cancer frequently appears years or decades after initial diagnosis and treatment.

Estrogen and progesterone receptors, present in some breast cancers, are nuclear hormone receptors that promote DNA replication and cell division when they are bound to the appropriate hormones. Thus, drugs that block these receptors may be useful in treating tumors with the receptors. About ⅔ of postmenopausal patients have an estrogen-receptor positive (ER+) tumor. Incidence of ER+ tumors is lower among premenopausal patients. Another cellular receptor is human epidermal growth factor receptor 2 (HER2) protein; its presence correlates with a poorer prognosis at any given stage of cancer.

Symptoms and Signs

Most breast cancers are discovered as a lump by the patient or during routine physical examination or mammography. Less commonly, the presenting symptom is breast pain or enlargement or a nondescript thickening in the breast. Paget's disease of the nipple presents with skin changes, including erythema, crusting, scaling, and discharge; these usually appear so benign that the patient ignores them, delaying diagnosis for a year or more. About 50% of patients with Paget's disease of the nipple have a palpable mass at presentation. A few patients with breast cancer present with signs of metastatic disease (eg, pathologic fracture, pulmonary dysfunction).

A common finding during physical examination is a dominant mass—a lump distinctly different from the surrounding breast tissue. Diffuse fibrotic changes in a quadrant of the breast, usually the upper outer quadrant, are more characteristic of benign disorders; a slightly firmer thickening in one breast but not the other may be a sign of cancer. More advanced breast cancers are characterized by fixation of the lump to the chest wall or to overlying skin, by satellite nodules or ulcers in the skin, or by exaggeration of the usual skin markings resulting from lymphedema (so-called peau d'orange). Matted or fixed axillary lymph nodes suggest tumor spread, as does supraclavicular or infraclavicular lymphadenopathy. Inflammatory breast cancer is characterized by diffuse inflammation and enlargement of the breast, often without a lump, and has a particularly aggressive course.

Diagnosis

Testing is required to differentiate benign lesions from cancer. Because early detection and treatment of breast cancer improves prognosis, this differentiation must be conclusive before evaluation is terminated.

If advanced cancer is suspected based on physical examination, biopsy should be done first; otherwise, the approach is as for breast lumps (see p. 2110). A prebiopsy bilateral mammogram may help delineate other areas that should be biopsied and provides a baseline for future reference. However, mammogram results should not alter the decision to perform a biopsy. Biopsy can be needle or incisional biopsy or, if the tumor is small, excisional biopsy. Any skin with the biopsy specimen should be examined because it may show cancer cells in dermal lymphatic vessels. Routinely, stereotactic biopsy (needle biopsy during mammography) or ultrasound-guided biopsy is being used to improve accuracy.

Evaluation after cancer diagnosis: Part of a positive biopsy specimen should be analyzed for estrogen and progesterone receptors and for HER2 protein. WBCs should be tested for *BRCA1* and *BRCA2* genes when family history includes multiple cases of early-onset breast cancer, when ovarian cancer develops in patients with a family history of breast or ovarian cancer, when breast and ovarian cancer occur in the same patient, when patients have Ashkenazi Jewish heritage, or when family history includes a single case of male breast cancer.

Chest x-ray, CBC, and liver function tests should be done to check for metastatic disease. Generally, measuring serum carcinoembryonic antigen (CEA), cancer antigen (CA) 15-3, CA 27-29, or a combination is not recommended because results have no effect on treatment or outcome. Bone scanning should be done if patients have tumors > 2 cm, musculoskeletal pain, lymphadenopathy, or elevated serum alkaline phosphatase or Ca levels. Abdominal CT is done if patients have abnormal liver function results, hepatomegaly, or locally advanced cancer with or without axillary lymph node involvement.

Grading and staging follow the TNM classification (see TABLE 253–2). Staging is refined during surgery, when regional lymph nodes can be evaluated.

Screening: Screening includes mammography, clinical breast examination (CBE) by health care practitioners, and monthly breast self-examination (BSE).

Mammography, done annually, reduces mortality rate by 25 to 35% in women ≥ 50 yr. However, there is considerable disagreement about screening for women 40 to 50 yr; recommendations include annual mammography (American Cancer Society), mammography every 1 to 2 yr (National Cancer Institute), and no periodic mammography (American College of Physicians).

CBE is usually part of routine annual care for women > 35; it can detect 7 to 10% of cancers that cannot be seen on a mammogram. In the US, CBE augments rather than replaces screening mammography. However, in some countries where mammography is considered too expensive, CBE is the sole screen; reports on its effectiveness in this role vary.

BSE has not been shown to reduce mortality rate but is widely practiced. Because a negative BSE may tempt some women to forego mammography or CBE, the need for these procedures is reinforced when BSE is taught.

Prognosis

Long-term prognosis depends on extent of lymph node involvement, number of axillary lymph nodes involved, size of primary tumor, tumor grade, stage, presence of estrogen and progesterone receptors, patient age, and presence of HER2 protein.

Nodal status correlates with disease-free and overall survival better than other prognostic factors. For node-negative patients, 10-yr disease-free survival rate is > 70%, and overall survival rate is > 80%. For node-positive patients, rates are about 25% and 40%, respectively.

Larger tumors are more likely to be node-positive and also confer a worse prognosis independent of nodal status. Patients with poorly differentiated tumors have a worse prognosis.

Patients with ER+ tumors have a somewhat better prognosis and are more likely to benefit from hormone therapy. Patients with progesterone receptors on a tumor may also have a better prognosis.

When the HER2 gene (*HER2/neu* [*erb-b2*]) is amplified, HER2 is overexpressed, increasing cell growth and reproduction and often resulting in more aggressive tumor cells. Overexpression of HER2 may be associated with high histologic grade, ER– tumors, greater proliferation, larger tumor size, and thus a poor prognosis.

For any given stage, patients with the *BRCA1* gene appear to have a worse prognosis than those with sporadic tumors, perhaps because they have a higher proportion of high-grade, hormone receptor-negative cancers. Patients with the *BRCA2* gene probably have the same prognosis as those without the genes if the tumors have similar characteristics. With either gene, risk of a 2nd cancer in remaining breast tissue is increased (to perhaps as high as 40%).

Treatment

For most patients, primary treatment is surgery, often with radiation therapy. Chemotherapy, hormone therapy, or both may also be used, depending on tumor and patient characteristics. For inflammatory or advanced

TABLE 253–2. STAGING AND SURVIVAL OF BREAST CANCER

STAGE	TUMOR	REGIONAL LYMPH NODE/ DISTANT METASTASIS	10-YR DISEASE-FREE SURVIVAL (%)*	
			No Treatment	Optimal Treatment
0	Tis	N0/M0	94	98
I	T1†	N0/M0	92	96
IIA	T0	N1/M0	80	90
	T1†	N1/M0	75	87
	T2	N0/M0	83	90
IIB	T2	N1/M0	60	80
	T3	N0/M0	50	75
		N1 (1–3 nodes)/M0	40	70
		N2 (4–9 nodes)/M0	30	65
		N2 (internal mammary nodes)/M0	30	60
IIIA	T0	N2/M0	50	75
	T1†	N2/M0	60	80
	T2	N2/M0	55	75
	T3	N1/M0	45	70
	T3	N2/M0	30	65
IIIB	T4	N0/M0	25	40
	T4	N1/M0	10	30
	T4	N2/M0	5	10
IIIC	Any T	N3/M0	5	10
IV	Any T	Any N/M1	5	10

*Data are for 60-yr-old women who have estrogen-receptor positive, intermediate nuclear grade, *HER2/neu*-negative cancer and who are in otherwise good health.

†T1 includes T1mic.

Tis = carcinoma in situ or Paget's disease of the nipple with no tumor (Paget's disease with a tumor is classified by tumor size); T1 = tumor < 2 cm; T1mic = microinvasion ≤ 0.1 cm; T2 = tumor > 2 but < 5 cm; T3 = tumor > 5 cm; T4 = any size with extension to chest wall, skin, or inflammatory cancer.

N0 = none; N1 = movable axillary nodes; N2 = axillary nodes fixed to each other or other structures; N3 = ipsilateral inframammary nodes.

M0 = none; M1 = present.

Adapted from the American Joint Committee on Cancer, *AJCC Cancer Staging Manual, Sixth Edition*. New York, Springer-Verlag, 2002.

breast cancer, primary treatment is systemic therapy, which, for inflammatory breast cancer, is followed by surgery and radiation therapy; surgery is usually not helpful for advanced cancer. Paget's disease of the nipple is treated as for other forms of breast cancer, although a very few patients can be treated successfully with local excision only.

Surgery: Most patients with DCIS are cured by simple mastectomy. However, more patients are being treated with wide excision alone, especially when the lesion is < 2.5 cm and histologic characteristics are favorable, or with wide excision plus radiation therapy when size and histologic characteristics are less favorable.

For patients with invasive cancer, survival rates do not differ significantly whether modified radical mastectomy (simple mastectomy plus lymph node dissection) or breast-conserving surgery (lumpectomy, wide excision, partial mastectomy, or quadrantectomy) plus radiation therapy is used. Thus, patient preference can guide choice of treatment within limits. The main advantage of breast-conserving surgery plus radiation therapy is cosmetic. In 15% of patients treated with breast-conserving surgery and radiation therapy, cosmetic results are excellent. However, need for total removal of the tumor with a tumor-free margin overrides cosmetic considerations. With both types of surgery, a lymph node dissection or node sampling should be done. Routine use of extensive procedures is not justified because the main value of lymph node removal is diagnostic, not therapeutic. However, results of frozen section analysis may change the extent of surgery needed. Some surgeons get prior agreement for more invasive surgery in case nodes are positive; others wake the patient and do a 2nd procedure if needed.

Some physicians use preoperative chemotherapy to shrink the tumor before removing it and applying radiation therapy; thus some patients who might otherwise have required mastectomy can have breast-conserving surgery. Early data suggest that this approach does not affect survival. Radiation therapy after mastectomy significantly reduces incidence of local recurrence on the chest wall and in regional lymph nodes and may improve overall survival in patients with primary tumors > 5 cm or with involvement of ≥ 4 axillary nodes. Adverse effects of radiation therapy are usually transient and mild.

Procedures for reconstruction include submuscular or subcutaneous (less common) placement of a silicone or saline implant, use of a tissue expander with delayed placement of the implant, muscle flap transfer using the latissimus dorsi or the lower rectus abdominis, and creation of a free flap by anastomosing the gluteus maximus to the internal mammary vessels. Free flap transfer is being increasingly used for DCIS.

After axillary dissection or radiation therapy, lymphatic drainage of the ipsilateral arm can be impaired, sometimes resulting in significant swelling due to lymphedema; magnitude of the effect is roughly proportional to the number of nodes removed. Venipuncture, BP measurement, and IV infusions are avoided on the affected side. A specially trained therapist must treat lymphedema. Special massage techniques once or twice daily may help drain fluid from congested areas toward functioning lymph basins; low-stretch bandaging is applied immediately after manual drainage, and patients should exercise daily as prescribed. After the lymphedema resolves, typically in 1 to 4 wk, patients continue daily exercise and overnight bandaging of the affected limb indefinitely.

Adjuvant systemic therapy: Patients with LCIS are treated with daily oral tamoxifen. If tamoxifen is unsuitable or refused, bilateral mastectomy may be considered.

For patients with invasive cancer, chemotherapy or hormone therapy is usually begun soon after surgery and continued for months or years; these therapies delay or prevent recurrence in almost all patients and prolong survival in some. However, some experts believe that these therapies are not necessary for tumors < 1 cm (particularly in postmenopausal patients) if lymph nodes are not involved because the prognosis is already excellent. Some experts begin adjuvant systemic therapy before surgery if tumors are > 5 cm.

Relative reduction in risk of recurrence and death associated with chemotherapy or hormone therapy is the same regardless of the clinical-pathologic stage of the cancer. Thus, absolute benefit is greater for patients with a greater risk of recurrence or death (ie, a 20% reduction reduces a 10% recurrence rate to 8% but a 50% rate to 40%). Adjuvant chemotherapy reduces annual odds of death on average by 25 to 35% for premenopausal patients; for postmenopausal patients, the reduction is about ½ of that (9 to 19%), and the absolute benefit in 10-yr survival is much smaller. Postmenopausal patients with ER– tumors benefit the most from adjuvant chemotherapy (see TABLE 253–3).

Combination chemotherapy regimens (eg, cyclophosphamide, methotrexate, plus 5-fluorouracil; doxorubicin plus cyclophosphamide) are more effective than a single drug. Regimens given for 4 to 6 mo are preferred; they are as effective as regimens given for 6 to 24 mo. Acute adverse effects depend on the regimen but usually include nausea, vomiting, mucositis, fatigue, alopecia, myelosuppression, and thrombocytopenia. Long-term adverse effects are infrequent with most regimens; death due to infection or bleeding is rare (< 0.2%). Whether increasing dose density (giving treatments more frequently) or adding a taxane (eg, docetaxel, paclitaxel) improves response or survival is uncertain.

TABLE 253–3. PREFERRED BREAST CANCER ADJUVANT SYSTEMIC THERAPY

AXILLARY LYMPH NODE	PREMENOPAUSAL		POSTMENOPAUSAL	
	ER+	ER–	ER+	ER–
Negative*	Chemotherapy plus tamoxifen	Chemotherapy	An aromatase inhibitor or tamoxifen with or without chemotherapy	Chemotherapy
Positive	Chemotherapy (with or without a taxane) plus tamoxifen	Chemotherapy (including a taxane)	Chemotherapy (with or without a taxane) plus an aromatase inhibitor or tamoxifen	Chemotherapy (including a taxane)

ER = estrogen receptor.

*Treatment of node-negative tumors also depends on tumor size and grade.

NOTE: For all protocols involving chemotherapy, enrollment in a clinical trial is often considered.

High-dose chemotherapy plus bone marrow or stem cell transplantation offers no therapeutic advantage over standard therapy and should not be used.

Hormone therapy includes tamoxifen and aromatase inhibitors. Tamoxifen competitively binds estrogen receptors. Aromatase inhibitors (anastrozole, exemestane, letrozole) block peripheral production of estrogen in postmenopausal women. Benefit of hormone therapy is greatest when tumors have estrogen and progesterone receptors, nearly as good when they have only estrogen receptors, minimal when they have only progesterone receptors, and absent when they have neither receptor. In patients with ER+ tumors, particularly low-risk tumors, hormone therapy may be used instead of chemotherapy. Aromatase inhibitors have recently been proven more effective than tamoxifen and are becoming the preferred treatment for early-stage breast cancer in receptor-positive postmenopausal patients. Adjuvant tamoxifen for 5 yr reduces annual odds of death by about 25% in premenopausal and postmenopausal women regardless of axillary lymph node involvement; treatment for 2 yr is not as effective, but treatment for > 5 yr has no advantage and may increase the likelihood that any recurrent cancer is tamoxifen-resistant. Letrozole may be used for postmenopausal women who have completed 5 yr of daily tamoxifen.

Tamoxifen can induce or exacerbate menopausal symptoms but reduces incidence of contralateral breast cancer and lowers serum cholesterol. Tamoxifen improves bone density in postmenopausal women, and there is some evidence of fracture reduction. Tamoxifen may reduce cardiovascular mortality risk. However, it significantly increases risk of developing endometrial cancer; reported incidence is 1% in postmenopausal women after 5 yr of use. Thus, if such women have spotting or bleeding, they must be evaluated for endometrial cancer (see p. 2121). Nonetheless, the improved survival for women with breast cancer far outweighs increased risk of death due to endometrial cancer. Unlike tamoxifen, aromatase inhibitors do not cause menopausal symptoms, but they may increase risk of osteoporosis.

Metastatic disease: Any indication of metastases should prompt immediate evaluation. Treatment of metastases increases median survival by only 3 to 6 mo, although relatively toxic therapies (eg, chemotherapy) may palliate symptoms and improve quality of life; the decision to undergo treatment is highly personal.

Choice of therapy depends on the hormone-receptor status of the tumor, length of the disease-free interval (from diagnosis to manifestation of metastases), number of metastatic sites and organs affected, and patient's menopausal status. Most patients with symptomatic metastatic disease are treated with systemic hormone therapy or chemotherapy. Radiation therapy alone may be used to treat isolated, symptomatic bone lesions or local skin recurrences not amenable to surgical resection. Radiation therapy is the most effective treatment for brain metastases, occasionally achieving long-term control. Patients with multiple metastatic sites outside the CNS should initially be given systemic therapy. There is no proof that treatment of asymptomatic metastases substantially increases survival, and it may reduce quality of life.

Hormone therapy is preferred over chemotherapy for patients with ER+ tumors, a disease-free interval of > 2 yr, or disease that is not life threatening. Tamoxifen is often used first in premenopausal women. Ovarian ablation by surgery, radiation therapy, or use of a luteinizing-releasing hormone agonist (eg, buserelin, goserelin, leuprolide) is a reasonable alternative. Some experts combine ovarian ablation with tamoxifen therapy. If the cancer initially responds to hormone therapy but progresses months or years later, additional forms of hormone therapy may be used sequentially until no further response is seen. Aromatase inhibitors are being increasingly used as primary hormone therapy in postmenopausal women.

The most effective cytotoxic drugs for treatment of metastatic breast cancer are capecitabine, doxorubicin (including its liposomal formulation), gemcitabine, the taxanes paclitaxel and docetaxel, and vinorelbine. Response rate to a combination of drugs is higher than that to a single drug, but survival is not improved and toxicity is increased. Thus, some oncologists use single drugs sequentially.

For tumors with amplification of *HER2/neu*, the humanized monoclonal antibody trastuzumab is effective in treating and controlling visceral metastatic sites. It is used alone or with hormone therapy or chemotherapy.

About 10% of patients with bone metastases eventually develop hypercalcemia, which can be treated with IV bisphosphonates (eg, pamidronate, zoledronate).

PHYLLODES TUMOR

Phyllodes tumor (cystosarcoma phyllodes) is a nonepithelial breast tumor that may be benign or malignant.

Tumors frequently are large (4 to 5 cm) at diagnosis. About ½ are malignant, accounting for < 1% of breast cancers. Between 20 and 35% of these tumors recur locally, and distant metastases occur in 10 to 20% of patients. Usual treatment is wide excision, but a mastectomy may be more appropriate if the mass is large or histology suggests cancer. Prognosis is good unless metastases are present.

254 GYNECOLOGIC TUMORS

Gynecologic cancers often involve the uterus, ovaries, cervix, vulva, vagina, fallopian tubes, or, usually secondarily, the peritoneum. The most common gynecologic cancer in the US is endometrial cancer, followed by ovarian cancer. Cervical cancer is not very common in developed countries because Papanicolaou (Pap) test screening is widely available and effective. Gestational trophoblastic disease is a gynecologic tumor that may behave aggressively whether malignant or not. Many gynecologic cancers manifest as pelvic masses (for diagnostic approach to pelvic masses, see p. 2065).

OVARIAN CANCER

Ovarian cancer is often fatal because it is usually advanced when diagnosed. Symptoms are usually absent in early stage and nonspecific in advanced stage. Evaluation usually includes ultrasonography, CT or MRI, and measurement of tumor markers (eg, cancer antigen 125). Diagnosis is by histologic analysis. Staging is surgical. Treatment requires hysterectomy, bilateral salpingo-oophorectomy, excision of as much involved tissue as possible, and, unless cancer is localized, chemotherapy.

In the US, ovarian cancer is the 2nd most common gynecologic cancer (affecting about 1/70) and the deadliest (1% of all women die of it); it is the 5th leading cause of cancer-related deaths in women. Incidence is higher in developed countries.

Etiology and Pathology

Ovarian cancer affects mainly perimenopausal and postmenopausal women. Nulliparity, delayed childbearing, and delayed menopause increase risk. Oral contraceptive use decreases risk.

A personal or family history of endometrial, breast, or colon cancer increases risk. Probably 5 to 10% of ovarian cancer cases are related to mutations in the autosomal dominant *BRCA* gene. XY gonadal dysgenesis predisposes to ovarian germ cell cancer.

Ovarian cancers are histologically diverse. At least 80% originate in the epithelium; 75% of these cancers are serous cystadenocarcinoma, and the rest include mucinous, endometrioid, transitional cell, clear cell, unclassified carcinomas, and Brenner tumor. The remaining 20% of ovarian cancers originate in primary ovarian germ cells or in sex cord and stromal cells or are metastases to the ovary (most commonly, from the breast or GI tract). Germ cell cancers usually occur in women < 30 and include dysgerminomas, immature teratomas, endodermal sinus tumors, embryonal carcinomas, choriocarcinomas, and polyembryomas. Stromal (sex cord–stromal) cancers include granulosa-theca cell tumors and Sertoli-Leydig cell tumors.

Ovarian cancer spreads by direct extension, exfoliation of cells into the peritoneal cavity (peritoneal seeding), lymphatic dissemination to the pelvis and around the aorta, or, less often, hematogenously to the liver or lungs.

Symptoms and Signs

Early cancer is usually asymptomatic; an adnexal mass, often solid, irregular, and fixed, may be discovered incidentally. Pelvic and rectovaginal examinations typically detect diffuse nodularity. A few women present with severe abdominal pain secondary to torsion of the ovarian mass (see p. 2097). Most women with advanced cancer present with nonspecific symptoms (eg, dyspepsia, bloating, early satiety, gas pains, backache). Later, pelvic pain, anemia, cachexia, and abdominal swelling due to ovarian enlargement or ascites usually occur. Germ cell or stromal tumors may have functional effects (eg, hyperthyroidism, feminization, virilization).

Diagnosis

Ovarian cancer is suspected in women with unexplained adnexal masses, unexplained abdominal bloating, changes in bowel habits, unintended weight loss, or abdominal pain. An ovarian mass is more likely to be cancer in older women. Benign functional cysts (see p. 2096) can simulate functional germ cell or stromal tumors in young women.

If cancer is suspected, ultrasonography is done first; findings that suggest cancer include a solid component, surface excrescences, size > 6 cm, irregular shape, and low vascular resistance on transvaginal Doppler flow studies. A pelvic mass plus ascites usually indicates ovarian cancer but sometimes indicates Meigs' syndrome (a benign fibroma with ascites and right hydrothorax). CT or MRI is usually done before surgery to determine extent of the cancer. Tumor markers, including the β subunit of human chorionic gonadotropin (β-hCG), LDH, α-fetoprotein, inhibin, and cancer antigen (CA) 125, are also measured. CA 125 is elevated in 80% of advanced epithelial ovarian cancers but may be mildly elevated in endometriosis, pelvic inflammatory disease, pregnancy, fibroids, peritoneal inflammation, or nonovarian peritoneal cancer. A mixed solid and cystic pelvic mass in postmenopausal women, especially if CA 125 is elevated, suggests ovarian cancer. Histologic analysis is mandatory for adnexal masses unless they appear benign. Benign-appearing masses include benign cystic teratomas (dermoid cysts), follicular cysts, or endometriomas. For masses that appear benign, ultrasonography is repeated after 6 wk. If women are not surgical candidates, samples are obtained by needle biopsy for masses or by needle aspiration for ascitic fluid.

Staging: Suspected or confirmed ovarian cancer is staged surgically (see TABLE 254–1). An abdominal midline incision that allows adequate access to the upper abdomen is required. All peritoneal surfaces, hemidiaphragms, and abdominal and pelvic viscera are inspected and palpated. Washings from the pelvis, abdominal gutters, and diaphragmatic recesses are obtained, and multiple biopsies of the peritoneum in the central and lateral pelvis and in the abdomen are done. For early-stage cancer, the infracolic omentum is removed, and pelvic and para-aortic lymph nodes are sampled.

Cancers are also graded histologically from 1 (least aggressive) to 3 (most aggressive).

Screening asymptomatic women using ultrasonography and serum CA 125 measure-

TABLE 254–1. SURGICAL STAGING OF OVARIAN CARCINOMA*

STAGE	DESCRIPTION
I	Tumor limited to the ovaries
IA	Tumor limited to one ovary; no tumor on the external surface, and capsule intact
IB	Tumor limited to both ovaries; no tumor on the external surface, and capsules intact
IC	Stage IA or IB but with tumor on the surface of one or both ovaries, with capsule ruptured, or with ascites or peritoneal washings containing malignant cells†
II	Tumor involving one or both ovaries with pelvic extension or metastases
IIA	Extension and/or metastases to the uterus, fallopian tubes, or both
IIB	Extension to other pelvic tissues
IIC	Stage IIA or IIB but with tumor on the surface of one or both ovaries, with capsule ruptured, or with ascites or peritoneal washings containing malignant cells†
III	Histologically confirmed peritoneal metastases outside the pelvis, superficial liver metastases, positive retroperitoneal or inguinal lymph nodes, or tumor limited to the true pelvis but with histologically verified malignant extension to the small intestine or omentum
IIIA	Gross tumor limited to the true pelvis with negative lymph nodes but with histologically confirmed microscopic tumor outside pelvis
IIIB	Histologically confirmed abdominal peritoneal metastases that extend beyond the pelvis and are < 2 cm in diameter and negative lymph nodes
IIIC	Abdominal peritoneal metastases that extend beyond the pelvis and are > 2 cm in diameter, positive retroperitoneal or inguinal lymph nodes, or both
IV	Distant metastases, including parenchymal liver metastases; if pleural effusion is present, cytologic test results must be positive to signify stage IV

*Based on staging established by the International Federation of Gynecology and Obstetrics (FIGO) and American Joint Committee on Cancer (AJCC), 1999, 2002.

†For stages IC and IIC, knowing whether capsule rupture was spontaneous or caused by the surgeon and whether the source of malignant cells was ascites or peritoneal washings helps determine prognosis.

ments can detect some cases of ovarian cancer but has not been shown to improve outcome, even for high-risk subgroups.

Prognosis and Treatment

The 5-yr survival rates with treatment are 70 to 100% with stage I, 50 to 70% with stage II, 15 to 35% with stage III, and 10 to 20% with stage IV. Prognosis is worse when tumor grade is higher or when surgery cannot remove all visibly involved tissue; then, prognosis is best when the involved tissue can be reduced to < 1 cm in diameter. With stages III and IV, recurrence rate is about 70%.

Hysterectomy and bilateral salpingo-oophorectomy are usually indicated. An exception is nonepithelial or low-grade unilateral epithelial cancer in young patients; fertility can be preserved by not removing the unaffected ovary and uterus. All visibly involved tissue is surgically removed if possible. If it cannot be removed completely, removing as much as possible (cytoreductive surgery) improves the efficacy of other therapies. Cytoreductive surgery usually includes infracolic omentectomy, sometimes with rectosigmoid resection (usually with primary reanastomosis), radical peritoneal stripping, resection of diaphragmatic peritoneum, or splenectomy.

Stage IA or B/grade 1 epithelial adenocarcinoma requires no postoperative therapy. Stage IA or B/grade 2 or 3 cancers and stage II cancers require 6 courses of chemotherapy (typically, paclitaxel and carboplatin).

Stage III or IV cancer requires 6 courses of similar chemotherapy. Intraperitoneal chemotherapy or high-dose chemotherapy with bone marrow transplantation is under study. Radiation therapy is used infrequently.

Even if chemotherapy results in a complete clinical response (ie, normal physical examination, normal serum CA 125, and negative CT scan of the abdomen and pelvis), about 50% of patients with stage III or IV cancer have residual tumor. Of patients with persistent elevation of CA 125, 90 to 95% have residual tumor.

If cancer recurs or progresses after effective chemotherapy, chemotherapy is restarted. Other useful drugs may include topotecan, liposomal doxorubicin, docetaxel, vinorelbine, gemcitabine, hexamethylmelamine, and oral etoposide.

Most patients with germ cell cancer or stage II or III stromal cancer are treated with combination chemotherapy, usually bleomycin, cisplatin, and etoposide.

FALLOPIAN TUBE CANCER

Fallopian tube cancer is usually adenocarcinoma, manifesting as an adnexal mass or as vague symptoms. Diagnosis, staging, and treatment are surgical.

Primary fallopian tube cancer is rare. Average age at diagnosis is 50 to 60. Risk factors include chronic salpingitis, other inflammatory disorders (eg, TB), and infertility.

Most (> 95%) fallopian tube cancers are papillary serous adenocarcinomas; a few are sarcomas. Spread, like that of ovarian cancer, is by direct extension, by peritoneal seeding, or through the lymphatics.

Most patients present with an adnexal mass or vague abdominal or pelvic symptoms (eg, abdominal discomfort, bloating, pain). A few patients present with hydrops tubae profluens (a triad of pelvic pain, copious watery discharge, and adnexal mass), which is more specific.

Imaging is typically done with CT scan. A distended solid adnexal mass and normal ovaries suggest fallopian tube cancer. If cancer is suspected, surgery is necessary for diagnosis, staging, and treatment. Staging (similar to that of ovarian cancer) requires washings from the pelvis, abdominal gutters, and diaphragmatic recesses; multiple pelvic and abdominal peritoneal biopsies; and pelvic and para-aortic lymph node dissection. Treatment includes total abdominal hysterectomy, bilateral salpingo-oophorectomy, and infracolic omentectomy. If cancer appears advanced, cytoreductive surgery is indicated.

Postoperative treatment is identical to that for ovarian cancer. External beam radiation is rarely indicated.

ENDOMETRIAL CANCER

Endometrial cancer is usually adenocarcinoma. Typically, postmenopausal vaginal bleeding occurs. Diagnosis is by biopsy. Staging is surgical. Treatment requires hysterectomy, bilateral salpingo-oophorectomy, usually pelvic and para-aortic lymph node dissection, and excision of all tissue likely to be involved. For advanced cancer, radiation, hormone, or cytotoxic therapy is usually indicated.

Endometrial cancer is more common in developed countries in which dietary fat is high. In the US, it is the 4th most common cancer in women, affecting 1 in 50.

Etiology and Pathology

Endometrial cancer affects mainly postmenopausal women, particularly those aged 50 to 65. Major risk factors are obesity, diabetes, and hypertension. Other risk factors include unopposed estrogen, tamoxifen use for > 5 yr, previous pelvic radiation therapy, and a personal or family history of breast or ovarian cancer. Unopposed estrogen (high circulating levels of estrogen with no or low levels of progesterone) may be associated with obesity, polycystic ovarian syndrome, nulliparity, late menopause, estrogen-producing tumors, anovulation (ovulatory dysfunction), and estrogen therapy without progesterone.

TABLE 254–2. STAGING OF ENDOMETRIAL CARCINOMA*

STAGE†	DEFINITION
I	Confined to the uterine corpus
IA	Tumor limited to endometrium
IB	Invasion of < ½ myometrium
IC	Invasion of > ½ myometrium
II	Involvement of the uterus and cervix but no extension outside of the uterus
IIA	Involvement of endocervical glands
IIB	Invasion of cervical stroma
III	Extension beyond the uterus but not beyond the true pelvis
IIIA	Invasion of serosa, adnexa, or both and/or positive peritoneal cytologic results
IIIB	Metastases to vagina
IIIC	Metastases to pelvic or para-aortic lymph nodes or both
IV	Involvement of the bladder or intestinal mucosa or distant metastases
IVA	Invasion of bladder or intestinal mucosa or both
IVB	Distant metastases, including intra-abdominal or inguinal lymph nodes or both

*Based on staging established by the International Federation of Gynecology and Obstetrics (FIGO) and American Joint Committee on Cancer (AJCC), 1989, 1992, and 1997. Endometrial cancer is usually surgically staged.

†For all but stage IVB, grade (G) indicates percentage of tumor with a nonsquamous or nonmorular solid growth pattern: G1 (≤ 5%), G2 (6–50%), or G3 (> 50%). Nuclear atypia excessive for the grade raises the grade of a G1 or G2 tumor by 1. In serous adenocarcinomas, clear cell adenocarcinomas, and squamous cell carcinomas, nuclear grading takes precedence. Adenocarcinomas with squamous differentiation are graded according to the nuclear grade of the glandular component.

Heredity contributes to endometrial cancer in about 6% of cases, usually in families with hereditary nonpolyposis colorectal cancer (HNPCC) syndrome.

Endometrial cancer is usually preceded by endometrial hyperplasia. Adenocarcinoma accounts for > 80% of endometrial cancers. Other types include papillary serous, clear cell, squamous, and mucinous carcinoma.

The cancer may spread from the surface of the uterine cavity to the cervical canal; through the myometrium to the serosa and into the peritoneal cavity; via the lumen of the fallopian tube to the ovary, broad ligament, and peritoneal surfaces; via the bloodstream, leading to distant metastases; or via the lymphatics. The higher (more undifferentiated) the grade of the tumor, the greater is the likelihood of deep myometrial invasion, pelvic or para-aortic lymph node metastases, or extrauterine spread.

Symptoms and Signs

Most (> 90%) women have abnormal uterine bleeding (eg, postmenopausal bleeding, premenopausal recurrent metrorrhagia); ⅓ of women with postmenopausal bleeding have endometrial cancer. A vaginal discharge may occur weeks or months before postmenopausal bleeding.

Diagnosis

Endometrial cancer is suspected in women with postmenopausal bleeding, in premenopausal women with abnormal bleeding, in postmenopausal women with a routine Pap test showing endometrial cells, and in any women with a routine Pap test showing atypical endometrial cells. If cancer is suspected, outpatient endometrial biopsy is done; it is > 90% accurate. If results are inconclusive or suggest cancer, inpatient fractional D & C with hysteroscopy is done. An alternative is transvaginal ultrasonography, which may help in diagnosis.

Once cancer is diagnosed, pretreatment evaluation includes serum electrolytes, kidney and liver function tests, CBC, chest x-ray, and ECG. If an abdominal mass or hepatomegaly is detected during physical examination, or liver function tests are abnormal, pelvic and abdominal CT are also done to check for extrauterine or metastatic cancer.

Staging: Staging is based on histologic differentiation (grade 1 [least aggressive] to 3 [most aggressive]) and extent of spread, including invasion depth, cervical involvement (glandular involvement vs stromal invasion), and extrauterine metastases (see TABLE 254–2). Staging is surgical and includes peritoneal fluid cytology, exploration of the abdomen and pelvis, and biopsy or excision of suspect extrauterine lesions. Pelvic and para-aortic lymph nodes are removed. Surgical staging is done traditionally via laparotomy but may be done via laparoscopy.

Prognosis, and Treatment

Prognosis is worse with higher-grade tumors, more extensive spread, and older patient age. Average 5-yr survival rates are 70 to 95% with stage I or II and 10 to 60% with stage III or IV. Overall, 63% of patients are cancer-free ≥ 5 yr after treatment.

If cancer appears to be stage I/grade 1 without deep myometrial invasion, the probability of unrecognized lymph node metastasis is < 2%. Treatment is usually total hysterectomy and bilateral salpingo-oophorectomy via laparotomy or laparoscopy. For grade 1 with deep myometrial invasion and grade 2 or 3, complete pelvic and para-aortic lymphadenectomy is also done.

Stage II or III cancer requires pelvic radiation therapy with or without chemotherapy. Treatment of stage III cancer must be individualized, but surgery is an option; generally patients who undergo combined surgery and radiation therapy have a better prognosis. Except in patients with bulky parametrial disease, a total abdominal hysterectomy and bilateral salpingo-oophorectomy should be performed. Treatment of stage IV is variable and patient dependent but typically involves a combination of surgery, radiation therapy, and chemotherapy. Occasionally, hormonal therapy should also be considered.

Hormone therapy with a progestin causes regression for up to 3 yr in 35 to 40% of patients. Pulmonary, vaginal, and mediastinal metastases may regress. Treatment continues as long as the response is favorable.

Several cytotoxic drugs (particularly doxorubicin and cisplatin; paclitaxel) are effective. With monthly regimens of doxorubicin 60 mg/m^2 plus cisplatin 60 mg/m^2 IV, overall response rate may be ≥ 50%.

Treatment of endometrial hyperplasia consists of progestins or surgery (eg, D & C), depending on the complexity of the lesion and the patient's desire to avoid hysterectomy.

UTERINE SARCOMAS

Uterine sarcomas are a group of disparate, highly malignant cancers developing from the uterine corpus.

Sarcomas account for < 5% of uterine cancers. Risk factors are similar to those for endometrial carcinoma (see p. 2121). The most common types are mixed mesodermal tumors (malignant mixed mullerian tumor, in which the sarcoma is mixed with adenocarcinoma), leiomyosarcomas, and endometrial stromal tumors.

Most sarcomas present with abnormal vaginal bleeding and, less commonly, pelvic pain or a palpable pelvic mass.

Symptoms usually prompt a transvaginal ultrasound and an endometrial biopsy or fractional D & C. Those in whom cancer is identified typically have CT or MRI preoperatively.

Stage I disease is confined to the corpus; stage II to the corpus and cervix; stage III is spread outside the uterus but confined to the pelvis; and stage IV is spread outside the true pelvis or into the mucosa of the bladder or rectum.

Prognosis is generally poorer than with endometrial cancer of similar stage; survival is generally poor when disease has spread beyond the uterus. In one study, 5-year survivals were 51%, 13%, 10%, and 3% for stages I through IV, respectively.

Treatment is total abdominal hysterectomy and bilateral salpingo-oophorectomy with complete exploration of the abdomen and biopsy of suspicious nodes; nodal dissection is prognostic but not therapeutic. Adjuvant radiation therapy is typically employed and appears to delay local recurrence but does not improve overall survival rate. Chemotherapeutic agents vary with tumor type; overall response is poor, although progestational agents are frequently effective for endometrial stromal tumors.

Recurrent disease occurs most commonly locally, in the abdomen, and the lungs.

GESTATIONAL TROPHOBLASTIC DISEASE

Gestational trophoblastic disease is proliferation of trophoblastic tissue in pregnant or recently pregnant women. Manifestations may include excessive uterine enlargement, vomiting, vaginal bleeding, and preeclampsia, particularly during early pregnancy. Diagnosis includes measurement of the β subunit of human chorionic gonadotropin and pelvic ultrasonography and confirmation by biopsy. Tumors are removed by D & C. If disease persists after removal, chemotherapy is indicated.

Gestational trophoblastic disease is a tumor originating from the trophoblast, which surrounds the blastocyst and develops into the chorion and amnion (see p. 2148). This disease can occur during or after an intrauterine or ectopic pregnancy. If the disease occurs during a pregnancy, spontaneous abortion, eclampsia, or fetal death typically occurs; the fetus rarely survives. Some forms are malignant; others are benign but behave aggressively.

Pathology

Classification is morphologic. A hydatidiform mole is an abnormal pregnancy in which villi become edematous (hydropic) and trophoblastic tissue proliferates. Chorioadenoma destruens (invasive mole) is local invasion of the myometrium by a hydatidiform mole. Choriocarcinoma is an invasive, usually widely metastatic tumor composed of malignant trophoblastic cells and lacking hydropic villi; most of these tumors develop after a hydatidiform mole. Placental site trophoblastic tumors, which are rare, consist of intermediate trophoblastic cells that persist after a term pregnancy. They may invade adjacent tissues or metastasize.

Hydatidiform moles are most common among women < 17 or > 35. They occur in about 1/2000 gestations in the US. For unknown reasons, incidence in Asiatic countries approaches 1/200. Most (> 80%) hydatidiform moles are benign and regress spontaneously. The rest may persist, tending to become invasive; 2 to 3% are followed by choriocarcinoma.

TABLE 254–3. NIH CRITERIA FOR POOR-PROGNOSIS METASTATIC GESTATIONAL TROPHOBLASTIC DISEASE

Criteria
Urinary hCG excretion > 100,000 IU in 24 h
Duration of disease > 4 mo (interval since prior pregnancy)
Brain or liver metastases
Disease after full-term pregnancy
Serum hCG > 40,000 mIU/mL
Failed prior chemotherapy
WHO score > 8

hCG = Human chorionic gonadotropin.

Symptoms, Signs, and Diagnosis

Initial manifestations of a hydatidiform mole suggest early pregnancy, but the uterus often becomes larger than expected within 10 to 16 wk gestation. Vaginal bleeding, lack of fetal movement, absent fetal heart sounds, and severe vomiting are common. Passage of grapelike tissue strongly suggests the diagnosis. Complications may include uterine infection, sepsis, hemorrhagic shock, and preeclampsia, which may occur during early pregnancy. Placental site trophoblastic tumors tend to cause bleeding. Choriocarcinoma usually manifests with symptoms due to metastases. Gestational trophoblastic disease does not impair fertility or predispose to prenatal or perinatal complications (eg, congenital malformations, spontaneous abortions).

If gestational trophoblastic disease is suspected, testing includes measurement of serum β subunit of human chorionic gonadotropin (β-hCG) and pelvic ultrasonography. Findings (eg, very high β-hCG levels) may suggest the diagnosis, but biopsy is required.

Treatment

Hydatidiform mole, invasive mole, and placental site trophoblastic tumor are evacuated by suction curettage. Alternatively, if childbearing is not planned, hysterectomy may be done.

After tumor removal, gestational trophoblastic disease is classified clinically to determine whether additional treatment is needed. (The clinical classification system does not correspond to the morphologic classification system.) A chest x-ray is taken, and serum β-hCG is measured. If the β-hCG level does not normalize within 10 wk, the disease is classified as persistent. Persistent disease requires CT of the brain, chest, abdomen, and pelvis. Results dictate whether disease is classified as nonmetastatic or metastatic. In metastatic disease, risk of death may be low or high (see TABLE 254–3).

Persistent disease is usually treated with chemotherapy. Treatment is considered successful if at least 3 consecutive serum β-hCG measurements at 1-wk intervals are normal. Typically, oral contraceptives (any is acceptable) are given for 6 to 12 mo; alternatively, any effective contraceptive method can be used. Nonmetastatic disease can be treated with a single chemotherapeutic drug (methotrexate or dactinomycin). Alternatively, hysterectomy is considered for patients > 40 or those desiring sterilization and may be required for those with severe infection or uncontrolled bleeding. If single-drug chemotherapy is ineffective, hysterectomy or multidrug chemotherapy is indicated. Virtually 100% of patients with nonmetastatic disease can be cured.

Low-risk metastatic disease is treated with single or multiple drug chemotherapy. High-risk metastatic disease requires aggressive multidrug chemotherapy. Cure rates are 90 to 95% for low-risk and 60 to 80% for high-risk disease.

Hydatidiform mole recurs in about 1% of subsequent pregnancies. Patients who have had a mole require ultrasonography early in subsequent pregnancies.

CERVICAL CANCER

Cervical cancer is usually a squamous cell carcinoma that is caused by human papillomavirus infection or an adenocarcinoma. Early cancer is asymptomatic; the 1st symptom of later cancer is usually postcoital vaginal bleeding. Diagnosis is by screening cervical Papanicolaou (Pap) test and biopsy. Staging is clinical. Treatment usually includes surgical resection, radiation therapy, and, unless cancer is localized, chemotherapy; if cancer is widely metastasized, treatment is primarily chemotherapy.

Cervical cancer is the 3rd most common gynecologic cancer and the 8th most common cancer among women in the US. Mean age at diagnosis is about 50, but the cancer can occur as early as age 20.

Cervical cancer results from cervical intraepithelial neoplasia (CIN), which appears to be caused by infection with human papillomavirus (HPV) type 16, 18, 31, 33, 35, or 39. Risk factors for cervical cancer include younger age at 1st intercourse, a high lifetime number of sex partners, and intercourse with men whose previous partners had cervical cancer. Other factors such as cigarette smoking and immunodeficiency also appear to contribute.

Pathology

CIN is graded as 1 (mild cervical dysplasia), 2 (moderate dysplasia), or 3 (severe dysplasia and carcinoma in situ). CIN 3 is unlikely to regress spontaneously; if untreated, it may, over months or years, penetrate the basement membrane, becoming invasive carcinoma.

About 80 to 85% of all cervical cancers are squamous cell carcinoma; most of the rest are adenocarcinomas. Sarcomas and small cell neuroendocrine tumors are rare.

Invasive cervical cancer usually spreads by direct extension into surrounding tissues or via the lymphatics to the pelvic and para-aortic lymph nodes. Hematogenous spread is possible.

Symptoms and Signs

CIN is usually asymptomatic. Early cervical cancer usually manifests as irregular vaginal bleeding; it is most often postcoital but may occur spontaneously between menses. Larger cancers are more likely to bleed spontaneously and may produce foul-smelling vaginal discharge or pelvic pain. More widespread cancer may produce obstructive uropathy, back pain, and leg swelling due to venous or lymphatic obstruction; examination may detect an exophytic necrotic tumor in the cervix.

Diagnosis

Cervical cancer is considered in women with visible cervical lesions, abnormal routine cervical Pap tests, or abnormal vaginal bleeding. Most CIN is evident on Pap tests, but about 50% of patients with cervical cancer have not had a Pap test for ≥ 10 yr. Patients at highest risk are the least likely to obtain regular preventive health care and to be tested regularly.

Reporting of cervical cytology results is standardized (see TABLE 254–4). Further evaluation is indicated if atypical or cancerous cells are found, particularly in women at risk. If there is no obvious cancer, colposcopy (examination of the vagina and cervix with a magnifying lens) can be used to identify areas that require biopsy. Colposcopy-directed biopsy is usually diagnostic. If not, cone biopsy (conization) is required; a cone of tissue is removed using a loop electrical excision procedure (LEEP), laser, or cold knife.

Staging: Cancers are clinically staged based on biopsy, physical examination, and chest x-ray results (see TABLE 254–5). If the stage is > IB1, CT or MRI of the abdomen and pelvis is also typically done to identify metastases, although results are not used for staging. Cystoscopy, sigmoidoscopy, and IV urography, when clinically indicated, may also be used for staging.

TABLE 254–4. BETHESDA CLASSIFICATION OF CERVICAL CYTOLOGY*

CATEGORY	SPECIFICS	COMMENT
Specimen type	Pap test, thin-layer (liquid-based), or other	Type of test is noted
Adequacy of the specimen	Satisfactory for evaluation	Any quality indicators (eg, endocervical/transformation zone component, partially obscuring blood, inflammation) are described
	Evaluated but unsatisfactory	Reason is specified
	Rejected for evaluation	Reason is specified
General categorization (optional)	Negative for intraepithelial lesion or cancer Epithelial cell abnormalities Other abnormalities	Findings are stated or described under Interpretation
Interpretation of negative (nonmalignant) abnormalities	Organisms	Possible findings include the following: *Trichomonas vaginalis* Fungi morphologically consistent with *Candida* sp Predominance of coccobacilli consistent with shift in vaginal flora suggesting bacterial vaginosis Bacteria morphologically consistent with *Actinomyces* sp Cellular changes associated with herpes simplex virus
	Other (reporting is optional)	Possible findings include the following: Reactive cellular changes associated with inflammation, radiation, or IUD use Presence of glandular cells after hysterectomy Atrophy
Interpretation of epithelial cell abnormalities	Squamous cell	Possible findings include the following: Atypical squamous cells of undetermined significance (ASC-US) Atypical squamous cells for which a high-grade lesion cannot be excluded (ASC-H) Low-grade squamous intraepithelial lesion encompassing HPV† infection or mild dysplasia (CIN 1) High-grade squamous intraepithelial lesion encompassing moderate (CIN 2) and severe dysplasia (CIN 3/CIS); whether the lesion has features suggesting invasion is noted Squamous cell carcinoma

TABLE 254–4. BETHESDA CLASSIFICATION OF CERVICAL CYTOLOGY*—Continued

CATEGORY	SPECIFICS	COMMENT
	Glandular cell	Possible findings include the following: Atypical cells: endocervical, endometrial, or glandular Atypical cells likely to be cancerous: endocervical or glandular Adenocarcinoma in situ: endocervical Adenocarcinoma: endocervical, endometrial, extrauterine, or NOS
Interpretation of other abnormalities	Endometrial cells (in a woman > 40)	Whether sample is negative for squamous intraepithelial lesion is specified
Other cancers	———	Type is specified

*Use of automated device for scanning should be reported, as should other tests (eg, HPV) and their results.

†Cellular changes of HPV infection—previously called koilocytosis, koilocytotic atypia, and condylomatous atypia—are included in the category of low-grade squamous intraepithelial lesion.

IUD = intrauterine device; HPV = human papillomavirus; CIN = cervical intraepithelial neoplasia; CIS = carcinoma in situ; NOS = not otherwise specified.

Adapted from the Bethesda System 2001, National Institutes of Health. www.bethesda2001.cancer.gov/terminology.html

When imaging tests suggest that pelvic or para-aortic lymph nodes are grossly enlarged (> 2 cm), surgical exploration, typically with a retroperitoneal approach, is occasionally indicated. Its sole purpose is to remove enlarged lymph nodes.

Prognosis and Treatment

In squamous cell carcinoma, distant metastases usually occur only when the cancer is advanced or recurrent. The 5-yr survival rates are 80 to 90% with stage I, 50 to 65% with stage II, 25 to 35% with stage III, and 0 to 15% with stage IV. Nearly 80% of recurrences manifest within 2 yr. Adverse prognostic factors include lymph node involvement, large tumor size and volume, deep cervical stromal invasion, parametrial invasion, vascular space invasion, and nonsquamous histology.

For patients with CIN or squamous cell carcinoma stage IA1, cone biopsy with LEEP, laser, or cold knife is usually sufficient treatment. Uncommonly, a hysterectomy is required.

If hysterectomy is done for stage IA1 cancer, simple (extrafascial) hysterectomy is usually sufficient when no adverse prognostic factors (nonsquamous histology or lymphatic or vascular invasion) are present because risk of recurrence and lymph node metastasis is < 1%. Pelvic lymph node dissection is not indicated. However, if adverse prognostic factors are present, radical hysterectomy is typically required; it includes bilateral pelvic lymphadenectomy and removal of all adjacent ligaments (cardinal, uterosacral) and parametria and the upper 2 cm of the vagina.

For stage IA2 to IIA, treatment may involve a radical hysterectomy or pelvic radiation therapy with concurrent chemotherapy. The 5-yr cure rates in stage IB or IIA are 85 to 90% with either treatment. Surgery provides additional staging data and preserves the ovaries. If extracervical spread is noted during surgery, postoperative radiation therapy may prevent local recurrence.

For patients with stage IIB to IVA cancer, radiation therapy is more suitable as primary therapy; radiation is also used for poor surgical candidates who would otherwise require hysterectomy. Surgical staging should be considered to determine whether para-aortic lymph nodes are involved and thus whether extended-field radiation therapy is indicated; a retroperitoneal approach is used. External beam radiation therapy shrinks the central tumor and treats regional lymph nodes; this therapy is followed by brachytherapy (local radioactive implants, usually using cesium)

TABLE 254–5. CLINICAL STAGING OF CERVICAL CARCINOMA*

STAGE	DESCRIPTION
0	Carcinoma in situ (CIN 3), intraepithelial carcinoma
I	Carcinoma strictly confined to the cervix (extension to the corpus should be disregarded)
IA	Preclinical carcinoma (diagnosed only by microscopy, with a depth of invasion < 5 mm from the surface)†
IA1	Measured invasion of stroma ≤ 3 mm in depth and ≤ 7 mm in width
IA2	Measured invasion of stroma > 3 mm and ≤ 5 mm in depth and ≤ 7 mm in width
IB	Clinically visible lesions confined to the cervix or preclinical lesions larger than those in stage IA2
IB1	Clinically visible lesions ≤ 4 cm
IB2	Clinically visible lesions > 4 cm
II	Extension beyond the cervix but not to the pelvic wall; involvement of the vagina but excluding the lower ⅓
IIA	No obvious parametrial involvement
IIB	Obvious parametrial involvement
III	Extension to the pelvic wall, with rectal examination detecting no cancer-free space between the tumor and pelvic wall; involvement of the lower ⅓ of the vagina; all cases with hydronephrosis or with a nonfunctioning kidney secondary to the carcinoma
IIIA	Extension to lower ⅓ of the vagina but not to the pelvic wall
IIIB	Extension to the pelvic wall, hydronephrosis, or a nonfunctioning kidney
IV	Extension beyond the true pelvis or clinical involvement of the bladder or rectal mucosa (bullous edema does not signify stage IV)
IVA	Spread to adjacent pelvic organs
IVB	Spread to distant organs

*Based on staging established by the International Federation of Gynecology and Obstetrics (FIGO) and American Joint Committee on Cancer (AJCC), 1995, 1996, 1997.

†Depth of invasion should be measured from the base of the epithelium (surface or glandular) from which it originates. Vascular space involvement (venous or lymphatic) should not alter staging.

to the cervix, which destroys the central tumor. Acute complications of radiation therapy (eg, radiation proctitis and cystitis) may occur. Occasionally, late complications (eg, vaginal stenosis, intestinal obstruction, rectovaginal and vesicovaginal fistula formation) occur.

For stages IIB to IVA, chemotherapy is usually given with radiation therapy, often to sensitize the tumor to radiation. Treatment is often ineffective for bulky and advanced-stage tumors.

Although stage IVA cancers are usually treated with radiation therapy initially, pelvic exenteration (excision of all pelvic organs) may be considered. If after radiation therapy, cancer remains but is confined to the central pelvis, exenteration is indicated and cures up to 50% of patients. The procedure may include a continent urostomy, low anterior rectal anastomosis without colostomy, omental carpet to close the pelvic floor (J-flap), and vaginal reconstruction with gracilis or rectus abdominis myocutaneous flaps.

For widely metastatic or recurrent cancer, chemotherapy is the primary treatment, but the resulting response is brief and occurs in only 15 to 25% of patients. Cisplatin is the most active drug and the current standard. Paclitaxel, topotecan, gemcitabine, and vinorelbine are under study for treatment of recurrent squamous cell carcinoma. Paclitaxel is also used to treat recurrent or metastatic nonsquamous cancer. Metastases outside the radiation field appear to respond better to chemotherapy than does previously irradiated pelvic cancer.

Prevention

Routine cervical Pap tests are recommended yearly, starting the year of 1st sexual intercourse or by age 18. Pap test and HPV test can be done simultaneously. If both are normal or if 3 consecutive Pap tests are normal, some physicians test at 2- to 3-yr intervals. Testing continues until patients are age 65 to 70, have normal results for 10 yr, or have a hysterectomy. Vaccination against HPV to prevent cervical cancer is under study. Sexually active women are advised that condoms should be used during intercourse to prevent spread of HPV.

VAGINAL CANCER

Vaginal cancer is usually a squamous cell carcinoma, most often occurring in women > 60. The most common symptom is abnormal vaginal bleeding. Diagnosis is by biopsy. Treatment for many small localized cancers is hysterectomy plus vaginectomy and lymph node dissection; radiation therapy is used for most others.

Vaginal cancer accounts for 1% of gynecologic cancers in the US. Average age at diagnosis is 60 to 65. Risk factors include human papillomavirus infection and cervical or vulvar cancer. Exposure to diethylstilbestrol in utero predisposes to clear cell adenocarcinoma of the vagina, which is rare; mean age at diagnosis is 19.

Most (95%) primary vaginal cancers are squamous cell carcinomas; others include primary and secondary adenocarcinomas, secondary squamous cell carcinomas (in older women), clear cell adenocarcinomas (in young women), and melanomas. The most common vaginal sarcoma, sarcoma botryoides (embryonal rhabdomyosarcoma), has a peak incidence at age 3.

Most vaginal cancers occur in the upper ⅓ of the posterior vaginal wall. They may spread by direct extension (into the local paravaginal tissues, bladder, or rectum), through inguinal lymph nodes from lesions in the lower vagina, through pelvic lymph nodes from lesions in the upper vagina, or hematogenously.

Symptoms and Signs

Most patients present with abnormal vaginal bleeding: postmenopausal, postcoital, or intermenstrual. Some also present with a watery vaginal discharge or dyspareunia. A few patients are asymptomatic, and the lesion is discovered during routine pelvic examination or evaluation of an abnormal Pap test. Vesicovaginal or rectovaginal fistulas are manifestations of advanced disease.

Diagnosis

Punch biopsy is usually diagnostic, but wide local excision is occasionally necessary. Cancers are staged clinically, based primarily on physical examination, endoscopy (ie, cystoscopy, proctoscopy), chest x-ray (for pulmonary metastases), and usually CT (for abdominal or pelvic metastases). Stage 0 is carcinoma in situ. Stage I tumors are limited to the vaginal wall. Stage II tumors involve subvaginal tissue. Stage III tumors extend to the pelvic wall. Stage IV tumors extend beyond the true pelvis or involve the bladder or rectal mucosa.

Prognosis and Treatment

The 5-yr survival rates are 65 to 70% with stage I, 47% with stage II, 30% with stage III, and 15 to 20% with stage IV. Prognosis is worse if the primary tumor is large or poorly differentiated.

Stage 0 tumors are treated with wide local excision only. Stage I tumors within the upper ⅓ of the vagina can be treated with radical hysterectomy, upper vaginectomy, and pelvic lymph node dissection. Most other primary tumors are treated with radiation therapy, usually a combination of external beam and brachytherapy. If radiation therapy is contraindicated because of vesicovaginal or rectovaginal fistulas, pelvic exenteration is done.

VULVAR CANCER

Vulvar cancer is usually a squamous cell skin cancer, most often occurring in elderly women. It usually manifests as a palpable

lesion. Diagnosis is by biopsy. Treatment includes excision and inguinal and femoral lymph node dissection.

Vulvar cancer accounts for about 3 to 4% of gynecologic cancers in the US. Average age at diagnosis is about 70, and incidence increases with age. Risk factors include vulvar intraepithelial neoplasia (VIN), human papillomavirus infection, heavy cigarette smoking, lichen sclerosus, squamous hyperplasia, squamous carcinoma of vagina or cervix, and chronic granulomatous diseases.

Pathology

VIN is a precursor to vulvar cancer. VIN may be multifocal. Sometimes adenocarcinoma of the vulva, breast, or Bartholin's glands also develops.

About 90% of vulvar cancers are squamous cell carcinomas; about 5% are melanomas. Others include adenocarcinomas and transitional cell, adenoid cystic, and adenosquamous carcinomas; all may originate in Bartholin's glands. Sarcomas and basal cell carcinomas with underlying adenocarcinoma also occur.

Vulvar cancer may spread by direct extension (eg, into the urethra, bladder, vagina, perineum, anus, or rectum), hematogenously, to the inguinal lymph nodes, or from the inguinal lymph nodes to the pelvic and para-aortic lymph nodes.

Symptoms and Signs

The most common presentation is a palpable vulvar lesion, frequently noticed by the woman or by a clinician during pelvic examination. Women often have a long history of pruritus. They may not present until cancer is advanced. The lesion may become necrotic or ulcerated, sometimes resulting in bleeding or a watery vaginal discharge. Melanomas may appear bluish black, pigmented, or papillary.

Diagnosis

Vulvar cancer may mimic sexually transmitted genital ulcers (see TABLE 194–2 on p. 1660), basal cell carcinoma, vulvar Paget's disease (a pale eczematoid lesion), Bartholin's gland cyst, or condyloma acuminatum. A dermal punch biopsy using a local anesthetic is usually diagnostic. Occasionally, wide local excision is necessary to differentiate VIN from cancer. Subtle lesions may be delineated by staining the vulva with toluidine blue or by using colposcopy.

Staging: Staging is based on tumor size and location and on regional lymph node spread as determined by lymph node dissection done as part of initial surgical treatment. Stage I tumors are ≤ 2 cm in all dimensions and confined to the vulva or perineum without nodal metastases. Stage II is the same except tumors are > 2 cm in any dimension. Stage III tumors spread to the adjacent lower urethra, vagina, or anus or metastasize to unilateral regional lymph nodes. Stage IV tumors invade the upper urethra, bladder mucosa, intestinal or rectal mucosa, pelvic bone, bilateral lymph nodes, or other distant tissues.

Prognosis and Treatment

Overall 5-yr survival rates are > 90% with stage I, 80% with stage II, 50 to 60% with stage III, and 15% with stage IV. Risk of lymph node spread is proportional to the tumor size and invasion depth. Melanomas metastasize frequently, depending mostly on invasion depth but also on tumor size.

Wide (≥ 2-cm margin) radical excision of the local tumor and a unilateral or bilateral inguinal and femoral lymph node dissection is necessary for cancers of all stages and is sufficient for stages I and II. For lateralized lesions ≤ 2 cm, unilateral hemivulvectomy and unilateral lymph node dissection can be used. Lesions near the midline and most lesions > 2 cm require bilateral lymph node dissection.

For stage III, lymph node dissection followed by postoperative external beam radiation therapy, often with chemotherapy (eg, 5-fluorouracil, cisplatin), is usually done before wide radical excision. The alternative is more radical or exenterative surgery. For stage IV, treatment is some combination of pelvic exenteration, radiation therapy, and systemic chemotherapy.

255 FAMILY PLANNING

A couple's decision to begin, prevent, or interrupt a pregnancy may be influenced by many medical factors, including maternal medical disorders, risks involved in pregnancy, and genetic evaluation. Often, religious, social, and other factors also affect family planning decisions; health care practitioners must be sensitive to these factors.

One or both members of a couple can use contraception to prevent pregnancy temporarily or sterilization to prevent pregnancy permanently. If contraception fails, abortion (termination of pregnancy) can be induced.

CONTRACEPTION

The contraceptive methods most commonly used in the US are (in order of popularity) oral contraceptives, condoms, withdrawal (coitus interruptus), periodic abstinence, progestin injections, spermicides, diaphragms, progestin subdermal implants, and intrauterine devices (IUDs). Over several years, pregnancy rates are < 1%/yr with methods unrelated to coitus (oral contraceptives, IUDs, progestin injections, subdermal progestin implants) and about 5%/yr with coitus-related methods (eg, condoms, diaphragms, spermicides, withdrawal); pregnancy rates tend to be higher during the 1st year, then decrease in later years as users become more facile and women's fertility decreases. In contrast, the pregnancy rate is 90%/1 yr with frequent, unprotected intercourse. Condoms are often preferred despite their relatively high failure rate because they protect against sexually transmitted diseases, especially HIV. Emergency contraception, done postcoitus, should not be used as a regular method of contraception.

ORAL CONTRACEPTIVES

Oral contraceptives (OCs) simulate ovarian hormones: They provide negative feedback to the hypothalamus; its release of gonadotropin-releasing hormone is inhibited, thus inhibiting pituitary release of the gonadotropins that stimulate ovulation. The endometrium becomes thin, and cervical mucus becomes thick and impervious to sperm.

An OC may be a combination of an estrogen and a progestin or a progestin alone. Most combination formulations are taken daily for 3 wk, then not taken during the 4th wk to allow for withdrawal bleeding. However, one formulation is taken daily for 12 wk, then not taken during the 13th wk, so that withdrawal bleeding occurs only 4 times/yr. Progestin alone is taken daily, often results in irregular bleeding, and may be less effective than combination OCs; progestin alone is not used unless estrogen is contraindicated—eg, during breastfeeding.

Combination formulations have similar efficacy; the pregnancy rate after 1 yr is < 0.3% with perfect use and about 8% with typical (ie, inconsistent) use. Low-dose formulations (20 to 35 μg of estrogen) are usually preferred to higher-dose formulations (50 μg of estrogen) because low-dose formulations appear equally effective and, except for a higher incidence of bleeding during the 1st few months of use, have fewer adverse effects.

Intermittently stopping OCs appears to have no benefit, so OCs can be taken continuously until menopause, which is indicated by an elevated follicle-stimulating hormone level. Combination OCs are not prescribed for women > 35 who smoke cigarettes or have other contraindications (see TABLE 255–1).

Adverse effects: OCs may cause breakthrough bleeding, which may resolve when the estrogen dose is increased, or amenorrhea, which may resolve when the progestin dose is decreased. In a few women, ovulation remains inhibited for a few months after they stop taking OCs. OCs do not adversely affect the outcome of pregnancy when conception occurs during or after their use.

Estrogens increase aldosterone production and cause Na retention, which can produce dose-related, reversible increases in BP and weight, up to about 2 kg; weight gain may be accompanied by bloating, edema, and breast tenderness. Most progestins used in OCs are related to 19-nortestosterone and are androgenic; norgestimate and desogestrel are less androgenic than levonorgestrel, norethindrone, norethindrone acetate, and ethynodiol diacetate. Androgenic effects may include acne, nervousness, and an anabolic effect resulting in weight gain. If a woman gains > 4.5 kg/yr, a less androgenic OC should be used. Drospirenone, a new progestin, is

TABLE 255–1. CONTRAINDICATIONS TO ORAL CONTRACEPTIVE USE

DEGREE	CONDITION
Absolute	Diabetes mellitus with vascular changes
	History of estrogen-dependent cancer, coronary artery disease, hepatic adenoma, idiopathic recurrent jaundice of pregnancy, stroke, thromboembolism, or deep venous thrombosis
	Hypertension if uncontrolled
	Immobilization of a lower extremity if prolonged and 1 mo before and after elective surgery
	Liver disorders if active
	Pregnancy
	Smoking after age 35
Relative	Amenorrhea with an undiagnosed cause
	Cigarette smoking if heavy in women < 35
	Depression
	Migraines with neurologic symptoms

related to spironolactone, not 19-nortestosterone; it is antiandrogenic and diuretic.

Incidence of deep vein thrombophlebitis and thromboembolism increases in relation to estrogen dose; formulations with 20 to 35 μg increase risk to about 3 to 4 times normal (but risk is still only about ½ the incidence during pregnancy). Varicose veins do not appear to further increase risk. Hypercoagulability is probably caused by increases in blood-clotting factors, particularly VII and X, and possibly increased platelet adhesion. If deep vein thrombophlebitis or pulmonary embolism is suspected, OCs should be stopped, pending results of diagnostic tests. OCs should be stopped 1 mo before elective major surgery and should not be restarted until 1 mo after major surgery.

Overall risk of breast cancer is slightly increased in women < 35 while they are taking OCs and for up to 10 yr after they stop. However, risk is not further increased in high-risk subgroups (eg, women with certain benign breast disorders or a family history of breast cancer). Also, in current and former OC users, risk of nonlocalized breast cancer is decreased. Risk of cervical cancer, mainly adenocarcinoma, is increased, particularly in women who have used OCs for > 5 yr; the reason is unknown. However, risk of cervical intraepithelial neoplasia, the precursor of cervical cancer, is not increased. Nonetheless, OC users should have an annual Papanicolaou (Pap) test.

CNS effects of OCs include nausea, vomiting, headache, depression, and sleep disturbances. Although increased stroke risk has been attributed to OCs, low-dose combination OCs do not appear to increase risk in healthy, normotensive, nonsmoking women. Nonetheless, if focal neurologic symptoms, aphasia, or other symptoms that may herald stroke develop, OCs should be stopped.

Although progestins may cause reversible, dose-related insulin resistance, use of current OCs, which have a low progestin dose, rarely results in hyperglycemia. Serum high density lipoprotein (HDL) cholesterol levels may decrease when OCs with a high progestin dose are used but usually increase when OCs with low progestin and estrogen doses are used. Most alterations in serum levels of other metabolites are not clinically significant. Thyroxine-binding globulin capacity may increase; free thyroxine levels, thyroid-stimulating hormone levels, and thyroid function are not affected. Levels of pyridoxine, folate, most other B vitamins, ascorbic acid, Ca, manganese, and zinc decrease; vitamin A levels increase.

OCs accelerate formation of existing gallstones but do not cause new stones to form. Thus, incidence of cholelithiasis increases during the 1st few years of OC use, then decreases. Women who develop idiopathic recurrent jaundice of pregnancy (cholestasis of pregnancy) may become jaundiced if they take OCs and should not use them. Rarely, benign hepatic adenomas that can rupture spontaneously develop. Incidence increases as duration of use and OC dose increase; adenomas usually regress spontaneously after the OC is stopped.

Melasma occurs in some women; it is accentuated by sunlight and disappears slowly after OCs are stopped. Because treatment is difficult (see p. 1003), OCs are stopped when melasma first appears. OCs do not increase risk of malignant melanoma.

Benefits: OCs decrease risk of endometrial and ovarian cancers by about 50% for

≥ 20 yr after OCs are stopped. They also decrease risk of benign ovarian tumors, abnormal uterine bleeding, dysmenorrhea, premenstrual syndrome, iron deficiency anemia, benign breast disorders, and functional ovarian cysts. Ectopic pregnancy and salpingitis, which can impair fertility, are also less likely.

Drug interactions: Although OCs can slow the metabolism of certain drugs (eg, meperidine), the effects are not clinically important.

Some drugs (eg, cyclophosphamide, rifampin) can induce liver enzymes that accelerate transformation of OCs to less biologically active metabolites; women who take these drugs should not be given OCs concurrently. Whether certain antibiotics (eg, penicillin, ampicillin, sulfonamides) and anticonvulsants (eg, phenytoin, phenobarbital) reduce the effectiveness of OCs is less clear. If therapeutic doses of antibiotics are prescribed, using a barrier method in addition to OCs may be prudent. Women who take anticonvulsants should use a 50-μg estrogen formulation because a lower dose often causes breakthrough bleeding.

Administration: Before OCs are started and annually thereafter, breast and pelvic examinations, liver palpation, and measurement of BP and weight are necessary. BP is also measured 3 mo after starting OCs. A Pap test is not routinely necessary for young women unless they are sexually active. If a woman has a history of a liver disorder, normal liver function must be documented before OCs are prescribed. Women at risk of diabetes (eg, those who have a family history or who have had high-birth-weight infants or unexplained fetal deaths in previous pregnancies) require annual blood glucose screening and a complete serum lipid profile (repeated annually if results are abnormal). Use of low-dose OCs is not contraindicated by abnormal glucose or lipid test results, except for triglycerides > 250 mg/dL.

When to start OCs after pregnancy is guided by when ovulation is expected. After an abortion, ovulation usually occurs after 2 to 4 wk and before the 1st menses; older gestational age predicts later ovulation. In women who have a term delivery and are not breastfeeding, ovulation can occasionally occur as early as 4 wk after delivery but usually not until after menses. In women who are breastfeeding, ovulation usually occurs ≥ 10 to 12 wk after delivery and after menses. After spontaneous or induced abortion of a fetus < 12 wk gestation, OCs are started immediately. If the fetus is 12 to 28 wk gestation, OCs are delayed 1 wk. If women deliver after 28 wk and are not breastfeeding, combination OCs are delayed 2 wk because they may enhance risk of thromboembolism, which normally increases postpartum. For women who are breastfeeding, progestin-only OCs are preferred because OCs that contain estrogen reduce the amount of milk produced as well as the protein and fat concentration in milk; progestin-only OCs are started a few days after delivery because they are not thrombogenic.

Barrier Contraceptives

Condom use is the only reversible male method other than withdrawal, which is probably much less effective. Condoms decrease risk of sexually transmitted diseases (only latex condoms can fully protect against HIV) and may prevent precancerous changes in the cervix. The condom is applied before penetration; the tip should extend about 1 cm beyond the penis to collect the ejaculate. During removal, care is taken to avoid spilling condom contents. A new condom is used for each act of coitus. Pregnancy rates in the 1st yr are 2% with perfect use but 15% with typical (ie, inconsistent) use. Adding a spermicide, which may be included in the condom's lubricant or inserted into the vagina, may lower these rates.

The diaphragm, a dome-shaped rubber cup with a flexible rim that fits over the cervix, is a barrier to sperm. Diaphragms are made in various sizes. A health care practitioner fits a diaphragm to a woman so that it is comfortable for her and her partner. After childbirth or a significant weight change, the woman is refitted. The diaphragm should remain in place for > 8 h after the last coitus. Spermicides should be used before each coitus in case the diaphragm is displaced. Pregnancy rates in the 1st yr are about 6% with perfect use but about 16% with typical use.

The cervical cap resembles the diaphragm but is smaller and more rigid. It comes in several sizes and is fitted by a health care practitioner. It can be left in place for 48 h. For nulliparous women, pregnancy rates in the 1st yr are 9% with perfect use and about 18% with typical use. Pregnancy rates for parous women are about twice as high because obtaining a secure fit is difficult.

Vaginal foams, creams, and suppositories provide a physical barrier to sperm and contain a spermicide, usually nonoxynol-9. They are combined with other barrier methods and are placed in the vagina before each coitus. These products appear to have similar efficacy. The contraceptive sponge, previously off the market, is once again available.

Periodic Abstinence

(Natural Family Planning)

Although the ovum can be fertilized for only a few hours after ovulation, sperm can fertilize an ovum for up to 5 days after coitus. Thus, periodic abstinence requires abstinence from coitus during the 5 days before ovulation. Ovulation occurs about 14 days before onset of menses.

The calendar rhythm method aims to predict ovulation solely by menstrual dates; this method is often inaccurate, even when menstrual cycles are regular. Duration of abstinence is determined by subtracting 18 days from the shortest of the previous 12 cycles and 11 days from the longest. For example, if cycles vary between 26 and 29 days, abstinence is required from days 8 through 18 of each cycle. The greater the variance in cycle length, the longer abstinence lasts.

Methods that incorporate better predictors of ovulation are more effective but require training and effort. Basal body temperature (measured daily before arising) increases by about 0.5° C, usually to > 37° C, after ovulation. Abstinence is required for > 72 h after the temperature increase. An increased amount of cervical mucus more accurately indicates ovulation. Coitus is restricted to every other day (so that semen is not confused with mucus) and is avoided completely from the time mucus quantity increases until 4 days after the quantity peaks. The symptothermal method relies on the combination of increase in temperature, appearance of cervical mucus, and symptoms of ovulation (eg, breast tenderness, bloating). Intercourse is avoided from the time cervical mucus appears watery until after temperature increases. It is the most effective method of periodic abstinence but still has a pregnancy rate of about 10%/yr.

Progestin Injections

Depot medroxyprogesterone acetate (DMPA) is a long-acting injectable formulation of medroxyprogesterone acetate. Pregnancy rates at 1 yr are 0.3% with perfect use and are slightly higher with typical use (ie, delays between injections).

To prevent ovulation, the injection must be given during the 1st 5 days of the menstrual cycle. The dose is 150 mg q 3 mo by deep gluteal or deltoid IM injection. The injection site is not massaged, ensuring slow absorption; levels are usually effective from 24 h to > 4 mo after injection. However, if the interval between injections is > 13 wk, a negative pregnancy test is required before giving the next injection.

The most common adverse effect is disruption of the menstrual cycle. In the 3 mo after the 1st DMPA injection, about 30% of women have amenorrhea. Another 30% have spotting or irregular bleeding (usually light) > 11 days/mo; anemia does not usually result. As use continues, bleeding and menses tend to decrease; after 2 yr, about 70% of women receiving DMPA have amenorrhea. Because DMPA has a long duration of action, ovulation may be delayed for up to 1 yr after the last injection; after ovulation occurs, fertility is usually rapidly restored.

Women typically gain 1.5 to 4 kg in the 1st yr of DMPA use and continue to gain weight thereafter. Usually, women who want to take DMPA are advised to decrease caloric intake and increase energy expenditure. Headache is a common reason for stopping DMPA; however, DMPA does not appear to increase incidence or severity of common headaches (eg, tension headaches, migraines). Mild, reversible, clinically insignificant deterioration of glucose tolerance and lipid profile may occur. Whether bone density is decreased is unclear; adolescents and young women using DMPA should ingest 1500 mg of Ca and 400 units of vitamin D daily. Unlike OCs, DMPA does not contribute to hypertension or thromboembolism.

DMPA does not appear to increase risk of breast, ovarian, or invasive cervical cancer. DMPA reduces risk of endometrial cancer and pelvic inflammatory disease. By stimulating erythropoiesis, DMPA reduces risk of iron deficiency anemia and, among women with sickle cell disease, risks of anemia and crises.

In the US, DMPA will soon be available in a low-dose (104-mg) sc formulation. Efficacy and safety are similar to those of IM injection, and the sc formulation may be better tolerated.

Transdermal and Intravaginal Steroid Contraceptives

A 20-cm^2 transdermal patch can deliver 150 µg of the progestin norelgestromin (the active metabolite of norgestimate) and 20 µg of ethinyl estradiol daily into the systemic circulation for 7 days; then, the patch is removed, and a new patch is applied to a different area of the skin. Steroid blood levels are much more constant than with OCs. After 3 patches, no patch is used for the 4th wk to allow withdrawal bleeding. Overall contraceptive efficacy, incidence of bleeding, and adverse effects are similar to those of OCs, but adherence may be better. The patch may be more likely to fail in overweight women.

Use of a flexible vaginal ring containing ethinyl estradiol and the progestin etonogestrel, which are absorbed through the vaginal epithelium, provides relatively constant blood levels. The ring is 58 mm in diameter and 4 mm thick. It is inserted and removed by the woman; it is left in place for 3 wk, then removed for 1 wk to allow withdrawal bleeding. Bleeding with the ring in place is uncommon. Contraceptive efficacy and adverse effects are similar to those of OCs, and adherence may be better.

Subdermal Implants

Progestin subdermal implants are available in some countries but not in the US. Polysiloxane capsules containing levonorgestrel are inserted subcutaneously through a small incision in the upper arm after a local anesthetic is used. Capsules are effective for 5 yr and are then removed. The cumulative pregnancy rate with one implantation is about 1% at 5 yr. A new, single-rod implant that releases etonogestrel at a rate of 50 μg/day is available in several countries. The implant provides excellent contraception for 3 yr.

The most common adverse effects are similar to those of other progestins (uterine bleeding, amenorrhea, headache, weight gain). Removing the capsules can be difficult because of surrounding fibrosis. After capsule removal, ovarian activity normalizes immediately.

Intrauterine Devices

Only about 1 million women in the US use intrauterine devices (IUDs), despite their advantages over OCs: IUDs are highly effective, have no systemic effects, and require only 1 contraceptive decision. IUDs induce endometrial inflammation, which attracts neutrophils; they render sperm ineffective. Persistent endometrial inflammation may prevent implantation if fertilization occurs, but if implantation occurs, an IUD does not cause abortion.

In the US, the levonorgestrel-releasing IUD (effective for 5 yr; cumulative pregnancy rate of 0.5%) and the copper-bearing T380A (effective for ≥ 10 yr; cumulative pregnancy rate of < 2%) are used. IUDs are inserted high in the fundus at any time during the cycle. Contraindications include pregnancy and untreated cervicitis or vaginitis. After IUD removal, fertility rate is normal after about 1 yr.

Adverse effects: During the 1st yr, 10 to 15% of women stop use; fewer stop thereafter. Of those who stop, > 50% do so because of bleeding and pain, which occur in about 15% of users during the 1st yr and 7% during the 2nd yr. Bleeding stops completely within 1 yr in 20%.

Spontaneous expulsion occurs in about 10% during the 1st yr (usually within the 1st few weeks) and in fewer women thereafter. Expulsion is more common among younger women and among nulligravidas. If another IUD is inserted, it is usually retained. Because about 20% of expulsions are unnoticed, a plastic string is attached to the IUD so that the user can check for its presence periodically.

Uterine perforation occurs in about 1/1000. Sometimes only the distal portion of the IUD penetrates; then over the next few months, uterine contractions force the IUD into the peritoneal cavity. Perforation is considered if a woman cannot feel the string but did not notice expulsion. If the string is not visible during pelvic examination, the uterine cavity is probed with a sound or biopsy instrument unless pregnancy is suspected. If the IUD cannot be felt, ultrasonography is done. If the IUD is not seen, an abdominal x-ray is taken to exclude intraperitoneal location. Intraperitoneal IUDs may cause intestinal adhesions. IUDs that have perforated the uterus are removed, often via laparoscopy.

Occasionally, salpingitis develops during the 1st mo because of contamination during insertion; risk is not high enough to warrant routine antibiotic prophylaxis. IUD strings do not provide access for bacteria. Pelvic infections that occur after 1 mo are sexually transmitted; unless severe, they can be treated with the IUD in place.

Intrauterine pregnancy that occurs with an IUD in place has an increased risk of spontaneous abortion (about 55%) and preterm delivery but not of congenital defects, fetal death, or pelvic infection during pregnancy. Risk of abortion decreases to 20% if the IUD is removed. IUDs decrease the absolute risk of ectopic pregnancy (by about 20 times). Nonetheless, if a woman becomes pregnant with an IUD in place, ectopic pregnancy, which occurs in about 5% of such pregnancies, must be ruled out (see p. 2192).

IUDs do not increase and may decrease risk of endometrial adenocarcinoma and cervical carcinoma.

Emergency Contraception

Emergency contraception is use of contraceptive hormones within 72 h of unprotected coitus. With emergency contraception, the pregnancy rate for a single act of unprotected coitus at midcycle decreases from about 8% to about 2%. The most commonly used regimen is 2 doses of levonorgestrel 0.75 mg taken 12 h apart. A single dose of mifepristone 600 mg (RU 486, a progesterone-receptor blocker) may be slightly more effective and may cause fewer adverse effects. Taking levonorgestrel 1.5 mg once seems to be equally effective. Another regimen—2 tablets, each containing ethinyl estradiol 50 μg and norgestrel 0.5 mg, followed by 2 more tablets 12 h later—has been used. The high estrogen load often causes nausea and may cause vomiting.

Inserting an IUD within 10 days of coitus is more expensive but more effective than hormone tablets; pregnancy rate is 0.1%.

STERILIZATION

In the US, $^1/_3$ of couples attempting to prevent pregnancy, particularly if the woman is > 30, choose sterilization with vasectomy or tubal ligation. Sterilization should be assumed to be permanent. However, reanastomosis and restoration of fertility is possible in 45 to 60% of men after vasectomy and in 50 to 80% of women after tubal ligation.

Vasectomy: The vasa deferentia are cut, and the cut ends are ligated or fulgurated. Vasectomy can be done in about 20 min with use of a local anesthetic. Sterility requires about 15 to 20 ejaculations after the operation and should be documented by 2 sperm-free ejaculates. Complications of vasectomy include hematoma (≤ 5%), sperm granulomas (inflammatory responses to sperm leakage), and spontaneous reanastomosis, which usually occurs shortly after the procedure.

Tubal ligation: The fallopian tubes are cut, and a segment is excised or the tubes are closed by ligation, fulguration, or various mechanical devices (plastic bands, spring-loaded clips). Sterilization using mechanical devices causes less tissue damage and thus may be more reversible. Via laparoscopy, tubal ligation can be done using a small periumbilical incision and a general or local anesthetic. Tubal ligation is often done immediately after or the day after delivery.

Microinserts with inner coils can be inserted via hysteroscopy to occlude the tubes. This procedure does not require incisions or cutting, clipping, or burning of the tubes.

Tubal occlusion, and thus sterility, is confirmed by hysterosalpingography done about 3 mo after the procedure. Pregnancy rates after successful occlusion are < 0.5% during the 1st yr and 1.5 to 2% after 10 yr. Rates are lower if the tube has been partly excised. With tubal ligation, mortality occurs in a few cases per 100,000, hemorrhage or intestinal injuries occur in about 0.5%, and other complications (eg, infarction, failure of occlusion) occur in up to about 5%. About 30% of pregnancies that occur after tubal ligation are ectopic.

INDUCED ABORTION

Induced abortion is legally available to about $^2/_3$ of women worldwide. In the US, abortion is legal in the 1st trimester (≤ 12 wk); after that, legality varies by state. In the US, about $^1/_2$ of pregnancies are unintended; about $^1/_2$ of these are terminated by elective abortion, with 90% during the 1st trimester.

Common methods of inducing abortion are instrumental evacuation through the vagina and medical induction (stimulation of uterine contractions). Uterine surgery (hysterotomy or hysterectomy) is a last resort that is usually avoided because mortality rates are higher. Hysterotomy also results in a uterine scar, which may rupture in subsequent pregnancies.

Gestational age, which usually dictates abortion method, is usually established by ultrasonography. $Rh_0(D)$ immune globulin, when indicated, is given to women with Rh-negative blood to prevent sensitization (see under Blood Products on p. 1136 and Erythroblastosis Fetalis on p. 2194). First-trimester abortions often require only local anesthesia; later abortions sometimes require general anesthesia.

Instrumental evacuation: Instrumental evacuation is used in 97% of all abortions and in virtually 100% of surgical abortions in pregnancies of < 12 wk.

At 4 to 6 wk, the uterus can be curetted gently via a cannula attached to a vacuum source. Because failure to terminate the pregnancy is more common in early than in later weeks, instrumental evacuation should usually not be done until a gestational sac is seen. Before this time, abortion is usually induced medically.

At 7 to 12 wk, dilation and curettage (D & C) is usually used; large-diameter suction cannulas are usually required, so the cervix must be dilated. Typically, progressively increasing sizes of tapered dilators are used. Cervical damage due to dilation can be prevented or minimized by using laminaria (dried seaweed stems) or other osmotic dilators, which can be inserted into the cervix and left for ≥ 4 h (usually overnight). They dilate the cervix by expanding or stimulating prostaglandin release.

At 12 to 18 wk, dilation and evacuation (D & E) is usually used. The cervix is dilated, usually with laminaria or other osmotic dilators and dilating instruments. Forceps are used to dismember and remove the fetus, and a suction cannula is used to aspirate the amniotic fluid, placenta, and fetal debris. D & E requires more skill than do other methods of instrumental evacuation.

Medical induction: Medical induction is possible using prostaglandins—vaginal prostaglandin E_2 (dinoprostone) suppositories, intravaginal prostaglandin E_1 analog (misoprostol) tablets, or IM injections of prostaglandin $F_{2\alpha}$ (dinoprost tromethamine). Two 100-μg intravaginal tablets of misoprostol q 12 h is nearly 90% successful within 48 h of treatment. Laminaria or other osmotic dilators used before medical induction usually shorten labor and decrease risk of cervicovaginal laceration. IV oxytocin accelerates induction by increasing the force of contractions and thus may result in laceration of the lower uterus.

Adverse effects of prostaglandins include nausea, vomiting, diarrhea, hyperthermia, facial flushing, vasovagal symptoms, bronchospasm, and decreased seizure threshold. In women with a severe kidney or liver disorder, activation of the drug may be decreased, so dose should be increased.

For up to 9 wk, mifepristone (RU 486), a progesterone-receptor blocker, followed by a vaginal prostaglandin is about 95% effective in terminating pregnancies. Methotrexate followed by misoprostol may also be used to terminate early pregnancy.

Complications

Complication rates with abortion (serious complications in < 1%; mortality in < 1 in 100,000) are higher than those with contraception, although the rates have decreased in the last few decades.Complication rates increase as gestational age increases. Serious early complications include perforation of the uterus (0.1%) or, less often, of the intestine or another organ by an instrument. Major hemorrhage (0.06%) may result from trauma or an atonic uterus. Laceration of the cervix (0.1 to 1%) ranges from superficial tenaculum tears to cervicovaginal tears, rarely with fistulas. General or local anesthesia rarely causes serious complications.

The most common delayed complications include bleeding and significant infection (0.1 to 2%), which usually occur simultaneously because placental fragments are retained, and thrombophlebitis. Mild inflammation is expected, but if infection is moderate or severe, peritonitis or sepsis may occur. Sterility may result from synechiae in the endometrial cavity or tubal fibrosis due to infection. Forceful dilation of the cervix in more advanced pregnancies may contribute to incompetent cervix. Elective abortion probably does not increase risks for the fetus or woman during subsequent pregnancies.

Psychologic complications do not typically occur but may occur in women who had psychologic symptoms before pregnancy, who terminated a desired pregnancy for medical reasons (maternal or fetal), who have considerable ambivalence about the abortion, who are adolescents, who had a late abortion, or who obtained an abortion illegally.

256 INFERTILITY

Infertility is inability of a couple to conceive after 1 yr of unprotected intercourse.

Overall, frequent, unprotected intercourse results in conception for 50% of couples within 3 mo, for 75% within 6 mo, and for 90% within 1 yr. Incidence of infertility is increasing, in part reflecting deferral of childbearing until women are older. Primary causes of infertility are sperm disorders (35% of couples), decreased ovarian reserve or ovulatory dysfunction (20%), tubal dysfunction and pelvic lesions (30%), abnormal cervical mucus (≤ 5%), and unidentified factors (10%). Inability to conceive often leads to feelings of frustration, anger, guilt, resentment, and inadequacy.

Couples wishing to conceive are encouraged to have frequent intercourse for the few days when ovulation is most likely, probably midway between menstrual cycles. Measuring morning body temperature daily can help determine when ovulation is occurring in women with regular menstrual cycles. A decrease suggests impending ovulation; an increase of ≥ 0.5° C suggests ovulation has just occurred. Commercially available luteinizing hormone (LH) prediction test kits, which identify the midcycle LH surge, can also help determine when ovulation occurs. Use of caffeine and tobacco, which can impair fertility, is discouraged.

Diagnosis begins with history, examination, and counseling of both partners. Men are evaluated for sperm disorders, and women for ovulatory and tubal dysfunction and pelvic lesions.

Support groups for couples (eg, American Fertility Association, RESOLVE) may help. If the likelihood of conceiving is low (usually after 2 yr of treatment), the clinician should mention adoption.

SPERM DISORDERS

Sperm disorders include defects in sperm production and emission. Diagnosis is by semen and genetic testing. The most effective treatment is usually in vitro fertilization via intracytoplasmic sperm injection.

Spermatogenesis occurs continuously. Each germ cell requires about 72 to 74 days to mature fully. Spermatogenesis is most efficient at 34° C. Within the seminiferous tubules, Sertoli cells regulate maturation, and Leydig cells produce the necessary testosterone. Fructose is normally produced in the seminal vesicles and secreted through the ejaculatory ducts. Sperm disorders may result in inadequate quantity of sperm—too few (oligospermia) or none (azoospermia)—or defects in sperm quality, such as abnormal motility or structure.

Etiology

Spermatogenesis can be impaired by heat, disorders (GU, endocrine, or genetic), drugs, or toxins (see TABLE 256–1), resulting in inadequate quantity or defective quality of sperm.

Causes of impaired sperm emission (obstructive azoospermia) include retrograde ejaculation into the bladder due to diabetes, neurologic dysfunction, retroperitoneal dissection (eg, for Hodgkin lymphoma), and prostatectomy. Other causes include obstruction of the vas deferens and congenital bilateral absence of the vas deferens or epididymis. Many affected men have mutations of the cystic fibrosis transmembrane conductance regulator (*CFTR*) gene, and almost all men with symptomatic cystic fibrosis have congenital bilateral absence of the vas deferens.

Men with microdeletions affecting the Y chromosome can develop oligospermia via various mechanisms, depending on the specific deletion. Another rare mechanism of infertility is destruction or inactivation of sperm by sperm antibodies, which are usually produced by the man.

Diagnosis

When couples are infertile, the man should always be evaluated for sperm disorders. History and physical examination focus on potential causes (eg, GU disorders). Normal volume of each testis is 20 to 25 mL. Semen analysis should be performed. If there is oligospermia or azoospermia, genetic testing, including standard karyotyping, PCR of tagged chromosomal sites (to detect microdeletions affecting Y chromosome), and evaluation for mutations of the *CFTR* gene, should be undertaken. The partner of a man with a *CFTR* gene mutation should also be tested to exclude cystic fibrosis carrier status before his sperm is used for reproduction.

Before semen testing, the man is asked to refrain from ejaculation for 2 to 3 days. Because sperm count varies, testing requires ≥ 2 specimens obtained ≥ 1 wk apart; each specimen is obtained by masturbation into a glass jar, preferably at the laboratory site. If this method is difficult, the man can use a condom at home; the condom must be free of lubricants and chemicals. After being at room temperature for 20 to 30 min, the ejaculate is evaluated for volume (normal 2 to 6 mL), viscosity (normally, beginning to liquefy within 30 min; completely liquefied within 1 h), gross and microscopic appearance (normally, opaque, cream-colored, 1 to 3 WBC/high-power field), pH (normal 7 to 8), sperm count (normal > 20 million/mL), sperm motility at 1 and 3 h (normal > 50% motile), percentage of sperm with normal morphology (normal > 14% using 1999 WHO strict criteria), and presence of fructose (indicating at least one ejaculatory duct is patent). Additional computer-assisted measures of sperm motility (eg, linear sperm velocity) are available; however, their correlation with fertility is unclear.

If a man without hypogonadism or congenital bilateral absence of the vas deferens has an ejaculate volume < 1 mL, urine is analyzed for sperm after ejaculation. A disproportionately large number of sperm in urine vs semen suggests retrograde ejaculation.

Specialized sperm tests, available at some infertility centers, may be considered if routine tests of both partners do not explain infertility and in vitro fertilization or gamete intrafallopian tube transfer is being contemplated. The immunobead test detects sperm antibodies, and the hypo-osmotic swelling test measures the structural integrity of sperm plasma membranes. The hemizona assay and sperm penetration assay determine the ability of sperm to fertilize the egg in vitro.

If necessary, testicular biopsy can distinguish between obstructive and nonobstructive azoospermia.

Treatment

Underlying GU disorders are treated. For men with sperm counts of 10 to 20 million/mL and no endocrine disorder, clomiphene citrate (25 to 50 mg po once/day taken 25 days/mo for 3 to 4 mo) can be tried. Clomiphene, an antiestrogen, may stimulate sperm production and increase sperm counts. However, whether it improves sperm motility or morphology is unclear, and increased fertility has not been confirmed.

If sperm count is < 10 million/mL or clomiphene is unsuccessful in men with normal sperm motility, the most effective treatment is usually in vitro fertilization with injections of single sperm into single eggs (ie, intracytoplasmic sperm injection). Alternatively, intrauterine insemination using washed semen samples and timed to coincide with ovulation is sometimes tried. Pregnancy is usually achieved by the 6th treatment cycle if it will occur at all.

Decreased number and viability of sperm may not preclude pregnancy. In such cases, fertility may be enhanced by controlled ovarian hyperstimulation of the woman plus artificial insemination or other assisted reproductive techniques (eg, in vitro fertilization, intracytoplasmic sperm injection).

TABLE 256–1. CAUSES OF IMPAIRED SPERMATOGENESIS

CONDITION	EXAMPLES
Endocrine disorders	Abnormalities of the hypothalamic-pituitary-gonadal axis Adrenal disorders Hyperprolactinemia Hypogonadism Hypothyroidism
Genetic disorders	Gonadal dysgenesis Klinefelter's syndrome Microdeletions of sections of the Y chromosome (in 10–15% of men with severely impaired spermatogenesis) Mutations of the cystic fibrosis transmembrane conductance regulator (*CFTR*) gene
GU disorders	Cryptorchidism Infections Injury Mumps orchitis Testicular atrophy Varicocele
Heat	Exposure to excessive heat within the last 3 mo Fever
Substances	Anabolic steroids Diethylstilbestrol Ethanol Recreational drugs (eg, opioids) Toxins

If the male partner cannot produce enough fertile sperm, a couple may consider insemination using donor sperm. Risk of AIDS and other sexually transmitted diseases is minimized by freezing donor sperm for ≥ 6 mo, after which donors are retested for infection before insemination proceeds.

ABNORMAL CERVICAL MUCUS

Abnormal cervical mucus may impair fertility by inhibiting penetration or increasing destruction of sperm.

Normally, cervical mucus is stimulated to change from thick and impenetrable to thin and stretchable by an increase in estradiol levels during the follicular phase of the menstrual cycle. Abnormal cervical mucus may remain impenetrable to sperm around the time of ovulation or may promote sperm destruction by facilitating influx of vaginal bacteria (eg, due to cervicitis) or, occasionally, by containing antibodies to sperm. Abnormal mucus rarely impairs fertility significantly, except in women with chronic cervicitis or cervical stenosis due to prior treatment for cervical intraepithelial neoplasia.

Women are examined to check for cervicitis and cervical stenosis. Unless they have one of these disorders, postcoital testing of cervical mucus, traditionally routine during infertility evaluation, is usually unnecessary.

DECREASED OVARIAN RESERVE

Decreased ovarian reserve is a decrease in the quantity or quality of oocytes leading to impaired fertility.

Ovarian reserve may begin to decrease at age 30 or even earlier and decreases rapidly after age 40. Ovarian lesions also decrease reserve. Although older age is a risk factor for decreased ovarian reserve, age and decreased ovarian reserve are each independent predictors of infertility and thus of a poorer response to fertility treatment.

Testing for decreased ovarian reserve is considered for women who are ≥ 35, who have had ovarian surgery, or who have responded poorly to treatments such as ovarian stimulation with exogenous gonadotropins. Follicle-stimulating hormone (FSH) levels > 10 mIU/mL or estradiol levels of < 80 pg/mL on day 3 of the menstrual cycle also suggest the diagnosis. Diagnosis can be made by giving the woman clomiphene 100 mg po once/day on days 5 to 9 of the menstrual cycle (clomiphene citrate challenge test). A dramatic increase in FSH and estradiol levels from day 3 to day 10 of the cycle indicates decreased reserve.

If women are > 42 or ovarian reserve is decreased, assisted reproduction using donor oocytes may be necessary.

OVULATORY DYSFUNCTION

Ovulatory dysfunction is abnormal, irregular, or absent ovulation. Menses are often irregular or absent. Diagnosis is often possible by history or can be confirmed by measurement of hormone levels or serial pelvic ultrasonography. Treatment is usually induction of ovulation with clomiphene or other drugs.

Chronic ovulatory dysfunction in premenopausal women is most commonly caused by polycystic ovary syndrome (PCOS—see p. 2078) but has many other causes, including hyperprolactinemia and hypothalamic dysfunction (eg, hypothalamic amenorrhea).

Symptoms, Signs, and Diagnosis

Ovulatory dysfunction is suspected if menses are absent, irregular, or not preceded by breast tenderness, lower abdominal bloating, or moodiness.

Measuring morning body temperature daily can help determine whether and when ovulation is occurring (see p. 2134). However, this method is often inaccurate and has an error margin of 2 days. More accurate methods include home testing kits, which detect an increase in urinary luteinizing hormone (LH) excretion 24 to 36 h before ovulation, and pelvic ultrasonography, which is used to monitor ovarian follicle diameter and rupture. Also, serum progesterone levels of ≥ 3 ng/mL (≥ 9.75 nmol/L) or elevated levels of one of its urinary metabolites, pregnanediol glucuronide (measured, if possible, 1 wk before onset of the next menstrual period), indicate that ovulation has just occurred.

Irregular ovulation should prompt evaluation for disorders of the pituitary, hypothalamus, or ovaries (eg, PCOS).

Treatment

Ovulation can usually be induced with drugs. Usually, chronic anovulation that is not due to hyperprolactinemia is initially treated with the antiestrogen clomiphene citrate. First, uterine bleeding, unless it has occurred spontaneously, is induced with medroxyprogesterone acetate 5 to 10 mg po once/day for 5 to 10 days. Clomiphene 50 mg po once/day is started on the 5th day after bleeding begins and given for 5 days. Ovulation usually occurs 5 to 10 days (mean 7 days) after the last day of clomiphene; if ovulation occurs, menses follows within 35 days of the prior bleeding episode. The daily dose can be increased by up to 50 mg every 2 cycles to a maximum of 200 mg/dose as needed to induce ovulation. Treatment is continued as needed for up to 4 ovulatory cycles.

Adverse effects of clomiphene include vasomotor flushes (10%), abdominal distention (6%), breast tenderness (2%), nausea (3%), visual symptoms (1 to 2%), and headaches (1 to 2%). Multifetal pregnancy (primarily twins) and ovarian hyperstimulation syndrome each occur in about 5%. Ovarian cysts are common. A previously suggested association between clomiphene taken for > 12 cycles and ovarian cancer has not been confirmed.

For patients with PCOS, most of whom also have insulin resistance, an insulin-sensitizing drug may be used first to induce ovulation. Drugs include metformin 750 to 1000 mg po bid (or 500 to about 750 mg po tid) or, less often, thiazolidinediones (eg, rosiglitazone, pioglitazone). If insulin sensitization is ineffective, clomiphene can be added.

For all women with ovulatory dysfunction that does not respond to clomiphene, human gonadotropins (ie, preparations that contain purified or recombinant follicle-stimulating hormone [FSH] and variable amounts of LH) can be used. Several IM and sc preparations with similar efficacy are available; they typically contain 75 IU of FSH activity with or without LH activity. They are usually given once/day, beginning on the 3rd to 5th day after induced or spontaneous bleeding; ideally, they stimulate maturation of 1 to 3 follicles, determined ultrasonographically, within 7 to 14 days. Ovulation is induced with human chorionic gonadotropin (hCG) 5000 to 10,000 IU IM after follicle maturation; criteria for induction may vary, but typically, at least one follicle should be > 16 mm in diameter. However, ovulation is not induced if women are at high risk of multifetal pregnancy or ovarian hyperstimulation syndrome. Risk factors include presence of > 3 follicles > 16 mm in diameter and preovulatory serum estradiol levels > 1500 pg/mL or possibly > 1000 pg/mL in women with several small ovarian follicles.

After gonadotropin therapy, 10 to 30% of successful pregnancies are multiple. Ovarian hyperstimulation syndrome occurs in 10 to 20% of patients; ovaries can become massively enlarged, and intravascular fluid volume shifts into the peritoneal space, causing potentially life-threatening ascites and hypovolemia.

Underlying disorders (eg, hyperprolactinemia—see p. 1188) are treated. If the cause is hypothalamic amenorrhea, gonadorelin acetate, a synthetic gonadotropin-releasing hormone (GnRH) given as a pulsatile IV infusion, can induce ovulation. Doses of 2.5 to 5.0 μg boluses (pulse doses) regularly q 60 to 90 min are most effective. Gonadorelin acetate is unlikely to cause multifetal pregnancy.

TUBAL DYSFUNCTION AND PELVIC LESIONS

Tubal dysfunction is fallopian tube obstruction or epithelial dysfunction that impairs zygote motility; pelvic lesions are structural abnormalities that can impede fertilization or implantation.

Tubal dysfunction can result from pelvic inflammatory disease, use of an intrauterine device, ruptured appendix, lower abdominal surgery leading to pelvic adhesions, inflammatory disorders (eg, TB), or ectopic pregnancy. Pelvic lesions such as intrauterine adhesions (Asherman's syndrome), fibroids obstructing the fallopian tubes or distorting the uterine cavity, and certain malformations can impede fertility, as can pelvic adhesions. Endometriosis can cause tubal, uterine, or other lesions that impair fertility.

All infertility evaluations include assessment of the fallopian tubes. Most often, hysterosalpingography (fluoroscopic imaging of the uterus and fallopian tubes after injection of a radiopaque agent into the uterus) is done 2 to 5 days after cessation of menstrual flow. Hysterosalpingography rarely indicates tubal patency falsely but often indicates tubal obstruction falsely. This test can also detect some pelvic and intrauterine lesions.

For unexplained reasons, fertility appears to be enhanced after hysterosalpingography if the test result is normal. Thus, in these cases, additional diagnostic tests of tubal function can be delayed for several cycles. Tubal lesions can be further evaluated with laparoscopy. Intrauterine and tubal lesions can be detected or further evaluated by sonohysterography (injection of isotonic fluid through the cervix into the uterus during ultrasonography) or hysteroscopy.

Diagnosis and treatment are often done simultaneously during laparoscopy or hysteroscopy. During laparoscopy, pelvic adhesions can be lysed, or pelvic endometriosis can be fulgurated or ablated by laser. Similarly, during hysteroscopy, adhesions can be lysed, and submucous fibroids and intrauterine polyps can be removed.

UNEXPLAINED INFERTILITY

Infertility is considered unexplained when semen in the man and ovulation and fallopian tubes in the woman are normal.

Fertility may be increased by stimulating development of multiple follicles (controlled ovarian hyperstimulation); the goal is inducing ovulation with > 1 oocyte (superovulation). First, for 3 to 4 menstrual cycles the woman is given clomiphene citrate and, to trigger ovulation, human chorionic gonadotropin (hCG). Intrauterine insemination is done within the next 2 days. If pregnancy does not result, the woman is given gonadotropins as for treatment of ovulatory dysfunction (see p. 2141), followed by hCG and by insemination within the next 2 days. Supplemental progesterone may be needed during the luteal phase. Start day in the cycle and gonadotropin dosage may vary, depending on the patient's age and ovarian reserve. With clomiphene and gonadotropin treatment, the pregnancy rate is 10 to 15%/cycle for the 1st 4 cycles. If pregnancy does not result after 4 cycles, assisted reproductive techniques are recommended. Controlled ovarian hyperstimulation may result in multifetal pregnancy.

ASSISTED REPRODUCTIVE TECHNIQUES

Assisted reproductive techniques involve manipulation of sperm and ova in vitro with the goal of producing an embryo.

Assisted reproductive techniques (ART) may result in multifetal pregnancy, but risk is less than that with controlled ovarian hyperstimulation. If risk of genetic defects is high, the embryo can often be tested for defects before implantation (see p. 2144).

In vitro fertilization (IVF) can be used to treat infertility due to oligospermia, sperm antibodies, tubal dysfunction, or endometriosis as well as unexplained infertility. The procedure includes controlled ovarian hyperstimulation, oocyte retrieval, fertilization, embryo culture, and embryo transfer. For ovarian hyperstimulation, clomiphene plus gonadotropins or gonadotropins alone can be used. A gonadotropin-releasing hormone (GnRH) agonist or antagonist is often given to prevent premature ovulation. After sufficient follicular growth, human chorionic gonadotropin (hCG) is given to induce final follicular maturation. About 34 h after hCG is given, oocytes are retrieved by direct needle puncture of the follicle, usually transvaginally with ultrasound guidance or less commonly laparoscopically. The oocytes are inseminated in vitro. The semen sample is typically washed several times with tissue culture medium and concentrated for motile sperm. Sperm are added, then the oocytes are cultured for about 2 to 5 days. Only 1 or a few of the resulting embryos are transferred to the uterine cavity, minimizing the chance of a multifetal pregnancy, the greatest risk of IVF. The number of embryos transferred is determined by the woman's age and likelihood of response to IVF. Other embryos may be frozen in liquid nitrogen for transfer in a subsequent cycle.

Gamete intrafallopian tube transfer (GIFT) is an alternative to IVF but is used infrequently, typically for women with unexplained infertility or with normal tubal function plus endometriosis. Multiple oocytes and sperm are obtained as for IVF but are transferred—transvaginally with ultrasound guidance or laparoscopically—to the distal fallopian tubes, where fertilization occurs. Success rates are about 25 to 35% at most infertility centers.

Intracytoplasmic sperm injection is useful when other techniques are not successful or unlikely to be so, or when a severe sperm disorder is present. Sperm are injected into the oocyte, bypassing these sperm abnormalities. The embryo is then cultured and transferred as for IVF. In 2002, over 52% of all ART cycles in the US involved intracytoplasmic sperm injection. Slightly more than 34% of ART cycles result in pregnancy, of which live births occur in 83%.

Other procedures include a combination of in vitro fertilization and GIFT, zygote intrafallopian tube transfer, use of donor oocytes, and transfer of frozen embryos to a surrogate mother. Some of these techniques raise moral and ethical issues (eg, rightful parentage in surrogate motherhood, selective reduction of the number of implanted embryos if multifetal pregnancy results).

257 PRENATAL GENETIC COUNSELING AND EVALUATION

(See also Ch. 327 on p. 2698.)

Counseling: Prenatal genetic counseling is provided for all prospective parents, ideally before conception, to assess risk factors for congenital disorders. Parents with risk factors are advised about possible outcomes and options for evaluation. If testing identifies a disorder, reproductive options are discussed; preconception options include contraception, artificial insemination if the man is a carrier, and oocyte donation if the woman is a carrier; postconception options include pregnancy termination and, in some cases, treatment (eg, dexamethasone to prevent virilization in a female fetus with 21-hydroxylase deficiency). Certain precautions to help prevent birth defects (eg, avoiding teratogens, taking supplemental folate—see p. 2152) are recommended for all women who are planning to become pregnant.

Information presented at genetic counseling should be as simple and jargon-free as possible to help anxious couples understand it. Frequent repetition may be necessary. Couples should be given time alone to formulate questions. Information is available on the internet (www.modimes.org) for many common problems (eg, advanced maternal age, recurrent spontaneous abortions, previous offspring with neural tube defects, previous offspring with trisomy).

Risk factors: Some risk of genetic abnormality exists in all pregnancies. Among live births, incidence is 0.5% for numeric or structural chromosomal disorders, 1% for single-gene (mendelian) disorders, and 1% for multiple-gene (polygenic) disorders. Among stillbirths, rates are higher. Most malformations involving a single organ system (eg, neural tube defects, most congenital heart defects) result from polygenic or multifactorial (ie, also influenced by environmental factors) inheritance.

Risk of having a fetus with a chromosomal disorder is increased for most couples who have had a previous fetus or infant with a chromosomal disorder (recognized or missed), except for a few specific types (eg, 45,X; triploidy; de novo chromosomal rearrangements). Chromosomal disorders are more likely to be present in fetuses that spontaneously abort during the 1st trimester (50 to 60%), in fetuses with a major malformation (30%), and in stillborns (5%). Rarely, a parent has a chromosomal disorder that increases risk of a chromosomal disorder in the fetus. Asymptomatic parental chromosomal disorders (eg, balanced abnormalities such as certain translocations and inversions) may not be suspected. A balanced parental chromosomal rearrangement should be suspected if couples have had recurrent spontaneous abortions, infertility, or a child with a malformation. For unclear reasons, risk of a fetal chromosomal disorder increases as maternal age increases. Among live births, the rate is about 0.2% at age 20, 0.5% at age 35, and 1.5% at age 40, increasing to 14% at age 49. Most chromosomal disorders due to older maternal age involve an extra chromosome (trisomy), particularly trisomy 21 (Down syndrome).

An autosomal dominant disorder is suspected if there is a family history in > 1 generation; autosomal disorders affect males and females equally. If one parent has an autosomal dominant disorder, risk is 50% that the disorder will be transmitted to an offspring. Paternal age > 50 increases risk of some spontaneous dominant mutations in offspring.

For an autosomal recessive disorder to be expressed, an offspring must receive the same mutant gene from both parents. Parents may be heterozygous (carriers) and, if so, are usually clinically normal. In such cases, offspring (male or female) are at a 25% risk of being homozygous for the mutant gene and thus affected, 50% are likely to be heterozygous, and 25% are likely to be genetically normal. If only siblings and no other relatives are affected, an autosomal recessive disorder should be suspected. Likelihood that both parents carry the same autosomal recessive trait is increased if they are consanguineous.

Because females have two X chromosomes and males have only one, X-linked recessive disorders are expressed in all males who carry the mutation. Such disorders are usually transmitted through clinically normal, heterozygous (carrier) females. Thus, for each son of a carrier female, risk of having the disorder is 50%, and for each daughter, risk of being a carrier is 50%. Affected males do not transmit the gene to their sons, but they transmit it to all their daughters, who thus are carriers. Unaffected males do not transmit the gene.

GENETIC EVALUATION

A screening history is part of routine prenatal care. The history is summarized as a pedigree (see FIG. 327–1 on p. 2700). Information should include the health status and presence of genetic disorders or carrier status of both parents, of 1st-degree relatives (parents, siblings, offspring), and of 2nd-degree relatives (aunts, uncles, grandparents), as well as ethnic and racial background and consanguineous matings. Outcomes of previous pregnancies are noted. If genetic disorders are suspected, relevant medical records must be reviewed.

Genetic screening tests are offered to parents at risk of being asymptomatic carriers for certain common mendelian disorders (see TABLE 257–1). Diagnostic tests for specific abnormalities are offered to parents when appropriate (see TABLE 257–2).

Between 15 and 20 wk gestation, pregnant women should be offered screening using multiple maternal serum markers (α-fetoprotein, β-human chorionic gonadotropin, estriol, inhibin A—see p. 2147) to detect neural tube defects, Down syndrome, and some other birth defects.

Fetal genetic diagnostic tests, unlike screening tests, are usually invasive and involve fetal risk. Genetic diagnostic tests are usually done via chorionic villus sampling, amniocentesis, or percutaneous umbilical blood sampling. These tests can detect all trisomies, many other chromosomal abnormalities, and > 100 mendelian abnormalities. Preimplantation diagnosis is not yet commonly used.

Ultrasonography

Some experts recommend conventional ultrasonography for all pregnant women. Others use ultrasonography only for specific indications, such as checking for suspected genetic or obstetric abnormalities or helping interpret abnormal maternal serum marker levels.

Ultrasonography is noninvasive and has no known risks to the woman or fetus. It can confirm gestational age, determine fetal viability, and detect multiple pregnancy. During the 2nd or 3rd trimester, ultrasonography may identify major malformations in the fetal intracranial structures, spine, heart, bladder, kidneys, stomach, thorax, abdominal wall, long bones, and umbilical cord. Although ultrasonography provides only structural information, some structural abnormalities strongly suggest genetic abnormalities. Multiple malformations may suggest a chromosomal disorder.

High-resolution ultrasonography may be indicated for couples with a family history of a congenital malformation (eg, congenital heart defects, cleft lip and palate, pyloric stenosis), particularly one that may be treated effectively before birth (eg, posterior urethral valves with megacystis) or at delivery (eg, diaphragmatic hernia). High-resolution ultrasonography may also be used if maternal serum marker levels are abnormal. High-resolution ultrasonography may allow detection of renal malformations (eg, renal agenesis [Potter's syndrome], polycystic kidney disease), lethal forms of short-limbed skeletal dysplasias (eg, thanatophoric skeletal dysplasia, achondrogenesis), gut malformations (eg, obstruction), diaphragmatic hernia, microcephalus, and hydrocephalus. If ultrasonography is done by skilled operators, sensitivity for major congenital malformations is high. However, some conditions (eg, oligohydramnios, maternal obesity, fetal

TABLE 257–1. GENETIC SCREENING FOR SOME ETHNIC GROUPS

ETHNIC GROUP	DISORDER	SCREENING TESTS	PRENATAL DIAGNOSIS
All	Cystic fibrosis*	DNA analysis of 25 *CFTR* mutations, which are present in ≥ 0.1% of the US population	CVS or amniocentesis for genotype determination†
Ashkenazi Jews‡	Canavan disease	DNA analysis to detect most common mutations	CVS or amniocentesis for DNA analysis
	Familial dysautonomia	DNA analysis to detect most common mutations	CVS or amniocentesis for DNA analysis
	Tay-Sachs disease	Measurement of serum hexosaminidase A to check for deficiency; possibly DNA analysis	CVS or amniocentesis for enzymatic assays or molecular analysis to check for hexosaminidase A; DNA analysis
Blacks	Sickle cell anemia	Screening tests for sickle cell hemoglobin, confirmatory hemoglobin electrophoresis	CVS or amniocentesis for genotype determination (direct DNA analysis)
Cajuns	Tay-Sachs	Measurement of serum hexosaminidase A to check for deficiency; possibly DNA analysis	CVS or amniocentesis for enzymatic assays or molecular analysis to check for hexosaminidase A
Mediterranean people	β-Thalassemia	MCV < 80%, followed by hemoglobin electrophoresis	CVS or amniocentesis for genotype determination (direct DNA analysis or linkage analysis)
Southeast Asians, Cambodians, Chinese, Filipinos, Laotians, Vietnamese	α-Thalassemia	MCV < 80%, followed by hemoglobin electrophoresis	CVS or amniocentesis for genotype determination (direct DNA analysis or linkage analysis)

*Should be offered to whites and Ashkenazi Jews; should be made available to other ethnic groups (eg, Asians, Hispanics, blacks).

† Definitive diagnosis is not always possible; sensitivity varies by ethnic group.

‡For Ashkenazi Jews, some experts also recommend screening for Gaucher's disease, Niemann-Pick disease type A, Fanconi's anemia (syndrome) group C, Bloom syndrome, and mucolipidosis IV. Most (90%) Jews are Ashkenazi; thus, Jews who do not know whether they are Ashkenazi should be screened.

CVS = chorionic villus sampling; MCV = mean corpuscular volume.

position) interfere with obtaining optimal images.

Amniocentesis

In amniocentesis, a needle is inserted transabdominally into the amniotic sac to withdraw amniotic fluid and fetal cells for testing, including measurement of chemical markers (eg, α-fetoprotein, acetylcholinesterase—see p. 2147). The safest time for amniocentesis is after 14 wk gestation. Immediately before amniocentesis, ultrasonography is done to assess fetal cardiac motion and determine gestational age, placental position, amniotic fluid location, and fetal number. If the mother has Rh-negative blood and is unsensitized, Rh_0(D) immune globulin 300 μg is given after the procedure to reduce the likelihood of sensitization (see p. 2195). Amniocentesis has traditionally been offered to

TABLE 257–2. INDICATIONS FOR FETAL GENETIC DIAGNOSTIC TESTS

INDICATION	COMMENT
Maternal age > 35 at expected delivery	
Recurrent previous spontaneous abortions	Chromosomal analysis may be indicated for parents
Chromosomal abnormality in a previous child	Chromosomal analysis may be indicated for parents
Paternal age > 50	Need for testing is controversial
Parental chromosomal disorder	Balanced parental chromosomal abnormalities may not require testing
Parental sex-linked mendelian disorder	
Autosomal recessive mendelian disorder diagnosed or suspected in both parents	
Levels of maternal serum markers* suggesting trisomy 21 or 18	Chorionic villus sampling, sometimes with ultrasound measurement of nuchal translucency, during the 1st trimester or amniocentesis during the 2nd trimester is done
Elevated maternal α-fetoprotein and indeterminate ultrasound results	Amniocentesis is done

*Measured during 1st or 2nd trimester.

pregnant women > 35 because their risk of having an infant with Down syndrome or another chromosomal abnormality is increased.

Occasionally, the amniotic fluid obtained is bloody. Usually, the blood does not affect amniotic cell growth and is maternal; however, if the blood is fetal, it may falsely elevate amniotic fluid α-fetoprotein level. Dark red or brown fluid indicates previous intra-amniotic bleeding and an increased risk of fetal loss. Green fluid, which usually results from meconium staining, does not appear to indicate increased risk of fetal loss.

Amniocentesis rarely results in significant maternal morbidity (eg, symptomatic amnionitis). With experienced operators, risk of fetal loss is about 0.2 to 0.3%. Vaginal spotting or amniotic fluid leakage, usually self-limited, occurs in 1 to 2% of women tested.

Chorionic Villus Sampling

In chorionic villus sampling (CVS), chorionic villi are aspirated into a syringe and cultured. CVS provides the same information about fetal genetic and chromosomal status as amniocentesis and has similar accuracy. However, CVS is done between 10 wk gestation and the end of the 1st trimester and thus provides earlier results. Therefore, if needed, pregnancy may be terminated earlier (and more safely and simply), or if results are normal, parental anxiety may be relieved earlier. Unlike amniocentesis, amniotic fluid is not obtained at the time of CVS and measurement of α-fetoprotein cannot be performed.

Depending on placental location (identified by ultrasonography), CVS can be done by passing a catheter through the cervix or by inserting a needle through the woman's abdominal wall. After CVS, $Rh_0(D)$ immune globulin 300 μg is given to Rh-negative unsensitized women.

Errors in diagnosis due to maternal cell contamination are rare. Detection of certain chromosomal abnormalities (eg, tetraploidy) may not reflect true fetal status but rather mosaicism confined to the placenta. Consultation with experts familiar with these abnormalities is advised. Rarely, subsequent amniocentesis is required to obtain additional information.

Rate of fetal loss due to CVS is similar to that of amniocentesis (ie, 0.2 to 0.3%). Transverse limb defects and oromandibular-limb hypogenesis have been attributed to CVS but are exceedingly rare if CVS is done after 10 wk gestation by an experienced operator.

Percutaneous Umbilical Blood Sampling

Fetal blood samples can be obtained by percutaneous puncture of the umbilical cord vein (funipuncture) via ultrasound guidance. Chromosome analysis can be completed in 48 to 72 h. This test is especially useful late in the 3rd trimester, particularly if fetal abnormalities are first suspected at this time. Procedure-related fetal loss rate is about 1%.

Preimplantation Diagnosis

Genetic diagnosis is sometimes possible before implantation; polar bodies from oocytes, blastomeres from 6- to 8-cell embryos, or a trophectoderm sample from the blastocyst is used. These tests are available only in specialized centers and are used primarily for couples with a high risk of certain mendelian disorders (eg, cystic fibrosis) or chromosomal abnormalities. Newer techniques may reduce costs and make such tests more widely available.

MATERNAL SERUM SCREENING

Maternal serum screening during the 2nd trimester is a noninvasive way to identify women at increased risk of having children with a neural tube defect (usually open spina bifida or anencephaly), Down syndrome, or trisomy 18. Screening should be offered to all pregnant women. When amniocentesis is recommended to test for fetal abnormalities, some women request serum screening before they agree to the procedure, so that risk of such abnormalities can be more precisely defined. Results are most accurate when the initial sample is obtained between 16 and 18 wk gestation, although screening can be done from about 15 to 20 wk. Normal values vary with gestational age. Corrections for maternal weight, diabetes mellitus, race, and other factors are necessary.

Maternal α-fetoprotein levels are measured first; elevated levels suggest open spina bifida, anencephaly, increased risk of pregnancy complications (eg, intrauterine growth restriction, abruptio placentae), or, occasionally, twins or other multifetal pregnancy. Closed spina bifida is usually not detected. Designating a cutoff value to determine whether further testing is warranted involves weighing the risk of missed abnormalities against the risk of complications from unnecessary testing. Usually, a cutoff value in the 95th to 98th percentile or 2.0 to 2.5 times the normal pregnancy median (multiples of the median, or MOM) is used. This value is about 80% sensitive for open spina bifida and 90% sensitive for anencephaly. When this value is used, amniocentesis is eventually required in 1 to 2% of women originally screened. Lower cutoff values increase sensitivity but decrease specificity, resulting in more amniocenteses.

If further testing is warranted, ultrasonography is the next step. It can confirm gestational age (which may be underestimated) or detect multiple gestation, fetal death, or congenital malformations. In some women, ultrasonography cannot identify a cause for elevated α-fetoprotein levels. Some experts believe that if high-resolution ultrasonography done by an experienced operator is normal, further testing is unnecessary. However, because this test occasionally misses neural tube defects, many experts recommend further testing regardless of ultrasonography results.

Subsequent testing includes amniocentesis and measurement of α-fetoprotein and acetylcholinesterase levels in amniotic fluid. Elevated α-fetoprotein in amniotic fluid suggests a neural tube defect, another malformation (eg, omphalocele, congenital nephrosis, cystic hygroma, gastroschisis, upper GI atresia), or contamination of the sample with fetal blood. Presence of acetylcholinesterase in amniotic fluid suggests a neural tube defect or another malformation. Elevated α-fetoprotein plus presence of acetylcholinesterase in amniotic fluid is virtually 100% sensitive for anencephaly and 90 to 95% sensitive for open spina bifida. High-resolution ultrasonography can detect most of these malformations. However, even if a malformation cannot be detected, abnormal amniotic fluid markers indicate that a malformation is likely, and parents should be informed.

During the 2nd trimester, maternal serum levels of α-fetoprotein, the β subunit of human chorionic gonadotropin (hCG), and unconjugated estriol (triple screening), adjusted for gestational age, are measured to refine estimates of Down syndrome risk. With triple screening, sensitivity for Down syndrome is about 65%, with a false-positive rate of about 5%. Some laboratories also measure inhibin A, increasing sensitivity to 75%. If screening suggests Down syndrome, ultrasonography is done to confirm gestational age, and risk is recalculated. If the original sample was drawn too early, another one must be drawn at the appropriate time. Amniocentesis is offered if risk exceeds the usual threshold for doing amniocentesis (1 in 270, which is about the same as risk when maternal age is > 35).

Triple screening can also detect risk of trisomy 18, indicated by low levels of all 3 serum markers. Sensitivity for trisomy 18 is 60 to 70%; false-positive rate is about 0.5%. Combining ultrasonography and serum screening increases sensitivity to about 80%.

Measurement of maternal serum free β-hCG and pregnancy-associated plasma protein A plus measurement of fetal nuchal translucency (by ultrasonography) is used to screen women in the 1st trimester for Down syndrome in the fetus. Sensitivity is about 80%; false-positive rate is about 5%. This screening method is being used increasingly in large centers; it provides information early so that a definitive diagnosis can be made with chorionic villus sampling.

258 CONCEPTION AND PRENATAL DEVELOPMENT

For conception (fertilization), a live sperm must unite with an ovum in a fallopian tube with normally functioning epithelium. Conception occurs just after ovulation, about 14 days after a menstrual period. At ovulation, cervical mucus becomes less viscid, facilitating rapid movement of sperm to the ovum, usually near the fimbriated end of the tube. Sperm may remain alive in the vagina for up to 3 days after intercourse.

The fertilized egg (zygote) divides repeatedly as it travels to the implantation site in the endometrium (usually near the fundus) over a period of 5 to 8 days. By the time of implantation, the zygote has become a layer of cells around a cavity, called a blastocyst. The blastocyst wall is 1 cell thick except for the embryonic pole, which is 3 or 4 cells thick. The embryonic pole, which becomes the embryo, implants first.

Amniotic sac and placenta: Within 1 or 2 days of implantation, a layer of cells (trophoblastic cells) develops around the blastocyst; the cells penetrate the endometrium, strengthening the attachment of the blastocyst. Trophoblastic cells develop into cytotrophoblast cells, which facilitate implantation and eventually formation of the placenta, and syncytial or syncytiotrophoblast cells, which produce chorionic gonadotropin by day 10 and other trophic hormones shortly thereafter. From the trophoblast develop an inner layer (amnion) and outer layer (chorion) of membranes; these membranes form the amniotic sac, which contains the conceptus (term used for derivatives of the zygote at any stage—see FIG. 258–1). When the sac is formed and the blastocyst cavity closes (by about 10 days), the conceptus is considered an embryo. The amniotic sac fills with fluid and expands with the growing embryo, filling the endometrial cavity by about 12 wk after conception; then, the amniotic sac is the only cavity remaining in the uterus.

The trophoblast also forms villi, which penetrate the uterus and develop into the placenta. The villi and placenta synthesize trophic hormones and provide arterial and venous exchange between the circulation of the conceptus and that of the mother. The placenta is fully formed by wk 18 to 20 but continues to grow, weighing about 500 g by term.

Embryo: Around day 10, 3 germ layers (ectoderm, mesoderm, endoderm) are usually distinct in the embryo. Then, the primitive streak, which becomes the neural tube, begins to develop. Around day 16, the cephalad portion of the mesoderm thickens, forming a central channel that develops into the heart and great vessels. The heart begins to pump plasma around day 20, and on the next day, fetal RBCs, which are immature and nucleated, appear. Fetal RBCs are soon replaced by mature RBCs, and blood vessels develop throughout the embryo. Eventually,

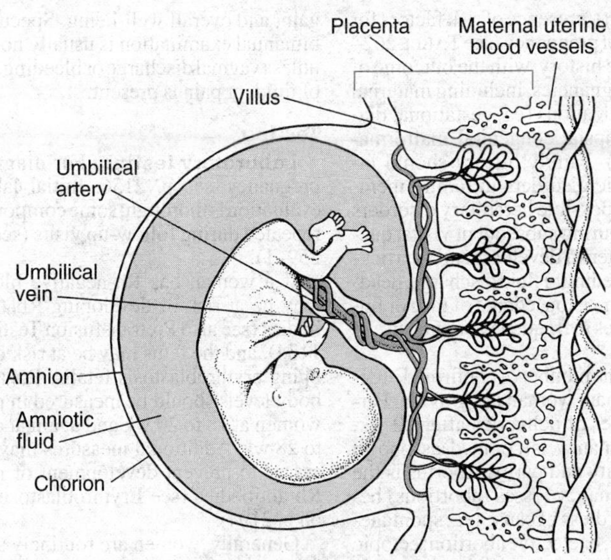

Fig. 258–1. Placenta and embryo at about 11 4/7 wk gestation. The embryo measures 4.2 cm.

the umbilical artery and vein develop, connecting the embryonic vessels with the placenta. Most organs form between 21 and 57 days after fertilization (between 5 and 10 wk gestation); however, the CNS continues to develop throughout pregnancy. Susceptibility to malformations induced by teratogens is highest when organs are forming.

259 APPROACH TO THE PREGNANT WOMAN AND PRENATAL CARE

Pregnant women require routine prenatal care to help ensure their health and the health of the fetus. Also, evaluation is often required for symptoms and signs of illness. Common symptoms that are often pregnancy-related include vaginal bleeding, pelvic pain, vomiting, and lower-extremity edema (for specific obstetric disorders, see Ch. 263 on p. 2191; for nonobstetric disorders in pregnant women, see Ch. 261 on p. 2167).

Ideally, women who are planning to become pregnant should see a physician before conception, so that they can be counseled about pregnancy risks and ways to reduce them. The initial routine prenatal visit should occur between 6 and 8 wk gestation. Follow-up visits should occur at about 4-wk intervals until 28 wk, at 2-wk intervals from 28 to 36 wk, and weekly thereafter until delivery. Prenatal care includes screening for disorders, taking measures to reduce fetal and maternal risks, and counseling.

History

During the initial visit, a full medical history is obtained. It includes previous and current disorders and drug use (therapeutic, social, and illicit), presence of risk factors for complications of pregnancy (see TABLE 262–1), and obstetric history, with the outcome of all previous pregnancies, including maternal and fetal complications (eg, gestational diabetes, preeclampsia, congenital malformations, stillbirth). Family history should include all chronic disorders in family members to identify possible hereditary disorders (see p. 2144). During subsequent visits, queries focus on interim developments, particularly vaginal bleeding or fluid discharge, headache, changes in vision, edema of face or fingers, and changes in frequency or intensity of fetal movement.

Gravidity is the number of confirmed pregnancies; a pregnant woman is a gravida. Parity is the number of deliveries after 20 wk. Multifetal pregnancy is counted as one in terms of gravidity and parity. Abortus is the number of pregnancy losses (abortions) before 20 wk regardless of cause (eg, spontaneous, therapeutic, or elective abortion; ectopic pregnancy). Sum of parity and abortus equals gravidity. Parity is often recorded as 4 numbers: number of term deliveries (after 37 wk), number of premature deliveries (> 20 and < 37 wk), number of abortions, and number of living children. Thus, a woman who is pregnant and has had one term delivery, one set of twins born at 32 wk, and 2 abortions is gravida 5, para 1-1-2-3.

Physical Examination

A full general examination, including height and weight, is done first. In the initial obstetric examination, speculum and bimanual pelvic examination is done, noting the presence of lesions or discharge as well as color and consistency of the cervix; also, fetal heart rate and, in patients presenting later in pregnancy, lie of the fetus are assessed (see FIG. 260–1 on p. 2163). Pelvic capacity can be estimated clinically by evaluating various measurements with the middle finger during bimanual examination. If the distance from the underside of the pubic symphysis to the sacral promontory is > 11.5 cm, the pelvic inlet is almost certainly adequate. Normally, distance between the ischial spines is ≥ 9 cm, length of the sacrospinous ligaments is 4 to ≥ 5 cm, and the subpubic arch is ≥ 90°.

During subsequent visits, BP and weight assessment is important. Obstetric examination focuses on uterine size, fundal height (in cm above the symphysis pubis), fetal heart rate and activity, and maternal diet, weight gain, and overall well-being. Speculum and bimanual examination is usually not needed unless vaginal discharge or bleeding, leakage of fluid, or pain is present.

Testing

Laboratory testing: For diagnosis of pregnancy, see p. 2156. Initial laboratory evaluation is thorough; some components are repeated during follow-up visits (see TABLE 259–1).

If a woman has Rh-negative blood, she may be at risk of developing $Rh_0(D)$ antibodies (see also Pretransfusion Testing on p. 1134), and the fetus may be at risk of developing erythroblastosis fetalis. $Rh_0(D)$ antibody levels should be measured in pregnant women at 18 to 20 wk and again at about 26 to 28 wk. Additional measures may be necessary to prevent development of maternal Rh antibodies (see Erythroblastosis Fetalis on p. 2194).

Generally, women are routinely screened for gestational diabetes between 24 and 28 wk. If women have risk factors for gestational diabetes, they are screened in the 1st trimester. Risk factors include gestational diabetes or a macrosomic neonate (weight > 4500 g at birth) in a previous pregnancy, unexplained fetal losses, a family history of diabetes, a history of persistent glucosuria, and body mass index (BMI) > 30 kg/m^2. Screening uses a 50-g, 1-h glucose tolerance test (see p. 2186).

Ultrasonography: Most obstetricians recommend at least one ultrasound examination during each pregnancy, ideally between 16 and 20 wk, when estimated delivery date (EDD) can still be confirmed fairly accurately and when placental location and fetal anatomy can be evaluated. Estimates of gestational age are based on measurements of fetal head circumference, biparietal diameter, abdominal circumference, and femur length. Measurement of fetal crown-rump length during the 1st trimester is particularly accurate in predicting EDD: to within about 5 days when measurements are made at < 12 wk gestation and within about 7 days at 12 to 15 wk. Ultrasound in the 3rd trimester is accurate for predicting EDD to within about 2 to 3 wk.

Specific indications for ultrasonography include investigation of abnormalities during the 1st trimester; need for detailed assessment of fetal anatomy; and detection of multifetal pregnancy, hydatidiform mole, polyhydramnios, placenta previa, and ectopic pregnancy. Other indications are determina-

TABLE 259–1. COMPONENTS OF ROUTINE PRENATAL EVALUATION

COMPONENT	INITIAL VISIT	FOLLOW-UP VISITS
Examination		
Height measurement	X	
Weight and BP measurement	X	X
Examination of thyroid, heart, lungs, breasts, abdomen, extremities, and optic fundus	X	
Examination of ankles for edema	X	X
Complete pelvic examination	X	
Examination to determine pelvic capacity	X	
Examination of uterus to determine size and fetal position[a]	X	X
Evaluation for fetal heart sounds[a]	X	X
Testing		
CBC[b]	X	
Serologic test for syphilis	X	
Hepatitis B serologic test (see p. 225)	X	
Cervical cultures for gonorrhea and chlamydia[c]	X	
Cervical Papanicolaou (Pap) test	X	
Rubella titer	X	
Urine culture	X	
Urine protein and glucose determination	X	X
Blood typing and $Rh_0(D)$ antibody levels[d]	X	
Genetic screening (see p. 2144)	X	
Diabetes screening[e]		X
Screening for TB (if at risk)	X	
Pelvic ultrasonography (not obtained routinely by all practitioners)[f]	X	

[a]Component may not be detectable depending on stage of pregnancy at presentation.
[b]Hct is repeated in 3rd trimester.
[c]For women at high risk, test is repeated at 36 wk.
[d]Repeated at 28 wk in Rh-negative women.
[e]Test is done only once: routinely at 28 wk; earlier in women at risk.
[f]Ideally, test is done in the 2nd trimester, between 16 and 20 wk.

tion of placental location, fetal position and size, and size of the uterus in relation to given gestational dates (too small or too large). Ultrasonography is also used for needle guidance during chorionic villus sampling, amniocentesis, and fetal transfusion. High-resolution ultrasonography includes techniques that maximize sensitivity for detecting fetal malformations.

If ultrasonography is needed during the 1st trimester (eg, to evaluate pain, bleeding, viability of pregnancy), use of an endovaginal transducer maximizes diagnostic accuracy; evidence of an intrauterine pregnancy (gestational sac or fetal pole) can be seen as early as 4 to 5 wk and is seen at 7 to 8 wk in > 95% of cases. With real-time ultrasonography, fetal movements and heart motion can be directly observed as early as 5 to 6 wk.

Other imaging: Conventional x-rays can induce spontaneous abortion or congenital malformations, particularly during early pregnancy. Risk is remote (up to about 1/million) with each x-ray of an extremity or of the neck, head, or chest if the uterus is shielded. Risk is higher with abdominal, pelvic, and lower back x-rays. Thus, for all women of childbearing age, an imaging test with less ionizing radiation (eg, ultrasonography) should be substituted when possible, or if x-rays are needed, the uterus should be shielded (because pregnancy is possible). Medically necessary x-rays or other imaging should not be postponed because of pregnancy. However, elective x-rays are postponed until after pregnancy.

Treatment

Problems identified during evaluation are managed. Women are counseled about exercise and diet, and nutritional supplements are prescribed. What to avoid, what to expect, and when to obtain further evaluation are explained. Couples are encouraged to attend childbirth classes.

Pregnant women with Rh-negative blood and thus at risk of developing $Rh_0(D)$ antibodies are given $Rh_0(D)$ immune globulin 300 μg IM after any significant vaginal bleeding or other sign of placental hemorrhage or separation (abruptio placentae), after a spontaneous or therapeutic abortion, after amniocentesis or chorionic villus sampling, prophylactically at 28 wk, and, if the neonate has $Rh_0(D)$-positive blood, after delivery.

Most pregnant women need a daily oral iron supplement of ferrous sulfate 300 mg or ferrous gluconate 450 mg, which may be better tolerated. Woman with anemia should take the supplements bid. All women should be given oral prenatal vitamins that contain folate 400 μg (0.4 mg), taken once/day; folate reduces risk of neural tube defects. For women who have had a fetus or infant with a neural tube defect, the recommended daily dose is 4000 μg (4 mg).

To provide nutrition for the fetus, most women require about 250 kcal extra daily; most should come from protein. If maternal weight gain is excessive (> 1.4 kg/mo during the early months) or inadequate (< 0.9 kg/mo), diet must be modified further. Weight-loss dieting during pregnancy is not recommended, even for morbidly obese women.

Pregnant women can continue to do moderate physical activities and exercise but should take care not to injure the abdomen. Sexual intercourse can be continued throughout pregnancy unless vaginal bleeding, pain, leakage of amniotic fluid, or uterine contractions occur.

Drugs and vitamins that are not medically indicated should be discouraged (see Drugs in Pregnancy on p. 2159). Vaccines for measles, mumps, rubella, and varicella should not be used during pregnancy (see p. 2160). The hepatitis B vaccine can be safely used if indicated, and the influenza vaccine is given to women who are in the 2nd or 3rd trimester during influenza season. Women should not use alcohol and tobacco and should avoid exposure to secondhand smoke. They should also avoid exposure to chemicals or paint fumes, direct handling of cat litter (due to risk of toxoplasmosis), prolonged temperature elevation (eg, in a hot tub or sauna), and exposure to people with active viral infections (eg, rubella, parvovirus infection [fifth disease], varicella). Women with substance abuse problems should be monitored by a specialist in high-risk pregnancy.

Women should be advised to seek evaluation for unusual headaches, visual disturbances, pelvic pain or cramping, vaginal bleeding, rupture of membranes, extreme swelling of the hands or face, diminished urine volume, any prolonged illness or infection, or persistent symptoms of labor. Multiparous women with a history of rapid labor should notify the physician at the 1st symptom of labor.

PELVIC PAIN DURING EARLY PREGNANCY

Disorders causing pelvic pain related to early pregnancy include spontaneous abortion, septic abortion, ruptured or unruptured ectopic pregnancy, and a ruptured corpus luteum cyst (an ovarian cyst at the site of ovum release). Nonobstetric disorders that should be considered include appendicitis, pyelonephritis, nephrolithiasis, musculoskeletal pain, irritable bowel syndrome, growth or degeneration of fibroids, and, rarely, pelvic inflammatory disease. Ectopic pregnancy can lead to hemorrhagic shock; septic abortion can lead to septic shock. Either should be treated with IV fluid resuscitation and other measures before and during evaluation.

Evaluation

Certain historical and examination findings may suggest causes of pregnancy-related pelvic pain (see TABLE 259–2). Nonobstetric disorders are evaluated as in nonpregnant women (see p. 2066).

History and examination: Risk factors for ectopic pregnancy include previous ectopic pregnancy, history of a sexually transmitted disease or pelvic inflammatory disease, current use of an intrauterine device, prior pelvic (particularly tubal) surgery, and smoking. A history of illicitly attempted termination of pregnancy or termination by an

TABLE 259–2. FINDINGS IN SOME DISORDERS CAUSING PELVIC PAIN RELATED TO EARLY PREGNANCY

FINDING	ECTOPIC PREGNANCY	SPONTANEOUS ABORTION	SEPTIC ABORTION	CORPUS LUTEAL CYST
Hemorrhagic shock out of proportion to external bleeding	Y*	N	N	N†
Septic shock	N	N	Y	N
Peritonitis	Y*	N	Y	Y*
Open cervical os or tissue passed through vagina	N	Y	Y	N
Purulent vaginal discharge	N	N	Y	N
Vaginal bleeding	Y	Y	Y	N
Colicky pain	N (usually)	Y	Y (early)	N
Adnexal mass	Y	N	N	Y
History of illicitly attempted abortion	N	N	Y	N

Y = finding is common or characteristic; N = finding is not characteristic.

*Ruptured.

†Unless ruptured and bleeding.

inexperienced practitioner suggests septic abortion, but absence of such a history does not exclude this diagnosis. Severe pain, particularly if worsened by movement, suggests peritonitis.

General and pelvic examinations are done. If the internal cervical os is open or if tissue has passed, spontaneous abortion is likely.

Testing: Pregnancy is confirmed (see p. 2156). If an obstetric cause is suspected, CBC, PT, PTT, fibrinogen level, and usually blood typing and screening or cross-matching are indicated. If the internal cervical os is open or if tissue has passed, further testing may be unnecessary unless septic abortion is suspected; then, blood cultures are obtained. If the os is closed and there is no evidence of tissue passage, ectopic pregnancy must be excluded; testing begins with quantitative measurement of the β subunit of human chorionic gonadotropin (β-hCG) and pelvic ultrasonography (see p. 2192). If hemorrhagic shock persists despite initial fluid resuscitation, ruptured ectopic pregnancy is presumed.

Treatment

Treatment is directed at the underlying disorder. Presumed ruptured ectopic pregnancy requires immediate laparoscopy or laparotomy.

VAGINAL BLEEDING DURING EARLY PREGNANCY

Vaginal bleeding occurs in about 20 to 30% of confirmed pregnancies during the first 20 wk; about ½ of these end in spontaneous abortion.

Etiology

Disorders that commonly cause vaginal bleeding during early pregnancy include ruptured or unruptured ectopic pregnancy (see p. 2192), spontaneous abortion (threatened, inevitable, incomplete, complete, or missed—see p. 2199), and, rarely, gestational trophoblastic disease (see p. 2123); for nonobstetric vaginal bleeding, see p. 2066. Ectopic pregnancy or disorders that cause copious vaginal bleeding can lead to hemorrhagic shock, which should be treated with IV fluid resuscitation and other measures before or during evaluation. If vaginal bleeding occurs, the pregnant woman must be evaluated.

Evaluation

History: Risk factors for ectopic pregnancy include previous ectopic pregnancy, history of any sexually transmitted disease or pelvic inflammatory disease, use of an intrauterine device, prior pelvic (particularly tubal) surgery, and smoking. Pain that resembles menstrual cramping suggests spontaneous abortion, as does passage of tissue or copious amounts of vaginal blood. Severe pain, particularly if worsened by movement, suggests peritonitis due to ruptured ectopic pregnancy.

Examination: Signs of peritonitis (eg, guarding, rigidity, rebound tenderness) suggest ruptured ectopic pregnancy. Pelvic examination includes evaluation for nonobstetric disorders that can cause vaginal bleeding (eg, trauma, vaginitis, cervicitis, cervical polyps). An open internal cervical os or passage of tissue indicates pregnancy-related bleeding, particularly spontaneous abortion. An adnexal mass suggests ectopic pregnancy. Uterine size that is much too large for gestational dates, hypertension, seizures, or hyperreflexia suggests gestational trophoblastic disease.

Testing: Pregnancy is verified (see p. 2156). If bleeding is minimal, blood typing and Rh testing are done to determine whether $Rh_0(D)$ immune globulin is needed (see Erythroblastosis Fetalis on p. 2194). If bleeding is significant, CBC and usually blood typing and cross-matching are indicated. If bleeding is severe, PT and PTT are determined.

If the os is closed and there is no evidence of tissue passage, threatened or missed abortion is possible, but ectopic pregnancy must be excluded. First, quantitative β subunit of human chorionic gonadotropin (β-hCG) is measured. If the woman is not in shock, transvaginal pelvic ultrasonography is done. If shock resolves after fluid resuscitation, pelvic ultrasonography may be done. If shock persists despite resuscitation or if ultrasound results suggest hemoperitoneum, ruptured ectopic pregnancy is assumed.

Treatment

Treatment is directed at the underlying disorder. If spontaneous abortion has occurred or appears inevitable, uterine evacuation (eg, D & C at 7 to 12 wk—see p. 2200) is indicated. Ruptured ectopic pregnancy is treated with immediate laparoscopy or laparotomy. Unruptured ectopic pregnancy may be treated with methotrexate or with salpingotomy or salpingectomy via laparoscopy or laparotomy.

VOMITING DURING EARLY PREGNANCY

Nausea and vomiting are common during pregnancy; they are thought to occur because estrogen levels increase rapidly. Although vomiting in the morning (morning sickness) is typical, nausea or vomiting can occur at any time. These symptoms are most common and most severe during the 1st trimester of pregnancy. Hyperemesis gravidarum (see p. 2195) is persistent pregnancy-induced vomiting that causes significant dehydration, often with electrolyte abnormalities or ketosis. Occasionally, prenatal vitamin preparations with iron cause nausea. Rarely, severe, persistent vomiting may result from hydatidiform mole. Vomiting can also result from many nonobstetric disorders.

Evaluation

Vomiting is less likely to be due to pregnancy if it begins after the 1st trimester of pregnancy. Vomiting is likely to be due to pregnancy if it lasts several days to weeks, abdominal pain is absent, and other apparent causes for vomiting are absent. If hyperemesis gravidarum is suspected, urine ketones are measured; if symptoms are particularly severe or persistent, serum electrolytes are measured. A normal intrauterine pregnancy should be confirmed to rule out hydatidiform mole. Other tests are done based on clinically suspected nonobstetric disorders.

Treatment

Pregnancy-induced vomiting may be relieved by drinking or eating frequently (5 or 6 small meals/day), but only small amounts of bland foods (eg, crackers, soft drinks, BRAT diet [*b*ananas, *r*ice, *a*pplesauce, dry *t*oast]) should be eaten. Eating before rising may help. If dehydration (eg, due to hyperemesis gravidarum) is suspected, normal saline or Ringer's lactate is given IV, and identified electrolyte abnormalities are corrected.

The antiemetics doxylamine (10 mg po at bedtime), metoclopramide (10 mg po or IV q 8 h as needed), ondansetron (8 mg po or IM q 12 h as needed), promethazine (12.5 to 25 mg po, IM, or rectally q 6 h as needed), and pyridoxine (vitamin B_6; 10 to 25 mg po tid as needed) are extensively used to relieve nausea and vomiting during the 1st trimester without evidence of adverse effects on the fetus; these drugs can be used safely throughout pregnancy. Ginger, acupuncture, motion sickness bands, and hypnosis may help, as may switching from prenatal vitamins to a children's chewable vitamin with folate.

LOWER-EXTREMITY EDEMA DURING LATE PREGNANCY

Lower-extremity edema is common during late pregnancy. Some edema results when the enlarged uterus intermittently compresses the inferior vena cava during recumbency, obstructing outflow from both femoral veins. Edema may result from deep venous thrombosis (DVT), which is more common during pregnancy because pregnancy is a hypercoagulable state and the woman may be less mobile. Edema may also result from preeclampsia (see p. 2197), which results from pregnancy-induced hypertension.

Evaluation

Evaluation aims to exclude DVT and preeclampsia. Physiologic edema is a diagnosis of exclusion.

History: Common risk factors for DVT include venous insufficiency, trauma, preexisting hypercoagulable disorders, cigarette smoking, immobility, and cancer. Common risk factors for preeclampsia include chronic hypertension, personal or family history of preeclampsia, age < 20, 1st pregnancy, multifetal pregnancy, diabetes, vascular disorders, and hydatidiform mole. Unilateral edema suggests DVT. Acute dyspnea may result from pulmonary embolism due to DVT. If edema involves the face or hands (eg, if a ring no longer fits its finger), preeclampsia should be considered (see p. 2197). Other clues suggesting preeclampsia include headache, acute right upper quadrant or epigastric pain, seizures, other focal or global neurologic deficits, visual field deficits, and a bleeding tendency.

Examination: BP is measured; hypertension (BP > 140/> 90 mm Hg) warrants evaluation for preeclampsia. Ocular fundic abnormalities, diffuse hyperreflexia, jaundice, petechiae, and purpura may indicate preeclampsia. Unilateral leg redness, warmth, and tenderness suggest DVT.

Testing: If preeclampsia is suspected, urine protein is assessed. Urine dipstick testing is used routinely, but if diagnosis is unclear, urine protein in a 24-h collection may be measured. Hypertension plus proteinuria indicates preeclampsia. Other tests are done based on the disorder clinically suspected.

Treatment

Physiologic edema can be reduced by intermittently lying on the left side, which moves the uterus off the inferior vena cava, and by wearing elastic support stockings.

VAGINAL BLEEDING DURING LATE PREGNANCY

The most worrisome causes of bleeding in late pregnancy are placenta previa (see p. 2196) and abruptio placentae (see p. 2191); either can result in hemorrhagic shock, which should be treated with IV fluid resuscitation and other measures before or during evaluation. Other obstetric causes include labor (with expulsion of a bloody mucus plug) and occult marginal placental separation. Disseminated intravascular coagulation (DIC) is an uncommon but significant complication of abruptio placentae. Because pelvic blood flow increases during late pregnancy, previously asymptomatic cervical and vaginal lesions (eg, polyps, ulcers) that are unrelated to pregnancy often bleed for the 1st time.

Evaluation

History: Risk factors for abruptio placentae include prior abruptio placentae, maternal age > 35, multiparity, hypertension, tobacco use, substance abuse (particularly of cocaine), abdominal trauma, maternal sickle cell anemia, thrombotic disorders, vasculitis, and other vascular disorders. Risk factors for placenta previa include multiparity, multifetal pregnancy, prior uterine surgery (particularly cesarean section), and other uterine abnormalities that can interfere with implantation (eg, fibroids). Placenta previa is usually recognized and diagnosed prenatally during routine ultrasonography (see p. 2196).

Dark, small-volume vaginal bleeding with moderate to severe uterine pain suggests abruptio placentae. Bright, large-volume vaginal bleeding with mild or minimal uterine pain suggests placenta previa.

Examination: Digital examination of the cervix should not be done until placenta previa has been excluded. Such examination can precipitate torrential bleeding in women with placenta previa. Speculum examination can be done but must be done very carefully.

However, if placenta previa is present, speculum examination rarely provides any information that would alter clinical management.

Signs of hemorrhagic shock or hypovolemia out of proportion to degree of vaginal bleeding suggest abruptio placentae, as do DIC and uterine irritability and tenderness.

Testing: If bleeding is minimal, blood typing and Rh testing are done to determine whether $Rh_0(D)$ immune globulin is needed (see Erythroblastosis Fetalis on p. 2194). If bleeding is significant, CBC, PT, PTT, blood typing, and cross-matching are indicated. If abruptio placentae is suspected, fibrinogen level and fibrin-split products are also measured to check for DIC.

Pelvic ultrasonography or fetal monitoring may be necessary, but testing should not delay obstetric consultation because immediate delivery may be indicated. Fetal distress out of proportion to vaginal bleeding suggests abruptio placentae.

Treatment

Hemorrhagic shock (see p. 562) and DIC (see p. 1084) are treated immediately. If hemorrhagic shock, DIC, abruptio placentae, or placenta previa are present, an obstetrician determines the method and timing of delivery.

TRAVEL DURING PREGNANCY

The safest time to travel during pregnancy is between 14 and 28 wk. Travel time should not exceed 5 or 6 h/day. Pregnant women should wear seat belts regardless of gestational dates and type of vehicle. Travel on airplanes is safe until 36 wk gestation.

260 NORMAL PREGNANCY, LABOR, AND DELIVERY

The earliest sign of pregnancy and the reason most pregnant women initially see a physician is missing a menstrual period. For sexually active women who are of reproductive age and have regular periods, missing a period for ≥ 1 wk is presumptive evidence of pregnancy.

Pregnancy is considered to last 266 days from the time of conception or 280 days from the 1st day of the last menstrual period if periods occur regularly every 28 days. Delivery date is estimated based on the last menstrual period. Delivery up to 2 wk earlier or later than the estimated date is normal.

Symptoms and Signs

Pregnancy may cause breasts to be engorged from increased levels of estrogen (primarily) and progesterone—an extension of premenstrual breast engorgement. Nausea, occasionally with vomiting, may occur from increased secretion of the β subunit of human chorionic gonadotropin (β-hCG) and estrogen by syncytial cells of the placenta, beginning 10 days after fertilization (see p. 2148). The corpus luteum in the ovary, stimulated by β-hCG, continues secreting large amounts of estrogen and progesterone to maintain the pregnancy. Many women become fatigued at this time, and a few women notice abdominal bloating very early.

Pelvic examination findings include a softer cervix and an irregularly softened, enlarged uterus. The cervix usually becomes bluish to purple, probably because blood supply to the uterus is increased. Around 12 wk gestation, the uterus extends above the true pelvis into the abdomen; at 20 wk, it reaches the umbilicus; and by 36 wk, the upper pole almost reaches the xiphoid process.

Diagnosis

Usually urine and occasionally blood tests are used to confirm or exclude pregnancy, often several days before a missed menstrual period or as early as several days after conception; both tests are accurate. Levels of β-hCG, which correlate with gestational age in normal pregnancies, can also be used to determine whether a fetus is growing normally. The best approach is to compare 2 serum β-hCG values, obtained 48 to 72 h apart and measured by the same laboratory. In a normal single pregnancy, β-hCG levels double about every 1.4 to 2.1 days during the 1st 60 days, then begin to decrease between 10 and 18 wk. Regular doubling of the β-hCG level during the 1st trimester strongly suggests normal growth.

Other accepted signs of pregnancy include presence of a gestational sac in the uterus, seen with ultrasonography typically at about 4 to 5 wk and typically corresponding to a serum β-hCG level of about 1500 mIU/mL (a yolk sac can usually be seen in the gestational sac by 5 wk); fetal heart motion, seen with real-time ultrasonography as early as 5 to 6 wk; fetal heart sounds, heard with Doppler ultrasonography as early as 8 to 10 wk if the uterus is accessible abdominally; and fetal movements felt by the examining physician after 20 wk. Pregnant women usually begin to feel fetal movement between 16 and 20 wk.

PHYSIOLOGY OF PREGNANCY

Pregnancy causes physiologic changes in all maternal organ systems; most return to normal after delivery. In general, the changes are more dramatic in multifetal than in single pregnancies.

Cardiovascular: Cardiac output (CO) increases 30 to 50%, beginning by 6 wk gestation and peaking between 16 and 28 wk (usually at about 24 wk). It remains elevated until after 30 wk, then may decrease slightly because the enlarging uterus partially obstructs the vena cava. During labor, CO increases another 30%. After delivery, the uterus contracts, and CO drops markedly to about 15 to 25% above normal, then slowly decreases over the next 3 to 4 wk until it reaches the prepregnancy level at about 6 wk postpartum. The increase in CO is due mainly to demands of the uteroplacental circulation; volume of the uteroplacental circulation increases markedly, and circulation within the intervillous space acts partly as an arteriovenous shunt. As the placenta and fetus develop, blood flow to the uterus must increase to about 1 L/min (20% of normal CO) at term. The needs of the skin (to regulate temperature) and kidneys (to excrete fetal wastes) account for some of the increased CO.

To increase CO, heart rate increases from the normal 70 to as high as 90 beats/min, and stroke volume increases. During the 2nd trimester, BP usually drops (and pulse pressure widens), even though CO and renin and angiotensin levels increase, because uteroplacental circulation expands (the placental intervillous space develops) and systemic vascular resistance decreases. Resistance decreases because blood viscosity and sensitivity to angiotensin decrease, probably mediated by vasodilating prostaglandins. During the 3rd trimester, BP may return to normal. With twins, CO increases more and diastolic BP is lower at 20 wk than with a single fetus.

Exercise increases CO, heart rate, O_2 consumption, and respiratory volume/min more during pregnancy than at other times. The hyperdynamic circulation of pregnancy increases frequency of functional murmurs and accentuates heart sounds. X-ray or ECG may show the heart displaced into a horizontal position, rotating to the left, with increased transverse diameter. Premature atrial and ventricular beats are common during pregnancy. All these changes are normal and should not be erroneously diagnosed as a heart disorder; they can usually be managed with reassurance alone. However, paroxysms of atrial tachycardia occur more frequently in pregnant women and may require prophylactic digitalization.

Hematologic: Total blood volume increases proportionally with CO, but the increase in plasma volume is greater (close to 50%) than that in RBC mass (about 25%); thus Hb is lowered by dilution, from about 13.3 to 12.1 g. With twins, total maternal blood volume increases more (closer to 60%, or an addition of ≥ 500 mL).

WBC count increases slightly to 9,000 to 12,000/μL. Marked leukocytosis (≥ 20,000/μL) occurs during labor and the 1st few days postpartum.

Iron requirements increase by a total of about 1 g during the entire pregnancy and are higher during the 2nd half of pregnancy—6 to 7 mg/day. The fetus and placenta use about 300 mg of iron, and the increased maternal RBC mass requires an additional 500 mg. Excretion accounts for 200 mg. Iron supplements are needed to prevent anemia because the amount absorbed from the diet and recruited from iron stores (average 300 to 500 mg) is usually insufficient to meet the demands of pregnancy.

Urinary: Changes in renal function parallel those in cardiac function. GFR increases 30 to 50%, peaks between 16 and 24 wk gestation, and remains at that level until nearly term, when it may decrease slightly because uterine pressure on the vena cava causes venous stasis in the lower extremities. Renal plasma flow increases proportionally. As a result, BUN decreases, usually to < 10 mg/dL (< 3.6 mmol urea/L), and creatinine levels decrease proportionally to 0.7 mg/dL (62 μmol/L). Marked dilation of the ureters (hydroureter) is caused by hormonal influences (predominantly progesterone) and by backup due to pressure from the enlarged uterus on the ureters, which can also cause hydronephrosis. Postpartum, the urinary collecting system may take as long as 12 wk to return to normal.

Postural changes affect renal function more during pregnancy than at other times; ie, the supine position increases renal function more, and upright positions decrease renal function more. Renal function also markedly increases in the lateral position; this position relieves the pressure that the enlarged uterus puts on the great vessels when pregnant women are supine. This positional increase in renal function is one reason pregnant women need to urinate frequently when trying to sleep.

Respiratory: Lung function changes partly because progesterone increases and partly because the enlarging uterus interferes with lung expansion. Progesterone signals the brain to lower CO_2 levels. To lower CO_2 levels, tidal and minute volume and respiratory rate increase, which increases plasma pH. O_2 consumption increases by about 20% to meet the increased metabolic needs of the fetus, placenta, and several maternal organs. Inspiratory and expiratory reserve, residual volume and capacity, and plasma P_{CO_2} decrease. Vital capacity and plasma P_{O_2} do not change. Thoracic circumference increases by about 10 cm. Considerable hyperemia and edema of the respiratory tract occur because CO increases. Occasionally, symptomatic nasopharyngeal obstruction and nasal stuffiness occur, eustachian tubes are transiently blocked, and tone and quality of voice change. Mild dyspnea during exertion is common, and deep respirations are more frequent.

GI and hepatobiliary: As pregnancy progresses, pressure from the enlarging uterus on the rectum and lower portion of the colon may cause constipation. GI motility decreases because elevated progesterone levels relax smooth muscle. Heartburn and belching are common, possibly resulting from delayed gastric emptying and gastroesophageal reflux due to relaxation of the lower esophageal sphincter and diaphragmatic hiatus. HCl production decreases; thus peptic ulcer disease is uncommon during pregnancy, and preexisting ulcers often become less severe.

Incidence of gallbladder disorders increases somewhat. Pregnancy subtly affects hepatic function, especially bile transport. Routine liver function test values are normal, but alkaline phosphatase levels increase progressively during the 3rd trimester and may be 2 to 3 times normal at term; the increase is due to placental production of this enzyme rather than hepatic dysfunction.

Endocrine: Pregnancy alters the function of most endocrine glands, partly because the placenta produces hormones and partly because most hormones circulate in protein-bound forms and protein binding increases during pregnancy.

The placenta produces a hormone (similar to thyroid-stimulating hormone) that stimulates the thyroid, causing hyperplasia, increased vascularity, and moderate enlargement. Estrogen stimulates hepatocytes, causing increased thyroid-binding globulin levels, so although total thyroxine levels may increase, levels of free thyroid hormones remain normal. The increase in thyroid function may resemble hyperthyroidism, with tachycardia, palpitations, excessive perspiration, and emotional instability. However, true hyperthyroidism occurs in only 0.08% of pregnancies.

The placenta produces corticotropin-releasing hormone (CRH), which stimulates maternal ACTH production. Increased ACTH levels increase levels of adrenal hormones, especially aldosterone and cortisol, and thus contribute to edema. Increased production of corticosteroids and increased placental production of progesterone lead to insulin resistance and an increased need for insulin, as does the stress of pregnancy and possibly the increased level of human placental lactogen. Insulinase, produced by the placenta, may also increase insulin requirements, so that many women with gestational diabetes develop more overt forms of diabetes (see pp. 1274 and 2170). The placenta produces melanocyte-stimulating hormone (MSH), which increases skin pigmentation late in pregnancy, and the β subunit of human chorionic gonadotropin (β-hCG), a trophic hormone that, like follicle-stimulating and luteinizing hormones, maintains the corpus luteum and thereby prevents ovulation.

The pituitary gland enlarges by about 135% during pregnancy. The maternal plasma prolactin level increases by 10-fold. Increased prolactin is related to an increase in thyrotropin-releasing hormone production, stimulated by estrogen. The primary function of increased prolactin is to ensure lactation. The level returns to normal postpartum, even in women who breastfeed.

Dermatologic: Increased levels of estrogens, progesterone, and MSH contribute to pigmentary changes, although exact pathogenesis is unknown. These changes include melasma (mask of pregnancy), which is a blotchy, brownish pigment over the forehead and malar eminences; darkening of the mammary areolae, axilla, and genitals; and the linea nigra, a dark line that appears down the midabdomen. Incidence of spider angiomas, usually only above the waist, and thin-walled, dilated capillaries, especially in the lower legs, increases.

DRUGS IN PREGNANCY

The most commonly used drugs include antiemetics, antacids, antihistamines, analgesics, antimicrobials, tranquilizers, hypnotics, diuretics, and social and illicit drugs. The FDA classifies drugs into 5 categories of safety for use during pregnancy (see TABLE 260–1). Few well-controlled studies of therapeutic drugs have been conducted in pregnant women. Most information about drug safety during pregnancy is derived from animal studies and uncontrolled studies in humans (eg, postmarketing reports). During pregnancy, drugs are often required to treat certain disorders (for selection, use, and adverse effects of specific drugs, see TABLE 261–2 on p. 2174). Despite widespread concern about drug safety, drug exposure, excluding alcohol, accounts for only 2 to 3% of all fetal congenital malformations; most malformations result from genetic, environmental, or unknown causes.

Not all maternal drugs cross the placenta to the fetus. Those that do can have a direct toxic or teratogenic effect (for known and suspected teratogens, see TABLE 260–2). Those that do not cross the placenta may still harm the fetus by constricting placental vessels and thus impairing gas and nutrient exchange; by producing severe uterine hypertonia resulting in anoxic injury; or by altering maternal physiology (eg, causing hypotension).

TABLE 260–1. FDA CATEGORIES OF DRUG SAFETY DURING PREGNANCY

CATEGORY	DESCRIPTION
A	Controlled human studies show no fetal risks; these drugs are the safest
B	Animal studies show no risk to the fetus and no controlled human studies have been conducted, or animal studies show a risk to the fetus but well-controlled human studies do not
C	No adequate animal or human studies have been conducted, or adverse fetal effects have been shown in animals but no human data are available
D	Evidence of human fetal risk exists, but benefits may outweigh risks in certain situations (eg, life-threatening disorders, serious disorders for which safer drugs cannot be used or are ineffective)
X	Proven fetal risks outweigh any possible benefit

Drugs diffuse across the placenta similarly to the way they cross other epithelial barriers (see Absorption on p. 2522). Whether and how quickly a drug crosses the placenta depend on the drug's mol wt, extent of its binding to another substance (eg, carrier protein), area available for exchange across the villi, and amount of drug metabolized by the placenta. Most drugs with a mol wt < 500 daltons readily cross the placenta and enter fetal circulation. Substances with a high mol wt (eg, protein-bound drugs) usually do not cross the placenta. The exception is immune globulin G, which is occasionally used to treat disorders such as fetal alloimmune thrombocytopenia. Generally, equilibration between maternal blood and fetal tissues takes at least 40 min.

A drug's effect on the fetus is determined largely by fetal age at exposure, drug potency, and drug dosage. Drugs given before the 20th day after fertilization may have an all-or-nothing effect, killing the embryo or not affecting it at all. Teratogenesis is not likely

TABLE 260–2. KNOWN OR SUSPECTED TERATOGENS

ACE inhibitors	Isotretinoin
Alcohol	Lithium
Aminopterin	Methimazole
Androgens	Methotrexate
Carbamazepine	Phenytoin
Coumarins	Radioactive iodine
Danazol	Tetracycline
Diethylstilbestrol	Trimethadione
Etretinate	Valproate

during this stage. It is more likely during organogenesis (between 14 and 56 days after fertilization). Drugs reaching the embryo at this stage may result in abortion, a sublethal gross anatomic defect (true teratogenic effect), or covert embryopathy (a permanent subtle metabolic or functional defect that may manifest later in life), or the drugs may have no measurable effect. Drugs given after organogenesis (in the 2nd and 3rd trimesters) are unlikely to be teratogenic, but they may alter growth and function of normally formed fetal organs and tissues.

Vaccines: Immunization is as effective in women who are pregnant as in those who are not. Influenza vaccine is recommended for all pregnant women in the 2nd or 3rd trimester during influenza season. Other vaccines should be reserved for situations in which the woman or fetus is at significant risk of exposure to a hazardous infection and risk of adverse effects from the vaccine is low. Vaccinations for cholera, hepatitis A and B, measles, mumps, plague, poliomyelitis, rabies, tetanus-diphtheria, typhoid, and yellow fever may be given during pregnancy if risk of infection is substantial. Live-virus vaccines should not be given to women who are or may be pregnant. Rubella vaccine, an attenuated live-virus vaccine, may cause subclinical placental and fetal infection. However, no defects in neonates have been attributed to rubella vaccine, and women vaccinated inadvertently during early pregnancy need not be advised to terminate pregnancy based solely on theoretical risk from the vaccine. Varicella is another attenuated live-virus vaccine that can potentially infect the fetus; risk is highest between 13 and 22 wk gestation. This vaccine is contraindicated during pregnancy.

Vitamin A: In the amount typically present in prenatal vitamins (5000 IU/day), vitamin A has not been associated with teratogenic risk. However, doses > 10,000 IU/day during early pregnancy may increase risk of congenital malformations.

Social and illicit drugs: Cigarette smoking and use of alcohol or cocaine during pregnancy can cause significant problems in fetuses and neonates (see p. 2189). Although marijuana's main metabolite can cross the placenta, recreational use of this drug does not consistently appear to increase risk of congenital malformations, fetal growth restriction, or postnatal neurobehavioral abnormalities. Many mothers of children with congenital heart defects used amphetamines during pregnancy, suggesting a possible teratogenic association.

Whether consuming large amounts of caffeine can increase risk of perinatal complications is unclear. Consuming caffeine in small amounts (eg, 1 cup of coffee/day) appears to pose little or no risk to the fetus, but some data, which did not account for tobacco or alcohol use, suggest that consuming large amounts (> 7 cups of coffee/day) increases risk of stillbirths, preterm deliveries, low birth weight, and spontaneous abortions. Decaffeinated beverages theoretically pose little risk to the fetus.

Use of the dietary sugar substitute aspartame during pregnancy is often questioned. The most common metabolite of aspartame, phenylalanine, is concentrated in the fetus by active placental transport; toxic levels may cause mental retardation. However, when ingestion is within the usual range, fetal phenylalanine levels are far below toxic levels. Thus, moderate ingestion of aspartame (eg, no more than 1 liter of diet soda per day) during pregnancy appears to pose little risk of fetal toxicity. However, in pregnant women with phenylketonuria (see p. 2460), intake of phenylalanine and thus aspartame is prohibited.

MANAGEMENT OF NORMAL LABOR

Labor consists of a series of rhythmic, involuntary, progressive contractions of the uterus that cause effacement (thinning) and dilation of the uterine cervix. The stimulus for labor is unknown, but digitally manipulating or mechanically stretching the cervix during examination enhances uterine contractile activity, most likely by stimulating release of oxytocin by the posterior pituitary gland. Normal labor usually begins within 2 wk (before or after) the estimated delivery date. In a 1st pregnancy, labor usually lasts a maximum of 12 to 14 h; subsequent labors are often shorter, averaging 6 to 8 h.

Stages of labor: There are 3 stages of labor.

The 1st stage—from onset of labor to full dilation of the cervix (about 10 cm)—has 2 phases, latent and active. During the latent phase, irregular contractions become progressively better coordinated, discomfort is minimal, and the cervix effaces and dilates to 4 cm. The latent phase is difficult to time precisely, and duration varies, averaging 8 ½ h in nulliparas and 5 h in multiparas; duration is considered abnormal if it lasts > 20 h in nulliparas or > 12 h in multiparas. During the active phase, the cervix becomes fully dilated, and the presenting part descends well into the midpelvis. On average, the active phase lasts 5 to 7 h in nulliparas and 2 to 4 h in multiparas. The cervix should dilate 1.2 cm/h in nulliparas and 1.5 cm/h in multiparas. Pelvic examinations are done every 2 to 3 h to evaluate labor progress. Lack of progress in dilation and descent of the presenting part may indicate dystocia (fetopelvic disproportion). If the membranes have not spontaneously ruptured, amniotomy (artificial rupture of membranes) is typically done during the active phase. As a result, labor may progress more rapidly, and meconium-stained amniotic fluid may be detected earlier. Amniotomy during this stage may be necessary for internal fetal monitoring to confirm fetal well-being. Women may begin to feel the urge to bear down as the presenting part descends into the pelvis. However, they should be discouraged from bearing down until the cervix is fully dilated so that they do not tear the cervix or waste energy.

The 2nd stage is the time from full cervical dilation to delivery of the fetus. On average, it lasts 2 h in nulliparas (median 50 min) and 1 h in multiparas (median 20 min). It may last another hour or more if conduction (epidural) analgesia or intense opioid sedation is used. For spontaneous delivery, women must supplement uterine contractions by expulsively bearing down.

Maternal heart rate and BP and fetal heart rate should be checked continuously by electronic monitoring or by auscultation during the 1st stage of labor (see p. 2164). In the 2nd stage, women should be attended constantly, and fetal heart sounds should be checked continuously or after every contraction. Uterine contractions may be monitored by palpation or electronically.

The 3rd stage of labor begins after delivery of the infant and ends with delivery of the placenta.

Before admission: Bloody show (a small amount of blood with mucous discharge from the cervix) may precede onset of labor by as much as 72 h. Labor begins with irregular contractions of varying intensity; they apparently soften (ripen) the cervix, which begins to efface and dilate. As labor progresses, contractions increase in duration, intensity, and frequency.

Occasionally, the membranes (amniotic and chorionic sac) rupture before labor begins, and amniotic fluid leaks through the cervix and vagina. Rupture of membranes at any stage before the onset of labor is called premature rupture of membranes (PROM—see p. 2204). Some women with PROM feel a gush of fluid from the vagina, followed by steady leaking. Further confirmation is not needed if during examination, fluid is seen leaking from the cervix. Confirmation of more subtle cases may require testing. For example, the pH of vaginal fluid may be tested with Nitrazine paper, which turns deep blue at a pH > 6.5 (pH of amniotic fluid: 7.0 to 7.6); false positives can occur if vaginal fluid contains blood or semen or if certain infections are present. A sample of the secretions from the posterior vaginal fornix or cervix may be obtained, placed on a slide, air dried, and viewed microscopically for ferning. Ferning (crystallization of NaCl in amniotic fluid) usually confirms rupture of membranes. If rupture is still unconfirmed, ultrasonography showing oligohydramnios (deficient amniotic fluid) provides further evidence suggesting rupture. Rarely, amniocentesis with instillation of dye is done to confirm rupture; dye detected in the vagina or on a tampon confirms rupture.

When a woman's membranes rupture, she should contact her physician immediately. About 80 to 90% of women with ruptured membranes at term and about 50% of women with preterm PROM go into labor spontaneously within 24 h; > 90% of women with PROM go into labor within 2 wk. The earlier the membranes rupture before 37 wk, the longer the delay between rupture and labor onset. If membranes rupture at term but labor does not start within several hours, labor is typically induced to lower risk of maternal and fetal infection.

Birthing options: Most women prefer hospital delivery, and most practitioners recommend it because unexpected maternal and fetal complications may occur during labor and delivery or postpartum. About 30% of hospital deliveries involve an obstetric complication (eg, laceration, postpartum hemorrhage). Complications include abruptio placentae (premature separation), nonreassuring fetal heart status, shoulder dystocia, need for emergency cesarean delivery, neonatal depression or abnormality, and maternal postpartum hemorrhage. Nonetheless, many women want a more homelike environment for delivery; in response, some hospitals provide birthing facilities with fewer formalities and rigid regulations but with emergency equipment and personnel available. Birthing centers may be freestanding or located in hospitals; care at either site is similar or identical. In some hospitals, certified nurse-midwives provide much of the care for low-risk pregnancies. Midwives work with a physician, who is continuously available for consultation and operative deliveries (eg, by forceps, vacuum extractor, or cesarean section). All birthing options should be discussed.

For many women, presence of the father or another support person during labor is helpful and should be encouraged. Moral support, encouragement, and expressions of affection decrease anxiety and make the process of labor less frightening and unpleasant. Childbirth education classes can prepare parents for a normal or complicated labor and delivery. Sharing the stresses of labor and the sight and sound of their own child tends to create strong bonds between the parents and between parents and child. The parents should be fully informed of any complications.

Admission: Typically, pregnant women are advised to go to the hospital if they believe their membranes have ruptured or if they are experiencing contractions lasting at least 30 sec and occurring regularly at intervals of about ≤ 6 min. Within an hour after presentation at a hospital, whether a woman is in labor can usually be determined based on occurrence of regular and sustained painful uterine contractions, bloody show, membrane rupture, and complete cervical effacement. If these criteria are not met, false labor may be tentatively diagnosed, and the pregnant woman is typically observed for a time and, if labor does not begin within several hours, sent home.

When pregnant women are admitted, their BP, heart and respiratory rates, temperature, and weight are recorded, and presence or absence of edema is noted. A urine specimen is collected for protein and glucose analysis, and blood is drawn for a CBC and blood typing. A physical examination is done. While examining the abdomen, the physician estimates size, position, and presentation of the fetus, using Leopold's maneuvers (see FIG. 260–1). The physician notes the presence and rate of fetal heart sounds. Preliminary estimates of the strength, frequency, and duration of contractions are also recorded. A helpful mnemonic device for evaluation is the 3 Ps: powers (contraction strength, frequency, and duration), passage (pelvic measurements), and passenger (eg, fetal size, position, heart rate pattern).

If labor is active and the pregnancy is at term, a labor-and-delivery nurse or a physician examines the vagina with 2 fingers of a gloved hand to evaluate progress of labor. If bleeding (particularly if heavy) is present, the examination is delayed until placental location is confirmed by ultrasonography. If bleeding results from placenta previa, vaginal examination can initiate severe hemorrhage. If labor is not active but membranes are ruptured, a speculum examination is done initially to document cervical dilation and effacement and to estimate station (location of the presenting part); however, digital examinations are delayed until the active phase of labor or problems (eg, decreased fetal heart sounds) occur. If the membranes have ruptured, any fetal meconium (producing greenish-brown discoloration) should be noted because it may be a sign of fetal stress. If labor is preterm (< 37 wk) or has not begun, only a sterile speculum examination should be done, and a culture should be taken for gonococci, chlamydiae, and group B streptococci.

Cervical dilation is recorded in centimeters as the diameter of a circle; 10 cm is considered complete. Effacement is estimated in percentages, from zero (no effacement) to 100% (complete thinning of the cervix). Cervical shortening may be recorded in centimeters using the normal, uneffaced average cervical length of 3.5 to 4.0 cm as a guide. Station is expressed in centimeters above or below the level of the ischial spines. Level of the is-

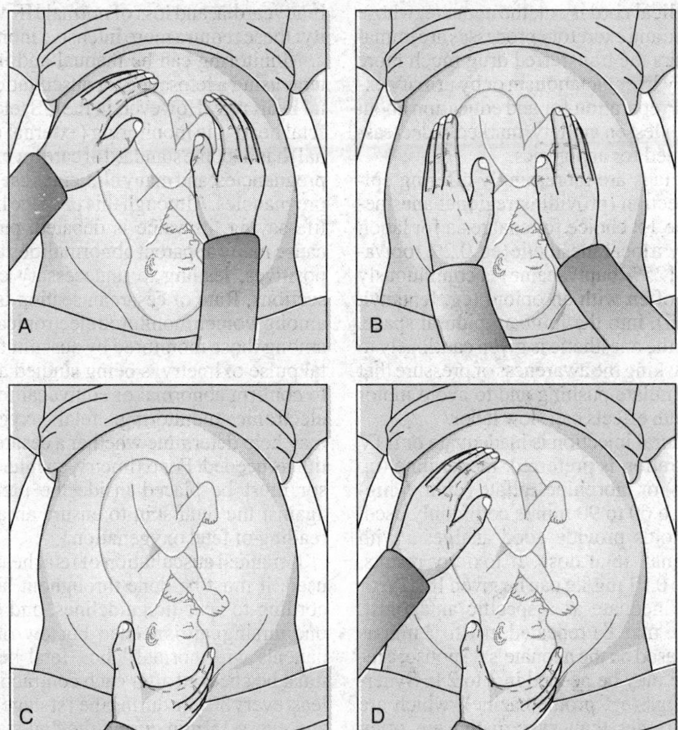

Fig. 260–1. Leopold maneuver. (A) The uterine fundus is palpated to determine which fetal part occupies the fundus. (B) Each side of the maternal abdomen is palpated to determine which side is fetal spine and which is the extremities. (C) The area above the symphysis pubis is palpated to locate the fetal presenting part and thus determine how far the fetus has descended and whether the fetus is engaged. (D) One hand applies pressure on the fundus while the index finger and thumb of the other hand palpate the presenting part to confirm presentation and engagement.

chial spines corresponds to 0 station; levels above (+) or below (−) the spines are recorded in cm increments. Fetal lie, position, and presentation are noted. Lie describes the relationship of the long axis of the fetus to that of the mother (longitudinal, oblique, transverse); presentation describes the part of the fetus at the cervical opening (eg, breech, vertex, shoulder). Position describes the relationship of the presenting part to the maternal pelvis (eg, occiput left anterior [OLA] for cephalic, sacrum right posterior [SRP] for breech).

Preparation for delivery: Women are admitted to the labor suite for frequent observation until delivery. If labor is active, they should receive little or nothing by mouth to prevent possible vomiting and aspiration during delivery or in case emergency delivery with general anesthesia is necessary. Enemas and shaving or clipping of vulvar hair are no longer indicated. An IV infusion of Ringer's lactate may be started, using a large-bore indwelling catheter inserted in a vein in the hand or forearm. During a normal labor of 6 to 10 h, women should be given 500 to 1000 mL of this solution. The infusion prevents dehydration during labor and subsequent hemoconcentration and maintains an adequate circulating blood volume. The catheter provides immediate access for drugs or blood if needed. Fluid preloading is also valuable if epidural or spinal anesthesia is to be used.

Analgesia: Analgesics may be given during labor as needed, but as little as possible should be given because they cross the placenta and may depress the neonate's breathing. Neonatal toxicity can occur because after the umbilical cord is cut, the neonate, whose metabolic and excretory processes are immature, clears the transferred drug much more slowly, by liver metabolism or by urinary excretion. Preparation for and education about childbirth lessen anxiety, markedly decreasing the need for analgesics.

Physicians are increasingly offering epidural injection (providing regional anesthesia) as the 1st choice for analgesia for labor. Typically, a local anesthetic (eg, 0.2% ropivacaine, 0.125% bupivacaine) is continuously infused, often with an opioid (eg, fentanyl, sufentanil), into the lumbar epidural space. Initially, the anesthetic is given cautiously to avoid masking the awareness of pressure that helps stimulate pushing and to avoid motor block; both effects can slow labor.

If epidural injection is inadequate or if IV administration is preferred, meperidine (up to 25 mg) or morphine sulfate (up to 5 mg) given IV q 60 to 90 min is commonly used. Both opioids provide good analgesia with only a small total dose. If toxicity results, naloxone 0.01 mg/kg can be given IM, IV, or sc to the neonate as a specific antagonist. Naloxone may be repeated in 1 to 2 min as needed based on the neonate's response; a repeat dose may be needed in 1 to 2 h. Synergistic drugs (eg, promethazine), which are additive rather than synergistic, are often used because they lessen nausea due to the opioid; small doses should be used because no antidote is available if an overdose is given or a problem develops. Thus, if more analgesia is needed, additional meperidine or morphine without synergistic drugs is preferred, or another analgesic method should be considered.

Fetal Monitoring

Fetal status must be monitored during labor. The main parameters are fetal heart rate and fetal heart rate variability, particularly in relationship to uterine contractions. Several patterns are recognized. One is considered normal and reassuring; the others are considered abnormal and nonreassuring. A normal pattern is a baseline heart rate (HR) of 120 to 160 beats/min that varies by 6 to 25 beats with movement or contractions, that accelerates appropriately for gestational age, and that does not decelerate during contractions. Patterns that indicate possible nonreassuring fetal heart status include late decelerations, variable decelerations, tachycardia, severe bradycardia, and loss of normal HR variability; these require more intensive monitoring.

Monitoring can be manual and intermittent, using a fetoscope for auscultation of fetal heart rate. However, in the US, electronic fetal heart rate monitoring (external or internal) has become standard of care for high-risk pregnancies, and many clinicians use it for all pregnancies. Although this practice has been life-saving, its value is debated, partly because many apparent abnormalities are false positives, leading to unnecessary cesarean sections. Rate of cesarean section is higher among women monitored electronically than among those monitored by auscultation. Fetal pulse oximetry is being studied as a way to confirm abnormal or equivocal results of electronic monitoring; fetal oxygenation may help determine whether a cesarean section is needed. For oximetry, an internal sensor must be placed inside the uterus and against the fetal skin to ensure an accurate reading of fetal oxygenation.

If manual auscultation of fetal heart rate is used, it must be done throughout labor according to specific guidelines, and one-on-one nursing care is needed. For low-risk pregnancies with normal labor, fetal heart rate must be checked after each contraction or at least every 30 min during the 1st stage of labor and every 15 min during the 2nd stage. For high-risk pregnancies, fetal heart rate must be checked every 15 min during the 1st stage and every 3 to 5 min during the 2nd stage. Listening for at least 1 to 2 min beginning at a contraction's peak is recommended. Periodic auscultation has a lower false-positive rate for abnormalities and incidence of intervention than continuous electronic monitoring, and it provides opportunities for more personal contact with women during labor. However, following the standard guidelines for auscultation is often difficult and may not be cost-effective. Also, unless done accurately, auscultation may not detect abnormalities.

For external electronic fetal heart rate monitoring, devices are applied to the maternal abdomen to record fetal heart sounds and uterine contractions. For internal monitoring, amniotic membranes must be ruptured. Then, leads are inserted through the cervix; an electrode is attached to the fetal scalp to monitor heart rate, and a catheter is placed in the uterine cavity to measure intrauterine pressure. Generally, external and internal monitoring are similarly reliable. External devices are used for women in normal labor; internal methods are used when external monitoring does not supply enough information about fetal well-being or uterine contraction intensity.

External fetal monitoring can be used to continuously record fetal heart rate and correlate it with fetal movements (called a nonstress test). A nonstress test is interpreted as nonreassuring if no accelerations occur during a 40-min period. External monitoring can be used similarly with a contraction stress test; fetal movements and heart rate are monitored during contractions induced by oxytocin (oxytocin challenge test) or breast stimulation or during spontaneous contractions. These tests are frequently used to monitor complicated or high-risk pregnancies (eg, complicated by maternal diabetes or hypertension or by prior stillbirth or fetal growth restriction).

If a problem is detected, intrauterine fetal resuscitation is tried; women may be given O_2 by tight non-rebreather face mask or rapid IV fluid infusion or may be positioned laterally. If fetal heart pattern does not improve in a reasonable period and delivery is not imminent, urgent delivery by cesarean section is needed.

MANAGEMENT OF NORMAL DELIVERY

Many obstetric units now use a combined labor, delivery, recovery, and postpartum room, so that the woman, support person, and neonate remain in the same room throughout their stay. Some units use a traditional labor room and separate delivery suite, to which the woman is transferred when delivery is imminent. The father or other support person should be offered the opportunity to accompany her. In the delivery room, the perineum is washed and draped, and the neonate delivered. After delivery, the woman may remain there or be transferred to a postpartum unit.

Anesthesia

Options include regional anesthesia, pudendal block, perineal infiltration, and general anesthesia. Local anesthetics and opioids are commonly used. These drugs pass through the placenta; thus, during the hour before delivery, such drugs should be given in small doses to avoid toxicity (eg, CNS depression and bradycardia) in the neonate. Opioids used alone do not provide adequate analgesia and so are most often used with anesthetics.

Regional anesthesia most commonly involves lumbar epidural injection of a local anesthetic (see p. 2164). Epidural injection is being increasingly used for delivery, including cesarean section, and has essentially replaced pudendal and paracervical blocks. The local anesthetics often used for epidural injection (eg, bupivacaine) have a longer duration of action and slower onset than those used for pudendal block (eg, lidocaine). Other forms of regional anesthesia include caudal injection (into the sacral canal), which is rarely used, and spinal injection (into the paraspinal subarachnoid space). Spinal injection may be used for cesarean section, but it is used less often for vaginal deliveries because it is short-lasting (preventing its use during labor) and has a small risk of spinal headache afterward. When spinal injection is used, patients must be constantly attended, and vital signs must be checked every 5 min to detect and treat possible hypotension.

Pudendal block, rarely used because of the widespread use of epidural analgesia, involves injecting a local anesthetic through the vaginal wall so that the anesthetic bathes the pudendal nerve as it crosses the ischial spine. This block anesthetizes the lower vagina, perineum, and posterior vulva; the anterior vulva, innervated by lumbar dermatomes, is not anesthetized. Pudendal block is a safe, simple method for uncomplicated spontaneous vaginal deliveries if women wish to bear down and push or if labor is advanced and there is no time for epidural injection.

Infiltration of the perineum with an anesthetic is commonly used, although this method is not as effective as a well-administered pudendal block.

Paracervical block is rarely appropriate for delivery because incidence of fetal bradycardia is > 15%. It is used mainly for 1st- or early 2nd-trimester abortion. The technique involves injecting 5 to 10 mL of 1% lidocaine at the 3 and 9 o'clock positions; the analgesic response is short-lasting.

General anesthesia with potent and volatile inhalation drugs (eg, isoflurane) can cause marked depression in mother and fetus; therefore, it is not recommended for routine delivery. Rarely, nitrous oxide 40% with O_2 may be used for analgesia during vaginal delivery as long as verbal contact with the woman is maintained. Thiopental, a hypnotic, is commonly given IV with other drugs (eg, succinylcholine, nitrous oxide plus O_2) for general anesthesia during cesarean delivery; used alone, thiopental provides inadequate analgesia. With thiopental, induction is rapid and recovery is prompt. It becomes concentrated in the fetal liver, preventing high levels in the CNS; high levels may cause neonatal depression. Diazepam is sometimes used; however, large doses given IV to pregnant women before delivery may result in hypotonia, hypothermia, low Apgar scores, impaired metabolic response to cold stress, and neurologic depression in neonates. Increased interest in preparation for childbirth has reduced the use of such drugs except for forceps, breech, or twin delivery and for cesarean section.

Delivery Procedures

A vaginal examination is done to determine position and station of the fetal head. When effacement is complete and the cervix is fully dilated, the woman is told to bear down and strain with each contraction to move the head through the pelvis and progressively dilate the vaginal introitus so that more and more of the head appears. When about 3 or 4 cm of the head is visible during a contraction in nulliparas (somewhat less in multiparas), the following maneuvers can facilitate delivery and reduce risk of perineal laceration. The clinician, if right-handed, places the left palm over the infant's head during a contraction to control and, if necessary, slightly slow progress. Simultaneously, the clinician places the curved fingers of the right hand against the dilating perineum, through which the infant's brow or chin is felt. To advance the head, the clinician can wrap a hand in towel and, with curved fingers, apply pressure against the underside of the brow or chin (modified Ritgen maneuver). The clinician controls the progress of the head to effect a slow, safe delivery.

Forceps or a vacuum extractor (see p. 2202) is often used for vaginal delivery when the 2nd stage of labor is likely to be prolonged (eg, because the mother is too exhausted to bear down adequately). Forceps may be required when epidural anesthesia precludes vigorous bearing down. Local anesthesia may not interfere with bearing down; thus, forceps or vacuum extractor is not usually needed unless complications develop. Indications for forceps and vacuum extractor are essentially the same.

An episiotomy is not routine and is done only if the perineum does not stretch adequately and is obstructing delivery, usually only for 1st deliveries at term. A local anesthetic can be infiltrated if epidural analgesia is inadequate. Episiotomy prevents excessive stretching and possible tearing of the perineal tissues, including anterior tears. The incision is easier to repair than a tear. The most common type is a midline incision made from the midpoint of the fourchette directly back toward the rectum. Extension into the rectal sphincter or rectum is a risk, but if recognized promptly, the extension can be repaired successfully and heals well. Tears or extensions into the rectum can usually be prevented by keeping the infant's head well flexed until the occipital prominence passes the subpubic arch. Episioproctotomy (intentionally cutting into the rectum) is not recommended because rectovaginal fistula is a risk. Another type of episiotomy is a mediolateral incision made from the midpoint of the fourchette at a 45° angle laterally on either side. This type usually does not extend into the sphincter or rectum, but it causes greater postoperative pain and takes longer to heal than midline episiotomy. Thus, for episiotomy, a midline cut is preferred. However, use of episiotomy is decreasing because extension or tearing into the sphincter or rectum is a concern.

After delivery of the head, the infant's body rotates so that the shoulders are in an anteroposterior position; gentle downward pressure on the head delivers the anterior shoulder under the symphysis. If the cord is tight around the neck, the cord may be clamped and cut. The head is gently lifted, the posterior shoulder slides over the perineum, and the rest of the body follows without difficulty. The nose, mouth, and pharynx are aspirated with a bulb syringe to remove mucus and fluids and help start respirations. The cord should be double-clamped and cut between the clamps, and a plastic clip should be applied. If fetal or neonatal compromise is suspected, a segment of umbilical cord is doubly clamped so that arterial blood gas analysis can be done. An arterial pH > 7.15 to 7.20 is considered normal. The infant is then placed in a warmed resuscitation bassinet or on the mother's abdomen.

After delivery of the infant, the clinician places a hand gently on the abdomen over the uterine fundus to detect contractions; placental separation usually occurs during the 1st or 2nd contraction, often with a gush of blood from behind the separating placenta. The mother can usually help deliver the placenta by bearing down. If she cannot and if substantial bleeding occurs, the placenta can usually be evacuated (expressed) by placing a hand on the abdomen and exerting firm downward pressure on the uterus; this procedure is done only if the uterus feels firm because pressure on a flaccid uterus can cause it to invert. If this procedure is not effective, the umbilical cord is held taut while a hand placed on the abdomen pushes upward on the firm uterus, away from the placenta; traction on the umbilical cord is avoided because it may invert the uterus. If the placenta has not been delivered within 45 to 60 min of delivery, manual removal may be necessary; the clinician inserts an entire hand into the uterine cavity, separating the placenta from its attachment, then extracts the placenta. In such cases, an abnormally adherent placenta (placenta accreta—see p. 2208) should be suspected.

The placenta should be examined for completeness because fragments left in the uterus can cause hemorrhage or infection later. If the placenta is incomplete, the uterine cavity should be explored manually. Some obstetricians routinely explore the uterus after each delivery. However, exploration is uncomfortable and is not routinely recommended. Immediately after delivery of the placenta, an oxytocic drug (oxytocin 10 units IM, or as an infusion of 20 units/1000 mL saline at 125 mL/h) is given to help the uterus contract firmly. Oxytocin should not be given as an IV bolus because cardiac arrhythmia may occur.

The cervix and vagina are inspected for lacerations, which, if present, are repaired, as is any episiotomy. Then if the mother and infant are recovering normally, they can begin bonding. Many mothers wish to begin breastfeeding soon after delivery, and this should be encouraged. Mother, infant, and father should remain together in a warm, private area for an hour or more to enhance parent-infant bonding. Then, the infant may be taken to the nursery or left with the mother depending on her wishes. For the 1st hour after delivery, the mother should be observed closely to make sure the uterus is contracting (detected by palpation during abdominal examination) and to check for bleeding, BP abnormalities, and general well-being. The time from delivery of the placenta to 4 h postpartum has been called the 4th stage of labor; most complications, especially hemorrhage (see p. 2208), occur at this time, and frequent observation is mandatory.

261 PREGNANCY COMPLICATED BY DISEASE

Nonobstetric disorders often complicate pregnancy; management sometimes differs from that in nonpregnant patients. Coordination of care between the obstetrician and medical specialist often helps.

ANEMIA IN PREGNANCY

Normally during pregnancy, erythroid hyperplasia of the marrow occurs, and RBC mass increases. However, a disproportionate increase in plasma volume results in hemodilution (hydremia of pregnancy): Hct decreases from between 38 and 45% in healthy women who are not pregnant to about 34% during late single pregnancy and to 30% in late multifetal pregnancy. Thus during pregnancy, anemia is defined as Hb < 10 g/dL (Hct < 30%). If Hb is < 11.5 g/dL at the onset of pregnancy, women may be treated prophylactically, because subsequent hemodilution usually reduces Hb to < 10 g/dL. Despite hemodilution, O_2-carrying capacity remains normal throughout pregnancy. Hct normally increases immediately after birth.

Anemia occurs in up to 80% of some groups. The most common causes are iron deficiency and folate deficiency.

Early symptoms are usually nonexistent or nonspecific (eg, fatigue, weakness, lightheadedness, mild dyspnea with exertion). Other symptoms and signs may include pallor and, if anemia is severe, tachycardia or hypotension.

Diagnosis begins with CBC; usually, if patients have anemia, subsequent testing is based on whether the MCV is low (< 79 fL) or high (> 100 fL). For microcytic anemias, evaluation includes testing for iron deficiency (measuring serum ferritin) and hemoglobinopathies (using hemoglobin electrophoresis). If these tests are nondiagnostic and there is no response to empiric treatment, consultation with a hematologist is usually warranted. Transfusion is usually indicated if severe constitutional symptoms (eg, lightheadedness, weakness, fatigue) or cardiopulmonary symptoms or signs (eg, dyspnea, tachycardia, tachypnea) are present; the decision is not based on the Hct.

Iron deficiency anemia: About 95% of anemia cases during pregnancy are due to iron deficiency (see p. 1036). The cause is usually inadequate dietary intake (especially in teenage girls), a previous pregnancy, or the normal recurrent loss of iron in menstrual blood (which approximates the amount normally ingested each month and thus prevents iron stores from building up). Typically, Hct is ≤ 30%, and MCV is < 79 fL. Decreased serum iron and ferritin and increased serum transferrin levels confirm the diagnosis.

One 325-mg ferrous sulfate tablet taken midmorning is usually effective. Higher or more frequent doses increase GI adverse effects, especially constipation, and one dose blocks absorption of the next dose, thereby reducing percentage intake. About 20% of pregnant women do not absorb enough supplemental oral iron; a few of them require parenteral therapy, usually iron dextran 100 mg IM every other day for a total of ≥ 1000 mg over 3 wk. Hct or Hb is measured weekly to determine response. If iron supplements are ineffective, folate deficiency should be suspected.

Neonates of mothers with iron deficiency anemia usually have a normal Hct but decreased total iron stores and a need for early dietary iron supplements.

Although the practice is controversial, iron supplements (usually ferrous sulfate 325 mg po once/day) are usually given routinely to pregnant women to prevent depletion of body iron stores and prevent the anemia that may result from abnormal bleeding or a subsequent pregnancy.

Folate deficiency anemia: Folate deficiency (see pp. 29 and 1044) increases risk of neural tube defects and possibly fetal alcohol syndrome. Deficiency occurs in 0.5 to 1.5% of pregnant women; macrocytic, megaloblastic anemia occurs if deficiency is moderate or severe. Rarely, severe anemia and glossitis occur. Folate deficiency is suspected if CBC shows macrocytic indexes or high RBC distribution width (RDW) anemia. Low serum folate levels confirm the diagnosis. Treatment is folate 1 mg po bid. Severe megaloblastic anemia may warrant bone marrow examination and further treatment in a hospital. For prevention, all pregnant women are given folate 0.4 mg po once/day. Women who have had a fetus with spina bifida should take 4.0 mg once/day, starting before conception.

HEMOGLOBINOPATHIES IN PREGNANCY

(See also sidebar 131–1 on p. 1054.)

During pregnancy, hemoglobinopathies, particularly sickle cell disease, Hb S-C disease, β-thalassemia disease, and α-thalassemia, can worsen maternal and perinatal outcomes (for genetic screening, see TABLE 257–1 on p. 2145).

Preexisting sickle cell disease, particularly if severe, increases risk of maternal infection (most often, pneumonia, UTIs, and endometritis), pregnancy-induced hypertension, heart failure, and pulmonary infarction. Fetal growth restriction, preterm delivery, and low birth weight are common. Anemia almost always becomes more severe as pregnancy progresses.

Treatment of sickle cell disease during pregnancy is complex. Painful crises should be treated aggressively. Prophylactic exchange transfusions to keep Hb A at ≥ 60% reduce risk of hemolytic crises and pulmonary complications, but they are not routinely recommended because they increase risk of transfusion reactions, hepatitis, HIV transmission, and blood group isoimmunization. Therapeutic transfusion is indicated for symptomatic anemia, heart failure, severe bacterial infection, and severe complications of labor and delivery (eg, bleeding, sepsis).

Hb S-C disease may first cause symptoms during pregnancy. The disease increases risk of pulmonary infarction by occasionally causing bony spicule embolization. Effects on the fetus are uncommon but, if they occur, often include fetal growth restriction. Sickle cell–β-thalassemia is similar to Hb S-C disease but is less common and more benign. α-Thalassemia does not cause maternal morbidity, but if the fetus is homozygous, hydrops and fetal death occur during the 2nd or early 3rd trimester.

ASTHMA IN PREGNANCY

The effect of pregnancy on asthma varies; deterioration is more common than improvement, but most pregnant women do not have severe attacks. The effect of asthma on pregnancy also varies, but risk of preterm delivery and fetal growth restriction is increased.

Pregnancy does not usually change treatment of asthma (see full discussion in Ch. 48 on p. 381). Inhaled bronchodilators and corticosteroid inhalers are 1st-line maintenance therapy. Theophylline is no longer recommended routinely during pregnancy. For an acute exacerbation, methylprednisolone 60 mg IV q 6 h for 24 to 48 h may be used, followed by oral prednisone in a tapering dose.

AUTOIMMUNE DISORDERS IN PREGNANCY

Autoimmune disorders are 5 times more common among women, and incidence tends to peak during reproductive years. Thus, these disorders commonly occur in pregnant women.

Systemic lupus erythematosus: SLE (see p. 266) may first appear during pregnancy; women who have had an unexplained 2nd-trimester stillbirth, a fetus with growth restriction, preterm delivery, or recurrent spontaneous abortions are often later diagnosed with SLE. The course of preexisting SLE during pregnancy cannot be predicted, but SLE may worsen, particularly immediately postpartum. Complications may include fetal growth restriction, preterm delivery due to preeclampsia, and congenital heart block due to maternal antibodies that cross the placenta. Significant preexisting renal or cardiac complications increase risk of maternal morbidity and mortality. Diffuse nephritis, hypertension, or the presence of circulating antiphospholipid antibodies increases risk of perinatal mortality. Women with anticardiolipin antibody (lupus anticoagulant), present in about 5 to 15% of women with SLE, have an increased risk of abortion, stillbirth, and maternal thromboembolic disorders.

Treatment may require prednisone; the lowest possible dose is used. However, 10 to 60 mg po once/day is often needed. Some patients are also treated with aspirin (81 mg po once/day) and prophylactic heparin (5,000 to 10,000 units bid sc). If the woman has severe, refractory SLE, the need to continue immunosuppressants (eg, hydroxychloroquine) during pregnancy is reviewed individually.

Rheumatoid arthritis (RA): RA (see p. 283) may begin during pregnancy or, even more often, the postpartum period. Preexisting RA generally abates during pregnancy. The fetus is not specifically affected, but delivery may be difficult if the woman's hip joints or lumbar spine is affected.

Myasthenia gravis (see p. 1899)**:** The course varies during pregnancy. Frequent acute myasthenic episodes may require increasing doses of anticholinesterase drugs (eg, neostigmine), which may produce symptoms of cholinergic excess (eg, abdominal pain, diarrhea, vomiting, increasing weakness); atropine may then be required. Sometimes myasthenia becomes refractory to standard therapy and requires corticosteroids or immunosuppressants. During labor, women may need assisted ventilation and are extremely sensitive to drugs that depress respiration (eg, sedatives, opioids, Mg). Because the IgG responsible for myasthenia crosses the placenta, transient myasthenia occurs in 20% of neonates, even more if mothers have not had a thymectomy.

Immune thrombocytopenic purpura (ITP): ITP (see p. 1068), mediated by maternal antiplatelet IgG, tends to worsen during pregnancy and increases risk of maternal morbidity. Corticosteroids reduce IgG levels and cause remission in most women, but improvement is sustained in only 50%. Immunosuppressive therapy and plasmapheresis further reduce IgG, increasing platelet counts. Rarely, splenectomy is required for refractory cases; it is best done during the 2nd trimester, when it causes sustained remission in about 80%. IV immune globulin increases platelets significantly but briefly, so that labor can be induced in women with low platelet counts. Platelet transfusions are indicated only when cesarean section is required and maternal platelet counts are < 50,000/μL.

Although IgG can cross the placenta, causing fetal and neonatal thrombocytopenia, it rarely occurs. Maternal antiplatelet antibody levels (measured by direct or indirect assay) cannot predict fetal involvement, and the fetus may be involved even when mothers have been treated with corticosteroids or previous splenectomy and do not have thrombocytopenia. Percutaneous umbilical blood sampling can be diagnostic. If fetal platelet count is < 50,000/μL, intracranial bleeding can occur during labor or delivery, and delivery by cesarean section is necessary.

CANCER IN PREGNANCY

(See also Ch. 254 on p. 2118.)

Pregnancy should not delay treatment of cancer. Treatment is similar to that in nonpregnant women except for rectal and gynecologic cancers.

Because embryonic tissues grow rapidly and have a high DNA turnover rate, they resemble cancer tissues and are thus very vulnerable to antineoplastic drugs. Many antimetabolites and alkylating drugs (eg, busulfan, chlorambucil, cyclophosphamide, 6-mercaptopurine, methotrexate) can cause fetal abnormalities. Methotrexate is particularly problematic; use during the 1st trimester increases risk of spontaneous abortion and, if the pregnancy continues, multiple congenital malformations. Although pregnancy often concludes successfully despite cancer treatment, risk of fetal injury due to treatment leads some women to choose abortion.

Rectal cancer: Rectal cancers may require hysterectomy to ensure complete tumor removal. If treatment occurs after 28 wk, cesarean section is done before hysterectomy to save the infant.

Cervical cancer: Pregnancy does not appear to worsen cervical cancer. Cervical cancer can develop during pregnancy, and an abnormal Papanicolaou (Pap) test should not be attributed to pregnancy. Abnormal Pap test are followed with colposcopy and directed biopsies when indicated. Usually, conization can be avoided. If biopsy shows mild dysplasia, normal delivery is possible, and follow-up evaluation can start 6 wk postpartum. Severe dysplasia or carcinoma in situ warrants further evaluation during pregnancy; colposcopy is usually accurate, but sometimes biopsy is necessary. For invasive cancer, some experts recommend that hysterectomy, depending on the stage of invasive disease, be done immediately after delivery. However, others recommend delaying treatment until 6 wk postpartum because risks due to hysterectomy are thought to be much greater at delivery because the blood supply to the pelvic organs is increased.

For microinvasive cancer (Federation of Gynecology and Obstetrics [FIGO] stage 0—see TABLE 254–5 on p. 2128), treatment is often deferred until after delivery because conservative options may be possible then. If invasive cancer (FIGO stage IA to IB) is diagnosed during early pregnancy, immediate therapy appropriate for the cancer is traditionally recommended. If invasive cancer is diagnosed after 20 wk and if the woman accepts the unquantified increase in risk, treatment can be deferred until into the 3rd trimester (eg, 32 wk) to maximize fetal maturity without prolonged delay. In certain cancers, chemotherapy may induce tumor regression, allowing the fetus to mature to a viable stage before definitive treatment (surgery or radiation). Delivery is usually by cesarean section, but vaginal delivery, although controversial, may be as safe.

Other gynecologic cancers: After 12 wk gestation, ovarian cancer is easily missed; then, the ovaries, with the uterus, rise out of the pelvis and are no longer easily palpable. Ovarian cancer during pregnancy may be fatal before completion of the pregnancy if very advanced disease exists. Affected women require bilateral oophorectomy as soon as possible. Endometrial and fallopian tube cancers rarely occur during pregnancy.

Leukemia and Hodgkin lymphoma: These disorders (see Chs. 142 on p. 1105 and 143 on p. 1116) are uncommon during pregnancy. Antineoplastic drugs typically used increase risk of fetal loss and congenital malformations. Because leukemias can become fatal rapidly, treatment occurs as soon as possible, without any significant delay to allow the fetus to mature. If Hodgkin lymphoma is confined to above the diaphragm, radiation therapy with the abdomen shielded may be used. If lymphoma is below the diaphragm, abortion may be recommended.

Breast cancer: Breast engorgement during pregnancy may make recognizing breast cancer difficult. Any solid or cystic breast mass should be evaluated.

DIABETES MELLITUS IN PREGNANCY

(See also Ch. 158 on p. 1274.)

Pregnancy aggravates preexisting type 1 (insulin-dependent) and type 2 (non–insulin-dependent) diabetes but does not appear to exacerbate diabetic retinopathy, nephropathy, or neuropathy. Also, gestational diabetes (diabetes that begins during pregnancy) can develop in overweight, hyperinsulinemic, insulin-resistant women or in thin, relatively insulin-deficient women. Gestational diabetes occurs in 1 to 3% of all pregnancies, but the rate may be much higher in certain groups (eg, Mexican Americans, American Indians, Asians, Indians, Pacific Islanders).

Diabetes during pregnancy increases fetal and maternal morbidity and mortality. Neonates are at risk of respiratory distress, hypoglycemia, hypocalcemia, hyperbilirubinemia, polycythemia, and hyperviscosity. Poor control of preexisting or gestational diabetes that occurs during organogenesis (up to about 10 wk gestation) increases risk of major congenital malformations. Gestational diabetes can result in fetal macrosomia (fetal weight > 4500 g at birth) even if plasma glucose is kept nearly normal.

Treatment

Preconception counseling and optimal control of diabetes before, during, and after pregnancy minimize maternal and fetal risks, including congenital malformations. Because malformations may develop before pregnancy is diagnosed, the need for constant, strict control of glucose levels is stressed to women who have diabetes and who are considering pregnancy (or not using contraception). Also, all pregnant women are screened for gestational diabetes (see p. 2150).

Risks are minimized by involving a diabetes team (eg, physicians, nurses, nutritionists, social workers) and a pediatrician; by promptly diagnosing and treating complications of pregnancy, no matter how trivial; by planning for delivery and having an experienced pediatrician present; and by ensuring that neonatal intensive care is available. In regional perinatal centers, specialists in management of diabetic complications are available.

During pregnancy: Treatment can vary, but some general management guidelines are useful (see TABLE 261–1). Women with type 1 or 2 should monitor their plasma glucose levels at home. During pregnancy, normal fasting plasma glucose levels are about 76 mg/dL (4.2 mmol/L); treatment aims to keep fasting plasma glucose levels at < 95 mg/dL and 2-h postprandial levels at ≤ 120 mg/dL (≤ 6.6 mmol/L). The goals are no wide plasma glucose fluctuations and glycosylated Hb (Hb A_{1c}) levels kept at < 8%.

Insulin is the drug of choice because it cannot cross the placenta and provides more predictable glucose control; it is used for types 1 and 2 diabetes. Human insulin is used if possible because it minimizes antibody formation. Insulin antibodies cross the placenta, but their effect on the fetus is unknown. In some women with long-standing type 1 diabetes, hypoglycemia does not trigger the normal release of counterregulatory hormones (catecholamines, glucagon, cortisol, and growth hormone); thus, too much insulin can trigger hypoglycemic coma without premonitory symptoms. All pregnant women with type 1 should have glucagon kits and be instructed (as should family members) in giving glucagon if severe hypoglycemia (indicated by unconsciousness, confusion, or plasma glucose levels < 40 mg/dL [< 2.2 mmol/L]) occurs.

Oral hypoglycemic drugs (eg, glyburide) are being increasingly used to manage diabetes in pregnant women because of the ease of administration (pills compared to injections), low cost, and single daily dosing. Several studies have demonstrated glyburide's safety in pregnancy and that it provides equivalent control compared to insulin for women with gestational diabetes. For women with pregestational type II diabetes, data on oral agents are scant; insulin is most often preferred. Those women on oral hypoglycemics during pregnancy may be continued postpartum while breastfeeding, but the infant should be closely monitored for signs of hypoglycemia.

Management of complications: Although diabetic retinopathy, nephropathy, and mild neuropathy do not contraindicate pregnancy, they require preconception counseling and close management before and during pregnancy.

Women with retinopathy require an ophthalmologic examination every trimester. If proliferative retinopathy is noted at the 1st prenatal visit, photocoagulation should be used as soon as possible to prevent progressive deterioration.

Nephropathy, particularly in women with renal transplants, predisposes to pregnancy-induced hypertension. Risk of preterm delivery is higher if maternal renal function is impaired or if transplantation was recent. Prognosis is best if delivery occurs ≥ 2 yr after transplantation.

Congenital malformations of major organs are predicted by elevated Hb A_{1c} levels at conception and during the 1st 8 wk of pregnancy. If the level is ≥ 8.5% during the 1st trimester, risk of congenital malformations is significantly increased, and targeted ultrasonography and fetal echocardiography are done during the 2nd trimester to check for malformations. If women with type 2 diabetes take oral hypoglycemic drugs during the 1st trimester, fetal risk of congenital malformations is unknown (see TABLE 261–2).

Labor and delivery: Timing of delivery depends on fetal well-being. Women are told to count fetal movements during a 60-min period daily (fetal kick count) and to report any sudden decreases to the obstetrician immediately. Nonstress testing is begun at 32 wk and,

TABLE 261–1. MANAGEMENT OF DIABETES MELLITUS DURING PREGNANCY

TYPE	CARE BEFORE CONCEPTION	PRENATAL CARE	LABOR AND DELIVERY
1*	Diabetes is controlled. Risk is lowest if Hb A_{1c} levels are ≤ 8% at conception.† Evaluation includes a 24-h urine collection (protein excretion and creatinine clearance) to check for renal complications, ophthalmologic examination to check for retinal complications, and ECG to check for cardiac complications.	Prenatal visits begin as soon as pregnancy is recognized. Frequency of visits is determined by degree of glycemic control. Diet should be individualized according to ADA guidelines and coordinated with insulin administration. Three meals and 3 snacks/day are recommended, with emphasis on consistent timing. Amount and type of insulin should be individualized. In the AM, ⅔ of total dose (60% NPH, 40% regular) is given; in the PM, ⅓ (50% NPH, 50% regular) is given.‡ Patients should be instructed in and perform home plasma-glucose monitoring. Hb A_{1c} level should be checked every trimester. Patients should be cautioned about the dangers of hypoglycemia during exercise and at night. Patient and family members should be instructed in glucagon administration. Fetal monitoring with nonstress tests, biophysical profiles, and kick counts should be done weekly from 32 wk to delivery (or earlier if indicated).	Vaginal delivery at term is possible if the patient has documented dating criteria and good glycemic control; amniocentesis may not be required. Cesarean section should be reserved for obstetrical indications or fetal macrosomia (> 4500 g), which increases the risk of shoulder dystocia. Delivery should occur by 38–40 wk. During delivery, a constant low-dose insulin infusion is usually preferred, and the usual sc administration of insulin is stopped. If delivery is induced, on the day before induction, the usual PM NPH insulin dose may be given. Continuing and postpartum diabetes care should be arranged. Postpartum insulin requirements may decrease by up to 50%.
2*	Weight loss is encouraged if BMI is > 27. Hyperglycemia is controlled.§ Risk is lowest if Hb A_{1c} levels are ≤ 8% at conception.† The diet should be low in fat, relatively high in complex carbohydrates, and high in fiber. Exercise is encouraged.	For overweight patients, diet and caloric intake are individualized and monitored to avoid weight gain of > 9 kg; daytime snacks are discouraged. Moderate walking after meals is recommended. Patients are instructed in and perform home plasma glucose monitoring. The 2-h postbreakfast plasma glucose level is checked weekly at clinic visits. Hb A_{1c} level should be checked every trimester. Amount and type of insulin is individualized. For obese patients, regular insulin is given before each meal. For patients who are not obese, ⅔ of total dose (60% NPH, 40% regular) is given in the AM; ⅓ (50% NPH, 50% regular) is given in the PM. Human insulin should be used.	Management is the same as for type 1.

TABLE 261–1. MANAGEMENT OF DIABETES MELLITUS DURING PREGNANCY—Continued

TYPE	CARE BEFORE CONCEPTION	PRENATAL CARE	LABOR AND DELIVERY
Gestational	Patients who have had gestational diabetes in previous pregnancies should try to reach a normal weight and engage in modest exercise. The diet should be low in fat, relatively high in complex carbohydrates, and high in fiber. Fasting plasma glucose and Hb A_{1c} levels should be checked.	Diet and caloric intake are individualized and monitored to prevent weight gain of > 9 kg. Obese patients are discouraged from daytime snacks. Moderate exercise after meals is recommended. Insulin therapy is reserved for persistent hyperglycemia (fasting plasma glucose > 95 mg/dL or 2-h postprandial plasma glucose > 120 mg/dL) despite a trial of dietary therapy for ≥ 2 wk. The amount and type of insulin should be individualized. For obese patients, regular insulin is taken before each meal. For nonobese patients, ⅔ of total dose (60% NPH, 40% regular) is taken in the AM; ⅓ (50% NPH, 50% regular) is taken in the PM. Fetal monitoring with nonstress tests, biophysical profiles, and kick counts should be done beginning at 32–34 wk (or earlier if indicated) and continuing until delivery for patients who require insulin.	Vaginal delivery at term is possible if patients have a well-documented delivery date and good diabetic control; amniocentesis may not be required. Cesarean section should be reserved for obstetric indications or fetal macrosomia (> 4500 g), which increases the risk of shoulder dystocia. Delivery should occur by 38–40 wk.

*Guidelines are only suggested; marked individual variations require appropriate adjustments.
†Normal values may differ depending on laboratory methods used.
‡Some hospital programs recommend up to 4 insulin injections daily. Continuous sc insulin infusion, which is labor-intensive, can sometimes be given in specialized diabetic research settings.
§Patients taking oral hypoglycemic drugs should stop them and use insulin to control plasma glucose levels; possible adverse effects of oral drugs on fetal development cannot be excluded.

Hb A_{1c} = glycosylated Hb; ADA = American Diabetes Association; NPH = neutral protamine Hagedorn; BMI = body mass index.

if nonreassuring, is followed by a biophysical profile (measurement of amniotic fluid and fetal muscle tone, movement, and breathing pattern). These tests and similar noninvasive prenatal fetal monitoring tests are often referred to as antenatal testing. Antenatal testing is initiated earlier if women have severe hypertension or a renal disorder or if fetal growth restriction is suspected. Amniocentesis to assess fetal lung maturity is often necessary in women with obstetric complications, inadequate prenatal care, an uncertain delivery date, or poor glucose control.

A spontaneous vaginal delivery at term is usually possible. If labor does not begin spontaneously by 38 to 40 wk, induction is necessary because of the increasing risk of stillbirth and shoulder dystocia. Dysfunctional labor, cephalopelvic disproportion, or risk of shoulder dystocia may make cesarean section necessary.

During labor and delivery, plasma glucose levels are best controlled using a continuous low-dose insulin infusion. If induction is planned, women eat their usual diet the day before and take their usual insulin dose. On

TABLE 261–2. DRUGS WITH ADVERSE EFFECTS DURING PREGNANCY

TYPE	EXAMPLES	ADVERSE EFFECTS	PREGNANCY SAFETY CATEGORY*
Antibacterials	Aminoglycosides	Ototoxicity (eg, damage to the fetal labyrinth), resulting in deafness	D
	Chloramphenicol	Gray baby syndrome In women or fetuses with G6PD deficiency, hemolysis	C
	Primaquine	In women or fetuses with G6PD deficiency, hemolysis	C
	Fluoroquinolones	Possibly arthralgia; theoretically, musculoskeletal defects (eg, impaired bone growth), but this effect has not been shown	C
	Sulfonamides (except sulfasalazine, which has minimal fetal risk)	When the drugs are given after about 34 wk gestation, neonatal jaundice and, without treatment, kernicterus In women or fetuses with G6PD deficiency, hemolysis	C
	Tetracycline	Slowed bone growth, enamel hypoplasia, permanent yellowing of the teeth, and increased susceptibility to cavities in offspring Occasionally, liver failure in pregnant women	D
Anticoagulants	Unfractionated heparin	When heparin is taken a long time (eg, > 6 mo), maternal osteoporosis and thrombocytopenia	C
	Low mol wt heparin	When heparin is taken a long time (eg, > 6 mo), maternal osteoporosis	B
	Warfarin	When warfarin is given during the 1st trimester, often fetal warfarin syndrome (eg, nasal hypoplasia, bone stippling, bilateral optic atrophy, various degrees of mental retardation) When the drug is given during the 2nd or 3rd trimester, optic atrophy, cataracts, mental retardation, microcephaly, microphthalmia, and fetal and maternal hemorrhage	X
Anticonvulsants	Carbamazepine	Hemorrhagic disease of the newborn Some risk of congenital malformations	D
	Phenobarbital	Hemorrhagic disease of the newborn Some risk of congenital malformations	D
	Phenytoin	Congenital malformations (eg, cleft lip, GU defects such as a narrowed or an incompletely formed urethra, cardiovascular defects) Hemorrhagic disease of the newborn	D

TABLE 261–2. DRUGS WITH ADVERSE EFFECTS DURING PREGNANCY—Continued

TYPE	EXAMPLES	ADVERSE EFFECTS	PREGNANCY SAFETY CATEGORY*
	Trimethadione	High risk of congenital malformations (eg, cleft palate; cardiac, craniofacial, hand, and abdominal defects); risk of spontaneous abortion Almost always contraindicated during pregnancy	D
	Valproate	Major congenital malformations (eg, meningomyelocele; cardiac, craniofacial, and limb defects)	D
Antivertigo drugs	Meclizine	Teratogenic in rodents, but this effect has not been proved in humans	B
Antihypertensives	ACE inhibitors (see Table 71–8 on p. 614)	When the drugs are given during the 2nd or 3rd trimester, fetal hypocalvaria and hypoperfusion, which can cause renal defects, renal failure, and the oligohydramnios sequence (oligohydramnios, craniofacial deformities, limb contractures, and hypoplastic lung development)	D
	β-Blockers	Fetal bradycardia, hypoglycemia, and possibly fetal growth restriction	C
	Thiazide diuretics	Prevention of normal maternal volume expansion, reducing placental perfusion and contributing to fetal growth restriction Neonatal hyponatremia, hypokalemia, and thrombocytopenia	D
Antineoplastic drugs	Actinomycin	Teratogenic in animals, but this effect has not been proved in humans	D
	Busulfan	Congenital malformations (eg, fetal growth restriction, mandibular hypoplasia, cleft palate, cranial dysostosis, spinal defects, ear defects, clubfoot)	D
	Chlorambucil	Same as those for busulfan	D
	Colchicine	Possibly congenital malformations and sperm abnormalities	D
	Cyclophosphamide	Same as those for busulfan	D
	Mercaptopurine	Same as those for busulfan	D
	Methotrexate	Same as those for busulfan	X
	Vinblastine	Teratogenic in animals, but this effect has not been proved in humans	D
	Vincristine	Teratogenic in animals, but this effect has not been proved in humans	D
Anxiolytics	Diazepam	When diazepam is given late in pregnancy, respiratory depression or a withdrawal syndrome that can cause neonatal irritability, tremors, and hyperreflexia	D

Table continues on the following page.

TABLE 261–2. DRUGS WITH ADVERSE EFFECTS DURING PREGNANCY—Continued

TYPE	EXAMPLES	ADVERSE EFFECTS	PREGNANCY SAFETY CATEGORY*
Hypoglycemic drugs (oral)	Chlorpropamide	Neonatal hypoglycemia	C
	Glyburide	Same as those for chlorpropamide	C
	Tolbutamide	Same as those for chlorpropamide	D
Lithium		Teratogenic Neonatal lethargy, hypotonia, poor feeding, hypothyroidism, goiter, and nephrogenic diabetes insipidus	D
Opioids		In neonates of women addicted to opioids, withdrawal symptoms 6 h to 8 days after birth With large doses given in the hour before delivery, possibly neonatal CNS depression and bradycardia	C
Retinoids	Isotretinoin	Congenital malformations, spontaneous abortion, mental retardation	X
Salicylates	Aspirin	Fetal kernicterus With large doses of the drugs, delayed onset of labor, premature closing of the fetal ductus arteriosus, jaundice, and occasionally maternal (intrapartum or postpartum) and neonatal hemorrhage When the drugs are taken late in pregnancy, oligohydramnios	D
	Others	Same as those for aspirin	D
Sex hormones	Danazol	When these drugs are given during the 1st 14 wk, masculinization of a female fetus's genitals (eg, pseudohermaphroditism), sometimes requiring surgery to correct	X
	Synthetic progestins (but not the low doses used in oral contraceptives)	Same as those for danazol	X
Thyroid drugs	Methimazole	Fetal goiter and neonatal scalp defects (aplasia cutis)	D
	Propylthiouracil	Fetal goiter	D
	Radioactive iodine (^{131}I)	Destruction of the fetal thyroid gland or, when the drug is given near the end of the 1st trimester, severe fetal hyperthyroidism	D
	Saturated solution of K iodide	Large fetal goiter, which may obstruct breathing in neonates	
	Triiodothyronine	Fetal goiter	D

TABLE 261–2. DRUGS WITH ADVERSE EFFECTS DURING PREGNANCY—Continued

TYPE	EXAMPLES	ADVERSE EFFECTS	PREGNANCY SAFETY CATEGORY*
Vaccines	Live-virus vaccines such as those for measles, mumps, rubella, polio, chickenpox, and yellow fever	With rubella vaccine, potential infection of the placenta and developing fetus; with other vaccines, potential but unknown risks	
Others	Naphthalene	In women or fetuses with G6PD deficiency, hemolysis	
	Vitamin K	In women or fetuses with G6PD deficiency, hemolysis	

*FDA pregnancy categories:

A: Studies in pregnant women show no risk.

B: Animal studies show no risk, but human data are insufficient; or, animal studies show toxicity, but human studies show no risk.

C: Animal studies show toxicity, human data are insufficient, but clinical benefit may exceed risk.

D: There is evidence of human risk, but clinical benefits may outweigh risk.

X: There is evidence of fetal abnormalities in humans, and risk exceeds benefits.

G6PD = glucose-6-phosphate dehydrogenase.

the morning of labor induction, breakfast and insulin are withheld, baseline fasting plasma glucose is measured, and an IV infusion of 5% dextrose in 0.45% saline solution is started at 125 mL/h, using an infusion pump. Initial insulin infusion rate is determined by capillary glucose level; initial insulin dose is 0 for a capillary level of < 80 mg/dL (< 4.4 mmol/L) or 0.5 units/h for a level of 80 to 100 mg/dL (4.4 to 5.5 mmol/L). Thereafter, insulin dose is increased by 0.5 units/h for each 40-mg/dL (2.2-mmol/L) increase in glucose level up to 2.5 units/h for levels > 220 mg/dL (> 12.2 mmol/L). Every hour during labor, the glucose level is measured at bedside, and the insulin dose is adjusted to keep the level at 70 to 120 mg/dL (3.8 to 6.6 mmol/L). If the glucose level is significantly elevated, additional bolus doses of insulin may be required. For spontaneous labor, the procedure is the same, except that if intermediate-acting insulin was taken in the previous 12 h, the insulin dose is decreased. For women who have fever, infection, or other complications and for obese women who have type 2 and have required > 100 units of insulin/day before pregnancy, the insulin dose is increased.

Postpartum: After delivery, loss of the placenta, which synthesizes large amounts of insulin antagonist hormones throughout pregnancy, decreases the insulin requirement immediately. Thus, women with gestational diabetes and many of those with type 2 require no insulin postpartum. For women with type 1, insulin requirements decrease dramatically but then gradually increase after about 72 h.

During the 1st 6 wk postpartum, the goal is tight glucose control. Glucose levels are checked before meals and at bedtime. Breastfeeding is not contraindicated but may result in hypoglycemia with oral hypoglycemics. Women who have had gestational diabetes should have a 2-h oral glucose tolerance test with 75 g of glucose at 6 to 12 wk postpartum to determine whether diabetes has resolved.

HEART DISORDERS IN PREGNANCY

Heart disorders account for about 10% of maternal obstetric deaths. In the US, because incidence of rheumatic heart disease has markedly declined, most heart problems during pregnancy result from congenital heart disease. Pregnancy is inadvisable for women with certain high-risk disorders (eg, pulmonary hypertension, severe valvular disorders, prior postpartum cardiomyopathy).

Pathophysiology

Pregnancy stresses the cardiovascular system, often worsening known heart disorders or unmasking occult heart disorders. Stresses include decreased Hb and increased blood volume, stroke volume, and eventually heart rate. Cardiac output increases by 30 to 50%. These changes become maximal between 28 and 34 wk gestation. During labor, cardiac output increases about 20% with each uterine contraction; other stresses include straining during the 2nd stage of labor and the increase in venous blood returning to the heart from the contracting uterus. Cardiovascular stresses do not return to prepregnancy levels until several weeks after delivery.

Symptoms and Signs

Findings resembling heart failure (eg, mild dyspnea, systolic murmurs, jugular venous distention, tachycardia, dependent edema, mild cardiomegaly seen on chest x-ray—see p. 652) typically occur during pregnancy. However, they may result from a heart disorder or from pregnancy itself. Diastolic or presystolic murmurs are more specific for heart disorders. Mild heart disorders may first become evident during pregnancy.

Heart failure can cause premature labor or arrhythmias. Risk of maternal or fetal death correlates with New York Heart Association functional classification, which is based on the amount of physical activity that causes symptoms of heart failure. Risk is not increased if symptoms do not occur with exertion (class I) or occur only with significant exertion (class II). Risk is increased if symptoms occur with mild exertion (class III) or with minimal or no exertion (class IV).

Diagnosis and Treatment

Diagnosis is usually clinical and by echocardiography.

Frequent prenatal visits, ample rest, avoidance of excessive weight gain and stress, and treatment of anemia are required. An anesthesiologist familiar with heart disorders in pregnancy should attend the labor. During labor, pain and anxiety are treated aggressively to minimize tachycardia. Women are closely monitored immediately postpartum and are followed for several weeks postpartum by a cardiologist.

Heart failure: Before women with class III or IV heart failure conceive, the disorder should be optimally treated medically and, if indicated (eg, if due to a valvular heart disorder), treated surgically.

Pregnant women with heart failure require hospitalization and bed rest. Those with class III heart failure may require digoxin 0.25 mg po once/day plus bed rest beginning at 20 wk. Cardiac glycosides (eg, digoxin, digitoxin) cross the placenta, but neonates (and children) are relatively resistant to their toxicity. Women with class IV heart failure may be advised to obtain early therapeutic abortion. ACE inhibitors are contraindicated because they may cause fetal renal damage. Other treatments for heart failure (eg, diuretics, nitrates, inotropes) may be continued during pregnancy depending on disease severity and fetal risk, as determined by a cardiologist and a perinatologist.

Arrhythmias: Atrial fibrillation may accompany cardiomyopathy or valvular lesions. Rate control is usually similar to that in nonpregnant patients, with β-blockers, Ca channel blockers, or digoxin (see p. 677). Certain antiarrhythmics (eg, amiodarone) should be avoided. In patients with new-onset atrial fibrillation or hemodynamic instability, cardioversion may be used to restore sinus rhythm. Anticoagulation may be required because the relative hypercoagulability during pregnancy makes atrial thrombi (and subsequent systemic or pulmonary embolization) more likely. Although neither standard heparin nor low mol wt heparins cross the placenta, low mol wt heparins have less risk of thrombocytopenia. Warfarin crosses the placenta and may cause fetal abnormalities (see TABLE 261–2), particularly during the 1st trimester. Warfarin use during the last month of pregnancy also has risks. Rapid reversal of warfarin's anticoagulant effects may be difficult and may be required due to fetal/neonatal intracranial hemorrhage resulting from birth trauma or due to maternal bleeding (eg, resulting from trauma or emergency cesarean delivery).

Management of acute supraventricular or ventricular tachycardia is the same as for nonpregnant patients.

Endocarditis prophylaxis: For pregnant patients with a structural heart disorder, indications and use of endocarditis prophylaxis for nonobstetric events are the same as for nonpregnant patients (see p. 729); those with rheumatic heart disease are given daily prophylaxis. Although rate of bacteremia with uncomplicated vaginal or caesarean delivery is low and routine prophylaxis is not recommended by the American College of Cardiology, many obstetricians give prophylactic antibiotics shortly before and after delivery for patients with valvular disease.

Valvular Stenosis and Insufficiency

Stenosis and regurgitation (insufficiency) in pregnancy most often affect the mitral and aortic valves. Pregnancy amplifies the murmurs of mitral and aortic stenosis but diminishes those of mitral and aortic regurgitation. During pregnancy, mild mitral or aortic regurgitation is usually easy to tolerate; stenosis is more difficult to tolerate and predisposes to maternal and fetal complications. Mitral stenosis is especially dangerous; the tachycardia, increased blood volume, and increased cardiac output during pregnancy interact with this disorder to increase pulmonary capillary pressure, causing pulmonary edema. Atrial fibrillation is also common.

Treatment

Ideally, valvular disorders are diagnosed and treated medically before conception; surgical correction is often recommended for severe disorders. Prophylactic antibiotics are required in certain situations (see p. 2178).

Mitral stenosis: Patients must be closely observed throughout pregnancy because mitral stenosis may rapidly become more severe. If required, valvotomy is relatively safe during pregnancy; however, open heart surgery increases fetal risk. During labor, conduction anesthesia (eg, epidural or spinal nerve block by a local anesthetic) is usually preferred.

Aortic stenosis: During labor, local anesthesia or, if necessary, general anesthesia, is preferred. Conduction anesthesia decreases filling pressures (preload), which may already be decreased by aortic stenosis. Straining, which can suddenly reduce filling pressures and impair cardiac output, is discouraged during the 2nd stage of labor; operative vaginal delivery may be preferred, if feasible. Cesarean section is done if indicated (see p. 2203).

Other Heart Disorders in Pregnancy

Mitral valve prolapse: This disorder occurs more frequently in younger women and tends to be familial. Mitral valve prolapse is usually an isolated abnormality but may cause some degree of mitral regurgitation or be accompanied by Marfan syndrome or an atrial septal defect. Women with mitral valve prolapse generally tolerate pregnancy well. The relative increase in ventricular size during normal pregnancy reduces the discrepancy between the disproportionately large mitral valve and the ventricle. Patients with mitral regurgitation may require prophylactic antibiotics during delivery. β-Blockers are indicated for recurrent arrhythmias. Rarely, thrombi and systemic emboli develop and require anticoagulation.

Congenital heart disease: For most asymptomatic patients, risk is not increased during pregnancy. However, patients with Eisenmenger's syndrome (now rare), primary pulmonary hypertension, or perhaps isolated pulmonary stenosis are predisposed, for unknown reasons, to sudden death during labor, during the postpartum period (the 6 wk after delivery), or after abortion at > 20 wk gestation. Thus, pregnancy is inadvisable. If patients become pregnant, they should be closely monitored with a pulmonary artery catheter and an arterial line during delivery. For patients with intracardiac shunts, the goal is to prevent right-to-left shunting by maintaining peripheral vascular resistance, and by minimizing pulmonary vascular resistance.

Patients with Marfan syndrome are at increased risk of aortic dissection and rupture of aortic aneurysms during pregnancy. Bed rest, avoidance of Valsalva maneuvers, and measurement of aortic diameter with echocardiography are required.

Peripartum cardiomyopathy: Heart failure with no identifiable cause (eg, MI, valvular disorder) can develop between the last month of pregnancy and 5 mo postpartum in patients without a previous heart disorder. Risk factors include multiparity, age ≥ 30, multifetal pregnancy, and preeclampsia. The 5-yr mortality rate is 50%. Recurrence is likely in subsequent pregnancies, particularly in patients with residual cardiac dysfunction; future pregnancies are therefore not recommended. Treatment is as for heart failure (see p. 2178).

HEPATIC DISORDERS IN PREGNANCY

Jaundice (see p. 191) may result from nonobstetric or obstetric conditions. Nonobstetric causes include drugs, acute cholecystitis, and biliary obstruction by gallstones. Gallstones appear to be more common during pregnancy, probably because bile lithogenicity is increased and gallbladder contractility is impaired. Obstetric causes include hyperemesis gravidarum (usually mild) and septic abortion; both cause hepatocellular injury and hemolysis.

Acute viral hepatitis: The most common cause of jaundice during pregnancy is acute viral hepatitis. It may predispose to preterm delivery but does not appear to be teratogenic. Acute viral hepatitis is generally mild, but hepatitis E, common in underdeveloped countries, may be severe. Hepatitis B virus may be transmitted to the neonate immediately after delivery or, less often, to the fetus transplacentally. Transmission is particularly likely if a woman is e-antigen–positive and is a chronic carrier of hepatitis B surface antigen (HBsAg) or if she has contracted hepatitis during the 3rd trimester. Affected neonates are more likely to develop subclinical hepatic dysfunction and become carriers than to develop clinical hepatitis. All pregnant women are tested for HBsAg to determine whether precautions against vertical transmission are needed (for prenatal prophylaxis with immune globulin and vaccination for neonates exposed to hepatitis B virus, see p. 2327).

Chronic active hepatitis: Chronic active hepatitis, especially with cirrhosis, impairs fertility. When pregnancy occurs, risk of spontaneous abortion and prematurity is increased, but risk of maternal mortality is not. Corticosteroids given for chronic active hepatitis can be continued during pregnancy because fetal risks have not been proved. Azathioprine and other immunosuppressants, despite fetal risks, are sometimes indicated for severe disease.

Cholestasis (pruritus) of pregnancy: This relatively common disorder apparently results from idiosyncratic exaggeration of normal bile stasis due to hormonal changes. Intense pruritus, the earliest symptom, develops during the 2nd or 3rd trimester; dark urine and jaundice sometimes follow. Acute pain and systemic symptoms are absent. The disorder usually resolves after delivery but tends to recur with each pregnancy or with use of oral contraceptives. For severe pruritus, oral cholestyramine 4 to 6 g bid or 3 to 4 g tid is usually effective. Bleeding due to hypoprothrombinemia occasionally develops but is readily reversed by vitamin K (phytonadione) 5 to 10 mg IM once/day for 2 to 3 days.

Fatty liver of pregnancy: This rare, poorly understood disorder occurs near term, sometimes with preeclampsia. Symptoms include acute nausea and vomiting, abdominal discomfort, and jaundice, followed in severe cases by rapidly progressive hepatocellular failure. Clinical and laboratory findings resemble those of fulminant viral hepatitis except that aminotransferase levels may be < 500 units/L and hyperuricemia may be present. Diagnosis is by clinical criteria, liver function tests, hepatitis serologic tests, and liver biopsy. Biopsy shows diffuse small droplets of fat in hepatocytes, usually with minimal apparent necrosis, but in some cases, findings are indistinguishable from viral hepatitis. Maternal and fetal mortality rates are high in severe cases. Depending on gestational age, prompt delivery or termination of pregnancy is usually advised, although whether either alters maternal outcome is unclear. Survivors recover completely and have no recurrences. A seemingly identical disorder may develop at any stage of pregnancy if high doses of tetracyclines are given IV.

Preeclampsia: Severe preeclampsia can cause hepatic fibrin deposition, necrosis, and hemorrhage that can result in abdominal pain, nausea, vomiting, and mild jaundice. Subcapsular hematoma with intra-abdominal hemorrhage occasionally occurs, most often in women with preeclampsia that progresses to the HELLP syndrome (*h*emolysis, *e*levated *l*iver enzymes, and *l*ow *p*latelet count—see p. 2197), and rarely causes the liver to rupture spontaneously; rupture is life threatening, and pathogenesis is unknown.

Chronic hepatic disorders: Pregnancy may temporarily worsen cholestasis in primary biliary cirrhosis and other cholestatic disorders, and the increased plasma volume during the 3rd trimester slightly increases risk of variceal hemorrhage in women with cirrhosis. However, pregnancy usually does not harm patients with a chronic hepatic disorder. Cesarean delivery is reserved for the usual obstetric indications.

HYPERTENSION IN PREGNANCY

(See also Ch. 71 on p. 604.)

Hypertension (BP ≥ 140/90 mm Hg) during pregnancy can be classified as chronic or gestational. Chronic hypertension is BP that is high before pregnancy or before 20 wk gestation. Chronic hypertension complicates about 1 to 5% of all pregnancies. Gestational hypertension develops after 20 wk gestation (typically after 37 wk) and remits by 6 wk postpartum; it occurs in about 5 to 10% of pregnancies, more commonly in multifetal pregnancy. Both types of hypertension increase risk of preeclampsia, eclampsia (see p. 2197), and other causes of maternal mortality or morbidity, including hypertensive encephalopathy, stroke, renal failure, left ventricular failure, and the HELLP syndrome (*h*emolysis, *e*levated *l*iver enzymes, and *l*ow *p*latelet count). Fetal mortality or morbidity increases because of decreased uteroplacental blood flow, which can cause vasospasm, growth restriction, hypoxia, and abruptio placentae. Outcomes are worse if hypertension is severe (BP > 180/100 mm Hg) or accompanied by renal insufficiency (eg, creatinine clearance < 60 mL/min, serum creatinine > 2 mg/dL [180 μmol/L]).

Diagnosis and Treatment

BP is measured routinely at prenatal visits. If severe hypertension occurs for the 1st time in pregnant women who do not have a multifetal pregnancy or gestational trophoblastic disease, tests to rule out renal artery stenosis, coarctation of the aorta, Cushing's syndrome, SLE, and pheochromocytoma should be considered (see p. 607).

Treatment of mild to moderate hypertension during pregnancy is controversial; the issue is whether and when risks of drug treatment outweigh risks of untreated disease. Because the uteroplacental circulation is maximally dilated and cannot autoregulate, decreasing maternal BP with drugs may acutely decrease uteroplacental blood flow. Diuretics reduce effective maternal circulating blood volume; consistent reduction increases risk of fetal growth restriction.

First-line drugs for hypertension during pregnancy include methyldopa, β-blockers, and Ca channel blockers. Initial methyldopa dose is 250 mg po bid, increased as needed to 2 g/day or sometimes more unless excessive somnolence, depression, and symptomatic orthostatic hypotension occur. The most commonly used β-blocker is labetalol (a β-blocker with some α_1-blocking effects), which can be used alone or with methyldopa when the maximum daily dose of methyldopa has been reached. Adverse effects of β-blockers include increased risk of fetal growth restriction, decreased maternal energy levels, and maternal depression (see TABLE 261–2). Ca channel blockers, usually extended-release nifedipine, may be preferred because it is given once/day (initial dose of 30 to 60 mg); adverse effects include headaches and pretibial edema. ACE inhibitors are contraindicated because risk of fetal urinary tract abnormalities is increased. Thiazide diuretics can adversely affect the fetus and should be avoided during pregnancy if possible.

If chronic hypertension is mild (140/90 to 150/100 mm Hg) and if BP is labile, drastically reduced physical activity often appears to decrease BP and improve fetal growth, making perinatal risks similar to those for patients without hypertension. However, if these conservative measures do not decrease BP, drug therapy is indicated.

If chronic hypertension is moderate (150/100 to 180/110 mm Hg), drug therapy is indicated: the drug or drugs used before pregnancy, methyldopa, a β-blocker, a Ca channel blocker, or a combination of these drugs. Patients must be taught to self-monitor BP and should have renal function testing every trimester. Fetal growth is monitored with monthly ultrasound examinations; antenatal testing begins at 32 wk. Delivery should occur by 38 wk or earlier if severe preeclampsia or fetal growth restriction is detected or fetal testing is nonreassuring.

If chronic hypertension is severe (≥ 180/110 mm Hg), immediate evaluation, including BUN and serum creatinine, creatinine clearance, total urinary protein, and funduscopy, is indicated. Risk of complications, both maternal (progression of end-organ dysfunction or preeclampsia) and fetal (prematurity, growth restriction, stillbirth) is increased significantly. If continuation of pregnancy is strongly desired despite the risk, several antihypertensives are often required. Hospitalization is also often required for much of the latter part of pregnancy. If the woman's condition worsens, pregnancy termination may be recommended.

INFECTIOUS DISEASE IN PREGNANCY

Most common maternal infections (eg, UTIs, skin and respiratory tract infections) are usually not serious problems during pregnancy, although some genital infections (bacterial vaginosis and genital herpes) affect labor or choice of delivery method. Thus, the main issue is usually use and safety of antimicrobial drugs. However, certain maternal infections can damage the fetus (see Ch. 279 on p. 2313 for congenital cytomegalovirus or herpes simplex virus infection, rubella, toxoplasmosis, hepatitis, or syphilis; see p. 2341 for HIV infection).

Bacterial vaginosis and possibly **genital chlamydial infection** predispose to premature rupture of the membranes and preterm labor. Tests for these infections are done during routine prenatal evaluations or if symptoms develop.

Genital herpes can be transmitted to the neonate during delivery, particularly if women have visible herpetic lesions or known infection with prodromal symptoms or if herpes infection first occurs during the late 3rd trimester (when the virus is likely to be excreted from the cervix at delivery). In such cases, delivery by cesarean section is preferred. If visible lesions or prodrome is absent, even in women with recurrent infections, risk is low, and vaginal delivery is possible. If women are asymptomatic, serial antepartum cultures do not help identify those at risk of transmission. If women have recurrent herpes infections during pregnancy but no other risk factors for transmission, delivery can sometimes be induced to occur between recurrences. When delivery is vaginal, cervical and neonatal herpesvirus cultures are done. Acyclovir (oral and topical) appears to be safe during pregnancy.

Antibacterials: Even more so than for other patients, antibacterials should not be given without strong evidence of a bacterial infection. Generally, penicillins, cephalosporins, macrolides, and sulfonamides are considered safe. Use of any antibacterial during pregnancy should be based on whether benefits outweigh risk, which varies by trimester (see TABLE 261–2 for specific adverse effects). Severity of the infection and other options for treatment are also considered.

Aminoglycosides may be used during pregnancy to treat pyelonephritis and chorioamnionitis, but treatment should be carefully monitored to avoid maternal or fetal damage.

Chloramphenicol, even in large doses, does not harm the fetus; however, neonates cannot adequately metabolize chloramphenicol, and the resulting high blood levels may lead to circulatory collapse (gray baby syndrome).

Use of metronidazole during the 1st trimester is controversial, but it is routinely used to treat bacterial vaginosis during the 2nd and 3rd trimesters. Fluoroquinolones are not used during pregnancy; they tend to have a high affinity for bone and cartilage and thus may have adverse musculoskeletal effects.

Long-acting sulfonamides cross the placenta and can displace bilirubin from binding sites. These drugs are often avoided after 34 wk gestation because neonatal kernicterus is a risk.

Tetracyclines cross the placenta and are concentrated and deposited in fetal bones and teeth, where they combine with Ca and impair development (see TABLE 261–2); they are not used from the middle to the end of pregnancy.

RENAL INSUFFICIENCY IN PREGNANCY

Pregnancy often does not worsen renal disorders; it seems to exacerbate noninfectious renal disorders only when uncontrolled hypertension coexists. However, usually, significant renal insufficiency (serum creatinine > 3 mg/dL [> 270 μmol/L] or BUN > 30 mg/dL [> 10.5 mmol urea/L]) before pregnancy prevents women from maintaining a pregnancy to term.

Treatment requires close consultation with a nephrologist. BP and weight are measured every 2 wk; BUN and creatinine levels plus creatinine clearance are measured often, at intervals dictated by severity and progression of disease. Furosemide is given only to control BP or excessive edema; some patients require other drugs to control BP. Women may be hospitalized after 28 wk gestation for bed rest, BP control, and close fetal monitoring. Which antenatal tests are done depends on the stage of pregnancy. Nonstress tests are usually done first, followed by an oxytocin challenge test or a biophysical profile if required. If results remain normal and reassuring, the pregnancy continues. Delivery is usually required before term because preeclampsia, fetal growth restriction, or uteroplacental insufficiency is detected. Sometimes amniocentesis to check fetal lung maturity can help determine when delivery should be done; a lecithin/sphingomyelin ratio > 2:1 or presence of phosphatidylglycerol indicates maturity. Cesarean section is very common, although vaginal delivery may be possible if the cervix is ripe and no impediments to vaginal delivery are evident.

SEIZURE DISORDERS IN PREGNANCY

Seizure disorders may impair fertility. Also, certain anticonvulsants may make oral contraceptives less effective, resulting in unintentional pregnancy.

If women get enough sleep and anticonvulsant levels are kept in the therapeutic range, seizure frequency does not usually increase during pregnancy, and pregnancy outcome is good; however, risks of preeclampsia, fetal growth restriction, and stillbirth are slightly increased. Generally, uncontrolled seizures are more harmful during pregnancy than is use of anticonvulsants; thus, the top priority of treatment during pregnancy is to control seizures. However, the minimum number of anticonvulsants in the lowest possible dose necessary to control seizures is used. Anticonvulsants slightly increase risk of congenital malformations and may tend to slightly decrease intelligence in offspring; mental retardation may be a risk. Risk of hemorrhagic disease of the newborn (erythroblastosis neonatorum) may be increased by in utero exposure to anticonvulsants (eg, phenytoin, carbamazepine, phenobarbital); however, if prenatal vitamins with vitamin D are taken and vitamin K is given to the neonate, hemorrhagic disease is rare.

Taken during pregnancy, phenobarbital may reduce the physiologic jaundice neonates commonly have, perhaps because the drug induces neonatal hepatic conjugating enzymes. Phenytoin is generally preferred.

All anticonvulsants increase the need for supplemental folate; 1 mg po is given once/day. Ideally, it is started before conception.

Vaginal delivery is usually preferred, but if women have repeated seizures during labor, cesarean section is indicated. Anticonvulsant levels can rapidly change postpartum and should be closely monitored then.

DISORDERS REQUIRING SURGERY DURING PREGNANCY

Certain disorders treated with surgery are difficult to diagnose during pregnancy. A high level of suspicion is required; assuming that all abdominal symptoms are pregnancy-related is an error. Surgery is tolerated well by pregnant women and the fetus when appropriate supportive care and anesthesia (maintaining BP and oxygenation at normal levels) are provided, so physicians should not be reluctant to operate; delaying treatment of an abdominal emergency is far more dangerous.

Appendicitis may occur during pregnancy but is more common immediately postpartum. Because the appendix rises in the abdomen as pregnancy progresses, pain and tenderness may not occur in the classic right lower quadrant location, and pain may be mild and cramping, mimicking pregnancy-related symptoms. Also, WBC count is normally somewhat elevated during pregnancy, making this test even less useful than usual. Serial clinical assessment and compression-graded ultrasonography are useful. Because diagnosis is often delayed, mortality rate from ruptured appendix is higher during pregnancy and particularly postpartum. Thus, if appendicitis is suspected, surgical evaluation (laparoscopy or laparotomy depending on the stage of pregnancy) should proceed without delay.

Benign ovarian cysts are common during pregnancy. Cysts that occur during the 1st 14 to 16 wk are often corpus luteal cysts, which spontaneously resolve. After 12 wk, cysts become difficult to palpate because the ovaries, with the uterus, rise out of the pelvis. Ovarian masses are evaluated first by ultrasonography (see p. 2096). Further evaluation (eg, excision) is delayed, if possible, until after 14 wk unless the cyst enlarges continuously, is tender, or has radiographic characteristics of cancer (eg, a solid component, surface excrescences, size > 6 cm, irregular shape). Adnexal torsion may occur (see p. 2097).

Gallbladder disease occurs occasionally and, if possible, is treated expectantly; if women do not improve, immediate surgery is needed.

Intestinal obstruction during pregnancy may cause intestinal gangrene with peritonitis and maternal or fetal morbidity or mortality. If pregnant women have symptoms and signs of intestinal obstruction and risk factors (eg, previous abdominal surgery, intra-abdominal infection), prompt exploratory laparotomy is indicated.

THROMBOEMBOLIC DISORDERS IN PREGNANCY

In the US, thromboembolic disorders—deep venous thrombosis (DVT—see p. 754) or pulmonary embolism (PE—see p. 412)—are a leading cause of maternal mortality. During pregnancy, risk is increased because venous capacitance and venous pressure in the legs are increased, resulting in stasis, and because pregnancy causes a degree of hypercoagulability. However, most thromboemboli develop postpartum and result from vascular trauma during delivery. Cesarean section also increases risk. Symptoms of thrombophlebitis or their absence do not accurately predict the diagnosis, disease severity, or risk of embolization. Thromboembolic disorders can occur without symptoms, with only minimal symptoms, or with significant symptoms. Also, calf edema, cramping, and tenderness, which may occur normally during pregnancy, may simulate Homans' sign.

Diagnosis and Treatment

Diagnosis of DVT is usually by Doppler ultrasonography. In the postpartum period, if Doppler ultrasonography and plethysmography are normal but iliac, ovarian, or other pelvic venous thrombosis is suspected, CT with contrast is used.

Diagnosis of PE is increasingly being made by helical CT rather than ventilation-perfusion scanning, because it involves less radiation and is equally sensitive. If the diagnosis of PE is uncertain, pulmonary angiography is required.

If DVT or PE is detected during pregnancy, the anticoagulant of choice is a low mol wt heparin (LMWH). LMWH, because of its molecular size, does not cross the placenta. It does not cause maternal osteoporosis or thrombocytopenia, which can result from prolonged (≥ 6 mo) use of unfractionated heparin. Warfarin crosses the placenta and may cause fetal abnormalities or death (see TABLE 261–2). Indications for thrombolysis during pregnancy are the same as for patients who are not pregnant. If PE recurs despite effective anticoagulation, surgery, usually placement of an inferior vena cava filter just distal to the renal vessels, is indicated.

If patients developed DVT or PE during a previous pregnancy or have an underlying thrombophilic disorder, they are treated with prophylactic LMWH 5000 units sc bid beginning at the first diagnosis of pregnancy and continuing until 6 wk postpartum.

THYROID DISORDERS IN PREGNANCY

(See also Ch. 152 on p. 1192.)

Thyroid disorders may predate or develop during pregnancy. Fetal effects vary with the disorder and drugs used for treatment. But generally, hyperthyroidism causes fetal growth restriction and stillbirth, and hypothyroidism causes intellectual deficits in offspring and miscarriage. The most common causes of maternal hypothyroidism are Hashimoto's thyroiditis and treatment of Graves' disease. If women have or have had a thyroid disorder, thyroid status should be closely monitored during and after pregnancy in the women and in the offspring.

Pregnancy does not change the symptoms of hypothyroidism and hyperthyroidism or the normal values and ranges of free serum thyroxine (T_4) and thyroid-stimulating hormone (TSH).

Graves' disease: Maternal Graves' disease is monitored clinically and with free T_4 and high-sensitivity TSH assays. Treatment varies. Usually, pregnant women are given the lowest possible dose of oral propylthiouracil (50 to 100 mg q 8 h). Therapeutic response occurs over 3 to 4 wk; then the dose is changed if needed. Propylthiouracil crosses the placenta and may cause goiter and hypothyroidism in the fetus. Simultaneous use of L-thyroxine or L-triiodothyronine is contraindicated because these hormones may mask the effects of excessive propylthiouracil in pregnant women and result in hypothyroidism in the fetus. Methimazole is an alternative to propylthiouracil. Graves' disease commonly improves during the 3rd trimester, often allowing dose reduction or discontinuation of the drug. Although very uncommon, in centers with experienced thyroid surgeons, a 2nd-trimester thyroidectomy may be considered after drug treatment restores euthyroidism. After thyroidectomy, women are given full replacement of L-thyroxine (0.15 to 0.2 mg/day), beginning 24 h later. Radioactive iodine (diagnostic or therapeutic) and iodide solutions are contraindicated during pregnancy because of adverse effects on the fetal thyroid gland. β-Blockers are used only for thyroid storm or severe maternal symptoms.

If pregnant women have or have had Graves' disease, fetal hyperthyroidism may develop. Whether these women are clinically euthyroid, hyperthyroid, or hypothyroid, thyroid-stimulating immunoglobulins (Igs) and thyroid-blocking Igs (if present) cross the placenta. Fetal thyroid function reflects the relative fetal levels of these stimulating and blocking Igs. Hyperthyroidism can cause fetal tachycardia (> 160 beats/min), growth restriction, and goiter, which can lead to decreased fetal swallowing, polyhydramnios, and preterm labor. Ultrasonography is used to evaluate fetal growth, thyroid gland, and heart.

Congenital Graves' disease: If pregnant women have taken propylthiouracil, congenital Graves' disease in the fetus may be masked until 7 to 10 days after birth, when the drug's effect subsides.

Maternal hypothyroidism: Women with mild to moderate hypothyroidism frequently have normal menstrual cycles and can become pregnant. During pregnancy, the usual dose of L-thyroxine is continued. As pregnancy progresses, minor dose adjustments may be necessary, ideally based on TSH measurement after several weeks. If hypothyroidism is first diagnosed during pregnancy, L-thyroxine is started at 0.1 mg po once/day.

Hashimoto's thyroiditis: Maternal immune suppression during pregnancy often ameliorates chronic thyroiditis; however, hypothyroidism or hyperthyroidism that requires treatment sometimes develops.

Acute (subacute) thyroiditis: Common during pregnancy, this disorder usually produces a tender goiter during or after a respiratory infection. Transient, symptomatic hyperthyroidism with elevated T_4 can occur, often resulting in misdiagnosis as Graves' disease. Usually, treatment is unnecessary.

Postpartum maternal thyroid dysfunction: Hypothyroid or hyperthyroid dysfunction occurs in 4 to 7% of women during the 1st 6 mo after delivery. Incidence seems to be higher among pregnant women with a goiter, Hashimoto's thyroiditis, a strong family history of autoimmune thyroid disorders, or type 1 (insulin-dependent) diabetes mellitus. In women with any of these risk factors, TSH and free serum T_4 levels should be checked in the 1st trimester and postpartum. Dysfunction is usually transient but may require treatment. After delivery, Graves' disease may recur transiently or persistently.

Painless thyroiditis with transient hyperthyroidism is a recently recognized postpartum, probably autoimmune, disorder. It develops abruptly in the 1st few weeks postpartum, results in a low radioactive iodine uptake, and is characterized by lymphocytic infiltration. Diagnosis is by symptoms, thyroid function tests, and by exclusion of other conditions. This disorder may persist, recur transiently, or progress.

URINARY TRACT INFECTION IN PREGNANCY

(See also p. 1968.)

UTI is common during pregnancy, apparently because of urinary stasis, which results from hormonal ureteral dilation, hormonal ureteral hypoperistalsis, and pressure of the expanding uterus against the ureters. Asymptomatic bacteriuria occurs in about 15% of pregnancies and sometimes progresses to symptomatic cystitis or pyelonephritis. Frank UTI is not always preceded by asymptomatic bacteriuria. Asymptomatic bacteriuria, UTI, and pyelonephritis increase risk of preterm labor and premature rupture of the membranes.

Urinalysis and culture at initial evaluation are routinely done to check for asymptomatic UTI. Diagnosis and treatment of symptomatic UTI is not changed by pregnancy, except drugs that may harm the fetus are avoided (see TABLE 261–2). Antibacterial drug selection is based on individual and local susceptibility and resistance patterns, but cephalexin, nitrofurantoin, or trimethoprim-sulfamethoxazole are usually good initial empiric choices. After treatment, proof-of-cure cultures are required. Women who have pyelonephritis or have had > 1 UTI may require suppressive therapy, usually with trimethoprim-sulfamethoxazole or nitrofurantoin, for the rest of the pregnancy. In women who have bacteriuria with or without UTI or pyelonephritis, urine should be cultured monthly.

262 HIGH-RISK PREGNANCY

In a high-risk (at-risk) pregnancy, the mother, fetus, or neonate is at increased risk of morbidity or mortality before or after delivery.

In the US, overall maternal mortality rate is 6/100,000 deliveries; incidence is 3 to 4 times higher in nonwhite women. The most common causes of death are hemorrhage, pregnancy-induced hypertension, pulmonary embolism, and infection.

Perinatal mortality rate in offspring is 11.5/1000 deliveries: 6.7/1000 are fetal, and 4.8/1000 are neonatal (age < 28 days). The most common causes of death are congenital malformations and preterm delivery.

Risk assessment is part of routine prenatal care. Risk is also assessed during or shortly after labor and at any time that events may modify risk status. Risk factors (see TABLE 262–1) are assessed systematically; each factor present increases overall risk. High-risk pregnancies require close monitoring and sometimes referral to a perinatal center. When referral is needed, transfer before rather than after delivery results in lower neonatal morbidity and mortality rates. The most common reasons for referral before delivery are preterm labor (often due to premature rupture of the membranes), pregnancy-induced hypertension, and hemorrhage.

RISK FACTORS

Risk factors include preexisting maternal disorders (see Ch. 261 on p. 2167), physical and social characteristics, age, problems in previous pregnancies (eg, spontaneous abortions), and problems that develop during the pregnancy (see Ch. 263 on p. 2191) or during labor and delivery (see Ch. 264 on p. 2202).

Hypertension: Pregnant women are considered to have chronic hypertension (CHTN) if hypertension was present before the pregnancy or if it develops before 20 wk of pregnancy. CHTN is differentiated from pregnancy-induced hypertension, which develops after 20 wk of pregnancy. In either case, hypertension is defined as systolic BP > 140 mm Hg or diastolic BP > 90 mm Hg on 2 occasions > 24 h apart. Hypertension increases risk of fetal growth restriction by decreasing uteroplacental blood flow. CHTN increases risk of preeclampsia to up to 50%. Poorly controlled hypertension increases risk of abruptio placentae by 2 to 10%.

Before attempting to conceive, women with hypertension should be counseled about the risks of pregnancy. If they become pregnant, prenatal care begins as early as possible and includes measurements of baseline renal function (eg, serum creatinine, BUN), funduscopic examination, and directed cardiovascular examination (auscultation, and sometimes with ECG, echocardiography, or both). Each trimester, 24-h urine protein, serum uric acid, serum creatinine, and Hct are measured. Ultrasonography to monitor fetal growth is done at 28 wk and every few weeks thereafter. Delayed growth is evaluated with multivessel Doppler testing by a maternal-fetal medicine specialist (for management of hypertension during pregnancy, see p. 2181).

Diabetes: Diabetes mellitus occurs in 3 to 5% of pregnancies, but incidence will probably increase as the incidence of obesity increases.

Pregnant women with preexisting insulin-dependent diabetes are at increased risk of pyelonephritis, ketoacidosis, pregnancy-induced hypertension, fetal death, major fetal malformations, fetal macrosomia (fetal weight > 4.5 kg), and, if vasculopathy is present, fetal growth restriction. Insulin requirements usually increase during pregnancy.

Women with gestational diabetes are at risk of hypertensive disorders and fetal macrosomia. Gestational diabetes is routinely screened for at 24 to 28 wk or, if women have risk factors, also during the 1st trimester. Risk factors include previous gestational diabetes, a macrosomic infant in a previous pregnancy, family history of non-insulin–dependent diabetes, unexplained fetal losses, and body mass index (BMI) > 30 kg/m^2. A 50-g, 1-h glucose tolerance test is used. If the result is 140 to 200 mg/dL, a 2-h glucose tolerance test is done (see TABLE 158–2 on p. 1275); if glucose is > 200 mg/dL or test results are abnormal, women are treated for the rest of the pregnancy with diet and, if necessary, insulin.

Good control of blood glucose during pregnancy almost eliminates the risk of adverse outcomes attributable to diabetes (for management of diabetes during pregnancy, see p. 2171).

TABLE 262–1. PREGNANCY RISK ASSESSMENT

CATEGORY	RISK FACTORS	SCORE*
Preexisting		
Cardiovascular and renal disorders	Moderate to severe preeclampsia	10
	Chronic hypertension	10
	Moderate to severe renal disorders	10
	Severe heart failure (class II–IV, NYHA classification)	10
	History of eclampsia	5
	History of pyelitis	5
	Mild heart failure (class I, NYHA classification)	5
	Mild preeclampsia	5
	Acute pyelonephritis	5
	History of cystitis	1
	Acute cystitis	1
	History of preeclampsia	1
Metabolic disorders	Insulin-dependent diabetes	10
	Previous endocrine ablation	10
	Thyroid disorders	5
	Prediabetes (diet-controlled gestational diabetes)	5
	Family history of diabetes	1
Obstetric history	Fetal exchange transfusion because of Rh incompatibility	10
	Stillbirth	10
	Postterm pregnancy (> 42 wk)	10
	Preterm newborn	10
	Small-for-gestational-age newborn	10
	Abnormal fetal position	10
	Polyhydramnios	10
	Multifetal pregnancy	10
	Neonatal death	10
	Cesarean section	5
	Habitual abortion	5
	Neonate > 4.5 kg	5
	Multiparity of > 5	5
	Seizure disorders or cerebral palsy	5
	Fetal malformations	1
Other disorders	Abnormal cervical cytologic findings	10
	Sickle cell disease	10
	Positive serologic results for STDs	5
	Severe anemia (Hb < 9 g/dL)	5
	History of TB or purified protein derivative injection site induration ≥ 10 mm	5
	Pulmonary disorders	5
	Mild anemia (Hb 9.0–10.9 g/dL)	1
Anatomic abnormalities	Uterine malformation	10
	Incompetent cervix	10
	Small pelvis	5
Maternal characteristics	Age ≥ 35 or ≤ 15 yr	5
	Weight < 45.5 or > 91 kg	5
	Emotional problem	1
Antepartum		
Exposure to teratogens	Viral infections	5
	Flu syndrome (severe)	5
	Excessive use of drugs	5
	Smoking ≥ 1 pack/day	1
	Alcohol (moderate)	1

Table continues on the following page.

TABLE 262–1. PREGNANCY RISK ASSESSMENT—Continued

CATEGORY	RISK FACTORS	SCORE*
Pregnancy complications	Rh sensitization only	5
	Vaginal spotting	5
Intrapartum		
Maternal	Moderate to severe preeclampsia	10
	Polyhydramnios or oligohydramnios	10
	Amnionitis	10
	Uterine rupture	10
	Postterm (> 42 wk)	10
	Mild preeclampsia	5
	Premature rupture of membranes > 12 h	5
	Preterm labor	5
	Primary dysfunctional labor	5
	Secondary arrest of dilation	5
	Meperidine > 300 mg	5
	Mg sulfate > 25 g	5
	Labor > 20 h	5
	Second stage > 2.5 h	5
	Clinical small pelvis	5
	Medical induction of labor	5
	Precipitous labor (< 3 h)	5
	Primary cesarean section	5
	Repeat cesarean section	5
	Elective induction of labor	1
	Prolonged latent phase	1
	Uterine tetany	1
	Oxytocin augmentation	1
Placental	Placenta previa	10
	Abruptio placentae	10
	Marginal separation	1
Fetal	Abnormal presentation (breech, brow, face) or transverse lie	10
	Multifetal pregnancy	10
	Fetal bradycardia > 30 min	10
	Breech delivery, total extraction	10
	Prolapsed cord	10
	Fetal weight < 2.5 kg	10
	Fetal acidosis pH ≤ 7.25 (stage I)	10
	Fetal tachycardia > 30 min	10
	Meconium-stained amniotic fluid (dark)	10
	Meconium-stained amniotic fluid (light)	5
	Operative delivery using forceps or vacuum extractor	5
	Breech delivery, spontaneous or assisted	5
	General anesthesia	5
	Outlet forceps	1
	Shoulder dystocia	1

*A score of 10 or more indicates a high risk.

NYHA = New York Heart Association; STDs = sexually transmitted diseases.

Sexually transmitted diseases (STDs—see Ch. 194 on p. 1650): Fetal syphilis in utero can cause fetal death, congenital malformations, and severe disability. Risk of transmission of HIV from woman to offspring in utero or perinatally is 30 to 50% within 6 mo (see pp. 1627 and 2341). During pregnancy, bacterial vaginosis, gonorrhea, and genital chlamydial infection increase risk of preterm labor and premature rupture of the membranes. Routine prenatal care includes screening tests for these infections at the 1st prenatal visit. Syphilis testing is repeated during pregnancy if risk continues and at delivery for all women. Pregnant women who have any of these infections are treated with antimicrobials.

Treatment of bacterial vaginosis, gonorrhea, or chlamydial infection may prolong the interval from rupture of the membranes to delivery and may improve fetal outcome by decreasing fetal inflammation. Treating HIV with zidovudine or nevirapine reduces risk of transmission by ⅔; risk is probably lower (< 2%) with a combination of 2 or 3 antivirals (see p. 2351). These drugs are recommended despite potential toxic effects in the fetus and woman.

Pyelonephritis: Pyelonephritis increases risk of premature rupture of the membranes, preterm labor, and infant acute respiratory distress syndrome. Pregnant women with pyelonephritis are hospitalized for evaluation and treatment, primarily with urine culture plus sensitivities, IV antibiotics (eg, a 3rd-generation cephalosporin with or without an aminoglycoside), antipyretics, and hydration. Pyelonephritis is the most common nonobstetric cause of hospitalization during pregnancy. Oral antibiotics specific to the causative organism are begun 24 to 48 h after fever resolves and continued until the total course of antibiotic therapy is 7 to 10 days. Prophylactic antibiotics (eg, nitrofurantoin, trimethoprim-sulfamethoxazole) with periodic urine cultures are continued for the rest of the pregnancy.

Acute surgical problems: Major surgery, particularly intra-abdominal, increases risk of preterm labor and fetal death. Also, physiologic changes of pregnancy make intra-abdominal disorders that require surgery (eg, appendicitis, cholecystitis, intestinal obstruction) difficult to recognize, often delaying diagnosis and thus worsening outcomes. After surgery, antibiotics and tocolytic drugs are given for 12 to 24 h. If nonemergency surgery is necessary during pregnancy, it is most safely done during the 2nd trimester.

Genital tract abnormalities: Structural abnormalities of the uterus and cervix (eg, uterine septum, bicornuate uterus) make fetal malpresentation, dysfunctional labor, and the need for cesarean section more likely. Uterine fibroids can cause placental abnormalities and may grow rapidly or degenerate during pregnancy; degeneration often causes severe pain and peritoneal signs. Cervical incompetence (see p. 2192) makes preterm delivery more likely. In women who have had full-thickness myomectomy, vaginal delivery may result in uterine rupture and thus should be avoided. Uterine abnormalities that lead to poor obstetric outcomes often require surgical correction, which is not done during pregnancy.

Maternal age: Teenagers, who account for 13% of all pregnancies, tend to neglect prenatal care. The result is an increased incidence of preeclampsia, preterm labor, and anemia, which often leads to fetal growth restriction.

In women > 35, the incidence of preeclampsia is increased, as is that of gestational diabetes, dysfunctional labor, abruptio placentae, stillbirth, and placenta previa. These women are also more likely to have preexisting disorders (eg, CHTN, diabetes). Because risk of fetal chromosomal abnormalities increases as maternal age increases, genetic testing should be considered (see p. 2144).

Maternal weight: Pregnant women whose BMI was < 19.8 kg/m^2 before pregnancy are considered underweight, which predisposes to low birth weight (< 2.5 kg) neonates. Such women are encouraged to gain about 12.5 to 18 kg during pregnancy.

Pregnant women whose BMI was > 29.0 kg/m^2 before pregnancy are considered overweight, making maternal hypertension and diabetes, postterm pregnancy, fetal macrosomia, and the need for cesarean section more likely. Such women are encouraged to limit weight gain during pregnancy to < 7 kg.

Exposure to teratogens: Common teratogens (agents that cause fetal malformation) include infections, drugs, and physical agents. Malformations are most likely to result if exposure occurs between the 2nd and 8th wk after conception (the 4th to 10th wk after the last menstrual period), when organs are forming. Other adverse pregnancy outcomes are also more likely. Pregnant women exposed to teratogens are counseled about increased risks and referred for detailed ultrasound evaluation to detect malformations.

Common infections that may be teratogenic include herpes simplex, viral hepatitis, rubella, varicella, syphilis, toxoplasmosis, and cytomegalovirus and coxsackievirus infections.

Commonly used drugs that may be teratogenic include alcohol, tobacco, and some anticonvulsants, antibiotics, and antihypertensives (see TABLE 260–2 on p. 2160).

Cigarette smoking is the most common addiction among pregnant women. Also, percentages of women who smoke and of those who smoke heavily appear to be increasing. Only 20% of smokers quit during pregnancy. Carbon monoxide and nicotine in cigarettes cause hypoxia and vasoconstriction, increasing risk of spontaneous abortion (fetal loss or delivery < 20 wk), fetal growth restriction (birth weight averaging 170 g less than that of neonates whose mothers do not smoke), abruptio placentae, placenta previa, premature rupture of the membranes, preterm birth, chorioamnionitis, and stillbirth. Neonates whose mothers smoke are also more likely to have anencephaly, congenital heart defects, orofacial clefts, sudden infant death syndrome, deficiencies in physical growth and intelligence, and behavioral problems. Smoking cessation or limitation reduces risks.

Alcohol is the most commonly used teratogen. Drinking alcohol during pregnancy increases risk of spontaneous abortion. Risk is probably related to amount of alcohol consumed, but no amount is known to be risk-free. Regular drinking decreases birth weight by about 1 to 1.3 kg. Binge drinking in particular, possibly as little as 45 mL of pure alcohol (equivalent to about 3 drinks) a day, can cause fetal alcohol syndrome. This syndrome occurs in 2.2/1000 live births; it includes fetal growth restriction, facial and cardiovascular defects, and neurologic dysfunction. It is a leading cause of mental retardation and can cause neonatal death due to failure to thrive.

Cocaine use has indirect risks (eg, maternal stroke or death during pregnancy). It also directly causes fetal vasoconstriction and hypoxia. Repeated use increases risk of spontaneous abortion, fetal growth restriction, abruptio placentae, preterm birth, stillbirth, and congenital malformations (eg, CNS, GU, and skeletal malformations; isolated atresias).

Although marijuana's main metabolite can cross the placenta, recreational use of marijuana use does not consistently appear to increase risk of congenital malformations, fetal growth restriction, or postnatal neurobehavioral abnormalities.

Prior stillbirth: Causes of stillbirth (fetal death > 20 wk) may be maternal, placental, or fetal (see p. 2201). Having had a stillbirth increases risk of fetal death in subsequent pregnancies. Fetal surveillance using antepartum testing (eg, nonstress testing, biophysical profile) is recommended. Treatment of maternal disorders (eg, CHTN, diabetes, infections) may lower risk of stillbirth in a current pregnancy.

Prior preterm delivery: Previous preterm delivery due to preterm labor increases risk of future preterm deliveries; if the previous preterm neonate weighed < 1.5 kg, risk of preterm delivery in the next pregnancy is 50%. Causes of preterm delivery include multifetal (multiple) pregnancy, preeclampsia or eclampsia, placental abnormalities, preterm rupture of the membranes (causing ascending uterine infection), pyelonephritis, some STDs, and spontaneous preterm labor. Women with prior preterm labor and delivery require ultrasound evaluation, including measurement of cervical length (see Cervical Incompetence on p. 2192), at 16 to 18 wk and should be monitored closely for pregnancy-induced hypertension. If symptoms of preterm labor develop, uterine contraction monitoring, testing for bacterial vaginosis, and fetal fibronectin measurement may identify women who need closer observation by their physician.

Prior neonate with a genetic or congenital disorder: Risk of a having a fetus with a chromosomal disorder is increased for most couples who have had a fetus or neonate with a chromosomal disorder (recognized or missed—see p. 2143). Recurrence risk for most genetic disorders is unknown. Most congenital malformations are multifactorial; risk of having a subsequent fetus with malformations is ≤ 1%. If couples have had a neonate with a genetic or chromosomal disorder, genetic screening is indicated. If couples have had a neonate with a congenital malformation, high-resolution ultrasonography and evaluation by a maternal-fetal medicine specialist is indicated.

Hydramnios (polyhydramnios) and oligohydramnios: Hydramnios (excess amniotic fluid) can lead to severe maternal shortness of breath and preterm labor. Risk factors include uncontrolled maternal diabetes, multifetal pregnancy, isoimmunization, and fetal malformations (eg, esophageal atresia, anencephaly, spina bifida).

Oligohydramnios (deficient amniotic fluid) often accompanies congenital malformations of the fetal urinary tract and severe fetal growth restriction (< 3rd percentile). Also, Potter's syndrome with pulmonary hypoplasia or fetal surface compression abnormalities may result, usually in the 2nd trimester, and cause fetal death.

Hydramnios and oligohydramnios are suspected if uterine size does not correspond to gestational date or may be discovered incidentally via ultrasonography, which is diagnostic.

Multifetal (multiple) pregnancy: Multifetal pregnancy increases risk of fetal growth restriction, preterm labor, abruptio placentae, congenital malformations, perinatal morbidity and mortality, and, after delivery, uterine atony and hemorrhage (see p. 2208). Multifetal pregnancy is detected during routine ultrasonography at 18 to 20 wk.

Prior birth injury: Birth of a neonate with a delivery-related injury (eg, cerebral palsy, developmental delay or trauma due to forceps or vacuum extractor delivery, shoulder dystocia with Erb-Duchenne paralysis) does not increase risk in future pregnancies. However, the prior delivery records should be assessed for modifiable risk factors that may have predisposed to the injury.

263 ABNORMALITIES OF PREGNANCY

Abnormalities that develop during pregnancy may be directly related to the pregnancy or not (for nonobstetric disorders, see Ch. 261 on p. 2167). Obstetric abnormalities increase the risk of morbidity or mortality for the woman, fetus, or neonate, as do such factors as maternal characteristics, problems in previous pregnancies, and drug use (see Ch. 262 on p. 2186).

ABRUPTIO PLACENTAE

Abruptio placentae is premature separation of a normally implanted placenta from the uterus during late pregnancy. Manifestations include vaginal bleeding, uterine pain and tenderness, hemorrhagic shock, and disseminated intravascular coagulation. Diagnosis is clinical and sometimes by ultrasonography. Treatment is bed rest for mild symptoms and prompt delivery for severe or persistent symptoms.

Abruptio placentae may involve any degree of placental separation, from a few millimeters to complete detachment. It results in bleeding into the decidua basalis behind the placenta (retroplacentally). Cause is unknown. Fetal ischemia can result. It can cause fetal death if it is acute and disrupts the bulk of uteroplacental blood flow; it can cause growth restriction if it is chronic and less extensive.

Risk factors include older maternal age, hypertension (pregnancy-induced or chronic), vasculitis, other vascular disorders, prior abruptio placentae, abdominal trauma, maternal thrombotic disorders, tobacco use, and particularly cocaine use. Abruptio placentae occurs in 0.4 to 1.5% of all pregnancies.

Symptoms and Signs

Abruptio placentae may result in blood exiting through the cervix (external hemorrhage) or remaining behind the placenta (concealed hemorrhage). Severity of symptoms and signs depends on degree of separation and blood loss. The uterus may be painful, tender, and irritable to palpation. Hemorrhagic shock may occur, as may signs of disseminated intravascular coagulation (DIC).

Diagnosis

Diagnosis is suggested by vaginal bleeding, uterine pain and tenderness, fetal distress, hemorrhagic shock, or DIC in late pregnancy, particularly if degree of tenderness or shock appears disproportionate to degree of vaginal bleeding. If bleeding occurs in late pregnancy, placenta previa, which has similar symptoms, must be ruled out before pelvic examination is done; examination may increase bleeding if placenta previa is present. Evaluation includes fetal heart monitoring, CBC, measurement of serum fibrinogen and fibrin-split products, and transabdominal pelvic ultrasonography. Fetal heart monitoring may detect a nonreassuring pattern or fetal death. Ultrasonography is insensitive; thus, diagnosis may ultimately be clinical.

Treatment

If bleeding does not threaten the life of the mother or fetus, if the fetal heart rate pattern is reassuring, and if the pregnancy is not near term, hospitalization and bed rest are advised; they may reduce the bleeding. If bleeding resolves, ambulation and usually hospital discharge are allowed. If bleeding continues, prompt delivery is indicated; method is chosen using criteria similar to that for preeclampsia or eclampsia (see p. 2197). Vaginal delivery accelerated by IV oxytocin or delivery by cesarean section is usually indicated, depending on the rapidity of maternal and fetal deterioration. Amniotomy (artificial rupture of membranes) is done early because it may accelerate delivery, preventing DIC. Treatment of complications (eg, shock, DIC) is supportive.

CERVICAL INCOMPETENCE

Cervical incompetence is painless cervical dilation resulting in delivery of a live fetus between 16 and 22 wk. Ultrasonography during the 2nd trimester may help assess risk. Treatment is reinforcing the cervical ring with suture material (cerclage).

In women with weak cervical tissue, the enlarging products of conception cause the cervix to dilate prematurely. Weakness may be congenital (eg, in Ehlers-Danlos syndrome) or secondary to cone biopsies (particularly when ≥ 1.7 to 2.0 cm of the cervix is removed), deep cervical lacerations, or previous excessive dilation with instruments. Additional risk factors include müllerian duct defects (eg, bicornuate or septate uterus), induction of ovulation (which often results in multifetal pregnancy), and ≥ 3 prior fetal losses during the 2nd trimester. Overall risk of recurrence of cervical incompetence is probably ≤ 30%. Risk is greatest for women with ≥ 3 prior 2nd-trimester fetal losses.

Diagnosis and Treatment

Cervical incompetence is diagnosed clinically. The increased use of routine second trimester transvaginal ultrasound has documented an inverse relationship between cervical length and preterm delivery; cervical shortening on ultrasound to < 2 cm is considered a risk factor.

Cerclage (reinforcement of the cervical ring with suture material) appears to prevent preterm delivery in patients with ≥ 3 prior 2nd-trimester fetal losses. For other patients, the procedure should probably be limited to those with a history suggesting cervical incompetence plus ultrasound demonstration of cervical shortening prior to 22 to 24 wk gestation; restricting cerclage to such patients does not appear to increase risk of preterm delivery and reduces the number of cerclages currently being done by ⅔. Evidence does not support use of cerclage simply for ultrasound-detected cervical shortening.

CHORIOAMNIONITIS

Chorioamnionitis is infection of the chorion and amnion, usually occurring near term.

Chorioamnionitis may result from an infection that ascends through the genital tract. Risk factors include premature rupture of membranes and prolonged labor. Consequences of chorioamnionitis include premature rupture of membranes and premature labor, and increased risk of neonatal pneumonia, bacteremia, meningitis, and death.

Diagnosis is suggested by fever occurring late in pregnancy. Fetal heart rate monitoring is required. Fetal heart rate increases during fever but, in the absence of chorioamnionitis, returns to baseline as fever resolves. Fetal tachycardia out of proportion to or in the absence of fever suggests chorioamnionitis.

Treatment is broad-spectrum antibiotics (eg, ampicillin plus gentamicin) plus delivery. Risk of chorioamnionitis is decreased by avoiding or minimizing digital pelvic examinations in patients with premature rupture of membranes (see p. 2204).

ECTOPIC PREGNANCY

In ectopic pregnancy, implantation occurs in a site other than the endometrial lining of the uterine cavity—in the fallopian tube, uterine interstitium, cervix, ovary, or abdominal or pelvic cavity. Ectopic pregnancies cannot be carried to term and eventually rupture or involute. Early symptoms and signs include pelvic pain, vaginal bleeding, and cervical motion tenderness. Syncope or hemorrhagic shock can occur with rupture. Diagnosis is by β-human chorionic gonadotropin measurement and ultrasonography. Treatment is with laparoscopic or open surgical resection or with IM methotrexate.

Incidence of ectopic pregnancy (overall, 2/100 diagnosed pregnancies) increases as maternal age increases. Other risk factors include prior pelvic inflammatory disease (particularly due to *Chlamydia trachomatis*), prior tubal surgery, prior ectopic pregnancy (10 to 25% recurrence risk), cigarette smoking, exposure to diethylstilbestrol, and prior induced abortion. Pregnancy is less likely to occur when an intrauterine device (IUD) is in place; however, about 5% of such pregnancies are ectopic. Simultaneous ectopic and intrauterine pregnancies occur in only 1/10,000 to 30,000 pregnancies but may be more common among women who have undergone ovulation induction or assisted reproductive techniques such as in vitro fertilization and gamete intrafallopian tube transfer (GIFT); in such cases, the reported ectopic pregnancy rate is ≤ 1%.

The most common site of ectopic implantation is a fallopian tube, followed by the uterine interstitium (cornua). Cervical, cesarean section scar, ovarian, abdominal, and pelvic pregnancies are rare. Rupture of an ectopic pregnancy results in bleeding that can be gradual, or rapid enough to produce hemorrhagic shock. Intraperitoneal blood eventually causes peritonitis.

Symptoms and Signs

Symptoms vary. Most patients have pelvic pain, sometimes crampy, vaginal bleeding, or both. Menses may or may not be delayed or missed. Rupture may be heralded by sudden, severe pain, followed by syncope or by symptoms and signs of hemorrhagic shock or peritonitis. Rapid hemorrhage is more likely in cornual ectopic pregnancies.

Cervical motion tenderness, unilateral or bilateral adnexal tenderness, or an adnexal mass may be present. The uterus may be slightly enlarged (but less than anticipated based on date of last menstrual period).

Diagnosis

Ectopic pregnancy is suspected in any female of reproductive age with pelvic pain, vaginal bleeding or unexplained syncope or hemorrhagic shock, regardless of sexual, contraceptive, and menstrual history. Findings of physical (including pelvic) examination are neither sensitive nor specific. Diagnosis requires measurement of the urine β subunit of human chorionic gonadotropin (β-hCG), which is about 99% sensitive for pregnancy (ectopic and otherwise). If urine β-hCG is negative and if clinical findings do not strongly suggest ectopic pregnancy, further evaluation is unnecessary unless symptoms recur or worsen. If urine β-hCG is positive or if clinical findings strongly suggest ectopic pregnancy, quantitative serum β-hCG and pelvic ultrasonography are indicated. If quantitative serum β-hCG is < 5 mIU/mL, ectopic pregnancy is excluded. If ultrasonography detects an intrauterine gestational sac, ectopic pregnancy is extremely unlikely except in women who have used assisted reproductive technologies; however, cornual and intraabdominal pregnancies may appear similar to intrauterine pregnancies. Ultrasonographic findings suggesting ectopic pregnancy (noted in 16 to 32%) include complex (mixed solid and cystic) masses, particularly in the adnexa; free fluid in the cul-de-sac; and absence of a uterine gestational sac on transvaginal views, particularly if the β-hCG level is > 1000 to 2000 mIU/mL. Absence of an intrauterine sac with a β-hCG level > 2000 mIU/mL strongly suggests an ectopic pregnancy. Use of transvaginal and color Doppler ultrasonography may improve detection rates.

If ectopic pregnancy appears unlikely and patients are stable, serum levels of β-hCG can be measured serially on an outpatient basis. Normally, the level doubles every 1.4 to 2.1 days up to 41 days; in ectopic pregnancy (and in abortions), levels may be lower than expected by dates and usually do not double as rapidly. If initial evaluation or serial β-hCG levels suggest ectopic pregnancy, diagnostic laparoscopy may be necessary for confirmation. Progesterone levels may be measured when the diagnosis is unclear; if they are ≤ 5 ng/mL, a viable intrauterine pregnancy is very unlikely.

Prognosis and Treatment

Untreated ectopic pregnancy is fatal to the fetus, but if treatment occurs before rupture, maternal death is very rare. In the US, ectopic pregnancy probably accounts for 9% of pregnancy-related maternal deaths.

Hemorrhagic shock is treated (see p. 562); such hemodynamically unstable patients require immediate laparotomy. For stable patients, treatment is usually laparoscopic surgery; sometimes laparotomy is required. If possible, salpingotomy, usually using cautery or laser, is done to conserve the tube, and the products of conception are evacuated. Salpingectomy is indicated when ectopic pregnancies recur or are > 5 cm, when the tubes are severely damaged, or when no future childbearing is planned. Only the irreversibly damaged portion of the tube is removed, maximizing the chance that tubal repair can restore fertility. The tube may or may not be repaired simultaneously. After a cornual pregnancy, the tube and ovary involved can usually be salvaged, but occasionally repair is impossible and hysterectomy is necessary.

If unruptured tubal pregnancies are ≤3.0 cm in diameter, no fetal heart activity is detected, and β-hCG level is < 5,000 mIU/mL ideally but < 15,000 mIU/mL certainly, women can be given a single dose of methotrexate 50 mg/m^2 IM. β-hCG measurement and ultrasonography are repeated on about days 4 and 7. If the β-hCG level does not decrease ≥ 15%, a 2nd dose of methotrexate or surgery is needed. About 10 to 30% of women treated with methotrexate eventually require a 2nd dose. Success rates with methotrexate are about 87%; 7% of women have serious complications (eg, rupture). Surgery is indicated when methotrexate is inappropriate (eg, β-hCG level > 15,000 mIU/mL) or ineffective.

ERYTHROBLASTOSIS FETALIS

Erythroblastosis fetalis is hemolytic anemia in the fetus or neonate caused by transplacental transmission of maternal antibodies to fetal RBCs. The disorder usually results from incompatibility between maternal and fetal blood groups, often Rh_0(D) antigens. Diagnosis begins with prenatal maternal antigenic and antibody screening and may require paternal screening, serial measurement of maternal antibody titers, and fetal testing. Treatment may involve intrauterine fetal transfusion or neonatal exchange transfusion. Prevention is Rh_0(D) immune globulin injection for women at risk.

Erythroblastosis fetalis classically results from Rh_0(D) incompatibility, which may develop when a woman with Rh-negative blood is impregnated by a man with Rh-positive blood and conceives a fetus with Rh-positive blood (see also p. 2272). Other fetomaternal incompatibilities that can cause erythroblastosis fetalis involve the Kell, Duffy, Kidd, MNSs, Lutheran, Diego, Xg, P, Ee, and Cc antigen systems, as well as other antigens. Incompatibilities of ABO blood types do not cause erythroblastosis fetalis.

Pathophysiology

Fetal RBCs move across the placenta to the maternal circulation throughout pregnancy. Movement is greatest at delivery or termination of pregnancy; in maternal abdominal trauma, fetomaternal hemorrhage may be marked. In women who have Rh-negative blood and are carrying a fetus with Rh-positive blood, fetal RBCs stimulate maternal antibody production against the Rh antigens (isoimmunization); the mechanism is the same when other antigen systems are involved.

In subsequent pregnancies, maternal antibodies cross the placenta and lyse fetal RBCs, causing anemia, hypoalbuminemia, and possibly high-output heart failure or fetal death. Anemia stimulates fetal bone marrow to produce and release immature RBCs (erythroblasts) into fetal peripheral circulation (erythroblastosis fetalis). Hemolysis results in elevated indirect bilirub in levels in neonates, which cause kernicterus in neonates (see p. 2278). Usually, isoimmunization does not cause symptoms in pregnant women.

Diagnosis and Treatment

At the 1st prenatal visit, all women are screened for blood and Rh type. If women have Rh-negative blood, the father's blood type and zygosity (if paternity is certain) are determined. If he has Rh-positive blood, maternal Rh antibody titers are measured at 26 to 28 wk. If titers are positive but < 1:32 (or below the value considered critical by the local blood bank), titers are measured more frequently. If titers are ≥ 1:32 (or above the local lab's crucial value), fetal middle cerebral artery blood flow is measured at intervals of 1 to 2 wk depending on titers and patient history; the purpose is to detect high-output heart failure. Elevated blood flow for gestational age should prompt percutaneous umbilical blood sampling (if anemia is strongly suspected) or biweekly spectrophotometric measurement of bilirubin levels in amniotic fluid (Δ OD450), obtained by amniocentesis. If paternity is reasonably certain and the father is likely to be heterozygous for Rh_0(D), the fetus' Rh type is determined from amniotic fluid cells. If fetal blood is Rh negative or if middle cerebral artery blood flow or amniotic bilirubin levels remain normal, pregnancy can continue to term untreated. If fetal blood is Rh positive or unknown and if middle cerebral artery flow or amniotic bilirubin levels are elevated, suggesting fetal anemia, the fetus can be given intravascular intrauterine blood transfusions by a specialist at an institution equipped to care for high-risk pregnancies. Transfusions occur every 1 to 2 wk until fetal lung maturity is confirmed (usually at 32 to 34 wk), when delivery should be performed. Corticosteroids should be given before the 1st transfusion if the pregnancy is ≥ 24 wk.

Delivery should be as atraumatic as possible. Manual removal of the placenta should be avoided because it may force fetal cells into maternal circulation. Neonates with erythroblastosis are immediately evaluated by a pediatrician to determine need for exchange transfusion (see p. 2270).

Prevention

Maternal sensitization and antibody production due to Rh incompatibility can be prevented by giving the woman Rh_0(D) immune globulin. This preparation contains high titers of anti-Rh antibodies, which neutralize Rh-positive fetal RBCs. Because fetomaternal transfer and likelihood of sensitization is greatest at termination of pregnancy, the preparation is given within 72 h of termination of each pregnancy, whether by delivery, abortion, or treatment of ectopic pregnancy. The standard dose is 300 μg. A rosette test can be used to rule out significant fetomaternal hemorrhage, and if results are positive, a Kleihauer-Betke (acid elution) test can measure the amount of fetal blood in the maternal circulation. If fetomaternal hemorrhage is massive (> 30 mL whole blood), additional injections (up to five 300-μg doses within 24 h) are necessary. Treatment at termination of pregnancy is occasionally ineffective because sensitization may have occurred earlier during pregnancy. Therefore, at about 28 wk, all pregnant women with Rh-negative blood and no known prior sensitization are also given a dose. Because giving Rh_0(D) immune globulin to sensitized women has no risks, the injection can be given when blood is drawn for titer measurement at 28 wk. Some experts recommend a 2nd dose if delivery has not occurred by 40 wk. Rh_0(D) immune globulin should also be given after any episode of vaginal bleeding and after amniocentesis or chorionic villus sampling. Anti-Rh antibodies persist for > 3 mo after one dose.

HERPES GESTATIONIS

(Pemphigoid Gestationis)

Herpes gestationis is a polymorphic vesicobullous eruption occurring during pregnancy or postpartum; it is not caused by herpesvirus. Diagnosis is clinical or by skin biopsy. Treatment is with topical or systemic corticosteroids.

Herpes gestationis appears to be an autoimmune phenomenon, probably caused by an IgG antibody directed against a 180 kD antigen in the basement membrane zone of the epidermis. Herpes gestationis occurs in 1/2,000 to 50,000 pregnancies; it usually begins during the 2nd or 3rd trimester or immediately postpartum. It recurs with subsequent pregnancies and after oral contraceptive use (in 25%). The fetus is affected about 10% of cases, presumably by transplacental antibodies.

Symptoms, Signs, and Diagnosis

The rash is very pruritic. Lesions often start on the abdomen, then become widespread. Initially, they are erythematous papules and plaques, often annular; subsequently, they form vesicles and bullae on the outer border and may cluster. The rash usually worsens during labor or immediately postpartum (in 75%), typically remitting within a few weeks or months. Neonates may have erythematous plaques or vesicles that resolve spontaneously in a few weeks.

Herpes gestationis may be confused clinically with several other pruritic eruptions of pregnancy, particularly pruritic urticarial papules and plaques of pregnancy. Direct immunofluorescence examination of perilesional skin is diagnostic.

Treatment

For mild symptoms, topical corticosteroids (eg, 0.1% triamcinolone acetonide cream up to 6 times/day) may be effective. Prednisone (eg, 40 mg po once/day) relieves moderate or severe pruritus and prevents new lesions; dose is tapered until few new lesions erupt, but it may need to be increased if symptoms become more severe (eg, during labor). Systemic corticosteroids given late in pregnancy do not seem to harm the fetus.

HYPEREMESIS GRAVIDARUM

Hyperemesis gravidarum is uncontrollable vomiting during pregnancy that results in dehydration and ketosis. Diagnosis is clinical and by measurement of urine ketones, serum electrolytes, and renal function. Treatment is with IV fluids, antiemetics, and temporary suspension of oral intake.

Pregnancy frequently causes nausea and vomiting; the cause appears to be rapidly increasing levels of estrogens or the β subunit of human chorionic gonadotropin (β-hCG). Most cases are morning sickness; ie, women continue to gain weight and do not become dehydrated. Hyperemesis gravidarum is distinguished from morning sickness by weight loss (> 5% of weight) and development of dehydration and ketoacidosis. Psychologic factors (eg, ambivalence, anxiety) may trigger hyperemesis gravidarum. Hyperemesis gravidarum that persists past 16 to 18 wk is uncommon but may seriously damage the liver, causing severe centrilobular necrosis, widespread fatty degeneration, Wernicke's encephalopathy, or esophageal rupture.

Diagnosis

If hyperemesis gravidarum is suspected, urine ketones, thyroid-stimulating hormone, serum electrolytes, AST, ALT, BUN, serum creatinine, Mg, P, and sometimes body weight are measured. Obstetric ultrasonography should be done to rule out hydatidiform mole and multifetal pregnancy. Other disorders that can cause vomiting and that may be hard to diagnose during pregnancy should be considered: eg, hepatitis, pyelonephritis, pancreatitis, intestinal obstruction, GI tract lesions, hyperthyroidism, gestational trophoblastic disease, and increased intracranial pressure. Tests for these disorders are done based on laboratory, clinical, or ultrasound findings.

Treatment

IV 0.9% normal saline solution with 5% dextrose is given, typically about 2 L over 2 h, the 1st liter containing 100 mg of thiamin; subsequent fluid rate requirements vary with patient response but may be as much as 1 L q 4 h or so for up to 3 days. This dose of thiamin should be given daily for 3 days. Electrolyte deficiencies are treated; K, Mg, and P are replaced as needed. Care must be taken not to correct low plasma Na levels too quickly as this can cause central pontine myelinolysis. At first, patients are given nothing by mouth. Vomiting that persists after initial fluid and electrolyte replacement is treated with an antiemetic (eg, pyridoxine 10 to 25 mg po tid; promethazine 12.5 to 25 mg po, IM, or rectally q 4 to 8 h; metoclopramide 5 to 10 mg IV or po q 8 h; ondansetron 8 mg po or IM q 12 h; prochlorperazine 5 to 10 mg po or IM q 3 to 4 h).

After dehydration and acute vomiting resolve, small amounts of oral liquids are given. Patients who cannot tolerate any oral fluids after IV rehydration and antiemetics may need to be hospitalized or given home IV therapy and take nothing by mouth for a longer period (sometimes several days or more). Once patients tolerate fluids, they can eat small, bland meals, and diet is expanded as tolerated. IV vitamin therapy is required initially and until vitamins can be taken by mouth. If treatment is ineffective, total parenteral nutrition or corticosteroids may be necessary. If progressive weight loss, jaundice, or persistent tachycardia occurs despite treatment, termination of the pregnancy should be considered.

PLACENTA PREVIA

Placenta previa is implantation of the placenta over or near the internal os of the cervix. Typically, bright red painless vaginal bleeding occurs during late pregnancy. Diagnosis is by transvaginal or abdominal ultrasonography. Treatment is bed rest for minor vaginal bleeding before 36 wk gestation or, after 36 wk or in refractory cases, immediate delivery, usually by cesarean section.

Placenta previa may be total (covering the internal os completely), partial (covering part of the os), or marginal (at the edge of the os), or the placenta may be low-lying (near the os without reaching it). Incidence of placenta previa is 1/200 deliveries. Risk factors include multiparity, prior cesarean delivery, uterine abnormalities that inhibit normal implantation (eg, fibroids), smoking, and multifetal pregnancy. If placenta previa occurs during early pregnancy, it usually resolves by 20 wk as the uterus enlarges.

Symptoms, Signs, and Diagnosis

Symptoms usually first occur in late pregnancy. Then, sudden, painless vaginal bleeding often begins; the blood may be bright red, and bleeding may be heavy, sometimes resulting in hemorrhagic shock. *If placenta previa is present, pelvic examination may increase bleeding, sometimes causing sudden, massive bleeding;* thus, *if* vaginal bleeding occurs after 20 wk, pelvic examination is contraindicated unless placenta previa is first ruled out by ultrasonography. Placenta previa frequently cannot be distinguished from abruptio placentae except by ultrasonography.

Transvaginal ultrasonography is an accurate, safe way to diagnose placenta previa.

Treatment

Treatment of minor vaginal bleeding before about 34 wk is hospitalization, bed rest, and avoidance of sexual intercourse, which can cause bleeding by initiating contractions or causing direct trauma. If bleeding stops, ambulation and usually hospital discharge are allowed. Delivery is indicated if bleeding is heavy, uncontrolled, or both or if fetal lungs are mature, usually at 36 wk. Delivery is almost always by cesarean section, but vaginal delivery may be possible for women with a low-lying placenta if the fetal head effectively compresses the placenta and labor is already advanced or if the pregnancy is < 23 wk and rapid delivery is expected. Hemorrhagic shock is treated (see p. 562).

PREECLAMPSIA AND ECLAMPSIA

Preeclampsia is pregnancy-induced hypertension plus proteinuria. Eclampsia is unexplained generalized seizures in patients with preeclampsia. Preeclampsia and eclampsia develop between 20 wk gestation and the end of the 1st wk postpartum. Diagnosis is clinical and by urine protein measurement. Treatment is with IV Mg sulfate and usually rapid delivery.

Preeclampsia affects 3 to 7% of pregnant women, usually primigravidas and women with preexisting hypertension (see p. 2180) or vascular disorders (eg, renal disorders, diabetic vasculopathy). Other risk factors may include maternal age < 20, a family history of preeclampsia, preeclampsia or poor outcome in previous pregnancies, multifetal pregnancy, obesity, and thrombotic disorders (eg, antiphospholipid antibody syndrome—p. 1082).

Preeclampsia develops during pregnancy and eclampsia usually does, but 25% of eclampsia cases develop postpartum, most often in the 1st 4 days. Untreated preeclampsia usually smolders for a variable time, then suddenly progresses to eclampsia, which occurs in 1/200 patients with preeclampsia. Untreated eclampsia is usually fatal.

Etiology

Cause and pathophysiology of preeclampsia and eclampsia are unknown. Factors may include poorly developed uterine placental spiral arterioles (which decrease uteroplacental blood flow in late pregnancy) and placental ischemia or infarction. Fetal growth restriction may result. Diffuse or multifocal vasospasm can result in ischemia, eventually damaging multiple organs, particularly the brain, kidneys, and liver. Contributors to vasospasm may include decreased prostacyclin (an endothelium-derived vasodilator), increased endothelin (an endothelium-derived vasoconstrictor), and increased soluble Flt-1 (a circulating receptor for vascular endothelial growth factor).

Lipid peroxidation of cell membranes induced by free radicals may contribute to preeclampsia. The coagulation system is activated, possibly secondary to endothelial cell dysfunction, leading to platelet activation. However, frank coagulopathy is rare unless abruptio placentae is also present.

Symptoms and Signs

Preeclampsia may be asymptomatic or may cause edema or excessive weight gain. Nondependent edema such as facial or hand swelling (the patient's ring may no longer fit her finger) is more specific than dependent edema. Other signs may include increased reflex reactivity, indicating neuromuscular irritability, which can progress to seizures (eclampsia). Petechiae may reflect a bleeding tendency. Severe preeclampsia may cause organ damage; manifestations may include headache, visual disturbances, confusion, epigastric or right upper quadrant abdominal pain (reflecting hepatic ischemia or capsular enlargement), nausea, vomiting, shortness of breath or dyspnea (reflecting pulmonary edema or acute respiratory distress syndrome [ARDS]), and oliguria (reflecting decreased plasma volume or ischemic acute tubular necrosis).

Diagnosis

Diagnosis is suggested by symptoms or presence of hypertension. Tests include urinalysis, CBC, platelet count, urate, liver function tests, and measurement of serum electrolytes, BUN, creatinine, creatine clearance, and 24-h urine protein. Preeclampsia is diagnosed when pregnant women have new-onset hypertension (BP ≥ 140/90 mm Hg) plus unexplained proteinuria of ≥ 1+ on dipstick on 2 occasions at least 4 h apart after 20 wk. Occasionally, tests detect the HELLP syndrome (*h*emolysis, *e*levated *l*iver function tests, and *l*ow *p*latelets).

Preeclampsia is classified as severe based on symptoms; other evidence of organ damage; presence of fetal growth restriction; and laboratory tests, including results that indicate HELLP syndrome, BP ≥ 160/110 mm Hg on 2 occasions ≥ 6 h apart, urine protein ≥ 5 g in a 24-h collection or ≥ 3+ in 2 samples obtained ≥ 4 h apart, and urine output < 500 mL in 24 h.

Treatment

Definitive treatment is delivery. For term pregnancy, immediate delivery after maternal stabilization is safest. For pregnancies < 37 wk, risk of early delivery is balanced against severity of the preeclampsia and response to treatment. Treatment aims to optimize maternal health, which usually optimizes fetal health. If preeclampsia is mild, outpatient treatment is possible; it includes strict bed rest, lying on the left side whenever possible, a normal salt intake, increased fluid intake, and evaluation every 2 or 3 days.

Patients with mild eclampsia that does not immediately abate, severe preeclampsia, or eclampsia require hospitalization; a few hours of stabilizing medical treatment to lower BP to 140 to 155/90 to 105 mm Hg, and to resolve seizures and reduce reflex reactivity; and then delivery. Exceptions include advanced prematurity when mild preeclampsia does not progress and severe preeclampsia that improves with hospitalization. Whether patients with mild preeclampsia always require Mg sulfate before delivery is controversial. Patients with severe preeclampsia require Mg sulfate as soon as diagnosis is made. When delivery is delayed before about 32 to 34 wk in patients who are not clinically deteriorating, corticosteroids are given for 48 h. Delivery is mandated at 34 wk or when deterioration of maternal or fetal status or documentation of fetal lung maturity occurs. Eclampsia always requires delivery after seizures and severe hypertension have been controlled. All hospitalized patients are checked frequently for seizures, symptoms of severe preeclampsia, and vaginal bleeding. BP, reflexes, and fetal heart rate are monitored continuously or several times a day.

Patients with severe preeclampsia or with eclampsia are often admitted to the ICU. Continued management by the obstetrician is mandatory. As part of stabilization, these patients are given IV Ringer's lactate or 0.9% normal saline solution at about 125 mL/h (to increase urine output) and IV Mg sulfate (to stop or prevent seizures and reduce reflex reactivity and BP). Mg sulfate 4 g IV over 20 min is followed by a constant IV infusion of about 1 to 3 g/h, with supplemental doses as necessary. Dose is adjusted based on the patient's reflexes, BP, and serum Mg levels (therapeutic range, 4 to 7 mEq/L). Patients with excess Mg levels (eg, with Mg levels > 10 mEq/L or a sudden decrease in reflex reactivity) or hypoventilation are treated with Ca gluconate 1 g IV. IV Mg sulfate may cause lethargy, hypotonia, and transient respiratory depression in neonates. However, serious neonatal complications are uncommon.

If Mg therapy is ineffective, phenytoin or valium can be given to stop seizures, and IV hydralazine or labetalol is given in a titrated dose to lower BP to 140 to 155/90 to 105 mm Hg. Persistent oliguria is treated with a fluid challenge, followed by furosemide 10 to 20 mg IV; *diuretics are not used otherwise*. If fluids plus furosemide are ineffective, determining intravascular volume and cardiac output with a Swan-Ganz catheter may be considered. Anuric patients with normovolemia may require renal vasodilators or dialysis.

The most efficient method of delivery should be used. If the cervix is favorable and rapid vaginal delivery seems feasible, a dilute IV infusion of oxytocin is given to accelerate labor; if labor is active, the membranes are ruptured. If the cervix is unfavorable and prompt vaginal delivery is unlikely, delivery by cesarean section is indicated. Preeclampsia and eclampsia, if not resolved before delivery, usually resolve rapidly afterward, beginning within 6 to 12 h. As patients gradually improve, ambulation is allowed. Patients should be evaluated every 1 to 2 wk postpartum with periodic BP measurement. If BP remains high after 8 wk postpartum, chronic hypertension should be considered.

PRURITIC URTICARIAL PAPULES AND PLAQUES OF PREGNANCY

Pruritic urticarial papules and plaques of pregnancy are pruritic eruptions that occur during 1/160 to 300 pregnancies; cause is unknown.

Lesions are intensely itchy, erythematous, solid, superficial, and elevated; some are surrounded by blanching, and some have minute vesicles in the center. Itching keeps most patients awake, but excoriation is uncommon. Lesions begin on the abdomen, frequently on striae atrophicae (stretch marks), and spread to the thighs, buttocks, and occasionally the arms; most patients have hundreds of lesions. Lesions develop during the 3rd trimester, most often in the last 2 to 3 wk and occasionally in the last few days. They usually resolve within 15 days after delivery. They may recur in up to 5% of subsequent pregnancies.

Diagnosis is clinical; differentiation from other pruritic eruptions may be difficult. Mild symptoms are treated with topical corticosteroids (eg, 0.1% triamcinolone acetonide cream up to 6 times/day). Rarely, more severe symptoms require systemic corticosteroids (eg, prednisone 40 mg po once/day, tapered as tolerated). Systemic corticosteroids given late in pregnancy do not seem to harm the fetus.

SPONTANEOUS ABORTION

(Miscarriage)

Spontaneous abortion is noninduced embryonic or fetal death or passage of products of conception before the 20th wk of pregnancy. Threatened abortion is vaginal bleeding occurring during this time frame and indicating that spontaneous abortion may occur. Diagnosis is by clinical criteria and ultrasonography. Treatment is usually with bed rest for threatened abortion and, if spontaneous abortion has occurred or appears unavoidable, uterine evacuation.

Death of the fetus or passage of products of conception (fetus and placenta) before 20 wk of pregnancy is considered abortion. Fetal death after 20 wk is considered late fetal death and, with delivery, is considered a stillbirth. Passage of a live fetus between 20 and 37 wk is considered preterm delivery (see p. 2205).

Abortions may be classified as early or late, spontaneous or induced for therapeutic or elective reasons (see p. 2136), threatened or inevitable, incomplete or complete, recurrent, missed, or septic (see TABLE 263–1).

About 20 to 30% of women with confirmed pregnancies bleed during the 1st 20 wk of pregnancy; ½ of these women spontaneously abort. Thus, incidence of spontaneous abortion is about 10 to 15% in confirmed pregnancies. Incidence in all pregnancies is probably higher because some very early abortions are mistaken for a late menstrual period.

TABLE 263–1. CLASSIFICATION OF ABORTION

TYPE	DEFINITION
Early	Abortion before 12 wk gestation
Late	Abortion between 12 and 20 wk gestation
Spontaneous	Abortion that is not induced
Induced	Termination of pregnancy for medical or elective reasons
Therapeutic	Termination of pregnancy to preserve the woman's life or health, or because of fetal death or malformations incompatible with life
Threatened	Vaginal bleeding occurring before 20 wk gestation without cervical dilation, which indicates that spontaneous abortion may occur
Inevitable	Vaginal bleeding or rupture of the membranes accompanied by dilation of the cervix
Incomplete	Expulsion of some products of conception
Complete	Expulsion of all products of conception
Recurrent (habitual)	Two or more consecutive spontaneous abortions
Missed	Undetected death of embryo or fetus that is not expelled and causes no bleeding (ie, blighted ovum, anembryonic pregnancy, or fetal demise)
Septic	Serious infection of the uterine contents during or shortly before or after an abortion

Etiology

Isolated spontaneous abortions may result from certain viruses—most notably cytomegalovirus, herpesvirus, parvovirus, and rubella virus—or from disorders that can cause sporadic or recurrent abortions (eg, chromosomal or mendelian abnormalities, luteal phase defects). Acquired and hereditary thrombophilias appear to cause abortions after ≥ 10 wk. Immunologic abnormalities and major trauma may be causes. Cause is often unknown. Subclinical thyroid disorders, well-controlled or subclinical diabetes mellitus, retroverted uterus, and minor trauma have not been shown to cause spontaneous abortions.

Symptoms and Signs

Symptoms include crampy pelvic pain, bleeding, and eventually expulsion of tissue. Late spontaneous abortion may begin with a gush of fluid when the membranes rupture. Hemorrhage is rarely massive. A dilated cervix indicates that abortion is inevitable.

If products of conception remain in the uterus after spontaneous abortion, vaginal bleeding may occur, usually after a delay. Infection may also develop, causing fever, pain, and sometimes sepsis.

Diagnosis

Diagnosis of threatened, inevitable, incomplete, or complete abortion is often possible based on clinical criteria (see TABLE 263–2) and a positive urine pregnancy test. However, ultrasonography and quantitative measurement of the serum β subunit of human chorionic gonadotropin (β-hCG) are usually done to exclude ectopic pregnancy, to differentiate among the different types of abortion, and to determine whether products of conception remain in the uterus (suggesting that abortion is incomplete rather than complete). However, results may be inconclusive, particularly during early pregnancy.

Missed abortion is suspected if the uterus does not progressively enlarge or if quantitative β-hCG is low for gestational age or does not double within 48 to 72 h. Missed abortion is confirmed if ultrasonography shows disappearance of previously detected embryonic or fetal cardiac activity or absence of such activity > 7 wk in a well-dated intrauterine pregnancy or when the fetal crown-rump length is > 5 mm using transvaginal ultrasonography. Testing to determine the cause of abortion is necessary if women have recurrent abortions (see p. 2201).

Treatment

Treatment of threatened abortion is bed rest, which may minimize bleeding and cramping; however, no evidence indicates that it prevents embryonic or fetal loss. If the cervix is dilated, avoidance of intercourse is often recommended to prevent infection; however, intercourse has not been shown to cause loss.

Treatment of inevitable, incomplete, or missed abortions is uterine evacuation or, at < 10 wk, waiting for spontaneous passage of the products of conception. Evacuation usually involves suction curettage at ≤ 12 wk; dilation and evacuation (at 12 to 23 wk); or medical induction (for women without prior uterine surgery) at > 16 to 23 wk (for treatment of late fetal death, see Stillbirth on p. 2201). The later the uterus is evacuated, the greater the likelihood of placental bleeding, uterine perforation by long bones of the fetus,

TABLE 263–2. CHARACTERISTIC SYMPTOMS AND SIGNS IN SPONTANEOUS ABORTIONS

TYPE OF ABORTION	VAGINAL BLEEDING	CERVICAL DILATION*	PASSAGE OF PRODUCTS OF CONCEPTION†
Threatened	Y	N	N
Inevitable	Y	Y	N
Incomplete	Y	Y	Y
Complete	Y	Y or N	Y
Missed	N	N	N

*Internal cervical os is open enough to admit a fingertip during digital examination.

†Products of conception may be visible in the vagina. Tissue examination is sometimes required to differentiate blood clots from tissue products of conception. Before the evaluation, products of conception may have been expelled without the patient recognizing it.

and difficulty dilating the cervix. These complications are reduced by preoperative use of osmotic cervical dilators (eg, laminaria), misoprostol, or mifepristone (RU 486). If complete abortion is suspected, uterine evacuation may be done routinely or only if bleeding or signs of infection develop, suggesting retained products of conception.

After an induced or spontaneous abortion, parents commonly feel grief and guilt. They are given emotional support and, in the case of spontaneous abortions, reassured that their actions were not the cause; formal counseling is rarely indicated.

RECURRENT ABORTION

(Habitual Abortion)

Recurrent abortion is ≥ 2 consecutive spontaneous abortions. Determining the cause may require extensive evaluation of both parents; some causes can be treated.

Etiology

Recurrent abortions usually result from disorders that cause intrauterine fetal damage, such as maternal or paternal chromosomal abnormalities (eg, balanced translocations). Chromosomal abnormalities may cause 50% of recurrent abortions, which are more common during early pregnancy; aneuploidy is involved in up to 80% of all spontaneous abortions occurring at < 10 wk gestation but in < 15% of those occurring at 20 wk. Other common causes may include maternal luteal phase defects (particularly at < 6 wk), overt endocrine disorders (eg, polycystic ovary syndrome, hypothyroidism, hyperthyroidism, poorly controlled diabetes mellitus), severe chronic renal disorders, immunologic abnormalities (eg, lupus anticoagulant, anticardiolipin antibodies, anti-β_2 glycoprotein I), and, particularly after 10 wk, inherited maternal thrombotic disorders (eg, activated protein C resistance; factor V Leiden and prothrombin 20210 gene mutation; hyperhomocysteinemia; deficiencies of antithrombin or protein Z, C, or S). Cervical incompetence and structural abnormalities of the uterine cavity (eg, polyps, fibroids, congenital malformations) may predispose to delivery at < 20 wk but do not necessarily cause intrauterine fetal damage.

Diagnosis and Treatment

Evaluation may be required to exclude possible genetic causes (see p. 2144). Other tests may include thyroid-stimulating hormone, as well as menstrual history, serum testosterone, fasting plasma glucose and insulin, and ultrasound to rule out polycystic ovary syndrome; BUN and creatinine if chronic renal disorder is suspected; serologic tests for immunologic causes; endometrial biopsies for luteal phase defects; and, if abortions occur after 10 wk, various tests for other thrombotic disorders (see Ch. 135 on p. 1080). Structural uterine abnormalities are evaluated by hysterosalpingography or sonohysterography. Cause cannot be determined in up to 50% of women.

Some causes can be treated. If the cause cannot be identified, the chance of a live birth in the next pregnancy is 35 to 85%.

SEPTIC ABORTION

Septic abortion is serious uterine infection during or shortly before or after an abortion.

Septic abortions usually result from induced abortions done by untrained practitioners using nonsterile techniques; they are much more common when induced abortion is illegal. Typical causative organisms include *Escherichia coli, Enterobacter aerogenes, Proteus vulgaris*, hemolytic streptococci, staphylococci, and some anaerobic organisms (eg, *Clostridium perfringens*).

Symptoms and signs are similar to those of pelvic inflammatory disease (eg, chills, fever, vaginal discharge, often peritonitis) and often those of threatened or incomplete abortion (eg, vaginal bleeding, cervical dilation, passage of products of conception). Septic shock may result, causing hypothermia, hypotension, oliguria, and respiratory distress. Sepsis due to *C. perfringens* may result in thrombocytopenia, ecchymoses, and findings of intravascular hemolysis (eg, anuria, anemia, jaundice, hemoglobinuria, hemosiderinuria).

Septic abortion is usually obvious clinically but must be confirmed by pregnancy testing and usually ultrasonography. Treatment is intensive antibiotic therapy (eg, clindamycin plus penicillin; ampicillin, gentamicin, plus clindamycin) plus uterine evacuation as soon as possible.

STILLBIRTH

Stillbirth is delivery of a dead fetus whose gestational age is > 20 wk.

Fetal death in late pregnancy may have maternal, placental, or fetal anatomic and genetic causes. Overall, the most common cause is abruptio placentae. Common maternal causes include uncontrolled diabetes mellitus, preeclampsia or eclampsia, sepsis, substance abuse, trauma, and hereditary thrombotic disorders. Placental causes include vasa previa, chorioamnionitis, umbilical cord accidents (eg, prolapse, knots) uteroplacental vascular insufficiency, twin-twin transfusion, and fetomaternal hemorrhage. The most common fetal causes are chromosomal abnormalities, single-gene disorders, infection, major congenital malformations (eg, of the heart or brain), alloimmune thrombocytopenia, fetal alloimmune or inherited anemia, and nonimmune hydrops fetalis.

If a fetus dies during late pregnancy or near term but remains in the uterus for weeks, disseminated intravascular coagulation may occur.

Tests to determine cause include fetal karyotype and autopsy, maternal platelet count, Kleihauer-Betke test, a thrombotic screen (eg, factor V Leiden, prothrombin 20210 mutation, protein C, S and Z levels, antithrombin activity, homocysteine level, antiphospholipid antibody screen), TORCH test (including IgG and IgM for *t*oxoplasmosis, *c*ytomegalovirus, *o*ther agents such as human parvovirus B19, *r*ubella, and *h*erpes simplex and varicella-zoster viruses), and rapid plasma reagin (RPR). Placental pathology should be evaluated. Often, cause cannot be determined.

Postdelivery management is similar to that for live birth. If dead fetus syndrome occurs, labor is induced (eg, with IV oxytocin infusion, sometimes preceded by a prostaglandin to make the cervix favorable—ie, open and effaced). After the products of conception are expelled, curettage may be needed to remove placental fragments.

Alternatively, a dilation and extraction (D&E) may be performed. In all cases, preabortion osmotic dilator cervical ripening should be used with or without misoprostol or RU 486 therapy.

Parents typically feel significant grief and require emotional support and sometimes formal counseling. Discussion of risks with future pregnancy is based on the stillbirth's cause.

264 ABNORMALITIES AND COMPLICATIONS OF LABOR AND DELIVERY

Abnormalities and complications of labor and delivery should be diagnosed and managed as early as possible. Most (eg, multifetal pregnancy, postdatism, postmaturity, premature rupture of membranes, some fetal dystocias) are usually evident before onset of labor. Some (eg, amniotic fluid embolism, some fetal dystocias, preterm labor, protracted labor, umbilical cord prolapse) develop or become evident during labor, often during early stages. Alternatives to spontaneous vaginal delivery may be needed. Some complications (eg, postpartum hemorrhage, inverted uterus) occur immediately after delivery of the fetus and around the time the placenta is delivered. For neonatal resuscitation and disorders of the birth process, see Ch. 272 on p. 2257; for meconium aspiration syndrome, see p. 2300.

ALTERNATIVES TO SPONTANEOUS DELIVERY

Abnormalities or difficulties in pregnancy or during labor and delivery can necessitate alternative delivery methods.

Forceps Delivery and Vacuum Extraction

Forceps and vacuum extractors are devices applied to the fetal head to extract the fetus through the birth canal.

Forceps delivery and vacuum extraction have essentially the same indications. Choice depends largely on user preference. Either procedure may be indicated when the 2nd stage of labor (from full cervical dilation until delivery of the fetus) is prolonged—eg, when the woman is exhausted or when epidural anesthesia prevents her from bearing down adequately. Other indications include fetal distress and some abnormal fetal presentations. These procedures are used when the station of the fetal head is low (≥ +2 cm); then, minimal force or rotation is required to deliver the head.

Contraindications for both procedures include a fetal head larger than the pelvic opening, incomplete dilation of the cervix, absence of engagement, and indeterminate fetal presentation or position. Major complications are maternal and fetal injuries, particularly if the operator is inexperienced.

Induction of Labor

Induction of labor is stimulation of uterine contractions, usually with oxytocin.

Indications: Induction of labor can be medically indicated (eg, for preeclampsia or eclampsia) or elective (to determine when delivery occurs). Before elective induction, fetal lung maturity must be assessed; if gestational age is < 39 wk, amniocentesis is done to determine lecithin/sphingomyelin ratio or other indexes of fetal lung maturity. Contraindications to induction include fundal uterine surgery, prior classical cesarean section, and hypertonic uterine dysfunction. Multiple prior uterine scars are a relative contraindication.

Technique: If the cervix is closed, long, and firm (unfavorable), drugs are given to cause the cervix to open and become effaced (favorable). Misoprostol 25 μg vaginally q 4 to 6 h may be effective. Contraindications to misoprostol include prior uterine surgery and cesarean section. Alternatives include prostaglandin E_2 given intracervically (0.5 mg) or as an intravaginal pessary (10 mg).

Once the cervix is favorable, labor is induced. Constant IV infusion of oxytocin is the safest, most effective method. Dose is 0.5 to 2 milliunits/min, increased by 0.5 to 2 milliunits q 15 to 30 min as needed to ensure strong contractions; uncommonly, > 20 milliunits/min is needed. With higher doses (>40 milliunits/min), excessive water retention may occur. Use of oxytocin must be supervised to prevent hypertonic uterine contractions, which may compromise the fetus. External fetal monitoring is routine, and internal monitoring may begin as soon as the membranes can be safely ruptured—usually, when the cervix is dilated 2 cm and the vertex is engaged.

Cesarean Section

Cesarean section is delivery by incision into the uterus.

About 15 to 25% of deliveries in the US are by cesarean section. This rate varies significantly between practices (and is much lower in most other countries).

Indications: Although morbidity and mortality rates of cesarean section are low, they are still several times higher than those of vaginal delivery; thus, cesarean section should be done only when it is safer for the woman or fetus than vaginal delivery. The most common specific indications are previous cesarean section, protracted labor, fetal dystocia (particularly breech presentation), and a nonreassuring fetal heart rate, which requires rapid delivery.

Many women are interested in elective cesarean section on demand. The rationale includes avoiding damage to the pelvic floor (and subsequent incontinence) and serious intrapartum fetal complications. However, such use is controversial and requires discussion between the woman and her physician. Many cesarean sections are done in women with previous cesarean sections because, for them, vaginal delivery increases risk of uterine rupture; however, risk of rupture with vaginal delivery is only about 1% overall (risk is higher for women who have had multiple cesarean sections or a vertical incision). Vaginal birth is successful in almost 75% of women who have had a single prior cesarean section and should be offered to those who have had a single prior cesarean section by lower uterine transverse incision. A trial of labor is often impractical because it requires the obstetrician, an anesthesiologist, and a surgical team to be available immediately.

Technique: During cesarean section, practitioners skilled in neonatal resuscitation should be available. The uterine incision can be classic or lower segment. A classic incision is made longitudinally in the anterior wall of the uterus, ascending to the fundus. This incision results in more blood loss than a lower-segment incision and is usually done only when placenta previa is present, fetal position is transverse, or the lower uterine segment is poorly developed. A lower-segment incision is made transversely or longitudinally in the thinned, elongated lower portion of the uterine body under the bladder reflection. A longitudinal lower-segment incision is used only for certain abnormal presentations and for excessively large fetuses. In such cases, a transverse incision can extend laterally into the uterine arteries, sometimes causing excessive blood loss.

MULTIFETAL PREGNANCY

Multifetal pregnancy is presence of > 1 fetus in the uterus.

Multifetal (multiple) pregnancy occurs in 1 of 70 to 80 deliveries. Risk factors include ovarian stimulation (usually with clomiphene or gonadotropins), assisted reproduction (eg, in vitro fertilization), prior multifetal pregnancy, and advanced maternal age. The overdistended uterus tends to stimulate early labor, causing preterm delivery (average gestation with twins, 36 wk). Fetal presentation may be abnormal. The uterus may contract after delivery of the 1st child, shearing away the placenta and increasing risk for the remaining fetuses. Sometimes uterine distention impairs postpartum uterine contraction, causing maternal hemorrhage.

Multifetal pregnancy is suspected if the uterus is large for dates and is evident on prenatal ultrasonography. Cesarean section is done when indicated (see p. 2203).

POSTDATISM

Postdatism is pregnancy of ≥ 42 wk.

Because dating is established by ultrasonography in most pregnancies, postdatism has become less common. In prolonged pregnancies (> 41 wk), risk of abnormal fetal growth, oligohydramnios, meconium in amniotic fluid, and fetal death is increased. Most experts recommend that nonstress testing and assessment of amniotic fluid volume or a biophysical profile (eg, assessment of amniotic fluid volume, fetal movement, breathing, and heart rate) be done at 41 wk. If either is abnormal, delivery is required. Many obstetricians induce labor (see p. 2203) in all pregnancies > 41 wk.

PREMATURE RUPTURE OF MEMBRANES

Rupture of the membranes before onset of labor is considered premature; it sometimes results in infection. Diagnosis is clinical. If fetal lungs are immature and infection is absent, treatment is bed rest plus delay of delivery with Mg sulfate and other tocolytic drugs as needed. If fetal lungs are mature or if fetal compromise or infection is present, treatment is expedited delivery (eg, by inducing labor).

Premature rupture of membranes (PROM) may occur at term or earlier (called preterm PROM). Preterm PROM predisposes to preterm delivery. PROM at any time increases risk of infection in the woman (chorioamnionitis), neonate (sepsis), or both; prolapse of the cord; and fetal complications, such as abnormal joint positioning and pulmonary hypoplasia, which may occur with PROM at < 24 wk. Group B streptococci are the most common cause of infection. Other organisms in the vagina may also cause infection.

The interval between PROM and onset of spontaneous labor (latent period) and delivery varies inversely with gestational age. At term, about 80% of women with PROM begin labor within 24 h; at 32 to 34 wk, mean latent period is about 4 days.

Symptoms, Signs, and Diagnosis

Unless complications occur, the only symptom is leakage or a sudden gush of fluid from the vagina. Fever, heavy vaginal discharge, abdominal pain, and fetal tachycardia, particularly if out of proportion to maternal temperature, strongly suggest infection.

Sterile speculum examination is done to verify PROM, estimate cervical dilation, collect amniotic fluid for culture and fetal maturity tests, and obtain cervical cultures. Digital pelvic examination, particularly multiple examinations, increases risk of infection and is best avoided. Diagnosis is assumed if amniotic fluid appears to be escaping from the cervix or if the fetal vernix or meconium is visible. Other less accurate indicators include vaginal fluid that ferns when dried on a glass slide or turns Nitrazine paper blue (indicating alkalinity, and hence amniotic fluid—normal vaginal fluid is acidic). Ultrasonography showing oligohydramnios suggests the diagnosis. Nonstress testing is done at least twice/wk if expectant management is used. In many hospitals, fetal monitoring is done daily while women are hospitalized. When gestational age is < 37 wk or unclear, fetal lung maturity can be assessed by amniotic fluid tests (eg, lecithin/sphingomyelin ratio); the sample may be obtained from the vagina or by amniocentesis.

Treatment

Management requires balancing risk of infection when delivery is delayed with risks due to fetal immaturity when delivery is immediate. No one strategy is correct, but generally, delivery should be prompt when there are signs of fetal compromise or infection (eg, persistently nonreassuring fetal testing results, uterine tenderness plus fever); otherwise, delivery can be delayed for a variable period if fetal lungs are still immature or if labor could start spontaneously (ie, later in the pregnancy). Some clinicians routinely induce labor when gestational age is > 34 wk.

When expectant management is used, bed rest is mandatory, and BP and temperature must be measured ≥ 3 times/day. Antibiotics, usually ampicillin and erythromycin, are given for 7 days; they lengthen the latent period and reduce risk of neonatal sepsis. Corticosteroids should be given to accelerate fetal lung maturity (see below) in pregnancies < 32 wk. Their use between 32 and 34 wk is controversial. If labor begins or persists before lungs are mature, Mg sulfate (see p. 2198) or another tocolytic (a drug that stops uterine contractions—see Preterm Labor, below) can be given. Use of tocolytics is also controversial.

PRETERM LABOR

Labor that begins before 37 wk gestation is considered preterm. Triggers include premature rupture of membranes, infection, and abnormalities of pregnancy. Diagnosis is clinical. Causes are identified. Treatment includes bed rest, tocolytic drugs (if labor persists), and corticosteroids (if gestational age is < 34 wk). Antistreptococcal antibiotics are given pending negative culture results.

Preterm labor may be triggered by premature rupture of membranes, chorioamnionitis (see p. 2192), or another ascending uterine infection; group B streptococci are the most common cause of such infections. Preterm labor may also be due to multifetal pregnancy, preeclampsia or eclampsia, placental abnormalities, pyelonephritis, or some sexually transmitted diseases; a cause may not be evident. Cervical culture and tests are done to check for causes suggested by clinical findings.

Treatment

Antibiotics effective against group B streptococci are given pending negative cervical cultures. Choices include penicillin G 5 million units IV followed by 2.5 million units q 4 h and, for penicillin-allergic patients, clindamycin 900 mg IV q 8 h. Preterm labor can be stopped in only about 25% of women with rupture of the membranes but can be stopped in 50% of those without it. Bed rest, hydration, and antibiotics may be sufficient. If the cervix dilates, tocolytics (drugs that stop uterine contractions) can usually delay labor for at least 48 h. Mg sulfate is the drug of choice and is well tolerated (see p. 2198). Terbutaline 0.25 mg sc (which may be repeated once in 30 min) is given q 4 h until contractions cease; maximum, 0.5 mg/4 h. Terbutaline is effective in 70 to 80% of women; women receiving the drug should be monitored for tachycardia. Maintenance with oral terbutaline is not effective. If the fetus is < 34 wk, the woman is given corticosteroids: betamethasone Na phosphate plus betamethasone acetate suspension 12 mg IM q 24 h for 2 doses or dexamethasone 6 mg IM q 12 h for 4 doses unless delivery is imminent. These corticosteroids accelerate maturation of fetal lungs and decrease risk of neonatal respiratory distress syndrome, intracranial bleeding, and mortality.

AMNIOTIC FLUID EMBOLISM

Amniotic fluid embolism is entrance of amniotic fluid and fetal cells into the maternal pulmonary circulation.

Amniotic fluid embolism is a rare obstetric emergency. It usually occurs during late pregnancy, typically during tumultuous labor and rupture of membranes but occasionally during a cesarean section. Amniotic fluid embolizes to the pulmonary circulation, causing tachycardia, hypotension, respiratory failure, and often rapid death, or, in survivors, disseminated intravascular coagulation. Autopsy may show fetal squamous cells and hair in the pulmonary circulation.

Diagnosis is clinical. Treatment is transfusion of RBCs and fresh frozen plasma (as needed to replace lost blood) and clotting factors as well as ventilatory and circulatory support, using inotropic drugs as needed.

FETAL DYSTOCIA

Fetal dystocia is abnormal fetal size or position resulting in difficult delivery. Diagnosis is by examination, ultrasonography, or response to augmentation of labor. Treatment is with physical maneuvers to reposition the fetus, forceps delivery, or cesarean section.

Fetal dystocia may occur when the fetus is too large for the pelvic opening (fetopelvic disproportion) or is abnormally positioned (eg, breech presentation, shoulder dystocia). Normal fetal presentation is vertex, with the occiput anterior.

Fetopelvic disproportion: Diagnosis is suggested by prenatal clinical estimates of pelvic dimensions (see p. 2150), ultrasonography, and protracted labor. If fetal weight is < 4500 g (in women without diabetes) and augmentation of labor restores normal progress, labor can safely continue. If progress is slow in the 2nd stage of labor, women are evaluated to determine whether delivery by forceps or vacuum extractor is safe and appropriate.

Occiput posterior presentation: The most common abnormal presentation is occiput posterior. The fetal neck is usually somewhat deflexed and thus a larger diameter of the head must pass through the pelvis. In face presentation, the head is hyperextended, and the chin may be posterior. Brow presentation usually converts spontaneously to occiput or face presentation. Many occiput posterior presentations require forceps delivery or cesarean section. If the chin is posterior in face presentation, cesarean section is necessary.

Breech presentation: The 2nd most common abnormal presentation is breech (buttocks before the head). In frank breech, the fetal hips are flexed, and the knees extended. In complete breech, the fetus seems to be sitting with hips and knees flexed. In single or double footling presentation, one or both legs are completely extended and present before the buttocks. Breech presentation is a problem primarily because the presenting part is a poor dilating wedge, which can cause the head to be trapped during delivery, often compressing the umbilical cord.

Umbilical cord compression may cause fetal hypoxemia. The fetal head is probably compressing the umbilical cord if the fetal umbilicus is visible at the introitus, particularly in primiparas whose pelvic tissues have not been dilated by previous deliveries. Breech presentation also increases risk of preterm delivery, fetal brachial plexus or spinal cord birth trauma, and perinatal death. Preventing complications is more effective and easier than treating them, so abnormal presentation must be identified before delivery. Cesarean section is usually done, although the external version maneuver can sometimes move the fetus to vertex presentation before labor, usually at 37 or 38 wk. The external version maneuver usually involves gently pressing on the maternal abdomen. A dose of a short-acting tocolytic (terbutaline 0.25 mg sc) may help. The success rate is about 50 to 60%.

Transverse lie: Fetal position is transverse, with the fetal long axis oblique or perpendicular rather than parallel to the maternal long axis. Shoulder-first presentation requires cesarean section unless the fetus is a 2nd twin.

Shoulder dystocia: In this infrequent condition, presentation is vertex, but the anterior fetal shoulder is lodged behind the symphysis pubis, preventing vaginal delivery. Risk factors include a large fetus and maternal obesity or diabetes mellitus. Shoulder dystocia is identified if the head, after passing through the cervix, appears to be pulled back tightly against the vulva (turtle sign). Asphyxiation can occur because the vaginal canal compresses the chest so that the fetus cannot breathe. Hypoxic injury can begin within 4 to 5 min.

Extra personnel are summoned to the room, and various maneuvers are tried sequentially, if needed, to disengage the anterior shoulder. (1) The woman's thighs are hyperflexed to widen the pelvic outlet (McRobert's maneuver), and suprapubic pressure is applied to rotate and dislodge the anterior shoulder. Fundal pressure is avoided because it may worsen the condition or cause uterine rupture. (2) The obstetrician inserts a hand into the posterior vagina and presses the posterior shoulder to rotate the fetus in whichever direction is easier (Wood's screw maneuver). (3) The posterior shoulder is pushed up toward the sacrum, and the obstetrician inserts a hand to flex the infant's elbow, grasps the infant's hand, and pulls it outside to deliver the infant's entire posterior arm. If all maneuvers are ineffective, the infant's head is flexed and pushed back into the vagina, and the infant is then delivered by cesarean section (Zavanelli maneuver).

PROTRACTED LABOR

Protracted labor is abnormally slow cervical dilation or fetal descent during active labor.

Active labor usually occurs after the cervix dilates to ≥ 4 cm. Normally, cervical dilation and descent of the head into the pelvis proceed at a rate of at least 1 cm/h and more quickly in multiparous women.

Etiology

Protracted labor may result from fetopelvic or fetomaternal disproportion (the fetus cannot fit through the maternal pelvis), which can occur because the maternal pelvis is abnormally small or because the fetus is abnormally large or abnormally positioned (fetal dystocia). Another cause is uterine contractions that are too weak or infrequent (hypotonic uterine dysfunction) or, occasionally, too strong or close together (hypertonic uterine dysfunction).

Diagnosis and Treatment

Diagnosis is clinical. The cause must be identified because it determines treatment. Assessing fetal and pelvic dimensions and fetal position (see p. 2150) can sometimes determine whether the cause is fetopelvic disproportion. For example, fetal weight > 5000 g suggests fetopelvic disproportion. Fetal weight > 4500 g in a diabetic patient would cause similar concern. Uterine dysfunction is diagnosed by evaluating the strength and frequency of contractions via palpation of the uterus or an intrauterine catheter.

Diagnosis is often based on response to treatment. If the 1st or 2nd stage of labor proceeds too slowly and fetal weight is < 5000 g, labor can be augmented with oxytocin, which is the treatment for hypotonic dysfunction. If normal progress is restored, labor can then proceed. If not, fetopelvic disproportion or intractable hypotonic dysfunction may be present, and delivery by cesarean section may be required. In the 2nd stage of labor, forceps or vacuum extraction may be appropriate after evaluation of fetal size, presentation, and station (≥ +2 cm) and evaluation of the maternal pelvis. Hypertonic uterine dysfunction is difficult to treat, but repositioning and analgesics may help.

UMBILICAL CORD PROLAPSE

Umbilical cord prolapse is abnormal position of the cord in front of the fetal presenting part, so that the fetus compresses the cord during labor, causing fetal hypoxemia.

The prolapsed umbilical cord may be contained within the uterus (occult) or may protrude into the vagina (overt). Both are uncommon.

In **occult prolapse,** the cord is often compressed by a shoulder or the head. A fetal heart rate pattern that suggests hypoxemia (eg, severe bradycardia, severe variable accelerations) may be the only clue. Changing the woman's position may relieve pressure on the cord; however, if the abnormal fetal heart rate pattern persists, immediate cesarean section is necessary.

Overt prolapse occurs with ruptured membranes and is more common with breech presentation or a transverse lie. Overt prolapse can also occur with vertex presentation, particularly if membranes rupture (spontaneously or iatrogenically) before the head is engaged. Treatment begins with gently lifting the presenting part and continuously holding it off the prolapsed cord to restore fetal blood flow while immediate cesarean delivery is done. Placing the woman in the knee-to-chest position and giving her terbutaline 0.25 mg IV once may help by reducing contractions.

INVERTED UTERUS

Inverted uterus is a rare medical emergency in which the corpus turns inside out and protrudes into the vagina or beyond the introitus.

The uterus is most commonly inverted when too much traction is applied to the umbilical cord in an attempt to deliver the placenta. Excessive pressure on the fundus during delivery of the placenta, a flaccid uterus, or placenta accreta (abnormally adherent placenta) can contribute.

Treatment of an inverted uterus is immediate manual reduction by pushing up on the fundus until the uterus is returned to its normal position. Because of discomfort, IV analgesics and sedatives are sometimes needed. Terbutaline 0.25 mg IV, nitroglycerin 50 μg IV, or inhalational anesthetics may also be needed.

If attempts to return the uterus are unsuccessful, a laparotomy may be necessary; the fundus is manipulated vaginally and abdominally to return it to its normal position. Once the uterus is in place, an oxytocin infusion should be started.

PLACENTA ACCRETA

Placenta accreta is an abnormally adherent placenta, resulting in delayed delivery of the placenta.

Placenta accreta occurs because the villi penetrate the uterine myometrium. It can result in incomplete expulsion of the placenta, hemorrhage, and infection. Risk factors include prior placental abnormality (eg, placenta previa), maternal age > 35, previous cesarean section or myomectomy, endometrial defects (eg, Asherman's syndrome), and fibroids. Incidence in women who have had placenta previa and ≥ 2 cesarean sections is almost 25%.

Placenta accreta can sometimes be diagnosed before delivery by ultrasonography or MRI. Then, preparations for cesarean hysterectomy are made. During delivery, the disorder is suspected if the placenta has not been delivered within 45 to 60 min of the infant's delivery. In such cases, laparotomy with preparation for large-volume hemorrhage is required. Hysterectomy is the safest procedure, but if keeping the uterus is important and hemorrhage is not massive, sometimes hysterectomy can be avoided by resection of the abnormal site (primarily when accreta is focal).

POSTPARTUM HEMORRHAGE

Postpartum hemorrhage is blood loss of > 500 mL during or immediately after the 3rd stage of labor. Diagnosis is clinical. Treatment is with uterine massage and IV oxytocin, sometimes supplemented by injections of 15-methyl prostaglandin $F_{2\alpha}$ or methylergonovine.

Postpartum hemorrhage commonly results from bleeding at the placental implantation site. Risk factors for bleeding at this site include uterine atony due to overdistention (caused by multifetal pregnancy, polyhydramnios, or an abnormally large fetus), prolonged or dysfunctional labor, grand multiparity (delivery of ≥ 5 viable fetuses), relaxant anesthetics, rapid labor, chorioamnionitis, and retention of placental tissue (eg, due to placenta accreta). Other possible causes of hemorrhage—lacerations of the genital tract, extension of an episiotomy, or uterine rupture—must also be considered. Uterine fibroids may contribute. Postpartum hemorrhage due to subinvolution (incomplete involution) of the placental site usually occurs early but may occur as late as 1 mo after delivery.

Treatment

Intravascular volume is replenished with 0.9% saline up to 2 L IV; blood transfusion is used if this volume of saline is inadequate. Hemostasis is attempted by bimanual uterine massage and IV oxytocin infusion, and the uterus is explored for lacerations and retained placental tissues. The cervix and vagina are also examined; lacerations are repaired. 15-Methyl prostaglandin $F_{2\alpha}$ 250 μg IM q 15 to 90 min up to 8 doses or methylergonovine 0.2 mg IM once (which may be followed by 0.2 mg po tid to qid for 1 wk) should be tried if excessive bleeding continues during oxytocin infusion; during cesarean section, these drugs may be injected directly into the myometrium. Prostaglandins should be avoided in women with asthma; methylergonovine should be avoided in women with hypertension. Sometimes misoprostol 800 to 1000 μg rectally can be used to increase uterine tone. If hemostasis cannot be achieved, hypogastric artery ligation or hysterectomy may be required.

Prevention

Predisposing conditions (eg, uterine fibroids, polyhydramnios, multifetal pregnancy), maternal coagulopathy, an unusual blood type, and history of puerperal hemorrhage are identified antepartum and, when possible, corrected. Careful, unhurried delivery with a minimum of intervention is always wise.

After placental separation, oxytocin 10 units IM or dilute oxytocin infusion (10 or 20 units in 1000 mL of an IV solution at 125 to 200 mL/h for 1 to 2 h) usually ensures uterine contraction and reduces blood loss. After the placenta is delivered, it is thoroughly examined for completeness; if it is incomplete, the uterus is manually explored and retained fragments are removed. Rarely, curettage is required. Uterine contraction and amount of vaginal bleeding must be observed for 1 h after completion of the 3rd stage of labor.

265 POSTPARTUM CARE

Clinical manifestations during the puerperium (6-wk period after delivery) generally reflect reversal of the physiologic changes that occurred during pregnancy. These changes are mild and temporary and should not be confused with pathologic conditions.

Within the 1st 24 h, the woman's pulse rate drops, and her temperature may be slightly elevated. Because WBCs increase during labor, marked leukocytosis (up to 20,000 to 30,000/μL) occurs in the 1st 24 h postpartum; WBC count returns to normal within 1 wk. Vaginal discharge is grossly bloody (lochia rubra) for 3 to 4 days; over the next 10 to 12 days, it changes to pale brown (lochia serosa) and finally to yellowish white (lochia alba). About 1 to 2 wk after delivery, eschar from the placental site sloughs off and bleeding occurs; bleeding is usually self-limited. Total blood loss is about 250 mL; comfortably fitting intravaginal tampons (changed frequently) or external pads may be used to absorb it. Tampons should not be used if they might inhibit healing of perineal or vaginal lacerations.

Urine temporarily increases in volume and may contain protein and sugar. Because blood volume is redistributed, Hct may fluctuate, although it tends to remain in the prepregnancy range if women do not hemorrhage. Plasma fibrinogen and ESR remain elevated during the 1st wk postpartum.

The uterus involutes progressively; after 5 to 7 days, it is firm and no longer tender, extending midway between the symphysis and umbilicus. By 2 wk, it is no longer palpable abdominally. Contractions of the involuting uterus, if painful (afterpains), may require analgesics.

Management in the Hospital

Risk of infection, hemorrhage, and pain must be minimized. The woman is typically observed for at least 1 h after the 3rd stage of labor, and the uterus is massaged periodically to ensure that it contracts and remains contracted, preventing excessive bleeding. If the uterus does not remain contracted with massage alone, oxytocin 10 units IM or a dilute oxytocin IV infusion (10 or 20 units/1000 mL of IV fluid) at 125 to 200 mL/h is given immediately after delivery of the placenta. The drug is continued until the uterus is firm; then it is decreased or stopped. Oxytocin should not be given as an IV bolus because severe hypotension may occur, subsequently increasing cardiac output. If general anesthesia was used for operative delivery (by forceps, vacuum extractor, or cesarean section), the woman is monitored (preferably in a recovery room or a labor, delivery, recovery, and postpartum room) for 2 to 3 h after delivery. For all women, O_2, type O-negative blood or blood tested for compatibility, and IV fluids must be available during the recovery period.

After the 1st 24 h, recovery is rapid. A regular diet should be offered as soon as the woman requests food. Full ambulation is encouraged as soon as possible. When to start an exercise routine depends on the woman; its safety depends on whether complications or disorders are present. Usually, exercises to strengthen abdominal muscles can be started once the discomfort of delivery (vaginal or cesarean) has subsided, typically within 1 day for women who deliver vaginally and later for those who deliver by cesarean section. Curl-ups, done in bed with the hips and knees flexed, tighten only abdominal muscles, usually without causing backache. If delivery was uncomplicated, showering and bathing are allowed, but vaginal douching is prohibited in the early puerperium. The vulva should be cleaned from front to back. Immediately after delivery, ice packs may help reduce pain and edema at the site of an episiotomy or repaired laceration; later, warm sitz baths several times a day can be used. Commonly used analgesics include codeine 30 to 60 mg, aspirin 650 mg, acetaminophen 650 mg, and ibuprofen 400 mg po q 4 to 6 h.

Urine retention, bladder overdistention, and catheterization should be avoided if possible. Rapid diuresis may occur, especially when oxytocin is stopped. Voiding must be encouraged and monitored to prevent asymptomatic bladder overfilling. A midline mass palpable in the suprapubic region or abnormal elevation of the uterine fundus above the umbilicus suggests bladder overdistention. If overdistention occurs, catheterization is necessary to promptly relieve discomfort and to prevent long-term urinary dysfunction. Women are encouraged to defecate before leaving the hospital, although with early discharge, this recommendation is often impractical. If defecation has not occurred within 3 days, a mild cathartic can be given. Maintaining good bowel function can prevent or help relieve existing hemorrhoids, which can be treated with warm sitz baths. Regional (spinal or epidural) anesthesia delays ambulation and may delay defecation and spontaneous urination.

A CBC to verify that women are not anemic is required before discharge only if peripartum blood loss was excessive. Women seronegative for rubella should be vaccinated against rubella on the day of discharge. If women with Rh-negative blood have an infant with Rh-positive blood but are not sensitized, they should be given Rh_0(D) immune globulin 300 μg IM within 72 h of delivery to prevent sensitization (see p. 2195).

The breasts may become painfully engorged during early lactation, when the amount of milk is beginning to increase. Breastfeeding helps reduce engorgement. If the woman is not going to breastfeed, firm support of the breasts can suppress lactation; gravity stimulates the let-down reflex and encourages milk flow. For many women, tight binding of the breasts, cold packs, and analgesics prn followed by firm support effectively control temporary symptoms while lactation is being suppressed.

Transient depression ("baby blues") is very common during the 1st week after delivery. Symptoms are typically mild and usually subside by 7 to 10 days. Treatment is supportive care and reassurance. Persistent symptoms, lack of interest in the infant, suicidal or homicidal thoughts, hallucinations, delusions, or psychotic behavior may require intensive counseling and antidepressants or antipsychotics. Women with a preexisting mental disorder are at high risk of recurrence or exacerbation during the puerperium and should be monitored closely.

Management at Home

The woman and infant can be discharged within 24 to 48 h postpartum; many family-centered obstetric units discharge them as early as 6 h postpartum if major anesthesia was not used and no complications occurred. Analgesics may be offered as necessary but should be limited if a woman is breastfeeding because most drugs are secreted in breast milk (see also p. 2227). Normal activities may be resumed as soon as the woman feels ready. Major problems are rare, but a home visit or close follow-up regimen is necessary.

Intercourse may be resumed as soon as desired and comfortable. However, a delay in sexual activity should be considered for those who need to heal a laceration or episiotomy repair. Pregnancy must be delayed for 1 mo if the woman was vaccinated against rubella at hospital discharge; also, preventing pregnancy for several months to allow complete recovery is in the woman's best interest. Because pregnancy is possible, contraception is required and can be started at discharge. If women are not breastfeeding, ovulation usually occurs about 4 wk postpartum, 2 wk before the 1st menses. However, conception may occur as early as 2 wk postpartum, so ovulation can occur earlier. Women who are breastfeeding tend to ovulate and menstruate later, usually at 10 to 12 wk postpartum, although a few ovulate and menstruate (and become pregnant) as quickly as those who are not breastfeeding.

Breastfeeding status affects choice of hormonal contraceptives. For breastfeeding women, progestin-only oral contraceptives, depot medroxyprogesterone acetate injections, and levonorgestrel implants are preferred because they do not affect milk production. Estrogen-progesterone contraceptives can interfere with milk production and should not be initiated until production is well established.

A diaphragm should be fitted only after complete involution of the uterus, at 6 to 8 wk; meanwhile, foams, jellies, and condoms should be used.

MASTITIS

Mastitis is painful inflammation of the breast, usually accompanied by infection.

Fever later in the puerperium is frequently due to mastitis. Symptoms include high fever, erythema, induration, tenderness, pain, swelling, and warmth to the touch.

Treatment includes encouragement of fluid intake and antibiotics aimed at *Staphylococcus aureus*, the most common causative pathogen. Examples are dicloxacillin 500 mg po q 6 h for 7 to 10 days and, for women allergic to penicillin, erythromycin 250 mg po q 6 h. If women do not improve and do not have an abscess, vancomycin 1 g IV q 12 h or cefotetan 1 to 2 g IV q 12 h to cover resistant organisms should be considered. Breastfeeding should be continued during treatment because treatment includes emptying the affected breast. Breast abscesses are very rare and are treated with incision, drainage, and antibiotics aimed at *S. aureus*.

PUERPERAL ENDOMETRITIS

Puerperal endometritis is uterine infection, typically caused by bacteria ascending from the lower genital or GI tract. Symptoms are abdominal tenderness and pain, fever, malaise, and sometimes discharge. Diagnosis is clinical, rarely aided by culture. Treatment is with broad-spectrum antibiotics (eg, clindamycin plus gentamycin).

Incidence of postpartum endometritis is affected mainly by the mode of delivery but also by patient characteristics. Postpartum endometritis occurs in 1 to 3% of normal vaginal deliveries, in 5 to 15% of scheduled caesarean deliveries (done before labor starts), and in 15 to 20% of unscheduled caesarean deliveries (done after labor starts).

Etiology and Pathophysiology

Endometritis may develop after chorioamnionitis during labor, or postpartum. Predisposing conditions include prolonged rupture of the membranes, internal fetal monitoring, prolonged labor, operative or traumatic delivery, repeated digital examination, young maternal age, low socioeconomic status, colonization of the lower genital tract, retention of placental fragments in the uterus, postpartum hemorrhage, and anemia.

Infection tends to be polymicrobial; the most common pathogens include gram-positive cocci (predominantly group B streptococci, *Staphylococcus epidermidis*, and *Enterococcus* sp), anaerobes (predominantly peptostreptococci, *Bacteroides* sp, and *Prevotella* sp), and gram-negative organisms (predominantly *Gardnerella vaginalis, Escherichia coli, Klebsiella pneumoniae*, and *Proteus mirabilis*).

Uncommonly, peritonitis, pelvic abscess, pelvic thrombophlebitis (with risk of pulmonary embolism), or a combination develop. Rarely, septic shock and its sequelae, including death, occur.

Symptoms and Signs

Typically, the 1st symptoms are lower abdominal pain and uterine tenderness, followed by fever—most commonly within the 1st 24 to 72 h postpartum. Chills, headache, malaise, and anorexia are common. Sometimes the only symptom is a low-grade fever.

Pallor, tachycardia, and leukocytosis usually occur, and the uterus is soft, large, and tender. Lochia may be decreased or profuse and malodorous. When parametria are affected, pain and pyrexia are severe; the large, tender uterus is indurated at the base of the broad ligaments, extending to the pelvic walls or posterior cul-de-sac. Pelvic abscess may present as a palpable mass separate from and adjacent to the uterus.

Diagnosis

Diagnosis may be apparent clinically, but other causes of fever and lower abdominal symptoms (eg, UTI, wound infection, pelvic thrombophlebitis) must be considered. Uterine tenderness is often difficult to distinguish from incisional tenderness in women who have had a cesarean section (or other operation).

Urinalysis and urine culture are usually required. Endometrial cultures are rarely indicated because specimens collected through the cervix are almost always contaminated by vaginal and cervical flora and because results are usually not available until after empiric therapy is underway. Endometrial cultures should be done only when endometritis is refractory to routine antibiotic regimens and no other cause of infection is obvious; sterile technique with a speculum is used to avoid vaginal contamination, and the sample is sent for aerobic and anaerobic cultures. Blood cultures are rarely indicated and should be done only when endometritis is refractory to routine antibiotic regimens or clinical findings suggest septicemia. If findings suggest abscess, imaging tests, usually CT, are done. Spiking fevers despite antibiotic therapy suggest pelvic thrombophlebitis, a clinical diagnosis of exclusion, occasionally helped by CT or MRI.

If patients have only low-grade fever, examination for other occult causes (eg, atelectasis, breast engorgement, UTI) is required. Endometrial infection is presumed if no other cause is apparent and the patient's temperature is ≥ 38° C on 2 successive days after the 1st 24 h postpartum. Fever due to breast engorgement tends to remain ≤ 39°C. If temperature abruptly rises after 2 or 3 days of low-grade fever, the cause is probably an infection.

Prevention and Treatment

Preventing or minimizing predisposing factors is essential. Appropriate hand washing should be encouraged. Vaginal delivery cannot be sterile, but aseptic techniques are used. Prophylactic antibiotics given when cesarean section is done can reduce risk of endometritis by up to ⅔ to ¾.

Treatment is a broad-spectrum antibiotic regimen given IV until the woman is afebrile for 48 h. The 1st-line choice is clindamycin 900 mg q 8 h plus gentamicin 1.5 mg/kg q 8 h or 5 mg/kg once/day; ampicillin 1 g q 6 h is added if enterococcal infection is suspected or if no improvement occurs by 48 h. Continuing treatment with oral antibiotics is not necessary.

PYELONEPHRITIS

Pyelonephritis is bacterial infection of the renal parenchyma.

Pyelonephritis may occur postpartum if bacteria ascend from the bladder. The infection may begin as asymptomatic bacteriuria during pregnancy and is sometimes associated with bladder catheterization to relieve urinary distention during and after labor. The causative organism is usually a type of coliform bacteria (eg, *Escherichia coli*). Symptoms include fever, flank pain, general malaise, and, occasionally, painful urination.

Initial treatment is ceftriaxone 1 to 2 g IV q 12 to 24 h or ampicillin 1 g IV q 6 h plus gentamicin 1.5 mg/kg IV q 8 h until the woman is afebrile for 48 h. Sensitivities with culture should be checked. Treatment is adjusted accordingly and continued for a total of 7 to 14 days; oral antibiotics are used after the initial IV antibiotics. Women should be encouraged to consume large amounts of liquids. A urine culture should be repeated 6 to 8 wk after delivery to verify cure. For all women with recurring episodes of pyelonephritis during or after pregnancy, contrast CT should be considered to look for calculi or congenital malformations.

SECTION 19
PEDIATRICS

INTRODUCTION

As children develop physiologically and emotionally, it is useful to define certain age-based groups. The following terminology is used in this section:

- Neonate (newborn): Birth to 1 mo
- Infant: 1 mo to 1 yr
- Young child: 1 yr through 4 yr
- Older child: 5 yr through 10 yr
- Adolescent: 11 yr through 17 to 19 yr

This section covers diseases and disorders unique to children (including those that may persist into adulthood) and those that have defining features different from adults. Pediatric diseases and disorders that are also prevalent in adults and manifest similarly (eg, pharyngitis, asthma, diabetes) are covered more fully elsewhere in THE MANUAL.

266 APPROACH TO THE CARE OF NORMAL INFANTS AND CHILDREN

Routine care for infants and children aims to promote healthy development through education, routine vaccination, and early detection and treatment of disease.

EVALUATION AND CARE OF THE NORMAL NEONATE

Hand washing is critical for all personnel to prevent transmission of infection. Active participation in the birth by both the mother and her partner facilitates adaptation of both to parenting.

The First Few Hours

Immediately at delivery, the neonate's respiratory effort, heart rate, color, tone, and reflex irritability should be assessed; all are key components of the Apgar score assigned at 1 and 5 min after birth (see TABLE 272–2 on p. 2261). Apgar scores between 8 and 10 indicate the neonate is making a smooth transition to extrauterine life; scores ≤ 7 at 5 min (particularly if sustained beyond 10 min) are linked to higher neonatal morbidity and mortality rates. Many normal neonates have cyanosis 1 min after birth that clears by 5 min. Cyanosis that does not clear may indicate congenital cardiopulmonary anomalies or CNS depression.

In addition to Apgar scoring, neonates should be evaluated for gross deformities (eg, clubfoot, polydactyly) and other important abnormalities such as heart murmurs. The evaluation should ideally be performed under a radiant warmer with the family close by.

Preventive interventions include administration into both eyes of an antimicrobial agent (eg, 1% silver nitrate solution 2 drops, 0.5% erythromycin 1 cm ribbon, 1% tetracycline 1 cm ribbon) to prevent gonococcal and chlamydial ophthalmia, and administration of vitamin K 1 mg IM to prevent hemorrhagic disease of the newborn.

Subsequently, the neonate is bathed, wrapped, and brought to the family. The head should be covered with a cap to prevent heat loss. Rooming-in and early breastfeeding should be encouraged so the family can get to know the baby and can receive guidance from staff during the hospital stay. Breastfeeding is more likely to be successful when the family is given frequent and adequate support.

The First Few Days

Physical examination: The neonate should undergo a thorough physical examination within 24 h. Performing the examination alongside the mother and family members allows the family to ask questions and the clinician to point out physical findings and provide anticipatory guidance.

Basic measurements include length, weight, and head circumference (see p. 2248). Length is measured from crown to heel; normal values are based on gestational age and should be plotted on a standard growth chart. When gestational age is uncertain or when the infant seems large or small for age, the gestational age can be precisely determined using physical and neuromuscular findings (see FIG. 266–1). These methods are typically accurate to ± 2 wk.

Many clinicians begin with examination of the heart and lungs when the infant is quiet. The examiner should identify the location where the heart sounds are loudest (to exclude dextrocardia). Normal heart rate is 100 to 160 beats/min. The rhythm should be regular, although an irregular rhythm from premature atrial or ventricular contractions is not uncommon. A murmur heard in the 1st 24 h is most commonly caused by a patent ductus arteriosus. Daily heart examination confirms the disappearance of this murmur, usually within 3 days. Femoral pulses are sought and compared with brachial pulses. A weak or delayed femoral pulse suggests aortic coarctation or other left ventricular outflow tract obstruction. Central cyanosis suggests congenital heart disease, pulmonary disease, or sepsis.

The respiratory system is evaluated by counting respirations over a full minute because breathing in neonates is irregular; normal rate is 40 to 60 breaths/min. The chest wall should be examined for symmetry, and lung sounds should be equal throughout. Grunting, nasal flaring, and retractions are signs of respiratory distress.

After cardiac and pulmonary evaluation, a systematic head to toe examination is

Neuromuscular Maturity

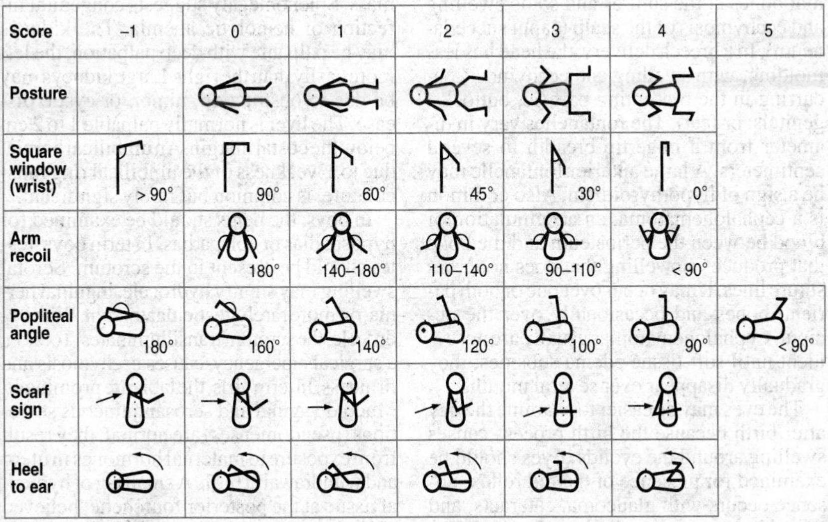

Score	−1	0	1	2	3	4	5
Posture							
Square window (wrist)	> 90°	90°	60°	45°	30°	0°	
Arm recoil		180°	140–180°	110–140°	90–110°	< 90°	
Popliteal angle	180°	160°	140°	120°	100°	90°	< 90°
Scarf sign							
Heel to ear							

Physical Maturity

Skin	Sticky, friable, transparent	Gelatinous, red, translucent	Smooth, pink; visible veins	Superficial peeling and/or rash; few veins	Cracking, pale areas; rare veins	Parchment, deep cracking; no vessels	Leathery, cracked, wrinkled
Lanugo	None	Sparse	Abundant	Thinning	Bald areas	Mostly bald	
Plantar surface	Heel-toe 40–50 mm: −1 < 40 mm: −2	> 50 mm, no crease	Faint red marks	Anterior transverse crease only	Creases anterior 2/3	Creases over entire sole	
Breast	Imperceptible	Barely perceptible	Flat areola, no bud	Stippled areola, 1–2 mm bud	Raised areola, 3–4 mm bud	Full areola, 5–10 mm bud	
Eye/Ear	Lids fused loosely: −1 tightly: −2	Lids open; pinna flat; stays folded	Slightly curved pinna; soft; slow recoil	Well curved pinna; soft but ready recoil	Formed and firm, instant recoil	Thick cartilage, ear stiff	
Genitals (male)	Scrotum flat, smooth	Scrotum empty, faint rugae	Testes in upper canal, rare rugae	Testes descending, few rugae	Testes down, good rugae	Testes pendulous, deep rugae	
Genitals (female)	Clitoris prominent, labia flat	Clitoris prominent, small labia minora	Clitoris prominent, enlarging minora	Majora and minora equally prominent	Majora large, minora small	Majora cover clitoris and minora	

Maturity Rating

Score	Weeks
−10	20
−5	22
0	24
5	26
10	28
15	30
20	32
25	34
30	36
35	38
40	40
45	42
50	44

Fig. 266–1. Assessment of gestational age—new Ballard score. Scores from neuromuscular and physical domains are added to obtain total score. (Adapted from Ballard JL, Khoury JC, Wedig K, et al: New Ballard score, expanded to include extremely premature infants. *The Journal of Pediatrics* 119(3);417–423, 1991; used with permission of the CV Mosby Company.)

performed. In a vertex delivery, the head is commonly molded with overriding of the cranial bones at the sutures and some swelling and ecchymosis of the scalp (caput succedaneum). In a breech delivery, the head has less molding, with swelling and ecchymosis occurring in the presenting part (ie, buttocks, genitals, or feet). The fontanelles vary in diameter from a fingertip breadth to several centimeters. A large anterior fontanelle may be a sign of hypothyroidism. Also common is a cephalohematoma, an accumulation of blood between the periosteum and the bone that produces a swelling that does not cross suture lines. It may occur over one or both parietal bones and occasionally over the occiput. Cephalohematomas usually are not evident until soft-tissue edema subsides; they gradually disappear over several months.

The eyes may be easier to examine the day after birth because the birth process causes swelling around the eyelids. Eyes should be examined for presence of the red reflex; absence occurs with glaucoma, cataracts, and retinoblastoma. Subconjunctival hemorrhages are common and caused by forces exerted during delivery.

Low-set ears may indicate genetic anomalies, including trisomy 21. The external auditory canal should be examined. Clinicians should look for external ear pits or tags, which are sometimes associated with hearing loss and kidney abnormalities.

The clinician should inspect and palpate the palate to detect a posterior palate defect. Some neonates are born with an epulis, a benign hamartoma of the gum, which if large enough can cause feeding difficulties and may obstruct the infant's airway. These lesions can be removed without recurrence. Neonates can also be born with primary or natal teeth. Natal teeth do not have roots and may need to be removed because they may fall out and be aspirated. Inclusion cysts called Epstein's pearls may occur on the roof of the mouth.

When examining the neck, the clinician must lift the chin to look for abnormalities such as cystic hygromas, goiters, or branchial arch remnants. Torticollis can be caused by a sternocleidomastoid hematoma from birth trauma.

The abdomen should be round and symmetric. A scaphoid abdomen may indicate a diaphragmatic hernia, through which intestines have migrated to the chest cavity in utero, sometimes causing pulmonary hypoplasia and postnatal respiratory distress. An asymmetric abdomen suggests an abdominal mass. Splenomegaly suggests congenital infection or hemolytic anemia. The kidneys may be palpable with deep palpation, the left more easily than the right. Large kidneys may be due to obstruction, tumor, or cystic disease. The liver is normally palpable 1 to 2 cm below the costal margin. An umbilical hernia, due to a weakness of the umbilical ring musculature, is common but rarely significant.

In boys, the penis should be examined for hypospadias or epispadias. In term boys, testes should be present in the scrotum. Scrotal swelling may signify hydrocele, inguinal hernia, or, more rarely, testicular torsion. With hydrocele, the scrotum transilluminates. Torsion, a surgical emergency, causes ecchymosis and firmness. In term girls, the labia are prominent. Mucoid vaginal and serosanguineous secretions (pseudomenses) are normal; they result from exposure to maternal hormones in utero and withdrawal at birth. A small tag of hymenal tissue at the posterior fourchette, believed to be due to maternal hormonal stimulation, is sometimes present but disappears over a few weeks. Ambiguous genitals (intersex) may be a consequence of several uncommon conditions (eg, congenital adrenal hyperplasia; 5α-reductase deficiency; Klinefelter's, Turner's, or Swyer syndrome); referral to an endocrinologist is indicated for evaluation and a discussion with the family about the benefits and risks of immediate vs delayed gender assignment.

Orthopedic examination focuses on detection of hip dysplasia. Risk factors for dysplasia include female sex, breech position in utero, twin gestation, and family history. The condition is assessed by using the Barlow or Ortolani maneuver. In the Ortolani maneuver, the neonate is placed on his back with his feet facing the examiner. With an index finger on the greater trochanter and a thumb on the lesser trochanter, the examiner first fully flexes the legs at the knees and hips, then fully abducts the legs while exerting pressure upward and inward until the knees touch the examining table. A palpable clunk of the femoral head with abduction signifies movement of an already dislocated femoral head into the acetabulum and constitutes a positive test for hip dysplasia.

The maneuver may be falsely negative in infants > 3 mo because of tighter hip muscles and ligaments. If the examination is equivocal or the infant is high risk (eg, girls who were in the breech position), hip ultrasonography should be done at 4 to 6 wk; some experts recommend screening ultrasonography at 4 to 6 wk for all infants with risk factors.

The neurologic examination includes an evaluation of the neonate's tone, level of alertness, movement of extremities, and reflexes. Typically, neonatal reflexes, including the Moro, suck, and rooting reflexes, are elicited. The Moro reflex, the neonate's response to startle, is elicited by pulling the arms slightly off the bed and releasing suddenly. In response, the neonate extends the arms with fingers extended, flexes the hips, and cries. The rooting reflex is elicited by stroking the neonate's cheek or lateral lip, which prompts the infant to turn the head toward the touch and open the mouth. The suck reflex can be elicited by using a pacifier or gloved finger. These reflexes are present for several months after birth and are markers of a normal peripheral nervous system.

A neonate's skin is usually ruddy; cyanosis of fingers and toes is common in the 1st few hours. Vernix caseosa covers most neonates > 24 wk gestation. Dryness and peeling often develop within days, especially at wrist and ankle creases. Petechiae may occur in areas experiencing trauma during delivery, such as the face, in a delivery where the face is the presenting part; however, neonates with diffuse petechiae should be evaluated for thrombocytopenia. Many neonates have erythema toxicum, a benign rash with an erythematous base and a white or yellow papule. This rash, which usually appears 24 h after birth, is scattered over the body and can last for up to 2 wk.

Screening: Screening recommendations vary by clinical context and state requirements.

Blood typing is indicated when the mother has type O or Rh-negative blood or when minor blood antigens are present because of the risk of hemolytic disease of the newborn (see p. 2194).

All neonates are evaluated for jaundice throughout the hospital stay and before discharge. The risk of hyperbilirubinemia is assessed using risk criteria, a measurement of bilirubin, or both (see also p. 2275). Bilirubin can be measured using transcutaneous or serum measurements. Many hospitals screen all neonates and use a predictive nomogram to establish the risk of extreme hyperbilirubinemia. Follow-up is based on age at discharge, predischarge bilirubin level, and risk of developing jaundice.

Most states test for specific inherited diseases (see p. 2458), including phenylketonuria, tyrosinemia, biotinidase deficiency, homocystinuria, maple syrup urine disease, galactosemia, congenital adrenal hyperplasia, sickle cell disease, and hypothyroidism. Some states also include testing for cystic fibrosis, disorders of fatty acid oxidation, and other organic acidemias.

HIV screening is required by some states and is otherwise indicated in children of mothers known to be HIV positive or those engaging in HIV high-risk behaviors.

Toxicology screening is indicated when there is a maternal history of drug use, unexplained placental abruption, or unexplained premature labor; the mother has had poor prenatal care; or the infant exhibits evidence of drug withdrawal.

Hearing screening varies by state; some screen only high-risk neonates (see TABLE 266–1), whereas others screen all. Initial screening often involves using a handheld device to test for echoes produced by healthy ears in response to soft clicks (otoacoustic emissions); if this test is abnormal, auditory brainstem response (ABR) testing is done. Some institutions use ABR testing as an initial screening test. Further testing by an audiologist may be needed.

TABLE 266–1. HIGH-RISK FACTORS FOR HEARING DEFICITS IN NEONATES

Birth weight < 1500 g
Apgar score ≤ 7 at 5 min
Serum bilirubin > 22 mg/dL (> 376 μmol/L) in a neonate whose birth weight is > 2000 g, or > 17 mg/dL (> 290 μmol/L) in a neonate < 2000 g
Perinatal anoxia or hypoxia
Neonatal sepsis or meningitis
Craniofacial abnormalities
Seizures or apneic spells
Congenital infections (rubella, syphilis, herpes simplex, cytomegalovirus, or toxoplasmosis)
Maternal exposure to aminoglycoside drugs
History of early hearing loss in a parent or close relative

Routine care and observation: Neonates are bathed once their temperature has stabilized at 37° C for 2 h. The umbilical cord clamp can be removed when the cord appears dry, usually at 24 h. The umbilical stump should be kept clean and dry to prevent infection. Some centers apply isopropyl alcohol several times a day or a single dose of triple dye, a bacteriostatic agent believed to decrease bacterial colonization of the cord. The cord should be observed daily for redness or drainage, because it is an entry portal for infection.

Circumcision can—if desired by the family—be safely performed using local anesthesia within the 1st few days of life. Circumcision should be delayed if there is displacement of the urethral meatus, hypospadias, or any other abnormality of the glans or penis, because the prepuce may be used later in plastic surgical repair; circumcision should not be performed if the neonate has hemophilia or another bleeding disorder, there is a family history of bleeding disorders, or the mother has taken anticoagulants or aspirin.

Most neonates lose 5 to 7% of their birth weight in the 1st few days of life, due primarily to urinary and insensible fluid losses and secondarily to passage of meconium, loss of vernix caseosa, and drying of the umbilical cord. In the 1st 2 days, urine may stain the diaper orange or pink because of urate crystals, which are normal and a result of urine concentration. Most neonates void within 24 h after birth; the average time of 1st void is 7 to 9 h after birth, and most void at least 2 times in the 2nd 24 h of life. A delay in voiding is more common in boys and may result from a tight foreskin; a male neonate's inability to void may indicate posterior urethral valves. Circumcision is usually delayed until at least the first void; failure to void within 12 h of the procedure may indicate a complication. If meconium has not been passed within 24 h, the clinician should consider evaluating the neonate for anatomic abnormalities, such as imperforate anus, Hirschsprung's disease, and cystic fibrosis, which can cause meconium ileus.

Hospital discharge: Neonates discharged within 48 h should be evaluated within 2 to 3 days to assess feeding success (breast or bottle), hydration, and jaundice (for those at increased risk). Follow-up for neonates discharged after 48 h should be based on risk factors, including those for jaundice and for breastfeeding difficulties.

NUTRITION

If the delivery was uncomplicated and the neonate is alert and healthy, the neonate can be brought to the mother for feeding immediately. Successful breastfeeding is enhanced by putting the neonate to the breast as soon as possible after delivery. Spitting mucus after feeding is common due to lax gastroesophageal smooth muscle but should subside within 48 h. If spitting mucus or emesis persists past 48 h, especially if it is bilious, complete evaluation of the upper GI and respiratory tracts is needed to detect congenital GI anomalies (see p. 2426).

Daily fluid and calorie requirements vary with age and are proportionately greater in neonates and infants than in older children and adults (see TABLES 266–2 and 266–3). Relative requirements for protein and energy (g or kcal/kg body weight) decline progressively from the end of infancy through adolescence (see TABLE 1–4 on p. 6), although absolute requirements increase. For example, protein requirements decrease from 1.2 g/kg/day at 1 yr to 0.9 g/kg/day at 18 yr, whereas mean relative energy requirements decrease from 100 kcal/kg at 1 yr to 40 kcal/kg in late adolescence. Nutritional recommendations are generally not evidence-based. Requirements for vitamins depend on the intake of calories, protein, fat, carbohydrate, and amino acids.

Feeding problems: Minor variations in day-to-day food intake are common and, although often of concern to parents, usually require only reassurance and guidance unless there are signs of disease or changes in growth parameters, particularly weight (changes in the child's percentile rank on standard growth curves are more significant than absolute changes).

Loss of > 5 to 7% of birth weight in the 1st wk indicates undernutrition. Birth weight should be regained by 2 wk, and a subsequent gain of about 20 to 30 g/day (1 oz/day) is expected for the 1st few months. Infants should double their birth weight by about 6 mo.

BREASTFEEDING

Breast milk is the nutrition of choice. The American Academy of Pediatrics (AAP) recommends exclusive breastfeeding for a minimum of 6 mo and introduction of appropriate solid food from 6 mo to 1 yr. Beyond 1 yr, breastfeeding continues for as long as both infant and mother desire, although after 1 yr, breastfeeding should complement a full diet of solid foods and fluids. To encourage breastfeeding, practitioners should begin discussions prenatally, mentioning the multiple advantages to the child (nutritional and cognitive; protection against infection, allergies, obesity, Crohn's disease, and diabetes) and mother (reduced fertility during lactation; more rapid return to normal prepartum condition [eg, uterine involution, weight loss]; protection against osteoporosis, obesity, and ovarian and premenopausal breast cancers).

In primiparas, milk production is fully established in 72 to 96 h, and in less time in multiparas. The first milk produced is colostrum, a high-calorie, high-protein, thin yellow fluid that is immunoprotective because it is rich in antibodies, lymphocytes, and macrophages, and also stimulates passage of meconium. Subsequent breast milk has a high lactose content, providing a readily available energy source compatible with neonatal enzymes; contains large amounts of vitamin E, which may help prevent anemia by increasing erythrocyte life span and is an important antioxidant; has a Ca:P ratio of 2:1, which prevents Ca-deficiency tetany; favorably changes the pH of stools and the intestinal flora, thus protecting against bacterial diarrhea; and transfers protective antibodies from mother to infant. Breast milk is also a natural source of ω-3 and ω-6 fatty acids. These substances and their very long-chain polyunsaturated derivatives (LC-PUFAS), arachidonic acid (ARA) and docosahexaenoic acid (DHA), are believed to contribute to the enhanced visual and cognitive outcomes of breastfed as compared with formula-fed infants. Breast milk also contains cholesterol and taurine, which are important to brain growth regardless of the mother's diet.

If the mother's diet is sufficiently diverse, no dietary or vitamin supplementation is needed for the mother or term breastfed infant, with the possible exception of vitamin D 200 units once/day beginning in the 1st 2 mo for all infants exclusively breastfed. Premature and dark-skinned infants and those with limited sunlight exposure (residence in northern climates) are especially at risk.

Infants < 6 mo should not be given additional water because of the risk of hyponatremia.

Technique: The mother should use whatever comfortable, relaxed position works best and should support her breast with her hand to ensure that it is centered in the infant's mouth, minimizing any soreness. The center of the infant's lower lip should be stimulated with the nipple so that rooting will occur and the mouth will open wide. The infant should be encouraged to take in as much of the breast and areola as possible, placing the lips 2.5 to 4 cm from the base of the nipple. The infant's tongue then compresses the nipple against the hard palate. Initially, it takes at least 2 min for the let-down reflex to occur. Volume of milk increases as the infant grows and stimulation from suckling increases. Feeding

TABLE 266–2. RANGE OF AVERAGE WATER REQUIREMENTS OF CHILDREN AT DIFFERENT AGES UNDER ORDINARY CONDITIONS

AGE	AVERAGE BODY Wt (kg)	TOTAL WATER IN 24 h (mL)	WATER/kg BODY Wt IN 24 h (mL)
3 days	3.0	250–300	80–100
10 days	3.2	400–500	125–150
3 mo	5.4	750–850	140–160
6 mo	7.3	950–1100	130–155
9 mo	8.6	1100–1250	125–145
1 yr	9.5	1150–1300	120–135
2 yr	11.8	1350–1500	115–125
4 yr	16.2	1600–1800	100–110
6 yr	20.0	1800–2000	90–100
10 yr	28.7	2000–2500	70–85
14 yr	45.0	2200–2700	50–60
18 yr	54.0	2200–2700	40–50

From Barness LA: Nutrition and nutritional disorders. In *Nelson Textbook of Pediatrics*, ed. 13, edited by RE Behrman, VC Vaughan III, and WE Nelson (Senior Editor). Philadelphia, WB Saunders Company, 1987, p. 115; used with permission.

TABLE 266–3. CALORIE REQUIREMENTS AT DIFFERENT AGES*

AGE	REQUIREMENT	
	kcal/lb/day	kcal/kg/day
< 6 mo	50–55	110–120
1 yr	45	95–100
15 yr	20	44

*When protein and calories are provided by breast milk that is completely digested and absorbed, the requirements between 3 mo and 9 mo of age may be lower.

duration is generally determined by the infant. Some women require a breast pump to increase or maintain milk production; in most women, a total of 90 min/day of breast pumping divided into 6 to 8 sessions produces enough milk for an infant not directly breastfeeding.

The infant should nurse on one breast until the breast softens and suckling slows or stops. The mother can then break suction with a finger before removing the infant from one breast and offering it the second. In the 1st days after birth, infants may only nurse on one side, in which case the mother should alternate sides with each feeding. If the infant tends to fall asleep before adequately nursing, the mother can remove the infant when suckling slows, burp the infant, and move the infant to the other side. This "switch" nursing keeps the infant awake for feedings and stimulates milk production in both breasts.

Mothers should be encouraged to feed on demand or about every 1½ to 3 h (8 to 12 feedings/day), a frequency that gradually diminishes over time; some newborns < 2500 g may need to feed even more frequently to prevent hypoglycemia. In the first few days, newborns may need to be wakened and stimulated. A schedule that allows the newborn to sleep as long as possible at night is usually best for both newborn and family.

Mothers who work outside the home can pump breast milk to maintain milk production while they are separated from their infants. Frequency varies but should approximate the infant's feeding schedule. Pumped breast milk should be immediately refrigerated if it is to be used within 48 h, and immediately frozen if it is to be used after 48 h. Refrigerated milk that is not used within 96 h should be discarded because of high risk of bacterial contamination. Frozen milk should be thawed by placing it in warm water; microwaving is not recommended.

Infant complications: The primary complication is underfeeding, which may lead to dehydration and hyperbilirubinemia. Risk factors for underfeeding include small or premature infants and mothers who are primiparous, who become ill, or who undergo difficult or operative deliveries. A rough assessment of feeding adequacy can be made by daily diaper counts; by 5 days of age, a normal neonate wets at least 6 diapers/day and soils 2 to 3 diapers/day; lower numbers suggest underhydration and undernutrition. Weight is also a reasonable parameter to follow (see p. 2224); failure to attain growth landmarks suggests undernutrition. Constant fussiness before age 6 wk, when colic may develop unrelated to hunger or thirst, may also indicate underfeeding. Dehydration should be suspected with decreases in vigor of the infant's cry and skin turgor; lethargy and sleepiness are extreme signs of dehydration and should prompt testing for hypernatremia.

Maternal complications: Common maternal complications include breast engorgement, sore nipples, plugged ducts, mastitis, and anxiety.

Breast engorgement, which occurs during early lactation and may last 24 to 48 h, may be minimized by early frequent feeding. A comfortable nursing brassiere worn 24 h/day can help, as can applying cool compresses after nursing and taking a mild analgesic (eg, ibuprofen). The mother may have to use massage and warm compresses and express her milk manually just before nursing to allow the infant to get the swollen areola into his mouth. Excessive expression of milk between feedings facilitates engorgement so expression should be done only enough to relieve discomfort.

For sore nipples, the infant's position should be checked; sometimes the infant draws in a lip and sucks it, which irritates the nipple. The mother can ease the lip out with her thumb. After feedings, she can express a little milk, letting the milk dry on the nipples. After nursing, cool compresses reduce engorgement and provide further relief.

Plugged ducts manifest as mildly tender lumps in the breasts of a lactating woman who shows no other systemic signs of illness. The lumps appear in different places and are not tender. Continued nursing ensures adequate emptying of the breast. Warm compresses and massage of the affected area before nursing may further aid emptying. Women may also alternate nursing positions, because different areas of the breast empty better depending on the infant's position at the breast. A good nursing brassiere is helpful, as regular brassieres with wire stays or constricting straps may contribute to milk stasis in a compressed area.

Mastitis is common and manifests as a tender, warm, swollen, wedge-shaped area of breast. It is caused by engorgement, blocking, or plugging of an area of the breast; infection may occur secondarily, most often with penicillin-resistant *Staphylococcus aureus* and less commonly with *Streptococcus* sp or *Escherichia coli.* With infection, fever ≥38.5° C, chills, and flu-like aching may develop. Diagnosis is by history and examination. Cell counts (WBCs > 10^6/mL) and cultures of breast milk (bacteria > 10^3/mL) may distinguish infectious from noninfectious mastitis. If symptoms are mild and present < 24 h, conservative management (milk removal via nursing or pumping, compresses, analgesics, supportive brassiere, and stress reduction) may be sufficient. If symptoms are not improving in 12 to 24 h or if the woman is acutely ill, antibiotics that are safe for nursing infants and effective against *S. aureus* (eg, dicloxacillin, cloxacillin, or cephalexin 500 mg po qid) should be started; duration of treatment is 10 to 14 days. Complications of delayed treatment are recurrence and abscess formation. Nursing may continue during treatment.

Maternal anxiety, frustration, and feelings of inadequacy may result from lack of experience with breastfeeding, mechanical difficulties holding the infant and getting the infant to latch on and suck, fatigue, difficulty assessing if nourishment is adequate, and postpartum physiologic changes. These factors and emotions are the most common reasons women choose to stop breastfeeding. Early follow-up with a pediatrician or consultation with a lactation specialist is helpful and effective for preventing early breastfeeding termination.

Drugs: Breastfeeding mothers should avoid taking drugs if possible. When drug therapy is necessary, the mother should avoid contraindicated drugs (see TABLE 266–4) and drugs that suppress lactation (eg, bromocriptine, levodopa, trazadone) and take the safest known alternative immediately after nursing or before the infant's longest sleep period; this strategy is less helpful with neonates who nurse frequently and exclusively. Knowledge of the adverse effects of most drugs comes from case reports and small studies. Safety of some (eg, acetaminophen, ibuprofen, cephalosporins, insulin) has been determined by extensive research, but others are considered safe only on the basis of the absence of case reports of adverse effects. Drugs with a long history of use are generally safer than newer drugs for which few data exist.

Weaning: Weaning can occur whenever the mother and infant mutually desire after 12 mo. Gradual weaning over weeks or months during the time solid food is introduced is most common; although some mothers and infants stop abruptly without problems, others continue nursing 1 or 2 times/day for 18 to 24 mo or longer. There is no correct schedule.

FORMULA FEEDING

The only acceptable alternative to breastfeeding in the 1st yr is formula; water can cause hyponatremia, and whole cow's milk is not nutritionally complete. Advantages of formula feeding include the ability to quantify the amount of nourishment and the ability of family members to participate in feedings. But all other factors being equal, these advantages are outweighed by the undisputed health benefits of breastfeeding.

Commercial infant formulas are available as powders, concentrated liquids, and prediluted (ready-to-feed) liquids; each contains vitamins, and most are supplemented with iron. Formula should be prepared with fluoridated water; fluoride drops (0.25 mg/day po) should be given after age 6 mo in areas where fluoridated water is unavailable and when using prediluted liquid formula, which is prepared with nonfluoridated water.

Choice of formula is based on infant need. Cow's milk–based formula is the standard choice unless fussiness, spitting up, or gas suggests sensitivity to cow's milk protein or lactose intolerance (rare in neonates), in which case a soy formula may be recommended. All soy formulas in the US are lactose free, but some infants allergic to cow's milk protein may also be allergic to soy protein, in which case a hydrolyzed (elemental) formula that may be derived from cow's milk, but which has triglycerides, proteins, and monosaccharides predigested to smaller, nonallergenic components, is indicated. Special carbohydrate-free formulas are also available. These formulas vary in vitamin content and preparation.

Bottle-fed infants are fed on demand, but because formula is digested slower than breast milk, they typically can go longer periods between feedings, initially every 3 to 4 h. Initial volumes of 15 to 60 mL (0.5 to 2 oz) can be increased gradually during the 1st wk of life up to 90 mL (3 oz) about 6 times/day, which supplies about 120 kcal/kg at 1 wk for a 3-kg infant.

SOLID FOODS

The WHO recommends exclusive breastfeeding for about 6 mo, with introduction of solid foods thereafter. Other organizations suggest introducing solid food between age

TABLE 266–4. DRUGS CONTRAINDICATED FOR BREASTFEEDING MOTHERS

DRUG CLASS	EXAMPLES	GENERAL CONCERN AND SPECIFIC EFFECTS
Anticoagulants	Dicumarol Warfarin	May be given cautiously, but very large doses may cause hemorrhage. (Heparin is not excreted in milk.)
Cytotoxics	Cyclophosphamide Cyclosporine Doxorubicin Methotrexate	Drugs may interfere with cellular metabolism of the nursing infant, causing possible immune suppression and neutropenia (cyclophosphamide and methotrexate); unknown effect on growth, unknown association with carcinogenesis
Psychoactive drugs	Anxiolytics (benzodiazepines [alprazolam diazepam, lorazepam, midazolam, prazepam, quazepam, temazepam], perphenazine) Antidepressants (tricyclic agents, SSRIs, bupropion) Antipsychotics (chlorpromazine, chlorprothixene, clozapine, haloperidol, mesoridazine, trifluoperazine)	Effect of most psychoactive drugs on infants is unknown, but drugs and metabolites appear in breast milk and in infant plasma and tissues and could conceivably alter short-term and long-term CNS function Fluoxetine is linked to colic, irritability, feeding and sleep disorders, slow weight gain Chlorpromazine may cause drowsiness and lethargy in infant and decline in developmental scores Haloperidol: Decline in developmental scores
Individual drugs detectable in breast milk that pose theoretical risk	Amiodarone	Possible hypothyroidism
	Chloramphenicol	Possible idiosyncratic bone marrow suppression
	Clofazimine	Potential for transfer of high percentage of maternal dose; possible increase in skin pigmentation
	Corticosteroids	When given to mother in large doses for weeks or months can achieve high concentrations in milk and risk suppressing growth and interfering with endogenous corticosteroid production in the infant
	Lamotrigine	Potential therapeutic serum concentrations in infant
	Metoclopramide	None described
	Metronidazole, tinidazole	In vitro mutagen; may discontinue breastfeeding for 12–24 h to allow excretion of dose when 2 g single-dose therapy given to mother; safe after 6 mo
	Sulfapyridine, sulfisoxazole	Caution in infant with jaundice or G6PD deficiency and ill, stressed, or premature infant

TABLE 266–4. DRUGS CONTRAINDICATED FOR BREASTFEEDING MOTHERS—Continued

DRUG CLASS	EXAMPLES	GENERAL CONCERN AND SPECIFIC EFFECTS
Individual drugs detectable in breast milk that have documented risk	Acebutolol	Hypotension, bradycardia, tachypnea
	Aminosalicylic acid	Diarrhea
	Atenolol	Cyanosis, bradycardia
	Bromocriptine	Suppresses lactation; may be hazardous to the mother
	Aspirin (salicylates)	Metabolic acidosis; with large maternal doses and sustained use, breastfed infants < 1 mo may achieve plasma concentrations that increase the risk of hyperbilirubinemia (salicylates compete for albumin-binding sites) and hemolysis in G6PD-deficient infants only
	Clemastine	Drowsiness, irritability, refusal to feed, high-pitched cry, neck stiffness
	Ergotamine	Vomiting, diarrhea, seizures (doses used in migraine medications)
	Estradiol	Withdrawal vaginal bleeding
	Iodides, iodine	Goiter
	Lithium	$\frac{1}{3}$ to $\frac{1}{2}$ therapeutic blood concentration in infants
	Phenobarbital	Sedation; infantile spasms after weaning, methemoglobinemia
	Phenytoin	Methemoglobinemia
	Primidone	Sedation, feeding problems
	Sulfasalazine (salicylazosulfapyridine)	Bloody diarrhea
	Nitrofurantoin, sulfapyridine, sulfisoxazole	Hemolysis in infants with G6PD deficiency; safe in others
Drugs of abuse*	Amphetamine	Irritability, poor sleeping pattern
	Alcohol	> 1 g/kg daily decreases milk ejection reflex; consumption of large amounts causes infant drowsiness, diaphoresis, deep sleep, weakness, decrease in linear growth, abnormal weight gain
	Cocaine	Cocaine intoxication: irritability, vomiting, diarrhea, tremulousness, seizures
	Heroin	Tremors, restlessness, vomiting, poor feeding
	Marijuana	Components can be measured in breast milk but effects uncertain
	Phencyclidine	Hallucinogen

*Effects of smoking are unclear; nicotine is detectable in breast milk, and smoking decreases breast milk production and infant weight gain, but also may decrease incidence of respiratory illness.

Data from Committee on Drugs of the American Pediatric Association: The transfer of drugs and other chemicals into human milk. *Pediatrics* 108(3):776–789, 2001.

4 mo and 6 mo while continuing breastfeeding or bottle-feeding. Before 4 mo, solid food is not needed nutritionally, and the extrusion reflex, in which the tongue pushes out anything placed in the mouth, makes feeding of solids difficult.

Initially, solid foods should be introduced after breastfeeding or bottle-feeding to ensure adequate nourishment. Iron-fortified rice cereal is traditionally the 1st food introduced because it is nonallergenic, easily digested, and a needed source of iron. It is generally recommended that one new, "single-ingredient" food be introduced per week so that food allergies can be identified. Foods need not be introduced in any specific order, though in general they can gradually be introduced by increasingly coarser textures, eg, from rice cereal to soft table food to chopped table food. Meat, pureed to prevent aspiration, is a good source of iron and zinc, both of which can be limited in the diet of an exclusively breastfed infant, and is therefore a good early complementary food. But vegetarian infants can get adequate iron from iron-fortified cereals and grains, peas, and dried beans, and adequate zinc from yeast-fermented whole-grain breads and fortified infant cereals.

Home preparations are equivalent to commercial foods, but commercial preparations of carrots, beets, turnips, collard greens, and spinach are preferable before 1 yr if available, because they are screened for high concentrations of nitrates, which are present when the vegetables are grown using water supplies contaminated by fertilizer and which can induce methemoglobinemia in young children. Eggs, peanuts, and cow's milk are generally avoided until the child is 1 yr to prevent food sensitivities. Honey should be withheld until 1 yr because of the risk of infant botulism. Foods that could obstruct the child's airway if aspirated should be avoided (eg, nuts, round candies), pureed (eg, meat), or cut into small pieces (eg, grapes). Nuts should be avoided until age 2 or 3 because they do not fully dissolve with mastication and small pieces can be aspirated with or without bronchial obstruction, causing pneumonia and other complications.

At or after 1 yr, the child can begin drinking whole cow's milk; reduced-fat milk is avoided until 2 yr, when the child's diet will essentially resemble that of the rest of the family. Parents should be advised to limit milk intake to 16 to 20 oz/day in young children; higher intake can reduce intake of other important sources of nutrition and contribute to iron deficiency.

Juice is a poor source of nutrition, contributes to dental caries, and should be limited to 4 to 6 oz/day or avoided altogether.

By about 1 yr, growth rate usually slows. Children require less food and may refuse it at some meals. Parents should be reassured and advised to assess a child's intake over a week rather than at a single meal or during a day. Underfeeding of solid food is only a concern when a child fails to achieve expected weights at an appropriate rate.

HEALTH SUPERVISION OF THE WELL CHILD

Well-child visits aim to prevent disease through routine vaccinations and education, detect and treat disease early, and guide parents to optimize the child's emotional and intellectual development. The American Academy of Pediatrics (AAP) has recommended preventive health care schedules (see FIG. 266–2) for children who have no significant health problems and who are growing and developing satisfactorily. Those who do not meet these criteria should have more frequent and intensive visits. If a child comes under care for the 1st time late on the schedule or if any items are not accomplished at the suggested age, the child should be brought up to date as soon as possible.

In addition to physical evaluation, providers should evaluate the child's intellectual and social development and parent-child interactions. These assessments can be made by taking a thorough history from parents and child, making direct observations, and sometimes seeking information from outside sources such as teachers and child care providers. Tools are available for office use to facilitate evaluation of intellectual and social development (see p. 2249).

Both physical examination and screening procedures are important parts of preventive health care in infants and children. Most parameters, such as weight, are included for all children, whereas others are applicable to selected patients, such as lead screening in 1- and 2-yr-olds.

PHYSICAL EXAMINATION

Growth: Length (crown-heel) or height (once the child can stand) and weight should be measured at each visit. Head circumference should be measured at each visit through 24 mo. The child's growth rate should be monitored using a growth curve with percentiles; evaluation of deviations in these parameters is discussed in Ch. 269 on p. 2248.

Blood pressure: Starting at age 3 yr, BP should be routinely checked by using an appropriate-sized cuff. The width of the inflatable rubber bag portion of the BP cuff should be about 40% of the circumference of the upper arm, and its length should cover 80 to 100% of the circumference. If no available cuff fits the criteria, it is better to use the larger cuff.

A child's systolic and diastolic BPs are considered normal if they are < 90th percentile; actual values for each percentile vary by gender, age, and size (as height percentile), so reference to published tables is essential. Systolic and diastolic BP measurements between the 90th and 95th percentiles should prompt continued observation and assessment of hypertensive risk factors. If measurements are consistently ≥ 95th percentile, the child should be considered hypertensive, and a cause should be determined.

Head: The most common abnormality is fluid in the middle ear (otitis media with effusion), manifesting as a change in the appearance of the tympanic membrane. Screening for hearing deficits is discussed below.

Eyes should be assessed at each visit for alignment (esotropia or exotropia); abnormalities in globe size suggesting congenital glaucoma; difference in pupil size, iris color, or both, suggesting Horner's syndrome, trauma, or neuroblastoma; and asymmetric pupils, which may be normal or represent an ocular, autonomic, or intracranial disorder. Absence or distortion of the red reflex suggests cataract or retinoblastoma.

Ptosis and eyelid hemangioma obscure vision and require attention. Infants born at < 32 wk gestation should be assessed by an ophthalmologist for evidence of retinopathy of prematurity (see p. 2268) and for refractive errors, which are more common. By 3 or 4 yr, vision testing by Snellen charts or newer testing machines can be performed. E charts are better than pictures; visual acuity of < 20/30 should be evaluated by an ophthalmologist.

Detection of dental caries is important, and referral to a dentist should be made if cavities are present, even in a child who has only deciduous teeth. Thrush is common in infants and not usually a sign of immunosuppression.

Heart: Auscultation is performed to identify new murmurs or rhythm disturbances; benign flow murmurs are common and need to be distinguished from pathologic murmurs. Palpation of the chest wall for the apical impulse may suggest cardiomegaly; palpation of asymmetric femoral pulses suggests aortic coarctation.

Abdomen: Palpation is repeated at every visit, because many masses, particularly Wilms' tumor and neuroblastoma, may be apparent only as the child grows. Stool often is palpable in the left lower quadrant.

Spine and extremities: Children old enough to stand should be screened for scoliosis with observations of posture, shoulder tip and scapular symmetry, torso list, and especially paraspinal asymmetry on forward bending (see p. 2381). Unequal leg length, adductor tightness, asymmetry of abduction or leg creases, or palpable, audible clunking of the femoral head as it slides into the hip socket are signs of developmental dysplasia of the hip. Toeing-in can result from adduction of the forefoot, tibial torsion, or femoral torsion. Only pronounced cases require therapy, and those children should be referred to an orthopedist.

Genital examination: All sexually active patients should be screened for sexually transmitted diseases; in girls, a pelvic examination is needed. Young women between the ages of 18 yr and 21 yr should be offered a pelvic examination and routine Papanicolaou test. Testicular and inguinal evaluation should be performed at every visit, specifically looking for undescended testes in infancy and early childhood, testicular masses in later adolescent years, and inguinal hernia at all ages.

SCREENING

Blood tests: To detect iron deficiency, Hct or Hb should be determined at age 9 to 12 mo for term infants, at age 5 to 6 mo for premature infants, and annually in menstruating adolescents. Testing for Hb S can be performed at age 6 to 9 mo (see p. 1055) if not performed as part of neonatal screening.

Recommendations for blood testing for lead exposure vary by state. In general, testing should be done between ages 9 mo and 1 yr in children at risk of exposure (those living in housing built before 1980) and be repeated at 24 mo. If the clinician is not sure of the child's risk, testing should be done. Levels > 10 μg/dL (> 0.48 μmol/L) pose a risk of neurologic damage (see p. 2668), although

AGE[5]	PRENATAL[1]	NEWBORN[2]	2–4 days[3]	By 1 mo	2 mo	4 mo	6 mo	9 mo	12 mo	15 mo	18 mo	24 mo	3 yr	4 yr	5 yr	6 yr	8 yr	10 yr	11 yr	12 yr	13 yr	14 yr	15 yr	16 yr	17 yr	18 yr	19 yr	20 yr	21 yr
	INFANCY[4]									**EARLY CHILDHOOD[4]**					**MIDDLE CHILDHOOD[4]**				**ADOLESCENCE[4]**										
HISTORY																													
Initial/Interval	•	•	•	•	•	•	•	•	•	•	•	•	•	•	•	•	•	•	•	•	•	•	•	•	•	•	•	•	•
MEASUREMENTS																													
Height and Weight		•	•	•	•	•	•	•	•	•	•	•	•	•	•	•	•	•	•	•	•	•	•	•	•	•	•	•	•
Head Circumference		•	•	•	•	•	•	•	•	•	•	•																	
Blood Pressure													•	•	•	•	•	•	•	•	•	•	•	•	•	•	•	•	•
SENSORY SCREENING																													
Vision		S	S	S	S	S	S	S	S	S	S	S	O[6]	O	O	O	O	O	S	O	S	S	O	S	S	O	S	S	S
Hearing		O[7]	S	S	S	S	S	S	S	S	S	S	S	O	O	O	O	O	S	O	S	S	O	S	S	O	S	S	S
DEVELOPMENTAL/ BEHAVIORAL ASSESSMENT[8]		•	•	•	•	•	•	•	•	•	•	•	•	•	•	•	•	•	•	•	•	•	•	•	•	•	•	•	•
PHYSICAL EXAMINATION[9]		•	•	•	•	•	•	•	•	•	•	•	•	•	•	•	•	•	•	•	•	•	•	•	•	•	•	•	•
PROCEDURES–GENERAL[10]																													
Hereditary/Metabolic Screening[11]		←	•	→																									
Immunization[12]		•	•	•	•	•	•	•	•	•	•	•	•	•	•	•	•	•	•	•	•	•	•	•	•	•	•	•	•
Hematocrit or Hemoglobin[13]								• →	→	* →	→	→	→	→	→				←	←	• 14	→	→	→	→	→	→	→	→
Urinalysis															•				←	←	←	←	←	• 15	→	→	→	→	→
PROCEDURES–PATIENTS AT RISK																													
Lead Screening[16]								* →	→			*																	
Tuberculin Test[17]									*	*	*	*	*	*	*	*	*	*	*	*	*	*	*	*	*	*	*	*	*
Cholesterol Screening[18]												*	*	*	*	*	*	*	*	*	*	*	*	*	*	*	*	*	*
STD Screening[19]																			*	*	*	*	*	*	*	*	*	*	*
Pelvic Exam[20]																			*	*	*	*	*	*	*	← *	* 20	*	* →
ANTICIPATORY GUIDANCE[21]	•	•	•	•	•	•	•	•	•	•	•	•	•	•	•	•	•	•	•	•	•	•	•	•	•	•	•	•	•
Injury Prevention[22]	•	•	•	•	•	•	•	•	•	•	•	•	•	•	•	•	•	•	•	•	•	•	•	•	•	•	•	•	•
Violence Prevention[23]	•	•	•	•	•	•	•	•	•	•	•	•	•	•	•	•	•	•	•	•	•	•	•	•	•	•	•	•	•
Sleep Positioning Counseling[24]	•	•	•	•	•	•	•																						
Nutrition Counseling[25]	•	•	•	•	•	•	•	•	•	•	•	•	•	•	•	•	•	•	•	•	•	•	•	•	•	•	•	•	•
DENTAL REFERRAL[26]									←	←	←	←	•																

Key: • = to be performed; * = to be performed for patients at risk; ←•→ = the range during which a service may be provided, with the dot indicating the preferred age

S = subjective, by history; O = objective, by a standard testing method

1. A prenatal visit is recommended for parents who are at high risk, for first-time parents, and for those who request a conference. The prenatal visit should include anticipatory guidance, pertinent medical history, and a discussion of benefits of breastfeeding and planned method of feeding per AAP statement "The Prenatal Visit" (1996).
2. Every infant should have a newborn evaluation after birth. Breastfeeding should be encouraged and instruction and support offered. Every breastfeeding infant should have an evaluation 48–72 h after discharge from the hospital to include weight, formal breastfeeding evaluation, encouragement, and instruction as recommended in the AAP statement "Breastfeeding and the Use of Human Milk" (1997).
3. For newborns discharged in less than 48 h after delivery per AAP statement "Hospital Stay for Healthy Term Newborns" (1995).
4. Developmental, psychosocial, and chronic disease issues for children and adolescents may require frequent counseling and treatment visits separate from preventive care visits.
5. If a child comes under care for the first time at any point on the schedule, or if any items are not accomplished at the suggested age, the schedule should be brought up to date at the earliest possible time.
6. If the patient is uncooperative, rescreen within 6 mo.
7. All newborns should be screened per the AAP Task Force on Newborn and Infant Hearing statement, "Newborn and Infant Hearing Loss: Detection and Intervention" (1999).
8. By history and appropriate physical examination: if suspicious, by specific objective developmental testing. Parenting skills should be fostered at every visit.
9. At each visit, a complete physical examination is essential, with infant totally unclothed, older child undressed and suitably draped.
10. These may be modified, depending upon entry point into schedule and individual need.
11. Metabolic screening (eg, thyroid, hemoglobinopathies, phenylketonuria [PKU], galactosemia) should be done according to state law.
12. Schedule(s) per the Committee on Infectious Diseases, published annually in the January edition of *Pediatrics*. Every visit should be an opportunity to update and complete a child's immunizations.
13. See AAP *Pediatric Nutrition Handbook* (1998) for a discussion of universal and selective screening options. Consider earlier screening for high-risk infants (eg, premature infants and low-birth-weight infants). See also "Recommendations to Prevent and Control Iron Deficiency in the United States," *MMWR*. 1998;47 (RR-3):1–29.

NB: Special chemical, immunologic, and endocrine testing is usually carried out upon specific indications. Testing other than newborn (eg, inborn errors of metabolism, sickle cell disease, etc.) is discretionary with the physician.

14. All menstruating adolescents should be screened annually.
15. Conduct dipstick urinalysis for leukocytes annually for sexually active male and female adolescents.
16. For children at risk of lead exposure, consult the AAP statement "Screening for Elevated Blood Levels" (1998). Additionally, screening should be done in accordance with state law where applicable.
17. TB testing per recommendations of the Committee on infectious Diseases, published in the current edition of *Red Book: Report of the Committee on Infectious Diseases*. Testing should be done upon recognition of high-risk factors.
18. Cholesterol screening for high-risk patients per AAP statement "Cholesterol in Childhood" (1998). If family history cannot be ascertained and other risk factors are present, screening should be at the discretion of the physician.
19. All sexually active patients should be screened for sexually transmitted diseases (STDs).
20. All sexually active females should have a pelvic examination. A pelvic examination and a routine Pap test should be offered as part of preventive health maintenance between the ages of 18 and 21 yr.
21. Age-appropriate discussion and counseling should be an integral part of each visit for care per the AAP *Guidelines for Health Supervision III* (1998).
22. From birth to age 12, refer to the AAP injury prevention program (TIPP®*) as described in *A Guide to Safety Counseling in Office Practice* (1994).
23. Violence prevention and management for all patients per AAP Statement "The Role of the Pediatrician in Youth Violence Prevention in Clinical Practice and at the Community Level" (1999).
24. Parents and caregivers should be advised to place healthy infants on their backs when putting them to sleep. Side positioning is a reasonable alternative but carries a slightly higher risk of SIDS. Consult the AAP statement "Positioning and Sudden Infant Death Syndrome (SIDS): Update" (1996).
25. Age-appropriate nutrition counseling should be an integral part of each visit per the AAP *Handbook of Nutrition* (1998).
26. Earlier initial dental examinations may be appropriate for some children. Subsequent examinations as prescribed by dentist.

The recommendations in this statement do not indicate an exclusive course of treatment or standard of medical care. Variations, taking into account individual circumstances, may be appropriate.

Fig. 266–2. Recommendations for preventive pediatric health care. Each child and family are unique; therefore, these recommendations are designed for the care of children who are receiving competent parenting, have no manifestations of any important health problems, and are growing and developing in satisfactory fashion. *Additional visits may become necessary* if circumstances suggest variations from normal.

These guidelines represent a consensus by the Committee on Practice and Ambulatory Medicine in consultation with national committees and sections of the American Academy of Pediatrics. The Committee emphasizes the great importance of *continuity of care* in comprehensive health supervision and the need to avoid *fragmentation of care*. (Reproduced with permission from *Pediatrics* 105(3):645–646, 2000. Copyright © 2000 by the American Academy of Pediatrics (AAP). See the AAP web site at www.aap.org/visit/prevent.htm for latest updates to recommended schedule.)

some experts question this threshold, believing that any lead in the system can be toxic.

Cholesterol screening is indicated for children > 2 yr who are at high risk because of family history. If other risk factors are present or family history is uncertain, testing is at the discretion of the physician.

Hearing (see also Ch. 85 on p. 781)**:** Parents may suspect a hearing deficit if their child ceases responding appropriately to noises or voices or does not understand or develop speech (see TABLE 266–5). Because hearing deficits impair language development, hearing problems must be remedied as early as possible. The clinician therefore should seek parental input about hearing at every visit during early childhood and be prepared to do formal testing or refer to an audiologist whenever there is any question of the child's ability to hear.

Audiometry can be performed in the primary care setting; most other audiologic procedures (electrophysiologic tests, eg, otoacoustic emission testing and brain stem auditory evoked response) should be done by an audiologist. Conventional audiometry can be used for children beginning at about age 3; young children also can be tested by observing their responses to sounds made through headphones, watching their attempts to localize the sound or complete a simple task. Tympanometry, another in-office procedure (see p. 787), can be used with a child of any age and is useful for determining middle ear function. Abnormal tympanograms often denote eustachian tube dysfunction or the presence of middle ear fluid that cannot be appreciated on otoscopic examination. Although pneumatic otoscopy is helpful in evaluating middle ear status, combining it with tympanometry is more informative than either procedure alone.

Other screening tests: Tuberculin testing should be performed when TB exposure is suspected, on all children born in developing countries, and on children of new immigrants from those countries. Sexually active adolescents should have dipstick analysis for leukocytes annually; some clinicians add urinary testing for *Chlamydia* infection.

TABLE 266–5. NORMAL HEARING IN THE VERY YOUNG CHILD*

AGE	EXPECTED RESPONSE
3 mo	Startles to a nearby loud sound, stirs or awakens from sleep when someone talks or makes a sound, is soothed by mother's voice
6 mo	Looks toward an interesting sound, turns when name is called, makes "moo," "ma," "da," "di" sounds to toys, and "coos" when listening to music
10 mo	Makes own sounds, imitates some sounds, understands "no" and "bye-bye"
18 mo	Understands many single words or commands, babbles in sentence-like patterns

*Children who do not pass these minimal performance standards or whose parents suspect there is a hearing loss at any age should be referred for testing.

VACCINATION

Vaccination follows a schedule recommended by the Centers for Disease Control and Prevention, the AAP, and the American Academy of Family Physicians (see FIG. 266–3). The latest recommendations can be obtained at www.cdc.gov/nip; vaccination status should be reassessed at every visit. Adolescents should receive tetanus boosters on schedule and are now recommended to receive meningococcal vaccine at age 11 to 12.

PREVENTION

Preventive counseling is part of every well-child visit and covers a broad spectrum of topics, from urging parents to have infants sleep on their backs to injury prevention, from nutritional advice to discussions of violence, firearms, and substance abuse.

Safety: Recommendations for injury prevention vary by age.

For infants from birth to 6 mo, safety recommendations focus on use of a rear-facing car seat, reduction of home water temperature < 49° C (< 120° F), prevention of falls, placing the infant to sleep on the back, and avoidance of foods and objects that the child can aspirate.

For infants from 6 to 12 mo, recommendations include continued car seat use (infants can face forward when the child reaches 9 kg [20 lb] and 1 yr of age, but rear-facing is still the safest position), avoidance of baby walkers, use of safety latches on cabinets, prevention of falls from changing tables and around stairs, and vigilant supervision of the child in bathtubs and while learning to walk.

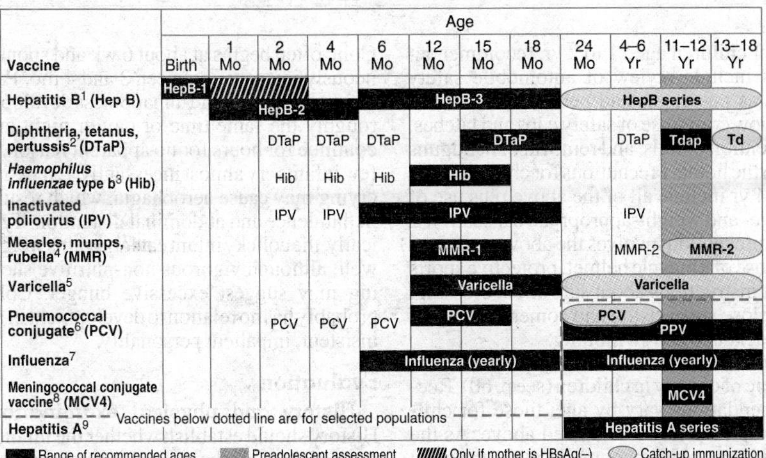

Age
Vaccine
Birth
1 Mo
2 Mo
4 Mo
6 Mo
12 Mo
15 Mo
18 Mo
24 Mo
4–6 Yr
11–12 Yr
13–18 Yr
Hepatitis B[1] (Hep B)
HepB-1
HepB-2
HepB-3
HepB series
Diphtheria, tetanus, pertussis[2] (DTaP)
DTaP
DTaP
DTaP
DTaP
DTaP
Tdap
Td
Haemophilus influenzae type b[3] (Hib)
Hib
Hib
Hib
Hib
Inactivated poliovirus (IPV)
IPV
IPV
IPV
IPV
Measles, mumps, rubella[4] (MMR)
MMR-1
MMR-2
MMR-2
Varicella[5]
Varicella
Varicella
Pneumococcal conjugate[6] (PCV)
PCV
PCV
PCV
PCV
PCV
PPV
Influenza[7]
Influenza (yearly)
Influenza (yearly)
Meningococcal conjugate vaccine[8] (MCV4)
MCV4
Vaccines below dotted line are for selected populations
Hepatitis A[9]
Hepatitis A series
Range of recommended ages
Preadolescent assessment
Only if mother is HBsAg(−)
Catch-up immunization

Tdap = tetanus, diphtheria, and petussis vaccine for adolescents; Td = tetanus-diphtheria toxoids; PPV = pneumococcal polysaccharide vaccine.

This schedule indicates the recommended ages for routine administration of currently licensed childhood vaccines, as of December 1, 2004, for children through age 18 yr. Any dose not administered at the recommended age should be administered at any subsequent visit when indicated and feasible.

(oval) Indicates age groups that warrant special effort to administer vaccines not previously administered. Additional vaccines may be licensed and recommended during the year. Licensed combination vaccines may be used whenever any components of the combination are indicated and other components of the vaccine are not contraindicated. Providers should consult the manufacturers' package inserts for detailed recommendations. Clinically significant adverse events that follow immunization should be reported to the Vaccine Adverse Event Reporting System (VAERS).

1. All infants should receive the 1st dose of HepB vaccine soon after birth and before hospital discharge; the 1st dose may also be administered by age 2 mo if the mother is hepatitis B surface antigen (HBsAg) negative. Only monovalent HepB may be used for the birth dose. Monovalent or combination vaccine containing HepB may be used to complete the series. Four doses of vaccine may be administered when a birth dose is given. The 2nd dose should be administered at least 4 wk after the 1st dose, except for combination vaccines, which cannot be administered before age 6 wk. The 3rd dose should be given at least 16 wk after the 1st dose and at least 8 wk after the 2nd dose. The last dose in the vaccination series (3rd or 4th dose) should not be administered before age 24 wk. **Infants born to HBsAg-positive mothers** should receive HepB and 0.5 mL of hepatitis B immune globulin (HBIG) at separate sites within 12 h of birth. The 2nd dose is recommended at age 1–2 mo. The final dose in the immunization series should not be administered before age 24 wk. These infants should be tested for HBsAg and antibody to HBsAg (anti-HBs) at age 9–15 mo. **Infants born to mothers whose HBsAg status is unknown** should receive the 1st dose of the HepB series within 12 h of birth. Maternal blood should be drawn as soon as possible to determine the mother's HBsAg status; if the HBsAg test is positive, the infant should receive HBIG as soon as possible (no later than age 1 wk). The 2nd dose is recommended at age 1–2 mo. The last dose in the immunization series should not be administered before age 24 wk.
2. The 4th dose of DTaP may be administered as early as age 12 mo provided 6 mo have elapsed since the 3rd dose and the child is unlikely to return at age 15–18 mo. Another dose should be given at age ≥ 4 yr. **Tetanus, diphtheria, and pertussis vaccine for adolescents (Tdap)** is recommended at age 11–12 yr if at least 5 yr have elapsed since the last dose of tetanus and diphtheria toxoid–containing vaccine. Subsequent routine Td boosters are recommended every 10 yr.
3. Three Hib conjugate vaccines are licensed for infant use. If PRP-OMP (PedvaxHIB® or ComVax® [Merck]) is administered at ages 2 and 4 mo, a dose at age 6 mo is not required. DTaP/Hib combination products should not be used for primary immunization in infants at ages 2, 4, or 6 mo but can be used as boosters after any Hib vaccine. The final dose in the series should be administered at age ≥ 12 mo.
4. The 2nd dose is recommended routinely at age 4–6 yr but may be administered during any visit, provided at least 4 wk have elapsed since the 1st dose and both doses are administered beginning at or after age 12 mo. Children who have not previously received the 2nd dose should complete the schedule by age 11–12 yr.
5. Varicella vaccine is recommended at any visit at or after age 12 mo for susceptible children (ie, those who lack a reliable history of chickenpox). Susceptible people aged ≥ 13 yr should receive 2 doses administered at least 4 wk apart.
6. The heptavalent **pneumococcal conjugate vaccine (PCV)** is recommended for all children aged 2–23 mo and for certain children aged 24–59 mo. The final dose in the series should be given at age ≥ 12 mo. **Pneumococcal polysaccharide vaccine (PPV)** is recommended in addition to PCV for certain high-risk groups. See *MMWR* 2000;49(RR-9):1–35.
7. Influenza vaccine is recommended annually for children aged ≥ 6 mo with certain risk factors (including but not limited to asthma, cardiac disease, sickle cell disease, HIV, and diabetes). In addition, healthy children aged 6–23 mo and close contacts of healthy children aged 0–23 mo are recommended to receive influenza vaccine because children in this age group are at substantially increased risk of influenza-related hospitalizations. Children receiving trivalent inactivated influenza vaccine (TIV) should be administered a dosage appropriate for their age (0.25 mL if aged 6–35 mo or 0.5 mL if aged ≥ 3 yr). Children aged ≤ 8 yr who are receiving influenza vaccine for the 1st time should receive 2 doses (separated by at least 4 wk for TIV and at least 6 wk for live attenuated influenza vaccine [LAIV]).
8. A tetravalent **meningococcal polysaccharide-protein conjugate vaccine (MCV4)** is recommended routinely at age 11–12 yr.
9. Hepatitis A vaccine is recommended for children and adolescents in selected states and regions and for certain high-risk groups; consult the local public health authority. Children and adolescents in these states, regions, and high-risk groups who have not been immunized against hepatitis A can begin the hepatitis A immunization series during any visit. The 2 doses in the series should be administered at least 6 mo apart. See *MMWR* 1999;48(RR12):1-37.

Fig. 266–3. Recommended childhood and adolescence immunization schedule. See www.cdc.gov/nip for latest updates to recommended schedule. (Adapted from the National Immunization Program, Centers for Disease Control and Prevention: 2005 Childhood and Adolescence Immunization Schedule.)

For children aged 1 to 2 yr, recommendations include review of automobile safety both as passenger and pedestrian, tying of window cords, use of safety caps and latches, prevention of falls, and removal of handguns from the home. Precautions for children aged 2 to 4 yr include all of the above plus use of an age- and weight-appropriate car seat. At ≥ 5 yr, prevention involves the above measures plus use of a bicycle helmet, protective sports gear, instructions about safe street crossing, and close supervision and sometimes use of life jackets when swimming.

Nutrition: Poor nutrition underlies the epidemic of obesity in children (see p. 60). Recommendations vary by age; those for children up to 2 yr are discussed above. As the child grows older, parents can allow the child some discretion in food choices, while keeping the diet within healthy parameters. The child should be guided away from frequent snacking and foods that are high in calories, salt, and sugar. Soda has been implicated as a major contributor to obesity.

Exercise: Physical inactivity also underlies the epidemic of obesity in children, and the benefits of exercise in maintaining good physical and emotional health should induce parents to make sure their children develop good habits early in life. In infancy and early childhood, children should be allowed to roam and explore in a safe environment under close supervision. Outdoor play should be encouraged from infancy.

As the child grows older, play becomes more complex, often evolving to formal school-based athletics. Parents should set good examples and encourage both informal and formal play, always keeping safety issues in mind and promoting healthy attitudes about sportsmanship and competition. Participation in sports and activities as a family provides children with exercise and has important psychologic and developmental benefits. Screening of children for sports participation is discussed on p. 2631.

Limits to television watching, which is linked directly to inactivity and obesity, should start at birth and be maintained throughout adolescence. Similar limits should be set for video games and noneducational computer time as the child grows older.

COLIC

Colic is paroxysms of crying and irritability in an infant. Although the term colic suggests an intestinal origin, etiology is unknown. Colic often begins at about 6 wk and spontaneously improves between 3 and 4 mo. Paroxysms of crying and unhappiness develop at roughly the same time of day or night and continue for hours for no apparent reason. A few infants cry almost incessantly. Excessive crying may cause aerophagia, which results in flatulence and abdominal distention. Typically, the colicky infant eats and gains weight well, although vigorous non-nutritive sucking may suggest excessive hunger. Colic probably has no relation to development of an insistent, impatient personality.

Evaluation

History and physical examination: History should establish whether the infant's crying is outside the normal range (up to 3 h/day in a 6-wk-old infant). Then it must distinguish colic from other causes of excessive crying, including fever, UTI, ear infection, and maltreatment. Thorough questioning may reveal that crying is not the chief concern but a symptom that the parents have used to justify their visiting the physician to present another problem—eg, concern over the death of a previous child or over their feelings of inability to cope with a new infant. A thorough physical examination typically detects no abnormalities but reassures parents that the doctor understands how stressful a colicky infant can be for parents.

Testing: No testing is necessary unless specific abnormalities are detected by history and examination.

Treatment

Parents should be reassured that the infant is healthy, that his irritability is not due to poor parenting, and that colic will resolve on its own with no long-term adverse effects. The infant who cries for short periods may respond to being held, rocked, or patted gently. An infant with a strong sucking urge who fusses soon after a feeding may need to suck more. If a bottle feeding takes < 15 to 20 min, nipples with smaller holes should be tried; a pacifier also may quiet the infant. A very active, restless infant may respond, paradoxically, to being swaddled tightly. An infant swing, music, and white noise (eg, from a vacuum cleaner, car engine, or clothes or hair dryer) may also be calming.

A milk-substitute formula may be tried briefly to ascertain whether milk intolerance exists, but frequent formula switching should be avoided. Sometimes in breastfed infants, removal of milk or another food from the mother's diet brings relief.

CONSTIPATION

Parents are often preoccupied with how and how often their children move their bowels, but most constipation has no serious consequences and should be a concern only when passing stools becomes painful and leads to further withholding of stools, or when constipation causes other symptoms.

In infants, bowel movements vary so much in frequency that it is difficult to define constipation. The same infant who generally has a bowel movement 4 times/day may, at other times, have one every 2 days. Most infants pass a hard, large stool with minimal discomfort, while some cry when passing a soft one. In general, signs of effort (eg, straining) do not signify constipation; infants only gradually develop the muscles to assist a bowel movement. In neonates, inability to pass meconium within 24 h suggests Hirschsprung's disease (see p. 2430). In infants, inability to pass stool for several days combined with other symptoms and signs, such as increase in abdominal girth and signs of pain, should raise suspicion of rare disorders (eg, Hirschsprung's disease or obstruction from a tumor).

In older children, constipation is defined as the passing of hard stools that cause discomfort and is most often caused by insufficient dietary fiber. The condition may be self-reinforcing, because discomfort while moving bowels causes further withholding of stool.

At any age, passage of hard stools can cause anal fissure. Fissures cause severe pain on defecation and the occasional passage of a small amount of bright red blood. Diagnosis of external fissures is by inspecting the anus; no assessment is necessary for internal fissures because treatment of constipation relieves symptoms. Most fissures heal quickly without intervention, but increased fluid intake and a stool softener may facilitate healing.

Evaluation

History: History focuses on frequency and consistency of stools, presence or absence of discomfort on defecation, presence or absence of blood, and composition of the diet, especially fluids and fiber. Reports of constipation going back to birth and refractory to conventional therapy suggest an anatomic defect, such as Hirschsprung's disease. Reports of painful defecation suggest an anal fissure. Reports of poor fluid intake suggest a dietary factor.

Physical examination: Examination focuses on the abdomen and anus. A distended abdomen or abdominal mass suggests a significant problem with stool retention, an obstruction, or rarely, a tumor. A crack or split in the anal skin establishes the diagnosis of an anal fissure. Finding hard stool at the end of the examining finger suggests that Hirschsprung's disease is not the problem.

Testing: Tests are ordered if history and examination suggest obstruction (as in Hirschsprung's disease) or tumor. Tests may include x-rays, CT scans, or MRI to define intra-abdominal masses, and rectal manometry and biopsy for Hirschsprung's disease.

Treatment

Most often, increases in dietary fluid and fiber (with whole grains, fruit, or supplements) are sufficient; temporarily reducing milk intake may help. Young children who are toilet trained often become distracted and typically do not sit long enough on the toilet to pass constipated stool. Parental guidance to sit longer and more frequently (eg, at least twice/day for 10 min after meals) establishes a routine that gives the child the opportunity to defecate fully. Stool softeners and laxatives (eg, senna 5 to 10 mL once/day for children < 6 yr and bid for those > 6 yr; Mg hydroxide 0.5 mL/kg once/day for children < 2 yr, 5 mL tid or 15 mL once/day for children 2 to 5 yr, 5 to 10 mL tid or 15 to 30 mL once/day for those 5 to 12 yr), as well as gentle enemas, are available and safe and can facilitate the process, though they may be required for several months before normal defecation returns permanently. In one regimen, laxatives or softeners are given for 2 to 3 wk, then every other day for 1 mo after initial catharsis, then daily for 1 to 2 wk if relapse occurs.

CRYING

Crying should be distinguished from colic (see p. 2236). Crying is the only means an infant has to signify distress. Causes may be mundane (eg, a neonate accustomed to the tight environment of the womb becoming frightened by unrestricted arm and leg movements) or serious (eg, ear infection, abdominal pain). Often there is no obvious cause. Persistent or prolonged crying, especially with signs of illness, requires a search for a cause. Crying almost always improves by 4 to 6 mo; when it does not, providers should suspect physical pain or tension within the family.

Evaluation

History: History focuses on the amount, timing, and quality of the crying as well as any signs of illness. Reports of fever or URI suggest possible otitis media. Reports of diarrhea or vomiting suggest pain from a GI process, ranging from gastroenteritis to more serious conditions. Reports of extreme parental frustration suggest tensions within the family that may be reflected in the infant's behavior.

Physical examination: Examination focuses on growth parameters and any signs of illness. Distorted or erythematous tympanic membranes suggest otitis media. Abdominal distention or masses suggest an intra-abdominal process causing pain. Fever and fussiness without an apparent cause may result from UTI.

Testing: In most cases, testing is unnecessary unless otherwise indicated by history and examination.

Treatment

The clinician's role in managing crying is to present explanations and options to parents, who can then try different strategies to diminish the child's crying. Approaches vary with cause and age. Infants are often comforted by swaddling, ambient noise, and movement, as in rocking or swinging in a swing. Both infants and older children often respond to a ride in the car. If parents and physician are convinced that there is no serious cause for the crying, the infant may be allowed to cry for a short period ("5-minute rule"), then parents comfort the infant and restart the clock. Often parents are relieved to know that they can let the infant cry, and often the infant will stop spontaneously before the prescribed period is over.

DIARRHEA

Frequent loose bowel movements (4 to 6/day) may occur in normal infants; they are of no concern unless anorexia, vomiting, weight loss, failure to gain weight, or passage of blood also occurs. Breastfed infants tend to have frequent bowel movements, especially if they are not receiving solid food. The significance of diarrhea in a child at any age differs if it is acute (< 2 wk) or chronic (> 2 wk).

Etiology

Acute diarrhea is most likely infectious, especially if onset is sudden or accompanied by vomiting, bloody stools, fever, anorexia, or listlessness. Diagnosis is clinical, and treatment is supportive until the condition resolves spontaneously.

Chronic diarrhea is usually more significant. Causes include gluten-induced enteropathy, cystic fibrosis, sugar malabsorption, and allergic gastroenteropathy. Inflammatory bowel disease and some infections (eg, with *Giardia*) can also cause chronic diarrhea.

With gluten-induced enteropathy (celiac sprue—see p. 144), the gluten fraction of wheat protein causes intestinal mucosal damage and malabsorption of dietary fats, resulting in malnutrition, anorexia, and bulky, foul-smelling stools. The change in stools starts when wheat and other gluten-containing foods are added.

With cystic fibrosis (see p. 2308), pancreatic insufficiency results in trypsin and lipase deficits, causing high fecal losses of protein and fats with consequent malnutrition and growth retardation. The stool is voluminous and often foul-smelling. Children who have cystic fibrosis often have respiratory problems and growth failure.

With sugar malabsorption, intestinal mucosal enzymes, such as lactase, which splits lactose to galactose and glucose, may be congenitally absent or temporarily deficient secondary to GI infection. Improvement after eliminating lactose (or other carbohydrates) from the diet or after substituting a lactose-free formula strongly suggests the diagnosis.

With allergic gastroenteropathy, cow's milk protein may cause diarrhea, often with vomiting and blood in the stools, but intolerance to the carbohydrate fraction of the ingested food should be suspected also. Symptoms often abate promptly when soy formula is substituted for cow's milk and return if cow's milk is reintroduced. Some infants intolerant of cow's milk are also intolerant of soy, so a formula that has had the protein predigested and does not contain the offending disaccharide may be needed. Spontaneous improvement usually occurs toward the end of the 1st yr.

Evaluation

History: History focuses on the quality and frequency of stools as well as accompanying signs and symptoms. Reports of vomiting or fever suggest GI infection. An accurate dietary history is critical. Reports of diarrhea beginning with the introduction of wheat cereal suggest celiac disease. Reports of variation in the stool pattern with certain elements of the diet suggest dietary intolerance. The persistent presence of blood in the stool mandates a careful search for more serious infection or GI disorder.

Physical examination: Examination focuses on overall appearance and signs of dehydration, growth parameters, and abdominal findings; poor growth suggests more serious disorders. Pulmonary status is also evaluated in children in whom cystic fibrosis is suspected.

Testing: Tests are ordered if history and examination suggest a chronic condition. Tests include electrolyte levels if there is dehydration; sweat Cl and Na levels for cystic fibrosis; cultures for viruses, bacteria, or parasites when infection appears to be present; and stool pH for disaccharide intolerance. Levels of certain antibodies are associated with celiac disease. Dietary manipulations can be diagnostic as well as therapeutic.

Treatment

Supportive care for acute diarrhea consists primarily of providing adequate oral (or rarely IV) rehydration (see p. 2293). Antimotility agents (eg, loperamide) are generally not recommended for infants and young children.

For chronic diarrhea, adequate nutrition must be maintained, particularly of fat-soluble vitamins. Specific treatments are indicated for certain causes (eg, gluten-free diet for those with celiac disease).

FEVER

Normal body temperature varies from person to person and throughout the day. As a working standard, fever is defined as a core body (rectal) temperature ≥ 38.0° C. Significance of fever depends on clinical context; some minor illnesses cause high fevers while some serious illnesses cause only mild temperature elevations.

Etiology

Nearly all acute fevers in infants and young children are caused by infection, most commonly viral respiratory or GI illness. Bacterial infections, typically otitis media, pneumonia, and UTI, are less common but occasionally very serious (eg, meningitis). Infants < 28 days are susceptible to perinatally acquired infection with group B *Streptococcus, Escherichia coli, Listeria monocytogenes*, and herpes simplex virus.

Children < 2 yr (particularly infants ≤ 3 mo) are at special risk of occult bacteremia (see p. 2353), defined as the presence of pathogenic bacteria in the blood of a febrile child who has no focal signs or symptoms. The most common causative organisms are *Streptococcus pneumoniae* and *Haemophilus influenzae*; vaccination against both of these is now widespread in the US and Europe, making occult bacteremia less common.

Rare, noninfectious causes of acute fevers include heat stroke and toxic ingestions (eg, anticholinergic agents). Some vaccinations can cause fever days (eg, pertussis) and even 1 or 2 wk (eg, measles) after administration. These fevers typically last from a few hours to a day. If the child is otherwise well, no evaluation is necessary. Teething does not cause fever.

Chronic fever suggests various potential causes, ranging from autoimmune disease (eg, juvenile RA, inflammatory bowel disease) to cancer (eg, leukemia, lymphoma), as well as chronic infections (eg, osteomyelitis, UTI). Hereditary periodic fevers are reviewed in Ch. 297 on p. 2475.

Evaluation

Evaluation varies by age group and focuses on identifying a source for infection or underlying noninfectious condition. Acute fever in an infant ≤ 3 mo requires a thorough evaluation regardless of other signs and symptoms because serious infection (eg, sepsis, meningitis) may occur without other manifestations.

History: For infants < 3 mo, history should focus on risks for sepsis, including maternal infection, prematurity, recent surgery, or known conditions such as HIV infection. In older children, history should focus on localizing symptoms and signs, vaccination history, recent exposures to infection (including family and caretaker infection), and other risk factors for infection, including indwelling medical devices (eg, catheters, ventriculoperitoneal shunts) and conditions predisposing to infection (eg, congenital heart disease, sickle cell anemia, neoplasm, immunodeficiency). A family history of autoimmune disease is relevant. Although there is no direct correlation between the height of fever and the seriousness of the cause, a temperature of 39°C puts children < 2 yr at higher risk for having occult bacteremia.

Physical examination: Appraisal of the child's overall appearance is critical. The febrile child who looks quite ill, especially when the temperature has come down, is a source of great concern and requires in-depth evaluation and continued observation. In all febrile children, careful attention should be paid to the tympanic membranes, throat, chest, abdomen, lymph nodes, neck flexibility, and skin. Petechiae or purpura often indicates serious infection.

Testing: All febrile children < 3 mo require WBC testing with a manual differential, blood cultures, and urinalysis and urine culture. Lumbar puncture is mandatory for children < 2 mo; opinions vary about the need for the test in children between 2 mo and 3 mo. Many providers also obtain a chest x-ray, and some obtain stool swabs for WBCs and stool cultures. Some clinicians add acute-phase reactants (eg, ESR, C-reactive protein, procalcitonin); however, although abnormalities on these tests are more common in serious bacterial illness, sensitivities and specificities are low, and use of these tests is under debate.

Febrile children between 3 mo and 24 mo who look well and can be watched carefully do not necessarily require laboratory testing. If there are signs or symptoms of specific infections, appropriate tests should be ordered (eg, chest x-ray when there is hypoxemia, dyspnea, or grunting; urinalysis and culture when there is foul-smelling urine). If the child looks ill but has no localizing signs, blood counts and cultures and urine tests should be considered as well as a lumbar puncture.

Testing in children > 24 mo is dictated by history and examination; screening blood cultures and WBC counts are not indicated.

Treatment

Symptomatic treatment of fever typically includes acetaminophen 10 to 15 mg/kg po or per rectum q 4 to 6 h (not to exceed 5 doses in 24 h) or ibuprofen 5 to 10 mg/kg q 6 to 8 h.

Definitive treatment of a clearly identified infection is site-specific. Management of fever without a clear source is determined by age, history, and screening test results.

Most experts treat infants ≤ 28 days with hospital admission and IV antibiotics to cover neonatal and community-acquired pathogens until results of screening tests are available. Current recommendations are for ceftriaxone (50 to 75 mg/kg q 24 h or 80 to 100 mg/kg q 24 h if cells are present in CSF) or cefotaxime (50 mg/kg q 6 h) plus ampicillin to cover *Listeria* and *Enterococcus*. Vancomycin (15 mg/kg q 6 h) can be added if penicillin-resistant *Streptococcus pneumoniae* is suspected, and acyclovir (20 mg/kg q 8 h) when herpes simplex is likely.

Criteria for managing febrile children between 3 and 24 mo are changing because of the effectiveness of vaccination on decreasing the incidence of occult bacteremia. Decisions about how intensive the testing should be, whether the child should receive antibiotics while cultures are pending, and whether management is conducted in the hospital or as an outpatient depend on the child's overall appearance, the family's reliability, and the presence or absence of risk factors for occult bacteremia. For detailed recommendations, see FIG. 280–2 on p. 2355.

Children > 24 mo require only symptomatic treatment.

SEPARATION AND STRANGER ANXIETY

Separation anxiety: Separation anxiety is crying when a parent leaves the room. It is normal starting at about 8 mo, peaks in intensity between 10 and 18 mo, and generally resolves by 24 mo. It should be distinguished from separation anxiety disorder (see p. 2498), which occurs later, at an age when such reaction is developmentally inappropriate; school (or preschool) refusal is a common manifestation.

Separation anxiety occurs at a time when infants start to become emotionally attached to their parents. Because they have no object permanence (incomplete memory and no sense of time), children fear that the departure of their parents is permanent. Separation anxiety resolves as the child develops a sense of memory and keeps an image of the parents in mind when they are gone and recalls that in the past the parents returned.

Parents should be advised not to limit or forego separations in response to separation anxiety; this could compromise the child's maturation and development. When parents leave the home (or leave the child at a child-care center), they should encourage the person with whom they are leaving the child to create distractions. The parent should then leave without responding at length to a child's crying. Parents should remain calm and reassuring and establish routines around separations to ease the child's anxiety. If the parents must momentarily go to another room in the home, they should call to the child while in the other room to reassure the child. This gradually teaches the child that parents are still present even though the child cannot see them. Separation anxiety may be worse when a child is hungry or tired, so feeding the child and letting him nap before leaving may also help.

Separation anxiety at the normal age causes no long-term harm to the child. Separation anxiety that lasts beyond age 2 may or may not be a problem depending on the extent to which it interferes with the child's development. It is normal for children to feel some fear upon leaving for preschool or kindergarten. This feeling should diminish with time. Rarely, excessive fear of separations inhibits a child from attending childcare or preschool or keeps him from playing normally with peers. This anxiety is probably abnormal (separation anxiety disorder—see p. 2498). In this case, the parents should seek medical attention for the child.

Stranger anxiety: Stranger anxiety is manifested by crying when an unfamiliar person approaches. It is normal starting at about 8 to 9 mo and usually abates by age 2 yr. Stranger anxiety is linked with the infant's developmental task of distinguishing the familiar from the unfamiliar. Both the duration and intensity of the anxiety vary greatly among children.

Some infants and young children show a strong preference for one parent over another at a given age, and grandparents may suddenly be viewed as strangers. Anticipating these occurrences during well child visits helps prevent misinterpretation of the infant's behavior. Comforting the child and avoiding overreaction to the behavior are usually the only therapy needed.

Common sense should dictate management. If a new sitter is coming, having that person spend some time with the family before the actual day makes sense. When the event arrives, having parents spend some time with the child and sitter before leaving is prudent. If grandparents are coming to watch the child for a few days while parents go away, they should arrive a day or two early. Similar techniques can be used in anticipation of hospitalization.

Stranger anxiety of pronounced intensity or extended duration may be a sign of more generalized anxiety and should prompt evaluation of the family situation, parenting techniques, and the child's overall emotional state.

SLEEPING

Sleep behaviors are culturally determined, and problems tend to be defined as behaviors that vary from accepted customs or norms. In cultures where children sleep separately from their parents in the same house, sleep problems are among the most common that parents and children face. Infants generally adapt to a day-night sleep schedule between 4 and 6 mo. Sleep problems beyond these ages take many forms, including difficulty falling asleep at night, frequent nighttime awakening, atypical daytime napping, and dependence on feeding or being held for sleep. These problems are related to parental expectations, the child's temperament and biologic rhythms, and child-parent interactions. Inborn biologic patterns are central to an infant's sleep patterns, whereas emotional factors and established habits become more important in the toddler and older child. In addition, sleep disturbances become common at 9 mo and again around 18 mo, when separation anxiety, increasing ability of the child to move independently and control his environment, long late-afternoon naps, overstimulating play before bedtime, and nightmares tend to become more common.

Evaluation

History: History focuses on the child's sleeping environment, consistency of bedtime, bedtime routines, and parental expectations. A detailed description of the child's average day can be useful. The history should probe for stressors in the child's life, such as difficulties in school, as well as exposure to unsettling television programs and caffeinated beverages (eg, sodas). Reports of inconsistent bedtimes, a noisy or chaotic environment, or frequent attempts by the child to manipulate parents by using sleep behaviors suggest the need for lifestyle changes. Extreme parental frustration suggests tension within the family or parents who are having difficulty being consistent and firm.

A sleep diary compiled over several nights may help identify unusual sleep patterns and sleep disorders (eg, sleepwalking, night terrors—see p. 1842). Careful questioning of older children and adolescents about school, friends, anxieties, depressive symptoms, and overall state of mind often reveals a source for a sleep problem.

Physical examination and testing: Examination and diagnostic testing generally yield little useful information.

Treatment

The clinician's role in treatment is to present explanations and options to parents, who must implement changes to get the child on an acceptable sleep schedule. Approaches vary with age and circumstances. Infants are often comforted by swaddling, ambient noise, and movement. However, always rocking the infant to sleep does not allow the infant to learn how to fall asleep on his own, which is an important developmental task. As a substitute for rocking, the parent can sit quietly by the crib until the infant falls asleep, and the infant eventually learns to be comforted and to fall asleep without being held. All children awaken during the night, but children who have been taught to fall asleep by themselves will usually settle themselves back to sleep. When a child is unable to get back to sleep, parents can check on the child to reassure themselves of the child's safety and to reassure the child, but the child should then be allowed to settle himself back to sleep.

In older children, a period of "winding down" with quiet activities such as reading at bedtime facilitates sleep. A consistent bedtime is important, and a fixed ritual is helpful for young children. Asking a fully verbal child to recount the events of the day often eliminates nightmares and waking. Encouraging exercise in the daytime, avoiding scary television programs and movies, and refusing to allow bedtime to become an element of manipulation also help prevent sleep problems. Stressful events (eg, moving, illness) may cause acute sleep problems in older children; reassurance and encouragement are always ultimately effective. Allowing the child to sleep in the parents' bed in such instances almost always prolongs rather than resolves the problem.

SPITTING UP AND VOMITING

Infants normally spit up small amounts (usually < 5 to 10 mL) during or soon after feedings, often when being burped; rapid feeding and swallowing of air may be a cause, though spitting up occurs even without these factors. It may be a sign of overfeeding. Occasional vomiting may also be normal, but persistent vomiting, especially if associated with poor growth, much more often signals a serious condition. Causes include serious infection (eg, sepsis, meningitis), gastroesophageal reflux, obstructive GI disorders such as pyloric stenosis or bowel obstruction (eg, from duodenal stenosis or volvulus), neurologic conditions (eg, meningitis, tumor or other space-occupying lesion), and metabolic disorders (eg, adrenogenital syndrome, galactosemia). In older children, vomiting often results from acute gastroenteritis or appendicitis.

Evaluation

History: History focuses on the frequency and estimated amount of vomiting, feeding pattern, stool frequency and consistency, urinary output, and presence of abdominal pain.

Because vomiting can be caused by many disorders, a careful review of systems should be done. The combination of vomiting and diarrhea suggests acute gastroenteritis. Fever suggests infection. Projectile vomiting suggests pyloric stenosis or other obstruction. Yellow or green (bile-stained) emesis suggests obstruction distal to the ampulla of Vater. Vomiting accompanied by extreme crying and absent or currant jelly stools can result from intussusception. Irritability, choking, and respiratory signs such as stridor may be manifestations of gastroesophageal reflux. A history of poor development or neurologic manifestations suggests a CNS disorder.

Physical examination: Examination focuses on overall appearance, signs of dehydration (eg, dry mucosa, tachycardia, lethargy), growth parameters, signs of developmental progress, and abdominal findings. Findings of poor weight gain or weight loss demand an intense search for a diagnosis. An epigastric mass or "olive" suggests pyloric stenosis. Abdominal distention or masses may represent obstructive lesions or tumors. An infant who is not showing appropriate developmental progress may have a CNS disorder. Abdominal tenderness suggests an inflammatory process.

Testing: No diagnostic testing is needed for an infant who is growing well and has no signs of disease. Tests should be ordered if history and examination suggest an underlying disorder and may include x-rays, CT scans, and MRI for lesions or tumors obstructing the GI tract; upper GI x-rays and pH probe for reflux; brain imaging for CNS disorders; cultures for infection; and specific blood chemistries for metabolic defects.

Treatment

Spitting up does not require treatment. When too-rapid feeding is a cause, treatment is use of bottles with firmer nipples and smaller holes, combined with more frequent burping.

Nonspecific treatment of vomiting involves ensuring adequate hydration (see p. 2293); those willing to take oral liquids may be given small, frequent amounts of electrolyte-containing fluids. IVs are rarely required. Antiemetics are not given to infants and young children because of concern about adverse effects. Specific treatment of vomiting is directed at the cause; gastroesophageal reflux responds to positioning of the head higher than the feet, thickened feedings, and sometimes acid-blocking and promotility drugs. Pyloric stenosis and other obstructive lesions require surgery.

TOILET TRAINING

Toilet training involves recognition of readiness for and implementation of the separate steps of toileting: discussion, undressing, eliminating, dressing again, flushing, and hand washing. Most children can be trained for bowel control between age 2 and 3 yr and for urinary control between age 3 and 4 yr. By age 5 yr, the average child can go to the toilet alone. Incontinence of urine (enuresis) or stool (encopresis) in a child ≥4 yr is discussed on p. 2480.

The key to successful toilet training is recognizing signs of readiness to train (usually at age 18 to 24 mo): the child can remain dry for several hours, shows interest in sitting on a potty chair and expresses visible signs of preparing to urinate or defecate, wants to be changed after either, has demonstrated the ability to place things where they belong, and can understand and carry out simple verbal commands. Approaches to toilet training must be consistent among all caregivers.

The timing method is the most common approach. Once the child has demonstrated readiness, the parent discusses with the child what will be happening, selecting words that the child can readily understand and say. The child is gradually introduced to the potty chair and briefly sits on it fully clothed; the child then practices taking the pants down, sitting on the potty chair for ≤5 or 10 min, and redressing. The purpose for the exercise is explained repeatedly and emphasized by placing wet or dirty diapers in the potty. Once this connection between the potty and elimination has been made, the parent should try to anticipate the child's need to eliminate and provide positive reinforcement for successful elimination. The child is also encouraged to practice using the potty whenever the need to eliminate is sensed. The child should also be taught about flushing and hand washing after each elimination. For the child with an unpredictable schedule, this type of plan is difficult, and training must be delayed until the child can anticipate elimination himself. Anger or punishment for accidents or lack of success is counterproductive.

A child who resists sitting on the potty should try again after a meal. If resistance continues for days, postponing toilet training for at least several weeks is the best strategy. Behavior modification with a reward given for successful toileting is one option; once the pattern is established, rewards are gradually withdrawn. Power struggles must be avoided because they often cause regression from any progress that has been made and may strain the parent-child relationship. Toilet-trained children may also regress during illness, emotional upset, or when they feel the need for more attention, such as when a new sibling arrives. Refusal to use the potty may also represent manipulation. In these situations, parents are advised to avoid pressuring the child, offer incentives, and if possible give the child more care and attention at times other than when toileting is involved.

267 APPROACH TO THE CARE OF ADOLESCENTS

Adolescence is a period from about 10 yr to the late teens or early 20s during which children undergo striking physical, intellectual, and emotional changes. Guiding people through this period is a challenge for parents as well as clinicians. Fortunately, most adolescents enjoy good physical health, but psychosocial problems are common as even normal individuals struggle with issues of identity, autonomy, sexuality, and relationships. "Who am I, where am I going, and how do I relate to all of these people in my life?" are constant preoccupations for most adolescents. Many unhealthy behaviors that begin during adolescence (eg, smoking, drug use, violence) eventually cause morbidity later in life.

Physical Growth

All organ systems and the body as a whole undergo major growth during adolescence; breasts in girls and genitals and body hair in both sexes undergo the most obvious changes. Even when this process goes normally, substantial emotional adjustments are required. If the timing is atypical, particularly in a boy whose physical development is delayed or a girl whose development occurs early, additional emotional stress is likely. Most boys who grow slowly have a constitutional delay and catch up eventually. Evaluation to exclude pathologic causes and reassurance are needed.

Guidance concerning nutrition, fitness, and lifestyle should be given to all adolescents, with special attention paid to the role of activities such as sports, the arts, social activities, and community service in the individual's life. Relative requirements for protein and energy (g or kcal/kg body weight) decline progressively from the end of infancy through adolescence (see TABLE 1–4 on p. 6), although absolute requirements increase. Protein requirements are 0.9 g/kg/day in late adolescence; mean relative energy requirements are 40 kcal/kg.

Sexuality

In addition to adapting to the bodily changes, the adolescent must become comfortable with the role of adult male or female and must put sexual urges, which can be very strong and sometimes frightening, into perspective. Relationships with one's own as well as the opposite sex must be defined; some adolescents struggle with the issue of sexual identity. Few elements of the human experience combine physical, intellectual, and emotional aspects as thoroughly as sexuality. Helping adolescents put sexuality into a healthy context, including issues of morality and the formation of a family, is extremely important.

Intellectual Growth

As the adolescent encounters schoolwork that is more complex, he begins to identify areas of strength and weakness. The weight of making decisions about one's future career gets increasingly heavy, and most adolescents do not have a clearly defined goal, although they gradually perceive spheres of interest and talent. Parents and clinicians must be aware of the adolescent's capabilities, help the young person formulate realistic expectations, and be prepared to identify impediments to learning that need remediation, such as learning disabilities, attention problems, or inappropriate learning environments.

Emotional Growth

The emotional aspect of growth is most trying, often taxing the patience of parents, teachers, and clinicians. Emotional lability is very common, as is frustration that arises from trying to grow in so many directions. A major area of conflict arises from the adolescent's desire for more freedom, which clashes with the parents' strong instincts to protect their children from harm. Communication within even stable families can be difficult and is worsened when families are divided or parents have emotional problems of their own. Clinicians can be of great help by offering adolescents and parents sensible, practical, supportive help while facilitating communication within the family.

Physical Problems

Although adolescents are susceptible to the same kinds of illness that afflict younger children, generally they are a healthy group. Adolescents should continue to receive vaccinations according to the recommended schedule (see FIG. 266–3 on p. 2235). Acne is extremely common and needs to be addressed because of its impact on self-esteem.

Trauma is very common in adolescence, with sports and motor vehicle injuries most frequent. Violence, sometimes involving weapons, is an everyday threat in certain adolescent groups.

Obesity is one of the most common reasons for visits to adolescent clinics. Most cases of obesity are due to eating more than is needed, often in conjunction with a sedentary life style. Genetic influences are common, and responsible genes are now being identified (see also Ch. 6 on p. 56). Determination of the body mass index (BMI) is recognized as an important aspect of physical assessment. Primary endocrine (eg, hyperadrenocorticism, hypothyroidism) or metabolic causes are uncommon. Hypothyroidism should be ruled out as a cause and should be suspected if height growth slows significantly. If the child is short and has hypertension, Cushing's syndrome should be considered. Type 2 diabetes mellitus is occurring with increasing frequency due to obesity in adolescents. Despite many therapeutic approaches, obesity is one of the most difficult and discouraging problems to treat, and long-term success rates remain low.

Infectious mononucleosis is particularly prevalent in adolescents. Sexually transmitted diseases become an important concern, and UTIs are common in girls. Some endocrine disorders, particularly thyroid disorders, are common in adolescents, as are menstrual abnormalities. Iron deficiency is relatively common in adolescent girls. Pregnancy also is not a rare occurrence and must be kept in mind when treating adolescent girls. Although not common, neoplastic diseases such as leukemia, lymphoma, bone cancers, and brain tumors also occur.

Psychosocial Disorders

Clinicians must be aware of the high frequency of psychosocial disorders that occur during this unsettled stage of life. Depression is common and should be looked for actively (see p. 2502). Suicide and especially suicidal gestures are common. Anxiety often manifests during adolescence (see p. 2496), as well as bipolar disease and problems with anger management. Adolescence is also a time when some people who will go on to develop some form of psychotic disorder experience their 1st psychotic break. Eating disorders, especially in girls, are common (see p. 1701). Some patients go to extraordinary lengths to hide an anorexic or bulimic state.

School problems, especially when related to learning or attention difficulties, can be dealt with by clinicians, who must work closely with school personnel and parents. Environmental changes and sometimes drug therapy can be of great help to struggling students.

A constant concern is substance abuse, which is a psychosocial problem with a strong physiologic component. Alcohol and cigarette use is extremely common, followed by marijuana and a long list of other substances available in all strata of society.

The clinician who has developed an open, trusting relationship with an adolescent often can identify these problems, can supply support and practical advice, and can get the adolescent to agree to more specialized care if necessary.

268 CARING FOR SICK CHILDREN AND THEIR FAMILIES

Illness and death cause emotional stresses on children and their families.

THE SICK NEONATE

Difficulties arise when a sick or premature infant must be taken away from the family after birth because of illness. The parents may not be able to see a critically ill infant during stabilization and may be separated from the infant because of transport to a different hospital. Some infants require prolonged separation from their families because of lengthy hospitalizations and treatments.

Many hospitals have recognized the importance of encouraging contact between infants and their families. In most places, parents are encouraged to visit, taking precautions to minimize the risk of spreading infections. Many hospitals have unlimited visiting hours for parents. Some hospitals have areas in which parents can stay for prolonged periods to be near their infants.

In most hospitals, parents are encouraged to interact with their sick infants as much as possible. *No neonate, even one on a respirator, is too ill for the parents to see and touch.* Parents are also encouraged to provide direct care for the infant as a way to get to know the infant and to prepare for taking the infant home. Some hospitals increase contact between parents and premature or sick infants by encouraging skin-to-skin contact; this may help parents feel more confident about taking care of their infants at home. Infants who experience skin-to-skin contact gain weight faster when compared with those who do not receive such care. Mothers can also provide breast milk directly or pumped to be given through a feeding tube.

When an infant has a birth defect, the parents should see the infant as soon after birth as possible, regardless of the medical condition. Otherwise, they may imagine the appearance and condition to be much worse than the reality. Intensive parental support is essential, with as many counseling sessions as are needed for parents to understand their infant's condition and recommended treatment and to accept the infant psychologically. To balance discussion of abnormalities, the physician should emphasize what is normal about the child and his potential.

When an infant dies without the parents having seen or touched him, the parents may later feel as though they never really had a child. Such parents have reported exaggerated feelings of emptiness and may develop prolonged depression because they could not mourn the loss of a "real infant." Parents who have not been able to see or hold their infants during life will usually be helped in the long term if allowed to do so after the infant has died. In all cases, follow-up visits with the physician and a social worker are helpful to review the circumstances of the infant's illness and death, answer questions that often arise later, and assess and alleviate feelings of guilt. The physician can also evaluate the parents' grieving process and provide appropriate guidance or a referral for more extensive support if necessary.

CHILDREN WITH CHRONIC HEALTH CONDITIONS

Chronic health conditions (both chronic illnesses and chronic physical disabilities) are generally defined as those conditions that last > 12 mo and are severe enough to create some limitations in usual activity. It has been estimated that chronic health conditions affect 10 to 30% of children, depending on the criteria. Examples of chronic illnesses include asthma, cystic fibrosis, congenital heart disease, diabetes mellitus, attention deficit hyperactivity disorder, and depression. Examples of chronic physical disabilities include meningomyelocele, hearing or visual impairments, cerebral palsy, and loss of limb function.

Effects on the child: Children with chronic health conditions may experience limitations in some activities; frequent pain or discomfort; abnormal growth and development; and more hospitalizations, outpatient visits, and medical treatments. Those with severe disabilities may be unable at times to participate in school and peer activities.

A child's response to a chronic health condition largely depends on his developmental stage when the condition occurs. Children with chronic conditions that appear in infancy will respond differently than children who develop conditions during adolescence. School-aged children may be most affected by the inability to attend school and form relationships with peers. Adolescents may struggle with their inability to achieve independence if they require assistance from parents and others for many of their daily needs; parents should encourage self-reliance within the adolescent's capability and avoid overprotection. Adolescents also find it particularly difficult to be viewed as different from their peers.

Health care practitioners can be advocates for appropriate hospital services for children with chronic health conditions. Age-appropriate playrooms can be set up and a school program initiated with the oversight of a trained child life specialist. Children can be encouraged to interact with peers whenever possible. All procedures and plans should be explained to the family and child whenever possible so the family knows what to expect during the hospitalization, thus relieving the anxiety that can be created by uncertainty.

Effects on the family: For the families, having a child who has a chronic health condition can lead to loss of their hope for an "ideal child," neglected siblings, major expense and time commitment, confusion caused by conflicting systems of health care management, lost opportunities (eg, family members providing primary care to the child and are therefore unable to return to work), and social isolation. Siblings may resent the extra attention the ill child receives. Such stress may cause family breakup, especially when there are preexisting difficulties with family function.

Conditions that affect the physical appearance of an infant (eg, cleft lip and palate or hydrocephalus) can affect the bond between these children and family or caretakers. Once the diagnosis of abnormality is made, parents may react with shock, denial, anger, sadness or depression, guilt, and anxiety. These reactions may occur at any time in the child's development, and each parent may be at a different stage of acceptance, making communication between them difficult. Parents may express their anger at the health care practitioner, or their denial may cause them to seek many opinions about their child's condition.

Care coordination: Without coordination of services, care will be crisis-oriented. Some services will be duplicated, while others will be neglected. Care coordination requires knowledge of the child's condition, his family, and the community in which he functions.

All professionals who care for children with chronic health conditions must ensure that someone is coordinating care. Sometimes the coordinator can be the child's parent. However, the systems that must be negotiated are often so complex that even the most capable parents need assistance. Other possible coordinators include the primary care physician, the subspecialty program staff, the community health nurse, and staff of the 3rd-party payer. Regardless of who coordinates services, the family and child must be partners in the process. In general, children from low-income families who have chronic conditions fare worse than others in part because of lack of access to health care and care coordination services. Some children with terminal illness benefit from hospice care.

DEATH AND DYING

Families often have difficulty dealing with an ill and dying child; children who are trying to make sense of the death of a friend or family member may have particular difficulty (see also Ch. 338 on p. 2762).

Death of a child: Most often the death of a child happens in the hospital or emergency department. Death can occur after a prolonged illness, such as cancer, or suddenly and unexpectedly, such as following injury or sudden infant death. The death of a child can be difficult for families to comprehend and accept. For parents, the death of a child means that they must give up their dreams and hopes for their child. The grieving process may also mean that they are unable to attend to the needs of other family members, including other children. Health care practitioners can help in the process by being available to the family for consultation and to provide comfort whenever possible. In some circumstances, referral to specialists skilled in working with families who have experienced the death of a child is appropriate.

Death of a family member or friend: Many children experience the death of a loved one. The way the child perceives the event (and hence the best response by parents and health care practitioners) is affected by the child's developmental level. Preschool children may have limited understanding of death. Relating the event to previous experience with a beloved pet may be helpful. Older children may be able to understand the event more easily. Death should never be equated with going to sleep and never waking up because the child may become fearful of sleeping.

Parents should discuss with health care practitioners whether to have children visit severely ill children or adults. Some children may express a specific desire to visit family members or friends who are dying. The child should be adequately prepared for such a visit so they will know what to expect. In the same way, adults often wonder whether to bring children to a funeral. This decision should be made individually, in consultation with the child whenever possible. When a child attends a funeral, a close friend or relative should accompany him to provide support throughout, and the child should be allowed to leave if necessary.

269 PHYSICAL GROWTH AND DEVELOPMENT

Physical growth is an increase in size; development is growth in function and capability. Both processes are highly dependent on genetic, nutritional, and environmental factors.

PHYSICAL GROWTH

(See also Failure to Thrive on p. 2395.)

Physical growth includes attainment of full height and appropriate weight and an increase in size of all organs (except lymphatic tissue, which decreases in size). Growth from birth to adolescence occurs in 2 distinct phases. The 1st phase (from birth to about age 1 to 2 yr) is one of rapid growth, although the rate of growth decreases over that period. In the 2nd stage (from about 2 yr to the onset of puberty), growth occurs in relatively constant annual increments. Puberty is the process of physical maturation from child to adult. Adolescence defines an age group; puberty occurs during adolescence. At puberty, a 2nd growth spurt occurs, affecting boys and girls slightly differently. All growth parameters can be charted on standard growth curves available from the Centers for Disease Control and Prevention at www.cdc.gov/growthcharts.

Length: Length is measured in children too young to stand; height is measured once the child can stand. In general, length in normal term infants increases about 30% by 5 mo and > 50% by 12 mo; infants grow 25 cm during the 1st yr; and height at 5 yr is about double birth length. In boys, $\frac{1}{2}$ the adult height is attained by about age 2; in girls, height at 19 mo is about $\frac{1}{2}$ the adult height.

Rate of change in height (height velocity) is a more sensitive measure of growth than time-specific height measures. In general, healthy term infants and children grow about 2.5 cm/mo between birth and 6 mo, 1.3 cm/mo from 7 to 12 mo, and about 7.6 cm/yr between 12 mo and 10 yr. Before 12 mo, height velocity varies and is due in part to perinatal factors (eg, prematurity). After 12 mo, height is mostly genetically determined, and height velocity stays constant until puberty; a child's height relative to peers tends to remain the same. Some small-for-gestational-age infants tend to be shorter throughout life than infants whose size is appropriate for their gestational age. Boys and girls demonstrate little difference in height and growth rate during infancy and childhood.

Extremities grow faster than the trunk, leading to a gradual change in relative proportions; the crown-to-pubis/pubis-to-heel ratio is 1.7 at birth, 1.5 at 12 mo, 1.2 at 5 yr, and 1.0 after 7 yr.

Peak height velocity is reached at 12.1 ± 0.9 yr in girls and at 14.1 ± 0.9 yr in boys. A growth spurt in boys occurs between ages 13 and $15\frac{1}{2}$; a gain of > 10 cm can be expected in the year of peak velocity. A growth spurt in girls begins at about age 11, may reach 4 cm in the year of peak velocity, and is almost completed by age $13\frac{1}{2}$. If puberty is delayed (see p. 2370), growth in height may slow considerably. If the delay is not pathologic, the adolescent growth spurt occurs later and growth catches up, with height crossing percentile lines until the child reaches a genetically determined stature. At age 18, almost 2.54 cm of growth remains for boys and slightly less for girls, for whom growth is 99% complete. In girls with true precocious puberty (prior to age $6\frac{1}{2}$), an early growth spurt occurs along with menarche at a young age and, ultimately, short stature because of early closure of growth plates.

Weight: Weight follows a similar pattern. Normal term neonates generally lose 5 to 8% of birth weight in the days after delivery but regain their birth weight within 2 wk. They then gain 14 to 28 g/day until 3 mo, then 4000 g between 3 and 12 mo, doubling their birth weight by 5 mo, tripling it by 12 mo, and almost quadrupling it by 2 yr. Between age 2 yr and puberty, weight increases 2 kg/yr. The recent epidemic of childhood obesity has involved markedly greater weight gain, even among very young children. In general, boys are heavier and taller than girls when growth is complete because boys have a longer prepubertal growth period, increased peak velocity during the pubertal growth spurt, and a longer adolescent growth spurt.

Head circumference: Head circumference reflects brain size and is routinely measured up to 2 yr. At birth, the brain is 25% of adult size, and head circumference averages 35 cm. Head circumference increases an average 1 cm/mo during the 1st year; growth is more rapid in the first 8 mo, and by 12 mo, the brain has completed $\frac{1}{2}$ its postnatal growth and is 75% of adult size. Head circumference increases 3.5 cm over the next 2 yr; by age 3 yr, the brain is 80% of adult size, 90% by age 7 yr.

Body composition: Body composition (proportions of body fat and water) changes and affects volume of distribution of drugs (see p. 2253). Proportion of fat increases rapidly from 13% at birth to 20 to 25% by 12 mo, accounting for the chubby appearance of most infants. Subsequently, a slow fall occurs until preadolescence, when body fat returns to about 13%. There is a slow rise again until the onset of puberty, when body fat may again fall, especially in boys. After puberty, the percentage generally stays stable in girls, while in boys there tends to be a slight decline.

Body water measured as a percentage of body weight is 70% at birth, dropping to 61% at 12 mo (about equal to the adult percentage). This change is fundamentally due to a decrease in ECF from 45% to 28% of body weight. ICF stays relatively constant. After age 12 mo, there is a slow and variable fall in ECF and rise in ICF to adult levels of about 20% and 40%, respectively. The relatively larger amount of body water, its high turnover rate, and the comparatively high surface losses (due to a proportionately large surface area) make infants more susceptible to fluid deprivation than older children and adults.

Tooth eruption: Tooth eruption is variable (see TABLE 269–1), primarily because of genetic factors. On average, normal infants should have 6 teeth by 12 mo, 12 teeth by 18 mo, 16 teeth by 2 yr, and all teeth (20) by 2½ yr; deciduous teeth are replaced by permanent teeth between the ages of 5 and 13 yr. Eruption of deciduous teeth is similar in both sexes; permanent teeth tend to appear earlier in girls. Tooth eruption may be delayed by familial patterns or by conditions such as rickets, hypopituitarism, hypothyroidism, or Down syndrome. Supernumerary teeth and congenital absence of teeth are probably normal variants.

TABLE 269–1. TOOTH ERUPTION TIMES

TEETH	NO.	AGE AT ERUPTION*
Deciduous (20 total)		
Lower central incisors	2	5–9 mo
Upper central incisors	2	8–12 mo
Upper lateral incisors	2	10–12 mo
Lower lateral incisors	2	12–15 mo
1st molars†	4	10–16 mo
Canines	4	16–20 mo
2nd molars†	4	20–30 mo
Permanent (32 total)		
1st molars†	4	5–7 yr
Incisors	8	6–8 yr
Bicuspids	8	9–12 yr
Canines	4	10–13 yr
2nd molars†	4	11–13 yr
3rd molars†	4	17–25 yr

*Varies greatly.

† Molars are numbered from the front to the back of the mouth (see FIG. 94–1 on p. 845).

DEVELOPMENT

(See also Ch. 299 on p. 2483.)

Development is often divided into specific domains, such as gross motor, fine motor, language, cognition, and social/emotional growth. These designations are useful, but substantial overlap exists. Studies have established average ages at which specific milestones are reached, as well as ranges of normality. In a normal child, progress within the different domains varies, as in the toddler who walks late but speaks in sentences early (see TABLE 269–2).

Environmental influences, ranging from nutrition to stimulation and from the impact of disease to the effects of psychologic factors, interact with genetic factors to determine the pace and pattern of development.

Assessment of development occurs constantly as parents, school personnel, and clinicians evaluate children. Many tools are available for monitoring development more specifically. The Denver Developmental Screening Test facilitates evaluation in several domains. The scoring sheet indicates the average ages for achieving certain milestones and nicely demonstrates the critical concept of a range of normality. Other tools can also be used (see TABLE 269–2).

Motor development: Motor development includes fine motor (eg, picking up small objects, drawing) and gross motor (eg, walking, climbing stairs) skills. It is a continuous process that depends on familial patterns, environmental factors (eg, when activity is limited by prolonged illness), and specific disorders (eg, cerebral palsy, mental retardation, muscular dystrophy). Children typically begin to

TABLE 269–2. DEVELOPMENTAL MILESTONES*

AGE	BEHAVIOR
Birth	Sleeps much of the time; sucks, clears airway, and responds with crying to discomforts and intrusions
4 wk	Brings hands toward eyes and mouth; moves head from side to side when lying on stomach; follows an object moved in an arch about 15 cm above face to the midline; responds to a noise in some way, such as startling, crying, or quieting; may turn toward familiar sounds and voices
6 wk	Regards objects in the line of vision, begins to smile when spoken to, lies flat on abdomen; head lags when pulled to a sitting position
3 mo	Holds head steady on sitting; raises head 45° when lying on stomach; opens and shuts hands; pushes down when feet are placed on a flat surface; swings at and reaches for dangling toys; follows an object moved in an arch above face from one side to the other; watches faces intently; smiles at sound of caretaker's voice; vocalizes sounds
5 to 6 mo	Holds head steady when upright; sits with support; rolls over, usually from stomach to back; supports himself in a standing position; reaches for objects; recognizes people at a distance; listens intently to human voices; smiles spontaneously; squeals in delight; babbles to toys
7 mo	Sits without support; bears some weight on legs when held upright; transfers objects from hand to hand; holds own bottle; looks for dropped object; responds to own name; responds to being told "no"; combines vowels and consonants to babble; moves body with excitement in anticipation of playing; plays peek-a-boo
9 mo	Sits well; crawls or creeps on hands and knees; pulls self up to standing position; works to get a toy that is out of reach; objects if toy is taken away; gets into a sitting position from stomach; stands holding on to someone or something; says "mama" or "dada" appropriately in reference to parents; plays pat-a-cake; waves bye-bye
12 mo	Walks by holding furniture ("cruising") or hands; may walk 1 or 2 steps without support; stands for a few moments at a time; drinks from a cup; speaks several words, helps dress self
18 mo	Walks well; can climb stairs holding on; turns several book pages at a time; speaks about 10 words; pulls toys on strings; partially feeds himself
2 yr	Runs well; climbs up and down stairs alone; turns single book pages; puts on simple clothing; makes 2- or 3-word sentences; verbalizes toilet needs
3 yr	Rides a tricycle; dresses well except for buttons and laces; counts to 10 and uses plurals; recognizes at least 3 colors; questions constantly; feeds himself well; about ½ of children can take care of toilet needs
4 yr	Alternates feet going up and down stairs; throws a ball overhand; hops on one foot; copies a cross; washes hands and face
5 yr	Skips; catches a bounced ball; copies a triangle; knows 4 colors; dresses and undresses without help

*The sequence is fairly consistent, but the timing of milestones varies; times above represent median values.

walk at 12 mo, can climb stairs at 21 mo, and run well at 2 yr, but the age at which these milestones are achieved by normal children varies widely. Motor development cannot be significantly accelerated by applying increased stimulation.

Language development: The ability to understand language precedes the ability to speak; children with few words usually can understand a great deal. Although delays in expressive speech are typically not accompanied by other developmental delays, all children with excessive language delays should be evaluated for the presence of other delays in development. Children who have delays in both receptive and expressive speech more often have additional developmental problems. Evaluation of any delay should start with an assessment of hearing. Most children who experience speech delay have normal intelligence. In contrast, children with accelerated speech development are often of above average intelligence.

Speech progresses from the utterance of vowel sounds (cooing) to the introduction of syllables that start with consonants (ba-ba-ba). Most children can say "Dada" and "Mama" specifically by 12 mo, use several words by 18 mo, and combine words into some sentences by 2 yr. The average 3-yr-old can carry on a conversation. These milestones are highly variable.

Cognitive and social/emotional development: Cognitive and social/emotional development refers to the intellectual and psychologic maturation of children as their physical development allows them to interact more with other people and the external world. There are multiple theories of these forms of development in children and adolescents; the oldest and most famous are those proposed by Freud, Piaget, and Erikson. All are based on clinical observations, but none has been tested in large groups of children. In general, these models are considered useful for describing aspects of development in some children, but none is universally applicable. Increasingly, appropriate attachments and nurturing in infancy and early childhood are recognized as critical factors in cognitive growth and emotional health. For example, reading to a child from an early age, providing intellectually stimulating experiences, and providing warm and nurturing relationships all have a major impact on growth in these domains. Intellect is appraised in young children by observations of language skills, curiosity, and problem-solving abilities. As the child becomes more verbal, intellectual functioning becomes easier to assess using a number of specialized clinical tools. Once the child starts school, he undergoes constant monitoring as part of the academic process.

Emotional growth and the acquisition of social skills are assessed by watching the child interact with others in everyday situations. When the child acquires speech, the understanding of his emotional state becomes much more accurate. As with intellect, emotional functioning can be delineated more precisely with specialized tools.

SEXUAL DEVELOPMENT

Sexual maturation generally proceeds in an established sequence in both sexes. The age at onset and rapidity of sexual development vary and are influenced by genetic and environmental factors. Sexual maturity begins earlier today than a century ago, probably because of improvements in nutrition, general health, and living conditions. The physiologic changes that underlie sexual maturation are discussed in Ch. 227 (see p. 1943) and Ch. 243 (see p. 2069).

In boys, sexual changes begin with growth of the scrotum and testes, followed by lengthening of the penis and growth of the seminal vesicles and prostate. Next, pubic hair appears. Axillary and facial hair appears about 2 yr after pubic hair. The growth spurt usually begins a year after the testes start growing. The median age for 1st ejaculation (between 12½ and 14 yr in the US) is affected by psychologic, cultural, and biologic factors. First ejaculation takes place about 1 yr after penis growth accelerates. Gynecomastia, usually in the form of breast buds, is common in young adolescent boys and usually resolves within several years.

In most girls, breast budding is the 1st visible sign of sexual maturation, followed closely by the initiation of the growth spurt. Shortly thereafter, pubic hair and axillary hair appear. Menarche generally occurs about 2 yr after onset of breast development and when growth in height slows after reaching its peak. Menarche occurs within a wide range, with most girls starting their periods at 12 or 13 yr. The stages of breast growth and pubic hair development can be detailed using Tanner's method (see Figs. 243–3 and 243–4 on pp. 2071 and 2072).

If the order of sexual changes is disturbed, growth may be abnormal, and the physician should consider pathologic reasons.

270 PRINCIPLES OF DRUG TREATMENT IN CHILDREN

Drug treatment in children differs from that in adults, most obviously because it is usually weight-based. Doses (and dosing intervals) differ because of age-related variations in drug absorption, distribution, metabolism, and elimination; children cannot safely receive an adult drug dose, nor can it be assumed that a child's dose is proportional to an adult's (eg, that a 7-kg child requires 1/10 the dose of a 70-kg adult). Most drugs have not been adequately studied in children, although legislation (the Best Pharmaceuticals for Children Act of 2001 and the Pediatric Research Equity Act of 2003) provides the statutory and regulatory authority to begin those studies.

Adverse effects and toxicity: Children are generally subject to the same adverse effects as adults (see p. 2533), but they have increased risk with certain drugs because of differences in pharmacokinetics or because of drug effects on growth and development. Common drugs with unique or higher risk of adverse effects in children are listed in TABLE 270–1.

Younger children are at especially high risk of accidental poisoning when they discover and take caregivers' vitamins or drugs. Infants are at risk for toxicity from drugs used by adults; toxicity can occur prenatally when they are exposed via placental transfer or postnatally through breast milk (numerous agents—see p. 2227 and TABLE 266–4 on p. 2228) or skin contact with caregivers who have recently applied certain topical drugs (eg, scopolamine for motion sickness, malathion for lice, diphenhydramine for poison ivy).

TABLE 270–1. DRUGS MANIFESTING UNUSUAL TOXICITY IN CHILDREN

DRUG	CLINICAL SYNDROME	MECHANISM	COMMENTS
Anesthetics (topical)	Cyanosis	Formation of methemoglobin (ferrous iron oxidized to ferric iron)	Incidence rare; examples of agents include benzocaine and a mixture of lidocaine and prilocaine
Ceftriaxone	Jaundice and kernicterus	Bilirubin displaced from albumin	Neonates only
Diphenoxylate	Respiratory depression, death	CNS depression (in immature CNS)	Overdose syndrome, usually seen in children < 2 yr
Fluoroquinolones	Cartilage toxicity	Unknown	Suspected on basis of animal studies but adverse effects in humans unproven
Hexachlorophene	Cystic brain lesions, death	Unknown	Topical disinfectant used to wash preterm infants; no longer used
Lindane (topical)	Seizures, CNS toxicity	Probably enhanced absorption in children	Use alternative agent in those < 50 kg
Prochlorperazine	Altered CNS function, extrapyramidal effects, opisthotonus, bulging fontanelles	Actions via multiple CNS receptors	Febrile and dehydrated infants especially at risk
Tetracycline	Discoloration and pitting of tooth enamel	Chelation with Ca in growing teeth	Restricted to children < 8 yr

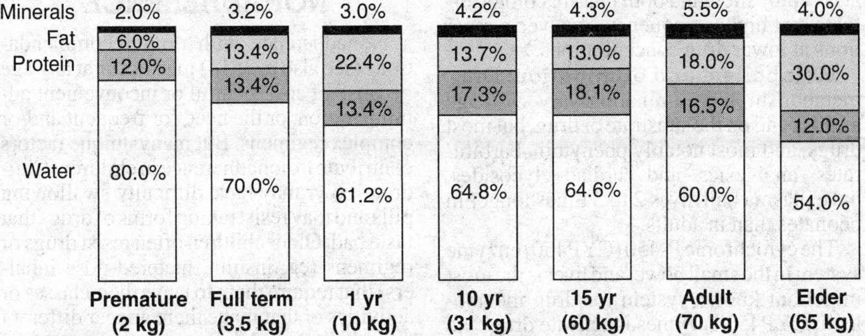

Fig. 270–1. Changes in body proportions of body composition with growth and aging. Adapted from Puig M: Body composition and growth. In *Nutrition in Pediatrics*, ed. 2, edited by WA Walker and JB Watkins. Hamilton, Ontario, BC Decker, 1996.

PHARMACOKINETICS

Pharmacokinetics refers to the processes of drug absorption, distribution, metabolism, and elimination (see p. 2520).

Absorption: Absorption from the GI tract is affected by gastric acid secretion, bile salt formation, gastric emptying time, intestinal motility, and microbial flora. All are reduced in neonates, and all may be reduced or increased in an ill child of any age. Reduced gastric acid secretion increases bioavailability of acid-labile drugs (eg, penicillin) and decreases bioavailability of weakly acidic drugs (eg, phenobarbital). Reduced bile salt formation decreases bioavailability of lipophilic drugs (eg, diazepam). Reduced gastric emptying and intestinal motility increase the time it takes to reach therapeutic concentrations when enteral drugs are given to infants < 3 mo. Drug-metabolizing enzymes present in the intestines of young infants are another cause of reduced drug absorption.

Injected drugs are often erratically absorbed because of variability in their chemical characteristics, differences in absorption by site of injection (IM or sc), variability in muscle mass among children, and illness (eg, compromised circulatory status). IM injections are generally avoided in children because of pain and the possibility of tissue damage, but when needed, water-soluble drugs are best because they do not precipitate at the injection site.

Transdermal absorption may be enhanced in neonates and young infants because the stratum corneum is thin and because the ratio of surface area to weight is much greater than for older children and adults. Skin disruptions (eg, abrasions, eczema, burns) increase absorption in children of any age.

Transrectal drug administration is generally appropriate only for emergencies when an IV route is not available (eg, use of rectal diazepam for status epilepticus). Site of placement of the drug within the rectal cavity may influence absorption because of the difference in venous drainage systems. Expulsion of the drug may also be enhanced in the young infant.

Absorption of drugs from the lung (eg, β-agonists for asthma, pulmonary surfactant for hyaline membrane disease) varies less by physiologic parameters and more by reliability of the delivery device and patient or caregiver technique.

Distribution: The volume of distribution of drugs in children changes with age because of changes in body composition (especially the extracellular and total body water spaces) and plasma protein binding.

Higher doses (per kilogram of body weight) of water-soluble drugs are required in younger children because a higher percentage of their body weight is water (see FIG. 270–1). Conversely, lower doses are required to avoid toxicity as children grow older because of the decline in water as a percentage of body weight.

Many drugs bind to proteins (primarily albumin, α_1-acid glycoprotein, and lipoproteins); protein binding limits distribution of free drug throughout the body. Albumin and total protein concentrations are lower in neonates but approach adult levels by 10 to 12 mo. Decreased protein binding in neonates is also due to qualitative differences in binding proteins and to competitive binding by molecules such as bilirubin and free fatty acids, which circulate in higher concentrations in neonates and infants. The net result may be increased free drug concentrations, greater drug availability at receptor sites, and both pharmacologic effects and higher frequency of adverse reactions at lower drug concentrations.

Metabolism and elimination: Drug metabolism and elimination vary with age and depend on the substrate or drug, but most drugs, and most notably phenytoin, barbiturates, analgesics, and cardiac glycosides, have plasma half-lives 2 to 3 times longer in neonates than in adults.

The cytochrome P-450 (CYP450) enzyme system in the small bowel and liver is the most important known system for drug metabolism; CYP450 enzymes inactivate drugs via oxidation, reduction, and hydrolysis (phase I metabolism) and via hydroxylation and conjugation (phase II metabolism). Phase I activity is reduced in neonates, increases progressively during the 1st 6 mo of life, exceeds adult rates by the 1st few years for some drugs, slows during adolescence, and usually attains adult rates by late puberty. However, adult rates of metabolism may be achieved for some drugs (eg, barbiturates, phenytoin) 2 to 4 wk postnatally. CYP450 activity can also be induced (reducing drug concentrations and effect) or inhibited (augmenting concentrations and effect) by coadministered drugs. Kidneys, lungs, and skin also play a role in the metabolism of some drugs, as do intestinal drug-metabolizing enzymes in neonates. Phase II metabolism varies considerably by substrate. Maturation of enzymes responsible for bilirubin and acetaminophen conjugation is delayed; enzymes responsible for morphine conjugation are fully mature even in preterm infants.

Drug metabolites are eliminated primarily through bile or the kidneys. Renal elimination depends on plasma protein binding, renal blood flow, GFR, and tubular secretion, all of which are altered in the 1st 2 yr of life. Renal plasma flow is low at birth (12 mL/min) and reaches adult levels of 140 mL/min by age 1 yr. Similarly, GFR is 2 to 4 mL/min at birth, increases to 8 to 20 mL/min by 2 to 3 days, and reaches adult levels of 120 mL/min by 3 to 5 mo.

Drug dosing: Because of the above factors, drug dosing in children < 12 yr is always a function of age, body weight, or both. This approach is practical but not ideal; even within a population of similar age and weight, drug requirements may differ because of maturational differences in absorption, metabolism, and elimination. Thus, when practical, dose adjustments should be based on plasma drug concentration. Unfortunately, this is not feasible for most drugs.

NONADHERENCE

Nonadherence with drug recommendations (see also p. 2514) may occur at any age because of cost, painful or inconvenient administration, or the need for frequent and/or complex regimens. But many unique factors contribute to nonadherence in children. Children < 6 yr may have difficulty swallowing pills and may resist taking forms of drugs that taste bad. Older children often resist drugs or regimens (eg, insulin, metered-dose inhalers) that require them to leave their classes or activities or that make them appear different from their peers. Adolescents may express rebellion and assert independence from parents by not taking their drugs. Parents or caregivers of younger children may only partially remember or understand the rationale and instructions for taking a drug, and their work schedules may preclude their being available to give children their scheduled doses. Some may wish to try folk or herbal remedies initially. Some caregivers have limited incomes and are forced to spend their money on other priorities, such as food; others have beliefs and attitudes that prevent them from giving children drugs.

To minimize nonadherence, a prescribing provider can do the following:

- Ascertain whether the patient or caregiver agrees with the diagnosis, perceives it as serious, and believes the treatment will work
- Correct misunderstandings and guide the patient or caregiver toward reliable sources of information
- Give written in addition to oral instructions in language the patient or caregiver can review and understand
- Make early follow-up telephone calls to families to answer residual questions
- Assess progress and remind the patient or caregiver of follow-up visits
- Review drug bottles at follow-up office visits for pill counts
- Educate the patient or caregiver about how to keep a daily symptom or drug diary.

Adolescents in particular need to feel in control of their illness and treatment and should be encouraged to communicate freely and to take as much responsibility as is possible for their own treatment. Regimens should be simplified (eg, synchronizing multiple drugs and minimizing the number of daily doses while maintaining efficacy) and matched to the patient's and caregivers' schedules. Critical aspects of the treatment should be emphasized (eg, taking the full course of an antibiotic). If lifestyle changes (eg, in diet or exercise) are also needed, such changes should be introduced incrementally over several visits, and realistic goals should be set (eg, to lose 1 of 14 kg [2 of 30 lb] by a 2-wk follow-up visit). Success in achieving a goal should be reinforced with praise, and only then should the next goal be added. For patients who require expensive long-term regimens, a list of pharmaceutical patient-assistance programs is available at www.needymeds.com.

271 PERINATAL PHYSIOLOGY

The transition from life in utero to life outside the womb involves multiple changes in physiology and function.

Bilirubin: Aged or damaged fetal RBCs are removed from the circulation by reticuloendothelial cells, which convert heme to bilirubin (1 g of Hb yields 35 mg of bilirubin). This bilirubin is transported to the liver, where it is transferred into hepatocytes. Glucuronyl transferase then conjugates the bilirubin with uridine diphosphoglucuronic acid (UDPGA) to form bilirubin diglucuronide (conjugated bilirubin), which is secreted actively into the bile ducts. Bilirubin diglucuronide makes its way into meconium in the GI tract but cannot be eliminated from the body, because the fetus does not normally pass stool. The enzyme β-glucuronidase, present in the fetus' small-bowel luminal brush border, is released into the intestinal lumen, where it deconjugates bilirubin glucuronide; free (unconjugated) bilirubin is then reabsorbed from the intestinal tract and reenters the fetal circulation. Fetal bilirubin is cleared from the circulation by placental transfer into the mother's plasma following a concentration gradient. The maternal liver then conjugates and excretes the fetal bilirubin.

At birth, the placenta is "lost," and although the neonate's liver continues to take up, conjugate, and excrete bilirubin into bile so it can be eliminated in the stool, the neonate lacks proper intestinal bacteria for oxidizing bilirubin to urobilinogen in the gut; consequently, unaltered bilirubin remains in the stool, imparting a typical bright-yellow color. Additionally, the neonate's GI tract (like that of the fetus) contains β-glucuronidase, which deconjugates some of the bilirubin. In many neonates, feedings produce the gastrocolic reflex, and bilirubin is excreted in stool before most of it can be deconjugated and reabsorbed. However in many others, the unconjugated bilirubin is reabsorbed and returned to the circulation from the intestinal lumen (enterohepatic circulation of bilirubin), contributing to physiologic hyperbilirubinemia and jaundice (see also p. 2275).

Cardiovascular: Fetal circulation is marked by right-to-left shunting of blood around unoxygenated lungs through a patent ductus arteriosus (connecting the pulmonary artery to the aorta) and foramen ovale (connecting the right and left atria). Shunting is encouraged by high pulmonary arteriolar resistance and relatively low resistance to blood flow in the systemic (including placental) circulation. About 90 to 95% of the right heart output bypasses the lungs and goes directly to the systemic circulation. The fetal ductus arteriosus is kept open by low fetal systemic PaO_2 (about 25 mm Hg) along with locally produced prostaglandins. The foramen ovale is kept open by differences in atrial pressures: left atrial pressure is relatively low because little blood is returned from the lungs, but right atrial pressure is relatively high because large volumes of blood return from the placenta.

Profound changes to this system occur after the first few breaths, resulting in increased pulmonary blood flow and closure of the foramen ovale. Pulmonary arteriolar resistance drops acutely as a result of vasodilation caused by lung expansion, increased PaO_2, and reduced $PaCO_2$. The elastic forces of the ribs and chest wall decrease pulmonary interstitial pressure, further enhancing blood flow through pulmonary capillaries.

As pulmonary blood flow is established, venous return from the lungs increases, raising left atrial pressure. Air breathing increases the PaO_2, which constricts the umbilical arteries. Placental blood flow is reduced or stops, reducing blood return to the right atrium. Thus, right atrial pressure decreases while left atrial pressure increases; as a result, the foramen ovale closes.

Soon after birth, systemic resistance becomes higher than pulmonary resistance, a reversal from the fetal state. Therefore, the direction of blood flow through the patent ductus arteriosus reverses, creating left-to-right shunting of blood (called transitional circulation). This state lasts from moments after birth (when the pulmonary blood flow increases and functional closure of the foramen ovale occurs) until about 24 to 72 h of age, when the ductus arteriosus usually closes. Blood entering the ductus and its vasa vasorum from the aorta has a high PO_2, which, along with alterations in prostaglandin metabolism, leads to constriction and closure of the ductus arteriosus. Once the ductus arteriosus closes, an adult-type circulation exists. The 2 ventricles now pump in series, and there are no major shunts between the pulmonary and systemic circulations.

During the days immediately after birth, a stressed neonate may revert to a fetal-type circulation. Asphyxia with hypoxia and hypercarbia causes the pulmonary arterioles to constrict and the ductus arteriosus to dilate, reversing the processes described above and resulting in right-to-left shunting through the now-patent ductus arteriosus, the reopened foramen ovale, or both. Consequently, the neonate becomes severely hypoxemic, a condition called persistent pulmonary hypertension or persistent fetal circulation (although there is no umbilical circulation). The goal of treatment is to reverse the conditions that produced pulmonary vasoconstriction.

Endocrine: The fetus depends completely on the maternal supply of glucose via the placenta and does not contribute to glucose production. The fetus begins to build a hepatic glycogen supply early in gestation, accumulating most glycogen stores during the 2nd half of the 3rd trimester. The neonate's glucose supply terminates when the umbilical cord is cut; concurrently, levels of circulating epinephrine, norepinephrine, and glucagon surge, while insulin levels decline. These changes stimulate gluconeogenesis and mobilization of hepatic glycogen stores. In healthy, term neonates, glucose levels reach a nadir 30 to 90 min after birth, after which neonates are typically able to maintain normal glucose homeostasis. Infants at highest risk for neonatal hypoglycemia include those with reduced glycogen stores (small-for-gestational-age and premature infants), critically ill infants with increased glucose catabolism, and infants of diabetic mothers (secondary to temporary fetal hyperinsulinemia).

Hemoglobin: In utero, RBC production is controlled exclusively by fetal erythropoietin produced in the liver; maternal erythropoietin does not cross the placenta. About 55 to 90% of fetal RBCs contain fetal Hb, which has high O_2 affinity. As a result, a high O_2 concentration gradient is maintained across the placenta, resulting in abundant O_2 transfer from the maternal to the fetal circulation. This increased O_2 affinity is less useful after birth, because fetal Hb gives up O_2 to tissues less readily, and it may be deleterious if severe pulmonary or cardiac disease with hypoxemia exists. The transition from fetal to adult Hb begins before birth; at delivery, the site of erythropoietin production changes from the liver to the kidney by an unknown mechanism. The abrupt increase in PaO_2 from about 25 to 30 mm Hg in the fetus to 90 to 95 mm Hg in the neonate just after delivery causes serum erythropoietin to fall, and RBC production shuts down between birth and about 6 to 8 wk, causing physiologic anemia and contributing to anemia of prematurity (see p. 2270).

Immunologic: At term, most immune mechanisms are not fully functional, more so with increasing prematurity. Thus, all neonates and young infants are immunodeficient relative to adults and are at increased risk for overwhelming infection. This risk is enhanced by prematurity, maternal illness, neonatal stress, and drugs (eg, immunosuppressants and anticonvulsants). The neonate's decreased immune response may explain the absence of localized clinical signs (eg, fever or meningismus) in the setting of infection.

In the fetus, phagocytic cells, present at the yolk sac stage of development, are critical for the inflammatory response that combats bacterial and fungal infection. Granulocytes and monocytes can be identified in the 2nd and 4th mo of gestation, respectively. Their level of function increases with gestational age but is still low at term.

At birth, the ultrastructure of neutrophils is normal, but in most neonates, chemotaxis of neutrophils and monocytes is decreased because of an intrinsic abnormality of cellular locomotion and adherence to surfaces. These functional deficits are more pronounced in premature infants.

By about the 14th wk of gestation, the thymus is functioning and producing lymphocytes. Also by 14 wk, T cells are present in the fetal liver and spleen, indicating that mature

T cells are established in the peripheral lymphoid organs by this age. The thymus is most active during fetal development and in early postnatal life. It grows rapidly in utero and is readily noted on chest x-ray in the healthy neonate, reaching a peak size at age 10 yr then involuting gradually over many years.

The number of T cells in the fetal circulation gradually increases during the 2nd trimester and reaches nearly normal levels by 30 to 32 wk gestation. At birth, the neonate has a relative T lymphocytosis compared to the adult. However, neonatal T cells do not function as effectively as adult T cells. For example, neonatal T cells may not respond adequately to antigens and may not produce cytokines.

B cells are present in fetal bone marrow, blood, liver, and spleen by the 12th wk of gestation. Trace amounts of IgM and IgG can be detected by the 20th wk and of IgA by the 30th wk; because the fetus is normally in an antigen-free environment, only small amounts of immunoglobulin (predominantly IgM) are produced in utero. Elevated levels of cord serum IgM indicate in utero antigen challenge, usually from congenital infection. Almost all IgG is acquired maternally from the placenta. After 22 wk gestation, placental transfer of IgG increases to reach maternal levels or greater at term. IgG levels at birth in premature infants are decreased relative to gestational age.

The passive transfer of maternal immunity from transplacental IgG and secretory IgA and antimicrobial factors in breast milk (eg, IgG, secretory IgA, WBCs, complement proteins, lysozyme, and lactoferrin) compensate for the neonate's immature immune system and confer immunity to many bacteria and viruses. Protective immune factors in breast milk coat the GI and upper respiratory tracts via mucosa-associated lymphoid tissue and prevent invasion of mucous membranes by respiratory and enteric pathogens.

Over time, passive immunity begins to wane, reaching a nadir when the infant is 3 to 6 mo old. Premature infants, in particular, may become profoundly hypogammaglobulinemic during the 1st 6 mo of life. By 1 yr, the IgG level rises to about 60% of average adult levels. IgA, IgM, IgD, and IgE, which do not cross the placenta and therefore are detectable only in trace amounts at birth, increase slowly during childhood. IgG, IgM, and IgA reach adult levels by about age 10 yr.

Pulmonary: Fetal lungs develop throughout gestation, and fairly well-developed alveoli are present by the 25th wk. The lungs continually produce fluid, a transudate from pulmonary capillaries plus surfactant secreted by type II pneumocytes. For normal gas exchange to occur at birth, pulmonary alveolar fluid and interstitial fluid must be cleared promptly by compression of the fetal thorax during delivery and by absorption of fluid into cells in the lung. Transient tachypnea of the newborn (see p. 2304) is probably caused by delay in this clearance process.

On delivery, when elastic recoil of ribs and strong inspiratory efforts draw air into the pulmonary tree, air-fluid interfaces are formed in alveoli. At the 1st breath, large amounts of surfactant are released into the air-fluid interfaces of infants ≥ 34 to 35 wk. Surfactant, a mixture of phospholipids (phosphatidylcholine, phosphatidyl glycerol, phosphatidylinositol), neutral lipids, and 3 surface active proteins all stored in lamellar inclusions in type II pneumocytes, reduces high surface tension, which would otherwise cause atelectasis and increase the work of breathing.

Before 34 to 35 wk gestation, surfactant is often not produced in sufficient quantities to prevent diffuse atelectasis, and respiratory distress syndrome develops (see p. 2303).

Renal: At birth, renal function is generally reduced, particularly in premature infants. GFR increases progressively during gestation, particularly during the 3rd trimester. By age 1 to 2 yr, GFR, urea clearance, and maximum tubular clearances have reached adult levels.

272 PERINATAL PROBLEMS

Extensive physiologic changes accompany the birth process, sometimes revealing conditions that posed no problem during intrauterine life. For that reason, a person with resuscitation skills must attend each birth. Each neonate is classified as premature, full-term, or postmature to help determine the risk for various complications.

Gestational age, the primary determinant of organ maturity, can be determined in the days

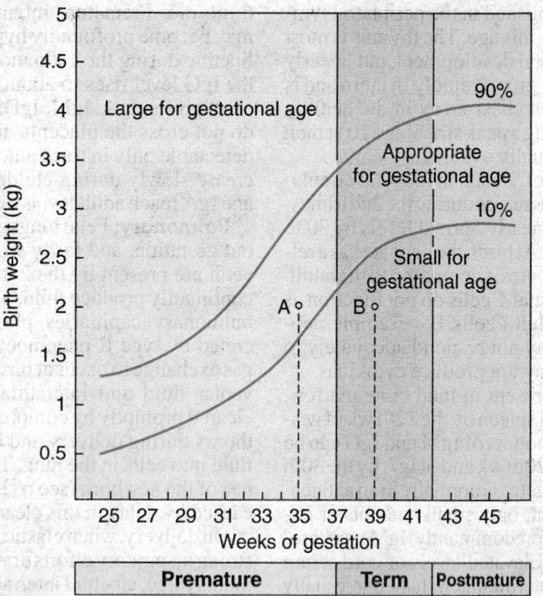

Fig. 272–1. Level of intrauterine growth based on birth weight and gestational age of liveborn, single, white infants. Point A represents a premature infant, while point B indicates an infant of similar birth weight who is mature but small for gestational age. The growth curves are representative of the 10th and 90th percentiles for all of the neonates in the sampling. (Adapted from Sweet AY: Classification of the low-birth-weight infant. In *Care of the High-Risk Neonate,* ed. 3, edited by MH Klaus and AA Fanaroff. Philadelphia, WB Saunders Company, 1986; used with permission.)

immediately after birth using the Ballard score (see FIG. 266–1 on p. 2221). Through plotting of weight vs gestational age (see FIG. 272–1), each infant is classified as small, appropriate, or large for gestational age. Head circumference and length are also plotted against gestational age (see FIG. 272–2). These parameters are influenced by genetic factors and intrauterine conditions. They also help to predict subsequent growth and development.

NEONATAL RESUSCITATION

About 10% of neonates require some degree of resuscitation at delivery. Causes are numerous (see TABLE 272–1), but most involve asphyxia or respiratory depression. Incidence rises significantly if birth weight is < 1500 g.

Assessment: The Apgar score assigns 0 to 2 points for each of 5 measures of neonatal health (Appearance, Pulse, Grimace, Activity, Respiration—see TABLE 272–2). Scores depend on physiologic maturity, maternal perinatal therapy, and fetal cardiorespiratory and neurologic conditions. A score of 7 to 10 at 5 min is considered normal; 4 to 6, intermediate; and 0 to 3, low. A low Apgar score is not *by itself* diagnostic of perinatal asphyxia but is associated with a risk of long-term neurologic dysfunction. An unduly prolonged (> 10 min) low Apgar score predicts increased risk of mortality in the 1st yr of life.

The earliest sign of asphyxia is acral cyanosis, followed by decreases in respiration, muscle tone, reflex response, and heart rate. Effective resuscitation leads initially to increased heart rate, followed by improved reflex response, color, respiration, and muscle tone. Evidence of intrapartum fetal distress, persistence of an Apgar score of 0 to 3 for > 5 min, an umbilical arterial blood pH < 7, and a sustained neonatal neurologic syndrome that includes hypotonia, coma, seizures, and evidence of multiorgan dysfunction are manifestations of perinatal asphyxia. The severity and prognosis of

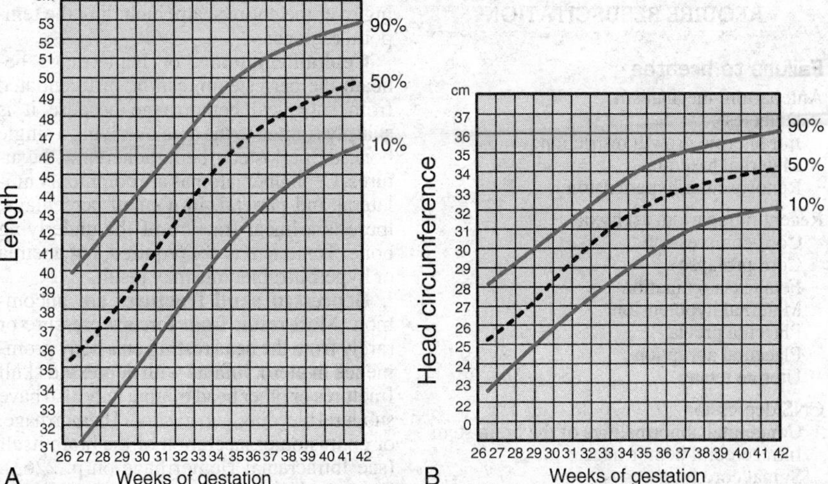

Fig. 272–2. Level of intrauterine growth based on gestational age, body length *(A)*, and head circumference *(B)* at birth. (Adapted from Lubchenco LC, Hansman C, Boyd E: Intrauterine growth in length and head circumference as estimated from live births at gestational ages from 26 to 42 weeks. *Pediatrics* 37:403, 1966; reproduced by permission of *Pediatrics*.)

posthypoxic encephalopathy can be estimated with the Sarnat classification (see TABLE 272–3) in conjunction with EEG, neuroradiologic imaging, and brain stem auditory and cortical evoked responses.

Resuscitation: Initial measures for all neonates include suctioning and tactile stimulation. Suctioning of the mouth, nose, and pharynx should be done before delivery of the thorax, especially in neonates delivered through meconium-stained amniotic fluid, and then performed intermittently, avoiding deep oropharyngeal suctioning. Suctioning requires appropriately sized catheters (see TABLE 64–4 on p. 540) and pressure limits of 100 mm Hg (136 cm H_2O). Tactile stimulation (eg, flicking the soles of the feet, rubbing the back) may be necessary to encourage regular, spontaneous breathing. Infants not responding with appropriate respirations and heart rate require O_2 administration, bag-mask ventilation, sometimes endotracheal intubation, and much less commonly, chest compressions (see also FIGS. 272–3 and 64–7 on p. 543).

The infant is quickly dried and placed supine under a preheated overhead warmer in the delivery room. The neck is supported in the neutral position with a rolled towel under the shoulders.

O_2 should be administered at 10 L/min through a face mask attached to a self-inflatable or anesthesia bag; if no mask is available, O_2 tubing may be placed adjacent the face and set to deliver 5 L/min. If spontaneous respirations are absent or heart rate is < 100 beats/min, respirations are assisted with the bag-mask. *Bradycardia in a distressed child is a sign of impending cardiac arrest; neonates tend to develop bradycardia with hypoxemia.* Advanced resuscitation techniques, including endotracheal intubation, and selection of equipment size, drugs and dosages, and CPR parameters are discussed in Ch. 64 on p. 524.

BIRTH INJURIES

The forces of labor and delivery occasionally cause physical injury to the infant. The incidence of neonatal injury from difficult or traumatic deliveries is decreasing due to increasing use of cesarean section in place of difficult versions, vacuum extractions, or mid- or high-forceps deliveries.

A traumatic delivery is anticipated when the mother has small pelvic measurements, when the infant seems large for gestational age (often the case with diabetic mothers), or when there is a breech or other abnormal presentation, especially in a primipara. In such situations, labor and the fetal condition should be monitored closely. If fetal distress

TABLE 272–1. PROBLEMS THAT MAY REQUIRE RESUSCITATION

Failure to breathe

Antepartum mechanism
- Diabetes
- Intrauterine growth restriction
- Maternal toxemia
- Renovascular hypertension

Recent intrapartum asphyxia
- Cord compression
- Cord prolapse
- Fetal exsanguination
- Maternal hypotension
- Placenta previa
- Placental abruption
- Uterine tetany

CNS depression
- Congenital abnormalities of the brain stem
- Intracerebral hemorrhage
- Spinal cord injury

Drugs
- Analgesics or hypnotics
- Anesthetics
- Magnesium
- Opioids, maternal drug abuse

Failure to expand the lungs

Airway obstruction
- Blood
- Meconium
- Mucus

Prematurity (respiratory distress syndrome)

Malformations involving the respiratory tract
- Agenesis
- Diaphragmatic hernia
- Hypoplasia
- Stenosis or atresia

is detected, the mother should be positioned on her side and given O_2. If fetal distress persists, an immediate cesarean section should be performed.

HEAD INJURIES

Head molding is common in vaginal delivery due to the high pressure exerted by uterine contractions on the infant's malleable cranium as it passes through the birth canal. This rarely causes problems or requires treatment.

Caput succedaneum is edema of the presenting portion of the scalp. It occurs when the area is forced against the uterine cervix. Subgaleal hemorrhage results from greater trauma and is characterized by a boggy feeling over the entire scalp, including the temporal regions.

Cephalhematoma, or hemorrhage beneath the periosteum, can be differentiated from subgaleal hemorrhage because it is sharply limited to the area overlying a single bone, the periosteum being adherent at the sutures. Cephalhematomas are commonly unilateral and parietal. In a small percentage, there is a linear fracture of the underlying bone. Treatment is not required, but anemia or hyperbilirubinemia may result.

Depressed skull fractures are uncommon. Most result from forceps pressure or rarely from the head resting on a bony prominence in utero. Infants with depressed skull fractures or other head trauma may also have subdural bleeding, subarachnoid hemorrhage, or contusion or laceration of the brain itself (see Intracranial Hemorrhage on p. 2263). Depressed skull fractures produce a palpable (and sometimes visible) step-off deformity, which must be differentiated from the palpable elevated periosteal rim occurring with cephalhematomas. CT scan is obtained to confirm the diagnosis and rule out complications. Neurosurgical elevation may be needed.

CRANIAL NERVE INJURY

The facial nerve is injured most often. Although frequently attributed to forceps pressure, most injuries probably result from pressure on the nerve in utero, which may be due to fetal positioning (eg, from the head lying against the shoulder, the sacral promontory, or a uterine fibroid).

Facial nerve injury usually occurs at or distal to its exit from the stylomastoid foramen and results in facial asymmetry, especially during crying. Identifying which side of the face is affected can be confusing, but the facial muscles on the side of the nerve injury cannot move. Injury can also occur to individual branches of the nerve, most often the mandibular. Another cause of facial asymmetry is mandibular asymmetry resulting from intrauterine pressure; in this case, muscle innervation is intact and both sides of the face can move. In mandibular asymmetry, the maxillary and the mandibular occlusal surfaces are not parallel, which differentiates it from a facial nerve injury. Testing or treatment is not needed for peripheral facial nerve injuries or mandibular asymmetry. They usually resolve by age 2 to 3 mo.

TABLE 272–2. APGAR SCORE

CRITERIA	MNEMONIC	SCORE* 0	1	2
Color	**A**ppearance	All blue, pale	Pink body, blue extremities	All pink
Heart rate	**P**ulse	Absent	< 100 beats/min	> 100 beats/min
Reflex response to nasal catheter/ tactile stimulation	**G**rimace	None	Grimace	Sneeze, cough
Muscle tone	**A**ctivity	Limp	Some flexion of extremities	Active
Respiration	**R**espiration	Absent	Irregular, slow	Good, crying

*A total score of 7–10 at 5 min is considered normal; 4–6, intermediate; and 0–3, low.

Brachial Plexus Injuries

Brachial plexus injuries follow stretching caused by shoulder dystocia, breech extraction, or hyperabduction of the neck in cephalic presentations. Injuries can be due to simple stretching, hemorrhage within a nerve, tearing of the nerve or root, or avulsion of the roots with accompanying cervical cord injury. Associated injuries (eg, fractures of the clavicle or humerus or subluxations of the shoulder or cervical spine) may occur.

Injuries of the upper brachial plexus (C5 to C6) affect muscles around the shoulder and elbow, whereas lesions of the lower plexus (C7 to C8 and T1) primarily affect muscles of the forearm and hand. The site and type of nerve root injury determine the prognosis.

Erb's palsy is an upper brachial plexus injury causing adduction and internal rotation of the shoulder with pronation of the forearm. Ipsilateral paralysis of the diaphragm is common. Treatment includes protecting the shoulder from excessive motion by immobilizing the arm across the upper abdomen and preventing contractures by passive range-of-motion exercises to involved joints performed gently every day starting at 1 wk of age.

Klumpke's palsy is a lower plexus injury resulting in paralysis of the hand and wrist, often with ipsilateral Horner's syndrome (miosis, ptosis, facial anhidrosis). Passive range-of-motion exercises are the only treatment needed.

Neither Erb's nor Klumpke's palsy usually produces demonstrable sensory loss, which suggests a tear or avulsion. These conditions usually improve rapidly, but deficits can persist. If a significant deficit persists > 3 mo, MRI is performed to determine the extent of injury to the plexus, roots, and cervical cord. Surgical exploration and repair have sometimes been helpful.

When the entire brachial plexus is injured, the involved upper extremity cannot move, and sensory loss is usually present. Ipsilateral pyramidal signs indicate spinal cord trauma; an MRI should be performed. The involved extremity's subsequent growth may be impaired. The prognosis for recovery is poor. Management may include neurosurgical exploration. Passive range-of-motion exercises can prevent contractures.

Other Peripheral Nerve Injuries

Injuries to other peripheral nerves (eg, the radial, sciatic, obturator) are rare in neonates and are usually not related to labor and delivery. They are usually secondary to a local traumatic event (eg, an injection in or near the sciatic nerve). Treatment includes placing the muscles antagonistic to those paralyzed at rest until recovery. Neurosurgical exploration of the nerve is seldom indicated. In most peripheral nerve injuries, recovery is complete.

Spinal Cord Injury

Spinal cord injury (see also p. 2583) is rare and involves variable degrees of cord disruption, often with hemorrhage. Complete disruption of the cord is very rare. Trauma usually occurs in breech deliveries after excess longitudinal traction to the spine. It can also follow hyperextension of the fetal neck in utero (the "flying fetus"). Injury usually affects

TABLE 272–3. CLINICAL STAGING OF POSTHYPOXIC ENCEPHALOPATHY

FACTOR	STAGE I (MILD)	STAGE II (MODERATE)	STAGE III (SEVERE)
Duration	< 24 h	2–14 days	Hours to weeks
Level of consciousness	Hyperalertness and irritability	Lethargy	Deep stupor or coma
Muscle tone	Normal	Hypotonia or proximal limb weakness	Flaccidity
Tendon reflexes	Increased	Increased	Depressed or absent
Myoclonus	Present	Present	Absent
Complex reflexes			
Sucking	Active	Weak	Absent
Moro response	Exaggerated	Incomplete	Absent
Grasping	Normal to exaggerated	Exaggerated	Absent
Oculocephalic (doll's eye)	Normal	Overreactive	Reduced or absent
Autonomic function			
Pupils	Dilated	Constricted	Variable or fixed
Respiration	Regular	Variable in rate and depth, periodic	Irregular apnea
Heart rate	Normal or tachycardic	Low resting < 120 beats/min	Bradycardia
Seizures	None	Common (70%)	Uncommon
EEG	Normal	Low voltage, periodic or paroxysmal, epileptiform activity	Periodic or isoelectric
Risk of death	< 1%	5%	> 60%
Risk of severe handicap	< 1%	20%	> 70%

Adapted from Sarnat HB, Sarnat MS: Neonatal encephalopathy following fetal distress. *Archives of Neurology* 33:696–705, 1975.

the lower cervical region (C5 to C7). When the injury is higher, lesions are generally fatal because respiration is completely compromised. Sometimes a click or snap is heard at delivery.

Spinal shock with flaccidity below the level of injury occurs initially. Usually, there is patchy retention of sensation or movement below the lesion. Spasticity develops within days or weeks. Breathing is diaphragmatic, because the phrenic nerve remains intact as it arises higher (C3 to C5) than the typical cord lesion. When the spinal cord lesion is complete, the intercostal and abdominal muscles become paralyzed and rectal and bladder sphincters cannot develop voluntary control. Sensation and sweating are lost below the involved level, which can cause fluctuations of body temperature with environmental changes.

An MRI of the cervical cord may demonstrate the lesion and excludes surgically treatable lesions, such as congenital tumors or hematomas pressing on the cord. The CSF is usually bloody.

With appropriate care, most infants survive for many years. The usual causes of death are recurring pneumonia and progressive loss of renal function. Treatment includes nursing care to prevent skin ulcerations, prompt treatment of urinary and respiratory infections,

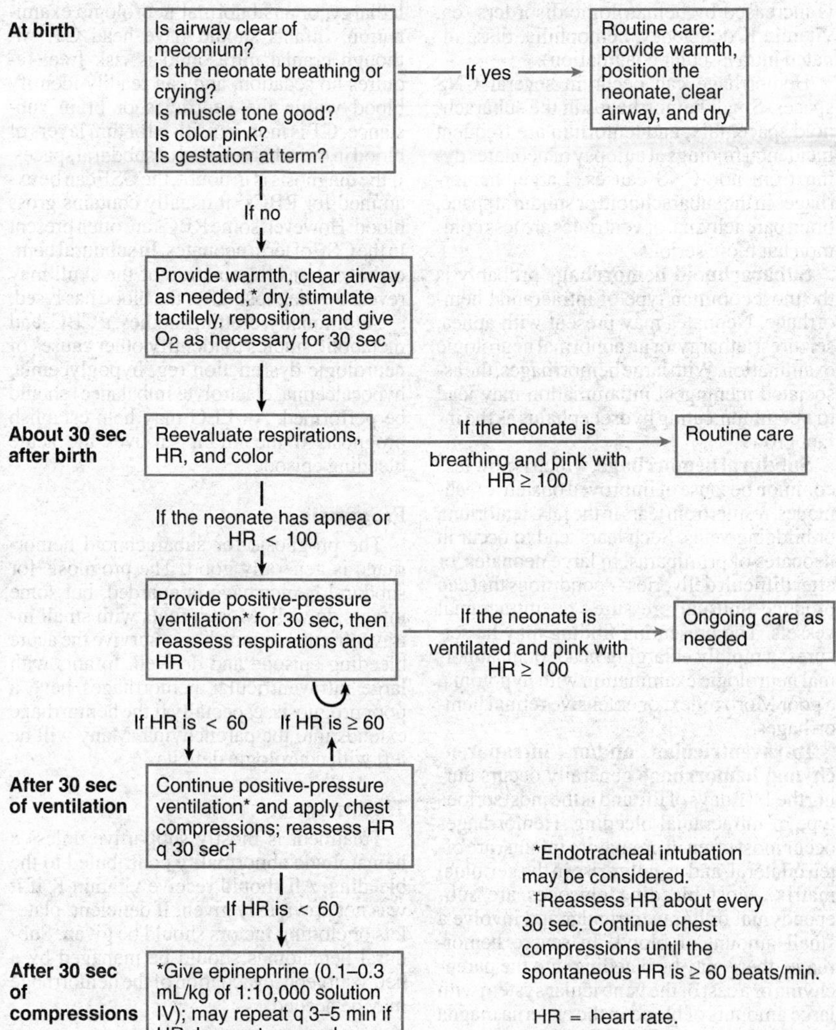

Fig. 272–3. Algorithm for resuscitation of neonates. (Adapted from *Neonatal Resuscitation Textbook*, ed. 4. American Academy of Pediatrics and American Heart Association, Appendix, pp. 6–7, 2000.)

and regular evaluations to identify obstructive uropathy early.

INTRACRANIAL HEMORRHAGE

Hemorrhage in or around the brain can occur in any neonate but is particularly common in those born prematurely; about 20% of premature infants < 1500 g have intracranial hemorrhage. Hypoxia-ischemia, variations in BP, and pressures exerted on the head during labor are major causes. The presence of the germinal matrix (a mass of embryonic cells lying over the caudate nucleus on the lateral wall of the lateral ventricles and present only in the fetus) makes hemorrhage more likely. Risk also is increased by hematologic disorders (eg, vitamin K deficiency, hemophilia, disseminated intravascular coagulation).

Hemorrhage can occur in several CNS spaces. Small hemorrhages in the subarachnoid space, falx, and tentorium are frequent incidental findings at autopsy of neonates dying from non-CNS causes. Larger hemorrhages in the subarachnoid or subdural space, brain parenchyma, or ventricles are less common but more serious.

Subarachnoid hemorrhage probably is the most common type of intracranial hemorrhage. Neonates may present with apnea, seizures, lethargy, or an abnormal neurologic examination. With large hemorrhages, the associated meningeal inflammation may lead to a communicating hydrocephalus as the infant grows.

Subdural hemorrhage, which is now less common because of improved obstetric techniques, results from tears in the falx, tentorium, or bridging veins. Such tears tend to occur in neonates of primiparas, in large neonates, or after difficult deliveries—conditions that can produce unusual pressures on intracranial vessels. The presenting finding may be seizures; a rapidly enlarging head; or an abnormal neurologic examination with hypotonia, a poor Moro reflex, or extensive retinal hemorrhages.

Intraventricular and/or intraparenchymal hemorrhage generally occurs during the 1st 3 days of life and is the most serious type of intracranial bleeding. Hemorrhages occur most often in premature infants, are often bilateral, and usually arise in the germinal matrix. Most bleeding episodes are subependymal or intraventricular and involve a small amount of blood. In severe hemorrhage, there may be bleeding into the parenchyma or a cast of the ventricular system with large amounts of blood in the cisterna magna and basal cisterns. Hypoxia-ischemia often precedes intraventricular and subarachnoid bleeding. Hypoxia-ischemia damages the capillary endothelium, impairs cerebral vascular autoregulation, and can increase cerebral blood flow and venous pressure, all of which make hemorrhage more likely. Most intraventricular hemorrhages are asymptomatic, but larger hemorrhages may cause apnea, cyanosis, or sudden collapse.

Diagnosis

Intracranial hemorrhage should be suspected in any neonate with apnea, seizures, lethargy, or an abnormal neurologic examination. Infants should have head CT. Although cranial ultrasound is risk free, requires no sedation, and can readily identify blood within the ventricles or brain substance, CT is more sensitive for thin layers of blood in the subarachnoid or subdural spaces. If the diagnosis is in doubt, the CSF can be examined for RBCs: it usually contains gross blood. However, some RBCs are often present in the CSF of term neonates. In subdural hemorrhage, transillumination of the skull may reveal the diagnosis after the blood has lysed.

Additionally, clotting studies, a CBC, and metabolic studies to identify other causes of neurologic dysfunction (eg, hypoglycemia, hypocalcemia, electrolyte imbalance) should be performed. An EEG may help establish prognosis if the infant survives the acute bleeding episode.

Prognosis

The prognosis for subarachnoid hemorrhage is generally good. The prognosis for subdural hemorrhage is guarded, but some infants do well. Most infants with small intraventricular hemorrhages survive the acute bleeding episode and do well. Infants with large intraventricular hemorrhages have a poor prognosis, especially if the hemorrhage extends into the parenchyma. Many will be left with neurologic deficits.

Treatment

Treatment is mostly supportive unless a hematologic abnormality contributed to the bleeding. All should receive vitamin K if it was not previously given. If deficient, platelets or clotting factors should be given. Subdural hematomas should be managed by a neurosurgeon; evacuation of the hemorrhage may be needed.

FRACTURES

Midclavicular fracture, the most common fracture during birth, occurs with shoulder dystocia and with normal, nontraumatic deliveries. Initially, the neonate is irritable and does not move the arm on the involved side either spontaneously or when the Moro reflex is elicited. Most clavicular fractures are greenstick and heal rapidly and uneventfully. A large callus forms at the fracture site within a week, and remodeling is completed within a month. Treatment consists of making a sling by pinning the shirt sleeve of the involved side to the opposite side of the infant's shirt.

The humerus and the femur may be fractured in difficult deliveries. Most of these are greenstick, mid-shaft fractures, and excellent remodeling of the bone usually follows, even if moderate angulation occurs initially. A long bone may be fractured through its epiphysis, but prognosis is excellent.

Soft-Tissue Injuries

All soft tissues are susceptible to injury during birth if they have been the presenting part or the fulcrum for the forces of uterine contraction. Edema and ecchymosis often follow injury, particularly of the periorbital and facial tissues in face presentations and of the scrotum or labia during breech deliveries. Breakdown of blood within the tissues and conversion of heme to bilirubin result whenever a hematoma develops. This added burden of bilirubin may produce sufficient neonatal hyperbilirubinemia to require phototherapy, and rarely, exchange transfusion (see p. 2278). No other treatment is needed.

HYPOTHERMIA

Hypothermia is a core temperature < 35 to 35.5° C. The condition may be purely environmental or represent intercurrent illness. Treatment is rewarming.

Etiology and Pathophysiology

Thermal equilibrium is affected by relative humidity, air flow, proximity of cold surfaces, and ambient air temperature. Neonates are particularly prone to rapid heat loss and consequent hypothermia because of a high surface area to weight ratio, which is particularly high in low-birth-weight neonates. Radiant heat loss occurs when bare skin is exposed to an environment containing objects of cooler temperature. Evaporative heat loss occurs when neonates are wet with amniotic fluid. Hypothermia also may be due to pathologic conditions that impair thermoregulation (eg, sepsis, intracranial hemorrhage).

Prolonged, unrecognized cold stress may divert calories to produce heat, impairing growth. Neonates respond to cooling by sympathetic nerve discharge of norepinephrine in the "brown fat." This specialized tissue of the neonate, located in the nape of the neck, between the scapulae, and around the kidneys and adrenals, responds by lipolysis followed by oxidation or re-esterification of the fatty acids that are released. These reactions produce heat locally, and a rich blood supply to the brown fat helps transfer this heat to the rest of the neonate's body. This reaction increases the metabolic rate and O_2 consumption 2- to 3-fold. Thus, in neonates with respiratory insufficiency (eg, the preterm infant with respiratory distress syndrome), cold stress may also result in tissue hypoxia and neurologic damage. Additionally, hypothermia can result in hypoglycemia, metabolic acidosis, and death.

Treatment and Prevention

Hypothermia is treated by rewarming in an incubator or under a radiant warmer. The neonate should be monitored and treated as needed for hypoglycemia, hypoxemia, and apnea. Underlying conditions such as sepsis or intracranial hemorrhage require specific treatment.

Hypothermia can be prevented by immediately drying the neonate and then swaddling him (including his head) in a warm blanket. If the neonate is exposed for resuscitation or observation, he should be placed under a radiant warmer. Sick neonates should be maintained in a neutral thermal environment to minimize the metabolic rate. The proper incubator temperature varies depending on the neonate's birth weight and postnatal age. Alternatively, heating can be adjusted with a servomechanism set to maintain skin temperature at 36.5° C.

LARGE-FOR-GESTATIONAL-AGE INFANT

Infants whose weight is > the 90th percentile for gestational age are classified as large for gestational age. The predominant cause is maternal diabetes. Complications include birth trauma, hypoglycemia, and hyperbilirubinemia.

Other than genetically determined size, the major cause of an infant's being large for gestational age (LGA) is maternal diabetes mellitus. The macrosomia results from the anabolic effects of high fetal insulin levels produced in response to excessive blood glucose during gestation. The less well controlled the mother's diabetes during pregnancy, the more severe is the fetal macrosomia. A rare nongenetic cause of macrosomia is Beckwith-Wiedemann syndrome (characterized by macrosomia, omphalocele, macroglossia, and hypoglycemia).

Symptoms, Signs, and Treatment

LGA infants are large, obese, and plethoric. These infants are often listless and limp and may feed poorly. Delivery complications can occur in any LGA infant. Metabolic and respiratory complications are specific to LGA infants of diabetic mothers.

Delivery complications: Because of the infant's large size, vaginal delivery may be difficult and occasionally results in birth injury. Shoulder dystocia, fractures of the clavicles or limbs, and perinatal asphyxia may occur. Therefore, cesarean section should be considered when the fetus is thought to be LGA, especially if the mother's pelvic measurements are at the lower end of normal.

Infants of diabetic mothers: These infants are very likely to become hypoglycemic in the first 1 to 2 h after delivery because of the state of hyperinsulinism and the sudden termination of maternal glucose when the umbilical cord is cut. Neonatal hypoglycemia can be prevented by close prenatal control of the mother's diabetes and by the prophylactic IV infusion of 10% glucose in water into the infant until early frequent feedings can be established. Blood glucose levels should be closely monitored by bedside testing during the transition period.

Hyperbilirubinemia (see also p. 2275) is common because of intolerance for oral feedings in the earliest days of life, which increases the enterohepatic circulation of bilirubin. Hyperbilirubinemia can also result from the infants' high Hct (another accompanying problem in infants of diabetic mothers).

Because surfactant production (and hence pulmonary maturation) may be delayed until late in gestation, respiratory distress syndrome may develop even if the infant is delivered only a few weeks prematurely. The lecithin/sphingomyelin ratio, and especially the presence of phosphatidyl glycerol, in amniotic fluid obtained by amniocentesis can evaluate fetal lung maturity and help determine the optimal time for safe delivery. Lung maturity can be assumed only if phosphatidyl glycerol is present. For treatment, see p. 2304.

POSTMATURE INFANT

A postmature infant is an infant born after 42 wk gestation.

The cause of postmaturity is generally unknown. Very rarely, it may be due to abnormalities that affect the fetal pituitary-adrenal axis (eg, anencephaly or adrenal agenesis).

Pathophysiology

Past term, the placenta involutes, and multiple infarcts and villous degeneration produce placental insufficiency syndrome. In this syndrome, the fetus receives inadequate nutrients from the mother, resulting in soft-tissue wasting. During labor, postmature infants are prone to develop asphyxia; meconium aspiration syndrome, which may be unusually severe because post-term amniotic fluid volume is decreased and the aspirated meconium is less diluted; and neonatal hypoglycemia due to insufficient glycogen stores at birth. Because anaerobic metabolism rapidly uses the remaining glycogen stores, hypoglycemia is exaggerated if perinatal asphyxia has occurred.

Symptoms, Signs, and Diagnosis

Postmature infants are alert and appear mature but have a decreased amount of soft-tissue mass, particularly subcutaneous fat. The skin may hang loosely on the extremities and is often dry and peeling. The fingernails and toenails are long. The nails and umbilical cord may be stained with meconium passed in utero. Diagnosis is by clinical appearance (see FIG. 266–1 on p. 2221) and estimated date of delivery.

Prognosis and Treatment

Prognosis and treatment depend on complications. Those with meconium aspiration may have chronic respiratory insufficiency and secondary pulmonary hypertension if untreated; surfactant replacement therapy is frequently helpful.

PREMATURE INFANT

A premature infant is an infant born before 37 wk gestation.

Full-term gestation is 40 wk. Infants born before 37 wk have an increased incidence of complications and mortality roughly proportional to the degree of prematurity. Preterm delivery is one of the chief causes of neonatal morbidity and mortality.

Previously, any infant weighing < 2.5 kg was termed premature. This definition is inappropriate because many neonates weighing < 2.5 kg are mature or postmature but small for gestational age; they have a different appearance and different problems. Infants < 2.5 kg at birth are considered low-birth-weight infants, and those < 1500 g are considered very low-birth-weight infants.

Etiology

The cause of premature labor and delivery, whether or not preceded by premature rupture of the membranes, is usually unknown. However, maternal history commonly shows low socioeconomic status; inadequate prenatal care; poor nutrition; poor education; unwed state; previous preterm birth; and intercurrent, untreated illness or infection (eg, bacterial vaginosis). Other risk factors include placental abruption and preeclampsia.

Symptoms, Signs, and Diagnosis

Findings on physical examination correlate with gestational age (see FIG. 266–1 on p. 2221). Prenatal ultrasound, if performed, also determines gestational age.

The premature infant is small, usually weighing < 2.5 kg, and tends to have thin, shiny, pink skin through which the underlying veins are easily seen. Little subcutaneous fat, hair, or external ear cartilage exists. Spontaneous activity and tone are reduced, and extremities are not held in the flexed position typical of term infants. In males, the scrotum may have few rugae, and the testes may be undescended. In females, the labia majora do not yet cover the labia minora. Reflexes develop at different times during gestation. The Moro reflex begins by 28 to 32 wk gestation and is well established by 37 wk. The palmar reflex starts at 28 wk and is well established by 32 wk. The tonic neck reflex starts at 35 wk and is most prominent at 1 mo post term.

Complications

Most complications relate to dysfunction of immature organ systems.

Lungs: Surfactant production is often inadequate to prevent alveolar collapse and atelectasis, which result in respiratory distress syndrome (see p. 2303).

CNS: Infants born before 34 wk gestation have inadequate coordination of sucking and swallowing reflexes and need to be fed intravenously or by gavage. Immaturity of the respiratory center in the brain stem results in apneic spells (central apnea—see p. 2297). Apnea may also result from hypopharyngeal obstruction alone (obstructive apnea). Both may be present (mixed apnea).

The periventricular germinal matrix (a mass of embryonic cells on the lateral wall of the lateral ventricles and present only in the fetus) is prone to hemorrhage, which may extend into the cerebral ventricles (intraventricular hemorrhage). Infarction of the periventricular white matter (periventricular leukomalacia) may also occur for reasons that are incompletely understood. Hypotension, inadequate or unstable brain perfusion, and BP peaks (as when fluid or colloid is given rapidly IV) may contribute to cerebral infarction or hemorrhage.

Infection: Sepsis (see p. 2333) or meningitis (see p. 2330) is about 4 times more likely. The increased likelihood results from indwelling intravascular catheters and endotracheal tubes, from areas of skin breakdown, and from markedly reduced serum immunoglobulin levels (see p. 2256).

Temperature regulation: Premature infants have an exceptionally large body surface area to mass ratio. Therefore, when exposed to temperatures below the neutral thermal environment (see also Hypothermia on p. 2265), they rapidly lose heat and have difficulty maintaining body temperature.

GI tract: The small stomach and immature sucking and swallowing reflexes hinder oral or NGT feedings and create a risk of aspiration. Necrotizing enterocolitis (see p. 2286) occurs more often.

Kidneys: Renal function is limited, so the concentrating and diluting limits of urine are decreased. Late metabolic acidosis and growth failure may result from the immature kidneys' inability to excrete fixed acids, which accumulate with high-protein formula feedings and as a result of bone growth. Na and HCO_3 are lost in the urine.

Metabolic problems: Hypoglycemia (see p. 2281) and hyperglycemia (see p. 2280) are discussed in Ch. 274.

Hyperbilirubinemia (see also p. 2275) occurs more commonly, and kernicterus may occur at serum bilirubin levels as low as 10 mg/dL (170 μmol/L) in small, sick, premature infants. The higher bilirubin levels may be partially due to inadequately developed hepatic excretion mechanisms, including deficiencies in the uptake of bilirubin from the serum, its hepatic conjugation to bilirubin diglucuronide, and its excretion into the biliary tree. Decreased intestinal motility enables more bilirubin diglucuronide to be deconjugated within the intestinal lumen by the luminal enzyme β-glucuronidase, thus permitting increased reabsorption of unconjugated bilirubin (enterohepatic circulation of bilirubin). Conversely, early feedings increase intestinal motility and reduce bilirubin reabsorption and can thereby significantly decrease the incidence and severity of physiologic jaundice. Uncommonly, delayed clamping of the umbilical cord increases the risk of significant hyperbilirubinemia by allowing the transfusion of a large RBC mass, thus increasing RBC breakdown and bilirubin production.

Prognosis and Treatment

Prognosis varies with presence and severity of complications, but usually survival rate improves greatly with increasing gestational age and birth weight. Survival rate for infants born with birth weights between 1250 g and 1500 g is about 95%.

Specific disorders are treated as discussed elsewhere in THE MANUAL. General supportive care is best provided in a neonatal ICU or special care nursery and involves careful attention to the thermal environment, using servo-controlled incubators; scrupulous adherence is paid to handwashing before and after all patient contact. Infants are continually monitored for apnea, bradycardia, and hypoxemia until 34 ½ or 35 wk gestation.

Parents should be encouraged to visit and interact with the infant as much as possible within the constraints of the infant's medical condition.

Feeding: Feeding should be by the nasogastric route until coordination of sucking, swallowing, and breathing is established at about 34 wk gestation, at which time breastfeeding is strongly encouraged. Most premature infants tolerate breast milk, which provides immunologic and nutritional factors that are absent in cow's milk formulas. However, breast milk does not provide sufficient Ca, phosphorus, and protein for very low-birth-weight infants (ie, < 1500 g), for whom it should be mixed with a breast milk fortifier. Alternatively, specific premature infant formulas that contain 20 to 24 kcal/oz (2.8 to 3.3 joules/mL) can be used.

In the initial 1 or 2 days, if adequate fluids and calories cannot be given by mouth or NGT because of the infant's condition, a 10% glucose solution with maintenance electrolytes is given IV to prevent dehydration and malnutrition. Continuous breast milk or formula feeding via NGT or nasojejunal tube can satisfactorily maintain caloric intake in small, sick, premature infants, especially those with respiratory distress or recurrent apneic spells. Feedings are begun with small amounts (eg, 1 to 2 mL q 3 to 6 h) to stimulate the GI tract. If tolerated, the volume and concentration of feedings are slowly increased over 7 to 10 days. In very small or critically sick infants, total parenteral hyperalimentation via a peripheral IV or a percutaneously or surgically placed central catheter may be required until full enteral feedings can be tolerated.

Prevention

The risk of preterm delivery can be reduced by ensuring that all women, especially those in high-risk groups, have access to early and appropriate prenatal care, including advice on the importance of avoiding alcohol, tobacco, and illicit drugs. The use of tocolytics to arrest premature labor and provide time for prenatal administration of corticosteroids to hasten lung maturation is discussed in Ch. 264 (see p. 2205).

RETINOPATHY OF PREMATURITY

(Retrolental Fibroplasia)

Retinopathy of prematurity is a bilateral disorder of abnormal retinal vascularization in premature infants, especially those of low-est birth weight. Outcomes range from normal vision to blindness. Diagnosis is by ophthalmoscopy. Treatment of severe disease may include cryotherapy or photocoagulation; other treatment is directed at complications (eg, retinal detachment).

The inner retinal blood vessels start growing about midpregnancy, but the retina is not fully vascularized until term. Retinopathy of prematurity (ROP) results if these vessels continue their growth in an abnormal pattern, forming a ridge of tissue between the vascularized central retina and the nonvascularized peripheral retina. In severe ROP, these new vessels invade the vitreous. Sometimes the entire vasculature of the eye becomes engorged ("plus" disease).

Susceptibility to ROP correlates with the proportion of retina that remains avascular at birth. More than 80% of neonates weighing < 1 kg at birth develop ROP. The percentage is higher when many medical complications exist. Administration of excessive (especially prolonged) O_2 increases the risk, but a safe level and duration of supplemental O_2 have not been determined; however, supplemental O_2 is often needed to adequately oxygenate the infant.

Diagnosis, Treatment, and Prevention

Diagnosis is made by ophthalmoscopic examination, which shows a line of demarcation and a ridge in mild cases and proliferation of retinal vessels in more severe cases. Because significant ROP is rare in appropriately managed infants weighing > 1500 g at birth, alternative diagnoses should be considered in these infants (eg, familial exudative retinopathy, Norrie's disease).

Abnormal vessel growth often subsides spontaneously but, in about 4% of survivors weighing < 1 kg at birth, progresses to produce retinal detachments and vision loss within 2 to 12 mo postpartum. Children with healed ROP have a higher incidence of myopia, strabismus, and amblyopia. A few children with moderate, healed ROP are left with cicatricial scars (eg, dragged retina or retinal folds) and are at risk for retinal detachments later in life; glaucoma and cataracts can also occur rarely in these patients.

In severe ROP, cryotherapy or laser photocoagulation to ablate the peripheral avascular retina reduces the incidence of retinal fold and detachment. Therefore, all high-risk infants should be examined by an ophthalmologist before 6 wk of age. Retinal vascularization must be followed at 1- to 2-wk intervals until the vessels have matured sufficiently. If retinal detachments occur in infancy, scleral buckling surgery or vitrectomy with lensectomy may be considered, but these procedures are late rescue efforts with low benefit.

Patients with residual scarring should be followed at least annually for life. Treatment of amblyopia and refractive errors in the 1st year optimizes vision. Infants with total retinal detachments should be monitored for secondary glaucoma and poor eye growth and referred to intervention programs for the visually impaired.

Prevention of premature birth is the best way to prevent ROP. After a preterm birth, O_2 should be supplemented only as needed to avoid hypoxia documented by ABG or pulse oximetry. Vitamin E and restricted light are not effective.

SMALL-FOR-GESTATIONAL-AGE INFANT

(Dysmaturity; Intrauterine Growth Restriction)

Infants whose weight is < the 10th percentile for gestational age are classified as small for gestational age. Complications include perinatal asphyxia, meconium aspiration, and hypoglycemia.

Etiology

An infant may be small at birth because of genetic factors. Nongenetic factors that can restrict intrauterine growth usually are not apparent before 32 to 34 wk gestation; these include placental insufficiency from maternal disease involving the small blood vessels (as in preeclampsia, primary hypertension, renal disease, or long-standing diabetes); placental involution accompanying postmaturity; and infectious agents such as cytomegalovirus, rubella virus, or *Toxoplasma gondii.* An infant may also be small for gestational age (SGA) if the mother is an opioid or cocaine addict or a heavy user of alcohol or, to a lesser degree, if she smoked cigarettes during pregnancy.

Symptoms and Signs

Despite their size, SGA infants have physical characteristics (eg, skin appearance, ear cartilage, sole creases) and behavior (eg, alertness, spontaneous activity, zest for feeding) similar to those of normal-sized infants of like gestational age.

If growth restriction is due to placental insufficiency and, therefore, malnutrition, the infant's weight is most affected, with a relative sparing of growth of the brain, cranium, and long bones (asymmetric growth restriction). In contrast, many genetic disorders and congenital infections cause symmetric growth restriction, in which height, weight, and head circumference are about equally affected.

Complications: Full-term SGA infants do not have the complications related to organ system immaturity that premature infants of similar size have. They are, however, at risk for perinatal asphyxia, meconium aspiration, and hypoglycemia.

Perinatal asphyxia is the most serious potential complication. It is a risk during labor if intrauterine growth restriction is due to placental insufficiency (with marginally adequate placental perfusion), because each uterine contraction slows or stops maternal placental perfusion by compressing the spiral arteries. Therefore, when placental insufficiency is suspected, the fetus should be assessed before labor and the fetal heart rate monitored during labor. If fetal compromise is detected, rapid delivery, often by cesarean section, is indicated.

Meconium aspiration may occur during perinatal asphyxia. SGA infants, especially those who are postmature, may pass meconium into the amniotic sac and begin deep gasping movements. The consequent aspiration is likely to result in meconium aspiration syndrome (often most severe in growth-restricted or postmature infants, because the meconium is contained in a smaller volume of amniotic fluid—see p. 2300).

Hypoglycemia often occurs in the early hours and days of life due to a lack of adequate glycogen stores (see p. 2281).

Polycythemia may occur when SGA fetuses experience chronic mild hypoxia due to placental insufficiency. Erythropoietin release is increased, leading to an increased rate of erythrocyte production. The neonate with polycythemia at birth appears ruddy and may be tachypneic or lethargic.

Prognosis and Treatment

If asphyxia can be avoided, neurologic prognosis is quite good.

Infants who are SGA because of genetic factors, congenital infection, or maternal drug use often have a worse prognosis, depending on the specific diagnosis. If intrauterine growth restriction is caused by chronic placental insufficiency, adequate nutrition may allow SGA infants to demonstrate remarkable "catch-up" growth after delivery.

Underlying conditions and complications are treated. There is no specific intervention for the SGA state, but prevention is aided by prenatal advice on the importance of avoiding alcohol, tobacco, and illicit drugs.

273 PERINATAL HEMATOLOGIC DISORDERS

Anemia and polycythemia are the most common hematologic disorders diagnosed at birth. Prenatal and perinatal changes in erythropoiesis are discussed in Ch. 271 (see p. 2255).

PERINATAL ANEMIA

(See also Ch. 129 on p. 1031.)

Anemia is Hb or Hct > 2 standard deviations below mean for age. Both Hb and Hct change rapidly as a neonate matures, so lower limits of normal also change. Variables such as gestational age (see TABLE 273–1), sampling site (capillary vs vein), and position of the neonate relative to the placenta before cord clamping (lower position causes blood to transfer in to the neonate; higher position causes blood to transfer out of the neonate) also affect test results.

Etiology

Anemia in neonates may be physiologic, or it may be caused by blood loss, decreased RBC production, or increased RBC destruction (hemolysis).

Physiologic anemia: Normal physiologic processes often cause normocytic-normochromic anemia in term and preterm infants. Physiologic anemias do not generally require extensive evaluation or treatment.

In term infants, the increase in oxygenation that occurs with normal breathing after birth causes an abrupt rise in tissue O_2 level, resulting in negative feedback on erythropoietin production and erythropoiesis. This reduction in erythropoiesis, as well as the shorter

TABLE 273–1. AGE-SPECIFIC VALUES FOR HEMOGLOBIN AND HEMATOCRIT

AGE	Hb (g/dL)	Hct (%)
28 wk gestation	14.5	45
32 wk gestation	15	47
Term	16.5	51
1–3 days	18.5	56
2 wk	16.6	53

lifespan (60 to 70 days vs 120 days in adults) of neonatal RBCs, causes Hb concentration to fall over the 1st 2 to 3 mo of life, usually no lower than 9.4 g/dL. Hb remains stable over the next several weeks, and then slowly rises in the 4th to 6th month secondary to renewed erythropoietin stimulation.

The same mechanism causes anemia in preterm infants during the 1st 4 to 12 wk, but lower erythropoietin production, shorter RBC life span (35 to 50 days), and more frequent phlebotomy contribute to a lower Hb nadir (8 to 10 g/dL). Infants < 32 wk gestation are most affected.

Blood loss: Anemia may develop because of prenatal, perinatal (at delivery), or postpartum hemorrhage. In neonates, blood volume is low (eg, preterm, 90 to 150 mL/kg; term, 78 to 86 mL/kg); therefore, acute loss of as little as 15 to 20 mL of blood may result in anemia. An infant with chronic blood loss can compensate physiologically and is typically more clinically stable than an infant with acute blood loss.

Prenatal hemorrhage may be caused by fetal-to-maternal hemorrhage, twin-to-twin transfusion, cord malformations, placental abnormalities, and diagnostic procedures. Fetal-to-maternal hemorrhage occurs spontaneously or as a result of maternal trauma, amniocentesis, external cephalic version, or placental tumor. It affects about 50% of pregnancies, although in most cases the volume of blood lost is extremely small (about 2 mL); "massive" blood loss, defined as > 30 mL, occurs in 3/1000 pregnancies. Twin-to-twin transfusion is the unequal sharing of blood supply between twins that affects 13 to 33% of monozygotic, monochorionic twin pregnancies. With significant blood transfer, the donor twin may become very anemic and develop heart failure, while the recipient may become polycythemic and develop hyperviscosity syndrome (see p. 2274). Cord malformations include velamentous insertion of the umbilical cord, vasa previa, or abdominal or placental insertion; mechanism of hemorrhage is by cord vessel shearing or rupture. The 2 important placental abnormalities causing hemorrhage are placenta previa and abruptio placentae. Diagnostic procedures causing hemorrhage include amniocentesis, chorionic villus sampling, and umbilical cord blood sampling.

Perinatal hemorrhage may be caused by precipitous delivery (ie, rapid, spontaneous delivery < 3 h after onset of labor, which causes hemorrhage due to umbilical cord tearing) and obstetrical accidents such as incision of the placenta during cesarean section. Cephalhematomas from procedures such as vacuum or forceps delivery are usually relatively harmless, but subgaleal bleeds can extend into soft tissue, sequestering sufficient blood volumes to result in anemia, hypotension, shock, and death. Far less often, rupture of the liver, spleen, or adrenal gland during delivery may lead to internal bleeding. Intraventricular hemorrhage in preterm infants (see p. 2263) as well as subarachnoid and subdural bleeding also can result in a significantly lowered Hct.

Hemorrhagic disease of the newborn (see full discussion under Vitamin K Deficiency on p. 45) is hemorrhage within a few days of a normal delivery caused by transient physiologic deficiency in vitamin K–dependent coagulation factors. Other possible causes of hemorrhage in the first few days of life are other coagulopathies (eg, hemophilia), disseminated intravascular coagulation from sepsis, vascular malformations, or prenatal maternal use of vitamin K antagonists (eg, phenytoin, warfarin, isoniazid).

Decreased RBC production: Defects in RBC production may be congenital or acquired.

Congenital defects are extremely rare, but Diamond-Blackfan and Fanconi's anemia are the most common.

Diamond-Blackfan anemia is characterized by lack of RBC precursors in bone marrow, macrocytic RBCs, lack of reticulocytes in peripheral blood, and lack of involvement of other blood cell lineages. It is often part of a syndrome of congenital anomalies including microcephaly, cleft palate, eye anomalies, thumb deformities, and web neck. Up to 25% of affected infants are anemic at birth, and low birth weight occurs in about 10%. It is thought to be caused by defective stem cell differentiation.

Fanconi's anemia is an autosomal recessive disorder of bone marrow progenitor cells that causes macrocytosis and reticulocytopenia with progressive failure of all hematopoietic cell lines. It is usually diagnosed after the neonatal period. The cause is a genetic defect that prevents cells from repairing damaged DNA or removing toxic free radicals that damage cells.

Other congenital anemias include Pearson's syndrome, a rare, multisystem disease involving mitochondrial defects that cause refractory sideroblastic anemia, pancytopenia, and variable hepatic, renal, and pancreatic insufficiency or failure; and congenital dyserythropoietic anemia, in which chronic anemia (typically macrocytic) results from ineffective or abnormal RBC production, and hemolysis caused by RBC abnormalities.

Acquired defects are those that occur after birth. The most common causes are infections (eg, malaria, rubella, syphilis, HIV, cytomegalovirus, adenovirus, bacterial sepsis) that impair RBC production in the bone marrow, and nutritional deficiency. Congenital parvovirus B19 infection may result in the absence of RBC production. Nutritional deficiencies of iron, copper, and folate and vitamins E and B_{12} may cause anemia in the early months of life but not usually at birth. The incidence of iron deficiency, the most common nutritional deficiency, is higher in less developed countries where it results from dietary insufficiency and exclusive and prolonged breastfeeding. Iron deficiency is common in neonates whose mothers have an iron deficit and in premature infants whose formula is not supplemented with iron; premature infants deplete iron stores by 10 to 14 wk if not supplemented.

Hemolysis: Hemolysis (see also p. 1045) may be immune-mediated or caused by RBC membrane disorders, enzyme deficiencies, hemoglobinopathies, or infection. All cause hyperbilirubinemia, which may cause jaundice and kernicterus (see p. 2278).

Immune-mediated hemolysis may occur when fetal RBCs with surface antigens (most commonly Rh and ABO blood antigens but also Kell, Duffy, and other minor group antigens) that differ from maternal RBC antigens enter the maternal circulation and stimulate production of IgG antibody directed against fetal RBCs. The most common scenario is that an Rh (D antigen)-negative mother becomes sensitized to the D antigen during her 1st pregnancy with an Rh-positive fetus; a 2nd Rh-positive pregnancy may then prompt an IgG response that may result in fetal and neonatal hemolysis (see full discussion under Erythroblastosis Fetalis on p. 2194). Intrauterine hemolysis may be severe enough to cause hydrops or death; postpartum, there may be significant anemia and hyperbilirubinemia with ongoing hemolysis secondary to persistent maternal IgG (half-life about 28 days). With widespread prophylactic use of anti-Rh D to prevent sensitization (see p. 2195), < 0.11% of pregnancies in Rh-negative women are affected. ABO incompatibility may cause hemolysis by a similar mechanism but rarely results in severe hemolysis requiring treatment; the immunoglobulin involved is predominantly IgM, which is incapable of crossing the placenta. Hemolysis from ABO incompatibility sometimes occurs in a 1st pregnancy if the mother has been previously sensitized by antigens in foods or bacteria.

RBC membrane disorders alter RBC shape and result in premature removal of RBCs from the circulation. The most common disorders are hereditary spherocytosis and hereditary elliptocytosis (see p. 1051).

Deficiencies of G6PD (see p. 1053) and pyruvate kinase (see Embden-Meyerhof Pathway Defects on p. 1052) are the most common enzyme disorders causing hemolysis.

Hemoglobinopathies are caused by deficiencies and structural abnormalities of globin chains. At birth, 55 to 90% of the neonate's hemoglobin is composed of 2 alpha and 2 gamma globin chains (fetal hemoglobin or Hb F [$\alpha^2\gamma^2$]). After birth, γ-chain production decreases (to < 2% by 2 to 4 yr of age) and β-chain production rises until adult hemoglobin (Hgb A [$\alpha^2\beta^2$]) becomes predominant. α-Thalassemia (see p. 1057) is a genetically inherited disorder of depressed α globin chain production and is the most common hemoglobinopathy causing anemia in the neonatal period. β-Thalassemia (see p. 1057) is an inherited decrease in β-chain production. Because β globin is naturally low at birth, β-thalassemia and structural abnormalities of the β globin chain (Hb S [sickle cell disease], Hb C) are rarely apparent at birth and symptoms do not appear until fetal Hb levels have fallen to sufficiently low levels at 3 to 4 mo.

Intrauterine infections by certain bacteria, viruses, fungi, and protozoa (most notably toxoplasmosis and malaria) also may trigger hemolytic anemia. In malaria, the *Plasmodium* parasite invades and ultimately ruptures the RBC. Immune-mediated destruction of parasitized RBCs and excess removal of nonparasitized cells occur. Associated bone marrow dyserythropoiesis results in inadequate compensatory erythropoiesis. Intravascular hemolysis, extravascular phagocytosis, and dyserythropoiesis can lead to anemia.

Symptoms and Signs

Symptoms and signs are similar regardless of the cause but vary with severity and rate of onset of the anemia. Neonates are generally pale and, if anemia is severe, have tachypnea, tachycardia, and sometimes a flow murmur; hypotension is present with acute blood loss. Jaundice may be present with hemolysis.

Evaluation

History: History should focus on maternal factors (eg, bleeding diatheses, hereditary RBC disorders, nutritional deficiencies, drugs), family history of hereditable disorders that cause neonatal anemia, and obstetric factors (eg, infections, vaginal bleeding, obstetrical interventions, mode of delivery, blood loss, treatment and appearance of the cord, placental pathology, fetal distress, number of fetuses). Nonspecific maternal factors may provide additional clues; splenectomy would indicate a possible history of hemolysis or autoimmune anemia, and cholecystectomy might indicate past hemolysis (producing excess bile and hence gallstones). Important neonatal factors include gestational age at delivery, age at presentation, sex, race, and ethnicity.

Physical examination: Tachycardia and hypotension suggest acute, significant blood loss. Jaundice suggests hemolysis, either systemic (from ABO incompatibility or G6PD deficiency) or localized (from breakdown of sequestered blood in cephalhematomas). Hepatosplenomegaly suggests either hemolysis or heart failure. Hematomas, ecchymoses, or petechiae suggest bleeding diathesis; congenital anomalies may suggest a bone marrow failure syndrome.

Testing: Anemia may be suspected prenatally if ultrasound shows hydrops fetalis, which is abnormal, excessive fluid in 2 or more body compartments (eg, pleura, peritoneum, pericardium); cardiac, hepatic, and splenic enlargement may be present.

After birth, if anemia is suspected, reticulocytes should be measured and the peripheral smear examined. The percentage of reticulocytes increases in anemia caused by blood loss or hemolysis, reflecting an appropriate bone marrow response; reticulocyte count is low when anemia is caused by acquired or congenital bone marrow dysfunction.

Whenever the reticulocyte count is elevated or normal, a direct antiglobulin test (DAT, or Coombs' test) should be obtained. If the DAT is positive, anemia is likely secondary to Rh, ABO, or other blood group incompatibility. If the DAT is negative, the RBC mean corpuscular volume (MCV) may prove helpful; a significantly low MCV suggests α-thalassemia or chronic intrauterine blood loss. With a normal or high MCV, peripheral blood smear may demonstrate abnormal RBC morphology compatible with a membrane disorder, microangiopathy, disseminated intravascular coagulation (DIC), or hemoglobinopathy. If the smear is normal, blood loss, enzyme deficiency, or infection should be considered and appropriate workup should ensue.

Fetal-to-maternal hemorrhage can be diagnosed by testing for fetal RBCs in maternal blood. The Kleihauer-Betke acid elution technique is the most frequently used test, but other tests include fluorescent antibody techniques and differential or mixed agglutination testing. In the Kleihauer-Betke technique, citric acid-phosphate buffer of pH 3.5 elutes hemoglobin from adult but not fetal RBCs; thus fetal RBCs stain with eosin and are visible on microscopy, whereas adult RBCs appear as red cell ghosts.

When the reticulocyte percentage is depressed, the infant should be evaluated for causes of bone marrow suppression with titers for viral infection (rubella, syphilis, HIV, cytomegalovirus, adenovirus), folate and vitamin B_{12} levels, and iron and copper levels.

Treatment

Need for treatment varies with degree of anemia and associated medical conditions; otherwise healthy term and preterm infants with mild anemia generally do not require treatment. Treatment is directed at the underlying diagnosis. Some patients require transfusion or exchange transfusion of packed RBCs.

Transfusion: Transfusion is indicated to treat severe anemia. Guidelines for when to transfuse vary, but one accepted set is:

- Hb ≤ 12 g/dL (Hct ≤ 36%) in the 1st 24 h of life
- ≥ 10% decrease in Hb in 1 wk
- ≥ 10% acute blood loss
- Hb ≤ 12 g/dL in a neonate requiring intensive care
- Hb ≤ 11 g/dL in a neonate with chronic O_2 dependency
- Hb ≤ 7 g/dL in a stable infant with late (ie, 4 to 6 wk) anemia

Before the 1st transfusion, if not already done, maternal and fetal blood should be screened for ABO and Rh types and the presence of atypical RBC antibodies, and a DAT should be performed on the infant's RBCs.

Blood for transfusion should be the same as or compatible with the neonate's ABO and Rh group and with any ABO or RBC antibody present in maternal or neonatal serum. Neonates produce RBC antibodies only rarely, so in cases where the need for transfusion persists, repeat antibody screening is usually not necessary until 4 mo of age.

Packed RBCs used for transfusion should be filtered (leukocyte depleted), irradiated, and given in aliquots of 5 to 15 mL/kg derived from a single donation; sequential transfusions from the same unit of blood minimize recipient exposure and transfusion complications.

Exchange transfusion: Exchange transfusion, in which blood from the neonate is removed in aliquots in sequence with packed RBC transfusion, is indicated for hemolytic anemia and some cases of severe anemia with heart failure. It decreases plasma antibody titers and bilirubin levels (when phototherapy fails) and minimizes fluid overload. Serious adverse events (eg, shock, pulmonary edema, or both caused by shifts in fluid balance) are common, so the procedure should be performed by experienced staff. Guidelines for when to begin exchange transfusion differ and are not evidence based.

Other treatments: Recombinant human erythropoietin is not routinely recommended, in part because it has not been shown to reduce transfusion requirements in the 1st 2 wk of life.

Iron administration is restricted to cases of repetitive blood loss (eg, hemorrhagic diathesis, GI bleeding, frequent phlebotomy). Oral iron supplements are preferred; parenteral iron sometimes causes anaphylaxis and should be pursued under guidance of a hematologist.

Treatment of more unusual causes of anemia is disorder specific (eg, corticosteroids in Diamond-Blackfan anemia, vitamin B_{12} for B_{12} deficiency).

PERINATAL POLYCYTHEMIA AND HYPERVISCOSITY SYNDROME

Polycythemia is an abnormal increase in RBC mass, defined in neonates as a venous Hct ≥ 65%; this can lead to hyperviscosity with sludging of blood within vessels and sometimes thrombosis. The main symptoms and signs of neonatal polycythemia are very ruddy complexion, feeding difficulties, lethargy, and seizures. Diagnosis is made clinically and with a spun Hct. The main symptoms and signs of hyperviscosity syndrome are cyanosis, jaundice, tachypnea, and renal failure. Treatment is with partial exchange transfusion.

The terms polycythemia and hyperviscosity are often used interchangeably but are not equivalent. Polycythemia is significant only because it increases risk for hyperviscosity syndrome. Hyperviscosity syndrome is symptoms and signs caused by sludging of blood within vessels. Sludging occurs because increased RBC mass causes a relative decrease in plasma volume and a relative increase in proteins and platelets.

Incidence of polycythemia ranges between 0.4% and 12%. Hyperviscosity occurs in 6.7% of neonates. Only 47% of infants with polycythemia exhibit hyperviscosity; 24% of infants with hyperviscosity have polycythemia.

Etiology

Dehydration causing relative hemoconcentration and an elevated Hct mimics polycythemia but RBC mass is not increased. Causes of true polycythemia include intrauterine hypoxia, placental transfusion, some congenital abnormalities (eg, cyanotic congenital heart disease, renovascular malformations, congenital adrenal hyperplasia), certain delivery procedures (eg, delayed cord clamping, holding neonate below the level of the mother before cord clamping, stripping the cord toward the neonate at delivery), maternal insulin-dependent diabetes, Down syndrome, Beckwith-Wiedemann syndrome, intrauterine growth restriction, twin-to-twin transfusion, and perinatal asphyxia. Premature infants rarely develop hyperviscosity syndrome.

Symptoms and Signs

Symptoms and signs of hyperviscosity syndrome are those of heart failure, thrombosis (cerebral and renal vessels), and CNS dysfunction, including tachypnea, respiratory distress, cyanosis, plethora, apnea, lethargy, irritability, hypotonia, tremulousness, seizures, and feeding problems. Renal vein thrombosis may also cause renal tubular damage and/or proteinuria.

Diagnosis

Diagnosis of polycythemia is by Hct; diagnosis of hyperviscosity syndrome is clinical. Capillary samples often overestimate Hct so a venous Hct, preferably spun, should be obtained before the diagnosis is made; most published studies of polycythemia use spun Hcts, which are generally higher than those obtained on automated counters. Laboratory measure of viscosity is not readily available.

Other laboratory abnormalities may include low blood glucose and Ca levels secondary to poor feeding, maternal diabetes, or both, and RBC lysis; thrombocytopenia (secondary to consumption with thrombosis); hyperbilirubinemia (from turnover of a higher number of RBCs); and reticulocytosis and increased peripheral nucleated RBCs (from increased erythropoiesis secondary to fetal hypoxia).

Treatment

Asymptomatic infants should be treated with IV hydration (see p. 2291). Symptomatic infants should undergo an isovolumic partial exchange transfusion to reduce the Hct to ≤ 55% and thereby decrease blood viscosity; blood is removed in 5 mL/kg (about 10 to 12 mL) aliquots and replaced with an equal volume of 0.9% saline. Asymptomatic infants whose Hct remains persistently > 70% despite hydration may also benefit from this procedure.

Although many studies show immediate measurable effects of partial exchange, the long-term benefits remain in question. Most studies have failed to document differences in long-term growth or neurodevelopment between children who received a partial exchange transfusion in the neonatal period and those who did not.

274 METABOLIC, ELECTROLYTE, AND TOXIC DISORDERS IN NEONATES

Inherited disorders of metabolism are discussed in Ch. 296 (see p. 2458). Electrolyte disorders also are discussed elsewhere in the manual.

HYPERBILIRUBINEMIA

Hyperbilirubinemia is an elevated serum bilirubin concentration; the threshold for an abnormal value varies by age and, in preterm infants, by health status. The primary sign is jaundice, but marked hyperbilirubinemia can cause kernicterus, a syndrome of neurologic damage. Diagnosis is obvious by examination and confirmed by measurement of serum bilirubin. Treatment depends on cause and degree of elevation; definitive treatments include phototherapy and exchange transfusion.

Etiology and Pathophysiology

TABLE 274–1 lists the causes of hyperbilirubinemia. In general, hyperbilirubinemia may be physiologic or pathologic and is always caused by increased production, decreased clearance, or increased enterohepatic circulation of bilirubin (see p. 2255). Most cases involve unconjugated hyperbilirubinemia, but liver dysfunction (eg, parenteral alimentation causing cholestasis, neonatal sepsis, severe erythroblastosis fetalis) may cause conjugated hyperbilirubinemia.

Physiologic hyperbilirubinemia occurs in almost all neonates. Shorter neonatal RBC life span increases bilirubin production; deficient conjugation decreases clearance; and low bacterial levels in the intestine combined with increased hydrolysis of conjugated bilirubin increase enterohepatic circulation. Bilirubin levels rise up to 18 mg/dL by 3 to 4 days of life (7 days in Asian infants) and fall thereafter.

Breastfeeding jaundice develops in ⅙ of breastfed infants in the 1st wk of life; breastfeeding increases enterohepatic circulation of bilirubin in some infants who have

TABLE 274–1. CAUSES OF NEONATAL HYPERBILIRUBINEMIA

MECHANISM	CAUSES
Overproduction	Breakdown of extravascular blood (eg, hematomas; petechiae; pulmonary, cerebral, or occult hemorrhage)
	Polycythemia due to maternofetal or fetofetal transfusion or delayed umbilical cord clamping
Overproduction due to hemolytic anemia	Certain drugs in neonates with G6PD deficiency (acetaminophen, alcohol, antimalarials, aspirin, bupivacaine, corticosteroids, diazepam, nitrofurantoin, oxytocin, penicillin, phenothiazine, and sulfonamides)
	Fetomaternal blood group incompatibility (eg, Rh, ABO)
	RBC enzyme deficiencies (eg, of G6PD or pyruvate kinase)
	Spherocytosis
	Thalassemias (α, β-δ)
	Vitamin K
Increased enterohepatic circulation	Breastfeeding
	Breastfeeding failure
	Drug-induced paralytic ileus (hexamethonium)
	Fasting or other cause for hypoperistalsis
	Hirschsprung's disease
	Intestinal atresia or stenosis, including annular pancreas
	Meconium ileus or meconium plug syndrome
	Pyloric stenosis*
	Swallowed blood
Undersecretion due to biliary obstruction	α_1-Antitrypsin deficiency*
	Biliary atresia*
	Choledochal cyst*
	Cystic fibrosis* (inspissated bile)
	Dubin-Johnson and Rotor's syndromes*
	Parenteral nutrition
	Tumor or band* (extrinsic obstruction)
Undersecretion due to metabolic-endocrine conditions	Crigler-Najjar syndrome (familial nonhemolytic jaundice types 1 and 2)
	Drugs and hormones
	Gilbert's disease
	Hypermethioninemia
	Hypopituitarism and anencephaly
	Hypothyroidism
	Lucey-Driscoll syndrome
	Maternal diabetes
	Prematurity
	Tyrosinosis
Mixed overproduction and undersecretion	Asphyxia
	Maternal diabetes
	Intrauterine infections

TABLE 274–1. CAUSES OF NEONATAL HYPERBILIRUBINEMIA—Continued

MECHANISM	CAUSES
Mixed overproduction and undersecretion (*continued*)	Cytomegalovirus inclusion disease Hepatitis Herpes simplex Respiratory distress syndrome Rubella Sepsis Severe erythroblastosis fetalis Syphilis Toxoplasmosis

*Jaundice may not occur in the neonatal period.
TORCH = toxoplasmosis, rubella, cytomegalovirus, herpes simplex virus.

Adapted from Poland RL, Ostrea EM Jr: Neonatal hyperbilirubinemia. In *Care of the High-Risk Neonate*, ed. 3, edited by MH Klaus and AA Fanaroff. Philadelphia, WB Saunders Company, 1986; used with permission.

decreased milk intake and who also have dehydration or low caloric intake.

Pathologic hyperbilirubinemia in term infants is bilirubinemia > 18 mg/dL that occurs in the 1st day or beyond the 1st wk of life or is caused by an abnormal process. The most common pathologic cause of increased bilirubin production is hemolytic anemia (see p. 2272), usually from blood type incompatibility; polycythemia (eg, from twin-to-twin transfusion) and hematomas are other causes. Conditions that decrease bilirubin clearance are genetic disorders that impair conjugation such as Crigler-Najjar and Gilbert syndromes (see p. 195).

Symptoms, Signs, and Diagnosis

Hyperbilirubinemia is asymptomatic but begins to cause jaundice at > 4 to 5 mg/dL (> 68 to 86 µmol/L). With increasing bilirubin levels, visible jaundice advances in a head-to-foot direction. Prolonged hyperbilirubinemia can cause kernicterus (see p. 2278).

Diagnosis is suspected by the infant's color and confirmed by measurement of serum bilirubin. A bilirubin concentration > 10 mg/dL (> 170 µmol/L) in preterm infants or > 18 mg/dL (> 308 µmol/L) in term infants warrants additional diagnostic testing, including Hct, blood smear, reticulocyte count, direct Coombs' test, total and direct serum bilirubin concentrations, and blood type and Rh group of the neonate and mother. Other tests, such as blood, urine, and CSF cultures to detect sepsis and measurement of RBC enzyme levels to detect unusual causes of hemolysis, may be indicated by the history, physical examination, or initial laboratory findings or by an initial bilirubin level > 25 mg/dL (428 µmol/L).

Breastfeeding jaundice, though suspected by history, is diagnosed by exclusion; it is important to consider other possible causes of hyperbilirubinemia that may require specific treatment (see also p. 2267).

Treatment

Physiologic jaundice usually is not clinically significant and resolves within 1 wk. Frequent formula feedings can reduce the incidence and severity of hyperbilirubinemia by increasing GI motility and frequency of stools, thereby minimizing the enterohepatic circulation of bilirubin. The type of formula does not appear important in increasing bilirubin excretion.

Breastfeeding jaundice may be prevented or reduced by increasing the frequency of feeds and minimizing the use of water to replace breast milk. In a term infant with early breastfeeding jaundice, if the bilirubin level continues to increase > 18 mg/dL, a temporary change from breast milk to formula feedings may be appropriate; phototherapy may also be indicated at higher levels. Stopping breastfeeding is necessary for only 1 or 2 days, and the mother should be encouraged to continue expressing breast milk regularly so she can resume nursing as soon as the neonate's bilirubin level starts to decline. She should also be assured that the hyperbilirubinemia has not caused any harm and that she may safely resume breastfeeding.

Definitive treatment involves phototherapy or exchange transfusion.

Phototherapy: Phototherapy is the use of light to photoisomerize bilirubin into forms that are more water-soluble and can be excreted rapidly by the liver without glucuronidation. It provides definitive treatment of hyperbilirubinemia and prevention of kernicterus. Phototherapy is an option when unconjugated bilirubin is > 12 mg/dL and may be indicated when unconjugated bilirubin is > 15 mg/dL at 25 to 48 h; 18 mg/dL at 49 to 72 h; and 20 mg/dL at > 72 h; it is not indicated for conjugated hyperbilirubinemia.

A standard phototherapy light configuration consists of overhead centrally placed blue bulbs and daylight fluorescent bulbs on each side of the infant. A double phototherapy light configuration consists of the same light configuration described above and a fiberoptic pad beneath the infant. Blue light is more effective than white, but blue light complicates detection of cyanosis, so broad-spectrum white light is also used. A clear acrylic shield placed between the phototherapy lights and the neonate screens out ultraviolet radiation, and the neonate is blindfolded to prevent eye damage (being cautious not to cause nasal obstruction). The light should be turned off and the blindfold removed during feedings. Because visible jaundice may disappear during phototherapy while serum bilirubin remains elevated, skin color cannot be used to evaluate jaundice severity. Blood taken for bilirubin determinations should be shielded from bright light, because bilirubin in the collection tubes may rapidly photo-oxidize.

Exchange transfusion: Exchange transfusion is indicated for severe hyperbilirubinemia, which most often occurs with hemolysis. Small amounts of blood are withdrawn and replaced through an umbilical vein catheter to remove partially hemolyzed and antibody-coated RBCs and replace them with uncoated donor RBCs. Only unconjugated hyperbilirubinemia can cause kernicterus, so if conjugated bilirubin is elevated, the level of unconjugated rather than total bilirubin is used to determine the need for exchange transfusion.

Specific indications are serum bilirubin ≥20 mg/dL at 24 to 48 h or ≥25 mg/dL at >48 h, failure of phototherapy to result in a 1- to 2-mg/dL decrease within 4 to 6 h of initiation, or at the 1st clinical signs of kernicterus regardless of bilirubin levels. If the serum bilirubin level is > 25 mg/dL when the infant is initially examined, preparation for an exchange transfusion should be made in case intensive phototherapy fails to lower the bilirubin level. An alternative approach uses the weight of the infant in grams divided by 100 to determine the bilirubin level (in mg/dL) at which exchange transfusion is indicated. Thus, a 1000- to 1500-g neonate would receive an exchange transfusion at a bilirubin level of 10 to 15 mg/dL, and a 1500- to 2000-g neonate at 15 to 20 mg/dL.

Most often, an exchange volume of 10 to 15 mL/kg of packed RBCs given over 2 to 4 h is used; an alternate is to give 2 successive aliquots of 10 mL/kg each over 1 to 2 h, for a total of 20 mL/kg. Goal is to reduce bilirubin by nearly 50%, with the knowledge that hyperbilirubinemia may rebound to about 60% of pretransfusion level within 1 to 2 h. It is also customary to lower the target level by 1 to 2 mg/dL in conditions that increase the risk of kernicterus (eg, fasting, sepsis, acidosis). Exchange transfusions may need to be repeated if bilirubin levels remain high.

Overall mortality is < 1% when performed by experienced personnel.

KERNICTERUS

(Bilirubin Encephalopathy)

Kernicterus is brain damage caused by unconjugated bilirubin deposition in basal ganglia and brain stem nuclei.

Normally, bilirubin bound to serum albumin stays in the intravascular space. However, bilirubin can cross the blood-brain barrier and cause kernicterus when serum bilirubin concentration is markedly elevated; serum albumin concentration is markedly low (eg, in preterm infants); or bilirubin is displaced from albumin by competitive binders (eg, sulfisoxazole, ceftriaxone, and aspirin; free fatty acids and hydrogen ions in fasting, septic, or acidotic infants).

In preterm infants, kernicterus may not produce recognizable clinical symptoms or signs. Early symptoms in term infants are lethargy, poor feeding, and vomiting. Opisthotonos, oculogyric crisis, seizures, and death may follow. Kernicterus may result in mental retardation, choreoathetoid cerebral palsy, sensorineural hearing loss, and paralysis of upward gaze later in childhood. It is unknown if minor degrees of kernicterus can produce less severe neurologic impairment (eg, perceptual-motor handicaps and learning disorders).

There is no reliable test to determine the risk of kernicterus, and the diagnosis is made presumptively. A definite diagnosis can be made only by autopsy.

There is no treatment once kernicterus develops; it can be prevented by treatment of hyperbilirubinemia (see p. 2277).

HYPERCALCEMIA

Hypercalcemia is total serum Ca > 12 mg/dL (3 mmol/L), or ionized Ca > 6 mg/dL (1.5 mmol/L). The most common cause is iatrogenic. GI signs may occur (anorexia, vomiting, constipation) and sometimes lethargy or seizures. Treatment is IV saline plus furosemide and sometimes bisphosphonates.

Etiology

The most common cause is iatrogenic, from excess Ca or vitamin D, or phosphate deprivation, which can result from prolonged feeding with incorrectly prepared formula or from dairy milk containing excess vitamin D. Other causes include maternal hypoparathyroidism, subcutaneous fat necrosis, parathyroid hyperplasia, abnormal renal function, Williams syndrome, and idiopathic. Williams syndrome includes supravalvular aortic stenosis, an elfin facies, and hypercalcemia of unknown pathophysiology; infants may also be small for gestational age, and hypercalcemia can be noted early in infancy, usually resolving by age 12 mo. Idiopathic neonatal hypercalcemia is a diagnosis of exclusion and is difficult to differentiate from Williams syndrome. Neonatal hyperparathyroidism is very rare. Subcutaneous fat necrosis may follow major trauma and causes hypercalcemia that usually resolves spontaneously. Maternal hypoparathyroidism or maternal hypocalcemia may cause secondary fetal hyperparathyroidism, with changes in fetal mineralization such as osteopenia.

Symptoms, Signs, and Diagnosis

Symptoms and signs may be noted when total serum Ca is > 12 mg/dL (> 3 mmol/L). These signs can include anorexia, GI reflux, vomiting, lethargy or seizures or generalized irritability, and hypertension. Other symptoms and signs include constipation, dehydration, feeding intolerance, and failure to thrive. With subcutaneous necrosis, firm purple nodules may be observed on trunk, buttocks, or legs.

Diagnosis is made by measuring total serum Ca concentration.

Treatment

Marked elevation of serum Ca may be treated with IV normal saline followed by furosemide and, when persistent, with corticosteroids and calcitonin. Bisphosphonates are also increasingly used in this context (eg, etidronate by mouth or pamidronate IV). Treatment of subcutaneous fat necrosis is with a low-Ca formula; fluids, furosemide, calcitonin, and corticosteroids are used as indicated by the degree of hypercalcemia. Fetal hypercalcemia from maternal hypoparathyroidism can be treated expectantly, because it usually resolves spontaneously within a few weeks. The treatment of chronic conditions includes a low-Ca, low-vitamin D formula.

HYPOCALCEMIA

Hypocalcemia is a serum total Ca concentration < 8 mg/dL (< 2 mmol/L) in term infants or < 7 mg/dL (< 1.75 mmol/L) in preterm infants. It is also defined as an ionized Ca level < 3.0 to 4.4 mg/dL (< 0.75 to 1.10 mmol/L), depending on the method (type of electrode) used. Signs include hypotonia, apnea, and tetany. Treatment is IV or oral Ca supplementation.

Etiology

Neonatal hypocalcemia may occur early (in the 1st 2 days of life) or late (> 3 days); late-onset hypocalcemia is rare. Some infants with congenital hypoparathyroidism (eg, from DiGeorge syndrome with agenesis or dysgenesis of the parathyroid glands [see p. 1343]) have both early and late (prolonged) hypocalcemia.

Risk factors for early hypocalcemia include prematurity, being small for gestational age, maternal diabetes, and perinatal asphyxia. Mechanisms vary. Normally, parathyroid hormone helps maintain normal Ca levels when the constant infusion of ionized Ca across the placenta is interrupted at birth. A transient, relative hypoparathyroidism may cause hypocalcemia in preterm and some small-for-gestational-age neonates, who have parathyroid glands that do not yet function adequately; and in infants of mothers with diabetes or hyperparathyroidism, because these women have higher-than-normal ionized Ca levels during pregnancy. Perinatal asphyxia may also increase serum calcitonin, which inhibits Ca release from bone and results in hypocalcemia. In other neonates, the normal phosphaturic renal response to parathyroid hormone is absent; the elevated phosphate (PO_4) leads to hypocalcemia.

The cause of late-onset hypocalcemia is usually infant ingestion of cow's milk or formula preparations with too high a PO_4 load; elevated serum PO_4 leads to hypocalcemia.

Symptoms, Signs, and Diagnosis

Symptoms and signs rarely occur unless total serum Ca is < 7 mg/dL (< 1.75 mmol/L) or the ionized Ca is < 3.0 mg/dL. Signs include hypotonia, tachycardia, tachypnea, apnea, poor feeding, jitteriness, tetany, and seizures. Similar symptoms may occur with hypoglycemia and opioid withdrawal.

Diagnosis is by measurement of serum total or ionized Ca; ionized Ca is the more physiologic measurement, because it obviates concerns about protein concentration and pH. Prolongation of the corrected QT interval (QT_c) on ECG also suggests hypocalcemia.

Treatment

Early-onset hypocalcemia ordinarily resolves in a few days, and asymptomatic neonates with serum Ca levels > 7 mg/dL (> 1.75 mmol/L) or ionized Ca > 3.5 mg/dL rarely require treatment. Those term infants with levels < 7 mg/dL (< 1.75 mmol/L) and preterm infants with Ca < 6 mg/dL (< 1.5 mmol/L) should be treated with 2 mL/kg of 10% Ca gluconate (200 mg/kg) by slow IV infusion over 30 min. Too-rapid infusion can cause bradycardia, so heart rate should be monitored during the infusion. The IV site should also be watched closely because tissue infiltration by a Ca solution is irritating and may cause local tissue damage or necrosis.

After acute correction of hypocalcemia, Ca gluconate may be mixed in the maintenance IV infusion and given continuously. Starting with 400 mg/kg/day of Ca gluconate, the dose may be increased gradually to 800 mg/kg/day, if needed, to prevent a recurrence. When oral feedings are begun, the formula may be supplemented with the same daily dose of Ca gluconate, if needed, by adding the 10% Ca gluconate solution into the day's formula. Supplementation is usually required for only a few days.

Treatment of late-onset hypocalcemia is addition of calcitriol or additional Ca to infant formula to provide a 4:1 molar ratio of Ca:PO_4 until normal Ca levels are maintained. Oral Ca preparations have a high sucrose content, which may lead to diarrhea in preterm infants.

HYPERGLYCEMIA

Hyperglycemia is a blood glucose concentration > 150 mg/dL (> 8.3 mmol/L).

Hyperglycemia in neonates is most often iatrogenic, caused by too-rapid IV infusions of glucose during the 1st few days of life in very low-birth-weight infants (< 1.5 kg). The other important cause is physiologic stress from surgery, hypoxia, respiratory distress syndrome, or sepsis; fungal sepsis poses a special risk. In premature infants, partially defective processing of proinsulin to insulin and relative insulin resistance may cause hyperglycemia. In addition, transient neonatal diabetes mellitus is a rare self-limited cause that usually occurs in small-for-gestational-age infants; corticosteroid administration may also result in transient hyperglycemia. Hyperglycemia is less common than hypoglycemia, but it is important because it increases morbidity and mortality of the underlying causes.

Symptoms and signs are those of the underlying condition; diagnosis is by serum glucose testing. Additional laboratory findings may include glycosuria and marked serum hyperosmolarity.

Treatment of iatrogenic hyperglycemia is reduction of IV dextrose concentration (eg, from 10 to 5%) or infusion rate; hyperglycemia persisting at low dextrose infusion rates (eg, 4 mg/kg/min) may indicate relative insulin deficiency or insulin resistance. Treatment of other causes is fast-acting insulin. One approach is to add insulin to an IV infusion of 10% dextrose at a uniform rate of 0.01 to 0.1 unit/kg/h, then titrate the rate until the glucose level is normalized. Another approach is to add insulin to a separate IV of 10% D/W given simultaneously with the maintenance IV infusion so that the insulin can be adjusted without changing the total infusion rate. Responses to insulin are unpredictable, and it is extremely important to monitor serum glucose levels and to titrate the insulin infusion rate carefully.

In transient neonatal diabetes mellitus, glucose levels and hydration should be carefully maintained until hyperglycemia resolves spontaneously, usually within a few weeks.

Any fluid or electrolytes lost through osmotic diuresis should be replaced.

HYPOGLYCEMIA

Hypoglycemia is a serum glucose concentration < 40 mg/dL (< 2.2 mmol/L) in term neonates or < 30 mg/dL (< 1.7 mmol/L) in preterm neonates. Risk factors include prematurity and perinatal asphyxia. The most common causes are deficient glycogen stores and hyperinsulinemia. Signs include tachycardia, cyanosis, seizures, and apnea. Diagnosis is suspected empirically and confirmed by glucose testing. Prognosis depends on the underlying condition. Treatment is enteral feeding or IV glucose.

Etiology

Hypoglycemia in neonates may be transient or persistent. Causes of transient hypoglycemia are inadequate substrate or immature enzyme function leading to deficient glycogen stores. Causes of persistent hypoglycemia include hyperinsulinism, defective counter-regulatory hormone release, and inherited disorders of metabolism (eg, glycogen storage diseases, disorders of gluconeogenesis, fatty acid oxidation disorders [see Ch. 296 on p. 2458]).

Deficiency of glycogen stores at birth is common in very low-birth-weight preterm infants, infants who are small for gestational age because of placental insufficiency, and infants who experience perinatal asphyxia. Anaerobic glycolysis consumes glycogen stores in these infants, and hypoglycemia may develop at any time in the 1st few days, especially if there is a prolonged interval between feedings or if nutritional intake is poor. A sustained input of exogenous glucose is therefore important to prevent hypoglycemia.

Transient hyperinsulinism most often occurs in infants of diabetic mothers and is inversely related to the degree of maternal diabetic control. It also commonly occurs in physiologically stressed infants who are small for gestational age. Less common causes include congenital hyperinsulinism (transmitted in both autosomal dominant and recessive fashion), severe erythroblastosis fetalis, and Beckwith-Wiedemann syndrome (in which islet cell hyperplasia accompanies features of macroglossia and umbilical hernia). Hyperinsulinemia characteristically results in a rapid fall in serum glucose in the 1st 1 to 2 h after birth when the continuous supply of glucose from the placenta is interrupted.

Hypoglycemia may also occur if an IV infusion of D/W is abruptly interrupted.

Symptoms, Signs, and Diagnosis

Many infants remain asymptomatic. Prolonged or severe hypoglycemia causes both adrenergic and neuroglycopenic signs. Adrenergic signs include diaphoresis, tachycardia, weakness, and shakiness or trembling. Neuroglycopenic signs include seizure, coma, cyanotic episodes, apnea, bradycardia or respiratory distress, and hypothermia. Listlessness, poor feeding, hypotonia, and tachypnea may occur. All signs are nonspecific and also occur in neonates who have experienced asphyxia, who have sepsis or hypocalcemia, or who are experiencing opioid withdrawal (see p. 2284). Therefore, at-risk patients with or without these signs require immediate bedside blood glucose check from a capillary sample. Abnormally low levels are confirmed by a venous sample.

Treatment

Most high-risk neonates are treated preventively. For example, infants of insulin-dependent diabetic women are often started at birth on a 10% dextrose infusion IV or given oral glucose, as are those who are sick, are extremely premature, or have respiratory distress. Other at-risk neonates who are not sick should be started on early, frequent formula feedings to provide carbohydrates.

Any neonate whose glucose falls ≤ 50 mg/dL should begin prompt treatment with enteral feeding or with an IV infusion of up to 12.5% D/W, 2 mL/kg over 10 min; higher concentrations of dextrose can be infused if necessary through a central catheter. The infusion should then continue at a rate that provides 4 to 8 mg/kg/min of glucose (ie, 10% D/W at about 2.5 to 5 mL/kg/h). Serum glucose levels must be monitored to guide adjustments in the infusion rate. Once the neonate's condition has improved, enteral feedings can gradually replace the IV infusion while the glucose concentration continues to be monitored. IV dextrose infusion should always be tapered, because sudden discontinuation can cause hypoglycemia.

If starting an IV infusion promptly in a hypoglycemic neonate is difficult, glucagon 100 to 300 μg/kg IM (maximum, 1 mg) usually raises the serum glucose rapidly, an effect that lasts 2 to 3 h, except in neonates with depleted glycogen stores. Hypoglycemia refractory to high rates of glucose infusion may be treated with hydrocortisone 2.5 mg/kg IM bid. If hypoglycemia is refractory to treatment, other causes (eg, sepsis) and possibly an endocrine evaluation for persistent hyperinsulinism and disorders of defective gluconeogenesis or glycogenolysis should be considered.

HYPERNATREMIA

(See also p. 1242.)

Hypernatremia is a serum Na concentration >150 mEq/L, usually from dehydration. Signs include lethargy and seizures. Treatment is cautious hydration with 0.45% saline solution.

Etiology and Pathophysiology

Hypernatremia develops when water is lost in excess of Na (hypernatremic dehydration), when Na intake exceeds Na losses (salt poisoning), or both.

Water loss in excess of Na intake is most commonly caused by diarrhea, vomiting, or high fever. It may also be caused by poor feeding in the early days of life (eg, when mother and infant are both learning to breastfeed) and may occur in very low-birth-weight (VLBW) infants born at 24 to 28 wk. In VLBW infants, insensible water losses through an immature, water-permeable stratum corneum combine with immature renal function and a reduced ability to produce concentrated urine to facilitate free water loss. Insensible water loss through the skin is also significantly increased by radiant warmers and phototherapy lights; exposed VLBW infants may require up to 250 mL/kg/day of water IV in the 1st few days, after which the stratum corneum develops and insensible water loss decreases.

Solute overload most commonly results from adding too much salt when preparing homemade infant formula or from administering hyperosmolar solutions. Fresh frozen plasma and human albumin contain Na and can contribute to hypernatremia when given repeatedly to very premature infants.

Symptoms, Signs, and Diagnosis

Symptoms and signs include lethargy, restlessness, hyperreflexia, spasticity, and seizures. Intracranial hemorrhage, venous sinus thrombosis, and acute renal tubular necrosis are major complications.

Diagnosis is suspected by symptoms and signs and confirmed by measuring serum Na concentration. Additional laboratory findings may include an increase in BUN, a modest increase in serum glucose, and, if serum K is low, a depression in the level of serum Ca.

Treatment

Treatment is with 5% dextrose/0.3% to 0.45% saline solution IV in volumes equal to the calculated fluid deficit (see p. 2291), given over 2 to 3 days to avoid a rapid fall in serum osmolality, which would cause rapid movement of water into cells and potentially lead to cerebral edema. The goal of treatment is to decrease serum Na by about 10 mEq/day. Body weight, serum electrolytes, and urine volume and specific gravity must be monitored regularly so that fluid administration can be adjusted appropriately. Once adequate urine output is demonstrated, K is added to provide maintenance requirements or replace urinary losses. Maintenance fluids should be provided concurrently.

Extreme hypernatremia (Na > 200 mEq/L) caused by salt poisoning should be treated with peritoneal dialysis, especially if poisoning causes a rapid rise in serum Na.

Prevention

Prevention requires attention to the volume and composition of unusual fluid losses and of solutions used to maintain homeostasis. In neonates and young infants, who are unable to signal thirst effectively and to replace losses voluntarily, the risk of dehydration is greatest. The composition of feedings whenever mixing is involved (eg, some infant formulas and concentrated preparations for tube feeding) requires particular attention, especially when the potential for developing dehydration is high, such as during episodes of diarrhea, poor fluid intake, vomiting, or high fever.

HYPONATREMIA

(See also p. 1237.)

Hyponatremia is a serum Na concentration < 135 mEq/L. Significant hyponatremia may cause seizures or coma. Treatment is cautious Na replacement with 0.9% saline; rarely 3% saline is required.

Etiology and Pathophysiology

The most frequent cause of hyponatremia is hypovolemic dehydration from vomiting or diarrhea (or both), when large GI losses are replaced with fluids that have little or no Na.

A less frequent cause is euvolemic hyponatremia from inappropriate ADH secretion and consequent water retention. Possible causes of inappropriate ADH include CNS tumors and infection. Also, overdilution of feeding formulas in infants can lead to water intoxication. Finally, hypervolemic hyponatremia occurs in the setting of water retention and excess Na retention, such as in heart failure or renal failure.

Symptoms, Signs, and Diagnosis

Symptoms and signs include nausea and vomiting, apathy, headache, seizures, and coma; other symptoms include cramps and weakness. Infants with hyponatremic dehydration may appear quite ill, because hyponatremia causes disproportionate reductions in ECF volume. Symptoms and signs are related to duration and degree of hyponatremia.

Diagnosis is suspected by symptoms and signs and by measuring serum Na concentration. In dehydration, an increase in BUN may be observed.

Treatment

Treatment is with 5% dextrose/0.45% to 0.9% saline solution IV in volumes equal to the calculated deficit, given over as many days as it takes to correct the Na concentration by no more than 10 to 12 mEq/L/day to avoid rapid fluid shifts in the brain. Patients with hypovolemic hyponatremia need volume expansion, using a solution containing salt to correct the Na deficit (10 to 12 mEq/kg of body weight or even 15 mEq/kg in young patients with severe hyponatremia) and include Na maintenance needs (3 mEq/kg/day in 5% dextrose solution). Patients with symptomatic hyponatremia (eg, lethargy, confusion) require emergency treatment with 3% saline to prevent seizure or coma. (For prevention, see under Hypernatremia on p. 2282.)

PRENATAL DRUG EXPOSURE

Alcohol and illicit drugs are toxic to the placenta and developing fetus and can cause congenital syndromes and withdrawal symptoms.

While exposure to some toxic substances does not imply illegal actions by the mother, some do. In any case, the home situation should be evaluated to determine if the infant will be safely cared for after discharge. With the supportive help of relatives, friends, and visiting nurses, the mother may be able to care for her infant. If not, foster home care or an alternative care plan may be best.

Alcohol: Alcohol exposure in utero can cause fetal alcohol syndrome (FAS), a variable constellation of physical and cognitive abnormalities. At birth, infants with FAS can be identified by small stature and a typical set of facial traits including microcephaly, microphthalmia, short palpebral fissures, epicanthal folds, a small or flat midface, a flat elongated philtrum, a thin upper lip, and a small chin. Abnormal palmar creases, cardiac defects, and joint contractures may also be evident. After birth, cognitive deficits become apparent. The most serious manifestation is severe mental retardation, thought to be a teratogenic effect of alcohol given the high number of retarded infants of alcoholic women; FAS may be the most common cause of noninherited mental retardation. No single physical or cognitive finding is pathognomonic; lesser degrees of alcohol use cause less severe manifestations, and the diagnosis of mild cases can be difficult because partial expression occurs. It is often difficult to distinguish the effects of alcohol on the developing fetus from those of other exposures (eg, tobacco, other drugs) and factors (eg, poor nutrition, lack of health care, violence) that affect women who drink excessively.

Diagnosis is given to infants with characteristic findings born to chronic alcoholics who drank during pregnancy.

Because it is unknown when during pregnancy alcohol is most likely to harm the fetus and whether there is a lower limit of alcohol use that is completely safe, pregnant women should be advised to avoid all alcohol intake. Siblings of an infant diagnosed with FAS should be examined for subtle manifestations of the disorder.

Barbiturates: Prolonged maternal abuse of barbiturates may cause neonatal drug withdrawal with jitteriness, irritability, and fussiness that often do not develop until 7 to 10 days postpartum, after the neonate has been discharged home. Sedation with phenobarbital 0.75 to 1.5 mg/kg po or IM q 6 h may be required and then tapered over a few days or weeks, depending on the duration of symptoms.

Cocaine: Cocaine inhibits reuptake of the neurotransmitters norepinephrine and epinephrine; it crosses the placenta and causes vasoconstriction and hypertension in the fetus. Cocaine abuse in pregnancy is associated with a higher rate of placental abruption and spontaneous abortion, perhaps caused by reduced maternal blood flow to the placental vascular bed; abruption may also lead to intrauterine fetal death or to neurologic damage if the infant survives. Neonates born to addicted mothers have low birth weight, reduced body length and head circumference, and lower Apgar scores. Cerebral infarcts may occur, and rare anomalies associated with prenatal cocaine use include limb amputations; GU malformations, including prune-belly syndrome; and intestinal atresia or necrosis. All are caused by vascular disruption, presumably secondary to local ischemia from the intense vasoconstriction of fetal arteries produced by cocaine. In addition, a pattern of mild neurobehavioral effects has also been observed, including decreases in attention and alertness, lower IQ, and impaired gross and fine motor skills.

Some neonates may show withdrawal symptoms if the mother used cocaine shortly before delivery, but symptoms are less common and less severe than for opioid withdrawal, and signs and treatment are the same.

Opioids: Opioid exposure in utero can cause withdrawal on delivery. The neonate of a woman addicted to opioids should be observed for withdrawal symptoms, which usually occur within 72 h after delivery. Characteristic signs of withdrawal include irritability, jitteriness, hypertonicity, vomiting, diarrhea, sweating, seizures, and hyperventilation that produces respiratory alkalosis. Prenatal benzodiazepine exposure may cause similar effects.

Mild withdrawal symptoms are treated by a few days of swaddling and soothing care to alleviate the physical overarousal and giving frequent feedings to reduce restlessness. With patience, most problems resolve in no more than a week. Severe symptoms can be controlled by diluting tincture of opium (which contains 10 mg morphine/mL) 25-fold with water and giving 2 drops (0.1 mL)/kg po q 4 h. The dose can be increased by 0.1 mL/kg q 4 h as needed. Phenobarbital 0.75 to 1.5 mg/kg po q 6 h may also control withdrawal symptoms. Treatment is tapered and stopped over several days or weeks as symptoms subside.

The incidence of SIDS is greater in infants born to opioid addicts but still is < 10/1000 infants, so routine use of home cardiorespiratory monitors is not recommended for these infants.

275 GASTROINTESTINAL DISORDERS IN NEONATES AND INFANTS

Infectious gastroenteritis is the most common pediatric GI disorder; about 1 billion episodes occur worldwide each year, most commonly in developing countries in children < 5 yr. Death due to dehydration occurs in 3 to 6 million cases/yr. In the US, 25 to 35 million cases occur annually, with 300 to 400 deaths. For a full discussion of causative agents, evaluation, and treatment, see Ch. 16 on p. 133. For dehydration and fluid therapy in children, see Ch. 276 on p. 2289.

HYPERTROPHIC PYLORIC STENOSIS

Hypertrophic pyloric stenosis is obstruction of the pyloric lumen due to pyloric muscular hypertrophy.

Hypertrophic pyloric stenosis may cause almost complete gastric outlet obstruction. It is more common in males by a 4:1 ratio. The exact etiology is uncertain, but a genetic component is likely because siblings and offspring of affected people are at increased risk. Proposed mechanisms include lack of neuronal nitric oxide synthase and abnormal innervation of the muscular layer. Infants exposed to erythromycin in the 1st few weeks of life are at significantly increased risk.

Symptoms develop between 2 and 6 wk of life. Projectile vomiting (without bile) occurs shortly after eating. Until dehydration sets in, the child feeds avidly and otherwise appears well, unlike many of those with vomiting due to systemic illness. Gastric peristaltic waves may be visible, crossing the epigastrium from left to right. A discrete, 2- to 3-cm, firm, movable olive-like pyloric mass is sometimes palpable deep in the right side of the epigastrium. With progression of illness, the child fails to gain weight, and signs of dehydration (see p. 2290) appear.

Diagnosis is by abdominal ultrasonography showing increased thickness of the pylorus (typically to ≥ 4 mm; normal, < 2 mm). If the diagnosis remains uncertain, ultrasonography can be repeated serially or an upper GI series obtained, which typically shows delayed gastric emptying and a "string sign" of a markedly narrowed, elongated pyloric lumen. In rare cases, upper endoscopy is required for confirmation. The classic electrolyte pattern of an infant with pyloric stenosis is that of hypochloremic metabolic alkalosis.

Initial treatment is directed at hydration and correcting electrolyte abnormalities. Definitive treatment is a longitudinal pyloromyotomy, which leaves the mucosa intact and separates the incised muscle fibers. Postoperatively, the infant usually tolerates feeding within a day.

INTUSSUSCEPTION

Intussusception is telescoping of one portion of the intestine (intussusceptum) into an adjacent segment (intussuscipiens), causing intestinal obstruction and sometimes intestinal ischemia.

Intussusception generally occurs between ages 3 mo and 3 yr, with 65% of cases occurring before age 1. It is the most common cause of intestinal obstruction in this age group, in whom it is usually idiopathic. In older children, there may be a "lead point," ie, a mass or other intestinal abnormality that triggers the telescoping; examples include polyps, lymphoma, Meckel's diverticulum, and Henoch-Schönlein purpura. Cystic fibrosis is also a risk factor.

The telescoping segments obstruct the intestine and ultimately impair blood flow, causing ischemia, gangrene, and perforation.

Symptoms and Signs

The initial symptoms are recurrent colicky abdominal pain that occurs q 15 to 20 min, often with vomiting. The child appears relatively well between episodes. Later, as intestinal ischemia develops, pain becomes steady, the child becomes lethargic, and mucosal hemorrhage causes heme-positive stool on rectal examination and sometimes spontaneous passage of a "currant jelly" stool. A palpable abdominal mass, described as sausage-shaped, is sometimes present. Perforation results in signs of peritonitis, with significant tenderness, guarding, and rigidity. Pallor, tachycardia, and diaphoresis indicate shock.

Diagnosis and Treatment

Studies and intervention must be performed urgently, because survival and likelihood of nonoperative reduction decrease significantly with time. Approach depends on clinical findings. Ill children with signs of peritonitis require fluid resuscitation (see p. 2291), broad-spectrum antibiotics (eg, ampicillin, gentamicin, clindamycin), nasogastric suction, and surgery. Others require imaging studies to confirm diagnosis and to treat the disorder.

Barium enema was once the preferred initial study because it is diagnostic and usually therapeutic; the pressure of the barium often reduces the telescoped segments. However, barium occasionally enters the peritoneum through a clinically unsuspected perforation and causes significant peritonitis. Thus, when available, ultrasound is preferred. If intussusception is confirmed, an air enema is used for reduction, which lessens the likelihood and consequences of perforation. Children are observed overnight after reduction to rule out occult perforation. If reduction is unsuccessful, immediate surgery is required. Without surgery, the recurrence rate is 10%.

MECONIUM ILEUS

Meconium ileus is obstruction of the terminal ileum by abnormally tenacious meconium; it almost universally occurs in neonates with cystic fibrosis. Meconium ileus accounts for up to ⅓ of neonatal small-bowel obstructions. Symptoms include emesis that may be bilious, abdominal distention, and failure to pass meconium. Diagnosis is based on clinical presentation and x-rays. Treatment is enemas with dilute contrast under fluoroscopy and surgery if enemas fail.

Meconium ileus is almost always an early manifestation of cystic fibrosis, which causes

GI secretions to be extremely viscid and adherent to the intestinal mucosa. Obstruction occurs at the level of the terminal ileum (unlike the colonic obstruction caused by meconium plug syndrome), typically occurs in utero, and may be diagnosed by prenatal ultrasound. Distal to the obstruction, the colon is narrow and empty or contains small amounts of desiccated meconium pellets. The relatively empty, small-caliber colon is called a microcolon.

About $1/2$ of the cases are complicated by malrotation, intestinal atresia, or perforation. The distended loops of small bowel may twist to form a volvulus in utero. If the intestine then loses its vascular supply and infarcts, sterile meconium peritonitis results. The infarcted intestinal loop may be resorbed, leaving an area or areas of intestinal atresia.

Symptoms and Signs

Unborn siblings of patients with cystic fibrosis or a neonate with any family history of cystic fibrosis should be monitored by ultrasound for meconium ileus q 6 wk. After birth, infants with meconium ileus usually have signs of intestinal obstruction—either a simple form with abdominal distention and obstipation or a more serious form with signs of peritonitis and respiratory distress. Loops of distended small bowel can sometimes be palpated through the abdominal wall and may feel characteristically doughy.

Diagnosis

Diagnosis is suspected in a neonate with signs of intestinal obstruction, particularly if a family history of cystic fibrosis exists. Patients should undergo abdominal x-rays, which show dilated intestinal loops and sometimes air-fluid levels. A "soap bubble" appearance due to small air bubbles mixed with the meconium is diagnostic of meconium ileus. If meconium peritonitis is present, calcified meconium flecks may line the peritoneal surfaces and even the scrotum. A barium enema reveals a microcolon with an obstruction in the terminal ileum.

Patients diagnosed with meconium ileus should be tested for cystic fibrosis (see p. 2308).

Treatment

Obstruction may be relieved in uncomplicated cases (eg, without perforation, volvulus, or atresia) by giving ≥ 1 enema with a dilute radiographic contrast medium plus *N*-acetylcysteine under fluoroscopy; hypertonic contrast material may cause large GI water losses requiring IV rehydration. If the enema does not relieve the obstruction, laparotomy is required. A double-barreled ileostomy with repeated *N*-acetylcysteine lavage of the proximal and distal loops is usually required to liquefy and remove the abnormal meconium.

Meconium Plug Syndrome

(Small Left Colon Syndrome)

Meconium plug syndrome is colonic obstruction caused by thick meconium.

Meconium plug syndrome usually occurs in infants who are otherwise healthy, but it is more common in infants of diabetic mothers and of toxemic mothers treated with Mg sulfate. Infants present in the 1st few days of life with failure to pass stools, abdominal distention, and vomiting. Thick, inspissated, rubbery meconium forms a cast of the colon, resulting in complete obstruction. A contrast enema with dilute meglumine diatrizoate outlines the meconium plug and usually separates the plug from the intestinal wall and expels it. Rarely, surgical decompression is required. Although most infants are healthy thereafter, diagnostic studies may be needed to rule out Hirschsprung's disease (see p. 2430) or cystic fibrosis (see p. 2309).

NECROTIZING ENTEROCOLITIS

Necrotizing enterocolitis is an acquired disease, primarily of preterm or sick neonates, characterized by mucosal or even deeper intestinal necrosis. Signs and symptoms include feeding intolerance, lethargy, temperature instability, ileus, bloating, bilious emesis, hematochezia, reducing substances in the stool, apnea, and sometimes signs of sepsis. Diagnosis is clinical and is confirmed by imaging studies. Treatment is primarily supportive and includes nasogastric suction, parenteral fluids, TPN, antibiotics, isolation in cases of infection, and, often, surgery.

Seventy-five percent of cases of necrotizing enterocolitis (NEC) occur in premature infants, particularly if prolonged rupture of the membranes with amnionitis or asphyxia occurred at birth. The incidence may also be higher in infants fed hypertonic formulas, in those who are small for gestational age, in those with cyanotic congenital heart disease, and in those who have undergone exchange transfusion.

Etiology and Pathophysiology

In infants who develop NEC, 3 intestinal factors are usually present: a preceding ischemic insult, bacterial colonization, and intraluminal substrate (ie, enteral feedings).

Etiology is not clear. It is believed that an ischemic insult damages the intestinal lining, leading to increased intestinal permeability and leaving the intestine susceptible to bacterial invasion. Once feedings are begun, ample substrate is present for proliferation of luminal bacteria, which can penetrate the damaged intestinal wall, producing hydrogen gas. The gas may collect within the intestinal wall (pneumatosis intestinalis) or enter the portal veins.

The initial ischemic insult may result from vasospasm of the mesenteric arteries, which can be produced by an anoxic insult triggering the primitive diving reflex that markedly diminishes intestinal blood flow. Intestinal ischemia may also result from low blood flow during an exchange transfusion, during sepsis, or from the use of hyperosmolar formulas. Similarly, congenital heart disease with reduced systemic blood flow or arterial O_2 desaturation may lead to intestinal hypoxia/ ischemia and predispose to NEC.

Necrosis begins in the mucosa and may progress to involve the full thickness of the intestinal wall, causing perforation with subsequent peritonitis and often free intra-abdominal air. Perforation occurs most commonly in the terminal ileum; the colon and the proximal small bowel are involved less frequently. Sepsis occurs in $\frac{1}{3}$ of infants, and death may occur.

NEC may occur as clusters of cases or as outbreaks in neonatal ICUs. Some clusters appear to be associated with specific organisms (eg, *Klebsiella, Escherichia coli,* coagulase-negative staphylococci), but often no specific pathogen is identified.

Symptoms, Signs, and Diagnosis

Infants may present with ileus manifested by abdominal distention, bilious gastric residuals (after feedings) that may progress to bilious emesis, or gross or microscopic blood in stool. Sepsis may be manifested by lethargy, temperature instability, increased apneic spells, and metabolic acidosis.

Screening the stools of enterally fed premature infants for occult blood or reducing substances may help diagnose NEC early. Early x-rays may be nonspecific and reveal only ileus. However, a fixed, dilated intestinal loop that does not change on repeated x-rays indicates NEC. X-ray signs diagnostic of NEC are pneumatosis intestinalis and portal vein gas. Pneumoperitoneum indicates bowel perforation and an urgent need for surgery.

Treatment and Prevention

The mortality rate is 20 to 40%. Aggressive support and judicious timing of surgical intervention maximize the chance of survival.

Nonsurgical support is sufficient in about 70% of cases. Feedings must be stopped immediately if NEC is suspected, and the intestine should be decompressed with a double-lumen nasogastric tube attached to intermittent suction. Appropriate colloid and crystalloid parenteral fluids must be given to support circulation, because extensive intestinal inflammation and peritonitis may lead to considerable 3rd-space fluid loss. TPN is needed for 14 to 21 days while the intestine heals. Systemic antibiotics should be started at once with a β-lactam antibiotic (ampicillin, ticarcillin) and an aminoglycoside. Additional anaerobic coverage (eg, clindamycin, metronidazole) may also be considered and should continue for 10 days (for dosage, see TABLE 279–1 on p. 2314). Because some outbreaks may be infectious, patient isolation should be considered, particularly if several cases occur within a short time.

The infant requires frequent reevaluation (eg, at least q 6 h) and serial abdominal x-rays, CBCs, platelet counts, and blood gases. Intestinal strictures are the most common long-term complication of NEC, occurring in 10 to 36% of infants who survive the initial event. Strictures are most commonly noted in the colon, especially on the left side. Resection of the stricture is then required.

Surgical intervention is needed in $\leq \frac{1}{3}$ of infants. Absolute indications are intestinal perforation (pneumoperitoneum), signs of peritonitis (absent intestinal sounds and diffuse guarding and tenderness or erythema and edema of the abdominal wall), or aspiration of purulent material from the peritoneal cavity by paracentesis. Surgery should be considered for an infant with NEC whose clinical and laboratory condition worsens despite nonsurgical support. During surgery, gangrenous bowel is resected, and ostomies are created. (Primary reanastomosis may be performed if the remaining intestine shows no signs of ischemia.) With resolution of sepsis and peritonitis, intestinal continuity can be reestablished several weeks or months later.

Risk may be decreased by delaying feedings for several days to weeks in tiny or sick premature infants while providing TPN; feedings are slowly advanced over weeks. However, in some studies this approach was not beneficial. The suggestion that breast milk offers protection is unproven. Recent evidence suggests that the use of probiotics may be beneficial in preventing NEC, but further studies are required before it can be recommended routinely.

NEONATAL CHOLESTASIS

Cholestasis is failure of bilirubin secretion, resulting in conjugated hyperbilirubinemia and jaundice. There are numerous causes, which are identified by laboratory testing, hepatobiliary scan, and, sometimes, liver biopsy and surgery. Treatment depends on cause.

Etiology

Cholestasis (see also p. 193) may result from extrahepatic or intrahepatic disorders, although some conditions overlap. The most common extrahepatic disorder is biliary atresia. There are numerous intrahepatic disorders, collectively termed the neonatal hepatitis syndrome.

Biliary atresia is obstruction of the biliary tree due to progressive sclerosis of the extrahepatic bile duct. In most cases, biliary atresia develops several weeks after birth, probably after inflammation and scarring of the extrahepatic (and sometimes intrahepatic) bile ducts. It is rarely present in premature infants or in neonates at birth. The cause of the inflammatory response is unknown, but infectious agents have been implicated.

Neonatal hepatitis syndrome (giant cell hepatitis) is an inflammatory condition of the newborn liver. It has numerous metabolic, infectious, and genetic causes; some cases are idiopathic. Metabolic diseases include α_1-antitrypsin deficiency, cystic fibrosis, neonatal iron storage disease, respiratory chain defects, and fatty acid oxidation defects. Infectious causes include congenital syphilis, echovirus, and some herpesviruses (simplex and cytomegalovirus); the hepatitis viruses are less common causes. There are also a number of less common genetic defects, such as Alagille syndrome and progressive familial intrahepatic cholestasis.

Pathophysiology

In cholestasis, the primary failure is of bilirubin excretion, resulting in excess conjugated bilirubin in the bloodstream and decreased bile salts in the GI tract. As a result of inadequate bile in the GI tract, there is malabsorption of fat and fat-soluble vitamins (A, D, E, and K) leading to vitamin deficiency, malnutrition, and growth failure.

Symptoms and Signs

Cholestasis typically is noted in the 1st 2 wk of life. Infants are jaundiced and often have dark urine (conjugated bilirubin), acholic stools, and hepatomegaly. If cholestasis persists, chronic pruritus is common, as are symptoms and signs of fat-soluble vitamin deficiency; progression on growth charts may show a decline. If the underlying disorder causes hepatic fibrosis and cirrhosis, portal hypertension with consequent ascites and upper GI bleeding from esophageal varices may develop.

Diagnosis

Any infant who is jaundiced after age 2 wk should be evaluated for cholestasis with measurement of total and direct bilirubin along with liver enzymes and other liver function tests, including albumin levels, PT, and PTT. Cholestasis is identified by an elevation in both total and direct bilirubin; once cholestasis is confirmed, further testing is required to determine the etiology. This evaluation includes tests for infectious causes (eg, toxoplasmosis, rubella, cytomegalovirus, herpesvirus, UTI, hepatitis B and C viruses) and a metabolic evaluation including urine for organic acids, serum for amino acids, α_1-antitrypsin phenotype, sweat test for cystic fibrosis, urine for reducing substances, and tests for galactosemia. If available, tests for bile salt defects can also be obtained. A hepatobiliary scan should also be performed; excretion of contrast into the intestine rules out biliary atresia, but lack of excretion can occur with both biliary atresia and severe neonatal hepatitis. An abdominal ultrasound can aid in assessing liver size and in attempting to visualize the gallbladder and common bile duct but is nonspecific. When no diagnosis has been made, a liver biopsy is generally performed relatively early on. Patients with biliary atresia typically have enlarged portal triads, bile duct proliferation, and increased fibrosis. Neonatal hepatitis is characterized by lobular disarray with multinucleated giant cells. Sometimes diagnosis remains unclear, and surgical exploration with operative cholangiography is required.

Prognosis and Treatment

Biliary atresia is progressive and if untreated results in liver failure, cirrhosis with portal hypertension by several months of age, and death by age 1 yr. Cholestasis due to neonatal hepatitis syndrome (particularly the idiopathic type) usually resolves slowly, but permanent liver damage may result and lead to death.

Initial treatment is supportive and consists primarily of nutritional therapy, including supplements of vitamins A, D, E, and K. For formula-fed infants, a formula that is high in medium-chain triglycerides should be used because it is absorbed better in the presence of bile salt deficiency. Administration of adequate calories is required; infants may need >130 calories/kg/day. In infants with some bile flow, ursodeoxycholic acid 10 to 15 mg/kg once/day or bid may relieve itching.

There is no specific therapy for neonatal hepatitis syndrome. Infants with presumed biliary atresia require surgical exploration with an intraoperative cholangiogram. If biliary atresia is confirmed, a portoenterostomy (Kasai procedure) should be performed. Ideally, this should be done in the 1st 1 to 2 mo of life. After this, the prognosis significantly worsens. Postoperatively, many patients have significant chronic problems, including persistent cholestasis, recurrent ascending cholangitis, and failure to thrive. Even with optimal therapy, many infants develop cirrhosis and require liver transplantation.

MISCELLANEOUS SURGICAL EMERGENCIES

Inguinal hernias (see p. 102) develop most often in male neonates, particularly if they are premature. About 10% of inguinal hernias are bilateral. Because inguinal hernias can become incarcerated, repair should be performed shortly after diagnosis. In contrast, umbilical hernias rarely become incarcerated, close spontaneously after several years, and do not ordinarily need surgical repair.

Gastric perforations in neonates are often spontaneous and may be due to a congenital defect in the stomach wall, usually along the greater curvature. The abdomen suddenly becomes distended, and massive pneumoperitoneum is seen on abdominal x-ray. Treatment with corticosteroids increases risk. Giving an H_2 blocker raises the gastric pH in premature infants and may reduce risk by inhibiting HCl production. Prognosis is usually good after surgical repair of the perforation.

Ileal perforation in premature infants has been reported after indomethacin has been given to close a patent ductus arteriosis. Ileal perforation is probably related to local ischemia resulting from vasoconstriction caused by indomethacin.

Mesenteric arterial occlusion from mural thrombi or emboli after high placement of an umbilical artery catheter is extremely rare but can cause extensive intestinal infarction requiring surgery and intestinal resection.

276 DEHYDRATION AND FLUID THERAPY

(See also Ch. 156 on p. 1233 and Hypernatremia and Hyponatremia on p. 2282.)

Unlike in adults, fluid management in children is based on weight and on specific guidelines, because children are more sensitive to fluid depletion (and excess). All guidelines are approximations; individualized adjustments based on close monitoring are essential.

DEHYDRATION

Dehydration is significant depletion of body water and, usually, of electrolytes. Symptoms and signs include thirst, lethargy, dry mucosa, decreased urine output, and, as the

degree of dehydration progresses, tachycardia, hypotension, and shock. Diagnosis is by history and physical examination. Treatment is with oral or IV replacement of fluid and electrolytes.

Dehydration, usually due to diarrhea, remains a major cause of morbidity and mortality in infants and young children worldwide. Infants are particularly susceptible to the ill effects of dehydration because of their greater baseline fluid requirements (due to a higher metabolic rate), higher evaporative losses (due to a higher ratio of surface area to volume), and inability to communicate thirst or seek fluid.

Etiology and Pathophysiology

Dehydration results from increased fluid loss, decreased fluid intake, or both.

The most common source of increased fluid loss is the GI tract from vomiting, diarrhea, or both (eg, gastroenteritis). Other sources are renal (eg, diabetic ketoacidosis), cutaneous (eg, excessive sweating, burns), and 3rd-space losses (eg, into the intestinal lumen in bowel obstruction). All types of lost fluid contain electrolytes in varying concentrations, so fluid loss is always accompanied by electrolyte loss.

Decreased fluid intake is common during serious illness of any kind and is particularly problematic when vomiting is present and during hot weather. It may also be a sign of neglect.

Symptoms, Signs, and Diagnosis

Symptoms and signs vary according to degree of deficit (see TABLE 276–1) and are affected by serum Na concentration: hemodynamic findings are exaggerated by hyponatremia and reduced by hypernatremia. In general, dehydration without hemodynamic changes is considered mild (about 5% body weight in infants and 3% in adolescents); tachycardia defines moderate dehydration (about 10% body weight in infants and 6% in adolescents); and hypotension with impaired perfusion defines severe dehydration (about 15% body weight in infants and 9% in adolescents). A more accurate method with acute dehydration is change in body weight; all short-term weight loss > 1%/day is presumed to represent fluid deficit. However, this method depends on knowing a precise, recent pre-illness weight. Parental estimates are usually inadequate; a 1-kg error in a 10-kg child causes a 10% error in the calculated percentage of dehydration—the difference between mild and severe dehydration.

Laboratory testing is generally reserved for moderately or severely ill children, in whom electrolyte disturbances (eg, hypernatremia, hypokalemia, metabolic acidosis) are more common. Other laboratory abnormalities include relative polycythemia from hemoconcentration, elevated BUN, and increased urine specific gravity.

TABLE 276–1. CLINICAL CORRELATES OF DEHYDRATION

	FLUID DEFICIT IN mL/kg (PERCENT BODY WT)*		
SEVERITY	**Infants**	**Adolescents**	**SIGNS**
Mild	50 (5%)	30 (3%)	Slightly dry buccal mucous membranes, increased thirst, slightly decreased urine output
Moderate	100 (10%)	50–60 (5–6%)	Dry buccal mucous membranes, tachycardia, little or no urine output, lethargy, sunken eyes and fontanelles, loss of skin turgor
Severe	150 (15%)	70–90 (5–9%)	Same as moderate plus a rapid, thready pulse; no tears, cyanosis; rapid breathing; delayed capillary refill; hypotension; mottled skin; coma

*Standard estimates for children between infancy and adolescence have not been established. For children between these age ranges, clinicians must estimate values between those for infants and those for adolescents based on clinical judgment.

Treatment

Treatment is best approached by considering separately the fluid resuscitation requirements, current deficit, ongoing losses, and maintenance requirements. The volume (eg, amount of fluid), composition, and rate of replacement may differ for each. Formulas and estimates used to determine treatment parameters provide a starting place, but treatment requires ongoing monitoring of vital signs, clinical appearance, urine output and specific gravity, weight, and sometimes serum electrolyte levels. Children with severe dehydration (eg, evidence of circulatory compromise) should receive fluids IV. Those unable or unwilling to drink or who have repetitive vomiting can receive fluid replacement IV, through an NGT, or sometimes orally through administration of frequently repeated small amounts (see p. 2293).

Resuscitation: Patients with signs of hypoperfusion should receive fluid resuscitation with boluses of isotonic fluid (eg, 0.9% saline or Ringer's lactate). The goal is to restore adequate circulating volume to restore BP and perfusion. The resuscitation phase should reduce moderate or severe dehydration to a deficit of about 8% of body weight. If dehydration is moderate, 20 mL/kg (2% body weight) is given IV over 20 to 30 min, reducing a 10% deficit to 8%. If dehydration is severe, 2 to 3 boluses of 20 mL/kg (2% body weight) will likely be required. The end point of the fluid resuscitation phase is restoration of peripheral perfusion and BP and return of increased heart rate toward normal.

Deficit replacement: Total deficit volume is estimated clinically as described above. Na deficits are generally about 80 mEq/L of fluid deficit, and K deficits are generally about 30 mEq/L of fluid deficit. The resuscitation phase should have reduced moderate or severe dehydration to a deficit of about 8% body weight; this remaining deficit can be replaced by providing 10 mL/kg (1% body weight)/h for 8 h. Because 0.45% saline has 77 mEq Na per liter, it is generally an appropriate fluid choice. K replacement (usually by adding 20 to 40 mEq K per liter of replacement fluid) should not begin until adequate urine output is established.

Dehydration with significant hypernatremia (eg, serum Na > 160 mEq/L) or hyponatremia (eg, serum Na < 120 mEq/L) requires special consideration to avoid complications (see pp. 2282–2283).

TABLE 276–2. ESTIMATED ELECTROLYTE DEFICITS BY CAUSE

CAUSE	SODIUM (mEq/L)	POTASSIUM (mEq/L)
Fasting and thirsting	50	10
Diarrhea		
Isotonic dehydration	80	80
Hypotonic dehydration	100	80
Hypertonic dehydration	20	10
Pyloric stenosis	80	100
Diabetic ketoacidosis	80	50

Ongoing losses: Volume of ongoing losses should be measured directly (eg, NGT, catheter, stool measurements) or estimated (eg, 10 mL/kg per diarrheal stool). Replacement should be milliliter for milliliter in time intervals appropriate for the rapidity and extent of the loss. Ongoing electrolyte losses can be estimated by source or cause (see TABLE 276–2). Urinary electrolyte losses vary with intake and disease process but can be measured if deficits fail to respond to replacement therapy.

Maintenance requirements: Fluid and electrolyte needs from basal metabolism must also be accounted for. Maintenance requirements are related to metabolic rate and affected by body temperature. Insensible losses (evaporative free water losses from the skin and respiratory tract in a ratio of 2:1) account for about ½ of maintenance needs.

Volume rarely must be exactly determined but generally should aim to provide an amount of water that does not require the kidney to significantly concentrate or dilute the urine. The most common estimate uses patient weight to calculate metabolic expenditure in kcal/24 h, which approximates fluid needs in mL/24 h (see TABLE 276–3). A simpler calculation (the Holliday-Segar formula) uses 3 weight classes (see TABLE 276–4). BSA derived from a nomogram (see FIG. 276–1) also can be used, allowing 1500 to 2000 mL/m^2/24 h. More complex calculations are rarely

TABLE 276–3. STANDARD BASAL METABOLIC RATES USED FOR CALCULATING MAINTENANCE FLUID REQUIREMENTS*

WEIGHT (kg)	kcal/24 h†, ‡		
	Male	Both Sexes	Female
3		140	
5		270	
7		400	
9		500	
11		600	
13		650	
15		710	
17		780	
19		830	
21		880	
25	1020		960
29	1120		1040
33	1210		1120
37	1300		1190
41	1350		1260
45	1410		1320
49	1470		1380
53	1530		1440
57	1590		1500
61	1640		1560

*Metabolic expenditure in kcal/24 h approximates maintenance fluid needs in mL/24 h.

†Add or subtract 12% to basal metabolic rate (general metabolic rate in kcal/24 h) for each degree C above or below rectal temperature of 37.8°C.

‡Add 0–30% to basal metabolic rate for usual activity; hypometabolic or hypermetabolic states require greater adjustments.

required. These volumes can be given as a separate simultaneous infusion, so that the rate of infusion replacing deficits and ongoing losses can be set and adjusted independent of rate of maintenance infusion.

Baseline estimates are affected by fever (increasing by 12% for each degree > 37.8° C), hypothermia, and activity (eg, increased for hyperthyroidism or status epilepticus, decreased for coma).

Composition differs from solutions used to replace deficits and ongoing losses. Patients require Na 3 mEq/100 kcal/24 h (3 mEq/100 mL/24 h) and K 2 mEq/100 kcal/24 h (2 mEq/100 mL/24 h). This need is met by using 0.2% to 0.3% saline with 20 mEq/L of K in a 5% dextrose solution (5% D/W). Other electrolytes (eg, Mg, Ca) are not routinely added. It is inappropriate to replace deficits and ongoing losses solely by increasing the amount or rate of maintenance fluids.

PRACTICAL EXAMPLE

A 7-mo-old infant has diarrhea for 3 days with weight loss from 10 kg to 9 kg. He is currently producing 1 diarrheal stool q 3 h and refusing to drink. Clinical findings of dry mucous membranes, poor skin turgor, markedly decreased urine output, and tachycardia with normal BP and capillary refill suggest 10% fluid deficit. Rectal temperature is 37°C; serum Na, 136 mEq/L; K, 4 mEq/L; Cl, 104 mEq/L; and HCO_3, 20 mEq/L.

Fluid volume is estimated by deficits, ongoing losses, and maintenance requirements.

The total fluid deficit given 1 kg weight loss = 1 L.

Ongoing diarrhea losses are measured as they occur by weighing the infant's diaper before application and after the diarrheal stool.

TABLE 276–4. HOLLIDAY-SEGAR FORMULA FOR MAINTENANCE FLUID REQUIREMENTS BY WEIGHT

WEIGHT	WATER		ELECTROLYTES ($mEq/L\ H_2O$)
	mL/day	mL/h	
0–10 kg	100/kg	4/kg	Na 30, K 20
11–20 kg	1000 + 50/kg for each kg >10	40 + 2/kg for each kg > 10	Na 30, K 20
> 20 kg	1500 + 20/kg for each kg > 20	60 + 1/kg for each kg > 20	Na 30, K 20

Baseline maintenance requirements by the weight-based Holliday-Segar method are 100 mL/kg × 10 kg = 1000 mL/day = 1000/24 or 40 mL/h.

Electrolyte losses from diarrhea (see TABLE 276–2) are an estimated 80 mEq of Na and 80 mEq of K.

Procedure

Resuscitation: The patient is given an initial bolus of Ringer's lactate 200 mL (20 mL/kg × 10 kg) over 30 min. This replaces 26 mEq of the estimated 80 mEq Na deficit.

Deficits: Residual fluid deficit is 800 mL (1000 initial minus 200 mL resuscitation), and Na deficit is 54 mEq (80 – 26 mEq). This is given over 8 h as 5% dextrose/0.45% saline at 100 mL/h. This replaces the Na deficit (0.8 L × 77 mEq Na/L = 62 mEq Na). When urine output is established, K is added at a concentration of 30 mEq/L (for safety reasons, no attempt is made to replace complete K deficit acutely).

Ongoing losses: Five percent dextrose/0.45% saline also is used to replace ongoing losses; volume and rate are determined by the amount of diarrhea.

Maintenance fluid: Five percent dextrose/0.2% saline is given at 40 mL/h with 20 mEq/L of K added when urine output is established. Alternatively, the deficit could be replaced during the initial 8 h followed by the entire day's maintenance fluid in the next 16 h (ie, 60 mL/h); 24 h of maintenance fluid given in 16 h reduces mathematically to a rate of 1.5 times the usual maintenance rate and obviates the need for simultaneous infusions (which may require 2 rate-controlling pumps).

ORAL REHYDRATION

Oral fluid therapy is effective, safe, convenient, and inexpensive compared with IV therapy. It should be used for children with mild to moderate dehydration who are accepting fluids orally unless prohibited by copious vomiting or underlying disorders (eg, surgical abdomen, intestinal obstruction).

Solutions: The oral rehydration solution should contain complex carbohydrate or 2% glucose and 50 to 90 mEq/L of Na. Sports drinks, soda, juice, and similar drinks do not meet these criteria and should not be used. They generally have too little Na and too much carbohydrate to take advantage of Na-glucose cotransport, and the osmotic effect of the excess carbohydrate may result in additional fluid loss.

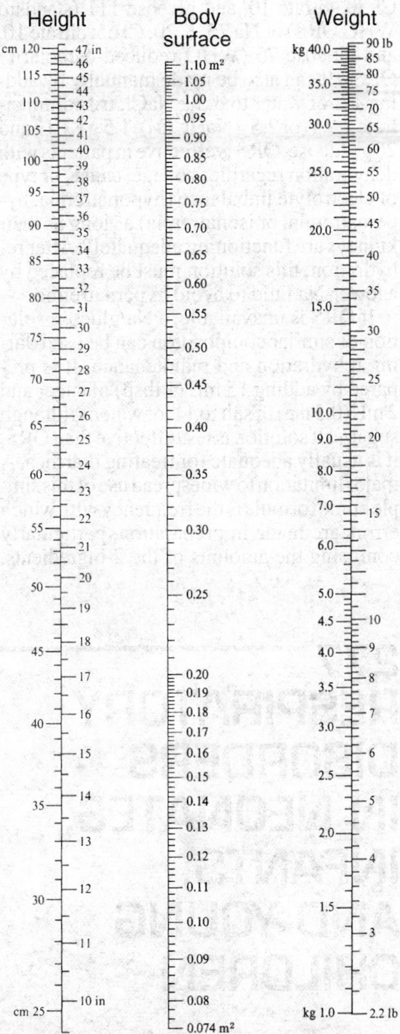

Fig. 276–1. Nomogram for calculating the body surface area of children. (Adapted from *Geigy Scientific Tables*, ed. 8, vol. 1, edited by C Lentner. Basle, Switzerland, Ciba-Geigy Ltd., 1981, pp. 226–227; used with permission.)

Oral rehydration solution (ORS) is recommended by the WHO and is widely available in the US without prescription. Most come as powders that are mixed with tap water. An ORS packet is dissolved in 1 L of water to produce a solution containing (in mmol/L) Na 90, K 20,

Cl 80, citrate 10, and glucose 111 (standard WHO ORS) or Na 75, K 20, Cl 65, citrate 10, and glucose 75 (WHO reduced-osmolarity ORS). It can also be made manually by adding 1 L of water to 3.5 g NaCl, trisodium citrate 2.9 g (or 2.5 g $NaHCO_3$), 1.5 g KCL, and 20 g glucose. ORS is effective in patients with dehydration regardless of age, cause, or type of electrolyte imbalance (hyponatremia, hypernatremia, or isonatremia) as long as their kidneys are functioning adequately. After rehydration, this solution must be replaced by a lower-Na fluid to avoid hypernatremia.

If ORS is unavailable, a Na/glucose solution of similar composition can be used during rehydration and maintenance. It is prepared by adding 15 mL (1 tbsp) of sugar and 2 mL (0.5 tsp) of salt to 1 L of water. Although sugar/salt solution is less effective than ORS, it is usually adequate for treating diarrhea. A major limitation to widespread use of this simple home formula is the frequency with which errors are made in preparation, particularly confusing the amounts of the 2 ingredients, such that 1 tbsp salt and ½ tsp sugar are used instead of 1 tbsp sugar and ½ tsp salt.

Administration: Generally, 50 mL/kg is given over 4 h for mild dehydration and 100 mL/kg for moderate. For each diarrheal stool, an additional 10 mL/kg (up to 240 mL) is given. After 4 h, the patient is reassessed. If signs of dehydration persist, the same volume is repeated. Patients with cholera may require many gallons of fluid/day.

Vomiting generally should not deter oral rehydration (absent bowel obstruction or other contraindication). Small, frequent amounts are used, starting with 5 mL q 5 min and increasing gradually as tolerated.

Once the deficit has been replaced, an oral maintenance solution containing less Na should be used. Children should eat an age-appropriate diet as soon as they have been rehydrated and are not vomiting. Infants may resume breastfeeding or formula. Infants with diarrhea who develop signs or symptoms of malabsorption (see p. 139) should be given lactose-free formula.

277 RESPIRATORY DISORDERS IN NEONATES, INFANTS, AND YOUNG CHILDREN

Respiratory distress in neonates and infants has multiple causes (see TABLE 277–1). Symptoms and signs vary and include nasal flaring; intercostal, subcostal, and suprasternal retractions; weak and/or irregular breathing; tachypnea and apneic spells; cyanosis, pallor, mottling, and/or delayed capillary refill; and hypotension. In neonates, symptoms and signs may be apparent immediately upon delivery or develop minutes or hours afterward.

Evaluation starts with a thorough history and physical examination. History in the neonate focuses on maternal and prenatal history, particularly gestational age, maternal infection or bleeding, meconium staining of amniotic fluid, and oligohydramnios or polyhydramnios. Physical examination focuses on the heart and lungs. Chest wall asymmetry or sunken abdomen suggests diaphragmatic hernia. Asymmetric breath sounds suggest pneumothorax, and a displaced left apical impulse and/or heart murmur suggests a congenital heart defect. Assessment of BP, femoral pulse, and capillary refill helps identify any concomitant circulatory compromise. In both neonates and infants, it is important to assess oxygenation and response to O_2 administration by pulse oximetry. Chest x-ray is also recommended.

There are several significant differences in the physiology of the respiratory system in infants compared with that of older children and adults. These differences include a more compliant collapsible chest wall, more reliance on diaphragmatic excursions over intercostal muscles, and collapsible extrathoracic airways; also, infants' smaller airway caliber gives increased airway resistance and increased tendency toward atelectasis. Yet, other principles of respiration are similar in adults and children.

TABLE 277–1. CAUSES OF RESPIRATORY DISTRESS IN NEONATES AND INFANTS

CATEGORY	CAUSE
Cardiac	**Right-to-left shunting with normal or increased pulmonary flow**: Transposition of the great vessels, total anomalous venous return, truncus arteriosus, hypoplastic left heart syndrome
	Right-to-left shunting with decreased pulmonary flow: Pulmonary atresia, tetralogy of Fallot, critical pulmonic stenosis, tricuspid atresia, single ventricle with pulmonic stenosis, Ebstein's anomaly, persistent fetal circulation/persistent pulmonary hypertension
Respiratory	**Upper tract**: Choanal atresia or stenosis, tracheobroncholaryngeal stenosis, compressive obstruction (eg, vascular ring), tracheoesophageal anomalies (eg, cleft, fistula)
	Lower tract: Respiratory distress syndrome, transient tachypnea of the newborn, meconium aspiration, pneumonia, sepsis, pneumothorax, congenital diaphragmatic hernia, pulmonary hypoplasia, cystic malformation of the lung, congenital deficiency of surfactant proteins B or C
Neurologic	Intracranial hemorrhage or hypertension, oversedation (infant or maternal), diaphragmatic paralysis, neuromuscular disease, seizure disorder
Hematologic	Methemoglobinemia, polycythemia, severe anemia
Miscellaneous	Hypoglycemia, blood loss, metabolic disorders (eg, acid-base disorders, hyperammonemia), hypovolemic shock

RESPIRATORY SUPPORT

Initial stabilization maneuvers include head positioning, suctioning of the mouth and nose, and tactile stimulation (see p. 2259), followed as needed by supplemental O_2, continuous positive airway pressure (CPAP), bag and mask ventilation, or mechanical ventilation. Infants who cannot be oxygenated by any of these means may require a full cardiac evaluation to exclude congenital heart disease and treatment with high frequency oscillatory ventilation, nitric oxide, and/or extracorporeal membrane oxygenation.

Oxygen: O_2 may be given using a nasal cannula, face mask, or O_2 hood, with O_2 concentration set to achieve a PaO_2 of 50 to 70 mm Hg in preterm infants and 50 to 80 mm Hg in term infants or an O_2 saturation of 88 to 94% in preterm infants and 92 to 96% in term infants. Lower PaO_2 in preterm infants provides almost full saturation of Hb, because fetal Hb has a higher affinity for O_2; maintaining higher PaO_2 may increase the risk of retinopathy of prematurity. No matter how O_2 is delivered, it should be warmed (36 to 37° C) and humidified to prevent secretions from cooling and drying and to prevent bronchospasm. An umbilical artery catheter (UAC) is usually placed for sampling ABGs in neonates who require fraction of inspired O_2 (FIO_2) ≥ 40%. If a UAC cannot be placed, a percutaneous radial artery catheter can be used for continuous BP monitoring and blood sampling.

Neonates who are unresponsive to these maneuvers may require fluid administration to improve cardiac output and are candidates for CPAP ventilation or bag and mask ventilation (40 to 60 breaths/min). If the infant does not oxygenate with or requires prolonged bag and mask ventilation, endotracheal intubation with mechanical ventilation is indicated, although very immature infants (eg, < 28 wk gestation or < 1000 g) are typically begun on ventilatory support immediately after delivery so that they can receive preventive surfactant therapy. Because bacterial sepsis is a common cause of respiratory distress in neonates, it is common practice to draw blood cultures and administer antibiotics to neonates with high O_2 requirements pending culture results.

Continuous positive airway pressure: CPAP delivers O_2 at a positive pressure, usually 5 to 7 cm H_2O, which keeps alveoli open and improves oxygenation by reducing the amount of blood shunted through atelectatic areas while the infant breathes spontaneously.

CPAP can be provided using nasal prongs and various types of apparatus to provide the positive pressure; it can also be given using an endotracheal tube connected to a conventional ventilator with the rate set to zero. CPAP is indicated when $FIO_2 \geq 40\%$ is required to maintain acceptable PaO_2 (50 to 70 mm Hg) in infants with respiratory diseases that are of limited duration (eg, diffuse atelectasis, mild respiratory distress syndrome, lung edema). In these children, CPAP may preempt the need for positive pressure ventilation.

Mechanical ventilation (see also p. 544): Endotracheal tubes 2.5 mm in diameter (the smallest) are typically used for infants < 1250 g; 3 mm for infants 1250 to 2500 g; and 3.5 mm for those > 2500 g. Intubation is safer if O_2 is insufflated into the infant's airway during the procedure. Orotracheal intubation is preferred; the tube should be inserted such that the 7-cm mark is at the lip for infants who weigh 1 kg; 8 cm for 2 kg; and 9 cm for 3 kg. The endotracheal tube is properly placed when its tip can be palpated through the anterior tracheal wall at the suprasternal notch. It should be positioned about halfway between the clavicles and the carina on chest x-ray, coinciding roughly with vertebral level T2. If position or patency is in doubt, the tube should be removed and the infant supported by bag and mask ventilation until a new tube is inserted. Acute deterioration of the infant's condition (sudden changes in oxygenation, ABGs, BP, or perfusion) should trigger suspicion of changes in the position and/or patency of the tube.

Ventilators can be set to deliver fixed pressures or volumes; can provide assist control (AC, in which the ventilator is triggered to deliver a full breath with each patient inspiration) or intermittent mandatory ventilation (IMV, in which the ventilator delivers a set number of breaths within a time period, and patients can take spontaneous breaths in between without triggering the ventilator); and can be normal or high frequency (delivering 400 to 900 breaths/min). No mode or type of ventilation is proven better than the other. Nevertheless, volume ventilators are considered useful for larger infants with varying pulmonary compliance or resistance (eg, in bronchopulmonary dysplasia), because delivering a set volume of gas with each breath ensures adequate ventilation; assist-control mode is often used for treatment of less severe pulmonary disease and in decreasing ventilator dependence while providing a small increase in airway pressure or a small volume of gas with each spontaneous breath; and high-frequency jet, oscillatory, and flow-interrupter ventilators are used in extremely premature infants (< 28 wk) and in some infants with air leaks, widespread atelectasis, or pulmonary edema.

Initial ventilator settings are estimated by judging the severity of respiratory impairment. Typical settings for an infant in moderate respiratory distress are $FIO_2 = 40\%$; inspiratory time (IT) = 0.4 sec; expiratory time = 1.1 sec; IMV or AC rate = 40 breaths/min; peak inspiratory pressure (PIP) = 15 cm H_2O for very low-birth-weight and up to 25 cm H_2O for near-term infants; and positive end-expiratory pressure (PEEP) = 5 cm H_2O. These settings are adjusted based on the infant's oxygenation, chest wall movement, breath sounds, and respiratory efforts along with the arterial or capillary blood gases.

$PaCO_2$ is lowered by increasing the minute ventilation through an increase in tidal volume (increasing PIP or decreasing PEEP) or an increase in rate. The PaO_2 is increased by increasing the FIO_2 or increasing the mean airway pressure (increasing PIP, PEEP, or rate or prolonging IT). Patient-triggered ventilation is often used to synchronize the positive pressure ventilator breaths with the onset of the patient's own spontaneous respirations. This appears to shorten the time on a ventilator and may reduce barotrauma. A pressure-sensitive air-filled balloon attached to a pressure transducer (Graseby capsule) taped to the infant's abdomen just below the xiphoid process can detect the onset of diaphragmatic contraction, or a flow or temperature sensor placed at the endotracheal tube adapter can detect the onset of a spontaneous inhalation.

Ventilator pressures or volumes should be as low as possible to prevent barotrauma and bronchopulmonary dysplasia; an elevated $PaCO_2$ is acceptable as long as pH remains ≥ 7.25 (permissive hypercapnia). Likewise, a PaO_2 as low as 40 mm Hg is acceptable if BP is normal and metabolic acidosis is not present.

Paralytics, sedation, and nitric oxide are adjunctive treatments used with mechanical ventilation in some patients. Paralytics (eg, vecuronium or pancuronium bromide 0.03 to 0.1 mg/kg IV q 1 to 2 h as needed [with pancuronium, a test dose of 0.02 mg/kg is recommended in neonates]) and sedatives (eg, fentanyl 1 to 4 μg/kg IV push q 2 to 4 h or midazolam 0.05 to 0.15 mg/kg IV over 5 min q 2 to 4 h) may facilitate endotracheal intubation and can help stabilize infants whose movements and spontaneous breathing prevent optimal ventilation. These agents should be used selectively, however, because paralyzed infants may need greater ventilator support, which can increase barotrauma. Inhaled nitric oxide 5 to 20 ppm may be used for refractory hypoxemia when pulmonary vasoconstriction is a contributor to hypoxia (eg, in idiopathic pulmonary hypertension, pneumonia, or congenital diaphragmatic hernia) and may prevent the need for extracorporeal membrane oxygenation (see below).

As respiratory status improves, the infant can be weaned from the ventilator by lowering the FIO_2, inspiratory pressure, and rate. Continuous-flow positive pressure ventilators permit the infant to breathe spontaneously against PEEP while the ventilator rate is progressively slowed. After the rate has been reduced to 10 breaths/min, the infant usually tolerates extubation. The final steps in ventilator weaning involve extubation, possibly support with nasal (or nasopharyngeal) CPAP, and, finally, use of a hood or nasal cannula to provide humidified O_2 or air.

Very low-birth-weight infants may benefit from the addition of a methylxanthine during the weaning process. Initial dosing for aminophylline is 5 mg/kg IV loading followed by a maintenance dose of 1.5 to 3 mg/kg IV q 8 h; for theophylline a 4 mg/kg loading dose is given orally or by gastric tube, followed by a maintenance dose of 2 mg/kg bid. Doses of both agents are adjusted as needed to maintain a blood theophylline level of 7 to 12 μg/mL (39 to 67 μmol/L). Methylxanthines are CNS-mediated respiratory stimulants that increase ventilatory effort and may reduce apneic and bradycardic episodes that may interfere with successful weaning. Corticosteroids, once used routinely for weaning and treatment of chronic lung disease, are no longer recommended in premature infants because risks (eg, impaired growth and neurodevelopmental delay) outweigh benefits. A possible exception is as a last resort in near-terminal illness, in which case parents should be fully informed of risks.

Complications of mechanical ventilation more common in neonates include asphyxia from endotracheal tube obstruction; ulceration, erosion, or narrowing of airway structures due to adjacent pressure; and bronchopulmonary dysplasia (see p. 2298).

Extracorporeal membrane oxygenation (ECMO): ECMO is a form of cardiopulmonary bypass used for infants who cannot be adequately oxygenated or ventilated with conventional ventilators. Eligibility criteria vary by center, but in general, infants should have reversible disease (eg, persistent pulmonary hypertension of the newborn, congenital diaphragmatic hernia, overwhelming pneumonia) and have been on mechanical ventilation < 7 days. After systemic heparinization, blood is circulated through large-diameter catheters from the internal jugular vein into a membrane oxygenator, which serves as an artificial lung to remove CO_2 and add O_2; oxygenated blood is then circulated back to the internal jugular vein (venovenous ECMO) or to the carotid artery (venoarterial ECMO). Venoarterial ECMO is used when circulatory in addition to ventilatory support is needed (eg, in overwhelming sepsis). Flow rates can be adjusted to obtain desired O_2 saturation and BP. ECMO is contraindicated in infants < 34 wk and/or < 2 kg because of the risk of intraventricular hemorrhage with systemic heparinization. Complications include thromboembolism, air embolization, neurologic (stroke, seizures) and hematologic (hemolysis, neutropenia, thrombocytopenia) problems, and cholestatic jaundice.

APNEA OF PREMATURITY

Apnea of prematurity is defined as respiratory pauses > 20 sec or airflow interruption and respiratory pauses < 20 sec associated with bradycardia (< 80 beats/min), central cyanosis, or O_2 saturation < 85% in infants born at < 37 wk gestation and with no underlying disorders causing apnea. Cause may be CNS immaturity (central) or airway obstruction. Diagnosis is by multichannel respiratory monitoring. Treatment is with respiratory stimulants for central apnea and head positioning for obstructive apnea. Prognosis is excellent; apnea resolves in most neonates by 37 wk.

About 25% of preterm infants have apnea of prematurity, which usually begins 2 to 3 days after birth and only rarely on the 1st day; apnea that develops > 14 days after birth in an otherwise healthy infant signifies a serious illness other than apnea of prematurity. Risk increases with earlier gestational age.

Etiology and Pathophysiology

Apnea of prematurity may be central, obstructive, or both; a mixed pattern is most common. Central apnea is caused by immaturity of medullary respiratory control centers; insufficient neural impulses from the respiratory centers in the medulla reach the respiratory muscles, and the infant stops breathing. Hypoxemia briefly stimulates respiratory efforts but, after a few seconds, suppresses respirations. Obstructive apnea is caused by obstructed airflow, either from neck flexion causing opposition of hypopharyngeal soft tissues or from nasal occlusion. Both types of apnea can cause hypoxemia, cyanosis, and bradycardia if the apnea is prolonged. Among infants dying of SIDS, 18% have a history of prematurity, but apnea of prematurity does not appear to be a precursor to SIDS.

Diagnosis

Diagnosis of apnea itself is occasionally made by observation alone, but high-risk infants are typically diagnosed by an apnea monitor worn for 5 to 7 days. Typical monitors use a chest band to detect chest wall movements and pulse oximetry to detect heart rate and O_2 saturation; nasal airflow must also be monitored if obstructive apnea is suspected. Apnea of prematurity is a diagnosis of exclusion. Other causes of apnea in neonates include hypoglycemia, hypocalcemia, sepsis, intracranial hemorrhage, and gastroesophageal reflux; these causes are sought with appropriate testing (see elsewhere in THE MANUAL).

High-risk infants who are not apneic and who are otherwise ready for discharge may be monitored at home. Parents need to be taught how to place the monitoring belt and leads; how to interpret the significance of alarms by assessing the infant's color and respirations; and how to intervene. They should also be instructed to keep a log of alarms and infant appearance and to contact medical providers if questions arise or apneic episodes occur. Many monitors store information, allowing providers to assess the type and frequency of events, compare them with events reported and logged by the parents, and determine if other treatment is needed or if monitoring can be stopped.

Prognosis and Treatment

Most preterm infants stop having apneic spells by the time they reach about 37 wk gestation; apnea may continue for weeks in infants born at extremely early gestational ages (eg, 23 to 27 wk). Mortality, treated or untreated, is probably negligible.

The infant's head should be kept in the midline and the neck in the neutral position or slightly extended to prevent upper airway obstruction. All premature infants, especially those with apnea of prematurity, are at risk of apnea, bradycardia, and O_2 desaturation while in a car seat and should undergo a car seat challenge test before discharge.

When apnea is noted, either by observation or monitor alarm, infants are stimulated, which may be all that is required; if breathing does not resume, bag-valve-mask or mouth-to-mouth-and-nose ventilation is provided (see p. 526). For infants at home, the physician is contacted if apnea occurred but ceased after stimulation; if intervention beyond stimulation is required, the infant should be rehospitalized and evaluated.

Respiratory stimulants are indicated for treatment of frequent or severe episodes, characterized by hypoxemia, cyanosis, and/or bradycardia. Caffeine is the safest and most commonly used drug. It can be given as caffeine base (loading dose 10 mg/kg followed by a maintenance dose of 2.5 mg/kg po q 24 h) or caffeine citrate, a caffeine salt which is 50% caffeine (loading dose 20 mg/kg followed by a maintenance dose of 5 mg/kg q 24 h). Other options include IV methylxanthines (aminophylline loading dose 6 to 7 mg/kg infused over 20 min followed by a maintenance dose of 1 to 3 mg/kg q 8 to 12 h [lower in younger, more premature infants] or theophylline loading dose 4 to 5 mg/kg followed by a maintenance dose of 1 to 2 mg/kg q 8 to 12 h), with doses adjusted to maintain a serum concentration of 6 to 12 μg/mL, and doxapram (0.5 to 2.0 mg/kg/h continuous IV infusion). Treatment continues until the neonate is 34 to 35 wk gestation and free from apnea requiring physical intervention for at least 5 to 7 days. Monitoring continues until the neonate is free of apnea requiring intervention for 5 to 10 days.

If apnea continues despite respiratory stimulants, the neonate may be given continuous positive airway pressure starting at 5 to 8 cm H_2O pressure. Intractable apneic spells require ventilator support. Discharge practices vary; some providers observe infants for 7 days after treatment has ended to ensure that apnea or bradycardia does not recur, whereas others discharge with theophylline if treatment appears effective.

BRONCHOPULMONARY DYSPLASIA

Bronchopulmonary dysplasia is chronic lung injury in premature infants caused by

supplemental O_2 and prolonged mechanical ventilation.

Bronchopulmonary dysplasia (BPD) is considered present when there is need for supplemental O_2 in premature infants at 36 wk gestation who do not have other conditions that require O_2 (eg, pneumonia, congenital heart disease). It is caused by high concentrations of inspired O_2 typically in patients on prolonged mechanical ventilation. Incidence increases with degree of prematurity; additional risk factors include pulmonary interstitial emphysema, high peak inspiratory pressures, increased airway resistance and pulmonary artery pressures, and male sex. BPD is typically suspected when a ventilated infant is unable to wean from O_2 therapy, mechanical ventilation, or both. Patients develop worsening hypoxemia, hypercapnia, and increasing O_2 requirements. Chest x-ray initially shows diffuse haziness due to accumulation of exudative fluid; appearance then becomes multicystic or spongelike, with alternating areas of emphysema, pulmonary scarring, and atelectasis. Alveolar epithelium may slough, and macrophages, neutrophils, and inflammatory mediators may be found in the tracheal aspirate.

Prognosis and Treatment

Prognosis varies with severity. Infants who still depend on mechanical ventilation at 36 wk gestation have a 20 to 30% mortality rate in infancy. Infants with BPD have a 3- to 4-fold increased rate of growth failure and neurodevelopmental problems. For several years, infants are at increased risk of lower respiratory tract infections (particularly viral) and may quickly develop respiratory decompensation if pulmonary infection occurs. The threshold for hospitalization should be low if signs of a respiratory infection or respiratory distress develop.

Treatment is supportive and includes nutritional supplementation, fluid restriction, diuretics, and perhaps inhaled bronchodilators. Respiratory infections must be diagnosed early and treated aggressively. Weaning from mechanical ventilation and supplemental O_2 should be accomplished as early as possible.

Feedings should achieve an intake of > 120 calories/kg/day; caloric requirements are increased because of the increased work of breathing and to aid lung healing and growth.

Because pulmonary congestion and edema may develop, daily fluid intake is often restricted to about 120 mL/kg/day. Diuretic therapy is sometimes used: chlorothiazide 10 to 20 mg/kg po bid plus spironolactone 1 to 3 mg/kg once/day or split into twice-daily doses. Furosemide (1 to 2 mg/kg IV or IM or 1 to 4 mg/kg po q 12 to 24 h for neonates and q 8 h for older infants) may be used for short periods, but prolonged use causes hypercalciuria with resultant osteoporosis, fractures, and renal calculi. Hydration and serum electrolytes should be monitored closely during diuretic therapy.

Weeks or months of additional ventilator support and/or supplemental O_2 may be required for advanced BPD. Ventilator pressures and fraction of inspired O_2 (FIO_2) should be reduced as rapidly as tolerated, but the infant should not be allowed to become hypoxemic. Arterial oxygenation should be continuously monitored with a pulse oximeter and maintained at ≥ 88% saturation. Respiratory acidosis may occur during ventilator weaning and treatment and is acceptable as long as the pH remains > 7.25 and the infant does not develop severe respiratory distress.

Passive immunoprophylaxis with palivizumab, a monoclonal antibody to respiratory syncytial virus (RSV), decreases RSV-related hospitalizations and ICU stays but is costly and is indicated primarily in high-risk infants (see p. 1600 for indications). During RSV season (November through April), children are given 15 mg/kg IM q 30 days until 6 mo after treatment of the acute illness. Infants > 6 mo should also be vaccinated against influenza.

Prevention

BPD often can be prevented by weaning infants to the lowest tolerated ventilator settings and completely off mechanical ventilation as soon as possible; early use of aminophylline as a respiratory stimulant may help preterm infants wean from intermittent mandatory ventilation. Prenatal corticosteroid administration, prophylactic surfactant administration in extremely low-birth-weight infants, early treatment of patent ductus arteriosus, and avoidance of large volumes of fluid also decrease BPD incidence and severity. When an infant cannot be weaned within the expected time, possible underlying conditions, including patent ductus arteriosus and nursery-acquired pneumonia, should be considered and treated.

MECONIUM ASPIRATION SYNDROME

Intrapartum meconium aspiration can cause chemical pneumonitis and mechanical bronchial obstruction producing a syndrome of respiratory distress. Findings include tachypnea, rales and rhonchi, and cyanosis or desaturation. Diagnosis is suspected when there is respiratory distress after delivery through meconium-tinged amniotic fluid and is confirmed by chest x-ray. Treatment is vigorous suction immediately on delivery before the neonate takes his 1st breath, followed by respiratory support as needed. Prognosis depends on the underlying physiologic stressors.

Etiology and Pathophysiology

Physiologic stress at the time of labor and delivery (eg, from hypoxia caused by umbilical cord compression or placental insufficiency or from infection) may cause the fetus to pass meconium into the amniotic fluid before delivery; meconium passage is noted in about 10 to 15% of births. During delivery, perhaps 5% of infants with meconium passage aspirate the meconium, triggering lung injury and respiratory distress, termed meconium aspiration syndrome. Postterm infants delivered through reduced amniotic fluid volume are at risk of more severe disease because the less dilute meconium is more likely to cause airway obstruction.

The mechanisms by which aspiration induces the clinical syndrome probably include nonspecific cytokine release, airway obstruction, surfactant inactivation, and/or chemical pneumonitis; the underlying physiologic stressors also may contribute. If complete bronchial obstruction occurs, atelectasis results; partial blockage leads to air trapping on expiration, resulting in hyperexpansion of the lungs and possibly pulmonary air leak (see p. 2302) with pneumomediastinum or pneumothorax. Continuing hypoxia may lead to persistent pulmonary hypertension of the newborn (see p. 2301).

Infants may also aspirate vernix caseosa, amniotic fluid, or blood of maternal or fetal origin during delivery and can develop respiratory distress and signs of aspiration pneumonia on chest x-ray. Treatment is supportive; if bacterial infection is suspected, cultures are taken and antibiotics begun.

Symptoms and Signs

Signs include tachypnea, nasal flaring, retractions, cyanosis or desaturation, rales, rhonchi, and greenish yellow staining of the umbilical cord, nail beds, or skin. Meconium staining may be visible in the oropharynx and (on intubation) in the larynx and trachea. Infants with air trapping may have a barrel-shaped chest and also symptoms and signs of pneumothorax, pulmonary interstitial emphysema, and pneumomediastinum (see pp. 2302–2303).

Diagnosis

Diagnosis is suspected when a neonate demonstrates respiratory distress in the setting of meconium-tinged amniotic fluid and is confirmed by chest x-ray demonstrating hyperinflation with variable areas of atelectasis and flattening of the diaphragm. Fluid may be seen in the lung fissures or pleural spaces, and air may be seen in the soft tissues or mediastinum. Because meconium may enhance bacterial growth and meconium aspiration syndrome is difficult to distinguish from bacterial pneumonia, cultures of blood and tracheal aspirate should also be obtained.

Prognosis and Treatment

Prognosis is generally good, although it varies with the underlying physiologic stressors; overall mortality is slightly increased. Infants with meconium aspiration syndrome may be at greater risk of asthma in later life.

Immediate treatment, indicated for all neonates delivered through meconium, is vigorous suctioning of the mouth and nasopharynx using a De Lee suction apparatus as soon as the head is delivered and before the neonate breathes and cries. If suction returns no meconium and the infant appears vigorous, observation without further intervention is appropriate. If the infant has labored or depressed respirations, poor muscle tone, or is bradycardic (< 100 beats/min), the trachea should be intubated with a 3.5- or 4.0-mm endotracheal tube. A meconium aspirator connected to a suction apparatus is attached directly to the endotracheal tube, which then serves as the suction catheter. Suction is maintained while the endotracheal tube is removed. Reintubation and continuous positive airway pressure are indicated for continued respiratory distress, followed by mechanical ventilation and admission to the neonatal ICU as needed. Because positive pressure ventilation enhances risk of pulmonary air-leak syndrome, regular evaluation (including physical examination and chest x-ray) is important to detect these complications; these should immediately be sought in any intubated infant whose BP, perfusion, or O_2 saturation suddenly worsens.

Additional treatments may include surfactant for mechanically ventilated infants with high O_2 requirements, which can decrease the need for extracorporeal membrane oxygenation, and antibiotics (usually ampicillin and an aminoglycoside). Treatment of airleak syndromes, a complication of air trapping, is discussed below.

PERSISTENT PULMONARY HYPERTENSION OF THE NEWBORN

Persistent pulmonary hypertension of the newborn is the persistence of or reversion to pulmonary arteriolar constriction, causing a severe reduction in pulmonary blood flow and right-to-left shunting. Symptoms and signs include tachypnea, retractions, and severe cyanosis or desaturation unresponsive to O_2. Diagnosis is by history, examination, chest x-ray, and response to O_2. Treatment is with O_2, alkalinization, inhaled nitric oxide, or, if medical therapy fails, extracorporeal membrane oxygenation.

Etiology and Pathophysiology

Persistent pulmonary hypertension of the newborn (PPHN) is a disorder of pulmonary vasculature that affects term or postterm infants. The most common causes involve perinatal asphyxia or hypoxia (a history of meconium staining of amniotic fluid or meconium in the trachea is common); hypoxia triggers reversion to or persistence of intense pulmonary arteriolar constriction, a normal state in the fetus. Additional causes include premature ductus arteriosus or foramen ovale closure, which increases fetal pulmonary blood flow and may be triggered by maternal NSAID use; polycythemia, which obstructs blood flow; congenital diaphragmatic hernia, in which the left lung is severely hypoplastic, forcing most of the pulmonary blood flow through the right lung; and neonatal sepsis, presumably from production of vasoconstrictive prostaglandins by activation of the cyclo-oxygenase pathway by bacterial phospholipids. Whatever the cause, elevated pressure in the pulmonary arteries causes abnormal smooth muscle development and hypertrophy in the walls of the small pulmonary arteries and arterioles and right-to-left shunting via the ductus arteriosus or a foramen ovale, resulting in intractable systemic hypoxemia.

Symptoms and Signs

Symptoms and signs include tachypnea, retractions, and severe cyanosis or desaturation unresponsive to supplemental O_2. In infants with a right-to-left shunt via a patent ductus arteriosus, oxygenation is higher in the right brachial artery than in the descending aorta; thus cyanosis may be differential, ie, O_2 saturation in the lower extremities is 5% lower than in the right upper extremity.

Diagnosis

Diagnosis should be suspected in any near-term infant with arterial hypoxemia and/or cyanosis, especially one with a suggestive history whose O_2 saturation does not improve with 100% O_2. Diagnosis is confirmed by echocardiogram, which can confirm the presence of elevated pressures in the pulmonary artery using Doppler interrogation and simultaneously excludes congenital heart disease. Lung fields on x-ray may be normal or may demonstrate changes due to the underlying cause (eg, meconium aspiration syndrome, neonatal pneumonia, congenital diaphragmatic hernia).

Prognosis and Treatment

An oxygenation index (mean airway pressure [cm H_2O] × fraction of inspired O_2 [FIO_2] × 100/PaO_2) > 40 predicts mortality of > 50%. Overall mortality ranges from 10 to 80% and is directly related to the oxygenation index but also varies with underlying disorder. However, many survivors (perhaps ⅓) exhibit developmental delay, hearing deficits, and/or functional disabilities. This rate of disability may be no different from that of other infants with severe illness.

Treatment with O_2, which is a potent pulmonary vasodilator, is begun immediately to prevent disease progression. O_2 is delivered via bag and mask or mechanical ventilation; mechanical distention of alveoli aids vasodilation. FIO_2 should initially be 1 but can be titrated downward to maintain PaO_2 between 50 and 90 mm Hg to minimize lung injury. Once PaO_2 is stabilized, weaning can be attempted by reducing FIO_2 in decrements of 2 to 3%, then reducing ventilator pressures; changes should be gradual, because a large drop in PaO_2 can cause recurrent pulmonary artery vasoconstriction. High-frequency oscillatory ventilation expands and ventilates the lungs while minimizing barotrauma and should be considered for infants with underlying lung disease in whom atelectasis and ventilation/perfusion (V/Q) mismatch may exacerbate the hypoxemia of PPHN.

Inhaled nitric oxide relaxes endothelial smooth muscle, dilating pulmonary arterioles, which increases pulmonary blood flow and rapidly improves oxygenation in as many as ½ of patients. Initial dose is 20 ppm, titrated downward by effect.

Extracorporeal membrane oxygenation (see p. 2297) may be used in patients with severe hypoxic respiratory failure defined by an oxygenation index > 35 to 40 despite maximum respiratory support.

Normal fluid, electrolyte, glucose, and Ca levels must be maintained. Infants should be kept in a neutral thermal environment and treated with antibiotics for possible sepsis until culture results are known.

PULMONARY AIR-LEAK SYNDROMES

Pulmonary air-leak syndromes involve dissection of air out of the normal pulmonary airspaces.

Air-leak syndromes include pulmonary interstitial emphysema, pneumomediastinum, pneumothorax, pneumopericardium, pneumoperitoneum, and subcutaneous emphysema. These syndromes occur in 1 to 2% of normal neonates, probably because large negative intrathoracic forces created when the neonate starts breathing occasionally disrupt alveolar epithelium, which allows air to move from the alveoli into extra-alveolar soft tissues or spaces. Air leak is more common and severe in infants with lung disease, who are at risk because of poor lung compliance and the need for high airway pressures (eg, in respiratory distress) or because of air trapping (eg, meconium aspiration syndrome), which leads to alveolar overdistention. Many affected neonates are asymptomatic; diagnosis is suspected clinically or because of deterioration in O_2 status and is confirmed by x-ray. Treatment varies by type of air leak but in ventilated infants always involves lowering inspiratory pressures to lowest tolerated settings. High-frequency ventilators may be helpful but are of unproven benefit.

Pulmonary interstitial emphysema: Pulmonary interstitial emphysema is leakage of air from alveoli into the pulmonary interstitium, lymphatics, or subpleural space. It usually occurs in infants with poor lung compliance, such as those with respiratory distress syndrome who are being treated with mechanical ventilation, but it may occur spontaneously. One or both lungs may be involved, and pathology may be focal or generalized within each lung. If dissection of air is widespread, respiratory status may acutely worsen because lung compliance is suddenly reduced.

Chest x-ray shows a variable number of cystic or linear lucencies in the lung fields. Some lucencies are elongated; others appear as enlarged subpleural cysts ranging from a few millimeters to several centimeters in diameter.

Pulmonary interstitial emphysema may resolve dramatically over 1 or 2 days or persist on x-ray for weeks. Some patients with severe respiratory disease and pulmonary interstitial emphysema develop bronchopulmonary dysplasia (BPD—see p. 2298), and the cystic changes of long-standing pulmonary interstitial emphysema then merge into the x-ray picture of BPD.

Treatment is generally supportive. If one lung is significantly more involved than the other, the infant may be laid down on the side of the lung with the more severe pulmonary interstitial emphysema; this will help to compress the lung with pulmonary interstitial emphysema, thereby decreasing air leakage and perhaps improving ventilation of the normal (elevated) lung. If one lung is very severely affected and the other is mildly affected or uninvolved, differential bronchial intubation and ventilation of the less-involved lung may also be attempted; total atelectasis of the nonintubated lung soon results. Because only one lung is now being ventilated, ventilator settings and fraction of inspired O_2 may need to be altered. After 24 to 48 h, the endotracheal tube is pulled back into the trachea, at which time the air leak may have stopped.

Pneumomediastinum: Pneumomediastinum is dissection of air into connective tissue of the mediastinum (see also p. 496); the air may further dissect into the subcutaneous tissues of the neck and scalp. Pneumomediastinum usually causes no symptoms or signs, though subcutaneous air causes crepitus. Diagnosis is by x-ray; in an anteroposterior view, air may form a lucency around the heart, whereas on a lateral view, air lifts the lobes of the thymus away from the cardiac silhouette (spinnaker sail sign). No treatment is usually needed, and the condition resolves spontaneously.

Pneumopericardium: Pneumopericardium is dissection of air into the pericardial sac. It affects mechanically ventilated infants almost exclusively. Most cases are asymptomatic, but if sufficient air accumulates, it can cause cardiac tamponade (see p. 732). Diagnosis is suspected if patients experience acute circulatory collapse and is confirmed by lucency around the heart on x-ray or by return of air on pericardiocentesis using a scalp vein needle. Treatment is pericardiocentesis followed by surgical insertion of a pericardial tube.

Pneumoperitoneum: Pneumoperitoneum is dissection of air into the peritoneum. It is generally not clinically significant but must be distinguished from pneumoperitoneum due to a ruptured abdominal viscus, which is a surgical emergency.

Pneumothorax: Pneumothorax is dissection of air into the pleural space; sufficient accumulation of air causes tension pneumothorax (see p. 496). Although sometimes asymptomatic, pneumothorax typically causes worsening of tachypnea, grunting, and cyanosis. Breath sounds decrease, and the chest enlarges on the affected side. Tension pneumothorax causes cardiovascular collapse.

Diagnosis is suspected by deterioration of respiratory status and/or by transillumination of the chest with a fiberoptic probe. Diagnosis is confirmed by chest x-ray or, in the case of tension pneumothorax, return of air during thoracentesis.

Most small pneumothoraces resolve spontaneously, but larger and tension pneumothoraces require evacuation of the air in the pleural cavity. In tension pneumothorax, a scalp vein needle or an angiocatheter and syringe can be used to temporarily evacuate free air from the pleural space. Definitive treatment is insertion of an 8 or 10 French chest tube attached to continuous suction. Follow-up auscultation, transillumination, and x-ray confirm that the tube is functioning properly.

RESPIRATORY DISTRESS SYNDROME

(Hyaline Membrane Disease)

Respiratory distress syndrome is caused by pulmonary surfactant deficiency in the lungs of neonates born at < 37 wk gestation. Risk increases with degree of prematurity. Symptoms and signs include grunting respirations, use of accessory muscles, and nasal flaring appearing soon after birth. Diagnosis is clinical; prenatal risk can be assessed with tests of fetal lung maturity. Treatment is surfactant therapy and supportive care.

Etiology and Pathophysiology

Pulmonary surfactant is a mixture of phospholipids and lipoproteins secreted by type II pneumocytes (see p. 2257); it diminishes the surface tension of the water film that lines alveoli, thereby decreasing the tendency of alveoli to collapse and the work required to inflate them.

With surfactant deficiency, the lungs become diffusely atelectatic, triggering inflammation and pulmonary edema. Because blood passing through the atelectatic portions of lung is not oxygenated (forming a right to left intrapulmonary shunt), the infant becomes hypoxemic. Lung compliance is decreased, thereby increasing the work of breathing. In severe cases, the diaphragm and intercostal muscles fatigue, and CO_2 retention and respiratory acidosis develop.

Surfactant is not produced in adequate amounts until relatively late in gestation; thus, risk of respiratory distress syndrome (RDS) increases with greater prematurity. Other risk factors include multifetal pregnancies and maternal diabetes. Risk decreases with fetal growth restriction, preeclampsia or eclampsia, maternal hypertension, prolonged rupture of membranes, and maternal corticosteroid use. Rare cases are hereditary, caused by mutations in surfactant protein (SP-B and SP-C) and ATP-binding cassette transporter *A3* (*ABCA3*) genes. Males and whites are at greater risk.

Symptoms and Signs

Symptoms and signs include rapid, labored, grunting respirations appearing immediately or within a few hours after delivery, with suprasternal and substernal retractions and flaring of the nasal alae. As atelectasis and respiratory failure progress, symptoms worsen, with cyanosis, lethargy, irregular breathing, and apnea.

Neonates weighing < 1000 g may have lungs so stiff that they are unable to initiate and/or sustain respirations in the delivery room.

Complications of RDS include intraventricular hemorrhage, periventricular white matter injury, tension pneumothorax, bronchopulmonary dysplasia, sepsis, and neonatal death. Intracranial complications have been linked to hypoxemia, hypercarbia, hypotension, swings in arterial BP, and low cerebral perfusion (see Intracranial Hemorrhage on p. 2263 and Hemorrhagic Shock and Encephalopathy Syndrome on p. 2398).

Diagnosis

Diagnosis is by clinical presentation, including recognition of risk factors; ABGs demonstrating hypoxemia and hypercapnia; and chest x-ray. Chest x-ray shows diffuse atelectasis classically described as having a ground-glass appearance with visible air bronchograms; appearance correlates loosely with clinical severity.

Differential diagnosis includes group B streptococcal pneumonia and sepsis, transient tachypnea of the newborn, persistent pulmonary hypertension, aspiration, pulmonary edema, and congenital cardiopulmonary anomalies. Patients typically require cultures of blood, CSF, and possibly tracheal aspirate. Clinical diagnosis of group B streptococcal pneumonia is extremely difficult; thus, antibiotics are usually started pending culture results.

RDS can be anticipated prenatally using tests of fetal lung maturity, which measure surfactant obtained by amniocentesis or collected from the vagina (if membranes have ruptured) and which can help determine the optimal timing of delivery. These are indicated for elective deliveries before 39 wk when fetal heart tones, human chorionic gonadotropin levels, and ultrasound measurements cannot confirm gestational age and for nonelective deliveries between 34 and 36 wk. Risk of RDS is low when lecithin/sphingomyelin ratio is > 2, phosphatidyl glycerol is present, foam stability index = 47, and/or surfactant/albumin ratio (measured by fluorescence polarization) is > 55 mg/g.

Treatment

Prognosis with treatment is excellent; mortality is < 10%. With adequate ventilatory support alone, surfactant production eventually begins, and once production begins, RDS resolves within 4 or 5 days, but severe hypoxemia in the meantime can result in multiple organ failure and death.

Specific treatment is intratracheal administration of surfactant; this requires endotracheal intubation, which may also be necessary to achieve adequate ventilation and oxygenation. Less premature infants (those > 1 kg) and those with lower O_2 requirements (fraction of inspired O_2 [FIO_2] < 40 to 50%) may respond well to supplemental O_2 alone.

Surfactant hastens recovery and decreases risk of pneumothorax, interstitial emphysema, intraventricular hemorrhage, bronchopulmonary dysplasia, and neonatal mortality in the hospital and at 1 yr. However, neonates who receive surfactant for established RDS have an increased risk of apnea of prematurity. Options for surfactant replacement include beractant (a lipid bovine lung extract supplemented with proteins B and C, colfosceril palmitate, palmitic acid, and tripalmitin) 100 mg/kg q 6 h prn up to 4 doses; poractant alfa (a modified porcine-derived minced lung extract containing phospholipids, neutral lipids, fatty acids, and surfactant-associated proteins B and C) 200 mg/kg followed by up to 2 doses of 100 mg/kg 12 h apart prn; and calfactant (a calf lung extract containing phospholipids, neutral lipids, fatty acids, and surfactant-associated proteins B and C) 105 mg/kg q 12 h up to 3 doses prn. Lung compliance can improve rapidly after administration; the ventilator peak inspiratory pressure may need to be rapidly lowered to reduce risk of a pulmonary air leak. Other ventilator parameters (eg, FIO_2, rate) may also need to be reduced.

Prevention

When a fetus must be delivered between 24 and 34 wk, giving 2 doses of betamethasone 12 mg 24 h apart or 4 doses of dexamethasone 6 mg IV or IM q 12 h to the mother at least 48 h before delivery induces fetal surfactant production and reduces the risk of RDS or decreases its severity (see also Preterm Labor on p. 2205).

TRANSIENT TACHYPNEA OF THE NEWBORN

(Neonatal Wet Lung Syndrome)

Transient tachypnea of the newborn is respiratory distress caused by delayed resorption of fetal lung fluid.

Transient tachypnea of the newborn affects premature infants, term infants delivered by cesarean section, and infants born with respiratory depression, all of whom have delayed clearance of fetal lung fluid. (Mechanisms for normal resorption of fetal lung fluid are described on p. 2257.) Maternal diabetes and asthma are also risk factors, for unknown reasons, and the disorder can occur in preterm infants with respiratory distress syndrome (RDS) and in term infants born through meconium-stained amniotic fluid.

Rapid respirations, grunting, and retractions begin soon after delivery, and cyanosis may develop. Chest x-ray shows hyperinflated lungs with streaky perihilar markings, giving the appearance of a shaggy heart border while the periphery of the lungs is clear. Fluid is often seen in the lung fissures.

Recovery usually occurs within 2 to 3 days. Treatment is supportive and involves giving O_2 by hood and monitoring ABGs or pulse oximetry. Rarely, extremely premature infants and/or those with neurologic depression at birth require continuous positive airway pressure and occasionally even mechanical ventilation.

BACTERIAL TRACHEITIS

(Pseudomembranous Croup)

Bacterial tracheitis is bacterial infection of the trachea.

Bacterial tracheitis is uncommon and can affect children of any age. *Staphylococcus aureus,* group A β-hemolytic streptococci, and *Haemophilus influenzae* type b are most frequently involved. Onset is acute and is characterized by respiratory stridor, high fever, and often copious purulent secretions. As in patients with epiglottitis, the child may have marked toxicity and respiratory distress that may progress rapidly and may require intubation.

Diagnosis is suspected clinically and can be confirmed by direct laryngoscopy, which reveals purulent secretions and inflammation in the subglottic area with a shaggy, purulent membrane or by lateral neck x-ray revealing subglottic narrowing that may be irregular as opposed to the symmetric tapering typical of croup.

Treatment in severe cases is the same as that of epiglottitis (see p. 821); whenever possible, endotracheal intubation should be performed in controlled circumstances by a person skilled in managing a pediatric airway (see p. 528). Initial antibiotics should cover *S. aureus*, streptococcal species, and *H. influenzae* type b; cefuroxime or an equivalent IV preparation may be appropriate empirically unless methicillin-resistant staphylococcus is prevalent in the community, in which case vancomycin should be used. Therapy for critically ill children should be guided by a consultant knowledgeable in local susceptibility patterns. Once definitive microbial diagnosis is made, coverage is narrowed and continued for ≥ 10 days.

Complications include bronchopneumonia, sepsis, and retropharyngeal cellulitis or abscess. Subglottic stenosis secondary to prolonged intubation is uncommon. Most children treated appropriately recover without sequelae.

BRONCHIOLITIS

Bronchiolitis is an acute viral infection of the lower respiratory tract affecting infants < 18 mo and characterized by respiratory distress, wheezing, and crackles. Diagnosis is suspected by history, including epidemic presentation; the primary cause, respiratory syncytial virus, can be identified with a rapid assay. Treatment is supportive with O_2 and hydration. Prognosis is generally excellent, but some patients develop apnea or respiratory failure.

Bronchiolitis often occurs in epidemics and mostly in children < 18 mo, with a peak incidence in infants < 6 mo. The annual incidence in the 1st yr of life is about 11 cases/100 children. Most cases occur between November and April, with a peak incidence during January and February.

Etiology and Pathophysiology

Most cases are caused by respiratory syncytial virus (RSV) and parainfluenza 3 virus infection; less frequent causes are influenza A and B, parainfluenza 1 and 2, metapneumovirus, and adenoviruses. Rhinoviruses, enteroviruses, measles virus, and *Mycoplasma pneumoniae* are uncommon causes.

The virus spreads from the upper respiratory tract to the medium and small bronchi and bronchioles, causing epithelial necrosis. The developing edema and exudate result in partial obstruction, which is most pronounced on expiration and leads to alveolar air trapping. Complete obstruction and absorption of the trapped air may lead to multiple areas of atelectasis.

Symptoms and Signs

Typically, an affected infant has URI symptoms with progressively increasing respiratory distress characterized by tachypnea, retractions, and a hacking cough. Young infants may present with recurrent apneic spells followed by more typical signs and symptoms over 24 to 48 h. Signs of distress may include circumoral cyanosis, deepening retractions, and audible wheezing. Fever is usually but not always present. Infants initially appear healthy and in no distress, despite tachypnea and retractions, but may become increasingly lethargic as the infection progresses. Dehydration may develop from vomiting and decreased oral intake. With fatigue, respirations may become more shallow and ineffective, leading to respiratory acidosis. Auscultation reveals wheezing, prolonged expiration, and, often, fine moist crackles. Many children have accompanying acute otitis media.

Diagnosis

Diagnosis is suspected by history, examination, and occurrence of the illness as part of an epidemic. Symptoms similar to bronchiolitis can result from asthma, which is more likely in a child > 18 mo of age, especially if previous episodes of wheezing and a family history of asthma have been documented. Gastric reflux with aspiration of gastric contents may also produce the clinical picture of bronchiolitis; multiple episodes in an infant may be a clue to this diagnosis. Foreign body aspiration occasionally causes wheezing and should be considered if the onset is sudden and not associated with manifestations of URI.

Patients suspected of having bronchiolitis should undergo pulse oximetry to evaluate oxygenation. No further testing is required for mild cases with normal O_2 levels, but in cases of hypoxemia, a chest x-ray supports the diagnosis, typically showing hyperinflated lungs, depressed diaphragm, and prominent hilar markings. Infiltrates may be present from atelectasis as well as RSV pneumonia, which is relatively common in infants with RSV bronchiolitis. RSV rapid antigen testing performed on a nasal swab or washing is diagnostic but not always necessary; it may be reserved for patients with illness severe enough to require hospitalization. Other laboratory testing is nonspecific; about ⅔ of the children have WBC counts of 10,000 to 15,000/μL. Most have 50 to 75% lymphocytes.

Prognosis and Treatment

Prognosis is excellent; most children recover in 3 to 5 days without sequelae, and mortality is < 1% when medical care is adequate. An increased incidence of asthma is suspected in children who had bronchiolitis in early childhood, but the association is controversial.

Treatment is supportive, and most children can be managed at home with hydration and comfort measures. Indications for hospitalization include accelerating respiratory distress, ill appearance (eg, cyanosis, lethargy, fatigue), apnea by history, and atelectasis by x-ray. Children with underlying conditions such as cardiac disease, immunodeficiency, or bronchopulmonary dysplasia, which put them at high risk of severe or complicated disease, should also be considered candidates for hospitalization. In hospitalized children, 30 to 40% O_2 delivered by tent or face mask is usually sufficient to maintain O_2 saturation > 90%. Endotracheal intubation is indicated for severe recurrent apnea, hypoxemia unresponsive to O_2 administration, or CO_2 retention or if the child cannot clear bronchial secretions.

Hydration may be maintained with frequent small feedings of clear liquids. For sicker children, fluids should be given IV initially, and the level of hydration should be monitored by urine output and specific gravity and by serum electrolyte determinations.

There is some evidence that systemic corticosteroids may be beneficial when given very early in the course of the illness or in patients with underlying corticosteroid-responsive conditions (eg, bronchopulmonary dysplasia, asthma), but benefit in most hospitalized infants is unproven.

Antibiotics should be withheld unless a secondary bacterial infection (a rare sequela) occurs. Bronchodilators are not uniformly effective, but a substantial subset of children may respond with short-term improvement. This is particularly true of infants who have wheezed previously. Hospital stays probably are not shortened.

Ribavirin, an antiviral drug active in vitro against RSV, influenza, and measles, is probably not effective clinically and is no longer recommended; it also is potentially toxic to hospital staff. RSV immune globulin has been tried but is probably ineffective.

Prevention of RSV infection by passive immunoprophylaxis with monoclonal antibody to RSV (palivizumab) decreases the frequency of hospitalization but is costly and is indicated primarily in high-risk infants (see p. 1600 for indications and dosage).

CROUP

Croup is acute inflammation of the upper and lower respiratory tracts caused most commonly by parainfluenza virus type 1 infection. It is characterized by a barking cough and inspiratory stridor. Diagnosis is usually obvious clinically but can be made by anteroposterior neck x-ray. Treatment is antipyretics, hydration, nebulized racemic epinephrine, and corticosteroids. Prognosis is excellent.

Etiology

Croup primarily affects children aged 6 mo to 3 yr. The parainfluenza viruses, especially type 1, are the major pathogens. Less common causes are respiratory syncytial virus (RSV) and influenza A and B viruses, followed by adenovirus, enterovirus, rhinovirus, and measles virus and *Mycoplasma pneumoniae.* Croup caused by influenza may be particularly severe and may occur in a broader age range of children.

Seasonal outbreaks are common: cases due to parainfluenza viruses tend to occur in the fall; those due to RSV and influenza viruses, in the winter and spring. Spread is usually through the air or by contact with infected secretions.

The infection produces inflammation of the larynx, trachea, bronchi, bronchioles, and lung parenchyma. Obstruction caused by swelling and inflammatory exudates develops and becomes pronounced in the subglottic region. Obstruction increases the work of breathing; rarely, tiring results in hypercapnia. Atelectasis may occur concurrently if the bronchioles become obstructed.

Symptoms and Signs

Croup is usually preceded by URI symptoms. A barking, often spasmodic, cough and hoarseness then occur, commonly at night; inspiratory stridor may be present as well. The child may awaken at night with respiratory distress, tachypnea, and retractions. In severe cases, cyanosis with increasingly shallow respirations may develop as the child tires.

The obvious respiratory distress and harsh inspiratory stridor are the most dramatic physical findings. Auscultation reveals prolonged inspiration and stridor, often with some expiratory rhonchi and wheezes. Rales also may be present. Breath sounds may be diminished with atelectasis. Fever is present in about ½ of patients. The child's condition may seem improved in the morning but worsen again at night.

Recurrent episodes are often called spasmodic croup. Allergy or airway reactivity may play a role in spasmodic croup, but the clinical manifestations cannot be differentiated from those of viral croup, and spasmodic croup is also usually initiated by a viral infection.

Diagnosis

Diagnosis is usually obvious by the barking nature of the cough. Similar inspiratory stridor can result from epiglottitis, bacterial tracheitis, foreign body, diphtheria, and retropharyngeal abscess. Epiglottitis (see p. 820), retropharyngeal abscess (see p. 822), and bacterial tracheitis (see p. 2305) have a more rapid onset and cause a more toxic appearance, odynophagia, and fewer upper respiratory tract symptoms. A foreign body may cause respiratory distress and a typical croupy cough, but fever and a preceding URI are absent. Diphtheria is excluded by a history of adequate immunization and confirmed by identification of the organism in viral cultures of scrapings from typical grayish diphtheritic membrane.

If the diagnosis is unclear, patients should have anteroposterior and lateral x-rays of neck and chest; subepiglottic narrowing (steeple sign) seen on anteroposterior neck x-ray supports the diagnosis. Seriously ill patients, in whom epiglottitis is a concern, should be examined in the operating room by appropriate specialists able to establish an airway (see p. 821). Patients should have pulse oximetry, and those with respiratory distress should have ABG measurement.

Prognosis and Treatment

The illness usually lasts 3 to 4 days and resolves spontaneously. A mildly ill child may be cared for at home with hydration and antipyretics. Keeping the child comfortable is important, because fatigue and crying can aggravate the condition. Humidification devices (eg, cold-steam vaporizers or humidifiers) may ameliorate upper airway drying.

Increasing or persistent respiratory distress, tachycardia, fatigue, cyanosis or hypoxemia, or dehydration indicates need for hospitalization. Pulse oximetry is helpful for assessing and monitoring severe cases. If O_2 saturation falls < 92%, humidified O_2 should be administered. A 30 to 40% inspired O_2 concentration is usually adequate. CO_2 retention ($PaCO_2$ > 45 mm Hg) generally indicates fatigue and the need for endotracheal intubation, as does inability to maintain oxygenation.

Nebulized racemic epinephrine 5 to 10 mg in 3 mL of saline q 2 h offers symptomatic improvement and relieves fatigue. However, the effects are transient; the course of the illness, the underlying viral infection, and the PaO_2 are not altered by its use; tachycardia and other adverse effects may occur.

High-dose dexamethasone (0.6 mg/kg IM or po once) may benefit patients hospitalized with moderate to severe croup. High-dose nebulized corticosteroids (budesonide 2 mg) have also been used but do not seem more effective. The value of corticosteroid treatment in outpatients has not been clearly demonstrated. Mist therapy is frequently used by families at home but has never been shown to be of important benefit.

The viruses that most commonly cause croup do not usually predispose to secondary bacterial infection, and antibiotics are rarely indicated.

278 CYSTIC FIBROSIS

Cystic fibrosis is an inherited disease of the exocrine glands affecting primarily the GI and respiratory systems. It leads to COPD, exocrine pancreatic insufficiency, and abnormally high sweat electrolytes. Diagnosis is by sweat test or identification of 2 cystic fibrosis mutations in patients with characteristic symptoms. Treatment is supportive through aggressive interdisciplinary care.

Cystic fibrosis (CF) is the most common life-shortening genetic disease in the white population. In the US, it occurs in about 1/3,300 white births, 1/15,300 black births, and 1/32,000 Asian-American births. Because of improved treatment and life expectancy, 40% of patients are adults.

CF is carried as an autosomal recessive trait by about 3% of the white population. The responsible gene has been localized on the long arm of chromosome 7q. It encodes a membrane-associated protein called the cystic fibrosis transmembrane regulator (CFTR). The most common gene mutation, ΔF_{508}, leads to absence of a phenylalanine residue at position 508 on the CFTR protein and occurs in about 70% of CF alleles; > 1200 less common mutations account for the remaining 30%. Although the exact function of CFTR is unknown, it appears to be part of a cAMP-regulated Cl channel, regulating Cl and Na transport across epithelial membranes. Heterozygotes may show subtle abnormalities of epithelial electrolyte transport but are clinically unaffected.

Pathophysiology

Nearly all exocrine glands are affected in varying distribution and degree of severity. Glands may

- Become obstructed by viscid or solid eosinophilic material in the lumen (pancreas, intestinal glands, intrahepatic bile ducts, gallbladder, submaxillary glands)
- Appear histologically abnormal and produce excessive secretions (tracheobronchial and Brunner's glands)
- Appear histologically normal but secrete excessive Na and Cl (sweat, parotid, and small salivary glands).

Infertility occurs in 98% of adult men secondary to maldevelopment of the vas deferens or to other forms of obstructive azoospermia. In women, fertility is decreased secondary to viscid cervical secretions, although many women with CF have carried pregnancies to term. However, the incidence of maternal complications and preterm births is increased.

Pulmonary: The lungs are generally histologically normal at birth. Pulmonary damage is probably initiated by diffuse obstruction in the small airways by abnormally thick mucus secretions. Bronchiolitis and mucopurulent plugging of the airways occur secondary to obstruction and infection. Bronchial changes are more common than parenchymal changes. Emphysema is not prominent. As the pulmonary process progresses, bronchial walls thicken; the airways fill with purulent, viscid secretions; areas of atelectasis develop; and hilar lymph nodes enlarge. Chronic hypoxemia results in muscular hypertrophy of the pulmonary arteries, pulmonary hypertension, and right ventricular hypertrophy. Much of the pulmonary damage may be caused by inflammation secondary to the release of proteases by neutrophils in the airways. Bronchoalveolar lavage fluid, even early in life, contains large numbers of neutrophils and increased concentrations of free neutrophil elastase, DNA, and IL-8.

Chronic pulmonary disease occurs almost universally and leads to episodic exacerbations with infection, inflammation, and progressive decline in pulmonary function. Early in the course, *Staphylococcus aureus* is the pathogen most often isolated from the respiratory tract, but as the disease progresses, *Pseudomonas aeruginosa* is most frequently isolated. A mucoid variant of *Pseudomonas* is uniquely associated with CF. Colonization with *Burkholderia cepacia* occurs in up to 7% of adult patients and may be associated with rapid pulmonary deterioration.

Symptoms and Signs

Meconium ileus due to obstruction of the ileum by viscid meconium may be the earliest sign (see p. 2285) and is present in 15 to 20% of affected neonates. It is often associated with volvulus, perforation, or atresia and, with rare exceptions, is followed by other CF signs. CF also may be associated with delayed neonatal passage of meconium and with the meconium plug syndrome (a transient form of distal intestinal obstruction secondary to one or more plugs of inspissated meconium in the anus or colon).

In infants without meconium ileus, disease onset may be heralded by a delay in regaining birth weight and inadequate weight gain at 4 to 6 wk of age.

Infants with CF who have been on soy protein formula or breast milk may develop hypoproteinemia with edema and anemia secondary to protein malabsorption.

Fifty percent of patients present with pulmonary manifestations, often beginning in infancy. Recurrent or chronic infections manifested by cough and wheezing are common. Cough is the most troublesome complaint, often accompanied by sputum, gagging, vomiting, and disturbed sleep. Intercostal retractions, use of accessory muscles of respiration, a barrel-chest deformity, digital clubbing, and cyanosis occur with disease progression. Upper respiratory tract involvement includes nasal polyposis and chronic or recurrent sinusitis. Adolescents may have retarded growth, delayed onset of puberty, and a declining tolerance for exercise. Pulmonary complications in adolescents and adults include pneumothorax, hemoptysis, and right heart failure secondary to pulmonary hypertension.

Pancreatic insufficiency is clinically apparent in 85 to 90% of children, usually early in life, and may be progressive. Manifestations include the frequent passage of bulky, foul-smelling, oily stools; abdominal protuberance; and poor growth pattern with decreased subcutaneous tissue and muscle mass despite a normal or voracious appetite. Rectal prolapse occurs in 20% of untreated infants and toddlers. Clinical manifestations may occur secondary to deficiency of fat-soluble vitamins.

Excessive sweating in hot weather or with fever may lead to episodes of hypotonic dehydration and circulatory failure. In arid climates, infants may present with chronic metabolic alkalosis. Salt crystal formation and a salty taste on the skin are highly suggestive of CF.

In patients ≥ 13 yr, type 1 diabetes develops in 17% and multilobular biliary cirrhosis with varices and portal hypertension develops in 5 to 6%. Chronic and/or recurrent abdominal pain may be related to intussusception, peptic ulcer disease, periappendiceal abscess, pancreatitis, gastroesophageal reflux, esophagitis, gallbladder disease, or episodes of partial intestinal obstruction secondary to abnormally viscid fecal contents. Other complications include osteopenia/osteoporosis and episodic arthralgias/arthritis.

Diagnosis

Diagnosis is suggested by characteristic clinical features and confirmed by a sweat test or identification of 2 known CF mutations. Diagnosis is usually confirmed in infancy or early childhood, but up to 10% of patients escape detection until adolescence or early adulthood.

The only reliable sweat test is the quantitative pilocarpine iontophoresis test: Localized sweating is stimulated pharmacologically with pilocarpine; the amount of sweat is measured, and its Cl concentration is determined. In patients with a suggestive clinical picture or a positive family history, a Cl concentration > 60 mEq/L confirms the diagnosis.

In infants, a Cl concentration > 30 mEq/L is highly suggestive of CF. False-negative results are rare (about 1:1000 patients with CF have sweat Cl < 50 mEq/L) but may occur in the presence of edema and hypoproteinemia or with collection of inadequate quantities of sweat. False-positive results are usually related to technical errors. Transient elevation of sweat Cl concentration can occur in association with psychosocial deprivation (child abuse, neglect) and in patients with anorexia nervosa. Although results are valid after the 1st 24 h of life, an adequate sweat sample (> 75 mg on filter paper or > 15 μL in microbore tubing) may be difficult to obtain before 3 to 4 wk of age. Although the sweat Cl concentration normally increases slightly with age, the test is still valid in adults.

A small subset of patients, labeled as having atypical CF, have chronic *Pseudomonas* bronchitis, normal pancreatic function, and normal or borderline sweat Cl concentrations. Normal pancreatic function occurs in patients with 1 or 2 "mild" CF mutations, whereas pancreatic insufficiency occurs only in patients with 2 "severe" mutations. Mutation testing is indicated in patients with clinical features of CF but normal or borderline sweat test results.

In a patient with ≥ 1 phenotypic features consistent with CF or with a history of CF in a sibling, diagnosis also can be confirmed by the identification of 2 known CF mutations.

Patients with CF have increased nasal transepithelial potential differences secondary to increased Na reabsorption across epithelium, which is relatively impermeable to Cl. This observation may be diagnostically useful when sweat Cl values are borderline or normal and 2 CF mutations are not identified.

The serum concentration of immunoreactive trypsin is elevated in neonates with CF. Measurement of this enzyme in conjunction with mutation analysis and sweat testing is the basis of neonatal screening programs carried out in many parts of the world.

In couples in which both partners are CF carriers (usually identified through having an affected child or through preconception/prenatal CF mutation screening), mutation testing can be used for preimplantation or prenatal diagnostic testing. It is now recommended in the US that carrier screening be part of routine preconception or prenatal obstetric care. Also, fetal ultrasound showing echogenic (hyperechoic) bowel predicts increased risk of CF; mutation testing should be offered in such cases.

In patients with pancreatic insufficiency, the duodenal fluid is abnormally viscid and shows absence or diminution of enzyme activity and decreased HCO_3^- concentration; stool trypsin and chymotrypsin are absent or diminished. The secretin-pancreozymin stimulation test is the gold standard for assessment of exocrine pancreatic function; however, it is invasive and technically difficult. Noninvasive, indirect assessment of pancreatic function can be accomplished by measuring 72-h fecal fat excretion or the concentration of human pancreatic elastase in stool. This latter measurement is valid even in the presence of exogenous pancreatic enzymes. About 40% of older patients have an oral glucose tolerance curve consistent with diabetes mellitus; abnormal glucose tolerance is secondary to reduced and delayed insulin response, and 17% of patients develop insulin-dependent diabetes mellitus.

Chest x-ray and high-resolution CT may demonstrate hyperinflation and bronchial wall thickening as the earliest findings. Subsequent changes include areas of infiltrate, atelectasis, and hilar adenopathy. With advanced disease, segmental or lobar atelectasis, cyst formation, bronchiectasis, and pulmonary artery and right ventricular enlargement occur. Branching, fingerlike opacifications that represent mucoid impaction of dilated bronchi are characteristic. In almost all cases, sinus x-rays and CT studies show persistent opacification of the paranasal sinuses.

Pulmonary function tests indicate hypoxemia; reduction in forced vital capacity (FVC), forced expiratory volume in 1 sec (FEV_1), forced expiratory flow between 25 and 75% expired volume (FEF_{25-75}), and FEV_1/FVC ratio; and an increase in residual volume and the ratio of residual volume to total lung capacity. Fifty percent of patients have evidence of reversible airway obstruction as evidenced by improvement in pulmonary function after aerosol administration of a bronchodilator.

Prognosis

The course is largely determined by the degree of pulmonary involvement. Deterioration is inevitable, leading to debilitation and eventual death, usually from a combination of respiratory failure and cor pulmonale. Prognosis has improved steadily over the past 5 decades, mainly because of aggressive treatment before the onset of irreversible pulmonary changes. Median survival in the US is to age 35 yr. Long-term survival is significantly better in patients without pancreatic insufficiency. Female sex, early colonization with mucoid *Pseudomonas,* presentation with respiratory symptoms, tobacco smoke exposure, and airway hyperreactivity are associated with a somewhat worse prognosis. The FEV_1, adjusted for age and sex, is the best predictor of mortality.

Treatment

Comprehensive and intensive therapy should be directed by an experienced physician working with an interdisciplinary team that includes other physicians, nurses, nutritionists, physical and respiratory therapists, counselors, pharmacists, and social workers. The goals of therapy are maintenance of adequate nutritional status, prevention or aggressive treatment of pulmonary and other complications, encouragement of physical activity, and provision of adequate psychosocial support. With appropriate support, most patients can make an age-appropriate adjustment at home and school. Despite myriad problems, the occupational and marital successes of patients are impressive.

Treatment of pulmonary problems centers on prevention of airway obstruction and prophylaxis against and control of pulmonary infection. Prophylaxis against pulmonary infections includes maintenance of pertussis, *Haemophilus influenzae*, varicella, *Streptococcus pneumoniae,* and measles immunity and annual influenza vaccination. In patients exposed to influenza, a neuraminidase inhibitor can be used prophylactically. Administration of palivizumab to infants with CF for prevention of respiratory syncytial virus infection has been shown to be safe, but efficacy has not been documented.

Chest physical therapy consisting of postural drainage, percussion, vibration, and assisted coughing is recommended at the 1st indication of pulmonary involvement (see p. 377). In older patients, alternative airway clearance techniques, such as active cycle of breathing, autogenic drainage, positive expiratory pressure devices, and mechanical vest therapy, may be effective. For reversible airway obstruction, bronchodilators may be given orally and/or by aerosol and corticosteroids by aerosol. O_2 therapy is indicated for patients with severe pulmonary insufficiency and hypoxemia.

Mechanical ventilation is generally not indicated for chronic respiratory failure. Its use should be restricted to patients with good baseline status in whom acute reversible respiratory complications develop, in association with pulmonary surgery, or in patients in whom lung transplantation is imminent. Noninvasive positive pressure ventilation nasally or by face mask also can be beneficial. IPPB devices should not be used because they may cause a pneumothorax. Oral expectorants are widely used, but few data support their efficacy. Cough suppressants should be discouraged. Long-term daily aerosol administration of dornase alfa (recombinant human deoxyribonuclease) has been shown to slow the rate of decline in pulmonary function and to decrease the frequency of severe respiratory tract exacerbations.

Pneumothorax can be treated with closed chest tube thoracostomy drainage. Open thoracotomy or thoracoscopy with resection of pleural blebs and sponge abrasion of the pleural surfaces is effective in treating recurrent pneumothoraces.

Massive or recurrent hemoptysis is treated by embolizing involved bronchial arteries.

Oral corticosteroids are indicated in infants with prolonged bronchiolitis and in patients with refractory bronchospasm, allergic bronchopulmonary aspergillosis, and inflammatory complications (eg, arthritis, vasculitis). Long-term use of alternate-day corticosteroid therapy can slow the decline in pulmonary function, but because of corticosteroid-related complications, it is not recommended for routine use. Patients receiving corticosteroids must be closely monitored for evidence of carbohydrate abnormalities and linear growth retardation.

Ibuprofen, when given at a dose sufficient to achieve a peak plasma concentration between 50 and 100 μg/mL over several years, has been shown to slow the rate of decline in pulmonary function, especially in children 5 to 13 yr. The appropriate dose must be individualized based on pharmacokinetic studies.

Antibiotics should be used in symptomatic patients to treat bacterial pathogens in the respiratory tract according to culture and sensitivity testing. Penicillinase-resistant penicillin (eg, cloxacillin or dicloxacillin) or a cephalosporin (eg, cephalexin) is the drug of choice for staphylococci. Erythromycin, amoxicillin-clavulanate, ampicillin, tetracycline, trimethoprim-sulfamethoxazole, or occasionally chloramphenicol may be used individually or in combination for protracted ambulatory therapy of pulmonary infection due to a variety of organisms. Fluoroquinolones are effective against sensitive strains of *Pseudomonas* and have been used safely in young children. For severe pulmonary exacerbations, especially in patients colonized with *Pseudomonas,* parenteral antibiotic therapy is advised, often requiring hospital admission but safely conducted at home in carefully selected patients. Combinations of an aminoglycoside (tobramycin, gentamicin) and an anti-*Pseudomonas* penicillin are given IV. IV administration of cephalosporins and monobactams with anti-*Pseudomonas* activity also may be useful. The usual starting dose of tobramycin or gentamicin is 2.5 to 3.5 mg/kg tid, but high doses (3.5 to 4 mg/kg tid) may be required to achieve acceptable serum concentrations (peak level 8 to 10 μg/mL [11 to 17 μmol/L], trough value of < 2 μg/mL [< 4 μmol/L]). Alternatively, tobramycin can be given safely and effectively in one daily dose (10 to 12 mg/kg). Because of enhanced renal clearance, large doses of some penicillins may be required to achieve adequate serum levels. The goal of treating pulmonary infections should be to improve the clinical status sufficiently so that continuous use of antibiotics is unnecessary. However, in patients who are colonized with *Pseudomonas*, long-term use of antibiotics may be indicated. In selected patients, alternate-month aerosol tobramycin therapy and oral azithromycin given 3 times/wk may be effective in improving or stabilizing pulmonary function and decreasing the frequency of pulmonary exacerbations.

In symptomatic patients who are chronically colonized with *Pseudomonas*, the role of antibiotic therapy is to improve clinical parameters and possibly reduce the bacterial burden in the airways. Eradication of *Pseudomonas* is not possible. It has been shown, however, that early antibiotic treatment around the time of initial airway colonization with nonmucoid strains of *Pseudomonas* may be effective in eradicating the organism for some period of time. Treatment strategies vary but usually consist of inhaled tobramycin or colistin, often in association with an oral fluoroquinolone.

Patients with symptomatic right heart failure should be treated with diuretics, salt restriction, and O_2.

Neonatal intestinal obstruction can sometimes be relieved by enemas containing a hyperosmolar or iso-osmolar radiopaque contrast material; otherwise, surgical enterostomy to flush out the viscid meconium in the intestinal lumen may be necessary. After the neonatal period, episodes of partial intestinal obstruction (distal intestinal obstruction syndrome) can be treated with enemas containing a hyperosmolar or iso-osmolar radiopaque contrast material or acetylcysteine, or by oral administration of a balanced intestinal lavage solution. A stool softener such as dioctyl sodium sulfosuccinate or lactulose may help prevent such episodes.

Pancreatic enzyme replacement should be given with all meals and snacks. The most effective enzyme preparations contain pancrelipase in pH-sensitive, enteric-coated microspheres or microtablets. Infants are usually started at a dose of 1000 to 2000 IU lipase per 120 mL of formula or per breastfeeding session. After infancy, weight-based dosing is used starting at 1000 IU lipase/kg/meal for children < 4 yr and at 500 IU lipase/kg/meal for those > 4 yr. Usually, half the standard dose is given with snacks. Doses > 2500 IU lipase/kg/meal or > 10,000 IU lipase/kg/day should be avoided because high enzyme dosages have been associated with fibrosing colonopathy. In patients with high enzyme requirements, use of an H_2 blocker or proton pump inhibitor may improve enzyme effectiveness.

Diet therapy includes sufficient calories and protein to promote normal growth—30 to 50% more than the usual recommended dietary allowances may be required (see TABLE 1–4 on p. 6) as well as a normal-to-high total fat intake to increase the caloric density of the diet; multivitamins in double the recommended daily allowance; supplemental vitamin E in water-miscible form; and salt supplementation during periods of thermal stress and increased sweating. Infants receiving broad-spectrum antibiotics and patients with liver disease and hemoptysis should be given supplemental vitamin K. Formulas containing protein hydrolysates and medium-chain triglycerides may be used instead of modified whole milk formulas for infants with severe pancreatic insufficiency. Glucose polymers and medium-chain triglyceride supplements can be used to increase caloric intake. In patients who fail to maintain adequate nutritional status, enteral supplementation via a nasogastric tube, gastrostomy, or jejunostomy may restore normal growth and stabilize pulmonary function (see p. 20). The use of appetite stimulants and/or androgens to enhance growth has not been shown to have significant advantages and is not usually recommended.

Surgery may be indicated for localized bronchiectasis or atelectasis that cannot be effectively treated with drugs, nasal polyps, chronic sinusitis, bleeding from esophageal varices secondary to portal hypertension, gallbladder disease, and intestinal obstruction due to a volvulus or an intussusception that cannot be medically reduced. Liver transplantations have been performed successfully in patients with end-stage liver disease. Bilateral cadaveric lung and live donor lobar transplantations have been performed successfully in patients with advanced cardiopulmonary disease.

End-of-life care: The patient and family deserve sensitive discussions of prognosis and preferences for care throughout the course, especially as the patient evidences more and more limited reserves. Most people facing the end of life with CF will be older adolescents or young adults and will be appropriately responsible for their own choices. Thus, they must know what is in store and what can be done. One mark of respect for the person who is living with CF is to ensure that he is given the information and opportunity to make life choices, including having a substantial hand in determining how and when to accept dying. Often, discussion of transplantation is needed. In considering transplantation, patients need to weigh the merits of longer survival with a transplant against the uncertainty of getting a transplant and the ongoing (but different) illness of living with an organ transplant.

Deteriorating patients need to discuss the eventuality of dying. Patients and their families need to know that most often dying is actually gentle and not profoundly symptomatic. Palliative care, including sufficient sedation, should be offered to ensure peaceful dying, when that is appropriate. One of the useful strategies for the patient to consider is to accept a time-limited trial of fully aggressive treatment when needed, but to agree in advance to parameters that should indicate when to stop aggressive measures and accept death.

279 INFECTIONS IN NEONATES

Neonatal infection can be acquired in utero transplacentally, through the birth canal during delivery (intrapartum), and from external sources after birth (postpartum).

In utero infection, which can occur any time before birth, results from overt or subclinical maternal infection. Consequences depend on the agent and timing of infection in gestation and include spontaneous abortion, intrauterine growth restriction, premature birth, stillbirth, congenital malformation (eg, rubella), and symptomatic neonatal infection (eg, toxoplasmosis, syphilis).

Intrapartum infection occurs from passage through an infected birth canal or by ascending infection if delivery is delayed after rupture of membranes. Common viral agents include herpes simplex, HIV, cytomegalovirus (CMV), and hepatitis B; these can less commonly be transmitted transplacentally. Bacterial agents include group B streptococci, enteric gram-negative organisms (primarily *Escherichia coli*), gonococci, and chlamydiae.

Postpartum infections are acquired from contact with an infected mother either directly (eg, TB, which also is sometimes transmitted in utero) or through breastfeeding (eg, HIV, CMV) or from contact with health care practitioners and the hospital environment (numerous organisms—see p. 2329).

Risk factors: Risk of contracting intra- and postpartum infection is inversely proportional to gestational age. Neonates are immunologically immature, with decreased PMN and monocyte function; premature infants are particularly so (see also p. 2256). Maternal IgG antibodies are actively transported across the placenta, but effective levels are not achieved until near term. IgM antibodies do not cross the placenta. Premature infants have decreased intrinsic antibody production and reduced complement activity. Premature infants are also more likely to require invasive procedures (eg, endotracheal intubation, prolonged IV access) that predispose to infection.

Antibacterial therapy: Drug selection is similar to that in adults (see p. 1408), because infecting organisms and their sensitivities are not specific to neonates. However, numerous factors, including age and weight, affect dose and frequency (see TABLES 279–1 and 279–2).

TABLE 279–1. RECOMMENDED DOSAGES OF SELECTED PARENTERAL ANTIBIOTICS FOR NEONATES

ANTIBIOTIC	ROUTE OF ADMINIS-TRATION	INDIVID-UAL DOSE	INTERVAL OF ADMINISTRATION						COMMENTS
			Body Weight < 1200 g		Body Weight 1200 – 1999 g		Body Weight ≥ 2000 g		
			Age		Age		Age		
			≤ 7 DAYS	8–28 DAYS	0–7 DAYS	≥ 8 DAYS	0–7 DAYS	≥ 8 DAYS	
Amikacin*	IV, IM	7.5–10 mg/kg	q 18–24 h	q 18–24 h	q 12–18 h	q 8–12 h	q 12 h	q 8 h	Monitor serum peak drug levels (peak = 20–30 µg/mL [34–43 µmol/L]); trough serum concentration should be < 10 µg/mL. Reduce dose for impaired renal function. Reduce frequency in very small, premature infants (q 18–24 h)
Amphotericin B†	IV	0.25–1 mg/kg	Dilute in 5% or 10 % D/W (do not use saline solution). Give a test dose of 0.1 mg/kg (maximum 1 mg) infused over 1 h to assess patient's febrile and hemodynamic response.‡ If no serious adverse effects are observed, a therapeutic dose of 0.4 mg/kg may be given the same day as the test dose. Infuse the dose over 2–4 h. The dose may be increased to a maximum of 1 mg/kg/day. Doses up to 1.5 mg/kg/day may be needed in select situations. After the patient improves, the dose may be given every other day until therapy is complete. Monitor K levels and hematologic and renal functions						
Ampicillin									IV as 15- to 30-min infusion
For meningitis	IV	50 mg/kg	q 12 h	q 12 h	q 12 h	q 8 h	q 8 h	q 6 h	
For other diseases	IV, IM	25 mg/kg	q 12 h	q 12 h	q 12 h	q 8 h	q 8 h	q 6 h	
Aztreonam	IV, IM	30 mg/kg	q 12 h	q 12 h	q 12 h	q 8 h	q 8 h	q 6 h	Limited data. For gram-negative bacilli only

Cefazolin‡	IV, IM	20 mg/kg	q 12 h	q 12 h	q 12 h	q 12 h	q 12 h	q 8 h	No primary indication. Limited data. Do not use for initial therapy of sepsis or meningitis
Cefotaxime	IV, IM	50 mg/kg	q 12 h	q 12 h	q 12 h	q 8 h	q 8–12 h	q 6–8 h	First-line therapy for neonatal meningitis
Ceftazidime	IV, IM	50 mg/kg	q 12 h	q 12 h	q 12 h	q 8 h	q 8 h	q 8 h	Ceftazidime penetrates well into inflamed meninges, and 70 to 90% of drug is excreted unchanged in urine
Ceftriaxone									Limited data. May cause biliary pseudolithiasis. May increase risk of bilirubin encephalopathy in jaundiced premature infants
For meningitis	IV, IM	50–75 mg/kg	q 24 h	q 24 h	q 12–24 h	q 12–24 h	q 12–24 h	q 12–24 h	
For other diseases	IV, IM	50 mg/kg	q 24 h	q 24 h	q 24 h	q 24 h	q 24 h	q 24 h	
Chloramphenicol	IV	25 mg/kg	q 24 h	q 24 h	q 24 h	q 24 h	q 24 h	q 12 h	Adjust doses by monitoring serum drug levels and hematologic parameters. For meningitis, desired peak = 15–25 µg/mL (46–77 µmol/L); for other infections, 10–20 µg/mL. Many clinicians monitor trough levels (for meningitis, 5–15 µg/mL; for other infections, 5–10 µg/mL)

Table continues on the following page.

TABLE 279–1. RECOMMENDED DOSAGES OF SELECTED PARENTERAL ANTIBIOTICS FOR NEONATES—Continued

			INTERVAL OF ADMINISTRATION						
			Body Weight < 1200 g		Body Weight 1200–1999 g		Body Weight ≥ 2000 g		
			Age		Age		Age		
ANTIBIOTIC	ROUTE OF ADMINISTRATION	INDIVIDUAL DOSE	≤ 7 DAYS	8–28 DAYS	0–7 DAYS	≥ 8 DAYS	0–7 DAYS	≥ 8 DAYS	COMMENTS
Clindamycin	IV, IM	5 mg/kg	q 12 h	q 12 h	q 12 h	q 8 h	q 8 h	q 6 h	For anaerobes and gram-positive cocci (not enterococci)
Gentamicin*	IV, IM	2.5 mg/kg	q 18–24 h	q 18–24 h	q 12–18 h	q 8–12 h	q 12 h	q 8 h	Monitor serum peak drug levels (peak = 5–10 µg/mL [10.4–20.9 µmol/L]). Trough serum concentration should be < 2 µg/mL. Reduce dose for impaired renal function. Reduce frequency (q 18–24 h) in very small, premature infants. Alternatively, in term infants, gentamicin 4 mg/kg q 24 h is an option
Imipenem	IV	20–25 mg/kg	q 18–24 h	q 18–24 h	q 12 h	q 12 h	q 12 h	q 8 h	Limited data

Kanamycin*	IV, IM	7.5–10 mg/kg	q 18–24 h	q 18–24 h	q 12–18 h	q 8–12 h	q 12 h	q 8 h	Monitor serum peak drug levels (peak = 20–30 µg/mL [31–52 µmol/L]); trough serum concentration should be < 10 µg/mL. Reduce dose for impaired renal function. Reduce frequency in very small, premature infants (q 18–24 h)
Methicillin									Rarely used; oxacillin and nafcillin are preferred. Monitor renal function
For meningitis or endocarditis	IV	50 mg/kg	q 12 h	q 12 h	q 12 h	q 8 h	q 8 h	q 6 h	
For other diseases	IV, IM	25 mg/kg	q 12 h	q 12 h	q 12 h	q 8 h	q 8 h	q 6 h	
Metronidazole	IV	7.5–15 mg/kg	q 24–48 h	q 24–48 h	q 24 h	q 12 h	q 12 h	q 12 h	Limited data. Give loading dose of 15 mg/kg. Subsequent dose 48 h later in preterm infants and 24 h later in full-term infants, then q 12 h
Mezlocillin	IV, IM	75 mg/kg	q 12 h	q 12 h	q 12 h	q 8 h	q 12 h	q 8 h	Limited data
Nafcillin									Monitor CBC and liver function
For meningitis or endocarditis	IV	50 mg/kg	q 12 h	q 12 h	q 12 h	q 8 h	q 8 h	q 6 h	
For other diseases	IV, IM	25 mg/kg	q 12 h	q 12 h	q 12 h	q 8 h	q 8 h	q 6 h	

Table continues on the following page.

TABLE 279–1. RECOMMENDED DOSAGES OF SELECTED PARENTERAL ANTIBIOTICS FOR NEONATES—Continued

ANTIBIOTIC	ROUTE OF ADMINISTRATION	INDIVIDUAL DOSE	INTERVAL OF ADMINISTRATION: Body Weight < 1200 g, Age ≤ 7 DAYS	Body Weight < 1200 g, Age 8–28 DAYS	Body Weight 1200 – 1999 g, Age 0–7 DAYS	Body Weight 1200 – 1999 g, Age ≥ 8 DAYS	Body Weight ≥ 2000 g, Age 0–7 DAYS	Body Weight ≥ 2000 g, Age ≥ 8 DAYS	COMMENTS
Netilmicin*	IV, IM	2.5 mg/kg	q 18–24 h	q 18–24	q 12–18 h	q 8–12 h	q 12 h	q 8 h	Monitor peak serum drug levels (peak = 5–10 μg/mL). Trough serum concentrations should be < 2 μg/mL. Reduce dose for impaired renal function. Reduce frequency in very small, premature infants (q 18 to 24 h)
Oxacillin									Oxacillin and nafcillin are preferred over methicillin for treatment of sensitive staphylococcal infections
For meningitis or endocarditis	IV	50 mg/kg	q 12 h	q 12 h	q 12 h	q 8 h	q 8 h	q 6 h	
For other diseases	IV, IM	25 mg/kg	q 12 h	q 12 h	q 12 h	q 8 h	q 8 h	q 6 h	
Penicillin G, aqueous									Maximum for group B streptococcal meningitis, 500,000 units/kg/day
For meningitis	IV	50,000–75,000 units/kg	q 12 h	q 12 h	q 12 h	q 8 h	q 8 h	q 6 h	
For other diseases	IV,IM	25,000 units/kg	q 12 h	q 12 h	q 12 h	q 8 h	q 8 h	q 6 h	

Penicillin G, procaine	IM	50,000 units/kg	Not recommended	Not recommended	q 24 h	q 24 h	q 24 h	q 24 h	CAUTION: Sterile abscess and procaine toxicity
Ticarcillin	IV, IM	75 mg/kg	q 12 h	q 12 h	q 12 h	q 8 h	q 8 h	q 6 h	No primary indication. Use in combination with aminoglycoside against *Pseudomonas aeruginosa*. Potential bleeding with renal failure
Tobramycin*	IV, IM	2.5 mg/kg	q 18–24 h	q 18–24 h	q 12–18 h	q 8–12 h	q 12 h	q 8 h	Monitor serum peak drug levels (peak = 5–10 µg/mL [11-21 µmol/L]); trough serum concentration should be < 2 µg/mL. Reduce dose in impaired renal function. Reduce frequency (q 18–24 h) in very small, premature infants
Vancomycin	IV	15 mg/kg loading dose, then 10–15 mg/kg	q 24 h	q 24 h	q 12–18 h	q 8–12 h	q 12 h	q 8 h	Limited data. Give by slow IV infusion, no less than 60 min. Monitoring serum concentrations for vancomycin is controversial (peak = 25–40 µg/mL [7–12.1 µmol/L]; trough = < 15 µg/mL [3 µmol/L]), adjust doses in renal failure. For premature infants < 1000 g, give 15 mg/kg q 24–36 h

*Sample to be obtained 30 min after a 30-min IV infusion.
†The need to administer a test dose of amphotericin B is controversial.
‡Does not cross the blood-brain barrier.

TABLE 279–2. RECOMMENDED DOSAGES OF SELECTED ORAL ANTIBIOTICS FOR NEONATES

ANTIBIOTIC	DOSAGE	INTERVAL	COMMENTS
Amoxicillin	15 mg/kg	q 8 h	Limited data
Cefaclor	15 mg/kg	q 8 h	Limited data
Clindamycin*	5 mg/kg	q 6–8 h	Limited data
Colistin	3–5 mg/kg	q 8 h	For gastroenteritis caused by enteropathogenic strains of *Escherichia coli*, and for prophylaxis of neonates at high risk for necrotizing enterocolitis, for 5 days. May be systemically absorbed in the presence of significant diarrhea. Unproven efficacy and safety
Erythromycin estolate	10 mg/kg	q 8 h	For chlamydial infections or pertussis
Erythromycin ethylsuccinate	12.5 mg/kg	q 6 h	For chlamydial infections or pertussis
Fluconazole	3–6 mg/kg	q 24 h	For candidal infections
Flucytosine	12.5–37.5 mg/kg	q 6 h	Limited data. Use only in combination with amphotericin B, to retard emergence of resistance
Neomycin	30–35 mg/kg	q 8 h	See Colistin
Rifampin†	10 mg/kg	q 24 h	For TB
	5 mg/kg	q 12 h	For meningococcus prophylaxis for 2 days
	10 mg/kg	q 24 h	For *Haemophilus influenzae* prophylaxis for 4 days

*The dose for neonates < 7 days who are < 2000 g is 5 mg/kg q 12 h.
†Serum levels in preterm infants should be monitored.

In neonates, the ECF constitutes up to 45% of total body weight, requiring relatively larger doses of certain antibiotics (eg, aminoglycosides) compared to adults. Lower serum albumin concentrations in premature infants may reduce antibiotic protein binding. Drugs that displace bilirubin from albumin (eg, sulfonamides, ceftriaxone) increase the risk of kernicterus.

Absence or deficiency of certain enzymes in neonates may prolong the half-life of certain antibiotics (chloramphenicol) and increase the risk of toxicity. Changes in GFR and renal tubular secretion during the 1st month of life necessitate dosing changes for other drugs (eg, penicillins, aminoglycosides, vancomycin).

CONGENITAL AND PERINATAL CYTOMEGALOVIRUS INFECTION

(See also Cytomegalovirus Infection on p. 1605.)

Cytomegalovirus infection may be acquired prenatally or perinatally. Signs at birth, if present, are intrauterine growth restriction, prematurity, microcephaly, jaundice, petechiae, hepatosplenomegaly, periventricular calcifications, chorioretinitis, and pneumonitis. Later in infancy, signs are pneumonia, hepatosplenomegaly, hepatitis, thrombocytopenia, and atypical lymphocytosis.

Diagnosis is by virus isolation or serology. Treatment is supportive. Parenteral ganciclovir can prevent hearing deterioration, but its use remains controversial.

Cytomegalovirus (CMV) is frequently isolated from neonates. Although most infants shedding this virus are asymptomatic, others have life-threatening illness and devastating long-term sequelae.

It is not known when a woman with primary CMV can safely conceive. Because risk to the fetus is difficult to assess, women who develop primary CMV during pregnancy should be counseled, but few experts recommend routine serologic testing for CMV before or during pregnancy in healthy women.

Etiology

Congenital CMV infection, which occurs in 0.2 to 2.2% of live births worldwide, may result from transplacental acquisition of either a primary or recurrent maternal infection. Clinically apparent disease in the neonate is much more likely to occur after a primary maternal exposure, particularly in the 1st half of pregnancy. In some higher socioeconomic groups in the US, 50% of young women lack antibody to CMV, making them susceptible to primary infection.

Perinatal CMV infection is acquired by exposure to infected cervical secretions, breast milk, or blood products. Maternal antibody is thought to be protective, and most exposed term infants are asymptomatic or not infected. In contrast, preterm infants (who lack antibody to CMV) can develop serious infection or death, particularly when transfused with CMV-positive blood. Efforts should be made to transfuse these infants with only CMV-negative blood or components.

Symptoms and Signs

Many women who become infected with CMV during pregnancy are asymptomatic, but some develop a mononucleosis-like illness.

About 10% of infants with congenital CMV infection are symptomatic at birth. Manifestations include intrauterine growth restriction, prematurity, microcephaly, jaundice, petechiae, hepatosplenomegaly, periventricular calcifications, chorioretinitis, and pneumonitis. Infants who acquire CMV after birth may develop pneumonia, hepatosplenomegaly, hepatitis, thrombocytopenia, and atypical lymphocytosis, especially if they are premature.

Diagnosis

Symptomatic congenital CMV infection must be distinguished from other congenital infections, including toxoplasmosis, rubella, and syphilis.

In neonates, viral culture is the primary diagnostic tool; maternal diagnosis can also be made by serologic testing (see p. 1606). Culture specimens should be refrigerated until inoculation on fibroblast cells. Congenital CMV is diagnosed if the virus is isolated from urine or other body fluids obtained within the 1st 2 wk of life. After 2 wk, positive cultures may indicate perinatal or congenital infection. Infants may shed CMV for several years after either type of infection.

A CBC and differential and liver function tests may be helpful. A cranial ultrasound or CT examination and an ophthalmologic evaluation should also be performed.

Prognosis and Treatment

Symptomatic neonates have a mortality rate of up to 30%, and 70 to 90% of survivors have some neurologic impairment, including hearing loss, mental retardation, and visual disturbances. In addition, 10% of asymptomatic neonates eventually develop neurologic sequelae. Because hearing defects are a concern, close monitoring after the neonatal period is needed.

No specific therapy is available. Ganciclovir decreases viral shedding in neonates with congenital CMV and prevents hearing deterioration at 6 mo. When therapy stops, the virus is again shed; therefore, its role in treatment remains controversial.

Prevention

Nonimmune pregnant women should attempt to limit exposure to the virus. For instance, because CMV infection is common in children attending day care centers, pregnant women should always wash their hands thoroughly after exposure to urine and respiratory secretions from children. Transfusion-associated perinatal CMV disease can be avoided by giving preterm neonates blood products from CMV-seronegative donors or products that have been treated to make them noninfectious. Development of a vaccine against CMV is under investigation.

CONGENITAL RUBELLA

(See also Rubella on p. 1646.)

Congenital rubella is a viral infection acquired from the mother during pregnancy. Signs

are multiple congenital anomalies that can result in fetal death. Diagnosis is by serology and viral culture. There is no specific treatment. Prevention is by routine vaccination.

Congenital rubella typically results from a primary maternal infection. Despite widespread vaccination, 10 to 20% of postpubertal people lack antibody.

Rubella is believed to invade the upper respiratory tract, with subsequent viremia and dissemination of virus to different sites, including the placenta. The fetus is at highest risk for developmental abnormalities when infected during the 1st 16 wk of gestation, particularly the 1st 8 to 10 wk. Early in gestation, the virus is thought to establish a chronic intrauterine infection. Its effects include endothelial damage to blood vessels, direct cytolysis of cells, and disruption of cellular mitosis.

Symptoms and Signs

Rubella in a pregnant woman may be asymptomatic or characterized by upper respiratory tract symptoms, fever, lymphadenopathy (especially in the suboccipital and posterior auricular areas), and a maculopapular rash. This illness may be followed by joint symptoms.

In the fetus there may be no effects, multiple anomalies, or death in utero. The most frequent abnormalities include intrauterine growth restriction, meningoencephalitis, cataracts, retinopathy, hearing loss, cardiac defects (patent ductus arteriosus and pulmonary artery stenosis), hepatosplenomegaly, and bone radiolucencies. Others are thrombocytopenia with purpura, dermal erythropoiesis resulting in bluish red skin lesions, adenopathy, and interstitial pneumonia. Close observation is needed to detect subsequent hearing loss, mental retardation, abnormal behavior, endocrinopathies, or a rare progressive encephalitis.

Diagnosis

Pregnant women routinely have a serum rubella titer measured early in pregnancy. Titer is repeated in seronegative women who develop symptoms or signs of rubella; diagnosis is made by seroconversion or a ≥4-fold rise between acute and convalescent titers. Virus may be cultured from nasopharyngeal swabs.

Infants suspected of having congenital rubella should have antibody titers and viral cultures. Persistence of rubella-specific IgG in the infant after 6 to 12 mo suggests congenital infection. Increased rubella-specific IgM antibodies also indicate rubella. Specimens from the nasopharynx, urine, CSF, buffy coat, and conjunctiva may grow virus; the laboratory should be notified that rubella virus is suspected. In a few centers, diagnoses can be made prenatally by isolating the virus from amniotic fluid, detecting rubella-specific IgM in fetal blood, or applying reverse transcriptase–PCR (RT-PCR) techniques to fetal blood or chorionic villus biopsy specimens.

Other tests include a CBC with differential, CSF analysis, and radiologic examination of the bones to detect characteristic radiolucencies. Thorough ophthalmologic and cardiac evaluation is also useful.

Treatment

No specific therapy is available for maternal or congenital rubella infection. Women exposed to rubella early in pregnancy should be informed of the potential risks to the fetus. Some experts recommend administering immune globulin (0.55 mL/kg IM) for exposure early in pregnancy, but this use does not guarantee prevention, and routine use is not recommended by the American Academy of Pediatrics.

Prevention

Rubella can easily be prevented by vaccination. In the US, infants should receive vaccination for rubella together with measles and mumps vaccinations at 12 to 15 mo of age and again at entry to grade school or junior high school (see FIG. 266–3 on p. 2235). Postpubertal females who are not known to be immune to rubella should be vaccinated. (CAUTION: *Rubella vaccination is contraindicated in immunodeficient or pregnant women.*) After vaccination, women should be advised not to become pregnant for 28 days. Efforts should also be made to screen and vaccinate high-risk groups, such as hospital and child care workers, military recruits, and college students.

CONGENITAL SYPHILIS

(See also Syphilis on p. 1657.)

Congenital syphilis is a multisystem infection caused by *Treponema pallidum* and transmitted to the fetus via the placenta. Early signs are characteristic skin lesions, lymphadenopathy, hepatosplenomegaly,

failure to thrive, blood-stained nasal discharge, perioral fissures, meningitis, choroiditis, hydrocephalus, seizures, mental retardation, osteochondritis, and pseudoparalysis. Later signs are gummatous ulcers, periosteal lesions, paresis, tabes, optic atrophy, interstitial keratitis, sensorineural deafness, and dental deformities. Diagnosis is clinical, confirmed by microscopy or serology. Treatment is penicillin.

Overall risk of transplacental infection of the fetus is about 60 to 80%. Untreated primary or secondary syphilis in the mother usually is transmitted, but latent or tertiary syphilis usually is not. As in adults, syphilis has early, latent, and late manifestations.

Symptoms and Signs

Many patients are asymptomatic and the disease remains latent throughout their lives.

Early congenital syphilis (birth through 1st few months of life) causes characteristic bullous eruptions or a macular, copper-colored rash on the palms and soles and papular lesions around the nose and mouth and in the diaper area. Generalized lymphadenopathy and hepatosplenomegaly often occur. The infant may fail to thrive and have a characteristic "old man" look, with fissured lesions around the mouth (rhagades) and a mucopurulent or blood-stained nasal discharge causing snuffles. A few infants develop meningitis, choroiditis, hydrocephalus, or seizures, and others may be mentally retarded. Within the 1st 3 mo of life, osteochondritis (chondroepiphysitis), especially of the long bones and ribs, may cause pseudoparalysis of the limbs with characteristic radiologic changes in the bones.

Late congenital syphilis usually does not manifest until after 2 yr of life and causes gummatous ulcers that tend to involve the nose, septum, and hard palate and periosteal lesions that result in saber shins and bossing of the frontal and parietal bones. Neurosyphilis is usually asymptomatic, but juvenile paresis and tabes may develop. Optic atrophy, sometimes leading to blindness, may occur. Interstitial keratitis, the most common eye lesion, frequently recurs, often resulting in corneal scarring. Sensorineural deafness, which is often progressive, may appear at any age. Hutchinson's incisors, mulberry molars, and maldevelopment of the maxilla resulting in "bulldog" facies are characteristic, if infrequent, sequelae.

Diagnosis

Early congenital syphilis: Diagnosis is usually suspected based on maternal serologic testing, which is routinely performed early in pregnancy, and often in the 3rd trimester and at delivery. Neonates of mothers with positive tests should have a thorough examination, darkfield microscopy of any skin or mucosal lesions, and a quantitative nontreponemal serum test (eg, rapid plasma reagin [RPR], venereal disease research laboratory [VDRL]); cord blood is not used for serum testing because results are less sensitive and specific. The placenta or umbilical cord should be analyzed using darkfield microscopy or fluorescent antibody staining. Infants with clinical signs of illness or suggestive serologic test results also should have lumbar puncture with CSF analysis for cell count, VDRL, and protein; CBC; liver function tests; and long-bone x-rays.

Diagnosis is confirmed by microscopic visualization of spirochetes in samples from the neonate or the placenta. Diagnosis based on neonatal serologic testing is complicated by the transplacental transfer of maternal IgG antibodies, which can cause a positive test in the absence of infection; however, a neonatal titer >4 times the maternal titer would not generally result from passive transfer, and diagnosis is considered confirmed or highly probable. Maternal disease acquired late in pregnancy may be transmitted before development of antibodies. Thus, in neonates with lower titers but typical clinical manifestations, syphilis is also considered highly probable. In neonates without signs of illness and low or (if maternal infection is diagnosed) negative serologic titers, syphilis is considered possible; subsequent approach depends on various maternal and neonatal factors (see Follow up on p. 2324). The utility of fluorescent assays for antitreponemal IgM, which is not transferred across the placenta, is controversial, but such assays have been used to detect neonatal infection.

Late congenital syphilis: Diagnosis is by clinical history, distinctive physical signs, and positive serologic tests (see also p. 1661). Hutchinson's triad of interstitial keratitis, Hutchinson's incisors, and 8th cranial nerve deafness is diagnostic. Sometimes the standard STS and *T. pallidum* immobilization test are negative, but the fluorescent treponemal antibody absorption test is usually positive. The diagnosis should be considered in cases of unexplained deafness, progressive intellectual deterioration, or keratitis.

Follow up: All seropositive infants and those whose mothers were seropositive should have VDRL or RPR titers q 2 to 3 mo until the test is nonreactive or the titer has decreased 4-fold. In uninfected and successfully treated infants, nontreponemal antibody titers are usually nonreactive by 6 mo. Passively acquired treponemal antibodies may be present for longer, perhaps 15 mo.

If VDRL or RPR remain reactive past 6 to 12 mo or titers increase, the infant should be reevaluated (including lumbar puncture for CSF analysis, and CBC with platelet count, long bone x-rays, and other tests as clinically indicated).

Treatment

Pregnant women: Pregnant women in the early stages of syphilis receive 2 doses of benzathine penicillin G (1.2 million units IM in each buttock q 1 wk). For later stages of syphilis or neurosyphilis, the appropriate regimen for nonpregnant patients should be followed (see p. 1662). Occasionally, a severe Jarisch-Herxheimer reaction occurs after such therapy, leading to spontaneous abortion. Patients allergic to penicillin may be desensitized and then treated with penicillin. RPR and VDRL tests become negative by 3 mo after adequate treatment in most patients and by 6 mo in nearly all patients. Erythromycin therapy is inadequate for both the mother and fetus and is not recommended. Tetracycline is *contraindicated.*

Early congenital syphilis: In confirmed or highly probable cases, 2002 CDC guidelines recommend aqueous penicillin G 50,000 units/kg IV q 12 h for the 1st 7 days of life, and q 8 h thereafter for a total of 10 days, or procaine penicillin G 50,000 units/kg IM once/day for 10 days. This regimen also is used for infants considered to have possible syphilis if the mother was untreated or her treatment status is unknown, she was treated ≤ 4 wk before delivery, or she was inadequately treated (a nonpenicillin regimen, or maternal titers did not decrease 4-fold).

Infants with possible syphilis whose mothers were adequately treated and who are clinically well can be given a single dose of benzathine penicillin 50,000 units/kg IM. If close follow up is assured, some clinicians instead obtain nontreponemal serology monthly for 3 mo, and at 6 mo, and treat with a full antibiotic course if titers rise or are positive at 6 mo.

Older infants and children with newly diagnosed congenital syphilis: The CSF should be examined before treatment starts. The CDC recommends that any child with late congenital syphilis be treated with aqueous crystalline penicillin G 50,000 to 75,000 units/kg IV q 4 to 6 h for 10 days. Many patients do not revert to seronegativity but do have a 4-fold decrease in titer of reagin (eg, VDRL) antibody. Interstitial keratitis is usually treated with corticosteroid and atropine drops in consultation with an ophthalmologist. Patients with nerve deafness may benefit from penicillin plus a corticosteroid such as prednisone 0.5 mg/kg po once/day for 1 wk, followed by 0.3 mg/kg once/day for 4 wk, after which the dose is gradually reduced over 2 to 3 mo. (Corticosteroids have not been critically evaluated in these conditions.) Contacts should be traced, and patients should be kept under long-term surveillance.

Prevention

Pregnant women should be routinely tested for syphilis and retested if they acquire other sexually transmitted diseases during pregnancy. In 99% of cases, adequate treatment during pregnancy cures both mother and fetus. However, in some cases, treatment late in pregnancy eliminates the infection but not some signs of syphilis that appear at birth.

When congenital syphilis is diagnosed, other family members should be examined regularly for physical and serologic evidence of infection. Retreatment of the mother in subsequent pregnancies is necessary only if serologic titers remain positive. Women who remain seropositive after adequate treatment may have been reinfected and should be retreated. A mother without lesions who is seronegative but who has had venereal exposure to a known patient with syphilis should be treated, because there is a 25 to 50% chance that she acquired syphilis.

CONGENITAL TOXOPLASMOSIS

(See also Toxoplasmosis on p. 1584.)

Congenital toxoplasmosis is caused by transplacental acquisition of *Toxoplasma gondii*. Signs, if present, are prematurity, intrauterine growth restriction, jaundice, hepatosplenomegaly, myocarditis, pneumonitis, rash, chorioretinitis, hydrocephalus,

intracranial calcifications, microcephaly, and seizures. Diagnosis is by serology. Treatment is with pyrimethamine, sulfadiazine, and leucovorin.

Toxoplasma gondii, a parasite found worldwide, causes congenital infection in about 1/10,000 to 80/10,000 births.

Etiology

With rare exception, congenital toxoplasmosis is due to a primary maternal infection during pregnancy. Infection with *T. gondii* occurs primarily from ingestion of inadequately cooked meat containing cysts, or ingestion of oocysts derived from cat feces. The rate of transmission to the fetus is higher in women infected later during pregnancy. However, those infected earlier in gestation generally have more severe disease. Overall, 30 to 40% of women infected during pregnancy will have a congenitally infected child.

Symptoms and Signs

Pregnant women infected with *T. gondii* generally do not have clinical manifestations. Similarly, infected neonates are usually asymptomatic at birth, but manifestations may include prematurity, intrauterine growth restriction, jaundice, hepatosplenomegaly, myocarditis, pneumonitis, and various rashes. Neurologic involvement, often prominent, includes chorioretinitis, hydrocephalus, intracranial calcifications, microcephaly, and seizures.

Diagnosis

Serology is important in diagnosing maternal and congenital infection; there are numerous tests, some of which are performed only in reference laboratories. The most reliable are the Sabin-Feldman dye test, the indirect fluorescent antibody (IFA) test, and the direct agglutination assay. Acute maternal infection is suggested by seroconversion or a ≥ 4-fold rise between acute and convalescent IgG titers. However, maternal IgG antibodies may be detectable in the infant through the 1st year. PCR analysis of fetal blood and amniotic fluid may prove a better method. Tests to isolate the organism include inoculation into mice and tissue culture.

In suspected congenital toxoplasmosis, serologic tests, MRI or CT imaging of the brain, CSF analysis, and a thorough eye examination by an ophthalmologist should be performed. CSF abnormalities include xanthochromia, pleocytosis, and increased protein concentration. The placenta is inspected for characteristic signs of *T. gondii* infection. Nonspecific laboratory findings include thrombocytopenia, lymphocytosis, monocytosis, eosinophilia, and elevated transaminases.

Prognosis and Treatment

Some have a fulminant course with early death, whereas others have long-term neurologic sequelae. Occasionally, neurologic manifestations (eg, chorioretinitis, mental retardation, deafness, seizures) develop years later in children who appeared normal at birth. Consequently, children with congenital toxoplasmosis should be closely monitored beyond the neonatal period.

Limited data suggest that treatment of infected women during pregnancy may be beneficial to the fetus. Spiramycin (available in the US from the FDA) has been used to prevent maternofetal transmission. Pyrimethamine and sulfonamides have been used later in gestation to treat the infected fetus.

Treatment of symptomatic and asymptomatic neonates may improve outcome. Therefore, treatment with pyrimethamine (initial loading dose of 2 mg/kg po once/day for 2 days followed by 1 mg/kg po once/day, maximum 25 mg), sulfadiazine (42.5 to 50 mg/kg po bid, maximum 4 g), and leucovorin (10 mg po 3 times/wk) is recommended. After the initial 6 mo of treatment, sulfadiazine and leucovorin are continued as previously, but the pyrimethamine is administered less frequently (only on Mon, Wed, and Fri). All treatment should be overseen by an expert. The use of corticosteroids is controversial and should be determined case by case.

Prevention

Pregnant women should avoid contact with cat litter boxes and other areas contaminated with cat feces. Meat should be thoroughly cooked before consumption, and hands should be washed after handling raw meat or unwashed produce. Women at risk for primary infection should be screened during pregnancy. Those infected during the 1st or 2nd trimester should be counseled regarding available treatments.

NEONATAL CONJUNCTIVITIS

(Ophthalmia Neonatorum)

Neonatal conjunctivitis is purulent ocular drainage due to a chemical irritant or a

pathogenic organism. Topical prevention is routine. Diagnosis is clinical and confirmed by laboratory testing. Treatment is with organism-specific antimicrobials.

Etiology

The major causes are, in decreasing order, chemical inflammation, bacterial infection, and viral infection (see also p. 889). Chemical conjunctivitis is generally secondary to the instillation of silver nitrate drops for ocular prophylaxis. Bacterial infection is acquired from infected mothers during passage through the birth canal. Chlamydial ophthalmia (caused by *Chlamydia trachomatis*) is the most common bacterial cause, occurring in 2 to 4% of births; it accounts for about 30 to 50% of conjunctivitis in neonates < 4 wk of age. The prevalence of maternal chlamydial infection ranges from 2 to 20%. About 30 to 50% of neonates born to acutely infected women develop conjunctivitis (and 5 to 20% develop pneumonia). Other bacteria, including *Streptococcus pneumoniae* and nontypeable *Haemophilus influenzae*, account for another 15% of cases. The incidence of gonorrheal ophthalmia (conjunctivitis due to *Neisseria gonorrhoeae*) in the US is 2 to 3/10,000 births. Isolation of bacteria other than *H. influenzae*, *S. pneumoniae*, and *N. gonorrhoeae*, including *Staphylococcus aureus,* usually represents colonization rather than infection. The major viral cause is herpes simplex virus (HSV) types 1 and 2 (herpetic keratoconjunctivitis).

Symptoms and Signs

Because they overlap in both presentation and onset, causes of neonatal conjunctivitis are difficult to distinguish clinically. Conjunctivae are injected, and discharge (watery or purulent) is present.

Chemical conjunctivitis secondary to silver nitrate usually appears within 6 to 8 h after instillation and disappears spontaneously within 48 to 96 h.

Chlamydial ophthalmia usually occurs 5 to 14 days after birth. It may range from mild conjunctivitis with minimal mucopurulent discharge to severe eyelid edema with copious drainage and pseudomembrane formation. Follicles are not present in the conjunctiva, as they are in older children and adults.

Gonorrheal ophthalmia produces an acute purulent conjunctivitis that appears 2 to 5 days after birth or earlier with premature rupture of membranes. The neonate has severe eyelid edema followed by chemosis and a profuse purulent exudate that may be under pressure. If untreated, corneal ulcerations and blindness may occur.

Conjunctivitis caused by other bacteria has a variable onset, ranging from 4 days to several weeks.

Herpetic keratoconjunctivitis can occur as an isolated infection or with disseminated or CNS infection. It can be mistaken for bacterial or chemical conjunctivitis, but the presence of dendritic keratitis is pathognomonic.

Diagnosis

Conjunctival material is Gram stained, cultured for gonorrhea (eg, on modified Thayer-Martin medium), and tested for chlamydia (eg, by direct immunofluorescence, enzyme-linked immunosorbent assay, nucleic acid amplification techniques—samples must contain cells). Conjunctival scrapings can also be examined with Giemsa stain; if blue intracytoplasmic inclusions are identified, chlamydial ophthalmia is confirmed. Viral culture is obtained only if viral infection is suspected by skin lesions or maternal infection.

Treatment

Neonates with conjunctivitis and maternal gonococcal infection or with gram-negative intracellular diplococci identified in conjunctival exudates should be treated with ceftriaxone before results of confirmatory tests.

In chlamydial ophthalmia, systemic therapy is the treatment of choice, because at least ½ of affected neonates also have nasopharyngeal infection and some develop chlamydial pneumonia. Erythromycin ethylsuccinate 12.5 mg/kg po q 6 h for 2 wk is recommended. Efficacy of this therapy is only 80%, so a 2nd treatment course may be needed.

A neonate with gonorrheal ophthalmia is hospitalized to observe for possible systemic gonococcal infection and given a single dose of ceftriaxone 25 to 50 mg/kg IM to a maximum dose of 125 mg (some clinicians use 100 mg/kg). Frequent saline irrigation of the eye prevents secretions from adhering. Topical antimicrobial ointments alone are ineffective.

Conjunctivitis due to other bacteria usually responds to topical ointments containing polymyxin plus bacitracin, erythromycin, or tetracycline.

Herpetic keratoconjunctivitis should be treated (with an ophthalmologist's consultation) with systemic acyclovir 20 mg/kg q 8 h for 14 to 21 days and topical 1% trifluridine ophthalmic drops or ointment, vidarabine 3% ointment, or 0.1% iododeoxyuridine q 2 to 3 h, with a maximum of 9 doses/24 h. Systemic therapy is important, because dissemination to the CNS and other organs can occur.

Corticosteroid-containing ointments may seriously exacerbate eye infections due to *C. trachomatis* and HSV and should be avoided.

Prevention

Routine use of 1% silver nitrate drops, 0.5% erythromycin, or 1% tetracycline ophthalmic ointments or drops instilled into each eye after delivery effectively prevents gonorrheal ophthalmia. However, none of these agents prevents chlamydial ophthalmia; povidone iodine 2.5% drops may be effective against chlamydia and is effective against gonococci but is not available in the US.

Neonates of mothers with untreated gonorrhea should receive a single injection of ceftriaxone 50 mg/kg IM or IV, up to 125 mg, and both mother and neonate should be screened for chlamydia infection.

NEONATAL HEPATITIS B VIRUS INFECTION

(See also Ch. 27 on p. 219.)

Neonatal hepatitis B virus infection is usually acquired during parturition. It is usually asymptomatic but can cause chronic subclinical disease. Symptomatic infection produces jaundice, lethargy, failure to thrive, abdominal distention, and clay-colored stools. Diagnosis is by serology. Severe illness may cause acute liver failure requiring liver transplantation. Less severe illness is treated supportively.

Of the recognized forms of primary viral hepatitis, only hepatitis B virus (HBV) is an important cause of neonatal hepatitis. Other viral infections (eg, cytomegalovirus, herpes simplex virus) may cause liver inflammation along with their other manifestations.

Etiology

HBV infection occurs during delivery from infected mothers. Maternal acute hepatitis B occurring within 2 to 3 mo of delivery has about a 70% risk of transmission, but disease occurring during the 1st or 2nd trimester has only about 5% risk. Risk of transmission is also high from asymptomatic hepatis B surface antigen (HBsAg) carriers with the e antigen (see p. 222). Carriers without the e antigen or with anti-HBe are less likely to transmit the disease.

Maternal-infant HBV transmission results primarily from maternal-fetal microtransfusions during labor or contact with infectious secretions in the birth canal. Transplacental transmission is unusual. Postpartum transmission occurs rarely through exposure to infectious maternal blood, saliva, stool, urine, or breast milk. Neonatal HBV infection may be an important viral reservoir in certain communities.

Symptoms, Signs, and Diagnosis

Most neonates with HBV infection are asymptomatic but develop chronic, subclinical hepatitis characterized by persistent HBsAg antigenemia and variably elevated transaminase activity. Many born to women with acute hepatitis B during pregnancy are of low birth weight, regardless of whether they are infected.

Infrequently, infected neonates develop acute hepatitis B, which is usually mild and self-limited. They develop jaundice, lethargy, failure to thrive, abdominal distention, and clay-colored stools. Occasionally, severe infection with hepatomegaly, ascites, and hyperbilirubinemia (primarily conjugated bilirubin) occurs. Rarely the disease is fulminant and even fatal. Fulminant disease occurs more often in neonates whose mothers are chronic carriers of hepatitis B.

Diagnosis is by serologic testing as discussed in Ch. 27 (see p. 224).

Prognosis and Treatment

Long-term prognosis is unknown, although HBsAg carriage early in life appears to increase the risk of subsequent liver disease (eg, chronic hepatitis, cirrhosis, hepatocellular carcinoma).

Symptomatic care and adequate nutrition are needed. Neither corticosteroids nor hepatitis B immune globulin (HBIG) is valuable. No therapy prevents the development of chronic, subclinical hepatitis, and because of the risk of developing significant disease, liver function should be monitored periodically.

Prevention

Pregnant women should be tested for HBsAg during an early prenatal visit. Failing that, they should be tested when admitted for delivery.

Neonates whose mothers are HBsAg-positive should be given 1 dose of HBIG

0.5 mL IM within 12 h of birth. Recombinant hepatitis B virus vaccine should be given IM in a series of 3 doses. (NOTE: Doses vary among proprietary vaccines.) The 1st dose is given concurrently with HBIG but at a different site. The 2nd and 3rd doses are given 1 to 2 mo and 6 mo, respectively, after the first. Testing for HBsAg and anti-HBs at 9 to 15 mo is recommended.

Particularly where hepatitis B infection is highly endemic or HBsAg screening of mothers is impractical, all neonates should be vaccinated.

Separating a neonate from its HBsAg-positive mother is not recommended, and breastfeeding does not appear to increase the risk of postpartum HBV transmission, particularly if HBIG and hepatitis B virus vaccine have been given. However, if a mother has cracked nipples, abscesses, or other breast pathology, breastfeeding could potentially transmit HBV.

NEONATAL HERPES SIMPLEX VIRUS INFECTION

(See also Herpes Simplex Virus Infections on p. 1606.)

Neonatal herpes simplex virus infection is usually transmitted during parturition. Signs are typically a vesicular eruption and subsequent disseminated disease. Diagnosis is by viral culture, histology, serology, or molecular biology. Treatment is with high-dose parenteral acyclovir and supportive care.

Neonatal herpes simplex virus (HSV) infection has high mortality and significant morbidity. Incidence estimates range from 1/3,000 to 1/20,000 births. HSV type 2 causes about 80% of cases; 20% are caused by HSV type 1.

HSV is usually transmitted during delivery through an infected maternal genital tract. Transplacental transmission of virus and hospital-acquired spread from one neonate to another by hospital personnel or family may account for about 15% of cases. Mothers of neonates with HSV infection tend to have no history or symptoms of genital infection at the time of delivery.

Symptoms and Signs

Manifestations generally occur between the 1st and 2nd wk of life but may not appear until as late as the 4th wk. Patients may present with local or disseminated disease. Skin vesicles are common in either form, occurring in about 55% overall. Those with no skin vesicles usually present with localized CNS disease. In patients with isolated skin or mucosal disease, progressive or more serious forms of disease frequently follow within 7 to 10 days if left untreated.

Neonates with localized disease can be divided into 2 groups. One group has encephalitis manifested by neurologic findings, CSF pleocytosis, and elevated protein concentration, with or without concomitant involvement of the skin, eyes, and mouth. The other group has only skin, eye, and mouth involvement and no evidence of CNS or organ disease.

Neonates with disseminated disease and visceral organ involvement have hepatitis, pneumonitis, and/or disseminated intravascular coagulation with or without encephalitis or skin disease.

Other signs, which can occur singly or in combination, include temperature instability, lethargy, hypotonia, respiratory distress, apnea, and seizures.

Diagnosis

Rapid diagnosis by viral culture or HSV PCR is essential. The most common site of retrieval is skin vesicles. The mouth, eyes, and CSF are also high-yield sites. In some with encephalitis, virus is found only in the brain. Diagnosis also can be made by neutralization with appropriate high-titer antiserum; immunofluorescence of lesion scrapings, particularly with use of monoclonal antibodies; and electron microscopy. If no diagnostic virology facilities are available, a Papanicolaou test of the lesion base may show characteristic multinucleated giant cells and intranuclear inclusions, but this procedure is less sensitive than culture, and false-positives also occur.

Prognosis

The mortality rate of untreated disseminated disease is 85%; among those with untreated local disease and encephalitis, it is about 50%. At least 95% of survivors have severe neurologic sequelae. Death is uncommon in those with local disease but without CNS or organ disease, except as the result of concomitant medical problems, but about 30% develop neurologic impairment, which may not manifest until 2 to 3 yr of age.

Treatment

Acyclovir decreases the mortality rate by 50% and increases the percentage of children who develop normally from 10 to 50%; dose is 20 mg/kg IV q 8 h for 14 to 21 days. Vigorous supportive therapy is required, including appropriate IV fluids, alimentation, respiratory support, correction of clotting abnormalities, and control of seizure disorders. Herpetic keratoconjunctivitis requires concomitant systemic acyclovir and topical therapy with a drug such as trifluridine (see p. 2326).

NEONATAL HOSPITAL-ACQUIRED INFECTION

Some infections are acquired after admission to the nursery rather than from the mother in utero or intrapartum. For some infections (eg, group B streptococci, herpes simplex virus [HSV]) it may not be clear whether the source is maternal or the hospital environment.

Hospital-acquired infection is primarily a problem for premature infants and for term infants with medical disorders requiring prolonged hospitalization. Healthy, term neonates have infection rates < 1%. For those in special care nurseries, the incidence increases as birth weight decreases. The rate is 7% for those 1251 to 1500 g, 18% for those 1001 to 1250 g, 33% for those 751 to 1000 g, and 48% for those 501 to 750 g.

Sepsis and pneumonia are the most common manifestations. Overall mortality rates are about 33%: for neonates whose birth weight is < 1000 g, 18 to 45%; and for those whose birth weight is > 2000 g, 2 to 12%.

Etiology

In term neonates, skin infection due to methicillin-sensitive *Staphylococcus aureus* is the most frequent hospital-acquired infection. Although nursery personnel who are *S. aureus* nasal carriers are potential sources of infection, colonized neonates are usually the reservoir. The umbilical stump and groin are most frequently colonized during the 1st few days of life, whereas the nares are more frequently colonized later. Often, infections do not manifest until the neonate is at home.

In very low-birth-weight (VLBW—< 1500 g) infants, gram-positive organisms cause about 70% of infections, the majority being with coagulase-negative staphylococci. Gram-negative organisms, including *Escherichia coli*, *Klebsiella*, *Pseudomonas*, *Enterobacter*, and *Serratia*, cause about 18%. Fungi (*Candida albicans* and *C. parapsilosis*) cause about 12%. Patterns of infection (and antibiotic resistance) vary among institutions and units and change with time. Intermittent "epidemics" sometimes occur as a particularly virulent organism colonizes a unit.

Infection is facilitated by the multiple invasive procedures VLBW infants undergo (eg, long-term arterial and venous catheterization, endotracheal intubation, continuous positive airway pressure, nasogastric or nasojejunal feeding tubes). The longer the stay in special care nurseries, and the more procedures performed, the higher the likelihood of infection.

Prevention

Bathing neonates with 3% hexachlorophene decreases frequency of *S. aureus* colonization, but this product can cause neurotoxicity, particularly in low-birth-weight infants, and is no longer used. The American Academy of Pediatrics recommends dry skin care, but this may result in high rates of colonization with *S. aureus*, and epidemics have occurred in some hospitals. During disease outbreaks, application of triple dye to the cord area or bacitracin or mupirocin ointment to the cord, nares, and circumcision site reduces colonization. Routine cultures of personnel or of the environment are not recommended.

Prevention of colonization and infection in special care nurseries requires provision of sufficient space (80 to 100 sq ft/infant in intensive care, 50 sq ft/infant in intermediate care, 6 ft between incubators or warmers, edge-to-edge in each direction) and personnel (nurse:patient ratio 1:1 to 1:2 in intensive care, 1:3 to 1:4 in intermediate care). Proper techniques are required, including placement and care of invasive devices and meticulous cleaning and disinfection or sterilization of equipment. Active surveillance for infection (not colonization) and monitoring of techniques are essential.

Other preventive measures include frequent hand washing, gowns, and gloves. Washing with alcohol preparations is more effective than soap and water. Forced-air incubators provide limited protective isolation; the exteriors and interiors of the units rapidly become heavily contaminated, and personnel are likely to contaminate their hands and forearms. Universal blood and body fluid precautions add further protection.

In an epidemic, establishing a cohort of diseased or colonized infants and assigning them a separate nursing staff are useful. Continuing surveillance for 1 mo after discharge is necessary to assess the adequacy of controls instituted to end an epidemic.

Prophylactic antimicrobial therapy is generally not effective, hastens development of resistant bacteria, and alters the balance of normal flora in the neonate. However, during a confirmed nursery epidemic, antibiotics against specific pathogens may be considered—eg, penicillin G for prophylaxis against group A streptococcal infection or oral colistin or neomycin for prophylaxis against enterotoxigenic or enteropathogenic *E. coli*.

Vaccination according to the routine schedule (see FIG. 266–3 on p. 2235) should be administered to any infant who is in the hospital at that time.

NEONATAL LISTERIOSIS

(See also Listeriosis on p. 1453.)

Neonatal listeriosis is acquired transplacentally or during or after parturition. Symptoms are those of sepsis. Diagnosis is by culture of mother and infant. Treatment is antibiotics, initially ampicillin plus an aminoglycoside.

Transplacental infection with *Listeria monocytogenes* can result in fetal dissemination with granuloma formation (eg, in the skin, liver, adrenal glands, lymphatic tissue, lungs, and brain), called granulomatosis infantisepticum. Aspiration or swallowing of amniotic fluid or vaginal secretions can lead to perinatal infection of the lungs, manifesting in the 1st several days of life with respiratory distress, shock, and a fulminant course. Acquisition in the hospital has occurred.

Symptoms and Signs

Infections in pregnant women may be asymptomatic or characterized by a primary bacteremia presenting as a nonspecific flu-like illness.

In the fetus and neonate, clinical presentation depends on the timing and route of infection. Abortion, premature delivery with amnionitis (with a characteristic brown, murky amniotic fluid), stillbirth, or neonatal sepsis is common. Infection may be apparent within hours or days of birth, or it may be delayed up to several weeks. Neonates with early-onset disease frequently are of low birth weight, have associated obstetric complications, and show evidence of sepsis with circulatory or respiratory insufficiency or both. Those with the delayed-onset form are full-term, previously well neonates presenting with meningitis or sepsis.

Diagnosis

Blood and cervix specimens should be obtained from any pregnant woman with a febrile disease and cultured for *L. monocytogenes*. A sick neonate whose mother has listeriosis should be evaluated for sepsis (see p. 2333), including cultures of the umbilical cord or peripheral blood vessels; the CSF, gastric aspirate, and meconium; the mother's lochia and exudates from cervix and vagina; and grossly diseased parts of the placenta. CSF examination may show a predominance of mononuclear cells. Gram-stained smears frequently are negative but may show pleomorphic, gram-variable coccobacillary forms, which should not be disregarded as diphtheroid contaminants. Serologic tests are not useful.

Prognosis and Treatment

Mortality, ranging from 10 to 50%, is higher in those with early-onset disease.

Initial treatment is with ampicillin plus an aminoglycoside (see also p. 1424). After clinical response is observed, the aminoglycoside is stopped. A 14-day course is usually satisfactory (21 days for meningitis), but the optimal duration is unknown. Other possible agents include ampicillin or penicillin with rifampin, trimethoprim-sulfamethoxazole, and imipenem, but these agents have not been well evaluated.

Neonates with sepsis require other measures (see p. 2336). In heavy infection, drainage/secretion precautions should be considered.

Prevention

Food products that may be contaminated by *L. monocytogenes* (eg, unpasteurized dairy products or raw vegetables exposed to cattle or sheep manure) should be avoided by pregnant women. Pregnant women who have previously given birth to infected infants should have cervical and stool cultures performed during the 3rd trimester to identify *L. monocytogenes* carrier state. Prophylactic treatment may then be given before delivery or intrapartum to prevent vertical transmission, but the usefulness of such treatment is unproven.

NEONATAL MENINGITIS

(See also Ch. 218 on p. 1858.)

Neonatal meningitis is inflammation of the meninges due to bacterial invasion in the 1st 90 days of life. Signs are those of sepsis,

CNS irritation—lethargy, seizures, vomiting, irritability, nuchal rigidity, a bulging or full fontanelle—and cranial nerve abnormalities. Diagnosis is by lumbar puncture. Treatment is with antibiotics.

Neonatal meningitis occurs in 2/10,000 full-term and 2/1,000 low-birth-weight (LBW) neonates, with a male predominance. It occurs in about 25% of neonates with sepsis and occasionally occurs in isolation.

Etiology

Group B streptococcus (GBS—predominantly type III), *Escherichia coli* (particularly those strains containing the K1 polysaccharide), and *Listeria monocytogenes* account for 75% of neonatal meningitis.

Enterococci, nonenterococcal group D streptococci, α-hemolytic streptococci, and other gram-negative enteric organisms (eg, *Klebsiella* sp, *Enterobacter* sp, *Citrobacter diversus*) also are important pathogens. *Haemophilus influenzae* type b, *Neisseria meningitidis*, and *Streptococcus pneumoniae* have been reported as causes.

Neonatal meningitis most frequently results from the bacteremia that occurs with neonatal sepsis; the higher the colony count in the blood culture, the higher is the risk for meningitis. Meningitis may also result from scalp lesions, particularly when developmental defects lead to communication between the skin surface and the subarachnoid space, which predisposes to thrombophlebitis of the diploic veins. Rarely, there is direct extension to the CNS from a contiguous otic focus (eg, otitis media).

Symptoms and Signs

Frequently, only those findings associated with neonatal sepsis (eg, temperature instability, respiratory distress, jaundice, apnea) are manifest. CNS signs (eg, lethargy, seizures [particularly focal], vomiting, irritability) more specifically suggest meningitis. A bulging or full fontanelle occurs in about 25% and nuchal rigidity in only 15%. Cranial nerve abnormalities (particularly those involving the 3rd, 6th, and 7th nerves) may also be present.

Meningitis due to GBS may occur in the 1st wk of life, accompanying early-onset neonatal sepsis and frequently presenting as a pneumonic illness. Usually, however, GBS meningitis occurs after this period (most commonly in the 1st 3 mo of life) as an isolated illness characterized by absence of antecedent obstetric or perinatal complications and the presence of more specific signs of meningitis (eg, fever, lethargy, seizures).

Ventriculitis frequently accompanies neonatal meningitis, particularly when caused by gram-negative enteric bacilli. Organisms that cause meningitis together with severe vasculitis, particularly *C. diversus* and *Enterobacter sakazakii*, are likely to produce cysts and abscesses. *Pseudomonas aeruginosa*, *E. coli* K1, and *Serratia* sp also may cause brain abscesses. An early clinical sign of brain abscess is increased intracranial pressure (ICP), commonly manifested by vomiting, a bulging fontanelle, and sometimes enlarging head size. Deterioration in an otherwise stable neonate with meningitis suggests progressive increased ICP increase from abscess or hydrocephalus, or rupture of an abscess into the ventricular system.

Diagnosis

Definitive diagnosis is made by CSF examination via lumbar puncture (LP), which should be performed in any neonate suspected of having sepsis or meningitis. However, LP can be difficult to perform in a neonate, and there is some risk for hypoxia. Poor clinical condition (eg, respiratory distress, shock, thrombocytopenia) makes LP risky. If LP is delayed, the neonate should be treated as though meningitis were present. Even when the clinical condition improves, the presence of inflammatory cells in CSF and abnormal chemistries days after illness onset can still suggest the diagnosis. A needle with a trocar should be used for LP to avoid introducing epithelial rests and subsequent development of epitheliomas. The CSF, even if bloody or acellular, should be cultured. About 15% of neonates with negative blood cultures have positive CSF cultures. LP should be repeated at 24 to 48 h if clinical response is questionable and at 72 h when gram-negative organisms are involved (to ensure sterilization). Some experts believe that a repeat LP at 24 h in neonates with GBS meningitis has prognostic value. LP should not be repeated at the end of therapy if the neonate is doing well.

Normal CSF values are controversial and age-related. In general, for LBW infants up to 4 wk of age, 40 WBCs/μL (½ of which may be PMNs), a protein level of 220 mg/dL, and a glucose level of 50 mg/dL (2.8 mmol/L) are considered the upper limits of normal. For term infants, these limits are 20 WBCs/μL (with ½ PMNs), a protein level of 170 mg/dL, and a glucose level of 50 mg/dL (2.8 mmol/L). The CSF glucose concentration depends largely on serum glucose concentration and may normally be as low as 20 to 30 mg/dL (1.1 to 1.7 mmol/L), therefore, serum glucose should be measured before LP so the ratio of CSF:serum glucose levels can be determined (< 50% is abnormal).

Ventriculitis is suspected in a neonate not responding appropriately to antimicrobial therapy. The diagnosis is made when a ventricular puncture yields a WBC count greater than that from the LP, Gram stain or culture is positive, ventricular pressure is increased, and ventricles are dilated. When ventriculitis or brain abscess is suspected, an MRI or CT scan with contrast may aid diagnosis.

Prognosis

Without treatment, the mortality rate from neonatal meningitis approaches 100%. With treatment, prognosis is determined by birth weight, organism, and clinical severity. Mortality rate for gram-negative neonatal meningitis is 20 to 30% and for gram-positive (eg, GBS), 10 to 20%. For organisms that produce vasculitis, meningitis, and brain abscess (necrotizing meningitis), the mortality rate may approach 75%. Neurologic sequelae (eg, hydrocephalus, hearing loss, mental retardation) develop in 20 to 50% of infants who survive, with a poorer prognosis when gram-negative enteric bacilli are the cause.

Prognosis also depends partly on the number of organisms present in CSF at diagnosis. The duration of positive CSF cultures correlates directly with the incidence of complications. In general, CSF cultures from neonates with GBS are usually sterilized within the 1st 24 h of antimicrobial therapy. Those from gram-negative bacillary meningitis remain positive for an average of 3 ½ days.

GBS meningitis has a mortality rate significantly lower than that of early-onset GBS sepsis.

Treatment

Empiric treatment is begun with ampicillin plus cefotaxime. Hospitalized neonates who previously received antibiotics (eg, for early-onset sepsis) may have resistant organisms; fungal disease may also be considered in a septic-appearing neonate after prolonged hospitalization. Until the diagnosis of meningitis is confirmed, ill neonates with hospital-acquired infection should initially receive vancomycin plus an aminoglycoside different from the one previously used, or a 3rd-generation cephalosporin (eg, cefotaxime). Antibiotics are adjusted when results of the LP are available and culture and sensitivities are known.

The recommended initial treatment for GBS meningitis in neonates < 1 wk of age is penicillin G 100,000 to 150,000 units/kg IV q 8 h or ampicillin 100 mg/kg IV q 8 h, plus gentamicin 2.5 mg/kg IV q 8 h. If clinical improvement occurs or sterilization of CSF is documented, gentamicin can be stopped.

For enterococci or *L. monocytogenes*, treatment is generally ampicillin plus gentamicin.

In gram-negative bacillary meningitis, treatment is difficult. The traditional regimen of ampicillin plus an aminoglycoside results in a 20 to 30% mortality rate, with a high rate of sequelae in survivors. A 3rd-generation cephalosporin (eg, cefotaxime) should be strongly considered in neonates with *proved* gram-negative meningitis (or sepsis) or those *convincingly* septic. If antibiotic resistance is a concern, both an aminoglycoside and a 3rd-generation cephalosporin may be used until sensitivities are known. However, these drugs are generally not used routinely, because certain gram-negative organisms are induced to produce β-lactamase by 3rd-generation cephalosporins, resulting in rapid development of resistance.

Parenteral therapy for gram-positive meningitis is given for a minimum of 14 days, and for complicated gram-positive or gram-negative meningitis, a minimum of 21 days.

Because meningitis may be considered part of the continuum of neonatal sepsis, the adjunctive measures used in treating neonatal sepsis (see p. 2338) should also be used in neonatal meningitis. Patients should be closely followed for neurologic complications during the 1st 2 yr of life.

NEONATAL PNEUMONIA

Neonatal pneumonia is lung infection in a neonate. Onset may be within hours of birth and part of a generalized sepsis syndrome, or after 7 days and confined to the lungs. Signs may be limited to respiratory distress or progress to shock and death. Diagnosis is by clinical and laboratory evaluation for sepsis. Treatment is initial broad-spectrum antibiotics changed to organism-specific drugs as soon as possible.

Early-onset pneumonia is part of generalized sepsis that presents at or within hours of birth. Late-onset pneumonia usually occurs after 7 days of age, most commonly in neonatal ICUs in infants who require prolonged endotracheal intubation because of lung disease.

Etiology

Organisms are acquired from the maternal genital tract or the nursery. These include gram-positive cocci (eg, groups A and B streptococci, *Staphylococcus aureus*) and gram-negative bacilli (eg, *Escherichia coli, Klebsiella* sp, and *Proteus* sp). In infants who have received broad-spectrum antibiotics, many other pathogens may be found, including *Pseudomonas, Citrobacter, Bacillus*, and *Serratia*.

Symptoms, Signs, and Diagnosis

Late-onset hospital-acquired pneumonia may begin gradually, with more secretions being suctioned from the endotracheal tube and higher ventilator settings. Other infants may be acutely ill, with temperature instability and neutropenia. New infiltrates may be visible on chest x-ray but may be difficult to recognize if the infant has severe bronchopulmonary dysplasia.

Evaluation includes cultures of blood and tracheal aspirate, chest x-ray, and pulse oximetry.

Treatment

Vancomycin and cefotaxime are the initial treatment of choice if methicillin-resistant *S. aureus* is suspected. Ceftazidime may be substituted for cefotaxime if *Pseudomonas* is a concern. More specific antibiotics are substituted after sensitivity results are available. General treatment is the same as that for neonatal sepsis (see p. 2336).

CHLAMYDIAL PNEUMONIA

Contamination with chlamydial organisms during delivery may result in development of chlamydial pneumonia at 2 to 12 wk. Infants are tachypneic but usually not critically ill and may also have conjunctivitis caused by the same organism. Eosinophilia may be present, and x-rays show bilateral interstitial infiltrates. Treatment with erythromycin leads to rapid resolution.

NEONATAL SEPSIS

(Sepsis Neonatorum)

(See also Ch. 68 on p. 566.)

Neonatal sepsis is invasive bacterial infection occurring in the 1st 90 days of life. Signs are multiple and include diminished spontaneous activity, less vigorous sucking, apnea, bradycardia, temperature instability, respiratory distress, vomiting, diarrhea, abdominal distention, jitteriness, seizures, and jaundice. Diagnosis is clinical, with extensive laboratory testing. Treatment is initially with ampicillin plus either gentamicin or cefotaxime, narrowed to organism-specific drugs as soon as possible.

Neonatal sepsis occurs in 0.5 to 8.0/1000 births. The highest rates occur in low-birth-weight (LBW) infants, those with depressed respiratory function at birth, and those with maternal perinatal risk factors. The risk is greater in males (2:1) and in neonates with congenital anomalies.

A neonate may be predisposed to sepsis by obstetric complications, eg, premature rupture of membranes (PROM) occurring ≥ 18 h before birth or maternal bleeding (placenta previa, abruptio placentae), toxemia, precipitous delivery, or maternal infection (particularly of the urinary tract or endometrium, most commonly manifested as maternal fever shortly before or during parturition).

Etiology

Early-onset sepsis (ie, within 7 days of birth) usually results from organisms acquired intrapartum. In > 50% of cases, early-onset sepsis appears within 6 h of birth, and most cases occur within 72 h. Late-onset sepsis (after 7 days) is often acquired from the environment (see Neonatal Hospital-Acquired Infection on p. 2329).

Group B streptococcus (GBS) and gram-negative enteric organisms (predominantly *Escherichia coli*) account for 70% of early-onset sepsis. Vaginal or rectal cultures of women at term may show GBS colonization rates of up to 30%. At least 35% of their infants also become colonized. The density of infant colonization determines the risk for invasive disease, which is 40 times higher with heavy colonization. Although only 1/100 of those colonized develop invasive disease due to GBS, > 50% of those present within the 1st 6 h of life. Nontypeable *Haemophilus influenzae* sepsis has been increasingly identified in neonates, especially premature neonates.

Other gram-negative enteric bacilli (eg, *Klebsiella* sp) and gram-positive organisms—*Listeria monocytogenes*, enterococci (eg, *Enterococcus faecalis, E. faecium*), group D streptococci (eg, *Streptococcus bovis*), α-hemolytic streptococci, and staphylococci—account for most other cases. *Streptococcus pneumoniae, H. influenzae* type b, and, less commonly, *Neisseria meningitidis* have been isolated. Asymptomatic gonorrhea occurs in 5 to 10% of pregnancies, so *N. gonorrhoeae* may be a pathogen.

Staphylococci account for 30 to 50% of late-onset cases and are most frequently due to intravascular devices (particularly umbilical artery or vein catheters). Isolation of *Enterobacter cloacae* or *E. sakazakii* from blood or CSF suggests contaminated feedings. Contaminated respiratory equipment is suspected in outbreaks of hospital-acquired *Pseudomonas aeruginosa* pneumonia or sepsis.

The role of anaerobes (particularly *Bacteroides fragilis*) remains unclear, although deaths have been attributed to *Bacteroides* bacteremia. Anaerobes may account for some culture-negative cases in which autopsy findings indicate sepsis.

Candida sp are increasingly important causes of late-onset sepsis, occurring in 12 to 13% of very LBW infants.

Certain viral infections (eg, disseminated herpes simplex, enterovirus, adenovirus, respiratory syncytial virus) may manifest as early- or late-onset sepsis.

Pathophysiology

The most important risk factor in late-onset sepsis is prolonged use of intravascular catheters. Others include associated illnesses (which may, however, be only a marker for the use of invasive procedures), exposure to antibiotics (which selects resistant bacterial strains), prolonged hospitalization, and contaminated equipment or IV or enteral solutions. Gram-positive organisms (eg, coagulase-negative staphylococci and *Staphylococcus aureus*) may be introduced from the environment. Gram-negative enteric bacteria are usually derived from the patient's endogenous flora, which may have been altered by antecedent antibiotic therapy or populated by resistant organisms transferred from the hands of personnel (the major means of spread) or contaminated equipment. Therefore, situations that increase exposure to these bacteria (eg, crowding, nurse:patient ratios > 1:1, inadequate hand washing) result in higher rate of hospital-acquired infection. Risk factor for *Candida* sp sepsis include prolonge (> 10 days) use of central IV catheters, hyperalimentation, use of antecedent antibiotics necrotizing enterocolitis, and previous surgery

Hematogenous and transplacental dissemination of maternal infection occurs i the transmission of certain viral (eg, rubella cytomegalovirus), protozoal (eg, *Toxoplasma gondii*), and treponemal (eg, *Treponema pallidum*) agents. A few bacterial pathogens (eg *L. monocytogenes, Mycobacterium tuberculosis*) may reach the fetus transplacentally but most are acquired by the ascending rout in utero or as the fetus passes through the colonized birth canal.

Though the intensity of maternal colonization is directly related to risk for invasiv disease in the neonate, many mothers wit low-density colonization give birth to infant with high-density colonization who ar therefore at risk. Amniotic fluid contaminated with meconium or vernix caseosa promotes growth of GBS and *E. coli.* Hence, th few organisms in the vaginal vault are able t proliferate rapidly after PROM, possibl contributing to this paradox. Organisms usually reach the bloodstream by fetal aspiratio or swallowing of contaminated amnioti fluid, leading to bacteremia. The ascendin route of infection helps to explain such phenomena as the high incidence of PROM i neonatal infections, the significance of adnexal inflammation (amnionitis is more commonly associated with neonatal sepsis than i central placentitis), the increased risk of infection in the twin closer to the birth canal and the bacteriologic characteristics of neonatal sepsis, which reflect the flora of the maternal vaginal vault.

Initial foci of infection can be in the paranasal sinuses, middle ear, lungs, or GI tract and may later disseminate to meninges, kidneys, bones, joints, peritoneum, and skin Pneumonia is the most common invasive bacterial infection after primary sepsis.

Symptoms and Signs

Early signs are frequently nonspecific and subtle and do not distinguish among organisms (including viral). Diminished spontaneous activity, less vigorous sucking, apnea, bradycardia, and temperature instability (hypo- or hyperthermia) are particularly common. Fever is present in only 10 to 50%

but, when sustained (eg > 1 h), generally indicates infection. Other symptoms and signs include respiratory distress, neurologic findings (eg, seizures, jitteriness), jaundice (especially occurring within the 1st 24 h without Rh or ABO blood group incompatibility and with a higher than expected direct bilirubin concentration), vomiting, diarrhea, and abdominal distention. Anaerobic infection is often indicated by foul-smelling amniotic fluid at birth.

Specific signs of an infected organ may pinpoint the primary or a metastatic site. Most neonates with early-onset GBS (and many with *L. monocytogenes*) infection present with respiratory distress that is difficult to distinguish from hyaline membrane disease. Periumbilical erythema, discharge, or bleeding without a hemorrhagic diathesis suggests omphalitis (infection prevents obliteration of the umbilical vessels). Coma, seizures, opisthotonos, or a bulging fontanelle suggests meningitis or brain abscess. Decreased spontaneous movement of an extremity and swelling, warmth, erythema, or tenderness over a joint indicates osteomyelitis or pyogenic arthritis. Unexplained abdominal distention may indicate peritonitis or necrotizing enterocolitis (particularly when accompanied by bloody diarrhea and fecal leukocytes). Cutaneous vesicles, mouth ulcers, and hepatosplenomegaly (particularly with disseminated intravascular coagulation [DIC]) can identify disseminated herpes simplex.

Early-onset GBS infection may manifest as a fulminating pneumonia. Often, obstetric complications (particularly prematurity, PROM, or chorioamnionitis) have occurred. In > 50% of neonates, GBS infection manifests within 6 h of birth; 45% have an Apgar score of < 5. Meningitis is frequently absent. In late-onset GBS infection (at 1 to 12 wk), meningitis is often present. Late-onset GBS infection is generally not associated with perinatal risk factors or demonstrable maternal cervical colonization and may be acquired postpartum.

Diagnosis

Early diagnosis is important and requires awareness of risk factors (particularly in LBW neonates) and a high index of suspicion when any neonate deviates from the norm in the 1st few weeks of life. Neonates with suspected sepsis, and those whose mother was thought to have chorioamnionitis, should have a CBC, differential with smear, platelet count, blood culture, urine culture, and lumbar puncture, if clinically feasible, as soon as possible. Those with respiratory symptoms require chest x-ray. Diagnosis is confirmed by isolation of a pathogen in culture. Other tests may have abnormal results but are not necessarily diagnostic.

For preterm neonates who appear well but whose mother received inadequate intrapartum antibiotics for GBS, the American Academy of Pediatrics recommends a limited evaluation (CBC and blood culture with at least 48-h observation).

CBC, differential, and smear: The normal WBC count in neonates varies, but values <4,000/μL or >25,000/μL are abnormal. The absolute band count is not sensitive enough to predict sepsis, but a ratio of immature:total PMNs of < 0.2 has a very high negative predictive value. A precipitous fall in a known absolute eosinophil count and morphologic changes in neutrophils (eg, toxic granulation, Döhle bodies, and intracytoplasmic vacuolization in noncitrated blood or ethylenediaminetetraacetic acid [EDTA]) suggest sepsis.

The platelet count may fall hours to days before the onset of clinical sepsis but more often remains elevated until a day or so after the neonate manifests illness. This fall is sometimes accompanied by other findings of DIC (eg, increased fibrin degradation products, decreased fibrinogen, prolonged INR).

Because of the large numbers of circulating bacteria, organisms can sometimes be seen in or associated with PMNs by applying Gram stain, methylene blue, or acridine orange to the buffy coat.

Lumbar puncture (LP): There is a risk of increasing hypoxia during an LP in an already hypoxemic neonate. Therefore, routine LP is not mandatory if the suspicion for sepsis is low. However, LP should be performed in a neonate with suspected sepsis as soon as he is able to tolerate the procedure (see also under Neonatal Meningitis on p. 2331). Supplemental O_2 is administered before and during LP to prevent hypoxia. Because GBS pneumonia manifesting in the 1st day of life can be confused with hyaline membrane disease, LP is often performed routinely in neonates suspected of having these diseases.

Blood cultures: Umbilical vessels are frequently contaminated by organisms on the umbilical stump, especially after a number of hours, so blood cultures from umbilical lines may not be reliable. Therefore, blood for culture should be obtained by venipuncture, preferably at 2 peripheral sites, each meticulously prepared by applying an iodine-containing liquid, then applying 95% alcohol, and finally allowing the site to dry. Blood should be cultured for both aerobic and anaerobic organisms. (*Bacteroides fragilis* requires special culture conditions, so the laboratory should be notified if this organism is a concern.) If catheter-associated sepsis is suspected, a culture should be obtained through the catheter as well as peripherally. In > 90% of positive bacterial blood cultures, growth occurs within 48 h of incubation; 50% of positive blood cultures contain > 50 colony-forming units (CFU)/mL. Because this bacteremia is high-density, a small amount of blood (eg, 1 mL) is usually sufficient for detecting organisms. Data on capillary blood cultures are insufficient to recommend them.

Candida sp grows in blood cultures and on blood agar plates, but if other fungi are suspected, a fungal culture medium should be used. For species other than *Candida,* fungal blood cultures may require 4 to 5 days of incubation before becoming positive and may be negative even in obviously disseminated disease. Proof of colonization (in mouth or stool or on skin) may be helpful before culture results are available. If disseminated candidiasis is suspected, indirect ophthalmoscopy with dilation of the pupils is done to identify retinal candidal lesions. Renal ultrasound is performed to detect renal mycetoma.

Urinalysis and culture: Urine should be obtained by catheterization or suprapubic aspiration, not by urine collection bags. Although only culture is diagnostic, a finding of > 5 WBCs/high-power field in the spun urine or any organisms in a fresh unspun gram-stained sample is presumptive evidence of a UTI. Absence of pyuria does not rule out UTI.

Other tests for infection and inflammation: Numerous tests are often abnormal in sepsis and have been evaluated as possible early markers. In general, however, sensitivities tend to be low until later in illness and specifities are suboptimal.

Counterimmunoelectrophoresis and latex agglutination tests detect antigen in body fluids (eg, CSF, concentrated urine); they can be used when antibiotic pretreatment renders culture results unreliable. They may also detect capsular polysaccharide antigen of GBS, *E. coli* K1, *N. meningitidis* type B, *S. pneumoniae,* and *H. influenzae* type b.

Acute-phase reactants are proteins produced by the liver under the influence of IL-1 when inflammation is present. The most valuable of these is quantitative C-reactive protein. A concentration of 1 mg/dL (measured by nephelometry) has both a false-positive and a false-negative rate of about 10%. Elevated levels occur within a day, peak at 2 to 3 days, and fall to normal within 5 to 10 days in neonates who recover.

The ESR is often elevated in sepsis. The micro-ESR correlates well with the standard Wintrobe method but has the same high false-negative rate (especially early in the course and with DIC) and a slow return to normal, well beyond the time of clinical cure. IL-6 and other inflammatory cytokines are being investigated as markers for sepsis.

Prognosis

The fatality rate is 2 to 4 times higher in LBW than in full-term infants. The overall mortality rate of early-onset sepsis is 15 to 40% (that of early-onset GBS infection is 2 to 30%) and of late-onset sepsis is 10 to 20% (that of late-onset GBS is about 2%).

Neonates who are both septic and granulocytopenic are less likely to survive, particularly if their bone marrow neutrophil storage pool (NSP) is depleted to < 7% of total nucleated cells (mortality rate, 75%). Since NSP levels may not be readily available, the peripheral blood immature:total (I:T) neutrophil ratio can approximate bone marrow NSP levels. I:T ratios of > 0.80 correlate with NSP depletion and death; such a ratio may identify patients who might benefit from granulocyte transfusion.

Treatment

Because sepsis may manifest with nonspecific clinical signs and its effects may be devastating, rapid empiric antibiotic therapy is recommended (see p. 1408); drugs are later adjusted according to sensitivities and the site of infection. If bacterial cultures show no growth by 48 h (although some pathogens may require 72 h) and the neonate appears well, antibiotics are stopped.

General supportive measures, including respiratory and hemodynamic management, are combined with antibiotic treatment.

Antibiotics: In early-onset sepsis, initial therapy should include ampicillin or penicillin G plus an aminoglycoside. Cefotaxime may be substituted for the aminoglycoside. If foul-smelling amniotic fluid is present at birth, therapy for anaerobes (eg, clindamycin, metronidazole) should be added. Antibi-

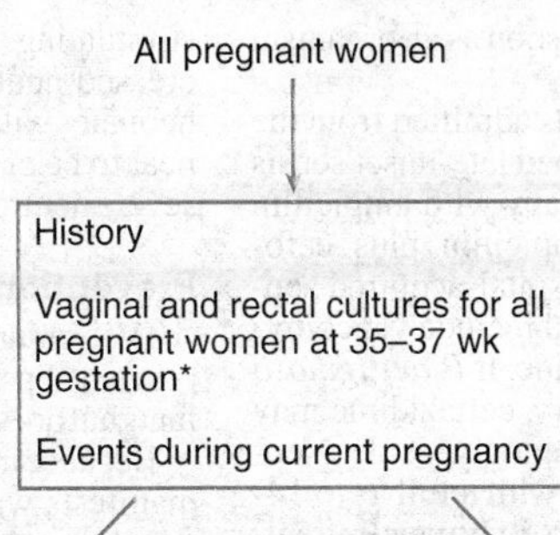

Previous infant with invasive disease due to GBS

GBS bacteriuria during current pregnancy

Positive screening culture for GBS during current pregnancy, unless delivery by cesarean section is planned and done before labor begins and membranes rupture

Unknown GBS status (because culture was not done or was incomplete or results are unknown) plus one of the following:

- Delivery occurring at < 37 wk gestation
- Membranes ruptured for ≥ 18 h, or at the start of labor or at membrane rupture if preterm delivery is highly likely
- Maternal intrapartum temperature of ≥ 38° C†

→ Prophylaxis

Negative screening culture for GBS during current pregnancy, regardless of intrapartum risk factors

Positive screening culture for GBS in a previous pregnancy, but culture during current pregnancy is negative

Cesarean section planned and done before labor begins and membranes rupture, regardless of GBS culture status

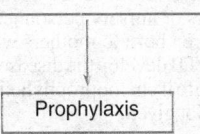

→ No Prophylaxis

*Prenatal screening for GBS with vaginal and rectal cultures is recommended for all pregnant women at 35–37 wk gestation, except for women who have had GBS bacteriuria during the current pregnancy or a previous infant who has had invasive disease due to GBS. Such women should routinely be given GBS prophylaxis.

†If amnionitis is suspected, broad-spectrum antibiotic therapy, including an antibiotic known to be effective against GBS, should replace GBS prophylaxis.

GBS = group B streptococcus.

Fig. 279–1. Indications for intrapartum antibiotic prophylaxis to prevent perinatal group B streptococcal disease. (Adapted from Schrag S, Gorwitz R, Fultz-Butts K, Schuchat A: Prevention of perinatal group B streptococcal disease. *Morbidity and Mortality Weekly Report* 51(RR-11): 1–22, 2002.)

otics may be changed as soon as an organism is identified.

Previously well infants admitted from the community with presumed late-onset sepsis should also receive therapy with ampicillin plus gentamicin or ampicillin plus cefotaxime. In late-onset hospital-acquired sepsis, initial therapy should include vancomycin plus an aminoglycoside. If *P. aeruginosa* is prevalent in the nursery, ceftazidime may be used instead of an aminoglycoside. Neonates previously treated with a full 7- to 14-day aminoglycoside course who need retreatment should receive a different aminoglycoside or a 3rd-generation cephalosporin.

If coagulase-negative staphylococci are suspected (eg, an indwelling catheter has been in place for > 72 h) or are isolated from blood or other normally sterile fluid and considered a pathogen, initial therapy for late-onset sepsis should include vancomycin. However, if the organism is sensitive to nafcillin, that drug should replace vancomycin. Removal of the presumptive source of the organism (usually an indwelling intravascular catheter) may be necessary to cure the infection, because coagulase-negative staphylococci may be protected by a glycocalix (covering slime that encourages adherence of organisms to the catheter).

Because *Candida* may take 2 to 3 days to grow in blood culture, initiation of amphotericin B therapy and removal of the infected catheter without positive blood or CSF cultures may be life saving.

Other treatment: Exchange transfusions have been used for severely ill (particularly hypotensive and metabolically acidotic) neonates. Their purported value is to increase levels of circulating immunoglobulins, decrease circulating endotoxin, increase Hb levels (with higher 2,3-diphosphoglycerate levels), and improve perfusion. However, no controlled prospective studies of their use have been conducted.

Fresh frozen plasma may help reverse the heat-stable and heat-labile opsonin deficiencies that occur in LBW neonates, but controlled studies of its use are unavailable, and transfusion-associated risks must be considered.

Granulocyte transfusions (see p. 1136) have been used in septic and granulocytopenic neonates but have not convincingly improved outcome.

Recombinant colony-stimulating factors (granulocyte colony-stimulating factor [G-CSF] and granulocyte-macrophage colony-stimulating factor [GM-CSF]) have increased neutrophil number and function in neonates with presumed sepsis, but do not appear to be of routine benefit in neonates with severe neutropenia; further study is required.

Prevention

IV immune globulin given at birth may prevent sepsis in certain high-risk LBW infants but does not help in established infection.

Because invasive disease due to GBS often manifests within the 1st 6 h of life, women who have previously given birth to an infant with GBS disease should receive intrapartum antibiotics, and women who have symptomatic or asymptomatic GBS bacteriuria during pregnancy should receive antibiotics at the time of diagnosis and intrapartum (see Fig. 279–1).

PERINATAL TUBERCULOSIS

(See also Tuberculosis on p. 1508.)

Tuberculosis can be acquired in the perinatal period. Symptoms and signs are nonspecific. Diagnosis is by culture and perhaps x-ray and biopsy. Treatment is with antituberculous drugs.

Infants may acquire tuberculosis (TB) by transplacental spread through the umbilical vein to the fetal liver, by aspiration or ingestion of infected amniotic fluid, or via airborne inoculation from close contacts (family members or nursery personnel). About 50% of children born to mothers with active pulmonary TB develop the disease during the 1st year of life if chemoprophylaxis or BCG vaccine is not given.

Symptoms, Signs, and Diagnosis

The clinical presentation of neonatal TB is nonspecific but is usually marked by multiple organ involvement. The neonate may look acutely or chronically ill. Fever, lethargy, respiratory distress, hepatosplenomegaly, or failure to thrive may indicate TB in a neonate with a history of exposure.

All neonates with suspected congenital TB should have chest x-ray and culture of tracheal aspirates, gastric washings, urine, and CSF for acid-fast bacilli. Skin testing is not extremely sensitive but should be performed; biopsy of the liver, lymph nodes, lung, or pleura may be needed to confirm diagnosis.

Well-appearing neonates whose mothers had a positive skin test but a negative chest x-ray and no evidence of active disease should have a skin test q 3 mo for 1 yr. If the test is positive, chest x-ray and cultures for acid-fast bacilli are obtained as above.

Treatment

Pregnant women with a positive tuberculin test: Because the hepatotoxicity of isoniazid (INH) is increased in pregnancy, and because the risk of contracting TB from a mother with a positive tuberculin test is greater for the neonate than for the fetus, INH use is deferred until the 3rd trimester unless the woman has active TB. Treatment is given for 9 mo, along with supplemental pyridoxine.

Infants with a positive tuberculin test: If there is no clinical or radiologic evidence of disease, the infant should receive INH 10 mg/kg po once/day for 9 mo and should be closely followed.

Pregnant women with active TB: INH, ethambutol, and rifampin use in recommended doses during pregnancy has not been shown to be teratogenic to the human fetus. The recommended initial treatment regimen in the US includes INH (300 mg po), ethambutol (15 to 25 mg/kg), and rifampin (600 mg po). All pregnant and breastfeeding women receiving INH should also take pyridoxine (25 mg po). All these drugs can be given once/day. The recommended duration of therapy is at least 9 mo unless the organism is drug-resistant, in which case an infectious disease consultation is recommended, and therapy may need to be extended to 18 mo. Streptomycin is potentially ototoxic to the developing fetus and should not be used early in pregnancy unless rifampin is contraindicated. If possible, other antituberculous drugs should be avoided because of teratogenicity (eg, ethionamide) or lack of clinical experience during pregnancy. Breastfeeding is not contraindicated for mothers receiving therapy who are not infective.

Asymptomatic infants of women with active TB: The infant usually is separated from the mother until effective treatment is under way or acid-fast stains of her sputum become negative (usually 2 to 12 wk). Family contacts should be investigated for undiagnosed TB before the infant goes home.

If compliance can be reasonably assured and the family is nontuberculous, the infant is started on a regimen of INH as above and sent home at the usual time. Skin testing should be performed at ages 3 and 6 mo. If the infant remains tuberculin-negative, INH is stopped and the infant is monitored with monthly to bimonthly clinical evaluations, and skin tests at 12 mo.

If compliance in a nontuberculous environment *cannot* be ensured, BCG vaccine may be considered for the infant, and INH therapy should be started as soon as possible. (Although INH inhibits the multiplication of BCG organisms, the combination of BCG vaccine and INH is supported by clinical trials and anecdotal reports.) BCG vaccination does not ensure against exposure to and development of tuberculous disease, but offers significant protection against serious and widespread invasion (eg, tuberculous meningitis). Infants should be monitored for development of tuberculous illness, particularly in the 1st year. (CAUTION: *BCG vaccine is contraindicated in immunosuppressed patients and those suspected of being infected with HIV.* However, in high-risk populations, the WHO recommends that asymptomatic HIV-infected infants receive BCG vaccine at birth or shortly thereafter.)

Neonates with active TB: The American Academy of Pediatrics recommends treatment once/day with INH (10 to 15 mg/kg po), rifampin (10 to 20 mg/kg po), pyrazinamide (20 to 40 mg/kg po), and streptomycin (20 to 40 mg/kg IM) for 2 mo, with INH and rifampin continued for another 10 mo. Alternatively, a 10-mo regimen of INH and rifampin twice/wk can be given after the 2-mo initial therapy. Depending on results of testing for resistance, capreomycin or kanamycin may be used instead of streptomycin. Breastfed infants should also receive pyridoxine supplementation.

When the CNS is involved, initial therapy also includes corticosteroids (prednisone 1 mg/kg po once/day for 6 to 8 wk, then gradually tapered). Therapy continues until all signs of meningitis have disappeared and cultures are negative on 2 successive lumbar punctures at least 1 wk apart. Therapy can then be continued with INH and rifampin once/day or twice/wk for another 10 mo.

TB in infants and children that is not congenitally acquired or disseminated; does not involve the CNS, bones, or joints; and results from drug-susceptible organisms can be treated effectively with a 6- to 9-mo (total) course of therapy. Organisms recovered from the infant or mother should be tested for drug sensitivity. Hematologic, hepatic, and otologic symptoms should be monitored frequently to determine response to therapy and drug toxicity. Frequent laboratory analysis is not usually necessary.

Directly observed therapy (DOT) is used to improve compliance and the success of therapy. Many anti-TB drugs are not available in pediatric dosages. Administering these drugs to children may be improved in settings with experienced personnel.

Prevention

Routine neonatal BCG vaccination is not indicated in developed countries but may curb the incidence of childhood TB or decrease its severity in populations at increased risk for infection.

280 INFECTIONS IN INFANTS AND CHILDREN

Infants and young children develop infections more frequently than do adults and older children. Infections may be present at birth (see p. 2313) but are more typically contracted afterward. A child's immune system is neither as mature nor as responsive as an adult's, perhaps because of hyporesponsiveness to T-cell–independent antigens, lower immunoglobulin concentrations, a greater proportion of naïve T and B cells compared to memory lymphocytes, or other factors. Children also are exposed to more pathogens from peers in daycare or school.

Many infectious illnesses that affect infants and children also occur in adults and are discussed elsewhere in THE MANUAL.

ERYTHEMA INFECTIOSUM

(Fifth Disease; Parvovirus B19 Infection)

Erythema infectiosum, acute infection with parvovirus B19, causes mild constitutional symptoms and a blotchy or maculopapular rash beginning on the cheeks and spreading primarily to exposed extremities. Diagnosis is clinical, and treatment is generally not needed.

The disease is caused by human parvovirus B19. It occurs mostly during the spring, commonly causing localized outbreaks every few years among children (particularly those 5 to 7 yr). Spread appears to be by respiratory droplets, with high rates of secondary infection among household contacts; infection can occur without symptoms or signs.

Parvovirus B19 causes transient suppression of erythropoiesis that is mild and asymptomatic except in patients with underlying hemoglobinopathies (eg, sickle cell disease) or other RBC disorders (eg, hereditary spherocytosis), who may develop transient aplastic crisis.

Symptoms and Signs

The incubation period is 4 to 14 days. Typical initial manifestations are nonspecific flu-like symptoms (eg, low-grade fever, slight malaise). Several days later, an indurated, confluent erythema appears over the cheeks ("slapped-cheek" appearance) and a symmetric rash appears that is most prominent on the arms, legs, and trunk, usually sparing the palms and soles. The rash is maculopapular, tending toward confluence; it forms reticular or lacy patterns of slightly raised, blotchy areas with central clearing, usually most prominent on exposed areas. The rash, and the entire illness, generally lasts 5 to 10 days. However, the rash may recur for several weeks, exacerbated by sunlight, exercise, heat, fever, or emotional stress. Mild joint pain and swelling (nonerosive arthritis) that may persist or recur for weeks to months sometimes occurs in adults.

Immunocompromised patients can develop protracted viremia (lasting 10 to 12 days), leading to severe anemia (chronic pure RBC aplasia). Erythema infectiosum can be transmitted transplacentally, sometimes resulting in stillbirth or severe fetal anemia with widespread edema (hydrops fetalis). However, about 1/2 of pregnant women are immune because of previous infection. The risk of fetal death is 5 to 9% after maternal infection, with risk greatest during the 2nd trimester.

Diagnosis and Treatment

The appearance and pattern of spread of the rash are the only diagnostic features; however, some enteroviruses may produce similar rashes. Rubella can be ruled out by serologic testing; an exposure history is also helpful. Serologic testing is not required in otherwise healthy children; however, in children with transient aplastic crisis or adults with arthropathy, the presence of IgM-specific antibody to parvovirus B19 in the late acute or early convalescent phase strongly supports the diagnosis. Parvovirus B19 viremia also can be detected by immunoprecipitation or molecular techniques, which are generally used for patients with transient aplastic crisis, immunocompromised patients with chronic pure RBC aplasia, and infants with hydrops fetalis or congenital infection.

Only symptomatic treatment is needed. IV immune globulin has been used to curtail viremia and increase erythropoiesis in immunocompromised patients with chronic RBC aplasia.

HUMAN IMMUNODEFICIENCY VIRUS INFECTION IN CHILDREN

(See also Ch. 192 on p. 1625.)

Human immunodeficiency virus infection (HIV) is caused by the retrovirus HIV-1 (and less commonly by the related retrovirus HIV-2). Infection leads to progressive immunologic deterioration and opportunistic infections and malignancies; the end stage is acquired immunodeficiency syndrome (AIDS). Diagnosis is by viral antibodies in children > 18 mo and viral PCR assay in those < 18 mo. Treatment is with combinations of antiretroviral agents.

The general natural history and pathophysiology of pediatric HIV infection is similar to that in adults; however, the method of infection, clinical presentations, and treatments often differ. HIV-infected children also have unique social integration issues (see sidebar 280–1).

Epidemiology

In the US, HIV probably occurred in children almost as early as in adults but was not clinically recognized for several years. Thus far, > 9300 cases have been reported in children and adolescents, representing only 1% of total cases.

More than 90% of US children acquired the infection from their mother, either before or around the time of birth (vertical transmission). Most of the remainder (including patients with hemophilia or other coagulation disorders) received contaminated blood or blood products. A few cases have resulted from sexual abuse. Fewer than 5% of cases have no clear source. Vertical transmission now accounts for almost all new cases in US preadolescents.

Worldwide, about 2.5 million children are alive with HIV infection (8% of the total caseload worldwide), and about 700,000 more children are infected each year (16% of all new infections). In sub-Saharan Africa, where the epidemic has been present longest, some prenatal clinics report that 25 to 40% of all women of childbearing age are seropositive for HIV. HIV infection is rapidly increasing in India, China, Southeast Asia, and some areas of Eastern Europe and Russia. About 500,000 children die of HIV infection worldwide each year.

Transmission: Infection risk for an infant born to an HIV-positive mother who did not receive antiretroviral therapy during pregnancy is estimated at 13 to 39%. Risk is greatest for infants born to mothers who seroconvert during pregnancy and for those with advanced disease, low peripheral $CD4^+$ T-lymphocyte counts, prolonged rupture of membranes, and high viral concentrations as evidenced by HIV p24 antigenemia, quantitative viral culture, or RNA concentration. In vaginal deliveries, a 1st-born twin is at greater risk than a 2nd-born twin, although this relationship may not hold true in developing countries.

Cesarean section may reduce the risk of transmission from mother to child. However, it is clear that mother-to-child transmission (MTCT) can be reduced significantly by giving antiretroviral therapy (including zidovudine [ZDV, AZT]) to the mother and neonate (see p. 2351). ZDV monotherapy reduces MTCT to about 8%; with current highly active antiretroviral therapy (HAART) regimens, the US MTCT rate is < 2%.

HIV has been detected in both the cellular and cell-free fractions of human breast milk. The incidence of transmission by breastfeeding is about 6/100 breastfed children/yr. Estimates of the overall risk of transmission through breastfeeding are 12 to 14%, reflecting varying durations of breastfeeding. Transmission by breastfeeding appears to be greatest in mothers with high plasma viral concentrations.

Sidebar 280–1. SOCIAL INTEGRATION OF HIV-INFECTED CHILDREN

Infection in a child affects the entire family. Serologic testing of siblings and parents is recommended. The physician must provide education and ongoing counseling.

The infected child should be taught good hygiene and behavior to reduce risk to others. How much he is told about the illness depends on age and maturity. Older children and adolescents should be made aware of their diagnosis and the possibility of sexual transmission and counseled appropriately. Families may be unwilling to share the diagnosis with people outside the immediate family because it can create social isolation. Feelings of guilt are common. Family members, including children, can become clinically depressed and require counseling.

Because HIV infection is not acquired through the typical types of contact that occur among children, eg, through saliva or tears, most HIV-infected children should be allowed to attend school without restrictions. Similarly, there are no inherent reasons to restrict foster care, adoptive placement, or childcare of HIV-infected children. Conditions that may pose an increased risk to others (eg, aggressive biting or the presence of exudative, weeping skin lesions that cannot be covered) may require special precautions.

The number of school personnel aware of the child's condition should be kept to the minimum needed to ensure proper care. The family has the right to inform the school, but people involved in the care and education of an infected child must respect the child's right to privacy. Disclosures of information should be only with the informed consent of the parents or legal guardians and age-appropriate assent of the child.

Acquisition of HIV during adolescence significantly contributes to the large number of cases in young adults. Routes of transmission in adolescents are similar to those for adults (see p. 1627), mostly unprotected sexual contact, and less commonly, injection drug use.

Classification: HIV infection causes a broad spectrum of disease, of which AIDS is the most severe. Epidemiologic classification schemes established by the Centers for Disease Control and Prevention (CDC) define the progression of clinical and immunologic decline. In children < 13 yr, clinical categories N, A, B, and C (defined by presence or absence of certain common opportunistic infections or malignancies) denote asymptomatic and mildly, moderately, and severely symptomatic HIV infection, respectively (see TABLE 280–1). Similarly, mild, moderate, and severe immunocompromise is denoted as category 1, 2, or 3, respectively; these are defined by age-specific $CD4^+$ T-lymphocyte counts (see TABLE 280–2). Thus, a child classified in stage B3 would have moderately advanced clinical symptoms and severe immunocompromise.

Symptoms and Signs

Infants infected perinatally usually are asymptomatic during the 1st few months of life. Although the median age at symptom onset is about 3 yr, some children remain asymptomatic for > 5 yr and, with appropriate antiretroviral (ARV) therapy, are expected to survive to adulthood. In the pre-ARV era, about 10 to 15% of children had rapid disease progression, with symptoms occurring in the 1st year of life and death occurring by 18 to 36 mo; these children were thought to have acquired HIV infection earlier in utero. Most children, however, probably acquire infection at or near birth and have slower disease progression (surviving beyond 5 yr even before ARV therapy was routinely used).

The most common manifestations of HIV infection in children include generalized lymphadenopathy, hepatomegaly, splenomegaly, failure to thrive, oral candidiasis, CNS disease (including developmental delay, which can be progressive), lymphoid interstitial pneumonitis, recurrent bacteremia, opportunistic infections, recurrent diarrhea, parotitis, cardiomyopathy, hepatitis, nephropathy, and malignancies.

Complications: *Pneumocystis jiroveci* (formerly *P. carinii*) pneumonia is the most common, serious, opportunistic infection in HIV-infected children and has high mortality. *Pneumocystis* pneumonia can occur as early as age 4 to 6 wk but occurs mostly in infants between age 3 and 6 mo who acquired infection before or at birth. Infants and children with *Pneumocystis* pneumonia characteristically develop a subacute, diffuse pneu-

TABLE 280–1. CLINICAL CATEGORIES FOR CHILDREN AGED < 13 YR WITH HIV INFECTION*

Category N: Not symptomatic

Children who have no symptoms or signs considered to be the result of HIV infection or have only 1 of the conditions listed in Category A

Category A: Mildly symptomatic

Children with ≥ 2 of the conditions listed below but none of the conditions listed in Categories B or C
Dermatitis
Hepatomegaly
Lymphadenopathy (≥ 0.5 cm at > 2 sites; bilateral = 1 site)
Parotitis
Recurrent or persistent upper respiratory tract infection, sinusitis, or otitis media
Splenomegaly

Category B: Moderately symptomatic

Children who have symptomatic conditions that are attributed to HIV infection beyond those listed in Category A but not among those listed in Category C. Examples of conditions in clinical Category B include but are not limited to:
Anemia (< 8 g/dL), neutropenia (< 1,000/μL), or thrombocytopenia (< 100,000/μL) persisting ≥ 30 days
Bacterial meningitis, pneumonia, or sepsis (single episode)
Candidiasis, oropharyngeal (thrush), persisting (> 2 mo) in children > 6 mo of age
Cardiomyopathy
Cytomegalovirus infection, with onset before 1 mo of age
Diarrhea, recurrent or chronic
Hepatitis
HSV stomatitis, recurrent (> 2 episodes within 1 yr)
HSV bronchitis, pneumonitis, or esophagitis with onset before 1 mo of age
Herpes zoster (shingles) involving at least 2 distinct episodes or > 1 dermatome
Leiomyosarcoma
Lymphoid interstitial pneumonitis or pulmonary lymphoid hyperplasia complex
Nephropathy
Nocardiosis
Persistent fever (lasting > 1 mo)
Toxoplasmosis, onset before 1 mo of age
Varicella, disseminated (complicated chickenpox)

Category C: Severely symptomatic

Serious bacterial infections, multiple or recurrent (ie, any combination of at least 2 culture-confirmed infections within a 2-yr period), of the following types: septicemia, pneumonia, meningitis, bone or joint infection, or abscess of an internal organ or body cavity (excluding otitis media, superficial skin or mucosal abscesses, and indwelling catheter-related infections)
Candidiasis, esophageal or pulmonary (bronchi, trachea, lungs)
Coccidioidomycosis, disseminated (at site other than or in addition to lungs or cervical or hilar lymph nodes)
Cryptococcosis, extrapulmonary
Cryptosporidiosis or isosporiasis with diarrhea persisting > 1 mo
Cytomegalovirus disease with onset of symptoms at age > 1 mo (at a site other than liver, spleen, or lymph nodes)
Encephalopathy (at least one of the following progressive findings present for at least 2 mo in the absence of a concurrent illness other than HIV infection that could explain the findings): (1) failure to attain or loss of developmental milestones or loss of intel-

Table continues on the following page.

TABLE 280-1. CLINICAL CATEGORIES FOR CHILDREN AGED < 13 YR WITH HIV INFECTION*—Continued

lectual ability, verified by standard developmental scale or neuropsychological tests; (2) impaired brain growth or acquired microcephaly demonstrated by head circumference measurements or brain atrophy demonstrated by CT or MRI (serial imaging is required for children < 2 yr); (3) acquired symmetric motor deficit manifested by ≥ 2 of the following: paresis, pathologic reflexes, ataxia, gait disturbance

HSV infection causing a mucocutaneous ulcer persisting for > 1 mo; or bronchitis, pneumonitis, or esophagitis for any duration affecting a child > 1 mo of age

Histoplasmosis, disseminated (at a site other than or in addition to lungs or cervical or hilar lymph nodes)

Kaposi's sarcoma

Lymphoma, primary, in brain

Lymphoma, small, noncleaved cell (Burkitt's), or immunoblastic, or large cell lymphoma of B-cell or unknown immunologic phenotype

Mycobacterium tuberculosis, disseminated or extrapulmonary

Mycobacterium, other species or unidentified species, disseminated (at a site other than or in addition to lungs, skin, or cervical or hilar lymph nodes)

Pneumocystis jiroveci (formerly *P. carinii*) pneumonia

Progressive multifocal leukoencephalopathy

Salmonella (nontyphoid) septicemia, recurrent

Toxoplasmosis of the brain with onset at >1 mo of age

Wasting syndrome in the absence of a concurrent illness other than HIV infection that could explain the following findings: (1) persistent weight loss > 10% of baseline *or* (2) downward crossing of at least 2 of the following percentile lines on the weight-for-age chart (eg, 95th, 75th, 50th, 25th, 5th) in a child ≥ 1 yr of age *or* (3) < 5th percentile on weight-for-height chart on 2 consecutive measurements ≥ 30 days apart *plus* (1) chronic diarrhea (ie, at least 2 loose stools per day for ≥ 30 days) *or* (2) documented fever (for ≥ 30 days, intermittent or constant)

HSV = Herpes simplex virus.

*The Categories form a unidirectional hierarchy such that a patient's illness proceeds from Category N to A to B to C. For example, if a child has hepatomegaly and lymphadenopathy (Category A) and develops persistent anemia, the child enters Category B. If the anemia eventually resolves (eg, with therapy), the child will remain classified as Category B. If *Pneumocystis* pneumonia develops, the child is reclassified in Category C. Similarly, immunologic categories form a unidirectional hierarchy; if a child with a $CD4^+$ count defining Category 2 experiences a rise in $CD4^+$ count with therapy such that the cells are increased enough to qualify for Category 1, the child nevertheless remains classified as Immunologic Category 2 (see TABLE 280-2).

Adapted from Centers for Disease Control and Prevention. 1994 Revised classification system for HIV infection in children less than 13 years of age; official authorized addenda: HIV infection codes and official guidelines for coding and reporting ICD-9-CM. *MMWR* 1994: 43 (No. RR-12), pp 1–19.

monitis with dyspnea at rest, tachypnea, O_2 desaturation, nonproductive cough, and fever (in contrast to non–HIV-infected immunocompromised children and adults, in whom onset is often more acute and fulminant).

Other common opportunistic infections include *Candida* esophagitis, disseminated cytomegalovirus infection, and chronic or disseminated herpes simplex and varicella-zoster virus infections and, less commonly, *Mycobacterium tuberculosis* and *Mycobacterium avium* complex infections, chronic enteritis caused by *Cryptosporidium* or other organisms, and disseminated or CNS cryptococcal or *Toxoplasma gondii* infection.

Malignancies in immunocompromised children with HIV infection are relatively uncommon, but leiomyosarcomas and certain lymphomas, including CNS lymphomas and non-Hodgkin B-cell lymphomas (Burkitt's type), occur much more often than in immunocompetent children. Kaposi's sarcoma is very rare in HIV-infected children.

Diagnosis

HIV-specific tests: In children > 18 mo, diagnosis is made using serum antibody tests (enzyme immunoassay [EIA] and confirmatory Western blot) as in adults. Only very rarely will an older HIV-infected child lack

TABLE 280–2. IMMUNOLOGIC CATEGORIES FOR CHILDREN < 13 YR WITH HIV INFECTION

IMMUNOLOGIC CATEGORIES	AGE-SPECIFIC CD4+ T-LYMPHOCYTE COUNTS AND AS PERCENTAGES OF TOTAL LYMPHOCYTE COUNTS					
	< 12 mo		1–5 yr		6–12 yr	
	CELLS/μL	%	CELLS/μL	%	CELLS/μL	%
1: No evidence of suppression	≥ 1500	≥ 25	≥ 1000	≥ 25	≥ 500	≥ 25
2: Evidence of moderate suppression	750–1499	15–24	500–999	15–24	200–499	15–24
3: Severe suppression	< 750	< 15	< 500	< 15	< 200	< 15

Adapted from Centers for Disease Control and Prevention. 1994 Revised classification system for HIV infection in children less than 13 years of age; official authorized addenda: HIV infection codes and official guidelines for coding and reporting ICD-9-CM. *MMWR* 1994: 43 (No. RR-12), pp. 1–19.

HIV antibody because of significant hypogammaglobulinemia.

Children < 18 mo retain maternal antibody, causing false-positive results on EIA, so diagnosis is made by HIV DNA PCR, which can diagnose about 30% of cases at birth and nearly 100% by 4 to 6 mo of age. HIV viral culture has acceptable sensitivity and specificity but is technically more demanding and hazardous and has been replaced by DNA PCR in most laboratories. HIV RNA PCR (the "viral load" assay used for monitoring efficacy of treatment) is probably as sensitive as DNA PCR in infants not exposed to ARV therapy. However, because of possible insensitivity in the presence of ARV therapy and possible nonspecificity of lower RNA concentrations, HIV RNA PCR is not recommended for diagnosis in infants. The modified p24 antigen assay is less sensitive than HIV DNA PCR and culture and should be used only if the latter are unavailable.

An initial DNA PCR test should be performed within the 1st 2 wk of life, at about 1 mo of age, and between 4 and 6 mo. A positive test should be confirmed immediately using the same or another test (eg, culture). If the serial DNA PCR tests are all negative, the child is considered uninfected with > 95% accuracy (in the absence of any AIDS-defining illness). Follow-up antibody tests (one EIA at > 18 mo or, alternatively, 2 EIAs performed between 6 and 18 mo) are obtained to exclude HIV infection and confirm seroreversion (loss of passively acquired HIV antibodies). If an infant < 18 mo with a positive antibody test but negative virologic tests develops an AIDS-defining illness (category C—see TABLE 280–1), HIV infection is diagnosed.

Newly available rapid tests for HIV antibody are derivatives of EIA assays that provide results within minutes to hours. They can be performed as point-of-care tests on oral secretions, whole blood, or serum. In the US, these tests are perhaps most useful in labor and delivery suites to test women of unknown HIV serostatus, thus allowing counseling, commencement of ARV therapy to prevent MTCT, and testing of the infant to be arranged during the birth visit. Similar advantages accrue in other episodic care settings (eg, emergency departments, sexually transmitted disease clinics) and in the developing world. Rapid assays require confirmatory tests, such as western blot testing. If expected HIV prevalence is low, even a specific rapid assay will yield mostly false positives (low positive predictive value by Bayes' theorem—(see p. 2706). However, if the expected probability of HIV (or seroprevalence) is high, the positive predictive value increases.

Before HIV testing of a child is performed, the mother or primary caregiver (and the child, if old enough) should be counseled about the possible psychosocial risks and benefits of testing. Written or oral consent should be obtained and recorded in the patient's chart, consistent with state, local, and hospital laws and regulations. Counseling and consent requirements should not deter testing if it is medically indicated; refusal of a patient or guardian to give consent does not relieve physicians of their professional and legal responsibilities, and sometimes authorization for testing must be obtained by other means (eg, court order). Test results should be discussed in person with the family, the primary caregiver, and, if old enough, the child; if the child is HIV-positive, appropriate counseling and subsequent follow-up care must be provided. In all cases, maintaining confidentiality is essential.

Children and adolescents meeting the criteria for AIDS must be reported to the appropriate public health department. In many states, HIV infection (before the development of AIDS) also must be reported.

Other tests: Infected children require T-helper $CD4^+$ and T-suppressor $CD8^+$ lymphocyte counts and measurement of plasma viral RNA concentration (viral load) to help determine degree of illness and prognosis. $CD4^+$ counts may be normal (eg, above the age-specific cutoffs of category 1 in TABLE 280–2) initially but fall eventually. $CD8^+$ counts usually increase initially and do not fall until late in the infection. These changes in cell populations result in a decrease in the $CD4^+$:$CD8^+$ cell ratio, a characteristic of HIV infection (although sometimes occurring in other infections). Plasma viral RNA concentrations in untreated children < 12 mo are typically very high (mean, about 200,000 RNA copies/mL). By 24 mo, viral concentrations in untreated children decrease (to a mean of about 40,000 RNA copies/mL). Although the wide range of HIV RNA concentrations in children make the data less predictive of morbidity and mortality than in adults, determining plasma viral concentrations in conjunction with $CD4^+$ counts still yields more accurate prognostic information than does determining either marker alone. Less expensive alternative surrogate markers such as total lymphocyte counts and serum albumin levels may also predict AIDS mortality in children, which may be useful in developing nations.

Although not routinely measured, serum immunoglobulin concentrations, particularly IgG and IgA, often are markedly elevated, but occasional children develop panhypogammaglobulinemia. Patients may be anergic to skin test antigens.

Prognosis

With appropriate HAART regimens, most perinatally infected children survive well beyond 5 yr. About 10 to 15% of untreated children from industrialized countries die before 4 yr, most of these before 18 mo of age. In developing countries, pediatric AIDS mortality is much greater during the 1st few years of life.

Opportunistic infections, particularly *Pneumocystis* pneumonia, progressive neurologic disease, and severe wasting, are associated with a poor prognosis; with *Pneumocystis* pneumonia, mortality ranges from 5 to 40% if treated and is almost 100% if untreated. Prognosis is also poor for those in whom virus is detected early (ie, by 7 days of life) or symptoms develop in the 1st year of life. However, since the advent of HAART and *P. jiroveci* antimicrobial prophylaxis (see p. 2352), the incidence of opportunistic infections and malignancies has dramatically decreased in children with good treatment adherence. Adolescents who acquire HIV infection have a slower progression of disease, similar to that of adults.

Treatment

There are nearly 2 dozen ARV drugs (see TABLE 280–3), including multidrug combination products, available in the US, each of which may have adverse effects and drug interactions with other ARV drugs or commonly used antibiotics, anticonvulsants, and sedatives. New ARV drugs, immunomodulators, and vaccines are under evaluation.

Standard treatment is with HAART, which uses combinations of drugs to maximize viral suppression and minimize selection of drug-resistant strains. Most commonly, HAART consists of a "backbone" of 2 nucleoside analog reverse transcriptase inhibitors (ZDV plus didanosine, ZDV plus lamivudine, or stavudine plus lamivudine) given in combination with either a protease inhibitor (nelfinavir, lopinavir/ritonavir, or others) or a non-nucleoside reverse transcriptase inhibitor (nevirapine or efavirenz). Other combinations (eg, ZDV, lamivudine, and abacavir; dual protease inhibitor regimens; tenofovir-containing regimens) are used, but fewer data are available to support their use as 1st-line regimens. Monotherapy or dual nucleoside reverse transcriptase inhibitor therapy alone (except for ZDV chemoprophylaxis in HIV-exposed infants) is discouraged. Because expert opinions on therapeutic strategies change rapidly, consultation with specialists is strongly advised. Continually updated clinical practice guidelines are

TABLE 280–3. DOSAGE AND ADMINISTRATION OF ANTIRETROVIRAL DRUGS FOR CHILDREN*

DRUG NAME	RECOMMENDED DOSAGE (ORAL)	ADVERSE EFFECTS
Nucleoside reverse transcriptase inhibitors (NRTIs)		
Abacavir (ABC)	< 13 yr: 8 mg/kg q 12 h ≥ 13 yr: 300 mg q 12 h or 600 mg q 24 h	*More common:* Nausea, vomiting, fever, headache, rash, anorexia *Less common:* ~ 5% hypersensitivity syndrome, fever, fatigue, malaise, nausea, vomiting, abdominal pain, lymphadenopathy, rash—mostly during 1st 6 wk of use. Do not rechallenge—risk of hypotension, death with rechallenge *Rare:* Pancreatitis, lactic acidosis, hepatomegaly with steatosis
Didanosine (ddI)	0-3 mo: 50 mg/m^2 q 12 h < 13 yr: 120 mg/m^2 q 12 h ≥ 13 yr, < 60 kg: tablet, 125 mg q 12 h; buffered powder, 167 mg q 12 h; enteric-coated capsule, 250 mg q 24 h ≥ 13 yr, ≥ 60 kg: tablet, 200 mg q 12 h; buffered powder, 250 mg q 12 h; enteric-coated capsule, 400 mg q 24 h	*More common:* Diarrhea, nausea, vomiting, headache *Less common:* Peripheral neuropathy, lactic acidosis, hepatomegaly with steatosis *Rare:* Pancreatitis, retinitis
Emtricitabine (FTC)	< 18 yr: unknown ≥ 18 yr: 200 mg q 24 h or 300 mg g 24 h	*More common:* Headache, nausea, diarrhea, rash, hyperpigmentation *Less common:* Lactic acidosis, hepatomegaly with steatosis
Lamivudine (3TC)	0–3 mo: 2 mg/kg q 12 h < 13 yr: 4 mg/kg q 12 h ≥ 13 yr: 150 mg q 12 h or 300 mg q 24 h	*More common:* Headache, fatigue, nausea, diarrhea, rash *Less common:* Pancreatitis, neutropenia, peripheral neuropathy, lactic acidosis, hepatomegaly with steatosis
Stavudine (d4T)	< 13 yr: 1 mg/kg q 12 h ≥ 13 yr: 30–40 mg q 12 h	*More common:* Headache, GI disturbances, rash *Less common:* Peripheral neuropathy, pancreatitis, lactic acidosis, hepatomegaly with steatosis
Tenofovir† (TDF)	< 18 yr: unknown ≥ 18 yr: 300 mg q 24 h	*More common:* Nausea, vomiting, diarrhea *Less common:* Lactic acidosis, hepatomegaly with steatosis
Zalcitabine (ddC)	< 13 yr: 0.01 mg/kg q 8 h ≥ 13 yr: 0.75 mg q 8 h	*More common:* Headache, GI disturbances, malaise *Less common:* Peripheral neuropathy, lactic acidosis, hepatomegaly with steatosis, pancreatitis, oral ulcers

Table continues on the following page.

TABLE 280–3. DOSAGE AND ADMINISTRATION OF ANTIRETROVIRAL DRUGS FOR CHILDREN*—Continued

DRUG NAME	RECOMMENDED DOSAGE (ORAL)	ADVERSE EFFECTS
Zidovudine (ZDV, AZT)	0–3 mo: 2 mg/kg q 6 h 3 mo–13 yr: 160 mg/m^2 q 8 h ≥ 13 yr: 300 mg q 12 h or 200 mg q 8 h	*More common:* Anemia, granulocytopenia, macrocytosis, headache *Less common:* Hepatotoxicity, myositis, myopathy *Rare:* Lactic acidosis, hepatomegaly with steatosis
NRTI combination products		
ZDV/3TC	300/150 mg q 12 h	See individual drug
ZDV/3TC/ABC	300/150/300 mg q 12 h	See individual drug
3TC/ABC	300/600 mg q 24 h	See individual drug
FTC/TDF	200/300 mg q 24 h	See individual drug
Non-nucleoside reverse transcriptase inhibitors (NNRTIs)		
Delavirdine (DLV)	< 13 yr: unknown ≥ 13 yr: 400 mg q 8 h	*More common:* Headache, GI disturbances, rash (including Stevens-Johnson syndrome), drug interactions
Efavirenz (EFV)	< 13 yr: 200–400 mg q 24 h ≥ 13 yr: 600 mg q 24 h	*More common:* Rash, CNS disturbances (mostly adults—somnolence, insomnia, abnormal dreams, confusion); teratogenic in primates; drug interactions
Nevirapine (NVP)	< 13 yr: 120–200 mg/m^2 q 12 h ≥ 13 yr: 200 mg q 12 h (dose escalation lead-in period reduces complications at all ages)	*More common:* Rash (including Stevens-Johnson syndrome), fever, nausea, headache, drug interactions *Less common:* Hepatic inflammation (rarely may be life threatening), especially in the presence of active hepatitis B, hepatitis C, pregnancy, hypersensitivity reactions
Protease inhibitors (PIs)		
Amprenavir (APV)	Capsule dosage form: 4–13 yr: 20 mg/kg q 12 h ≥ 13 yr: 1200 mg q 12 h Oral suspension: 22.5 mg/kg q 12 h	*More common:* Nausea, vomiting, diarrhea, circumoral paresthesias *Less common:* Rash (including Stevens-Johnson syndrome), fat redistribution, lipid abnormalities *Rare:* Diabetes mellitus, hyperglycemia, vitamin E toxicity (contained in capsules and syrup), propylene glycol toxicity in young children (contained in syrup); theoretical risk of allergy in sulfonamide-sensitive patients

TABLE 280–3. DOSAGE AND ADMINISTRATION OF ANTIRETROVIRAL DRUGS FOR CHILDREN*—Continued

DRUG NAME	RECOMMENDED DOSAGE (ORAL)	ADVERSE EFFECTS
Atazanavir (ATV)	< 13 yr: unknown ≥ 13 yr: 400 mg q 24 h or 300 mg q 24 h with ritonavir (RTV) 100 mg q 24 h as pharmacokinetic booster	*More common:* Asymptomatic indirect hyperbilirubinemia (30%), jaundice (10%), headache, arthralgia, nausea, vomiting, diarrhea, insomnia *Less common:* PR interval prolongation on ECG *Rare:* Hepatitis, hyperglycemia, diabetes mellitus
Indinavir (IDV)	< 13 yr: unknown ≥ 13 yr: 800 mg q 8 h	*More common:* Nausea, headache, asymptomatic indirect hyperbilirubinemia (10%), drug interactions, crystalluria *Less common:* Nephrolithiasis (4%, especially if not adequately hydrated), fat redistribution, lipid abnormalities *Rare:* Pancreatitis, hepatitis, ketoacidosis, diabetes mellitus, hemolytic anemia
Lopinavir/ritonavir (LPV/r)	< 13 yr: 10–12 mg/kg lopinavir q 12 h ≥ 13 yr: 400 mg lopinavir q 12 h (LPV is coformulated with a small amount of RTV as a pharmacokinetic booster)	*More common:* Nausea, vomiting, diarrhea, headache, rash *Less common:* Fat redistribution, lipid abnormalities *Rare:* Pancreatitis, hepatitis, hyperglycemia, ketoacidosis, diabetes mellitus
Nelfinavir (NFV)	< 13 yr: 50–55 mg/kg q 12 h or 30 mg/kg q 8 h ≥ 13 yr: 1250 mg q 12 h	*More common:* Diarrhea, some drug interactions *Less common:* Abdominal pain, rash, fat redistribution, lipid abnormalities *Rare:* Pancreatitis, hepatitis, ketoacidosis, diabetes mellitus
Ritonavir (RTV)	< 13 yr: 400 mg/m^2 q 12 h ≥ 13 yr: 600 mg q 12 h (dose escalation lead-in period reduces complications at all ages)	*More common:* Nausea, vomiting, diarrhea, anorexia, headache; multiple drug interactions *Less common:* Circumoral paresthesias, fat redistribution, lipid abnormalities *Rare:* Pancreatitis, hepatitis, ketoacidosis, diabetes mellitus
Saquinavir (SQV)	< 13 yr: unknown ≥ 13 yr: 1000 mg q 12 h with either ritonavir (RTV) 100 mg q 12 h or lopinavir/ritonavir (LPV/r) 400 mg q 12 h as a pharmacokinetic booster	*More common:* Nausea, vomiting, diarrhea, anorexia, headache, rash; some drug interactions *Less common:* Fat redistribution, lipid abnormalities *Rare:* Pancreatitis, hepatitis, ketoacidosis, diabetes mellitus

Table continues on the following page.

TABLE 280–3. DOSAGE AND ADMINISTRATION OF ANTIRETROVIRAL DRUGS FOR CHILDREN*—Continued

DRUG NAME	RECOMMENDED DOSAGE (ORAL)	ADVERSE EFFECTS
Fusion inhibitor		
Enfuvirtide (T20)	< 13 yr: 2 mg/kg sc q 12 h ≥ 13 yr: 90 mg sc q 12 h (NOTE: An oral preparation is not available.)	*More common:* ~ 98% local injection site reaction (pain, discomfort, induration, erythema, nodules, ecchymosis) *Rare:* Hypersensitivity reaction

*Listed are the most commonly suggested doses (including infant doses where known) and notable adverse effects; other doses, drug interactions, and adverse effects are possible. For additional information, see Working Group on Antiretroviral Therapy and Medical Management of the HIV-Infected Child convened by the National Pediatric and Family HIV Resource Center, Health Resources and Services Administration (HRSA), and the National Institutes of Health (NIH). Guidelines for the Use of Antiretroviral Agents in Pediatric HIV Infection (March 24, 2005 version). Available at http://www.aidsinfo.nih.gov.

†TDF is functionally grouped within NRTIs but actually is a nucleotide reverse transcriptase inhibitor (NtRTI) by chemical structure.

available at several web sites, the most useful among them being www.aidsinfo.nih.gov, www.hivguidelines.org, and www.unaids.org.

Therapy will be successful only if the family and child are able to adhere to a possibly complex medical regimen. Nonadherence not only leads to failure to control HIV, but also selects drug-resistant HIV strains, which reduces future therapeutic choices. Barriers to adherence should be addressed before initiation of therapy. These include availability and palatability of pills or suspensions; drug interactions with current therapy; pharmacokinetic factors such as need to administer some drugs with food or in the fasted state; the fact that children depend on others to administer drugs (and HIV-infected parents may have problems with remembering their own drugs); and for adolescents, denial or fear of their infection, distrust of the medical establishment, and lack of family support.

Indications: Initiation of ARV therapy depends on virologic, immunologic, and clinical criteria; authorities differ on these. The goal is to suppress HIV replication (as measured by plasma HIV RNA PCR viral load) and maintain or achieve age-normal $CD4^+$ counts and percentages.

ARV therapy is recommended for all children > 12 mo of age with severe clinical or immunologic disease (clinical category C or immunologic category 3—see TABLES 280–1 and 280–2), regardless of the plasma HIV RNA viral load. Therapy is considered for mildly to moderately symptomatic children > 12 mo of age (clinical categories A or B, or immunologic category 2) and those who have plasma HIV RNA viral loads of > 100,000 copies/mL. Some experts use lower thresholds (eg, > 50,000 HIV RNA viral copies/mL or $CD4^+$ percentage of 15 to 20%). Children with no evidence of clinical disease or immunosuppression (category N1) may be followed closely without ARV therapy if their plasma HIV RNA is < 50,000 to 100,000 copies/mL.

Therapy should be given to all clinically symptomatic or immunosuppressed children < 12 mo of age (clinical categories A, B, C or immunologic categories 2 or 3) regardless of plasma HIV RNA viral load. Many experts treat asymptomatic infants < 12 mo (category N1) because HIV infection tends to progress rapidly in the 1st year of life.

Monitoring: Clinical and laboratory monitoring are important for identifying drug toxicity and therapeutic failure. Physical examination and monitoring of CBC, HIV RNA viral load, and lymphocyte subsets should be done q 3 to 4 mo; serum chemistry values, including liver enzymes, lipid profiles, and amylase and lipase levels, should be monitored once/yr to twice/yr at minimum.

Vaccination in symptomatic HIV infection: In general, live-virus (eg, oral poliovirus, varicella) vaccines and live-bacterial (eg, BCG) vaccines should not be given to children with AIDS or other manifestations of advanced HIV infection indicative of immunosuppression. An exception is measles-mumps-rubella vaccine in patients who are not severely immunocompromised (ie, not in category 3); this vaccine should be given at age 12 mo to enhance the likelihood of an immune response, ie, before the immune system deteriorates, if possible. The 2nd dose may be administered as soon as 4 wk later to attempt to induce seroconversion as early as possible. If the risk of exposure to measles is increased, such as during an outbreak, the vaccine should be given at an earlier age, such as at 6 to 9 mo.

Other childhood vaccines, eg, diphtheria and tetanus toxoids combined with acellular pertussis vaccine (DTaP), hepatitis B, *Haemophilus influenzae* type b and *Streptococcus pneumoniae* conjugates, and inactivated poliovirus (IPV), are given according to the usual immunization schedule (see FIG. 266–3 on p. 2235). Pneumococcal polysaccharide vaccine at 2 yr and annual inactivated influenza vaccination beginning at age 6 mo also are recommended.

Because children with symptomatic HIV infection generally have poor immunologic responses to vaccines, when they are exposed to a vaccine-preventable disease such as measles or tetanus, they should be considered susceptible, regardless of the history of vaccination. Therefore, if indicated, they should receive passive immunization with immune globulin. Immune globulin also should be given to any nonimmunized household member who is exposed to measles.

Vaccination in asymptomatic HIV infection: Such children should receive DTaP, IPV, *H. influenzae* type b and *S. pneumoniae* conjugates, hepatitis B, and measles-mumps-rubella vaccines, according to the usual immunization schedules. Although oral poliovirus vaccine (OPV) has been given to these patients without adverse effects, the live polioviruses in OPV can be excreted and transmitted to immunosuppressed contacts, creating an increased risk for paralytic poliomyelitis caused by vaccine virus infection (this is no longer a consideration in areas such as the US in which only IPV is used).

Varicella vaccine is safe and recommended in patients with early HIV infection (categories N1 or A1). Because HIV-infected children ≥ 2 yr are at increased risk of invasive pneumococcal infection, they should receive pneumococcal polysaccharide vaccination at age 2 yr (in addition to the infant series of pneumococcal conjugate vaccination). Revaccination once after 3 to 5 yr is recommended. Inactivated influenza vaccination should be administered annually for HIV-infected children ≥ 6 mo of age.

In the US and in areas of low TB prevalence, BCG vaccine is not recommended. However, in developing countries where TB prevalence is high, the WHO recommends that BCG be given to all infants at birth if they are asymptomatic, regardless of maternal HIV infection. Some cases of disseminated BCG infection in severely immunocompromised AIDS patients have been reported.

Passive immunization after exposure to measles, tetanus, and varicella is advisable.

Vaccination for seronegative children living with a patient with symptomatic HIV infection: Such children, as well as seropositive ones, should receive IPV vaccine rather than OPV. Measles-mumps-rubella vaccine may be given because these vaccine viruses are not transmitted. To reduce the risk of transmission of influenza to patients with symptomatic HIV infection, annual influenza vaccination (inactivated or live) is indicated for household contacts.

Varicella vaccination of seronegative siblings and susceptible adult caregivers of HIV-infected children is strongly encouraged to prevent acquisition of the wild-type varicella-zoster infection, which can cause severe disease in immunocompromised hosts; however, person-to-person transmission of the varicella vaccine virus does occur rarely.

Prevention

For postexposure prevention, see p. 1639.

Prevention of perinatal transmission: Appropriate prenatal ARV therapy attempts to optimize maternal health, interrupt MTCT, and minimize in utero drug toxicity. In the US and countries where ARV agents are available and the infrastructure for HIV diagnostic testing exists, treatment with ARV drugs is standard for all HIV-infected pregnant women (see also p. 1639). In HIV-infected women not previously receiving ARV agents who do not meet adult criteria for HAART, ZDV is administered orally 300 mg bid beginning at 14 to 34 wk gestation and is continued throughout pregnancy and is given IV during labor 2 mg/kg for the 1st hour and then 1 mg/kg/h until delivery. ZDV 2 mg/kg po qid is administered to the neonate for the 1st 6 wk of life. Women whose clinical or immunologic status does not meet treatment criteria for HAART are nevertheless recommended to initiate HAART if the viral load is > 1000 copies/mL. In the immediate postpartum period, a decision can be made whether to continue maternal therapy. Women whose clinical or immunologic status meets treatment criteria (see p. 1635) are given a multiple-drug regimen, preferably including ZDV.

Pregnancy is not a contraindication to HAART regimens, although the pregnant woman and her health care provider should discuss the possible benefits and risks of such therapy and the absence of definitive safety data. ZDV monotherapy reduces MTCT from 25% to 8%; many ARV combinations are also effective. With current HAART regimens, the US MTCT rate is < 2%. Thus, although the final decision to accept ARV therapy remains with the pregnant woman, it should be stressed that the proven benefits of therapy appear to outweigh the theoretical risks of fetal toxicity.

Most experts believe that HIV-infected women already receiving combination ARV therapy who become pregnant should continue that therapy, even during the 1st trimester; an alternative is to stop all therapy until the beginning of the 2nd trimester and resume at that time.

To reduce MTCT from HIV-infected pregnant women who are in labor but have had no prior therapy (or even for neonates delivered to untreated HIV-infected women), clinicians have used both ARV combinations and cesarean delivery. Rapid HIV testing of pregnant women who present in labor without documentation of their HIV serostatus may allow immediate institution of such measures. An expert in pediatric or maternal HIV infection should be immediately consulted in this situation.

Breastfeeding (or donating to milk banks) should be strongly discouraged in HIV-infected women in countries where safe and affordable alternative sources of feeding are readily available. However, in countries where infectious diseases and malnutrition are important causes of early childhood mortality and safe, affordable infant formula is not available, the protection from mortality risks of respiratory and GI infections afforded by breastfeeding may counterbalance the risk of HIV transmission. In these developing countries, the WHO recommends that mothers continue to breastfeed.

Prevention of adolescent transmission: Because adolescents are at special risk for HIV infection, they should receive education, have access to HIV testing, and know their serostatus. Education should include information about transmission, implications of infection, and strategies for prevention, including abstaining from high-risk behaviors and engaging in safe sex practices (correct and consistent use of condoms) for those who are sexually active.

Efforts should be targeted at adolescents at high risk of HIV infection. Informed consent is necessary for testing and the release of information regarding serostatus. Decisions regarding disclosure of HIV status to a sex partner without the patient's consent should be based on the likelihood that the partner is at risk, whether the partner has reasonable cause to suspect the risk and to take precautions, whether there is a legal requirement to withhold or disclose such information, and the possible effects of such disclosure on future relationships.

Prevention of opportunistic infections: Prophylaxis against *Pneumocystis* pneumonia is indicated for HIV-infected children with significant immunocompromise (ie, immunologic category 3). Generally, chemoprophylaxis is continued for life, although older adolescents and children on HAART with immune reconstitution (ie, immune category 1 or 2 for several months) may be able to stop prophylaxis as long as they remain in category 1 or 2. At present, lifelong chemoprophylaxis, regardless of the $CD4^+$ count, is recommended for those surviving an episode of *Pneumocystis* pneumonia. *Pneumocystis* prophylaxis also is recommended for all HIV-exposed infants born to HIV-infected women beginning at 4 to 6 wk of age. Prophylaxis may be stopped when HIV has been reasonably excluded by serial HIV PCR or culture. The drug of choice is trimethoprim-sulfamethoxazole (TMP-SMX) 75 mg TMP/375 mg SMX/m^2 po bid on 3 consecutive days/wk (eg, Monday-Tuesday-Wednesday); alternative schedules include the same total dose once/day for 3 days/wk, or bid every day of the week or on alternate days. For patients ≥ 5 yr who cannot tolerate TMP-SMX, aerosolized pentamidine (300 mg via specially designed inhaler) may be given once/mo. IV pentamidine has also been used but appears to be less effective and potentially more toxic. Another alternative, especially for those < 5 yr, is daily oral dapsone (2 mg/kg, not to exceed 100 mg). Other drugs that may be useful include pyrimethamine with dapsone, pyrimethamine-sulfadoxine, and oral atovaquone. However, experience with these drugs is very limited, and they should be considered only when the recommended regimens are not tolerated or cannot be used.

For prophylaxis against *Mycobacterium avium* complex infections in children ≥ 6 yr with $CD4^+$ counts < 50/μL (or children 2 to

6 yr with $CD4^+$ counts < 75/μL, 1 to 2 yr < 500/μL, or < 1 yr < 750/μL), weekly azithromycin or daily clarithromycin is the drug of choice, and daily rifabutin is an alternative. Data are limited on the use of prophylaxis for other opportunistic infections, such as cytomegalovirus, fungal disease, and toxoplasmic encephalitis.

OCCULT BACTEREMIA

Occult bacteremia is the presence of bacteria in the bloodstream of febrile young children who have no apparent foci of infection and look well. Diagnosis is by blood culture and exclusion of focal infection. Treatment is with antibiotics, either in the hospital or as outpatients; select children are treated pending blood culture results.

About 3% (range 2 to 10%) of children aged 1 to 36 mo with a febrile illness (temperature ≥ 39° C) and no localizing abnormalities have bacteremia, which is hence considered occult. Of these, about 5 to 10% develop focal bacterial infections (eg, septic arthritis, osteomyelitis, meningitis) or sepsis (see pp. 566 and 2333), which could be minimized by early identification and treatment of the bacteremia. The likelihood of progression to serious focal illness depends on the cause: 7 to 25% for *Haemophilus influenzae* type b (Hib) bacteremia but 4 to 6% for *Streptococcus pneumoniae* bacteremia.

Organisms: In the 1980s, 80% of occult bacteremia cases were caused by *Streptococcus pneumoniae*. The remainder was caused by Hib (10%), *Neisseria meningitidis* (5%), and others (predominantly *Staphylococcus aureus* and *Salmonella* sp). In the US, since the 1990s, routine Hib conjugate vaccination in infancy essentially eliminated Hib bacteremia. More recent routine use of the *S. pneumoniae* conjugate vaccine in infancy has reduced invasive pneumococcal disease in young children by > 66%, and increased use is expected to essentially eliminate the problem. When meningococcal conjugate vaccines are proven effective in this age group and licensed, the vast majority of occult bacteremia will be prevented.

Symptoms, Signs, and Diagnosis

The major symptom is fever; by definition, children with apparent focal disease (eg, cough, dyspnea, and pulmonary crackles suggesting pneumonia; skin erythema suggesting cellulitis or septic arthritis) are excluded. A toxic appearance (eg, limp and listless, lethargy, signs of poor perfusion, cyanosis, marked hypoventilation or hyperventilation) suggests sepsis or septic shock; bacteremia in such children is not classified as occult. However, early sepsis can be difficult to distinguish from occult bacteremia.

Diagnosis requires blood culture; typically one sample is obtained, and results are available within 24 h. Urinalysis and examination of the stool for leukocytes (if diarrhea is present) will help to identify specific infections and stratify risk. Recommendations regarding selection of children for testing and choice of tests vary with age, temperature, and clinical appearance (see Figs. 280–1 and 280–2); the goal is to minimize testing without missing bacteremia. These recommendations are sensitive but relatively nonspecific, making them much more effective in identifying children at low risk of infection who can be treated expectantly rather than in identifying children with true bacteremia.

CBC usually shows an elevated WBC count; however, only about 10% of children with WBC counts of > 15,000/μL are bacteremic, so specificity is low. Acute-phase reactants (eg, ESR, C-reactive protein) are used by some clinicians but add little information; however, in combination with elevated procalcitonin levels, acute-phase reactants may be more specific for serious illness. In children < 3 mo, band counts > 1,500/μL and either low (< 5,000) or high (>15,000) WBC counts may indicate bacteremia.

Prognosis and Treatment

Children who receive antibiotics before bacteremia is confirmed by blood culture appear less likely to develop focal infections, although data are inconsistent. However, because of the low overall incidence of bacteremia, many children would receive unnecessary treatment if all who were tested were empirically treated. One common system for management before culture results (see Figs. 280–1 and 280–2) minimizes antibiotic use in most febrile infants and children who do not have serious bacterial infection and provides antibiotics promptly to the few who need them. Nevertheless, some authorities prefer to hospitalize all febrile infants < 1 to 2 mo of age and administer parenteral antibiotics (eg, ceftriaxone) pending results of blood, urine, and CSF cultures.

All children are reexamined in 24 to 48 h. Those with persistent fever or positive blood or urine cultures have further cultures obtained and are admitted for evaluation of possible sepsis and administration of parenteral antibiotics. Those who are afebrile and well

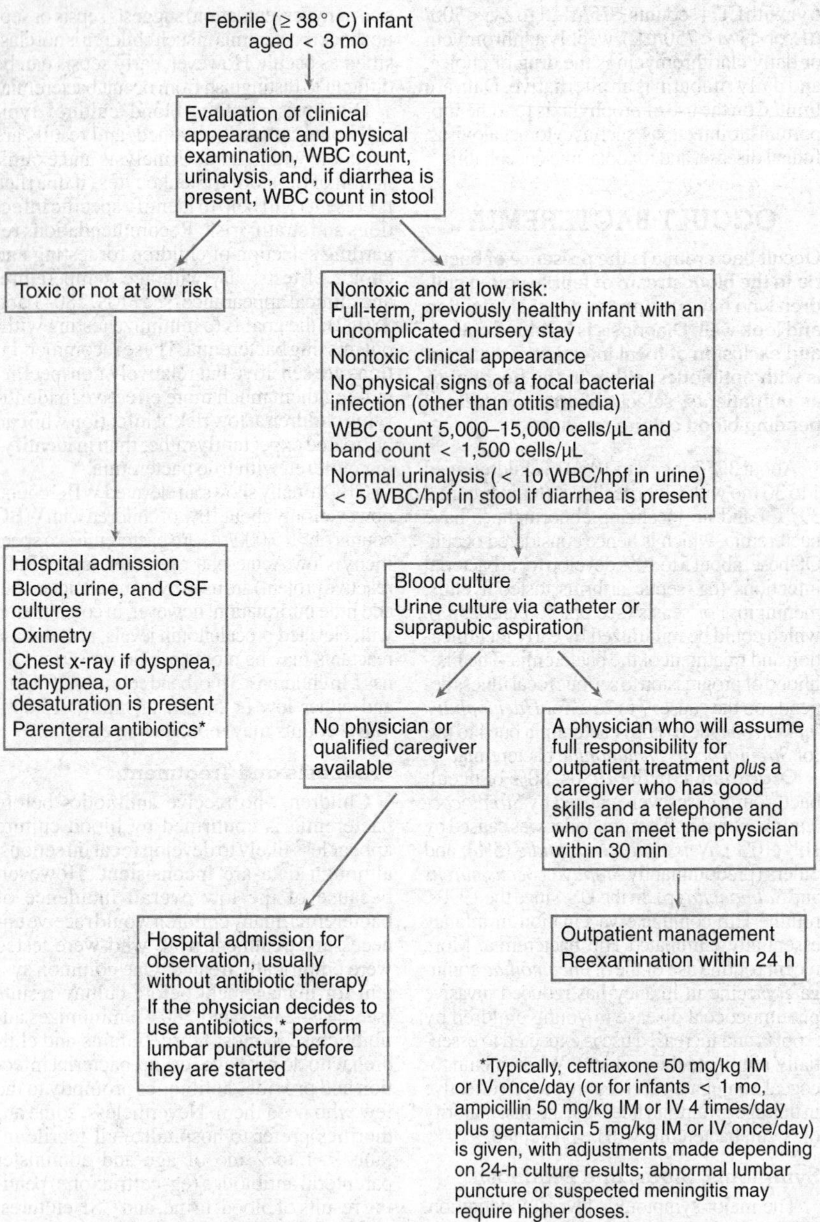

Fig. 280–1. Evaluation and management of the febrile infant aged < 3 mo. hpf = high-power field. (See also Ch. 279 on p. 2313.)

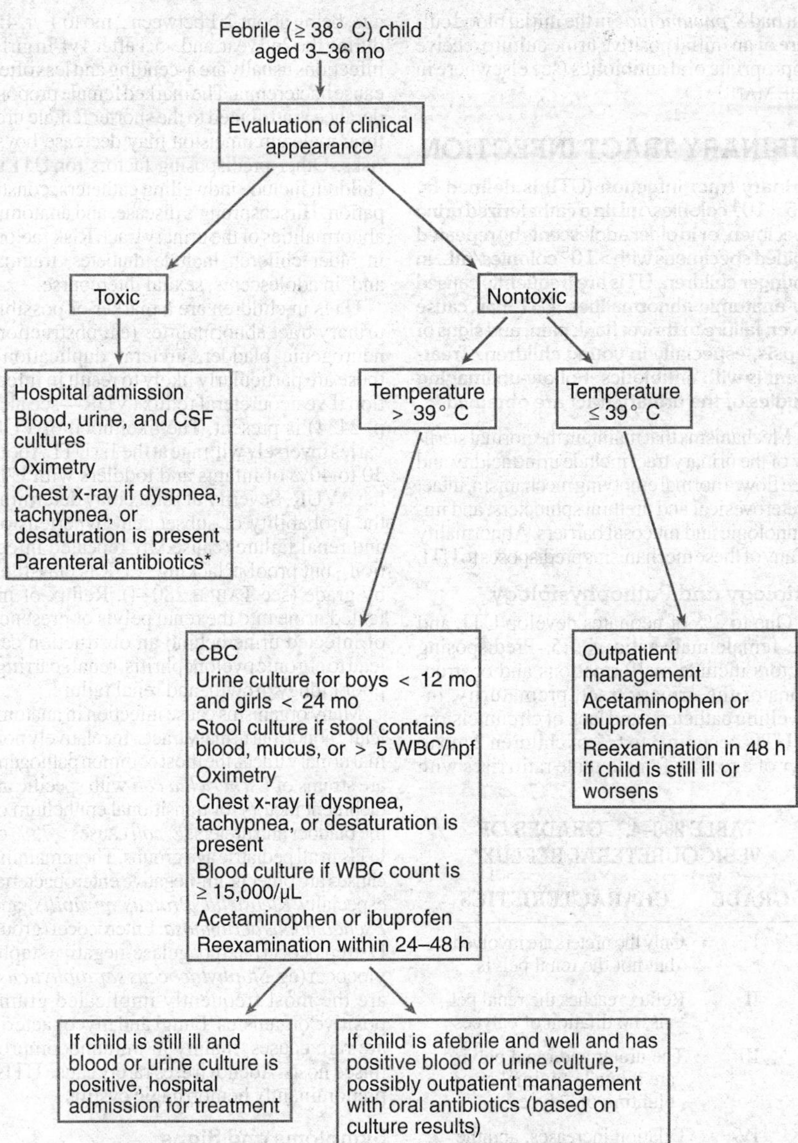

Fig. 280–2. Evaluation and management of the febrile child aged 3 to 36 mo. hpf = high-power field.

but had *S. pneumoniae* in the initial blood culture or an initial positive urine culture receive appropriate oral antibiotics (see elsewhere in THE MANUAL).

URINARY TRACT INFECTION

Urinary tract infection (UTI) is defined by > 5 × 10⁴ colonies/mL in a catheterized urine specimen, or in older adolescents by repeated voided specimens with > 10⁵ colonies/mL. In younger children, UTIs are frequently caused by anatomic abnormalities. UTI may cause fever, failure to thrive, flank pain, and signs of sepsis, especially in young children. Treatment is with antibiotics. Follow-up imaging studies of the urinary tract are obtained.

Mechanisms that maintain the normal sterility of the urinary tract include urine acidity and free flow, a normal emptying mechanism, intact ureterovesical and urethral sphincters, and immunologic and mucosal barriers. Abnormality of any of these mechanisms predisposes to UTI.

Etiology and Pathophysiology

One to 2% of neonates develop UTI, and the female:male ratio is 1:5. Predisposing factors include malformations and obstructions of the urinary tract, prematurity, indwelling catheters, and lack of circumcision.

UTIs occur in 3 to 6% of children 2 mo to 2 yr of age. The female:male ratio rises with age, being about 2:1 between 2 mo to 1 yr, 4:1 during the 2nd year, and > 5:1 after 4 yr. In girls, infections usually are ascending and less often cause bacteremia. The marked female preponderance is attributed to the shorter female urethra; male circumcision may decrease boys' risks. Other predisposing factors for UTI in children include indwelling catheters, constipation, Hirschsprung's disease, and anatomic abnormalities of the urinary tract. Risk factors in older children include diabetes, trauma, and, in adolescents, sexual intercourse.

UTIs in children are a marker of possible urinary tract abnormalities (eg, obstruction, neurogenic bladder, ureteral duplication); these are particularly likely to result in infection if vesicoureteral reflux (VUR—see also p. 2434) is present. The likelihood of VUR varies inversely with age at the 1st UTI. About 30 to 40% of infants and toddlers with UTI have VUR. Severity of reflux may determine the probability of subsequent hypertension and renal failure (caused by repeated infection), but proof is lacking. VUR is classified by grade (see TABLE 280–4). Reflux of infected urine into the renal pelvis or presence of infected urine behind an obstruction can lead to chronic pyelonephritis, renal scarring, poor kidney growth, and renal failure.

Many organisms cause infection in anatomically abnormal urinary tracts. In relatively normal urinary tracts, the most common pathogens are strains of *Escherichia coli* with specific attachment factors for transitional epithelium of the bladder and ureters. *E. coli* causes > 75% of UTIs in all pediatric age groups. The remaining causes are other gram-negative enterobacteria, especially *Klebsiella, Proteus mirabilis*, and *Pseudomonas aeruginosa*. Enterococci (group D streptococci) and coagulase-negative staphylococci (eg, *Staphylococcus saprophyticus*) are the most frequently implicated gram-positive organisms. Fungi and mycobacteria are rare causes, mainly in immunocompromised hosts. Adenoviruses rarely cause UTIs, predominantly hemorrhagic cystitis.

TABLE 280–4. GRADES OF VESICOURETERAL REFLUX*

GRADE	CHARACTERISTICS
I	Only the ureters are involved, but not the renal pelvis
II	Reflux reaches the renal pelvis; no dilation of calyces
III	The ureter and renal pelvis are dilated; minimal or no blunting of calyces
IV	Dilation increases, and the sharp angle of the calyceal fornices is obliterated
V	The ureter, pelvis, and calices are grossly dilated; papillary impressions frequently are absent

*As defined by the International Reflux Study Committee.

Symptoms and Signs

In neonates, symptoms and signs are nonspecific and include poor feeding, diarrhea, failure to thrive, vomiting, mild jaundice, lethargy, fever, and hypothermia. Neonatal sepsis (see p. 2333) may develop.

Infants and toddlers may also present with poorly localizing signs, such as fever, GI symptoms (eg, vomiting, diarrhea, abdominal pain), or foul-smelling urine.

In children > 2 yr, the more classic picture of cystitis or pyelonephritis can occur. Symptoms of cystitis include dysuria, frequency, hematuria, urinary retention, suprapubic pain, urgency, pruritus, incontinence, foul-smelling urine, and enuresis. Symptoms of pyelonephritis include high fever, chills, and costovertebral pain and tenderness.

Findings suggesting associated urinary tract abnormalities include abdominal masses, enlarged kidneys, urethral abnormalities, and signs of lower spinal malformations. Diminished force of the urinary stream may be the only clue to obstruction or neurogenic bladder.

Diagnosis

Urine tests: Diagnosis requires demonstration by culture of significant bacteriuria in properly collected urine. Most clinicians obtain urine by transurethral catheterization in infants and young children, reserving suprapubic aspiration of the bladder for boys with moderate to severe phimosis. Both procedures require technical expertise, but catheterization is less invasive, slightly safer, and has sensitivity of 95% and specificity of 99% compared with suprapubic aspiration. Bagged specimens are unreliable and should not be used for diagnosis.

If urine is obtained by suprapubic aspiration, the presence of any bacteria is significant. In a catheterized specimen, $> 5 \times 10^4$ colonies/mL commonly defines UTI. Clean-catch, midstream-voided specimens are significant when colony counts of a single pathogen (ie, not the total count of "mixed flora") are $> 10^5$/mL. Urine should be examined and cultured as soon as possible or stored at 4° C if a delay of > 10 min is expected. Occasionally, UTI may be present despite colony counts lower than the above guidelines, possibly because of prior antibiotic therapy, very dilute urine (specific gravity < 1.003), or obstruction to the flow of grossly infected urine. Sterile cultures generally rule out UTI unless the child is receiving antibiotics or the urine is contaminated with antibacterial skin cleansing agents.

Microscopic examination of urine is useful but not definitive. Pyuria (> 5 to 10 WBCs/high-power field in spun urine sediment) is about 70% sensitive for UTI. A WBC count (using a hemocytometer) > 10/μL in unspun urine has sensitivity of 90% but is not used by many laboratories. Presence of bacteria on Gram stain of spun or unspun urine is about 80% sensitive. Specificity of microscopy also is about 80%.

Dipstick tests on urine to detect bacteria (nitrite test) or leukocytes (leukocyte esterase test) are typically performed; if either is positive, the diagnostic sensitivity for UTI is about 93%. The specificity of the nitrite test is quite high; a positive result on a freshly voided specimen is highly predictive of UTI. Specificity of leukocyte esterase is much lower.

Differentiating an upper from a lower UTI can be difficult. High fever, costovertebral angle tenderness, and gross pyuria with casts indicate pyelonephritis. However, many children without these symptoms and signs have an upper UTI. Tests to distinguish upper from lower infection are not indicated in most clinical settings, because treatment is not altered.

Blood tests: A CBC and tests for inflammation (ESR, C-reactive protein) may help diagnose infection in those with borderline urine findings. Some authorities measure serum BUN and creatinine during a 1st UTI. Blood cultures are appropriate for infants with UTIs and for children > 1 to 2 yr who appear toxic.

Urinary tract imaging: Many major renal or urologic anomalies now are diagnosed in utero by routine prenatal ultrasonography. However, the high incidence of anatomic anomalies still warrants imaging the urinary tracts of all children 2 mo to 2 yr of age after a 1st UTI. If a 1st UTI occurs at ≥ 2 yr, most authorities recommend imaging; however, some physicians postpone imaging until after a 2nd UTI in girls > 2 yr of age. Options include voiding cystourethrogram (VCUG), radionuclide cystogram (RNC) with technetium 99m pertechnetate, and ultrasound.

VCUG and RNC are better than ultrasound for detecting VUR and anatomic abnormalities. RNC delivers about 1% of the gonadal radiation of VCUG; it is sensitive in detecting VUR, and some recommend it as the initial test. However, most authorities prefer the better anatomic definition of contrast VCUG as the initial test, using RNC in follow up to determine when VUR has resolved. Low-dose radiographic equipment has narrowed the gap in radiation between the contrast VCUG and RNC. These tests are recommended at the earliest convenient time after clinical response, typically toward the end of therapy, when bladder reactivity has resolved and urine sterility has been regained. If imaging is not scheduled until after therapy is due to be completed, the child should continue antibiotics at prophylactic doses until VUR is excluded.

Ultrasound helps exclude obstruction and hydronephrosis and is typically done within a week of diagnosing UTI in infants, especially if they do not respond quickly to antimicrobials. Otherwise, ultrasonography can be delayed until VCUG is done.

Prognosis

Properly managed children rarely progress to renal failure unless they have uncorrectable urinary tract abnormalities. However, repeated infection, particularly in the presence of VUR, may cause renal scarring, which may lead to hypertension and end-stage renal disease. High-grade VUR has a 4- to 6-fold greater rate of long-term renal scarring than low-grade VUR and an 8- to 10-fold greater rate than in children without VUR. Extreme scarring after VUR leads to end-stage renal disease in 3 to 10% of patients, although these data are likely biased because affected children may also have other renal abnormalities.

Treatment

Treatment aims to eliminate the acute infection, prevent urosepsis, and preserve renal parenchymal function. Antibiotics are begun presumptively in all toxic-appearing children and in nontoxic children with likely UTI (positive leukocyte esterase or nitrite, or microscopy showing pyuria or bacteriuria). Others can await culture results.

In infants 2 mo to 2 yr with toxicity, dehydration, or inability to retain oral intake, parenteral antibiotics are used, typically a 3rd-generation cephalosporin (eg, ceftriaxone 75 mg/kg IV/IM q 24 h or cefotaxime 50 mg/kg IV q 6 h). A 1st-generation cephalosporin (eg, cefazolin) may be used if typical local pathogens are known to be sensitive. Aminoglycosides (eg, gentamicin), although potentially nephrotoxic, are useful to treat potentially resistant gram-negative bacilli such as *Pseudomonas* in complex UTIs (eg, urinary tract abnormalities, presence of indwelling catheters, recurrent UTIs). If blood cultures are negative and clinical response is good, an appropriate oral antibiotic (eg, a cephalosporin, trimethoprim-sulfamethoxazole [TMP-SMX], or amoxicillin) selected on the basis of antimicrobial sensitivities can be used to complete a 10- to 14-day course. A poor clinical response suggests a resistant organism or an obstructive lesion and warrants urgent evaluation with ultrasonography and repeat urine culture.

In nontoxic, nondehydrated infants and children who are able to retain oral intake, oral antibiotics may be given initially. The drug of choice is TMP-SMX, 3 to 6 mg/kg (of TMP component) bid. Alternatives include cephalosporins such as cefdinir 7 mg/kg bid, cefprozil 15 mg/kg bid, cefixime 4 mg/kg bid, and cephalexin 12.5 to 25 mg/kg qid. Therapy is changed based on the results of cultures and antimicrobial sensitivities. Treatment is generally for > 10 days, although many older children with uncomplicated UTI can be treated for 7 days. Urine culture is repeated 2 to 3 days after therapy starts if efficacy is not clinically apparent.

Vesicoureteral reflux: Children with grades I to III VUR can be followed clinically and given antibiotic prophylaxis; about 13%/yr resolve. Although it is generally thought that antibiotic prophylaxis reduces recurrences and prevents kidney damage, few long-term data are available. Drugs include nitrofurantoin 2 mg/kg po once/day or TMP-SMX 2 mg/kg po (of TMP component) once/day, usually given at bedtime. If grade IV or grade V VUR or a major renal abnormality is detected, prophylactic antibiotics are used; surgery is often needed because ≤ 5%/yr resolve.

281 RHEUMATIC FEVER

Rheumatic fever is a nonsuppurative, acute inflammatory complication of group A streptococcal infection, causing combinations of arthritis, carditis, subcutaneous nodules, erythema marginatum, and chorea. Diagnosis is based on applying the Jones criteria to information from history, examination, and laboratory testing. Treatment includes aspirin or other NSAIDs, corticosteroids during severe carditis, and antimicrobials to eradicate residual streptococcal infection and prevent reinfection.

A first episode of acute rheumatic fever (ARF) occurs most often between 5 and 15 yr and is uncommon before 3 and after 21 yr. Testing for group A streptococcal (GAS) infection for primary prevention of rheumatic fever is therefore usually not necessary in patients younger than 3 yr with pharyngitis. In the US, incidence is < 1/100,000. The attack rate (percentage of patients with untreated GAS pharyngitis who develop ARF) varies from 0.4 to 3.0%. Higher attack rates occur with certain streptococcal M protein serotypes and a stronger host immune response. In patients with a prior episode of ARF, the attack rate in untreated GAS pharyngitis approaches 50%, underscoring the importance of long-term antistreptococcal prophylaxis. Incidence has declined in most developed countries but remains high in the underdeveloped world. However, more recent local outbreaks of ARF suggest that more virulent (rheumatogenic) strains of streptococci may have returned to the US. The prevalence of chronic rheumatic heart disease is uncertain because criteria are not standardized and autopsy is not performed routinely.

Etiology and Pathophysiology

GAS infection is the etiologic precursor of ARF, but host and environmental factors are important. GAS M proteins share epitopes (antigenic-determinant sites that are recognized by antibodies) with proteins found in synovium, heart muscle, and heart valve, suggesting that molecular mimicry contributes to the arthritis, carditis, and valvular damage. Genetic host risk factors include the D8/17 B-cell antigen and certain class II histocompatibility antigens. Malnutrition, overcrowding, and lower socioeconomic status predispose to streptococcal infections and subsequent episodes of rheumatic fever.

The joints, heart, skin, and CNS are most often affected. Pathology varies by site.

Joints: Joint involvement manifests as nonspecific inflammation in a synovial biopsy specimen, sometimes with small foci resembling Aschoff bodies (granulomatous collections of leukocytes, myocytes, and interstitial collagen).

Heart: Cardiac involvement manifests as carditis, which can involve myocardium, endocardium, and pericardium, and is sometimes followed years later by chronic rheumatic heart disease (eg, primarily valvular stenosis, but can also include regurgitation, arrhythmias, and ventricular dysfunction). Aschoff bodies often develop in the myocardium and other parts of the heart. Fibrinous nonspecific pericarditis, sometimes with effusion, occurs only in patients with endocardial inflammation and usually subsides without permanent damage. Characteristic and potentially dangerous valve changes may occur. Acute interstitial valvulitis may cause valvular edema. Left untreated, valve thickening, fusion, and retraction or other destruction of leaflets and cusps may result, leading to stenosis or insufficiency. Similarly, chordae tendineae can shorten, thicken, or fuse, adding to regurgitation of damaged valves or producing regurgitation of an otherwise unaffected valve. Dilation of valve rings may also cause regurgitation. The mitral, aortic, tricuspid, and pulmonic valves are affected, in order of decreasing frequency. Regurgitation and stenosis are the usual effects on the mitral and tricuspid valves; the aortic valve generally becomes regurgitant initially and stenotic much later.

Skin: Subcutaneous nodules are indistinguishable from those of RA but on biopsy show features resembling Aschoff bodies. Erythema marginatum differs histologically from other skin lesions with similar macroscopic appearance, eg, the rash of systemic-onset juvenile rheumatoid arthritis (JRA), Henoch-Schönlein purpura, erythema chronicum migrans, and erythema multiforme. Perivascular neutrophilic and mononuclear infiltrates of the dermis occur.

CNS: Sydenham chorea, the form of chorea that occurs with ARF, manifests in the CNS as hyperperfusion and increased metabolism in the basal ganglia. Increased levels of antineuronal antibodies have also been demonstrated.

Symptoms and Signs

An initial episode of symptoms occurs typically about 2 to 4 wk after the streptococcal infection. The 5 major manifestations of ARF (see TABLE 281–1), occurring alone or in combination, produce many clinical patterns.

Joints: Migratory polyarthritis is the most common manifestation, occurring in about 70% of children; it is often accompanied by fever. Occasionally monarthritis occurs. Joints become extremely painful and tender and may also be red, hot, and swollen. Ankles, knees, elbows, and wrists are usually involved. Shoulders, hips, and small joints of the hands and feet also may be involved, but almost never alone. If vertebral joints are affected, other disease should be suspected.

Arthralgia-like symptoms may be due to nonspecific myalgia or tenodynia in the periarticular zone; tenosynovitis may develop at the site of muscle insertions. Joint pain and

TABLE 281–1. MODIFIED JONES CRITERIA FOR A FIRST EPISODE*

Major manifestations
Carditis
Chorea
Erythema marginatum
Polyarthritis
Subcutaneous nodules
Minor manifestations
Arthralgia
Elevated ESR or C-reactive protein
Fever
Prolonged PR interval (on ECG)

*Diagnosis of acute rheumatic fever requires either 2 major or 1 major and 2 minor manifestations, and evidence of group A streptococcal infection (elevated or rising antistreptococcal antibody titer [eg, antistreptolysin-O, anti-DNase B], positive throat culture, or positive rapid antigen test).

Adapted from Guidelines for the diagnosis of rheumatic fever. Jones criteria, 1992 update. Special Writing Group of the Committee on Rheumatic Fever, Endocarditis, and Kawasaki Disease of the Council on Cardiovascular Disease in the Young of the American Heart Association. *JAMA* 268(15):2069–2073, 1992.

fever usually subside within 2 wk and seldom last > 1 mo.

Heart: Carditis can occur alone or in combination with pericardial rub, murmurs, cardiac enlargement, or heart failure. In the 1st episode of ARF, carditis occurs in about 50%. A patient may seek medical attention for high fever, chest pain, or if heart failure produces respiratory, peripheral, or abdominal manifestations. In about 50% of cases, cardiac damage (ie, valve dysfunction) occurs much later.

Murmurs are common and usually evident early. The soft diastolic blow of aortic regurgitation and the presystolic murmur of mitral stenosis may be difficult to detect. Murmurs often persist indefinitely. If no worsening occurs during the next 2 to 3 wk, new manifestations of carditis seldom follow. ARF typically does not produce chronic, smoldering carditis. Scars left by acute valvular damage may contract and change, and secondary hemodynamic difficulties may develop in the myocardium without persistence of acute inflammation.

Heart failure from the combination of carditis and valvular dysfunction may produce dyspnea without rales, nausea and vomiting, a right upper quadrant or epigastric ache, and a hacking, nonproductive cough.

Skin: Cutaneous and subcutaneous features are uncommon and almost never occur alone, usually developing in a patient who already has carditis, arthritis, or chorea. Fever and other systemic manifestations such as anorexia and malaise can be prominent but are not specific. Subcutaneous nodules, which occur most frequently on the extensor surfaces of large joints, usually coexist with arthritis and carditis. About 2% of children with ARF have nodules. Ordinarily, the nodules are painless, transitory, and responsive to the treatment of joint or heart inflammation.

Erythema marginatum is a serpiginous, flat or slightly raised, nonscarring, and painless rash. About 2% of children have this rash. It sometimes lasts < 1 day. Its appearance is often delayed after the inciting streptococcal infection; it may appear with or after the other manifestations of rheumatic inflammation.

CNS: Sydenham's chorea occurs in about 10% of children. It may develop along with other manifestations but frequently arises after the other manifestations have subsided. Onset of chorea is typically insidious and may be preceded by inappropriate laughing or crying. Chorea consists of rapid and irregular jerking movements that may begin in the hands but often becomes generalized, involving the feet and face. Associated motor symptoms include loss of fine motor control, weakness, and hypotonia. Obsessive-compulsive behavior develops in many patients.

Other: Lethargy, malaise, and fatigue often occur and may be caused by heart failure. Other manifestations may include abdominal pain and anorexia, either because of the hepatic mechanism described for heart failure or from concomitant mesenteric adenitis. Because of the fever, elevated WBC count, and abdominal guarding, the situation may resemble acute appendicitis, particularly when other rheumatic manifestations are absent. Epistaxis occurs in about 4% of children with an initial episode and 9% of those with a recurrence.

Prolonged episodes of ARF (> 8 mo) occur in about 5% of patients, with spontaneous recurrences of inflammation (clinical and laboratory manifestations) unrelated to intervening streptococcal infection or to cessation of anti-inflammatory therapy. Recurrences usually mimic the initial episode.

Diagnosis

Diagnosis of a first episode of ARF is based on the modified Jones criteria (see TABLE 281–1); 2 major criteria or 1 major and 2 minor criteria are required, along with evidence of preceding GAS infection. The Jones criteria should not be used to establish a recurrence.

A preceding streptococcal infection is suggested by a recent history of pharyngitis and confirmed by a positive throat culture, an increase in the antistreptolysin O titer, or a positive rapid GAS antigen test. Recent scarlet fever is highly suggestive. Throat cultures and rapid antigen tests are often negative by the time ARF manifests, whereas titers of antistreptolysin O and other antibodies typically are peaking. Only 80% of children with a prior infection have a significantly elevated antistreptolysin O titer; anti-DNase B antibody level should be obtained in such cases.

Joint aspiration may be needed to exclude other causes, such as infection. The fluid is usually cloudy and yellow, with an elevated WBC count composed primarily of neutrophils; culture is negative. Complement levels are usually normal or slightly decreased, compared with decreased levels in other inflammatory arthritides.

Baseline ECG and echocardiogram are performed at the time of diagnosis. Normal cardiac troponin I levels in children exclude prominent myocardial damage. ECG abnormalities such as PR prolongation do not correlate with other evidence of carditis. Only 35% of children with ARF have a prolonged PR interval. Other ECG abnormalities may be due to pericarditis, enlargement of ventricles or atria, or arrhythmias. Echocardiography can detect evidence of carditis in many patients. Chest x-rays are not routinely performed but can detect cardiomegaly, a common manifestation of carditis in ARF. Biopsy of a subcutaneous nodule can aid in early diagnosis, especially when other major clinical manifestations are absent. Rheumatic carditis must be distinguished from congenital heart disease and endocardial fibroelastosis; echocardiography or coronary angiography can be used to verify difficult diagnoses.

ESR and serum C-reactive protein (CRP) are sensitive but not specific. The ESR is often >120 mm/h. CRP is often >2 mg/dL; because it rises and falls faster than ESR, a normal CRP may confirm the absence of inflammation in a patient with prolonged ESR elevation after acute symptoms have subsided. In the absence of carditis, ESR usually returns to normal within 3 mo. Evidence of acute inflammation, including ESR, usually subsides within 5 mo in uncomplicated carditis. The WBC count reaches 12,000 to 20,000/μL and may go higher with corticosteroid therapy.

The differential diagnosis includes JRA (especially systemic-onset JRA and, less so, polyarticular JRA), Lyme disease, reactive arthritis, arthropathy of sickle cell disease, leukemia or other malignancy, SLE, embolic bacterial endocarditis, serum sickness, Kawasaki disease, drug reactions, and gonococcal arthritis. These are frequently distinguished by history or specific laboratory tests. The absence of an antecedent GAS infection, the diurnal variation of the fever, evanescent skin rash, and prolonged symptomatic joint inflammation usually distinguish systemic-onset JRA from ARF.

Prognosis

Prognosis depends mostly on the severity of the initial carditis. Patients with severe carditis during the first episode may have residual heart disease that is often worsened by the rheumatic fever recurrences to which they are particularly susceptible. Murmurs eventually disappear in about ½ of patients whose acute episodes were manifested by mild carditis without major cardiac enlargement or decompensation. Risk of recurrent inflammation is intermediate, between the low risk of those without carditis and the high risk of those with a history of severe carditis, but recurrences may cause or worsen permanent cardiac damage. Patients who did not have carditis are less likely to have recurrences and are unlikely to develop carditis if ARF recurs. Sydenham chorea usually lasts several months and resolves completely in most patients, but about ⅓ of patients have recurrences. All other manifestations subside without residual effects.

Treatment

The primary goals are suppression of inflammation and relief of acute symptoms, eradication of GAS infection, and prophylaxis against future infection to prevent recurrent heart disease.

Patients should generally limit their activities if symptomatic with arthritis, chorea, or heart failure. In the absence of carditis, no physical restrictions are needed after the initial episode subsides. In asymptomatic patients with carditis, strict bed rest has no proven value.

Aspirin controls fever and pain from arthritis and carditis. The dose is titrated upward until clinical effectiveness is attained or toxicity supervenes. The starting dose for children and adolescents is 15 mg/kg po qid. If not effective overnight, the dosage is increased to 22.5 mg/kg qid the next day and 30 mg/kg qid on the next. Salicylate toxicity is manifested by tinnitus, headache, or hyperpnea and may not appear until after ≥ 1 wk. Salicylate levels are measured only to manage toxicity. Enteric-coated, buffered, or complex salicylate molecules provide no advantage. Other NSAIDs can be used. For example, naproxen, 7.5 to 10 mg/kg po bid, is as effective as aspirin. If a therapeutic effect has not occurred after the 4th day, which is sometimes the case if carditis or arthritis is severe, NSAIDs should be abandoned in favor of a corticosteroid.

Prednisone 0.25 to 1 mg/kg po bid (or 0.125 to 0.5 mg po qid) up to 60 mg/day is recommended. If inflammation is not suppressed after 2 days, a corticosteroid pulse of methylprednisolone succinate (30 mg/kg IV once/day, maximum 1 g/day, for 3 successive days) may be given. Oral corticosteroids are given until ESR has remained normal for ≥ 1 wk and then are tapered at the rate of 5 mg q 2 days. To prevent worsening of inflammation during the corticosteroid taper, NSAIDs are begun simultaneously and continued until 2 wk after the corticosteroid has been stopped. Laboratory tests are used to monitor disease activity and response to treatment. Inflammatory markers such as ESR and CRP are the best indicators of therapeutic response.

Recurrences of cardiac inflammation (indicated by fever or chest pain) may subside spontaneously, but NSAIDs or corticosteroids should be resumed for heart failure uncontrolled by cardiotonic drugs. In patients with prolonged, recurrent episodes of carditis, immunosuppressive drugs may also be effective. Although useful in the acute episode, NSAIDS and corticosteroids do not prevent or reduce long-term valve damage.

Although poststreptococcal inflammation is well developed by the time ARF is detected, antibiotics are used to eradicate any lingering organisms and to prevent reinfection. Appropriate regimens for the treatment of acute infection are described under Streptococcal and Enterococcal Infections on p. 1444.

Antistreptococcal prophylaxis should be maintained continuously after the initial episode of ARF to prevent recurrences (see TABLE 281–2). Antibiotics taken orally are just as effective as those given by injection, and the oral route is usually recommended because the injections are painful and require clinic visits and observation for postinjection reactions. The optimal duration of antistreptococcal prophylaxis is uncertain. Children without carditis should receive prophylaxis for 5 yr or up to age 21 (if the patient turns 21 before 5 yr of prophylaxis is completed). The American Academy of Pediatrics recommends that those with carditis without evidence of residual heart damage receive prophylaxis for 10 yr. Children with carditis and evidence of residual heart damage should receive prophylaxis for > 10 yr; many experts recommend that such patients continue prophylaxis indefinitely. Some experts believe prophylaxis should be life long in all patients with chorea and should continue in all patients who have close contact with young children, owing to their high rate of GAS carriage.

In patients with known or suspected rheumatic valvular disease who have not remained on prophylactic antibiotics, short-term prophy-

TABLE 281–2. RECOMMENDED PROPHYLAXIS AGAINST RECURRENT GROUP A STREPTOCOCCAL INFECTION

PATIENT PARAMETER	DRUG	DOSE
Standard	Penicillin G benzathine	1.2 million units IM q 3–4 wk* ≤ 27 kg: 600,000 units IM q 3–4 wk*
Alternatives	Penicillin V **or**	250 mg po bid
	Sulfadiazine	≤ 27 kg: 500 mg po once/day > 27 kg: 1 g po once/day
Allergic to penicillin and sulfadiazine	Erythromycin	250 mg po bid

*In developing countries, IM prophylaxis q 3 wk is superior to q 4 wk.

laxis against bacterial endocarditis should be instituted for dental or oral surgical procedures likely to cause gingival bleeding, upper respiratory tract surgery, and surgery or instrumentation of the GU and lower GI tracts (see TABLES 77–3, 77–4, and 77–5 on pp. 730–731).

POSTSTREPTOCOCCAL REACTIVE ARTHRITIS

Poststreptococcal reactive arthritis is development of arthritis after group A streptococcal infection in patients who do not meet the criteria for acute rheumatic fever.

Poststreptococcal reactive arthritis may represent an attenuated variant of ARF. Compared with the arthritis of ARF, poststreptococcal reactive arthritis typically involves fewer joints, is less migratory but more protracted, and responds less to aspirin. It can be treated with other NSAIDs (eg, ibuprofen, naproxen, tolmetin). Although clinical practice for secondary prevention of cardiac involvement varies greatly, it is reasonable to give antistreptococcal prophylaxis for 1 yr and then to repeat the echocardiogram. If cardiac lesions are detected by echocardiogram, long-term prophylaxis is indicated.

282 ENDOCRINE AND METABOLIC DISORDERS IN CHILDREN

(See also Hypopituitarism in Children Resulting in Short Stature on p. 1183.)

Some endocrine and metabolic disorders occur mostly in children; others occur in children and adults.

CONGENITAL GOITER

Congenital goiter is a diffuse or nodular enlargement of the thyroid gland present at birth. Thyroid hormone secretion may be decreased, increased, or normal. Diagnosis is by confirming thyroid size with ultrasonography. Treatment is thyroid hormone replacement when hypothyroidism is the cause. Surgery is indicated when breathing or swallowing is impaired.

Etiology

Congenital goiters may be caused by dyshormonogenesis (abnormal thyroid hormone production), transplacental passage of maternal antibodies, or transplacental passage of goitrogens. Some causes are hereditary.

Dyshormonogenesis: Genetic defects in thyroid hormone production result in increased levels of thyroid-stimulating hormone (TSH), which in turn can cause congenital goiter. There are 4 main types of dyshormonogenesis.

Type 1 is caused by a defect in iodide transport secondary to altered synthesis of a cell surface protein necessary for transport.

Type 2 is caused by one of several defects in thyroid iodination mechanisms. The enzyme peroxidase, necessary for iodine organification, may be absent (resulting in goitrous cretinism) or dysfunctional. Another defect may impair hydrogen peroxide generation. Children with Pendred's syndrome have mild hypothyroidism or euthyroidism, goiter, and sensorineural hearing loss due to an abnormal transport protein (pendrin) involved in iodine transport and also cochlear function.

Type 3 is caused by complete or partial deiodination defects of monoiodotyrosine and diiodotyrosine in thyroglobulin.

Type 4 is caused by one of several defects in thyroglobulin synthesis, usually via X-linked inheritance. This condition does not cause clinical hypothyroidism. It is, however, characterized by a very low level of total serum thyroxine (T_4) but normal levels of free T_4 and TSH.

Transplacental passage of maternal antibodies: Women with an autoimmune thyroid disorder produce antibodies that may cross the placenta. Depending on the disorder, the antibodies either block TSH receptors, producing hypothyroidism, or stimulate them, producing hyperthyroidism. Typically, in affected infants, the change in hormone secretion and the associated goiter resolve spontaneously within 3 to 6 mo.

Transplacental passage of goitrogens: Goitrogens such as amiodarone or antithyroid drugs (eg, propylthiouracil, methimazole) can cross the placenta, sometimes causing hypothyroidism and rarely causing goiter.

Symptoms and Signs

The most common presentation is firm, nontender enlargement of the thyroid. Enlargement is most often diffuse but can be nodular. It may be noticeable at birth or detected later. In some patients, enlargement is not directly observable but continued growth can cause deviation or compression of the trachea, compromising breathing and swallowing. Many children with goiters are euthyroid, but some present with hypothyroidism or hyperthyroidism.

Diagnosis and Treatment

If the diagnosis is suspected, thyroid size is typically assessed by ultrasonography. TSH is checked.

Hypothyroidism is treated with thyroid hormone. Goiters that compromise breathing and swallowing can be treated surgically.

HYPOTHYROIDISM

Hypothyroidism is thyroid hormone deficiency. Symptoms in infants include poor feeding and growth failure; symptoms in older children and adolescents are similar to those of adults but also include growth failure, delayed puberty, or both (see p. 1197). Diagnosis is by thyroid function testing (eg, serum thyroxine, thyroid-stimulating hormone). Treatment is thyroid hormone replacement.

Hypothyroidism during infancy and early childhood: Hypothyroidism in infants and young children may be congenital or neonatal. Congenital hypothyroidism occurs in about 1/4000 live births. Most congenital cases are sporadic, but about 10 to 20% are inherited. The most frequent cause of congenital hypothyroidism is dysgenesis, either absence (agenesis) or underdevelopment (thyroid hypoplasia) of the thyroid gland. About 10% of congenital hypothyroidism results from dyshormonogenesis (abnormal thyroid hormone production) of which there are 4 types (see p. 2363). Rarely in the US but commonly in certain developing countries, hypothyroidism results from maternal iodine deficiency. Rarely, transplacental transfer of antibodies, goitrogens (eg, amiodarone), or antithyroid drugs (eg, propylthiouracil, methimazole) cause transient hypothyroidism.

Symptoms and signs differ from those in adults. If iodine deficiency occurs very early during pregnancy, infants may present with endemic cretinism (a syndrome involving deaf-mutism), mental retardation, and spasticity. Most other hypothyroid infants initially have few if any symptoms or signs because some maternal thyroid hormone crosses the placenta. However, after the maternal thyroid hormone is metabolized, if the underlying cause of hypothyroidism persists and hypothyroidism remains undiagnosed or untreated, it usually slows CNS development moderately to severely and may be accompanied by low muscle tone, prolonged hyperbilirubinemia, umbilical hernia, respiratory distress, macroglossia, large fontanelles, poor feeding, and hoarse crying. Rarely, delayed diagnosis and treatment of severe hypothyroidism lead to mental retardation and short stature.

Routine screening of neonates detects hypothyroidism before clinical signs are evident. If screening is positive, thyroid function tests, including serum thyroxine (T_4), free T_4, and thyroid-stimulating hormone (TSH), are indicated.

Most cases require lifelong thyroid hormone replacement. Treatment with L-thyroxine 10 to 15 g/kg po once/day must be started immediately and be closely monitored. This dose is intended to rapidly normalize serum T_4 and should then be adjusted to maintain serum T_4 level between 10 and 15 μg/dL during infancy. After age 1 yr, the usual dose is 5 to 6 μg/kg po once/day, titrated to maintain serum T_4 and TSH levels within the normal range for age. In most treated infants, motor and mental development is normal. Severe congenital hypothyroidism, even when treated promptly, may still cause subtle developmental problems and neurosensory hearing loss. Hearing loss may be so mild that initial screening misses it. Retesting after infancy is advised to detect subtle hearing loss, which may interfere with language acquisition. Thyroxine-binding globulin deficiency, detected by screening that relies primarily on T_4 measurement, does not require treatment because affected infants are euthyroid.

Hypothyroidism during later childhood and adolescence: Usually, the cause is autoimmune thyroiditis (Hashimoto's thyroiditis). Some symptoms and signs are similar to those of adults (eg, weight gain; constipation; coarse, dry hair; sallow, cool, or mottled coarse skin). Signs specific to children are growth retardation, delayed skeletal maturation, and usually delayed puberty. Treatment with L-thyroxine is 5 to 6 μg/kg po once/day; the dose is decreased to 2 to 3 μg/kg po once/day in adolescents and titrated to maintain serum T_4 and TSH levels within the normal range.

HYPERTHYROIDISM

Hyperthyroidism is excessive thyroid hormone production. Diagnosis is by thyroid function testing (eg, free serum thyroxine, thyroid-stimulating hormone). Treatment is with propylthiouracil or methimazole.

Hyperthyroidism during infancy: Hyperthyroidism is rare in infants but potentially life-threatening. It develops in fetuses of women with current or prior Graves' disease who have elevated titers of thyroid-stimulating immunoglobulins (TSI), which overstimulate thyroid hormone production by binding to thyroid-stimulating hormone (TSH) receptors in the thyroid gland. These antibodies cross the placenta and cause thyroid hyperfunction in the fetus (intrauterine Graves' disease), which can result in fetal death or premature birth. Because infants clear the antibodies after birth, neonatal Graves' disease is usually transient. However, because the clearance rate varies, duration of neonatal Graves' disease varies.

Symptoms and signs include irritability, feeding problems, hypertension, tachycardia, exophthalmos, goiter, frontal bossing, and microcephaly. Other early findings are failure to thrive, vomiting, and diarrhea. Affected infants almost always recover within 6 mo; the course is rarely longer. Persistent hyperthyroidism may result in craniosynostosis (premature fusion of the cranial sutures), impaired intellect, growth failure, short stature, and hyperactivity later in childhood. Mortality rate may reach 10 to 15%.

Diagnosis is suspected in infants whose mothers have Graves' disease and high titers of stimulatory antibodies (TSI) and is confirmed by measuring free serum thyroxine (T_4) and TSH. Infants are given an antithyroid drug (eg, propylthiouracil 1.7 to 3.3 mg/kg po tid, methimazole 0.17 to 0.33 mg/kg po tid), sometimes with a β-blocker (eg, propranolol 0.8 mg/kg po tid), to treat symptoms. Treatment must be monitored closely and discontinued as soon as the disease has run its course (for treatment of Graves' disease during pregnancy, see p. 2184).

Hyperthyroidism during childhood and adolescence: Graves' disease is the usual cause; it is characterized by diffuse goiter, thyrotoxicosis, and, rarely, infiltrative ophthalmopathy. Diagnosis and treatment are similar to those in adults (see p. 1195).

CONGENITAL ADRENAL HYPERPLASIA

(Adrenogenital Syndrome; Adrenal Virilism)

Congenital adrenal hyperplasia is a group of genetic disorders, each characterized by inadequate synthesis of cortisol, aldosterone, or both.

In the various forms of congenital adrenal hyperplasia, production of cortisol (a glucocorticoid), aldosterone (a mineralocorticoid), or both is impaired because of an autosomal recessive genetic defect in one of the adrenal enzymes involved in synthesizing adrenal steroid hormones from cholesterol. The enzyme may be absent or deficient, completely or partially disabling synthesis of cortisol, aldosterone, or both. In the forms in which cortisol synthesis is absent or decreased, ACTH (corticotropin) release, normally suppressed by cortisol, is excessive. In the most common forms, 21-hydroxylase deficiency and 11β-hydroxylase deficiency, precursors proximal to the enzyme block accumulate and are shunted into adrenal androgens. The consequent excess androgen secretion causes varying degrees of virilization in external genitals of affected female fetuses; no defects are discernible in external genitals of male fetuses. In some less common forms affecting enzymes other than 21-hydroxylase and 11β-hydroxylase, the enzyme block impairs androgen synthesis. As a result, virilization of male fetuses is inadequate, but no defect is discernible in female fetuses.

21-HYDROXYLASE DEFICIENCY

21-Hydroxylase (CYP21A2) deficiency causes defective conversion of adrenal precursors to cortisol, and in some cases to aldosterone, resulting in virilization and sometimes severe hyponatremia and hyperkalemia. Diagnosis is by measurement of cortisol, its precursors, and adrenal andro-

gens, sometimes after ACTH administration. Treatment is with a glucocorticoid plus, if needed, a mineralocorticoid and, for some female patients with genital ambiguity, surgical reconstruction.

21-Hydroxylase deficiency causes 90% of all cases of congenital adrenal hyperplasia. Incidence ranges from 1/10,000 to 1/15,000 live births. The deficiency completely or partially blocks conversion of adrenal precursors into cortisol and aldosterone, resulting in increased levels of progesterone, 17-hydroxyprogesterone, dehydroepiandrosterone (DHEA, a weak androgen that masculinizes affected female infants), and androstenedione. Plasma deoxycorticosterone, deoxycortisol, cortisol, and aldosterone levels are low or absent.

Complete 21-hydroxylase deficiency, the salt-wasting form, accounts for 70% of 21-hydroxylase deficiency cases. The salt-wasting form (sometimes called the classic form of congenital adrenal hyperplasia) is the most severe form of 21-hydroxylase deficiency; aldosterone is not secreted and salt is lost, leading to hyponatremia, hyperkalemia, and increased plasma renin activity. Partial 21-hydroxylase deficiency causes a less severe, non–salt-losing form, in which aldosterone levels are normal or only slightly decreased.

Symptoms and Signs

The salt-wasting form causes hyponatremia (sometimes severe), hyperkalemia, and hypotension as well as virilization. If undiagnosed and untreated, this form can lead to life-threatening adrenal crisis, with vomiting, diarrhea, hypoglycemia, hypovolemia, and shock.

Very young female infants with the salt-wasting form will have ambiguous external genitals, with clitoral enlargement, fusion of the labia majora, and a urogenital sinus rather than distinct urethral and vaginal openings. Male infants typically have normal sexual development. When the enzyme deficiency is much milder, neonates have little or no virilization, but androgen excess manifests later with early appearance of pubic hair and increase in growth velocity in both sexes, clitoral enlargement in girls, and penile enlargement and earlier deepening of voice in boys.

In affected females, especially those with the salt-wasting form, reproductive function may be impaired as they reach adulthood; they may have labial fusion and anovulatory cycles or amenorrhea. Some males with the salt-wasting form are fertile as adults, but others have Leydig cell dysfunction, decreased testosterone, and impaired spermatogenesis. Most affected males with the non–salt-losing form, even if untreated, are fertile, but in some, spermatogenesis is impaired. Individuals with the non–salt-losing form are normotensive.

Diagnosis

Prenatal screening and diagnosis (and experimental treatment) are possible; *CYP21* genes are analyzed if risk is high (eg, the fetus has an affected sibling with the genetic defect). Carrier status (heterozygosity) can be determined in children and adults.

In neonates, serum levels of 17-hydroxyprogesterone are measured in the dried blood on filter paper of the newborn screen. If levels are elevated compared with age-adjusted norms, the diagnosis must be confirmed by identifying low blood levels of deoxycortisol, cortisol, deoxycorticosterone, corticosterone, progesterone, and 17-hydroxyprogesterone and by identifying high levels of DHEA and androstenedione, measured in whole blood from the neonate. Rarely, the diagnosis is uncertain, and levels of these hormones must be measured before and 60 min after ACTH is administered (ACTH or cosyntropin stimulation test). In patients who develop symptoms later, ACTH stimulation testing may help, but genotyping may be required. In children with the salt-wasting form, deoxycorticosterone, corticosterone, and aldosterone levels are low, and renin levels are high. Levels of urinary metabolites of cortisol precursors (eg, pregnanetriol) and androgen precursors (eg, 17-ketosteroids) are also high, but rarely necessary for the diagnosis.

Treatment

For adrenal crisis in infants, urgent therapy with IV fluids is needed. Stress doses of hydrocortisone (100 mg/m^2/day) are given by continuous IV infusion; the dose is reduced over several weeks to a more physiologic replacement dose. Stress doses of hydrocortisone are also given to prevent adrenal crisis if the salt-wasting form is suspected.

Maintenance treatment is corticosteroids as replacement for deficient steroids (typically, oral hydrocortisone 5 to 8 mg/m^2 tid or prednisone 1.5 to 2 mg/m^2 bid). Dexamethasone is used only in postpubertal adolescents and adults. Cortisone acetate 18 to 36 mg/m^2 IM q 3 days may be used in infants when oral therapy is unreliable. Response to therapy is monitored in infants q 3 mo and in children aged > 12 mo q 3 to 4 mo. Overtreatment with a corticosteroid results in iatrogenic Cushing's disease, causing obesity, subnormal growth, and delayed skeletal maturation. Undertreatment results in inability to suppress ACTH with consequent hyperandrogenism, causing virilization and supranormal growth velocity in children and, eventually, premature termination of growth and short stature. Monitoring involves measuring serum 17-hydroxyprogesterone and DHEA or androstenedione, as well as assessing growth velocity and skeletal maturation each year.

Maintenance treatment for the salt-wasting form, in addition to corticosteroids, is mineralocorticoid replacement for restoration of Na and K homeostasis. Oral fludrocortisone (usually 0.1 mg once/day, range 0.05 to 0.3 mg) is given if salt loss occurs. Infants often require supplemental oral salt for about 1 yr. Close monitoring during therapy is critical.

Affected female infants may require surgical reconstruction with reduction clitoroplasty and construction of a vaginal opening. Often, further surgery is required during adulthood, but with appropriate care and attention to psychosexual issues, a normal sex life and fertility may be expected.

For prenatal treatment, a corticosteroid (usually dexamethasone) is given to the pregnant mother to suppress fetal pituitary secretion of ACTH and thus reduce or prevent masculinization of affected female fetuses. Treatment, which is experimental, must begin in the 1st several weeks of gestation.

11β-Hydroxylase Deficiency

11β-Hydroxylase (CYP11B1) deficiency involves defective conversion of adrenal precursors, resulting in virilization, hypernatremia, hypokalemia, and hypertension. Diagnosis is by measurement of cortisol, its precursors, and adrenal androgens and sometimes by measuring 11-deoxycortisol and 11-deoxycorticosterone after ACTH administration. Treatment is with a corticosteroid.

11β-Hydroxylase deficiency causes about 5% of all cases of congenital adrenal hyperplasia. Conversion of 11-deoxycortisol to cortisol and 11-deoxycorticosterone to corticosterone is partially blocked, leading to increased levels of ACTH and overproduction of 11-deoxycortisol, 11-deoxycorticosterone (which has mineralocorticoid activity), and adrenal androgens.

Symptoms and Signs

Female neonates may present with genital ambiguity, including clitoral enlargement, labial fusion, and a urogenital sinus. Male neonates usually appear normal, but some present with penile enlargement. Some children present later, with sexual precocity or, in females, menstrual irregularities and hirsutism. Salt retention with hypernatremia, hypertension, and hypokalemic alkalosis may result from increased mineralocorticoid activity.

Diagnosis and Treatment

Prenatal diagnosis is not available. Plasma levels in neonates are determined for 11-deoxycortisol, 11-deoxycorticosterone, adrenal androgens, and renin; urinary levels of tetrahydro-11-deoxycortisol, tetrahydro-11-deoxycortisone, 17-hydroxycorticosteroids, and 17-ketosteroids are measured. Diagnosis is established by increased levels. If the diagnosis is uncertain, levels of 11-deoxycortisol and 11-deoxycorticosterone are measured before and 60 min after ACTH stimulation. In affected adolescents, basal plasma levels may be normal so ACTH stimulation is recommended.

Treatment is cortisol replacement, typically with hydrocortisone 5 to 8 mg/m^2 tid, which reduces ACTH secretion and reduces levels of 11-deoxycorticosterone and adrenal androgens to normal. Mineralocorticoid replacement is usually not necessary for restoration of Na and K homeostasis but may be required in the neonate or during severe stress. Response to treatment should be monitored, typically by measuring serum 11-deoxycortisol, DHEA, and androstenedione and by assessing growth velocity and skeletal maturation. BP should be monitored in patients who presented with hypertension.

Affected female infants may require surgical reconstruction with reduction clitoroplasty and construction of a vaginal opening. Often, further surgery is required in adulthood, but with appropriate care and attention to psychosexual issues, a normal sex life and fertility may be expected.

MALE HYPOGONADISM IN CHILDREN

(See also p. 1944.)

Male hypogonadism is decreased production of testosterone, sperm, or both or, rarely, decreased response to testosterone,

resulting in delayed puberty, reproductive insufficiency, or both. Diagnosis is by measurement of serum testosterone, luteinizing hormone, and follicle-stimulating hormone and by stimulation tests with human chorionic gonadotropin or gonadotropin-releasing hormone. Treatment depends on cause.

Classification

There are 3 types of hypogonadism: primary, secondary, and a type caused by defective androgen action, primarily due to defective androgen receptor activity.

Primary: In primary (hypergonadotropic) hypogonadism, damage to the Leydig cells impairs testosterone production, damages the seminiferous tubules, or does both; oligospermia or azoospermia and elevated gonadotropins result. The most common cause is Klinefelter's syndrome; other causes are gonadal dysgenesis (rare), cryptorchidism, bilateral anorchia, Leydig cell aplasia, Noonan's syndrome, and myotonic dystrophy. Rare causes include orchitis due to mumps, which is becoming even rarer as immunization rates increase; testicular torsion; and trauma.

Klinefelter's syndrome is seminiferous tubule dysgenesis associated with the 47,XXY karyotype, in which an extra X chromosome is acquired through maternal or, to a lesser extent, paternal meiotic nondisjunction (see also p. 2454). The syndrome is usually identified at puberty, when inadequate sexual development is noted, or later, when infertility is investigated. Diagnosis is based on elevated gonadotropin levels and low to low-normal testosterone levels.

Gonadal dysgenesis occurs in hermaphroditism, which is rare.

In **cryptorchidism,** one or both testes are undescended (see p. 2436). Etiology is usually unknown. Sperm counts may be slightly low if one testis is undescended but are almost always very low if both are undescended.

In **bilateral anorchia (vanishing testes syndrome),** the testes were presumably present but were resorbed before or after birth. External genitals and wolffian structures are normal, but müllerian duct structures are lacking. Thus, testicular tissue must have been present during the 1st 12 wk of embryogenesis because testicular differentiation occurred and testosterone and müllerian-inhibiting factor were produced.

In **Leydig cell aplasia,** congenital absence of Leydig cells causes male pseudohermaphroditism with ambiguous external genitals. Although wolffian ducts develop to some extent, testosterone production is insufficient to induce normal male differentiation of the external genitals. Müllerian ducts are absent because of normal production of müllerian-inhibiting hormone by Sertoli cells. Gonadotropin levels are high with low testosterone levels.

Noonan's syndrome may occur sporadically or as an autosomal dominant disorder. Phenotypic abnormalities include hyperelasticity of the skin, hypertelorism, ptosis, low-set ears, short stature, shortened 4th metacarpals, high-arched palate, and primarily right-sided cardiovascular abnormalities (eg, pulmonic valve stenosis, atrial septal defect). Testes are often small or cryptorchid. Testosterone levels may be low with high gonadotropin levels.

Defective androgen synthesis is caused by enzyme defects that impair androgen synthesis, which may occur in any of the pathways leading from cholesterol to dihydrotestosterone. These congenital problems may occur in congenital adrenal hyperplasia when the same enzyme defect occurs in the adrenal glands and the testes, resulting in defective androgen activity and ambiguous external genitals (ie, male pseudohermaphroditism) of varying degrees.

Secondary: Causes of secondary hypogonadism include panhypopituitarism, hypothalamic pituitary tumors, isolated gonadotropin deficiency, Kallmann syndrome, Laurence-Moon syndrome, constitutional delay of puberty, isolated luteinizing hormone deficiency, Prader-Willi syndrome, and functional and acquired disorders of the CNS (eg, trauma, infection). Several acute disorders and chronic systemic disorders (eg, chronic renal insufficiency, anorexia nervosa) may lead to hypogonadotropic hypogonadism, which resolves after recovery from the underlying disorder. Relative hypogonadism is becoming more common among long-term survivors of childhood cancers treated with craniospinal irradiation. Chemotherapy with alkylating drugs may lead to testicular damage and relative hypogonadism.

Panhypopituitarism may occur congenitally or anatomically (eg, in septo-optic dysplasia or Dandy-Walker malformation), causing deficiency of hypothalamic-releasing factors or pituitary hormones. Acquired hypopituitarism may result from tumors, neoplasia, their treatment, vascular disorders, infiltrative disorders (eg, sarcoidosis, Langerhans' cell histiocytosis), infections (eg, encephalitis, meningitis), or trauma. Hypopituitarism in childhood may cause delayed growth, hypothyroidism, diabetes insipidus, hypoadrenalism, and lack of sexual development when puberty is expected. Hormone deficiencies, whether originating in the anterior or posterior pituitary, may be varied and multiple.

Kallmann syndrome is characterized by anosmia due to aplasia or hypoplasia of the olfactory lobes and by hypogonadism due to deficiency of hypothalamic gonadotropin-releasing hormone (GnRH). It occurs when fetal GnRH neurosecretory neurons do not migrate from the olfactory placode to the hypothalamus. The genetic defect is known; inheritance is usually X-linked. Other manifestations include microphallus, cryptorchidism, midline defects, and unilateral kidney agenesis.

Laurence-Moon syndrome is characterized by obesity, mental retardation, retinitis pigmentosa, and polydactyly.

Constitutional delay of puberty is absence of pubertal development in boys ≥ 14 yr. Many have a family history of delayed sexual development in a parent or sibling. Most affected boys have some evidence of sexual maturation by age 18 yr or have a skeletal age of at least 12 yr (the average age at which testicular enlargement is first noted). Typically, stature is usually short during childhood, adolescence, or both but ultimately reaches normal range. Growth velocity is nearly normal, and growth pattern parallels the lower percentile curves of the growth chart; the pubertal growth spurt is delayed. When skeletal age is plotted on the growth curve, it essentially equals the percentile curve of the genetic target. Diagnosis is by exclusion of growth hormone deficiency, hypothyroidism, and hypogonadism (whether primary or due to gonadotropin deficiency).

Isolated luteinizing hormone (LH) deficiency (fertile eunuch syndrome) is monotropic loss of LH secretion in boys; follicle-stimulating hormone (FSH) levels are normal. At puberty, growth of the testes is normal because most testicular volume consists of seminiferous tubules, which respond to FSH. Spermatogenesis may occur as tubular development proceeds. However, absence of LH results in Leydig cell atrophy and testosterone deficiency. Therefore, patients do not develop normal secondary sexual characteristics, but they continue to grow, reaching eunuchoidal proportions because the epiphyses do not close.

Prader-Willi syndrome is characterized by diminished fetal activity, failure to thrive during early childhood, obesity during childhood and adolescence, muscular hypotonia, mental retardation, and hypogonadotropic hypogonadism. The syndrome is caused by deletion or disruption of a gene or genes on the proximal long arm of paternal chromosome 15 or by uniparental disomy of maternal chromosome 15. Failure to thrive due to hypotonia and feeding difficulties during infancy usually resolves after age 6 to 12 mo. From 12 to 18 mo onward, uncontrollable hyperphagia causes excessive weight gain and psychologic problems; plethoric obesity becomes the most striking feature. Rapid weight gain continues into adulthood; stature remains short. Features include emotional lability, poor gross motor skills, facial abnormalities (eg, a narrow bitemporal dimension, almond-shaped eyes, a mouth with thin upper lips and down-turned corners), and skeletal abnormalities (eg, scoliosis, kyphosis, osteopenia). Hands and feet are small. Other features include cryptorchidism and a hypoplastic penis and scrotum.

Symptoms and Signs

Clinical presentation depends on whether, when, and how testosterone and sperm production are affected. For presentation in adulthood, see p. 1944.

If androgen deficiency or defects in androgen activity occur during the 1st trimester (< 12 wk gestation), differentiation of internal wolffian ducts and external genitals is inadequate. Presentation may range from ambiguous external genitals (ie, male pseudohermaphroditism) to normal-appearing female external genitals. Androgen deficiency during the 2nd and 3rd trimesters may cause a microphallus and partially or completely undescended testes.

Androgen deficiency that develops early in childhood has few consequences, but if it occurs when puberty is expected, secondary sexual development is impaired. Such patients have poor muscle development, a high-pitched voice, inadequate phallic and testicular growth, a small scrotum, sparse pubic and axillary hair, and absent body hair. They may develop gynecomastia and grow to eunuchoidal body proportions (arm span exceeds height by 5 cm; pubic to floor length exceeds crown to pubic length by > 5 cm) because fusion of the epiphyses is delayed and long bone growth continues.

Diagnosis

Diagnosis is often suspected based on developmental abnormalities or delayed puberty but requires confirmation by testing, including measurement of testosterone, LH, and FSH. LH and FSH levels are more sensitive than testosterone levels, especially for detecting primary hypogonadism.

LH and FSH levels also help determine whether hypogonadism is primary or secondary: High levels, even with low-normal testosterone levels, indicate primary hypogonadism, and levels that are low or lower than expected for the testosterone level indicate secondary hypogonadism. In boys with short stature, delayed pubertal development, low testosterone, and low FSH and LH levels may indicate constitutional delay. Elevated serum FSH levels with normal serum testosterone and LH levels typically indicate impaired spermatogenesis but not impaired testosterone production. In primary hypogonadism, it is important to determine the karyotype to investigate for Klinefelter's syndrome.

Measurement of testosterone, FSH, and LH for diagnosis of hypogonadism requires an understanding of how the levels vary. Before puberty, serum testosterone levels are < 20 ng/dL (< 0.7 nmol/L) and in adulthood, levels are > 300 to 1200 mg/dL. Serum testosterone secretion is primarily circadian. In the 2nd half of puberty, levels are higher at night than during the day. A single sample can establish that circulating testosterone levels are normal. Because 98% of testosterone is bound to carrier proteins in serum (testosterone-binding globulin), alterations in these protein levels alter total testosterone levels.

For LH and FSH levels, 3 blood samples should be taken at 20-min intervals. This approach maximizes the likelihood of detecting LH pulsations, which occur at 90- to 120-min intervals. Serum LH and FSH levels are usually < 5 mIU/mL before puberty and fluctuate between 5 and 20 mIU/mL during the 2nd half of puberty and into adulthood.

The human chorionic gonadotropin (hCG) stimulation test is done to assess the presence and secretory ability of testicular tissue; hCG 100 IU/kg is given to children. hCG stimulates Leydig cells, as does LH, with which it shares a structural subunit, and stimulates testicular production of testosterone. Testosterone levels should double after 3 to 4 days.

The GnRH stimulation test is performed in boys to distinguish between hypothalamic dysfunction and pituitary dysfunction as the cause of hypogonadotropic hypogonadism. GnRH 2.5 μg/kg or leuprolide acetate 500 μg is rapidly injected IV. The injection directly stimulates the pituitary to secrete LH and FSH, which are measured q 20 to 30 min for 2 h. Throughout childhood and into early puberty, response to GnRH is predominantly an increase in FSH with little or no increase in LH. During puberty, LH and FSH respond more or less equally (by doubling or tripling). An inadequate to absent increase in FSH and LH may indicate hypopituitarism.

Treatment

Cryptorchidism is corrected early to obviate concerns about cancer developing in later adulthood and to prevent testicular torsion (see p. 2437).

For secondary hypogonadism, any underlying pituitary or hypothalamic disorder is treated. Overall, the goal is to provide androgen replacement starting with a low dose and progressively increasing the dose over 18 to 24 mo.

Adolescents with androgen deficiency should be given long-acting injectable testosterone enanthate or cypionate 50 mg q 2 to 4 wk; the dose is increased up to 200 mg over 18 to 24 mo. A transdermal patch or gel may be used instead.

Treatment of Kallmann syndrome with hCG can correct cryptorchidism and establish fertility. Pulsatile GnRH therapy given subcutaneously by a portable pump leads to endogenous sex steroid secretion, progressive virilization, and even fertility.

In isolated LH deficiency, testosterone, via conversion to estrogen by aromatase, induces normal epiphyseal closure.

DELAYED PUBERTY

Delayed puberty is absence of sexual maturation at the expected time.

Delayed puberty may result from constitutional delay (see p. 2369), which often occurs in adolescents with a family history of delayed growth. Prepubertal growth velocity is normal, but skeletal maturation and adolescent growth spurt are delayed; sexual maturation is delayed but normal. Other causes include Turner's syndrome in girls, Klinefelter's syndrome in boys, CNS disorders (eg, pituitary tumors that reduce gonadotropin secretion), certain chronic disorders (eg, diabetes mellitus, renal disorders, cystic fibrosis), and excess physical activity, especially in girls.

In boys, delayed puberty is diagnosed if no testicular enlargement occurs by age 14, if no pubic hair appears by age 15, or if > 5 yr elapse between initial and complete growth of the genitals. In girls, delayed puberty is diagnosed if no breast development occurs by age 13, if no pubic hair appears by age 14, if > 5 yr elapse between the beginning of breast growth and menarche, or if menstruation does not occur by age 16. Short stature may indicate delayed puberty in either sex. Although many children seem to be starting puberty earlier than in past years, there are no indications that the criteria for delayed puberty should change.

Constitutional delay of puberty is more prevalent in boys. Girls with severe pubertal delay should be investigated for primary amenorrhea. If boys show no sign of pubertal development or of skeletal maturation beyond 11 to 12 yr by age 15, they may be given a 4- to 8-mo course of IM testosterone enanthate 50 mg once/mo. These low doses induce puberty with some degree of virilization and do not jeopardize adult height potential.

PRECOCIOUS PUBERTY

Precocious puberty is onset of sexual maturation before age 8 in girls or age 9 in boys. Diagnosis is by comparison with population standards, x-ray of the left hand and wrist to assess skeletal maturation and check for accelerated bone growth, and measurement of serum levels of gonadotropins and gonadal and adrenal steroids. Treatment depends on the cause.

The definition of precocious puberty depends on reliable population standards for onset of puberty (ie, when pubertal milestones occur); because onset seems to be occurring earlier in the US, these standards are being reevaluated. Almost 8 to 10% of white girls, almost 30% of black girls, and an intermediate percentage of Hispanic girls reach early puberty at age 8. The lower limit of normal puberty may be 7 yr for white girls and 6 yr for black girls. The mean age for early breast development is about 10 yr for white girls and 9 yr for black girls (range 8 to 13 yr). The mean age for pubic hair growth is 9 to 10.5 yr for both groups. These findings imply that guidelines for evaluating disorders that cause precocious puberty can be interpreted more leniently if children are otherwise healthy and are not at risk of not reaching their full adult height potential.

In girls, the 1st pubertal milestone is typically breast development (thelarche), followed soon after by appearance of pubic hair (pubarche) and axillary hair and later by the 1st menstrual period (menarche). In boys, the 1st pubertal milestone is typically testicular growth, followed by penile growth and appearance of pubic and axillary hair. In both sexes, appearance of pubic and axillary hair is called adrenarche.

Precocious puberty can be divided into 2 types: gonadotropin-releasing hormone (GnRH)–dependent (central) or GnRH-independent (peripheral). GnRH-dependent precocious puberty is 5 to 10 times more frequent in girls; in boys, GnRH-dependent and GnRH-independent precocious puberty occur with similar frequency. In GnRH-dependent precocious puberty, the hypothalamic-pituitary axis is activated, resulting in enlargement and maturation of the gonads, development of secondary sexual characteristics, and spermatogenesis or oogenesis. In GnRH-independent precocious puberty, secondary sexual characteristics result from high circulating levels of androgens or estrogens, without activation of the hypothalamic-pituitary axis.

Precocious puberty may also be classified by whether gonadarche or adrenarche occurs. In girls, gonadarche includes breast development, change in body habitus, growth of the uterus, and eventually menarche. In boys, gonadarche includes testicular enlargement; phallic growth; appearance of pubic, facial, and axillary hair; adult body odor; and facial skin oiliness or acne.

Premature appearance of only one specific pubertal milestone is generally considered a benign variant of development. Examples are precocious appearance of pubic and axillary hair before age 8 in girls and age 9 in boys, and precocious onset of breast development before age 8 in girls.

Etiology

GnRH-dependent precocious puberty: In most affected girls ≥ 4 yr, a specific cause cannot be identified. However, many girls < 4 yr have a CNS lesion. Most (60%) affected boys have an identifiable underlying lesion. Such lesions include intracranial tumors, especially of the hypothalamus (hamartoma, rarely craniopharyngioma) or pineal gland region (teratoma, pinealoma). Neurofibromatosis and a few other rare disorders have also been linked to precocious puberty.

GnRH-independent precocious puberty: Follicular ovarian cysts cause most cases; other causes include granulosa-theca cell tumors, adrenal enzyme defects, and McCune-Albright syndrome (a triad of follicular cysts, polyostotic fibrous dysplasia, and café-au-lait spots). Causes of GnRH-independent precocious puberty in boys include certain enzyme defects, familial male gonadotropin-independent precocity (due to an activating mutation of the gene for luteinizing hormone [LH] receptors), testosterone-producing testicular tumors, and occasionally McCune-Albright syndrome.

Rarely in girls and boys, pseudoprecocious puberty results from pituitary adenomas that secrete gonadotropins.

Symptoms, Signs, and Diagnosis

In boys, facial, axillary, and pubic hair appears and the penis grows, with or without enlargement of testes. In girls, breasts develop, and pubic hair, axillary hair, or both appear. Girls may begin to menstruate. Body odor, acne, and behavior changes may develop in either sex. Height growth is initially rapid in both sexes, but premature closure of the epiphyses results in short adult stature. Testicular or ovarian enlargement occurs in precocious puberty but is usually absent in isolated precocious adrenarche.

Diagnosis is clinical. X-rays of the left hand and wrist are done to assess skeletal maturation and check for accelerated bone growth. Unless history and examination suggest an abnormality, no further evaluation is required for children with pubertal milestones that are within 1 yr of population standards or for girls and boys with precocious adrenarche and girls with precocious thelarche as long as x-rays confirm that bone growth is not accelerated.

When further evaluation is necessary, the following serum hormones may be measured: β-human chorionic gonadotropin, estradiol, testosterone, dehydroepiandrosterone, 17-hydroxyprogesterone, LH, follicle-stimulating hormone (FSH), and prolactin. Pelvic and adrenal ultrasonography and MRI or CT of the brain may be done.

A GnRH stimulation test (see p. 2370) confirms a diagnosis of GnRH-independent precocious puberty when gonadotropin responses to exogenous GnRH are prepubertal in boys or girls with no tumor or other obvious cause of early sexual development. If the response is pubertal, CNS lesions must be excluded.

Treatment

If pubertal milestones are within 1 yr of population standards, reassurance and regular reexamination are sufficient. Treatment is not needed for premature adrenarche or thelarche, but regular reexamination is warranted to check for later development of precocious puberty. For GnRH-dependent precocious puberty, pituitary LH and FSH secretion can be suppressed until normal puberty begins with the GnRH agonist leuprolide acetate 0.2 to 0.3 mg/kg (minimum, 7.5 mg) IM q 4 wk. Responses to treatment must be monitored, and drug dosages modified accordingly.

If GnRH-independent precocious puberty in boys is due to familial male gonadotropin-independent precocity or McCune-Albright syndrome, androgen antagonists (eg, spironolactone) ameliorate the effects of excess androgen. The antifungal drug ketoconazole reduces testosterone in boys with familial male gonadotropin-independent precocity. Testolactone, an aromatase inhibitor, reduces serum estradiol and effectively treats girls with McCune-Albright syndrome; alternatively, tamoxifen, an estrogen antagonist, may be beneficial.

If GnRH-independent precocious puberty is due to a hormone-producing tumor (eg, granulosa-theca cell tumors in girls, testicular tumors in boys), such tumor should be excised. However, girls require extended follow-up to check for recurrence in the contralateral ovary.

283 NEUROLOGIC DISORDERS IN CHILDREN

Congenital neurologic anomalies are discussed in Ch. 292 (see p. 2441). Seizures are discussed in Ch. 214 (see p. 1822); meningitis, in Ch. 218 (see p. 1858) and Ch. 279 (see p. 2330).

CEREBRAL PALSY SYNDROMES

Cerebral palsy refers to nonprogressive syndromes characterized by impaired voluntary movement or posture and resulting from prenatal developmental malformations or perinatal or postnatal CNS damage. Syndromes manifest before age 5 yr. Diagnosis is clinical. Treatment may include physical and occupational therapy, braces, drug therapy or botulinum toxin injections, orthopedic surgery, intrathecal baclofen, or, in certain cases, dorsal rhizotomy.

Cerebral palsy (CP) is a group of syndromes that causes nonprogressive spasticity, ataxia, or involuntary movements; it is not a specific disorder or single syndrome. CP syndromes occur in 0.1 to 0.2% of children and affect up to 15% of premature infants.

Etiology

Etiology is multifactorial, and a specific cause is often hard to establish. Prematurity, in utero disorders, neonatal encephalopathy, and kernicterus often contribute. Perinatal factors (eg, perinatal asphyxia, stroke, CNS infections) probably cause 15 to 20% of cases. Common associations include spastic diplegia after premature birth, spastic quadriparesis after perinatal asphyxia, and athetoid and dystonic forms after perinatal asphyxia or kernicterus. CNS trauma or a severe systemic disorder (eg, stroke, meningitis, sepsis, dehydration) during early childhood may also cause a CP syndrome.

Symptoms and Signs

There are 4 main categories: spastic, athetoid, ataxic, and mixed depending on which parts of the CNS are damaged. Before the specific syndrome develops, symptoms include lagging motor development and often persistent infantile reflex patterns, hyperreflexia, and altered muscle tone.

Associated problems are present in about 25% of patients, most often in those with spasticity. Strabismus and other visual defects may occur. Children with athetosis due to kernicterus commonly have nerve deafness and upward gaze paralysis. Many children with spastic hemiplegia or paraplegia have normal intelligence; children with spastic quadriplegia and mixed forms may have disabling mental retardation.

Spastic syndromes occur in > 70% of cases. Spasticity is a state of resistance to passive range of motion; resistance increases with increasing speed of that motion. It is due to upper motor neuron involvement and may mildly or severely affect motor function. These syndromes may produce hemiplegia, quadriplegia, diplegia, or paraplegia. Usually in affected limbs, deep tendon reflexes are increased, muscles are hypertonic, and voluntary movements are weak and poorly coordinated. Joint contractures develop, and joints may become misaligned. A scissors gait and toe walking are typical. In mild cases, impairment may occur only during certain activities (eg, running). Corticobulbar impairment of oral, lingual, and palatal movement, with consequent dysarthria, commonly occurs with quadriplegia.

Athetoid or dyskinetic syndromes occur in about 20% of cases and result from basal ganglia involvement. The syndromes are defined by slow, writhing, involuntary movements of the proximal extremities and trunk (athetoid movements) often activated by attempts at voluntary movement or by excitement. Abrupt, jerky, distal movements (choreic movements) may also occur. Movements increase with emotional tension and disappear during sleep. Dysarthria occurs and is often severe.

Ataxic syndromes occur in < 5% of cases and result from involvement of the cerebellum or its pathways. Weakness, incoordination, and intention tremor produce unsteadiness, a wide-based gait, and difficulty with rapid or fine movements.

Mixed forms are common—most often, spasticity and athetosis.

Diagnosis

CP can rarely be confirmed during early infancy, and the specific syndrome often cannot be characterized until age 2 yr. High-risk children (eg, those with evidence of asphyxia, stroke, periventricular abnormalities seen on cranial ultrasonography in premature infants, jaundice, meningitis, neonatal seizures, hypertonia, hypotonia, or reflex suppression) should be followed closely.

If CP is suspected, cranial MRI is done; it detects abnormalities in most cases.

CP should be differentiated from progressive hereditary neurologic disorders and disorders requiring surgical or other specific neurologic treatments. Ataxic forms are particularly hard to distinguish, and in many children with ataxia, a progressive cerebellar degenerative disorder is ultimately identified as the cause. Athetosis, self-mutilation, and hyperuricemia in boys indicate Lesch-Nyhan syndrome (see p. 2473). Cutaneous or ocular abnormalities may indicate tuberous sclerosis, neurofibromatosis, ataxia-telangiectasia, von Hippel-Lindau disease, or Sturge-Weber syndrome. Infantile spinal muscular atrophy and muscular dystrophies associated with hypotonia and hyporeflexia usually lack signs of cerebral disease. Adrenoleukodystrophy begins later in childhood.

Laboratory tests can exclude certain progressive storage disorders that involve the motor system (eg, Tay-Sachs disease, metachromatic leukodystrophy, mucopolysaccharidoses). Other progressive disorders (eg, infantile neuroaxonal dystrophy) may be suggested by nerve conduction studies and electromyography but must be diagnosed clinically or pathologically. Children with pronounced mental retardation and symmetric motor abnormalities should be evaluated for amino acid and other metabolic abnormalities (see p. 2458).

Prognosis and Treatment

Most children survive to adulthood. Severe limitations in sucking and swallowing, which may require feeding by gastrostomy tube, decrease likelihood of survival. The goal is for children to develop maximal independence within the limits of their motor and associated deficits; with appropriate management, many children, especially those with spastic paraplegia or hemiplegia, can lead near-normal lives.

Physical therapy and occupational therapy for stretching, strengthening, and facilitating good movement patterns are usually used first. Bracing, drug therapy, and surgery are used to treat spasticity. Botulinum toxin may be injected into muscles to decrease their uneven pull at joints and to prevent fixed contractures. Drugs such as baclofen, benzodiazepines (eg, diazepam), tizanidine, and sometimes dantrolene may diminish spasticity. Orthopedic surgery (eg, muscle-tendon release) may help reduce restricted joint motion or misalignment. Intrathecal baclofen (via subcutaneous pump and catheter) is the most effective treatment for severe spasticity. Selective dorsal rhizotomy may help a few children who were premature if spasticity affects primarily the legs and cognitive abilities are good.

When intellectual and physical limitations are not severe, children should attend mainstream schools. However, some children will require varying degrees of lifelong supervision and assistance. Speech training or other forms of facilitated communication may be required. Even severely affected children can benefit from training in activities of daily living (eg, washing, dressing, feeding), which increases their independence and self-esteem and greatly reduces the burden for family members or other caretakers.

Parents of a child with chronic limitations need assistance and guidance in understanding the child's status and potential and in dealing with their own feelings of guilt, anger, denial, and sadness (see p. 2246). Such children reach their maximal potential only with stable, sensible parental care and the assistance of public and private agencies (eg, community health agencies, vocational rehabilitation organizations, lay health organizations such as the United Cerebral Palsy Association).

FEBRILE SEIZURES

Febrile seizures occur in children < 6 yr with body temperature > 38°C and no previous afebrile seizures and that have no other identifiable cause. Diagnosis is clinical after exclusion of other causes. Treatment of seizures lasting < 15 min is supportive. Seizures lasting ≥ 15 min are treated with IV lorazepam and, if persistent, IV fosphenytoin. Maintenance drug therapy is usually not indicated.

Febrile seizures occur in about 2 to 5% of children < 6 yr; most occur at age 6 to 18 mo. Simple febrile seizures last < 15 min and have no focal features, and if they occur in a series, total duration is < 30 min. Complex febrile seizures last > 15 min, have focal features or postictal paresis, or occur in a series with a total duration of > 30 min. Most (> 90%) febrile seizures are simple.

Febrile seizures occur during bacterial or viral infections. They also sometimes occur after certain vaccinations such as diphtheria, tetanus toxoid, and pertussis or measles, mumps, and rubella. Genetic and familial factors may increase susceptibility to febrile seizures. Monozygotic twins have a much higher concordance rate than dizygotic twins.

Symptoms, Signs, and Diagnosis

Often, febrile seizures occur during the initial rapid rise in body temperature, and most develop within 24 h of fever onset. Typically, seizures are generalized; most are clonic, but some manifest as periods of atonic or tonic posturing.

Seizures are diagnosed as febrile after exclusion of other causes. A fever also may trigger seizures in a child with previous afebrile seizures; such events are not termed "febrile seizures" because the child has already demonstrated a tendency to seizures. If children are < 6 mo of age, have meningeal signs or signs of CNS depression, or have seizures after several days of febrile illness, CSF should be analyzed to rule out meningitis and encephalitis. Sometimes, laboratory tests for metabolic abnormalities or disorders should be done. Plasma glucose, Na, Ca, Mg, P, and liver and kidney function tests are done if the history includes recent vomiting, diarrhea, or impaired fluid intake; if there are signs of dehydration or edema; or if a complex febrile seizure occurs. Cranial CT or MRI should be done if examination detects focal features or if there are signs of increased intracranial pressure. EEG typically does not identify specific abnormalities or help predict recurrent seizures; it is not recommended after an initial simple febrile seizure in children with a normal neurologic examination. EEG should be considered after complex or recurrent febrile seizures.

Prognosis and Treatment

Overall recurrence rate is about 35%. Risk of recurrence is higher if children are < 1 yr of age when the initial seizure occurs or have 1st-degree relatives who have had febrile seizures. Risk of developing an afebrile seizure disorder after experiencing febrile seizures is about 2 to 5%.

Treatment is supportive if seizures last < 15 min. Seizures lasting > 15 min require drugs to end them, with careful monitoring of circulatory and respiratory status. Intubation may be necessary if response is not immediate and the seizure persists.

Drug therapy is usually IV, with a short-acting benzodiazepine (eg, lorazepam 0.05 to 0.1 mg/kg repeated q 5 min for up to 3 doses). Fosphenytoin 15 to 20 mg PE (phenytoin equivalents)/kg may be given over 15 min if the seizure persists. Diazepam rectal gel 0.5 mg/kg may be given once and repeated in 20 min if lorazepam cannot be given IV.

Maintenance drug therapy to prevent recurrent febrile seizures or development of afebrile seizures is usually not indicated unless multiple or prolonged episodes have occurred.

NEONATAL SEIZURE DISORDERS

(See also Ch. 214 on p. 1822.)

Neonatal seizures are abnormal electrical discharges in the CNS of neonates usually manifesting as stereotyped muscular activity or autonomic changes. Diagnosis is confirmed by EEG; testing for causative conditions is indicated. Treatment depends on cause.

Seizures occur in up to 1.4% of term infants and 20% of premature infants. Seizures may be a serious neonatal problem and require immediate evaluation. Most neonatal seizures are focal, probably because in neonates generalization of the electrical activity is impeded by lack of myelination and incomplete formation of dendrites and synapses in the brain. Some neonates undergoing EEG for assessment of symptoms of encephalopathy (eg, hypoactivity, decreased responsiveness) are found to have clinically silent seizures (epileptiform electrical activity during an EEG but without any visible seizure activity). Occasionally, clinically silent electrical activity is continuous and persists for > 20 min; at that point, it is defined as electrical status epilepticus.

Etiology

The abnormal CNS electrical discharge may be caused by a primary intracranial process (eg, meningitis, ischemic stroke, encephalitis, intracranial hemorrhage, tumor) or may be secondary to a systemic problem (eg, hypoxia-ischemia, hypoglycemia, hypocalcemia, hyponatremia). Seizures resulting from an intracranial process usually cannot be differentiated from seizures resulting from a systemic problem by their clinical features (eg, focal vs generalized).

Hypoxia-ischemia, the most common cause of neonatal seizures, may occur before, during, or after delivery. Such seizures may be severe and difficult to treat, but they tend to abate after about 3 to 4 days.

Ischemic stroke is more likely in neonates with polycythemia or with thrombophilia due to a genetic disorder but may also occur without any risk factors. Stroke typically occurs in the middle cerebral artery distribution or watershed zones. Seizures resulting from stroke tend to be focal and may cause apnea.

Infections such as meningitis and sepsis may cause seizures; in such cases, seizures are usually accompanied by other symptoms and signs. Group B streptococcus and gram-negative bacteria are common causes of such infections in neonates. Encephalitis due to cytomegalovirus, herpes simplex virus, rubella virus, *Treponema pallidum,* or *Toxoplasma gondii* can also cause seizures.

Hypoglycemia is common among neonates whose mothers have diabetes, who are small for gestational age, or who have hypoxia-ischemia or other stresses. Seizures due to hypoglycemia tend to be focal and variable. Prolonged or recurrent hypoglycemia may permanently affect the CNS.

Intracranial hemorrhage, including subarachnoid, intracerebral, and intraventricular hemorrhage, may cause seizures. Intraventricular hemorrhage, which occurs in premature infants, results from bleeding in the germinal matrix (a region adjacent to the ventricles that gives rise to neurons and glial cells during development).

Hypernatremia or **hyponatremia** may cause seizures. Hypernatremia can result from accidental oral or IV NaCl overload. Hyponatremia can result from dilution (when too much water is given po or IV) or may follow Na loss in stool or urine.

Hypocalcemia (serum Ca level < 7.5 mg/dL [< 1.87 mmol/L]) is usually accompanied by a serum P level of > 3 mg/dL (> 0.95 mmol/L) and can also be asymptomatic. Risk factors for hypocalcemia include prematurity and a difficult birth.

Hypomagnesemia is a rare cause of seizures, which may occur when the serum Mg level is < 1.4 mEq/L (< 0.7 mmol/L). Hypomagnesemia often occurs with hypocalcemia and should be considered in neonates with hypocalcemia if seizures continue after adequate Ca therapy.

Inborn errors of metabolism (eg, amino or organic aciduria) can cause neonatal seizures. Rarely, pyridoxine deficiency or dependency causes seizures; it is readily treated.

Other causes include CNS malformations. Maternal substance abuse (eg, cocaine, heroin, diazepam) is an increasingly common problem; seizures can occur with acute withdrawal after birth. Neonatal seizures may be familial; some have genetic causes.

Symptoms and Signs

Neonatal seizures are usually focal and may be difficult to recognize. Migratory clonic jerks of extremities, alternating hemi-seizures, or primitive subcortical seizures (which cause respiratory arrest, chewing movements, persistent eye deviations or nystagmoid movements, episodic changes in muscle tone) are common. Generalized tonic-clonic seizures are uncommon.

Clinically silent electrical seizure activity is often present after a hypoxic-ischemic insult including perinatal asphyxia or stroke and in neonates with CNS infections.

Jitteriness (alternating contraction and relaxation of opposing muscles in the extremities) must be distinguished from true seizure activity. Jitteriness is usually stimulus-induced and can be stopped by holding the extremity still. Seizures occur spontaneously, and motor activity is felt even when the limb is held still.

Diagnosis

Evaluation begins with a detailed family history and a physical examination. EEG (waking and sleep) is essential, especially when it is difficult to determine whether the neonate is having seizures; EEG is also helpful for monitoring response to treatment. EEG should capture periods of active and quiet sleep and thus may require ≥ 2 h of recording. A normal EEG with expected variation during sleep is a good prognostic sign; an EEG with diffuse severe abnormalities (eg, suppressed voltage or burst suppression pattern) is a poor one.

Other tests should include pulse oximetry; measurement of plasma glucose, Na, K, Cl, HCO_3, Ca, and Mg; and lumbar puncture for CSF analysis (cell count and differential, glucose, protein) and culture. Urine and blood cultures are obtained. The need for other metabolic tests (eg, arterial pH, blood gases, serum bilirubin, urine amino or organic acids) or tests for commonly abused drugs (passed to the neonate transplacentally or by breast-feeding) depends on the clinical situation.

Most infants should have a head CT because it can detect intracranial bleeding and some brain malformations. Cranial ultrasonography may detect intraventricular bleeding but not subarachnoid bleeding; it may be preferred as a bedside test for very sick infants who cannot be moved to radiology. Diffusion-weighted MRI may detect ischemic tissue within a few hours but is usually done after the 2nd day to look for parenchymal damage.

Prognosis

About 50% of neonates with seizures due to hypoxia-ischemia develop normally. Most neonates with seizures due to subarachnoid hemorrhage, hypocalcemia, or hyponatremia do well. Those with severe intraventricular hemorrhage have a high morbidity rate. For idiopathic seizures or seizures due to malformations, earlier onset is associated with higher morbidity and mortality rates.

Whether neonatal seizures cause damage beyond that caused by the underlying disorder is unknown, although there is concern that the metabolic stress of prolonged nerve cell firing during lengthy seizures may cause additional brain damage. When caused by hypoxia-ischemia, stroke, or infection, neonates may have a series of seizures, but seizures typically abate after about 3 to 4 days; they may recur months to years later if brain damage has occurred. Seizures from other causes may be more persistent in the neonatal period.

Treatment

Treatment focuses primarily on the underlying disorder and secondarily on seizures.

For low plasma glucose, 10% dextrose 2 mL/kg IV is given, and plasma glucose level is monitored; additional infusions are given as needed. For hypocalcemia, 10% Ca gluconate 1 mL/kg IV (9 mg/kg of elemental Ca) is given; this dose can be repeated for persistent hypocalcemic seizures. Rate of Ca gluconate infusion should not exceed 50 mg/min; continuous cardiac monitoring is necessary during the infusion. Extravasation should be avoided because skin may slough. For hypomagnesemia, 0.2 mL/kg of a 50% Mg sulfate solution is given IM. Bacterial infections are treated with antibiotics.

Anticonvulsants are used unless seizures stop quickly after correction of hypoglycemia, hypocalcemia, hypomagnesemia, hyponatremia, hypernatremia, or other underlying disorders. Phenobarbital is the drug of choice; a loading dose of 20 mg/kg IV is given. If seizures continue, 5 mg/kg can be given q 30 min until seizures cease or until a maximum of 40 mg/kg is given. Maintenance therapy is started about 12 h later at 1.5 to 2 mg/kg bid and increased to 2.5 mg/kg bid based on clinical or EEG response or serum drug levels. Phenobarbital is continued IV, especially if seizures are frequent or prolonged. When seizures are controlled, phenobarbital can be given orally. Therapeutic serum levels of phenobarbital are 15 to 40 μg/mL (65 to 170 μmol/L).

If a 2nd drug is needed, fosphenytoin or phenytoin is used. The loading dose is 20 mg PE (phenytoin equivalents)/kg IV. It is given over 15 min to avoid hypotension or arrhythmias. A maintenance dose is then started at 2 to 3 mg/kg q 12 h and adjusted based on clinical response or serum levels. Therapeutic serum levels for phenytoin are 10 to 20 μg/mL (40 to 80 μmol/L).

Lorazepam 0.1 mg/kg IV may be used for resistant seizures and repeated at 5- to 10-min intervals, up to 3 doses in any 8-h period.

Neonates given IV anticonvulsants are closely observed; overmedication may result in respiratory depression.

NEUROFIBROMATOSIS

Neurofibromatosis is an autosomal dominant disorder producing tumors along the course of nerves and occasionally resulting in marked soft tissue or bony deformity. Diagnosis is clinical. There is no specific treatment, but tumors can be removed surgically.

Neurofibromatosis has 2 forms. Type 1 (von Recklinghausen's disease) is most prevalent, causing neurologic, cutaneous, and sometimes orthopedic manifestations. Type 2 accounts for 10% of cases, manifesting primarily as congenital bilateral acoustic neuroma.

Neurofibromas are benign tumors consisting of Schwann cells and neural fibroblasts. Peripheral neurofibromas develop anywhere along the course of peripheral nerves. Most appear during adolescence. There are 4 types. Cutaneous neurofibromas are soft and fleshy; subcutaneous neurofibromas are firm and nodular. Nodular plexiform neurofibromas may involve spinal nerve roots, typically growing through an intervertebral foramen to produce intraspinal and extraspinal masses (dumbbell tumor). The intraspinal part may compress the spinal cord. Diffuse plexiform neurofibromas can be disfiguring and may produce deficits distal to the neuroma. Plexiform neurofibromas can undergo malignant transformation. There are 2 types of central (cranial nerve) neurofibromas: optic gliomas, which may cause progressive blindness, and acoustic neuromas (vestibular schwannomas), which may cause dizziness, ataxia, deafness, and tinnitus. Optic gliomas occur in type 1 neurofibromatosis, whereas acoustic neuromas occur in type 2 neurofibromatosis.

Symptoms and Signs

Type 1: With type 1, most patients are asymptomatic and identified during routine examination, examination for cosmetic complaints, or when evaluating a positive family history. Some present with neurologic symptoms or bony abnormalities. In > 90%, characteristic skin lesions are apparent at birth or develop during infancy. Lesions are medium-brown (café-au-lait), freckle-like macules, distributed most commonly over the trunk, pelvis, and flexor creases of elbows and knees. During late childhood, flesh-colored cutaneous tumors of various sizes and shapes appear, ranging in number from several to thousands. Rarely, plexiform neuromas (subcutaneous nodules or amorphous overgrowth of underlying bone or Schwann cells) develop, producing an irregularly thickened, distorted structure with grotesque deformities.

Neurologic symptoms are varied but relate to location and number of neurofibromas. Skeletal anomalies include fibrous dysplasia, subperiosteal bone cysts, vertebral scalloping, scoliosis, thinning of the long-bone cortex, pseudarthrosis, and absence of the greater wing of the sphenoid bone (posterior orbital wall), with consequent pulsating exophthalmos. An optic glioma and Lisch nodules (iris hamartomas) occur in some patients. Some children have learning problems and slightly larger heads.

Type 2: In type 2, bilateral acoustic neuromas develop and become symptomatic in childhood or early adulthood. They cause hearing loss and unsteadiness, and sometimes headache or facial weakness. Bilateral 8th cranial (vestibulocochlear) nerve masses may be present. Family members may have gliomas, meningiomas, or schwannomas.

Diagnosis and Treatment

Diagnosis is clinical (see TABLE 283–1). CT or MRI may detect 8th cranial nerve masses in type 2; MRI may show focal density changes in type 1. Genetic testing is not routinely available.

No general treatment is available. Neurofibromas that produce severe symptoms may

TABLE 283–1. DIAGNOSING NEUROFIBROMATOSIS

TYPE	CRITERIA
1	Two or more of the following must be present:
	≥ 6 café-au-lait macules with a diameter at the widest point of > 5 mm in prepubertal patients and > 15 mm in postpubertal patients
	≥ 2 neurofibromas of any type or 1 plexiform neurofibroma
	Freckling in the axillary or inguinal region
	Optic glioma
	≥ 2 Lisch nodules (iris hamartomas)
	A distinctive osseous lesion (eg, sphenoid dysplasia or thinning of long-bone cortex), with or without pseudarthrosis
	A parent, sibling, or child with diagnosed type 1 neurofibromatosis
2	One of the following must be present:
	Bilateral 8th nerve masses seen with CT or MRI
	A parent, sibling, or child with type 2 neurofibromatosis and either a unilateral 8th nerve mass or any 2 of the following: neurofibroma, meningioma, glioma, schwannoma, or juvenile posterior subcapsular lenticular opacity

Adapted from Martuza RL, Eldredge R: Neurofibromatosis 2 (bilateral acoustic neurofibromatosis). Reprinted by permission of *The New England Journal of Medicine* 318:684–688, 1988.

require surgical removal or irradiation, although surgery may obliterate function of the involved nerve. Genetic counseling is advisable. If either parent has neurofibromatosis, risk to subsequent offspring is 50%; if neither has it, subsequent risk is unclear because new mutations are common.

TOURETTE'S SYNDROME

(Gilles de la Tourette's Syndrome)

Tourette's syndrome is a hereditary tic disorder that begins in childhood. Symptoms include simple, complex, and vocal tics. Diagnosis is clinical. Treatment may include clonidine or antipsychotics.

Tourette's syndrome is probably autosomal dominant with variable penetrance; the specific genetic abnormality is unknown. Male:female ratio is 3:1. Simple transient tics and Tourette's syndrome form a continuum or spectrum.

Symptoms and Signs

The movement disorder may begin with simple tics (eg, facial grimacing, head jerking, blinking, sniffing) that progress to multiple complex tics, including respiratory and vocal ones (eg, loud, irritating vocalizations; snorting). Vocal tics may begin as grunting or barking noises and evolve into compulsive utterances that are often loud or shrill. Patients may voluntarily suppress tics for seconds or minutes. Coprolalia (involuntary scatologic or obscene utterances) occurs in a few patients. Severe tics and coprolalia are physically and socially disabling. Echolalia (immediate repetition of one's own or another person's words or phrases) is common.

Diagnosis

Diagnosis is clinical. To differentiate Tourette's syndrome from transient tics, physicians may have to monitor patients over time. Comorbid disorders (eg, attention-deficit/hyperactivity disorder, obsessive-compulsive disorder, learning disabilities) are common and may add to the patient's burden.

Treatment

Clonidine 0.05 to 0.1 mg po tid or qid is effective in some patients. Adverse effects of fatigue may limit dosage; hypotension is uncommon. Antipsychotics (eg, risperidone 0.25 mg to 1 mg po bid or tid, haloperidol 0.5 to 2 mg po bid or tid, pimozide 1 to 2 mg po bid, olanzapine 2.5 mg to 5 mg once/day) may be required. The lowest dose required to make tics tolerable is used; doses are tapered as tics wane. Adverse effects of dysphoria, parkinsonism, akathisia, and tardive dyskinesia may limit use of antipsychotics; using lower daytime doses and higher bedtime doses may decrease adverse effects.

TUBEROUS SCLEROSIS

Tuberous sclerosis is a dominantly inherited genetic disorder in which tumors (usually hamartomas) affect multiple organs.

Children with tuberous sclerosis (TS or TS complex) have tumors of multiple organs. If either parent has TS, there is a 50% chance a child will have it. New mutations, however, account for most new cases. TS may affect the heart, eyes, lungs, and skin.

Symptoms and Signs

Affected children may have epilepsy, mental retardation, autism, learning disorders, or behavioral problems. Infants may present with a type of seizure called infantile spasms (see p. 1825). Many children have kidney tumors, usually angiomyolipomas, which can cause hypertension and cystic kidney disease. Renal carcinoma can also occur. Some children also have cardiac rhabdomyomas. Brain tubers (gyral enlargements) and tumors, usually astrocytomas, can occur. Retinal patches are common.

Skin findings include initially pale, ash leaf–shaped macules, which develop in infancy or early childhood; angiofibromas of the face (adenoma sebaceum), which develop in later childhood; congenital shagreen patches (raised lesions that have an orange-peel consistency and usually appear on the back); subcutaneous nodules; café-au-lait spots; and subungual fibromas, which can develop any time in childhood or early adulthood.

Diagnosis

Cardiac or cranial manifestations may be visible on prenatal ultrasounds. Retinal patches may be visible with funduscopy. MRI or ultrasound of the affected organs is necessary for confirmation. Specific genetic testing is available.

Prognosis and Treatment

Prognosis depends on symptom severity. Infants with mild symptoms generally do well and live long, productive lives, whereas infants with more severe symptoms may have serious disabilities. Regardless of severity, most children show continued developmental progress. Occasionally, neurologic degeneration may occur and requires investigation.

Treatment is symptomatic and may include anticonvulsants, or even brain surgery, for seizures. Skin lesions may be removed with dermabrasion or laser techniques. Drugs may be used for neurobehavioral problems and hypertension caused by renal problems, and surgery may be used to remove growing tumors. Genetic counseling is indicated for adolescents and adults of childbearing age.

284 BONE AND CONNECTIVE TISSUE DISORDERS IN CHILDREN

Many bone and connective tissue disorders, particularly those affecting lower extremities, result from the dramatic changes that occur in a growing child's musculoskeletal system. These disorders may resolve or worsen with continued growth. Other bone and connective tissue disorders may be inherited or acquired. For congenital abnormalities, see Ch. 288 on p. 2421; for Juvenile Rheumatoid Arthritis, see Ch. 34 on p. 289.

CONGENITAL HYPOPHOSPHATASIA

Congenital hypophosphatasia is absence or low levels of serum alkaline phosphatase due to mutations in the gene encoding tissue nonspecific alkaline phosphatase.

Because serum alkaline phosphatase is absent or decreased, Ca is not diffusely deposited in bones, causing low bone density and hypercalcemia. Vomiting, inability to gain weight, and enlargement of the epiphyses (similar to that in rickets) usually occur. Patients who survive infancy have bony deformities and short stature, but mental development is normal. No treatment is effective, but infusions of alkaline phosphatase and bone marrow transplantation have limited roles. NSAIDs reduce bone pain.

CUTIS LAXA

Cutis laxa is characterized by lax skin hanging in loose folds. Diagnosis is clinical. There is no specific treatment, but plastic surgery is sometimes done.

Two hereditary forms (one autosomal dominant, one autosomal recessive) are relatively benign. Another autosomal recessive form causes potentially lethal cardiovascular, respiratory, and GI complications.

Rarely, acquired cutis laxa occurs in infants after a febrile illness or after exposure to a specific drug (eg, hypersensitivity reaction to penicillin, fetal exposure to penicillamine). In children or adolescents, cutis laxa usually develops after a severe illness involving fever, polyserositis, or erythema multiforme. In adults, it may develop insidiously. The underlying defect is unknown, but fragmented elastin is present in all forms.

Symptoms and Signs

In hereditary forms, dermal laxity may be present at birth or develop later; it occurs wherever the skin is normally loose and hanging in folds, most obviously on the face. Affected children have mournful or Churchillian facies and a hooked nose. The benign autosomal recessive form causes developmental retardation and joint laxity. GI tract hernias and diverticula are common. If the disorder is severe, progressive pulmonary emphysema may precipitate cor pulmonale.

Diagnosis and Treatment

Diagnosis is clinical. Typical cutis laxa can be distinguished from Ehlers-Danlos syndrome because dermal fragility and articular hypermobility are absent. Other disorders sometimes cause localized areas of loose skin: In Turner's syndrome, lax skinfolds at the base of an affected girl's neck tighten and resemble webbing as she ages; in neurofibromatosis, unilateral pendular plexiform neuromas occasionally develop, but their configuration and texture distinguish them from cutis laxa.

There is no specific treatment. Plastic surgery considerably improves appearance in patients with hereditary cutis laxa but is less successful in those with acquired cutis laxa. Healing is usually uncomplicated, but dermal laxity may recur. Extracutaneous complications are treated appropriately.

EHLERS-DANLOS SYNDROME

Ehlers-Danlos syndrome is a hereditary collagen disorder characterized by articular hypermobility, dermal hyperelasticity, and widespread tissue fragility. Diagnosis is clinical. Treatment is supportive.

Inheritance is usually autosomal dominant, but Ehlers-Danlos syndrome is heterogeneous: Different gene mutations affect the amount, structure, or assembly of different collagens. There are 5 major types plus several rare or hard-to-classify types.

Symptoms, Signs, and Diagnosis

Symptoms and signs vary widely. Skin can be stretched several centimeters but returns to normal when released. Wide papyraceous scars often overlie bony prominences, particularly elbows, knees, and shins; scarring is less severe in the hypermobility type. Molluscoid pseudotumors (fleshy outgrowths) frequently form on top of scars or at pressure points. Extent of joint hypermobility varies but may be marked in the arthrochalasis, classical, and hypermobility types. Bleeding tendency is rare, although the vascular type is characterized by vascular rupture and bruising. Subcutaneous calcified spherules may be palpated or seen on x-rays.

Minor trauma may cause wide gaping wounds but little bleeding; surgical wound closure may be difficult because sutures tend to tear out of the fragile tissue. Surgical complications occur because of deep tissue fragility. Sclera may be fragile, leading to perforation of the globe in the ocular-kyphoscoliotic type.

Bland synovial effusions, sprains, and dislocations occur frequently. Spinal kyphoscoliosis occurs in 25% of patients (especially those with the ocular-kyphoscoliotic type), thoracic deformity in 20%, and talipes equinovarum in 5%. About 90% of affected adults have pes planus (flat feet). Congenital hip dislocation occurs in 1% (the arthrochalasis type is characterized by bilateral congenital hip dislocation).

GI hernias and diverticula are common. Rarely, portions of the GI tract spontaneously hemorrhage and perforate, and dissecting aortic aneurysm and large arteries spontaneously rupture. In pregnant women, tissue extensibility may cause premature birth; if the fetus is affected, fetal membrane is fragile, sometimes resulting in early rupture. Maternal tissue fragility may complicate episiotomy or cesarean section. Antenatal, perinatal, and postnatal bleeding may occur. Other potentially serious complications include arteriovenous fistula, ruptured viscus, and pneumothorax or pneumohemothorax.

Although genetic and biochemical tests are available for some types, diagnosis is still largely based on clinical evaluation using major and minor criteria, which distinguish among the different types.

Prognosis and Treatment

Life span is usually normal. Potentially lethal complications occur in certain types (eg, arterial rupture in the vascular type).

There is no specific treatment. Trauma should be minimized. Protective clothing and padding may help. If surgery is done, hemostasis must be meticulous. Wounds are carefully sutured, and tissue tension is avoided. Obstetric supervision during pregnancy and delivery is mandatory. Genetic counseling should be provided.

IDIOPATHIC SCOLIOSIS

Idiopathic scoliosis is lateral curvature of the spine.

Idiopathic scoliosis can be detected in 2 to 3% of children aged 10 to 16 yr; 60 to 80% are girls.

Symptoms and Signs

Scoliosis may first be suspected when one shoulder seems higher than the other or when clothes do not hang straight, but it is often detected during routine physical examination. Patients may initially report fatigue in the lumbar region after prolonged sitting or standing. Muscular backaches in areas of strain (eg, in the lumbosacral angle) may follow.

Diagnosis and Treatment

The curve is most pronounced when patients bend forward. Most curves are convex to the right in the thoracic area and to the left in the lumbar area, so that the right shoulder is higher than the left. X-ray examination should include standing anteroposterior and lateral views of the spine.

The greater the curve, the greater the likelihood that it will progress after the skeleton matures. Curves > 10° are considered significant. Prognosis depends on site and severity of the curve and age at symptom onset. Significant intervention is required in < 10% of patients.

Prompt referral to an orthopedist is indicated. Moderate curves (20 to 40°) are treated conservatively (eg, with a cast or Milwaukee brace) to prevent further deformity. Severe curves (> 40°) can often be ameliorated surgically (eg, spinal fusion with rod placement). Scoliosis and its treatment often interfere with an adolescent's self-image and self-esteem. Counseling or psychotherapy may be needed.

KNEE PAIN

Knee pain with swelling over the tibial tubercle in adolescents is usually due to Osgood-Schlatter disease (see p. 2387). Chondromalacia patellae (softening of the patellar articular cartilage) often causes more generalized knee pain, without swelling, especially when climbing or descending stairs, playing sports that exert an axial load on the knees, or sitting for a long time. This disorder probably results from angular or rotational changes in the leg that unbalance elements of the quadriceps and cause patellar misalignment during movement. Knee pain with infrapatellar tendon tenderness in physically active children is most likely caused by infrapatellar tendinitis (jumper's knee), an overuse syndrome that usually occurs in figure skaters and basketball or volleyball players.

Acute pain from chondromalacia patellae and infrapatellar tendinitis is treated by applying ice and taking analgesics. Children with chondromalacia patellae or infrapatellar tendinitis should avoid pain-producing activities (typically, those that involve bending the knee) for several days. Persistent or recurrent pain from chondromalacia patellae can often be relieved by arthroscopic smoothing of the patella's undersurface.

MARFAN SYNDROME

Marfan syndrome consists of connective tissue anomalies resulting in ocular, skeletal, and cardiovascular abnormalities (eg, dilation of ascending aorta, which can lead to aortic dissection). Diagnosis is clinical. Treatment may include prophylactic β-blockers to slow dilation of the ascending aorta or prophylactic aortic surgery.

Inheritance is autosomal dominant. The basic biomolecular defect results from mutations in *FBN-1*, the gene encoding the glycoprotein fibrillin-1, which is the main component of microfibrils and helps anchor cells to the extracellular matrix. The principal structural defect involves the aortic media. Uncommon variants result from mutations in the gene encoding fibrillin-2.

Symptoms and Signs

Severity varies greatly. Patients are taller than average for age and family; arm span exceeds height. Arachnodactyly (disproportionately long, thin digits) is noticeable, often by the thumb sign (the distal phalanx of the thumb protrudes beyond the edge of the clenched fist). Sternum deformity—pectus carinatum (outward displacement) or pectus excavatum (inward displacement)—is common, as are joint hyperextensibility, genu recurvatum (backward curvature of the legs at the knees), flat feet, kyphoscoliosis, and diaphragmatic and inguinal hernias. Subcutaneous fat usually is sparse. The palate is often high-arched.

Ocular findings include ectopia lentis (subluxation or upward dislocation of the lens) and iridodonesis (tremulousness of the iris). The margin of the dislocated lens can often be seen through the undilated pupil. High-grade myopia may be present, and spontaneous retinal detachment sometimes occurs.

Most severe complications result from pathologic changes in the aortic root and ascending aorta. The aortic media is affected preferentially in areas subject to the greatest hemodynamic stress. The aorta progressively dilates or acutely dissects, beginning in the coronary sinuses, sometimes before age 10 yr. The aortic root dilates in 50% of children and 60 to 80% of adults and can cause aortic regurgitation. Bacterial endocarditis may develop. Redundant cusps and chordae tendineae may lead to mitral valve prolapse or regurgitation, producing systolic clicks and a late systolic murmur. Cystic lung disease and recurrent spontaneous pneumothorax may occur.

Manifestations in patients with mutation of the gene encoding fibrillin-2 include congenital contractural arachnodactyly, joint hypermobility, and external ear malformations.

Diagnosis

Diagnosis can be difficult because many patients have few typical symptoms and signs and no specific histologic or biochemical changes. Considering this variability, diagnostic criteria are based on constellations of clinical findings and family and genetic history (see TABLE 284–1). Nonetheless, diagnosis is uncertain in many partial cases of Marfan syndrome. Homocystinuria can partially mimic Marfan syndrome but can be differentiated by detecting homocystine in the urine. Prenatal diagnosis by linkage analysis of the *FBN1* gene mutation is hampered by poor genotype/phenotype correlation.

Treatment

Treatment focuses on prevention and treatment of complications. For very tall girls, inducing precocious puberty by age 10 with estrogens and progesterone may reduce potential adult height. All patients should routinely be given β-blockers (eg, atenolol, propranolol) to help prevent cardiovascular complications. These drugs lower myocardial contractility and pulse pressure and reduce progression of aortic root dilation and risk of dissection. Prophylactic surgery is offered if aortic diameter is > 5 cm (less in children). Pregnant women are at especially high risk of aortic complications; elective aortic repair before conception should be discussed. Bacterial endocarditis prophylaxis is indicated before invasive dental and GI procedures (see TABLES 77–3, 77–4, and 77–5 on pp. 730–731).

Cardiovascular, skeletal, and ocular findings should be re-evaluated annually. Together, these measures can improve quality of life and reduce mortality risk; life expectancy has increased from 33 yr in the early 1970s to 61 yr in 1996. Appropriate genetic counseling is indicated.

NAIL-PATELLA SYNDROME

(Osteo-Onychodysplasia; Arthro-Onychodysplasia; Onycho-Osteodysplasia)

Nail-patella syndrome is a rare inherited disorder of mesenchymal tissue characterized by abnormalities of bones, joints, fingernails and toenails, and kidneys.

Nail-patella syndrome is an autosomal dominant disorder caused by a mutation in the homeobox gene *LMX1B*. It encodes a transcription factor that plays important roles in vertebrate limb and kidney development.

There is bilateral hypoplasia or absence of the patella, subluxation of the radial head at the elbows, and bilateral accessory iliac horns. Fingernails and toenails are absent or hypoplastic, with pitting and ridges.

Renal dysfunction occurs in up to 50% of patients due to focal, segmental glomerular deposits of IgM and C3. Proteinuria is the most common manifestation, but about 30% of those with renal involvement slowly progress to renal failure.

Diagnosis is suggested clinically; sometimes renal biopsy is indicated, which is diagnostic. *LMX1B* mutation analysis is possible, including for prenatal diagnosis, but the type of mutation does not usually predict clinical severity. There is no specific treatment, but when indicated, kidney transplantation has been successful without evidence of recurrent disease in the graft.

OSTEOCHONDRODYSPLASIAS

(Genetic Skeletal Dysplasias)

Osteochondrodysplasias involve abnormal bone or cartilage growth leading to skeletal maldevelopment, often short-limbed dwarfism. Diagnosis is by physical examination, x-rays, and, in some cases, genetic testing. Treatment is surgical.

In most types of osteochondrodysplasia, the basic defect is unknown; abnormal type II collagen is implicated in a few rare types.

TABLE 284–1. DIAGNOSTIC CRITERIA FOR MARFAN SYNDROME (GHENT NOSOLOGY)

ORGAN SYSTEM	MAJOR CRITERIA	MINOR CRITERIA	NEEDED FOR INVOLVEMENT
Cardiovascular	One of the following: Dilation of ascending aorta and sinuses of Valsalva Aortic dissection	Mitral valve prolapse Annulus mitralis calcification in patients < 40 yr Pulmonary artery dilation Descending or abdominal aorta dilation or dissection in patients < 50 yr	One major or 1 minor criterion
Dura	Lumbosacral dural ectasia (detected by MRI or CT)	N/A	One major criterion
Family/genetic history	First-degree relative with Marfan syndrome Presence of the *FBN1* mutation known to cause Marfan syndrome	N/A	One major criterion*
Musculoskeletal	Four of the following: Pectus carinatum Pectus excavatum requiring surgery Arm span/height ratio > 1.05 or upper segment/lower segment ratio < 0.86 (in adults) Wrist and thumb signs Scoliosis > 20° or spondylolisthesis Elbow extension < 170° Pes planus Protrusio acetabuli	Typical facies (dolichocephaly, malar hypoplasia, enophthalmos, retrognathia, down-slanting palpebral fissures) Joint hypermobility Pectus excavatum not requiring surgery High-arched palate with crowded teeth	Two of the 8 components comprising the major criteria or 1 of these plus 2 minor criteria
Ocular	Ectopia lentis (lens dislocation)	Myopia Flat cornea Iris or ciliary muscle hypoplasia	Two minor criteria
Pulmonary	N/A	Pneumothorax Apical blebs (seen on chest x-ray)	One minor criterion
Skin	N/A	Atrophic striae not secondary to pregnancy or weight change Recurrent or incisional hernia	One minor criterion

See table footnote on the following page.

Dwarfism is markedly short stature (adult height < 4 ft 10 in) frequently associated with disproportionate growth of trunk and extremities. Achondroplasia is the most common and best-known type of short-limbed dwarfism, but there are many other distinct types, which differ widely in genetic background, course, and prognosis (see TABLE 284–2). Lethal short-limbed dwarfism (thanatophoric dysplasia) causes severe chest wall deformities and respiratory failure in neonates, resulting in death.

Diagnosis and Treatment

Characteristic radiographic changes may be diagnostic. A whole-body x-ray of every affected neonate, even if stillborn, should be taken because diagnostic precision is essential for predicting prognosis. Prenatal diagnosis by fetoscopy or ultrasonography is possible in some cases (eg, when fetal limb shortening is severe). Standard laboratory tests do not help, but molecular diagnosis is feasible for achondroplasia (due to *FGFR3* mutation) and disorders associated with defects in the *DTDST* gene (eg, diastrophic dysplasia, multiple epiphyseal dysplasia, atelosteogenesis type 2, achondrogenesis 1B).

For some nonlethal types, surgery (eg, prosthetic hip replacement) may help improve function. Hypoplasia of the odontoid process can predispose to subluxation of the 1st and 2nd cervical vertebrae and compression of the spinal cord. Therefore, the odontoid process should be evaluated preoperatively, and if it is abnormal, the patient's head should be carefully supported when hyperextended for endotracheal intubation during anesthesia.

Because the inheritance pattern in most types is known, genetic counseling can be effective. Organizations such as Little People of America (www.lpaonline.org) provide resources for affected people and act as advocates on their behalf. Similar societies are active in other countries.

OSTEOCHONDROSES

Osteochondroses are noninflammatory, noninfectious derangements of bony growth at various ossification centers occurring during their greatest developmental activity and affecting the epiphyses.

Etiology is unknown, and inheritance is complex. Osteochondroses differ in their anatomic distribution, course, and prognosis; they typically cause pain and have important orthopedic implications. Rare osteochondroses and the involved bones include Freiberg's disease (head of 2nd metatarsal), Panner's disease (capitulum), Blount disease (proximal tibia), Sever's disease (calcaneus), and Sindling-Larsen-Johansson syndrome (patella).

KÖHLER'S BONE DISEASE

Köhler's bone disease is osteochondrosis of the tarsal navicular bone.

Köhler's bone disease is rare, affects children aged 3 to 5 yr (more commonly boys), and is unilateral. The foot becomes swollen and painful; tenderness is maximal over the medial longitudinal arch. Weight bearing and walking increase discomfort, and gait is disturbed. On x-rays, the navicular bone is initially flattened and sclerotic

---

*Family/genetic history is considered contributory.

N/A = not applicable.

If family/genetic history is not contributory, index case diagnosis requires major criteria in 2 organ systems and involvement in a 3rd. Alternatively, if a mutation known to cause Marfan syndrome is present, index case diagnosis requires 1 major criterion in 1 organ system and involvement in a 2nd. Diagnosis of an index case's relative requires 1 major criterion in family history, 1 major criterion in 1 organ system, and involvement in a 2nd. Minor criteria are used only to score organ system involvement and in themselves do not count toward the diagnosis.

Adapted from De Paepe A, Devereux RB, Dietz HC, et el: Revised criteria for Marfan syndrome. *American Journal of Medical Genetics* 62:417–426, 1996; Loeys B, Nuytinck L, Delvaux I, De Bie S, De Paepe A: Genotype and phenotype analysis of 171 patients referred for molecular study of the fibrillin-1 gene *FBN1* because of suspected Marfan syndrome. *Archives of Internal Medicine* 161:2447–2454, 2001.

TABLE 248–2. TYPES OF OSTEOCHONDRODYSPLASTIC DWARFISM

DISORDER	SYMPTOMS AND SIGNS	USUAL MODE OF INHERITANCE	REPORTED CASES
Achondroplasia	Bulky forehead, saddle nose, lumbar lordosis, bowlegs	AD	Common
Chondrodysplasia punctata	Variable extraskeletal manifestations; radiographic epiphyseal stippling in infancy from calcifications	See below	See below
Chondrodysplasia punctata, rhizomelic form	Marked proximal limb shortening; death during infancy	AR	30
Chondrodysplasia punctata, Conradi-Hünermann form	Mild asymmetric limb shortening; benign	AD or XL dominant	100
Chondroectodermal dysplasia (Ellis-van Creveld syndrome)	Distal limb shortening, postaxial polydactyly, structural cardiac defects	AR	100
Diastrophic dysplasia	Severe dwarfism with rigid hitchhiker thumb and fixed talipes equinovarum	AR	200
Hypochondroplasia	Symptoms of achondroplasia but milder	AD	100
Mesomelic dysplasia*	Predominantly, shortening of the forearms and shanks; normal facies and spine	AD or AR	50
Metaphyseal chondrodysplasia†	In some forms, malabsorption, neutropenia, thymolymphopenia	AR or AD	200
Multiple epiphyseal dysplasia	Mild dwarfism, normal spine and facies, sometimes stubby digits, hip dysplasia (often as 1st symptom); very heterogeneous	AD	Common
Pseudoachondroplasia	Normal facies, various degrees of dwarfism and kyphoscoliosis; heterogeneous	AD or AR	200
Spondyloepiphyseal dysplasia	Predominantly, kyphoscoliosis; sometimes myopia and a flat facies; heterogeneous	AD, AR, or XL	100

*There are several eponymous forms (eg, Nievergelt, Langer).
†There are many different eponymous forms (eg, Jansen, Schmid, McKusick).

AD = autosomal dominant; AR = autosomal recessive; XL = X-linked.

and later becomes fragmented, before reossification. X-rays comparing the affected with the unaffected side help assess progression.

The course is chronic, but the disease rarely persists ≥ 2 yr. Rest, pain relief, and avoiding excessive weight bearing are required. In acute cases, a few weeks in a below-knee walking plaster cast, well molded under the longitudinal arch, may help.

LEGG-CALVÉ-PERTHES DISEASE

Legg-Calvé-Perthes disease is idiopathic aseptic necrosis of the femoral capital epiphysis.

Legg-Calvé-Perthes disease is the most common osteochondrosis, has a maximum incidence at age 5 to 10 yr, is more common among boys, and is usually unilateral. About 10% of cases are familial. Characteristic symptoms are pain in the hip joint and gait disturbance; onset is gradual, and progression is slow. Joint movements are limited, and thigh muscles may become wasted.

Diagnosis and Treatment

Diagnosis is suspected based on symptoms. Bone scan or MRI should be done to confirm the diagnosis. X-rays initially may not be useful, because they can be normal or show minimal flattening. Later x-rays can show fragmentation of the femoral head, which contains areas of lucency and sclerosis.

In bilateral or familial cases, a skeletal survey to exclude hereditary skeletal disorders, particularly multiple epiphyseal dysplasia, is mandatory because prognosis and optimal management differ. Hypothyroidism, sickle cell anemia, and trauma must also be excluded.

Without treatment, the course is usually prolonged but self-limited (usually 2 to 3 yr). When the disease eventually becomes quiescent, residual distortion of the femoral head and acetabulum predisposes to secondary degenerative osteoarthritis. With treatment, sequelae are less severe.

Orthopedic treatment includes prolonged bed rest, mobile traction, slings, and abduction plaster casts and splints to contain the femoral head. Some experts advocate subtrochanteric osteotomy with internal fixation and early ambulation.

Osgood-Schlatter Disease

Osgood-Schlatter disease is osteochondrosis of the tibial tubercle.

Osgood-Schlatter disease occurs between ages 10 and 15 yr, is more common among boys, and is usually unilateral. Etiology is thought to be trauma due to excessive traction by the patellar tendon on its immature epiphyseal insertion. Characteristic symptoms are pain, swelling, and tenderness over the tibial tubercle at the patellar tendon insertion. There is no systemic disturbance.

Diagnosis and Treatment

Diagnosis is by examination. Lateral knee x-rays show fragmentation of the tibial tubercle. However, x-rays are not needed unless pain and swelling extend beyond the area over the tibial tubercle or unless pain is accompanied by redness and warmth. In such cases, x-rays are useful to rule out injuries or acute inflammatory conditions.

Resolution is usually spontaneous within weeks or months. Usually, taking analgesics and avoiding excessive exercise, especially deep knee bending, are the only necessary measures. Complete avoidance of sports is unnecessary. Rarely, immobilization in plaster, intralesional injection of hydrocortisone, surgical removal of loose bodies (eg, ossicles, avulsed fragments of bone), drilling, and grafting are required.

Scheuermann's Disease

Scheuermann's disease causes localized changes in vertebral bodies leading to backache and kyphosis.

Scheuermann's disease manifests in adolescence, is relatively common, and is slightly more common among boys. It probably represents a group of diseases with similar symptoms, but etiology and pathogenesis are uncertain. It may result from osteochondritis of the upper and lower cartilaginous vertebral end plates or trauma. Some cases are familial.

Most patients present with a round-shouldered posture and persistent low-grade backache. Some have an appearance similar to people with Marfan syndrome; trunk and limb length are disproportionate. Normal thoracic kyphosis is increased diffusely or locally.

Diagnosis and Treatment

Some cases are recognized during routine screening for spinal deformity at school. Lateral spinal x-rays confirm the diagnosis by showing anterior wedging of the vertebral bodies, usually in the lower thoracic and upper lumbar regions. Later, the end plates become irregular and sclerotic. Spinal misalignment is predominantly kyphotic but is sometimes partly scoliotic. In atypical cases, generalized skeletal dysplasia must be excluded by radiographic skeletal survey and spinal TB must be excluded by CT/MRI.

The course is mild but long, often lasting several years (although duration varies greatly). Trivial spinal misalignment often persists after the disorder has become quiescent.

Mild, nonprogressive disease can be treated by reducing weight-bearing stress and by avoiding strenuous activity. Occasionally, when kyphosis is more severe, a spinal brace or rest with recumbency on a rigid bed is indicated. Rarely, progressive cases require surgical stabilization and correction of misalignment.

OSTEOGENESIS IMPERFECTA

Osteogenesis imperfecta is a hereditary collagen disorder causing diffuse abnormal fragility of bone and sometimes accompanied by sensorineural hearing loss, blue sclerae, dentinogenesis imperfecta, and joint hypermobility.

There are 4 main types of osteogenesis imperfecta; types I and IV are autosomal dominant, whereas types II and III are autosomal recessive. Other types are rare. Diagnosis is usually clinical, but there are no standardized criteria. Analysis of type I procollagen (a structural component of bones, ligaments, and tendons) from cultured fibroblasts (from a skin biopsy) or sequence analysis of the *COL1A1* and *COL1A2* genes can be used when clinical diagnosis is unreliable.

Type I is the mildest. Symptoms and signs in some patients are limited to blue sclerae (due to a deficiency in connective tissue allowing the underlying vessels to show through) and musculoskeletal pain due to joint hypermobility.

Type II (neonatal lethal type or osteogenesis imperfecta congenita) is the most severe. Multiple congenital fractures result in shortened extremities. Sclerae are blue. Some infants also have hearing loss, presumably due to otosclerosis caused by abnormal connective tissue around the auditory ossicles. The skull is soft and, when palpated, feels like a bag of bones. Because the skull is soft, trauma during delivery may cause intracranial hemorrhage and stillbirth, or neonates may die suddenly during the 1st few days or weeks of life.

Types III and IV are intermediate in severity. Survival rate is high. Accurate diagnosis is important because these patients may benefit from treatment. IV bisphosphonates (eg, pamidronate, 0.25 to 1 mg/kg once/day for 3 days, repeated as needed q 2 to 6 mo) can increase bone density and decrease bone pain and fracture frequency. Preliminary evidence suggests that oral alendronate (1 mg/kg, 20 mg maximum) is also effective. Orthopedic surgery, physical therapy, and occupational therapy help prevent fractures and improve function.

OSTEOPETROSES

(Marble Bones)

Osteopetroses are characterized by increased bone density and skeletal modeling abnormalities.

Osteopetroses can be categorized based on whether sclerosis or defective skeletal modeling predominates. Some types are comparatively benign; others are progressive and fatal. Bony overgrowth sometimes severely distorts the face. Malocclusion of the teeth may require specialized orthodontic measures. Surgical decompression may be required to relieve elevated intracranial pressure or to release a trapped facial or auditory nerve.

Craniotubular Dysplasias

Craniotubular dysplasias involve minor osteosclerosis with normal skeletal modeling.

Metaphyseal dysplasia (Pyle's disease): This rare, autosomal recessive disorder is often confused semantically with craniometaphyseal dysplasia (see below). Affected people are clinically normal, apart from genu valgum, although scoliosis and bone fragility occasionally occur.

Diagnosis is usually made when x-rays are taken for an unrelated reason. Radiographic changes are striking. Long bones are undermodeled, and bony cortices are generally thin. Tubular leg bones have gross Erlenmeyer flask flaring, particularly in the distal femur. Pelvic bones and thoracic cage are expanded. However, the skull is virtually spared.

Craniometaphyseal dysplasia: In this autosomal dominant disorder, paranasal bossing develops during infancy, and progressive expansion and thickening of the skull and mandible distort the jaw and face. The encroaching bone entraps cranial nerves, causing dysfunction. Malocclusion of the teeth may be troublesome; partial sinus obliteration predisposes to recurrent nasorespiratory infection. Height and general health are normal, but progressive elevation of intracranial pressure is a rare, serious complication.

Radiographic changes are age-related and usually evident by age 5 yr. Sclerosis is the main feature in the skull. Long bones have widened metaphyses, appearing club shaped, particularly at the distal femur. However, these changes are much less severe than those in Pyle's disease. The spine and pelvis are unaffected.

Frontometaphyseal dysplasia: This disorder has distinct autosomal dominant and X-linked forms; it becomes evident during early childhood. The supraorbital ridge is prominent, resembling a knight's visor. The mandible is hypoplastic with anterior constriction; dental anomalies are common. Deafness develops during adulthood because sclerosis narrows the internal acoustic foramina and middle ear. Long leg bones are moderately bowed. Progressive contractures in the digits may simulate RA. Height and general health are normal.

On x-rays, bony overgrowth of the frontal region is obvious; patchy sclerosis occurs in the cranial vault. Vertebral bodies are dysplastic but not sclerotic. Iliac crests are abruptly flared and pelvic inlet distorted. Femoral capital epiphyses are flattened, with expansion of the femoral heads and coxa valga (hip deformity). Finger bones are undermodeled, with erosion and loss of joint space. Corrective surgery is indicated for severely disfiguring deformities or those causing orthopedic problems.

Craniotubular Hyperostoses

Craniotubular hyperostoses are bony overgrowths that alter contour and increase skeletal density.

Endosteal hyperostosis (van Buchem's syndrome): Endosteal hyperostosis is usually inherited as autosomal recessive. Overgrowth and distortion of the mandible and brow become evident during midchildhood. Subsequently, cranial nerves become entrapped, leading to facial palsy and deafness. Life span is not compromised, stature is normal, and bones are not fragile. X-rays show widening and sclerosis of the calvaria, cranial base, and mandible. Diaphyseal endosteum in the tubular bones is thickened. Surgical decompression of entrapped nerves may be helpful.

Sclerosteosis: Sclerosteosis, an autosomal recessive disorder, is most common among Afrikaners of South Africa. Overgrowth and sclerosis of the skeleton, particularly of the skull, develop during early childhood. Height and weight are often excessive. Initial symptoms and signs may include deafness and facial palsy due to cranial nerve entrapment. Distortion of facies, apparent by age 10 yr, eventually becomes severe. Cutaneous or bony syndactyly of the 2nd and 3rd fingers distinguishes sclerosteosis from other forms of craniotubular hyperostoses. Predominant radiographic features are gross widening and sclerosis of the calvaria and mandible. Vertebral bodies are spared, although their pedicles are dense. Pelvic bones are sclerotic but have normal contours. Long bones have sclerosed, hyperostotic cortices and undermodeled shafts. Surgery to relieve intracranial pressure may help.

Diaphyseal dysplasia (Camurati-Engelmann disease): Diaphyseal dysplasia, an autosomal dominant disorder, manifests during midchildhood with muscular pain, weakness, and wasting, typically in the legs. These symptoms usually resolve by age 30. Cranial nerve compression and elevated intracranial pressure occasionally occur. Some patients are severely handicapped; others are virtually asymptomatic. The predominant radiographic feature is marked thickening of the periosteal and medullary surfaces of the diaphyseal cortices of the long bones, but findings vary. Medullary canals and external bone contours are irregular. The extremities and axial skeleton usually are spared. Rarely, the skull is involved, with calvarial widening and basal sclerosis. Corticosteroids may help relieve bone pain and improve muscle strength.

Osteosclerosis

Osteosclerosis is abnormal hardening of bone that involves increased skeletal density with little disturbance of modeling.

Osteopetrosis with delayed manifestations (Albers-Schönberg disease): This type is autosomal dominant, benign, and delayed (tarda), manifesting during childhood, adolescence, or young adulthood. It is relatively common and has a wide geographic and ethnic distribution. Affected people may be asymptomatic; general health is usually unimpaired. However, facial palsy, deafness, and mild anemia may occur.

The skeleton usually is radiologically normal at birth. However, bone sclerosis becomes increasingly apparent as children age, and diagnosis is typically based on x-rays taken for unrelated reasons. Bony involvement is widespread but patchy. The calvaria is dense, and sinuses may be obliterated. Sclerosis of the vertebral end plate produces the characteristic rugby-shirt appearance (horizontal banding). Some patients require transfusion or splenectomy to treat anemia.

Osteopetrosis with precocious manifestations: This type of osteopetrosis is autosomal recessive, malignant, and congenital, manifesting during infancy. It is uncommon, frequently lethal, and often due to a mutation in the osteoclast-associated gene *TCIRG1*. Bony overgrowth causes marrow dysfunction. Initial symptoms include failure to thrive, spontaneous bruising, abnormal bleeding, and anemia. Palsies of the 2nd, 3rd, and 7th cranial nerves and hepatosplenomegaly occur later. Death due to bone marrow failure (anemia, overwhelming infection, or hemorrhage) usually occurs in the 1st year of life.

General increased bone density is the predominant feature on x-rays. Penetrated x-rays of long bones show transverse bands in the metaphyseal regions and longitudinal striations in the shafts. As the disorder progresses, the ends of the long bones, particularly the proximal humerus and distal femur, become flask-shaped. Characteristic endobones (bone within a bone) form in the vertebrae, pelvis, and tubular bones. The skull becomes thickened, and the spine has a rugby-shirt appearance.

Bone marrow transplantation with HLA-identical sibling grafts has had excellent results. However, prognosis is poor with HLA-mismatched grafts. Prednisone, calcitriol, and interferon-γ are effective in some cases.

Osteopetrosis with renal tubular acidosis: This type is autosomal recessive. It causes weakness, stunted stature, and failure to thrive. Bones appear dense on x-rays, and cerebral calcifications are seen; renal tubular acidosis (RTA) is present, and RBC carbonic anhydrase activity is decreased. The genetic defect involves mutations of the carbonic anhydrase II gene. Bone marrow transplant cures the osteopetrosis but has no effect on the RTA. Maintenance therapy consists of bicarbonate and electrolyte supplementation to correct renal losses.

Pyknodysostosis: In this autosomal recessive disorder, short stature becomes evident in early childhood; adult height is ≤ 150 cm (5 ft). Other manifestations, including an enlarged skull, short and broad hands and feet, dystrophic nails, and blue sclerae (due to a deficiency in connective tissue allowing the underlying vessels to show through), are usually recognized during infancy. Affected people resemble each other closely; they have a small face, a receding chin, and carious, misplaced teeth. The cranium bulges, and the anterior fontanelle remains patent. Terminal phalanges are short, and fingernails are dysplastic. Pathologic fractures are a complication.

Bone sclerosis appears on x-rays during childhood, but neither bone striations nor endobones are seen. Facial bones and paranasal sinuses are hypoplastic, and the mandibular angle is obtuse. Clavicles may be gracile, and their lateral portions underdeveloped; distal phalanges are rudimentary. Plastic surgery has been used to correct severe deformities of the face and jaw.

SLIPPED CAPITAL FEMORAL EPIPHYSIS

Slipped capital femoral epiphysis is movement of the femoral neck upward and forward on the femoral epiphysis.

Slipped capital femoral epiphysis (SCFE) usually occurs in early adolescence and preferentially affects boys. Obesity is a significant risk factor. Genetic factors also contribute. SCFE is bilateral in ⅕ of patients, and unilateral SCFE becomes bilateral in up to ⅔ of patients. Exact cause is unknown but probably relates to weakening of the physis (growth plate), which can result from trauma, hormonal changes, inflammation, or increased shearing forces due to obesity.

Symptoms and Signs

Onset is usually insidious, and symptoms are associated with stage of slippage. The 1st symptom may be hip stiffness that abates with rest; it is followed by a limp, then hip pain that radiates down the anteromedial thigh to the knee. Up to 15% of patients present with knee or thigh pain, and the true problem (hip) may be missed until slippage worsens. Early hip examination may detect neither pain nor limitation of movement. In more advanced stages, findings may include pain during movement of the affected hip, with limited flexion, abduction, and medial rotation; knee pain without specific knee abnormalities; and a limp. The affected leg is externally rotated. If blood supply to the area is compromised, avascular necrosis and collapse of the epiphysis may occur.

Diagnosis and Treatment

Because treatment of advanced slippage is difficult, early diagnosis is vital. Anteroposterior and frog-leg lateral x-rays of both hips are taken. X-rays show widening of the epiphyseal line or apparent posterior and inferior displacement of the femoral head. Ultrasonography and MRI are also useful, especially if x-rays are normal.

SCFE usually progresses; it requires surgery as soon as it is diagnosed. Patients should not bear weight on the affected leg until SCFE has been ruled out or treated. Surgical treatment consists of screw fixation through the epiphysis.

285 PEDIATRIC CANCERS

Childhood cancers include many that also occur in adults. Some of these cancers are discussed elsewhere in THE MANUAL (eg, leukemias on p. 1105, bone cancers on p. 347, and brain cancers on p. 1916). Others exclusive to children are described below.

NEUROBLASTOMA

Neuroblastoma is a cancer arising in the adrenal gland or less often from the extra-adrenal sympathetic chain, including the retroperitoneum, chest, and neck. Diagnosis is based on biopsy. Treatment may include surgical resection, chemotherapy, radiation therapy, and high-dose chemotherapy with stem cell transplantation.

Neuroblastoma is the most common cancer in infants. Almost 90% of cases present in children < 5 yr. There are numerous different cytogenetic abnormalities on several chromosomes that can result in neuroblastoma; in 1 to 2%, abnormalities appear to be inherited. Some markers (eg, N-*myc* oncogene, hyperdiploidy) correlate with progression and prognosis.

About 65% begin in the abdomen and 15 to 20% begin in the thorax; the rest arise from the neck, pelvis, or other sites. Neuroblastoma occurs very rarely as a primary CNS cancer.

Most neuroblastomas produce catecholamines, which can be detected as elevated levels of urinary catecholamine breakdown products. Ganglioneuroma is a fully differentiated, benign variant of neuroblastoma.

About 40 to 50% of children have localized or regional disease at diagnosis; 50 to 60% have metastases at diagnosis.

Symptoms and Signs

Symptoms and signs depend on the site of the primary cancer and the pattern of disease spread. The most common symptoms are abdominal pain, discomfort, and fullness due to an abdominal mass. Some children present with bone pain from widespread bony metastases. Periorbital ecchymosis and proptosis may occur with retrobulbar metastasis. Liver metastases, especially in infants, may cause abdominal distention and respiratory problems. Occasionally, pallor (anemia), petechiae (thrombocytopenia), and leukopenia develop due to bone marrow metastases. Other less common sites of metastasis include the skin and brain. Hemorrhage and necrosis into the tumor may occur. Children occasionally present with focal neurologic deficits or paralysis due to direct extension of the cancer into the spinal canal. They may also present with paraneoplastic syndromes (see p. 1150) such as cerebellar ataxia, opsoclonus-myoclonus, watery diarrhea, or hypertension.

Diagnosis

Routine prenatal ultrasound occasionally detects neuroblastoma. Patients presenting with abdominal symptoms or a mass should have ultrasound or CT. Diagnosis is then confirmed by biopsy of any identified mass. Alternatively, diagnosis can be confirmed by the presence of characteristic cancer cells in a bone marrow aspirate or core biopsy, along with elevated urinary catecholamine intermediates. Urinary vanillylmandelic acid (VMA), homovanillic acid (HVA), or both are elevated in ≥ 90 to 95% of patients. A 24-h urine collection can be used, although a spot urine test is usually sufficient. Neuroblastomas must be differentiated from Wilms' tumor, other renal masses, rhabdomyosarcoma, hepatoblastoma, lymphoma, and tumors of genital origin.

The following should be performed to evaluate for metastases: bone marrow aspirates and core biopsies from multiple sites (typically, both iliac crests), skeletal survey, bone scan or ^{131}I-metaiodobenzylguanidine (MBIG) scan, and abdominal and chest CT or MRI. Cranial imaging with CT or MRI is indicated if symptoms or signs are suggestive of brain metastases. When the cancer is resected, a portion should be analyzed for DNA index (a quantitative measure of chromosome content) and amplification of the N-*myc* oncogene to determine prognosis and intensity of therapy.

Prognosis and Treatment

Prognosis is better for children with low-risk disease (age < 1 yr, lack of amplification of the N-*myc* oncogene, and lower stage [localized] disease). Chemotherapy (typical agents: vincristine, cyclophosphamide, doxorubicin, cisplatin, carboplatin, ifosfamide, and etoposide) is usually necessary for children with intermediate risk disease (disease that has spread regionally but lacks amplification of the N-*myc* oncogene). High-dose chemotherapy with stem cell transplantation and *cis*-retinoic acid are frequently used for children with high-risk disease (age ≥ 1 yr with metastatic disease and/or amplification of the N-*myc* oncogene). Radiation therapy is sometimes needed for children with intermediate or high-risk disease.

RETINOBLASTOMA

Retinoblastoma is a cancer arising from the immature retina. Symptoms and signs commonly include leukocoria (a white reflex from the pupil) and strabismus, and less often, inflammation and impaired vision. Diagnosis is based on ophthalmoscopic examination and ultrasound, CT, or MRI. Treatment of smaller cancers and bilateral disease may include photocoagulation, cryotherapy, and radiation therapy. Treatment of larger cancers is enucleation. Chemotherapy is sometimes used to reduce cancer volume and for cancers that have spread beyond the eye.

Retinoblastoma occurs in 1/15,000 to 1/30,000 live births and represents about 2% of childhood cancers. Most cases present in children < 2 yr, with < 5% of cases diagnosed in those > 5 yr. The disease is sometimes hereditary. About 25% of patients have bilateral disease, which is always heritable. Another 15% of patients have heritable unilateral disease, and the remaining 60% have nonheritable unilateral disease. The pathogenesis of inheritance appears to involve mutational deactivation of both alleles of a retinoblastoma suppressor gene located on chromosome 13q14. In the heritable form, a germline mutation alters one allele in all cells and a later somatic mutation alters the other allele in the child's retinal cells (the 2nd hit in this "2 hit" model), resulting in the cancer. The nonheritable form likely involves somatic mutation of both alleles in a retinal cell.

Symptoms, Signs, and Diagnosis

Diagnosis is usually made when a white reflex from the pupil (leukocoria, sometimes referred to as cat's-eye pupil) or strabismus is investigated. Much less often, patients present with inflammation of the eye or impaired vision. Rarely, the cancer has already spread, via the optic nerve or the choroid, or hematogenously, resulting in an orbital or soft-tissue mass, headache, anorexia, or vomiting.

Both fundi must be closely examined by indirect ophthalmoscopy with the pupils widely dilated and the child under general anesthesia. The cancers appear as single or multiple gray-white elevations in the retina; cancer seeds may be visible in the vitreous. Diagnosis is usually confirmed by orbital ultrasound or CT. In almost all cancers, calcification can be detected by CT. However, if the optic nerve appears abnormal during ophthalmoscopy, MRI is better for finding cancer extension into the optic nerve or choroid. Whenever extraocular spread is suspected, testing should include a bone scan, a bone marrow aspirate and biopsy, and lumbar puncture.

Children who have a parent or sibling with a history of retinoblastoma should be evaluated by an ophthalmologist shortly after birth and then every 4 mo until age 4 yr. Patients with retinoblastoma should undergo molecular genetic testing, and if a germline mutation is identified, parents should undergo testing for detection of the same mutation. Subsequent offspring of parents found to have the germline mutation should undergo the same genetic testing and regular ophthalmologic examination. Recombinant DNA probes may be useful for detecting asymptomatic carriers.

Prognosis and Treatment

If treated when the cancer is intraocular, > 90% of patients can be cured. The prognosis for metastatic disease is poor. Patients with hereditary retinoblastoma have an increased incidence of 2nd malignancies, about 50% of which arise within the irradiated area. These malignancies can include sarcomas and malignant melanoma. Within 30 yr of diagnosis, 70% have developed a 2nd malignancy.

Unilateral retinoblastoma is managed by enucleation with removal of as much of the optic nerve as possible. For those with bilateral disease, vision usually can be preserved. Options include bilateral photocoagulation or unilateral enucleation and photocoagulation, cryotherapy, or radiation therapy of the other eye. Radiation therapy is by external beam or, for very small cancers, attachment of a radioactive plaque to the eye wall in close proximity to the cancer (brachytherapy). Systemic chemotherapy, such as carboplatin and etoposide or cyclophosphamide and vincristine, may be helpful to reduce the size of large cancers or when the disease has disseminated beyond the eye. However, chemotherapy alone can seldom cure this disease. Ophthalmologic reexamination of both eyes and retreatment, if necessary, are required at 2- to 4-mo intervals.

RHABDOMYOSARCOMA

Rhabdomyosarcoma is a cancer arising from embryonal mesenchymal cells that have potential to differentiate into skeletal muscle cells. It can arise from almost any type of muscle tissue in any location, resulting in highly variable clinical manifestations. Cancers are typically detected by CT or MRI, and diagnosis is confirmed by biopsy. Treatment involves surgery, radiation therapy, and chemotherapy.

Rhabdomyosarcoma is the 3rd most common extra-CNS cancer in children (after Wilms' tumor and neuroblastoma). Nonetheless, it accounts for only 3 to 4% of all childhood cancers. The incidence of rhabdomyosarcoma in children is 4.3/million/yr. Two thirds of cancers are diagnosed in children < 7 yr. The disease is more common in whites than blacks (largely due to a lower frequency in black girls) and is slightly more common in boys than girls.

There are 2 major histologic subtypes: the embryonal variant is characterized by loss of heterozygosity on chromosome 11p15.5, and the alveolar subtype is associated with a translocation involving *PAX3* or *PAX7*, regulators of transcription during neuromuscular development (chromosome 2;13 or 1;13 translocation). Although rhabdomyosarcoma can occur almost anywhere in the body, the disease has predilection for several sites. The most common are the head and neck region (usually in the orbit or nasopharyngeal passages), accounting for 35 to 40% of primary cancers, the GU system (usually bladder, prostate, vagina) in 25% of cases, and the extremities in 20% of cases. Fewer than 25% of children present with metastatic disease.

Symptoms and Signs

Children do not typically have systemic symptoms such as fever, night sweats, or weight loss. In general, children present with a firm, palpable mass or with organ dysfunction due to impingement of the organ by the cancer.

Orbital and nasopharyngeal cancers are most common in school-aged children. Orbital cancers may cause tearing, eye pain, or proptosis. Nasopharyngeal cavity cancers may cause nasal congestion, change in voice, or mucopurulent discharge.

GU cancers usually occur in infants and toddlers; they cause abdominal pain, a palpable abdominal mass, difficulty urinating, and hematuria. Extremity cancers are most common in adolescents; they present as firm, indiscrete masses anywhere on the arms or legs. Metastases occur frequently with extremity cancers, especially in the lung, bone marrow, and lymph nodes, and usually do not cause symptoms.

Diagnosis

Masses are evaluated by CT scan, although head and neck lesions are often better defined by MRI. Diagnosis is confirmed by biopsy or excision of the mass. The standard metastatic evaluation includes a chest CT scan, a bone scan, and a bone marrow aspiration and biopsy.

Prognosis and Treatment

Prognosis is based on cancer location (eg, head and GU cancers have a better prognosis), extent of resection, and occurrence of metastasis. Other important prognostic factors are age (more favorable in younger children) and histology (embryonal histology is associated with a better outcome than alveolar histology). Combinations of these prognostic factors place children in 1 of 3 risk categories: low, intermediate, or high. Treatment intensifies with each risk category, and overall survival ranges from > 90% in children with low-risk disease to < 50% in children with high-risk disease.

Treatment consists of surgery, radiation therapy, and chemotherapy. Complete excision of the primary cancer is recommended when it can safely be done. Because the cancer is so sensitive to chemotherapy and radiation therapy, aggressive resection is discouraged if it may result in organ damage or dysfunction. Children in all risk categories are treated with chemotherapy; the most commonly used agents are vincristine, actinomycin D, cyclophosphamide, doxorubicin, ifosfamide, and etoposide. Radiation therapy is generally reserved for children with residual cancer after surgery and for children with intermediate and high-risk disease.

WILMS' TUMOR

(Nephroblastoma)

Wilms' tumor is an embryonal cancer of the kidney composed of blastemal, stromal, and epithelial elements. Genetic abnormalities have been implicated in the pathogenesis, but familial inheritance accounts for only 1 to 2% of cases. Diagnosis is made by ultrasound and abdominal CT scan and confirmed by biopsy. Treatment may include surgical resection, chemotherapy, and radiation therapy.

Wilms' tumor usually presents in children < 5 yr but occasionally in older children and rarely in adults. Wilms' tumor accounts for about 6% of cancers in children < 15 yr. Bilateral synchronous tumors occur in about 4% of cases, with bilateral disease more common in very young children, especially girls. A chromosomal deletion of *WT1*, the Wilms' tumor suppressor gene, has been identified in some cases. Other associated genetic abnormalities include deletion of *WT2* (a 2nd Wilms' tumor suppressor gene), deletion of chromosome 16, and duplication of chromosome 12.

About 10% of cases manifest other congenital abnormalities, especially GU abnormalities, but also commonly hemihypertrophy (asymmetry of the body). WAGR syndrome is the combination of Wilms' tumor (with *WT1* deletion), aniridia, GU malformations (eg, renal hypoplasia, cystic disease, hypospadias, cryptorchidism), and mental retardation.

Symptoms and Signs

The most frequent presentation is a painless, palpable abdominal mass. Less frequent findings include abdominal pain, hematuria, fever, anorexia, nausea, and vomiting. Hematuria (occurring in 15 to 20%) indicates invasion of the collecting system. Hypertension may occur if compression of the renal pedicle or renal parenchyma causes ischemia.

Diagnosis

Abdominal ultrasound determines the cystic or solid nature of the mass and whether the renal vein or vena cava is involved. Abdominal CT is needed to determine the extent of the tumor and spread to regional lymph nodes, the contralateral kidney, or liver. The diagnosis is confirmed by biopsy of the mass. Renal arteriography, vena cavography, retrograde urography, or excretory urography seldom is required. Chest x-ray (and possibly chest CT) is needed to detect metastatic pulmonary involvement at initial diagnosis.

Prognosis and Treatment

Prognosis depends on histology (favorable or unfavorable), the stage at diagnosis, and the patient's age (younger is better). The outcome for children with Wilms' tumor is excellent. Cure rates for lower stage disease (localized to the kidney) range from 85 to 95%. Even children with more advanced disease fare well, with cure rates ranging from 60% (unfavorable histology) to 90% (favorable histology). Recurrences do occur, typically within 2 yr of diagnosis. Cure is possible in children with recurrent cancer. Outcome after recurrence is better in children who presented initially with lower stage disease, whose tumors recur at a site that has not been irradiated, who relapse > 1 yr after presentation, and who receive less intensive treatment initially.

The National Wilms' Tumor Study Group has established staging criteria and guidelines for treatment. Prompt surgical exploration of potentially resectable lesions is indicated, with examination of the contralateral kidney. If the cancer is unilateral and limited to the kidney or if extension is minimal, complete resection by nephrectomy is performed, followed by treatment with vincristine and actinomycin D. If a unilateral cancer has spread extensively or if the disease is bilateral, chemotherapy with actinomycin D and vincristine, with or without radiation therapy, is used. Children with more advanced disease also receive doxorubicin. Other frequently used drugs include cyclophosphamide, ifosfamide, and etoposide. Children with very large nonresectable tumors or bilateral tumors are candidates for chemotherapy followed by reevaluation and possibly resection.

286 MISCELLANEOUS DISORDERS IN INFANTS AND CHILDREN

FAILURE TO THRIVE

Failure to thrive is weight consistently below the 3rd to the 5th percentile for age, progressive decrease in weight to below the 3rd to the 5th percentile, or a decrease in the percentile rank of 2 major growth parameters in a short period. The cause may be an identified medical condition or related to environmental factors. Both types relate to inadequate nutrition. Treatment aims to restore proper nutrition.

Etiology and Pathophysiology

The physiologic basis for failure to thrive (FTT) of any etiology is inadequate nutrition.

Organic FTT: Growth failure is due to an acute or chronic disorder that interferes with nutrient intake, absorption, metabolism, or excretion or that increases energy requirements (see TABLE 286–1). Illness of any organ system can be a cause.

Nonorganic FTT: Up to 80% of children with growth failure do not have an apparent growth-inhibiting (organic) disorder; growth failure occurs because of environmental neglect (eg, lack of food) or stimulus deprivation.

Lack of food may be due to impoverishment, poor understanding of feeding techniques, improperly prepared formula (eg, overdiluting formula to "stretch" it because of financial difficulties), or an inadequate supply of breast milk (eg, because the mother is under stress, exhausted, or poorly nourished).

Nonorganic FTT is often a complex of disordered interaction between a child and caregiver. In some cases, the psychologic basis of nonorganic FTT appears similar to that of "hospitalism," a syndrome observed in infants who have depression secondary to stimulus deprivation. The unstimulated child becomes depressed, apathetic, and ultimately anorexic. Stimulation may be lacking because the caregiver is depressed or apathetic, has poor

TABLE 286–1. SOME CAUSES OF ORGANIC FAILURE TO THRIVE

MECHANISM	DISORDER
Decreased nutrient intake	Cleft lip or palate CNS disorder Gastroesophageal reflux Pyloric stenosis Rumination
Malabsorption	Celiac disease Cystic fibrosis Disaccharidase (eg, lactase) deficiency
Impaired metabolism	Fructose intolerance Inborn errors of metabolism Galactose-1-phosphate uridyl transferase deficiency ("classic" galactosemia)
Increased excretion	Diabetes mellitus Proteinuria
Increased energy requirements	Bronchopulmonary dysplasia Cystic fibrosis Heart failure Hyperthyroidism

parenting skills, is anxious about or unfulfilled by the caregiving role, feels hostile toward the child, or is responding to real or perceived external stresses (eg, demands of other children in large or chaotic families, marital dysfunction, a significant loss, financial difficulties).

Poor caregiving does not fully account for all cases of nonorganic FTT. The child's temperament, capacities, and responses help shape caregiver nurturance patterns. Common scenarios involve parent-child mismatches, in which the child's demands, although not pathologic, cannot be adequately met by the parents, who might, however, do well with a child who has different needs or even with the same child under different circumstances.

Mixed FTT: In mixed FTT, organic and nonorganic causes can overlap; those with organic disorders also have disturbed environments or dysfunctional parental interactions. Likewise, those with severe undernutrition from nonorganic FTT can develop organic medical problems.

Diagnosis

Children with organic FTT may present at any age depending on the underlying disorder. Most children with nonorganic FTT manifest growth failure before age 1 yr and many by age 6 mo. Age should be plotted against weight, height, and head size. Until premature infants reach 2 yr, age should be corrected for gestation.

Weight is the most sensitive indicator of nutritional status. Reduced linear growth usually indicates more severe, prolonged malnutrition. Because the brain is preferentially spared in protein-energy malnutrition (see p. 15), reduced growth in head circumference

TABLE 286–2. ESSENTIALS OF THE HISTORY FOR FAILURE TO THRIVE

ITEM	COMMENTS
Growth chart	Measurements, including those obtained at birth if possible, should be examined to determine the trend in growth rate. Because of wide normal variations, diagnosis of failure to thrive should not be based on a single measurement, except when malnutrition is obvious
Diet history (3 days)	Diet history should be detailed, including feeding schedule and techniques for the preparation and feeding of formula or adequacy of breast milk supply. As soon as possible, the parents should be observed feeding the infant to evaluate their technique and the infant's vigor of sucking. An infant who tires easily may have underlying exercise intolerance. Enthusiastic burping or rapid rocking during feeding may result in excessive regurgitation or even vomiting. A disinterested parent may be depressed or apathetic, suggesting a psychosocial environment that is lacking stimulation for and interaction with the infant
Assessment of the child's elimination pattern	Abnormal losses through urine, stool, or emesis are investigated to detect underlying renal disease, malabsorption syndrome, pyloric stenosis, or gastroesophageal reflux
Medical history, birth history	Of concern is any evidence of intrauterine growth restriction or prematurity with growth delay that has not been compensated; of developmental delay; of unusual, prolonged, or chronic infections (eg, TB, parasitic, HIV); of neurologic, cardiac, pulmonary, or renal disease; of illness, hospitalization; and of possible food intolerance
Family history	Included is information about familial growth patterns, especially in parents and siblings; the occurrence of diseases known to affect growth (eg, cystic fibrosis); and a parent's recent physical or psychiatric illness resulting in inability to provide consistent stimulation and nurturance
Social history	Attention is focused on family composition, socioeconomic status, desire for pregnancy with and acceptance of this child, and stresses (eg, job changes, family moves, separation, divorce, deaths, other losses)

occurs late and indicates very severe or long-standing malnutrition.

Usually, when growth failure is noted, a history (including diet history—see TABLE 286–2) is obtained, diet counseling is provided, and the child's weight is monitored frequently. A child who does not gain weight satisfactorily in spite of outpatient assessment and intervention is usually admitted to the hospital so that all necessary observations can be made and diagnostic tests performed quickly. Without historic or physical evidence of a specific underlying etiology for growth failure, no single clinical feature or test can reliably distinguish organic from nonorganic FTT. Because nonorganic FTT is not a diagnosis of exclusion, the physician should simultaneously search for an underlying physical problem and for personal, family, and child-family characteristics that support a psychosocial etiology. Optimally, evaluation is multidisciplinary, involving a physician, a nurse, a social worker, a nutritionist, an expert in child development, and often a psychiatrist or psychologist. The child's feeding behaviors with health care practitioners and with the parents must be observed, whether the setting is inpatient or outpatient.

Engaging the parents as co-investigators is essential. It helps foster their self-esteem and avoids blaming those who may already feel frustrated or guilty because of a perceived inability to nurture their child. The family should be encouraged to visit as often and as long as possible. Staff members should make them feel welcome, support their attempts to feed the child, and provide toys and ideas that promote parent-child play and other interactions. Staff members should avoid any comments implying parental inadequacy, irresponsibility, or other fault as the cause of FTT. However, parental adequacy and sense of responsibility should be evaluated. Suspected neglect or abuse must be reported to social services, but in many instances, referral for preventive services that are targeted to meet the family's needs for support and education (eg, additional food stamps, more accessible child care, parenting classes) is more appropriate.

During hospitalization, the child's interaction with people in the environment is closely observed, and evidence of self-stimulatory behaviors (eg, rocking, head banging) is noted. Some children with nonorganic FTT have been described as hypervigilant and wary of close contact with people, preferring interactions with inanimate objects if they interact at all. Although nonorganic FTT is more consistent with neglectful than abusive parenting, the child should be examined closely for evidence of abuse (see p. 2507). A screening test of developmental level should be performed and, if indicated, followed with more sophisticated assessment.

Testing: Extensive laboratory tests are usually nonproductive. If a thorough history or physical examination does not indicate a particular cause, most experts recommend limiting screening tests to a CBC with differential, an ESR, BUN or serum creatinine level, urinalysis (including ability to concentrate and acidify), urine culture, and examination of the stool for pH, reducing substances, odor, color, consistency, and fat content. Depending on prevalence of specific disorders in the community, blood lead level, HIV, or TB testing may be warranted.

Other tests that are sometimes appropriate include electrolyte concentrations if the child has a history of significant vomiting or diarrhea; a thyroxine level if growth in height is more severely affected than growth in weight; and a sweat test if the child has a history of recurrent upper or lower respiratory tract disease, a salty taste when kissed, a ravenous appetite, foul-smelling bulky stools, hepatomegaly, or a family history of cystic fibrosis. Investigation for infectious diseases should be reserved for children with evidence of infection (eg, fever, vomiting, cough, diarrhea). Radiologic investigation should be reserved for children with evidence of anatomic or functional pathology (eg, pyloric stenosis, gastroesophageal reflux).

Prognosis

Prognosis with organic FTT depends on the cause. With nonorganic FTT, 50 to 75% of children > 1 yr achieve a stable weight > 3rd percentile. Cognitive function, especially verbal skills, remains below the normal range in about 1/3; children who develop FTT before 1 yr of age are at high risk, and those diagnosed at < 6 mo of age—when the rate of postnatal brain growth is maximal—are at highest risk. General behavioral problems, identified by teachers or mental health professionals, occur in about 50%. Problems specifically related to eating (eg, pickiness, slowness) or elimination tend to occur in a similar proportion of children, usually those with other behavioral or personality disturbances.

Treatment

Treatment aims to provide sufficient health and environmental resources to promote satisfactory growth. A nutritious diet containing adequate calories for catch-up growth (about 150% of normal caloric requirement) and individualized medical and social supports are usually necessary. Ability to gain weight in the hospital does not always differentiate infants with nonorganic FTT from those with organic FTT; all children grow when given sufficient nutrition. However, some children with nonorganic FTT lose weight in the hospital, highlighting the complexity of this condition.

For children with organic or mixed FTT, the underlying disorder should be treated quickly. For children with apparent nonorganic FTT or mixed FTT, management includes provision of education and emotional support to correct problems interfering with the parent-child relationship. Because long-term social support or psychiatric treatment is often required, the evaluation team may be able only to define the family's needs, provide initial instruction and support, and institute appropriate referrals to community agencies. The parents should understand why the referrals are being made and, if options exist, should participate in decisions concerning which agencies will be involved. If the child is hospitalized in a tertiary care center, the referring physician should be consulted regarding local agencies and the level of expertise available in the community.

A predischarge planning conference involving hospital-based personnel, representatives from the community agencies that will provide follow-up services, and the child's primary physician is ideal. Areas of responsibility and lines of accountability must be clearly defined, preferably in writing, and distributed to everyone involved. The parents should be invited to a summary session after the conference so that they can meet the community workers, ask questions, and arrange follow-up appointments.

In some cases, the child must be placed in foster care. If the child is expected to eventually return to the biologic parents, parenting skill training and psychologic counseling must be provided for them. Their child's progress must be monitored scrupulously. Return to the biologic parents should be based on the parents' demonstrated ability to care for the child adequately, not only on the passage of time.

HEMORRHAGIC SHOCK AND ENCEPHALOPATHY SYNDROME

Hemorrhagic shock and encephalopathy syndrome is an extremely rare disease characterized by acute onset of severe shock, coagulopathy, encephalopathy, and hepatic and renal dysfunction in previously healthy children, resulting in death or catastrophic neurologic outcome.

Hemorrhagic shock and encephalopathy syndrome (HSES) occurs predominantly in infants aged 3 to 8 mo (median age, 5 mo) but was reported in a 15-yr-old. HSES resembles heatstroke, with extremely high temperature and multiple organ dysfunction, but the cause is unknown. Overwrapping of infants who have febrile illness has been suggested, but evidence is slim. Other theories include a reaction to intestinal or environmental toxins, pancreatic release of trypsin, or an unidentified virus or bacterium. Diffuse cerebral edema with herniation and focal hemorrhages and infarcts in the cerebral cortex and other organs are common. The lungs and myocardium are not primarily involved.

Symptoms and Signs

A prodrome of fever, upper respiratory tract symptoms, or vomiting and diarrhea occurs in most patients. The major features are an acute onset of encephalopathy, cerebral edema (manifested as seizures, coma, and hypotonia), and severe shock (ie, hypotension and poor perfusion). Other common features include hyperpyrexia (up to 43.9° C rectally), bloody or watery diarrhea, disseminated intravascular coagulation (DIC), myoglobinuria, and rhabdomyolysis.

Diagnosis

Similar symptoms can result from sepsis, Reye's syndrome, and hemolytic-uremic syndrome. Patients require laboratory evaluation including blood and urine culture, ABG, CBC, electrolytes, BUN, creatinine, PT/PTT, and liver function tests. Multiple abnormalities include metabolic acidosis, elevated liver transaminases, acute renal failure, thrombocytopenia, falling Hct, leukocytosis, hypoglycemia, and hyperkalemia. Bacteriologic and viral cultures are negative. Diagnosis is by exclusion.

Prognosis and Treatment

In all series, >60% of patients died, and ≥70% of survivors had severe neurologic sequelae.

Treatment is entirely supportive. Infusions of large volumes of isotonic solutions and blood products (fresh frozen plasma, albumin, whole blood, packed RBCs) along with inotropic support (eg, dopamine, epinephrine) are necessary to maintain circulation. Marked temperature elevation (eg, > 39° C) requires external cooling (see p. 2609). Increased intracranial pressure from cerebral edema requires intubation and hyperventilation. DIC often progresses despite use of fresh frozen plasma.

KAWASAKI DISEASE

Kawasaki disease is a vasculitis, sometimes involving the coronary arteries, that tends to occur in infants and children between ages 1 and 8 yr. It is characterized by prolonged fever, exanthem, conjunctivitis, mucous membrane inflammation, and lymphadenopathy. Coronary artery aneurysms may develop and rupture or cause MI. Diagnosis is by clinical criteria; once the disease is diagnosed, echocardiography is performed. Treatment is aspirin and IV immune globulin. Coronary thrombosis may require fibrinolysis or percutaneous interventions.

Kawasaki disease (KD) is a vasculitis of medium-sized arteries, most significantly the coronary arteries, which are involved in about 20% of untreated patients. Early manifestations include acute myocarditis with heart failure, arrhythmias, endocarditis, and pericarditis. Coronary artery aneurysms may subsequently form. Giant coronary artery aneurysms (>8 mm internal diameter on echocardiogram), though rare, have the greatest risk of producing cardiac tamponade, thrombosis, or infarction. KD is the leading cause of acquired heart disease in children. Extravascular tissue may also become inflamed, including the upper respiratory tract, pancreas, biliary tract, and kidneys.

The etiology is unknown, but the epidemiology and clinical presentation suggest an infection or an abnormal immunologic response to an infection in genetically predisposed children. Children of Japanese descent have a particularly high incidence, but KD occurs worldwide. In the US, 3000 to 5000 cases occur annually. The male:female ratio is about 1.5:1. Eighty percent of patients are < 5 yr (peak, 18 to 24 mo). Cases in teenagers, adults, and infants < 4 mo are rare. Cases occur year-round, but most often in spring or winter. Clusters have been reported in communities without clear evidence of person-to-person spread. About 2% of patients have recurrences, typically months to years later.

Symptoms and Signs

The illness tends to progress in stages, beginning with fever lasting at least 5 days, usually remittent and > 39° C, associated with irritability, occasional lethargy, or intermittent colicky abdominal pain. Usually within a day or two of fever onset, bilateral bulbar conjunctival injection appears without exudate. Within 5 days, a polymorphous, erythematous macular rash appears, primarily over the trunk, often with accentuation in the perineal region. The rash may be urticarial, morbilliform, erythema multiforme, or scarlatiniform. It is accompanied by injected pharynx; reddened, dry, fissured lips; and a red strawberry tongue. During the 1st week, pallor of the proximal portion of the fingernails or toenails (leukonychia partialis) may occur. Erythema or a purple-red discoloration and variable edema of the palms and soles usually appear on about the 3rd to 5th day. Although edema may be slight, it is often tense, hard, and nonpitting. Periungual, palmar, and plantar and perineal desquamation begins on about the 10th day. The superficial layer of the skin sometimes comes off in large casts, revealing new normal skin. Tender, nonsuppurative cervical lymphadenopathy (≥ 1 node, ≥ 1.5 cm in size) is present throughout the course in about 50% of patients. The illness may last from 2 to 12 wk or longer. Incomplete or atypical cases can occur, especially in younger infants, who have higher risk of developing coronary artery disease. These findings manifest in about 90% of patients.

Other less specific findings indicate involvement of many systems. Arthritis or arthralgias (mainly involving large joints) occur in about ⅓ of patients. Other clinical features include urethritis, aseptic meningitis, hepatitis, otitis, vomiting, diarrhea, hydrops of the gallbladder, and anterior uveitis.

Cardiac manifestations usually begin in the subacute phase of the syndrome about 1 to 4 wk after onset, as the rash, fever, and other early acute clinical symptoms begin to subside.

Diagnosis

Diagnosis is by clinical criteria (see TABLE 286–3). Similar symptoms can result from

TABLE 286–3. CRITERIA FOR DIAGNOSIS OF KAWASAKI DISEASE

Diagnosis is made if fever of ≥ 5 days has occurred and 4 of the following 5 criteria are noted:

1. Bilateral nonexudative conjunctival injection
2. Changes in the lips, tongue, or oral mucosa (injection, drying, fissuring, red strawberry tongue)
3. Changes in the peripheral extremities (edema, erythema, desquamation)
4. Polymorphous truncal exanthem
5. Cervical lymphadenopathy (at least one node ≥ 1.5 cm in diameter)

scarlet fever, staphylococcal exfoliative syndromes, measles, drug reactions, and juvenile RA; less common mimics are leptospirosis and Rocky Mountain spotted fever.

Laboratory tests are not diagnostic but may be obtained to exclude other disorders. Patients generally undergo CBC, antinuclear antibody (ANA), rheumatoid factor (RF), ESR, and throat and blood culture. Leukocytosis, often with a marked increase in immature cells, is common acutely. Other hematologic findings include a mild normocytic anemia, thrombocytosis (≥ 450,000/μL) in the 2nd or 3rd wk of illness, and elevated ESR or C-reactive protein. ANA, RF, and cultures are negative. Other abnormalities, depending on the organ systems involved, include sterile pyuria, elevated liver enzymes, proteinuria, and CSF pleocytosis.

Consultation with a pediatric cardiologist is important. At diagnosis, ECG and echocardiography are performed; because abnormalities may not appear until later, these tests are repeated at 2 to 3 wk, 6 to 8 wk, and perhaps at 6 to 12 mo after onset. ECG may show arrhythmias, decreased voltage, or left ventricular hypertrophy. Echocardiography should detect coronary artery aneurysms, valvular regurgitation, pericarditis, or myocarditis. Coronary arteriography is occasionally useful in patients with aneurysms and abnormal stress testing.

Prognosis

Without therapy, mortality may approach 1%, usually occurring within 6 wk of onset. The mortality rate is < 0.01% in the US with adequate therapy. Long duration of fever increases cardiac risk. Deaths most commonly result from cardiac complications and can be sudden and unpredictable: > 50% occur within 1 mo of onset, 75% within 2 mo, and 95% within 6 mo but may occur as long as 10 yr later. Effective therapy reduces acute symptoms and, more importantly, the incidence of coronary artery aneurysms from 20% to < 5%. In the absence of coronary artery disease, the prognosis for complete recovery is excellent. About ⅔ of coronary aneurysms regress within 1 yr, although it is unknown whether residual coronary stenosis remains. Giant coronary aneurysms are less likely to regress and require more intensive follow-up and therapy.

Treatment

Children should be treated by or in close consultation with an experienced pediatric cardiologist and/or pediatric infectious disease specialist. Therapy is started as soon as possible, optimally within the 1st 10 days of illness, with a combination of high-dose immune globulin IV (IGIV), a single dose of 2 g/kg given over 10 to 12 h, and oral high-dose aspirin, 20 to 25 mg/kg po qid. The aspirin dose is reduced to 3 to 5 mg/kg once/day after the child has been afebrile for 4 to 5 days; some authorities prefer to continue high-dose aspirin until the 14th day of illness. Aspirin metabolism is erratic during acute KD, which partially explains the high dose requirements. Some authorities monitor serum aspirin levels during high-dose therapy, especially if therapy is given for 14 days.

Most patients have a brisk response over the 1st 24 h of therapy. A small fraction continues to be ill with fever for several days and requires repeated dosing with IGIV. An alternative regimen, which may lead to slightly slower resolution of symptoms but may benefit those with cardiac dysfunction who could not tolerate the volume of a 2 g/kg IGIV infusion, is IGIV 400 mg/kg once/day for 4 days (again in combination with high-dose aspirin). The efficacy of IGIV/aspirin therapy when begun > 10 days after onset of illness is unknown, but therapy should still be considered.

After the child has improved for 4 to 5 days, aspirin 3 to 5 mg/kg/day is continued for at least 8 wk after onset until repeated echocardiographic testing is completed. If there are no coronary artery aneurysms and signs of inflammation are absent (demonstrated by normalization of ESR and platelets), aspirin may be stopped. Because of its antithrombotic effect, aspirin is continued indefinitely for children with coronary artery abnormalities. Children with giant coronary aneurysms may require additional anticoagulant therapy (eg, warfarin, dipyridamole).

Children who receive IGIV therapy may have a lower response rate to live viral vaccines. Thus, measles-mumps-rubella vaccine should generally be delayed for 11 mo after IGIV administration, and varicella vaccine should be delayed for ≥ 11 mo. If the risk of measles exposure is high, vaccination should proceed, but revaccination (or serologic testing) should be performed 11 mo later.

A small risk of Reye's syndrome exists in children receiving long-term aspirin during outbreaks of influenza or varicella; thus, annual influenza vaccination is indicated for children (≥ 6 mo of age) receiving long-term aspirin therapy. Further, parents of children receiving aspirin should be instructed to contact their child's physician promptly if the child is exposed to or develops symptoms of influenza or varicella. Temporary interruption of aspirin may be considered (with substitution of dipyridamole for children with documented aneurysms).

PROGERIA

(Hutchinson-Gilford syndrome)

Progeria is a rare syndrome of accelerated aging that manifests early in childhood and causes premature death.

Progeria is caused by a sporadic mutation in the *LMNA* gene that codes for a protein (lamin A) which provides the molecular scaffolding of cell nuclei. Defective protein leads to nuclear instability from cell division and early death of every body cell.

Symptoms and signs develop within 2 yr and include growth failure, craniofacial abnormalities (eg, craniofacial disproportion, micrognathia, beaked nose), and physical changes of aging (eg, wrinkled skin, balding). Diagnosis is usually obvious by appearance but must be distinguished from segmental progerias (eg, acrogeria, metageria) and other causes of growth failure. Median age at death is 12 yr; cause is coronary artery and cerebrovascular disease. Of note is that other problems associated with normal aging (eg, increased cancer risk, degenerative arthritis) are not present. There is no known treatment.

Premature aging is a feature of other rare progeroid syndromes, including Werner's syndrome (premature aging after puberty with hair thinning and development of conditions of old age [eg, cataracts, diabetes, osteoporosis, atherosclerosis]) and Rothmund-Thomson syndrome (premature aging with increased susceptibility to cancer). Both are caused by gene mutations leading to defective RecQ DNA helicases, which normally repair DNA. Cockayne syndrome is an autosomal recessive disease caused by mutation in the *ERCC8* gene, which is important in DNA excision repair. Clinical features include severe growth failure, cachectic appearance, retinopathy, hypertension, renal failure, skin photosensitivity, and mental retardation. Neonatal progeroid (Wiedemann-Rautenstrauch) syndrome is a recessively inherited syndrome of aging causing death by 2 yr. Other syndromes (eg, Down, Ehlers-Danlos) occasionally have progeroid features.

REYE'S SYNDROME

Reye's syndrome is a rare form of acute encephalopathy and fatty infiltration of the liver that tends to follow some acute viral infections, particularly when salicylates are used. Diagnosis is clinical. Treatment is supportive.

The cause of Reye's syndrome is unknown, but many cases seem to follow infection with influenza A or B or varicella. Using salicylates during such illness increases the risk by as much as 35-fold. This finding has led to a marked decrease in salicylate use in the US since the mid-1980s (except when specifically indicated such as in juvenile RA and Kawasaki disease), and a corresponding decrease in the incidence of Reye's from several hundred annual cases to < 20. The syndrome occurs almost exclusively in children < 18 yr. In the US, most cases occur in late fall and winter.

The disease affects mitochondrial function, causing disturbance in fatty acid and carnitine metabolism. Pathophysiology is similar to a number of inherited metabolic disorders.

Symptoms and Signs

The disease varies greatly in severity but is characteristically biphasic. Initial viral symptoms (URI or sometimes chickenpox) are followed in 5 to 7 days by pernicious nausea and vomiting and a sudden change in mental status. The changes in mental status may vary from a mild amnesia and lethargy to intermittent episodes of disorientation and agitation, which can progress rapidly to deepening stages of coma manifested by progressive unresponsiveness, decorticate and decerebrate posturing, seizures, flaccidity, fixed dilated pupils, and respiratory arrest. Focal neurologic findings are usually not present. Hepatomegaly occurs in about 40% of cases, but jaundice is absent.

Complications include electrolyte and fluid disturbances, increased intracranial pressure (ICP), diabetes insipidus, syndrome of inappropriate ADH secretion, hypotension, arrhythmias, bleeding diatheses (especially GI), pancreatitis, respiratory insufficiency, hyperammonemia, aspiration pneumonia, and poor temperature regulation.

Diagnosis

Reye's syndrome should be suspected in any child exhibiting the acute onset of an encephalopathy (without known heavy metal or toxin exposure) and pernicious vomiting associated with hepatic dysfunction. Liver biopsy provides the definitive diagnosis, showing microvesicular, fatty changes, and is especially useful in sporadic cases and in children < 2 yr. The diagnosis may also be made when the typical clinical findings and history are associated with the following laboratory findings: increased liver transaminases (AST, ALT > 3 times normal), normal bilirubin, increased blood ammonia level, and prolonged PT. CSF examination usually shows increased pressure, < 8 to 10 WBCs/μL, and normal protein levels; the CSF glutamine level may be elevated. Hypoglycemia and hypoglycorrhachia occur in 15% of cases, especially in children < 4 yr; they should be screened for metabolic disease. The condition is staged from I to V according to severity.

Signs of metabolic derangement include elevated serum amino acid levels, acid-base disturbances (usually with hyperventilation, mixed respiratory alkalosis–metabolic acidosis), osmolar changes, hypernatremia, hypokalemia, and hypophosphatemia.

Differential diagnosis includes other causes of coma and hepatic dysfunction, such as sepsis or hyperthermia (especially in infants); potentially treatable inborn abnormalities of urea synthesis (eg, ornithine transcarbamylase deficiency) or of fatty acid oxidation (eg, systemic carnitine deficiency, medium chain acyl-CoA dehydrogenase deficiency); phosphorus or carbon tetrachloride intoxication; acute encephalopathy caused by salicylism or other drugs (eg, valproate) or poisons; viral encephalitis or meningoencephalitis; and acute hepatitis. Illnesses such as idiopathic steatosis of pregnancy and tetracycline liver toxicity may show similar light microscopic findings.

Prognosis

Outcome is related to the duration of cerebral dysfunction, severity and rate of progression of coma, severity of the increased ICP, and degree of blood ammonia elevation. Progression from stage I to higher stages is likely when the initial blood ammonia level is > 100 μg/dL (> 60 μmol/L) and the PT is ≥ 3 sec longer than that of the control. In fatal cases, the mean time from hospitalization to death is 4 days. Fatality rates average 21% but range from < 2% among patients in stage I to > 80% in patients in stage IV or V. Prognosis for survivors usually is good, and recurrences are rare. However, the incidence of neurologic sequelae (mental retardation, seizure disorders, cranial nerve palsies, motor dysfunction) is as high as 30% among those who developed seizures or decerebrate posturing during illness.

Treatment

Treatment is supportive, with particular attention paid to control of ICP and to blood glucose, because glycogen depletion is common. Treatment of elevated ICP includes intubation, hyperventilation, fluid restriction of 1500 mL/m²/day, elevating the head of bed, and osmotic diuretics. Infusion of 10 or 15% dextrose is common to maintain euglycemia. Coagulopathy may require fresh frozen plasma or vitamin K. Other treatments (eg, exchange transfusion, hemodialysis, and induction of deep coma with the use of barbiturates) have not been proved effective but are sometimes used.

SUDDEN INFANT DEATH SYNDROME

Sudden infant death syndrome is the sudden and unexpected death of an infant or young child between 2 wk and 1 yr of age in which a thorough postmortem examination fails to show cause.

Sudden infant death syndrome (SIDS) is the most common cause of death between 2 wk and 1 yr of age, accounting for 35 to 55% of all deaths in this age group. Distribution is worldwide, occurring in 1.5/1000 births in the US. Peak incidence is between the 2nd and 4th mo of life. Many risk factors for SIDS (see TABLE 286–4) apply to non-SIDS infant deaths as well. Almost all SIDS deaths occur when the infant is thought to be sleeping.

Etiology

The cause is unknown, although it is most likely due to dysfunction of neural cardiorespiratory control mechanisms. The dysfunction may be intermittent or transient, and multiple mechanisms are probably involved. Fewer than 5% of SIDS victims have been noted to have episodes of prolonged apnea before their death, so the overlap between the SIDS population and infants with recurrent prolonged apnea is very small. Many studies link a prone (on stomach) sleeping position with increased risk of SIDS. Other risk factors include soft bedding (eg, lamb's wool), waterbed mattresses, smoking in the home, and an overheated environment.

Diagnosis

The diagnosis, while largely one of exclusion, cannot be made without an adequate autopsy to rule out other causes of sudden, unexpected death (eg, intracranial hemorrhage, meningitis, myocarditis).

Management

Parents who have lost a child to SIDS are grief-stricken and unprepared for the tragedy. Because no definitive cause can be found for their child's death, they usually have excessive guilt feelings, which may be aggravated by investigations conducted by police, social workers, or others. Family members require support not only during the days immediately after the infant's death, but for at least several months to help them with their grief and dispel guilt feelings. Such support includes, whenever possible, an immediate home visit to observe the circumstances in which SIDS occurred and to inform and counsel the parents concerning the cause of death.

Autopsy should be performed quickly. As soon as the preliminary results are known (usually within 12 h), they should be communicated to the parents. Some clinicians advise a series of home or office visits over the 1st month to continue the earlier discussions, answer questions, and give the family the final (microscopic) autopsy results. At the last meeting, it is appropriate to discuss the parents' adjustment to their loss, especially their attitude toward having other children. Much of the counseling and support can be complemented by specially trained nurses or by lay people who have themselves experienced the tragedy of and adjustment to SIDS (eg, members of a local chapter of the National Foundation for Sudden Infant Death Syndrome or of the International Guild for Infant Survival).

TABLE 286–4. RISK FACTORS FOR SUDDEN INFANT DEATH SYNDROME

Cold temperatures/winter months
Episodes of apnea requiring resuscitation
Low birth weight
Lower socioeconomic group
Maternal age < 20 yr
Maternal drug use during pregnancy
Maternal smoking during pregnancy
Overheating (blankets, hot room)
Prematurity
Recent illness
Sibling of a SIDS victim
Soft bedding

Prevention

The American Academy of Pediatrics recommends that infants be placed supine (on back) for sleep unless other medical conditions prevent this. The incidence of SIDS increases with overheating (clothing, blankets, hot room) and in cold weather. Thus, every effort should be made to avoid an overheated or an overly cold environment, to avoid overwrapping the infant, and to remove soft bedding, such as sheepskin, pillows, stuffed toys/animals, and comforters, from the crib. Mothers should avoid smoking during pregnancy, and infants should not be exposed to smoke. Parents should not have the infant in the parents' bed.

287 CONGENITAL CARDIOVASCULAR ANOMALIES

(See also Ch. 76 on p. 708.)

Congenital anomalies of the heart and blood vessels arise during the 1st 10 wk of embryonic development and are present at birth. The incidence is 1/120 live births; estimated risk is 2 to 3% in children with an affected 1st-degree relative.

About 5% of patients have a chromosomal abnormality (eg, trisomy 13, 18, or 21, Turner's syndrome); other anomalies may be part of a genetic syndrome (eg, Holt-Oram syndrome). Other possible causes are maternal illnesses (eg, diabetes mellitus, SLE, rubella), environmental exposure (eg, to thalidomide, isotretinoin, or alcohol [fetal alcohol syndrome]), or a combination. Usually, no specific cause is identified.

TABLE 287–1. CLASSIFICATION OF CONGENITAL HEART ANOMALIES*

CLASSIFICATION	EXAMPLE
Cyanotic	Tetralogy of Fallot
	Transposition of the great arteries
	Tricuspid atresia
	Pulmonary atresia
	Hypoplastic left heart syndrome
	Persistent truncus arteriosus
Acyanotic	
Left-to-right shunt	Ventricular septal defect
	Atrial septal defect
	Patent ductus arteriosus
	Atrioventricular septal defect
Obstructive	Pulmonic stenosis
	Aortic stenosis
	Aortic coarctation

*In decreasing order of frequency.

Pathophysiology

Congenital heart anomalies are classified as acyanotic or cyanotic, and acyanotic anomalies are classified as left-to-right shunts or obstructive lesions (see TABLE 287–1). Some anomalies, particularly when severe, may cause heart failure (HF).

Left-to-right shunts: Oxygenated blood from the left heart (left atrium or left ventricle) or the aorta shunts to the right heart (right atrium or right ventricle) or the pulmonary artery through an abnormal opening between the 2 sides. Blood flows from left to right initially because BPs are normally higher on the left side. The additional blood on the right side increases pulmonary blood flow and pulmonary artery pressure to a varying degree. The greater the increase, the more severe the symptoms; a small left-to-right shunt is usually asymptomatic.

High-pressure shunts (those at the ventricular or great artery level) become apparent several days to a few weeks after birth; low-pressure shunts (atrial septal defects) become apparent considerably later. If untreated, elevated pulmonary artery pressure may lead to Eisenmenger's syndrome (see p. 2420). A large left-to-right shunt (eg, large ventricular septal defect [VSD], patent ductus arteriosus) decreases lung compliance, leading to frequent lower respiratory tract infections.

Obstructive lesions: Blood flow is obstructed without shunting, causing a pressure gradient across the obstruction. The resulting pressure overload proximal to the obstruction may cause ventricular hypertrophy and HF. The principal manifestation is a heart murmur, which results from turbulent flow through the obstructed (stenotic) point. Examples are congenital aortic stenosis, which accounts for 3 to 6% of congenital heart anomalies, and congenital pulmonary stenosis, which accounts for 8 to 12% (for both, see Ch. 76 on p. 708).

Cyanotic heart anomalies: Varying amounts of deoxygenated venous blood are shunted to the left heart, reducing systemic arterial O_2 saturation. If there is > 5 g/dL of deoxygenated Hb, cyanosis (bluish discoloration of the skin, mucous membranes, and nails) results. Detection of cyanosis may be delayed in infants with dark pigmentation. Complications of persistent cyanosis include polycythemia, clubbing, thromboembolism, bleeding disorders, and hyperuricemia.

Hypercyanotic spells frequently occur in infants with tetralogy of Fallot (see p. 2414).

Depending on the anomaly, pulmonary blood flow may be increased (often resulting in HF), normal, or reduced (manifesting with severe cyanosis). Heart murmurs are variably audible and are not specific.

Heart failure: Some congenital heart anomalies (eg, bicuspid aortic valve, mild aortic stenosis) do not significantly alter hemodynamics. Others cause pressure or volume overload, sometimes producing HF. HF occurs when cardiac output is insufficient to meet the body's metabolic needs or when the heart cannot adequately dispose of venous return, causing pulmonary congestion (in left ventricular failure), edema primarily in dependent tissues and abdominal viscera (in right ventricular failure), or both (see p. 652). HF in infants and children has many causes other than heart anomalies (see TABLE 287–2).

Symptoms and Signs

Manifestations of the various heart anomalies are limited to several common ones (eg, murmurs, cyanosis, HF). Less commonly, chest pain, diminished or impalpable pulses, circulatory shock, and arrhythmias are present.

Most left-to-right shunts and obstructive lesions produce systolic murmurs. Systolic murmurs and thrills are most prominent at the surface closest to their point of origin, making location diagnostically helpful. Increased flow across the pulmonary or aortic valve produces a midsystolic (ejection systolic) murmur. Regurgitant flow through an atrioventricular valve or flow across a VSD produces a holosystolic (pansystolic) murmur, possibly obscuring heart sounds as its intensity increases. Patent ductus arteriosus produces a continuous murmur that is uninterrupted by the 2nd heart sound (S_2) because blood flows through the ductus during systole and diastole.

In infants, signs of HF include tachycardia, tachypnea, dyspnea with feeding, diaphoresis, restlessness, and irritability. Dyspnea with feeding causes inadequate intake and poor growth, which may be worsened by increased metabolic demands in HF and frequent respiratory tract infections. Hepatomegaly is common except with some left-to-right shunts. However, in contrast to adults and older children, most infants do not have distended neck veins and dependent edema, although they occasionally have edema in the periorbital area. Findings in older children with HF are similar to those in adults (see p. 656).

In neonates, circulatory shock may be the 1st manifestation of certain anomalies (eg, hypoplastic left heart syndrome, critical aortic or pulmonic stenosis, coarctation of the aorta). Patients appear extremely ill and have cold extremities, diminished pulses, low BP, and reduced response to stimuli.

Chest pain may be the 1st symptom in infants with a coronary artery anomaly or in older children with severe aortic or pulmonic stenosis. Eisenmenger's syndrome may also cause chest pain.

Diagnosis

Diagnosis is suggested by the presence of heart murmurs, HF, or cyanosis, usually during the 1st few months of life. Cyanosis due to heart defects should be distinguished from that due to other disorders (eg, various respiratory disorders, CNS depression, hypothermia, hypoglycemia, hypocalcemia, sepsis). Pulse oximetry, ECG, and chest x-ray are required. Echocardiography usually confirms the diagnosis. Cardiac catheterization and angiocardiography may be needed to confirm the diagnosis or to assess severity of the anomaly before surgery.

Treatment

Specific anomalies are treated, sometimes with surgery. Medical treatment of HF is similar to that in adults; it may include a diuretic (eg, furosemide 0.5 to 1.0 mg/kg po bid or tid), an ACE inhibitor (eg, captopril 0.1 to 0.3 mg/kg po tid), digoxin (dose varies by age; see TABLE 287–3), and salt restriction.

Because HF increases metabolic demands but makes feeding more difficult, enhanced caloric content feedings are recommended. Some patients require nasogastric or gastrostomy feedings to maintain growth. If these measures do not result in weight gain, surgical repair of the anomaly is indicated.

Acute severe HF in neonates or infants is a medical emergency. Vascular access should be established via an umbilical venous catheter to administer a diuretic (eg, furosemide or ethacrynic acid 1 mg/kg, repeated in 4 to 6 h) and to infuse inotropic drugs (dobutamine 5 to 15 μg/kg/min) and drugs that reduce afterload (nitroprusside 0.5 to 3.0 μg/kg/min IV; hydralazine 0.1 to 0.5 mg/kg IV or IM repeated in 4 to 6 h). Humidified O_2 should be given by croupette, mask, or nasal prongs with adequate FIO_2 to prevent cyanosis and

TABLE 287–2. COMMON CAUSES OF HEART FAILURE IN CHILDREN

AGE AT ONSET	CAUSES
In utero (uncommon)	Chronic anemia with subsequent volume overload
	Myocardial dysfunction secondary to myocarditis
	Sustained intrauterine tachycardia
Birth through 1st few days	Any of the above
	Critical aortic or pulmonic stenosis
	Hypoplastic left heart syndrome
	Intrauterine or neonatal paroxysmal supraventricular tachycardia
	Large systemic arteriovenous fistulas
	Metabolic disorders (eg, hypoglycemia, hypothermia, severe metabolic acidosis)
	Perinatal asphyxia with myocardial damage
	Severe intrauterine anemia (hydrops fetalis)
	Severe tricuspid or pulmonary insufficiency related to hypoxia
Up to 1 mo	Any of the above
	Anomalous pulmonary venous drainage, particularly with pulmonary vein obstruction
	Coarctation of aorta, with or without associated abnormalities
	Complete heart block associated with structural heart anomalies
	Left-to-right shunts in premature infants (eg, patent ductus arteriosus)
	Systemic arteriovenous fistulas
	Transposition of great arteries
Infancy (especially 6 to 8 wk)	Anomalous pulmonary venous return
	Bronchopulmonary dysplasia (right ventricular failure)
	Complete atrioventricular septal defects
	Patent ductus arteriosus
	Persistent truncus arteriosus
	Rare metabolic disorders (eg, glycogen storage disease)
	Single ventricle
	Supraventricular tachycardia
	Ventricular septal defect
Childhood	Acute cor pulmonale (caused by upper airway obstructions such as large tonsils)
	Acute rheumatic fever with carditis
	Acute severe hypertension (with acute glomerulonephritis)
	Bacterial endocarditis
	Chronic anemia (severe)
	Dilated congestive cardiomyopathy
	Nutritional deficiencies
	Valvular heart disorders due to rheumatic fever
	Viral myocarditis
	Volume overload in a noncardiac disorder

TABLE 287–3. ORAL DIGOXIN DOSAGE IN CHILDREN*

AGE	DIGITALIZING DOSE (μg/kg)	MAINTENANCE DOSE† (μg/kg bid)
Preterm neonates	20	2.5
Term neonates	30	4–5
1 mo–2 yr	40–50	5–6
2–10 yr	30–40	4–5
> 10 yr	10–15	1.25–2.5

*The IV dose is 75% of the oral dose.

†The maintenance dose is 25% of the digitalizing dose, given in 2 divided doses.

All doses based on ideal body weight.

The digitalizing dose is usually only necessary when treating arrhythmias or acute congestive heart failure. The total digitalizing dose is usually given over 24 h with ½ the dose given twice separated by 8- to 12-h intervals with ECG monitoring.

alleviate respiratory distress; when possible, FIO_2 should be kept < 40% to prevent pulmonary epithelial damage. A cardiac chair position may benefit small infants and children; this position reduces upward pressure into the thorax exerted by abdominal organs and thus reduces work required for breathing.

Need for prophylaxis against infective endocarditis depends on the specific anomaly.

ATRIAL SEPTAL DEFECT

(Ostium Secundum Defect)

An atrial septal defect is one or more openings in the interatrial septum, producing a left-to-right shunt, pulmonary hypertension, and heart failure. Symptoms and signs include exercise intolerance, dyspnea, fatigue, and atrial arrhythmias. A soft midsystolic murmur at the upper left sternal border is common. Diagnosis is by echocardiography. Treatment is surgical or catheter-based repair. Endocarditis prophylaxis is not usually required.

Atrial septal defects (ASDs) account for about 6 to 10% of cases of congenital heart disease. Most cases are isolated and sporadic, but some are part of a genetic syndrome (eg, mutations of chromosome 5, Holt-Oram syndrome).

ASDs can be classified by location: ostium secundum (defect in the fossa ovalis—in the center [or middle] part of the atrial septum), sinus venosus (defect in the posterior aspect of the septum, near the superior vena cava or inferior vena cava), or ostium primum (defect in the anteroinferior aspect of the septum, a form of endocardial cushion defect [atrioventricular septal defect—see p. 2410]).

To understand hemodynamic changes seen in ASD (and other anomalies), see Fig. 287–1 for normal hemodynamic data. In ASD, shunting is left to right initially (see Fig. 287–2). Most small ASDs close spontaneously during the 1st few years of life. However, persistent, large shunts result in right atrial and ventricular volume overload, pulmonary artery hypertension, elevated pulmonary vascular resistance, and right ventricular hypertrophy. Atrial fibrillation may occur later. Ultimately, the increase in right-sided pressure may result in a bidirectional atrial shunt with cyanosis during adulthood (see Eisenmenger's Syndrome on p. 2420).

Symptoms and Signs

Most small ASDs are asymptomatic. Larger shunts may cause exercise intolerance, dyspnea during exertion, fatigue, and atrial arrhythmias sometimes with palpitations. Passage of microemboli from the venous circulation across the ASD (paradoxical embolization), often associated with arrhythmias, may lead to cerebral or systemic thromboembolic disorders. Rarely, when an ASD is undiagnosed or untreated, Eisenmenger's syndrome develops.

Auscultation typically reveals a grade 2 to 3/6 midsystolic (or ejection systolic) murmur and a widely split, fixed S_2 at the upper left sternal border in children. A large left-to-right atrial shunt may produce a low-pitched diastolic murmur (due to increased tricuspid flow) at the left lower sternal border. These findings may be absent in infants, even those who have a large defect. A prominent right ventricular cardiac impulse may be present.

Diagnosis

Diagnosis is suggested by cardiac examination, chest x-rays, and ECG and confirmed by 2-dimensional echocardiography with color flow and Doppler studies.

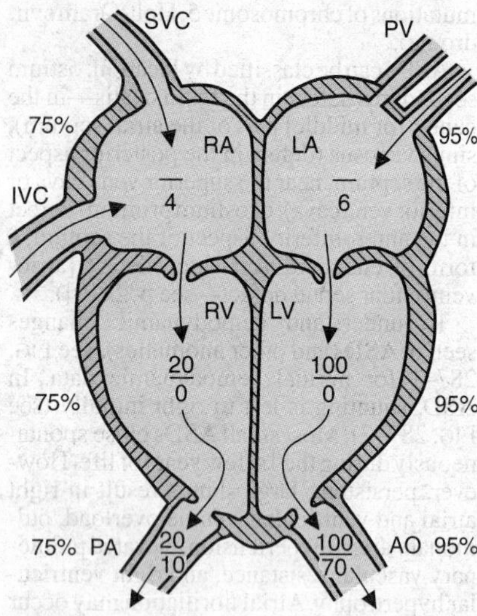

Fig. 287–1. Normal circulation with representative right and left heart pressures (in mm Hg). Representative right heart O_2 saturation = 75%; representative left heart O_2 saturation = 95%. Atrial pressures are mean pressures. AO = aorta; IVC = inferior vena cava; LA = left atrium; LV = left ventricle; PA = pulmonary artery; PV = pulmonary veins; RA = right atrium; RV = right ventricle; SVC = superior vena cava.

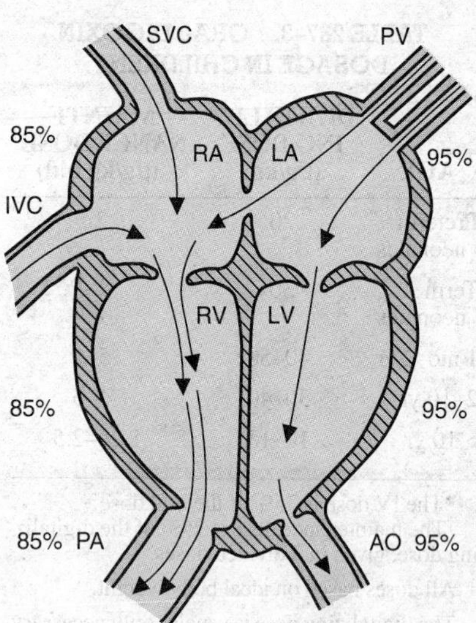

Fig. 287–2. In atrial septal defect, pulmonary blood flow and RA and RV volume are increased. AO = aorta; IVC = inferior vena cava; LA = left atrium; LV = left ventricle; PA = pulmonary artery; PV = pulmonary veins; RA = right atrium; RV = right ventricle; SVC = superior vena cava.

With a significant shunt, ECG may show right axis deviation, right ventricular hypertrophy, or right bundle branch block (with rSR′ pattern in V_1). Chest x-rays show cardiomegaly with dilation of the right atrium and right ventricle, a prominent main pulmonary artery segment, and increased pulmonary vascular markings.

Cardiac catheterization is not usually necessary unless additional associated anomalies are suspected.

Treatment

Most small ostium secundum ASDs (< 3 mm) close spontaneously; about 80% of those between 3 mm and 8 mm close spontaneously by age 18 mo. However, ostium primum and sinus venosus ASDs do not close spontaneously.

Asymptomatic children with a small shunt require annual echocardiography. Because these children are at risk of paradoxical systemic embolization, some centers recommend a catheter-delivered closure device (eg, Amplatzer Septal Occluder, Cardio-Seal device) even for small ASDs. However, these devices are not suitable for primum or sinus venosus defects because these defects are near important structures.

Patients with moderate to large defects (eg, pulmonary to systemic flow ratio > 1.5:1) should have the ASD closed, typically between age 2 to 6 yr. Closure devices are preferred when appropriate anatomic characteristics are present and the defect is < 13 mm in diameter. Otherwise, surgical repair is indicated. If ASDs are repaired during childhood, perioperative mortality rate approaches 0, and long-term survival rates approach those of the general population. Before repair, patients with large shunts and heart failure should be treated with diuretics, digoxin, and ACE inhibitors.

Patients with primum ASD require endocarditis prophylaxis (see TABLES 77–3, 77–4, and 77–5 on pp. 730–731); those with secundum or sinus venosus ASD do not.

VENTRICULAR SEPTAL DEFECT

A ventricular septal defect is one or more openings in the interventricular septum, producing a shunt between ventricles. Large defects result in a significant left-to-right shunt and produce dyspnea with feeding and poor growth. A loud, harsh, holosystolic murmur at the lower left sternal border is common. Recurrent respiratory infections and heart failure may develop. Diagnosis is by echocardiography. Defects may close spontaneously during infancy or require surgical repair. Endocarditis prophylaxis is recommended.

Ventricular septal defect (VSD—see FIG. 287–3) is the 2nd most common congenital heart anomaly after bicuspid aortic valve, accounting for 15 to 20%. It can occur alone or with other congenital anomalies (eg, tetralogy of Fallot, complete atrioventricular septal defects, transposition of the great arteries).

VSDs are classified by location: membranous (perimembranous), trabecular muscular, outlet (supracristal or subpulmonary), or inlet defects. Membranous defects (70 to 80%) involve varying amounts of muscular tissue adjacent to the membranous septum (thus called perimembranous defects); the most common type occurs immediately below the aortic valve. Trabecular muscular defects (5 to 20%) occur in the middle portion of the muscular septum. Outlet defects (5 to 7% in the US; about 30% in Far Eastern countries) occur in the ventricular septum under the pulmonary valve. Inlet defects (5 to 8%) occur posterior to the septal leaflet of the tricuspid valve.

Magnitude of the shunt depends primarily on defect size; larger defects result in a larger left-to-right shunt. Over time, a large shunt causes pulmonary artery hypertension, elevated pulmonary artery vascular resistance, right ventricular pressure overload, and right ventricular hypertrophy. Ultimately, the increased pulmonary vascular resistance causes shunt direction to reverse (from the right to the left ventricle), leading to Eisenmenger's syndrome (see p. 2420).

Small defects produce a relatively small left-to-right shunt; the pulmonary artery pressure is normal or only slightly increased. Heart failure (HF) and Eisenmenger's syndrome do not develop.

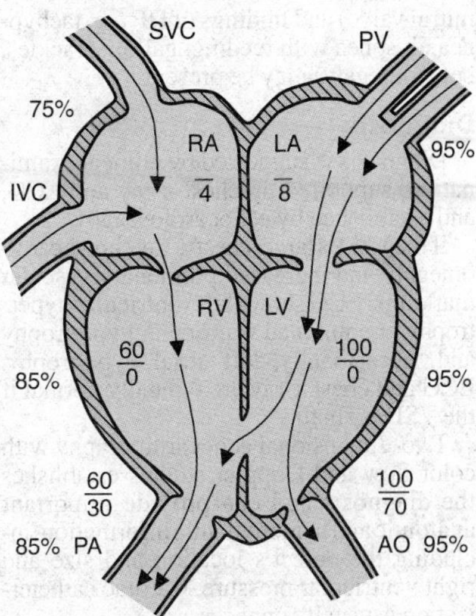

Fig. 287–3. In ventricular septal defect, pulmonary blood flow and LA and LV volumes are increased. Atrial pressures are mean pressures. RV pressure and O_2 saturation are positively related to defect size. AO = aorta; IVC = inferior vena cava; LA = left atrium; LV = left ventricle; PA = pulmonary artery; PV = pulmonary veins; RA = right atrium; RV = right ventricle; SVC = superior vena cava.

Symptoms and Signs

Symptoms depend on defect size and magnitude of the left-to-right shunt. Children with a small VSD are typically asymptomatic and grow and develop normally. In those with a larger defect, symptoms of HF (eg, poor weight gain, fatigue after feeding) appear at age 4 to 6 wk. Frequent lower respiratory tract infections may occur. Eventually, untreated patients may develop symptoms of Eisenmenger's syndrome.

Small VSDs typically produce a grade 3 to 4/6 holosystolic murmur (with or without thrill) at the lower left sternal border; it is audible shortly after birth. The precordium may be mildly hyperactive, but S_2 is normally split and has normal intensity.

Larger VSDs produce a similarly loud holosystolic murmur that is present by age 2 to 3 wk. S_2 is usually narrowly split with an accentuated pulmonary component. An apical diastolic rumble (due to overflow through the mitral valve) and findings of HF (eg, tachypnea, dyspnea with feeding, gallop, crackles, hepatomegaly) may be present.

Diagnosis

Diagnosis is suggested by clinical examination, supported by chest x-ray and ECG, and established by echocardiography.

If the VSD is large, chest x-ray shows cardiomegaly and increased pulmonary vascular markings. ECG shows left ventricular hypertrophy or combined ventricular hypertrophy and, occasionally, left atrial hypertrophy. ECG and chest x-ray are typically normal if the VSD is small.

Two-dimensional echocardiography with color flow and Doppler studies establishes the diagnosis and can provide important anatomic and hemodynamic information, including the defect's location and size and right ventricular pressure. Cardiac catheterization is usually unnecessary.

Treatment

Small VSDs, particularly muscular septal defects, often close spontaneously during the 1st few years of life. A small defect that remains open does not require medical or surgical therapy.

Moderate-sized defects are less likely to close spontaneously. Diuretics, digoxin, and ACE inhibitors are indicated before surgery if HF develops. If infants do not respond to medical treatment or have large shunts (with pulmonary to systemic flow ratio ≥ 2:1), surgical repair may be done during the 1st few months of life. Current surgical mortality rate is 2 to 5%. Surgical complications may include residual ventricular shunt, right bundle branch block, complete heart block, and ventricular arrhythmias.

All patients with a VSD, regardless of size, should be given endocarditis prophylaxis with antibiotics (see TABLE 77–4 on p. 730) before dental or surgical procedures that are likely to produce bacteremia.

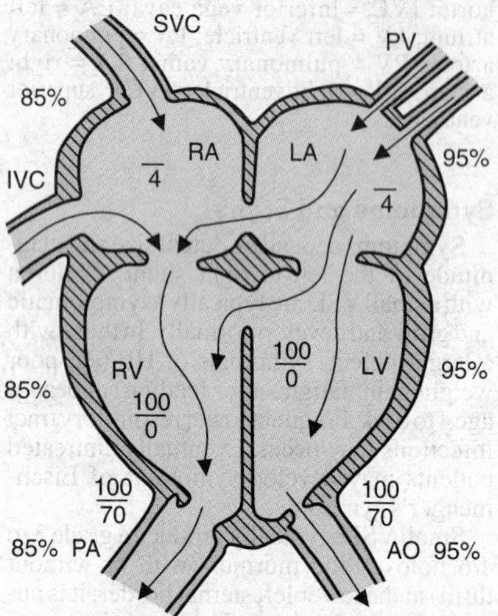

Fig. 287–4. In atrioventricular septal defect, pulmonary blood flow, chamber volume (all), and often pulmonary vascular resistance are increased. Atrial pressures are mean pressures. AO = aorta; IVC = inferior vena cava; LA = left atrium; LV = left ventricle; PA = pulmonary artery; PV = pulmonary veins; RA = right atrium; RV = right ventricle; SVC = superior vena cava.

ATRIOVENTRICULAR SEPTAL DEFECT

(Atrioventricular Canal Defect; Endocardial Cushion Defect; Persistent Ostium Primum)

Atrioventricular (AV) septal defect consists of primum type atrial septal defect with AV valve malformation, with or without a ventricular septal defect. These defects result from maldevelopment of the endocardial cushions. Defects may be asymptomatic if small. If large, they may cause heart failure, with dyspnea with feeding, poor growth, tachypnea, diaphoresis, or arrhythmias. A single loud S_2 and heart murmur are common. Diagnosis is by echocardiography or cardiac catheterization. Treatment is surgical repair for moderate to severe cases. Endocarditis prophylaxis is recommended.

AV septal defect accounts for about 5% of congenital heart anomalies. It may be complete or partial; 30% of patients with the complete form have Down syndrome. AV septal defect is also common in patients with asplenia or polysplenia syndrome.

Complete AV septal defect (see FIG. 287–4) consists of a large ostium primum atrial septal defect (ASD, in which the defect is in the anteroinferior aspect of the septum), an inlet ventricular septal defect (VSD), and a common AV valve orifice with regurgitation. A left-to-right shunt occurs at the atrial and ventricular levels; AV valve regurgitation may be significant, sometimes producing a direct left ventricle-to-right atrial shunt. These abnormalities result in enlargement of all 4 cardiac chambers. Over time, the increase in pulmonary blood flow, pulmonary artery pressure, and pulmonary vascular resistance may lead to reversal of shunt direction with cyanosis and Eisenmenger's syndrome (see p. 2420).

Partial AV septal defect consists of an ostium primum ASD, 2 separate AV valve openings, and a cleft in the mitral valve. The ventricular septum is intact. Hemodynamic abnormalities are similar to those of ostium secundum ASD.

Symptoms and Signs

Complete AV septal defect with a large left-to-right shunt produces signs of heart failure (HF—tachypnea, dyspnea with feeding, poor weight gain, diaphoresis) by age 4 to 6 wk. Pulmonary vascular obstructive disease (Eisenmenger's syndrome) may begin to develop before age 1 yr, especially in children with Down syndrome. Smaller defects with little or no AV valve regurgitation may be asymptomatic during childhood.

Partial AV septal defect is asymptomatic during childhood if mitral regurgitation is mild or absent. However, symptoms (eg, exercise intolerance, fatigue, palpitations) may develop during adolescence. Infants with moderate or severe mitral regurgitation often have signs of HF.

Physical examination in children with complete AV septal defect detects an active precordium because of volume and pressure overload. A single loud S_2 and a grade 3 to 4/6 holosystolic murmur are audible. Most children with a partial defect have wide splitting of the S_2 and a midsystolic (or ejection systolic) murmur audible at the upper left sternal border. A mid-diastolic rumble may be present at the lower left sternal border when the atrial shunt is large. A cleft in the AV valve produces the blowing apical murmur of mitral regurgitation.

Cardiac findings in children with the partial form are the same as those described for secundum ASD (see p. 2407); if mitral regurgitation coexists, there will also be an early systolic murmur at the apex.

Diagnosis

Diagnosis is suggested by clinical examination, supported by chest x-ray and ECG, and established by 2-dimensional echocardiography with color flow and Doppler studies.

Chest x-ray shows cardiomegaly with right atrial enlargement, biventricular enlargement, a prominent main pulmonary artery segment, and increased pulmonary vascular markings.

ECG shows a superiorly directed QRS axis, a counterclockwise QRS loop in the vectorcardiogram, frequent 1st-degree AV block, left or right ventricular hypertrophy or both, occasional right atrial hypertrophy, and right bundle branch block.

Cardiac catheterization is not usually necessary unless anatomy must be further characterized before surgical repair.

Treatment

Complete AV septal defect should be repaired before age 1 yr (in many centers as early as age 3 to 4 mo) to prevent development of Eisenmenger's syndrome, especially in infants with Down syndrome. In patients with 2 suitably sized ventricles and no additional defects, the primum ASD and inlet VSD are closed and the AV valve is reconstructed into 2 trileaflet valves. For a single-stage complete repair, mortality rate is 5 to 10%. Surgical complications include complete heart block (3%) and mitral regurgitation (7%). Pulmonary artery banding is no longer recommended unless associated abnormalities make complete repair high risk. For asymptomatic patients with a partial defect, elective surgery is done at age 1 to 2 yr. Surgical mortality rate is about 3%.

For patients with large shunts and HF, diuretics, digoxin, and ACE inhibitors are indicated before surgery.

All patients with AV septal defect should be given endocarditis prophylaxis (see TABLE 77–4 on p. 730) before dental or surgical procedures that are likely to produce bacteremia.

PATENT DUCTUS ARTERIOSUS

Patent ductus arteriosus (PDA) is a persistence of the fetal connection (ductus arteriosus) between the aorta and pulmonary artery after birth, resulting in a left-to-right shunt. Symptoms may include failure to thrive, poor feeding, tachycardia, and tachypnea. A continuous machine-like murmur in the upper left sternal border is common. Diagnosis is by echocardiography. Administration of

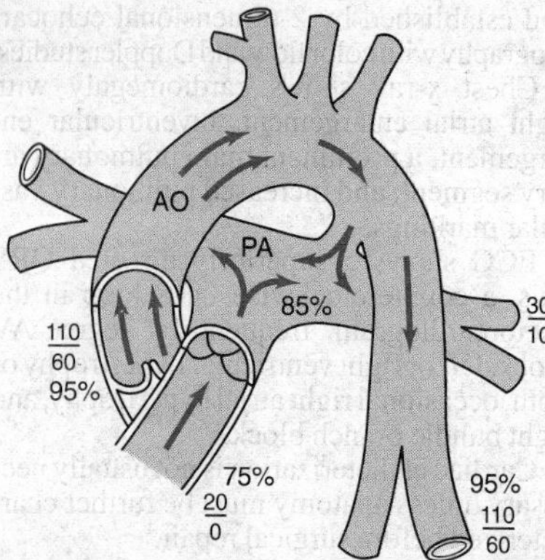

Fig. 287–5. In patent ductus arteriosus, pulmonary blood flow, LA and LV volumes, and ascending AO volume are increased. AO = aorta; LA = left atrium; LV = left ventricle; PA = pulmonary artery.

indomethacin with or without fluid restriction may be tried in premature infants with a significant shunt but not in term infants with PDA. If the connection persists, surgical or catheter-based correction is indicated. Endocarditis prophylaxis is recommended before and for 6 to 12 mo after correction.

Patent ductus arteriosus (PDA) accounts for 5 to 10% of congenital heart anomalies; the male:female ratio is 1:3. PDA is very common among premature infants (in 45% with birth weight < 1750 g; in about 80% with birth weight < 1200 g). Significant PDA causes heart failure (HF) in 15% of premature infants with birth weight < 1750 g and in 40 to 50% of those with birth weight < 1500 g.

The ductus arteriosus is a normal connection between the pulmonary artery and aorta; it is necessary for proper fetal circulation. At birth, the rise in PaO_2 and decline in prostaglandin concentration cause closure of the ductus arteriosus, typically within the 1st 10 to 15 h of life. If this normal process does not occur, PDA results (see FIG. 287–5).

Physiologic consequences depend on ductal size. A small ductus rarely produces symptoms. A large (and short) ductus causes a large left-to-right shunt. Over time, a large shunt results in pulmonary artery hypertension and elevated pulmonary vascular resistance, ultimately leading to Eisenmenger's syndrome (see p. 2420).

Symptoms and Signs

Clinical presentation depends on PDA size and gestational age at delivery. Infants and children with a small PDA are generally asymptomatic; infants with a large PDA present with signs of HF (eg, failure to thrive, poor feeding, tachypnea, dyspnea with feeding, tachycardia). Premature infants may present with respiratory distress, apnea, or other serious complications (eg, necrotizing enterocolitis). Signs of HF occur earlier in premature infants than in full-term infants and may be more severe.

Most children with a small PDA have normal heart sounds and peripheral pulses. A grade 1 to 3/6 continuous machinery murmur is heard best in the upper left sternal border.

Full-term infants with significant PDA shunt have full or bounding peripheral pulses with a wide pulse pressure. A grade 1 to 3/6 continuous machinery murmur is characteristic. A gallop rhythm may be audible if HF develops.

Premature infants with significant shunt have bounding pulses and a hyperdynamic precordium. A heart murmur occurs in the pulmonary area; the murmur may be continuous, systolic with a short diastolic component, or only systolic. Some infants have no audible heart murmur.

Diagnosis

Diagnosis is suggested by clinical examination, supported by chest x-rays and ECG, and established by 2-dimensional echocardiography with color flow and Doppler studies.

Chest x-ray and ECG are typically normal if the PDA is small. If the shunt is significant, chest x-rays show prominence of the left atrium, left ventricle, and ascending aorta and increased pulmonary vascular markings; ECG may show left ventricular hypertrophy. Cardiac catheterization is not usually necessary.

TABLE 287–4. INDOMETHACIN DOSING GUIDELINES (mg/kg)

AGE AT DOSE 1	DOSE 1	DOSE 2	DOSE 3
< 48 h	0.2	0.1	0.1
2–7 days	0.2	0.2	0.2
> 7 days	0.2	0.25	0.25

Treatment

In premature infants with compromised respiratory status, the PDA can sometimes be closed by using a prostaglandin synthesis inhibitor (eg, indomethacin [see TABLE 287–4 for doses] IV q 12 h for 3 doses; or ibuprofen 10 mg/kg po followed by 2 doses of 5 mg/kg at 24-h intervals) with or without fluid restriction. If this treatment is ineffective, surgical ligation is indicated.

In full-term infants, indomethacin is usually ineffective. For a large PDA, surgical ligation and division are typically done electively at age 6 mo to 3 yr. If HF develops, surgery can be done earlier after medical management for HF. Nonsurgical options for PDA closure include various catheter-delivered occlusion devices (percutaneous coil occlusion, Amplatzer duct occluder, Rashkind umbrella device). These techniques have become the treatment of choice in children > 1 yr. Outcomes after PDA closure are excellent.

Before and for 6 to 12 mo after surgical or catheter-based PDA closure, all patients require endocarditis prophylaxis (see TABLE 77–4 on p. 730) before dental or surgical procedures. Patients with a residual shunt require prophylaxis indefinitely.

COARCTATION OF THE AORTA

Coarctation of the aorta is localized narrowing of the aortic lumen that results in upper-extremity hypertension, left ventricular hypertrophy, and malperfusion of the abdominal organs and lower extremities. Symptoms vary with the anomaly's severity and range from headache, chest pain, cold extremities, fatigue, and leg claudication to fulminant heart failure and shock. A soft bruit may be heard over the coarctation site. Diagnosis is by echocardiography or by CT or MR angiography. Treatment is balloon angioplasty with stent placement, or surgical correction. Endocarditis prophylaxis is recommended.

Coarctation of the aorta accounts for 8 to 10% of congenital heart anomalies. It occurs in 10 to 20% of patients with Turner's syndrome. The male:female ratio is 2:1.

Coarctation of the aorta usually occurs at the proximal thoracic aorta just beyond the left subclavian artery. It rarely involves the abdominal aorta. Coarctation may occur alone or with various other congenital anomalies (eg, bicuspid aortic valve, ventricular septal defect, aortic stenosis, patent ductus arteriosus, mitral valve disorders, intracerebral aneurysm).

Physiologic consequences include increased left ventricular pressure overload, left ventricular hypertrophy, overperfusion of the upper part of the body including the brain, and malperfusion of the abdominal organs and lower extremities.

Symptoms and Signs

If coarctation is significant, circulatory shock with renal insufficiency (oliguria or anuria) and metabolic acidosis may develop during the neonatal period and may mimic findings of other systemic disorders such as sepsis.

Less severe coarctation may be asymptomatic during infancy. Subtle symptoms (eg, headache; chest pain, fatigue, and leg claudication during physical activities) may be present as children age. Hypertension is often present, but heart failure (HF) rarely develops after the neonatal period. Rarely, intracerebral aneurysms rupture, resulting in subarachnoid or intracerebral hemorrhage.

Typical physical examination findings include hypertension in the upper extremities, diminished or delayed femoral pulses, and low or unobtainable arterial BP in the lower extremities. A grade 2 to 3/6 ejection systolic murmur is best heard in the left interscapular area. Dilated intercostal collateral arteries may produce a continuous murmur in the intercostal spaces. Affected females may have Turner's syndrome, a congenital disorder producing lymphedema of the feet, webbed neck, squarely shaped chest, cubitus valgus, and widely spaced nipples.

Untreated coarctation may result in left ventricular failure, rupture of the aorta, intracranial hemorrhage, hypertensive encephalopathy, and hypertensive cardiovascular disease during adulthood.

Diagnosis

Diagnosis is suggested by clinical examination (including BP measurement in all 4 extremities), supported by chest x-rays and ECG, and established by 2-dimensional echocardiography with color flow and Doppler studies or with CT or MR angiography.

Chest x-ray shows coarctation as a "3" sign in the upper left mediastinal shadow. Heart size is normal unless HF supervenes. Dilated intercostal collateral arteries may erode the 3rd to 8th ribs, making the ribs notched, but notching is seldom seen before age 5 yr.

ECG usually shows left ventricular hypertrophy but may be normal. In neonates and small infants, ECG usually shows right ventricular hypertrophy or right bundle branch block rather than left ventricular hypertrophy.

Treatment

Symptomatic neonates require cardiopulmonary stabilization with infusion of prostaglandin E_1 (0.05 to 0.10 μg/kg/min—may titrate up to 0.4 μg/kg/min, then back down to lowest effective dose) to reopen the constricted ductus arteriosus. Then, pulmonary artery blood can perfuse the descending aorta through the ductus, improving systemic perfusion and reversing metabolic acidosis. Short-acting inotropic drugs (eg, dopamine, dobutamine), diuretics, and O_2 are used to treat HF.

Before surgery, hypertension may be treated with β-blockers; ACE inhibitors should be avoided. After surgery, hypertension can be treated with β-blockers, ACE inhibitors, or angiotensin II receptor blockers.

The preferred definitive treatment is controversial. Some centers prefer balloon angioplasty with or without stent placement, but others prefer surgical correction and reserve the balloon procedure for recoarctation after surgical correction. Initial success rate after balloon angioplasty is 80 to 90%; subsequent catheterization can dilate the stent as children grow.

Surgical options include resection and end-to-end anastomosis, patch aortoplasty, and left subclavian flap aortoplasty. Choice depends on anatomy and center preference. Surgical mortality rate is < 5% for symptomatic infants and < 1% for older children. Residual coarctation is common (6 to 33%). Rarely, paraplegia results from cross-clamping of the aorta during surgery.

All patients should be given endocarditis prophylaxis (see TABLE 77–4 on p. 730) before dental or surgical procedures that are likely to produce bacteremia, regardless of whether surgical correction has been done.

TETRALOGY OF FALLOT

Tetralogy of Fallot consists of 4 congenital anomalies: a large ventricular septal defect, right ventricular outflow obstruction, right ventricular hypertrophy, and over-riding of the aorta. Symptoms include cyanosis, dyspnea with feeding, poor growth, and tet spells (sudden, potentially lethal episodes of severe cyanosis). A harsh systolic murmur at the left upper sternal border with a single S_2 is common. Diagnosis is by echocardiography or cardiac catheterization. Definitive treatment is surgical repair. Endocarditis prophylaxis is recommended.

Tetralogy of Fallot (see FIG. 287–6) accounts for 7 to 10% of congenital heart anomalies. Anomalies other than the 4 listed above are frequently present; they include right aortic arch (25%), abnormal coronary artery anatomy (5%), stenosis of the pulmonary artery branches, presence of aorticopulmonary collateral vessels, patent ductus arteriosus, complete atrioventricular septal defect, and aortic valve regurgitation.

The ventricular septal defect (VSD) is typically large; thus, systolic pressures in the right and left ventricles (and in the aorta) are the same. Pathophysiology depends on degree of right ventricular outflow obstruction. A mild obstruction may produce a left-to-right shunt through the VSD; a severe obstruction produces a right-to-left shunt, resulting in low systemic arterial saturation (cyanosis) that is unresponsive to supplemental O_2.

In some patients with tetralogy of Fallot, sudden episodes of profound cyanosis ("tet spell") may occur, which may be lethal. A spell may be triggered by any event that slightly decreases O_2 saturation (eg, crying, defecating) or that suddenly decreases systemic vascular resistance (eg, playing, kicking legs when awakening) or by sudden onset of tachycardia or hypovolemia. A vicious circle may develop: The initial fall in arterial Po_2 stimulates the respiratory center and produces hyperpnea. Hyperpnea increases systemic venous return to the right ventricle by making the negative thoracic pump more efficient. In the presence of a fixed right ventricular outflow obstruction or decreased systemic vascular resistance, the increased systemic venous return to the right ventricle goes out the aorta, further decreasing arterial O_2 saturation and thus creating the vicious circle of the hypoxic spell.

Symptoms and Signs

Neonates with severe right ventricular outflow obstruction (or atresia) have severe cyanosis and dyspnea with feeding with poor weight gain. But those with minimal obstruction may not have cyanosis at rest.

Tet spells may be precipitated by activity and are characterized by paroxysms of hyperpnea (rapid and deep respirations), irritability and prolonged crying, increasing cyanosis, and decreasing intensity of the heart murmur. The spells occur most often in young infants; peak incidence is age 2 to 4 mo. A severe spell may lead to limpness, seizures, and occasionally death. During play, some toddlers may intermittently squat, a position that decreases systemic venous return, possibly increases systemic vascular resistance, and thus raises arterial O_2 saturation.

Auscultation detects a harsh grade 3 to 5/6 midsystolic murmur at the left upper sternal border (due to pulmonary stenosis rather than the VSD). S_2 is often single because the pulmonary component is markedly reduced. A prominent right ventricular impulse and a systolic thrill may be present.

Diagnosis

Diagnosis is suggested by history and clinical examination, supported by chest x-ray and ECG, and established by 2-dimensional echocardiography with color flow and Doppler studies.

Chest x-rays show a boot-shaped heart with a concave main pulmonary artery segment and diminished pulmonary vascular markings. A right aortic arch is present in 25%. ECG shows right ventricular hypertrophy and may also show right atrial hypertrophy. Cardiac catheterization is often indicated before surgery to detect concomitant abnormalities that may complicate surgical repair.

Treatment

Neonates with severe cyanosis due to ductal constriction are given an infusion of prostaglandin E_1 (0.05 to 0.1 μg/kg/min IV) to reopen the ductus arteriosus.

Treatment of tet spells consists of placing infants in a knee-chest position (older children usually squat spontaneously and do not develop tet spells) and administering morphine 0.1 to 0.2 mg/kg IM. IV fluids are used for volume expansion. If these measures do not control the spell, systemic BP can be increased with phenylephrine 0.02 mg/kg IV or ketamine 0.5 to 3 mg/kg IV or 2 to 3 mg/kg IM; ketamine is also sedating. Propranolol 0.25 to 1.0 mg/kg po q 6 h may prevent recurrences. Supplemental O_2 has a limited benefit.

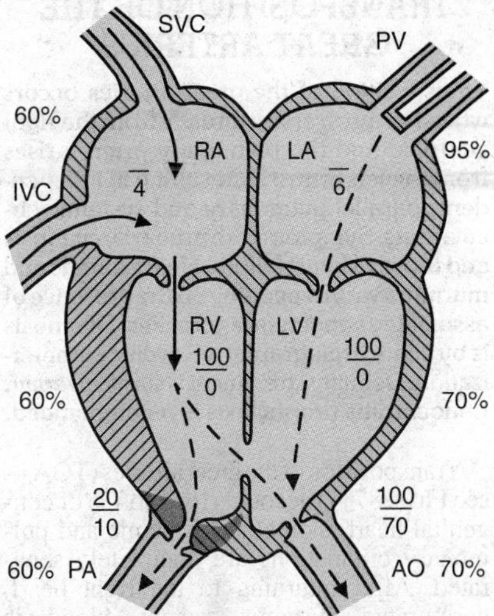

Fig. 287–6. In tetralogy of Fallot, pulmonary blood flow is decreased, the RV is hypertrophied, and unoxygenated blood enters the AO. Systolic pressures in the RV, LV, and AO are identical. Level of arterial desaturation is related to severity of the RV outflow tract obstruction. Atrial pressures are mean pressures. AO = aorta; IVC = inferior vena cava; LA = left atrium; LV = left ventricle; PA = pulmonary artery; PV = pulmonary veins; RA = right atrium; RV = right ventricle; SVC = superior vena cava.

Palliative surgery can be done in patients who are not ideal surgical candidates for complete repair or in some patients with tet spells. In the most popular procedure, a modified Blalock-Taussig shunt, the subclavian artery is connected to the ipsilateral pulmonary artery with a synthetic graft.

Complete repair consists of patch closure of the VSD and widening of the right ventricular outflow tract. Surgery is usually done electively during the 1st yr of life but, if symptoms are present, can be done any time after age 3 to 4 mo. Perioperative mortality rate is < 3% for uncomplicated tetralogy of Fallot. For untreated patients, survival rates are 55% at 5 yr and 30% at 10 yr.

All patients should be given endocarditis prophylaxis (see TABLE 77–4 on p. 730) before dental or surgical procedures that are likely to produce bacteremia, regardless of whether surgical repair has been done.

TRANSPOSITION OF THE GREAT ARTERIES

Transposition of the great arteries occurs when the aorta arises directly from the right ventricle and the pulmonary artery arises from the left ventricle, resulting in independent, parallel pulmonary and systemic circulations. Symptoms are primarily cyanosis and those of heart failure. Heart sounds and murmurs vary depending on the presence of associated congenital anomalies. Diagnosis is by echocardiography or cardiac catheterization. Definitive treatment is surgical repair. Endocarditis prophylaxis is recommended.

Transposition of the great arteries (TGA—see FIG. 287–7) accounts for 5 to 7% of congenital heart anomalies. Systemic and pulmonary circulations are completely separated. After returning to the right heart, desaturated systemic venous blood is pumped into the systemic circulation without being oxygenated in the lungs; oxygenated blood entering the left heart goes back to the lungs rather than to the rest of the body. This

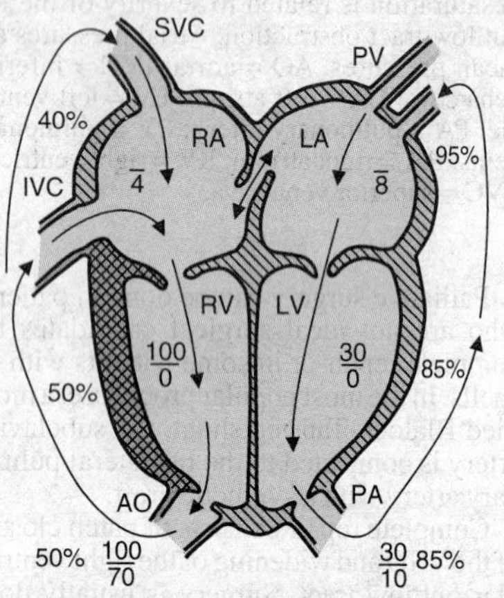

Fig. 287–7. In transposition of the great arteries, unoxygenated blood returning to the right heart enters the AO, producing severe cyanosis. Oxygenated blood returning to the LA enters the pulmonary circulation again. The RV is hypertrophied, and the foramen ovale permits minimal mixing. Atrial pressures are mean pressures. AO = aorta; IVC = inferior vena cava; LA = left atrium; LV = left ventricle; PA = pulmonary artery; PV = pulmonary veins; RA = right atrium; RV = right ventricle; SVC = superior vena cava.

anomaly is not compatible with life unless desaturated and oxygenated blood can mix through openings at one or more levels (eg, atrial, ventricular, or great artery level).

About 30 to 40% of patients have a ventricular septal defect (VSD); 5% have subpulmonary stenosis.

Symptoms and Signs

Severe cyanosis occurs within hours of birth, progressing rapidly to metabolic acidosis secondary to poor tissue oxygenation. Patients with a large VSD, a patent ductus arteriosus, or both are less cyanotic, but symptoms and signs of heart failure (eg, tachypnea, dyspnea, tachycardia, diaphoresis, inability to gain weight) may develop during the 1st 3 to 6 wk of life.

Except for generalized cyanosis, physical examination is usually unremarkable. Heart murmurs may be absent unless associated anomalies are present. S_2 is single and loud.

Diagnosis

Diagnosis is suspected clinically, supported by chest x-ray and ECG, and established by 2-dimensional echocardiography with color flow and Doppler studies.

On chest x-ray, the cardiac shadow may have the classic egg-on-a-string appearance with a narrow upper mediastinum. ECG shows right ventricular hypertrophy but may be normal during the 1st few days of life.

Cardiac catheterization is not usually necessary for diagnosis unless anatomy must be further characterized before surgical repair.

Treatment

Initially, prostaglandin E_1 (0.05 to 0.1 μg/kg/min IV) is infused to prevent closure of the ductus arteriosus. Metabolic acidosis is corrected via infusion of Na bicarbonate. Pulmonary edema and respiratory failure may require intubation and mechanical ventilation.

For severely hypoxemic neonates, cardiac catheterization and balloon atrial septostomy (Rashkind's procedure) can immediately improve systemic arterial saturation. A balloon-tipped catheter is advanced into the left atrium through the patent foramen ovale. The balloon is inflated with diluted radiopaque dye and abruptly withdrawn to the right atrium, using fluoroscopic or echocardiographic monitoring, to create a large opening in the atrial septum.

Definitive repair is the arterial switch operation (Jantene operation), typically done during the 1st 2 wk of life. The proximal portions of the great arteries are transected; the coronary arteries are transplanted to the proximal pulmonary artery, and the great arteries are connected to the correct ventricles, correcting the anomaly. Survival rate after surgery is > 90% at 1 yr and 5 yr. Presence of associated anomalies (eg, pulmonary stenosis, VSD) requires staged surgery.

All patients should be given endocarditis prophylaxis (see TABLE 77–4 on p. 730) before dental or surgical procedures that are likely to produce bacteremia.

TRICUSPID ATRESIA

Tricuspid atresia is absence of the tricuspid valve accompanied by a hypoplastic right ventricle. Associated anomalies are common and include atrial septal defect, ventricular septal defect, patent ductus arteriosus, and transposition of the great arteries. Symptoms include cyanosis and those of heart failure. S_2 is single, and murmurs depend on the presence of the associated anomalies. Diagnosis is by echocardiography or cardiac catheterization. Definitive treatment is surgical repair. Endocarditis prophylaxis is recommended.

Tricuspid atresia accounts for 1 to 3% of congenital heart anomalies. In the most common type (about 50%), a ventricular septal defect (VSD) and pulmonary stenosis are present, and pulmonary blood flow is decreased. A right-to-left shunt occurs at the atrial level, causing cyanosis. In another 30%, the great arteries are transposed, with a normal pulmonary valve, and pulmonary blood flow comes directly from the left ventricle, typically resulting in heart failure (HF).

Symptoms and Signs

Infants usually have severe cyanosis at birth. Signs of HF (tachypnea, dyspnea with feeding, poor weight gain, diaphoresis) may appear by age 4 to 6 wk.

Physical examination usually detects a single S_2 and a grade 2 to 3/6 holosystolic or early systolic murmur of a VSD at the lower left sternal border. A systolic murmur of pulmonary stenosis or a continuous murmur of patent ductus arteriosus may be present in the upper left sternal border. A systolic thrill is rarely palpable if pulmonary stenosis is present. An apical diastolic rumble is rarely audible if pulmonary blood flow is increased. Long-standing cyanosis may result in clubbing.

Diagnosis

Diagnosis is suspected clinically, supported by chest x-ray and ECG, and established by 2-dimensional echocardiography with color flow and Doppler studies.

In the most common form, chest x-rays show normal or slightly increased heart size, right atrial enlargement, and decreased pulmonary vascular markings. Occasionally, the cardiac silhouette resembles that of tetralogy of Fallot (with a boot-shaped heart and concave pulmonary artery segment). Pulmonary vascular markings may be increased and cardiomegaly present in infants with transposition of the great arteries. ECG characteristically shows left superior QRS axis (between 0° and −90°) and left ventricular hypertrophy. Right atrial hypertrophy or combined atrial hypertrophy is also common.

Cardiac catheterization is usually necessary to further characterize the anatomy before surgical repair.

Treatment

In severely cyanotic neonates, prostaglandin E_1 (beginning at 0.05 to 0.1 μg/kg/min IV) is infused to prevent closure of the ductus arteriosus or to reopen the constricted ductus before planned cardiac catheterization or surgical repair.

Balloon atrial septostomy (Rashkind's procedure) may be done as part of the initial catheterization to improve the right-to-left atrial shunt when the interatrial communication is inadequate. Some infants with transposition of the great arteries and signs of HF require medical treatment (eg, diuretics, digoxin, ACE inhibitors—see p. 2405).

Definitive repair requires staged operations: soon after birth, a Blalock-Taussig shunt (connection of a systemic and a pulmonary artery by a Gore-Tex tube); at age 4 to 8 mo, a bidirectional Glenn shunt (anastomosis between the superior vena cava and right pulmonary artery) or the hemi-Fontan procedure (diversion of blood from the superior vena cava to the central portion of the pulmonary artery through an anastomosis between the right atrial appendage and pulmonary artery and a patch sewed in the upper part of the right atrium); and by age 2 yr, a modified Fontan procedure. This approach has increased early survival rates to > 90%; survival rates are 85% at 1 mo, 80% at 5 yr, and 70% at 10 yr.

All patients should be given endocarditis prophylaxis (see TABLE 77–4 on p. 730) before dental or surgical procedures that are likely to produce bacteremia, regardless of whether surgical repair has been done.

HYPOPLASTIC LEFT HEART SYNDROME

Hypoplastic left heart syndrome consists of hypoplasia of the left ventricle and ascending aorta, maldevelopment of the aortic and mitral valves, an atrial septal defect, and a large patent ductus arteriosus. Unless normal closure of the patent ductus arteriosus is prevented with prostaglandin infusion, cardiogenic shock and death ensue. A loud single S_2 and nonspecific systolic murmur are common. Diagnosis is by emergency echocardiography or cardiac catheterization. Definitive treatment is staged surgical correction or heart transplantation. Endocarditis prophylaxis is recommended.

Hypoplastic left heart syndrome accounts for 1% of congenital heart anomalies. Oxygenated blood coming into the left atrium from the lungs cannot enter the hypoplastic left ventricle. Instead, it crosses through an atrial communication into the right heart, where it mixes with desaturated blood. This relatively desaturated blood exits the right ventricle through the pulmonary artery to the lungs and through the ductus arteriosus to the systemic circulation. Systemic blood flow is maintained only through the right-to-left ductal shunt; immediate survival thus depends on patency of the ductus arteriosus.

Symptoms and Signs

Symptoms appear when the ductus arteriosus begins to close during the 1st 24 to 48 h of life. Subsequently, symptoms of cardiogenic shock (eg, tachypnea, dyspnea, weak pulse, pallor, cyanosis, hypothermia, metabolic acidosis, lethargy, oliguria or anuria) develop. When systemic circulation is compromised, coronary and cerebral perfusion may be reduced, leading to symptoms of myocardial or cerebral ischemia. If the ductus arteriosus is not reopened, death rapidly ensues.

Physical examination detects vasoconstriction in the extremities and bluish gray skin color (due to cyanosis and poor perfusion). S_2 is loud and single. Occasionally, a soft nonspecific systolic murmur is present. Severe metabolic acidosis out of proportion to the P_{O_2} and P_{CO_2} is characteristic.

Diagnosis

Diagnosis is suspected clinically and confirmed by emergency echocardiography with color flow and Doppler studies. Cardiac catheterization is usually required to further characterize the anatomy before surgery.

Chest x-ray shows cardiomegaly and pulmonary venous congestion or pulmonary edema. ECG almost always shows right ventricular hypertrophy.

Treatment

All affected infants should be stabilized immediately in a neonatal intensive care unit. Vascular access should be established, usually via an umbilical venous catheter; then prostaglandin E_1 (PGE_1; beginning at 0.05 to 0.1 µg/kg/min IV) is infused to prevent closure of the ductus arteriosus or to reopen a constricted ductus. Neonates usually require intubation and mechanical ventilation. Metabolic acidosis is corrected via infusion of Na bicarbonate. Severely ill neonates with cardiogenic shock may require inotropic drugs and diuretics to improve cardiac function and control volume status.

Survival ultimately requires staged operations that enable the right ventricle to function as the systemic ventricle. The 1st stage, done during the 1st wk of life, is the Norwood procedure. The main pulmonary artery is divided, the distal stump is closed with a patch, and the ductus arteriosus is ligated. Then, a right-sided Blalock-Taussig shunt or right ventricular-pulmonary artery conduit (Sano modification) is done; the atrial septum is enlarged, and the proximal pulmonary artery and hypoplastic aorta are connected with an aortic or pulmonary artery allograft to create a neoaorta. Stage 2, done 6 mo later, consists of a bidirectional Glenn operation (end-to-side connection of the superior vena cava to the right pulmonary artery) or a hemi-Fontan procedure (see Tricuspid Atresia on p. 2417) is done. The 3rd stage, done about 12 mo after the 2nd, is a modified Fontan procedure; blood from the inferior vena cava is directed to the pulmonary circulation, completely bypassing the right ventricle. Survival rate is 75% after stage 1, 95% after stage 2, and 90% after stage 3. Survival rate is 70% at 5 yr after surgical correction. Many survivors have neurodevelopmental disabilities, which may be due to preexisting developmental abnormalities of the CNS rather than the surgery.

In some centers, heart transplantation is the procedure of choice; however, PGE_1 infusion must be continued until a donor heart is available. Also, availability of donor hearts is very limited; about 20% of infants die while waiting for one. The 5-yr survival rates after transplantation and after multistage surgery are similar. After heart transplantation, immunosuppressants are required. These drugs make patients more susceptible to infections and cause pathologic changes in the coronary arteries of the transplanted heart in > 50% of patients over a 5-yr period. The only known treatment for allograft coronary artery disease is retransplantation.

All patients should be given endocarditis prophylaxis (see TABLE 77–4 on p. 730) before dental or surgical procedures that are likely to produce bacteremia.

PERSISTENT TRUNCUS ARTERIOSUS

Persistent truncus arteriosus occurs when, during fetal development, the primitive truncus does not divide into the pulmonary artery and aorta, resulting in a single large arterial trunk that overlies a large, perimembranous, infundibular ventricular septal defect. Consequently, a mixture of oxygenated and deoxygenated blood enters systemic, pulmonary, and coronary circulations. Symptoms include cyanosis, poor feeding, diaphoresis, and tachypnea. A normal S_1 and a loud single S_2 are common; murmurs may vary. Diagnosis is by echocardiography or cardiac catheterization. Medical treatment for heart failure is typically followed by surgical repair. Endocarditis prophylaxis is recommended.

Persistent truncus arteriosus accounts for 1 to 2% of congenital heart anomalies. About 35% of patients have DiGeorge syndrome or velocardiofacial syndrome. There are 4 types. In type I, the main pulmonary artery arises from the truncus, then divides into the right and left pulmonary arteries. In types II and III, the right and left pulmonary arteries arise separately from the posterior and lateral aspects of the truncus, respectively. In type IV, arteries arising in the descending aorta supply the lungs; this type is now considered a severe form of tetralogy of Fallot.

Other anomalies (eg, truncal valve insufficiency, coronary artery anomalies, atrioventricular septal defect, double aortic arch) may be present and may contribute to the high surgical mortality rate.

Physiologic consequences of type I include mild cyanosis, heart failure (HF), and significant pulmonary overcirculation. In types II and III, cyanosis is more noticeable and HF is infrequent because pulmonary blood flow is normal or only slightly increased.

Symptoms and Signs

Neonates with type I present with mild cyanosis and symptoms and signs of HF (tachypnea, poor feeding, diaphoresis) in the 1st few weeks of life. Neonates with type II or III present with more noticeable cyanosis, but HF is less likely to develop.

Physical examination may detect a hyperdynamic precordium, increased pulse pressure, a loud and single S_2, and an ejection click. A grade 2 to 4/6 holosystolic murmur is audible along the left sternal border. A mid-diastolic mitral flow murmur may be audible at the apex when pulmonary blood flow is increased. With truncal valve insufficiency, a high-pitched diastolic decrescendo murmur is audible over the mid left sternal border.

Diagnosis

Diagnosis is suspected clinically, supported by chest x-ray and ECG, and established by 2-dimensional echocardiography with color flow and Doppler studies. Cardiac catheterization is often necessary to delineate associated anomalies before surgery.

Chest x-rays show varying degrees of cardiomegaly with increased pulmonary vascular markings, right aortic arch (in about 30%), and relatively high position of pulmonary arteries. ECG commonly shows combined ventricular hypertrophy. Substantial pulmonary overcirculation may produce evidence of left atrial hypertrophy.

Treatment

HF is treated vigorously with diuretics, digoxin, and ACE inhibitors, followed by early surgical repair. IV prostaglandin infusion is not beneficial.

Surgical management consists of complete primary repair. The ventricular septal defect is closed so that the left ventricle ejects into the truncal artery. A conduit with or without a valve is placed between the right ventricle and the confluence of the pulmonary arteries. Surgical mortality rate is 10 to 30%.

All patients require endocarditis prophylaxis (see TABLE 77–4 on p. 730) before dental or surgical procedures that are likely to produce bacteremia.

EISENMENGER'S SYNDROME

(Pulmonary Vascular Obstructive Disease)

Eisenmenger's syndrome is a complication of uncorrected congenital heart anomalies that produce left-to-right shunting. Increased pulmonary resistance often develops over time, reversing left-to-right shunting to right-to-left shunting. Deoxygenated blood enters the systemic circulation, causing symptoms of hypoxia. Murmurs and heart sounds depend on the underlying anomaly. Diagnosis is by echocardiography or cardiac catheterization. Treatment is generally supportive, but heart and lung transplantation may be an option when symptoms are severe. Endocarditis prophylaxis is recommended.

Congenital heart anomalies that, if untreated, result in Eisenmenger's syndrome include ventricular septal defect, atrioventricular canal defect, atrial septal defect, persistent truncus arteriosus, and transposition of the great arteries. In the US, incidence has markedly decreased because of early diagnosis and definitive repair of the causative anomaly.

Right-to-left shunting due to Eisenmenger's syndrome results in cyanosis and its complications. Systemic desaturation leads to clubbing of fingers and toes, secondary polycythemia, hyperviscosity, and sequelae of increased RBC turnover (eg, hyperuricemia causing gout, hyperbilirubinemia causing cholelithiasis, iron deficiency with or without anemia).

Symptoms and Signs

Symptoms usually do not occur until age 20 to 40 yr; they include cyanosis, syncope, dyspnea during exertion, fatigue, chest pain, palpitations, atrial and ventricular arrhythmias, and rarely right HF (hepatomegaly, peripheral edema, jugular venous distention). Hemoptysis is a late symptom. Signs of cerebral embolic phenomena or endocarditis may develop.

Secondary polycythemia commonly causes symptoms (eg, slurred speech, visual problems, headaches, increased fatigue, or signs of thromboembolic disorders). Abdominal pain may result from cholelithiasis.

Physical examination detects central cyanosis and digital clubbing. Rarely, signs of right ventricular failure (see p. 2405) may be present. A holosystolic murmur of tricuspid regurgitation may be present at the lower left sternal border. An early diastolic decrescendo murmur of pulmonary insufficiency may be audible along the left sternal border. A loud, single S_2 is a constant finding; an ejection click is common. Scoliosis is present in about ⅓ of patients.

Diagnosis

Diagnosis is suspected by history of uncorrected cardiac anomalies, supported by chest x-rays and ECG, and established by 2-dimensional echocardiography with color flow and Doppler studies or cardiac catheterization.

Laboratory testing shows polycythemia with Hct > 55%. Increased RBC turnover may be reflected as an iron deficiency state (eg, microcythemia), hyperuricemia, and hyperbilirubinemia.

Chest x-rays usually show prominent central pulmonary arteries, peripheral pulmonary pruning, and right heart enlargement. ECG shows right ventricular hypertrophy and, occasionally, right atrial hypertrophy.

Treatment

Ideally, corrective operations should have been done earlier to prevent Eisenmenger's syndrome. There is no specific treatment once the syndrome develops, but drugs that may lower pulmonary artery pressure are being studied. They include prostacyclin antagonists (treprostinol, epoprostenol), endothelin antagonists (bosentan), and nitric oxide enhancers (sildenafil).

Supportive treatment includes avoidance of conditions that may exacerbate the syndrome (eg, pregnancy, volume depletion, isometric exercise, high altitudes) and use of supplemental O_2. Polycythemia can be treated by cautious phlebotomy to lower Hct to 50 to 60% plus simultaneous volume replacement with normal saline. Hyperuricemia can be treated with allopurinol 300 mg po once/day. Aspirin 81 mg po once/day is indicated to prevent thrombotic complications.

Life expectancy depends on type and severity of the underlying congenital anomaly and ranges from 20 to 50 yr; median age at death is 37 yr. However, low exercise tolerance and secondary complications severely limit quality of life.

Heart and lung transplantation may be an option but is reserved for patients with severe symptoms. Long-term survival after transplantation is not promising.

All patients should be given endocarditis prophylaxis (see TABLE 77–4 on p. 730) before dental or surgical procedures that are likely to produce bacteremia.

COMPLEX AND RARE ABNORMALITIES

Complex and rare cyanotic heart anomalies include single ventricle with or without pulmonary stenosis, pulmonary atresia with an intact ventricular septum, and double outlet right ventricle. Diagnosis is by echocardiography; cardiac catheterization and angiography are usually indicated to delineate the exact anatomy before surgery.

Initially, surgical management involves ensuring adequate pulmonary blood flow via a systemic-to-pulmonary artery anastomosis (eg, Blalock-Taussig shunt) and protecting the pulmonary vascular bed via pulmonary artery banding. Later, the Fontan procedure can be used as definitive treatment to make a functioning ventricle the systemic ventricle.

Rare noncyanotic abnormalities include congenital complete heart block, congenital metabolic errors usually leading to severe acidosis and secondary myocardial dysfunction, and prolonged QT syndrome with risks of severe and possibly fatal arrhythmia.

288 CONGENITAL CRANIOFACIAL AND MUSCULOSKELETAL ABNORMALITIES

Many craniofacial and musculoskeletal abnormalities occur only at a single, specific site. They may be a deformity (alteration in shape due to unusual pressure and malpositioning, eg, clubfoot) or a malformation (an error in normal organ or tissue development, eg, anencephaly). Both deformities and malformations affect function. Some abnormalities (eg, arthrogryposis multiplex congenita) affect multiple sites.

ARTHROGRYPOSIS MULTIPLEX CONGENITA

(Multiple Congenital Contractures)

Arthrogryposis multiplex congenita is characterized by multiple joint contractures (especially of the upper limbs and neck) and amyoplasia, typically without other serious congenital abnormalities. Intelligence is relatively normal.

Any condition that impairs in utero movement (eg, uterine malformations, multiple gestations, oligohydramnios) can result in arthrogryposis multiplex congenita (AMC). AMC is not genetic, although in some genetic disorders (eg, spinal muscular atrophy type I, trisomy 18), incidence of arthrogryposis is increased. AMC can result from neurogenic, myopathic, or connective tissue disorders. Congenital myopathies, anterior horn cell disorders, and maternal myasthenia gravis have been proposed as causes of the associated amyoplasia.

Symptoms and Signs

Deformities are prominent at birth. AMC is not progressive; however, the condition that causes it (eg, muscular dystrophy) may be. Affected joints are contracted in flexion or extension. Shoulders are usually adducted and internally rotated, the elbows extended, and the wrists and digits flexed. Hips may be dislocated and are usually slightly flexed. Knees are extended; feet are often in the equinovarus position. Leg muscles are usually hypoplastic, and limbs tend to be tubular and featureless. Soft-tissue webbing sometimes occurs over ventral aspects of the flexed joints. The spine may be scoliotic. Except for slenderness of the long bones, the skeleton is radiographically normal. Physical disabilities may be severe. Intelligence is usually unimpaired or mildly abnormal.

Other abnormalities that rarely accompany arthrogryposis include microcephaly, cleft palate, cryptorchidism, and cardiac and urinary tract abnormalities.

Diagnosis and Treatment

Evaluation should include a thorough assessment for associated abnormalities. Electromyography and muscle biopsy are useful to diagnose neuropathic and myopathic disorders. Muscle biopsy typically shows amyoplasia, with fatty and fibrous replacement of tissues.

Early orthopedic and physical therapy evaluations are indicated. Joint manipulation during the first few months of life may produce considerable improvement. Orthotics may help. Surgery may be needed later to align the angle of ankylosis, but mobility is rarely enhanced. Muscle transfers (eg, surgically moving the triceps so that it can flex the elbow) may improve function. Many children do remarkably well; ⅔ are ambulatory after treatment.

CONGENITAL AMPUTATIONS

Congenital amputations are transverse or longitudinal limb deficiencies due to primary intrauterine growth inhibition or secondary intrauterine destruction of normal embryonic tissues.

Congenital amputations are missing or incomplete limbs at birth. Etiology is often unclear, but teratogenic agents (eg, thalidomide) and amniotic bands are known causes.

In transverse deficiencies, all elements beyond a certain level are absent, and the limb resembles an amputation stump. For example, in proximal femoral focal deficiency, the proximal femur and acetabulum do not develop; degree of deficiency varies. Longitudinal deficiencies involve specific maldevelopments (eg, complete or partial absence of the radius, fibula, or tibia). They may result from a syndrome such as VACTERL (formerly VATER: *v*ertebral anomalies, *a*nal atresia, *c*ardiac malformations, *t*racheo*e*sophageal fistula, *r*enal anomalies, and *l*imb anomalies [eg, radial aplasia]). Infants with transverse or longitudinal limb deficiencies may also have hypoplastic or bifid bones, synostoses, duplications, dislocations, or other bony defects. One or more limbs may be affected, and type of defect may be different in each limb. CNS abnormalities are rare. X-rays are essential to determine which bones are involved.

Treatment consists mainly of prosthetic devices, which are most valuable for lower-limb deficiencies or for completely or almost completely absent upper limbs. If any activity in an arm or hand exists, no matter how great the malformation, functioning capacity must be thoroughly assessed before a prosthesis or operation is recommended. Therapeutic amputation of any limb or portion of a limb should be considered only after evaluating the functional and psychologic implications of the loss and when essential for fitting a prosthesis.

An upper-limb prosthesis should be designed to serve as many needs as possible so that the number of devices is kept to a minimum. Children use a prosthesis most successfully when it is fitted early and becomes an integral part of their body and body image during the developmental years. Devices used during infancy should be as simple and durable as possible; eg, a hook rather than a bioelectric arm. With effective orthopedic and ancillary support, most children with congenital amputations lead normal lives.

CRANIOFACIAL ABNORMALITIES

Various craniofacial abnormalities result from maldevelopment of the 1st and 2nd visceral arches, which form facial bones and ears during the 2nd mo of gestation. These deformities include cleft lip and cleft palate; Treacher Collins (mandibulofacial dysostosis), Goldenhar's (oculoauriculovertebral dysplasia or hemifacial microsomia), Waardenburg's, and Pierre Robin syndromes; hypertelorism; and external and middle ear deformities (see TABLE 288–1). Most infants with craniofacial abnormalities have normal intelligence.

Cleft palate and cleft lip: The most common 1st arch deformities are cleft palate and cleft lip, which occur in 1/700 to 800 births. Both environmental and genetic factors are thought to contribute. Prenatal maternal use of tobacco and alcohol may increase risk. Having one affected child increases risk of having a second one. Folic acid, taken just

TABLE 288–1. COMMON CRANIOFACIAL SYNDROMES

SYNDROME	TYPICAL FINDINGS
Waardenburg's syndrome	Deafness, partial albinism (white forelock usually), heterochromic iris, laterally displaced medial canthi
Pierre Robin syndrome	Micrognathia with glossoptosis, mandibular hypoplasia, cleft soft palate
Treacher Collins syndrome	Malformed external ear, mandibular and malar hypoplasia, antimongoloid slant of the palpebral fissures, coloboma of the lower eyelid, conductive hearing loss
Goldenhar's syndrome (oculoauriculovertebral dysplasia)	Facial asymmetry, unilateral malformed external ear with preauricular tags and sinuses, conductive hearing loss, microphthalmia, epibulbar lipodermoid, macrostomia with mandibular hypoplasia, vertebral abnormalities
Velocardiofacial syndrome	Cleft palate, hypernasal speech, cardiac abnormalities, typical facies, learning disabilities

before becoming pregnant and through the 1st trimester, decreases the risk.

The cleft may vary from involvement of only the soft palate to a complete fissure of the soft and hard palates, the alveolar process of the maxilla, and the lip. The mildest form is a bifid uvula. An isolated cleft lip can occur.

A cleft palate interferes with feeding and speech development. Goals of treatment are to ensure normal feeding, speech, and maxillofacial growth and to avoid formation of fistulas. Early treatment, depending on the specific abnormality, consists of specially designed bottle nipples (to facilitate flow) or dental appliances (to occlude the cleft so suckling can occur) and a feeder that can be squeezed to deliver formula. Ultimate treatment is surgical closure; however, timing of surgery, which may interfere with growth centers around the premaxilla, is somewhat controversial. For a cleft palate, a 2-stage procedure is often done. The cleft lip and soft palate are repaired during infancy (at age 3 to 6 mo). Then, the residual hard palate cleft is repaired at age 15 to 18 mo. Surgery can result in significant improvement, but if deformities are severe or treatment is inadequate, patients may be left with a nasal voice, compromised appearance, and a tendency to regurgitate. Dental and orthodontic treatment, speech therapy, and counseling may be required.

Deformities characterized by a small mandible: Pierre Robin syndrome and Treacher Collins syndrome are characterized by glossoptosis (a tongue that falls to the back of the throat) and respiratory problems as well as micrognathia (a small mandible). A cleft palate as well as conductive hearing loss may be present. Feeding can be difficult, and sometimes cyanosis develops because the tongue is posterior and may obstruct the pharynx. Prone positioning during feeding may help, but uncoordinated swallowing may require nasogastric gavage feedings or a gastrostomy tube. If cyanosis or respiratory problems persist, tracheostomy or surgery to affix the tongue in a forward position (eg, sewing it to the inner lower lip) may be required. Otologic evaluation is indicated.

Agenesis of the jaw: Congenital absence of the condyloid process (and sometimes the coronoid process, the ramus, and parts of the mandibular body) is a severe malformation. The mandible deviates to the affected side, resulting in severe malocclusion; the unaffected side is elongated and flattened. Abnormalities of the external, middle, and inner ear; temporal bone; parotid gland; masticatory muscles; and facial nerve often coexist.

X-rays of the mandible and temporomandibular joint show the degree of underdevelopment and distinguish agenesis from other conditions that result in similar facial deformities but do not involve severe structural loss.

Treatment consists of reconstruction with autogenous bone grafting (costochondral graft) and is done promptly to limit progression of facial deformity. Often, mentoplasty, onlay grafts of bone and cartilage, and soft-tissue flaps and grafts further improve facial symmetry. Distraction osteogenesis is being increasingly used; an osteotomy is done, and a distraction (separator) device is attached to both pieces. Over time, the distance between the 2 pieces is widened, and new bone grows in between to enlarge the bone. Orthodontic treatment in early adolescence helps correct malocclusion.

Congenital ear malformations: Malformed pinna (microtia) and external auditory canal atresia, which causes conductive hearing loss, involve the external ear. These malformations, which frequently coexist, are often identified at or soon after birth. Occasionally, school-based screening tests identify a partially occluded external auditory canal in children with a normal pinna.

Hearing tests (see p. 785) and CT of the temporal bone are necessary to evaluate possible additional bony malformations. Treatment can include surgery and a bone-conduction hearing aid, depending on whether the malformation is unilateral or bilateral; whether it affects hearing, learning, and social development; and whether complications (eg, facial nerve involvement, cholesteatoma, otitis media) are present. Surgery may include pinna reconstruction, the creation of an external auditory canal, tympanic membrane, and ossicles, or both.

HIP, LEG, AND FOOT ABNORMALITIES

Developmental dysplasia of the hip (formerly congenital dislocation of the hip): Dysplasia is abnormal development of the hip joint, leading to subluxation or dislocation. It is more common among infants with breech presentation, especially females. It seems to result from laxity of the ligaments around the joint or from in utero positioning. Dysplasia can be unilateral or bilateral. Asymmetric skin creases in the thigh and groin are common, but such creases also occur in infants without hip dysplasia. If dysplasia remains undetected and untreated, the affected leg eventually becomes shorter, and the hip may become painful. Abduction of the hip is often impaired, due to adductor spasm.

Two screening procedures commonly are used. In the Ortolani maneuver, the thigh of the hip being tested is abducted and gently pulled anteriorly. Instability is indicated by the palpable, sometimes audible, clunk of the femoral head moving over the posterior rim of the acetabulum and relocating in the cavity. Next, in the Barlow maneuver, the hip is adducted while the thigh is pushed posteriorly. A clunk indicates that the head of the femur is moving out of the acetabulum. Also, a difference in knee height when the child is prone with hips flexed, knees bent, and feet on the examining table (Galeazzi sign) suggests dysplasia, especially unilateral. Somewhat later, subluxation or dislocation is indicated by inability to completely abduct the thigh when the hip and knee are flexed; abduction is impeded by adductor spasm, which is often present even if the hip is not actually dislocated at the time of examination. Minor benign clicks are commonly detected. Although clicks usually disappear within 1 or 2 mo, they should be checked regularly. Because bilateral dysplasia may be difficult to detect at birth, periodic testing for limited hip abduction during the 1st year of life is advised.

All female neonates who were in breech position require ultrasonography of the hips to rule out dysplasia. For all other infants, imaging is required when any abnormality is suspected during examination. Hip ultrasonography can accurately establish the diagnosis early. Hip x-rays are helpful after the bones have started to ossify, typically after age 3 or 4 mo.

Early treatment is critical. With any delay, the potential for correction without surgery decreases steadily. The hip usually can be reduced immediately after birth, and with growth, the acetabulum can form a nearly normal joint. Treatment is with devices, most commonly the Pavlik harness, which holds the affected hips abducted and externally rotated. The Frejka pillow and other splints may help. Padded diapers are not effective.

Femoral torsion (twisting): The femoral head may be twisted. Torsion may be either internal (femoral anteversion; knees pointing toward each other with toes in) or external (femoral retroversion; knees pointing in opposite directions) and is common among neonates. At birth, internal torsion can be as much as 40° and still be normal. External torsion can also be prominent at birth and still be normal.

Children with internal torsion may regularly sit in the W position or sleep in a prone position with legs extended or flexed and internally rotated. These children probably assume this position because it is more comfortable. The W sitting position was thought to worsen the torsion, but there is little evidence that the position should be discouraged or avoided. By adolescence, internal torsion tends to gradually decrease to about 15° without intervention.

External torsion may occur if in utero forces result in an abduction or external rotation soft-tissue positioning. If external torsion is prominent at birth, a thorough check (including x-rays or ultrasonography) for hip dislocation is indicated. External torsion typically corrects spontaneously, especially after children begin to stand and walk, but orthopedic referral is needed when excessive torsion persists after 8 yr.

Genu varum and valgum: The 2 major types of knee or femoral-tibial angular deformities are genu varum (bowlegs) and genu valgum (knock-knees). Untreated, both can cause osteoarthritis of the knee in adulthood.

Genu varum is common among toddlers and usually resolves spontaneously by age 18 mo. If it persists or becomes more severe, Blount disease (progressive tibial osteochondrosis) should be suspected. Early diagnosis of Blount disease is difficult, because x-rays may be normal. Rickets also should be ruled out. Early use of a Danish night splint can be effective, but osteotomy is often needed.

Genu valgum is less common and, even if severe, usually resolves spontaneously by age 9 yr. Skeletal dysplasia or hypophosphatasia should be excluded. If marked deformity persists after age 10 yr, surgical stapling of the medial distal femoral epiphysis is indicated.

Knee dislocation: Anterior knee dislocation with hyperextension is rare at birth but requires emergency treatment. It may occur with Larsen's syndrome, which consists of multiple congenital dislocations (eg, elbows, hips, knees), clubfoot, and characteristic face (eg, prominent forehead, depressed nasal bridge, wide-spaced eyes) or with arthrogryposis (see p. 2421). The dislocation may be related to muscle imbalance (if myelodysplasia or arthrogryposis is present) or intrauterine positioning. Ipsilateral hip dislocation often coexists.

If the infant is otherwise normal, immediate treatment with daily passive flexion movements and splinting in flexion usually results in a functional knee.

Tibial torsion: Tibial torsion can be external (lateral) or internal (medial) twisting. External torsion occurs normally with growth: from 0° at birth to 20° by adulthood. External torsion is rarely a problem. However, tibial bowing with a narrow sclerotic intramedullary canal (Blount disease), seen on x-ray, has a high risk of fracture and pseudarthrosis and requires a protective orthosis. Tibial bowing also may be due to rickets.

Internal torsion is common at birth, but it typically resolves with growth. However, an excessive degree of torsion may indicate a neuromuscular problem. Persistent, excessive torsion can lead to toeing-in and bowlegs.

Talipes equinovarus: Sometimes called clubfoot, talipes equinovarus is characterized by plantar flexion, inward tilting of the heel (from the midline of the leg), and adduction of the forefoot (medial deviation away from the leg's vertical axis). It results from an abnormality of the talus. It occurs in about2 of every 1000 births, is bilateral in up to 50% of affected children, and may occur alone or as part of a syndrome. Deformities that result from in utero positioning can be distinguished from talipes equinovarus clubfoot because they can be easily corrected passively.

Treatment requires orthopedic care, which consists initially of repeated cast applications, taping, or use of malleable splints to normalize the foot's position. If casting is not successful and the abnormality is severe, surgery may be required. Optimally, surgery is done before 12 mo, while the tarsal bones are still cartilaginous.

Talipes calcaneovalgus: The foot is flat or convex and dorsiflexed, with the heel turned outward. The foot can easily be approximated against the lower tibia. Early treatment with a cast (to place the foot in the equinovarus position) or with corrective braces is usually successful.

Metatarsus adductus: The forefoot turns toward the midline. The foot may be supinated at rest. Usually, the foot can be passively abducted and everted beyond the neutral position when the sole is stimulated. Occasionally, an affected foot is rigid, not correcting to neutral. The deformity usually resolves without treatment during the 1st year of life. If it does not, casting or surgery (abductory midfoot osteotomy) is required.

Metatarsus varus: The plantar surface of the foot is turned inward, so that the arch is raised. This deformity usually results from in utero positioning. It typically does not resolve after birth and may require corrective casting.

MUSCLE ABNORMALITIES

Individual muscles or groups of muscles may be absent at birth.

Partial or complete agenesis of the pectoralis major is common and occurs alone or with ipsilateral hand abnormalities, as Poland's syndrome. Poland's syndrome may be associated with Möbius' syndrome (paralysis of the lower cranial nerves, especially the 6th, 7th, and 12th), which is linked to autism.

In prune-belly syndrome (see also p. 2437), one or more layers of the abdominal musculature are absent at birth; this often occurs with severe GU abnormalities, particularly hydronephrosis. Incidence is highest in male infants, who often also have undescended testes. Malformations involving the feet and rectum also often coexist. Prognosis is guarded, even with early relief of urinary tract obstruction.

NECK AND BACK ABNORMALITIES

Congenital torticollis: The head becomes tilted at or soon after birth. The most common cause is neck injury during delivery. Torticollis that develops within the 1st few days or weeks of life may result from hematoma, fibrosis, and contracture of the sternocleidomastoid (SCM) muscle. A nontender mass may be noted in the SCM, usually in the midsegment.

Other causes include spinal abnormalities, such as Klippel-Feil syndrome (fusion of the cervical vertebrae, short neck, and low hairline, often with urinary tract abnormalities) or atlanto-occipital fusion. CNS tumors, bulbar palsies, and ocular dysfunction are common neurologic causes but are rarely present at birth (see also Spasmodic Torticollis on p. 326). Fractures, dislocations, or subluxations of the cervical spine (especially C1 and C2) or odontoid abnormalities are rare but serious causes; permanent neurologic damage may result from spinal cord injury. Cervical imaging should be done to exclude bony causes, which may require stabilization. When torticollis is due to birth trauma, frequent passive SCM stretching (rotating the head and stretching the neck laterally to the opposite side) is indicated. Injections of botulinum toxin into the SCM may help in refractory cases. Untreated torticollis may lead to plagiocephaly and asymmetrical facies.

Vertebral defects: Examples are idiopathic scoliosis (see p. 2381), which is rarely apparent at birth, and isolated vertebral defects (eg, hemivertebrae, wedge or butterfly vertebrae), which are more common. Vertebral defects should be suspected when posterior midline cutaneous, renal, or congenital lower-limb abnormalities exist. Some syndromes such as VACTERL (formerly VATER; *v*ertebral anomalies, *a*nal atresia, *c*ardiac malformations, *t*racheo*e*sophageal fistula, *r*enal anomalies, and *l*imb anomalies [eg, radial aplasia]) include vertebral defects. As children grow, the spinal curve caused by a vertebral defect or defects can progress rapidly; therefore, the spine should be monitored closely. Braces or body jackets, which may have to be worn 18 h/day, are often necessary initially. Surgery may be needed if the curvature progresses. Because renal abnormalities commonly coexist, renal ultrasonography is indicated for initial screening.

289 CONGENITAL GASTROINTESTINAL ANOMALIES

Most congenital GI anomalies result in some type of intestinal obstruction, frequently presenting with feeding difficulties, distention, and emesis at birth or within 1 or 2 days. Infants with GI malformations have a high mortality rate, ranging from 10 to 40%; the highest rate occurs in those with congenital diaphragmatic hernia. A common type of anomaly is atresia, in which a segment of the GI tract fails to form or develop normally. The most common type is esophageal atresia, followed by that in the jejunoileal region and in the duodenum.

Immediate management includes bowel decompression (by continuous nasogastric suction to prevent emesis, which can lead to aspiration pneumonia or further abdominal distention with respiratory embarrassment) and referral to a center for neonatal surgery.

Also vital are maintenance of body temperature, prevention of hypoglycemia with 10% dextrose and electrolytes IV, and prevention or treatment of acidosis and infections so that the infant is in optimal condition for surgery.

Because about 1/3 of infants with a GI malformation have another congenital anomaly, such infants should be evaluated for malformations of other organ systems, especially of the CNS, heart, and kidneys.

HIGH ALIMENTARY TRACT OBSTRUCTION

Esophageal, gastric, duodenal, and sometimes jejunal obstruction should be considered when excess amniotic fluid (polyhydramnios) is diagnosed, because such obstructions prevent the fetus from swallowing and absorbing amniotic fluid (jejunal obstruction is discussed on p. 2429). An NGT should be passed into the neonate's stomach immediately after delivery. Finding large amounts of fluid in the stomach, especially if bile-stained, supports the diagnosis of upper GI obstruction, whereas inability to pass the NGT into the stomach suggests esophageal atresia. Diaphragmatic hernia sometimes causes high alimentary tract obstruction.

Esophageal Atresia

Esophageal atresia is incomplete formation of the esophagus, frequently associated with tracheoesophageal fistula. Diagnosis is by failure to pass an NGT. Treatment is surgical repair.

Esophageal atresia is the most common GI atresia. There are 5 major types of esophageal atresia. The most common (85%) is a blind upper esophagus with a fistula between the lower esophageal segment and the trachea. The next most common (8%) is pure esophageal atresia without a fistula. The remainder are due to an "H type" fistula between the trachea and the esophagus with an intact esophagus (4%), esophageal atresia with proximal fistula with the trachea (1%), and esophageal atresia with 2 fistulas (1%).

Characteristic signs are excessive secretions, coughing and cyanosis after attempts at feeding, and aspiration pneumonia. Esophageal atresia with a distal fistula leads to abdominal distention because, as the infant cries, air from the trachea is forced through the fistula into the lower esophagus and stomach.

Diagnosis

Diagnosis is suggested by inability to pass an NGT into the stomach. A radiopaque catheter determines the location of the atresia on x-ray. In atypical cases, a small amount of water-soluble contrast material may be needed to define the anatomy under fluoroscopy. The contrast material should be quickly aspirated back because its entrance into the lungs can cause a chemical pneumonitis. This procedure should be done only by a trained radiologist at the center where neonatal surgery will be performed.

Treatment

Preoperative management aims to get the infant into optimal condition for surgery and prevent aspiration pneumonia, which makes surgical correction more hazardous. Oral feedings are withheld. Continuous suction with a double-lumen catheter in the upper esophageal pouch prevents aspiration of swallowed saliva. The infant should be positioned prone with the head elevated 30 to 40° and with the right side down to facilitate gastric emptying and minimize the risk of aspirating gastric acid through the fistula. If definitive repair must be deferred because of extreme prematurity, aspiration pneumonia, or other congenital malformations, gastrostomy is done to decompress the stomach. Suction through the gastrostomy tube then reduces the risk that gastric contents will reflux through the fistula into the tracheobronchial tree.

When the infant's condition is stable, extrapleural surgical repair of the esophageal atresia and closure of the tracheoesophageal fistula can be performed. Occasionally, interposing a segment of colon between the esophageal segments may be required.

The most common acute complications are leakage at the anastomosis site and stricture formation. Feeding difficulties are common after successful surgical repair because of poor motility of the distal esophageal segment, which predisposes the infant to gastroesophageal reflux. If medical management for reflux fails, a Nissen fundoplication may be required.

Diaphragmatic Hernia

Diaphragmatic hernia is protrusion of abdominal contents into the thorax through a defect in the diaphragm. Lung compression may cause persistent pulmonary hypertension. Diagnosis is by chest x-ray. Treatment is surgical repair.

Diaphragmatic hernia usually occurs in the posterolateral portion of the diaphragm (Bochdalek's hernia) and is on the left side in 90% of cases. Loops of small and large bowel, stomach, liver, and spleen may protrude into the hemithorax on the involved side. If the hernia is large, the lung on the affected left side will be hypoplastic. After delivery, as the neonate cries and swallows air, the loops of intestine quickly fill with air and rapidly enlarge, causing further acute respiratory embarrassment as the heart and mediastinal structures are pushed to the right, compressing the more normal right lung. Respiratory distress is immediate in severe cases. A scaphoid abdomen (due to displacement of abdominal viscera into the chest) is likely. Bowel sounds (and an absence of breath sounds) may be heard over the involved hemithorax. In less severe cases, mild respiratory difficulty develops a few hours or days later as abdominal contents progressively herniate through a smaller diaphragmatic defect.

Other pulmonary consequences include underdevelopment of the pulmonary vasculature, resulting in an elevation of pulmonary vascular resistance and hence pulmonary hypertension. Persistent pulmonary hypertension (see p. 2301) leads to right-to-left shunting at the level of the foramen ovale or through a patent ductus arteriosus, which prevents adequate oxygenation even with O_2 supplementation or mechanical ventilation. Persistent pulmonary hypertension is the major cause of death among infants with congenital diaphragmatic hernia.

Diagnosis

Sometimes diagnosis is by prenatal ultrasound. After delivery, diagnosis is by chest x-ray showing intestine protruding into the chest. In a large defect, there are numerous air-filled loops of intestine filling the hemithorax and contralateral displacement of the heart and mediastinal structures. If the x-ray is taken immediately after delivery before the neonate has swallowed air, the abdominal contents appear as an opaque airless mass in the hemithorax.

Treatment

The neonate should be immediately endotracheally intubated and ventilated in the delivery room; bag-and-mask ventilation may fill the intrathoracic viscera with air and worsen respiratory compromise. Continuous nasogastric suction with a double-lumen tube prevents swallowed air from progressing through the GI tract and causing further lung compression. Sometimes paralytic drugs are needed to prevent swallowing of air. Surgery is required to replace the intestine in the abdomen and to close the diaphragmatic defect.

Severe persistent pulmonary hypertension requires stabilization before surgery with IV $NaHCO_3$ and inhaled nitric oxide, which may help dilate the pulmonary arteries and improve systemic oxygenation. Some neonates benefit from extracorporeal membrane oxygenation (ECMO—see p. 2297), although neonates with extreme pulmonary hypoplasia still do not survive. Successful transport of a critically ill neonate with congenital diaphragmatic hernia and persistent pulmonary hypertension is very difficult. Therefore, if diaphragmatic hernia is diagnosed by prenatal ultrasound, delivery at a pediatric center with ECMO facilities is prudent.

Duodenal Obstruction

The duodenum can be obstructed by atresia, stenosis, and pressure from an extrinsic mass.

Duodenal atresia is the 3rd most common atresia of the GI tract (1:6,000 to 10,000 live births). Duodenal atresia is due to the failure of canalization of the embryonic duodenum. About 25% of infants with duodenal atresia have Down syndrome. Malrotation of the intestine frequently occurs, as do other congenital anomalies. Infants with duodenal atresia present with polyhydramnios, feeding difficulties, and emesis that may be bilious. The diagnosis is suspected by symptoms and classic "double-bubble" x-ray findings—one bubble is in the stomach and the other in the proximal duodenum; little to no air is in the distal gut. An upper GI series provides definitive diagnosis but must be performed carefully to avoid aspiration. Once the disorder is suspected, infants should receive nothing by mouth, and an NGT should be placed to decompress the stomach. Surgery is the definitive therapy.

Duodenal stenosis occurs less commonly than duodenal atresia but presents in a similar fashion and requires surgery. It too is frequently associated with Down syndrome.

Choledochal cyst or **annular pancreas** may obstruct the duodenum by extrinsic pressure. Infants with choledochal cyst classically present with a triad of abdominal pain, mass, and jaundice. If the cyst is large, it may also present with variable degrees of duodenal obstruction. Choledochal cyst is most commonly diagnosed with ultrasound. Treatment is surgical and requires complete excision of the cyst because of the risk of developing cancer in the cyst remnants. Annular pancreas is a rare congenital anomaly in which pancreatic tissue encircles the 2nd portion of the duodenum, causing duodenal obstruction; presentation is usually during the neonatal period but may be delayed until adulthood. The diagnosis can be suggested on upper GI series and more definitively made with a CT scan. Treatment is surgical.

JEJUNOILEAL AND LARGE-BOWEL OBSTRUCTION

(See also Meconium Ileus on p. 2285 and Meconium Plug Syndrome on p. 2286.)

Obstruction of the jejunum and ileum can occur as the result of jejunoileal atresia, malrotation, intestinal duplication, or meconium ileus. Large-bowel obstruction is typically due to Hirschsprung's disease, meconium plug syndrome, and colonic or anal atresia.

In 75% of cases, no history of maternal polyhydramnios exists because much of the swallowed amniotic fluid can be absorbed from the intestine proximal to the obstruction. These disorders, other than malrotation, intestinal duplication, and Hirschsprung's disease, typically manifest in the 1st few days of life with feeding problems, abdominal distention, and emesis that may be bilious or fecal. The neonate may pass a small amount of meconium initially but thereafter does not pass stools. Malrotation, intestinal duplication, and Hirschsprung's disease can manifest in the 1st several days of life or years later.

The general diagnostic approach and preoperative management include giving nothing by mouth, placing an NGT to prevent further bowel distention or possible aspiration of vomitus, correcting fluid and electrolyte disturbances, taking a plain film x-ray, and then performing a contrast enema to delineate the anatomy (the enema may also relieve obstruction in meconium plug syndrome or meconium ileus). For Hirschsprung's disease, a rectal biopsy is needed.

Jejunoileal Atresia

Jejunoileal atresia is incomplete formation of the jejunum, usually from an ischemic insult.

There are 5 major types of jejunoileal atresia. Type I consists of a membrane completely occluding the lumen with the intestine intact. Type II is a gap in the intestine with a fibrous cord between the proximal and distal segments of intestine. Type IIIA is a gap without any connection between the segments. Type IIIB is jejunal atresia with absence of the distal superior mesenteric artery; the distal small bowel is coiled like an apple peel, and the gut is short. Type IV consists of multiple atretic segments.

Neonates with jejunoileal atresia usually present late during day 1 or on day 2 with increasing abdominal distention, failure to pass stools, and, finally, regurgitated feedings. Plain x-rays of the abdomen may reveal dilated loops of small bowel with air-fluid levels and a paucity of air in the colon and rectum.

Preoperative management consists of placing an NGT, giving nothing by mouth, and providing IV fluids. Surgery is the definitive therapy. At surgery, the entire intestine should be inspected to be sure multiple areas of atresia are not present. The atretic portion is resected, usually with a primary anastomosis. If the proximal portion of the ileum is extremely dilated and difficult to anastomose to the distal, unused part of the intestine, it is sometimes safer to perform a double-barreled ileostomy and defer anastomosis until the caliber of the distended proximal intestine has diminished.

Prognosis is based on the length of remaining small bowel and the presence of the ileocecal valve. Infants who subsequently develop short bowel syndrome require TPN for extended periods. They should be provided continuous enteral feedings to promote gut adaptation, maximize absorption, and minimize the use of TPN. Infants should also be provided small amounts of nutrition by mouth to maintain sucking and swallowing.

Malrotation of the Bowel

Bowel malrotation is failure of the bowel to assume its normal place in the abdomen during intrauterine development.

During embryonic development, the primitive bowel protrudes from the abdominal cavity. As it returns to the abdomen, the large bowel normally rotates counterclockwise, with the cecum coming to rest in the right lower quadrant. Incomplete rotation, in which the cecum ends up elsewhere (usually in the right upper quadrant or midepigastrium), may cause bowel obstruction from retroperitoneal bands that stretch across the duodenum or from a volvulus of the small bowel, which, lacking its normal peritoneal attachment, twists on its narrow, stalk-like mesentery.

Patients with malrotation can present in infancy or in adulthood with acute abdominal pain and bilious emesis, with an acute volvulus, with typical reflux symptoms, or with chronic abdominal pain. Bilious emesis in an infant is an emergency and should be evaluated immediately to make sure the infant does not have malrotation and a midgut volvulus; untreated, the risk of bowel infarction and subsequent short bowel syndrome or death is high.

Plain films of the abdomen should be done immediately. If they show dilated small bowel and/or a paucity of bowel gas distal to the duodenum suggesting a midgut volvulus, further diagnosis and treatment must be done emergently. Barium enema typically identifies malrotation by showing the cecum outside the right lower quadrant. If the diagnosis remains uncertain, an upper GI series can be done cautiously.

The presence of malrotation and midgut volvulus is an emergency requiring immediate surgery, which consists of Ladd's procedure with lysis of the peritoneal bands and relief of the midgut volvulus.

INTESTINAL DUPLICATION

Intestinal duplications are tubular structures attached to the intestines and sharing a common blood supply; their lining resembles that of the GI tract.

Intestinal duplications are uncommon. The most common site of duplication is the jejunum and ileum followed by the esophagus, stomach, colon, and duodenum. Colonic duplication is often associated with anomalies of the urogenital system. Intestinal duplications usually manifest in the 1st 2 yr of life. Duplications can be asymptomatic or cause obstructive symptoms, chronic pain, or abdominal mass. If they are detected, treatment is surgical with complete resection of the duplicated portion.

HIRSCHSPRUNG'S DISEASE

(Congenital Megacolon)

Hirschsprung's disease is a congenital anomaly of innervation of the lower intestine, usually limited to the colon, resulting in partial or total functional obstruction. Symptoms are obstipation and distention. Diagnosis is by barium enema and biopsy. Treatment is surgical.

Hirschsprung's disease is caused by congenital absence of Meissner's and Auerbach's autonomic plexus in the intestinal wall. It is usually limited to the distal colon but can involve the entire colon or even the entire large and small bowel. Peristalsis in the involved segment is absent or abnormal, resulting in continuous smooth muscle spasm and partial or complete obstruction with accumulation of intestinal contents and massive dilation of the more proximal, normally innervated intestine. "Skip lesions" almost never occur.

Symptoms and Signs

Patients most commonly present early in life; 15% in the 1st month, 60% by age 1 yr, and 85% by age 4 yr. The infant presents with obstipation, abdominal distention, and, finally, vomiting as in other forms of distal bowel obstruction. Occasionally, infants with ultra-short segment aganglionosis have only mild or intermittent constipation, often with intervening bouts of mild diarrhea, resulting in delay in diagnosis. In older infants, symptoms and signs may include anorexia, lack of a physiologic urge to defecate, and, on examination, an empty rectum with stool palpable higher up in the colon. The child also may fail to thrive.

Diagnosis

Diagnosis should be made as soon as possible. The longer the disease goes untreated, the greater the chance of developing Hirschsprung's enterocolitis (toxic megacolon), which may be fulminant and fatal (see p. 2431). Most cases can be diagnosed in early infancy.

Initial approach is typically with barium enema or sometimes rectal suction biopsy. Barium enema may show a transition in diameter between the dilated, normally innervated colon proximal to the narrowed distal segment (which lacks normal innervation). Barium enema should be done without prior preparation, which can dilate the abnormal segment rendering the test nondiagnostic. Because characteristic findings may not be present in the neonatal period, a 24-h post-evacuation film should be obtained; if the colon is still filled with barium, Hirschsprung's disease is likely. A rectal suction biopsy can disclose the absence of ganglion cells. Acetylcholinesterase staining can be performed to highlight the enlarged nerve trunks. Some centers also have the capability of performing rectal manometrics, which can reveal abnormal innervation. Definitive diagnosis requires a full-thickness biopsy of the rectum.

Treatment

Treatment in the neonate has typically involved a colostomy proximal to the aganglionic segment to decompress the colon and allow the child to grow before the 2nd stage of the procedure. Later resection of the entire aganglionic portion of the colon and a pull-through procedure was performed. However, a number of centers now perform one-stage procedures in the neonatal period.

After definitive repair, the prognosis is good, although a number of infants have chronic dysmotility with constipation and/or obstructive problems.

Hirschsprung's Enterocolitis

(Toxic Megacolon)

Hirschsprung's enterocolitis is a life-threatening complication of Hirschsprung's disease resulting in a grossly enlarged colon, often followed by sepsis and shock.

The etiology of Hirschsprung's enterocolitis appears to be marked proximal dilatation secondary to obstruction, with thinning of the colonic wall, bacterial overgrowth, and translocation of gut bacteria. Shock can develop and death can follow rapidly. Close monitoring of infants with Hirschsprung's disease is therefore essential.

Hirschsprung's enterocolitis occurs most commonly in the 1st several months of life before surgical correction but can occur postoperatively. Infants present with fever, abdominal distention, diarrhea (which may be bloody), and, subsequently, obstipation.

Initial treatment is supportive with fluid resuscitation, decompression with an NGT and rectal tube, and broad-spectrum antibiotics to include anaerobic coverage (eg, a combination of ampicillin, gentamicin, and clindamycin). Some experts advocate saline enemas to clean out the colon, but this must be done carefully so as not to increase colonic pressure and cause perforation. Surgery is the definitive treatment, as noted above.

Anal Atresia

Anal atresia is an imperforate anus.

A fistula often extends from the anal pouch to the perineum or the urethra in males and to the vagina, the fourchette, or, rarely, the bladder in females. The blind anus and the skin of the perineum may be several centimeters apart or separated by just a thin membrane of skin covering the anal opening.

Anal atresia is obvious on routine physical examination of the neonate because the anus is not patent. Should the diagnosis be missed and the neonate be fed, signs of distal bowel obstruction soon develop.

The urine should be filtered and examined for meconium, indicating the presence of a fistula to the urinary tract. Plain x-rays and "fistulograms" with the neonate in a lateral prone position can define the level of the lesion. A cutaneous fistula generally indicates low atresia. In such cases, definitive repair using a perineal approach is possible. If no perineal fistula exists, a high lesion is likely.

Definitive repair is usually deferred until the infant is older and the structures to be repaired are larger. Until then, a colostomy is done to relieve the obstruction.

DEFECTS IN ABDOMINAL WALL CLOSURE

Several congenital defects involve the abdominal wall, allowing protrusion of the viscera.

Omphalocele

An omphalocele is a protrusion of abdominal viscera from a midline defect at the base of the umbilicus.

In omphalocele, the herniated viscera are covered by a thin membrane and may be small (only a few loops of intestine) or may contain most of the abdominal viscera (intestine, stomach, and liver). Immediate dangers are drying of the viscera, hypothermia and dehydration from evaporation of water from the exposed viscera, and infection of the peritoneal surfaces. Infants with omphalocele have a very high incidence of other congenital anomalies, including bowel atresia; chromosomal abnormalities, such as Down syndrome; and cardiac and renal anomalies, which must be identified and evaluated before surgical correction.

At delivery, the exposed viscera should be immediately covered with sterile saline-soaked sponges and then with an occlusive dressing to maintain sterility and prevent evaporation. Placing the neonate's body in a sterile bowel bag containing warm sterile saline also stops evaporation from the exposed viscera.

The infant is evaluated for associated anomalies before going to surgery. Primary closure is performed when feasible. With a large omphalocele, the abdominal cavity may be too small to accommodate the viscera. In this case, the viscera are covered by a pouch or "silo" of polymeric silicone sheeting, which is progressively reduced in size over several days as the abdominal capacity slowly increases, until all of the viscera are enclosed within the abdominal cavity.

Gastroschisis

Gastroschisis is protrusion of the abdominal viscera through an abdominal wall defect, usually to the right of the umbilical cord insertion.

In gastroschisis, unlike omphalocele, there is no membranous covering over the intestine, which is markedly edematous and erythematous and is often enclosed in a fibrin mat. These findings indicate long-standing inflammation from the intestine being directly exposed to amniotic fluid (ie, chemical peritonitis). Infants with gastroschisis have low incidence of associated congenital anomalies other than malrotation. Surgery is similar to that for omphalocele. It often takes several weeks before GI function recovers and oral feedings can be given; occasionally, infants have long-term problems caused by abnormal intestinal motility.

290 CONGENITAL RENAL AND GENITOURINARY ANOMALIES

Congenital anatomic anomalies of the GU tract are more common than those of any other organ system. Urinary tract anomalies predispose to many complications, including infection, obstruction, stasis, calculus formation, and impaired renal function. Genital anomalies may cause sexual dysfunction or impaired fertility. Treatment of GU anomalies is often surgical.

Some congenital renal anomalies (eg, autosomal dominant polycystic kidney disease and medullary cystic disease [see Ch. 232 on p. 1975] and hereditary nephritis [see p. 1997]) typically do not manifest until adulthood.

RENAL ANOMALIES

Renal agenesis: Bilateral renal agenesis as part of a syndrome of oligohydramnios, pulmonary hypoplasia, and extremity and facial anomalies (classic Potter's syndrome) is fatal within minutes to hours.

Unilateral renal agenesis is not uncommon and usually is accompanied by ureteral agenesis with absence of the ipsilateral trigone and ureteral orifice. No treatment is necessary; compensatory hypertrophy of the solitary kidney maintains normal renal function.

Autosomal recessive polycystic kidney disease: Incidence is 1/10,000 births; autosomal dominant polycystic kidney disease is much more common and is discussed on p. 1978. Autosomal recessive disease affects both kidneys and the liver. Kidneys are usually greatly enlarged and contain small cysts; renal failure is common in childhood. The liver is enlarged and has periportal fibrosis, bile duct proliferation, and scattered cysts; the remainder of the hepatic parenchyma is normal. Fibrosis produces portal hypertension by age 5 to 10 yr, but hepatic function is normal or minimally impaired.

Disease severity and progression vary. Severe disease may manifest prenatally or soon after birth or in early childhood with renal-related symptoms; less severely affected patients present in late childhood or adolescence with hepatic-related symptoms.

Affected neonates have a protuberant abdomen with huge, firm, smooth, symmetric kidneys. Severely affected neonates commonly have pulmonary hypoplasia secondary to the in utero effects of renal dysfunction and oligohydramnios.

In patients aged 5 to 10 yr, signs of portal hypertension, such as esophageal and gastric varices and hypersplenism, occur. If the patient presents in adolescence, nephromegaly is less marked, renal insufficiency may be mild to moderate, and the major symptoms are those related to portal hypertension.

Diagnosis may be difficult, especially without a family history. Ultrasonography may demonstrate renal or hepatic cysts; definitive diagnosis may require biopsy. Ultrasonography in late pregnancy usually allows presumptive in utero diagnosis.

Many neonates die in the 1st few days or weeks of life from pulmonary insufficiency. Most who survive develop progressive renal failure often requiring renal replacement therapy. Experience with renal transplantation with or without hepatic transplantation is limited. When transplantation is done, hypersplenism must be controlled (see p. 1091) to obviate difficulty with hypersplenism-induced leukopenia, which increases the risk of systemic infection. Portal hypertension may be treated by portacaval or splenorenal shunts, which reduce morbidity but not mortality.

Duplication anomalies: Supernumerary collecting systems may be unilateral or bilateral and may involve the renal pelvis and ureters (accessory renal pelvis, double or triple pelvis and ureter), calyx, or ureteral orifice. Duplex kidney, a single renal mass with > 1 collecting system, differs from a fused kidney, which involves fusion of 2 renal parenchymal masses. Some duplication anomalies have ureteral ectopy with or without ureterocele. Management depends on the anatomy and function of each separately drained segment. Surgery may be needed to correct obstruction or vesicoureteral reflux.

Fusion anomalies: With fusion anomalies, the kidneys are joined, but the ureters enter the bladder on each side. These anomalies increase the risk of ureteropelvic junction obstruction, vesicoureteral reflux, congenital renal cystic dysplasia (see p. 1975), and injury from anterior abdominal trauma.

Horseshoe kidney, the most common fusion anomaly, occurs when renal parenchyma on each side of the vertebral column is joined at the corresponding (usually lower) poles; an isthmus of renal parenchyma or fibrous tissue joins at the midline. The ureters course medially and anteriorly over this isthmus and generally drain well. Obstruction, if present, is usually secondary to insertion of the ureters high in the renal pelvis. Pyeloplasty relieves the obstruction and can be done without resecting the isthmus.

Crossed fused renal ectopia is the 2nd most common fusion anomaly. The renal parenchyma (representing both kidneys) is on one side of the vertebral column. One of the ureters crosses the midline and enters the bladder on the side opposite the kidneys. When ureteropelvic junction obstruction is present, pyeloplasty is the treatment of choice.

Fused pelvic kidney (pancake kidney) is much less common. A single pelvic kidney is served by 2 collecting systems and ureters. If obstruction is present, reconstruction is needed.

Malrotation: Malrotation is usually of little clinical significance. Ultrasonography often demonstrates hydronephrosis, but diagnosis is best made with IVU, which identifies an axis shift and defines the collecting system anatomy.

Multicystic dysplastic kidney: In this condition, a nonfunctioning renal unit consists of noncommunicating cysts with intervening solid tissue composed of fibrosis, primitive tubules, and foci of cartilage. Usually, ureteral atresia is also present. Uncommonly, the kidney develops tumors or infection, and hypertension may develop. Most experts recommend observation, although some advocate removing these kidneys, especially if solid tissue is extensive or unusual appearing on ultrasonography.

Renal dysplasia: In renal dysplasia, a histologic diagnosis, the renal vasculature, tubules, collecting ducts, or drainage apparatus develops abnormally. Diagnosis is by biopsy. If dysplasia is segmental, treatment is often unnecessary. If dysplasia is extensive, renal dysfunction may necessitate nephrologic care, including renal replacement therapy.

Renal ectopia: Renal ectopia, abnormal renal location, usually results when a kidney fails to ascend from its origin in the true pelvis; a rare exception occurs with a superiorly ascended (thoracic) kidney. Pelvic ectopia increases the incidence of ureteropelvic junction obstruction, vesicoureteral reflux, and multicystic renal dysplasia. Obstruction is corrected surgically. Severe reflux can be corrected surgically when indicated (if causing hypertension, recurrent infections, or renal growth retardation).

Renal hypoplasia: Hypoplasia usually occurs because inadequate ureteral bud branching causes an underdeveloped, small kidney with histologically normal nephrons. If hypoplasia is segmental, hypertension can occur, and ablative surgery may be needed.

URETERAL ANOMALIES

Ureteral anomalies frequently occur with renal anomalies but may occur independently. Complications include obstruction and infection and calculus formation from urinary stasis. Urinary incontinence occurs if the ureter bypasses the bladder and terminates in the urethra, perineum, or vagina. Diagnosis typically involves ultrasonography and voiding cystourethrography; some conditions may present on routine fetal ultrasonography. Treatments are surgical.

Duplication anomalies: Partial or complete duplication of one or both ureters may occur with duplication of the ipsilateral renal pelvis. The ureter from the upper pole of the kidney opens at a more caudal location than the orifice of the lower pole ureter. Ectopia or stenosis of one or both orifices, vesicoureteral reflux into the lower ureter or both ureters, and ureterocele may occur. Surgery may be necessary if there is obstruction, vesicoureteral reflux, or urinary incontinence.

Ectopic orifices: Malpositioned openings of single or duplicated ureters may occur on the lateral bladder wall, distally along the trigone, in the bladder neck, in the female urethra distal to the sphincter (leading to continuous incontinence), in the genital system (prostate and seminal vesicle in the male, uterus or vagina in the female), or externally. Lateral ectopic orifices frequently lead to vesicoureteral reflux, whereas distal ectopic orifices more often cause obstruction and incontinence. Surgery is needed for obstruction and incontinence and sometimes for vesicoureteral reflux.

Retrocaval ureter: Anomalous development of the vena cava (pre-ureteric vena cava) allows the infrarenal vena cava to form anterior to the ureter (usually the right); a retrocaval ureter on the left occurs only with persistence of the left cardinal vein system or with complete situs inversus. Retrocaval ureter can cause ureteral obstruction. For significant ureteral obstruction, the ureter is surgically divided with uretero-ureteral anastomosis anterior to the vena cava or iliac vessel.

Stenosis: Narrowing may occur at any location in the ureter, most frequently at the ureteropelvic junction and less commonly at the ureterovesical junction (primary megaureter). Consequences include infection, hematuria, and obstruction. Stenoses often diminish as the child grows. In primary megaureter, ureteral tapering and reimplantation may be needed when dilation increases or infection or obstruction occurs.

Ureterocele: Prolapse of the lower end of the ureter into the bladder with pinpoint obstruction may produce progressive ureterectasis, hydronephrosis, infection, occasional calculus formation, and impaired renal function. Treatment options include endoscopic transurethral incision and open repair.

When a ureterocele involves the upper pole of duplex ureters, treatment depends on function in that renal segment, because of the significant incidence of renal dysplasia. Removal of the affected renal segment and ureter may be preferable to obstruction repair if no segmental renal function is found or if significant renal dysplasia is suspected.

Vesicoureteral reflux: Reflux is retrograde passage of urine from the bladder back into the collecting system. It is most often due to congenital anomalous development of the ureterovesical junction. Incomplete development of the intramural ureteral tunnel causes failure of the normal flap valve mechanism at the ureterovesical junction that permits reflux of bladder urine into the ureter and renal pelvis. Reflux can occur even when the tunnel is ordinarily sufficient if bladder outlet obstruction increases intravesical pressures.

Reflux of urine from the bladder into the ureter may damage the upper urinary tract by bacterial infection and occasionally by increased hydrostatic pressure. Bacteria in the lower urinary tract can easily be transmitted by reflux to the upper tract, leading to recurrent parenchymal infection with potential scarring and renal dysfunction. Chronically elevated emptying pressures (> 40 cm H_2O) and increased bladder volume and pressure often cause progressive kidney damage, even without infection or reflux.

Symptoms and signs are typically those of UTI; these may include fever, abdominal or flank pain, dysuria or flank pain with voiding, frequency, and urgency. Pyuria, hematuria, proteinuria, and bacteriuria may be present on urinalysis.

Tests for reflux include filling and voiding cystourethrogram (which is best to diagnose bladder outlet obstruction) and radioisotope cystogram. Renal ultrasonography evaluates for size, hydronephrosis, and scarring. Renal cortical involvement with acute infection or scarring is precisely delineated with succimer (dimercaptosuccinic acid) nuclear scans, when indicated. Urodynamic studies may demonstrate elevated filling and voiding pressures in the bladder.

Vesicoureteral reflux is usually mild to moderate (with little or no calyceal dilatation—see grading system in TABLE 280–4 on p. 2356) and often resolves spontaneously over months to several years while daily antibacterial prophylaxis (eg, with trimethoprim-sulfamethoxazole, amoxicillin, nitrofurantoin, sulfisoxazole) is maintained. Reflux accompanied by high-pressure storage of urine in the bladder or high intravesical pressures with voiding is treated by lowering bladder pressures with drugs (eg, oxybutynin), behavioral modification using perineal electromyography, or both. Reflux with complications (eg, infection, impaired renal growth, renal scarring) is treated with endoscopic subtrigonal injection of a bulking agent or ureteral reimplantation. Obstruction is also surgically repaired.

BLADDER ANOMALIES

Congenital urinary bladder anomalies often occur without other GU abnormalities. They may cause infection, retention, incontinence, and reflux. Symptomatic anomalies may require surgery.

Bladder diverticula: Bladder diverticula predispose to UTIs and may coexist with vesicoureteral reflux. They are usually discovered during evaluation of recurrent UTIs in young children. Diagnosis is by voiding cystourethrography. Surgical removal of diverticula and reconstruction of the bladder wall may be needed.

Exstrophy: The bladder is open suprapubically, and urine drips from the opening rather than through the urethra. The bladder mucosa is continuous with the abdominal skin, and the pubic bones are separated. Despite the seriousness of the deformity, normal renal function usually is maintained. The bladder can usually be reconstructed and returned to the pelvis, although vesicoureteral reflux invariably occurs and is managed as needed. Continent urinary diversion may be used to treat a bladder reservoir that fails to expand sufficiently or has sphincter insufficiency. Reconstruction of the genitals is required.

Megacystis syndrome: Megacystis syndrome, a large, thin-walled, smooth bladder without evident outlet obstruction that usually occurs in girls, is poorly understood. The syndrome may be a manifestation of a primary myoneural defect, especially when intestinal obstruction (megacystis-microcolon, intestinal hypoperistalsis syndrome) is also present. Symptoms are related to UTIs, and vesicoureteral reflux is common. Ultrasonography with the bladder empty may disclose normal-appearing upper tracts, but voiding cystourethrography may show reflux with massive upper tract dilation. Ureteral reimplantation may be effective, although some patients benefit from antibacterial prophylaxis, timed voiding with behavioral modification, intermittent catheterization, or a combination.

PENILE AND URETHRAL ANOMALIES

Congenital anomalies of the urethra in boys usually involve anatomic abnormalities of the penis and vice versa; in girls, they may exist without other external genital abnormalities. Surgical repair is needed when function is impaired or cosmetic correction is desired.

Chordee: Chordee is ventral or rotational curvature of the penis, which is most apparent with erection and caused by fibrous tissue along the usual course of the corpus spongiosum. It is often associated with hypospadias.

Epispadias: The urethra opens on the dorsum of the glans or penile shaft, or at the penopubic junction. In girls, the urethra opens between the clitoris and labia or in the abdomen. Epispadias can be partial (in 15%) or complete; the most severe form occurs with bladder exstrophy (see above). Symptoms and signs are those of incontinence, reflux, and UTIs. Treatment is surgical. In partial epispadias, prognosis for continence with treatment is good. In the complete form, surgical reconstruction of the penis alone may lead to persistent incontinence; bladder outlet reconstruction is required to achieve complete urinary control.

Hypospadias: Hypospadias is caused by failure of tubularization and fusion of the urethral groove. It almost always occurs in boys, in whom the urethra opens onto the underside of the penile shaft, at the penoscrotal junction, between the scrotal folds, or in the perineum. The foreskin fails to become circumferential and appears as a dorsal hood. Hypospadias is frequently associated with chordee.

Prognosis for functional and cosmetic correction is good. Outpatient surgery at about 6 mo of age involves construction of a neourethra using penile shaft skin or foreskin and repair of the chordee.

Hypospadias is extremely rare in girls; the urethra opens into the vaginal introitus.

Phimosis and paraphimosis: Phimosis, the most common penile abnormality, is constriction of the foreskin with inability to retract over the glans; it may be congenital or acquired (see full discussion on p. 2039). Paraphimosis is inability of the retracted constricting foreskin to be reduced distally over the glans.

Topical corticosteroids and gentle stretching may help resolve phimosis; some require circumcision.

Other penile anomalies: Less common anomalies include penile agenesis, duplication, and lymphedema. Many anomalies also involve urethral abnormality, or other anomalies, such as exstrophy. Treatment of most anomalies is surgical and may include complete removal of the genitals with sex reassignment.

Microphallus results from androgen deficiency or insensitivity; in boys with deficiency, treatment is testosterone supplementation.

Urethral meatal stenosis: Most commonly acquired after newborn circumcision in boys, urethral meatal stenosis is occasionally congenital and associated with hypospadias. Meatotomy is needed for a significantly deflected stream or for a pinpoint stream.

Urethral stricture: Urethral stricture causes obstruction along some part of the length of the urethra. It almost always occurs in boys, is usually acquired, and typically results from a crush injury after straddle trauma. Congenital urethral stricture may manifest similarly to urethral valves and be diagnosed by prenatal ultrasound, or postnatally by symptoms and signs of outlet obstruction or patent urachus and confirmed by retrograde urethrogram. Initial management is often with endoscopic urethrotomy, although open urethroplasty may be necessary.

Urethral valves: In boys, folds in the posterior urethra may act as valves impairing urine flow. Urethral valves can cause urinary hesitancy and a weak urinary stream, UTI, overflow incontinence, myogenic bladder malfunction, vesicoureteral reflux, upper urinary tract damage, and renal insufficiency. They occasionally occur with a patent urachus. Diagnosis is often made by routine prenatal ultrasonography; cases suspected postnatally are confirmed by voiding cystourethrography. Surgery (usually via endoscopy) is done at time of diagnosis to prevent progressive renal deterioration.

A much less common entity, diverticulum of the anterior urethra, may act as a valve (anterior urethral valve) and is also treated endoscopically.

VAGINAL ANOMALIES

Most congenital anomalies of the vagina are rare. Vaginal anomalies include vaginal agenesis, obstruction, duplication, and fusion. Duplication and fusion anomalies have numerous manifestations (eg, as 2 uteri, 2 cervices, and 2 vaginas, or 2 uteri with 1 cervix and 1 vagina). Girls may also have urogenital sinus anomalies, in which urinary and genital tracts open into a common channel, and cloacal anomalies, in which urinary, genital, and anorectal tracts open into a common channel.

Diagnosis of most is by physical examination, ultrasonography, and retrograde contrast studies. Duplication and fusion anomalies may not require treatment, but others require surgical correction.

TESTICULAR AND SCROTAL ANOMALIES

Rare anomalies include scrotal agenesis, hypoplasia, ectopia, or hemangioma; penoscrotal transposition; and bifid scrotum. More commonly, boys are born with congenital hydrocele or undescended testes (cryptorchidism). For testicular torsion, see p. 2042.

Congenital hydrocele: A congenital hydrocele is a collection of fluid in the scrotum. It may be isolated or may communicate with the abdominal cavity through a patent processus vaginalis, a potential hernia space. Hydrocele manifests as a painless, enlarged scrotum. The condition may resolve spontaneously but usually requires repair if it persists after 6 to 9 mo or if it enlarges.

Cryptorchidism: Failure of 1 or both testes to descend into the scrotum affects about 3% of term infants and up to 30% of preterm infants; ⅔ of undescended testes will spontaneously descend within the 1st 4 mo of life. Normally, the testes develop at 7 to 8 wk gestation and remain cephalad to the internal inguinal ring until about 28 wk, when they begin their descent into the scrotum guided by condensed mesenchyma (the gubernaculum). Onset of descent is mediated by hormonal (eg, androgens, müllerian-inhibiting factor), physical (eg, gubernacular regression, intra-abdominal pressure), and environmental (eg, maternal exposure to estrogenic or antiandrogenic substances) factors, but undescended testes are almost always idiopathic. About 10% of cases are bilateral; suspicion should be high for female virilization from congenital adrenal hyperplasia in phenotypic boys with bilateral, nonpalpable, undescended testes at birth (especially if associated with hypospadias).

Undescended testes may cause subfertility and are associated with testicular carcinoma, mainly in the undescended testis and particularly with intra-abdominal malposition. However, in patients with one undescended testis, 10% of cancers develop on the normal side. In untreated cases of intra-abdominal testes, testicular torsion may occur, manifesting as an acute abdomen. Almost all who present with an undescended testis at birth also have an inguinal hernia (patent processus).

In about 80% of cases, the scrotum is empty at birth; in the remainder of cases, a testis is palpable in the scrotum at birth but appears to ascend with linear growth because of an ectopic gubernacular attachment that restrains it from following the normal "descent" of the scrotum. A true undescended testis remains in the inguinal canal along the path of descent or is less commonly present in the abdominal cavity or retroperitoneum. An ectopic testis lies outside the normal course of descent (eg, suprapubically, in the superficial inguinal pouch, within the perineum, or along the inner aspect of the thigh). Undescended and ectopic testes must be distinguished from hypermobile (retractile) testes, which are present in the scrotum but easily retract into the inguinal canal.

Diagnosis is by physical examination; a warm environment, warm examiner's hands, and a relaxed patient are important to avoid stimulating testicular retraction. In those with a unilateral nonpalpable testis, a descended testis that is larger than expected suggests an atrophic undescended testis; confirmation requires abdominal laparoscopy. For bilateral nonpalpable testes, a human chorionic gonadotropin (hCG) stimulation test is done. Patients receive injections of hCG 2000 IU IM once/day for 3 to 4 days; blood levels of testosterone, luteinizing hormone (LH), and follicle-stimulating hormone (FSH) are obtained before and testosterone levels within 24 h of the final injection. Those with bilateral cryptorchidism should respond by producing testosterone, whereas those without testes (including genotypic females) produce none. In addition, basal levels of FSH and possibly LH are elevated.

In ⅔ of boys, the testis spontaneously descends by 3 to 4 mo, resulting in prevalence of about 0.8% requiring treatment.

For a palpable undescended testis, treatment is surgical orchiopexy, in which the testis is brought into the scrotum and sutured into place; the associated inguinal hernia also is repaired. For nonpalpable undescended testis, abdominal laparoscopy is done; if the testis is located, it is surgically fixed in place, or if it is atrophic, the tissue is removed. Surgery should be done at about 6 mo of age because early intervention improves fertility potential and may reduce cancer risk. Atrophic undescended testes are likely the result of prenatal testicular torsion.

hCG 250 to 1000 IU IM 2 or 3 times/wk for up to 6 wk may stimulate local testosterone production and precipitate testicular descent, either complete or enough to make the testis palpable, increase its blood supply, or both, making surgery easier.

No intervention is needed for a retractile testis as long as the spermatic cord length is sufficient to allow the testis to rest in a dependent scrotal position without traction when the cremasteric reflex is not stimulated. Hypermobility usually resolves without treatment by puberty when increased testicular size makes retraction more difficult.

PRUNE-BELLY SYNDROME

(Triad Syndrome)

Prune-belly syndrome consists of abdominal muscle deficiency, urinary tract abnormalities, and intra-abdominal undescended testes.

The name prune-belly syndrome derives from the characteristic wrinkled appearance of the abdominal wall in neonates. The cause of this congenital syndrome, which occurs primarily but not exclusively in males, is unclear. Urinary abnormalities may include hydronephrosis, megaureters, vesicoureteral reflux, and urethral abnormalities. Severe cases may involve renal failure, bronchopulmonary dysplasia, and stillbirth.

Diagnosis is often made on routine prenatal ultrasonography. Further evaluation includes voiding cystourethrography, ultrasonography, and isotope renography.

Urinary tract abnormalities may require open surgical reconstruction; orchidopexy can be done at the same time. If no urinary intervention is necessary, laparoscopic orchidopexy is done in childhood.

291 RENAL TRANSPORT ABNORMALITIES

Defects in renal tubular transport can lead to a number of metabolic disorders, some of which are serious.

CYSTINURIA

Cystinuria is an inherited defect of the renal tubules in which resorption of the amino acid cystine is impaired, urinary excretion is increased, and cystine stones form in the urinary tract. Symptoms are colic from stones and perhaps urinary infection or the sequelae of renal failure. Diagnosis is by measurement of cystine excretion in the urine. Treatment is with increased fluid intake and alkalinization of the urine.

Cystinuria is inherited as an autosomal recessive trait. Heterozygotes may excrete increased quantities of cystine in the urine but seldom enough to form stones.

Pathophysiology

The primary defect is diminished renal tubular resorption of cystine, which increases cystine concentration in the urine. Cystine is poorly soluble in acidic urine, so that when its urinary concentration exceeds its solubility, crystals precipitate and stones form.

Resorption of dibasic amino acids (lysine, ornithine, arginine) is also impaired, which causes no problems because these amino acids have an alternative transport system separate from that shared with cystine. Furthermore, they are more soluble than cystine in urine, and their increased excretion does not result in crystal or stone formation. Their absorption (and that of cystine) is also decreased in the small bowel.

Symptoms, Signs, and Diagnosis

Symptoms, most commonly renal colic, usually appear between ages 10 and 30. UTI and renal failure due to obstruction may develop.

Radiopaque cystine stones form in the renal pelvis or bladder. Staghorn stones are common. Cystine may appear in the urine as yellow-brown hexagonal crystals. Excessive cystine in the urine may be detected with the nitroprusside cyanide test. Diagnosis is confirmed by observing a cystine excretion of > 400 mg/day (normal, < 30 mg/day).

Prognosis and Treatment

Eventually, end-stage renal disease usually develops. Decreasing the urinary concentration of cystine decreases renal toxicity. This is accomplished by increasing urine volume. Fluid intake must be sufficient to provide a urine flow rate of 3 to 4 L/day. Hydration is particularly important at night when urinary pH drops. Alkalinization of the urine to pH > 7.4 with $NaHCO_3$ or $KHCO_3$ 1 mEq/kg po bid to tid and acetazolamide 5 mg/kg (up to 250 mg) po at bedtime increases the solubility of cystine significantly. When high fluid intake and alkalinization do not reduce stone formation, other drugs may be tried. Penicillamine (7.5 mg/kg qid and 250 mg to 1 g po qid in older children) is effective, but toxicity limits its usefulness. About ½ of all patients develop some toxic manifestation, such as fever, rash, arthralgias, or, less commonly, nephrotic syndrome, pancytopenia, or SLE-like reaction. Captopril (0.3 mg/kg po tid) is not as effective as penicillamine but is much less toxic.

FANCONI SYNDROME

Fanconi syndrome consists of multiple defects in renal proximal tubular reabsorption, producing glucosuria, phosphaturia, generalized aminoaciduria, and HCO_3 wasting. Symptoms in children are failure to thrive, growth retardation, and rickets. Symptoms in adults are osteomalacia and muscle weakness. Diagnosis is by demonstrating glucosuria, phosphaturia, and aminoaciduria. Treatment is HCO_3 replacement and measures directed at renal failure.

Etiology

Hereditary Fanconi syndrome usually accompanies another genetic disorder, particularly cystinosis. Fanconi syndrome may also accompany Wilson's disease, hereditary fructose intolerance, galactosemia, glycogen storage disease, Lowe syndrome, and tyrosinemia. Inheritance patterns vary with the associated disorder.

Acquired Fanconi syndrome may be caused by various drugs, including certain cancer chemotherapy agents (eg, ifosfamide, streptozocin), antiretrovirals (eg, didanosine, cidofovir), and outdated tetracycline. All of these drugs are nephrotoxic. It also may occur with renal transplantation, multiple myeloma, amyloidosis, intoxication with heavy metals or other chemical agents, or vitamin D deficiency.

Pathophysiology, Symptoms, and Signs

Various defects of proximal tubular transport function occur, including impaired resorption of glucose, phosphate, amino acids, HCO_3, uric acid, water, K, and Na. The aminoaciduria is generalized, and, unlike cystinuria, increased cystine excretion is a minor component. The basic pathophysiologic abnormality is unknown but may involve a mitochondrial disturbance. Low values of serum phosphate cause rickets, which is worsened by decreased proximal tubular conversion of vitamin D to its active form.

In hereditary Fanconi syndrome, the chief clinical features—proximal tubular acidosis, hypophosphatemic rickets, hypokalemia, polyuria, and polydipsia—usually appear in infancy.

When Fanconi syndrome occurs because of cystinosis, failure to thrive and growth retardation are common. The retinas show patchy depigmentation. Interstitial nephritis develops, leading to progressive renal failure that may be fatal before adolescence.

In acquired Fanconi syndrome, adults present with the laboratory abnormalities of renal tubular acidosis (proximal type II), hypophosphatemia, and hypokalemia. They may present with symptoms of bone disease (osteomalacia) and muscle weakness.

Diagnosis and Treatment

Diagnosis is made by demonstrating the abnormalities of renal function, particularly glucosuria (in the presence of normal serum glucose), phosphaturia, and aminoaciduria. In cystinosis, slit-lamp examination may show cystine crystals in the cornea.

Other than removing the offending nephrotoxin, there is no specific treatment. Acidosis may be lessened by giving tablets or solutions of Na or K HCO_3 or citrate, eg, Shohl's solution (Na citrate and citric acid; 1 mL is equivalent to 1 mmol of HCO_3) given 1 mEq/kg bid to tid or 5 to 15 mL after meals and at bedtime. K depletion may require replacement therapy with a K-containing salt. Hypophosphatemic rickets can be treated as described below. Renal transplantation has been successful in treating renal failure. However, when cystinosis is the underlying disease, progressive damage may continue in other organs and eventually result in death.

HARTNUP DISEASE

Hartnup disease is a rare disease due to abnormal absorption and excretion of tryptophan and other amino acids. Symptoms are rash, CNS abnormalities, short stature, headache, and collapsing or fainting. Diagnosis is by high urinary content of tryptophan and other amino acids. Prevention is with niacinamide or niacin, and attacks are treated with nicotinamide.

Hartnup disease is inherited as an autosomal recessive trait. Small-bowel malabsorption of tryptophan, phenylalanine, methionine, and other monoaminomonocarboxylic amino acids occurs. Accumulation of unabsorbed amino acids in the GI tract increases their metabolism by bacterial flora. Some tryptophan degradation products, including indoles, kynurenine, and serotonin, are absorbed by the intestine and appear in the urine. Renal amino acid resorption is also defective, causing a generalized aminoaciduria involving all neutral amino acids except proline and hydroxyproline. Conversion of tryptophan to niacinamide is also defective.

Symptoms, Signs, and Diagnosis

Poor nutritional intake nearly always precedes appearance of symptoms. Symptoms and signs are due to niacinamide deficiency and resemble those of pellagra (see p. 31), particularly the rash on parts of the body exposed to the sun. Neurologic manifestations include cerebellar ataxia and mental abnormalities. Mental retardation, short stature, headache, and collapsing or fainting are common. Although the disorder is present from birth, symptoms may manifest in infancy, childhood, or early adulthood. Symptoms may be precipitated by sunlight, fever, drugs, or other stresses.

Diagnosis is made by demonstrating the characteristic amino acid excretion pattern in the urine. Indoles and other tryptophan degradation products in the urine provide supplementary evidence of the disease.

Treatment

Prognosis is good, and frequency of attacks usually diminishes with aging. Attacks can be prevented by maintaining good nutrition and supplementing the diet with niacin or niacinamide 50 to 100 mg po tid. Attacks may be treated with nicotinamide 20 mg po once/day.

HYPOPHOSPHATEMIC RICKETS

(Vitamin D–Resistant Rickets)

Hypophosphatemic rickets is a disorder characterized by hypophosphatemia, defective intestinal absorption of Ca, and rickets or osteomalacia unresponsive to vitamin D. It is usually hereditary. Symptoms are bone pain, fractures, and growth abnormalities. Diagnosis is by serum phosphate, alkaline phosphatase, and 1,25-dihydroxyvitamin D_3 levels. Treatment is oral phosphate plus calcitriol.

Familial hypophosphatemic rickets is inherited as an X-linked dominant trait. Sporadic acquired cases sometimes are associated with benign mesenchymal tumors (oncogenic rickets).

The observed abnormality is decreased proximal renal tubular resorption of phosphate, resulting in hypophosphatemia. This defect is due to a circulating factor and is associated with a primary abnormality in osteoblast function. Decreased intestinal Ca and phosphate absorption also occurs. Deficient bone mineralization is due to low phosphate levels and osteoblast dysfunction rather than to the low Ca and elevated parathyroid hormone (PTH) levels in Ca-deficient rickets (see p. 41). Because 1,25-dihydroxyvitamin D_3 levels are normal to slightly low, a defect in conversion is presumed; hypophosphatemia would normally cause elevated 1,25-dihydroxyvitamin D_3 levels.

Symptoms, Signs, and Diagnosis

The disease manifests as a spectrum of abnormalities, from hypophosphatemia alone to growth retardation and short stature to severe rickets or osteomalacia. Children usually present after they begin walking, with bowing of the legs and other bone deformities, pseudofractures, bone pain, and short stature. Bony outgrowth at muscle attachments may limit motion. Rickets of the spine or pelvis, dental enamel defects, and tetany that occur in dietary vitamin D deficiency are rarely present in hypophosphatemic rickets.

Patients should undergo measurement of serum levels of Ca, phosphate, alkaline phosphatase, 1,25-dihydroxyvitamin D_3, and PTH, and of urinary phosphate. Serum phosphate levels are depressed, but urinary phosphate excretion is large. Serum Ca and PTH are normal, and alkaline phosphatase often is elevated. In Ca-deficient rickets, hypocalcemia is present, hypophosphatemia is mild or absent, and urinary phosphate is not elevated.

Treatment

Treatment consists of phosphate 10 mg/kg po qid as neutral phosphate solution or tablets. Because this phosphate may cause hyperparathyroidism, vitamin D is given as calcitriol, initially 0.005 to 0.01 μg/kg po once/day, then 0.015 to 0.03 μg/kg once/day as maintenance. Increase in plasma phosphate and decrease in alkaline phosphatase concentrations, healing of rickets, and improvement of growth rate occur. Hypercalcemia, hypercalciuria, and nephrocalcinosis with reduced renal function may complicate treatment. In adults with oncogenic rickets, dramatic improvement has followed removal of the small cell mesenchymal tumor that produces a humoral factor that decreases proximal renal tubular resorption of phosphate.

292 CONGENITAL NEUROLOGIC ANOMALIES

Some of the most serious neurologic anomalies (eg, anencephaly, encephalocele, spina bifida) develop in the first 2 mo of gestation and represent defects in neural tube formation (dysraphism). Others, such as lissencephaly, result from problems with neuronal migration, which occurs between 9 and 24 wk of gestation. Hydranencephaly and porencephaly are secondary to destructive processes that occur after the brain has formed. Some anomalies (eg, meningocele) are relatively benign.

Amniocentesis (see p. 2145) and ultrasonography (see p. 2144) permit accurate in utero detection of many malformations. Parents need psychologic support when a malformation is detected and also genetic counseling, because the risk of having a subsequent child with such a malformation is high.

In women who have had a fetus or infant with a neural tube defect, folate (folic acid) supplementation (4 mg/day) beginning 3 mo before conception and during the 1st trimester reduces the risk for such defects in future pregnancies by 75%. All women of child-bearing age who have not had a fetus or infant with a neural tube defect should consume at least 400 μg/day of folate through diet or by taking a supplement (some experts recommend 800 μg/day to further reduce risk) and continue doing so during the 1st trimester. Although such supplementation reduces the risk of having a child with a neural tube defect, the degree of risk reduction is less than in women with a prior history of an affected fetus or infant.

BRAIN ANOMALIES

Congenital brain anomalies usually cause severe neurologic deficits; some may be fatal.

HYDROCEPHALUS

Hydrocephalus is ventricular enlargement with excessive CSF. Manifestations include an enlarged head and brain atrophy. Increased cranial pressure causes irritability and bulging fontanelles in infants. Diagnosis is by ultrasonography in neonates and by CT or MRI in older infants. Treatment usually is with a ventricular shunt procedure.

Hydrocephalus is the most common cause of abnormally large heads in neonates. It results from either obstruction of CSF flow (obstructive hydrocephalus) or impaired resorption (communicating hydrocephalus). Obstruction most often occurs in the aqueduct of Sylvius but sometimes at the outlets of the 4th ventricle (Luschka and Magendie foramina). Impaired resorption in the subarachnoid spaces usually results from meningeal inflammation, secondary either to infection or to blood in the subarachnoid space (eg, in the premature infant who has intraventricular hemorrhage).

Obstructive hydrocephalus can be caused by Dandy-Walker malformation or Chiari II type (formerly Arnold-Chiari) malformation. Dandy-Walker malformation is progressive cystic enlargement of the 4th ventricle. In Chiari II type malformation, which frequently occurs with spina bifida (see p. 2443) and syringomyelia (see p. 1915), severe elongation of the cerebellar tonsils causes them to protrude through the foramen magnum, with beaking of the colliculi and thickening of the upper cervical spinal cord.

Symptoms and Signs

Neurologic findings depend on whether intracranial pressure is increased, symptoms of which include headache (or irritability in infants), high-pitched cry, vomiting, lethargy, strabismus or decreased vision, and bulging fontanelle (in infants). Papilledema is a late sign of increased intracranial pressure; initial absence is not reassuring. Consequences of chronically increased pressure may include precocious puberty in girls, learning disorders (eg, difficulties with attention, information processing, memory), and impaired executive function (eg, problems with conceptualizing, abstracting, generalizing, reasoning, and organizing and planning information for problem-solving).

Diagnosis

Diagnosis is often made by prenatal ultrasound. After birth, diagnosis is suspected if routine examination reveals an increased head circumference; infants may have a bulging fontanelle or widely separated cranial sutures. Similar findings can result from intracranial, space-occupying lesions (eg, subdural hematomas, porencephalic cysts, tumors). Macrocephaly may result from an underlying brain problem (eg, Alexander or Canavan disease), or it may be benign, in which excessive CSF surrounds a normal brain. Patients suspected of having hydrocephalus require cranial imaging by CT, MRI, or ultrasonography. Cranial CT or ultrasonography (if the anterior fontanelle is open) is used to follow progression of hydrocephalus once an anatomic diagnosis has been made. If seizures occur, an EEG may be helpful.

Treatment

Treatment depends on etiology, severity, and whether hydrocephalus is progressive (ie, size of the ventricles increases over time relative to the size of the brain). Progressive hydrocephalus usually requires a ventricular shunt. To temporarily reduce CSF pressure in infants, ventricular taps or serial lumbar punctures (if the hydrocephalus is communicating) may be used.

The type of ventricular shunt used depends on the neurosurgeon's experience, although ventriculoperitoneal shunts produce fewer complications than ventriculoatrial shunts. Any shunt has a risk of infection. After the shunt is placed, head circumference and development are assessed, and imaging is performed periodically. Shunt obstruction can be a medical emergency; children present with symptoms and signs of suddenly increased intracranial pressure such as headache, vomiting, lethargy, irritability, esotropia, or paralysis of upward gaze. Seizures may occur. If the obstruction is gradual, more subtle symptoms and signs can occur, such as irritability, poor school performance, and lethargy, which may be mistaken for depression.

Although some children cease to need the shunt as they age, determining the appropriate time for removal (which may cause bleeding and trauma) is difficult. Thus, shunts are rarely removed. Fetal surgery to treat congenital hydrocephalus has not been successful.

Other Brain Anomalies

Anencephaly: Anencephaly is absence of the cerebral hemispheres. The absent brain is sometimes replaced by malformed cystic neural tissue, which may be exposed or covered with skin. Parts of the brain stem and spinal cord may be missing or malformed. Infants are stillborn or die within days or weeks. Treatment is supportive.

Encephalocele: Encephalocele is a protrusion of nervous tissue and meninges through a skull defect. The defect is caused by incomplete closure of the cranial vault (cranium bifidum). Encephaloceles usually occur in the midline and protrude anywhere along a line from the occiput to the nasal passages but can be present asymmetrically in the frontal or parietal regions. Small encephaloceles may resemble cephalhematomas, but x-rays show a bony skull defect at their base. Hydrocephalus (see p. 2441) often occurs with encephalocele. About 50% of affected infants have other congenital anomalies.

Prognosis, which depends on the location and size of the lesion, is usually good. Most encephaloceles can be repaired. Even large ones often contain mostly heterotopic nervous tissue, which can be removed without worsening functional ability. When other serious malformations coexist, the decision to repair may be more difficult.

Malformed cerebral hemispheres: Cerebral hemispheres may be large, small, or asymmetric; the gyri may be absent, unusually large, or multiple and small; and microscopic sections of normal-appearing brain may show disorganization of the normal laminar neuronal arrangement. Microcephaly, moderate to severe motor and mental retardation, and epilepsy often occur with these defects. Treatment is supportive, including anticonvulsants, if needed, to control seizures.

Holoprosencephaly occurs when the embryonic prosencephalon does not undergo segmentation and cleavage. The anterior midline brain, cranium, and face are abnormal. This malformation may be caused by defects of the *sonic hedgehog* gene. Severely affected fetuses may die before birth. Treatment is supportive.

Lissencephaly consists of an abnormally thick cortex, reduced or abnormal lamination, and diffuse neuronal heterotopia. It is caused by abnormal neuronal migration, the process by which immature neurons attach to radial glia and move from their points of origin near the ventricle to the cerebral surface. Several single-gene defects may cause this anomaly (eg, *LIS1*). Affected infants may have mental retardation, muscle spasms, and seizures. Treatment is supportive, but many children die before age 2 yr.

Polymicrogyria, in which the gyri are small and overabundant, is believed to arise from injuries occurring between 17 wk and 26 wk gestation. It can cause mental retardation and seizures. Treatment is supportive.

Porencephaly: Porencephaly is a cyst or cavity in a cerebral hemisphere that communicates with a ventricle. It may develop pre- or postnatally. The defect may be caused by a developmental anomaly, inflammatory disease, or a vascular accident such as intraventricular hemorrhage with parenchymal extension. Neurologic examination is usually abnormal. Diagnosis is confirmed by cranial CT, MRI, or ultrasonography. Progressive hydrocephalus occurs rarely with porencephaly. Prognosis is variable; a few patients develop only minor neurologic signs and have normal intelligence. Treatment is supportive.

Hydranencephaly is an extreme form of porencephaly in which the cerebral hemispheres are almost totally absent. Usually, the cerebellum and brain stem are formed normally, and the basal ganglia are intact. The meninges, bones, and skin over the cranial vault are normal. Often hydranencephaly is diagnosed by prenatal ultrasonography. Neurologic examination is usually abnormal, and the infant does not develop normally. Externally, the head may appear normal, but when transilluminated, light shines completely through. CT or ultrasound confirms the diagnosis. Treatment is supportive, with shunting if head growth is excessive.

Schizencephaly, which many classify as a form of porencephaly, results from formation of abnormal slits, or clefts, in the cerebral hemispheres. Unlike porencephalies, however, which are thought to be the result of brain injury, schizencephaly is thought to represent a defect in neuronal migration and is thus a true malformation. Treatment is supportive.

Septo-optic dysplasia: Septo-optic dysplasia (de Morsier syndrome) is a malformation of the front of the brain that occurs toward the end of the 1st mo of gestation and includes optic nerve hypoplasia, absence of the septum pellucidum (the membranes that separate the front of the 2 lateral ventricles), and pituitary deficiencies. Although the cause may be multiple, abnormalities of one particular gene (*HESX1*) have been found in some patients with septo-optic dysplasia.

Symptoms may include decreased visual acuity in one or both eyes, nystagmus, strabismus, and endocrine dysfunction (including growth hormone deficiency, hypothyroidism, adrenal insufficiency, diabetes insipidus, and hypogonadism). Seizures may occur. Although some children have normal intelligence, others have learning disabilities, mental retardation, cerebral palsy, or other developmental delay. Diagnosis is by MRI. All children diagnosed with this disorder should be screened for endocrine and developmental dysfunction. Treatment is supportive.

SPINA BIFIDA

Spina bifida is defective closure of the vertebral column. Although the cause is not known, low folate levels during pregnancy increase risk. Some cases are asymptomatic, and others cause severe neurologic dysfunction below the lesion. Open spina bifida can be diagnosed prenatally by ultrasound or suggested by elevated α-fetoprotein levels in maternal serum and amniotic fluid. After birth, a lesion is typically visible on the back. Treatment is usually surgical.

Spina bifida is one of the most serious neural tube defects compatible with prolonged life. It is most common in the lower thoracic, lumbar, or sacral region and usually extends for 3 to 6 vertebral segments. Severity ranges from occult, in which there are no apparent anomalies, to protruding sacs (spina bifida cystica), to a completely open spine (rachischisis) with severe neurologic disability and death.

In occult spina bifida, anomalies of the skin overlying the lower back (typically in the lumbosacral area) occur; these include sinus tracts that have no visible bottom, are above the lower sacral area, or are not in the midline; hyperpigmented areas; and tufts of hair. These children often have anomalies in the underlying portion of the spinal cord, such as lipomas and tethering (in which the cord has an abnormal attachment).

In spina bifida cystica, the protruding sac can contain meninges (meningocele), spinal cord (myelocele), or both (meningomyelocele). In a meningomyelocele, the sac usually consists of meninges with a central neural plaque. If not well covered with skin, the sac can easily rupture, increasing the risk of meningitis.

Hydrocephalus is common and may be related to Chiari II type malformations (see p. 2441) or aqueductal stenosis. Other congenital anomalies, such as abnormal migration of neuronal cells in the brain, syringomyelia, and soft-tissue masses, may be present.

Symptoms and Signs

Many children with minor defects are asymptomatic. When the spinal cord or lumbosacral nerve roots are involved, as is usual, varying degrees of paralysis affect all muscles below the lesion. Lack of muscle innervation also leads to atrophy of the legs and decreased rectal tone. Because paralysis occurs in the fetus, orthopedic problems may be present at birth (eg, clubfoot, arthrogryposis of the legs, dislocated hip). Kyphosis is sometimes present and can hinder surgical closure and prevent the patient from lying supine.

Paralysis also impairs bladder function, leading to urine reflux, which can cause hydronephrosis, frequent UTIs, and, ultimately, kidney damage.

Diagnosis

Spinal cord imaging, with ultrasonography or MRI, is essential; even children with minimal cutaneous findings may have underlying spinal abnormalities. Plain x-rays of the spine, hips, and, if they are malformed, lower extremities are obtained along with cranial imaging by using ultrasonography, CT, or MRI.

Once the diagnosis of spina bifida is made, urinary tract evaluation is essential and includes urinalysis, urine culture, BUN and creatinine determination, and ultrasonography. Measurement of the bladder capacity and pressure at which urine refluxes into the urethra can determine prognosis and intervention. Need for further testing, such as urodynamics and voiding cystourethrogram, depends on previous findings and associated anomalies.

Prognosis

Prognosis varies by the level of cord involvement and the number and severity of associated anomalies. Prognosis is poorest for patients with higher cord levels (eg, thoracic) or who have kyphosis, hydrocephalus, early hydronephrosis, and associated congenital anomalies. With proper care, however, many children do well. Loss of renal function and shunt complications are the usual causes of death in older patients.

Treatment and Prevention

Without rapid surgical treatment, neurologic damage can progress. Treatment requires a united effort by specialists from several disciplines; neurosurgical, urologic, orthopedic, pediatric, and social service evaluations are initially important. It is important to assess the type, vertebral segment, and extent of the lesion; the infant's health status; and associated anomalies. Prior to intervention, discussion with the family should ascertain the family's strengths, desires, and resources, and community resources, including availability of ongoing care.

A meningomyelocele identified at birth is covered immediately with a sterile dressing. If the meningomyelocele is leaking CSF, antibiotics are started to prevent meningitis. Neurosurgical repair of a meningomyelocele or an open spine typically is performed within the 1st 72 h after birth to reduce the risk of meningeal or ventricular infection. If the lesion is large or is in a difficult location, plastic surgeons may be consulted to ensure adequate closure.

Hydrocephalus may require a shunt procedure in the neonatal period. Kidney function must be followed closely, and UTI should be treated promptly. Obstructive uropathy at either the bladder outlet or ureteral level must be treated vigorously to prevent infection. Orthopedic care should begin early. If a clubfoot is present, a cast is applied. Hip joints are checked for dislocation. Affected children should be monitored for development of scoliosis, pathologic fractures, pressure sores, and muscle weakness and spasm.

Folate supplementation in women beginning 3 mo before conception and during the 1st trimester reduces the risk for neural tube defects (see p. 2441).

293 EYE DEFECTS AND CONDITIONS IN CHILDREN

Defects and conditions can affect any part of the eye. They often affect vision, and some can result in blindness if not adequately treated. Other defects and conditions that affect vision during childhood are discussed elsewhere in THE MANUAL (see Ch. 101 on p. 888, Ch. 102 on p. 895, and Ch. 219 on p. 1867).

AMBLYOPIA

Amblyopia is functional reduction in visual acuity of an eye caused by disuse during visual development. Blindness can occur in the affected eye if amblyopia is not detected and treated before age 8 yr. Diagnosis is based on detecting a difference in visual acuity between the 2 eyes. Treatment depends on the cause.

Amblyopia affects about 2 to 3% of children and almost always develops before age 2.

The brain must simultaneously receive a clear image from each eye. Amblyopia results when there is persistent interference with the image from one eye but not the other. The visual cortex suppresses the image from the affected eye.

There are 3 causes. Strabismus (see p. 2446) can cause amblyopia because misalignment of the eyes results in different retinal images being sent to the visual cortex. Similarly, anisometropia (inequality of refraction in the 2 eyes, most often from astigmatism, myopia, or hyperopia) results in different retinal images, with the image from the eye with the greater refractive error being less well focused. Obstruction of the visual axis at some point between the surface of the eye and the retina (eg, by a cataract) interferes with or completely disrupts formation of a retinal image in the affected eye.

Symptoms and Signs

Children rarely complain of unilateral vision loss. Very young children either do not notice or are unable to express awareness that their vision differs in one eye compared with the other. Some older children may report impaired vision in the affected eye or exhibit poor depth perception. When strabismus is the cause, deviation of gaze may be noticeable to others. A cataract causing occlusion of the visual axis may go unnoticed.

Diagnosis

Screening for amblyopia (and strabismus) is recommended for all children before starting school, optimally around age 3 yr. Photoscreening is one approach for screening very young children and children with learning and developmental disorders who are unable to undergo subjective testing. Photoscreening involves use of a camera to record images of pupillary reflexes during fixation on a visual target and red reflexes in response to light; the images are then compared for symmetry. Screening in older children consists of acuity testing with figures (eg, tumbling E figures, Allen cards, or the HOTV figures) or Snellen eye charts.

Identifying the underlying cause requires additional testing. Strabismus can be confirmed with the cover test or the cover-uncover test (see p. 2447). Anisometropia can be confirmed by performing a refraction to assess the refractive power of each eye. Obstruction of the visual axis can be confirmed by ophthalmoscopy or slit-lamp examination.

Prognosis and Treatment

Amblyopia may become irreversible if not diagnosed and treated before age 8, a time at which the visual system will have matured. Most of those identified and treated before age 5 have some vision improvement. Earlier treatment increases the likelihood of complete vision recovery. Recurrence is possible in certain cases until the visual system matures.

Treatment should be under the direction of an ophthalmologist. Any underlying causes must be treated (eg, eyeglasses or contact lenses to correct refractive error, removal of a cataract). Use of the amblyopic eye is then encouraged by patching the better eye or by administering atropinic drops into the better eye to provide a visual advantage to the amblyopic eye. Adherence to treatment is better with drop therapy. Maintenance treatment for prevention of recurrences may be recommended after improvement has stabilized, until a child is about 8 to 10.

CONGENITAL CATARACT

(Infantile Cataract)

Congenital cataract is a lens opacity that is present at birth or shortly after birth.

Congenital cataracts may be sporadic, or they may be caused by chromosomal anomalies, metabolic disease (eg, galactosemia), or intrauterine infection (eg, rubella) or other maternal disease during pregnancy. Cataracts may be nuclear, or they may involve the lens material underneath the anterior or posterior lens capsule. They may be unilateral or bilateral. They may not be noticed unless the red reflex is checked or unless ophthalmoscopy is performed at birth. As with other cataracts, the lens opacity obscures vision. Cataracts may obscure the view of the optic disk and vessels and should be evaluated by an ophthalmologist.

Removal of a cataract within 17 wk after birth permits development of vision and cortical visual pathways. Cataracts are removed by aspirating them through a small incision. In many children, an intraocular lens may be implanted. Postoperative visual correction with eyeglasses, contact lenses, or both is usually required to achieve good vision.

After a unilateral cataract is removed, the quality of the image in the treated eye is inferior to that of the other eye (assuming the other eye is normal). Because the better eye is preferred, the brain suppresses the poorer-quality image, and amblyopia (see p. 2445) develops. Thus, effective amblyopia therapy is necessary for the treated eye to develop normal sight. Some children are unable to attain good visual acuity. In contrast, children with bilateral cataract removal in which image quality is similar in both eyes more frequently develop equal vision in both eyes.

Some cataracts are partial (posterior lenticonus) and opacify during the 1st decade of life. Eyes with partial cataracts will have a better visual outcome.

PRIMARY INFANTILE GLAUCOMA

(Infantile Glaucoma; Congenital Glaucoma; Buphthalmos)

Primary infantile glaucoma is a rare defect in the iridocorneal filtration angle of the anterior chamber that causes a relative obstruction of egress of aqueous fluid from the eye, which increases intraocular pressure.

The disorder occurs in infants and young children and may be unilateral (40%) or bilateral (60%). Intraocular pressure increases above the normal range (10 to 22 mm Hg). The eye becomes enlarged; the large-diameter (normal is < 12 mm) cornea is thinned and sometimes cloudy. If untreated, corneal clouding progresses, the optic nerve is damaged (as evidenced clinically by optic nerve cupping), and blindness may occur. Early surgical intervention (goniotomy, trabeculotomy, trabeculectomy) is the mainstay of treatment.

Glaucoma can also occur after trauma or intraocular surgery or be associated with aniridia or Lowe or Sturge-Weber syndrome. In such cases, it is called secondary glaucoma.

STRABISMUS

Strabismus is misalignment of the eyes, which produces deviation from the parallelism of normal gaze. Diagnosis is clinical, including observation of the corneal light reflex and use of a cover test. Treatment may include correction of visual impairment with patching and corrective lenses, alignment by corrective lenses, and surgery.

Strabismus occurs in about 3% of children. Strabismus rarely results from retinoblastoma or other serious ocular defects or from neurologic disease. Left untreated, about 50% of children with strabismus have some visual loss due to amblyopia (see p. 2445).

Several varieties of strabismus have been described, based on direction of deviation, specific conditions under which deviation occurs, and whether deviation is constant or intermittent. Description of these varieties requires definition of several terms.

The prefixes eso- and exo- refer to nasal and temporal deviations, respectively. The prefixes hyper- and hypo- refer to upward and downward deviations, respectively. Manifest deviations, detectable with both eyes open so that vision is binocular, are designated as tropia, and latent deviation, detectable only when one eye is covered so that vision is monocular, is designated as phoria. Tropia can be constant or intermittent. Tropia may involve only one eye, or it may involve both eyes. Deviations that are the same (amplitude or degree of misalignment remains the same) in all gaze directions are designated as comitant, whereas deviations that vary (amplitude or degree of misalignment changes) depending on gaze direction are referred to as incomitant.

Etiology

Strabismus may be congenital (the term infantile is preferred, because detection of strabismus at birth is uncommon, and infantile permits inclusion of varieties that develop within the 1st 6 mo of life) or acquired (includes those that develop after 6 mo).

Risk factors for infantile strabismus include family history (1st- or 2nd-degree relative), genetic disorders (Down and Crouzon syndromes), prenatal drug exposure (including alcohol), prematurity or low birth weight, congenital eye defects, and cerebral palsy.

Acquired strabismus can develop acutely or gradually. Risk factors for acquired strabismus include tumors (eg, retinoblastoma, head trauma), neurologic conditions (eg, cerebral palsy; spina bifida; palsy of the 3rd, 4th, or 5th cranial nerves), viral infections (eg, encephalitis, meningitis), and acquired eye defects. Specific causes vary depending on the type of deviation.

Esotropia is commonly infantile. Infantile esotropia is considered idiopathic, although an anomaly of fusion is the suspected cause. Accommodative esotropia, a common variety of acquired esotropia, develops between 2 and 4 yr and is associated with hyperopia. Sensory esotropia occurs when severe visual loss (due to conditions such as cataracts, optic nerve anomalies, or tumors) interferes with the brain's effort to maintain ocular alignment.

Esotropia can be paralytic, so designated because the cause is a 6th (abducens) cranial nerve palsy, but it is an uncommon cause. Esotropia can also be a component of a syndrome. Duane's syndrome (congenital absence of the abducens nucleus with anomalous innervation of the lateral rectus extraocular muscle by the 3rd [oculomotor] cranial nerve) and Möbius' syndrome (anomalies of multiple cranial nerves) are specific examples.

Exotropia may be intermittent and idiopathic. Less often, exotropia is constant and paralytic, as with 3rd cranial nerve palsy.

Hypertropia can be paralytic, caused by 4th (trochlear) cranial nerve palsy that occurs congenitally or after head trauma, or less commonly, as a result of palsy of the 3rd cranial nerve.

Hypotropia can be restrictive, caused by mechanical restriction of full movement of the globe rather than neurologic interference with eye movement. For example, restrictive hypotropia can result from a blowout fracture of the orbit floor or walls. Less commonly, restrictive hypotropia can be caused by Graves' ophthalmopathy. Third cranial nerve palsy and Brown's syndrome (congenital or acquired tightness and restriction of the superior oblique muscle tendon) are other uncommon causes.

Symptoms and Signs

Unless severe, phorias rarely cause symptoms.

Tropias sometimes result in symptoms. For example, torticollis may develop to compensate for the brain's difficulty in fusing images from misaligned eyes and to reduce diplopia. Some children with tropias have normal and equal visual acuity. However, amblyopia frequently develops with tropias; it is due to cortical suppression of the image in the deviating eye to avoid confusion and diplopia.

Diagnosis

Strabismus can be detected during well-child checkups. History should include questions about family history of amblyopia or strabismus and, if family or caregivers have noticed deviation of gaze, questions about when the deviation began, when it is present, and whether there is a preference for using one eye for fixation. Physical examination should include an assessment of visual acuity, pupil reactivity, and the extent of extraocular movements. Neurologic examination, particularly of the cranial nerves, is important.

The corneal light reflex test is a good screening test, but it is not very sensitive for detecting small deviations. The child looks at a light and the light reflection (reflex) from the pupil is observed; normally, the reflex appears symmetric (ie, in the same location on each pupil). The light reflex for an exotropic eye is nasal to the pupillary center, whereas the reflex for an esotropic eye is temporal to the pupillary center.

When performing the alternate cover test, the child is asked to fixate on an object. One eye is then covered while the other is observed for movement. No movement should be detected if the eyes are properly aligned, but strabismus is present if the unoccluded eye shifts to establish fixation once the other eye, which had fixed on the object, is occluded. The test is then repeated on the other eye.

In a variation of the cover test, called the cover-uncover test, the patient is asked to fix on an object while the examiner alternately covers and uncovers one eye and then the other, back and forth. An eye with a latent strabismus shifts position when it is uncovered. In exotropia, the eye that was covered turns *in* to fixate; in esotropia, it turns *out* to fixate. Tropia can be quantified by using prisms positioned such that the deviating eye need not move to fixate. The power of the prism used to prevent deviation quantifies the tropia and provides a measurement of the magnitude of misalignment of the visual axes. The unit of measurement used by ophthalmologists is the prism diopter.

Strabismus should be distinguished from pseudostrabismus, which is the appearance of esotropia in a child with good visual acuity in both eyes but a wide nasal bridge or broad epicanthal folds that obscure much of the white sclera nasally when looking laterally. The light reflex and cover tests are normal in a child with pseudostrabismus.

Prognosis and Treatment

Strabismus should not be ignored on the assumption that it will be outgrown. Permanent vision loss can occur if strabismus and its attendant amblyopia are not treated before age 4 to 6 yr.

Treatment aims to equalize vision and then align the eyes. Children with amblyopia require patching or penalization of the normal eye; improved vision offers a better prognosis for development of binocular vision and for stability if surgery is performed. Patching is not, however, a treatment for strabismus. Eyeglasses or contact lenses are sometimes used if the amount of refractive error is significant enough to interfere with fusion, especially in children with accommodative esotropia. Topical miotic agents, such as echothiophate iodide 0.125%, may facilitate accommodation in children with accommodative esotropia. Orthoptic eye exercises can help correct intermittent exotropia and convergence insufficiency.

Surgery is generally performed when nonsurgical methods are unsuccessful in aligning the eyes satisfactorily. Surgery consists of loosening (recession) and tightening (resection) procedures, most often involving the rectus muscles. Surgery is typically performed in an outpatient setting. Rates for successful realignment usually exceed 80%. The most common complications are overcorrection or undercorrection and recurrence of the strabismus later in life. Rare complications include infection, excessive bleeding, and vision loss.

294 CHROMOSOMAL ANOMALIES

Karyotype describes the full set of chromosomes in a person's cells; genotype describes the genetic constitution determined by the karyotype; and phenotype describes the person's biochemical, physiologic, and physical makeup as determined by the genotype and environmental factors (see p. 2698).

Chromosomal anomalies cause various disorders. Those affecting autosomes (the paired chromosomes that are alike in males and females) are more common than those affecting sex chromosomes. Specific anomalies include trisomies, translocations, deletions and duplications of various chromosomes or parts of chromosomes, and mosaicisms.

Diagnosis

Circulating blood lymphocytes are used for chromosomal analysis, except prenatally, when amniocytes are usually used (see p. 2145). Cells are cultured with phytohemagglutinin to stimulate cell division. Colchicine is added to arrest mitosis during metaphase, when each chromosome has replicated into 2 chromatids attached at the centromere. Cells are then stained. Chromosomes from single cells are photographed, their images cut out of the print, and pasted onto a piece of paper, forming a karyotype. Computer imaging also can produce a visual display of the chromosomes.

Chromosome staining is routinely performed by G (Giemsa)- or Q (fluorescent)-banding stain techniques. DNA probes with fluorescent tags help locate specific genes or DNA sequences on the chromosomes. Fluorescent in situ hybridization (FISH) is used to identify gene organization and chromosomal anomalies.

Each arm of a chromosome is divided into 1 to 4 major regions, each demarcated into several bands by staining. Each band, positively or negatively stained, is given a number, which increases as the distance from the centromere increases. For example, 1q23 designates the chromosome (1), the long arm (q), the 2nd region distal to the centromere (2), and the 3rd band (3) in that region.

DOWN SYNDROME

(Trisomy 21; Trisomy G)

Down syndrome is an anomaly of chromosome 21, causing mental retardation, microcephaly, short stature, and characteristic facies. Diagnosis is suggested by physical anomalies and abnormal development and confirmed by karyotype analysis. Treatment depends on specific manifestations and anomalies.

Overall incidence among live births is about 1/800, but varies markedly depending on maternal age: for mothers < 20 yr, the incidence is about 1/2000; for mothers > 40 yr, it rises to about 1/40. However, because most births occur to younger women, just 20% of infants with Down syndrome are born to mothers > 35 yr.

Etiology

In about 95% of cases, there is an extra whole chromosome 21 (trisomy 21), which is almost always maternally derived. Some people with Down syndrome have only 46 chromosomes, but a piece of an additional chromosome 21 has been translocated to another chromosome. The most common translocation is t(14;21), in which a piece of an additional chromosome 21 is attached to chromosome 14. In about ½ the cases, both parents have normal karyotypes, indicating a de novo translocation. In the other ½, 1 parent (almost always the mother), although phenotypically normal, has only 45 chromosomes, 1 of which is t(14;21). Theoretically, the chance that a carrier mother will have a Down syndrome child is 1:3, but for unknown reasons the actual risk is lower (about 1:10). If the father is the carrier, the risk is only 1:20. The next most common translocation is t(21;22). In these cases, carrier mothers have about a 1:10 risk of having a Down syndrome child; the risk is less for carrier fathers.

Down syndrome mosaicism presumably results from nondisjunction during cell division in the embryo. Most affected people have 2 cell lines, 1 with 46 and 1 with 47 chromosomes. The prognosis for intelligence probably depends on the proportion of trisomy 21 cells in the brain. A few people with mosaic Down syndrome have barely recognizable clinical signs and normal intelligence. If a parent has germ-line mosaicism for trisomy 21, an increased risk exists for a 2nd affected child.

Symptoms and Signs

Affected neonates tend to be placid, rarely cry, and demonstrate muscular hypotonia. Most have a flat facial profile (particularly flattening of the bridge of the nose), although some appear normal at birth and then develop characteristic facial features during infancy. A flattened occiput, microcephaly, and extra skin around the back of the neck are common. The outer sides of the eyes are slanted upward, and epicanthal folds at the inner corners usually are present. Brushfield's spots (gray to white spots resembling grains of salt around the periphery of the iris) usually are visible and disappear during the 1st 12 mo. The mouth is often held open because of a large, protruding, furrowed tongue that lacks the central fissure. The ears are often small and rounded. The hands are short and broad and often have a simian crease (a single, palmar crease). The fingers are short, with clinodactyly (incurving) of the 5th digit, which often has only 2 phalanges. The feet may have a wide gap between the 1st and 2nd toes, and a plantar furrow often extends backward on the foot. Hands and feet show characteristic dermatoglyphics.

About 40% of affected neonates have congenital heart disease; ventricular septal defect and atrioventricular canal (endocardial cushion defect) are most common. Incidence of almost all other congenital anomalies, particularly duodenal atresia, is increased. Many people with Down syndrome develop thyroid disease (most often hypothyroidism).

As affected children grow, retardation of physical and mental development quickly becomes apparent. Stature is short, and the mean intelligence quotient (IQ) is about 50.

The aging process seems to be accelerated. The median age at death is 49; however, many reach their 50s or 60s. Life expectancy is decreased primarily by heart disease and to a lesser degree by increased susceptibility to infections and acute myelocytic leukemia.

Additionally, as they age, people with Down syndrome may develop hearing and vision problems. Many people develop clinical signs of Alzheimer's disease at an early age, and at autopsy, brains of adults with Down syndrome show typical microscopic findings.

Affected women have a 50% chance that their fetus will also have Down syndrome. However, many affected fetuses abort spontaneously. Men with Down syndrome are infertile except for those who are mosaic.

Diagnosis

Diagnosis may be suspected prenatally based on physical anomalies detected by fetal ultrasound, or by abnormal levels (eg, low α-fetoprotein or unconjugated estriol, high human chorionic gonadotropin) on maternal serum screening, and confirmed by amniocentesis with karyotyping. Diagnosis in neonates is based on physical anomalies and confirmed by karyotype analysis.

Treatment

Treatment depends on specific manifestations. The underlying disorder cannot be treated. Treatment should also include genetic counseling for the family, social support, and educational programming appropriate for the level of intellectual functioning (see Mental Retardation on p. 2491). Some congenital cardiac anomalies are repaired surgically. Hypothyroidism is treated with thyroid hormone replacement.

TRISOMY 18

(Edwards' Syndrome; Trisomy E)

Trisomy 18 is caused by an extra chromosome 18 and usually consists of mental retardation, small birth size, and many developmental anomalies, including severe microcephaly, prominent occiput, low-set malformed ears, and a characteristic pinched facial appearance.

Trisomy 18 occurs in 1/6000 live births, but spontaneous abortions are common. More than 95% of affected children have complete trisomy 18. The extra chromosome is almost always maternally derived, and advanced maternal age increases risk. The female:male ratio is 3:1.

Symptoms and Signs

A history of feeble fetal activity, polyhydramnios, a small placenta, and a single umbilical artery often exists. Size at birth is markedly small for gestational age, with hypotonia and marked hypoplasia of skeletal muscle and subcutaneous fat. The cry is weak, and response to sound is decreased. The orbital ridges are hypoplastic, the palpebral fissures short, the mouth and jaw small—all of which give the face a pinched appearance. Microcephaly, prominent occiput, low-set malformed ears, narrow pelvis, and a short sternum are common. A clenched fist with the index finger overlapping the 3rd and 4th fingers usually occurs. The distal crease on the 5th finger is often absent, and there is a low-arch dermal ridge pattern on the fingertips. The fingernails are hypoplastic, and the big toe is shortened and frequently dorsiflexed. Clubfeet and rocker-bottom feet are common. Severe congenital heart disease is common, especially patent ductus arteriosus and ventricular septal defects. Anomalies of lungs, diaphragm, GI tract, abdominal wall, kidneys, and ureters are frequent. Hernias and/or diastasis recti abdominis, cryptorchidism, and redundant skinfolds (particularly over the back of the neck) also are common.

Diagnosis and Treatment

Diagnosis may be suspected prenatally by abnormalities on ultrasound or maternal serum screening and postnatally by appearance. Confirmation in both cases is by karyotyping. Karyotyping may be suspected by intrauterine growth restriction, multiple congenital anomalies, and abnormal maternal serum screening.

More than 50% die within the 1st week; < 10% are still alive at 1 yr. Those who survive have marked developmental delay and disability. No specific treatment is available.

TRISOMY 13

(Patau's Syndrome; Trisomy D)

Trisomy 13 is caused by an extra chromosome 13 and consists of abnormal forebrain, midface, and eye development; severe mental retardation; and small birth size.

Trisomy 13 occurs in about 1/10,000 live births; about 80% of cases are complete trisomy 13. Advanced maternal age increases the likelihood, and the extra chromosome is usually maternally derived.

Infants tend to be small for gestational age. Midline anomalies (eg, scalp defects and dermal sinuses) are characteristic. Holoprosencephaly (failure of the forebrain to divide properly) is common. Concurrent facial anomalies can include cleft lip and cleft palate. Microphthalmia, colobomas (fissures) of the iris, and retinal dysplasia are also common. Supraorbital ridges are shallow, and palpebral fissures usually are slanted. The ears are abnormally shaped and usually low-set. Deafness is common. Loose folds of skin often present over the back of the neck. Simian crease (a single, palmar crease), polydactyly, and hyperconvex narrow fingernails are also common. About 80% of cases have severe congenital cardiovascular anomalies; dextrocardia is common. Genitals are frequently abnormal in both sexes; cryptorchidism and an abnormal scrotum occur in boys, and a bicornuate uterus occurs in girls. Apneic spells in early infancy are frequent. Mental retardation is severe.

Diagnosis and Treatment

Diagnosis may be suspected prenatally by abnormalities on ultrasound (eg, intrauterine growth restriction) or maternal serum screening, and postnatally by appearance. Confirmation in both cases is by karyotyping.

Most patients (80%) are so severely affected that they die before age 1 mo; < 10% survive longer than 1 yr.

CHROMOSOMAL DELETION SYNDROMES

Chromosomal deletion syndromes result from loss of parts of chromosomes. They tend to cause severe congenital anomalies and markedly retarded mental and physical development. Chromosomal deletion syndromes are rarely suspected prenatally but may be incidentally discovered at that time if karyotyping is done for other reasons. Postnatal diagnosis is suspected by clinical appearance and confirmed by karyotyping and other genetic analysis.

5p-Deletion (cri du chat syndrome): Deletion of the end of the short arm of chromosome 5 (5p) is characterized by a high-pitched, mewing cry, closely resembling the cry of a kitten, which is heard in the immediate neonatal period, lasts several weeks, and then disappears. Affected neonates are of low birth weight, hypotonic, and have microcephaly, a round face with wide-set eyes, downward slanting of the palpebral fissures (with or without epicanthal folds), strabismus, and a broad-based nose. The ears are low-set, abnormally shaped, and frequently have narrow external auditory canals and preauricular tags. Syndactyly, hypertelorism, and heart anomalies occur often. Mental and physical development is markedly retarded. Many affected children survive into adulthood but are very disabled.

4p-Deletion (Wolf-Hirschhorn syndrome): Deletion of the short arm of chromosome 4 (4p) results in profound mental retardation. Manifestations also may include a broad or beaked nose, midline scalp defects, ptosis and colobomas, cleft palate, delayed bone development, and, in boys, hypospadias and cryptorchidism. Many affected children die during infancy; the relatively few who survive into their 20s are severely handicapped and prone to infections and epilepsy.

Contiguous gene syndromes: These include micro- and submicroscopic deletions of contiguous genes on particular parts of many chromosomes; small duplications of chromosomes also occur. The effects of duplications, however, are usually milder than deletions. Almost all cases are sporadic; however, mildly affected parents, as in some 22q11.21 deletions, can pass on the syndrome. Numerous syndromes have been identified, with widely varying manifestations (see TABLE 294–1). Deletions and duplications are often detectable by using fluorescent probes and other techniques. Sometimes deletions and duplications cannot be shown cytogenetically, but their presence can be confirmed by DNA probes specific to the deleted area.

Telomeric deletions: These are small and often submicroscopic and may occur at either end of a chromosome. Phenotypic changes may be minimal. Telomeric deletions may account for many cases of nonspecific mental retardation in which the affected person has mildly dysmorphic features.

SEX CHROMOSOME ANOMALIES

Sex chromosome anomalies may involve aneuploidy, partial deletions or duplications of sex chromosomes, or mosaicisms.

Sex chromosome anomalies are common and produce syndromes that include a range

TABLE 294–1. EXAMPLES OF CONTIGUOUS GENE SYNDROMES

SYNDROME	CHROMOSOMAL DELETION	DESCRIPTION
Alagille syndrome	20p.12	Cholestasis, bile duct paucity, cardiac anomalies, pulmonary artery stenoses, butterfly vertebrae, posterior embryotoxon of the eye
Angelman's syndrome	Maternal chromosome at 15q11	Seizures, puppet-like ataxia, outbursts of laughter, hand flapping, severe mental retardation
DiGeorge syndrome (DiGeorge anomaly, velocardiofacial syndrome, pharyngeal pouch syndrome, thymic aplasia—see p. 1343)	22q11.21	Hypoplasia or lack of thymus and parathyroids; often heart anomalies, cleft palate, mental retardation, and psychiatric problems
Langer-Giedion syndrome (trichorhinophalangeal syndrome type II)	8q24.1	Exostosis, cone epiphyses, sparse hair, bulbous nose, mental retardation
Miller-Dieker syndrome	17p13.3	Lissencephaly; short, upturned nose; severe growth retardation; seizures; severe mental retardation
Prader-Willi syndrome (see p. 2369)	Paternal chromosome at 15q11	Hypotonic neonate, obesity, hypogonadism, small hands and feet, mental retardation
Rubinstein-Taybi syndrome	16p13–	Broad thumbs and large toes, prominent nose and columella, mental retardation
Smith-Magenis syndrome	17p11.2	Brachycephaly, midfacial hypoplasia, prognathism, hoarse voice, short stature, mental retardation
Williams syndrome	7q11.23	Aortic stenosis, mental retardation, elfin facies, transient hypercalcemia in infants

of congenital and developmental anomalies. They are rarely suspected prenatally but may be incidentally discovered at that time if karyotyping is done for other reasons. They are often hard to recognize at birth and may not be diagnosed until puberty.

X chromosome anomalies are relatively benign, compared with analogous autosomal anomalies. Females with 3 X chromosomes are often normal physically and mentally and are fertile. In contrast, all known autosomal trisomies have devastating effects. Similarly, the absence of 1 X chromosome, although it leads to a specific syndrome (Turner's syndrome), is relatively benign, whereas the absence of an autosome is invariably lethal.

Lyon hypothesis (X-inactivation): Females have 2 loci for every X-linked gene, as compared with males' single locus. This imbalance would seem to produce a genetic "dosage" problem. However, according to the Lyon hypothesis, 1 of the two X chromosomes in each female somatic cell is genetically inactivated early in embryonic life (on or about day 16). In fact, no matter how many X chromosomes are present, all but 1 are inactivated. However, recent molecular genetic studies have demonstrated that some genes on the inactivated X chromosome (or chromosomes) remain functional, and these few are essential to normal female development. The Barr body, or sex chromatin mass within the nuclei of female somatic cells, represents the inactivated X chromosome. *XIST* is the gene responsible for inactivating the genes of the X chromosome.

Whether the maternal or paternal X is inactivated is a random event within each cell at the time of inactivation; that same X then remains inactive in all descendant cells. Thus, all females are mosaics, with some cells having an active maternal X and others an active paternal X.

Sometimes, random statistical distribution of inactivation in the relatively small number of cells present at the time of inactivation results in a particular descendant tissue having a preponderance of active maternal or paternal X (skewed inactivation). Skewed inactivation may account for the occasional manifestation of minor symptoms in females who are heterozygous for X-linked disorders such as hemophilia and muscular dystrophy (all would presumably be asymptomatic if they had a 50:50 distribution of active X chromosomes). Skewed inactivation also may occur by post-inactivation selection.

TURNER'S SYNDROME

(Bonnevie-Ullrich Syndrome)

Turner's syndrome results from complete or partial absence of 1 of the 2 sex chromosomes, producing a phenotypic female. Diagnosis is based on clinical findings and confirmed by karyotype analysis. Treatment depends on manifestations and may include surgery for cardiac anomalies, and often growth hormone therapy for short stature and estrogen replacement for pubertal failure.

Turner's syndrome occurs in about 1/4000 live female births and is the most common sex chromosome anomaly in females. However, 99% of 45,X conceptions abort spontaneously.

About 50% of affected girls have a 45,X karyotype; about 80% have lost the paternal X. Most of the other 50% are mosaics (eg, 45,X/46,XX or 45,X/47,XXX). Among mosaic individuals, phenotype may vary from that of typical Turner's syndrome to normal. Occasionally, affected girls have 1 normal X and 1 X that has formed a ring chromosome; for this formation to happen, a piece must be lost from both the short and long arms of the abnormal X. Some affected girls have 1 normal X and 1 long arm isochromosome formed by the loss of short arms and development of a chromosome consisting of 2 long arms of the X chromosome. These girls tend to have many of the phenotypic features of Turner's syndrome; thus, deletion of the X chromosome's short arm seems to play an important role in producing the phenotype.

Symptoms and Signs

Many neonates are very mildly affected; however, some present with marked dorsal lymphedema of the hands and feet and with lymphedema or loose folds of skin over the back of the neck. Other frequent anomalies include a webbed neck and a broad chest with widely spaced and inverted nipples. Affected girls have short stature compared with family members. Less common findings include a low hairline on the back of the neck, ptosis, multiple pigmented nevi, short 4th metacarpals and metatarsals, prominent finger pads with whorls in the dermatoglyphics on the ends of the fingers, and hypoplasia of the nails. Increased carrying angle at the elbow occurs.

Common cardiac anomalies include coarctation of the aorta and bicuspid aortic valve. Hypertension frequently occurs with aging even without coarctation. Renal anomalies and hemangiomas are frequent. Occasionally, telangiectasia occurs in the GI tract, with resultant GI bleeding or protein loss.

Gonadal dysgenesis (ovaries are replaced by bilateral streaks of fibrous stroma and are devoid of developing ova) occurs in 90%, resulting in the inability to go through puberty, develop breast tissue, or begin menses. However, 5 to 10% of affected girls do go through menarche spontaneously, and, very rarely, affected women are fertile and have children.

Mental retardation is rare, but many have some diminution of certain perceptual abilities and thus score poorly on performance tests and in mathematics, even though they score average or above in the verbal components of intelligence tests.

Diagnosis

In neonates, diagnosis may be suspected based on presence of lymphedema or a webbed neck. In the absence of these findings, some children are diagnosed later, based on short stature, lack of pubertal development, and amenorrhea. Diagnosis is confirmed by karyotype analysis. Echocardiography or MRI is indicated to detect cardiac anomalies.

Cytogenetic analysis and Y-specific probe studies are obtained for all people with gonadal dysgenesis to rule out mosaicism with a Y-bearing cell line (eg, 45,X/46,XY). These people are usually phenotypic females who have variable features of Turner's syndrome.

They are at high risk for gonadal malignancy, especially gonadoblastoma, and should have the gonads removed prophylactically as soon as the diagnosis is made.

Treatment

There is no specific treatment for the underlying genetic condition. Coarctation of the aorta is usually repaired surgically. Other cardiac anomalies are monitored and repaired as needed. Lymphedema can usually be controlled with support hosiery.

Recombinant human growth hormone therapy may be initiated if height is < 5th percentile, beginning with 0.05 mg/kg sc once/day. Estrogen replacement is usually needed to initiate puberty and is typically given at age 12 to 13 as conjugated estrogens 0.3 mg po or micronized estradiol 0.5 mg once/day. Thereafter, birth control pills with a progestin are given to maintain secondary sexual characteristics. Growth hormone can be given with estrogen replacement until epiphyses are fused, at which time growth hormone is discontinued. Continuation of estrogen replacement helps establish optimal bone density and skeletal development.

KLINEFELTER'S SYNDROME (47,XXY)

Klinefelter's syndrome is ≥ 2 X chromosomes plus 1 Y, resulting in a phenotypic male.

Klinefelter's syndrome occurs in about 1/800 live male births. The extra X chromosome is maternally derived in 60% of cases.

Affected boys tend to be tall, with disproportionately long arms and legs. They often have small, firm testes, and about 30% develop gynecomastia. Puberty usually occurs at the normal age, but often facial hair growth is light. There is a predisposition for learning disorders, and many have lower verbal IQ, auditory processing, and reading. Clinical variation is great, and many 47,XXY males have normal appearance and intellect. Many are diagnosed during an infertility workup (probably all 47,XXY males are sterile). Testicular development varies from hyalinized nonfunctional tubules to some production of spermatozoa; urinary excretion of follicle-stimulating hormone is frequently increased.

Mosaicism occurs in 15% of cases. These men may be fertile. Some affected men have 3, 4, and even 5 X chromosomes along with the Y. As the number of X chromosomes increases, the severity of mental retardation and of malformations also increases.

47,XYY SYNDROME

47,XYY syndrome is 2 Y chromosomes and 1 X, resulting in a phenotypic male.

The 47,XYY syndrome occurs in about 1/1000 live male births. Affected boys tend to be taller than average and have a 10- to 15-point IQ reduction compared with family members. There are few physical problems. Minor behavior disorders, hyperactivity, attention deficit disorder, and learning disorders are more common.

OTHER X CHROMOSOME ANOMALIES

About 1/1000 apparently normal females have 47,XXX karyotype. Physical anomalies are rare. Menstrual irregularity and infertility sometimes occur. Affected girls may have mildly impaired intellect and may have more school problems than siblings. Advanced maternal age increases risk of the triple X anomaly, and the extra X chromosome is usually maternally derived.

Although rare, 48,XXXX and 49,XXXXX females exist. There is no consistent phenotype. The risk of mental retardation and congenital anomalies increases markedly when there are > 3 X chromosomes. The genetic imbalance in early embryonic life before X-inactivation may cause anomalous development.

295 INHERITED MUSCULAR DISORDERS

Inherited metabolic disorders affecting the muscles, such as disorders of mitochondrial oxidative phosphorylation and glycogen storage diseases, are discussed in Ch. 296 on p. 2458.

MUSCULAR DYSTROPHIES

Muscular dystrophies are inherited, progressive muscle disorders resulting from defects in one or more genes needed for normal muscle function. They are distinguished by the selective distribution of weakness and the specific nature of the genetic abnormality involved.

Duchenne's dystrophy is the most common and important form of muscular dystrophy. Becker's dystrophy, although closely related, has a later onset and produces milder symptoms. Other forms include Emery-Dreifuss dystrophy, myotonic dystrophy, limb-girdle dystrophy, facioscapulohumeral dystrophy, and congenital dystrophies.

DUCHENNE'S AND BECKER'S DYSTROPHIES

Duchenne's and Becker's dystrophies are X-linked recessive disorders characterized by progressive proximal muscle weakness caused by muscle fiber degeneration. Becker's dystrophy has later onset and produces milder symptoms. Diagnosis is suggested clinically and confirmed by analysis of the protein product (dystrophin) of the mutated gene. Treatment focuses on maintaining function through physical therapy and the use of braces and orthotics; prednisone is given to some patients experiencing severe functional decline.

Duchenne's and Becker's dystrophies are caused by mutations at the Xp21 locus. In Duchenne's dystrophy, this mutation results in the absence of dystrophin, a protein in the muscle cell membrane. In Becker's dystrophy, the mutation results in production of abnormal dystrophin or less dystrophin. Duchenne's dystrophy affects 1/3000 live male births; Becker's dystrophy, 1/30,000 live male births.

Symptoms and Signs

Duchenne's dystrophy manifests typically between ages 2 and 3 yr. Weakness affects proximal muscles, typically in the lower limbs initially. Children frequently demonstrate a waddling gait, toe walking, and lordosis. They fall frequently and have difficulty running, jumping, climbing stairs, and rising from the floor. Progression of weakness is steady, and limb flexion contractures and scoliosis develop. Firm pseudohypertrophy (fatty and fibrous replacement of certain enlarged muscle groups, notably the calves) develops. Most patients are confined to a wheelchair by age 12 and die of respiratory complications by age 20. Cardiac involvement is usually asymptomatic, although 90% of patients have ECG abnormalities. One third have mild, nonprogressive intellectual impairment that affects verbal ability more than performance.

Becker's dystrophy typically becomes symptomatic much later and is milder. Ambulation is usually preserved until at least age 15, and many patients remain ambulatory into adulthood. Most affected patients survive into their 30s and 40s.

Diagnosis

Diagnosis is suspected by characteristic clinical findings, age at onset, and family history suggestive of X-linked recessive inheritance. Myopathic changes are noted on electromyography (rapidly recruited, short, low-amplitude motor unit potentials) and muscle biopsy (necrosis and marked variation in muscle fiber size). CK levels are elevated to up to 100 times normal.

Diagnosis is confirmed by analysis of dystrophin with immunostaining. Dystrophin is undetectable in patients with Duchenne's dystrophy; in patients with Becker's dystrophy, dystrophin is typically abnormal (lower molecular weight) or present in low concentration. Mutation analysis of DNA from peripheral blood leukocytes can also be confirmatory by identifying abnormalities in the dystrophin gene (deletions or duplications in about 65% and point mutations in about 25% of patients).

Carrier detection and prenatal diagnosis are possible using conventional studies (pedigree analysis, CK determinations, fetal sex determination) combined with recombinant DNA analysis and dystrophin immunostaining of muscle tissue.

Treatment

No specific treatment exists. Moderate exercise is encouraged for as long as possible. Passive exercises may extend the period of ambulation. Ankle-foot orthoses help prevent flexion during sleep. Leg braces may temporarily help preserve ambulation or standing. Obesity should be avoided; caloric requirements are likely to be less than normal. Genetic counseling is indicated (see p. 2143).

Daily prednisone does not produce significant long-term clinical improvement, but it possibly slows the course of the disease. No consensus on long-term effectiveness exists. Gene therapy is not yet available. Corrective surgery is sometimes needed. Respiratory insufficiency may be treated with noninvasive ventilatory support (eg, nasal mask—see p. 547). Elective tracheostomy is gaining acceptance, allowing patients to live into their 20s.

OTHER FORMS OF MUSCULAR DYSTROPHY

Emery-Dreifuss dystrophy: Emery-Dreifuss dystrophy can be inherited as an autosomal dominant, autosomal recessive (the rarest), or X-linked recessive disorder. The overall incidence is unknown. Females can be carriers, but only males are affected clinically by X-linked inheritance. Genes associated with Emery-Dreifuss dystrophy encode for certain nuclear membrane proteins; lamin A/C (autosomal), and emerin (X-linked).

Muscle weakness and wasting can begin any time before age 20 and commonly affect the biceps and triceps and, less often, distal leg muscles. The heart is frequently involved, with atrial paralysis, conduction abnormalities (atrioventricular block), cardiomyopathy, and a high likelihood of sudden death.

Diagnosis is indicated by clinical findings, age at onset, and family history; supported by mildly increased serum CK levels and myopathic features on electromyography and muscle biopsy; and confirmed by DNA testing.

Treatment involves therapy to prevent contractures. Cardiac pacemakers are sometimes lifesaving in patients with abnormal conduction.

Myotonic dystrophy: Myotonic dystrophy, the most common form of muscular dystrophy among whites, affects about 30/100,000 live male and female births. Inheritance is autosomal dominant with variable penetrance. Two genetic loci—DM 1 and DM 2—cause the abnormality. Symptoms and signs begin during adolescence or young adulthood and include myotonia (delayed relaxation after muscle contraction), weakness and wasting of distal limb muscles (especially in the hand) and facial muscles (ptosis is especially common), and cardiomyopathy. Mental retardation, cataracts, and endocrine disorders can also occur.

Diagnosis is indicated by characteristic clinical findings, age at onset, and family history and confirmed by DNA testing. Treatment includes braces for foot drop and drug therapy for control of myotonia (eg, mexiletine 75 to 150 mg po bid or tid).

Limb-girdle dystrophy: Limb-girdle dystrophy has several subtypes, some autosomal recessive and some autosomal dominant. The overall incidence is unknown. Males and females are affected equally. Several chromosomal loci have been identified for autosomal dominant (5q [no known gene product]) and recessive (2q, 4q [beta-sarcoglycan], 13q [gamma-sarcoglycan], 15q [calpain, a Ca-activated protease], and 17q [alpha-sarcoglycan, or adhalin]) forms. Structural (dystrophin-associated glycoproteins) or nonstructural (eg, proteases) proteins can be affected.

Symptoms involve weakness in a limb girdle and proximal limb distribution. Onset of symptoms ranges from early childhood to adulthood; autosomal recessive cases tend to have childhood onset and primarily have a pelvic girdle distribution.

Diagnosis is indicated by characteristic clinical findings, age at onset, and family history. For autosomal recessive cases, DNA testing and muscle biopsy are diagnostic; DNA testing for autosomal dominant disease is not readily available.

Treatment focuses on prevention of contractures.

Facioscapulohumeral dystrophy: Facioscapulohumeral dystrophy is an autosomal dominant disorder characterized by weakness of the facial muscles and shoulder girdle, usually beginning at age 7 to 20. An infantile variety, characterized by facial, shoulder, and hip girdle weakness, is rapidly progressive. A classic variety has onset during adolescence or young adulthood and is characterized by slow progression and difficulty in whistling, closing the eyes, and raising the arms (due to weakness of the scapular stabilizer muscles). Life expectancy is normal.

Diagnosis is indicated by characteristic clinical findings, age at onset, and family history and confirmed by DNA testing.

Treatment consists of physical therapy.

Congenital muscular dystrophy: Congenital muscular dystrophy is not a single disorder but instead refers to muscular dystrophy evident at birth, occurring from any of several rare forms of muscular dystrophy. The diagnosis is suspected in any "floppy" neonate but must be distinguished from congenital myopathy by muscle biopsy.

Treatment consists of physical therapy, which may help preserve function.

CONGENITAL MYOPATHIES

Congenital myopathy is a term sometimes applied to hundreds of distinct neuromuscular disorders that may be present at birth, but it is usually reserved for a group of rare inherited primary muscle disorders that cause hypotonia and weakness at birth or during the neonatal period and, in some cases, delayed motor development later in childhood.

The 5 most common types of congenital myopathy are nemaline myopathy, myotubular myopathy, central core myopathy, congenital fiber type disproportion, and multicore myopathy. They are distinguished primarily by their histologic features, symptoms, and prognosis. Diagnosis is indicated by characteristic clinical findings and confirmed by muscle biopsy. Treatment consists of physical therapy, which may help preserve function.

Nemaline myopathy: Nemaline myopathy can be autosomal dominant or recessive and result from various mutations on different chromosomes. Nemaline myopathy may be severe, moderate, or mild in neonates. Severely affected patients may experience weakness of respiratory muscles and respiratory failure. Moderate disease produces progressive weakness in muscles of the face, neck, trunk, and feet, but life expectancy may be nearly normal. Mild disease is nonprogressive, and life expectancy is normal.

Myotubular myopathy: Myotubular myopathy is autosomal or X-linked. The more common autosomal variation produces mild weakness and hypotonia in both sexes. The X-linked variation affects males and results in severe skeletal muscle weakness and hypotonia, facial weakness, impaired swallowing, and respiratory muscle weakness and respiratory failure.

Central core myopathy: Inheritance is autosomal dominant. Most affected patients develop hypotonia and mild proximal muscle weakness as neonates. Many also have facial weakness. Weakness is nonprogressive, and life expectancy is normal. However, patients are at higher risk of developing malignant hyperthermia (the gene associated with central core myopathy is also associated with increased susceptibility to malignant hyperthermia).

Congenital fiber type disproportion: Congenital fiber type disproportion is inherited, but the pattern is poorly understood. Hypotonia and weakness of the face, neck, trunk, and limbs are often accompanied by skeletal abnormalities and dysmorphic features. Most affected children improve with age, but a small percentage develops respiratory failure.

Multicore myopathy: Multicore myopathy is usually autosomal recessive but may be autosomal dominant. Infants typically present with proximal weakness, but some children present later with generalized weakness. Progression is highly variable.

FAMILIAL PERIODIC PARALYSIS

Familial periodic paralysis is a rare autosomal condition characterized by episodes of flaccid paralysis with loss of deep tendon reflexes and failure of muscle to respond to electrical stimulation. There are 3 forms: hyperkalemic, hypokalemic, and normokalemic. Diagnosis is indicated by history and confirmed by provoking an episode (by administering glucose and insulin to produce hypokalemia or KCl to produce hyperkalemia). Treatment depends on the form.

The hypokalemic form of familial periodic paralysis is due to genetic mutation in the dihydropyridine receptor–associated Ca channel gene. The hyperkalemic form is due to mutations in the gene that encodes the α-subunit of the skeletal muscle Na channel (SCN4A). The cause of the normokalemic form is unclear; in some instances it may result from a mutation in a gene that encodes Na channels.

Symptoms and Signs

In the hypokalemic form, episodes usually begin before age 16. The day after vigorous exercise, the patient often awakens with weakness, which may be mild and limited to certain muscle groups or may affect all 4 limbs. Episodes are precipitated by carbohydrate-rich meals. Ocular, bulbar, and respiratory muscles are spared. Consciousness is not altered. Serum and urine K are decreased. Weakness lasts up to 24 h.

In the hyperkalemic form, episodes often begin at an earlier age and usually are shorter, more frequent, and less severe. Episodes are precipitated by exercise after meals or by fasting. Myotonia (delayed relaxation after muscle contraction) is common. Eyelid myotonia may be the only symptom.

In the normokalemic form, affected patients are sensitive to K ingestion and experience episodes of mild weakness occurring without any change in serum K.

Diagnosis and Treatment

The best diagnostic indicator is a history of typical episodes. If measured during an episode, serum K may be abnormal. Episodes can sometimes be provoked by administering dextrose and insulin (hypokalemic form) or KCl (hyperkalemic form), but only experienced physicians should attempt this procedure, because respiratory paralysis or cardiac conduction abnormalities may occur with provoked episodes.

Episodes of hypokalemic paralysis are managed by administering KCl 2 to 10 g in an unsweetened oral solution or administering K IV. Following a low-carbohydrate, low-Na diet; avoiding strenuous activity or alcohol after periods of rest; and taking acetazolamide 250 to 2000 mg po once/day may help prevent hypokalemic episodes.

At onset, mild episodes of hyperkalemic paralysis are aborted by light exercise and a 2 g/kg carbohydrate load. An established episode requires thiazides, acetazolamide, or inhaled β-agonists. Severe attacks require Ca gluconate, or insulin and dextrose IV. Regularly ingesting carbohydrate-rich, low-K meals and avoiding fasting and strenuous activity after meals and exposure to cold help prevent hyperkalemic episodes.

In the normokalemic form, large doses of Na improve the weakness. Dextrose has no effect. Attacks may be prevented by avoiding resting after exercise, excess alcohol, and cold exposure.

296 INHERITED DISORDERS OF METABOLISM

Most inherited disorders (also called inborn errors) of metabolism are caused by mutations in genes that code for enzymes; enzyme deficiency or inactivity leads to accumulation of substrate precursors or metabolites or to deficiencies of the enzyme's products. Hundreds of disorders exist, and most are extremely rare; they are typically grouped by the affected substrate (eg, carbohydrates, amino acids, fatty acids).

Most states routinely test all neonates for specific inherited disorders of metabolism and other conditions (see p. 2223), including phenylketonuria, tyrosinemia, biotinidase deficiency, homocystinuria, maple syrup urine disease, and galactosemia. Some states also include testing for disorders of fatty acid oxidation and other organic acidemias.

Metabolic defects that primarily cause disease in adults (eg, gout, porphyria), are organ-specific (eg, Wilson's disease, congenital adrenal hypoplasia), or are common (eg, cystic fibrosis, hemochromatosis) are discussed elsewhere in THE MANUAL. Inherited disorders of lipoprotein metabolism are listed in TABLE 159–3 on p. 1298.

APPROACH TO THE PATIENT WITH A SUSPECTED INHERITED DISORDER OF METABOLISM

Most inherited disorders (inborn errors) of metabolism are rare, and therefore their diagnosis requires a high index of suspicion. Timely diagnosis leads to early treatment and may help avoid acute and chronic complications, developmental compromise, and even death.

Evaluation

Symptoms and signs tend to be nonspecific and are more often caused by something other than an inherited disorder of metabolism (eg, infection); these more likely causes should also be investigated.

History and physical examination: Disorders presenting in the neonatal period tend to be more serious; manifestations of many of the disorders typically include lethargy, poor feeding, vomiting, and seizures. Disorders with later presentation tend to affect growth and development, but vomiting, seizures, and weakness also may appear.

Growth delay suggests decreased anabolism or increased catabolism and may be due to decreased availability of energy-generating substrates (eg, in glycogen storage disease [GSD]) or inefficient energy or protein use (eg, in organic acidemias or urea cycle defects).

Developmental delay may reflect chronic energy deficit in the brain (eg, pyruvate dehydrogenase deficiency), decreased supply of needed carbohydrates that are non-energy substrates for the brain (eg, lack of uridine-5′-diphosphate-galactose [UDP-galactose] in untreated galactosemia), or chronic amino acid deficit in the brain (eg, tyrosine deficiency in phenylketonuria).

Neuromuscular symptoms, such as seizures, muscle weakness, hypotonia, myoclonus, and muscle pain, and strokes or coma may suggest acute energy deficit in the brain (eg, hypoglycemic seizures in GSD type I, strokes in mitochondrial oxidative phosphorylation defects) or muscle (eg, muscle weakness in muscle forms of GSD). Neuromuscular symptoms may also reflect accumulation of toxic compounds in the brain (eg, hyperammonemic coma in urea cycle defects) or tissue breakdown (eg, rhabdomyolysis and myoglobinuria in patients with long-chain hydroxyacyl dehydrogenase deficiency or muscle forms of GSD).

Autonomic symptoms can result from hypoglycemia caused by increased glucose consumption or decreased glucose production (eg, vomiting, diaphoresis, pallor, and tachycardia in GSD or hereditary fructose intolerance) or from metabolic acidosis (eg, vomiting and Kussmaul respirations in organic acidemias). Some conditions cause both (ie, in propionic acidemia, accumulation of acyl-CoAs inhibits gluconeogenesis, thus causing hypoglycemia, and also causes metabolic acidosis).

Nonphysiologic jaundice after the neonatal period usually reflects intrinsic hepatic disease but may be due to inherited disorders of metabolism (eg, untreated galactosemia, hereditary fructose intolerance, tyrosinemia type I).

Unusual odors in body fluids reflect accumulation of specific compounds (eg, "sweaty feet" odor in isovaleric acidemia, smoky-sweet odor in maple syrup urine disease, mousy or musty odor in phenylketonuria, boiled cabbage odor in tyrosinemia).

Urine changes color when exposed to air in some disorders (eg, darkish brown in alkaptonuria, purplish brown in porphyria).

Organomegaly may reflect a failure in substrate degradation resulting in substrate accumulation within the organ cells (eg, hepatomegaly in hepatic forms of GSD and many lysosomal storage diseases, cardiomegaly in GSD type II). Eye changes include cataracts in galactokinase deficiency or classic galactosemia, and ophthalmoplegia and retinal degeneration in oxidative phosphorylation defects.

Testing: When an inherited disorder of metabolism is suspected, evaluation proceeds with simple metabolic screening tests, typically glucose, electrolytes, CBC, liver function tests, ammonia levels, and urinalysis.

Glucose measurement detects hypoglycemia or hyperglycemia; measurement may have to be timed relative to meals (eg, fasting hypoglycemia in GSD).

Electrolyte measurement detects metabolic acidosis and presence or absence of an anion gap; metabolic acidosis may need to be corroborated by ABG measurements. Non-anion gap acidosis occurs in inborn errors that cause renal tubular damage (eg, galactosemia, tyrosinemia type I). Anion gap acidosis occurs in inborn errors in which accumulation of titratable acids is typical, such as methylmalonic and propionic acidemias; it can also be caused by lactic acidosis (eg, in pyruvate decarboxylase deficiency or mitochondrial oxidative phosphorylation defects). When the anion gap is elevated, lactate and pyruvate levels should be obtained. An increase in the lactate:pyruvate ratio distinguishes oxidative phosphorylation defects from disorders of pyruvate metabolism, in which the lactate:pyruvate ratio remains normal.

CBC and smear detect hemolysis caused by RBC energy deficits or WBC defects (eg, in some pentose phosphate pathway disorders and GSD type Ib) and cytopenia caused by metabolite accumulation (eg, neutropenia in propionic acidemia due to propionyl CoA accumulation).

Liver function tests detect hepatocellular damage, dysfunction, or both (eg, in untreated galactosemia, hereditary fructose intolerance, or tyrosinemia type I).

Ammonia levels are elevated in urea cycle defects and organic acidemias.

Urinalysis detects ketonuria (present in some GSDs and maple syrup urine disease); absence of ketones in the presence of acidosis suggests a fatty acid oxidation defect.

When one or more of the above simple screening tests supports an inherited disorder of metabolism, more specific tests may be indicated. Carbohydrate metabolites, mucopolysaccharides, and amino and organic acids can be measured directly by chromatography and mass spectrometry. Common tests include quantitative plasma amino acids, urine organic acids, plasma acylcarnitine profile, and urine acylglycine profile; these have replaced earlier nonspecific screening tests.

Confirmatory tests also may include biopsy (eg, liver biopsy to distinguish hepatic forms of GSDs from other disorders associated with hepatomegaly, muscle biopsy to detect ragged red fibers in mitochondrial myopathy); enzyme studies (eg, using blood and skin cells to diagnose lysosomal storage diseases); and DNA studies, which identify gene mutations that cause disease. DNA testing can be done on almost all cells (except RBCs and platelets), thus avoiding the need for tissue biopsies; however, sensitivity for any given disease is often suboptimal because not all mutations that cause disease have been characterized.

Challenge testing is used judiciously to detect symptoms, signs, or measurable biochemical abnormalities not detectable in the normal state. The need for challenge testing has diminished with the availability of highly sensitive metabolite detection methods, but it is still occasionally used. Examples include fasting tests (eg, to provoke hypoglycemia in hepatic forms of GSD); provocative tests (eg, fructose challenge to trigger symptoms in hereditary fructose intolerance, glucagon challenge in hepatic forms of GSD [failure to observe hyperglycemia suggests disease]); and physiologic challenge (eg, exercise stress testing to elicit lactic acid production and other deformities in muscle forms of GSD). Challenge tests are often associated with an element of risk, so they must be performed under well-controlled conditions with a clear plan for reversing symptoms and signs.

AMINO ACID AND ORGANIC ACID METABOLISM DISORDERS

Defects of amino acid transport in the renal tubule are discussed in Ch. 291 on p. 2438.

PHENYLKETONURIA

Phenylketonuria is a clinical syndrome of mental retardation with cognitive and behavioral abnormalities caused by elevated serum phenylalanine. The primary cause is deficient phenylalanine hydroxylase activity. Diagnosis is by detecting high phenylalanine levels and normal or low tyrosine levels. Treatment is lifelong dietary phenylalanine restriction. Prognosis is excellent with treatment.

Phenylketonuria (PKU) is most common in all white populations and relatively less common among Ashkenazi Jews, Chinese, and blacks. Inheritance is autosomal recessive; incidence is about 1/10,000 births among whites.

Excess dietary phenylalanine (ie, that not used for protein synthesis) is normally converted to tyrosine by phenylalanine hydroxylase; tetrahydrobiopterin (BH4) is an essential cofactor for this reaction. When one of several gene mutations results in deficiency or absence of phenylalanine hydroxylase, dietary phenylalanine accumulates; the brain is the main organ affected, possibly due to disturbance of myelination. Some of the excess phenylalanine is metabolized to phenylketones, which are excreted in the urine, giving rise to the term phenylketonuria. The degree of enzyme deficiency, and hence severity of hyperphenylalaninemia, varies among patients depending on the specific mutation.

Variant forms: Although nearly all cases (98 to 99%) of PKU result from phenylalanine hydroxylase deficiency, phenylalanine also can accumulate if BH4 is not synthesized because of deficiencies of dihydrobiopterin synthase or not regenerated because of deficiencies of dihydropteridine reductase. Additionally, because BH4 is also a cofactor for tyrosine hydroxylase, which is involved in the synthesis of dopamine and serotonin, BH4 deficiency alters synthesis of neurotransmitters, causing neurologic symptoms independently of phenylalanine accumulation.

Symptoms and Signs

Most children are normal at birth but develop symptoms and signs slowly over several months as phenylalanine accumulates. The hallmark of untreated PKU is severe mental retardation. Children also manifest extreme hyperactivity, gait disturbance, and psychoses and often exhibit an unpleasant, mousy body odor caused by phenylacetic acid (a breakdown product of phenylalanine) in urine and sweat. Patients also tend to have a lighter skin, hair, and eye color than unaffected family members, and some may develop a rash similar to infantile eczema.

Diagnosis

In the US and many developed countries, all neonates are screened for PKU 24 to 48 h after birth with one of several blood tests; abnormal results are confirmed by directly measuring phenylalanine levels. In classic PKU, patients often have phenylalanine levels > 20 mg/dL (1.2 mM/L). Those with partial deficiencies typically have levels < 8 to 10 mg/dL while on a normal diet (levels > 6 mg/dl require treatment); distinction from classic PKU requires a liver phenylalanine hydroxylase activity assay demonstrating activity between 5% and 15% of normal or a mutation analysis identifying mild mutations in the gene. BH4 deficiency is distinguished from other forms of PKU by elevated concentrations of biopterin or neopterin in urine, blood, CSF, or all 3; recognition is important because standard PKU treatment will not prevent neurologic damage.

Children in families with a positive family history can be diagnosed prenatally by using direct mutation studies after chorionic villus sampling or amniocentesis.

Prognosis and Treatment

Adequate treatment begun in the first days of life prevents all manifestations of disease. Treatment begun after 2 to 3 yr may be effective only in controlling the extreme hyperactivity and intractable seizures. Children born to mothers with poorly controlled PKU (ie, they have high phenylalanine levels) during pregnancy are at high risk for microcephaly and developmental deficit.

Treatment is lifelong dietary phenylalanine restriction. All natural protein contains about 4% phenylalanine, therefore dietary staples include low-protein natural foods (eg, fruits, vegetables, certain cereals); protein hydrolysates treated to remove phenylalanine; and phenylalanine-free elemental amino acid mixtures. Examples of commercially available phenylalanine-free products include XPhe products (XP Analog for infants, XP Maxamaid for children 1 to 8 yr, XP Maxamum for children > 8 yr); Phenex I and II; Phenyl-Free I and II; PKU-1, -2, and -3; PhenylAde (varieties); Loflex; and Plexy10. Some phenylalanine is required for growth and metabolism; this is supplied by measured quantities of natural protein from milk or low-protein foods.

Frequent monitoring of plasma phenylalanine levels is required; recommended targets are between 2 mg/dL and 4 mg/dL (120 to 240 μmol/L) for children < 12 yr and between 2 mg/dL and 10 mg/dL (120 to 600 μmol/L) for children > 12 yr. Dietary planning and management need to be initiated in women of childbearing age before pregnancy to ensure a good outcome for the child.

For those with BH4 deficiency, treatment also includes tetrahydrobiopterin 1 to 5 mg/kg po tid; levodopa, carbidopa, and 5-OH tryptophan; and folinic acid 10 to 20 mg po once/day in cases of dihydropteridine reductase deficiency. However, treatment goals and approach are the same as those for PKU.

Disorders of Tyrosine Metabolism

Tyrosine is a precursor of several neurotransmitters (eg, dopamine, norepinephrine, epinephrine), hormones (eg, thyroxine), and melanin; deficiencies of enzymes involved in its metabolism lead to a variety of syndromes.

Transient tyrosinemia of the newborn: Transient immaturity of metabolic enzymes, particularly 4-hydroxyphenylpyruvic acid dioxygenase, sometimes leads to elevated plasma tyrosine levels (usually in premature infants, particularly those receiving high-protein diets); metabolites may show up on routine neonatal screening for PKU. Most patients are asymptomatic, but some demonstrate lethargy and poor feeding. Tyrosinemia is distinguished from PKU by elevated plasma tyrosine levels.

Most resolves spontaneously. Symptomatic patients should have dietary tyrosine restriction (2 g/kg/day) and vitamin C 200 to 400 mg po once/day.

Tyrosinemia type I: This disorder is an autosomal recessive trait caused by deficiency of fumarylacetoacetate hydroxylase, an enzyme important for tyrosine metabolism. Disease may manifest as fulminant liver failure in the neonatal period or as indolent subclinical hepatitis, painful peripheral neuropathy, and renal tubular disorders (eg, normal anion gap metabolic acidosis, hypophosphatemia, vitamin D–resistant rickets) in older infants and children. Long-term survivors have an increased risk of liver cancer.

Diagnosis is suggested by elevated plasma levels of tyrosine; it is confirmed by a high level of succinylacetone in plasma or urine and by low fumarylacetoacetate hydroxylase activity in blood cells or liver biopsy specimens. Treatment with 2(2-nitro-4-trifluoromethylbenzoyl)-1,3-cyclo-hexanedione (NTBC) is effective in acute episodes and slows progression. A diet low in phenylalanine and tyrosine is recommended. Liver transplantation is effective.

Tyrosinemia type II: This is a rare autosomal recessive disorder caused by tyrosine transaminase deficiency. Accumulation of tyrosine causes cutaneous and corneal ulcers. Secondary elevation of phenylalanine, though mild, may cause neuropsychiatric abnormalities if not treated. Diagnosis is by elevation of tyrosine in plasma, absence of succinylacetone in plasma or urine, and by measurement of decreased enzyme activity in liver biopsy. This disease is easily treated with mild to moderate restriction of dietary phenylalanine and tyrosine.

Alkaptonuria: This is a rare autosomal recessive disorder caused by homogentisic acid oxidase deficiency; homogentisic acid oxidation products accumulate in and darken skin, and crystals precipitate in joints. The condition is usually diagnosed in adults and causes dark skin pigmentation (ochronosis) and arthritis. Urine turns dark when exposed to air because of oxidation products of homogentisic acid. Diagnosis is by finding elevated urinary levels of homogentisic acid (> 4 to 8 g/24 h). There is no effective treatment, but ascorbic acid 1 g po once/day may diminish pigment deposition by increasing renal excretion of homogentisic acid.

Oculocutaneous albinism: Tyrosinase deficiency results in absence of skin and retinal pigmentation, causing a much increased risk for skin cancer and considerable visual loss. Nystagmus is often present, and photophobia is common (see also Albinism on p. 1002).

Disorders of Branched-Chain Amino Acid Metabolism

Valine, leucine, and isoleucine are branched-chain amino acids; deficiency of enzymes involved in their metabolism leads to accumulation of organic acids with severe metabolic acidosis.

Maple syrup urine disease: This is a group of autosomal recessive disorders caused by deficiency of one or more subunits of a decarboxylase active in the 2nd step of branched-chain amino acid catabolism. Although quite rare, incidence is significant (perhaps 1/200 births) in Amish and Mennonite populations.

Clinical manifestations include body fluid odor that resembles maple syrup (particularly strong in cerumen) and overwhelming illness in the 1st days of life, beginning with vomiting and lethargy, and progressing to seizures, coma, and death if untreated. Patients with milder forms of the disease may manifest symptoms only during stress (eg, infection, surgery).

Biochemical findings are profound ketonemia and acidemia. Diagnosis is by finding elevated plasma levels of branched-chain amino acids (particularly leucine).

Acutely, treatment with peritoneal dialysis or hemodialysis may be required, along with IV hydration and nutrition (including high-dose dextrose). Long-term management is restriction of dietary branched-chain amino acids; however, small amounts are required for normal metabolic function. Thiamin is a cofactor for the decarboxylation, and some patients respond favorably to high-dose thiamin (up to 200 mg po once/day).

Isovaleric acidemia: The 3rd step of leucine metabolism is the conversion of isovaleryl CoA to 3-methylcrotonyl CoA, a dehydrogenation step. Deficiency of this dehydrogenase results in isovaleric acidemia, also known as "sweaty feet" syndrome, because accumulated isovaleric acid emits an odor that smells like sweat.

Clinical manifestations of the acute form occur in the 1st few days of life with poor feeding, vomiting, and respiratory distress as patients develop profound anion gap metabolic acidosis, hypoglycemia, and hyperammonemia. Bone marrow suppression often occurs. A chronic intermittent form may not present for several months or years.

Diagnosis is made by detecting elevated levels of isovaleric acid and its metabolites in blood or urine. Acute treatment is with IV hydration and nutrition (including high-dose dextrose) and measures to increase isovaleric acid clearance; glycine and carnitine may help increase excretion. If these measures are insufficient, exchange transfusion and peritoneal dialysis may be needed. Long-term treatment is with dietary leucine restriction and continuation of glycine and carnitine supplements. Prognosis is excellent with treatment.

Propionic acidemia: Deficiency of propionyl CoA carboxylase, the enzyme responsible for metabolizing propionic acid to methylmalonate, causes propionic acid accumulation. Illness begins in the 1st days or weeks of life with poor feeding, vomiting, and respiratory distress due to profound anion gap metabolic acidosis, hypoglycemia, and hyperammonemia. Seizures may occur, and bone marrow suppression is common. Physiologic stresses may trigger recurrent attacks. Survivors may have mental retardation and neurologic abnormalities. Propionic acidemia can also be seen as part of multiple carboxylase deficiency, biotin deficiency, or biotinidase deficiency.

Diagnosis is suggested by elevated levels of propionic acid metabolites, including methylcitrate and tiglate and their glycine conjugates in blood and urine, and confirmed by measuring propionyl CoA carboxylase activity in WBCs or cultured fibroblasts. Acute treatment is with IV hydration (including high-dose dextrose) and nutrition; carnitine may be helpful. If these measures are insufficient, peritoneal dialysis or hemodialysis may be needed. Long-term treatment is dietary restriction of precursor amino acids and odd-chain fatty acids and possibly continuation of carnitine supplementation. A few patients respond to high-dose biotin because it is a cofactor for propionyl CoA and other carboxylases.

Methylmalonic acidemia: This disorder is caused by deficiency of methylmalonyl CoA mutase, which converts methylmalonyl CoA (a product of the propionyl CoA carboxylation) into succinyl CoA. Adenosylcobalamin, a metabolite of vitamin B_{12}, is a cofactor; its deficiency also may cause methylmalonic acidemia (and also homocystinuria and megaloblastic anemia). Methylmalonic acid accumulates. Age of onset, clinical manifestations, and treatment are similar to those of propionic acidemia except that cobalamin, instead of biotin, may be helpful for some patients.

Disorders of Methionine Metabolism

A number of defects in methionine metabolism lead to accumulation of homocysteine (and its dimer, homocystine) with adverse effects including thrombotic tendency, lens dislocation, and CNS and skeletal abnormalities.

Homocysteine is an intermediate in methionine metabolism; it is either remethylated to regenerate methionine or combined with serine in a series of transsulfuration reactions to form cystathionine and then cysteine. Cysteine is then metabolized to sulfite, taurine, and glutathione. Various defects in remethylation or transsulfuration can cause homocysteine to accumulate, resulting in disease.

The first step in methionine metabolism is its conversion to adenosylmethionine; this requires the enzyme methionine adenosyltransferase. Deficiency of this enzyme results in methionine elevation, which is not clinically significant except that it causes false-positive neonatal screens for homocystinuria.

Classic homocystinuria: This disorder is caused by an autosomal recessive deficiency of cystathionine β-synthase, which catalyzes cystathionine formation from homocysteine and serine. Homocysteine accumulates and dimerizes to form the disulfide homocystine, which is excreted in the urine. Because remethylation is intact, some of the additional homocysteine is converted to methionine, which accumulates in the blood. Excess homocysteine predisposes to thrombosis and has adverse effects on connective tissue (perhaps involving fibrillin), particularly the eyes and skeleton; adverse neurologic effects may be due to thrombosis or a direct effect.

Arterial and venous thromboembolic phenomena can occur at any age. Many develop ectopia lentis (lens subluxation), mental retardation, and osteoporosis. Patients can have a marfanoid habitus even though they are not usually tall.

Diagnosis is by neonatal screening for elevated serum methionine; elevated total plasma homocysteine levels are confirmatory. Enzymatic assay in skin fibroblasts can also be done. Treatment is a low-methionine diet, combined with high-dose pyridoxine (a cystathionine synthetase cofactor) 100 to 500 mg po once/day. Because about ½ of patients respond to high-dose pyridoxine alone, some clinicians do not restrict methionine intake in these patients. Betaine (trimethylglycine), which enhances remethylation, can also help lower homocysteine; dose is 100 to 125 mg/kg po bid. Folate 500 to 1000 μg once/day is also given. With early treatment, intellectual outcome is normal or near normal.

Other forms of homocystinuria: Various defects in the remethylation process can result in homocystinuria. Defects include deficiencies of methionine synthase (MS) and MS reductase (MSR), delivery of methylcobalamin and adenosylcobalamin, and deficiency of methylenetetrahydrofolate reductase (MTHFR, which is required to generate the 5-methyltetrahydrofolate needed for the methionine synthase reaction). Because there is no methionine elevation in these forms of homocystinuria, they are not detected by neonatal screening.

Clinical manifestations are similar to other forms of homocystinuria. In addition, MS and MSR deficiencies are accompanied by neurologic deficits and megaloblastic anemia. Clinical manifestation of MTHFR deficiency is variable, including mental retardation, psychosis, weakness, ataxia, and spasticity.

Diagnosis of MS and MSR deficiencies is suggested by homocystinuria and megaloblastic anemia and confirmed by DNA testing. Those with cobalamin defects will have megaloblastic anemia and methylmalonic acidemia. MTHFR deficiency is diagnosed by DNA testing.

Treatment is by replacement of hydroxycobalamin 1 mg IM once/day (for patients with MS, MSR, and cobalamin defects) and folate in supplementation similar to characteristic homocystinuria.

Cystathioninuria: This disorder is caused by deficiency of cystathionase, which converts cystathionine to cysteine. Cystathionine accumulation results in increased urinary excretion but no clinical symptoms.

Sulfite oxidase deficiency: Sulfite oxidase converts sulfite to sulfate in the last step of cysteine and methionine degradation; it requires a molybdenum cofactor. Deficiency of either the enzyme or the cofactor causes similar disease; inheritance for both is autosomal recessive. In its most severe form, clinical manifestations appear in neonates and include seizures, hypotonia, and myoclonus, progressing to early death. Patients with milder forms may present similarly to cerebral palsy (see p. 2373) and may have choreiform movements. Diagnosis is suggested by elevated urinary sulfite and confirmed by measuring enzyme levels in fibroblasts and cofactor levels in liver biopsy specimens. Treatment is supportive.

Urea Cycle Disorders

Urea cycle disorders are characterized by hyperammonemia under catabolic or protein-loading conditions.

Primary urea cycle disorders (UCDs) include carbamoyl phosphate synthase (CPS) deficiency, ornithine transcarbamylase (OTC) deficiency, argininosuccinate synthetase deficiency (citrullinemia), argininosuccinate lyase deficiency (argininosuccinic aciduria), and arginase deficiency (argininemia). In addition, N-acetylglutamate synthetase (NAGS) deficiency has been reported. The more "proximal" the enzyme deficiency is, the more severe the hyperammonemia; thus, disease severity in descending order is NAGS deficiency, CPS deficiency, OTC deficiency, citrullinemia, argininosuccinic aciduria, and argininemia.

Inheritance for all UCDs is autosomal recessive, except for OTC deficiency, which is X-linked.

Symptoms and Signs

Clinical manifestations range from mild (eg, failure to thrive, mental retardation, episodic hyperammonemia) to severe (eg, altered mental status, coma, death). Manifestations in females with OTC deficiency range from growth failure, developmental delay, psychiatric abnormalities, and episodic (especially postpartum) hyperammonemia, to a phenotype similar to that of affected males.

Diagnosis and Treatment

Diagnosis is based on amino acid profiles. For example, elevated ornithine indicates CPS deficiency or OTC deficiency, whereas elevated citrulline indicates citrullinemia.

To distinguish between CPS deficiency and OTC deficiency, orotic acid measurement is helpful because accumulation of carbamoyl phosphate in OTC deficiency results in its alternative metabolism to orotic acid.

Treatment is dietary protein restriction that still provides adequate amino acids for growth, development, and normal protein turnover. Arginine has become a staple of treatment. It supplies adequate urea cycle intermediates to encourage the incorporation of more nitrogen moieties into urea cycle intermediates, each of which is readily excretable. Arginine is also a positive regulator of acetylglutamate synthesis. Recent studies suggest that oral citrulline is more effective than arginine in patients with OTC deficiency. Additional treatment is with Na benzoate, phenylbutyrate, or phenylacetate, which by conjugating glycine (Na benzoate) and glutamine (phenylbutyrate and phenylacetate) provides a “nitrogen sink.” Despite these therapeutic advances, many UCDs remain difficult to treat, and liver transplantation is eventually required for many patients.

CARBOHYDRATE METABOLISM DISORDERS

Glycogen Storage Diseases

Glycogen storage diseases are caused by deficiencies of enzymes involved in glycogen synthesis or breakdown; the deficiencies may occur in the liver or muscles and cause hypoglycemia or deposition of abnormal amounts or types of glycogen (or its intermediate metabolites) in tissues.

Inheritance for glycogen storage diseases (GSDs) is autosomal recessive except for GSD type VIII/IX, which is X-linked. Incidence is estimated at about 1/25,000 births, which may be an underestimate because milder subclinical forms may be undiagnosed.

Age of onset, clinical manifestations, and severity vary by type, but symptoms and signs are most commonly those of hypoglycemia and myopathy. Diagnosis is suspected by history, examination, and detection of glycogen and intermediate metabolites in tissues by MRI or biopsy.

Diagnosis is confirmed by significant decrease of enzyme activity in liver (types I, III, VI, and VIII/IX), muscle (types IIb, III, VII, and VIII/IX), skin fibroblasts (types IIa and IV), or RBCs (type VII) or by lack of an increase in venous lactate with forearm activity/ischemia (types V and VII). Prognosis and treatment vary by type, but treatment typically includes dietary supplementation with cornstarch to provide a sustained source of glucose for the hepatic forms of GSD and exercise avoidance for the muscle forms.

Defects in glycolysis (rare) may cause syndromes similar to GSDs. Deficiencies of phosphoglycerate kinase, phosphoglycerate mutase, and lactate dehydrogenase mimic the myopathies of GSD types V and VII; deficiencies of glucose transport protein 2 (Fanconi-Bickel syndrome) mimic the hepatopathy of other GSD types (eg, I, III, IV, VI).

Galactosemia

Galactosemia is caused by inherited deficiencies in enzymes that convert galactose to glucose. Symptoms and signs include hepatic and renal dysfunction, cognitive deficits, cataracts, and premature ovarian failure. Diagnosis is by enzyme analysis of RBCs. Treatment is dietary elimination of galactose. Physical prognosis is good with treatment, but cognitive and performance parameters are often subnormal.

Galactose is found in dairy products, fruits, and vegetables; autosomal recessive enzyme deficiencies cause 3 clinical syndromes.

Galactose-1-phosphate uridyl transferase deficiency: This deficiency causes classic galactosemia. Incidence is 1/62,000 births; carrier frequency is 1/125. Infants become anorectic and jaundiced within a few days or weeks of consuming breast milk or lactose-containing formula. Vomiting, hepatomegaly, poor growth, lethargy, diarrhea, and septicemia (usually *Escherichia coli*) develop, as does renal dysfunction (eg, proteinuria, aminoaciduria, Fanconi syndrome), leading to metabolic acidosis and edema. Hemolytic anemia may also occur. Without treatment, children remain short and develop cognitive, speech, gait, and balance deficits in their teenage years; many also have cataracts, osteomalacia (caused by hypercalciuria), and premature ovarian failure. Patients with the Duarte variant have a much milder phenotype.

Galactokinase deficiency: Patients develop cataracts from production of galactitol, which osmotically damages lens fibers; idiopathic intracranial hypertension (pseudotumor cerebri) is rare. Incidence is 1/40,000 births.

Uridine diphosphate galactose 4-epimerase deficiency: There are benign and severe phenotypes. Incidence of the benign form is 1/23,000 births in Japan; no incidence data are available for the more severe form. The benign form is restricted to RBCs and WBCs and causes no clinical abnormalities. The severe form causes a syndrome indistinguishable from classic galactosemia, although sometimes with hearing loss.

Diagnosis and Treatment

Diagnosis is suggested clinically and supported by elevated galactose levels and the presence of reducing substances other than glucose (eg, galactose, galactose 1-phosphate) in the urine; it is confirmed by enzyme analysis of RBCs, hepatic tissue, or both. Most states require that neonates be screened for galactose-1-phosphate uridyl transferase deficiency.

Treatment is elimination of all sources of galactose in the diet, most notably lactose, which is a source of galactose present in all dairy products, including milk-based infant formulas and a sweetener used in many foods. A lactose-free diet prevents acute toxicity and reverses some manifestations (eg, cataracts) but may not prevent neurocognitive deficits. Many patients require supplemental Ca and vitamins. For patients with epimerase deficiency, some galactose intake is critical to ensure a supply of uridine-5′-diphosphate-galactose (UDP-galactose) for various metabolic processes.

Disorders of Fructose Metabolism

Deficiency of enzymes that metabolize fructose may be asymptomatic or cause hypoglycemia.

Fructose is a monosaccharide that is present in high concentrations in fruit and honey and is a constituent of sucrose and sorbitol.

Fructose 1-phosphate aldolase (aldolase B) deficiency: This deficiency causes the clinical syndrome of hereditary fructose intolerance. Inheritance is autosomal recessive; incidence is estimated at 1/20,000 births. Infants are healthy until they ingest fructose; fructose 1-phosphate then accumulates, causing hypoglycemia, nausea and vomiting, abdominal pain, sweating, tremors, confusion, lethargy, seizures, and coma. Prolonged ingestion may cause cirrhosis, mental deterioration, and proximal renal tubular acidosis with urinary loss of phosphate and glucose.

Diagnosis is suggested by symptoms in relation to recent fructose intake and is confirmed by enzyme analysis of liver biopsy tissue or by induction of hypoglycemia by fructose infusion, 200 mg/kg IV. Diagnosis and identification of heterozygous carriers of the mutated gene can also be made by direct DNA analysis. Short-term treatment is glucose for hypoglycemia; long-term treatment is exclusion of dietary fructose, sucrose, and sorbitol. Many patients develop a natural aversion to fructose-containing food. Prognosis is excellent with treatment.

Fructokinase deficiency: This deficiency causes benign elevation of blood and urine fructose levels (benign fructosuria). Inheritance is autosomal recessive; incidence is about 1/130,000 births. The condition is asymptomatic and diagnosed accidentally when a nonglucose reducing substance is detected in urine.

Deficiency of fructose-1,6-bisphosphatase: This deficiency compromises gluconeogenesis and results in fasting hypoglycemia, ketosis, and acidosis. This deficiency can be fatal in neonates. Inheritance is autosomal recessive; incidence is unknown. Febrile illness can trigger episodes. Acute treatment is oral or IV glucose. Tolerance to fasting generally improves with age.

Disorders of Pyruvate Metabolism

Inability to metabolize pyruvate causes lactic acidosis and a variety of CNS abnormalities.

Pyruvate is an important substrate in carbohydrate metabolism.

Pyruvate dehydrogenase deficiency: Pyruvate dehydrogenase is a multi-enzyme complex responsible for the generation of acetyl CoA from pyruvate for the Krebs cycle. Deficiency results in elevation of pyruvate and thus elevation of lactic acid levels. Inheritance is X-linked or autosomal recessive.

Clinical manifestations vary in severity but include lactic acidosis and CNS malformations and other postnatal changes, including cystic lesions of the cerebral cortex, brain stem, and basal ganglia; ataxia; and psychomotor retardation. Diagnosis is confirmed by enzyme analysis of skin fibroblasts, DNA testing, or both. There is no clearly effective treatment, although a low-carbohydrate or ketogenic diet and dietary thiamin supplementation have been beneficial for some patients.

Pyruvate carboxylase deficiency: Pyruvate carboxylase is an enzyme important for gluconeogenesis from pyruvate and alanine generated in muscle. Deficiency may be primary, or secondary to deficiency of holocarboxylase synthetase, biotin, or biotinidase; inheritance for both is autosomal recessive and both result in lactic acidosis.

Primary deficiency incidence is < 1/250,000 births but may be higher in certain American Indian populations. Psychomotor retardation with seizures and spasticity are the major clinical manifestations. Laboratory abnormalities include hyperammonemia; lactic acidosis; ketoacidosis; elevated levels of plasma lysine, citrulline, alanine, and proline; and increased excretion of α-ketoglutarate. Diagnosis is confirmed by enzyme analysis of cultured skin fibroblasts.

Secondary deficiency is clinically similar, with failure to thrive, seizures, and other organic aciduria.

There is no effective treatment, but selected patients with primary deficiency and all those with secondary deficiencies should be given biotin supplementation 5 to 20 mg po once/day.

Other Disorders of Carbohydrate Metabolism

Phosphoenolpyruvate carboxykinase deficiency impairs gluconeogenesis and results in symptoms and signs similar to the hepatic forms of GSD but without hepatic glycogen accumulation.

Other deficiencies include those of glycolytic enzymes or enzymes in the pentose phosphate pathway. Common examples are pyruvate kinase deficiency (see p. 1052) and glucose-6-phosphate dehydrogenase (G6PD) deficiency (see p. 1053), both of which may result in hemolytic anemia. Wernicke-Korsakoff syndrome (see p. 33) is caused by a partial deficiency of transketolase, which is an enzyme for the pentose phosphate pathway that requires thiamin as a cofactor.

FATTY ACID AND GLYCEROL METABOLISM DISORDERS

Fatty acids are the preferred energy source for the heart and an important energy source for skeletal muscle during prolonged exertion. Also, during fasting, the bulk of the body's energy needs must be supplied by fat metabolism. Using fat as an energy source requires catabolizing adipose tissue into free fatty acid and glycerol. The free fatty acid is metabolized in the liver and peripheral tissue via β-oxidation into acetyl CoA; the glycerol is used by the liver for triglyceride synthesis or for gluconeogenesis. Primary disorders of carnitine are discussed in Ch. 2 (see p. 19), but secondary carnitine deficiency is a secondary biochemical feature of many organic acidemias and fatty acid oxidation defects.

Disorders of the β-Oxidation Cycle

There are numerous inherited defects in these processes, which typically manifest during fasting with hypoglycemia and acidosis; some cause cardiomyopathy and muscle weakness.

Acetyl CoA is generated from fatty acids through repeated β-oxidation cycles. Sets of 4 enzymes (an acyl dehydrogenase, a hydratase, a hydroxyacyl dehydrogenase, and a lyase) specific for different chain lengths (very long chain, long chain, medium chain, and short chain) are required to catabolize a long chain fatty acid completely. Inheritance for all fatty acid oxidation defects is autosomal recessive.

Medium-chain acyl dehydrogenase deficiency (MCADD): This is the most common defect in the β-oxidation cycle and has been incorporated into expanded neonatal screening in many states.

Clinical manifestations typically begin after 2 to 3 mo of age and usually follow fasting (as little as 12 h). Patients have vomiting and lethargy that may progress rapidly to seizures, coma, and sometimes death (which can also appear as SIDS). During attacks, patients have hypoglycemia, hyperammonemia, and unexpectedly low urinary and plasma ketones. Metabolic acidosis is often present but may be a late manifestation.

Diagnosis is by presence of abnormal metabolites in blood or urine or by demonstration of enzyme deficiency in cultured fibroblasts; however, DNA testing can confirm most cases.

Treatment of acute attacks is with 10% dextrose IV at 1 to 5 times the maintenance rate (see p. 2291); some clinicians also advocate carnitine supplementation during acute episodes.

Prevention is a low-fat, high-carbohydrate diet and avoidance of prolonged fasting. Cornstarch therapy is often used to provide a margin of safety during overnight fasting.

Long-chain hydroxyacyl-CoA dehydrogenase deficiency (LCHADD): This is the 2nd most common fatty acid oxidation defect. It shares many features of MCADD, but patients may also have cardiomyopathy; rhabdomyolysis, massive creatine kinase elevations, and myoglobinuria with muscle exertion; peripheral neuropathy; and abnormal liver function. Mothers with an LCHADD fetus often have HELLP syndrome (*h*emolysis, *e*levated *l*iver enzymes, *l*ow *p*latelets—see p. 2197) during pregnancy.

Diagnosis is based on the presence of excess long-chain hydroxy acids on organic acid analysis and on the presence of their carnitine conjugates in an acylcarnitine profile or glycine conjugates in an acylglycine profile. It can be confirmed by enzyme study in skin fibroblasts. Treatment during acute exacerbations includes hydration, high-dose glucose, bed rest, urine alkalinization, and carnitine supplementation. Long-term treatment includes a high-carbohydrate diet, medium-chain triglyceride supplementation, and avoidance of fasting and strenuous exercise.

Very long-chain acyl-coA dehydrogenase deficiency (VLCADD): This deficiency is similar to LCHADD but is commonly associated with significant cardiomyopathy.

Glutaric acidemia type II: A defect in the transfer of electrons from the coenzyme of fatty acyl dehydrogenases to the electronic transport chain affects reactions involving fatty acids of all chain lengths (multiple acyl-coA dehydrogenase deficiency); oxidation of several amino acids is also affected. Clinical manifestations thus include fasting hypoglycemia, severe metabolic acidosis, and hyperammonemia. Diagnosis is by increased ethylmalonic, glutaric, 2- and 3-hydroxyglutaric, and other dicarboxylic acids in organic acid analysis, and glutaryl and isovaleryl and other acylcarnitines in tandem mass spectrometry studies. Enzyme deficiencies in skin fibroblasts can be confirmatory. Treatment is similar to that for MCADD, except that riboflavin may be effective in some patients.

DISORDERS OF GLYCEROL METABOLISM

Glycerol is converted to glycerol-3-phosphate by the hepatic enzyme glycerol kinase; deficiency results in episodic vomiting, lethargy, and hypotonia.

Glycerol kinase deficiency is X-linked; many with this deficiency also have a chromosomal deletion that extends beyond the glycerol kinase gene into the contiguous gene region, which contains the genes for congenital adrenal hypoplasia and Duchenne's muscular dystrophy. Thus, patients with glycerol kinase deficiency may have one or more of these disease entities.

Symptoms begin at any age and are usually accompanied by acidosis, hypoglycemia, and elevated blood and urine levels of glycerol. Treatment is with a low-fat diet, but glucocorticoid replacement is critical for those with adrenal hypoplasia.

LYSOSOMAL STORAGE DISORDERS

Lysosomal enzymes break down macromolecules, either those from the cell itself (eg, when cellular structural components are being recycled) or those acquired outside the cell. Inherited defects or deficiencies of lysosomal enzymes (or other lysosomal components) can result in accumulation of undegraded metabolites. Because there are numerous specific deficiencies, storage diseases are usually grouped biochemically by the accumulated metabolite. Subgroups include mucopolysaccharidoses, sphingolipidoses (lipidoses), and mucolipidoses. The most important are the mucopolysaccharidoses and sphingolipidoses. Type 2 glycogenosis is a lysosomal storage disorder, but most glycogenoses are not.

Because reticuloendothelial cells (eg, in the spleen) are rich in lysosomes, such tissues are involved in a number of lysosomal storage disorders, but generally, tissues richest in the substrate are most affected. Thus the brain, which is rich in gangliosides, is particularly affected by gangliosidoses, whereas mucopolysaccharidoses affect many tissues because mucopolysaccharides are present throughout the body.

Mucopolysaccharidoses: Mucopolysaccharidoses (MPS) are inherited deficiencies of enzymes involved in glycosaminoglycan breakdown. Glycosaminoglycans (previously termed mucopolysaccharides) are polysaccharides abundant on cell surfaces and in extracellular matrix and structures. Enzyme deficiencies that prevent glycosaminoglycan breakdown cause accumulation of glycosaminoglycan fragments in lysosomes and cause extensive bone, soft tissue, and CNS changes. Inheritance is usually autosomal recessive (except for MPS type II).

Age at presentation, clinical manifestations, and severity vary by type. Common manifestations include coarse facial features, neurodevelopmental delays and regression, joint contractures, organomegaly, stiff hair, progressive respiratory insufficiency (from airway obstruction and sleep apnea), cardiac valvular disease, skeletal changes, and cervical vertebral subluxation.

Diagnosis is suggested by history, physical examination, bone abnormalities (eg, dysostosis multiplex) found during skeletal survey, and elevated total and fractionated urinary glycosaminoglycans. Diagnosis is confirmed by enzyme analysis of cultured fibroblasts (prenatal) or peripheral WBCs (postnatal). Additional testing is required to monitor organ-specific changes (eg, echocardiogram for valvular disease, audiometry for hearing changes).

Treatment of MPS type I (Hurler's disease) is enzyme replacement with α-L-iduronidase, which effectively halts progression and reverses all non-CNS complications of the disease. Hematopoietic stem cell (HSC) transplantation has also shown promise in early studies but is ineffective for CNS disease. The combination of enzyme replacement and HSC transplantation is under study.

Sphingolipidoses: Sphingolipids are normal lipid components of cell membranes; they accumulate in lysosomes and cause extensive neuronal, bone, and other changes when enzyme deficiencies prevent their breakdown. Although incidence is low, carrier rate of some forms is high. Gaucher's disease is the most common sphingolipidosis. Others include Niemann-Pick, Tay-Sachs, Sandhoff's, Fabry's, Krabbe's, and cholesteryl ester storage diseases and metachromatic leukodystrophy.

Gaucher's Disease

Gaucher's disease is a sphingolipidosis resulting from glucocerebrosidase deficiency, causing deposition of glucocerebroside and related compounds. Symptoms and signs vary by type but are most commonly hepatosplenomegaly or CNS changes. Diagnosis is by enzyme analysis of WBCs.

Glucocerebrosidase normally hydrolyzes glucocerebroside to glucose and ceramide. Genetic defects of the enzyme cause glucocerebroside accumulation in tissue macrophages through phagocytosis, forming Gaucher's cells. Accumulation of Gaucher's cells in the perivascular spaces in the brain causes gliosis in the neuronopathic forms. There are 3 types, which vary in epidemiology, enzyme activity, and manifestations.

Type I (non-neuronopathic) is most common (90% of all patients). Residual enzyme activity is highest. Ashkenazi Jews are at greatest risk; 1:12 is a carrier. Onset ranges from age 2 yr to late adulthood. Symptoms and signs include splenohepatomegaly, bone disease (eg, osteopenia, pain crises, osteolytic lesions with fractures), growth failure, delayed puberty, ecchymoses, and pingueculae. Epistaxis and ecchymoses resulting from thrombocytopenia are common. X-rays show flaring of the ends of the long bones (Erlenmeyer flask deformity) and cortical thinning.

Type II (acute neuronopathic) is rarest, and residual enzyme activity in this type is lowest. Onset occurs during infancy. Symptoms and signs are progressive neurologic deterioration (eg, rigidity, seizures) and death by age 2 yr.

Type III (subacute neuronopathic) falls between types I and II in incidence, enzyme activity, and clinical severity. Onset occurs at any time during childhood. Clinical manifestations vary by subtype and include progressive dementia and ataxia (IIIa), bone and visceral involvement (IIIb), and supranuclear palsies with corneal opacities (IIIc). Patients who survive to adolescence may live for many years.

Diagnosis and Treatment

Diagnosis is by enzyme analysis of WBCs. Carriers are detected, and types are distinguished by mutation analysis. Although biopsy is unnecessary, Gaucher's cells—lipid-laden tissue macrophages in the liver, spleen, lymph nodes, or bone marrow that have a wrinkled tissue-paper appearance—are diagnostic.

Enzyme replacement with placental or recombinant glucocerebrosidase is effective in types I and III; there is no treatment for type II disease. The enzyme is modified for efficient delivery to lysosomes. Patients receiving enzyme replacement require routine Hb and platelet monitoring; routine assessment of spleen and liver volume by CT or MRI; and routine assessment of bone disease by skeletal survey, dual-energy x-ray absorptiometry scanning, or MRI.

Miglustat (100 mg po tid), a glucosylceramide synthase inhibitor, reduces glucocerebroside concentration (the substrate for glucocerebrosidase) and is an alternative for patients unable to receive enzyme replacement.

Splenectomy may be helpful for patients with anemia, leukopenia, or thrombocytopenia or when spleen size causes discomfort. Patients with anemia may also need blood transfusions.

Bone marrow or stem cell transplantation provides a definitive cure but is considered a last resort because of substantial morbidity and mortality.

NIEMANN-PICK DISEASE

Niemann-Pick disease is a sphingolipidosis caused by deficient sphingomyelinase activity, resulting in accumulation of sphingomyelin (ceramide phosphorylcholine) in reticuloendothelial cells.

Niemann-Pick disease inheritance is autosomal recessive and appears most often in Ashkenazi Jews; 2 types, A and B, exist. Type C Niemann-Pick disease is an unrelated enzymatic defect involving abnormal cholesterol storage.

Type A patients have < 5% of normal sphingomyelinase activity. The disease is characterized by hepatosplenomegaly, failure to thrive, and rapidly progressive neurodegeneration. Death occurs by age 2 or 3 yr.

Type B patients have sphingomyelinase activity within 5 to 10% of normal. Type B is more variable clinically than type A. Hepatosplenomegaly and lymphadenopathy may occur. Pancytopenia is common. Most patients with type B have little or no neurologic involvement and survive into adulthood; they may be clinically indistinguishable from those with type I Gaucher's disease. In severe cases of type B, progressive pulmonary infiltrates cause major complications.

Diagnosis and Treatment

Both types are usually suspected by history and examination, most notably hepatosplenomegaly. Diagnosis can be confirmed by sphingomyelinase assay on WBCs and can be made prenatally by using amniocentesis or chorionic villus sampling. Bone marrow or stem cell transplantation is under investigation as a potential treatment option.

TAY-SACHS DISEASE AND SANDHOFF'S DISEASE

Tay-Sachs disease and Sandhoff's disease are sphingolipidoses caused by hexosaminidase deficiency that produces severe neurologic symptoms and early death.

Gangliosides are complex sphingolipids present in the brain. There are 2 major forms, GM_1 and GM_2, both of which may be involved in lysosomal storage disorders; there are 2 main types of GM_2 gangliosidosis, each of which can be caused by numerous different mutations.

Tay-Sachs disease: Deficiency of hexosaminidase A results in accumulation of GM_2 in the brain. Inheritance is autosomal recessive; the most common mutations are carried by 1/27 normal adults of Eastern European (Ashkenazi) Jewish origin, although other mutations cluster in some French-Canadian and Cajun populations.

Children with Tay-Sachs disease start missing developmental milestones after age 6 mo and develop progressive cognitive and motor deterioration resulting in seizures, mental retardation, paralysis, and death by age 5 yr. A cherry-red macular spot is common.

Diagnosis is clinical and can be confirmed by enzyme assay. In the absence of effective treatment, management has focused on screening adults of childbearing age in high-risk populations to identify carriers (by way of enzyme activity and mutation testing) combined with genetic counseling.

Sandhoff's disease: There is a combined hexosaminidase A and B deficiency. Clinical manifestations include progressive cerebral degeneration beginning at 6 mo, accompanied by blindness, cherry-red macular spot, and hyperacusis. It is almost indistinguishable from Tay-Sachs disease in course, diagnosis, and management, except that there is visceral involvement (hepatomegaly and bone change) and no ethnic association.

KRABBE'S DISEASE

Krabbe's disease is a sphingolipidosis that causes retardation, paralysis, blindness, deafness, and pseudobulbar palsy, progressing to death.

Krabbe's disease (galactosylceramide lipidosis, globoid cell leukodystrophy) is caused by an autosomal recessive galactocerebroside β-galactosidase deficiency. It affects infants and is characterized by retardation, paralysis, blindness, deafness, and pseudobulbar palsy, progressing to death. Diagnosis is by detecting enzyme deficiency in WBCs or cultured skin fibroblasts. No effective treatment exists. Prenatal testing is available.

Metachromatic Leukodystrophy

Metachromatic leukodystrophy is a sphingolipidosis caused by arylsulfatase A deficiency, which produces progressive paralysis and dementia resulting in death by age 10 yr.

In metachromatic leukodystrophy (sulfatide lipidosis), arylsulfatase A deficiency causes metachromatic lipids to accumulate in the white matter of the CNS, peripheral nerves, kidney, spleen, and other visceral organs; accumulation in the nervous system causes central and peripheral demyelination. Numerous mutations exist; patients vary in age at onset and speed of progression.

The infantile form is characterized by progressive paralysis and dementia usually beginning before age 4 yr and resulting in death about 5 yr after onset of symptoms. The juvenile form manifests between 4 yr and 16 yr of age with gait disturbance, intellectual impairment, and findings of peripheral neuropathy. Contrary to the infantile form, deep tendon reflexes are usually brisk. There is also a milder adult form. Diagnosis is suggested clinically and by findings of decreased nerve conduction velocity; it is confirmed by detecting enzyme deficiency in WBCs or cultured skin fibroblasts. There is no effective treatment.

Fabry's Disease

Fabry's disease is a sphingolipidosis caused by deficiency of α-galactosidase A, which produces angiokeratomas, acroparesthesias, corneal opacities, recurrent febrile episodes, and renal or heart failure.

Fabry's disease (angiokeratoma corporis diffusum) is an X-linked deficiency of the lysosomal enzyme α-galactosidase A, which is needed for normal trihexosylceramide catabolism. Glycolipid (globotriaosylceramide) accumulates in many tissues (eg, vascular endothelium, lymph vessels, heart, kidney).

Diagnosis in males is clinical, based on appearance of typical skin lesions (angiokeratomas) over the lower trunk and by characteristic features of peripheral neuropathy (causing recurrent burning pain in the extremities), corneal opacities, and recurrent febrile episodes. Death results from renal failure or cardiac or cerebral complications of hypertension or other vascular disease. Heterozygous females are usually asymptomatic but may have an attenuated form of disease often characterized by corneal opacities.

Diagnosis is by assay of galactosidase activity—prenatally in amniocytes or chorionic villi and postnatally in serum or WBCs. Treatment is enzyme replacement with recombinant α-galactosidase A (agalsidase beta) combined with supportive measures for fever and pain. Kidney transplantation is effective for treating renal failure.

Cholesteryl Ester Storage Disease and Wolman's Disease

Cholesteryl ester storage disease and Wolman's disease are sphingolipidoses caused by lysosomal acid lipase deficiency resulting in hyperlipidemia and hepatomegaly.

These are rare, autosomal recessive disorders that result in accumulation of cholesteryl esters and triglycerides, mainly in lysosomes of histiocytes, resulting in foam cells in the liver, spleen, lymph nodes, and other tissues. Serum LDL is usually elevated.

Wolman's disease is the more severe form, manifesting in the 1st weeks of life with poor feeding, vomiting, and abdominal distention secondary to hepatosplenomegaly; infants usually die within 6 mo.

Cholesteryl ester storage disease is less severe and may not manifest until later in life, even adulthood, at which time hepatomegaly may be detected; premature atherosclerosis, often severe, may develop.

Diagnosis is based on clinical features and demonstration of acid lipase deficiency in liver biopsy specimens or cultured skin fibroblasts, lymphocytes, or other tissues. Prenatal diagnosis is based on the absence of acid lipase activity in cultured chorionic villi.

There is no proven treatment, but statins reduce plasma LDL levels, and cholestyramine combined with a low-cholesterol diet has reportedly improved other signs.

MITOCHONDRIAL OXIDATIVE PHOSPHORYLATION DISORDERS

Impairment of oxidative phosphorylation often, but not always, causes lactic acidosis, particularly affecting the CNS, retina, and muscle.

Cellular respiration (oxidative phosphorylation) occurs in the mitochondria, where a series of enzymes catalyze the transfer of electrons to molecular oxygen and the generation of energy-storing ATP. Mitochondrial or nuclear genetic defects involving enzymes used in this process impair cellular respiration, decreasing the ATP:ADP ratio. Tissues with a high energy demand (eg, brain, nerves, retina, skeletal and cardiac muscle) are particularly vulnerable. The most common clinical manifestations are seizures, hypotonia, ophthalmoplegia, stroke-like episodes, muscle weakness, and cardiomyopathy.

Biochemically, there is profound lactic acidosis because the NADH:NAD ratio increases, shifting the equilibrium of the lactate dehydrogenase reaction toward lactate. The increase in the lactate:pyruvate ratio distinguishes oxidative phosphorylation defects from other genetic causes of lactic acidosis such as pyruvate carboxylase or pyruvate dehydrogenase deficiency, in which the lactate:pyruvate ratio remains normal. A large number of oxidative phosphorylation defects have been described; only the most common ones are outlined here, along with their distinguishing features.

Mitochondrial mutations and variants have also been implicated in a number of diseases of aging (eg, Parkinson's disease, Alzheimer's disease, diabetes, deafness, cancer).

Leber's hereditary optic neuropathy (LHON): This is a disease with acute or subacute bilateral central vision loss caused by retinal degeneration. Onset usually occurs in the patient's 20s or 30s but can occur from childhood to adulthood. Male:female ratio is 4:1. Many mutations have been defined, but 3 common ones account for 90% of those in European patients. LHON pedigrees usually show a pattern of maternal inheritance typical of mitochondrial disorders.

Mitochondrial encephalomyopathy, lactic acidosis, and stroke-like episodes (MELAS): Mutations in the mitochondrial *tRNA^leu^* gene cause this progressive neurodegenerative disease characterized by repeated episodes of "chemical strokes," myopathy, and lactic acidosis. In many cases, cells contain both wild-type and mutant mitochondrial DNA (heteroplasmy); thus, expression is variable.

Myoclonic epilepsy with ragged-red fibers (MERRF): This is a progressive disease characterized by uncontrolled muscle contractions (myoclonic seizures), dementia, ataxia, and myopathy, which shows ragged-red fibers (indicating mitochondrial proliferation) with specialized stains when biopsied. Mutations are in the mitochondrial *tRNA^lys^* gene. Heteroplasmy is common; thus, expression is variable.

Kearns-Sayre syndrome and chronic progressive external ophthalmoplegia (CPEO): These disorders are characterized by ophthalmoplegia, ptosis, atypical retinitis pigmentosa, ragged-red fiber myopathy, ataxia, deafness, and cardiomyopathy typically occurring before age 20 yr. Most mutations involve contiguous deletion/duplication of part of the mitochondrial tRNA and other protein-coding genes.

Neurogenic muscle atrophy and retinitis pigmentosa (NARP) and Leigh disease: Pigmentary retinopathy in the presence of neuromuscular degeneration and Leigh disease (subacute necrotizing encephalopathy characterized by ataxias and basal ganglia degeneration) is a genetically heterogeneous syndrome. Mutations can be seen in the *ATP6* gene of the mitochondrial genomes.

PEROXISOMAL DISORDERS

Peroxisomes are intracellular organelles that contain enzymes for β-oxidation. These enzymes overlap in function with those in mitochondria, with the exception that mitochondria lack enzymes to metabolize very long-chain fatty acids (VLCFA), those 20 to 26 carbons in length. Therefore, peroxisomal disorders generally manifest with elevated VLCFA levels (except rhizomelic chondrodysplasia). Although VLCFA levels may help screen for these disorders, other assays are also required (plasma levels of phytanic, pristanic, and pipecolic acids; RBC plasmalogen levels).

There are 2 types of peroxisomal disorders: those with defective peroxisome formation and those with defects in single peroxisomal enzymes. X-linked adrenoleukodystrophy is the most common peroxisomal disorder (incidence 1/17,000 births); all others are autosomal recessive, with a combined incidence of about 1/50,000 births.

Zellweger syndrome (ZS), neonatal adrenoleukodystrophy, and infantile Refsum's disease (IRD): These are 3 expressions of a disease continuum, from most (ZS) to least (IRD) severe. The responsible genetic defect occurs in 1 of at least 11 genes involved in peroxisomal formation or protein import (the *PEX* gene family).

Manifestations include facial dysmorphism, CNS malformations, demyelination, neonatal seizures, hypotonia, hepatomegaly, cystic kidneys, short limbs with stippled epiphyses (chondrodysplasia punctata), cataracts, retinopathy, hearing deficit, psychomotor delay, and peripheral neuropathy. Diagnosis is by demonstrating elevated blood levels of VLCFA, phytanic acid, bile acid intermediates, and pipecolic acid. Experimental treatment with docosahexaenoic acid (DHA—levels of which are reduced in patients with disorders of peroxisome formation) has shown some promise.

Rhizomelic chondrodysplasia punctata: This defect of peroxisomal biogenesis is caused by *PEX7* gene mutations and characterized by skeletal changes that include midface hypoplasia, strikingly short proximal limbs, frontal bossing, small nares, cataracts, ichthyosis, and profound psychomotor retardation. Vertebral clefts are also common. Diagnosis is by x-ray findings, serum elevation of phytanic acid, and low RBC plasmalogen levels; VLCFA levels are normal. There is no effective treatment.

X-linked adrenoleukodystrophy: This disorder is caused by deficiency of the peroxisomal membrane transporter ALDP, coded for by the gene *ABCD1*.

The cerebral form affects 40% of patients. Onset occurs between age 4 and 8 yr, and symptoms of attention deficit progress over time to severe behavioral problems; dementia; and vision, hearing, and motor deficits, causing total disability and death 2 to 3 yr after diagnosis. Milder adolescent and adult forms have also been described.

About 45% of patients have a milder form called adrenomyeloneuropathy (AMN); onset occurs in the 20s or 30s, with progressive paraparesis, and sphincter and sexual disturbance. About ⅓ of these patients also develop cerebral symptoms.

Patients with any form may also develop adrenal insufficiency; about 15% have isolated Addison's disease without neurologic involvement.

Diagnosis is confirmed by isolated elevation of VLCFA. Bone marrow or stem cell transplantation may help stabilize symptoms in selected cases. Adrenal steroid replacement is needed for patients with adrenal insufficiency. Dietary supplement with a 4:1 mixture of glyceryl trioleate and glyceryl trierucate (Lorenzo's oil) can normalize plasma VLCFA levels and may be beneficial in some cases but is under study.

Classic Refsum's disease: Genetic deficiency of a single peroxisomal enzyme, phytanoyl-CoA hydroxylase, which catalyzes metabolism of phytanic acid (a common dietary plant component), causes phytanic acid accumulation.

Clinical manifestations include progressive peripheral neuropathy, impaired vision from retinitis pigmentosa, hearing deficit, anosmia, cardiomyopathy and conduction defects, and ichthyosis. Onset is usually in the 20s. Diagnosis is confirmed by elevation of serum phytanic acid and decreased levels of pristanic acid (phytanic acid elevation is accompanied by pristanic acid elevation in several other peroxisomal disorders).

Treatment is dietary restriction of phytanic acid (< 10 mg/day), which can be effective in preventing or delaying symptoms when started before symptom onset.

PURINE AND PYRIMIDINE METABOLISM DISORDERS

Purines are key components of cellular energy systems (eg, ATP, NAD), signaling (eg, GTP, cAMP, cGMP), and, along with pyrimidines, RNA and DNA production. Purines and pyrimidines may be synthesized de novo or recycled by a salvage pathway from normal catabolism. The end product of complete catabolism of purines is uric acid; catabolism of pyrimidines produces citric acid cycle intermediates.

Disorders of Purine Salvage

Lesch-Nyhan syndrome: This is a rare, X-linked, recessive disorder caused by deficiency of hypoxanthine-guanine phosphoribosyl transferase (HPRT); degree of deficiency (and hence manifestations) vary with the specific mutation. HPRT deficiency results in failure of the salvage pathway for hypoxanthine and guanine. These purines are instead degraded to uric acid. Additionally, a decrease in inositol monophosphate and guanosyl monophosphate leads to an increase in conversion of 5-phosphoribosyl-1-pyrophosphate (PRPP) to 5-phosphoribosylamine, which further exacerbates uric acid overproduction. Hyperuricemia predisposes to gout and its complications. Patients also have a number of cognitive and behavioral dysfunctions, etiology of which is unclear; they do not appear related to uric acid.

The disease usually manifests between 3 mo and 12 mo of age with the appearance of orange sandy precipitate (xanthine) in the urine; it progresses to CNS involvement with mental retardation, spastic cerebral palsy, involuntary movements, and self-mutilating behavior (particularly biting). Later, chronic hyperuricemia causes symptoms of gout (eg, urolithiasis, nephropathy, gouty arthritis, tophi).

Diagnosis is suggested by the combination of dystonia, retardation, and self-mutilation. Serum uric acid levels are usually elevated, but confirmation by HPRT enzyme assay is usually done.

CNS dysfunction has no known treatment; management is supportive. Self-mutilation may require physical restraint, dental extraction, and sometimes drug therapy; a variety of agents has been used. Hyperuricemia is treated with a low-purine diet (eg, avoiding organ meats, beans, sardines) and allopurinol, a xanthine oxidase inhibitor (the last enzyme in the purine catabolic pathway). Allopurinol prevents conversion of accumulated hypoxanthine to uric acid; because hypoxanthine is highly soluble, it is excreted.

Adenine phosphoribosyltransferase deficiency: This is a rare autosomal recessive disorder that results in the inability to salvage adenine for purine synthesis. Accumulated adenine is oxidized to 2,8-dihyroxyadenine, which precipitates in the urinary tract, causing problems similar to those of uric acid nephropathy (eg, renal colic, frequent infections, and, if diagnosed late, renal failure). Onset can occur at any age.

Diagnosis is by demonstrating elevated levels of 2,8-dihyroxyadenine, 8-hyroxyadenine, and adenine in urine and confirmed by enzyme assay; serum uric acid is normal.

Treatment is with dietary purine restriction, high fluid intake, and avoidance of urine alkalinization. Allopurinol can prevent oxidation of adenine; renal transplantation may be needed for end-stage renal disease.

Disorders of Purine Nucleotide Synthesis

Phosphoribosylpyrophosphate synthetase superactivity: This is an X-linked, recessive disorder that causes purine overproduction. Excess purine is degraded, resulting in hyperuricemia and gout, and neurologic and developmental abnormalities. Diagnosis is by enzyme studies on RBCs and cultured skin fibroblasts. Treatment is with allopurinol and a low-purine diet.

Adenylosuccinase deficiency: This is an autosomal recessive disorder causing profound mental retardation, autistic behavior, and seizures. Diagnosis is by identifying elevated levels of succinylaminoimidazole carboxamide riboside and succinyladenosine in CSF and urine. There is no effective treatment.

Disorders of Purine Catabolism

Myoadenylate deaminase deficiency (or muscle adenosine monophosphate deaminase deficiency): This enzyme converts AMP to inosine and ammonia. Deficiency may be asymptomatic or it may cause exercise-induced myalgias or cramping; expression seems to be variable because, despite the high frequency of the mutant allele (10 to 14%), the frequency of the muscle phenotype is quite low in patients homozygous for the mutant allele. When symptomatic patients exercise, they do not accumulate ammonia or inosine monophosphate as do normal people; this is how the disorder is diagnosed. Treatment is exercise modulation as appropriate.

Adenosine deaminase deficiency: Adenosine deaminase converts adenosine and deoxyadenosine to inosine and deoxyinosine, which are further broken down and excreted. Enzyme deficiency (from 1 of > 60 known mutations) results in accumulation of adenosine, which is converted to its ribonucleotide and deoxyribonucleotide (dATP) forms by cellular kinases. The dATP increase results in inhibition of ribonucleotide reductase and underproduction of other deoxyribonucleotides. DNA replication is compromised as a result. Immune cells are especially sensitive to this defect; adenosine deaminase deficiency causes one form of severe combined immunodeficiency (see p. 1345). Diagnosis is by low RBC and WBC enzyme activity. Treatment is by bone marrow or stem cell transplantation and enzyme replacement therapy. Somatic cell gene therapy is being evaluated as well.

Purine nucleoside phosphorylase deficiency: This rare, autosomal recessive deficiency is characterized by immunodeficiency with severe T-cell dysfunction and often neurologic symptoms. Manifestations are lymphopenia, thymic deficiency, recurrent infections, and hypouricemia. Many have developmental delay, ataxia, or spasticity. Diagnosis is by low enzyme activity in RBCs. Treatment is with bone marrow or stem cell transplantation.

Xanthine oxidase deficiency: This enzyme catalyzes uric acid production from xanthine and hypoxanthine. Deficiency causes buildup of xanthine, which may precipitate in the urine, causing symptomatic stones with hematuria, urinary colic, and UTIs. Diagnosis is by low plasma uric acid and high urine and plasma hypoxanthine and xanthine. Enzyme determination requires liver or intestinal mucosal biopsy and is rarely indicated. Treatment is high fluid intake to minimize likelihood of stone formation and allopurinol in some patients.

Disorders of Pyrimidine Metabolism

Uridine monophosphate synthase deficiency (hereditary orotic aciduria): This enzyme catalyzes orotate phosphoribosyltransferase and orotidine-5′-monophosphate decarboxylase reactions. With deficiency, orotic acid accumulates, causing clinical manifestations of megaloblastic anemia, orotic crystalluria and nephropathy, cardiac malformations, strabismus, and recurrent infections.

Diagnosis is by enzyme assay in a variety of tissues. Treatment is with oral uridine supplementation.

297 HEREDITARY PERIODIC FEVER SYNDROMES

Hereditary periodic fever syndromes are inherited disorders characterized by recurrent fever and other symptoms in the absence of secondary causes. Most patients develop symptoms during childhood; < 10% develop symptoms after age 18. Disorders best characterized are familial Mediterranean fever, hyper-IgD syndrome, and tumor necrosis factor (TNF) receptor–associated periodic syndrome; others include Muckle-Wells syndrome (periodic fever, urticaria, arthralgia, deafness, and risk of late-onset renal amyloidosis); familial cold autoinflammatory syndrome (fever, rash, arthralgia, and conjunctivitis triggered by cold ambient temperatures); and PFAPA (periodic fever, aphthous stomatitis, pharyngitis, and cervical adenitis).

FAMILIAL MEDITERRANEAN FEVER

Familial Mediterranean fever is an inherited disorder characterized by recurrent bouts of fever and peritonitis, sometimes with pleuritis, skin lesions, arthritis, and, very rarely, pericarditis. Renal amyloidosis may develop, which may lead to renal failure. Descendants of inhabitants of the Mediterranean basin are most affected. Diagnosis is largely clinical, although genetic testing is available. Treatment with prophylactic colchicine prevents acute attacks as well as renal amyloidosis in most patients. Prognosis is excellent with treatment.

Familial Mediterranean fever (FMF) is a disease of people with genetic origins in the Mediterranean basin, predominantly Sephardic Jews, North African Arabs, Armenians, Turks, Greeks, and Italians. However, cases have occurred in enough other groups (eg, Ashkenazi Jews, Cubans, Belgians) to caution against excluding the diagnosis solely on the basis of ancestry. About 50% of patients have a family history of the disorder, usually involving siblings.

Etiology

FMF is caused by mutations in the *MEFV* gene on the short arm of chromosome 16 and is inherited in an autosomal-recessive manner. The *MEFV* gene normally codes a protein (called pyrin or marenostrin) expressed in circulating neutrophils. Its presumed action is to blunt the inflammatory response, possibly by inhibiting neutrophil activation and chemotaxis. Gene mutations cause defective pyrin molecules; it is hypothesized that minor, unknown triggers to inflammation that are normally checked by intact pyrin cannot be suppressed by the altered protein. The clinical consequence is spontaneous bouts of neutrophil-predominant inflammation in the abdominal cavity as well as at other sites.

Symptoms and Signs

Onset is usually between the ages of 5 and 15 yr but may be much later or earlier, even during infancy. Attacks have no regular pattern of recurrence and vary in the same patient. They usually last 24 to 72 h, but some last ≥ 1 wk. Frequency ranges from 2 attacks/wk to 1 attack/yr (most commonly once every 2 to 6 wk). Severity and frequency tend to decrease during pregnancy and with amyloidosis. Spontaneous remissions may last years.

Fever as high as 40° C, usually accompanied by peritonitis, is the major manifestation. Abdominal pain (usually starting in one quadrant and spreading to the whole abdomen) occurs in about 95% of patients and can vary in severity with each attack. Decreased bowel sounds, distention, guarding, and rebound tenderness are likely to occur at the peak of an attack and cannot be differentiated from a perforated viscus on physical examination. Consequently, many patients undergo urgent laparotomy before the correct diagnosis is made. With diaphragmatic involvement, splinting of the chest and pain in one or both shoulders may occur.

Other manifestations include acute pleurisy (in 30%); arthritis (in 25%), usually involving the knee, ankle, and hip; an erysipelas-like rash of the lower leg; and scrotal swelling and pain caused by inflammation of the tunica vaginalis of the testis. Pericarditis occurs very rarely. However, the pleural, synovial, and skin manifestations of FMF vary in frequency among different populations and are less frequently encountered in the US than elsewhere.

The most significant long-term complication of FMF is chronic renal failure caused by deposition of amyloid protein in the kidneys. Amyloid deposition may also occur in the GI tract, liver, spleen, heart, testes, and thyroid.

Diagnosis

Diagnosis is mainly clinical, but genetic testing is now available and is particularly useful in the evaluation of atypical cases. Nonspecific findings include elevated WBCs with neutrophil predominance, ESR, C-reactive protein, and fibrinogen. Urinary excretion of > 0.5 g protein/24 h suggests renal amyloidosis. Differential diagnosis includes acute intermittent porphyria, hereditary angioedema with abdominal attacks, relapsing pancreatitis, and other hereditary relapsing fevers.

Prognosis and Treatment

Despite the severity of symptoms during acute attacks, most patients recover swiftly and remain free of illness until their next attack. Widespread use of prophylactic colchicine has led to a dramatic reduction in the incidence of amyloidosis and subsequent renal failure.

Prophylactic colchicine 0.6 mg po bid (some patients require qid dosing and others a single daily dose) provides complete remission or distinct improvement in about 85% of patients. For patients with infrequent attacks that involve a prodromal phase, colchicine can be reserved until initial symptoms occur and then begun at 0.6 mg po q 1 h for 4 h, then q 2 h for 4 h, then q 12 h for 48 h. Initiation of colchicine at the peak of an attack, even if delivered IV, is unlikely to be beneficial. Children often require adult dosages to achieve effective prophylaxis. Colchicine does not add to the increased risk of infertility and miscarriage among affected women, nor does it increase the number of teratogenic events when taken during pregnancy.

Lack of response to colchicine is often caused by poor adherence to the drug regimen, but a correlation has also been noted between poor response and diminished colchicine concentration in circulating monocytes. Weekly IV colchicine may reduce attack frequency and severity in nonresponders. Untested alternatives in nonresponders include interferon-α 3 to 10 million units sc, prazosin 3 mg po bid, and thalidomide.

Opioids are sometimes needed for pain relief but should be administered prudently to avoid addiction.

HYPER-IgD SYNDROME

Hyper-IgD syndrome is a rare hereditary disorder in which recurring attacks of chills and fever begin during the 1st yr of life. Episodes usually last 4 to 6 days and may be triggered by physiologic stress, such as vaccination or minor trauma. There is no known treatment.

Hyper-IgD syndrome clusters in children of Dutch, French, and other Northern European ancestry and is caused by mutations in the gene coding mevalonate kinase, an enzyme important for cholesterol synthesis. The mechanism by which this abnormality produces the clinical syndrome is unknown.

Symptoms besides chills include abdominal pain, vomiting or diarrhea, headache, and arthralgias. Signs besides fever include cervical lymphadenopathy, hepatosplenomegaly, arthritis, skin lesions (maculopapular rash, petechiae, or purpura), and orogenital aphthous ulcers.

Diagnosis is by history, examination, and serum IgD level > 100 IU/mL. Nonspecific abnormalities include leukocytosis and elevated acute-phase reactants during fever; specific but insensitive findings include elevated urinary neopterin and mevalonic acid.

There are no known treatments to prevent attacks. Patients can expect to have recurrent bouts of fever throughout their lives, although episodes tend to diminish in frequency after adolescence.

TNF RECEPTOR–ASSOCIATED PERIODIC SYNDROME

(Familial Hibernian Fever)

Tumor necrosis factor (TNF) receptor–associated periodic syndrome is a hereditary disorder causing recurrent fever and painful, migratory myalgias with tender overlying erythema. Levels of type 1 TNF receptors are low. Treatment is with corticosteroids and etanercept.

TNF receptor–associated periodic syndrome was described in a family of Irish and Scottish pedigree but has been reported to occur in many different ethnic groups. The cause is mutations in the gene coding the TNF receptor. Defective shedding of this receptor is presumed to cause unchecked TNF signaling with resultant inflammation.

Attacks of this rare disorder usually begin before age 20. They may last from 1 to 2 days to > 1 wk. The most prominent features of an attack are muscle pain and swelling in the extremities. Other symptoms may include headache, abdominal pain, diarrhea or constipation, nausea, painful conjunctivitis, joint pains, rash, and testicular pain. Males are prone to develop inguinal hernias. Amyloidosis involving the kidneys has been reported in a minority of families.

Diagnosis is by history, examination, and low levels of type 1 TNF receptor (< 1 ng/mL) when measured between attacks. Nonspecific findings include neutrophilia, elevated acute-phase reactants, and polyclonal gammopathy during attacks. Patients should be screened regularly for proteinuria.

The prognosis is good with treatment but is more guarded in cases of renal amyloidosis. Attacks can be effectively treated with prednisone in doses of at least 20 mg po once/day. Increasing dosage may be needed over time. Early therapeutic experience with etanercept, which binds and inactivates TNF, has been promising. Recommended dosage is 0.4 mg/kg sc for children and 25 mg sc for adults, twice/wk.

298 BEHAVIORAL CONCERNS AND PROBLEMS

Many behaviors exhibited by children or adolescents concern parents or other adults. Behaviors or behavioral patterns become clinically significant if they are frequent or persistent and maladaptive (eg, interfere with emotional maturation or social and cognitive functioning). Severe behavioral problems may be classified as mental disorders (eg, oppositional defiant disorder or conduct disorder—see p. 2505). Prevalence rates vary according to how behavioral problems are defined and measured.

Evaluation

Diagnosis consists of a multistep behavioral assessment. Concerns with infants and young children generally involve bodily function (eg, eating, eliminating, sleeping), whereas in older children and adolescents interpersonal behavioral concerns (eg, activity level, disobedience, aggression) predominate.

Problem identification: A behavioral problem may manifest alarmingly and abruptly as a single incident (eg, setting a fire, fighting at school). More often, problems manifest gradually and identification involves gathering information over time. Behavior is best assessed in the context of the child's physical and mental development, general health, temperament (eg, difficult, easygoing), and relationships with parents and caregivers.

Direct observation of parent-child interaction during an office visit provides valuable clues, including parental response to behaviors. These observations are supplemented, whenever possible, by information from others, including relatives, teachers, and school nurses.

Interviewing parents or caregivers provides a chronology of the child's activities during a typical day. Parents are asked to provide examples of events that precede and follow the specific behavior. Parents also are asked for their interpretation of typical age-related behaviors, expectations for the child, level of parenting interest, support (eg, social, emotional, financial) for fulfilling their parenting role, and relationship with the rest of their family.

Problem interpretation: Some "problems" represent unrealistic parental expectations (eg, that a 2-yr-old will pick up toys without help). Parents misinterpret other normal, age-related behaviors, such as oppositional behavior (eg, refusal to follow an adult's request or rule) in a 2-yr-old, as problematic.

The child's history may include factors thought to increase the likelihood of developing behavioral problems, such as exposure to toxins, complications during pregnancy, or occurrence of a serious illness in the family. Poor quality of parent-infant interactions (eg, disinterested parents) contributes to subsequent problems. Well-meaning parental reactions to a problem may worsen it (eg, overprotecting a fearful, clinging child or giving in to a manipulative child).

In young children, some problems represent a circular behavioral pattern in which negative parental reaction to a child's behavior causes an adverse response from the child, which in turn leads to continued negative parental reaction. In circular behavioral patterns, children often respond to stress and emotional discomfort with stubbornness, back talk, aggressiveness, and temper outbursts rather than with crying. In the most common circular behavioral pattern, a parent reacts to an aggressive and resistant child by scolding, yelling, and spanking; the child then escalates the behaviors that led to the parent's initial response, and the parent reacts more forcefully.

In older children and adolescents, behavioral problems may arise as independence is sought from parental rules and supervision. Such problems must be distinguished from occasional errors in judgment.

Treatment

Once a behavioral problem has been identified and its etiology investigated, early intervention is desirable because behaviors are more difficult to change the longer they exist.

The clinician reassures parents that the child is physically well (eg, that the child's misbehavior is not a manifestation of physical illness). By identifying with parental frustrations and pointing out the prevalence of behavioral problems, the clinician can often allay parental guilt and facilitate exploration of possible sources and treatment of problems. For simple problems, parental education, reassurance, and a few specific suggestions often are sufficient. Parents can be reminded of the importance of spending at least 15 to 20 min/day in a pleasurable activity with the child. Parents also can be encouraged to regularly spend time away from the child. For some problems, however, parents benefit from additional strategies for disciplining children and modifying behavior.

The clinician can encourage parents to limit the child's dependency-seeking and manipulative behavior so that mutual respect is reestablished. Desired and undesired behavior should be clearly defined. Consistent rules and limits should be established, and parents need to track compliance on an ongoing basis and provide appropriate rewards for success and consequences for inappropriate behavior. Positive reinforcement for appropriate behavior is a powerful tool with no adverse effects. Parents should try to minimize anger when enforcing rules and increase positive contact with the child (eg, "catch the child being good").

TABLE 298–1. TIME-OUT PROCEDURE

This disciplinary technique is best used when children are aware that their actions are incorrect or unacceptable; typically this is not the case until age 2 yr. Care should be taken when this technique is used in group settings like daycare, because it can result in harmful humiliation.

The technique can be applied when a child misbehaves in a way that is known to result in a time-out.

- The misbehavior is explained to the child, who is told to sit in the time-out chair or is led there if necessary.
- The child should sit in the chair 1 min for each year of age (maximum, 5 min).
- A child who gets up from the chair before the allotted time is returned to the chair, and the time-out is restarted. A child who gets up repeatedly may need to be held in the chair (not in one's lap). Talking and eye contact are avoided.
- If the child stays in the chair but does not quiet down before the allotted time, the time-out is restarted.
- When it is time for the child to get up, the caregiver asks the reason for the time-out without anger and nagging. A child who does not recall the correct reason is briefly reminded.

Soon after the time-out, the caregiver should praise the child's good behavior, which may be easier to achieve if the child is started in a new activity far from the scene of the inappropriate behavior.

Ineffective discipline may result in inappropriate behavior. Scolding or physical punishment may briefly control a child's behavior but eventually may decrease the child's sense of security and self-esteem. Threats to leave or send the child away are damaging.

A time-out procedure (see TABLE 298–1), in which the child must sit alone in a dull place (a corner or room other than the child's bedroom, with no television or toys, which is not dark or scary) for a brief period, is a good approach to altering unacceptable behavior. Time-outs are learning processes for the child and are best used for one inappropriate behavior or a few at one time.

The circular behavioral pattern may be interrupted if parents ignore behavior that does not disturb others (eg, refusal to eat) and use distraction or temporary isolation to limit behavior that cannot be ignored (public tantrums).

A behavioral problem that does not change in 3 to 4 mo should be reevaluated; mental health consultation may be indicated.

BREATH-HOLDING SPELLS

A breath-holding spell is an episode in which the child stops breathing involuntarily and loses consciousness for a short period immediately after a frightening or emotionally upsetting event or after a painful experience.

Breath-holding spells occur in 5% of otherwise healthy children. They usually begin at age 2. They disappear by age 4 in 50% of children and by age 8 in about 83% of children. The remainder may continue to have spells into adulthood. Breath-holding spells are either cyanotic or pallid. The cyanotic form, the most common, often occurs as part of a temper tantrum or in response to a scolding or other upsetting event. The pallid form typically follows a painful experience, such as falling and banging the head, but can follow frightening or startling events. Both forms are involuntary and readily distinguished from uncommon brief periods of voluntary breath-holding by stubborn children, who invariably resume normal breathing after getting what they want or upon becoming uncomfortable when they fail to get what they want.

During a cyanotic episode, the child holds his breath (without necessarily being aware he is doing so) until he loses consciousness. Typically, the child cries out, exhales, and stops breathing. Shortly afterward, the child begins to turn blue and unconsciousness ensues. A brief seizure may occur. After a few seconds, breathing resumes and normal skin color and consciousness return. It may be possible to interrupt a spell by placing a cold rag on the child's face at onset. Despite the episode's frightening nature, parents must try to avoid reinforcing the initiating behavior. As the child recovers, parents should continue to enforce household rules; the child cannot be given free reign of the house just because the spell occurred with a temper tantrum. Distracting the child and avoiding situations that lead to tantrums are good strategies.

During a pallid episode, vagal stimulation severely slows the heart rate. The child stops breathing, rapidly loses consciousness, and becomes pale and limp. If the spell lasts more than a few seconds, muscle tone increases, and a seizure and incontinence may occur. After the spell, the heart speeds up again, breathing restarts, and consciousness returns without any treatment. Because this form is rare, further diagnostic evaluation and treatment may be needed if the spells occur often.

EATING PROBLEMS

Eating problems range from age-appropriate variability in appetite to serious or even life-threatening eating disorders (see p. 1701) such as anorexia nervosa, bulimia nervosa, and binge-eating. Parents of 2- to 8-yr-olds are often concerned that a child is not eating enough or eating too much, eating the wrong foods, refusing to eat certain foods, or engaging in inappropriate mealtime behavior (eg, sneaking food to a pet, throwing or intentionally dropping food).

Assessment includes problem frequency, duration, and intensity. Height and weight are measured. Children should be assessed more thoroughly for serious eating disorders if they voice persistent concerns about their appearance or weight, if their weight decreases, or if their weight begins to increase at a noticeably faster rate than their previous growth rate. However, most eating problems do not persist long enough to interfere with growth and development. If the child appears well and growth is within an acceptable range, parents should be reassured and encouraged to minimize conflict and coercion related to eating. Prolonged and excessive parental concern may in fact contribute to subsequent eating disorders. Attempts to force-feed are unlikely to increase intake; the child may hold food in his mouth or vomit. Parents should offer meals while sitting at a table with the family, without distractions such as television or pets, and show little emotion when putting the food in front of the child. Food should be removed in 20 to 30 min without comment about what is or is not eaten. The child should participate in cleaning up any food that is thrown or intentionally dropped on the floor. These techniques, along with restricting between-meal eating to one morning and one afternoon snack, usually restore the relationship among appetite, the amount eaten, and the child's nutritional needs.

TEMPER TANTRUMS

A temper tantrum is a violent emotional outburst, usually in response to frustration.

Temper tantrums usually appear toward the end of the 1st yr, are most common at age 2 ("terrible twos") to 4, and are infrequent after age 5. If tantrums are frequent after age 5, they may persist throughout childhood.

Causes include frustration, tiredness, and hunger. Children may also have temper tantrums to seek attention, obtain something, or avoid doing something. Parents often blame themselves for temper tantrums (because of imagined poor parenting) when the actual cause is often a combination of the child's personality, immediate circumstances, and developmentally normal behavior. An underlying mental, physical, or social problem rarely may be the cause but is likely only if tantrums last > 15 min or occur multiple times each day.

Temper tantrums may involve shouting, screaming, crying, thrashing about, rolling on the floor, stomping, and throwing things. The child may become red in the face and hit or kick. Some children may voluntarily hold their breath for a few seconds and then resume normal breathing (unlike breath-holding spells—see p. 2479).

To stop a tantrum, parents should ask the child simply and firmly to do so. If the child does not stop and if the behavior is sufficiently disruptive, the child may have to be removed physically from the situation. At this point, a time-out can be very effective (see TABLE 298–1).

TOILETING PROBLEMS

Most children are trained for bowel control at age 2 to 3 yr and for urinary control at age 3 to 4 yr (see Toilet Training on p. 2243). By age 5 yr, the average child can go to the toilet alone.

Nocturnal Enuresis

Nocturnal enuresis is urinary incontinence during sleep.

Primary nocturnal enuresis (failure to have developed bedtime bladder control) affects 30% of children at age 4, 10% at age 6, 3% at age 12, and 1% at age 18. It is more common in boys, seems to be familial, and is sometimes associated with sleep disorders (see p. 1834). Enuresis usually represents only a delay in maturation that resolves with time.

Diagnosis

Only 1 to 2% of patients have an organic etiology (see also Incontinence in Children on p. 1960), usually a UTI. Infection can be excluded by urinalysis and urine culture. Rare causes—congenital anomalies, sacral nerve disorders, diabetes mellitus or insipidus, a pelvic mass—can be excluded by a thorough history and physical examination. Nocturnal enuresis accompanied by daytime urinary symptoms (eg, frequency, urgency, or incontinence) may indicate the need for renal ultrasonography, IVU, cystourethrography, or urologic consultation. Secondary nocturnal enuresis, in which previous bedtime control is lost, usually is due to a psychologically stressful event or condition. The chance of an organic etiology (eg, UTI, diabetes mellitus) is greater than in primary nocturnal enuresis. Additional testing or consultation is indicated when secondary nocturnal enuresis is accompanied by daytime urinary symptoms or by bowel symptoms such as constipation or encopresis.

Treatment

Most cases without an organic cause resolve spontaneously before age 6; treatment is not recommended. The spontaneous resolution rate after age 6 is 15%/yr. Psychological consequences that can occur (eg, embarrassment) make treatment considerations most compelling after age 6.

Initial counseling to demystify nocturnal enuresis is helpful. The child is counseled about the etiology and prognosis of enuresis, the aim of which is to remove blame and guilt. The child assumes an active role, including talking to the physician, urinating before going to bed, recording wet and dry nights, and changing wet clothing and bedding himself. The child should not consume fluids during the 2 to 3 h before bedtime, and caffeinated beverages should be strictly limited. Positive reinforcement is given for dry nights (eg, a star calendar, other age-appropriate rewards).

In addition to counseling, enuresis alarms are effective and often recommended simultaneously. Two studies involving 5- to 15-yr-olds reported a 70% cure rate with only a 10 to 15% relapse rate. These alarms are easy to set up, are affordable, and are triggered by a few drops of urine. The disadvantage is the time required for complete success: In the 1st few weeks, the child awakens after full voiding; in the next few weeks, partial inhibition of urination is achieved; and, eventually, the child awakens with a conditioned response to bladder contractions before urination occurs. The alarm should not be discontinued until 3 wk after the last wetting episode.

Drug therapy can be effective in patients unresponsive to counseling and alarms. Short-term treatment (4 to 6 wk) with desmopressin acetate nasal spray (a synthetic analog of ADH) is typically used in patients ≥ 6 yr with persistent, frequent nocturnal enuresis. Recommended initial dosage is one spray in each nostril (total, 20 µg) at bedtime. If effective, the dose can sometimes be reduced to one spray only (10 µg); if ineffective, the dose can be increased to 2 sprays in each nostril (total, 40 µg). Adverse reactions are infrequent, particularly at recommended doses, but may include headache, nausea, nasal congestion, nosebleed, sore throat, cough, flushing, and mild abdominal cramps.

Imipramine and other tricyclics are no longer recommended as 1st-line therapy because of adverse effects (eg, agranulocytosis); potentially life-threatening, accidental excessive ingestion; and the greater long-term success rate of alarms. If other modalities fail and the family strongly favors treatment, imipramine may be used (10 to 25 mg po at bedtime and increased at weekly intervals by 25 mg to a maximum dose of 50 mg in children 6 to 12 yr and 75 mg in children > 12 yr). If imipramine is likely to succeed, a response usually occurs in the 1st week of treatment, which is advantageous, particularly if a rapid response is important to the family and child. Once the child has no enuresis for 1 mo, the drug should be tapered for 2 to 4 wk and stopped. Relapses are very common, reducing the long-term cure rate to 25%. If relapse occurs, a 3-mo course may be tried. Blood counts to detect agranulocytosis, a rare occurrence, should be done q 2 to 4 wk during treatment.

ENCOPRESIS

Encopresis is voluntary or involuntary passage of stool in inappropriate places in a child > 4 yr.

Encopresis is repetitive fecal incontinence in children > 4 who do not have an organic defect or illness. It occurs in about 3% of 4-yr-olds and 1% of 5-yr-olds. Stool retention and overflow due to chronic constipation (see p. 2237) is most often the cause; likelihood of occurrence is highest at milestones such as toilet training or starting school. Rarely, however, encopresis occurs without retention or constipation.

Most physical causes are apparent on history and physical examination; in their absence, testing is usually not indicated.

Treatment

Initial treatment involves educating the parents and child about the physiology of encopresis, removing blame from the child, and diffusing the emotional reactions of those involved.

If history and physical examination rule out specific pathologic diagnoses, the bowel should be emptied by using a laxative such as Mg hydroxide or polyethylene glycol. Maintenance of regular bowel movements is most likely achieved by implementing dietary, environmental, and behavioral changes (modifications of toileting habits). A high-roughage diet should be provided, but the child should not be coerced to eat it. The child should sit on the toilet at consistent times twice/day for 10 min at most (after meals is probably best). Intermittent, short-term use of laxatives is sometimes needed. If this regimen fails, further evaluation of diet and bowel movement patterns is indicated.

VIOLENCE

Children and adolescents may engage in occasional physical confrontations, but most do not develop a sustained pattern of violent behavior or engage in violent crime. Those who become violent before puberty may be higher risks for committing crimes.

Violent behavior is increasingly common in children and adolescents. Almost 10% of students in middle or junior high school and high school report being victims of bullying. In 2001, almost 20% of high school students in the US reported carrying a weapon at least once during the month before they were surveyed as part of a study on youth risks.

Despite growing interest in the possibility of a relationship between violent behavior and genetic defects or chromosomal anomalies, there is minimal evidence for such a relationship. However, several risks have been associated with violent behavior, including being subjected to violent discipline, engaging in alcohol and drug abuse, and gang involvement. There seems to be a relationship between violence and access to firearms, exposure to violence through media, and exposure to child abuse and domestic violence. Children who are bullied may reach a breaking point, at which time they strike back with potentially dangerous or catastrophic results.

Bullying is intentional infliction of psychologic or physical damage on less powerful children. Bullying can take several forms, including persistent teasing, threats, intimidation, harassment, and even violent assaults. Cyber-bullying is a newly described form in which bullies use e-mail and instant messaging to convey threats. Bullies act in order to inflate their sense of self-worth. Bullies often report that bullying creates feelings of power and control. Both bullies and their victims are at risk for poor outcomes. Victims often tell no one about being bullied due to feelings of helplessness, shame, and fear of retaliation. Victims are at risk for physical injury, poor self-esteem, anxiety, depression, and school absence. Bullies are more likely to be incarcerated; they are less likely to remain in school, be employed, or have stable relationships as adults.

Participation in gangs has been linked with violent behavior. Youth gangs are self-formed associations of ≥ 3 members, typically ages 13 to 24. Gangs usually adopt a name and identifying symbols, such as a particular style of clothing, the use of certain hand signs, or graffiti. Some gangs require prospective members to perform random acts of violence before membership is granted. Increasing youth gang violence has been blamed at least in part on gang involvement in drug distribution and drug use, particularly crack cocaine. Use of firearms is a frequent feature of gang violence.

Prevention should begin in early childhood. In young children, violence-free discipline may be effective. Limiting access to weapons and exposure to violence through media and video games may help. In school-age children, measures to create and maintain a safe school environment are needed. Victims should be encouraged to discuss problems with parents, school authorities, and their doctor. In older children and adolescents, emphasis should be placed on teaching strategies for avoidance of high-risk situations (eg, places or settings where others have weapons, or are using alcohol or drugs) and for reacting to or defusing tense situations.

299 LEARNING AND DEVELOPMENTAL DISORDERS

Developmental disorders (including attention-deficit/hyperactivity disorder, autism spectrum disorders, learning disabilities, and mental retardation) are neurologically based conditions that can interfere with the acquisition, retention, or application of specific skills or sets of information. They may involve dysfunction in attention, memory, perception, language, problem-solving, or social interaction.

ATTENTION-DEFICIT/HYPERACTIVITY DISORDER

Attention-deficit/hyperactivity disorder (ADHD) is a syndrome of inattention, hyperactivity, and impulsivity. The 3 types of ADHD are predominantly inattentive, predominantly hyperactive-impulsive, and combined. Diagnosis is made by clinical criteria. Treatment usually includes drug therapy with stimulant drugs, behavioral therapy, and educational interventions.

Attention-deficit/hyperactivity disorder (ADHD) has been classified as a developmental disorder, although increasingly it is considered a disruptive behavior disorder. ADHD affects an estimated 3 to 10% of school-aged children. However, many experts think ADHD is overdiagnosed, largely because criteria are applied inaccurately. According to the *Diagnostic and Statistical Manual,* Fourth Edition (DSM-IV), there are 3 types: predominantly inattentive, predominantly hyperactive-impulsive, and combined. The predominantly hyperactive-impulsive type occurs 2 to 9 times more frequently in boys, although the predominantly inattentive type occurs with about equal frequency in both sexes. ADHD tends to run in families.

ADHD has no known single, specific cause. Potential causes include genetic, biochemical, sensorimotor, physiologic, and behavioral factors. Some risk factors include birth weight < 1000 g, head trauma, and lead exposure, as well as prenatal exposures to alcohol, tobacco, and cocaine. Fewer than 5% of children with ADHD have other symptoms and signs of neurologic damage. Increasing evidence implicates abnormalities in dopaminergic and noradrenergic systems with decreased activity or stimulation in upper brain stem and frontal-midbrain tracts.

Symptoms and Signs

Onset often occurs before age 4 and invariably before age 7. The peak age for diagnosis is between age 8 and 10; however, those with the predominantly inattentive type may not be diagnosed until after adolescence.

Core symptoms and signs of ADHD are inattention, hyperactivity, and impulsivity (see TABLE 299–1) that are more pronounced than expected for the child's developmental level; impaired academic or social function is common.

Inattention tends to appear when a child is involved in tasks that require vigilance, rapid reaction time, visual and perceptual search, and systematic and sustained listening. Inattention and impulsivity impede development of academic skills and thinking and reasoning strategies, motivation for school, and adjustment to social demands. Children who have predominantly inattentive ADHD tend to be hands-on learners who have difficulty in passive-learning situations that require continuous performance and task completion. Overall, about 30% of children with ADHD have learning disabilities.

TABLE 299–1. DSM-IV SYMPTOM CRITERIA FOR ADHD*

SYMPTOM CLASS	SPECIFIC SYMPTOM
Inattention	Does not pay attention to details
	Has difficulty sustaining attention at school
	Does not seem to listen when spoken to
	Does not follow through on instructions or finish tasks
	Has difficulty organizing tasks and activities
	Avoids, dislikes, or is reluctant to engage in tasks that require sustained mental effort
	Often loses things
	Is easily distracted
	Is forgetful
Hyperactivity	Often fidgets with hands or feet or squirms
	Often leaves seat in classroom or elsewhere
	Often runs about or climbs excessively
	Has difficulty playing quietly
	Often on the go, acting as if driven by a motor
	Often talks excessively
Impulsivity	Often blurts out answers before questions are completed
	Often has difficulty awaiting turn
	Often interrupts or intrudes on others

ADHD = attention-deficit/hyperactivity disorder.

*Diagnosis by DSM-IV criteria requires that symptom criteria must be present in at least 2 situations and present before age 7. Diagnosis of the predominantly inattentive type requires at least 6 of the 9 possible symptoms of inattention. Diagnosis of the hyperactive-impulsive type requires at least 6 of the 9 possible symptoms of hyperactivity and impulsivity. Diagnosis of the combined type requires at least 6 symptoms each of inattention and hyperactivity-impulsivity.

Behavioral history can reveal low frustration tolerance, opposition, temper tantrums, aggressiveness, poor social skills and peer relationships, sleep disturbances, anxiety, dysphoria, depression, and mood swings. Although there are no specific physical examination or laboratory findings associated with ADHD, symptoms and signs can include motor incoordination or clumsiness; nonlocalized, "soft" neurologic findings; and perceptual-motor dysfunctions.

The American Academy of Pediatrics has published guidelines for the diagnosis and treatment of ADHD.

Diagnosis

Diagnosis is clinical and is based on comprehensive medical, developmental, educational, and psychologic evaluations.

DSM-IV diagnostic criteria include 9 symptoms and signs of inattention, 6 of hyperactivity, and 3 of impulsivity (see TABLE 299–1); diagnosis using these criteria requires that symptoms and signs occur in at least 2 situations (eg, home and school) and be present before age 7. Diagnosis of the predominantly inattentive type requires at least 6 of the 9 possible symptoms and signs of inattention. Diagnosis of the hyperactive-impulsive type requires at least 6 of the 9 possible symptoms and signs of hyperactivity and impulsivity. Diagnosis of the combined type requires at least 6 symptoms and signs each of inattention and hyperactivity-impulsivity.

Differentiating between ADHD and other conditions can be challenging. Over-diagnosis must be avoided, and other conditions must be properly identified. Many ADHD signs expressed during the preschool years could also indicate communication problems that can occur in other developmental disorders (eg, pervasive developmental disorders) or in certain learning disorders, anxiety, depression, or behavioral disorders (eg, conduct disorder). During later childhood, however, ADHD signs become more qualitatively distinct; such children often exhibit continuous movement of the lower extremities, motor impersistence (eg, purposeless movement and fidgeting of hands), impulsive talking, and a seeming lack of awareness of their environment.

Medical assessment focuses on identifying potentially treatable conditions that may contribute to or worsen symptoms and signs.

Developmental assessment focuses on determining the onset and course of symptoms and signs. Educational assessment focuses on documenting core symptoms and signs; it may involve reviewing educational records and the use of rating scales or checklists. However, rating scales and checklists alone often cannot distinguish ADHD from other developmental disorders or from behavioral disorders.

Prognosis

Traditional classrooms and academic activities often exacerbate symptoms and signs in children with untreated or inadequately treated ADHD. Social and emotional immaturity may be persistent. Poor acceptance by peers and loneliness tend to increase with age and with the obvious display of symptoms. Substance abuse may result if ADHD is not identified and treated.

Although hyperactivity symptoms and signs tend to diminish with age, adolescents and adults may display residual difficulties. Coexisting low intelligence, aggressiveness, social and interpersonal problems, and parental psychopathology are predictors of poor outcomes in adolescence and adulthood. Problems in adolescence and adulthood manifest predominantly as academic failure, low self-esteem, and difficulty learning appropriate social behavior. Adolescents and adults who have predominately impulsive ADHD may have an increased incidence of personality trait disorders and antisocial behavior; many continue to display impulsivity, restlessness, and poor social skills. People with ADHD seem to adjust better to work than to academic and home situations.

Treatment

Randomized, controlled studies show behavioral therapy alone is less effective than therapy with stimulant drugs alone; combination therapy has mixed results. Although correction of the underlying neurophysiologic differences of patients with ADHD does not occur with drug therapy, drugs are effective in alleviating ADHD symptoms and they do permit participation in activities previously inaccessible because of poor attention and impulsivity. Drugs often interrupt the cycle of inappropriate behavior, enhancing behavioral and academic interventions, motivation, and self-esteem. Treatment of adults follows similar principles, but drug selection and dosing are still being worked out.

Drugs: Stimulant preparations that include methylphenidate or dextroamphetamine are most widely used. Response varies greatly, and dosage depends on the severity of the behavior and the child's ability to tolerate the drug.

Methylphenidate is usually started as 5 mg po once/day (immediate-release form), which is then increased weekly, usually to about 5 mg tid. A typical starting dose of dextroamphetamine (either alone or in combination with amphetamine) is 2.5 mg po once/day in children < 6, which can then be titrated up to 2.5 mg bid. In children > 6, the starting dose of dextroamphetamine is typically 5 mg po once/day, which can then be increased to 5 mg bid. Dose titration should balance effectiveness against adverse effects. In general, dextroamphetamine doses are about ⅔ those of methylphenidate preparations. For either methylphenidate or dextroamphetamine, once an optimal dosage is reached, an equivalent dosage of the same drug in a sustained-release form is often substituted to avoid the need for drug administration in school. Learning often is enhanced at low doses, but improvement in behavior often requires higher doses.

Dosing schedules of stimulant drugs can be adjusted to cover specific days and times (eg, during school hours and while doing homework). Drug holidays should be tried on weekends, holidays, or during summer vacations. Placebo periods (for 5 to 10 school days to ensure reliability of observations) are recommended to determine whether the drugs are still needed.

Common adverse effects of stimulant drugs include sleep disturbances (eg, insomnia), depression, headache, stomachache, appetite suppression, and elevated heart rate and BP. Some studies have shown slowing of growth over 2 yr of stimulant drug use, but it remains unclear whether slowing persists over longer periods of use. Some patients who are sensitive to stimulant drug effects will appear over-focused or dulled; decreasing the stimulant drug dosage or trying a different drug may be helpful.

Atomoxetine, a selective norepinephrine reuptake inhibitor, is also used. The drug is effective, but data are mixed regarding its efficacy compared to stimulant drugs. Many children experience nausea, sedation, irritability, and temper tantrums; rarely, severe liver toxicity and suicidal ideation have occurred. Atomoxetine should not be considered a 1st-line drug. A typical starting dose is 0.5 mg/kg po once/day, titrated weekly to 1.2 mg/kg. The long half-life allows once-daily dosing but requires continuous use to be effective. The maximum daily dosage is 60 mg.

Antidepressants such as bupropion, α-2 agonists such as clonidine and guanfacine, and other psychoactive drugs are sometimes used in cases of stimulant drug ineffectiveness or unacceptable adverse effects, but they are less effective and are not recommended as 1st-line drugs. Pemoline is no longer recommended.

Behavioral management: Counseling, including cognitive-behavioral therapy (eg, goal-setting, self-monitoring, modeling, role-playing), is often effective and helps the child understand ADHD. Structure and routines are essential.

Classroom behavior is often improved by environmental control of noise and visual stimulation, appropriate task length, novelty, coaching, and teacher proximity.

When difficulties persist at home, parents should be encouraged to seek additional professional assistance and training in behavior management techniques. Adding incentives and token rewards reinforces behavior management and is often effective. Children with ADHD in whom hyperactivity and poor impulse control predominate are often helped at home when structure, consistent parenting techniques, and well-defined limits are established.

Elimination diets, megavitamin treatments, use of antioxidants or other compounds, and nutritional and biochemical interventions (eg, administration of petrochemicals) have had the least effect. The value of biofeedback is unsubstantiated. Most studies have shown minimal change in behavior and no sustained benefit.

AUTISM SPECTRUM DISORDERS

Autism is a neurodevelopmental disorder characterized by impaired social interaction and communication, repetitive and stereotyped patterns of behavior, and uneven intellectual development often with mental retardation. Symptoms begin in early childhood. The cause in most children is unknown, although evidence supports a genetic component; in some, autism may be caused by a medical condition. Diagnosis is based on developmental history and observation. Treatment consists of behavioral management and sometimes drug therapy.

Autism, a neurodevelopmental disorder, is the most common of the disorders called pervasive developmental disorders (PDDs—see TABLE 299–2). Given the wide clinical variability of these conditions, many people also refer to PDDs as "autism spectrum disorders." Estimates of prevalence range from 5/10,000 to 50/1000. Autism is 2 to 4 times more common in boys. In the past decade, there has been a rapid rise in the diagnosis of autism spectrum disorders, partially because of changes in diagnostic criteria.

Etiology

Most cases of autism spectrum disorders are unrelated to diseases that affect the brain. However, some cases have occurred with congenital rubella syndrome, cytomegalic inclusion disease, phenylketonuria, and fragile X syndrome.

Strong evidence supports a genetic component. Parents of one child with a PDD have a risk 50 to 100 times greater of having a subsequent child with a PDD. The concordance rate of autism is high in monozygotic twins. Research on families has suggested several potential target gene areas, including those related to neurotransmitter receptors (GABA) and CNS structural control (*HOX* genes). Environmental causes (including vaccination and various diets) have been suspected but are unproven.

Abnormalities of brain structure and function probably underlie much of the pathogenesis of autism. Some children with autism have enlarged ventricles, some have hypoplasia of the cerebellar vermis, and others have abnormalities of brainstem nuclei.

Symptoms, Signs, and Diagnosis

Autism usually manifests in the 1st yr of life and always by age 3. The disorder is characterized by atypical interaction (ie, lack of attachment, inability to cuddle or to form reciprocal relationships, avoidance of eye gaze), insistence on sameness (ie, resistance to change, rituals, intense attachment to familiar objects, repetitive acts), speech and language problems (ranging from total muteness to delayed onset of speech to markedly idiosyncratic use of language), and uneven intellectual performance. Some affected children injure themselves. About 25% of affected children experience a documented loss of previously acquired skills.

TABLE 299–2. PERVASIVE DEVELOPMENTAL DISORDERS SPECTRUM

SUBTYPE	CHARACTERISTICS
Asperger's syndrome	Language and cognition generally better than in autism; socially isolated and often viewed as odd or eccentric; clumsiness; repetitive patterns of behavior, interests, and activities; atypical sensory responses (eg, exquisite sensitivity to noises, food odors or tastes, or clothing textures); pragmatic deficits (eg, extremely concrete use of language or difficulty recognizing irony or jokes)
Autism (autistic disorder)	Onset before age 3 yr; impaired social interaction and communication; repetitive stereotyped behavior; some degree of mental retardation in most cases; in some cases severe regression of language and sociability occurs between 18 and 24 mo
Childhood disintegrative disorder	After 2 yr of normal growth, a marked regression occurs in at least 2 of the following: social skills, language, bladder and bowel control, motor skills; can eventually become more severe than is typical in autism; other behaviors may mimic autism or childhood schizophrenia
Pervasive developmental disorder not otherwise specified	Does not meet criteria for any of other subtypes yet exhibits a wide range of cognitive and behavioral problems and impairment in social interactions; less severe than autism
Rett syndrome	Affects development after initial 6-mo period of normal development; deceleration of head growth; severe mental retardation; impaired social interaction; loss of speech and purposeful use of hands (results in "hand-wringing stereotypy"); seizures, autistic features, ataxia; affects almost exclusively girls (caused by mutation in *MECP2* gene on Xq28)

Current theory holds that a fundamental problem in autism spectrum disorders is "mind blindness," the inability to imagine what another person might be thinking. This difficulty is thought to result in interaction abnormalities that in turn lead to abnormal language development. One of the earliest and most sensitive markers for autism is a 1-yr-old child's inability to point communicatively at objects. It is theorized that the child cannot imagine that another person would understand what was being indicated; instead, the child indicates wants only by physically touching the desired object or using the adult's hand as a tool.

Nonfocal neurologic findings include poorly coordinated gait and stereotyped motor movements. Seizures occur in 20 to 40% of these children (particularly those with an intelligence quotient [IQ] < 50).

Diagnosis is made clinically and usually requires evidence of impairment of social interaction and communication, and presence of restricted, repetitive, stereotyped behaviors or interests. Screening tests include the Social Communication Questionnaire, the M-CHAT, and others. Formal "gold standard" diagnostic tests such as the Autism Diagnostic Observation Schedule (ADOS), based on DSM-IV criteria, are usually administered by psychologists. Children with autism are difficult to test; they usually do better on performance items than verbal items in IQ tests and may show instances of age-appropriate performance despite retardation in most areas. Nonetheless, an IQ test administered by an experienced examiner often can provide a useful predictor of outcome.

Treatment

Treatment is usually multidisciplinary, and recent studies show measurable benefits from intensive, behaviorally based approaches that encourage interaction and meaningful communication. Psychologists and educators typically focus on behavioral

TABLE 299–3. COMMON LEARNING DISORDERS

DISORDER	MANIFESTATION
Dyslexia	Problems with reading
Phonologic dyslexia	Problems with sound analysis and memory
Surface dyslexia	Problems with visual recognition of forms and structures of words
Dysgraphia	Problems with spelling, written expression, or handwriting
Dyscalculia	Problems with mathematics and difficulties with problem-solving
Ageometria	Problems due to disturbances in mathematical reasoning
Anarithmia	Disturbances in basic concept formation and inability to acquire computational skills
Dysnomia	Difficulty recalling words and information from memory on demand

analysis and then match behavioral management strategies to the person's specific behavioral problems at home and at school. Speech and language therapy should begin early and use a range of media, including signing, picture exchange, and speech. Physical and occupational therapists plan and implement strategies to help affected children compensate for specific deficits in motor function and motor planning. SSRIs may improve control of ritualistic behaviors. Antipsychotics and mood stabilizers such as valproate may help control self-injurious behavior.

LEARNING DISABILITIES

Learning disabilities are conditions that cause a discrepancy between potential and actual levels of academic performance as predicted by the person's intellectual abilities. Learning disabilities involve impairments or difficulties in concentration or attention, language development, or visual and aural information processing. Diagnosis includes intellectual, educational, speech and language, medical, and psychologic evaluations. Treatment consists primarily of educational management and sometimes medical, behavioral, and psychologic therapy.

Specific learning disabilities affect the ability to understand or use spoken or written language, do mathematical calculations, coordinate movements, or focus attention on a task. These disabilities include problems in reading, mathematics, spelling, written expression or handwriting, and understanding or using verbal and nonverbal language (see TABLE 299–3). Most learning disabilities are complex or mixed, with deficits in more than one system.

Although the number of children with learning disabilities is unknown, about 5% of the school-age population in the US receives special educational services for learning disabilities. Among affected children, boys outnumber girls 5:1.

Learning disabilities may be congenital or acquired. No single cause has been defined, but neurologic deficits are evident or presumed. Genetic influences are often implicated. Other possible causes include maternal illness or toxic drug use during pregnancy, complications during pregnancy or delivery (eg, spotting, toxemia, prolonged labor, precipitous delivery), and neonatal problems (eg, prematurity, low birth weight, severe jaundice, perinatal asphyxia, postmaturity, respiratory distress). Potential postnatal factors include exposure to environmental toxins (eg, lead), CNS infections, cancers and their treatments, trauma, malnutrition, and severe social isolation or deprivation.

Symptoms and Signs

Children with learning disabilities typically have at least average intelligence, although such disabilities can occur in those with lower cognitive function as well. Symptoms and signs of severe disabilities tend to manifest at an early age. Mild to moderate learning disabilities are usually not recognized until school age, when the rigors of academic learning are encountered. Affected children may have trouble learning the alphabet and may be delayed in paired associative learning (eg, color-naming, labeling, counting, letter-naming). Speech perception may be limited, language may be learned at a slower rate, and vocabulary may be decreased. Affected children may not understand what is read; may have very messy handwriting or hold a pencil awkwardly; may have trouble organizing or beginning tasks or retelling a story in sequential order; or may confuse math symbols and misread numbers.

Disturbances or delays in expressive language or listening comprehension are predictors of academic problems beyond the preschool years. Memory may be defective, including short- and long-term memory, memory use (eg, rehearsal), and verbal recall or retrieval. Problems may occur in conceptualizing, abstracting, generalizing, reasoning, and organizing and planning information for problem solving. Visual perception and auditory processing problems may occur, including difficulties in spatial cognition and orientation (eg, object localization, spatial memory, awareness of position and place), visual attention and memory, and sound discrimination and analysis.

Some children with learning disabilities may have difficulty following social conventions (eg, taking turns, standing too close to the listener, not understanding jokes); these are often components of mild autism spectrum disorders as well (see p. 2486). Short attention span, motor restlessness, fine motor problems (eg, poor printing and copying), and variability in performance and behavior over time are other early signs. Difficulties with impulse control, non-goal–directed behavior and overactivity, discipline problems, aggressiveness, withdrawal and avoidance behavior, excessive shyness, and excessive fear may occur. As noted above, learning disabilities and attention-deficit/hyperactivity disorder (ADHD) often occur together.

Diagnosis

Children with learning disabilities are typically identified when a discrepancy is recognized between their academic potential and their academic performance. Speech and language, intellectual, educational, medical, and psychologic evaluations are necessary for determining deficiencies in skills and cognitive processes. Social and emotional-behavioral evaluations are also necessary for planning treatment and monitoring progress.

Intellectual evaluation typically includes verbal and nonverbal intelligence testing and is usually performed by school personnel. Psychoeducational testing may be helpful in describing the child's preferred manner of processing information (eg, holistically or analytically, visually or aurally). Neuropsychologic assessment is particularly useful in children with known CNS injury or illness to map those areas of the brain that correspond to specific functional strengths and weaknesses. Speech and language evaluations establish integrity of comprehension and language use, phonologic processing, and verbal memory.

Teachers' observations of classroom behavior and academic performance are essential. Reading evaluations measure abilities in word-decoding and recognition, comprehension, and fluency. Writing samples should be obtained to evaluate spelling, syntax, and fluency of ideas. Mathematical ability should be assessed in terms of computation skills, knowledge of operations, and understanding of concepts.

Medical evaluation includes a detailed family history, the child's medical history, a physical examination, and a neurologic or neurodevelopmental examination to look for underlying disorders. Although infrequent, physical abnormalities and neurologic signs may indicate medically treatable causes of learning disabilities. Gross motor coordination problems may indicate neurologic deficits or neurodevelopmental delays. Developmental level is evaluated according to standardized criteria.

Psychologic evaluation identifies ADHD, conduct disorder, anxiety disorders, depression, and poor self-esteem, which frequently accompany and must be differentiated from learning disabilities. Attitude toward school, motivation, peer relationships, and self-confidence is assessed.

Treatment

Treatment centers on educational management but may also involve medical, behavioral, and psychologic therapy. Effective teaching programs may take a remedial, compensatory, or strategic (ie, teaching the child how to learn) approach. A mismatch of instructional method to a child's learning disability and learning preference aggravates the disability.

Some children require specialized instruction in only one area while continuing to attend regular classes. Other children need separate and intense educational programs. Optimally, and as required by US law, affected children should participate as much as possible in inclusive classes with peers who do not have learning disabilities.

Drugs minimally affect academic achievement, intelligence, and general learning ability, although certain drugs (eg, stimulants, such as methylphenidate and several amphetamine preparations—see p. 2485) may enhance attention and concentration, allowing the child to respond more efficiently to instruction. Many popular remedies and therapies (eg, eliminating food additives, using antioxidants or megadoses of vitamins, patterning by sensory stimulation and passive movement, sensory integrative therapy through postural exercises, auditory nerve training, optometric training to remedy visual-perceptual and sensorimotor coordination processes) are unproven.

DYSLEXIA

Dyslexia describes a general term for primary reading disorder. Diagnosis is based on intellectual, educational, speech and language, medical, and psychologic evaluations. Treatment is primarily educational management, consisting of instruction in word recognition and component skills.

No definition of dyslexia is universally accepted; thus incidence is undetermined. An estimated 15% of public school children receive special instruction for reading problems, of which about ½ may have persistent reading disabilities. Dyslexia is identified more often in boys than girls, but gender is not a proven risk factor for developing dyslexia.

Etiology and Pathophysiology

Phonologic processing problems produce deficits in discrimination, blending, memory, and analysis of sounds. Dyslexia may affect both production and understanding of written language, which is often restricted further by problems with auditory memory, speech production, and naming or word-finding. Underlying weaknesses in verbal language are often present.

Dyslexia tends to run in families. Children with a family history of reading or learning difficulties are at higher risk. Because changes have been identified in the brains of people with dyslexia, experts believe dyslexia results predominantly from cortical dysfunction stemming from congenital neurodevelopmental abnormalities. Lesions affecting the integration or interactions of specific brain functions are suspected. Most researchers concur that dyslexia is left hemisphere–related and linked to dysfunctions in brain areas responsible for language association (Wernicke's motor speech area) and sound and speech production (Broca's area) and in the interconnection of these areas via the fasciculus arcuatus. Dysfunctions or defects in the angular gyrus, the medial occipital area, and the right hemisphere produce word recognition problems.

The inability to learn derivational rules of printed language is often considered part of dyslexia. Affected children may have difficulty determining root words or word stems and determining which letters in words follow others.

Reading problems other than dyslexia are usually caused by difficulties in language comprehension or low cognitive ability. Visual-perceptual problems and abnormal eye movements are not dyslexia. However, these problems can interfere further with word learning.

Symptoms and Signs

Dyslexia may manifest as delayed language production; speech articulation difficulties; and difficulties remembering the names of letters, numbers, and colors. Children with phonologic processing problems often have difficulty blending sounds, rhyming words, identifying the positions of sounds in words, and segmenting words into pronounceable components. They may reverse the order of sounds in words. Delay or hesitation in choosing words, substituting words, or naming letters and pictures is often an early sign. Short-term auditory memory and auditory sequencing difficulties are common.

Fewer than 20% of children with dyslexia have difficulties with the visual demands of reading. However, some confuse letters and words with similar configurations or have difficulty visually selecting or identifying letter patterns and clusters (sound-symbol association) in words. Reversals or visual confusions can occur, most often because of retention or retrieval difficulties that cause affected children to forget or confuse the names of letters and words that have similar structures; subsequently, *d* becomes *b*, *m* becomes *w*, *h* becomes *n*, *was* becomes *saw*, *on* becomes *no*. Such reversals are normal in children < 8 yr, however.

Diagnosis

Most children with dyslexia are not identified until kindergarten or 1st grade, when they encounter symbolic learning. Children with a history of delayed language acquisition or use, who are not accelerating in word learning by the end of 1st grade, or who are not reading at the level expected for their verbal or intellectual abilities at any grade level should be evaluated. Often, the best diagnostic indicator is the child's inability to respond to traditional or typical reading approaches during 1st grade, although wide variation in reading skills can still be seen at this level. Demonstration of phonologic processing problems is essential for diagnosis.

Children suspected of having dyslexia should undergo reading, speech and language, auditory, cognitive, and psychologic evaluations to identify their functional strengths and weaknesses and their preferred learning styles. Such evaluations can be requested of school staff by the child's teacher or family based on the Individuals with Disabilities Education Act (IDEA), a US special education law. Evaluation findings then guide the most effective instructional approach.

Comprehensive reading evaluations test word recognition and analysis, fluency, reading or listening comprehension, and level of understanding of vocabulary and the reading process.

Speech, language, and auditory evaluations assess spoken language and deficits in processing phonemes (sound elements) of spoken language. Receptive and expressive language functions are also assessed. Cognitive abilities (eg, attention, memory, reasoning) are tested.

Psychologic evaluations address emotional concerns that can exacerbate a reading disability. A complete family history of mental disorders and emotional problems is obtained.

The physician should ensure that the child's vision and hearing are normal, either through office-based screening or referral for formal audiologic or vision testing. Neurologic evaluations may help detect secondary features (eg, neurodevelopmental immaturity or minor neurologic abnormalities) and rule out other disorders (eg, seizures).

Treatment

Although dyslexia is a lifelong problem, many children develop functional reading skills. However, other children never reach adequate literacy.

Treatment consists of educational interventions, including direct and indirect instruction in word recognition and component skills. Direct instruction includes teaching specific phonics skills separate from other reading instruction. Indirect instruction includes integrating phonics skills into reading programs. Instruction may teach reading from a whole-word or whole-language approach or by following a hierarchy of skills from the sound unit to the word to the sentence. Multisensory approaches that include whole-word learning and the integration of visual, auditory, and tactual procedures to teach sounds, words, and sentences are then recommended.

Component skills instruction consists of teaching children to blend sounds to form words, segment words into word parts, and identify the positions of sounds in words. Component skills for reading comprehension include identifying the main idea, answering questions, isolating facts and details, and reading inferentially. Many children benefit from using a computer to help isolate words within text samples or for word processing of written work.

Other treatments (eg, optometric training, perceptual training, auditory integration training) and drug therapies are unproven and not recommended.

MENTAL RETARDATION

Mental retardation is characterized by significantly subaverage intellectual functioning (often expressed as an intelligence quotient < 70 to 75) combined with limitations of > 2 of the following: communication, self-direction, social skills, self-care, use of community resources, and maintenance of personal safety. Management consists of education, family counseling, and social support.

Basing severity on intelligence quotient (IQ) alone (eg, mild, 52 to 70 or 75; moderate, 36 to 51; severe, 20 to 35; and profound, < 20) is inadequate. Classification must also account for the level of support needed, ranging from intermittent to ongoing high-level support for all activities. Such an approach focuses on a person's strengths and weaknesses, relating them to the demands of the person's environment and the expectations and attitudes of the family and community.

About 3% of the population functions at IQ of < 70, which is least 2 standard deviations below the mean IQ of the general population

(IQ of < 100); if the need for support is considered, only about 1% of the population has severe mental retardation (MR). Severe MR occurs in families from all socioeconomic groups and educational levels. Less severe MR (requiring intermittent or limited support) occurs most often in lower socioeconomic groups, paralleling with observations that IQ correlates best with success in school and socioeconomic status rather than specific organic factors. Nevertheless, recent studies suggest that genetic factors even play roles in milder cognitive disabilities.

Etiology

Intelligence is both genetically and environmentally determined. Children born to parents with MR are at increased risk for a range of developmental disabilities, but clear genetic transmission of MR is unusual. Although advances in genetics have increased the likelihood of identifying the cause of a person's intellectual disability, in 60 to 80% of cases a specific cause still cannot be identified. A cause is most likely to be identified in severe cases. Deficits in language and personal-social skills may be due to emotional problems, environmental deprivation, learning disorders, or deafness rather than MR.

Prenatal: A number of chromosomal anomalies and genetic metabolic and neurologic disorders can cause MR (see TABLE 299–4).

Congenital infections that can cause MR include rubella virus, cytomegalovirus, *Toxoplasma gondii*, *Treponema pallidum*, and HIV.

Prenatal drug and toxin exposure (see p. 2159) can cause MR. Fetal alcohol syndrome (see also p. 2283) is the most common of these conditions. Anticonvulsants such as phenytoin or valproate, chemotherapy drugs, radiation exposure, lead, and methylmercury are also causes. Severe malnutrition during pregnancy may affect fetal brain development, resulting in MR.

Perinatal: Complications related to prematurity, CNS bleeding, periventricular leukomalacia, breech or high forceps delivery, multiple births, placenta previa, preeclampsia, and perinatal asphyxia may increase the risk of MR. The risk is increased in small-for-gestational-age infants; intellectual impairment and decreased weight share the same cause. Very low- and extremely low-birth-weight infants have variably increased chances of having MR, depending on gestational age, perinatal events, and quality of care.

TABLE 299–4. CHROMOSOMAL AND GENETIC CAUSES OF MENTAL RETARDATION*

CHROMOSOMAL ABNORMALITIES	GENETIC METABOLIC DISORDERS	GENETIC NEUROLOGIC DISORDERS
Cri du chat syndrome	Autosomal recessive disorders:	Autosomal dominant disorders:
Down syndrome	Aminoacidurias and acidemias	Myotonic dystrophy
Fragile X syndrome	Peroxisomal disorders:	Neurofibromatosis
Klinefelter's syndrome	Galactosemia	Tuberous sclerosis
Mosaicisms	Maple syrup urine disease	Autosomal recessive disorders:
Trisomy 13 (Patau's syndrome)	Phenylketonuria	Primary microcephaly
Trisomy 18 (Edwards' syndrome)	Lysosomal defects:	
Turner's syndrome	Gaucher's disease	
	Hurler's syndrome (mucopolysaccharidosis)	
	Niemann-Pick disease	
	Tay-Sachs disease	
	X-linked recessive disorders:	
	Lesch-Nyhan syndrome (hyperuricemia)	
	Hunter's syndrome (a variant of mucopolysaccharidosis)	
	Lowe's oculocerebrorenal syndrome	

*This is a partial list of disorders.

Postnatal: Malnutrition and environmental deprivation (lack of physical, emotional, and cognitive support required for growth, development, and social adaptation) during infancy and early childhood may be the most common causes of MR worldwide. Viral and bacterial encephalitides (including AIDS-associated neuroencephalopathy) and meningitides, poisoning (eg, lead, mercury), severe malnutrition, and accidents that cause severe head injuries or asphyxia may result in MR.

Symptoms and Signs

The primary manifestations are delayed intellectual development, immature behavior, and limited self-care skills. Some children with mild MR may not develop recognizable symptoms until preschool age. However, early identification is common in those with moderate to severe MR and in those in whom MR is accompanied by physical abnormalities or signs of a condition (eg, cerebral palsy) that may be associated with a particular cause of MR (eg, perinatal asphyxia). Delayed development is usually apparent by preschool age. Among older children, hallmark features are a low IQ combined with limitations in adaptive behavior skills. Although developmental patterns may vary, it is much more common for children with MR to experience slow progress than developmental arrest.

Some children may have cerebral palsy or other motor deficits, language delays, or hearing loss. Such motor or sensory impairments can mimic cognitive impairment but are not in themselves causes of it. As children mature, some develop anxiety or depression if they are socially rejected by other children or if they are disturbed by the realization that others see them as different and deficient. Well-managed, inclusive school programs can help maximize social integration, thereby minimizing such emotional responses. Behavioral disorders are the reason for most psychiatric referrals and out-of-home placements for people with MR. Behavior problems are often situational, and precipitating factors can usually be found. Factors that predispose to unacceptable behavior include lack of training in socially responsible behavior, inconsistent discipline, reinforcement of faulty behavior, impaired ability to communicate, and discomfort from coexisting physical problems and mental health disorders such as depression or anxiety. In institutional settings, overcrowding, understaffing, and lack of activities contribute.

Diagnosis

For suspected cases, development and intelligence are assessed, typically by early intervention or school staff. Standardized intelligence tests can measure subaverage intellectual ability but are subject to error, and results should be questioned when they do not match clinical findings; illness, motor or sensory impairments, language barriers, or cultural differences may hamper a child's test performance. Such tests also have a middle-class bias but are generally reasonable in appraising intellectual ability in children, particularly in older ones. Developmental screening tests such as the Ages and Stages Questionnaire or the Parents' Evaluation of Developmental Status (PEDS) provide gross assessments of development for young children and can be administered by a physician or others. Such measures should be used only for screening and not as substitutes for standardized intelligence tests, which should be administered by qualified psychologists. A neurodevelopmental assessment should be initiated as soon as developmental delays are suspected. A developmental pediatrician or pediatric neurologist should investigate all cases of moderate to severe developmental delays, progressive disability, neuromuscular deterioration, or suspected seizure disorders.

Establishing MR is followed by efforts to determine a cause. Accurate determination of the cause may provide a developmental prognosis, suggest plans for educational and training programs, help in genetic counseling, and relieve parental guilt. History (including perinatal, developmental, neurologic, and familial) may identify causes. An algorithm for the diagnostic evaluation of the child with MR (global developmental delay) has been proposed by the Child Neurology Society. Cranial imaging (eg, MRI) can demonstrate CNS malformations (as seen in neurodermatoses such as neurofibromatosis or tuberous sclerosis), treatable hydrocephalus, or more severe brain malformations such as schizencephaly. Genetic tests may help identify disorders such as Down syndrome (trisomy 21) via standard karyotyping, 5p-deletion (cri du chat syndrome) or DiGeorge syndrome (chromosome 22q deletion) via fluorescent in situ hybridization (FISH), or fragile X syndrome via direct DNA studies.

Genetic metabolic disorders may be suggested by their clinical manifestations (eg, failure to thrive, lethargy, vomiting, seizures, hypotonia, hepatosplenomegaly, coarse facial

TABLE 299–5. TESTS FOR SOME CAUSES OF MENTAL RETARDATION

SUSPECTED CAUSE	INDICATED TESTS
Single major anomaly or multiple minor anomalies, family history of retardation	Chromosomal analysis Cranial CT and/or MRI*
Failure to thrive, idiopathic hypotonia, genetic metabolic disorders	HIV screen in high-risk infants Nutritional and psychosocial history Urine and/or blood amino acid and enzyme studies for storage diseases or peroxisomal disorders Muscle enzymes SMA 12/60 Bone age, skeletal x-rays
Seizures	EEG Cranial CT and/or MRI* Blood Ca, phosphorus, magnesium, amino acids, glucose, and lead levels
Cranial abnormalities (eg, premature closure of the sutures, microcephaly, macrocephaly, craniostenosis, hydrocephalus), cerebral atrophy, cerebral malformations, CNS hemorrhage, tumor, intracranial calcifications due to toxoplasmosis, cytomegalovirus infection, or tuberous sclerosis	Cranial CT and/or MRI* TORCH screen Urine culture for virus Chromosomal analysis

*After neurologic consultation.
SMA = sequential multiple analyzer; TORCH = toxoplasmosis, rubella, cytomegalovirus, herpes.

features, abnormal urinary odor, macroglossia). Isolated delays in sitting or walking (gross motor skills) and in pincer grasp, drawing, or writing (fine motor skills) may indicate a neuromuscular disorder. Specific laboratory tests are performed depending on the suspected cause (see TABLE 299–5). Visual and auditory assessments should be performed at an early age, and screening for lead poisoning is often appropriate.

Prognosis and Treatment

Treatment and support needs depend on social competence and cognitive function. Referral to an early intervention program during infancy may prevent or decrease the severity of disability resulting from a perinatal insult. Realistic methods of caring for the child must be established.

Family support and counseling are crucial. As soon as MR is confirmed or strongly suspected, the parents should be informed and given ample time to discuss causes, effects, prognosis, education and training of the child, and the importance of balancing known prognostic risks against negative self-fulfilling prophecies in which diminished expectations result in poor functional outcomes later in life. Sensitive ongoing counseling is essential for family adaptation. If the family's physician cannot provide coordination and counseling, the child and family should be referred to a center with a multidisciplinary team that evaluates and serves children with MR; however, the family's physician should provide continuing medical care and advice.

A comprehensive, individualized program is developed with the help of appropriate specialists, including educators. Neurologists or developmental pediatricians, orthopedists, physical therapists, and occupational therapists assist in managing comorbidities in children with motor deficits. Speech pathologists and audiologists help with language delays or with a suspected hearing loss. Nutritionists can help with treatment of malnutrition and social workers can help reduce environmental deprivation. Affected children with concomitant mental health disorders such as depression may be given appropriate psychoactive drugs in dosages similar to those used in children without MR. The use of psychoactive drugs without behavioral therapy and environmental changes is rarely helpful.

Every effort should be made to have the child live at home or in a community-based residence. Although the presence of a child with MR in the home can be disruptive, it can also be extremely rewarding. The family may benefit from psychologic support and help with daily care provided by daycare centers, homemakers, and respite services. The living environment must encourage independence and reinforce learning of skills needed to accomplish this goal. Whenever possible, a child with MR should attend an appropriately adapted daycare center or school with peers who are not mentally retarded. The Individuals with Disabilities Education Act (IDEA), a US special education law, stipulates that all children with disabilities should receive appropriate educational opportunities and programming in the least restrictive and most inclusive environments. As people with MR reach adulthood, an array of supportive living and work settings is available. Large residential institutions are being replaced by small group or individual residences matched to the affected person's functional abilities and needs.

Many people with mild to moderate MR can support themselves, can live independently, and can be successful at jobs that require basic intellectual skills. Life expectancy may be shortened, depending on the etiology of the disability, but health care is improving long-term health outcomes for people with all types of developmental disabilities. People with severe MR are likely to require life-long support. The more severe the retardation and the greater the immobility, the higher is the mortality risk.

Prevention

Genetic counseling (see also p. 2143) may help high-risk couples understand possible risks. If a child has MR, evaluation of the etiology can provide the family with appropriate risk information for future pregnancies.

High-risk couples who choose to have children often undergo prenatal testing, which enables a couple to consider pregnancy termination and subsequent family planning. Amniocentesis or chorionic villus sampling may detect inherited metabolic and chromosomal disorders, carrier states, and CNS malformations (eg, neural tube defects, anencephaly). Ultrasonography may also identify CNS defects. Maternal serum α-fetoprotein is a helpful screen for neural tube defects, Down syndrome, and other abnormalities. Amniocentesis is indicated for all pregnant women > 35 yr (because their risk of having an infant with Down syndrome is increased) and for women with family histories of inborn metabolic disorders.

Rubella vaccine has all but eliminated congenital rubella as a cause. A vaccine for cytomegalovirus infection is being sought. Continuing improvements in and increased availability of obstetric and neonatal care and the use of exchange transfusion and $Rh_0(D)$ immune globulin to prevent hemolytic disease of the newborn have reduced the incidence of MR; the increase in survival of very-low-birth-weight infants has kept the prevalence constant.

300 MENTAL DISORDERS IN CHILDREN AND ADOLESCENTS

Although it is sometimes assumed that childhood and adolescence are times of carefree bliss, as many as 20% of children and adolescents have one or more diagnosable mental disorders. Most of these disorders may be viewed as exaggerations or distortions of normal behaviors and emotions.

Like adults, children and adolescents are temperamentally variable; some are shy and reticent, others socially exuberant, some methodical and cautious, still others are impulsive and careless. Whether a child is behaving like a typical child or has a disorder is determined by the presence of impairment and distress related to the symptoms at hand. For example, a 12-yr-old girl may be frightened by the prospect of delivering a book report in front of her class. This fear would not be viewed as social phobia unless her fears were severe enough to cause clinically significant impairments and distress.

There is much overlap between the symptoms of many disorders and the challenging behaviors and emotions of normal children. Thus, many of the strategies useful for addressing behavioral problems in children (see p. 2478) can also be applied to children with mental disorders. Furthermore, appropriate management of childhood behavioral problems may prevent temperamentally vulnerable children from developing a full-blown disorder.

The most common mental disorders of childhood and adolescence fall into 4 broad categories: anxiety disorders, schizophrenia, mood disorders (primarily depression), and disruptive behavioral disorders. However, more often than not, children and adolescents have symptoms and problems that cut across diagnostic boundaries.

Evaluation

Assessment of mental complaints or symptoms in children and adolescents differs from assessment in adults in 3 important respects. First, the developmental context is critically important in children. Behaviors that are normal at a young age may be indicative of serious mental illness at an older age. Second, children exist in the context of a family system, and that system has a profound impact on the child's symptoms and behaviors; a normal child living in a family troubled by domestic violence and substance abuse may superficially appear to have one or more mental disorders. Third, children often do not have the cognitive and linguistic sophistication needed to accurately describe their symptoms. Thus, the clinician must rely very heavily on direct observation, corroborated by the observations of others, such as parents and teachers.

In many cases, the child's developmental progress creates concerns that are difficult to separate from those resulting from a mental disorder. These concerns often arise because of poor academic progress, delays in language acquisition, and deficits in social skills. In such cases, formal developmental and neuropsychologic testing should be part of the evaluation process.

Because of these factors, the evaluation of a child with a mental disorder is typically more complex than a comparable evaluation of an adult. Fortunately, most cases are not severe and can be competently managed by a thoughtful primary care provider. However, severe cases are best managed in consultation with a child and adolescent psychiatry specialist.

ANXIETY DISORDERS

Some measure of anxiety is a normal aspect of development. For example, most toddlers become fearful when separated from their mother, especially in unfamiliar surroundings. Fears of the dark, monsters, bugs, and spiders are common in 3- to 4-yr-olds. Shy children may initially react to new situations with fear or withdrawal. Fears of injury and death are more common in older children. Older children and adolescents often become anxious when giving a book report in front of their classmates. Such difficulties should not be viewed as evidence of a disorder. However, when these otherwise normal manifestations of anxiety become so exaggerated that functioning becomes greatly impaired or severe distress is endured, an anxiety disorder should be considered.

About 10 to 15% of children experience an anxiety disorder (eg, generalized, separation, and social phobia disorders; obsessive-compulsive disorder; specific phobia; panic disorder; acute and posttraumatic stress disorders) at some point during childhood. Common to all anxiety disorders is a state of fear, worry, or dread that greatly impairs the child's ability to function normally and is disproportionate to the circumstances at hand.

The etiology of anxiety disorders seems to have a genetic basis but is heavily modified by psychosocial experience; the heritability is polygenetic and only a small number of the specific genes have been characterized thus far. Anxious parents tend to have anxious children, which has the unfortunate potential of making the child's problems worse than they otherwise might be. Even a normal child has difficulty remaining calm and composed in the presence of an anxious parent, and this is all the more challenging for a child who is genetically predisposed to anxiety. In as many as 30% of cases, it is helpful to treat parental anxiety in conjunction with the child's anxiety (see p. 1673 for treatment of anxiety in adults).

Symptoms, Signs, and Diagnosis

Perhaps the most common manifestation is school refusal. "School refusal" has largely supplanted the term "school phobia." Actual fear of school is exceedingly rare. Most children who refuse to go to school probably have separation anxiety, social phobia, panic, or a combination of all three. School refusal is also occasionally seen in children with specific phobia.

Some children complain directly about their anxiety, describing it in terms of worries, eg, "I am worried that I will never see you again" (separation anxiety) or "I am worried the kids will laugh at me" (social phobia). However, most children instead couch their discomfort in terms of somatic complaints: "I cannot go to school because I have a stomachache." Such a complaint can lead to some confusion because the child is often telling the truth. An upset stomach, nausea, and headaches often develop in children with anxiety.

Diagnosis varies according to the specific anxiety disorder.

Prognosis and Treatment

Prognosis depends on severity, availability of competent treatment, and the child's resiliency. In most cases, children struggle with anxiety symptoms into adulthood and beyond. However, with early treatment, many children learn how to control their anxiety.

Childhood anxiety disorders are treated with behavioral therapy (using principles of exposure and response prevention), sometimes in conjunction with drug therapy. With behavioral therapy, the child is systematically exposed to the anxiety-provoking situation in a graded fashion. By helping the child to remain in the anxiety-provoking situation (response prevention), the child gradually becomes desensitized and the anxiety is diminished. Behavioral therapy is most effective when an experienced therapist knowledgeable in child development individualizes these principles.

In mild cases, behavioral therapy alone is usually sufficient, but drug therapy may be needed in more severe cases or when access to an experienced child behavior therapist is limited. SSRIs are the usual 1st choice when drug therapy is needed (see TABLE 300–1).

Most children tolerate SSRIs without difficulty. Occasionally, upset stomach, diarrhea, or insomnia may occur. Some children exhibit behavioral side effects (BSE) that include activation and disinhibition (see Depressive Disorders on p. 2502). A few children do not tolerate SSRIs and, for them, serotonergic tricyclic antidepressants such as clomi-

TABLE 300–1. SSRIs FOR TREATING OLDER CHILDREN AND ADOLESCENTS

DRUG	STARTING DOSE	MAINTENANCE DOSE	COMMENTS/PRECAUTIONS*
Citalopram	20 mg once/day	40 mg once/day	Very similar to escitalopram
Escitalopram	10 mg once/day	20 mg once/day	Most selective SSRI
Fluoxetine	10 mg once/day	40 mg once/day	Long half-life; most activating SSRI; accumulation of active metabolites may occur in some patients
Fluvoxamine	50 mg once/day	100 mg bid	May elevate caffeine and other xanthine levels
Paroxetine	10 mg once/day	50 mg once/day or in divided doses	Most sedating SSRI; withdrawal effects may occur in some patients
Sertraline	25 mg once/day	50 mg once/day or in divided doses	FDA-approved for OCD to age 6

OCD = obsessive-compulsive disorder.

*Behavioral side effects (BSEs) such as disinhibition and behavioral activation can occur. Mild to moderate BSEs are common; patients usually respond to a downward adjustment in drug dose or a change to a different drug. In rare instances, severe BSEs such as aggressiveness or suicidality may appear. BSEs are idiosyncratic and may appear with any antidepressant and at any time during treatment. As a result, children and adolescents taking such drugs must be closely monitored.

Dose ranges are approximate. There is considerable individual variability in both therapeutic response and adverse effects; starting dose is increased only if needed. This table is not a substitute for the full prescribing information.

pramine or imipramine are useful alternatives; for both of these drugs, 25 mg po given at bedtime is a typical starting dose that often gives a satisfactory response. When higher doses are needed, serum drug levels should be monitored as well as ECGs. Tricyclic levels should generally not exceed 225 ng/mL, because higher levels are associated with an increased risk of adverse effects with little increased therapeutic benefit. Because of variability in drug absorption and metabolism, the dose needed to achieve these levels varies greatly. In some cases, dividing the single bedtime dose into a 2- or 3-dose regimen may be needed to reduce adverse effects.

Generalized Anxiety Disorder

Generalized anxiety disorder is a persistent state of heightened anxiety and apprehension characterized by excessive worrying, fear, and dread. Physical symptoms can include tremor, sweating, multiple somatic complaints, and exhaustion. Diagnosis is by history. Treatment is behavioral therapy, sometimes combined with drug therapy.

Generalized anxiety disorder (GAD) is diagnosed in children and adolescents who have prominent and impairing anxiety symptoms that are not focused enough to meet criteria for a specific disorder such as social phobia or panic disorder. In addition, GAD is an appropriate diagnosis for children who have a specific anxiety disorder, such as separation anxiety, but also have other significant anxiety symptoms above and beyond those of the specific anxiety disorder.

Occasionally, GAD can be confused with attention-deficit/hyperactivity disorder (ADHD—see p. 2483). Children who are diffusely anxious often have difficulty paying attention, and their anxiety can also result in psychomotor agitation (ie, hyperactivity). A key difference is that children with ADHD tend to be no more prone to worries than children without ADHD, whereas children with GAD have many distressing worries.

Because of the diffuse focus of symptoms, GAD is especially challenging to treat with behavioral therapy. Relaxation training is often more appropriate. Patients who have severe GAD or who do not respond to psychotherapeutic interventions may need anxiolytics. As with other anxiety disorders, SSRIs (see TABLE 300–1) are typically the drugs of choice. Buspirone is a useful alternative, especially for children who do not tolerate SSRIs; starting dose is 5 mg po bid and may be gradually increased to 30 mg bid (or 20 mg tid) as tolerated. GI distress or headache may be limiting factors in dosage escalation.

Social Phobia

(Social Anxiety Disorder)

Social phobia is a persistent fear of embarrassment, ridicule, or humiliation in social settings. Typically, affected children avoid situations that might provoke social scrutiny (such as school). Diagnosis is by history. Treatment is behavioral therapy; in severe cases, SSRIs are used.

School refusal is often the initial presentation of social phobia, particularly in adolescents. Complaints often have a somatic focus (eg, "My stomach hurts," "I have a headache"). In some cases, there is a history of many doctor appointments and medical evaluations in response to these somatic complaints. Affected children are terrified that they will humiliate themselves in front of their peers by giving the wrong answer, saying something inappropriate, becoming embarrassed, or even vomiting. In some cases, social phobia emerges after an unfortunate and embarrassing incident. In severe cases, children may refuse to talk on the telephone or even refuse to leave the house.

Behavioral therapy is the cornerstone of treatment. The child should not be allowed to miss school. Absence serves only to make the child even more reluctant to attend school.

Not all children and adolescents are sufficiently motivated to participate in behavioral therapy; others simply may not have an adequate response. For these children, an anxiolytic such as one of the SSRIs may be very helpful (see TABLE 300–1). Treatment with an SSRI may reduce anxiety enough to facilitate the child's participation in behavioral therapy.

Separation Anxiety Disorder

Separation anxiety disorder is a persistent, intense, and developmentally inappropriate fear of separation from a major attachment figure (usually the mother). Affected children desperately attempt to avoid such separations. When separation is forced, these children are distressfully preoccupied with reunification. Diagnosis is by history. Treatment is behavioral therapy for the child and family; in severe cases, SSRIs are used.

Separation anxiety is a normal emotion in children between about age 8 and 24 mo (see p. 2240); it typically resolves as children develop a sense of object permanence and realize their parents will return. In some children, separation anxiety persists beyond this time, or returns later, and may be severe enough to be considered a disorder.

Symptoms and Signs

Like social phobia, separation anxiety disorder often presents as school (or preschool) refusal. However, separation anxiety disorder commonly occurs in younger children and is rare after puberty. Separation anxiety is often compounded by the mother's own anxiety symptoms. Her own anxiety exacerbates the child's anxiety, leading to a vicious circle that can only be interrupted by sensitive and appropriate treatment of both the mother and child simultaneously.

Dramatic scenes typically occur at the time of separation; when separated, the child fixates on reunification with the attachment figure (typically the mother) and is often worried that she might have been harmed (eg, in a car accident, by a serious illness). The child also may refuse to sleep alone and may even insist on always being in the same room as the attachment figure. Separation scenes are typically painful for both mother and child. The child often wails and pleads with such desperation that the mother is unable to leave, which results in protracted scenes that are yet more difficult to interrupt. The child often develops somatic complaints.

The child's demeanor is often normal when the mother is present. This normal demeanor can sometimes give a false impression that the problem is of minor consequence.

Diagnosis and Treatment

Diagnosis is by history and by observation of separation scenarios.

Treatment is with behavioral therapy in which regular separations are systematically enforced. The goodbye scenes should be kept as brief as possible, and the child's mother should be coached to react to protestations matter-of-factly. Assisting the child in forming an attachment to one of the adults in the preschool or school setting may be helpful. In extreme cases, the child may benefit from an anxiolytic such as one of the SSRIs (see TABLE 300–1). However, separation anxiety disorder often affects children as young as 3 yr, and experience with these drugs in the very young is limited.

Successfully treated children are prone to relapses after holidays and breaks from school. Because of these relapses, it is often wise to plan regular separations during these periods to help the child remain accustomed to being away from the mother.

OBSESSIVE-COMPULSIVE DISORDER

Obsessive-compulsive disorder is characterized by obsessions, compulsions, or both. The obsessions and compulsions cause great distress and interfere with academic or social functioning. Diagnosis is by history. Treatment is behavioral therapy and SSRIs.

Most cases of obsessive-compulsive disorder (OCD) have no clear etiology. However, a few cases are thought to be associated with group A β-hemolytic streptococcal infections. This syndrome is called pediatric autoimmune neuropsychiatric disorder associated with streptococcus (PANDAS). PANDAS should be considered in all children with a sudden onset of severe OCD-like symptoms, because early antibiotic treatment may prevent or attenuate long-lasting impairment. This is currently an area of active research, and if PANDAS is suspected, consultation with a specialist is strongly recommended.

Symptoms and Signs

Typically, OCD has a gradual, insidious onset. Most children initially hide their symptoms and report struggling with symptoms years before a definitive diagnosis is made.

Obsessions are typically experienced as worries or fears of harm, eg, contracting a deadly disease, sinning and going to hell, or some form of injury to themselves or others. Compulsions are deliberate volitional acts, usually done for the purpose of neutralizing or offsetting obsessional fears, eg, checking behaviors; excessive washing, counting, arranging; and many more. The connection between the obsessions and compulsions may have an element of logic, eg, hand washing to avoid disease. In other cases, the relationship may be illogical and idiosyncratic, eg, counting to 50 over and over to prevent grandpa from having a heart attack.

Most children have some awareness that their obsessions and compulsions are abnormal. Many affected children are embarrassed and secretive. Raw, chapped hands may be the presentation for children who compulsively wash. Another common symptom is excessively long periods of time in the bathroom. Schoolwork may be done very slowly (because of an obsession about mistakes) or may be replete with corrections. Parents may note that the child engages in repetitive or odd behaviors such as checking door locks, chewing food a certain number of times, or avoiding touching certain things.

These children make frequent and tedious requests for reassurance, sometimes dozens or even hundreds of times per day. Some examples of reassurance seeking include questions such as, "Do you think I have a fever? Could we have a tornado? Do you think the car will start? What if we're late? What if the milk is sour? What if a burglar comes?"

Prognosis and Treatment

In about 5% of cases, the disorder remits after a few years and treatment can be discontinued. Remaining cases tend to be chronic, but normal functioning can be maintained with ongoing treatment. About 5% of children are resistant to treatment and remain greatly impaired.

In the vast majority of cases not associated with streptococcal infection, treatment is usually a combination of behavioral therapy and an SSRI. If appropriate services are available and the child is highly motivated, behavioral therapy alone may be adequate treatment.

Panic Disorder and Agoraphobia

Panic disorder is present when a child has recurrent, frequent (at least once/wk) panic attacks. Panic attacks are discrete spells lasting about 20 min during which the child experiences somatic or cognitive symptoms. Panic disorder can occur with or without agoraphobia. Agoraphobia is a persistent fear of being trapped in situations or places without a way to escape easily and without help. Diagnosis is by history. Treatment is with benzodiazepines or SSRIs and behavioral therapy.

Panic disorder is rare in prepubertal children compared to adolescents. TABLE 196–2 on p. 1675 lists symptoms of a panic attack. Because many panic symptoms are somatic in nature, many children undergo medical assessments before panic disorder is suspected. This diagnosis is further complicated in children who have a concurrent medical illness, especially asthma; a panic attack can trigger an asthma attack and vice versa. Panic attacks also can occur in the context of other anxiety disorders such as OCD or separation anxiety.

Panic attacks usually develop spontaneously, but over time, children begin to attribute them to certain situations and environments. Affected children then attempt to avoid those situations, which can lead to agoraphobia. Agoraphobia is diagnosed when the child's avoidance behaviors are of such a degree that they greatly impair normal functioning, such as going to school, visiting the mall, or doing other typical activities.

In adult panic disorder, concerns about future attacks, the implications of the attacks, and changes in behavior are important features of the diagnostic criteria. Children and younger adolescents usually lack the sufficient insight and forethought necessary to evolve these additional manifestations. Behavioral changes, when they occur, typically involve avoiding circumstances or situations related (in the child's belief) to the panic attack.

Diagnosis

In most cases, a physical examination should be done to rule out medical causes of somatic symptoms. Careful screening is needed for other anxiety disorders, such as OCD or social phobia, because any one of these disorders may be the primary problem and the panic attacks a secondary symptom.

Prognosis and Treatment

Prognosis for panic disorder with or without agoraphobia in children and adolescents is good with treatment. Without treatment, adolescents may drop out of school, withdraw from society, and become reclusive and suicidal. Panic disorder often waxes and wanes in severity without any discernible reason. Some patients experience long periods of spontaneous symptom remission, only to experience a relapse years later.

Treatment is usually a combination of drug therapy and behavioral therapy. In children, it is difficult to even begin behavioral therapy until the panic attacks have been controlled by drug therapy. Benzodiazepines are the most effective drugs for controlling panic attacks, but SSRIs are often preferred because benzodiazepines are sedating and may greatly impair learning and memory. However, SSRIs do not work quickly, and a short course of a benzodiazepine (eg, lorazepam 0.5 to 2.0 mg po tid) may be helpful until the SSRI is effective.

Behavioral therapy is especially useful for agoraphobia symptoms. These symptoms rarely respond to drugs, because children often continue to fear they might have a panic attack, even long after their panic has been well controlled by drug therapy.

Acute and Posttraumatic Stress Disorders

Acute stress disorder (ASD) is a brief period (about 1 mo) of intrusive recollections (eg, flashbacks and nightmares), dissociation, avoidance, and anxiety occurring within 1 mo of a traumatic incident. Posttraumatic stress disorder (PTSD) produces recurring, intrusive recollections of an overwhelming traumatic incident that persist > 1 mo, as well as emotional numbing and hyperarousal. Diagnosis is by history and examination. Treatment is behavioral therapy, SSRIs, and antiadrenergic agents.

Because of differences in vulnerability and temperament, not all children who are exposed to a severe traumatic event develop a disorder. Traumatic events commonly associated with these disorders include assaults, sexual assaults, car accidents, dog attacks, and injuries (especially burns). In young children, domestic violence is the most common cause of PTSD.

Symptoms, Signs, and Diagnosis

ASD and PTSD are closely related and are distinguished primarily by duration of symptoms; ASD is diagnosed within 1 mo of the traumatic event and PTSD only after 1 mo has passed and symptoms have persisted. Also, a child with ASD is typically "in a daze" and may seem dissociated from everyday surroundings.

Intrusive recollections cause these children to re-experience the traumatic event. The most dramatic kind of recollection is a flashback. Flashbacks may be spontaneous but are most commonly triggered by something associated with the original trauma. For example, the sight of a dog may trigger a flashback in children who experienced a dog attack. During a flashback, these children may be in a terrified state and unaware of their current surroundings while desperately searching for a way to hide or escape; they may temporarily lose touch with reality and believe they are in grave danger. Some children experience nightmares. With other kinds of reexperiencing (eg, thoughts, mental images, recollections), these children maintain awareness of current surroundings, although they may still be greatly distressed.

"Emotional numbing" describes a group of symptoms that includes general lack of interest, social withdrawal, and a subjective sense of feeling "numb." The child may develop a foreshortened expectation of the future, eg, "I will not live to see 20."

Hyperarousal symptoms include a sense of jitteriness, exaggerated startle response, and difficulty relaxing. Sleep may be disrupted and complicated by frequent nightmares.

Diagnosis of ASD and PTSD is based on history of severely frightening and horrifying trauma followed by the onset of reexperiencing, emotional numbing, and hyperarousal. These symptoms must be severe enough to cause impairment or distress. In a few cases, the onset of symptoms of PTSD may be delayed months or even years after the traumatic incident.

Prognosis and Treatment

Prognosis for ASD is much better than for PTSD but both benefit from early treatment. The severity of the trauma, associated physical injuries, and the underlying resiliency of the child and family all affect the final outcome.

SSRIs are often helpful in reducing the emotional numbing and replaying symptoms but are less effective for hyperarousal. Antiadrenergic agents (eg, clonidine, guanfacine, prazosin) may be helpful for hyperarousal symptoms, but supportive data are preliminary. Supportive psychotherapy may be helpful in children who have adjustment issues associated with trauma, such as disfigurement from burns. Behavioral therapy can be useful for systematic desensitizing against triggers that replay symptoms.

CHILDHOOD SCHIZOPHRENIA

(See also p. 1722.)

Schizophrenia is defined as the presence of hallucinations and delusions causing considerable psychosocial dysfunction and lasting ≥ 6 mo.

Onset of schizophrenia is typically from mid-adolescence to the mid-20s. Features in adolescents and young adults are quite similar (see full discussion on p. 1723). Schizophrenia in prepubertal children is extremely rare; features are usually similar to those in adolescents and adults, but delusions and visual hallucinations (which may be more common in children) may be less elaborate.

Sudden-onset psychosis in a young child should always be treated as a medical emergency with a thorough medical assessment to search for a physiologic cause of the mental status change (eg, Wilson's disease, the porphyrias, HIV infection, brain trauma).

DEPRESSIVE DISORDERS

(See also p. 1704.)

Depressive disorders in children and adolescents are characterized by a pervasive and abnormal mood state consisting of sadness or irritability that is severe or persistent enough to interfere with functioning or cause considerable distress. Decreased interest or pleasure in activities may be as or even more apparent than the mood abnormalities. Diagnosis is by history and examination. Treatment is with antidepressants, psychotherapy, or both.

Major depression occurs in as many as 2% of children and 5% of adolescents. Rates for other depressive disorders are unknown. The exact cause of depression in children and adolescents is unknown, but in adults, it is believed to result from the interactions of genetically determined risk factors and environmental stress (particularly early life deprivation and loss).

Symptoms and Signs

The basic manifestations of childhood depression are similar to those seen in adults but are related to typical concerns of children, such as schoolwork and play. Children may be unable to explain inner feelings or moods. Depression should be considered when a previously well-performing youth does poorly in school, withdraws from society, or commits delinquent acts.

Common symptoms include a sad appearance, excessive irritability, apathy and withdrawal, reduced capacity for pleasure (often expressed as profound boredom), feeling rejected and unloved, somatic complaints (eg, headaches, abdominal pain, insomnia), and persistent self-blame. Others include anorexia, weight loss (or failure to achieve expected weight gain), sleep disruption (including nightmares), despondency, and suicidal ideation. The irritability associated with childhood depression may manifest as overactivity and aggressive, antisocial behavior.

Mood disorders can occur in children with mental retardation but may manifest as somatic symptoms and behavioral disturbances.

Diagnosis

Diagnosis is based on symptoms and signs. A careful review of the history and appropriate laboratory studies are needed to exclude drug abuse and physical disorders such as infectious mononucleosis and thyroid disease. History should address causative factors such as domestic violence, sexual abuse and exploitation, and drug adverse effects. Questions about suicidal behavior (eg, ideation, gestures, attempts) should be asked.

Other mental disorders that can cause depressive symptoms must also be considered, including anxiety and bipolar disorders. Some children who go on to develop a bipolar disorder or schizophrenia present initially with major depression.

Prognosis and Treatment

Major depression in adolescents is a risk factor for academic failure, substance abuse, and suicidal behavior (see p. 2506). Untreated, major depression may remit in 6 to 12 mo, but recurrences are common. Furthermore, while they are depressed, children and adolescents tend to fall far behind academically, lose important peer relationships, and are at increased risk for substance abuse.

Evaluation of the family and social setting is required to identify stresses that may have precipitated depression. Appropriate measures directed at the family and school must accompany direct treatment of the child to enhance continued functioning and provide appropriate educational accommodations. Brief hospitalization may be necessary in acute crises, especially when suicidal behavior is identified.

Treatment response in adolescent depression generally parallels that of adult depression. In most adult depression studies, a combination of psychotherapy and antidepressants greatly outperforms either modality used alone. The situation in preadolescent depression is much less clear. Most clinicians opt for a course of psychotherapy in younger children unless the depression is severe or has not previously responded to psychotherapy. In the more severe cases, antidepressants may provide a useful adjunct to psychotherapy.

Usually, an SSRI (see TABLE 300–1) is the 1st-line choice when an antidepressant is indicated. Children should be closely monitored for the emergence of behavioral side effects (see footnote in TABLE 300–1), such as disinhibition and behavioral activation. Adult-based research has suggested that antidepressants that act on both the serotonergic and adrenergic/dopaminergic systems may be modestly more effective; however, such drugs (eg, duloxetine, venlafaxine, mirtazapine; certain tricyclics, particularly clomipramine) also tend to have more adverse effects. Such drugs may be especially useful in treatment-resistant cases. Nonserotonergic antidepressants such as bupropion and desipramine may also be combined with an SSRI to enhance efficacy.

As in adults, relapse and recurrence are common. Children and adolescents should remain in treatment for at least 1 yr after symptoms have remitted. Most experts now agree that children who have experienced ≥ 2 episodes of major depression should be treated indefinitely.

BIPOLAR DISORDER

Bipolar disorder is characterized by alternating periods of manic, depressed, and normal mood states, each lasting for weeks to months at a time. In recent years, the label "bipolar" has also been applied to prepubertal children disabled by intense, unstable moods. In these young children, however, the mood states last from moments to days. In both cases, diagnosis is by history and mental status examination; treatment is a combination of mood stabilizers (eg, lithium, certain anti-epilepsy and antipsychotic drugs), psychotherapy, and psychosocial support.

Bipolar disorder typically begins during mid-adolescence to the mid-20s. In many cases, the initial manifestation is one or more episodes of depression; about 1/3 of children who experience an episode of severe depression before puberty will "convert" to bipolar disorder during their adolescent or early adult years.

Symptoms, Signs, and Diagnosis

The hallmark of bipolar disorder is the manic episode. During a manic episode, the adolescent's mood may be either very positive or hyperirritable and often alternates depending on social circumstances. Speech is rapid and pressured, sleep is decreased, and self-esteem is inflated. Mania may reach psychotic proportions, eg, "I have become one with God." Judgment may be severely impaired, and the adolescent may engage in risky behaviors such as promiscuous sex or reckless driving.

In recent years, the term "bipolar" has been applied to prepubertal children with unstable, intense moods. This is controversial and an area of active research. These children experience dramatic mood states, but the duration of these mood states is much shorter, often lasting only a few moments. Onset is characteristically insidious, and history is typically that the child has always been very temperamental and difficult to manage.

A number of medical conditions and drug intoxication must be ruled out with the appropriate medical assessment, including a toxicology screen for both drugs of abuse (eg, amphetamines, cocaine, phencyclidines) and environmental toxins (eg, lead). The interviewer should also search for precipitating events, such as severe psychologic stress, including sexual abuse or incest.

Prognosis and Treatment

Prognosis for adolescent-onset bipolar disorder is variable. Patients who have mild to moderate symptoms, who have a good response to treatment, and who remain compliant and cooperative with treatment have an excellent prognosis. All too often, however, treatment response is incomplete, and adolescents are notoriously noncompliant with medications. The long-term prognosis for these patients is not as good. At present, little is known about the long-term prognosis of young children diagnosed with bipolar disorder based on highly unstable and intense moods.

For both adolescents and young children, mood stabilizers treat the manic or agitated phase of the illness while psychotherapy and antidepressants treat the depressive periods. Mood stabilizers roughly fall into 3 categories: mood-stabilizing anti-epilepsy drugs, mood-stabilizing antipsychotics, and lithium (see TABLE 300–2). All mood stabilizers have a potential to produce troubling and even dangerous adverse effects. Because of this potential, treatment must be individualized. Furthermore, drugs that are highly successful during the initial stabilization period may be unacceptable for maintenance because of adverse effects, most notably weight

TABLE 300–2. SELECTED DRUGS FOR BIPOLAR DISORDER

DRUG	SYMPTOM INDICATION	STARTING DOSE*	MAINTENANCE DOSE*	NOTES
Lithium	Acute and maintenance	300 mg bid	300–1200 mg bid	Dose titrated to a blood level of 0.8–1.2 mEq/L
Antipsychotics				
Chlorpromazine	Acute mania	10 mg once/day	50–300 bid	Rarely used because newer drugs have a more favorable adverse effect profile
Olanzapine	Acute mania	5 mg once/day	Up to 7.5 mg bid	Weight gain may be a limiting adverse effect in some patients
Risperidone	Acute mania	1 mg once/day	Up to 3 mg bid	Higher doses increase the risk of neurologic adverse effects
Quetiapine	Acute mania	25 mg bid	Up to 200 mg bid	Sedation may limit dose increases
Olanzapine/fluoxetine fixed combination	Bipolar depression	6 mg/25 mg once/day	Up to 12 mg/50 mg once/day	Limited experience in children
Aripiprazole	Acute mania	5 mg once/day	Up to 30 mg once/day	Very limited experience in children
Ziprasidone	Acute mania	20 mg bid	Up to 80 mg bid	Very limited experience in children
Antiepileptics				
Divalproex	Acute mania	250 mg bid	Up to 30 mg/kg bid in divided doses	Dose titrated to a blood level of 50–125 μg/mL
Lamotrigine	Maintenance	25 mg once/day	Up to 100 mg bid	Dosing guidelines in the package insert should be followed closely
Carbamazepine	Acute mania and mixed	200 mg bid	Up to 600 mg bid	Because of metabolic enzyme induction, dose adjustments may be necessary

* Dose ranges are approximate. There is considerable individual variability in both therapeutic response and adverse effects. This table is not a substitute for the full prescribing information.

NOTE: These drugs carry a small but serious risk for a wide variety of major adverse effects. Therefore, benefits must be carefully weighed against the potential risks.

gain. Antidepressants are usually used in conjunction with a mood stabilizer, because they may trigger a "switch" from depression to mania.

DISRUPTIVE BEHAVIORAL DISORDERS

These disorders are so-named because affected children tend to disrupt those around them, including family members, school staff, and peers. The most common disruptive behavioral disorder is attention-deficit/hyperactivity disorder (see p. 2483).

Oppositional Defiant Disorder

Oppositional defiant disorder is a recurrent or persistent pattern of negative, defiant, or even hostile behavior directed at authority figures. Diagnosis is by history. Treatment is individual psychotherapy combined with family or caretaker therapy. Occasionally, drugs may be used to reduce irritability.

Prevalence estimates vary widely because the diagnostic criteria are highly subjective; prevalence of oppositional defiant disorder (ODD) may be as high as 15% of children and adolescents. Before puberty, affected boys greatly outnumber girls; after puberty, the difference narrows.

Although ODD is sometimes viewed as a "mild version" of conduct disorder, only superficial similarities exist between the 2 disorders. The hallmark of ODD is an interpersonal style characterized by irritability and defiance. A child with a conduct disorder, however, seemingly lacks a conscience and repeatedly violates the rights of others—sometimes without any evidence of irritability. The etiology of ODD is unknown, but it is probably most common in children from families in which the adults model loud, argumentative, interpersonal conflicts. This diagnosis should not be viewed as a circumscribed disorder but rather as an indication of underlying problems that may require further investigation and treatment.

Symptoms, Signs, and Diagnosis

Children with ODD tend to lose their temper easily and repeatedly, argue with adults, frequently defy adults, refuse to obey rules, deliberately annoy people, blame others for their own mistakes or misbehavior, be easily annoyed and angered, and be spiteful or vindictive. ODD is diagnosed if a child has had ≥ 4 of these symptoms for at least 6 mo. The symptoms must also be severe and disruptive. Caution must be taken to avoid incorrectly diagnosing ODD in response to the mild to moderate oppositional behaviors demonstrated periodically by nearly all children and adolescents.

ODD-like symptoms are often seen in children with untreated attention-deficit/hyperactivity disorder (ADHD). ODD-like symptoms often resolve when ADHD is adequately treated. Additionally, childhood major depressive disorder (MDD) may be mistaken for ODD, because in some children with MDD, the predominant mood is irritability rather than sadness (an important distinction between childhood and adult MDD). Because irritability is also the hallmark of ODD, MDD in these children is identified by the presence of anhedonia and neurovegetative symptoms (eg, sleep and appetite disruption); these symptoms are easily overlooked in children.

Prognosis and Treatment

Prognosis depends on identifying and successfully treating underlying mood disorders, family dysfunction, and ADHD. Even without treatment, most cases of ODD gradually improve over time.

Initially, the treatment of choice is a rewards-based behavior modification program designed to shape the child's behaviors in a more socially appropriate direction. In addition, many of these children lack social skills and can benefit from group-based, skills-building therapy. Sometimes, drugs used for depressive disorders (see p. 2502) may be beneficial.

Conduct Disorder

Conduct disorder is a recurrent or persistent pattern of behavior that violates the rights of others or major age-appropriate societal norms or rules. Diagnosis is by history. No treatment has been proven effective, and many children require considerable supervision.

The prevalence of some level of conduct disorder (CD) is about 10%. Onset is usually in late childhood or early adolescence, and the disorder is much more common in boys than girls. The etiology is likely a complex interplay of genetic and environmental factors.

Parents of adolescents with CD often have engaged in substance abuse and antisocial behaviors, and frequently have been diagnosed with ADHD, mood disorders, schizophrenia, or antisocial personality disorder. However, CD can occur in children from high-functioning, healthy families.

Symptoms, Signs, and Diagnosis

Children or adolescents with CD lack sensitivity to the feelings and well-being of others and sometimes misperceive the behavior of others as threatening. They may demonstrate aggression by bullying and making threats, brandishing or using a weapon, committing acts of physical cruelty, or forcing someone into sexual activity, all with little or no feelings of remorse. In some cases their aggression and cruelty is directed at animals. These children or adolescents may engage in destruction of property, deceit, and theft. They tolerate frustration poorly and are commonly reckless, violating rules and parental prohibitions (eg, by running away from home, being frequently truant from school). Aberrant behaviors differ between the sexes: Boys tend to fight, steal, and vandalize; girls are likely to lie, run away, and engage in prostitution. Both genders are likely to use and abuse illicit drugs and have difficulties in school. Suicidal ideation is common, and suicide attempts must be taken seriously.

CD is diagnosed if the child or adolescent has demonstrated ≥ 3 of the above findings in the previous 12 mo, and at least 1 in the previous 6 mo. The symptoms or behaviors must be significant enough to impair functioning in relationships, at school, or at work.

Prognosis and Treatment

Most youth with CD cease their disruptive behaviors in early adulthood, but about ⅓ of cases persist. Of these, many meet criteria for antisocial personality disorder. Early onset is associated with a poorer prognosis. Some develop subsequent mood or anxiety disorders, somatoform and substance-related disorders, and early adult-onset psychotic disorders. Children and adolescents with CD tend to have higher rates of physical and other mental disorders.

Treating comorbid disorders with drug therapy and psychotherapy may improve the patient's self-esteem and self-control and ultimately improve control of CD. Moralization and dire admonitions are ineffective and should be avoided. Individual psychotherapy, including cognitive therapy and behavior modification, may help. Often, only separation from a damaging environment and external discipline and consistent behavioral management systems offer hope of success.

SUICIDAL BEHAVIOR

(See also p. 1741.)

Youth suicide rates have declined in recent years after more than a decade of steady increase. The reasons for the previous increase and the recent decline remain unclear. It has been proposed that the more liberal use of antidepressants may be partially responsible for the recent decline in this statistic, although there is growing suspicion that certain antidepressants increase the risk of suicidal behavior. Nonetheless, suicide is the 2nd or 3rd leading cause of death in 15- to 19-yr-olds and remains a considerable public health concern.

Risk factors: These vary by age. More than ½ of adolescent suicidal behaviors stem from depression. Other predisposing factors include a history of suicide in family members or close friends, a recent death in the family, substance abuse, and conduct disorder (see p. 2505). More immediate precipitating factors can include loss of self-esteem (eg, resulting from family arguments, a humiliating disciplinary episode, pregnancy, school failure); loss of a boyfriend or girlfriend; and loss of familiar surroundings (eg, school, neighborhood, friends) due to a geographic move. Other factors may be a lack of structure and boundaries, leading to an overwhelming feeling of lack of direction, or intense parental pressure to succeed accompanied by the feeling of falling short of expectations. A frequent motive for a suicide attempt is the effort to manipulate or punish others with the fantasy "You will be sorry after I am dead." A rise in suicides is seen after a well-publicized suicide (eg, of a rock star) and among self-identified populations (eg, a high school, a college dormitory), indicating the power of suggestion. Early community intervention to support youths in such circumstances may be helpful.

Treatment

Every suicide attempt is a serious matter that requires thoughtful and appropriate intervention. Once the immediate threat to life has been removed, a decision has to be made regarding the need for hospitalization. This need depends on the balance between the degree of risk and the family's capacity to provide support. Hospitalization (even on an open medical or pediatric ward with special-duty nursing) is the surest form of short-term protection and usually is indicated if depression, psychosis, or both are suspected.

Lethality of suicidal intent can be assessed by the degree of forethought evidenced (eg, writing a suicide note), the method used (firearms are more lethal than pills), the degree of self-injury sustained, and the circumstances or immediate precipitating factors surrounding the attempt.

Drug therapy may be indicated for any underlying disorder (eg, depression, bipolar or impulse disorder, psychosis) but cannot prevent suicide. Indeed, antidepressant use may increase the risk of suicide in some adolescents. Drugs should be carefully monitored and supplied in sublethal amounts. Psychiatric referral is most successful if continuity with the primary caretaker occurs. Rebuilding morale and restoring emotional equilibrium within the family are essential. A negative or unsupportive parental response is a serious concern and may suggest a need for a more intensive intervention such as out-of-home placement. If the family shows love and concern, a positive outcome is most likely.

Prevention

Suicidal incidents often are preceded by behavioral changes (eg, despondent mood, low self-esteem, sleep and appetite disturbances, inability to concentrate, truancy from school, somatic complaints, and suicidal preoccupation), which often bring the child or adolescent to the physician's office. Statements such as "I wish I had never been born" or "I would like to go to sleep and never wake up" should be taken seriously as possible indications of suicidal intent. A suicidal threat or attempt represents an important communication about the intensity of experienced despair. Early recognition of the risk factors mentioned above may help prevent a suicide attempt. In responding to these early cues, or when confronted with threatened or attempted suicide or severe risk-taking behavior, vigorous intervention is appropriate. Patients should be directly questioned about their unhappy or self-destructive feelings; such direct questioning may diminish suicide risk. The physician should not provide unfounded reassurance, which can undermine the physician's credibility and further lower the patient's self-esteem.

SELF-INJURIOUS BEHAVIOR

In recent years, many communities have seen a virtual epidemic of self-injurious behaviors that are sometimes confused with suicidal intentions. These behaviors include superficial scratching and cutting, burning the skin with cigarettes or curling irons, crude ballpoint pen tattoos, and many others. In some communities, these behaviors suddenly sweep through a high school in fad-like fashion and then gradually diminish over time.

In many instances, these behaviors are not indicative of suicidality but instead are the adolescent's effort to establish autonomy, identify with a peer group, or provocatively gain parental attention. Even when these behaviors are not an expression of suicidality, they are serious and warrant intervention. Such behaviors suggest the adolescent is in great distress and are often associated with illicit substance abuse.

All self-injurious behaviors should be evaluated by a clinician experienced in working with troubled adolescents to assess whether suicidality is an issue and to diagnose the underlying distress leading to the self-injurious behaviors.

301 CHILD MALTREATMENT

Child maltreatment is behavior toward a child that is outside the norms of conduct and entails substantial risk of causing physical or emotional harm. Four types of maltreatment are generally recognized: physical abuse, sexual abuse, emotional abuse (psychologic abuse), and neglect. The causes of child maltreatment are varied and not well understood. Abuse and neglect are often associated with physical injuries, delayed growth and development, and mental

problems. Diagnosis is based on history and physical examination. Management includes documentation and treatment of any injuries and urgent physical and mental conditions, mandatory reporting to appropriate state agencies, and sometimes hospitalization or other steps such as foster care to keep the child safe.

In 2002, 1.8 million cases of child abuse and neglect were reported in the US, of which about 896,000 were confirmed. Both sexes are affected equally.

About 1400 children died in the US from maltreatment in 2002, about ¾ of whom were < 4 yr. One third of the fatalities were attributed to neglect. Children from birth to age 3 yr had the highest rate of victimization (16/1000 children). More than ½ of all reports to Child Protective Services were made by professionals who are mandated to report maltreatment (eg, educators, law enforcement personnel, social services personnel, legal professionals, day care providers, medical or mental health personnel, foster care providers).

Of confirmed cases in the US in 2002, 60.2% involved neglect (including medical neglect); 18.6%, physical abuse; 9.9%, sexual abuse; and 6.5%, emotional abuse. In addition, 18.9% experienced other types of maltreatment, such as abandonment and congenital drug addictions. Many children were victims of multiple types of maltreatment. In confirmed cases of abuse or neglect in 2002, > 80% of the perpetrators were parents; 58% of perpetrators were women.

Classification

Different forms often coexist, and overlap is considerable.

Physical abuse: Physical abuse is inflicting physical harm or engaging in actions that create a high risk of harm. Specific forms include shaking, dropping, striking, biting, and burning (eg, by scalding or touching with cigarettes). Severe corporal punishment constitutes physical abuse, but this may be culturally defined. Abuse is the most common cause of serious head injury in infants. In toddlers, abdominal injury is common.

Infants and toddlers are the most vulnerable (perhaps because perpetrators know they cannot complain), with risk declining in the early school years and increasing again in adolescence.

Sexual abuse: Any action with a child that is done for the sexual gratification of an adult or significantly older child constitutes sexual abuse (see also Pedophilia on p. 1735). Forms of sexual abuse include intercourse, which is oral, anal, or vaginal penetration; molestation, which is genital contact without intercourse; and nonspecific forms, which do not involve physical contact, including exposure, showing sexual material to a child, and forcing a child to participate in a sex act with another child or to participate in the making of sexual material.

Sexual abuse does not include sexual play, in which children close in age (typically considered < 4 yr apart) view or touch each other's genital area without force or coercion.

Emotional abuse: Emotional abuse is infliction of emotional harm through the use of words or actions. Specific forms include berating a child by yelling or screaming, spurning by belittling the child's abilities and achievements, intimidating and terrorizing with threats, and exploiting or corrupting by encouraging deviant or criminal behavior. Emotional abuse can also occur when words or actions are omitted or withheld, in essence becoming emotional neglect (eg, ignoring or rejecting a child or isolating him from interaction with other children or adults).

Neglect: Neglect is the failure to provide for or meet a child's basic physical, emotional, educational, and medical needs. Neglect differs from abuse in that it usually occurs without intent to harm. Physical neglect includes failure to provide adequate food, clothing, shelter, supervision, and protection from potential harm. Emotional neglect is failure to provide affection or love or other kinds of emotional support. Educational neglect is failure to enroll a child in school, ensure attendance at school, or provide home schooling. Medical neglect is failure to ensure that a child receives appropriate preventive care, such as vaccines or needed treatment for injuries or physical or mental disorders.

Etiology

Abuse: Generally, abuse can be attributed to a breakdown of impulse control in the parent or caregiver. Several factors contribute.

Parental characteristics and personality features can play a role. The parent's own childhood may have lacked affection and warmth, may not have been conducive to the development of adequate self-esteem or emotional maturity, and in most cases also included other forms of abuse. Abusive parents may look toward their children as a source of unlimited and unconditional affection and the support that they never received. As a result, they may have unrealistic expectations of what their child can supply for them; they are frustrated easily and lose control; and they may be unable to give what they never experienced. Drug or alcohol use may provoke impulsive and uncontrolled behaviors toward the child. Parental mental disorders may increase the risk, and in some cases abuse occurs while a parent is psychotic.

Irritable, demanding, or hyperactive children may provoke parents' tempers, as may a developmentally or physically disabled child, who often is more dependent. Sometimes, strong emotional ties do not develop between parents and premature or sick infants separated from parents early in infancy or with biologically unrelated children (eg, stepchildren), increasing the risk of abuse.

Situational stress may precipitate abuse, particularly when emotional support of relatives, friends, neighbors, or peers is unavailable.

Physical abuse, emotional abuse, and neglect are associated with poverty and lower socioeconomic status. However, all types of abuse, including sexual abuse, occur across the spectrum of socioeconomic groups. The risk of sexual abuse is increased in children who have several caregivers or a caregiver with several sex partners.

Neglect: Neglect often occurs in impoverished families in which parents also have mental disorders (typically depression or schizophrenia), drug or alcohol abuse, or limited intellectual capacity. Desertion by a father who is unable or unwilling to assert a controlling influence in the family may precipitate neglect. Children of cocaine-using mothers are particularly at risk of desertion.

Symptoms and Signs

Symptoms and signs depend on the nature and duration of the abuse or neglect.

Physical abuse: Skin lesions are common and may include handprints or oval fingertip marks from slapping or grabbing and shaking; long, bandlike ecchymoses from belt whipping or narrow arcuate bruises from extension cord whipping; multiple small round burns from cigarettes; symmetric scald burns of upper or lower extremities or buttocks from intentional immersion; bite marks; and thickened skin or scarring at the corners of the mouth from being gagged. Patchy alopecia can result from hair pulling.

Fractures frequently associated with physical abuse include rib fractures, vertebral fractures, long bone and digit fractures in nonambulatory children, and metaphyseal fractures. Confusion and localizing neurologic abnormalities can occur with CNS injuries. Infants subjected to violent shaking may be comatose or stuporous from brain injury yet lack visible signs of injury (with the common exception of retinal hemorrhage). Traumatic injury to organs within the chest or abdominal region may also occur without visible signs.

Children who are frequently abused are often fearful and irritable and sleep poorly. They may appear depressed or anxious. Violent or suicidal behavior may occur.

Sexual abuse: In most cases, children do not freely disclose sexual abuse and rarely exhibit behavioral or physical signs of sexual abuse. In some cases, abrupt or extreme changes in behavior may occur. Aggressiveness or withdrawal may develop, as may phobias or sleep disturbances. Some sexually abused children act in ways that are sexually inappropriate for their age. Physical signs of sexual abuse may include difficulty in walking or sitting; bruises or tears around the genitals, rectum, or mouth; vaginal discharge or pruritus; or a sexually transmitted disease. If a disclosure is made, it is generally delayed, sometimes days to years. After a delay of a few days to 2 wk, the genitals may be normal or may reveal healed, subtle hymen changes.

Emotional abuse: In early infancy, emotional abuse may blunt emotional expressiveness and decrease interest in the environment. Emotional abuse commonly results in failure to thrive and is often misdiagnosed as mental retardation or physical illness. Delayed development of social and language skills often results from inadequate parental stimulation and interaction. Emotionally abused children may be insecure, anxious, distrustful, superficial in interpersonal relationships, passive, and overly concerned with pleasing adults. Children who are spurned may have very low self-esteem. Children who are terrorized or threatened may seem fearful and withdrawn. The emotional effect on children usually becomes obvious at school age, when difficulties develop in forming relationships with teachers and peers. Often, emotional effects are appreciated only after the child has been placed in another environment or after aberrant behaviors abate and are replaced by more acceptable behaviors.

Children who are exploited may commit crimes or abuse alcohol or drugs.

Neglect: Malnutrition, fatigue, lack of hygiene or appropriate clothing, and failure to thrive are common signs due to inadequate provision of food, clothing, or shelter. Stunted growth and death from starvation or exposure may occur.

Diagnosis

Evaluation of injuries and nutritional deficiencies is discussed elsewhere in THE MANUAL. Recognition of maltreatment as the cause can be difficult, and a high index of suspicion must be maintained. Diagnosis of inflicted acute head trauma is commonly missed when it occurs in 2-parent households with median-level incomes.

Sometimes direct questions provide an answer. Children who have been maltreated may describe the events and the perpetrator, but some children, particularly those who have been sexually abused, may be sworn to secrecy, threatened, or so traumatized that they are reluctant to speak (and may even deny abuse when specifically questioned). The child should be interviewed alone in a relaxed manner, with open-ended questions; yes-or-no questions ("Did daddy do this?" "Did he touch you here?") can easily sculpt an untrue history in young children.

Examination includes observation of interactions between the victim and possible perpetrators whenever possible. Documentation of the history and physical examination should be as comprehensive and accurate as possible, including recording of exact quotes from the history and photographs of injuries.

Physical abuse: Both history and physical examination provide clues suggestive of maltreatment. Features suggestive of abuse on history are parental reluctance or inability to give a history of injury; a history that is inconsistent with the injury (eg, bruises on the backs of the legs attributed to a fall) or apparent stage of resolution (eg, old injuries described as recent); a history that varies depending on the information source; a history of injury that is incompatible with the child's stage of development (eg, injuries ascribed to a fall downstairs in an infant too young to crawl); an inappropriate response by the parents to the severity of the injury—either overly concerned or unconcerned; and delay in reporting the injury.

Major indicators of abuse on examination are atypical injuries and injuries incompatible with stated history. Childhood injuries resulting from falls are typically solitary and on the forehead, chin or mouth, or extensor surfaces of the extremities, particularly elbows, knees, forearms, and shins. Bruises on the back, buttocks, and the back of the legs are extremely rare from falls. Fractures, apart from clavicular fracture and distal radius (Colles') fracture, are less common in typical falls during play or down stairs. No fractures are pathognomonic of abuse, but classic metaphyseal lesions, rib fractures (especially posterior and 1st rib), and depressed or multiple skull fractures from apparently minor trauma, scapular fractures, sternal fractures, and spinous processes fractures should raise concern.

Physical abuse should be considered when an infant who is not walking has a serious injury. Young infants with minor injuries to the face should be further evaluated. The younger infant may appear to be perfectly normal or sleeping despite significant brain trauma, and inflicted acute head trauma in infants should be part of the differential diagnosis of every lethargic infant. Other hints are multiple injuries at different stages of resolution or development; cutaneous lesions specific for particular sources of injury; and repeated injury, which is suggestive of abuse or inadequate supervision.

Retinal hemorrhage occurs in 65 to 95% of shaken babies and is quite rare in accidental head trauma. It also may occur from childbirth and persist for up to 4 wk.

Children < 2 yr with possible physical abuse should undergo a skeletal survey for evidence of previous bony injuries (fractures in various stages of healing or subperiosteal elevations in long bones). Surveys are sometimes obtained on children aged 2 to 5 yr but are generally not helpful for those > 5 yr. The standard survey includes anteroposterior (AP) views of the skull and chest, lateral views of the spine and long bones, AP views of the pelvis, and AP and oblique views of the hands. Physical disorders causing multiple fractures include osteogenesis imperfecta and congenital syphilis.

Sexual abuse: Sexually transmitted disease (STD) of any sort in a child < 12 yr must be considered the result of sexual abuse until proven otherwise. When a child has been sexually abused, behavioral change (eg, irritability, fearfulness, insomnia) may be the only clue initially. If sexual abuse is suspected, the perioral and rectal areas and the external genitals must be examined for evidence of injury.

If the suspected abuse is thought to have occurred recently, hair samples and swabs of body fluids are obtained for legal evidence (see p. 2105). An examination involving use of a magnifying light source with a camera, such as with a specially equipped colposcope, may be helpful for documentation for legal purposes.

Emotional abuse and neglect: Evaluation focuses on general appearance and behavior to determine whether the child is failing to develop normally. Teachers and social workers are often the first to recognize neglect. The physician may notice a pattern of missed appointments and vaccinations that are not up-to-date. Medical neglect of life-threatening, chronic diseases, such as reactive airways dysfunction syndrome or diabetes, can lead to a subsequent increase in office or emergency department visits and poor compliance with recommended drugs.

Treatment

Treatment first addresses urgent medical needs (including possible STDs) and the child's immediate safety. Ultimately, treatment is directed at long-standing disturbed patterns of personal interaction. In both abuse and neglect situations, families should be approached in a helping rather than a punitive manner.

Immediate safety: Physicians and other professionals in contact with children (eg, nurses, teachers, day care workers, police) are required by law in all states to report incidents of suspected abuse or neglect. Every state has its own laws. Members of the general public are encouraged, but not mandated, to report suspected abuse. Any person who makes a report of abuse based on reasonable cause and in good faith is immune from criminal and civil liability. A mandated reporter who fails to make a report can be subject to criminal and civil penalties. The reports are made to Child Protective Services or another appropriate child protection agency. Health professionals should, but are not required to, tell parents that a report is being made pursuant to the law and that they will be contacted, interviewed, and possibly visited at their home. In some cases, the health professional may determine that informing the parent before police or other agency assistance is available creates greater risk of injury to the child. Under those circumstances, the health professional may choose to delay informing the parent or caregiver.

Representatives of child protective agencies and social workers can help the physician determine likelihood of subsequent harm and thus identify the best immediate disposition for the child. Options include protective hospitalization, placement with relatives or in temporary housing (sometimes a whole family is moved out of an abusive partner's home), temporary foster care, and going home with prompt social service follow-up. The physician plays an important role in working with community agencies to advocate for the best and safest disposition for the child.

Follow-up: A source of primary medical care is fundamental. However, the families of abused and neglected children frequently relocate, making continuity of care difficult. Broken appointments are common; outreach and home visits by social workers or a public health nurse may be needed to relay the patient's progress to all concerned.

A close review of the family setting, prior contacts with various community service agencies, and the parents' needs is essential. A social worker can conduct such reviews and help with interviews and family counseling. Social workers also provide tangible assistance to the parents in obtaining public assistance and day care and homemaker services (which can relieve a parent under stress, allowing a few hours each day for relaxation) and coordinating mental health services for parents. Periodic or ongoing social work contact usually is needed.

Parent-aide programs, which employ trained nonprofessionals to relate closely to abusive and negligent parents, are available in some communities. Other parent support groups also have been successful.

Sex offenses may have lasting effects on the child's development and sexual adaptation, particularly among older children and adolescents. Counseling or psychotherapy for the child and the adults concerned may lessen these effects.

Removal from the home: Although emergency temporary removal from the home until evaluation is complete and safety ensured is not uncommon, the ultimate goal of Child Protective Services is to keep the child with his family in a safe, healthy environment. If the above interventions do not ensure this, consideration must be made for long-term removal and possibly termination of parental rights. This significant step requires a court petition, presented by the legal counsel of the appropriate welfare department. The procedure varies from state to state but usually entails family court testimony by a physician. When the court decides in favor of removing the child from the home, a disposition is arranged. The family's physician should participate in this disposition planning; if not, his agreement and consent to the disposition should be sought. While the child is in temporary placement, the physician should, if possible, maintain contact with the parents and ensure that adequate efforts are being made to help them. Occasionally, children are reabused while in foster care. The physician should be alert to this possibility. The physician's input is integral to the decision for reuniting the child and parents. As the dynamics of the family setting improve, the child may be able to return to the parents' care. However, recurrences of abuse are common.

Prevention

Prevention of maltreatment should be a part of every well-child office visit through education of parents or caregivers and referrals for appropriate community services of identified at-risk families. Parents who have been victims of abuse or neglect may be at risk of abusing their own children. Such parents often verbalize anxiety about their abusive background and are amenable to assistance. First-time parents and teenage parents as well as parents with several children < 5 yr are also at risk. Often, maternal risk factors for abuse are identified prenatally, eg, a mother who does not seek prenatal care, smokes, abuses drugs, or has a history of domestic violence. Medical problems during pregnancy, delivery, or early infancy that may affect the infant's health can weaken parent-infant bonding (see also p. 2245). During such times it is important to elicit the parents' feelings about their own inadequacies and the infant's well-being. How well can they tolerate an infant with many needs or health demands? Do the parents give moral and physical support to each other? Are there relatives or friends to help in times of need? The care provider who is alert to clues and able to provide support in such settings goes a long way toward preventing tragic events.

FEMALE GENITAL MUTILATION

Female genital mutilation is practiced routinely in parts of Africa (usually northern or central Africa), where it is deeply ingrained as part of some cultures. Women who experience sexual pleasure are considered impossible to control, are shunned, and cannot be married.

The average age of girls who undergo mutilation is 7 yr, and mutilation is done without anesthesia. Mutilation may be limited to partial clitoral excision. Infibulation, the most extreme form, is removal of the clitoris and labia, usually followed by suturing of the remaining tissue closed except for a 1- to 2-cm opening for menses and urine. The legs are often bound together for weeks afterward. Traditionally, infibulated females are cut open on their wedding night.

Sequelae of genital mutilation may include operative or postoperative bleeding and infection (including tetanus). For infibulated females, recurrent urinary or gynecologic infection and scarring are possible; they have increased susceptibility to AIDS, and childbirth may result in fatal hemorrhage. Psychologic sequelae may be severe.

Female genital mutilation may be decreasing due to the influence of religious leaders who have spoken out against the practice and growing opposition in some communities.

SECTION 20
CLINICAL PHARMACOLOGY

302 CONCEPTS IN PHARMACOTHERAPY

Drugs are selected based on characteristics of the drug (eg, efficacy, safety profile, route of administration, route of elimination, dosing frequency, cost) and of the patient (eg, age, sex, likelihood of pregnancy, ethnicity, other genetic determinants). Risks and benefits of the drug are also assessed; every drug poses some risk. Response to a drug depends partly on the patient's characteristics and behaviors (eg, consumption of foods or supplements, adherence to a dosing regimen), coexistence of other disorders, and use of other drugs. Drug errors (eg, prescribing an inappropriate drug, misreading a prescription, administering a drug incorrectly) can also affect response.

ADHERENCE TO A DRUG REGIMEN

Adherence (compliance) is the degree to which a patient follows a treatment regimen. For drugs, adherence requires that the prescription be obtained promptly and the drug be taken as prescribed in terms of dose, dosing interval, and duration of treatment. Patients should be told that if they stop or alter the way they take a drug, they should alert their physician, but they rarely do so.

Only about 1/2 of patients who leave a physician's office with a prescription take the drug as directed. The most common reasons for nonadherence are frequent dosing, denial of illness, poor comprehension of the benefits of taking the drug, and cost. Many other reasons contribute to nonadherence (see TABLE 302–1).

Children are less likely than adults to follow a treatment regimen. Adherence is worst with chronic disorders requiring complex, long-term treatment (eg, juvenile diabetes, asthma). Parents may not clearly understand prescription instructions and, within 15 min, forget about 1/2 the information given by the physician.

The elderly follow treatment regimens as well as other adults. However, factors that decrease adherence (eg, inadequate finances, use of multiple drugs or drugs that must be taken several times a day) are more common among the elderly. Cognitive impairment may further decrease adherence. Sometimes a prescriber must be creative, picking a drug that is easier to use, even if otherwise it may not be the first choice. For example, some antihypertensives (eg, clonidine) may be given by a patch that can be replaced by a visiting nurse or a family member.

The most obvious result of nonadherence is that the disorder may not be relieved or cured. Nonadherence is estimated to result in 125,000 deaths due to cardiovascular disorders each year in the US. If patients took their drugs as directed, up to 23% of nursing home admissions, 10% of hospital admissions, many physician visits, many diagnostic tests, and many unnecessary treatments could be avoided.

Pharmacists and nurses may detect and help solve adherence problems. For example, a pharmacist may note that a patient does not obtain refills or that a prescription is being refilled too soon. In reviewing prescription

TABLE 302–1. CAUSES OF NONADHERENCE

SOURCE	CAUSE
Patient	Apathy
	Concern about taking drugs (eg, adverse effects, addiction)
	Denial of the disorder or its significance
	Financial concerns
	Forgetfulness
	Misunderstanding of prescribing instructions
	No faith in the drug's efficacy
	Physical difficulties (eg, with swallowing tablets or capsules, opening bottles, or getting prescriptions filled)
	Reduction, fluctuation, or disappearance of symptoms
Drug	Adverse effects (real or imagined)
	Complex regimen (eg, frequent dosing, many drugs)
	Inconvenient or restrictive precautions (eg, no alcohol or cheese)
	Similar appearance of drugs
	Unpleasant taste or smell

directions with the patient, a pharmacist or nurse may uncover a patient's misunderstandings or fears and alleviate them. Doctors can alter complicated or frequent dosing or substitute safe, effective, but less expensive drugs. Communication among all health care practitioners that provide care for a patient is important.

DRUG ERRORS

Drug errors contribute to morbidity. They are estimated to cost the US health care system up to $177 billion (depending on definitions) annually. Drug errors may involve:

- The wrong choice of a drug or a prescription for the wrong dose, frequency, or duration
- An error in reading the prescription by the pharmacist so that the wrong drug or dose is dispensed
- Incorrect instructions to the patient
- Incorrect administration by a health care practitioner or patient
- Incorrect storage of a drug by the pharmacist or patient, altering the drug's potency
- Use of outdated drug, altering the drug's potency
- Confusion of the patient so that the drug is taken incorrectly
- Unscrupulous replacement of a drug with an inferior, diluted, or inactive product

Errors in prescribing are common, especially for certain populations. The elderly (see Ch. 306, especially TABLE 306–3 on p. 2538), women of childbearing age, and children are particularly at risk. Drug interactions particularly affect those taking many drugs. To minimize risk, a physician should know all drugs being taken—including those prescribed by others and OTC drugs—and keep a complete problem list.

Prescriptions must be written as clearly as possible. The names of some drugs are similar and cause confusion if not written clearly. Changing some traditional but easily confused notations may also help reduce errors. For example, "qd" (once/day) may be confused with "qid" (4 times/day). Writing "once/day" is preferred.

Drugs may be administered incorrectly, especially in institutions. A drug may be given to the wrong patient, at the wrong time, or by the wrong route. Certain drugs must be given slowly when given IV, and some drugs cannot be given simultaneously. When an error is recognized, it should be reported immediately to a physician, and a pharmacist should be consulted.

A pharmacist should store drugs to ensure their potency. Mail-order pharmacies should follow procedures to ensure proper transportation. Storage by patients is often suboptimal. If stored incorrectly, drugs are likely to decrease in potency long before the stated expiration date. Labeling should clearly state whether a drug needs to be stored in the refrigerator or kept cool, needs to be kept out of excessive heat or sun, or otherwise requires special storage. On the other hand, unnecessary precautions decrease adherence and waste patient time. For example, unopened insulin should be refrigerated, but a bottle in use can be stored safely outside the refrigerator for a relatively long time if not exposed to excessive heat and sun.

Use of outdated drugs is common. For some drugs (eg, aspirin, tetracycline), risk of harm is great when outdated drug is used. Prescriptions should be written and filled for only as much drug as is likely to be used before expiration.

Most commonly, drug error results from a patient's confusion about how to take drugs. Patients may take the wrong drug or dose. Dosing instructions for each drug, including why the drug has been prescribed, should be completely explained to patients. They should be advised to ask their pharmacist for additional advice about taking their drugs. Packaging should be convenient but safe. If children are not likely to have access to the drug and patients may have difficulty opening the packaging, packaging that is not childproof should be used.

DRUG INTERACTIONS

Drug interactions are changes in a drug's effects due to recent or concurrent use of another drug or drugs (drug-drug interactions) or due to ingestion of food (drug-nutrient interactions—see p. 8).

A drug interaction may increase or decrease the effects of one or both drugs. Clinically significant interactions are often predictable and usually undesired. Adverse effects or therapeutic failure may result.

TABLE 302–2. SOME DRUGS WITH POTENTIALLY SERIOUS DRUG INTERACTIONS*

MECHANISM	EXAMPLES
Narrow margin of safety†	Antiarrhythmic drugs (eg, quinidine) Antineoplastic drugs (eg, methotrexate) Digoxin Lithium Theophylline Warfarin
Extensive metabolism by certain hepatic enzymes	Alprazolam Amitriptyline Atorvastatin Carbamazepine Clozapine Corticosteroids Cyclosporine Diazepam Imipramine Lovastatin Midazolam Olanzapine Phenytoin Protease inhibitors Sildenafil Simvastatin Tacrolimus Tadalafil Theophylline Triazolam Vardenafil Warfarin
Inhibition of certain hepatic enzymes	Cimetidine Ciprofloxacin Clarithromycin Diltiazem Erythromycin Fluconazole Fluoxetine Fluvoxamine Itraconazole Ketoconazole Nefazodone Paroxetine Ritonavir Telithromycin
Induction of certain hepatic enzymes	Barbiturates (eg, phenobarbital) Carbamazepine Phenytoin Rifabutin Rifampin St. John's wort

*Any drug to be used concurrently with one of these drugs should be thoroughly evaluated for possible drug interactions.

†Even when used alone, these drugs may have serious adverse effects. Concurrent use of another drug that increases the action of these drugs further increases risk of adverse effects.

In therapeutic duplication, 2 drugs with similar properties are taken at the same time and have additive effects. For example, taking a benzodiazepine for anxiety and another benzodiazepine at bedtime for insomnia may have a cumulative effect, leading to toxicity.

Drug interactions involve pharmacodynamics or pharmacokinetics. In pharmacodynamic interactions, one drug alters the sensitivity or responsiveness of tissues to another drug by having the same (agonistic) or a blocking (antagonistic) effect. These effects usually occur at the receptor level but may occur intracellularly.

In pharmacokinetic interactions, a drug usually alters absorption, distribution, protein binding, metabolism, or excretion of another drug. Thus, the amount and persistence of available drug at receptor sites change. Pharmacokinetic interactions alter magnitude and duration, not type, of effect. They are often predicted based on knowledge of the individual drugs or detected by monitoring drug concentrations or clinical signs.

Minimizing drug interactions: Prescribers should know all drugs taken by patients, including drugs prescribed by other prescribers and all OTC drugs, herbal products, and nutritional supplements. Asking patients relevant questions about diet and alcohol consumption may be appropriate. The fewest drugs in the lowest doses for the shortest possible time should be prescribed. The effects, desired and undesired, of all drugs taken should be determined because these effects usually include the spectrum of drug interactions. If possible, drugs with a wide margin of error should be used. Patients should be observed and monitored for adverse events, particularly after a change in treatment; some interactions (eg, effects that are influenced by enzyme induction) may take ≥ 1 wk to appear. Drug interactions should be considered as a possible cause of any unexpected problems. When unexpected clinical responses occur, prescribers should determine serum concentrations of selected drugs being taken, consult the literature or an expert in drug interactions, and adjust the dosage until the desired effect is obtained. If dosage adjustment is ineffective, the drug should be replaced by one that does not interact with other drugs being taken.

PHARMACOGENETICS

Pharmacogenetics concerns variations in drug response due to genetic makeup.

The activity of drug-metabolizing enzymes often varies widely among healthy people, making metabolism highly variable. Drug elimination rates vary up to 40-fold. Genetic factors and aging appear to account for most of these variations.

Pharmacogenetic variation (eg, in acetylation, hydrolysis, oxidation, or drug-metabolizing enzymes) can have clinical consequences (see TABLE 302–3). For example, patients who metabolize certain drugs rapidly may require higher, more frequent doses to achieve therapeutic concentrations; patients who metabolize certain drugs slowly may need lower, less frequent doses to avoid toxicity, particularly for drugs with a narrow margin of safety. However, most genetic differences cannot be predicted before drug administration. Also, many environmental and developmental factors can interact with each other and with genetic factors to affect drug response (see FIG. 302–1).

Malignant hyperthermia: A life-threatening elevation in body temperature can result from a hypermetabolic response to concurrent use of a depolarizing muscle relaxant (usually succinylcholine) and a potent, volatile inhalational general anesthetic (eg, halothane

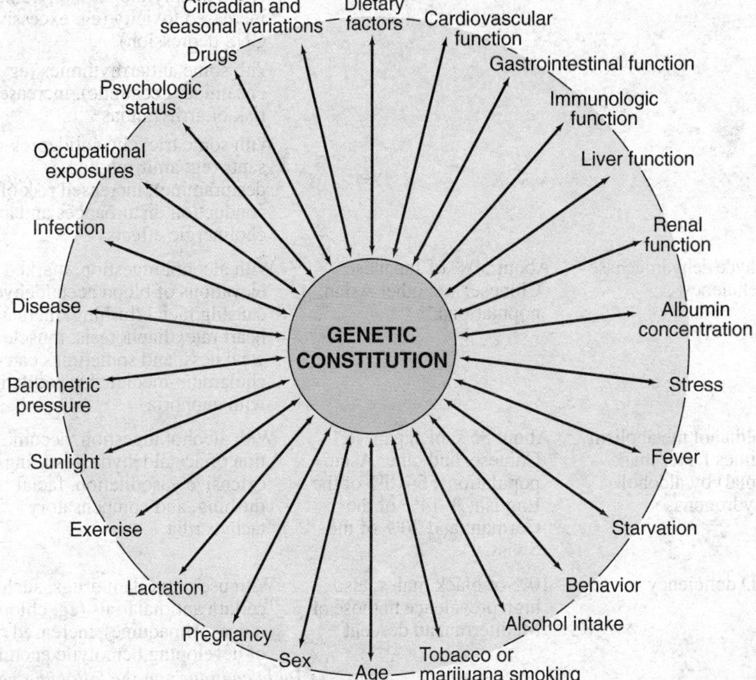

Fig. 302–1. Genetic, environmental, and developmental factors that can interact, causing variations in drug response among patients.

TABLE 302–3. EXAMPLES OF PHARMACOGENETIC VARIATIONS

VARIATION	INCIDENCE	EFFECTS
Slow acetylation (drug inactivation by hepatic *N*-acetyltransferase)	About 50% of the US population	Increased susceptibility to adverse effects of drugs that are acetylated (eg, with isoniazid, peripheral neuritis; with hydralazine or procainamide, lupus)
Fast acetylation	—	Need for higher or more frequent doses of drugs that are acetylated (eg, isoniazid) to obtain the desired therapeutic response
Plasma pseudocholinesterase deficiency	About 1/1500 people	Decreased succinylcholine inactivation With conventional succinylcholine doses, prolonged paralysis of the respiratory muscles and sometimes persistent apnea requiring mechanical ventilation until the drug can be eliminated by alternate pathways
Reduced hydroxylation	—	With metoprolol or timolol, an unusually large therapeutic response to β-receptor blockade With nortriptyline or phenytoin, increased toxicity (eg, excessive CNS depression) With some antiarrhythmics (eg, encainide, flecainide), increased risk of arrhythmias With some tricyclic antidepressants (eg, amitriptyline, desipramine), increased risk of conduction disturbances and anticholinergic effects
Aldehyde dehydrogenase-2 deficiency	About 50% of Japanese, Chinese, and other Asian populations	With alcohol ingestion, marked elevations of blood acetaldehyde, causing facial flushing, increased heart rate, diaphoresis, muscle weakness, and sometimes catecholamine-mediated vasodilation with euphoria
Fast ethanol metabolism (5 times faster than normal) by alcohol dehydrogenase	About 85% of Japanese, Chinese, and other Asian populations; 5–10% of the English; 9–14% of the German; and 20% of the Swiss	With alcohol ingestion, accumulation of acetaldehyde, resulting in extensive vasodilation, facial flushing, and compensatory tachycardia
G6PD deficiency	10% of black males; also high prevalence in those of Mediterranean descent	With use of oxidant drugs, such as certain antimalarials (eg, chloroquine, primaquine), increased risk of developing hemolytic anemia

Table continues on the following page.

TABLE 302–3. EXAMPLES OF PHARMACOGENETIC VARIATIONS—Continued

VARIATION	INCIDENCE	EFFECTS
RBC glutathione synthetase deficiency	Much rarer than G6PD deficiency	With use of oxidant drugs, increased risk of developing hemolytic anemia With such drugs as acetaminophen and nitrofurantoin, increased risk of liver damage if RBC glutathione synthetase levels in hepatocytes are low
Reduced warfarin activity*	—	Because anticoagulant activity after usual therapeutic doses of warfarin is substantially reduced, potential need for a dose many times higher than usual to produce the desired effect

*Reduced activity may be due to a genetically controlled reduction in binding affinity of the warfarin receptor; biotransformation of warfarin is normal in affected people.

G6PD = glucose-6-phosphate dehydrogenase.

[most commonly], isoflurane, sevoflurane). This drug combination produces a similar reaction in some patients with muscular dystrophy and myotonia.

Malignant hyperthermia affects about 1/20,000 people. Inheritance for susceptibility is autosomal dominant. The mechanism may be related to halothane-induced potentiation of Ca activity in the sarcoplasmic reticulum of skeletal muscle; in susceptible patients, this tissue is hyperreactive to Ca. As a result, Ca-induced biochemical reactions are accelerated, causing severe muscle contractions and elevating metabolic rate.

Malignant hyperthermia may develop during anesthesia or the early postoperative period. Clinical presentation varies, depending on the drug used and the patient's susceptibility. Muscular rigidity is often the first sign, followed by tachycardia, other arrhythmias, acidosis, shock, and hyperthermia. Hyperkalemia, respiratory and metabolic acidosis, hypocalcemia, CK elevation, myoglobinemia, and coagulation abnormalities (particularly disseminated intravascular coagulation) can develop. Treatment with dantrolene (starting with 2.5 mg/kg IV) must be initiated immediately after symptoms develop.

PLACEBOS

Placebos are inactive substances, most often used in controlled studies for comparison with presumably active drugs.

Effects: Placebos, although often considered inert and harmless, may have substantial effects—good and bad. They may help patients with many physical and mental disorders. But placebos may also produce nausea, headache, dizziness, sleepiness, insomnia, fatigue, depression, numbness, hallucinations, itching, vomiting, tremor, tachycardia, diarrhea, pallor, rashes, hives, ataxia, and edema.

Some people have characteristics of drug addiction to a placebo: a tendency to increase the dose, a compulsive desire to take the substance, and an abstinence syndrome when they are deprived of it.

All effects of placebos appear to be related to anticipation (usually, that the drug will work) or to spontaneous change. Spontaneous change, whether improvement, deterioration, or an entirely new problem (eg, headache, rash), may be mistakenly attributed to a placebo.

Correlations between personality characteristics and response to placebos have not been well established. However, people who have dependent personalities and who want to please their physicians may be more likely to report beneficial effects; those with histrionic personalities may be more likely to report any effect, good or bad (see p. 1719).

Uses: In clinical studies comparing an active drug with a placebo, effects of placebo must be subtracted from those of the drug. The active drug must perform significantly better than the placebo to demonstrate efficacy. In some studies, placebo relieves the disorder in > 50% of patients, making demonstration of the active drug's efficacy difficult.

A placebo may be used with the patient's consent to examine the patient's need for a potentially toxic drug—eg, to determine whether a patient with chronic pain is benefiting from a potentially addictive analgesic. However, obtaining consent is likely to undermine the placebo effect. The problem is solved by blindly alternating active drug and placebo.

Rarely, when the prescriber determines that an active drug is not needed, placebos may be prescribed without a patient's knowledge to relieve symptoms or meet the patient's demands for treatment. Such use of a placebo may damage the physician-patient relationship and may make misinterpreting the patient's response more likely. If response to a placebo is positive, a physician may unjustifiably conclude that symptoms are not due to a physical disorder or that they are psychologically exaggerated. Thus, physicians are more likely to prescribe vitamins or vitamin B_{12} injections, which are often tantamount to placebos.

DRUG DEVELOPMENT

Promising compounds can be identified by screening molecules for biologic activity, often via computer modeling or by understanding disease mechanisms, and then trying to create molecules that affect those mechanisms.

During **early development**, potentially useful compounds are studied in animals to evaluate desired effects and toxicity. Compounds that appear effective and safe are candidates for human studies. A protocol describing the clinical study must be approved by an appropriate institutional research board (IRB) and the FDA, which then issues an investigational new drug (IND) exemption permit. At this point, the patent time period for the compound begins, which usually provides the owner with exclusive rights for the next 20 yr; however, the drug cannot be sold until FDA approved.

Phase 1 evaluates safety and toxicity in humans. Different amounts of the compound are given to a small number (often 20 to 80) of healthy, young, usually male volunteers to determine the dose at which toxicity first appears.

Phase 2 determines whether the compound is active against the target disorder. The compound is given to up to about 100 patients for treatment or prevention of the target disorder. An additional goal is to determine an optimal dose-response range.

Phase 3 evaluates the drug's effect in larger (often 100s to 1000s), more heterogeneous populations in an attempt to duplicate the drug's proposed clinical use. This phase also compares the drug with existing treatments, a placebo, or both. Studies may involve many practicing physicians and multiple research sites. The purpose is to verify efficacy and detect effects—good and bad—that may not have been observed during phases 1 and 2.

When sufficient data have been collected to justify and request approval of the drug, a new drug application (NDA) is submitted to the FDA. The process from early development to approval of a drug often takes ≥ 10 yr. Only 2% of drug candidates enter human studies (phase 1), and only 20% that enter phase 1 are approved for marketing as new drugs.

Phase 4 studies occur after the drug is approved and marketed. They are ongoing and involve large populations. Often, special subpopulations (eg, pregnant women, children, the elderly) are studied. Phase 4 also includes ongoing reporting of adverse effects.

303 PHARMACOKINETICS

Pharmacokinetics, sometimes described as what the body does to a drug, refers to the movement of drug into, through, and out of the body—the time course of its absorption, bioavailability, distribution, metabolism, and excretion. Pharmacodynamics (see p. 2530), described as what a drug does to the body, involves receptor binding, postreceptor effects, and chemical interactions. Drug pharmacokinetics determines the onset, duration, and intensity of a drug's effect. Formulas relating these processes summarize the pharmacokinetic behavior of most drugs (see TABLE 303–1).

TABLE 303–1. FORMULAS DEFINING BASIC PHARMACOKINETIC PARAMETERS

CATEGORY	PARAMETER	FORMULA
Absorption	Absorption rate constant	Rate of drug absorption ÷ Amount of drug remaining to be absorbed
	Bioavailability	Amount of drug absorbed ÷ Drug dose
Distribution	Apparent volume of distribution	Amount of drug in body ÷ Plasma drug concentration
	Unbound fraction	Plasma concentration of unbound drug ÷ Plasma drug concentration
Elimination	Rate of elimination	Renal excretion + Extrarenal (usually metabolic) elimination
	Clearance	Rate of drug elimination ÷ Plasma drug concentration
	Renal clearance	Rate of renal excretion of drug ÷ Plasma drug concentration
	Metabolic clearance	Rate of drug metabolism ÷ Plasma drug concentration
	Fraction excreted unchanged	Rate of renal excretion of drug ÷ Rate of drug elimination
	Elimination rate constant	Rate of drug elimination ÷ Amount of drug in body Clearance ÷ Volume of distribution
	Biologic half-life	0.693 ÷ Elimination rate constant

Pharmacokinetics of a drug depends on patient-related factors as well as on the drug's chemical properties. Some patient-related factors (eg, genetic makeup, sex, age) can be used to predict pharmacologic response of populations. For example, the half-life of some drugs, especially those that require both metabolism and excretion, may be remarkably long in the elderly (see FIG. 303–1). Other factors are related to individual physiology. The effects of some individual factors (eg, renal failure, obesity, hepatic failure, dehydration) can be reasonably predicted, but other factors are idiosyncratic and thus have

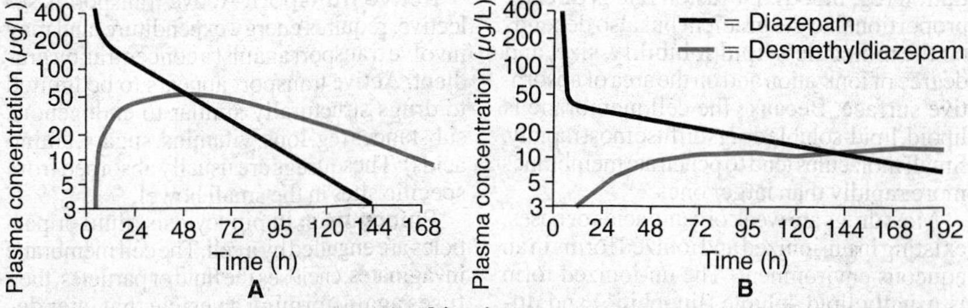

Fig. 303–1. Comparison of pharmacokinetic outcomes for diazepam in a younger man (A) and an older man (B). Diazepam is metabolized in the liver to desmethyldiazepam through P-450 enzymes. Desmethyldiazepam is an active sedative, which is excreted by the kidneys. 0 = time of dosing. (Adapted from Greenblatt DJ et al: Diazepam disposition determinants. *Clinical Pharmacology and Therapeutics* 27(3):304, 1980.)

unpredictable effects. Because of individual differences, drug administration must be based on each patient's needs—traditionally, by empirically adjusting dosage until the therapeutic objective is met. This approach is frequently inadequate because it can delay optimal response or result in adverse effects. Knowledge of pharmacokinetic principles helps prescribers adjust dosage more accurately and rapidly.

ABSORPTION

Drug absorption is determined by the drug's physicochemical properties, formulation, and route of administration. Dosage forms (eg, tablets, capsules, solutions), consisting of the drug plus other ingredients, are formulated to be given by various routes (eg, oral, buccal, sublingual, rectal, parenteral, topical, inhalational). Drugs must be in solution to be absorbed. Thus, solid forms (eg, tablets) must be able to disintegrate and deaggregate.

Unless given IV, a drug must cross several semipermeable cell membranes before it reaches the systemic circulation. Cell membranes are biologic barriers that selectively inhibit passage of drug molecules. The membranes are composed primarily of a bimolecular lipid matrix, which determines membrane permeability characteristics. Drugs may cross cell membranes by passive diffusion, facilitated passive diffusion, active transport, or pinocytosis. Sometimes various globular proteins embedded in the matrix function as receptors and help transport molecules across the membrane.

Passive diffusion: Drugs diffuse across a cell membrane from a region of high concentration (eg, GI fluids) to one of low concentration (eg, blood). Diffusion rate is directly proportional to the gradient but also depends on the molecule's lipid solubility, size, and degree of ionization and on the area of absorptive surface. Because the cell membrane is lipoid, lipid-soluble drugs diffuse most rapidly. Small molecules tend to penetrate membranes more rapidly than larger ones.

Most drugs are weak organic acids or bases, existing in un-ionized and ionized forms in an aqueous environment. The un-ionized form is usually lipid soluble (lipophilic) and diffuses readily across cell membranes. The ionized form has low lipid solubility (but high water solubility—hydrophilic) and high electrical resistance and thus cannot penetrate cell membranes easily. The proportion of the un-ionized form present (and thus the drug's ability to cross a membrane) is determined by the pH and the drug's pK_a. The pK_a is the pH at which concentrations of ionized and un-ionized forms are equal. When the pH is lower than the pK_a, the un-ionized form of a weak acid predominates, but the ionized form of a weak base predominates. Thus, in plasma (pH 7.4), the ratio of un-ionized to ionized forms for a weak acid (eg, with a pK_a of 4.4) is 1:1000; in gastric fluid (pH 1.4), the ratio is reversed (1000:1). Therefore, when a weak acid is given orally, most of the drug in the stomach is un-ionized, favoring diffusion through the gastric mucosa. For a weak base with a pK_a of 4.4, the outcome is reversed; most of the drug in the stomach is ionized. Theoretically, weakly acidic drugs (eg, aspirin) are more readily absorbed from an acid medium (stomach) than are weakly basic drugs (eg, quinidine). However, whether a drug is acidic or basic, most absorption occurs in the small bowel because the surface area is larger and membranes are more permeable (see Oral Administration on p. 2523).

Facilitated passive diffusion: Certain molecules with low lipid solubility (eg, glucose) penetrate membranes more rapidly than expected. One theory is facilitated passive diffusion: A carrier molecule in the membrane combines reversibly with the substrate molecule outside the cell membrane, and the carrier-substrate complex diffuses rapidly across the membrane, releasing the substrate at the interior surface. In such cases, the membrane transports only substrates with a relatively specific molecular configuration, and the availability of carriers limits the process. The process does not require energy expenditure, and transport against a concentration gradient cannot occur.

Active transport: Active transport is selective, requires energy expenditure, and may involve transport against a concentration gradient. Active transport appears to be limited to drugs structurally similar to endogenous substances (eg, ions, vitamins, sugars, amino acids). These drugs are usually absorbed from specific sites in the small bowel.

Pinocytosis: In pinocytosis, fluid or particles are engulfed by a cell. The cell membrane invaginates, encloses the fluid or particles, then fuses again, forming a vesicle that later detaches and moves to the cell interior. Energy expenditure is required. Pinocytosis probably plays a small role in drug transport, except for protein drugs.

Oral Administration

To be absorbed, a drug given orally must survive encounters with low pH and numerous GI secretions, including potentially degrading enzymes. Peptide drugs (eg, insulin) are particularly susceptible to degradation and are not used orally. Absorption of oral drugs involves transport across membranes of the epithelial cells in the GI tract. Absorption is affected by differences in luminal pH along the GI tract, surface area per luminal volume, blood perfusion, the presence of bile and mucus, and the nature of epithelial membranes.

The oral mucosa has a thin epithelium and rich vascularity, which favor absorption; however, contact is usually too brief for substantial absorption. A drug placed between the gums and cheek (buccal administration) or under the tongue (sublingual administration) is retained longer, enhancing absorption.

The stomach has a relatively large epithelial surface, but its thick mucous layer and short transit time limit absorption. Because most absorption occurs in the small bowel, gastric emptying is often the rate-limiting step. Food, especially fatty food, slows gastric emptying (and rate of drug absorption), explaining why taking some drugs on an empty stomach speeds absorption. Drugs that affect gastric emptying (eg, parasympatholytic drugs) affect the absorption rate of other drugs. Food may enhance the extent of absorption for poorly soluble drugs (eg, griseofulvin), reduce it for drugs degraded in the stomach (eg, penicillin G), or have little or no effect.

The small bowel has the largest surface area for drug absorption in the GI tract, and its membranes are more permeable than those in the stomach. For these reasons, most drugs are absorbed primarily in the small bowel, and acids, despite their ability as un-ionized drug to readily cross membranes, are absorbed faster in the bowel than in the stomach. The intraluminal pH is 4 to 5 in the duodenum but becomes progressively more alkaline, approaching 8 in the lower ileum. GI microflora may reduce absorption. Decreased blood flow (eg, in shock) may lower the concentration gradient across the intestinal mucosa and reduce absorption by passive diffusion.

Intestinal transit time can influence drug absorption, particularly for drugs that are absorbed by active transport (eg, B vitamins), that dissolve slowly (eg, griseofulvin), or that are polar (ie, with low lipid solubility; eg, many antibiotics).

Most drugs are given orally as tablets or capsules primarily for convenience, economy, stability, and patient acceptance. Because solid drug forms must dissolve before absorption can occur, dissolution rate determines availability of the drug for absorption. Dissolution, if slower than absorption, becomes the rate-limiting step. Manipulating the formulation (eg, the drug's form as salt, crystal, or hydrate) can change the dissolution rate and thus control overall absorption.

Parenteral Administration

Drugs given IV directly enter the systemic circulation. However, drugs injected IM or sc must cross one or more biologic membranes to reach the systemic circulation. If protein drugs with a molecular mass > 20,000 g/mole are injected IM or sc, movement across capillary membranes is so slow that most absorption occurs via the lymphatic system. In such cases, drug delivery to systemic circulation is slow and often incomplete because of 1st-pass metabolism by proteolytic enzymes in the lymphatics.

Perfusion (blood flow/gram of tissue) greatly affects capillary absorption of small molecules injected IM or sc. Thus, injection site can affect absorption rate. Absorption after IM or sc injection may be delayed or erratic for salts of poorly soluble bases and acids (eg, parenteral form of phenytoin).

Controlled-Release Forms

Controlled-release forms are designed to reduce dosing frequency for drugs with a short elimination half-life and duration of effect. These forms also limit fluctuation in plasma drug concentration, providing a more uniform therapeutic effect. Absorption rate is slowed by coating drug particles with wax or other water-insoluble material, by embedding the drug in a matrix that releases it slowly during transit through the GI tract, or by complexing the drug with ion-exchange resins. Most absorption of these forms occurs in the large bowel. Crushing or otherwise disturbing a controlled-release pill can often be dangerous.

Transdermal controlled-release forms are designed to release the drug for extended periods, sometimes for several days. Drugs for transdermal delivery must have suitable skin penetration characteristics and high potency because the penetration rate and area of application are limited.

Many nonintravenous parenteral forms are designed to sustain plasma drug concentrations. Absorption of antimicrobials can be extended by using their relatively insoluble salt form (eg, penicillin G benzathine) injected IM. For other drugs, suspensions or solutions in nonaqueous vehicles (eg, crystalline suspensions for insulin) are designed to delay absorption.

BIOAVAILABILITY

Bioavailability refers to the extent to and rate at which the active moiety (drug or metabolite) enters systemic circulation, thereby accessing the site of action.

Bioavailability of a drug is largely determined by the properties of the dosage form (which depend partly on its design and manufacture), rather than by the drug's physicochemical properties, which determine absorption potential. Differences in bioavailability among formulations of a given drug can have clinical significance; thus, knowing whether drug formulations are equivalent is essential.

Chemical equivalence indicates that drug products contain the same compound in the same amount and meet current official standards; however, inactive ingredients in drug products may differ. Bioequivalence indicates that the drug products, when given to the same patient in the same dosage regimen, result in equivalent concentrations of drug in plasma and tissues. Therapeutic equivalence indicates that drug products, when given to the same patient in the same dosage regimen, have the same therapeutic and adverse effects. Bioequivalent products are expected to be therapeutically equivalent. Therapeutic nonequivalence (eg, more adverse effects, less efficacy) is usually discovered during long-term treatment when patients who are stabilized on one formulation are given a nonequivalent substitute.

Sometimes therapeutic equivalence is possible despite differences in bioavailability. For example, the therapeutic index (ratio of the minimum toxic concentration to the median effective concentration) of penicillin is so wide that efficacy and safety are usually not affected by the moderate differences in plasma concentration due to bioavailability differences in penicillin products. In contrast, for drugs with a relatively narrow therapeutic index, bioavailability differences may cause substantial therapeutic nonequivalence.

Causes of low bioavailability: Orally administered drugs must pass through the intestinal wall and then through the portal circulation to the liver; both are common sites of 1st-pass metabolism (metabolism of a drug before it reaches systemic circulation). Thus, many drugs may be metabolized before adequate plasma concentrations are reached. Low bioavailability is most common with oral dosage forms of poorly water-soluble, slowly absorbed drugs.

Insufficient time for absorption in the GI tract is a common cause of low bioavailability. If the drug does not dissolve readily or cannot penetrate the epithelial membrane (eg, if it is highly ionized and polar), time at the absorption site may be insufficient. In such cases, bioavailability tends to be highly variable as well as low.

Age, sex, physical activity, genetic phenotype, stress, disorders (eg, achlorhydria, malabsorption syndromes), or previous GI surgery can also affect drug bioavailability.

Chemical reactions that reduce absorption can reduce bioavailability. They include formation of a complex (eg, between tetracycline and polyvalent metal ions), hydrolysis by gastric acid or digestive enzymes (eg, penicillin and chloramphenicol palmitate hydrolysis), conjugation in the intestinal wall (eg, sulfoconjugation of isoproterenol), adsorption to other drugs (eg, of digoxin to cholestyramine), and metabolism by luminal microflora.

Assessing bioavailability: Bioavailability is usually assessed by determining the maximum (peak) plasma drug concentration, peak time (when maximum plasma drug concentration occurs), and area under the plasma concentration–time curve (AUC—see FIG. 303–2). Plasma drug concentration increases with extent of absorption; the peak is reached when drug elimination rate equals absorption rate. Bioavailability determinations based on the peak plasma concentration can be misleading because drug elimination begins as soon as the drug enters the bloodstream. Peak time is the most widely used general index of absorption rate; the slower the absorption, the later the peak time.

AUC is the most reliable measure of bioavailability. AUC is directly proportional to the total amount of unchanged drug that reaches systemic circulation. Drug products may be considered bioequivalent in extent and rate of absorption if their plasma concentration curves are essentially superimposable.

For drugs excreted primarily unchanged in urine, bioavailability can be estimated by

cleavage (oxidation, reduction, hydrolysis); these reactions are nonsynthetic. Phase II reactions involve conjugation with an endogenous substance (eg, glucuronic acid, sulfate, glycine); these reactions are synthetic. Metabolites formed in synthetic reactions are more polar and more readily excreted by the kidneys (in urine) and the liver (in bile) than those formed in nonsynthetic reactions. Some drugs undergo only phase I or phase II reactions; thus, phase numbers reflect functional rather than sequential classification.

Rate: For almost all drugs, the metabolism rate in any given pathway has an upper limit (capacity limitation). However, at therapeutic concentrations of most drugs, usually only a small fraction of the metabolizing enzyme's sites are occupied, and the metabolism rate increases with drug concentration. In such cases, called 1st-order elimination (or kinetics), the metabolism rate of the drug is a constant fraction of the drug remaining in the body (rather than a constant amount of drug per hour); ie, the drug has a specific half-life. For example, if 500 mg is present in the body at time zero, after metabolism, 250 mg may be present at 1 h and 125 mg at 2 h (illustrating a half-life of 1 h). However, when most of the enzyme sites are occupied, metabolism occurs at its maximal rate and does not change in proportion to drug concentration; ie, a fixed amount of drug is metabolized per unit time (zero-order kinetics). In this case, if 500 mg is present in the body at time zero, after metabolism, 450 mg may be present at 1 h and 400 mg at 2 h (illustrating a maximal clearance of 50 mg/h and no specific half-life). As drug concentration increases, metabolism shifts from 1st-order to zero-order kinetics.

Cytochrome P-450: The most important enzyme system of phase I metabolism is cytochrome P-450, a microsomal superfamily of isoenzymes that catalyze the oxidation of many drugs. The electrons are supplied by NADPH (cytochrome P-450 reductase, a flavoprotein that transfers electrons from NADPH (the reduced form of nicotinamide-adenine dinucleotide phosphate) to cytochrome P-450. Cytochrome P-450 enzymes can be induced or inhibited by many drugs and substances, helping explain many drug interactions in which one drug enhances the toxicity or reduces the therapeutic effect of another drug. For examples of drugs that interact with specific enzymes, see TABLE 303–2 (see also Drug Interactions on p. 2515).

With aging, the liver's capacity for metabolism through the cytochrome P-450 enzyme system is reduced by ≥30% because liver volume and hepatic flow are decreased. Thus, drugs that are metabolized through this system reach higher levels and have prolonged half-lives in the elderly (see FIG. 303–1). Because neonates have partially developed liver microsomal enzyme systems, they also have difficulty metabolizing many drugs.

Conjugation: Glucuronidation, the most common phase II reaction, is the only one that occurs in the liver microsomal enzyme system. Glucuronides are secreted in bile and eliminated in urine. Thus, conjugation makes most drugs more soluble and easily excreted by the kidneys. Amino acid conjugation with glutamine or glycine produces conjugates that are readily excreted in urine but not extensively secreted in bile. Aging does not affect glucuronidation. However, in neonates, conversion to glucuronide is slower, sometimes with serious effects.

Conjugation may also occur through acetylation or sulfoconjugation. Sulfate esters are polar and readily excreted in urine. Aging does not affect these processes.

EXCRETION

The kidneys, which excrete water-soluble substances, are the principal organs of excretion. The biliary system contributes to excretion to the degree that drug is not reabsorbed from the GI tract. Generally, the contribution of intestine, saliva, sweat, breast milk, and lungs to excretion is small, except for exhalation of volatile anesthetics. Excretion via breast milk, although not important to the mother, may affect the breastfeeding infant (see TABLE 266–4 on p. 2228).

Hepatic metabolism often makes drugs more polar and thus more water soluble. The resulting metabolites are then more readily excreted.

Renal excretion: Renal filtration accounts for most drug excretion. About $1/5$ of the plasma reaching the glomerulus is filtered through pores in the glomerular endothelium; nearly all water and most electrolytes are passively and actively reabsorbed from the renal tubules back into the circulation. However, polar compounds, which include most drug metabolites, cannot diffuse back into the circulation and are excreted unless a specific transport mechanism exists for their reabsorption

TABLE 303–2. SOME SUBSTANCES THAT INTERACT WITH CYTOCHROME P-450 ENZYMES

ENZYME	SUBSTRATES	INHIBITORS	INDUCERS
CYP1A2	Acetaminophen Caffeine Estradiol Lidocaine Tacrine Theophylline Verapamil *(R)*-Warfarin	Cimetidine Ciprofloxacin Erythromycin Isoniazid Tacrine	Charcoal-broiled beef Cigarette smoke Omeprazole Phenobarbital Rifampin
CYP2C9	Diclofenac Phenytoin Piroxicam Tetrahydrocannabinol Tolbutamide *(S)*-Warfarin	Amiodarone Cimetidine Fluconazole Lovastatin Sulfaphenazole Sulfinpyrazone	Phenobarbital Other barbiturates Phenytoin Rifampin
CYP2C19	Diazepam Hexobarbital *(S)*-Mephenytoin Omeprazole Pentamidine Propranolol *(R)*-Warfarin	Felbamate Fluoxetine Fluvoxamine Omeprazole Tranylcypromine	Carbamazepine Phenobarbital Rifampin
CYP2D6	Codeine Debrisoquine Dextromethorphan Encainide Haloperidol Metoprolol Mexiletine Paroxetine Phenothiazines Propranolol Risperidone Sertraline Tricyclic antidepressants Venlafaxine	Amiodarone Cimetidine Fluoxetine Fluvoxamine Mibefradil Omeprazole Propoxyphene Quinidine Sertraline	Carbamazepine
CYP2E1	Acetaminophen Alcohol	Disulfiram	Alcohol Isoniazid
CYP3A4	Amiodarone Amlopidine Clarithromycin Cyclosporine Erythromycin Lovastatin Nifedipine Tamoxifen Terfenadine Verapamil *(R)*-Warfarin	Amiodarone Cimetidine Cisapride Clarithromycin Cyclophosphamide Delavirdine Diazepam Diltiazem Erythromycin Fluoxetine Fluvoxamine Grapefruit juice Indinavir	Carbamazepine Phenobarbital Phenytoin Rifampin

Table continues on the following page.

TABLE 303–2. SOME SUBSTANCES THAT INTERACT WITH CYTOCHROME P-450 ENZYMES—Continued

ENZYME	SUBSTRATES	INHIBITORS	INDUCERS
CYP3A4 (*Continued*)		Itraconazole Ketoconazole Loratadine Mibefradil Metronidazole Nefazodone Nelfinavir Propoxyphene Tacrolimus Troleandomycin Verapamil	

(eg, as for glucose, ascorbic acid, and B vitamins). With aging, renal drug excretion decreases (see Ch. 306 and TABLE 306–1 on p. 2536); at age 80, clearance is typically reduced to ½ of what it was at age 30.

The principles of transmembrane passage govern renal handling of drugs. Drugs bound to plasma proteins remain in the circulation; only unbound drug is contained in the glomerular filtrate. Un-ionized forms of drugs and their metabolites tend to be reabsorbed readily from tubular fluids.

Urine pH, which varies from 4.5 to 8.0, may markedly affect drug reabsorption and excretion by determining whether a weak acid or base is in an un-ionized or ionized form (see p. 2522). Acidification of urine increases reabsorption and decreases excretion of weak acids and decreases reabsorption of weak bases. Alkalinization of urine has the opposite effect. In some cases of overdose, these principles are used to enhance the excretion of weak bases or acids; eg, urine is alkalinized to enhance excretion of acetylsalicylic acid. The extent to which changes in urinary pH alter the rate of drug elimination depends on the contribution of the renal route to total elimination, the polarity of the un-ionized form, and the molecule's degree of ionization.

Active tubular secretion in the proximal tubule is important in the elimination of many drugs. This energy-dependent process may be blocked by metabolic inhibitors. When drug concentration is high, secretory transport can reach an upper limit (transport maximum); each substance has a characteristic transport maximum.

Anions and cations are handled by separate transport mechanisms. Normally, the anion secretory system eliminates metabolites conjugated with glycine, sulfate, or glucuronic acid. Anions (weak acids) compete with each other for secretion. This competition can be used therapeutically; eg, probenecid blocks the normally rapid tubular secretion of penicillin, resulting in higher plasma penicillin concentrations for a longer time. In the cation transport system, cations or organic bases (eg, pramipexole, dofetilide) are secreted by the renal tubules; this process can be inhibited by cimetidine, trimethoprim, prochlorperazine, megestrol, or ketoconazole.

Biliary excretion: Some drugs and their metabolites are extensively excreted in bile. Because they are transported across the biliary epithelium against a concentration gradient, active secretory transport is required. When plasma drug concentrations are high, secretory transport may approach an upper limit (transport maximum). Substances with similar physicochemical properties may compete for excretion.

Drugs with a mol wt > 300 g/mole and with both polar and lipophilic groups are more likely to be excreted in bile; smaller molecules are generally excreted only in negligible amounts. Conjugation, particularly with glucuronic acid, facilitates biliary excretion.

In the enterohepatic cycle, a drug secreted in bile is reabsorbed into the circulation from the intestine. Biliary excretion eliminates substances from the body only to the extent that enterohepatic cycling is incomplete—when some of the secreted drug is not reabsorbed from the intestine.

304 PHARMACODYNAMICS

Pharmacodynamics, sometimes described as what a drug does to the body, involves receptor binding (including receptor sensitivity), postreceptor effects, and chemical interactions. Pharmacodynamics, with pharmacokinetics (what the body does to a drug—see p. 2520), helps explain drug effects.

A drug's pharmacodynamics can be affected by physiologic changes due to disorders, aging, or other drugs. Disorders that affect pharmacodynamic responses include genetic mutations, thyrotoxicosis, undernutrition, myasthenia gravis, and some forms of insulin-resistant diabetes mellitus. These disorders can change receptor binding, alter the level of binding proteins, or decrease receptor sensitivity. Aging tends to affect pharmacodynamic responses through alterations in receptor binding or in postreceptor response (see TABLE 306–2 on p. 2537). Pharmacodynamic drug-drug interactions result in competition for receptor binding sites or alter postreceptor response.

DRUG-RECEPTOR INTERACTIONS

Receptors are macromolecules involved in chemical signaling between and within cells; they may be located on the cell surface membrane or within the cytoplasm (see TABLE 304–1). Activated receptors directly or indirectly regulate cellular biochemical processes (eg, ion conductance, protein phosphorylation, DNA transcription). Molecules (eg, drugs, hormones, neurotransmitters) that bind to a receptor are called ligands. A ligand may activate or inactivate a receptor; activation may either increase or decrease a particular cell function. Each ligand may interact with multiple receptor subtypes. Few if any drugs are absolutely specific for one receptor or subtype, but most have relative selectivity. Selectivity is the degree to which a drug acts on a given site relative to other sites; selectivity relates largely to physicochemical binding of the drug to cellular receptors.

A drug's ability to affect a given receptor is related to the drug's affinity (probability of the drug occupying a receptor at any given instant) and intrinsic efficacy (intrinsic activity—degree to which a ligand activates receptors and leads to cellular response). A drug's affinity and activity are determined by its chemical structure.

Physiologic functions (eg, contraction, secretion) are usually regulated by multiple receptor-mediated mechanisms, and several steps (eg, receptor-coupling, multiple intracellular 2nd messenger substances) may be interposed between the initial molecular drug-receptor interaction and ultimate tissue or organ response. Thus, several dissimilar drug molecules can often be used to produce a desired response.

Ability to bind to a receptor is influenced by external factors as well as by intracellular regulatory mechanisms. Baseline receptor density and the efficiency of stimulus-response mechanisms vary from tissue to tissue. Drugs, aging, genetic mutations, and disorders can increase (up-regulate) or decrease (down-regulate) the number and binding affinity of receptors. For example, clonidine down-regulates α_2-receptors; thus, rapid withdrawal of clonidine can produce hypertensive crisis. Chronic therapy with β-blockers up-regulates β-receptor density; thus, severe hypertension or tachycardia can result from abrupt withdrawal. Receptor up-regulation and down-regulation affect adaptation to drugs (eg, desensitization, tachyphylaxis, tolerance, acquired resistance, postwithdrawal supersensitivity).

Ligands bind to precise molecular regions, called recognition sites, on receptor macromolecules. The binding site for a drug may be the same as or different from that of an endogenous agonist (hormone or neurotransmitter). Agonists that bind to an adjacent or a different site are sometimes called allosteric agonists. Nonspecific drug binding also occurs—ie, at molecular sites not designated as receptors (eg, plasma proteins).

Agonists and antagonists: Agonist drugs activate receptors to produce the desired response. Conventional agonists increase the proportion of activated receptors. Inverse agonists stabilize the receptor in its inactive conformation and act similarly to competitive antagonists (see p. 2531). Many hormones, neurotransmitters (eg, acetylcholine, histamine, norepinephrine), and drugs (eg, morphine, phenylephrine, isoproterenol) act as agonists.

Antagonists prevent receptor activation. Preventing activation has many effects.

TABLE 304–1. SOME TYPES OF PHYSIOLOGIC AND DRUG-RECEPTOR PROTEINS

TYPE	STRUCTURE	CELLULAR LOCATION	EXAMPLES
Multisubunit ion channels	Out; In; Cell membrane; Ion flux	Cell surface transmembrane	Acetylcholine (nicotinic) $GABA_A$ Glutamate Glycine
G-protein–coupled receptors	Out; In; Cell membrane; G protein; GTP; GDP	Cell surface transmembrane	Acetylcholine (muscarinic) α- and β-Adrenergic receptor proteins Eicosanoids
Protein kinases	Binding Site; Out; In; Cell membrane; Catalysis	Cell surface transmembrane	Growth factors Insulin Peptide hormones
Transcription factors	Nucleus; Ligand; Cytosol; Receptor; Activation/suppression of DNA transcription	Cytoplasm	Steroid hormones Thyroid hormone Vitamin D

GABA = γ-aminobutyric acid; GTP = guanosine triphosphate; GDP = guanosine diphosphate.

Antagonist drugs increase cellular function if they block the action of a substance that normally decreases cellular function. Antagonist drugs decrease cellular function if they block the action of a substance that normally increases cellular function.

Receptor antagonists can be classified as reversible or irreversible. Reversible antagonists readily dissociate from their receptor; irreversible antagonists form a stable, permanent or nearly permanent chemical bond with their receptor (eg, in alkylation). Pseudo-irreversible antagonists slowly dissociate from their receptor.

In competitive antagonism, binding of the antagonist to the receptor prevents binding of the agonist to the receptor. In noncompetitive antagonism, agonist and antagonist can be bound simultaneously, but antagonist binding reduces or prevents the action of the agonist. In reversible competitive antagonism, agonist and antagonist form short-lasting bonds with the receptor, and steady state between agonist, antagonist, and receptor is reached. Such antagonism can be overcome by increasing the concentration of the agonist. For example, naloxone (an opioid receptor antagonist that is structurally similar to morphine), when given shortly before or after morphine, blocks morphine's effects. However, competitive antagonism by naloxone can be overcome by giving more morphine.

Structural analogs of agonist molecules frequently have agonist and antagonist properties; such drugs are called partial (low-efficacy) agonists, or agonist-antagonists. For example, pentazocine activates opioid receptors but blocks their activation by other opioids. Thus, pentazocine provides opioid effects but blunts the effects of another opioid if the opioid is given while pentazocine is still bound. A drug that acts as a partial agonist in one tissue may act as a full agonist in another.

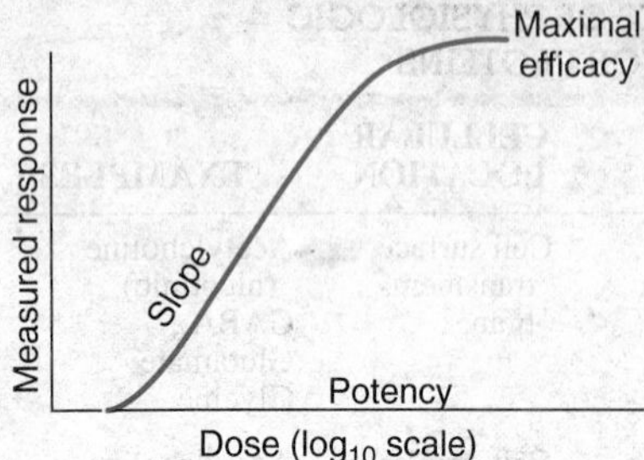

Fig. 304–1. Hypothetical dose-response curve.

CHEMICAL INTERACTIONS

Some drugs produce effects without altering cellular function and without binding to a receptor. For example, most antacids decrease gastric acidity through simple chemical reactions; antacids are bases that chemically interact with acids to produce neutral salts. The primary action of cholestyramine, a bile acid sequestrant, is to bind bile acids in the GI tract.

DOSE-RESPONSE RELATIONSHIPS

Regardless of how a drug effect occurs—through binding or chemical interaction—the concentration of the drug at the site of action controls the effect. However, response to concentration may be complex and is often nonlinear. The relationship between the drug dose, regardless of route used, and the drug concentration at the cellular level is even more complex (see Ch. 303 on p. 2520).

Dose-response data are typically graphed with the dose or dose function (eg, log_{10} dose) on the x-axis and the measured effect (response) on the y-axis. Because a drug effect is a function of dose and time, such a graph depicts the dose-response relationship independent of time. Measured effects are frequently recorded as maxima at time of peak effect or under steady-state conditions (eg, during continuous IV infusion). Drug effects may be quantified at the level of molecule, cell, tissue, organ, organ system, or organism.

A hypothetical dose-response curve has features that vary (see FIG. 304–1): potency (location of curve along the dose axis), maximal efficacy or ceiling effect (greatest attainable response), and slope (change in response per unit dose). Biologic variation (variation in magnitude of response among test subjects in the same population given the same dose of drug) also occurs. Graphing dose-response curves of drugs studied under identical conditions can help compare the pharmacologic profiles of the drugs (see FIG. 304–2). This information helps determine the dose necessary to achieve the desired effect. Dose-response, which involves the principles of pharmacokinetics and pharmacodynamics, determines the required dose and frequency as well as the therapeutic index for a drug in a population. The therapeutic index (ratio of the minimum toxic concentration to the median effective concentration) helps determine the efficacy and safety of a drug. However, these features differ by population and are affected by patient-related factors (eg, pregnancy [see p. 2159] and age [see p. 2534]).

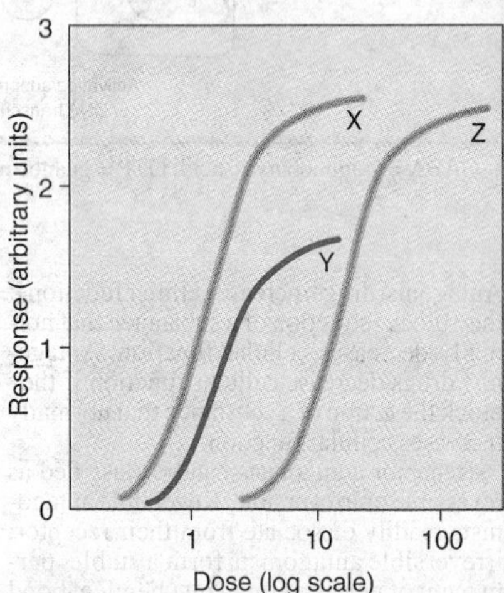

Fig. 304–2. Comparison of dose-response curves for drugs X, Y, and Z. Drug X has greater biologic activity per dosing equivalent and is thus more potent than drug Y or Z. Drugs X and Z have equal efficacy, indicated by their maximal attainable response (ceiling effect). Drug Y is more potent than drug Z, but its maximal efficacy is lower.

305 ADVERSE DRUG REACTIONS

Adverse drug reaction (ADR, or adverse drug effect) is a broad term referring to unwanted, uncomfortable, or dangerous effects that a drug may have. ADRs can be considered a form of toxicity; however, toxicity is most commonly applied to effects of overingestion (accidental or intentional—see p. 2651) or to elevated blood levels or enhanced drug effects that occur during appropriate use (eg, when drug metabolism is temporarily inhibited by a disorder or another drug). Side effect is an imprecise term often used to refer to a drug's unintended effects that occur within the therapeutic range. Because all drugs have the potential for ADRs, risk-benefit analysis (analyzing the likelihood of benefit vs risk of ADRs) is necessary whenever a drug is prescribed.

In the US, 3 to 7% of all hospitalizations are due to ADRs. ADRs occur during 10 to 20% of hospitalizations, about 10 to 20% of which are severe. Incidence of death due to ADRs is unknown; suggested rates of 0.5 to 0.9% may be falsely high because many of the patients included had serious and complex disorders.

Incidence and severity of ADRs vary by patient characteristics (eg, age, sex, ethnicity, coexisting disorders, genetic or geographic factors) and by drug factors (eg, type of drug, administration route, treatment duration, dosage, bioavailability). Incidence is probably higher and ADRS are more severe in the elderly (see p. 2536), although age per se may not be the primary cause. The contribution of prescribing and adherence errors to the incidence of ADRs is unclear (see p. 2514).

Etiology

Most ADRs are dose-related; others are allergic or idiosyncratic. Dose-related ADRs are usually predictable; ADRs unrelated to dose are usually unpredictable.

Dose-related ADRs are particularly a concern when drugs have a narrow therapeutic index (eg, hemorrhage with oral anticoagulants). ADRs may result from decreased drug clearance in patients with impaired renal or hepatic function or from drug-drug interactions.

Allergic ADRs are not dose-related and require prior exposure. Allergies develop when a drug acts as an antigen or allergen. After a patient is sensitized, subsequent exposure to the drug produces one of several different types of allergic reaction (see p. 1361). Clinical history and appropriate skin tests can sometimes help predict allergic ADRs.

Idiosyncrasy is an imprecise term used to classify unexpected ADRs that are not dose-related or allergic. They occur in a small percentage of patients given a drug. Idiosyncrasy has been defined as a genetically determined abnormal response to a drug, but not all idiosyncratic reactions have a pharmacogenetic cause. The term may become obsolete as specific mechanisms of ADRs become known.

Symptoms and Signs

ADRs are usually classified as mild, moderate, severe, or lethal (see TABLE 305–1). Symptoms and signs may manifest soon after the 1st dose or only after chronic use. They may obviously result from drug use or be too subtle to identify as drug-related. In the elderly, subtle ADRs can cause functional deterioration, changes in mental status, failure to thrive, loss of appetite, confusion, and depression.

Allergic ADRs typically occur soon after a drug is taken but generally do not occur after the 1st dose; typically, they occur when the drug

TABLE 305–1. CLASSIFICATION OF ADVERSE DRUG REACTIONS

SEVERITY	DESCRIPTION
Mild	No antidote or treatment is required; hospitalization is not prolonged
Moderate	A change in treatment (eg, modified dosage, addition of a drug), but not necessarily discontinuation of the drug, is required; hospitalization may be prolonged, or specific treatment may be required
Severe	An ADR is potentially life threatening and requires discontinuation of the drug and specific treatment of the ADR
Lethal	An ADR directly or indirectly contributes to a patient's death

is given after an initial exposure. Symptoms include itching, rash, fixed-drug eruption, upper or lower airway edema with difficulty breathing, and hypotension.

Idiosyncratic ADRs can produce almost any symptom or sign and usually cannot be predicted.

Diagnosis

Symptoms that occur soon after a drug is taken are often easily connected with use of a drug. However, diagnosing symptoms due to chronic drug use requires a significant level of suspicion and is often complicated. Stopping a drug is sometimes necessary but is difficult if the drug is essential and does not have an acceptable substitute. When proof of the relationship between drug and symptoms is important, rechallenge should be considered, except in the case of serious allergic reactions.

Physicians should report most suspected ADRs to MedWatch (the FDA's ADR monitoring program), which is an early alert system. Only through such reporting can unexpected ADRs be identified and investigated. MedWatch also monitors changes in the nature and frequency of ADRs. Forms for and information about reporting ADRs are available in the *Physicians' Desk Reference, AMA Drug Evaluations,* and *FDA Drug Bulletin* (mailed to all physicians at least yearly) and at www.fda.gov/medwatch; forms may also be obtained by calling 800-FDA-1088. Nurses, pharmacists, and other health care practitioners should also report ADRs.

Prevention and Treatment

Prevention of ADRs requires familiarity with the drug and potential reactions to it. Computer-based analysis should be used to check for potential drug interactions; analysis should be repeated whenever drugs are changed or added. Drugs and initial dosage must be carefully selected for the elderly (see Ch. 306, below). If patients develop nonspecific symptoms, ADRs should always be considered before beginning symptomatic treatment.

For dose-related ADRs, modifying the dose or eliminating or reducing precipitating factors may suffice. Increasing the rate of drug elimination is rarely necessary. For allergic and idiosyncratic ADRs, the drug usually should be withdrawn and not tried again. Switching to a different drug class is often required for allergic ADRs and sometimes required for dose-related ADRs.

306 DRUG THERAPY IN THE ELDERLY

Providing safe, effective drug therapy is one of the greatest challenges in geriatrics. The elderly use more drugs than any other age group and have many chronic disorders that affect drug response. Acute or chronic disorders can further deplete the already diminished physiologic reserves of the elderly, increasing their risk of adverse drug effects. Aging also alters pharmacodynamics and pharmacokinetics and thus affects the choice, dose, and frequency of use of many drugs. For the elderly, drug therapy is further complicated because they may be unable to obtain or afford drugs or adhere to complex drug regimens.

Prevalence of prescription drug use among ambulatory adults increases substantially with aging. Among people ≥ 65, > 90% use ≥ 1 drug/week, > 40% use ≥ 5 different drugs/week, and 12% use ≥ 10 different drugs/week. Women take more drugs, particularly psychoactive and arthritis drugs. Drug use is greatest among the frail elderly, hospitalized patients, and nursing home residents; typically, a nursing home resident is given 7 to 8 different drugs on a regular basis.

When prescribed and used appropriately, most drugs can benefit the elderly. Drugs are critical for prevention and treatment of acute and chronic disorders. Many directly modulate disease; others control symptoms that reduce quality of life. However, the elderly are at substantial risk of having adverse drug effects (see pp. 2533 and 2536). Among ambulatory people ≥ 65, adverse drug events occur at a rate of about 50 events/1000 person-years; nearly 30% of these events result from drug errors, predominantly in drug prescribing and monitoring, as well as lack of patient adherence. For optimal drug therapy in the elderly, benefits must be maximized while risks are minimized.

Polypharmacy (concurrent use of many drugs) alone does not accurately gauge appropriateness of therapy because the elderly often have many disorders requiring treatment; however, the elderly often use unnecessary drugs, prescribed for minor symptoms that are best treated nonpharmacologically. Use of unnecessary drugs (eg, analgesics, antibiotics, H_2 blockers, hypnotics, laxatives) increases cost and may lead to avoidable toxicity.

Some drugs are underused in the elderly. Examples are drugs to treat depression, pain, heart failure, incontinence and to prevent glaucoma, influenza, and pneumococcal infections.

PHARMACOKINETICS IN THE ELDERLY

Pharmacokinetics (see p. 2520) is best defined as what the body does to the drug; it includes absorption, distribution across body compartments, metabolism, and excretion. With aging, the metabolism and excretion of many drugs decrease, and the physiologic changes of aging require dose adjustment for some drugs. Toxicity may accumulate slowly because levels of chronically used drugs tend to increase for about 6 half-lives. For example, certain benzodiazepines (diazepam, flurazepam, chlordiazepoxide) have half-lives of up to 96 h in many elderly patients; signs of toxicity may not appear until days or weeks after therapy is started.

Absorption: Despite an age-related decrease in small-bowel surface area and an increase in gastric pH, changes in drug absorption tend to be trivial and clinically inconsequential.

Distribution: With aging, the body's fat compartment increases, and the water compartment decreases. Increased fat increases the volume of distribution for highly lipophilic drugs (eg, diazepam) and may increase their elimination half-lives.

Serum albumin decreases and α_1-acid glycoprotein increases with aging, but the clinical effect of these changes on serum drug binding is unclear. In patients with an acute disorder or undernutrition, rapid reductions in serum albumin may enhance drug effects because serum levels of unbound drug may increase.

Hepatic metabolism: Overall hepatic metabolism of many drugs through the cytochrome P-450 enzyme system decreases with aging. For drugs with decreased hepatic metabolism (see TABLE 306–1), clearance typically decreases 30 to 40%. Theoretically, maintenance drug doses should be decreased by this percentage; however, rate of drug metabolism varies greatly from person to person, and individual titration is required.

Hepatic clearance of drugs with multistage metabolism (nonsynthetic and synthetic reactions) is more likely to be prolonged in the elderly (see also Metabolism on p. 2526). Usually, age does not greatly affect clearance of drugs that are metabolized by conjugation, typically with glucuronic acid.

Renal elimination: After age 30, creatinine clearance decreases an average of 8 mL/min/1.73 m^2/decade; however, interindividual variation in the decline with aging is substantial. Serum creatinine levels often remain within normal limits despite a decrease in GFR because the elderly have less muscle mass and thus produce less creatinine. Decreases in tubular function parallel those in glomerular function.

These changes decrease renal elimination of some drugs (see TABLE 306–1). Clinical implications depend on the extent that renal elimination contributes to total systemic elimination and on the drug's therapeutic index (ratio of maximum tolerated dose to minimum effective dose). Creatinine clearance (measured or estimated using computer programs or a formula—see p. 1934) is used to guide drug dose. Because renal function is dynamic, maintenance doses of drugs should be adjusted when patients become ill, dehydrated, or have recently recovered from dehydration.

PHARMACODYNAMICS IN THE ELDERLY

Pharmacodynamics is defined as what the drug does to the body or the response of the body to the drug; it is affected by receptor binding, postreceptor effects, and chemical interactions (see p. 2530). The effects of similar drug concentrations at the site of action (sensitivity) may be greater or smaller than those in younger people (see TABLE 306–2). Differences may be due to changes in drug-receptor interaction, in postreceptor events, or in adaptive homeostatic responses and, among frail patients, are often due to organ pathology.

Elderly patients are particularly sensitive to anticholinergic drug effects. Many drugs

TABLE 306–1. EFFECT OF AGING ON DRUG METABOLISM* AND ELIMINATION

CLASS OR CATEGORY	DECREASED HEPATIC METABOLISM	DECREASED RENAL ELIMINATION
Analgesics and anti-inflammatory drugs	Dextropropoxyphene Ibuprofen Meperidine Morphine Naproxen	—
Antibiotics	—	Amikacin Ciprofloxacin Gentamicin Nitrofurantoin Streptomycin Tobramycin
Cardiovascular drugs	Amlodipine Diltiazem Lidocaine† Nifedipine Propranolol Quinidine Theophylline Verapamil	*N*-Acetylprocainamide Captopril Digoxin Enalapril Lisinopril Procainamide Quinapril
Diuretics	—	Amiloride Furosemide Hydrochlorothiazide Triamterene
Psychoactive drugs	Alprazolam† Chlordiazepoxide Desipramine† Diazepam Imipramine Nortriptyline Trazodone Triazolam†	Risperidone
Others	Levodopa	Amantadine Chlorpropamide Cimetidine Lithium Ranitidine

*When aging's effect on hepatic metabolism of a drug is controversial, effects reported in the majority of studies are listed.

†The effect occurs in men but not in women.

(eg, tricyclic antidepressants, most nonselective antihistamines, some antipsychotic drugs, many OTC hypnotics and cold preparations) are anticholinergic. The elderly, most notably those with dementia, are particularly prone to CNS adverse effects of such drugs and may develop confusion and somnolence. Anticholinergic drugs also commonly cause constipation, urinary retention (especially in elderly men with benign prostatic hyperplasia), blurred vision, orthostatic hypotension, and dry mouth.

ADVERSE DRUG EFFECTS IN THE ELDERLY

The elderly are at increased risk of adverse effects with certain drugs (see TABLE 306–3). Increased risk may result from age-related changes in pharmacokinetics or pharmacodynamics. Risk of an adverse effect increases exponentially with the number of drugs used, partly because multiple drug therapy reflects the presence of many diseases and

TABLE 306–2. EFFECT OF AGING ON DRUG RESPONSE

CLASS	DRUG	ACTION	EFFECT OF AGING
Analgesics	Aspirin	Acute gastroduodenal mucosal damage	↔
	Morphine	Acute analgesic effect	↑
	Pentazocine	Analgesic effect	↑
Anticoagulants	Heparin	PTT	↔
	Warfarin	PT	↑
Bronchodilators	Albuterol	Bronchodilation	↓
	Ipratropium	Bronchodilation	↔
Cardiovascular drugs	Adenosine	Minute ventilation and heart rate response	↔
		Venodilation	↔
	Angiotensin II receptor blockers	Decreased BP	↑
	Diltiazem	Acute antihypertensive effect	↑
	Dopamine	Increased creatinine clearance	↓
	Enalapril	Acute antihypertensive effect	↑
	Felodipine	Antihypertensive effect	↑
	Histamine	Venodilation	↔
	Isoproterenol	Increased heart rate	↓
		Increased ejection fraction	↓
		Venodilation	↓
	Nitroglycerin	Venodilation	↔
	Norepinephrine	Acute vasoconstriction	↔
	Phenylephrine	Acute venoconstriction	↔
		Acute hypertensive effect	↔
	Prazosin	Acute antihypertensive effect	↔
	Propranolol	Decreased heart rate	↔
	Timolol	Decreased heart rate	↔
	Verapamil	Acute antihypertensive effect	↑
Diuretics	Bumetanide	Increased urine flow and Na excretion	↓
	Furosemide	Latency and size of peak diuretic response	↓
Oral hypoglycemics	Glyburide	Chronic hypoglycemic effect	↔
	Tolbutamide	Acute hypoglycemic effect	↓
Psychoactive drugs	Diazepam	Sedation	↑↑
	Diphenhydramine	Psychomotor function	↑
	Haloperidol	Acute sedation	↑
	Midazolam	EEG activity	↑
		Sedation	↑
	Temazepam	Postural sway	↑
		Psychomotor effect	↑
		Sedation	↑
	Thiopental	Anesthesia	↔
	Triazolam	Sedation	↔
Others	Atropine	Impaired gastric emptying	↔
	Levodopa	Adverse effects	↑
	Metoclopramide	Sedation	↔

↔ = unchanged; ↑ = increased; ↓ = decreased.

Adapted from Cusack BJ, Vestal RE: Clinical pharmacology: Special considerations in the elderly. In *Practice of Geriatric Medicine*, edited by E Calkins, PJ Davis, and AB Ford. Philadelphia, WB Saunders Company, 1986, pp. 115–136; used with permission.

TABLE 306–3. HIGH-RISK DRUGS IN THE ELDERLY (BASED ON BEERS CRITERIA)

CLASS	DRUG	PRESCRIBING CONCERN
Analgesics	Indomethacin	Of available NSAIDs, indomethacin has the most CNS adverse effects and therefore should be avoided in the elderly
	Ketorolac	Immediate and long-term use should be avoided in the elderly because many have asymptomatic GI disorders
	Meperidine	Meperidine is not an effective oral analgesic and has many disadvantages compared with other opioids. It should be avoided in the elderly
	Non–COX-selective NSAIDs (naproxen, oxaprozin, and piroxicam)	Long-term use of the maximum dosage may cause GI bleeding, renal failure, hypertension, and heart failure
	Pentazocine	Pentazocine is an opioid analgesic that has more CNS adverse effects (eg, confusion, hallucinations) more commonly than other opioids; it is a mixed agonist/antagonist. For both reasons, it should usually be avoided in the elderly
	Propoxyphene and combination products	Propoxyphene should usually be avoided in the elderly. It has few analgesic advantages over acetaminophen but has the adverse effects of other opioids
Antidepressants	Cyclic antidepressants (eg, amitriptyline, doxepin)	Because of strong anticholinergic and sedating effects, amitriptyline or doxepin is rarely the antidepressant of choice for the elderly
	Fluoxetine (taken daily)	Fluoxetine has a long half-life, may cause excessive CNS stimulation and sleep disturbances, and may increase agitation. Safer alternative SSRIs exist
Antihistamines	Chlorpheniramine Cyproheptadine Dexchlorpheniramine Diphenhydramine Hydroxyzine Orphenadrine Promethazine Tripelennamine	All OTC and many prescription antihistamines have potent anticholinergic properties. Antihistamines are commonly included with other drugs in cough and cold preparations. However, many cough and cold preparations without antihistamines are available; they are safer alternatives for the elderly
Antipsychotics	Mesoridazine Thioridazine	Risk of CNS and extrapyramidal adverse effects is increased
Cardiovascular drugs	Amiodarone	Adverse effects include QTc prolongation and risk of provoking torsades de pointes
	Clonidine	Adverse effects include orthostatic hypotension and CNS effects
	Digoxin	Because renal clearance of digoxin is decreased in the elderly, doses should rarely exceed 0.125 mg/day, unless the patient is monitored
	Dipyridamole	Dipyridamole frequently causes orthostatic hypotension in the elderly. It has proved beneficial only in patients with artificial heart valves. If possible, it should be avoided in the elderly

TABLE 306–3. HIGH-RISK DRUGS IN THE ELDERLY (BASED ON BEERS CRITERIA)—Continued

CLASS	DRUG	PRESCRIBING CONCERN
	Disopyramide	Of all antiarrhythmics, disopyramide is the most potent negative inotrope and therefore may induce heart failure in the elderly. It is also strongly anticholinergic. Other antiarrhythmics, when needed, should be used
	Doxazosin	Adverse effects include hypotension, dry mouth, and urinary problems
	Ethacrynic acid	Adverse effects include hypertension and fluid imbalances
	Guanethidine Guanadrel	Adverse effects include orthostatic hypotension
	Methyldopa	Methyldopa may cause bradycardia and exacerbate depression in the elderly. Alternate treatments for hypertension are generally preferred
	Nifedipine (short-acting)	Adverse effects include hypotension, constipation, and reflex tachycardia
	Reserpine	Doses > 0.25 mg pose unnecessary risks in the elderly by inducing depression, impotence, sedation, and orthostatic hypotension. Safer alternatives exist
	Ticlopidine	Ticlopidine is no better than aspirin in preventing clotting and is considerably more toxic. It should be used only as a 2nd-line drug in the elderly
GI antispasmodics	Belladonna alkaloids Clidinium/chlordiazepoxide Dicyclomine Hyoscyamine Propantheline	GI antispasmodics are highly anticholinergic and usually produce substantial toxicity in the elderly. Efficacy at doses tolerated by the elderly is questionable. All of these drugs are best avoided in the elderly, especially for long-term use
Hypoglycemics	Chlorpropamide	Chlorpropamide has a prolonged half-life in the elderly and can cause prolonged, serious hypoglycemia. It is the only oral hypoglycemic that causes SIADH. It should be avoided in the elderly
Laxatives (stimulant)	Bisacodyl Cascara Neoloid except when used with opioids	Stimulant laxatives may exacerbate bowel dysfunction
Muscle relaxants	Carisoprodol Chlorzoxazone Cyclobenzaprine Metaxalone Methocarbamol Oxybutynin	Most muscle relaxants and antispasmodics are poorly tolerated by the elderly, resulting in anticholinergic effects, sedation, and weakness. Efficacy at doses tolerated by the elderly is questionable. If possible, they should not be used in the elderly
Sedative-hypnotics	Alprazolam* 2 mg Lorazepam 3 mg Oxazepam 60 mg Temazepam 15 mg Triazolam 0.25 mg	Because sensitivity to benzodiazepines is increased in the elderly, smaller doses may be effective as well as safer; total daily doses should rarely exceed those listed

Table continues on the following page.

TABLE 306–3. HIGH-RISK DRUGS IN THE ELDERLY (BASED ON BEERS CRITERIA)—Continued

CLASS	DRUG	PRESCRIBING CONCERN
	Barbiturates (except phenobarbital)	Barbiturates cause more adverse effects in the elderly than most other sedative-hypnotics and are highly addictive. They should not be started as new therapy in the elderly except to control seizures
	Chlordiazepoxide Chlordiazepoxide/amitriptyline Clorazepate Clidinium/chlordiazepoxide Diazepam Flurazepam Halazepam Nitrazepam Quazepam	These long-acting benzodiazepines have a long half-life in the elderly (often days), causing prolonged sedation and increasing risk of falls and fractures. Short- or intermediate-acting benzodiazepines are preferred if a benzodiazepine is required
	Diphenhydramine	Diphenhydramine is potently anticholinergic and usually should not be used as a hypnotic in the elderly. When used to treat or prevent allergic reactions, it should be used in the smallest possible dose and with great caution
	Meprobamate	Meprobamate is a highly addictive and sedating anxiolytic. It should be avoided in the elderly. Those using it for long periods may become addicted, and the drug may need to be withdrawn slowly
Other	Amphetamines and anorexics	These drugs may cause dependence, hypertension, angina, and MI. Amphetamines (except methylphenidate) have CNS stimulant adverse effects
	Cimetidine	Cimetidine has CNS adverse effects, including confusion
	Cyclandelate Ergot mesylates	These drugs in the doses studied have not been shown to be effective for treatment of dementia or any other disorder
	Desiccated thyroid	Cardiac effects are a concern. Safer alternatives exist
	Estrogens only (oral)	Evidence suggests that estrogens increase risk of breast and endometrial cancer and may increase risk of pulmonary embolism, stroke, and coronary artery disease in older women
	Ferrous sulfate	Doses > 325 mg/day do not substantially increase total absorption and are more likely to cause constipation
	Isoxsuprine	Isoxsuprine is not effective in the elderly
	Methyltestosterone	Adverse effects include benign prostatic hypertrophy and cardiac problems
	Mineral oil	Mineral oil may result in aspiration
	Nitrofurantoin	Nitrofurantoin is ineffective in patients with moderate to severe renal insufficiency; peripheral neuropathy may occur due to metabolites

Table continues on the following page.

TABLE 306–3. HIGH-RISK DRUGS IN THE ELDERLY (BASED ON BEERS CRITERIA)—Continued

CLASS	DRUG	PRESCRIBING CONCERN
	Trimethobenzamide	Trimethobenzamide is one of the least effective antiemetics and can have extrapyramidal adverse effects. When possible, it should be avoided in the elderly

*Doses of alprazolam may be higher when used to treat panic disorders.

SIADH = syndrome of inappropriate antidiuretic hormone secretion.

Adapted from Fick DM et al: Updating the Beers criteria for potentially inappropriate medication use in older adults. *Archives of Internal Medicine* 163:2716–2724, 2003.

increases risk of drug-disease and drug-drug interactions.

Drug-disease interactions (exacerbation of a disease by a drug given for another reason) can occur in any age group but are especially important in the elderly, who are more likely to have multiple disorders. Distinguishing often subtle adverse drug effects from the effects of disease is difficult (see TABLE 306–4). Anticholinergic drugs are a common cause of such interactions.

Drug-drug interactions are myriad, but there appear to be few differences in drug-drug interactions in the elderly. However, induction of drug metabolism by dichloralphenazone, glutethimide, and rifampin may be decreased in the elderly. Concurrent use of more than one drug with similar toxicity can increase the risk or severity of adverse effects.

CONSIDERATIONS FOR EFFECTIVE DRUG THERAPY IN THE ELDERLY

The prescribing cascade begins when an adverse drug effect is misinterpreted as a new disorder. In response, another drug is prescribed, and patients may develop additional adverse effects related to the second, unnecessary drug. Additional adverse effects may also be misinterpreted as a new disorder and treated unnecessarily, and so on. In elderly patients, prescribers should always consider the possibility that a new symptom or sign is due to drug therapy.

Doses must often be reduced, although dose requirements vary considerably from person to person. In general, starting doses of about $\frac{1}{3}$ to $\frac{1}{2}$ the usual adult dose are indicated for drugs with a low therapeutic index and when a condition may be exacerbated by a drug. However, titrating the dose upward as tolerated is essential to providing maximal therapeutic benefit for the elderly.

Adherence (compliance) is affected by many factors but not by age per se. However, about 40% of elderly patients do not take drugs as directed, usually taking less than prescribed (underadherence). Causes are the same as for younger adults (see p. 2514). In addition, financial and physical constraints may make purchasing drugs difficult, dementia may make taking drugs difficult, and lack of information may lead to errors. Taking drugs can be facilitated by easy-access containers, containers equipped with reminder alarms, containers filled by daily drug needs, or reminder phone calls.

DRUG CATEGORIES OF CONCERN IN THE ELDERLY

Some drug categories (eg, analgesics, anticoagulants, antihypertensives, antiparkinsonian drugs, diuretics, hypoglycemic drugs, psychoactive drugs) pose special risks for elderly patients.

Analgesics: NSAIDs are widely used; several are available without prescription. Serious adverse effects include peptic ulceration and upper GI bleeding; risk is increased when an NSAID is begun and when dose is increased. Risk of upper GI bleeding increases when NSAIDs are given with warfarin or aspirin. NSAIDs may increase risk of cardiovascular events and can cause fluid retention. Selective COX-2 inhibitors (coxibs) cause less GI irritation and platelet inhibition than

TABLE 306–4. DRUG-DISEASE INTERACTIONS IN THE ELDERLY

DISEASE	DRUGS	POSSIBLE ADVERSE EFFECTS
Bladder outflow obstruction	Anticholinergic drugs Antihistamines Antidepressants Decongestants Flavoxate GI antispasmodics Muscle relaxants Oxybutynin Tolterodine	Impaired outflow leading to urinary retention
Clotting disorders	Aspirin Clopidogrel Dipyridamole NSAIDs Ticlopidine	Prolonged clotting time due to inhibition of platelet aggregation, resulting in increased risk of bleeding
Arrhythmias	Tricyclic antidepressants	Heart block, proarrhythmic effect, QT interval changes
COPD	Benzodiazepines (long-acting) Propranolol	CNS adverse effects, respiratory depression
Chronic renal impairment	Aminoglycosides NSAIDs Radiopaque dyes	Acute renal failure
Constipation	Anticholinergic drugs Ca channel blockers Tricyclic antidepressants	Exacerbation of constipation
Dementia	Amantadine Anticholinergic drugs Anticonvulsants Antispasmodics Barbiturates Levodopa Muscle relaxants Psychoactive drugs	Increased confusion, delirium
Depression	Alcohol Benzodiazepines (long-acting) β-Blockers Central-acting antihypertensives Corticosteroids	Precipitation or exacerbation of depression
Diabetes	Diuretics	Hyperglycemia
Falls	Benzodiazepines Tricyclic antidepressants	Increased risk of falls
Glaucoma	Anticholinergic drugs	Exacerbation of glaucoma
Heart failure	Diltiazem Disopyramide Verapamil	Exacerbation of heart failure
Hypertension	Amphetamines NSAIDs Phenylpropanolamine Pseudoephedrine	Increased BP

TABLE 306–4. DRUG-DISEASE INTERACTIONS IN THE ELDERLY—Continued

DISEASE	DRUGS	POSSIBLE ADVERSE EFFECTS
Hypokalemia	Digoxin	Cardiac toxicity
Incontinence	α-Blockers Anticholinergics Benzodiazepines (long-acting) Tricyclic antidepressants	Polyuria, exacerbation of stress incontinence
Obesity	Olanzapine	Increased appetite, weight gain
Orthostatic hypotension	Antihypertensives Antipsychotics Diuretics Levodopa Tricyclic antidepressants	Dizziness, falls, syncope
Osteopenia	Corticosteroids	Fractures
Parkinson's disease	Antipsychotics (conventional) Metoclopramide Tacrine	Exacerbation of symptoms
Peptic ulcer disease	Anticoagulants NSAIDs	Upper GI bleeding
Prostate disease	α-Agonists Anticholinergic drugs	Urinary retention
Seizure disorders	Bupropion Chlorpromazine Clozapine Meperidine Thioridazine Thiothixene	Lowering of seizure threshold
Undernutrition	CNS stimulants (dextroamphetamine, fluoxetine, methylphenidate, methamphetamine, pemoline)	Decreased appetite

Adapted from Fick DM et al: Updating the Beers criteria for potentially inappropriate medication use in older adults. *Archives of Internal Medicine* 163:2716–2724, 2003.

other NSAIDs. Nonetheless, coxibs have a risk of GI bleeding, especially in patients taking warfarin or aspirin (even at low dose) and in those who have had GI events. Coxibs, as a class, appear to increase risk of cardiovascular events, but that risk may vary by drug; their use should be approached cautiously. Coxibs have renal effects comparable to those of other NSAIDs. Monitoring serum creatinine is necessary, especially in patients with other risk factors (eg, heart failure, renal impairment, cirrhosis with ascites, volume depletion, diuretic use).

Anticoagulants: Aging does not alter the pharmacokinetics of warfarin but may increase sensitivity to its anticoagulant effect. Careful dosing and scrupulous monitoring can largely overcome the increased risk of bleeding in elderly patients taking warfarin.

Antihypertensives: In many elderly patients, lower starting doses of antihypertensives may be necessary to reduce risk of adverse effects; however, for most elderly patients with hypertension, achieving BP goals requires standard doses and multidrug therapy. Initially, a thiazide-type diuretic is usually given alone or with one of the other classes (ACE inhibitors, angiotensin II receptor blockers, β-blockers, Ca channel blockers) shown to be beneficial. Short-acting dihydropyridines (eg, nifedipine) may increase mortality risk and should not be used.

Antiparkinsonian drugs: Levodopa clearance is reduced in elderly patients, who are also more susceptible to orthostatic hypotension and confusion. Therefore, elderly patients should be given a lower starting dose of levodopa and carefully monitored for adverse effects (see also p. 1883). Patients who become confused while taking levodopa may also not tolerate newer dopamine agonists (eg, bromocriptine, pergolide, pramipexole, ropinirole). Because elderly patients with parkinsonism may be cognitively impaired, anticholinergic drugs should be avoided.

Digoxin: Digoxin clearance decreases an average of 50% in elderly patients with normal serum creatinine levels. Therefore, maintenance doses should be started low (0.125 mg/day) and adjusted according to response and serum digoxin levels. Digoxin must be used with caution in patients with heart failure. In men with heart failure and a left ventricular ejection fraction of ≤ 45%, serum digoxin levels > 0.8 ng/mL are associated with increased mortality risk. Among women with heart failure and depressed left ventricular function, digoxin, regardless of serum level, is associated with increased mortality risk.

Diuretics: Lower doses of thiazide diuretics (eg, hydrochlorothiazide or chlorthalidone 12.5 to 25 mg) can effectively control hypertension in many elderly patients and have less risk of hypokalemia and hyperglycemia (see also p. 609). Thus, K supplements may be required less often. K-sparing diuretics should be used with caution in the elderly; the K level must be carefully monitored, particularly when these diuretics are given with ACE inhibitors.

Antihyperglycemics: Doses of antihyperglycemics should be titrated carefully in patients with diabetes mellitus. Risk of hypoglycemia due to sulfonylureas may increase with aging. Chlorpropamide is not recommended because elderly patients are at increased risk of hyponatremia due to syndrome of inappropriate antidiuretic hormone secretion (SIADH) and because the drug's long duration of action is dangerous if adverse effects or hypoglycemia occurs. Risk of hypoglycemia is greater with glyburide than with other oral antihyperglycemics.

Metformin, a biguanide excreted by the kidneys, increases peripheral tissue sensitivity to insulin and can be effective given alone or with sulfonylureas. Risk of lactic acidosis, a rare but serious complication, increases with degree of renal impairment and with patient age. Heart failure is a contraindication.

Psychoactive drugs: In nonpsychotic, agitated patients, antipsychotics control symptoms only marginally better than do placebos. Antipsychotics can reduce paranoia but may worsen confusion (see also p. 1727). Elderly patients, especially women, are at increased risk of tardive dyskinesia, which is often irreversible. The FDA has issued a warning regarding the use of atypical antipsychotics in the treatment of behavioral disorders in elderly patients with dementia. A review of placebo-controlled studies has shown a higher death rate associated with their use. Sedation, orthostatic hypotension, anticholinergic effects, and akathisia (subjective motor restlessness) can occur in up to 20% of elderly patients taking an antipsychotic, and drug-induced parkinsonism can persist for up to 6 to 9 mo after stopping the drug. Antipsychotic drugs should be reserved for psychosis. When an antipsychotic is used, the starting dose should be about ¼ the usual starting adult dose and should be increased gradually. Extrapyramidal dysfunction can develop when atypical antipsychotics (eg, olanzapine, quetiapine, risperidone) are used, especially at higher doses. Clinical trial data relating to dosing, efficacy, and safety of these drugs in the elderly are limited; thus, dose reduction is prudent.

Use of anxiolytics and hypnotics can be problematic. Treatable causes of insomnia should be sought and managed before using hypnotics (see also p. 1837). Nonbenzodiazepine hypnotics (eg, the imidazopyridines, alpidem and zolpidem) are options for treating insomnia in the elderly if nonpharmacologic measures (eg, avoiding caffeinated beverages, limiting daytime napping, modifying bedtime) are ineffective. These drugs bind mainly to a benzodiazepine receptor subtype. Imidazopyridines disturb the sleep pattern less than benzodiazepines and have a more rapid onset, fewer rebound effects, and less potential for dependence. Longer-acting benzodiazepines (eg, clonazepam, diazepam, flurazepam) should be avoided because they are likely to accumulate and have adverse effects (eg, drowsiness, impaired memory, impaired balance leading to falls and fractures). Duration of anxiolytic or hypnotic therapy should be limited if possible because tolerance and dependence may develop; withdrawal may lead to rebound anxiety and insomnia. Short- or intermediate-acting benzodiazepines with half-lives < 24 h (eg, alprazolam, lorazepam, oxazepam, temazepam) may be preferable to long-acting benzodiazepines, but these drugs may also have adverse effects, including those that lead to falls and fractures. Antihistamines (eg, diphenhydramine, hydroxyzine) are not recommended as anxiolytics or hypnotics because they have anticholinergic effects.

Buspirone, a partial serotonin agonist, can be effective for general anxiety disorder; elderly patients tolerate doses up to 30 mg/day well. The slow onset of anxiolytic action (up to 2 to 3 wk) can be a disadvantage in urgent cases.

Of antidepressants, SSRIs and mixed serotonin/dopamine reuptake inhibitors are generally preferred. These drugs appear to be as effective as tricyclic antidepressants and cause less toxicity. A possible disadvantage of fluoxetine is the long elimination half-life, especially of its active metabolite. Paroxetine is more sedating than other SSRIs, has anticholinergic effects, and, like some other SSRIs, can inhibit hepatic cytochrome P-450 2D6 enzyme activity, possibly impairing the metabolism of several drugs, including some antipsychotics, antiarrhythmics, and tricyclic antidepressants. Sertraline is more activating; diarrhea is a common adverse effect. Doses of these drugs should be reduced by up to 50%. Many SSRIs are available, but data on their use in the elderly are sparse. Tricyclic antidepressants are effective but should rarely be used in the elderly because safer alternatives exist.

SECTION 21
INJURIES; POISONING

307 APPROACH TO THE TRAUMA PATIENT

Injury is the number one cause of death for people aged 1 to 44. In the US, there were 160,000 trauma deaths in 2001, about ⅔ being accidental. Of intentional injury deaths, about 60% were due to self-harm. In addition to deaths, injury results in about 40 million emergency department visits annually.

The most seriously injured patients benefit from treatment in designated trauma centers, hospitals that have special staffing and protocols to provide immediate care to critically injured patients. Criteria for such designation (and for the necessity of transport to them) vary by state but usually follow guidelines of the American College of Surgeons' Committee on Trauma.

Many traumatic injuries (eg, burns, fractures, dislocations, sprains) are discussed elsewhere in THE MANUAL.

Etiology and Pathophysiology

Of the myriad ways people are injured, most can be categorized as blunt or penetrating. Blunt injury involves a forceful impact (eg, blow, kick, strike with object, fall, motor vehicle collision, blast). Penetrating injury involves breach of the skin by an object (eg, knife, broken glass) or projectile (eg, bullet, shrapnel from explosion).

Other injury types include thermal and chemical burns, toxic inhalations or ingestions, and radiation injury. These and other specific injuries (eg, fractures [see p. 2559], spinal cord injury [see p. 2579], head injury [see p. 2572]) are discussed elsewhere in THE MANUAL.

All injuries, by definition, produce direct tissue damage, the nature and extent depending on the anatomic site, mechanism, and intensity of trauma. Severe direct tissue damage (eg, to the heart, brain, spinal cord) is responsible for most immediate trauma deaths.

Patients surviving the initial insult may develop indirect injury effects. Disruption of blood vessels produces hemorrhage, which may be external (and hence visible) or internal, either confined within an organ as a contusion or hematoma, or as free hemorrhage into a body compartment (eg, peritoneal cavity, thorax). Small amounts of hemorrhage (ie, < 10% of blood volume) are tolerated well by most patients. Larger amounts cause progressive declines in BP and organ perfusion (shock—see full discussion on p. 559), leading to cellular dysfunction, organ failure, and eventually death. Hemorrhagic shock causes most short-term (ie, within hours) deaths, and multiple organ failure from prolonged shock causes many of the near-term (ie, first 14 days) deaths. Additional near-term deaths result from infection because of disruption of normal anatomic barriers.

Evaluation and Treatment

This chapter mostly addresses care in the emergency department rather than emergency care delivered at the accident site. Evaluation and treatment are performed simultaneously, beginning with systems that pose the most immediate threat to life if damaged. *Attending to dramatic but not deadly injuries (eg, open lower extremity fracture, finger amputations) before evaluating immediate life threats can be a fatal mistake.* As in cardiac resuscitation, a helpful mnemonic is "A, B, C, D." Systems are rapidly examined for major abnormalities; a more detailed examination (secondary survey) is performed after stabilization.

Airway: Airway patency is threatened by blood clots in the oropharynx and soft-tissue laxity caused by obtundation (eg, from head injury, shock, intoxication). These are readily visible on direct inspection of the mouth; having the patient speak can rapidly confirm an adequate airway.

Blood and foreign material are removed by suction or manually. Obtunded patients whose airway is in doubt and those with significant oropharyngeal injury require endotracheal intubation, usually with pharmacologic adjuncts for paralysis and sedation (see p. 528).

Breathing: Adequate ventilation is threatened by decreased central respiratory drive (from head injury, intoxication, shock) or by chest injury (eg, hemo- or pneumothorax, multiple rib fractures, pulmonary contusion).

Adequacy of air exchange is usually apparent on auscultation. Tension pneumothorax (see p. 497) may cause the trachea to deviate to the side opposite the injury, with decreased breath sounds and sometimes distended neck veins. The chest wall is palpated for obvious rib fractures and presence of subcutaneous air (sometimes the only finding with pneumothorax).

Pneumothorax is decompressed by chest tube (see p. 498) and must be excluded before initiating positive-pressure ventilation (which may markedly enlarge a pneumothorax and convert it to a tension pneumothorax). Inadequate ventilation is treated with endotracheal intubation and mechanical ventilation.

Circulation: Significant external hemorrhage can occur from any major vessel but is always apparent. Life-threatening internal hemorrhage is often less obvious. However, this volume of hemorrhage can occur in only a few body compartments: the chest, abdomen, and soft tissues of the pelvis or thigh (eg, from pelvis or femur fracture).

Pulse and BP are assessed, and signs of shock are noted (eg, dusky color, diaphoresis, altered mental status). Abdominal distention and tenderness, pelvis instability, or thigh deformity and instability are often present when internal hemorrhage in those areas is large enough to be life threatening.

External hemorrhage is controlled by direct pressure. Two large-bore (eg, 14- or 16-gauge) IVs are started with 0.9% saline or Ringer's lactate; rapid infusion of 1 to 2 L (20 mL/kg for children) is given for signs of shock and hypovolemia (see p. 562). Patients in whom there is strong clinical suspicion of major intra-abdominal hemorrhage may require immediate laparotomy.

Disability: Neurologic function is evaluated for major deficits involving the brain and spinal cord. The Glasgow Coma Scale (GCS—see TABLE 310–1 on p. 2574 and, for infants and children, TABLE 310–2 on p. 2575) and pupillary response screen for major intracranial injury. Gross motor movement and sensation in each extremity screen for major spinal cord injury. The cervical spine is palpated for tenderness and deformity and stabilized in a rigid collar if injury cannot be excluded. With careful manual stabilization of the head and neck, the patient is "log rolled" onto a side to allow palpation of the thoracic and lumbar spine and rectal examination to check tone (decreased tone indicates possible cord injury) and presence of blood. In the US, most patients arriving by ambulance are immobilized on a long, rigid board for ease of transport and to stabilize possible spinal fractures. If examination reveals no sign of spinal injury, patients are taken off the board because it is quite uncomfortable and pressure ulcers are possible within a few hours.

Secondary survey: After immediate life threats are assessed and stabilized, a more thorough evaluation is performed, and a focused history is obtained. If only limited conversation is possible, an "AMPLE" history covers essential information: *A*llergies, *M*edications, *P*ast medical history, *L*ast meal, and *E*vents of the injury.

After the patient is completely undressed, the examination generally proceeds from head to toe; it includes all orifices and a more detailed look at areas examined in the initial survey. All soft tissues are inspected for lesions and swelling, all bones are palpated for tenderness, and range of motion is assessed in joints (unless there is obvious fracture or deformity).

A urinary catheter is usually placed in seriously injured and obtunded patients provided there is no evidence of urethral injury (eg, blood at the meatus, ecchymosis of the perineum, high-riding prostate). Seriously injured patients often also have a nasogastric tube placed, provided there is no major midface trauma (rare reports exist of intracranial tube insertion through a cribriform plate fracture).

Open wounds are covered with sterile dressings, but cleansing and repair are deferred until completion of evaluation and treatment of more serious injuries. Major clinically apparent dislocations with marked deformity or neurovascular compromise are reduced immediately. Obvious or suspected fractures are splinted pending imaging.

Testing: Imaging tests are the cornerstone; laboratory tests are generally ancillary. Patients with penetrating trauma typically have focal injuries that can limit necessary imaging to the obviously involved region(s). Blunt trauma, particularly when significant deceleration is involved (eg, fall, motor vehicle collision), can affect any part of the body, and imaging is used more liberally. Such patients typically have x-ray of the chest, cervical spine, and pelvis unless they are awake and alert, completely lacking in symptoms or findings suggesting injury to those areas, and have no "distracting" injuries (eg, femur fracture) that might keep them from complaining about injuries elsewhere. These imaging tests are directed at life threats that may not be clinically obvious. Chest x-ray can identify airway disruption, lung injury, and pneumothorax and can suggest thoracic aorta tears (eg, by mediastinal widening).

Identification of intra-abdominal injury is essential. Previously, diagnostic peritoneal lavage was used, in which a peritoneal dialysis catheter was inserted through the abdominal wall into the peritoneal cavity and 1 L of 0.9% saline was run in and allowed to drain back out. Finding > 100,000 RBCs/mL of effluent is very sensitive for the presence of abdominal injury. However, this test is invasive, and many of the injuries so diagnosed do not require operative repair, so many clinicians now use ultrasound, CT, or both to better delineate the nature and extent of injury. These tests also have the advantage of being repeatable if the patient's condition changes.

Head CT is typically obtained for patients with altered mental status or focal neurologic abnormalities and for those who sustained loss of consciousness (some clinicians feel that patients with a brief loss of consciousness who are completely alert and neurologically intact do not require CT). Imaging is obtained more liberally in children < 2 yr with scalp hematoma, the elderly, and patients taking anticoagulants.

Plain x-rays are obtained of any suspected fractures. Other imaging tests are obtained for specific indications (eg, angiography to diagnose and sometimes embolize vascular injury; CT to better delineate spinal, pelvic, or complex joint fractures).

Useful laboratory tests include ABGs for P_{O_2} and base deficit, urine examined for blood, CBC to establish a baseline to monitor ongoing hemorrhage, and type and crossmatch for possible blood transfusion. Measures of perfusion (serum lactate, sublingual pCO_2) may help identify early or partially treated shock states. Other reflexively obtained tests (eg, electrolytes and other chemistries, coagulation studies) are unlikely to be of use barring relevant medical history. Toxicology screening (eg, blood alcohol, urine drug screen) is often performed; these tests rarely change immediate management but can help identify substance abuse causative of injury, allowing intervention to prevent subsequent trauma.

Patients with suspicion of significant blunt chest injury have ECG to diagnose myocardial injury and possible consequent arrhythmias. Those with abnormalities usually have blood levels of cardiac markers measured and sometimes echocardiography (see p. 592).

308 LACERATIONS

Care of lacerations enables prompt healing, minimizes risk of infection, and optimizes cosmetic result.

Physiology

Healing begins immediately after injury with coagulation and introduction of WBCs; neutrophils and monocytes remove debris (including devitalized tissue) and bacteria. Monocytes also encourage fibroblast replication and neovascularization. Fibroblasts deposit collagen, typically beginning within 48 h and reaching a maximum in about 7 days. Collagen deposition is essentially complete in 1 mo, but collagen fiber strength builds more slowly as fibers undergo crosslinking. Wound tensile strength is only about 20% of ultimate by 3 wk, 60% by 4 mo, and maximum at 1 yr; strength never becomes equivalent to the undamaged state.

Epithelial cells from the wound edge migrate across the wound shortly after injury. In a surgically repaired wound (healing by primary intention), they form an effective protective barrier to water and bacteria in 24 to 48 h and resemble normal epidermis within 5 days. In a wound that is not repaired (ie, heals by secondary intention), epithelialization is prolonged proportionally to the defect size.

There are static forces on the skin from its natural elasticity and the underlying muscles (see FIG. 308–1). Because scar tissue is not as strong as adjacent undamaged skin, these forces tend to widen scars, sometimes resulting in a cosmetically unacceptable appearance after apparently adequate wound closure. Scar widening is particularly likely when the forces are perpendicular to the wound edge. This tendency (and resultant scar stress) is readily observed in the fresh wound; gaping edges indicate perpendicular tension, and relatively well approximated edges indicate parallel forces.

Scars tend to be red and prominent for about 8 wk. As collagen remodeling occurs, the scar shrinks and loses its erythema. In some

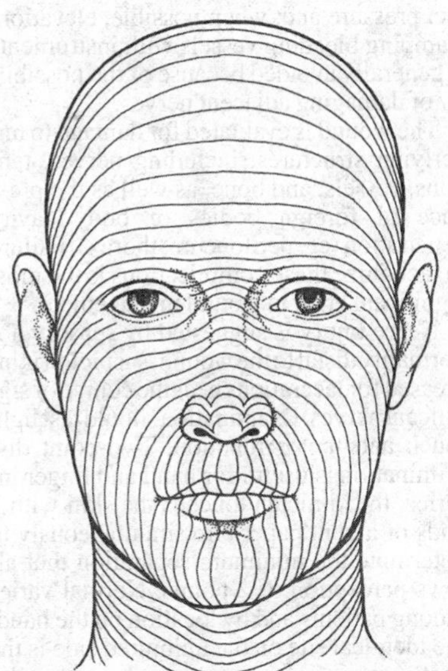

Fig. 308–1. Representative skin tension lines. Direction of force is along each line. Cuts perpendicular to these lines are thus under greatest tension and most likely to widen.

patients, however, the scar hypertrophies, becoming unsightly and raised. Keloids are hypertrophic scars that extend beyond the limits of the original wound (see p. 1018).

The main factors interfering with wound healing involve tissue ischemia, infection, or both. These occur for numerous reasons. Circulation can be impaired by disease (eg, diabetes, arterial insufficiency), features of the injury (eg, a crush-type injury, which damages the microvasculature), and factors in the repair such as overly tight sutures and perhaps use of a vasoconstrictor with the local anesthetic. Lower extremities are generally at greatest risk of circulatory problems. Wound hematoma, foreign material (including subcutaneous suture material), delayed treatment (> 6 h for lower extremities; > 12 to 18 h for face and scalp), and significant wound contamination predispose to bacterial proliferation. Bite wounds (see p. 2638) are usually heavily contaminated.

Evaluation

The clinician must first find and treat serious injury (see p. 2549) before focusing on skin lacerations, however dramatic. Actively bleeding wounds require hemostasis before evaluation. Hemostasis is best obtained by direct pressure and, when possible, elevation; clamping bleeding vessels with instruments is generally avoided because of the possibility of damaging adjacent nerves.

The wound is evaluated for damage to underlying structures, including nerves, tendons, vessels, and bone, as well as the presence of foreign bodies or body cavity penetration (eg, peritoneum, thorax). Failure to recognize these complications is the most significant error in wound management.

Nerve injury is suggested by sensory abnormality distal to the wound; suspicion is increased for lacerations near the course of significant nerves. Examination should test light touch and motor function. Two-point discrimination is useful for hand and finger injuries; the clinician touches the skin with 2 ends of a bent paper clip simultaneously to determine the minimum separation that allows perception of 2 points. Normal varies among patients and by location on the hand; the identical site on the uninjured side is the best control.

Tendon injury is suspected in any laceration over the course of a tendon. Complete tendon laceration usually produces a resting deformity (eg, foot drop from Achilles laceration, loss of normal resting finger flexion with digital flexor laceration) because forces from antagonist muscles are unopposed. Resting deformity does not occur with partial tendon laceration, which may present with only pain or relative weakness on strength testing or be discovered only on exploration of the wound.

Serious injury to vascular structures is suggested by pallor, decreased pulses, or perhaps slowed capillary refill distal to the laceration (all compared with the uninjured side).

Bone is occasionally injured, particularly after penetrating trauma (eg, stab wound, bite), or when injury occurs over a bony prominence. If the mechanism or location of injury is concerning, plain x-rays are taken to rule out fracture.

Foreign bodies are sometimes present in wounds, depending on the mechanism; wounds involving glass are likely to have foreign bodies, lacerations from sharp metal rarely do, and wounds involving other substances are of intermediate risk. Although not very sensitive, a patient's complaint of feeling a foreign body is fairly specific and should not be ignored. Imaging studies are recommended for all wounds involving glass and for others if a foreign body is suspected because of mechanism or inability to examine the wound's full depth. If glass or inorganic material (eg, stones, metal fragments) is involved, plain x-rays are taken; glass bits as small as 1 mm can be seen. Organic materials (eg, wood splinters, plastic) are rarely detected on plain x-ray (although the outline of larger objects may be visible by their displacement of normal tissue); various other modalities have been used, including xerography, ultrasonography, CT, and MRI. None of these is 100% sensitive, but CT may offer the best balance between accuracy and practicality. A high index of suspicion and careful exploration of all wounds are always appropriate.

Penetration of the abdominal or thoracic cavity should be considered in any wound over those locations in which the bottom of the laceration is not clearly visible. Wounds should *not* be blindly probed; blind probing is unreliable and may cause further injury. Patients with suspected thoracic lacerations require a chest x-ray initially, with a repeat film after 6 h of observation; any slowly developing pneumothorax should be visible by that time. In patients with abdominal lacerations, local anesthesia facilitates exploration (lacerations can be extended horizontally if necessary). Patients with wounds penetrating the fascia should be observed in the hospital; sometimes abdominal CT is used to identify hemoperitoneum.

Treatment

Treatment involves cleansing, local anesthesia, exploration, debridement, and closure. Tissue should be handled as gently as possible.

Cleansing: Both the wound and the surrounding skin are cleaned. Subepidermal tissue in the wound is relatively delicate and should not be exposed to harsh substances (eg, full-strength povidone iodine, chlorhexidine, hydrogen peroxide) and vigorous scrubbing.

Removing hair from laceration edges is not necessary for wound hygiene but can make markedly hairy areas (eg, scalp) easier to work on. If necessary, hair is removed by clipping with scissors, not shaving; razors create microtrauma, allowing skin pathogens to enter and increasing risk of infection. Hair is clipped before wound irrigation so that any clipped hair entering the wound is removed. Eyebrows are never trimmed because the hair-skin border is needed for proper alignment of wound edges.

Although wound cleansing is not particularly painful, local anesthesia (see below) is usually administered first, except for heavily contaminated wounds; these are best initially cleansed with running tap water and mild soap before local anesthesia administration. Tap water is clean, free of typical wound pathogens, and used in this manner does not seem to increase risk of infection. Wounds are then cleansed by a high-velocity stream of liquid, and sometimes scrubbed with a fine-pore sponge; brushes and rough materials are avoided. An appropriate irrigation stream can be created using a 20- or 35-mL syringe with a 20-gauge needle or IV catheter attached. Sterile 0.9% saline is an effective irrigant; specialized surfactant irrigants are costly and of doubtful additional benefit. If bacterial contamination is of particular concern (eg, bites, old wounds, organic debris), povidone iodine solution diluted 1:10 in 0.9% saline is beneficial and is not harmful to tissues at this concentration. The volume necessary varies. Irrigation continues until visible contamination is removed and at least 100 to 300 mL has been applied (more for large wounds).

Painting the skin with povidone iodine before suturing may reduce skin flora, but the substance should not be introduced into the wound.

Local anesthesia: Generally, injectable local anesthetics are used, but topical agents are beneficial in certain cases.

Common injectable agents are lidocaine 0.5, 1, and 2%, and bupivacaine 0.25 and 0.5%, both from the amide group of local anesthetics; the ester group includes procaine, tetracaine, and benzocaine. Lidocaine is more commonly used. Bupivacaine has a slightly slower onset (several minutes vs almost immediate) and a significantly longer duration (2 to 4 h vs 30 to 60 min). Duration of action of both can be prolonged by adding epinephrine 1:100,000, a vasoconstrictor. Because vasoconstriction may impair wound defenses, epinephrine is generally used only for wounds in highly vascular areas (eg, face, scalp); to prevent tissue ischemia, it is avoided in lower extremities and other distal parts (eg, nose, ears, fingers, penis).

Maximum dose of lidocaine is 3 to 5 mg/kg (1% solution = 1 g/100 mL = 10 mg/mL), that of bupivacaine is 2.5 mg/kg. Addition of epinephrine increases the allowable dose of lidocaine to 7 mg/kg, and of bupivacaine to 3.5 mg/kg.

Adverse reactions to local anesthetics include allergic reactions (hives and, occasionally, anaphylaxis—(see p. 1360) and sympathomimetic effects from epinephrine (eg, palpitations, tachycardia). True allergic reaction is rare, particularly to amide anesthetics; many patient-reported events represent anxiety or vagal reactions. Furthermore, allergic reactions are often due to methylparaben, the preservative used in multidose vials of anesthetic. If the offending agent can be identified, an agent from another class (eg, ester instead of amide) can be used. Otherwise, a test dose of 0.1 mL preservative-free (single-dose vial) lidocaine can be given intradermally; if there is no reaction in 30 min, that agent can be used.

Topical anesthesia avoids injection and is completely painless, which is of benefit in children and fearful adults. Two admixtures are common. TAC contains tetracaine 0.5%, epinephrine (adrenaline) 1:2000, and cocaine 11.8%. LET is lidocaine 2 to 4%, epinephrine 1:2000, and tetracaine 0.5 to 2%. A cotton dental pledget (or cotton ball) the length of the wound soaked in several milliliters of the solution and placed within the wound for 30 min usually provides adequate anesthesia; sometimes supplemental injectable anesthetic is required. Because of the presence of vasoconstrictors, the solutions are used mainly on the face and scalp, avoiding the ears, tip of nose, and distal extremities. Very rare deaths have occurred from mucosal absorption of cocaine, so it is not applied near the lips or eyes; LET appears safer.

Exploration: The full extent of the wound is explored to look for foreign material and possible tendon injury. Foreign material may best be discerned by palpating gently with the tip of a blunt forceps, feeling for a characteristic click. Deep wounds near a major artery should be explored in the operating room by a surgeon.

Debridement: Debridement uses a scalpel, scissors, or both to remove dead and devitalized tissue and sometimes firmly adherent wound contamination (eg, grease, paint). It is *not* used to convert irregular wounds to straight lines. Macerated or ragged wound edges are excised; usually 1 to 2 mm is sufficient. Sharply beveled wound edges are sometimes trimmed so that they are perpendicular.

Closure: Decision to close a wound depends on wound location, age, cause, degree of contamination, and patient risk factors.

Most wounds can be closed immediately (primary closure). This is appropriate for clean wounds < 6 to 8 h old (< 18 to 24 h for face and scalp wounds) without signs of infection.

Many other wounds can be closed after several days (delayed primary closure). This is appropriate for wounds > 6 to 8 h old, particularly if signs of inflammation have begun, and those of any age with significant contamination, particularly if organic debris is involved. The threshold for using delayed primary closure is lowered for patients with risk factors for poor healing. At initial presentation, anesthesia, exploration, and debridement are carried out as for all wounds (if not more thoroughly), but the wound is loosely packed with moist gauze. The dressing is changed at least daily and evaluated for closure after 3 to 5 days. If there are no signs of infection, the laceration is closed by standard techniques (see below). "Loosely" closing such wounds initially is ineffective and inappropriate because the wound edges nonetheless seal shut.

Some wounds should not be closed. These include cat bites, any type of bite to hands or feet (see also p. 2638), puncture wounds, and high-velocity missile wounds.

Materials and methods: Traditionally, sutures have been used for laceration repair, but metal staples, adhesive strips, and liquid tissue adhesives are now used for certain wounds. Whatever the material used, preliminary wound care is the same; a common error is to perform cursory exploration and no debridement because a noninvasive closure not requiring local anesthesia is planned.

Staples are quick and easy to apply and, because there is minimal foreign material in the skin, are less likely to cause infection than sutures. However, they are suited mainly for straight, smooth cuts with perpendicular edges in areas of low skin tension and no particular cosmetic significance. Successful application usually requires 2 people, one to approximate and evert skin edges with forceps and the other to operate the stapler; inadequate edge eversion is the most common error.

Tissue adhesives in the US contain octylcyanoacrylate. It hardens within a minute; is strong, nontoxic, and waterproof; and has some antibacterial properties. However, adhesive should not be allowed into the wound. Infectious complications are very unlikely, and good cosmetic results are possible. Adhesive is best for simple, regular lacerations; it is not suited for wounds under tension. In wounds requiring debridement, subcutaneous suturing, or exploration under local anesthesia, the advantages of decreased pain and time are minimized. As with stapling, adhesives usually require a 2nd person to hold the skin edges together while the adhesive is applied. Three or 4 layers are applied for maximum strength. The adhesive sloughs spontaneously in about a week. Excess or inadvertently applied adhesive is removed with any petrolatum-based ointment or, in areas away from the eyes or open wounds, acetone.

Adhesive strips are probably the quickest repair method and have a very low infection rate. They are useful for the same type wounds as tissue adhesives, with the same limitations. Additionally, use on lax tissue (eg, dorsum of hand) is difficult as edges tend to invert. Adhesive strips are particularly advantageous for lacerations in an extremity that is to be casted (thus blocking appropriate suture removal). Skin must be dry before application. Many clinicians apply tincture of benzoin to boost adhesion. Strips may be removed by the patient.

Sutures are the best choice for irregular or complex lacerations, areas of loose skin, areas under tension, and other wounds requiring subcutaneous closure. Because sutures can serve as an entry site for bacteria and there

TABLE 308–1. SUTURE MATERIALS

CATEGORY	MATERIAL	COMMENTS
Nonabsorbable		Preferred for cutaneous repair
Monofilament		
	Nylon	Strong, stiff, moderately hard to work with
	Polypropylene	Poorest knot security, most difficult to work with
	Polybutester	Somewhat elastic, so lengthens with wound edema and contracts as edema resolves
Braided		
	Polyester	Low reactivity; not preferred to monofilament for cutaneous use
	Silk	Soft; easy to work with; good knot security; high tissue reactivity. Generally limited to mouth, lips, eyelids, intraoral, where patient comfort is significantly better
Absorbable		Preferred for subcutaneous sutures
Monofilament		
	Polydioxanone	Very strong and long lasting (absorption, 180 days); stiffer, more difficult to handle than other absorbable sutures
Natural		
	Gut, chromic gut	From sheep intima. Weak; poor knot security; rapidly absorbed (1 wk); high tissue reactivity. Not preferred
Braided		Easy handling; good knot security; mild reactivity
	Polyglycolic acid	Original absorbable; most strength gone in 1 wk
	Polyglactic acid	Probably current preference

is a significant amount of foreign material under the skin, they have the highest rate of infection. Suture materials are generally classified as monofilament vs braided, and absorbable vs nonabsorbable. Characteristics and uses vary (see TABLE 308–1); generally, absorbable material is used for subcutaneous stitches, and nonabsorbable is used for cutaneous ones. Braided material generally poses slightly higher risk of infection than does monofilament but is soft and easy to handle and has good knot security.

Suture technique: The goal is to closely approximate skin margins, evert the edges, and eliminate dead space while minimizing tension of individual sutures and the amount of subcutaneous material.

Sutures may be placed and tied individually (interrupted sutures) or be continuous (running suture). They may be completely buried under the skin (subcutaneous—sc) or enter and exit the skin to be tied externally (percutaneous—pc).

If the wound is gaping, sc suturing is typically used initially (see FIG. 308–2); the resultant narrow epidermal gap is then closed by pc sutures. For wounds on the face, any gaping past 2 to 3 mm may benefit from sc suturing (not used in nose and eyelids); in other body areas, a wider gap is acceptable. Interrupted sutures using size 4-0 or 5-0 (smaller numbers indicate thicker material) braided absorbable material (eg, polyglactic acid) are most common. They are placed with the knot at the bottom of the wound to avoid a palpable lump and must not be too tight. A running sc suture (subcuticular) is sometimes used in cosmetic repairs.

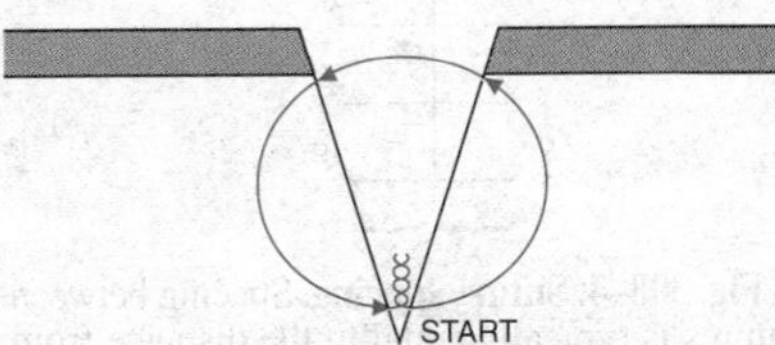

Fig. 308–2. Simple subcutaneous suture. The suture begins and ends at the bottom of the wound so that the knot is deeply buried.

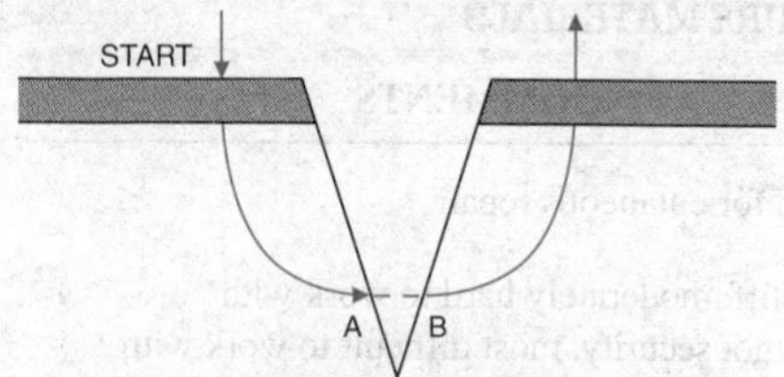

Fig. 308–3. Simple cutaneous suture. The suture begins and ends equidistant from the wound margins. Points A and B are at the same depth.

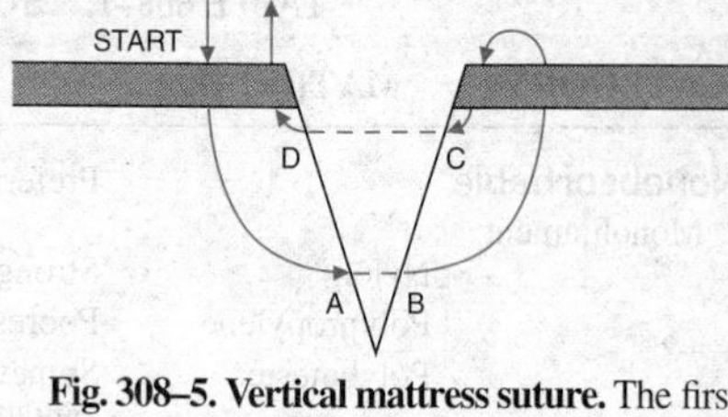

Fig. 308–5. Vertical mattress suture. The first pass of the needle is the same as a large simple suture, but instead of tying off, another smaller bite is taken back across the wound to end on the starting side. Both ends are pulled up to approximate the wound. Points A and B must be at the same depth, as must points C and D; this gives proper vertical alignment.

Epidermal closure is typically with simple, interrupted sutures (see FIG. 308–3) of nonabsorbable monofilament (eg, nylon). Areas over large joints and the scalp receive size 3-0, the face receives 6-0, and most other areas receive 4-0 or 5-0. Sutures are placed about as deep as they are wide and are spaced as far apart as the distance from the needle entry point to wound edge (see FIG. 308–4). Small "bites" are used for cosmetic repair and thin tissues, typically 1 to 3 mm from the wound edge. For other repairs, wider bites are used, varying with the tissue thickness.

A vertical mattress suture (see FIG. 308–5) is sometimes used instead of a layered closure, provided skin tension is not marked; it also helps ensure proper edge eversion in loose tissue. A running suture (see FIG. 308–6) is quicker to place than interrupted sutures and can be used when wound edges are well aligned.

In all cases, epidermal closure must precisely realign edges horizontally using natural skin landmarks (folds, creases, lip margins). Vertical alignment is equally important to avoid a step-off deformity. Excess tension following closure is evidenced by indenting of the skin or a "sausage link" appearance. Such a repair should be redone, adding sc sutures, additional pc sutures, or both as needed.

Aftercare: Tetanus vaccination is given if necessary (see TABLE 178–1 on p. 1506). Antibiotic ointment is not clearly necessary but appears to cause no harm and is believed by some to be beneficial; however, it is not used over tissue adhesive or adhesive strips. Prophylactic systemic antibiotics are not indicated except in certain bite wounds (see p. 2638), wounds involving tendons, bones, or joints, and possibly intraoral lacerations and massively contaminated wounds. If deemed necessary, antibiotics are given as early as possible and preferably parenterally for the first dose.

Excess movement of the affected area interferes with healing. Bulky dressings are used to immobilize fingers and hands. Patients with distal lower extremity lacerations (other than minor) should stay off their feet for several days; crutches may be helpful.

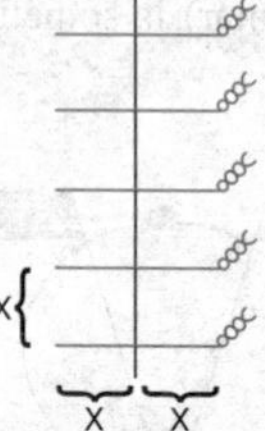

Fig. 308–4. Suture spacing. Spacing between sutures is typically equal to the distance from needle entry to wound margin. Sutures should enter and exit at an equal distance from the wound margin.

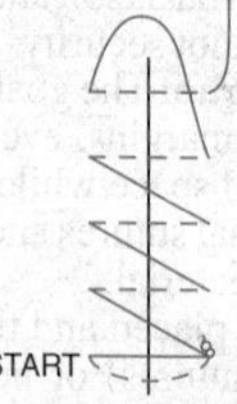

Fig. 308–6. Running suture. It begins with a simple suture at one end of the wound. The tail is cut without the needle, and suturing is continued. Sutures are snugged up as they are done, except for the last one, which is left as a loop. The tail is tied to the loop.

The wound is kept clean and dry; dressings are removed in 48 h and the wound inspected. A reliable patient may inspect minor, clean lacerations, but physician examination is preferable for higher risk wounds and in unreliable patients.

Wound infection occurs in 2 to 5% of lacerations; steadily increasing pain is often the earliest manifestation, and initial signs are redness and swelling. Systemic antibiotics effective against skin flora are begun; cephalexin 500 mg po qid (penicillin 500 mg po qid for oral infection) is typically used. Infection beginning > 5 to 7 days later suggests retained foreign body.

After 48 h, well-healing wounds can be cleansed gently of residual secretions with water or half-strength hydrogen peroxide (this can be done earlier and more frequently in facial wounds that are initially left uncovered) and can be left open. Brief wetting in the shower is safe, but prolonged soaking is avoided.

Closure material (except for tissue adhesive) is removed after various intervals depending on location. For facial lacerations, sutures are removed in 3 to 5 days to prevent cross-hatching and visible needle entrance marks; some clinicians apply adhesive strips to bolster the wound for a few more days. Sutures and staples on the torso and upper extremities are removed in 7 to 10 days. Those on the extensor surface of the elbow, knee, and anywhere below the knee should remain for 10 to 12 days.

Abrasions

Abrasions are skin scrapes that do not fully penetrate the epidermis.

Abrasions are evaluated, cleansed, and debrided similarly to lacerations. They are harder to anesthetize, however, which is particularly problematic when large amounts of dirt, stones, or glass are embedded as is frequently the case; regional block or IV sedation may be needed. After thoroughly removing all debris, antibiotic ointment (eg, bacitracin) and a nonadherent gauze dressing can be applied. Other commercial wound dressings may be used, the goals being to keep the wound from drying out, as this interferes with reepithelialization, and to keep the dressing from adhering.

309 FRACTURES, DISLOCATIONS, AND SPRAINS

Musculoskeletal injuries include fractures, joint dislocations, ligament sprains, muscle strains, and tendon injuries. Injuries may be open (in communication with a skin wound) or closed. Some injuries can cause rapid blood loss that is sometimes internal. Fat embolism (see p. 414) is a life-threatening but preventable complication of long-bone fractures. Fractures may injure nerves, including the spinal cord (see p. 2579).

Complications that threaten limb viability or cause permanent limb dysfunction occur in a small percentage of extremity injuries. The greatest threat to a limb is from injuries that impair vascular supply, primarily by direct injury to arteries or occasionally to veins. Closed injuries can cause ischemia by arterial disruption, as can occur in posterior knee dislocations, hip dislocations, and displaced supracondylar humeral fractures. Certain injuries can cause compartment syndrome (increased tissue pressure within a tight fascial compartment, impairing vascular supply and tissue perfusion). A penetrating injury may sever a peripheral nerve. A blunt, closed injury may result in neuropraxia (bruised peripheral nerve) or axonotmesis (crushed nerve), which is more severe. Dislocation (complete separation of the bones in a joint) may cause vascular and neural injuries, particularly if reduction (realignment of fracture fragments or dislocated joints) is delayed. Infection can result from open injuries. Closed and uncomplicated fractures, sprains, strains, and tendon tears least commonly result in serious complications.

Evaluation

This section describes evaluation in the emergency department, not on site. First, patients are evaluated for vascular and neurologic injuries and damage to internal organs.

Patients with pelvic or femoral fractures especially are evaluated for hemorrhagic shock (see p. 561) from occult blood loss. If patients have symptoms or signs of ischemia (eg, absent pulses, marked pallor, coolness distal to the injury) or injuries likely to involve arteries, arteriography helps assess arterial injury. Pain out of proportion to the apparent severity of the injury or pain that steadily worsens in the first hours to days immediately after injury suggests compartment syndrome; compartmental pressure is then measured (see p. 2567). Motor or sensory deficits suggest neurologic injury, and paresthesias or sensory deficits alone suggest neuropraxia. Motor plus sensory deficits suggest axonotmesis.

Examination includes inspection for deformity, swelling, ecchymoses, decreased or abnormal motion, and palpation for tenderness, crepitus, and gross instability. Deformity suggests dislocation, subluxation (partial separation), or fracture. Localized bone tenderness and crepitus suggest fracture. Gross joint instability suggests dislocation or severe sprain. Ligamentous tenderness suggests sprain. If sprain is suspected, joint stability is evaluated by stress testing (see p. 2569); however, if fracture is suspected, stress testing is deferred until x-rays exclude fracture. Tendon tenderness, dysfunction, or palpable defects suggest tendon tears. Attention to certain areas during examination can help detect commonly missed injuries (see TABLE 309–1).

Imaging: Plain x-rays show primarily bone and thus are useful for diagnosing most fractures as well as dislocations and subluxations that have not spontaneously reduced. X-rays are usually indicated for a suspected fracture or dislocation unless diagnosis of fracture would not alter treatment (eg, for most injuries of toes 2 through 5, which are treated symptomatically whether a fracture is present or not). Plain x-rays and other imaging studies should include at least 2 views taken from different planes (usually 1 anteroposterior and 1 lateral view).

CT or MRI can be used to better delineate fractures (eg, complex pelvic fractures)

TABLE 309–1. EXAMINATION FOR SOME COMMONLY MISSED INJURIES

SYMPTOM	FINDING	INJURY
Shoulder pain	Restriction of passive external rotation with the elbow flexed	Posterior shoulder (glenohumeral) dislocation
	Inability to maintain and hold a position at 90° of abduction when slight downward pressure is applied (drop-arm test)	Rotator cuff tear
	Tenderness with palpation of sternoclavicular joint	Sternoclavicular joint injury
Wrist pain or swelling	Tenderness with palpation of the anatomic snuffbox (located just distal to the radius, between the extensor pollicis longus, extensor pollicis brevis, and abductor pollicis longus tendons)	Scaphoid fracture
	Tenderness over the lunate fossa (in the wrist at the base of the 3rd metacarpal) and pain with axial compression of the 3rd metacarpal	Lunate fracture
Hip pain	Pain with passive hip rotation when the knee is flexed; inability to flex hip	Subcapital hip fracture
Knee pain in a child or an adolescent	Pain with passive hip rotation when the knee is flexed	Hip injury (eg, slipped capital femoral epiphysis [see p. 2386], Legg-Calvé-Perthes disease [see p. 2390])
Knee pain or swelling	Weak active knee extension	Quadriceps tendon rupture; patellar tendon rupture

identified on plain x-rays and to check for fractures suspected despite negative plain x-rays (common with subcapital hip fractures). MRI can also be done to diagnose complex sprains (including complete rupture of a ligament) and other soft-tissue injuries (eg, meniscal tears, cartilaginous injuries). Arteriography may be necessary for suspected arterial injuries (eg, some popliteal artery injuries). Nerve conduction studies may be indicated for nerve injuries.

Treatment

This section describes treatment in the emergency department, not on site. Hemorrhagic shock is treated. Injuries to arteries are repaired surgically unless they affect only small arteries with good collateral circulation. Severed nerves are surgically repaired; initial treatment of neuropraxia and axonotmesis is usually observation, supportive measures, and sometimes physical therapy.

Most injuries, particularly grossly unstable ones, are immobilized immediately by splinting (immobilization with a nonrigid or noncircumferential device) to prevent further soft-tissue injury by unstable injuries and to decrease pain. In patients with long-bone fractures, splinting may prevent fat embolism. Pain is treated, typically with opioids (see p. 1772). Definitive treatment often involves reduction, which usually requires analgesia or sedation. Closed reduction (without skin incision) is done when possible; if not, open reduction (with skin incision) is done. Closed reduction of fractures is usually maintained by casting; some dislocations require only a splint or sling. Open reduction is usually maintained by various surgical hardware (eg, pins, screws, plates, external fixators).

Local care: Patients who have soft-tissue injuries, with or without musculoskeletal injuries, benefit from RICE (rest, ice, compression, elevation) therapy. Rest prevents further injury and may accelerate healing. Ice, enclosed in a plastic bag or towel and applied intermittently during the first 24 to 48 h (for 15 to 20 min, as often as possible), minimizes swelling and pain. Compression, via a splint, an elastic bandage, or, particularly, a Jones compression dressing (multiple elastic bandages separated by fabric), helps minimize swelling and pain. Elevating the injured limb above the heart for the first 2 days, in a way that allows gravity to help drain edema fluid, also minimizes swelling. After 48 h, periodic application of warmth (eg, a heating pad) for 15 to 20 min may relieve pain and speed healing.

Immobilization: Immobilization facilitates healing by preventing further injury and is helpful except for very rapidly healing injuries. Joints proximal and distal to the injury should be immobilized.

A cast is usually applied. Rarely, significant swelling develops under a cast, contributing to compartment syndrome (see p. 2567). Sometimes, if significant swelling is thought likely, a cast is cut through from end to end medially and laterally (bivalved). Patients with casts should be given written instructions (eg, to keep the cast dry; never to put an object inside the cast; to seek medical care at once if an odor emanates from within the cast or if they have a fever, which may indicate infection). Good hygiene is important. Casts made of plaster must be kept dry.

A splint (see FIG. 309–1) can be used to immobilize some stable injuries. A splint allows patients to apply ice and to move more and does not contribute to compartment syndrome.

Immobilization with bed rest, which is occasionally required for fractures (eg, some pelvic fractures), can cause problems (eg, deep venous thrombosis, UTI). Immobilization of a single joint can also cause problems (eg, contractures, muscle atrophy). Some rapidly healing injuries are best treated with resumption of active motion within the first few days or weeks (early mobilization); this approach may minimize contractures and muscle atrophy, thus accelerating functional recovery.

FRACTURES

(See p. 306 for vertebral compression fractures; p. 858 for dental fractures; p. 2579 for spinal fractures; pp. 2584 and 2585 for fractures of the temporal bone, jaw and contiguous structures, and nose; p. 2637 for metatarsal stress fractures; p. 2588 for orbital fractures; and p. 2264 for fractures that occur during birth.)

Fractures are cracks in bones. Symptoms include pain, swelling, ecchymosis, crepitus, deformity, and abnormal motion. Occasional complications include fat embolism, arterial injury, compartment syndrome, nerve injuries, and infection. Fracture diagnosis is by clinical criteria and usually plain x-rays. Treatment involves analgesics, immobilization, and sometimes surgery.

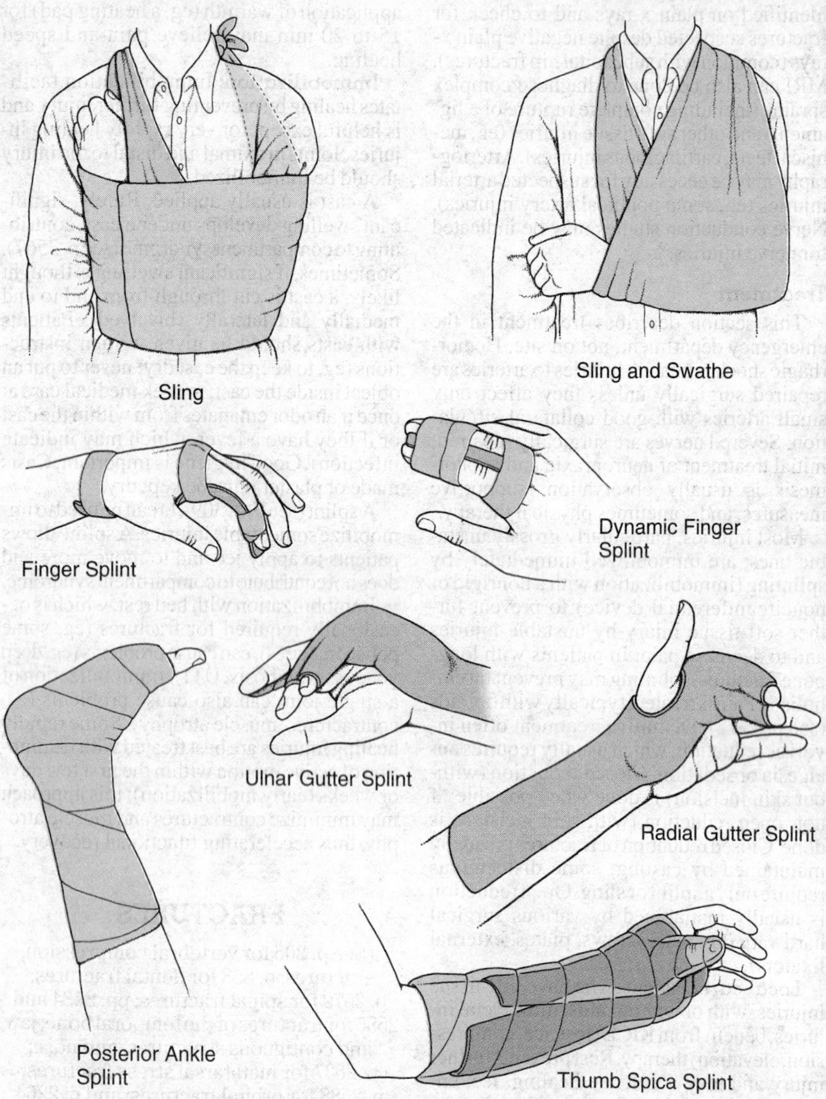

Fig. 309–1. Joint immobilization as acute treatment: some commonly used techniques.

Most fractures result from a single application of significant force to otherwise normal bone. Pathologic fractures result from application of mild or minimal force to a bone weakened by cancer or another disorder. Stress fractures (eg, metatarsal stress fracture—see p. 2637) result from repetitive application of force.

Pathophysiology

If Ca and vitamin D levels are adequate and bone tissue is healthy, fractures heal within weeks or months via remodeling: New tissue (callus) is produced within weeks, and bone reshapes at variable rates during the first weeks or months. Ultimately, optimal remodeling requires gradual resumption of normal joint motion. However, remodeling can be disrupted and refracture can occur if application of force or joint motion occurs prematurely; thus, immobilization is usually needed.

Serious complications are unusual. Arterial injuries occur occasionally in closed supracondylar fractures of the humerus and femur but are rare in other closed fractures. Compartment syndrome or nerve injury may occur. Open fractures predispose to bone infection (see p. 317), which can be intractable. Fractures of long bones may release enough fat (and other marrow contents) that embolizes through the veins to the lungs to cause respiratory complications (see p. 414). Fractures that extend into joints usually disrupt the articular cartilage; misaligned articular cartilage tends to scar, causing osteoarthritis and impairing joint motion.

Symptoms, Signs, and Diagnosis

Pain is usually immediate. Swelling increases for several hours. Both usually begin to resolve after 12 to 24 h; worsening pain after this period suggests compartment syndrome. Other symptoms and signs may include bone tenderness, ecchymosis, decreased or abnormal motion, deformity, and crepitus.

Patients with findings suggesting fracture are examined for ischemia, compartment syndrome, and nerve injury. If a wound is close to a fracture, open fracture is assumed. Fractures are diagnosed by imaging, beginning with plain x-rays. If there is no obvious fracture line, bone density, trabecular pattern, and cortical margins are examined for subtle clues to fracture. If plain x-rays do not show a fracture that is strongly suspected or if more precise detail is needed to guide treatment, MRI or CT is done. Some experts recommend imaging the joints proximal and distal to the fracture.

A fracture's appearance on x-rays can be described precisely using 5 terms: type of fracture line (see Fig. 309–2), location of fracture line, angulation, displacement (see Fig. 309–3), and open or closed. Location may be the bone's head (sometimes involving the articular surface), neck, or shaft (proximal, middle, or distal third).

Treatment

Immediate treatment includes analgesics and, for suspected unstable or fractures of long bones, splinting. Suspected open fractures require sterile wound dressings, tetanus prophylaxis, and broad-spectrum antibiotics (eg, combination of a 2nd-generation cephalosporin and an aminoglycoside).

If rotational malalignment or significant angulation or displacement occurs, it is corrected with reduction. Exceptions include some diaphyseal fractures in children. In these fractures, remodeling gradually corrects some types of significant angulation, and end-to-end realignment of fractured bone fragments can stimulate bone growth, which may then be excessive.

Surgical treatment may consist of fixation of fracture fragments using hardware (open reduction and internal fixation, or ORIF). In general, ORIF is indicated when an intra-articular fracture is displaced (to precisely align the joint cartilage), when ORIF has been shown to yield better results for a particular type of fracture, when closed treatment was ineffective, or when the fracture traverses a cancerous lesion (because normal bone healing does not occur). Because ORIF provides early structural stability, which facilitates mobilization, ORIF is also indicated when prolonged immobility, which is required for callus formation and remodeling, is undesirable (eg, in hip fractures). Surgical treatment is required when injury to a major vessel is suspected (for vessel repair), when the fracture is open (for irrigation and debridement to prevent infection), or when closed reduction is unsuccessful (for open reduction and sometimes ORIF).

Fractures, whether they require reduction, surgery, or neither, are typically immobilized, as are the proximal and distal joints. Usually, a cast is applied for weeks or months, but a splint may be used instead, particularly for fractures that heal faster when mobilized early. Home care for fractures includes supportive measures such as RICE therapy (rest, ice, compression, elevation—see p. 2559).

Patients are told to seek care immediately if symptoms of compartment syndrome occur (see p. 2567).

Specific Fractures

Stress fractures: Stress fractures are small and result from repetitive forces; they occur most often in the metatarsals (usually in runners—see p. 2637), followed by the fibula and tibia. Symptoms include gradual onset of intermittent pain that worsens with weight bearing and eventually becomes constant. Sometimes swelling occurs. Examina-

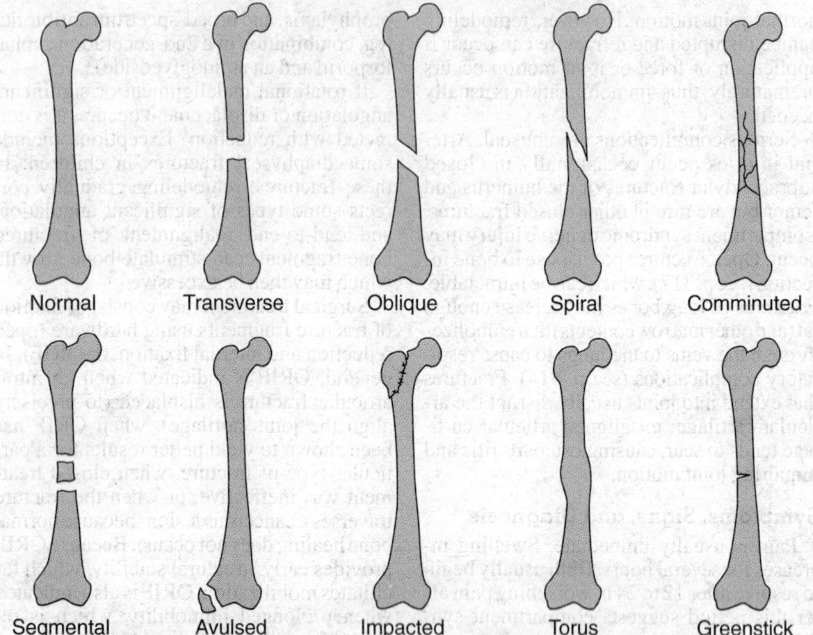

Fig. 309–2. Common types of fracture lines. Transverse fractures are perpendicular to the long axis of bone. Oblique fractures are not. Spiral fractures imply a rotatory mechanism; they are differentiated from oblique fractures by a component parallel to the long axis of bone in at least 1 view. Comminuted fractures have > 2 bone fragments. Comminuted fractures include segmental and avulsion fractures; avulsion fractures are caused by a tendon dislodging a bone fragment. Impacted fractures shorten bone; they may be visible as a focal abnormal density in trabeculae or irregularities in bone cortex. Childhood fractures include torus fractures, which involve buckling of the bone cortex, and greenstick fractures, which are cracks in only 1 side of the cortex.

tion detects localized bone tenderness. Plain x-rays are done but may be falsely negative at first. Many such fractures are treated presumptively, and plain x-ray is repeated 1 to 2 wk later when callus may be visible. Treatment is rest, elevation, analgesics, and sometimes immobilization. CT or MRI is rarely needed.

Growth plate fractures: Bone grows as tissue is added proximally by the growth (epiphyseal) plate, which is bordered by the metaphysis proximally and the epiphysis distally. The age at which the growth plate closes and bone growth ceases varies according to the bone, but the growth plate is closed in all bones by the end of puberty.

The growth plate is the most fragile part of the bone and thus is usually the 1st structure disrupted when force is applied. Growth plate fractures are classified by the Salter-Harris system (see FIG. 309–4). Disruption of future bone growth is common with types III, IV, and V and uncommon with types I and II.

Growth plate fractures are suspected in children with localized growth plate tenderness. These fractures are clinically differentiated from contusions by circumferential tenderness. In fracture types I and V, x-rays may be normal. If so, these fractures can sometimes be differentiated by injury mechanism (distraction [separation in longitudinal axis] vs compression). Closed treatment is usually sufficient for types I and II; ORIF is often required for types III and IV. Patients with type V injuries should be referred to a pediatric orthopedist because such injuries almost always lead to growth abnormalities.

Rib fractures: Typically, rib fractures result from blunt injury to the chest wall, usually involving a strong force (eg, from high-speed deceleration, a baseball bat, or a fall); however, sometimes in the elderly, only mild or moderate force (eg, in a minor fall) is required. Concomitant injuries may include aortic, subclavian, or cardiac injuries (uncommon but can occur with major deceleration, particularly if rib 1 or 2 is fractured); splenic or abdominal injuries (with fractures of any of ribs 7 through 12); pulmonary contusion; pneumothorax; and other tracheobronchial injuries (uncommon).

Pain is severe, is aggravated by coughing or deep breathing, and lasts for several weeks. Inspiratory splinting (incomplete inspiration

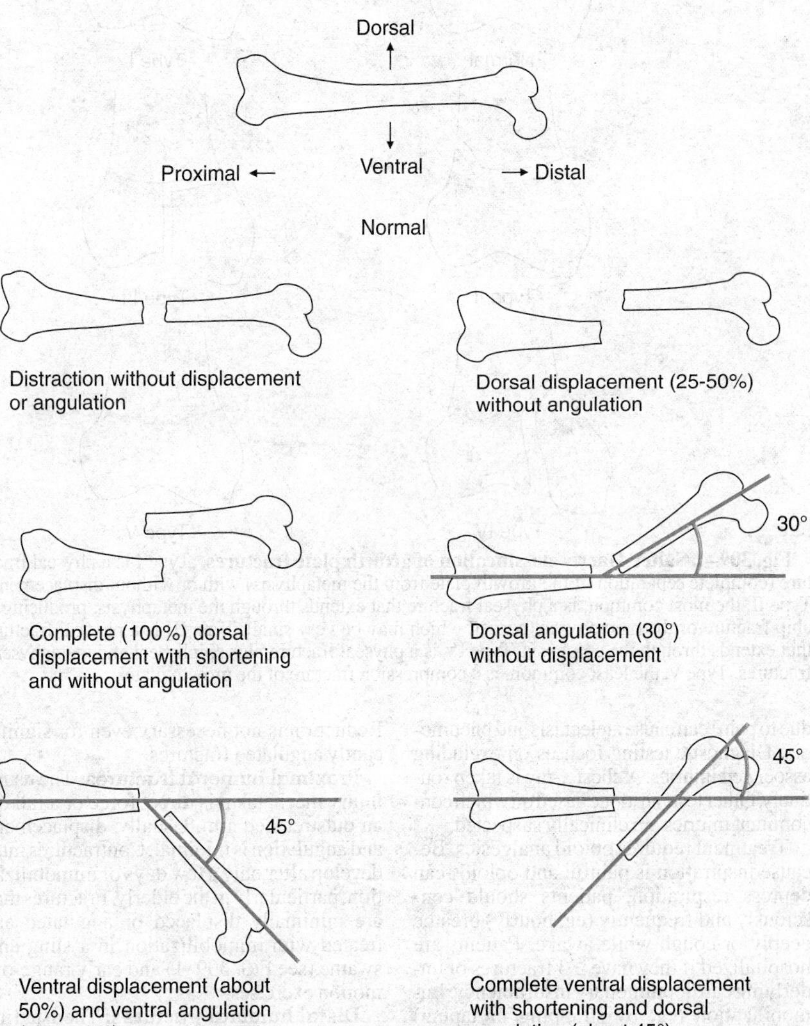

Fig. 309–3. Spatial relationship between fracture fragments. Distraction, displacement, angulation, or shortening (overriding) may occur. Distraction is separation in the longitudinal axis. Displacement is the degree to which the fractured ends are out of alignment with each other; it is described in millimeters or bone width percentage. Angulation is the angle of the distal fragment measured from the proximal fragment. Displacement and angulation may occur in the ventral-dorsal plane, lateral-medial plane, or both.

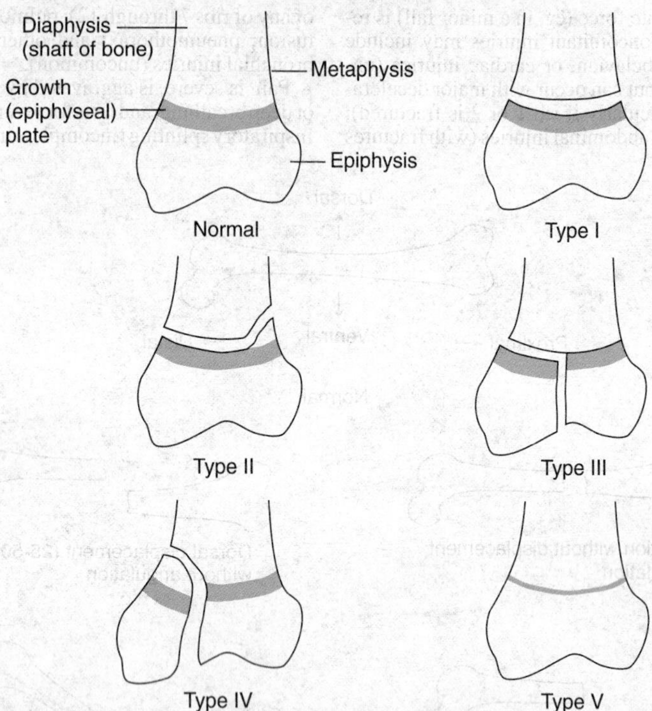

Fig. 309–4. Salter-Harris classification of growth plate fractures. Type I is a physeal fracture (complete separation of the growth plate from the metaphysis) with or without displacement. Type II, the most common, is a physeal fracture that extends through the metaphysis, producing a chip fracture of the metaphyseal corner, which may be very small. Type III is a physeal fracture that extends through the epiphysis. Type IV is a physeal fracture plus epiphyseal and metaphyseal fractures. Type V, the least common, is a compression fracture of the growth plate.

due to pain) can cause atelectasis and pneumonia. Diagnostic testing focuses on excluding associated injuries. A chest x-ray is taken routinely. Other tests are done based on which concomitant injuries are clinically suspected.

Treatment requires opioid analgesics. Because inspiration is painful and opioids can depress respiration, patients should consciously and frequently (eg, hourly) breathe deeply or cough while awake. Patients are hospitalized if they have ≥ 3 fractures or underlying cardiopulmonary insufficiency. Immobilization (eg, by strapping or taping) should usually be avoided; it constricts respiration and may predispose to atelectasis and pneumonia.

Clavicle fractures: The usual injury mechanism is a fall on an outstretched arm or a direct blow. About 80% involve the middle $\frac{1}{3}$ of the bone and are immobilized with a sling. Reduction is not necessary even for significantly angulated fractures.

Proximal humeral fractures: The usual injury mechanism is direct force or a fall on an outstretched arm. Usually, displacement and angulation is minimal. Contractures may develop after only a few days of immobilization, particularly in the elderly. Fractures that are minimally displaced or angulated are treated with immobilization in a sling and swathe (see FIG. 309–1) and early range-of-motion exercises.

Distal humeral fractures: The usual injury mechanism is direct force or a fall on an outstretched arm. The brachial artery or radial nerve may be damaged, even if the fracture is not displaced. Angulation must be corrected, and ORIF is often necessary.

Radial head fractures: The usual injury mechanism is a fall on an outstretched arm.

The radial head is palpable as a structure on the lateral elbow that rotates during pronation and supination. Routine anteroposterior and lateral x-rays usually show a joint effusion but often do not show the fracture. Patients with localized radial head tenderness and effusion require oblique views (which are more sensitive for fracture) or presumptive treatment of a fracture. Treatment of fractures with only minimal angulation and minimal displacement is a splint with the elbow flexed 90° or a sling. Starting range-of-motion exercises 10 days after the injury maximizes joint flexibility.

Distal radial fractures: The usual injury mechanism is wrist hyperextension. Dorsally displaced or angulated fractures (sometimes called Colles' fractures) are common. Treatment is reduction and immobilization at 15 to 30° of wrist extension. ORIF is necessary if the joint is disrupted.

Metacarpal neck fractures (except thumb): The usual injury mechanism is an axial load (eg, a punch with a clenched fist). If wounds are near the metacarpophalangeal joint, contamination with human oral flora should be suspected, and measures to prevent infection are required (see p. 2638). Reduction is necessary for fractures of the 2nd and 3rd metacarpals but is unnecessary for dorsal or volar angulation of < 35° for the 4th metacarpal or of 45° for the 5th metacarpal. Treatment is a splint (eg, an ulnar gutter splint for fractures of the 4th or 5th metacarpal—see FIG. 309–1).

Scaphoid (navicular) fractures: The usual injury mechanism is wrist hyperextension. Avascular necrosis is a common complication and can cause disabling, degenerative arthritis of the wrist. Fracture signs include pain with axial compression of the thumb, pain with wrist supination against resistance, and, particularly, tenderness in the anatomic snuffbox with ulnar wrist deviation. The anatomic snuffbox is palpated just distal to the radius, between the extensor pollicis longus, extensor pollicis brevis, and abductor pollicis longus tendons. The initial plain x-ray is often normal. Patients with suspected fractures require MRI, which is more sensitive, or treatment of fracture with a thumb spica splint pending follow-up plain x-ray in 1 to 2 wk; rarely, this x-ray is falsely normal.

Fingertip (tuft) fractures: Fingertip fractures involve the tuft of the distal phalanx and usually result from a crush injury. Subungual (beneath the nail) hematoma usually occurs and produces a blue-black, tender bruise, which may elevate the nail; hematoma indicates a nail bed laceration. Most fingertip fractures are treated symptomatically with a protective covering (eg, commercially available aluminum and foam splint material) wrapped around the fingertip. Subungual hematomas can be drained, relieving pain, by puncturing the nail (trephination), usually with an 18-gauge needle in a rotatory motion or, if no nail polish is on the nail, with an electrocautery device. If trephination is done gently and rapidly, anesthesia is often unnecessary. Large displaced fractures are repaired surgically. Hyperesthesia frequently persists long after a large fracture has healed and requires desensitization therapy.

Pelvic fractures: Compression of the symphysis pubis or simultaneous compression of both anterior superior iliac spines is often painful, particularly in severe fractures. For pelvic fractures, CT is more sensitive than plain x-rays.

Stable fractures do not disrupt the pelvic ring. Some (eg, symphyseal or pubic ramus fractures) result from minor injuries (eg, household falls), especially in patients with osteoporosis. Treatment is often symptomatic, particularly if patients can walk unaided.

Unstable fractures disrupt the pelvic ring in 2 places; disruptions can be fractures within bones or separations between the fibrous unions joining different bones (syndesmoses). Unstable fractures usually result from severe forces (eg, high-speed motor vehicle collisions). Intestinal injuries may occur. Concomitant GU injuries (eg, urethral or bladder tears) are common, particularly with anterior pelvic fractures. Vascular injuries may occur and cause hemorrhagic shock, especially with posterior pelvic fractures. Mortality rate is high. Initial evaluation and treatment are directed at associated injuries. The fracture often requires surgical repair.

Hip fractures: Hip fractures are most common among the elderly, particularly those with osteoporosis (mostly women—see p. 305). The most common hip fractures involve the femoral neck (subcapital fractures) or extend from the greater to the lesser trochanter (intertrochanteric fractures).

Subcapital fractures may be small or large stress fractures. They may result from minimal force (eg, walking); further fracture or displacement may occur secondary to a fall after the initial fracture. Patients with small fractures may be ambulatory and have only minor pain. However, such patients may be unable to flex the entire lower extremity forcefully with the knee extended. Passive hip rotation with the knee flexed aggravates the pain, helping to differentiate hip fracture from extra-articular disorders such as trochanteric bursitis. Patients with larger or more displaced fractures have more severely limited hip motion or leg shortening and external rotation.

Plain x-rays are occasionally normal if fractures are small; if a fracture is still suspected, MRI or, if MRI is unavailable or contraindicated, CT is done. Treatment is usually surgical repair (typically ORIF) and early ambulation for patients who are expected to resume walking and have no contraindication to surgery; prolonged bed rest should usually be avoided in elderly patients.

Intertrochanteric fractures usually result from falls or direct blows. Patients have tenderness, ecchymosis, and swelling over the hip, usually with leg shortening and external rotation. Plain x-rays are usually diagnostic. Treatment is usually ORIF and early mobilization.

Femoral shaft fractures: The usual injury mechanism is severe direct force or an axial load to the flexed knee. Blood loss up to 1.5 L/fracture is possible. Treatment is immediate splinting, then ORIF.

Ankle fractures: The ankle structures form a ring that connects the tibia and fibula to the talus. Four structures bind and stabilize the ring: 2 bones (medial malleolus of the tibia and lateral malleolus of the fibula) and 2 ligament complexes (medially, the deltoid ligament; laterally, mainly the anterior and posterior talofibular ligaments and calcaneofibular ligament—see FIG. 309–5).

Ankle fractures are common and can result from multiple injury mechanisms. Fractures that disrupt the ring in one place often disrupt it in another (eg, if only one bone is fractured, a ligament is often simultaneously and severely torn). If fractures disrupt any combination of ≥ 2 of the structures stabilizing the ankle ring, the ankle is unstable; surgery may be required, and prognosis is guarded. Stable ankle fractures without other indications for surgery can usually be treated with cast immobilization for 6 wk; prognosis is good.

Fractures of the 2nd metatarsal bone base with dislocation (Lisfranc's fracture-dislocation): The usual mechanism is a fall on a foot in plantar flexion. Disruption of the tarsometatarsal joint should be suspected even if it is not visible on plain x-rays. A plain x-ray may show only a fracture at the base of the 2nd metatarsal or chip fractures of the cuneiform. Dislocations often spontaneously reduce, but immediate referral for closed reduction requiring general anesthesia may be warranted.

Fractures of the 5th metatarsal bone base (dancer's fracture): The usual injury mechanism is a twist or crush injury. These fractures usually heal relatively quickly; nonunion is uncommon. Treatment is a protective walking shoe.

Fractures of the 5th metatarsal bone diaphysis (Jones fracture): The usual injury mechanism is a crush injury. These fractures are less common than those of the metatarsal bone base, and delayed union or

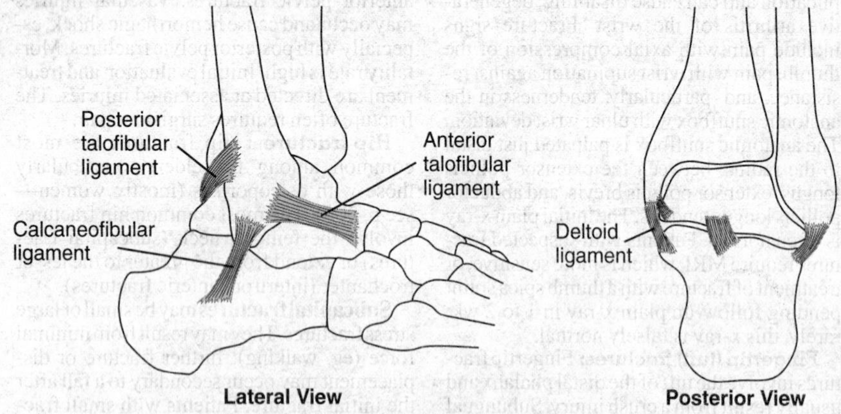

Fig. 309–5. Ligaments of the ankle.

nonunion occurs more commonly. Treatment is a cast that immobilizes the ankle.

Toe fractures: The usual injury mechanism is a crush injury. Unless rotational deformity or joint involvement is suspected or the proximal phalanx of the great toe is injured, x-rays are usually unnecessary. Treatment is taping the injured toe to an adjacent toe (dynamic splinting or buddy taping).

COMPARTMENT SYNDROME

Compartment syndrome is increased tissue pressure within a tight fascial compartment, resulting in tissue ischemia. The earliest symptom is pain out of proportion to the degree of injury. Diagnosis is by measurement of compartmental pressure. Treatment is fasciotomy.

Compartment syndrome is a self-perpetuating cascade of events. It begins with the tissue edema that normally occurs after injury (eg, due to soft-tissue swelling or a hematoma). If this edema occurs within a fascial compartment, typically in the anterior or posterior compartments of the leg, there is little room for tissue expansion, so interstitial (compartmental) pressure increases. As compartmental pressure exceeds about 20 mm Hg, cellular perfusion slows and may ultimately cease. (NOTE: Because 20 mm Hg is much lower than arterial pressure, cellular flow can be occluded well before pulses disappear.) Resultant tissue ischemia further worsens edema in a vicious circle. As ischemia progresses, muscles become necrotic, threatening loss of limb and, if untreated, death. Compartment syndrome can also result from tissue ischemia due to arterial injury.

Common causes include fractures, severe contusions, and, rarely, snakebites, casts, and other rigid enclosures that limit swelling and thus increase compartmental pressure.

Compartment syndrome usually occurs in the anterior lower leg. The earliest symptom is worsening pain. It is typically out of proportion to the degree of apparent injury and is exacerbated by passive stretching of the muscles within the compartment (eg, for the anterior leg compartment, by passive toe flexion, which stretches the toe extensor muscles). Later findings are the other "5 P's" of tissue ischemia (pain, paresthesias, paralysis, pallor, and pulselessness); compartments may be tense to palpation.

Diagnosis is by measuring compartmental pressure (normal, ≤ 20 mm Hg), usually with a commercially available wick catheter. Pressures of 20 to 40 mm Hg can sometimes be treated conservatively with analgesics, elevation, and splinting; casts are removed or bivalved. Pressures > 40 mm Hg usually require immediate fasciotomy to relieve pressure.

Diagnosis must be made and treatment started before pallor or pulselessness develop, indicating necrosis. If necrosis occurs, amputation may be needed. Necrosis can lead to rhabdomyolysis and infections.

DISLOCATIONS

(See also p. 328 for neck and back malalignment, p. 328 for atlantoaxial subluxation, and p. 858 for mandibular dislocation.)

Dislocations are complete separations of the bone ends that normally articulate to form a joint; subluxations are partial separations.

The most commonly dislocated extremity joint is the glenohumeral (shoulder). Arterial and nerve injuries, although uncommon, are a risk with dislocations (eg, of the knee, elbow, or hip), particularly those that are not rapidly reduced.

Symptoms and signs include pain, swelling, deformity, and inability to move. Diagnosis is by plain x-rays. Treatment is usually closed reduction as soon as possible; it requires sedation and analgesia or, occasionally, general anesthesia. Neurovascular assessment is done before and after reduction. If closed reduction is ineffective, open reduction is necessary.

SPECIFIC DISLOCATIONS

Glenohumeral (shoulder) dislocations: Glenohumeral dislocations are anterior in ≥ 95% of patients; the cause is abduction and external rotation of the humerus. Often, the axillary nerve is injured, or the greater tuberosity is fractured, particularly in patients > 45. The acromion is prominent; the humeral head is displaced anteriorly and inferiorly and cannot be palpated in its usual position. Axillary nerve sensation over the lateral deltoid is tested. Treatment is usually closed reduction with conscious sedation. The traction-countertraction technique is

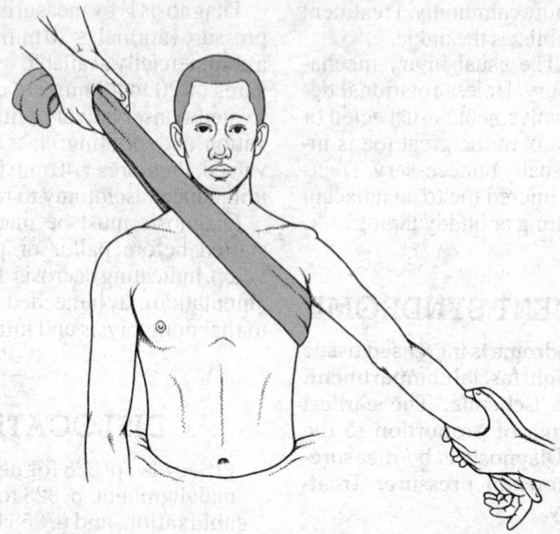

Fig. 309–6. Traction-countertraction technique for reducing anterior shoulder dislocations. The patient lies on a stretcher, and its wheels are locked. An assistant pulls on a folded sheet wrapped around the patient's chest. A 2nd practitioner pulls the affected limb down and laterally 45°. After the humerus is dislodged, slight lateral traction on the upper humerus may be needed.

one of many commonly used methods of reduction (see FIG. 309–6). After reduction, the joint is immobilized immediately with a sling and swathe (see FIG. 309–1).

Occasionally, dislocation is posterior—a commonly missed injury (see TABLE 309–1)—or inferior (luxatio erecta). In patients with luxatio erecta, the brachial artery or brachial plexus is often also injured.

Elbow dislocations: Most elbow dislocations result from a fall on an extended, abducted arm. They are common and usually posterior. Associated injuries may include fractures, injuries to the ulnar or median nerve, and possibly injury to the brachial artery. The joint is usually flexed about 45°, and the olecranon is prominent and posterior to the humeral epicondyles; however, these anatomic relationships may be difficult to determine because of swelling. Reduction is usually with sustained, gentle traction after sedation and analgesia.

Radial head subluxations (nursemaid's elbow): In adults, the radial head is wider than the radial neck; consequently, the head cannot fit through ligaments that tightly surround the neck. However, in toddlers (about 2 to 3 yr), the radial head is no wider than the radial neck and can easily slip through these ligaments (radial head subluxation). Subluxation results from traction on the forearm as when a reluctant toddler is pulled forward; however, many caregivers do not remember doing so. Symptoms may include pain and tenderness; however, many toddlers cannot describe their symptoms and simply avoid moving the affected elbow (pseudoparalysis). Plain x-rays are normal and considered unnecessary by some experts unless an alternate diagnosis is clinically suspected. Reduction may be diagnostic and therapeutic. The elbow is completely extended and supinated, then flexed, usually without sedation or analgesia. Children may start to move the elbow after about 20 min. Immobilization is unnecessary.

Proximal interphalangeal (PIP) joint dislocations: PIP joint dislocations are common. Dorsal dislocations, which are more common than volar, are usually due to hyperextension, sometimes displacing the volar joint structures intra-articularly. Volar dislocations can rupture the central slip of the extensor tendon, causing boutonnière deformity (see p. 331). Dislocations usually cause obvious deformities. A lateral x-ray should be taken with the affected digit visibly separated from the others.

For most dislocations, closed reduction using digital block anesthesia is done; axial traction and volar force are used for dorsal dislocations, and dorsal force is used for volar dislocations. Dorsal dislocations are splinted at 15° of flexion for 3 wk. Volar dislocations are splinted at extension for 1 to 2 wk. Some dorsal dislocations require open reduction.

Hip dislocations: Most are posterior and result from a severe posteriorly directed force to the knee with the knee and hip flexed (eg, against a car dashboard). Complications may include arterial injury (particularly if the dislocation is anterior) with subsequent avascular necrosis of the femoral head and sciatic nerve injury. Treatment is reduction as soon as possible, followed by bed rest or joint immobilization.

Knee (tibiofemoral) dislocations: Most anterior dislocations result from hyperextension; most posterior dislocations result from a posteriorly directed force to the proximal tibia with the knee slightly flexed. Many dislocations spontaneously reduce before medical evaluation, resulting in gross instability of the knee. The popliteal artery is often injured, even if ischemia is not evident. *Angiography is indicated for every patient with a knee dislocation or with gross instability.* Treatment is immediate reduction and surgical repair.

Lateral patellar dislocations: The usual injury mechanism is quadriceps contraction plus flexion and external tibial rotation. Most patients have an underlying chronic patellofemoral abnormality. Many dislocations spontaneously reduce before medical evaluation. Treatment is reduction; with the hip flexed, the patella is gently moved medially while the knee is extended. Reduction is followed by a cylindrical leg cast or surgical repair.

SPRAINS, STRAINS, AND TENDON TEARS

Tears may occur in ligaments (sprains), in muscles (strains), or in tendons. Tears may be graded as minimal (1st degree), moderate to severe (2nd degree), or complete (3rd degree). Third-degree sprains may result in joint instability and are differentiated from 2nd-degree sprains by stress testing. Third-degree tendon tears disrupt muscle function. Treatment of all tears includes analgesics, immobilization, and, for some 3rd-degree sprains and tendon tears, surgical repair.

Sprains commonly involve the acromioclavicular joint, proximal interphalangeal joint, knee (see p. 2570), and ankle; tendon tears commonly involve the knee extensor mechanism and Achilles tendon. Various muscles are commonly strained. Sprains, strains, and tendon tears cause pain, tenderness, and usually swelling. Second-degree sprains are very painful when stretched. Third-degree sprains often cause joint instability because ligaments that stabilize joints may be disrupted. In 3rd-degree tendon tears, the muscle cannot move the bone normally attached to it by the tendon; a tendon defect may be palpable.

Bedside stress testing involves passively opening the joint in a direction other than the normal range of motion (stressing) to detect joint instability; this test helps differentiate between 2nd- and 3rd-degree sprains. Because muscle spasm during acutely painful injuries may mask joint instability, the surrounding muscles are relaxed as much as possible, and examinations are repeated, with slightly more force each time. Findings are compared with those for the opposite, normal side. With 2nd-degree sprains, stress is painful, and joint opening is limited. With 3rd-degree sprains, stress is less painful because the ligament is completely torn and is not being stretched, and joint opening is less limited. If muscle spasm is severe, the examination should be repeated after injection of a local anesthetic, after use of systemic analgesia or sedation, or after a few days, when the spasm has subsided.

Treatment of all tears includes RICE (rest, ice, compression, elevation—see p. 2559) therapy and, if necessary, analgesics. First-degree tears are usually best treated with early mobilization. Mild 2nd-degree tears are often immobilized with a sling or splint for a few days. Severe 2nd-degree and some 3rd-degree sprains and tendon tears are immobilized for days or weeks, sometimes with a cast. Many 3rd-degree sprains and tendon tears require surgical repair.

SPECIFIC SPRAINS AND TENDON TEARS

Acromioclavicular joint sprains (separation): The usual injury mechanism is a fall on the point of a shoulder or on an outstretched arm. Severe sprains tear the coracoclavicular ligament, displacing the clavicle upward from the acromion. Treatment is immobilization (eg, with a sling) and early mobility exercises. Some severe sprains are surgically repaired.

Ulnar collateral ligament sprains (gamekeeper's thumb): The usual injury mechanism is lateral deviation of the thumb. Stress testing involves radial deviation of the thumb, which requires digital block anesthesia. Treatment is immobilization with a thumb spica splint; if maximum possible radial deviation is > 20° than that in the opposite thumb, then surgical repair is necessary.

Ankle sprains: The most important ankle ligaments are the strong deltoid (medial) and the anterior and posterior talofibular and calcaneofibular (lateral—see FIG. 309–5). Ankle sprains are very common, typically resulting from turning the foot inward (inversion); inversion tears the lateral ligaments, usually beginning with the anterior talofibular ligament. Severe 2nd- and 3rd-degree sprains often cause chronic joint buckling and instability and predispose to additional sprains. Ankle sprains cause pain and swelling, which are usually maximal at the anterolateral ankle. Third-degree sprains often cause more diffuse pain and swelling (sometimes egg-shaped).

Ankle x-rays are done to exclude significant fractures in patients with any of the following: age > 55, inability to bear weight immediately after the injury plus inability to take 4 steps when first examined, or bone tenderness at the posterior edge or tip of either malleolus. The ankle anterior drawer test assesses stability of the anterior talofibular ligament, helping differentiate between 2nd- and 3rd-degree lateral sprains. Patients are sitting or supine with the knee at least slightly flexed; one of the examiner's hands prevents forward movement of the anterior distal tibia while the other hand cups the heel, pulling it anteriorly. First-degree sprains are treated with RICE therapy and early weight bearing. Second-degree sprains are treated with RICE therapy and immobilization of the ankle in a neutral position with a posterior splint, followed by mobilization within a few days for mild sprains or longer for severe sprains. Third-degree sprains may require surgical repair. If differentiation between severe 2nd- and 3rd-degree sprains is impossible (eg, due to muscle spasm or pain), MRI may be done, or immobilization may be tried and evaluation repeated after a few days.

Occasionally, the deltoid ligament is sprained during eversion, often with simultaneous fracture of the fibular head.

Achilles tendon tears: The usual injury mechanism is ankle dorsiflexion, particularly if the tendon is taut. When the calf is squeezed with the patient prone (Simmonds test), passive ankle plantar flexion is decreased. Partial tears are often missed. Treatment of complete tears is usually emergency surgical repair. Treatment of incomplete tears and some complete tears is a posterior ankle splint with the ankle in plantar flexion for 4 wk.

KNEE SPRAINS AND MENISCAL INJURIES

Knee trauma commonly causes sprains of the external (medial and lateral collateral) or internal (anterior and posterior cruciate) ligaments or injures the menisci. Symptoms include pain, effusion, instability (with severe sprains), and locking (with some meniscal injuries). Diagnosis is by physical examination and sometimes MRI or arthroscopy. Treatment is RICE (rest, ice, compression, elevation) therapy and, for severe injuries, casting or surgical repair.

Structures that are located mainly outside of the joint and that help stabilize the knee include muscles (eg, quadriceps, semimembranosus), their insertions (eg, pes anserinus), and extracapsular ligaments. The lateral collateral ligament is extracapsular; the medial (tibial) collateral ligament has a superficial extracapsular portion and a deep portion that is part of the joint capsule.

Knee joint structures that provide stabilization include the joint capsule and the posterior and highly vascular anterior cruciate ligaments. The medial and lateral menisci are intra-articular cartilaginous structures that provide shock absorption and limited joint stabilization (see FIG. 309–7).

The most commonly injured knee structures are the medial collateral and anterior cruciate ligaments. The most common mechanism for ligamentous knee injuries is an inward, medial force accompanied usually by some external rotation and flexion (as when being tackled in football). In such cases, the medial collateral ligament is usually injured first, followed by the anterior cruciate ligament, then the medial meniscus. The next most common mechanism is an outward force, often injuring the lateral collateral ligament, anterior cruciate ligament, or both.

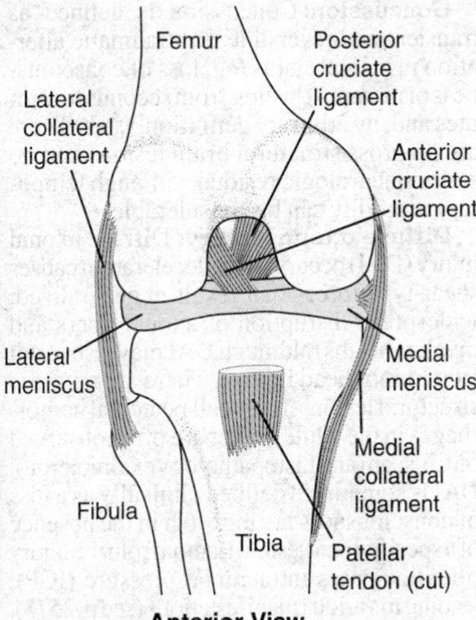

Fig. 309–7. Ligaments of the knee.

Anterior or posterior forces and hyperextension typically injure the cruciate ligaments. Weight bearing and rotation at the time of injury predispose to meniscal injuries.

Symptoms and Signs

Swelling and muscle spasm progress over the first few hours. With 2nd-degree sprains, pain is typically moderate or severe. With 3rd-degree sprains, pain may be mild, and surprisingly, some patients can walk unaided. An audible pop is uncommon; it suggests an anterior cruciate tear. An effusion suggests injury to the anterior cruciate and possibly other intra-articular structures. However, in severe 3rd-degree tears of the medial collateral ligament or anterior cruciate, no effusion may be apparent because these tears result in an open joint capsule and blood can exit the joint. Location of maximum tenderness often corresponds to the injured structure; medial meniscal injuries cause tenderness in the medial joint plane (joint line tenderness), and lateral meniscal injuries cause tenderness in the lateral joint plane. These injuries also cause swelling and sometimes restrict passive motion (called locking).

Diagnosis

A spontaneously reduced knee dislocation should be suspected in patients with gross instability; immediate angiography should be done. Otherwise, the knee is fully examined first. Knee extension is assessed.

Other injuries can be assessed with various maneuvers. For the Apley test, the examiner flexes the prone patient's knee 90°. Pain during compression and knee rotation suggests a meniscal injury; pain during distraction and knee rotation suggests a ligamentous or joint capsule injury. For assessment of the medial and lateral collateral ligaments, the patient is examined supine, with the knee flexed about 20° and the hamstring muscles relaxed. The examiner puts one hand over the side of the knee opposite the ligament being tested. With the other hand, the examiner cups the heel and bends the lower leg outward to test the medial collateral ligament or inward to test the lateral collateral ligament. Moderate instability after acute injury suggests that a meniscus or cruciate ligament is torn as well as the collateral ligament. Lachman's test is the most sensitive physical test for acute anterior cruciate ligament tears; the examiner supports the recumbent patient's thigh and calf, and the patient's knee is flexed 20°. Excessive passive anterior motion of the tibia from the femur suggests a significant tear.

If stress testing is difficult (eg, due to pain or muscle spasm), patients require reexamination after local anesthetic injection or systemic analgesia and sedation, follow-up examination after 2 to 3 days (after swelling and spasm have subsided), or MRI or arthroscopy. If severe injury cannot be excluded clinically, MRI or arthroscopy is done.

Treatment

Draining large effusions (see FIG. 31–3 on p. 255) may decrease pain and spasm. Most 1st-degree and mild or moderate 2nd-degree injuries can be treated initially with RICE therapy and immobilization of the knee at 20° of flexion with a commercially available knee immobilizer or splint. Most 3rd-degree and severe 2nd-degree sprains and most meniscal injuries require casting for ≥ 6 wk. However, some 3rd-degree injuries of the medial collateral ligament, anterior cruciate ligament, and menisci require arthroscopic surgical repair.

310 TRAUMATIC BRAIN INJURY

Traumatic brain injury is physical injury to brain tissue that temporarily or permanently impairs brain function. Diagnosis is suspected clinically and confirmed by imaging (primarily CT, although MRI is sometimes of additional value). Treatment initially consists of support of respiration, oxygenation, and BP to prevent additional injury and subsequently may include surgery and rehabilitation.

In the US, about 1.4 million people/yr sustain traumatic brain injury (TBI); of these, about 50,000 people die and about 80,000 survivors have resultant disability. Causes include motor vehicle crashes and other transportation-related causes (eg, bicycle crashes, collisions with pedestrians), falls (especially in older adults and young children), assaults, and sports activities.

Pathology

Head injuries can cause various types of structural damage. Structural changes may be gross or microscopic, depending on the mechanism and forces involved; patients with less severe injuries may have no gross structural damage. Clinical manifestations vary markedly in severity and consequences. Injuries are commonly categorized as open or closed.

Open injuries involve penetration of the scalp and skull (and usually the meninges and underlying brain tissue). They typically involve bullets or sharp objects, but a skull fracture with overlying laceration due to severe blunt force is also considered an open injury.

Closed injuries typically occur when the head is struck, strikes an object, or is shaken violently, causing rapid brain acceleration and deceleration. Acceleration or deceleration can injure tissue at the point of impact (coup), at its opposite pole (contrecoup), or diffusely; the frontal and temporal lobes are particularly vulnerable. Axons, blood vessels, or both can be sheared or torn. Blood vessels that are disrupted leak, producing contusions, intracerebral or subarachnoid hemorrhages, and hematomas (epidural and subdural).

Concussion: Concussion is defined as transient and reversible posttraumatic alteration in mental status (eg, loss of consciousness or memory) lasting from seconds to minutes and, by arbitrary definition, < 6 h. There are no gross structural brain lesions and no serious neurologic residua, although temporary disability can be considerable.

Diffuse axonal injury: Diffuse axonal injury (DAI) occurs when deceleration causes shear-type forces that result in generalized, widespread disruption of axonal fibers and myelin sheaths (although DAI may also result from minor head injury). There are no gross structural lesions, but small petechial hemorrhages in the white matter are often observed on CT scan (and histopathology examination). DAI is sometimes defined clinically as a loss of consciousness lasting > 6 h in the absence of a specific focal lesion. Edema from the injury often increases intracranial pressure (ICP), leading to various manifestations (see p. 2573). DAI is typically the underlying injury in shaken baby syndrome.

Brain contusions: Contusions (bruises of the brain) can occur with open (including penetrating) or closed injuries and can impair a wide range of brain functions, depending on contusion size and location. Larger contusions may cause widespread brain edema and increase ICP.

Hematomas: Hematomas (collections of blood in or around the brain) can occur with penetrating or closed injuries and may be epidural, subdural, or intracerebral. Subarachnoid hemorrhage (SAH—bleeding into the subarachnoid space—see p. 1798) is common in TBI.

A subdural hematoma is blood between the dura mater and the pia-arachnoid mater. Acute subdural hematomas, which are often caused by laceration of brain or cortical veins or avulsion of bridging veins between cortex and dural sinuses, often occur after falls or motor vehicle crashes. Edema may occur as the hematoma compresses brain tissue, resulting in signs of increased ICP (see p. 2574). Mortality and morbidity can be significant.

A chronic subdural hematoma may appear and produce symptoms gradually over several weeks after trauma. These hematomas occur more often in elderly patients (especially those taking antiplatelet drugs or anticoagulants), who may consider the head injury relatively trivial or may have even forgotten it. In contrast to acute subdural hematoma, edema and increased ICP are unusual.

Epidural hematomas (blood between the skull and dura mater) are less common than subdural hematomas. Epidural hematomas are usually caused by arterial bleeding, classically due to damage to the middle meningeal artery by a temporal bone fracture. Without intervention, patients with large or arterial epidural hematomas may rapidly deteriorate and die. Small, venous epidural hematomas are rarely lethal.

Intracerebral hematomas (collections of blood within the brain itself) often result from coalescence of contusions; thus, the distinction between contusion and intracerebral hematoma is not well defined. Increased ICP, herniation, and brain stem failure can subsequently develop, especially with hematomas in the temporal lobes or cerebellum.

Skull fractures: Penetrating injuries by definition involve fractures. Closed injuries may also cause skull fractures, which may be linear, depressed, or comminuted. Although serious and even fatal TBI may occur without skull fracture, the presence of a fracture suggests that significant force was involved. Fractures in patients with diffuse head trauma indicate increased risk of intracranial injury. In contrast, fractures due to focal head trauma (eg, being hit with a small object) do not necessarily suggest high risk of intracranial injury. Also, a simple linear skull fracture is not usually high risk unless there is neurologic impairment or the fracture occurs in an infant.

Depressed fractures have the highest risk of tearing the dura, damaging the underlying brain, or both.

If temporal bone fractures cross the area of the middle meningeal artery, an epidural hematoma is likely. Fractures crossing one of the major dural sinuses may cause significant hemorrhage and venous epidural or venous subdural hematoma. Fractures that involve the carotid canal can result in carotid artery dissection.

Because the occipital bone and base of the skull (basilar bones) are thick and strong, fractures in these areas indicate a high-intensity impact. Basilar skull fractures that extend into the petrous part of the temporal bone often damage middle and inner ear structures and can impair facial, acoustic, and vestibular nerve function.

In infants, the meninges may become trapped in a linear skull fracture with subsequent development of a leptomeningeal cyst and growth of the original fracture (growing fracture).

Pathophysiology

Brain function may be immediately impaired by direct damage (eg, crush, laceration) of brain tissue. Further damage may occur shortly thereafter from the cascade of events triggered by the initial injury.

TBI of any sort can produce edema in the damaged tissues. The cranial vault is fixed in size (constrained by the skull) and almost completely filled by noncompressible fluid (CSF) and minimally compressible brain tissue; consequently, any swelling from edema, hemorrhage, or hematoma has nowhere to expand and thus increases ICP. Cerebral blood flow is proportional to the cerebral perfusion pressure (CPP), which is the difference between mean arterial pressure (MAP) and mean ICP. Thus, as ICP increases (or MAP decreases), CPP decreases, and when it is below about 50 mm Hg, brain tissue may become ischemic. This mechanism may produce ischemia at a local level when compression from focal edema or hematoma compromises blood flow in the region of the lesion. Ischemia and edema then trigger release of excitatory neurotransmitters and free radicals, causing further edema, which further increases ICP. Systemic complications from trauma (eg, hypotension, hypoxia) can also contribute to cerebral ischemia and are often called secondary brain insults.

Excessive ICP initially causes global cerebral dysfunction. If excessive ICP is unrelieved, it can push brain tissue across the tentorium or through the foramen magnum, causing herniation (see p. 1800), which significantly increases morbidity and mortality risk. Also, if ICP increases to equal MAP, CPP becomes zero, resulting in complete brain ischemia, which rapidly leads to brain death; absent cranial blood flow can be used as one criterion for brain death (see p. 1806).

Symptoms and Signs

Initially, most patients with TBI lose consciousness (usually for seconds or minutes), although with minor injuries, some have only confusion or amnesia (amnesia is usually retrograde and lasts for seconds to a few hours). Young children may simply become irritable. Some patients have seizures, often within the 1st hour or day. After these initial symptoms, patients may be fully awake and alert, or consciousness and function may be altered to some degree, from mild confusion to stupor to coma. Duration of unconsciousness and

TABLE 310–1. GLASGOW COMA SCALE*

AREA ASSESSED	RESPONSE	POINTS
Eye opening	Open spontaneously; open with blinking at baseline	4
	Open to verbal command, speech, or shouting	3
	Open in response to pain applied to the limbs or sternum	2
	None	1
Verbal	Oriented	5
	Confused conversation, but able to answer questions	4
	Inappropriate responses; words discernible	3
	Incomprehensible speech	2
	None	1
Motor	Obeys commands for movement	6
	Responds to pain with purposeful movement	5
	Withdraws from pain stimuli	4
	Responds to pain with abnormal (spastic) flexion (decorticate posture)	3
	Responds to pain with abnormal (rigid) extension (decerebrate posture)	2
	None	1

*Combined scores < 8 are typically regarded as coma.

Adapted from Teasdale G, Jennett B: Assessment of coma and impaired consciousness. A practical scale. *Lancet* 2:81–84; 1974.

severity of obtundation are roughly proportional to injury severity but are not specific. The Glasgow Coma Scale (GCS—see TABLE 310–1) is a quick, reproducible scoring system to be used during the initial examination to estimate severity of TBI. It is based on alertness (as evidenced by eye opening) and best motor and best verbal responses. A score of 3 indicates potentially fatal damage, especially if both pupils fail to respond to light and oculovestibular responses are absent. Higher initial scores tend to predict better recovery. By convention, the severity of head injury is initially defined by the GCS (GCS score of 14 or 15 is mild TBI; GCS score of 9 to 13 is moderate TBI; GCS score of 3 to 8 is severe TBI); however, the severity and prognosis are predicted more accurately by also considering CT scan findings and other factors. Some patients with initially moderate TBI and a few patients with initially mild TBI deteriorate. For infants and young children, the Modified Glasgow Coma Scale for Infants and Children is used (see TABLE 310–2).

Symptoms of epidural hematoma usually develop within minutes to several hours after the injury and consist of increasing headache, decreased level of consciousness, hemiparesis, and pupillary dilation with loss of light reactivity. Some patients lose consciousness, followed by a transient lucid interval, then subsequent neurologic deterioration.

Markedly increased ICP classically manifests as a combination of hypertension, bradycardia, and respiratory depression (Cushing's triad). Vomiting may occur but is nonspecific. Severe diffuse brain injury or markedly increased ICP may produce decorticate or decerebrate posturing. Both are bad prognostic signs.

Transtentorial herniation (see p. 1800) may result in coma, unilaterally or bilaterally dilated and unreactive pupils, hemiplegia (usually on the side opposite a unilaterally dilated pupil), hypertension, bradycardia, and respiratory depression (slow and irregular).

Basilar skull fracture may result in drainage of CSF from the nose (CSF rhinorrhea) or ear (CSF otorrhea), blood behind the tympanic membrane (hemotympanum) or in the external ear canal if the tympanic membrane has been ruptured, and ecchymosis behind the ear (Battle's sign) or in the periorbital area (raccoon eyes). Loss of smell, hearing, or facial nerve function sometimes occurs immediately or after a delay. Other fractures of the cranial vault are sometimes palpable, particularly through a scalp laceration, as a depression or step-off deformity. However, blood under the galea aponeurotica may mimic such a step-off deformity.

Patients with chronic subdural hematomas may present with increasing daily headache, fluctuating drowsiness or confusion (which may mimic early dementia), and mild-to-moderate hemiparesis.

Long-term symptoms: Amnesia may persist and be both retrograde and anterograde. Postconcussion syndrome, which commonly follows a significant concussion, includes headache, dizziness, fatigue, difficulty concentrating, variable amnesia, depression, apathy, and anxiety. Commonly smell (and thus taste), sometimes hearing, or rarely vision is altered or lost. Symptoms usually resolve spontaneously over weeks to months.

A range of cognitive and neuropsychiatric deficits can persist after severe and even moderate TBI, particularly if structural damage was significant. Common problems include amnesia, behavioral changes (eg, agitation, impulsivity, disinhibition, lack of motivation), emotional lability, sleep disturbances, and decreased intellectual function. Late seizures

TABLE 310–2. MODIFIED GLASGOW COMA SCALE FOR INFANTS AND CHILDREN

AREA ASSESSED	INFANTS	CHILDREN	SCORE*
Eye opening	Open spontaneously	Open spontaneously	4
	Open in response to verbal stimuli	Open in response to verbal stimuli	3
	Open in response to pain only	Open in response to pain only	2
	No response	No response	1
Verbal response	Coos and babbles	Oriented, appropriate	5
	Irritable cries	Confused	4
	Cries in response to pain	Inappropriate words	3
	Moans in response to pain	Incomprehensible words or nonspecific sounds	2
	No response	No response	1
Motor response†	Moves spontaneously and purposefully	Obeys commands	6
	Withdraws to touch	Localizes painful stimulus	5
	Withdraws in response to pain	Withdraws in response to pain	4
	Responds to pain with decorticate posturing (abnormal flexion)	Responds to pain with flexion	3
	Responds to pain with decerebrate posturing (abnormal extension)	Responds to pain with extension	2
	No response	No response	1

*Score ≤ 12 suggests a severe head injury. Score < 8 suggests need for intubation and ventilation. Score ≤ 6 suggests need for intracranial pressure monitoring.

†If the patient is intubated, unconscious, or preverbal, the most important part of this scale is motor response. This section should be carefully evaluated.

Adapted from Davis RJ et al: Head and spinal cord injury. In *Textbook of Pediatric Intensive Care,* edited by MC Rogers. Baltimore, Williams & Wilkins, 1987; James H, Anas N, Perkin RM: *Brain Insults in Infants and Children.* New York, Grune & Stratton, 1985; and Morray JP et al: Coma scale for use in brain-injured children. *Critical Care Medicine* 12:1018, 1984.

(> 7 days after the injury) develop in a small percentage of patients, often weeks, months, or even years later. Spastic motor impairment, gait and balance disturbances, ataxia, and sensory losses may occur.

A persistent vegetative state (see p. 1805) may follow a TBI that destroys forebrain cognitive functions but spares the brain stem. The capacity for self-aware mental activity is absent; however, autonomic and motor reflexes and normal sleep-wake cycles are preserved. Few patients recover normal neurologic function when a persistent vegetative state lasts for 3 mo after injury, and almost none recover after 6 mo.

Neurologic function tends to improve for at least 2 yr to a few yr after TBI, most rapidly during the initial 6 mo.

Diagnosis

An initial overall assessment of injuries should be done (see p. 2549); diagnosis and treatment occur simultaneously in seriously injured patients.

A rapid, focused neurologic evaluation is part of the initial assessment, including assessment of the components of the GCS, adequacy of the airway and breathing, and oculomotor activity. Patients are ideally assessed before paralytics and opioids are given. Patients are reassessed at frequent intervals (eg, q 15 to 30 min initially, then q 1 h after stabilization). Subsequent improvement or deterioration helps estimate injury severity and prognosis. Complete neurologic examination is done as soon as the patient is sufficiently stable. Children should be examined carefully for retinal hemorrhages, which may indicate shaken baby syndrome. Funduscopic examination in adults is insensitive for TBI and often difficult to perform.

Diagnosis of concussion is clinical, but imaging can help establish the gross condition of the brain and identify hematomas. Imaging should always be done in patients with impaired consciousness, GCS score < 15, focal neurologic findings, persistent vomiting, seizures, or clinically suspected fractures. However, many clinicians obtain a CT scan for all patients with more than a trivial head injury, because the clinical and medicolegal consequences of missing a hematoma are severe.

CT is the best choice for initial imaging; it can detect skull fractures (thin cuts are obtained to reveal clinically suspected basilar skull fractures, which may otherwise not be visible), hematomas, contusions, and sometimes DAI. Although plain x-rays can detect some skull fractures, they cannot help assess the brain and are seldom used. MRI may be useful later in the clinical course to detect more subtle contusions and DAI; it is usually more sensitive than CT for diagnosis of very small acute or isodense subacute and isodense chronic subdural hematomas. Angiography is occasionally used when vascular injury is suspected or when CT findings are inconsistent with physical examination findings.

Prognosis

In the US, adults with severe TBI who are treated have a mortality rate of about 25 to 33%; mortality is lower with higher GCS scores. Mortality rates are lower in children ≥5 yr (≤10% with a GCS score of 5 to 7). Children overall do better than adults with a comparable injury.

The vast majority of patients with mild TBI retain good neurologic function. With moderate or severe TBI, the prognosis is not as good but is much better than is generally believed. The most commonly used scale to assess outcome in TBI patients is the Glasgow Outcome Scale. On this scale, the possible outcomes are good recovery (defined by the absence of new neurologic deficits), moderate disability (defined by new neurologic deficits in a patient capable of self-care), severe disability (defined by a patient incapable of self-care), vegetative (defined by a patient with no cognitive function), and death. Over 50% of adults with severe TBI have a good recovery or moderate disability. In adults with severe TBI, recovery occurs most rapidly within the initial 6 mo; smaller improvements continue for perhaps as long as a few years. Children have a better immediate recovery from TBI regardless of severity and continue to improve for a longer period of time.

Cognitive deficits, with impaired concentration, attention, and memory, and various personality changes are a more common cause of disability in social relations and employment than are specific motor or sensory impairments. Posttraumatic anosmia and acute traumatic blindness seldom resolve after 3 to 4 mo. Hemiparesis and aphasia usually abate, except in the elderly.

Treatment

Multiple noncranial injuries, which are likely with motor vehicle crashes and falls, often require simultaneous treatment. For initial resuscitation of trauma patients, see p. 2549.

At the injury scene,a clear airway is secured and external bleeding is controlled before the patient is moved. Particular care is taken to avoid displacement of the spine or other bones to protect the spinal cord and blood vessels. Proper immobilization should be maintained with a cervical collar and long spine board until stability of the entire spine has been established by appropriate examination and imaging (see p. 2581). After the initial rapid neurologic assessment, pain should be relieved with a short-acting opioid (eg, fentanyl).

In the hospital, after quick initial evaluation, neurologic findings (GCS and pupillary reaction), BP, pulse, and temperature should be recorded frequently for several hours because any deterioration demands prompt attention. Serial GCS and CT results stratify injury severity within the categories defined by GCS, which helps guide treatment.

The cornerstone of management for all patients is maintenance of adequate pulmonary gas exchange and brain perfusion to avoid secondary brain insult. Aggressive early management of hypoxia, hypercapnia, hypotension, and increased ICP helps avoid secondary complications. Other complications to check for and prevent include hyperthermia, hyponatremia, hyperglycemia, and fluid imbalance.

Bleeding from injuries (external and internal) is rapidly controlled as required, and intravascular volume is promptly replaced with the appropriate fluid (0.9% saline or sometimes blood transfusion) to maintain cerebral perfusion. Hypotonic fluids (especially 5% D/W) are contraindicated because they contain excess free water. Fever is controlled.

Mild injury: Injury is mild (by GCS score) in 80% of patients who have TBI and present to an emergency department. If there is brief or no loss of consciousness and if patients have stable vital signs, a normal head CT scan, and normal mental and neurologic function, they may be discharged home provided family members or friends can observe them closely for an additional 24 h. These observers are instructed to return patients to the hospital if any of the following develop: decreased level of consciousness, focal neurologic deficits, worsening headache, vomiting, or deterioration of mental function.

Patients who have minimal or no neurologic changes but have minor abnormalities on head CT should be admitted for observation and follow-up CT.

Moderate and severe injury: Injury is moderate in 10% of patients who have TBI and present to an emergency department. They often do not require intubation and mechanical ventilation (unless other injuries are present) or ICP monitoring. However, because deterioration is possible, these patients should be admitted and observed even if head CT is normal.

Injury is severe in 10% of patients who have TBI and present to an emergency department. They are admitted to a critical care unit. Because usually airway protective reflexes are impaired and ICP is increased, patients are intubated endotracheally while measures are taken to avoid increasing ICP. Close monitoring using the GCS and pupillary response should continue, and CT scan is repeated.

Increased intracranial pressure: Patients with TBI who require airway support or mechanical ventilation undergo oral rather than nasotracheal intubation (see Ch. 65 on p. 544), which is more likely to increase ICP. Appropriate drugs should be used in a controlled, efficient way to minimize the increase in ICP that may occur with intubation via either route—eg, some clinicians recommend giving lidocaine 1.5 mg/kg IV 1 to 2 min before giving the paralytic. Succinylcholine 1 mg/kg IV is typically used as a paralytic. Etomidate is a good choice for an induction agent because it has minimal effects on BP; IV dose in adults is 0.3 mg/kg (or 20 mg for an average-sized adult) and in children is 0.2 to 0.3 mg/kg. Alternatively, if hypotension is absent and unlikely and if propofol is more readily available, intubation can be done using 0.2 to 1.5 mg/kg.

Pulse oximetry and ABGs (if possible, end-tidal CO_2) should be used to assess adequacy of oxygenation and ventilation. The goal is a normal $PaCO_2$ level (38 to 42 mm Hg). Previously, prophylactic hyperventilation ($PaCO_2$ 25 to 35 mm Hg) was recommended. However, although this lower $PaCO_2$ reduces ICP by causing cerebral vasoconstriction, it also decreases cerebral perfusion and thus may produce ischemia. Therefore, hyperventilation is used only within the first several hours to treat increased ICP unresponsive to other measures, only to achieve $PaCO_2$ of 30 to 35 mm Hg, and only for short periods (see p. 2578).

In patients with severe TBI who cannot follow simple commands, especially those with an abnormal head CT scan, ICP and CPP monitoring (see p.516) and control are recommended. The goal is to maintain ICP at < 20 mm Hg and CPP at 50 to 70 mm Hg. Cerebral venous drainage can be enhanced (thus lowering ICP) by elevating the head of the bed to 30° and by keeping the patient's head in a midline position. If a ventricular catheter is in place, CSF drainage can lower ICP.

Preventing agitation, excessive muscular activity (eg, from delirium), and pain can also help prevent increases in ICP. For sedation, propofol is often used in adults (contraindicated in children) because it has quick onset and duration of action; dose is 0.3 mg/kg/h continuous IV infusion, titrated gradually upward as needed (up to 3 mg/kg/h). An initial bolus is not used. The most common adverse effect is hypotension. Prolonged use at high doses can cause pancreatitis. Benzodiazepines (eg, midazolam, lorazepam) can also be used for sedation. Antipsychotics can delay recovery and should be avoided if possible. For delirium, haloperidol may be used for a few days; delirium that lasts longer can be treated with trazodone, gabapentin, valproate preparations, or quetiapine, although it is not clear that these drugs are better than haloperidol. Rarely, paralytics may be needed; if so, adequate sedation must be ensured because agitation can no longer be assessed clinically. Opioids are often needed for adequate pain control.

Patients should be kept euvolemic and normosmolar or slightly hyperosmolar (target serum osmolality 295 to 320 mOsm/kg). Osmotic diuretics (eg, mannitol) may be given IV to lower ICP and maintain serum osmolality. However, they should be reserved for patients whose condition is deteriorating or used preoperatively for patients with hematomas. Mannitol 20% solution is given 0.5 to 1 g/kg IV over 15 to 30 min and repeated in a dose ranging from 0.25 to 0.5 g/kg given as often as needed (usually q 6 to 8 h); it lowers ICP for a few hours. Mannitol must be used cautiously in patients with severe coronary artery disease, heart failure, renal insufficiency, or pulmonary vascular congestion because mannitol rapidly expands intravascular volume. Because osmotic diuretics increase renal excretion of water relative to Na, prolonged use of mannitol may also result in water depletion and hypernatremia. Furosemide 1 mg/kg IV is also helpful to decrease total body water, particularly when the transient hypervolemia associated with mannitol is to be avoided. Fluid and electrolyte balance should be monitored closely while osmotic diuretics are used. A 3% saline solution is being studied as another potential osmotic agent to control ICP.

Hyperventilation (eg, to a $PaCO_2$ of 30 to 35 mm Hg) may be necessary briefly when increased ICP is refractory to other modulating strategies. An alternative treatment for intractable increased ICP is decompressive craniotomy. For this procedure, a bone flap is removed (to be replaced later), and duraplasty is done to allow outward brain swelling.

Another treatment for intractable increased ICP is pentobarbital coma. Coma is induced by giving pentobarbital 10 mg/kg over 30 min, 5 mg/kg/h for 3 doses, then 1 mg/kg/h. The dose may be adjusted to suppress bursts of EEG activity, which is continuously monitored. Hypotension is common and managed by giving fluids and, if necessary, vasopressors.

Therapeutic systemic hypothermia has not proved helpful. Corticosteroids are not useful to control ICP and are not recommended; they were associated with a worse outcome in a recent multinational study.

Seizures: Prolonged seizures, which can worsen brain damage and increase ICP, should be prevented if possible and treated promptly when they occur. In patients with significant structural injury (eg, larger contusions or hematomas, brain laceration, depressed skull fracture) or a GCS score < 10, a prophylactic anticonvulsant should be considered. If phenytoin is used, a loading dose of 20 mg/kg IV is given (at a maximum rate of 50 mg/min to prevent cardiovascular adverse effects such as hypotension and bradycardia). The starting maintenance IV dose for adults is 2 to 2.7 mg/kg tid; children require higher doses (up to 5 mg/kg bid for children < 4 yr). Serum levels should be measured to adjust the dose. Duration of treatment varies and depends on the type of injury and EEG results. If no seizures develop within 1 wk, anticonvulsants should be stopped because their value in preventing future seizures is not established. Newer anticonvulsants are under study.

Skull fractures: Aligned closed fractures require no specific treatment. Depressed fractures sometimes require surgery to elevate fragments, manage lacerated cortical vessels, repair dura mater, and debride injured brain. Open fractures require debridement. Use of antibiotic prophylaxis is controversial because of limited data on its efficacy and the concern that it encourages drug-resistant strains.

Surgery: Intracranial hematomas may require surgical evacuation of blood. Prompt evacuation of the hematoma can prevent or treat brain shift and compression; early neurosurgical consultation is mandatory. However, many hematomas do not require surgical removal. Small intracerebral hematomas rarely require surgery. Patients with small subdural hematomas can often be treated without surgery. Factors that suggest a need for surgery include a midline brain shift of > 5 mm, compression of the basal cisterns, and worsening neurologic examination findings. Chronic subdural hematomas may require surgical drainage but much less urgently than acute subdural hematomas. Large or arterial epidural hematomas are treated surgically, but small venous epidural hematomas can be followed with serial CT scans.

Rehabilitation: When neurologic deficits persist, rehabilitation is needed. Brain injury support groups may provide assistance to the families of brain-injured patients.

Occurrence and duration of coma after a TBI are strong predictors of rehabilitation needs; of patients whose coma exceeds 24 h, 50% have major persistent neurologic sequelae, and 2 to 6% remain in a persistent vegetative state at 6 mo. For patients who survive the initial hospitalization, a prolonged period of rehabilitation, particularly in cognitive and emotional areas, is often required, and rehabilitation services should be planned early.

Rehabilitation is best provided through a team approach that combines physical, occupational, and speech therapy; skill-building activities; and counseling to meet the patient's social and emotional needs (see also p. 2756).

311 SPINAL TRAUMA

Trauma to the spine may produce injuries involving the spinal cord, vertebrae, or both. Occasionally, the spinal nerves are affected (see p. 1901). The anatomy of the spinal column is reviewed in Ch. 224 on p. 1908.

Etiology and Pathophysiology

Cord injury: During a typical year, there are > 10,000 spinal cord injuries in the US. Nearly 40% occur in motor vehicle collisions (also called motor vehicle accidents), and 25% result from violent encounters. The remainder is attributed to falls, sports, and work-related accidents. More than 80% of patients are male.

Spinal cord injuries occur when direct physical force damages the vertebrae, ligaments, or disks of the spinal column causing bruising, crushing, or tearing of spinal cord tissue; and when the spinal cord is penetrated (eg, by a gunshot or a knife wound). Such injuries can also produce vascular injury with resultant ischemia or hematoma (typically extradural), leading to further damage. All forms of injury can cause spinal cord edema, further decreasing blood flow and oxygenation. Damage may be mediated by excessive release of neurotransmitters from damaged cells, an inflammatory immune response with release of cytokines, accumulation of free radicals, and apoptosis.

Vertebral injury: Bony injuries include fractures and dislocations. Fractures may involve the vertebral body, lamina, pedicles, and spinous and transverse processes. Dislocations typically involve the facets. Subluxation involves ligament rupture without bony injury. In the neck, fractures of the posterior elements and dislocations can damage the vertebral arteries, causing a stroke-like syndrome.

Unstable vertebral injuries are those in which bony and ligamentous integrity is disrupted sufficiently that free movement can occur, potentially compressing the spinal cord or its vascular supply and resulting in marked worsening of neurologic function or pain. Such vertebral movement may occur even with a shift in patient position (eg, for ambulance transport, during initial evaluation). Stable fractures are able to resist such movement.

Specific injuries typically vary with mechanism of trauma. Flexion injuries can produce wedge fractures of the vertebral body or

TABLE 311–1. EFFECTS OF SPINAL CORD INJURY BY LOCATION

LOCATION OF INJURY*	POSSIBLE EFFECTS†
Above C5	Respiratory paralysis and often death
At or above C4 to C5	Complete quadriplegia
Between C5 and C6	Paralysis of legs, but arm abduction and flexion possible
Between C6 and C7	Paralysis of legs, wrists, and hands, but shoulder movement and elbow flexion usually possible
Above T1	With transverse lesions, miotic pupils
Between T11 and T12	Paralysis of leg muscles above and below the knee
At T12 to L1	Paralysis below the knee
Cauda equina	Hyporeflexic or areflexic paresis of the lower extremities and usually pain and hyperesthesia in the distribution of the nerve roots
At S3 to S5 or conus medullaris at L1	Complete loss of bowel and bladder control

*Abbreviations refer to vertebrae; the cord is shorter than the spine, so that moving down the spine, the cord segments and vertebral levels are increasingly out of alignment.

†Priapism, reduced rectal tone, and changes in reflexes may occur with injury at any level.

spinous process fractures; greater flexion force may cause bilateral facet dislocation, or if occurring at the C1-C2 level, odontoid fracture and/or atlantooccipital or atlantoaxial subluxation. Rotational injury can cause unilateral facet dislocation. Extension injury can cause posterior neural arch fracture. Compression injuries can cause burst fracture of vertebral bodies.

Cauda equina injury: The lower tip of the spinal cord (conus medullaris) is usually at the L1 vertebra level. Spinal nerves below this level comprise the cauda equina. Spinal injuries below this level thus do not produce typical findings of cord injury (see also p. 1910).

Symptoms and Signs

The cardinal sign of cord injury is a discrete injury level in which neurologic function above the injury is intact, and function below the injury is absent or markedly diminished. Specific manifestations depend on the exact level (see TABLE 311–1) and whether cord injury is complete or partial.

Vertebral injury, as with other fractures and dislocations, typically is painful, but patients who are distracted by other painful injuries (eg, long bone fractures) or whose level of consciousness is altered by intoxicants or head injury may not complain of pain.

Complete cord injury: Transection leads to immediate, complete, flaccid paralysis (including loss of anal sphincter tone), loss of all sensation and reflex activity, and autonomic dysfunction below the level of the injury.

High cervical injury (at or above C5) affects the muscles controlling respiration, causing respiratory insufficiency; ventilator dependence may occur, especially for injuries at or above C3. Autonomic dysfunction from cervical injury can result in bradycardia and hypotension, termed spinal neurogenic shock (see p. 560); unlike in other forms of shock, the skin remains warm and dry. Arrhythmias and BP instability may develop. Pneumonia is a frequent cause of death in people with a high spinal cord injury, especially in those who are ventilator dependent.

Flaccid paralysis gradually changes over hours or days to spastic paralysis due to exaggeration of the normal stretch reflexes resulting from loss of descending inhibition. Later, if the lumbosacral cord is intact, flexor muscle spasms appear, and deep tendon reflexes and autonomic reflexes return.

Partial cord injury: Partial motor and sensory loss occurs, which may be permanent or temporary depending on the etiology; function may be lost briefly due to concussion or more lastingly due to a contusion or laceration. Sometimes with a cord concussion, however, rapid swelling of the cord results in total neurologic dysfunction resembling complete cord transection. Termed spinal shock (not to be confused with spinal neurogenic shock), symptoms resolve over one to several days; residual disability often remains.

Manifestations depend on which portion of the cord is involved; several discrete syndromes are recognized.

Brown-Séquard syndrome results from hemisection of the cord. Patients have ipsilateral spastic paralysis and loss of postural sense below the lesion, and contralateral loss of pain and thermal sense.

Anterior cord syndrome results from direct injury to the anterior spinal cord or to the anterior spinal artery. Patients lose motor and pain sensation bilaterally below the lesion. Posterior cord function (vibration, proprioception) is intact.

Central cord syndrome usually occurs in patients with a narrowed spinal canal (congenital or degenerative) after a hyperextension injury. Motor function in the arms is impaired to a greater extent than that in the legs. If the posterior columns are affected, posture, vibration, and light touch are lost. If the spinothalamic tracts are affected, pain, temperature, and, often, light or deep touch are lost.

Hemorrhage in the spinal cord from trauma (hematomyelia) is usually confined to the cervical central gray matter, resulting in signs of lower motor neuron damage (muscle weakness and wasting, fasciculations, and diminished tendon reflexes in the arms), which is usually permanent. Motor weakness is often proximal and accompanied by selective impairment of pain and temperature sensation.

Cauda equina lesions: Motor and/or sensory loss is likely to be partial. Sensation is usually diminished in the perineal region ("saddle anesthesia"). Anal sphincter tone is lax. Bowel and bladder function impairment may involve incontinence or retention. Men may have erectile dysfunction, and women diminished sexual response.

Complications: Sequelae depend on the severity and level of the injury. Breathing may be impaired if the injury is at or above the C5 segment; reduced mobility increases the risk of blood clots and pressure sores. Disabling spasticity may develop. Autonomic dysreflexia may occur in response to triggering events such as pain or pressure on the body. Chronic neurogenic pain may manifest as burning or stinging.

Diagnosis

Spinal cord injuries with trauma are not always obvious. Injury to the spine and spinal cord must be considered in patients with injuries that involve the head, pelvic fractures, penetrating injuries in the area of the spine, in most motor vehicle collisions, and in any injuries related to falling from heights or diving into water.

Motor function is tested in all extremities. Sensation testing should involve both light touch (posterior column function), pinprick (anterior spinothalamic tract), and position sense. Identification of the sensory level is best done by testing from distal to proximal and by testing thoracic roots on the back to avoid being misled by the cervical cape. Priapism may occur in the acute phase of spinal cord injury and indicates spinal cord damage. Rectal tone may be decreased, and lower-limb reflexes may be exuberant or diminished.

Plain x-rays are taken of any possibly injured areas; CT scans are obtained of abnormal areas and those of high clinical suspicion. Some trauma centers use CT as primary imaging for spinal trauma. MRI helps identify the type and location of cord injury. Manifestations of injury may be characterized using the ASIA (American Spinal Injury Association) Impairment Scale or a similar instrument (see TABLE 311–2).

Prognosis and Treatment

Transected or degenerated nerves in the cord do not recover, and functional damage is permanent. Compressed nerve tissue can recover its function. Return of a movement or sensation during the 1st week after injury heralds a favorable recovery; dysfunction remaining after 6 mo is likely to be permanent.

Immediate care: After stabilization of the airway, breathing, and circulation (see p. 2549), the goal is to prevent secondary injury to the spine or spinal cord. In unstable injuries, flexion or extension of the spine can contuse or transect the cord. Thus, when injury victims are moved, inappropriate han-

TABLE 311–2. SPINAL INJURY IMPAIRMENT SCALE*

LEVEL	IMPAIRMENT
A = Complete	No motor or sensory function, including in the sacral segments S4–S5
B = Incomplete	Sensory but not motor function is preserved below the neurologic level and includes the sacral segments S4—S5
C = Incomplete	Motor function is preserved below the neurologic level, and > ½ of key muscles below neurologic level have a muscle grade < 3
D = Incomplete	Motor function is preserved below the neurologic level, and at least ½ of key muscles below the neurologic level have a muscle grade = 3
E = Normal	Motor and sensory function are normal

*According to the American Spinal Injury Association.

dling can precipitate paraplegia, quadriplegia, or even death from spinal injury. Patients who may have a spinal injury should be moved en bloc and transported on a firm, flat backboard or similar surface, with padding to stabilize their position without excessive pressure. A rigid collar should be used to immobilize the cervical spine. Patients with thoracic or lumbar spine injuries can be carried prone or supine; those with cervical cord damage that could induce respiratory difficulties should be carried supine, with attention to maintaining a patent airway and avoiding chest constriction. Transfer to a trauma center is desirable.

Medical care should be directed at avoiding hypoxia and hypotension, both of which can further stress the injured cord. In high cervical segment injuries, intubation and respiratory support is usually needed; in-line stabilization should be applied during intubation.

Large doses of corticosteroids, started within 8 h after spinal cord injury, may improve the outcome. Methylprednisolone 30 mg/kg IV over 1 h, followed by 5.4 mg/kg/h for the next 23 h is recommended. Injuries are treated with rest, analgesics, and muscle-relaxing drugs with or without surgery until swelling and local pain have subsided. Additional general treatment for trauma patients is discussed on p. 2549.

Unstable injuries are immobilized until bone and soft tissues have healed to ensure proper alignment; surgery with fusion and internal fixation is sometimes needed. In complete injury, surgery aims to stabilize the spine to allow early mobilization. The return of useful neurologic function below the level of the injury is unlikely. In contrast, patients with incomplete cord injuries can have significant neurologic improvement after decompression. The timing of surgery in incomplete lesions is debatable. Early surgery (eg, within 24 h) may have a better neurologic outcome and allows for earlier mobilization and rehabilitation.

Nursing care includes preventing urinary and pulmonary infections and pressure sores—eg, by moving the paralyzed patient q 2 h (on a Stryker frame when necessary). Deep venous thrombosis prophylaxis is required. An inferior vena cava filter could be considered in immobile patients.

Long-term care: Drugs effectively control spasticity in some patients. Oral agents such as baclofen 5 mg po tid (maximum, 80 mg during a 24-h period) and tizanidine 4 mg po tid (maximum, 36 mg during a 24-h period) are typically used for spasticity associated with spinal cord injury. Intrathecal baclofen 50 to 100 μg once/day may be considered in patients in whom oral drugs are ineffective.

Rehabilitation is needed to help people recover as fully as possible (see p. 2756). Rehabilitation, best provided through a team approach, combines physical therapies, skill-building activities, and counseling to meet social and emotional needs. The rehabilitation team is best directed by a physician with training and expertise in rehabilitation (physiatrist); it usually includes nurses, social workers, nutritionists, psychologists, physical and occupational therapists, recreational therapists, and vocational counselors (see also Ch. 336 on p. 2748).

Physical therapy focuses on exercises for muscle strengthening and appropriate use of assistive devices such as braces, a walker, or a wheelchair that may be needed to improve mobility. Strategies for controlling spasticity, autonomic dysreflexia, and neurogenic pain are taught. Occupational therapy focuses on redeveloping fine motor skills. Bladder and bowel management programs teach toileting techniques, which may require intermittent catheterization. A bowel regimen, involving timed stimulation with laxatives, is often needed.

Vocational rehabilitation involves assessing both fine and gross motor skills, as well as cognitive capabilities, to determine the likelihood for meaningful employment. The vocational specialist then helps identify possible work sites and determines need for assistive equipment and workplace modifications. Recreation therapists use a similar approach in identifying and facilitating participation in hobbies, athletics, and other activities.

Emotional care aims to combat the depersonalization and the almost unavoidable depression that occur after losing control of the body. Emotional care is fundamental to the success of all other components of rehabilitation and must be accompanied by efforts to educate the patient and encourage active involvement of family and friends.

Investigational treatments are under study to promote nerve regeneration. Such treatments include injections of autologous, incubated macrophages; epidurally administered BA-210, an experimental drug that may be neuroprotective and stimulate nerve growth; and HP-184 for treatment of chronic spinal cord injury.

Spinal Cord Injury in Children

Although children < 10 yr have the lowest rate of spinal cord injuries, such injuries are not rare. Any child that has been in a motor vehicle collision, fallen from a height ≥ 3 m, or has had a submersion injury should be assumed to have a spinal cord injury until examination and imaging studies prove otherwise.

In children < 8 yr, cervical spine injuries occur most commonly above C4; in those > 8 yr, injuries at C5 to C8 are more common. Of increasing importance has been the recognition of *S*pinal *C*ord *I*njury *W*ithout evidence *O*f *R*adiologic *A*bnormality (SCIWORA). This type of injury occurs almost exclusively in children and is related to direct spinal cord traction, spinal cord concussion, and vascular injury.

Treatment is similar to that in adults, with immobilization and attention to the adequacy of oxygenation, ventilation, and circulation, and may include high-dose corticosteroids (same weight-based dose). Children with significant spinal cord trauma should be transferred to a pediatric trauma center as soon as possible.

312 FACIAL TRAUMA

Patients with trauma to the face and head require evaluation of all structures; injuries often occur in combination (see p. 858 for dental trauma, p. 802 for tympanic membrane trauma, and p. 2586 for eye trauma).

EXTERNAL EAR TRAUMA

Trauma to the external ear may result in hematoma, laceration, avulsion, or fracture.

Blunt trauma to the pinna may cause a subperichondrial hematoma; the accumulation of blood between the perichondrium and cartilage renders the pinna a shapeless, reddish purple mass. Because the perichondrium supplies blood to the cartilage, infection, abscess formation, or avascular necrosis of the cartilage may follow. The resultant destruction causes the cauliflower ear characteristic of wrestlers and boxers. Treatment consists of evacuating the clot through an incision and preventing reaccumulation of the hematoma with through-and-through ear sutures over dental gauze rolls or insertion of a Penrose drain plus a pressure dressing to keep the cartilage close to its blood supply. Because these injuries are prone to infection, an oral antibiotic effective against staphylococci (eg, cephalexin 500 mg tid) is given for 5 days.

If lacerations of the pinna penetrate the cartilage and skin on both sides, the skin margins are sutured; then, the cartilage is splinted externally with benzoin-impregnated cotton, and a protective dressing is applied. Sutures should not extend into the cartilage. Oral antibiotics are given as above.

Complete or partial avulsions are repaired by an otolaryngologist or plastic surgeon.

Forceful blows to the mandible may be transmitted to the anterior wall of the ear canal (posterior wall of the glenoid fossa). Displaced fragments from a fractured anterior wall may cause stenosis of the canal and must be reduced or removed surgically under general anesthesia.

FRACTURES OF THE JAW AND CONTIGUOUS STRUCTURES

Blunt facial trauma can fracture the jaw and other bones of the midface.

Fractures of the jaw are suspected in patients with a new malocclusion or focal swelling and tenderness over a segment of the mandible. Some fractures result in palpable instability. Fractures of the mandibular condyle usually cause preauricular pain, swelling, and limited opening of the mouth. With a unilateral condylar fracture, the jaw deviates to the affected side when the mouth is opened.

Fractures of the midface, which includes the area from the superior orbital rim to the maxillary teeth, can cause irregularity in the smooth contour of the cheeks, malar eminences, zygomatic arch, or orbital rims, as well as infraorbital anesthesia. Enophthalmos and diplopia suggest orbital floor fracture. The Le Fort classification (see FIG. 312–1) can be used to describe maxillary fractures. Brain injury and fractured cervical vertebrae are possible when trauma has been severe enough to fracture facial bones. In major impact injuries, hemorrhage and edema due to a facial fracture may compromise the airway.

A panoramic dental x-ray is preferred for an isolated mandibular fracture. Plain x-rays (posteroanterior, oblique, occlusal, Water's, and Towne views) may screen for facial fracture, but if available, CT should be used; CT is recommended when fracture is seen on plain x-rays.

Treatment

An orotracheal airway may be required to maintain airway patency in patients with hemorrhage, edema, or major tissue disruption (see p. 527). Definitive facial fracture management is complex and may include internal fixation.

Fractures through a tooth socket are open fractures. They require antibiotic prophylaxis given orally as a liquid or parenterally.

For a fractured mandible, treatment is intermaxillary fixation or rigid open fixation. If fixation is available within the 1st few hours after injury, closure of any lip or oral lacerations should be delayed until the fracture has been reduced. For intermaxillary fixation, arch bars are attached to the teeth of each jaw and then wired to each other after correct occlusion has been established. Patients should always carry wire cutters in case of vomiting. Eating is restricted to liquids, pureed foods, and supplements. Because only the outer surfaces of the teeth can be brushed, a 60-sec rinse with 30 mL of chlorhexidine 0.12% every morning and evening controls plaque formation, infection, and halitosis. Jaw-opening exercises usually help restore function after fixation is discontinued.

Condylar fractures may require only 2 wk of external fixation. However, severely displaced,

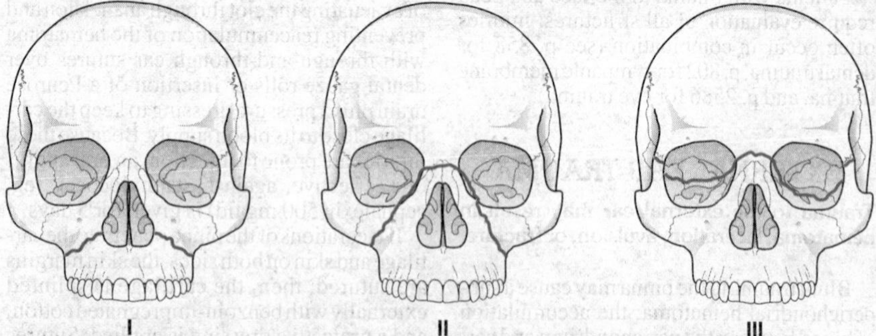

Fig. 312–1. Le Fort classification of midface fractures. I: only the lower maxilla; II: the infraorbital rim; III: complete detachment of the midface from the skull.

bilaterally fractured condyles may require open reduction and fixation. Condylar fracture in children should not be rigidly immobilized because ankylosis and abnormal facial development may result. Elastic fixation for 5 days is usually sufficient.

FRACTURES OF THE NOSE

Fractures of the nasal bones or cartilaginous injury may result in swelling, point tenderness, hypermobility, crepitus, epistaxis, and periorbital bruising. Diagnosis is usually clinical. Treatment may include reduction, stabilization through internal packing, and splinting.

The nasal bones are the most frequently fractured facial bones because of their central location and protrusion. Depending on the mechanism of injury, fractures of the maxilla, orbit, or cribriform plate and injury to the nasolacrimal ducts may also occur.

Complications include cosmetic deformity and functional obstruction. Septal hematoma may lead to avascular or septic necrosis of the cartilage with resultant deformity. Cribriform plate fracture can lead to meningitis or brain abscess.

Symptoms and Signs

Facial trauma resulting in epistaxis may indicate a nasal fracture. Other symptoms and signs include obvious or subtle nasal deformity, swelling, point tenderness, crepitus, and instability. Lacerations, ecchymosis (nasal and periorbital), septal deviation, and nasal obstruction may be present. Septal hematoma appears as a purplish bulge on the septum. CSF rhinorrhea appears as clear drainage but may be mixed with blood, making it difficult to identify.

Diagnosis and Treatment

Diagnosis is based on physical examination. Plain x-rays of an uncomplicated nasal fracture are not helpful because their sensitivity and specificity are poor. If other facial fractures or complications are suspected, CT of facial bones is done.

Immediate treatment includes symptomatic control with ice and analgesics. Reduction is needed only for fractures causing clinically visible deformity or nasal airway obstruction. The end-point of reduction is determined by clinical appearance or improved airway. Therefore, reduction is usually deferred for 3 to 5 days after injury to allow swelling to subside. Nasal fractures in adults may be reduced after a local anesthetic is given; children require general anesthesia. A blunt elevator is passed through the nares and placed under the depressed nasal bone, which is lifted anteriorly and laterally while pressure is applied to the other side of the nose to bring the nasal dorsum to the midline. The nose may be stabilized with internal packing (consisting of antibiotic-impregnated strip gauze) placed high within the nasal vestibule, as well as with external splinting. Internal packing is left in place for 4 to 7 days; external splinting is left for 7 to 14 days.

Cartilaginous injuries often do not require reduction. In the rare circumstance that a deformity persists after swelling subsides, a reduction and splinting under local anesthesia are usually sufficient.

Septal hematomas must be immediately incised and drained to prevent infection and cartilage necrosis. Septal fractures are difficult to hold in position and often require septal surgery later.

TEMPORAL BONE FRACTURES

Temporal bone fractures can occur after severe blunt trauma to the head and sometimes involve structures of the ear, causing hearing loss or facial paralysis.

Temporal bone fractures are suggested by Battle's sign (postauricular ecchymosis) and bleeding from the ear. Bleeding may come from the middle ear through a ruptured tympanic membrane or from a fracture line in the ear canal. A hemotympanum makes the tympanic membrane appear blue-black. CSF otorrhea indicates a communication between the middle ear and the subarachnoid space. Longitudinal fractures can extend through the middle ear and rupture the tympanic membrane; they cause facial paralysis in 15% of cases and rarely cause sensorineural hearing loss. Delayed-onset complete facial paralysis usually indicates edema within an intact nerve. Conductive hearing loss may occur secondary to disruption of the ossicular chain. Transverse fractures cross the fallopian canal and cochlea and nearly always cause facial paralysis and permanent sensorineural hearing loss.

Diagnosis and Treatment

If a temporal bone fracture is suspected, immediate CT of the head with special attention to the temporal bone is recommended. Audiometry is required for all patients with a temporal bone fracture, although it does not have to be performed immediately. The Weber and Rinne tuning fork tests during physical examination can differentiate between conductive and sensorineural hearing loss.

Treatment is based on managing facial nerve injury, hearing loss, and CSF leakage. Immediate complete facial paralysis usually indicates a severed facial nerve, which requires surgical exploration and end-to-end re-anastomosis. Delayed-onset complete facial paralysis almost always resolves with conservative management, including use of a corticosteroid taper. Incomplete facial palsy, whether immediate or delayed in onset, almost always resolves with conservative management.

Conductive hearing loss requires ossicular chain reconstruction several weeks to months after the injury. Good results can be expected. When sensorineural hearing loss occurs, it is typically permanent, and there are no medical or surgical therapies available to improve hearing. However, in the rare case of fluctuating sensorineural hearing loss, an exploratory tympanotomy to search for a perilymph fistula may be indicated.

Patients who have a temporal bone fracture and CSF otorrhea should be hospitalized because of risk of meningitis. The leak usually stops spontaneously within a few days, although a lumbar drain or surgical closure of the defect is occasionally required.

313 EYE INJURIES

(See also Retinal Detachment on p. 919.)

Common causes of eye injury include domestic accidents (eg, during hammering or exposure to household chemicals or cleaners), assault, car battery explosions, sporting injuries (including air- or paint pellet-gun injuries), and motor vehicle accidents (including air-bag injuries). Injury may be to the eyeball (globe), surrounding soft tissues (including muscles, nerves, and tendons), or bones of the eye socket.

General evaluation should include tests of vision; range of extraocular motion; pupillary responses; intraocular pressure determination; visual fields to confrontation; depth of anterior chamber; location and depth of lid and conjunctival lacerations and of foreign bodies; and presence of anterior chamber or vitreous hemorrhage, cataract, or red reflex. If an orbital fracture or foreign body is suspected, CT is performed.

Use of eye guards, goggles, or special eyeglasses, such as those constructed of polycarbonate lenses in a wrap-around polyamide frame, is a simple precaution that greatly reduces the risk of injury.

BURNS

Lid burns: These should be cleansed thoroughly with sterile isotonic saline solution followed by application of an antimicrobial ointment (eg, bacitracin bid).

Chemical burns: Burns of the cornea and conjunctiva can be serious, particularly when strong acid or alkali is involved.

Burns should be immediately irrigated with copious amounts of water or with 0.9% saline if available. The eye may be anesthetized with 1 drop of proparacaine 0.5%, but irrigation should not be delayed and should last for at least 30 min. In acid and alkali burns, some suggest 1 to 2 h of irrigation, whereas others recommend that the pH of conjunctiva be measured with nitrazine paper and irrigation continued until pH is normal.

After irrigation, the conjunctival fornices should be swept with a swab to remove trapped particles. Using double eversion, the superior fornices are examined for chemical embedded in the tissue.

Chemical iritis is treated by instilling a long-acting cycloplegic (eg, a single dose of atropine 1% solution). Corneal epithelial defects are treated by applying an antibiotic ointment (eg, ciprofloxacin 0.3%). Topical anesthetics should be avoided after initial irrigation; significant pain may be treated with acetaminophen with or without oxycodone.

Severe chemical burns require treatment by an ophthalmologist to save vision and prevent major complications such as uveitis, perforation of the globe, and lid deformities. Patients with significant redness of the eye, avascular areas of conjunctiva, or loss of conjunctival or corneal epithelium as demonstrated by fluorescein staining should be examined by an ophthalmologist within 24 h.

CORNEAL ABRASIONS AND FOREIGN BODIES

Corneal abrasions are self-limited, superficial epithelial defects.

The most common conjunctival and corneal injuries are foreign bodies and abrasions. Improper use of contact lenses can damage the cornea. Superficial foreign bodies often spontaneously exit the cornea in the tear film, occasionally leaving a residual abrasion, but other foreign bodies remain on or within the eye. Intraocular penetration can occur with seemingly minor trauma, particularly with foreign bodies resulting from high-speed machines (eg, drills, saws), hammering, or explosions. Infection rarely follows a corneal injury.

Symptoms, Signs, and Diagnosis

Symptoms and signs of abrasion or foreign body include pain, tearing, redness, and discharge. Vision is rarely affected (other than by tearing).

After an anesthetic (eg, 2 drops of proparacaine 0.5%) is instilled onto the conjunctiva, each lid is everted, and the entire conjunctiva and cornea are inspected with a binocular lens (loupe) or a slit lamp. Fluorescein staining (see p. 870) with cobalt light illumination renders abrasions and nonmetallic foreign bodies more apparent. Patients with a high-risk intraocular injury or (more rarely) visible globe perforation undergo CT to rule out intraocular foreign body.

Treatment

After instillation of an anesthetic into the conjunctiva, conjunctival foreign bodies can be removed by irrigation or lifted out with a moist sterile cotton applicator. A corneal foreign body that cannot be dislodged by irrigation may be lifted out carefully on the point of a sterile spud or of a 25- or 27-gauge hypodermic needle under loupe or, preferably, slit-lamp magnification. Steel or iron foreign bodies remaining on the cornea for more than a few hours may leave a rust ring on the cornea that also requires removal under slit-lamp magnification by scraping or using a low-speed rotary burr.

For all abrasions, an antibiotic ointment (eg, bacitracin/polymyxin B or a fluoroquinolone qid for 3 to 5 days) is used. Contact lens wearers with corneal abrasions require an antibiotic with optimal antipseudomonal coverage (eg, ciprofloxacin 0.3% ointment qid). For larger abrasions (eg, area > 10 mm^2) accompanied by symptoms (ie, pain), the pupil also is dilated with a short-acting cycloplegic (eg, 1 drop cyclopentolate 1% or homatropine 5%). Eye patches are usually not used, particularly for an abrasion caused by a contact lens or an object that may be contaminated with soil or vegetation. Topical NSAIDs, such as ketorolac 0.5% qid prn, can be used for 1 to 2 days to lessen discomfort. Ophthalmic corticosteroids tend to promote the growth of fungi and herpes simplex virus and are contraindicated.

The corneal epithelium regenerates rapidly; even large abrasions heal within 1 to 3 days. A contact lens should not be worn for 7 to 14 days. Follow-up examination by an ophthalmologist 1 or 2 days after injury is wise, especially if a foreign body was removed with a needle or spud.

Intraocular foreign bodies require immediate surgical treatment by an ophthalmologist. Before surgery, the pupil is often dilated with 1 drop of cyclopentolate 1% and 1 drop of phenylephrine 2.5% to allow examination of the crystalline lens, vitreous, and retina. Systemic and topical antimicrobials are indicated, eg, gentamicin 1 mg/kg IV q 8 h (if kidney function is adequate), in combination with cefazolin 1 g IV q 6 h and gentamicin 0.3% ophthalmic solution 1 drop hourly. Ointment should be avoided if the globe is lacerated. A protective shield (such as a Fox shield or the bottom third of a paper cup) is placed and taped over the eye to avoid inadvertent pressure that could extrude ocular contents through the penetration site.

CONTUSIONS AND LACERATIONS

Consequences of blunt trauma to the eye range from eyelid to orbital injury.

Eyelids: Eyelid contusions (black eyes) are more cosmetically than clinically significant, though corneal injuries may sometimes accompany them and should not be overlooked. Uncomplicated contusions are treated with ice packs to inhibit swelling during the first 24 to 48 h, followed by hot compresses to aid absorption of the hematoma.

Minor lid lacerations not involving the lid margin or tarsal plate may be repaired with nylon (or, in children, plain gut) 6-0 or 7-0 sutures. Lid-margin lacerations are best repaired by an ophthalmic surgeon to ensure accurate apposition and to avoid a notch in the contour. Major lid lacerations, which include those of the medial portion of the lower lid (possibly involving the lacrimal canaliculus), through-and-through lacerations, and those exposing orbital fat or involving the tarsal plate, should also be repaired by an ophthalmic surgeon.

Globe: Trauma may cause conjunctival, anterior chamber, and vitreous hemorrhage; retinal hemorrhage or detachment; laceration of the iris; cataract; dislocated lens; glaucoma; and rupture. Evaluation can be difficult with massive lid edema or laceration. Nonetheless, because immediate surgical treatment is required for some conditions, the lid is opened, taking care not to exert inward pressure, and as complete an examination as possible is conducted. At a minimum, visual acuity, pupillary responses, extraocular movements, anterior chamber depth or hemorrhage, and presence of red reflex are noted. An analgesic or anxiolytic may facilitate examination. Gentle and careful use of eyelid retractors or an eyelid speculum makes it possible to open the lids. Emergency treatment that can be given before an ophthalmologist is available consists of dilating the pupil with 1 drop of cyclopentolate 1% and 1 drop of phenylephrine 2.5%, applying a protective shield (see p. 2587), and combating possible infection with local and systemic antimicrobials as discussed for intraocular foreign bodies above. If the globe is lacerated, topical antibiotics should be instilled in the form of drops only, because ointment entering the globe is undesirable. Because fungal contamination of open wounds is dangerous, corticosteroids are contraindicated until after wounds are closed surgically. Very rarely, after laceration of the globe, the uninjured, contralateral eye becomes inflamed (sympathetic ophthalmia—see p. 915) and may lose vision to the point of blindness unless treated. The mechanism is an autoimmune reaction; corticosteroid drops can prevent the process.

Anterior chamber hemorrhage (hyphema): This injury requires immediate attention by an ophthalmologist. It may be followed by recurrent bleeding, glaucoma, and blood staining of the cornea, any of which may result in permanent vision loss. Symptoms are of associated injuries unless the hyphema is large enough to obstruct vision. Direct inspection typically reveals layering of blood or the presence of clot or both in the anterior chamber. Layering is seen as a meniscus-like blood level in the lower part of the anterior chamber. Microhyphema, a less severe form, may be detectable by direct inspection as haziness in the anterior chamber or by slit-lamp examination as suspended RBCs.

The patient is placed on bed rest with the head elevated 30 degrees and given an eye shield to protect the eye from further trauma (as described on p. 2587). Patients who are at high risk of recurrent bleeding (eg, those with large hyphemas, bleeding diatheses, anticoagulant use, sickle cell disease), who have intraocular pressure (IOP) that is difficult to control, or who are likely to be noncompliant may be hospitalized. Oral and topical NSAIDs are contraindicated because they may contribute to recurrent bleeding. IOP can rise acutely (within hours, usually in patients with sickle cell disease or trait) or months to years later. Thus, IOP is monitored daily for several days and then regularly over subsequent weeks and months and if symptoms develop (eg, eye ache, decreased vision, nausea—similar to acute angle-closure glaucoma). If pressure rises, timolol 0.5% bid, brimonidine 0.2% or 0.15% bid, or both are given. Response to treatment is determined by pressure, often checked q 1 or 2 h until controlled or until a significant rate of reduction is demonstrated; thereafter, it is usually checked once or twice daily. Mydriatic drops (eg, atropine 1% tid for 5 days) and topical corticosteroids (eg, prednisolone acetate 1% 4 to 8 times/day for 2 to 3 wk are often given. Administration of aminocaproic acid 50 to 100 mg/kg po q 4 h (not exceeding 30 g/day) for 5 days may reduce recurrent bleeding. The nonophthalmologist should not use miotic or mydriatic drugs in these cases. Rarely, recurrent bleeding with secondary glaucoma requires surgical evacuation of the blood.

Blowout fracture: Blowout fracture occurs when blunt trauma forces the orbital contents through the most fragile portion of the orbital wall, typically the floor. Medial and roof fractures also can occur. Symptoms include double vision, enophthalmos, inferiorly displaced globe, numbness of the cheek and upper lip (from infraorbital nerve injury), or subcutaneous emphysema. Nosebleed, lid edema, and ecchymosis may occur. Diagnosis is best made by CT scan. If diplopia or cosmetically unacceptable enophthalmos persists beyond 2 wk, surgical repair is indicated.

Posttraumatic Iridocyclitis

(Traumatic Anterior Uveitis; Traumatic Iritis)

Posttraumatic iridocyclitis is an inflammatory reaction of the uvea and iris, typically developing within 3 days of blunt eye trauma.

Symptoms of posttraumatic iridocyclitis include tearing, throbbing pain and redness of the eye, photophobia, and blurred vision. Diagnosis is by history, symptoms, and slit-lamp examination, which typically reveals flare (due to an increase in protein content of the aqueous humor from the inflammatory exudate) and WBCs in the anterior chamber. Treatment involves a cycloplegic (eg, 1 drop scopolamine 0.25% tid, cyclopentolate 1% tid, or homatropine 5% tid). Topical corticosteroids (eg, prednisolone acetate 1% 4 to 8 times/day) are often used to shorten symptom duration.

314 GENITOURINARY TRACT TRAUMA

The GU tract can be injured by blunt trauma (eg, motor vehicle collisions, falls) or penetrating trauma (eg, gunshot or stab wounds). Many injuries are caused during surgical procedures. Symptoms and signs are often subtle or nonspecific; therefore, diagnosis requires a high level of suspicion. Whenever urinalysis shows any hematuria in the setting of trauma, GU injury should be presumed until proven otherwise. Imaging studies, usually contrast-enhanced CT, are typically used to make a diagnosis. See Ch. 307 (p. 2548) for general evaluation of the trauma patient.

BLADDER TRAUMA

Bladder injuries can be caused by blunt or penetrating trauma. Both may cause rupture; blunt trauma may simply cause contusions (damage to the bladder wall without urinary leakage). Rupture can be intraperitoneal, extraperitoneal, or both. Intraperitoneal rupture usually involves the bladder dome; it often occurs when the bladder is distended at the time of trauma and is the most common bladder injury in children because the bladder lies in the abdomen. Extraperitoneal rupture is most common in adults and usually occurs with pelvic fractures or penetrating trauma. Complications of bladder trauma include infection, incontinence, and bladder instability. Associated intra-abdominal and pelvic injuries are common because of the magnitude of force required to injure the well-protected bladder.

Symptoms, Signs, and Diagnosis

Symptoms may include suprapubic pain and inability to void; signs may include suprapubic tenderness, distention, and in the case of intraperitoneal rupture, absent bowel sounds and peritoneal signs. Diagnosis is suspected by history, physical examination, and hematuria on urinalysis. Confirmation is by retrograde cystography using plain film x-rays or CT; plain film x-rays are accurate, but CT also helps delineate associated injuries (eg, pelvic fracture).

Treatment

All penetrating trauma and intraperitoneal ruptures from blunt trauma require surgical exploration and repair. Contusions require no surgical intervention, but catheterization is indicated if gross blood or bladder neck displacement from pelvic hematoma makes voiding difficult. Extraperitoneal ruptures can be treated by catheter drainage alone if urine is draining freely and the injury does not involve the bladder neck, in which case surgical exploration and repair are required.

Mortality rate is about 20%, usually due to associated, severe injuries.

GENITAL TRAUMA

Nearly all genital trauma occurs in men and includes injury to the testicle, scrotum, and penis. Genital mutilation of women by removing the clitoris, which is done in some cultures, is considered by many to be a form of genital trauma and is considered by some to be a form of child abuse (see p. 2512).

Most testicular injuries result from blunt trauma; penetrating testicular injuries are less common. Blunt trauma may cause hematoma, or if severe, testicular rupture.

Scrotal injury may be caused by infections, burns, and avulsions.

Penile injuries have diverse mechanisms. Zipper injuries may be most common. Penile fractures, which are ruptures of the corpus cavernosum, occur most often during sexual activity; urethral injury may also be present. Amputations (usually self-inflicted or from clothing trapped by heavy machinery) and strangulations (usually from constricting penile rings used to enhance erections) are additional mechanisms. Penetrating injuries, including animal bites and gunshot wounds, are less common and typically also involve the urethra.

Fournier's gangrene may be a complication of injury. Both aerobic and anaerobic bacteria are responsible. Contributing conditions include alcohol abuse, diabetes mellitus, prolonged bed rest in debilitated patients, immunocompromise, and chronic urethral catheterization. Complications of genital injuries include erectile dysfunction, infection, tissue loss, and urethral scarring.

Symptoms, Signs, and Diagnosis

Testicular and scrotal injury may cause no symptoms or signs or manifest with swelling and tenderness. Hematocele, which manifests as a painful palpable mass, may develop with rupture of the tunica albuginea; ecchymosis of the groin and perineum may develop if the tunica vaginalis ruptures. Penile fracture manifests with marked swelling and ecchymosis, and sometimes palpable and visible deformity. Necrotizing scrotal infections initially present with pain, swelling, and fever; they progress rapidly.

Diagnosis of external scrotal and penile injury is made clinically. Diagnosis of testicular injury is made by scrotal ultrasound. A urethral x-ray (retrograde urethrogram) should be done for any patient with penile trauma because of the high incidence of coexisting urethral injury.

The clinical course of necrotizing scrotal infections is rapidly progressive with skin necrosis and even septic shock. Diagnosis is made on physical examination. Early on, the scrotum appears erythematous, swollen, and tender, which can rapidly progress to blistering, discoloration, and crepitus. In the early stages, patients often have systemic symptoms of sepsis that appear disproportionate to the appearance of the scrotal skin.

Treatment

Patients with penetrating testicular injuries or testicular rupture should be surgically explored and repaired; those with findings suggesting rupture but with negative scrotal ultrasound also should be explored. Similarly, all penile ruptures and penetrating injuries should be surgically explored and the defects repaired. Penile amputations should be repaired by microsurgical reimplantation if the amputated segment is viable. For zipper injury, local anesthetic is injected and one attempt may be made to unzip the zipper after mineral oil lubrication. If this attempt is unsuccessful, a sturdy wire cutter is used to cut the median bar on the top of the zipper slider, which connects its front and back plates; then the slider falls off, and the two sides of the zipper come apart readily.

Management of necrotizing scrotal infections is more complicated. Patients with these infections should be started on broad-spectrum IV antibiotics; the affected areas should be generously debrided in the operating room. Urinary or fecal diversion is often needed. Scrotal reconstruction should be attempted only after the infection has been thoroughly controlled.

RENAL TRAUMA

Renal injuries most often involve parenchymal lacerations, but the collecting system and vasculature also may be disrupted. Most injuries result from blunt trauma. Five grades of injury are defined (see TABLE 314–1). Other visceral injuries (eg, hepatic, splenic, small bowel, colon, mesenteric, gastric) coexist in up to 40% of patients.

Symptoms, Signs, and Diagnosis

Diagnosis should be suspected in any patient with penetrating injury between mid chest and lower abdomen and in those with significant deceleration injury or a direct blow to the flank. Hematuria strongly suggests renal injury; other indicators include seat-belt marks, diffuse abdominal tenderness, flank contusions, and lower rib fractures.

Laboratory testing should include Hct and urinalysis. Because degree of hematuria does not predict injury severity, contrast-enhanced CT imaging is often used to determine grade of renal injury and identify accompanying intraabdominal trauma and complications, including retroperitoneal hemorrhage and urinary extravasation. For blunt trauma, patients with microscopic hematuria may have renal contusions or minor lacerations, but these almost never require imaging or surgical repair. CT should be done whenever the trauma involves a fall from a great height or a high-speed motor vehicle collision or if the patient has gross hematuria, microscopic hematuria with hypotension, or flank hematoma. For penetrating trauma, CT should be done for patients with any hematuria. Rarely, angiography is indicated to assess persistent or prolonged bleeding and may be combined with selective arterial embolization.

Treatment

Most blunt renal injuries, including nearly all minor and many high-grade injuries, can be safely treated without surgery. Patients require strict bed rest until gross hematuria has resolved. Surgical repair is required for those with persistent bleeding, expanding perinephric hematoma, and for some with urinary extravasation. Penetrating trauma usually requires surgical exploration, although waiting may be appropriate for patients in whom renal injury has been accurately staged by CT, BP is stable, and no associated intra-abdominal injuries need operation.

URETERAL TRAUMA

Noniatrogenic ureteral injury accounts for only about 1% of all GU trauma. It usually results from gunshot wounds and rarely from stab wounds; in children, avulsion injuries are more common. Complications include ureteral stricture, obstruction, or both; peritoneal or retroperitoneal urinary leakage; and fistula (eg, ureterovaginal, ureterocutaneous) formation.

TABLE 314–1. GRADES OF RENAL INJURY

GRADE	INJURY
1	Renal contusion; non-expanding subcapsular hematoma
2	Laceration < 1 cm in depth sparing the renal medulla and collecting system; non-expanding retroperitoneal hematoma
3	Laceration > 1 cm sparing the collecting system
4	Laceration > 1 cm involving the collecting system; renal vessel injury with hemorrhage
5	Shattered kidney or avulsed renal vessels

Diagnosis is suspected by history and requires a high index of suspicion, because symptoms are nonspecific and hematuria is absent in ≥ 30% of patients. Diagnosis is confirmed by imaging (eg, CT with radiocontrast, IV urogram), exploratory surgery, or both. Flank pain and fever are the main manifestations.

All injuries require intervention. A diverting percutaneous nephrostomy tube or cystoscopic placement of a ureteral stent is often sufficient for minor injuries (eg, contusions or partial transections). Complete transections or avulsion injuries typically require reconstructive techniques, including ureteral reimplantation, primary ureteral anastomosis, anterior bladder flap, ileal interposition, and, as last resort, autotransplantation.

URETHRAL TRAUMA

Urethral injury usually occurs in men. Most major urethral trauma is due to blunt trauma. Penetrating, isolated urethral trauma is less common; it may result from inserting objects into the urethra during sexual activity or because of psychiatric illness.

Urethral injuries are classified as contusions, partial disruptions, or complete disruptions, and they may be posterior or anterior. Posterior urethral injuries are usually caused by the shearing force of pelvic fractures.

Anterior urethral injuries are often consequences of a perineal straddle injury. Penetrating and iatrogenic trauma and injuries may be anterior or posterior.

Complications include stricture formation, infection, erectile dysfunction, and incontinence.

Blood at the urethral meatus is the most important sign of a urethral injury. Additional signs include perineal, scrotal, and penile ecchymosis, edema, or both, and a high-riding prostate on rectal examination. Diagnosis is confirmed by retrograde urethrography. Urethral catheterization should not be attempted until urethrography is done.

Treatment

Contusions can be safely treated with 10 days of indwelling transurethral catheterization. Partial disruptions are best treated with suprapubic catheter placement; however, in select cases of posterior partial disruptions, primary urethral realignment using catheterization may be attempted.

Complete disruptions are treated with drainage via suprapubic cystostomy. This option is simplest and can be used safely in all patients. Definitive surgery is deferred for about 3 mo until the urethral scar tissue has stabilized and the patient has recovered from any associated injuries.

315 BURNS

(See also p. 2586 for ocular burns and p. 2663 for caustic ingestions.)

Burns are injuries of skin or other tissue caused by thermal, radiation, chemical, or electrical contact. Burns are classified by depth (1st degree, partial thickness, and full thickness) and percentage of total body surface area (BSA) involved. Complications include hypovolemic shock, rhabdomyolysis, infection, scarring, and joint contractures. Patients with large burns (> 15% BSA) require fluid resuscitation. Treatments for burn wounds include topical antibacterials, regular cleaning, elevation, and sometimes skin grafting. Burns of joints require range-of-motion exercises and splinting.

Burns cause about 3000 deaths/yr in the US and about 1 million emergency department visits.

Etiology and Pathophysiology

Thermal burns may result from any external heat source (flame, liquids, solid objects, or gases). Fires may also result in toxic inhalation (see sidebar 315–1 and Carbon Monoxide Poisoning on p. 2662).

Radiation burns most commonly result from prolonged exposure to solar ultraviolet radiation (sunburn) but may result from prolonged or intense exposure to other sources of ultraviolet radiation (eg, tanning beds) or from exposure to sources of x-ray or other nonsolar radiation.

Chemical burns may result from strong acids, strong alkalis (eg, lye, cement), phenols, cresols, mustard gas, or phosphorus. Skin and deeper tissue necrosis due to these agents may progress over several hours.

Electrical burns (see also p. 2597) result from the electrical generation of heat; they may cause extensive deep tissue damage despite minimal apparent cutaneous injury.

Events associated with the burn (eg, jumping from a burning building, being struck by debris, motor vehicle collision) may cause other injuries.

Burns cause protein denaturation and thus coagulation necrosis. Around the coagulated burned tissue, platelets aggregate, vessels constrict, and marginally perfused tissue (known as the zone of stasis) can necrose. Around the zone of stasis, tissue is hyperemic and inflamed. Damage to the normal epidermal barrier allows bacterial invasion and external fluid leakage; damaged tissues often become edematous, further enhancing volume loss. Heat loss can be significant because thermoregulation of the damaged dermis is impaired and because fluid leakage increases evaporative heat loss.

Depth: Burns are classified by depth of skin affected. First-degree burns are limited to the epidermis. Partial-thickness (2nd-degree) burns involve part of the dermis and are subdivided into superficial and deep. Superficial partial-thickness burns involve the upper ½ of the dermis. These burns heal within 2 to 3 wk.

Sidebar 315–1. SMOKE INHALATION

Burns and smoke inhalation often occur together but may occur separately. When smoke is inhaled, toxic products of combustion and sometimes heat injure airway tissues. Heat usually burns only upper airways because incoming gas usually delivers the full heat load to the upper airways. A common exception is steam, which often burns lower airways. Many toxic chemicals produced in routine house fires (eg, hydrogen chloride, phosgene, sulfur dioxide, toxic aldehydes, ammonia) irritate and injure lower airways and sometimes upper airways. Some toxic products of combustion, usually carbon monoxide or cyanide (see p. 2662), impair cellular respiration systemically.

Upper airway injury usually produces symptoms within minutes but occasionally over several hours; upper airway edema may cause stridor. Lower airway injury usually causes symptoms (eg, shortness of breath, wheezing, sometimes coughing or chest pain) over 24 h.

Smoke inhalation is suspected in patients with respiratory symptoms, a history of prolonged confinement in a burning environment, or carbonaceous sputum. Perioral burns and singed nasal hairs may also be clues, unless they have resulted from flash burns (eg, from lighting a gas grill). Diagnosis of upper airway injury is by endoscopy (laryngoscopy or bronchoscopy) that is adequate to see the upper airways and trachea fully and that shows edema or soot in the airways; however, injury occasionally develops after an early normal study. Endoscopy is done as soon as possible, usually with a flexible fiberoptic scope. Diagnosis of lower airway injury is by chest x-ray and oximetry or ABGs; the diagnosis may not be evident for about 24 h.

All patients at risk of smoke inhalation injury are given 100% O_2 by face mask pending diagnosis. Patients with airway obstruction or respiratory failure require endotracheal intubation or another artificial airway and mechanical ventilation (see p. 546). Patients with edema or significant soot in the upper airways require intubation as soon as possible because intubation becomes more difficult as edema increases. Patients with lower airway injury may require supplemental O_2, bronchodilators, and other supportive measures.

Healing occurs from epidermal cells lining sweat gland ducts and hair; these cells grow to the surface, then migrate across the surface to meet cells from neighboring glands and follicles. Burns that heal within 2 to 3 wk rarely scar unless they become infected. Deep partial-thickness burns involve the bottom ½ of the dermis and take ≥ 3 wk to heal; usually, healing occurs only from hair follicles. Scarring is common. Full-thickness (3rd-degree) burns extend through the entire dermis and into the underlying fat. Healing occurs only from the periphery; these burns, unless small, require skin grafting.

Complications

Systemic: The greater the percentage of BSA involved, the greater the risk of developing systemic complications. Risk factors for severe systemic complications and mortality include burns of > 40% of BSA, age > 60 yr or < 2 yr, and presence of simultaneous major trauma or smoke inhalation.

The most common systemic complications are hypovolemia and infection. Hypovolemia, causing hypoperfusion of burned tissue and sometimes shock, can result from fluid losses due to burns that are deep or that involve large parts of the body surface. Hypoperfusion of burned tissue also may result from direct damage to blood vessels or from vasoconstriction secondary to hypovolemia. Infection, even in small burns, is a common cause of sepsis and mortality, as well as local complications. Impaired host defenses and devitalized tissue enhance bacterial invasion and growth. The most common pathogens are streptococci and staphylococci during the 1st few days and gram-negative bacteria after 5 to 7 days; however, flora are always mixed.

Metabolic abnormalities may include hypoalbuminemia that is partly due to hemodilution (secondary to replacement fluids) and partly due to protein loss into the extravascular space through damaged capillaries. Hypoalbuminemia and hemodilution contribute to hypocalcemia, but ionized Ca usually remains normal. Other dilutional electrolyte deficiencies can develop; they include hypomagnesemia, hypophosphatemia, and, particularly in patients taking K-wasting diuretics, hypokalemia. However, extensive tissue destruction may produce hyperkalemia. Metabolic acidosis may result from shock. Rhabdomyolysis or hemolysis can result from deep thermal or electrical burns of muscle or from muscle ischemia due to constricting eschars (see below). Rhabdomyolysis causing myoglobinuria or hemolysis causing hemoglobinuria can lead to acute tubular necrosis.

Hypothermia may result from large volumes of cool IV fluids and extensive exposure of body surfaces to a cool emergency department environment, particularly in patients with extensive burns. Ventricular arrhythmias may develop secondary to electrolyte abnormalities, shock, metabolic acidosis, sometimes hypothermia, and, in patients with smoke inhalation, hypoxia. Ileus is common after extensive burns.

Local: Full-thickness circumferential burns can produce constricting eschars. Constricting eschars around the limbs can cause local ischemia, and those around the thorax can compromise respiration.

Spontaneous healing of deep burns causes excessive granulation tissue, resulting in scarring and contractures; if the burn is located near joints or in the hands, feet, or perineum, function can be severely impaired. Infection can increase scarring. Keloids form in some patients with burns, especially in black patients.

Symptoms and Signs

First-degree burns are red, blanch markedly and widely with light pressure, and are painful and tender. Vesicles or bullae do not develop.

Superficial partial-thickness burns blanch with pressure and are painful and tender. Vesicles or bullae develop within 24 h. The bases of vesicles and bullae are pink and subsequently develop a fibrinous exudate.

Deep partial-thickness burns may be white, red, or mottled red and white. They do not blanch and are less painful and tender than more superficial burns. A pinprick is often interpreted as pressure rather than as a prick. Vesicles or bullae may develop; these burns are usually dry.

Full-thickness burns may be white and pliable, black and charred, brown and leathery, or bright red because of fixed Hb in the subdermal region. Pale full-thickness burns may simulate normal skin except the skin does not blanch to pressure. Full-thickness burns are usually anesthetic or hypoesthetic. Hairs can be pulled easily from their follicles. Vesicles and bullae usually do not develop. Sometimes features that differentiate full-thickness from deep partial-thickness burns take a few days to develop.

Diagnosis

Because findings evolve rapidly, burns are examined as soon as patients are stable. Location and depth of burned areas are recorded on a burn diagram. Burns with an appearance compatible with both deep partial-thickness and full-thickness are assumed to be full-thickness until differentiation is possible. The percentage of BSA involved is calculated; only partial- and full-thickness burns are included in this calculation. For adults, the percentage BSA for parts of the body is estimated by the rule of nines (see FIG. 315–1A); for smaller scattered burns, estimates can be based on the size of the patient's palmar hand surface, which is about 1% of BSA. Children have large heads and small thighs, so the percentage BSA is more accurately estimated using the Lund-Browder chart (see FIG. 315–1B).

If patients require hospitalization (see p. 2596), Hb and Hct, serum electrolytes, BUN, creatinine, albumin, protein, phosphate, and ionized Ca should be measured; ECG, urinalysis for myoglobin, and chest x-ray are also required. Myoglobinuria is suggested by urine that is grossly dark or that tests positive for blood on dipstick in the absence of microscopic RBCs. These tests are repeated as needed.

Infection is suggested by wound exudate, impaired wound healing, or systemic evidence of infection (eg, fever, leukocytosis). If the diagnosis is unclear, infection can be confirmed by biopsy; cultures from wound surface or exudate are unreliable.

Treatment

Initial treatment: Treatment begins in the prehospital setting. The 1st priorities are the same as for any injured patient: ABC (airway, breathing, and circulation). An airway is provided, ventilation is supported, and possible associated smoke inhalation is treated with 100% O_2 (see sidebar 315–1). Ongoing burning is extinguished, and smoldering and hot material is removed. All clothing is removed. Chemicals, except powders, are flushed with water; powders should be brushed off before

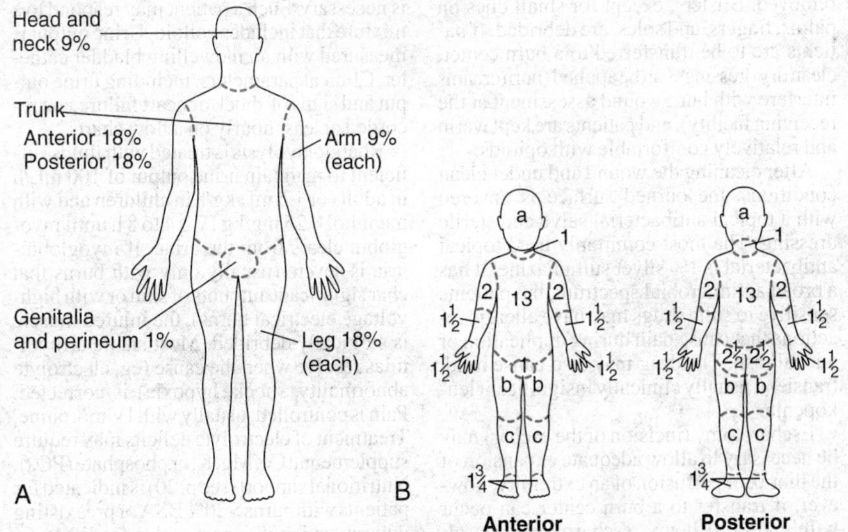

Relative percentage of body surface area (% BSA) affected by growth

Body Part	Age				
	0 yr	1 yr	5 yr	10 yr	15 yr
a = 1/2 of head	9 1/2	8 1/2	6 1/2	5 1/2	4 1/2
b = 1/2 of 1 thigh	2 3/4	3 1/4	4	4 1/4	4 1/2
c = 1/2 of 1 lower leg	2 1/2	2 1/2	2 3/4	3	3 1/4

Fig. 315–1. (A) Rule of nines (for adults) and (B) Lund-Browder chart (for children) for estimating extent of burns. (Redrawn from Artz CP, JA Moncrief: *The Treatment of Burns*, ed. 2. Philadelphia, WB Saunders Company, 1969; used with permission.)

wetting. Burns caused by acids, alkalis, or organic compounds (eg, phenols, cresols) are flushed with copious amounts of water continuously for at least 20 min after nothing of the original solution seems to remain.

IV fluids are given to patients in shock or with burns > 15% BSA. A 14- to 16-gauge venous cannula is placed in 1 or 2 peripheral veins through unburned skin if possible. Venous cutdown, which has a high risk of infection, is avoided.

Initial fluid resuscitation is guided by treatment of clinically evident shock (see p. 564). If shock is absent, fluid administration aims to replace the deficit and supply maintenance fluids. The Parkland formula is used to estimate the fluid volume needed to replace the deficit; it specifies 3 mL/kg/% BSA of crystalloid (lactated Ringer's solution) over the 1st 24 h (eg, in a person who weighs 70 kg and has a 40% BSA burn, 3 mL×70×40=8400 mL in the 1st 24 h). Half of this amount is given over the 1st 8 h after the estimated time of injury; the rest is given over the next 16 h. Some clinicians give colloid during the 2nd day to patients who have larger burns, are very young or old, or have heart disease.

Hypothermia is treated (see p. 2611), and pain is relieved. Opioids are always given IV. A tetanus toxoid booster (0.5 mL sc or IM) is given to patients previously fully vaccinated and who have not received a booster within the past 5 yr; patients whose booster was more remote or who had not received a full vaccine series are given tetanus immune globulin 250 units IM and concomitant active vaccination (see p. 1506).

Small burns are sometimes immersed early in cold water for relief, but there is no evidence that this measure limits depth of the burn. After analgesia, the wound is cleaned with soap and water, and all loose debris is removed. Blisters, except for small ones on palms, fingers, and soles, are debrided. If patients are to be transferred to a burn center, clean dry dressings can be applied (burn creams interfere with burn wound assessment at the receiving facility), and patients are kept warm and relatively comfortable with opioids.

After cleaning the wound and under clean conditions, the burned surface is covered with a topical antibacterial salve and sterile dressing. The most commonly used topical antibacterial is 1% silver sulfadiazine. It has a broad antimicrobial spectrum, but patients sensitive to sulfa drugs may have allergic reactions that cause pain during application or a local rash. The drug may also cause mild, transient, usually clinically insignificant leukopenia.

Escharotomy (incision of the eschar) may be necessary to allow adequate expansion of the thorax or perfusion of an extremity; however, if transfer to a burn center can occur within several hours, escharotomy can almost always be deferred until then.

Prophylactic antibiotics are not given.

After initial treatment and stabilization, the need for hospitalization is assessed. Inpatient treatment, optimally at a burn center, is needed for full-thickness burns > 1% BSA; partial-thickness burns > 5% BSA; any burns > 10% BSA; and partial-thickness or deeper burns of the hands, face, feet, or perineum. Hospitalization may be necessary if patients are < 2 yr or > 60 yr or if adherence to home care measures is likely to be poor or difficult (eg, if continuous elevation of the hands or feet is difficult at home). Many experts recommend that all burns, except for 1st-degree burns < 1% BSA, be treated by experienced physicians and that brief inpatient care be strongly considered for all burns > 2% BSA. Maintaining adequate analgesia and exercise can be difficult for many patients and caregivers.

Ongoing fluid needs and systemic complications: Fluids are given and systemic complications are treated with supportive measures for as long as necessary. Ongoing fluid needs are estimated more by clinical response than by formulas. Goals include avoiding shock, maintaining satisfactory urine output, and avoiding fluid overload and heart failure. Satisfactory urine output is ≥ 30 mL/h (0.5 mL/kg/h) in adults and 1 mL/kg/h in children. If a patient's urine output is inadequate despite administration of a large volume of crystalloid, consultation with a burn center is necessary. Such a patient may respond to a mixture that includes colloid. Urine output is measured with an indwelling bladder catheter. Clinical parameters, including urine output and signs of shock or heart failure, are recorded at least hourly on a flow chart.

Rhabdomyolysis is treated with fluids sufficient to maintain urine output of 100 mL/h in adults or 1.5 mL/kg/h in children and with mannitol 0.25 mg/kg IV q 4 to 8 h until myoglobin clears from the urine. If myoglobinuria is severe (usually only with burns that char significant amounts of skin or with high-voltage electrical burns), the injured muscle is surgically debrided. Most stable arrhythmias resolve when the cause (eg, electrolyte abnormality, shock, hypoxia) is corrected. Pain is controlled, usually with IV morphine. Treatment of electrolyte deficits may require supplemental Ca, Mg, K, or phosphate (PO_4). Nutritional support (see p. 20) is indicated for patients with burns > 20% BSA or preexisting undernutrition. Support with a feeding tube begins as soon as possible. Parenteral support is rarely necessary.

Initial empiric antibiotic treatment for apparent infection during the 1st 7 days should cover staphylococci and streptococci (eg, with nafcillin). Infection that develops after 7 days is treated with a more broad-spectrum antibiotic that covers gram-positive and gram-negative bacteria. Antibiotic selection is subsequently adjusted based on culture and sensitivity results.

Dressing changes: Dressings are usually changed daily. The burn is cleaned completely, and all residual topical antibacterial is removed with water. Then, the wound is debrided if necessary, and a new layer of topical antibacterial is applied; a dressing is applied lightly to keep the salve from running. Until swelling subsides, burned extremities, especially the legs and hands, are elevated above heart level whenever possible.

Surgery: Surgery is indicated for burns that are not expected to heal within 3 wk, which includes most deep partial-thickness and all full-thickness burns. Eschars are removed as soon as possible, ideally within 7 days, to help prevent sepsis and facilitate early wound grafting, which shortens hospitalization and improves the functional result. If burns are extensive and life threatening, the largest eschars are removed first to accomplish early closure of as much burn area as possible. Such burns should be treated only in burn centers. The order in which eschars are removed depends on the preferences of an experienced burn surgeon.

After excision, grafting proceeds, ideally using partial-thickness autografts (the patient's skin), which are permanent. Autografts can be transplanted as sheets (solid pieces of skin) or meshed grafts (sheets of donor skin that are stretched to cover a larger area by making multiple, regularly spaced, small incisions). Meshed grafts are used in areas where appearance is not a concern when burns are > 20% BSA and donor skin is scarce. Meshed grafts heal with an uneven gridlike appearance, sometimes with excessive hypertrophic scarring. When burns are > 40% BSA and the supply of autograft material appears insufficient, an artificial dermal regeneration template can be used. Although less desirable, allografts (viable skin usually from cadaver donors) can be used; they are rejected, sometimes within 10 to 14 days, and ultimately must be replaced with autografts.

Physical therapy: Physical therapy is begun at admission to help minimize scarring and contractures, particularly for body surfaces with high skin tension and frequent movement (eg, face, chest, hands, joints, upper legs). Active and passive range-of-motion exercises become easier as the initial edema subsides; they are done once or twice/day until skin is grafted. After grafting, exercises are usually suspended for 5 days, then resumed. Joints affected by partial- or full-thickness burns are splinted in functional positions as soon as possible and kept splinted continuously (except during exercise) until the graft has been placed and healing has occurred.

Outpatient treatment: Outpatient treatment includes keeping burns clean and, to the extent possible, keeping the affected body part elevated. Salve dressings are used and are changed as for inpatients. Outpatient follow-up visits are scheduled as needed depending on burn severity (eg, for very minor burns, initial visit within 24 h, then subsequent visits every 5 to 7 days). Visits include debridement if indicated, reassessment of burn depth, and evaluation of the need for physical therapy and grafting. Infection is suggested by fever, purulent discharge, ascending lymphangitis, pain that increases after the 1st 24 h, and increasing blanching or tender erythema. Outpatient treatment is acceptable for minor cellulitis in healthy patients aged 2 to 60 yr; hospitalization is indicated for other infections.

316 ELECTRICAL AND LIGHTNING INJURIES

Electricity may be from manmade sources (eg, from high- or low-voltage power lines) or atmospheric (lightning).

ELECTRICAL INJURIES

Electrical injury is damage caused by manmade electrical current passing through the body. Symptoms may include skin burns, damage to internal organs and other soft tissues, cardiac arrhythmias, and respiratory arrest. Diagnosis is by clinical criteria and selective laboratory testing. Treatment is supportive, with aggressive care for severe injuries.

Although accidental electrical injuries encountered in the home (eg, touching an electrical outlet or getting shocked by a small appliance) rarely result in significant injury or sequelae, accidental exposure to high voltage causes about 400 deaths annually in the US.

Pathophysiology

Traditional teaching is that the severity of electrical injury depends on Kouwenhoven's 6 factors: type of current (direct [DC] or alternating [AC]), voltage and amperage (both are measures of current strength), duration of exposure (longer exposure increases injury severity), body resistance, and pathway of current (which determines the specific tissue damaged). However, electrical field strength, a newer concept, seems to predict injury severity more accurately.

Kouwenhoven's factors: AC changes direction frequently; it is the current usually supplied by household electrical outlets in the US and Europe. DC flows in the same direction constantly; it is the current supplied by batteries. Defibrillators and cardioverters usually deliver DC current. How AC affects the body depends largely on frequency. Low-frequency (50- to 60-Hz) AC is used in US (60 Hz) and European (50 Hz) households; it can be more dangerous than high-frequency AC and is 3 to 5 times more dangerous than DC of the same voltage and amperage. Low-frequency AC produces extended muscle contraction (tetany), which may freeze the hand to the current's source, prolonging exposure. DC is most likely to cause a single convulsive contraction, which often forces the victim away from the current's source.

Usually, for both AC and DC, the higher the voltage (V) and amperage, the greater the ensuing electrical injury (for the same duration of exposure). Household current in the US is 110 V (standard electrical outlet) to 220 V (large appliance, such as a dryer). High-voltage (> 500 V) currents tend to cause deep burns, and low-voltage (110 to 220 V) currents tend to cause muscle tetany and freezing to the current's source. The threshold for perceiving DC current entering the hand is about 5 to 10 milliamperes (mA); for AC at 60 Hz, the threshold is about 1 to 10 mA. The maximum amperage that can cause flexors of the arm to contract but that allows release of the hand from the current's source is called the let-go current. Let-go current varies with weight and muscle mass. For an average 70-kg man, let-go current is about 75 mA for DC and about 15 mA for AC.

Low-voltage 60-Hz AC traveling through the chest for a fraction of a second can cause ventricular fibrillation at amperage as low as 60 to 100 mA; for DC, about 300 to 500 mA are required. If current has a direct pathway to the heart (eg, via a cardiac catheter or pacemaker electrodes), < 1 mA (AC or DC) can cause ventricular fibrillation.

Amount of dissipated heat energy equals amperage^2 × resistance × time; thus, for any given current and duration, tissue with the highest resistance tends to suffer the most damage. Body resistance (measured in ohms/cm^2) is provided primarily by the skin. Skin thickness and dryness increase resistance; dry, well-keratinized, intact skin averages 20,000 to 30,000 ohms/cm^2. For a thickly calloused palm or sole, resistance may be 2 to 3 million ohms/cm^2; for moist, thin skin, resistance is about 500 ohms/cm^2. Resistance for punctured skin (eg, cut, abrasion, needle puncture) or moist mucous membranes (eg, mouth, rectum, vagina) may be as low as 200 to 300 ohms/cm^2. If skin resistance is high, much electrical energy may be dissipated at the skin, resulting in large skin burns at entry and exit points but less internal damage. If skin resistance is low, skin burns are less extensive or absent, but more electrical energy may be dissipated in internal organs. Thus, the absence of external burns does not predict the absence of electrical injury, and the severity of external burns does not predict the severity of electrical injury.

Damage to internal tissues depends also on their resistance and additionally on current density (current per unit area; energy is concentrated when the same current flows through a smaller area). For example, as electrical energy flows in an arm (primarily through lower-resistance tissues, eg, muscle, vessels, nerves), current density increases at joints because a significant proportion of the joint's cross-sectional area consists of higher-resistance tissues (eg, bone, tendon), which decreases the area of lower-resistance tissue; thus, damage to the lower-resistance tissues tends to be most severe at joints.

The current's pathway through the body determines which structures are injured. Because AC current continually reverses direction, the commonly used terms "entry" and "exit" are inappropriate; "source" and "ground" are most precise. The hand is the most common source point, followed by the head. The foot is the most common ground point. Current traveling between arm and arm or between arm and foot is likely to traverse the heart, possibly causing arrhythmia. This current tends to be more dangerous than current traveling from one foot to the other. Current to the head may damage the CNS.

Electrical field strength: Electrical field strength determines the degree of tissue injury. For instance, 20,000 volts (20 kV) applied to a 6-ft (about 2 m) man from his head to ground result in a field strength of about 10 kV/m. Similarly, 110 volts, if applied only to 1 cm (eg, across a toddler's lip), result in a similar field strength of 11 kV/m; this is why such a "low-voltage" injury can cause the same severity of tissue injury as some high-voltage injuries applied to a larger area. Conversely, when considering voltage rather than electrical field strength, minor or trivial electrical injuries may be classified as high voltage. For example, the shock received from shuffling across a carpet in the winter involves thousands of volts.

Pathology: Application of low electrical field strength produces an immediate, unpleasant feeling (being "shocked") but seldom results in serious or permanent injury. Application of high electrical field strength may cause thermal or electrochemical damage to internal tissues. Damage may include hemolysis, protein coagulation, coagulation necrosis of muscle and other tissues, vascular thrombosis, dehydration, and muscle and tendon avulsion. High electrical field strength injuries may result in massive edema, which, as veins coagulate and muscles swell, results in compartment syndromes. Massive edema may also cause hypovolemia and hypotension. Muscle destruction may result in rhabdomyolysis and myoglobinuria. Myoglobinuria, hypovolemia, and hypotension increase risk of acute renal failure. Electrolyte disturbances can also occur. The consequences of organ dysfunction do not always correlate with the amount of tissue destroyed (eg, ventricular fibrillation may occur with relatively little tissue destruction).

Symptoms and Signs

Burns may be sharply demarcated on the skin even when current penetrates irregularly into deeper tissues. Severe involuntary muscular contractions, seizures, ventricular fibrillation, or respiratory arrest due to CNS damage or muscle paralysis may occur. Brain or nerve damage may result in various neurologic deficits. Cardiac arrest may occur without burns in bathtub accidents (when a wet [grounded] person contacts a 110-V circuit—eg, from a hairdryer or radio).

Toddlers who bite or suck on extension cords can burn their mouth and lips. Such burns may cause cosmetic deformities and impair growth of the teeth, mandible, and maxilla. Labial artery hemorrhage, which results when the eschar separates 5 to 10 days after injury, occurs in up to 10% of these toddlers.

An electrical shock can cause powerful muscle contractions or falls (eg, from a ladder or roof), resulting in dislocations (electrical shock is one of the few causes of posterior shoulder dislocation), vertebral or other fractures, injuries to internal organs, and loss of consciousness.

Diagnosis and Treatment

The first priority is to break contact between victim and current source. Shutting off the current is best (eg, by throwing a circuit breaker or switch, by disconnecting the device from its electrical outlet). If the current cannot be shut off rapidly, the victim is removed from contact with the current. If the current is low voltage, rescuers should first well-insulate themselves, then knock the victim free or use an insulating material (eg, cloth, dry wood, rubber, leather belt) to pull the victim free. CAUTION: *If power lines could be high voltage, no attempts to disengage the victim should be made until the power is shut off.* High- and low-voltage power lines are not always easily differentiated, particularly outdoors.

The victim, once free, is assessed for cardiac and respiratory arrest (see p. 524). Next, shock, which may result from trauma or massive burns, is treated (see p. 562). After initial resuscitation, patients are examined from head to toe.

Asymptomatic patients who are not pregnant, have no known heart disorders, and who have had only brief exposure to household current usually have no significant internal or external injuries. They can be discharged.

For other patients, ECG, CBC, measurement of cardiac enzymes, and urinalysis (especially to check for myoglobin) should be considered. Cardiac monitoring for 6 to 12 h is indicated for patients with arrhythmias, chest pain, any suggestion of cardiac damage, and possibly for patients who are pregnant or have known heart disorders. Patients with impaired consciousness may require CT or MRI.

The pain of an electrical burn is treated by the judicious titration of IV opioids. For myoglobinuria, alkalinizing the urine and maintaining adequate urine output (about 100 mL/h in adults and 1.5 mL/kg/h in children) decreases the risk of renal failure. Standard burn fluid resuscitation formulas, which are based on the extent of skin burns, underestimate the fluid requirement in electrical burns; thus, such formulas are not used. Surgical debridement of large amounts of muscle tissue may help to decrease myoglobinuric renal failure.

Appropriate tetanus prophylaxis and topical burn wound care are required (see p. 2594). All patients with significant electrical burns should be referred to a specialized burn unit. Children with lip burns should be referred to a pedodontist or oral surgeon familiar with such injuries.

Prevention

Electrical devices that touch or may be touched by the body should be properly insulted, grounded, and incorporated into circuits containing protective circuit-breaking equipment. Ground-fault circuit breakers, which trip when as little as 5 mA of current leaks to ground, are effective and readily available.

LIGHTNING INJURIES

Lightning injuries include cardiac arrest, loss of consciousness, and temporary or permanent neurologic deficits; serious burns and internal tissue injury are rare. Diagnosis is clinical; evaluation requires ECG and cardiac monitoring. Treatment is supportive.

Lightning strikes cause about 50 to 75 deaths and several times more injuries annually in the US. Lightning tends to strike tall objects. It can strike a victim directly, or the current can be transferred to the victim through the ground or a nearby object. Lightning can also travel from outdoor power or electrical lines to indoor electrical equipment or telephone lines. The force may throw the victim several yards.

Although lightning current contains a large amount of energy, it flows for an extremely brief period (1/10,000 to 1/1000 sec). Thus, it rarely, if ever, causes serious cutaneous wounds and seldom causes rhabdomyolysis or serious internal tissue damage, unlike high-voltage and high-current electrical injury from manmade sources. Occasionally, patients have intracranial hemorrhage.

Symptoms and Signs

The electrical charge can affect the heart, causing asystole or other arrhythmias, or the brain, causing loss of consciousness, acute confusion, or amnesia.

Keraunoparalysis is paralysis and mottling, coldness, and pulselessness of the lower and sometimes upper extremities with motor and sensory deficits; the cause is sympathetic nervous system instability. Keraunoparalysis is common and usually resolves within several hours, although some degree of permanent paresis occasionally results. Other manifestations of lightning injury may include minor skin burns in a punctate or feathered, branched pattern, tympanic membrane perforation, and cataracts. Neurologic problems may include confusion, cognitive deficits, and peripheral neuropathy. Neuropsychologic problems (eg, sleep disturbances, anxiety) may occur. Cardiopulmonary arrest at the time of the strike is the most common cause of death. Cognitive deficits, pain syndromes, and sympathetic nervous system damage are the most common long-term sequelae.

Diagnosis and Treatment

Lightning injuries are often witnessed but also should be suspected when people found outside during or after storms have amnesia or are unconscious. Cardiopulmonary resuscitation is initiated for cardiac or respiratory arrest or both. All patients are hospitalized; ECG and cardiac monitoring are done. QT prolongation may be present, and occasionally arrhythmias appear after > 24 h. Cardiac enzymes are measured for patients with chest pain, abnormal ECGs, or altered mental status. Patients with initially abnormal or later deteriorating mental status or focal brain deficits require a brain CT or MRI.

Supportive care is provided. Fluids are usually restricted to minimize potential brain edema.

Prevention

Preventing lightning strikes involves following lightning safety guidelines, knowing the weather forecast, and having an escape plan involving evacuation to a safer area and enough time to reach it. If thunder is heard or the interval between lightning and thunder is < 30 sec, people should seek shelter and remain there until ≥ 30 min after the last lightning or thunder. Large, habitable buildings or enclosed vehicles are safest. When indoors during an electrical storm, people should avoid plumbing and electrical appliances, stay away from windows and doors, and not use a hard-wired telephone or computer. If unable to get indoors during an electrical storm, people should avoid high ground, tall objects, open spaces, and water.

317 RADIATION INJURY

Ionizing radiation injures tissues variably depending on the type of radiation and amount and extent of exposure. Symptoms may be local (eg, burns) or systemic (eg, acute radiation sickness). Diagnosis is by history of exposure and sometimes use of Geiger or alpha counters. Treatment is by reverse isolation and (when indicated) decontamination but is otherwise largely supportive. Uptake inhibitors or chelating agents may be useful for treatment of internal contamination with specific radionuclides. Prognosis is estimated by measuring the lymphocyte count during the initial 24 to 72 h.

Radiation refers to high-energy electromagnetic waves (x-rays, gamma rays) or particles (alpha particles, beta particles, neutrons) emitted by radioactive elements or man-made sources (eg, x-ray and radiation therapy equipment).

Alpha particles are helium nuclei emitted by various radionuclides (eg, plutonium, radium, uranium) that cannot penetrate skin beyond a shallow depth (< 0.1 mm). Beta particles are high-energy electrons that are emitted from the nuclei of unstable atoms (eg, cesium-137, iodine-131). These particles can penetrate more deeply into skin (1 to 2 cm) and cause both epithelial and subepithelial damage. Neutrons are electrically neutral particles ejected from the nucleus of some radioactive atoms and produced in nuclear reactions (eg, reactors, linear accelerators); they can penetrate deeply into tissues (>2 cm), where they collide with stable atoms, resulting in emission of alpha and beta particles and gamma radiation. Gamma radiation and x-rays are high-energy electromagnetic radiation (ie, photons) that can travel many centimeters into human tissue.

Because of these characteristics, alpha and beta particles cause the most damage when radioactive elements that emit them are within (internal contamination) or directly on the body; only tissue in close proximity to the element is affected. Gamma rays and x-rays can cause damage at a great distance from their source and are typically responsible for acute radiation syndromes (see p. 2602).

Measurement: Units of measurement include the roentgen, gray, and sievert. The roentgen (R) represents the intensity of x- or gamma radiation in air. The gray (Gy) is the amount of that energy absorbed by tissue. Because biologic damage per Gy varies with radiation type (it is higher for neutrons and alpha particles), the dose in Gy is corrected by a quality factor; the resulting unit is the sievert (Sv). The Gy and Sv have replaced the rad and rem (Gy = 100 rad; Sv = 100 rem) in current nomenclature and are essentially equal when describing gamma or beta radiation.

Exposure: The 2 main types of radiation exposure are contamination and irradiation. Many radiation incidents involve both.

Contamination is contact with and retention of radioactive material, usually as a dust or liquid. External contamination is on skin or clothing, from which it can fall or be rubbed off, contaminating other people and objects. Radioactive material also can be absorbed through the lungs, GI tract, or breaks in the skin (internal contamination). Absorbed material is transported to various sites in the body (eg, bone marrow), where it continues to release radiation until it is removed or decays. Internal contamination is more difficult to remove.

Irradiation is exposure to penetrating radiation but not radioactive material (ie, no contamination is involved). Typically, gamma rays and x-rays are involved. Irradiation can involve the whole body, which can result in systemic symptoms and radiation syndromes (see p. 2602), or a small part of the body (eg, from therapeutic radiation), which can result in focal symptoms.

Sources: People are constantly exposed to low levels of natural radiation (background radiation). Background radiation includes cosmic radiation, much of which is blocked by the atmosphere; thus, exposure is greater for people living at high altitudes and during airplane flights. Radioactive elements, particularly radon gas, are also present in many rocks and minerals. These elements end up in various substances, including food and construction materials. Radon exposure typically accounts for about ⅔ of the total dose of naturally occurring radiation.

People are also exposed to radiation from man-made sources, including from nuclear weapons (eg, during testing) and various medical tests and treatments. The average person receives a total of about 3 to 4 mSv/yr

TABLE 317–1. AVERAGE ANNUAL RADIATION EXPOSURE IN THE US

SOURCE	DOSE (millisieverts)
Naturally occurring sources	
Radon gas	2.00
Other terrestrial sources	0.28
Radiation from outer space	0.27
Natural internal radio-active elements	0.39
Subtotal	**2.94**
Man-made sources	
Diagnostic x-rays (for average person)	0.39
Nuclear medicine	0.14
Consumer products	0.10
Fallout from weapons testing	< 0.01
Nuclear industry	< 0.01
Subtotal	**0.63**
Total Annual Exposure	**3.6**
Other sources of exposure	
Airline travel	0.005/h of flight
Dental x-rays	0.09
Chest x-ray	0.10
Barium enema	8.75

from natural and man-made sources (see TABLE 317–1).

Radiation has escaped from nuclear power plants, including the Three Mile Island plant in Pennsylvania in 1979 and at Chernobyl in Ukraine in 1986. Exposure from Three Mile Island was minimal; people living within 1.6 km of the plant received only about 0.08 mSv. However, people living near the Chernobyl plant were exposed to about 430 mSv of radiation. More than 30 people died, many more were injured, and radiation from that accident reached other parts of Europe, Asia, and the US. In total, excluding Chernobyl, radiation exposure from reactors in the first 40 yr of nuclear energy use has resulted in 35 serious exposures with 10 deaths, none of which were associated with commercial power plants. Other significant events include the detonation of the atomic bombs over Japan in August 1945, which caused > 100,000 deaths from the immediate blast and hundreds of thousands more deaths from radiation illness and other associated injuries.

Intentional radiation exposure through terrorist activities is a concern. Possible scenarios range from limited dispersal of radioactive substances without explosives to dispersal using conventional explosives ("dirty bombs") to attacks on nuclear reactors and detonation of nuclear weapons.

Pathophysiology

Ionizing radiation damages mRNA, DNA, and proteins directly and by generation of highly reactive free radicals. Large doses of ionizing radiation cause cell death, whereas lower doses interfere with cell proliferation. Damage to other cellular components can result in progressive hypoplasia, atrophy, and eventually fibrosis. Genetic damage may result in malignant transformation or a transmissible genetic defect.

Tissues that normally undergo continual and rapid renewal are particularly vulnerable to radiation. Most sensitive are lymphoid cells, followed by (in descending order) gonads, proliferating bone marrow cells, intestinal epithelial cells, epidermis, hepatic cells, epithelium of lung alveoli and biliary passages, kidney epithelial cells, endothelial cells (pleura and peritoneum), nerve cells, bone cells, and muscle and connective tissue cells.

The precise dose at which toxic effects occur depends on the time course of exposure, ie, a single rapid dose of several Gy is more damaging than the same dose given over weeks or months. Dose response also depends on the amount of body area exposed. Significant illness is certain, and fatalities occur after whole-body irradiation with > 4.5 Gy; however, 10s of Gy can be tolerated well when delivered over a long period to a small area of tissue (eg, for cancer therapy).

Children are more susceptible to radiation injury because they have a higher rate of cellular proliferation and a higher number of future cell divisions.

Symptoms and Signs

Manifestations depend on whether radiation exposure involves the whole body (acute radiation syndrome) or a focal area.

Acute radiation syndromes: Several distinct syndromes occur after whole-body radiation. These syndromes have 3 different phases: a prodromal phase (0 to 2 days after exposure) with lethargy, nausea, and vomiting; a latent asymptomatic phase (1 to 20 days after exposure); and a phase of overt systemic illness (2 to 60 days after exposure) classified by the main organ system affected. The higher the radiation dose, the more severe and rapid is the progression. The symptoms and time course are fairly consistent for a given dose of radiation; thus, they can be used to estimate the radiation exposure.

The cerebral syndrome, produced by extremely high whole-body doses of radiation (> 10 Gy), is always fatal. The prodrome develops within minutes to 1 h of exposure. There is little or no latent phase, and patients develop tremors, seizures, ataxia, cerebral edema, and death within hours to 1 or 2 days.

The GI syndrome is produced by whole-body doses of ≥ 4 Gy and is dominated by effects on the GI tract. Prodromal symptoms, often marked, develop within 2 to 12 h and resolve within 2 days. During the latent period of 4 to 5 days, GI mucosal cells die; cell death is followed by intractable nausea, vomiting, and diarrhea, which lead to severe dehydration and electrolyte imbalances, diminished plasma volume, and vascular collapse. Bowel necrosis may also occur, predisposing to bacteremia and sepsis. Death is common. Survivors also have the hematopoietic syndrome.

The hematopoietic syndrome is produced by whole-body doses of > 2 Gy. A mild prodrome may begin after 6 to 12 h, lasting 24 to 36 h. Bone marrow cells are affected immediately, resulting initially in lymphopenia (maximal within 24 to 36 h). However, the patient remains asymptomatic during a latent period of > 1 wk as marrow production falls. Various infections result from neutropenia (most prominent at 2 to 4 wk) and decreased antibody production, and petechiae and mucosal bleeding result from thrombocytopenia, which develops within 3 to 4 wk and may persist for months. Anemia develops slowly, because preexisting RBCs have a longer lifespan than WBCs and platelets. Survivors have an increased incidence of leukemias.

Focal injury: Radiation to nearly any organ can produce both acute and chronic adverse effects. In most patients, these adverse effects result from therapeutic radiation (see TABLE 317–2 and also Radiation Therapy on p. 1158).

Diagnosis

After acute radiation exposure, laboratory evaluation includes blood chemistries, urinalysis, and CBC with differential. Type and compatibility testing and blood for HLA typing should be obtained in the event that transfusion or hematopoietic stem cell transplantation is

TABLE 317–2. FOCAL RADIATION INJURY*

TISSUE EXPOSED	ADVERSE EFFECTS
Brain	See p. 1920
Cardiovascular	Chest pain, radiation pericarditis, radiation myocarditis
Dermatologic	Local erythema with intense burning or tingling, xerosis, keratosis, telangiectasis, vesiculation, hair loss (within 5 to 21 days of exposure) Dose > 5 Gy: Wet gangrene, ulceration Long-term effects: Progressive fibrosis, squamous cell carcinoma
Gonads	Dose ≤ 0.01 to 0.015 Gy: Depressed spermatogenesis, amenorrhea, decreased libido Dose 5–6 Gy: Sterility
Head and neck	Mucositis, odynophagia, thyroid carcinoma
Musculoskeletal	Myopathy, neoplastic changes, osteosarcoma
Ophthalmic	Dose 0.2 Gy: Cataract
Pulmonary	Radiation pneumonitis Dose > 30 Gy: Sometimes-fatal pulmonary fibrosis
Renal	Decreased GFR, decreased renal tubular function High doses (6 mo to 1 yr latent period): Proteinuria, renal insufficiency, anemia, hypertension Cumulative dose > 20 Gy in < 5 wk: Radiation fibrosis, oliguric renal failure
Spinal cord	Dose > 50 Gy: Myelopathy, neurologic dysfunction
Fetus	Growth restriction, congenital malformations, in-born errors of metabolism, cancer, fetal demise

*Typically from therapeutic radiation.

TABLE 317–3. RELATIONSHIP BETWEEN LYMPHOCYTE COUNT AT 48 H, RADIATION DOSE,* AND PROGNOSIS

LOWEST LYMPHOCYTE COUNT (CELLS/μL)	RADIATION DOSE (Gy)	PROGNOSIS
1500 (normal)	0.4	Excellent
1000–1499	0.5–1.9	Good
500–999	2.0–3.9	Fair
100–499	4.0–7.9	Poor
< 100	8.0	Almost always fatal

*Whole-body irradiation (approximate dose).

Adapted from Mettler FA Jr, Voelz GL: Major radiation exposure—what to expect and how to respond. *New England Journal of Medicine* 346:1554–1561, 2002.

necessary. The lymphocyte count should be obtained 24, 48, and 72 h after exposure to estimate the initial radiation dose and prognosis (see TABLE 317–3). CBC is repeated weekly to monitor marrow activity and as needed based on the clinical course.

Contamination: When radionuclides are involved, the entire body is surveyed with a Geiger counter to identify external contamination. Additionally, to detect possible internal contamination, the nares, ears, mouth, and wounds are wiped with moistened swabs that are then tested with the counter. Urine, feces, and emesis should also be tested for radioactivity.

Prognosis

Without medical care, the LD_{50} (dose fatal to 50% of patients within 60 days) for whole-body radiation is about 4 Gy; ≥ 6 Gy exposure is nearly always fatal. With < 6 Gy, survival is possible and is inversely related to total dose. Time to death is also inversely proportional to dose (and hence symptoms). Death results within hours to a few days in the cerebral syndrome and usually within 3 to 10 days in the GI syndrome. In the hematopoietic syndrome, death may occur within 2 to 4 wk because of a supervening infection or within 3 to 6 wk because of massive hemorrhage. Patients exposed to whole-body doses < 2 Gy should fully recover within 1 mo, although long-term sequelae (eg, cancer) may occur.

With medical care, the LD_{50} is about 6 Gy and occasional patients have survived up to 10 Gy.

Treatment

Radiation exposure may be accompanied by physical injuries (eg, from blast or fall); *associated trauma is more immediately life threatening than radiation exposure and must be treated expeditiously* (see p. 2549). Trauma resuscitation of the seriously injured must not be delayed awaiting special radiation management equipment and personnel. Standard universal precautions as routinely used in trauma care adequately protect the resuscitation team.

Hospitalization: Accrediting agencies mandate that all hospitals have protocols and that personnel have training to deal with radioactive contamination. Identification of radioactive contamination on a patient should prompt his isolation in a designated area, decontamination, and notification of the hospital radiation safety officer, public health officials, hazardous material teams, and law enforcement agencies as appropriate to investigate the source of radioactivity.

Treatment area surfaces may be covered with plastic sheeting to aid in facility decontamination; this preparation should never take precedence over provision of medical stabilization. Waste receptacles (labeled "Caution, Radioactive Material"), sample containers, and Geiger counters should be readily available. All equipment that has come into contact with the room or with the patient (including ambulance equipment) should remain isolated until lack of contamination has been verified.

Personnel should wear caps, masks, gowns, gloves, and shoe covers, and all openings in protective gear should be sealed with tape. Used gear should be placed in specially marked bags or containers. Dosimeter badges should be worn to monitor radiation exposure. Personnel may be rotated to minimize exposure, and pregnant personnel should be excluded from the treatment area.

Decontamination: After isolation in the designated area, clothes are removed carefully to minimize the spread of contamination and placed in appropriately marked containers. Clothing removal eliminates about 90% of external contamination. Contaminated skin surface is washed with lukewarm water and mild detergent until radioactivity counts are equal to about 2 times background or until successive washings do not significantly reduce contamination levels. All wounds are covered during washing to prevent the introduction of radioactive material. Scrubbing may be firm but should not abrade the skin. Special attention is usually required for fingernails and skinfolds. Special chelating solutions containing ethylenediaminetetraacetic acid are not necessary.

Wounds are checked with Geiger counters and irrigated until counts normalize; debridement is sometimes necessary to remove embedded material. Foreign bodies should be disposed of in lead containers.

Ingested radioactive material should be removed promptly by induced vomiting or lavage if exposure is recent. Frequent mouth rinsing with saline or dilute hydrogen peroxide is indicated for oral contamination. Eye exposure should be decontaminated by directing a stream of water or saline laterally to avoid contaminating the nasolacrimal duct.

Other, more specific measures to reduce internal contamination depend on the specific radionuclide involved; consultation with a specialist is recommended. If there is exposure to radioiodine (which should be presumed after a reactor incident or nuclear detonation), the patient should be given K iodide (KI) as soon as possible; its effectiveness diminishes significantly within several hours after exposure. KI can be given either in tablet form or as a supersaturated solution (dosage: adult, 130 mg; age 3 to 18 yr, 65 mg; age 1 to 36 mo, 32 mg; age < 1 mo, 16 mg). Various chelating agents are available for treating internal contamination with other radioactive substances: supersaturated K (radioactive iodine), Ca or zinc diethylenetriamine penta-acetate (plutonium-239 or yttrium-90), Prussian blue (cesium-137, rubidium-82, thallium-201), or oral Ca or aluminum phosphate solutions (radioactive strontium).

Decontamination is not necessary for patients who have been irradiated by an external source and are uncontaminated.

Specific management: Symptomatic treatment is given as needed and includes managing shock and anoxia, relieving pain and anxiety, and giving sedatives (lorazepam 1 to 2 mg IV prn) to control seizures, antiemetics (metoclopramide 10 to 20 mg IV q 4 to 6 h; prochlorperazine 5 to 10 mg IV q 4 to 6 h; ondansetron 4 to 8 mg IV q 8 to 12 h) to control vomiting, and antidiarrheal agents (kaolin/pectin 30 to 60 mL po with each loose stool; loperamide 4 mg po initially, then 2 mg po with each loose stool) for diarrhea.

There is no specific treatment for the cerebral syndrome. It is universally fatal; care should address patient comfort.

The GI syndrome is treated with aggressive fluid resuscitation and electrolyte replacement. Parenteral nutrition should be initiated to promote bowel rest. If the patient is febrile, broad-spectrum antibiotics (eg, imipenem 500 mg IV q 6 h) should be initiated immediately. However, septic shock from overwhelming infection remains the most likely cause of death.

Management of the hematopoietic syndrome is similar to that of marrow hypoplasia and pancytopenia of any cause (see Aplastic Anemia on p. 1041). Blood products should be transfused to treat anemia and thrombocytopenia, and hematopoietic growth factors (granulocyte colony-stimulating factor and granulocyte macrophage colony-stimulating factor) and broad-spectrum antibiotics should be given to treat neutropenia and neutropenic fever, respectively (see p. 1062). Neutropenic patients should also be placed in reverse isolation. With radiation doses > 4 Gy, the probability of bone marrow recovery is poor, and hematopoietic growth factors should be given as soon as possible. Stem cell transplants have had limited success but should be considered for exposure > 7 to 8 Gy (see p. 1371).

Aside from regular monitoring for signs of disease (eg, ophthalmic examination for cataracts, thyroid function studies for thyroid disease), there is no specific monitoring or treatment for specific organ injury. Radiation-induced cancer is treated in the same way as a similar spontaneous cancer.

Prevention

Protection from radiation exposure is accomplished through minimizing the time of exposure, maximizing the distance from the source, and using shielding. Shielding from a known discrete radioactive source can be reasonably achieved (eg, with lead aprons or commercially available transparent shields); however, shielding from most radionuclide contamination from large-scale disasters (eg, nuclear accident or attack) is not feasible. Thus, if at all possible after radiation release, evacuation of the area of exposure should be undertaken, with evacuation lasting 1 wk if the anticipated dose is > 0.05 Gy and permanent resettlement if the lifetime dose is expected to be > 1 Gy. When evacuation is not possible, taking shelter in a concrete or metal structure (eg, basement) can confer some protection.

People living within 16 km (10 miles) of a nuclear power plant should have ready access to KI tablets. These can be obtained from local pharmacies and some public health agencies. Many drugs and chemicals (eg, sulfhydryl compounds) increase survival rate in animals if given before irradiation. However, none are practical for humans.

All personnel working with radioactivity should wear dosimeter badges and be monitored for signs of excessive radiation exposure. The standard occupational limit is 0.05 Gy/yr. For emergency medical personnel, recommended dosage limits include 0.05 Gy for any non-lifesaving events and 0.25 Gy for any lifesaving event.

318 HEAT ILLNESS

Exposure to warm environments affects many physiologic functions and may cause dehydration. Most people experience mild but uncomfortable symptoms; however, effects may range from cramps and edema to syncope, heat exhaustion, and heat stroke. Core temperature is elevated in some types of heat illness. Those with dehydration (see pp. 1233 and 2289) may have tachycardia, tachypnea, and orthostatic hypotension. CNS dysfunction suggests heat stroke, the most serious disorder; confusion and lethargy may further impair the ability to escape the heat and rehydrate.

Pathophysiology

Heat input comes from the environment and metabolism. Heat output occurs through the skin by radiation, evaporation (eg, via sweat), and convection; the contribution of each of these mechanisms varies with environmental temperature and humidity. Radiation predominates at room temperature, but as environmental temperature approaches body temperature, evaporation becomes more important, providing essentially 100% of cooling at > 35° C. However, high humidity greatly limits evaporative cooling (see Heatstroke, on p. 2608).

Heat output is modulated by changes in cutaneous blood flow and sweat production. Cutaneous blood flow is 200 to 250 mL/min at normal temperatures but increases to 7 to 8 L/min with heat stress, requiring a marked increase in cardiac output. Also, heat stress increases sweat production from negligible to > 2 L/h; thus, significant dehydration can occur rapidly. Because sweat contains electrolytes, electrolyte loss may be substantial. However, prolonged exposure triggers physiologic changes to accommodate heat load (acclimatization); for example, sweat Na levels are 40 to 100 mEq/L in unacclimatized people but decrease to 10 to 70 mEq/L in acclimatized people.

The body can compensate for large variations in heat load, but significant or prolonged exposure to heat increases core temperature. Modest, transient core temperature elevations are tolerable, but severe elevations (typically > 41° C) lead to protein denaturation and, especially during hard work in the heat, release of inflammatory cytokines (eg, tumor necrosis factor-α, IL-1β). As a result, cellular dysfunction occurs and the inflammatory cascade is activated, leading to malfunction of most organs and activation of the coagulation cascade. These pathophysiologic processes are similar to those of multiple organ dysfunction syndrome (see p. 560), which follows prolonged shock.

Compensatory mechanisms include an acute-phase response by other cytokines that moderate the inflammatory response (eg, by stimulating production of proteins that decrease production of free radicals and inhibit release of proteolytic enzymes). Also, increased core temperature triggers expression of heat-shock proteins. These proteins transiently enhance heat tolerance by poorly understood mechanisms (eg, possibly by preventing protein denaturation) and by regulation of cardiovascular responses. With prolonged or extreme temperature elevation, compensatory mechanisms are overwhelmed or malfunction, allowing inflammation and multiple organ dysfunction syndrome to occur.

Etiology

Heat disorders are caused by some combination of increased heat input and decreased output. Clinical effects are exacerbated by inability to tolerate increased cardiovascular demands, dehydration, electrolyte disturbance, and use of certain drugs. The elderly and the very young and people with cardiovascular disorders or electrolyte depletion (eg, due to diuretic use) are at highest risk.

Excess heat input typically results from strenuous exertion, high environmental temperatures, or both. Medical disorders (eg, hyperthyroidism, neuroleptic malignant syndrome) and use of stimulant drugs (eg, amphetamines, cocaine, methylenedioxymethamphetamine [MDMA or Ecstasy]) can increase heat production.

Cooling is impaired by heavy clothing (particularly protective gear for workers and athletes), obesity, high humidity, and anything that impairs sweating or evaporation of sweat. Sweating can be impaired by skin disorders (eg, heat rash, extensive psoriasis or eczema, scleroderma) and use of anticholinergic drugs (eg, phenothiazines, antihistamines, drugs used to treat parkinsonism).

Prevention

Common sense is the best prevention. During excessively hot weather, the elderly and the young should not remain in unventilated residences without air-conditioning. Children should not be left in automobiles in the hot sun. If possible, strenuous exertion in a very hot environment or an inadequately ventilated space should be avoided, and heavy, insulating clothing should not be worn.

Weight loss after exercise or work is used to monitor dehydration; people who lose 2 to 3% of their body weight should be reminded to drink extra fluids and should be within 1 kg of starting weight before the next day's exposure. If people lose > 4%, activity should be limited for 1 day.

If exertion in the heat is unavoidable, fluid (often lost imperceptibly in very hot, very dry air) should be replaced by frequently drinking water, and evaporation should be facilitated by wearing open-mesh clothing or by using fans. Thirst is a poor indicator of dehydration during exertion; fluids should be drunk every few hours regardless of thirst. However, overhydration must be avoided; significant hyponatremia (see p. 1237) has occurred in endurance athletes who drink very frequently during exercise. Plain water is adequate for hydration during most activity; cool water is absorbed more readily. Special hydrating solutions (eg, sports drinks) are not required, but their flavoring enhances consumption, and their modest salt content is helpful if fluid requirements are high. Drinking fluids and consuming generously salted foods should be encouraged. Laborers or others who sweat heavily can lose ≥ 20 g of salt/day, making heat cramps more likely; such people need to replace the Na loss with drink and food. A palatable drink providing about 20 mmol of salt/L may be prepared by adding a rounded teaspoon of table salt to 5 gallons of any Kool-Aid–like drink. People on low-salt diets should increase salt intake.

Successively and incrementally increasing the level and amount of work done in the heat eventually results in acclimatization, which enables people to work safely at temperatures that were previously intolerable or life threatening. Progressing from 15 min/day of moderate activity (enough to stimulate sweating) during a hot time of day to 90 min of vigorous activity over 10 to 14 days is typically adequate. Acclimatization markedly increases the amount of sweat (and hence cooling) produced at a given level of exertion and markedly decreases the electrolyte content of sweat. Acclimatization significantly decreases risk of a heat illness.

HEAT CRAMPS

Heat cramps are exertion-induced contractions that occur during or after exertion in the heat.

Although exertion may induce cramps during cool weather, such cramps are not heat related and probably reflect lack of fitness. In contrast, heat cramps can occur in physically fit people who sweat profusely and replace lost water but not salt, thereby causing hyponatremia. Heat cramps are common among manual laborers (eg, engine room personnel, steel workers, miners), basic military trainees, and athletes.

Cramping is abrupt, usually occurring in muscles of the extremities. Severe pain and carpopedal spasm may incapacitate the hands and feet. Temperature is normal, and other findings are unremarkable. The cramp usually lasts minutes to hours.

Cramps may be relieved immediately by firm passive stretching of the involved muscle (eg, plantar dorsiflexion for a calf cramp). Fluids and electrolytes should be replenished orally (1 L water containing 10 g [2 level tsp] salt) or IV (1 L 0.9% saline solution).

Adequate conditioning, acclimatization, and appropriate management of salt balance help prevent cramps.

HEAT EXHAUSTION

Heat exhaustion is a non–life-threatening clinical syndrome of weakness, malaise, nausea, syncope, and other nonspecific symptoms caused by heat exposure. Thermoregulation is not impaired.

Heat exhaustion is caused by water and electrolyte imbalance due to heat exposure, with or without exertion.

Symptoms are often vague, and patients may not realize that heat is the cause. Symptoms may include weakness, dizziness, headache, nausea, and sometimes vomiting. Syncope due to standing for long periods in the heat (heat syncope) is common and may mimic cardiovascular disorders. On examination, patients appear tired and are usually sweaty and tachycardic. Mental status is typically normal, unlike in heatstroke. Temperature is usually normal and, when elevated, does not exceed 40° C.

Diagnosis is clinical and requires exclusion of other possible causes (eg, hypoglycemia, acute coronary syndrome, various infections). Laboratory testing is required only if needed to rule out such disorders.

Treatment involves removing patients to a cool environment, having them lie flat, and giving IV fluid and electrolyte replacement therapy, typically using 0.9% saline solution; oral rehydration does not provide sufficient electrolytes. Rate and volume of rehydration are guided by age, underlying disorders, and clinical response. Replacement of 1 to 2 L at 500 mL/h is often adequate. Elderly patients and patients with heart disorders may require only slightly lower rates; patients with suspected hypovolemia may require higher rates initially. External cooling measures (see p. 2609) are not required. Rarely, severe heat exhaustion after hard work may be complicated by rhabdomyolysis, myoglobinuria, acute renal failure, and disseminated intravascular coagulation.

HEATSTROKE

Heatstroke is hyperthermia accompanied by a systemic inflammatory response causing multiple organ dysfunction and often death. Symptoms include temperature > 40° C and altered mental status; sweating is often absent. Diagnosis is clinical. Treatment is rapid external cooling, IV fluid resuscitation, and support as needed for organ failure.

Heatstroke occurs when thermoregulatory mechanisms do not function and core temperature increases substantially. Inflammatory cytokines are activated, and multiple organ failure may develop. Endotoxin from GI flora also may play a role. Organ failure may occur in the CNS, skeletal muscle (rhabdomyolysis), liver, kidneys, lungs (acute respiratory distress syndrome), and heart. The coagulation cascade is activated, sometimes causing disseminated intravascular coagulation. Hyperkalemia and hypoglycemia may occur.

There are 2 variants: classic and exertional. Classic heatstroke takes 2 to 3 days of exposure to develop. It occurs during summer heat waves, typically in older, sedentary people with no air-conditioning and often with limited access to fluids. Classic heatstroke caused the large number of deaths in Europe during the exceptionally hot summer of 2003.

Exertional heatstroke occurs abruptly in healthy active people (eg, athletes, military recruits, factory workers). Intense exertion in a hot environment causes a sudden massive heat load that the body cannot modulate. Rhabdomyolysis is common; renal failure and coagulopathy are somewhat more likely and severe.

A syndrome similar to heatstroke may occur after using certain drugs (eg, cocaine, phencyclidine [PCP], amphetamines, monoamine oxide inhibitors). Usually, an overdose is required, but exertion and environmental conditions can be additive. Malignant hyperthermia (see p. 2517) can result from exposure to some anesthetics and antipsychotics; this genetic disorder has a high mortality rate.

Symptoms and Signs

Global CNS dysfunction is the hallmark, ranging from confusion to delirium, seizures, and coma. Tachycardia, even when the patient is supine, and tachypnea are common. In classic heatstroke, the skin is hot and dry. In exertional heatstroke, sweating is relatively common. In both, temperature is > 40° C and may be > 46° C.

Diagnosis

Diagnosis is usually clear from a history of exertion and environmental heat; however, when conditions reported are less extreme, acute infection (eg, sepsis, meningitis) and toxic shock must be excluded. Drugs that may have caused the episode should be considered.

Laboratory testing includes CBC, PT, PTT, electrolytes, BUN, creatinine, Ca, CPK, and hepatic profile to evaluate organ function. A urethral catheter is placed to obtain urine, which is checked for occult blood by dipstick, and to monitor output. A urine drug screen may be helpful. Tests to detect myoglobin are unnecessary. Continual monitoring of core temperature, usually by rectal or esophageal probe, is desired.

Prognosis and Treatment

Mortality rate is significant but varies markedly with age, underlying disorders, maximum temperature, and, most importantly, duration of hyperthermia and promptness of cooling. About 20% of survivors have residual brain damage. In some patients, renal insufficiency persists. Temperature may be labile for weeks.

The importance of rapid recognition and effective, aggressive cooling cannot be overemphasized. Cooling methods that do not cause shivering or cutaneous vasoconstriction are preferred, although ice-soaked towels and ice water immersion are effective. Evaporative cooling is comfortable and convenient and considered the most rapid method by some experts. During the process, patients are continually wetted with water, and the skin is fanned and vigorously massaged to promote blood flow. A spray hose and larger fans are best and may be used for large groups of people in the field. Comfortable, tepid (eg, 30° C) water is adequate because evaporation causes cooling; cold or ice water is not needed. Cool water immersion in a pond or stream can also be used in the field. Ice packs applied to the axillae and groin can be used but not as the sole cooling method. In life-threatening cases, literally packing a patient in ice, with close monitoring, has been advocated to rapidly reduce core temperature.

IV hydration with 0.9% saline solution is begun (as described on p. 2608). Organ failure and rhabdomyolysis are treated (see elsewhere in THE MANUAL). Injectable benzodiazepines (eg, lorazepam or diazepam) may be used to prevent agitation and seizures (which increase heat production); seizures may occur during cooling. Because vomiting and aspiration of gastric contents are possible, measures to protect the airway may be required. Severely agitated patients may require paralysis and mechanical ventilation.

Platelets and fresh-frozen plasma may be required for severe disseminated intravascular coagulation. IV $NaHCO_3$ to alkalinize the urine may help prevent nephrotoxicity if myoglobinuria is present. IV Ca salts may be necessary to treat hyperkalemic cardiotoxicity. Vasoconstrictors used to treat hypotension may reduce cutaneous blood flow and decrease heat loss. Hemodialysis may be required. Antipyretics (eg, acetaminophen) are of no value. Dantrolene is used to treat anesthetic-induced malignant hyperthermia but has no proven benefit for other causes of severe hyperthermia.

319 COLD INJURY

Exposure to cold may cause decreased body temperature (hypothermia) and focal soft-tissue injury. Tissue injury with freezing is frostbite. Tissue injury without freezing includes frostnip, immersion foot, and chilblains. Treatment is rewarming.

Susceptibility to cold injury is increased by exhaustion, hunger, dehydration, hypoxia, impaired cardiovascular function, and contact with moisture or metal. The elderly, the very young, and people intoxicated with drugs or alcohol are particularly at risk. The elderly often have diminished temperature sensation and impaired mobility and communication, resulting in a tendency to remain in an overly cool environment. These impairments, combined with diminished subcutaneous fat, contribute to hypothermia in the elderly—sometimes even indoors in cool rooms. The very young have similarly diminished mobility and communication and have an increased surface area/mass ratio, which enhances heat loss. Intoxicated people who lose consciousness in a cold environment are likely to become hypothermic.

Prevention is crucial. Several layers of warm clothing and protection against moisture and wind are important even when the weather does not seem to threaten cold injury. Clothing that remains insulating when wet (eg, made of wool or polypropylene) should be worn. Gloves and socks should be kept as dry as possible; insulated boots that do not impede circulation should be worn in very cold weather. A warm head covering is particularly important because 30% of heat is lost from the head. Consuming ample fluids and food helps sustain metabolic heat production. Paying attention to when body parts become cold or numb and immediately warming them may prevent cold injury.

NONFREEZING TISSUE INJURIES

Acute or chronic injuries without freezing of tissue may result from cold exposure.

Frostnip: The mildest cold injury is frostnip. Affected areas are numb, swollen, and red. Treatment is rewarming, which causes pain and itching. Rarely, mild hypersensitivity to cold persists for months to years.

Immersion (trench) foot: Prolonged exposure to wet cold can cause immersion foot. Peripheral nerves and the vasculature are usually injured; muscle and skin tissue may be injured in severe cases.

Initially, the foot is pale, edematous, clammy, cold, and numb; tissue maceration may occur if patients walk extensively. Rewarming causes hyperemia, pain, and often hypersensitivity to light touch, which persist for 6 to 10 wk. Skin may ulcerate, or a black eschar may develop. Autonomic dysfunction is common, with increased or decreased sweating, vasomotor changes, and local hypersensitivity to temperature change. Muscle atrophy and dysesthesia or anesthesia may occur and become chronic.

Immersion foot can be prevented by not wearing tight-fitting boots, keeping feet and boots dry, and changing socks frequently. Immediate treatment is rewarming in 40 to 42° C water, followed by sterile dressings. Chronic neuropathic symptoms are difficult to treat; amitriptyline may be tried (see Neuropathic Pain on p. 1779).

Chilblains (pernio): Localized areas of erythema, swelling, and pruritus result from repeated exposure to dry cold; the mechanism is unclear. Blistering or ulceration may occur. Chilblains most commonly affects the fingers and pretibial area and is self-limited. Occasionally, symptoms recur.

Pernio is often used to refer to a vasculitic disorder most common among young females with a history of Raynaud's phenomenon. Endothelial and neuronal damage results in vascular hypersensitivity to cold and sympathetic instability. Nifedipine 20 mg po tid may be effective for refractory pernio. Sympatholytic drugs may also help.

FROSTBITE

Frostbite is injury due to freezing of tissue. Initial presentation may be deceptively benign. Skin may appear white or blistered and is numb; rewarming causes substantial pain. Gangrene may develop. Treatment is rewarming in warm (40 to 42° C) water and local care. Severely damaged tissue may autoamputate. Surgical amputation is occasionally necessary, but a decision, often guided by imaging results, should usually be delayed until several months after injury.

Frostbite usually occurs in extreme cold, especially at high altitude, and is aggravated by hypothermia. Distal extremities and exposed skin are affected most often.

Ice crystals form within or between tissue cells, essentially freezing the tissue and causing cell death. Adjacent unfrozen areas are at risk because local vasoconstriction and thrombosis can cause ischemic damage. With reperfusion during rewarming, inflammatory cytokines (eg, thromboxanes, prostaglandins) are released, exacerbating tissue injury.

Symptoms and Signs

The affected area is cold, hard, white, and numb; when warmed, it becomes blotchy red, swollen, and painful. Blisters form within 4 to 6 h, but the full extent of injury may not be apparent for several days. Blisters filled with clear serum indicate superficial damage; blood-filled, proximal blisters indicate deep damage and likely tissue loss. Superficial damage heals without residual tissue loss. Freezing of deep tissue causes dry gangrene with a hard black carapace over healthy tissue; wet gangrene, which is gray, edematous, and soft, is less common. Wet gangrene may become infected, but dry gangrene is unlikely to do so. Depth of tissue loss depends on duration and depth of freezing. Severely damaged tissue may autoamputate. All degrees of frostbite may produce long-term neuropathic symptoms: sensitivity to cold, excessive sweating, faulty nail growth, and numbness (symptoms resembling those of complex regional pain syndrome [see p. 1780], although any relationship is speculative).

Treatment

In the field, frostbitten extremities should be rewarmed rapidly by totally immersing the affected area in water that is tolerably warm to the touch (≤ 40.5° C). Because the area is numb, rewarming with an uncontrolled dry heat source (eg, fire, heating pad) risks burns. Rubbing may further damage tissue and is avoided. The longer an area remains frozen, the greater the ultimate damage may be. However, thawing the feet is inadvisable if a patient must walk any distance to receive care because thawed tissue is particularly sensitive to the trauma of walking and, if refrozen, will be more severely damaged than if left frozen. If thawing must be delayed, the frozen area is gently cleaned, dried, and protected in sterile compresses; patients are given analgesics, if available, and the whole body is kept warm.

Once in the hospital, extremities are rapidly rewarmed in large containers of circulating water kept at ≤ 40.5° C; 15 to 30 min is usually adequate. Thawing is often ended prematurely because pain may be severe during rewarming. Parenteral analgesics, including opioids, may be used. Patients are encouraged to move the affected part gently during thawing. Large, clear blisters are left intact. Hemorrhagic blisters are also left intact to avoid secondary desiccation of deep dermal layers. Broken vesicles are debrided.

Anti-inflammatory measures (eg, topical aloe vera q 6 h, ibuprofen 400 mg po q 8 h) probably help. Affected areas are left open to warm air, and extremities are elevated to decrease edema. Anticoagulants, IV low mol wt dextran, and intra-arterial vasodilators (eg, reserpine, tolazoline) have no proven clinical benefit. Phenoxybenzamine (10 to 60 mg po once/day), a long-acting α-blocker, may theoretically decrease vasospasm and improve blood flow.

Preventing infection is fundamental. If wet gangrene is present, broad-spectrum antibiotics are used. Tetanus toxoid is given if vaccination is not up to date.

Adequate nutrition is important to sustain metabolic heat production.

Imaging tests (eg, radionuclide scanning, MRI, microwave thermography, laser-Doppler flowmetry, angiography) can help assess circulation, determine tissue viability, and thus guide treatment. MRI and particularly magnetic resonance angiography (MRA) may establish the line of demarcation before clinical demarcation and thus make earlier surgical debridement or amputation possible. However, whether earlier surgery improves long-term outcome is unclear. Usually, surgery is delayed as long as possible because the black carapace is often shed, leaving viable tissue. "Freeze in January, operate in July" is an old adage. Patients with severe frostbite are warned that many weeks of observation may be required before demarcation and the extent of tissue loss become apparent.

Whirlpool baths at 37° C 3 times/day followed by gentle drying, rest, and time are the best long-term management. No totally effective treatment for the long-lasting symptoms of frostbite (eg, numbness, hypersensitivity to cold) is known, although chemical or surgical sympathectomy may be useful for late neuropathic symptoms.

HYPOTHERMIA

Hypothermia is a core body temperature < 35° C. Symptoms progress from shivering and lethargy to confusion, coma, and death. Mild hypothermia requires a warm environment and insulating blankets (passive rewarming). Severe hypothermia requires active rewarming of the body surface (eg, with forced-air warming systems, radiant sources, heating pads) or core (eg, body cavity lavage, extracorporeal blood rewarming).

Hypothermia results when body heat loss exceeds body heat production. Hypothermia is most common during cold weather or immersion in cold water, but it may occur in warm climates when people lie immobile on a cool surface (eg, when they are intoxicated) or after very prolonged immersion in swimming-temperature water (eg, 20 to 24° C).

Primary hypothermia causes about 600 deaths each year in the US. Hypothermia also has a significant and underrecognized effect on mortality risk in cardiovascular and neurologic disorders.

Etiology and Pathophysiology

Immobility, wet clothing, windchill, and lying on a cold surface increase risk of hypothermia. Conditions that cause loss of consciousness, immobility, or both (eg, trauma, hypoglycemia, seizure disorders, stroke, drug or alcohol intoxication) are common predisposing factors.

Hypothermia slows all physiologic functions, including cardiovascular and respiratory systems, nerve conduction, mental acuity, neuromuscular reaction time, and metabolic rate. Thermoregulation ceases below about 30° C; the body must then depend on an external heat source for rewarming. Renal cell dysfunction and decreased levels of ADH lead to production of a large volume of dilute urine (cold diuresis). Diuresis plus fluid leakage into the interstitial tissues causes hypovolemia. Vasoconstriction, which occurs with hypothermia, may mask hypovolemia, which then manifests as sudden shock or cardiac arrest during rewarming (rewarming collapse) when peripheral vasculature dilates.

Immersion in cold water can trigger the diving reflex, which involves reflex vasoconstriction in visceral muscles; blood is shunted to essential organs (eg, heart, brain). The reflex is most pronounced in small children and may help protect them. Also, hypothermia due to total immersion in near-freezing water may protect the brain from hypoxia by decreasing metabolic demands. The decreased demand probably accounts for the occasional survival after prolonged cardiac arrest due to extreme hypothermia.

Symptoms and Signs

Intense shivering occurs initially, but it ceases below about 31° C, allowing body temperature to drop more precipitously. CNS dysfunction progresses as body temperature decreases; people do not sense the cold. Lethargy and clumsiness are followed by confusion, irritability, sometimes hallucinations, and eventually coma. Pupils may become unreactive. Respirations and heartbeat slow and ultimately cease. Initially, sinus bradycardia and slow atrial fibrillation are present; the terminal rhythm is ventricular fibrillation or asystole. However, these rhythms are potentially less ominous than in normothermia.

Diagnosis

Diagnosis is by rectal temperature. Electronic thermometers are preferred because standard mercury thermometers have a lower limit of 34° C and even though low-temperature mercury thermometers are available. Esophageal probes and thermistors in pulmonary artery catheters are most accurate but are usually not immediately available.

Causes are sought. Laboratory tests include CBC, glucose, electrolytes, BUN, creatinine, and ABGs. ABGs are not corrected for low temperature. ECG typically shows J (Osborn) waves (see FIG. 319–1) and interval prolongation (PR, QRS, QT), although these findings are not always present. If the cause is unclear, alcohol level is measured, and drug screening and thyroid function tests are done. Sepsis and occult head or skeletal trauma must be considered.

Prognosis and Treatment

Patients who have been immersed in icy water for 1 h or (rarely) longer have been successfully rewarmed without permanent brain damage (see p. 2618), even when core temperature was 13.7° C or when pupils were unreactive. Outcome is difficult to predict and cannot be based on the Glasgow Coma Scale. Grave prognostic markers include evidence of cell lysis (hyperkalemia > 10 mEq/L) and

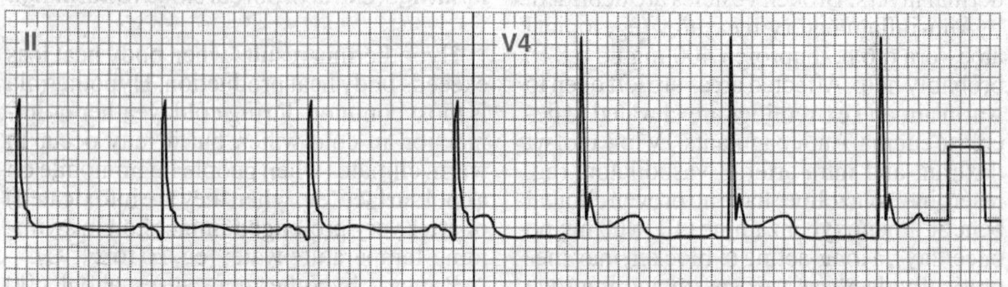

Fig. 319–1. Abnormal ECG showing J (Osborn) waves (V4).

intravascular thrombosis (fibrinogen < 50 mg/dL). For a given degree and duration of hypothermia, children are more likely to recover than adults.

The first priority is to prevent further heat loss by removing wet clothing, wrapping the patient in blankets, and covering the patient's head. Subsequent measures depend on how severe hypothermia is and whether cardiovascular instability or cardiac arrest is present. Returning patients to a normal temperature is less urgent in hypothermia than in severe hyperthermia. For stable patients, elevation of core temperature by 1° C/h is acceptable.

If hypothermia is mild and thermoregulation is present (indicated by shivering and temperature typically 31 to 35° C), insulation with heated blankets and warm fluids to drink are adequate.

Fluid resuscitation is essential for hypovolemia. Patients are given 1 to 2 L of 0.9% saline solution (20 mL/kg for children) IV; it is heated if possible to 45° C. More is given as needed to maintain perfusion.

Active rewarming is required if patients have cardiovascular instability, temperature < 32.2° C, endocrinologic insufficiency, or hypothermia secondary to trauma, toxins, or disorders. If body temperature is at the warmer end of the range, external rewarming with heating pads or forced hot air enclosures may be used. Patients with lower temperatures, particularly those with low BP or cardiac arrest, require core rewarming. One option is lavage of the peritoneal and thoracic cavities with heated lavage fluid or 0.9% saline solution. Heated arteriovenous or venovenous circuits (as in hemodialysis) are more effective but logistically difficult. Cardiopulmonary bypass (using a heart-lung machine) is the quickest effective method. These extracorporeal measures require a prearranged protocol with appropriate specialists.

CPR is not done if patients have a perfusing rhythm, even if pulses are not palpable; fluids and rewarming proceed as above. Hypotension and bradycardia are expected when core temperature is low and, if due solely to hypothermia, need not be aggressively treated. Patients with ventricular fibrillation or asystole require cardiopulmonary resuscitation. Chest compressions and endotracheal intubation are done. Defibrillation is difficult if body temperature is low; 1 or 2 attempts may be made, but if they are ineffective, further attempts are deferred until temperature reaches > 28° C. Advanced life support should be continued until temperature reaches 32° C unless obviously lethal injuries or disorders are present. However, advanced cardiac life-support drugs (eg, antiarrhythmics, vasopressors, inotropes) are usually not given. Low-dose dopamine (1 to 5 μg/kg/min) or other catecholamine infusions are typically reserved for patients who have disproportionately severe hypotension and who do not respond to crystalloid resuscitation and rewarming. Severe hyperkalemia (> 10 mEq/L) during resuscitation typically indicates a fatal outcome and can guide resuscitative efforts.

320 ALTITUDE SICKNESS

Altitude sickness includes several related syndromes caused by decreased O_2 availability at high altitudes. Acute mountain sickness (AMS), the mildest form, is headache plus one or more systemic manifestations. High-altitude cerebral edema (HACE) is encephalopathy in people with AMS. High-altitude pulmonary edema (HAPE) is a form of noncardiogenic pulmonary edema causing severe dyspnea and hypoxemia. Minor forms of AMS may occur in recreational hikers and skiers. Diagnosis is clinical. Treatment of mild AMS is with analgesics and acetazolamide. Severe syndromes require descent and supplemental O_2 if available. In addition, dexamethasone may be useful for HACE, and nifedipine may be useful for HAPE.

As altitude increases, atmospheric pressure decreases while the percentage of O_2 in air remains constant; thus, the partial pressure of O_2 decreases with altitude and, at 5800 m (19,000 ft), is about ½ that at sea level.

Most people can ascend to 1500 to 2000 m (5000 to 6500 ft) in 1 day without problems, but about 20% who ascend to 2500 m (8000 ft) and 40% who ascend to 3000 m (10,000 ft) develop some form of altitude sickness (AS). Rate of ascent, maximum altitude reached, and sleeping altitude influence the likelihood of developing the disorder.

Risk factors: Effects of high altitude vary greatly. But generally, risk is increased by exertion and perhaps cold and is greater in people who have had previous AS and in those who live at low altitude (< 900 m [< 3000 ft]). Young children and young adults are probably more susceptible. Disorders such as diabetes, coronary artery disease, and mild COPD are not risk factors for AS, but hypoxia may adversely affect these disorders. Physical fitness is not protective.

Pathophysiology

Acute hypoxia (eg, as occurs during rapid ascent to high altitude in an unpressurized aircraft) alters CNS function within minutes. However, AS results from the body's neurohumoral and hemodynamic responses to hypoxia and develops over hours to days.

The CNS and lungs are primarily affected. In both, elevated capillary pressure, capillary leakage, and consequent edema formation probably occur.

In the lungs, hypoxia-induced elevation of pulmonary artery pressure causes interstitial and alveolar pulmonary edema, resulting in impaired oxygenation. Small-vessel hypoxic vasoconstriction is patchy, causing overperfusion with elevated pressure, capillary wall damage, and capillary leakage in less constricted areas. Various additional mechanisms have been proposed; they include sympathetic overactivity, endothelial dysfunction, decreased alveolar nitric oxide (perhaps due to decreased nitric oxide synthase), and a defect in the amiloride-sensitive Na channel. Some of these factors may have a genetic component.

Pathophysiology in the CNS is less clear but may involve a combination of hypoxia-induced cerebral vasodilation, alteration of the blood-brain barrier, and Na and water retention producing cerebral edema. One hypothesis is that patients with a low ratio of CSF to brain volume are less able to tolerate swelling (ie, by displacement of CSF) and thus are more likely to develop AS. The roles of atrial natriuretic peptide, aldosterone, renin, and angiotensin are unclear.

Acclimatization: Acclimatization is an integrated series of responses that gradually restores tissue oxygenation toward normal in people exposed to altitude. However, in spite of acclimatization, all people at high altitude have tissue hypoxia. Most people acclimatize to altitudes of up to 3000 m (10,000 ft) in a few days. The higher the altitude, the longer full acclimatization takes. However, no one can fully acclimatize to long-term residence at > 5100 m (> 17,000 ft).

Features of acclimatization include sustained hyperventilation, which increases tissue oxygenation but also causes respiratory alkalosis. Alkalosis normalizes within days as HCO_3 is excreted in urine; as pH normalizes, ventilation can increase further. Cardiac output increases initially; RBC mass and tolerance for aerobic work also increase. After many generations at altitude, some ethnic groups have adapted in slightly different ways.

Symptoms, Signs, and Diagnosis

The various clinical forms of AS are not separate entities but parts of a spectrum in which one or more forms may be present in different degrees.

Acute mountain sickness (AMS): This form is by far the most common and may develop at altitudes as low as 2000 m (6500 ft). It is probably due to mild cerebral edema and is characterized by headache plus at least one of the following: fatigue, GI symptoms (anorexia, nausea, vomiting), dizziness, and sleep disturbance. Exertion aggravates the symptoms. Symptoms typically develop 6 to 10 h after ascent and subside in 24 to 48 h, but they occasionally evolve into HAPE, HACE, or both. Diagnosis is clinical; laboratory tests are nonspecific and usually unnecessary. AMS is common at ski resorts, and some people affected by it mistakenly attribute it to excessive alcohol intake (hangover) or a viral illness.

High-altitude cerebral edema (HACE): Marked cerebral edema manifests as headache and diffuse encephalopathy with confusion, drowsiness, stupor, and coma. Gait ataxia is a reliable early warning sign. Seizures and focal deficits (eg, cranial nerve palsy, hemiplegia) are less common. Papilledema and retinal hemorrhage may be present but are not necessary for diagnosis. Coma and death may occur within a few hours. HACE can usually be differentiated from other causes of coma (eg, infection, ketoacidosis) by the history. In addition, fever and nuchal rigidity are absent, and blood and CSF studies are normal.

High-altitude pulmonary edema (HAPE): HAPE usually develops 24 to 96 h after rapid ascent to > 2500 m (> 8000 ft) and is responsible for most deaths due to AS. Respiratory infections, even minor ones, appear to increase risk. HAPE is more common among men (unlike other forms of AS). Longtime high-altitude residents can develop HAPE when they return after a brief stay at low altitude.

Initially, patients have dyspnea, decreased exertion tolerance, and dry cough. Pink or bloody sputum and respiratory distress are later findings. On examination, cyanosis, tachycardia, tachypnea, and low-grade fever (< 38.5° C) are common. Focal or diffuse rales (sometimes audible without a stethoscope) are usually present. Hypoxemia is often severe, with pulse oximetry showing 40 to 70% saturation. If obtained, chest x-ray shows a normal-sized heart and patchy lung edema (often middle or lower lobes), unlike what is seen in heart failure. HAPE may worsen rapidly; coma and death may occur within hours.

Other disorders: Peripheral and facial edema is common at high altitude. Headache, without other symptoms of AMS, is frequent.

Retinal hemorrhages may develop at altitudes as low as 2700 m (9000 ft) and are common at > 5000 m (> 16,000 ft). They are usually asymptomatic unless they occur in the macular region; they resolve rapidly without sequelae.

People who have had radial keratotomy may have significant visual disturbances at altitudes > 5000 m (> 16,000 ft) or even as low as 3000 m (10,000 ft). These alarming symptoms disappear rapidly after descent.

Chronic mountain sickness (Monge's disease) is an uncommon disorder that affects longtime high-altitude residents; it is characterized by fatigue, dyspnea, aches and pains, excessive polycythemia, and occasionally thromboembolism. The disorder often involves alveolar hypoventilation. Patients should descend to low altitude; recovery is slow, and return to high altitude may cause recurrence. Repeated phlebotomy can reduce polycythemia, but polycythemia may recur.

Treatment

AMS: Patients should halt ascent and reduce exertion until symptoms resolve. Other treatment includes fluids, analgesics for headache, and a light diet. For severe symptoms, descent of 500 to 1000 m (1650 to 3200 ft) is usually rapidly effective. Acetazolamide 250 mg po bid may relieve symptoms and improve sleep.

HAPE and HACE: Patients should descend to low altitude immediately. If descent is delayed, patients should rest and be given O_2. If descent is impossible, O_2, drugs, and pressurization in a portable hyperbaric bag help buy time but are not substitutes for descent.

For HAPE, nifedipine 20 mg sublingually followed by a 30-mg slow-release tablet lowers pulmonary artery pressure and is beneficial. Diuretics (eg, furosemide) are contraindicated. The heart is normal in HAPE, and digitalis is of no value. When promptly treated by descent, patients usually recover from HAPE within 24 to 48 h. People who have had one episode of HAPE are likely to have another and should be so warned.

For HACE (and severe AMS), dexamethasone 4 to 8 mg initially, followed by 4 mg q 6 h, may help. It may be given po, sc, IM, or IV. Acetazolamide 250 mg po bid may be added.

Prevention

Drinking extra water is important because breathing large volumes of dry air at altitude greatly increases water loss, and dehydration with some degree of hypovolemia aggravates symptoms. Additional salt should be avoided. Alcohol seems to worsen AMS and reduces nocturnal ventilation, thus accentuating sleep disturbance. Eating frequent small meals that are high in easily digested carbohydrates (eg, fruits, jams, starches) is recommended for the 1st few days. Although physical fitness enables greater exertion at altitude, it does not protect against any form of AS.

Ascent: Graded ascent is essential for activity at > 2500 m (> 8000 ft). Sleeping on the 1st night should be at < 2500 to 3000 m (8,000 to 10,000 ft), and climbers should sleep at that altitude for 2 to 3 nights if subsequent higher sleeping altitudes are planned. Each day thereafter, sleeping altitude can be increased by about 300 m (1000 ft), although higher day hikes are acceptable with return to the lower level for sleep. Climbers vary in ability to ascend without developing symptoms; a climbing party should be paced for its slowest member.

Acclimatization reverses quickly. After descent to low levels for more than a few days, acclimatized climbers should once more follow a graded ascent.

Drugs: Acetazolamide 125 mg q 8 h reduces the incidence of AMS. Sustained-release capsules (500 mg once/day) are also available.

Acetazolamide can be started on the day of the ascent; it acts by inhibiting carbonic anhydrase and thus increasing ventilation. Acetazolamide 125 mg po at bedtime reduces the amount of periodic breathing (almost universal during sleep at high altitude), thus limiting sharp falls in blood O_2. Acetazolamide should not be given to patients allergic to sulfa drugs. Analogs of acetazolamide offer no advantage. Acetazolamide may cause numbness and paresthesias of the fingers; these symptoms are benign but can be annoying. Carbonated drinks taste flat to people taking acetazolamide.

Low-flow O_2 during sleep at altitude is effective but inconvenient and may pose logistic difficulties.

Patients who have had a previous episode of HAPE should consider prophylaxis with sustained-release nifedipine 20 to 30 mg po bid. Inhaled β-agonists may also be effective.

Analgesics may prevent high-altitude headache. Dexamethasone is not recommended for prevention.

321 MOTION SICKNESS

Motion sickness is a symptom complex that usually includes nausea, often accompanied by vague abdominal discomfort, vomiting, dizziness, and related symptoms; it is caused by repetitive angular and linear acceleration and deceleration. Behavioral change and drug therapy can help prevent or control symptoms.

Individual susceptibility to motion sickness varies greatly. However, motion sickness is more common in women, and incidence ranges from < 1% on airplanes to nearly 100% on ships in rough seas and upon becoming weightless during space travel.

Excessive stimulation of the vestibular apparatus by motion is the primary cause. Afferent pathways from the labyrinth to the vomiting center in the medulla are undefined, but motion sickness occurs only when the 8th cranial nerve and cerebellar vestibular tracts are intact. Movement via any form of transportation can produce excessive vestibular stimulation, including ship, motor vehicle, train, plane, spacecraft, and playground or amusement park ride. Motion sickness can also occur when there is conflicting vestibular, visual, and proprioceptive input; when the pattern of motion differs from that previously experienced; and when motion is expected yet not experienced (eg, when viewing motion on a television or movie screen). Visual stimuli (eg, a moving horizon), poor ventilation (with fumes, smoke, or carbon monoxide), and emotional factors (eg, fear, anxiety) may act with motion to precipitate an episode.

In the space adaptation syndrome (motion sickness during space travel), weightlessness (zero gravity) is an etiologic factor. This syndrome reduces the efficiency of astronauts during the first few days of space flight, but adaptation occurs over several days.

Symptoms, Signs, and Diagnosis

Nausea and vague abdominal discomfort are characteristic. Vomiting may also occur. These symptoms may be preceded by yawning, hyperventilation, salivation, pallor, profuse cold sweating, and somnolence. Other symptoms include aerophagia, dizziness, headache, fatigue, weakness, and inability to concentrate. Pain, shortness of breath, and visual and speech disturbances are absent. With prolonged exposure to motion, the patient may adapt. However, symptoms may recur if motion increases or after a short respite.

Prolonged motion sickness with vomiting may rarely lead to dehydration with hypotension, inanition, and depression. Motion sickness can be serious in patients with other illnesses.

The diagnosis is clinical and usually straightforward. Occasionally, cerebrovascular events, such as stroke or transient ischemic event, may mimic motion sickness.

Treatment and Prevention

Several interventions are available, and all are more effective when used for prevention than when used after symptoms develop. People prone to motion sickness should take prophylactic drugs before symptoms start.

Scopolamine is available as a prescription transdermal patch or in oral form. The patch is a good choice for longer trips because after being applied behind the ear at least 4 h before travel (optimally 8 to 12 h), it is effective for up to 72 h as it releases about 1 mg. The oral form of scopolamine is given as 0.4 mg to 0.8 mg 1 h before travel and then q 8 h as needed. Adverse effects, which include drowsiness, blurred vision, dry mouth, and bradycardia, occur less commonly with patches. Inadvertent contamination of the eye with patch residue may cause a fixed and widely dilated pupil. Additional adverse effects of scopolamine in the elderly can include confusion, hallucinations, and urinary retention. Scopolamine is contraindicated in people who are at risk of angle-closure glaucoma. Scopolamine can be used by children > 12 yr in the same dosages as for adults. Use in children < 12 yr is probably safe but is not recommended.

Alternatively, beginning 1 h before departure, susceptible people may be given nonprescription dimenhydrinate, diphenhydramine, or meclizine 25 to 50 mg po qid (dimenhydrinate for children 2 to 6 yr, 12.5 to 25 mg q 6 to 8 h, maximum 75 mg/day; for children 6 to 12 yr, 25 to 50 mg q 6 to 8 h, maximum 150 mg/day); promethazine 25 to 50 mg po bid (for children < 12 yr, 0.5 mg/kg bid); or cyclizine 50 mg po qid (for children 6 to 12 yr, 25 mg tid) to minimize vagal-mediated GI symptoms. However, all of these drugs are anticholinergic and can cause adverse effects, especially in the elderly.

If vomiting occurs, an antiemetic can be given rectally or parenterally to be effective. If vomiting is prolonged, IV fluids and electrolytes may be required for replacement and maintenance.

Some nondrug therapies are unproven but may be helpful. These include use of wristbands that apply acupressure and wristbands that apply electrical stimulation. Both can be safely used by people of all ages. Ginger (1 to 2 g) may help prevent motion sickness.

Susceptible people should minimize exposure by positioning themselves where motion is the least (eg, in the middle of a ship close to water level, over the wings in an airplane). If traveling in a motor vehicle, driving or riding in the front passenger seat is best. Whatever the form of transportation, rear-facing seats should be avoided. A supine or semirecumbent position with the head supported is best. Adequate ventilation helps prevent symptoms. Reading should be avoided. Keeping the axis of vision at a 45° angle above the horizon and whenever possible focusing on stationary objects help reduce susceptibility. Alcoholic beverages and overeating before or during travel increase the likelihood of motion sickness. Small amounts of fluids and bland food should be consumed frequently during extended travel; some people find that dry crackers and carbonated beverages, especially ginger ale, are best. If air travel time is short, food and fluids should be avoided. In the space adaptation syndrome, movement, which aggravates the symptoms, should be avoided.

322 NEAR DROWNING

Near drowning is suffocation in water that does not result in death; it does result in hypoxia due to aspiration or laryngospasm. Sequelae of hypoxia may include brain damage and multiple organ failure. Patients are evaluated with chest x-ray and oximetry or ABGs. Treatment is supportive, including reversal of cardiac and respiratory arrest, hypoxia, hypoventilation, and hypothermia.

Drowning, or fatal suffocation in water, is the 7th most common cause of accidental death in the US overall and the 2nd most common cause in children ages 1 to 14 yr. Rates are highest for those < 4 yr and for children from African American, immigrant, and impoverished families. Risk factors for people of all ages include alcohol or drug use and conditions that cause temporary incapacitation (eg, seizure, hypoglycemia, stroke, MI). Near drowning is common in pools, hot tubs, natural water settings, and, among infants and toddlers, in toilets, bathtubs, buckets of water, and cleaning fluids. For every drowning death, about 4 near drownings that result in hospitalization occur.

Pathophysiology

Hypoxia is the major insult in near drowning, affecting the brain, heart, and other tissues; respiratory followed by cardiac arrest may occur. Brain hypoxia may cause cerebral edema and, occasionally, permanent neurologic sequelae. Generalized tissue hypoxia may cause metabolic acidosis. Immediate hypoxia results from aspiration of fluid or gastric contents, acute reflex laryngospasm, or both. Lung injury from aspiration or hypoxia itself may cause delayed hypoxia. Aspiration, particularly with particulate matter or chemicals, may cause chemical pneumonitis (occasionally primary, or secondary to bacterial pneumonia) and may impair alveolar secretion of surfactant, resulting in patchy atelectasis. Extensive atelectasis may make the affected areas of the lungs stiff, noncompliant, and poorly ventilated, potentially causing respiratory failure (see pp. 548 and 556) with hypercapnia and respiratory acidosis. Perfusion of poorly ventilated areas of the lungs (V/Q mismatch) worsens hypoxia. Alveolar hypoxia may cause noncardiogenic pulmonary edema.

Laryngospasm often limits the volume of fluid aspirated; however, large volumes of water are occasionally aspirated in near drowning and may change electrolyte concentrations and blood volume. Seawater may increase Na and Cl slightly. In contrast, large quantities of fresh water can decrease electrolyte concentration significantly, increase blood volume, and cause hemolysis.

Skeletal, soft tissue, head, and internal injuries may occur. People who dive into shallow water may sustain cervical and other spine injuries (which may be the cause of drowning). Exposure to cold water induces systemic hypothermia (see p. 2611), which can be a significant problem. However, hypothermia can also be protective by stimulating the diving reflex, slowing the heartbeat, and constricting the peripheral arteries, shunting oxygenated blood away from the extremities and the gut to the heart and brain. Also, hypothermia decreases the O_2 needs of tissues, possibly prolonging survival and delaying the onset of hypoxic tissue damage. The diving reflex and the overall clinically protective effects of cold water are usually greatest in young children.

Symptoms, Signs, and Diagnosis

Children who are unable to swim may become submerged in < 1 min, more rapidly than adults. After rescue, anxiety, vomiting, wheezing, and altered consciousness are common. Patients may have respiratory failure with tachypnea, retractions, or cyanosis. Sometimes, respiratory symptoms are delayed until several hours after submersion.

Most people are found in or near water, making the diagnosis obvious clinically. Resuscitation may need to precede completion of the diagnostic assessment. Cervical spine injury is assumed, and the spine is immobilized in patients who have altered consciousness or whose mechanism of injury involves diving. Procedures to remove water from the lungs are generally not helpful. Secondary head injury and conditions that may have contributed to drowning (eg, hypoglycemia, stroke, MI) are considered.

All patients undergo assessment of oxygenation by oximetry or, if there are respiratory symptoms or signs, ABG and chest x-ray. Because respiratory symptoms may be delayed, even asymptomatic patients are transported to the hospital and observed for several hours. In patients with symptoms or a history of prolonged submersion, core body temperature is measured, ECG and serum electrolytes are obtained, and continuous oximetry and cardiac monitoring are done. Patients with possible cervical spine injury undergo cervical spine imaging (see p. 2581). Patients with altered consciousness undergo head CT. Any other suspected predisposing or secondary conditions are evaluated with appropriate testing (eg, rapid blood glucose, ECG). In patients with pulmonary infiltrates, bacterial pneumonia is differentiated from chemical pneumonitis using blood cultures and sputum Gram stain and culture.

Prognosis and Treatment

Factors that increase the chance of surviving submersion without permanent injury are a briefer duration of submersion; colder water temperature; younger age; absence of underlying medical conditions, secondary trauma, and aspiration of particulate matter or chemicals; and, most importantly, more rapid institution of resuscitation. Survival may be possible in cold water submersion that lasts > 1 h, especially among children; thus, even patients with prolonged submersion are vigorously resuscitated.

Treatment aims to correct cardiac arrest, hypoxia, hypoventilation, hypothermia, and other physiologic insults. If the patient is apneic, rescue breathing is started immediately—in the water, if necessary. If spinal immobilization is necessary, it is done in a neutral position and rescue breathing is performed using a jaw thrust without head tilt or chin lift. If necessary, cardiac compression is started followed by advanced cardiac life support (see p. 532); oxygenation, endotracheal intubation, or both are performed as soon as possible. Hypothermic patients are warmed as soon as possible (see p. 2612).

All hypoxic or moderately symptomatic patients are hospitalized. In the hospital, supportive treatment continues, aimed primarily at achieving acceptable arterial O_2 and CO_2 levels. Mechanical ventilation may be necessary. One hundred percent O_2 is given; the concentration is titrated lower based on the ABG results. Positive end-expiratory pressure (see p. 547) or intermittent positive pressure ventilation may be necessary to help expand or maintain patency of alveoli to maintain adequate oxygenation; pulmonary support may be necessary for hours or days. Nebulized β_2-agonists may help reduce bronchospasm and wheezing. Patients with bacterial pneumonia are treated with antibiotics directed at organisms identified or suspected based on results of sputum analysis or blood cultures. Corticosteroids are not used.

Fluids or electrolytes are rarely required to correct significant electrolyte imbalances. Fluid restriction is rarely indicated, even if pulmonary or cerebral edema occurs. For prolonged brain hypoxia, treatment is similar to that for brain hypoxia after cardiac arrest (see Neurologic Support on p. 539).

Patients with mild symptoms and normal oxygenation can be observed in the emergency department for several hours. If symptoms resolve and oxygenation remains normal, they can be discharged with instructions to return if symptoms recur.

Prevention

Use of alcohol or drugs, a major risk factor, should be avoided before and during swimming, boating, and when supervising children around water.

Swimmers should be accompanied by an experienced swimmer or swim only in guarded areas. Swimming should stop if the person looks or feels very cold, because hypothermia may impair judgment. Ocean swimmers should learn to escape rip currents by swimming parallel to the beach rather than toward the beach.

Children must wear flotation devices when in or near water. They must be supervised by an adult when around water, including beaches, pools, and ponds; infants and toddlers should also be supervised, ideally within arm's length, when near toilets and bathtubs. Adults should remove water from containers such as pails and buckets immediately after use. Swimming pools should be surrounded with a locked fence ≥ 1.5 m in height.

When in boats, wearing flotation devices is encouraged for all people and required for non-swimmers and small children. The debilitated, the elderly, and people with seizure disorders or other medical conditions that can alter consciousness require particular care when swimming or boating.

Community swimming areas need to be supervised by trained lifeguards. Comprehensive community prevention programs should target high-risk groups, teach children to swim as early as possible, and teach as many adolescents and adults CPR as possible.

323 INJURY DURING DIVING OR WORK IN COMPRESSED AIR

More than 1000 diving-related injuries occur annually in the US; > 10% are fatal. Similar injuries can befall workers in tunnels or caissons, in which pressurized air is used to exclude water from work sites. Many injuries are related to high pressure, which, at depth or in a caisson, results from the water weight above plus the atmospheric pressure at the surface. At a depth of 33 ft (10 m), seawater exerts a pressure equivalent to standard sea level atmospheric pressure, which is 14.7 lb/sq in, 760 mm Hg, or 1 atmosphere absolute (atm abs); thus, the total pressure at that depth is 2 atm abs. Every additional 33 ft of descent adds 1 atm.

The volume of gases in body compartments is inversely related to external pressure; an increase or a decrease in gas volume due to pressure change exerts direct physical forces that can disrupt various body tissues (barotrauma). The amount of gas dissolved in the bloodstream increases as ambient pressure increases. Increased gas content can cause injury directly (eg, nitrogen narcosis, O_2 toxicity) or indirectly during ascent when decompression of the supersaturated bloodstream releases N_2 bubbles (decompression sickness). Arterial gas embolism can result from barotrauma or decompression. For other diving-related injuries (eg, drowning, hypothermia, trauma), see elsewhere in THE MANUAL.

Physicians caring for patients with diving or compressed air injuries may contact the Divers Alert Network (919-684-8111; www.diversalertnetwork.org).

BAROTRAUMA

Barotrauma is tissue injury caused by a pressure-related change in body compartment gas volume; it affects air-containing areas, including lungs, ears, sinuses, GI tract, air spaces in tooth fillings, and space contained by the diving face mask. Symptoms may include ear pain, vertigo, hearing loss, sinus pain, epistaxis, and abdominal pain. Dyspnea and loss of consciousness are life threatening and may result from alveolar rupture and pneumothorax. Diagnosis is clinical but sometimes requires imaging tests. Treatment generally is supportive but may include decongestants and analgesics for ear and sinus barotrauma or O_2 and chest tube placement for pneumothorax. If arterial gas embolism accompanies lung barotrauma, recompression therapy (in a hyperbaric chamber) is needed. Proper diving safety techniques and prophylactic use of decongestants may reduce incidence of barotrauma.

Barotrauma risk is greatest from the surface to 30 ft; risk is increased by any condition that can interfere with equilibration of pressure (eg, sinus congestion, eustachian tube blockage, structural anomaly, infection) in the air-containing spaces of the body. Ear barotrauma constitutes about ⅔ of all diving injuries. If a diver inspires even a single breath of air or other gas at depth and does not let it escape freely during ascent, the expanding gas may overinflate the lungs.

Symptoms, Signs, and Diagnosis

Manifestations depend on the affected area; all occur almost immediately when pressure changes. Some nonfatal disorders, if they occur at depth, may be disabling or disorienting and thus lead to drowning. Diagnosis is primarily clinical; imaging tests can sometimes confirm it.

Pulmonary barotrauma: During very deep breath-hold diving, compression of the lungs during descent may rarely lead to a decrease in volume below residual volume, causing mucosal edema, vascular engorgement, and hemorrhage, which manifest clinically as dyspnea and hemoptysis on ascent.

When people are breathing compressed air, an increase in lung volume due to ascending too rapidly or not exhaling properly can cause overexpansion and alveolar rupture, leading to pneumothorax (causing dyspnea, chest pain, and unilateral decrease in breath sounds) or pneumomediastinum (causing sensation of fullness in the chest, neck pain, pleuritic chest pain that may radiate to the shoulders, dyspnea, coughing, hoarseness, and dysphagia). Tension pneumothorax, although rare with barotrauma, can cause hypotension, distended neck veins, hyperresonance to percussion, and tracheal deviation. If pneumomediastinum occurs, crepitation in the neck, due to associated subcutaneous emphysema, may be present, and a crackling sound may be heard over the heart during systole (Hamman's sign). Alveolar rupture often allows air into the pulmonary venous circulation with subsequent arterial gas embolism (see p. 2622).

The above symptoms require a neurologic examination to look for signs of cerebral injury due to gas embolism. If no neurologic injury is found, upright chest x-ray is done to look for signs of pneumothorax or pneumomediastinum (radiolucent band along the cardiac border). If chest x-ray is negative but there is strong clinical suspicion, helical CT, which may be more sensitive than plain film x-rays, may be diagnostic.

Ear barotrauma (ear squeeze): Diving can affect the external, middle, and inner ear. Typically, the diver experiences ear fullness and pain during descent; if pressure is not quickly equilibrated, middle ear hemorrhage or tympanic membrane rupture may occur. On examination of the ear canal, the tympanic membrane may show congestion, hemotympanum, and lack of mobility during air insufflation with a pneumatic otoscope; conduction hearing loss is usually present.

Inner ear barotrauma often involves rupture of the round or oval window, which causes tinnitus, sensorineural hearing loss, vertigo, nausea, and vomiting. The resulting labyrinthine fistula and perilymph leakage can permanently damage the inner ear. Patients should be referred for formal audiometry. Neurologic examination should focus on vestibular testing (see p. 780).

Sinus barotrauma (sinus squeeze): Barotrauma most often affects the frontal sinuses, followed by the ethmoid and maxillary sinuses. Divers experience mild pressure to severe pain, with a feeling of congestion in the involved sinus compartments during ascent or descent and sometimes epistaxis. Pain can be severe, sometimes accompanied by facial tenderness on palpation. Rarely, the sinus may rupture and cause pneumocephalus with facial or oral pain, nausea, vertigo, or headache. Physical examination may detect tenderness in the sinuses or nasal hemorrhage. Diagnosis is clinical. Imaging (eg, plain x-rays, CT) is not necessary, although CT is useful if sinus rupture is suspected.

Dental barotrauma (tooth squeeze): During descent or ascent, pressure in the air spaces at the roots of infected teeth or adjacent to fillings can change rapidly and cause pain or tooth damage. The affected tooth may be tender when percussed with a tongue blade. Diagnosis is primarily clinical.

Mask barotrauma (mask squeeze): If the pressure in the space behind the face mask is not equalized during descent, the resulting relative vacuum can lead to local pain, conjunctival hemorrhage, and ecchymosed skin where the mask touches the face. Diagnosis is clinical.

Eye barotrauma (eye squeeze): Small air bubbles trapped behind hard contact lenses can damage the eye and cause soreness, decreased visual acuity, and a halo effect around lights. Diagnosis is clinical, but a screening ophthalmic examination should be done to rule out other causes.

GI barotrauma (gut squeeze): Breathing improperly from a regulator or using ear and sinus pressure-equalization techniques may cause divers to swallow small amounts of air during a dive. This air expands during ascent, causing abdominal fullness, cramps, pain, belching, and flatulence; these symptoms are self-limited and require no testing. GI rupture rarely occurs, manifesting with severe abdominal pain and tenderness with rebound and guarding. If these signs are present, immediate upright abdominal and chest x-rays or CT are done to detect free air.

Prognosis and Treatment

Most barotrauma injuries resolve spontaneously and require only symptomatic treatment and outpatient follow-up. Potentially life-threatening barotrauma emergencies are those involving alveolar or GI rupture, particularly in patients who present with neurologic symptoms, pneumothorax, peritoneal signs, or abnormal vital signs. Initial stabilizing treatment includes high-flow 100% O_2, IV access, and intubation if respiratory failure is considered imminent. Positive pressure ventilation may cause or exacerbate pneumothorax.

Patients with neurologic symptoms or other evidence of arterial gas embolism are immediately transported to a recompression chamber for treatment (see p. 2626). If patients with suspected pneumothorax are hemodynamically unstable or have signs of tension pneumothorax, immediate chest decompression (see p. 498) is done with a large-bore needle placed into the 2nd intercostal space in the midclavicular line, followed by tube thoracostomy. If a smaller pneumothorax is present and there is no sign of hemodynamic or respiratory instability, the pneumothorax may resolve when high-flow 100% O_2 is given for 24 to 48 h. If this treatment is ineffective or if a larger pneumothorax is present, tube thoracostomy is done (see p. 380).

No specific treatment is required for pneumomediastinum; symptoms usually resolve spontaneously within hours to days. After a few hours of observation, most patients can be treated as outpatients; high-flow 100% O_2 is recommended to hasten resorption of extra-alveolar gas in these patients. Rarely, mediastinotomy is required to relieve tension pneumomediastinum.

Patients with GI rupture require aggressive fluid resuscitation, broad-spectrum antibiotic therapy (eg, imipenem 500 mg IV q 6 h), and immediate surgical consultation for possible exploratory laparotomy.

Medical treatment for sinus and middle ear barotrauma is identical. Decongestants (oxymetazoline 0.05%, 2 sprays each nostril bid for 3 to 5 days; pseudoephedrine 60 to 120 mg po bid to qid up to a maximum of 240 mg/day for 3 to 5 days) can open occluded chambers. Severe cases can be treated with nasal corticosteroids. Performing the Valsalva maneuver immediately after nasal spray therapy may help distribute the decongestant into the occluded chamber. Pain can be controlled with NSAIDs or opioids. If bleeding or evidence of effusion is present, antibiotics are given (eg, amoxicillin 500 mg po q 12 h for 10 days; trimethoprim-sulfamethoxazole 1 double-strength tablet po bid for 10 days). For middle ear barotrauma, some physicians also advocate a short course of oral corticosteroids (prednisone 60 mg po once/day for 6 days, then tapered over 7 to 10 days).

Surgery (eg, tympanotomy for direct repair of a ruptured round or oval window, myringotomy to drain fluid from the middle ear, sinus decompression) may be necessary for serious inner or middle ear or sinus injuries. Referral to an otorhinolaryngologist is indicated for severe or persistent symptoms.

Prevention

Ear barotrauma may be avoided by frequently swallowing or exhaling against pinched nostrils to open the eustachian tubes and equalize pressure between the middle ear and the environment. Pressure within the face mask is equalized by exhaling from the nose into the mask. Pressure behind ear plugs and goggles cannot be equalized, so these devices should not be used for diving. Also, prophylaxis with pseudoephedrine (60 to 120 mg po bid or qid up to a maximum of 240 mg/day), beginning 12 to 24 h before a dive, can reduce the incidence of ear and sinus barotrauma. Diving should not be done if congestion does not resolve or if a URI or uncontrolled allergic rhinitis is present.

Patients with pulmonary blebs, Marfan syndrome, or COPD are at very high risk of pneumothorax and should not dive or work in areas of compressed air. Patients with asthma may be at risk of lung barotrauma, but many with asthma can dive safely after they are evaluated and treated appropriately.

Patients treated for diving-related injuries should not return to diving until they have consulted with a diving medicine specialist.

For prevention of other diving injuries, see p. 2627.

ARTERIAL GAS EMBOLISM

(Air Embolism)

Arterial gas embolism is a potentially catastrophic event that occurs when gas bubbles enter or form in the arterial vasculature and occlude blood flow, causing organ ischemia. Arterial gas embolism can cause CNS injury with rapid loss of consciousness, other CNS manifestations, or both; it also may affect other organs. Diagnosis is clinical and may be corroborated by imaging tests. Treatment is immediate recompression.

Gas emboli may enter the arterial circulation from ruptured alveoli after lung barotrauma, from within the arterial circulation itself in severe decompression sickness, or may migrate from the venous circulation (venous gas embolism) either via a right-to-left shunt (patent foramen ovale, atrial septal defect) or by overwhelming the filtering capacity of the lungs. Venous gas embolism that does not enter the arterial circulation is less serious. Although cerebral embolism is considered the most serious manifestation, arterial gas embolism can cause significant ischemia in other organs (eg, spinal cord, heart, skin, kidneys, spleen, GI tract).

Symptoms and Signs

Symptoms occur within a few minutes of surfacing and may include altered mental status, hemiparesis, focal motor or sensory deficits, seizures, loss of consciousness, apnea, and shock; death may follow. Signs of pulmonary barotrauma (see p. 2620) or type II decompression sickness (see p. 2624) may also be present.

Other symptoms may result from arterial gas embolism in coronary arteries (eg, arrhythmias, MI, cardiac arrest), skin (eg, cyanotic marbling of the skin, focal pallor of the tongue), or kidneys (eg, hematuria, proteinuria, renal failure).

Diagnosis

Diagnosis is primarily clinical, with a high level of suspicion if a diver loses consciousness during or immediately after ascent. Confirming the diagnosis is difficult because air may be reabsorbed from the affected artery before testing. However, imaging techniques that can corroborate the diagnosis include echocardiography (showing air in the ventricles), ventilation-perfusion scan (showing results consistent with pulmonary emboli), chest CT angiography (showing air in the pulmonary veins), and head CT (showing intraparenchymal gas and diffuse edema). Sometimes decompression sickness is similar (for a comparison of features, see TABLE 323–1).

Treatment

A diver thought to have gas embolism should be recompressed promptly (see p. 2626).

TABLE 323–1. COMPARISON OF GAS EMBOLISM AND DECOMPRESSION SICKNESS

FEATURE	GAS EMBOLISM	DECOMPRESSION SICKNESS
Symptoms and signs	Common: Unconsciousness, often with seizures (*any unconscious diver should be assumed to have gas embolism and should be recompressed promptly*) Less common: Milder cerebral manifestations, mediastinal or subcutaneous emphysema, and pneumothorax	Extremely variable—the bends (pain, most often in or near a joint), neurologic manifestations of almost any type or degree, and the chokes (respiratory distress followed by circulatory collapse—*an extreme emergency*), occurring alone or with other symptoms
Onset	Sudden onset during or shortly after surfacing	Gradual or sudden onset after surfacing or up to 24 h after dives* of > 33 ft (> 10 m) or hyperbaric exposures of > 2 atm abs
Proximate cause	Usual: Breath holding or airway obstruction during ascent, even from a few feet of depth, or decompression from increased pressure	Usual: Diving or hyperbaric exposure beyond no-stop limits and without appropriate decompression stops Occasional: Diving or hyperbaric exposure within no-stop limits or with appropriate decompression stops; low-pressure exposure (eg, loss of cabin pressure in aircraft at altitude)
Mechanism	Usual: Overinflation of lungs causing entry of free gas into pulmonary vessels followed by embolization of cerebral vessels Occasional: Pulmonary, cardiac, or systemic circulatory obstruction by free gas from any source	Formation of bubbles from excess dissolved gas in blood or tissue when external pressure decreases
Emergency treatment	Essential emergency care (eg, airway patency, hemostasis, cardiopulmonary resuscitation) Prompt transport to nearest recompression chamber Horizontal position 100% O_2 by close-fitting mask Fluids orally if patient is conscious; otherwise, IV	Same

atm abs = atmospheres absolute.

*Repeat dives are frequently involved.

Transport to a recompression chamber takes precedence over nonessential procedures. Transport by air may be justified if it saves significant time, but exposure to reduced pressure at altitude must be minimized.

Before transport, high-flow 100% O_2 enhances N_2 washout by widening the N_2 pressure gradient between the lungs and the circulation, thus accelerating reabsorption of embolic bubbles. Patients should remain in a supine position. Mechanical ventilation, vasopressors, and volume resuscitation are used as needed. Placing patients in the left lateral decubitus position (Durant's maneuver) or Trendelenburg position is no longer recommended.

DECOMPRESSION SICKNESS

(Caisson Disease; The Bends)

Decompression sickness occurs when rapid pressure reduction (eg, during ascent from a dive, exit from a caisson or hyperbaric chamber, or ascent to altitude) causes gas previously dissolved in blood or tissues to form bubbles in blood vessels. Symptoms typically include pain, neurologic symptoms, or both. Severe cases can be fatal. Diagnosis is clinical. Definitive treatment is recompression therapy. Proper diving techniques are essential for prevention.

Henry's law states that the solubility of a gas in a liquid is directly proportional to the pressure exerted on the gas and liquid. Thus, the amount of inert gases (eg, N_2, helium) taken up in the blood and tissues increases at higher pressure. During ascent, when the surrounding pressure decreases, bubbles may form. The liberated gas bubbles can arise in any tissue and cause local symptoms, or they can travel via the blood to distant organs. Bubbles cause symptoms by blocking vessels, rupturing or compressing tissue, or activating clotting and inflammatory cascades. Because N_2 dissolves readily in fat, tissues with a high lipid content (eg, in the CNS) are particularly susceptible.

Decompression sickness occurs in about 2 to 4/10,000 dives. Risk factors include cold-temperature dives, stress, fatigue, asthma, dehydration, obesity, older age, exercise, flying after diving, rapid ascents, and prolonged or deep dives. Because excess N_2 remains dissolved in body tissues for at least 12 h after each dive, repeated dives within 1 day require special techniques to determine proper decompression procedures and are most likely to cause decompression sickness.

Classification: Generally, there are 2 types. Type I, which involves muscles, skin, and lymphatics, is milder and not typically life threatening. Type II is serious, is sometimes life threatening, and affects various organ systems. The spinal cord is especially vulnerable; other vulnerable areas include the brain, respiratory system (eg, pulmonary emboli), and circulatory system (eg, heart failure, cardiogenic shock). "The bends" refers to local joint or muscle pain due to decompression sickness but is often used as a synonym for any component of the disorder.

Symptoms and Signs

Severe symptoms may manifest within minutes of surfacing, but in most patients, symptoms begin gradually, sometimes with a prodrome of malaise, fatigue, anorexia, and headache. Symptoms occur within 1 h of surfacing in about 50% of patients and by 6 h in 90%. Rarely, symptoms can manifest 24 to 48 h after surfacing, particularly after exposure to altitude after diving.

Type I decompression sickness typically causes progressively worsening pain in the joints (typically elbows and shoulders), back, and muscles; the pain intensifies during movement and is described as "deep" and "boring." Other symptoms include lymphadenopathy, skin mottling, itching, and rash.

Type II decompression sickness typically manifests with paresis, numbness and tingling, neuropraxia, difficulty urinating, and loss of bowel or bladder control. Headache and fatigue may be present but are nonspecific. Dizziness, tinnitus, and hearing loss may result if the inner ear is affected. Severe symptoms include seizures, slurred speech, vision loss, confusion, and coma. Death can occur. The chokes (respiratory decompression sickness) is a rare but grave manifestation; symptoms include shortness of breath, chest pain, and cough. Massive bubble embolization of the pulmonary vascular tree can result in rapid circulatory collapse and death.

Dysbaric osteonecrosis is a late manifestation of decompression sickness. It is an insidious form of aseptic bone necrosis caused by prolonged or closely repeated exposures to pressurized areas (typically in people working in compressed air and in deep commercial rather than recreational divers). Deterioration of shoulder and hip articular surfaces can cause chronic pain and severe disability.

Diagnosis

Diagnosis is clinical. CT and MRI may show brain or spinal cord abnormalities but are not sensitive, and treatment should usually begin based on clinical suspicion. Sometimes arterial gas embolism is similar (for a comparison of features, see TABLE 323–1).

For dysbaric osteonecrosis, plain x-rays may show joint degeneration, which cannot be distinguished from that caused by other joint disorders; MRI is usually diagnostic.

Treatment

About 80% of patients recover completely.

Initially, high-flow 100% O_2 enhances N_2 washout by widening the N_2 pressure gradient between the lungs and the circulation, thus accelerating reabsorption of embolic bubbles.

Recompression therapy (see p. 2626) is indicated for all patients except perhaps those whose symptoms are limited to itching, skin mottling, and fatigue; they should be observed for deterioration. Other patients are transported to a suitable recompression facility. Because time to treatment is a main determinant of outcome, transport should not be delayed even in cases that appear mild or for performance of nonessential procedures. If air evacuation is required, low altitude (eg, ground-level cabin pressure or < 2000 ft [< 609 m] in unpressurized aircraft) is preferred. Commercial airlines typically have a cabin pressure equivalent to 8000 ft (2438 m), which may exacerbate symptoms. Flying in commercial aircraft shortly after a dive can precipitate symptoms.

Prevention

Significant bubble formation can usually be avoided by limiting the depth and duration of dives to a range that does not need decompression stops during ascent (called no-stop limits) or by ascending with decompression stops as specified in published guidelines (eg, the decompression table in the *US Navy Diving Manual*; see www.diverlink.com/library/usn). Many divers now wear a portable dive computer that continually tracks depth and time at depth and calculates a decompression schedule. Also, many divers make a safety stop for a few minutes at about 15 ft (4.6 m) below the surface.

However, about 50% of cases develop after appropriately identified no-stop dives, and the incidence of decompression sickness has not decreased despite widespread use of dive computers. The reason may be that published tables and computer programs do not completely account for the variation in risk factors among divers or that people do not obey the recommendations precisely.

GAS TOXICITY

Various physiologic (eg, O_2, N_2, CO_2) and nonphysiologic (eg, carbon monoxide) gases can cause symptoms during diving.

O_2 toxicity: O_2 toxicity typically occurs when the partial pressure of O_2 reaches 1.6 atmospheres, equivalent to about 200-ft depth when air is breathed. Symptoms include paresthesias, focal seizures, vertigo, nausea, vomiting, and constricted vision. About 10% of patients have generalized seizures or syncope, which typically results in drowning.

Nitrogen narcosis: When compressed air is breathed at depths of > 100 ft (> 30 m), the elevated partial pressure of N_2 exerts an anesthetic-like effect similar to that of nitrous oxide. Nitrogen narcosis ("rapture of the deep") causes symptoms and signs similar to those of alcohol intoxication (eg, impaired intellectual and neuromuscular performance, changes in behavior and personality). Impairment of judgment can lead to drowning. Hallucinations and loss of consciousness can occur at depths of > 300 ft (> 91 m).

Because divers recover rapidly during ascent, diagnosis is clinical. Treatment entails immediate but controlled ascent. Nitrogen narcosis can be prevented by using helium to dilute O_2 for deep diving because helium lacks the anesthetic properties of N_2. However, using pure helium/O_2 mixtures increases the risk of developing high-pressure neurologic syndrome (see p. 2626).

CO_2 poisoning: Hypoventilation may be caused by inadequate respiratory effort, a tight wetsuit, overexertion, regulator malfunction, deep diving, or air supply contamination by exhaled gases. Hypoventilation can increase blood CO_2 levels and cause shortness of breath and sedation. Severe cases can cause nausea, vomiting, dizziness, headache, rapid breathing, flushing, confusion, seizures, and loss of consciousness.

Mild cases are suspected if divers frequently have dive-related headaches or low air-use rates. Hypoventilation usually resolves during ascent; thus, ABG testing after a dive typically does not detect any increase in CO_2 levels. Treatment is gradual ascent and termination of the diving exercise or correction of the precipitating cause.

Carbon monoxide poisoning (see also p. 2662)**:** Carbon monoxide can enter a diver's air if the air compressor intake valve is placed too close to engine exhaust or if the lubricating oil in a malfunctioning compressor becomes hot enough to partially combust ("flashing"), producing carbon monoxide.

Symptoms include nausea, headache, weakness, clumsiness, and mental changes. Severe cases can cause seizures, syncope, or coma. Diagnosis is by detecting an elevated carboxyhemoglobin (COHb) level in blood; pulse oximetry readings are nondiagnostic and usually normal because pulse oximeters cannot distinguish between oxyhemoglobin and COHb. The diver's air supply can be tested for carbon monoxide.

Treatment is with high-flow 100% O_2, best given via a nonrebreather mask, which decreases the half-life of COHb from 4 to 8 h in room air to 40 to 80 min. For severe cases, hyperbaric O_2 therapy is indicated to improve tissue oxygenation and further decrease the half-life of COHb to 15 to 30 min.

High-pressure neurologic syndrome: A poorly understood syndrome of neuromuscular and cerebral abnormalities can develop at ≥ 600 ft (≥ 180 m), particularly when the diver is compressed rapidly while breathing helium/O_2 mixtures. Symptoms include nausea, vomiting, fine tremors, incoordination, dizziness, fatigue, somnolence, myoclonic jerking, stomach cramps, and decrements in intellectual and psychomotor performance. Diagnosis is clinical.

RECOMPRESSION THERAPY

(Hyperbaric O_2 Therapy)

Recompression therapy is administration of 100% O_2 for several hours in a sealed chamber pressurized to > 1 atm, gradually lowered to atmospheric pressure. In divers, this therapy is used primarily for decompression sickness and arterial gas embolism. A shorter time to start of therapy is associated with a better patient outcome. Untreated pneumothorax requires chest tube placement before or during recompression therapy.

The goals of recompression therapy are to increase O_2 solubility and delivery, increase N_2 washout, decrease gas bubble size, and, for the rare case of diving-related carbon monoxide poisoning, decrease the half-life of carboxyhemoglobin and reduce ischemia. Hyperbaric O_2 therapy is also used for several general medical disorders unrelated to diving (see TABLE 323–2).

Because recompression is relatively well tolerated, it should be started if there is any likelihood that it would promote recovery; recompression may help even if started up to 48 h after surfacing.

TABLE 323–2. HYPERBARIC O_2 THERAPY*

SUPPORTING EVIDENCE	DISORDERS
Good	Arterial gas embolism
	Carbon monoxide poisoning (severe)
	Clostridial infection
	Decompression sickness
	Osteoradionecrosis
	Poorly healing skin grafts
Some	Anemia (severe) with hemorrhagic shock
	Burns
	Intracranial abscess with actinomycosis
	Necrotizing fasciitis
	Radiation soft-tissue injury
	Refractory osteomyelitis
	Traumatic crush injury and compartment syndrome
	Wound healing in ischemic limbs
Little or none	Dementia
	Multiple sclerosis

*Hyperbaric O_2 therapy (HBO) is the mainstay of treatment for diving-related decompression injury and arterial gas embolism. It is also tried for many conditions, including medical disorders, but its efficacy is more strongly established for some conditions than others. Relative contraindications include chronic lung disorders, sinus problems, seizure disorders, and claustrophobia. Pregnancy is not a contraindication. In the US, HBO chambers can be located by calling the Divers Alert Network (919-684-8111; www.diversalertnetwork.org).

Recompression chambers are either multiplace, with space for one or more patients on a gurney and for a medical attendant, or monoplace, with space for only a patient. Although monoplace chambers are less expensive, a patient cannot be accessed during recompression; their use for critically ill patients, who may require intervention, can be risky.

Information regarding the location of the nearest recompression chamber, the most rapid means of reaching it, and the most appropriate source to consult by telephone should be known by most divers, medical staff members, and rescue and police personnel in popular diving areas. Such information is also available from the Divers Alert Network

TABLE 323–3. SPECIFIC MEDICAL CONTRAINDICATIONS TO DIVING

CONTRAINDICATION	SPECIFIC EXAMPLES OR ADVERSE EFFECTS
Lung disorder	Active asthma, COPD, cystic fibrosis, bronchiectasis, interstitial lung disease, history of spontaneous pneumothorax
Cardiovascular disorder	History of significant ventricular arrhythmias, intracardiac shunt, heart failure, significant coronary artery disease
Psychologic disorder	Panic or phobia
Structural disorder	Unrepaired inguinal hernia
Neurologic disorder	Seizure disorder, syncope
Metabolic disorder	Insulin-dependent diabetes mellitus, gross obesity
No equilibration of gases between body compartments	Lung cysts, perforated tympanic membrane, upper respiratory infection, allergic rhinitis
Pregnancy	Increase in incidence of birth defects and fetal death
Habitual air-swallowing	GI overinflation during ascent due to swallowing pressurized air at depth
Poor exercise tolerance	—
Severe gastroesophageal reflux	Aggravated by loss of gravity effect on abdomen when submerged
Children < 10 yr	—

(919-684-8111; www.diversalertnetwork.org) 24 h/day; the Undersea and Hyperbaric Medical Society (www.uhms.org) is another invaluable information source.

Recompression protocols: Pressure and duration of treatment ("dive") are usually decided by a hyperbaric medicine specialist at the recompression facility. Treatments are given once or twice/day for 45 to 300 min until symptoms abate; 5- to 10-min air breaks are added to reduce risk of O_2 toxicity. Chamber pressure is usually maintained between 2.5 and 3.0 atm, but patients with life-threatening neurologic symptoms due to gas embolism may begin with an excursion to 6 atm to rapidly compress cerebral gas bubbles.

Although recompression therapy is usually done with 100% O_2 or compressed air, special gas mixtures (eg, helium/O_2 or N_2/O_2 in nonatmospheric proportions) may be indicated if the diver used an unusual gas mixture or if depth or duration of the dive was extraordinary. Specific protocol tables for treatment are included in the *US Navy Diving Manual* (see www.diverlink.com/library/usn).

Patients with residual neurologic deficits should be given repetitive, intermittent hyperbaric treatments and may require several days to reach maximum improvement.

Complications and contraindications: Recompression therapy can cause problems similar to those that occur with barotrauma (see p. 2620), including reversible myopia and ear and sinus barotrauma. Rarely, pulmonary barotrauma, pulmonary O_2 toxicity, hypoglycemia, or seizures result. Patients with a history of a seizure disorder, pneumothorax, or chest surgery are at highest risk of complications related to barotrauma or CNS O_2 toxicity. Sedatives and opioids may obscure symptoms and cause respiratory insufficiency; they should be avoided or used only in the lowest effective doses.

Relative contraindications include obstructive lung disorders, upper respiratory or sinus infections, recent ear surgery or injury, fever, and claustrophobia.

DIVING PRECAUTIONS AND PREVENTION OF DIVING INJURIES

Diving is a relatively safe recreational activity for healthy people who have been appropriately trained and educated. Diving safety courses offered by national diving organizations are widely available.

Diving safety: Incidence of barotrauma can be decreased through active equalization of various air spaces, including the face mask (by blowing out air from the nose into the mask) and the middle ear (by yawning, swallowing, or performing a Valsalva maneuver). Divers should avoid holding their breath and breathe normally during ascent, which should be no faster than 0.5 to 1 ft/sec, a rate that allows for gradual offloading of N_2 and emptying of air-filled spaces (eg, lungs, sinuses). Current recommendations also include a 3- to 5-min safety stop at 15 ft (4.6 m) for further equilibration. Also, divers should not fly for 15 to 18 h after diving.

Divers should be aware of and avoid certain diving conditions (eg, poor visibility, currents requiring excessive effort). Cold temperatures are a particular hazard because hypothermia can develop rapidly and affect judgment and dexterity or induce fatal cardiac arrhythmias in susceptible people. Diving alone is not recommended.

Illicit drugs and alcohol in any amount may have unpredictable or unanticipated effects at depth and should be strictly avoided. Prescription drugs rarely interfere with recreational diving, but if the disorder being treated is a contraindication to diving, the dive should not be pursued.

Contraindications to diving: Because diving can involve heavy exertion, divers should not have a significant cardiovascular or pulmonary disorder and should have above-average aerobic capacity. Disorders that can impair consciousness, alertness, or judgment generally prohibit diving. If there is any doubt as to whether diving is contraindicated by a specific disorder, a recognized expert should be consulted. For specific diving contraindications, see TABLE 323–3.

324 EXERCISE AND SPORTS INJURY

Regular exercise enhances health and sense of well-being. However, injury, particularly overuse injury, is a risk for people who exercise regularly. (For musculoskeletal injuries not particularly associated with sports, see Ch. 309 on p. 2557.)

EXERCISE

Exercise stimulates tissue change and adaptation, whereas rest and recovery allow such change and adaptation to occur. Recovery from exercise is as important as the exercise stimulus. Regular physical activity decreases the incidence of the major causes of death, improves functional status for sports and activities of daily living, and protects against injury. Specific exercises are also commonly prescribed to rehabilitate patients after MI, major surgery, and musculoskeletal injury. Regardless of indication, recommendations for exercise should be based on 2 principles:

- Goals for activity should be specific to the patient, accounting for motivation, needs, physical ability, and psychology, to maximize the likelihood of patient participation and desired outcome.
- Activity should be prescribed in a proper dose to achieve a desired effect; an exercise stimulus should be sufficient for the body to adapt to a higher state of function but not so great that it causes injury. Following the principle of diminishing returns, more activity is not always better; too little or too much may prevent achievement of desired outcomes.

A prescription for exercise should specify intensity (level of exertion), volume (amount of activity in a session), frequency (number of exercise sessions), and progressive overload (either the amount of increase in one or more of these elements over time, or the actual load). The balance of these elements depends on individual tolerance and physiologic principles (eg, as intensity increases, volume and frequency may need to decrease, whereas as volume increases, intensity may need to decrease). Intensity, volume, and frequency can be increased concurrently but only to a point because human tolerance to strain is finite. The objective is to discover the appropriate amount of exercise for optimal benefit in the context of patient goals. Fixed and traditional recommendations (eg, 3 sets of 10 to 12 repetitions, running 30 min 3 times/wk) are suboptimal and do not address individual and specific requirements.

Stretching and flexibility: Flexibility is important for safe, comfortable performance of physical activities. Specific flexibility exercises involve slowly and steadily stretching muscle groups without jerking or bouncing; these exercises can be performed before or after other forms of training or as a program itself, as occurs in yoga and Pilates sessions. Although stretching before exercise enhances mental preparedness, there is no evidence that stretching decreases risk of injury. However, there is no need to discourage preactivity stretching if patients enjoy it. General warming-up (eg, with low-intensity simulation of the exercise to be performed, jogging on the spot, calisthenics, or other light activities that increase core temperature) appears to be more effective than stretching for facilitating safe exercise. Stretching after exercise may be preferred because tissues stretch more effectively when warmed; this may be beneficial in strength training to improve range of motion and help relax muscles.

Aerobic exercise: Aerobic exercise is continuous, rhythmic physical activity that is maintained for a significant period; exertion occurs at a level that can be supported by aerobic metabolism (although brief periods of more intense exertion triggering anaerobic metabolism may be interspersed) continuously for at least 5 min as a starting point and increased slowly over time. Aerobic conditioning increases maximal O_2 uptake and cardiac output (mainly an increase in stroke volume), decreases resting heart rate, and reduces cardiac and all-cause mortality; however, too much activity causes excessive wear on the body and increases cellular oxidation. Examples of aerobic exercise include running, jogging, fast walking, swimming, bicycling, rowing, kayaking, skating, cross-country skiing, and using aerobic exercise machines (eg, treadmill, stair-climbing or elliptical machines).

Aerobic metabolism starts within 2 min of beginning activity, but more sustained effort is needed to achieve health benefits. The usual recommendation is to exercise ≥ 30 min/day at least 3 times/wk with a 5-min warm-up and a 5-min cool-down period, but this recommendation is based on convenience as much as evidence. Optimal aerobic conditioning can occur with as little as 10 to 15 min of activity per session 2 to 3 times/wk if interval cycling is used. In interval cycling, a person alternates short periods of moderate activity with intense exertion; in one regimen, about 90 sec of moderate activity (60 to 80% maximum heart rate [HR_{max}]) is alternated with about 20 to 30 sec of all-out sprint-type work (85 to 95% HR_{max} or as hard as the person can exert for that time). This regimen is more strenuous on joints and tissues and so should be implemented sporadically or alternated with more conventional, lower to moderate intensity exercise methods.

Resistance training machines or free weights can be used for aerobic exercise as long as a sufficient number of repetitions are done, rest between repetitions is minimal (20 to 60 sec), and intensity of effort is relatively high. In circuit training, the large muscles (of the legs, hips, back, and chest) are exercised followed by the smaller muscles (of the shoulders, arms, abdomen, and neck). Circuit training of only 15 to 20 min benefits the cardiovascular system more than jogging or using aerobic exercise machines for the same time because the workout is more intense.

Volume of aerobic exercise is graded simply by duration. Intensity is guided by heart rate. Target heart rate for appropriate intensity is 60 to 85% of a person's HR_{max} (the heart rate at peak O_2 consumption [VO_{2peak}], or the rate beyond which aerobic metabolism can no longer be sustained because O_2 is lacking and anaerobic metabolism begins). HR_{max} can be directly measured, or calculated as

$$HR_{max} = 220 - \text{age}$$

Alternatively, the Karvonen formula can be used to calculate target heart rate:

$$\text{Target heart rate} = [(0.50 \text{ to } 0.85) \times (HR_{max} - HR_{resting})] + HR_{resting}$$

However, the more athletic or deconditioned compared to average, the less accurate these formulas, making metabolic/VO_2 testing more valuable.

Chronologic should be distinguished from biologic age. Patients of any age who are less accustomed to aerobic exercise (less conditioned) reach the target heart rate much sooner and with less effort, necessitating briefer exercise periods, at least initially. Obese patients may be deconditioned and must move a larger body weight, causing heart rate to increase much faster and to a greater extent with less vigorous activity than in thinner people. Disorders and some drugs (eg, β-blockers) also modify the relationship between age and heart rate. For these groups, a target of 50 to 60% of HR_{max} is probably sufficient, at least initially.

Strength training: Strength (resistance) training involves forceful muscular contraction against a load—typically provided by free or machine weights. Such training increases muscle strength, endurance, and size and improves functional ability and aerobic performance; cardiovascular endurance and flexibility increase concurrently.

Volume typically is categorized in terms of amount of weight lifted and numbers of sets and repetitions. However, an equally important parameter is tension time, the total duration of lifting and lowering the weight in one set. Appropriate tension time may be about 60 sec for moderate conditioning and 90 to 120 sec for injury rehabilitation. For increasing strength, tension time is more important than number of repetitions, which can vary within tension time by technique and set duration. When a patient can achieve at least 60-sec tension time with good technique, resistance (weight) can be increased so that a tension time of at least 60 sec is tolerable at the next weight level. Number of sets is determined by intensity of the training.

Intensity is generally a subjective measure of perceived effort and how close a person comes to muscular fatigue in a given set (or exhaustion in a workout). Intensity may be characterized objectively by the amount of weight lifted expressed as a percentage of the person's maximum for one repetition (1 RM) of a given exercise; ie, for a person who can deadlift at most 100 kg one time, 75 kg is 75% RM. Generally, lifting < 30 to 40% RM provides minimal strength gain, although aerobic conditioning may occur with sufficient tension time and effort. Intensity is limited by patient motivation and tolerance; for many patients undergoing rehabilitation, discomfort, pain, and exercise inexperience result in less effort than may be possible or tolerated, so that more sets are required to derive equal benefit. However, continual high-intensity training is counterproductive, even for trained athletes; exercising to fatigue is not necessary to benefit significantly from strength training. Training intensity should vary on a regular basis to provide both a mental and physical hiatus.

Good technique is important for safety and involves avoidance of jerking or dropping weights, which can cause minor tissue injury due to sudden force, and controlled breathing, which prevents dizziness (and in extreme cases, fainting) that can occur with the Valsalva maneuver. Patients should exhale while lifting a weight and inhale when lowering a weight. If a movement is slow, such as lowering a weight for ≥ 5 sec, patients may need to breathe in and out more than once, but breathing should still be coordinated so that a final breath is taken in just before the lifting phase and released during lifting. BP increases during resistance training but returns to normal quickly after exercise; the increase is minimal when breathing technique is correct, no matter how hard a person exerts.

Balance training: Balance training involves challenging one's center of gravity by undertaking exercises in unstable environments, such as standing on one leg or using balance or wobble boards. Although specialized balance training can help some people with impaired proprioception, it often is misused to prevent falls in the elderly. For most elderly patients, a program of flexibility and strengthening exercises in a controlled environment (eg, slow movements using resistance exercise machines or rubber bands) is more effective. Such a program develops strength around the joints and helps patients hold body positions more effectively while standing and walking. If a person has difficulty standing and walking because of poor balance, more challenging balance tasks (eg, standing on a wobble board) are simply likely to facilitate injury and are contraindicated.

Hydration: Proper hydration is important, particularly when exertion is prolonged or in a hot environment. People should be well-hydrated prior to activity, drink fluids regularly during extended exertion, and replace any deficit remaining after activity. During exertion, about 120 to 240 mL ($\frac{1}{2}$ to 1 cup) q 15 to 20 min is reasonable depending on heat and exertion level; however, overhydration, which can cause hyponatremia and consequent seizures is to be avoided. Fluid deficit following exertion is calculated by comparing pre- and post-exercise body weight and replaced on a one-for-one basis (ie, 1 L for each kg lost, or 2 cups/lb). In most cases plain water is acceptable. Electrolyte-containing sports drinks may be preferred. However fluids with a carbohydrate content of >8% will cause a decrease in gastric emptying, accompanied by a slower fluid absorption rate. Often it is best to mix plain water with sports drinks at a 50:50 ratio to allow faster absorption of the glucose and electrolytes. Patients with findings suggesting heat illness (see p. 2606) or dehydration may require oral or IV electrolyte replacement.

SCREENING FOR SPORTS PARTICIPATION

(See also Ch. 82 on p. 766.)

Screening for all children and adults should include a thorough history and physical examination (including BP, and supine and standing cardiac auscultation). These measures aim to identify the rare, apparently healthy, young patient at high risk of life-threatening cardiac events (eg, those with hypertrophic cardiomyopathy or other structural heart disorders); a more practical objective is to facilitate participation by identifying existing injuries and disorders, optimizing treatments, and removing unnecessary restrictions.

Two at-risk populations are commonly overlooked: Boys who physically mature late are at greater risk of injury in contact sports with larger and stronger children, and overweight or obese people who participate in activities that require high agility are at greater risk of injury from sudden stops and starts because of their excess body weight.

Adolescents and young adults should be asked about use of illicit and performance-enhancing drugs (see www.usantidoping.org). In females, screening should detect delayed onset of menarche and presence of the female athlete triad (eating disorders, amenorrhea or other menstrual dysfunction, and diminished bone mineral density), which is becoming more common as more adolescent and young women engage in overly intensive physical activity and overly zealous loss of body fat.

Older adults beginning exercise should be asked about previous diagnosis of or symptoms suggesting coronary artery disease or arrhythmia and about arthritic disorders, particularly those involving major weight-bearing joints (eg, knees, ankles, hips). Other specific concerns are elevated serum cholesterol, obesity, hypertension, and a family history of coronary artery disease.

There are almost no absolute contraindications to sports participation. Exceptions in children include myocarditis, which increases risk of sudden cardiac death; acute splenic enlargement because splenic rupture is a risk; fever, which decreases exercise tolerance, increases risk of heat-related disorders, and may be a sign of serious illness; and possibly diarrhea because dehydration is a risk. Exceptions in adults include angina pectoris and recent (within 6 wk) MI. Contraindications are more commonly relative and lead to recommendations for precautions or for participation in some sports rather than others. For example, people with a history of multiple concussions should participate in noncollision sports; males with a single testis should wear a protective cup for most contact sports; people at risk of heat intolerance and dehydration (eg, those with diabetes or cystic fibrosis) should hydrate frequently during activity; and those with suboptimal seizure control should avoid swimming, weight lifting, and sports such as archery and riflery because of risk to others.

APPROACH TO SPORTS INJURIES

Sports participation always has a risk of injury. Most injuries (eg, fractures and dislocations—see p. 2557; concussions—see p. 2572) are not unique to athletics and can occur with routine activities or accidents (see also elsewhere in THE MANUAL).

Generally, mechanisms of sports injury can be divided into overuse, blunt trauma, and acute soft-tissue sprains and strains. For fractures and dislocations, see Ch. 309 on p. 2557.

Overuse is one of the most common causes of athletic injury; it can traumatize muscle, tendons, cartilage, ligaments, bursae, fascia, and bone in any combination. Risk of overuse injury depends on complex interactions between individual and extrinsic factors. Individual factors include muscle weakness and inflexibility, joint laxity, previous injury, bone malalignment, and limb asymmetries. Extrinsic factors include training errors (eg, exercise without sufficient recovery time, excess load, building one group of muscles without training the opposing group, and extensive use of the same movement patterns), environmental conditions (eg, excessive running on banked tracks or crowned roads), and training equipment characteristics (eg, unusual or unaccustomed motions, such as that on an elliptical trainer). Runners most often sustain injury after too rapidly increasing their intensity or length of workouts. Swimmers may be least prone to overuse injuries because buoyancy has protective effects, although they still are at risk, particularly in the shoulders, from which most movement occurs.

Blunt athletic trauma causes contusions, concussions, fractures, and other injuries. Mechanisms usually involve high-impact collisions with other athletes or objects (eg, being tackled in football or checked into the sideboards in hockey), falls, and direct blows (eg, in boxing and the martial arts).

Sprains and strains typically occur with sudden, forceful exertion, most commonly during running, particularly with sudden changes of direction. Such injuries also are common in strength training, when a person quickly drops or yanks at the load rather than moving slowly and smoothly.

Symptoms, Signs, and Diagnosis

Injury always causes pain, which ranges from mild to severe. Signs may be absent or may include any combination of soft-tissue edema, erythema, warmth, point tenderness, ecchymosis, and loss of mobility.

Diagnosis should include a thorough history and physical examination. History should focus on the motions and physical stresses of the activity, past injuries, timing of pain onset, and extent and duration of pain before, during, and after activity. Diagnostic testing (eg, x-ray, CT, MRI, bone scans) and referral to a specialist may be required.

Treatment

Immediate treatment of most acute sports injuries is rest, ice, compression, and elevation (RICE). Rest prevents further injury. Ice (or a commercial cold pack if correctly used; these packs can damage the skin) causes vasoconstriction and reduces soft-tissue swelling, inflammation, and pain. Compression and elevation reduce edema and pain. An elastic bandage can be wrapped around a tightly closed plastic bag containing ice to keep it in place; the bandage should not be wrapped too firmly which may cause swelling. Ice and elevation of the injured extremity should be used periodically throughout the initial 24 h after the acute injury.

Pain control usually involves use of NSAIDs. However, if pain persists after 72 h, referral to a specialist is recommended. For persistent pain, oral or injectable corticosteroids are sometimes used; they should be given only by a specialist and when necessary because corticosteroids can delay soft-tissue healing and sometimes weaken injured tendons and muscles.

In general, injured athletes should avoid the specific activity that caused the injury until after healing occurs; however, to minimize deconditioning, they can cross-train (ie, perform different or related exercises that do not cause reinjury or pain). Resumption of full activity should be gradual once pain subsides. Athletes should be placed in a graduated program to restore flexibility, strength, and endurance. They also need to feel psychologically ready before reengaging in an activity at full capacity and may benefit from motivational counseling.

Prevention

Exercise itself helps prevent injuries because tissues become more resilient and tolerant of the forces they experience during vigorous activities. Initially, exercise should be low in intensity to strengthen weak muscles, tendons, and ligaments. General warming up raises muscle temperature and makes muscles more pliable, stronger, and more resistant to injury; it also improves workout performance by enhancing mental and physical preparedness. Stretching elongates muscles so that they can develop greater force, although doing warm-up exercises with light weights also has the same effect. Cooling down can prevent dizziness and syncope after aerobic exercise and helps remove metabolic/exercise byproducts, such as lactic acid, from muscles and the bloodstream. Cooling down also helps decrease heart rate slowly and gradually to near-resting levels—an important effect for patients with heart disorders; cooling down does not prevent muscular soreness, which is caused by damage to muscle fibers, in subsequent days.

Injury due to excessive pronation (turning in or inversion of the foot during weight bearing) can be prevented with use of shoe inserts or orthotics (flexible or semirigid).

ROTATOR CUFF INJURY

Rotator cuff injury includes strain, tendinitis, and partial or complete tears.

The rotator cuff, consisting of the supraspinatus, infraspinatus, teres minor, and subscapularis (SITS) muscles, helps stabilize the humerus in the glenoid fossa of the scapula during many athletic overhead arm motions (eg, pitching, swimming, weightlifting, serving in racket sports). Disorders can involve strain, tendinitis, or a partial or complete tear.

Tendinitis typically results from impingement of the supraspinatus tendon between the humeral head and coracoacromial arch (the acromion, acromioclavicular joint, coracoid process, and coracoacromial ligament). This tendon is thought to be particularly susceptible because it has an undervascularized region near its insertion on the greater tuberosity. The resultant inflammatory reaction and edema further narrow the subacromial space, accelerating the process. If the process is not interrupted, tendinitis, fibrosis, and sometimes partial or complete tear may result. Degenerative rotator cuff tendinitis is common among older (> 40 yr) nonathletes for the same reason. Subacromial (subdeltoid) bursitis commonly results from rotator cuff injury.

Symptoms, Signs, and Diagnosis

Symptoms of bursitis include shoulder pain, especially with overhead activity, and weakness. The pain usually is worse between 80° and 120° (painful arc of motion) of shoulder abduction or flexion and is usually minimal or absent at < 80° or > 120°. Signs vary by severity. Incomplete tendon tears and tendinitis produce similar symptoms.

Diagnosis is by history and physical examination. The rotator cuff cannot be palpated directly, but it can be assessed indirectly by maneuvers that test specific muscles; significant pain or weakness is considered a positive result.

The supraspinatus is assessed by having the patient resist downward pressure on the arms held in forward flexion with the thumbs pointing downward ("empty can" test).

The infraspinatus and teres minor are assessed by having the patient resist external rotation pressure with the arms held at the sides with elbows flexed to 90°; this position isolates rotator cuff muscle function from that of other muscles such as the deltoid. Weakness during this test suggests significant rotator cuff dysfunction (eg, a complete tear).

The subscapularis is assessed by having the patient resist internal rotation pressure or by having the patient place the back of the hand on the back and then try to lift the hand off (lift-off test).

Other tests include the Apley scratch test, Neer test, and Hawkins test. The Apley scratch test checks shoulder range of motion by having the patient attempt to touch the opposite scapula: Reaching overhead, behind the neck, and to the opposite scapula with the tips of the fingers tests abduction and external rotation; reaching under, behind the back, and across to the opposite scapula with the back of the hand tests adduction and internal rotation. The Neer test checks for impingement of the rotator cuff tendons under the coracoacromial arch; it is done by placing the patient's arm in forced flexion (arm lifted overhead) with the arm fully pronated. The Hawkins test also checks for impingement; it is done by elevating the patient's arm to 90° while forcibly rotating the shoulder internally.

The acromioclavicular and sternoclavicular joints, cervical spine, biceps tendon, and scapula should be palpated to check for any tenderness or deformity and to exclude problems associated with those areas.

The neck always should be examined as part of any shoulder evaluation because pain can be referred to the shoulder from the cervical spine (particularly with C5 radiculopathy).

Suspected rotator cuff injury can be further evaluated with MRI, arthroscopy, or both.

Treatment

In most cases, rest and strengthening exercises are sufficient. Surgery may be necessary if the injury is severe (eg, a complete tear), particularly in a younger patient.

GLENOID LABRAL TEAR

The glenoid labrum usually tears as a result of a specific trauma such as a fall onto an outstretched arm. It causes pain during motion. Treatment is with physical therapy and sometimes surgery.

The shoulder (unlike the hip or elbow) is an inherently unstable joint; it has been likened to a golf ball sitting on a tee. To enhance structural stability, the glenoid (anatomically, a very shallow socket) is deepened by the labrum, which is a rubbery, fibrocartilaginous material attached around the lip of the glenoid. This structure can tear during athletics, especially during throwing sports, or as a result of blunt trauma when falling and landing on an outstretched upper extremity.

Diagnosis is usually based on the presence of pain deep in the shoulder during movement, especially when pitching a baseball.

This discomfort may be accompanied by a painful clicking sensation and a feeling of catching. A thorough shoulder and neck physical examination should be done initially, but referral to a specialist is frequently needed because more sophisticated diagnostic tests (eg, contrast-enhanced MRI) are often the only way to definitively identify the pathology.

If symptoms do not improve with physical therapy, and the diagnosis has been confirmed by MRI, surgical debridement or repair is the treatment of choice. This is usually done arthroscopically.

LATERAL EPICONDYLITIS

(Tennis Elbow)

Lateral epicondylitis results from inflammation and microtearing of fibers in the extensor tendons of the forearm; symptoms include pain at the lateral epicondyle of the elbow, which can radiate into the forearm.

Theories about the pathophysiology of lateral epicondylitis include nonathletic and occupational activities that require repetitive and forceful forearm supination and pronation, as well as overuse or weakness (or both) of the extensor carpi radialis brevis and longus muscles of the forearm, which originate from the lateral epicondyle of the elbow. For example, during a backhand return in racket sports such as tennis, the elbow and wrist are extended, and the extensor tendons, particularly the extensor carpi radialis brevis, can be damaged when they roll over the lateral epicondyle and radial head. Contributing factors include poor technique, weak shoulder and wrist muscles, a racket strung too tightly, an undersized grip, hitting heavy wet balls, and hitting off-center on the racket.

In resistance trainees, lateral epicondylitis is most noticeable during arm curls and various rowing and chin-up exercises for the back muscles, particularly when the hands are pronated. Injuries often are caused by overuse (too much activity or performing the same movements too often) or by muscle imbalance between the forearm extensors and flexors.

Symptoms, Signs, and Diagnosis

Pain initially occurs in the extensor tendons when the wrist is extended against resistance (eg, as in manual screw driving or hitting a backhand shot with a racket). Pain can extend from the lateral epicondyle to the mid forearm; with time, subperiosteal hemorrhage, calcification, spur formation on the lateral epicondyle, and, most importantly, tendon degeneration can occur.

Pain along the common extensor tendon when the fingers are extended against resistance and the elbow is held straight is diagnostic. Alternatively, the diagnosis is confirmed if the same pain occurs during the following maneuver: The patient sits on a chair with the elbow held straight, arm on a table, and hand held palm downward; the examiner places a hand firmly on top of that of the patient, who tries to raise the hand by bending the wrist.

Treatment

Treatment involves a 2-phase approach. Initially, rest, ice, NSAIDs, and stretching are used, occasionally with a cortisone injection into the painful area around the tendon. When the pain subsides, gentle resistive exercises of the extensor and flexor muscles in the forearm are done followed by eccentric and concentric resistive exercises. Activity that hurts when the wrist is extended or pronated should be avoided. Use of a tennis elbow brace is often advised. Adjusting the fit and type of racket used can also help prevent further injury.

Although surgery is not usually needed, surgical techniques to treat lateral epicondylitis involve removing scar and degenerative tissue from the involved extensor tendons at the elbow.

MEDIAL EPICONDYLITIS

(Golfer's Elbow)

Medial epicondylitis is inflammation of the flexor pronator muscle mass originating at the medial epicondyle of the elbow; it is much less common than lateral epicondylitis.

Medial epicondylitis is caused by any activity that places a valgus force on the elbow, as occurs during pitching, playing golf, serving a tennis ball (particularly with top spin, with a racket that is too heavy or too tightly strung or has an undersized grip, or with heavy balls), and throwing a javelin. Nonathletic activities that may cause medial epicondylitis include bricklaying, hammering, and typing.

Symptoms, Signs, and Diagnosis

The patient reports pain in the flexor pronator tendons (attached to the medial epicondyle) and in the medial epicondyle when the wrist is flexed or pronated against resistance.

To confirm the diagnosis, the examiner has the patient sit in a chair with the forearm resting on a table and the hand supinated. The patient tries to raise the fist by bending the wrist while the examiner holds it down. Pain on the medial epicondyle and in the flexor pronator tendons is diagnostic.

Treatment

Treatment is similar to that of lateral epicondylitis (see p. 2634). The patient should avoid any activity that causes pain when flexing or pronating the wrist. Initially, rest, ice, NSAIDs, and stretching are used, occasionally with a cortisone injection into the painful area around the tendon. When pain subsides, gentle resistive exercises of the extensor and flexor muscles of the forearm are done, followed by eccentric and concentric resistive exercises.

In general, surgery is considered only after 6 to 12 mo of failed conservative management. Surgical techniques to treat medial epicondylitis involve removing scar tissue and reattaching damaged tissues.

PIRIFORMIS SYNDROME

Piriformis syndrome is compression of the sciatic nerve by the piriformis muscle, causing pain.

The piriformis muscle extends from the pelvic surface of the sacrum to the upper border of the greater trochanter of the femur. During running or sitting, this muscle can compress the sciatic nerve at the site where it emerges from under the piriformis to pass over the hip rotator muscles.

Symptoms and Signs

A chronic nagging ache, pain, tingling, or numbness starts in the buttocks and can extend along the course of the sciatic nerve, down the entire back of the thigh and calf, and sometimes into the foot. Pain is usually chronic and worsens when the piriformis is pressed against the sciatic nerve (eg, while sitting on a toilet, a car seat, or a narrow bicycle seat or while running). Unlike piriformis pain, lumbar disk compression of the sciatic nerve (sciatica—see p. 327) is usually associated with low back pain, in addition to sciatic pain down the lower extremity.

Diagnosis

Diagnosis is by physical examination. Pain with forceful internal rotation of the flexed thigh (Freiberg's maneuver), abduction of the affected leg while sitting (Pace's maneuver), raising of the knee several centimeters off the table while lying on a table on the side of the unaffected leg (Beatty's maneuver), or pressure into the buttocks where the sciatic nerve crosses the piriformis muscle while the patient slowly bends to the floor (Mirkin test) is diagnostic. Imaging is not useful except to rule out other causes of sciatic compression. Differentiation from a lumbar disk disorder is sometimes difficult, and referral to a specialist may be needed.

Treatment

The patient should temporarily stop running, bicycling, or doing any activity that elicits pain. A patient whose pain is aggravated by sitting should stand up immediately or, if unable to do so, change positions to raise the painful area from the seat. Specific stretching exercises for the posterior hip and piriformis can be beneficial. Surgery is rarely warranted. A carefully directed corticosteroid injection near the site where the piriformis muscle crosses the sciatic nerve often helps.

ANTERIOR KNEE PAIN

Anterior knee pain is common among athletes.

Etiology

There are many causes, particularly in runners. Causes include subluxation of the patella (when bending the knee) during running; chondromalacia of the patella (softening of the knee cap cartilage—see p. 2382), which is one of the more common causes among younger running athletes; intra-articular pathology, such as meniscal tears and plicae (infolding of the normal synovial lining of the knee); fat pad inflammation; patellar tendinitis; stress fractures of the tibia; and malalignment of the lower

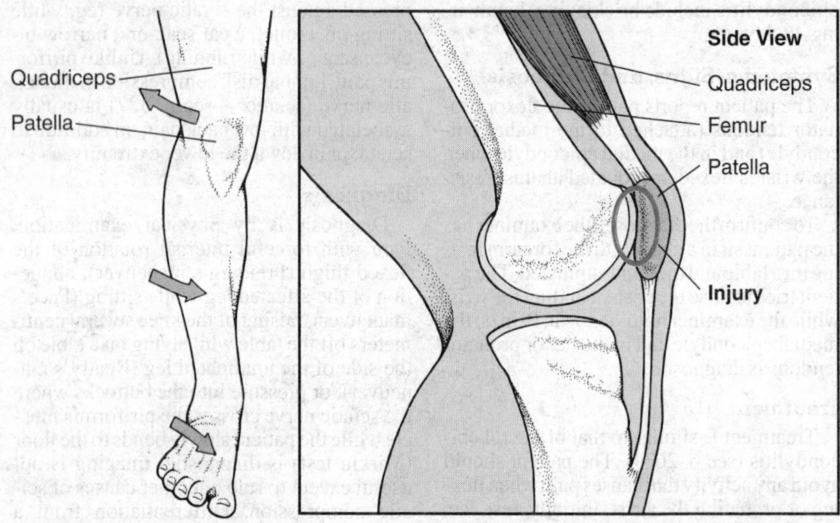

Fig. 324–1. Overpronation and patellofemoral syndrome. Overpronation of the foot causes the lower leg to twist inward, pulling the kneecap inward, while the quadriceps pulls the kneecap outward. As a result, the patella subluxates laterally and rubs against the lateral condyle of the femur, resulting in pain.

extremities. Knee pain may represent referred pain from the lumbar spine or hip or result from foot problems (eg, overpronation—see Fig. 324–1).

Evaluation

Diagnosis requires a thorough review of the injured athlete's training program, including a history of symptom onset and aggravating factors, and a complete lower-extremity examination (for knee examination, see p. 2570).

Chondromalacia is suggested by pain in the knee after running, especially on hills, and pain and stiffness after sitting for any length of time (positive movie sign). On examination, pain is typically reproduced by compression of the patella against the femur.

Treatment

Treatment of chondromalacia includes quadriceps strengthening exerciseswith balanced strengthening exercises for the hamstrings, use of arch supports if excessive pronation is a possible contributor, and use of NSAIDs.

For patellar subluxation, use of patella-stabilizing pads or braces may be necessary, especially in sports that require rapid, agile movements in various planes (eg, basketball, tennis).

SHIN SPLINTS

The term shin splints refers to nonspecific pain that occurs in the lower legs during running.

Repetitive impact forces during jogging or running often cause shin pain. Such pain sometimes results from a specific injury (eg, tibial stress fracture, exercise-induced compartment syndrome, tibial periostitis, excessive foot pronation), but often an exact cause cannot be identified. In such cases, the term "shin splints" is used.

Symptoms, Signs, and Diagnosis

Shin splint pain can occur in the anterior or posterior aspect of the leg and typically begins at the start of running activity but then lessens as running continues. Pain that persists during rest suggests another cause, such as stress fracture of the tibia.

On examination, severe point tenderness is usually present over the anterior compartment muscles and sometimes is accompanied by palpable bone pain.

X-rays are usually unremarkable, regardless of the cause. If a stress fracture is suspected, a bone scan may be necessary. Exercise-induced compartment syndrome is diagnosed by using a specialized manometer to document increased intra-compartmental pressure after exercise.

Treatment

Running must be stopped until it causes no pain. Early treatment is ice, NSAIDs, and stretching of the anterior and posterior calf muscles. During the rest phase of treatment, deconditioning can be minimized by encouraging the athlete to use cross-training techniques that do not require repetitive weight-bearing activity.

Once symptoms have resolved, it is advised that a return to running be gradual. Wearing supportive shoes with rigid heel counters and arch supports sometimes helps support the foot and ankle during running and can aid recovery and prevent further symptoms. Avoiding running on hard surfaces (eg, cement roads) can also help. Exercising the front of the calves by dorsiflexing the ankle against resistance (eg, rubber bands) increases function and helps prevent shin splints.

ACHILLES TENDON INJURY

Achilles tendon injuries include inflammation of the paratenon and partial or complete tears.

The calf muscle attaches to the calcaneus via the Achilles tendon. During running, the calf muscles help with the lift-off phase of gait. Repetitive forces from running combined with insufficient recovery time can initially cause inflammation in the paratenon (fatty areolar tissue that separates the Achilles tendon from its sheath). A complete tear of the Achilles tendon is a serious injury, usually resulting from sudden, forceful stress.

Symptoms, Signs, and Diagnosis

The primary symptom of Achilles tendon inflammation is pain in the back of the heel, which initially increases when exercise is begun and often lessens as exercise continues. A complete tear causes sudden, severe pain and prohibits normal ambulation.

On examination, an inflamed Achilles tendon is tender when squeezed between the fingers. With a complete tear, a defect along the course of the tendon is palpable, and squeezing the calf muscle does not cause the normally expected plantar flexion (a positive Thompson test).

Treatment

Tendon inflammation can be treated by placing a heel lift in the shoes and by instructing the athlete to do stretching exercises for the calf muscles. Ice and NSAIDs should also be used. The patient should avoid uphill and downhill running until the tendon is not painful. A torn tendon requires surgical repair.

METATARSAL STRESS FRACTURE

Metatarsal stress fractures involve the metatarsal shafts and are caused by repetitive weight-bearing stress.

Stress fractures do not result from a discrete injury (eg, fall, blow) but occur after repeated stress. Metatarsal stress fractures (march fractures) usually occur in runners and in poorly conditioned patients who walk long distances carrying a load (eg, new recruit soldiers); they most commonly occur in the 2nd metatarsal. Risk factors include a cavus foot (high arch), shoes with inadequate shock-absorbing qualities, and osteoporosis; these fractures also may be a sign of the female athlete triad (amenorrhea, eating disorder, and osteoporosis).

Symptoms, Signs, and Diagnosis

Forefoot pain that occurs after a long or intense workout, then disappears shortly after stopping exercise is the typical initial presentation. With subsequent exercise, onset of pain is progressively earlier, and pain may become so severe that it prohibits exercise and persists even when the patient is not bearing weight.

Standard x-rays are recommended but may be normal until a callus forms 2 to 3 wk after the injury. Often, technetium diphosphonate bone scanning is necessary for definitive diagnosis. Women with recurrent stress fractures may have osteoporosis and should undergo dual-energy x-ray absorptiometry (see p. 306).

Treatment

Treatment includes reduction of weight bearing on the involved foot with initial use of crutches and a wooden shoe or other commercially available supportive shoe or boot. Casts are rarely needed; if applied, they should be left on for only 1 to 2 wk because they can cause significant muscle atrophy and delay rehabilitation. Healing usually takes 3 to 12 wk

325 BITES AND STINGS

Bites and stings cause about 100 deaths/year in the US, and > 90,000 are reported annually to poison control centers; many more occur that are not reported. All patients with bites and stings should receive appropriate tetanus prophylaxis (see TABLE 178–1 on p. 1506).

HUMAN AND MAMMAL BITES

(For rat bites, see p. 1481.)

Human and mammal (mostly dog and cat, but also squirrel, gerbil, rabbit, guinea pig, and monkey) bites are common and occasionally cause significant morbidity and disability. The hands, extremities, and face are most frequently affected, although human bites can occasionally involve breasts and genitals.

In addition to tissue trauma, infection from the biting organism's oral flora is a major concern. Human bites can theoretically transmit viral hepatitis and HIV. Bites to the hand (see also p. 332) carry a higher risk of infection, specifically cellulitis, tenosynovitis, septic arthritis, and osteomyelitis, compared to other bite sites; this higher risk is particularly a concern in human bites resulting from a clenched-fist strike to the mouth ("fight bite"). Human bites to sites other than the hand have not been proven to carry a greater risk for infection than bites from other mammals. Rabies, a risk with certain mammal bites, is discussed on p. 1855.

Diagnosis

Wounds are evaluated for damage to underlying structures (eg, nerves, vasculature, tendons, bone) and for foreign bodies, as in any other wound (see p. 2552). Evaluation should focus on careful assessment of function and the extent of the bite. Wounds over or near joints should be examined in the position in which they were inflicted (eg, with fist clenched) and explored under sterile conditions to assess tendon, bone, and joint involvement and to detect retained foreign bodies. Culturing fresh wounds is not valuable for targeting antimicrobial therapy, but infected wounds should be cultured. Screening victims of human bites for hepatitis or HIV is recommended only if the attacker is known or suspected to be seropositive.

Treatment

Hospitalization is indicated when infection or loss of function is evident at presentation, when the wound has damaged or threatens deep structures, and when close follow up would be difficult. Priorities of treatment include wound cleaning, debridement, closure, and infection prophylaxis.

Wound care: Wounds should first be cleaned with a mild antibacterial soap and water (non-sterile water is sufficient), then pressure irrigated with copious volumes of saline solution using a syringe and IV catheter. A dilute povidone-iodine solution (10:1 with 0.9% saline) may also be used, but pressure irrigation with saline best decontaminates the wound. A local anesthetic should be used as needed. Dead and devitalized tissue is debrided.

Wound closure practices vary. Many wounds should initially be left open, including puncture-type wounds; wounds to the hands, feet, perineum, or genitals; wounds greater than several hours old; wounds that are heavily contaminated, markedly edematous, show signs of inflammation, or involve deeper structures (eg, tendon, cartilage, bone); wounds from human bites; and wounds occurring in a contaminated environment (eg, marine, field, sewers). In addition, wound resolution in immunocompromised patients may be better with delayed closure. Other wounds (ie, fresh, cutaneous lacerations) can usually be closed after proper wound hygiene. If there is any question, results with delayed primary closure are comparable to those with primary closure, so little is lost by leaving the wound open initially.

Hand bites should be wrapped in sterile gauze, splinted in position of function (slight wrist extension, metacarpophalangeal joint and finger flexion), and continuously elevated. Facial bites may require reconstructive surgery given the cosmetic sensitivity of the area and the potential for scarring.

Infection prophylaxis: Thorough wound cleaning often suffices to prevent infection. No consensus exists on indications for antibiotics. The drugs will not prevent infection in heavily contaminated or improperly cleaned wounds; however, many practitioners prescribe prophylactic antibiotics for bites to the hand and some other bites. For human and dog bites, the preferred drug for prophylaxis and treatment is amoxicillin-clavulanate

500 to 875 mg po bid for 3 (prophylaxis) or 5 to 7 (treatment) days for outpatients. Ampicillin-sulbactam 1.5 to 3.0 g IV q 6 h is a reasonable empiric choice for inpatients; it covers α-hemolytic streptococci, *Staphylococcus aureus*, and *Eikenella corrodens*, the organisms most commonly cultured from human bites, and the *Pasteurella* species (*P. canis* and *P. multocida*) and *Capnocytophaga canimorsus* found in dog bites. For cat bites, a fluoroquinolone (eg, ciprofloxacin 500 mg po bid for 5 to 7 days) for prophylaxis and treatment is recommended because of the prevalence of *P. multocida*. (*Bartonella henselae* is also transmitted by cat bites and is discussed on p. 1455.) Alternatives for penicillin-allergic patients are clarithromycin 500 mg po bid for 7 to 10 days or clindamycin 150 to 300 mg po qid for 7 to 10 days. Squirrel, gerbil, rabbit, and guinea pig bites rarely become infected but can be treated like cat bites.

Victims of human bites should also receive postexposure prophylaxis for viral hepatitis (see p. 226) and HIV (see p. 1639) as indicated by victim and attacker serostatus.

Infected wounds: Clinical infections are treated initially with empiric antibiotics chosen by biting species as above. Culture results should guide subsequent therapy. Debridement, suture removal, soaking, splinting, elevation, and IV antibiotics may be appropriate depending on the specific infection and clinical scenario. Joint infections and osteomyelitis may require prolonged IV antibiotic therapy and orthopedic consultation.

Monkey bites, usually restricted in the US to animal laboratory workers, carry a small risk of herpes simiae virus infection, which causes vesicular skin lesions at the inoculation site and can progress to an often-fatal encephalitis. Treatment is with IV acyclovir.

INSECT STINGS

Stinging insects are members of the order Hymenoptera of the class Insecta. Major subgroups are apids (eg, honeybees, bumblebees), vespids (eg, wasps, yellow jackets, hornets), and formicids (eg, non-winged fire ants).

Apids usually do not sting unless provoked; however, Africanized honeybees (killer bees), migrants from South America that reside in some southern US states, are especially aggressive when agitated. Apids typically sting once and dislodge their barbed stinger into the wound, which introduces venom and kills the insect. Melittin is thought to be the main pain-inducing component of the venom. The venom of Africanized honeybees is no more potent than that of other honeybees but causes more severe consequences, because these insects attack in swarms and inflict multiple stings, increasing the dose of venom. In the US, bee stings cause 3 to 4 times more deaths than do venomous snakebites.

Vespid stingers have few barbs and do not stay in the skin, so these insects can inflict multiple stings. The venom contains phospholipase, hyaluronidases, and a protein termed antigen 5, which is the most allergenic. Although vespids also avoid stinging unless provoked, they nest close to humans, so provocative encounters are more frequent. Yellow jackets are the major cause of allergic reactions to insect stings in the US.

Fire ants are found in the Southern US, particularly in the Gulf region, where in urban areas they may sting as many as 40% of the population. There are several species, but *Solenopsis invicta* predominates and is responsible for an increasing number of allergic reactions. The ant bites to anchor itself to its victim and stings repeatedly as it rotates its body in an arc around the bite, producing a characteristic central bite partially encircled by a reddened sting line. The venom has hemolytic, cytolytic, antimicrobial, and insecticidal properties; 3 or 4 small aqueous protein fractions are probably responsible for allergic reactions.

Hymenoptera venoms cause local toxic reactions in all people and allergic reactions only in those previously sensitized. Severity depends on the dose of venom and degree of previous sensitization. Victims of swarm attacks and those with high venom-specific IgE levels are most at risk of anaphylaxis; many children never outgrow the risk. The average unsensitized person can safely tolerate 22 stings/kg (10 stings/lb) body weight; thus, the average adult can withstand > 1000 stings, whereas 500 stings can kill a child.

Symptoms and Signs

Local apid and vespid reactions are immediate burning, transient pain, and itching, with a few-centimeter area of erythema, swelling, and induration. Swelling and erythema usually peak at 48 h, can persist for a week, and can involve an entire extremity. This local chemical cellulitis is often confused with secondary cellulitis, which is more painful and uncommon after envenomation. Allergic reactions may manifest with urticaria, angioedema, bronchospasm, refractory hypotension, or a combination; swelling alone is not a manifestation of allergic reaction.

Symptoms and signs of a fire ant (formicid) sting are immediate pain followed by a wheal and flare lesion, which often resolves within 45 min and gives rise to a sterile pustule, which breaks down within 30 to 70 h. The lesion sometimes becomes infected and can lead to sepsis. In some cases, an edematous, erythematous, and pruritic lesion, rather than a pustule, develops. Anaphylaxis due to fire ant stings probably occurs in < 1% of patients. Mononeuritis and seizures have been reported.

Treatment

Stingers, if present, should be removed as quickly as possible without concern for removal method. An ice cube placed over the sting as soon as possible, H_1 blockers, and oral NSAIDs reduce pain. Allergic reactions are treated with antihistamines; anaphylaxis is treated with epinephrine with IV fluids and vasopressors if necessary (see p. 1360).

People with known hypersensitivity to stings should carry a kit containing a prefilled syringe of epinephrine and seek medical care immediately at the onset of systemic symptoms.

Prevention

People who have had anaphylaxis or positive venom skin test results and are at risk for subsequent stings should receive immunotherapy regardless of age or time since anaphylaxis. Venom immunotherapy (see also IMM03) is highly effective, reducing the chance of recurrent anaphylaxis from 50% to about 10% after 2 yr of therapy and to about 2% after 3 to 5 yr of therapy. Children who receive venom immunotherapy have a significantly lower risk of systemic reaction to stings 10 to 20 yr after treatment. Venom immunotherapy seems to be safe for use during pregnancy. Desensitization is advised and can be carried out using single-venom therapy. After initial immunotherapy, maintenance doses may be needed for up to 5 yr.

MARINE BITES AND STINGS

(See p. 2665 for fish poisonings [eg, scombroid, ciguatera, fugu] and paralytic shellfish poisoning.)

Some marine bites and stings are toxic; all create wounds at risk for infection with marine organisms, most notably *Vibrio* and *Aeromonas* spp and *Mycobacterium marinarum.* Shark bites result in jagged lacerations with near-total or total amputations and should be treated as for other major traumas (see p. 2549).

CNIDARIA (COELENTERATES)

Cnidaria—corals, sea anemones, jellyfish (including sea nettles), and hydroids (eg, Portuguese man-of-war)—are responsible for more envenomations than any other marine animal. However, of the 9000 species, only about 100 are toxic to humans. Cnidaria have multiple, highly developed stinging units (nematocysts) on their tentacles that can penetrate human skin; one tentacle may fire thousands of nematocysts into the skin on contact.

Lesions vary with the type of Cnidaria. Usually, lesions initially appear as small, linear, papular eruptions that develop rapidly in one or several discontinuous lines, at times surrounded by a raised erythematous zone. Pain is immediate and may be severe; itching is common. The papules may vesiculate and proceed to pustulation, hemorrhage, and desquamation. Systemic manifestations include weakness, nausea, headache, muscle pain and spasms, lacrimation and nasal discharge, increased perspiration, changes in pulse rate, and pleuritic chest pain.

In North American waters, the Portuguese man-of-war has caused several deaths. In Indo-Pacific waters, members of the Cubomedusae order, particularly the sea wasp (*Chironex fleckeri*) and the box jellyfish (*Chiropsalmus quadrigatus*), are most dangerous and have caused several deaths.

To arrest the stinging of the embedded nematocysts, vinegar is applied to box jellyfish stings and Portuguese man-of-war stings, and baking soda in a 50:50 slurry to sea nettle injuries. Fresh water may activate undischarged nematocysts. The tentacles are removed immediately; if possible a forceps is used and the hand is double-gloved. Symptoms are treated supportively. Analgesia with an NSAID or other analgesic can be used for minor stings if needed; opioids are preferred for severe pain. Painful muscle spasms may be treated with benzodiazepines. IV fluids and epinephrine can be used as initial empiric treatment for the few cases in which shock develops. Antivenom is available for the stings of *C. fleckeri* and box jellyfish but is of no value for North American species.

Seabather's eruption is a stinging, pruritic, maculopapular rash that affects swimmers in some Atlantic locales (eg, Florida, Caribbean, Long Island). It is caused by bites from the larvae of the sea anemone *Edwardsiella lineata.* The rash is typically worse where bathing suits press closest to the skin. Symptoms and signs resolve with washing off the larvae.

Stingrays

Stingrays once caused about 750 stings/year along North American coasts; the present incidence is unknown, and most cases are not reported. Venom is contained in the one or more spines on the dorsum of the animal's tail. Injuries usually occur when an unwary swimmer wading in ocean surf, bay, or backwater steps on a stingray buried in the sand and provokes it to thrust its tail upward and forward, driving the dorsal spine (or spines) into the victim's foot or leg. The integumentary sheath surrounding the spine ruptures, and the venom escapes into the victim's tissues, causing immediate severe pain. Although often limited to the injured area, the pain may spread rapidly, reaching its greatest intensity in <90 min; in most cases, pain gradually diminishes over 6 to 48 h, but may occasionally last days or weeks. Syncope, weakness, nausea, and anxiety are common and may be due, in part, to peripheral vasodilation. Lymphangitis, vomiting, diarrhea, sweating, generalized cramps, inguinal or axillary pain, and respiratory distress have been reported.

The wound is usually jagged, bleeds freely, and is often contaminated with parts of the integumentary sheath. The edges of the wound are often discolored, and some localized tissue destruction may occur. Generally, some swelling and edema are present. Open wounds are subject to infection.

Injuries to an extremity should be irrigated with salt water. An attempt should be made to remove the integumentary sheath if it can be seen. The extremity should then be submerged for 30 to 90 min in water as hot as the patient can tolerate without injury, which inactivates the venom. The wound should be reexamined for remnants of the sheath and debrided; local anesthesia may be given as needed. Patients stung on the trunk should undergo closer evaluation for puncture of viscera. Treatment of systemic manifestations is supportive. Tetanus prophylaxis should be given, and the injured extremity should be elevated for several days. Use of antibiotics and surgical wound closure may be necessary.

Mollusks

Mollusks include cones (including cone snails), octopi, and bivalves. *Conus californicus* is the only known dangerous cone in North American waters. Its sting produces localized pain, swelling, redness, and numbness that rarely progresses to shock. Treatment is largely supportive. Local measures seem to be of little value, and reports that local injection of epinephrine and neostigmine are helpful are unproven. Severe *Conus* stings may require mechanical ventilation and measures to reverse shock.

Cone snails are a rare cause of marine envenomation among divers and shell collectors in the Indian and Pacific oceans. The snail injects its venom through a harpoon-like tooth when aggressively handled (eg, during shell cleaning or when placed in a pocket). The venom contains multiple neurotoxins that block ion channels and neurotransmitter receptors, resulting in paralysis that is usually reversible but has resulted in some deaths. Treatment is supportive and may include local pressure immobilization, immersion in hot water, and tetanus prophylaxis. Severe cases may require respiratory support.

The bites of North American octopi are rarely serious. Bites from the blue-ringed octopus, most common in Australian waters, causes tetrodotoxin envenomation with local anesthesia, neuromuscular paralysis, and respiratory failure; treatment is supportive.

Sea Urchins

Most sea urchin injuries result when spines break off in the skin and cause local tissue reactions. Without treatment, the spines can migrate into deeper tissues, causing a granulomatous nodular lesion, or they may wedge against bone or nerve. Joint and muscle pain and dermatitis may also occur. A few sea urchins (eg, *Globiferous pedicellariae*) have venom organs with calcareous jaws that can penetrate human skin, but injuries are rare.

Diagnosis is usually obvious by history. A bluish discoloration at the entry site may help locate the spine. X-rays can help when the location is not obvious on examination. Treatment is immediate removal. Vinegar dissolves most superficial spines; soaking the wound in vinegar several times a day, applying a wet vinegar compress, or both may be sufficient. Rarely, a small incision must be made to extract the spine; care must be taken because the spine is very fragile. A spine that has migrated into deeper tissues may require surgical removal. Once spines are removed, pain may continue for days; pain beyond 5 to 7 days should trigger suspicion for infection or a retained foreign body.

G. pedicellariae stings are treated by washing the area and applying a mentholated balm.

MITE BITES

There are multiple kinds of biting mites. Chiggers are probably the most common. Chiggers are mite larvae that are ubiquitous outdoors except in arid regions; they bite, feed in the skin, then fall off. Outside the US, chiggers may carry *Rickettsia tsutsugamushi* (see p. 1493). They do not burrow into the skin, but their small size means that they are not readily seen on the skin surface.

Common mite species that bite and burrow into the skin include *Sarcoptes scabiei*, which causes scabies (see p. 995), and *Demodex* mites. *Demodex* mites cause a scabies-like dermatitis (sometimes referred to as mange) that occurs almost exclusively in animals and are a possible etiologic agent in rosacea.

Dermatitis is caused by mites that occasionally bite humans but are ordinarily ectoparasites of birds, rodents, or pets and by mites associated with plant materials or stored food or feed. Bird mites may bite people who handle live poultry or pet birds or who have bird's nests on their homes. Rodent mites from cats, dogs (especially puppies), and rabbits and swine mange mites (*S. scabiei* var *suis*) from pig farms or pet pigs may also bite humans.

The straw itch mite (*Pyemotes tritici*) is often associated with seeds, straw, hay, or other plant material; it is parasitic on soft-bodied insects that are (or have been) present in such materials. These mites often bite people who handle the infested items; granary workers, those who handle grass seeds or grass hay, and those who make dried plant arrangements are most at risk.

Several species of mites associated with stored grain products, cheese, and other foods do not bite but cause allergic dermatitis or grocer's itch because people become sensitized to allergens on the mites or their waste products.

House dust mites do not bite but feed on sloughed skin cells in pillows and mattresses and on floors (especially on carpets). They are significant because many people develop pulmonary hypersensitivity to allergens in exoskeletons and feces.

Symptoms and Signs

Most bites cause some version of pruritic dermatitis; pruritus from chigger bites is especially intense. Diagnosis of non-burrowing mite bites is presumptive based on the patient's history (eg, living, working, and recreational environments) and physical examination; the mites themselves are rarely found because they fall off after biting, the skin reaction is usually delayed, and most patients seek a physician's assistance only after several days. Lesions caused by different mites are usually indistinguishable and may superficially resemble other skin conditions (eg, other insect bites, contact dermatitis, folliculitis). Diagnosis of burrowing mites can be confirmed by skin biopsy.

Treatment

Treatment of non-burrowing mite bites is symptomatic; topical corticosteroids or oral antihistamines are used as needed to control pruritus until hypersensitivity reaction resolves. Through discussion of possible sources, the physician can help the patient avoid repeated exposure to mites. Treatment of *Demodex* bites is with veterinary consultation. See p. 997 for treatment of scabies, p. 386 for treatment of respiratory hypersensitivity, and p. 1353 for treatment of other systemic allergic reactions.

SCORPION STINGS

Although all scorpions in North America sting, most are relatively harmless; the stings usually cause only localized pain with minimal swelling, some lymphangitis with regional lymphadenopathy, and increased skin temperature and tenderness around the wound.

A significant exception is the bark scorpion (*Centruroides sculpturatus*, also known as *C. exilicauda*), found in Arizona, New Mexico, and the California side of the Colorado River. This species is venomous and can cause more serious injury and illness. Initial symptoms are immediate pain and sometimes numbness or tingling over the involved part. Swelling is usually absent, and there are few skin changes. Serious symptoms, most common in children, include restlessness; muscle spasms; abnormal and random head, neck, and eye movements; anxiety and agitation; and sialorrhea and diaphoresis. In adults, tachycardia, hypertension, increased respirations, weakness, muscle spasms, and fasciculations may predominate. Respiratory difficulties rarely occur in both age groups. *C. sculpturatus* stings have resulted in death in children < 6 yr and in hypersensitive people.

Diagnosis and Treatment

Diagnosis is obvious from the history, but several species of scorpions kept as exotic pets in the US (known by names that falsely suggest toxicity, such as yellow death stalker and black death scorpion) are similar in appearance to foreign species with dangerously toxic venom. However, the actual species of pet scorpion is seldom known by the stinging victim or, if provided, may be unreliable. Stings should be treated as potentially dangerous until signs or lack of signs indicates otherwise.

Treatment of nonvenomous scorpion stings is nonspecific; an ice pack over the wound and oral NSAIDs reduce pain. Treatment of venomous *Centruroides* stings is bedrest; benzodiazepines for muscle spasms; and IV drugs as needed to control hypertension, agitation, and pain. Patients are kept npo for 8 to 12 h after the bite. Antivenom, available only in Arizona, should be given in an ICU setting in all severe cases and to those unresponsive to supportive care, particularly children. Information on availability and dosing may be obtained by contacting a regional poison control center.

SNAKEBITES

Of about 3000 snake species throughout the world, only about 15% worldwide and 20% in the US are dangerous to humans because of venom or toxic salivary secretions (see TABLE 325–1). At least one species of venomous snake is native to every state in the US except Alaska, Maine, and Hawaii. Almost all are crotalines (also called pit vipers because of pit-like depressions on either side of the head that are heat-sensing organs), consisting of rattlesnakes, copperheads, and cottonmouths (water moccasins). Between 7000 and 8000 venomous snakebites occur annually. Rattlesnakes account for the majority of bites and almost all deaths. Copperheads and, to a lesser extent, cottonmouths account for most other venomous bites. Coral snakes (elapids) and imported species (in zoos, schools, snake farms, and amateur and

TABLE 325–1. SIGNIFICANT VENOMOUS SNAKES BY REGION

GEOGRAPHIC REGION	SNAKES
Africa	Puff adder Gaboon viper Burrowing asp Natal black snake Boomslang Bird snake Mole viper Mamba
Asia	Asiatic pit vipers Russell's viper Red-necked keelback Malaysian pit viper Krait King cobra
Australia	Taipan Tiger snake King brown snake Death adder Red-bellied black snake
Central and South America	Rattlesnake Fer-de-lance Bushmaster Coral snake Palm pit viper Cantil pit viper
Europe	Adder Asp viper Nose horned viper Ottoman viper Blunt nose viper
Indo-Pacific	Sea snakes Sea kraits
Middle East	Saw scaled viper Horned or desert vipers Burrowing asp Natal black snake Mole vipers Egyptian cobra Sinai desert snake Palestinian viper
North America	Rattlesnake (eg, diamondback, sidewinder, timber, prairie, Mojave) Copperhead Cottonmouth (water moccasin) Coral snakes

professional collections) account for < 1% of all bites. Most victims are males between 17 yr and 27 yr, of whom 50% are intoxicated and deliberately handled or molested the snake. Most bites occur on the upper extremities. Only 5 to 6 deaths occur annually. Risks for death include age extremes, handling of captive snakes (rather than wild encounters), delay in treatment, and undertreatment.

Pathophysiology

Snake venoms are complex substances, chiefly proteins, with enzymatic activity. Although enzymes play an important role, lethal properties of venom can be due to certain smaller polypeptides. Most venom components appear to bind to multiple physiologic receptors, and attempts to classify venom as toxic to a specific system (eg, neurotoxin, hemotoxin, cardiotoxin, myotoxin) are misleading and can lead to errors in clinical judgment.

The venom of most North American pit vipers produces local effects and coagulopathy and other systemic effects. Results may include local tissue damage; vascular defects; hemolysis; a disseminated intravascular coagulation (DIC)–like (defibrination) syndrome; and pulmonary, cardiac, renal, and neurologic defects. Venom alters capillary membrane permeability, causing extravasation of electrolytes, albumin, and RBCs through vessel walls into the envenomated site. This process may occur in the lungs, myocardium, kidneys, peritoneum, and, rarely, the CNS. Initially, edema, hypoalbuminemia, and hemoconcentration occur. Later, blood and fluids pool in the microcirculation, causing hypotension, lactic acidemia, shock, and, in severe cases, multisystem organ failure. Effective circulating blood volume falls and may contribute to cardiac and renal failure. Clinically significant thrombocytopenia (platelet count < 20,000/μL) is common in severe rattlesnake bites and may occur alone or in combination with other coagulopathies. Venom-induced intravascular clotting may trigger defibrination syndrome, resulting in epistaxis, gingival bleeding, hematemesis, hematuria, internal hemorrhage, as well as spontaneous bleeding at the bite site and venipuncture sites. Renal failure may result from severe hypotension, hemolysis, rhabdomyolysis, nephrotoxic venom effects, or a DIC-like syndrome. Proteinuria, hemoglobinuria, and myoglobinuria may occur in severe rattlesnake bites. The venom of most North American pit vipers produces very minor changes in neuromuscular conduction, except for Mojave and Eastern diamondback rattlesnake venom, which may cause serious neurologic deficits.

Coral snake venom contains primarily neurotoxic components, which result in a presynaptic neuromuscular blockade, potentially causing respiratory paralysis. The lack of significant proteolytic enzyme activity accounts for the paucity of symptoms and signs at the bite site.

Symptoms and Signs

A snakebite, whether from a venomous or nonvenomous snake, usually causes terror, often with autonomic manifestations (eg, nausea, vomiting, tachycardia, diarrhea, diaphoresis), which may be difficult to distinguish from systemic manifestations of envenomation.

Nonvenomous snakebites cause only local symptoms and signs, usually pain and 2 to 4 rows of scratches from the snake's upper jaw at the bite site.

Symptoms and signs of envenomation may be local, systemic, coagulopathic, or a combination, depending on degree of envenomation and species of snake.

Pit viper: About 25% of pit viper bites are dry (venom is not deposited), and no systemic symptoms or signs develop. Local signs include fang mark(s) and scratch(es). If envenomation has occurred, edema and erythema or ecchymosis at the bite site and adjacent tissues will occur, usually within 30 to 60 min. Edema progresses rapidly and may involve the entire extremity within hours. Lymphangitis and enlarged, tender regional lymph nodes may develop; temperature increases over the bite area. In moderate or severe envenomations (see Diagnosis on p. 2645), ecchymosis is common and may appear at and around the bite site within 3 to 6 h. Ecchymosis is most severe after bites by Eastern and Western diamondbacks; cottonmouths; and prairie, Pacific, and timber rattlesnakes. Ecchymosis is less common after copperhead and Mojave rattlesnake bites. The skin around the bite may appear tense and discolored. Bullae, serous, hemorrhagic, or both, usually appear at the bite site within 8 h. Edema resulting from North American rattlesnake envenomations is usually limited to dermal and subcutaneous tissues, although severe envenomation rarely produces edema in subfascial tissue, causing compartment syndrome (defined as compartment pressures ≥ 30 mm Hg over 1 h). Necrosis around the bite site is common after rattlesnake envenomations. Most venom effects on soft tissues peak within 2 to 4 days.

Systemic manifestations of envenomation include nausea, vomiting, diaphoresis, anxiety, confusion, spontaneous bleeding, fever, hypotension, and shock. Some rattlesnake bite victims develop a rubbery, minty, or metallic taste in their mouth. The venom of most North American pit vipers produces minor neuromuscular conduction changes, including generalized weakness and paresthesias and muscle fasciculations. Some patients may have alterations in mental status. Venom of Mojave and Eastern diamondback rattlesnakes may cause serious neurologic deficits, including respiratory depression. Rattlesnake envenomations may induce various coagulation abnormalities, including thrombocytopenia, prolongation of PT (measured by the INR) or activated PTT, hypofibrinogenemia, elevated fibrin degradation products, or a combination of these disorders, resembling a DIC-like (defibrination) syndrome. Thrombocytopenia is usually the first manifestation and may be asymptomatic or, in the presence of a multicomponent coagulopathy, cause spontaneous bleeding. Victims with coagulopathy typically hemorrhage from the bite site or from mucous membranes, hematemesis, hematochezia, hematuria, or a combination. A rise in Hct is an early finding secondary to hemoconcentration. Later, Hct may fall as a result of fluid replacement and blood loss from the DIC-like syndrome. In severe cases, hemolysis may cause a rapid fall in Hct.

Coral snake: Pain and swelling may be minimal or absent and are often transitory. The absence of local symptoms and signs may erroneously suggest a dry bite, producing a false sense of security for both victim and clinician. Weakness of the bitten extremity may become evident within several hours. Systemic neuromuscular manifestations may be delayed for 12 h and include weakness and lethargy; altered sensorium, including euphoria and drowsiness; cranial nerve palsies causing ptosis, diplopia, blurred vision, dysarthria, and dysphagia; increased salivation; muscle flaccidity; and respiratory distress or failure. Once the neurotoxic venom effects manifest, they are difficult to reverse and may last 3 to 6 days. Untreated patients may die of respiratory failure. Mechanical ventilation may be necessary.

Diagnosis

Definitive diagnosis requires positive identification of the snake along with clinical manifestations of envenomation. History should include the time of bite, description of snake, type of field therapy, underlying medical conditions, allergy to horse or sheep products, and history of previous venomous snakebite(s) and therapy. A complete physical examination should be performed, including baseline measurements of limb circumference proximal and distal to the bite site.

Patients often cannot recall details of the snake's appearance; however, pit vipers differ from nonvenomous snakes by their arrowhead-shaped heads, elliptical pupils, heat-sensing pits between the eyes and nose, retractable fangs, and a single row of subcaudal plates extending from the anal plate on the underside of the tail.

Coral snakes in the US have round pupils and black snouts but lack facial pits. They have blunt- or cigar-shaped heads and alternating bands of red, yellow (cream), and black, often causing them to be mistaken for the common nonvenomous scarlet king snake, which has alternating bands of red, black, and yellow ("red on yellow, kill a fellow," "red on black, venom lack"). Coral snakes have short, fixed fangs and inject venom through successive chewing movements. Fang marks are suggestive but not conclusive; rattlesnakes may leave single or double fang marks or other teeth marks, whereas bites by nonvenomous snakes usually show multiple superficial teeth marks. However, the number of teeth marks and bite sites may vary because snakes may strike and bite multiple times.

A dry pit viper bite is diagnosed when no symptoms or signs of envenomation appear over 8 h.

Severity of envenomation depends on the size and species of the snake (rattlesnakes > cottonmouths > copperheads); the amount of venom injected; the number of bites; the location and depth of the bite (eg, envenomation in bites to the head and trunk tends to be more severe than in bites to the extremities); the age, size, and health of the victim; the time elapsed before treatment; and the victim's susceptibility (response) to the venom.

Severity of envenomation can be graded as minimal, moderate, or severe, based on the most severe of the local findings, systemic symptoms and signs, coagulation parameters, and laboratory results (see TABLE 325–2).

TABLE 325–2. SEVERITY OF PIT VIPER ENVENOMATION

GRADE	DESCRIPTION
Minimal	Changes at bite site only; no systemic symptoms, signs, or laboratory findings
Moderate	Changes extend beyond the bite site; non–life-threatening systemic symptoms and signs (eg, nausea, vomiting, paresthesias); mildly abnormal coagulation or laboratory changes without clinically significant bleeding
Severe	Changes involving the entire extremity; severe systemic symptoms and signs (eg, hypotension, dyspnea, shock); markedly abnormal coagulation and laboratory changes with clinically significant bleeding

Grading should be determined by the most severe symptom, sign, or laboratory finding.

Envenomation may progress rapidly from minimal to severe and must be continually reassessed.

Treatment

General approach: In the field, the victim should move or be moved beyond the snake's striking distance. The victim should avoid exertion and be reassured, kept warm, and rapidly transported to the nearest medical facility. A bitten extremity should be loosely immobilized in a functional position just below heart level, and all rings, watches, and constrictive clothing should be removed. Pressure immobilization to delay systemic absorption of venom (eg, by wrapping crepe bandages around the limb) may be appropriate for coral snake bites but is not recommended in the US, where most bites are from pit vipers; pressure immobilization may cause arterial insufficiency and necrosis. First responders should support airway and breathing, administer O_2, and establish IV access in an unaffected extremity while transporting the victim as quickly as possible to the nearest medical facility. All other out-of-hospital interventions (eg, tourniquets, topical preparations, suction by mouth or with a device with or without incision, cryotherapy, electrical shock) are of no proven benefit, may be harmful, and may delay appropriate treatment. However, tourniquets that are already placed, unless causing limb-threatening ischemia, should remain in place until the patient is transported to the hospital and envenomation excluded or definitive treatment initiated.

In the emergency department, primary attention should be given to establishing or maintaining an airway, breathing, and circulation. Circumferential extremity measurements should be performed on arrival and every 15 to 20 min until local progression subsides; it is also useful to outline the margins of local edema with an indelible marker to assess progression of local envenomation. All but trivial pit viper bites require a baseline CBC (including platelets), coagulation profile (eg, PT, PTT, fibrinogen), fibrin degradation products, and urinalysis, as well as measurement of electrolytes, BUN, and creatinine. For moderate and severe envenomations, patients require blood typing and cross matching; ECG and chest x-ray; and CK tests, usually every 4 h for the 1st 12 h and then daily or as governed by the patient's status. In coral snake bites, neurotoxic venom effects require monitoring of O_2 saturation and baseline and serial pulmonary function tests (eg, peak flow, vital capacity).

All pit viper bite victims should be observed closely in the emergency department or ICU for at least 8 h. Patients without evidence of envenomation after 8 h may be sent home after adequate wound care (see p. 2647). Coral snake bite victims should be monitored for at least 12 h in an intensive care setting in the event that respiratory paralysis develops. Envenomation initially assessed as mild may progress to severe within several hours. Without close monitoring and appropriate treatment, the patient could die.

Treatment may include respiratory support, benzodiazepines for anxiety and sedation, opioids for pain, and fluid replacement and vasopressor support for shock. Most coagulopathies respond to sufficient quantities of neutralizing antivenom. Transfusions (eg, packed RBCs, fresh frozen plasma, cryoprecipitate, platelets) may be required but should not be given before the patient has received adequate quantities of neutralizing antivenom. Tracheostomy may be needed if trismus, laryngeal spasm, or excessive salivation is present.

Antivenom: Along with aggressive supportive care, antivenom is the mainstay of treatment for patients with moderate to severe envenomations.

For pit viper envenomation, equine-derived antivenom has been largely replaced by ovine-derived Crotalidae polyvalent immune FAb antivenom (purified FAb fragments of IgG harvested from pit viper venom–immunized sheep). The effectiveness of the equine-derived antivenom is time and dose related; it is most effective within 4 h of the envenomation and less effective after 12 h, although it may reverse coagulopathies after 24 h. Recent case reports suggest that Crotalidae polyvalent immune FAb may not be affected by time and dose and may be effective even when started 24 h after envenomation. Crotalidae polyvalent immune FAb is also safer than equine-derived antivenom, although it can still cause acute (cutaneous or anaphylactic) reactions and delayed hypersensitivity reactions (serum sickness). Serum sickness develops in up to 16% of patients 1 to 3 wk after administration of the FAb product. A loading dose of 4 to 6 vials of reconstituted Crotalidae polyvalent immune FAb diluted in 250 mL of normal saline should be infused slowly at 20 to 50 mL/h for the 1st 10 min, then, if no adverse reactions occur, the remainder is infused over the next hour; the same dose can be repeated 2 times as needed to control symptoms, reverse coagulopathies, or correct physiologic parameters. In children, the dose is not decreased (eg, based on weight or size). Measuring the circumference of the involved extremity at 3 points proximal to the bite and measuring the advancing border of edema every 15 to 30 min can guide decisions about the need for additional doses. Once control is achieved, a 2-vial dose in 250 mL saline is given at 6, 12, and 18 h to prevent recurrence of limb swelling and other venom effects.

Cottonmouth envenomation may require smaller doses. Antivenom is usually unnecessary for copperhead and pygmy rattlesnake bites, except in children, the elderly, and patients with underlying medical conditions (eg, diabetes mellitus, coronary artery disease).

For coral snake envenomation, equine-derived polyvalent coral snake antivenom is given at a dose of 5 vials for suspected envenomation and an additional 10 to 15 vials if symptoms develop. Dose is similar in adults and children.

In cases where equine-derived antivenom is required, skin testing for sensitivity to horse serum is controversial. Skin testing has no predictive value for development of acute hypersensitivity reactions, and a negative result does not completely preclude an immediate hypersensitivity reaction. However if the skin test result is positive and the envenomation is considered life- or limb-threatening, H_1 and H_2 blockers should be given before antivenom administration in a critical care setting equipped to treat anaphylaxis. Early anaphylactoid reactions to antivenom are common and usually result from too-rapid infusion; treatment is temporary discontinuation of the infusion and treatment with epinephrine, H_1 and H_2 blockers, and IV fluid depending on severity. Usually, antivenom can be resumed after diluting the antivenom further and infusing it at a slower rate. Serum sickness is common and manifests 7 to 21 days after treatment as fever, rash, malaise, urticaria, arthralgia, and lymphadenopathy (see p. 1362). Treatment is H_1 blockers and a tapering course of oral corticosteroids.

Adjunctive measures: Patients should receive tetanus prophylaxis (toxoid and sometimes Ig) as suggested by history (see TABLE 178–1 on p. 1506). Snakebites rarely become infected, and antibiotics are indicated only for clinical evidence of infection. If necessary, options include a 1st-generation cephalosporin (eg, oral cephalexin, IV cefazolin) or a broad-spectrum penicillin (eg, oral amoxicillin/clavulanate, IV ampicillin/sulbactam). Subsequent antibiotic choices should be based on culture and sensitivity results from wound cultures.

Bite wounds should be treated like other puncture wounds by cleaning and dressing the area. For limb bites, the extremity is splinted in a functional position and elevated. Wounds should be examined and cleaned daily and covered with a sterile dressing. Surgical debridement of blebs, bloody vesicles, or superficial necrosis should be carried out between days 3 and 10 and may need to be done in stages. Sterile whirlpool may be indicated for wound debridement and physical therapy. Fasciotomy for compartment syndrome is rarely necessary but is an option when compartment pressure rises ≥ 30 mm Hg over 1 h; causes severe vascular compromise; and is unresponsive to limb elevation, mannitol 1 to 2 g/kg IV, and antivenom. Joint motion, muscle strength, sensation, and girth should be evaluated within 2 days of the bite. To avoid contractures, immobilization is interrupted by frequent periods of gentle exercise, progressing from passive to active.

Regional poison control centers and zoos are excellent resources when dealing with snakebites, including those by nonnative snakes. These facilities maintain a list of physicians trained in snakebite care as well as the *Antivenin Index,* published and periodically updated by the American Zoo and Aquarium Association and the American Association of Poison Control Centers, which catalogs the location and number of vials of antivenom available for all native venomous snakes and most exotic species. A national help line is available at 800-222-1222.

OTHER REPTILE BITES

Other reptile bites of significance include those of venomous lizards, alligators and crocodiles, and iguanas.

Venomous lizards include the Gila monster (*Heloderma suspectum*), found in the Southwestern US and Mexico, and the beaded lizard (*H. horridum*) of Mexico. Their complex venom contains serotonin, arginine esterase, hyaluronidase, phospholipase A_2, and one or more salivary kallikreins but lacks neurotoxic components or coagulopathic enzymes. Bites are rarely fatal. When they bite, venomous lizards clamp on firmly and chew the venom into the victim. Symptoms and signs include intense pain, swelling and edema, ecchymosis, lymphangitis, and lymphadenopathy. Systemic manifestations, including weakness, sweating, thirst, headache, and tinnitus, may develop in moderate or severe cases. Cardiovascular collapse occurs rarely. The clinical course is similar to that of a minimal to moderate envenomation by a larger species of rattlesnake. Treatment in the field involves removing the lizard with pliers, by applying a flame to the lizard's chin, or by immersing the animal entirely underwater. In a hospital setting, treatment is supportive and similar to that for pit viper envenomation; no antivenom is available. The wound should be probed with a small needle for broken or shed teeth and then cleaned. Prophylactic antibiotics are usually not recommended.

Alligator and crocodile bites usually result from handling, although native encounters rarely occur. Bites are not venomous, are notable for a high frequency of *Aeromonas* sp soft-tissue infections, and are generally treated as major trauma. Wounds are irrigated and debrided and then undergo delayed primary closure or are allowed to heal by secondary intention. Patients are treated preventively with clindamycin and trimethoprim-sulfamethoxazole (1st choice) or tetracycline.

Iguana bites and claw injuries are becoming more frequent as more are kept as pets. Wounds are superficial, and treatment is local. Soft-tissue infection is uncommon, but *Salmonella* is a notable pathogen when infection occurs and can be treated with a fluoroquinolone antibiotic.

SPIDER BITES

Almost all of the 30,000 species of spiders are venomous. However, the fangs of most species are too short or too fragile to penetrate the skin. Serious systemic reactions most frequently occur with bites from brown (eg, violin, fiddleback, brown recluse—*Loxosceles* sp) spiders and black widow (*Latrodectus* sp) spiders. Brown spiders are found in the Midwest and South Central US, sparing the coastal and Canadian border states, except when imported through clothing or luggage. Widow spiders are found throughout the US. Several venomous species (eg, *Pamphobeteus*, *Cupiennius*, *Phoneutria*) are not native to the US but may be imported on produce or other materials or through commercial trade in spiders as novelty pets.

Only a few spider venoms have been studied in detail. Of greatest significance are those having necrotizing (brown and some house spiders) and neurotoxic (widow spiders) venom components. The most toxic component of widow spider venom seems to be a peptide that affects neuromuscular transmission. The specific fraction of brown spider venom that produces the characteristic necrotic lesion has not been isolated.

Symptoms and Signs

Brown spider bites are most common in the US. Some bites are painless initially, but pain, which can be severe and involve the entire extremity, develops within 30 to 60 min in all cases. The bite area becomes erythematous and ecchymotic and may be pruritic.

Generalized pruritus may also be present. A central bleb forms at the bite site, often surrounded by an irregular ecchymotic area ("bull's eye" lesion). The lesion may mimic pyoderma gangrenosum. The central bleb becomes larger, fills with blood, ruptures, and leaves an ulcer over which a black eschar forms and eventually sloughs. Most bites leave minimal residual scarring but some can leave a large tissue defect, which may involve muscle. Loxoscelism, a venom-induced systemic syndrome, may not be detected until 24 to 72 h after the bite and is uncommon. Systemic effects (eg, fever, chills, nausea and vomiting, arthralgias, myalgias, generalized rash, seizures, hypotension, disseminated intravascular coagulation, thrombocytopenia, hemolysis, renal failure) are responsible for all reported fatalities.

Widow spider bites usually cause an immediate, sharp, stinging sensation. Within 1 h of envenomation, there may be progression to local pain, diaphoresis, erythema, and piloerection at the bite site. The pain may be described as dull and numbing and may be disproportionate to the clinical signs. Latrodectism, a systemic syndrome caused by neurotoxic venom components, manifests as restlessness, anxiety, sweating, headache, dizziness, nausea and vomiting, hypertension, salivation, weakness, diffuse erythematous rash, pruritus, ptosis, eyelid and extremity edema, respiratory distress, increased skin temperature over the affected area, and cramping pain and muscular rigidity in the abdomen, shoulders, chest, and back. Abdominal pain may be severe and mimic an acute surgical abdomen. Latrodectism is very uncommon and most likely develops in patients at age extremes and those with underlying, chronic medical conditions. Death is extremely rare. Symptoms decline over 1 to 3 days, but residual spasms, paresthesias, agitation, and weakness may persist for weeks to months.

Tarantula bites are extremely rare and nonvenomous, but agitation of the spider may cause it to throw needle-like hairs; the hairs act as foreign bodies in skin or eyes, and can trigger mast cell degranulation and an anaphylactoid reaction (eg, urticaria, angioedema, bronchospasm, hypotension) in sensitized people, usually pet owners who handle the spider daily.

Diagnosis

Spider bites are often falsely suspected by patients. Diagnosis is typically suspected based on history and physical signs, but confirmation is rare because it requires a witness to the biting, recovery and identification of the spider, and exclusion of other causes. Conditions that mimic spider bites include ant, flea, bedbug, tick, mite, fly, and Reduviid bug (eg, assassin, wheel, kissing bugs) bites; skin disorders (eg, toxic epidermal necrolysis, erythema chronicum migrans, erythema nodosum, sporotrichosis, chronic herpes simplex, or periarteritis nodosa); infectious sources (eg, disseminated gonococcal infection, septic emboli in endocarditis or IV drug use, cutaneous anthrax, methicillin-resistant *Staphylococcus aureus* skin abscess); trauma (eg, subcutaneous drug injection, self-inflicted injuries); and anxiety disorder, panic attack, or both. Severe cases of latrodectism may mimic acute abdomen, rabies, or tetanus. Spiders are identified by location and markings. Widow spiders live outdoors in protected spaces (eg, rock piles, firewood cords, hay bales, outhouses) and have a red or orange hourglass marking on the ventral abdomen. Brown spiders live indoors in protected spaces (eg, in clothing, behind furniture, under baseboards) and have a fiddle- or violin-like marking on the cephalothorax.

Treatment

Treatment common to all spider bites includes wound cleaning, ice to reduce pain, extremity elevation, tetanus prophylaxis, and observation. Most local reactions respond to these measures alone. Ulcerating lesions should be cleaned daily and debrided as needed; topical antibiotic ointment (eg, polymyxin-bacitracin-neomycin) may be used. Urticarial lesions can be treated with antihistamines, topical corticosteroids, or both. The necrotic lesions seen in brown recluse spider bites should be cleaned and bandaged. Dapsone 100 mg po once/day until inflammation subsides has been used by some physicians when necrotic areas are > 2 cm, but benefits are unproven. Local injection of corticosteroids is of no value. Surgical excision, if necessary, should be delayed until the area of necrosis is fully demarcated, a process that may take weeks.

Systemic manifestations of widow spider bites are initially treated supportively. Myalgias and muscle spasms from widow spider bites respond poorly to muscle relaxants and opioid analgesics. A 10% Ca gluconate bolus given slowly IV in increments of 2 to 3 mL as needed may relieve pain briefly but requires continuous cardiac monitoring. Patients < 16 yr or > 60 yr, those with hypertension and those with symptoms of severe envenomation should be hospitalized. Equine-derived antivenom is available for patients with severe latrodectism. It must be given within 30 min; response can be dramatic. The dose for children and adults is 1 vial (6000 units) IV in 10 to 50 mL of normal saline usually over 3 to 15 min. The manufacturer recommends skin testing before administering the antivenom; however, skin testing does not always predict adverse reactions (eg, acute anaphylaxis).

TICK BITES

(See also p. 1478 [Lyme disease], Ch. 177 on p. 1488, and p. 1571 [Babesiosis].)

Most tick bites in the US are from various species of Ixodidae, which attach and feed for several days if not removed.

Tick bites most often occur in spring and summer and are painless. The vast majority are uncomplicated and do not transmit disease; they often cause a red papule at the bite site and may induce hypersensitivity or granulomatous foreign body reactions. The bites of *Ornithodoros coriaceus* ticks (pajaroello) cause local vesiculation, pustulation with rupture, ulceration, and eschar, with varying degrees of local swelling and pain. Similar reactions have occurred from bites of other ticks.

Treatment

Ticks should be removed as soon as possible to reduce the cutaneous immune response and the likelihood of disease transmission. If the patient presents with the tick still attached, the best method of extracting the tick and all of its mouth parts from the skin is by using a blunt forceps with medium-sized, curved tips. The forceps should be placed parallel to the skin to grasp the tick's mouth parts firmly as close to the skin as possible. Care should be taken to avoid puncturing the patient's skin and the tick's body. The forceps should be pulled slowly and steadily, directly away from the skin without twisting. Curved-tip forceps are best because the outer curve can be laid against the skin while the handle remains far enough from the skin to grasp easily. Tick mouth parts that remain in the skin and are readily visible should be carefully removed. However, if the presence of mouth parts is questionable, attempts at surgical removal may cause more tissue trauma than would occur if the parts are left in the skin; leaving mouth parts in the skin does not affect disease transmission and, at most, prolongs irritation. Other methods of tick removal, such as burning it with a match (which can damage the patient's tissues) or covering it with petroleum jelly (which is ineffective), are not recommended.

After tick removal, an antiseptic should be applied. The tick's degree of engorgement indicates its duration of attachment. If local swelling and discoloration are present, an oral antihistamine may be helpful. Although rarely practical, the tick may be saved for laboratory analysis to detect etiologic agents of tick-borne disease in the geographic area where the patient acquired the tick. Antibiotic prophylaxis for tick-transmitted infection is usually not recommended, but some experts recommend Lyme disease prophylaxis (single-dose doxycycline 200 mg po) for Ixodidae bites in areas of high Lyme disease prevalence (see p. 1481).

Pajaroello tick lesions should be cleaned, soaked in 1:20 Burow's solution, and debrided when necessary. Corticosteroids are of value in severe cases. Infections are common during the ulcer stage but rarely require more than local antiseptic measures.

Tick Paralysis

Tick paralysis is a rare, ascending flaccid paralysis that occurs when toxin-secreting Ixodidae ticks bite and remain attached for several days.

In North America, some species of *Dermacentor* and *Amblyomma* cause tick paralysis from a neurotoxin secreted in tick saliva. The toxin is not present in tick saliva during early stages of feeding, so paralysis occurs only when a tick has fed for several days or more. A single tick can cause paralysis, especially if it is attached to the back of the skull or near the spine, but multiple ticks should be sought over the entire body surface.

Symptoms and signs include anorexia, lethargy, muscle weakness, impaired coordination, nystagmus, and ascending flaccid paralysis. Bulbar or respiratory paralysis may develop. Differential diagnosis includes Guillain-Barré syndrome, botulism, myasthenia gravis, hypokalemia, and spinal cord tumor. The paralysis is rapidly reversible on removal of the tick (or ticks). If breathing is impaired, O_2 therapy or respiratory assistance may be needed.

OTHER ARTHROPOD BITES

The more common biting non-tick arthropods in the US include sand flies, horseflies, deerflies, blackflies, stable flies, mosquitoes, fleas, lice (see P. 994), bedbugs, and certain water bugs. All of these arthropods, except wheel bugs and water bugs, also suck blood, but none are venomous.

Arthropod saliva composition varies considerably, and the lesions produced by bites vary from small papules to large ulcers with swelling and acute pain. Dermatitis may also occur. Most serious consequences result from hypersensitivity reactions or infection; in sensitized people, they can be fatal. Flea allergens may trigger respiratory allergy even without a bite in some people.

The location and pattern of wheals and lesions is sometimes diagnostic of the bite source. For example, blackfly bites are usually on the neck, ears, and face; flea bites may be numerous, mostly on the feet and legs; and bedbug bites often occur in linear patterns, most commonly on the torso.

The bite should be cleaned, and an antihistamine or corticosteroid cream should be applied for itching. Severe hypersensitivity reactions should be treated (see P. 1360).

326 POISONING

Accidental poisoning and intentional self-poisoning result in many emergency department visits and a few deaths. (For effects of alcohol and illicit drug use, see Ch. 198 on p. 1683.)

GENERAL PRINCIPLES

Poisoning is contact with a substance that results in toxicity. Symptoms vary, but certain common syndromes may suggest particular classes of poisons. Diagnosis is primarily clinical, but for some poisonings, blood and urine tests can help. Treatment is supportive for most poisonings; specific antidotes are necessary for a few. Prevention includes labeling drug containers clearly and keeping poisons out of the reach of children.

Most poisonings are dose-related. Toxicity may result from exposure to excess amounts of normally nontoxic substances. Some poisonings occur from exposure to substances that are poisonous at all doses. Poisoning is distinguished from hypersensitivity and idiosyncratic reactions, which are unpredictable and not dose-related, and from intolerance, which is a toxic reaction to a usually nontoxic dose of a substance.

Poisoning is commonly due to ingestion but can result from injection, inhalation, or exposure of body surfaces (eg, skin, eye, mucous membrane). Many commonly ingested nonfood substances are generally nontoxic (see TABLE 326–1); however, almost any substance can be toxic if ingested in excessive amounts.

Accidental poisoning is common among young children, who are curious and ingest items indiscriminately despite noxious tastes and odors; usually, only a single substance is involved. Poisoning is also common among older children, adolescents, and adults attempting suicide; multiple drugs, including alcohol, acetaminophen, and other OTC drugs, may be involved. Accidental poisoning may occur in the elderly because of confusion, poor eyesight, mental impairment, or multiple prescriptions of the same drug by different physicians.

Occasionally, people are poisoned by someone who intends to kill or disable them (eg, to rape or rob them). Drugs used to disable (eg, scopolamine, benzodiazepines, γ-hydroxybutyrate) tend to have sedative or amnestic properties or both. Rarely, parents, who may have some medical knowledge, poison their children because of unclear psychiatric reasons or a desire to cause illness and thus gain medical attention (a disorder called Munchausen syndrome by proxy—see P. 1739).

Most poisons are metabolized, pass through the GI tract, or are excreted. Occasionally,

TABLE 326–1. SUBSTANCES USUALLY NOT DANGEROUS WHEN INGESTED*

Adhesives	Magnesium silicate (antacid)
Barium sulfate	Matches
Bathtub toys (floating)	Methylcellulose
Blackboard chalk (Ca carbonate)	Mineral oil (if not aspirated)
Candles (insect-repellent type may be toxic)	Modeling clay and other modeling compounds
Carbowax (polyethylene glycol)	Paraffin, chlorinated
Carboxymethylcellulose (dehydrating material packed with drugs, film, and other products)	Pencil lead (graphite)
Castor oil	Pepper, black (except inhaled in mass)
Cetyl alcohol	Petrolatum jelly
Contraceptives	Polyethylene glycols
Crayons (children's; marked A.P., C.P., or C.S. 130–46)	Polyethylene glycol stearate
Dichloral (herbicide)	Polysorbate
Dry cell battery (alkaline)	Putty
Glycerol	Shaving cream
Glyceryl monostearate	Silica (silicon dioxide)
Graphite	Spermaceti
Gums (eg, acacia, agar, ghatti)	Stearic acid
Ink (amount in one ballpoint pen)	Sweeteners
Iodide salts	Talc (except when inhaled)
Kaolin	Tallow
Lanolin	Thermometer fluid (including liquid mercury)
Linoleic acid	Titanium oxide
Linseed oil (not boiled)	Triacetin (glyceryl triacetate)
Lipstick	Vitamins, children's multiple with or without iron
	Vitamins, multiple without iron

*This table is intended only as a guide; substances may be combined with phenol, petroleum distillate vehicles, or other toxic chemicals. A poison control center should be consulted for up-to-date information. Almost any substance can be toxic if ingested in sufficient amounts.

tablets (eg, aspirin, iron, enteric-coated drugs) form large concretions (bezoars) in the GI tract, where they tend to remain, continuing to be absorbed and causing toxicity.

Symptoms and Signs

Symptoms and signs vary depending on the substance (see TABLE 326–8). Also, different patients poisoned with the same substance may present with very different symptoms. However, 6 clusters of symptoms (toxic syndromes, or toxidromes) occur commonly and may suggest particular classes of substances (see TABLE 326–2). Patients who ingest multiple substances are less likely to have symptoms characteristic of a single substance.

Symptoms typically begin soon after contact but, with certain poisons, are delayed. The delay may occur because a metabolite is toxic rather than the parent substance (eg, methanol, ethylene glycol, hepatotoxins). Ingestion of hepatotoxins (eg, acetaminophen, iron, *Amanita phalloides* mushrooms) may cause acute hepatic failure that occurs one to a few days later. With metals or hydrocarbon solvents, symptoms typically occur only after chronic exposure to the toxin.

Ingested toxins generally cause systemic symptoms. Caustics and corrosive liquids damage mainly the mucous membranes of the GI tract, causing stomatitis, enteritis, or perforation. Some toxins (eg, alcohol, hydrocarbons) cause characteristic breath odors. Skin contact with toxins can cause various acute cutaneous symptoms (eg, rashes, pain, blistering); chronic exposure may cause dermatitis. Inhaled toxins are likely to cause

TABLE 326–2. COMMON TOXIC SYNDROMES (TOXIDROMES)

SYNDROME	SYMPTOMS	COMMON CAUSES
Anticholinergic	Tachycardia, hyperthermia, mydriasis, warm and dry skin, urinary retention, ileus, delirium ("mad as a hatter, blind as a bat, red as a beet, hot as a hare, and dry as a bone"*)	Antihistamines Atropine Belladonna alkaloids Jimson weed Mushrooms (some) Psychoactive drugs (many) Scopolamine Tricyclic antidepressants
Cholinergic, muscarinic	SLUDGE syndrome (*s*alivation, *l*acrimation, *u*rination, *d*efecation, *G*I cramps, and *e*mesis), miosis, bronchorrhea, wheezing, bradycardia	Carbamates Mushrooms (some) Organophosphates Physostigmine Pilocarpine Pyridostigmine
Cholinergic, nicotinic	Tachycardia, hypertension, fasciculations, abdominal pain, paresis	Black widow spider bites Carbamates Insecticides (some) Nicotine
Opioid	Hypoventilation, hypotension, miosis, sedation, possibly hypothermia	Opioids (eg, diphenoxylate, fentanyl, heroin, methadone, morphine, pentazocine, propoxyphene)
Sympathomimetic	Tachycardia, hypertension, mydriasis, agitation, seizures, diaphoresis, hyperthermia, psychosis (after chronic use)	Amphetamines Caffeine Cocaine Ephedrine MDMA (Ecstasy) Phenylpropanolamine Theophylline
Withdrawal	Tachycardia, hypertension, mydriasis, diaphoresis, agitation, restlessness, seizures, hyperreflexia, piloerection, yawning, abdominal cramps, lacrimation, hallucinations	Withdrawal of any of the following: Alcohol Barbiturates Benzodiazepines Opioids Sedatives (some)

*From Carroll L: *Alice in Wonderland*.
MDMA = methylenedioxymethamphetamine.

symptoms of upper airway injury if they are water soluble and symptoms of lower airway (lung parenchyma) injury and noncardiogenic pulmonary edema if they are less water soluble. Eye contact with toxins (solid, liquid, or vapor) may damage the cornea and lens, causing eye pain, redness, and loss of vision.

Some substances (eg, cocaine, phencyclidine, amphetamine) can cause severe agitation, which can result in hyperthermia, acidosis, and rhabdomyolysis.

Diagnosis

The first step of diagnosis is to assess the overall status of the patient. Severe poisoning may require rapid intervention to treat cardiopulmonary collapse.

Poisoning may be known at presentation. It should be suspected if patients have unexplained symptoms, especially altered consciousness. If purposeful self-poisoning occurs in adults, multiple substances should be suspected.

History is often the most valuable tool. Because many patients (eg, preverbal children, suicidal or psychotic adults, patients with altered consciousness) cannot provide reliable information, friends, relatives, and rescue personnel should be questioned. Even seemingly reliable patients may incorrectly report the amount or time of ingestion. When possible, the patient's living quarters should be inspected for clues (eg, partially empty pill containers, evidence of recreational drug use). Pharmacy and medical records may provide useful information. In potential workplace poisonings, coworkers and supervisors should be questioned. All industrial chemicals must have a material safety data sheet (MSDS) readily available at the workplace; the MSDS provides detailed information about toxicity and any specific treatment.

In the US, Europe, and parts of Asia and South America, information about household and industrial chemicals can be obtained from poison control centers. Consultation with the centers is encouraged because ingredients, first-aid measures, and antidotes printed on product containers are occasionally inaccurate or outdated. Also, the container may have been replaced, or the package tampered with. Poison control centers may be able to help identify unknown pills based on their appearance. The centers have ready access to toxicologists. The telephone number of the nearest center is often listed with other emergency numbers in the front of the local telephone book; the number is also available from the telephone operator or, in the US, by dialing 1-800-222-1222.

Physical examination sometimes detects signs suggesting particular types of substances (eg, toxidromes, breath odor, needle tracks suggesting IV drug use, stigmas of chronic alcohol use).

Even if a patient is known to be poisoned, altered consciousness may have other causes (eg, CNS infection, head trauma, hypoglycemia, stroke, hepatic encephalopathy, Wernicke's encephalopathy), which should also be considered. Attempted suicide must always be considered in older children, adolescents, and adults who have ingested a drug. After such patients are stabilized, psychiatric intervention should be considered.

Testing: In most cases, laboratory testing provides limited help. Standard, readily available tests to identify common drugs of abuse (often called, "toxic screens") are qualitative, not quantitative. These tests may provide false results, and they check for only a limited number of substances. Also, the presence of a drug of abuse does not necessarily indicate that the drug caused the patient's symptoms or signs.

For most substances, blood levels cannot be easily determined or do not help guide treatment. For a few substances (eg, acetaminophen, aspirin, carbon monoxide, digoxin, ethylene glycol, iron, lithium, methanol, phenobarbital, phenytoin, theophylline), blood levels may help guide treatment. Many authorities recommend measuring acetaminophen levels in all patients with mixed ingestions because acetaminophen ingestion is common, is often asymptomatic during the early stages, and can cause serious delayed toxicity that can be prevented by an antidote. For some substances, other blood tests (eg, PT/INR for warfarin overdose, methemoglobin levels for certain substances) may help guide treatment. For patients who have altered consciousness or abnormal vital signs or who have ingested certain substances, tests should include serum electrolytes, BUN, serum creatinine, serum osmolality, plasma glucose, and ABGs. Other tests may be indicated for specific substances.

For certain poisonings (eg, due to iron, lead, arsenic, other metals, or to packets of cocaine or other illicit drugs ingested by so-called body packers), plain abdominal x-rays may show the presence and location of ingested substances. X-rays are also indicated for patients with serious symptoms possibly due to poisoning with an unknown substance.

For poisonings with drugs that have cardiovascular effects or with an unknown substance, ECG and cardiac monitoring are indicated.

If blood levels of a substance or symptoms of toxicity increase after initially decreasing or persist for an unusually long time, a bezoar, a sustained-release preparation, or reexposure (eg, repeated covert exposure to a recreationally used drug) should be suspected.

Treatment

Seriously poisoned patients may require ventilation or treatment of cardiovascular collapse. Those with impaired consciousness may require continuous monitoring or restraints. The discussion of treatment for specific poisonings, below and in TABLES 326–3, 326–4, and 326–8, is general and does not include specific complexities and details. Consultation with a poison control center is recommended for any poisonings except the mildest and most routine.

TABLE 326–3. COMMON SPECIFIC ANTIDOTES

TOXIN	ANTIDOTE
Acetaminophen	*N*-Acetylcysteine
Anticholinergics	Physostigmine*
Benzodiazepines	Flumazenil*
β-Blockers	Glucagon
Ca channel blockers	Ca IV insulin in high doses with IV glucose
Carbamates	Atropine Protopam
Digitalis glycosides (digoxin, digitoxin, oleander, foxglove)	Digoxin-specific Fab fragments
Ethylene glycol	Ethanol Fomepizole
Heavy metals	Chelating drugs (see TABLE 326–4)
Iron	Deferoxamine
Isoniazid	Pyridoxine (vitamin B_6)
Methanol	Ethanol Fomepizole
Methemoglobin-forming agents (eg, aniline dyes, some local anesthetics, nitrates, nitrites, phenacetin, sulfonamides)	Methylene blue
Opioids	Naloxone
Organophosphates	Atropine Pralidoxime
Tricyclic antidepressants	$NaHCO_3$

*Use is controversial.

Fab = fractionated antibodies.

Initial stabilization: Treatment of any systemic poisoning begins with airway, breathing, and circulatory stabilization (see p. 532).

If patients have apnea or compromised airways (eg, foreign material in the oropharynx, decreased gag reflex), an endotracheal tube should be inserted. If patients have respiratory depression or hypoxia, supplemental O_2 or mechanical ventilation should be provided as needed.

In patients with apnea, IV naloxone (2 mg in adults; 0.1 mg/kg in children) should be tried while airway support is maintained. In opioid addicts, naloxone may precipitate withdrawal, but withdrawal is preferable to apnea. If respiratory depression persists despite use of naloxone, endotracheal intubation and continuous mechanical ventilation are required. If naloxone relieves respiratory depression, patients are monitored; if respiratory depression recurs, patients can be treated with another bolus of IV naloxone or mechanical ventilation. Using continuous naloxone infusion to maintain respiratory drive is controversial.

If patients have altered consciousness, plasma glucose should be measured immediately at bedside, or IV dextrose (50 mL of a 50% solution for adults; 2 to 4 mL/kg of a 25% solution for children) should be given empirically. For adults with suspected thiamin deficiency (eg, alcoholics, malnourished patients), thiamin 100 mg IV is given with or before glucose.

Hypotension is treated with IV fluids. If fluids are ineffective, invasive hemodynamic monitoring may be necessary to guide fluid and vasopressor therapy. The 1st-choice vasopressor for most poison-induced hypotension is norepinephrine 0.5 to 1 μg/min IV infusion, but treatment should not be delayed if another vasopressor is more immediately available.

Topical decontamination: Any body surface (including the eyes) exposed to a toxin is flushed with large amounts of water or saline. Contaminated clothing, including shoes and socks, and jewelry should be removed.

Activated charcoal: Charcoal is usually given, particularly when multiple or unknown substances have been ingested. Use of charcoal adds little risk unless patients are at risk of vomiting and aspiration, but its use may not substantially reduce overall morbidity or mortality. When used, charcoal is given as soon as possible. Activated charcoal adsorbs most toxins because of its molecular configuration and large surface area. Multiple doses of activated charcoal may be effective for substances that undergo enterohepatic recirculation (eg, phenobarbital, theophylline) and for sustained-release preparations. Charcoal may be given at 4- to 6-h intervals for serious poisoning with such substances unless bowel sounds are hypoactive. Charcoal is ineffective for caustics, alcohols, and simple

TABLE 326–4. GUIDELINES FOR CHELATION THERAPY

CHELATING DRUG*	METAL	DOSAGE†
Dimercaprol, 10% in oil	Antimony Arsenic Bismuth Chromates‡ Chromic acid‡ Chromium trioxide‡ Copper salts Gold Mercury Nickel Tungsten Zinc salts	3–4 mg/kg via deep IM injection q 4 h on day 1, 2 mg/kg IM q 4 h on day 2, 3 mg/kg IM q 6 h on day 3, then 3 mg/kg IM q 12 h for 7–10 days until recovery
Edetate Ca disodium (Ca disodium edathamil), diluted to ≤ 3%	Cadmium Lead Zinc Zinc salts	25–35 mg/kg IV slowly (over 1 h) q 12 h for 5–7 days, followed by 7 days without the drug; then repeated
Penicillamine	Arsenic Copper salts Gold Lead Mercury‡ Nickel Zinc salts	20–30 mg/kg/day in 3–4 divided doses (usual starting dose is 250 mg qid) to a maximum adult dose of 2 g/day
Succimer	Arsenic, occupational exposure in adults Bismuth Lead if children have blood lead levels > 45 μg/dL (> 2.15 μmol/L) Lead, occupational exposure in adults Mercury, occupational exposure in adults	10 mg/kg po q 8 h for 5 days, then 10 mg/kg po q 12 h for 14 days

*Iron and thallium salts are not chelated effectively by these drugs; each has its own chelating drug (see iron and thallium salts in TABLES 326–3 and 326–8).
† Dosages depend on type and severity of poisoning.
‡Chelating drug of choice.

ions (eg, cyanide, iron, other metals, lithium). The recommended dose is 5 to 10 times that of the suspected toxin ingested. However, because the amount of toxin ingested is usually unknown, the usual dose is 1 to 2 g/kg, which is about 10 to 25 g for children < 5 yr and 50 to 100 g for older children and adults. Charcoal is given as a slurry in water or soft drinks. It may be unpalatable and results in vomiting in 30% of patients; administration via a gastric tube should be considered. Activated charcoal should probably be used without sorbitol or other cathartics, which have no clear benefit and can cause dehydration and electrolyte abnormalities.

Gastric emptying: Gastric emptying, which used to be well-accepted and seems intuitively beneficial, is not routinely done. It does not clearly reduce overall morbidity or mortality and has risks. Gastric emptying is considered if it can be done within 1 h of a life-threatening ingestion. However, many poisonings manifest too late, and whether a poisoning is life threatening is not always clear. Thus, gastric emptying is seldom indicated and, if a caustic substance has been ingested, is contraindicated (see p. 2663).

If gastric emptying is used, gastric lavage is the preferred method. Syrup of ipecac has unpredictable effects, often causes prolonged vomiting, and may not remove substantial amounts of poison from the stomach. Gastric lavage may cause complications such as epistaxis, aspiration, or, rarely, oropharyngeal or esophageal injury.

For gastric lavage, tap water is instilled and withdrawn from the stomach with a tube. The largest tube possible (usually > 36 French for adults or 24 French for children) is used so that tablet fragments can be retrieved. If patients have altered consciousness or a weak gag reflex, endotracheal intubation should be done before lavage to prevent aspiration. Patients are placed in the left lateral decubitus position to prevent aspiration, and the tube is inserted orally. Because lavage sometimes forces substances farther into the GI tract, a 25-g dose of charcoal is instilled through the tube first. Then aliquots (about 3 mL/kg) of tap water are instilled, and the gastric contents are withdrawn by gravity or syringe. Lavage continues until the withdrawn fluids appear free of the substance; usually, 500 to 3000 mL of fluid must be instilled. After lavage, a 2nd 25-g dose of charcoal is instilled.

Whole-bowel irrigation: This procedure flushes the GI tract and theoretically decreases GI transit time for pills and tablets. Irrigation has not been proved to reduce morbidity or mortality. Irrigation is indicated for some serious poisonings due to sustained-release preparations or substances that are not adsorbed by charcoal (eg, heavy metals), for drug packets (eg, latex-coated packets of heroin or cocaine ingested by body packers), or for a suspected bezoar. A commercially prepared solution of polyethylene glycol (which is nonabsorbable) and electrolytes is given at a rate of 1 to 2 L/h for adults or at 25 to 40 mL/kg/h for children until the rectal effluent is clear; this process may require many hours or even days. The solution is usually given via a gastric tube, although some motivated patients can drink these large volumes.

Alkaline diuresis: Alkaline diuresis enhances elimination of weak acids (eg, salicylates, phenobarbital). A solution made by combining 1 L of 5% D/W with 3 50-mEq ampules of $NaHCO_3$ and 20 to 40 mEq of K can be given at a rate of 250 mL/h in adults and 2 to 3 mL/kg/h in children. Urine pH is kept at > 8.0. Hypernatremia, alkalemia, and fluid overload may occur but are usually not serious. However, alkaline diuresis is contraindicated in patients with renal insufficiency.

Dialysis: Common toxins that may require dialysis or hemoperfusion include ethylene glycol, lithium, methanol, salicylates, and theophylline. These therapies are less useful if the poison is a large or charged (polar) molecule, has a large volume of distribution (ie, if it is stored in fatty tissue), or is extensively bound to tissue protein (as with digoxin, phencyclidine, phenothiazines, or tricyclic antidepressants). The need for dialysis is usually determined by both laboratory values and clinical status. Methods of dialysis include hemodialysis, peritoneal dialysis, and lipid dialysis (which removes lipid-soluble substances from the blood), as well as hemoperfusion (which more rapidly and efficiently clears specific poisons—see Ch. 234 on p. 1989).

Specific antidotes: For the most commonly used antidotes, see TABLE 326–3. Chelating drugs are used for poisoning with heavy metals and occasionally with other drugs (see TABLE 326–4).

Ongoing supportive measures: Most symptoms (eg, agitation, sedation, coma, cerebral edema, hypertension, arrhythmias, renal failure, hypoglycemia) are treated with the usual supportive measures (see elsewhere in THE MANUAL). Drug-induced hypotension and arrhythmias may not respond to the usual drug treatments. For refractory hypotension, dopamine, epinephrine, other vasopressors, an intra-aortic balloon pump, or even extracorporeal circulatory support may be considered. For refractory arrhythmias, cardiac pacing may be necessary. Often, torsades de pointes can be treated with Mg sulfate 2 to 4 g IV, overdrive pacing, or a titrated isoproterenol infusion. Seizures are first treated with benzodiazepines; phenobarbital or phenytoin can also be used. Severe agitation must be controlled; benzodiazepines in large doses, other potent sedatives (eg, propofol), or, in extreme cases, induction of paralysis and mechanical ventilation may be required. Hyperthermia is treated with physical cooling measures rather than with antipyretics. Organ failure may ultimately require kidney or liver transplantation.

Hospital admission: General indications for hospital admission include altered consciousness, persistently abnormal vital signs, and predicted delayed toxicity. For example, admission is considered if patients have ingested sustained-release preparations, particularly of drugs with potentially serious effects, such as cardiovascular drugs. If there are no other reasons for admission and if symptoms are gone after patients have been observed for 4 to 6 h, most patients can be discharged; however, if ingestion was intentional, patients require a psychiatric evaluation.

Prevention

In the US, widespread use of child-resistant containers with safety caps has greatly reduced the number of poisoning deaths in children < 5 yr. Limiting the amount of OTC analgesics in a single container reduces the severity of poisonings, particularly with acetaminophen, aspirin, or ibuprofen. Preventive measures also include clearly labeling household products and prescription drugs, storing drugs and toxic substances in cabinets that are locked and inaccessible to children, promptly flushing expired drugs down the toilet, and using carbon monoxide detectors. Public education measures to encourage storage of substances in their original containers (eg, not placing insecticide in drink bottles) are important. Use of imprint identifications on solid drugs helps prevent confusion and errors by patients, pharmacists, and health care practitioners.

ACETAMINOPHEN POISONING

Acetaminophen poisoning can cause gastroenteritis within hours and hepatotoxicity 1 to 3 days after ingestion. Severity of hepatotoxicity after a single acute overdose is predicted by serum acetaminophen levels. Treatment is with N-acetylcysteine to prevent or minimize hepatotoxicity.

Acetaminophen is contained in > 100 products sold OTC; they include many children's preparations in liquid, tablet, and capsule form and many cough and cold preparations. Many prescription drugs also contain acetaminophen. Consequently, acetaminophen overdose is common.

The principal toxic metabolite of acetaminophen, *N*-acetyl-*p*-benzoquinone imine (NAPQI), is produced by the hepatic cytochrome P-450 enzyme system; glutathione stores in the liver detoxify this metabolite. An acute overdose depletes glutathione stores in the liver. As a result, NAPQI accumulates, causing hepatocellular necrosis and possibly damage to other organs (eg, kidneys, pancreas). Theoretically, alcoholic liver disease or undernutrition could increase risk of toxicity because hepatic enzyme preconditioning may increase formation of NAPQI and because undernutrition (also common among alcoholics) reduces hepatic glutathione stores. However, whether the risk is actually increased is unclear. Acute alcohol ingestion may be protective because hepatic P-450 enzymes preferentially metabolize ethanol and thus cannot produce toxic NAPQI.

To cause toxicity, an acute overdose must total ≥ 150 mg/kg (about 7.5 g in adults) within 24 h.

Chronic excessive use or repeated overdoses cause hepatotoxicity in a few patients. Usually, chronic overdose is not an attempt at self-injury but instead results from taking inappropriately high doses to treat pain.

Symptoms, Signs, and Diagnosis

Single acute overdose: Mild poisoning may not cause symptoms, and when present, symptoms are usually minor until ≥ 48 h after ingestion. Symptoms, which occur in 4 stages (see TABLE 326–5), include anorexia, nausea, vomiting, and right upper quadrant abdominal pain. AST, ALT, and, if poisoning is severe, bilirubin and INR may be elevated. AST levels > 1000 IU/L are more likely to result from acetaminophen poisoning than from chronic hepatitis or alcoholic liver disease. Renal failure and pancreatitis may occur, occasionally without hepatic failure. After > 5 days, hepatotoxicity resolves or progresses to multiple organ failure, which can be fatal.

Acetaminophen overdose should be considered in all patients with nonaccidental ingestions that may be attempts at suicide because acetaminophen overdose is common. Also, it often causes minimal symptoms during the early stages, is potentially lethal but is treatable, and may not be reported by suicidal or obtunded patients.

Likelihood and severity of hepatotoxicity can be predicted by the amount ingested or, more accurately, by the serum acetaminophen level. If the time of ingestion is known, the Rumack-Matthew nomogram (see FIG. 326–1) is used to estimate likelihood of hepatotoxicity; if the time is unknown, the nomogram cannot be used. For a single acute overdose of traditional acetaminophen or rapid-relief acetaminophen (which is absorbed 7 to 8 min faster), levels are measured ≥ 4 h after ingestion

TABLE 326–5. STAGES OF ACETAMINOPHEN POISONING

STAGE	TIME POST-INGESTION	DESCRIPTION
I	0 to 24 h	Anorexia, nausea, and vomiting
II	24 to 72 h	Right upper quadrant abdominal pain (common); AST, ALT, and, if poisoning is severe, bilirubin and PT (usually reported as the INR) sometimes elevated
III	72 to 96 h	Vomiting and symptoms of hepatic failure; AST, ALT, bilirubin, and INR peak; sometimes renal failure and pancreatitis
IV	> 5 days	Resolution of hepatotoxicity or progression to multiple organ failure (sometimes fatal)

and plotted on the nomogram. A level ≤ 150 μg/mL (≤ 990 μmol/L) and absence of toxic symptoms indicate that hepatotoxicity is very unlikely. Higher levels indicate possible hepatotoxicity. For a single acute overdose with extended-relief acetaminophen (which has 2 peak serum levels about 4 h apart), acetaminophen levels are measured ≥ 4 h after ingestion and 4 h later; if either level is above the Rumack-Matthew line of toxicity, treatment is required.

Chronic overdose: Symptoms may be absent or may include any of those that occur with acute overdose. The Rumack-Matthew nomogram cannot be used, but likelihood of clinically significant hepatotoxicity can be estimated based on AST, ALT, and serum acetaminophen levels. If AST and ALT are normal (< 50 IU/L) and the acetaminophen level is < 10 μg/mL, significant hepatotoxicity is very unlikely. If AST and ALT are normal but the acetaminophen level is ≥ 10 μg/mL, significant hepatotoxicity is possible; AST and ALT are remeasured after 24 h. If repeat AST and ALT are normal, significant hepatotoxicity is unlikely; if they are high, significant hepatotoxicity is assumed. If initial AST and ALT are high, regardless of the acetaminophen level, significant hepatotoxicity is assumed.

Prognosis

With appropriate treatment, mortality is uncommon. Poor prognostic indicators at 24 to 48 h postingestion include pH < 7.3 after adequate resuscitation, INR > 3, serum creatinine > 2.6, hepatic encephalopathy grade III (confusion and somnolence) or grade IV (stupor and coma), hypoglycemia, and thrombocytopenia. Acute acetaminophen toxicity does not predispose patients to cirrhosis.

Treatment

Activated charcoal is given if acetaminophen is likely to still remain in the GI tract.

N-Acetylcysteine is an antidote for acetaminophen poisoning. This drug is a glutathione precursor that decreases acetaminophen toxicity by increasing hepatic glutathione stores and possibly via other mechanisms.

For acute poisoning, *N*-acetylcysteine is given if hepatotoxicity is likely based on acetaminophen dose or serum level. The drug is most effective if given within 8 h of acetaminophen ingestion.

For chronic poisoning, *N*-acetylcysteine is given for the 1st 24 h if hepatotoxicity is possible (if AST and ALT are normal and acetaminophen level is initially elevated). If repeat AST and ALT (after 24 h) are normal, *N*-acetylcysteine is stopped; if repeat levels are high, they are remeasured daily, and *N*-acetylcysteine is continued until levels are normal. If hepatotoxicity is likely (especially if initial AST and ALT are high), a full course of *N*-acetylcysteine is given.

N-Acetylcysteine is equally effective given IV or po. IV therapy is given as a continuous infusion. A loading dose of 150 mg/kg in 200 mL of 5% D/W given over 15 min is followed by maintenance doses of 50 mg/kg in 500 mL of 5% D/W given over 4 h, then 100 mg/kg in 1000 mL of 5% D/W given over 16 h. For children, dosing may need to be adjusted to decrease the total volume of fluid delivered; consultation with a poison control center is recommended.

The loading dose of oral *N*-acetylcysteine is 140 mg/kg. This dose is followed by 17 additional doses of 70 mg/kg q 4 h. Oral acetylcysteine is unpalatable; it is given diluted 1:4 in a carbonated beverage or fruit

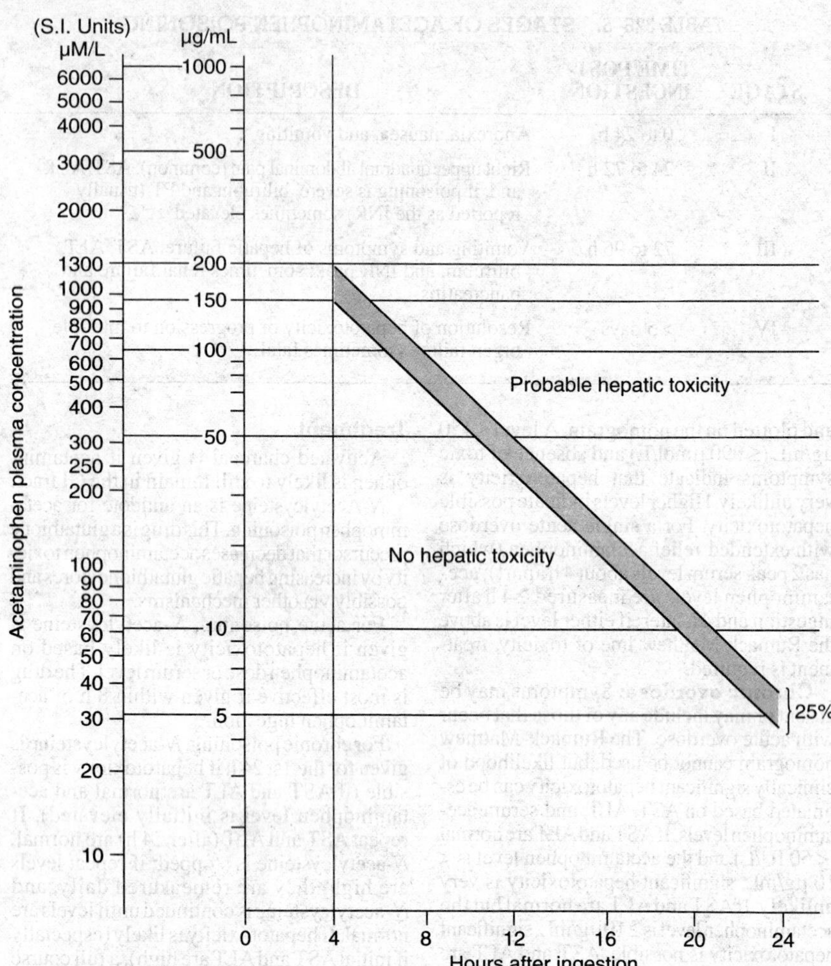

Fig. 326–1. Rumack-Matthew nomogram for single acute acetaminophen poisoning. Semilogarithmic plot of plasma acetaminophen levels vs time. *Cautions for use of this chart:* (1) The time coordinates refer to time of ingestion. (2) Serum levels drawn before 4 h may not represent peak levels. (3) The graph should be used only in relation to a single acute ingestion. (4) The lower solid line 25% below the standard nomogram is included to allow for possible errors in acetaminophen plasma assays and estimated time from ingestion of an overdose. (Adapted from Rumack BH, Matthew H: Acetaminophen poisoning and toxicity. *Pediatrics* 55(6): 871–876, 1975; reproduced by permission of *Pediatrics*.)

juice and may still cause vomiting. If vomiting occurs, an antiemetic can be used; if vomiting occurs within 1 h of a dose, the dose is repeated.

Hepatic failure is treated supportively. Patients with fulminant hepatic failure may require liver transplantation.

ASPIRIN AND OTHER SALICYLATE POISONING

(Salicylism)

Salicylate poisoning can cause vomiting, tinnitus, confusion, hyperthermia, respiratory alkalosis, metabolic acidosis, and multiple

organ failure. Diagnosis is clinical, supplemented by measurement of the anion gap, ABGs, and serum salicylate levels. Treatment is with activated charcoal and alkaline diuresis or hemodialysis.

Acute ingestion of > 150 mg/kg can cause severe toxicity. Salicylate tablets may form bezoars, prolonging absorption and toxicity. Chronic toxicity can occur after several days of high therapeutic doses; it is common, often undiagnosed, and often more serious than acute toxicity. Chronic toxicity tends to occur in elderly patients.

The most concentrated and toxic form of salicylate is oil of wintergreen (methyl salicylate, a component of some liniments and solutions used in hot vaporizers); ingestion of < 5 mL can kill a young child. Any exposure should be considered serious.

Pathophysiology

Salicylates impair cellular respiration by uncoupling oxidative phosphorylation. They stimulate respiratory centers in the medulla, producing primary respiratory alkalosis, which is often unrecognized in young children. Salicylates simultaneously and independently produce primary metabolic acidosis. Eventually, as salicylates disappear from the blood, enter the cells, and poison mitochondria, metabolic acidosis becomes the primary acid-base abnormality.

Salicylate poisoning also causes ketosis, fever, and, even when systemic hypoglycemia is absent, low brain glucose levels. Renal Na, K, and water loss and increased but imperceptible respiratory water loss due to hyperventilation lead to dehydration.

Salicylates are weak acids that cross cell membranes relatively easily; thus, they are more toxic when blood pH is low. Dehydration, hyperthermia, and chronic ingestion increase salicylate toxicity because they result in greater distribution of salicylate to tissues. Excretion of salicylates increases when urine pH increases.

Symptoms and Signs

With acute overdose, early symptoms include nausea, vomiting, tinnitus, and hyperventilation. Later symptoms include hyperactivity, fever, confusion, and seizures. Rhabdomyolysis, acute renal failure, and respiratory failure may eventually develop. Hyperactivity may quickly turn to lethargy; hyperventilation (with respiratory alkalosis) changes to hypoventilation (with mixed respiratory and metabolic acidosis) and respiratory failure.

With chronic overdose, symptoms and signs tend to be nonspecific and vary greatly. They include subtle confusion, changes in mental status, fever, hypoxia, noncardiogenic pulmonary edema, dehydration, lactic acidosis, and hypotension.

Diagnosis

Salicylate poisoning is suspected in patients with a history of a single acute overdose or repeated ingestions of therapeutic doses (particularly in patients with fever and dehydration), in patients with unexplained metabolic acidosis, and in elderly patients with unexplained confusion and fever. If poisoning is suspected, serum salicylate (drawn at least a few hours after ingestion), urine pH, ABGs, serum electrolytes, serum creatinine, plasma glucose, and BUN are measured. If rhabdomyolysis is suspected, serum CK and urine myoglobin are measured.

Significant salicylate toxicity is suggested by serum levels much higher than therapeutic (therapeutic range, 10 to 20 mg/dL), particularly 6 h after ingestion (when absorption is usually almost complete), and by acidemia plus ABG results compatible with salicylate poisoning. Usually, ABGs suggest primary respiratory alkalosis during the 1st few hours after ingestion; later, they suggest compensated metabolic acidosis or mixed metabolic acidosis/respiratory alkalosis. Eventually, usually as salicylate levels decrease, poorly compensated or uncompensated metabolic acidosis is the primary finding. If respiratory failure occurs, ABGs suggest combined metabolic and respiratory acidosis, and chest x-ray shows diffuse pulmonary infiltrates. Plasma glucose levels may be normal, low, or high. Serial salicylate levels help determine whether absorption is continuing; ABGs should always be determined simultaneously. Increased serum CK and urine myoglobin levels suggest rhabdomyolysis.

Treatment

Activated charcoal is given as soon as possible and, if bowel sounds are present, may be repeated q 4 h until charcoal appears in the stool.

After volume and electrolyte abnormalities are corrected, alkaline diuresis can be used to increase urine pH, ideally to ≥ 8. Alkaline diuresis is indicated for patients with any symptoms of poisoning and should not be delayed until salicylate levels are determined. This intervention is safe and exponentially increases salicylate excretion. Because hypokalemia may interfere with alkaline diuresis, patients are given a solution consisting of 1 L of 5% D/W, 3 50-mEq ampules of $NaHCO_3$, and 40 mEq of KCl at 1.5 to 2 times the maintenance IV fluid rate. Serum K is monitored.

Drugs that increase urinary HCO_3 (eg, acetazolamide) should be avoided because they worsen metabolic acidosis and decrease blood pH. Drugs that decrease respiratory drive should be avoided if possible because they may impair hyperventilation and respiratory alkalosis, decreasing blood pH.

Fever can be treated with physical measures such as external cooling (see p. 2609). Seizures are treated with benzodiazepines. In patients with rhabdomyolysis, alkaline diuresis may help prevent renal failure.

Hemodialysis may be required to enhance salicylate elimination in patients with severe neurologic impairment, renal or respiratory insufficiency, acidemia despite other measures, or very high serum salicylate levels (> 100 mg/dL [> 7.25 mmol/L] with acute overdose or > 60 mg/dL [> 4.35 mmol/L] with chronic overdose).

CARBON MONOXIDE POISONING

Carbon monoxide poisoning causes acute symptoms such as headache, nausea, weakness, angina, dyspnea, loss of consciousness, and coma. Neuropsychiatric symptoms may develop weeks later. Diagnosis is by carboxyhemoglobin levels and ABGs, including measured O_2 saturation. Treatment is with supplemental O_2. Prevention is often possible with household carbon monoxide detectors.

Carbon monoxide (CO) poisoning, one of the most common fatal poisonings, occurs by inhalation. CO is a colorless, odorless gas that results from incomplete combustion of hydrocarbons. Common sources of CO in poisonings include house fires and improperly vented automobiles, furnaces, hot water heaters, wood- or charcoal-burning stoves, and kerosene heaters. CO is produced when natural gas (methane or propane) burns. Inhaling tobacco smoke results in CO in the blood but not enough to cause poisoning. The elimination half-life of CO is about 4.5 h with inhalation of room air, 1.5 h with 100% O_2, and 20 min with 3 atmospheres (pressure) of O_2 (as in a hyperbaric chamber—see p. 2626).

Mechanisms of CO toxicity are not completely understood. They appear to involve displacement of O_2 from Hb (because CO has greater affinity for Hb than does O_2), shifting of the O_2-Hb dissociation curve to the left (decreasing release of O_2 from Hb to tissues—see FIG. 46–4), and inhibition of mitochondrial respiration. Direct toxic effects on brain tissue are possible.

Symptoms and Signs

Symptoms tend to correlate well with the patient's peak blood carboxyhemoglobin levels. Many symptoms are nonspecific. Headache and nausea can begin when levels are 10 to 20%. Levels > 20% commonly cause vague dizziness, generalized weakness, difficulty concentrating, and impaired judgment. Levels > 30% commonly cause dyspnea during exertion, chest pain (in patients with coronary artery disease), and confusion. Higher levels can cause syncope, seizures, and obtundation. Hypotension, coma, respiratory failure, and death may occur, usually when levels are > 60%.

Patients may also have many other symptoms, including visual deficits, abdominal pain, and focal neurologic deficits. If poisoning is severe, neuropsychiatric symptoms and signs can develop weeks after exposure. Because CO poisoning often results from house fires, patients may have concomitant airway injuries (see sidebar 315–1 on p. 2593), which may increase risk of respiratory failure.

Diagnosis

Because symptoms can be vague, nonspecific, and variable, the diagnosis is easily missed. Many cases of mild poisoning with nonspecific symptoms are mistaken for viral syndromes. Physicians must maintain a high level of suspicion. If people from the same dwelling, particularly a heated dwelling, experience nonspecific symptoms, CO exposure should be considered.

If CO poisoning is suspected, the carboxyhemoglobin level is measured with a CO-oximeter; venous samples can be used because arteriovenous differences are trivial. ABGs are not measured routinely. ABGs and pulse oximetry, alone or combined, are inadequate for diagnosis of CO poisoning because O_2 saturation reported in ABGs represents dissolved O_2 and is thus unaffected by carboxyhemoglobin concentration; furthermore, the pulse oximeter cannot differentiate normal hemoglobin from carboxyhemoglobin and thus provides a falsely elevated oxyhemoglobin reading. Although elevated carboxyhemoglobin levels are clear evidence of poisoning, levels may be falsely low because they decrease rapidly after CO exposure ends, particularly in patients treated with supplemental O_2 (eg, in an ambulance). Metabolic acidosis can be a clue to the diagnosis. Other tests may help evaluate specific symptoms (eg, ECG for chest pain, CT for neurologic symptoms).

Prevention and Treatment

Prevention involves checking sources of indoor combustion to make sure they are correctly installed and vented to the outdoors. Exhaust pipes should be inspected periodically for leaks. CO detectors should be installed because they provide early warning that CO is free in a dwelling's atmosphere. If CO is suspected in a dwelling, windows should be opened, and the dwelling should be evacuated and evaluated for the source of CO.

Patients should be removed from the source of CO and stabilized as necessary. They are given 100% O_2 (by nonrebreather mask) and treated supportively. Hyperbaric oxygen therapy should be considered for patients who have life-threatening cardiopulmonary complications, ongoing chest pain, altered consciousness, loss of consciousness (no matter how brief), or a carboxyhemoglobin level > 25% and for pregnant patients. Patients are placed in a chamber at 2 to 3 atmospheres of O_2. Hyperbaric O_2 therapy may decrease the incidence of delayed neuropsychiatric symptoms. However, this therapy may cause barotrauma and, because therapy is not available at most hospitals, may require transfer of patients, who may not be stable; also, a chamber may not be available locally. Evidence for efficacy of hyperbaric O_2 therapy is somewhat inconclusive. A poison control center or hyperbaric specialist should be consulted.

CAUSTIC INGESTION

Caustics (strong acids and alkalis), when ingested, burn upper GI tract tissues, sometimes resulting in esophageal or gastric perforation. Symptoms may include drooling, dysphagia, and pain in the mouth, chest, or stomach; strictures may develop later. Diagnostic endoscopy may be required. Treatment is supportive. Gastric emptying and activated charcoal are contraindicated. Perforation is treated surgically.

Common sources of caustics include solid and liquid drain and toilet bowl cleaners. Industrial products are usually more concentrated than household products and thus tend to be more damaging.

Acids cause coagulation necrosis; an eschar forms, limiting further damage. Acids tend to affect the stomach more than the esophagus. Alkalis cause rapid liquefaction necrosis; no eschar forms, and damage continues until the alkali is neutralized or diluted. Alkalis tend to affect the esophagus more than the stomach, but ingestion of large quantities severely affects both.

Solid products tend to leave particles that stick to and burn tissues, discouraging further ingestion and causing localized damage. Because liquid preparations do not stick, larger quantities are easily ingested, and damage may be widespread. Liquids may also be aspirated, leading to upper airway injury.

Symptoms, Signs, and Diagnosis

Initial symptoms include drooling and dysphagia. In severe cases, pain and sometimes bleeding develop immediately in the mouth, throat, chest, or abdomen. Airway burns may cause coughing, tachypnea, or stridor.

Swollen, erythematous tissue may be visible intraorally; however, caustic liquids may produce no intraoral burns despite serious injury farther down the GI tract. Esophageal perforation may result in mediastinitis, with severe chest pain, tachycardia, fever, tachypnea, and shock. Gastric perforation may result in peritonitis. Esophageal or gastric perforation may occur within hours, after weeks, or anytime in between. Esophageal strictures can develop over weeks, even if initial symptoms were mild and treatment was adequate.

Because the presence or absence of intraoral burns does not reliably indicate whether the esophagus and stomach are burned, meticulous endoscopy is indicated to check for the presence and severity of esophageal and gastric burns when symptoms or history suggests more than trivial ingestion.

Treatment

Treatment is supportive. CAUTION: *Gastric emptying by emesis or lavage is contraindicated* because it can reexpose the upper GI tract to the caustic. Attempts to neutralize a caustic acid by correcting pH with an alkaline substance (and vice versa) are contraindicated because severe exothermic reactions may result. Activated charcoal is contraindicated because it may infiltrate burned tissue and interfere with endoscopic evaluation.

Oral fluids are started when they can be tolerated. Esophageal or gastric perforation is treated with antibiotics and surgery (see p. 100). IV corticosteroids and prophylactic antibiotics are not recommended. Strictures are treated with bougienage or, if they are severe or unresponsive, with esophageal bypass by colonic interposition.

CHEMICAL FOOD POISONING

Chemical food poisoning is caused by eating plants or animals that contain a naturally occurring toxin.

Chemical food poisoning often involves mushrooms, poisonous plants, or marine animals. Activated charcoal may be useful. Complications (eg, gastroenteritis, dehydration, renal or hepatic failure, respiratory insufficiency) are treated supportively.

Mushrooms: Numerous species when ingested cause toxicity. Differentiating them in the wild is difficult, even for highly knowledgeable people; folklore rules for differentiating toxic and nontoxic species are unreliable. If patients have eaten an unidentified mushroom, identifying the species can help determine specific treatment. However, because an experienced mycologist is seldom available for immediate consultation, treatment of patients who become ill after mushroom ingestion is usually guided by symptoms. If a sample of the mushroom, uningested or from the patient's emesis, is available, it can be sent to a mycologist for analysis.

All toxic mushrooms cause vomiting and abdominal pain; other manifestations vary significantly by mushroom type. Generally, mushrooms that cause symptoms early (within 2 h) are less dangerous than those that cause symptoms later (usually after 6 h).

Mushrooms that cause early GI symptoms (eg, *Chlorophyllum molybdites*, the little brown mushrooms that often grow in lawns) cause gastroenteritis, sometimes with headaches or myalgias. Diarrhea is occasionally bloody. Symptoms usually resolve within 24 h.

Mushrooms that cause early neurologic symptoms include hallucinogenic mushrooms, which are usually ingested recreationally because they contain psilocybin, a hallucinogen. The most common are members of the *Psilocybe* genus, but some other genera contain psilocybin. Symptoms begin within 15 to 30 min and include euphoria, enhanced imagination, and hallucinations. Tachycardia and hypertension are common, and hyperpyrexia occurs in some children; however, serious consequences are rare. Treatment occasionally involves sedation (eg, with benzodiazepines).

Mushrooms that cause early muscarinic symptoms include members of the *Inocybe* and *Clitocybe* genera. Symptoms may include the SLUDGE syndrome (see TABLE 326–2), miosis, bronchorrhea, bradycardia, diaphoresis, wheezing, and fasciculations. Symptoms are usually mild, begin within 30 min, and resolve within 12 h. Atropine may be given to treat severe muscarinic symptoms (eg, wheezing, bradycardia).

Mushrooms that cause delayed GI symptoms include members of the *Amanita, Gyromitra*, and *Cortinarius* genera. The most toxic *Amanita* mushroom is *Amanita phalloides*, which causes 95% of mushroom poisoning deaths. Initial gastroenteritis, which may occur 6 to 12 h after ingestion, can be severe; hypoglycemia can occur. Initial symptoms abate for a few days; then, hepatic and sometimes renal failure develops. Initial care involves close monitoring for hypoglycemia and possibly repeated doses of activated charcoal. Treatment of hepatic failure may require liver transplantation; other specific treatments (eg, *N*-acetylcysteine, high-dose penicillin, silibinin) are unproven.

Gyromitra mushrooms can cause hypoglycemia simultaneously with or shortly after gastroenteritis. Other manifestations may include CNS toxicity (eg, seizures) and, after a few days, hepatorenal syndrome. Initial care involves close monitoring for hypoglycemia and possibly repeated doses of activated charcoal. Neurologic symptoms are treated with pyridoxine 25 mg/kg (maximum daily dose of 25 g); hepatic failure is treated supportively.

Most *Cortinarius* mushrooms are endogenous to Europe. Gastroenteritis may last for

3 days. Renal failure, with symptoms of flank pain and decreased urine output, may occur 3 to 20 days after ingestion. Renal failure often resolves spontaneously.

Poisonous plants: A few commonly grown plants are poisonous. Highly toxic and potentially fatal plants include castor bean, jequirity bean, poison hemlock, and water hemlock, as well as oleander and foxglove, which contain digitalis glycosides (see TABLE 326–6). Few plant poisonings have specific antidotes.

Castor bean contains ricin, an extremely concentrated poison, but in a relatively impervious shell; thus, the bean must be chewed to release the toxin. Jequirity bean also has a concentrated cellular poison, which can cause death after swallowing or, in children, after chewing only 1 bean. Symptoms of either poisoning may include delayed gastroenteritis, sometimes severe and hemorrhagic, followed by delirium, seizures, coma, and death. Whole-bowel irrigation should be considered; it aims to remove all beans ingested.

Oleander, foxglove, and the similar but less toxic lily of the valley can cause gastroenteritis, confusion, hyperkalemia, and arrhythmias. The serum digoxin level can confirm ingestion but is not useful as quantitative information. K levels are closely monitored. Hyperkalemia may respond only to hemodialysis. Ca is not recommended for arrhythmias. Digoxin-specific Fab (fractionated antibody) fragments have been used to treat ventricular arrhythmias.

Hemlock poisoning can cause symptoms within 15 min. Poison hemlock has nicotinic effects, beginning with dry mouth and progressing to tachycardia, tremors, diaphoresis, mydriasis, seizures, and muscle paresis. Rhabdomyolysis and bradycardia may occur. Water hemlock appears to enhance γ-aminobutyric acid (GABA) activity. Symptoms may include gastroenteritis, delirium, refractory seizures, and coma.

Fish: There are 3 common types of fish poisoning.

Ciguatera poisoning may result from eating any of > 400 species of fish from the tropical reefs of Florida, the West Indies, or the Pacific, where a dinoflagellate produces a toxin that accumulates in the flesh of the fish. Older fish and large fish (eg, grouper, snapper, kingfish) contain more toxin. No known processing procedures, including cooking, are protective, and flavor is unaffected. Symptoms may begin 2 to 8 h after eating. Abdominal cramps, nausea, vomiting, and diarrhea last 6 to 17 h; then, pruritus, paresthesias, headache, myalgia, reversal of hot and cold sensation, and face pain may occur. For months afterward, unusual sensory phenomena and nervousness may cause debilitation. IV mannitol has been suggested as a treatment, but no clear benefit has been shown.

Scombroid poisoning is caused by high histamine levels in fish flesh due to bacterial decomposition after the fish is caught. Commonly affected species include tuna, mackerel, bonito, skipjack, and mahimahi. The fish may taste peppery or bitter. Facial flushing and possibly nausea, vomiting, epigastric pain, and urticaria occur within a few minutes of eating and resolve within 24 h. Symptoms are often mistaken for those of a seafood allergy. Unlike other fish poisonings, this poisoning can be prevented by properly storing the fish after it is caught. Treatment may include H_1 and H_2 blockers.

Tetrodotoxin poisoning is most commonly due to eating the puffer fish (fugu), a sushi delicacy, but > 100 fresh and salt water species contain tetrodotoxin. Symptoms are similar to those of ciguatera poisoning; potentially fatal respiratory paralysis can also occur. The toxin cannot be destroyed by cooking or freezing.

Shellfish: Paralytic shellfish poisoning can occur from June to October, especially on the Pacific and New England coasts, when mussels, clams, oysters, and scallops are contaminated by the poisonous dinoflagellate responsible for red tide. This dinoflagellate produces the neurotoxin saxitoxin, which is resistant to cooking. Circumoral paresthesias occur 5 to 30 min after eating. Nausea, vomiting, and abdominal cramps then develop, followed by muscle weakness. Untreated respiratory paralysis may be fatal; for survivors, recovery is usually complete.

HYDROCARBON POISONING

Hydrocarbon poisoning may result from ingestion or inhalation. Ingestion, most common among children < 5 yr, can result in aspiration pneumonitis. Inhalation, most common among adolescents, can result in ventricular fibrillation, usually without warning symptoms. Diagnosis of pneumonitis is by clinical criteria, chest x-ray, and oximetry. Gastric emptying is contraindicated because aspiration is a risk. Treatment is supportive.

TABLE 326–6. MODERATELY POISONOUS PLANTS

PLANT	SYMPTOMS	TREATMENT
Aloe spp	Gastroenteritis, nephritis, skin irritation	Supportive care and irrigation with soap and water
Azalea	Cholinergic symptoms	Supportive care and atropine
Cactus spp	Infection, granuloma formation	Removal of spines
Caladium spp	Oral mucosal damage due to Ca oxalate crystals in leaves	Supportive care and demulsification (eg, with milk or ice cream)
Capsicum spp (peppers)	Mucous membrane irritation and swelling	Supportive care, irrigation, and possibly demulsification
Colchicine (autumn crocus, meadow saffron, glory lily)	Delayed gastroenteritis, multiple organ failure	Supportive care and colchicine-specific Fab fragments*
Deadly nightshade	Anticholinergic symptoms, hallucinations	Supportive care; for severe hyperthermia or seizures, possibly physostigmine
Dumbcane (dieffenbachia)	Oral mucosal damage due to Ca oxalate crystals in leaves	Supportive care and demulsification (eg, with milk or ice cream)
Fava beans	In patients with G6PD deficiency, gastroenteritis, fever, headache, hemolytic anemia	Supportive care; for severe anemia and poisoning, consideration of exchange transfusion
Green potato and potato sprout	Gastroenteritis, hallucinations, delirium	Supportive care
Holly berries	Gastroenteritis	Supportive care
Jimsonweed	Anticholinergic symptoms, hallucinations	Supportive care; for severe hyperthermia or seizures, possibly physostigmine
Lily of the valley	Hyperkalemia, arrhythmias	See discussion of digitalis preparations on p. 662
Mistletoe	Gastroenteritis	Supportive care
Nettle	Local stinging and burning	Supportive care
Nightshade, common or woody	Gastroenteritis, hallucinations, delirium	Supportive care
Philodendron spp	Oral mucosal damage due to Ca oxalate crystals in leaves	Supportive care and demulsification (eg, with milk or ice cream)
Poinsettia	Minor mucous membrane irritation	Unnecessary
Poison ivy	Dermatitis	See Ch.114 on p. 954
Pokeweed	Mucous membrane irritation, gastroenteritis	Supportive care
Pothos	Oral mucosal damage due to Ca oxalate crystals in leaves	Supportive care and demulsification (eg, with milk or ice cream)
Yew	Gastroenteritis; rarely, seizures, arrhythmias, coma	Supportive care

*Not available outside France.

Fab = fractionated antibodies.

Ingestion of hydrocarbons, such as petroleum distillates (eg, gasoline, kerosene, mineral oil, lamp oil, paint thinners), results in minimal systemic effects but can cause severe aspiration pneumonitis. Toxic potential depends mainly on viscosity, measured in Saybolt seconds universal (SSU). Hydrocarbon liquids with low viscosity (SSU < 60), such as gasoline and mineral oil, can spread rapidly over large surface areas and are more likely to cause aspiration pneumonitis than are hydrocarbons with SSU > 60, such as tar. Hydrocarbons, if ingested in large amounts, may be absorbed systemically and cause CNS or hepatic toxicity, which is more likely with halogenated hydrocarbons (eg, carbon tetrachloride, trichloroethylene).

Recreational inhalation of halogenated hydrocarbons (eg, paint, solvents, cleaning sprays, gasoline, fluorocarbons used as refrigerants or propellants in aerosols), called huffing or bagging, is common among adolescents. It can cause euphoria and mental status changes and can sensitize the heart to endogenous catecholamines. Fatal ventricular arrhythmias may result; they usually occur without premonitory palpitations or other warning, often when patients are startled or chased.

Symptoms, Signs, and Diagnosis

After ingestion of even a very small amount of liquid hydrocarbon, patients initially cough, choke, and may vomit. Young children may have cyanosis, hold their breath, and cough persistently. Older children and adults may report burning in the stomach. Aspiration pneumonitis produces hypoxia and respiratory distress. Symptoms and signs of pneumonitis may develop a few hours before infiltrates are visible on x-ray. Substantial systemic absorption, particularly of a halogenated hydrocarbon, may cause lethargy, coma, and seizures. Nonfatal pneumonitis usually resolves in about 1 wk; mineral or lamp oil ingestion usually takes 5 to 6 wk to resolve. Arrhythmias usually occur before presentation and are unlikely to recur after presentation unless patients have excessive agitation.

If patients are too obtunded to provide a history, hydrocarbon exposure may be suspected if their breath or clothing has an odor or if a container is found near them. Paint residue on the hands or around the mouth may suggest recent paint sniffing. Diagnosis of aspiration pneumonitis is by symptoms and signs as well as by chest x-ray and oximetry, which are done about 6 h after ingestion, or sooner if symptoms are severe. If respiratory failure is suspected, ABGs are measured.

Treatment

Any contaminated clothing is removed, and the skin is washed. CAUTION: *Gastric emptying, which increases risk of aspiration, is contraindicated.* Charcoal is not recommended. Patients who do not have aspiration pneumonitis or other symptoms after 4 to 6 h are discharged. Patients who have symptoms are admitted and treated supportively; antibiotics and corticosteroids are not indicated.

IRON POISONING

Iron poisoning is the leading cause of poisoning deaths in children. Symptoms begin with acute gastroenteritis, followed by a quiescent period, then shock and hepatic failure. Diagnosis is by measuring serum iron, detecting radiopaque iron tablets in the GI tract, or detecting unexplained metabolic acidosis in patients with other findings suggesting iron poisoning. Treatment of a substantial ingestion is usually whole-bowel irrigation and chelation therapy with IV deferoxamine.

Many commonly used OTC preparations contain iron. Of the many iron compounds used in OTC and prescription preparations, the most common are ferrous sulfate (20% elemental iron), ferrous gluconate (12% elemental iron), and ferrous fumarate (33% elemental iron). To children, iron tablets may look like candy. Prenatal multivitamins are the source of iron in most lethal ingestions among children. Children's chewable multivitamins with iron usually have such small amounts that toxicity rarely occurs.

Iron is toxic to the GI, cardiovascular, and central nervous systems. Specific mechanisms are unclear, but excess free iron is inserted into enzymatic processes and interferes with oxidative phosphorylation, producing metabolic acidosis. Iron also catalyzes free radical formation, acts as an oxidizer, and, when plasma protein binding is saturated, combines with water to form iron hydroxide and free H^+ ions, compounding the metabolic acidosis. Coagulopathy may appear early because of interference with the coagulation cascade and later because of liver injury. Up to 20 mg/kg of elemental iron is not toxic; 20 to 60 mg/kg is mildly to moderately toxic, and > 60 mg/kg can cause severe symptoms and morbidity.

TABLE 326–7. STAGES OF IRON POISONING

STAGE	TIME POST-INGESTION	DESCRIPTION
1	Within 6 h	Vomiting, hematemesis, explosive diarrhea, irritability, abdominal pain, and lethargy If toxicity is severe, tachypnea, tachycardia, hypotension, coma, and metabolic acidosis
2	Within 6–48 h	Up to 24 h of apparent improvement (latent period)
3	12–48 h	Shock, seizures, fever, coagulopathy, and metabolic acidosis
4	2–5 days	Hepatic failure, jaundice, coagulopathy, and hypoglycemia
5	2–5 wk	Gastric outlet or duodenal obstruction secondary to scarring

Symptoms, Signs, and Diagnosis

Symptoms occur in 5 stages (see TABLE 326–7); however, symptoms and their progression vary significantly. The severity of stage 1 symptoms usually reflects the overall severity of poisoning; late-stage symptoms develop only if stage 1 symptoms are moderate or severe.

Iron poisoning should be considered in mixed ingestions (because iron is ubiquitous) and in small children with access to iron and unexplained metabolic acidosis or severe or hemorrhagic gastroenteritis. Because children often share, siblings and playmates of small children who have ingested iron should be evaluated.

Abdominal x-ray is usually recommended to confirm ingestion; it detects intact iron tablets or iron concretions but misses chewed and dissolved tablets, liquid iron preparations, and iron in multivitamin preparations. Serum iron, electrolytes, and pH are determined 3 to 4 h after ingestion. Toxicity is assumed if suspected ingestion is accompanied by vomiting and abdominal pain, serum iron levels > 350 μg/dL (63 μmol/L), iron visible on x-ray, or unexplained metabolic acidosis. These iron levels may indicate toxicity; however, iron levels alone do not predict toxicity accurately. Total iron binding capacity (TIBC) is often inaccurate and not helpful in diagnosing serious poisoning and is not recommended. The most accurate approach is to serially measure levels of serum iron, HCO_3, and pH (with calculation of the anion gap); these findings are then evaluated together, and results are correlated with the patient's clinical status. For example, toxicity is suggested by increasing iron levels, metabolic acidosis, worsening symptoms, or, more typically, some combination of these findings.

Prognosis and Treatment

If no symptoms develop within the 1st 6 h after ingestion, risk of serious toxicity is minimal. If shock and coma develop within the 1st 6 h, the mortality rate is about 10%.

If radiopaque tablets are visible on abdominal x-ray, whole-bowel irrigation with polyethylene glycol 1 to 2 L/h for adults or 24 to 40 mL/kg/h for children is done until no iron is visible on repeat abdominal x-ray. Gastric lavage is usually not helpful because vomiting tends to empty the stomach more efficiently. Activated charcoal does not adsorb iron and should be used only if other toxins were also ingested.

All patients with more than mild gastroenteritis are hospitalized. Patients with severe toxicity (metabolic acidosis, shock, severe gastroenteritis, or serum iron level > 500 μg/dL) are treated with IV deferoxamine to chelate free serum iron. Deferoxamine is infused at rates up to 15 mg/kg/h IV, titrated until hypotension occurs. Because both deferoxamine and iron poisoning can decrease BP, patients receiving deferoxamine require IV hydration.

LEAD POISONING

(Plumbism)

Lead poisoning often causes minimal symptoms at first but can cause acute encephalopathy or irreversible organ damage, commonly resulting in cognitive deficits in children. Diagnosis is by whole blood lead level. Treatment involves stopping lead exposure and sometimes using chelation therapy with succimer or edetate Ca disodium, with or without dimercaprol.

Leaded paint was commonly used until 1960, used to some degree until the early

1970s, and mostly eliminated in 1978; thus, for a significant number of older housing units, leaded paint still poses some hazard. Lead poisoning is usually caused by direct ingestion of leaded paint chips (from cracked, peeling paint). During home remodeling, patients may be exposed to significant amounts of aerosolized lead in the form of particles scraped or sanded off during surface preparation for repainting. Improperly lead-glazed ceramic ware, common outside the US, can leach lead, particularly when it comes in contact with acidic substances (eg, fruits, cola drinks, tomatoes, wine cider). Lead-contaminated moonshine whiskey and folk remedies are possible sources, as are occasional lead foreign objects in the stomach or tissues (eg, bullets, curtain or fishing weights). Bullets lodged in soft tissues may increase blood lead levels, but that process takes years to occur. Occupational exposure can occur during battery manufacture and recycling, bronzing, brass making, glassmaking, pipe cutting, soldering and welding, smelting, or working with pottery or pigments. Certain ethnic cosmetic products and imported herbal products and medicinal herbs contain lead and have caused cluster outbreaks of lead poisoning in immigrant communities. Fumes of leaded gasoline (in countries other than the US) recreationally inhaled for CNS effects may cause lead poisoning.

Symptoms and Signs

Lead poisoning is most often a chronic disorder and may not cause acute symptoms. With or without acute symptoms, poisoning eventually has irreversible effects (eg, cognitive deficits, peripheral neuropathy, progressive renal dysfunction).

Risk of cognitive deficits increases when the whole blood lead level (PbB) is ≥ 10 μg/dL (≥ 0.48 μmol/L) for an extended period, although the cutoff may be even lower. Other symptoms (eg, abdominal cramping, constipation, tremors, mood changes) may occur if PbB is > 50 μg/dL (> 2.4 μmol/L). Encephalopathy is likely if PbB is > 100 μg/dL (> 4.8 μmol/L).

In children, acute lead poisoning may cause irritability, decreased attentiveness, and acute encephalopathy. Cerebral edema develops over 1 to 5 days, producing persistent and forceful vomiting, ataxic gait, seizures, altered consciousness, and, finally, intractable seizures and coma. Encephalopathy may be preceded by several weeks of irritability and decreased play activity. Chronic lead poisoning in children may cause mental retardation, seizure disorders, aggressive behavior disorders, developmental regression, chronic abdominal pain, and anemia.

Adults with occupational exposure characteristically develop symptoms (eg, personality changes, headache, abdominal pain, neuropathy) over several weeks or longer. Encephalopathy is unusual.

Children and adults may develop anemia because lead interferes with the normal formation of Hb. Children and adults who inhale tetra-ethyl or tetra-methyl lead (in leaded gasoline) may develop toxic psychosis in addition to more characteristic symptoms of lead poisoning.

Diagnosis

Lead poisoning is suspected in patients with characteristic symptoms; however, because symptoms are often nonspecific, diagnosis is often delayed. Evaluation includes CBC and measurement of serum electrolytes, BUN, serum creatinine, plasma glucose, and PbB levels. An abdominal x-ray should be taken to look for lead particles, which are radiopaque. X-rays of long bones are taken in children. Horizontal, metaphyseal lead bands representing lack of RBC remodeling and increased Ca deposition in the zones of provisional calcification in children's long bones are somewhat specific for poisoning with lead or other heavy metals but are insensitive. Normocytic or microcytic anemia suggests lead toxicity, particularly when the reticulocyte count is elevated or RBC basophilic stippling occurs; however, sensitivity and specificity are limited. Diagnosis is definitive if the PbB level is ≥ 10 μg/dL.

Because measuring PbB is not always possible and can be expensive, other preliminary or screening tests for lead poisoning can be used. Capillary blood testing for lead is accurate, inexpensive, and quick. All positive tests should be confirmed with PbB. The erythrocyte protoporphyrin (also called zinc protoporphyrin or free erythrocyte protoporphyrin) test is often inaccurate and now is seldom used.

The edetate Ca disodium ($CaNa_2EDTA$) mobilization test, previously used for diagnosis and treatment, is considered obsolete by most toxicologists and is usually not done.

Treatment

For all patients, the source of lead is eliminated. If lead chips are visible on abdominal x-ray, whole-bowel irrigation with a polyethylene glycol electrolyte solution at 1000 to 2000 mL/h for adults or 25 to 40 mL/kg/h for children is done until repeat x-ray shows no lead. If the cause is bullets, surgical removal should be considered. Children with PbB > 70 μg/dL (> 3.40 μmol/L) and all patients with neurologic symptoms should be hospitalized. Patients with acute encephalopathy are admitted to an ICU.

Chelating drugs (eg, succimer [*meso*-2,3-dimercaptosuccinic acid], $CaNa_2EDTA$, dimercaprol [British antilewisite, or BAL]) can be given to bind lead into forms that can be excreted. *Chelation should be supervised by an experienced toxicologist.* Chelation is indicated for adults with symptoms of poisoning plus PbB > 70 μg/dL and for children with encephalopathy or PbB > 45 μg/dL (> 2.15 μmol/L). Liver and kidney disorders are relative contraindications for chelating drugs. Chelating drugs should not be given to any patient with ongoing exposure to lead because chelation can increase GI absorption of lead. Chelation removes only relatively small amounts of metal. If total body burden of lead is very large, multiple chelations over many years may be required.

Patients with encephalopathy are treated with dimercaprol 75 mg/m^2 (or 4 mg/kg) IM q 4 h and $CaNa_2EDTA$ 1000 to 1500 mg/m^2 IV (infusion) once/day. The 1st dose of dimercaprol should precede the 1st dose of $CaNa_2EDTA$ by at least 4 h to prevent redistribution of lead into the brain. Dimercaprol may be stopped after the first few doses depending on lead levels and symptom severity. Dimercaprol-$CaNa_2EDTA$ combination therapy is given for 5 days, followed by a 3-day washout period; then the need for continued chelation is reassessed.

Patients without encephalopathy are usually treated with succimer 10 mg/kg po q 8 h for 5 days, followed by 10 mg/kg po q 12 h for 14 days. If these patients have symptoms, they can alternatively be treated for 5 days with dimercaprol 50 mg/m^2 via deep IM injection q 4 h plus $CaNa_2EDTA$ 1000 mg/m^2 IV once/day.

Dimercaprol, which can cause vomiting, is given with parenteral or oral fluids. Dimercaprol can also cause pain at the injection site, numerous systemic symptoms, and, in patients with G6PD deficiency, moderate to severe acute intravascular hemolysis. This drug should not be given concurrently with iron supplements. Dimercaprol is formulated with peanut derivatives and thus is contraindicated in patients with known or suspected peanut allergy.

$CaNa_2EDTA$ can cause thrombophlebitis, which can be prevented by giving the drug IV, not IM, and by using an IV concentration of < 0.5%. Before beginning treatment with $CaNa_2EDTA$, adequate urine flow must be confirmed. Serious reactions to $CaNa_2EDTA$ include renal insufficiency, proteinuria, microscopic hematuria, fever, and diarrhea. Renal toxicity, which is dose-related, is usually reversible. Adverse effects of $CaNa_2EDTA$ are probably due to zinc depletion.

Common adverse effects of succimer include rash, GI symptoms (eg, anorexia, nausea, vomiting, diarrhea, metallic taste), and transient elevations of liver enzymes.

Patients with PbB > 10 μg/dL should be monitored closely, and they or their parents should be taught how to reduce their exposure to lead.

Prevention

Patients at risk should be screened by measuring PbB. Measures that reduce risk of household poisoning include regular hand washing, regular washing of children's toys and pacifiers, and regular cleaning of household surfaces; drinking water, household paint (except in houses built after 1978), and ceramic ware made outside the US should be tested for lead. Adults exposed to lead dust at work should use appropriate personal protective equipment, change their clothing and shoes before coming home, and shower before going to bed.

TABLE 326–8. SYMPTOMS AND TREATMENT OF SPECIFIC POISONS

POISON*	SYMPTOMS	TREATMENT
ACE inhibitors	Angioedema, hypotension	Charcoal, supportive care; for angioedema, epinephrine, antihistamines, or corticosteroids possibly effective
Acephate	See Organophosphates	—
Acetaminophen	See Acetaminophen Poisoning on p. 2658	—
Acetanilid Aniline dyes and oil Chloroaniline Phenacetin (acetophenetidin, phenylacetamide)	Cyanosis due to formation of methemoglobin and sulfhemoglobin, dyspnea, weakness, vertigo, angina, rashes and urticaria, vomiting, delirium, depression, respiratory and circulatory failure	Ingestion: Charcoal; then as for inhalation Skin contact: Clothing removed and area washed with copious soap and water; then as for inhalation Inhalation: O_2, respiratory support; blood transfusion; for severe cyanosis, methylene blue 1–2 mg/kg IV
Acetic acid	Low concentration: Mild mucosal irritation High concentration: See caustic ingestion	Supportive care with irrigation and dilution
Acetone Ketones Model airplane glues or cements Nail polish remover	Ingestion: As for inhalation, except direct pulmonary effect Inhalation: Bronchial irritation, pneumonia (pulmonary congestion and edema, decreased respiration, dyspnea), drunkenness, stupor, ketosis, cardiac arrhythmias	Removal from source, respiratory support, O_2 and fluids, correction of metabolic acidosis
Acetonitrile Cosmetic nail adhesive	Converted to cyanide, with usual symptoms and signs	See Cyanides
Acetophenetidin	See Acetanilid	—
Acetylene gas	See Carbon monoxide	
Acetylsalicylic acid	See Aspirin and Other Salicylate Poisoning on p. 2660	—
Acids and alkalis	See specific acids and alkalis (eg, Boric acid, Fluorides) and Caustic Ingestion on p. 2663 or, for eye or skin contact, see pp. 2586 and 2592, respectively.	—
Airplane glues or cements (model-building)	See Acetone, Benzene (toluene), Petroleum distillates	—
Alcohol, ethyl (ethanol) Brandy Whiskey Other liquors	Emotional lability, impaired coordination, flushing, nausea, vomiting, stupor to coma, respiratory depression	Supportive care, IV glucose to prevent hypoglycemia
Alcohol, isopropyl Rubbing alcohol	Dizziness, incoordination, stupor to coma, gastroenteritis, hemorrhagic gastritis, hypotension; *no* retinal injury or acidosis	Supportive care, IV glucose, correction of dehydration and electrolyte abnormalities; for gastritis, IV H_2 blockers or proton pump inhibitors

Table continues on the following page.

TABLE 326–8. SYMPTOMS AND TREATMENT OF SPECIFIC POISONS—Continued

POISON*	SYMPTOMS	TREATMENT
Alcohol, methyl (methanol, wood alcohol) Antifreeze Paint solvent Solid canned fuel Varnish	High toxicity with 60–250 mL (2–8 oz) in adults or 8–10 mL (2 tsp) in children; latency period 12–18 h; headache, weakness, leg cramps, vertigo, seizures, retinal injury, dimmed vision, acidosis, decreased respiration	Fomepizole (15 mg/kg, then 10 mg/kg q 12 h); alternatively, 10% ethanol/5% D/W IV; initial ethanol loading dose 10 mL/kg over 1 h, then 1–2 mL/kg/h to maintain a blood ethanol level of 100 mg/dL (22 mmol/L); hemodialysis (which is definitive treatment)
Aldrin	See Chlorinated hydrocarbons	—
Alkalis	See Acids and alkalis	—
Alphaprodine	See Opioids	—
Aminophylline Caffeine Theophylline	Wakefulness, restlessness, anorexia, vomiting, dehydration, seizures, tachycardia; in adults, greater toxicity after acute overdose added to chronic intake	Ingestion: Charcoal, discontinuation of drug, measurement of blood theophylline level, phenobarbital or diazepam for seizures, parenteral fluids, maintenance of BP; if serum level > 50–100 mg/L (> 278–555 μmol/L) or if acidosis, seizures, or coma is present, possibly dialysis; for patients without asthma, possibly β-blocker (eg, esmolol)
Amitriptyline	See Tricyclic antidepressants	—
Ammonia gas (anhydrous ammonia [NH_3])	Irritation of eyes and respiratory tract, cough, choking, abdominal pain	Flushing of eyes for 15 min with tap water or saline; if severe toxicity, positive pressure O_2 to manage pulmonary edema; respiratory support
Ammonia water (ammonium hydroxide [NH_4OH])	See Caustic Ingestion on p. 2663	—
Ammoniated mercury (NH_2HgCl)	See Mercury	—
Ammonium carbonate ($[NH_4]_2CO_3$)	See Caustic Ingestion on p. 2663	—
Ammonium fluoride (NH_4F)	See Fluorides	—
Amobarbital	See Barbiturates	—
Amphetamines Amphetamine sulfate or phosphate Dextroamphetamine Methamphetamine Phenmetrazine	Increased activity, exhilaration, talkativeness, insomnia, irritability, exaggerated reflexes, anorexia, diaphoresis, tachyarrhythmia, anginal chest pain, psychotic-like states, inability to concentrate or sit still, paranoia	Charcoal possibly effective long after ingestion because of recycling via enterohepatic circulation, benzodiazepines for sedation and seizures, reduction of external stimuli, external cooling, prevention of cerebral edema; in patients without asthma, β-blockers possibly helpful but rarely necessary

TABLE 326–8. SYMPTOMS AND TREATMENT OF SPECIFIC POISONS—Continued

POISON*	SYMPTOMS	TREATMENT
Amyl nitrite	See Nitrites	—
Aniline	See Acetanilid	—
Anticoagulants Dicumarol Superwarfarins Warfarin	Increased PT/INR after repeated ingestions	Observation for single ingestion; for repeated chronic ingestions, measurement of PT/INR to determine if vitamin K therapy is needed
Antidepressants	See Bupropion, Mirtazapine, Selective serotonin reuptake inhibitors, Trazodone, Tricyclic antidepressants, and Venlafaxine	—
Antifreeze	See Alcohol, methyl; Ethylene glycol	—
Antihistamines	Anticholinergic symptoms (tachycardia, hyperthermia, mydriasis, warm and dry skin, urinary retention, ileus, delirium)	Consideration of physostigmine 0.5–2.0 mg in adults or 0.02 mg/kg in children IV (slowly) for diagnostic testing or for treatment of severe symptoms refractory to sedation (CAUTION: seizures—see Physostigmine)
Antihyperglycemic drugs, oral	See Hypoglycemic drugs, oral	—
Antimony	See Arsenic	—
Antineoplastic drugs Methotrexate Mercaptopurine Vincristine > 50 Others	Effects on hematopoiesis, nausea, vomiting, specific acute vs chronic effects depending on drug	Supportive care, leucovorin rescue, observation for postacute problems (> 24–48 h)
Antipsychotic drugs (conventional) Chlorpromazine Fluphenazine Haloperidol Loxapine Mesoridazine Molindone Perphenazine Pimozide Prochlorperazine Thioridazine Thiothixene Trifluoperazine Triflupromazine	A wide range of symptoms (eg, sedation, seizures, excitement, coma, dystonia, hypotension, tachycardia, ventricular arrhythmias or torsades de pointes, anticholinergic effects, hyperthermia or hypothermia)	Diphenhydramine or benztropine for dystonia; norepinephrine for hypotension refractory to fluids; consideration of alkalinization for ventricular arrhythmias
Antipsychotic drugs (2nd-generation) Clozapine Olanzapine Quetiapine Risperidone Ziprasidone	CNS depression (particularly with olanzapine), miosis, anticholinergic effects, hypotension, dystonia, QT prolongation (occasionally), fatal bone marrow suppression (rare)	Diphenhydramine or benztropine for dystonia; norepinephrine for hypotension refractory to fluids; consideration of alkalinization for ventricular arrhythmias

Table continues on the following page.

TABLE 326–8. SYMPTOMS AND TREATMENT OF SPECIFIC POISONS—Continued

POISON*	SYMPTOMS	TREATMENT
Ant poison	See Arsenic (sodium arsenate), Borates	—
Arsenic Donovan's solution Fowler's solution Herbicides Paris green Pesticides Selenium Sodium arsenate Antimony Stibophen Tartar emetic	Throat constriction, dysphagia, burning GI pain, vomiting, diarrhea, GI hemorrhage, dehydration, pulmonary edema, renal failure, liver failure	Chelation with penicillamine, dimercaprol for patients who cannot take oral drugs, hydration, treatment of shock and pain
Arsine gas	Acute hemolytic anemia	Transfusions, diuresis
Artificial bitter almond oil	See Cyanide	—
Asphalt	See Petroleum distillates	—
Aspirin	See Aspirin and Other Salicylate Poisoning on p. 2660	—
Atropine	See Belladonna	—
Automobile exhaust	See Carbon monoxide	—
Barbiturates Amobarbital Meprobamate Pentobarbital Phenobarbital Secobarbital	Bradycardia, hypothermia, confusion, delirium, loss of corneal reflex, respiratory failure, drowsiness, ataxia, coma	Charcoal up to 24 h after ingestion, supportive care, forced alkaline diuresis for phenobarbital (to aid in elimination); for severe cases, hemodialysis
Barium compounds (soluble) Barium acetate Barium carbonate Barium chloride Barium hydroxide Barium nitrate Barium sulfide Depilatories Explosives Fireworks Rat poisons	Vomiting, abdominal pain, diarrhea, tremors, seizures, colic, hypertension, cardiac arrest, dyspnea and cyanosis, ventricular fibrillation, severe hypokalemia, skeletal muscle weakness	KCl 10–15 mEq/h IV; Na or Mg sulfate 60 g po to precipitate barium in stomach, then possible gastric lavage; diazepam to control seizures; O_2 for dyspnea and cyanosis
Belladonna Atropine Hyoscyamine Hyoscyamus Scopolamine (hyoscine) Stramonium	Anticholinergic symptoms (tachycardia, hyperthermia, mydriasis, warm and dry skin, urinary retention, ileus, delirium)	Consideration of physostigmine 0.5–2.0 mg in adults or 0.02 mg/kg in children IV (slowly) for diagnostic testing or for treatment of severe symptoms refractory to sedation (rarely needed) (CAUTION: seizures—see Physostigmine)

TABLE 326–8. SYMPTOMS AND TREATMENT OF SPECIFIC POISONS—Continued

POISON*	SYMPTOMS	TREATMENT
Benzene Benzol Hydrocarbons Model airplane glue Toluene Toluol Xylene	Dizziness, weakness, headache, euphoria, nausea, vomiting, ventricular arrhythmia, paralysis, seizures With chronic poisoning, aplastic anemia, hypokalemia, leukemia, CNS depression	Decontamination with water, avoiding vomiting and aspiration; O_2; respiratory support; ECG monitoring (ventricular fibrillation can occur early); diazepam to control seizures; blood transfusion for severe anemia; replacement of potassium as necessary; *epinephrine is contraindicated*
γ-Benzene hexachloride Benzene hexachloride Hexachlorocyclohexane Lindane	Irritability, CNS excitation, muscle spasms, atonia, clonic and tonic seizures, respiratory failure, pulmonary edema, nausea, vomiting, obtundation, coma	Supportive care, diazepam to control seizures, activated charcoal after airway control
Benzine (benzin)	See Petroleum distillates	—
Benzodiazepines Chlordiazepoxide Diazepam Flurazepam	Sedation to coma, particularly if drugs are accompanied by alcohol; hypotension	Airway control, IV fluids and vasopressors for hypotension; avoidance of flumazenil (CAUTION: *If tricyclic antidepressants are involved, flumazenil may precipitate seizures; in patients dependent on benzodiazepines, flumazenil may precipitate withdrawal*)
Benzol	See Benzene	—
Beta-blockers	Hypotension, bradycardia, seizures, cardiac arrhythmias, hypoglycemia, altered mental status	Close monitoring and attention to airway maintenance; for symptomatic patients, consideration of dopamine, epinephrine, other vasopressors, glucagon 3–5 mg IV followed by infusion, $CaCl_2$, IV insulin and glucose, cardiac pacing, and intra-aortic balloon pump
Bichloride of mercury	See Mercury	—
Bichromates	See Chromic acid	—
Bidrin (dicrotophos)	See Organophosphates	—
Bifenthrin	See Pyrethroids	—
Bishydroxycoumarin	See Warfarin	—
Bismuth compounds	Acute: Abdominal pain, oliguria, acute renal failure Chronic: Poor absorption, ulcerative stomatitis, anorexia, progressive encephalopathy	Respiratory support, consideration of chelation with dimercaprol and succimer (see TABLE 326–4)
Bitter almond oil	See Cyanides	—
Bleach, chlorine	See Hypochlorites	—
β-Blockers	See Beta-blockers	—

Table continues on the following page.

TABLE 326–8. SYMPTOMS AND TREATMENT OF SPECIFIC POISONS—Continued

POISON*	SYMPTOMS	TREATMENT
Boric acid	Nausea, vomiting, diarrhea, hemorrhagic gastroenteritis, weakness, lethargy, CNS depression, seizures, "boiled lobster" rash, shock	Removal from skin, prevention or treatment of electrolyte abnormalities and shock, control of seizures; for severe poisoning (rare), dialysis
Brandy	See Alcohol, ethyl	—
Bromates	Vomiting, diarrhea, epigastric pain, acidosis, deafness	Supportive care, thiosulfate to reduce bromate to less toxic bromide, hemodialysis for renal failure
Bromides	Nausea, vomiting, rash (may be acneiform), slurred speech, ataxia, confusion, psychotic behavior, coma, paralysis	Discontinuation of drug, hydration and NaCl IV to promote diuresis, furosemide 10 mg q 6 h; for severe poisoning, hemodialysis
Bromine	Highly corrosive; with exposure to liquid or vapor, skin and mucous membrane burns	Aggressive decontamination, supportive care
Bupropion HCl	Respiratory depression, ataxia, seizures	Charcoal, benzodiazepines, supportive care
Butyl nitrate	See Nitrites	
Cadmium Solder	Severe gastric cramps, vomiting, diarrhea, dry throat, cough, dyspnea, headache, shock, coma, brown urine, renal failure	Dilution with milk or albumin, respiratory support, hydration, intermittent positive pressure breathing for pulmonary edema, edetate Ca disodium (see TABLE 326–4); *dimercaprol contraindicated*
Caffeine	See Aminophylline	—
Calcium channel blockers Diltiazem Nifedipine Verapamil Others	Nausea, vomiting, confusion, bradycardia, hypotension, total cardiovascular collapse	Consideration of whole-bowel irrigation for sustained-release preparations; consideration of $CaCl_2$ (25–50 mg/kg [about 1–3 mL of 10% solution]) or 3 times as much Ca gluconate IV with additional amounts as needed, pacemaker, or intra-aortic balloon pump for hypotension or severe arrhythmias; possible consideration of regular insulin 10–100 units IV and 50–100 mL 50% dextrose plus 50–100 mL/h 10% dextrose IV infusion
Calomel	See Mercury	—
Camphor Camphorated oils	Camphor odor on breath, headache, confusion, delirium, hallucinations, seizures, coma	Diazepam to prevent and treat seizures, respiratory support
Canned fuel, solid	See Alcohol, methyl	—

TABLE 326–8. SYMPTOMS AND TREATMENT OF SPECIFIC POISONS—Continued

POISON*	SYMPTOMS	TREATMENT
Cantharides Cantharidin Spanish fly	Irritated skin and mucous membranes, skin vesicles, nausea, vomiting, bloody diarrhea, burning pain in back and urethra, respiratory depression, seizures, coma, abortion, menorrhagia	Avoidance of all oils, respiratory support, treatment of seizures, maintenance of fluid balance, no specific antidote
Carbamates Aldicarb Bendiocarb Benomyl Carbaryl Carbofuran Fenothiocarb Methiocarb Methomyl Oxamyl Propoxur	Slightly to highly toxic effects; similar to those of organophosphates except cholinesterase inhibition is not permanent	See Organophosphates
Carbamazepine	Progressive CNS depression, seizures (occasional), cardiac arrhythmia (rare)	Supportive care after decontamination, heart rate monitoring
Carbolic acid	See Phenols	—
Carbonates (ammonium, potassium, sodium)	See Caustic Ingestion on p. 2663	—
Carbon bisulfide	See Carbon disulfide	—
Carbon dioxide	Dyspnea, weakness, tinnitus, palpitations, asphyxia	Respiratory support, O_2
Carbon disulfide Carbon bisulfide	Garlic-breath odor, irritability, weakness, mania, narcosis, delirium, mydriasis, blindness, parkinsonism, seizures, coma, paralysis, respiratory failure	Washing of skin, O_2, diazepam sedation, respiratory and circulatory support
Carbon monoxide Acetylene gas Automobile exhaust Coal gas Furnace gas Illuminating gas Marsh gas	Variable toxicity depending on length of exposure, concentration inhaled, and respiratory and circulatory rates; various symptoms depending on % carboxyhemoglobin in blood; headache, vertigo, vomiting, dyspnea, confusion, dilated pupils, seizures, coma	100% O_2 by mask, respiratory support if needed, immediate measurement of carboxyhemoglobin level; if carboxyhemoglobin is > about 25%, hyperbaric O_2 (see text) possibly effective
Carbon tetrachloride (sometimes used in chemical manufacturing) Cleaning fluids (nonflammable)	Nausea, vomiting, abdominal pain, headache, confusion, visual disturbances, CNS depression, ventricular fibrillation, renal injury, hepatic injury, cirrhosis	Washing of skin, O_2, respiratory support, monitoring of renal and hepatic function and appropriate treatment
Carbonyl iron	See Iron	—
Caustic soda (sodium hydroxide)	See Caustic Ingestion on p. 2663	—

Table continues on the following page.

TABLE 326–8. SYMPTOMS AND TREATMENT OF SPECIFIC POISONS—Continued

POISON*	SYMPTOMS	TREATMENT
Chloral hydrate Chloral amide	Drowsiness, confusion, shock, coma, respiratory depression, renal injury, hepatic injury	Respiratory support, assessment of concomitant ingestions, β-blockers for ventricular arrhythmias
Chlorates Nitrates Permanent wave neutralizers	Vomiting, nausea, diarrhea, cyanosis (methemoglobin), toxic nephritis, shock, seizures, CNS depression, coma, jaundice	Methylene blue for methemoglobinemia, 10% thiosulfate to reduce chlorate to the less toxic chloride, transfusion for severe cyanosis, ascorbic acid, treatment of shock, O_2; for complex cases, possibly dialysis
Chlordane	See Chlorinated hydrocarbons	—
Chlorethoxyfos	See Organophosphates	—
Chlorinated and other halogenated hydrocarbons Aldrin Benzene hexachloride Chlordane Chlorothalonil DDD (2-dichlorethane) DDT (chlorophenothane) Dicofol Dieldrin Dienochlor Dilan Endosulfan Endrin Heptachlor Lindane Methoxychlor Perchlordecone Prolan Toxaphene Other chlorinated organic insecticides and industrial compounds	Slightly toxic effects (eg, with methoxychlor) to highly toxic effects (eg, with dieldrin); vomiting (early or delayed), paresthesias, malaise, coarse tremors, seizures, pulmonary edema, ventricular fibrillation, respiratory failure	Diazepam or phenobarbital to prevent and control tremors and seizures, cautious use of epinephrine, avoidance of sudden stimuli, parenteral fluids, monitoring for renal and hepatic failure
Chlorinated lime	See Chlorine	—
Chlorine (see also Hypochlorites) Chlorinated lime Chlorine water Tear gas	Ingestion: Irritation, corrosion of mouth and GI tract, possible ulceration or perforation, abdominal pain, tachycardia, prostration, circulatory collapse Inhalation: Severe respiratory and ocular irritation, glottal spasm, cough, choking, vomiting, pulmonary edema, cyanosis	Ingestion: Dilution with water or milk, treatment of shock Inhalation: O_2, respiratory support, observation for and treatment of pulmonary edema
Chloroaniline	See Acetanilid	—

TABLE 326–8. SYMPTOMS AND TREATMENT OF SPECIFIC POISONS—Continued

POISON*	SYMPTOMS	TREATMENT
Chloroform Ether Nitrous oxide Trichloromethane	Drowsiness, coma; with nitrous oxide, delirium	Ingestion: Observation for renal and hepatic damage; respiratory, cardiac, and circulatory support Inhalation: Respiratory, cardiac, and circulatory support
Chlorothalonil	See Chlorinated hydrocarbons	—
Chlorothion	See Organophosphates	—
Chlorpromazine	See Phenothiazines	—
Chlorpyrifos	See Organophosphates	—
Chromates	See Chromic acid	—
Chromic acid Bichromates Chromates Chromium trioxide	Corrosive effects due to oxidation, ulcerated and perforated nasal septum, severe gastroenteritis, shock, vertigo, coma, nephritis	Dilution with milk or water, cautious use of fluids and electrolytes to support renal function, consideration of *N*-acetylcysteine and ascorbic acid to convert hexavalent to the less toxic trivalent compound
Chromium	Irritation of skin and mucous membranes	Thorough washing with water and 10% ascorbic acid solution for 15 min
Chromium trioxide	See Chromic acid	—
Cimetidine; ranitidine	Slight dryness and drowsiness, possible altered metabolism of concomitant drugs	No specific antidote available; focus on metabolism of other drugs
Clonidine	Bradycardia, sedation, periodic apnea, hypotension, hypothermia	Supportive care; vasopressors; naloxone 5 µg/kg up to 2–20 mg, repeated prn, to possibly reduce sedation
Coal gas	See Carbon monoxide	—
Cobalt	Tachycardia, tachypnea and hypoxia after inhalation, skin and mucous membrane irritation, glomerulonephritis, hypothyroidism (rare)	Supportive care, decontamination with water and soap
Cobaltous chloride	See Cobalt	—
Cocaine†	Stimulation then depression, nausea, vomiting, loss of self-control, anxiety, hallucinations, sweating, hyperthermia, seizures, MI (rare)	Diazepam for excitation (primary treatment), O_2, respiratory and circulatory support if needed, IV $NaHCO_3$, extremely cautious use of IV esmolol for arrhythmias, observation for myocardial or pulmonary disorder (usually before emergency department arrival), external cooling for hyperthermia
Codeine	See Opioids	—

Table continues on the following page.

TABLE 326–8. SYMPTOMS AND TREATMENT OF SPECIFIC POISONS—Continued

POISON*	SYMPTOMS	TREATMENT
Copper	See Copper salts	—
Copper salts Cupric sulfate, acetate, or subacetate Cuprous chloride or oxide Zinc salts	Vomiting, burning sensation, metallic taste, diarrhea, pain, shock, jaundice, anuria, seizures	Penicillamine or dimercaprol (see TABLE 326–4), electrolyte and fluid balance, respiratory support, monitoring of GI tract, treatment of shock, control of seizures, monitoring for hepatic and renal failure
Corrosive sublimate (mercuric chloride)	See Mercury	—
Coumaphos	See Organophosphates	—
Creosote, cresols	See Phenols	—
Cyanides Bitter almond oil Hydrocyanic acid Nitroprusside Potassium cyanide Prussic acid Sodium cyanide Wild cherry syrup	Tachycardia, headache, drowsiness, hypotension, coma, rapid severe acidosis, seizures, death, possibly bitter almond odor in breath, bright red venous blood; *very rapidly lethal* (1–15 min)	*Speed essential*. For inhalation, removal from source. For both inhalation and ingestion exposures, 100% O_2; respiratory support; inhalation of amyl nitrite 0.2 mL (1 ampule) for 30 sec of each min; 3% Na nitrite 10 mL at 2.5–5 mL/min IV (in children, 10 mg/kg), then 25% Na thiosulfate 25–50 mL at 2.5–5 mL/min IV (Lilly cyanide kit); treatment repeated if symptoms recur; consideration of hydroxocobalamin 5 g IV
Cyfluthrin	See Pyrethroids	—
Cypermethrin	See Pyrethroids	—
DDD (2-dichlorethane)	See Chlorinated hydrocarbons	—
DDT (chlorophenothane)	See Chlorinated hydrocarbons	—
Demeton	See Organophosphates	—
Deodorizers, household	See Naphthalene, Paradichlorobenzene	—
Depilatories	See Barium compounds	—
Desipramine	See Tricyclic antidepressants	—
Detergent powders	See Caustic Ingestion on p. 2663	—
Dextroamphetamine	See Amphetamines	—
Diazinon	See Organophosphates	—
Dichlorvos	See Organophosphates	—
Dicofol	See Chlorinated hydrocarbons	—
Dicumarol	See Warfarin	—
Dieldrin	See Chlorinated hydrocarbons	—
Dienochlor	See Chlorinated hydrocarbons	—

TABLE 326–8. SYMPTOMS AND TREATMENT OF SPECIFIC POISONS—Continued

POISON*	SYMPTOMS	TREATMENT
Diethylene glycol	See Ethylene glycol	—
Digitalis, digitoxin, digoxin	See discussion of digitalis preparations on p. 662	—
Dilan	See Chlorinated hydrocarbons	—
Dimethoate	See Organophosphates	—
Dinitrobenzene	See Nitrobenzene	—
Dinitro-*o*-cresol Herbicides Pesticides	Fatigue, thirst, flushing, nausea, vomiting, abdominal pain, hyperpyrexia, tachycardia, loss of consciousness, dyspnea, respiratory arrest, skin absorption	Fluid therapy, O_2, renal and hepatic toxicity anticipated, no specific antidote, detergents to rinse skin
Diphenoxylate with atropine	Lethargy, nystagmus, pinpoint pupils, tachycardia, coma, respiratory depression (NOTE: Toxicity may be delayed up to 12 h)	Activated charcoal, naloxone, careful monitoring of all children for 12–18 h if ingestion is verified, supportive care
Diquat	See Paraquat	—
Dishwasher detergents	See Caustic Ingestion on p. 2663	—
Disulfoton	See Organophosphates	—
Diuretics, mercurial	See Mercury	—
Donovan's solution	See Arsenic	—
Doxepin	See Tricyclic antidepressants	—
Drain cleaners	See Caustic Ingestion on p. 2663	—
Endosulfan	See Chlorinated hydrocarbons	—
Endrin	See Chlorinated hydrocarbons	—
Ergot derivatives	Thirst, diarrhea, vomiting, lightheadedness, burning feet, increased heart rate and BP, cardiovascular collapse, seizures, hypotension, coma, abortion, gangrene of feet, cataracts	Benzodiazepine or a short-acting barbiturate for seizures; for peripheral ischemia, heparin plus phentolamine 5–10 mg in 10 mL normal saline sc or nitroprusside 1–2 µg/kg/min IV; for coronary vasospasm, IV nitroglycerin and nifedipine
Eserine	See Physostigmine	—
Esfenvalerate	See Pyrethroids	—
Ethanol	See Alcohol, ethyl	—
Ether	See Chloroform	—
Ethion	See Organophosphates	—
Ethyl alcohol	See Alcohol, ethyl	—
Ethyl biscoumacetate	See Warfarin	—

Table continues on the following page.

TABLE 326–8. SYMPTOMS AND TREATMENT OF SPECIFIC POISONS—Continued

POISON*	SYMPTOMS	TREATMENT
Ethylene glycol Diethylene glycol Permanent antifreeze	Ingestion: Inebriation but no alcohol odor on breath, nausea, vomiting; later, carpopedal spasm, lumbar pain, oxalate crystalluria, oliguria progressing to anuria and acute renal failure, respiratory distress, seizures, coma Eye contact: Iridocyclitis	Ingestion: Respiratory support, correction of electrolyte imbalance (anion gap), consideration of correcting acidemia, ethanol (see treatment of methyl alcohol) or fomepizole 15 mg/kg IV (loading dose) followed by 10 mg/kg IV q 12 h; definitive treatment is hemodialysis Eye contact: Flushing of eyes
Explosives	See Barium compounds (fireworks), Nitrogen oxides	—
Famphur	See Organophosphates	—
Fava bean (favism)	See TABLE 326–5	—
Fenthion	See Organophosphates	—
Ferric salts	See Iron	—
Ferrous salts (eg, gluconate, sulfate)	See Iron	—
Fireworks	See Barium compounds	—
Fluorides Ammonium fluoride Fluorine Hydrofluoric acid Rat poisons Roach poisons Sodium fluoride Soluble fluorides generally	Ingestion: Salty or soapy taste; with large doses: tremors, seizures, CNS depression, shock, renal failure Skin and mucosal contact: Painful superficial or deep burns Inhalation: Intense eye and nasal irritation, headache, dyspnea, sense of suffocation, glottal edema, pulmonary edema, bronchitis, pneumonia, mediastinal and subcutaneous emphysema due to bleb rupture	Ingestion: Dilution with milk or water, IV glucose and saline, 10% Ca gluconate 10 mL IV (in children, 1 mL/kg) or 10% $CaCl_2$ 1–2 mL/kg IV, monitoring for cardiac irritability, treatment of shock and dehydration Skin and mucosal contact: Copious flushing with water, debridement of white tissue, sometimes injection of 10% Ca gluconate locally but may be given intra-arterially, application of Ca gluconate or Ca carbonate paste Inhalation: O_2, respiratory support, prednisone for chemical pneumonitis (in adults, 15–40 mg bid), management of pulmonary edema
Fluvalinate	See Pyrethroids	—
Formaldehyde Formalin (NOTE: May contain methyl alcohol)	Ingestion: Oral and gastric pain, nausea, vomiting, hematemesis, shock, hematuria, anuria, coma, respiratory failure Skin contact: Irritation, coagulation necrosis (with high concentrations), dermatitis, hypersensitivity Inhalation: Eye, nose, and respiratory tract irritation; laryngeal spasm and edema; dysphagia; bronchitis; pneumonia	Ingestion: Dilution with water or milk; treatment of shock, $NaHCO_3$ to correct acidosis, respiratory support, observation for perforations Skin contact: Washing with copious soap and water Inhalation: Flushing of eyes with saline, O_2, respiratory support

TABLE 326–8. SYMPTOMS AND TREATMENT OF SPECIFIC POISONS—Continued

POISON*	SYMPTOMS	TREATMENT
Fowler's solution	See Arsenic	—
Fuel, canned	See Alcohol, methyl	—
Fuel oil	See Petroleum distillates	—
Furnace gas	See Carbon monoxide	—
Gas	See Ammonia gas, Carbon monoxide (acetylene gas, automobile exhaust, coal gas, furnace gas, illuminating gas, marsh gas), Chlorine (tear gas), Hydrogen sulfide (sewer gas, volatile hydrides), Organophosphates (nerve gas)	—
Gasoline	See Petroleum distillates	—
Glues, model airplane	See Acetone, Benzene (toluene), Petroleum distillates	—
Glutethimide	Drowsiness, areflexia, mydriasis, hypotension, respiratory depression, coma	Activated charcoal, respiratory support, maintenance of fluid and electrolyte balance, hemodialysis possibly helpful, treatment of shock
Gold salts	See gold in TABLE 326–4 and gold compounds under Treatment of RA on p. 288	—
Guaiacol	See Phenols	—
H_2 blockers (eg, cimetidine, ranitidine)	Minor GI problems, possibly altered levels of other drugs	Nonspecific supportive measures
Heptachlor	See Chlorinated hydrocarbons	—
Herbicides	See Arsenic, Dinitro-*o*-cresol	—
Heroin	See Opioids	—
Hexachlorocyclohexane	See γ-Benzene hexachloride	—
Hexaethyltetraphosphate	See Organophosphates	—
Histamine-2 blockers	See H_2 blockers	—
Hydrides, volatile	See Hydrogen sulfide	—
Hydrocarbons	See Benzene	—
Hydrocarbons, chlorinated	See Chlorinated hydrocarbons	—
Hydrocarbons, halogenated	See Chlorinated hydrocarbons	—
Hydrochloric acid	See Caustic Ingestion on p. 2663	—
Hydrocodone	See Opioids	—
Hydrocyanic acid	See Cyanides	—
Hydrofluoric acid	See Fluorides	—
Hydrogen chloride or fluoride	See Nitrogen oxides	—

Table continues on the following page.

TABLE 326–8. SYMPTOMS AND TREATMENT OF SPECIFIC POISONS—Continued

POISON*	SYMPTOMS	TREATMENT
Hydrogen sulfide Alkali sulfides Phosphine Sewer gas Volatile hydrides	"Gas eye" (subacute keratoconjunctivitis), lacrimation and burning, cough, dyspnea, pulmonary edema, caustic skin burns, erythema, pain, profuse salivation, nausea, vomiting, diarrhea, confusion, vertigo, sudden collapse, unconsciousness	O_2, respiratory support
Hyoscine (scopolamine) Hyoscyamine Hyoscyamus	See Belladonna	—
Hypochlorites Bleach, chlorine Javelle water	Usually mild pain and inflammation of oral and GI mucosa; cough, dyspnea, vomiting, skin vesicles	Dilution with milk for usual 6% household preparations (little else required); treatment of shock; if concentrated forms have been ingested, esophagoscopy
Hypoglycemic drugs, oral Chlorpropamide Glipizide	Hypoglycemia, diaphoresis, lethargy, confusion	Admission to the hospital, IV dextrose as needed, frequent feeding (not just sugar) plus careful observation of behavior and periodic measurement of plasma glucose; for persistent hypoglycemia, consideration of octreotide 50–75 μg sc
Illuminating gas	See Carbon monoxide	—
Imipramine	See Tricyclic antidepressants	—
Insecticides	See Chlorinated hydrocarbons, Organophosphates, Paradichlorobenzene, Pyrethroids	—
Iodine	Burning pain in mouth and esophagus, brown-stained mucous membranes, laryngeal edema, vomiting, abdominal pain, diarrhea, shock, nephritis, circulatory collapse	Milk, starch, or flour po; early airway support; fluid and electrolytes; treatment of shock; early, aggressive airway management
Iodoform Triiodomethane	Dermatitis, vomiting, cerebral depression, excitation, coma, respiratory difficulty	Ingestion: Dilution with milk or water, respiratory support Skin contact: Washing with $NaHCO_3$ or alcohol
Iron Carbonyl iron (see Carbon monoxide) Ferric salts Ferrous salts Ferrous gluconate Ferrous sulfate Vitamins with iron (NOTE: Children's chewables with iron are remarkably safe)	Vomiting, upper abdominal pain, pallor, cyanosis, diarrhea, drowsiness, shock; possible toxicity if > 20 mg/kg of elemental iron is ingested	For serum iron > 400–500 μg/dL (> 72–90 μmol/L) at 3–6 h plus GI symptoms, deferoxamine IV infusion starting at 15 mg/kg/h and titrated to BP

TABLE 326–8. SYMPTOMS AND TREATMENT OF SPECIFIC POISONS—Continued

POISON*	SYMPTOMS	TREATMENT
Isofenfos	See Organophosphates	—
Isoniazid	CNS stimulation, seizures, obtundation, coma	Pyridoxine IV for seizures, mg for mg ingested or, if amount ingested is unknown, 5 g IV; $NaHCO_3$ for acidosis
Isopropyl alcohol	See Alcohol, isopropyl	—
Javelle water	See Hypochlorites	—
Kerosene	See Petroleum distillates	—
Ketones	See Acetone	—
Lambda-cyhalothrin	See Pyrethroids	—
Lead Lead salts Solder Some paints and painted surfaces	Acute ingestion: Thirst, burning abdominal pain, vomiting, diarrhea, CNS symptoms as below Acute inhalation: Insomnia, headache, ataxia, mania, seizures Chronic exposure: Anemia, peripheral neuropathy, confusion, lead encephalopathy	See Lead Poisoning on p. 2668
Lead, tetraethyl	Vapor inhalation, skin absorption, or ingestion: CNS symptoms (insomnia, restlessness, ataxia, delusions, mania, seizures)	Supportive care, diazepam to control seizures, fluid and electrolytes, elimination of source
Lime, chlorinated	See Chlorine	—
Lindane	See γ-Benzene hexachloride, Chlorinated hydrocarbons	—
Liquor	See Alcohol, ethyl	—
Lithium salts	Nausea, vomiting, diarrhea, tremors, drowsiness, diabetes insipidus, ataxia, seizures	Acute: Hydration, diazepam, possibly dialysis for end-organ damage or serum lithium level > 4 mEq/L Chronic: Dialysis if symptoms are severe
Lye (sodium hydroxide)	See Caustic Ingestion on p. 2663	—
Lysergic acid diethylamide (LSD)	Confusion, hallucinations, hyperexcitability, coma, flashbacks	Supportive care, benzodiazepines; for severe agitation, haloperidol 2 to 10 mg IV or IM in adults (repeated as necessary)
Malathion	See Organophosphates	—
Manganese	See Potassium permanganate	—
Marsh gas	See Carbon monoxide	—
Meperidine	See Opioids	—
Meprobamate	See Barbiturates	—

Table continues on the following page.

TABLE 326–8. SYMPTOMS AND TREATMENT OF SPECIFIC POISONS—Continued

POISON*	SYMPTOMS	TREATMENT
Mercury All mercury compounds Ammoniated mercury Bichloride of mercury Calomel Corrosive sublimate Diuretics, mercurial Mercuric chloride Mercury vapor Merthiolate	Acute: Severe gastroenteritis, burning mouth pain, salivation, abdominal pain, vomiting, colitis, nephrosis, anuria, uremia; skin burns from alkyl and phenyl mercurials Chronic: Gingivitis, mental disturbance, neurologic deficits Mercury vapor: Severe pneumonitis	Consideration of gastric lavage, activated charcoal, penicillamine (or succimer—see TABLE 326–4), maintenance of fluid and electrolyte balance, hemodialysis for renal failure, observation for GI perforation Skin contact: Soap and water for scrubbing Lungs: Supportive care
Merthiolate (thimerosal)	See Mercury—usually nontoxic	—
Metaldehyde Slug bait	Nausea, vomiting, retching, abdominal pain, muscular rigidity, hyperventilation, seizures, coma	Supportive care, diazepam
Metals	See specific metals	See TABLE 326–4
Methadone	See Opioids	—
Methamphetamine	See Amphetamines	—
Methanol	See Alcohol, methyl	—
Methidathion	See Organophosphates	—
Methoxychlor	See Chlorinated hydrocarbons	—
Methyl alcohol	See Alcohol, methyl	—
Methyl parathion	See Organophosphates	—
Methyl salicylate	See Aspirin and Other Salicylate Poisoning on p. 2660	—
Mineral spirits	See Petroleum distillates	—
Mirtazapine	Usually benign; most commonly, sedation, confusion, tachycardia	Observation for ≥ 8 h
Model airplane glues, solvents	See Acetone, Benzene, Petroleum distillates	—
Monoamine oxidase (MAO) inhibitors Isocarboxazid Phenelzine Selegiline Tranyl-cypromine	Nonspecific and highly variable symptoms, which are often delayed 6–24 h; sympathomimetic toxidromes, headache, nausea, dystonia, hallucinations, nystagmus, fasciculations, diarrhea, seizures, agitation, muscle rigidity; hypotension and bradycardia may be ominous	Consideration of gastric decontamination, supportive care
Monosodium glutamate	Burning sensations throughout the body, facial pressure, anxiety, chest pain (Chinese restaurant syndrome)	Supportive care
Morphine	See Opioids	—

TABLE 326–8. SYMPTOMS AND TREATMENT OF SPECIFIC POISONS—Continued

POISON*	SYMPTOMS	TREATMENT
Moth balls, crystals, or repellent cakes	See Naphthalene, Paradichlorobenzene	—
Mushrooms, poisonous	See Chemical Food Poisoning on p. 2664	—
Nail polish remover	See Acetone	—
Naled	See Organophosphates	—
Naphtha	See Petroleum distillates	—
Naphthalene (see also Paradichlorobenzene) Deodorizer cakes Moth balls, crystals, or repellent cakes	Ingestion: Abdominal cramps, nausea, vomiting, headache, confusion, dysuria, intravascular hemolysis, seizures, hemolytic anemia in people with G6PD deficiency Skin contact: Dermatitis, corneal ulceration Inhalation: Headache, confusion, vomiting, dyspnea	Ingestion: Blood transfusion for severe hemolysis, urine alkalinization for hemoglobinuria, benzodiazepines to control seizures Skin contact: Clothing removed if formerly stored with naphthalene moth balls, flushing of skin and eyes
Naphthols	See Phenols	—
Narcotics	See Opioids	—
Nefazodone	See Trazodone	—
Neostigmine	See Physostigmine	—
Nerve gas agents	See Organophosphates	—
Nickel	Hypersensitivity dermatitis; with chronic inhalation, pulmonary inflammation	Removal from source of nickel; irrigation with water
Nickel carbonyl	Pneumonitis, cyanosis, delirium, seizures (see also Nickel)	Removal from source, decontamination, consideration of disulfiram to treat severe toxicity.
Nicotine	See Tobacco	—
Nitrates	See Chlorates	—
Nitric acid	See Caustic Ingestion on p. 2663	—
Nitrites Amyl nitrite Butyl nitrite Nitroglycerin Potassium nitrite Sodium nitrite	Methemoglobinemia, cyanosis, anoxia, GI disturbance, vomiting, headache, dizziness, hypotension, respiratory failure, coma	O_2; for methemoglobinemia, 1% methylene blue 1–2 mg/kg slowly IV
Nitrobenzene Artificial bitter almond oil Dinitrobenzene	Bitter almond odor (suggests cyanides), drowsiness, headache, vomiting, ataxia, nystagmus, brown urine, convulsive movements, delirium, cyanosis, coma, respiratory arrest	See Acetanilid

Table continues on the following page.

TABLE 326–8. SYMPTOMS AND TREATMENT OF SPECIFIC POISONS—Continued

POISON*	SYMPTOMS	TREATMENT
Nitrogen oxides (see also Chlorine, Fluorides, Hydrogen sulfide, Sulfur dioxide, and Ch. 57) Air contaminants that form atmospheric oxidants and that were liberated from missile fuels, explosives, or agricultural wastes Cobaltous chloride Hydrogen chloride Hydrogen fluoride	Delayed onset of symptoms with nitrogen oxides unless heavy concentration; fatigue, cough, dyspnea, pulmonary edema; later, bronchitis, pneumonia	Bed rest; O_2 as soon as symptoms develop; for excessive pulmonary foam: suction, postural drainage, tracheotomy; prednisone 30–80 mg/day in adults and dexamethasone 1 mg/m^2 BSA in children to possibly prevent pulmonary fibrosis
Nitroglycerin	See Nitrites	—
Nitroprusside	See Cyanides	—
Nitrous oxide	See Chloroform	—
NSAIDs Ibuprofen	Nausea, vomiting, CNS toxicity (eg, seizures with massive overdoses)	Clinical observation, supportive care
Nortriptyline	See Tricyclic antidepressants	—
Octamethyl pyrophosphoramide	See Organophosphates	—
Oil of wintergreen	See Aspirin and Other Salicylate Poisoning on p. 2660	—
Oils	See Acetanilid (aniline oil), Petroleum distillates (fuel oil, lubricating oils)	—
Opioids (see also Opioids in Ch. 198) Alphaprodine Codeine Fentanyl Heroin Hydrocodone Meperidine Methadone Morphine Opium Oxycodone Propoxyphene	Pinpoint pupils, drowsiness, shallow respirations, spasticity, respiratory failure	Charcoal, respiratory support, naloxone IV as required to awaken patients and improve respiration, IV fluids to support circulation
Opium	See Opioids	—
Organophosphates Acephate Bidrin Chlorethoxyfos Chlorothion Chlorpyrifos Coumaphos	Nausea, vomiting, abdominal cramping, excessive salivation, increased pulmonary secretion, headache, rhinorrhea, blurred vision, miosis, slurred speech, mental confusion, difficulty breathing, frothing at the mouth,	Removal of clothing; flushing and washing of skin; for increased secretions, atropine 2 mg in adults or 0.01–0.05 mg/kg in children IV or IM q 15–60 min, repeated prn (massive amounts may be necessary);

TABLE 326–8. SYMPTOMS AND TREATMENT OF SPECIFIC POISONS—Continued

POISON*	SYMPTOMS	TREATMENT
Organophosphates (cont'd) Demeton Diazinon Dichlorvos Dimethoate Disulfoton Ethion Famphur Fenthion Hexaethyltetraphosphate Isofenfos Malathion Methidathion Methyl parathion Naled Nerve gas agents Octamethyl pyrophosphoramide Oxydemeton-methyl Parathion Phorate Phosdrin Phosmet Pirimiphos-methyl Temefos Tetrachlorvinphos Trichlorfon Turbufos	coma; absorption via skin, inhalation, or ingestion	pralidoxime chloride 1–2 g in adults or 20–40 mg/kg in children IV over 15–30 min, repeated in 1 h if needed; O_2; respiratory support; correction of dehydration For attendants, avoidance of self-contamination
Oxalic acid Oxalates	Burning pain in throat, vomiting, intense pain, hypotension, tetany, shock, glottal and renal damage, oxaluria	Milk or Ca lactate, 10% Ca gluconate 10–20 mL IV, pain control, saline IV for shock, observation for glottal edema and stricture
Oxycodone	See Opioids	—
Oxydemeton-methyl	See Organophosphates	—
Paints	See Lead	—
Paint solvents	See Alcohol, methyl; Petroleum distillates (mineral spirits); Turpentine	—
Paradichlorobenzene Insecticides Moth repellents Pesticides Toilet bowl deodorizers	Abdominal pain, nausea, vomiting, diarrhea, seizures, tetany (rare)	Fluid replacement, diazepam to control seizures
Paraldehyde	Acetic acid odor on breath, incoherence, miosis, depressed respiration, coma	O_2, respiratory support
Paraquat (a strong corrosive) Diquat	Immediate: GI pain and vomiting Within 24 h: Respiratory failure (but no pulmonary problems with diquat)	Activated charcoal, fuller's earth, limited O_2, consultation with poison control center or manufacturer

Table continues on the following page.

TABLE 326–8. SYMPTOMS AND TREATMENT OF SPECIFIC POISONS—Continued

POISON*	SYMPTOMS	TREATMENT
Parathion	See Organophosphates	—
Paris green	See Arsenic	—
Pentobarbital	See Barbiturates	—
Perchlordecone	See Chlorinated hydrocarbons	—
Permanent wave neutralizers	See Chlorates	—
Permethrin	See Pyrethroids	—
Pesticides	See Arsenic, Barium compounds, Chlorinated hydrocarbons, Dinitro-*o*-cresol, Fluorides, Organophosphates, Paradichlorobenzene, Phosphorus, Pyrethroids, Thallium salts, Warfarin	—
Petroleum distillates (see also Hydrocarbon Poisoning on p. 2665) Asphalt Benzine (benzin) Fuel oil Gasoline Kerosene Lubricating oils Mineral spirits Model airplane glue Naphtha Petroleum ether Tar	Ingestion: Burning throat and stomach, vomiting, diarrhea, pneumonia only if aspiration has occurred Vapor inhalation: Euphoria, burning in chest, headache, nausea, weakness, CNS depression, confusion, dyspnea, tachypnea, rales, possibly myocardial sensitization to catecholamines (which can result in cardiac arrhythmias) Aspiration: Early acute pulmonary changes	Because major problems result from aspiration (not GI absorption), gastric evacuation usually not warranted; supportive care for pulmonary edema; O_2; respiratory support
Phenacetin	See Acetanilid	—
Phencyclidine (PCP)	Inattentiveness with eyes open, agitation, violent behavior, unconsciousness, tachycardia, hypertension	Quiet environment; for sedation, benzodiazepines
Phenmetrazine	See Amphetamines	—
Phenobarbital	See Barbiturates	—
Phenols Carbolic acid Creosote Cresols Guaiacol Naphthols	Corrosive effects; mucous membrane burns; pallor; weakness; shock; seizures in children; pulmonary edema; smoky urine; respiratory, cardiac, and circulatory failure	Removal of clothing, washing of external burns with water, activated charcoal, pain relief, O_2, respiratory support, correction of fluid imbalance, observation for esophageal stricture (rare)
Phenothiazines Chlorpromazine Prochlorperazine Promazine Trifluoperazine	Extrapyramidal symptoms (ataxia, muscular and carpopedal spasms, torticollis), usually idiosyncratic; if overdose, dry mouth, drowsiness, seizures, coma, respiratory depression	Diphenhydramine 2–3 mg/kg IV or IM for extrapyramidal symptoms, diazepam to control seizures
Phenylpropanolamine	Nervousness, irritability, bradycardia, hypertension plus other sympathomimetic effects	Supportive care, diazepam, phentolamine 5 mg or nitroprussides for hypertension

TABLE 326–8. SYMPTOMS AND TREATMENT OF SPECIFIC POISONS—Continued

POISON*	SYMPTOMS	TREATMENT
Phorate	See Organophosphates	—
Phosdrin	See Organophosphates	—
Phosmet	See Organophosphates	—
Phosphine	See Hydrogen sulfide	—
Phosphoric acid	See Caustic Ingestion on p. 2663	—
Phosphorus (yellow or white) Rat poisons Roach powders (NOTE: Red phosphorus is unabsorbable and nontoxic)	Stage 1: Garlicky taste, garlic-breath odor, local irritation, skin and throat burns, nausea, vomiting, diarrhea, corrosion of mucous membranes Stage 2: Symptom-free 8 h to several days Stage 3: Nausea, vomiting, diarrhea, liver enlargement, jaundice, hemorrhages, renal damage, seizures, coma Toxicity enhanced by alcohol, fats, or digestible oils	Protection of patient and attendant from vomitus and feces; GI lavage with dilute K permanganate (1:5000) or hydrogen peroxide (eg, 1–2%), which may change phosphorus to nontoxic oxides; if phosphorus is embedded in skin, submersion of patient's body in water; irrigation with dilute K permanganate or cupric sulfate (250 mg in 250 mL of water) recommended by some experts; mineral oil 100 mL (applied topically to prevent absorption), repeated in 2 h; prevention of shock; meticulous surgical debridement, 5% $NaHCO_3$ plus 3% cupric sulfate plus 1% hydroxyethyl cellulose as a paste applied to exposed skin, which is thoroughly washed off after 30 min (prolonged contact with cupric sulfate may result in copper poisoning)
Physostigmine Eserine Neostigmine Pilocarpine *Pilocarpus* genus	Dizziness, weakness, vomiting, cramping pain, bradycardia, possibly seizures, agitation	Atropine sulfate 0.6–1 mg in adults or 0.01 mg/kg in children sc or IV, repeated prn; a benzodiazepine for sedation
Pilocarpine	See Physostigmine	—
Pilocarpus genus	See Physostigmine	—
Pirimiphos-methyl	See Organophosphates	—
Potash (potassium hydroxide or potassium carbonate)	See Acids and alkalis	—
Potassium cyanide	See Cyanides	—
Potassium nitrite	See Nitrites	—
Potassium permanganate	Brown discoloration and burns of oral mucosa, glottal edema, hypotension, renal involvement	Dilution with water or milk, consideration of early endoscopy, maintenance of fluid balance

Table continues on the following page.

TABLE 326–8. SYMPTOMS AND TREATMENT OF SPECIFIC POISONS—Continued

POISON*	SYMPTOMS	TREATMENT
Prochlorperazine	See Phenothiazines	—
Prolan	See Chlorinated hydrocarbons	—
Promazine	See Phenothiazines	—
Propoxyphene	See Opioids	—
Protriptyline	See Tricyclic antidepressants	—
Prussic acid	See Cyanides	—
Pyrethrin	See Pyrethroids	—
Pyrethroids Bifenthrin Cyfluthrin Cypermethrin Esfenvalerate Fluvalinate Lambda-cyhalothrin Permethrin Pyrethrin Resmethrin Sumithrin Tefluthrin Tetramethrin	Allergic response (including anaphylactic reactions and skin sensitivity) in sensitive people; otherwise, low toxicity unless vehicle is a petroleum distillate	Thorough washing of skin, symptomatic and supportive care
Ranitidine	See Cimetidine	—
Rat poisons	See Barium compounds, Fluorides, Phosphorus, Thallium salts, Warfarin	—
Resmethrin	See Pyrethroids	—
Resorcinol (resorcin)	Vomiting, dizziness, tinnitus, chills, tremor, delirium, seizures, respiratory depression, coma, methemoglobinemia	Respiratory support, methylene blue for methemoglobinemia
Roach poisons	See Fluorides, Phosphorus, Thallium salts	—
Rubbing alcohol	See Alcohol, isopropyl	—
Salicylates	See Aspirin and Other Salicylate Poisoning on p. 2660	—
Salicylic acid	See Aspirin and Other Salicylate Poisoning on p. 2660	—
Scopolamine (hyoscine)	See Belladonna	—
Secobarbital	See Barbiturates	—
Selective serotonin reuptake inhibitors (SSRIs) Citalopram Fluoxetine Fluvoxamine Paroxetine Sertraline	Fatality (rare); commonly, sedation, vomiting, tremor, tachycardia; possibly, seizures, hallucinations, hypotension, serotonin syndrome; with citalopram, QRS prolongation possible	Airway protection; consideration of alkalinization for QRS widening; admission of patients who have symptoms > 6 h after ingestion

TABLE 326–8. SYMPTOMS AND TREATMENT OF SPECIFIC POISONS—Continued

POISON*	SYMPTOMS	TREATMENT
Selenium	See Arsenic, Thallium salts	—
Sewer gas	See Hydrogen sulfide	—
Silver salts Silver nitrate	Stained lips (white, brown, then black), gastroenteritis, shock, vertigo, seizures	Control of pain, diazepam to control seizures
Smog	See Sulfur dioxide	—
Soda, caustic (sodium hydroxide)	See Caustic Ingestion on p. 2663	—
Sodium carbonate	See Acids and alkalis	—
Sodium cyanide	See Cyanides	—
Sodium fluoride	See Fluorides	—
Sodium hydroxide	See Caustic Ingestion on p. 2663	—
Sodium nitrite	See Nitrites	—
Sodium salicylate	See Aspirin and Other Salicylate Poisoning on p. 2660	—
Solder	See Cadmium, Lead	—
Stibophen	See Arsenic	—
Stramonium	See Belladonna	—
Strychnine	Restlessness, hyperacuity of hearing, vision, and tactile sensation; violent myoclonus that simulates generalized seizures but with intact mental status, caused by minor stimuli; complete muscle relaxation between apparent seizures; perspiration; respiratory arrest	Isolation and restricted stimulation to prevent seizures, activated charcoal po, IV diazepam, respiratory support; for severe seizures, neuromuscular blockade and mechanical ventilatory support
Sulfur dioxide Smog	Respiratory tract irritation, sneezing, cough, dyspnea, pulmonary edema	Removal from contaminated area, O_2, positive pressure breathing, respiratory support
Sulfuric acid	See Caustic Ingestion on p. 2663	—
Sumithrin	See Pyrethroids	—
Syrup of wild cherry	See Cyanides	—
Tar	See Petroleum distillates	—
Tartar emetic	See Arsenic	—
Tear gas	See Chlorine	—
Tefluthrin	See Pyrethroids	—
Temefos	See Organophosphates	—
Tetrachlorvinphos	See Organophosphates	—
Tetraethyl lead	See Lead, tetraethyl	—
Tetramethrin	See Pyrethroids	—

Table continues on the following page.

TABLE 326–8. SYMPTOMS AND TREATMENT OF SPECIFIC POISONS—Continued

POISON*	SYMPTOMS	TREATMENT
Thallium salts (formerly used in ant, rat, and roach poisons) Selenium	Abdominal pain (colic), vomiting (may be bloody), diarrhea (may be bloody), stomatitis, excessive salivation, tremors, leg pains, paresthesias, polyneuritis, ocular and facial palsy, delirium, seizures, respiratory failure, loss of hair about 3 wk after poisoning	Treatment of shock, supportive care, diazepam to control seizures, activated charcoal (which effectively binds thallium and interrupts enterohepatic circulation), Prussian blue 60 mg/kg qid via NGT(same purpose as charcoal), chelation therapy with dimercaprol (used with varying success), avoidance of penicillamine and diethyldithiocarbamate (which may redistribute thallium into the CNS), consultation with poison control center for latest information advisable
Theophylline	See Aminophylline	—
Thyroxine	Usually asymptomatic; rarely, increasing irritability progressing to thyroid storm in 5–7 days	Emesis, observation at home, diazepam, possibly antithyroid preparations and propranolol *only* if symptoms occur
Tobacco Nicotine	Excitement, confusion, muscular twitching, weakness, abdominal cramps, generalized myoclonus, CNS depression, rapid respirations, palpitations, cardiovascular collapse, coma, respiratory failure	Activated charcoal, respiratory support, O_2, diazepam for seizures, thorough washing of skin if contaminated
Toilet bowl cleaners, deodorizers	See Caustic Ingestion on p. 2663; Paradichlorobenzene	—
Toluene, toluol	See Benzene	—
Toxaphene	See Chlorinated hydrocarbons	—
Trazodone Nefazodone	CNS depression, orthostatic hypotension, seizures, QRS prolongation (but torsades de pointes is rare), hypotension (rare)	Airway protection; for hypotension refractory to fluids, norepinephrine
Trichlorfon	See Organophosphates	—
Trichloromethane	See Chloroform	—
Tricyclic antidepressants Amitriptyline Desipramine Doxepin Imipramine Nortriptyline Protriptyline	Anticholinergic effects (eg, blurred vision, urinary hesitation), CNS effects (eg, drowsiness, stupor, coma, ataxia, restlessness, agitation, hyperactive reflexes, muscle rigidity, seizures), cardiovascular effects (tachycardia, other arrhythmias, bundle branch block, QRS widening, impaired conduction,	Symptomatic treatment and supportive care; charcoal; monitoring of vital signs and ECG; maintenance of airway; $NaHCO_3$ as a rapid IV injection (0.5–2 mEq/kg), repeated periodically to narrow the QRS, prevent arrhythmias, and maintain blood pH > 7.45 (constant infusion may be

TABLE 326–8. SYMPTOMS AND TREATMENT OF SPECIFIC POISONS—Continued

POISON*	SYMPTOMS	TREATMENT
Tricyclic antidepressants (cont'd)	heart failure), respiratory depression, hypotension, shock, vomiting, hyperpyrexia, mydriasis, diaphoresis	needed); diazepam to control seizures; vasopressors (eg, norepinephrine) to maintain BP
Trifluoperazine	See Phenothiazines	—
Triiodomethane	See Iodoform	—
Tungsten	See TABLE 326–4	—
Turbufos	See Organophosphates	—
Turpentine Paint solvent Varnish	Turpentine odor, burning oral and abdominal pain, coughing, choking, respiratory failure, nephritis	Respiratory support, O_2, control of pain, monitoring of renal function
Valproate	Progressive CNS and respiratory depression	Respiratory and cardiovascular supportive measures, monitoring of liver function
Varnish	See Alcohol, methyl; Turpentine	—
Venlafaxine	Fatality (rare); possibly sedation, seizures, QRS prolongation, sympathomimetic symptoms (tremor, mydriasis, tachycardia, hypertension, diaphoresis), hypotension	Observation for ≥ 6 h; for QRS prolongation, consideration of alkalinization
Vitamins with iron	See Iron	—
Warfarin (sometimes used in pesticides) Bishydroxycoumarin Dicumarol Ethyl biscoumacetate Superwarfarins (sometimes used in pesticides)	Single ingestion not serious; with multiple overdoses, coagulopathy	For hemorrhagic manifestations, vitamin K_1 (phytonadione—see p. 46) until INR is normal, transfusion with fresh blood if necessary
Whiskey	See Alcohol, ethyl	—
Wild cherry syrup	See Cyanides	—
Wintergreen oil	See Aspirin and Other Salicylate Poisoning on p. 2660	—
Wood alcohol	See Alcohol, methyl	—
Xylene	See Benzene	—
Zinc	See TABLE 326–4	—
Zinc salts	See Copper salts	—

* Inclusion of one poison with another (eg, toluene with benzene) in a single row indicates that the terms are synonymous, that the poisons are chemically related, or that one poison is an ingredient or impurity of the other.

†Physicians should be aware of people who smuggle plastic bags of cocaine in the GI tract (so-called packers) or in the mouth, rectum, or vagina (so-called stuffers).

SECTION 22
SPECIAL SUBJECTS

327 GENERAL PRINCIPLES OF MEDICAL GENETICS

Human development depends on genetic and environmental factors. Genetic information is carried in the DNA of the chromosomes and mitochondria.

Genotype is a person's genetic makeup; the term can refer to genetic makeup in its entirety or at one location (locus) on a chromosome. Karyotype is the full set of chromosomes in a person's cells.

The concepts of genotype and phenotype are closely related but not identical. Phenotype is the expression or manifestation of the genotype that occurs over time together with environmental effects. Phenotype manifests as traits. A trait may be as simple as the color of the eyes or as complex as susceptibility to diabetes. If a trait is dominant, its expression requires only one copy of the dominant gene. If a trait is recessive, its expression requires 2 copies of the recessive gene.

Expression of a trait may involve only one gene at one locus; these traits (called mendelian traits) are inherited in recognizable patterns. For other traits, expression involves more than one gene and is more complex. For still others, expression involves more than one gene and interaction with environmental factors; these interactions do not always produce clearly recognizable patterns of expression or inheritance. Expression of the genes responsible for recognizable traits is further complicated by mitochondrial and nontraditional patterns of inheritance.

Genes (20,000 to 30,000 in humans) are carried by chromosomes and mitochondria. In humans, somatic (nongerm) cells normally have 46 chromosomes in 23 pairs. Each pair consists of one chromosome from the mother and one from the father. Twenty-two of the pairs, the autosomes, are usually homologous (identical in size, shape, and position and number of genes). One pair, the sex chromosomes (X and Y), determines a person's sex. Women have 2 X chromosomes (which are homologous) in every somatic cell nucleus; men have one X and one Y chromosome (which are heterologous). The X chromosome carries genes responsible for many hereditary traits; the small, differently shaped Y chromosome carries genes that initiate male sex differentiation, as well as other genes. Germ cells (egg and sperm) undergo meiosis, which reduces the number of chromosomes to 23—½ that of somatic cells (46). Thus, when an egg is fertilized by a sperm at conception, the normal number of 46 chromosomes is reconstituted. In meiosis, the genetic information inherited from a person's mother and father is recombined through crossing over (exchange between homologous chromosomes).

Genes, the basic units of heredity, are arranged linearly along the DNA of chromosomes; each gene has a specific locus on the chromosomes. The number and arrangement of loci on homologous chromosomes are usually identical. However, a specific gene may have minor structural variations (polymorphisms). The genes that occupy the same locus on each chromosome of a pair (one inherited from the mother and one from the father) are called alleles. Each gene consists of a specific nucleotide sequence; 2 alleles may have slightly different or the same nucleotide sequences. A person with a pair of identical alleles for a particular gene is a homozygote; a person with a pair of nonidentical alleles is a heterozygote.

Gene structure is only part of the complex biologic interactions that ultimately result in gene expression. Other factors include control elements (promoters and enhancers), coding sequences (exons), intervening sequences that are located between exons and do not code for proteins (introns), and termination signals.

Expressivity and penetrance: A gene's phenotypic expression (expressivity) may be influenced by the environment and by other genes so that people with the same gene vary in phenotype. Penetrance is the degree to which a gene results in expression of a trait. For some traits, a clinical abnormality cannot be detected in some carriers (called nonpenetrance); however, the unaffected carrier of the abnormal allele can pass it to children, who may have all of the abnormalities. In such cases, the pedigree appears to skip a generation. However, some cases of apparent nonpenetrance are due to the examiner's unfamiliarity with or failure to recognize minor manifestations of the disorder. Cases with minimal expression are sometimes called a "forme fruste" of the disorder.

Pleiotropy: A single-gene defect may produce abnormalities in multiple organ systems. For example, osteogenesis imperfecta (a connective tissue disorder that often results from abnormalities in a collagen gene) may cause fragile bones, deafness, bluish whites of the eyes, dysplastic teeth, hypermobile joints, and heart valve abnormalities (see also p. 2388).

Sex-limited inheritance: A trait that appears in only one sex is called sex-limited. Sex-limited inheritance differs from X-linked inheritance, which refers to traits carried on the X chromosome. Sex-limited inheritance, perhaps more correctly called sex-influenced inheritance, refers to special cases in which sex hormones and other physiologic differences between males and females alter the expressivity and penetrance of a gene. For example, premature baldness is an autosomal dominant trait, but presumably because of female sex hormones, baldness is rarely expressed in females and then usually only after menopause.

Mutations: Mutations are spontaneous changes in genetic information (DNA); new mutations thus produce a trait de novo within a family pedigree. For example, about 80% of people with achondroplastic dwarfism (an autosomal dominant trait) have no family history of dwarfism and thus represent new mutations. In achondroplasia, mutations occur at a very specific place in the gene; for many other traits, new mutations may occur at many different places in the gene (or even at different genes). In general, unaffected parents are not at increased risk of having additional affected children with an autosomal dominant disorder, but a few normal-appearing parents have had 2 or even 3 children with typical dominant achondroplastic dwarfism. The explanation is a germline mutation, which occurs early in the embryonic life of a normal-appearing parent, when only a handful of germ cell precursors are present. The cell possessing the new mutation can then contribute many cells to the developing gonad. The existence of germline mutations has been confirmed via molecular studies of the gene mutation in parents and children.

GENETIC SCREENING

Genetic screening may be used in populations at risk of a particular genetic disorder. Genetic screening is appropriate only when genetic inheritance patterns of a disorder are understood; when effective therapy is available; and when screening tests are valid, reliable, appropriately sensitive and specific, noninvasive, and safe. Prevalence in a defined population must be high enough to justify the cost of screening.

Genetic screening may aim to identify heterozygotes carrying a gene for a recessive disorder but not expressing it (eg, Ashkenazi Jews for Tay-Sachs disease, blacks for sickle cell anemia, several ethnic groups for thalassemia—see TABLE 257–1 on p. 2145). If a heterozygote's mate is also a heterozygote, the couple is at risk of having an affected child.

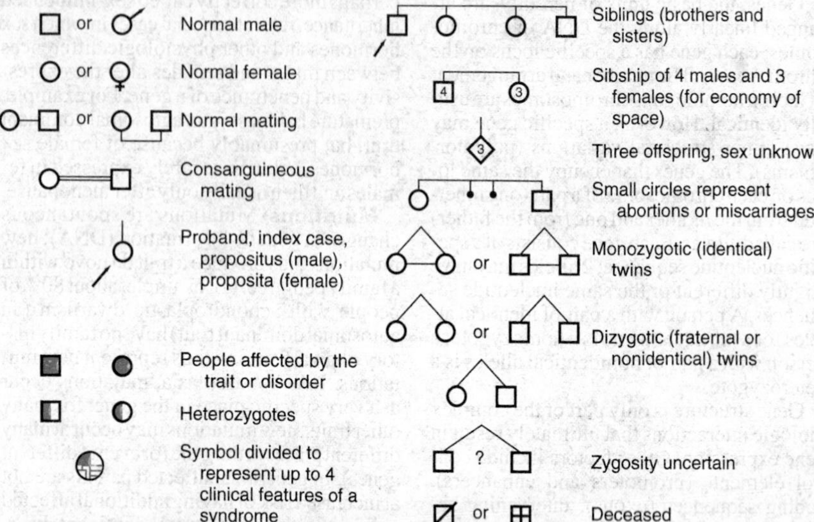

Fig. 327–1. Symbols for constructing a family pedigree. In the pedigree, symbols for each generation in the family are placed in a row, numbered with Roman numerals, starting with the older generation at the top and ending with the most recent at the bottom (see FIGS. 327–2 to 327–5). Within each generation, people are numbered from left to right with Arabic numerals. Siblings are usually listed by age, with the oldest on the left. Thus, each member of the pedigree can be identified by 2 numbers (eg, II, 4). A spouse is also assigned an identifying number.

Screening may be appropriate before symptoms begin if people have a family history of a dominantly inherited disorder that manifests later in life (eg, Huntington's disease, breast cancer). Screening defines risks for a person, who can then make appropriate plans. If identified as a carrier, the person can also make informed decisions about procreation.

Prenatal screening may involve amniocentesis, chorionic villus sampling, umbilical cord blood sampling, maternal blood sampling, maternal serum screening, or fetal visualization (see Ch. 257 on p. 2143). Common reasons for prenatal screening include maternal age > 35, a family history of a disorder that can be diagnosed via prenatal techniques, abnormal maternal serum screening results, and certain symptoms during pregnancy.

Screening in neonates allows prophylaxis (special diet or replacement therapy) for phenylketonuria, galactosemia, and hypothyroidism.

Construction of a family pedigree: The family pedigree (family tree) is commonly used in genetic counseling. It uses conventional symbols to represent family members and pertinent health information about them (see FIG. 327–1). Some familial disorders with identical phenotypes have several patterns of inheritance.

MITOCHONDRIAL DNA ABNORMALITIES

Mitochondria contain a unique circular chromosome that codes for 13 proteins, various RNAs, and several regulating enzymes. However, > 90% of mitochondrial proteins are coded by nuclear genes. Each cell has several hundred mitochondria in its cytoplasm.

Mitochondrial disorders (see also p. 2472) can be due to mitochondrial or nuclear DNA abnormalities (eg, deletions, duplications, mutations). High-energy tissues (eg, muscle, heart, brain) are particularly at risk of malfunction due to mitochondrial abnormalities. Patterns of tissue involvement correlate with particular mitochondrial DNA abnormalities (see TABLE 327–1). Mitochondrial abnormalities occur in many common disorders

TABLE 327–1. MITOCHONDRIAL DISORDERS

DISORDER	DESCRIPTION
Chronic progressive external ophthalmoplegia	Progressive paralysis of the extraocular muscles usually preceded by bilateral, symmetrical, progressive ptosis that begins months to years earlier
Kearns-Sayre syndrome	A multisystem variant of chronic progressive external ophthalmoplegia that also includes heart block, retinitis pigmentosa, and CNS degeneration
Leber's hereditary optic neuropathy	Variable but often devastating bilateral visual loss that often occurs in adolescents and that is due to a point mutation in mitochondrial DNA
MERRF syndrome	*M*yoclonic *e*pilepsy, *r*agged *r*ed *f*ibers, dementia, ataxia, and myopathy
MELAS syndrome	*M*itochondrial *e*ncephalomyopathy, *l*actic *a*cidosis, and *s*trokelike episodes
Pearson's syndrome	Sideroblastic anemia, pancreatic insufficiency, and progressive liver disease that begins in the 1st few months of life and is frequently fatal in infants

such as some types of Parkinson's disease (which may involve large mitochondrial deletions in the cells of the basal ganglia) and many types of muscle disorders.

Maternal inheritance characterizes abnormalities of mitochondrial DNA. For practical purposes, all mitochondria are inherited from the cytoplasm of the egg; thus, all offspring of an affected female are at risk of inheriting the abnormality, but no offspring of an affected male are at risk. Variability in clinical manifestations is the rule and may be due in part to variable mixtures of inherited mutant and normal mitochondrial genomes (heteroplasmy) within cells and tissues.

SINGLE-GENE DEFECTS

Genetic disorders determined by a single gene (mendelian disorders) are easiest to analyze and the most fully studied. Many specific disorders have been described. Single-gene defects may be autosomal or X-linked, dominant or recessive.

AUTOSOMAL DOMINANT

Only one abnormal allele of a gene is needed to express an autosomal dominant trait; ie, heterozygotes and homozygotes for the abnormal gene are affected. A typical pedigree of an autosomal dominant trait is shown in FIG. 327–2.

In general, the following rules apply:

- An affected person has an affected parent.
- A heterozygous affected parent and an unaffected parent have, on average, an equal number of affected and unaffected children; ie, risk of occurrence for each child of an affected person is 50%.
- Unaffected children of an affected parent do not transmit the trait to their descendents.
- Males and females are equally likely to be affected.

AUTOSOMAL RECESSIVE

Two copies of an abnormal allele are needed to express an autosomal recessive trait. A typical pedigree is shown in FIG. 327–3. In certain populations, the percentage of heterozygotes (carriers) is high because of a founder effect (ie, the group started with few members, one of whom was a carrier) or because carriers have a selective advantage (eg, heterozygosity for sickle cell anemia protects against malaria).

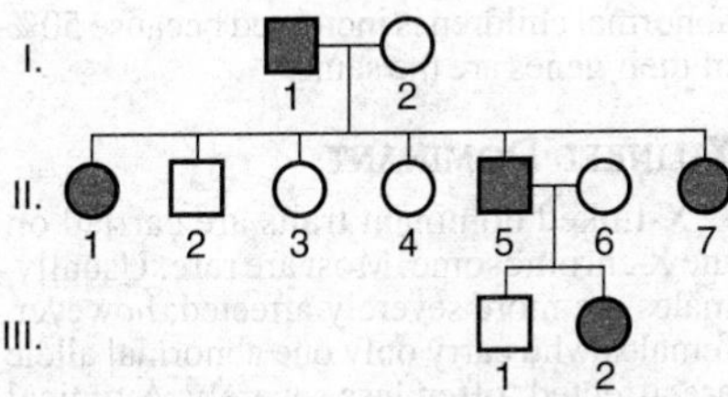

Fig. 327–2. Autosomal dominant inheritance.

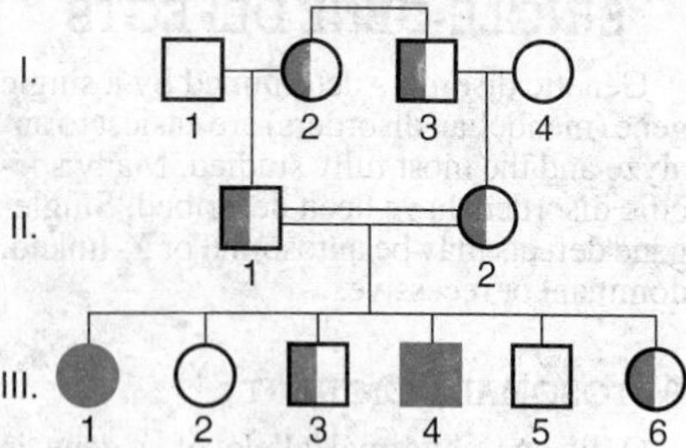

Fig. 327–3. Autosomal recessive inheritance and consanguineous mating.

In general, the following rules of inheritance apply:

- If normal parents have an affected child, both parents are heterozygotes, and on average, $\frac{1}{4}$ of their children are affected, $\frac{1}{2}$ are heterozygotes, and $\frac{1}{4}$ are normal.
- All children of an affected person and a genotypically normal person are phenotypically normal heterozygotes.
- On average, $\frac{1}{2}$ the children of an affected person and a heterozygote are affected, and $\frac{1}{2}$ are heterozygotes.
- All children of 2 affected people are affected.
- Males and females are equally likely to be affected.
- Heterozygotes are phenotypically normal but carry the trait. If the trait is caused by a defect of a specific protein (eg, an enzyme), heterozygotes usually have a reduced amount of that protein. If the mutation is known, molecular genetic techniques can identify heterozygous phenotypically normal people.

Relatives are more likely to carry the same mutant allele, so mating between close relatives (consanguinity) increases the likelihood of having affected children. In parent-child or brother-sister unions, risk of having abnormal children is increased because 50% of their genes are the same.

X-LINKED DOMINANT

X-linked dominant traits are carried on the X chromosome. Most are rare. Usually, males are more severely affected; however, females who carry only one abnormal allele are affected, often less severely. A typical pedigree is shown in FIG. 327–4.

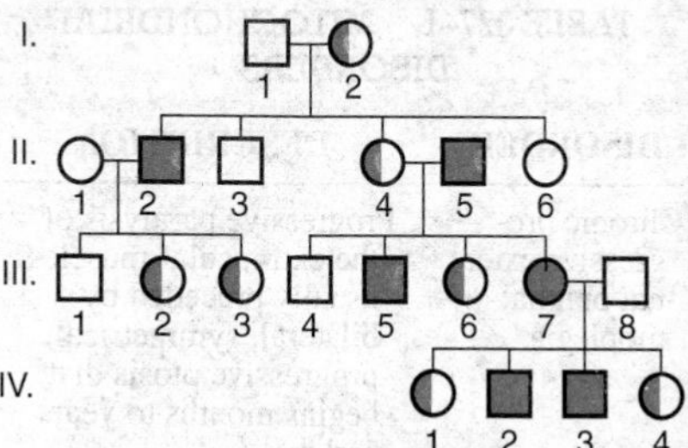

Fig. 327–4. X-linked dominant inheritance.

In general, the following rules of inheritance apply:

- Affected males transmit the trait to all of their daughters but not to their sons (male-to-male transmission does not occur); however, if an affected male is married to an affected female, as in FIG. 327–4, they may have an affected son.
- Affected heterozygous females transmit the trait to $\frac{1}{2}$ of their children, regardless of sex.
- Affected homozygous females transmit the trait to all of their children.
- Twice as many affected females as males have the trait unless it is lethal in males.

X-linked dominant inheritance may be difficult to differentiate from autosomal dominant inheritance without use of molecular probes. Large pedigrees are required, with particular attention to children of affected males, because male-to-male transmission rules out X-linkage (males pass only their Y chromosomes to their sons). Some X-linked dominant disorders are lethal in males.

X-LINKED RECESSIVE

X-linked recessive traits are carried on the X chromosome. A typical pedigree is shown in FIG. 327–5.

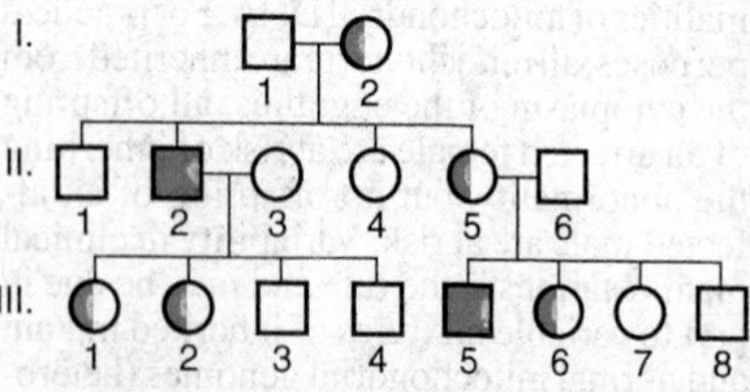

Fig. 327–5. X-linked recessive inheritance.

In general, the following rules of inheritance apply:

- Nearly all affected people are male.
- Heterozygous females are usually phenotypically normal but, as carriers, may transmit the trait to their children (however, the trait may represent a new mutation in an affected male).
- An affected male never transmits the trait to his sons.
- All daughters of an affected male are carriers.
- A carrier female transmits the trait to ½ of her sons.
- No daughters of a carrier female have the trait (unless they also inherit the trait, such as color blindness, from their father), but ½ are carriers.

An affected female usually has the abnormal gene on both X chromosomes (homozygote) for it to be expressed; ie, she has an affected father and a mother who is heterozygous or homozygous for the mutant gene.

Occasionally, females who are heterozygous for X-linked mutations show some expression, but they are rarely affected as severely as males who are hemizygous (having only one of a pair of genes). Heterozygous females can be affected if a structural chromosomal rearrangement (eg, X-autosome translocation, missing or deleted X chromosome) or skewed X inactivation occurs. X inactivation occurs early in development; usually, it involves the random but equal inactivation of the maternally or paternally inherited X chromosome. Occasionally, however, most of the inactivation occurs to the X chromosome from one parent; this is called skewed X inactivation.

CODOMINANT

In codominant inheritance, the phenotype of heterozygotes is distinct from that of either homozygote. Each allele at a genetic locus usually has a detectable effect. For example, codominance is recognized in blood group antigens (eg, AB, MN), WBC antigens (eg, DR4, DR3), serum proteins with different electrophoretic mobility (eg, albumin, haptoglobulin), and enzyme activities (eg, of paraoxonase).

MULTIFACTORIAL INHERITANCE

Many traits (eg, height) are distributed along a bell-shaped curve (normal distribution); this distribution is compatible with multigene determination of the trait. Each gene adds to or subtracts from the trait independently of other genes. In this distribution, few people are at the extremes and many are in the middle because people are unlikely to inherit multiple factors acting in the same direction. Environmental factors, each adding to or subtracting from the final result, contribute to the normalcy of distribution.

Many relatively common congenital anomalies and familial disorders result from multifactorial inheritance. In an affected person, the disorder represents the sum of genetic and environmental influences. Risk of occurrence of such a trait is much higher in 1st-degree relatives (who share 50% of the affected person's genes) than in more distant relatives, who are likely to inherit only a few high-liability genes.

Common disorders with multifactorial causes include hypertension, arteriosclerotic heart disease, diabetes mellitus, cancer, neural tube defects, and arthritis. Many specific genes are being identified. Genetically determined predisposing factors, including a family history and biochemical and molecular parameters, can identify people who are at risk and are likely to benefit from preventive measures.

NONTRADITIONAL INHERITANCE

Mosaicism: Mosaicism is the presence of ≥ 2 cell lines differing in genotype or karyotype but derived from one zygote. Mutations are likely to occur during cell division in any large multicellular organism. Each time a cell divides, 4 or 5 changes are estimated to occur in the genome. Thus, any large multicellular organism has subclones of cells that have a slightly different genetic makeup. These somatic mutations (mutations during mitotic cell division) may not lead to an identifiable trait or disease but may be recognized as disorders in which patchy changes occur. For example, McCune-Albright syndrome causes patchy dysplastic changes in the bone, endocrine gland abnormalities, patchy pigmentary changes, and occasionally heart or liver abnormalities. Occurrence of the McCune-Albright mutation in all cells would cause early death; however, mosaic individuals survive because normal tissue supports the abnormal tissue. Occasionally, a parent with a single-gene disorder seems to have a mild form but is actually a mosaic; offspring may be more severely affected if they receive a germ cell with the mutant allele and thus have the abnormality in every cell. Chromosomal mosaicism occurs in some embryos and can be detected in the placenta using chorionic villus sampling. Most chromosomally abnormal embryos and fetuses abort spontaneously. However, the presence of normal cells during early development may support certain chromosomal abnormalities, allowing offspring to be born alive.

Genomic imprinting: Genomic imprinting is the differential expression of genetic material depending on whether it has been inherited from the father or mother. The difference in expression results from differential gene activation. Genomic imprinting is tissue-specific and time-in-development–specific. Biallelic or biparental expression of alleles may occur in some tissues, and uniparental expression occurs in other tissues. Depending on whether the genetic change is paternally or maternally inherited, a different syndrome may be produced if a gene is genomically imprinted. Genomic imprinting must be considered in disorders that appear to skip a generation.

Uniparental disomy: Uniparental disomy occurs when 2 chromosomes of a pair are inherited from only one parent. It is very rare and is thought to involve trisomy rescue; ie, the zygote started off as a trisomy and one of the 3 chromosomes was lost, leading to uniparental disomy in ⅓ of cases. Imprinting effects may occur because genetic information from the other parent is absent. Also, if duplicates of the same chromosome (isodisomy) are present and carry an abnormal allele for an autosomal recessive disorder, affected people can have an autosomal recessive disorder even though only one parent is a carrier.

Triplet (trinucleotide) repeat disorders: A triplet of nucleotides often occurs and is sometimes repeated many times. Occasionally, the number of triplets within a gene increases from one generation to the next (a normal gene has relatively few tandem triplet repeats). When the gene is transmitted from one generation to the next or sometimes as cells divide within the body, the triplet repeat can expand and enlarge, stopping the gene from functioning normally. Expansion is detected by molecular studies. This type of genetic change is unusual but occurs in several disorders (eg, myotonic dystrophy, fragile X mental retardation), particularly those involving the CNS (eg, Huntington's disease).

Anticipation: Anticipation occurs when a disorder has an earlier age of onset and is expressed more severely in each successive generation. Anticipation may occur when a parent is a mosaic and the child has the full mutation in all cells. It may also occur in triplet repeat expansion when the number of repeats and thus the severity of phenotype increase with each generation.

GENE THERAPY

Therapy for genetic disorders is often similar to therapy for other disorders. Special diets can eliminate compounds that are toxic to patients (eg, in phenylketonuria or homocystinuria). Vitamins or other agents can improve a biochemical pathway and thus reduce toxic levels of a compound; for example, folic acid reduces homocysteine levels in people with 5,10-methylene tetrahydrofolate reductase polymorphism. Therapy may involve replacing a deficient compound or blocking an overactive pathway. Fetuses can sometimes be treated by treating the mother (eg, corticosteroids for congenital virilizing adrenal hypoplasia) or by using in utero cellular therapy (eg, stem cell transplantation). Neonates with a genetic disorder may be candidates for stem cell or organ transplantation.

Gene therapy may involve insertion of normal copies of a gene into the cells of people with a specific genetic disorder. Trials of somatic gene therapy have been undertaken for very severe genetic disorders (eg, adenosine deaminase deficiency). Germline gene therapy may involve correcting an abnormality in the genes of sperm or egg; however, use of this therapy raises ethical issues. Gene therapy may also involve turning off genes (eg, by antisense DNA).

328 CLINICAL DECISION MAKING

Clinicians must choose from among a large number of tests and interpret a huge variety of clinical data while facing pressure to decrease uncertainty, risks to patients, and costs. A clinician must decide what information to gather, which tests to order, how to interpret and integrate this information into diagnostic hypotheses, and what treatments to give—a topic known as "clinical decision making."

CLINICAL RULES

Traditionally, clinical decision making has followed logical "if...then..." rules (eg, if a patient is febrile and neutropenic, then institute broad-spectrum antibiotics). Such rules can be made explicit and presented as guidelines or algorithms. Such guidelines have gained increasing popularity but should be applied only to patients who fall within the specific clinical context explicitly described by the algorithm.

However, most patients have some feature that distinguishes them from the groups presented in such formal guidelines. Guidelines cannot adequately represent variations among patients with different demographics, comorbidities, and histories. Guidelines can aid in the management of many clinical problems, but the clinician must always use appropriate clinical judgment and interpret conflicting data that fall between the rules. To incorporate uncertainty and the relative value of potential outcomes into clinical decision making and to follow the logic and principles underlying how clinical decisions are made, clinicians must understand the basics of probability.

Formalizing the decision-making process forces clinicians to confront the assumptions and uncertainties that underlie decisions. Although clinicians make complex decisions and informally weigh the risks and benefits of various options in straightforward or common situations, sometimes the amount of information they must consider exceeds their cognitive abilities. Mathematical computations can assist clinical decision making and, even when exact numbers are unavailable, can better define clinical probabilities and their logical relations.

REASONING WITH PROBABILITIES

Clinicians often generate a list of possible causes to better understand a patient's symptoms or signs—the differential diagnosis. Some causes are more or less likely; clinicians often use vague terms such as "highly likely," "improbable," and "cannot rule out" to describe the likelihood of disease. Both clinicians and patients often misinterpret such semiquantitative terms. Imprecise terminology can be clarified by using explicit quantities called probabilities.

The probability of a disease (or event) occurring in a patient whose clinical information is unknown is the frequency with which the disease or event occurs in a population. Probabilities range from 0.0 (impossible) to 1.0 (certain) and are often expressed as the proportion in 100 patients (ie, percentages ranging from 0 to 100). When only 2 states (eg, disease and no disease) are considered, probabilities can sometimes be better understood by considering the ratio of affected to unaffected patients (ie, the odds of disease vs no disease). Thus, a probability of 0.2 (20%) corresponds to odds of 0.2/0.8 (20%/80%) or 0.25 (sometimes expressed as 1 in 4). Odds (Ω) and probabilities (p) can be converted one to the other, as $\Omega = p/(1-p)$ or $p = \Omega/(1+\Omega)$. Rounding very small probabilities to 0, which excludes all possibility of disease (sometimes done in implicit clinical reasoning), can lead to erroneous conclusions when quantitative reasoning is used.

DIAGNOSTIC TESTING

Clinicians use laboratory tests to help them make choices. Test results may help reduce uncertainty, make a diagnosis (diagnostic testing), or identify patients who are likely to have occult disease (screening). However, test results may increase uncertainty if the tests poorly discriminate between patients with and patients without disease, if the test results are at variance with the clinical picture, or if test results are improperly integrated into the clinical context.

Laboratory tests are imperfect and may mistakenly identify some people who do not have a specific disease as having the disease (false-positive result) or may mistakenly identify some affected people as not having the disease (false-negative result). A test's ability to correctly include or exclude disease depends on how likely a person is to have a disease (prior probability, see below) and the sensitivity and specificity of the test (see below).

In addition to the risk of providing misleading information, laboratory tests consume limited resources, may delay treatment, may induce unnecessary treatment or cause necessary treatment to be withheld, and may place the patient at risk for an adverse event from the test itself.

Although a single test can provide information about a variety of diseases, a test is often used to establish the presence or absence of only one disease. Similarly, many tests provide a quantitative result (eg, blood sugar 120 mg/dL) or one of several results (eg, exercise ECG with < 1, 1 to 2, > 2 mm ST-segment depression) that are defined as positive only when they meet or exceed some established criterion or cutoff point. Such cutoff points can be based on statistics or can be adjusted to reflect the burdens of false-positive and false-negative results. When laboratory tests are used to establish that disease is present or absent and the test results can be only positive or negative, a test's sensitivity and specificity can be defined.

Sensitivity is the likelihood of a positive test result in patients with the disease; it measures how well the test detects the disease. The false-negative rate is the complement of sensitivity (ie, the false-negative rate plus the sensitivity = 100%).

Specificity is the likelihood of a negative test result in patients without the disease; it measures how well the test excludes disease. The false-positive rate is the complement of specificity.

Conditional probability is the probability that a disease (or event) will occur if another event, test result, or condition is present. Sensitivity and specificity are special types of conditional probabilities, in this case whether a positive or negative result will occur if the disease is present or absent, as defined by some gold standard (often based on histologic, microbiologic, or radiographic criteria that define the presence or absence of disease).

Prior (or pre-test) probability is the likelihood that a patient has a condition or disease before the test result is known. Prior probability is based on clinical judgment: how strongly do the symptoms and signs suggest the disease is present, what in a patient's history and risk factors support the diagnosis, and how common is the disease in a representative population?

Post-test probability is the likelihood the condition or disease is present after the test results are known. The extent to which the test results change assessment of the probability of disease depends on the test's sensitivity and specificity.

Multiple Screening Tests

Patients often must consider whether to be screened for occult disease. The premises of screening are that early detection of disease can improve outcomes in patients with occult disease and that the false-positive results that often occur during screening do not create a burden that exceeds the benefit of early detection. With the expanding array of screening tests available, the implications of a panel of such tests must be considered. For example, a test with a specificity of 95% will result in 5% of patients without the target disease having a false-positive result. If 2 different screening tests were done, each concerning a different occult disease, in a patient who actually has neither disease, the chance that both tests will be negative is 95% × 95%, or 90%; there would be a 10% chance of at least one false-positive result. If 3 different screening tests for 3 unrelated diseases were done, the chance that all 3 would be negative would be 95% × 95% × 95%, or 86%; corresponding to a 14% chance of at least one false-positive result. If 12 different tests for 12 different diseases were done, the chance of at least one false-positive result is 46%! This underscores the need for caution when deciding on a panel of screening tests and interpreting the results.

BAYES' THEOREM

When interpreting a test result, the clinician converts a pre-test or prior probability of disease into the appropriate post-test or posterior probability. Clinicians must use their best judgment—from all clinical data available—to assign reasonable estimates of pre-test probabilities. To illustrate this process in a clinical context, consider a 25-yr-old woman who presents with dysuria. Assume that the clinician thought the probability of UTI was moderately low (30%) based on the patient's history and physical examination. Before sending the patient's urine for microscopic examination of the sediment and for culture, the clinician does a dipstick leukocyte esterase test, which has a positive result. To determine the post-test probability of UTI, the clinician must know the sensitivity (71%) and specificity (85%) of the test. FIG. 328–1 considers 100,000 women similar to this patient, of whom 30% (30,000) have UTI and 70% (70,000) do not. Test results will be positive in 21,300 (71%, the test's sensitivity) of the women with UTI and in 10,500 (15%, the test's false-positive rate) of the women without UTI. Of the 31,800 women from the original cohort with positive test results (whether true positive or false positive), 21,300 (67%) actually have UTI. Thus, the posterior or revised probability of UTI after a positive leukocyte esterase test result is 67%, making the diagnosis more likely than not but not certain. The positive result has not provided certainty but has made the diagnosis far more likely.

What if the test result had been negative? Of the 68,200 women with negative test results (whether true negative or false negative), 8,700 (13%) will actually have UTI. Thus, the posterior or revised probability of UTI after a negative leukocyte esterase test result is 13%, making the diagnosis less likely but still possible.

These calculations are shown in TABLE 328–1. To illustrate how this table can be used to revise probabilities, consider a 2nd woman with dysuria and frequency, but no vaginal discharge or irritation, who has had frequent UTIs in the past; assume that her prior probability of UTI is high, say 77%. The upper half of TABLE 328–1 interprets a positive leukocyte esterase test result in this woman; the lower half interprets a negative test result. Although the sensitivity (71%) and specificity (85%) of the test are unchanged from the values in the first example, a positive test result increases the probability of UTI to 94%, or almost certain, and a negative result decreases it to only 54%, or just a bit more likely than not.

The process of using the pre-test probability of disease and the test characteristics to calculate the post-test probability is called Bayes' theorem or bayesian revision. Bayes' theorem can be expressed as an equation, but a flowchart (see FIG. 328–1) or tabular approach (see TABLE 328–1) is easier to use and less subject to error.

When several tests must be interpreted, Bayes' theorem can be applied sequentially

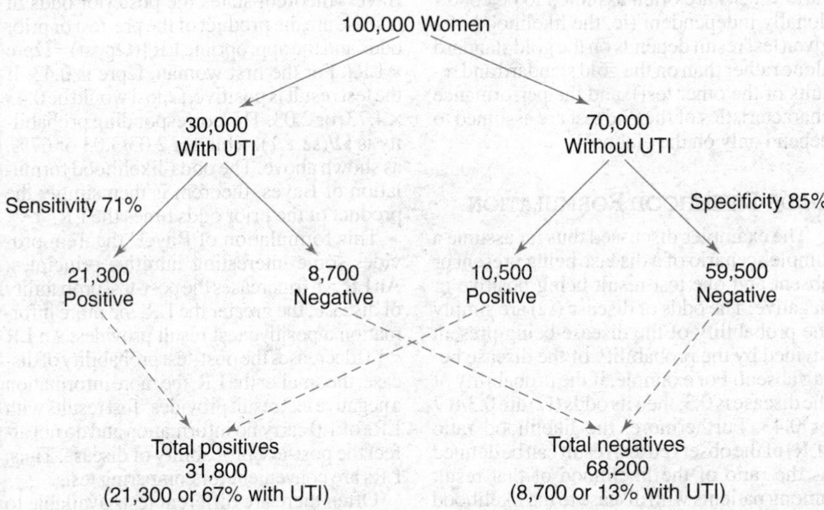

Fig. 328–1. Interpretation of leukocyte esterase test result in a woman with a 30% prior probability of a UTI, simulating a cohort of 100,000 identical women.

TABLE 328–1. INTERPRETATION OF A LEUKOCYTE ESTERASE TEST RESULT IN A WOMAN WITH A HIGH (77%) PRIOR PROBABILITY OF UTI

A DIAGNOSIS	B* PRIOR PROBABIL-ITY (%)	C* CONDITIONAL PROBABILITY OF RESULT (%)	D PRODUCT (B × C)	E POSTERIOR PROBABILITY† (%)
		Positive Result		
UTI	77	71	5467	94
No UTI	22	15	330	6
			Total = 5797	
		Negative Result		
UTI	77	29	2233	54
No UTI	22	85	1870	46
			Total = 4103	

*The entries in columns B and C can be in any convenient scale (eg, probabilities, percentages, cases/1000), and the scale for each column can be different.

†The row-wise product divided by the total of column D.

by using the posterior probability of one test as the prior probability for the next test. The conditional probability used for interpreting subsequent test results must be based on the gold standard for diagnosis and on the observed results of the preceding test. When such data are unavailable, the results of the various tests are often assumed to be conditionally independent (ie, the likelihood of a given test result depends on the gold standard alone rather than on the gold standard and results of the other test), and the performance characteristics of the 2nd test are assumed to depend only on the diagnosis.

ODDS-LIKELIHOOD FORMULATION

The examples discussed thus far assume a simple scenario of a disease being present or absent and one test result being positive or negative. The odds of disease (Ω) are simply the probability of the disease being present divided by the probability of the disease being absent. For example, if the probability of the disease is 0.3, then its odds (Ω) are 0.3/0.7 or 0.43. Furthermore, the likelihood ratio (LR) of the observed test result can be defined as the ratio of the likelihood of that result among patients with disease to the likelihood among patients without disease. That is, the LR for a positive result (LRpos) equals the true-positive rate divided by the false-positive rate. Similarly, the LR for a negative result (LRneg) equals the false-negative rate divided by the true-negative rate. For example, if the sensitivity and specificity are 71% and 85%, as above, then LRpos equals 0.71/0.15 or 4.73 and LRneg equals 0.29/0.85 or 0.34.

The odds-likelihood formulation of Bayes' theorem states the posterior odds of disease are the product of the pre-test or prior odds and the appropriate LR [(Ωpost) = Ωpre × LR]. For the first woman, Ωpre is 0.43. If the test result is positive, Ωpost would be 0.43 × 4.73, or 2.03. The corresponding probability is Ω/(Ω + 1), which is 2.03/3.03 or 67%, as shown above. The odds-likelihood formulation of Bayes' theorem is then simply the product of the prior odds times the LR.

This formulation of Bayes' theorem provides some interesting intuitive principles. An LR > 1.0 increases the post-test probability of disease; the greater the LR, the more information a positive test result provides. An LR < 1.0 decreases the post-test probability of disease; the smaller the LR, the more information a negative test result provides. Test results with LRs of 1.0 carry no information and do not affect the post-test probability of disease. Thus, LRs are convenient for comparing tests.

Often there are different tests available to screen for the same disease. Whether a test that has higher sensitivity or specificity is used depends on the consequences of a false-positive

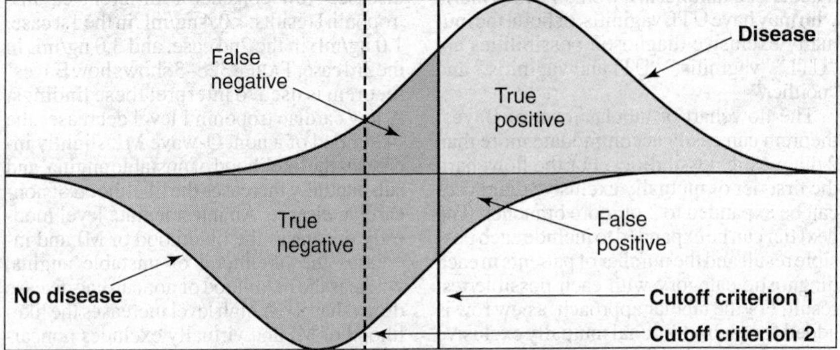

Fig. 328–2. Distributions of test results. Patients with disease are shown in the upper distribution; patients without disease are shown in the lower distribution. The relationship between a test's true-positive and false-positive rates (for different criteria or cutoff points) can be displayed as a receiver-operator characteristic (ROC) curve. The area beneath such a curve corresponds to the discriminatory power of the test.

or false-negative test result as well as the pretest probability of disease. For example, in testing for a serious disease for which an efficacious treatment is available (eg, coronary heart disease), one would be willing to tolerate more false positives (lower specificity) than false negatives (lower sensitivity). Among populations with a higher prevalence of disease, the positive predictive value of a screening test will increase; as prevalence decreases, the post-test or posterior probability of a positive result decreases. Therefore, when screening for disease in high-risk populations, tests with a higher sensitivity are preferred over those with a higher specificity because they are better at ruling out disease (fewer false negatives). On the other hand, in low-risk populations or for diseases for which therapy has lower benefit or higher risk, tests with a higher specificity are preferred.

Defining a Positive Test Result

For Bayes' theorem (or even the terms "sensitivity" and "specificity") to be used, every possible result of a diagnostic test must be classified as positive or negative. When a test is not inherently positive or negative, the laboratory (or whoever describes the test's performance) establishes a criterion for positivity such that all results beyond that criterion are defined as positive and vice versa. Two overlapping distributions of results are transected by a criterion or cutoff line (see Fig. 328–2). The region beneath the distribution of results for patients with disease that lies above (to the right of) the criterion corresponds to the test's true-positive rate (ie, its sensitivity); the region that lies below (to the left of) the criterion corresponds to the false-negative rate. For the distribution of results for patients without disease, these 2 regions correspond to the false-positive rate and the true-negative rate (ie, its specificity), respectively. For the overlapping portion of the 2 distributions (eg, patients with and without disease), changing the criterion or cutoff line affects sensitivity and specificity but in opposite directions. Sensitivity and specificity cannot both be improved by changing the cutoff line, but rather only by improving the discrimination of the test itself.

Multiple Diagnostic Possibilities

Bayes' theorem can also help interpret clinical information in situations in which more than 2 diagnostic possibilities (ie, disease present and disease absent) exist. Reasoning explicitly is increasingly important when the diagnostic task becomes more complex. The only requirements for bayesian interpretation are that all diagnostic possibilities be considered and assigned a prior probability and that all be mutually exclusive (ie, only one of the listed possibilities can be present). Combinations must be explicitly listed. For example, in a woman with dysuria who may have UTI, vaginitis, or both, the mutually exclusive diagnostic possibilities are "UTI," "vaginitis," "UTI and vaginitis," and "neither."

The flowchart or tabular form of Bayes' theorem can easily accommodate more than 2 diagnostic possibilities. For the flowchart, the first tier of mutually exclusive diagnoses can be expanded to 3 or more branches. The next tier can be expanded to include each possible result and the number of patients in each diagnostic category with each possible test result. For the tabular approach, a new row is added for each additional mutually exclusive diagnosis considered, and a section is added for each possible test result.

For example, cardiac troponin I levels can help evaluate a 59-yr-old man with a history of diabetes and hypertension who presents to the emergency room with new-onset chest pain that occurred at rest 5 h ago. ECGs show no ST-segment elevations or Q waves; T waves are inverted anteriorly. Diagnostic possibilities include a non–Q-wave MI, unstable angina, and noncardiac disease. A serum cardiac troponin I level can help differentiate these diagnoses. Very high cardiac troponin I levels occur most often in patients with MI, intermediate levels occur in patients with unstable angina, and very low levels occur in patients with noncardiac disease. Mathematical analysis improves understanding of the implications of a test result. Assume that the conditional probabilities are those shown in TABLE 328–2. For each diagnosis, the sum of the conditional probabilities is 100% because all possible results are listed.

After clinical evaluation (ie, history, physical examination, ECG), assume that the probability is 25% for non–Q-wave MI, 70% for unstable angina, and 5% for noncardiac disease. Now consider 3 different cardiac troponin I results: < 0.4 ng/mL in the 1st case, 1.0 ng/mL in the 2nd case, and 3.0 ng/mL in the 3rd case. TABLE 328–3 shows how Bayes' theorem is used to interpret these findings. A low cardiac troponin I level decreases the likelihood of a non–Q-wave MI, slightly increases the likelihood of unstable angina, and substantially increases the likelihood of noncardiac disease. An intermediate level modestly decreases the likelihood of MI and increases the likelihood of unstable angina, whereas the likelihood of noncardiac disease drops sharply. A high level increases the likelihood of MI and virtually excludes noncardiac disease.

DETERMINING A THRESHOLD FOR TREATING

After evaluation, a clinician must decide whether to initiate or withhold treatment or gather more information about the diagnosis (eg, by doing additional diagnostic tests). However, in some situations, further information cannot be obtained and a decision about treatment must be made (see FIG. 328–3).

The expected value of each strategy (ie, treatment or no treatment) is a linear function of the probability of disease. The clinician must also consider the likelihood that the treatment will be successful and whether the patient can tolerate the treatment. The treatment threshold (RxT, the probability of disease above which the patient should be treated) can be expressed in terms of the benefit/risk ratio (B/R) of treatment: RxT = 1/(B/R + 1). It follows that if the benefit of treatment is very large compared with the risk (eg, giving an antibiotic to a diabetic patient who may have a cellulitis), the B/R becomes

TABLE 328–2. CARDIAC TROPONIN I LEVELS IN ACUTE ISCHEMIC HEART DISEASE

	PROBABILITY			
DIAGNOSIS	cTnI < 0.4 ng/mL (%)	cTnI = 0.4–2.5 ng/mL (%)	cTnI > 2.5 ng/mL (%)	TOTAL (%)
Non–Q-wave MI	25	40	35	100
Unstable angina	40	55	5	100
Noncardiac disease	96	3.9	0.1	100

cTnI = cardiac troponin level.

TABLE 328–3. INTERPRETATION OF CARDIAC TROPONIN I RESULTS USING BAYES' THEOREM

A DIAGNOSIS	B PRIOR PROBABILITY (%)	C CONDITIONAL PROBABILITY OF RESULT (%)	D PRODUCT (B × C)	E POSTERIOR PROBABILITY (%)*
		cTnI < 0.4 ng/mL		
Non–Q-wave MI	25	25.0	625.0	16.0
Unstable angina	70	40.0	2800.0	71.7
Noncardiac disease	5	96.0	480.0	12.3
			Total = 3905.0	
		cTnI = 1.0 ng/mL		
Non–Q-wave MI	25	40.0	1000.0	20.5
Unstable angina	70	55.0	3850.0	79.1
Noncardiac disease	5	3.9	19.5	0.4
			Total = 4869.5	
		cTnI = 3.0 ng/mL		
Non–Q-wave MI	25	35.0	875.0	71.40
Unstable angina	70	5.0	350.0	28.56
Noncardiac disease	5	0.1	0.5	0.04
			Total = 1225.5	

cTnI = cardiac troponin I level.

*The row-wise product divided by the total of column D.

very large and the RxT very low, perhaps 0.2 (ie, treatment may be appropriate even at relatively low pre-test probabilities of disease). However, if the benefit of treatment is very small compared with the risk (eg, chemotherapy for pancreatic cancer), the B/R is small and the RxT is near 1 (ie, treatment is preferred over no treatment only if disease is highly probable). Finally, if the benefit of treatment (in patients with disease) equals the risk (in patients without disease), the B/R is 1.0, and the RxT is 0.5. In other words, only patients who are more likely than not to have disease (ie, probability > 50%) should be treated. The treatment threshold divides the probability domain into 2 strategic regions based on how likely it is the patient has the disease.

For example, in a patient with coronary artery disease and ECG evidence of previous MI who develops symptoms consistent with a new MI, how high should the clinical likelihood of acute MI be for thrombolytic therapy to be given, assuming the choice is based on short-term mortality? For anterior MI, assume that mortality rate without thrombolytic therapy is 12%, which falls to only 9% if thrombolytic therapy is given within 4 h of the onset of symptoms (ie, B is 3% [12% − 9%]). Further assume that the frequency of intracranial hemorrhage with thrombolytic therapy is 1% (R) and that all patients who sustain an intracranial hemorrhage die. Then, the B/R is 3/1 and the RxT is 1/(3 + 1), or treatment should be given if the probability of acute MI is > 25%. If the likelihood of the disease is expressed as its odds (Ω), then the treatment threshold as odds (RxT-O) is simply R/B or 0.33, which when represented as a probability is 0.33/(0.33 + 1) or again 0.25.

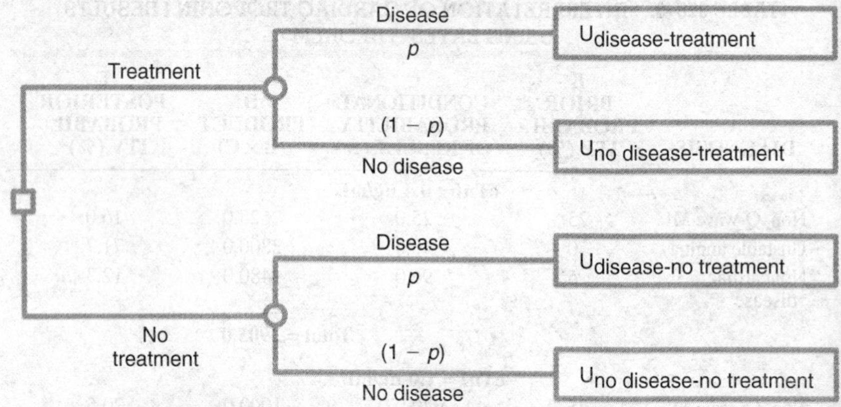

Fig. 328–3. Decision tree about whether to treat when no test is available. When the problem is limited to a single disease and a single treatment in patients with the disease, the utility of giving treatment is denoted as $U_{\text{disease-treatment}}$, the utility of withholding treatment as $U_{\text{disease-no treatment}}$, and the differences in these utilities as the benefit of treatment (B). In patients without the disease, the utility of withholding treatment is denoted as $U_{\text{no disease-no treatment}}$, the utility of giving treatment as $U_{\text{no disease-treatment}}$, and the differences in these utilities as the risk of treatment (R). Benefit is defined in patients with the disease; risk is defined in patients without the disease.

DETERMINING A THRESHOLD FOR PERFORMING A TEST

Laboratory tests or imaging studies should generally be done only if their results will affect management. In many cases, a positive test result implies a decision to treat, and a negative result implies withholding treatment. There are 2 threshold probabilities (TestT, the testing threshold and TestRxT, the test-treatment threshold) that create 3 different probabilities ranges (see FIG. 328–4). If the probability of disease is lower than the TestT (see above), then the laboratory test and treatment should generally be withheld; if the probability of disease is higher than the TestRxT, the laboratory test should not be done and treatment should be given empirically. Only if the probability of disease falls between TestT and TestRxT should the laboratory test be done. These thresholds depend on the benefits (B) and risks (R) of treatment, the test's sensitivity and specificity, and the risk, if any, of the test.

For a test that can only be positive or negative and that has no adverse effects, the TestT equals

$$\frac{[(1 - \text{specificity}) \times R]}{\{[(1 - \text{specificity}) \times R] + [\text{sensitivity} \times B]\}}$$

and the TestRxT equals

$$\frac{(\text{specificity} \times R)}{\{(\text{specificity} \times R) + [(1 - \text{sensitivity}) \times B]\}}$$

For example, should a rapid echocardiogram be done before giving thrombolytic therapy to a patient with a previous MI but without a previous echocardiogram for comparison? Assume that the sensitivity of the echocardiogram in diagnosing a new MI is 60% and the specificity is 70% and that the benefit of thrombolytic therapy is 3% and the risk is 1%. In this case, the TestT equals (30% × 1%)/[(30% × 1%) + (60% × 3%)], or 14%, and the TestRxT equals (70% × 1%)/[(70% × 1%) + (40% × 3%)], or 37% (compared with the calculated RxT of 25%, 1/[B/R + 1], when no test was available). An urgent echocardiogram would be appropriate only when the probability of an acute MI is between 14% and 37%. If the likelihood of the disease is expressed as its odds (Ω), then the TestT as odds (TestT-O) is simply (R/B) × (1/likelihood ratio for a positive result [LRpos]) and the TestRxT as odds (TestRxT-O) is simply (R/B) × (1/LR for a negative result [LRneg]). Here, R/B is 0.33, LRpos is 0.6/0.3 or 2, and LRneg is 0.4/0.7 or 0.57, so TestT-O is 0.33/2 or 0.17 and TestRxT-O is 0.33/0.57 or 0.58, which correspond to probabilities of 14% and 37%, as above.

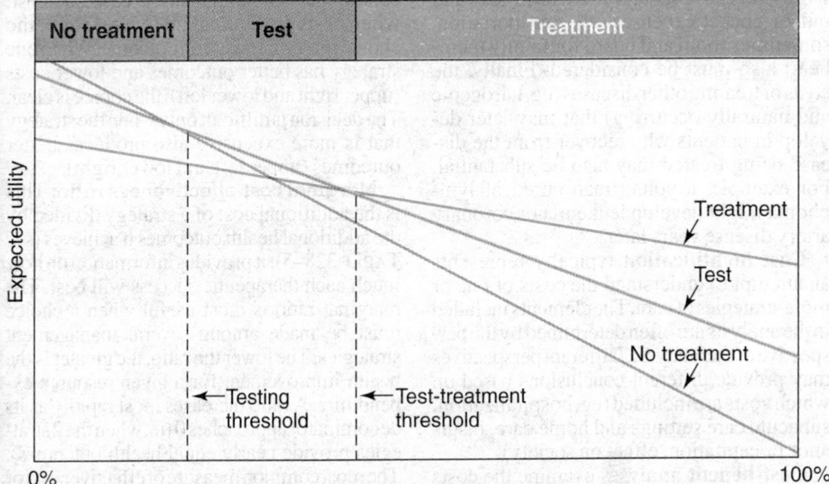

Fig. 328–4. One-way sensitivity analysis of testing threshold tree. In deciding whether to treat, test, or withhold treatment, the top panel illustrates strategic regions according to the probability of disease (the abscissa). The ordinate represents the expected utility of each strategy. If the probability of disease is lower than the testing threshold, treatment should be withheld; if the probability of disease is higher than the test-treatment threshold, treatment should be given. If the probability of disease falls between the 2 thresholds, further testing is indicated.

In cases in which the test itself poses risk, the numerator of the equation for TestT is increased by the risk of the test, and the numerator of the equation for the TestRxT is decreased by the risk of the test; both are measured on the same scale used to express the benefit and risk of treatment. Thus, the effect of decreasing a test's sensitivity and specificity or increasing its risk is to narrow the range of probabilities of disease at which testing is the best strategy. Improving the test's ability to discriminate or decreasing its risk will broaden the range of probabilities over which testing is the best strategy.

NUMBER NEEDED TO TREAT OR HARM

To gain a rapid picture of the benefit (B) or harm of a given treatment, it is sometimes useful to calculate the number of people that would need to be treated to save or lose one life. That number is simply the reciprocal of the difference in absolute (not relative) risk (R). Considering again the example of thrombolytic therapy for an acute MI, the absolute risk difference is 12% – 9%, or 3% (B), so the number needed to treat (NNT) is 1/0.03 or 33. In the setting of an acute MI, one would need to treat 33 patients with thrombolytic therapy to save one life. On the other hand, the absolute risk difference for an intracranial hemorrhage is 1% (R), so the number needed to harm (NNH) is 1/0.01 or 100. One would need to give 100 patients thrombolytic therapy to cause one fatal intracranial hemorrhage. These simple calculations do not weigh the relative value of the benefit and the harm, but the NNT and the NNH can provide a useful snapshot of benefits and risks.

ECONOMIC ANALYSES

Given limited societal and personal resources and restrictions under health insurance, cost considerations have become more relevant in clinical decision making. Limited resources should not be wasted. For example, when a screening test is used to identify patients with a disease that occurs at a low prevalence (eg, ovarian cancer), the costs (and perhaps the risks) of pursuing positive results that turn out to be false positives can exceed the costs of evaluating and treating patients who actually have the disease. From a societal perspective, costs such as time lost from work (for patients and their families) and out-of-pocket expenses (eg, transportation, sometimes room and board for family members) also must be considered. Finally, the costs of treating other diseases (eg, iatrogenic and naturally occurring) that may later develop in patients who recover from the disease being treated may also be substantial. For example, a young man cured of lymphoma might develop leukemia or coronary artery disease years later.

Cost identification typically represents an attempt to understand the costs of one or more strategies of care. The elements included in the analysis are often determined by the perspective of the analysis. Different perspectives may provide different conclusions based on which costs are included (eg, hospitalization, subacute care settings and home care, insurance or capitation, effect on society).

Cost-benefit analyses examine the costs and health benefits of management on an economic scale, often translating health benefits into perceived dollar equivalents. Such analyses can determine whether a given strategy saves resources or requires the net expenditure of resources. In the latter cases, such analyses do not indicate whether the expenditures are worthwhile. The magnitude of the gain or loss often depends on the number of people considered and how long they are included in the analysis and on assumptions about the economic value of improved health.

Cost-effectiveness analyses track medical costs and health outcomes separately. Both outcome measures can be strongly affected by the perspective and duration of the analysis and by the underlying assumptions made about the analysis. Comparing the costs and health outcomes of 2 management strategies results in 1 of 9 pairings (see TABLE 328–4). When health outcomes are equivalent (center column), the choice should be based on cost; when costs are equivalent (center row), the choice should be based on outcome. When one strategy has better outcomes and lower costs (upper right and lower left), the choice is clear. The decision is difficult only when the strategy that is more expensive also produces better outcomes (upper left and lower right).

Marginal cost-effectiveness ratio: This is the additional cost of a strategy divided by the additional health outcomes it achieves (see TABLE 328–5); it provides information on how much each therapeutic success will cost. The marginal ratio is most useful when a choice must be made among several management strategies. The lower the ratio, the greater is the health improvement for a given resource expenditure. A ratio increases most rapidly as its denominator approaches 0 (ie, when the 2 strategies provide nearly equal health outcomes). The most common measure of effectiveness for policy analyses is the quality-adjusted life year, making the units of the corresponding marginal cost-effectiveness ratio additional dollars spent per quality-adjusted life year gained. However, the marginal cost-effectiveness ratio has been criticized because elderly patients or patients with life-limiting comorbidities have a smaller potential gain in survival from a treatment and therefore have a higher or less advantageous cost-effectiveness ratio. A marginal cost-effectiveness ratio can be calculated (see TABLE 328–5) by first ordering the strategies by increasing cost (column B), associating each with effectiveness (column C), calculating the marginal cost (column D) and marginal effectiveness (column E), and, finally, calculating the marginal ratio (column F).

For example, consider no antiarrhythmic therapy vs an implantable cardioverter defibrillator (ICD) for patients who have survived several months after an acute anterior MI and

TABLE 328–4. COST-EFFECTIVENESS COMPARISON OF MANAGEMENT STRATEGIES A AND B

	HEALTH OUTCOME		
COST	A > B	A = B	A < B
A > B	Calculate marginal cost-effectiveness ratio*	B less expensive: choose B	B dominates A: choose B
A = B	A better outcome: choose A	Makes no difference	B better outcome: choose B
A < B	A dominates B: choose A	A less expensive: choose A	Calculate marginal cost-effectiveness ratio*

*See TABLE 328–5.

TABLE 328-5. CALCULATING A MARGINAL COST-EFFECTIVENESS RATIO

A STRATEGY	B COST ($)	C EFFECTIVENESS (QALY)	D MARGINAL COST ($)	E MARGINAL EFFECTIVENESS (QALY)	F MARGINAL COST-EFFECTIVENESS RATIO ($/QALY)
		ANALYSIS 1 (2 STRATEGIES)			
No antiarrhythmic therapy	78,300	7.42			
ICD	131,400	7.87	53,100	0.45	118,000
		ANALYSIS 2 (3 STRATEGIES)			
No antiarrhythmic therapy	78,300	7.42			
Amiodarone	96,800	7.69	18,500	0.27	68,519
ICD	131,400	7.87	34,600	0.18	192,222

QALY = quality-adjusted life year; ICD = implantable cardioverter defibrillator.

who have a mildly depressed ejection fraction (between 0.3 and 0.4). Using a prophylactic ICD increases life expectancy but at an additional cost of $53,100, based on the cost of the device and professional fees; initial hospitalization; and ongoing therapy, including physician visits, laboratory tests, drugs, re-hospitalizations for ICD-related complications, and replacement of ICD generator or leads. Prophylactic ICD enhances survival at a cost of $118,000 per quality-adjusted life year compared to no antiarrhythmic therapy (see TABLE 328-5, Analysis 1).

Now assume a 3rd strategy, prophylactic amiodarone therapy, is available. It is less expensive but also less effective than ICD. The effect of adding the 3rd intermediate strategy is noteworthy (see TABLE 328-5, Analysis 2): the marginal cost-effectiveness ratio of amiodarone is lower ($68,519 per quality-adjusted life year gained) than that for an ICD calculated above, but the existence of an intermediate cost strategy with partial effectiveness increases ICD's marginal cost-effectiveness ratio from $118,000 to $192,222 per quality-adjusted life year gained. This analysis would suggest that an expensive therapy such as an ICD be used selectively in subpopulations expected to reap the greatest benefit.

329 PRINCIPLES OF RADIOLOGIC IMAGING

COMPUTED TOMOGRAPHY

CT uses an x-ray tube–detector assembly that rotates around the patient to obtain multiple point images of specific depth (tomograms), which are digitized and transformed into cross-sectional images. CT provides 2- and 3-dimensional information not available from plain radiography and with much higher contrast resolution. As a result, CT has become the standard for imaging most intracranial, head and neck, intrathoracic, and intra-abdominal structures.

Early CT scanners used a single x-ray detector, and the patient moved through the scanner incrementally, pausing for each scan.

This method has been largely replaced by helical CT: The patient continuously moves through the scanner, which continuously rotates and takes images. Helical CT greatly reduces imaging time and slice thickness. Use of multidetector scanners (4 to 64 rows of x-ray detectors) further reduces imaging time and provides slice thickness of < 1 mm.

With this amount of imaging data, images can be reconstructed in almost any plane (as is done in MRI) and can be used to construct 3-dimensional images while maintaining diagnostic image resolution. Clinical applications include CT angiography (eg, in evaluation for pulmonary embolism) and cardiac imaging (eg, coronary angiography, evaluation for coronary artery calcification). Electron-beam CT, another type of fast CT, can also be used to evaluate coronary artery calcification.

CT images may be obtained with or without contrast. Noncontrast CT can detect acute hemorrhage (which appears bright white) and characterize bone fractures. Contrast CT uses IV or oral contrast or both. IV contrast, similar to that used in plain radiography, is used to image tumors, infection, inflammation, and trauma in soft tissues and to assess the vascular system, as in suspected cases of pulmonary embolism, aortic aneurysm, or aortic dissection. Excretion of contrast via the kidneys allows evaluation of the GU system. For contrast reactions and their treatment, see p. 2718.

Oral contrast is used for abdominal imaging; it helps distinguish intestinal from surrounding structures. Standard oral contrast is barium-based, but iodine-based contrast can be used when intestinal perforation is suspected (eg, in trauma); low-osmolar contrast should be used when risk of aspiration is high.

Radiation exposure is an important consideration when CT is used. The radiation dose from typical abdominal CT is 200 to 300 times that from a typical chest x-ray. CT now accounts for most man-made radiation exposure in the general population and for > ⅔ of overall medical radiation exposure. This degree of exposure is not trivial, and lifetime radiation risk for children undergoing CT is predicted to be much higher than that for adults. Therefore, for each patient, the benefit of each CT examination must be weighed carefully against the risks.

MAGNETIC RESONANCE IMAGING

MRI produces images by using a magnetic field to induce changes in proton spin within tissues. Normally, the magnetic axes of multiple protons within tissues are randomly aligned. When surrounded by a strong magnetic field, as in an MRI machine, the magnetic axes align along the field. Application of a radiofrequency pulse causes the axes of all protons to momentarily align against the field in a high-energy state; some protons then relax back to their baseline state within the magnetic field. The magnitude and rate of energy release that occurs with return to baseline alignment (T1 relaxation) and with the wobbling (precession) of protons during the process (T2 relaxation) are recorded as spatially localized signal intensities by a coil (antenna). These intensities are used to produce images. The relative signal intensity (brightness) of tissues on an MR image is determined by multiple factors, including the radiofrequency pulse and gradient waveforms used to obtain the image, intrinsic T1 and T2 tissue characteristics, and tissue proton density.

Pulse sequences are computer programs that control the radiofrequency pulse and gradient waveforms, which determine how an image is weighted and how various tissues appear. Images can be T1-weighted, T2-weighted, or proton density–weighted. For example, fat appears bright (high signal intensity) on T1-weighted images and relatively dark (low signal intensity) on T2-weighted images; water and fluids appear as intermediate signal intensity on T1-weighted images and bright on T2-weighted images. T1-weighted images optimally show normal soft-tissue anatomy (fat planes are well seen as high signal intensity) and fat (eg, to confirm a fat-containing mass). T2-weighted images optimally show fluid and pathology (eg, tumors, inflammation, trauma). In practice, T1- and T2-weighted images provide complementary information, so both are important for characterizing pathology.

Contrast may be used to highlight vascular structures (magnetic resonance angiography) and to help characterize inflammation and tumors. The most commonly used agents are gadolinium derivatives, which have magnetic properties that affect proton relaxation times. Gadolinium agents can cause headache, nausea, pain and sensation of cold at the injection site, taste distortion, dizziness, vasodilation, and reduced threshold for seizures; serious contrast reactions are rare and much less common than those with iodinated contrast agents.

MRI is preferred to CT when soft-tissue contrast resolution is important—eg, to evaluate intracranial, spinal, or spinal cord abnormalities or to evaluate suspected musculoskeletal tumors, inflammation, trauma, or internal joint derangement (imaging of intra-articular structures may include injection of a gadolinium agent into a joint). MRI also helps in evaluation of hepatic abnormalities (eg, tumors) and female reproductive organs.

The primary relative contraindication to MRI is the presence of implanted material that can be affected by powerful magnetic fields. These materials include ferromagnetic metal (containing iron), magnetically activated or electronically controlled medical devices (eg, pacemakers, implantable cardioverter defibrillators, cochlear implants), and nonferromagnetic metal electronically conductive wires or materials (eg, pacemaker wires, certain pulmonary artery catheters). Ferromagnetic material may be displaced by the strong magnetic field and injure a nearby organ; displacement is more likely if the material has been present < 6 wk (before scar tissue forms). Ferromagnetic material can also cause imaging artifacts. Magnetically activated medical devices may malfunction. In conductive materials, magnetic fields may induce current, which, in turn, may produce heat. The MRI compatibility of a device or object may be specific to the type of device, components, or manufacturer (see www.mrisafety.com); testing is usually required. Also, MRI machines of different magnetic field strengths have different effects on materials, so safety in one machine does not ensure safety in another.

The MRI magnetic field is very strong and always on. Thus, a ferromagnetic object (eg, an oxygen tank, some IV poles) at the entrance of the scanning room may be pulled into the magnet bore at high velocity; a patient may be injured, and separating the object from the magnet may be impossible.

The MRI machine is a tight, enclosed space and can trigger claustrophobia even in patients without preexisting phobias or anxiety. Also, some obese patients do not fit on the table or within the machine. Premedication with an anxiolytic (eg, alprazolam or lorazepam 1 to 2 mg po) 15 to 30 min before scanning is effective for most anxious patients.

Several unique MRI techniques are used for specific indications.

Gradient echo is a pulse sequence used for fast imaging (eg, magnetic resonance angiography). Moving blood and CSF generate strong signals.

Echo planar imaging is an ultrafast technique used for diffusion, perfusion, and functional imaging of the brain.

PLAIN RADIOGRAPHY

In plain radiography, an x-ray beam is generated and passed through a patient to a piece of film or a detector that registers the amount of radiation received, producing an image. Soft tissues differ in ability to attenuate x-ray photons (density); as density increases, the corresponding section of the image appears whiter (more radiopaque). The range of densities, from most to least dense, is represented by metal (white [radiopaque]), bone cortex (less white), fat (gray), muscle and fluid (much darker gray), and air or gas (black [radiolucent]).

Radiography is typically the first imaging method indicated to evaluate the extremities, chest, or abdomen because these areas have important structures with densities that may differ from those of adjacent tissues. Thus, radiography is a 1st-line test for detecting fractures (bone is well seen because it is adjacent to gray soft tissues), pneumonia (consolidation of soft tissue and inflammatory exudate are well seen when surrounded by air), and intestinal obstruction (dilated, air-filled loops of intestine are well seen because density of air differs from that of surrounding soft tissue).

When the density of adjacent tissues is similar, radiopaque contrast (see p. 2718) is often added to one tissue or structure to differentiate it from its surroundings. Structures typically requiring addition of contrast to enhance their visibility include blood vessels and the lumina of the GI tract, biliary system, and GU system. Gas may be used to distend the lower GI tract and make it visible.

Fluoroscopy is similar to radiography except it involves a continuous x-ray beam, which makes moving structures or objects visible. It is most often used with contrast agents (eg, in swallowing studies or coronary artery catheterization) or during medical procedures to identify placement of a lead, catheter, or needle (eg, in electrophysiologic testing or percutaneous coronary interventions).

POSITRON EMISSION TOMOGRAPHY

PET uses compounds containing radionuclides that decay by releasing a positron (β+), the antimatter equivalent of an electron. The released positron combines with an electron and produces 2 photons whose paths are 180° apart. Ring detector systems encircling the positron-emitting source simultaneously detect the 2 photons to localize the source. By incorporating positron-emitting radionuclides into metabolically active compounds, PET can provide information about tissue function as well as structure.

Fluorine-18 [^{18}F]–labeled deoxyglucose (FDG) is used most commonly in clinical PET imaging. FDG is an analog of glucose, and its uptake is proportional to glucose metabolic rates. Relative glucose metabolic rate is expressed as the standardized uptake value (SUV) and calculated by dividing the uptake by the injected dose divided by the patient's body weight. Because the half-life of FDG is short (110 min), rapid shipment must be arranged with the manufacturer, who requires a cyclotron to produce it.

Indications for PET include testing for myocardial hibernation in patients considered for coronary artery bypass graft surgery or heart transplantation and testing to distinguish metastasis from necrosis and fibrosis in the enlarged lymph nodes of cancer patients. PET is also used to evaluate pulmonary nodules and determine whether they are metabolically active and to evaluate lung cancer, colorectal cancer, esophageal cancer, head and neck cancer, lymphoma, and melanoma. CT can be combined with PET to correlate morphologic and functional data.

RADIOGRAPHIC CONTRAST AND CONTRAST REACTIONS

Most contrast used in radiography and fluoroscopy is iodine-based; iodine attenuates x-rays and is radiopaque, providing excellent contrast against soft-tissue backgrounds. Contrast agents may be ionic (high osmolar) or nonionic. Ionic contrast agents should not be used for myelography or in injections that may enter the spinal canal (because neurotoxic effects are a risk) or the bronchial tree (because pulmonary edema is a risk). Nonionic contrast agents may be low osmolar (which is still hyperosmolar relative to blood) or iso-osmolar. Nonionic low-osmolar contrast agents are now routinely used at many institutions because they cause fewer contrast-related problems, such as allergic-type reactions and contrast nephropathy (renal damage after IV contrast administration—for full discussion, including treatment and prevention, see p. 2016).

Allergic-type contrast reactions: These reactions may be mild (eg, nausea, flushing, itching); moderate (eg, urticaria, vomiting, chills and rigors); or severe (eg, anaphylactoid reactions, bronchospasm, laryngeal edema, hypotension, tachycardia or bradycardia, cardiopulmonary arrest, seizures), potentially resulting in death. The mechanism is unknown; risk factors include a previous allergic-type reaction, asthma, and other allergies.

Treatment begins with cessation of contrast infusion. Mild and moderate reactions typically respond to diphenhydramine 25 to 50 mg IV. Treatment of severe reactions depends on the type of reaction and may include leg elevation, oxygen, epinephrine, IV fluids, and possibly atropine (for bradycardia).

If patients are at risk of contrast reactions, imaging methods that do not require iodine-based contrast should be used. If contrast must be used, a nonionic agent should be used, and patients should be premedicated with prednisone (50 mg po 13 h, 7 h, and 1 h before injection of contrast) and diphenhydramine (50 mg po or IM 1 h before the injection). Patients who require imaging urgently can be given hydrocortisone 200 mg IV q 4 h until imaging is completed plus diphenhydramine (as above).

RADIONUCLIDE SCANNING

A radionuclide is an unstable isotope that becomes more stable by releasing energy as radiation (called nuclear decay). This radiation can include particulate emission (see Positron Emission Tomography on p. 2717) or γ-ray photons. Radiation produced by radionuclides may be used in imaging and in specific situations to treat disorders (eg, thyroid disorders).

A radionuclide can also be combined with different stable compounds to form a radiopharmaceutical that localizes to a particular anatomic or diseased structure. For example, a radionuclide combined with a diphosphonate is used to image the skeleton and check for bone metastasis or infection; radionuclide-labeled WBCs are used to identify inflammation; and labeled RBCs are used to localize lower GI bleeding. Labeled sulfur colloid is taken up by the liver, spleen, and bone marrow. Labeled iminodiacetic acid derivatives are used to image the biliary system and check for biliary obstruction and gallbladder disorders. Other clinical nuclear medicine techniques are used to image the cerebrovascular system, thyroid gland, cardiovascular system, respiratory system, GU system, and tumors.

Various types of cameras are used. An Anger (gamma) camera uses a crystal to convert photons emitted by the radionuclide into an image. Whole-body cameras are used for bone scans; portable cameras are also available. Single-photon emission computed tomography (SPECT) imaging uses a rotating camera and computer algorithms to produce images that allow 3-dimensional localization of radionuclide uptake, similar to a CT image.

ULTRASONOGRAPHY

Ultrasonography uses high-frequency sound waves generated by electrical stimulation of a piezoelectric crystal to image soft tissues. A transducer sends and receives sound waves; scattering, refraction, and attenuation of the waves by body structures influence the intensity of the reflected waves, which are converted back into electrical signals. This information can be displayed in several ways.

A-mode ultrasonography is the simplest display mode; electrical signals are recorded as spikes. The vertical axis of the display shows the echo amplitude, and the horizontal axis shows depth. This type of ultrasonography is used for ophthalmologic scanning.

B-mode (gray-scale) ultrasonography is the type most often used in diagnostic imaging; electrical signals are displayed as a 2-dimensional image. B-mode is commonly used to evaluate the developing fetus and multiple organs including the liver, spleen, kidneys, thyroid gland, testes, breasts, and prostate gland. Advantages of B-mode ultrasonography over CT or MRI include greater portability, lower cost, improved accessibility, and, compared with CT, lack of ionizing radiation.

M-mode ultrasonography is used to image moving structures; electrical signals reflected by the moving structures are converted into waves displayed continuously across a longitudinal axis. M-mode is used primarily for assessment of fetal heartbeat and in cardiac imaging, most notably of valvular disorders.

Doppler ultrasonography is used to assess blood flow. Changes in frequency of sound waves reflected from the moving source are converted into information about blood flow direction and velocity; the information can be displayed graphically as a spectral waveform or as a cross-sectional image with color indicating velocity. By convention, red indicates flow toward and blue indicates flow away from the transducer.

Duplex ultrasonography combines gray-scale (2-dimensional) imaging and Doppler techniques.

330 COMPLEMENTARY AND ALTERNATIVE MEDICINE

(See also Ch. 331 on p. 2724.)

Complementary and alternative medicine (CAM) includes various healing approaches and therapies that originate from around the world and that are not based on conventional Western medicine. These therapies are called alternative medicine when they are used alone and complementary medicine when they are used with conventional medicine. Integrative medicine refers to the use of all appropriate therapeutic approaches (conventional and alternative) in a framework that focuses on the whole person and reaffirms the relationship between health care practitioner and patient. For simplicity, the term alternative medicine is used in the rest of this chapter.

Alternative medicine includes therapies and health care practices not widely taught in most medical schools; however, many such practices are popular, and some are used in hospitals and reimbursed by insurance companies. An increasing number of patients in Western countries are exploring alternative medicine. In the US in 2002, 36% of people ≥ 18 yr used some form of alternative medicine; when prayer specifically for health reasons is included as part of alternative medicine, the percentage increases to 62%.

Although the distinction between conventional and alternative medicine is not always easy to determine, a basic philosophic difference exists. Conventional medicine generally defines health as the absence of disease; disease is usually thought to result from isolated factors (eg, pathogens, biochemical imbalances), and treatment often involves drugs or surgery. Alternative medicine often defines health as a balance of body systems—physical, emotional, and spiritual—involving the whole patient; ie, the approach is holistic. Disease is thought to result from disharmony and imbalances between body systems. Theories are based more on energy pathways and function than on anatomy and structural organization. Treatment often involves strengthening the body's own defenses and restoring these balances and energy flows.

Patients are most likely to seek alternative medicine for conditions such as chronic low back pain, stress, migraine headaches, menopausal symptoms, cancer, and arthritis. Some patients seek alternative medicine when conventional medicine offers little hope, especially at the end of life.

In 1992, the Office of Alternative Medicine within the National Institutes of Health (NIH) was formed to research the effectiveness and safety of alternative therapies. In 1999, this office became the National Center for Complementary and Alternative Medicine (NCCAM; see www.nccam.nih.gov/).

Some alternative therapies have been shown to be effective for specific conditions. However, these therapies are often applied more broadly without evidence of effectiveness. Some alternative therapies have been proved ineffective, and their use cannot be advocated. Others cannot be explained by modern scientific principles. Most forms of alternative medicine have not been thoroughly evaluated; however, lack of proof is not equivalent to proven ineffectiveness.

The safety record of many complementary therapies is good. However, some alternative therapies have the potential for harm. Using an alternative approach instead of a proven conventional approach has the greatest risk but is rarely done.

Because the FDA regulates medicinal herbs and drugs differently, manufacturers of medicinal herb products do not have to prove safety despite the fact that many herbs contain substances with significant pharmacologic activity. Alternative therapies that involve manipulation of the body or other nonchemical interventions can also cause harm. For most types of alternative medicine, potential harm has not been established or excluded; however, in some cases, potential harm has been shown but is widely discounted by proponents.

Alternative medicine can be categorized in many ways; each relies on underlying theories about the origins of disease or factors that contribute to disease. Five categories of alternative medicine are generally recognized (see TABLE 330–1): alternative medical systems, mind-body techniques, biologically based treatments, manipulative and body-based methods, and energy therapies. The name of many therapies only partially describes their components.

ALTERNATIVE MEDICAL SYSTEMS

Alternative medical systems are complete systems of diagnosis and practice.

Ayurveda: Ayurveda, the traditional medical system of India, originated > 4000 yr ago. It is based on the theory that disease results from an imbalance of the body's life force (prana). The balance of prana is determined by equilibrium of the 3 bodily qualities (doshas): vata, pitta, and kapha. Most people have a dominant dosha; the specific balance is unique to each person. Ayurveda uses herbs, massage, yoga, and therapeutic elimination—typically with enemas, oil massages, or nasal lavage—to restore balance within the body and with nature.

Homeopathy: Developed in Germany in the late 1700s, homeopathy is based on the principle that like cures like. A substance that, when given in large doses, causes a set of symptoms is believed to cure the same symptoms when it is given in minute doses.

Remedies used in homeopathy are derived from naturally occurring substances, such as plant extracts and minerals. Extremely low concentrations are prepared in a specific way. The more dilute the homeopathic medicine, the stronger it is considered to be.

Traditional scientists can find no scientific explanation for how the diluted remedies used in homeopathy could cure disease. Some solutions are so dilute that they con-

TABLE 330–1. TYPES OF COMPLEMENTARY AND ALTERNATIVE MEDICINE

SELECTED THERAPIES	DESCRIPTION
Alternative medical systems	
Ayurveda	The traditional medical system of India, originating > 4000 yr ago, uses herbs, massage, yoga, and therapeutic elimination to restore balance within the body and with nature. It is based on balancing the 3 bodily qualities (doshas): vata, pitta, and kapha
Homeopathy	Developed in Germany during the late 1700s, homeopathy is a system of medicine based on the law of similars: A substance that, when given in large doses, causes a set of symptoms can purportedly cure the same symptoms when it is given in minute doses
Naturopathy	Founded on the healing power of nature, this system uses a combination of therapies, including acupuncture, counseling, exercise therapy, herbal medicine, homeopathy, hydrotherapy, natural childbirth, nutrition, physical medicine, and stress management
Traditional Chinese medicine	Originating in China > 2000 yr ago, this system uses acupuncture, herbs, massage, and meditative exercise (qi gong) to restore balance within the body and with nature. It is based on the 8 principles of yin and yang, which manifest in the body as hot and cold, internal and external, and deficiency and excess
Mind-body techniques	
Biofeedback	Mechanical devices are used to provide information about physiologic signals (eg, BP, muscle activity) and to teach patients methods of regulating these processes through intention
Guided imagery	Mental images are used to promote relaxation or wellness or to promote healing of a particular condition (eg, cancer, psychologic trauma). The images can involve any of the senses and may be self-directed or guided by the practitioner
Hypnotherapy	Patients are put into a state of attentive and focused concentration. They become absorbed in the images presented by the hypnotherapist and can be relatively unaware, but not entirely unconscious, of their surroundings; they tend not to register experiences as a part of their conscious awareness
Meditation	Mediation is intentional self-regulation of attention or a systematic mental focus on particular aspects of inner or outer experience. Most meditation practices were developed in a religious or spiritual context; their ultimate goal was some type of spiritual growth, personal transformation, or transcendental experience. However, some practitioners suggest that as a health care intervention, meditation may be effective regardless of a person's cultural or religious background
Relaxation techniques	These techniques are specifically designed to elicit a psychophysiologic state of hypoarousal. They may be aimed at reducing sympathetic nervous system activity and BP, easing muscle tension, slowing metabolic processes, or altering brain wave activity
Biologically based treatments	
Diet therapies	Specialized dietary regimens (eg, Gerson therapy, Kelley regimen, macrobiotic diet, Ornish diet, Pritikin diet) are used to treat or prevent a specific disease (eg, cancer, cardiovascular disorders) or to generally promote health

Table continues on the following page.

TABLE 330–1. TYPES OF COMPLEMENTARY AND ALTERNATIVE MEDICINE—Continued

SELECTED THERAPIES	DESCRIPTION
Biologic therapies	Substances (eg, shark cartilage) or molecules (eg, *S*-adenylosyl-L-methionine [SAMe], glucosamine) naturally occurring in animals are used to treat disease
Herbalism	Plants are used to treat disease and promote health
Orthomolecular therapies	Molecules normally found in the body (eg, hormones, vitamins, nutrients) are used to treat disease and promote health
Manipulative and body-based methods	
Chiropractic	Chiropractic is based on the relationship between structure of the spine and function of the nervous system; bones and joints are manipulated to restore balance to the body
Massage	Tissues are manipulated to promote wellness and to reduce pain and stress
Postural reeducation	Movement and touch are used to help patients relearn healthy posture. Techniques include Alexander, Feldenkrais, and Trager. Therapies seek to release habitual, harmful ways of holding the body by focusing on awareness through movement
Reflexology	Manual pressure is applied to specific areas of the foot that theoretically correspond to different organs or systems of the body
Rolfing	The fascia are manipulated and stretched to reestablish healthy bone and muscle alignment
Energy therapies	
External qi gong	In this subset of Chinese medical qi gong practice, master healers use the energy of their own biofield to bring the patient's energy into balance
Magnets	Magnets are placed on the body to reduce pain
Pulsed electrical field	Injured body parts are placed in an induced electrical field to facilitate healing
Reiki	In this technique of Japanese origin, practitioners channel energy through their body and into a patient's body to promote healing
Therapeutic touch	This technique is often referred to as laying on of hands, even though actual touch is not required; it uses the therapist's healing energy to identify and repair imbalances in a patient's biofield

tain no molecules of the "active" ingredient. However, homeopathy has few risks; rarely, an allergic or toxic reaction occurs.

Naturopathy: This therapy began as a formal health care system in the US during the early 1900s. Founded on the healing power of nature, naturopathy emphasizes prevention and treatment of disease through a healthy lifestyle, treatment of the whole patient, and use of the body's natural healing abilities. This system also focuses on finding the cause of a disease rather than merely treating symptoms. Some of this system's principles are not that different from those of modern Western medicine.

Naturopathy uses a combination of therapies, including acupuncture, counseling, exercise therapy, herbal medicine, homeopathy, hydrotherapy, natural childbirth, nutrition, physical medicine, and guided imagery.

Traditional Chinese medicine: Originating > 2000 yr ago, traditional Chinese medicine is based on the theory that disease results from improper flow of the life force (qi). Qi is restored by balancing the opposing forces of yin and yang, which manifest in the body as heat and cold, external and internal, and deficiency and excess. Various practices (eg, acupuncture, herbal remedies, massage, meditation) are used to preserve and restore health.

Acupuncture, a therapy within traditional Chinese medicine, is one of the most widely accepted alternative therapies in the Western world. Specific points on the body are stimulated, usually by inserting thin needles into the skin and underlying tissues. Sometimes additional stimulation is added by using a very low voltage electrical current, by twisting the needle, or by warming the needle. Stimulating these specific points is believed to unblock the flow of qi along energy pathways (meridians) and thus restore balance between yin and yang. The procedure is not painful but may cause a tingling sensation. A variation of acupuncture, called acupressure, uses localized massage instead of needles to stimulate acupuncture points. Acupuncturists are licensed to practice after receiving 3000 h of training and passing a state board examination; some medical doctors, often pain specialists, perform acupuncture after about 300 h of training. Licensure varies by state. Research has shown that acupuncture releases various neurotransmitters (eg, endorphins) that act as natural painkillers. Reasonable evidence supports the effectiveness of acupuncture as a pain reliever, an antinauseant, and an antiemetic. However, acupuncture is ineffective for smoking cessation and weight loss. Adverse effects are rare if the procedure is done correctly. Worsening of symptoms (usually temporary) and fainting are the most common. Infection is extremely rare; most practitioners use disposable needles.

MIND-BODY TECHNIQUES

Mind-body techniques are based on the theory that mental and emotional factors influence physical health through a system of mainly neuronal and hormonal connections throughout the body. Behavioral, psychologic, social, and spiritual techniques are used to preserve health and to prevent or cure disease (see TABLE 330–1).

Because scientific evidence supporting the benefits of mind-body techniques is abundant, many of these approaches are now considered mainstream. Techniques such as biofeedback, guided imagery, hypnotherapy, meditation, and relaxation are used in the treatment of coronary artery disease, headaches, insomnia, and incontinence and as aids during childbirth. These techniques are also used to help patients cope with disease-related and treatment-related symptoms of cancer and to prepare patients for surgery. Use of mind-body techniques in patients with arthritis, asthma, hypertension, pain, or tinnitus has been less successful.

Biofeedback: For this technique, electronic devices are used to provide information to patients about biologic functions (eg, heart rate, BP, muscle activity). Patients can then use this information to relax, thereby lessening the effects of conditions such as pain, stress, insomnia, and headaches.

Hypnotherapy: This alternative therapy is derived from Western practice. Patients are put into an advanced state of relaxation. They become absorbed in the images presented by the hypnotherapist and are relatively unaware, but not entirely unconscious, of their surroundings and the experiences they are undergoing. Hypnosis is used to treat pain syndromes and conversion disorders and has been used with some success to manage smoking cessation and weight loss. Some patients learn to hypnotize themselves.

BIOLOGICALLY BASED TREATMENTS

Biologically based treatments use naturally occurring substances and include biologic and diet therapies, herbalism (see TABLE 330–1), and orthomolecular medicine.

Orthomolecular medicine: This therapy, also called megavitamin therapy, uses high-dose combinations of vitamins, minerals, and amino acids that normally occur in the body to treat specific conditions. Some of the more common orthomolecular treatments use shark cartilage to treat cancer, chelation therapy to remove toxic materials from the bloodstream and to treat cardiovascular disorders, and essential fatty acids and vitamins to treat attention-deficit hyperactivity disorder and other mental disorders.

MANIPULATIVE AND BODY-BASED METHODS

Manipulative and body-based methods include chiropractic, massage therapy, postural reeducation, reflexology, and rolfing (see TABLE 330–1).

Chiropractic: In chiropractic, the relationship between the structure of the spine and function of the nervous system is thought to be the key to maintaining or restoring health. The main method for achieving balance is spinal manipulation.

Chiropractic is often useful in treating low back pain, headaches, and nerve impingement syndromes. Generally, however, the effect of manipulation on conditions not directly related to the musculoskeletal system has not been established. Serious complications resulting from spinal manipulation (eg, low back pain, damage to cervical nerves, damage to arteries in the neck) are rare.

Massage therapy: Body tissues are manipulated to promote wellness and reduce pain and stress. The therapeutic value of massage for many musculoskeletal symptoms and stress is widely accepted. Massage has been shown to help relieve muscle soreness, pain due to back injuries, and fibromyalgia and to help relieve anxiety in cancer patients. Massage therapy is also effective in treating low birth weight infants, preventing injury to the mother's genitals during childbirth, relieving chronic constipation, and controlling asthma.

Reflexology, a variant of massage therapy, relies on manual pressure applied to specific areas of the foot; these areas are believed to correspond to different organs or body systems via meridians. Stimulation of these areas is believed to eliminate the blockage of energy responsible for pain or disease in the corresponding body part.

ENERGY THERAPIES

Energy therapies usually focus on energy fields thought to exist in and around the body (biofields). All energy therapies are based on the belief that a universal life force or subtle energy resides in and around the body.

Energy therapy may rely on magnetic (alternating- or direct-current) fields. Magnets, in particular, are a popular treatment for various musculoskeletal conditions, although multiple studies have shown no effectiveness, especially for pain relief, one of their most common applications.

Therapeutic touch, often referred to as laying on of hands, uses the therapist's healing energy to identify and repair imbalances in a patient's biofield. Reiki, which originated in Japan, is a similar technique; in Reiki, practitioners channel energy through their hands and into the patient's body to promote healing. Practitioners are thought to have special healing powers, which are required for these treatments.

331 DIETARY SUPPLEMENTS

(See also Ch. 330 on p. 2719.)

The Dietary Supplement Health Education Act (DSHEA) of 1994 defines a dietary supplement as any product (except tobacco)—in pill, capsule, tablet, or liquid form—containing a vitamin, mineral, herb, amino acid, or other known dietary substance that is intended as a supplement to the normal diet. The act requires that the product label identify the product as a dietary supplement and notify the consumer that the claims for the supplement have not been evaluated by the FDA; the label must also list each ingredient by name, quantity, and total weight and identify plant parts from which ingredients are derived (see the DSHEA at http://www.fda.gov/opacom/laws/dshea.html). Manufacturers are permitted to make claims about the product's structure and function (eg, good for urinary tract health) but cannot make or imply claims for the product as a drug or therapy (eg, treats UTIs).

Dietary supplements are the most commonly used of all complementary and alternative therapies, primarily because they are widely available and can be bought without consulting a professional health practitioner. Most patients who use dietary supplements assume that they are good for health generally, are safe and effective for treating specific conditions, or both, because such supplements are natural (ie, derived from plants or animals) and because some are supported by centuries of use in traditional systems of medicine. However, the FDA regulates dietary supplements differently from drugs. The FDA regulates only quality control and good manufacturing processes but does not ensure standardization of the active ingredients. They are slowly moving in this direction, however. Also, the FDA does not require manufacturers of dietary supplements to prove safety or efficacy (although supplements must have a history of safety). Most supplements have not been rigorously studied. For most, evidence suggesting safety or efficacy comes from traditional use, in vitro studies, certain case reports, and animal studies. However, a few supplements (eg, fish oil, chondroitin/glucosamine, saw palmetto) are now proven to be safe and useful complements to standard drugs. Evidence concerning the safety and efficacy of dietary supplements is increasing rapidly as more and more clinically based studies are being done. Information about such studies is available at the National Institutes of Health's National Center for Complementary and Alternative Medicine (NCCAM) web site (www.nccam.nih.gov/clinicaltrials/).

Lack of regulation and government monitoring also means that supplements are not monitored to ensure that they contain the ingredients or amount of active ingredient the manufacturer claims they contain. The supplement may have unlisted ingredients, which may be inert or harmful, or it may contain variable amounts of active ingredients, especially when whole herbs are ground or made into extracts. Consumers are at risk of getting less, more, or, in some cases, none of the active ingredient, if the active ingredient is even known. Most herbal products are mixtures of several substances, and which ingredient is the most active is not always known. Some supplements have been standardized and may include a designation of standardization on the label.

Additional areas of concern include use of dietary supplements instead of conventional drugs, stability of supplements (especially herbal products) once manufactured, toxicity in children and the elderly, and interactions between supplements and drugs. Most information about these concerns comes from sporadic individual reports of interactions (see TABLE 331–1) and some references.

Despite these concerns, many patients strongly believe in the benefits of supplements and continue to use them with or without a physician's involvement. Patients may not think to disclose or may wish to conceal their use of dietary supplements. For this reason, the outpatient history should periodically include explicit questions about past and new use of complementary and alternative therapies, including dietary supplements. Many physicians incorporate some supplement use into their practice; their reasons include proven benefit of the supplement, a desire to ensure that supplements are used safely by patients who will use supplements anyway, and the physician's belief that the supplements are safe and effective. There are few data to guide patient counseling regarding supplement safety. But some experts believe that the overall number of problems due to dietary supplements are rare compared with the overall number of doses taken and that the product, if correctly manufactured, is likely to be safe. As a result, these experts advise purchase of supplements from a well-known manufacturer, and many recommend buying supplements made in Germany because there they are regulated as drugs and thus oversight is stricter than in the US.

The following supplements are ones that are most popular, are effective, or have some questions about their safety. More complete information is available through the NCCAM web site (www.nccam.nih.gov/).

BLACK COHOSH

Black cohosh is a plant rhizome (underground stem) that can be ingested directly in powdered form or extracted into tablet or liquid form. The rhizome contains no phytoestrogens that can account for its purported estrogen-like effects, but it contains small amounts of anti-inflammatory compounds, including salicylic acid.

Claims: Black cohosh is said to be useful for menopausal symptoms (hot flushes, mood lability, tachycardia, vaginal dryness) and for arthralgias in RA or osteoarthritis.

Adverse effects: Headaches, dizziness, diaphoresis, and hypotension (if high doses are taken) may occur. Theoretically, black cohosh is contraindicated in patients with aspirin sensitivity.

CHAMOMILE

The flower of chamomile is dried and drunk as a tea or used topically as an extract.

TABLE 331–1. SOME POSSIBLE DIETARY SUPPLEMENT–DRUG INTERACTIONS*

DIETARY SUPPLEMENT	AFFECTED DRUGS	INTERACTION
Chamomile	Barbiturates and other sedatives	May intensify or prolong effects of sedatives because its volatile oils have additive effects
	Iron supplements	May reduce iron absorption via tannins in the plant
	Warfarin	May increase risk of bleeding because chamomile contains phytocoumarins, which may have additive effects
Echinacea	Drugs metabolized by cytochrome P-450 enzymes (eg, amiodarone, anabolic steroids, ketoconazole, methotrexate)	If taken with another these drugs, may increase risk of hepatotoxicity by slowing their metabolism
	Immunosuppressants (eg, corticosteroids, cyclosporine)	May lessen immunosuppressive effects via T-cell stimulation
Feverfew	Antimigraine drugs (eg, ergotamine, methysergide—see TABLE 216–2 on p. 1846)	May increase heart rate and BP because it has additive vasoconstrictive effects; may augment effects of methysergide
	Antiplatelet drugs	May increase risk of bleeding because feverfew inhibits platelet aggregation (has additive effects)
	Iron supplements	May reduce iron absorption via tannins in the plant
	NSAIDs (see p. 1771)	Feverfew's efficacy in preventing and managing migraine headaches is reduced by NSAIDs
	Warfarin	May increase risk of bleeding because warfarin may have additive effects
Garlic	Antihypertensives	May augment antihypertensive effect
	Antiplatelet drugs	May increase risk of bleeding because these drugs negate garlic's inhibition of platelet aggregation and fibrinolytic effects
	Protease inhibitors (eg, saquinavir)	Blood level of protease inhibitors reduced by garlic
	Warfarin	May increase risk of bleeding by augmenting warfarin's anticoagulant effects
Ginger	Antiplatelet drugs	May increase risk of bleeding by augmenting inhibition of platelet aggregation
	Warfarin	May increase risk of bleeding by augmenting warfarin's anticoagulant effects
Ginkgo	Anticonvulsants (eg, phenytoin)	May reduce efficacy of anticonvulsants because contaminants in ginkgo preparations may reduce anticonvulsant effects

TABLE 331–1. SOME POSSIBLE DIETARY SUPPLEMENT–DRUG INTERACTIONS*—Continued

DIETARY SUPPLEMENT	AFFECTED DRUGS	INTERACTION
	Aspirin and other NSAIDs	May increase risk of bleeding by augmenting inhibition of antiplatelet aggregation
	Warfarin	May increase risk of bleeding by augmenting warfarin's anticoagulant effects
Ginseng	Antihyperglycemic drugs (eg, glipizide)	May intensify effects of these drugs, causing hypoglycemia
	Aspirin and other NSAIDs	May increase risk of bleeding by augmenting inhibition of antiplatelet aggregation
	Corticosteroids	May intensify adverse effects of corticosteroids because ginseng has anti-inflammatory effects
	Digoxin	May increase digoxin levels
	Estrogens	May intensify adverse effects of estrogen
	MAOIs (eg, tranylcypromine)	Can cause headache, tremors, and manic episodes
	Warfarin	May increase risk of bleeding by augmenting warfarin's anticoagulant effects
Goldenseal	Warfarin and heparin	May oppose effects of warfarin and heparin, increasing risk of thromboembolism
Milk thistle	Antihyperglycemic drugs	May intensify effects of these drugs, causing hypoglycemia
	Indinavir	May interfere with metabolizing enzymes, lowering blood level of indinavir
Saw palmetto	Estrogens (eg, oral contraceptives)	May augment effects of these drugs
St. John's wort	Cyclosporine	May reduce blood level of cyclosporine, increasing risk of organ transplant rejection
	Digoxin	May reduce blood level of digoxin, making it less effective, with potentially dangerous results
	Iron supplements	May reduce iron absorption
	MAOIs	May augment effects of MAOIs, possibly causing very high BP requiring emergency treatment
	Non-nucleoside reverse transcriptase inhibitors	Increases metabolism of these drugs, reducing their efficacy
	Oral contraceptives	Increases metabolism of these drugs, reducing their efficacy
	Protease inhibitors	May reduce blood level of protease inhibitors, reducing their efficacy
	SSRIs (eg, fluoxetine, paroxetine, sertraline)	May augment effects of these drugs

Table continues on the following page.

TABLE 331–1. SOME POSSIBLE DIETARY SUPPLEMENT–DRUG INTERACTIONS*—Continued

DIETARY SUPPLEMENT	AFFECTED DRUGS	INTERACTION
	Tricyclic antidepressants	May augment effects of these drugs
	Warfarin	May reduce blood level of warfarin, increasing risk of thromboembolism
Valerian	Barbiturates	May intensify effects of barbiturates, causing excessive sedation

*Caution is required when dietary supplements are used because these products are not standardized and thus vary considerably and because information about their use is continually changing. The theoretical status of many published interactions does not obviate the need for cautious use. Before prescribing any drug, health care practitioners should ask patients whether they are taking dietary supplements and, if so, which ones. Practitioners must identify any potential adverse interactions of drugs and supplements taken by a patient, then determine appropriate drugs and dosages.

MAOIs = Monoamine oxidase inhibitors.

Claims: Chamomile tea is said to reduce inflammation and fever, to be a mild sedative, to relieve stomach cramps and indigestion, and to promote healing of gastric ulcers. Chamomile extract applied topically in a compress is said to soothe irritated skin.

Adverse effects: Chamomile is generally safe. It may interact with alcohol and sedatives (eg, barbiturates). Some people are allergic to pollen in chamomile products.

CHONDROITIN SULFATE

Chondroitin sulfate is a glycosaminoglycan, a natural component of cartilage. It is extracted from shark or cow cartilage or manufactured synthetically. It is frequently combined with glucosamine.

Claims: Chondroitin sulfate is used to treat osteoarthritis. Scientific evidence supports its use for reducing joint pain, improving joint mobility, and reducing doses of conventional anti-inflammatory drugs when it is taken for 6 to 24 mo. Effects over longer periods are unclear. Mechanism is unknown. Dose is 600 mg po once/day to 400 mg po tid.

Adverse effects: No serious effects have been reported.

CHROMIUM PICOLINATE

Chromium, a mineral, is required in small quantities for carbohydrate and fat metabolism. Dietary sources include carrots, potatoes, broccoli, whole grains, and molasses. Picolinate is a by-product of tryptophan that is paired with chromium in supplements because it is said to help the body absorb chromium more efficiently.

Claims: Chromium picolinate is said to promote weight loss, build muscle, reduce body fat, lower cholesterol and triglyceride levels, and enhance insulin function. Chromium is necessary for the action of insulin on cells. Some evidence supports its use in patients with diabetes, but not all patients respond; chromium is no substitute for standard lifestyle changes and drugs in the treatment of diabetes.

Adverse effects: Some evidence suggests that chromium picolinate damages chromosomes and may cause cancer. Some forms of chromium may contribute to GI irritation and ulcers.

COENZYME Q10

Coenzyme Q10 (ubiquinone) is an antioxidant that is also a cofactor for mitochondrial ATP generation.

Claims: Coenzyme Q10 is said to be useful because of its antioxidant effect and role in energy metabolism. Specific claims include an anticancer effect mediated by immune stimulation, decreased insulin requirements in patients with diabetes, slowed progression of Parkinson's disease, efficacy in treatment of heart failure, and protection against anthracycline cardiotoxicity.

Adverse effects: Coenzyme Q10 may decrease response to warfarin. There are case reports of GI symptoms (abdominal pain, nausea, and vomiting) and CNS symptoms (dizziness, photophobia, irritability, and headache).

CREATINE

Phosphocreatine is a compound stored in muscle; it donates phosphate to ADP and thereby rapidly replenishes ATP during anaerobic muscle contraction. It is synthesized endogenously in the liver from arginine, glycine, and methionine; dietary sources are milk, steak, and some fish.

Claims: Creatine is said to improve physical and athletic performance and to reduce fatigue. Some evidence suggests creatine is effective at increasing work performed in a short maximal effort (eg, sprinting, weightlifting). It has proven therapeutic use in muscle phosphorylase deficiency (glycogen storage disease type V [McArdle disease]) and gyrate atrophy of the choroid and retina; early data also suggest possible effects in Parkinson's disease and amyotrophic lateral sclerosis.

Adverse effects: Creatine may cause weight gain, possibly because of an increase in muscle mass, and spurious increases in serum creatinine levels. Minor GI symptoms, dehydration, electrolyte imbalance, and muscle cramps have been reported anecdotally.

DEHYDROEPIANDROSTERONE

Dehydroepiandrosterone (DHEA) is a steroid produced by the adrenal gland and is a precursor of estrogens and androgens. Effects on the body are similar to those of testosterone. DHEA can also be synthesized from precursors in the Mexican yam; this form is the most commonly available.

Claims: DHEA supplements are said to improve mood, energy, sense of well-being, and the ability to function well under stress. They are also said to improve athletic performance, stimulate the immune system, deepen nightly sleep, lower cholesterol levels, decrease body fat, build muscles, reverse aging, improve brain function in patients with Alzheimer's disease, and increase libido.

Adverse effects: Adverse effects are unknown. There are theoretical risks of gynecomastia in men, hirsutism in women, and stimulation of prostate and breast cancer. There is a case report of mania.

ECHINACEA

Echinacea, a North American wildflower, contains a variety of biologically active substances.

Claims: Echinacea is said to stimulate the immune system. When taken at the start of a cold, it is said to shorten the duration of cold symptoms. Well-designed studies have not supported this effect. Topical preparations are used to promote wound healing.

Adverse effects: Most adverse effects are mild and transitory; they include dizziness, fatigue, headache, and GI symptoms. No other adverse effects are known. Theoretically, echinacea is contraindicated in patients with autoimmune disorders, multiple sclerosis, AIDS, TB, and organ transplants because it may stimulate T cells. Echinacea inhibits some cytochrome P-450 enzymes and stimulates others; it can therefore potentially interact with drugs metabolized by the same enzymes (eg, anabolic steroids, azole antifungals, methotrexate). Allergic reactions are possible in patients with pollen allergies.

FEVERFEW

Feverfew is a bushy perennial herb. Parthenolide and glycosides are thought to be the components responsible for its purported anti-inflammatory effects and relaxant effects on smooth muscle.

Claims: Feverfew is thought to be effective in the prevention of migraine headaches. It is also said to be useful for relieving menstrual pain, asthma, and arthritis. In vitro, feverfew inhibits platelet aggregation.

Adverse effects: Mouth ulcers, contact dermatitis, dysgeusia, and mild GI symptoms may occur. Abrupt discontinuation may worsen migraines and cause nervousness and insomnia. Feverfew is contraindicated in pregnant women; theoretically, it is contraindicated in patients taking antimigraine drugs, iron supplements, NSAIDs, antiplatelet drugs, or warfarin.

FISH OIL

Fish oil may be extracted directly or concentrated and put in capsule form. Active ingredients are ω-3 fatty acids (eicosapentaenoic acid [EPA] and docosahexaenoic acid [DHA]).

Claims: Fish oil is used for prevention and treatment of atherosclerotic cardiovascular disease. Strong scientific evidence suggests that EPA/DHA 800 to 1500 mg/day reduces risk of MI and death due to arrhythmia in patients who have preexisting coronary artery disease and are taking conventional drugs. It also reduces triglycerides in a dose-dependent way (25 to 40% with EPA/DHA 4 g/day) and slightly lowers BP (2 to 4 mm Hg with EPA/DHA > 3 g/day). Mechanisms are probably multiple but unknown. Benefits are suspected but not yet proven for primary prevention of atherosclerotic cardiovascular disease, treatment of RA, and prevention of cyclosporine nephrotoxicity.

Adverse effects: Fishy eructation, nausea, and diarrhea may occur. Risk of bleeding increases with EPA/DHA > 3 g/day. Concerns about mercury contamination are not substantiated in laboratory testing.

GARLIC

Garlic bulbs are extracted and made into tablet form; the major active ingredient is allicin, an amino acid by-product.

Claims: Garlic is said to have favorable effects on several cardiac risk factors, including reduction of BP and serum lipid and glucose levels; garlic inhibits platelets in vitro. Garlic is also thought to protect against laryngeal, gastric, colorectal, and endometrial cancer and adenomatous colorectal polyps.

Adverse effects: Breath and body smell and nausea may occur; high doses may cause burning in the mouth, esophagus, and stomach. Theoretically, garlic is contraindicated in patients who have bleeding diatheses or who take antihypertensives, antiplatelet drugs, or warfarin; garlic can reduce serum saquinavir levels.

GINGER

Ginger root is extracted and made into tablet form; active ingredients include gingerols (which give ginger its flavor and odor) and shogaols.

Claims: Ginger is said to be an effective antiemetic, especially for nausea due to motion sickness or pregnancy, and to relieve intestinal cramps. Ginger is also used as an anti-inflammatory and analgesic. It may have antibacterial properties and antiplatelet effects in vitro, but data are inconsistent.

Adverse effects: Nausea, dyspepsia, and dysgeusia are possible. Theoretically, ginger is contraindicated in patients who have bleeding diatheses or who take antiplatelet drugs or warfarin.

GINKGO

Ginkgo (*Ginkgo biloba*) is prepared from leaves of the ginkgo tree; active ingredients are believed to be terpene ginkgolides and flavonoids. Cooked ginkgo seeds are eaten in Asia and are available in Asian food shops in the US; because the seeds do not contain ginkgolides and flavonoids, they do not have therapeutic effects.

Claims: Strong scientific evidence supports use of ginkgo for symptomatic relief of claudication, although exercise and cilostazol may be more effective. Ginkgo may be useful for some deficits in patients with dementia, although data are conflicting and any real effect is likely to be modest. Further scientific substantiation is required for claims that ginkgo is effective for treating vertigo, headache, tinnitus, depression, premenstrual dysphoria, and erectile and other sexual dysfunction and that it can prevent memory loss.

Adverse effects: Nausea, dyspepsia, headache, dizziness, and heart palpitations may occur. Ginkgo may interact with aspirin, other NSAIDs (see p. 1771), and warfarin and may reduce the efficacy of anticonvulsants. Contact with the fruit pulp, which may be encountered under female ginkgo trees (planted for ornamental purposes), can cause severe dermatitis.

GINSENG

Ginseng is a family of plants. Dietary supplements are derived from American or Asian ginseng; Siberian ginseng does not contain the ingredients believed to be active in the 2 forms used in supplements. Ginseng can be taken as fresh or dried roots, extracts, solutions, capsules, tablets, sodas, and teas or used as cosmetics. Active ingredients in American ginseng are panaxosides (saponin glycosides). Active ingredients in Asian ginseng are ginsenosides (triterpenoid glycosides).

Claims: Ginseng is said to enhance physical (including sexual) and mental performance and to have adaptogenic effects (eg, to increase energy and resistance to the harmful effects of stress and aging). Other claims include reduction in plasma glucose levels; increases in high density lipoprotein (HDL), Hb, and protein levels; stimulation of the immune system; and anticancer, cardiotonic, endocrine, CNS, and estrogenic effects.

Adverse effects: Nervousness and excitability may occur but decrease after the first few days. Ability to concentrate may decrease, and plasma glucose may become abnormally low (causing hypoglycemia). Because ginseng has an estrogen-like effect, women who are pregnant or breastfeeding should not take it, nor should children. Occasionally, there are reports of more serious effects, such as asthma attacks, increased BP, palpitations, and, in postmenopausal women, uterine bleeding. To many people, ginseng tastes unpleasant.

Ginseng can interact with antihyperglycemic drugs, aspirin, other NSAIDs, corticosteroids, digoxin, estrogens, monoamine oxidase inhibitors, and warfarin.

GLUCOSAMINE SULFATE

Glucosamine sulfate is a precursor of multiple cartilage constituents. It is extracted from chitin (in shells of crabs, oysters, and shrimp) and is taken in tablet or capsule form, often combined with chondroitin sulfate (see p. 2728).

Claims: Strong scientific evidence supports use of glucosamine sulfate for treatment of mild to moderate osteoarthritis of the knee. Its role in the treatment of more severe knee osteoarthritis and osteoarthritis in other locations is less well defined. Some evidence suggests it has both analgesic and disease-modifying effects. Mechanism is unknown but may be related to improved glycosaminoglycan synthesis as a result of the sulfate moiety. Dose is 500 mg po tid.

Adverse effects: Allergy (in patients who have shellfish allergy and take forms extracted from shellfish), dyspepsia, fatigue, insomnia, headache, photosensitivity, and nail changes may occur.

GOLDENSEAL

Goldenseal, an endangered US plant, is related to the buttercup. Its active components are hydrastine and berberine, which have antiseptic and antidiarrheal activity.

Claims: Goldenseal is used as an antiseptic wash for mouth sores, inflamed and sore eyes, and irritated skin and as a douche for vaginal infections. It has been combined with echinacea as a cold remedy, but the efficacy of goldenseal as a cold remedy has not been proved. Goldenseal is also used as a remedy for indigestion and diarrhea. In 2 relatively well-designed studies, berberine isolated from goldenseal reduced diarrhea.

Adverse effects: Goldenseal can have many adverse effects, including nausea, anxiety, dyspepsia, uterine contractions, jaundice in neonates, and worsening of hypertension. If taken in large amounts, goldenseal can cause seizures and respiratory failure and may affect contraction of the heart. Goldenseal may interact with warfarin. Women who are pregnant or breastfeeding, neonates, and people who have seizure disorders or problems with blood clotting should not take goldenseal. Berberine may reduce the anticoagulant effect of heparin.

GREEN TEA

Green tea is made from the dried leaves of an evergreen shrub native to Asia. It may be drunk or ingested in extracted tablet or capsule form. It has multiple components that are thought to have antioxidant and anticancer effects. Green tea contains caffeine, but many extracts have been decaffeinated.

Claims: Green tea is said to have multiple health benefits; it has been used for cancer prevention, weight loss, serum lipid reduction, prevention of coronary artery disease, memory enhancement, relief of osteoarthritis pain, treatment of menopausal symptoms, and longevity.

Adverse effects: Adverse effects are related to effects of caffeine. They include insomnia, anxiety, tachycardia, and mild tremor.

KAVA

Kava comes from the root of a shrub (*Piper methysticum*) that grows in the South Pacific. It is ingested as a tea or in capsule form. Active ingredients are thought to be kavalactones.

Claims: Strong scientific evidence supports use of kava as an anxiolytic and sleep aid. Mechanism is unknown. Dose is 100 mg of standardized extract tid.

Adverse effects: Reports of hepatic toxicity and failure in Europe have led the FDA to mandate a warning label on kava products, and safety is under continuing surveillance. When kava is prepared traditionally (as tea) and used in high doses (>6 to 12 g/day of dried root) or over long periods (up to 6 wk), there have been reports of scaly skin rash (kava dermopathy), blood changes (macrocytosis, leukopenia), and neurologic changes (torticollis, oculogyric crisis, worsening of Parkinson's disease, movement disorders). Also, kava may prolong the effect of other sedatives (eg, barbiturates) and affect driving or other activities requiring alertness.

MELATONIN

Melatonin, a hormone produced by the pineal gland, regulates circadian rhythms. It is derived from animals or can be manufactured synthetically.

Claims: Some scientific evidence supports use of melatonin to minimize the effects of jet lag, especially in people traveling eastward over 2 to 5 time zones (see the Cochrane review's abstract on melatonin for the prevention and treatment of jet lag).

Standard dosage is not established and ranges from 0.5 to 5 mg po taken 1 h before usual bedtime on the day of travel and 2 to 4 nights after arrival. Evidence supporting use of melatonin as a sleep aid in adults and children with neuropsychiatric disorders (eg, pervasive developmental disorders) is less strong.

Adverse effects: Hangover drowsiness, headache, and transient depression may occur. Melatonin may worsen depression. Theoretically, prion infection from products derived from neurologic tissues of animals is a risk.

MILK THISTLE

Milk thistle is a purple-flowered plant; its sap and seeds contain the active ingredient silymarin, a potent antioxidant.

Claims: Milk thistle is believed to be a treatment for cirrhosis and to protect the liver from viral hepatitis, the damaging effects of alcohol, and hepatotoxic drugs. In vitro, silymarin increases levels of intrahepatic glutathione, an antioxidant important for detoxification.

Adverse effects: No serious effects have been reported. Milk thistle may intensify the effects of antihyperglycemic drugs and may interfere with indinavir therapy.

S-ADENOSYL-L-METHIONINE

S-adenosyl-L-methionine (SAMe) is a derivative of methionine and a cofactor for multiple synthetic pathways.

Claims: SAMe is said to be effective for treatment of depression, osteoarthritis, and liver disorders. It is a platelet inhibitor in vitro.

Adverse effects: No serious adverse effects have been reported. SAMe is contraindicated in patients with bipolar disorder because SAMe can precipitate manic episodes.

SAW PALMETTO

Saw palmetto berries contain the plant's active ingredients, which are unidentified but which appear to inhibit 5α-reductase. The berries can be used to make a tea, or they can be extracted into tablets, capsules, or a liquid preparation. Most formulations evaluated in clinical studies are hexane extracts of saw palmetto berries, which are 80 to 90% essential fatty acids and phytosterols.

Claims: Strong scientific evidence supports use of saw palmetto to treat symptoms of benign prostatic hyperplasia; no evidence suggests it reverses the hyperplasia. Mechanism is unknown but may be inhibition of conversion of testosterone to dihydrotestosterone. Dose is 320 mg once/day or 160 mg bid.

Adverse effects: Headache and diarrhea may occur, but no other serious adverse effects have been reported. Saw palmetto may interact with estrogens.

ST. JOHN'S WORT

The flowers of St. John's wort contain its biologically active ingredients hypericin and hyperforin.

Claims: Strong scientific evidence supports use of St. John's wort for treatment of patients with mild to moderate depression and without suicidal ideation. Mechanism is unknown, but St. John's wort may increase CNS serotonin and, in very high doses, acts like a monoamine oxidase inhibitor (MAOI). Dose is 300 to 600 mg po once/day of a preparation standardized to 0.2 to 0.3% hypericin, to 1 to 4% hyperforin, or to both (usually). St. John's wort is also said to be useful for treating HIV infection but has proven adverse interactions with protease inhibitors and nonnucleoside reverse transcriptase inhibitors (NNRTIs).

Adverse effects: Photosensitivity, dry mouth, constipation, dizziness, confusion, and mania (in patients with bipolar disorder) may occur. St. John's wort is contraindicated in pregnant women. Potential adverse interactions occur with cyclosporine, digoxin, iron supplements, MAOIs, NNRTIs, oral contraceptives, protease inhibitors, SSRIs, tricyclic antidepressants, and warfarin.

VALERIAN

Valerian is an herb; the root contains active ingredients, including valepotriates and pungent odiferous oils.

Claims: Valerian is used as a sedative and sleep aid and is especially popular in Europe.

Adverse effects: Valerian may prolong the effect of other sedatives (eg, barbiturates) and affect driving or other activities requiring alertness.

ZINC

Zinc, a mineral, is required in small quantities for multiple metabolic processes. Dietary sources include oysters, beef, and fortified cereals.

Claims: Some experts believe that when taken soon after cold symptoms develop, zinc taken as zinc gluconate or acetate lozenges can shorten the course of the common cold. There is stronger evidence that in developing countries, supplements containing zinc 20 mg and iron taken once/wk reduce mortality in infants who have diarrhea and respiratory infection. There is also strong evidence that supplements containing zinc 80 mg and antioxidants taken once/day slow progression of moderate to severe atrophic (dry form) age-related maculopathy in elderly people.

Adverse effects: Zinc is generally safe, but toxicity can develop if high doses are used (see p. 56).

332 SMOKING CESSATION

Nicotine is a highly addictive drug found in tobacco and is a major component of cigarette smoke. This drug stimulates the brain reward system activated during pleasurable activities in a manner similar to that of most other addictive drugs (see p. 1683). People smoke to feed their nicotine addiction but simultaneously inhale hundreds of carcinogens, noxious gases, and chemical additives that are a part of cigarette smoke. These components are responsible for the multiple health consequences of smoking.

Epidemiology

Smoking: The percentage of people in the US who smoke cigarettes has declined since 1964, when the Surgeon General first publicized the link between smoking and ill health. Nevertheless, about 45 million adults (nearly 23%) still smoke. Smoking is most prevalent in men, people with < 12 yr of education, people living at or below the poverty income level, non-Hispanic whites, non-Hispanic blacks, American Indians, and Alaska natives. Smoking is least common among Asian Americans.

Most smokers start during childhood. Children as young as 10 yr experiment with cigarettes. Over 2000 start daily, 31% before age 16 and over ½ before age 18, and age of initiation continues to decrease. Risk factors for childhood initiation include parental, peer, and role model (eg, celebrity) smoking; poor school performance; high-risk behavior (eg, excessive dieting among boys or girls, physical fighting, drunk driving); and poor problem-solving abilities.

Smoking harms nearly every organ in the body and is, as of 2000, the leading cause of mortality in the US, accounting for an estimated 435,000 deaths/yr. About ½ of all current smokers will die prematurely of a disease directly caused by smoking, losing 10 to 14 yr of life (7 min/cigarette) on average. Sixty-five percent of smoking-attributable deaths are from ischemic heart disease, lung cancer, and chronic lung disease; the rest are from noncardiac vascular diseases (eg, stroke, aortic aneurysm), other cancers (eg, bladder, cervical, esophageal, kidney, laryngeal, oropharyngeal, pancreatic, stomach, throat), pneumonia, and perinatal conditions (eg, preterm birth, low birth weight, SIDS). In addition, smoking is a risk factor for other conditions that convey profound morbidity and disability, such as acute myelocytic leukemia, frequent URIs, cataracts, reproductive effects (eg, infertility, spontaneous abortion, ectopic pregnancy, premature menopause), and periodontitis.

Quitting: More than 70% of smokers present to a primary care setting every year, yet only a minority leaves having received counseling and medications to assist them in quitting. Most smokers < 18 yr believe they will not be smoking in 5 yr, and over ½ report having tried to quit in the previous year. However, longitudinal studies show that 73% of daily smokers in high school remain daily smokers 5 to 6 yr later.

Passive smoking: Passive exposure to cigarette smoke (secondhand smoke, environmental tobacco smoke) has grave health implications for children and adults. Risks to neonates, infants, and children include low birth weight, SIDS, asthma and other related respiratory illnesses, and otitis media. Children exposed to cigarette smoke lose more school days to illness than non-exposed children. Smoking-related fires kill 80 children each year and injure almost 300 more; they are the leading cause of deaths resulting from unintentional fires in the US. Treating children for smoking-related illnesses is estimated to cost $4.6 billion/yr. In addition, 43,000 children each year lose one or more caretakers who die from smoking-related diseases.

Exposure in adults is linked to the same neoplastic, respiratory, and cardiovascular diseases that threaten active smokers. Overall, secondhand smoke is estimated to be responsible for 50,000 to 60,000 deaths each year in the US. These findings have led 6 states and municipalities across the US to ban smoking within workplaces in an effort to protect the health of workers and others from the substantive risks of environmental tobacco smoke.

Symptoms and Signs

Smoking cessation often causes intense withdrawal symptoms, primarily a craving for cigarettes but also anxiety, depression (mostly mild, sometimes major), inability to concentrate, irritability, restlessness, insomnia, drowsiness, impatience, hunger, tremor, sweating, dizziness, headaches, and digestive disturbances. These symptoms are worst in the 1st wk and subside within 3 to 4 wk, but many patients resume smoking as symptoms peak. An average weight gain of 4 to 5 kg is common and is another reason for recidivism. Smokers with ulcerative colitis often experience an exacerbation soon after quitting.

Treatment

The addiction and withdrawal symptoms are powerful enough that, even with knowledge of the many health risks, many smokers thinking of quitting are often unwilling to try, and those attempting to quit are often unsuccessful. A minority quits permanently in initial attempts, but most go on to smoke for many years, cycling through multiple periods of relapse and remission. The optimal evidence-based approach to patients, particularly those unwilling to quit or those who have not yet considered quitting, should be guided by the same principles that guide chronic disease management, namely:

- Continually assessing and monitoring smoking status
- Setting realistic goals, including those that fall short of total smoking cessation, such as temporary abstinence and reduction in consumption (smoking reduction can increase motivation to quit, particularly when combined with nicotine replacement therapy)
- Using different interventions (or combinations) for different patients as needed

Effective interventions require 3 core components: counseling, drug therapy (in patients without contraindications), and consistent identification of and intervention with smokers.

The counseling approach for children is similar to that for adults. Children should be screened for smoking and risk factors by age 10. Parents should be advised to maintain smoke-free households and to communicate the expectation to their children that they will remain nonsmokers. Cognitive-behavioral therapy that involves establishing awareness of tobacco use, providing motivations to quit, preparing to quit, and providing strategies to maintain abstinence after cessation are effective in treating nicotine-dependent adolescents. Alternative approaches to smoking cessation, such as hypnosis and acupuncture, have been inadequately studied and cannot be recommended for routine use.

Counseling: Counseling efforts begin with the 5 *A*'s: *a*sk at every visit if a patient smokes and document the response; *a*dvise all smokers to quit in clear, strong language they will understand; *a*ssess a smoker's willingness to quit within the next 30 days; *a*ssist those willing to make a quit attempt with brief counseling and medications; and *a*rrange a follow-up, preferably within the 1st wk of the quit date.

For smokers willing to quit, clinicians should establish a quit date, preferably within 2 wk, and stress that total abstinence is better than reduction. Past quitting experiences can be reviewed to identify what helped and what did not, and smoking triggers or challenges to quitting should be planned for in advance. For example, alcohol use is associated with relapse, so alcohol restriction or abstinence should be discussed. In addition, quitting is more difficult with another smoker in the household; spouses and housemates can be encouraged to quit together. In general, patients should be instructed to develop social support among family and friends for their quit attempt, and clinicians should reinforce their availability and assistance in support of the attempt. Although these counseling strategies make good sense and provide important patient support, little scientific evidence supports their use in preventing relapse.

About 40 states in the US have telephone quitlines that can provide additional support to smokers trying to quit. Phone numbers for these can be obtained locally or from the American Cancer Society (1-800-ACS-2345; www.cancer.org).

Drugs: Drugs proven effective and safe for smoking cessation include bupropion SR and nicotine (in the form of gum, lozenge, inhaler, nasal spray, or patch; see TABLE 332–1). Some evidence suggests bupropion is more effective than nicotine replacement. All forms of nicotine are equivalent as monotherapy, but the combination of a nicotine patch with gum or nasal spray increases long-term abstinence compared to any one form alone. Nortriptyline 25 to 75 mg po at bedtime may be an effective 2nd-line alternative for smokers with depression. Drug choice is guided by the clinician's familiarity with the drug, patient preference and previous experience (positive or negative), and contraindications.

Contraindications to bupropion include a history of seizures, eating disorder, and MAO inhibitor use within 2 wk. Nicotine replacement should be used cautiously in patients with certain cardiovascular risks (those within 2 wk of an MI, with serious arrhythmias, or with serious angina). Nicotine gum is contraindicated in patients with temporomandibular joint syndrome, and nicotine patches are contraindicated in patients with severe topical sensitization. All these drugs should be used cautiously, if at all, in pregnant and breastfeeding women and adolescents and, because nicotine toxicity is possible and evidence of benefit is lacking, in patients who smoke < 10 cigarettes/day. These drugs delay but do not prevent weight gain.

Despite their proven efficacy, smoking cessation drugs are used by < 25% of smokers attempting to quit. Reasons include low rates of insurance coverage, clinician concerns about the safety of simultaneous smoking and nicotine replacement, and discouragement because of past unsuccessful quit attempts.

Therapies under investigation for smoking cessation include a vaccine that intercepts nicotine before the nicotine reaches its specific receptors and rimonabant, a cannabinoid CB1 receptor antagonist.

Prognosis

More than 90% of the about 20 million smokers in the US who try to quit each year relapse within days, weeks, or months. Almost ½ report having tried to quit in the last year, usually by using a "cold turkey" or other approach that did not work. Success rates are 20 to 30% among smokers who use cessation counseling or drugs.

Other Kinds of Tobacco

Cigarette smoking is the most harmful form of tobacco use, although pipe, cigar, and smokeless tobacco use results in similar ominous consequences. Exclusive pipe smoking is relatively rare in the US (< 1% of people ≥ 12 yr), although it has increased among middle and high school students since 1999. About 5.4% of persons > 12 yr smoke cigars. Although this percentage has declined since 2000, people < 18 yr comprise the largest group of new cigar smokers. Risks of pipe and cigar smoking include cardiovascular disease;

TABLE 332–1. DRUG THERAPIES FOR SMOKING CESSATION

DRUG THERAPY	DOSAGE	DURATION	ADVERSE EFFECTS	COMMENTS
Bupropion SR	150 mg every morning for 3 days, then 150 mg twice/day (begin treatment 1–2 wk before quitting)	7–12 wk initially; may continue up to 6 mo	Insomnia; dry mouth	Prescription only; contraindicated with history of seizure, eating disorder, MAO inhibitor use within past 2 wk
Nicotine gum	If smoking 1–24 cigarettes/day, 2 mg gum (up to 24 pieces/day) If smoking 25 + cigarettes/day, 4 mg gum (up to 24 pieces/day)	Up to 12 wk	Mouth soreness; dyspepsia	OTC only
Nicotine lozenge	If smoking > 30 min after waking, 2 mg; if smoking < 30 min after waking, 4 mg Schedule for both dosage strengths is 1 q 1–2 h for wk 1–6; 1 q 2–4 h for wk 7–9; 1 q 4–8 h for wk 10–12	Up to 12 wk	Nausea; insomnia	OTC only
Nicotine inhaler	6–16 cartridges/day for wk 1–12, then taper down over next 6–12 wk	3–6 mo	Local irritation of mouth and throat	Prescription only
Nicotine nasal spray	8–40 doses/day 1 dose = 2 sprays	14 wk	Nasal irritation	Prescription only
Nicotine patch	21 mg/24 h for 6 wk, then 14 mg/24 h for 2 wk, then 7 mg/24 h for 2 wk If smoking > 10 cigarettes/day, start with 21-mg dose; if smoking < 10 cigarettes/day, start with 14-mg dose or	10 wk	Local skin reaction; insomnia	OTC and prescription
	15 mg/16 h if smoking > 10 cigarettes/day	6 wk		

COPD; cancers of the oral cavity, lung, larynx, esophagus, colon, pancreas; and periodontal disease and tooth loss.

About 3.3% of persons ≥ 12 yr use smokeless tobacco (chewing tobacco and snuff). Toxicity of smokeless tobacco varies by brand. Risks include cardiovascular disease, oral disorders (eg, cancers, gum recession, gingivitis, periodontitis and its consequences), and teratogenicity. Smoking cessation for smokeless tobacco users and pipe and cigar smokers is accomplished similarly as that for cigarette smokers. Success rates are higher among smokeless tobacco users. However, success rates for pipe and cigar smokers are not well documented and are impacted by concurrent use of cigarettes and whether or not smokers inhale.

333 MEDICAL ASPECTS OF TRAVEL

Planning and preparation reduce medical risks of travel. Travelers should carry their medications, extra eyeglasses or other corrective lenses (as well as a current written prescription for either), and hearing-aid batteries in a carry-on bag in case their checked baggage is delayed, lost, or stolen. Medications should be kept in their original labeled containers. Travelers who need to carry opioids, syringes, or large amounts of medication should have a prescription or verifying letter from a physician to avoid possible security or customs complications. A medical record summary (including ECG for those with significant cardiac history) is invaluable if a traveler becomes ill. Travelers subject to disabling illness (eg, epilepsy) or those with chronic disease should wear a medical identification bracelet or necklace.

AIR TRAVEL

Air travel can cause or worsen certain medical problems. Those with severe heart disease or recent MI (4 wk for uncomplicated MI, 6 wk for complicated MI), unstable angina, and severe pulmonary disease should not fly, because the partial pressure of O_2 in passenger jets is reduced at altitude to the equivalent of an altitude of 6000 to 8000 ft (1830 to 2440 m), resulting in a PaO_2 of about 70 mm Hg. When flying is essential, supplemental O_2 may be arranged for in advance with the airline. Those with extreme immunodeficiency and highly contagious infections should not fly because of exposure risk to self and others. Those with an immobilized jaw (unless the appliance is fitted with a special quick-release device) also should not fly, because air sickness may cause vomiting.

Most implanted cardiac devices, including pacemakers and cardioverter defibrillators, are effectively shielded from interference from security devices. However, the metal content of some of these devices, as well as certain orthopedic prostheses and braces, may trigger a security alarm; a physician's letter should be carried to avoid security difficulties. People with implanted bone growth stimulators or insulin pumps should not pass through metal detectors or be screened by hand wands.

People with very specific dietary and medical needs should plan carefully and carry their own food and supplies. With several days' notice, all airlines departing from or arriving in the US (and most others) can make reasonable efforts to accommodate passengers with physical handicaps and special needs, including those who require O_2 therapy. Wheelchairs can be accommodated on all US airlines and most foreign ones, but advance notice is advisable. Some airlines accept passengers requiring more highly specialized equipment (eg, IV fluids, respirators) provided that appropriate personnel accompany the passenger and arrangements have been made in advance. If travelers cannot be accommodated on a commercial aircraft because of severe illness, air ambulance service is necessary.

During a flight, any health care practitioner among the passengers may be asked to help fellow passengers who become ill. Additionally, most commercial aircrafts carry first-aid equipment, including an automatic external cardioverter defibrillator and limited medical supplies. Airline personnel are receiving more first-aid training now than in the past.

Further information about air travel may be obtained from the medical department of major airlines or from the Federal Aviation Administration (www.cami.jccbi.gov/aam-400/PassengerHandS.htm).

Barometric pressure changes: Untreated dental problems or dental work may become painful when air pressure changes. In commercial airplanes and jet aircraft, free air in body cavities expands by about 25%; this expansion may aggravate certain medical conditions. People with upper respiratory inflammation or allergic rhinitis may develop obstructed eustachian tubes or sinus ostia, which may cause, respectively, barotitis media and barosinusitis. Frequent yawning or closed-nose swallowing during descent, using decongestant nasal sprays, or using antihistamines before or during flight often prevents or relieves these conditions.

Air travel is contraindicated for patients who have or are likely to develop pneumothorax (eg, who have large pulmonary blebs or cavities) and for those in whom air or gas is trapped (eg, those with an incarcerated bowel, < 10 days after chest or abdominal surgery, or intraocular gas injection), because even modest expansion may cause pain or tissue damage. Patients with a colostomy should wear a large bag and expect frequent filling due to expansion of intestinal gas.

Children: Children < 7 days of age should not fly. Children are particularly susceptible to barotitis media and should be given fluids or food during descent to encourage swallowing, which can equalize pressures. Infants can be breastfed or given a bottle or pacifier. Precautions applied to adults are the same for children with chronic disease (eg, congenital heart disease, chronic lung disease, anemia).

Circadian dysrhythmia (jet lag—see also p. 1839**):** Rapid travel across multiple time zones disrupts the normal circadian rhythm. Because bright sunlight resets the internal clock, exposure to bright late-afternoon light delays the onset of normal sleep time, and early-morning light advances the biologic clock, so that sleep time is earlier than usual. Melatonin, a hormone secreted by the pineal gland, may provide a "time-of-night cue" (see p. 2732). If those traveling east across several time zones take melatonin 0.5 to 5 mg po in the evening of their day of arrival, their sleep time may be earlier. However, large placebo-controlled trials of melatonin are lacking. Melatonin's effectiveness depends on coordinating its therapy with the destination's time pattern.

Some therapeutic regimens must be altered to compensate for circadian dysrhythmia. For example, insulin dosage and timing may require modification depending on the number of time zones traversed, time spent at destination, available food, and activity; glucose must be monitored frequently. Regimens may require modification based on elapsed rather than local time.

Decreased O_2 tension: In general, anyone who can walk 50 m or climb one flight of stairs and whose disease is stable can tolerate normal passenger jet cabin conditions without additional O_2. However, problems may arise for travelers with moderate or severe pulmonary disease (eg, asthma, COPD, cystic fibrosis), heart failure, anemia with Hb < 8.5 g/dL, severe angina pectoris, sickle cell disease (but not trait), and some congenital heart diseases. Such patients can usually fly safely with specially designed continuous O_2 equipment, which must be provided by the airline. Mild ankle edema due to venous stasis commonly develops during long flights and should not be confused with heart failure. Smoking can aggravate mild hypoxia and should be avoided before flying. Hypoxia and fatigue may increase the effects of alcohol.

Low cabin humidity: Dehydration may develop because of very low cabin humidity. It can be avoided with adequate fluid intake and alcohol avoidance. Contact lens wearers should instill artificial tears frequently to avoid corneal irritation resulting from low cabin humidity.

Pregnancy: Uncomplicated pregnancy through 36 wk is not a contraindication to air travel; high-risk pregnancies must be individually evaluated. Flight during the 9th mo usually requires a physician's written approval dated within 72 h of departure and indicating expected delivery date. Seatbelts should be worn below the abdomen, across the hips.

Psychologic stress: Hypnosis and behavior modification have benefited some people with fear of flying and claustrophobia. Fearful passengers may also benefit from a short-acting anxiolytic taken before and, depending on duration, during flight. Hyperventilation commonly simulates heart disease and may cause tetany-like symptoms or altered awareness. Psychotic tendencies may become more acute and troublesome during flight. Patients with violent or unpredictable tendencies must be accompanied by an attendant and appropriately sedated.

Restricted mobility: Deep venous thrombosis may develop in anyone sitting for long periods and may result in a pulmonary embolus. Those with a history of venous disease, pregnant women, and women taking oral contraceptives are at increased risk. Frequent (every 1 to 2 h) ambulation, short-movement exercises while seated, and proper hydration are recommended; however, studies demonstrating benefit from these measures are lacking.

Turbulence: Turbulence may cause motion sickness (see p. 2616) or injury. While seated, passengers should keep their seatbelts fastened at all times.

FOREIGN TRAVEL

About 1/30 people traveling abroad requires emergency care. Illness in a foreign country may involve significant difficulties. Many

TABLE 333–1. USEFUL CONTACTS FOR THOSE TRAVELING ABROAD

ORGANIZATION	PHONE NUMBERS	WEB SITE
International Association for Medical Assistance to Travelers	US: (716) 754-4883 (Niagara Falls, NY) Canada: (519) 836-0102 (Guelph, Ontario); (416) 652-0137 Toronto, Ontario)	http://www.iamat.org
Centers for Disease Control and Prevention (CDC)	US: Toll-free (877) FYI TRIP (877-394-8747) (404) 639-3311 (Atlanta, GA)	http://www.cdc.gov/travel
CDC Malaria Hotline	US: (770) 488-7788; after hours, (770) 488-7100	http://www.cdc.gov/malaria
US Department of State (Overseas Citizens Services)	US: (888) 407-4747 (Washington, DC)	http://www.travel.state.gov
World Health Organization (WHO)	International: (+41 22)-791-2111 (Geneva, Switzerland)	http://www.who.int/en/

insurance plans, including Medicare, are not valid in foreign countries; overseas hospitals often require a substantial cash deposit for nonresidents, regardless of insurance. Travel insurance plans, including some that arrange for emergency evacuation, are available through travel agencies and some major credit card companies. Directories listing English-speaking physicians in foreign countries, US consulates who may assist in obtaining emergency medical services, and information on foreign travel risks are available (see TABLE 333–1).

Immunizations: Some countries require specific immunizations, some of which must be given weeks to months before departure. General travel and up-to-date immunization information and malaria chemoprophylaxis requirements are available from the Centers for Disease Control and Prevention.

Injury and death: Road traffic accidents are the most frequent cause of death of non-elderly international travelers. Travelers should use seat belts whenever possible and a helmet when cycling. Travelers should avoid motorcycles and mopeds and avoid riding on bus roofs or in open truck beds. To prevent drowning, another common cause of death while abroad, travelers should avoid beaches with turbulent surf and avoid swimming after drinking alcoholic beverages.

Traveler's diarrhea (see also p. 137): Traveler's diarrhea (TD) is the most common health problem in international travelers. Although TD is usually a self-limited illness, typically resolving in 5 days, 3 to 10% of travelers with TD may have symptoms lasting longer than 2 wk, and up to 3% of travelers have TD lasting over 30 days. TD lasting < 1 wk requires no workup. For persistent TD, a laboratory workup is performed (see p. 79). Self-initiated treatment is with an appropriate antibiotic (eg, a fluoroquinolone for most destinations, a macrolide such as azithromycin for Southeast Asia), loperamide, and replacement fluids.

Problems after returning home: Some diseases become evident months after a traveler has returned home; a travel history with exposure risks is useful for patients who present with a puzzling illness. Malaria (see p. 1576), hepatitis A and B (see p. 219), typhoid fever (see p. 1470), sexually transmitted diseases (see p. 1650), including HIV infection (see p. 1625), amebiasis (see p. 1565), and meningitis (see p. 1858) are the most commonly acquired dangerous diseases.

334 SYNDROMES OF UNCERTAIN ORIGIN

Many patients suffer greatly from syndromes for which no specific cause has been identified. Some physicians think these syndromes have psychologic causes, but many physicians and most patients with these syndromes reject that idea. Some data—often incomplete, inconsistent, or contradictory—suggest a physical cause, although the exact cause remains uncertain. The causative or contributory role of psychologic pathology is also uncertain.

Some patients have scattered, apparently unrelated symptoms that do not form a recognizable syndrome. With better definitions, case recognition may improve; further study of patients with such symptoms is needed to clarify symptom etiology and the clinical significance of these syndromes, to develop appropriate diagnostic strategies, and to define optimum care.

The evaluating physician's first responsibility is to obtain a thorough history, including history of exposure to potentially noxious substances, and to exclude specific, potentially treatable causes. Often, there is little guidance as to what testing is appropriate, but the physician must avoid tests that are inappropriate or not clearly indicated. If no treatable cause is identified after the evaluation, supportive, empathic follow-up is required. A physician should be aware that many patients with such syndromes turn to alternative and complementary medical practices in their search for relief.

CHRONIC FATIGUE SYNDROME

Chronic fatigue syndrome is defined as longstanding, severe, disabling fatigue without demonstrable muscle weakness. Underlying disorders that could explain the fatigue are absent. Depression, anxiety, and other psychologic diagnoses are typically absent. Treatment is rest and psychologic support, often including antidepressants.

This definition of chronic fatigue syndrome (CFS) has several variants, and heterogeneity among patients who meet the criteria of this definition is considerable. Prevalence is impossible to state precisely; it varies from 7 to 38/100,000 people. Prevalence may vary because of differences in diagnostic evaluation, physician-patient attitudes, social acceptability, risk of exposure to an infectious or toxic agent, or definition and case finding. CFS occurs slightly more often in females. In office-based studies, prevalence is highest among whites. However, community surveys indicate a higher prevalence among blacks, Hispanics, and American Indians than among whites.

Etiology and Pathophysiology

Etiology is controversial, and the precise cause remains unknown. Psychologic factors may be the cause in an unknown percentage of cases; however, CFS seems to be distinct from typical depression, anxiety, or other psychologic disorders. A chronic viral infection has been proposed as a cause because many patients relate onset of CFS to an event similar to influenza or mononucleosis. Epstein-Barr virus has also been proposed as a cause, but immunologic markers of exposure do not appear to be sensitive or specific. Other possible but unproven viral causes include enteroviruses, human herpesvirus 6, and human T-cell lymphotropic virus. Allergic reactions have also been proposed; about 65% of patients report previous allergies, and the rate of cutaneous reactivity to inhalants or foods is 25 to 50% higher in this group than in the general population.

Various immunologic abnormalities have been reported; they include low levels of IgG, decreased lymphocytic proliferation, low interferon-γ levels in response to mitogens, and poor cytotoxicity of natural killer cells. Some patients have abnormal IgG, with circulating autoantibodies and immune complexes. Many other immunologic abnormalities have been studied; none provides adequate sensitivity and specificity for defining the syndrome. Additionally, no consistent or readily reproducible pattern of immunologic abnormalities has been identified.

Other proposed mechanisms include neuroendocrine abnormalities, abnormal levels of neurotransmitters, inadequate cerebral circulation, and elevated levels of ACE.

Data indicate that relatives of patients with CFS have an increased risk of developing the syndrome, suggesting a familial or genetic component.

Symptoms, Signs, and Diagnosis

Onset is usually abrupt, and many patients report an initial viral-like illness with swollen lymph nodes, extreme fatigue, fever, and upper respiratory symptoms. The main symptom is severe fatigue (usually for ≥6 mo) that interferes with daily activities (see TABLE 334–1 for other symptoms).

Usually, no signs of muscle weakness, arthritis, neuropathy, or organomegaly are present. However, some definitions require the presence of low-grade fever, nonexudative pharyngitis, or palpable or tender lymph nodes.

Because the cause is unknown, diagnosis is by clinical criteria (see TABLE 334–1). Further evaluation aims to exclude treatable disorders. A reasonable assessment includes CBC and measurement of electrolytes, ESR, and thyroid-stimulating hormone. In some cases, chest x-ray and tests for antinuclear antibody, rheumatoid factor, hepatitis, and HIV should be added. Other viral antibody and other expensive tests are unlikely to shed light on the diagnosis or cause. Obvious depression or severe anxiety excludes the diagnosis of CFS.

TABLE 334–1. DIAGNOSTIC CRITERIA FOR CHRONIC FATIGUE SYNDROME

Unexplained, persistent, or relapsing chronic fatigue that is new or has a definite onset; that is not due to ongoing exertion; that is not substantially alleviated by rest; and that substantially reduces occupational, educational, social, or personal activities

At least 4 of the following for ≥6 mo*:
- Impaired short-term memory (self-reported) severe enough to substantially reduce occupational, educational, social, or personal activities
- Sore throat
- Low-grade fever
- Tender, enlarged, painful cervical or axillary lymph nodes
- Muscle pain
- Abdominal pain
- Multijoint pain without joint swelling or tenderness (arthralgia)
- Headaches that are new in type, pattern, or severity
- Unrefreshing sleep
- Postexertional malaise lasting >24 h
- Cognitive difficulties (especially with concentrating and sleeping)

*Must not predate the fatigue.

Data from the Centers for Disease Control and Prevention, the National Institutes of Health, and the International Chronic Fatigue Study Group.

Treatment

Nonsedating antidepressants are commonly prescribed, although their value is undetermined. Antiviral treatments with acyclovir and amantadine do not appear effective. Studies of immunologic treatments, including high-dose immune globulins, dialyzable WBC extract, amphigen, interferons, isoprinosine, and corticosteroids, have been inconclusive and mostly disappointing. Dietary supplements and high-dose vitamins are commonly used, but their usefulness has not been substantiated. Psychologic intervention (eg, individual or group therapy) may help some patients. Formal, structured physical rehabilitation programs may help. Persistent or prolonged rest should be firmly discouraged because it can worsen deconditioning and promote progressive frailty.

MULTIPLE CHEMICAL SENSITIVITY SYNDROME

(Idiopathic Environmental Intolerance)

Multiple chemical sensitivity syndrome is characterized by recurrent, nonspecific symptoms attributed to low-level exposure to chemically unrelated substances commonly occurring in the environment. Symptoms are numerous, often involving multiple organ systems, but physical findings are unremarkable. Diagnosis is by exclusion. Treatment is psychologic support and avoidance of perceived triggers, although triggers can rarely be defined.

No universally accepted definition exists, but multiple chemical sensitivity syndrome is generally defined as the development of multiple symptoms attributed to exposure to any number of identifiable or unidentifiable chemical substances (inhaled, touched, or ingested) in the absence of clinically detectable organ dysfunction or related physical signs.

Many theories—immunologic and nonimmunologic—have been proposed. These theories are all hampered by lack of a consistent dose response to proposed causative substances; ie, symptoms may not be replicated after exposure to high levels of a substance that previously, at much lower levels, seemed to provoke a reaction. Similarly, consistent objective evidence of systemic inflammation, cytokine excess, or immune system activation in relation to symptoms is lacking. Many physicians consider the etiology to be psychologic, probably a form of somatization disorder (see p. 1740). Others suggest that the syndrome is a type ofpanic attack or agoraphobia (see p. 1674). Some facets of the syndrome resemble the no-longer-used psychologic diagnosis of neurasthenia.

Although measurable biologic abnormalities (eg, decreased levels of B cells, elevated levels of IgE) are rare, some patients have such abnormalities. However, these abnormalities appear without a consistent pattern, and their significance is uncertain.

Symptoms (eg, tachycardia, chest pain, sweating, shortness of breath, fatigue, flushing, dizziness, nausea, choking, trembling, numbness, coughing, hoarseness, difficulty concentrating) are numerous and usually involve more than one organ system. Most patients present with a long list of suspected agents, self-identified or identified by a physician during previous testing. Such patients often go to great lengths to avoid these agents by changing residence and employment, avoiding all foods containing "chemicals," sometimes wearing masks in public, or avoiding public settings altogether. Physical examination is characteristically unremarkable.

Diagnosis initially involves exclusion of demonstrable allergies and other known disorders with similar presentation (eg, atopic disorders such as asthma, allergic rhinitis, food allergies, and angioedema). Atopic disorders are excluded based on a typical clinical history, skin-prick testing, serum assays of specific IgE, or all three. Consultation with an allergy specialist may be necessary.

Despite an uncertain cause-and-effect relationship, treatment is usually aimed at avoiding the suspected precipitating agents, which may be difficult because many are ubiquitous. However, social isolation and costly and highly disruptive avoidance behaviors should be discouraged. Psychologic evaluation and intervention may help, but characteristically many patients resist this approach. However, the point of this approach is not to demonstrate that the cause is psychologic but rather to help patients cope with their suffering.

335 CARE OF THE SURGICAL PATIENT

Care of surgical patients often involves nonsurgical consultants (eg, internists, general practitioners), who may be asked to provide preoperative risk assessment (sometimes requested as medical clearance), to manage complex medical conditions, and to advise about antibiotic therapy. Psychiatric consultation may be needed to assess capacity or help deal with underlying psychiatric problems that can interfere with recovery. Elderly patients may benefit from involvement of an interdisciplinary geriatric team, which may need to involve social workers, therapists, ethicists, and others.

PREOPERATIVE EVALUATION

If an emergency procedure is required, preoperative evaluation must be rapid and is thus limited. In other cases, the surgical team may consult an internist to obtain a formal preoperative evaluation, which helps minimize risk by identifying correctable abnormalities and by determining whether additional monitoring is needed or whether a procedure should be delayed so that an underlying disorder (eg, hypertension, hyperglycemia, hematologic abnormalities) can be stabilized.

Routine preoperative evaluation varies substantially from patient to patient, depending on the patient's age and general health and risks of the procedure. Usually, evaluation requires a relevant history, including information about allergies, prior use of anesthetics, bleeding abnormalities, risk factors for thromboembolism, infections, and any cardiopulmonary symptoms. If an indwelling catheter may be needed, patients should be asked about prior urinary retention or prostate surgery. Physical examination should include not only areas affected by the surgical procedure but also the cardiopulmonary system and a search for any signs of ongoing infection (eg, upper respiratory tract or skin). When spinal anesthesia is likely, patients should be evaluated for scoliosis and other anatomic back abnormalities that may complicate lumbar puncture. Any cognitive dysfunction, especially in elderly patients who will be given a general anesthetic, should be noted. Preexisting dysfunction may become more apparent postoperatively and, if undetected beforehand, may be misinterpreted as a surgical complication.

Testing: Laboratory evaluation usually includes a CBC and urinalysis (glucose, protein, and cells). Serum electrolytes and creatinine and plasma glucose are measured unless patients are extremely healthy and the procedure is considered very low risk. Liver enzymes may be measured depending on the patient's history. If a general anesthetic is to be used, a recent chest x-ray is typically obtained, although its usefulness is limited.

If patients have a chronic pulmonary disorder, pulmonary function testing before surgery may provide information useful to perioperative management. Patients with poorly controlled coronary artery disease may need additional tests (eg, stress testing, coronary angiography) before surgery.

Surgical risk factors: Surgical risk varies with the procedure and patient risk factors. Risk is highest with heart or lung surgery, prostatectomy, and major orthopedic procedures (eg, hip replacement). Some clinicians quantify patient risk factors using published criteria (see TABLE 335–1). Older age alone does not significantly increase risk of a complication but is associated with greater morbidity if a complication occurs. Chronic disorders and associated morbidity predict postoperative complications better than does age alone. Older age is not an absolute contraindication to surgery.

Several preoperative factors dramatically increase surgical risk. Among the most serious are unstable angina, recent MI, and poorly controlled heart failure. When a heart disorder cannot be corrected before surgery, intraoperative and sometimes preoperative monitoring with Swann-Ganz catheterization may be advised.

Incidental infections (eg, UTIs) should be treated with antibiotics but should not delay surgery. However, if prosthetic material is

TABLE 335–1. CARDIAC RISK INDEX IN NONCARDIAC SURGERY

CRITERIA	FINDING	POINTS*
Age (yr)	>70	5
Cardiac status	MI within 6 mo	10
	Ventricular gallop or jugular venous distention (signs of heart failure)	11
	Significant aortic stenosis	3
	Arrhythmia other than sinus or premature atrial contractions	7
	≥5 premature ventricular contractions/min	7
General medical condition	Po_2 < 60 mm Hg, Pco_2 > 50 mm Hg, K < 3 mmol/L, HCO_3 <20 mmol/L, BUN > 50 mg/dL, serum creatinine > 3 mg/dL, elevated AST, a chronic liver disorder, or bedbound	3
Type of surgery needed	Emergency surgery	4
	Intraperitoneal, intrathoracic, or aortic surgery	3

*Risk is based on the total number of points:
Level I: 0–5
Level II: 6–12
Level III: 13–25
Level IV: >25

Adapted from Goldman L et al: Multifactorial index of cardiac risk in noncardiac surgical procedures. *New England Journal of Medicine* 297:845–850, 1977.

being implanted, patients should be free of infection before surgery if possible.

Fluid and electrolyte imbalance should be corrected before surgery if possible. Dehydration should be treated with IV normal saline because BP tends to fall when anesthesia is induced. K deficiencies should be corrected to reduce risk of arrhythmias.

Undernutrition (see p. 10) increases surgical risk. Serum albumin < 2.8 g/dL increases morbidity. If an operation can be delayed for several weeks, sometimes nutritional deficiencies are correctable. Usually, the patient's calorie and protein intake should be increased during the perioperative period. Obesity is unlikely to be correctable in the time available.

PERIOPERATIVE MANAGEMENT

Usually, an anesthesiologist reviews a patient's drugs and stipulates which ones should be taken on the day of surgery. Such a review is necessary because some drugs interact with general anesthetics.

On the day of surgery, patients with insulin-dependent diabetes are typically given $\frac{1}{3}$ of their usual insulin dose in the morning. Those who take oral drugs are given $\frac{1}{2}$ of their usual dose. If possible, surgery is performed early in the day. The anesthesiologist monitors plasma glucose during surgery and gives additional insulin or dextrose as needed (see p. 1289); close monitoring with fingerstick testing continues throughout the perioperative period.

Many other drugs, especially cardiovascular drugs, including antihypertensives, should be continued throughout the perioperative period. Most oral drugs can be given with a small sip of water on the day of surgery. Others may have to be given parenterally or delayed until after surgery. In patients with a seizure disorder, anticonvulsant levels should be measured preoperatively.

Patients who are taking corticosteroids (mineralocorticoids or glucocorticoids) or have taken them within the previous 3 to 6 mo should be given supplemental doses of these drugs in case perioperative stress (eg, fluid shifts, hypotension) causes adrenal suppression.

Anticoagulants (eg, warfarin) and antiplatelet drugs (eg, aspirin) are usually stopped 5 to 7 days before surgery. However, if the procedure has a low risk of bleeding, an anticoagulant may be continued even on the day of the procedure, although risk of postoperative bleeding is slightly increased.

Patients who are dependent on drugs or alcohol may experience withdrawal during the perioperative period. Alcoholics should be given prophylactic, long-acting benzodiazepines (eg, chlordiazepoxide, diazepam, oxazepam) starting at admission. Opioid addicts may be given opioid analgesics to prevent withdrawal; they may require larger doses than patients who are not addicted. Rarely, opioid addicts require methadone to prevent withdrawal during the perioperative period.

Smokers are advised to stop smoking as early as possible before any procedure involving the chest or abdomen. Several weeks of smoking cessation are required for ciliary mechanisms to recover. An incentive inspirometer should be used before and after surgery.

Before intubation, dentures must be removed. Ideally, before patients are moved from the preanesthetic holding area, they should give dentures to a family member. Patients with a deviated septum or another airway abnormality should be evaluated by an anesthesiologist before surgery requiring intubation.

OUTPATIENT PROCEDURES

Many surgical procedures are performed in outpatient settings. Patients are evaluated (eg, with laboratory tests—see p. 2742) one to several days before the procedure.

The general rule is for patients to have no oral intake after midnight the night before surgery. For certain GI procedures, cleansing enemas or oral solutions must be started 1 to 2 days before surgery. When prophylactic antibiotics are needed before a procedure, the initial dose must be given within 1 h before the surgical incision.

If sedatives (eg, opioids, benzodiazepines) are used during an outpatient procedure, patients should not leave the hospital unaccompanied. Even after anesthetic effects have worn off, patients are likely to be weak and have subtle residual effects that make driving inadvisable; many patients require opioids for pain. Elderly patients may be temporarily disoriented because of the combined effects of anesthesia and surgical stress.

ANTIBIOTIC PROPHYLAXIS

Most surgical procedures do not require prophylactic or postoperative antibiotics. However, certain patient- and procedure-related factors alter the risk-benefit ratio in favor of prophylactic use.

Patient-related factors include valvular heart disorders and immunosuppression. Procedures with higher risk involve areas where bacterial seeding is likely (mouth, GI tract, respiratory tract, GU tract). In so-called clean (likely to be sterile) procedures, prophylaxis is beneficial generally only when prosthetic material or devices are being inserted or when the consequence of infection is known to be serious (eg, mediastinitis after coronary artery bypass grafting).

Drug choice is based on the bacteria most likely to contaminate the wound during a specific procedure. For commonly recommended regimens by procedure, see TABLE 335–2. Prophylaxis usually begins immediately before the procedure. Antibiotics may be given po or IV, depending on the procedure. The need for additional doses after the procedure is controversial (see TABLE 335–2), but for clean operations, no additional doses are needed. Postoperative prophylaxis is continued > 24 h only when an active infection is detected during surgery; antibiotics are then considered treatment, not prophylaxis.

POSTOPERATIVE CARE

Postoperative care begins in the recovery room and continues throughout the recovery period. Critical concerns are airway clearance, pain control, mental status, and wound healing. Preventing urinary retention, constipation, deep venous thrombosis, and BP variability (high or low) is also important. For patients with diabetes, plasma glucose levels are closely monitored by finger-stick testing q 1 to 4 h until patients are awake and eating, as glycemic control improves outcome.

Airway: Most patients are extubated before leaving the operating room and rapidly clear secretions from their airway. Patients should not leave the recovery room until they can clear and protect their airway (unless they are going to an ICU). After intubation, patients with normal lungs and trachea may have a mild cough for 24 h after extubation; for smokers and patients with a history of bronchitis, postextubation coughing lasts longer. Most patients who have been intubated, especially smokers and patients with a lung disorder, benefit from an incentive inspirometer.

Postoperative dyspnea may be caused by pain secondary to chest or abdominal incisions or by hypoxemia (see also p. 520). Hypoxemia is usually secondary to pulmonary dysfunction; oversedation sometimes causes hypoxemia in which the sensation of dyspnea is masked by the sedation. Pulmonary dysfunction is often due to atelectasis; fluid overload and heart failure must be considered, especially in patients with a history of heart failure. Whether dyspnea is hypoxic or nonhypoxic must be determined by pulse oximetry and sometimes ABGs; chest x-ray can help differentiate fluid overload from atelectasis.

Hypoxic dyspnea is treated with oxygen; nonhypoxic dyspnea may be treated with anxiolytics or analgesics.

Pain: Pain control may be necessary as soon as patients are conscious (see p. 1771). Opioids are typically the 1st-line choice and can be given orally or parenterally. Often, oxycodone/acetaminophen 2 tablets po q 4 to 6 h or morphine 2 to 4 mg IV q 3 h is given as a starting dose, which is subsequently adjusted as needed. With less frequent dosing, breakthrough pain, which should be avoided, is possible. For more severe pain, IV patient-controlled, on-demand dosing is best (see p. 1775). If patients do not have a renal disorder or a history of GI bleeding, giving NSAIDs at regular intervals may reduce breakthrough pain, allowing the opioid dosage to be reduced.

Mental status: All patients are briefly confused when they come out of anesthesia. The elderly, especially those with dementia, are at risk of postoperative delirium, which can delay discharge and increase risk of death. Risk of delirium is high when anticholinergic drugs are used. They are sometimes used before or during surgery to decrease upper airway secretions, but they should be avoided whenever possible. Opioids, given postoperatively, may also cause delirium, as can high doses of H_2 blockers. The mental status of elderly patients should be assessed frequently during the postoperative period. If delirium occurs, oxygenation should be assessed, and all nonessential drugs should be stopped. Patients should be mobilized as they are able, and any electrolyte or fluid imbalances should be corrected.

Wound care: Wound care should be meticulous. The surgeon must individualize care of each wound. Typically, dry sterile bandages are used. The site should be checked twice/day, if possible, for signs of infection (eg, increasing pain, erythema, drainage). If they occur, wound drainage, systemic antibiotics, or

TABLE 335–2. ANTIMICROBIAL PROPHYLAXIS FOR SURGERY

CATEGORY	PROCEDURE	ADULT DOSAGE*
Abdominal	Gastroduodenal surgery in patients with hemorrhage, cancer, obstruction, or other high-risk features	Cefazolin 1–2 g IV preoperatively *or* Clindamycin 600 mg plus gentamicin 120 mg IV preoperatively
	Gastric bypass	Cefazolin 1–2 g IV preoperatively
	Percutaneous gastrostomy	Cefazolin 1–2 g IV preoperatively
	Biliary tract (including ERCP) in patients who have acute symptoms, jaundice, or other high-risk features or who have had previous surgery	Cefazolin 1–2 g IV preoperatively *or* Gentamicin 80 mg IV preoperatively and q 8 h for 3 doses
	Appendectomy (without perforation)	Cefoxitin, cefotetan, or cefmetazole 1–2 g IV preoperatively and q 6 h for 3 doses *or* Metronidazole 500 mg plus gentamicin 1.5 mg/kg preoperatively
	Colorectal surgery, elective	Neomycin 1 g plus erythromycin base 1 g po at 1, 2, and 11 PM on the day before surgery ± parenteral drugs listed below for emergency surgery
	Colorectal surgery, emergency	Cefoxitin, cefotetan, or cefmetazole 2 g IV preoperatively and q 4 h for 3 doses *or* Metronidazole 500 mg IV plus gentamicin 1.7 mg/kg IV preoperatively and q 8 h for 3 doses
Cardiac	Median sternotomy, coronary artery bypass graft surgery, valve surgery, or pacemaker insertion	Cefazolin 2 g preoperatively and q 4–6 h intraoperatively *or* Cefuroxime 1.5 g IV preoperatively and q 4–6 h intraoperatively *or* Vancomycin 1 g preoperatively
Neurosurgery	Craniotomy, high-risk only (eg, reexplorations, microsurgery, entry into sinuses or nasopharynx)	Vancomycin 1g IV plus gentamicin 1.5 mg/kg IV preoperatively *or* Cefazolin 1 g IV preoperatively
	CSF shunt placement—only in hospitals with high infection rates (15–20%)	Trimethoprim 160 mg IV plus sulfamethoxazole 800 mg IV preoperatively and q 12 h for 3 doses *or* Vancomycin 10 mg plus gentamicin 3 mg injected into a cerebral ventricle
Noncardiac thoracic	Pneumonectomy, lobectomy, other resections, or esophageal surgery	Cefazolin 1–2 g IV preoperatively and q 6 h for 24 h *or* Vancomycin 1 g IV preoperatively
Obstetric-gynecologic	Cesarean section, high-risk only (eg, premature rupture of membranes)	Cefazolin 1 g IV after clamping cord and q 6 h for 2 doses

TABLE 335–2. ANTIMICROBIAL PROPHYLAXIS FOR SURGERY—Continued

CATEGORY	PROCEDURE	ADULT DOSAGE*
	Abortion, 2nd-trimester instillation	Cefazolin 1 g IV preoperatively and q 6 h for 2 doses
	Abortion, 1st trimester in patients with a history of pelvic inflammatory disease, gonorrhea, or multiple partners	Penicillin G 1–2 million units IV preoperatively and 3 h later *or* Doxycycline 100 mg po before the procedure and 200 mg 1/2 h afterward
	Hysterectomy, vaginal or abdominal	Cefazolin 1 g IV preoperatively and q 6 h for 2 doses *or* Doxycycline 200 mg IV preoperatively
Ophthalmic	Extraction of lens, with or without insertion of prosthesis	Gentamicin, tobramycin, or neomycin-gramicidin-polymyxin B drops over 2–24 h plus cefazolin 100 mg subconjunctivally at the end of the procedure
Orthopedic	Arthroplasty, including replacements	Cefazolin 1–2 g IV preoperatively and q 6 h for 3 doses *or* Vancomycin 1 g IV preoperatively
	Open reduction of fractures	Cefazolin 1 g IV preoperatively and q 6 h for 3 doses
	Lower-extremity amputation (nonischemic)	Cefoxitin 2 g IV preoperatively and q 6 h for 4 doses
Otolaryngologic	Major head and neck surgery involving mucosa of the oral cavity or pharynx	Cefazolin 1–2 g IV preoperatively and q 8 h for 2 doses *or* Clindamycin 600–900 mg IV ± gentamicin 1.5 mg/kg IV preoperatively and q 8 h for 2 doses
Urologic	Prostatectomy if bacteriuria is present	Cefazolin 1 g IV preoperatively or another drug selected based on susceptibility tests
	Penile prosthesis insertion	Cefazolin 1 g IV preoperatively
Vascular	Lower-extremity or abdominal arterial surgery or lower-extremity amputation for ischemia	Cefazolin 1–2 g IV preoperatively and q 6 h for 24 h *or* Vancomycin 1 g IV preoperatively and 12 h after the procedure

*Drugs, dosages, routes, and frequencies given represent current expert recommendations. Cefazolin remains highly favored because of its spectrum of bactericidal activity, long half-life, low cost, and low toxicity. Alternatives are primarily for patients with β-lactam allergies.

± = with or without.

Adapted from Kernodle DS, Kaiser AB: Postoperative infections and antimicrobial prophylaxis. In *Principles and Practice of Infectious Diseases*, ed 5, edited by GL Mandell, JE Bennett, and R Dolin. New York, Churchill Livingstone, 2000, pp. 3186–3187 and from Antimicrobial prophylaxis in surgery. *The Medical Letter* 37:79–82, 1995.

both may be required. Topical antibiotics are usually not helpful. A drain tube, if present, must be monitored for quantity and quality of the fluid collected. Sutures, skin staples, and other closures are usually left in place 7 days to 3 wk, depending on the site and the patient. Face and neck wounds may be superficially healed in 3 days; wounds on the lower extremities may take weeks to heal to a similar degree.

Deep venous thrombosis (DVT) prophylaxis: Risk of DVT after surgery is small but significant. Surgery itself increases coagulability and often requires prolonged immobility, another risk factor for DVT (see Chs. 50 and 81). Prophylaxis for DVT usually begins in the operating room (see TABLE 50–4 on p. 421). Alternatively, heparin may be started shortly after surgery, when risk of bleeding has decreased. Patients should begin moving their limbs as soon as it is safe for them to do so.

Other issues: Certain types of surgery require additional precautions. For example, hip surgery requires that patients be moved and positioned so that the hip does not dislocate. Any physician moving such patients for any reason, including auscultation of the lungs, must know the positioning protocol to avoid doing harm; often, a nurse is the best instructor.

Urinary retention and constipation are common after surgery. Causes include use of anticholinergic or opioid drugs, immobility, and decreased oral intake. Patients must be monitored for urinary retention. If patients have a distended bladder and are uncomfortable or if they have not urinated for 6 to 8 h after surgery, straight catheterization is typically necessary, although Credé's maneuver sometimes helps. Chronic retention is best treated by avoiding causative drugs and by having patients sit up as often as possible. Bethanechol 5 to 10 mg can be tried in patients unlikely to have any bladder obstruction and who have not had a laparotomy; doses can be repeated every hour up to a maximum of 50 mg/day. Sometimes a Foley catheter is needed, especially if patients have a history of retention or a large initial output after straight catheterization. Constipation is treated by avoiding causative drugs and, if patients have not had GI surgery, by giving stimulant laxatives (eg, bisacodyl, senna, cascara). Stool softeners (eg, docusate) do not help.

Prolonged bed rest causes loss of muscle mass (sarcopenia) and strength in all patients. With complete bed rest, young adults lose about 1% of muscle mass/day, but the elderly lose up to 5%/day because growth hormone levels decrease with aging. Avoiding sarcopenia is essential to recovery. Thus, as soon as safety allows, patients should sit up in bed, transfer, stand, and exercise as much as is safe for their surgical and medical condition.

336 REHABILITATION

Rehabilitation aims to facilitate recovery from loss of function. Loss may be due to fracture, amputation, stroke or another neurologic disorder, arthritis, cardiac impairment, or prolonged deconditioning (eg, after some disorders and surgical procedures). Rehabilitation may involve physical, occupational, and speech therapy; psychologic counseling; and social services. For some patients, the goal is complete recovery with full, unrestricted function; for others, it is recovery of the ability to perform as many activities of daily living (ADLs) as possible. Results of rehabilitation depend on the nature of the loss and the patient's motivation. Progress may be slow for elderly patients and for patients who lack muscle strength or motivation.

Rehabilitation may begin in an acute care hospital, but such hospitals rarely have intensive rehabilitation programs. Rehabilitation hospitals usually provide the most extensive and intensive care; they should be considered for patients who have good potential for recovery and can participate in and tolerate aggressive therapy (generally, ≥ 3 h/day). Many nursing homes have less intensive programs (generally, 1 to 3 h/day, up to 5 days/wk) and thus are better suited to patients less able to tolerate therapy (eg, frail or elderly patients). Less varied and less frequent rehabilitation programs may be offered in outpatient settings or at home and are appropriate for many patients. However, outpatient rehabilitation can be intensive (several hours/day up to 5 days/wk).

TABLE 336–1. NORMAL VALUES FOR RANGE OF MOTION OF JOINTS*

JOINT	MOTION	RANGE (°)
Hip	Flexion	0–125
	Extension	115–0
	Hyperextension†	0–15
	Abduction	0–45
	Adduction	45–0
	Lateral rotation	0–45
	Medial rotation	0–45
Knee	Flexion	0–130
	Extension	120–0
Ankle	Plantar flexion	0–50
	Dorsiflexion	0–20
Foot	Inversion	0–35
	Eversion	0–25
Metatarsophalangeal joints	Flexion	0–30
	Extension	0–80
Interphalangeal joints of toes	Flexion	0–50
	Extension	50–0
Shoulder	Flexion to 90°	0–90
	Extension	0–50
	Abduction to 90°	0–90
	Adduction	90–0
	Lateral rotation	0–90
	Medial rotation	0–90
Elbow	Flexion	0–160
	Extension	145–0
	Pronation	0–90
	Supination	0–90
Wrist	Flexion	0–90
	Extension	0–70
	Abduction	0–25
	Adduction	0–65
Metacarpophalangeal joints	Abduction	0–25
	Adduction	20–0
	Flexion	0–90
	Extension	0–30
Interphalangeal proximal joints of fingers	Flexion	0–120
	Extension	120–0
Interphalangeal distal joints of fingers	Flexion	0–80
	Extension	80–0
Metacarpophalangeal joint of thumb	Abduction	0–50
	Adduction	40–0
	Flexion	0–70
	Extension	60–0
Interphalangeal joint of thumb	Flexion	0–90
	Extension	90–0

*Ranges are for people of all ages. Age-specific ranges have not been established; however, values are typically lower in fully functional elderly people than in younger people.

†Extension beyond midline.

To initiate formal rehabilitation therapy, a physician must write a referral/prescription to a physiatrist, therapist, or rehabilitation center. The referral/prescription should state the diagnosis and goal of therapy. The diagnosis may be specific (eg, after left-sided stroke, residual right-sided deficits in upper and lower extremities) or functional (eg, generalized weakness due to bed rest). Goals should be as specific as possible (eg, training to use a prosthetic limb, maximizing general muscle strength and overall endurance). Although vague instructions (eg, "physical therapy to evaluate and treat") are often accepted, they are not optimal. Physicians unfamiliar with writing referrals for rehabilitation can consult a therapist, physiatrist, or orthopedic surgeon.

An interdisciplinary approach is best because disability can lead to various problems (eg, depression, lack of motivation to regain lost function, financial problems). Thus, patients may require psychologic intervention and help from social workers. Also, family members may need help learning how to adjust to the patient's disability and to help the patient.

Initial evaluation sets goals for restoring functions needed to perform ADLs, which include caring for self (eg, grooming, bathing, dressing, feeding, toileting), cooking, cleaning, shopping, managing drugs, managing finances, using the telephone, and traveling. The referring physician and rehabilitation team determine which activities are achievable and which are essential for the patient's independence. Once ADL function is maximized, goals that can help improve quality of life are added.

Patients improve at different rates. Some courses of therapy last only a few weeks; others last longer. Some patients who have completed initial therapy need additional therapy.

PHYSICAL THERAPY

Physical therapy aims to improve joint and muscle function (eg, range of motion) and thus improve the patient's ability to stand, balance, walk, and climb stairs. For example, physical therapy is usually used to train lower-extremity amputees.

Limited range of motion impairs function and tends to cause pain (for normal values, see TABLE 336–1). Range-of-motion exercises stretches stiff joints. Stretching is usually most effective and least painful when tissue temperature is raised to about 43° C (see p. 2753).

Active range-of-motion exercise is used when patients can exercise without assistance;

TABLE 336–2. GRADES OF MUSCLE STRENGTH

GRADE	DESCRIPTION
5 or N	Full range of motion against gravity and full resistance for the patient's size, age, and sex
N–	Slight weakness
G+	Moderate weakness
4 or G	Movement against gravity and moderate resistance at least 10 times without fatigue
F+	Movement against gravity several times or mild resistance one time
3 or F	Full range against gravity
F–	Movement against gravity and complete range of motion one time
P+	Full range of motion with gravity eliminated but some resistance applied
2 or P	Full range of motion with gravity eliminated
P–	Incomplete range of motion with gravity eliminated
1 or T	Evidence of contraction (visible or palpable) but no joint movement
0	No palpable or visible contraction and no joint movement

N = normal; G = good; F = fair; P = poor; T = trace.

patients must move their limbs themselves. Active assistive range-of-motion exercise is used when muscles are weak or when joint movement causes discomfort; patients must move their limbs, but a therapist helps them do so. Passive range-of-motion exercise is used when patients cannot actively participate in exercise; no effort is required from patients.

Many exercises aim to improve muscle strength (for grading muscle strength, see TABLE 336–2). Muscle strength may be increased with progressive resistive exercise. When a muscle is very weak, gravity alone is sufficient resistance. When muscle strength becomes fair, additional manual or mechanical resistance (eg, weights, spring tension) is needed.

General conditioning exercises combine various exercises to treat the effects of debilitation, prolonged bed rest, or immobilization. The goals are to reestablish hemodynamic balance, increase cardiorespiratory capacity, and maintain range of motion and muscle strength.

Proprioceptive neuromuscular facilitation helps promote neuromuscular activity in patients who have upper motor neuron damage with spasticity. For example, applying strong resistance to the left elbow flexor (biceps) of patients with right hemiplegia causes the hemiplegic biceps to contract, flexing the right elbow.

Coordination exercises improve motor skills by repeating a movement that works more than one joint and muscle simultaneously.

Before proceeding to ambulation exercises, patients must be able to balance in a standing position. Balancing exercise is usually done using parallel bars with a therapist standing in front of or directly behind the patient. While holding the bars, patients shift weight from side to side and from forward to backward. Once patients can balance safely, they can proceed to ambulation exercises.

Ambulation is often the main goal of rehabilitation. If individual muscles are weak or spastic, an orthosis (eg, a brace) may be used (see p. 2751). Ambulation exercises are commonly started using parallel bars; as patients progress, they use a walker, crutches, or cane and then walk without devices. Some patients wear an assistive belt used by the therapist to help prevent falls. Anyone assisting patients with ambulation should know how to correctly support them (see FIG. 336–1).

Transfer training is particularly important after a hip fracture, amputation, or stroke. Transferring safely is critical to remaining at home. Patients who cannot transfer independently from bed to chair, chair to commode, or chair to a standing position usually require attendants 24 h/day. Adjusting the heights of commodes and chairs may help; sometimes assistive devices are useful.

OCCUPATIONAL THERAPY

Occupational therapy focuses on self-care activities and improvement of fine motor coordination of muscles and joints, particularly in the upper extremities. Occupational

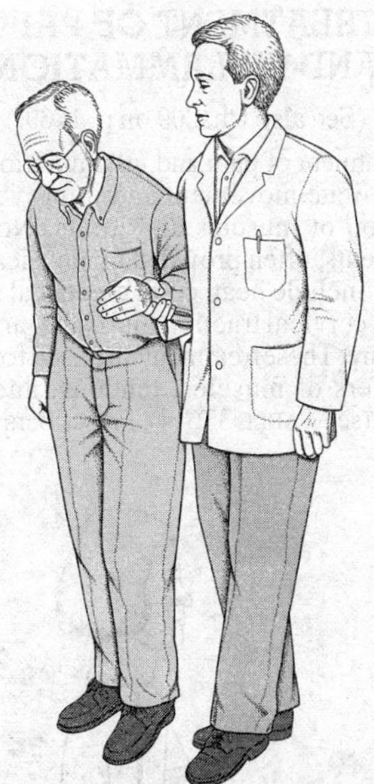

Fig. 336–1. Supporting a patient during ambulation. Aides should place one arm under that of the patient, gently grasp the patient's forearm, and lock their arm firmly under the patient's axilla. Thus, if the patient starts to fall, the aide can provide support at the patient's shoulder. If a patient is wearing a waist belt, the aide uses his free hand to grasp the belt.

therapy develops a patient's ability to handle everyday objects as they are intended for use. After observing a patient's performance, the therapist may identify various assistive devices that can help the patient perform many activities of daily living. Most occupational therapists can select wheelchairs appropriate for the patient's needs and provide training for upper-extremity amputees. Occupational therapists may construct and fit devices to prevent contractures and treat other functional disorders. Occupational therapists may also assess a patient's home for hazards and make recommendations to ensure that self-care activities can be done safely.

THERAPEUTIC AND ASSISTIVE DEVICES

Orthoses provide support for damaged joints, ligaments, tendons, muscles, and bones. Most are customized to a patient's needs and anatomy. Orthoses designed to fit into shoes may shift the patient's weight to different parts of the foot to compensate for lost function, prevent deformity or injury, help bear weight, or relieve pain, as well as provide support.

Walking aids include walkers, crutches, and canes (see FIG. 336–2). They help with weight bearing, balance, or both. Each device has advantages and disadvantages, and each is available in several models. After evaluation, a therapist should choose the one that provides the best combination of stability and freedom for the patient (see TABLE 336–3). Most physicians are unfamiliar with how to prescribe such device, but they should know how to fit crutches (see FIG. 336–3).

Wheelchairs provide mobility to patients who cannot walk. Some models are designed to be self-propelled and to provide stability

TABLE 336–3. AMBULATION AIDS

CHARACTERISTIC	WALKER	CRUTCHES	CANES
Stability	Very good	Good	Least stable
Walking speed	Slowest	Slow	Can be fast
Use on steps	None	Training needed	Easy
Strength of arms required for use	Normal	Moderate strength	Normal
Number of hands required for use	2	Usually 2	Usually 1
Possibility of carrying objects	Requires attachment of basket	None	Possible
Cost	Most expensive	Relatively inexpensive	Least expensive

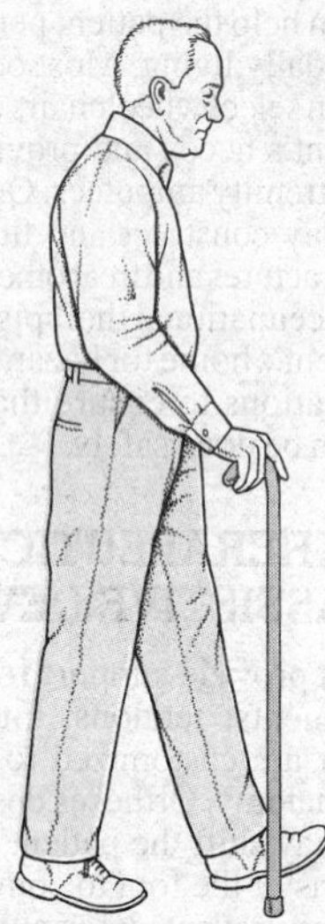

Fig. 336–2. Correct cane height. The patient's elbow should be bent at slightly less than 45° when maximum force is applied.

for traveling over uneven ground and up and down curbs. Other models are designed to be pushed by an assistant; they provide less stability and speed. Wheelchairs are available with various features. For athletic patients with impaired lower extremities but good upper body strength, racing wheelchairs are available. A one-arm–drive or hemi-height wheelchair may be suitable for hemiplegic patients with good coordination. If patients have little or no arm function, a motorized wheelchair is prescribed. Wheelchairs for quadriplegics may have chin or mouth (sip and puff) controls and built-in ventilators.

Prostheses are artificial limbs designed to replace lower or upper extremities after amputation. Technical innovations have greatly improved the comfort and functionality of prostheses. Many prostheses can be cosmetically altered to appear natural. A prosthetist should be consulted early to help patients understand the many options in prosthetic design, which should meet the patient's needs and safety requirements. Many patients can expect to regain considerable function. Physical therapy should be started even before the prosthesis is fitted; therapy should continue until patients can function with the new limb.

TREATMENT OF PAIN AND INFLAMMATION

(See also Ch. 209 on p. 1769.)

Treatment of pain and inflammation aims to facilitate movement and improve coordination of muscles and joints. Nondrug treatments, often provided by physical therapists, include heat, cold, electrical stimulation, cervical traction, massage, and acupuncture. These treatments are used for many disorders of muscles, tendons, and ligaments (see TABLE 336–4). Prescribers should

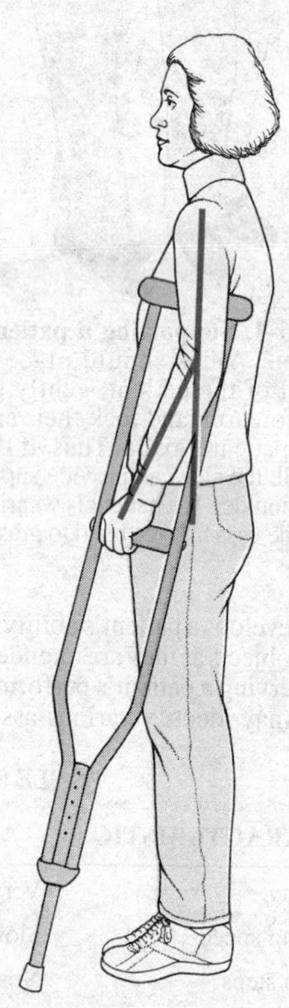

Fig. 336–3. Fitting crutches. Patients should wear the type of shoes usually worn, stand erect, and look straight ahead with the shoulders relaxed. For a correct fit, the end of each crutch should be placed about 5 cm from the side of the shoe and about 15 cm in front of the toe, and the top of the crutch should be about 2 to 3 finger widths (about 5 cm) below the axilla. The hand grip should be adjusted so that the elbow bends 20 to 30°.

include the diagnosis, type of treatment (eg, ultrasound, hot pack), location of application (eg, right shoulder, low back), frequency (eg, once/day, every other day), and duration (eg, 10 days, 1 wk). More detail (eg, dosage, duration of individual treatments) is unnecessary because therapists make such decisions. If physicians are unsure of which treatment is needed, they can consult a physical therapist.

Heat: Heat provides temporary relief in subacute and chronic traumatic and inflammatory disorders (eg, sprains, strains, fibrositis, tenosynovitis, muscle spasm, myositis, back pain, whiplash injuries, various forms of arthritis, arthralgia, neuralgia). Heat increases blood flow and the extensibility of connective tissue; heat also decreases joint stiffness, pain, and muscle spasm and helps relieve inflammation, edema, and exudates. Heat application may be superficial or deep. Intensity and duration of the physiologic effects depend mainly on tissue temperature, rate of temperature elevation, and area treated.

Infrared heat is applied with a lamp, usually for 20 min/day. Contraindications include any advanced heart disorder, peripheral vascular disease, impaired skin sensation (particularly to temperature and pain), and significant hepatic or renal insufficiency. Precautions must be taken to avoid burns.

Hot packs are cotton cloth containers filled with silicate gel; they are boiled in water or warmed in a microwave oven, then applied to the skin. The packs must not be too hot. Wrapping the packs in several layers of towels helps protect the skin from burns. Contraindications are the same as for infrared heat.

For a paraffin bath, the affected area is dipped in, immersed in, or painted with melted wax that has been heated to 49° C. The heat can be retained by wrapping the affected area with towels for 20 min. Paraffin is usually applied to small joints—typically, by dipping or immersion for a hand and by painting for a knee or an elbow. Paraffin should not be applied to open wounds or used on patients allergic to it.

Hydrotherapy may be used to enhance wound healing. Agitated warm water stimulates blood flow and debrides burns and wounds. This treatment is often given in a Hubbard tank (a large industrial whirlpool) with water heated to 35.5 to 37.7° C. Total immersion in water heated to 37.7 to 40° C may

TABLE 336–4. INDICATIONS FOR NONDRUG PAIN TREATMENTS

TREATMENT	INDICATIONS
Heat (eg, infrared heat, hot packs, paraffin bath, hydrotherapy)	Arthralgia Arthritis (various forms) Back pain Fibrositis Muscle spasm Myositis Neuralgia Sprains Strains Tenosynovitis Whiplash injuries
Diathermy (short wave or microwave)	Pain due to pelvic infections Pain due to sinusitis (acute or chronic) Pain due to urinary calculi
Ultrasound	Bone injuries Bursitis Complex regional pain syndrome Contractures Osteoarthritis Tendinitis
Cold	Inflammation (acute) Low back pain (acute) Muscle spasm Myofascial pain Traumatic pain
Transcutaneous electrical nerve stimulation (TENS)	Neuralgia, musculoskeletal pain, peripheral vascular disease
Cervical traction	Disk prolapse pain Neck pain (chronic) due to cervical spondylosis Torticollis Whiplash injuries
Massage	Arthritis* Bruises Bursitis* Cerebral palsy* Contracted tissues Fibrositis* Fractures Hemiplegia* Joint injuries Low back pain* Multiple sclerosis* Neuritis* Paraplegia* Periarthritis* Peripheral nerve injuries Quadriplegia* Sprain Strain
Acupuncture†	Pain (chronic) Stroke (to enhance rehabilitation)

*Massage should be considered.
†Acupuncture is used with other treatments.

also help relax muscles and relieve pain. Hydrotherapy is particularly useful with range-of-motion exercises.

Short wave diathermy is therapeutic heating of tissues using oscillating high-frequency electromagnetic fields. It is applied with capacitor plates or inductive coil applicators. Short wave diathermyis rarely very effective; however, it is sometimes used to treat the pain of urinary calculi, pelvic infections, or acute and chronic sinusitis. Contraindications include cancer, hemorrhagic disorders, peripheral vascular disease, loss of sensation, and nonremovable prostheses, pacemakers, or electrophysiologic braces. (CAUTION: *Short wave diathermy cannot be used if patients have metal implants in or near the area to be treated.*)

Microwave diathermy is simpler to apply and more comfortable than short wave diathermy, and output can be adjusted more accurately. Microwave diathermy provides deeper heat without undue heating of the skin because microwaves (a form of electromagnetic radiation) are selectively absorbed in tissues with a high water content (eg, muscles). With a direct-contact applicator, 915-MHz microwave diathermy heats muscles uniformly. Indications and contraindications are the same as for short wave diathermy.

Ultrasound uses high-frequency sound waves to penetrate deep (4 to 10 cm) into the tissue; its effects are thermal, mechanical, chemical, and biologic. It is indicated for tendinitis, bursitis, contractures, osteoarthritis, bone injuries, and complex regional pain syndrome. Ultrasound should not be applied to ischemic tissue, anesthetized areas, or areas of acute infection nor be used to treat hemorrhagic diathesis or cancer. Also, it should not be applied over the eyes, brain, spinal cord, ears, heart, reproductive organs, brachial plexus, or bones that are healing.

Cold: The choice between heat and cold therapies is often empiric. When heat does not work, cold is applied. However, for acute injury or pain, cold seems to be better than heat. Cold may help relieve muscle spasm, myofascial or traumatic pain, acute low back pain, and acute inflammation; cold may also help induce some local anesthesia. Cold is usually used during the first few hours or the day after an injury; consequently, it is seldom used in physical therapy.

Cold may be applied locally using an ice bag, a cold pack, or volatile fluids (eg, ethyl chloride, vapocoolant spray), which cool by evaporation. The spread of cold on the skin depends on the thickness of the epidermis, underlying fat and muscle, water content of the tissue, and rate of blood flow. Care must be taken to avoid tissue damage and hypothermia. Cold should not be applied over poorly perfused areas.

Electrical stimulation: Transcutaneous electrical nerve stimulation (TENS) uses low current at low-frequency oscillation to relieve pain. Patients feel a gentle tingling sensation without increased muscle tension. Depending on the severity of pain, 20 min to a few hours of stimulation may be applied several times daily. Often, patients are taught to use the TENS device and decide when to apply treatment. Because TENS may cause arrhythmia, it is contraindicated in patients with any advanced heart disorder or a pacemaker. It should not be applied over the eyes.

Cervical traction: Cervical traction is often indicated for chronic neck pain due to cervical spondylosis, disk prolapse, whiplash injuries, or torticollis. Vertical traction (with patients in a sitting position) is more effective than horizontal traction (with patients lying in bed). Motorized intermittent rhythmic traction with 7.5 to 10 kg is most effective. For best results, traction should be applied with the patient's neck flexed 15 to 20°. Generally, hyperextension of the neck should be avoided because it may increase nerve root compression in the intervertebral foramina. Traction is usually combined with other physical therapy, including exercises and manual stretching.

Massage: Massage may mobilize contracted tissues, relieve pain, and reduce swelling and induration associated with trauma (eg, fracture, joint injury, sprain, strain, bruise, peripheral nerve injury). Massage should be considered for low back pain, arthritis, periarthritis, bursitis, neuritis, fibrositis, hemiplegia, paraplegia, quadriplegia, multiple sclerosis, and cerebral palsy. It should not be used to treat infections or thrombophlebitis. Only a licensed massage therapist should perform massage for treatment of an injury.

Acupuncture: Thin needles are inserted through the skin at specific body sites, frequently far from the site of pain (see p. 2723). Acupuncture is sometimes used with other treatments to manage chronic pain and to enhance rehabilitation after stroke.

REHABILITATION FOR SOME SPECIFIC PROBLEMS

Blindness: Patients are taught to rely more on the other senses, to develop specific skills, and to use devices for the blind (eg, Braille, cane, reading machine). Therapy aims to help restore psychologic security and help patients deal with and influence the attitudes of others. Therapy varies depending on the way vision was lost (suddenly or slowly and progressively), extent of vision loss, the patient's functional needs, and coexisting deficits. For example, patients with peripheral neuropathy and diminished tactile sensation in the fingers may have difficulty reading Braille. Many blind people need psychologic counseling (usually cognitive-behavioral therapy) to help them better cope with their condition.

For ambulation, therapy may involve learning to use a cane; canes used by the blind are usually white and longer and thinner than ordinary canes. People who use a wheelchair are taught to use one arm to operate the wheelchair and the other to use a cane. People who prefer to use a trained dog instead of a cane are taught to handle and care for the dog. When walking with a sighted person, a blind person can hold onto the bent elbow of the sighted person, rather than use an ambulation aid. The sighted person should not lead the blind person by the hand.

Speech problems: Speech therapists can identify the most effective methods of communication for patients who have aphasia, dysarthria, or verbal apraxia or who have undergone laryngectomy. Patients with expressive aphasia may use a letter or picture board. Breathing and muscle control plus repetition exercises may help patients with mild to moderate dysarthria or apraxia. Those with severe dysarthria or apraxia may use an electronic device with a keyboard and message display (print or screen). After laryngectomy, patients require a new way to produce a voice (eg, by an electrolarynx—see p. 841).

Cardiovascular disorders: Rehabilitation may benefit some patients who have coronary artery disease or heart failure or who have had a recent MI or coronary artery bypass surgery, particularly those who could perform activities of daily living independently and walk before the event. Cardiac rehabilitation aims to help patients maintain or regain independence (see p. 652).

Typically, rehabilitation begins with light activities and progresses; ECG monitoring is often used. When patients are able, they are taken by wheelchair to a physical therapy gym. Exercise may involve walking, a treadmill, or a stationary bicycle. When patients tolerate these exercises well, they progress to stair-climbing. If shortness of breath, light-headedness, or chest pain occurs during exercise, the exercise should be stopped immediately, and cardiac status should be reassessed. Before hospital discharge, patients are assessed so that an appropriate postdischarge rehabilitation program or exercise regimen can be recommended.

Stroke: Rehabilitation aims to preserve or improve range of motion, muscle strength, bowel and bladder function, and functional and cognitive abilities. Specific programs are based on the patient's social situation (eg, prospects of returning to home or work), ability to participate in a rehabilitation program supervised by nurses and therapists, learning ability, motivation, and coping skills. As soon as patients are medically stable, rehabilitation should begin to prevent secondary disabilities (eg, contractures, pressure ulcers) and help prevent depression. Patients can safely begin sitting up once they are fully conscious and neurologic deficits are no longer progressing, usually ≤ 48 h after the stroke.

Resistive exercise for hemiplegic extremities may increase spasticity and thus is controversial. A gait abnormality in hemiplegic patients is caused by many factors (eg, muscle weakness, spasticity, distorted body image) and is thus difficult to correct. Also, attempts to correct gait often increase spasticity, may result in muscle fatigue, and may increase the already high risk of falls, which often result in a hip fracture; functional prognosis of hemiplegic patients with a hip fracture is very poor. Consequently, as long as hemiplegic patients can walk safely and comfortably, gait correction should not be tried.

Leg amputation: Rehabilitation teaches ambulation skills; it includes exercises to improve general conditioning and balance, to stretch the hip and knee, to strengthen all extremities, and to help patients tolerate the prosthesis. As soon as patients are medically stable, rehabilitation should be started to help prevent secondary disabilities. Flexion contracture of the hip or knee may develop rapidly, making fitting and using the prosthesis difficult; contractures can be prevented with extension braces made by occupational therapists. Exercise assists the natural process of shrinking that must occur before a prosthesis can be used. All stumps must be tapered, so an elastic stump shrinker or elastic bandages are applied and maintained on a 24-h basis. Physical therapists teach amputees how to care for the stump and how to recognize the earliest signs of skin breakdown.

Phantom limb sensation, a painless awareness of the amputated limb possibly accompanied by tingling, is experienced by some new amputees. This sensation may last several months or years but usually disappears without treatment. Phantom limb pain is less common and can be severe and difficult to control. Some experts think it is more likely to occur if the patient had a painful condition before amputation or if pain was not adequately controlled intraoperatively and postoperatively. Various treatments, such as simultaneous exercise of amputated and contralateral limbs, massage of the stump, finger percussion of the stump, use of mechanical devices (eg, a vibrator), and ultrasound, are reportedly effective. Drugs (eg, gabapentin) may help.

The most common cause of stump pain is a poorly fitted prosthetic socket. Other common causes are neuroma and spur formation at the amputated end of the bone. An amputation neuroma is usually palpable. Daily ultrasound treatment for 5 to 10 sessions may be most effective. Other treatments include injection of corticosteroids or analgesics into the neuroma or the surrounding area, cryotherapy, and continuous tight bandaging of the stump. Surgical resection often has disappointing results. Spurs may be diagnosed by palpation and x-ray. The only effective treatment of a spur is surgical resection.

Head injury: The term head injury is often used interchangeably with traumatic brain injury (TBI—see p. 2572). Abnormalities vary and may include muscle weakness, spasticity, incoordination, and ataxia; cognitive dysfunction (eg, memory loss, loss of problem-solving skills, language and visual disturbances) is common.

Early intervention by rehabilitation specialists is indispensable for maximal functional recovery. Such intervention includes prevention of secondary disabilities (eg, pressure ulcers, joint contractures), prevention of pneumonia, and family education. As early as possible, rehabilitation specialists should evaluate patients to establish baseline findings. Later, before starting rehabilitation therapy, patients should be reevaluated; these findings are compared with baseline findings to help prioritize treatment. Patients with severe cognitive dysfunction require extensive cognitive therapy.

Spinal cord injury: Specific rehabilitation therapy varies depending on the patient's abnormalities, which depend on the level and extent (partial or complete) of the injury (see Ch. 311 and TABLE 311–1 on p. 2580). Complete transsection causes flaccid paralysis; partial transsection causes spastic paralysis of muscles innervated by the affected segment. A patient's functional capacity depends on the level of injury (see p. 1909) and the development of complications (eg, joint contractures, pressure ulcers, pneumonia).

The affected area must be immobilized surgically or nonsurgically as soon as possible and throughout the acute phase. During the acute phase, daily routine care should include measures to prevent contractures, pressure ulcers, and pneumonia; all measures needed to prevent other complications (eg, orthostatic hypotension, atelectasis, deep venous thrombosis, pulmonary embolism) should also be taken. Placing patients on a tilt table and increasing the angle gradually toward the upright position may help reestablish hemodynamic balance. Compression stockings, an elastic bandage, or an abdominal binder may prevent orthostatic hypotension.

Minor injuries: Rehabilitation may be needed after minor injuries (eg, sprains, isolated distal extremity fractures).

337 GERIATRIC MEDICINE

Geriatrics refers to medical care for the elderly, an age group that is not easy to define precisely; "older people" is sometimes preferred but is equally imprecise. Gerontology is the study of aging, including biologic, sociologic, and psychologic changes.

Most age-related biologic functions peak before age 30 and gradually decline linearly thereafter (see TABLE 337–1); the decline may be critical during stress, but it generally has little or no effect on daily activities. Therefore, disorders, rather than normal aging, are the primary cause of functional loss during old age. Also, in many cases, the declines that occur with aging may be due at least partly to lifestyle, behavior, diet, or environment and thus can be modified. For example, aerobic exercise can prevent or partially reverse declines in maximal exercise capacity (O_2 consumption per unit time, or $V{O_2}max$), muscle strength, and glucose tolerance in healthy but sedentary older people. The unmodifiable effects of aging may be less dramatic than thought, and healthier, more vigorous aging may be possible for many people.

Demographics: Around 1900 in the US, people > 65 accounted for 4% of the population; now, they account for > 13% (37 million, with a net gain of > 1000/day). In 2026, when post–World War II baby boomers begin to reach age 80, estimates suggest that > 20% (almost 80 million) will be > 65. The mean age of those > 65 is now a little over 75, and the proportion of those > 85 is predicted to continue to increase.

For men, life expectancy is 16 yr at age 65 and 9 yr at age 75. For women, life expectancy is 19 yr at age 65 and 12 yr at age 75. Overall, women live about 5 yr longer than men, probably because of genetic, biologic, and environmental factors. These differences in survival have not changed, despite changes in women's lifestyle (eg, increased smoking, increased stress). Maximum human life span (estimated at 110 to 120 yr) has increased modestly compared with the substantial increase in average life expectancy during this century but continues to increase without slowing of the rate. People > 65 are in better health than their predecessors and remain healthier longer. Because of these improvements in health, decline tends to be most dramatic in the oldest old.

Approach to the elderly patient: The elderly have different, often more complicated, health care needs. On average, an elderly patient has 6 diagnosable disorders, and the primary care physician is often unaware of some of them. A disorder in one organ system can weaken another system, exacerbating the deterioration of both and leading to disability, dependence, and, without intervention, death. Multiple disorders complicate diagnosis and treatment, and the effects of the disorders are magnified by social disadvantage (eg, isolation) and poverty (as patients outlive their resources and supportive peers).

Certain common geriatric symptoms (eg, dizziness, syncope, falling, mobility problems, weight or appetite loss) require particular attention because they may result from disorders of multiple organ systems. Also, physicians should use the history, physical examination, and simple laboratory tests to actively screen elderly patients for disorders that occur only or commonly in the elderly (see TABLE 337–2); many of these disorders are often missed and can be more easily treated when diagnosed early. Common treatable disorders include vitamin B_{12} deficiency, iron deficiency anemia, hypothyroidism, heart failure, GI bleeding, diabetes mellitus, foot disorders interfering with mobility, oral disorders interfering with eating, hearing and vision abnormalities, dementia, and depression. In the elderly, these disorders are often diagnosed late or missed or, if noticed, may be erroneously attributed to aging. Prescription and OTC drug use should be reviewed frequently, particularly for drug interactions and use of drugs considered inappropriate for the elderly (see p. 2534); computer-based management is more efficient when multiple drugs are used. Early detection of disorders or potential drug interactions results in early intervention, which can prevent deterioration and improve quality of life often through relatively minor, inexpensive interventions (eg, lifestyle changes).

Caring for elderly patients with multiple disorders requires good diagnostic, analytic, and interpersonal skills. Often, early diagnosis depends on the clinician's familiarity with the patient's behavior and history, including mental status. Commonly, the first signs of a

TABLE 337–1. SELECTED PHYSIOLOGIC AGE-RELATED CHANGES

AFFECTED ORGAN OR SYSTEM	PHYSIOLOGIC CHANGE	CLINICAL MANIFESTATIONS
Body composition	↓Lean body mass ↓Muscular mass ↓Creatinine production ↓Skeletal mass ↓Total body water ↑ Percentage adipose tissue (until age 60, then ↓until death)	Changes in drug levels ↓Strength Tendency toward dehydration
Cells	DNA damage and ↓DNA repair capacity ↓Oxidative capacity Accelerated cell senescence ↑ Fibrosis Lipofuscin accumulation	↑ Cancer risk
CNS	↓Number of dopamine receptors ↑ α-Adrenergic responses ↑ Muscarinic parasympathetic responses	Tendency to parkinsonian symptoms (eg, ↑ muscle tone, ↓arm swing)
Ears	Loss of high-frequency hearing	↓Ability to recognize speech
Endocrine system	Menopause, ↓estrogen and progesterone secretion ↓Testosterone secretion ↓Growth hormone secretion ↓Vitamin D absorption and activation ↑ Incidence of thyroid abnormalities ↑ Incidence of diabetes (↓insulin sensitivity or ↑ insulin resistance) ↑ Bone mineral loss ↑ Secretion of ADH in response to osmolar stimuli	↓Muscle mass ↓Bone mass ↑ Fracture risk Vaginal dryness Changes in skin Water intoxication
Eyes	↓Lens flexibility ↑ Time for pupillary reflexes (constriction, dilation) ↑ Incidence of cataracts	Presbyopia ↑ Glare and difficulty adjusting to changes in lighting ↓Visual acuity
GI tract	↓Splanchnic blood flow ↑ Transit time	Tendency toward constipation and diarrhea
Heart	↓Intrinsic heart rate and maximal heart rate Blunted baroreflex Cardiac acceleration ↓Diastolic relaxation ↑ Atrioventricular conduction time ↑ Atrial and ventricular ectopy	Tendency toward syncope ↓Ejection fraction
Immune system	↓T-cell function ↓B-cell function	Tendency toward some infections and possibly cancer ↓Antibody response to immunization or infection but ↑ autoantibodies

TABLE 337–1. SELECTED PHYSIOLOGIC AGE-RELATED CHANGES—Continued

AFFECTED ORGAN OR SYSTEM	PHYSIOLOGIC CHANGE	CLINICAL MANIFESTATIONS
Joints	Degeneration of cartilaginous tissues Fibrosis ↓Elasticity	Tightening of joints Tendency toward osteoarthritis
Kidneys	↓Renal blood flow ↓Renal mass ↓Glomerular filtration ↓Renal tubular secretion and reabsorption ↓Ability to excrete a free-water load	Changes in drug levels with ↑ risk of adverse drug effects Tendency toward dehydration
Liver	↓Hepatic mass ↓Hepatic blood flow ↓Activity of P-450 enzyme system	Changes in drug levels
Nose	↓Smell	↓Taste and consequent ↓appetite ↑Likelihood (slightly) of nosebleeds
Peripheral nervous system	↓Baroreflex responses ↓β-Adrenergic responsiveness and number of receptors ↓Signal transduction ↓Muscarinic parasympathetic responses Preserved α-adrenergic responses	Tendency toward syncope ↓Response to β-blockers Exaggerated response to anticholinergic drugs
Pulmonary system	↓Vital capacity ↓Lung elasticity (compliance) ↑Residual volume ↓FEV_1 ↑ V/Q mismatch	↑Likelihood of shortness of breath during vigorous exercise if people are normally sedentary or if exercise is done at high altitudes ↑Risk of death due to pneumonia ↑Risk of serious complications for patients with a pulmonary disorder
Vasculature	↓Endothelin-dependent vasodilation ↑ Peripheral resistance	Tendency toward hypertension

↓ = decreased; ↑ = increased; FEV_1 = forced expiratory volume in 1 sec; V/Q = ventilation/perfusion.

Adapted from the Institute of Medicine: *Pharmacokinetics and Drug Interactions in the Elderly Workshop.* Washington DC, National Academy Press, 1997, pp. 8–9.

physical disorder, often at a treatable stage, are mental or emotional. If clinicians are unaware of this possibility and attribute these signs to dementia, diagnosis and treatment can be delayed.

If patients have multiple disorders, treatments (eg, bed rest, surgery, drugs) must be well integrated and monitored to avoid iatrogenic consequences. With complete bed rest, elderly patients can lose 5 to 6% of muscle mass and strength each day (sarcopenia), and the effects of bed rest alone can ultimately result in death. Treating one disorder without treating associated disorders may accelerate decline.

Interdisciplinary care: For the above reasons, many elderly patients require interdisciplinary care—coordinated care, typically by physicians, nurses, pharmacists, and sometimes dietitians, physical and occupational therapists, and social workers. For the oldest patients and those with complex conditions, care is usually best managed by a geriatrician. Occasionally, an ethicist or hospice physician is needed. Interdisciplinary care aims to ensure that patients move safely and easily from one place of care to another and from one health care practitioner to another. It also aims to ensure that the most qualified health care practitioner provides care for each problem and that care is not duplicated. Interdisciplinary care is not available everywhere.

TABLE 337–2. DISORDERS COMMON AMONG THE ELDERLY

FREQUENCY	DISORDERS
Almost exclusive in the elderly	Accidental hypothermia Normal-pressure hydrocephalus Urinary incontinence
More common in the elderly than among other age groups	Basal cell carcinoma Chronic lymphocytic leukemia Degenerative osteoarthritis Dementia Diabetic hyperosmolar nonketotic coma Falls Herpes zoster Hip fracture Monoclonal gammopathies Osteoporosis Parkinsonism Polymyalgia rheumatica Pressure ulcers Prostate cancer Stroke Temporal arteritis (giant cell arteritis)

HEALTH CARE DELIVERY

Because the elderly tend to have multiple disorders and may have social or functional problems, they use a disproportionately large amount of health care resources. In the US, they account for > 40% of acute hospital bed days, buy > 30% of prescription and 40% of OTC drugs, and use 33% of the > $1.4 trillion health budget and > 75% of the federal health budget.

Sometimes the elderly unintentionally delay delivery of health care. Many elderly people believe that not feeling well is a natural, unavoidable part of aging. Thus, they often do not tell a physician about symptoms that may indicate serious but treatable disorders, although they may tell family members. Depression (which is common), the cumulative losses of old age, and discomfort due to a disorder may make the elderly less interested in regaining health. Patients with impaired cognition may have difficulty describing problems, impeding the physician's evaluation. Also, the elderly may be reluctant to seek care because they fear hospitalization, which they may associate with dying.

Care may be delivered in various settings, including a physician's office, the patient's home, an assisted living facility, a board-and-care facility, a nursing home, a hospital, and a hospice facility. Coordination of this care, especially across multiple settings for a particular patient, is called continuity of care. In general, the lowest, least restrictive level of care suitable to a person's needs should be used. This approach conserves financial resources and helps preserve the person's independence and functioning.

Home care: Home care is most commonly used after hospital discharge, but hospitalization is not a prerequisite. Usually, home care is indicated when patients need monitoring, education, adjustment of drugs, dressing changes, and limited physical therapy. In general, home care is not suitable for patients who need assistance > 0.5 to 1 h 3 times/wk, although special arrangements can sometimes be made. Nurses provide services under the supervision of a physician, who consults with them as changes in care are needed. Few people with a serious, chronic disorder can afford full home care even though most would prefer to remain at home. Medicare covers some home care services in certain circumstances, which depend on the Medicare option chosen. Services include personal care; part-time skilled nursing care; physical, occupational, and speech therapy; social services; durable medical equipment; and medical supplies. Private insurance policies may be purchased to cover long-term home care.

Nursing home care: The term nursing home refers specifically to a skilled nursing facility. In the US, nursing home care cost $21 billion in 1980 and $70 billion in 2000. In 2000, nursing home beds outnumbered acute hospital beds. In the US, people > 65 occupy 90% of 1.7 million nursing home beds. However, < 5% of people > 65 live in nursing homes or other institutions; about 10 yr ago, the percentage was almost 6%. The decrease results from increased use of assisted living facilities and home health care; use of both depends substantially on informal caregiving.

About 45% of people > 65 spend some time in a nursing home; of these, > 50% stay > 1 yr, and a minority of these will die there. However, twice as many functionally dependent elderly live in the community as in nursing homes, and 25% of the community-dwelling elderly have no living relatives. Special attention to health and health care needs of the community-dwelling elderly could add quality and years to their lives and limit costs by preventing institutionalization.

The Program of All-Inclusive Care for the Elderly (PACE) is a successful Medicare program that combines funds from Medicare and Medicaid. PACE is designed for eligible elderly people who meet criteria for nursing home admission. PACE funds are used to enable enrollees to live at home as long as possible.

A nursing home may be needed temporarily to facilitate recovery from an acute disorder, especially hip fracture, MI, or stroke. In such cases, a nursing home that can provide services relevant to the patient's needs (eg, high-quality physical therapy or rehabilitation) should be chosen. Nursing homes vary in services provided and in quality.

The most common reasons for long-term nursing home care are incontinence, dementia, and immobility. Certain problems (eg, decline in functional ability, undernutrition, weight loss, pressure ulcers, incontinence, constipation, infections, depression, use of multiple drugs) commonly develop or worsen in residents of nursing homes but sometimes can be prevented with attentive care.

Hospitalization: Only seriously ill elderly patients should be hospitalized. Hospitalization itself poses risks to elderly patients because of confinement, immobility, diagnostic testing, and treatments (including drugs). When patients are transferred to or from a hospital, drugs are likely to be added or changed, leading to a higher risk of adverse effects. For example, if a drug that a patient has been taking is not on the hospital formulary, a hospital physician may substitute another drug without paying enough attention to possible differences requiring adjustments. Or, if a patient does not take the drug as prescribed at home, giving the drug correctly in the hospital may result in adverse effects. Most seriously, a useful, effective drug may be inadvertently omitted at admission or discharge. In the hospital, elderly patients frequently experience nighttime confusion (sundowning), fall, fracture a bone with no identifiable trauma, or become unable to walk; many develop pressure ulcers, urinary incontinence, fecal impaction, and urinary retention. Convalescence may be prolonged.

Hospice care: Hospices provide care for the dying (see p. 2763). The goal is to alleviate symptoms and keep people comfortable rather than to cure a disorder. Medicare covers hospice care only for people with < 6 mo life expectancy; hospice care replaces the usual Medicare benefit package, although hospitalization is still covered. Hospice care can be provided in the home, a nursing home, or a separate inpatient facility. In the US, hospice care tends to be started very late in fatal disorders, especially for disorders other than cancer (eg, Alzheimer's disease, heart failure, chronic lung disorders).

UNUSUAL PRESENTATIONS IN THE ELDERLY

The elderly often do not have the characteristic symptoms and signs of a disorder but instead tend to have one or more nonspecific manifestations, called geriatric syndromes (eg, falling, incontinence, dizziness, acute confusion, syncope, worsening dementia, weight loss, failure to thrive). These syndromes are multifactorial in origin; nonetheless, patients may improve when only some of the precipitating factors are corrected.

During old age, many common conditions (eg, heart failure, unstable angina, pulmonary embolism, alcohol abuse, systemic infections, pneumonia, acute abdomen, depression, adverse drug effects) may manifest without the typical or classic features. Depression is the most common affective disorder among community-dwelling elderly but is no more common than among younger people. However, it is more common among the institutionalized elderly.

338 THE DYING PATIENT

(See also pp. 2247and 2768.)

Helping patients and family members find comfort in the experience of dying is often more important than adhering to medical routines or correcting symptomless physiologic abnormalities. However, distressing symptoms should be prevented or relieved as effectively as possible. Preventing suffering is also important. Suffering is a global perception of distress due to factors that, together, undermine quality of life (eg, pain; physical impairment; psychologic disturbances; social, family, financial, and spiritual concerns).

People differ in what they consider important, especially when facing death. Some people search for closure: They reach out to friends and family to share time and to express love; they complete projects important to their lives; and they tie up loose ends. Often, with appropriate support, people die at a time and in a way that allows them to experience a satisfying close. Other people cannot accept their imminent mortality and avoid such closure. For some, life is to be prolonged, even at the cost of pain, marked confusion, or severe respiratory distress. For others, quality of life is the overarching concern: They prefer comfort measures rather than prolonged disability and struggle.

Accommodating patient preferences as much as possible is essential when planning care. Patients who fear pain or confusion more than death should be treated differently from those who cherish every moment of life, regardless of its quality. Health care practitioners should know local laws and institutional policy governing living wills, durable powers of attorney, and procedures for forgoing resuscitation and hospitalization; such knowledge helps them ensure that patients' wishes are followed when they are no longer able to direct their own care.

Supportive care may be the only realistic goal for a dying patient. Medical management of troubling symptoms can enable patients and family members to avoid needless suffering and to share valuable time. However, to say that a patient's care has changed from curative to supportive or from treatment to palliation is an oversimplification of a complex decision process.

Many patients ask whether the time until death can be predicted. Often, such estimates are incorrect, particularly for disorders in which death tends to come suddenly, without reliable warning signs (eg, for heart failure or emphysema). For other disorders (eg, commonly cancer), recognizable changes may presage death by several weeks or months. Many people live for months or years in a very fragile state of health. Family support, advance care planning, focus on relieving symptoms and maximizing function, and attention to spiritual issues are appropriate throughout this time, and much is lost by postponing these issues until death is clearly imminent.

Effective care for dying patients usually involves a team because no one caregiver is available 24 h/day and because the skills and perspectives of several disciplines are needed. Palliative care or hospice teams anticipate potential problems and make appropriate arrangements, such as obtaining supplies or opioids in anticipation of a potential emergency. When death is imminent, an experienced team member can comfort family members and may prevent an inappropriate call to the emergency medical system. Dying patients often have spiritual needs that should be recognized, acknowledged, and addressed.

Managing death: The physician should prepare family members for death far in advance. Preparation includes discussion of the likely course and a reasonable range of possible complications with their time course. Patients should be told that their disorder is likely to cause death (even when the time frame is unclear); when death becomes imminent, they should be told. A health care practitioner must not assume that patients or family members understand the fatal nature of certain disorders (even metastatic cancer) or that they recognize when the patient is nearing death. Initial discussions should be honest and sensitive to the language and culture of patients and family members. The physician should not delay full disclosure too long because doing so can give patients and family members false hope and reduce the opportunity for attending to spiritual and family concerns.

Many patients and family members benefit from making plans based on their priorities and preferences for the different courses provided by various end-of-life treatments (see

p. 2768). At some point, virtually every dying patient should have a do-not-resuscitate (DNR) order written in the medical record, and all clinicians in every setting should abide by that decision. Other important decisions about medical care (eg, whether patients are to be hospitalized or use a ventilator) should also be made and recorded. Often, specific actions are required to implement these decisions (eg, to have the needed drugs at home).

Family members should be told about the changes that may occur in the patient's body directly before and after death. They should not be surprised by irregular breathing, cool extremities, confusion, a purplish skin color, or somnolence in the last hours.

Some patients close to death develop noisy bronchial congestion or palatal relaxation, commonly known as the death rattle. If this symptom distresses family members, scopolamine or diphenhydramine (see p. 2766) can dry the patient's secretions and reduce the noise. Also, CNS irritability, with agitation and restlessness, may develop; it can be relieved with a sedative.

If a patient is expected to die at home, family members should be told whom to call (eg, physician, hospice nurse) and whom not to call (eg, ambulance service). They should also be told how to obtain legal advice and to arrange burial or cremation services. Religious practices may affect how the body is cared for and usually should be discussed before death with the patient, family members, or both.

The last moments of a patient's life can have a lasting effect on family members, friends, and caregivers. The patient should be in an area that is peaceful, quiet, and physically comfortable. Any stains or tubes on the bed should be covered, and odors should be masked. Family members should be encouraged to maintain physical contact, such as holding hands, with the patient. If desired by the patient and family members, the presence of friends and clergy should be encouraged. Accommodation should be made for spiritual, cultural, ethnic, or personal rites of passage desired by the patient and family members.

After death: A physician, nurse, or other authorized person should make the official determination of death as quickly as possible to reduce the family's anxiety and uncertainty. Family members or funeral directors should be provided with a completed death certificate as quickly as possible. Even when death was expected, physicians may need to report the death to the coroner or police.

Physicians, nurses, and other health care practitioners should respond to the psychologic needs of family members and provide appropriate counseling, a comfortable environment where family members can grieve together, and adequate time for them to be with the body. Friends, neighbors, and clergy may be able to help provide support. Health care practitioners should be sensitive to cultural differences in behavior at the time of death.

Organ donation, if appropriate, should be discussed before death or immediately after death; such discussions are sometimes mandated by law. The attending physician should know how to arrange for organ donation and autopsy, even for patients who die at home or in a nursing home. Autopsy should be readily available regardless of where the death occurred. The decision about having an autopsy can be discussed before or just after death. Usually, a health care practitioner who has had previous contact with family members should discuss autopsy with family members. This discussion should not be left to a covering physician or house officer.

HOSPICE CARE

Hospice is a concept as well as a program of care. It is specifically designed to minimize suffering for dying patients and their family members. In the US, hospice is the only widely available comprehensive service to support very sick people at home. Philosophically, it forgoes most diagnostic testing and life-prolonging treatments in favor of symptom relief, education of patients and family members about appropriate care, and comfort care.

Hospice is always interdisciplinary, relying on physicians, nurses, and attendants (eg, home health aides). Pharmacists, nutritionists, and therapists may also be involved. Care may be provided at home, in a nursing home, or in another care facility; usually, hospitals and rehabilitation centers do not provide such care. Hospice programs differ substantially in the services they readily provide and in treatments and devices they support and use. Which kind of hospice care is best depends on the needs and wishes of patients and family members, financial considerations, and local availability.

Hospice care can provide most necessary medical treatments. Nurses can oversee drug use and maintain O_2 therapy and IV lines needed to provide analgesics or other drugs. Physicians who work in the hospice program can see patients as needed and communicate with nurses regularly.

Hospice also provides psychologic support and counseling to patients and family members. As part of that effort, hospice care workers should prepare family members for death by describing what is likely to happen near the time of death. They should tell family members what to do when the patient dies, whom to call, and whom not to call.

Most patients ill enough to require hospice also require some assistance with daily activities (eg, dressing, bathing, preparing food), and some may be completely dependent. If family members and friends are unable to provide this care, home attendants may be engaged. However, these services are usually not covered by hospice programs; private funds may be needed.

Medicare or insurance pays for most home hospice services, but usually only after a physician certifies that a patient has a terminal disorder and that life expectancy in the usual course of the disorder is < 6 mo.

Physicians are often reluctant to use hospice because a treatable condition outside of the hospice program's capabilities may develop. Because patients can leave hospice at any time and re-enroll later, this reluctance is not useful. Rather, early hospice enrollment may be a good way to provide comprehensive supportive care at home when such care is needed.

SOCIETAL CONCERNS

Financial concerns: Financial coverage for care of dying patients is problematic. Medicare regulations restrict payment for many aspects of supportive care. Not all patients qualify for hospice care, and physicians are often reluctant to certify the 6-mo prognosis required for coverage. Sometimes the need for skilled nursing care can justify Medicare payment to a nursing home for short-term, high-cost, terminally ill patients. Physicians should know financing options and the financial effects of choices and discuss these issues with patients or family members.

Legal and ethical concerns (see also p. 2768)**:** Many health care practitioners worry that medical treatments intended to relieve pain or other suffering can hasten death, but such treatments rarely do. If medical care is good, questions of assisted suicide or other wrongdoing are rare. Typically, criminal law does not differentiate between intentional and unintentional crime, although motivation commonly affects the penalty. However, even if dyspnea is relieved only by doses of opioids that may also hasten death, the resulting death is not considered wrongful.

Assisting with suicide remains a criminal act in most states, but the laws vary substantially and are rarely invoked. Directly providing a dying patient with lethal drugs and instructions for using them could be grounds for prosecution in most states but is specifically authorized in Oregon. Charges of homicide rather than charges of assisting with suicide are more likely if the patient's interests are not carefully advocated, if the patient lacks capacity or is severely functionally impaired just before death, if documentation is sparse, or if the prosecutor's electoral base is expected to approve such charges. Physicians who manage symptoms vigorously and forgo life-sustaining treatment need to document decision making carefully, to provide care in a reputable setting, and to be willing to discuss these issues honestly and sensitively with patients, other practitioners, and the public. Physicians should avoid any treatment that is conventionally considered a means of homicide (eg, lethal injection), even if the intention is to relieve suffering.

SYMPTOM CONTROL IN THE DYING

Physical and mental distress is common during terminal disorders. Patients commonly fear that their suffering will be protracted and that no one will control it. Relief of discomfort enables patients to focus on living as fully as possible and on confronting the issues presented by the approach of death.

Symptom control should be based on etiology when possible. For example, vomiting due to hypercalcemia is treated differently from that due to elevated intracranial pressure. However, diagnosing the cause of a symptom may be inappropriate if testing is burdensome or risky or if specific treatment (eg, major surgery) has already been ruled out. For dying patients, comfort measures, including nonspecific treatment or a short sequential trial of empiric treatments, are often better than an exhaustive diagnostic evaluation.

Because one symptom can have many causes and may respond differently to treatment as the patient's condition deteriorates, treatments must be closely monitored and repeatedly reevaluated. Drug overdosage or underdosage must be avoided, especially as worsening physiology causes changes in drug disposition.

When survival is expected to be brief, symptom severity frequently dictates initial treatment. Sometimes the fear that a symptom will worsen can be more crippling than the symptom itself, and reassurance that effective treatment is available may be all a patient needs. Other times, a symptom is so severe and the diagnostic alternatives are so nonspecific that immediate symptom suppression is indicated.

Pain (see also p. 1769)**:** About ½ of patients dying of cancer have severe pain. Yet, only ½ of these patients receive reliable pain relief. Many patients dying of organ system failure and dementia also have severe pain. Sometimes pain could be controlled but persists because patients, family members, and physicians have misconceptions about pain and the drugs (especially opioids) that can control it, resulting in significant underdosing.

Patients perceive pain differently, depending on whether other factors (eg, fatigue, insomnia, anxiety, depression, nausea) are present. Analgesic choice depends largely on pain intensity and cause, which can be determined only by talking with and observing patients. All pain can be relieved by an appropriately potent drug at sufficient dosage, although this treatment may also produce sedation or confusion. Commonly used drugs are aspirin, acetaminophen, or NSAIDs for mild pain; codeine or oxycodone for moderate pain; and hydromorphone, morphine, or fentanyl for severe pain (see p. 1771).

In terminal disorders, oral administration of opioids is most convenient and cost effective. Rectal administration provides slower absorption but with very little 1st-pass effect; morphine suppositories or pills may be given rectally at the same dose used for oral forms and then titrated as needed. IV or sc administration of opioids is preferred to IM injections, which are painful and result in variable absorption. Long-acting opioids are best for long-lasting pain. When opioids are indicated, the physician should prescribe them in adequate dosage and on a continuous basis to prevent pain. Unreasonable concerns by the public and by health care practitioners about addiction often tragically limit appropriate use of opioids. Pharmacologic dependence may result from regular use but causes no problems in dying patients except the need to avoid inadvertent withdrawal. Addictive behaviors are rare and usually easy to control.

Adverse effects of opioids include nausea, sedation, confusion, constipation, and respiratory depression. Constipation should be treated prophylactically (see p. 2767). Patients usually develop substantial tolerance to the respiratory depressant and sedative effects of morphine but much less tolerance to the analgesic and constipating effects. Opioids may also cause myoclonus, agitated delirium, hyperalgesia, and seizures. These effects may result from accumulation of toxic metabolites and usually resolve when another opioid is substituted.

When a stable opioid dose becomes inadequate, increasing the dose by 1.5 to 2.0 times the previous dose is reasonable. Usually, serious respiratory depression does not occur unless the dose is much more than twice the previously tolerated dose.

Use of adjunctive drugs for pain control often increases comfort and allows the opioid dosage and consequent adverse effects to be reduced. Corticosteroids are widely used in the terminally ill to reduce the pain of inflammation and swelling. Tricyclic antidepressants (eg, nortriptyline, doxepin) help manage neuropathic pain (see p. 1779); doxepin provides sedation as well. Gabapentin 300 to 1200 mg po tid helps relieve neuropathic pain. Methadone is effective for refractory or neuropathic pain; however, its kinetics vary, and it requires close monitoring. Benzodiazepines are useful for patients whose pain is worsened by anxiety.

For severe localized pain, regional nerve blocks, done by an anesthesiologist experienced in pain management, may provide relief with few adverse effects. Various nerve-blocking techniques may be used. Indwelling epidural or intrathecal catheters may be placed to provide continuous infusion of analgesics, often mixed with anesthetic drugs.

Pain-modification techniques (eg, guided mental imagery, hypnosis, acupuncture, relaxation) help some patients (see p. 2723). Counseling for stress and anxiety may be very helpful, as may spiritual support from a chaplain.

Dyspnea: Dyspnea is one of the most feared symptoms and probably the most distressing to dying patients. Its causes may be treatable. For example, antibiotics for pneumonia or thoracentesis for a pleural effusion may be appropriate. However, if death is imminent, such measures are not necessary; patients can be made comfortable without invasive or aggressive measures, regardless of the cause of dyspnea.

Initially, O_2 helps correct hypoxemia. Even when its benefit is no longer certain, O_2 may continue to be psychologically comforting to patients and family members. It is usually most comfortable when given by nasal cannula.

Morphine 2 to 10 mg sublingually or 2 to 4 mg sc q 2 to 4 h prn helps reduce breathlessness. Low-dose morphine may blunt the medullary response to CO_2 retention or O_2 decline, reducing dyspnea and decreasing anxiety without causing significant respiratory depression. If patients are already taking typical doses of opioids for pain, doses for respiratory symptoms must be much higher.

Airway congestion is best managed with drugs that dry secretions (eg, topical scopolamine gel 0.25 to 0.5 mg q 8 to 12 h, hyoscyamine 0.125 mg sublingually q 8 h, diphenhydramine 10 to 50 mg IM q 4 to 6 h prn).

Nebulized saline may be used to treat patients with viscous secretions. Bronchospasm and bronchial inflammation may be treated with nebulized albuterol and oral or injectable corticosteroids.

Benzodiazepines often help relieve anxiety associated with dyspnea. Useful nondrug measures include providing a cool draft from an open window or fan and maintaining a calming presence.

Anorexia: Anorexia and marked weight loss are common among dying patients. For family members, accepting the patient's poor oral intake is often difficult because it means accepting that the patient is dying. Patients should be offered their favorite foods whenever possible. Conditions that may cause poor intake and can be easily treated—gastritis, constipation, oral candidiasis, pain, and nausea—should be treated. Some patients benefit from appetite stimulants such as oral corticosteroids (dexamethasone 2 to 8 mg bid or prednisone 10 to 30 mg once/day) or megestrol 160 to 480 mg po once/day. However, if a patient is close to death, family members should be counseled that neither food nor hydration is necessary to maintain the patient's comfort.

IV fluids, TPN, and tube feedings do not prolong the life of dying patients. All of these measures seem to increase discomfort and may hasten death. In dying patients who are fed artificially, incidence of pulmonary congestion and pneumonia is increased. Artificial hydration may worsen edema and pain associated with inflammation. Conversely, dehydration and ketosis due to caloric restriction are associated with analgesic effects and absence of discomfort. The only reported discomfort due to dehydration near death is xerostomia, which is easily relieved with oral swabs or ice chips.

Family members should be gently told that the patient is dying and that food does not help the patient's strength nor substantially delay death; they should be reassured that the patient does not suffer from having little or no intake. Suggesting specific tasks (eg, providing favorite foods, small portions, and foods that are easy to swallow) and other ways to show caring and love can help family members.

Even debilitated and cachectic patients may live for several weeks after all food and hydration is stopped. Family members should be told that stopping fluids will not result in the patient's immediate death and ordinarily does not hasten death. Supportive care, including good oral hygiene, is imperative for patient comfort during this time. Oral hygiene (brushing the teeth, swabbing the oral cavity, applying lip salve, and providing ice chips for xerostomia) is a valuable part of care that family members can provide for the dying patient.

Nausea and vomiting: Many seriously ill patients experience nausea, frequently without vomiting. Nausea may be exacerbated by GI problems (eg, constipation, gastritis), metabolic abnormalities (eg, hypercalcemia, uremia), drug adverse effects, increased intracranial pressure secondary to cerebral cancer, and psychosocial stress. Treatment should be guided by the likely cause; eg, NSAIDs are stopped, gastritis is treated with H_2 blockers, and patients with known or suspected brain metastases are treated with a trial of corticosteroids. If nausea is due to gastric distention and reflux, metoclopramide (po or sc) is useful because it increases gastric tone and contractions while relaxing the pyloric sphincter.

If no cause for mild nausea is identified, patients may benefit from nonspecific treatment with a phenothiazine (eg, promethazine 25 mg po qid; prochlorperazine 10 mg po before meals or, for patients who cannot take oral drugs, 25 mg rectally bid). Anticholinergic drugs such as scopolamine and the antihistamines meclizine and diphenhydramine prevent recurrent nausea in many patients. Combining lower doses of the above drugs often improves efficacy. Second-line drugs for intractable nausea include haloperidol, started at 1 mg po or sc q 6 to 8 h, then titrated to as much as 15 mg/day. The 5-HT_3 antagonists ondansetron and granisetron often dramatically relieve chemotherapy-induced nausea. They are 2nd-line drugs for more complex causes of nausea in dying patients.

Nausea and pain due to intestinal obstruction are common among patients with widespread abdominal cancer. Generally, IV fluids and nasogastric suction are not useful in hospice care. Symptoms of nausea, pain, and intestinal spasm may be controlled with hyoscyamine 0.125 to 0.25 mg q 4 h sublingually or sc, scopolamine 1.5 mg topically, morphine given sc or rectally, or any of the other above antiemetics. Octreotide 150 μg sc or IV q 12 h inhibits GI secretions and dramatically reduces nausea and painful distention. Given with antiemetics, octreotide usually eliminates the need for nasogastric suctioning. Corticosteroids (eg, dexamethasone 4 to 6 mg IV, IM, or rectally tid) may decrease obstructive inflammation at the tumor site and temporarily relieve the obstruction. IV fluids may exacerbate obstructive edema.

Constipation: Constipation is common among dying patients because of inactivity, use of opioids and anticholinergic drugs, and decreased intake of fluids and dietary fiber. Laxatives help prevent fecal impaction, especially in patients receiving opioids. All patients should be asked about bowel function. Most patients do well on a twice/day regimen of stool softener (eg, docusate) plus a mild stimulant laxative (eg, casanthranol, senna). If stimulant laxatives cause cramping discomfort, patients may respond to increased doses of docusate alone or an osmotic laxative, such as lactulose or sorbitol (which is much cheaper and equally effective) started at 15 to 30 mL po bid and titrated to effect.

Soft fecal impaction may be treated with a bisacodyl suppository or saline enema. For a hard fecal impaction, a mineral oil enema may be given, possibly with an oral benzodiazepine (eg, lorazepam) or an analgesic, followed by digital disimpaction. After disimpaction, patients should be placed on a rigorous bowel regimen to avoid recurrence. Regular bowel movements are essential to the comfort of dying patients, at least until the last day or two.

Pressure ulcers: Many dying patients are immobile, poorly nourished, incontinent, and cachectic and thus are at risk of pressure ulcers (see also p. 1011). Prevention requires relieving pressure by rotating patients q 2 h; a specialized mattress or continuously inflated air-suspension bed may be used. Incontinent patients should be kept as dry as possible. Generally, use of an indwelling catheter, with its inconvenience and risk of infection, is justified only when bedding changes cause pain or when patients or family members strongly prefer it.

Confusion: Mental changes that can accompany the terminal stage of a disorder may distress patients and family members; however, patients are often unaware of them. Confusion (delirium) is common; causes include drugs, hypoxia, metabolic disturbances, and intrinsic CNS disorders. If the cause can be determined, simple treatment may be worthwhile provided it enables patients to communicate more meaningfully with family members and friends. Patients who are comfortable and less aware of their surroundings may do better with no treatment. When possible, the physician should ascertain the preferences of patients and family members and use them to guide treatment.

Simple causes of confusion and agitation should be sought. Agitation and restlessness often result from urinary retention, which resolves promptly with urinary catheterization. Confusion in debilitated patients is worsened by sleep deprivation. Agitated patients may benefit from benzodiazepines; however, benzodiazepines may also cause confusion. Poorly controlled pain may cause insomnia or agitation. If pain has been appropriately controlled, a nighttime sedative may help.

Family members and visitors may help lessen confusion by frequently holding the patient's hand and repeating where the patient is and what is happening. Patients with severe terminal agitation resistant to other measures may respond best to barbiturates; family members should be involved in the decision to use these drugs. Pentobarbital, a rapid-onset, short-acting barbiturate, may be given as 100 to 200 mg IM q 4 h prn. Phenobarbital, which is longer-acting, may be given po, sc, or rectally. Midazolam, a short-acting benzodiazepine, is often effective.

Depression: Most dying patients experience some depressive symptoms. Providing psychologic support and allowing patients to express concerns and feelings are usually the best approach. A skilled social worker, physician, nurse, or chaplain can help with these concerns.

A trial of antidepressants is often appropriate for patients who have persistent, clinically significant depression. SSRIs are useful for patients likely to live beyond the 4 wk usually needed for onset of the antidepressant effect. Depressed patients with anxiety and insomnia may benefit from a sedating tricyclic antidepressant given at bedtime. For patients who are withdrawn or who have vegetative signs (see 1805), methylphenidate may be started at 2.5 mg po once/day and increased to 2.5 to 5 mg bid (given at breakfast and lunch) as necessary. Methylphenidate (same dose) is sometimes used to provide a few days or weeks of increased energy for patients who are fatigued or somnolent because of analgesics. Methylphenidate has a rapid effect but may precipitate agitation. Because its duration of action is short, adverse effects are also short-lived.

Stress: A few people approach death peacefully, but more patients and family members experience stress. Death is particularly stressful when interpersonal conflicts keep patients and family members from sharing their last moments together in peace. Such conflicts can lead to excessive guilt or inability to grieve in survivors and can cause anguish in patients. A family member who is caring for a dying patient at home may experience physical and emotional stress. Usually, stress in patients and family members is best treated with compassion, information, counseling, and sometimes brief psychotherapy. Social services may be needed to relieve caregiver burden. Sedatives should be used sparingly and briefly.

When a partner dies, the survivor may be overwhelmed by having to make decisions about legal or financial matters or to manage the household. For an elderly couple, the death of one may reveal the survivor's cognitive impairment, for which the deceased partner had compensated. Physicians should identify such high-risk situations, usually with the help of social workers, so that they can mobilize the resources needed to prevent undue suffering and dysfunction.

Grief: Grieving is a normal process that usually begins before an anticipated death. For patients, grief often starts with denial caused by fears about loss of control, separation, suffering, an uncertain future, and loss of self. Staff members can help patients accept their prognosis by listening to their concerns, helping them understand that they can control important elements of their lives, explaining how the disorder will worsen and how death will come, and assuring them that their physical symptoms will be controlled.

Family members may need support in expressing grief. Any health care team member who has come to know the patient and family members can help them through this process and direct them to professional services if needed. Physicians and other team members need to develop regular procedures that ensure follow-up of grieving family members.

339 MEDICOLEGAL ISSUES

Medicine today is practiced within an expanding and evolving system of legal rights and obligations, patient protections, health care financing regulation, and standards of care. Thus, medical care can involve significant legal issues, including advance directives, capacity of patients to make health care decisions, confidentiality of medical information, and malpractice liability.

ADVANCE DIRECTIVES

Two types of legal documents extend personal control over medical care when a patient loses capacity to make health care decisions: a living will and a durable power of attorney for health care. Both documents are called advance directives because they direct, in advance of incapacitation, preferences for medical care to be carried out during any period when the patient can no longer effectively communicate those decisions. An advance directive cannot be completed after a patient becomes mentally incapacitated, and it does not become effective until after incapacity has been determined. If no advance directive has been prepared, a surrogate (see p. 2771) must be appointed to take control of medical care decisions and provide substituted judgment.

Living will: A living will expresses a patient's preferences for medical care (it is called a living will because it is in effect while the person is alive). In some states, the document is called a directive to doctors. State laws vary greatly regarding living wills.

A living will allows a person to express any preferences for medical care, from no interventions to maximum care. Preferences should be written as specifically as possible to provide clarity to health care practitioners. A living will cannot, however, compel health care practitioners to provide medical care that is medically or ethically unwarranted.

To be valid, a living will must comply with state law. Some states require that living wills be written in a fairly standardized way. Others are more flexible, permitting any language as long as the document is appropriately signed and witnessed. In most states, a health care practitioner involved in the patient's care cannot be a witness. A document that does not comply with state law requirements for statutory living wills may still serve as a valid communication of a patient's wishes as long as it is an authentic expression of the patient's wishes.

Living wills go into effect upon (1) the loss of ability to make health care decisions and (2) the existence of a medical condition specified in the directive—typically a terminal condition, permanent vegetative state, or the end-stage of a chronic condition. Often, state law provides a process for confirming and documenting the loss of decisional capacity and the medical condition.

Durable power of attorney for health care: This is a document in which one person (the principal) names another person (the agent, proxy, or the attorney-in-fact) to make decisions about health care and *only* health care. A power is *durable* if it remains legally in force, even when the principal becomes mentally incapable of making a health care decision or if it goes into effect at the point of incapacity. The latter is called a "springing" power.

While a living will states a person's specific preferences regarding medical treatment, a durable power of attorney for health care designates an agent to make health care decisions. The agent is granted the power to discuss medical alternatives with the doctors and make a decision if an accident or illness incapacitates the person. In most states, a health care practitioner involved in the care of the patient cannot serve as his attorney-in-fact for health care matters, unless the practitioner is a close relative. The durable power of attorney for health care can include a living will provision but should do so only as guidance for the agent, rather than as a binding instruction.

The use of the durable power of attorney for health care is especially critical for unmarried couples, same-sex partners, friends, or other individuals considered legally unrelated who wish to grant each other the legal authority to make health care decisions and to ensure rights of visitation and access to medical information.

Ideally, doctors should obtain a copy of a patient's living will and durable power of attorney for health care, review its contents with the patient if possible, and make it part of the medical record.

CAPACITY AND COMPETENCY

Historically, "incapacity" was considered primarily a clinical finding, and "incompetency" was considered a legal finding. That distinction is no longer firmly recognized; most state laws now use "incapacity" rather than "incompetency," although the terms are frequently used interchangeably. The key distinction now is between clinical incapacity and legal incapacity to make a health care decision.

Patients who have clinical and legal capacity have the right to make health care decisions, including refusal of medically necessary care, even if death may result from refusal. Patients who lack either capacity cannot make health care decisions.

Clinical capacity: Clinical capacity to make health care decisions is the ability to understand the significant benefits and risks of proposed health care, to understand possible alternative treatments, and to make and communicate a health care decision. Health care practitioners determine this type of capacity clinically and document the determination process. The courts may become involved only when the determination itself or another aspect of the process is challenged.

Clinical capacity is determined for specific health care decisions and thus is limited to those decisions. The level of clinical capacity needed to make a health care decision depends on the complexity of that decision. Capacity may be intermittent, variable, and affected by the environment. Patients who are intoxicated, delirious, comatose, severely depressed, agitated, or otherwise impaired are likely to lack the capacity to make health care decisions but may later regain that capacity. Patients with some level of diminished capacity, even those with fairly severe cognitive deficits, may still possess enough capacity to make a health care decision, depending on the complexity of the decision.

For patients who lack clinical capacity, health care practitioners must obtain consent from an agent or proxy under the patient's durable power of attorney for health care or from another legally authorized surrogate (see p. 2771), unless urgent or emergency care is needed (eg, for unconscious patients after an acute event). In such cases, if there is no surrogate, the doctrine of presumed consent applies: Patients are presumed to consent to any necessary treatment. Ignoring the decision of patients with capacity or accepting the decision of patients without capacity is unethical and risks civil liability.

Legal capacity: Legal capacity (also called competency) is a legal status; it cannot be determined by health care practitioners. In the US, people aged ≥ 18 yr are automatically considered legally capable of making health care decisions for themselves. Emancipated minors are persons below the age of majority (usually 18) who are also considered legally capable; the definition of this group varies by state but generally includes minors who are married or in the armed forces or who have obtained a court decree of emancipation.

A person remains legally capable until a judge with appropriate jurisdiction declares him legally incapacitated with respect to some or all areas of functioning. The legal requirements for declaring legal incapacity vary by state. However, substantiation of all of the following is typically required: a disabling condition (eg, mental retardation, a mental or physical disorder, dementia, altered consciousness, chronic use of drugs); inability to receive and evaluate information or to make or communicate decisions; and inability to meet essential requirements of physical health, safety, or self-care without protective intervention.

When a person is declared legally incapacitated, the court appoints a guardian or conservator to make legally binding decisions for the person in the range of matters directed by the court. Courts can also direct or approve specific decisions that are disputed. If the issue is in dispute, physicians may seek a court's determination of legal capacity, or physicians may be asked to testify or provide supporting documentation for a hearing to determine legal capacity.

CONFIDENTIALITY AND HIPPA

Traditionally, ethical medical care has always included the need to keep patients' medical information confidential. However, the Health Information Portability and Accountability Act (HIPAA—see www.hhs.gov/ocr/hipaa) has codified that responsibility for health care providers. In HIPAA, "health care providers" includes health plans, health care clearinghouses, and health care practitioners who electronically conduct financial and administrative transactions (eg, enrollment, billing, and eligibility verification). Key provisions of HIPAA involve the following areas.

Access to medical records: Generally, patients should be able to see and obtain copies of their medical records and request corrections if they identify errors and mistakes.

Notice of privacy practices: Health care providers must provide a notice about their possible uses of personal medical information and about patient rights under the new privacy regulation.

Limits on use of personal medical information: HIPAA limits how health care providers may use individually identifiable (protected) health information. The act does not restrict physicians, nurses, and other providers from sharing information needed to treat their patients. However, providers may use or share only the minimum amount of protected information needed for a particular purpose. In most other situations, personal health information may not be used for purposes unrelated to health care. For example, a patient must sign a specific authorization before a health care provider can release medical information to a life insurer, a bank, a marketing firm, or another outside business for purposes unrelated to the patient's health care.

Marketing: HIPAA limits the use of patient information for marketing purposes. A patient's specific authorization must be obtained before disclosing information for marketing. However, health care providers can freely communicate with patients about treatment options and other health-related information, including disease-management programs.

Confidential communications: A patient can request that health care providers take reasonable steps to ensure that their communications with the patient are confidential. For example, patients could ask a physician to call their office rather than home. Nonetheless, unless the patient objects, providers can share medical information with a patient's immediate family members or close personal friend if the information relates directly to that person's involvement with the patient's care or payment for care. Providers are expected to exercise professional judgment. For purposes of the privacy rule, an authorized personal representative of the patient (eg, a proxy appointed in a power of attorney for health care or a state-authorized decision-making surrogate) should be treated the same as the patient. Thus, the representative has the same access to information and may exercise the same rights regarding confidentiality of information. Nevertheless, providers may restrict information or access if there are reasonable concerns about domestic violence, abuse, or neglect by the representative.

Complaints: Consumers may file complaints about compliance with these privacy practices. Complaints can be made directly to the health care practitioner or to the Office for Civil Rights in the US Department of Health and Human Services. Patients do not have a right to file a private lawsuit under HIPAA. There are civil and criminal penalties for misuse of personal health information; however, such penalties should not worry health care providers who, in good faith, make reasonable attempts to comply.

INFORMED CONSENT

Consent of the patient is a prerequisite for any medical intervention. However, that consent often does not need to be expressed. For emergency care, consent is normally presumed. For interventions considered routine and unlikely to cause harm (eg, routine phlebotomy, placement of an IV line), circumstances are typically considered to imply consent. For example, by holding out their arm, patients manifest consent to receive certain interventions. For more invasive or risky interventions, express informed consent is always required.

To give informed consent, patients must have legal and clinical capacity. Health care practitioners obtaining informed consent must be qualified to explain the risks and benefits of the intervention, as described below, and to answer appropriate questions. The law requires that health care practitioners take reasonable steps to adequately communicate with patients who do not speak English or who have other communication barriers.

Ethical and legal authorities generally agree that health care practitioners are obligated to ensure, at a minimum, that patients understand their current medical status, including its likely course if no treatment is pursued; potentially helpful treatments, including a description and explanation of potential risks and benefits; and usually, the practitioner's professional opinion as to the best alternative. Uncertainties associated with each of these elements should also be discussed. Generally, these discussions are noted in the medical record, and a document describing the discussion is signed by the patient.

MEDICAL MALPRACTICE

Patients can sue health care practitioners if they feel they have been injured. However, successful medical malpractice lawsuits require proof of all of the following:

- The care provided was below the ordinary standard of care that would be provided by similar health care practitioners under similar circumstances
- A professional relationship existed between the health care practitioner and the injured party
- The patient was harmed because of the deviation from the standard of care

Concern about lawsuits sometimes makes physicians act in ways that are not in the best interest of their patients. For example, physicians may order tests or treatments that are not medically necessary just because patients request them. However, such an approach is not required by law, may not protect against lawsuits, and is generally considered excessive and inappropriate. The best defense against malpractice lawsuits appears to be providing excellent medical care and building close, trusting, collaborative relationships with patients.

SURROGATE DECISION MAKING

When patients lack capacity to consent to or to refuse medical treatment, health care practitioners must rely on an authorized surrogate for consent, unless urgent or emergency care is needed. If adults already have a court-appointed guardian with authority to make health care decisions, the guardian is the authorized surrogate. If patients who lack capacity have a durable power of attorney for health care, the agent or proxy appointed by that document is authorized to make health care decisions within the scope of authority granted by the document. Generally, specific instructions that are given in a living will, health care declaration, or other advance directive executed by patients while competent can also be relied upon.

If the decision of an authorized agent or proxy appears to conflict directly with instructions in a living will, the outcome depends on the scope of discretion given to the agent or proxy. Normally, the durable power of attorney for health care confers broad decision-making discretion on the agent. Nevertheless, the health care practitioner should determine whether the document gives the agent broad discretion beyond the written instructions or limits the agent to the written instructions; legal advice may be needed.

Patient choice is not limitless. For example, health care practitioners are not required to provide medically inappropriate or futile treatment. However, sometimes there are legitimate differences of opinion regarding what is inappropriate or futile. Physicians do not have to act against their conscience but may have a responsibility to try to transfer a patient to another physician or institution of the patient's choice.

If patients have no authorized surrogate, health care practitioners usually rely on the next of kin or even a close friend; however, the exact scope of authority and the priority of permissible surrogates varies by state. Typically, the order of priority is a spouse (or domestic partner in jurisdictions that recognize the status), an adult child, a parent, a sibling, then possibly other relatives or a close friend. If more than one person has the same priority (eg, several adult children), consensus is preferred, but some states allow health care practitioners to rely on a majority decision.

If a patient's decision-making capacity, a surrogate's authority, or the ethical or legal appropriateness of a particular treatment decision is disputed, consultation with an institutional ethics committee or similar body is advisable. If an ethically and legally sound resolution cannot be found, health care practitioners may need to request court review. Many institutions make the ethics committee available on short notice (eg, in 1 or 2 days); judicial review is typically more time consuming. When immediate decisions are medically required, the doctrine of presumed consent applies (see p. 2770).

For most nonemergency medical decisions affecting minors, medical care cannot proceed without a parent's or guardian's consent. The parent's or guardian's decision can be overridden only if a court determines that the decision constitutes neglect or abuse of the minor. In some states, minors can consent to certain medical treatments (eg, treatment of sexually transmitted diseases, prescriptions for birth control, abortion) without parental permission. Individual state law must be consulted.

APPENDIX I

READY REFERENCE GUIDES

In the US, most laboratory test results are reported in what are termed conventional units; the rest of the world reports results in *Système International d'Unités* (SI) or international units (IU). The unit basis for SI is updated periodically by a panel.

Many SI units are the same as units used in the US system; however, SI units for concentrations are not. SI concentrations are reported as moles (mol) or decimal fractions of a mole (eg, millimole, micromole) per unit volume in liters (L). Conventional units are reported as mass (eg, grams, milligrams) or chemical equivalency (eg, milliequivalents) per unit volume, which may be in liters or decimal fractions of liters (eg, deciliters, milliliters). Results reported in amount per 100 mL (1 dL) are sometimes expressed as percent (eg, 10 mg/dL may be written as 10 mg%).

Moles, milligrams, and milliequivalents: A mole is an Avogadro's number (6.023×10^{23}) of elementary entities (eg, atoms, ions, molecules); the mass of 1 mole of a substance is its atomic weight in grams (eg, 1 mole of sodium = 23 g, 1 mole of calcium = 40 g). Similarly, the mass of a given quantity of substance divided by its atomic weight gives the number of moles (eg, 20 g sodium = 20/23, or 0.87, mol).

An equivalent is a unit that integrates charge and moles; 1 equivalent represents one mole of charges and is calculated by multiplying the number of moles of charged particles in a substance times the valence of that substance. Thus, for ions with a +1 or −1 charge (eg, Na^+, K^+, Cl^-), 1 mole is 1 equivalent ($1 \times 1 = 1$); for ions with a +2 or −2 charge (eg, Ca^{2+}), 1/2 mole is 1 equivalent ($1/2 \times 2 = 1$), and so forth for other valence values. A milliequivalent (mEq) is 1/1000 of an equivalent.

The following can be used to convert between mEq, mg, and mmol:

$$\text{mEq} = \text{mg/formula wt} \times \text{valence} = \text{mmol} \times \text{valence}$$
$$\text{mg} = \text{mEq} \times \text{formula wt/valence} = \text{mmol} \times \text{formula wt}$$
$$\text{mmol} = \text{mg/formula wt} = \text{mEq/valence}$$

(NOTE: Formula wt = atomic or molecular wt.)

Alternatively, conversion tables are available in print and on the Internet (eg, at www.merckvetmanual.com/mvm/htm/bc/reftbl08.htm).

METRIC SYSTEM

UNIT	EQUIVALENT SUBUNIT
Mass	
1 kilogram (kg)	1000 grams (10^3 g)
1 gram (g)	1000 milligrams (10^3 mg)
1 milligram (mg)	1000 micrograms (10^{-3} g)
1 microgram (µg)	1000 nanograms (10^{-6} g)
1 nanogram (ng)	1000 picograms (pg; 10^{-9} g)
Volume	
1 liter (L)	1000 milliliters (mL)
1 liter (L)	1000 cubic centimeters (cc)

METRIC–NONMETRIC EQUIVALENTS

METRIC UNIT	EQUIVALENT NONMETRIC UNIT*
Liquid	
30 milliliters (mL)	1 fluid ounce (oz)
250 mL	8+ fluid oz
500 mL	1+ pint
1000 mL (1 liter)	1+ quart
Weight	
65 mg	1 grain (gr)
28.35 g	1 oz
1 kg	2.2 pounds (lb)
Linear	
1 millimeter (mm)	0.04 inch (in)
1 centimeter (cm)	0.4 in
2.54 cm	1 in
1 meter (m)	39.37 in
Household	
4 mL	1 teaspoon (tsp)
5 mL	1 teaspoon, medical
8 mL	1 dessert spoon
15 mL	1 tablespoon (tbsp—1/2 fluid oz)
240 mL	1 cup (8 fluid oz)

*Approximate.

ATOMIC WEIGHT OF SOME ELEMENTS IMPORTANT IN MEDICINE

ELEMENT	SYMBOL	ATOMIC WEIGHT*
Hydrogen	H	1
Carbon	C	12
Nitrogen	N	14
Oxygen	O	16
Sodium	Na	23
Magnesium	Mg	24
Phosphorus	P	31
Chlorine	Cl	35.5
Potassium	K	39
Calcium	Ca	40

*Approximate.

CENTIGRADE–FAHRENHEIT EQUIVALENTS*

APPLICATION	°C	°F
Freezing for water at sea level	0	32
Clinical range	36.0	96.8
	36.5	97.7
	37.0	98.6
	37.5	99.5
	38.0	100.4
	38.5	101.3
	39.0	102.2
	39.5	103.1
	40.0	104.0
	40.5	104.9
	41.0	105.8
	41.5	106.7
	42.0	107.6
Pasteurization (holding),† 30 min at	62.8	145.0
Pasteurization (flash),† 15 sec at	71.7	161.0
Boiling for water at sea level	100.0	212.0

*Conversion:
To convert °F to °C, subtract 32, then multiply by 5/9 or 0.555.
To convert °C to °F, multiply by 9/5 or 1.8, then add 32.

†According to the FDA Code of Federal Regulations, 1991.

APPENDIX II

TRADE NAMES OF SOME COMMONLY USED DRUGS

Throughout THE MANUAL, generic (nonproprietary) names for drugs are used whenever possible. Most prescription drugs have trade names (also called proprietary, brand, or specialty names) to distinguish them as being produced and marketed by a particular manufacturer. In the US, these names are usually registered as trademarks with the Patent Office, which confers certain legal rights with respect to their use. A trade name may be registered for a product containing a single active ingredient (with or without additives) or ≥ 2 active ingredients (combination drugs). A chemical substance marketed by several manufacturers may have several trade names. A drug may be marketed under different trade names in different countries.

Trade names are found in many publications and are used extensively in clinical medicine. For convenience, the following table lists trade names for most drugs mentioned in THE MANUAL, primarily those marketed in the US. The table is not all-inclusive and does not list every trade name for each drug. A few drugs in the table are investigational and may subsequently be approved by the FDA. Inclusion of a drug does not indicate approval of its use for any indication, nor does it imply efficacy or safety of its action. Inclusion of a trade name indicates neither endorsement nor preference by THE MANUAL.

TRADE NAMES OF SOME COMMONLY USED DRUGS

GENERIC NAME	TRADE NAMES
bacavir	ZIAGEN
bciximab	REOPRO
carbose	PRECOSE
cetazolamide	DIAMOX
cetylcysteine	MUCOMYST
cyclovir	ZOVIRAX
dalimumab	HUMIRA
denosine	ADENOCARD
lbuterol	PROVENTIL, VENTOLIN
lbuterol/ipratropium	COMBIVENT, DUONEB
lendronate	FOSAMAX
lfuzosin	UROXATRAL
llopurinol	ZYLOPRIM
lmotriptan	AXERT
lprazolam	XANAX
lprostadil	CAVERJECT, EDEX, MUSE
lteplase	ACTIVASE
mantadine	SYMMETREL
mikacin	AMIKIN
miloride	MIDAMOR
minocaproic acid	AMICAR
minophylline	SOMOPHYLLIN
miodarone	CORDARONE
mitriptyline	ELAVIL, ENDEP
mlodipine	NORVASC
moxapine	ASENDIN
moxicillin	AMOXIL, TRIMOX
moxicillin/clavulanate	AUGMENTIN
mphotericin B	ABELCET, AMBISOME, AMPHOCIN, AMPHOTEC, FUNGIZONE
mpicillin	OMNIPEN, PRINCIPEN
mpicillin/sulbactam	UNASYN

GENERIC NAME	TRADE NAMES
Amprenavir	AGENERASE
Amrinone	INOCOR
Anastrozole	ARIMIDEX
Aprepitant	EMEND
Aripiprazole	ABILIFY
Asparaginase	ELSPAR
Atazanavir	REYATAZ
Atenolol	TENORMIN
Atomoxetine	STRATTERA
Atorvastatin	LIPITOR
Atovaquone	MEPRON
Azathioprine	IMURAN
Azithromycin	ZITHROMAX
Aztreonam	AZACTAM
Baclofen	LIORESAL
Beclomethasone	BECLOVENT, BECONASE
Benazepril	LOTENSIN
Benzonatate	TESSALON
Benztropine	COGENTIN
Betamethasone	CELESTONE, DIPROLENE, LUXIQ, MAXIVATE, VALISONE
Betaxolol	BETOPTIC, KERLONE
Bethanechol	DUVOID, URECHOLINE
Bisacodyl	DULCOLAX
Bisoprolol	ZEBETA
Bleomycin	BLENOXANE
Bosentan	TRACLEER
Bretylium	BRETYLOL
Brimonidine	ALPHAGAN
Bromocriptine	PARLODEL
Brompheniramine	DIMETANE
Budesonide	PULMICORT, RHINOCORT

GENERIC NAME	TRADE NAMES
Bumetanide	BUMEX
Bupropion	WELLBUTRIN, ZYBAN
Buspirone	BUSPAR
Busulfan	MYLERAN
Butorphanol	STADOL
Calcitonin-salmon	CALCIMAR, MIACALCIN
Calcitriol	ROCALTROL
Candesartan	ATACAND
Capecitabine	XELODA
Capreomycin	CAPASTAT
Captopril	CAPOTEN
Carbamazepine	TEGRETOL
Carbenicillin	GEOCILLIN
Carbidopa-levodopa	SINEMET
Carisoprodol	SOMA
Carvedilol	COREG
Caspofungin	CANCIDAS
Cefaclor	CECLOR
Cefadroxil	DURICEF
Cefazolin	ANCEF, KEFZOL
Cefixime	SUPRAX
Cefoperazone	CEFOBID
Cefotaxime	CLAFORAN
Cefotetan	CEFOTAN
Cefoxitin	MEFOXIN
Cefprozil	CEFZIL
Ceftazidime	FORTAZ, TAZICEF
Ceftriaxone	ROCEPHIN
Cefuroxime	CEFTIN, ZINACEF
Celecoxib	CELEBREX
Cephalexin	KEFLEX, KEFTAB
Cetuximab	ERBITUX
Chloral hydrate	NOCTEC
Chlorambucil	LEUKERAN
Chlordiazepoxide	LIBRIUM

GENERIC NAME	TRADE NAMES
Chlorpheniramine	CHLOR-TRIMETON
Chlorpromazine	THORAZINE
Chlorpropamide	DIABINESE
Chlorthalidone	HYGROTON
Cholestyramine	QUESTRAN
Cidofovir	VISTIDE
Cilostazol	PLETAL
Cimetidine	TAGAMET
Ciprofloxacin	CILOXAN, CIPR
Cisplatin	PLATINOL
Clarithromycin	BIAXIN
Clemastine	TAVIST
Clindamycin	CLEOCIN
Clomiphene	CLOMID
Clomipramine	ANAFRANIL
Clonazepam	KLONOPIN
Clonidine	CATAPRES
Clopidogrel	PLAVIX
Clorazepate	TRANXENE
Clozapine	CLOZARIL
Colestipol	COLESTID
Cosyntropin	CORTROSYN
Cromolyn	CROLOM, INTAL NASALCROM
Cyclobenzaprine	FLEXERIL
Cyclophosphamide	CYTOXAN
Cyclosporine	NEORAL, SANDIMMUNE
Cyproheptadine	PERIACTIN
Cytarabine	CYTOSAR-U
Dacarbazine	DTIC-DOME
Dactinomycin	COSMEGEN
Dalteparin	FRAGMIN
Danazol	DANOCRINE
Dantrolene	DANTRIUM
Daptomycin	CUBICIN
Darbepoetin	ARANESP
Daunorubicin	CERUBIDINE

GENERIC NAME	TRADE NAMES
eferoxamine	DESFERAL
elavirdine	RESCRIPTOR
esipramine	NORPRAMIN
esmopressin	DDAVP, STIMATE
examethasone	DECADRON, DEXASONE, HEXADROL
exmethylphenidate	FOCALIN
extromethorphan	BENYLIN DM, DELSYM, DEXALONE
iazepam	VALIUM
iclofenac	CATAFLAM, VOLTAREN
iclofenac/misoprostol	ARTHROTEC
icloxacillin	DYCILL, DYNAPEN, PATHOCIL
icyclomine	BENTYL
idanosine	VIDEX
iflunisal	DOLOBID
igoxin	DIGITEK, LANOXIN
iltiazem	CARDIZEM, CARTIA, DILACOR
iphenhydramine	BENADRYL, NYTOL
iphenoxylate/atropine	LOMOTIL
ipivefrin	PROPINE
ipyridamole/aspirin	AGGRENOX
isopyramide	NORPACE
ivalproex	DEPAKOTE
obutamine	DOBUTREX
ocetaxel	TAXOTERE
ocusate	COLACE, SURFAK
olasetron	ANZEMET
onepezil	ARICEPT
opamine	INTROPIN
ornase alfa	PULMOZYME
orzolamide	TRUSOPT

GENERIC NAME	TRADE NAMES
Doxazosin	CARDURA
Doxepin	SINEQUAN, ZONALON
Doxorubicin	ADRIAMYCIN
Doxycycline	PERIOSTAT, VIBRAMYCIN
Dronabinol	MARINOL
Droperidol	INAPSINE
Drotrecogin alfa	XIGRIS
Duloxetine	CYMBALTA
Efavirenz	SUSTIVA
Eletriptan	RELPAX
Emtricitabine	EMTRIVA
Emtricitabine/tenofovir	TRUVADA
Enalapril	VASOTEC
Enfuvirtide	FUZEON
Enoxaparin	LOVENOX
Entacapone	COMTAN
Eplerenone	INSPRA
Epoetin alfa	EPOGEN, PROCRIT
Epoprostenol	FLOLAN
Eprosartan	TEVETEN
Eptifibatide	INTEGRILIN
Ergocalciferol	DRISDOL
Ertapenem	INVANZ
Escitalopram	LEXAPRO
Esmolol	BREVIBLOC
Esomeprazole	NEXIUM
Estazolam	PROSOM
Estrogens, conjugated	PREMARIN
Etanercept	ENBREL
Etidronate	DIDRONEL
Etodolac	LODINE
Etomidate	AMIDATE
Etoposide	ETOPOPHOS, VEPESID
Ezetimibe	ZETIA
Famciclovir	FAMVIR

GENERIC NAME	TRADE NAMES
Famotidine	PEPCID
Felodipine	PLENDIL
Fentanyl	ACTIQ, DURAGESIC, SUBLIMAZE
Fexofenadine	ALLEGRA
Filgrastim	NEUPOGEN
Finasteride	PROPECIA, PROSCAR
Flecainide	TAMBOCOR
Fluconazole	DIFLUCAN
Flucytosine	ANCOBON
Fludarabine	FLUDARA
Fludrocortisone	FLORINEF
Flunisolide	NASALIDE
Fluocinonide	LIDEX
Fluorouracil	ADRUCIL
Fluoxetine	PROZAC, SARAFEM
Fluoxymesterone	HALOTESTIN
Flurazepam	DALMANE
Flurbiprofen	ANSAID, OCUFEN
Fluvastatin	LESCOL
Fluvoxamine	LUVOX
Fosamprenavir	LEXIVA
Foscarnet	FOSCAVIR
Fosfomycin	MONUROL
Fosinopril	MONOPRIL
Frovatriptan	FROVA
Furosemide	LASIX
Gabapentin	NEURONTIN
Galantamine	REMINYL
Ganciclovir	CYTOVENE
Gemcitabine	GEMZAR
Gemifloxacin	FACTIVE
Gemfibrozil	LOPID
Gentamicin	GARAMYCIN
Glimepiride	AMARYL
Glipizide	GLUCOTROL

GENERIC NAME	TRADE NAMES
Glyburide	DIABETA, GLYNASE, MICRONASE
Goserelin	ZOLADEX
Granisetron	KYTRIL
Griseofulvin	FULVICIN, GRIFULVIN V, GRISACTIN
Guaifenesin	ROBITUSSIN
Guanabenz	WYTENSIN
Guanadrel	HYLOREL
Guanethidine	ISMELIN
Guanfacine	TENEX
Haloperidol	HALDOL
Hydralazine	APRESOLINE
Hydrochlorothiazide	ESIDRIX, HYDRODIURIL
Hydrocortisone	CORTEF, SOLU-CORTEF
Hydromorphone	DILAUDID
Hydroxychloroquine	PLAQUENIL
Hydroxyprogesterone	DELALUTIN
Hydroxyurea	HYDREA
Hydroxyzine	ATARAX, VISTARIL
Ibuprofen	ADVIL, MOTRIN, NUPRIN
Ifosfamide	IFEX, MITOXANA
Imatinib	GLEEVEC
Imipenem/cilastatin	PRIMAXIN
Imipramine	TOFRANIL
Indapamide	LOZOL
Indinavir	CRIXIVAN
Indomethacin	INDOCIN
Infliximab	REMICADE
Insulin	HUMULIN, NOVOLIN
Insulin aspart	NOVOLOG
Insulin glargine	LANTUS
Insulin lispro	HUMALOG
Ipratropium	ATROVENT

GENERIC NAME	TRADE NAMES
rbesartan	AVAPRO
rinotecan	CAMPTOSAR
ron dextran	IMFERON
ron sucrose	VENOFER
soetharine	BRONKOSOL
soniazid	INH, NYDRAZID
soproterenol	ISUPREL
sosorbide dinitrate	ISORDIL, SORBITRATE
sosorbide mononitrate	IMDUR, ISMO, MONOKET
sotretinoin	ACCUTANE
sradipine	DYNACIRC
traconazole	SPORANOX
Ketoconazole	NIZORAL
Ketoprofen	ORUDIS, ORUVAIL
Ketorolac	TORADOL
abetalol	NORMODYNE, TRANDATE
actulose	CEPHULAC, CHRONULAC, KRISTALOSE
amivudine	EPIVIR
amotrigine	LAMICTAL
ansoprazole	PREVACID
atanoprost	XALATAN
eflunomide	ARAVA
epirudin	REFLUDAN
euprolide	LUPRON
evalbuterol	XOPENEX
evallorphan	LORFAN
evamisole	ERGAMISOL
evetiracetam	KEPPRA
evodopa	DOPAR, LARODOPA
Levothyroxine (T_4)	LEVOXYL, SYNTHROID
Lidocaine	XYLOCAINE
Lindane	KWELL
Linezolid	ZYVOX

GENERIC NAME	TRADE NAMES
Liothyronine (T_3)	CYTOMEL
Liotrix	THYROLAR
Lisinopril	PRINIVIL, ZESTRIL
Lithium	ESKALITH, LITHOBID, LITHONATE
Lomefloxacin	MAXAQUIN
Lomustine	CEENU
Loperamide	IMODIUM
Loratadine	ALAVERT, CLARITIN
Lorazepam	ATIVAN
Losartan	COZAAR
Mebendazole	VERMOX
Mechlorethamine	MUSTARGEN
Meclizine	ANTIVERT, BONINE
Meclofenamate	MECLOMEN
Medroxyprogesterone	PROVERA
Mefenamic acid	PONSTEL
Megestrol	MEGACE
Meloxicam	MOBIC
Melphalan	ALKERAN
Memantine	NAMENDA
Meperidine	DEMEROL
Meprobamate	EQUANIL, MILTOWN
Mercaptopurine	PURINETHOL
Meropenem	MERREM
Mesalamine	ASACOL, ROWASA
Mesna	MESNEX
Mesoridazine	SERENTIL
Metaraminol	ARAMINE
Metaxalone	SKELAXIN
Metformin	GLUCOPHAGE
Methadone	DOLOPHINE
Methimazole	TAPAZOLE
Methocarbamol	ROBAXIN

GENERIC NAME	TRADE NAMES
Methotrexate	RHEUMATREX
Methyldopa	ALDOMET
Methylphenidate	CONCERTA, RITALIN
Methylprednisolone	MEDROL
Methyltestosterone	ORETON
Methysergide	SANSERT
Metoclopramide	REGLAN
Metolazone	ZAROXOLYN
Metoprolol	LOPRESSOR, TOPROL
Metronidazole	FLAGYL
Mexiletine	MEXITIL
Miconazole	MICATIN, MONISTAT
Milrinone	PRIMACOR
Minocycline	MINOCIN
Minoxidil	LONITEN, ROGAINE
Mirtazapine	REMERON
Misoprostol	CYTOTEC
Mitomycin	MUTAMYCIN
Modafinil	PROVIGIL
Mometasone	NASONEX
Montelukast	SINGULAIR
Morphine	AVINZA, DEPODUR, KADIAN, MS CONTIN, MSIR, ROXANOL
Moxalactam	MOXAM
Moxifloxacin	AVELOX
Mupirocin	BACTROBAN
Mycophenolate mofetil	CELLCEPT
Nabumetone	RELAFEN
Nadolol	CORGARD
Nafcillin	UNIPEN
Nalbuphine	NUBAIN
Nalidixic acid	NEGGRAM
Naloxone	NARCAN
Naltrexone	REVIA

GENERIC NAME	TRADE NAMES
Nandrolone	DURABOLIN
Naproxen	ALEVE, NAPROSYN
Naratriptan	AMERGE
Nedocromil	TILADE
Nefazodone	SERZONE
Nelfinavir	VIRACEPT
Neostigmine	PROSTIGMIN
Nesiritide	NATRECOR
Nevirapine	VIRAMUNE
Niacin	NIACOR, NIASPAN, SLO-NIACIN
Niacin/lovastatin	ADVICOR
Nicardipine	CARDENE
Nicotine	COMMIT, NICORETTE, NICOTROL
Nifedipine	ADALAT, PROCARDIA
Nimodipine	NIMOTOP
Nitrofurantoin	FURADANTIN, MACROBID, MACRODANTIN
Nitroglycerin	NITRO-BID, NITRO-DUR, NITROL, NITROQUICK
Nitroprusside	NIPRIDE
Nizatidine	AXID
Norepinephrine	LEVOPHED
Norfloxacin	NOROXIN
Nortriptyline	AVENTYL
Nystatin	MYCOSTATIN, NILSTAT
Octreotide	SANDOSTATIN
Ofloxacin	FLOXIN
Olanzapine	ZYPREXA
Olmesartan	BENICAR
Olopatadine	PATANOL
Omeprazole	PRILOSEC
Ondansetron	ZOFRAN

GENERIC NAME	TRADE NAMES
Oseltamivir	TAMIFLU
Oxacillin	BACTOCILL, PROSTAPHLIN
Oxaliplatin	ELOXATIN
Oxandrolone	OXANDRIN
Oxaprozin	DAYPRO
Oxazepam	SERAX
Oxcarbazepine	TRILEPTAL
Oxybutynin	DITROPAN
Oxycodone	OXYCONTIN, OXYIR
Oxymetazoline	AFRIN, DURATION
Oxytocin	PITOCIN, SYNTOCINON
Paclitaxel	TAXOL
Pamidronate	AREDIA
Pancrelipase	PANCREASE, VIOKASE
Pancuronium	PAVULON
Pantoprazole	PROTONIX
Papaverine	PAVABID
Paroxetine	PAXIL
Pegfilgrastim	NEULASTA
Penciclovir	DENAVIR
Penicillamine	CUPRIMINE
Penicillin G	BICILLIN, DURACILLIN
Penicillin V potassium	PEN-VEE, V-CILLIN K
Pentamidine	NEBUPENT, PENTAM 300
Pentazocine	TALWIN
Pentobarbital	NEMBUTAL
Pentoxifylline	TRENTAL
Pergolide	PERMAX
Perphenazine	TRILAFON
Phenazopyridine	PYRIDIUM
Phenelzine	NARDIL
Phenmetrazine	PRELUDIN
Phenobarbital	LUMINAL

GENERIC NAME	TRADE NAMES
Phenylephrine	NEO-SYNEPHRINE
Phenytoin	DILANTIN
Phytonadione	MEPHYTON
Pimecrolimus	ELIDEL
Pindolol	VISKEN
Pioglitazone	ACTOS
Piperacillin	PIPRACIL
Piperacillin/tazobactam	ZOSYN
Pipobroman	VERCYTE
Pirbuterol	MAXAIR
Piroxicam	FELDENE
Plicamycin	MITHRACIN
Pravastatin	PRAVACHOL
Prazepam	CENTRAX
Prazosin	MINIPRESS
Prednisolone	ORAPRED, PRELONE
Prednisone	DELTASONE
Primidone	MYSOLINE
Procainamide	PROCAN SR, PRONESTYL
Procarbazine	MATULANE
Prochlorperazine	COMPAZINE
Promethazine	PHENERGAN
Propafenone	RYTHMOL
Propantheline	PRO-BANTHINE
Propoxyphene	DARVON, DOLENE
Propoxyphene/acetaminophen	DARVOCET
Propranolol	INDERAL
Pseudoephedrine	AFRINOL, SUDAFED
Pyridostigmine	MESTINON
Pyrimethamine	DARAPRIM
Quazepam	DORAL
Quetiapine	SEROQUEL
Quinapril	ACCUPRIL
Quinidine	CARDIOQUIN, QUINAGLUTE

GENERIC NAME	TRADE NAMES
Quinupristin/dalfopristin	SYNERCID
Raloxifene	EVISTA
Ramipril	ALTACE
Ranitidine	ZANTAC
Remifentanil	ULTIVA
Reteplase	RETAVASE
Ribavirin	VIRAZOLE
Rifabutin	MYCOBUTIN
Rifampin	RIFADIN, RIMACTANE
Rimantadine	FLUMADINE
Risedronate	ACTONEL
Risperidone	RISPERDAL
Ritodrine	YUTOPAR
Ritonavir	NORVIR
Rituximab	RITUXAN
Rizatriptan	MAXALT
Rosiglitazone	AVANDIA
Salmeterol	SEREVENT
Salmeterol/fluticasone	ADVAIR
Salsalate	DISALCID, SALFLEX
Saquinavir	FORTOVASE, INVIRASE
Sargramostim	LEUKINE
Scopolamine	TRANSDERM-SCOP
Secobarbital	SECONAL
Selegiline	ELDEPRYL
Selenium	SELSUN
Sertraline	ZOLOFT
Sibutramine	MERIDIA
Sildenafil	VIAGRA
Silver sulfadiazine	SILVADENE
Simethicone	MYLICON
Simvastatin	ZOCOR
Sirolimus	RAPAMUNE
Somatropin	HUMATROPE
Sotalol	BETAPACE
Spironolactone	ALDACTONE
Stavudine	ZERIT
Sucralfate	CARAFATE
Sufentanil	SUFENTA
Sulfamethoxazole	GANTANOL
Sulfasalazine	AZULFIDINE
Sulindac	CLINORIL
Sumatriptan	IMITREX
Tacrine	COGNEX
Tacrolimus	PROGRAF
Tadalafil	CIALIS
Tamoxifen	NOLVADEX
Tamsulosin	FLOMAX
Tegaserod	ZELNORM
Telithromycin	KETEK
Telmisartan	MICARDIS
Temazepam	RESTORIL
Tenecteplase	TNKASE
Tenofovir	VIREAD
Terazosin	HYTRIN
Terbutaline	BRETHINE, BRICANYL
Testosterone	DELATESTRYL
Tetracycline	ACHROMYCIN V, TETRACYN, TETREX
Theophylline	ELIXOPHYLLIN, THEO-DUR
Thioridazine	MELLARIL
Thiothixene	NAVANE
Thyrotropin	THYTROPAR
Ticarcillin	TICAR
Ticlopidine	TICLID
Timolol	BLOCADREN, TIMOPTIC
Tinzaparin	INNOHEP
Tiotropium	SPIRIVA
Tobramycin	NEBCIN, TOBI, TOBREX
Tolbutamide	ORINASE
Tolmetin	TOLECTIN

GENERIC NAME	TRADE NAMES
Tolnaftate	TINACTIN
Tolterodine	DETROL
Topiramate	TOPAMAX
Topotecan	HYCAMTIN
Torsemide	DEMADEX
Tramadol	ULTRAM
Trandolapril	MAVIK
Tranylcypromine	PARNATE
Trastuzumab	HERCEPTIN
Travoprost	TRAVATAN
Trazodone	DESYREL
Tretinoin	RETIN-A
Triacetin	ENZACTIN
Triamcinolone	ARISTOCORT, KENACORT, KENALOG, NASACORT
Triamterene	DYRENIUM
Triamterene/hydrochlorothiazide	DYAZIDE, MAXIDE
Triazolam	HALCION
Trifluoperazine	STELAZINE
Trimethobenzamide	TIGAN
Trimethoprim	PROLOPRIM, TRIMPEX
Trimethoprim-sulfamethoxazole (cotrimoxazole)	BACTRIM, SEPTRA
Unoprostone	RESCULA
Ursodiol	ACTIGALL
Valacyclovir	VALTREX
Valganciclovir	VALCYTE
Valproic acid	DEPAKENE
Valsartan	DIOVAN
Vancomycin	VANCOCIN
Vardenafil	LEVITRA
Vasopressin	PITRESSIN
Venlafaxine	EFFEXOR
Verapamil	CALAN, ISOPTIN
Vinblastine	VELBAN
Vincristine	ONCOVIN
Vinorelbine	NAVELBINE
Voriconazole	VFEND
Warfarin	COUMADIN
Zafirlukast	ACCOLATE
Zalcitabine	HIVID
Zaleplon	SONATA
Zidovudine	RETROVIR
Ziprasidone	GEODON
Zoledronic acid	ZOMETA
Zolmitriptan	ZOMIG
Zolpidem	AMBIEN
Zonisamide	ZONEGRAN

INDEX

NOTE: Page numbers followed by *f* refer to illustrations; page numbers followed by *sb* refer to sidebars; page numbers followed by *t* refer to tables. Page numbers in boldface indicate a major discussion of a topic.

D

H

I

J

K

L

Q

S

T

V

W

X

Y

Z

The Eighteenth Edition of THE MERCK MANUAL is set in 9-point Times Roman, with section and chapter titles in Eurostile Demi and text headings in Memphis Bold. The index is set in 8 1/2-point Times Roman. The original draft was produced using Microsoft Word XP at the editorial offices of the Merck Manuals Department in Blue Bell, Pennsylvania and transmitted to Nesbitt Graphics, Inc., in Fort Washington, Pennsylvania, where it was electronically assembled into pages using Adobe FrameMaker. The book was printed by web offset on 20-pound paper at National Publishing Company, a subsidiary of Courier Corporation, in Philadelphia, Pennsylvania.